Nelson Textbook of

PEDIATRICS

Nelson Textbook of PEDIATRICS

19th Edition

Robert M. Kliegman, MD
Professor and Chair
Department of Pediatrics
Medical College of Wisconsin
Pediatrician-in-Chief
Pamela and Leslie Muma Chair in Pediatrics
Children's Hospital of Wisconsin
Executive Vice President
Children's Research Institute
Milwaukee, Wisconsin

Bonita F. Stanton, MD
Professor and Schotanus Family Endowed Chair of Pediatrics
Pediatrician-in-Chief
Carman and Ann Adams Department of Pediatrics
Children's Hospital of Michigan
Wayne State University School of Medicine
Detroit, Michigan

Nina F. Schor, MD, PhD
William H. Eilinger Professor and Chair
Department of Pediatrics
Professor
Department of Neurology
Pediatrician-in-Chief
Golisano Children's Hospital
University of Rochester Medical Center
Rochester, New York

Joseph W. St. Geme III, MD
James B. Duke Professor and Chair
Department of Pediatrics
Duke University School of Medicine
Chief Medical Officer
Duke Children's Hospital and Health Center
Durham, North Carolina

Richard E. Behrman, MD
Nonprofit Healthcare and Educational
Consultants to Medical Institutions
Santa Barbara, California

ELSEVIER
SAUNDERS

ELSEVIER
SAUNDERS

1600 John F. Kennedy Blvd.
Ste 1800
Philadelphia, PA 19103-2899

NELSON TEXTBOOK OF PEDIATRICS, NINETEENTH EDITION
INTERNATIONAL EDITION

ISBN: 978-1-4377-0755-7
ISBN: 978-0-8089-2420-3

Notices

Knowledge and best practice in this field are constantly changing. As new research and experience broaden our understanding, changes in research methods, professional practices, or medical treatment may become necessary.

Practitioners and researchers must always rely on their own experience and knowledge in evaluating and using any information, methods, compounds, or experiments described herein. In using such information or methods they should be mindful of their own safety and the safety of others, including parties for whom they have a professional responsibility.

With respect to any drug or pharmaceutical products identified, readers are advised to check the most current information provided (i) on procedures featured or (ii) by the manufacturer of each product to be administered, to verify the recommended dose or formula, the method and duration of administration, and contraindications. It is the responsibility of practitioners, relying on their own experience and knowledge of their patients, to make diagnoses, to determine dosages and the best treatment for each individual patient, and to take all appropriate safety precautions.

To the fullest extent of the law, neither the Publisher nor the authors, contributors, or editors, assume any liability for any injury and/or damage to persons or property as a matter of products liability, negligence or otherwise, or from any use or operation of any methods, products, instructions, or ideas contained in the material herein.

Library of Congress Cataloging-in-Publication Data

Nelson textbook of pediatrics. — 19th ed. / [edited by] Robert M. Kliegman ... [et al.].
p. ; cm.
Textbook of pediatrics
Includes bibliographical references and index.
ISBN 978-1-4377-0755-7 (hardcover : alk. paper) 1. Pediatrics. I. Kliegman, Robert. II. Nelson, Waldo E. (Waldo Emerson), 1898-1997. Textbook of pediatrics. III. Title: Textbook of pediatrics.
[DNLM: 1. Pediatrics. WS 100]
RJ45.N4 2011
618.92—dc22

2011009671

Publishing Director: Judith Fletcher
Senior Developmental Editor: Jennifer Shreiner
Publishing Services Manager: Patricia Tannian
Senior Project Manager: Kristine Feeherty
Design Direction: Lou Forgione

Printed in the United States of America

Last digit is the print number: 9 8 7 6 5 4 3 2 1

This edition is dedicated to the leadership, mentorship, and editorial wisdom of Richard E. Behrman. Dick's monumental commitment to the field of pediatrics spans more than five decades as an editor, teacher, researcher, and clinician and has contributed greatly to the growth of the profession and the improved health and well-being of children across the globe. We are privileged to work with Dick and are grateful to him for his steadfast counsel and guidance.

Contributors

Jon S. Abramson, MD
Chair, Department of Pediatrics, Wake Forest University School of Medicine, Winston-Salem, North Carolina
Streptococcus pneumoniae *(Pneumococcus)*

Mark J. Abzug, MD
Professor, Department of Pediatrics-Infectious Diseases, University of Colorado School of Medicine, The Children's Hospital, Aurora, Colorado
Nonpolio Enteroviruses

John J. Aiken, MD, FACS, FAAP
Associate Professor of Surgery, Division of Pediatric General and Thoracic Surgery, Medical College of Wisconsin, Milwaukee, Wisconsin
Acute Appendicitis; Inguinal Hernias; Epigastric Hernia

H. Hesham A-kader, MD, MSc
Professor, Department of Pediatrics; Chief, Pediatric Gastroenterology, Hepatology and Nutrition; The University of Arizona, Tucson, Arizona
Neonatal Cholestasis

Prof. Cezmi A. Akdis, MD
Director, Swiss Institute of Allergy and Asthma Research (SIAF), Davos, Switzerland
Allergy and the Immunologic Basis of Atopic Disease

Harold Alderman, MS, PhD
Development Research Group, The World Bank, Washington, District of Columbia
Nutrition, Food Security, and Health

Ramin Alemzadeh, MD
Professor of Pediatrics, Department of Pediatrics, Medical College of Wisconsin, MACC Fund Research Center, Milwaukee, Wisconsin
Diabetes Mellitus

Evaline A. Alessandrini, MD, MSCE
Director, Quality Scholars Program in Health Care Transformation, Divisions of Health Policy/Clinical Effectiveness and Emergency Medicine, Cincinnati Children's Hospital Medical Center; Professor, Department of Pediatrics, University of Cincinnati College of Medicine, Cincinnati, Ohio
Outcomes and Risk Adjustment

Omar Ali, MD
Assistant Professor, Department of Pediatrics, Medical College of Wisconsin, Milwaukee, Wisconsin
Hypofunction of the Testes; Pseudoprecocity Resulting from Tumors of the Testes; Gynecomastia; Diabetes Mellitus

Namasivayam Ambalavanan, MBBS, MD
Associate Professor, Division of Neonatology, Departments of Pediatrics, Cell Biology, and Pathology, University of Alabama at Birmingham, Birmingham, Alabama
Nervous System Disorders; Respiratory Tract Disorders; Digestive System Disorders

Karl E. Anderson, MD, FACP
Professor, Departments of Preventive Medicine and Community Health, Internal Medicine and Pharmacology and Toxicology, University of Texas Medical Branch, Galveston, Texas
The Porphyrias

Peter M. Anderson, MD, PhD
Professor, University of Texas MD Anderson Cancer Center, Houston, Texas
Wilms Tumor; Other Pediatric Renal Tumors

Kelly K. Anthony, PhD
Assistant Professor, Durham Child Development and Behavioral Health Clinic and Department of Psychiatry and Behavioral Sciences, Duke University Medical Center, Durham, North Carolina
Musculoskeletal Pain Syndromes

Alia Y. Antoon, MD
Chief of Pediatrics, Shriners Hospital for Children; Assistant Clinical Professor, Harvard Medical School, Boston, Massachusetts
Burn Injuries; Cold Injuries

Stacy P. Ardoin, MD, MS
Assistant Professor of Clinical Medicine, Ohio State University and Nationwide Children's Hospital, Columbus, Ohio
Systemic Lupus Erythematosus; Vasculitis Syndromes

Carola A.S. Arndt, MD
Professor of Pediatrics, Pediatric Hematology-Oncology, Mayo Clinic, Rochester, Minnesota
Soft Tissue Sarcomas; Neoplasms of Bone

Stephen S. Arnon, MD
Founder and Chief, Infant Botulism Treatment and Prevention Program, Center for Infectious Diseases, California Department of Public Health, Richmond, California
Botulism (Clostridium botulinum); *Tetanus* (Clostridium tetani)

Stephen C. Aronoff, MD
Waldo E. Nelson Professor and Chairman, Department of Pediatrics, Temple University School of Medicine, Philadelphia, Pennsylvania
Cryptococcus neoformans; *Histoplasmosis* (Histoplasma capsulatum); Paracoccidioides brasiliensis; *Sporotrichosis* (Sporothrix schenckii); *Zygomycosis (Mucormycosis); Primary Amebic Meningoencephalitis; Nonbacterial Food Poisoning*

David M. Asher, MD
Chief, Laboratory of Bacterial and Transmissible Spongiform Encephalopathy Agents, Office of Blood Research and Review, Center for Biologics Evaluation and Research (CBER), U.S. Food and Drug Administration, Rockville, Maryland
Transmissible Spongiform Encephalopathies

Barbara L. Asselin, MD
Associate Professor of Pediatrics and Oncology, Golisano Children's Hospital at Strong Pediatrics, Rochester, New York
Epidemiology of Childhood and Adolescent Cancer

Joann L. Ater, MD
Professor, Division of Pediatrics, University of Texas MD Anderson Cancer Center, Houston, Texas
Brain Tumors in Childhood; Neuroblastoma

Dan Atkins, MD
Associate Professor of Pediatrics, University of Colorado School of Medicine; Professor of Pediatrics, Director, Ambulatory Pediatrics, National Jewish Health, Denver, Colorado
Diagnosis of Allergic Disease; Principles of Treatment of Allergic Disease; Urticaria (Hives) and Angioedema

Erika F. Augustine, MD
Senior Instructor of Neurology, Division of Child Neurology, University of Rochester Medical Center, Rochester, New York
Movement Disorders

Marilyn Augustyn, MD
Director, Division of Developmental and Behavioral Pediatrics, Department of Pediatrics, Boston Medical Center, Boston, Massachusetts
Impact of Violence on Children

Ellis D. Avner, MD
Director, Children's Research Institute; Associate Dean for Research, Departments of Pediatrics and Physiology, Medical College of Wisconsin, Milwaukee, Wisconsin
Introduction to Glomerular Diseases; Glomerulonephritis Associated with Infections; Membranous Glomerulopathy; Membranoproliferative Glomerulonephritis; Glomerulonephritis Associated with Systemic Lupus Erythematosus; Henoch-Schönlein Purpura Nephritis; Rapidly Progressive (Crescentic) Glomerulonephritis; Goodpasture Disease; Hemolytic-Uremic Syndrome; Upper Urinary Tract Causes of Hematuria; Hematologic Diseases Causing Hematuria; Anatomic Abnormalities Associated with Hematuria; Lower Urinary Tract Causes of Hematuria; Introduction to the Child with Proteinuria; Transient Proteinuria; Orthostatic (Postural) Proteinuria; Fixed Proteinuria; Nephrotic Syndrome; Tubular Function; Renal Tubular Acidosis; Nephrogenic Diabetes Insipidus; Bartter and Gitelman Syndromes and Other Inherited Tubular Transport Abnormalities; Tubulointerstitial Nephritis; Toxic Nephropathy; Cortical Necrosis; Renal Failure

Parvin H. Azimi, MD
Director, Infectious Diseases, Children's Hospital and Research Center at Oakland; Clinical Professor of Pediatrics, University of California, San Francisco, California
Chancroid (Haemophilus ducreyi)

Carlos A. Bacino, MD
Genetics Service Chief, Texas Children's Hospital; Associate Professor of Genetics, Department of Molecular and Human Genetics, Baylor College of Medicine and Texas Children's Hospital, Houston, Texas
Cytogenetics

Robert N. Baldassano, MD
Colman Family Chair in Pediatric Inflammatory Bowel Disease; Professor, University of Pennsylvania, School of Medicine; Director, Center for Pediatric Inflammatory Bowel Disease, The Children's Hospital of Philadelphia, Philadelphia, Pennsylvania
Inflammatory Bowel Disease; Eosinophilic Gastroenteritis

Christina Bales, MD
Fellow, Division of Gastroenterology, Hepatology, and Nutrition, The Children's Hospital of Philadelphia, Philadelphia, Pennsylvania
Intestinal Atresia, Stenosis, and Malrotation

William F. Balistreri, MD
Director Emeritus, Pediatric Liver Care Center; Medical Director Emeritus, Liver Transplantation, Dorothy M.M. Kersten Professor of Pediatrics, Division of Gastroenterology, Hepatology and Nutrition at Cincinnati Children's Hospital Medical Center, University of Cincinnati College of Medicine, Cincinnati, Ohio
Morphogenesis of the Liver and Biliary System; Manifestations of Liver Disease; Neonatal Cholestasis; Metabolic Diseases of the Liver; Viral Hepatitis; Liver Disease Associated with Systemic Disorders; Mitochondrial Hepatopathies

Robert S. Baltimore, MD
Professor of Pediatrics and of Epidemiology and Public Health, Department of Pediatrics, Section of Pediatric Infectious Disease, Yale University School of Medicine, New Haven, Connecticut
Listeria monocytogenes; Pseudomonas aeruginosa; Burkholderia; Stenotrophomonas

Manisha Balwani, MD, MS
Assistant Professor, Department of Genetics and Genomic Sciences, Mount Sinai School of Medicine, New York, New York
The Porphyrias

Shahida Baqar, PhD
Head, Immunology Branch, Infectious Diseases Directorate, Enteric Diseases Department, Naval Medical Research Center, Silver Spring, Maryland
Campylobacter

Christine E. Barron, MD
Assistant Professor, Department of Pediatrics, Warren Alpert Medical School at Brown University, Rhode Island Hospital, Providence, Rhode Island
Adolescent Rape

Dorsey M. Bass, MD
Associate Professor of Pediatrics, Department of Pediatrics, Stanford University School of Medicine, Division of Pediatric Gastroenterology, Palo Alto, California
Rotaviruses, Caliciviruses, and Astroviruses

Mark L. Batshaw, MD
Chief Academic Officer, Children's National Medical Center, Chairman of Pediatrics and Associate Dean for Academic Affairs, George Washington University School of Medicine, Washington, District of Columbia
Intellectual Disability

Richard E. Behrman, MD
Emeritus Professor of Pediatrics and Dean, Case Western Reserve University School of Medicine; Clinical Professor of Pediatrics, University of California, San Francisco, and George Washington University, Washington, District of Columbia; Director, Non-Profit Health Care and Educational Consultants, Santa Barbara, California
Overview of Pediatrics

Michael J. Bell, MD
Associate Professor of Critical Care Medicine, Neurological Surgery and Pediatrics; Director, Pediatric Neurocritical Care; Director, Pediatric Neurotrauma Center; Associate Director, Safar Center of Resuscitation Research, University of Pittsburgh School of Medicine, Pittsburgh, Pennsylvania
Neurologic Emergencies and Stabilization

John W. Belmont, MD, PhD
Professor, Department of Molecular and Human Genetics, and Pediatrics, Baylor College of Medicine, Houston, Texas
Genetics of Common Disorders

Daniel K. Benjamin, Jr., MD, MPH, PhD
Professor of Pediatrics, Duke University; Chief, Division of Quantitative Sciences; Director, DCRI Clinical Research Fellowship Program, Duke University Health System, Durham, North Carolina
Principles of Antifungal Therapy; Candida

Michael J. Bennett, PhD, FRCPath, FACB, DABCC
Professor of Pathology & Laboratory Medicine, University of Pennsylvania; Evelyn Willing Bromley Endowed Chair in Clinical Laboratories & Pathology; Director, Metabolic Disease Laboratory, The Children's Hospital of Philadelphia, Philadelphia, Pennsylvania
Defects in Metabolism of Liquids

Daniel Bernstein, MD
Chief, Division of Pediatric Cardiology; Director, Children's Heart Center, Lucile Packard Children's Hospital at Stanford; Alfred Woodley Salter and Mabel G. Salter Professor of Pediatrics, Stanford University, Palo Alto, California
Cardiac Development; The Fetal to Neonatal Circulatory Transition; History and Physical Examination; Laboratory Evaluation; Epidemiology and Genetic Basis of Congenital Heart Disease; Evaluation of the Infant or Child with Congenital Heart Disease; Acyanotic Congenital Heart Disease: The Left-to-Right Shunt Lesions; Acyanotic Congenital Heart Disease: The Obstructive Lesions; Acyanotic Heart Disease: Regurgitant Lesions; Cyanotic Congenital Heart Disease: Evaluation of the Critically Ill Neonate with Cyanosis and Respiratory Distress; Cyanotic Congenital Heart Lesions: Lesions Associated with Decreased Pulmonary Blood Flow; Cyanotic Congenital Heart Disease: Lesions Associated with Increased Pulmonary Blood Flow; Other Congenital Heart and Vascular Malformations; Pulmonary Hypertension; General Principles of Treatment of Congenital Heart Disease; Infective Endocarditis; Rheumatic Heart Disease; Heart Failure; Pediatric Heart and Heart-Lung Transplantation; Diseases of the Blood Vessels (Aneurysms and Fistulas)

Jatinder Bhatia, MD, FAAP
Professor and Chief, Division of Neonatology; Vice Chair for Clinical Research, Medical College of Georgia, Augusta, Georgia
Feeding Healthy Infants, Children, and Adolescents

Zulfiqar Ahmed Bhutta, MD, PhD
Husein Lalji Dewraj Professor & Founding Chair, Division of Women & Child Health, Aga Khan University, Karachi, Pakistan
Salmonella; *Acute Gastroenteritis in Children*

Leslie G. Biesecker, MD
Chief, Genetic Disease Research Branch, National Human Genome Research Institute, National Institutes of Health, Bethesda, Maryland
Dysmorphology

James Birmingham, MD
Clinical Assistant Professor, Michigan State University College of Human Medicine; Division Chief, Helen Devos Pediatric Rheumatology; Adult and Pediatric Rheumatologist, West Michigan Rheumatology, PLLC, Grand Rapids, Michigan
Ankylosing Spondylitis and Other Spondyloarthritides; Reactive and Postinfectious Arthritis

Samra S. Blanchard, MD
Associate Professor of Pediatrics; Division Head, Department of Pediatric Gastroenterology, University of Maryland, School of Medicine, Baltimore, Maryland
Peptic Ulcer Disease in Children

Ronald Blanton, MD, MSC
Professor, Center for Global Health and Diseases, Case Western Reserve University School of Medicine, Cleveland, Ohio
Adult Tapeworm Infections; Cysticercosis; Echinococcosis (Echinococcus granulosus *and* Echinococcus multilocularis)

Archie Bleyer, MD
Clinical Research Professor, Radiation Medicine, Oregon Health & Science University, Portland, Oregon
Principles of Treatment; The Leukemias

C.D.R. Lynelle M. Boamah, MD, MEd, FAAP
Staff Pediatric Gastroenterologist; Assistant Pediatric Program Director, Naval Medical Center San Diego, San Diego, California
Manifestations of Liver Disease

Steven R. Boas, MD
Associate Professor, Department of Pediatrics, Northwestern University Feinberg School of Medicine; Medical Director, Cystic Fibrosis Center of Chicago, Chicago, Illinois
Emphysema and Overinflation; α_1-Antitrypsin Deficiency and Emphysema; Other Distal Airway Diseases; Skeletal Diseases Influencing Pulmonary Function

Thomas F. Boat, MD
Professor of Pediatrics, Cincinnati Children's Hospital Medical Center; Executive Associate Dean for Clinical Affairs, University of Cincinnati College of Medicine, Cincinnati, Ohio
Chronic or Recurrent Respiratory Symptoms

Walter Bockting, PhD
Associate Professor, Department of Family Medicine and Community Health; Coordinator of Transgender Health Services, Program in Human Sexuality, University of Minnesota Medical School, Minneapolis, Minnesota
Adolescent Development

Mark Boguniewicz, MD
Professor, Department of Pediatrics, Division of Pediatric Allergy-Immunology, National Jewish Health and University of Colorado School of Medicine, Aurora, Colorado
Ocular Allergies; Adverse Reactions to Drugs

Daniel J. Bonthius, MD, PhD
Professor, Departments of Pediatrics and Neurology, University of Iowa School of Medicine, Iowa City, Iowa
Lymphocytic Choriomeningitis Virus

Laurence A. Boxer, MD
Henry and Mala Dorfman Family Professor of Pediatric Hematology/Oncology, University of Michigan School of Medicine, Ann Arbor, Michigan
Neutrophils; Eosinophils; Disorders of Phagocyte Function; Leukopenia; Leukocytosis

Amanda M. Brandow, DO, MS
Assistant Professor of Pediatrics, Department of Pediatrics, Section of Hematology/Oncology/Bone Marrow Transplantation, Medical College of Wisconsin, and Children's Research Institute of the Children's Hospital of Wisconsin, Milwaukee, Wisconsin
Polycythemia; Secondary Polycythemia; Anatomy and Function of the Spleen; Splenomegaly; Hyposplenism, Splenic Trauma, and Splenectomy

David Branski, MD
Professor and Chair of Pediatrics, The Hebrew University-Hadassah School of Medicine, Jerusalem, Israel
Disorders of Malabsorption; Chronic Diarrhea

David T. Breault, MD, PhD
Division of Endocrinology, Children's Hospital Boston, Boston, Massachusetts
Diabetes Insipidus; Other Abnormalities of Arginine Vasopressin Metabolism and Action

Rebecca H. Buckley, MD
J. Buren Sidbury Professor of Pediatrics, Professor of Immunology, Departments of Pediatrics and Immunology, Duke University Medical Center, Durham, North Carolina
Evaluation of Suspected Immunodeficiency; T Lymphocytes, B Lymphocytes, and Natural Killer Cells; Primary Defects of Antibody Production; Primary Defects of Cellular Immunity; Primary Combined Antibody and Cellular Immunodeficiencies

Cynthia Etzler Budek, MS, APN/NP, CPNP-AC/PC
Pediatric Nurse Practitioner, Transitional Care Unit/Pulmonary Habilitation Program, Children's Memorial Hospital, Chicago, Illinois
Chronic Respiratory Insufficiency

E. Stephen Buescher, MD
Professor of Pediatrics, Department of Pediatrics, Eastern Virginia Medical School, Norfolk, Virginia
Diphtheria (Corynebacterium diphtheriae)

Gale R. Burstein, MD, MPH, FSAHM
Clinical Associate Professor, Department of Pediatrics, State University of New York at Buffalo School of Medicine and Biomedical Sciences, Adolescent Medicine, Buffalo, New York
The Epidemiology of Adolescent Health Problems; Delivery of Health Care to Adolescents; Sexually Transmitted Infections

Amaya Lopez Bustinduy, MD
Pediatric Infectious Diseases Fellow, Department of Pediatrics, Division of Infectious Diseases, Rainbow Babies & Children's Hospital, University Hospitals of Cleveland, Case Western Reserve University School of Medicine, Cleveland, Ohio
Schistosomiasis (Schistosoma); *Flukes (Liver, Lung, and Intestinal)*

Mitchell S. Cairo, MD
Chief, Division of Pediatric Blood and Marrow Transplantation; Professor of Pediatrics, Medicine, Pathology and Cell Biology, Morgan Stanley Children's Hospital of New York–Presbyterian, Columbia University, New York, New York
Lymphoma

Bruce M. Camitta, MD
Rebecca Jean Slye Professor, Department of Pediatrics, Hematology/Oncology, Medical College of Wisconsin, Midwest Center for Cancer and Blood Disorders, Milwaukee, Wisconsin
Polycythemia; Secondary Polycythemia; Anatomy and Function of the Spleen; Splenomegaly; Hyposplenism, Splenic Trauma, and Splenectomy; Anatomy and Function of the Lymphatic System; Abnormalities of Lymphatic Vessels; Lymphadenopathy

Angela Jean Peck Campbell, MD, MPH
Assistant Professor, Department of Pediatrics, Division of Infectious Diseases, University of Washington, Seattle Children's Hospital, Seattle, Washington
Parainfluenza Viruses

Rebecca G. Carey, MD, MS
Assistant Professor of Pediatrics, Tufts University, Attending Maine Medical Center, Division of Pediatric Gastroenterology, Portland, Maine
Metabolic Diseases of the Liver; Mitochondrial Hepatopathies

Waldemar A. Carlo, MD
Edwin M. Dixon Professor of Pediatrics; Director, Division of Neonatology, University of Alabama, Birmingham Hospital, Birmingham, Alabama
Overview of Mortality and Morbidity; The Newborn Infant; High-Risk Pregnancies; The Fetus; The High-Risk Infant; Clinical Manifestations of Diseases in the Newborn Period; Nervous System Disorders; Delivery Room Emergencies; Respiratory Tract Disorders; Digestive System Disorders; Blood Disorders; Genitourinary System; The Umbilicus; Metabolic Disturbances

Robert B. Carrigan, MD
The Children's Hospital of Philadelphia, Philadelphia, Pennsylvania
The Upper Limb

Mary T. Caserta, MD
Associate Professor of Pediatrics, Department of Pediatrics, Division of Infectious Diseases; Director, Pediatric Infectious Diseases Fellowship, University of Rochester Medical Center, Rochester, New York
Roseola (Human Herpesviruses 6 and 7); Human Herpesvirus 8

Ellen Gould Chadwick, MD
Irene Heinz Given and John LaPorte Given Professor of Pediatrics, Feinberg School of Medicine, Northwestern University; Associate Director, Section of Pediatric, Adolescent and Maternal HIV Infection, Division of Infectious Diseases, Children's Memorial Hospital, Chicago, Illinois
Acquired Immunodeficiency Syndrome (Human Immunodeficiency Virus)

Lisa J. Chamberlain, MD, MPH
Assistant Professor of Pediatrics, Division of General Pediatrics, Stanford University School of Medicine, Palo Alto, California
Chronic Illness in Childhood

Jennifer I. Chapman, MD
Attending, Pediatric Emergency Medicine, PEM Fellowship Director; Assistant Professor of Pediatrics, Children's National Medical Center, George Washington University School of Medicine, Washington, District of Columbia
Principles Applicable to the Developing World

Ira M. Cheifetz, MD, FCCM, FAARC
Professor of Pediatrics; Chief, Pediatric Critical Care Medicine; Medical Director, Pediatric ICU; Medical Director, Pediatric Respiratory Care & ECMO Programs, Duke Children's Hospital, Durham, North Carolina
Pediatric Emergencies and Resuscitation; Shock

Wassim Chemaitilly, MD
Assistant Professor of Pediatrics, Pediatric Endocrinology, University of Pittsburgh, Pittsburgh, Pennsylvania
Physiology of Puberty; Disorders of Pubertal Development

Sharon F. Chen, MD, MS
Instructor, Department of Pediatrics, Stanford University School of Medicine, Stanford, California; Attending Physician, Division of Pediatric Infectious Diseases, Lucile Packard Children's Hospital, Palo Alto, California
Principles of Antiparasitic Therapy

Yuan-Tsong Chen, MD, PhD
Professor, Department of Pediatrics, Genetics, Duke University Medical Center, Durham, North Carolina
Defects in Metabolism of Carbohydrates

Russell W. Chesney, MD
Le Bonheur Professor and Chair, Department of Pediatrics, University of Tennessee Health Science Center, Le Bonheur Children's Medical Center, Memphis, Tennessee
Renal Tubular Acidosis; Bone Structure, Growth, and Hormonal Regulation; Primary Chondrodystrophy (Metaphyseal Dysplasia); Hypophosphatasia; Hyperphosphatasia; Osteoporosis

Jennifer A. Chiriboga, PhD
Pediatric and School Psychologist; Assistant Professor of School Psychology, Duquesne University, Pittsburgh, Pennsylvania
Anxiety Disorders

Robert D. Christensen, MD
Director, Neonatology Research, Intermountain Healthcare; Director, Neonatology, Urban North Region, Intermountain Healthcare, McKay-Dee Hospital, Ogden, Utah
Development of the Hematopoietic System

Andrew Chu, MD
Fellow, Division of Gastroenterology, Hepatology & Nutrition, The Children's Hospital of Philadelphia, Philadelphia, Pennsylvania
Superior Mesenteric Artery Syndrome (Wilkie Syndrome, Cast Syndrome, Arteriomesenteric Duodenal Compression Syndrome); Ileus, Adhesions, Intussusception, and Closed-Loop Obstructions

Michael J. Chusid, MD
Professor and Chief, Pediatric Infectious Diseases, Medical College of Wisconsin, Milwaukee, Wisconsin
Infection Prevention and Control; Other Anaerobic Infections

Theodore J. Cieslak, MD
Colonel, Medical Corps, USA; Department of Defense Liaison Officer, Centers for Disease Control and Prevention, Atlanta, Georgia
Biologic and Chemical Terrorism

Jeff A. Clark, MD
Associate Professor of Pediatrics, Wayne State University School of Medicine; Associate Director PICU, Children's Hospital of Michigan, Detroit, Michigan
Respiratory Distress and Failure

Thomas G. Cleary, MD
Professor of Epidemiology, Center for Infectious Diseases, University of Texas School of Public Health, University of Texas Health Science Center—Houston, Houston, Texas
Shigella; Escherichia coli

John David Clemens, MD
Director-General, International Vaccine Institute, Kwanak, Seoul, Korea
International Immunization Practices

Joanna S. Cohen, MD
Assistant Professor of Pediatrics and Emergency Medicine, Children's National Medical Center, Washington, District of Columbia
Care of Abrasions and Minor Lacerations

Mitchell B. Cohen, MD
Professor and Vice-Chair of Pediatrics; Director, Gastroenterology, Hepatology, and Nutrition, Department of Pediatrics, Cincinnati Children's Hospital Medical Center, Cincinnati, Ohio
Clostridium difficile *Infection*

Pinchas Cohen, MD
Professor and Chief, UCLA—Pediatric Endocrinology, Los Angeles, California
Hyperpituitarism, Tall Stature, and Overgrowth Syndromes

Michael Cohen-Wolkowiez, MD
Assistant Professor, Department of Pediatrics, Duke Clinical Research Institute, Durham, North Carolina
Principles of Antifungal Therapy

Robert A. Colbert, MD, PhD
Senior Investigator; Chief, Pediatric Translational Research Branch, NIAMS, National Institutes of Health, DHHS, Bethesda, Maryland
Ankylosing Spondylitis and Other Spondyloarthritides; Reactive and Postinfectious Arthritis

F. Sessions Cole, MD
Park J. White, MD, Professor of Pediatrics; Assistant Vice Chancellor for Children's Health; Director, Division of Newborn Medicine, St. Louis Children's Hospital, St. Louis, Missouri
Pulmonary Alveolar Proteinosis; Inherited Disorders of Surfactant Metabolism

Joanna C.M. Cole, PhD
Clinical Psychologist, Department of Child and Adolescent Psychiatry; Director of Child Psychology Training, Boston Medical Center, Boston University School of Medicine, Boston, Massachusetts
Suicide and Attempted Suicide

John L. Colombo, MD
Pediatric Pulmonology and Nebraska Cystic Fibrosis Center, University of Nebraska Medical Center and Children's Hospital, Omaha, Nebraska
Aspiration Syndromes; Chronic Recurrent Aspiration

Amber R. Cooper, MD, MSCI
Assistant Professor, Department of Obstetrics and Gynecology, Division of Reproductive Endocrinology and Infertility, Washington University School of Medicine in St. Louis, St. Louis, Missouri
Vulvovaginal and Müllerian Anomalies

Ronina A. Covar, MD
Associate Professor, Department of Pediatrics, National Jewish Health, Denver, Colorado
Childhood Asthma

Barbara Cromer, MD
Professor of Pediatrics, Case Western Reserve University School of Medicine, Department of Pediatrics, MetroHealth Medical Center, Cleveland, Ohio
Adolescent Development; Delivery of Health Care to Adolescents; The Breast; Menstrual Problems; Contraception

James E. Crowe, Jr., MD
Professor, Department of Pediatrics, Microbiology, and Immunology, Vanderbilt University Medical Center, Nashville, Tennessee
Respiratory Syncytial Virus; Human Metapneumovirus

Natoshia Raishevich Cunningham, MS
Doctoral Candidate, Clinical Psychology, Virginia Polytechnic Institute and State University, Cincinnati, Ohio
Attention-Deficit/Hyperactivity Disorder

Steven J. Czinn, MD
Professor and Chair, Department of Pediatrics, University of Maryland School of Medicine, Baltimore, Maryland
Peptic Ulcer Disease in Children

Toni Darville, MD
Chief, Division of Infectious Diseases, Professor of Pediatrics and Immunology, Children's Hospital of Pittsburgh at UPMC, Pittsburgh, Pennsylvania
Neisseria gonorrhoeae *(Gonococcus)*

Robert S. Daum, MD, CM
Professor of Pediatrics, Microbiology, and Molecular Medicine, The University of Chicago Medical Center, Department of Pediatrics, Section of Infectious Diseases, Chicago, Illinois
Haemophilus influenzae

Richard S. Davidson, MD
Associate Professor of Orthopaedic Surgery, The Children's Hospital of Philadelphia, Philadelphia, Pennsylvania
The Foot and Toes; Leg-Length Discrepancy; Arthrogryposis

H. Dele Davies, MD, MS, MHCM
Professor and Chair, Department of Pediatrics and Human Development, Michigan State University, East Lansing, Michigan
Chancroid (Haemophilus ducreyi); *Syphilis* (Treponema pallidum); *Nonvenereal Treponemal Infections*; Leptospira; *Relapsing Fever* (Borrelia)

Peter S. Dayan, MD, MSc
Associate Director and Fellowship Director, Division of Pediatric Emergency Medicine, Morgan Stanley Children's Hospital of New York–Presbyterian, New York, New York
Acute Care of the Victim of Multiple Trauma

Michael R. DeBaun, MD, MPH
Professor of Pediatrics and Medicine, J.C. Peterson Professor, Vice Chair for Clinical Research, Pediatrics Director, Vanderbilt-Meharry Center of Excellence in Sickle Cell Disease, Vanderbilt University, Nashville, Tennessee
Hemoglobinopathies

Guenet H. Degaffe, MD
Fellow—PGY 6, Department of Pediatric Infectious Diseases, University of Texas Houston Medical School, Department of Pediatrics, Houston, Texas
Aeromonas *and* Plesiomonas

David R. DeMaso, MD
Psychiatrist-in-Chief and Chairman of Psychiatry, Children's Hospital Boston; The Leon Eisenberg Chair in Psychiatry, Children's Hospital Boston; Professor of Psychiatry and Pediatrics, Harvard Medical School, Boston, Massachusetts
Assessment and Interviewing; Psychologic Treatment of Children and Adolescents; Psychosomatic Illness; Rumination, Pica, and Elimination (Enuresis, Encopresis) Disorders; Habit and Tic Disorders; Mood Disorders; Suicide and Attempted Suicide; Disruptive Behavioral Disorders; Pervasive Developmental Disorders and Childhood Psychosis

Mark R. Denison, MD
Professor of Pediatrics, Microbiology and Immunology, Vanderbilt University Medical Center, Nashville, Tennessee
Coronaviruses

Arlene E. Dent, MD, PhD
Assistant Professor, Case Western Reserve University School of Medicine, Rainbow Babies & Children's Hospital, Pediatric Infectious Diseases, RBC, Center for Global Health & Diseases, Cleveland, Ohio
Ascariasis (Ascaris lumbricoides); *Trichuriasis* (Trichuris trichiura); *Enterobiasis* (Enterobius vermicularis); *Strongyloidiasis* (Strongyloides stercoralis); *Lymphatic Filariasis* (Brugia malayi, Brugia timori, *and* Wuchereria bancrofti); *Other Tissue Nematodes; Toxocariasis (Visceral and Ocular Larva Migrans); Trichinosis* (Trichinella spiralis)

Nirupama K. DeSilva, MD
Assistant Professor, Resident Program Director; Director, Pediatric and Adolescent Gynecology, University of Oklahoma-Tulsa, Tulsa, Oklahoma
Breast Concerns

Robert J. Desnick, PhD, MD
Dean for Genetics and Genomics; Professor and Chairman, Department of Genetics and Genomic Sciences, Mount Sinai School of Medicine; Physician-in-Chief, Department of Medical Genetics and Genomics, The Mount Sinai Hospital, New York, New York
Defects in Metabolism of Lipids; Defects in Metabolism of Carbohydrates; The Porphyrias

Gabrielle deVeber, MD
Professor of Paediatrics, University of Toronto; Senior Scientist, Hospital for Sick Children Research Institute; Director, Children's Stroke Program and Staff Neurologist, Division of Neurology, Hospital for Sick Children, Toronto, Ontario, Canada
Pediatric Stroke Syndromes

Esi Morgan DeWitt, MD, MSCE
Assistant Professor, Division of Pediatric Rheumatology, Division of Health Policy and Clinical Effectiveness, Cincinnati Children's Hospital Medical Center, Cincinnati, Ohio
Treatment of Rheumatic Diseases; Sarcoidosis

Chetan Anil Dhamne, MD
Fellow, Pediatric Hematology Oncology, University of Texas MD Anderson Cancer Center, Houston, Texas
Neoplasms of the Kidney

Prof. Anil Dhawan, MD, FRCPCH
Professor of Paediatric Hepatology, Pediatric Liver, GI, and Nutrition Centre, King's College London School of Medicine, King's College Hospital NSH Foundation Trust, Denmark Hill, London
Liver and Biliary Disorders Causing Malabsorption

Harry Dietz III, MD
Victor A. McKusick Professor of Medicine and Genetics, Department of Pediatrics, Institute of Genetic Medicine; Investigator, Howard Hughes Medical Institute, Johns Hopkins University School of Medicine, Baltimore, Maryland
Marfan Syndrome

Lydia J. Donoghue, MD
CHM Department of Pediatric Surgery, Wayne State University, Detroit, Michigan
Tumors of the Digestive Tract

Patricia A. Donohoue, MD
Professor and Chief of Pediatric Endocrinology and Diabetes, Department of Pediatrics, Medical College of Wisconsin, Milwaukee, Wisconsin
Development and Function of the Gonads; Hypofunction of the Testes; Pseudoprecocity Resulting from Tumors of the Testes; Gynecomastia; Hypofunction of the Ovaries; Pseudoprecocity Due to Lesions of the Ovary; Disorders of Sex Development

Mary K. Donovan, RN, CS, PNP
Pediatric Nurse Practitioner, Shriners Hospital for Children, Shriners Burns Hospital, Boston, Massachusetts
Burn Injuries; Cold Injuries

John P. Dormans, MD
Professor of Orthopedic Surgery, Department of Orthopedics, University of Pennsylvania, The Children's Hospital of Philadelphia, Philadelphia, Pennsylvania
Growth and Development; Evaluation of the Child; The Hip; The Spine; The Neck; Common Fractures

Daniel A. Doyle, MD
Associate Professor of Pediatrics, Thomas Jefferson University, Philadelphia, Pennsylvania; Staff Endocrinologist, Alfred I. duPont Hospital for Children, Wilmington, Delaware
Hormones and Peptides of Calcium Homeostasis and Bone Metabolism; Hypoparathyroidism; Pseudohypoparathyroidism (Albright Hereditary Osteodystrophy); Hyperparathyroidism

Jefferson Doyle, MBBChir, MHS, MA(Oxon)
Post-Doctoral Fellow, Institute of Genetic Medicine, Johns Hopkins University School of Medicine, Baltimore, Maryland
Marfan Syndrome

Stephen C. Dreskin, MD, PhD
Professor of Medicine and Immunology, Division of Allergy and Clinical Immunology, University of Colorado School of Medicine, Aurora, Colorado
Urticaria (Hives) and Angioedema

Denis S. Drummond, MD, FRCS(C)
The Children's Hospital of Philadelphia, Professor of Orthopaedic Surgery, University of Pennsylvania, Philadelphia, Pennsylvania
Arthrogryposis

Howard Dubowitz, MD, MS
Professor of Pediatrics; Director, Center for Families; Chief, Division of Child Protection, Department of Pediatrics, University of Maryland School of Medicine, Baltimore, Maryland
Abused and Neglected Children

J. Stephen Dumler, MD
Professor, Division of Medical Microbiology, Department of Pathology, Johns Hopkins University School of Medicine, Johns Hopkins Hospital, Baltimore, Maryland
Spotted Fever and Transitional Group Rickettsioses; Scrub Typhus (Orientia tsutsugamushi); *Typhus Group Rickettsioses; Ehrlichioses and Anaplasmosis; Q Fever* (Coxiella burnetii)

Janet Duncan, RN, MSN, CPNP, CPON
Nursing Director, Pediatric Palliative Care Division, Children's Hospital Boston and Dana-Farber Cancer Institute, Boston, Massachusetts
Pediatric Palliative Care

Paula M. Duncan, MD
Professor, Department of Pediatrics, University of Vermont, Burlington, Vermont
Maximizing Children's Health: Screening, Anticipatory Guidance, and Counseling

LauraLe Dyner, MD
Assistant Professor, Lucile Packard Children's Hospital at Stanford, Stanford University, Palo Alto, California
Central Nervous System Infections; Brain Abscess

Michael G. Earing, MD
Associate Professor of Internal Medicine and Pediatrics, Divisions of Adult Cardiovascular Medicine and Pediatric Cardiology, Children's Hospital of Wisconsin, Medical College of Wisconsin, Milwaukee, Wisconsin
Congenital Heart Disease in Adults

Elizabeth A. Edgerton, MD, MPH, FAAP
Division of Emergency Medicine, Children's National Medical Center, Washington, District of Columbia
Interfacility Transport of the Seriously Ill or Injured Pediatric Patient

Marie Egan, MD
Associate Professor, Departments of Pediatrics and Cellular and Molecular Physiology, Yale School of Medicine, New Haven, Connecticut
Cystic Fibrosis

Jack S. Elder, MD
Associate Director, Vattikuti Urology Institute; Chief of Urology, Henry Ford Health System, Department of Urology, Children's Hospital of Michigan, Detroit, Michigan; Clinical Professor of Urology, Case Western Reserve University School of Medicine, Cleveland, Ohio
Congenital Anomalies and Dysgenesis of the Kidneys; Urinary Tract Infections; Vesicoureteral Reflux; Obstruction of the Urinary Tract; Anomalies of the Bladder; Neuropathic Bladder; Voiding Dysfunction; Anomalies of the Penis and Urethra; Disorders and Anomalies of the Scrotal Contents; Trauma to the Genitourinary Tract; Urinary Lithiasis

Sara B. Eleoff, MD
Clinical Instructor in Pediatrics, University of Rochester School of Medicine and Dentistry, Rochester, New York
Foster and Kinship Care

Dianne S. Elfenbein, MD
Professor of Pediatrics, Clinical Educator, St. Louis University School of Medicine; Director of Adolescent Medicine, Cardinal Glennon Children's Medical Center, Department of Pediatrics, St. Louis, Missouri
Adolescent Pregnancy

Stephen C. Eppes, MD
Professor of Pediatrics, Jefferson Medical College; Division Chief, Pediatric Infectious Diseases, Alfred I. duPont Hospital for Children, Wilmington, Delaware
Lyme Disease (Borrelia burgdorferi)

Michele Burns Ewald, MD
Assistant Professor of Pediatrics, Harvard Medical School, Pediatric Emergency Medicine/Toxicology, Children's Hospital Boston, Boston, Massachusetts
Poisonings

Jessica K. Fairley, MD
Fellow, Division of Infectious Diseases and HIV Medicine, Case Western Reserve University School of Medicine, University Hospitals Case Medical Center, Cleveland, Ohio
Health Advice for Children Traveling Internationally

Susan Feigelman, MD
Associate Professor, Department of Pediatrics, University of Maryland School of Medicine, Baltimore, Maryland
Overview and Assessment of Variability; The First Year; The Second Year; The Preschool Years; Middle Childhood

Marianne E. Felice, MD
Professor and Chair, Department of Pediatrics, University of Massachusetts Medical School; Physician-in-Chief, UMass Memorial Children's Medical Center, Worcester, Massachusetts
Adolescent Pregnancy; Adolescent Rape

Eric I. Felner, MD, MSCR
Associate Professor of Pediatrics, Division of Pediatric Endocrinology, Children's Healthcare of Atlanta (CHOA); Director, Pediatric Endocrinology Fellowship Program, Emory University School of Medicine; Adjunct Associate Professor of Chemical and Biomolecular Engineering, School of Chemical and Biomolecular Engineering, Georgia Institute of Technology, Atlanta, Georgia
Hormones of the Hypothalamus and Pituitary; Hypopituitarism

Edward Fels, MD
Pediatric and Adult Rheumatology, Rheumatology Associates, P.A., Portland, Maine
Vasculitis Syndromes

Thomas Ferkol, MD
Professor of Pediatrics, Cell Biology and Physiology, Washington University School of Medicine in St. Louis, St. Louis, Missouri
Primary Ciliary Dyskinesia (Immotile Cilia Syndrome)

Jonathan D. Finder, MD
Professor of Pediatrics, University of Pittsburgh School of Medicine; Clinical Director, Division of Pulmonology Medicine, Children's Hospital of Pittsburgh, Pittsburgh, Pennsylvania
Bronchomalacia and Tracheomalacia; Congenital Disorders of the Lung

Kristin N. Fiorino, MD
Assistant Professor, Division of Gastroenterology, Hepatology and Nutrition, The Children's Hospital of Philadelphia, Philadelphia, Pennsylvania
Motility Disorders and Hirschsprung Disease

David M. Fleece, MD
Associate Professor of Clinical Pediatrics, Pediatrics, Temple University School of Medicine, Philadelphia, Pennsylvania
Sporotrichosis (Sporothrix schenckii)

Patricia M. Flynn, MD
Member, Department of Infectious Diseases, St. Jude Children's Research Hospital; Professor, Departments of Pediatrics and Preventive Medicine, University of Tennessee Health Science Center, Memphis, Tennessee
Infection Associated with Medical Devices; Cryptosporidium, Isospora, Cyclospora, *and Microsporidia*

Joel A. Forman, MD
Associate Professor, Departments of Pediatrics and Preventive Medicine; Vice-Chair for Education and Residency Program Director, Department of Pediatrics, Mount Sinai School of Medicine, New York, New York
Chemical Pollutants

Michael M. Frank, MD
Samuel L. Katz Professor of Pediatrics, Professor of Medicine and Immunology, Duke University Medical Center, Durham, North Carolina
Urticaria (Hives) and Angioedema

Melvin H. Freedman, MD, FRCPC, FAAP
Professor Emeritus, Department of Pediatrics, University of Toronto Faculty of Medicine; Honorary Consultant, Hematology-Oncology, Hospital for Sick Children, Toronto, Ontario, Canada
The Inherited Pancytopenias

Melissa Frei-Jones, MD, MSCI
Assistant Professor of Pediatrics, University of Texas Health Science Center at San Antonio, Division of Hematology-Oncology, CHRISTUS Santa Rosa Children's Hospital, San Antonio, Texas
Hemoglobinopathies

Jared E. Friedman, MD
New York State/American Program, Sackler School of Medicine, Tel Aviv University, Tel Aviv, Israel
Leg-Length Discrepancy

Sheila Gahagan, MD, MPH
Professor and Chief, Child Development and Community Health, Martin Stein Endowed Chair, Developmental-Behavioral Pediatrics, University of California, San Diego, California; Research Scientist, Center for Human Growth and Development, University of Michigan, Ann Arbor, Michigan
Overweight and Obesity

Paula Gardiner, MD, MPH
Assistant Professor, Department of Family Medicine, Boston University Medical Center, Boston, Massachusetts
Herbs, Complementary Therapies, and Integrative Medicine

Luigi Garibaldi, MD
Professor of Pediatrics; Clinical Director, Division of Pediatric Endocrinology, Children's Hospital of the University of Pittsburgh Medical Center, Pittsburgh, Pennsylvania
Physiology of Puberty; Disorders of Pubertal Development

Gregory M. Gauthier, MD, MS
Assistant Professor (CHS), Department of Medicine, Section of Infectious Diseases, University of Wisconsin–Madison, Madison, Wisconsin
Blastomycosis (Blastomyces dermatitidis)

Abraham Gedalia, MD
Professor & Chief, Division of Pediatric Rheumatology, Department of Pediatrics, Children's Hospital of New Orleans, New Orleans, Louisiana
Behçet Disease; Sjögren Syndrome; Hereditary Periodic Fever Syndromes; Amyloidosis

Matthew J. Gelmini, LRT, RRT
Respiratory Care, Children's Hospital of Michigan, Detroit, Michigan
Long-Term Mechanical Ventilation in the Acutely Ill Child

Michael A. Gerber, MD
Cincinnati Children's Hospital Medical Center, Division of Infectious Diseases, Cincinnati, Ohio
Group A Streptococcus; Non–Group A or B Streptococci

K. Michael Gibson, PhD, FACMG
Professor and Chair, Department of Biological Sciences, Michigan Technological University, Houghton, Michigan
Genetic Disorders of Neurotransmitters

Mark Gibson, MD
Obstetrics and Gynecology, University of Utah School of Medicine, Salt Lake City, Utah
Polycystic Ovary Syndrome and Hirsutism

Francis Gigliotti, MD
Professor of Pediatrics, Chief of Infectious Diseases; Associate Chair for Academic Affairs, Department of Pediatrics, Infectious Diseases, Microbiology and Immunology, University of Rochester Medical Center, Rochester, New York
Pneumocystis jirovecii

Walter S. Gilliam, PhD
Associate Professor in Child Psychiatry and Psychology, Yale School of Medicine, Child Study Center, New Haven, Connecticut
Child Care: How Pediatricians Can Support Children and Families

Janet R. Gilsdorf, MD
Robert P. Kelch Research Professor and Director, Pediatric Infectious Diseases, University of Michigan Medical Center, Ann Arbor, Michigan
Neisseria meningitidis *(Meningococcus)*

Charles M. Ginsburg, MD
Marilyn R. Corrigan Distinguished Chair in Pediatric Research; Senior Associate Dean, University of Texas, Southwestern Medical Center, Dallas, Texas
Animal and Human Bites

Frances P. Glascoe, MD, PhD
Department of Pediatrics, Vanderbilt University, Mertztown, Pennsylvania
Developmental-Behavioral Screening and Surveillance

Donald A. Goldmann, MD
Professor of Pediatrics, Harvard Medical School; Professor of Immunology and Infectious Diseases, and Epidemiology, Harvard School of Public Health; Senior Associate in Infectious Diseases, Children's Hospital Boston, Boston, Massachusetts
Diagnostic Microbiology

Denise M. Goodman, MD, MS
Division of Critical Care Medicine, Children's Memorial Hospital, Northwestern University Feinberg School of Medicine, Chicago, Illinois
Wheezing, Bronchiolitis, and Bronchitis

Marc H. Gorelick, MD, MSCE
Professor and Chief, Pediatric Emergency Medicine, Medical College of Wisconsin, Children's Corporate Center, Milwaukee, Wisconsin
Evaluation of the Sick Child in the Office and Clinic

Gary J. Gosselin, MD
Instructor in Psychiatry, Harvard Medical School; Medical Director, Inpatient Psychiatry, Children's Hospital, Boston, Massachusetts
Habit and Tic Disorders; Pervasive Developmental Disorders and Childhood Psychosis

Jane M. Gould, MD
Attending Physician/Hospital Epidemiologist/Assistant Professor of Pediatrics, Pediatrics/Section of Infectious Diseases, Drexel University School of Medicine/St. Christopher's Hospital for Children, Philadelphia, Pennsylvania
Cryptococcus neoformans; *Histoplasmosis* (Histoplasma capsulatum); Paracoccidioides brasiliensis; *Zygomycosis (Mucormycosis)*

Olivier Goulet, MD, PhD
Professor of Pediatrics, Pediatric Gastroenterology-Hepatology and Nutrition, Reference Center for Rare Digestive Diseases, Intestinal Failure Rehabilitation Center, Hôpital Necker-Enfants Malades/AP-HP, University of Paris V—René Descartes, Paris, France
Other Malabsorptive Syndromes

Dan M. Granoff, MD
Clorox Endowed Chair for Immunobiology and Vaccine Development, Senior Research Scientist and Director, Center for Immunobiology and Vaccine Development, Children's Hospital Oakland Research Institute, Oakland, California
Neisseria meningitidis *(Meningococcus)*

Michael Green, MD, MPH
Professor of Pediatrics, Surgery and Clinical & Translational Science, University of Pittsburgh School of Medicine, Division of Infectious Diseases, Children's Hospital of Pittsburgh, Pittsburgh, Pennsylvania
Infections in Immunocompromised Persons

Thomas P. Green, MD
Founder's Board Centennial Professor and Chair, Department of Pediatrics, Northwestern University Medical School, Children's Memorial Hospital, Chicago, Illinois
Diagnostic Approach to Respiratory Disease; Chronic or Recurrent Respiratory Symptoms; Pulmonary Edema

Larry A. Greenbaum, MD, PhD
Director, Division of Pediatric Nephrology, Emory University and Children's Healthcare of Atlanta, Atlanta, Georgia
Rickets and Hypervitaminosis D; Vitamin E Deficiency; Vitamin K Deficiency; Micronutrient Mineral Deficiencies; Electrolyte and Acid-Base Disorders; Maintenance and Replacement Therapy; Deficit Therapy

Marie Michelle Grino, MD
Pediatrics, University of Texas Medical Branch, Department of Pediatrics, Galveston, Texas
Aspartic Acid (Canavan Disease)

Andrew B. Grossman, MD
Clinical Assistant Professor of Pediatrics, University of Pennsylvania School of Medicine; Attending Physician, Division of GI, Hepatology, and Nutrition, The Children's Hospital of Philadelphia, Philadelphia, Pennsylvania
Inflammatory Bowel Disease; Eosinophilic Gastroenteritis

David C. Grossman, MD, MPH
Senior Investigator, Group Health Research Institute; Professor, Health Services; Adjunct Professor, Pediatrics, University of Washington, Seattle, Washington
Injury Control

Alfredo Guarino, MD
Professor of Pediatrics, University of Naples "Federico II"; Chief, Division of Infectious Disease, Department of Pediatrics, University of Naples "Federico II," Naples, Italy
Chronic Diarrhea

Lisa R. Hackney, MD
Assistant Professor of Pediatrics, University of Rochester Medical Center, Pediatric Hematology/Oncology, Rochester, New York
Hereditary Stomatocytosis; Enzymatic Defects

Gabriel G. Haddad, MD
Chairman, Department of Pediatrics; Professor of Pediatrics & Neurosciences; Physician-in-Chief & Chief Scientific Officer, Rady Children's Hospital-San Diego, Department of Pediatrics, University of California, San Diego, California
Diagnostic Approach to Respiratory Disease

Joseph Haddad, Jr., MD
Director, Pediatric Otolaryngology/Head & Neck Surgery, Morgan Stanley Children's Hospital of New York–Presbyterian, New York, New York
Congenital Disorders of the Nose; Acquired Disorders of the Nose; Nasal Polyps; General Considerations and Evaluation; Hearing Loss; Congenital Malformations; External Otitis (Otitis Externa); The Inner Ear and Diseases of the Bony Labyrinth; Traumatic Injuries of the Ear and Temporal Bone; Tumors of the Ear and Temporal Bone

Joseph F. Hagan, Jr., MD, FAAP
Clinical Professor in Pediatrics, University of Vermont College of Medicine; Hagan and Rinehart Pediatricians, PLLC, Burlington, Vermont
Maximizing Children's Health: Screening, Anticipatory Guidance, and Counseling

Scott B. Halstead, MD
Director, Supportive Research and Development, Pediatric Dengue Vaccine Initiative, International Vaccine Institute, Seoul, Korea
Arboviral Encephalitis in North America; Arboviral Encephalitis outside North America; Dengue Fever and Dengue Hemorrhagic Fever; Yellow Fever; Other Viral Hemorrhagic Fevers; Hantavirus Pulmonary Syndrome

Margaret R. Hammerschlag, MD
Professor of Pediatrics and Medicine; Director, Division of Pediatric Infectious Diseases, SUNY Downstate Medical Center, Brooklyn, New York
Chlamydophila pneumoniae; Chlamydia trachomatis; *Psittacosis* (Chlamydophila psittaci)

Aaron Hamvas, MD
Professor, Department of Pediatrics, Washington University School of Medicine in St. Louis, St. Louis Children's Hospital, St. Louis, Missouri
Pulmonary Alveolar Proteinosis; Inherited Disorders of Surfactant Metabolism

James C. Harris, MD
Professor of Psychiatry and Behavioral Sciences, Pediatrics, and Mental Hygiene; Director, Developmental Neuropsychiatry, Department of Psychiatry and Behavioral Sciences, Johns Hopkins Medical Institutions, Baltimore, Maryland
Disorders of Purine and Pyrimidine Metabolism

Mary E. Hartman, MD, MPH
Assistant Professor of Pediatrics, Pediatrics/Pediatric Critical Care Medicine, Duke Children's Hospital, Duke University Medical Center, Durham, North Carolina
Pediatric Emergencies and Resuscitation

David B. Haslam, MD
Associate Professor of Pediatrics and Molecular Microbiology, Division of Infectious Diseases, Washington University School of Medicine in St. Louis, St. Louis, Missouri
Enterococcus

Fern R. Hauck, MD, MS
Professor of Family Medicine and Public Health Sciences; Director, International Family Medicine Clinic, Department of Family Medicine and Public Health Sciences, University of Virginia Health System, Charlottesville, Virginia
Sudden Infant Death Syndrome

Gregory F. Hayden, MD
Professor, Department of Pediatrics, University of Virginia School of Medicine; Attending Physician, University of Virginia Children's Hospital, Charlottesville, Virginia
The Common Cold; Acute Pharyngitis

Jacqueline T. Hecht, MS, PhD
Professor and Vice Chair for Research, Department of Pediatrics, University of Texas Medical School at Houston, Houston, Texas
General Considerations; Disorders Involving Cartilage Matrix Proteins; Disorders Involving Transmembrane Receptors; Disorders Involving Ion Transporters; Disorders Involving Transcription Factors; Disorders Involving Defective Bone Resorption; Disorders for Which Defects Are Poorly Understood or Unknown

Sabrina M. Heidemann, MD
Professor of Pediatrics, Wayne State University, Detroit, Michigan
Respiratory Pathophysiology and Regulation

J. Owen Hendley, MD
Professor of Pediatrics, Department of Pediatrics, University of Virginia Health System, Charlottesville, Virginia
Sinusitis; Retropharyngeal Abscess, Lateral Pharyngeal (Parapharyngeal) Abscess, and Peritonsillar Cellulitis/Abscess

Fred M. Henretig, MD
Professor, Pediatrics and Emergency Medicine, The Children's Hospital of Philadelphia, Division of Emergency Medicine, Philadelphia, Pennsylvania
Biologic and Chemical Terrorism

Gloria P. Heresi, MD
Professor, Pediatric Infectious Diseases, The University of Texas Health Science Center, Houston, Texas
Campylobacter; Yersinia; Aeromonas *and* Plesiomonas

Andrew D. Hershey, MD, PhD, FAHS
Professor of Pediatrics and Neurology, University of Cincinnati; Director, Headache Center; Associate Director, Neurology Research, Cincinnati Children's Hospital Medical Center, University of Cincinnati, College of Medicine, Cincinnati, Ohio
Headaches

Cynthia E. Herzog, MD
Professor, Division of Pediatrics, University of Texas MD Anderson Cancer Center, Houston, Texas
Retinoblastoma; Gonadal and Germ Cell Neoplasms; Neoplasms of the Liver; Benign Vascular Tumors; Rare Tumors

Jessica Hochberg, MD
Assistant Professor of Pediatrics, New York Medical College, Maria Ferari Children's Hospital, Valhalla, New York
Lymphoma

Lauren D. Holinger, MD, FAAP, FACS
Professor, Department of Otolaryngology—Head and Neck Surgery, Northwestern University Feinberg School of Medicine; Paul H. Holinger, MD, Professor, Head, Division of Otolaryngology, Department of Surgery, The Children's Memorial Hospital, Chicago, Illinois
Congenital Anomalies of the Larynx, Trachea, and Bronchi; Foreign Bodies of the Airway; Laryngotracheal Stenosis and Subglottic Stenosis; Neoplasms of the Larynx, Trachea, and Bronchi

Jeffrey D. Hord, MD
Director, Pediatric Hematology/Oncology; Professor of Pediatrics, NEOUCOMP, Akron, Ohio
The Acquired Pancytopenias

B. David Horn, MD
Assistant Professor of Clinical Orthopaedic Surgery, University of Pennsylvania School of Medicine, Division of Orthopaedic Surgery, Philadelphia, Pennsylvania
The Hip

William A. Horton, MD
Director of Research, Shriners Hospital for Children; Professor of Molecular & Medical Genetics, Oregon Health & Sciences University, Portland, Oregon
General Considerations; Disorders Involving Cartilage Matrix Proteins; Disorders Involving Transmembrane Receptors; Disorders Involving Ion Transporters; Disorders Involving Transcription Factors; Disorders Involving Defective Bone Resorption; Disorders for Which Defects Are Poorly Understood or Unknown

Harish S. Hosalkar, MD
Attending Orthopedic Surgeon, Clinical Professor of Orthopedic Surgery, School of Medicine, UCSD; Co-Director of International Center for Pediatric and Adolescent Hip Disorders; Director Hip Research Program, Pediatric Hip and Trauma Specialist, AONA Faculty for Pediatric Orthopedic Trauma, Rady Children's Hospital, UCSD, San Diego, California
The Foot and Toes; Arthrogryposis

Hidekazu Hosono, MD
Pediatric Endocrinology Fellow, UCLA-Mattel Children's Hospital, Los Angeles, California
Hyperpituitarism, Tall Stature, and Overgrowth Syndromes

Peter J. Hotez, MD, PhD
Distinguished Research Professor & Chair, Department of Microbiology, Immunology, and Tropical Medicine, George Washington University, Washington, District of Columbia
*Hookworms (*Necator americanus *and* Ancylostoma *spp.)*

Michelle S. Howenstine, MD
Professor of Clinical Pediatrics, Section of Pediatric Pulmonology, Critical Care and Pediatric Allergy; Center Director, Cystic Fibrosis Center, James Whitcomb Riley Hospital for Children, Indianapolis, Indiana
Interstitial Lung Diseases

Heather G. Huddleston, MD
Assistant Professor, University of California, San Francisco, Division of Reproductive Endocrine and Infertility, Department of Obstetrics, Gynecology and Reproductive Sciences, San Francisco, California
Polycystic Ovary Syndrome and Hirsutism

Vicki Huff, PhD
Professor, Department of Genetics, The University of Texas MD Anderson Cancer Center, Houston, Texas
Neoplasms of the Kidney

Denise Hug, MD
Assistant Professor of Ophthalmology, University of Missouri–Kansas City School of Medicine, Kansas City, Missouri
Growth and Development; Examination of the Eye; Abnormalities of Refraction and Accommodation; Disorders of Vision; Abnormalities of Pupil and Iris; Disorders of Eye Movement and Alignment; Abnormalities of the Lids; Disorders of the Lacrimal System; Disorders of the Conjunctiva; Abnormalities of the Cornea; Abnormalities of the Lens; Disorders of the Uveal Tract; Disorders of the Retina and Vitreous; Abnormalities of the Optic Nerve; Childhood Glaucoma; Orbital Abnormalities; Orbital Infections; Injuries to the Eye

Winston W. Huh, MD
Assistant Professor of Pediatrics, University of Texas MD Anderson Cancer Center, Division of Pediatrics, Houston, Texas
Gonadal and Germ Cell Neoplasms

Carl E. Hunt, MD
Research Professor of Pediatrics, Uniformed Services University of the Health Sciences, Chevy Chase, Maryland
Sudden Infant Death Syndrome

Anna Klaudia Hunter, MD
Fellow, Department of Pediatrics, Division of Pediatric Gastroenterology, Hepatology and Nutrition, Children's Hospital of Philadelphia, Philadelphia, Pennsylvania
Pyloric Stenosis and Other Congenital Anomalies of the Stomach

Patricia Ibeziako, MD
Director, Pediatric Psychiatry Consultation Service, Children's Hospital Boston; Instructor in Psychiatry, Harvard Medical School, Boston, Massachusetts
Psychosomatic Illness

Richard F. Jacobs, MD, FAAP
Robert H. Fiser, Jr., M.D. Endowed Chair in Pediatrics; Professor and Chair, Department of Pediatrics, University of Arkansas for Medical Sciences, Arkansas Children's Hospital, Little Rock, Arkansas
Actinomyces; Nocardia; *Tularemia* (Francisella tularensis); Brucella

Peter Jensen, MD
President and CEO, The REACH Institute; New York, New York; Co-Director, Division of Child Psychiatry & Psychology, The Mayo Clinic, Rochester, Minnesota
Attention-Deficit/Hyperactivity Disorder

Hal B. Jenson, MD, MBA
Chief Academic Officer, Baystate Medical Center; Professor of Pediatrics, and Dean, Western Campus of Tufts University School of Medicine, Springfield, Massachusetts
Chronic Fatigue Syndrome; Epstein-Barr Virus; Human T-Lymphotropic Viruses (1 and 2)

Chandy C. John, MD
Director, Center for Global Pediatrics; Professor of Pediatrics and Medicine, University of Minnesota Medical School, Minneapolis, Minnesota
Health Advice for Children Traveling Internationally; Giardiasis and Balantidiasis; Malaria (Plasmodium)

Michael V. Johnston, MD
Professor of Neurology, Pediatrics and Physical Medicine and Rehabilitation, Johns Hopkins University School of Medicine; Blum-Moser Chair for Pediatric Neurology, Kennedy Krieger Institute, Baltimore, Maryland
Congenital Anomalies of the Central Nervous System; Encephalopathies

Richard B. Johnston, Jr., MD
Professor of Pediatrics; Associate Dean for Research Development, University of Colorado School of Medicine—National Jewish Health, Aurora, Colorado
Monocytes, Macrophages, and Dendritic Cells; The Complement System; Disorders of the Complement System

Bridgette L. Jones, MD
Assistant Professor of Pediatrics, Pediatric Clinical Pharmacology and Allergy/Asthma/Immunology, Children's Mercy Hospital and Clinics, University of Missouri–Kansas City School of Medicine, Kansas City, Missouri
Principles of Drug Therapy

James F. Jones, MD
Research Medical Officer/Chronic Viral Diseases Branch, Division of High-Consequence Pathogens and Pathology, National Center for Emerging and Infectious Diseases, Centers for Disease Control and Prevention, Atlanta, Georgia
Chronic Fatigue Syndrome

Marsha Joselow, BS, MFA, MSW
LICSW, Social Worker; Social Work Fellowship Director, Pediatric Advanced Care Team, Children's Hospital Boston and Dana-Farber Cancer Institute, Boston, Massachusetts
Pediatric Palliative Care

Anupama Kalaskar, MD
Pediatric Infectious Disease Fellow, Department of Pediatrics, University of Texas Health Science Center at Houston, Houston, Texas
Yersinia

Linda Kaljee, PhD
Associate Professor, The Carman and Ann Adams Department of Pediatrics, Wayne State University, School of Medicine, Detroit, Michigan
Cultural Issues in Pediatric Care

Deepak Kamat, MD, PhD, FAAP
Professor and Vice Chair of Education, Department of Pediatrics, Wayne State University School of Medicine, Children's Hospital of Michigan, Detroit, Michigan
Fever; Fever without a Focus

Alvina R. Kansra, MD
Assistant Professor, Division of Endocrinology, Diabetes and Metabolism, Department of Pediatrics, Medical College of Wisconsin, Milwaukee, Wisconsin
Hypofunction of the Ovaries; Pseudoprecocity Due to Lesions of the Ovary

Sheldon L. Kaplan, MD
Professor and Vice-Chairman for Clinical Affairs; Head, Section of Infectious Diseases, Department of Pediatrics, Baylor College of Medicine; Chief, Infectious Disease Service, Texas Children's Hospital, Houston, Texas
Osteomyelitis; Septic Arthritis

Emily R. Katz, MD
Assistant Professor of Psychiatry and Human Behavior (Clinical), Alpert Medical School, Brown University; Director, Child and Adolescent Psychiatry, Consultation/Liaison Service, Hasbro Children's Hospital/Rhode Island Hospital, Providence, Rhode Island
Rumination, Pica, and Elimination (Enuresis, Encopresis) Disorders

James W. Kazura, MD
Professor of International Health and Medicine, Center for Global Health and Diseases, Case Western Reserve University School of Medicine, Cleveland, Ohio
Ascariasis (Ascaris lumbricoides); *Trichuriasis* (Trichuris trichiura); *Enterobiasis* (Enterobius vermicularis); *Strongyloidiasis* (Strongyloides stercoralis); *Lymphatic Filariasis* (Brugia malayi, Brugia timori, *and* Wuchereria bancrofti); *Other Tissue Nematodes; Toxocariasis (Visceral and Ocular Larva Migrans); Trichinosis* (Trichinella spiralis)

Virginia Keane, MD
Associate Professor of Pediatrics, University of Maryland School of Medicine, Baltimore, Maryland
Assessment of Growth

Gregory L. Kearns, PharmD, PhD
Marion Merrell Dow/Missouri Chair of Medical Research; Professor of Pediatrics and Pharmacology, University of Missouri–Kansas City; Chairman, Department of Medical Research; Associate Chairman, Department of Pediatrics; Director, Pediatric Pharmacology Research Unit, Children's Mercy Hospitals and Clinics, Kansas City, Missouri
Principles of Drug Therapy

Desmond P. Kelly, MD
Medical Director, Division of Developmental-Behavioral Pediatrics; Vice Chair for Academics, Children's Hospital, Greenville Hospital System; GHS Professor of Clinical Pediatrics, University of South Carolina School of Medicine, Columbia, South Carolina
Neurodevelopmental Function and Dysfunction in the School-Aged Child

Judith Kelsen, MD
Attending, Pediatric Gastroenterology, The Children's Hospital of Philadelphia, Philadelphia, Pennsylvania
Foreign Bodies and Bezoars

Kathi J. Kemper, MD, MPH, FAAP
Caryl J. Guth Chair for Complementary and Integrative Medicine; Professor, Pediatrics and Public Health Sciences, Wake Forest University School of Medicine, Winston-Salem, North Carolina
Herbs, Complementary Therapies, and Integrative Medicine

Melissa Kennedy, MD
Clinical Fellow, Pediatric Gastroenterology, Hepatology, and Nutrition, The Children's Hospital of Philadelphia, Philadelphia, Pennsylvania
Intestinal Atresia, Stenosis, and Malrotation; Intestinal Duplications, Meckel Diverticulum, and Other Remnants of the Omphalomesenteric Duct; Ileus, Adhesions, Intussusception, and Closed-Loop Obstructions; Malformations; Ascites

Eitan Kerem, MD
Professor and Chair, Department of Pediatrics, Hadassah University Medical Center, Jerusalem, Israel
Impact of Violence on Children

Joseph E. Kerschner, MD, FACS, FAAP
CEO, Children's Specialty Group; Senior Associate Dean of Clinical Affairs, Medical College of Wisconsin (MCW); Executive Vice President, Children's Hospital and Health System; Professor and Interim Chair, Department of Otolaryngology (MCW), Children's Hospital of Wisconsin, Milwaukee, Wisconsin
Otitis Media

Seema Khan, MBBS
Associate Professor of Pediatrics, Thomas Jefferson University, Philadelphia, Pennsylvania; Division of Gastroenterology, Nemours/Alfred I. duPont Hospital for Children, Wilmington, Delaware
Embryology, Anatomy, and Function of the Esophagus; Congenital Anomalies; Obstructing and Motility Disorders of the Esophagus; Dysmotility; Hiatal Hernia; Gastroesophageal Reflux Disease; Eosinophilic Esophagitis and Non-GERD Esophagitis; Esophageal Perforation; Esophageal Varices; Ingestions

Young-Jee Kim, MD
Associate Professor of Pediatrics, Section of Pediatric Pulmonology, Riley Hospital for Children, Indianapolis, Indiana
Interstitial Lung Diseases

Charles H. King, MD
Professor of International Health, Center for Global Health and Diseases, Case Western Reserve University School of Medicine, Cleveland, Ohio
Schistosomiasis (Schistosoma); *Flukes (Liver, Lung, and Intestinal)*

Stephen L. Kinsman, MD
Associate Professor of Neurology, Pediatric Neurology, Department of Neurosciences, Medical University of South Carolina, Charleston, South Carolina
Congenital Anomalies of the Central Nervous System

Adam Kirton, MD, MSc, FRCPC
Director, Calgary Pediatric Stroke Program; Assistant Professor of Pediatrics and Clinical Neuroscience, Faculty of Medicine, University of Calgary; Pediatric Neurologist, Alberta Children's Hospital, Calgary, Alberta, Canada
Pediatric Stroke Syndromes

Priya S. Kishnani, MD
Professor of Pediatrics, Division Chief, Medical Genetics, Duke University Medical Center, Durham, North Carolina
Defects in Metabolism of Carbohydrates

Nora T. Kizer, MD
Gynecologic Oncology Fellow, Division of Gynecologic Oncology, Washington University School of Medicine in St. Louis, St. Louis, Missouri
Neoplasms and Adolescent Screening for Human Papilloma Virus

Martin B. Kleiman, MD
Ryan White Professor of Pediatrics, Indiana University School of Medicine, Riley Children's Hospital, Indianapolis, Indiana
Coccidioidomycosis (Coccidioides species)

Bruce L. Klein, MD
Chief, Division of Transport Medicine, Children's National Medical Center, Washington, District of Columbia
Emergency Medical Services for Children; Acute Care of the Victim of Multiple Trauma

Bruce S. Klein, MD
Gerard B. Odell Professor, Pediatrics, Medicine and Medical Microbiology and Immunology, University of Wisconsin-Madison, Madison, Wisconsin
Blastomycosis (Blastomyces dermatitidis)

Michael D. Klein, MD
Arvin I. Philippart Endowed Chair in Pediatric Surgical Research; Professor of Surgery, Wayne State University, Children's Hospital of Michigan, Detroit, Michigan
Anorectal Malformations; Tumors of the Digestive Tract

Robert M. Kliegman, MD
Professor and Chair, Department of Pediatrics, Medical College of Wisconsin; Pediatrician-in-Chief, Pamela and Leslie Muma Chair in Pediatrics, Children's Hospital of Wisconsin; Executive Vice President, Children's Research Institute, Milwaukee, Wisconsin
Psychosis Associated with Epilepsy; Dysfluency (Stuttering, Stammering); Cholestasis; Liver Abscess

William C. Koch, MD, FAAP, FIDSA
Associate Professor of Pediatrics, Division of Infectious Diseases, Virginia Commonwealth University School of Medicine; Attending Physician, VCU Children's Medical Center, Medical College of Virginia Hospitals, Richmond, Virginia
Parvovirus B19

Patrick M. Kochanek, MD
Director, Safar Center for Resuscitation Research; Professor and Vice Chairman, Department of Critical Care Medicine; Professor of Anesthesiology, Clinical and Translational Science, and Pediatrics, University of Pittsburgh School of Medicine, Pittsburgh, Pennsylvania
Neurologic Emergencies and Stabilization

Eric Kodish, MD
F.J. O'Neill Professor and Chairman, Department of Bioethics, The Cleveland Clinic Foundation; Professor of Pediatrics, Lerner College of Medicine, Cleveland, Ohio
Ethics in Pediatric Care

Stephan A. Kohlhoff, MD
Assistant Professor, Department of Pediatrics, SUNY Downstate Medical Center, Brooklyn, New York
Chlamydophila pneumoniae; *Psittacosis* (Chlamydophila psittaci)

Elliot J. Krane, MD
Professor of Pediatrics and Anesthesia, Stanford University School of Medicine; Chief, Pediatric Pain Management Service, Lucile Packard Children's Hospital at Stanford, Stanford, California
Pediatric Pain Management

Peter J. Krause, MD
Senior Research Scientist, Yale School of Public Health, New Haven, Connecticut
Malaria (Plasmodium); *Babesiosis* (Babesia)

Richard E. Kreipe, MD
Professor, Division of Adolescent Medicine, Department of Pediatrics, Golisano Children's Hospital, University of Rochester School of Medicine, Rochester, New York
Eating Disorders

Steven E. Krug, MD
Professor of Pediatrics, Northwestern University Feinberg School of Medicine; Head, Division of Emergency Medicine, Children's Memorial Hospital, Chicago, Illinois
Emergency Medical Services for Children

John F. Kuttesch, Jr., MD, PhD
Director of Clinical Research, Division of Pediatric Hematology/Oncology and Stem Cell Transplantation, Penn State Hershey Children's Hospital; Professor of Pediatrics, Pennsylvania State University College of Medicine, Hershey, Pennsylvania
Brain Tumors in Childhood

Jennifer M. Kwon, MD, MPH
Associate Professor of Neurology and Pediatrics, University of Rochester Medical Center, Rochester, New York
Neurodegenerative Disorders of Childhood

Catherine S. Lachenauer, MD
Assistant Professor of Pediatrics, Harvard Medical School; Associate in Medicine, Division of Infectious Diseases, Children's Hospital Boston, Boston, Massachusetts
Group B Streptococcus

Stephan Ladisch, MD
Bosworth Chair in Cancer Biology, Center for Cancer and Immunology Research, Children's Research Institute; Children's National Medical Center and Vice Chair, Department of Pediatrics; Professor of Pediatrics and Biochemistry/Molecular Biology, George Washington University School of Medicine, Washington, District of Columbia
Histiocytosis Syndromes of Childhood

Stephen LaFranchi, MD
Professor, Department of Pediatrics, Oregon Health & Science University, Portland, Oregon
Thyroid Development and Physiology; Defects of Thyroxine-Binding Globulin; Hypothyroidism; Thyroiditis; Goiter; Hyperthyroidism; Carcinoma of the Thyroid

Oren Lakser, MD
Assistant Professor of Pediatrics, Medical College of Wisconsin; Pediatric Pulmonologist, Children's Physician Group—Illinois, Gurnee, Illinois
Parenchymal Disease with Prominent Hypersensitivity, Eosinophilic Infiltration, or Toxin-Mediated Injury; Bronchiectasis; Pulmonary Abscess

Marc B. Lande, MD, MPH
Associate Professor, Pediatric Nephrology, University of Rochester, School of Medicine and Dentistry, Rochester, New York
Systemic Hypertension

Philip J. Landrigan, MD, MSc
Ethel H. Wise Professor and Chairman, Department of Preventive Medicine; Professor of Pediatrics; Director, Children's Environmental Health Center; Dean for Global Health, Mount Sinai School of Medicine, New York, New York
Chemical Pollutants

Gregory L. Landry, MD
Professor, Department of Pediatrics, University of Wisconsin School of Medicine and Public Health, Madison, Wisconsin
Epidemiology and Prevention of Injuries; Management of Musculoskeletal Injury; Head and Neck Injuries; Heat Injuries; Female Athletes: Menstrual Problems and the Risk of Osteopenia; Performance-Enhancing Aids; Specific Sports and Associated Injuries

Wendy G. Lane, MD, MPH
Assistant Professor, Department of Epidemiology and Preventive Medicine and Department of Pediatrics, University of Maryland School of Medicine, Baltimore, Maryland
Abused and Neglected Children

Philip S. LaRussa, MD
Professor of Clinical Pediatrics, College of Physicians and Surgeons, Columbia University, New York, New York
Varicella-Zoster Virus Infections

Brendan Lee, MD, PhD
Professor, Department of Molecular and Human Genetics, Baylor College of Medicine; Houston, Texas; Investigator, Howard Hughes Medical Institute, Chevy Chase, Maryland
Integration of Genetics into Pediatric Practice; The Genetic Approach in Pediatric Medicine; The Human Genome; Patterns of Genetic Transmission; Cytogenetics; Genetics of Common Disorders

Chul Lee, PhD
Professor, Department of Preventive Medicine and Community Health, The University of Texas Medical Branch, Galveston, Texas
The Porphyrias

K. Jane Lee, MD, MA
Assistant Professor of Pediatrics, Medical College of Wisconsin, Milwaukee, Wisconsin
Brain Death

J. Steven Leeder, PharmD, PhD
Marion Merrell Dow/Missouri Endowed Chair in Pediatric Clinical Pharmacology; Chief, Division of Clinical Pharmacology and Medical Toxicology, Children's Mercy Hospital, Kansas City, Missouri
Pediatric Pharmacogenetics, Pharmacogenomics, and Pharmacoproteomics

Rebecca K. Lehman, MD
Instructor of Neurology & Pediatrics, University of Rochester Medical Center, Division of Child Neurology, Strong Memorial Hospital, Rochester, New York
Neurologic Evaluation

Michael J. Lentze, MD
Professor of Pediatrics, Zentrum für Kinderheilkunde, University Hospitals Bonn/Germany, Bonn, Germany
Disorders of Malabsorption

Norma B. Lerner, MD, MPH
Chief, Section of Hematology, St. Christopher's Hospital for Children, Philadelphia, Pennsylvania
The Anemias; Congenital Hypoplastic Anemia (Diamond-Blackfan Anemia); Pearson's Syndrome; Acquired Pure Red Blood Cell Anemia; Anemia of Chronic Disease and Renal Disease; Congenital Dyserythropoietic Anemias; Physiologic Anemia of Infancy; Megaloblastic Anemias; Iron-Deficiency Anemia

Steven Lestrud, MD
Department of Pediatrics, Feinberg School of Medicine, Northwestern University, Chicago, Illinois
Bronchopulmonary Dysplasia

Donald Y.M. Leung, MD, PhD
Professor of Pediatrics, University of Colorado Medical School; Edelstein Family Chair of Pediatric Allergy-Immunology, National Jewish Health, Denver, Colorado
Allergy and the Immunologic Basis of Atopic Disease; Diagnosis of Allergic Disease; Principles of Treatment of Allergic Disease; Allergic Rhinitis; Childhood Asthma; Atopic Dermatitis (Atopic Eczema); Insect Allergy; Ocular Allergies; Urticaria (Hives) and Angioedema; Anaphylaxis; Serum Sickness; Adverse Reactions to Foods; Adverse Reactions to Drugs

Chris A. Liacouras, MD
Professor of Pediatrics, Division of Gastroenterology, Hepatology and Nutrition, The Children's Hospital of Philadelphia, The University of Pennsylvania School of Medicine, Philadelphia, Pennsylvania
Normal Digestive Tract Phenomena; Major Symptoms and Signs of Digestive Tract Disorders; Normal Development, Structure, and Function; Pyloric Stenosis and Other Congenital Anomalies of the Stomach; Intestinal Atresia, Stenosis, and Malrotation; Intestinal Duplications, Meckel Diverticulum, and Other Remnants of the Omphalomesenteric Duct; Motility Disorders and Hirschsprung Disease; Ileus, Adhesions, Intussusception, and Closed-Loop Obstructions; Foreign Bodies and Bezoars; Functional Abdominal Pain (Nonorganic Chronic Abdominal Pain); Malformations; Ascites

Susanne Liewer, PharmD, BCOP
Assistant Professor, Adjunct Title Series, Division of Pharmacy Practice & Science, University of Kansas School of Pharmacy; Assistant Clinical Professor, Adjunct Title Series, Division of Pharmacy Practice & Science, University of Missouri–Kansas City School of Pharmacy; Clinical Pharmacy Manager, Clinical Pharmacy Specialist, Stem Cell Transplant, Children's Mercy Hospital, Kansas City, Missouri
Principles of Drug Therapy

Andrew H. Liu, MD
Associate Professor, Department of Pediatrics, National Jewish Health, University of Colorado School of Medicine, Aurora, Colorado
Childhood Asthma

Stanley F. Lo, PhD
Associate Professor, Pediatric Pathology, Children's Hospital of Wisconsin, Milwaukee, Wisconsin
Laboratory Testing in Infants and Children; Reference Intervals for Laboratory Tests and Procedures

Franco Locatelli, MD
Full Professor of Pediatrics, IRCCS Ospedale Bambino Gesù, University of Pavia, Rome, Italy
Principles and Clinical Indications; HSCT from Alternative Sources and Donors; Graft Versus Host Disease (GVHD) and Rejection; Infectious Complications of HSCT; Late Effects of HSCT

Sarah S. Long, MD
Professor of Pediatrics, Drexel University College of Medicine; Chief, Section of Infectious Diseases, St. Christopher's Hospital for Children, Philadelphia, Pennsylvania
Pertussis (Bordetella pertussis *and* Bordetella parapertussis)

Anna Lena Lopez, MD, MPH, FAAP
Director, Scientific Affairs, Asia-Pacific, Pfizer, Inc., Hong Kong
Cholera

Steven V. Lossef, MD
Associate Professor of Radiology; Director, Pediatric Interventional Radiology, Children's National Medical Center, Washington, District of Columbia
Pleurisy, Pleural Effusions, and Empyema; Pneumothorax; Hydrothorax; Hemothorax; Chylothorax

Jennifer A. Lowry, MD
Division of Clinical Pharmacology and Medical Toxicology, Children's Mercy Hospital; Assistant Professor, Department of Pediatrics, University of Missouri–Kansas City School of Medicine, Kansas City, Missouri
Principles of Drug Therapy

Kerith Lucco, MD
Clinical Instructor, Obstetrics, Gynecology and Reproductive Sciences, UCSF, San Francisco General Hospital; Volunteer Clinical Faculty, UCSF, San Francisco General Hospital, San Francisco, California
History and Physical Examination

G. Reid Lyon, PhD
Distinguished Professor and Chairman, Department of Education Policy and Leadership, Southern Methodist University; Distinguished Scientist in Cognition and Neuroscience, Center for Brain Health, University of Texas, Dallas, Texas
Dyslexia

Prashant V. Mahajan, MD, MPH, MBA
Division Chief and Research Director, Pediatric Emergency Medicine; Associate Professor of Pediatrics and Emergency Medicine, Carman and Ann Adams Department of Pediatrics, Children's Hospital of Michigan, Detroit, Michigan
Heavy Metal Intoxication

Akhil Maheshwari, MD
Associate Professor of Pediatrics; Director, Division of Neonatology, Department of Pediatrics, University of Illinois at Chicago, Chicago, Illinois
Respiratory Tract Disorders; Digestive System Disorders; Blood Disorders

Joseph A. Majzoub, MD
Professor of Pediatrics and Medicine, Harvard Medical School; Chief, Division of Endocrinology, Children's Hospital Boston, Boston, Massachusetts
Diabetes Insipidus; Other Abnormalities of Arginine Vasopressin Metabolism and Action

Asim Maqbool, MD
Assistant Professor of Pediatrics, Gastroenterology, Hepatology and Nutrition, The Children's Hospital of Philadelphia, University of Pennsylvania School of Medicine, Philadelphia, Pennsylvania
Nutritional Requirements

Ashley M. Maranich, MD
Staff, Pediatric Infectious Disease, San Antonio Military Medical Consortium, San Antonio, Texas
Malassezia

Mona Marin, MD
Medical Epidemiologist, Division of Viral Diseases, National Center for Immunization and Respiratory Diseases, Centers for Disease Control and Prevention, Atlanta, Georgia
Varicella-Zoster Virus Infections

Joan C. Marini, MD, PhD
Chief, Bone and Extracellular Matrix Branch, National Institute for Child Health and Development, National Institutes of Health, Bethesda, Maryland
Osteogenesis Imperfecta

Morri Markowitz, MD
Professor of Pediatrics, Albert Einstein College of Medicine; Clinical Director, Division of Pediatric Environmental Sciences, The Children's Hospital at Montefiore, Albert Einstein College of Medicine, Bronx, New York
Lead Poisoning

Kevin P. Marks, MD
General Pediatrician, PeaceHealth Medical Group; Assistant Clinical Professor, Oregon Health & Sciences University School of Medicine, Eugene, Oregon
Developmental-Behavioral Screening and Surveillance

Stacene R. Maroushek, MD, PhD, MPH
Assistant Professor of Pediatrics, Pediatric Infectious Diseases and General Pediatrics, Hennepin County Medical Center, Minneapolis, Minnesota
Adoption; Principles of Antimycobacterial Therapy

Wilbert H. Mason, MD, MPH
Chief Medical Quality Officer; Former Head, Division of Infectious Diseases, Children's Hospital of Los Angeles, Los Angeles, California
Measles; Rubella; Mumps

Christopher Mastropietro, MD
Assistant Professor of Pediatrics, Wayne State University, Carman and Ann Adams Department of Pediatrics, Division of Critical Care, Children's Hospital of Michigan, Detroit, Michigan
Mechanical Ventilation

Kimberlee M. Matalon, MD, PhD
Professor of Pediatrics, Biochemistry and Molecular Biology, University of Texas Medical Branch, Galveston, Texas
Aspartic Acid (Canavan Disease)

Reuben K. Matalon, MD, PhD
Professor of Pediatrics and Genetics, University of Texas Children's Hospital, Galveston, Texas
Aspartic Acid (Canavan Disease)

Robert Mazor, MD
Clinical Assistant Professor of Pediatrics, Division of Critical Care Medicine, Seattle Children's Hospital, Seattle, Washington
Pulmonary Edema

Susanna A. McColley, MD
Head, Division of Pulmonary Medicine; Director, Cystic Fibrosis Center, Northwestern University Feinberg School of Medicine, Children's Memorial Hospital, Chicago, Illinois
Pulmonary Tumors; Extrapulmonary Diseases with Pulmonary Manifestations

Margaret M. McGovern, MD, PhD
Professor and Chair, Department of Pediatrics, Stony Brook University Medical Center, Stony Brook, New York
Defects in Metabolism of Lipids; Defects in Metabolism of Carbohydrates

Heather S. McLean, MD
Assistant Professor, Division of Hospital and Emergency Medicine, Department of Pediatrics, Duke University Medical Center, Durham, North Carolina
Failure to Thrive

Rima McLeod, MD
Professor, Departments of Surgery (Visual Sciences) and Pediatrics (Infectious Diseases); Committees on Molecular Medicine, Immunology and Genetics, and Institute of Genomics and Systems Biology, University of Chicago, Chicago, Illinois
Toxoplasmosis (Toxoplasma gondii)

Peter C. Melby, MD
Director, Center for Tropical Diseases; Professor, Internal Medicine (Infectious Diseases), Microbiology and Immunology, and Pathology, University of Texas Medical Branch, Galveston, Texas
Leishmaniasis (Leishmania)

Joseph John Melvin, DO, JD
Assistant Professor, Child Neurology, Alfred I. DuPont Hospital for Children: Nemours Foundation, Wilmington, Delaware
Phenylalanine

Diane F. Merritt, MD
Professor, Obstetrics and Gynecology, Washington University School of Medicine in St. Louis, St. Louis, Missouri
History and Physical Examination; Vulvovaginitis; Bleeding; Breast Concerns; Neoplasms and Adolescent Screening for Human Papilloma Virus; Vulvovaginal and Müllerian Anomalies

Ethan A. Mezoff, MD
Research Associate, Division of Pediatric Gastroenterology, Hepatology, and Nutrition, Cincinnati Children's Hospital Medical Center, Cincinnati, Ohio
Clostridium difficile *Infection*

Marian G. Michaels, MD, MPH
Professor, Pediatrics and Surgery, Division of Pediatric Infectious Diseases, University of Pittsburgh School of Medicine, Children's Hospital of Pittsburgh, Pittsburgh, Pennsylvania
Infections in Immunocompromised Persons

Alexander G. Miethke, MD
Assistant Professor of Pediatrics, Division of Gastroenterology, Hepatology and Nutrition, Cincinnati Children's Hospital Medical Center, Cincinnati, Ohio
Morphogenesis of the Liver and Biliary System

Mohamad A. Mikati, MD
Wilburt C. Davison Distinguished Professor of Pediatrics; Professor of Neurobiology; Chief, Division of Pediatric Neurology, Duke University Medical Center, Durham, North Carolina
Seizures in Childhood; Conditions That Mimic Seizures

Henry Milgrom, MD
Professor, Department of Pediatrics, University of Colorado School of Medicine, National Jewish Health, Aurora, Colorado
Allergic Rhinitis

E. Kathryn Miller, MD, MPH
Assistant Professor, Pediatric Allergy and Immunology, Vanderbilt Children's Hospital, Nashville, Tennessee
Rhinoviruses

Jonathan W. Mink, MD, PhD
Professor, Departments of Neurology, Neurobiology and Anatomy, Brain and Cognitive Sciences, and Pediatrics, University of Rochester Medical Center, Rochester, New York
Movement Disorders

Grant A. Mitchell, MD
Professor, Division of Medical Genetics, Department of Pediatrics, CHU Sainte-Justine, University of Montreal, Montreal, Quebec, Canada
Tyrosine

Robert R. Montgomery, MD
Program Director, TS Zimmerman Program for the Molecular and Clinical Biology of VWD; Senior Investigator, Blood Research Institute; Professor of Pediatric Hematology, Department of Pediatrics, Medical College of Wisconsin, Milwaukee, Wisconsin
Hemostasis; Hereditary Clotting Factor Deficiencies (Bleeding Disorders); von Willebrand Disease; Postneonatal Vitamin K Deficiency; Liver Disease; Acquired Inhibitors of Coagulation; Disseminated Intravascular Coagulation; Platelet and Blood Vessel Disorders

Joseph G. Morelli, MD
Professor of Dermatology and Pediatrics, University of Colorado School of Medicine; Section Head, Pediatric Dermatology, The Children's Hospital, Aurora, Colorado
Morphology of the Skin; Evaluation of the Patient; Principles of Therapy; Diseases of the Neonate; Cutaneous Defects; Ectodermal Dysplasias; Vascular Disorders; Cutaneous Nevi; Hyperpigmented Lesions; Hypopigmented Lesions; Vesiculobullous Disorders; Eczematous Disorders; Photosensitivity; Disorders of Keratinization; Diseases of the Dermis; Diseases of Subcutaneous Tissue; Disorders of the Sweat Glands; Disorders of Hair; Disorders of the Nails; Disorders of the Mucous Membranes; Cutaneous Fungal Infections; Cutaneous Viral Infections; Arthropod Bites and Infestations; Acne; Tumors of the Skin; Nutritional Dermatoses

Anna-Barbara Moscicki, MD
Professor of Pediatrics; Associate Director, Division of Adolescent Medicine, University of California, San Francisco, California
Human Papillomaviruses

Hugo W. Moser, MD†
Professor of Neurology and Pediatrics, Johns Hopkins University; Director of Neurogenetics Research, Kennedy Krieger Institute, Johns Hopkins University School of Medicine, Baltimore, Maryland
Defects in Metabolism of Lipids

Kathryn D. Moyer, MD
Pediatric gastroenterologist, NW Pediatric Gastroenterology, LLC, Portland, Oregon
Liver Disease Associated with Systemic Disorders

James R. Murphy, PhD
Professor, Department of Pediatrics, University of Texas Health Science Center, Houston, Texas
Campylobacter; Yersinia; Aeromonas *and* Plesiomonas

Timothy F. Murphy, MD
UB Distinguished Professor, Departments of Medicine and Microbiology, University at Buffalo, State University of New York, Buffalo, New York
Moraxella catarrhalis

†Deceased.

Thomas S. Murray, MD, PhD
Assistant Professor, Yale University School of Medicine, Departments of Pediatrics and Laboratory Medicine, Sections of Infectious Disease and Medical Microbiology, New Haven, Connecticut
Pseudomonas, Burkholderia, *and* Stenotrophomonas

Mindo J. Natale, PsyD
Senior Staff Psychologist; Director of Training; Pediatric, Adolescent and Sports Medicine; Neuropsychologist, Department of Pediatric Services, Division of Psychology; Developmental-Behavioral Pediatrics, Greenville Hospital System Children's Hospital; Assistant Professor of Clinical Pediatrics, University of South Carolina School of Medicine, Greenville, South Carolina
Neurodevelopmental Function and Dysfunction in the School-Aged Child

William A. Neal, MD
James H. Walker Chair of Pediatric Cardiology, West Virginia University, Morgantown, West Virginia
Defects in Metabolism of Lipids

Jayne Ness, MD, PhD
Associate Professor of Pediatrics, Division of Pediatric Neurology, University of Alabama at Birmingham, Children's Hospital of Alabama, Birmingham, Alabama
Demyelinating Disorders of the CNS

Kathleen A. Neville, MD, MS
Associate Professor of Pediatrics, Divisions of Pediatric Clinical Pharmacology and Medical Toxicology and Pediatric Hematology/Oncology, Children's Mercy Hospitals and Clinics, Kansas City, Missouri
Pediatric Pharmacogenetics, Pharmacogenomics, and Pharmacoproteomics

Mary A. Nevin, MD, FAAP
Attending Physician, Pulmonary Medicine, Children's Memorial Hospital, Chicago, Illinois; Assistant Professor of Pediatrics, Northwestern Feinberg School of Medicine, Chicago, Illinois
Pulmonary Hemosiderosis; Pulmonary Embolism, Infarction, and Hemorrhage

Jane W. Newburger, MD, MPH
Commonwealth Professor of Pediatrics, Harvard Medical School; Associate Chief for Academic Affairs, Department of Cardiology, Boston, Massachusetts
Kawasaki Disease

Peter E. Newburger, MD
Ali and John Pierce Professor of Pediatric Hematology/Oncology; Vice Chair for Research, Department of Pediatrics, University of Massachusetts Medical School, Worcester, Massachusetts
Neutrophils; Eosinophils; Disorders of Phagocyte Function; Leukopenia; Leukocytosis

Linda S. Nield, MD
Associate Professor of Pediatrics, West Virginia University School of Medicine, Morgantown, West Virginia
Fever; Fever without a Focus

Zehava Noah, MD
Associate Professor, Department of Pediatrics, Northwestern University Feinberg School of Medicine, Children's Memorial Hospital, Chicago, Illinois
Chronic Severe Respiratory Insufficiency

Lawrence M. Nogee, MD
Professor of Pediatrics, Division of Neonatology, Johns Hopkins University School of Medicine, The Johns Hopkins Hospital, Baltimore, Maryland
Pulmonary Alveolar Proteinosis; Inherited Disorders of Surfactant Metabolism

Robert L. Norris, MD
Professor of Surgery, Emergency Medicine, Stanford University Medical Center, Palo Alto, California
Envenomations

Stephen K. Obaro, MD, PhD, FWACP, FRCPCH, FAAP
Associate Professor of Pediatrics, Division of Pediatric Infectious Disease, Department of Pediatrics and Human Development, College of Human Medicine, Michigan State University, East Lansing, Michigan
Nonvenereal Treponemal Infections; Relapsing Fever (Borrelia)

Makram Obeid, MD
Child Neurology Resident, Division of Pediatric Neurology, Department of Neurology, College of Physicians and Surgeons, Columbia University, New York, New York
Conditions That Mimic Seizures

Theresa J. Ochoa, MD
Assistant Professor of Pediatrics, Universidad Peruana Cayetano Heredia, Lima, Peru; Assistant Professor of Epidemiology, University of Texas School of Public Health, Houston, Texas
Shigella; Escherichia coli

Katherine A. O'Donnell, MD
Instructor in Pediatrics, Harvard Medical School; Attending Physician, Medical Toxicology and Hospitalist Services, Children's Hospital Boston, Boston, Massachusetts
Poisonings

Robin K. Ohls, MD
Professor of Pediatrics; Director of Pediatric Integration, CTSC, University of New Mexico, Albuquerque, New Mexico
Development of the Hematopoietic System

Jean-Marie Okwo-Bele, MD, MPH
Director, Immunization, Vaccines and Biologicals Department, World Health Organization, Geneva, Switzerland
Immunization Practices

Keith T. Oldham, MD
Professor and Chief, Division of Pediatric Surgery, Medical College of Wisconsin; Marie Z. Uihlein Chair and Surgeon-in-Chief, Children's Hospital of Wisconsin, Milwaukee, Wisconsin
Acute Appendicitis; Inguinal Hernias; Epigastric Hernia

Scott E. Olitsky, MD
Professor, Section of Ophthalmology, University of Missouri–Kansas City School of Medicine, Kansas City, Missouri
Growth and Development; Examination of the Eye; Abnormalities of Refraction and Accommodation; Disorders of Vision; Abnormalities of Pupil and Iris; Disorders of Eye Movement and Alignment; Abnormalities of the Lids; Disorders of the Lacrimal System; Disorders of the Conjunctiva; Abnormalities of the Cornea; Abnormalities of the Lens; Disorders of the Uveal Tract; Disorders of the Retina and Vitreous; Abnormalities of the Optic Nerve; Childhood Glaucoma; Orbital Abnormalities; Orbital Infections; Injuries to the Eye

John Olsson, MD
Brody School of Medicine, East Carolina University, Greenville, North Carolina
The Newborn

Susan R. Orenstein, MD
Professor Emerita, Pediatric Gastroenterology, University of Pittsburgh School of Medicine, Pittsburgh, Pennsylvania
Embryology, Anatomy, and Function of the Esophagus; Congenital Anomalies; Obstructing and Motility Disorders of the Esophagus; Dysmotility; Hiatal Hernia; Gastroesophageal Reflux Disease; Eosinophilic Esophagitis and Non-GERD Esophagitis; Esophageal Perforation; Esophageal Varices; Ingestions

Walter A. Orenstein, MD, D.Sc. (Hon)
Deputy Director for Immunization Programs, Vaccine Delivery, Global Health Program, Bill & Melinda Gates Foundation, Seattle, Washington
Immunization Practices

Judith A. Owens, MD, MPH
Director, Pediatric Sleep Disorders Clinic, Department of Pediatrics, Hasbro Children's Hospital, Providence, Rhode Island
Sleep Medicine

Charles H. Packman, MD
Clinical Professor of Medicine, University of North Carolina School of Medicine; Chief, Hematology-Oncology Division, Carolinas Medical Center, Charlotte, North Carolina
Hemolytic Anemias Resulting from Extracellular Factors—Immune Hemolytic Anemias

Michael J. Painter, MD
Division of Child Neurology, Children's Hospital of Pittsburgh, Pittsburgh, Pennsylvania
Progeria

Priya Pais, MBBS, MS
Assistant Professor, Pediatric Nephrology, Department of Pediatrics, Medical College of Wisconsin, Wauwatosa, Wisconsin
Lower Urinary Tract Causes of Hematuria; Introduction to the Child with Proteinuria; Fixed Proteinuria; Nephrotic Syndrome; Cortical Necrosis

Cynthia G. Pan, MD
Professor of Pediatrics; Section Head, Pediatric Nephrology, Medical College of Wisconsin; Medical Director, Pediatric Dialysis and Transplant Services, Children's Hospital of Wisconsin, Milwaukee, Wisconsin
Introduction to Glomerular Diseases; Clinical Evaluation of the Child with Hematuria; Isolated Glomerular Disease with Recurrent Gross Hematuria; Glomerulonephritis Associated with Infections; Glomerulonephritis Associated with Systemic Lupus Erythematosus

Vijay Pannikar, MD
Former Team Leader, WHO Global Leprosy Programme, Bangalore, Karnataka, India
Hansen Disease (Mycobacterium leprae)

Diane E. Pappas, MD, JD
Associate Professor of Pediatrics, University of Virginia School of Medicine, Charlottesville, Virginia
Sinusitis; Retropharyngeal Abscess, Lateral Pharyngeal (Parapharyngeal) Abscess, and Peritonsillar Cellulitis/Abscess

Anjali Parish, MD
Assistant Professor of Pediatrics, Division of Neonatology, Medical College of Georgia, Augusta, Georgia
Feeding Healthy Infants, Children, and Adolescents

John S. Parks, MD, PhD
Professor, Department of Pediatrics, Emory University School of Medicine, Decatur, Georgia
Hormones of the Hypothalamus and Pituitary; Hypopituitarism

Laura A. Parks, MD
Assistant Professor, Department of Obstetrics and Gynecology, Washington University School of Medicine in St. Louis, St. Louis, Missouri
Bleeding

Maria Jevitz Patterson, MD, PhD
Professor, Departments of Microbiology/Molecular Genetics and Pediatrics, Michigan State University, East Lansing, Michigan
Syphilis (Treponema pallidum)

Pallavi P. Patwari, MD
Assistant Professor of Pediatrics at Northwestern University Feinberg School of Medicine; Assistant Director, Center for Autonomic Medicine in Pediatrics (C.A.M.P.), Children's Memorial Hospital, Chicago, Illinois
Chronic Respiratory Insufficiency

Timothy R. Peters, MD
Assistant Professor of Pediatrics, Wake Forest University School of Medicine, Winston-Salem, North Carolina
Streptococcus pneumoniae *(Pneumococcus)*

Larry K. Pickering, MD, FAAP
Senior Advisor to the Director, National Center for Immunization and Respiratory Diseases; Executive Secretary, Advisory Committee on Immunization Practices, Centers for Disease Control and Prevention, Atlanta, Georgia
Immunization Practices

Misha L. Pless, MD
Associate Professor of Neurology, Harvard Medical School; Chief, Divisions of Neuro-ophthalmology and General Neurology, Massachusetts General Hospital, Boston, Massachusetts
Pseudotumor Cerebri

Laura S. Plummer, MD
Assistant Professor, University of Missouri–Kansas City; Clinical Assistant Professor, Kansas University, Department of Ophthalmology, Children's Mercy Hospitals and Clinics, Kansas City, Missouri
Growth and Development; Examination of the Eye; Abnormalities of Refraction and Accommodation; Disorders of Vision; Abnormalities of Pupil and Iris; Disorders of Eye Movement and Alignment; Abnormalities of the Lids; Disorders of the Lacrimal System; Disorders of the Conjunctiva; Abnormalities of the Cornea; Abnormalities of the Lens; Disorders of the Uveal Tract; Disorders of the Retina and Vitreous; Abnormalities of the Optic Nerve; Childhood Glaucoma; Orbital Abnormalities; Orbital Infections; Injuries to the Eye

Craig C. Porter, MD
Professor and Vice Chair for Faculty, Department of Pediatrics, Division of Nephrology, Medical College of Wisconsin, Milwaukee, Wisconsin
Upper Urinary Tract Causes of Hematuria; Hematologic Diseases Causing Hematuria; Anatomic Abnormalities Associated with Hematuria; Transient Proteinuria; Orthostatic (Postural) Proteinuria; Tubulointerstitial Nephritis; Toxic Nephropathy

Dwight A. Powell, MD
Professor of Pediatrics, The Ohio State University College of Medicine, Nationwide Children's Hospital, Columbus, Ohio
Hansen Disease (Mycobacterium leprae); Mycoplasma pneumoniae; *Genital Mycoplasmas* (Mycoplasma hominis, Mycoplasma genitalium, *and* Ureaplasma urealyticum)

David T. Price, MD
Pediatrics/Hospital and Emergency Medicine, Duke University Health System, Durham, North Carolina
Failure to Thrive

Charles G. Prober, MD
Professor of Pediatrics, Microbiology & Immunology; Senior Associate Dean, Medical Education, Stanford University School of Medicine, Stanford, California
Central Nervous System Infections; Brain Abscess

Linda Quan, MD
Professor, Division of Emergency Medicine, Department of Pediatrics, University of Washington School of Medicine, Seattle, Washington
Drowning and Submersion Injury

Elisabeth H. Quint, MD
Clinical Professor, Department of Obstetrics and Gynecology, University of Michigan Health System, Ann Arbor, Michigan
Gynecologic Care for Girls with Special Needs

C. Egla Rabinovich, MD, MPH
Associate Professor of Pediatrics; Co-Chief, Division of Pediatric Rheumatology, Pediatrics/Rheumatology, Duke University Health System, Durham, North Carolina
Evaluation of Suspected Rheumatic Disease; Treatment of Rheumatic Diseases; Juvenile Idiopathic Arthritis; Scleroderma and Raynaud Phenomenon

Leslie J. Raffini, MD, MSCE
Assistant Professor of Pediatrics, University of Pennsylvania School of Medicine; Medical Director, Hemostasis and Thrombosis Center, Children's Hospital of Philadelphia, Philadelphia, Pennsylvania
Hemostasis; Hereditary Predisposition to Thrombosis; Thrombotic Disorders in Children; Anticoagulant and Thrombolytic Therapy; Disseminated Intravascular Coagulation

Denia Ramirez-Montealegre, MD, MPH, PhD
Pediatric Neurology Chief Resident, Department of Neurology, Division of Child Neurology, University of Rochester Medical Center, Rochester, New York
Movement Disorders

Giuseppe Raviola, MD
Instructor in Psychiatry, Harvard Medical School; Director, Patient Safety and Quality, Department of Psychiatry, Children's Hospital Boston, Boston, Massachusetts
Pervasive Developmental Disorders and Childhood Psychosis

Ann M. Reed, MD
Professor of Pediatrics; Chair, Pediatric Rheumatology, Mayo Clinic, Rochester, Minnesota
Juvenile Dermatomyositis

Harold L. Rekate, MD
Chairman, Division of Pediatric Neurosciences, Barrow Neurological Institute; St. Joseph's Hospital and Medical Center, Phoenix, Arizona
Spinal Cord Disorders

Megan E. Reller, MD, MPH
Assistant Professor of Pathology, Division of Medical Microbiology, Department of Pathology, Johns Hopkins University School of Medicine, Baltimore, Maryland
Spotted Fever and Transitional Group Rickettsioses; Scrub Typhus (Orientia tsutsugamushi); *Typhus Group Rickettsioses; Ehrlichioses and Anaplasmosis; Q Fever* (Coxiella burnetii)

Gary Remafedi, MD, MPH
Professor of Pediatrics, University of Minnesota; Director, Youth and AIDS Projects, Minneapolis, Minnesota
Adolescent Homosexuality

Jorge D. Reyes, MD
Professor of Surgery, University of Washington; Chief of the Division of Transplantation Surgery, University of Washington Medical Center; Chief of Pediatric Transplantation, Seattle Children's Hospital, Seattle, Washington
Intestinal Transplantation in Children with Intestinal Failure; Liver Transplantation

Geoffrey Rezvani, MD
Assistant Professor, Department of Pediatrics, Drexel University College of Medicine; Section of Endocrinology, Diabetes and Metabolism, St. Christopher's Hospital for Children, Philadelphia, Pennsylvania
An Approach to Inborn Errors of Metabolism

Iraj Rezvani, MD
Professor of Pediatrics (Emeritus), Temple University School of Medicine; Adjunct Professor of Pediatrics, Drexel University College of Medicine, Section of Pediatric Endocrinology and Metabolism, St. Christopher's Hospital for Children, Philadelphia, Pennsylvania
An Approach to Inborn Errors of Metabolism; Defects in Metabolism of Amino Acids

A. Kim Ritchey, MD
Chief, Division of Pediatric Hematology/Oncology, Children's Hospital of Pittsburgh of UPMC; Professor of Pediatrics; Vice Chair for Clinical Affairs, Department of Pediatrics, University of Pittsburgh School of Medicine, Pittsburgh, Pennsylvania
Principles of Diagnosis; Principles of Treatment; The Leukemias

Frederick P. Rivara, MD, MPH
Children's Hospital Guild Endowed Chair, Professor of Pediatrics; Adjunct Professor of Epidemiology, University of Washington, Seattle, Washington
Maximizing Children's Health Screening, Anticipatory Guidance, and Counseling

Angela Byun Robinson, MD, MPH
Assistant Professor, Pediatric Rheumatology, Rainbow Babies & Children's Hospital, Cleveland, Ohio
Juvenile Dermatomyositis; Miscellaneous Conditions Associated with Arthritis

Luise E. Rogg, MD, PhD
Fellow, Pediatric Infectious Diseases, Duke University Medical Center, Department of Pediatrics, Division of Pediatric Infectious Diseases, Durham, North Carolina
Aspergillus

Genie E. Roosevelt, MD, MPH
Associate Professor of Pediatrics, Section of Emergency Medicine, University of Colorado School of Medicine, Aurora, Colorado
Acute Inflammatory Upper Airway Obstruction (Croup, Epiglottitis, Laryngitis, and Bacterial Tracheitis)

David R. Rosenberg, MD
Miriam L. Hamburger Endowed Chair of Child Psychiatry, Children's Hospital of Michigan and Wayne State University; Professor and Chief of Child Psychiatry and Psychology, Wayne State University, Detroit, Michigan
Anxiety Disorders

Melissa Beth Rosenberg, MD
Assistant Professor, Michigan State University, College of Osteopathic Medicine, Department of Pediatrics, East Lansing, Michigan
Leptospira

David S. Rosenblatt, MD
Chair, Department of Human Genetics; Professor of Human Genetics, Pediatrics and Medicine, McGill University, Montreal, Quebec, Canada
Defects in Metabolism of Amino Acids

Cindy Ganis Roskind, MD
Assistant Clinical Professor of Pediatrics, Pediatric Emergency Medicine, Columbia University College of Physicians and Surgeons, New York, New York
Acute Care of the Victim of Multiple Trauma

Mary M. Rotar, RN, BSN, CIC
Infection Prevention and Control Coordinator, Children's Hospital of Wisconsin, Milwaukee, Wisconsin
Infection Prevention and Control

Ranna A. Rozenfeld, MD
Associate Professor of Pediatrics, Northwestern University Feinberg School of Medicine, Children's Memorial Hospital, Chicago, Illinois
Atelectasis

Sarah Zieber Rush, MD
Assistant Professor of Pediatrics, The University of Colorado Denver, Center for Cancer and Blood Disorders, The Children's Hospital, Aurora, Colorado
Brain Tumors in Childhood

Colleen A. Ryan, MD
Attending, Child and Adolescent Psychiatry Inpatient Service, Children's Hospital Boston; Instructor, Harvard Medical School, Boston, Massachusetts
Habit and Tic Disorders

Prof. H.P.S. Sachdev, MD, Hon. FRCPCH
Senior Consultant Pediatrics and Clinical Epidemiology, Sitaram Bhartia Institute of Science and Research, New Delhi, India; Adjunct Professor, Division of Population Health, St. John's Research Institute, St. John's National Academy of Health Sciences, Bangalore, India
Vitamin B Complex Deficiencies and Excess; Vitamin C (Ascorbic Acid)

Ramesh C. Sachdeva, MD, PhD, FAAP, FCCM
Professor of Pediatrics (Critical Care and Sleep Medicine), Medical College of Wisconsin; Corporate Vice President and Chief Quality Officer, Children's Hospital and Health System, Milwaukee, Wisconsin
Quality and Safety in Health Care for Children

Mustafa Sahin, MD, PhD
Department of Neurology, Children's Hospital Boston, Boston, Massachusetts
Neurocutaneous Syndromes

Robert A. Salata, MD
Professor and Executive Vice Chair, Department of Medicine; Chief, Division of Infectious Diseases and HIV Medicine, Case Western Reserve University, University Hospitals Case Medical Center, Cleveland, Ohio
Amebiasis; Trichomoniasis (Trichomonas vaginalis); *African Trypanosomiasis (Sleeping Sickness;* Trypanosoma brucei *Complex); American Trypanosomiasis (Chagas Disease*; Trypanosoma cruzi)

Denise A. Salerno, MD
Professor of Pediatrics; Pediatric Clerkship Director; Associate Chair for Undergraduate Education, Department of Pediatrics, Temple University School of Medicine, Philadelphia, Pennsylvania
Nonbacterial Food Poisoning

Edsel Maurice T. Salvana, MD, DTM&H (Diploma in Tropical Medicine and Hygiene)
Associate Professor of Medicine, Section of Infectious Diseases, Department of Medicine, Philippine General Hospital, University of the Philippines Manila; Research Faculty, Institute of Molecular Biology and Biotechnology, National Institutes of Health, University of the Philippines Manila, Manila, Philippines
Amebiasis; Trichomoniasis (Trichomonas vaginalis); *African Trypanosomiasis (Sleeping Sickness;* Trypanosoma brucei *Complex); American Trypanosomiasis (Chagas Disease;* Trypanosoma cruzi)

Hugh A. Sampson, MD
Kurt Hirschhorn Professor of Pediatrics; Dean for Translational Biomedical Sciences; Director, Jaffe Food Allergy Institute, Mount Sinai School of Medicine, New York, New York
Anaphylaxis; Adverse Reactions to Foods

Thomas J. Sandora, MD, MPH
Hospital Epidemiologist; Medical Director of Infection Prevention and Control, Division of Infectious Diseases, Children's Hospital Boston; Assistant Professor of Pediatrics, Harvard Medical School, Boston, Massachusetts
Community-Acquired Pneumonia

Tracy Sandritter, PharmD
Clinical Pharmacy Specialist, Personalized Medicine, Children's Mercy Hospitals and Clinics; Adjunct Associate Clinical Professor, University of Missouri–Kansas City School of Pharmacy, Kansas City, Missouri
Principles of Drug Therapy

Wudbhav N. Sankar, MD
Assistant Professor of Orthopaedic Surgery, University of Pennsylvania School of Medicine; Attending Physician, The Children's Hospital of Philadelphia, Philadelphia, Pennsylvania
The Hip

Ajit Ashok Sarnaik, MD
Staff Intensivist, Children's Hospital of Michigan; Assistant Professor of Pediatrics, Wayne State University School of Medicine, Detroit, Michigan
Respiratory Distress and Failure

Ashok P. Sarnaik, MD
Chief, Critical Care Medicine, Children's Hospital of Michigan; Professor of Pediatrics, Wayne State University School of Medicine, Detroit, Michigan
Respiratory Distress and Failure; Respiratory Pathophysiology and Regulation; Regulation of Respiration

Harvey B. Sarnat, MS, MD, FRCPC
Professor of Paediatrics, Pathology, (Neuropathology) and Clinical Neurosciences, Divisions of Paediatric Neurology and Neuropathology, University of Calgary, Faculty of Medicine, Alberta Children's Hospital, Calgary, Alberta, Canada
Evaluation and Investigation; Developmental Disorders of Muscle; Muscular Dystrophies; Endocrine and Toxic Myopathies; Metabolic Myopathies; Disorders of Neuromuscular Transmission and of Motor Neurons; Hereditary Motor-Sensory Neuropathies; Toxic Neuropathies; Autonomic Neuropathies; Guillain-Barré Syndrome; Bell Palsy

Minnie M. Sarwal, MD, FRCP, PhD, DCH
Professor, Pediatrics and Immunology; Medical Director, Pediatric Kidney Transplant, Stanford University, Palo Alto, California
Renal Transplantation

Mary Saunders, MD
Assistant Professor, Department of Pediatrics, Emergency Medicine, Medical College of Wisconsin, Milwaukee, Wisconsin
Evaluation of the Sick Child in the Office and Clinic

Laura E. Schanberg, MD
Professor of Pediatrics; Co-Chief, Division of Pediatric Rheumatology, Duke University Medical Center, Durham, North Carolina
Treatment of Rheumatic Diseases; Systemic Lupus Erythematosus; Musculoskeletal Pain Syndromes

Mark R. Schleiss, MD
American Legion Chair of Pediatrics; Director, Division of Infectious Diseases and Immunology; Associate Head for Research, Department of Pediatrics, University of Minnesota School of Medicine, Center for Infectious Diseases and Microbiology Translational Research, Minneapolis, Minnesota
Principles of Antibacterial Therapy; Principles of Antiviral Therapy; Principles of Antiparasitic Therapy

Nina F. Schor, MD, PhD
William H. Eilinger Professor and Chair, Department of Pediatrics; Professor, Department of Neurology; Pediatrician-in-Chief, Golisano Children's Hospital, University of Rochester Medical Center, Rochester, New York
Neurologic Evaluation; Neuromyelitis Optica; Acute Disseminated Encephalomyelitis (ADEM)

Bill J. Schroeder, DO
Clinical Assistant Professor, Emergency Medicine/Pediatric Emergency Medicine, University of Illinois at Chicago, Advocate Christ Hospital/Hope Children's Hospital, Oak Lawn, Illinois
Envenomations

Robert L. Schum, PhD
Professor, Department of Pediatrics, Medical College of Wisconsin; Clinical Psychologist, Child Development Center, Children's Hospital of Wisconsin, Milwaukee, Wisconsin
Language Development and Communication Disorders

Gordon E. Schutze, MD, FAAP
Professor of Pediatrics, Vice-Chairman for Educational Affairs, Department of Pediatrics, Section of Retrovirology; Vice President, Baylor International Pediatric AIDS Initiative at Texas Children's Hospital, Baylor College of Medicine, Houston, Texas
Actinomyces; Nocardia; *Tularemia* (Francisella tularensis); Brucella

Daryl A. Scott, MD, PhD
Assistant Professor, Department of Molecular and Human Genetics, Baylor College of Medicine, Houston, Texas
The Genetic Approach in Pediatric Medicine; The Human Genome; Patterns of Genetic Transmission

J. Paul Scott, MD
Professor, Department of Pediatrics, Medical College of Wisconsin, BloodCenter of Wisconsin, Milwaukee, Wisconsin
Hemostasis; Hereditary Clotting Factor Deficiencies (Bleeding Disorders); von Willebrand Disease; Hereditary Predisposition to Thrombosis; Thrombotic Disorders in Children; Postneonatal Vitamin K Deficiency; Liver Disease; Acquired Inhibitors of Coagulation; Disseminated Intravascular Coagulation; Platelet and Blood Vessel Disorders

Theodore C. Sectish, MD
Program Director, Children's Hospital Boston; Associate Professor, Harvard Medical School; Executive Director, Federation of Pediatric Organizations, Boston, Massachusetts
Community-Acquired Pneumonia

George B. Segel, MD
Professor of Pediatrics and Medicine, Department of Pediatrics, University of Rochester Medical Center, Rochester, New York
Definitions and Classification of Hemolytic Anemias; Hereditary Spherocytosis; Hereditary Elliptocytosis; Hereditary Stomatocytosis; Other Membrane Defects; Enzymatic Defects; Hemolytic Anemias Resulting from Extracellular Factors—Immune Hemolytic Anemias; Hemolytic Anemias Secondary to Other Extracellular Factors

Kriti Sehgal, BA
Clinical Research Coordinator, Department of Orthopaedics, The Children's Hospital of Philadelphia, Philadelphia, Pennsylvania
Growth and Development; Evaluation of the Child; Torsional and Angular Deformities; The Knee; Common Fractures

Ernest G. Seidman, MDCM, FRCPC, FACG
Professor of Medicine and Pediatrics, Canada Research Chair in Immune Mediated Gastrointestinal Disorders; Bruce Kaufman Endowed Chair in IBD at McGill Digestivelab, Research Institute of McGill University Health Centre, Montreal, Quebec, Canada
Disorders of Malabsorption

Janet R. Serwint, MD
Professor of Pediatrics; Director of Pediatric Resident Education, Johns Hopkins University School of Medicine, Baltimore, Maryland
Loss, Separation, and Bereavement

Dheeraj Shah, MD (Pediatrics), DNB (Pediatrics), MNAMS
Associate Professor, Department of Pediatrics, University College of Medical Sciences (University of Delhi) and Guru Tegh Bahadur Hospital, Delhi, India
Vitamin B Complex Deficiencies and Excess; Vitamin C (Ascorbic Acid)

Prof. Raanan Shamir, MD
Chairman, Institute of Gastroenterology, Nutrition and Liver Diseases, Schneider Children's Medical Center of Israel; Professor of Pediatrics, Sackler Faculty of Medicine, Tel-Aviv University, Petach-Tikva, Israel
Disorders of Malabsorption

Bruce K. Shapiro, MD
The Arnold J. Capute, MD, MPH Chair in Neurodevelopmental Disabilities; Professor of Pediatrics, Johns Hopkins University School of Medicine; Vice President, Training, Kennedy Krieger Institute, Baltimore, Maryland
Intellectual Disability

Richard J. Shaw, MB, BS
Professor of Psychiatry and Pediatrics, Stanford University School of Medicine; Medical Director, Pediatric Psychosomatic Medicine Service, Lucile Packard Children's Hospital at Stanford, Stanford, California
Psychosomatic Illness

Bennett A. Shaywitz, MD
The Charles and Helen Schwab Professor in Dyslexia and Learning Development, Pediatrics and Neurology, Yale University School of Medicine, New Haven, Connecticut
Dyslexia

Sally E. Shaywitz, MD
The Audrey G. Ratner Professor in Learning Development, Department of Pediatrics, Yale University School of Medicine, New Haven, Connecticut
Dyslexia

Meera Shekar, Bsc, Msc, PhD
Lead Health and Nutrition Specialist, World Bank, Human Development Network, Washington, District of Columbia
Nutrition, Food Security, and Health

Elena Shephard, MD, MPH
Assistant Professor of Pediatrics, Seattle Children's Hospital, Seattle, Washington
Drowning and Submersion Injury

Philip M. Sherman, MD, FRCPC
Professor of Paediatrics, Microbiology, and Dentistry, Hospital for Sick Children, University of Toronto; Canada Research Chair in Gastrointestinal Disease, Toronto, Ontario, Canada
Disorders of Malabsorption

Benjamin L. Shneider, MD
Professor of Pediatrics, University of Pittsburgh School of Medicine; Director of Pediatric Hepatology, Children's Hospital of Pittsburgh of UPMC, Pittsburgh, Pennsylvania
Autoimmune Hepatitis

Scott H. Sicherer, MD
Professor of Pediatrics, Jaffe Food Allergy Institute, Mount Sinai School of Medicine, New York, New York
Insect Allergy; Serum Sickness

Richard Sills, MD
Professor of Pediatrics; Director, Pediatric Hematology/Oncology, Upstate Medical University, Syracuse, New York
Iron-Deficiency Anemia; Other Microcytic Anemias

Mark D. Simms, MD, MPH
Chief, Section of Child Development, Department of Pediatrics, Medical College of Wisconsin; Medical Director, Child Development Center, Children's Hospital of Wisconsin, Milwaukee, Wisconsin
Language Development and Communication Disorders; Adoption

Eric A.F. Simões, MBBS, DCH, MD
Professor of Pediatrics, Division of Infectious Diseases, The Children's Hospital, Aurora, Colorado
Polioviruses

Thomas L. Slovis, MD
Professor of Radiology and Pediatrics, Children's Hospital of Michigan, Wayne State University Medical School, Detroit, Michigan
Biologic Effects of Radiation on Children

P. Brian Smith, MD, MPH, MHS
Assistant Professor, Department of Pediatrics, Duke University Medical Center, Duke Clinical Research Institute, Durham, North Carolina
Candida

Mary Beth F. Son, MD
Instructor in Pediatrics, Harvard Medical School, Boston, Massachusetts
Kawasaki Disease

Laura Stout Sosinsky, PhD
Assistant Professor, Department of Psychology, Fordham University, Bronx, New York
Child Care: How Pediatricians Can Support Children and Families

Joseph D. Spahn, MD
Associate Professor Pediatrics, Department of Pediatrics, National Jewish Health, Denver, Colorado
Childhood Asthma

Mark A. Sperling, MD
Professor of Pediatrics, Division of Endocrinology, Children's Hospital of Pittsburgh, Pittsburgh, Pennsylvania
Hypoglycemia

Robert Spicer, MD
Professor of Pediatrics, University of Cincinnati; Medical Director, Cardiac Transplantation; Director, Cardiology Fellowship Program; Director, Pediatric Cardiology Training Program, Cincinnati Children's Hospital, Cincinnati, Ohio
Diseases of the Myocardium; Diseases of the Pericardium; Tumors of the Heart

David A. Spiegel, MD
Pediatric Orthopaedic Surgeon, Division of Orthopaedic Surgery, The Children's Hospital of Philadelphia; Assistant Professor of Orthopaedic Surgery, University of Pennsylvania School of Medicine, Philadelphia, Pennsylvania
The Foot and Toes; The Spine; The Neck

Helen Spoudeas, MD, MBBS, DRCOG, FRCP, FRCPCH
Consultant/Honorary Senior Lecturer in Paediatric/Adolescent Neuroendocrinology at London Centre for Paediatric and Adolescent Endocrinology, Great Ormond Street and University College Hospitals, Neuroendocrine Division, London, United Kingdom
Chronic Diarrhea

Jürgen Spranger, MD
Professor, Im Fuchsberg, Sinzheim, Germany
Mucopolysaccharidoses

Rajasree Sreedharan, MD, MBBS
Assistant Professor, Medical College of Wisconsin, Pediatric Nephrology, Wauwatosa, Wisconsin
Tubular Function; Renal Tubular Acidosis; Nephrogenic Diabetes Insipidus; Bartter and Gitelman Syndromes and Other Inherited Tubular Transport Abnormalities; Renal Failure

Raman Sreedharan, MD, DCH, MRCPCH
Attending Physician, Division of Gastroenterology, Hepatology and Nutrition, The Children's Hospital of Philadelphia; Clinical Assistant Professor of Pediatrics, University of Pennsylvania School of Medicine, Philadelphia, Pennsylvania
Major Symptoms and Signs of Digestive Tract Disorders; Functional Abdominal Pain (Nonorganic Chronic Abdominal Pain)

Shawn J. Stafford, MD, FAAP
Assistant Clinical Professor, Pediatric Surgery, University of Arizona School of Medicine, Arizona Pediatric Surgery, Tucson, Arizona
Surgical Conditions of the Anus and Rectum

Margaret M. Stager, MD
Interim Chairman, Department of Pediatrics; Associate Professor of Pediatrics, Division of Adolescent Medicine, Case Western Reserve University School of Medicine, MetroHealth Medical Center, Cleveland, Ohio
Violent Behavior; Substance Abuse

Sergio Stagno, MD
Katharine Reynolds Ireland Distinguished Professor and Chairman, Department of Pediatrics, University of Alabama at Birmingham, Birmingham, Alabama
Cytomegalovirus

Virginia A. Stallings, MD
Professor of Pediatrics, University of Pennsylvania School of Medicine; Cortner Endowed Chair in Pediatric Gastroenterology; Director, Office of Faculty Development, Research Institute; Director, Nutrition Center, The Children's Hospital of Philadelphia, Philadelphia, Pennsylvania
Nutritional Requirements; Feeding Healthy Infants, Children, and Adolescents

Lawrence R. Stanberry, MD, PhD
Reuben S. Carpentier Professor and Chairman, Department of Pediatrics, Columbia University College of Physicians and Surgeons, New York, New York
Herpes Simplex Virus

Charles A. Stanley, MD
Professor of Pediatrics, The Children's Hospital of Philadelphia, Philadelphia, Pennsylvania
Defects in Metabolism of Lipids

Bonita F. Stanton, MD
Professor and Schotanus Family Endowed Chair of Pediatrics, Pediatrician-in-Chief, Carman and Ann Adams Department of Pediatrics, Children's Hospital of Michigan, Wayne State University School of Medicine, Detroit, Michigan
Overview of Pediatrics; Cultural Issues in Pediatric Care

Jeffrey R. Starke, MD
Professor of Pediatrics, Department of Pediatrics, Baylor College of Medicine, Texas Children's Hospital, Houston, Texas
Tuberculosis (Mycobacterium tuberculosis)

Merrill Stass-Isern, MD
Associate Clinical Professor, Department of Ophthalmology, Children's Mercy Hospitals and Clinics, University of Missouri–Kansas City, Kansas City, Missouri
Growth and Development; Examination of the Eye; Abnormalities of Refraction and Accommodation; Disorders of Vision; Abnormalities of Pupil and Iris; Disorders of Eye Movement and Alignment; Abnormalities of the Lids; Disorders of the Lacrimal System; Disorders of the Conjunctiva; Abnormalities of the Cornea; Abnormalities of the Lens; Disorders of the Uveal Tract; Disorders of the Retina and Vitreous; Abnormalities of the Optic Nerve; Childhood Glaucoma; Orbital Abnormalities; Orbital Infections; Injuries to the Eye

Barbara W. Stechenberg, MD
Chief, Pediatric Infectious Diseases; Pediatrics Program Director, Baystate Children's Hospital; Professor of Pediatrics, Tufts University School of Medicine, Springfield, Massachusetts
Bartonella

Leonard D. Stein, MD
Professor of Pediatrics, Division of Allergy, Immunology, Rheumatology and Infectious Diseases, The University of North Carolina at Chapel Hill, Chapel Hill, North Carolina
Miscellaneous Conditions Associated with Arthritis

William J. Steinbach, MD
Associate Professor of Pediatrics, Molecular Genetics and Microbiology, Division of Pediatric Infectious Diseases, Duke University Medical Center, Durham, North Carolina
Principles of Antifungal Therapy; Aspergillus

Nicolas Stettler, MD, MSCE
Associate Professor of Pediatrics and Epidemiology, Division of Gastroenterology, Hepatology, and Nutrition, The Children's Hospital of Philadelphia, Philadelphia, Pennsylvania
Nutritional Requirements; Feeding Healthy Infants, Children, and Adolescents

Barbara J. Stoll, MD
George W. Brumley, Jr., Professor and Chair, Department of Pediatrics, Emory University School of Medicine, Atlanta, Georgia
Infections of the Neonatal Infant

Gregory A. Storch, MD
Ruth L. Siteman Professor of Pediatrics, Washington University School of Medicine in St. Louis, St. Louis, Missouri
Polyomaviruses

Ronald G. Strauss, MD
Professor Emeritus, Departments of Pathology and Pediatrics, University of Iowa College of Medicine, Coralville, Iowa
Red Blood Cell Transfusions and Erythropoietin Therapy; Platelet Transfusions; Neutrophil (Granulocyte) Transfusions; Plasma Transfusions; Risks of Blood Transfusions

Frederick J. Suchy, MD
Professor of Pediatrics; Vice Chair for Research; Chief of Pediatric Hepatology, Jack and Lucy Clark Department of Pediatrics, Mount Sinai School of Medicine, Mount Sinai Kravis Children's Hospital, New York, New York
Autoimmune Hepatitis; Drug- and Toxin-Induced Liver Injury; Fulminant Hepatic Failure; Cystic Diseases of the Biliary Tract and Liver; Diseases of the Gallbladder; Portal Hypertension and Varices

Karen Summar, MD, MS
Medical Director, Jane and Richard Thomas Center for Down Syndrome, Cincinnati Children's Hospital Medical Center; Assistant Professor of Pediatrics, University of Cincinnati, Cincinnati, Ohio
Cytogenetics

Moira Szilagyi, MD, PhD
Associate Professor of Pediatrics, University of Rochester; Medical Director, Starlight Pediatrics, Monroe County Health Department, Rochester, New York
Foster and Kinship Care

Norman Tinanoff, DDS, MS
Professor and Chair, Department of Health Promotion and Policy, University of Maryland Dental School, Baltimore, Maryland
Development and Developmental Anomalies of the Teeth; Disorders of the Oral Cavity Associated with Other Conditions; Malocclusion; Cleft Lip and Palate; Syndromes with Oral Manifestations; Dental Caries; Periodontal Diseases; Dental Trauma; Common Lesions of the Oral Soft Tissues; Diseases of the Salivary Glands and Jaws; Diagnostic Radiology in Dental Assessment

James K. Todd, MD
Professor of Pediatrics, Microbiology and Epidemiology, University of Colorado School of Medicine and Colorado School of Public Health, Jules Amer Chair of Community Pediatrics; Director of Epidemiology, The Children's Hospital, Aurora, Colorado
Staphylococcus

Lucy S. Tompkins, MD, PhD
Lucy Becker Professor of Medicine (Infectious Diseases); Professor of Microbiology and Immunology, Stanford University School of Medicine, Stanford University Medical Center, Stanford, California
Legionella

Richard L. Tower II, MD, MS
Assistant Professor of Pediatrics, Pediatrics, Hematology/Oncology/BMT Section, Medical College of Wisconsin, Milwaukee, Wisconsin
Anatomy and Function of the Lymphatic System; Abnormalities of Lymphatic Vessels; Lymphadenopathy

Prof. Riccardo Troncone
Professor of Pediatrics, Head, European Laboratory for the Investigation of Food-Induced Diseases, University Federico II, Naples, Italy
Disorders of Malabsorption

Amanda A. Trott, MD
Resident, Department of Pediatrics, University of Texas Medical Branch, Galveston, Texas
Defects in Metabolism of Amino Acids

David G. Tubergen, MD
Medical Director, Host Program, MD Anderson Physicians Network, University of Texas MD Anderson Cancer Center, Houston, Texas
The Leukemias

David A. Turner, MD
Associate Director, Pediatric Critical Care Fellowship Program; Medical Instructor, Department of Pediatrics, Division of Pediatric Critical Care Medicine, Duke University Medical Center, Durham, North Carolina
Shock

Ronald B. Turner, MD
Associate Dean for Clinical Research; Professor of Pediatrics, University of Virginia School of Medicine, Charlottesville, Virginia
The Common Cold; Acute Pharyngitis

Christina Ullrich, MD, MPH
Attending Physician in Pediatric Hematology/Oncology and Pediatric Palliative Care, Children's Hospital Boston/Dana-Farber Cancer Institute; Instructor in Pediatrics, Harvard Medical School, Boston, Massachusetts
Pediatric Palliative Care

George F. Van Hare, MD
Louis Larrick Ward Professor of Pediatrics, Washington University in St. Louis; Director, Pediatric Cardiology, St. Louis Children's Hospital, St. Louis, Missouri
Disturbances of Rate and Rhythm of the Heart; Sudden Death

Jakko van Ingen, MD, PhD
National Tuberculosis Reference Laboratory, National Institute of Public Health and the Environment, Bilthoven, The Netherlands; Department of Pulmonary Diseases, Radboud University Nijmegen Medical Center, Nijmegen, The Netherlands
Nontuberculous Mycobacteria

Heather A. Van Mater, MD, MS
Assistant Professor, Department of Pediatrics, Division of Pediatric Rheumatology, Duke University, Durham, North Carolina
Juvenile Idiopathic Arthritis; Scleroderma and Raynaud Phenomenon

Prof. Dr. Dick van Soolingen
Head of the Tuberculosis Reference Laboratory, National Institute for Public Health and the Environment, Bilthoven, The Netherlands; Department of Pulmonary Diseases and Medical Microbiology, Radboud University Nijmegen Medical Centre, Nijmegen, The Netherlands
Nontuberculous Mycobacteria

Scott K. Van Why, MD
Professor of Pediatrics, Medical College of Wisconsin, Wauwatosa, Wisconsin
Membranous Glomerulopathy; Membranoproliferative Glomerulonephritis; Henoch-Schönlein Purpura Nephritis; Rapidly Progressive (Crescentic) Glomerulonephritis; Goodpasture Disease; Hemolytic-Uremic Syndrome

Pankhuree Vandana, MD
Second Year Fellow, Child and Adolescent Psychiatry, Department of Child and Adolescent Psychiatry, Feinberg School of Medicine/Northwestern University/Children's Memorial Hospital, Chicago, Illinois
Anxiety Disorders

Douglas Vanderbilt, MD
Assistant Professor of Clinical Pediatrics, Keck School of Medicine, University of Southern California; Children's Hospital Los Angeles Developmental-Behavioral Pediatrics Fellowship Director, Los Angeles, California
Impact of Violence on Children

Jon A. Vanderhoof, MD
Lecturer in Pediatrics, Harvard Medical School; Professor Emeritus, Pediatrics, University of Nebraska College of Medicine, Omaha, Nebraska
Disorders of Malabsorption

Andrea Velardi, MD
Professor of Hematology, Division of Hematology and Clinical Immunology, University of Perugia, Perugia, Italy
Principles and Clinical Indications; HSCT from Alternative Sources and Donors; Graft Versus Host Disease (GVHD) and Rejection; Infectious Complications of HSCT; Late Effects of HSCT

Elliott Vichinsky, MD
Medical Director, Department of Hematology/Oncology; Adjunct Professor UCSF, Oakland, California
Hemoglobinopathies

Linda A. Waggoner-Fountain, MD, MEd
Associate Professor of Pediatrics, Division of Infectious Diseases, University of Virginia, Charlottesville, Virginia
Child Care and Communicable Diseases

Steven G. Waguespack, MD, FAAP, FACE
Associate Professor, Department of Endocrine Neoplasia and Hormonal Disorders, Department of Pediatrics, University of Texas MD Anderson Cancer Center, Houston, Texas
Rare Tumors

David M. Walker, MD
Assistant Professor, Pediatrics (Emergency Medicine), Yale University School of Medicine; Clinical Instructor, Pediatric Nurse Practitioner Program, Yale University School of Nursing; Attending Physician, Pediatric Emergency Department, Yale-New Haven Children's Hospital, New Haven, Connecticut
Emergency Medical Services for Children

Heather J. Walter, MD, MPH
Professor of Psychiatry and Pediatrics, Vice-Chair of Psychiatry, Boston University School of Medicine; Chief, Child and Adolescent Psychiatry, Boston Medical Center, Boston, Massachusetts
Assessment and Interviewing; Psychologic Treatment of Children and Adolescents; Mood Disorders; Suicide and Attempted Suicide; Disruptive Behavioral Disorders; Pervasive Developmental Disorders and Childhood Psychosis

Stephanie Ware, MD, PhD
Associate Professor of Pediatrics, Department of Pediatrics, Cincinnati Children's Hospital Medical Center, University of Cincinnati College of Medicine, Cincinnati, Ohio
Diseases of the Myocardium; Diseases of the Pericardium; Tumors of the Heart

Kimberly Danieli Watts, MD, MS
Instructor of Pediatrics, Northwestern University Feinberg School of Medicine; Attending, Division of Pulmonary Medicine, Children's Memorial Hospital, Chicago, Illinois
Wheezing, Bronchiolitis, and Bronchitis

Ian M. Waxman, MD
Medical Officer, U.S. Food and Drug Administration, Bethesda, Maryland
Lymphoma

Debra E. Weese-Mayer, MD
Professor of Pediatrics at Northwestern University Feinberg School of Medicine; Director, Center for Autonomic Medicine in Pediatrics (C.A.M.P.), Children's Memorial Hospital, Chicago, Illinois
Chronic Respiratory Insufficiency

Kathryn Weise, MD, MA
Program Director, Cleveland Fellowship in Advanced Bioethics, Department of Bioethics, Cleveland Clinic, Cleveland, Ohio
Ethics in Pediatric Care

Martin E. Weisse, MD
Chief, Department of Pediatrics, Tripler Army Medical Center, Honolulu, Hawaii; Professor of Pediatrics, Uniformed Services University, F. Edward Hebert School of Medicine, Bethesda, Maryland
Malassezia; *Primary Amebic Meningoencephalitis*

Lawrence Wells, MD
Assistant Professor of Orthopaedic Surgery, University of Pennsylvania School of Medicine; Attending Orthopedic Surgeon, The Children's Hospital of Philadelphia, Philadelphia, Pennsylvania
Growth and Development; Evaluation of the Child; Torsional and Angular Deformities; The Knee; The Hip; Common Fractures

Jessica Wen, MD
Fellow, The Children's Hospital of Philadelphia/University of Pennsylvania, Division of Gastroenterology, Philadelphia, Pennsylvania
Ascites; Peritonitis

Steven L. Werlin, MD
Professor, Department of Pediatrics (Gastroenterology), The Medical College of Wisconsin, Milwaukee, Wisconsin
Embryology, Anatomy, and Physiology; Pancreatic Function Tests; Disorders of the Exocrine Pancreas; Treatment of Pancreatic Insufficiency; Pancreatitis; Pseudocyst of the Pancreas; Pancreatic Tumors

Michael R. Wessels, MD
John F. Enders Professor of Pediatrics and Professor of Medicine, Harvard Medical School; Chief, Division of Infectious Diseases, Children's Hospital Boston, Boston, Massachusetts
Group B Streptococcus

Ralph F. Wetmore, MD
Chief, Division of Otolaryngology, The Children's Hospital of Philadelphia; E. Mortimer Newlin Professor of Pediatric Otolaryngology, University of Pennsylvania School of Medicine, Philadelphia, Pennsylvania
Tonsils and Adenoids

Randall C. Wetzel, MB, BS, MBA, MRCS, LRCP, FAAP, FCCM
Chair, Department of Anesthesiology, Critical Care Medicine, Children's Hospital of Los Angeles, Los Angeles, California
Anesthesia, Perioperative Care, and Sedation

Isaiah D. Wexler, MD, PhD
Associate Professor, Department of Pediatrics, Hadassah University Medical Center, Jerusalem, Israel
Impact of Violence on Children

Perrin C. White, MD
Professor of Pediatrics, UT Southwestern Medical Center; Director of Pediatric Endocrinology, Division of Pediatric Endocrinology, University of Texas Southwestern Medical Center, Dallas, Texas
Physiology of the Adrenal Gland; Adrenocortical Insufficiency; Congenital Adrenal Hyperplasia and Related Disorders; Cushing Syndrome; Primary Aldosteronism; Adrenocortical Tumors; Pheochromocytoma; Adrenal Masses

John V. Williams, MD
Assistant Professor, Pediatric Infectious Disease, Microbiology and Immunology, Vanderbilt University, Nashville, Tennessee
Adenoviruses; Rhinoviruses

Rodney E. Willoughby, Jr., MD
Professor, Pediatric Infectious Diseases, Medical College of Wisconsin, Children's Corporate Center, Milwaukee, Wisconsin
Rabies

Samantha L. Wilson, PhD
Assistant Professor, Medical College of Wisconsin; Member, Children's Specialty Group, Brookfield, Wisconsin
Adoption

Glenna B. Winnie, MD
Director, The Pediatric Sleep Center, Fairfax Neonatal Associates, Fairfax, Virginia
Emphysema and Overinflation; α_1-Antitrypsin Deficiency and Emphysema; Pleurisy, Pleural Effusions, and Empyema; Pneumothorax; Pneumomediastinum; Hydrothorax; Hemothorax; Chylothorax

Paul H. Wise, MD, MPH
Richard E. Behrman Professor of Child Health and Society; Professor of Pediatrics, Centers for Policy, Outcomes and Prevention/Health Policy/Primary Care and Outcomes Research, Stanford University, Stanford, California
Chronic Illness in Childhood

Laila Woc-Colburn, MD
Assistant Professor, Section of Infectious Diseases, Department of Medicine, Baylor College of Medicine, Houston, Texas
American Trypanosomiasis (Chagas Disease; Trypanosoma cruzi)

Joanne Wolfe, MD, MPH
Director, Pediatric Palliative Care, Children's Hospital Boston; Division Chief, Pediatric Palliative Care Service, Department of Psychosocial Oncology and Palliative Care, Dana-Farber Cancer Institute, Boston, Massachusetts
Pediatric Palliative Care

Cynthia J. Wong, MD
Clinical Assistant Professor, Stanford University School of Medicine, Stanford, California
Renal Transplantation

Laura L. Worth, MD, PhD
Associate Professor in the Division of Pediatrics Center, Medical Director for the Children's Cancer Hospital at The University of Texas MD Anderson Cancer Center, Houston, Texas
Molecular and Cellular Biology of Cancer

Joseph L. Wright, MD, MPH
Senior Vice President; Professor of Pediatrics (Vice Chair), Emergency Medicine and Health Policy, Children's National Medical Center, Washington, District of Columbia
Emergency Medical Services for Children

Peter F. Wright, MD
Professor of Pediatrics, Division of Infectious Disease and International Health, Dartmouth Medical School, Lebanon, New Hampshire
Influenza Viruses; Parainfluenza Viruses

Terry W. Wright, PhD
Associate Professor, Pediatrics and Microbiology and Immunology, University of Rochester School of Medicine, Rochester, New York
Pneumocystis jirovecii

Eveline Y. Wu, MD
Fellow, Pediatric Rheumatology and Allergy and Immunology, Duke University Medical Center, Durham, North Carolina
Juvenile Idiopathic Arthritis; Sarcoidosis

Anthony Wynshaw-Boris, MD, PhD
Charles J. Epstein Professor of Human Genetics and Pediatrics; Chief, Division of Medical Genetics, Department of Pediatrics and Institute of Human Genetics, University of California, San Francisco, School of Medicine, San Francisco, California
Dysmorphology

Nada Yazigi, MD
Associate Professor of Clinical Pediatrics, University of Cincinnati Medical School, Division of Gastroenterology, Hepatology and Nutrition, Cincinnati Children's Medical Center, Cincinnati, Ohio
Viral Hepatitis

Ram Yogev, MD
Professor, Department of Pediatrics, Northwestern University Medical School; Deputy Director for Clinical Research—Clinical Sciences, Children's Memorial Hospital, Chicago, Illinois
Acquired Immunodeficiency Syndrome (Human Immunodeficiency Virus)

Marc Yudkoff, MD
W.T. Grant Professor of Pediatrics, University of Pennsylvania School of Medicine; Chief, Division of Child Development, Rehabilitation and Metabolic Disease, The Children's Hospital of Philadelphia, Philadelphia, Pennsylvania
Defects in Metabolism of Amino Acids

Peter E. Zage, MD
Assistant Professor, Division of Pediatrics, University of Texas MD Anderson Cancer Center, Houston, Texas
Neuroblastoma; Retinoblastoma

Anita K.M. Zaidi, MBBS, SM, FAAP
A. Sultan Jamal Professor of Pediatrics and Child Health, and Microbiology; Chair, Department of Pediatrics and Child Health, Aga Khan University, Karachi, Pakistan
Diagnostic Microbiology

Lonnie K. Zeltzer, MD
Director, Pediatric Pain Program; Professor of Pediatrics, Anesthesiology, Psychiatry and Biobehavioral Sciences, David Geffen School of Medicine at UCLA, Los Angeles, California
Pediatric Pain Management

Maija H. Zile, PhD
Professor, Department of Food Science and Human Nutrition, Michigan State University, East Lansing, Michigan
Vitamin A Deficiencies and Excess

Prof. Dr. Peter Zimmer
Abt. Allgemeine Pädiatrie und Neonatologie, Zentrum für Kinderheilkunde und Jugendmedizin, Universitätsklinikum Gießen und Marburg GmbH, Justus-Liebig-Universität, Feulgenstr, Gießen, Germany
Disorders of Malabsorption

Barry Zuckerman, MD
Joel and Barbara Alpert Professor and Chair, Department of Pediatrics, Boston University School of Medicine, Boston Medical Center, Boston, Massachusetts
Impact of Violence on Children

Preface

The publication of the 19th edition of *Nelson Textbook of Pediatrics* combines an important synthesis of clinical pediatrics with the major advances in genomics, diagnosis, imaging, and therapeutics. The 19th edition continues to represent the "state of the art" on the care of the normal and ill neonate, child, or adolescent by presenting both evidence-based medicine and astute clinical experiences from leading international authors.

The promise that translational medicine will improve the lives of all children is greater than ever. Knowledge of human development, behavior, and diseases from the molecular to sociologic levels is increasing at fantastic rates. This has led to greater understanding of health and illness in children, as well as to substantial improvements in health quality for those who have access to health care. These exciting scientific advances also provide hope to effectively address new and emerging diseases threatening children and their families.

Unfortunately, many children throughout the world have not benefited from the significant advances in the prevention and treatment of health-related problems, primarily because of a lack of political will and misplaced priorities. Additionally, many children are at substantial risk from the adverse effects of poverty, war, and bioterrorism. In order for our increasing knowledge to benefit all children and youth, medical advances and good clinical practice must always be coupled with effective advocacy.

This new edition of *Nelson Textbook of Pediatrics* attempts to provide the essential information that practitioners, house staff, medical students, and other care providers involved in pediatric health care throughout the world need to understand to effectively address the enormous range of biologic, psychologic, and social problems that our children and youth may face. Our goal is to be comprehensive yet concise and reader friendly, embracing both the new advances in science as well as the time-honored art of pediatric practice.

The 19th edition is reorganized and revised from the previous edition. There are the additions of new diseases and new chapters, as well as substantial expansion or significant modification of others. In addition, many more tables, photographs, imaging studies, and illustrative figures, as well as up-to-date references, have been added. Every subject has been scrutinized for updating and improvement in its exposition and usefulness to pediatric health care providers. Although to an ill child and his or her family and physician, even the rarest disorder is of central importance, all health problems cannot possibly be covered with the same degree of detail in one general textbook of pediatrics. Thus, leading articles and subspecialty texts are referenced and should be consulted when more information is desired. In addition, to include as much information as possible and to take advantage of advances in providing background, pathophysiology, and literature citations, we have placed even more material on the website accompanying the printed text. This permits an unlimited ability to provide more detailed and updated information through our associated electronic media. Text vital to the care of children remains printed, but additional material will be provided to the reader at *www.expertconsult.com*, including links to Gold Standard's premier online formulary for the most current information available on drugs and dosing.

The outstanding value of the 19th edition of the textbook is due to its expert and authoritative contributors. We are all indebted to these dedicated authors for their hard work, knowledge, thoughtfulness, and good judgment. Our sincere appreciation also goes to Judy Fletcher and Jennifer Shreiner at Elsevier and to Carolyn Redman at the Pediatric Department of the Medical College of Wisconsin. We have all worked hard to produce an edition that will be helpful to those who provide care for children and youth and to those desiring to know more about children's health worldwide.

In this edition we have had informal assistance from many faculty and house staff of the departments of pediatrics at the Medical College of Wisconsin, Wayne State University School of Medicine, Duke University School of Medicine, and University of Rochester School of Medicine. The help of these individuals and of the many practicing pediatricians from around the world who have taken the time to offer thoughtful feedback and suggestions is always greatly appreciated and helpful.

Last and certainly not least, we especially wish to thank our families for their patience and understanding without which this textbook would not have been possible.

Robert M. Kliegman, MD
Bonita F. Stanton, MD
Joseph W. St. Geme III, MD
Nina F. Schor, MD, PhD

Contents

PART I

The Field of Pediatrics

Chapter 1 **Overview of Pediatrics** 1
Bonita F. Stanton and Richard E. Behrman

Chapter 2 **Quality and Safety in Health Care for Children** 13
Ramesh C. Sachdeva

Chapter 3 **Ethics in Pediatric Care** 13
Eric Kodish and Kathryn Weise

Chapter 4 **Cultural Issues in Pediatric Care** 13
Linda Kaljee and Bonita F. Stanton

Chapter 5 **Maximizing Children's Health: Screening, Anticipatory Guidance, and Counseling** 13
Joseph F. Hagan, Jr. and Paula M. Duncan

5.1 **Injury Control** 17
Frederick P. Rivara and David C. Grossman

PART II

Growth, Development, and Behavior

Chapter 6 **Overview and Assessment of Variability** 26
Susan Feigelman

6.1 **Assessment of Fetal Growth and Development** 26
Susan Feigelman

Chapter 7 **The Newborn** 26
John Olsson

Chapter 8 **The First Year** 26
Susan Feigelman

Chapter 9 **The Second Year** 31
Susan Feigelman

Chapter 10 **The Preschool Years** 33
Susan Feigelman

Chapter 11 **Middle Childhood** 36
Susan Feigelman

Chapter 12 **Adolesence** 39

Chapter 13 **Assessment of Growth** 39
Virginia Keane

Chapter 14 **Developmental-Behavioral Screening and Surveillance** 39
Frances P. Glascoe and Kevin P. Marks

Chapter 15 **Child Care: How Pediatricians Can Support Children and Families** 45
Laura Stout Sosinsky and Walter S. Gilliam

Chapter 16 **Loss, Separation, and Bereavement** 45
Janet R. Serwint

Chapter 17 **Sleep Medicine** 46
Judith A. Owens

PART III

Behavioral and Psychiatric Disorders

Chapter 18 **Assessment and Interviewing** 56
Heather J. Walter and David R. DeMaso

Chapter 19 **Psychologic Treatment of Children and Adolescents** 60
David R. DeMaso and Heather J. Walter

19.1 **Psychopharmacology** 60
David R. DeMaso and Heather J. Walter

19.2 **Psychotherapy** 65
David R. DeMaso and Heather J. Walter

19.3 **Psychiatric Hospitalization** 66
David R. DeMaso and Heather J. Walter

Chapter 20 **Psychosomatic Illness** 67
Patricia Ibeziako, Richard J. Shaw, and David R. DeMaso

Chapter 21 **Rumination, Pica, and Elimination (Enuresis, Encopresis) Disorders** 70

21.1 **Rumination Disorder** 70
Emily R. Katz and David R. DeMaso

21.2 **Pica** 71
Emily R. Katz and David R. DeMaso

21.3 **Enuresis (Bed-Wetting)** 71
Emily R. Katz and David R. DeMaso

21.4 **Encopresis** 73
Emily R. Katz and David R. DeMaso

Chapter 22 **Habit and Tic Disorders** 75
Colleen A. Ryan, Gary J. Gosselin, and David R. DeMaso

Chapter 23 **Anxiety Disorders** 77
David R. Rosenberg, Pankhuree Vandana, and Jennifer A. Chiriboga

Chapter 24 **Mood Disorders** 82
Heather J. Walter and David R. DeMaso

24.1 **Major Depression** 82
Heather J. Walter and David R. DeMaso

24.2 **Bipolar Disorder** 85
Heather J. Walter and David R. DeMaso

24.3 **Dysthymic Disorder** 87
Heather J. Walter and David R. DeMaso

Chapter 25 **Suicide and Attempted Suicide** 87
Joanna C.M. Cole, Heather J. Walter, and David R. DeMaso

Chapter 26 **Eating Disorders** 90
Richard E. Kreipe

Chapter 27 **Disruptive Behavioral Disorders** 96
Heather J. Walter and David R. DeMaso

27.1 **Age-Specific Behavioral Disturbances** 99
Heather J. Walter and David R. DeMaso

Chapter 28 **Pervasive Developmental Disorders and Childhood Psychosis** 100
Giuseppe Raviola, Gary J. Gosselin, Heather J. Walter, and David R. DeMaso
28.1 **Autistic Disorder** 100
Giuseppe Raviola, Gary J. Gosselin, Heather J. Walter, and David R. DeMaso
28.2 **Asperger's Disorder** 106
Giuseppe Raviola, Gary J. Gosselin, Heather J. Walter, and David R. DeMaso
28.3 **Childhood Disintegrative Disorder** 106
Giuseppe Raviola, Gary J. Gosselin, Heather J. Walter, and David R. DeMaso
28.4 **Childhood Schizophrenia** 106
Giuseppe Raviola, Gary J. Gosselin, Heather J. Walter, and David R. DeMaso
28.5 **Psychosis Associated with Epilepsy** 106
Robert M. Kliegman
28.6 **Acute Phobic Hallucinations of Childhood** 106
Giuseppe Raviola, Gary J. Gosselin, Heather J. Walter, and David R. DeMaso

PART IV
Learning Disorders

Chapter 29 **Neurodevelopmental Function and Dysfunction in the School-Aged Child** 108
Desmond P. Kelly and Mindo J. Natale
Chapter 30 **Attention-Deficit/Hyperactivity Disorder** 108
Natoshia Raishevich Cunningham and Peter Jensen
Chapter 31 **Dyslexia** 112
G. Reid Lyon, Sally E. Shaywitz, and Bennett A. Shaywitz
Chapter 32 **Language Development and Communication Disorders** 114
Mark D. Simms and Robert L. Schum
32.1 **Dysfluency (Stuttering, Stammering)** 122
Robert M. Kliegman
Chapter 33 **Intellectual Disability** 122
Bruce K. Shapiro and Mark L. Batshaw

PART V
Children with Special Needs

Chapter 34 **Adoption** 130
Mark D. Simms and Samantha L. Wilson
34.1 **Medical Evaluation of Immigrant (Foreign-Born) Children for Infectious Diseases** 132
Stacene R. Maroushek
Chapter 35 **Foster and Kinship Care** 134
Moira Szilagyi and Sara B. Eleoff
Chapter 36 **Impact of Violence on Children** 135
Marilyn Augustyn and Barry Zuckerman
36.1 **Bullying and School Violence** 135
Douglas Vanderbilt and Marilyn Augustyn
36.2 **Effects of War on Children** 135
Isaiah D. Wexler and Eitan Kerem
Chapter 37 **Abused and Neglected Children** 135
Howard Dubowitz and Wendy G. Lane
37.1 **Sexual Abuse** 142
Howard Dubowitz and Wendy G. Lane
37.2 **Factitious Disorder by Proxy (Munchausen Syndrome by Proxy)** 146
Howard Dubowitz and Wendy G. Lane
Chapter 38 **Failure to Thrive** 147
Heather S. McLean and David T. Price
Chapter 39 **Chronic Illness in Childhood** 149
Lisa J. Chamberlain and Paul H. Wise
Chapter 40 **Pediatric Palliative Care** 149
Christina Ullrich, Janet Duncan, Marsha Joselow, and Joanne Wolfe

PART VI
Nutrition

Chapter 41 **Nutritional Requirements** 160
Asim Maqbool, Nicolas Stettler, and Virginia A. Stallings
Chapter 42 **Feeding Healthy Infants, Children, and Adolescents** 160
Nicolas Stettler, Jatinder Bhatia, Anjali Parish, and Virginia A. Stallings
Chapter 43 **Nutrition, Food Security, and Health** 170
Harold Alderman and Meera Shekar
Chapter 44 **Overweight and Obesity** 179
Sheila Gahagan
Chapter 45 **Vitamin A Deficiencies and Excess** 188
Maija H. Zile
Chapter 46 **Vitamin B Complex Deficiency and Excess** 191
H.P.S. Sachdev and Dheeraj Shah
46.1 **Thiamine (Vitamin B_1)** 191
H.P.S. Sachdev and Dheeraj Shah
46.2 **Riboflavin (Vitamin B_2)** 192
H.P.S. Sachdev and Dheeraj Shah
46.3 **Niacin (Vitamin B_3)** 193
H.P.S. Sachdev and Dheeraj Shah
46.4 **Vitamin B_6 (Pyridoxine)** 195
H.P.S. Sachdev and Dheeraj Shah
46.5 **Biotin** 196
H.P.S. Sachdev and Dheeraj Shah
46.6 **Folate** 196
H.P.S. Sachdev and Dheeraj Shah
46.7 **Vitamin B_{12} (Cobalamin)** 197
H.P.S. Sachdev and Dheeraj Shah
Chapter 47 **Vitamin C (Ascorbic Acid)** 198
Dheeraj Shah and H.P.S. Sachdev
Chapter 48 **Rickets and Hypervitaminosis D** 200
Larry A. Greenbaum
Chapter 49 **Vitamin E Deficiency** 209
Larry A. Greenbaum
Chapter 50 **Vitamin K Deficiency** 209
Larry A. Greenbaum
Chapter 51 **Micronutrient Mineral Deficiencies** 211
Larry A. Greenbaum

PART VII
Pathophysiology of Body Fluids and Fluid Therapy

Chapter 52 **Electrolyte and Acid-Base Disorders** 212
Larry A. Greenbaum
52.1 **Composition of Body Fluids** 212
Larry A. Greenbaum
52.2 **Regulation of Osmolality and Volume** 212
Larry A. Greenbaum
52.3 **Sodium** 212
Larry A. Greenbaum
52.4 **Potassium** 219
Larry A. Greenbaum
52.5 **Magnesium** 224
Larry A. Greenbaum
52.6 **Phosphorus** 225
Larry A. Greenbaum
52.7 **Acid-Base Balance** 229
Larry A. Greenbaum

Chapter 53 **Maintenance and Replacement Therapy** 242
Larry A. Greenbaum

Chapter 54 **Deficit Therapy** 245
Larry A. Greenbaum

Chapter 55 **Fluid and Electrolyte Treatment of Specific Disorders** 249

PART VIII
Pediatric Drug Therapy

Chapter 56 **Pediatric Pharmacogenetics, Pharmacogenomics, and Pharmacoproteomics** 250
Kathleen A. Neville and J. Steven Leeder

Chapter 57 **Principles of Drug Therapy** 250
Jennifer A. Lowry, Bridgette L. Jones, Tracy Sandritter, Susanne Liewer, and Gregory L. Kearns

Chapter 58 **Poisonings** 250
Katherine A. O'Donnell and Michele Burns Ewald

Chapter 59 **Herbs, Complementary Therapies, and Integrative Medicine** 270
Paula Gardiner and Kathi J. Kemper

PART IX
The Acutely Ill Child

Chapter 60 **Evaluation of the Sick Child in the Office and Clinic** 275
Mary Saunders and Marc H. Gorelick

Chapter 61 **Emergency Medical Services for Children** 278
Joseph L. Wright and Steven E. Krug
61.1 **Interfacility Transport of the Seriously Ill or Injured Pediatric Patient** 278
Elizabeth A. Edgerton and Bruce L. Klein
61.2 **Outcomes and Risk Adjustment** 278
Evaline A. Alessandrini
61.3 **Principles Applicable to the Developing World** 278
Jennifer I. Chapman and David M. Walker

Chapter 62 **Pediatric Emergencies and Resuscitation** 279
Mary E. Hartman and Ira M. Cheifetz

Chapter 63 **Neurologic Emergencies and Stabilization** 296
Patrick M. Kochanek and Michael J. Bell
63.1 **Brain Death** 304
K. Jane Lee

Chapter 64 **Shock** 305
David A. Turner and Ira M. Cheifetz

Chapter 65 **Respiratory Distress and Failure** 314
Ashok P. Sarnaik and Jeff A. Clark
65.1 **Mechanical Ventilation** 321
Ashok P. Sarnaik and Christopher Mastropietro
65.2 **Long-Term Mechanical Ventilation** 329
Ajit Ashok Sarnaik, Matthew J. Gelmini, and Ashok P. Sarnaik

Chapter 66 **Acute Care of the Victim of Multiple Trauma** 333
Cindy Ganis Roskind, Peter S. Dayan, and Bruce L. Klein
66.1 **Care of Abrasions and Minor Lacerations** 340
Joanna S. Cohen and Bruce L. Klein

Chapter 67 **Drowning and Submersion Injury** 341
Elena Shephard and Linda Quan

Chapter 68 **Burn Injuries** 349
Alia Y. Antoon and Mary K. Donovan

Chapter 69 **Cold Injuries** 357
Alia Y. Antoon and Mary K. Donovan

Chapter 70 **Anesthesia, Perioperative Care, and Sedation** 359
Randall C. Wetzel
70.1 **Sedation and Procedural Pain** 360
Randall C. Wetzel
70.2 **Anesthetic Neurotoxicity** 360
Randall C. Wetzel

Chapter 71 **Pediatric Pain Management** 360
Lonnie K. Zeltzer and Elliot J. Krane

PART X
Human Genetics

Chapter 72 **Integration of Genetics into Pediatric Practice** 376
Brendan Lee
72.1 **Genetic Counseling** 377
Brendan Lee
72.2 **Management and Treatment of Genetic Disorders** 379
Brendan Lee

Chapter 73 **The Genetic Approach in Pediatric Medicine** 380
Daryl A. Scott and Brendan Lee

Chapter 74 **The Human Genome** 383
Daryl A. Scott and Brendan Lee

Chapter 75 **Patterns of Genetic Transmission** 383
Daryl A. Scott and Brendan Lee

Chapter 76 **Cytogenetics** 394
Carlos A. Bacino and Brendan Lee

76.1 **Methods of Chromosome Analysis** 394
Carlos A. Bacino and Brendan Lee

76.2 **Down Syndrome and Other Abnormalities of Chromosome Number** 399
Karen Summar and Brendan Lee

76.3 **Abnormalities of Chromosome Structure** 404
Carlos A. Bacino and Brendan Lee

76.4 **Sex Chromosome Aneuploidy** 408
Carlos A. Bacino and Brendan Lee

76.5 **Fragile Chromosome Sites** 411
Carlos A. Bacino and Brendan Lee

76.6 **Mosaicism** 412
Carlos A. Bacino and Brendan Lee

76.7 **Chromosome Instability Syndromes** 412
Carlos A. Bacino and Brendan Lee

76.8 **Uniparental Disomy and Imprinting** 412
Carlos A. Bacino and Brendan Lee

Chapter 77 **Genetics of Common Disorders** 414
John W. Belmont and Brendan Lee

77.1 **Major Genetic Approaches to the Study of Common Pediatric Disorders** 414
John W. Belmont and Brendan Lee

77.2 **Current Understanding of Genetics of Common Disorders in Children** 415

PART XI

Genetic Disorders of Metabolism

Chapter 78 **An Approach to Inborn Errors of Metabolism** 416
Iraj Rezvani and Geoffrey Rezvani

Chapter 79 **Defects in Metabolism of Amino Acids** 418

79.1 **Phenylalanine** 418
Iraj Rezvani and Joseph John Melvin

79.2 **Tyrosine** 422
Grant A. Mitchell and Iraj Rezvani

79.3 **Methionine** 425
Iraj Rezvani and David S. Rosenblatt

79.4 **Cysteine/Cystine** 429
Iraj Rezvani

79.5 **Tryptophan** 429
Iraj Rezvani

79.6 **Valine, Leucine, Isoleucine, and Related Organic Acidemias** 430
Iraj Rezvani and David S. Rosenblatt

79.7 **Glycine** 438
Iraj Rezvani

79.8 **Serine** 442
Iraj Rezvani

79.9 **Proline** 442
Iraj Rezvani

79.10 **Glutamic Acid** 443
Iraj Rezvani

79.11 **Genetic Disorders of Neurotransmitters** 445
Iraj Rezvani and K. Michael Gibson

79.12 **Urea Cycle and Hyperammonemia (Arginine, Citrulline, Ornithine)** 447
Iraj Rezvani and Marc Yudkoff

79.13 **Histidine** 453
Iraj Rezvani

79.14 **Lysine** 453
Iraj Rezvani

79.15 **Aspartic Acid (Canavan Disease)** 455
Amanda A. Trott, Kimberlee M. Matalon, Marie Michelle Grino, and Reuben K. Matalon

Chapter 80 **Defects in Metabolism of Lipids** 456

80.1 **Disorders of Mitochondrial Fatty Acid β-Oxidation** 456
Charles A. Stanley and Michael J. Bennett

80.2 **Disorders of Very Long Chain Fatty Acids** 462
Hugo W. Moser

80.3 **Disorders of Lipoprotein Metabolism and Transport** 470
William A. Neal

80.4 **Lipidoses (Lysosomal Storage Disorders)** 482
Margaret M. McGovern and Robert J. Desnick

80.5 **Mucolipidoses** 491
Margaret M. McGovern and Robert J. Desnick

Chapter 81 **Defects in Metabolism of Carbohydrates** 492
Priya S. Kishnani and Yuan-Tsong Chen

81.1 **Glycogen Storage Diseases** 492
Priya S. Kishnani and Yuan-Tsong Chen

81.2 **Defects in Galactose Metabolism** 502
Priya S. Kishnani and Yuan-Tsong Chen

81.3 **Defects in Fructose Metabolism** 503
Priya S. Kishnani and Yuan-Tsong Chen

81.4 **Defects in Intermediary Carbohydrate Metabolism Associated with Lactic Acidosis** 503
Priya S. Kishnani and Yuan-Tsong Chen

81.5 **Defects in Pentose Metabolism** 509
Priya S. Kishnani and Yuan-Tsong Chen

81.6 **Disorders of Glycoprotein Degradation and Structure** 509
Margaret M. Mcgovern and Robert J. Desnick

Chapter 82 **Mucopolysaccharidoses** 509
Jürgen Spranger

Chapter 83 **Disorders of Purine and Pyrimidine Metabolism** 516
James C. Harris

Chapter 84 **Progeria** 516
Michael J. Painter

Chapter 85 **The Porphyrias** 517
Karl E. Anderson, Chul Lee, Manisha Balwani, and Robert J. Desnick

Chapter 86 **Hypoglycemia** 517
Mark A. Sperling

PART XII

The Fetus and the Neonatal Infant

Chapter 87 **Overview of Mortality and Morbidity** 532
Waldemar A. Carlo

Chapter 88 **The Newborn Infant** 532
Waldemar A. Carlo

88.1 History in Neonatal Pediatrics 532
88.2 Physical Examination of the Newborn Infant 532
Waldemar A. Carlo
88.3 Routine Delivery Room and Initial Care 536
Waldemar A. Carlo
88.4 Nursery Care 538
Waldemar A. Carlo
88.5 Parent-Infant Bonding 538
Waldemar A. Carlo

Chapter 89 High-Risk Pregnancies 540
Waldemar A. Carlo

Chapter 90 The Fetus 541
Waldemar A. Carlo
90.1 Fetal Growth and Maturity 541
Waldemar A. Carlo
90.2 Fetal Distress 541
Waldemar A. Carlo
90.3 Maternal Disease and the Fetus 545
Waldemar A. Carlo
90.4 Maternal Medication and Toxin Exposure and the Fetus 546
Waldemar A. Carlo
90.5 Teratogens 547
Waldemar A. Carlo
90.6 Radiation 548
Waldemar A. Carlo
90.7 Intrauterine Diagnosis of Fetal Disease 548
Waldemar A. Carlo
90.8 Treatment and Prevention of Fetal Disease 550
Waldemar A. Carlo

Chapter 91 The High-Risk Infant 552
Waldemar A. Carlo
91.1 Multiple Gestation Pregnancies 553
Waldemar A. Carlo
91.2 Prematurity and Intrauterine Growth Restriction 555
Waldemar A. Carlo
91.3 Post-Term Infants 564
Waldemar A. Carlo
91.4 Large-for-Gestational-Age Infants 564
Waldemar A. Carlo
91.5 Infant Transport 564
Waldemar A. Carlo

Chapter 92 Clinical Manifestations of Diseases in the Newborn Period 564
Waldemar A. Carlo

Chapter 93 Nervous System Disorders 565
Waldemar A. Carlo
93.1 The Cranium 565
Waldemar A. Carlo
93.2 Traumatic, Epidural, Subdural, and Subarachnoid Hemorrhage 566
Waldemar A. Carlo
93.3 Intracranial-Intraventricular Hemorrhage and Periventricular Leukomalacia 566
Waldemar A. Carlo
93.4 Brain Injury from Inflammation, Infection, and Medications 568
Waldemar A. Carlo
93.5 Hypoxic-Ischemic Encephalopathy 569
Namasivayam Ambalavanan and Waldemar A. Carlo
93.6 Spine and Spinal Cord 573
Waldemar A. Carlo
93.7 Peripheral Nerve Injuries 573
Waldemar A. Carlo

Chapter 94 Delivery Room Emergencies 575
Waldemar A. Carlo

Chapter 95 Respiratory Tract Disorders 579
Waldemar A. Carlo
95.1 Transition to Pulmonary Respiration 579
Waldemar A. Carlo
95.2 Apnea 580
Waldemar A. Carlo
95.3 Respiratory Distress Syndrome (Hyaline Membrane Disease) 581
Waldemar A. Carlo and Namasivayam Ambalavanan
95.4 Transient Tachypnea of the Newborn 590
Namasivayam Ambalavanan and Waldemar A. Carlo
95.5 Aspiration of Foreign Material (Fetal Aspiration Syndrome, Aspiration Pneumonia) 590
Waldemar A. Carlo
95.6 Meconium Aspiration 590
Namasivayam Ambalavanan and Waldemar A. Carlo
95.7 Persistent Pulmonary Hypertension of the Newborn (Persistent Fetal Circulation) 592
Namasivayam Ambalavanan and Waldemar A. Carlo
95.8 Diaphragmatic Hernia 594
Akhil Maheshwari and Waldemar A. Carlo
95.9 Foramen of Morgagni Hernia 597
Akhil Maheshwari and Waldemar A. Carlo
95.10 Paraesophageal Hernia 597
Akhil Maheshwari and Waldemar A. Carlo
95.11 Eventration 597
Akhil Maheshwari and Waldemar A. Carlo
95.12 Extrapulmonary Air Leaks (Pneumothorax, Pneumomediastinum, Pulmonary Interstitial Emphysema, Pneumopericardium) 597
Waldemar A. Carlo
95.13 Pulmonary Hemorrhage 599
Namasivayam Ambalavanan and Waldemar A. Carlo

Chapter 96 Digestive System Disorders 600
Akhil Maheshwari and Waldemar A. Carlo
96.1 Meconium Ileus in Cystic Fibrosis 601
Akhil Maheshwari and Waldemar A. Carlo
96.2 Neonatal Necrotizing Enterocolitis 601
Akhil Maheshwari and Waldemar A. Carlo
96.3 Jaundice and Hyperbilirubinemia in the Newborn 603
Namasivayam Ambalavanan and Waldemar A. Carlo
96.4 Kernicterus 608
Namasivayam Ambalavanan and Waldemar A. Carlo

Chapter 97 Blood Disorders 612
97.1 Anemia in the Newborn Infant 612
Akhil Maheshwari and Waldemar A. Carlo
97.2 Hemolytic Disease of the Newborn (Erythroblastosis Fetalis) 615
Akhil Maheshwari and Waldemar A. Carlo
97.3 Plethora in the Newborn Infant (Polycythemia) 619
Akhil Maheshwari and Waldemar A. Carlo

97.4 Hemorrhage in the Newborn Infant 620
Akhil Maheshwari and Waldemar A. Carlo

Chapter 98 **Genitourinary System** 621
Waldemar A. Carlo

Chapter 99 **The Umbilicus** 622
Waldemar A. Carlo

Chapter 100 **Metabolic Disturbances** 622
Waldemar A. Carlo

100.1 Maternal Selective Serotonin Reuptake Inhibitors and Neonatal Behavioral Syndromes 625
Waldemar A. Carlo

100.2 Fetal Alcohol Syndrome 625
Waldemar A. Carlo

Chapter 101 **The Endocrine System** 627
Waldemar A. Carlo

101.1 Infants of Diabetic Mothers 627
Waldemar A. Carlo

Chapter 102 **Dysmorphology** 629
Anthony Wynshaw-Boris and Leslie G. Biesecker

Chapter 103 **Infections of the Neonatal Infant** 629

103.1 Pathogenesis and Epidemiology 629
Barbara J. Stoll

103.2 Modes of Transmission and Pathogenesis 629
Barbara J. Stoll

103.3 Immunity 631
Barbara J. Stoll

103.4 Etiology of Fetal and Neonatal Infection 632
Barbara J. Stoll

103.5 Epidemiology of Early- and Late-Onset Neonatal Infections 633
Barbara J. Stoll

103.6 Clinical Manifestations of Transplacental Intrauterine Infections 636
Barbara J. Stoll

103.7 Diagnosis 639
Barbara J. Stoll

103.8 Treatment 644
Barbara J. Stoll

103.9 Complications and Prognosis 646
Barbara J. Stoll

103.10 Prevention 647
Barbara J. Stoll

PART XIII
Adolescent Medicine

Chapter 104 **Adolescent Development** 649

104.1 Adolescent Physical and Social Development 649
Barbara Cromer

104.2 Sexual Identity Development 654
Walter Bockting

104.3 Adolescent Homosexuality 658
Gary Remafedi

Chapter 105 **The Epidemiology of Adolescent Health Problems** 660
Gale R. Burstein

Chapter 106 **Delivery of Health Care to Adolescents** 663
Gale R. Burstein and Barbara Cromer

106.1 Legal Issues 664
Gale R. Burstein

106.2 Screening Procedures 665
Gale R. Burstein

106.3 Health Enhancement 667
Gale R. Burstein

106.4 Transitioning to Adult Care 667
Barbara Cromer

Chapter 107 **Violent Behavior** 667
Margaret M. Stager

Chapter 108 **Substance Abuse** 671
Margaret M. Stager

108.1 Alcohol 678
Margaret M. Stager

108.2 Tobacco 679
Margaret M. Stager

108.3 Marijuana 680
Margaret M. Stager

108.4 Inhalants 681
Margaret M. Stager

108.5 Hallucinogens 682
Margaret M. Stager

108.6 Cocaine 683
Margaret M. Stager

108.7 Amphetamines 683
Margaret M. Stager

108.8 Opiates 684
Margaret M. Stager

108.9 Anabolic Steroids 685

Chapter 109 **The Breast** 685
Barbara Cromer

Chapter 110 **Menstrual Problems** 685
Barbara Cromer

110.1 Amenorrhea 686
Barbara Cromer

110.2 Abnormal Uterine Bleeding 688
Barbara Cromer

110.3 Dysmenorrhea 690
Barbara Cromer

110.4 Premenstrual Syndrome 691
Barbara Cromer

Chapter 111 **Contraception** 692
Barbara Cromer

111.1 Barrier Methods 694
Barbara Cromer

111.2 Spermicides 694
Barbara Cromer

111.3 Combination Methods 696
Barbara Cromer

111.4 Hormonal Methods 696
Barbara Cromer

111.5 Emergency Contraception 698
Barbara Cromer

111.6 Intrauterine Devices 699
Barbara Cromer

Chapter 112 **Adolescent Pregnancy** 699
Dianne S. Elfenbein and Marianne E. Felice

Chapter 113 **Adolescent Rape** 702
Christine E. Barron and Marianne E. Felice

Chapter 114 **Sexually Transmitted Infections** 705
Gale R. Burstein

Chapter 115 **Chronic Fatigue Syndrome** 714
James F. Jones and Hal B. Jenson

PART XIV
Immunology

Section 1 **EVALUATION OF THE IMMUNE SYSTEM** 715

Chapter 116 **Evaluation of Suspected Immunodeficiency** 715
Rebecca H. Buckley

Section 2 **The T-, B-, AND NK-CELL SYSTEMS** 722

Chapter 117 **T Lymphocytes, B Lymphocytes, and Natural Killer Cells** 722
Rebecca H. Buckley

Chapter 118 **Primary Defects of Antibody Production** 722
Rebecca H. Buckley

118.1 **Treatment of B-Cell Defects** 727
Rebecca H. Buckley

Chapter 119 **Primary Defects of Cellular Immunity** 728
Rebecca H. Buckley

Chapter 120 **Primary Combined Antibody and Cellular Immunodeficiencies** 730
Rebecca H. Buckley

120.1 **Severe Combined Immunodeficiency (SCID)** 730
Rebecca H. Buckley

120.2 **Combined Immunodeficiency (CID)** 733
Rebecca H. Buckley

120.3 **Defects of Innate Immunity** 735
Rebecca H. Buckley

120.4 **Treatment of Cellular or Combined Immunodeficiency** 736
Rebecca H. Buckley

120.5 **Immune Dysregulation with Autoimmunity or Lymphoproliferation** 737
Rebecca H. Buckley

Section 3 **THE PHAGOCYTIC SYSTEM** 739

Chapter 121 **Neutrophils** 739
Peter E. Newburger and Laurence A. Boxer

Chapter 122 **Monocytes, Macrophages, and Dendritic Cells** 739
Richard B. Johnston, Jr.

Chapter 123 **Eosinophils** 739
Laurence A. Boxer and Peter E. Newburger

Chapter 124 **Disorders of Phagocyte Function** 741
Laurence A. Boxer and Peter E. Newburger

Chapter 125 **Leukopenia** 746
Peter E. Newburger and Laurence A. Boxer

Chapter 126 **Leukocytosis** 752
Laurence A. Boxer and Peter E. Newburger

Section 4 **THE COMPLEMENT SYSTEM** 753

Chapter 127 **The Complement System** 753
Richard B. Johnston, Jr.

Chapter 128 **Disorders of the Complement System** 753

128.1 **Evaluation of the Complement System** 753
Richard B. Johnston, Jr.

128.2 **Genetic Deficiencies of Complement Components** 753
Richard B. Johnston, Jr.

128.3 **Deficiencies of Plasma, Membrane, or Serosal Complement Control Proteins** 755
Richard B. Johnston, Jr.

128.4 **Secondary Disorders of Complement** 755
Richard B. Johnston, Jr.

128.5 **Treatment of Complement Disorders** 756
Richard B. Johnston, Jr.

Section 5 **HEMATOPOIETIC STEM CELL TRANSPLANTATION** 757

Chapter 129 **Principles and Clinical Indications** 757
Andrea Velardi and Franco Locatelli

Chapter 130 **HSCT from Alternative Sources and Donors** 760
Andrea Velardi and Franco Locatelli

Chapter 131 **Graft Versus Host Disease (GVHD) and Rejection** 760
Andrea Velardi and Franco Locatelli

Chapter 132 **Infectious Complications of HSCT** 762
Andrea Velardi and Franco Locatelli

Chapter 133 **Late Effects of HSCT** 763
Andrea Velardi and Franco Locatelli

PART XV
Allergic Disorders

Chapter 134 **Allergy and the Immunologic Basis of Atopic Disease** 764
Donald Y.M. Leung and Cezmi A. Akdis

Chapter 135 **Diagnosis of Allergic Disease** 764
Dan Atkins and Donald Y.M. Leung

Chapter 136 **Principles of Treatment of Allergic Disease** 768
Dan Atkins and Donald Y.M. Leung

Chapter 137 **Allergic Rhinitis** 775
Henry Milgrom and Donald Y.M. Leung

Chapter 138 **Childhood Asthma** 780
Andrew H. Liu, Ronina A. Covar, Joseph D. Spahn, and Donald Y.M. Leung

Chapter 139 **Atopic Dermatitis (Atopic Eczema)** 801
Donald Y.M. Leung

Chapter 140 **Insect Allergy** 807
Scott H. Sicherer and Donald Y.M. Leung

Chapter 141 **Ocular Allergies** 809
Mark Boguniewicz and Donald Y.M. Leung

Chapter 142 **Urticaria (Hives) and Angioedema** 811
Dan Atkins, Michael M. Frank, Stephen C. Dreskin, and Donald Y.M. Leung

Chapter 143 **Anaphylaxis** 816
Hugh A. Sampson and Donald Y.M. Leung

Chapter 144 **Serum Sickness** 819
Scott H. Sicherer and Donald Y.M. Leung

Chapter 145 **Adverse Reactions to Foods** 820
Hugh A. Sampson and Donald Y.M. Leung

Chapter 146 **Adverse Reactions to Drugs** 824
Mark Boguniewicz and Donald Y.M. Leung

PART XVI
Rheumatic Diseases of Childhood

Chapter 147 **Evaluation of Suspected Rheumatic Disease** 829
C. Egla Rabinovich

Chapter 148 **Treatment of Rheumatic Diseases** 829
Esi Morgan DeWitt, Laura E. Schanberg, and C. Egla Rabinovich

Chapter 149 **Juvenile Idiopathic Arthritis** 829
Eveline Y. Wu, Heather A. Van Mater, and C. Egla Rabinovich

Chapter 150 **Ankylosing Spondylitis and Other Spondyloarthritides** 839
James Birmingham and Robert A. Colbert

Chapter 151 **Reactive and Postinfectious Arthritis** 839
James Birmingham and Robert A. Colbert

Chapter 152 **Systemic Lupus Erythematosus** 841
Stacy P. Ardoin and Laura E. Schanberg

152.1 **Neonatal Lupus** 845
Stacy P. Ardoin and Laura E. Schanberg

Chapter 153 **Juvenile Dermatomyositis** 846
Angela Byun Robinson and Ann M. Reed

Chapter 154 **Scleroderma and Raynaud Phenomenon** 850
Heather A. Van Mater and C. Egla Rabinovich

Chapter 155 **Behçet Disease** 853
Abraham Gedalia

Chapter 156 **Sjögren Syndrome** 854
Abraham Gedalia

Chapter 157 **Hereditary Periodic Fever Syndromes** 855
Abraham Gedalia

Chapter 158 **Amyloidosis** 860
Abraham Gedalia

Chapter 159 **Sarcoidosis** 860
Eveline Y. Wu and Esi Morgan DeWitt

Chapter 160 **Kawasaki Disease** 862
Mary Beth F. Son and Jane W. Newburger

Chapter 161 **Vasculitis Syndromes** 867
Stacy P. Ardoin and Edward Fels

161.1 **Henoch-Schönlein Purpura** 868
Stacy P. Ardoin and Edward Fels

161.2 **Takayasu Arteritis** 871
Stacy P. Ardoin and Edward Fels

161.3 **Polyarteritis Nodosa and Cutaneous Polyarteritis Nodosa** 872
Stacy P. Ardoin and Edward Fels

161.4 **ANCA-Associated Vasculitis** 874
Stacy P. Ardoin and Edward Fels

161.5 **Other Vasculitis Syndromes** 876
Stacy P. Ardoin and Edward Fels

Chapter 162 **Musculoskeletal Pain Syndromes** 876
Kelly K. Anthony and Laura E. Schanberg

162.1 **Fibromyalgia** 878
Kelly K. Anthony and Laura E. Schanberg

162.2 **Complex Regional Pain Syndrome** 879
Kelly K. Anthony and Laura E. Schanberg

162.3 **Erythromelalgia** 880
Laura E. Schanberg

Chapter 163 **Miscellaneous Conditions Associated with Arthritis** 880
Angela Byun Robinson and Leonard D. Stein

PART XVII
Infectious Diseases

Section 1 **GENERAL CONSIDERATIONS** 881

Chapter 164 **Diagnostic Microbiology** 881
Anita K.M. Zaidi and Donald A. Goldmann

Section 2 **PREVENTIVE MEASURES**

Chapter 165 **Immunization Practices** 881
Walter A. Orenstein and Larry K. Pickering

165.1 **International Immunization Practices** 893
Jean-Marie Okwo-Bele and John David Clemens

Chapter 166 **Infection Prevention and Control** 895
Michael J. Chusid and Mary M. Rotar

Chapter 167 **Child Care and Communicable Diseases** 895
Linda A. Waggoner-Fountain

Chapter 168 **Health Advice for Children Traveling Internationally** 896
Jessica K. Fairley and Chandy C. John

Chapter 169 **Fever** 896
Linda S. Nield and Deepak Kamat

Chapter 170 **Fever without a Focus** 896
Linda S. Nield and Deepak Kamat

Chapter 171 **Infections in Immunocompromised Persons** 902
Marian G. Michaels and Michael Green

171.1 **Infections Occurring with Primary Immunodeficiencies** 902
Marian G. Michaels and Michael Green

171.2 **Infections Occurring with Acquired Immunodeficiencies** 903
Marian G. Michaels and Michael Green

171.3 **Prevention of Infection in Immunocompromised Persons** 903
Marian G. Michaels and Michael Green

Chapter 172 **Infection Associated with Medical Devices** 903
Patricia M. Flynn

Section 3 **ANTIBIOTIC THERAPY** 903

Chapter 173 **Principles of Antibacterial Therapy** 903
Mark R. Schleiss

Section 4 **GRAM-POSITIVE BACTERIAL INFECTIONS** 903

Chapter 174 ***Staphylococcus*** 903
James K. Todd

174.1 ***Staphylococcus aureus*** 904
James K. Todd

174.2 **Toxic Shock Syndrome** 908
James K. Todd

174.3 **Coagulase-Negative Staphylococci** 909
James K. Todd

Chapter 175 ***Streptococcus pneumoniae*** **(Pneumococcus)** 910
Timothy R. Peters and Jon S. Abramson

Chapter 176 **Group A Streptococcus** 914
Michael A. Gerber

176.1 **Rheumatic Fever** 920
Michael A. Gerber

Chapter 177 **Group B Streptococcus** 925
Catherine S. Lachenauer and Michael R. Wessels

Chapter 178 **Non–Group A or B Streptococci** 928
Michael A. Gerber

Chapter 179 ***Enterococcus*** 928
David B. Haslam

Chapter 180 **Diphtheria *(Corynebacterium diphtheriae)*** 929
E. Stephen Buescher

Chapter 181 ***Listeria monocytogenes*** 929
Robert S. Baltimore

Chapter 182 ***Actinomyces*** 929
Richard F. Jacobs and Gordon E. Schutze

Chapter 183 ***Nocardia*** 929
Richard F. Jacobs and Gordon E. Schutze

Section 5 **GRAM-NEGATIVE BACTERIAL INFECTIONS** 929

Chapter 184 ***Neisseria meningitidis*** **(Meningococcus)** 929
Dan M. Granoff and Janet R. Gilsdorf

Chapter 185 ***Neisseria gonorrhoeae*** **(Gonococcus)** 935
Toni Darville

Chapter 186 ***Haemophilus influenzae*** 940
Robert S. Daum

Chapter 187 **Chancroid *(Haemophilus ducreyi)*** 944
H. Dele Davies and Parvin H. Azimi

Chapter 188 ***Moraxella catarrhalis*** 944
Timothy F. Murphy

Chapter 189 **Pertussis (*Bordetella pertussis* and *Bordetella parapertussis*)** 944
Sarah S. Long

Chapter 190 ***Salmonella*** 948
Zulfiqar Ahmed Bhutta

190.1 **Nontyphoidal Salmonellosis** 949
Zulfiqar Ahmed Bhutta

190.2 **Enteric Fever (Typhoid Fever)** 954
Zulfiqar Ahmed Bhutta

Chapter 191 ***Shigella*** 959
Theresa J. Ochoa and Thomas G. Cleary

Chapter 192 ***Escherichia coli*** 961
Theresa J. Ochoa and Thomas G. Cleary

Chapter 193 **Cholera** 965
Anna Lena Lopez

Chapter 194 ***Campylobacter*** 968
Gloria P. Heresi, Shahida Baqar, and James R. Murphy

Chapter 195 ***Yersinia*** 971
Anupama Kalaskar, Gloria P. Heresi, and James R. Murphy

195.1 ***Yersinia enterocolitica*** 971
Anupama Kalaskar, Gloria P. Heresi, and James R. Murphy

195.2 ***Yersinia pseudotuberculosis*** 972
Anupama Kalaskar, Gloria P. Heresi, and James R. Murphy

195.3 **Plague *(Yersinia pestis)*** 973
Anupama Kalaskar, Gloria P. Heresi, and James R. Murphy

Chapter 196 ***Aeromonas*** **and** ***Plesiomonas*** 974
Guenet H. Degaffe, Gloria P. Heresi, and James R. Murphy

196.1 ***Aeromonas*** 974
Guenet H. Degaffe, Gloria P. Heresi, and James R. Murphy

196.2 ***Plesiomonas shigelloides*** 974
Guenet H. Degaffe, Gloria P. Heresi, and James R. Murphy

Chapter 197 ***Pseudomonas, Burkholderia,*** **and** ***Stenotrophomonas*** 975

197.1 ***Pseudomonas aeruginosa*** 975
Thomas S. Murray and Robert S. Baltimore

197.2 ***Burkholderia*** 977
Thomas S. Murray and Robert S. Baltimore

197.3 ***Stenotrophomonas*** 977
Thomas S. Murray and Robert S. Baltimore

Chapter 198 **Tularemia *(Francisella tularensis)*** 978
Gordon E. Schutze and Richard F. Jacobs

Chapter 199 ***Brucella*** 980
Gordon E. Schutze and Richard F. Jacobs

Chapter 200 ***Legionella*** 982
Lucy S. Tompkins

Chapter 201 ***Bartonella*** 982
Barbara W. Stechenberg

201.1 **Bartonellosis *(Bartonella bacilliformis)*** 982
Barbara W. Stechenberg

201.2 **Cat-Scratch Disease *(Bartonella henselae)*** 983
Barbara W. Stechenberg

201.3 **Trench Fever *(Bartonella quintana)*** 986
Barbara W. Stechenberg

201.4 **Bacillary Angiomatosis and Bacillary Peliosis Hepatis (*Bartonella henselae* and *Bartonella quintana*)** 986
Barbara W. Stechenberg

Section 6 **ANAEROBIC BACTERIAL INFECTIONS** 987

Chapter 202 **Botulism *(Clostridium botulinum)*** 987
Stephen S. Arnon

Chapter 203 **Tetanus *(Clostridium tetani)*** 991
Stephen S. Arnon

Chapter 204 ***Clostridium difficile* Infection** 994
Ethan A. Mezoff and Mitchell B. Cohen

Chapter 205 **Other Anaerobic Infections** 995
Michael J. Chusid

Section 7 **MYCOBACTERIAL INFECTIONS** 996

Chapter 206 **Principles of Antimycobacterial Therapy** 996
Stacene R. Maroushek

Chapter 207 **Tuberculosis *(Mycobacterium tuberculosis)*** 996
Jeffrey R. Starke

Chapter 208 **Hansen Disease *(Mycobacterium leprae)*** 1011
Dwight A. Powell and Vijay Pannikar

Chapter 209 **Nontuberculous Mycobacteria** 1011
Jakko van Ingen and Dick van Soolingen

Section 8 **SPIROCHETAL INFECTIONS** 1016

Chapter 210 **Syphilis *(Treponema pallidum)*** 1016
Maria Jevitz Patterson and H. Dele Davies

Chapter 211 **Nonvenereal Treponemal Infections** 1023
Stephen K. Obaro and H. Dele Davies

211.1 **Yaws *(Treponema pertenue)*** 1023
Stephen K. Obaro and H. Dele Davies

211.2 **Bejel (Endemic Syphilis; *Treponema pallidum* subspecies *endemicum*)** 1023
Stephen K. Obaro and H. Dele Davies

211.3 **Pinta *(Treponema carateum)*** 1023
Stephen K. Obaro and H. Dele Davies

Chapter 212 ***Leptospira*** 1023
H. Dele Davies and Melissa Beth Rosenberg

Chapter 213 **Relapsing Fever *(Borrelia)*** 1025
H. Dele Davies and Stephen K. Obaro

Chapter 214 **Lyme Disease *(Borrelia burgdorferi)*** 1025
Stephen C. Eppes

Section 9 **MYCOPLASMAL INFECTIONS** 1029

Chapter 215 ***Mycoplasma pneumoniae*** 1029
Dwight A. Powell

Chapter 216 **Genital Mycoplasmas *(Mycoplasma hominis, Mycoplasma genitalium,* and *Ureaplasma urealyticum)*** 1032
Dwight A. Powell

Section 10 **CHLAMYDIAL INFECTIONS** 1033

Chapter 217 ***Chlamydophila pneumoniae*** 1033
Stephan A. Kohlhoff and Margaret R. Hammerschlag

Chapter 218 ***Chlamydia trachomatis*** 1035
Margaret R. Hammerschlag

218.1 **Trachoma** 1035
Margaret R. Hammerschlag

218.2 **Genital Tract Infections** 1035
Margaret R. Hammerschlag

218.3 **Conjunctivitis and Pneumonia in Newborns** 1037
Margaret R. Hammerschlag

218.4 **Lymphogranuloma Venereum** 1037
Margaret R. Hammerschlag

Chapter 219 **Psittacosis *(Chlamydophila psittaci)*** 1038
Stephan A. Kohlhoff and Margaret R. Hammerschlag

Section 11 **RICKETTSIAL INFECTIONS** 1038

Chapter 220 **Spotted Fever and Transitional Group Rickettsioses** 1038
Megan E. Reller and J. Stephen Dumler

220.1 **Rocky Mountain Spotted Fever *(Rickettsia rickettsii)*** 1038
Megan E. Reller and J. Stephen Dumler

220.2 **Mediterranean Spotted Fever or Boutonneuse Fever *(Rickettsia conorii)*** 1043
Megan E. Reller and J. Stephen Dumler

220.3 **Rickettsialpox *(Rickettsia akari)*** 1044
Megan E. Reller and J. Stephen Dumler

Chapter 221 **Scrub Typhus *(Orientia tsutsugamushi)*** 1045
Megan E. Reller and J. Stephen Dumler

Chapter 222 **Typhus Group Rickettsioses** 1046
Megan E. Reller and J. Stephen Dumler

222.1 **Murine Typhus *(Rickettsia typhi)*** 1046
Megan E. Reller and J. Stephen Dumler

222.2 **Epidemic Typhus *(Rickettsia prowazekii)*** 1047
Megan E. Reller and J. Stephen Dumler

Chapter 223 **Ehrlichioses and Anaplasmosis** 1048
Megan E. Reller and J. Stephen Dumler

Chapter 224 **Q Fever *(Coxiella burnetii)*** 1051
Megan E. Reller and J. Stephen Dumler

Section 12 **FUNGAL INFECTIONS** 1053

Chapter 225 **Principles of Antifungal Therapy** 1053
William J. Steinbach, Michael Cohen-Wolkowiez, and Daniel K. Benjamin, Jr.

Chapter 226 ***Candida*** 1053
P. Brian Smith and Daniel K. Benjamin, Jr.

226.1 **Neonatal Infections** 1053
P. Brian Smith and Daniel K. Benjamin, Jr.

226.2 **Infections in Immunocompetent Children and Adolescents** 1054
P. Brian Smith and Daniel K. Benjamin, Jr.

226.3 **Infections in Immunocompromised Children and Adolescents** 1055
P. Brian Smith and Daniel K. Benjamin, Jr.

226.4 **Chronic Mucocutaneous Candidiasis** 1056
P. Brian Smith and Daniel K. Benjamin, Jr.

Chapter 227 ***Cryptococcus neoformans*** 1056
Jane M. Gould and Stephen C. Aronoff

Chapter 228 ***Malassezia*** 1058
Martin E. Weisse and Ashley M. Maranich

Chapter 229 ***Aspergillus*** 1058
Luise E. Rogg and William J. Steinbach

229.1 **Allergic Disease (Hypersensitivity Syndromes)** 1058
Luise E. Rogg and William J. Steinbach

229.2 **Saprophytic (Noninvasive) Syndromes** 1059
Luise E. Rogg and William J. Steinbach

229.3 **Invasive Disease** 1060
Luise E. Rogg and William J. Steinbach

Chapter 230 **Histoplasmosis *(Histoplasma capsulatum)*** 1062
Jane M. Gould and Stephen C. Aronoff

Chapter 231 **Blastomycosis (*Blastomyces dermatitidis*)** 1064
Gregory M. Gauthier and Bruce S. Klein

Chapter 232 **Coccidioidomycosis (*Coccidioides* Species)** 1065
Martin B. Kleiman

Chapter 233 ***Paracoccidioides brasiliensis*** 1068
Jane M. Gould and Stephen C. Aronoff

Chapter 234 **Sporotrichosis *(Sporothrix schenckii)*** 1068
David M. Fleece and Stephen C. Aronoff

Chapter 235 **Zygomycosis (Mucormycosis)** 1069
Jane M. Gould and Stephen C. Aronoff

Chapter 236 ***Pneumocystis jirovecii*** 1069
Francis Gigliotti and Terry W. Wright

Section 13 **VIRAL INFECTIONS** 1069

Chapter 237 **Principles of Antiviral Therapy** 1069
Mark R. Schleiss

Chapter 238 **Measles** 1069
Wilbert H. Mason

Chapter 239 **Rubella** 1075
Wilbert H. Mason

Chapter 240 **Mumps** 1078
Wilbert H. Mason

Chapter 241 **Polioviruses** 1081
Eric A.F. Simões

Chapter 242 **Nonpolio Enteroviruses** 1088
Mark J. Abzug

Chapter 243 **Parvovirus B19** 1094
William C. Koch

Chapter 244 **Herpes Simplex Virus** 1097
Lawrence R. Stanberry

Chapter 245 **Varicella-Zoster Virus Infections** 1104
Philip S. LaRussa and Mona Marin

Chapter 246 **Epstein-Barr Virus** 1110
Hal B. Jenson

Chapter 247 **Cytomegalovirus** 1115
Sergio Stagno

Chapter 248 **Roseola (Human Herpes Viruses 6 and 7)** 1117
Mary T. Caserta

Chapter 249 **Human Herpesvirus 8** 1121
Mary T. Caserta

Chapter 250 **Influenza Viruses** 1121
Peter F. Wright

Chapter 251 **Parainfluenza Viruses** 1125
Angela Jean Peck Campbell and Peter F. Wright

Chapter 252 **Respiratory Syncytial Virus** 1126
James E. Crowe, Jr.

Chapter 253 **Human Metapneumovirus** 1129
James E. Crowe, Jr.

Chapter 254 **Adenoviruses** 1131
John V. Williams

Chapter 255 **Rhinoviruses** 1133
E. Kathryn Miller and John V. Williams

Chapter 256 **Coronaviruses** 1134
Mark R. Denison

256.1 **Severe Acute Respiratory Syndrome–Associated Coronavirus** 1134
Mark R. Denison

Chapter 257 **Rotaviruses, Caliciviruses, and Astroviruses** 1134
Dorsey M. Bass

Chapter 258 **Human Papillomaviruses** 1137
Anna-Barbara Moscicki

Chapter 259 **Arboviral Encephalitis in North America** 1141
Scott B. Halstead

Chapter 260 **Arboviral Encephalitis outside North America** 1144
Scott B. Halstead

260.1 **Venezuelan Equine Encephalitis** 1144
Scott B. Halstead

260.2 **Japanese Encephalitis** 1145
Scott B. Halstead

260.3 **Tick-Borne Encephalitis** 1146
Scott B. Halstead

Chapter 261 **Dengue Fever and Dengue Hemorrhagic Fever** 1147
Scott B. Halstead

Chapter 262 **Yellow Fever** 1150
Scott B. Halstead

Chapter 263 **Other Viral Hemorrhagic Fevers** 1150
Scott B. Halstead

Chapter 264 **Lymphocytic Choriomeningitis Virus** 1153
Daniel J. Bonthius

Chapter 265 **Hantavirus Pulmonary Syndrome** 1154
Scott B. Halstead

Chapter 266 **Rabies** 1154
Rodney E. Willoughby, Jr.

Chapter 267 **Polyomaviruses** 1157
Gregory A. Storch

Chapter 268 **Acquired Immunodeficiency Syndrome (Human Immunodeficiency Virus)** 1157
Ram Yogev and Ellen Gould Chadwick

Chapter 269 **Human T-Lymphotropic Viruses (1 and 2)** 1177
Hal B. Jenson

Chapter 270 **Transmissible Spongiform Encephalopathies** 1177
David M. Asher

Section 14 **ANTIPARASITIC THERAPY** 1177

Chapter 271 **Principles of Antiparasitic Therapy** 1177
Mark R. Schleiss and Sharon F. Chen

Section 15 **PROTOZOAN DISEASES** 1178

Chapter 272 **Primary Amebic Meningoencephalitis** 1178
Martin E. Weisse and Stephen C. Aronoff

Chapter 273 **Amebiasis** 1178
Edsel Maurice T. Salvana and Robert A. Salata

Chapter 274 **Giardiasis and Balantidiasis** 1180
274.1 ***Giardia lamblia*** 1180
Chandy C. John
274.2 **Balantidiasis** 1183
Chandy C. John

Chapter 275 ***Cryptosporidium, Isospora, Cyclospora,* and Microsporidia** 1183
Patricia M. Flynn

Chapter 276 **Trichomoniasis *(Trichomonas vaginalis)*** 1185
Edsel Maurice T. Salvana and Robert A. Salata

Chapter 277 **Leishmaniasis *(Leishmania)*** 1186
Peter C. Melby

Chapter 278 **African Trypanosomiasis (Sleeping Sickness; *Trypanosoma brucei* Complex)** 1190
Edsel Maurice T. Salvana and Robert A. Salata

Chapter 279 **American Trypanosomiasis (Chagas Disease; *Trypanosoma cruzi*)** 1193
Edsel Maurice T. Salvana, Laila Woc-Colburn, and Robert A. Salata

Chapter 280 **Malaria *(Plasmodium)*** 1198
Chandy C. John and Peter J. Krause

Chapter 281 **Babesiosis *(Babesia)*** 1207
Peter J. Krause

Chapter 282 **Toxoplasmosis *(Toxoplasma gondii)*** 1208
Rima McLeod

Section 16 **HELMINTHIC DISEASES** 1217

Chapter 283 **Ascariasis *(Ascaris lumbricoides)*** 1217
Arlene E. Dent and James W. Kazura

Chapter 284 **Hookworms (*Necator americanus* and *Ancylostoma* spp.)** 1218
Peter J. Hotez
284.1 **Cutaneous Larva Migrans** 1220
Peter J. Hotez

Chapter 285 **Trichuriasis *(Trichuris trichiura)*** 1221
Arlene E. Dent and James W. Kazura

Chapter 286 **Enterobiasis *(Enterobius vermicularis)*** 1222
Arlene E. Dent and James W. Kazura

Chapter 287 **Strongyloidiasis *(Strongyloides stercoralis)*** 1223
Arlene E. Dent and James W. Kazura

Chapter 288 **Lymphatic Filariasis (*Brugia malayi, Brugia timori,* and *Wuchereria bancrofti*)** 1224
Arlene E. Dent and James W. Kazura

Chapter 289 **Other Tissue Nematodes** 1225
Arlene E. Dent and James W. Kazura

Chapter 290 **Toxocariasis (Visceral and Ocular Larva Migrans)** 1227
Arlene E. Dent and James W. Kazura

Chapter 291 **Trichinosis *(Trichinella spiralis)*** 1229
Arlene E. Dent and James W. Kazura

Chapter 292 **Schistosomiasis *(Schistosoma)*** 1230
Charles H. King and Amaya Lopez Bustinduy

Chapter 293 **Flukes (Liver, Lung, and Intestinal)** 1231
Charles H. King and Amaya Lopez Bustinduy

Chapter 294 **Adult Tapeworm Infections** 1232
Ronald Blanton

Chapter 295 **Cysticercosis** 1234
Ronald Blanton

Chapter 296 **Echinococcosis (*Echinococcus granulosus* and *Echinococcus multilocularis*)** 1237
Ronald Blanton

PART XVIII

The Digestive System

Section 1 **CLINICAL MANIFESTATIONS OF GASTROINTESTINAL DISEASE** 1240

Chapter 297 **Normal Digestive Tract Phenomena** 1240
Chris A. Liacouras

Chapter 298 **Major Symptoms and Signs of Digestive Tract Disorders** 1240
Raman Sreedharan and Chris A. Liacouras

Section 2 **THE ORAL CAVITY** 1249

Chapter 299 **Development and Developmental Anomalies of the Teeth** 1249
Norman Tinanoff

Chapter 300 **Disorders of the Oral Cavity Associated with Other Conditions** 1251
Norman Tinanoff

Chapter 301 **Malocclusion** 1252
Norman Tinanoff

Chapter 302 **Cleft Lip and Palate** 1252
Norman Tinanoff

Chapter 303 **Syndromes with Oral Manifestations** 1253
Norman Tinanoff

Chapter 304 **Dental Caries** 1254
Norman Tinanoff

Chapter 305 **Periodontal Diseases** 1257
Norman Tinanoff

Chapter 306 **Dental Trauma** 1258
Norman Tinanoff

Chapter 307 **Common Lesions of the Oral Soft Tissues** 1259
Norman Tinanoff

Chapter 308 **Diseases of the Salivary Glands and Jaws** 1261
Norman Tinanoff

Chapter 309 **Diagnostic Radiology in Dental Assessment** 1261
Norman Tinanoff

Section 3 **THE ESOPHAGUS** 1261

Chapter 310 **Embryology, Anatomy, and Function of the Esophagus** 1261
Seema Khan and Susan R. Orenstein

310.1 **Common Clinical Manifestations and Diagnostic Aids** 1261
Seema Khan and Susan R. Orenstein

Chapter 311 **Congenital Anomalies** 1262

311.1 **Esophageal Atresia and Tracheoesophageal Fistula** 1262
Seema Khan and Susan R. Orenstein

311.2 **Laryngotracheoesophageal Clefts** 1263
Seema Khan and Susan R. Orenstein

Chapter 312 **Obstructing and Motility Disorders of the Esophagus** 1263
Seema Khan and Susan R. Orenstein

Chapter 313 **Dysmotility** 1264
Seema Khan and Susan R. Orenstein

Chapter 314 **Hiatal Hernia** 1265
Seema Khan and Susan R. Orenstein

Chapter 315 **Gastroesophageal Reflux Disease** 1266
Seema Khan and Susan R. Orenstein

315.1 **Complications of Gastroesophageal Reflux Disease** 1269
Seema Khan and Susan R. Orenstein

Chapter 316 **Eosinophilic Esophagitis and Non-GERD Esophagitis** 1270
Seema Khan and Susan R. Orenstein

Chapter 317 **Esophageal Perforation** 1271
Seema Khan and Susan R. Orenstein

Chapter 318 **Esophageal Varices** 1271
Seema Khan and Susan R. Orenstein

Chapter 319 **Ingestions** 1271

319.1 **Foreign Bodies in the Esophagus** 1271
Seema Khan and Susan R. Orenstein

319.2 **Caustic Ingestions** 1272
Seema Khan and Susan R. Orenstein

Section 4 **STOMACH AND INTESTINES** 1273

Chapter 320 **Normal Development, Structure, and Function** 1273
Chris A. Liacouras

Chapter 321 **Pyloric Stenosis and Other Congenital Anomalies of the Stomach** 1274

321.1 **Hypertrophic Pyloric Stenosis** 1274
Anna Klaudia Hunter and Chris A. Liacouras

321.2 **Congenital Gastric Outlet Obstruction** 1275
Chris A. Liacouras

321.3 **Gastric Duplication** 1276
Anna Klaudia Hunter and Chris A. Liacouras

321.4 **Gastric Volvulus** 1276
Anna Klaudia Hunter and Chris A. Liacouras

321.5 **Hypertrophic Gastropathy** 1276
Anna Klaudia Hunter and Chris A. Liacouras

Chapter 322 **Intestinal Atresia, Stenosis, and Malrotation** 1277
Christina Bales and Chris A. Liacouras

322.1 **Duodenal Obstruction** 1277
Christina Bales and Chris A. Liacouras

322.2 **Jejunal and Ileal Atresia and Obstruction** 1278
Christina Bales and Chris A. Liacouras

322.3 **Malrotation** 1280
Melissa Kennedy and Chris A. Liacouras

Chapter 323 **Intestinal Duplications, Meckel Diverticulum, and Other Remnants of the Omphalomesenteric Duct** 1281

323.1 **Intestinal Duplication** 1281
Chris A. Liacouras

323.2 **Meckel Diverticulum and Other Remnants of the Omphalomesenteric Duct** 1281
Melissa Kennedy and Chris A. Liacouras

Chapter 324 **Motility Disorders and Hirschsprung Disease** 1283

324.1 **Chronic Intestinal Pseudo-Obstruction** 1283
Kristin N. Fiorino and Chris A. Liacouras

324.2 **Functional Constipation** 1284
Kristin N. Fiorino and Chris A. Liacouras

324.3 **Congenital Aganglionic Megacolon (Hirschsprung Disease)** 1284
Kristin Fiorino and Chris A. Liacouras

324.4 **Intestinal Neuronal Dysplasia** 1287
Kristin N. Fiorino and Chris A. Liacouras

324.5 **Superior Mesenteric Artery Syndrome (Wilkie Syndrome, Cast Syndrome, Arteriomesenteric Duodenal Compression Syndrome)** 1287
Andrew Chu and Chris A. Liacouras

Chapter 325 **Ileus, Adhesions, Intussusception, and Closed-Loop Obstructions** 1287

325.1 **Ileus** 1287
Andrew Chu and Chris A. Liacouras

325.2 **Adhesions** 1287
Andrew Chu and Chris A. Liacouras

325.3 **Intussusception** 1287
Melissa Kennedy and Chris A. Liacouras

325.4 **Closed-Loop Obstructions** 1289
Andrew Chu and Chris A. Liacouras

Chapter 326 **Foreign Bodies and Bezoars** 1290

326.1 **Foreign Bodies in the Stomach and Intestine** 1290
Judith Kelsen and Chris A. Liacouras

326.2 **Bezoars** 1291
Judith Kelsen and Chris A. Liacouras

Chapter 327 **Peptic Ulcer Disease in Children** 1291
Samra S. Blanchard and Steven J. Czinn

327.1 **Zollinger-Ellison Syndrome** 1294
Samra S. Blanchard and Steven J. Czinn

Chapter 328 **Inflammatory Bowel Disease** 1294
Andrew B. Grossman and Robert N. Baldassano

328.1 **Chronic Ulcerative Colitis** 1295
Andrew B. Grossman and Robert N. Baldassano
328.2 **Crohn Disease (Regional Enteritis, Regional Ileitis, Granulomatous Colitis)** 1300
Andrew B. Grossman and Robert N. Baldassano

Chapter 329 **Eosinophilic Gastroenteritis** 1304
Andrew B. Grossman and Robert N. Baldassano

Chapter 330 **Disorders of Malabsorption** 1304
David Branski
330.1 **Evaluation of Children with Suspected Intestinal Malabsorption** 1306
Michael J. Lentze and David Branski
330.2 **Gluten-Sensitive Enteropathy (Celiac Disease)** 1308
David Branski and Riccardo Troncone
330.3 **Other Malabsorptive Syndromes** 1311
Philip M. Sherman, David Branski, and Olivier Goulet
330.4 **Intestinal Infections and Infestations Associated with Malabsorption** 1313
David Branski and Raanan Shamir
330.5 **Immunodeficiency Disorders** 1314
Ernest G. Seidman and David Branski
330.6 **Immunoproliferative Small Intestinal Disease** 1315
Ernest G. Seidman and David Branski
330.7 **Short Bowel Syndrome** 1315
Jon A. Vanderhoof and David Branski
330.8 **Chronic Malnutrition** 1317
Raanan Shamir and David Branski
330.9 **Enzyme Deficiencies** 1317
Michael J. Lentze and David Branski
330.10 **Liver and Biliary Disorders Causing Malabsorption** 1319
Anil Dhawan and David Branski
330.11 **Rare Inborn Defects Causing Malabsorption** 1319
Peter Zimmer and David Branski
330.12 **Malabsorption in Eosinophilic Gastroenteritis** 1322
Ernest G. Seidman and David Branski
330.13 **Malabsorption in Inflammatory Bowel Disease** 1322
Ernest G. Seidman and David Branski

Chapter 331 **Intestinal Transplantation in Children with Intestinal Failure** 1322
Jorge D. Reyes

Chapter 332 **Acute Gastroenteritis in Children** 1323
Zulfiqar Ahmed Bhutta
332.1 **Traveler's Diarrhea** 1338
Zulfiqar Ahmed Bhutta

Chapter 333 **Chronic Diarrhea** 1339
Alfredo Guarino and David Branski
333.1 **Diarrhea from Neuroendocrine Tumors** 1346
Helen Spoudeas and David Branski

Chapter 334 **Functional Abdominal Pain (Nonorganic Chronic Abdominal Pain)** 1346
Raman Sreedharan and Chris A. Liacouras

Chapter 335 **Acute Appendicitis** 1349
John J. Aiken and Keith T. Oldham

Chapter 336 **Surgical Conditions of the Anus and Rectum** 1355
336.1 **Anorectal Malformations** 1355
Shawn J. Stafford and Michael D. Klein
336.2 **Anal Fissure** 1359
Shawn J. Stafford and Michael D. Klein
336.3 **Perianal Abscess and Fistula** 1359
Shawn J. Stafford and Michael D. Klein
336.4 **Hemorrhoids** 1360
Shawn J. Stafford and Michael D. Klein
336.5 **Rectal Mucosal Prolapse** 1361
Shawn J. Stafford and Michael D. Klein
336.6 **Pilonidal Sinus and Abscess** 1362
Shawn J. Stafford and Michael D. Klein

Chapter 337 **Tumors of the Digestive Tract** 1362
Lydia J. Donoghue and Michael D. Klein

Chapter 338 **Inguinal Hernias** 1362
John J. Aiken and Keith T. Oldham

Section 5 **EXOCRINE PANCREAS** 1368

Chapter 339 **Embryology, Anatomy, and Physiology** 1368
Steven L. Werlin
339.1 **Anatomic Abnormalities** 1368
Steven L. Werlin
339.2 **Physiology** 1368
Steven L. Werlin

Chapter 340 **Pancreatic Function Tests** 1369
Steven L. Werlin

Chapter 341 **Disorders of the Exocrine Pancreas** 1369
Steven L. Werlin

Chapter 342 **Treatment of Pancreatic Insufficiency** 1369
Steven L. Werlin

Chapter 343 **Pancreatitis** 1370
343.1 **Acute Pancreatitis** 1370
Steven L. Werlin
343.2 **Chronic Pancreatitis** 1372
Steven L. Werlin

Chapter 344 **Pseudocyst of the Pancreas** 1373
Steven L. Werlin

Chapter 345 **Pancreatic Tumors** 1374
Steven L. Werlin

Section 6 **THE LIVER AND BILIARY SYSTEM** 1374

Chapter 346 **Morphogenesis of the Liver and Biliary System** 1374
Alexander G. Miethke and William F. Balistreri

Chapter 347 **Manifestations of Liver Disease** 1374
Lynelle M. Boamah and William F. Balistreri
347.1 **Evaluation of Patients with Possible Liver Dysfunction** 1378
Lynelle M. Boamah and William F. Balistreri

Chapter 348 **Cholestasis** 1381
348.1 **Neonatal Cholestasis** 1381
H. Hesham A-kader and William F. Balistreri

348.2 Cholestasis in the Older Child 1388
Robert M. Kliegman

Chapter 349 **Metabolic Diseases of the Liver** 1388
William F. Balistreri and Rebecca G. Carey

349.1 Inherited Deficient Conjugation of Bilirubin (Familial Nonhemolytic Unconjugated Hyperbilirubinemia) 1389
Rebecca G. Carey and William F. Balistreri

349.2 Wilson Disease 1391
William F. Balistreri and Rebecca G. Carey

349.3 Indian Childhood Cirrhosis 1392
William F. Balistreri and Rebecca G. Carey

349.4 Neonatal Iron Storage Disease 1392
Rebecca G. Carey and William F. Balistreri

349.5 Miscellaneous Metabolic Diseases of the Liver 1393
William F. Balistreri and Rebecca G. Carey

Chapter 350 **Viral Hepatitis** 1393
Nada Yazigi and William F. Balistreri

Chapter 351 **Liver Abscess** 1404
Robert M. Kliegman

Chapter 352 **Liver Disease Associated with Systemic Disorders** 1405
Kathryn D. Moyer and William F. Balistreri

Chapter 353 **Mitochondrial Hepatopathies** 1405
Rebecca G. Carey and William F. Balistreri

Chapter 354 **Autoimmune Hepatitis** 1408
Benjamin L. Shneider and Frederick J. Suchy

Chapter 355 **Drug- and Toxin-Induced Liver Injury** 1410
Frederick J. Suchy

Chapter 356 **Fulminant Hepatic Failure** 1412
Frederick J. Suchy

Chapter 357 **Cystic Diseases of the Biliary Tract and Liver** 1415
Frederick J. Suchy

Chapter 358 **Diseases of the Gallbladder** 1415
Frederick J. Suchy

Chapter 359 **Portal Hypertension and Varices** 1415
Frederick J. Suchy

Chapter 360 **Liver Transplantation** 1415
Jorge D. Reyes

Section 7 **PERITONEUM** 1416

Chapter 361 **Malformations** 1416
Melissa Kennedy and Chris A. Liacouras

Chapter 362 **Ascites** 1416
Melissa Kennedy and Chris A. Liacouras

362.1 Chylous Ascites 1416
Jessica Wen and Chris A. Liacouras

Chapter 363 **Peritonitis** 1416
Jessica Wen and Chris A. Liacouras

363.1 Acute Primary Peritonitis 1416
Jessica Wen and Chris A. Liacouras

363.2 Acute Secondary Peritonitis 1417
Jessica Wen and Chris A. Liacouras

363.3 Acute Secondary Localized Peritonitis (Peritoneal Abscess) 1417
Jessica Wen and Chris A. Liacouras

Chapter 364 **Epigastric Hernia** 1418
John J. Aiken and Keith T. Oldham

364.1 Incisional Hernia 1418
John J. Aiken and Keith T. Oldham

PART XIX
Respiratory System

Section 1 **DEVELOPMENT AND FUNCTION** 1419

Chapter 365 **Respiratory Pathophysiology and Regulation** 1419
Ashok P. Sarnaik and Sabrina M. Heidemann

365.1 Lung Volumes and Capacities in Health and Disease 1419
Ashok P. Sarnaik and Sabrina M. Heidemann

365.2 Chest Wall 1419
Ashok P. Sarnaik and Sabrina M. Heidemann

365.3 Pulmonary Mechanics and Work of Breathing in Health and Disease 1419
Ashok P. Sarnaik and Sabrina M. Heidemann

365.4 Airway Dynamics in Health and Disease 1420
Ashok P. Sarnaik and Sabrina M. Heidemann

365.5 Interpretation of Clinical Signs to Localize the Site of Pathology 1420
Ashok P. Sarnaik and Sabrina M. Heidemann

365.6 Ventilation-Perfusion Relationship in Health and Disease 1420
Ashok P. Sarnaik and Sabrina M. Heidemann

365.7 Gas Exchange in Health and Disease 1420
Ashok P. Sarnaik and Sabrina M. Heidemann

365.8 Interpretation of Blood Gases 1420
Ashok P. Sarnaik and Sabrina M. Heidemann

365.9 Pulmonary Vasculature in Health and Disease 1421
Ashok P. Sarnaik and Sabrina M. Heidemann

365.10 Immune Response of the Lung to Injury 1421
Ashok P. Sarnaik and Sabrina M. Heidemann

365.11 Regulation of Respiration 1421
Ashok P. Sarnaik and Sabrina M. Heidemann

Chapter 366 **Diagnostic Approach to Respiratory Disease** 1421
Gabriel G. Haddad and Thomas P. Green

Chapter 367 **Sudden Infant Death Syndrome** 1421
Carl E. Hunt and Fern R. Hauck

Section 2 **DISORDERS OF THE RESPIRATORY TRACT** 1429

Chapter 368 **Congenital Disorders of the Nose** 1429
Joseph Haddad, Jr.

Chapter 369 **Acquired Disorders of the Nose** 1431
Joseph Haddad, Jr.

369.1 Foreign Body 1431
Joseph Haddad, Jr.

369.2 Epistaxis 1432
Joseph Haddad, Jr.

Chapter 370 **Nasal Polyps** 1433
Joseph Haddad, Jr.

Chapter 371 **The Common Cold** 1434
Ronald B. Turner and Gregory F. Hayden

Chapter 372 **Sinusitis** 1436
Diane E. Pappas and J. Owen Hendley

Chapter 373 **Acute Pharyngitis** 1439
Gregory F. Hayden and Ronald B. Turner

Chapter 374 **Retropharyngeal Abscess, Lateral Pharyngeal (Parapharyngeal) Abscess, and Peritonsillar Cellulitis/Abscess** 1440
Diane E. Pappas and J. Owen Hendley

Chapter 375 **Tonsils and Adenoids** 1442
Ralph F. Wetmore

Chapter 376 **Chronic or Recurrent Respiratory Symptoms** 1445
Thomas F. Boat and Thomas P. Green

Chapter 377 **Acute Inflammatory Upper Airway Obstruction (Croup, Epiglottitis, Laryngitis, and Bacterial Tracheitis)** 1445
Genie E. Roosevelt

377.1 **Infectious Upper Airway Obstruction** 1445
Genie E. Roosevelt

377.2 **Bacterial Tracheitis** 1449
Genie E. Roosevelt

Chapter 378 **Congenital Anomalies of the Larynx, Trachea, and Bronchi** 1450
Lauren D. Holinger

378.1 **Laryngomalacia** 1450
Lauren D. Holinger

378.2 **Congenital Subglottic Stenosis** 1451
Lauren D. Holinger

378.3 **Vocal Cord Paralysis** 1451
Lauren D. Holinger

378.4 **Congenital Laryngeal Webs and Atresia** 1451
Lauren D. Holinger

378.5 **Congenital Subglottic Hemangioma** 1451
Lauren D. Holinger

378.6 **Laryngoceles and Saccular Cysts** 1451
Lauren D. Holinger

378.7 **Posterior Laryngeal Cleft and Laryngotracheoesophageal Cleft** 1452
Lauren D. Holinger

378.8 **Vascular and Cardiac Anomalies** 1452
Lauren D. Holinger

378.9 **Tracheal Stenoses, Webs, and Atresia** 1452
Lauren D. Holinger

378.10 **Foregut Cysts** 1452
Lauren D. Holinger

378.11 **Tracheomalacia and Bronchomalacia** 1452

Chapter 379 **Foreign Bodies of the Airway** 1453
Lauren D. Holinger

379.1 **Laryngeal Foreign Bodies** 1454
Lauren D. Holinger

379.2 **Tracheal Foreign Bodies** 1454
Lauren D. Holinger

379.3 **Bronchial Foreign Bodies** 1454
Lauren D. Holinger

Chapter 380 **Laryngotracheal Stenosis and Subglottic Stenosis** 1454
Lauren D. Holinger

380.1 **Congenital Subglottic Stenosis** 1454
Lauren D. Holinger

380.2 **Acquired Laryngotracheal Stenosis** 1454
Lauren D. Holinger

Chapter 381 **Bronchomalacia and Tracheomalacia** 1455
Jonathan D. Finder

Chapter 382 **Neoplasms of the Larynx, Trachea, and Bronchi** 1455

382.1 **Vocal Nodules** 1455
Lauren D. Holinger

382.2 **Recurrent Respiratory Papillomatosis** 1455
Lauren D. Holinger

382.3 **Congenital Subglottic Hemangioma** 1455
Lauren D. Holinger

382.4 **Vascular Anomalies** 1455
Lauren D. Holinger

382.5 **Other Laryngeal Neoplasms** 1455
Lauren D. Holinger

382.6 **Tracheal Neoplasms** 1456
Lauren D. Holinger

382.7 **Bronchial Tumors** 1456
Lauren D. Holinger

Chapter 383 **Wheezing, Bronchiolitis, and Bronchitis** 1456

383.1 **Wheezing in Infants: Bronchiolitis** 1456
Kimberly Danieli Watts and Denise M. Goodman

383.2 **Bronchitis** 1459
Denise M. Goodman

Chapter 384 **Emphysema and Overinflation** 1460
Steven R. Boas and Glenna B. Winnie

Chapter 385 **α_1-Antitrypsin Deficiency and Emphysema** 1462
Glenna B. Winnie and Steven R. Boas

Chapter 386 **Other Distal Airway Diseases** 1463

386.1 **Bronchiolitis Obliterans** 1463
Steven R. Boas

386.2 **Follicular Bronchitis** 1463
Steven R. Boas

386.3 **Pulmonary Alveolar Microlithiasis** 1463
Steven R. Boas

Chapter 387 **Congenital Disorders of the Lung** 1463

387.1 **Pulmonary Agenesis and Aplasia** 1463
Jonathan D. Finder

387.2 **Pulmonary Hypoplasia** 1464
Jonathan D. Finder

387.3 **Cystic Adenomatoid Malformation** 1464
Jonathan D. Finder

387.4 **Pulmonary Sequestration** 1465
Jonathan D. Finder

387.5 **Bronchogenic Cysts** 1466
Jonathan D. Finder

387.6 **Congenital Pulmonary Lymphangiectasia** 1467
Jonathan D. Finder

387.7 **Lung Hernia** 1467
Jonathan D. Finder

387.8 **Other Congenital Malformations of the Lung** 1467
Jonathan D. Finder

Chapter 388 **Pulmonary Edema** 1468
Robert Mazor and Thomas P. Green

Chapter 389 **Aspiration Syndromes** 1469
John L. Colombo

Chapter 390 **Chronic Recurrent Aspiration** 1471
John L. Colombo

Chapter 391 **Parenchymal Disease with Prominent Hypersensitivity, Eosinophilic Infiltration, or Toxin-Mediated Injury** 1473

391.1 **Hypersensitivity to Inhaled Materials** 1473
Oren Lakser

391.2 **Silo Filler Disease** 1474
Oren Lakser

391.3 **Paraquat Lung** 1474
Oren Lakser

391.4 **Eosinophilic Lung Disease** 1474
Oren Lakser

Chapter 392 **Community-Acquired Pneumonia** 1474
Thomas J. Sandora and Theodore C. Sectish

Chapter 393 **Bronchiectasis** 1479
Oren Lakser

Chapter 394 **Pulmonary Abscess** 1480
Oren Lakser

Chapter 395 **Cystic Fibrosis** 1481
Marie Egan

Chapter 396 **Primary Ciliary Dyskinesia (Immotile Cilia Syndrome)** 1497
Thomas Ferkol

Chapter 397 **Interstitial Lung Diseases** 1497
Young-Jee Kim and Michelle S. Howenstine

Chapter 398 **Pulmonary Alveolar Proteinosis** 1497
Aaron Hamvas, Lawrence M. Nogee, and F. Sessions Cole

Chapter 399 **Inherited Disorders of Surfactant Metabolism** 1497
Aaron Hamvas, Lawrence M. Nogee, and F. Sessions Cole

Chapter 400 **Pulmonary Hemosiderosis** 1498
Mary A. Nevin

Chapter 401 **Pulmonary Embolism, Infarction, and Hemorrhage** 1500

401.1 **Pulmonary Embolus and Infarction** 1500
Mary A. Nevin

401.2 **Pulmonary Hemorrhage and Hemoptysis** 1503
Mary A. Nevin

Chapter 402 **Atelectasis** 1504
Ranna A. Rozenfeld

Chapter 403 **Pulmonary Tumors** 1504
Susanna A. McColley

Chapter 404 **Pleurisy, Pleural Effusions, and Empyema** 1505
Glenna B. Winnie and Steven V. Lossef

404.1 **Dry or Plastic Pleurisy (Pleural Effusion)** 1505
Glenna B. Winnie and Steven V. Lossef

404.2 **Serofibrinous or Serosanguineous Pleurisy (Pleural Effusion)** 1506
Glenna B. Winnie and Steven V. Lossef

404.3 **Purulent Pleurisy or Empyema** 1507
Glenna B. Winnie and Steven V. Lossef

Chapter 405 **Pneumothorax** 1509
Glenna B. Winnie and Steven V. Lossef

Chapter 406 **Pneumomediastinum** 1512
Glenna B. Winnie

Chapter 407 **Hydrothorax** 1513
Glenna B. Winnie and Steven V. Lossef

Chapter 408 **Hemothorax** 1513
Glenna B. Winnie and Steven V. Lossef

Chapter 409 **Chylothorax** 1514
Glenna B. Winnie and Steven V. Lossef

Chapter 410 **Bronchopulmonary Dysplasia** 1516
Steven Lestrud

Chapter 411 **Skeletal Diseases Influencing Pulmonary Function** 1516
Steven R. Boas

411.1 **Pectus Excavatum (Funnel Chest)** 1516
Steven R. Boas

411.2 **Pectus Carinatum and Sternal Clefts** 1517
Steven R. Boas

411.3 **Asphyxiating Thoracic Dystrophy (Thoracic-Pelvic-Phalangeal Dystrophy)** 1517
Steven R. Boas

411.4 **Achondroplasia** 1517
Steven R. Boas

411.5 **Kyphoscoliosis: Adolescent Idiopathic Scoliosis and Congenital Scoliosis** 1518
Steven R. Boas

411.6 **Congenital Rib Anomalies** 1518
Steven R. Boas

Chapter 412 **Chronic Severe Respiratory Insufficiency** 1519
Zehava Noah and Cynthia Etzler Budek

412.1 **Neuromuscular Diseases** 1519
Zehava Noah and Cynthia Etzler Budek

412.2 **Congenital Central Hypoventilation Syndrome** 1520
Zehava Noah, Cynthia Etzler Budek, Pallavi P. Patwari, and Debra E. Weese-Mayer

412.3 **Other Conditions** 1522
Zehava Noah and Cynthia Etzler Budek

412.4 **Long-Term Mechanical Ventilation** 1524
Zehava Noah and Cynthia Etzler Budek

Chapter 413 **Extrapulmonary Diseases with Pulmonary Manifestations** 1526
Susanna A. McColley

PART XX
The Cardiovascular System

Section 1 **DEVELOPMENTAL BIOLOGY OF THE CARDIOVASCULAR SYSTEM** 1527

Chapter 414 **Cardiac Development** 1527
Daniel Bernstein

414.1 **Early Cardiac Morphogenesis** 1527
Daniel Bernstein

414.2 **Cardiac Looping** 1527
Daniel Bernstein

414.3 **Cardiac Septation** 1527
Daniel Bernstein

414.4 Aortic Arch Development 1527
Daniel Bernstein
414.5 Cardiac Differentiation 1528
Daniel Bernstein
414.6 Developmental Changes in Cardiac Function 1528
Daniel Bernstein

Chapter 415 **The Fetal to Neonatal Circulatory Transition** 1529
415.1 The Fetal Circulation 1529
Daniel Bernstein
415.2 The Transitional Circulation 1529
Daniel Bernstein
415.3 The Neonatal Circulation 1529
Daniel Bernstein
415.4 Persistent Pulmonary Hypertension of the Neonate (Persistence of Fetal Circulatory Pathways) 1529

Section 2 **EVALUATION OF THE CARDIOVASCULAR SYSTEM** 1529

Chapter 416 **History and Physical Examination** 1529
Daniel Bernstein

Chapter 417 **Laboratory Evaluation** 1537
417.1 Radiologic Assessment 1537
Daniel Bernstein
417.2 Electrocardiography 1537
Daniel Bernstein
417.3 Hematologic Data 1541
Daniel Bernstein
417.4 Echocardiography 1541
Daniel Bernstein
417.5 Exercise Testing 1545
Daniel Bernstein
417.6 MRI, MRA, CT, and Radionuclide Studies 1545
Daniel Bernstein
417.7 Diagnostic and Interventional Cardiac Catheterization 1546
Daniel Bernstein

Section 3 **CONGENITAL HEART DISEASE** 1549

Chapter 418 **Epidemiology and Genetic Basis of Congenital Heart Disease** 1549
Daniel Bernstein

Chapter 419 **Evaluation of the Infant or Child with Congenital Heart Disease** 1549
Daniel Bernstein

Chapter 420 **Acyanotic Congenital Heart Disease: The Left-to-Right Shunt Lesions** 1551
420.1 Atrial Septal Defect 1551
Daniel Bernstein
420.2 Ostium Secundum Defect 1551
Daniel Bernstein
420.3 Sinus Venosus Atrial Septal Defect 1553
Daniel Bernstein
420.4 Partial Anomalous Pulmonary Venous Return 1553
Daniel Bernstein
420.5 Atrioventricular Septal Defects (Ostium Primum and Atrioventricular Canal or Endocardial Cushion Defects) 1554
Daniel Bernstein
420.6 Ventricular Septal Defect 1556
Daniel Bernstein
420.7 Supracristal Ventricular Septal Defect with Aortic Insufficiency 1559
Daniel Bernstein
420.8 Patent Ductus Arteriosus 1559
Daniel Bernstein
420.9 Aorticopulmonary Window Defect 1561
Daniel Bernstein
420.10 Coronary-Cameral Fistula 1561
Daniel Bernstein
420.11 Ruptured Sinus of Valsalva Aneurysm 1561
Daniel Bernstein

Chapter 421 **Acyanotic Congenital Heart Disease: The Obstructive Lesions** 1561
421.1 Pulmonary Valve Stenosis with Intact Ventricular Septum 1561
Daniel Bernstein
421.2 Infundibular Pulmonary Stenosis and Double-Chamber Right Ventricle 1564
Daniel Bernstein
421.3 Pulmonary Stenosis in Combination with an Intracardiac Shunt 1564
Daniel Bernstein
421.4 Peripheral Pulmonary Stenosis 1564
Daniel Bernstein
421.5 Aortic Stenosis 1565
Daniel Bernstein
421.6 Coarctation of the Aorta 1567
Daniel Bernstein
421.7 Coarctation with Ventricular Septal Defect 1570
Daniel Bernstein
421.8 Coarctation with Other Cardiac Anomalies and Interrupted Aortic Arch 1570
Daniel Bernstein
421.9 Congenital Mitral Stenosis 1570
Daniel Bernstein
421.10 Pulmonary Venous Hypertension 1570
Daniel Bernstein

Chapter 422 **Acyanotic Congenital Heart Disease: Regurgitant Lesions** 1571
422.1 Pulmonary Valvular Insufficiency and Congenital Absence of the Pulmonary Valve 1571
Daniel Bernstein
422.2 Congenital Mitral Insufficiency 1571
Daniel Bernstein
422.3 Mitral Valve Prolapse 1572
Daniel Bernstein
422.4 Tricuspid Regurgitation 1572
Daniel Bernstein

Chapter 423 **Cyanotic Congenital Heart Disease: Evaluation of the Critically Ill Neonate with Cyanosis and Respiratory Distress** 1572
Daniel Bernstein

Chapter 424 **Cyanotic Congenital Heart Lesions: Lesions Associated with Decreased Pulmonary Blood Flow** 1573
424.1 Tetralogy of Fallot 1573
Daniel Bernstein

424.2 **Tetralogy of Fallot with Pulmonary Atresia** 1578
Daniel Bernstein
424.3 **Pulmonary Atresia with Intact Ventricular Septum** 1578
Daniel Bernstein
424.4 **Tricuspid Atresia** 1580
Daniel Bernstein
424.5 **Double-Outlet Right Ventricle** 1582
Daniel Bernstein
424.6 **Transposition of the Great Arteries with Ventricular Septal Defect and Pulmonary Stenosis** 1582
Daniel Bernstein
424.7 **Ebstein Anomaly of the Tricuspid Valve** 1583
Daniel Bernstein

Chapter 425 **Cyanotic Congenital Heart Disease: Lesions Associated with Increased Pulmonary Blood Flow** 1585
425.1 **D-Transposition of the Great Arteries** 1585
Daniel Bernstein
425.2 **D-Transposition of the Great Arteries with Intact Ventricular Septum** 1585
Daniel Bernstein
425.3 **Transposition of the Great Arteries with Ventricular Septal Defect** 1587
Daniel Bernstein
425.4 **L-Transposition of the Great Arteries (Corrected Transposition)** 1587
Daniel Bernstein
425.5 **Double-Outlet Right Ventricle without Pulmonary Stenosis** 1588
Daniel Bernstein
425.6 **Double-Outlet Right Ventricle with Malposition of the Great Arteries (Taussig-Bing Anomaly)** 1588
Daniel Bernstein
425.7 **Total Anomalous Pulmonary Venous Return** 1589
Daniel Bernstein
425.8 **Truncus Arteriosus** 1590
Daniel Bernstein
425.9 **Single Ventricle (Double-Inlet Ventricle, Univentricular Heart)** 1592
Daniel Bernstein
425.10 **Hypoplastic Left Heart Syndrome** 1592
Daniel Bernstein
425.11 **Abnormal Positions of the Heart and the Heterotaxy Syndromes (Asplenia, Polysplenia)** 1595
Daniel Bernstein

Chapter 426 **Other Congenital Heart and Vascular Malformations** 1596
426.1 **Anomalies of the Aortic Arch** 1596
Daniel Bernstein
426.2 **Anomalous Origin of the Coronary Arteries** 1598
Daniel Bernstein
426.3 **Pulmonary Arteriovenous Fistula** 1599
Daniel Bernstein
426.4 **Ectopia Cordis** 1599
Daniel Bernstein
426.5 **Diverticulum of the Left Ventricle** 1599
Daniel Bernstein

Chapter 427 **Pulmonary Hypertension** 1600
427.1 **Primary Pulmonary Hypertension** 1600
Daniel Bernstein
427.2 **Pulmonary Vascular Disease (Eisenmenger Syndrome)** 1601
Daniel Bernstein

Chapter 428 **General Principles of Treatment of Congenital Heart Disease** 1602
Daniel Bernstein
428.1 **Congenital Heart Disease in Adults** 1605
Michael G. Earing

Section 4 **CARDIAC ARRHYTHMIAS** 1610

Chapter 429 **Disturbances of Rate and Rhythm of the Heart** 1610
George F. Van Hare
429.1 **Principles of Antiarrhythmic Therapy** 1610
George F. Van Hare
429.2 **Sinus Arrhythmias and Extrasystoles** 1610
George F. Van Hare
429.3 **Supraventricular Tachycardia** 1613
George F. Van Hare
429.4 **Ventricular Tachyarrhythmias** 1616
George F. Van Hare
429.5 **Long Q-T Syndromes** 1616
George F. Van Hare
429.6 **Sinus Node Dysfunction** 1618
George F. Van Hare
429.7 **AV Block** 1618
George F. Van Hare

Chapter 430 **Sudden Death** 1619
George F. Van Hare

Section 5 **ACQUIRED HEART DISEASE** 1622

Chapter 431 **Infective Endocarditis** 1622
Daniel Bernstein

Chapter 432 **Rheumatic Heart Disease** 1626
Daniel Bernstein

Section 6 **DISEASES OF THE MYOCARDIUM AND PERICARDIUM** 1628

Chapter 433 **Diseases of the Myocardium** 1628
Robert Spicer and Stephanie Ware
433.1 **Dilated Cardiomyopathy** 1630
Robert Spicer and Stephanie Ware
433.2 **Hypertrophic Cardiomyopathy** 1631
Robert Spicer and Stephanie Ware
433.3 **Restrictive Cardiomyopathy** 1633
Robert Spicer and Stephanie Ware
433.4 **Left Ventricular Noncompaction, Arrhythmogenic Right Ventricular Cardiomyopathy, and Endocardial Fibroelastosis** 1633
Robert Spicer and Stephanie Ware
433.5 **Myocarditis** 1634
Robert Spicer and Stephanie Ware

Chapter 434 **Diseases of the Pericardium** 1635
Robert Spicer and Stephanie Ware
434.1 **Acute Pericarditis** 1636
Robert Spicer and Stephanie Ware

434.2 Constrictive Pericarditis 1637
Robert Spicer and Stephanie Ware

Chapter 435 Tumors of the Heart 1637
Robert Spicer and Stephanie Ware

Section 7 CARDIAC THERAPEUTICS 1638

Chapter 436 Heart Failure 1638
Daniel Bernstein

436.1 Cardiogenic Shock 1638
Daniel Bernstein

Chapter 437 Pediatric Heart and Heart-Lung Transplantation 1638

437.1 Pediatric Heart Transplantation 1638
Daniel Bernstein

437.2 Heart-Lung and Lung Transplantation 1638
Daniel Bernstein

Section 8 DISEASES OF THE PERIPHERAL VASCULAR SYSTEM 1638

Chapter 438 Diseases of the Blood Vessels (Aneurysms and Fistulas) 1638

438.1 Kawasaki Disease 1638
Daniel Bernstein

438.2 Arteriovenous Fistulas 1638
Daniel Bernstein

Chapter 439 Systemic Hypertension 1639
Marc B. Lande

PART XXI
Diseases of the Blood

Section 1 THE HEMATOPOIETIC SYSTEM 1648

Chapter 440 Development of the Hematopoietic System 1648
Robert D. Christensen and Robin K. Ohls

Chapter 441 The Anemias 1648
Norma B. Lerner

Section 2 ANEMIAS OF INADEQUATE PRODUCTION 1650

Chapter 442 Congenital Hypoplastic Anemia (Diamond-Blackfan Anemia) 1650
Norma B. Lerner

Chapter 443 Pearson's Syndrome 1652
Norma B. Lerner

Chapter 444 Acquired Pure Red Blood Cell Anemia 1652
Norma B. Lerner

Chapter 445 Anemia of Chronic Disease and Renal Disease 1653

445.1 Anemia of Chronic Disease 1653
Norma B. Lerner

445.2 Anemia of Renal Disease 1653
Norma B. Lerner

Chapter 446 Congenital Dyserythropoietic Anemias 1654
Norma B. Lerner

Chapter 447 Physiologic Anemia of Infancy 1654
Norma B. Lerner

Chapter 448 Megaloblastic Anemias 1655
Norma B. Lerner

448.1 Folic Acid Deficiency 1655
Norma B. Lerner

448.2 Vitamin B_{12} (Cobalamin) Deficiency 1655
Norma B. Lerner

448.3 Other Rare Megaloblastic Anemias 1655
Norma B. Lerner

Chapter 449 Iron-Deficiency Anemia 1655
Norma B. Lerner and Richard Sills

Chapter 450 Other Microcytic Anemias 1658
Richard Sills

Section 3 HEMOLYTIC ANEMIAS 1659

Chapter 451 Definitions and Classification of Hemolytic Anemias 1659
George B. Segel

Chapter 452 Hereditary Spherocytosis 1659
George B. Segel

Chapter 453 Hereditary Elliptocytosis 1662
George B. Segel

Chapter 454 Hereditary Stomatocytosis 1662
George B. Segel and Lisa R. Hackney

Chapter 455 Other Membrane Defects 1662
George B. Segel

Chapter 456 Hemoglobinopathies 1662
Michael R. DeBaun, Melissa Frei-Jones, and Elliott Vichinsky

456.1 Sickle Cell Disease 1663
Michael R. DeBaun, Melissa Frei-Jones, and Elliott Vichinsky

456.2 Sickle Cell Trait (Hemoglobin AS) 1670
Michael R. DeBaun, Melissa Frei-Jones, and Elliott Vichinsky

456.3 Other Hemoglobinopathies 1670
Michael R. DeBaun, Melissa Frei-Jones, and Elliott Vichinsky

456.4 Unstable Hemoglobin Disorders 1670
Michael R. DeBaun, Melissa Frei-Jones, and Elliott Vichinsky

456.5 Abnormal Hemoglobins with Increased Oxygen Affinity 1671
Michael R. DeBaun, Melissa Frei-Jones, and Elliott Vichinsky

456.6 Abnormal Hemoglobins Causing Cyanosis 1672
Michael R. DeBaun, Melissa Frei-Jones, and Elliott Vichinsky

456.7 Hereditary Methemoglobinemia 1672
Michael R. DeBaun, Melissa Frei-Jones, and Elliott Vichinsky

456.8 Syndromes of Hereditary Persistence of Fetal Hemoglobin 1673
Michael R. DeBaun, Melissa Frei-Jones, and Elliott Vichinsky

456.9 Thalassemia Syndromes 1674
Michael R. DeBaun, Melissa Frei-Jones, and Elliott Vichinsky

Chapter 457 **Enzymatic Defects** 1677
457.1 **Pyruvate Kinase Deficiency** 1677
George B. Segel
457.2 **Other Glycolytic Enzyme Deficiencies** 1677
George B. Segel
457.3 **Glucose-6-Phosphate Dehydrogenase Deficiency and Related Deficiencies** 1678
George B. Segel and Lisa R. Hackney

Chapter 458 **Hemolytic Anemias Resulting from Extracellular Factors—Immune Hemolytic Anemias** 1680
George B. Segel and Charles H. Packman

Chapter 459 **Hemolytic Anemias Secondary to Other Extracellular Factors** 1683
George B. Segel

Section 4 **POLYCYTHEMIA (ERYTHROCYTOSIS)** 1683

Chapter 460 **Polycythemia** 1683
Amanda M. Brandow and Bruce M. Camitta

Chapter 461 **Secondary Polycythemia** 1683
Amanda M. Brandow and Bruce M. Camitta

Section 5 **THE PANCYTOPENIAS** 1684

Chapter 462 **The Inherited Pancytopenias** 1684
Melvin H. Freedman

Chapter 463 **The Acquired Pancytopenias** 1691
Jeffrey D. Hord

Section 6 **BLOOD COMPONENT TRANSFUSIONS** 1692

Chapter 464 **Red Blood Cell Transfusions and Erythropoietin Therapy** 1692
Ronald G. Strauss

Chapter 465 **Platelet Transfusions** 1693
Ronald G. Strauss

Chapter 466 **Neutrophil (Granulocyte) Transfusions** 1693
Ronald G. Strauss

Chapter 467 **Plasma Transfusions** 1693
Ronald G. Strauss

Chapter 468 **Risks of Blood Transfusions** 1693
Ronald G. Strauss

Section 7 **HEMORRHAGIC AND THROMBOTIC DISEASES** 1693

Chapter 469 **Hemostasis** 1693
J. Paul Scott, Leslie J. Raffini, and Robert R. Montgomery
469.1 **Clinical and Laboratory Evaluation of Hemostasis** 1695
J. Paul Scott, Leslie J. Raffini, and Robert R. Montgomery

Chapter 470 **Hereditary Clotting Factor Deficiencies (Bleeding Disorders)** 1699
J. Paul Scott and Robert R. Montgomery
470.1 **Factor VIII or Factor IX Deficiency (Hemophilia A or B)** 1699
J. Paul Scott and Robert R. Montgomery
470.2 **Factor XI Deficiency (Hemophilia C)** 1702
J. Paul Scott and Robert R. Montgomery
470.3 **Deficiencies of the Contact Factors (Nonbleeding Disorders)** 1703
J. Paul Scott and Robert R. Montgomery
470.4 **Factor VII Deficiency** 1703
J. Paul Scott and Robert R. Montgomery
470.5 **Factor X Deficiency** 1703
J. Paul Scott and Robert R. Montgomery
470.6 **Prothrombin (Factor II) Deficiency** 1703
J. Paul Scott and Robert R. Montgomery
470.7 **Factor V Deficiency** 1703
J. Paul Scott and Robert R. Montgomery
470.8 **Combined Deficiency of Factors V and VIII** 1704
J. Paul Scott and Robert R. Montgomery
470.9 **Fibrinogen (Factor I) Deficiency** 1704
J. Paul Scott and Robert R. Montgomery
470.10 **Factor XIII Deficiency (Fibrin-Stabilizing Factor or Transglutaminase Deficiency)** 1704
J. Paul Scott and Robert R. Montgomery
470.11 **Antiplasmin or Plasminogen Activator Inhibitor Deficiency** 1704
J. Paul Scott and Robert R. Montgomery

Chapter 471 **von Willebrand Disease** 1704
Robert R. Montgomery and J. Paul Scott

Chapter 472 **Hereditary Predisposition to Thrombosis** 1707
Leslie J. Raffini and J. Paul Scott

Chapter 473 **Thrombotic Disorders in Children** 1709
Leslie J. Raffini and J. Paul Scott
473.1 **Anticoagulant and Thrombolytic Therapy** 1711
Leslie J. Raffini and J. Paul Scott

Chapter 474 **Postneonatal Vitamin K Deficiency** 1712
J. Paul Scott and Robert R. Montgomery

Chapter 475 **Liver Disease** 1712
J. Paul Scott and Robert R. Montgomery

Chapter 476 **Acquired Inhibitors of Coagulation** 1712
J. Paul Scott and Robert R. Montgomery

Chapter 477 **Disseminated Intravascular Coagulation** 1713
J. Paul Scott, Leslie J. Raffini, and Robert R. Montgomery

Chapter 478 **Platelet and Blood Vessel Disorders** 1714
J. Paul Scott and Robert R. Montgomery
478.1 **Idiopathic (Autoimmune) Thrombocytopenic Purpura** 1714
J. Paul Scott and Robert R. Montgomery
478.2 **Drug-Induced Thrombocytopenia** 1718
J. Paul Scott and Robert R. Montgomery
478.3 **Nonimmune Platelet Destruction** 1718
J. Paul Scott and Robert R. Montgomery
478.4 **Hemolytic-Uremic Syndrome** 1718
J. Paul Scott and Robert R. Montgomery
478.5 **Thrombotic Thrombocytopenic Purpura** 1718
J. Paul Scott and Robert R. Montgomery
478.6 **Kasabach-Merritt Syndrome** 1719
J. Paul Scott and Robert R. Montgomery
478.7 **Sequestration** 1719
J. Paul Scott and Robert R. Montgomery

478.8 Congenital Thrombocytopenic Syndromes 1719
J. Paul Scott and Robert R. Montgomery
478.9 Neonatal Thrombocytopenia 1720
J. Paul Scott and Robert R. Montgomery
478.10 Thrombocytopenia Due to Acquired Disorders Causing Decreased Production 1721
J. Paul Scott and Robert R. Montgomery
478.11 Platelet Function Disorders 1721
J. Paul Scott and Robert R. Montgomery
478.12 Acquired Disorders of Platelet Function 1721
J. Paul Scott and Robert R. Montgomery
478.13 Congenital Abnormalities of Platelet Function 1721
J. Paul Scott and Robert R. Montgomery
478.14 Disorders of the Blood Vessels 1722
J. Paul Scott and Robert R. Montgomery

Section 8 THE SPLEEN 1723

Chapter 479 Anatomy and Function of the Spleen 1723
Amanda M. Brandow and Bruce M. Camitta

Chapter 480 Splenomegaly 1723
Amanda M. Brandow and Bruce M. Camitta

Chapter 481 Hyposplenism, Splenic Trauma, and Splenectomy 1723
Amanda M. Brandow and Bruce C. Camitta

Section 9 THE LYMPHATIC SYSTEM 1723

Chapter 482 Anatomy and Function of the Lymphatic System 1723
Richard L. Tower II and Bruce M. Camitta

Chapter 483 Abnormalities of Lymphatic Vessels 1724
Richard L. Tower II and Bruce M. Camitta

Chapter 484 Lymphadenopathy 1724
Richard L. Tower II and Bruce M. Camitta
484.1 Kikuchi-Fujimoto Disease (Histiocytic Necrotizing Lymphadenitis) 1724
Richard L. Tower II and Bruce M. Camitta
484.2 Sinus Histiocytosis with Massive Lymphadenopathy (Rosai-Dorfman Disease) 1724
Richard L. Tower II and Bruce M. Camitta
484.3 Castleman Disease 1724
Richard L. Tower II and Bruce M. Camitta

PART XXII
Cancer and Benign Tumors

Chapter 485 Epidemiology of Childhood and Adolescent Cancer 1725
Barbara L. Asselin

Chapter 486 Molecular and Cellular Biology of Cancer 1728
Laura L. Worth

Chapter 487 Principles of Diagnosis 1728
A. Kim Ritchey

Chapter 488 Principles of Treatment 1731
Archie Bleyer and A. Kim Ritchey

Chapter 489 The Leukemias 1732
David G. Tubergen, Archie Bleyer, and A. Kim Ritchey
489.1 Acute Lymphoblastic Leukemia 1732
David G. Tubergen, Archie Bleyer, and A. Kim Ritchey
489.2 Acute Myelogenous Leukemia 1737
David G. Tubergen, Archie Bleyer, and A. Kim Ritchey
489.3 Down Syndrome and Acute Leukemia and Transient Myeloproliferative Disorder 1738
David G. Tubergen, Archie Bleyer, and A. Kim Ritchey
489.4 Chronic Myelogenous Leukemia 1738
David G. Tubergen, Archie Bleyer, and A. Kim Ritchey
489.5 Juvenile Myelomonocytic Leukemia 1739
David G. Tubergen, Archie Bleyer, and A. Kim Ritchey
489.6 Infant Leukemia 1739
David G. Tubergen, Archie Bleyer, and A. Kim Ritchey

Chapter 490 Lymphoma 1739
Ian M. Waxman, Jessica Hochberg, and Mitchell S. Cairo
490.1 Hodgkin Lymphoma 1739
Ian M. Waxman, Jessica Hochberg, and Mitchell S. Cairo
490.2 Non-Hodgkin Lymphoma 1743
Ian M. Waxman, Jessica Hochberg, and Mitchell S. Cairo
490.3 Late Effects in Children and Adolescents with Lymphoma 1746
Ian M. Waxman, Jessica Hochberg, and Mitchell S. Cairo

Chapter 491 Brain Tumors in Childhood 1746
John F. Kuttesch, Jr., Sarah Zieber Rush, and Joann L. Ater

Chapter 492 Neuroblastoma 1753
Peter E. Zage and Joann L. Ater

Chapter 493 Neoplasms of the Kidney 1757
493.1 Wilms Tumor 1757
Peter M. Anderson, Chetan Anil Dhamne, and Vicki Huff
493.2 Other Pediatric Renal Tumors 1760
Peter M. Anderson, Chetan Anil Dhamne, and Vicki Huff

Chapter 494 Soft Tissue Sarcomas 1760
Carola A.S. Arndt

Chapter 495 Neoplasms of Bone 1763
495.1 Malignant Tumors of Bone 1763
Carola A.S. Arndt
495.2 Benign Tumors and Tumor-like Processes of Bone 1766
Carola A.S. Arndt

Chapter 496 Retinoblastoma 1768
Peter E. Zage and Cynthia E. Herzog

Chapter 497 Gonadal and Germ Cell Neoplasms 1769
Cynthia E. Herzog and Winston W. Huh

Chapter 498 Neoplasms of the Liver 1771
Cynthia E. Herzog

Chapter 499 **Benign Vascular Tumors** 1772
499.1 **Hemangiomas** 1772
Cynthia E. Herzog
499.2 **Lymphangiomas and Cystic Hygromas** 1772
Cynthia E. Herzog

Chapter 500 **Rare Tumors** 1772
500.1 **Thyroid Tumors** 1772
Steven G. Waguespack
500.2 **Melanoma** 1772
Cynthia E. Herzog
500.3 **Nasopharyngeal Carcinoma** 1773
Cynthia E. Herzog
500.4 **Adenocarcinoma of the Colon and Rectum** 1773
Cynthia E. Herzog
500.5 **Adrenal Tumors** 1773
Steven G. Waguespack
500.6 **Desmoplastic Small Round Cell Tumor** 1773
Cynthia E. Herzog

Chapter 501 **Histiocytosis Syndromes of Childhood** 1773
Stephan Ladisch
501.1 **Class I Histiocytoses** 1774
Stephan Ladisch
501.2 **Class II Histiocytoses: Hemophagocytic Lymphohistiocytosis (HLH)** 1776
Stephan Ladisch
501.3 **Class III Histiocytoses** 1777
Stephan Ladisch

PART XXIII
Nephrology

Section 1 **GLOMERULAR DISEASE** 1778

Chapter 502 **Introduction to Glomerular Diseases** 1778
502.1 **Anatomy of the Glomerulus** 1778
Cynthia G. Pan and Ellis D. Avner
502.2 **Glomerular Filtration** 1778
Cynthia G. Pan and Ellis D. Avner
502.3 **Glomerular Diseases** 1778
Cynthia G. Pan and Ellis D. Avner

Section 2 **CONDITIONS PARTICULARLY ASSOCIATED WITH HEMATURIA** 1778

Chapter 503 **Clinical Evaluation of the Child with Hematuria** 1778
Cynthia G. Pan and Ellis D. Avner

Chapter 504 **Isolated Glomerular Diseases with Recurrent Gross Hematuria** 1781
Cynthia G. Pan and Ellis D. Avner
504.1 **Immunoglobulin A Nephropathy (Berger Nephropathy)** 1781
Cynthia G. Pan and Ellis D. Avner
504.2 **Alport Syndrome** 1782
Cynthia G. Pan and Ellis D. Avner
504.3 **Thin Basement Membrane Disease** 1783
Cynthia G. Pan and Ellis D. Avner

Chapter 505 **Glomerulonephritis Associated with Infections** 1783
505.1 **Acute Poststreptococcal Glomerulonephritis** 1783
Cynthia G. Pan and Ellis D. Avner
505.2 **Other Chronic Infections** 1785
Cynthia G. Pan and Ellis D. Avner

Chapter 506 **Membranous Glomerulopathy** 1786
Scott K. Van Why and Ellis D. Avner

Chapter 507 **Membranoproliferative Glomerulonephritis** 1787
Scott K. Van Why and Ellis D. Avner

Chapter 508 **Glomerulonephritis Associated with Systemic Lupus Erythematosus** 1788
Cynthia G. Pan and Ellis D. Avner

Chapter 509 **Henoch-Schönlein Purpura Nephritis** 1789
Scott K. Van Why and Ellis D. Avner

Chapter 510 **Rapidly Progressive (Crescentic) Glomerulonephritis** 1789
Scott K. Van Why and Ellis D. Avner

Chapter 511 **Goodpasture Disease** 1790
Scott K. Van Why and Ellis D. Avner

Chapter 512 **Hemolytic-Uremic Syndrome** 1791
Scott K. Van Why and Ellis D. Avner

Chapter 513 **Upper Urinary Tract Causes of Hematuria** 1794
513.1 **Interstitial Nephritis** 1794
513.2 **Toxic Nephropathy** 1794
513.3 **Cortical Necrosis** 1794
513.4 **Pyelonephritis** 1794
513.5 **Nephrocalcinosis** 1794
513.6 **Vascular Abnormalities** 1794
Craig C. Porter and Ellis D. Avner
513.7 **Renal Vein Thrombosis** 1794
Craig C. Porter and Ellis D. Avner
513.8 **Idiopathic Hypercalciuria** 1795
Craig C. Porter and Ellis D. Avner

Chapter 514 **Hematologic Diseases Causing Hematuria** 1795
514.1 **Sickle Cell Nephropathy** 1795
Craig C. Porter and Ellis D. Avner
514.2 **Coagulopathies and Thrombocytopenia** 1796
Craig C. Porter and Ellis D. Avner

Chapter 515 **Anatomic Abnormalities Associated with Hematuria** 1796
515.1 **Congenital Anomalies** 1796
Craig C. Porter and Ellis D. Avner
515.2 **Autosomal Recessive Polycystic Kidney Disease** 1796
Craig C. Porter and Ellis D. Avner
515.3 **Autosomal Dominant Polycystic Kidney Disease** 1798
Craig C. Porter and Ellis D. Avner
515.4 **Trauma** 1799
Craig C. Porter and Ellis D. Avner
515.5 **Renal Tumors** 1799

Chapter 516 **Lower Urinary Tract Causes of Hematuria** 1799
516.1 **Infectious Causes of Cystitis and Urethritis** 1799
Priya Pais and Ellis D. Avner
516.2 **Hemorrhagic Cystitis** 1799
Priya Pais and Ellis D. Avner
516.3 **Vigorous Exercise** 1799
Priya Pais and Ellis D. Avner

Section 3 **CONDITIONS PARTICULARLY ASSOCIATED WITH PROTEINURIA** 1799

Chapter 517 **Introduction to the Child with Proteinuria** 1799
Priya Pais and Ellis D. Avner

Chapter 518 **Transient Proteinuria** 1800
Craig C. Porter and Ellis D. Avner

Chapter 519 **Orthostatic (Postural) Proteinuria** 1800
Craig C. Porter and Ellis D. Avner

Chapter 520 **Fixed Proteinuria** 1800
Priya Pais and Ellis D. Avner
520.1 **Glomerular Proteinuria** 1801
Priya Pais and Ellis D. Avner
520.2 **Tubular Proteinuria** 1801
Priya Pais and Ellis D. Avner

Chapter 521 **Nephrotic Syndrome** 1801
Priya Pais and Ellis D. Avner
521.1 **Idiopathic Nephrotic Syndrome** 1804
Priya Pais and Ellis D. Avner
521.2 **Secondary Nephrotic Syndrome** 1806
Priya Pais and Ellis D. Avner
521.3 **Congenital Nephrotic Syndrome** 1807
Priya Pais and Ellis D. Avner

Section 4 **TUBULAR DISORDERS** 1807

Chapter 522 **Tubular Function** 1807
Rajasree Sreedharan and Ellis D. Avner

Chapter 523 **Renal Tubular Acidosis** 1808
Rajasree Sreedharan and Ellis D. Avner
523.1 **Proximal (Type II) Renal Tubular Acidosis** 1808
Rajasree Sreedharan and Ellis D. Avner
523.2 **Distal (Type I) Renal Tubular Acidosis** 1810
Rajasree Sreedharan and Ellis D. Avner
523.3 **Hyperkalemic (Type IV) Renal Tubular Acidosis** 1810
Rajasree Sreedharan and Ellis D. Avner
523.4 **Rickets Associated with Renal Tubular Acidosis** 1811
Russell W. Chesney

Chapter 524 **Nephrogenic Diabetes Insipidus** 1812
Rajasree Sreedharan and Ellis D. Avner

Chapter 525 **Bartter and Gitelman Syndromes and Other Inherited Tubular Transport Abnormalities** 1813
525.1 **Bartter Syndrome** 1813
Rajasree Sreedharan and Ellis D. Avner
525.2 **Gitelman Syndrome** 1814
Rajasree Sreedharan and Ellis D. Avner
525.3 **Other Inherited Tubular Transport Abnormalities** 1814
Rajasree Sreedharan and Ellis D. Avner

Chapter 526 **Tubulointerstitial Nephritis** 1814
Craig C. Porter and Ellis D. Avner

Section 5 **TOXIC NEPHROPATHIES—RENAL FAILURE** 1816

Chapter 527 **Toxic Nephropathy** 1816
Craig C. Porter and Ellis D. Avner

Chapter 528 **Cortical Necrosis** 1818
Priya Pais and Ellis D. Avner

Chapter 529 **Renal Failure** 1818
529.1 **Acute Renal Failure** 1818
Rajasree Sreedharan and Ellis D. Avner
529.2 **Chronic Kidney Disease** 1822
Rajasree Sreedharan and Ellis D. Avner
529.3 **End-Stage Renal Disease** 1825
Rajasree Sreedharan and Ellis D. Avner

Chapter 530 **Renal Transplantation** 1826
Minnie M. Sarwal and Cynthia J. Wong

PART XXIV
Urologic Disorders in Infants and Children

Chapter 531 **Congenital Anomalies and Dysgenesis of the Kidneys** 1827
Jack S. Elder

Chapter 532 **Urinary Tract Infections** 1829
Jack S. Elder

Chapter 533 **Vesicoureteral Reflux** 1834
Jack S. Elder

Chapter 534 **Obstruction of the Urinary Tract** 1838
Jack S. Elder

Chapter 535 **Anomalies of the Bladder** 1847
Jack S. Elder

Chapter 536 **Neuropathic Bladder** 1847
Jack S. Elder

Chapter 537 **Voiding Dysfunction** 1847
Jack S. Elder

Chapter 538 **Anomalies of the Penis and Urethra** 1852
Jack S. Elder

Chapter 539 **Disorders and Anomalies of the Scrotal Contents** 1858
Jack S. Elder

Chapter 540 **Trauma to the Genitourinary Tract** 1864
Jack S. Elder

Chapter 541 **Urinary Lithiasis** 1864
Jack S. Elder

PART XXV
Gynecologic Problems of Childhood

Chapter 542 **History and Physical Examination** 1865
Kerith Lucco and Diane F. Merritt

Chapter 543 **Vulvovaginitis** 1865
Diane F. Merritt

Chapter 544 **Bleeding** 1869
Laura A. Parks and Diane F. Merritt

Chapter 545 **Breast Concerns** 1870
Nirupama K. DeSilva and Diane F. Merritt

Chapter 546 **Polycystic Ovary Syndrome and Hirsutism** 1870
Mark Gibson and Heather G. Huddleston

Chapter 547 **Neoplasms and Adolescent Screening for Human Papilloma Virus** 1870
Nora T. Kizer and Diane F. Merritt

Chapter 548 **Vulvovaginal and Müllerian Anomalies** 1874
Amber R. Cooper and Diane F. Merritt

Chapter 549 **Gynecologic Care for Girls with Special Needs** 1874
Elisabeth H. Quint

PART XXVI
The Endocrine System

Section 1 **DISORDERS OF THE HYPOTHALAMUS AND PITUITARY GLAND** 1876

Chapter 550 **Hormones of the Hypothalamus and Pituitary** 1876
John S. Parks and Eric I. Felner

Chapter 551 **Hypopituitarism** 1876
John S. Parks and Eric I. Felner

Chapter 552 **Diabetes Insipidus** 1881
David T. Breault and Joseph A. Majzoub

Chapter 553 **Other Abnormalities of Arginine Vasopressin Metabolism and Action** 1884
David T. Breault and Joseph A. Majzoub

Chapter 554 **Hyperpituitarism, Tall Stature, and Overgrowth Syndromes** 1886
Hidekazu Hosono and Pinchas Cohen

Chapter 555 **Physiology of Puberty** 1886
Luigi Garibaldi and Wassim Chemaitilly

Chapter 556 **Disorders of Pubertal Development** 1886
Luigi Garibaldi and Wassim Chemaitilly

556.1 **Central Precocious Puberty** 1887
Luigi Garibaldi and Wassim Chemaitilly

556.2 **Precocious Puberty Resulting from Organic Brain Lesions** 1889
Luigi Garibaldi and Wassim Chemaitilly

556.3 **Precocious Puberty Following Irradiation of the Brain** 1890
Luigi Garibaldi and Wassim Chemaitilly

556.4 **Syndrome of Precocious Puberty and Hypothyroidism** 1891
Luigi Garibaldi and Wassim Chemaitilly

556.5 **Gonadotropin-Secreting Tumors** 1891
Luigi Garibaldi and Wassim Chemaitilly

556.6 **McCune-Albright Syndrome (Precocious Puberty with Polyostotic Fibrous Dysplasia and Abnormal Pigmentation)** 1891
Luigi Garibaldi and Wassim Chemaitilly

556.7 **Familial Male Gonadotropin-Independent Precocious Puberty** 1892
Luigi Garibaldi and Wassim Chemaitilly

556.8 **Incomplete (Partial) Precocious Development** 1893
Luigi Garibaldi and Wassim Chemaitilly

556.9 **Medicational Precocity** 1894
Luigi Garibaldi and Wassim Chemaitilly

Section 2 **DISORDERS OF THE THYROID GLAND** 1894

Chapter 557 **Thyroid Development and Physiology** 1894
Stephen LaFranchi

557.1 **Thyroid Hormone Studies** 1894
Stephen LaFranchi

Chapter 558 **Defects of Thyroxine-Binding Globulin** 1894
Stephen LaFranchi

Chapter 559 **Hypothyroidism** 1895
Stephen LeFranchi

Chapter 560 **Thyroiditis** 1903
Stephen LaFranchi

Chapter 561 **Goiter** 1905
Stephen LaFranchi

561.1 **Congenital Goiter** 1905
Stephen LaFranchi

561.2 **Intratracheal Goiter** 1906
Stephen LaFranchi

561.3 **Endemic Goiter and Cretinism** 1906
Stephen LaFranchi

561.4 **Acquired Goiter** 1908
Stephen LaFranchi

Chapter 562 **Hyperthyroidism** 1909
Stephen LaFranchi

562.1 **Graves Disease** 1909
Stephen LaFranchi

562.2 **Congenital Hyperthyroidism** 1913
Stephen LaFranchi

Chapter 563 **Carcinoma of the Thyroid** 1914
Stephen LaFranchi

563.1 **Solitary Thyroid Nodule** 1915
Stephen LaFranchi

563.2 **Medullary Thyroid Carcinoma** 1915
Stephen LaFranchi

Section 3 **DISORDERS OF THE PARATHYROID GLAND** 1916

Chapter 564 **Hormones and Peptides of Calcium Homeostasis and Bone Metabolism** 1916
Daniel A. Doyle

Chapter 565 **Hypoparathyroidism** 1916
Daniel A. Doyle

Chapter 566 **Pseudohypoparathyroidism (Albright Hereditary Osteodystrophy)** 1919
Daniel A. Doyle

Chapter 567 **Hyperparathyroidism** 1920
Daniel A. Doyle
567.1 **Other Causes of Hypercalcemia** 1922
Daniel A. Doyle

Section 4 **DISORDERS OF THE ADRENAL GLAND** 1923

Chapter 568 **Physiology of the Adrenal Gland** 1923
568.1 **Histology and Embryology** 1923
Perrin C. White
568.2 **Adrenal Steroid Biosynthesis** 1923
Perrin C. White
568.3 **Regulation of the Adrenal Cortex** 1923
Perrin C. White
568.4 **Adrenal Steroid Hormone Actions** 1923
Perrin C. White
568.5 **Adrenal Medulla** 1923
Perrin C. White

Chapter 569 **Adrenocortical Insufficiency** 1924
Perrin C. White
569.1 **Primary Adrenal Insufficiency** 1924
Perrin C. White
569.2 **Secondary Adrenal Insufficiency** 1929
Perrin C. White
569.3 **Adrenal Insufficiency in the Critical Care Setting** 1930
Perrin C. White

Chapter 570 **Congenital Adrenal Hyperplasia and Related Disorders** 1930
Perrin C. White
570.1 **Congenital Adrenal Hyperplasia Due to 21-Hydroxylase Deficiency** 1930
Perrin C. White
570.2 **Congenital Adrenal Hyperplasia Due to 11β-Hydroxylase Deficiency** 1935
Perrin C. White
570.3 **Congenital Adrenal Hyperplasia Due to 3β-Hydroxysteroid Dehydrogenase Deficiency** 1936
Perrin C. White
570.4 **Congenital Adrenal Hyperplasia Due to 17-Hydroxylase Deficiency** 1936
Perrin C. White
570.5 **Lipoid Adrenal Hyperplasia** 1937
Perrin C. White
570.6 **Deficiency of P450 Oxidoreductase (Antley-Bixler Syndrome)** 1937
Perrin C. White
570.7 **Aldosterone Synthase Deficiency** 1938
Perrin C. White
570.8 **Glucocorticoid-Suppressible Hyperaldosteronism** 1938
Perrin C. White

Chapter 571 **Cushing Syndrome** 1939
Perrin C. White

Chapter 572 **Primary Aldosteronism** 1941
Perrin C. White

Chapter 573 **Adrenocortical Tumors** 1941
Perrin C. White
573.1 **Virilizing Adrenocortical and Feminizing Adrenal Tumors** 1941
Perrin C. White

Chapter 574 **Pheochromocytoma** 1941
Perrin C. White

Chapter 575 **Adrenal Masses** 1943
575.1 **Adrenal Incidentaloma** 1943
Perrin C. White
575.2 **Adrenal Calcification** 1943
Perrin C. White

Section 5 **DISORDERS OF THE GONADS** 1943

Chapter 576 **Development and Function of the Gonads** 1943
Patricia A. Donohoue

Chapter 577 **Hypofunction of the Testes** 1943
Omar Ali and Patricia A. Donohoue
577.1 **Hypergonadotropic Hypogonadism in the Male (Primary Hypogonadism)** 1944
Omar Ali and Patricia A. Donohoue
577.2 **Hypogonadotropic Hypogonadism in the Male (Secondary Hypogonadism)** 1948
Omar Ali and Patricia A. Donohoue

Chapter 578 **Pseudoprecocity Resulting from Tumors of the Testes** 1950
Omar Ali and Patricia A. Donohoue

Chapter 579 **Gynecomastia** 1950
Omar Ali and Patricia A. Donohoue

Chapter 580 **Hypofunction of the Ovaries** 1951
Alvina R. Kansra and Patricia A. Donohoue
580.1 **Hypergonadotropic Hypogonadism in the Female (Primary Hypogonadism)** 1951
Alvina R. Kansra and Patricia A. Donohoue
580.2 **Hypogonadotropic Hypogonadism in the Female (Secondary Hypogonadism)** 1956
Alvina R. Kansra and Patricia A. Donohoue

Chapter 581 **Pseudoprecocity Due to Lesions of the Ovary** 1957
Alvina R. Kansra and Patricia A. Donohoue

Chapter 582 **Disorders of Sex Development** 1958
Patricia A. Donohoue
582.1 **46,XX DSD** 1961
Patricia A. Donohoue
582.2 **46,XY DSD** 1962
Patricia A. Donohoue
582.3 **Ovotesticular DSD** 1967
Patricia A. Donohoue

Section 6 **DIABETES MELLITUS IN CHILDREN** 1968

Chapter 583 **Diabetes Mellitus** 1968
583.1 **Introduction and Classification** 1968
Ramin Alemzadeh and Omar Ali
583.2 **Type 1 Diabetes Mellitus (Immune Mediated)** 1969
Ramin Alemzadeh and Omar Ali
583.3 **Type 2 Diabetes Mellitus** 1990
Ramin Alemzadeh and Omar Ali
583.4 **Other Specific Types of Diabetes** 1993
Ramin Alemzadeh and Omar Ali

PART XXVII
The Nervous System

Chapter 584 **Neurologic Evaluation** 1998
Rebecca K. Lehman and Nina F. Schor

Chapter 585 **Congenital Anomalies of the Central Nervous System** 1998
Stephen L. Kinsman and Michael V. Johnston

585.1 **Neural Tube Defects** 1998
Stephen L. Kinsman and Michael V. Johnston

585.2 **Spina Bifida Occulta (Occult Spinal Dysraphism)** 1999
Stephen L. Kinsman and Michael V. Johnston

585.3 **Meningocele** 1999
Stephen L. Kinsman and Michael V. Johnston

585.4 **Myelomeningocele** 2000
Stephen L. Kinsman and Michael V. Johnston

585.5 **Encephalocele** 2002
Stephen L. Kinsman and Michael V. Johnston

585.6 **Anencephaly** 2003
Stephen L. Kinsman and Michael V. Johnston

585.7 **Disorders of Neuronal Migration** 2003
Stephen L. Kinsman and Michael V. Johnston

585.8 **Agenesis of the Corpus Callosum** 2005
Stephen L. Kinsman and Michael V. Johnston

585.9 **Agenesis of the Cranial Nerves and Dysgenesis of the Posterior Fossa** 2006
Stephen L. Kinsman and Michael V. Johnston

585.10 **Microcephaly** 2007
Stephen L. Kinsman and Michael V. Johnston

585.11 **Hydrocephalus** 2008
Stephen L. Kinsman and Michael V. Johnston

585.12 **Craniosynostosis** 2011
Stephen L. Kinsman and Michael V. Johnston

Chapter 586 **Seizures in Childhood** 2013
Mohamad A. Mikati

586.1 **Febrile Seizures** 2017
Mohamad A. Mikati

586.2 **Unprovoked Seizures** 2019
Mohamad A. Mikati

586.3 **Partial Seizures and Related Epilepsy Syndromes** 2021
Mohamad A. Mikati

586.4 **Generalized Seizures and Related Epilepsy Syndromes** 2023
Mohamad A. Mikati

586.5 **Mechanisms of Seizures** 2024
Mohamad A. Mikati

586.6 **Treatment of Seizures and Epilepsy** 2025
Mohamad A. Mikati

586.7 **Neonatal Seizures** 2033
Mohamad A. Mikati

586.8 **Status Epilepticus** 2037
Mohamad A. Mikati

Chapter 587 **Conditions That Mimic Seizures** 2039
Mohamad A. Mikati and Makram Obeid

Chapter 588 **Headaches** 2039
Andrew D. Hershey

588.1 **Migraine** 2040
Andrew D. Hershey

588.2 **Secondary Headaches** 2045
Andrew D. Hershey

588.3 **Tension-Type Headaches** 2046
Andrew D. Hershey

Chapter 589 **Neurocutaneous Syndromes** 2046
Mustafa Sahin

589.1 **Neurofibromatosis** 2046
Mustafa Sahin

589.2 **Tuberous Sclerosis** 2049
Mustafa Sahin

589.3 **Sturge-Weber Syndrome** 2051
Mustafa Sahin

589.4 **Von Hippel–Lindau Disease** 2052
Mustafa Sahin

589.5 **Linear Nevus Syndrome** 2052
Mustafa Sahin

589.6 **PHACE Syndrome** 2052
Mustafa Sahin

589.7 **Incontinentia Pigmenti** 2052
Mustafa Sahin

Chapter 590 **Movement Disorders** 2053
Erika F. Augustine and Jonathan W. Mink

590.1 **Ataxias** 2053
Denia Ramirez-Montealegre and Jonathan W. Mink

590.2 **Chorea, Athetosis, Tremor** 2055
Denia Ramirez-Montealegre and Jonathan W. Mink

590.3 **Dystonia** 2058
Denia Ramirez-Montealegre and Jonathan W. Mink

Chapter 591 **Encephalopathies** 2061
Michael V. Johnston

591.1 **Cerebral Palsy** 2061
Michael V. Johnston

591.2 **Mitochondrial Encephalomyopathies** 2065
Michael V. Johnston

591.3 **Other Encephalopathies** 2068
Michael V. Johnston

Chapter 592 **Neurodegenerative Disorders of Childhood** 2069
Jennifer M. Kwon

592.1 **Sphingolipidoses** 2069
Jennifer M. Kwon

592.2 **Neuronal Ceroid Lipofuscinoses** 2073
Jennifer M. Kwon

592.3 **Adrenoleukodystrophy** 2073
Jennifer M. Kwon

592.4 **Sialidosis** 2074
Jennifer M. Kwon

592.5 **Miscellaneous Disorders** 2074
Jennifer M. Kwon

Chapter 593 **Demyelinating Disorders of the CNS** 2076
Jayne Ness

593.1 **Multiple Sclerosis** 2076
Jayne Ness

593.2 **Neuromyelitis Optica** 2077
Nina F. Schor

593.3 **Acute Disseminated Encephalomyelitis (ADEM)** 2079
Nina F. Schor

Chapter 594 **Pediatric Stroke Syndromes** 2080
Adam Kirton and Gabrielle deVeber
594.1 **Arterial Ischemic Stroke (AIS)** 2080
Adam Kirton and Gabrielle deVeber
594.2 **Cerebral Sinovenous Thrombosis (CSVT)** 2082
Adam Kirton and Gabrielle deVeber
594.3 **Hemorrhagic Stroke (HS)** 2084
Adam Kirton and Gabrielle deVeber
594.4 **Differential Diagnosis of Strokelike Events** 2085
Adam Kirton and Gabrielle deVeber

Chapter 595 **Central Nervous System Infections** 2086
Charles G. Prober and LauraLe Dyner
595.1 **Acute Bacterial Meningitis Beyond the Neonatal Period** 2087
Charles G. Prober and LauraLe Dyner
595.2 **Viral Meningoencephalitis** 2095
Charles G. Prober and LauraLe Dyner
595.3 **Eosinophilic Meningitis** 2097
Charles G. Prober and LauraLe Dyner

Chapter 596 **Brain Abscess** 2098
Charles G. Prober and LauraLe Dyner

Chapter 597 **Pseudotumor Cerebri** 2099
Misha L. Pless

Chapter 598 **Spinal Cord Disorders** 2101
598.1 **Tethered Cord** 2101
Harold L. Rekate
598.2 **Diastematomyelia** 2102
Harold L. Rekate
598.3 **Syringomyelia** 2103
Harold L. Rekate
598.4 **Spinal Cord Tumors** 2104
Harold L. Rekate
598.5 **Spinal Cord Injuries in Children** 2106
Harold L. Rekate
598.6 **Transverse Myelitis** 2107
Harold L. Rekate
598.7 **Spinal Arteriovenous Malformations** 2107
Harold L. Rekate

PART XXVIII
Neuromuscular Disorders

Chapter 599 **Evaluation and Investigation** 2109
Harvey B. Sarnat

Chapter 600 **Developmental Disorders of Muscle** 2112
Harvey B. Sarnat
600.1 **Myotubular Myopathy** 2113
Harvey B. Sarnat
600.2 **Congenital Muscle Fiber-Type Disproportion** 2115
Harvey B. Sarnat
600.3 **Nemaline Rod Myopathy** 2116
Harvey B. Sarnat
600.4 **Central Core, Minicore, and Multicore Myopathies** 2117
Harvey B. Sarnat
600.5 **Myofibrillar Myopathies** 2117
Harvey B. Sarnat
600.6 **Brain Malformations and Muscle Development** 2118
Harvey B. Sarnat
600.7 **Amyoplasia** 2118
Harvey B. Sarnat
600.8 **Muscular Dysgenesis (Proteus Syndrome Myopathy)** 2118
Harvey B. Sarnat
600.9 **Benign Congenital Hypotonia** 2118
Harvey B. Sarnat
600.10 **Arthrogryposis** 2119
Harvey B. Sarnat

Chapter 601 **Muscular Dystrophies** 2119
Harvey B. Sarnat
601.1 **Duchenne and Becker Muscular Dystrophies** 2119
Harvey B. Sarnat
601.2 **Emery-Dreifuss Muscular Dystrophy** 2123
Harvey B. Sarnat
601.3 **Myotonic Muscular Dystrophy** 2123
Harvey B. Sarnat
601.4 **Limb-Girdle Muscular Dystrophies** 2126
Harvey B. Sarnat
601.5 **Facioscapulohumeral Muscular Dystrophy** 2126
Harvey B. Sarnat
601.6 **Congenital Muscular Dystrophy** 2127
Harvey B. Sarnat

Chapter 602 **Endocrine and Toxic Myopathies** 2129
Harvey B. Sarnat

Chapter 603 **Metabolic Myopathies** 2130
Harvey B. Sarnat
603.1 **Periodic Paralyses (Potassium-Related)** 2130
Harvey B. Sarnat
603.2 **Malignant Hyperthermia** 2130
Harvey B. Sarnat
603.3 **Glycogenoses** 2131
Harvey B. Sarnat
603.4 **Mitochondrial Myopathies** 2131
Harvey B. Sarnat
603.5 **Lipid Myopathies** 2132
Harvey B. Sarnat
603.6 **Vitamin E Deficiency Myopathy** 2132
Harvey B. Sarnat

Chapter 604 **Disorders of Neuromuscular Transmission and of Motor Neurons** 2132
604.1 **Myasthenia Gravis** 2132
Harvey B. Sarnat
604.2 **Spinal Muscular Atrophies** 2136
Harvey B. Sarnat
604.3 **Other Motor Neuron Diseases** 2138
Harvey B. Sarnat

Chapter 605 **Hereditary Motor-Sensory Neuropathies** 2138
Harvey B. Sarnat
605.1 **Peroneal Muscular Atrophy (Charcot-Marie-Tooth Disease; HMSN Type I)** 2138
Harvey B. Sarnat
605.2 **Peroneal Muscular Atrophy (Axonal Type)** 2139
Harvey B. Sarnat
605.3 **Déjerine-Sottas Disease (HMSN Type III)** 2139
Harvey B. Sarnat
605.4 **Roussy-Lévy Syndrome** 2139
Harvey B. Sarnat

605.5 **Refsum Disease** 2139
Harvey B. Sarnat

605.6 **Fabry Disease** 2139
Harvey B. Sarnat

605.7 **Giant Axonal Neuropathy** 2140
Harvey B. Sarnat

605.8 **Congenital Hypomyelinating Neuropathy** 2140
Harvey B. Sarnat

605.9 **Tomaculous (Hypermyelinating) Neuropathy; Hereditary Neuropathy with Liability to Pressure Palsies** 2140
Harvey B. Sarnat

605.10 **Leukodystrophies** 2140
Harvey B. Sarnat

Chapter 606 **Toxic Neuropathies** 2140
Harvey B. Sarnat

Chapter 607 **Autonomic Neuropathies** 2141
Harvey B. Sarnat

607.1 **Familial Dysautonomia** 2141
Harvey B. Sarnat

607.2 **Other Autonomic Neuropathies** 2143
Harvey B. Sarnat

Chapter 608 **Guillain-Barré Syndrome** 2143
Harvey B. Sarnat

Chapter 609 **Bell Palsy** 2146
Harvey B. Sarnat

PART XXIX
Disorders of the Eye

Chapter 610 **Growth and Development** 2148
Scott E. Olitsky, Denise Hug, Laura S. Plummer, and Merrill Stass-Isern

Chapter 611 **Examination of the Eye** 2148
Scott E. Olitsky, Denise Hug, Laura S. Plummer, and Merrill Stass-Isern

Chapter 612 **Abnormalities of Refraction and Accommodation** 2150
Scott E. Olitsky, Denise Hug, Laura S. Plummer, and Merrill Stass-Isern

Chapter 613 **Disorders of Vision** 2152
Scott E. Olitsky, Denise Hug, Laura S. Plummer, and Merrill Stass-Isern

Chapter 614 **Abnormalities of Pupil and Iris** 2154
Scott E. Olitsky, Denise Hug, Laura S. Plummer, and Merrill Stass-Isern

Chapter 615 **Disorders of Eye Movement and Alignment** 2157
Scott E. Olitsky, Denise Hug, Laura S. Plummer, and Merrill Stass-Isern

Chapter 616 **Abnormalities of the Lids** 2163
Scott E. Olitsky, Denise Hug, Laura S. Plummer, and Merrill Stass-Isern

Chapter 617 **Disorders of the Lacrimal System** 2165
Scott E. Olitsky, Denise Hug, Laura S. Plummer, and Merrill Stass-Isern

Chapter 618 **Disorders of the Conjunctiva** 2166
Scott E. Olitsky, Denise Hug, Laura S. Plummer, and Merrill Stass-Isern

Chapter 619 **Abnormalities of the Cornea** 2169
Scott E. Olitsky, Denise Hug, Laura S. Plummer, and Merrill Stass-Isern

Chapter 620 **Abnormalities of the Lens** 2169
Scott E. Olitsky, Denise Hug, Laura S. Plummer, and Merrill Stass-Isern

Chapter 621 **Disorders of the Uveal Tract** 2172
Scott E. Olitsky, Denise Hug, Laura S. Plummer, and Merrill Stass-Isern

Chapter 622 **Disorders of the Retina and Vitreous** 2174
Scott E. Olitsky, Denise Hug, Laura S. Plummer, and Merrill Stass-Isern

Chapter 623 **Abnormalities of the Optic Nerve** 2181
Scott E. Olitsky, Denise Hug, Laura S. Plummer, and Merrill Stass-Isern

Chapter 624 **Childhood Glaucoma** 2181
Scott E. Olitsky, Denise Hug, Laura S. Plummer, and Merrill Stass-Isern

Chapter 625 **Orbital Abnormalities** 2181
Scott E. Olitsky, Denise Hug, Laura S. Plummer, and Merrill Stass-Isern

Chapter 626 **Orbital Infections** 2182
Scott E. Olitsky, Denise Hug, Laura S. Plummer, and Merrill Stass-Isern

Chapter 627 **Injuries to the Eye** 2184
Scott E. Olitsky, Denise Hug, Laura S. Plummer, and Merrill Stass-Isern

PART XXX
The Ear

Chapter 628 **General Considerations and Evaluation** 2188
Joseph Haddad, Jr.

Chapter 629 **Hearing Loss** 2188
Joseph Haddad, Jr.

Chapter 630 **Congenital Malformations** 2196
Joseph Haddad, Jr.

Chapter 631 **External Otitis (Otitis Externa)** 2196
Joseph Haddad, Jr.

Chapter 632 **Otitis Media** 2199
Joseph E. Kerschner

Chapter 633 **The Inner Ear and Diseases of the Bony Labyrinth** 2213
Joseph Haddad, Jr.

Chapter 634 **Traumatic Injuries of the Ear and Temporal Bone** 2213
Joseph Haddad, Jr.

Chapter 635 **Tumors of the Ear and Temporal Bone** 2214
Joseph Haddad, Jr.

PART XXXI
The Skin

Chapter 636 **Morphology of the Skin** 2215
Joseph G. Morelli

Chapter 637 **Evaluation of the Patient** 2215
Joseph G. Morelli
637.1 **Cutaneous Manifestations of Systemic Diseases** 2215
Joseph G. Morelli
637.2 **Multisystem Medication Reactions** 2215
Joseph G. Morelli

Chapter 638 **Principles of Therapy** 2215
Joseph G. Morelli

Chapter 639 **Diseases of the Neonate** 2218
Joseph G. Morelli

Chapter 640 **Cutaneous Defects** 2220
Joseph G. Morelli

Chapter 641 **Ectodermal Dysplasias** 2222
Joseph G. Morelli

Chapter 642 **Vascular Disorders** 2223
Joseph G. Morelli

Chapter 643 **Cutaneous Nevi** 2231
Joseph G. Morelli

Chapter 644 **Hyperpigmented Lesions** 2236
Joseph G. Morelli

Chapter 645 **Hypopigmented Lesions** 2238
Joseph G. Morelli

Chapter 646 **Vesiculobullous Disorders** 2241
Joseph G. Morelli
646.1 **Erythema Multiforme** 2241
Joseph G. Morelli
646.2 **Stevens-Johnson Syndrome** 2242
Joseph G. Morelli
646.3 **Toxic Epidermal Necrolysis** 2243
Joseph G. Morelli
646.4 **Mechanobullous Disorders** 2244
Joseph G. Morelli
646.5 **Pemphigus** 2247
Joseph G. Morelli
646.6 **Dermatitis Herpetiformis** 2248
Joseph G. Morelli
646.7 **Linear IgA Dermatosis (Chronic Bullous Dermatosis of Childhood)** 2249
Joseph G. Morelli

Chapter 647 **Eczematous Disorders** 2249
Joseph G. Morelli
647.1 **Contact Dermatitis** 2250
Joseph G. Morelli
647.2 **Nummular Eczema** 2252
Joseph G. Morelli
647.3 **Pityriasis Alba** 2252
Joseph G. Morelli
647.4 **Lichen Simplex Chronicus** 2252
Joseph G. Morelli
647.5 **Vesicular Hand and Foot Dermatitis (Dyshidrotic Eczema, Dyshidrosis, Pompholyx)** 2253
Joseph G. Morelli
647.6 **Seborrheic Dermatitis** 2253
Joseph G. Morelli

Chapter 648 **Photosensitivity** 2254
Joseph G. Morelli

Chapter 649 **Diseases of the Epidermis** 2259
649.1 **Psoriasis** 2259
Joseph G. Morelli
649.2 **Pityriasis Lichenoides** 2260
Joseph G. Morelli
649.3 **Keratosis Pilaris** 2261
Joseph G. Morelli
649.4 **Lichen Spinulosus** 2261
Joseph G. Morelli
649.5 **Pityriasis Rosea** 2262
Joseph G. Morelli
649.6 **Pityriasis Rubra Pilaris** 2262
Joseph G. Morelli
649.7 **Darier Disease (Keratosis Follicularis)** 2263
Joseph G. Morelli
649.8 **Lichen Nitidus** 2263
Joseph G. Morelli
649.9 **Lichen Striatus** 2264
Joseph G. Morelli
649.10 **Lichen Planus** 2264
Joseph G. Morelli
649.11 **Porokeratosis** 2265
Joseph G. Morelli
649.12 **Papular Acrodermatitis of Childhood (Gianotti-Crosti Syndrome)** 2266
Joseph G. Morelli
649.13 **Acanthosis Nigricans** 2266
Joseph G. Morelli

Chapter 650 **Disorders of Keratinization** 2267
Joseph G. Morelli

Chapter 651 **Diseases of the Dermis** 2273
Joseph G. Morelli

Chapter 652 **Diseases of Subcutaneous Tissue** 2282
Joseph G. Morelli
652.1 **Panniculitis and Erythema Nodosum** 2282
Joseph G. Morelli
652.2 **Lipodystrophy** 2285
Joseph G. Morelli

Chapter 653 **Disorders of the Sweat Glands** 2286
Joseph G. Morelli

Chapter 654 **Disorders of Hair** 2289
Joseph G. Morelli

Chapter 655 **Disorders of the Nails** 2293
Joseph G. Morelli

Chapter 656 **Disorders of the Mucous Membranes** 2297
Joseph G. Morelli

Chapter 657 **Cutaneous Bacterial Infections** 2299
657.1 **Impetigo** 2299
Joseph G. Morelli
657.2 **Subcutaneous Tissue Infections** 2300
Joseph G. Morelli
657.3 **Staphylococcal Scalded Skin Syndrome (Ritter Disease)** 2302
Joseph G. Morelli
657.4 **Ecthyma** 2303
Joseph G. Morelli

657.5 Other Cutaneous Bacterial Infections 2304
Joseph G. Morelli

Chapter 658 **Cutaneous Fungal Infections** 2309
Joseph G. Morelli

Chapter 659 **Cutaneous Viral Infections** 2315
Joseph G. Morelli

Chapter 660 **Arthropod Bites and Infestations** 2317

660.1 Arthropod Bites 2317
Joseph G. Morelli

660.2 Scabies 2319
Joseph G. Morelli

660.3 Pediculosis 2321
Joseph G. Morelli

660.4 Seabather's Eruption 2322
Joseph G. Morelli

Chapter 661 **Acne** 2322
Joseph G. Morelli

Chapter 662 **Tumors of the Skin** 2328
Joseph G. Morelli

Chapter 663 **Nutritional Dermatoses** 2328
Joseph G. Morelli

PART XXXII
Bone and Joint Disorders

Section 1 **ORTHOPEDIC PROBLEMS** 2331

Chapter 664 **Growth and Development** 2331
Lawrence Wells, Kriti Sehgal, and John P. Dormans

Chapter 665 **Evaluation of the Child** 2331
Lawrence Wells, Kriti Sehgal, and John P. Dormans

Chapter 666 **The Foot and Toes** 2335
Harish S. Hosalkar, David A. Spiegel, and Richard S. Davidson

666.1 Metatarsus Adductus 2335
Harish S. Hosalkar, David A. Spiegel, and Richard S. Davidson

666.2 Calcaneovalgus Feet 2336
Harish S. Hosalkar, David A. Spiegel, and Richard S. Davidson

666.3 Talipes Equinovarus (Clubfoot) 2336
Harish S. Hosalkar, David A. Spiegel, and Richard S. Davidson

666.4 Congenital Vertical Talus 2337
Harish S. Hosalkar, David A. Spiegel, and Richard S. Davidson

666.5 Hypermobile Pes Planus (Flexible Flatfeet) 2338
Harish S. Hosalkar, David A. Spiegel, and Richard S. Davidson

666.6 Tarsal Coalition 2339
Harish S. Hosalkar, David A. Spiegel, and Richard S. Davidson

666.7 Cavus Feet 2340
Harish S. Hosalkar, David A. Spiegel, and Richard S. Davidson

666.8 Osteochondroses and Apophysitis 2340
Harish S. Hosalkar, David A. Spiegel, and Richard S. Davidson

666.9 Puncture Wounds of the Foot 2341
Harish S. Hosalkar, David A. Spiegel, and Richard S. Davidson

666.10 Toe Deformities 2341
Harish S. Hosalkar, David A. Spiegel, and Richard S. Davidson

666.11 Painful Foot 2344
Harish S. Hosalkar, David A. Spiegel, and Richard S. Davidson

666.12 Shoes 2344
Harish S. Hosalkar, David A. Spiegel, and Richard S. Davidson

Chapter 667 **Torsional and Angular Deformities** 2344

667.1 Normal Limb Development 2344
Lawrence Wells and Kriti Sehgal

667.2 Evaluation 2344
Lawrence Wells and Kriti Sehgal

667.3 Torsional Deformities 2347
Lawrence Wells and Kriti Sehgal

667.4 Coronal Plane Deformities 2348
Lawrence Wells and Kriti Sehgal

667.5 Congenital Angular Deformities of the Tibia and Fibula 2350
Lawrence Wells and Kriti Sehgal

Chapter 668 **Leg-Length Discrepancy** 2351
Jared E. Friedman and Richard S. Davidson

Chapter 669 **The Knee** 2351
Lawrence Wells and Kriti Sehgal

669.1 Discoid Lateral Meniscus 2352
Lawrence Wells and Kriti Sehgal

669.2 Popliteal Cysts (Baker Cysts) 2352
Lawrence Wells and Kriti Sehgal

669.3 Osteochondritis Dissecans 2353
Lawrence Wells and Kriti Sehgal

669.4 Osgood-Schlatter Disease 2353
Lawrence Wells and Kriti Sehgal

669.5 Idiopathic Adolescent Anterior Knee Pain Syndrome 2354
Lawrence Wells and Kriti Sehgal

669.6 Patellar Subluxation and Dislocation 2354
Lawrence Wells and Kriti Sehgal

Chapter 670 **The Hip** 2355
Wudbhav N. Sankar, B. David Horn, Lawrence Wells, and John P. Dormans

670.1 Developmental Dysplasia of the Hip 2356
Wudbhav N. Sankar, B. David Horn, Lawrence Wells, and John P. Dormans

670.2 Transient Monoarticular Synovitis (Toxic Synovitis) 2360
Wudbhav N. Sankar, B. David Horn, Lawrence Wells, and John P. Dormans

670.3 Legg-Calvé-Perthes Disease 2361
Wudbhav N. Sankar, B. David Horn, Lawrence Wells, and John P. Dormans

670.4 Slipped Capital Femoral Epiphysis 2363
Wudbhav N. Sankar, B. David Horn, Lawrence Wells, and John P. Dormans

Chapter 671 **The Spine** 2365
David A. Spiegel and John P. Dormans

671.1 Idiopathic Scoliosis 2365
David A. Spiegel and John P. Dormans
671.2 Congenital Scoliosis 2368
David A. Spiegel and John P. Dormans
671.3 Neuromuscular Scoliosis, Genetic Syndromes, and Compensatory Scoliosis 2370
David A. Spiegel and John P. Dormans
671.4 Kyphosis (Round Back) 2371
David A. Spiegel and John P. Dormans
671.5 Back Pain in Children 2373
David A. Spiegel and John P. Dormans
671.6 Spondylolysis and Spondylolisthesis 2374
David A. Spiegel and John P. Dormans
671.7 Disk Space Infection 2376
David A. Spiegel and John P. Dormans
671.8 Intervertebral Disk Herniation and Slipped Vertebral Apophysis 2377
David A. Spiegel and John P. Dormans
671.9 Tumors 2377
David A. Spiegel and John P. Dormans

Chapter 672 **The Neck** 2377
672.1 Torticollis 2377
David A. Spiegel and John P. Dormans
672.2 Klippel-Feil Syndrome 2379
David A. Spiegel and John P. Dormans
672.3 Cervical Anomalies and Instabilities 2380
David A. Spiegel and John P. Dormans

Chapter 673 **The Upper Limb** 2383
Robert B. Carrigan

Chapter 674 **Arthrogryposis** 2387
Harish S. Hosalkar, Denis S. Drummond, and Richard S. Davidson

Chapter 675 **Common Fractures** 2387
Lawrence Wells, Kriti Sehgal, and John P. Dormans
675.1 Unique Characteristics of Pediatric Fractures 2388
Lawrence Wells, Kriti Sehgal, and John P. Dormans
675.2 Pediatric Fracture Patterns 2389
Lawrence Wells, Kriti Sehgal, and John P. Dormans
675.3 Upper Extremity Fractures 2390
Lawrence Wells, Kriti Sehgal, and John P. Dormans
675.4 Fractures of Lower Extremity 2392
Lawrence Wells, Kriti Sehgal, and John P. Dormans
675.5 Operative Treatment 2393
Lawrence Wells, Kriti Sehgal, and John P. Dormans
675.6 Complications of Fractures in Children 2394
Lawrence Wells, Kriti Sehgal, and John P. Dormans
675.7 Outcomes Assessment 2394
Lawrence Wells, Kriti Sehgal, and John P. Dormans

Chapter 676 **Osteomyelitis** 2394
Sheldon L. Kaplan

Chapter 677 **Septic Arthritis** 2398
Sheldon L. Kaplan

Section 2 **SPORTS MEDICINE** 2401

Chapter 678 **Epidemiology and Prevention of Injuries** 2401
Gregory L. Landry

Chapter 679 **Management of Musculoskeletal Injury** 2406
Gregory L. Landry
679.1 Growth Plate Injuries 2408
Gregory L. Landry
679.2 Shoulder Injuries 2409
Gregory L. Landry
679.3 Elbow Injuries 2410
Gregory L. Landry
679.4 Low Back Injuries 2412
Gregory L. Landry
679.5 Hip and Pelvis Injuries 2413
Gregory L. Landry
679.6 Knee Injuries 2414
Gregory L. Landry
679.7 Lower Leg Pain: Shin Splints, Stress Fractures, and Chronic Compartment Syndrome 2416
Gregory L. Landry
679.8 Ankle Injuries 2417
Gregory L. Landry
679.9 Foot Injuries 2418
Gregory L. Landry

Chapter 680 **Head and Neck Injuries** 2418
Gregory L. Landry

Chapter 681 **Heat Injuries** 2420
Gregory L. Landry

Chapter 682 **Female Athletes: Menstrual Problems and the Risk of Osteopenia** 2421
Gregory L. Landry

Chapter 683 **Performance-Enhancing Aids** 2422
Gregory L. Landry

Chapter 684 **Specific Sports and Associated Injuries** 2423
Gregory L. Landry

Section 3 **THE SKELETAL DYSPLASIAS** 2424

Chapter 685 **General Considerations** 2424
William A. Horton and Jacqueline T. Hecht

Chapter 686 **Disorders Involving Cartilage Matrix Proteins** 2424
William A. Horton and Jacqueline T. Hecht

Chapter 687 **Disorders Involving Transmembrane Receptors** 2428
William A. Horton and Jacqueline T. Hecht

Chapter 688 **Disorders Involving Ion Transporters** 2430
William A. Horton and Jacqueline T. Hecht

Chapter 689 **Disorders Involving Transcription Factors** 2431
William A. Horton and Jacqueline T. Hecht

Chapter 690 **Disorders Involving Defective Bone Resorption** 2432
William A. Horton and Jacqueline T. Hecht

Chapter 691 **Disorders for Which Defects Are Poorly Understood or Unknown** 2433
William A. Horton and Jacqueline T. Hecht

Chapter 692 **Osteogenesis Imperfecta** 2437
Joan C. Marini

Chapter 693 **Marfan Syndrome** 2440
Jefferson Doyle and Harry Dietz III

Section 4 **METABOLIC BONE DISEASE** 2446

Chapter 694 **Bone Structure, Growth, and Hormonal Regulation** 2446
Russell W. Chesney

Chapter 695 **Primary Chondrodystrophy (Metaphyseal Dysplasia)** 2446
Russell W. Chesney

Chapter 696 **Hypophosphatasia** 2446
Russell W. Chesney

Chapter 697 **Hyperphosphatasia** 2446
Russell W. Chesney

Chapter 698 **Osteoporosis** 2446
Russell W. Chesney

PART XXXIII

Environmental Health Hazards

Chapter 699 **Biologic Effects of Radiation on Children** 2448
Thomas L. Slovis

Chapter 700 **Chemical Pollutants** 2448
Philip J. Landrigan and Joel A. Forman

Chapter 701 **Heavy Metal Intoxication** 2448
Prashant V. Mahajan

Chapter 702 **Lead Poisoning** 2448
Morri Markowitz

Chapter 703 **Nonbacterial Food Poisoning** 2454

703.1 **Mushroom Poisoning** 2454
Denise A. Salerno and Stephen C. Aronoff

703.2 **Solanine Poisoning** 2454
Denise A. Salerno and Stephen C. Aronoff

703.3 **Seafood Poisoning** 2454
Denise A. Salerno and Stephen C. Aronoff

703.4 **Melamine Poisoning** 2454
Denise A. Salerno and Stephen C. Aronoff

Chapter 704 **Biologic and Chemical Terrorism** 2454
Theodore J. Cieslak and Fred M. Henretig

Chapter 705 **Animal and Human Bites** 2454
Charles M. Ginsburg

705.1 **Rat Bite Fever** 2457
Charles M. Ginsburg

705.2 **Monkeypox** 2459
Charles M. Ginsburg

Chapter 706 **Envenomations** 2460
Bill J. Schroeder and Robert L. Norris

PART XXXIV

Laboratory Medicine

Chapter 707 **Laboratory Testing in Infants and Children** 2466
Stanley F. Lo

Chapter 708 **Reference Intervals for Laboratory Tests and Procedures** 2466
Stanley F. Lo

Nelson Textbook of PEDIATRICS

PART I The Field of Pediatrics

Chapter 1
Overview of Pediatrics

Bonita F. Stanton and Richard E. Behrman

Children are the world's most important resource. Pediatrics is the sole discipline concerned with all aspects of the well-being of infants, children, and adolescents, including their health; their physical, mental, and psychologic growth and development; and their opportunity to achieve full potential as adults. Pediatricians must be concerned not only with particular organ systems and biologic processes, but also with environmental and social influences, which have a major impact on the physical, emotional, and mental health and social well-being of children and their families.

Pediatricians must be advocates for the individual child and for all children, irrespective of culture, religion, gender, race, or ethnicity or of local, state, or national boundaries. Children cannot advocate for themselves. The more politically, economically, or socially disenfranchised a population or a nation is, the greater the need for advocacy for children by the profession whose entire purpose is to advance the well-being of children. The young are often among the most vulnerable or disadvantaged in society and, thus, their needs require special attention. As divides between nations blur through advanced transportation and communication, through globalization of the economy, and through modern means of warfare and as the categorization of countries into "developed" or "industrialized" and "developing" or "low income" break down due to uneven advances within and across countries, a global perspective for the field of pediatrics becomes both a reality and a necessity.

The world population is growing at the rate of 1.14%/yr, with that of the USA growing at 0.88%/yr. Worldwide children younger than age 15 yr account for 1.8 billion (28%) of the world's 6.4 billion persons; in the USA, children younger than age 18 yr constitute approximately one quarter of the population.

In 2006, there were an estimated 133 million births worldwide, 124 million (92%) of which were in developing countries and 4.3 million (3%) of which were in the USA.

SCOPE AND HISTORY OF PEDIATRICS AND VITAL STATISTICS

More than a century ago, pediatrics emerged as a medical specialty in response to increasing awareness that the health problems of children differ from those of adults and that a child's response to illness and stress varies with age. In 1959, the United Nations issued the Declaration of the Rights of the Child, articulating the universal presumption that children everywhere have fundamental needs and rights. Virtually all nations have practicing pediatricians and most medical schools across the globe have departments of pediatrics or child health.

The health problems of children and youth vary widely between and within populations in the nations of the world depending on a number of often interrelated factors. These factors include (1) economic considerations (economic disparities); (2) educational, social, and cultural considerations; (3) the prevalence and ecology of infectious agents and their hosts; (4) climate and geography; (5) agricultural resources and practices (nutritional resources); (6) stage of industrialization and urbanization; (7) the gene frequencies for some disorders; and (8) the health and social welfare infrastructure available within these countries. Health problems are not restricted to single nations and are not limited by country boundaries; the interrelation of health issues across the globe has achieved widespread recognition in the wake of the SARS (severe acute respiratory syndrome) and AIDS epidemics, expansions in the pandemics of cholera and West Nile virus, war and bioterrorism, the tsunami of 2004, and the global recession beginning in 2008.

Reducing Child Mortality

Despite global interconnectedness, child health priorities continue to reflect local politics, resources, and needs. The state of health of any community must be defined by the incidence of illness and by data from studies that show the changes that occur with time and in response to programs of prevention, case finding, therapy, and surveillance. To ensure that the needs of children and adults across the globe were not obscured by local needs, in 2000 the international community established 8 Millennium Development Goals (MDGs) to be achieved by 2015 (*www.countdown2015mnch.org*). Although all 8 MDGs impact child well-being, MDG 4 ("Reduce by two-thirds, between 1990 and 2015, the under-five mortality rate") is exclusively focused on children. Globally, there has been a 23% reduction in under-5 mortality since 1990 (from 93 to 72 deaths per 1,000 live births), with a 40% reduction in developed countries (10 to 6) but only a 21% reduction in the least developed countries (180 to 142). In 62 countries progress was inadequate to meet the goals and 27 countries (including most of those in sub-Saharan Africa) made no progress or declined between 1990 and 2006. There were nearly 13 million under-5 deaths in 1990; 2006 marked the 1st year that there were fewer than 10 million deaths (9.7 million) with a further decrease to 9.0 million in 2007 and 8.8 million in 2008. However, overall progress has not been on target to reach the goal (Fig. 1-1).

In the late 19th century in the USA, 200 of every 1,000 children born alive died before the age of 1 yr of conditions such as diarrhea, pneumonia, measles, diphtheria, and whooping cough. In developing countries today, the leading causes of death remains diarrhea, pneumonia, malaria, and measles with much of the reductions in mortality that have occurred resulting from effective vaccine programs, oral rehydration therapy, early diagnosis and treatment of pneumonia, and, treated mosquito nets.

Neonatal (<1 mo) death contributes substantially to the under-5 mortality rate, growing in proportion as the under-5 death rate decreases. Globally, the neonatal mortality rate of 28 per 1,000 live births represents 62% of the infant mortality rate of 45 per 1,000 live births and 43% of the under-5 death rate of 72. The proportion of neonatal deaths in industrialized countries is higher (60% of infant deaths and 50% of under-5 mortality) than in the least developed countries (49% of infant deaths and 31% of under-5 deaths). In populations with the highest child mortality rates, however, just over 20% of all child deaths occurred in the neonatal period, but in countries with mortality rates <35/1,000 live births, >50% of child deaths were in neonates.

Across the globe, there are significant variations in infant mortality rates by nation, by region, by economic status, and by level of industrial development, the categorizations employed by the World Bank and the United Nations (Table 1-1). Most of the decline in infant mortality in the USA and other industrialized countries since 1970 is attributable to a decrease in the birthweight-specific infant mortality rate related to neonatal intensive care, not to the prevention of low-birthweight births

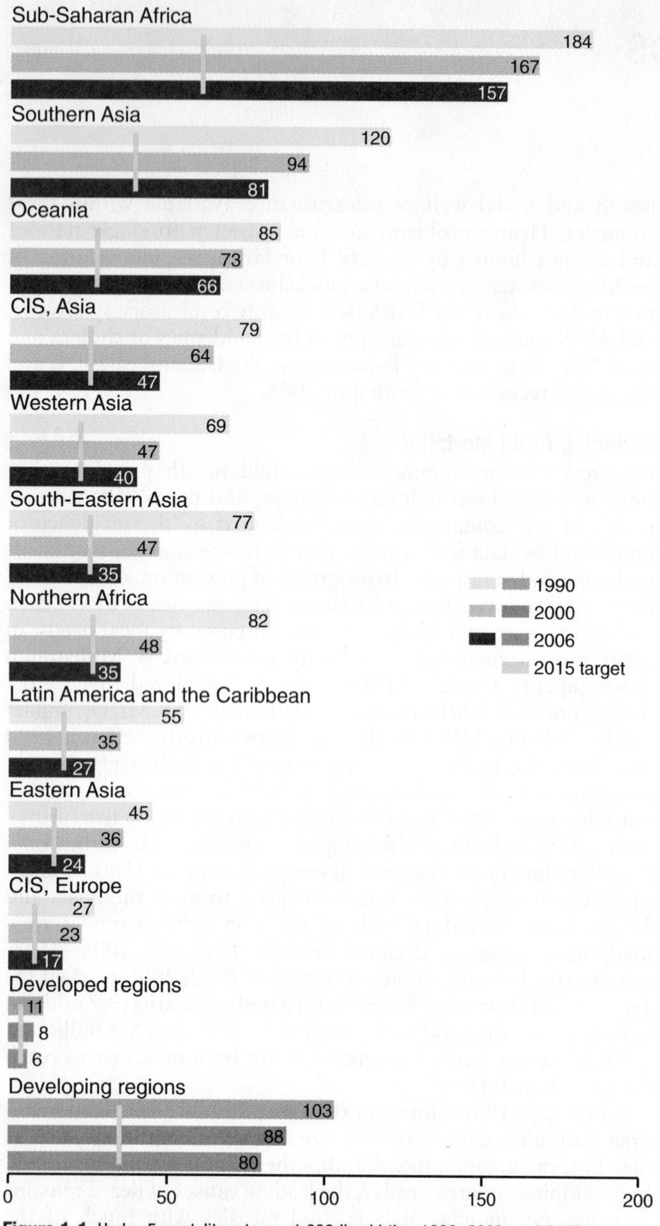

Figure 1-1 Under-5 mortality rate per 1,000 live births, 1990, 2000, and 2006. CIS, Commonwealth of Independent States (formerly the USSR). (From United Nations: *The millennium development goals report 2008,* New York, 2008, United Nations, p 20.)

(Chapter 87). The majority of deaths of infants younger than 1 yr of age occur in the 1st 28 days of life, most of these in the 1st 7 days; moreover, a large proportion of the deaths in the 1st 7 days occur on the 1st day. An increasing number of severely ill infants born at very low birthweight survive the neonatal period, however, and die later in infancy of neonatal disease, its sequelae, or its complications (Tables 1-2 through 1-4).

Causes of death vary by developmental status of the nation. In the USA, the 3 leading causes of death among infants were congenital anomalies, disorders related to gestation and low birthweight, and sudden infant death (Table 1-5). By contrast, in developing countries, the majority of infant deaths result from infectious diseases; even in the neonatal period, 24% of deaths are caused by severe infections and 7% by tetanus. In developing countries, 29% of neonatal deaths are due to birth asphyxia and 24% due to complications of prematurity.

In the majority of countries, the most robust predictor of infant mortality is a poor level of maternal education (and therefore another of the MDG addresses the need for universal access to primary schooling for girls). Other maternal risk characteristics, such as unmarried status, adolescence, and high parity, correlate with increased risk of postneonatal mortality and morbidity and low birthweight.

Health Among Postinfancy Children

A profound improvement in child health within industrialized nations occurred in the 20th century with the introduction of antibacterial disinfectants, antibiotic agents, and vaccines. Efforts to control infectious diseases were complemented by better understanding of nutrition. In the USA, Canada, and parts of Europe, new and continuing discoveries in these areas led to establishment of public well child clinics for low-income families. Although the timing of control of infectious disease was uneven around the globe, this focus on control was accompanied by significant decreases in morbidity and mortality in all countries. The smallpox eradication program of the 1970s resulted in the global eradication of smallpox in 1977. The introduction in the 1970s of the Expanded Program of Immunizations (universal vaccination against polio, diphtheria, measles, tuberculosis, tetanus, and pertussis) by the World Health Organization (WHO) and United Nations Children's Fund (UNICEF) has resulted in an estimated annual reduction of 1 to 2 million deaths per year globally. Recognizing the importance of prevention of infectious diseases to the health of children, several countries among the 50 currently ranked by the World Bank as among the poorest nations (per capita income <$750/yr) have invested heavily in infectious disease control through the development of internal vaccine production capability. As diarrheal diseases continued through the mid-1970s to account for ≈25% of infant and childhood deaths in the nonindustrialized countries (~4 million deaths per year at that time), attention turned to the development and utilization of oral resuscitation fluids to sustain children through potentially life-threatening episodes of acute diarrheal diseases. Oral rehydration solutions are largely credited with the current reduction of diarrheal deaths annually to 1.5 million.

In the later 20th century, with improved control of infectious diseases (including the elimination of polio in the Western hemisphere) through both prevention and treatment, pediatric medicine in industrialized nations increasingly turned its attention to a broad spectrum of conditions. These included both potentially lethal conditions and temporarily or permanently handicapping conditions; among these disorders were leukemia, cystic fibrosis, diseases of the newborn infant, congenital heart disease, mental retardation, genetic defects, rheumatic diseases, renal diseases, and metabolic and endocrine disorders. Thus, in industrialized nations, the end of the 20th century and 1st decade of the 21st century have been marked by accelerated understanding of new approaches to the management of many disorders as a consequence of advances in molecular biology, genetics, and immunology.

Increasing attention has also been given to behavioral and social aspects of child health, ranging from re-examination of child-rearing practices to creation of major programs aimed at prevention and management of abuse and neglect of infants and children. Developmental psychologists, child psychiatrists, neuroscientists, sociologists, anthropologists, ethnologists, and others have brought us new insights into human potential, including new views of the importance of the environmental circumstances during pregnancy, surrounding birth, and in the early years of child rearing. The later 20th century witnessed the beginning of nearly universal acceptance by pediatric professional societies of attention to normal development, child rearing, and psychosocial disorders across the continents. In the last decade, irrespective of level of industrialization, nations have developed programs addressing not only causes of mortality and physical morbidity (such as infectious diseases and protein-calorie malnutrition), but also factors leading to decreased cognition and thwarted psychosocial development, including punitive child-rearing practices,

Table 1-1 CHILD HEALTH INDICATORS WORLDWIDE BY REGION

	MORTALITY RATE BY YR PER 1,000 LIVE BIRTHS Under-5			Infant Mortality			Gross National per Capita Income 2008	Life Expectancy at Birth 2008	Primary School Attendance 2003-2008
	1960	1990	2008	1960	1990	2008			
Sub-Saharan Africa	278	187	144	185	111	86	$1,109	52 yr	65%
Eastern and Southern Africa		165	120		102	76	$1,409	53 yr	71%
West and Central Africa		208	169		119	96	$833	51 yr	61%
Middle East and North Africa	249	79	43	157	58	33	$3,942	70 yr	84%
South Asia	244	123	76	148	87	57	$1,001	64 yr	81%
East Asia and Pacific	208	55	28	137	41	22	$3,136	72 yr	95%
Latin America and Caribbean	153	55	23	102	43	19	$6,888	74 yr	93%
CEE/CIS	112	53	23	83	43	20	$6,992	69 yr	93%
Industrialized countries	39	10	6	32	9	5	$40,772	80 yr	95%
Developing countries	224	103	72	142	70	49	$2,778	67 yr	83%
Least developed countries	278	180	129	171	113	82	$583	57 yr	66%
World	198	93	65	127	64	45	$8,633	69 yr	84%

Adapted from UNICEF: *The state of the world's children 2005: childhood under threat,* New York, 2004, UNICEF, Table 1, pp 108 and 117; and The State of The World's Children, Special Edition, Statistical Tables, 2009. Table 1, page 11.
CEE/CIS, Central and Eastern Europe/Commonwealth of Independent States (formerly the USSR).

Table 1-2 DEATH RATES FOR ALL CAUSES, BY SEX, RACE, AND AGE: UNITED STATES, SELECTED YEARS 1960 AND 2005

	1960 White	1960 Black	2005 White	2005 Black
MALE				
Under 1 yr	2,694.1	5,306.8	640.0	1,437.2
1-4 yr	104.9	208.5	30.9	46.7
5-14 yr	52.7	75.1	17.1	27.0
15-24 yr	143.7	212.0	110.4	172.1
FEMALE				
Under 1 yr	2,007.7	4,162.2	515.3	1,179.7
1-4 yr	85.2	173.3	22.9	36.7
5-14 yr	34.7	53.8	12.8	19.4
15-24 yr	54.9	107.5	41.5	51.2

Adapted from National Center for Health Statistics: *Health, United States, 2007: with chartbook on trends in the health of Americans,* Hyattsville, MD, 2007, U.S. Department of Health and Human Services, Table 35, pp 1–3, selected years 1960 and 2005.

Table 1-3 DEATHS RATES FOR ALL CAUSES AMONG CHILDREN AND YOUNG ADULTS ACCORDING TO SEX, RACE, HISPANIC ORIGIN, AND AGE: 2006

	DEATHS PER 100,000 RESIDENT POPULATION Under 1 yr	1-4 yr	5-14 yr	15-24 yr
All persons	692.7	28.4	15.3	82.1
Male	757.6	30.5	17.5	119.1
Female	624.7	26.2	12.9	42.8
MALES				
White	635.9	27.5	16.4	111.7
Black male (African-American)	1387.0	46.8	24.9	171.1
American Indian or Alaska Native	1,066.6	58.1	16.8	153.2
Asian or Pacific Islander	478.0	18.6	11.4	60.8
Hispanic or Latino	642.1	28.8	16.0	118.8
White not Hispanic or Latino	625.7	26.8	16.2	107.9
FEMALES				
White	519.1	23.4	12.0	41.8
Black (African-American)	1194.9	39.5	17.3	51.1
American Indian or Alaska Native	689.9	51.7	17.0	63.2
Asian or Pacific Islander	368.6	21.3	10.3	25.6
Hispanic or Latino	542.5	23.9	11.8	34.5
White not Hispanic or Latino	505.4	23.2	11.9	43.1

Adapted from Heron MP, Hoyert DL, Xu J, et al: Deaths: preliminary data for 2006, *Natl Vital Stat Rep* 56(16):1–52, 2008.

child labor, undernutrition, war, and poor schooling. Obesity is recognized as a major health risk not only in industrialized nations, but increasingly in transitional countries. Progress at the turn of the 21st century in unraveling the human genome offers for the 1st time the realization that significant genetic screening, individualized pharmacotherapy, and genetic manipulation will be a part of routine pediatric treatment and prevention practices in the future. The prevention implications of the genome project give rise to the possibility of reducing costs for the care of illness but also increase concerns about privacy issues (Chapter 3).

Although local famines and disasters, and regional and national wars have periodically disrupted the general trend for global improvement in child health indices, it was not until the advent of the AIDS epidemic in the later 20th century that the 1st substantial global erosion of progress in child health outcomes occurred. This erosion has resulted in ever-widening gaps between childhood health indices in sub-Saharan Africa compared to the rest of the world. From 1990 to 2002, life expectancy in sub-Saharan Africa decreased from 50 yr to 46 yr; although, as of 2008, it had returned to 52 yrs. Increasing rates of tuberculosis and continued problems with pandemics such as cholera further challenge many of these nations. Strains of drug-resistant malaria are also a major concern in isolated areas around the world, but 90% of malarial deaths (the majority among children) are occurring in sub-Saharan Africa. Diseases once confined to limited geographic niches, including West Nile virus, and diseases previously uncommon among humans, such as the avian flu virus, increased awareness of the interconnectedness of health around the world. Formerly perceived as a problem of industrialized nations, motor vehicle crashes are now a major cause of mortality in developing countries as well.

Enormous disparities exist in childhood mortality rates across the globe (see Table 1-1). Among the ~8.7 million childhood deaths occurring worldwide, ≈50% occur in sub-Saharan Africa, home to <10% of the world's population. Fifty percent of the world's childhood deaths are occurring in 6 nations; 90% of childhood deaths are occurring in only 42 of the world's 192 nations. In 2008, the USA had an under-5 mortality rate of 8/1,000 live births. Forty-two nations had under-5 mortality rates

Table 1-4 INFANT, NEONATAL, AND POSTNATAL DEATHS AND MORTALITY RATES BY SPECIFIED RACE OR ORIGIN OF MOTHER: USA, 2005

RACE OF MOTHER	LIVE BIRTHS	MORTALITY RATE PER 1,000 LIVE BIRTHS		
		Infant	Neonatal	Postnatal
All races	4,138,573	6.86	4.54	2.32
White	3,229,494	5.73	3.77	1.96
Black or African American	633,152	13.26	8.92	4.33
American Indian or Alaska Native	44,815	8.06	4.04	4.02
Asian or Pacific Islander	231,112	4.89	3.37	1.51
Hispanic or Latino	985,513	5.62	3.86	1.76
Mexican	693,202	5.53	3.78	1.75
Puerto Rican	63,341	8.30	5.95	2.37
Cuban	16,064	4.42	3.05	1.37
Central and South American	151,202	4.68	3.23	1.46
Other and unknown Hispanic or Latino	61,704	6.43	4.31	2.14
Not Hispanic or Latino				
White	2,279,959	5.76	3.71	2.05
Black or African American	583,764	13.63	9.13	4.50

Adapted from Mathews TJ, MacDorman MF. Infant mortality statistics from the 2005 period linked birth/infant death data set, *Natl Vital Stat Rep* 57(2):1–32, 2008.

lower than that of the USA, with Singapore, Finland, Luxembourg, Iceland, and Sweden having the lowest rates at 3/1,000. The comparable child mortality rate in sub-Saharan Africa was 144/1,000 live births. As of 2008, Afghanistan has the highest under-5 mortality rate of 257/1,000 live births, followed by Angola at 220/1,000 live births and Chad at 209/1,000 live births. In 1990 Afghanistan and Angola had an under-5 mortality rate of 260/1,000 live births, showing minimal improvement over 2 decades. Causes of under-5 mortality differ markedly between developed and developing nations. In developing countries, 66% of all deaths resulted from infectious and parasitic diseases. Among the 42 countries having 90% of childhood deaths, diarrheal disease accounted for 22% of deaths, pneumonia 21%, malaria 9%, AIDS 3%, and measles 1%. Neonatal causes contributed to 33%. The contribution for AIDS varies greatly by country, being responsible for a substantial proportion of deaths in some countries and negligible amounts in others. Likewise, there is substantial co-occurrence of infections; a child may die with HIV, malaria, measles, and pneumonia. Infectious diseases are still responsible for much of the mortality in developing countries. In the USA, pneumonia (and influenza) accounted for only 2% of under-5 deaths, with only negligible contributions from diarrhea and malaria. Unintentional injury is the most common cause of death among U.S. children ages 1-5 yr, accounting for about 33% of deaths, followed by congenital anomalies (11%), malignant neoplasms (8%), and homicides (7%). Other causes accounted for <5% of total mortality within this age group (see Table 1-5). Although unintentional injuries in developing countries are proportionately less important causes of mortality than in developed countries, their absolute rates and their contributions to morbidity are substantially greater.

Morbidities Among Children

It is important to examine morbidities as well as mortality. Adequately addressing special health care needs is important in all countries both to minimize loss of life and to maximize the potential of each individual.

In the USA, ≈70% of all pediatric hospital bed days are for chronic illnesses; 80% of pediatric health expenditures are for 20% of children. In 2006, about 13.9% of U.S. children were reported to have special health care needs; 21.8 percent of households with children had ≥1 child with a special health care need (Chapter 39). Significantly more poor children and minority children have special health care needs. Although there are multiple chronic conditions and the prevalence of these disorders vary by population, 2 of these morbidities—obesity and asthma—have a substantial and increasing presence worldwide and are associated with substantial health consequences and costs. In the USA, ~25% of children and adolescents are overweight, representing a 2.3- to 3.3-fold increase over the past 25 yr. Similar rates have been reported from Australia and multiple countries in Europe, Egypt, Chile, Peru, and Mexico (Chapter 44).

Also increasing in prevalence among industrialized nations and in middle- and low-income nations with substantial urbanization are rates of asthma. In the mid-1990s, the USA reported an annual prevalence rate of wheezing of 57.8/1,000 among children ages 0-4 yr and 74.4/1,000 among youth ages 5-15 yr, approximately 2-fold higher than comparable prevalence rates in 1980. In 2007, the Centers for Disease Control and Prevention (CDC) estimated that 9% of U.S. children have asthma, including 19.2% of Puerto Rican and 12.7% of non-Hispanic black children. The International Study of Asthma and Allergies in Childhood has conducted a systematic review of asthma prevalence, with compelling evidence for a substantial global burden of childhood asthma, although rates vary substantially between and within countries. The highest annual prevalence rates are in the United Kingdom, Australia, New Zealand, and Ireland, with the lowest rates in Eastern European countries, Indonesia, China, Taiwan, India, and Ethiopia (Chapter 138).

Chronic cognitive morbidities represent another substantial problem. Although different diagnostic criteria have been applied, attention-deficit/hyperactivity disorder (ADHD) has been identified in 5-12% of children in countries across the globe. Rates exceeding 10% have been reported in the USA, New Zealand, Australia, Spain, Italy, Colombia, and Great Britain. Variations in cultural tolerance and/or differences in screening approaches or tools may account for some of the differences in prevalence of the disorder by country, but genetic and gene-environmental interactions may also play a role. Despite variations in rate, the condition is universal. Beyond the personal and familial stress caused by the disorder, costs to the educational system are considerable. It is estimated that in 2010 the U.S. drug treatment costs for ADHD will exceed $4 billion. In developing countries without resources for special education, these children are unlikely to fulfill their academic potential (Chapter 30).

Mental retardation affects ≈1-3% of children in the USA, with ~80% of these children having mild retardation. Rates are severalfold higher among very low birthweight infants, although data from European cerebral palsy (CP) registries has revealed a significant decrease in the prevalence of CP in very low birthweight infants, from 60.6 per 1,000 live births in 1980 to 39.5 per 1,000 live births in 1996. In the USA, there is substantial variation in rates of mild retardation by socioeconomic status (9-fold higher in the lowest compared to the highest socioeconomic stratum) but relatively equivalent rates of severe retardation. A similar income-related distribution is found in other countries, including some of the most impoverished countries such as Bangladesh. Lower overall rates have been reported in some countries, including countries ranging from Saudi Arabia to Sweden to China; the difference is primarily in the prevalence of mild retardation (Chapter 33).

The prevalence of post-traumatic stress disorder (PTSD) varies considerably around the globe, but in children with substantial exposure to violence, the rates may be very high. After the attacks on the World Trade Center towers and the Pentagon in 2001, 33% of U.S. children had experienced 1 or more symptoms of PTSD. One half of Palestinian children experience at least 1 significant lifetime trauma and >33% (66% of those experiencing

Table 1-5 LEADING CAUSES OF DEATH AND NUMBERS OF DEATHS, ACCORDING TO AGE: UNITED STATES 2005

AGE AND RANK ORDER	CAUSE OF DEATH	NUMBER	PERCENT OF TOTAL DEATHS
Under 1 yr	All causes	27,936	100.0
	Congenital malformations, deformations, and chromosomal abnormalities	5,622	20.1
	Disorders related to short gestation and low birthweight, not elsewhere classified	4,642	16.6
	Sudden infant death syndrome	2,246	8.0
	Newborn affected by maternal complications of pregnancy	1,715	6.1
	Accidents	1,052	3.8
	Newborn affected by complications of placenta, cord, and membranes	1,042	3.7
	Respiratory distress of newborn	875	3.1
	Bacterial sepsis of newborn	827	3.0
	Neonatal hemorrhage	616	2.2
	Diseases of the circulatory system	593	2.1
	All other causes	8,706	31.2
1-4 yr	All causes	4,785	100.0
	Accidents	1,641	34.3
	Congenital malformations, deformations, and chromosomal abnormalities	569	11.9
	Malignant neoplasms	399	8.3
	Assault	377	7.9
	Diseases of heart	187	3.9
	Influenza and pneumonia	119	2.5
	Septicemia	84	1.8
	Certain conditions originating in the perinatal period	61	1.3
	In situ neoplasms, benign neoplasms, and neoplasms of uncertain or unknown behavior	53	1.1
	Chronic lower respiratory diseases	48	1.0
	All other causes	1,247	26.1
5-9 yr	All causes	2,888	100.0
	Accidents	1,126	39.0
	Malignant neoplasms	526	18.2
	Congenital malformations, deformations, and chromosomal abnormalities	205	7.1
	Assault	122	4.2
	Diseases of heart	83	2.9
	Chronic lower respiratory diseases	46	1.6
	In situ neoplasms, benign neoplasms, and neoplasms of uncertain or unknown behavior	41	1.4
	Septicemia	38	1.3
	Cerebrovascular diseases	34	1.2
	Influenza and pneumonia	33	1.1
	All other causes	634	22.0
10-14 yr	All causes	3,946	100.0
	Accidents	1,540	39.0
	Malignant neoplasms	493	12.5
	Intentional self-harm	283	7.2
	Assault	207	5.2
	Congenital malformations, deformations, and chromosomal abnormalities	184	4.7
	Diseases of heart	162	4.1
	Chronic lower respiratory diseases	74	1.9
	Influenza and pneumonia	49	1.2
	In situ neoplasms, benign neoplasms, and neoplasms of uncertain or unknown behavior	43	1.1
	Cerebrovascular diseases	43	1.1
	All other causes	868	22.0
15-19 yr	All causes	13,706	100.0
	Accidents	6,825	49.8
	Assault	1,932	14.1
	Intentional self-harm	1,700	12.4
	Malignant neoplasms	731	5.3
	Diseases of heart	366	2.7
	Congenital malformations, deformations, and chromosomal abnormalities	257	1.9
	Cerebrovascular diseases	69	0.5
	Influenza and pneumonia	67	0.5
	Chronic lower respiratory diseases	85	0.6
	In situ neoplasms, benign neoplasms, and neoplasms of uncertain or unknown behavior	50	0.4
	Anemias	50	0.4
	All other causes	1,574	11.5
20-24 yr	All causes	19,715	100.0
	Accidents	8,624	43.7
	Assault	3,153	16.0
	Intentional self-harm	2,616	13.3
	Malignant neoplasms	978	5.0
	Diseases of heart	672	3.4
	Congenital malformations, deformations, and chromosomal abnormalities	226	1.1
	Human immunodeficiency virus	160	0.8
	Cerebrovascular diseases	142	0.7
	Pregnancy, childbirth, and the puerperium	131	0.7
	Influenza and pneumonia	118	0.6
	All other causes	2,895	14.7

Adapted from National Center for Health Statistics: Health, United States, 2007: with chartbook on trends in the health of Americans, Hyattsville, MD, 2007, U.S. Department of Health and Human Services.

trauma) meet the criteria of PTSD. Natural disasters such as the tsunami of 2004 and the Haitian and Chilean earthquakes and Pakistani floods of 2010; war, including those in Afghanistan, Sudan, and Iraq; and urban violence all leave their indelible marks on the minds of children.

SPECIAL RISK POPULATIONS

In addition to the enormous differences in infant and child health between regions and nations, within countries there are substantial variations in morbidity and mortality rates by socioeconomic class and ethnicity. Most children at special risk need a nurturing environment but have had their futures compromised by actions or policies arising from their families, schools, communities, nations, or the international community. These problems have several causes, whether the end result is homeless children, runaway children, children in foster care, or children in other disadvantaged groups. The most effective preventive approach involves alleviation of poverty, inadequate parenting, discrimination, violence, poor housing, and poor education. Optimal care of these children requires reducing barriers to health care with organized programs, multidiscipline teams, and special financing.

Children in Poverty

Family income is central to the health and well-being of children. Children living in poor families, especially those located in poor communities, are much more likely than children living in upper- or middle-class families to experience material deprivation and poor health, die during childhood, score lower on standardized tests, be retained in a grade or drop out of school, have out-of-wedlock births, experience violent crime, end up as poor adults, and suffer other undesirable outcomes. In 2008, 20.7% of U.S. children <18 yr (21% of those less than 6 yr) lived in poverty (defined as income <$21,756/yr for a family of 4), a rate among the highest of developed countries. Seven percent lived in extreme poverty. The poverty rates are higher for children than adults and are highest for infants and toddlers. Children who are poor have higher than average rates of death and illness from almost all causes (exceptions being suicide and motor vehicle crashes, which are most common among white, non-poor children). Many factors associated with poverty are responsible for these illnesses; crowding, poor hygiene and health care, poor diet, environmental pollution, poor education, and stress.

Similar poverty-linked disparities may exist in countries with very high infant mortality rates (sub-Saharan Africa). In the low-income developing countries, the rate of infant mortality among the poorest quintile of the population is more than twice that of the wealthiest quintile (Fig. 1-2).

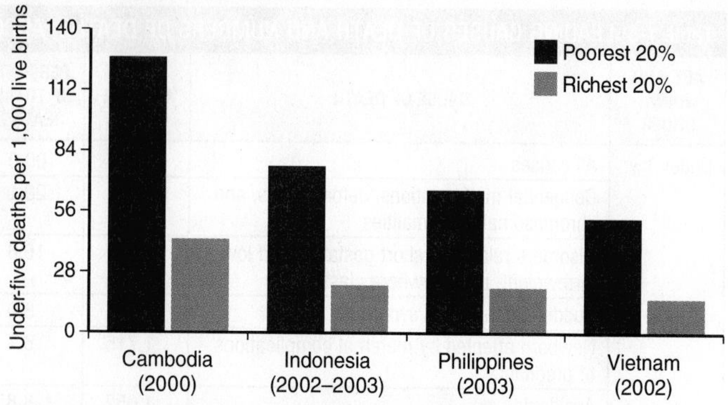

Figure 1-2 Poor children across South-Eastern Asia are much more likely to die before age 5 than their wealthier peers. (From World Health Organization: *World health statistics 2007,* Geneva, 2007, World Health Organization, p 74; and United Nations Development Programme: *Human Development Report 2007/08: fighting climate change: human solidarity in a divided world,* New York, 2007, United Nations Development Programme, p 255.)

Poverty and economic loss diminish the capacity of parents to be supportive, consistent, and involved with their children. Clinicians at all times but especially in the context of a national or global recession need to be especially alert to the development and behavior of children whose parents have lost their jobs or who live in permanent poverty. Fathers who become unemployed frequently develop psychosomatic symptoms, and their children often develop similar symptoms. Young children who grew up in the Great Depression in the USA and whose parents were subject to acute poverty suffered more than older children, especially if the older ones were able to take on responsibilities for helping the family economically. Such responsibilities during adolescence seem to give purpose and direction to an adolescent's life. The younger children, faced with parental depression and unable to do anything to help, suffered a higher frequency of illness and a diminished capacity to lead productive lives even as adults.

Pediatricians and other child health workers have a responsibility both to mitigate the effects of poverty on their patients and to contribute to efforts to reduce the number of children living in poverty. Clinicians should ask parents about their economic resources, adverse changes in their financial situation, and the family's attempts to cope. Encouraging concrete methods of coping, suggesting ways to reduce stressful social circumstances while increasing social networks that are supportive, and referring patients and their families to appropriate welfare, job training, and family agencies can significantly improve the health and functioning of children at risk when their families live in poverty. In many cases, special services, especially social services, need to be added to the traditional medical services; outreach is required to find and encourage parents to use health services and bring their children into the health care system. Pediatricians also have the responsibility to contribute to and advocate for safety net services for impoverished children within and outside the boundaries of their own country. An increasing number of programs are available to help children of greatest need worldwide, such as Project Smile, CARE, Project Hope, and Doctors without Borders.

Children of Immigrants and Racial Minority Groups Including U.S. Native Americans

Eleven percent of the U.S. population is foreign-born; 1 of every 5 children lives in an immigrant family. The USA is experiencing a wave of immigration larger than that occurring in the early 20th century. There has been an increase in immigration from China, India, Southeast Asia, Mexico, the Dominican Republic, and the former Soviet Union nations. Until the mid-20th century, emigrants to the USA were primarily white and from Europe. Such individuals now represent only about 10% of immigrants; the remainder are overwhelmingly of color and from throughout the world. Although immigrants in the USA have faced discrimination and oppression throughout history, the potential for such discrimination is compounded by the racial differences represented in the current immigrant pool. In the USA, about 240,000 children legally immigrate each year, and an estimated 50,000/yr enter the country illegally, although these numbers have been declining in the wake of the 2008 recession. Immigrants comprise >15% of the population in >50 countries, including many Western European countries.

The immigrant population constitutes a substantial proportion of the low-wage labor market. Immigrants represent 14% of all U.S. workers but 20% of low-wage workers. Immigrants are twice as likely as U.S.–born citizens to earn less than minimum wage. The poverty rate of children in immigrant families is 50% greater than in U.S.–born families, with 50% of immigrant children compared to 33% of children in U.S.–born families being below the 200% poverty level. Contributing to the lack of access to higher salaried jobs is the lack of proficiency in English (≈66% of immigrants) and the lack of education (40% have not completed high school). In the past decade, about 9 million immigrants attained permanent residency status. There may be 850,000-1,000,000 illegal immigrant children.

Families of different origins obviously bring different health problems and different cultural backgrounds, which influence health practices and use of medical care. To provide appropriate services, clinicians need to understand these influences (Chapter 4). For example, the high prevalence of hepatitis among women from Southeast Asia makes use of hepatitis B vaccine essential for their newborns. Children from Southeast Asia and South America have growth patterns that are generally below the norms established for children of Western European origin, as well as high rates of hepatitis, parasitic diseases, and nutritional deficiencies and high degrees of psychosocial stress. Foreign-born children may surpass American-born children in some health outcomes, but their health deteriorates as they become acculturated (Chapter 4).

Refugee children who escape from war or political violence and whose families have been subjected to extreme stress represent a subset of immigrant children who have faced severe trauma. These children have a particularly high incidence of mental and behavioral problems (Chapter 23).

"Linguistically isolated households," in which no one older than 14 yr of age speaks English, often present significant obstacles to providing quality health care to children because of difficulties in understanding and communicating basic concerns and instructions, avoiding compromising privacy and confidentiality interests, and obtaining informed consent (Chapter 4).

The USA is home to multiple minority populations, including the 2 largest groups, Latinos and African-Americans. The nonwhite minority groups will constitute >50% of the U.S. population by 2050 (Chapter 4). Nonwhite children in the USA disproportionately experience adverse child health outcomes (see Tables 1-2 through 1-4). Infants that are born to African-American mothers experience low birthweight and infant mortality rates twice those with white mothers (Chapter 87). Rates of these 2 adverse health outcomes are also substantially higher among some groups of Hispanic infants and children, although there is great variation by country of origin. The rates are particularly high among those of Puerto Rican descent (≈1.5 times the rates for white infants). In 2006, the overall infant mortality rate was 6.7/1,000 live births, whereas that for non-Hispanic African-America infants was 13.6; for Native Americans, 8.1; and for Puerto Ricans, 8.3. Mexicans, Asians, Pacific Islanders, Central and South Americans, and Cubans were below the national average. Latino, Native American, and African-American children are substantially more likely to live in poverty than are white children.

There are ≈2.5 million Native Americans (4.1 million in combination with other races/ethnicities) and 558 federally recognized tribes. With 840,000 children (1.4 million in combination), the Native American population has a much higher proportion of children (34%) than does the remainder of the U.S. population (26%). About 60% of Native Americans live in urban areas, not on or near native lands. Like their minority immigrant counterparts, they have faced social and economic discrimination. The unemployment and poverty levels of Native Americans are, respectively, 3-fold and 4-fold that of the white population, and far fewer Native Americans graduate from high school or go to college. The rate of low birthweight among Native Americans is more than the white rate but less than the black rate. The neonatal and the postneonatal mortality rates are higher for Native Americans living in urban areas than for urban white Americans. Deaths in the 1st yr of life due to sudden infant death syndrome, pneumonia, and influenza are higher than the average in the USA, whereas deaths due to congenital anomalies, respiratory distress syndrome, and disorders relating to short gestation and low birthweight are similar.

Unintended injury deaths among Native Americans occur at twice the rate for other U.S. populations; deaths due to malignant neoplasms are lower. During adolescence and young adulthood, suicide and homicide are the 2nd and 3rd causes of death in this population and occur at about twice the rates of the rest of the population. There may be significant underreporting of deaths of Native American children.

As many as 75% of Native American children have recurrent otitis media and high rates of hearing loss, resulting in learning problems. Tuberculosis and gastroenteritis, formerly much more common among Native Americans, now occur at about the national average. Psychosocial problems are more prevalent in these populations than in the general population: depression, alcoholism, drug abuse, out-of-wedlock teenage pregnancy, school failure and dropout, and child abuse and neglect.

Most other nations have indigenous populations who are subjected to discrimination, social and economic sanctions, and/or physical maltreatment and who demonstrate the poorest child health outcomes. An estimated 300 million indigenous persons live in 70 countries (50% in Asia) and speak ≈4,000 languages. Such children endure lower vaccination rates, lower school entry and higher dropout rates, higher rates of poverty, and lower access to justice. Indigenous children in Latin America account for 66% of the deaths of children younger than age 2 yr.

In the USA, existing programs for meeting child health problems are not available to all families in need, with gaps between eligibility for public support and parents' ability to pay for services. Needed services for immigrants are often either nonexistent or fragmented among programs, agencies, or policies. Programs are often poorly coordinated, and the data collection is inadequate.

Children of Migrant Workers

Families facing economic, social, or political hardship have been forced to leave their land and homes in search of better opportunities; such migrations are often within a country or between neighboring countries. Both industrialized and developing countries experience these migrations.

In the USA, there are an estimated 3-5 million migrant and seasonal farm workers and their families. The eastern migration is primarily from Florida, whereas the western migration comes from Texas, other border states, and Mexico. Many children travel with their parents and experience poor housing, frequent moves, and a socioeconomic system controlled by a crew boss who arranges the jobs, provides transportation, and often, together with the farm owners, provides food, alcohol, and drugs under a "company store" system that leaves migrant families with little money or in debt. Children often go without schooling; medical care is usually limited.

The medical problems of children of migrant farm workers are similar to those of children of homeless families: increased frequency of infections (including HIV), trauma, poor nutrition, poor dental care, low immunization rates, exposures to animals and toxic chemicals, anemia, and developmental delays.

Among the most substantial migrant populations in the world is China's "floating population," an estimated 100 million (almost 10% of China's population) of rural to urban migrants. The rapidly growing urban versus rural income gradient and a relaxation of restrictions on movement in the country has fueled this influx of rural residents who arrive in China's urban areas without health, education, or employment benefits for themselves or their children. Similar patterns are seen in many countries in Asia, Africa, and South America. In most of these countries there are few legal or social programs to aid the families or their children, spawning massive squatter settlements without provisions for water, sanitation, education, or basic health needs. Government policies vary worldwide, but in some instances their response to such communities is to bulldoze the settlements and imprison or deport the residents.

Homeless Children

Families with children are the fastest growing segment of the homeless population in the USA. Children make up over 35% of the homeless population, over 40% of whom are under age 5 yr, with an estimated 100,000 children living in shelters on a given night and about 500,000 homeless each year. Many homeless are not in shelters (living in the street or with extended families), and thus these figures are low estimates. The population of homeless children has been increasing as a consequence of more families with children living in poverty or near poverty, fewer available affordable dwellings for these families, decreasing public assistance programs for the non-elderly poor, and the rising prevalence of substance abuse.

Homeless children have an increased frequency of illness, including intestinal infections, anemia, neurologic disorders, seizures, behavioral disorders, mental illness, and dental problems, as well as increased frequency of trauma and substance abuse. Homeless children are admitted to U.S. hospitals at a much higher rate than the national average. They have higher school failure rates, and the likelihood of their being victims of abuse and neglect is much higher. In 1 study, 50% of such children were found to have psychosocial problems, such as developmental delays, severe depression, or learning disorders. The increased frequency of maternal psychosocial problems, especially depression, in homeless households has a significant untoward impact on the mental and physical health of these children. Because families tend to break apart under the strain of poverty and homelessness, many homeless children end up in foster care. If their families remain intact, frequent moves make it very difficult for them to receive continuity of medical care.

Homelessness exists worldwide. There are an estimated 3 million people in the 15 countries of the European Union who do not have a permanent home while in Canada there are 200,000-300,000 homeless. In some nations in Latin America, Asia, and Africa, the distinction between rural-to-urban migrants and homelessness is blurred.

Provision of adequate housing, job retraining for the parents, and mental health and social services are necessary to prevent homelessness from occurring. Physicians can have an important role in motivating society to adopt the social policies that will prevent homelessness from occurring by educating policymakers that these homeless children are at greater risk of becoming burdens both to themselves and to society if their special health needs are not met.

Runaway and Thrown-Away Children

The number of runaway and thrown-away children and youths in the USA is estimated at about 500,000; several hundred thousand of these children have no secure and safe place to stay. Teenagers make up most of both groups. The usual definition of a runaway is a youth younger than 18 yr who is gone for at least 1 night from his or her home without parental permission. Most runaways leave home only once, stay overnight with friends, and have no contact with the police or other agencies. This group is no different from their "healthy" peers in psychologic status. A smaller but unknown number become multiple or permanent "runners" and are significantly different from the one-time runners.

Thrown-aways include children told directly to leave the household, children who have been away from home and are not allowed to return, abandoned or deserted children, and children who run away but whose caretakers make no effort to recover them or do not appear to care if they return. The same constellation of causes common to many of the other special-risk groups is characteristic of permanent runaways, including environmental problems (family dysfunction, abuse, poverty) and personal problems of the young person (poor impulse control, psychopathology, substance abuse, or school failure). Thrown-aways experience more violence and conflicts in their families.

In the USA, it is a minority of runaway youths who become homeless street people. These youths have a high frequency of problem behaviors, with 75% engaging in some type of criminal activity and 50% engaging in prostitution. A majority of permanent runaways have serious mental problems; more than 33% are the product of families who engage in repeated physical and sexual abuse (Chapter 37). These children also have a high frequency of medical problems, including hepatitis, sexually transmitted infections, and drug abuse. Although runaways often distrust most social agencies, they will come to and use medical services. Medical care may become the point of re-entry into mainstream society and the path to needed services. U.S. parents who seek a physician's advice about a runaway child should be asked about the child's history of running away, the presence of family dysfunction, and personal aspects of the child's development. If the youth contacts the physician, the latter should examine the youth and assess his or her health status, as well as willingness to return home. If it is not feasible for the youth to return home, foster care, a group home, or an independent living arrangement should be sought by referral to a social worker or a social agency. Although legal considerations involved in the treatment of homeless minor adolescents may be significant, most states, through their "Good Samaritan" laws and definitions of emancipated minors, authorize treatment of homeless youths. Legal barriers should not be used as an excuse to refuse medical care to runaway or thrown-away youths.

The issue of runaway youths is very complex in many developing nations, where in many instances the youth may be orphaned and/or leaving situations of forced sex or other abusive situations. It is estimated that there are tens of millions of such youth worldwide. Natural disasters such as the 2010 earthquake devastating Haiti also contribute to growing numbers of orphaned children. In 2007, there were an estimated 11-15 million HIV orphans in Africa; this number is estimated to grow to as high as 20 million by 2010. With school attendance <50% in many parts of sub-Saharan Africa, children who are orphaned are 17% less likely to attend school. Humanitarian and international organizations have begun to focus on this very vulnerable group of youths across the globe. Rates are often uncertain, and in many countries, these children have not even been recognized as an at-risk group, so great is the social chaos and so massive are the unmet needs.

Children Directly Affected By War (Chapter 36.2)

Since the end of the Second World War, there have been ~250 major wars (defined as armed combat with over 1,000 casualties), the majority of which have been civil wars. Many of these conflicts have lasted over a decade; Angola has been engaged in civil war for nearly 3 decades. Sixteen of the world's poorest 20 countries have endured a civil war in the past 15 yr. In modern wars, 70-80% of casualties are among women and children. Direct mortality and morbidity to children account for only a portion of war's destructive impact on children. In 1996 the United Nations commissioned a report addressing the full consequences of war on children entitled "Promotion and Protection of the Rights of Children: Impact of Armed Conflict on Children" including (1) the disruption of basic educational and child health pediatric care and services; (2) hardships endured as a result of refugee status; (3) the abuse of the 250,000 to 300,000 children under age 18 yr who are soldiers; and (4) the impact on children when 1 or both parents are deployed to serve.

Inherent Strengths in Vulnerable Children and Interventions

By age 20-30 yr, many children in the USA and other developed countries who were at special risk will have made moderate successes of their lives. Teenage mothers and children who were born prematurely or in poverty demonstrate that, by this age, the majority have made the transition to stable marriages and jobs and are accepted by their communities as responsible citizens. As the numbers of risk factors increases for an individual, however, the odds for a successful adulthood decline.

Certain biologic characteristics are associated with success, such as being born with an accepting temperament. Avoidance of additional social risks is even more important. Premature infants or preadolescent boys with conduct disorders and poor reading skills, who must also face a broken family, poverty, frequent moves, and family violence, are at much greater risk than children with only 1 of these risks. Perhaps most important are the protective buffers that have been found to enhance children's resilience because these can be aided by an effective health care system and community. Children generally do better if they can gain social support, either from family members or from a nonjudgmental adult outside the family, especially an older mentor or peer. Providers of medical services should develop ways to "prescribe" supportive "other" persons for children who are at risk. Promotion of self-esteem and self-efficacy is a central factor in protection against risks. It is essential to promote competence in some area of these children's lives. Prediction of the consequences of risk is never 100% accurate. However, the confidence that, even without aid, many such children will achieve a good outcome by age 30 yr does not justify ignoring or withholding services from them in early life.

A team is needed because it is rare for 1 individual to be able to provide the multiple services needed for high-risk children. Successful programs are characterized by at least 1 caring person who can make personal contact with these children and their families. Most successful programs are relatively small (or are large programs divided into small units) and nonbureaucratic but are intensive, comprehensive, and flexible. They work not only with the individual, but also with the family, school, community, and at broader societal levels. Generally, the earlier the programs are started, in terms of the age of the children involved, the better is the chance of success. It is also important for services to be continued over a long period.

The Challenge to Pediatricians

Concerns about the aforementioned problems of children throughout the world have generated 3 sets of goals. The *1st set* includes that all families have access to adequate perinatal, preschool, and family-planning services; that international and national governmental activities be effectively coordinated at the global, regional, national, and local levels; that services be so organized that they reach populations at special risk; that there be no insurmountable or inequitable financial barriers to adequate care; that the health care of children have continuity from prenatal through adolescent age periods; and that every family ultimately have access to all necessary services, including developmental, dental, genetic, and mental health services. A *2nd set* of goals addresses the need for reducing unintended injuries and environmental risks, for meeting nutritional needs, and for health education aimed at fostering health-promoting lifestyles. A *3rd set* of goals covers the need for research in biomedical and behavioral science, in fundamentals of bioscience and human biology, and in the particular problems of mothers and children.

The unfinished business in the quest for physical, mental, and social health in the community is illustrated by the disparities with which deaths due to disease, injuries, and violence are distributed among white, black, and Hispanic children in the USA and between and within nations. Homicide is a major cause of adolescent deaths and has increased in rate among the very young, in whom the increase may, in part, represent the more accurate identification of child abuse (Chapter 37). Among adolescents, homicide may reflect unresolved social tensions, substance abuse (cocaine, crack), and an unhealthy preoccupation with violence in our society (Part III and Chapters 36, 107, and 108).

PATTERNS OF HEALTH CARE

In 2005, children younger than 15 yr made ≈211 million patient visits to U.S. physicians' offices and hospital outpatient departments. This represents 34.8 visits per 100 children per year, up from 25.3 in 1995. Pediatricians report an average of 50 preventive care visits per week, 33% for infants. The visits average 17-20 min, increasing in length as children become adolescents. The principal diagnoses, accounting for ≈40% of these visits, are well child visits (15%), middle-ear infections (12%), and injuries (10%). Ambulatory visits by children and youth decrease with age. The opposite occurs with adults. Nonwhite children are more likely than white children to use hospital facilities (including the emergency room) for their ambulatory care; the number of well child visits annually is almost 80% higher among white infants than black infants. Children with private insurance are more likely than children with public insurance who, in turn, are more likely than uninsured children to receive non–emergency room care. Insurance coverage increases outpatient utilization and receipt of preventive care by approximately 1 visit per year for children.

In the USA, between 70 and 90 children per 1,000 children are hospitalized per year. White children are less likely to be hospitalized than black or Hispanic children, but more likely than Asian children. Poor children are nearly twice as likely as nonpoor children to be hospitalized. Insurance coverage also appears to reduce hospital admissions that are potentially manageable in an ambulatory setting.

Health care utilization differs significantly among nations. In most countries, however, hospitals are sources of both routine and intensive child care, with medical and surgical services that may range from immunization and developmental counseling to open heart surgery and renal transplantation. In most countries, clinical conditions and procedures requiring intensive care are also likely to be clustered in university-affiliated centers serving as regional resources—if these resources exist.

In the USA, the hospitalization rates for children (excluding newborn infants) are less than those of adults younger than 65 yr of age, except in the 1st yr of life. The rate of hospitalization and lengths of hospital stay have declined significantly for children and adults in the past decade. Children represent <7% of the total acute hospital discharges; in children's hospitals, ≈70% of admissions are for chronic conditions, and 10-12% of pediatric hospitalizations are related to birth defects and genetic diseases.

Patterns of health care vary widely around the globe, reflecting differences in the geography and wealth of the country, the priority placed on health care vs other competing needs and interests, philosophy regarding prevention vs curative care, and the balance between child health and adult health care needs. The significant declines in infant and child mortality enjoyed in many of the developing countries in the past 3 decades have occurred in the context of support from international agencies like UNICEF, WHO, and the World Bank; bilateral donors (the aid provided from 1 country to another); and nongovernmental agencies to develop integrated, universal primary pediatric care with an emphasis on primary (vaccination) and selected secondary (oral rehydration solution [ORS], treatment of pneumonia and malaria) prevention strategies.

PLANNING AND IMPLEMENTING A SYSTEM OF CARE

Through much of the 20th century, pediatricians were primarily focused on the treatment and prevention of physical illness and disorders. Currently, physicians caring for children, especially those in developed countries, have been increasingly called on to advise in the management of disturbed behavior of children and adolescents or problematic relationships between child and parent, child and school, or child and community. The medical problems of children are often intimately related to problems of mental and social health. There is also an increasing concern about disparities in how the benefits of what we know about child health reach various groups of children. In both developed and developing nations, the health of children lags far behind what it could be if the means and will to apply current knowledge were focused on the health of children. The children most at risk are disproportionately represented among ethnic minority groups. Pediatricians have a responsibility to address these problems aggressively.

Linked with these views of the broad scope of pediatric concern is the concept that access to at least a basic level of quality services to promote health and treat illness is a right of every person. Among children in the USA, having health insurance is strongly associated with access to primary care. The failure of health services and health benefits to reach all children who need them has led to re-examination of the design of health care systems in many countries, but unresolved problems remain in most health care systems, such as the maldistribution of physicians, institutional unresponsiveness to the perceived needs of the individual, failure of medical services to adjust to the need and convenience of patients, and deficiencies in health education. Efforts to make the delivery of health care more efficient and effective have led imaginative pediatricians to create new categories of health care providers, such as pediatric nurse practitioners in industrialized nations and trained birth attendants in developing countries, and to participate in new organizations for providing care to children, such as various managed care arrangements.

New insights into the needs of children have reshaped the child health care system in other ways. Growing understanding of the need of infants for certain qualities of stimulation and care has led to revision of the care of newborn infants (Chapters 7 and 88) and of procedures leading to an adoption or to placement with foster families (Chapters 34 and 35). For handicapped children, the massive centralized institutions of past years are being replaced by community-centered arrangements offering a better opportunity for these children to achieve their maximum potential.

Without question, the U.S. Patient Protection and Affordable Care Act passed in 2010 will impact the organization of health care. In particular, the new relationships expected between physicians and hospital systems through Accountable Care Organizations (ACOs) should streamline patient access.

Health Services for At-Risk Populations

Adverse health outcomes are not evenly distributed among all children, but are concentrated in certain high-risk populations. At-risk populations may require additional, targeted, or special programs designed to be effective with unique populations. All nations, regardless of wealth and level of industrialization, have subgroups of children at particular risk, requiring additional services.

In the USA, the largest vulnerable group is children living in poverty, representing about 14% of U.S. children. Substantial proportions of children in other industrialized countries are also living in poverty. The approach to addressing the needs of this group in the USA has been the establishment of a targeted insurance program, Medicaid, which became law in 1965 as a jointly funded cooperative venture between the federal and state governments to assist states in the provision of adequate medical care to eligible needy persons. The federal statute identifies >25 different eligibility categories for which federal funds are available. These statutory categories can be classified into 5 broad coverage groups: children, pregnant women, adults in families with dependent children, individuals with disabilities, and individuals ≥65 yr old. Pediatric care in the USA is highly dependent on Medicaid; however, only a relatively small proportion of the Medicaid funds actually go to child health, with the remainder serving older adults. Following broad national guidelines, each state establishes its own eligibility standards; determines the type, amount, duration, and scope of services; sets the rate of payment for services; and administers its own program. Although Medicaid has made great strides in enrolling low-income children, significant numbers of children remain uninsured. From 1988 to 1998, the proportion of children insured through Medicaid increased from 15.6% to 19.8%, but the percentage of children without health insurance increased from 13.1% to 15.4%. Minority children were disproportionately among those without insurance. The Balanced Budget Act of 1997 created a new children's health insurance program called the State Children's Health Insurance Program (SCHIP). This program gave each state permission to offer health insurance for children, up to age 19 yr, who are not already insured. SCHIP is a state-administered program and each state sets its own guidelines regarding eligibility and services. There is great variation by state, but in many states, the SCHIP program has begun to reduce racial inequities in access to health care for children. In 2009, the percent of children without insurance had decreased to 9%.

Many industrialized nations have adapted different "safety net" systems to assure adequate coverage of all youth. Many of these programs provide health insurance for all children, regardless of income, hoping to avoid problems with children losing insurance coverage and access to health care due to changes in eligibility by providing a single form of insurance that all providers accept. The response of developing countries to the issue of universal access to care for children has been uneven, with some providing no safety net, but many having limited universal or safety net services.

To address the special needs of Native Americans in the USA, the Indian Health Service, established in 1954, has been the responsibility of the Public Health Service, but the 1975 Indian Self-Determination Act gave tribes the option of managing Native American health services in their communities. The Indian Health Service is managed through local administrative units, and some tribes contract outside the Indian Health Service for health care. Much of the emphasis is on adult services: treatment for alcoholism, nutrition and dietetic counseling, and public health nursing services. There are also >40 urban programs for Native Americans, with an emphasis on increasing access of this population to existing health services, providing special social services, and developing self-help groups. In an effort to accommodate traditional Western medical, psychologic, and social services to the Native American cultures, such programs include the "Talking Circle," the "Sweat Lodge," and other interventions based on Native American culture (Chapter 4). The efficacy of any of these programs, especially those to prevent and treat the sociopsychologic problems particular to Native Americans, has not been determined.

Recognizing the health needs of migrants in the USA, the U.S. Public Health Service initiated in 1964 the Migrant Health Program to provide funds for local groups to organize medical care for migrant families. Many migrant health projects that were initially staffed by part-time providers and were open for only part of the year have been transformed into community health care centers that provide services not only for migrants but also for other local residents. In 2001, the ≈400 Migrant Health Centers served >650,000 migrant and seasonal farm workers; >85% were people of color. Health services for migrant farm workers often need to be organized separately from existing primary care programs because the families are migratory. Special record-keeping systems that link the health care provided during winter months in the south with the care provided during the migratory season in the north are difficult to maintain in ordinary group practices or individual physicians' offices. Outreach programs that take medical care to the often remote farm sites are necessary, and specially organized Head Start, early education, and remedial education programs should also be provided. Approaches in other countries have also focused on business initiatives for migrant populations to enable them to overcome the cycle of financial dependency on their migratory lifestyle.

The USA has spent >$12 billion through the 1987 McKinney-Vento Act to provide emergency food, shelter, and health care; to finance help for young runaways; to aid homeless people in making their way back into the housing market; and to place homeless children in school. Mobile vans, with a team consisting of a physician, nurse, social worker, and welfare worker, have been shown to provide effective comprehensive care, ensure delivery of immunizations, link the children to school health services, and bring the children and their families into a stable relationship with the conventional medical system. Special record-keeping systems have been introduced to enhance continuity and to provide a record of care once the family has moved to a permanent location. Because of the high frequency of developmental delays in this group, linkage of preschool homeless children to Head Start programs is an especially important service. The Runaway Youth Act, Title III of the Juvenile Justice and Delinquency Prevention Act of 1974 (Public Law 93-414) and its amended version (Public Law 95-509) have supported shelters and provide a toll-free 24 hr telephone number (1-800-621-4000) for youths who wish to contact their parents or request help after having run away.

In Belgium, Finland, the Netherlands, Portugal, and Spain, the right to housing has been incorporated into the national constitutions. The Finnish government has devised a multifaceted response to the problem, including house building, social welfare and health care services, and the obligation to provide a home of minimum standards for every homeless person. The number of homeless in Finland has been reduced by 50%.

COSTS OF HEALTH CARE

The growth of high technology, the increasing number of people older than 65 yr, the redesign of health institutions (particularly with respect to the needs for and the uses of personnel), the public's demand for medical services, the increase in administrative bureaucracies, and the manner in which the costs of health care are paid have driven the costs of health care in the USA up to a point at which they represent a significant proportion of the gross national product. Although children (0-18 yr) represent about 25% of the population, they account for only about 12% of the health care expenditures, or about 60% of adult per capita expenditures. Efforts to contain costs have led to revisions of the way in which physicians and hospitals are paid for services. Limits have been set on the fees for some services, capitated prepayment and various managed care systems flourish, a program of reimbursement (diagnosis-related groups [DRGs]) based on the diagnosis rather than on the particular services rendered to an individual patient has been implemented, and a relative value scale for varying rates of payment among different physician services has been instituted. These and other changes in the system of financing health services raise important ethical, quality of care, and professional issues for pediatricians to address (Chapter 3).

Health care costs have been better contained in most other industrialized nations, the majority of which also enjoy lower childhood mortality rates than does the USA.

Evaluation of Health Care

The shaping of health care systems to meet the needs of children and their families requires accurate statistical data and difficult decisions in setting priorities. Along with growing concerns about the design and cost of health care systems and the ability to distribute health services equitably has come increasing concern about the quality of health care and about its efficiency and effectiveness. There are large local and regional variations among similar populations of children in the rates of use of procedures and technology and of hospital admissions. These variations require continuing evaluation and explanation in terms of the actual impact of medical and surgical services on health status and the outcome of illness.

The Institute of Medicine (IOM) issued a report, "Crossing the Quality Chasm: A New Health System for the 21st Century" in 2001. This report, challenging American physicians to renew efforts to focus not just on access and cost, but also on quality of care, has been furthered in several pediatric initiatives, including but not limited to: specific initiatives for monitoring child health outlined in the IOM report "Children's Health, the Nation's Wealth"; challenge/demonstration grants funded by the Robert Wood Johnson Foundation; and the National Initiative for Children's Healthcare Quality. Importantly, each of these initiatives is calling for the establishment of measurable standards for assessment of quality of care and for the establishment of routine plans for periodic reassessment thereof. Efforts have been initiated at some medical centers to establish evidence-based clinical pathways for disorders (such as asthma) where there exists sound evidence to advise these guidelines. Pediatricians have developed tools to evaluate the content and delivery of pediatric preventive "anticipatory guidance," the cornerstone of modern pediatrics (Chapter 5).

Consistent with the increased focus on quality and lifelong learning, the Residency Review and Redesign in Pediatrics (R3P) project involving a broad-based pediatric constituency led by the American Board of Pediatrics, was undertaken to ensure that pediatric residency training meets the health care and well-being needs of children in the 21st century. The R3P and the follow-on program, the Initiative for Innovation in Pediatric Education (IIPE), are calling for a transformation of residency training that focuses on continuous evaluation, adaptation to the differing and changing needs of children, and the recognition that continued training throughout a pediatrician's professional career will be necessary if the field of pediatrics is to best meet the needs of children. Increased attention is also being focused on the importance of providing pediatricians with the skills to communicate effectively with parents and patients and understanding the responsibilities of professionalism. These efforts are having an impact, with evidence that 66% of children are receiving good or excellent preventive care with no disparities according to race or income level. The increased focus on quality improvement in pediatric practice is reflected in the pediatric residency training competency requirements of practice-based learning and improvement and system-based practice.

THE INFORMATION EXPLOSION OF THE 21ST CENTURY

Currently there are over 5,000 journals and 1 million papers listed on PubMed. With globalization, pediatricians in settings around the world must be familiar with health and disease and health practices across the globe. In earlier years, new information in any field of medicine was easily accessible through a relatively small number of journals, texts, or monographs. Today, relevant information is so widely dispersed among the many journals that elaborate electronic data systems are necessary to make it accessible. To access 100% of the randomized clinical trials published each year requires access to over 2,000 journals.

The Internet is revolutionizing access to medical knowledge in developing and transitional countries. Previously, medical schools in these settings were highly dependent on slow and often unpredictable mail systems to connect them with medical advances, new directions in medical practice, and medical colleagues in general. Now, many of the same schools have immediate access to hundreds of journals and their professional counterparts across the globe.

There is no touchstone through which physicians can ensure that the process of their own continuing education will keep them abreast of advancing knowledge in the field, but they must find a way to base their decisions on the best available scientific evidence if they are to discharge their responsibility to their patients. An essential element of this process may be for physicians to take an active role, such as participating in medical student and resident education. Efforts in continuing self-education will also be fostered if clinical problems can be made a stimulus for a review of standard literature, alone or in consultation with an appropriate colleague or consultant. This continuing review will do much to identify those inconsistencies or contradictions that will indicate, in the ultimate best interest of patients that things are not what they seem or have been said to be. These difficulties may be exacerbated by commercially sponsored education programs and research projects that may, on occasion, put profit before the patient's best interests. Physicians still learn most from their patients, but this will not be the case if they fall into the easy habit of accepting their patients' problems casually or at face value because the problems appear to be simple.

The tools that physicians must use in dealing with the problems of children and their families fall into 3 main categories: *cognitive* (up-to-date factual information about diagnostic and therapeutic issues, available on recall or easily found in readily accessible sources, and the ability to relate this information to the pathophysiology of their patients in the context of individual biologic variability); *interpersonal* or *manual* (the ability to carry out a productive interview, execute a reliable physical examination, perform a deft venipuncture, or manage cardiac arrest or resuscitation of a depressed newborn infant); and *attitudinal* (the

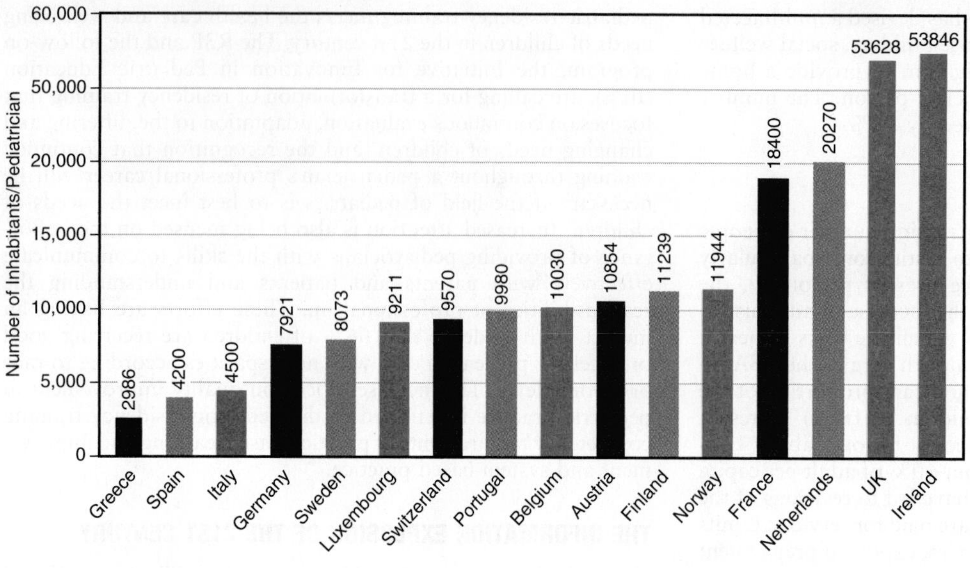

Figure 1-3 European differences in health care delivery system: numbers of inhabitants per pediatrician. (Courtesy of Alfred Tenore, President, European Board of Pediatrics.)

physician's unselfish commitment to the fullest possible implementation of knowledge and skills on behalf of children and their families in an atmosphere of empathic sensitivity and concern). With regard to this last category, it is important that children participate with their families in informed decision-making about their own health care in a manner appropriate to their stage of development and the nature of the particular health problem.

The workaday needs of professional persons for knowledge and skills in care of children vary widely. Primary care physicians need depth in developmental concepts and in the ability to organize an effective system for achieving quality and continuity in assessing and planning for health care during the entire period of growth. They may often have little or no need for immediate recall of esoterica. On the other hand, consultants or subspecialists not only need a comfortable grasp of both common and uncommon facts within their field and perhaps within related fields, but also must be able to cope with controversial issues with flexibility that will permit adaptation of various points of view to the best interest of their unique patient.

At whatever level of care (primary, secondary, or tertiary) or in whatever position (student, pediatric nurse practitioner, resident pediatrician, practitioner of pediatrics or family medicine, or pediatric or other subspecialists), professional persons dealing with children must be able to identify their roles of the moment and their levels of engagement with a child's problem; each must determine whether his or her experience and other resources at hand are adequate to deal with this problem and must be ready to seek other help when they are not. Among the necessary resources are general textbooks, more detailed monographs in subspecialty areas, selected journals, Internet materials, audiovisual aids, and, above all, colleagues with exceptional or complementary experience and expertise. The intercommunication of all these levels of engagement with medical and health problems of children offers the best hope of bringing us closer to the goal of providing the opportunity for all children to achieve their maximum potential.

ORGANIZATION OF THE PROFESSION AND THE GROWTH OF SPECIALIZATION

The 20th century witnessed the formation of professional societies of pediatricians around the globe. Some of these societies, such as the European Board of Pediatrics and the American Board of Pediatrics (ABP) and the, are concerned with education and the awarding of credentials certifying competence and the continuing maintenance of competence as a pediatrician and/or a pediatric subspecialist to the public. In 2010, the ABP reported that there were ≈96,514 board-certified pediatricians. Among those presenting for 1st time certification to the ABP in 2003, 80% were American Medical Graduates (20% were International Medical Graduates) and 63% were women. Other societies are primarily concerned with organizing members of the profession in their country or region to dedicate their efforts and resources toward children. In the USA, the American Academy of Pediatrics (AAP) currently has a membership of ≈60,000 child health specialists in both academic and private practice. Most general pediatricians in the USA enter private practice; ≈66% are in group practices, 5% enter solo practice, and 5% work in a health maintenance organization. There is an increasing shortage of primary care pediatricians, particularly those skilled to take care of children with chronic conditions and special needs. The AAP provides a variety of continuing educational services to pediatricians in multiple national and regional settings and tracks the professional activities and practices of its members. A comparable group in India, the Indian Academy of Pediatrics, was formed in 1963, and now has ~16,500 members and 16 subspecialty chapters. Likewise, the Pakistani Pediatrics Association was founded in 1967, the Malaysian Pediatric Association was started in 1985, and the Canadian Pediatric Society was founded in 1922. Established in 1974, the Asian Pacific Pediatric Association includes 20 member pediatric societies from throughout eastern Asia, and the International Pediatric Association established in 1910 includes 144 national pediatric societies from 139 countries, 10 regional pediatric societies, and 11 international pediatric specialty societies. The European Academy of Pediatrics is the pediatric specialist organization for the member countries of the European Union and the European Free Trade Association, and the Pediatric Council of the Arab Board of Medical Specializations is the comparable institution for 19 of the world's Arab nations These societies represent but a few of the many national and regional pediatric professional organizations around the world who seek to identify and bring treatments and approaches supporting child well-being to pediatricians worldwide.

The amount of information relevant to child health care is rapidly expanding, and no person can become master of it all. Physicians are increasingly dependent on one another for the highest quality of care for their patients. About 25% of pediatricians in the USA claim an area of special knowledge and skill, including 20,138 who have board certification in 1 of the 13 pediatric subspecialties with board certification. Each year about

10% of the ≈3,000 pediatric residents training in the USA are enrolled in a dual residency training program that will lead to eligibility for board certification in both pediatrics and internal medicine.

The growth of specialization within pediatrics has taken a number of different forms: interests in problems of age groups of children have created neonatology and adolescent medicine; interests in organ systems have created pediatric cardiology, neurology, child abuse, child development, allergy, hematology, nephrology, gastroenterology, child psychiatry, pulmonology, endocrinology, rheumatology, and specialization in metabolism and genetics; interests in the health care system have created pediatricians devoted to ambulatory care, emergency care, and intensive care; and, finally, multidisciplinary subspecialties have grown up around the problems of handicapped children, to which pediatrics, neurology, psychiatry, psychology, nursing, physical and occupational therapy, special education, speech therapy, audiology, and nutrition all make essential contributions. This growth of specialization has been most conspicuous in university-affiliated departments of pediatrics and medical centers for children. There is growing concern in the USA regarding the shortage of pediatric subspecialists in virtually all of the subspecialty areas and especially in rural states. This results in long waits for patients.

In the USA, most subspecialists practice in academic settings or children's hospitals. Likewise, specialists are growing in number in other industrialized countries and in developing nations that are becoming industrialized. Reflecting the diverse cultures, organization of medical care, economic circumstances and the history of medicine within each of the ~200 countries across the globe, is the great diversity in role of pediatricians within the health care delivery system to children in each country; Figure 1-3 illustrates the result variations in pediatricians per population among European nations.

BIBLIOGRAPHY

Please visit the Nelson Textbook of Pediatrics *website at www.expertconsult.com for the complete bibliography.*

Chapter 2
Quality and Safety in Health Care for Children

Ramesh C. Sachdeva

THE NEED FOR QUALITY IMPROVEMENT

There is a significant quality gap between known and recommended evidence-based care, and the actual care that is delivered. Adults receive recommended care slightly higher than 50% of the time and children receive recommended care only about 46% of the time. This quality gap exists due to a chasm between knowledge and practice—a chasm made wider by variations in practice and disparities in care from doctor to doctor, institution to institution, geographic region to geographic region, and socioeconomic group to socioeconomic group.

For the full continuation of this chapter, please visit the Nelson Textbook of Pediatrics *website at www.expertconsult.com.*

Chapter 3
Ethics in Pediatric Care

Eric Kodish and Kathryn Weise

Pediatric ethics is a branch of bioethics that analyzes moral aspects of decisions made relating to the health care of children. In general terms, the **autonomy** driven framework of adult medical ethics is replaced by a **beneficent** paternalism (or parentalism) in pediatrics. Pediatric ethics is distinctive because the pediatric clinician has an independent fiduciary obligation to act in a younger child's **best interest** that takes moral precedence over the wishes of the child's parent(s). For older children, the concept of **assent** suggests that the voice of the patient must be heard. These factors create the possibility of conflict among child, parent, and clinician. The approach to the ethical issues that arise in pediatric practice must include respect for parental responsibility and authority balanced with a child's developing capacity and autonomy. Heterogeneity of social, cultural, and religious views about the role of children adds complexity. Children are both vulnerable and resilient, and represent the future of our society.

For the full continuation of this chapter, please visit the Nelson Textbook of Pediatrics *website at www.expertconsult.com.*

Chapter 4
Cultural Issues in Pediatric Care

Linda Kaljee and Bonita F. Stanton

Pediatricians live and work in a multicultural world. Among the world's 6 billion people residing in >200 countries, >6,000 languages are spoken. As the global population becomes more mobile and integrated, ethnic and economic diversity increases in all countries; from 1970 to 2000, the foreign-born population in the USA increased 3-fold. In the 2000 U.S. census, 25-30% of Americans self-identified as belonging to an ethnic or racial minority group. One or both parents of approximately 17 million children in the USA are foreign-born; 1 of every 5 children lives in an immigrant family. Whereas in 1920, 97% of immigrant families in the USA were from Europe or Canada; in 2000, 84% of U.S. immigrant children were from Latin America or Asia. Nonwhite children are projected to outnumber white children in the USA by the year 2030. Increased migration and diversity in the migrant pool is not limited to the USA; immigrants account for over 15% of the population in >50 nations.

For the full continuation of this chapter, please visit the Nelson Textbook of Pediatrics *website at www.expertconsult.com.*

Chapter 5
Maximizing Children's Health: Screening, Anticipatory Guidance, and Counseling

Joseph F. Hagan, Jr. and Paula M. Duncan

The care of well infants, children, and adolescents is an essential prevention effort for children and youth worldwide. The constantly changing tableau of a child's development lends added value to regular and periodic encounters between children and their families and practitioners of pediatric health care. Health supervision visits from birth to age 21 yr are the platform for a young person's health care: well care is provided in the medical home, fostering strong relationships between clinic or practice and child and family, and assisting in the provision of appropriate surveillance, screening, and sick care.

The evolution of this preventive health care approach is derived from the long-standing view that the science of pediatrics is a science of health and development. To assure the optimal health of the developing child, pediatric care in the USA and other countries evolved into regularly scheduled visits to assure adequate nutrition, detect and immunize against infectious diseases, and observe the child's development. Immunization, nutrition assessment, and developmental assessment remain essential elements of the well child health supervision visit, but changes in the population's health have led to the addition of other components to the content of today's well child encounter. Preventive care for children and youth offers greater opportunity for health cost savings.

It is axiomatic that a healthy economy requires educated and healthy workers. For children to have a successful educational experience, they must have both physical and emotional health. Educational success is also tied to early childhood developmental competence. Thus health supervision well child care plays a vital role in promoting adult health, a concept endorsed by business leaders.

Adversity impairs development and adverse factors in life experience increase the risk of disease. Adults who experienced abuse, violence, or other stressors as children have an increased risk for depression, heart disease, and other morbidities. Biology informs us that stress leads to increased heart rate and blood pressure, and increased levels of inflammatory cytokines, cortisol, and other stress hormones, all of which impair brain activity, immune status, and cardiovascular function. There is a causal model for preventable childhood events adversely affecting health.

PERIODICITY

The frequency and content for well child care activities are derived from expert consensus, both from federal agencies and professional organizations such as the American Academy of Pediatrics (AAP), and from evidence-based practice, when available. The Recommendations for Preventive Pediatric Health Care or Periodicity Schedule (Fig. 5-1) is a compilation of recommendations listed by age-based visits. It is intended to guide practitioners of pediatric primary care to perform certain services and make observations at age-specific visits.

GUIDELINES

Comprehensive guides for care of well infants, children, and adolescents have been developed, based on the Periodicity Schedule, which expand and further recommend how practitioners might accomplish the tasks outlined in the Periodicity Schedule. In the USA, the current guideline standard is *The Bright Futures Guidelines for Health Supervision of Infants, Children, and Adolescents*, 3rd Edition. These guidelines were developed by the AAP under the leadership of the Maternal Child Health Bureau of the U.S. Department of Health and Human Services, in collaboration with the National Association of Pediatric Nurse Practitioners, the American Academy of Family Physicians, the American Medical Association, the American Academy of Pediatric Dentistry, Family Voices, and others. This subsumes previous guidelines and is consistent with the AAP and *Bright Futures* Periodicity Schedule (see Fig. 5-1).

TASKS OF WELL CHILD CARE

The well child encounter has unique contributions for promoting the physical and emotional well-being of children and youth. Child health professionals, including pediatricians, family medicine physicians, nurse practitioners, and physician assistants, take advantage of the opportunity the well child visits provide to elicit parental questions and concerns, gather relevant family and individual health information, perform a physical examination, and initiate screening tests.

The tasks of each well child visit include:

- Disease detection
- Disease prevention
- Health promotion
- Anticipatory guidance

To achieve these outcomes, health care professionals employ techniques to screen for disease, screen for risk of disease, and provide advice about healthy behaviors. These activities lead to the formulation of appropriate anticipatory guidance and health advice.

Clinical detection of disease in the well child encounter is accomplished by both surveillance and screening. In well child care, surveillance occurs in every health encounter and is enhanced by the opportunity for repeated visits and observations with advancing developmental stages. It relies on the experience of a skilled clinician over time. Screening is a more formal process utilizing some form of tool, which has been validated and has known sensitivity and specificity. For example, anemia surveillance is accomplished through taking a dietary history and seeking signs of anemia in the physical examination. Anemia screening is done by hematocrit or hemoglobin tests. Developmental surveillance relies on the observations of parents and the watchful eyes of providers of pediatric health care who are experienced in child development. Developmental screening utilizes a structured developmental screening tool or approach by personnel trained in its use or in the scoring and interpretation of parent report questionnaires.

The 2nd essential action of the well child encounter, *disease prevention,* may include both *primary prevention* activities applied to a whole population and *secondary prevention* activities aimed at patients with specific factors of risk. For example, counseling about reducing fat intake is appropriate for all children and families. Counseling is intensified for overweight and obese youth or in the presence of a family history of hyperlipidemia and its sequelae. The child and adolescent health care professional needs to individualize disease prevention strategies to the community, as well as to the specific family and patient.

Health promotion and **anticipatory guidance** activities distinguish the well child health supervision visit from all other encounters with the health care system. Disease detection and disease prevention activities are germane to all interactions of children with physicians and other health care providers, but health promotion and anticipatory guidance shift the focus to wellness and to the strengths of the family, for example, what is being done well and how this might be improved. This approach is an opportunity to help the family address relationship issues, broach important safety topics, access community services, and engage with extended family, school, neighborhood, and church.

It is not possible to cover all the topics suggested by comprehensive guidelines such as *Bright Futures* in the average 18 min well child visit. Child health professionals must prioritize the most important topics to cover. Consideration should be given to a discussion of:

- The agenda the parent or child brings to the health supervision visit
- The topics where evidence suggests counseling is effective in behavioral change
- The topics where there is a clear rationale for the issue's critical importance to health, for example, sleep environment to prevent sudden infant death syndrome (SIDS) or attention to diet and physical activity
- A summary of the child's progress in emotional and social development, physical growth, and strengths
- Issues that address the questions, concerns, or specific health problems relevant to the individual family
- Community-specific problems that could significantly impact the child's health; for example, neighborhood violence from which children need protection or absence of bike paths that would promote activity

American Academy of Pediatrics
DEDICATED TO THE HEALTH OF ALL CHILDREN™

Recommendations for Preventive Pediatric Health Care

Bright Futures/American Academy of Pediatrics

Bright Futures.
prevention and health promotion for infants, children, adolescents, and their families™

Each child and family is unique; therefore, these **Recommendations for Preventive Pediatric Health Care** are designed for the care of children who are receiving competent parenting, have no manifestations of any important health problems, and are growing and developing in satisfactory fashion. **Additional visits may become necessary** if circumstances suggest variations from normal.

Developmental, psychosocial, and chronic disease issues for children and adolescents may require frequent counseling and treatment visits separate from preventive care visits.

These guidelines represent a consensus by the American Academy of Pediatrics (AAP) and Bright Futures. The AAP continues to emphasize the great importance of **continuity of care** in comprehensive health supervision and the need to avoid **fragmentation of care.**

The recommendations in this statement do not indicate an exclusive course of treatment or standard of medical care. Variations, taking into account individual circumstances, may be appropriate.

	INFANCY								EARLY CHILDHOOD						
AGE[1]	PRENATAL[2]	NEWBORN[3]	3–5 d[4]	By 1 mo	2 mo	4 mo	6 mo	9 mo	12 m	15 mo	18 mo	24 mo	30 mo	3 y	4 y
HISTORY															
Initial/Interval	●	●	●	●	●	●	●	●	●	●	●	●	●	●	●
MEASUREMENTS															
Length/Height and Weight		●	●	●	●	●	●	●	●	●	●	●	●	●	●
Head Circumference		●	●	●	●	●	●	●	●	●	●	●			
Weight for Length		●	●	●	●	●	●	●	●	●	●				
Body Mass Index												●	●	●	●
Blood Pressure[5]		★	★	★	★	★	★	★	★	★	★	★	★	●	●
SENSORY SCREENING															
Vision		★	★	★	★	★	★	★	★	★	★	★	★	●[6]	●
Hearing		●[7]	★	★	★	★	★	★	★	★	★	★	★	★	●
DEVELOPMENTAL/BEHAVIORAL ASSESSMENT															
Developmental Screening[8]								●			●		●		
Autism Screening[9]											●	●			
Developmental Surveillance[8]		●	●	●	●	●	●		●	●		●		●	●
Psychosocial/Behavioral Assessment		●	●	●	●	●	●	●	●	●	●	●	●	●	●
Alcohol and Drug Use Assessment															
PHYSICAL EXAMINATION[10]		●	●	●	●	●	●	●	●	●	●	●	●	●	●
PROCEDURES[11]															
Newborn Metabolic/Hemoglobin Screening[12]		←—	●	——	—→										
Immunization[13]		●	●	●	●	●	●	●	●	●	●	●	●	●	●
Hematocrit or Hemoglobin[14]						★			●		★	★		★	★
Lead Screening[15]							★	★	● or ★[16]		★	● or ★[16]		★	★
Tuberculin Test[17]				★			★		★		★	★		★	★
Dyslipidemia Screening[18]												★			★
STI Screening[19]															
Cervical Dysplasia Screening[20]															
ORAL HEALTH[21]							★	★	● or ★[21]		● or ★[21]	● or ★[21]	● or ★[21]	●[22]	
ANTICIPATORY GUIDANCE[23]	●	●	●	●	●	●	●	●	●	●	●	●	●	●	●

	MIDDLE CHILDHOOD						ADOLESCENCE										
AGE[1]	5 y	6 y	7 y	8 y	9 y	10 y	11 y	12 y	13 y	14 y	15 y	16 y	17 y	18 y	19 y	20 y	21 y
HISTORY																	
Initial/Interval	●	●	●	●	●	●	●	●	●	●	●	●	●	●	●	●	●
MEASUREMENTS																	
Length/Height and Weight	●	●	●	●	●	●	●	●	●	●	●	●	●	●	●	●	●
Head Circumference																	
Weight for Length																	
Body Mass Index	●	●	●	●	●	●	●	●	●	●	●	●	●	●	●	●	●
Blood Pressure[5]	●	●	●	●	●	●	●	●	●	●	●	●	●	●	●	●	●
SENSORY SCREENING																	
Vision	●	●	★	●	★	●	★	●	★	★	●	★	★	●	★	★	★
Hearing	●	●	★	●	★	●	★	★	★	★	★	★	★	★	★	★	★
DEVELOPMENTAL/BEHAVIORAL ASSESSMENT																	
Developmental Screening[8]																	
Autism Screening[9]																	
Developmental Surveillance[8]	●	●	●	●	●	●	●	●	●	●	●	●	●	●	●	●	●
Psychosocial/Behavioral Assessment	●	●	●	●	●	●	●	●	●	●	●	●	●	●	●	●	●
Alcohol and Drug Use Assessment							★	★	★	★	★	★	★	★	★	★	★
PHYSICAL EXAMINATION[10]	●	●	●	●	●	●	●	●	●	●	●	●	●	●	●	●	●
PROCEDURES[11]																	
Newborn Metabolic/Hemoglobin Screening[12]																	
Immunization[13]	●	●	●	●	●	●	●	●	●	●	●	●	●	●	●	●	●
Hematocrit or Hemoglobin[14]	★	★	★	★	★	★	★	★	★	★	★	★	★	★	★	★	★
Lead Screening[15]	★	★															
Tuberculin Test[17]	★	★	★	★	★	★	★	★	★	★	★	★	★	★	★	★	★
Dyslipidemia Screening[18]		★		★		★	★	★	★	★	★	★	★	←—	——	●	—→
STI Screening[19]							★	★	★	★	★	★	★	★	★	★	★
Cervical Dysplasia Screening[20]							★	★	★	★	★	★	★	★	★	★	★
ORAL HEALTH[21]		●[22]															
ANTICIPATORY GUIDANCE[23]	●	●	●	●	●	●	●	●	●	●	●	●	●	●	●	●	●

1. If a child comes under care for the first time at any point on the schedule, or if any items are not accomplished at the suggested age, the schedule should be brought up to date at the earliest possible time.
2. A prenatal visit is recommended for parents who are at high risk, for first-time parents, and for those who request a conference. The prenatal visit should include anticipatory guidance, pertinent medical history, and a discussion of benefits of breastfeeding and planned method of feeding per AAP statement "The Prenatal Visit" (2001) [URL: http://aappolicy.aappublications.org/cgi/content/full/pediatrics;107/6/1456].
3. Every infant should have a newborn evaluation after birth, breastfeeding encouraged, and instruction and support offered.
4. Every infant should have an evaluation within 3 to 5 days of birth and within 48 to 72 hours after discharge from the hospital, to include evaluation for feeding and jaundice. Breastfeeding infants should receive formal breastfeeding evaluation, encouragement, and instruction as recommended in AAP statement "Breastfeeding and the Use of Human Milk" (2005) [URL: http://aappolicy.aappublications.org/cgi/content/full/pediatrics;115/2/496]. For newborns discharged in less than 48 hours after delivery, the infant must be examined within 48 hours of discharge per AAP statement "Hospital Stay for Healthy Term Newborns" (2004) [URL: http://aappolicy.aappublications.org/cgi/content/full/pediatrics;113/5/1434].
5. Blood pressure measurement in infants and children with specific risk conditions should be performed at visits before age 3 years.
6. If the patient is uncooperative, rescreen within 6 months per the AAP statement "Eye Examination in Infants, Children, and Young Adults by Pediatricians" (2007) [URL: http://aappolicy.aappublications.org/cgi/content/full/pediatrics;111/4/902].
7. All newborns should be screened per AAP statement "Year 2000 Position Statement: Principles and Guidelines for Early Hearing Detection and Intervention Programs " (2000) [URL: http://aappolicy.aappublications.org/cgi/content/full/pediatrics;106/4/798]. Joint Committee on Infant Hearing. Year 2007 position statement: principles and guidelines for early hearing detection and intervention programs. *Pediatrics.* 2007;120:898–921.
8. AAP Council on Children With Disabilities, AAP Section on Developmental Behavioral Pediatrics, AAP Bright Futures Steering Committee, AAP Medical Home Initiatives for Children With Special Needs Project Advisory Committee. Identifying infants and young children with developmental disorders in the medical home: an algorithm for developmental surveillance and screening. *Pediatrics.* 2006;118:405–420 [URL: http://aappolicy.aappublications.org/cgi/content/full/pediatrics;118/1/405].
9. Gupta VB, Hyman SL, Johnson CP, et al. Identifying children with autism early? *Pediatrics.* 2007;119:152–153 [URL: http://pediatrics.aappublications.org/cgi/content/full/119/1/152].
10. At each visit, age-appropriate physical examination is essential, with infant totally unclothed, older child undressed and suitably draped.
11. These may be modified, depending on entry point into schedule and individual need.
12. Newborn metabolic and hemoglobinopathy screening should be done according to state law. Results should be reviewed at visits and appropriate retesting or referral done as needed.
13. Schedules per the Committee on Infectious Diseases, published annually in the January issue of *Pediatrics.* Every visit should be an opportunity to update and complete a child's immunizations.
14. See AAP *Pediatric Nutrition Handbook,* 5th Edition (2003) for a discussion of universal and selective screening options. See also Recommendations to prevent and control iron deficiency in the United States. *MMWR.* 1998;47(RR-3):1–36.
15. For children at risk of lead exposure, consult the AAP statement "Lead Exposure in Children: Prevention, Detection, and Management" (2005) [URL: http://aappolicy.aappublications.org/cgi/content/full/pediatrics;116/4/1036]. Additionally, screening should be done in accordance with state law where applicable.
16. Perform risk assessments or screens as appropriate, based on universal screening requirements for patients with Medicaid or high prevalence areas.
17. Tuberculosis testing per recommendations of the Committee on Infectious Diseases, published in the current edition of *Red Book: Report of the Committee on Infectious Diseases.* Testing should be done on recognition of high-risk factors.
18. "Third Report of the National Cholesterol Education Program (NCEP) Expert Panel on Detection, Evaluation, and Treatment of High Blood Cholesterol in Adults (Adult Treatment Panel III) Final Report" (2002) [URL: http://circ.ahajournals.org/cgi/content/full/106/25/3143] and "The Expert Committee Recommendations on the Assessment, Prevention, and Treatment of Child and Adolescent Overweight and Obesity." Supplement to *Pediatrics.* In press.
19. All sexually active patients should be screened for sexually transmitted infections (STIs).
20. All sexually active girls should have screening for cervical dysplasia as part of a pelvic examination beginning within 3 years of onset of sexual activity or age 21 (whichever comes first).
21. Referral to dental home, if available. Otherwise, administer oral health risk assessment. If the primary water source is deficient in fluoride, consider oral fluoride supplementation.
22. At the visits for 3 years and 6 years of age, it should be determined whether the patient has a dental home. If the patient does not have a dental home, a referral should be made to one. If the primary water source is deficient in fluoride, consider oral fluoride supplementation.
23. Refer to the specific guidance by age as listed in Bright Futures Guidelines. (Hagan JF, Shaw JS, Duncan PM, eds. *Bright Futures: Guidelines for Health Supervision of Infants, Children, and Adolescents.* 3rd ed. Elk Grove Village, IL: American Academy of Pediatrics; 2008.)

KEY

● = to be performed ★ = risk assessment to be performed, with appropriate action to follow, if positive ←●→ = range during which a service may be provided, with the symbol indicating the preferred age

Figure 5-1 Recommendations for Preventive Pediatric Health Care. (From Bright Futures/American Academy of Pediatrics. Copyright 2008, American Academy of Pediatrics, Elk Grove Village, Illinois.)

It is important to note that this approach is directed at all children, including those with special health needs. Children with special health needs are no different from other children in their need for guidance about healthy nutrition, physical activity, progress in school, connection with friends, a healthy sense of self-efficacy, and avoidance of risk-taking behaviors. The coordination of specialty consultation, medication monitoring, and functional assessment, which should occur in their periodic visits, needs to be balanced with a discussion of the child's unique ways of accomplishing the emotional, social, and developmental tasks of childhood and adolescence.

INFANCY AND EARLY CHILDHOOD

Nutrition, physical activity, sleep, safety, and emotional, social, and physical growth along with parental well-being are critical for all children. For each well child visit, there are topics that are specific to individual children based on their age, family situation, chronic health condition, or a parental concern, for example, sleep environment to prevent SIDS, activities to lose weight, and fences around swimming pools. Attention should also be focused on the family milieu, for example, screening for parental depression (especially maternal postpartum depression) and other mental illness, family violence, substance abuse, nutritional inadequacy, or lack of housing. These issues are essential to the care of young children.

Answering parents' questions is 1 of the most important priorities of the well child visit. Promoting family-centered care and partnership with parents increases the ability to elicit parent concerns, especially about their child's development, learning, and behavior. It is important to identify children with developmental disorders as early as possible. Developmental surveillance at every visit combined with a structured developmental screening and autism screening at some visits is a way to improve diagnosis, especially for some of the more subtle language delays or autism spectrum disorders where early intervention is believed to be associated with reduced morbidity.

MIDDLE CHILDHOOD AND ADOLESCENCE

As the child enters school-aged years, additional considerations emerge. Attention to developing autonomy requires fostering a clinician-patient relationship separate from the clinician-child-family relationship with increasing needs for privacy and confidentiality as the child ages.

The 6 health behaviors that are most important in adolescent and adult morbidity and mortality are: nutrition, physical activity; sexuality related behavior; tobacco, alcohol, and other drug use; behaviors that contribute to unintentional and intentional injuries; and violence. Emotional well-being with attention to the developmental tasks of adolescence (competence at school and other activities, connection to friends and family, autonomy, empathy, and a sense of self-worth), as well as early diagnosis and treatment of mental health problems, are of equal importance.

OFFICE INTERVENTION FOR BEHAVIORAL AND MENTAL HEALTH ISSUES

Twenty percent of primary care encounters with children are for a behavioral or mental health problem, or are sickness visits complicated by a mental health issue. Pediatricians need increased knowledge for diagnosis, treatment, and referral criteria for attention-deficit/hyperactivity disorder (ADHD) (Chapter 30), depression (Chapter 24), anxiety (Chapter 23), and conduct disorder (Chapter 27), as well as an understanding of the pharmacology of the frequently prescribed psychotropic medications. Encouragement of behavioral change is also an important responsibility of the clinician. Motivational interviewing provides a structured approach that has been designed to help patients and parents identify the discrepancy between their desire for health and their behavioral choices. It also allows the clinician to use proven strategies that lead to a patient-initiated plan for change.

STRENGTH-BASED APPROACHES AND FRAMEWORK

Questions about school or extracurricular accomplishments or competent personal characteristics should be integrated into the content of the well child visit. This often sets a positive context for the visit, deepens the partnership with the family, and acknowledges the child's healthy development. This facilitates discussing social-emotional development with children and their parents. There is a strong relationship between appropriate social-emotional development (e.g., children's strong connection to their family, social friends, and mentors; competence; empathy; and appropriate autonomy) and decreased participation in all the risk behaviors of adolescence (related to drugs, sex, and violence). An organized approach to the identification and encouragement of a child's strengths during health supervision visits provides both the child and parent with an understanding of how to promote healthy achievement of the developmental tasks of childhood and adolescence. Children with special health needs often have a different timetable, but they have an equal need to be encouraged to develop strong family and peer connections, competence in a variety of arenas, ways to do things for others, and appropriate independent decision-making.

OFFICE SYSTEM CHANGE FOR QUALITY IMPROVEMENT

Some of the office strategies to improve the preventive services delivered to children and youth include screening schedules and parent handouts, flow sheets, registries, and the use of parent and youth previsit questionnaires. Such tools are available in *The Bright Futures Guidelines, 3rd Edition, Toolkit.* These efforts are part of a larger national effort that is built on a coordinated team approach in the office setting and the use of continuous measurement for improvement.

EVIDENCE

The clinical encounter with the well child is guideline- and recommendation-driven and requires the integration of clinician goals, family needs, and community realities in seeking better health for the child. Few well child care activities have been evaluated for efficacy, yet these activities are highly valued; lack of evidence is not the same as lack of benefit. The rationale for well child care activities is a balance of evidence from research, clinical practice guidelines, professional recommendations, expert opinion, experience, habit, intuition, and preferences or values. Clinical or counseling decisions and recommendations may also be based on legislation (seat belts), on common sense measures not likely to be studied experimentally (lowering water heater temperatures), or on the basis of relational evidence (television watching associated with violent behavior in young children). Most important, sound clinical and counseling decisions are responsive to family needs and desires, and support "patient-centered decision-making."

CARING FOR THE CHILD AND YOUTH IN THE CONTEXT OF THE FAMILY AND COMMUNITY

A successful primary care practice for children incorporates families, is family centered, and embraces the concept of the medical home. A medical home is defined by the AAP as primary care that is accessible, continuous, comprehensive, family centered, coordinated, compassionate, and culturally effective. In a medical home, a pediatrician works in partnership with the family and patient to assure that all medical and nonmedical needs of the child are met. Through this partnership, the child health care professional helps the family/patient access and coordinate specialty care, educational services, out-of-home care, family support, and other public and private community services that are important to the overall health of the child and family.

Ideally, health promotion activities occur not only in the medical home, but also in partnership with community members and other health and education professionals. This rests on a clear understanding of the important role that the community plays in supporting healthy behaviors among families. Communities where children and families feel safe and valued, and have access to positive activities and relationships, provide the important base that the health care professional can build on and refer to for needed services that support health but are outside the realm of the health care system or primary care medical home. It is important for the medical home and community agencies to identify mutual resources, communicate well with families and each other, and partner in designing service delivery systems. This interaction is the practice of community pediatrics, whose unique feature is its concern for all of the population: those who remain well but need preventive services, those who have symptoms but do not receive effective care, and those who do seek medical care either in a physician's office or in a hospital.

BIBLIOGRAPHY

Please visit the Nelson Textbook of Pediatrics *website at www.expertconsult.com for the complete bibliography.*

5.1 Injury Control

Frederick P. Rivara and David C. Grossman

Injuries are the most common cause of death during childhood and adolescence beyond the 1st few mo of life and represent 1 of the most important causes of preventable pediatric morbidity and mortality (Figs. 5-2 and 5-3). The identification of risk factors for injuries has led to the development of successful programs for prevention and control. Strategies for injury prevention and control should be pursued by the pediatrician in the office, emergency department, hospital, and community setting.

INJURY CONTROL

The term **accident prevention** has been replaced by **injury control.** The word **accident** implies an event occurring by chance, without pattern or predictability. In fact, most injuries occur under fairly predictable circumstances to high-risk children and families. *Accident* connotes a random event that cannot be prevented. The use of the term **injury** promotes an awareness of a medical condition with defined risk and protective factors that can be used to define prevention strategies.

The reduction of morbidity and mortality from injuries can be accomplished not only through primary prevention (averting the event or injury in the first place), but also through secondary and tertiary prevention. The latter 2 approaches include appropriate emergency medical services for injured children; regionalized trauma care for the child with multiple injuries, severe burns, or head injury; and specialized pediatric rehabilitation services that attempt to return children to their previous level of functioning. This broadened scope of prevention is more properly described by the term *injury control.*

This expanded definition also encompasses intentional injuries (assaults, self-inflicted injuries). These injuries are important in adolescents and young adults, and in some populations, they rank 1st or 2nd as causes of death in these age groups. Many of the same principles of injury control can be applied to these problems; limiting access to firearms may reduce both unintentional shootings and suicides.

SCOPE OF THE PROBLEM

Mortality

In the USA, injuries cause 42% of deaths among 1-4 yr old children and 3 times more deaths than the next leading cause, congenital anomalies. For the rest of childhood and adolescence up to the age of 19 yr, 65% of deaths are due to injuries, more than all other causes combined. In 2006, injuries caused 17,252 deaths (21 deaths per 100,000) among individuals 19 yr old and younger in the USA (Table 5-1), resulting in more years of potential life lost than any other cause.

Table 5-1 INJURY DEATHS IN THE USA, 2006*

CAUSE OF DEATH	YOUNGER THAN 1 YR	1-4 YR	5-9 YR	10-14 YR	15-19 YR	0-19 YR
ALL CAUSES	**28,527**	**4,631**	**2,735**	**3,414**	**13,739**	**53,046**
ALL INJURIES	**1,576**	**2,028**	**1,218**	**1,709**	**10,722**	**17,252**
All unintentional	1,668	1,610	1,044	1,214	6,659	11,674
Motor vehicle occupant	82	179	191	311	2,448	3,211
Pedestrian	5	139	112	133	268	657
Other motor vehicle, unspecified	51	150	173	187	1,834	2,395
Drowning	51	458	142	114	312	1,077
Fire and burn	28	202	118	64	83	495
Poisoning	16	27	18	40	738	839
Bicycle	0	1	34	50	46	131
Firearm	0	13	18	23	100	154
Fall	23	26	17	21	81	180
Suffocation	843	57	50	58	76	1,164
All intentional	336	366	152	457	3,846	5,157
Suicide	0	0	3	216	1,555	1,772
Firearm suicide	0	0	0	62	701	763
Homicide	336	366	149	241	2,291	3,383
Firearm homicide	6	46	62	175	1,940	2,229
Undetermined intent	114	52	22	37	181	406

*Injury data from Centers for Disease Control and Prevention: Web-based Injury Statistics Query and Reporting System (WISQARS) (website). National Center for Injury Prevention and Control, Centers for Disease Control and Prevention (producer). www.cdc.gov/injury/wisqars/index.html. Accessed May 23, 2009.

	Age groups				
Rank	<1	1-4	5-9	10-14	15-24
1	Congenital anomalies 5,785	Unintentional injury 1,588	Unintentional injury 965	Unintentional injury 1,229	Unintentional injury 15,897
2	Short gestation 4,857	Congenital anomalies 546	Malignant neoplasms 480	Malignant neoplasms 479	Homicide 5,551
3	SIDS 2,453	Homicide 398	Congenital anomalies 196	Homicide 213	Suicide 4,140
4	Maternal pregnancy comp. 1,769	Malignant neoplasms 364	Homicide 133	Suicide 180	Malignant neoplasms 1,653
5	Unintentional injury 1,285	Heart disease 173	Heart disease 110	Congenital anomalies 178	Heart disease 1,084
6	Placenta cord membranes 1,135	Influenza & pneumonia 109	Chronic low. respiratory disease 54	Heart disease 131	Congenital anomalies 402
7	Bacterial sepsis 820	Septicemia 78	Influenza & pneumonia 48	Chronic low. respiratory disease 64	Cerebro-vascular 195
8	Respiratory distress 789	Perinatal period 70	Benign neoplasms 41	Influenza & pneumonia 55	Diabetes mellitus 168
9	Circulatory system disease 624	Benign neoplasms 59	Cerebro-vascular 38	Cerebro-vascular 45	Influenza & pneumonia 163
10	Neonatal hemorrhage 597	Chronic low. respiratory disease 57	Septicemia 36	Benign neoplasms 43	Three tied* 160

* The three causes are: Complicated pregnancy, HIV, Septicemia

Figure 5-2 Ten leading causes of death by age group, USA, 2007. (Modified from National Vital Statistics System, National Center for Health Statistics, CDC. Produced by Office of Statistics and Programming, National Center for Injury Prevention and Control, CDC: *10 leading causes of death by age group, United States—2007* [PDF]. www.cdc.gov/injury/wisqars/pdf/Death_by_Age_2007-a.pdf. Accessed November 1, 2010.)

	Age groups				
Rank	<1	1-4	5-9	10-14	15-24
1	Unintentional fall 125,097	Unintentional fall 878,612	Unintentional fall 639,091	Unintentional fall 607,635	Unintentional struck by/ against 1,031,192
2	Unintentional struck by/ against 37,010	Unintentional struck by/ against 371,404	Unintentional struck by/ against 399,995	Unintentional struck by/ against 583,948	Unintentional fall 918,574
3	Unintentional other bite/sting 13,092	Unintentional other bite/sting 134,920	Unintentional cut/pierce 106,907	Unintentional overexertion 283,813	Unintentional MV occupant 743,738
4	Unintentional foreign body 11,035	Unintentional foreign body 123,369	Unintentional other bite/sting 83,107	Unintentional cut/pierce 135,610	Unintentional overexertion 735,400
5	Unintentional fire/burn 9,101	Unintentional cut/pierce 81,571	Unintentional pedal cyclist 80,743	Unintentional pedal cyclist 108,016	Other assault* struck by/ against 475,386
6	Unintentional other specified 8,271	Unintentional overexertion 78,018	Unintentional overexertion 75,796	Unintentional unknown/ unspecified 100,842	Unintentional cut/pierce 452,297
7	Unintentional unknown/ unspecified 6,722	Unintentional other specified 69,043	Unintentional MV occupant 57,236	Unintentional MV occupant 75,969	Unintentional other specified 203,484
8	Unintentional cut/pierce 5,916	Unintentional fire/burn 50,708	Unintentional foreign body 56,624	Other assault* struck by/ against 73,372	Unintentional unknown/ unspecified 191,276
9	Unintentional inhalation/ suffocation 4,975	Unintentional unknown/ unspecified 45,071	Unintentional other transport 45,158	Unintentional other transport 57,597	Unintentional other bite/sting 167,310
10	Unintentional MV occupant 4,818	Unintentional Dog bite 38,214	Unintentional unknown/ unspecified 41,967	Unintentional other bite/sting 52,489	Unintentional other transport 125,828

* The "other assault" catagory includes all assaults that are **not** classified as sexual assault. It represents the majority of assaults.

Figure 5-3 National estimates of the 10 leading causes of nonfatal injuries treated in hospital emergency departments, USA, 2008. (Modified from NEISS All Injury Program operated by the Consumer Product Safety Commission [CPSC]. Produced by Office of Statistics and Programming, National Center for Injury Prevention and Control, CDC: *National estimates of the 10 leading causes of nonfatal injuries treated in hospital emergency departments, United States—2008* [PDF]. www.cdc.gov/injury/wisqars/pdf/Nonfatal_2008-a.pdf. Accessed November 1, 2010.)

Motor vehicle injuries lead the list of injury deaths at all ages during childhood and adolescence, even in children younger than 1 yr of age. In children and adults, motor vehicle **occupant** injuries account for the majority of these deaths. During adolescence, occupant injuries are the leading cause of injury death, accounting for >50% of unintentional trauma mortality in this age group.

Drowning ranks 2nd overall as a cause of unintentional trauma deaths, with peaks in the preschool and later teenage years (Chapter 67). In some areas of the USA, drowning is the leading cause of death from trauma for preschool-aged children. The causes of drowning deaths vary with age and geographic area. In young children, bathtub and swimming pool drowning predominate, whereas in older children and adolescents, drowning occurs predominantly in natural bodies of water while the victim is swimming or boating.

Fire and burn deaths account for 4% of all unintentional trauma deaths and 8% in those younger than 5 yr of age (Chapter 68). Most of these are due to house fires; deaths are caused by smoke inhalation and asphyxiation rather than severe burns. Children and the elderly are at greatest risk for these deaths because of difficulty in escaping from burning buildings.

Suffocation accounts for approximately 73% of all unintentional deaths in children younger than 1 yr of age. The majority of these deaths result from choking on food items, such as hot dogs, candy, grapes, and nuts. Nonfood items that can cause choking include undersized infant pacifiers, small balls, and latex balloons.

Homicide is the 3rd leading cause of injury death in children 1-4 yr of age and the 2nd leading cause of injury death in adolescents (15-19 yr old). Homicide in the pediatric age group falls into 2 patterns: infantile and adolescent. Infantile homicide involves children younger than the age of 5 yr and represents child abuse (Chapter 37). The perpetrator is usually a caretaker; death is generally the result of blunt trauma to the head and/or abdomen. The adolescent pattern of homicide involves peers and acquaintances and is due to firearms in >80% of cases. The majority of these deaths involve handguns. Children between these 2 age groups experience homicides of both types.

Suicide is rare in children younger than age 10 yr; only 1% of all suicides occur in children younger than age 15 yr. The suicide rate increases markedly after the age of 10 yr, with the result that suicide is now the 3rd leading cause of death for 15-19 yr olds. Native American teenagers are at the highest risk, followed by white males; black females have the lowest rate of suicide in this age group. Approximately one half of teenage suicides involve firearms (Chapter 25).

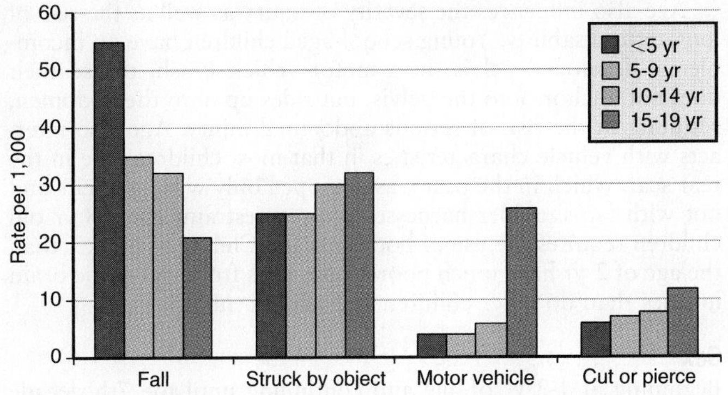

Figure 5-4 Emergency department visit rates for leading 1st-listed causes of injury by age, USA, 1993-1994. (Data from Centers for Disease Control and Prevention, National Center for Health Statistics, and National Hospital Ambulatory Medical Case Survey.)

Nonfatal Injuries

Mortality statistics reflect only a small portion of the effects of childhood injuries. Approximately 11% of children and adolescents receive medical care for an injury each year in hospital emergency departments, and at least an equal number are treated in physicians' offices. Of these, 2% require inpatient care and 55% have at least short-term temporary disability as a result of their injuries.

The distribution of these nonfatal injuries is very different from that of fatal trauma (Fig. 5-4). Falls are the leading cause of both emergency department visits and hospitalizations. Bicycle-related trauma is the most common type of sports and recreational injury, accounting for approximately 300,000 emergency department visits annually. Nonfatal injuries, such as anoxic encephalopathy from near-drowning, scarring and disfigurement from burns, and persistent neurologic deficits from head injury, may be associated with severe morbidity, leading to substantial changes in the quality of life for victims and their families.

Global Child Injuries

It is important to understand that child injuries are a global public health issue and that prevention efforts are necessary in low, middle, and high income countries. Nearly 1 million children and adolescents die from injuries and violence each year, and more than 90% of these deaths are in low and middle income countries. As child mortality undergoes an "epidemiologic transition" due to better control of infectious diseases and malnutrition, injuries have and will increasingly become the leading cause of death for children in the developing world as it now is in all industrialized countries. Drowning is now the 5th most common cause of death for 5-9 yr old children globally, and in some countries, such as Bangladesh, it is the leading cause of death from all causes in this age group. An estimated 1 billion people do not currently have access to roads; as industrialization and motorization spreads, the incidence of motor vehicle crashes, injuries, and fatalities will climb. The rate of child injury death in low- and middle-income countries is 3-fold higher than that in high income countries, and reflects both a higher incidence of many types of injuries as well as a much higher case-fatality ratio in those injured because of a lack of emergency and surgical care. As in high-income countries, prevention of child injuries and consequent morbidity and mortality is feasible with multifaceted approaches, many of which are low cost and of proven effectiveness.

PRINCIPLES OF INJURY CONTROL

At one time injury prevention centered on attempts to pinpoint the innate characteristics of a child that result in greater frequency of injury. Most discount the theory of the *accident-prone child*. Although longitudinal studies have demonstrated an association between hyperactivity and impulsivity and increased rates of injury, the sensitivity and specificity of these traits for injury are extremely low. The concept of *accident proneness* is, in fact, counterproductive in that it shifts attention away from potentially more modifiable factors, such as product design or the environment. It is more appropriate to examine the physical and social environment of children with frequent rates of injury than to try to identify particular personality traits or temperaments, which are difficult to modify. Children at high risk for injury are likely to be relatively poorly supervised, to have disorganized or stressed families, and to live in hazardous environments.

Table 5-2 INJURY PREVENTION TOPICS FOR ANTICIPATORY GUIDANCE BY THE PEDIATRICIAN

NEWBORN
Car seats
Tap water temperature
Smoke detectors
INFANT
Car seats
Tap water temperature
Bath safety
TODDLER AND PRESCHOOLER
Car seats
Pedestrian skills training
Water safety
Childproof caps on medicines and household poisons
PRIMARY SCHOOL CHILD
Pedestrian skills training
Water skills training
Seat belts
Bicycle helmets
Removal of firearms from home
MIDDLE SCHOOL CHILD
Seat belts
Removal of firearms from home
Pedestrian skills training
HIGH SCHOOL AND OLDER ADOLESCENT
Seat belts
Alcohol and drug use, especially while driving, boating, and swimming
Occupational injuries
Removal of firearms from home

Efforts to control injuries include education or persuasion, changes in product design, and modification of the social and physical environment. Efforts to persuade individuals, particularly parents, to change their behaviors have constituted the greater part of injury control efforts. Speaking with parents specifically about using child car seat restraints and bicycle helmets, installing smoke detectors, and checking the tap water temperature is likely to be more successful than offering well-meaning but too-general advice about supervising the child closely, being careful, and "childproofing" the home. This information should be geared to the developmental stage of the child and presented in moderate doses in the form of anticipatory guidance at well-child visits. Important topics to discuss at each developmental stage are shown in Table 5-2.

The most successful injury prevention strategies generally are those involving changes in product design, as shown in Table 5-3. These passive interventions protect all individuals in the population, regardless of cooperation or level of skill, and are likely to be more successful than active measures that require repeated behavior change by the parent or child. However, for some types of injuries, effective passive interventions are not available or feasible; we must rely heavily on attempts to change the behavior of individuals. Turning down the water heater temperature, installing smoke detectors, and using child-resistant caps on medicines and household products are examples of effective product

Table 5-3 INJURY CONTROL INTERVENTIONS

PRODUCT MODIFICATION	ENVIRONMENTAL MODIFICATION	EDUCATION
Child-resistant caps	Cabinet locks	Anticipatory guidance
Airbags	Roadway design	Public service announcements
Fire-safe cigarettes	Smoke detectors	School safety programs

modifications. Many interventions require both active and passive measures. Smoke detectors provide passive protection when fully functional, but behavior change is required to ensure annual battery changes and proper testing.

Modification of the environment often requires greater changes than individual product modification, but may be very effective in reducing injuries. Safe roadway design, decreased traffic volume and speed limits in neighborhoods, and elimination of guns from households are examples of such interventions. Included in this concept are changes in the social environment through legislation, such as laws mandating child seat restraint and seatbelt use, bicycle helmet use, and graduated driver licensing laws.

Prevention campaigns combining 2 or more of these approaches have been particularly effective in reducing injuries. The classic example is the combination of legislation and education to increase child seat restraint and seatbelt use; other examples are programs to promote bike helmet use among school-aged children and improvements in occupant protection in motor vehicles.

RISK FACTORS FOR CHILDHOOD INJURIES

Major factors associated with an increased risk of injuries to children include age, sex, race and ethnicity, socioeconomic status, rural-urban location, and the environment.

Age

Toddlers are at the greatest risk for burns, drowning, and falling. As these children acquire mobility and exploratory behavior, poisonings become another risk. Young school-aged children are at greatest risk for pedestrian injuries, bicycle-related injuries (the most serious of which usually involve motor vehicles), motor vehicle occupant injuries, burns, and drowning. During the teenage years, there is a markedly increased risk from motor vehicle occupant trauma, a continued risk from drowning and burns, and the new risk of intentional trauma. Work-related injuries associated with child labor, especially for 14-16 yr olds, are an additional risk.

Injuries occurring at a particular age represent a window of vulnerability during which a child or an adolescent encounters a new task or hazard that he or she may not have the developmental skills to handle successfully. Toddlers do not have the judgment to know that medications can be poisonous or that some houseplants are not to be eaten; they do not understand the hazard presented by a swimming pool or an open 2nd-story window. For young children, parents may inadvertently set up this mismatch between the skills of the child and the demands of the task. A walker converts an infant into a mobile toddler and greatly increases contact with hazards. Many parents expect young school-aged children to walk home from school, the playground, or the local candy store, tasks for which most children are not developmentally ready. Likewise, the lack of skills and experience to handle many tasks during the teenage years contributes to an increased risk of injuries, particularly motor vehicle injuries. The high rate of motor vehicle crashes among 15-17 yr old teens is caused in part by inexperience, but also appears to reflect their level of development and maturity. Alcohol and other drugs often add to these limitations.

Age also influences the severity of injury as well as the risk of long-term disability. Young school-aged children have an incompletely developed pelvis. In a motor vehicle crash, the seatbelt does not anchor onto the pelvis, but rides up onto the abdomen, resulting in the risk of serious abdominal injury. Age also interacts with vehicle characteristics in that most children ride in the rear seat, which in the past was equipped only with lap belts and not with lap-shoulder harnesses. Proper restraint for 4-8 yr old children requires the use of booster seats. Children younger than the age of 2 yr have much poorer outcomes from traumatic brain injuries than do older children and adolescents.

Sex

Beginning at 1-2 yr of age and continuing until the 7th decade of life, males have higher rates of injury than females. During childhood, this does not appear to be due to developmental differences between the sexes, differences in coordination, or differences in muscle strength. Variation in exposure to risk may account for the male predominance in some types of injuries. Although boys in all age groups have higher rates of bicycle-related injuries, adjusting for exposure reduces this excess rate. Boys may have higher rates of injuries because they use bicycles more frequently or for more hours. Sex differences in rates of pedestrian injuries do not appear to be caused by differences in the amount of walking, but rather reflect differences in behavior between young girls and boys. Greater risk-taking behavior, combined with greater frequency of alcohol use, may lead to the disproportionately high rate of motor vehicle crashes among teenage males.

Race and Ethnicity

African-Americans have higher rates of injuries than whites, whereas Asians have lower rates; rates for Hispanics are intermediate between those for African-Americans and those for whites. Native Americans have the highest death rate from unintentional injuries. These discrepancies are even more pronounced for some injuries. The homicide rate for African-Americans age 15-19 yr was 37.8/100,000 in 2006, compared with 10.2/100,000 for American Indians and Alaskan Natives and 5.5/100,000 for whites. The suicide rate for Native American youth is 2.5 times the rate for whites and nearly 5-fold greater than that for African-Americans. The rate of fire and burn deaths in African-American preschool children is more than 3 times higher than that for whites: 2.8/100,000 compared with 0.9/100,000, respectively.

These disparities appear to be primarily related to poverty, the educational status of parents, and the presence of hazardous environments, rather than to race. Homicide rates among African-Americans are nearly equivalent to those among whites, when adjusted for socioeconomic status. It is important to understand racial disparities in injury rates, but inappropriate to ascribe the etiology of these differences to race or ethnicity.

Socioeconomic Status

Poverty is one of the most important risk factors for childhood injury. Mortality from fires, motor vehicle crashes, and drowning is 2-4 times higher in poor children. Death rates among both African-Americans and whites have an inverse relationship to income level: the higher the income level, the lower the death rate. Native Americans have especially high rates. Other factors are single-parent families, teenage mothers, multiple care providers, family stress, and multiple siblings; these are primarily a function of poverty rather than independent risk factors.

Rural-Urban Location

Injury rates are generally higher in rural than in urban areas. Homicide rates are higher in urban areas, as is violent crime in general. Case fatality from injury is generally twice as high in rural areas than in urban areas, reflecting both the increased severity of some injuries (such as motor vehicle crashes occurring at higher speeds) and poorer access to emergency medical services and definitive trauma care in rural areas. Some injuries are unique to rural areas, such as agricultural injuries to children and adolescents.

Environment

Poverty increases the risk of injury to children, at least in part through its effect on the environment. Children who are poor are at increased risk for injury because they are exposed to more hazards in their living environments. They may live in poor housing, which is more likely to be dilapidated and less likely to be protected by smoke detectors. The roads in their neighborhoods are more likely to be major thoroughfares. Their neighborhoods are more likely to experience higher levels of violence, and they are more likely to be victims of assault than are children and adolescents living in the suburbs. The focus on the environment is also important because it directs attention away from relatively immutable factors, such as family dynamics, poverty, and race, and directs efforts toward factors that can be changed through interventions.

MECHANISMS OF INJURY

Motor Vehicle Injuries

Motor vehicle injuries are the leading cause of serious and fatal injuries for individuals of all ages. Among adolescents ages 14-19 yr, motor vehicle crashes alone account for 37% of all deaths in 2006, including deaths from natural causes. Large and sustained reductions in motor vehicle crash injuries can be accomplished by identifiable interventions.

OCCUPANTS Injuries to passenger vehicle occupants are the predominant cause of motor vehicle deaths among children and adolescents, with the exception of the 5-9 yr old group, in whom pedestrian injuries make up the largest proportion. The peak injury and death rate for both males and females in the pediatric age group occurs between 15 and 19 yr of age (see Table 5-1). Proper restraint use in vehicles is the single most effective method for preventing serious or fatal injury. The recommended restraints at different ages are shown in Table 5-4. Examples of car safety seats are noted in Figure 5-5.

Much attention has been given to child occupants younger than 8 yr of age. Use of child restraint devices, infant car seats, and booster seats can be expected to reduce fatalities by 71% and the risk of serious injuries by 67% in this age group. All 50 states and the District of Columbia have laws mandating their use, though the upper age limit for booster seat requirements varies by state. Physician reinforcement of the positive benefits of child seat restraints has been successful in improving parent acceptance. Pediatricians should point out to parents that toddlers who normally ride restrained behave better during car trips than children who ride unrestrained.

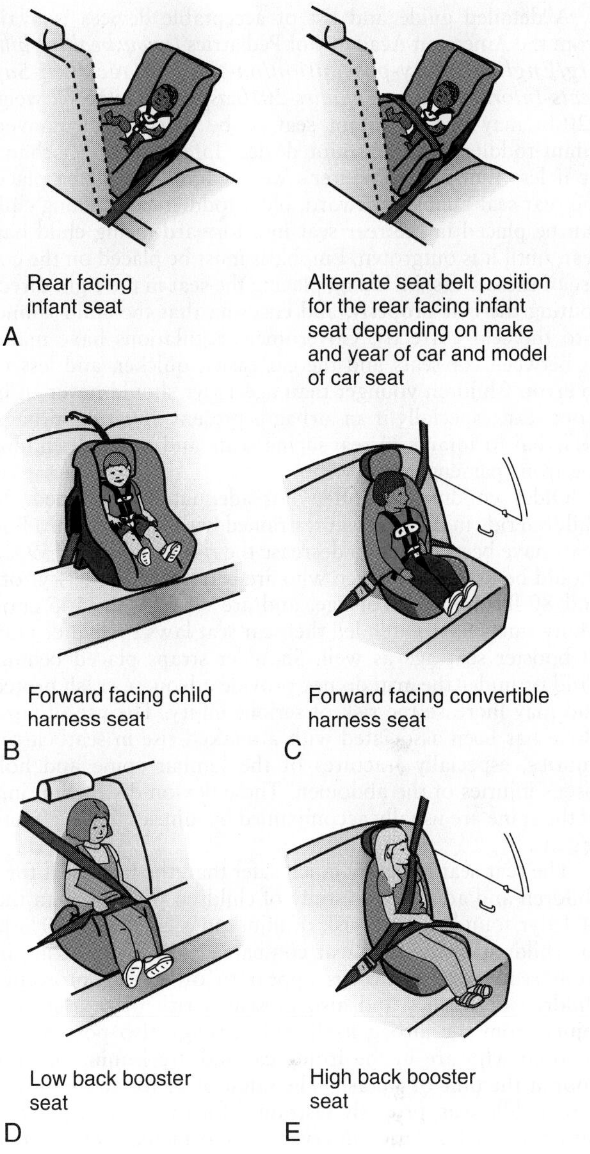

Figure 5-5 Car safety seats. *A,* Rear-facing infant seat. *B,* Forward-facing child harness seat. *C,* Forward-facing convertible harness seat. *D,* Low-back booster seat. *E,* High-back booster seat. (From Ebel BE, Grossman DC: Crash proof kids? An overview of current motor vehicle child occupant safety strategies, *Curr Probl Pediatr Adolesc Health Care* 33:33–64, 2003. Source: NHTSA; graphics courtesy of Transportation Safety Training Center, Virginia Commonwealth University: *Types of child safety seats* [website]. www.nhtsa.dot.gov/people/injury/childps/safetycheck/typeseats/index.htm. Accessed November 1, 2010.)

Table 5-4 RECOMMENDED CHILD RESTRAINT METHODS

	INFANTS	TODDLERS (1-4 yr)	YOUNG CHILDREN
Recommended age/weight requirements	Birth to 2 yr or below weight limit of seat	Older than 2 yr	>40 lb and under 4′ 9″; generally between 4 and 8 yr of age, 40-80 lb
Type of seat	Infant only or rear-facing convertible	Convertible/forward-facing harness seat	Belt positioning booster seat
Seat position	Rear-facing only	Can be rear-facing until 30 lb if seat allows; generally forward-facing	Forward-facing
Notes	Children should use rear-facing seat until 1 yr and at least 20 lb	Harness straps should be at or above shoulder level	Belt positioning booster seats must be used with both lap and shoulder belts
	Harness straps should be at or below shoulder level	Most seats require top slot for forward-facing use	Make sure the lap belt fits low and tightly across the lap/upper thigh area and the shoulder belt fits snugly, crossing the chest and shoulder to avoid abdominal injuries

Modified from Ebel BE, Grossman DC: Crash proof kids? An overview of current motor vehicle child occupant safety strategies, *Curr Probl Pediatr Adolesc Health Care* 33:33–64, 2003; and Durbin DR; Committee on Injury, Violence, and Poison Prevention: Child passenger safety, *Pediatrics* 127:788–793, 2011. See also NHTSA 4 Steps for Kids. www.nhtsq.gov/Driving+Safety/Child+Safety/4+Steps+for+Kids.

A detailed guide and list of acceptable devices is available from the American Academy of Pediatrics (*www.healthychildren.org/English/safety-prevention/on-the-go/pages/Car-Safety-Seats-Information-for-Families-2010.aspx*). Children weighing <20 lb may use an infant seat or be placed in a convertible infant-toddler child restraint device. Infants younger than 2 yr or if less than manufacturer's weight limit should be placed in the rear seat facing backward; older toddlers and young children can be placed in the rear seat in a forward-facing child harness seat, until it is outgrown. Emphasis must be placed on the correct use of these seats, including placing the seat in the right direction, routing the belt properly, and ensuring that the child is buckled into the seat correctly. Government regulations have made the fit between car seats and the car easier, quicker, and less prone to error. Children younger than age 13 yr should never sit in the front seat, especially if an airbag is present. Inflating airbags can be lethal to infants in rear-facing seats and to small children in the front passenger seat.

Older children are often not adequately restrained. Many children ride in the rear seat restrained with lap belts only. Booster seats have been shown to decrease the risk of injury by 59%, and should be used by children who are between 40 lb (≈4 yr of age) and 80 lb, are <8 yr of age, and are <4 ft, 9 in (145 cm) tall. Many states have extended their car seat laws to include children of booster seat age as well. Shoulder straps placed behind the child or under the arm do not provide adequate crash protection and may increase the risk of serious injury. The use of lap belts alone has been associated with a marked rise in seatbelt-related injuries, especially fractures of the lumbar spine and hollow-viscus injuries of the abdomen. These flexion-distraction injuries of the spine are usually accompanied by injuries to the abdominal organs.

The rear seat is clearly much safer than the front seat for both children and adults. One study of children younger than the age of 15 yr found that the risk of injury in a crash was 70% lower for children in the rear seat compared with those sitting in the front seat. Frontal airbags appear to offer little protection to children in crashes and also present a risk of serious or fatal injury from the airbag itself. Side airbags also pose a risk for children who are in the front seat and are leaning against the door at the time of a crash. The safest place for children is in the rear middle seat, properly restrained for their age and size. Educational and legislative interventions to increase the number of children traveling in the rear seat have been successful.

Transportation of premature infants presents special problems. The possibility of oxygen desaturation, sometimes associated with bradycardia, among premature infants while in child seat restraints has led the AAP to recommend monitoring of infants born at <37 wk of gestational age in the seat before discharge and the use of oxygen or alternative restraints for infants who experience desaturation or bradycardia, such as seats that can be reclined and used as a car bed. Monitoring in the neonatal intensive care unit should be done for 60-90 min. Car seats should only be used for travel and not as a general use infant seat around the home.

Children riding in the back of pickup trucks are at special risk for injury because of the possibility of ejection from the truck and resultant serious head injury. They are also at increased risk for carbon monoxide poisoning from faulty exhaust systems.

TEENAGE DRIVERS Drivers aged 15-17 yr of age have more than twice the rate of collisions compared with motorists 18 yr of age and older. Formal driver education courses for young drivers appear to be ineffective as a primary means of decreasing the number of collisions, and in fact may increase risk by allowing younger teens to drive. The risk of serious injury and mortality is directly related to the speed at the time of the crash and inversely related to the size of the vehicle. Small, fast cars greatly increase the risk of a fatal outcome in the event of a crash.

The number of passengers traveling with teen drivers influences the risk of a crash. The risk of death for 17 yr old drivers is 50% greater when driving with 1 passenger compared with driving alone; this risk is 2.6-fold higher with 2 passengers and 3-fold higher with 3 or more passengers. The risk is also increased if the driver is male and the passengers are younger than age 30 yr.

Teens driving at night are overrepresented in crashes and fatal crashes, with nighttime crashes accounting for >33% of teen motor vehicle fatalities. Almost 50% of fatal crashes involving drivers younger than age 18 yr occur in the 4 hr before or after midnight. Teens are 5-10 times more likely to be in a fatal crash while driving at night compared with driving during the day. The difficulty of driving at night combined with the inexperience of teen drivers appears to be a deadly combination.

Graduated licensing laws (GLL) consist of a series of steps over a designated period before a teen can get full, unrestricted driving privileges. In a 3-stage graduated license, the student driver must first pass vision and knowledge-based tests. This is followed by obtaining a learner's permit and once a specific age has been achieved and driving skills advanced, the student driver is eligible to take the driving test. Once given the provisional license, the new driver will have a specified time to do low-risk driving. GLLs usually place initial restrictions on the number of passengers (especially teenaged) allowed in the vehicle and restrict driving during nighttime. There is a decrease in the number of crashes of 20-40% among the youngest drivers in states with a graduated licensing system. Elements of graduated licensing programs have been adopted by many states. Driver's education classes do not consistently reduce motor vehicle crashes.

Alcohol use is a major cause of motor vehicle trauma among adolescents. The combination of inexperience in driving and inexperience with alcohol is particularly dangerous. Approximately 20% of all deaths from motor vehicle crashes in this age group are the result of alcohol intoxication, with impairment of driving seen at blood alcohol concentrations as low as 0.05 g/dL. Approximately 30% of adolescents report riding with a driver who had been drinking and about 10% report driving after drinking. All states have adopted a zero tolerance policy, which defines any measurable alcohol content as legal intoxication, to adolescent drinking while driving. All adolescent motor vehicle injury victims should have their blood alcohol concentration measured in the emergency department and be screened for high-risk alcohol use with a validated screening test (such as the CRAFFT or AUDIT screening tools) to identify those with alcohol abuse problems (Chapter 108.1). Individuals who have evidence of alcohol abuse should not leave the emergency department or hospital without plans for appropriate alcohol abuse treatment. Interventions for problem drinking can be effective in decreasing the risk of subsequent motor vehicle crashes. Even brief interventions in the emergency department using motivational interviewing can be successful in decreasing adolescent problem drinking.

ALL-TERRAIN VEHICLES All-terrain vehicles (ATVs) in many parts of the country are an important cause of injuries to children and adolescents. These vehicles can attain high speeds and are prone to rollover because of the high center of gravity. Orthopedic and head injuries are the most common serious injuries seen among children involved in ATV crashes. Helmets can significantly decrease the risk and severity of head injuries among ATV riders, but current use is very low. Unfortunately, voluntary industry efforts to decrease the risk of injuries appear to have had little effect in making ATVs safer. The AAP recommends that children younger than 16 yr should not ride on ATVs.

Bicycle Injuries

Each year in the USA, approximately 170 children and adolescents die of injuries incurred while riding bicycles, and another 300,000 are treated in emergency departments, making bicycle-related injuries one of the most common reasons that children with trauma visit emergency departments. The majority of severe and fatal bicycle injuries involve head trauma. A logical step in the prevention of these head injuries is the use of helmets. Helmets are very effective, reducing the risk of head injury by 85% and the risk of brain injury by 88%. Helmets also reduce injuries to the mid and upper face by as much as 65%. Pediatricians can be effective advocates for the use of bicycle helmets and should incorporate this advice into their anticipatory guidance schedules for parents and children. Appropriate helmets are those with a firm polystyrene liner that fit properly on the child's head. Parents should avoid buying a larger helmet to give the child "growing room."

Promotion of helmet use can and should be extended beyond the pediatrician's office. Community education programs spearheaded by coalitions of physicians, educators, bicycle clubs, and community service organizations have been successful in promoting the use of bicycle helmets to children across the socioeconomic spectrum, resulting in helmet use rates of 60% or more with a concomitant reduction in the number of head injuries. Passage of bicycle helmet laws also leads to increased helmet use.

Consideration should also be given to other types of preventive activities, although the evidence supporting their effectiveness is limited. Bicycle paths are a logical method for separating bicycles and motor vehicles.

Pedestrian Injuries

Pedestrian injuries are one of the most common causes of traumatic death for children of ages 5-9 yr in the USA and in most industrialized countries. Although case fatality rates are <5%, serious nonfatal injuries constitute a much larger problem, resulting in 50,000 emergency department visits annually for children and adolescents. Pedestrian injuries are the most important cause of traumatic coma in children and a frequent cause of serious lower extremity fractures, particularly in school-aged children.

Most injuries occur during the day, with a peak in the after-school period. Improved lighting or reflective clothing would, therefore, be expected to prevent few injuries. Surprisingly, approximately 30% of pedestrian injuries occur while the individual is in a marked crosswalk, perhaps reflecting a false sense of security and decreased vigilance in these areas. The risk of pedestrian injury is greater in neighborhoods with high traffic volumes, speeds greater than ≈25 mph, absence of play space adjacent to the home, household crowding, and low socioeconomic status.

One important risk factor for childhood pedestrian injuries is the developmental level of the child. Children younger than age 5 yr are at risk for being run over in the driveway. Few children younger than 9 or 10 yr of age have the developmental skills to successfully negotiate traffic 100% of the time. Young children have poor ability to judge the distance and speed of traffic and are easily distracted by playmates or other factors in the environment. Many parents are not aware of this potential mismatch between the abilities of the young school-aged child and the skills needed to cross streets safely.

Prevention of pedestrian injuries is difficult, but should consist of a multifaceted approach. Education of the child in pedestrian safety should be initiated at an early age by the parents and continue into the school-age years. Younger children should be taught never to cross streets when alone; older children should be taught (and practice how) to negotiate quiet streets with little traffic. Major streets should not be crossed alone until the child is 10 yr of age or older.

Legislation and police enforcement are important components of any campaign to reduce pedestrian injuries. Right-turn-on-red laws increase the hazard to pedestrians. In many cities, few drivers stop for pedestrians in crosswalks, a special hazard for young children. Engineering changes in roadway design are extremely important as passive prevention measures. Most important are measures to slow the speed of traffic and to route traffic away from schools and residential areas; these efforts are endorsed by parents and can decrease the risk of injuries and death by 10-35%. Other modifications include networks of 1-way streets, proper placement of transit or school bus stops, sidewalks in urban and suburban areas, edge stripping in rural areas to delineate the edge of the road, and curb parking regulations. Comprehensive traffic "calming" schemes using these strategies have been very successful in reducing child pedestrian injuries in Sweden, the Netherlands, Germany, and increasingly, the USA.

Ski- and Snowboard-Related Injuries

One area of recreation and sport that has improved in recent years has been the increasing use of helmets in snow sports such as skiing and snowboarding. Head injuries are the most common cause of death in these sports and helmets appear to be able to reduce the risk of head injury by 50% or more in most studies. Use of helmets does not result in skiers or snow boarders taking more risks and should be encouraged in all snow sports.

Fire- and Burn-Related Injuries (Chapter 68)

Fire- and burn-related injuries are the 5th most common cause of unintentional injury death in the USA, with approximately 3,800 fire and burn deaths occurring each year to people of all ages. For both injuries and deaths, the 1st decade of life is the period of highest risk. The likelihood of burn injury is strongly related to low socioeconomic status, with the highest rates among the poor, the less educated, and those living in mobile homes. Burns are much more frequent among males than among females. Among children 10-14 yr of age with burns involving flammable substances, males are burned 8 times more frequently than females.

One of the earliest effective interventions involved using nonflammable fabrics. Flame burns resulting from ignition of clothing were a common, serious burn injury, especially in small children. At least 30% of those injuries involved infant sleepwear. Such burns averaged 30% of the body surface, requiring hospitalization for an average of 70 days. In 1967, the Federal Flammable Fabrics Act was passed, requiring children's sleepwear to be flame-retardant. As a result of this and similar state legislation, clothing ignition burns in small children now account for only a small fraction of burns in children. Parents should not circumvent these protective regulations by using cotton T-shirts for infant and child sleepwear.

Another hazard modification resulting in substantial reduction of injury involves scald burns due to tap water. Scalds account for 40% of burn injuries in children requiring hospitalization, and a substantial proportion of these scald burns involve tap water. Scalds from hot liquids and foods are the most common reason for a burn admission to the hospital in children younger than age 5 yr. Avoiding the use of electric kettles or frying pans with long cords, avoiding the use of baby walkers, avoiding drinking hot tea or coffee while holding an infant, and keeping children away from pots cooking on the stove will help to prevent many of these injuries. Unlike those with flame burns, children with scalds generally do not die; many children have long hospitalizations, multiple surgical procedures, and severe disfigurement. The risk of full-thickness burns increases geometrically at water temperatures >125°F. At 150°F, a full-thickness burn will be produced in adult skin in 2 sec. A simple and effective preventive maneuver is to lower the water heater temperature to 125°F (51.6°C). At this setting, dishwashers and washing machines operate effectively, but the risk of serious scald injury is greatly reduced. New water heaters are usually preset at this lower temperature.

Fireworks are a seasonal injury, and >40% of those injured by fireworks are children younger than 15 yr of age. Community restrictions on certain types of fireworks and adult supervision of the use of all fireworks have been effective in decreasing burns, amputations, and ocular injuries caused by these devices.

More than 80% of all fire deaths in the USA occur in private dwellings. Of these deaths, 60% are caused by smoke asphyxiation and not by flame burns. Smoke detectors are an inexpensive but highly effective method of preventing the majority of these deaths. Two major types of detectors are available: ionization and photoelectric detectors. Ionization detectors are more sensitive to flames and photoelectric devices to smoke. Photoelectric detectors placed near cooking areas appear to have a lower rate of false alarms than ionization detectors and are less likely to be intentionally disabled by families. Detectors should be placed on every level of the home and outside of every bedroom. Physicians can increase parental smoke detector use by offering information on smoke detectors in their offices.

Cigarettes are estimated to cause 45% of all fires and 22-56% of deaths from house fires. The combination of smoking and alcohol use appears to be particularly lethal. Most cigarettes made in the USA contain additives in both the paper and the tobacco that allow them to burn for as long as 28 min, even if left unattended. Fire-safe, or self-extinguishing, cigarettes have been mandated in 32 states and all Canadian provinces, which will prevent thousands of deaths and injuries in North America.

Some burns result from fire setting by children or adolescents. In young children, this usually represents exploratory play. However, such behavior in older children and adolescents may signify a serious conduct disorder and warrants careful psychiatric and family evaluation. More than 50% of adolescent fire setters will be involved in repeat incidents.

Poisoning (Chapter 58)

Deaths caused by unintentional poisoning among younger children have decreased dramatically over the past 2 decades, particularly among children younger than 5 yr of age. In 1970 when the Poison Packaging Prevention Act was passed, 226 poisoning deaths of children younger than age 5 yr occurred compared with only 34 in 2007. Poisoning prevention demonstrates the effectiveness of passive strategies, including the use of child-resistant packaging and limited doses per container. The Poison Packaging Prevention Act currently includes 28 categories of household products and drugs. This law has been remarkably effective in reducing poisoning deaths and hospitalizations. Nevertheless, ingestions by children younger than 6 yr account for 50% of all calls to poison control centers in the USA. The most common substances ingested by young children are cosmetics, cleaning agents, analgesics, topical medications, and cough and cold preparations. In contrast, analgesics, cough and cold preparations, antidepressants, and carbon monoxide were responsible for most deaths in children younger than 6 yr. Among poisoning fatalities of adolescents, almost one half were classified as suicides and one third were attributed to intentional abuse. Over the past 15 yr, there has been a sharp rise in the rate of deaths from unintentional poisoning deaths among adolescents and young adults. In 2006, these deaths accounted for 9% of all deaths among 15-24 yr olds, and 18% of all injury deaths. This trend has been associated with an increased rate of opioid prescribing for chronic pain and other conditions.

Difficulty using child-resistant containers by adults is an important cause of poisoning in young children today. A survey by the U.S. Centers for Disease Control and Prevention found that 18.5% of households in which poisoning occurred in children younger than 5 yr of age had replaced the child-resistant closure and 65% of the packaging used did not work properly. Nearly 20% of ingestions occur from drugs owned by grandparents, a group that has difficulty using traditional child-resistant containers. There is a need for better child-resistant closures that do not require manual dexterity or strength greater than the capabilities of older adults.

Poison control centers serve as the frontline for managing poisonous ingestions in the USA; efforts to educate parents about the role of poison control centers can increase their use and the cost-effective management of ingestions. Poison control centers can be reached anywhere in the nation by dialing 1-800-222-1222.

Drowning (Chapter 67)

In 2006, 1,139 drownings (1.4 deaths per 100,000) primarily associated with recreational activities, occurred among children and adolescents in the USA. Among children ages 1-9 yr, drowning ranks 2nd only to motor vehicle injury as a cause of traumatic death. It is estimated that an additional 3447 near-drownings resulted in an emergency department visit in 2007. Because of spinal cord damage, diving headfirst into shallow water accounts for the most serious aquatic injuries. Of the estimated 700 spinal cord injuries resulting from aquatic activities each year, the majority result in permanent paralysis.

The proportion of drowning deaths occurring in pools varies by region of the country. In Los Angeles, CA, one half of all drownings take place in residential pools, a rate similar to that in other areas with large numbers of pools. Children younger than 5 yr of age do not understand the consequences of falling into deep water and usually do not call for help. A majority of child victims drown during lapses in adult supervision. Clearly, the most effective way to prevent childhood pool drowning is through circumferential fencing. To give the greatest protection, these barriers should restrict entry to the pool from the yard and residence, use self-closing and self-latching gates, be at least 5 ft high, and have no vertical openings more than 4 in wide. Ordinances to require appropriate fencing have been demonstrated to be effective. Swimming lessons have long thought to be protective against drowning, though evidence has been lacking. One recent national case control study estimated that formal lessons were associated with an 88% reduction in the risk of drowning among 1-4 yr old children.

Among adolescents and young adults, alcohol and drug use has been found to be involved in nearly 50% of all drowning deaths. The risk of drowning while boating is increased 10-50 times with alcohol intoxication, both because of the risk of falling overboard and the increased risk of drowning if drunk while submerged. The restriction of the sale and consumption of alcoholic beverages in boating, pool, harbor, marina, and beach areas may combat this dangerous combination of activities. More restrictive licensing of boat owners should also be considered.

Personal flotation devices (PFDs) are believed to be an important device to protect children from drowning. Although the exact protective effect of PFDs is unknown, a study by the U.S. Coast Guard showed that although only 7% of boats involved in mishaps lacked available PFDs, they accounted for 29% of boating fatalities. All children and adolescents should wear a PFD when boating in open water.

The risk of bathtub drowning is markedly increased in poorly supervised toddlers and in children with a seizure disorder, including older children and adolescents. Older children with seizure disorders should be instructed to shower instead of using a bathtub and younger children need careful, constant supervision while bathing.

Firearm Injuries

Injuries to children and adolescents involving firearms occur in 3 different situations: unintentional injury, suicide attempt, and assault. The injury induced may be fatal or may result in permanent sequelae.

Unintentional firearm injuries and deaths have continued to decrease and account for only a small fraction of all firearm injuries among children and adolescents. The majority of these deaths occur to teens during hunting or recreational activities. **Suicide** is the 3rd most common cause of trauma death in both male and female teenagers. During the 1950s to 1970, suicide rates for children and adolescents more than doubled; firearm suicide rates peaked in 1994 and decreased by 58% from this peak in 2006. It remains the most common means of suicide in males of all ages. The difference in the rate of suicide between males and females is related less to the number of attempts than to the method. Women die less often in suicide attempts, partly because they use less lethal means (mainly drugs) and perhaps have a lower degree of intent. The use of firearms in a suicidal act usually converts an attempt into a fatality.

Homicides are 2nd only to motor vehicle crashes among causes of death in teenagers older than the age of 15 yr. In 2006, 3,418 children and adolescents were homicide victims; nonwhite teenagers accounted for 56% of the total, making homicides the most common cause of death among nonwhite teenagers. In 2006, 88% of homicides among teenage males involved firearms, the majority of which are handguns.

In the USA, approximately 35% of households own guns. Handguns account for approximately 20% of the firearms in use today, yet they are involved in 80% of criminal and other firearm misuse. Home ownership of guns increases the risk of adolescent suicide 3- to 10-fold and the risk of adolescent homicide up to 4-fold. In homes with guns, the risk to the occupants is far greater than the chance that the gun will be used against an intruder; for every death occurring in self-defense, there may be 1.3 unintentional deaths, 4.6 homicides, and 37 suicides.

Of all firearms, handguns pose the greatest risk to children and adolescents. Access to handguns by adolescents is surprisingly common and is not restricted to those involved in gang or criminal activity. Stricter approaches to reduce youth access to handguns, rather than all firearms, would appear to be the most appropriate focus of efforts to reduce shooting injuries in children and adolescents.

Locking and unloading guns as well as storing ammunition locked in a different location substantially reduces the risk of a suicide or unintentional firearm injury among youth by up to 73%. Because up to 50% of homes have at least 1 firearm stored unsafely, 1 potential approach to reducing these injuries could focus on improving household firearm storage practices where children and youth reside or visit. The evidence regarding the effectiveness of office-based counseling to influence firearm storage practice is mixed.

Adolescents with mental health conditions and alcoholism are at particularly high risk for firearm injury. In the absence of conclusive evidence, physicians should continue to work with families to eliminate access to guns in these households.

Falls

Falls are the leading cause of nonfatal injury in children up to age 15 yr and the 2nd leading cause of nonfatal injury in 15-19 yr olds. Altogether, there were more than 2 million falls that led to emergency department visits in 2007 alone for children and adolescents; approximately 1.5% of these visits led to a hospitalization. Relatively little is known about the epidemiology of falls. One reason is that in the *International Classification of Diseases*, 9th edition, the codes for external cause of injury are relatively nonspecific and do not describe mechanisms with sufficient detail. There have been relatively few in-depth analytic studies of falls, except in particular circumstances, such as playground injuries. Strategies to prevent falls depend on the environmental circumstances and social context in which they occur. Window falls have been successfully prevented with the use of devices that prevent egress, and injuries from playground falls can be mitigated through the use of proper surfacing, such as woodchips or other soft, energy-absorbing materials. Alcohol may also contribute to falls among teenagers, and these injuries can be reduced by general strategies to reduce teen alcohol use.

Violence

Although the current rates of homicide are much lower than they were at their peak in the late 1980s and early 1990s, the problem of violence is still large. The origins of violence occur during childhood. Adults who commit violent acts usually have a history of violent behavior during childhood or adolescence. Longitudinal studies following groups of individuals from birth have found that aggression occurs among infants and that most children learn to control this aggression early in childhood. Children who later become violent adolescents and adults do not learn to control this aggressive behavior.

The most successful interventions for violence are those occurring early in life. These include home visits by nurses beginning in the prenatal period and continuing for the 1st few years of life to provide support and guidance to parents, especially parents without other resources. Early childhood education starting at age 3 yr has been shown to be effective in improving school success, keeping children in school, and decreasing the chance that the child will be a delinquent adolescent. School-based interventions, including curricula to increase the social skills of children and improve the parenting skills of caregivers, have long-term effects on violence and risk-taking behavior. Early identification of behavior problems by primary care pediatricians can best be accomplished through the routine use of formal screening tools. Interventions in adolescence, such as family therapy, multisystemic therapy, and therapeutic foster care, can decrease problem behavior and a subsequent decline into delinquency and violence.

PSYCHOSOCIAL CONSEQUENCES OF INJURIES

Many children and their parents have substantial psychosocial sequelae from trauma. Studies in adults indicate that 10-40% of hospitalized injured patients will have post-traumatic stress disorder (PTSD; Chapter 23). Among injured children involved in motor vehicle crashes, 90% of families will have symptoms of acute stress disorder after the crash, although the diagnosis of acute stress disorder is not predictive of later PTSD. Standardized questionnaires that collect data from the child, the parents, and the medical record at the time of initial injury can serve as useful screening tests for later development of PTSD. Early mental health intervention, with close follow-up, is important for the treatment of PTSD and for minimizing its effect on the child and family.

BIBLIOGRAPHY

Please visit the Nelson Textbook of Pediatrics *website at www.expertconsult.com for the complete bibliography.*

PART II Growth, Development, and Behavior

Chapter 6
Overview and Assessment of Variability
Susan Feigelman

The goal of pediatric care is to optimize the growth and development of each child. Pediatricians need to understand normal growth, development, and behavior in order to monitor children's progress, identify delays or abnormalities in development, obtain needed services, and counsel parents. In addition to clinical experience and personal knowledge, effective practice requires familiarity with major theoretical perspectives and evidence-based strategies for optimizing growth and development. To target factors that increase or decrease risk, pediatricians need to understand how biologic and social forces interact within the parent-child relationship, within the family, and between the family and the larger society. Growth is an indicator of overall well-being, status of chronic disease, and interpersonal and psychologic stress. By monitoring children and families over time, pediatricians can observe the interrelationships between physical growth and cognitive, motor, and emotional development. Observation is enhanced by familiarity with developmental theory and understanding of developmental models which describe normal patterns of behavior and provide guidance for prevention of behavior problems. Effective pediatricians also recognize how they can work with families and children to bring about healthy behaviors and behavioral change.

For the full continuation of this chapter, please visit the Nelson Textbook of Pediatrics *website at www.expertconsult.com.*

6.1 Assessment of Fetal Growth and Development
Susan Feigelman

The most dramatic events in growth and development occur before birth and involve the transformation of a fertilized egg into an embryo and a fetus, the elaboration of the nervous system, and the emergence of behavior in utero. The psychologic changes occurring in the parents during the gestation profoundly impact the lives of all members of the family. The developing fetus is affected by such social and environmental influences as maternal undernutrition; alcohol, cigarette, and drug use (both legal and illicit); and psychologic trauma. The complex interplay between these forces and the somatic and neurologic transformations occurring in the fetus influence growth and behavior at birth, through infancy, and potentially throughout the individual's life.

For the full continuation of this chapter, please visit the Nelson Textbook of Pediatrics *website at www.expertconsult.com.*

Chapter 7
The Newborn
John Olsson

The **newborn (neonatal) period** begins at birth (regardless of gestational age) and includes the 1st mo of life. During this time, marked physiologic transitions occur in all organ systems, and the infant learns to respond to many forms of external stimuli. Because infants thrive physically and psychologically only in the context of their social relationships, any description of the newborn's developmental status has to include consideration of the parents' role as well.

For the full continuation of this chapter, please visit the Nelson Textbook of Pediatrics *website at www.expertconsult.com.*

Chapter 8
The First Year
Susan Feigelman

Advances in imaging permit us to understand the anatomic and physiologic correlates of the physical growth, maturation, acquisition of competence, and psychologic reorganization that characterizes infancy and radically change the infant's behavior and social relationships. Some activities previously thought to be "primitive" or "reflexive" result from complex systems. Swallowing, rather than a simple reflex, results from a complex highly coordinated process involving multiple levels of neural control distributed among several physiologic systems whose nature and relationships mature throughout the 1st year of life. Substantial learning of the basic tools of language (phonology, word segmentation) occurs during infancy. Speech processing in older individuals requires defined and precise neuronal networks; imaging studies have revealed that the infant brain possesses a structural and functional organization similar to that of adults, leading to the belief that structural neurologic processing of speech may guide infants to discover the properties of his or her native language. Myelination of the cortex begins at 8 mo gestation and is nearly complete by age 2 yr; much of this process occurs during infancy. Given the importance of iron and other nutrients in myelination, adequate stores throughout infancy are critical (Chapter 42). Inadequate dietary intake, insufficient interactions with caregivers, or both may alter experience-dependent processes that are critical to brain structure development and function during infancy. Although some of these processes may be delayed, as the periods of plasticity close during the rapid developmental changes occurring in infancy, more permanent deficits may result.

The infant acquires new competences in all developmental domains. The concept of developmental trajectories recognizes that complex skills build on simpler ones; it is also important to realize how development in each domain affects functioning in all of the others. Physical growth parameters and normal ranges for attainable weight, length, and head circumference are found in the Centers for Disease Control and Prevention growth charts (see Figs. 9-1 and 9-2 on the *Nelson Textbook of Pediatrics* website at www.expertconsult.com). Table 8-1 presents an overview of key milestones by domain; Table 8-2 presents similar information arranged by age. Table 8-3 presents age at time of appearance on x-ray of centers of ossification. Parents often seek information about "normal development" during this period and should be directed to reliable sources, including the American Academy of Pediatrics website (*www.AAP.org*).

AGE 0-2 MONTHS

Myelination begins prenatally at 30 wk gestation. In the full term infant, it is present by the time of birth in the dorsal brainstem,

Table 8-1 DEVELOPMENTAL MILESTONES IN THE FIRST 2 YR OF LIFE

MILESTONE	AVERAGE AGE OF ATTAINMENT (MO)	DEVELOPMENTAL IMPLICATIONS
GROSS MOTOR		
Holds head steady while sitting	2	Allows more visual interaction
Pulls to sit, with no head lag	3	Muscle tone
Brings hands together in midline	3	Self-discovery of hands
Asymmetric tonic neck reflex gone	4	Can inspect hands in midline
Sits without support	6	Increasing exploration
Rolls back to stomach	6.5	Truncal flexion, risk of falls
Walks alone	12	Exploration, control of proximity to parents
Runs	16	Supervision more difficult
FINE MOTOR		
Grasps rattle	3.5	Object use
Reaches for objects	4	Visuomotor coordination
Palmar grasp gone	4	Voluntary release
Transfers object hand to hand	5.5	Comparison of objects
Thumb-finger grasp	8	Able to explore small objects
Turns pages of book	12	Increasing autonomy during book time
Scribbles	13	Visuomotor coordination
Builds tower of 2 cubes	15	Uses objects in combination
Builds tower of 6 cubes	22	Requires visual, gross, and fine motor coordination
COMMUNICATION AND LANGUAGE		
Smiles in response to face, voice	1.5	More active social participant
Monosyllabic babble	6	Experimentation with sound, tactile sense
Inhibits to "no"	7	Response to tone (nonverbal)
Follows one-step command with gesture	7	Nonverbal communication
Follows one-step command without gesture	10	Verbal receptive language (e.g., "Give it to me")
Says "mama" or "dada"	10	Expressive language
Points to objects	10	Interactive communication
Speaks first real word	12	Beginning of labeling
Speaks 4-6 words	15	Acquisition of object and personal names
Speaks 10-15 words	18	Acquisition of object and personal names
Speaks 2-word sentences (e.g., "Mommy shoe")	19	Beginning grammaticization, corresponds with 50 word vocabulary
COGNITIVE		
Stares momentarily at spot where object disappeared	2	Lack of object permanence (out of sight, out of mind [e.g., yarn ball dropped])
Stares at own hand	4	Self-discovery, cause and effect
Bangs 2 cubes	8	Active comparison of objects
Uncovers toy (after seeing it hidden)	8	Object permanence
Egocentric symbolic play (e.g., pretends to drink from cup)	12	Beginning symbolic thought
Uses stick to reach toy	17	Able to link actions to solve problems
Pretend play with doll (e.g., gives doll bottle)	17	Symbolic thought

cerebellar peduncles, and posterior limb of the internal capsule. The cerebellar white matter acquires myelin by 1 mo of age and is well myelinated by 3 mo of age. The subcortical white matter of the parietal, posterior frontal, temporal, and calcarine cortex is partially myelinated by 3 mo of age. In this period, the infant experiences tremendous growth. Physiologic changes allow the establishment of effective feeding routines and a predictable sleep-wake cycle. The social interactions that occur as parents and infants accomplish these tasks lay the foundation for cognitive and emotional development.

Physical Development

A newborn's weight may initially decrease 10% below birthweight in the 1st wk as a result of excretion of excess extravascular fluid and limited nutritional intake. Nutrition improves as colostrum is replaced by higher-fat breast milk, as infants learn to latch on and suck more efficiently, and as mothers become more comfortable with feeding techniques. Infants regain or exceed birthweight by 2 wk of age and should grow at approximately 30 g (1 oz)/day during the 1st mo (see Table 13-1). This is the period of fastest postnatal growth. Limb movements consist largely of uncontrolled writhing, with apparently purposeless opening and closing of the hands. Smiling occurs involuntarily. Eye gaze, head turning, and sucking are under better control and thus can be used to demonstrate infant perception and cognition. An infant's preferential turning toward the mother's voice is evidence of recognition memory.

Six behavioral states have been described (Chapter 7). Initially, sleep and wakefulness are evenly distributed throughout the 24-hr day (Fig. 8-1). Neurologic maturation accounts for the consolidation of sleep into blocks of 5 or 6 hr at night, with brief awake, feeding periods. Learning also occurs; infants whose parents are consistently more interactive and stimulating during the day learn to concentrate their sleeping during the night.

Cognitive Development

Infants can differentiate among patterns, colors, and consonants. They can recognize facial expressions (smiles) as similar, even when they appear on different faces. They also can match abstract properties of stimuli, such as contour, intensity, or temporal pattern, across sensory modalities. Infants at 2 mo of age can discriminate rhythmic patterns in native vs non-native language. Infants appear to seek stimuli actively, as though satisfying an innate need to make sense of the world. These phenomena point to the integration of sensory inputs in the central nervous system. Caretaking activities provide visual, tactile, olfactory, and auditory stimuli; all of these support the development of cognition. Infants habituate to the familiar, attending less to repeated stimuli and increasing their attention to novel stimuli.

Emotional Development

The infant is dependent on the environment to meet his or her needs. The consistent availability of a trusted adult to meet the infant's urgent needs creates the conditions for secure attachment. Basic trust vs mistrust, the first of Erikson's psychosocial stages (Chapter 6), depends on attachment and reciprocal maternal bonding. Crying occurs in response to stimuli that may be obvious (a soiled diaper), but are often obscure. Infants who are consistently picked up and held in response to distress cry less at 1 yr and show less aggressive behavior at 2 yr. Cross-cultural studies show that in societies in which infants are carried close to the mother, babies cry less than in societies in which babies are only periodically carried. Crying normally peaks at about 6 wk of age, when healthy infants may cry up to 3 hr/day, then decreases to 1 hr or less by 3 mo.

The emotional significance of any experience depends on both the individual child's temperament and the parent's responses (see Table 6-1); differing feeding schedules produce differing reactions. Hunger generates increasing tension; as the urgency

Table 8-2 EMERGING PATTERNS OF BEHAVIOR DURING THE 1ST YEAR OF LIFE*

NEONATAL PERIOD (1ST 4 WK)	
Prone:	Lies in flexed attitude; turns head from side to side; head sags on ventral suspension
Supine:	Generally flexed and a little stiff
Visual:	May fixate face on light in line of vision; "doll's-eye" movement of eyes on turning of the body
Reflex:	Moro response active; stepping and placing reflexes; grasp reflex active
Social:	Visual preference for human face
AT 1 MO	
Prone:	Legs more extended; holds chin up; turns head; head lifted momentarily to plane of body on ventral suspension
Supine:	Tonic neck posture predominates; supple and relaxed; head lags when pulled to sitting position
Visual:	Watches person; follows moving object
Social:	Body movements in cadence with voice of other in social contact; beginning to smile
AT 2 MO	
Prone:	Raises head slightly farther; head sustained in plane of body on ventral suspension
Supine:	Tonic neck posture predominates; head lags when pulled to sitting position
Visual:	Follows moving object 180 degrees
Social:	Smiles on social contact; listens to voice and coos
AT 3 MO	
Prone:	Lifts head and chest with arms extended; head above plane of body on ventral suspension
Supine:	Tonic neck posture predominates; reaches toward and misses objects; waves at toy
Sitting:	Head lag partially compensated when pulled to sitting position; early head control with bobbing motion; back rounded
Reflex:	Typical Moro response has not persisted; makes defensive movements or selective withdrawal reactions
Social:	Sustained social contact; listens to music; says "aah, ngah"
AT 4 MO	
Prone:	Lifts head and chest, with head in approximately vertical axis; legs extended
Supine:	Symmetric posture predominates, hands in midline; reaches and grasps objects and brings them to mouth
Sitting:	No head lag when pulled to sitting position; head steady, tipped forward; enjoys sitting with full truncal support
Standing:	When held erect, pushes with feet
Adaptive:	Sees pellet, but makes no move to reach for it
Social:	Laughs out loud; may show displeasure if social contact is broken; excited at sight of food
AT 7 MO	
Prone:	Rolls over; pivots; crawls or creep-crawls (Knobloch)
Supine:	Lifts head; rolls over; squirms
Sitting:	Sits briefly, with support of pelvis; leans forward on hands; back rounded
Standing:	May support most of weight; bounces actively
Adaptive:	Reaches out for and grasps large object; transfers objects from hand to hand; grasp uses radial palm; rakes at pellet
Language:	Forms polysyllabic vowel sounds
Social:	Prefers mother; babbles; enjoys mirror; responds to changes in emotional content of social contact
AT 10 MO	
Sitting:	Sits up alone and indefinitely without support, with back straight
Standing:	Pulls to standing position; "cruises" or walks holding on to furniture
Motor:	Creeps or crawls
Adaptive:	Grasps objects with thumb and forefinger; pokes at things with forefinger; picks up pellet with assisted pincer movement; uncovers hidden toy; attempts to retrieve dropped object; releases object grasped by other person
Language:	Repetitive consonant sounds ("mama," "dada")
Social:	Responds to sound of name; plays peek-a-boo or pat-a-cake; waves bye-bye
AT 1 YR	
Motor:	Walks with one hand held (48 wk); rises independently, takes several steps (Knobloch)
Adaptive:	Picks up pellet with unassisted pincer movement of forefinger and thumb; releases object to other person on request or gesture
Language:	Says a few words besides "mama," "dada"
Social:	Plays simple ball game; makes postural adjustment to dressing

*Data are derived from those of Gesell (as revised by Knobloch), Shirley, Provence, Wolf, Bailey, and others.
From Knobloch H, Stevens F, Malone AF: *Manual of developmental diagnosis,* Hagerstown, MD, 1980, Harper & Row.

peaks, the infant cries, the parent offers the breast or bottle and the tension dissipates. Infants fed "on demand" consistently experience this link between their distress, the arrival of the parent, and relief from hunger. Most infants fed on a fixed schedule quickly adapt their hunger cycle to the schedule. Those who cannot because they are temperamentally prone to irregular biologic rhythms experience periods of unrelieved hunger as well as unwanted feedings when they already feel full. Similarly, infants who are fed at the parents' convenience, with neither attention to the infant's hunger cues nor a fixed schedule may not consistently experience feeding as the pleasurable reduction of tension. These infants often show increased irritability and physiologic instability (spitting, diarrhea, poor weight gain) as well as later behavioral problems.

Table 8-3 TIME OF APPEARANCE IN X-RAYS OF CENTERS OF OSSIFICATION IN INFANCY AND CHILDHOOD

BOYS—AGE AT APPEARANCE*	BONES AND EPIPHYSEAL CENTERS	GIRLS—AGE AT APPEARANCE*
HUMERUS, HEAD		
3 wk		3 wk
CARPAL BONES		
2 mo ± 2 mo	Capitate	2 mo ± 2 mo
3 mo ± 2 mo	Hamate	2 mo ± 2 mo
30 mo ± 16 mo	Triangular†	21 mo ± 14 mo
42 mo ± 19 mo	Lunate†	34 mo ± 13 mo
67 mo ± 19 mo	Trapezium†	47 mo ± 14 mo
69 mo ± 15 mo	Trapezoid†	49 mo ± 12 mo
66 mo ± 15 mo	Scaphoid†	51 mo ± 12 mo
No standards available	Pisiform†	No standards available
METACARPAL BONES		
18 mo ± 5 mo	II	12 mo ± 3 mo
20 mo ± 5 mo	III	13 mo ± 3 mo
23 mo ± 6 mo	IV	15 mo ± 4 mo
26 mo ± 7 mo	V	16 mo ± 5 mo
32 mo ± 9 mo	I	18 mo ± 5 mo
FINGERS (EPIPHYSES)		
16 mo ± 4 mo	Proximal phalanx, 3rd finger	10 mo ± 3 mo
16 mo ± 4 mo	Proximal phalanx, 2nd finger	11 mo ± 3 mo
17 mo ± 5 mo	Proximal phalanx, 4th finger	11 mo ± 3 mo
19 mo ± 7 mo	Distal phalanx, 1st finger	12 mo ± 4 mo
21 mo ± 5 mo	Proximal phalanx, 5th finger	14 mo ± 4 mo
24 mo ± 6 mo	Middle phalanx, 3rd finger	15 mo ± 5 mo
24 mo ± 6 mo	Middle phalanx, 4th finger	15 mo ± 5 mo
26 mo ± 6 mo	Middle phalanx, 2nd finger	16 mo ± 5 mo
28 mo ± 6 mo	Distal phalanx, 3rd finger	18 mo ± 4 mo
28 mo ± 6 mo	Distal phalanx, 4th finger	18 mo ± 5 mo
32 mo ± 7 mo	Proximal phalanx, 1st finger	20 mo ± 5 mo
37 mo ± 9 mo	Distal phalanx, 5th finger	23 mo ± 6 mo
37 mo ± 8 mo	Distal phalanx, 2nd finger	23 mo ± 6 mo
39 mo ± 10 mo	Middle phalanx, 5th finger	22 mo ± 7 mo
152 mo ± 18 mo	Sesamoid (adductor pollicis)	121 mo ± 13 mo
HIP AND KNEE		
Usually present at birth	Femur, distal	Usually present at birth
Usually present at birth	Tibia, proximal	Usually present at birth
4 mo ± 2 mo	Femur, head	4 mo ± 2 mo
46 mo ± 11 mo	Patella	29 mo ± 7 mo
FOOT AND ANKLE‡		

Values represent mean ± standard deviation, when applicable.
*To nearest month.
†Except for the capitate and hamate bones, the variability of carpal centers is too great to make them very useful clinically.
‡Standards for the foot are available, but normal variation is wide, including some familial variants, so this area is of little clinical use.
The norms present a composite of published data from the Fels Research Institute, Yellow Springs, OH (Pyle SI, Sontag L: *AJR Am J Roentgenol* 49:102, 1943), and unpublished data from the Brush Foundation, Case Western Reserve University, Cleveland, OH, and the Harvard School of Public Health, Boston, MA. Compiled by Lieb, Buehl, and Pyle.

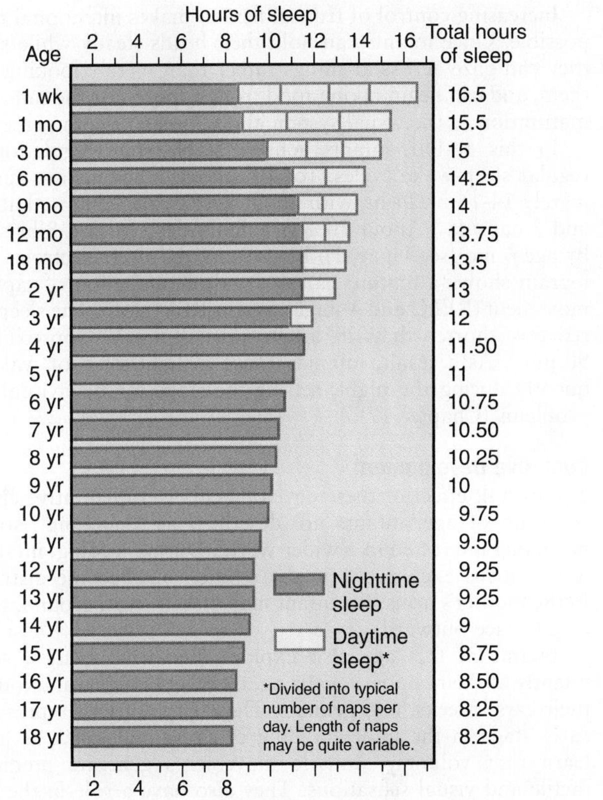

Figure 8-1 Typical sleep requirements in children. (From Ferber R: *Solve your child's sleep problems,* New York, 1985, Simon & Schuster.)

Implications for Parents and Pediatricians

Success or failure in establishing feeding and sleep cycles determines parents' feelings of efficacy. When things go well, the parents' anxiety and ambivalence, as well as the exhaustion of the early weeks, decrease. Infant issues (colic) or familial conflict will prevent this from occurring. With physical recovery from delivery and endocrinologic normalization, the mild postpartum depression that affects many mothers passes. If the mother continues to feel sad, overwhelmed, and anxious, the possibility of moderate to severe postpartum depression, found in 10% of postpartum women, needs to be considered. Major **depression** that arises during pregnancy or in the postpartum period threatens the mother-child relationship and is a risk factor for later cognitive and behavioral problems. The pediatrician may be the first professional to encounter the depressed mother and should be instrumental in assisting her in seeking treatment (Chapter 7).

AGE 2-6 MONTHS

At about 2 mo, the emergence of voluntary (social) smiles and increasing eye contact mark a change in the parent-child relationship, heightening the parents' sense of being loved reciprocally. During the next months, an infant's range of motor and social control and cognitive engagement increases dramatically. Mutual regulation takes the form of complex social interchanges, resulting in strong mutual attachment and enjoyment. Parents are less fatigued.

Physical Development

Between 3 and 4 mo of age, the rate of growth slows to approximately 20 g/day (see Table 13-1; see Figs. 9-1 and 9-2 on the *Nelson Textbook of Pediatrics* website at www.expertconsult.com). By 4 mo, birthweight is doubled. Early reflexes that limited voluntary movement recede. Disappearance of the asymmetric tonic neck reflex means that infants can begin to examine objects in the midline and manipulate them with both hands (Chapter 584). Waning of the early grasp reflex allows infants both to hold objects and to let them go voluntarily. A novel object may elicit purposeful, although inefficient, reaching. The quality of spontaneous movements also changes, from larger writhing to smaller, circular movements that have been described as "fidgety." Abnormal or absent fidgety movements may constitute a risk factor for later neurologic abnormalities.

Increasing control of truncal flexion makes intentional rolling possible. Once infants can hold their heads steady while sitting, they can gaze across at things rather than merely looking up at them, and can begin taking food from a spoon. At the same time, maturation of the visual system allows greater depth perception.

In this period, infants achieve stable state regulation and regular sleep-wake cycles. Total sleep requirements are approximately 14-16 hr/24 hr, with about 9-10 hr concentrated at night and 2 naps/day. About 70% of infants sleep for a 6-8 hr stretch by age 6 mo (see Fig. 8-1). By 4-6 mo, the sleep electroencephalogram shows a mature pattern, with demarcation of rapid eye movement (REM) and 4 stages of non-REM sleep. The sleep cycle remains shorter than in adults (50-60 min vs approximately 90 min). As a result, infants arouse to light sleep or wake frequently during the night, setting the stage for behavioral sleep problems (Chapter 17).

Cognitive Development

The overall effect of these developments is a qualitative change. At 4 mo of age, infants are described as "hatching" socially, becoming interested in a wider world. During feeding, infants no longer focus exclusively on the mother, but become distracted. In the mother's arms, the infant may literally turn around, preferring to face outward.

Infants at this age also explore their own bodies, staring intently at their hands, vocalizing, blowing bubbles, and touching their ears, cheeks, and genitals. These explorations represent an early stage in the understanding of cause and effect as infants learn that voluntary muscle movements generate predictable tactile and visual sensations. They also have a role in the emergence of a sense of self, separate from the mother. This is the first stage of personality development. Infants come to associate certain sensations through frequent repetition. The proprioceptive feeling of holding up the hand and wiggling the fingers always accompanies the sight of the fingers moving. Such self sensations are consistently linked and reproducible at will. In contrast, sensations that are associated with "other" occur with less regularity and in varying combinations. The sound, smell, and feel of the mother sometimes appear promptly in response to crying, but sometimes do not. The satisfaction that the mother or another loving adult provides continues the process of attachment.

Emotional Development and Communication

Babies interact with increasing sophistication and range. The primary emotions of anger, joy, interest, fear, disgust, and surprise appear in appropriate contexts as distinct facial expressions. When face-to-face, the infant and a trusted adult can match affective expressions (smiling or surprise) about 30% of the time. Initiating games (facial imitation, singing, hand games) increases social development. Such face-to-face behavior reveals the infant's ability to share emotional states, the first step in the development of communication. Infants of depressed parents show a different pattern, spending less time in coordinated movement with their parents and making fewer efforts to re-engage. Rather than anger, they show sadness and a loss of energy when the parents continue to be unavailable.

Implications for Parents and Pediatricians

Motor and sensory maturation makes infants at 3-6 mo exciting and interactive. Some parents experience their 4 mo old child's outward turning as a rejection, secretly fearing that their infants no longer love them. For most parents, this is a happy period. Most parents excitedly report that they can hold conversations with their infants, taking turns vocalizing and listening. Pediatricians share in the enjoyment, as the baby coos, makes eye contact, and moves rhythmically. If this visit does not feel joyful and relaxed, causes such as social stress, family dysfunction, parental mental illness, or problems in the infant-parent relationship should be considered. Parents can be reassured that responding to an infant's emotional needs cannot spoil him or her. Giving vaccines and drawing blood while the child is seated on the parent's lap or nursing at the breast increases pain tolerance.

AGE 6-12 MONTHS

With achievement of the sitting position, increased mobility, and new skills to explore the world around them, 6-12 mo old infants show advances in cognitive understanding and communication, and there are new tensions around the themes of attachment and separation. Infants develop will and intentions, characteristics that most parents welcome, but still find challenging to manage.

Physical Development

Growth slows more (see Table 13-1; see Figs. 9-1 and 9-2 on the *Nelson Textbook of Pediatrics* website at www.expertconsult.com). By the 1st birthday, birthweight has tripled, length has increased by 50%, and head circumference has increased by 10 cm. The ability to sit unsupported (6-7 mo) and to pivot while sitting (around 9-10 mo) provides increasing opportunities to manipulate several objects at a time and to experiment with novel combinations of objects. These explorations are aided by the emergence of a thumb-finger grasp (8-9 mo) and a neat pincer grasp by 12 mo. Many infants begin crawling and pulling to stand around 8 mo, followed by cruising. Some walk by 1 yr. Motor achievements correlate with increasing myelinization and cerebellar growth. These gross motor skills expand infants' exploratory range and create new physical dangers as well as opportunities for learning. Tooth eruption occurs, usually starting with the mandibular central incisors. Tooth development reflects skeletal maturation and bone age, although there is wide individual variation (see Table 8-3 and Chapter 299).

Cognitive Development

The 6 mo old infant has discovered his hands and will soon learn to manipulate objects. At first, everything goes into the mouth. In time, novel objects are picked up, inspected, passed from hand to hand, banged, dropped, and then mouthed. Each action represents a nonverbal idea about what things are for (in Piagetian terms, a *schema*; Chapter 6). The complexity of an infant's play, how many different schemata are brought to bear, is a useful index of cognitive development at this age. The pleasure, persistence, and energy with which infants tackle these challenges suggest the existence of an intrinsic drive or mastery motivation. Mastery behavior occurs when infants feel secure; those with less secure attachments show limited experimentation and less competence.

A major milestone is the achievement at about 9 mo of **object permanence** (constancy), the understanding that objects continue to exist, even when not seen. At 4-7 mo of age, infants look down for a yarn ball that has been dropped but quickly give up if it is not seen. With object constancy, infants persist in searching. They will find objects hidden under a cloth or behind the examiner's back. Peek-a-boo brings unlimited pleasure as the child magically brings back the other player. Events seem to occur as a result of the child's own activities.

Emotional Development

The advent of object permanence corresponds with qualitative changes in social and communicative development. Infants look back and forth between an approaching stranger and a parent, and may cling or cry anxiously, demonstrating **stranger anxiety**. Separations often become more difficult. Infants who have been sleeping through the night for months begin to awaken regularly and cry, as though remembering that the parents are in the next room.

A new demand for autonomy also emerges. Poor weight gain at this age often reflects a struggle between an infant's emerging independence and parent's control of the feeding situation. Use of the 2-spoon method of feeding (1 for the child and 1 for the parent), finger foods, and a high chair with a tray table can avert potential problems. Tantrums make their first appearance as the drives for autonomy and mastery come in conflict with parental controls and the infants' still-limited abilities.

Communication

Infants at 7 mo of age are adept at nonverbal communication, expressing a range of emotions and responding to vocal tone and facial expressions. Around 9 mo of age, infants become aware that emotions can be shared between people; they show parents toys as a way of sharing their happy feelings. Between 8 and 10 mo of age, babbling takes on a new complexity, with many syllables ("ba-da-ma") and inflections that mimic the native language. Infants now lose the ability to distinguish between vocal sounds that are undifferentiated in their native language. Social interaction (attentive adults taking turns vocalizing with the infant) profoundly influences the acquisition and production of new sounds. The first true word (i.e., a sound used consistently to refer to a specific object or person) appears in concert with an infant's discovery of object permanence. Picture books now provide an ideal context for verbal language acquisition. With a familiar book as a shared focus of attention, a parent and child engage in repeated cycles of pointing and labeling, with elaboration and feedback by the parent.

Implications for Parents and Pediatricians

With the developmental reorganization that occurs around 9 mo of age, previously resolved issues of feeding and sleeping re-emerge. Pediatricians can prepare parents at the 6 mo visit so that these problems can be understood as the result of developmental progress and not regression. Parents should be encouraged to plan ahead for necessary, and inevitable, separations (e.g., baby sitter, daycare). Routine preparations may make these separations easier. Introduction of a **transitional object** may allow the infant to self-comfort in the parents' absence. The object cannot have any potential for asphyxiation or strangulation.

Infants' wariness of strangers often makes the 9 mo examination difficult, particularly if the infant is temperamentally prone to react negatively to unfamiliar situations. Initially, the pediatrician should avoid direct eye contact with the child. Time spent talking with the parent and introducing the child to a small, washable toy will be rewarded with more cooperation. The examination can be continued on the parent's lap when feasible.

BIBLIOGRAPHY

Please visit the Nelson Textbook of Pediatrics *website at* *www.expertconsult.com* *for the complete bibliography.*

Chapter 9
The Second Year

Susan Feigelman

The child's sense of self and others are shaped by the skills emerging in the 2nd yr of life. Although the ability to walk allows separation and newly found independence; the child continues to need secure attachment to the parents. At approximately 18 mo of age, the emergence of symbolic thought and language causes a reorganization of behavior, with implications across many developmental domains.

AGE 12-18 MONTHS

Physical Development

Toddlers have relatively short legs and long torsos, with exaggerated lumbar lordosis and protruding abdomens. Although slower than in the 1st yr, considerable brain growth occurs in the 2nd yr; this growth and continuing myelinization, results in an increase in head circumference of 2 cm over the year.

Most children begin to walk independently near their 1st birthday; some do not walk until 15 mo of age. Early walking is not associated with advanced development in other domains. Infants initially toddle with a wide-based gait, with the knees bent and the arms flexed at the elbow; the entire torso rotates with each stride; the toes may point in or out, and the feet strike the floor flat. The appearance is that of genu varus (bowleg). Subsequent refinement leads to greater steadiness and energy efficiency. After several months of practice, the center of gravity shifts back and the torso stays more stable, while the knees extend and the arms swing at the sides for balance. The feet are held in better alignment, and the child is able to stop, pivot, and stoop without toppling over (Chapters 664 and 665).

Cognitive Development

Exploration of the environment increases in parallel with improved dexterity (reaching, grasping, releasing) and mobility. Learning follows the precepts of Piaget's sensory-motor stage (Chapter 6). Toddlers manipulate objects in novel ways to create interesting effects, such as stacking blocks or putting things into a computer disk drive. Playthings are also more likely to be used for their intended purposes (combs for hair, cups for drinking). Imitation of parents and older children is an important mode of learning. Make-believe (symbolic) play centers on the child's own body (pretending to drink from an empty cup) (Table 9-1; also see Table 8-1).

Emotional Development

Infants who are approaching the developmental milestone of taking their first steps may be irritable. Once they start walking, their predominant mood changes markedly. Toddlers are described as "intoxicated" or "giddy" with their new ability and with the power to control the distance between themselves and their parents. Exploring toddlers orbit around their parents, moving away and then returning for a reassuring touch before moving away again. A securely attached child will use the parent as a secure base from which to explore independently. Proud of her or his accomplishments, the child illustrates Erikson's stage of autonomy and separation (Chapter 6). The toddler who is overly controlled and discouraged from active exploration will feel doubt, shame, anger, and insecurity. All children will experience tantrums, reflecting their inability to delay gratification, suppress or displace anger, or verbally communicate their emotional states. The quality of the maternal-child relationship may moderate negative effects of child care arrangements when parents work.

Linguistic Development

Receptive language precedes expressive language. By the time infants speak their first words around 12 mo of age, they already respond appropriately to several simple statements, such as "no," "bye-bye," and "give me." By 15 mo, the average child points to major body parts and uses 4-6 words spontaneously and correctly. Toddlers also enjoy **polysyllabic** jargoning (see Tables 8-1 and 9-1), but do not seem upset that no one understands. Most communication of wants and ideas continues to be nonverbal.

Implications for Parents and Pediatricians

Parents may express concern about poor food intake as growth slows. The growth chart should provide reassurance. Parents who cannot recall any other milestone tend to remember when their child began to walk, perhaps because of the symbolic significance of walking as an act of independence. All toddlers should be encouraged to explore their environments; a child's ability to wander out of sight also increases the risks of injury and the need for supervision.

Table 9-1 EMERGING PATTERNS OF BEHAVIOR FROM 1 TO 5 YR OF AGE*

15 MO	
Motor:	Walks alone; crawls up stairs
Adaptive:	Makes tower of 3 cubes; makes a line with crayon; inserts raisin in bottle
Language:	Jargon; follows simple commands; may name a familiar object (e.g., ball); responds to his/her name
Social:	Indicates some desires or needs by pointing; hugs parents
18 MO	
Motor:	Runs stiffly; sits on small chair; walks up stairs with one hand held; explores drawers and wastebaskets
Adaptive:	Makes tower of 4 cubes; imitates scribbling; imitates vertical stroke; dumps raisin from bottle
Language:	10 words (average); names pictures; identifies one or more parts of body
Social:	Feeds self; seeks help when in trouble; may complain when wet or soiled; kisses parent with pucker
24 MO	
Motor:	Runs well, walks up and down stairs, one step at a time; opens doors; climbs on furniture; jumps
Adaptive:	Makes tower of 7 cubes (6 at 21 mo); scribbles in circular pattern; imitates horizontal stroke; folds paper once imitatively
Language:	Puts 3 words together (subject, verb, object)
Social:	Handles spoon well; often tells about immediate experiences; helps to undress; listens to stories when shown pictures
30 MO	
Motor:	Goes up stairs alternating feet
Adaptive:	Makes tower of 9 cubes; makes vertical and horizontal strokes, but generally will not join them to make cross; imitates circular stroke, forming closed figure
Language:	Refers to self by pronoun "I"; knows full name
Social:	Helps put things away; pretends in play
36 MO	
Motor:	Rides tricycle; stands momentarily on one foot
Adaptive:	Makes tower of 10 cubes; imitates construction of "bridge" of 3 cubes; copies circle; imitates cross
Language:	Knows age and sex; counts 3 objects correctly; repeats 3 numbers or a sentence of 6 syllables; most of speech intelligible to strangers
Social:	Plays simple games (in "parallel" with other children); helps in dressing (unbuttons clothing and puts on shoes); washes hands
48 MO	
Motor:	Hops on one foot; throws ball overhand; uses scissors to cut out pictures; climbs well
Adaptive:	Copies bridge from model; imitates construction of "gate" of 5 cubes; copies cross and square; draws man with 2 to 4 parts besides head; identifies longer of 2 lines
Language:	Counts 4 pennies accurately; tells story
Social:	Plays with several children, with beginning of social interaction and role-playing; goes to toilet alone
60 MO	
Motor:	Skips
Adaptive:	Draws triangle from copy; names heavier of 2 weights
Language:	Names 4 colors; repeats sentence of 10 syllables; counts 10 pennies correctly
Social:	Dresses and undresses; asks questions about meaning of words; engages in domestic role-playing

*Data derived from those of Gesell (as revised by Knobloch), Shirley, Provence, Wolf, Bailey, and others. After 5 yr, the Stanford-Binet, Wechsler-Bellevue, and other scales offer the most precise estimates of developmental level. To have their greatest value, they should be administered only by an experienced and qualified person.

In the office setting, many toddlers are comfortable exploring the examination room, but cling to the parents under the stress of the examination. Performing most of the physical examination in the parent's lap may help allay fears of separation. Infants who become more, not less, distressed in their parents' arms or who avoid their parents at times of stress may be insecurely attached. Young children who, when distressed, turn to strangers rather than parents for comfort are particularly worrisome. The conflicts between independence and security manifest in issues of discipline, temper tantrums, toilet training, and changing feeding behaviors. Parents should be counseled on these matters within the framework of normal development.

AGE 18-24 MONTHS

Physical Development

Motor development is incremental at this age, with improvements in balance and agility and the emergence of running and stair climbing. Height and weight increase at a steady rate during this year, with a gain of 5 in and 5 lb. By 24 mo, children are about ½ of their ultimate adult height. Head growth slows slightly. Ninety percent of adult head circumference is achieved by age 2 yr, with just an additional 5 cm gain over the next few years (Figs. 9-1 and 9-2 on the *Nelson Textbook of Pediatrics* website at www.expertconsult.com; see also Table 13-1).

Cognitive Development

At approximately 18 mo of age, several cognitive changes come together to mark the conclusion of the sensory-motor period. These can be observed during self-initiated play. Object permanence is firmly established; toddlers anticipate where an object will end up, even though the object was not visible while it was being moved. Cause and effect are better understood, and toddlers demonstrate flexibility in problem solving (e.g., using a stick to obtain a toy that is out of reach, figuring out how to wind a mechanical toy). Symbolic transformations in play are no longer tied to the toddler's own body, so that a doll can be "fed" from an empty plate. Like the reorganization that occurs at 9 mo, the cognitive changes at 18 mo correlate with important changes in the emotional and linguistic domains (see Table 9-1).

Emotional Development

In many children, the relative independence of the preceding period gives way to increased clinginess around 18 mo. This stage, described as "rapprochement," may be a reaction to growing awareness of the possibility of separation. Many parents report that they cannot go anywhere without having a small child attached to them. **Separation anxiety** will be manifest at bedtime. Many children use a special blanket or stuffed toy as a **transitional object,** which functions as a symbol of the absent parent. The transitional object remains important until the transition to symbolic thought has been completed and the symbolic presence of the parent has been fully internalized. Despite the attachment to the parent, the child's use of "no" is a way of declaring independence. Individual differences in temperament, in both the child and the parents play a critical role in determining the balance of conflict vs cooperation in the parent-child relationship. As effective language emerges, conflicts become less frequent.

Self-conscious awareness and internalized standards of behavior first appear at this age. Toddlers looking in a mirror will, for the first time, reach for their own face rather than the mirror image if they notice something unusual on their nose. They begin to recognize when toys are broken and may hand them to their parents to fix. When tempted to touch a forbidden object, they may tell themselves "no, no." Language becomes a means of impulse control, early reasoning, and connection between ideas. This is the very beginning of the formation of a conscience. The fact that they often go on to touch the object anyway demonstrates the relative weakness of internalized inhibitions at this stage.

Linguistic Development

Perhaps the most dramatic developments in this period are linguistic. Labeling of objects coincides with the advent of symbolic thought. After the realization that words can stand for things occurs, a child's vocabulary balloons from 10-15 words at 18 mo to between 50 and 100 at 2 yr. After acquiring a vocabulary of about 50 words, toddlers begin to combine them to make simple sentences, the beginning of grammar. At this stage, toddlers understand **2-step commands,** such as "Give me the ball and then get your shoes." Language also gives the toddler a sense of control over the surroundings, as in "night-night" or "bye-bye." The emergence of verbal language marks the end of the sensory-motor period. As toddlers learn to use symbols to express ideas and solve problems, the need for cognition based on direct sensation and motor manipulation wanes.

Implications for Parents and Pediatricians

With children's increasing mobility, physical limits on their explorations become less effective; words become increasingly important for behavior control as well as cognition. Children with delayed language acquisition often have greater behavior problems and frustrations due to problems with communication. Language development is facilitated when parents and caregivers use clear, simple sentences; ask questions; and respond to children's incomplete sentences and gestural communication with the appropriate words. Television viewing decreases parent-child verbal interactions, whereas looking at picture books together provides an ideal context for language development.

In the office setting, certain procedures may lessen the child's **stranger anxiety.** Avoid direct eye contact initially. Perform as much of the examination as feasible with the child on the parent's lap. Pediatricians can help parents understand the resurgence of problems with separation and the appearance of a treasured blanket or teddy bear as a developmental phenomenon. Parents must understand the importance of exploration. Rather than limiting movement, parents should place toddlers in safe environments or substitute 1 activity for another. Methods of discipline, including corporal punishment, should be discussed; effective alternatives will usually be appreciated. Helping parents to understand and adapt to their children's different temperamental styles can constitute an important intervention (see Table 6-1). Developing daily routines is helpful to all children at this age. Rigidity in those routines reflects a need for mastery over a changing environment.

BIBLIOGRAPHY

Please visit the Nelson Textbook of Pediatrics *website at www.expertconsult.com for the complete bibliography.*

Chapter 10
The Preschool Years

Susan Feigelman

The critical milestones for children ages 2 to 5 yr are the emergence of language and exposure of children to an expanding social sphere. As toddlers, children learn to walk away and come back to the secure adult or parent. As preschoolers, they explore emotional separation, alternating between stubborn opposition and cheerful compliance, between bold exploration and clinging dependence. Increasing time spent in classrooms and playgrounds challenges a child's ability to adapt to new rules and relationships. Preschool children know that they can do more than ever before, but they also are increasingly cognizant of the constraints imposed on them by the adult world and their own limited abilities.

PHYSICAL DEVELOPMENT

Somatic and brain growth slows by the end of the 2nd yr of life, with corresponding decreases in nutritional requirements and appetite, and the emergence of "picky" eating habits (see Table 13-1). Increases of ~2 kg (4-5 lb) in weight and 7-8 cm (2-3 in) in height per yr are expected. Birthweight quadruples by 2½ yr of age. An average 4 yr old weighs 40 lb and is 40 in tall. The head will grow only an additional 5 cm between ages 3 and 18 yr. Current growth charts, with growth parameters, can be found on the Centers for Disease Control and Prevention website (*www.cdc.gov/nchs*) and in Chapter 13. Children with early adiposity rebound (increase in body mass index) are at increased risk for adult obesity.

Growth of sexual organs is commensurate with somatic growth. The preschooler has genu valgum (knock-knees) and mild pes planus (flatfoot). The torso slims as the legs lengthen. Physical energy peaks, and the need for sleep declines to 11-13 hr/24 hr, with the child eventually dropping the nap (see Fig. 8-1). Visual acuity reaches 20/30 by age 3 yr and 20/20 by age 4 yr. All 20 primary teeth have erupted by 3 yr of age (Chapter 299).

Most children walk with a mature gait and run steadily before the end of their 3rd yr (see Table 9-1). Beyond this basic level, there is wide variation in ability as the range of motor activities expands to include throwing, catching, and kicking balls; riding on bicycles; climbing on playground structures; dancing; and other complex pattern behaviors. Stylistic features of gross motor activity, such as tempo, intensity, and cautiousness, also vary significantly. Although toddlers may walk with different styles, toe walking should not persist.

The effects of such individual differences on cognitive and emotional development depend in part on the demands of the social environment. Energetic, coordinated children may thrive emotionally with parents or teachers who encourage physical activity; lower-energy, more cerebral children may thrive with adults who value quiet play.

Handedness is usually established by the 3rd yr. Frustration may result from attempts to change children's hand preference. Variations in fine motor development reflect both individual proclivities and different opportunities for learning. Children who are seldom allowed to use crayons, for example, develop a mature pencil grasp later.

Bowel and bladder control emerge during this period, with "readiness" for toileting having large individual and cultural variation. Girls tend to train faster and earlier than boys. Bedwetting is normal up to age 4 yr in girls and age 5 yr in boys (Chapter 21.3). Many children master toileting with ease, particularly once they are able to verbalize their bodily needs. For others, toilet training can involve a protracted power struggle. Refusal to defecate in the toilet or potty is relatively common and can lead to constipation and parental frustration. Defusing the issue with a temporary cessation of training (and a return to diapers) often allows toilet mastery to proceed.

Implications for Parents and Pediatricians

The normal decrease in appetite at this age may cause parental concern about nutrition; growth charts should reassure parents that the child's intake is adequate. Children normally modulate their food intake to match their somatic needs according to feelings of hunger and satiety. Daily intake fluctuates, at times widely, but intake during the period of a week is relatively stable. Parents should provide a predictable eating schedule, with 3 meals and 2 snacks per day, allowing the child to choose how much to eat.

Highly active children face increased risks of injury, and parents should be counseled about safety precautions. Parental concerns about possible hyperactivity may reflect inappropriate expectations, heightened fears, or true overactivity. Children who engage in impulsive activity with no apparent regard for personal safety should be evaluated further.

LANGUAGE, COGNITION, AND PLAY

These three domains all involve symbolic function, a mode of dealing with the world that emerges during the preschool period.

Language

Language development occurs most rapidly between 2 and 5 yr of age. Vocabulary increases from 50-100 words to more than 2,000. Sentence structure advances from telegraphic phrases ("Baby cry") to sentences incorporating all of the major grammatical components. As a rule of thumb, between the ages of 2 and 5 yr, the number of words in a typical sentence equals the child's age (2 by age 2 yr, 3 by age 3 yr, and so on). By 21 mo to 2 yr, most children are using possessives ("My ball"), progressives (the "-ing" construction, as in "I playing"), questions, and negatives. By age 4 yr, most children can count to 4 and use the past tense; by age 5 yr, they can use the future tense. Children do not use figurative speech; they will only comprehend the literal meaning of words. Referring to an object as "light as a feather" may produce a quizzical look on a child.

It is important to distinguish between *speech* (the production of intelligible sounds) and *language,* which refers to the underlying mental act. Language includes both expressive and receptive functions. Receptive language (understanding) varies less in its rate of acquisition than does expressive language; therefore, it has greater prognostic importance (Chapters 14 and 32).

Language acquisition depends critically on environmental input. Key determinants include the amount and variety of speech directed toward children and the frequency with which adults ask questions and encourage verbalization. Children raised in poverty typically perform lower on measures of language development compared to children from economically advantaged families.

Although experience influences the rate of language development, many linguists believe that the basic mechanism for language learning is "hard-wired" in the brain. Children do not simply imitate adult speech; they abstract the complex rules of grammar from the ambient language, generating implicit hypotheses. Evidence for the existence of such implicit rules comes from analysis of grammatical errors, such as the overgeneralized use of "-s" to signify the plural and "-ed" to signify the past ("We seed lots of mouses.").

Language is linked to both cognitive and emotional development. Language delays may be the first indication that a child has mental retardation, has an autism spectrum disorder, or has been maltreated. Language plays a critical part in the regulation of behavior through internalized "private speech" in which a child repeats adult prohibitions, first audibly and then mentally. Language also allows children to express feelings, such as anger or frustration, without acting them out; consequently, language-delayed children show higher rates of tantrums and other externalizing behaviors.

Preschool language development lays the foundation for later success in school. Approximately 35% of children in the USA may enter school lacking the language skills that are the prerequisites for acquiring literacy. Children from socially and economically disadvantaged backgrounds have an increased risk of school problems, making early detection, along with referral and enrichment, important. Although children typically learn to read and write in elementary school, critical foundations for literacy are established during the preschool years. Through repeated early exposure to written words, children learn about the uses of writing (telling stories or sending messages) and about its form (left to right, top to bottom). Early errors in writing, like errors in speaking, reveal that literacy acquisition is an active process involving the generation and revision of hypotheses. Programs such as Head Start are especially important for improving language skills for children from bilingual homes. (Such parents should be reassured that although bilingual children do initially lag behind their monolingual peers in acquiring language over time, they learn the differing rules governing both languages. Bilingual children do not follow the same course of language development as monolingual children, but create a different system of language cues. Several cognitive advantages have been repeatedly demonstrated among bilingual compared to monolingual children.)

Picture books have a special role not only in familiarizing young children with the printed word but also in the development of verbal language. Children's vocabulary and receptive language improve when their parents consistently read to them. Reading aloud with a young child is an interactive process in which a parent repeatedly focuses the child's attention on a particular picture, asks questions, and then gives the child feedback. The elements of shared attention, active participation, immediate feedback, repetition, and graduated difficulty make such routines ideal for language learning. Programs in which physicians provide books to preschool children have shown improvement in language skills among the children.

The period of rapid language acquisition is also when **developmental dysfluency** and **stuttering** are most likely to emerge; these can be traced to activation of the cortical motor, sensory, and cerebellar areas. Common difficulties include pauses and repetitions of initial sounds. Stress or excitement exacerbates these difficulties, which generally resolve on their own. Although 5% of preschool children will stutter, it will resolve in 80% by age 8 yr. Children with stuttering should be referred for evaluation if it is severe, persistent, or associated with anxiety, or if parental concern is elicited. **Treatment** includes guidance to parents to reduce pressures associated with speaking.

Cognition

The preschool period corresponds to Piaget's preoperational (prelogical) stage, characterized by **magical thinking, egocentrism,** and **thinking that is dominated by perception,** not abstraction (see Table 6-2). Magical thinking includes confusing coincidence with causality, animism (attributing motivations to inanimate objects and events), and unrealistic beliefs about the power of wishes. A child might believe that people cause it to rain by carrying umbrellas, that the sun goes down because it is tired, or that feeling resentment toward a sibling can actually make that sibling sick. Egocentrism refers to a child's inability to take another's point of view and does not connote selfishness. A child might try to comfort an adult who is upset by bringing him or her a favorite stuffed animal. After 2 yr of age, the child develops a concept of herself or himself as an individual and senses the need to feel "whole."

Piaget demonstrated the dominance of perception over logic. In one experiment, water is poured back and forth between a tall, thin vase and a low, wide dish, and children are asked which container has more water. Invariably, they choose the one that looks larger (usually the tall vase), even when the examiner points out that no water has been added or taken away. Such misunderstandings reflect young children's developing hypotheses about the nature of the world as well as their difficulty in attending simultaneously to multiple aspects of a situation.

Recent work indicating that preschool children do have the ability to understand some causal relationships has modified our understanding of the ability of preschool children to engage in some abstract thinking.

Play

Maria Montessori considered play to be the work of childhood, but she did not lend credence to the importance of fantasy and imagination (symbolic play). Play involves learning, physical activity, socialization with peers, and practicing adult roles. Play increases in complexity and imagination, from simple imitation of common experiences, such as shopping and putting baby to bed (2 or 3 yr of age), to more extended scenarios involving singular events, such as going to the zoo or going on a trip (3 or 4 yr of age), to the creation of scenarios that have only been imagined, such as flying to the moon (4 or 5 yr of age). By age 3 yr, cooperative play is seen in activities such as building a tower of blocks together; later, more structured role-play activity, as in playing house, is seen. Play also becomes increasingly governed by rules, from early rules about asking (rather than taking) and sharing (2 or 3 yr of age), to rules that change from moment to moment, according to the desires of the players (4 and 5 yr of age), to the beginning of the recognition of rules as relatively immutable (5 yr of age and beyond).

Play also allows for resolution of conflicts and anxiety and for creative outlets. Children can vent anger safely (spanking a doll), take on superpowers (dinosaur and superhero play), and obtain things that are denied in real life (a make-believe friend or stuffed animal). Creativity is particularly apparent in drawing, painting, and other artistic activities. Themes and emotions that emerge in a child's drawings often reflect the emotional issues of greatest importance for the child.

Difficulty distinguishing fantasy from reality colors a child's perception of what he or she views in the media, through programming and advertising. One fourth of young children have a television set in their bedroom and watch many hours of television per week, and much of what they view is violent. Attitudes about violence are formed early, and early exposure has been associated with later behavior problems.

Implications for Parents and Pediatricians

The significance of language as a target for assessment and intervention cannot be overestimated because of its central role as an indicator of cognitive and emotional development and a key factor in behavioral regulation and later school success. As language emerges, parents can support emotional development by using words that describe the child's feeling states ("You sound angry right now.") and urging the child to use words to express, rather than act out, feelings. Active imaginations will come into play when children offer explanations for misbehavior. A parent's best way of dealing with untruths is to address the event, not the child, and have the child participate in making things right.

Parents should have a regular time each day for reading or looking at books with their children. Programs such as Reach Out and Read, in which pediatricians give out picture books along with appropriate guidance during primary care visits, have been effective in increasing reading aloud and thereby promoting language development, particularly in lower-income families. Television and similar media should be limited to 2 hr/day of quality programming, and parents should be watching the programs with their children and debriefing their young children afterward. At-risk children, particularly those living in poverty, can better meet future school challenges if they have early high-quality experiences, such as Head Start.

Preoperational thinking constrains how children understand experiences of illness and treatment. Children begin to understand that bodies have "insides" and "outsides." Children should be given simple, concrete explanations for medical procedures and given some control over procedures if possible. Children should be reassured that they are not to blame when receiving a vaccine or venipuncture. An adhesive bandage will help to make the body whole again in a child's mind.

The active imagination that fuels play and the magical, animist thinking characteristic of preoperational cognition can also generate intense fears. More than 80% of parents report at least 1 fear in their preschool children. Refusal to take baths or to sit on the toilet may arise from the fear of being washed or flushed away, reflecting a child's immature appreciation of relative size. Attempts to demonstrate rationally that there are no monsters in the closet often fail, inasmuch as the fear arises from prerational thinking. However, this same thinking allows parents to be endowed with magical powers that can banish the monsters with "monster spray" or a night light. Parents should acknowledge the fears, offer reassurance and a sense of security, and give the child some sense of control over the situation. Use of the Draw-a-Person, in which a child is asked to draw the best person he or she can, may help elucidate a child's viewpoint.

EMOTIONAL AND MORAL DEVELOPMENT

Emotional challenges facing preschool children include accepting limits while maintaining a sense of self-direction, reining in aggressive and sexual impulses, and interacting with a widening circle of adults and peers. At 2 yr of age, behavioral limits are predominantly external; by 5 yr of age, these controls need to be internalized if a child is to function in a typical classroom. Success in achieving this goal relies on prior emotional development, particularly the ability to use internalized images of trusted adults to provide a secure environment in times of stress. The love a child feels for important adults is the main incentive for the development of self-control.

Children learn what behaviors are acceptable and how much power they wield vis-à-vis important adults by testing limits. Testing increases when it elicits attention, even though that attention is often negative, and when limits are inconsistent. Testing often arouses parental anger or inappropriate solicitude as a child struggles to separate, and it gives rise to a corresponding parental challenge: letting go. Excessively tight limits can undermine a child's sense of initiative, whereas overly loose limits can provoke anxiety in a child who feels that no one is in control.

Control is a central issue. Young children cannot control many aspects of their lives, including where they go, how long they stay, and what they take home from the store. They are also prone to lose internal control, that is, to have temper tantrums. Fear, overtiredness, inconsistent expectations, or physical discomfort can also evoke tantrums. Tantrums normally appear toward the end of the 1st yr of life and peak in prevalence between 2 and 4 yr of age. Tantrums lasting more than 15 min or regularly occurring more than 3 times/day may reflect underlying medical, emotional, or social problems.

Preschool children normally experience complicated feelings toward their parents that can include strong attachment and possessiveness toward the parent of the opposite sex, jealousy and resentment of the other parent, and fear that these negative feelings might lead to abandonment. These emotions, most of which are beyond a child's ability to comprehend or verbalize, often find expression in highly labile moods. The resolution of this crisis (a process extending over years) involves a child's unspoken decision to identify with the parents rather than compete with them. Play and language foster the development of emotional controls by allowing children to express emotions and role-play.

Curiosity about genitals and adult sexual organs is normal, as is masturbation. Excessive masturbation interfering with normal activity, acting out sexual intercourse, extreme modesty, or mimicry of adult seductive behavior all suggests the possibility of sexual abuse or inappropriate exposure (Chapter 37.1). Modesty appears gradually between 4 and 6 yr of age, with wide variations among cultures and families. Parents should begin to teach children about "private" areas before school entry.

Moral thinking is constrained by a child's cognitive level and language abilities, but develops as the child continues her or his identity with the parents. Beginning before the 2nd birthday, the child's sense of right and wrong stems from the desire to earn approval from the parents and avoid negative consequences. The child's impulses are tempered by external forces; she or he has not yet internalized societal rules or a sense of justice and fairness. Over time, as the child internalizes parental admonitions, words are substituted for aggressive behaviors. Finally, the child accepts personal responsibility. Actions will be viewed by damage caused, not by intent. Empathic responses to others' distress arise during the 2nd yr of life, but the ability to consider another child's point of view remains limited throughout this period. In keeping with a child's inability to focus on more than 1 aspect of a situation at a time, fairness is taken to mean equal treatment, regardless of circumstance. A 4 yr old will acknowledge the importance of taking turns, but will complain if he didn't get enough time. Rules tend to be absolute, with guilt assigned for bad outcomes, regardless of intentions.

Implications for Parents and Pediatricians

The importance of the preschooler's sense of control over his or her body and surroundings has implications for practice. Preparing the patient by letting the child know how the visit will proceed is reassuring. Tell the child what will happen, but don't ask permission unless you are willing to deal with a "no" answer. A brief introduction to "private parts" is warranted before the genital examination.

The visit of the 4 or 5 yr old should be entertaining, because of the child's ability to communicate, as well as his or her natural curiosity. Physicians should realize that all children are occasionally difficult. Guidance emphasizing appropriate expectations for behavioral and emotional development and acknowledging normal parental feelings of anger, guilt, and confusion should be part of all visits at this time. Parents should be queried about daily routines and their expectations of child behavior. Providing children with choices (all options being acceptable to the parent) and encouraging independence in self-care activities (feeding, dressing, and bathing) will reduce conflicts.

Although some cultures condone the use of corporal punishment for disciplining of young children, it is not an effective means of behavioral control. As children habituate to repeated spanking, parents have to spank ever harder to get the desired response, increasing the risk of serious injury. Sufficiently harsh punishment may inhibit undesired behaviors, but at great psychologic cost. Children mimic the corporal punishment that they receive, and it is common for preschool children to strike their parents or other children. Whereas spanking is the use of force, externally applied, to produce behavior change, **discipline** is the process that allows the child to internalize controls on behavior. Alternative discipline strategies should be offered, such as the "countdown," along with consistent limit setting, clear communication of rules, and frequent approval. Discipline should be immediate, specific to the behavior, and time-limited. Time-out for approximately 1 min/yr of age is very effective. A kitchen timer allows the parent to step back from the situation; the child is free when the timer rings.

BIBLIOGRAPHY

Please visit the Nelson Textbook of Pediatrics *website at* *www.expertconsult.com* *for the complete bibliography.*

Chapter 11
Middle Childhood

Susan Feigelman

Middle childhood (6-11 yr of age), previously referred to as *latency*, is the period during which children increasingly separate from parents and seek acceptance from teachers, other adults, and peers. Self-esteem becomes a central issue, as children develop the cognitive ability to consider their own self-evaluations and their perception of how others see them. For the first time, they are judged according to their ability to produce socially valued outputs, such as getting good grades, playing a musical instrument, or hitting home runs. Children are under pressure to conform to the style and ideals of the peer group.

PHYSICAL DEVELOPMENT

Growth during the period averages 3-3.5 kg (7 lb) and 6-7 cm (2.5 in) per year (see Figs. 9-1 and 9-2 on the *Nelson Textbook of Pediatrics* website at www.expertconsult.com). Growth occurs **discontinuously**, in 3-6 irregularly timed spurts each year, but varies both within and among individuals. The head grows only 2-3 cm in circumference throughout the entire period, reflecting a slowing of brain growth. Myelinization is complete by 7 yr of age. Body habitus is more erect than previously, with long legs compared with the torso.

Growth of the midface and lower face occurs gradually. Loss of deciduous (baby) teeth is a more dramatic sign of maturation, beginning around 6 yr of age. Replacement with adult teeth occurs at a rate of about 4 per year, so that by age 9 yr, children will have 8 permanent incisors and 4 permanent molars. Premolars erupt by 11-12 yr of age (Chapter 299). Lymphoid tissues hypertrophy, often giving rise to impressive tonsils and adenoids.

Muscular strength, coordination, and stamina increase progressively, as does the ability to perform complex movements, such as dancing or shooting baskets. Such higher-order motor skills are the result of both maturation and training; the degree of accomplishment reflects wide variability in innate skill, interest, and opportunity.

There has been a general decline in physical fitness among school-aged children. Sedentary habits at this age are associated with increased lifetime risk of obesity and cardiovascular disease (Chapter 44). The number of overweight children and the degree of overweight are both increasing; although the proportion of overweight children of all ages has increased over the last half century, this rate has increased over four-fold among children ages 6-11 yr (Table 11-1). Only 8% of middle and junior high schools require daily physical education class. One quarter of youth do not engage in any free-time physical activity, whereas the recommendation is for 1 hr of physical activity per day.

Perceptions of body image develop early during this period; children as young as 5 and 6 yr express dissatisfaction with their body image; by ages 8 and 9 yr many of these youth report

Table 11-1 PERCENT OVERWEIGHT INDIVIDUALS AMONG CHILDREN AND ADOLESCENTS AGES 2-19 YR, FOR SELECTED YR 1963-1965 THROUGH 1999-2002

AGE (YEARS)	NHANES 1963-1965 1966-1970	NHANES 1971-1974	NHANES 1976-1980	NHANES 1988-1994	NHANES 1999-2000	NHANES 2001-2002	NHANES 2003-2004
2-5	—	5	5	7.2	10.3	10.6	13.9
6-11	4.2	4	6.5	11.3	15.1	16.3	18.8
12-19	4.6	6.1	5	10.5	14.8	16.7	17.4

From National Center for Health Statistics and Monitoring the Nation's Health: *Fact sheet, Table 1* (website). http://www.cdc.gov/nchs/data/hestats/overweight/overweight_child_03.htm#Table1.

trying to diet, often using ill-advised regimens. Loss of control (binge) eating occurs among approximately 6% of children of this age.

Prior to puberty, the sensitivity of the hypothalamus and the pituitary changes, leading to increased gonadotropin synthesis. For most children, the sexual organs remain physically immature, but interest in gender differences and sexual behavior remains active in many children and increases progressively until puberty. Although this is a period when sexual drives are limited, masturbation is common, and children may be interested in differences between genders. Though still somewhat controversial, there is growing consensus that breast development and menarche are occurring at an earlier age among girls in the USA. Rates of maturation differ by geography, ethnicity, and country. These differences in maturation have implications for differing expectations of others about them based on sexual maturation.

Implications for Parents and Pediatricians

Middle childhood is generally a time of excellent health. However, children have variable sizes, shapes, and abilities. Children of this age compare themselves with others, eliciting feelings about their physical attributes and abilities. Fears of being "defective" can lead to avoidance of situations in which physical differences might be revealed, such as gym class or medical examinations. Children with actual physical disabilities may face special stresses. Medical, social, and psychologic risks tend to occur together.

Children should be asked about regular physical activity. Participation in organized sports or other organized activities can foster skill, teamwork, and fitness, as well as a sense of accomplishment, but pressure to compete when the activity is no longer enjoyable has negative effects. Prepubertal children should not engage in high-stress, high-impact sports, such as power lifting or tackle football, because skeletal immaturity increases the risk of injury.

COGNITIVE DEVELOPMENT

The thinking of early elementary school-aged children differs qualitatively from that of preschool children. In place of magical, egocentric, and perception-bound cognition, school-aged children increasingly apply rules based on observable phenomena, factor in multiple dimensions and points of view, and interpret their perceptions using physical laws. Piaget documented this shift from *"preoperational"* to *"concrete logical operations."* When 5 yr olds watch a ball of clay being rolled into a snake, they might insist that the snake has "more" because it is longer. In contrast, 7 yr olds typically reply that the ball and the snake must weigh the same because nothing has been added or taken away or because the snake is both longer and thinner. This cognitive reorganization occurs at different rates in different contexts. In the context of social interactions with siblings, young children often demonstrate an ability to understand alternate points of view long before they demonstrate that ability in their thinking about the physical world. Understanding time and space constructs occurs in the later part of this period.

The concept of **"school readiness"** is controversial. There is no consensus on whether there is a defined set of skills needed for success on school entry, and whether certain skills predict later achievement. By age 5 yr, most children have the ability to learn in a school setting, as long as the setting is sufficiently flexible to support children with a variety of developmental achievements. Rather than delaying school entry, high quality early education programs may be the key to ultimate school success. Separation anxiety, or school refusal, is common in the early school years.

School makes increasing cognitive demands on the child. Mastery of the elementary curriculum requires that a large number of perceptual, cognitive, and language processes work efficiently (Table 11-2), and children are expected to attend to many inputs at once. The first 2 to 3 yr of elementary school is devoted to acquiring the fundamentals: reading, writing, and basic mathematics skills. By 3rd grade, children need to be able to sustain attention through a 45 min period and the curriculum requires more complex tasks. The goal of reading a paragraph is no longer to decode the words, but to understand the content; the goal of writing is no longer spelling or penmanship, but composition. The volume of work increases along with the complexity.

Cognitive abilities interact with a wide array of attitudinal and emotional factors in determining classroom performance. These factors include external rewards (eagerness to please adults and

Table 11-2 SELECTED PERCEPTUAL, COGNITIVE, AND LANGUAGE PROCESSES REQUIRED FOR ELEMENTARY SCHOOL SUCCESS

PROCESS	DESCRIPTION	ASSOCIATED PROBLEMS
PERCEPTUAL		
Visual analysis	Ability to break a complex figure into components and understand their spatial relationships	Persistent letter confusion (e.g., between *b*, *d*, and *g*); difficulty with basic reading and writing and limited "sight" vocabulary
Proprioception and motor control	Ability to obtain information about body position by feel and unconsciously program complex movements	Poor handwriting, requiring inordinate effort, often with overly tight pencil grasp; special difficulty with timed tasks
Phonologic processing	Ability to perceive differences between similar sounding words and to break down words into constituent sounds	Delayed receptive language skill; attention and behavior problems secondary to not understanding directions; delayed acquisition of letter-sound correlations (phonetics)
COGNITIVE		
Long-term memory, both storage and recall	Ability to acquire skills that are "automatic" (i.e., accessible without conscious thought)	Delayed mastery of the alphabet (reading and writing letters); slow handwriting; inability to progress beyond basic mathematics
Selective attention	Ability to attend to important stimuli and ignore distractions	Difficulty following multistep instructions, completing assignments, and behaving well; problems with peer interaction
Sequencing	Ability to remember things in order; facility with time concepts	Difficulty organizing assignments, planning, spelling, and telling time
LANGUAGE		
Receptive language	Ability to comprehend complex constructions, function words (e.g., if, when, only, except), nuances of speech, and extended blocks of language (e.g., paragraphs)	Difficulty following directions; wandering attention during lessons and stories; problems with reading comprehension; problems with peer relationships
Expressive language	Ability to recall required words effortlessly (word finding), control meanings by varying position and word endings, and construct meaningful paragraphs and stories	Difficulty expressing feelings and using words for self-defense, with resulting frustration and physical acting out; struggling during "circle time" and in language-based subjects (e.g., English)

approval from peers) and internal rewards (competitiveness, willingness to work for a delayed reward, belief in one's abilities, and ability to risk trying when success is not ensured). Success predisposes to success, whereas failure impacts self-esteem and reduces self-efficacy, diminishing a child's ability to take future risks.

Children's intellectual activity extends beyond the classroom. Beginning in the 3rd or 4th grade, children increasingly enjoy strategy games and wordplay (puns and insults) that exercise their growing cognitive and linguistic mastery. Many become experts on subjects of their own choosing, such as sports trivia, or develop hobbies, such as special card collections. Others become avid readers or take on artistic pursuits. Whereas board and card games were once the usual leisure time activity of youth, video and computer games currently fill this need.

Implications for Parents and Pediatricians

Concrete operations allow children to understand simple explanations for illnesses and necessary treatments, although they may revert to prelogical thinking when under stress. A child with pneumonia may be able to explain about white cells fighting the "germs" in the lungs, but still secretly harbors the belief that the sickness is a punishment for disobedience.

As children are faced with more abstract concepts, academic and classroom behavior problems emerge and come to the pediatrician's attention. Referrals may be made to the school for remediation or to community resources (medical or psychologic) when appropriate. The causes may be one or more of the following: deficits in perception (vision and hearing); specific learning disabilities; global cognitive delay (mental retardation); primary attention deficit; and attention deficits secondary to family dysfunction, depression, anxiety, or chronic illness (Chapters 14 and 29). Children whose learning style does not fit the classroom culture may have academic difficulties and need assessment before failure sets in. Simply having a child repeat a failed grade rarely has any beneficial effect and often seriously undercuts the child's self-esteem. In addition to finding the problem areas, identifying each child's strengths is important. Educational approaches that value a wide range of talents ("multiple intelligences") beyond the traditional ones of reading, writing, and mathematics may allow more children to succeed.

The change in cognition allows the child to understand "if/when" clauses. Increased responsibilities and expectations accompany increased rights and privileges. Discipline strategies should move toward negotiation and a clear understanding of consequences, including removal of privileges for infringements.

SOCIAL, EMOTIONAL, AND MORAL DEVELOPMENT

Social and Emotional Development

In this period energy is directed toward creativity and productivity. The central Ericksonian psychosocial issue, the crisis between industry and inferiority, guides social and emotional development. Changes occur in three spheres: the home, the school, and the neighborhood. Of these, the home and family remain the most influential. Increasing independence is marked by the 1st sleepover at a friend's house and the 1st time at overnight camp. Parents should make demands for effort in school and extracurricular activities, celebrate successes, and offer unconditional acceptance when failures occur. Regular chores, associated with an allowance, provide an opportunity for children to contribute to family functioning and learn the value of money. These responsibilities may be a testing ground for psychologic separation, leading to conflict. Siblings have critical roles as competitors, loyal supporters, and role models.

The beginning of school coincides with a child's further separation from the family and the increasing importance of teacher and peer relationships. Social groups tend to be same-sex, with frequent changing of membership, contributing to a child's growing social development and competence. Popularity, a central ingredient of self-esteem, may be won through possessions (having the latest electronic gadgets or the right clothes) as well as through personal attractiveness, accomplishments, and actual social skills. Children are aware of racial differences and are beginning to form opinions about racial groups that impact their relationships.

Some children conform readily to the peer norms and enjoy easy social success. Those who adopt individualistic styles or have visible differences may be teased. Such children may be painfully aware that they are different, or they may be puzzled by their lack of popularity. Children with deficits in social skills may go to extreme lengths to win acceptance, only to meet with repeated failure. Attributions conferred by peers, such as funny, stupid, bad, or fat, may become incorporated into a child's self-image and affect the child's personality, as well as school performance. Parents may have their greatest effect indirectly, through actions that change the peer group (moving to a new community or insisting on involvement in structured after-school activities).

In the neighborhood, real dangers, such as busy streets, bullies, and strangers, tax school-aged children's common sense and resourcefulness. Interactions with peers without close adult supervision call on increasing conflict resolution or pugilistic skills. Media exposure to adult materialism, sexuality, and violence may be frightening, reinforcing children's feeling of powerlessness in the larger world. Compensatory fantasies of being powerful may fuel the fascination with heroes and superheroes. A balance between fantasy and an appropriate ability to negotiate real-world challenges indicates healthy emotional development.

Moral Development

By the age of 5 or 6 yr, the child has developed a conscience, meaning that he or she has internalized the rules of the society. She or he can distinguish right from wrong, but may take context and motivation into account. Children will adopt family and community values, seeking approval of peers, parents, and other adult role models. Social conventions are important, even though the reason behind some rules may not be understood. Initially, children have a rigid sense of morality, relying on clear rules for themselves and others. By age 10 yr, most children understand fairness as reciprocity (treat others as you wish to be treated).

Implications for Parents and Pediatricians

Children need unconditional support as well as realistic demands as they venture into a world that is often frightening. A daily query from parents over the dinner table or at bedtime about the good and bad things that happened during the child's day may uncover problems early. Parents may have difficulty allowing the child independence or may exert excessive pressure on their children to achieve academic or competitive success. Children who struggle to meet such expectations may have behavior problems or psychosomatic complaints.

Many children face stressors that exceed the normal challenges of separation and success in school and the neighborhood. Divorce affects nearly 50% of children. Domestic violence, parental substance abuse, and other mental health problems may also impair a child's ability to use home as a secure base for refueling emotional energies. In many neighborhoods, random violence makes the normal development of independence extremely dangerous. Older children may join gangs as a means of self-protection and a way to attain recognition and belong to a cohesive group. Children who bully others, and/or are victims of bullying, should be evaluated, since this behavior is associated with mood disorders, family problems, and school adjustment problems. Parents should reduce exposure to hazards where possible. Due to the risk of unintentional firearm injuries to children, parents should be encouraged to ask parents of playmates whether a gun is kept in their home and, if so, how it is secured. The high prevalence of adjustment disorders among school-aged children attests to the effects of such overwhelming stressors on development.

Pediatrician visits are infrequent in this period; therefore, each visit is an opportunity to assess children's functioning in all contexts (home, school, neighborhood). Maladaptive behaviors, both internalizing and externalizing, occur when stress in any of these environments overwhelms the child's coping responses. Due to continuous exposure and the strong influence of media (programming and advertisements) on children's beliefs and attitudes, parents must be alert to exposures from the television and Internet. An average American youth spends over 6 hr/day with a variety of media, and ⅔ of these children have a television in their bedrooms. Parents should be advised to remove the television from their children's rooms, limit viewing to 2 hr/day, and monitor what programs children watch. The Draw-a-Person (for ages 3-10 yr, with instructions to "draw a complete person") and Kinetic Family Drawing (beginning at age 5 yr, with instructions to "draw a picture of everyone in your family doing something") are useful office tools to assess a child's functioning.

BIBLIOGRAPHY

Please visit the Nelson Textbook of Pediatrics *website at www.expertconsult.com for the complete bibliography.*

Chapter 12
Adolesence

See Part XIII, Chapter 104 on Adolescent Development.

Chapter 13
Assessment of Growth

Virginia Keane

A critical component of pediatric health surveillance is the assessment of a child's growth. Growth results from the interaction of genetics, health, and nutrition. Many biophysiologic and psychosocial problems can adversely affect growth, and aberrant growth may be the first sign of an underlying problem. The most powerful tool in growth assessment is the growth chart (see Figs. 9-1, 9-2, and 13-1 on the *Nelson Textbook of Pediatrics* website at www.expertconsult.com) used in combination with accurate measurements of height, weight, head circumference, and calculation of the body mass index (BMI).

For the full continuation of this chapter, please visit the Nelson Textbook of Pediatrics *website at www.expertconsult.com.*

Chapter 14
Developmental-Behavioral Screening and Surveillance

Frances P. Glascoe and Kevin P. Marks

Developmental-behavioral problems are the most common conditions of childhood and adolescence. When combined with school failure and high school drop-out rates, prevalence reaches 1 in 4 to 1 in 5 children. In inner-city low-income settings, drop-out rates often reach as high as 50%. If intervention is instituted prior to school entrance, many problems can be prevented, and all can be ameliorated. The Individuals with Disabilities Education Act (IDEA) coupled with the Head Start Act ensure a free national system to locate and treat young children deemed at risk for developmental-behavioral problems or who have established delays. Early intervention depends on early detection performed by primary care providers.

Many young children at risk for school failure lack measurable delays but have markers in the form of multiple psychosocial risk factors that are strong predictors of future problems. Measurable delays are common in children with a history of abuse or neglect. High-risk psychosocial factors are frequently found in foster children and warrant an automatic referral (no screen required) to an IDEA program. Other psychosocial risks include parents with less than a high school education, parental mental health problems (depression or anxiety), housing and food instability, ethnic or linguistic minority, ≥3 children in the home, or an authoritarian parenting style (e.g., highly directive, rarely engaging verbally in children's unique interests, punitive). Such risks, with or without apparent delays, often result in children being held back in grade, dropping out of high school, teen pregnancy, unemployment, drug abuse, or criminality. Early intervention reverses this cycle. Access to programs such as Head Start/Early Head Start for most children with psychosocial risk factors is based on federal poverty guidelines. Families often need parent training mental health referrals, housing, and social work services. Older children with risk factors, benefit from drop-out prevention assistance, including after-school tutoring, Boys and Girls Club, summer academic programs, and mentoring.

Of children with measurable delays or disabilities, the most common (and least well-identified) condition is speech-language impairment (17.5% at 30-36 mo) (Chapter 32), Other common conditions are social-emotional disorders (9.5-14.2%), attention-deficit/hyperactivity disorder (7.8%) (Chapter 30), learning disabilities (6.5%), intellectual disabilities (1.2%) (Chapter 33), and autism spectrum disorders (0.6-1.1%) (Chapter 28). Less common conditions include cerebral palsy (physical impairments) (0.23%) (Chapter 591.1), hearing impairment (0.12%), vision impairment (0.8%) (Chapter 613), and other forms of health or physical impairments (e.g., Down syndrome, fragile X syndrome, traumatic brain injury). Early detection of emerging deficits among very young children typically requires clinicians to screen with tools proven to be accurate.

Despite the serious long-term consequences of delays and disabilities, at young ages, children's problems are often so subtle that clinical judgment is ineffective. In addition, many children with developmental deficits present with behavior problems first. In all cases and at all well visits, screening with accurate tools is the only way to identify problems, discern developmental from behavioral/mental health issues, and thus make wise decisions about needed referrals.

Very young children with delays, (i.e., birth to 3 yr of age) do not require a specific diagnosis to receive IDEA services. They are eligible under *developmental delay*, defined as a 25% departure from typical performance in ≥2 developmental domains (e.g., receptive language, expressive language, fine motor, gross motor, social-emotional, cognitive/pre-academic, and behavior). Primary care providers need not make a diagnosis in very young children but instead should focus on detection and referral to IDEA programs. Nevertheless, clinicians can simultaneously refer to subspecialty services, particularly when autism spectrum disorder is suspected. Children over the age of 3 yr are served and tested by the public schools psychologists, and speech-language pathologists will define disabilities more discretely.

EARLY DETECTION IN PRIMARY CARE

Only about 25% of children with developmental delays are detected prior to school entrance, meaning that most children with problems will have missed opportunities for early intervention. Although clinicians are effective at detecting severe disabilities associated with congenital, metabolic, or genetic abnormalities, providers are far less adept at discerning the more common conditions because these typically lack overt dysmorphology.

Reasons for underdetection in primary care include (1) dependence on nonstandard administration of standardized screens (including selected items from longer measures) and informal milestones checklists; both approaches lack proof of validity and criteria for making accurate decisions; (2) failure to continually check on developmental progress; (3) clinical judgment (because it tends to depend heavily on dysmorphology and organicity, which are not present in the majority of children with disabilities); (4) requirement of repeated screening test failure before making a referral (due to lack of awareness that quality screening measures are highly reliable and that a repeated screen is likely to yield identical results); (5) false optimism about outcome (children rarely outgrow developmental problems in the absence of intervention); (6) discomfort at delivering difficult news; (7) lack of familiarity with tools effective for busy primary care settings; and (8) problematic reimbursement for screening services (generally due to insurance non-reimbursement policies or ineffective use of procedure codes).

To improve better detection in primary care, the American Academy of Pediatrics recommends developmental screening and surveillance at well visits. **Developmental screening** refers to the administration of brief, standardized, and validated instruments that have been researched for their *sensitivity* in detecting children with probable problems and *specificity* in determining when children probably do not have problems. Standards for screening test accuracy are 70-80% sensitivity and specificity. Although these figures are low compared to standards for most medical screens, developmental problems develop over time. Repeated screening is expected to compensate for underdetection of what is essentially a "moving target." Over-referrals are less concerning because research shows that most children with false-positive screens, while ineligible for special education services, are nevertheless in need of remedial programs (e.g., Head Start, after-school tutoring, summer school, and quality preschool or day care), due to psychosocial risk factors, including poverty and limited maternal education and below-average performance in the better predictors of school success (i.e., language, intelligence, and academic/pre-academic skills).

In addition to repeated developmental screening, physicians are also encouraged to practice developmental surveillance at each well visit. **Developmental surveillance** provides a context for screening results and involves scrutinizing family functioning and risk factors, observing longitudinally child behavior and developmental skills, eliciting and attending to parents' concerns, and deploying knowledge of children's medical history. Information obtained through surveillance should never be used to override a positive screening test result, but it can be used to elevate suspicions about negative screening results. Surveillance is essential for determining service needs and for selecting optimal methods to help parents promote positive development through written materials, hands-on parent training, and/or social work services.

Screening and surveillance must use quality measures to ensure accurate detection. Fortunately, many tools serve both functions. Table 14-1 shows a range of screens useful for early detection of developmental and behavioral problems including autism spectrum disorders. Because well visits are brief and have enormous agendas (physical exams, immunizations, anticipatory guidance, safety and injury prevention counseling, and developmental promotion), tools relying on information from parents are ideal because they can be completed in advance of appointments, online, or in waiting or exam rooms.

Table 14-2 provides a step-by-step process of evidence-based screening and surveillance. The sequence is based on the American Academy of Pediatrics 2006 policy statement (with enhancements added to the referral and follow-up process).

RESOURCES FOR SCREENING, NONMEDICAL REFERRAL, AND DEVELOPMENTAL PROMOTION

American Academy of Pediatrics' Section on Developmental and Behavioral Pediatrics provides information on screening, rationale, implementation, etc. *www.dbpeds.org*

National Early Childhood Technical Assistance Center provides links to early intervention and public school services in each state, region, and community. *www.nectac.org*

Websites with information on coding, reimbursement, advocacy assistance with denied claims. *www.coding.aap.org and www.pedstest.com*

Guidance on establishing a medical home for children with special needs. *www.medicalhomeinfo.org*

American Academy of Pediatrics, policy statement on developmental screening and surveillance. *http://aappolicy.aappublications.org*

Centers for Disease Control and Prevention, Using Developmental Screening to Improve Children's Health: offers information on the value of screening with links to research and services, and wall charts on milestones. *www.cdc.gov/ncbddd/actearly*

Guidelines and information on Bright Futures guidelines for providing comprehensive health supervision services, case-based learning examples, etc. *www.brightfutures.org*

Slide shows and other materials for teaching screening measures, a trial of online developmental-behavioral and autism screens, parent education handouts, and an early detection discussion list. *www.pedstest.com*

Implementation guidance and research, with an excellent video of pediatricians and a hospital administrator at Harvard University showing opinions about screening before and after implementing a quality tool. *www.developmentalscreening.org and www.pedstest.com*

Help locating Head Start and Early Head Start programs. *www.ehsnrc.org*

Find quality preschool and day care programs. *www.childcareaware.org and www.naeyc.org*

Information on parent training programs and the YWCA. *www.patnc.org and www.ywca.org*

Help locating mental health services. *www.mentalhealth.org*

Find services and information about autistic spectrum disorders. *www.firstsigns.org.*

Downloadable parenting information handouts. *www.kidshealth.org*

Locate social services addressing domestic violence, housing and food instability, child abuse and neglect, adoption, state, and local services, etc. *www.acf.hhs.gov*

Reach Out and Read (parenting information and guidance for providers on how to implement this highly effective approach to in-office developmental promotion). *www.reachoutandread.org*

BIBLIOGRAPHY

Please visit the Nelson Textbook of Pediatrics *website at www.expertconsult.com for the complete bibliography.*

Table 14-1 TOOLS FOR DEVELOPMENTAL-BEHAVIORAL SCREENING AND SURVEILLANCE

The following chart is a list of measures meeting standards for screening test accuracy, meaning that they correctly identify, at all ages, at least 70-80% of children with disabilities while also correctly identifying at least 70-80% children without disabilities. All listed measures were standardized on national samples, proven to be reliable, and validated against a range of diagnostic measures and diagnosed conditions. Not included are measures such as the Denver-II that fail to meet psychometric standards (limited standardization, absent validation, problematic sensitivity and specificity).

The first column provides publication information and the cost of purchasing a specimen set. The "Description" column provides information on alternative ways, if available, to administer measures (e.g., waiting rooms). The "Accuracy" column shows the percentage of patients with and without problems identified correctly. The "Time Frame/Costs" column shows the costs of materials per visit, along with the costs of professional time (using an average salary of $50 per hour) needed to administer each measure, but does not include time needed for generating referral letters. For parent-report tools, administration time reflects not only scoring of test results, but also the relationship between each test's reading level and the percentage of parents with less than a high school education (who may or may not be able to complete measures in waiting rooms due to literacy problems and thus will need interview administrations).

BEHAVIORAL AND/OR DEVELOPMENTAL SCREENS RELYING ON INFORMATION FROM PARENTS	AGE RANGE	DESCRIPTION	SCORING	ACCURACY	TIME FRAME/COSTS*
Parents' Evaluations of Developmental Status (PEDS). (2010). PEDS*Test*.com, LLC, 1013 Austin Court, Nolensville, TN 37135 Phone: 615-776-4121; fax: 615-776-4119 http://www.pedstest.com ($36.00) **Electronic offerings:** see electronic options below. **Training options:** training is freely offered via downloadable slide shows with notes, case examples, and handouts, website discussion list (covering all screens), training modules, short videos, e-mail/phone consultation with research/training staff.	0-8 yr	10 questions eliciting parents' concerns in English, Spanish, Vietnamese, and many other languages. Written at the 4th-5th grade level. Determines when to refer, provide a second screen, provide patient education, or monitor development, behavior/emotional, and academic progress. Provides longitudinal surveillance and triage.	Identifies when to: Refer and what types of referrals are needed; Advise parents; Monitor vigilantly; Screen further (or refer for screening); or Reassure.	**By age:** Sensitivity: 74-79% Specificity: 70-80% **By disabilities**, i.e., learning, intellectual, language, mental health, and autism spectrum disorders (ASDs): Sensitivity: 71-87%	Scoring Time: 1 min. Scoring Cost: $1.00 Materials: $0.39 **Total (Self-Report): $1.39** Interview Time: 2 min. Interview Cost: $2.00 Scoring/Materials: $1.39 **Total (Interview): $3.39**
PEDS: Developmental Milestones (DM) (Screening Version) PEDS*Test*.com, LLC. 1013 Austin Court, Nolensville, TN 37135 Phone: 615-776-4121; fax: 615-776-4119 http://www.pedstest.com ($275.00). **Electronic offerings:** see below. **Training options:** training is freely offered via downloadable slide shows with notes, case examples, and handouts, website discussion list (covering all screens), training modules, short videos, e-mail/phone consultation with research/training staff.	0-8 yr	PEDS:DM consists of 6-8 items at each age level (spanning the well visit schedule). Each item taps a different domain (fine/gross motor, self-help, academics, expressive/receptive language, social-emotional). Items are administered by parents or professionals (by interview or hands-on). Forms are laminated and marked with a grease pencil. It can be used to complement PEDS or stand alone. Written at the 2nd grade level. A longitudinal score form tracks performance. Supplemental surveillance measures focused on the American Academy of Pediatrics 2006 statement are included (see descriptions below): the M-CHAT, Family Psychosocial Screen, Pictorial PSC-17, the SWILS, the Vanderbilt attention-deficit/hyperactivity disorder (ADHD) Scale, and the Brigance Parent-Child Interactions Scale. In English, Spanish, and Taiwanese.	Pass/fail cutoffs tied to performance above and below the 16th percentile for each item and its domain.	**By age:** Sensitivity: 70-94% Specificity: 77-93% **By developmental domain:** Sensitivity: 75-87% Specificity: 71-88%	Scoring Time: 1 min Scoring Cost: $1.00 Materials: $0.02 **Total (Self-Report): $1.02** If interview, time: 3 min Interview Cost: $3.00 If hands-on, time: 4 min Hands-on Cost: $4.00 Scoring/Materials: $1.02 **Total (Interview): $4.02** **Total (Direct Admin): $5.02**
Ages and Stages Questionnaire-3 (ASQ-3) (2009). Paul H. Brookes Publishing, Inc., PO Box 10624, Baltimore, MD 21285 (1-800-638-3775). ($249.95 each for English or Spanish) www.agesandstages.com. **Electronic offerings:** see electronic options below. **Training options:** purchasable videos, case examples, e-mail support, and live training at a cost.	1 mo-66 mo	Parents indicate children's developmental skills on 30 or so items plus overall concerns. The ASQ has a different form (5-8 pages) for each age interval. Written at the 4th-6th grade level per the user's manual. Can be used in mass mail-outs for child find programs. Manual contains detailed instructions for organizing child-find programs and includes activity handouts for parents. The ASQ-3 is available in English, Spanish, French, and Korean with additional translations underway.	Cutoff scores set at 2 SDs below the mean, in 5 developmental domains. Includes typical (above cutoff), monitoring (near cutoff), and refer (below cutoff) zones.	**By age:** Sensitivity: 82-89% Specificity:77-92% **By domain:** Sensitivity: 83% Specificity: 91% **By disabilities,** i.e., cerebral palsy, visual and hearing impairment: Sensitivity: 87% Specificity: 82%	Scoring Time: 2 min Scoring Cost: $2.00 Materials: ~$0.36 **Total (Self-Report): $2.36** Interview Time: 12 min. Interview Cost: $12.00 Scoring/Materials: $2.36 **Total (Interview): $14.36**
AUTISM-SPECIFIC SCREENING					
Note: The American Academy of Pediatrics recommends ASD screening at 18 mo and again at 24-30 mo. Nevertheless, the following measure should not be used as the sole screen for all children, because it will not accurately detect the more common disabilities of childhood, i.e., language impairment, intellectual disabilities, and learning disabilities. Narrow-band tools should always be administered along with a broad-band tool, such as those listed previously.					

Continued

Table 14-1 TOOLS FOR DEVELOPMENTAL-BEHAVIORAL SCREENING AND SURVEILLANCE—cont'd

BEHAVIORAL AND/OR DEVELOPMENTAL SCREENS RELYING ON INFORMATION FROM PARENTS	AGE RANGE	DESCRIPTION	SCORING	ACCURACY	TIME FRAME/COSTS*
Modified Checklist for Autism in Toddlers (M-CHAT) (1999). Free download at www.mchatscreen.com Included in the PEDS:DM (www.pedstest.com). **Electronic offerings:** see below. **Training options:** none.	16-48 mo	Parent report of 23 yes/no questions and written at 4th-6th grade reading level. Screens for ASD. Downloadable scoring template and .xls files for automated scoring. Available in multiple languages. If M-CHAT is failed, then the M-CHAT Follow-Up Interview is strongly recommended by its authors. This is because 6-10% of children fail the M-CHAT at the 18- and 24-month well-visits, which leads to a high over-referral rate for an expensive comprehensive ASD evaluation.	Pass/fail scores based on failing at least 2 critical items, or 3 or more noncritical items.	**By age and by disability,** i.e., ASDs: Sensitivity: 90% Specificity: 99% However, future validity studies are pending.	Scoring Time: 1 min (manual scoring with a transparent sheet) Scoring Costs: $1.00 Materials: $0.06 **Total (Self-Report): $1.06** Interview Time: 5 min (excluding follow-up on any failed items) Interview Cost: $5.00 Scoring/Materials: $1.06 **Total (Interview): $6.06**
SCREENS FOR OLDER CHILDREN					
These screens focus on academic skills and mental health, including ADHD screening. The shorter ones, such as the SWILS and PSC, are suitable for primary care.					
Safety Word Inventory and Literacy Screener (SWILS). PEDS*Test*.com, LLC. Items courtesy of Curriculum Associates, Inc. The SWILS is included (laminated) in PEDS:DM (www.pedstest.com). **Electronic offerings:** none. **Training options:** slide shows, email consultation at www.pedstest.com.	6-14 yr	Children are asked (by parents or professionals) to read 29 common safety words (e.g., High Voltage, Wait, Poison) aloud. The number of correctly read words is compared to a cutoff score. Results predict performance in math, written language, and a range of reading skills. Test content may serve as a springboard to injury prevention counseling and can be used to screen for parental literacy. Because even non-English speakers living in the USA need to read safety words in English, the measure is available only in English.	Single cutoff score indicating the need for a referral.	**By age/academic deficits,** Sensitivity: 73-88% Specificity: 77-88%	Administration/Scoring time: ~7 min Admin/Scoring Costs: ~$7.00 Materials: laminated: $0.00/ photocopy: $.06 **Total (Direct Admin): = ~$7.00-7.06**
Pediatric Symptom Checklist (PSC). http://psc.partners.org The Pictorial PSC (PPSC) is useful with low-income Spanish-speaking families. Its 17-item factorial version (facilitates screening for ADHD, internalizing and externalizing disorders) is included (laminated) in the PEDS:DM (www.pedstest.com). **Electronic offerings:** none. **Training options:** slide shows, email consultation at www.pedstest.com.	4-16 yr	35 vs. 17 short statements of problem behaviors including both externalizing (conduct) and internalizing (depression, anxiety, adjustment, etc.). Uses parent-report or youth self-report. The PSC/PPSC in their 17-item versions produces cutoffs for attentional, internalizing, and externalizing problems. Readability is ~ 2nd grade. In English, Spanish, Portuguese, Chinese, Dutch, Filippino, French, Somali, and several other languages. Last standardized in 1998.	Single refer/no refer score. Cutoffs scores also available for attention, internalizing, and externalizing problems. No questionable category.	**PSC/PPSC by disability,** i.e., mental health disorders of any kind, across numerous studies: Sensitivity: 80-95% Sensitivity: 68-100% **PSC-17/PPSC-17 by specific disability,** i.e., ADHD: Sensitivity: 58% Specificity: 91% Internalizing Disorders: Sensitivity: 52-73% Specificity: 74% Externalizing Disorders: Sensitivity: 62% Specificity: 89%	Scoring Time: 3 min Scoring Cost: $3.00 Materials: laminated: $0.00/ photocopy~$0.06 **Total (Self-Report): $3.00-$3.06** Interview Time: 3 min Interview Cost: $3.00 Materials/Scoring: $3.00-$3.06 **Total (Interview): $6.00-$6.06**

FAMILY PSYCHOSOCIAL SCREENING					
Family Psychosocial Screening (FPS). Kemper KJ, Kelleher KJ: *Family psychosocial screening: instruments and techniques.* Included in PEDS:DM and downloadable at http://www.pedstest.com. **Electronic offerings:** none. **Training options:** none.	Parents of all ages	A 2-page clinic measure of psychosocial risk factors associated with developmental problems, often used for clinic intake. More than 4 risk factors are associated with developmental delays. The FPS also includes: a) a 4-item screen for parental history of physical abuse as a child; b) a 6-item measure of parental substance abuse; c) a 4-item screen for domestic violence; and d) a 3-item measure of maternal depression. Can be used along with the Brigance Parent-Child Interactions Scale to view parenting risk and resilience. More than 4 psychosocial risk factors are associated with developmental delays. Readability is 4th grade. In English and Spanish.	Refer/no refer scores for each risk factor. Also has guides to referring and resource lists.	**By condition,** i.e., parental depression, substance abuse, etc.: Sensitivity: >90% Specificity: >90%	Scoring Time: 3 min Scoring Cost: $3.00 Material Costs: $0.00 (laminated)/$0.06 (photocopied) **Total (Self-Report): $3.00-$3.06** Interview Time: 15 min Interview Cost: $15.00 Scoring/Materials $.3.00-$3.06 **Total (Interview): $18.00-$18.06**

ELECTRONIC RECORDS OPTIONS FOR SCREENING WITH QUALITY TOOLS (INCLUDING ONLINE AND OTHER DIGITAL APPROACHES TO ADMINISTRATION AND SCORING)

Essential Definitions Are:

- **Keyboards (including iPad-type tools):** users can type in text-based answers to questions
- **Touch-screens applications:** hopefully self-explanatory, but these often allow parents to also listen to questions and response options, thus reducing literacy demands. Other than touching the screen to select multiple choice responses, actual text cannot be entered.
- **Online:** meaning an Internet connection; preferably high speed is needed
- **CD-ROM:** offline but still electronic, and requiring installation on the user's computer
- **Parent portal:** applications (typically web-based and thus online) where parents can complete measures but do not see results. Rather, these are sent to a different office computer for inclusion in the medical record/sharing results.
- **Webcasts/webinars:** either live or constantly available on publishers' websites. Live webcasts are generally translated into webinars (a few days after a live webcast) and thus become videos/audios, usually freely available on demand.

COMPANY	TRAINING/SUPPORT OPTIONS	DESCRIPTION AND PRICING
CHADIS (http://www.chadis.com) PEDS, ASQ, M-CHAT, and other measures online for touch-screen, tablet PCs, keyboards, and parent portal methods). Spanish language version coming soon.	Downloadable guides, live training at exhibits, and other training services on request.	CHADIS also includes decision support for a large range of other measures, both diagnostic and parent/family focused, such as the Vanderbilt ADHD Diagnostic Rating Scale, and various parental depression inventories. CHADIS offers integration with existing electronic health records. Works with a range of equipment/applications, and automatically generates reports. Pricing is ~$2.00 per use.
PEDSTest.com. LLC (www.pedstest.com/online) PEDS, M-CHAT, PEDS:DM online for keyboard and parent portal (PEDS:DM in Spanish and other translations coming soon).	Slide shows, website FAQs, email support, online videos, discussion list	This site offers PEDS, PEDS:DM, and the M-CHAT for applications for keyboards (including iPad) allowing for actual comments from parents. Offers a parent portal (wherein families do not see the results), etc. Scoring is automated as are summary reports for parents, referral letters when needed, and ICD-9/procedure codes. HL-7 integration with electronic records is available as is data export and aggregate views of records. $2.06-$2.75 per use (depending on volume).
Brookes Publishing (www.agesandstages.com) (ASQ/ASQ:SE via CD-ROM installed on keyboard computers, along with web-based scoring service.)	Live training, online training, purchasable training videos, email listserv	ASQ on a CD-ROM enables users to click answers and receive an automated score. The software offers aggregation of results, report writing templates, and progress tracking.
Patient Tools (www.patienttools.com) (PEDS, M-CHAT, ASQ, ASQ:SE and others measures online for tablet PCs.) Coming soon.	Webcasts/webinars, live support by phone, email	Patient Tools plans to offer the ASQ, ASQ:SE, M-CHAT, the Vanderbilt ADHD Scales, and a wide range of behavioral/mental health measures for adolescents and adults. A parent portal approach is available via Survey Tablets. Equipment including docking stations is rented, lease-purchased, or purchased ($74.00-$1,320) after which $58.00/mo is the ongoing cost of hosting, data storage, telephone, technical and installation support.

Disclosure: This table was compiled and vetted in collaboration with many researchers, clinicians, and test authors, without regard to the latter's potential financial interests in products mentioned.

*Publisher pricing and salary costs often change.

Table 14-2 COMBINING SCREENING AND SURVEILLANCE: A PRACTICE ALGORITHM

1. ENSURE A MEDICAL HOME.
Timely, equitable access to care logically correlates to well child care compliance rates and therefore, developmental delay identification rates. Children with developmental and behavioral problems or special health care needs use health care services at >2× the rate of other patients. Visits are often complex due to the need to make referrals, locate information from prior visits and services, make follow-up appointments, and coordi nate with other providers. The AAP's medical home model (*www.medicalhomeinfo.org*) is an essential guide to organizing practices to ensure continuity and coordination of care and to best meet the needs of children with disabilities and their families.

2. REVIEW MEDICAL CHART FOR HEALTH RISK FACTORS.
Consider potentially harmful exposures including radiation or medications, infectious illnesses, fever, addictive substances, trauma, and results of neonatal screens, including phenylketonuria, congenital hypothyroidism, and numerous other metabolic conditions. The perinatal history includes birthweight, gestational age, Apgar scores, and any medical complications (Chapter 88.1). Postnatal medical factors that are sometimes overlooked include failure to thrive, abnormal growth curves for head circumference, neurological (e.g., seizure) disorders, endocrine disorders, amblyopia or other significant forms of visual impairment, chronic respiratory or allergic illness, conductive or sensorineural hearing impairment, congenital heart disease, iron deficiency anemia, head trauma, and sleep disorders (particularly obstructive sleep apnea [Chapter 17]). In most states, children are automatically eligible for early intervention if their conditions have a well-established association with developmental delay (e.g., Down syndrome, birthweight <1500 g).

3. IDENTIFY AND MONITOR PSYCHOSOCIAL RISK AND PROTECTIVE FACTORS.
Risk factors include parents with less than a high school education, parental mental health or substance abuse problems, 4 or more children in the home, single parent, poverty, frequent household moves, limited social support, parental history of abuse as a child, ethnic minority, and problematic parenting style. The latter is often observable during encounters (e.g., parents who don't talk much to their children, tend to bark orders at them, talk to their children only when they are crying, etc.). Four or more risk factors tend to plunge developmental status into the below average range and suggest the need for enrichment or remedial programs such as Head Start/Early Head Start regardless of screening results. All children with a history of abuse or neglect should be referred automatically for early intervention. An initial visit standardized intake measure, such as the Family Psychosocial Screen (see Table 14-1), followed by readministration of its 2-item parental depression screen and any other of its imbedded measures (e.g., substance abuse, housing and food instability) in the 2nd year of life. When a concerning psychosocial screen occurs, the next step is to provide an appropriate community referral (e.g., mental health provider, domestic violence shelter, parenting or postpartum depression support group) and to contact (via a phone call or a courtesy copy note) the parent's primary care provider. If parental suicidal/homicidal ideation or psychosis is identified, consider that a medical emergency. Not only does psychosocial screening allow for higher quality surveillance, it's an early opportunity to ameliorate or prevent a future delay.

Protective (also called resilience) factors focus almost exclusively on positive parenting styles. These behaviors are often observable (e.g., when parents actively and age-appropriately teach children new things, label objects of interest, share books, and converse with their child [including back-and-forth sound play in infancy, playing peek-a-boo, etc.]). Identifying other positive parenting behaviors usually requires questioning (e.g., whether parents talk with children at meals and perceive their child as soothable and interested in conversing). PEDS:DM (described in Table 14-1) includes a validated parent-child interactions questionnaire. Trigger questions from the Bright Futures initiative are also helpful (http://www.brightfutures.org).

4. ELICIT AND ADDRESS PARENTS' CONCERNS.
Informal questions to parents are rarely effective at eliciting developmental-behavioral concerns. In addition, informal questions do not render the decision support providers need in order to recognize what type of intervention is needed. It is best to use a standardized, validated tool such as PEDS that not only offers questions proven to enhance parent-professional communication, but also an evidence-based algorithm for helping professionals determine when to refer, advise, monitor more carefully, screen further, or reassure. PEDS also functions as both a screening and surveillance measure.

5. ADMINISTER AND SCORE DEVELOPMENTAL-BEHAVIORAL SCREENING TEST(S) FOCUSED ON MILESTONES.
Because surveillance requires monitoring milestones, and because the AAP recommends formal screening at specific visits, both screening and surveillance can be accomplished simultaneously via measures such as PEDS:DM or Ages and Stages Questionnaire (see Table 14-1). These measures offer longitudinal progress tracking and evidence-based cutoff scores. Such screens are needed at 9, 18, 24-30 months *and at annual well visits thereafter.* An autism-specific screen should be added at 18 months and again at 24 months (e.g., M-CHAT [Modified Checklist for Autism in Toddlers]). Use of previsit, parent-completed tools is particularly efficient. When a parent-report screen is completed and scored before the visit, clinicians are better able to collaborate with families during encounters, determine the optimal content for developmental promotion, refine the physical exam (and any subsequent subspecialty referrals), and incorporate information about psychosocial risk and resilience factors into quality decision-making about needed intervention services. Administration options may include online parent portals, paper/pencil in waiting rooms, and interview at weigh-in or by nursing staff.

6. IF INDICATED, ADMINISTER (OR REFER FOR) ADDITIONAL MENTAL HEALTH SCREENS.
Whenever a child performs poorly on broad-band screens or when parents' concerns about behavior or social-emotional concerns persist, the AAP recommends use of focused measures of mental health (meaning social-emotional and behavioral issues). The overlap between developmental and mental health problems is considerable; about 1 in 3 children with developmental problems also have emotional difficulties. PEDS and the PEDS:DM provide brief indicators, but more in-depth measures such as the Ages and Stages Questionnaire: Social-Emotional are helpful. See www.aap.org/mentalhealth for more information and additional tool options. When time is limited, parents can be given measures to take home in preparation for a follow-up appointment. Alternatively, referrals for mental health screening can be made to services funded by the IDEA including early intervention and public schools special education (see Resources for Screening, Nonmedical Referral, and Developmental Promotion). Such programs are prepared to administer mental health screens and other detailed assessments without charge to families.

7. PROVIDE PHYSICAL EXAMINATION AND CLINICAL OBSERVATION.
Points of particular importance include growth parameters and head shape and circumference, facial and other body dysmorphology, eye findings (e.g., cataracts in various inborn errors of metabolism), vascular markings, and signs of neurocutaneous disorders (café-au-lait spots in neurofibromatosis, hypopigmented macules in tuberous sclerosis). Vision and hearing screening should occur per the AAP's guidelines. Examine closely for findings consistent with abuse/neglect (e.g., geometrically shaped bruises). A neurological exam (Chapter 584), along with careful observation of the child's behavior and the parent-child interaction, is a key part to any developmental evaluation. Does the parent interact appropriately with the child or does something "not feel right" during your exam? Does the child behave age-appropriately around the parent? Is there a concern about the child being over or under attached to the parent? (See Step 3.)

8. WHEN INDICATED, PLAN AND REFER FOR ADDITIONAL MEDICAL TESTS.
Vision and hearing screening are needed, not only routinely but additionally when developmental-behavioral screening tests indicate probable problems. Many IDEA services cannot begin testing unless these are documented in referral letters. With young children, referrals to audiologists may be needed (depending on office equipment and child compliance). Iron deficiency and lead poisoning are common contributors to developmental delays and are easily detected through screening. Electroencephalograms and neuroimaging are not routinely indicated but might be used if there is clinical suspicion of a seizure disorder, hydrocephalus, micro- or macrocephaly, encephalopathy, neurofibromatosis, tuberous sclerosis, brain tumor, or other neurological problem (not including autism). Extreme handedness at an early age and persistence of fisting after 4 months is another indicator of potential neuron migration disorders requiring imaging. Uncommonly, surveillance may indicate a need for additional metabolic screens, such as serum electrolytes and glucose, venous blood gas, serum ammonia, urine glycosaminoglycans, endocrine screens (e.g., TSH, free T4), genetic testing (chromosomal analysis, DNA for fragile X, etc.), or screens for an infectious disease (e.g., HIV antibody testing [Chapter 268], TORCH infection testing [Chapter 103]). Due to the need to discern which tests are needed, referral to a developmental-behavioral or neurodevelopmental pediatrician is wise.

Table 14-2 COMBINING SCREENING AND SURVEILLANCE: A PRACTICE ALGORITHM—cont'd
9. EXPLAIN SCREENING RESULTS TO PARENTS. The primary medical provider should present the screening results to parents in person. Results should be explained in a positive manner (e.g., "There is much we can do to help.") with emphasis on available community services and how these optimize a child's (and family's) outcome. Providers' first-hand experience with community services is essential for understanding what intervention programs do and for adequately describing them to families. It is advisable to use euphemistic terms for diagnosis, because the specific condition may not be known (e.g., "developmental delay," "behind other children," "seems to be having difficulties with…."), and because determining a final diagnosis is not needed for enrollment in intervention. Asking the parents if they know any families with children who have developmental differences may be helpful in understanding any strong reaction to the information being presented. Offers to re-explain findings to other family members may be needed.
10. MAKE REFERRALS FOR NONMEDICAL INTERVENTIONS AND FOLLOWING UP. Making appointments for families, wherever possible, increases the likelihood of follow through. Referrals should always start with IDEA programs (www.nectac.org). Services are free to parents, provided under federal and state law within 30-40 school days from the time of referral, and generally provide high quality therapies, evaluations, remediation programs or high quality preschool for those with psychosocial risk factors (or when further evaluation reveals the screening results were false-positive). Referral forms or letters, which target the areas of concern, help IDEA programs to better assess and track children. To expedite assessments and eligibility placements, parental signatures should be obtained to release information back and forth between the medical provider and the IDEA program. Some children will be automatically eligible for services based on a condition highly likely to result in a developmental delay (e.g., Down syndrome, birth weight <1500 g). Referral forms or letters should include suggestions for the types of evaluations needed (e.g., speech-language therapy, occupational and physical therapy, social-emotional assessment, intelligence testing, academics) and documentation of hearing and vision status, because IDEA programs require this information before providing evaluations. If referrals seem needed for autism-specific evaluations or mental health services, refer for these separately but do not defer referrals to IDEA services in the interim. Many specialized evaluations and interventions have lengthy waiting lists (e.g., 9-12 months). Children need prompt services through IDEA while they wait.
11. REVIEW REPORTS AND OTHER FEEDBACK FROM REFERRAL SOURCES AND FOLLOW UP WITH FAMILIES. Surveillance does not end after a referral. Not all families follow through with clinicians' recommendations for services. Some parents wish to try at-home interventions. Other parents get "cold feet" and may be deterred by differing opinions from relatives and spouses (e.g., "His father was just like that"; "It is a phase. She'll grow out of it."). A follow-up appointment in 3-4 months is helpful for encouraging families, and, if needed, at least advising parents to visit the programs recommended. Reassessing parents' concerns is also helpful because when parents have multiple concerns, they are more likely to seek intervention programs. Note that ambiguous concerns such as "I think he's doing better" still convey substantial risk. When families have followed through with recommendations, clinicians should carefully review (and, when indicated, take action on) reports from the IDEA programs and other subspecialists. These reports may include recommendations for specific services (e.g., speech-language, occupational or physical therapy), and some states require physician authorization. IDEA programs should ideally give feedback to clinicians about whether the child followed up on the referral (hence the value of a two-way consent form). Was the child lost to follow-up, screened out, placed on a monitoring list, or made eligible for services? When children have not qualified for services, providers should make referrals to Head Start, quality daycare/preschool or parent training (and establish a vigilant plan for rescreening because, if delays persist, children may qualify for IDEA programs in the future). Clinicians should also establish communication preferences with intervention programs (e.g., by email, fax, or telephone [including available hours]) and the preferences for the kind of information to be sent (e.g., evaluation reports, individual education plans, etc.).
12. PROVIDE DEVELOPMENTAL-BEHAVIORAL PROMOTION. When screening and surveillance methods do not identify a need for nonmedical interventions, the need to address "the normal problems of normal children" remains. All parents need advice about typical problems (e.g., toilet training, temper tantrums). All parents need to be encouraged to promote their child's language and preacademic/academic development. This is most easily accomplished with written patient education materials, by encouraging parents to visit websites with quality information, participating in Reach and Read, or by parent training classes, group well visits, or social work services. A well-organized system for filing and retrieving parent-focused materials is essential (see Table 15-2). Follow up with families, in 6-8 weeks to assess the effectiveness of promotion activities, especially in-office advice about behavior and social skills. If less than successful, encourage parents to engage in more intensive services (e.g., parenting classes, family therapy). Information and referral resources are listed under Resources for Screening, Nonmedical Referral, and Developmental Promotion.

AAP, American Academy of Pediatrics; IDEA, Individuals with Disabilities Education Act; PEDS:DM, Parents' Evaluations of Developmental Status: Developmental Milestones.

Chapter 15
Child Care: How Pediatricians Can Support Children and Families
Laura Stout Sosinsky and Walter S. Gilliam

With increasing movement of women into the workplace across the globe, child care is a primary developmental context for millions of young children. Child-care providers play a major role in the day-to-day safety, health, and developmental well-being of young children. Given the large proportion of young children in child-care settings, child-care providers are an important potential ally to parents and pediatricians. The provision of child care is complex, with enormous variation across the globe. Child care is affected by many factors including maternal leave policies. The U.S. federal leave program allows for 12 weeks of unpaid job-protected leave during pregnancy or after childbirth, but companies with <50 employees, part-time employees, and those working in informal labor markets are exempt. By contrast, according to the national leave programs in Norway and Sweden, mothers may receive up to 42 and 52 weeks, respectively, of paid benefits after the birth of an infant. Countries vary in terms of the proportion of children being cared for by the extended family. Pediatricians need to understand how child care is structured and utilized in their country or region to appreciate the challenges parents face in finding and accessing high-quality child care and the challenges child-care providers face in maintaining a physically and developmentally healthy environment.

For the full continuation of this chapter, please visit the Nelson Textbook of Pediatrics *website at www.expertconsult.com.*

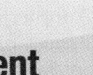

Chapter 16
Loss, Separation, and Bereavement
Janet R. Serwint

All children will experience involuntary separations from illness and/or death of loved ones at some time in their lives. Parents and children may turn to their pediatrician and other health care professionals for help following various types of personal losses. Relatively brief separations of children from their parents, such as vacations, usually produce minor transient effects, but more enduring and frequent separation may cause sequelae. The potential impact of each event must be considered in light of the age and stage of development of the child, the particular relationship with the absent person, and the nature of the situation. As a trustworthy, familiar resource, pediatricians are uniquely positioned to offer information, support, and guidance, and to facilitate coping.

For the full continuation of this chapter, please visit the Nelson Textbook of Pediatrics *website at www.expertconsult.com.*

Chapter 17
Sleep Medicine

Judith A. Owens

INTRODUCTION

Sleep regulation involves the simultaneous operation of two basic highly coupled processes that govern sleep and wakefulness (the "two process" sleep system). The **homeostatic process** ("Process S"), primarily regulates the length and depth of sleep, and may be related to the accumulation of adenosine and other sleep-promoting chemicals ("somnogens"), such as cytokines, during prolonged periods of wakefulness. This sleep pressure appears to build more quickly in infants and young children, thus limiting the duration of sustained wakefulness during the day and necessitating periods of daytime sleep (i.e., naps). The endogenous **circadian rhythm** ("Process C"), influences the internal organization of sleep and timing and duration of daily sleep-wake cycles, and govern predictable patterns of alertness throughout the 24 hr day. The "master circadian clock" that controls sleep-wake patterns is located in the suprachiasmatic nucleus (SCN) in the ventral hypothalamus; other "circadian clocks" govern the timing of multiple other physiologic systems in the body (e.g., cardiovascular reactivity, hormone levels, renal and pulmonary functions). Because the human circadian clock is actually slightly longer than 24 hr, intrinsic circadian rhythms must are synchronized or "entrained" to the 24 hr day cycle by environmental cues called **zeitgebers.** The most powerful of these zeitgebers is the light–dark cycle; light signals are transmitted to the SCN via the circadian photoreceptor system within the retina (functionally and anatomically separate from the visual system), which switch the body's production of the hormone melatonin off (light) or on (dark) by the pineal gland. Circadian rhythms are also synchronized by other external time cues, such as timing of meals and alarm clocks.

The relative level of sleepiness (sleep propensity) or alertness existing at any given time during a 24 hr period is partially determined by the duration and quality of previous sleep, as well as time awake since the last sleep period (the homeostatic or "sleep drive"). Interacting with this "sleep homeostat" is the 24 hr cyclic pattern or rhythm characterized by clock-dependent periods of maximum sleepiness ("circadian troughs") and maximum alertness ("circadian nadirs"). There are 2 periods of maximum sleepiness, 1 in the late afternoon (3:00-5:00 PM) and one toward the end of the night (3:00-5:00 AM), and 2 periods of maximum alertness, 1 in mid-morning and 1 in the evening, just prior to sleep onset (the so-called second wind).

Another basic principle of sleep physiology relates to the consequences of the failure to meet basic sleep needs, termed insufficient/inadequate sleep or **sleep loss.** Adequate sleep is a biologic imperative that appears necessary for sustaining life as well as for optimal functioning. Slow-wave sleep (SWS) appears to be the most "restorative" form of sleep and rapid eye movement (REM) sleep appears not only to be involved in vital cognitive functions, such as the consolidation of memory, but to be an integral component of the growth and development of the central nervous system (CNS). Adequate amounts of both of these sleep stages are necessary for optimal learning. Partial sleep loss (sleep restriction) on a chronic basis accumulates in what is termed a **sleep debt** and produces deficits equivalent to those seen under conditions of total sleep deprivation. If the sleep debt becomes large enough and is not voluntarily paid back (by obtaining adequate recovery sleep), the body may respond by overriding voluntary control of wakefulness, resulting in periods of decreased alertness, dozing off, and napping, that is excessive daytime sleepiness. The sleep-deprived individual may also experience very brief (several seconds) repeated daytime microsleeps of which he or she may be completely unaware, but which nonetheless may result in significant lapses in attention and vigilance. There is also a relationship between the amount of sleep restriction and performance, with decreased performance correlating with decreased sleep.

Both insufficient quantity and poor quality of sleep in children and adolescents usually result in excessive daytime sleepiness and decreased daytime alertness levels. Sleepiness may be recognizable as drowsiness, yawning, and other classic "sleepy behaviors," but can also be manifested as mood disturbance, including complaints of moodiness, irritability, emotional lability, depression, and anger; fatigue and daytime lethargy, including increased somatic complaints (headaches, muscle aches); cognitive impairment, including problems with memory, attention, concentration, decision-making, and problem solving; daytime behavior problems, including overactivity, impulsivity, and noncompliance; and academic problems, including chronic tardiness related to insufficient sleep and school failure resulting from chronic daytime sleepiness.

To evaluate sleep problems, it is important to have an understanding of what constitutes "normal" sleep in children and adolescents. Sleep disturbances, as well as many characteristics of sleep itself, have some distinctly different features in children from sleep and sleep disorders in adults. In addition, changes in sleep architecture and the evolution of sleep patterns and behaviors reflect the physiologic/chronobiologic, developmental, and social/environmental changes that are occurring across childhood. These trends may be summarized as the gradual assumption of more adult sleep patterns as children mature:

- A decline in the average 24 hr sleep duration from infancy through adolescence, which involves a decrease in both diurnal and nocturnal sleep amounts. There is a dramatic decline in daytime sleep (scheduled napping) by 5 yr, with a less marked and more gradual continued decrease in nocturnal sleep amounts into late adolescence.
- A dramatic decrease in the proportion of REM sleep from birth (50% of sleep) through early childhood into adulthood (25-30%), and a similar initial predominance of SWS that peaks in early childhood, drops off abruptly after puberty (40-60% decline), and then further decreases over the life span. This SWS preponderance in early life has clinical significance; the high prevalence of partial arousal parasomnias (sleepwalking and sleep terrors) in preschool and early school-aged children is related to the relative increased proportion of SWS in this age group.
- Due to the lengthening of the nocturnal ultradian sleep cycle, a concomitant decrease in the number of end-of-cycle arousals across the nocturnal sleep period occurs.
- A gradual shift to a later bedtime and sleep onset time that begins in middle childhood and accelerates in early to mid-adolescence.
- Irregularity of sleep/wake patterns characterized by increasingly larger discrepancies between school night and non–school night bedtimes and wake times, and increased weekend oversleep that typically begins in middle childhood and peaks in adolescence.

Normal developmental changes in children's sleep are found in Table 17-1.

COMMON SLEEP DISORDERS

Most sleep problems in children may be broadly conceptualized as resulting from either inadequate duration of sleep for age and sleep needs (insufficient sleep quantity) or disruption and fragmentation of sleep (poor sleep quality) as a result of frequent, repetitive, and brief arousals during sleep. Less common causes

Table 17-1 NORMAL DEVELOPMENTAL CHANGES IN CHILDREN'S SLEEP

AGE CATEGORY	SLEEP DURATION AND SLEEP PATTERNS	ADDITIONAL SLEEP ISSUES	SLEEP DISORDERS
Newborn (0-2 mo)	Total sleep: 10-19 hr per 24 r (average = 13-14.5 hr), may be higher in premature babies Bottle-fed babies generally sleep for longer periods (2-5 hr bouts) than breast-fed babies (1-3 hr) Sleep periods are separated by 1-2 hr awake. No established nocturnal/diurnal pattern in the 1st few wk; sleep is evenly distributed throughout the day and night, averaging 8.5 hr at night and 5.75 hr during the day	The American Academy of Pediatrics issued a formal recommendation in 2005 advocating against bed sharing in the first year of life, instead encouraging proximate but separate sleeping surfaces for mother and infant. Safe sleep practices for infants: Place the baby on his or her back to sleep at night and during nap times. Place the baby on a firm mattress with a well-fitting sheet in a safety-approved crib. Do not use pillows or comforters Cribs should not have corner posts over $\frac{1}{16}$ in high or decorative cut-outs. Make sure the baby's face and head stay uncovered and clear of blankets and other coverings during sleep.	Most sleep issues that are perceived as problematic at this stage represent a discrepancy between parental expectations and developmentally appropriate sleep behaviors. Newborns who are noted by parents to be extremely fussy and persistently difficult to console are more likely to have underlying medical issues, such as colic, gastroesophageal reflux, and formula intolerance.
Infant (2-12 mo)	Total sleep: average is 12-13 hr (note that there is great individual variability in sleep times during infancy) Nighttime: average is 9-10 hr Naps: average is 3-4 hr	Sleep regulation or self-soothing involves the infant's ability to negotiate the sleep-wake transition, both at sleep onset and following normal awakenings throughout the night. The capacity to self-soothe begins to develop in the 1st 12 wk of life, and is a reflection of both neurodevelopmental maturation and learning. Sleep consolidation, or "sleeping through the night," is usually defined by parents as a continuous sleep episode without the need for parental intervention (e.g., feeding, soothing) from the child's bedtime through the early morning. Infants develop the ability to consolidate sleep between 6 wk to 3 mo	Behavioral insomnia of childhood; sleep onset association type Sleep-related rhythmic movements (head banging, body rocking)
Toddler (1-3 yr)	Total sleep: average is 11-13 hr Nighttime: average is 9.5-10.5 hr Naps: average is 2-3 hr; decrease from 2 naps to 1 at average age of 18 mo	Cognitive, motor, social, language developmental issues impact on sleep Nighttime fears develop; transitional objects, bedtime routines important	Behavioral insomnia of childhood, sleep onset association type Behavioral insomnia of childhood, limit setting type
Preschool (3-5 yr)	Nighttime: average is 9-10 hr Naps decrease from 1 nap to no nap Overall, 26% of 4 yr olds and just 15% of 5 yr olds nap	Persistent co-sleeping tends to be highly associated with sleep problems in this age group Sleep problems may become chronic	Behavioral insomnia of childhood, limit setting type Sleepwalking Sleep terrors Nighttime fears/nightmares Obstructive sleep apnea
Middle childhood (6-12 hr)	9-11 hr	School and behavior problems may be related to sleep problems Media and electronics, such as television, computer, video games, and the Internet compete increasingly for sleep time Irregularity of sleep–wake schedules reflects increasing discrepancy between school and nonschool night bedtimes and waketimes	Nightmares Obstructive sleep apnea Insufficient sleep
Adolescence (>12 yr)	Average sleep duration 7-7.5 hr; only 20% of adolescents overall get the recommended 9-9.25 hr of sleep Later bedtimes; increased discrepancy sleep patterns weekdays/weekends	Puberty-mediated phase delay (later sleep onset and wake times), relative to sleep-wake cycles in middle childhood Earlier required wake times Environmental competing priorities for sleep	Insufficient sleep Delayed sleep phase disorder Narcolepsy Restless legs syndrome/periodic limb movement disorder

of sleep disturbance in childhood involve inappropriate timing of the sleep period (as occurs in circadian rhythm disturbances), or primary disorders of excessive daytime sleepiness (central hypersomnias such as narcolepsy). Insufficient sleep is usually the result of difficulty initiating (delayed sleep onset) and/or maintaining sleep (prolonged night wakings), but, especially in older children and adolescents, may also represent a conscious lifestyle decision to sacrifice sleep in favor of competing priorities, such as homework and social activities. The underlying causes of sleep onset delay/prolonged night wakings or sleep fragmentation may in turn be related to primarily behavioral factors (bedtime resistance resulting in shortened sleep duration) and/or medical causes (obstructive sleep apnea causing frequent, brief arousals).

It should be noted that certain pediatric populations are relatively more vulnerable to acute or chronic sleep problems. These include children with medical problems, including chronic illnesses, such as cystic fibrosis, asthma, and rheumatoid arthritis, and acute illnesses, such as otitis media; children taking medications or ingesting substances with stimulant (e.g., psychostimulants, caffeine), sleep-disrupting (e.g., corticosteroids), or daytime sedating (some anticonvulsants, α-agonists) properties; hospitalized children; and children with a variety of psychiatric disorders, including attention-deficit/hyperactivity disorder (ADHD), depression, bipolar disorder, and anxiety disorders. Children with neurodevelopmental disorders may be more prone to nocturnal seizures, as well as other sleep disruptions, and children with blindness, mental retardation, some chromosomal syndromes (Smith-Magenis, fragile X), and autism spectrum disorders are at increased risk for severe sleep onset difficulty and night wakings, as well as circadian rhythm disturbances.

Insomnia of Childhood

Insomnia may be broadly defined as repeated difficulty initiating and/or maintaining sleep that occurs despite age-appropriate time and opportunity for sleep. These sleep complaints must also result in some degree of impairment in daytime functioning for the child and/or family, which may range from fatigue, irritability, lack of energy, and mild cognitive impairment to effects on mood, school performance, and quality of life. Insomnia complaints may be of a short-term and transient nature (usually related to an acute event), or may be characterized as long-term and chronic. Insomnia is a set of *symptoms* with a large number of possible etiologies (e.g., pain, medication, medical and psychiatric conditions, learned behaviors) and not as a *diagnosis* per se. Insomnia, like many behavioral issues in children, is often primarily defined by parental concerns rather than by objective criteria, and therefore should be viewed in the context of family (i.e., maternal depression, stress), child (i.e., temperament, developmental level), and environmental (i.e., cultural practices, sleeping space) considerations.

One of the most common sleep disorders found in infants and toddlers is **behavioral insomnia of childhood, sleep onset association type.** In this disorder, the child learns to fall asleep only under certain conditions or associations which typically require parental presence, such as being rocked or fed, and does not develop the ability to self-soothe. During the night, when the child experiences the type of brief arousal that normally occurs at the end of a sleep cycle (every 60-90 minutes in infants) or awakens for other reasons, he or she is not able to get back to sleep without those same conditions being present. The infant then "signals" the parent by crying (or coming into the parents' bedroom, if the child is no longer in a crib) until the necessary associations are provided. The problem is one of prolonged night waking resulting in insufficient sleep (for both child and parent).

Management of night wakings should include establishment of a set sleep schedule and bedtime routine, and implementation of a behavioral program. The treatment approach typically involves a program of rapid withdrawal (extinction) or more gradual withdrawal (graduated extinction) of parental assistance at sleep onset and during the night. Extinction ("cry it out") involves putting the child to bed at a designated bedtime, "drowsy but awake," and then systematically ignoring the child until a set time the next morning. Although it has considerable empirical support, extinction is often not an acceptable choice for families. Graduated extinction involves weaning the child from dependence on parental presence with periodic "checks" by the parents at successively longer intervals during the sleep-wake transition; the exact amount of time is determined by the parents' tolerance for crying and the child's temperament. The goal is to allow the infant or child to develop skills in self-soothing during the night, as well as at bedtime. In older infants, the introduction of more appropriate sleep associations that will be readily available to the child during the night (transitional objects, such as a blanket or toy), in addition to positive reinforcement (i.e., stickers for remaining in bed), is often beneficial. If the child has become habituated to awaken for nighttime feedings ("learned hunger"), then these feedings should be slowly eliminated. Parents must be consistent in applying behavioral programs to avoid inadvertent, intermittent reinforcement of night wakings; they should also be forewarned that crying behavior often temporarily escalates at the beginning of treatment ("post-extinction burst").

Bedtime problems, including stalling and refusing to go to bed, are more common in preschool-aged and older children. Sleep disturbances of this type generally fall within the diagnostic category known as **behavioral insomnia of childhood, limit setting type,** and are often the result of parental difficulties in setting limits and managing behavior, including the inability or unwillingness to set consistent bedtime rules and enforce a regular bedtime, and may be exacerbated by the child's oppositional behavior. In some cases the child's resistance at bedtime is due to an underlying problem in falling asleep that is caused by other factors (medical conditions, such as asthma or medication use; a sleep disorder, such as restless legs syndrome; or anxiety) or a mismatch between the child's intrinsic circadian rhythm ("night owl") and parental expectations.

Successful treatment of limit setting sleep disorder generally involves a combination of parent education regarding appropriate limit setting, decreased parental attention for bedtime-delaying behavior, establishment of bedtime routines, and positive reinforcement (sticker charts) for appropriate behavior at bedtime; other behavioral management strategies that have empirical support include bedtime fading (temporarily setting the bedtime closer to the actual sleep onset time and then gradually advancing the bedtime to an earlier target bedtime). Older children may benefit from being taught relaxation techniques to help themselves fall asleep more readily. Following the principles of sleep hygiene for children is essential (Table 17-2).

When the insomnia is not primarily a result of parent behavior or secondary to another sleep disturbance, or to a psychiatric or medical problem, it is referred to as **psychophysiologic or primary insomnia,** also sometimes called "learned insomnia." Primary insomnia usually occurs largely in adolescents and is characterized by a combination of learned sleep-preventing associations and heightened physiologic arousal resulting in a complaint of sleeplessness and decreased daytime functioning. A hallmark of primary insomnia is excessive worry about sleep and an exaggerated concern of the potential daytime consequences. The physiologic arousal can be in the form of cognitive hypervigilance, such as "racing" thoughts; in many individuals with insomnia an increased baseline level of arousal is further intensified by this secondary anxiety about sleeplessness. Treatment usually involves educating the adolescent about the principles of sleep hygiene (Table 17-3), institution of a consistent sleep-wake schedule, avoidance of daytime napping, instructions to use the bed for sleep only and to get out of bed if unable to fall asleep (stimulus control), restricting time in bed to the actual time asleep (sleep restriction), addressing maladaptive cognitions about sleep, and teaching relaxation techniques to reduce anxiety. Hypnotic medications are rarely needed.

Table 17-2 BASIC PRINCIPLES OF SLEEP HYGIENE FOR CHILDREN

1. **Have a set bedtime and bedtime routine** for your child.
2. **Bedtime and wake-up time should be about the same time on school nights and non-school nights.** There should not be more than about an hour difference from one day to another.
3. **Make the hour before bed shared quiet time.** Avoid high-energy activities, such as rough play, and stimulating activities, such as watching television or playing computer games, just before bed.
4. **Don't send your child to bed hungry.** A *light* snack (such as milk and cookies) before bed is a good idea. Heavy meals within an hour or two of bedtime, however, may interfere with sleep.
5. **Avoid products containing caffeine for at least several hours before bedtime.** These include caffeinated sodas, coffee, tea, and chocolate.
6. **Make sure your child spends time outside every day** whenever possible and is involved in regular exercise.
7. **Keep your child's bedroom quiet and dark.** A low-level night light is acceptable for children who find completely dark rooms frightening.
8. **Keep your child's bedroom at a comfortable temperature** during the night (<75°F).
9. **Don't use your child's bedroom for time-out or punishment.**
10. **Keep the television set out of your child's bedroom.** Children can easily develop the bad habit of "needing" the television to fall asleep. It's also much more difficult to control your child's viewing if the set is in the bedroom.

Table 17-3 BASIC PRINCIPLES OF SLEEP HYGIENE FOR ADOLESCENTS

1. **Wake up and go to bed at about the same time** every night. Bedtime and wake-up time should not differ from school to non-school nights by more than approximately an hour.
2. **Avoid sleeping in on weekends** to "catch up" on sleep. This makes it more likely that you will have problems falling asleep.
3. If you take **naps**, they should be **short** (no more than an hour) and **scheduled in the early to midafternoon**. However, if you have a problem with falling asleep at night, **napping** during the day may make it worse and should be avoided.
4. **Spend time outside** every day. Exposure to sunlight helps to keep your body's internal clock on track.
5. **Exercise regularly.** Exercise may help you fall asleep and sleep more deeply.
6. **Use your bed for sleeping only.** Don't study, read, listen to music, watch television, etc., on your bed.
7. Make the 30-60 minutes before a **quiet or wind-down time**. Relaxing, calm, enjoyable activities, such as reading a book or listening to calm music, help your body and mind slow down enough to let you get to sleep. Don't study, watch exciting/scary movies, exercise, or get involved in "energizing" activities just before bed.
8. Eat regular meals and **don't go to bed hungry**. A light snack before bed is a good idea; eating a full meal in the hour before bed is not.
9. **Avoid** eating or drinking products containing **caffeine** from dinner time on. These include caffeinated sodas, coffee, tea, and chocolate.
10. **Do not use alcohol.** Alcohol disrupts sleep and may cause you to awaken throughout the night.
11. **Smoking disturbs sleep.** Don't smoke at least one hour before bed (and preferably, not at all!).
12. Don't use **sleeping pills, melatonin**, or other **over-the-counter sleep aids** to help you sleep unless specifically recommended by your doctor. These can be dangerous, and the sleep problems often return when you stop taking the medicine.

Obstructive Sleep Apnea

Sleep-disordered breathing (SDB) in children encompasses a broad spectrum of respiratory disorders that occur exclusively in or are exacerbated by sleep, and includes primary snoring and upper airway resistance syndrome, as well as apnea of prematurity and central apnea. **Obstructive sleep apnea (OSA)**, the most important clinical entity within the SDB spectrum, is a respiratory disorder that is characterized by repeated episodes of prolonged upper airway obstruction during sleep despite continued or increased respiratory effort, resulting in complete (apnea) or partial (hypopnea; ≥50% reduction in airflow) cessation of airflow at the nose and/or mouth, as well as in disrupted sleep. Both intermittent hypoxia and the multiple arousals resulting from these obstructive events likely contribute to significant metabolic, cardiovascular, and neurocognitive/neurobehavioral morbidity.

Primary snoring is defined as snoring without associated ventilatory abnormalities (e.g., apneas or hypopneas, hypoxemia, hypercapnia) or respiratory-related arousals, and is a manifestation of the vibrations of the oropharyngeal soft tissue walls that occur when an individual attempts to breathe against increased upper airway resistance during sleep. Children with primary snoring may still have subtle breathing abnormalities during sleep, including evidence of increased respiratory effort, which in turn may be associated with adverse neurodevelopmental outcomes.

ETIOLOGY In general terms, OSA results from an anatomically or functionally narrowed upper airway; this typically involves some combination of decreased upper airway patency (upper airway obstruction and/or decreased upper airway diameter), increased upper airway collapsibility (reduced pharyngeal muscle tone), and decreased drive to breathe in the face of reduced upper airway patency (reduced central ventilatory drive) (Table 17-4). Upper airway obstruction varies in degree and level (i.e., nose, nasopharynx/oropharynx, hypopharynx) and is most commonly due to adenotonsillar hypertrophy, although tonsillar size does not necessarily correlate with degree of obstruction, especially in older children. Other causes of airway obstruction include allergies associated with chronic rhinitis/nasal obstruction; craniofacial abnormalities, including hypoplasia/displacement of the maxilla and mandible; gastroesophageal reflux with resulting pharyngeal reactive edema; nasal septal deviation; and velopharyngeal flap cleft palate repair. Reduced upper airway tone may result from neuromuscular diseases, including hypotonic cerebral palsy and muscular dystrophies, or hypothyroidism. Reduced central ventilatory drive may be present in some children with Arnold-Chiari malformation and meningomyelocele. In other situations, the etiology is mixed; individuals with Down syndrome, by virtue of their facial anatomy, hypotonia, macroglossia, and central adiposity, as well as the increased incidence of hypothyroidism, are at particularly high risk for OSA, with some estimates of as great as 70% prevalence.

Table 17-4 ANATOMIC FACTORS THAT PREDISPOSE TO OBSTRUCTIVE SLEEP APNEA AND HYPOVENTILATION IN CHILDREN

NOSE
Anterior nasal stenosis
Choanal stenosis/atresia
Deviated nasal septum
Seasonal or perennial rhinitis
Nasal polyps, foreign body, hematoma, mass lesion
NASOPHARYNGEAL AND OROPHARYNGEAL
Adenotonsillar hypertrophy
Macroglossia
Cystic hygroma
Velopharyngeal flap repair
Cleft palate repair
Pharyngeal mass lesion
CRANIOFACIAL
Micrognathia/retrognathia
Midface hypoplasia (e.g., trisomy 21, Crouzon, Apert syndrome)
Mandibular hypoplasia (Pierre Robin sequence, Treacher Collins, Cornelia de Lange)
Craniofacial trauma
Skeletal and storage diseases
Achondroplasia
Storage diseases (e.g., glycogen, Hunter, Hurler syndrome)

Although many children with OSA are of normal weight, an increasingly large percentage are overweight or obese, and many of these children are school-aged and younger. There is a significant correlation between weight and SDB (habitual snoring, OSA, central apneas). While adenotonsillar hypertrophy also plays an important etiologic role in overweight/obese children with OSA, mechanical factors related to an increase in the amount of adipose tissue in the throat (pharyngeal fat pads), neck (increased neck circumference), and chest wall and abdomen can create increased upper airway resistance, worsen gas exchange, and increased work of breathing, particularly in the supine position and during REM sleep. There may be a component of blunted central ventilatory drive in response to hypoxia/hypercapnia and hypoventilation as well, particularly in children with morbid or syndrome-based (Prader-Willi) obesity. Overweight and obese children and adolescents are at a particularly high risk for metabolic and cardiovascular complications of SDB, such as insulin resistance and systemic hypertension; morbidly obese children may also be at increased risk for postoperative complications following adenotonsillectomy.

EPIDEMIOLOGY Overall prevalence of parent-reported snoring in the pediatric population is about 8%; "always" snoring is reported in 1.5-6%, and "often" snoring in 3-15%. When defined by parent-reported symptoms, the prevalence of OSA is 4-11%. The prevalence of pediatric OSA as documented by overnight sleep studies utilizing ventilatory monitoring procedures (e.g., in-lab PSG, home studies) is 1-4% overall, with a reported range of 0.1-13%. Prevalence is also affected by the demographic characteristics, such as age (increased prevalence between 2 and 8 yr), gender (more common in boys, especially after puberty), race/ethnicity (increased prevalence in African-American and Asian children), and family history of OSA.

PATHOGENESIS The upregulation of inflammatory pathways, as indicated by an increase in peripheral markers of inflammation such as C-reactive protein (CRP), appear to be linked to metabolic dysfunction (e.g., insulin resistance, dyslipidemia) in both obese and non-obese children with OSA. Both systemic inflammation and arousal-mediated increases in sympathetic autonomic nervous system activity with altered vasomotor tone may be key contributors to increased cardiovascular risk in both adults and children with OSA. Mechanical stress on the upper airway induced by chronic snoring may also result in both local mucosal inflammation of adenotonsillar tissues and subsequent upregulation of inflammatory molecules, most notably leukotrienes. Another potential mechanism that may mediate cardiovascular sequelae in both adults and children with OSA is altered endothelial function.

Although yet to be fully elucidated, one of the primary mechanisms by which OSA is believed to exert negative influences on cognitive function appears to involve repeated episodic arousals from sleep leading to sleep fragmentation and resulting sleepiness. An equally important role may be intermittent hypoxia that leads directly to systemic inflammatory vascular changes in the brain. Levels of inflammatory markers such as CRP and cytokine IL-6 are elevated in children with OSA and are also associated with cognitive dysfunction.

CLINICAL MANIFESTATIONS The clinical manifestations of OSA may be divided into sleep-related and daytime symptoms. The most common nocturnal manifestations of OSA in children and adolescents are loud, frequent, and disruptive snoring, breathing pauses, choking or gasping arousals, restless sleep, and nocturnal diaphoresis. Many children who snore do not have OSA, but very few children with OSA do not snore. Most children, like adults, tend to have more frequent and more severe obstructive events in REM sleep and when sleeping in the supine position. Children with OSA may adopt unusual sleeping positions, keeping their necks hyperextended in order to maintain airway patency. Frequent arousals associated with obstruction may result in nocturnal awakenings, but are more likely to cause fragmented sleep.

Daytime symptoms of OSA include mouth breathing and dry mouth, chronic nasal congestion/rhinorrhea, hyponasal speech, morning headaches, difficulty swallowing, and poor appetite. Children with OSA may have secondary enuresis, most likely as a result of the disruption of the normal nocturnal pattern of antidiuretic hormone secretion. Partial arousal parasomnias (sleepwalking and sleep terrors) may occur more frequently in children with OSA, related to the frequent associated arousals and an increased percentage of delta sleep, or SWS.

One of the most important but frequently overlooked sequelae of OSA in children is the effect on mood, behavior, learning, and academic functioning. The neurobehavioral consequences of OSA in children include daytime sleepiness with drowsiness, difficulty in morning waking, and unplanned napping or dozing off during activities, although evidence of frank hypersomnolence tends to be less common in children compared to adults with OSA. Mood changes include increased irritability, mood instability and emotional dysregulation, low frustration tolerance, and depression/anxiety. Behavioral issues include both "internalizing" (i.e., increased somatic complaints and social withdrawal) and "externalizing" behaviors, including aggression, impulsivity, hyperactivity, oppositional behavior, and conduct problems. There is a substantial overlap between the clinical impairments associated with OSA and the diagnostic criteria for ADHD, including inattention, poor concentration, and distractibility (Chapter 30). There also appears to be a selective impact of OSA specifically on "executive functions," which include cognitive flexibility, task initiation, self-monitoring, planning, organization, and self-regulation of affect and arousal; executive function deficits are also a hallmark of ADHD.

Studies that have looked at changes in behavior and neuropsychologic functioning in children following treatment (usually adenotonsillectomy) for OSA have largely documented significant improvement in outcomes, in both the short and long term, of OSA syndrome post-treatment, including daytime sleepiness, mood, behavior, academics, and quality of life. Many studies have failed to find a dose-dependent relationship between OSA in children and specific neurobehavioral/neurocognitive deficits, suggesting that other factors may influence neurocognitive outcomes, including individual genetic susceptibility, environmental influences such as passive smoking exposure, and co-morbid conditions, such as obesity, shortened sleep duration, and the presence of other sleep disorders.

DIAGNOSIS The American Academy of Pediatrics clinical practice guidelines provide excellent information for the evaluation and management of uncomplicated childhood OSA (Table 17-5). There are no physical examination findings that are truly pathognomonic for OSA, and most healthy children with OSA appear normal; certain physical examination findings may suggest OSA. Growth parameters may be abnormal (obesity or, less commonly, failure to thrive), and there may be evidence of chronic nasal obstruction (hyponasal speech, mouth breathing, septal deviation, "adenoidal facies"), as well as signs of atopic disease (i.e., "allergic shiners"). Oropharyngeal examination may reveal enlarged tonsils, excess soft tissue in the posterior pharynx, and a narrowed posterior pharyngeal space. Any abnormalities of the facial structure, such as retrognathia and/or micrognathia, midfacial hypoplasia, best appreciated by inspection of the lateral facial profile, increase the likelihood of OSA and should be noted. In very severe cases, there may be evidence of pulmonary hypertension, right-sided heart failure, and cor pulmonale; systemic hypertension, unlike in adults, is relatively uncommon.

Because no combination of clinical history and physical findings can accurately predict which children with snoring have OSA, the gold standard for diagnosing OSA remains an overnight **polysomnogram** (PSG).

An overnight PSG is a technician-supervised, monitored study that documents physiologic variables during sleep; sleep staging, arousal measurement, cardiovascular parameters, and body movements (electroencephology, electrooculography, chin and leg electromyography, ECG, body position sensors, and video recording), and a combination of breathing monitors

Table 17-5 AMERICAN ACADEMY OF PEDIATRICS CLINICAL PRACTICE GUIDELINES FOR OBSTRUCTIVE SLEEP APNEA SYNDROME (APRIL 2002)

All children should be screened for snoring.
Complex high-risk patients should be referred to a specialist.
Patients with cardiorespiratory failure cannot await elective evaluation.
Diagnostic evaluation is useful in discriminating between primary snoring and obstructive sleep apnea syndrome, the gold standard being polysomnography.
Adenotonsillectomy is the first line of treatment for most children, and continuous positive airway pressure (CPAP) is an option for those who are not candidates for surgery or do not respond to surgery.
High-risk patients should be monitored as inpatients postoperatively.
Patients should be re-evaluated postoperatively to determine whether additional treatment is required.

(oronasal thermal sensor and nasal air pressure transducer for airflow), chest/abdominal monitors (e.g., inductance plethysmography for respiratory effort, pulse oximeter for O_2 saturation, end-tidal or transcutaneous CO_2 for hypercarbia, snore microphone). The polysomnographic parameter most commonly used in evaluating for sleep disordered breathing is the apnea/hypopnea index (AHI), which indicates the number of apneic and hypopneic events per hr of sleep. It should be noted that currently there are no universally accepted polysomnographic normal reference values and parameters for diagnosing OSA in children, and it is still unclear which parameters best predict morbidity. Normal preschool and early school-aged children may have a total AHI of less than 1.5, and this is the most widely used cutoff value for OSA in children 12 yr and below; in adolescents, the adult cutoff of an AHI ≥5 is generally used. In cases in which the AHI is between 1 and 5 obstructive events per hour, clinical judgment regarding risk factors for SDB, evidence of daytime sequelae, and the technical quality of the overnight sleep study should determine further management.

TREATMENT There are presently no universally accepted guidelines regarding the indications for treatment of pediatric SDB (i.e., including primary snoring and OSA). Current recommendations largely emphasize weighing what is known about the potential cardiovascular, metabolic, and neurocognitive sequelae of SDB in children in combination with the individual health care professional's clinical judgment. The decision of whether and how to treat OSA specifically in children is contingent on a number of parameters, including severity (nocturnal symptoms, daytime sequelae, sleep study results), duration of disease, and individual patient variables such as age, co-morbid conditions, and underlying etiologic factors. In the case of moderate to severe disease (AHI >10), the decision to treat is usually straightforward, and most pediatric sleep experts recommend that any child with an apnea index >5 should be treated.

In the majority of cases of pediatric OSA, adenotonsillectomy is the first-line treatment in any child with significant adenotonsillar hypertrophy, even in the presence of additional risk factors such as obesity. Adenotonsillectomy in uncomplicated cases generally (70-90% of children) results in complete resolution of symptoms; regrowth of adenoidal tissue after surgical removal occurs in some cases. Groups considered high-risk include young children (<3 yr old), as well as those with severe OSA documented on polysomnography, significant clinical sequelae of OSA (e.g., failure to thrive), or associated medical conditions, such as craniofacial syndromes, morbid obesity, and hypotonia. All patients should be re-evaluated postoperatively to determine whether additional evaluation and/or treatment are required. If there are significant residual risk factors (e.g., obesity) or continued symptoms of OSA, a follow-up sleep study at least 6 wk post-adenotonsillectomy may be indicated.

Additional treatment measures that may be appropriate include weight loss, positional therapy (attaching a firm object, such as a tennis ball, to the back of a sleep garment to prevent the child from sleeping in the supine position), and aggressive treatment of additional risk factors when present, such as asthma, seasonal allergies, and gastroesophageal reflux; there is some evidence that intranasal corticosteroids and leukotriene inhibitors may be helpful in mild OSA. Other surgical procedures, such as uvulopharyngopalatoplasty, and maxillofacial surgery (mandibular distraction osteogenesis and maxillomandibular advancement), are seldom performed in children but may be indicated in selected cases. Oral appliances, such as mandibular advancing devices and tongue retainers, are typically considered for adolescents in whom facial bone growth is largely complete.

Continuous or bilevel positive airway pressure (nasal CPAP or BiPAP) is the most common treatment for OSA in adults and can be used successfully in children and adolescents. CPAP delivers humidified, warmed air through an interface (mask, nasal pillows) that, under pressure, effectively "splints" the upper airway open. Optimal pressure settings (that abolish or significantly reduce respiratory events without increasing arousals or central apneas) are determined in the sleep lab during a full night CPAP titration. Efficacy studies at the current pressure and retitrations should be conducted periodically with long-term use (every 6 mo in young children and at least yearly or with significant weight changes in older children and adolescents). CPAP may be recommended if removing the adenoids and tonsils is not indicated, if there is residual disease following adenotonsillectomy, or if there are major risk factors that are not amenable to treatment with surgery (obesity, hypotonia).

Parasomnias

Parasomnias are defined as episodic nocturnal behaviors that often involve cognitive disorientation and autonomic and skeletal muscle disturbance. Parasomnias may be further characterized as occurring primarily during NREM sleep (partial arousal parasomnias) or in association with REM sleep, including nightmares, hypnogogic hallucinations, and sleep paralysis; other common parasomnias include sleep-talking. Sleep-related movement disorders, including restless legs syndrome/periodic limb movement disorder (RLS/PLMD) and rhythmic movement disorder (head banging, body rocking), are reviewed in a separate section below.

ETIOLOGY Partial arousal parasomnias, which include **sleepwalking, sleep terrors**, and **confusional arousals** are more common in preschool and school-aged children because of the relatively higher percentage of SWS in younger children. Any factor that is associated with an increase in the relative percentage of SWS (certain medications, previous sleep deprivation) may increase the frequency of events in a predisposed child. There appears to be a genetic predisposition for both sleepwalking and night terrors. In contrast, nightmares, which are much more common than the partial arousal parasomnias but are often confused with them, are concentrated in the last third of the night, when REM sleep is most prominent. Partial arousal parasomnias may also be difficult to distinguish from nocturnal seizures. Table 17-6 summarizes similarities and differences among these nocturnal arousal events.

EPIDEMIOLOGY Many children (15-40%) **sleepwalk** on at least one occasion; the prevalence of children who regularly sleepwalk is approximately 17%, and 3-4% have frequent episodes. Sleepwalking may persist into adulthood, with the prevalence in adults of about 4%. The prevalence is approximately 10 times greater in children with a family history of sleepwalking. Approximately 1-6% of children experience **sleep terrors**, primarily during the preschool and elementary school years, and the age of onset is usually between 4 and 12 yr. Because of the common genetic predisposition, the prevalence of sleep terrors in children who sleepwalk is about 10%. Although sleep terrors can occur at any age from infancy through adulthood, most individuals outgrow sleep terrors by adolescence. Confusional arousals commonly co-occur with sleepwalking and sleep terrors; prevalence rates have been estimated to be upwards of 15% in children ages 3-13 yr.

CLINICAL MANIFESTATIONS The partial arousal parasomnias have several features in common. Because they typically occur at the transition out of "deep" or SWS, partial arousal parasomnias have clinical features of both the awake (ambulation, vocalizations) and the sleeping (high arousal threshold, unresponsiveness to the environment) states; there is usually amnesia for the events. The typical timing of partial arousal parasomnias during the first few hours of sleep is related to the predominance of SWS in the first third of the night; the duration is typically a few minutes (sleep terrors) to an hour (confusional arousals). Sleep terrors are sudden in onset and characteristically involve a high degree of autonomic arousal (i.e., tachycardia, dilated pupils), while

Table 17-6 DIFFERENTIATION OF EPISODIC NOCTURNAL PHENOMENA

CHARACTERISTICS	PARTIAL AROUSAL PARASOMNIAS	NIGHTMARES	NOCTURNAL SEIZURES
Sleep stage	SWS	REM	Non-REM > Wake > REM
Timing during night	First third	Last third	Variable; often at sleep-wake transition
Level autonomic arousal	Low/high/medium	Mild to high	Variable
Arousal threshold	High	Low	Low
Recall of event	None or fragmentary	Vivid	Not usual
Daytime sleepiness	None	+/–	Often
Incontinence, tongue biting, drooling, stereotypy, postictal behavior	No	No	Yes
Multiple episodes per night	Rare	Occasional	More common
Increased by sleep deprivation	Yes	Sometimes	+/–
PSG	Indicated if atypical features	Not indicated	Indicated if atypical features; requires extended EEG montage
Family history	Common	Rare	Variable

EEG, electroencephalography; PSG, polysomnography; REM, rapid eye movement; SWS, slow-wave sleep.

confusional arousals typically arise more gradually from sleep, may involve thrashing around but usually not displacement from bed, and are often accompanied by slow mentation on arousal from sleep ("sleep inertia"). Sleepwalking may be associated with safety concerns (e.g., falling out of windows, wandering outside). Avoidance of, or increased agitation with, comforting by parents or attempts at awakening are also common features of all partial arousal parasomnias.

TREATMENT Management of partial arousal parasomnias involves some combination of parental education and reassurance, good sleep hygiene, and avoidance of exacerbating factors such as sleep deprivation and caffeine. Particularly in the case of sleepwalking, it is important to institute safety precautions such as use of gates in doorways and at the top of staircases, locking of outside doors and windows, and installation of parent notification systems such as bedroom door alarms. Scheduled awakenings, a behavioral intervention that involve having the parent wake the child approximately 15 to 30 min before the time of night that the first parasomnia episode is most likely to be successful in situations in which partial arousal episodes occur on a nightly basis. Pharmacotherapy is rarely necessary, but may be indicated in cases of frequent or severe episodes, high risk of injury, violent behavior, or serious disruption to the family; the primary pharmacologic agents used are potent SWS suppressants, primarily benzodiazepines and tricyclic antidepressants.

Sleep-Related Movement Disorders: Restless Legs Syndrome/Periodic Limb Movement Disorder and Rhythmic Movements

Restless legs syndrome (RLS) is a neurologic, primarily sensory disorder, characterized by uncomfortable sensations in the lower extremities that are accompanied by an almost irresistible urge to move the legs. The sensations are usually at least partially relieved by movement, including walking, stretching, and rubbing, but only as long as the motion continues. RLS is a clinical diagnosis that is based on the presence of these key symptoms. **Periodic limb movement disorder** (PLMD) is characterized by periodic, repetitive, brief (0.5-10 sec), and highly stereotyped limb jerks typically occurring at 20 to 40 sec intervals. These movements occur primarily during sleep, most commonly occur in the legs, and frequently consist of rhythmic extension of the big toe and dorsiflexion at the ankle. The diagnosis of **periodic limb movements** (PLMs) requires overnight polysomnography to document the characteristic limb movements with anterior tibialis EMG leads.

ETIOLOGY "Early-onset" RLS (i.e., onset of symptoms before 35-40 yr of age), often termed "primary" RLS, appears to have a particularly strong genetic component. Variants of the *PTPRD* gene are associated with RLS. Low serum iron levels in both adults and children may be an important etiologic factor for the presence and severity of both RLS symptoms and PLMs. As a marker of decreased iron stores, serum ferritin levels in both children and adults with RLS are frequently low. The underlying mechanism that has been postulated is related to the role of iron as a cofactor of tyrosine hydroxylase in a rate-limiting step of the synthesis of dopamine; in turn, dopaminergic dysfunction has been implicated as playing a key role particularly in the genesis of the sensory component of RLS, as well as in PLMD. Certain medical conditions, including diabetes mellitus, end-stage renal disease, cancer, rheumatoid arthritis, hypothyroidism, and pregnancy, may also be associated with RLS/PLMD, as are specific medications (i.e., antihistamines such as diphenhydramine, antidepressants, and H-2 blockers such as cimetidine) and substances (e.g., caffeine).

EPIDEMIOLOGY Previous studies have found prevalence rates of RLS in the pediatric population ranging from 1-6%; the percent of 8-17 yr olds meeting criteria for "definite" RLS is approximately 2%. Prevalence rates of PLMs greater than 5 per hour in clinical populations of children referred for sleep studies range from 5-27%; in survey studies of PLM symptoms, rates are 8-12%. Several studies in referral populations have found that PLMs occur in as much as one fourth of children diagnosed with ADHD.

CLINICAL MANIFESTATIONS In addition to the sensory component and the urge to move the legs, most RLS episodes begin or are exacerbated by rest or inactivity, such as lying in bed to fall asleep or riding in a car for prolonged periods. A unique feature of RLS is that the timing of symptoms also appears to have a circadian component, in that they often peak in the evening hours. Some children may complain of "growing pains," although this is considered a nonspecific feature. Because RLS symptoms are usually worse in the evening, bedtime struggles and difficulty falling asleep are 2 of the most common presenting complaints. In contrast to patients with RLS, individuals with PLMs are usually unaware of these movements; these movements may result in arousals during sleep and consequent significant sleep disruption. Parents of children with RLS/PLMD may complain that their child is a restless sleeper, moves around or even falls out of bed during the night.

TREATMENT The decision of whether and how to treat RLS depends on the level of severity (intensity, frequency, and periodicity) of sensory symptoms, the degree of interference with sleep, and the impact of daytime sequelae in a particular child or adolescent. With PLMs, for an index (PLMs per hr) less than 5, usually no treatment is recommended; for an index over 5, the decision to specifically treat PLMs should be based on the presence or absence of nocturnal symptoms (restless or nonrestorative sleep) and daytime clinical sequelae. A reasonable initial approach would be to promote good sleep hygiene (including restricting caffeine) and instituting iron supplements in children if serum ferritin levels are low (<50); the recommended dose of ferrous sulfate is typically in the range of 4-6 mg/kg/day for a duration of 3-6 mo. Medications that increase dopamine levels in the CNS, such as ropinirole and pramipexole, have been found to be effective in relieving RLS/PLMD symptoms in adults; data in children are extremely limited.

Sleep-related rhythmic movements, including head banging, body rocking, and head rolling, are characterized by repetitive, stereotyped, and rhythmic movements or behaviors that involve large muscle groups. These behaviors typically occur with the transition at sleep at bedtime, but also at nap times and following nighttime arousals. Children typically engage in these behaviors as a means of soothing themselves to (or back to) sleep; they are much more common in the 1st yr of life and usually disappear by 4 yr of age. In most instances, rhythmic movement behaviors are benign, because sleep is not significantly disrupted as a result of these movements and associated significant injury is rare. These behaviors typically occur in normally developing children, and in the vast majority of cases their presence does not indicate that there is some underlying neurological or psychological problem. Usually, the most important aspect in management of sleep-related rhythmic movements is reassurance to the family that this behavior is normal, common, benign, and self-limited.

Narcolepsy

Hypersomnia is a clinical term that is used to describe a group of disorders characterized by recurrent episodes of **excessive daytime sleepiness (EDS)**, reduced baseline alertness, and/or prolonged nighttime sleep periods that interfere with normal daily functioning. It is important to recognize that there are many potential causes of EDS, which may be broadly grouped as "extrinsic" (e.g., secondary to insufficient and/or fragmented sleep) or "intrinsic" (e.g., resulting from an increased need for sleep). **Narcolepsy** is a chronic lifelong CNS disorder, typically presenting in adolescence and early adulthood, that is characterized by profound daytime sleepiness and resultant significant functional impairment. Other symptoms frequently associated with narcolepsy, cataplexy, hypnogogic/hypnopompic hallucinations, and sleep paralysis, may be conceptualized as representing the "intrusion" of REM sleep features into the waking state.

ETIOLOGY There is a specific deficit in the hypothalamic orexin/hypocretin neurotransmitter system in the genesis of narcolepsy with cataplexy. The underlying pathogenesis of narcolepsy involves selective loss of cells that secrete hypocretin/orexin in the lateral hypothalamus; it has been postulated that autoimmune mechanisms, possibly triggered by viral infections, in combination with a genetic predisposition and environmental factors, may be involved. Human leukocyte antigen testing also shows a strong association with narcolepsy; however, the vast majority of individuals with this antigen do not have narcolepsy. Although the majority of cases of narcolepsy are considered idiopathic, "secondary" narcolepsy with cataplexy may also result from CNS insults.

EPIDEMIOLOGY The prevalence of narcolepsy is reported to be between 3 and 16 per 10,000, with the prevalence of narcolepsy with cataplexy approximately 0.2-0.5/10,000. The risk of developing narcolepsy with cataplexy in a first-degree relative of a narcoleptic patient is estimated at 1-2%; this represents an increase of 10- to 40-fold compared to the general population.

CLINICAL MANIFESTATIONS AND DIAGNOSIS The typical onset of symptoms of narcolepsy is in adolescence and early adulthood, although symptoms may initially present in school-aged and even younger children. The early manifestations of narcolepsy are often ignored, misinterpreted, or misdiagnosed as other medical, neurologic, and psychiatric conditions, and the appropriate diagnosis is frequently delayed for a number of years.

The most prominent clinical manifestation of narcolepsy is profound daytime sleepiness, characterized by both an increased baseline level of daytime drowsiness and by the repeated occurrence of sudden and unpredictable sleep episodes. These "**sleep attacks**" are often described as "irresistible" in that the child or adolescent is unable to stay awake despite considerable effort, and they occur even in the context of normally stimulating activities (e.g., during meals, in the middle of a conversation). Very brief (several seconds) sleep attacks may also occur in which the individual may "stare off," appear unresponsive, or continue to engage in an ongoing activity (automatic behavior). **Cateplexy** is considered pathognomonic for narcolepsy. Cataplexy is rarely the first symptom of narcolepsy, but it often develops within the 1st year of the onset of EDS. It is described as an abrupt, bilateral, partial or complete loss of muscle tone, classically triggered by an intense positive emotion (e.g., laughter, surprise). The cataplectic attacks are typically brief (seconds to minutes), and fully reversible, with complete recovery of normal tone when the episode ends. **Hypnogogic/hypnopompic hallucinations** involve vivid visual, auditory, and sometimes tactile sensory experiences occurring during transitions between sleep and wakefulness, primarily at sleep onset (hypnogogic) and sleep offset (hypnopompic). **Sleep paralysis** is the inability to move or speak for a few seconds or minutes at sleep onset or offset, and often accompanies the hallucinations. Other symptoms associated with narcolepsy include disrupted nocturnal sleep, inattention, and behavioral and mood issues.

Overnight polysomnography followed by a multiple sleep latency test (MSLT) are strongly recommended components of the evaluation of a patient with profound unexplained daytime sleepiness or suspected narcolepsy. The purpose of the overnight PSG is to evaluate for primary sleep disorders, such as OSA that may cause EDS. The MSLT involves a series of 5 opportunities to nap (20 min long), during which narcoleptics demonstrate a pathologically shortened sleep onset latency as well as periods of REM sleep occurring immediately after sleep onset.

TREATMENT An individualized narcolepsy treatment plan usually involves education, good sleep hygiene, behavioral changes, and medication. Scheduled naps may be helpful. Medications such as psychostimulants and modafinil are often prescribed to control the EDS. The goal should be to allow the fullest possible return of normal functioning in school, at home, and in social situations. Medications such as tricyclic antidepressants and serotonin reuptake inhibitors may also be used to control the REM-associated phenomena, such as cataplexy, hypnogogic hallucinations, and sleep paralysis.

Delayed Sleep Phase Disorder

Delayed sleep phase disorder (DSPD), a circadian rhythm disorder, involves a significant, persistent, and intractable phase shift in sleep-wake schedule (later sleep onset and wake time) that conflicts with the individual's normal school, work, and/or lifestyle demands. DSPD may occur at any age, but is most common in adolescents and young adults.

ETIOLOGY Individuals with DSPD often start out as night owls; that is, they have an underlying predisposition or circadian preference for staying up late at night and sleeping late in the morning, especially on weekends, holidays, and summer vacations. The underlying pathophysiology of DSPD is still unknown, although some authors have theorized that it involves an intrinsic abnormality in the circadian oscillators that govern the timing of the sleep period.

EPIDEMIOLOGY Studies indicate that DSPD affects approximately 7-16% of adolescents.

CLINICAL MANIFESTATIONS The most common clinical presentation is sleep initiation insomnia when the individual attempts to fall asleep at a "socially acceptable" desired bedtime, accompanied by extreme difficulty getting up in the morning even for desired activities, and daytime sleepiness. Sleep maintenance is generally not problematic, and no sleep onset insomnia is experienced if bedtime coincides with the preferred sleep onset time (e.g., on weekends, school vacations). School tardiness and frequent absenteeism are often present.

TREATMENT The goal in the treatment of DSPD is basically 2-fold: first, shifting the sleep-wake schedule to an earlier time, and second, maintaining the new schedule. Gradual advancement of bedtime in the evening and rise time in the morning typically involves shifting bedtime/wake time earlier by 15-30 min increments; more significant phase delays (difference between

Table 17-7 BEARS SLEEP SCREENING ALGORITHM

The BEARS instrument is divided into 5 major sleep domains, providing a comprehensive screen for the major sleep disorders affecting children 2-18 years old. Each sleep domain has a set of age-appropriate "trigger questions" for use in the clinical interview.

B = Bedtime problems
E = Excessive daytime sleepiness
A = Awakenings during the night
R = Regularity and duration of sleep
S = Snoring

EXAMPLES OF DEVELOPMENTALLY APPROPRIATE TRIGGER QUESTIONS

	TODDLER/PRESCHOOL CHILD (2-5 YR)	SCHOOL-AGED CHILD (6-12 YR)	ADOLESCENT (13-18 YR)
1. **B**edtime problems	Does your child have any problems going to bed? Falling asleep?	Does your child have any problems at bedtime? (P) Do you any problems going to bed? (C)	Do you have any problems falling asleep at bedtime? (C)
2. **E**xcessive daytime sleepiness	Does your child seem overtired or sleepy a lot during the day? Does she still take naps?	Does your child have difficulty waking in the morning, seem sleepy during the day, or take naps? (P) Do you feel tired a lot? (C)	Do you feel sleepy a lot during the day? In school? While driving? (C)
3. **A**wakenings during the night	Does your child wake up a lot at night?	Does your child seem to wake up a lot at night? Any sleepwalking or nightmares? (P) Do you wake up a lot at night? Do you have trouble getting back to sleep? (C)	Do you wake up a lot at night? Do you have trouble getting back to sleep? (C)
4. **R**egularity and duration of sleep	Does your child have a regular bedtime and wake time? What are they?	What time does your child go to bed and get up on school days? Weekends? Do you think he is getting enough sleep? (P)	What time do you usually go to bed on school nights? Weekends? How much sleep do you usually get? (C)
5. **S**noring	Does your child snore a lot or have difficulty breathing at night?	Does your child have loud or nightly snoring or any breathing difficulties at night? (P)	Does your teenager snore loudly or nightly? (P)

C, child; P, parent.

current sleep onset and desired bedtime) may require "chronotherapy," which involves delaying bedtime and wake time by 2-3 hr daily to every other day. Exposure to light in the morning (either natural light or a "light box") and avoidance of evening light exposure are often beneficial. Exogenous oral melatonin supplementation may also be used; larger doses (i.e., 5 mg) are typically given at bedtime, but some studies have suggested that physiologic doses of oral melatonin (0.3-0.5 mg) administered in the afternoon or early evening (i.e., 5-7 hr before the habitual sleep onset time) seem to be most effective in advancing the sleep phase.

HEALTH SUPERVISION

It is especially important for pediatricians to both screen for and recognize sleep disorders in children and adolescents during health encounters. The well child visit is an opportunity to educate parents about normal sleep in children and to teach strategies to prevent sleep problems from developing (primary prevention) or from becoming chronic, if problems already exist (secondary prevention). Developmentally appropriate screening for sleep disturbances should take place in the context of every well child visit and should include a range of potential sleep problems; one simple sleep screening algorithm, the "BEARS," is outlined in Table 17-7. Because parents may not always be aware of sleep problems, especially in older children and adolescents, it is also important to question the child directly about sleep concerns. The recognition and evaluation of sleep problems in children requires both an understanding of the association between sleep disturbances and daytime consequences, such as irritability, inattention, and poor impulse control, and familiarity with the developmentally appropriate differential diagnoses of common presenting sleep complaints (difficulty initiating and maintaining sleep, episodic nocturnal events). An assessment of sleep patterns and possible sleep problems should be part of the initial evaluation of every child presenting with behavioral and/or academic problems, especially ADHD.

Effective preventive measures include educating parents of newborns about normal sleep amounts and patterns. The ability to regulate sleep, or control internal states of arousal to fall asleep at bedtime and to fall back asleep during the night, begins to develop in the first 12 wk of life. Thus, it is important to recommend that parents put their 2-4 mo old infants to bed "drowsy but awake" to avoid dependence on parental presence at sleep onset and to foster the infants' ability to self-soothe. Other important sleep issues include discussing the importance of regular bedtimes, bedtime routines, and transitional objects for toddlers, and providing parents and children with basic information about good "sleep hygiene" and adequate sleep amounts.

The cultural and family context within which sleep problems in children occur should be considered. Co-sleeping of infants and parents is a common and accepted practice in many ethnic groups, including African-Americans, Hispanics, and Southeast Asians. The goal of independent self-soothing in young infants may not be shared by these families. On the other hand, the institution of co-sleeping by parents as an attempt to address a child's underlying sleep problem, rather than as a lifestyle choice, is likely to yield only a temporary respite from the problem and may set the stage for more significant sleep issues.

EVALUATION OF PEDIATRIC SLEEP PROBLEMS

The clinical evaluation of a child presenting with a sleep problem involves obtaining a careful medical history to assess for potential medical causes of sleep disturbances, such as allergies, concomitant medications, and acute or chronic pain conditions. A developmental history is important because of the aforementioned frequent association of sleep problems with developmental delays and autism spectrum disorders. Assessment of the child's current level of functioning (school, home) is a key part of evaluating possible mood, behavioral, and neurocognitive sequelae of sleep problems. Current sleep patterns, including the usual sleep duration and sleep-wake schedule, are often best assessed with a sleep diary, in which parents record daily sleep behaviors for an extended period. A review of sleep habits, such as bedtime routines, daily caffeine intake, and the sleeping environment (e.g., temperature, noise level) may reveal environmental factors that contribute to the sleep problems. Nocturnal symptoms that may be indicative of a medically based sleep disorder, such as OSA (loud snoring, choking or gasping, sweating) or PLMs (restless sleep, repetitive kicking movements), should be elicited. An overnight sleep study is seldom warranted in the evaluation of a child with sleep problems unless there are symptoms suggestive of OSA or periodic leg movements, unusual features of episodic nocturnal events, or daytime sleepiness that is unexplained.

BIBLIOGRAPHY

Please visit the Nelson Textbook of Pediatrics *website at www.expertconsult.com for the complete bibliography.*

PART III Behavioral and Psychiatric Disorders

Chapter 18
Assessment and Interviewing

Heather J. Walter and David R. DeMaso

In children, mental illness is more prevalent than leukemia, diabetes, and AIDS combined. In 2006 in the USA, more money (8.9 billion dollars) was spent on mental disorders than on any other childhood illness, including asthma, trauma, upper respiratory infections, and infectious diseases. Although nearly 1 in 10 youths suffers from a psychiatric disorder severe enough to cause significant impairment, 75% to 80% do not receive needed mental health services. Untreated psychiatric disorders are associated with significant adverse sequelae, including increased morbidity and mortality, failure to achieve life's developmental tasks, cross-generational transmission of disadvantage, and substantial costs to society. Psychiatric disorders negatively affect the course of physical illness, adherence to treatment regimens, and use of medical resources. The strong heterotypic and homotypic continuity into adulthood of pediatric psychiatric disorders further underscores the importance of early identification and treatment.

AIMS OF ASSESSMENT

The aims of the psychosocial assessment in the pediatric setting are to determine whether there are signs and symptoms of cognitive, developmental, emotional, behavioral, or social difficulties and to characterize these signs and symptoms sufficiently to determine their appropriate management. The focus of the assessment varies with the nature of the presenting problem and the clinical setting. Under emergency circumstances, the focus may be limited to an assessment of dangerousness to self or others for the purpose of determining the appropriate level of care. In routine circumstances (well child visits), the focus may be broader, involving a screen for symptoms and functional impairment in all major psychosocial domains. The challenge for the pediatric practitioner will be to determine as accurately as possible whether the presenting signs and symptoms are likely to meet criteria for a psychiatric disorder and whether the severity and complexity of the disorder suggests referral to a mental health specialist or management in the pediatric setting.

PRESENTING PROBLEMS

Infants are brought to clinical attention because of concerns about failure to gain weight and length, poor social responsiveness, problems with eating and sleep regulation, relative lack of vocalization, apathy or disinterest, and response to strangers that is excessively fearful or overly familiar. Psychiatric disorders most commonly diagnosed during this period are feeding and reactive attachment disorders.

Toddlers are assessed for concerns about sleep problems, extreme misbehavior, extreme shyness, inflexible adherence to routine, language delay, motor hyperactivity, difficulty separating from parents, struggles over toilet training or new foods, and testing limits. Developmental delays and more subtle physiologic, sensory, and motor processing problems can be presented as concerns. Problems with goodness of fit between the child's temperament and the parents' expectations can create relationship difficulties that also require assessment. Psychiatric disorders most commonly diagnosed during this period are pervasive developmental and reactive attachment disorders.

Presenting problems in *preschoolers* include elimination difficulties, sibling jealousy, lack of friends, self-destructive impulsiveness, multiple fears, nightmares, refusal to follow directions, somatization, speech that is difficult to understand, and temper tantrums. Psychiatric disorders most commonly diagnosed in this period are pervasive developmental, communication, disruptive behavior, anxiety, and sleep disorders.

Older children are brought to clinical attention because of concerns about angry mood, depression, bedwetting, overactivity, impulsiveness, distractibility, learning problems, arguing, defiance, nightmares, school refusal, bullying or being bullied, worries and fears, somatization, communication problems, tics, and withdrawal or isolation. Psychiatric disorders most commonly diagnosed during this period are attention, disruptive behavior, anxiety (separation anxiety, selective mutism, generalized anxiety), elimination, somatoform, learning, and tic disorders.

Adolescents are assessed for concerns about the family situation, experimentation with sexuality and drugs, delinquency and gang involvement, friendship patterns, issues of independence, identity formation, self-esteem, and morality. Psychiatric disorders most commonly diagnosed during this period are anxiety (panic, social anxiety), depression, bipolar, psychotic, drug use, and eating disorders.

GENERAL PRINCIPLES OF THE PSYCHOSOCIAL INTERVIEW

Psychosocial interviewing in the context of a routine pediatric visit requires adequate time and privacy. The purpose of this line of inquiry should be explained to the child and parents ("to make sure things are going OK at home, at school, and with friends"), along with the limits of confidentiality. Thereafter, the first goal of the interview is to build rapport with both the child and the parents.

With the parents, this rapport is grounded in respect for the parents' knowledge of their child, their role as the central influence in their child's life, and their desire to make a better life for their child. Parents often feel anxious or guilty because they believe that problems in a child imply that their parenting skills are inadequate. In addition, parents' experiences of their own childhood influence the meaning a parent places on a child's feelings and behavior. A good working alliance allows mutual discovery of the past as it is active in the present and permits potential distortions to be modified more readily. Developmentally appropriate overtures can facilitate rapport with the child. Examples include playing peek-a-boo with an infant, racing toy cars with a preschooler, commenting on sports with a child who is wearing a baseball cap, and discussing music with a teenager who is wearing a rock t-shirt.

After an overture with the child, it is helpful to begin with family-centered interviewing, in which the parent is invited to present any psychosocial concerns (development, thinking, feelings, behavior, peer relationships) about the child. With adolescent patients, it is important to conduct a separate interview to give the adolescent an opportunity to confirm or refute the parent's presentation and to present the problem from his or her perspective. Following the family's undirected presentation of the primary problem, it is important to shift to direct questioning to clarify the duration, frequency, and severity of symptoms, associated distress or functional impairment, and the developmental and environmental context in which the symptoms occur.

Because of the high degree of comorbidity of psychosocial problems in children, after eliciting the presenting problem the pediatric practitioner should then briefly screen for problems in all of the major developmentally appropriate categories of cognitive, developmental, emotional, behavioral, and social disturbance, including problems with mood, anxiety, attention, behavior, thinking and perception, substance use, social relatedness, eating, elimination, development, language, and learning. This can be preceded by a transition statement such as "Now I'd like to ask about some other issues that I ask all parents and kids about."

A useful guide for this area of inquiry is provided by the "11 Action Signs" (Table 18-1), which was designed to give frontline clinicians the tools needed to recognize early symptoms of mental disorders. Functional impairment can be assessed by inquiring about symptoms and function in the major life domains, including home and family, school, peers, and community. These domains are included in the HEADSS (home, education, activities, drugs, sexuality, suicide/depression) interview guide, often used in the screening of adolescents (Table 18-2).

The nature and severity of the presenting problem(s) can be further characterized through the use of a standardized self-, parent-, or teacher-informant rating scale (Table 18-3 gives a sample of scales in the public domain). A rating scale is a type of measure that provides a relatively rapid assessment of a specific construct with an easily derived numerical score that is readily interpreted. The use of rating scales can ensure systematic coverage of relevant symptoms, quantify symptom severity, and document a baseline against which treatment effects can be measured.

Table 18-1 MENTAL HEALTH ACTION SIGNS

- Feeling very sad or withdrawn for more than 2 weeks
- Seriously trying to harm or kill yourself, or making plans to do so
- Sudden overwhelming fear for no reason, sometimes with a racing heart or fast breathing
- Involvement in many fights, using a weapon, or wanting to badly hurt others
- Severe out-of-control behavior that can hurt yourself or others
- Not eating, throwing up, or using laxatives to make yourself lose weight
- Intense worries or fears that get in the way of your daily activities
- Extreme difficulty in concentrating or staying still that puts you in physical danger or causes school failure
- Repeated use of drugs or alcohol
- Severe mood swings that cause problems in relationships
- Drastic changes in your behavior or personality

From The Action Signs Project, Center for the Advancement of Children's Mental Health at Columbia University.

Table 18-2 HEADSS SCREENING INTERVIEW FOR TAKING A RAPID PSYCHOSOCIAL HISTORY

PARENT INTERVIEW

- Home
  - How well does the family get along with each other?
- Education
  - How well does your child do in school?
- Activities
  - What does your child like to do?
  - Does your child do anything that has you really concerned?
  - How does your child get along with peers?
- Drugs
  - Has your child used drugs or alcohol?
- Sexuality
  - Are there any issues regarding sexuality or sexual activity that are of concern to you?
- Suicide/Depression
  - Has your child ever been treated for an emotional problem?
  - Has your child ever intentionally tried to hurt him/herself or made threats to others?

ADOLESCENT INTERVIEW

- Home
  - How do you get along with your parents?
- Education
  - How do you like school and your teachers?
  - How well do you do in school?
- Activities
  - Do you have a best friend or group of good friends?
  - What do you like to do?
- Drugs
  - Have you used drugs or alcohol?
- Sexuality
  - Are there any issues regarding sexuality or sexual activity that are of concern to you?
- Suicide/Depression
  - Everyone feels sad or angry some of the time. How about you?
  - Did you ever feel so upset that you wished you were not alive or so angry you wanted to hurt someone else badly?

From Cohen E, MacKenzie RG, Yates GL: HEADSS, a psychosocial risk assessment instrument: implications for designing effective intervention programs for runaway youth, *J Adolesc Health* 12:539–544, 1991.

Table 18-3 SELECTED LIST OF MENTAL HEALTH RATING SCALES IN THE PUBLIC DOMAIN

INSTRUMENTS	FOR AGES (YEARS)	INFORMANT: NUMBER OF ITEMS	TIME TO COMPLETE (MINUTES)	AVAILABLE AT
BROAD BAND				
Pediatric Symptom Checklist (PSC)	6-16	Parent: 35	5-10	*www.brightfutures.org*
SNAP-IV Rating Scale	6-18	Parent, Teacher: 90	10	*www.adhd.net*
Strengths & Difficulties Questionnaire (SDQ)	3-17	Parent, Teacher, Child: 25	5	*www.sdqinfo.com*
NARROW BAND				
Anxiety				
Self-Report for Childhood Anxiety Related Emotional Disorders (SCARED)	8+	Parent, Child: 41	5	*www.wpic.pitt.edu/research*
Attention and Behavior				
Vanderbilt ADHD Diagnostic Rating Scale	6-12	Parent: 55 Teacher: 43	10	*www.brightfutures.org*
Autism				
Modified Checklist for Autism in Toddlers (M-CHAT)	16-30 months	Parent: 23	5-10	*www.firstsigns.org*
Depression				
Center for Epidemiological Studies Depression Scale for Children (CES-DC)	6-17	Child: 20	5	*www.brightfutures.org*

Clinical experience and methodologic studies suggest that parents and teachers are more likely than the child to report externalizing problems (disruptive, impulsive, overactive, or antisocial behavior). Children may be more likely to report anxious or depressive feelings, including suicidal thoughts and acts, of which the parents may be unaware. Functional impairment also can be assessed with self -and other-rating scales. Although concerns have been raised about children's competence as self-reporters (because of limitations in linguistic skills; self-reflection; emotional awareness; ability to monitor behavior, thoughts, and feelings; and tendency toward social desirability), children and adolescents can be reliable and valid self-reporters.

Clinicians are encouraged to become familiar with the psychometric characteristics and appropriate use of at least one broad-based measure of psychosocial problems, such as the Strengths and Difficulties Questionnaire (SDQ), the Pediatric Symptom Checklist (PSC) (Fig. 18-1), or the Swanson, Nolan, and Pelham–IV (SNAP-IV). If the interview or broad-based rating scale suggests difficulties in one or more specific symptom areas, the clinician can follow with a psychometrically sound, appropriate narrow-based instrument such as the Modified Checklist for Autism in Toddlers (M-CHAT), the Vanderbilt ADHD Diagnostic Rating Scale for attention and behavior problems, the Center for Epidemiological Studies Depression Scale for Children (CES-DC) for depression, or the Screen for Child Anxiety Related Emotional Disorders (SCARED) for anxiety.

Children and adolescents scoring above standardized cutpoints in most cases should be referred to a qualified mental health professional for assessment and treatment, because scores in this range are highly correlated with clinically significant psychiatric disorders. Youths scoring just below or slightly above cutpoints (e.g., subsyndromal or mild mood, anxiety, or disruptive behavior disorders) may be appropriate for management in the pediatric setting, as may youths scoring well above cutpoints for certain biologically based disorders (e.g., attention-deficit/hyperactivity).

The safety of the child in the context of the home and community is of paramount importance. The interview should sensitively assess whether the child has been exposed to any frightening events, including parental arguing or domestic violence, abuse or neglect, or community violence, whether the child shows any indication of depression or suicidality, or whether the child (if age-appropriate) has been involved in any risky behavior, including running away, staying out without permission, truancy, gang involvement, experimentation with substances, and unprotected sexuality. The interview also should assess the capacity of the parents to adequately provide for the child's physical, emotional, and social needs or whether parental capacity has been diminished by psychiatric disorder, family dysfunction, or the sequelae of disadvantaged socioeconomic status. Any indications of threats to the child's safety should be immediately followed by thorough assessment and protective action.

INDICATIONS FOR REFERRAL

There is variability in the level of confidence pediatric practitioners perceive in diagnosing psychosocial problems in children and adolescents. Pediatricians who have familiarity with psychiatric diagnostic criteria as presented in the *Diagnostic and Statistical Manual of Mental Disorders, Fourth Edition, Primary Care* (DSM-IV-PC) may feel confident diagnosing certain disorders, particularly those with a strong biological base (e.g., attention-deficit/hyperactivity disorder, autistic disorder, enuresis, encopresis, anorexia). The disorders about which pediatric practitioners might have less diagnostic confidence include the disruptive behavior, mood, anxiety, psychotic, and substance-use disorders. Pediatricians should refer to a qualified mental health practitioner whenever they experience diagnostic uncertainty with a child who has distressing or functionally impairing psychosocial symptoms. Children who upon initial assessment are found to have indicators of dangerousness always should be referred to a qualified mental health professional.

PSYCHIATRIC DIAGNOSTIC EVALUATION

The objectives of the psychiatric diagnostic evaluation of the child and adolescent are to determine whether psychopathology or developmental risk is present and if so, to establish an explanatory formulation and a differential diagnosis, and to determine whether treatment is indicated and if so, to develop a treatment plan and facilitate the parents' and child's involvement in the plan. The aims of the diagnostic evaluation are to clarify the reasons for the referral; to obtain an accurate accounting of the child's developmental functioning and the nature and extent of the child's psychosocial difficulties, functional impairment, and subjective distress; and to identify potential individual, family, or environmental factors that might account for, influence, or ameliorate these difficulties. The issues relevant to diagnosis and treatment planning can span genetic, constitutional, and temperamental factors; individual psychodynamics; cognitive, language, and social skills; family patterns of interaction and child-rearing practices; and community, school, and socioeconomic influences.

The focus of the evaluation is developmental; it seeks to describe the child's functioning in various realms and to assess the child's adaptation in these areas relative to that expected for the child's age and phase of development. The developmental perspective extends beyond current difficulties to vulnerabilities that can affect future development and as such are important targets for preventive intervention. Vulnerabilities may include subthreshold or subsyndromal difficulties that, especially when manifold, often are accompanied by significant distress or impairment and as such are important as potential harbingers of future problems.

Throughout the assessment, the clinician focuses on identifying a realistic balance of vulnerabilities and strengths in the child, in the parents, and in the parent-child interactions. From this strength-based approach, over time a hopeful family narrative is co-constructed to frame the child's current developmental progress and predict his or her ongoing progress within the scope of current risk and protective factors.

Although the scope of the evaluation will vary with the clinical circumstance, the full **psychiatric diagnostic evaluation** has 6 major components: the presenting problem; a review of psychiatric symptoms and risk status; a developmental history; a full mental status examination; a biopsychosocial formulation and multiaxial diagnosis; and a treatment plan. For infants and young children, the presenting problem and historical information is derived from parents and other informants. As children mature, they become increasingly important contributors to the information base, and they become the primary source of information in later adolescence. Information relevant to formulation and differential diagnosis is derived in multiple ways, including directive and nondirective questioning, interactive play, and observation of the child alone and together with the caregiver(s).

The **explication of the presenting problem** includes information about onset, duration, frequency, and severity of symptoms, associated distress and/or functional impairment, and predisposing, precipitating, or perpetuating contextual factors. The **symptom review** assesses potential comorbidity in the major domains of child and adolescent psychopathology, including problems with attention; anger; disruptive behavior; antisocial behavior; substance use; depressed, irritable, or manic mood; anxiety; eating; elimination; psychosis; development, language, or learning; and the details of prior psychiatric treatment. This review also includes a careful assessment of risk status, including suicidality, homicidality, and involvement in risky behavior or situations.

BRIGHT FUTURES TOOL FOR PROFESSIONALS

Pediatric Symptom Checklist (PSC)

Emotional and physical health go together in children. Because parents are often the first to notice a problem with their child's behavior, emotions, or learning, you may help your child get the best care possible by answering these questions. Please indicate which statement best describes your child.

Please mark under the heading that best decribes your child:

		Never	Sometimes	Often
1. Complains of aches and pains	1	____	____	____
2. Spends more time alone	2	____	____	____
3. Tires easily, has little energy	3	____	____	____
4. Fidgety, unable to sit still	4	____	____	____
5. Has trouble with teacher	5	____	____	____
6. Less interested in school	6	____	____	____
7. Acts as if driven by a motor	7	____	____	____
8. Daydreams too much	8	____	____	____
9. Distracted easily	9	____	____	____
10. Is afraid of new situations	10	____	____	____
11. Feels sad, unhappy	11	____	____	____
12. Is irritable, angry	12	____	____	____
13. Feels hopeless	13	____	____	____
14. Has trouble concentrating	14	____	____	____
15. Less interested in friends	15	____	____	____
16. Fights with other children	16	____	____	____
17. Absent from school	17	____	____	____
18. School grades dropping	18	____	____	____
19. Is down on him- or herself	19	____	____	____
20. Visits the doctor with doctor finding nothing wrong	20	____	____	____
21. Has trouble sleeping	21	____	____	____
22. Worries a lot	22	____	____	____
23. Wants to be with you more than before	23	____	____	____
24. Feels he or she is bad	24	____	____	____
25. Takes unnecessary risks	25	____	____	____
26. Gets hurt frequently	26	____	____	____
27. Seems to be having less fun	27	____	____	____
28. Acts younger than children his or her age	28	____	____	____
29. Dose not listen to rules	29	____	____	____
30. Does not show feelings	30	____	____	____
31. Does not understand other people's feelings	31	____	____	____
32. Teases others	32	____	____	____
33. Blames others for his or her troubles	33	____	____	____
34. Takes things that do not belong to him or her	34	____	____	____
35. Refuses to share	35	____	____	____

Total score______________

Does your child have any emotional or behavioral problems for which she or he needs help? ( ) N ( ) Y
Are there any services that you would like your child to receive for these problems? ( ) N ( ) Y

If yes, what services?____

Figure 18-1 Pediatric Symptom Checklist. (From Green M, Palfrey JS, editors: *Bright futures: guidelines of the health supervision of infants, children, and adolescents*, ed 2, revised, Arlington, VA, 2002, National Center for Education in Maternal and Child Health.)

The **developmental history** includes information about the circumstances of conception, pregnancy, or adoption; physical development and medical history; cognitive and linguistic abilities and school achievement; emotional development and temperament; conscience and values; interests, hobbies, talents, and avocations; family constellation, functioning, and relationships; family medical and psychiatry history; community and culture; peer relationships; stressful or traumatic exposures; and strengths. The **mental status examination** assesses appearance, relatedness, cognition, communication, mood, affective expression, behavior, memory, orientation, and perception.

The evaluation culminates in a **biopsychosocial formulation and differential diagnosis.** The formulation is derived from an assessment of vulnerabilities and strengths in the biologic, psychologic, and social domains and serves to identify targets for intervention and treatment. In the biologic domain, major vulnerabilities include a family history of psychiatric disorder and personality or behavior problems and a personal history of pre-, peri-, or postnatal insults; cognitive or linguistic impairments; physical illness; and a difficult temperament. In the psychologic domain, major vulnerabilities include failure to achieve developmental tasks, maladaptive coping skills, and immature defensive styles. In the social domain, major vulnerabilities include parental incapacity, unskilled parenting, family dysfunction, social isolation, poor social skills, unfavorable school setting, unsupportive community structures, and sociodemographic disadvantage. Major strengths include cognitive and linguistic capability; physical health and attractiveness; stable, moderate temperamental characteristics; and stable and supportive parenting, family, peer, and community structures.

The diagnosis must be made in accordance with the nomenclature in the *Diagnostic and Statistical Manual of Mental Disorders, Fourth Edition, Text Revision* (DSM-IV-TR). This nomenclature categorizes cross-sectional phenomenology into discrete clinical syndromes and seeks to improve diagnostic accuracy at the expense of theories of causation and dimensional presentations. Mental health clinicians use a multiaxial scheme to (along with the formulation) approximate a complete picture of the child. The diagnoses are coded on Axis I. Axis II and Axis III allow the developmental and medical disturbances to be brought into focus. Axis IV permits a similar consideration for social dimensions of stress. Axis V gives a numeric description of overall level of functioning on a scale from 1 (persistent risk of self-harm) to 100 (superior functioning in a wide range of activities with no symptoms).

The psychiatric diagnostic evaluation culminates in a **treatment plan** that brings the broad array of targeted psychosocial interventions to the service of the child. Diagnoses drive the choice of evidence-based psychotherapeutic and psychopharmacologic treatments. The formulation drives the selection of interventions targeted at biologic, psychologic, and social vulnerabilities and strengths. Many of these treatments and interventions are described in the succeeding chapters.

SPECIAL CONSIDERATIONS IN THE DIAGNOSTIC EVALUATION OF INFANTS AND YOUNG CHILDREN

Psychiatric evaluation of infants and young children includes the domains of physiology, temperament, motor behavior, affective behavior, social behavior, and communication. Although much of the information in these domains will be derived from parent report, much also can be gleaned from nonverbal behavior and observation of the parent-child interaction. Observations should include predominant affective tone of parent and child (positive, negative, apathetic); involvement in the situation (curiosity, disinterest); social responsiveness (mutuality of gaze, auditory responsiveness); and reactions to transitions (including separation).

A screen for maternal depression is critical at this stage, as is an assessment of the mother's (or other caregiver's) ability to rapidly respond on a contingent basis to the child's expressed needs, regulate the child's rapid shifts of emotion and behavior, and provide a stimulus shelter to prevent the child from being overwhelmed.

Standardized screening instruments (e.g., Bayley Scales of Infant Development) designed for this age group can be helpful in systematizing the evaluation. In addition, the Infant, Toddler and Preschool Mental Status Exam (ITP-MSE) is a reference tool that describes how traditional categories of the mental status exam can be adapted to observations of young children. Additional categories, including sensory and state regulation, have been added that reflect important areas of development in young children.

Diagnostic systems that are more age-appropriate than DSM-IV-TR have been developed for infants and young children. These systems include the *Research Diagnostic Criteria—Preschool Age* (RDC-PA) and the *Zero to Three Diagnostic Classification of Mental Health and Developmental Disorders of Infancy and Early Childhood-Revised* (DC: 0-3R). The DC: 0-3R includes relationship classification that assesses the range of interactional adaptation in each parent-child relationship and regulation disorders of sensory processing that identify a range of constitutionally and maturationally based sensory reactivity patterns, motor patterns, and behavior patterns that together can dysregulate a child internally and with his or her interactions with caregivers.

BIBLIOGRAPHY

Please visit the Nelson Textbook of Pediatrics *website at* *www.expertconsult.com* *for the complete bibliography.*

Chapter 19
Psychologic Treatment of Children and Adolescents

David R. DeMaso and Heather J. Walter

Barriers that prevent children and their families from obtaining needed mental health services include stigma, shortages of mental health professionals, inadequate coverage of mental health services in public and private health insurance programs, inadequately trained clinicians, and fragmented service delivery systems. Pediatric practitioners are gatekeepers to children's mental health services and increasingly are the primary providers of these services when specialized mental health care is not available.

The provision of supportive counseling, anticipatory guidance, and parent psychoeducation (Chapter 5) combined with medication management of noncomplex attention-deficit/hyperactivity disorder (ADHD) and pervasive developmental disorders are commonly undertaken in the medical home. Youngsters with complex and co-occurring psychiatric illnesses require intervention from specially trained mental health clinicians.

BIBLIOGRAPHY

Please visit the Nelson Textbook of Pediatrics *website at* *www.expertconsult.com* *for the complete bibliography.*

19.1 Psychopharmacology

David R. DeMaso and Heather J. Walter

Safety and efficacy data are available for the use of *single* psychotropic medications for the treatment of a number of childhood psychiatric disorders, including depressive, obsessive-compulsive, attention-deficit/hyperactivity, anxiety (including

Table 19-1 CLINICAL APPROACH TO PSYCHOPHARMACOLOGIC TREATMENT

Identify and assess target symptoms
- Patient, parent, caregiver interviews to assess symptom intensity, duration, exacerbating or ameliorating factors, time trends, and degree of interference with functioning
- Consider input from school staff and other caretakers
- Consider self-report, parent, and teacher rating scales

Search for medical factors that may be causing or exacerbating target symptoms
- Consider sources of pain or discomfort
- Consider other general medical condition causes or contributors
- Consider medication causes or contributors

Complete any medical tests that have a bearing on treatment course

Consider psychotropic medication on the basis of presence of:
- Evidence that target symptoms are interfering substantially with psychosocial functioning
- Research evidence that target symptoms and/or psychiatric diagnoses are amenable to pharmacologic intervention
- Suboptimal response to available psychotherapy interventions and/or environmental changes

Choose a medication on the basis of:
- Likely efficacy for the specific target symptoms and/or psychiatric diagnoses
- Potential adverse side effects
- Practical considerations such as formulations available, dosing schedule, costs, etc.
- Informed consent from parent or guardian and assent from patient

Establish a plan for monitoring effects
- Identify outcome measure
- Discuss time course of expected effects
- Arrange follow-up visits, telephone contact, and/or rating scales accordingly
- Outline a plan regarding what might be tried if there is a negative or suboptimal response or to address additional target symptoms
- Obtain baseline laboratory data if necessary for the drug being prescribed and plan for appropriate monitoring

Explore the reasonable dosage range for a single medication for an adequate length of time before changing to or adding a different medication

Monitor for adverse effects systematically

Consider careful withdrawal of medication after 6-12 months of therapy to determine if it is still needed

Modified from Myers SM, Johnson CP, American Academy of Pediatrics Council on Children with Disabilities: Management of children with autism spectrum disorders, *Pediatrics* 120:1162–1182, 2007.

separation anxiety, social phobia, generalized anxiety), bipolar, and tic disorders. There also is evidence supporting the use of psychotropic medications for aggression and serious problems with impulse control in disruptive behavior and pervasive developmental disorders.

The evidence for treatment using multiple psychotropic medications at the same time is much smaller. Combinations of medications are used to address complex comorbid conditions, manage side effects, increase treatment response, and/or address symptoms hypothesized to be associated with multiple underlying neurotransmitter abnormalities (e.g., dopamine agonists for hyperactivity and serotonin agonists for anxiety).

To ensure safe and appropriate use of psychotropic medications, prescribers should follow best practice principles that underlie medication prescribing (Table 19-1). The use of medication involves a series of interconnected steps including performing an assessment, deciding on treatment and a monitoring plan, obtaining treatment assent or consent, and implementing treatment. Cognitive, emotional, and/or behavior symptoms are targets for medication intervention when there is no response to available evidence-based psychosocial interventions, there is a significant risk of harm, and/or there is significant functional impairment. Commonly encountered target symptom domains include agitation, anxiety, depression, hyperactivity, inattention, impulsivity, mania, and psychosis (Table 19-2).

Table 19-2 TARGET SYMPTOM APPROACH TO PSYCHOPHARMACOLOGIC MANAGEMENT

TARGET SYMPTOM	MEDICATION CONSIDERATIONS
Agitation	Atypical antipsychotic Typical antipsychotic Anxiolytic (e.g., benzodiazepine)
Anxiety	Antidepressant Anxiolytic
Depression	Antidepressant
Hyperactivity, inattention, impulsivity	Atomoxetine, bupropion, stimulant
Mania	Atypical antipsychotic Mood stabilizer
Psychosis	Atypical antipsychotic

Modified from Shaw RJ, DeMaso DR: *Clinical manual of pediatric psychosomatic medicine: mental health consultation with physically ill children and adolescents,* Washington, DC, 2006, American Psychiatric Press, p 306.

STIMULANTS

Stimulants are sympathomimetic drugs that act both in the central nervous system and peripherally by enhancing dopaminergic and noradrenergic transmission (Table 19-3). These medications are used to treat ADHD (Chapter 30) and in some cases as an adjunct in the treatment of depression and for fatigue or malaise associated with chronic physical illnesses. There is a range of stimulant options including those with short half-lives (typically 4 hr) and those with long half-lives (8-12 hr). The most commonly reported side effects are appetite suppression and sleep disturbances. Irritability, headaches, stomachaches, lethargy, hallucinations, and fatigue have also been reported. Anorexia and weight loss have been noted with controversy about their impact on ultimate growth in height.

Sudden death has been reported in association with the use of stimulants in children with structural cardiac abnormalities. This has led to the recommendation to avoid stimulants in patients with these abnormalities. Currently, no routine pretreatment cardiology evaluation is indicated unless the patient has a cardiac disorder and/or symptoms.

Atomoxetine is a selective inhibitor of presynaptic norepinephrine transporters; it increases dopamine and norepinephrine in the prefrontal cortex. It is effective in treating ADHD for 24 hr despite a plasma half-life of 4 hr. Common side effects include sedation, fatigue, somnolence, decreased appetite, weight loss, nausea, upset stomach, abdominal pain, and dizziness along with nonclinical increases in heart rate and blood pressure. In ADHD treatment studies, atomoxetine has had effect sizes of 0.6 to 0.7, compared to the 0.9 effect size with stimulants.

ANTIDEPRESSANTS

Antidepressant drugs act on pre- and postsynaptic receptors affecting the release and reuptake of brain neurotransmitters, including norepinephrine, serotonin, and dopamine (Table 19-4). These medications have been useful in the treatment of depressive, anxiety, and obsessive-compulsive disorders.

The selective serotonin reuptake inhibitors (SSRIs) are the first line of medication treatment for anxiety and depressive disorders; the evidence supports a higher degree of efficacy for anxiety compared to depression. They have a large margin of safety with no cardiovascular effects. Side effects include irritability, insomnia, appetite changes, gastrointestinal symptoms, headaches, diaphoresis, restlessness, and sexual dysfunction (Chapter 58). Withdrawal symptoms are more common in short-acting SSRIs. Behavioral activation and suicidal thoughts have been reported. This has led to recommendations for close monitoring for these adverse effects, especially in the 1st wks of treatment.

Table 19-3 MEDICATIONS FOR ADHD SYMPTOMS

NAME	FDA APPROVED (AGE RANGE IN YEARS)	TARGET SYMPTOMS	USUAL DAILY DOSAGE	SUGGESTED TOP END OF DAILY DOSAGE RANGE
STIMULANTS				
Long Acting				
Methylphenidate (Concerta)	ADHD (6-17)	Inattention Hyperactivity Impulsivity	Child: 18-54 mg Teen: 18-72 mg	108 mg (teen)
Dexmethylphenidate (Focalin XR)	ADHD (6-17)	Inattention Hyperactivity Impulsivity	5-30 mg	50 mg
Amphetamine combination (Adderall XR)	ADHD (6-17)	Inattention Hyperactivity Impulsivity	5-30 mg	60 mg (>100 lb)
Dextroamphetamine (Dexedrine Spansule)	ADHD (3-17)	Inattention Hyperactivity Impulsivity	5-40 mg	60 mg (>100 lb)
Intermediate Acting				
Methylphenidate (Metadate ER, Metadate CD, Methylin ER, Ritalin LA, Ritalin SR)	ADHD (6-17)	Inattention Hyperactivity Impulsivity	10-60 mg	100 mg (>100 lb)
Short Acting				
Dexmethylphenidate (Focalin)	ADHD (6-17)	Inattention Hyperactivity Impulsivity	2.5-20 mg	50 mg
Methylphenidate (Ritalin, Methylin)	ADHD (6-17)	Inattention Hyperactivity Impulsivity	5-60 mg	100 mg (>100 lb)
Amphetamine combination (Adderall)	ADHD (3-17)	Inattention Hyperactivity Impulsivity	2.5-40 mg	60 mg (>100 lb)
Dextroamphetamine (Dexedrine)	ADHD (3-17)	Inattention Hyperactivity Impulsivity	2.5-40 mg	60 mg (>100 lb)
SEROTONIN-NOREPINEPHRINE REUPTAKE INHIBITOR				
Atomoxetine (Strattera)	ADHD (6-17)	Inattention Hyperactivity Impulsivity	10-100 mg	100 mg

ADHD, attention-deficit/hyperactivity disorder.

The tricyclic antidepressants (TCAs) have mixed mechanisms of action (e.g., clomipramine is primarily serotonergic; imipramine is both noradrenergic and serotoninergic). With the advent of the SSRIs, the lack of efficacy studies (particularly in depression), and more serious side effects, the use of TCAs in children has declined. They continue to be used in the treatment of some anxiety disorders (particularly obsessive-compulsive disorder) and, unlike the SSRIs, can be helpful in pain disorders. They have a narrow therapeutic index, with overdoses being potentially fatal (Chapter 58). Anticholinergic symptoms (e.g., dry mouth, blurred vision, and constipation) are the most common side effects. TCAs can have cardiac conduction effects in doses higher than 3.5 mg/kg. Blood pressure and electrocardiographic monitoring is indicated at doses above this level.

The atypical antidepressants include bupropion, venlafaxine, and trazodone (see Table 19-4); they are second-line medications for anxiety and depressive disorders. Bupropion has also been used for smoking cessation and ADHD. Bupropion appears to have an indirect mixed agonist effect on dopamine and norepinephrine transmission. Common side effects include irritability, nausea, anorexia, headache, and insomnia. Venlafaxine has both serotonergic and noradrenergic properties. Side effects are similar to SSRIs, including irritability, insomnia, headaches, anorexia, nervousness, dizziness, and blood pressure changes. Trazodone also has a mixed mechanism of action, with serotonergic and anti-α-adrenergic properties. Sedation is its most common side effect, leading to its common use for insomnia.

Anxiolytic agents (including lorazepam, clonazepam, buspirone, and hydroxyzine) have all been effectively used for acute situational anxiety (see Table 19-4). Their efficacy as chronic medication is poorer, particularly when used as a monotherapy agent.

ANTIPSYCHOTICS

Based on their mechanism of action, antipsychotic medication can be divided into typical (blocking dopamine D_2 receptor) and atypical (mixed dopaminergic and serotoninergic ($5\text{-}HT_2$) activity) agents (Table 19-5).

The atypical antipsychotics have relatively strong antagonistic interactions with $5\text{-}HT_2$ receptors and perhaps more variable activity at central adrenergic, cholinergic, and histaminic sites, which might account for varying side effects noted among these agents. These medications have an evidence base for the treatment of psychotic disorders, moderate to severe agitation, and increasingly for monotherapy in bipolar disorder. Risperidone and aripiprazole are two of the most commonly used medications in this class.

The atypical antipsychotics have significant side effects including extrapyramidal symptoms (e.g., restlessness and dyskinesias), weight gain, metabolic syndrome, diabetes, hyperprolactinemia, hematologic adverse effects (e.g., leukopenia or neutropenia), seizures, hepatotoxicity, neuroleptic malignant syndrome, and cardiovascular effects. For all atypical antipsychotics, body mass

Table 19-4 MEDICATIONS FOR DEPRESSION AND ANXIETY SYMPTOMS

NAME	FDA APPROVED (AGE RANGE IN YEARS)	TARGET SYMPTOMS	USUAL DAILY DOSAGE	SUGGESTED TOP END OF DAILY DOSAGE
SELECTIVE SEROTONIN REUPTAKE INHIBITORS				
Citalopram (Celexa)	None	Depression Anxiety OCD	10-40 mg	40 mg
Escitalopram (Lexapro)	Depression (12-17)	Depression Anxiety OCD	5-20 mg	20 mg
Fluoxetine (Prozac)	Depression (8-17) OCD (7-17)	Depression Anxiety OCD	10-60 mg	60 mg
Sertraline (Zoloft)	OCD (6-17)	Depression Anxiety OCD	25-200 mg	200 mg
TRICYCLIC ANTIDEPRESSANTS				
Clomipramine (Anafranil)	OCD (10-17)	OCD	25-100 mg	200 mg
Imipramine (Tofranil)	Enuresis (6-17)	Enuresis	25 mg	6-12 yr: 50 mg 12-17 yr: 75 mg
ATYPICAL ANTIDEPRESSANTS				
Bupropion (Wellbutrin)	None	Depression ADHD	75-450 mg	450 mg
Venlafaxine (Effexor)	None	Depression Anxiety	75-375 mg	375 mg
Trazodone	None	Depression Sleep	Depression: 25-150 mg Sleep: 25-100 mg	Depression: 400 mg Sleep: 100 mg
ANXIOLYTIC AGENTS				
Lorazepam (Ativan)	Anxiety (12-17)	Acute anxiety	0.25-2 mg/dose	2 mg/dose
Clonazepam (Klonopin)	None	Anxiety	0.5-1 mg	4 mg
Buspirone (BuSpar)	None	Anxiety	5-30 mg	50 mg
Hydroxyzine (Atarax, Vistaril)	Anxiety	Anxiety	50-100 mg	6-12 yr: 100 mg >12 yr: 600 mg

ADHD, attention-deficit/hyperactivity disorder; OCD, obsessive-compulsive disorder.

index, blood pressure, fasting blood glucose, fasting lipid profiles, and abnormal movements should be closely monitored. If there is a family or personal history suggestive of cardiac disease, electrocardiograms should also be monitored.

Haloperidol is a high-potency butyrophenone that is the typical antipsychotic most commonly used. This medication is useful in psychosis, Tourette's disorder, and severe agitation. Side effects include anticholinergic effects, weight gain, drowsiness, and extrapyramidal symptoms (dystonia, rigidity, tremor, and akathisia). There is a risk of tardive dyskinesia with chronic administration.

α-ADRENERGIC AGENTS

The α-adrenergic agents (clonidine and guanfacine) are presynaptic adrenergic agonists that appear to stimulate inhibitory presynaptic autoreceptors in the central nervous system. Although most commonly used in Tourette's disorder and ADHD, these agents may be useful in controlling aggression, particularly in patients with developmental disorders (see Table 19-5). Sedation, hypotension, dry mouth, depression, and confusion are potential side effects. Abrupt withdrawal can result in rebound hypertension. Guanfacine appears to be less sedating and to have a longer duration of action than clonidine.

MOOD STABILIZERS

Several medications have been shown to be potentially helpful in children experiencing significant mood instability and/or mania, although the evidence base is sparse (Table 19-6).

Lithium's mechanism of action is not well understood, though proposed theories relate to neurotransmission, endocrine effects, circadian rhythm, and cellular processes. Common side effects include polyuria and polydipsia and central nervous system symptoms (tremor, somnolence, and memory impairment). Periodic monitoring of lithium levels along with thyroid and renal function is needed. Lithium serum levels of 0.8-1.2 mEq/L are targeted for acute episodes and 0.6-0.9 mEq/L are targeted for maintenance therapy.

Valproic acid is an anticonvulsant with some evidence supporting its use in the treatment of mania. The therapeutic plasma concentration range is 50-100 μg/mL. Common side effects include sedation, gastrointestinal symptoms, and hair thinning. Idiosyncratic bone marrow suppression and liver toxicity have been reported, necessitating monitoring of blood counts as well as liver and kidney function. Lamotrigine is another anticonvulsant that may be useful in the treatment of adolescent bipolar depression. It has been associated with potentially life-threatening Stevens-Johnson syndrome.

MEDICATION USE IN PHYSICAL ILLNESS

There are special considerations in the use of psychotropic medications with physically ill children. Between 80% and 95% of psychotropic medications are protein bound, with the exceptions being lithium (0%), methylphenidate (10-30%), venlafaxine (25-30%), gabapentin (0-3%), and topiramate (9-17%). As a result, psychotropic levels may be directly affected because albumin binding is reduced in many physical illnesses. Metabolism is primarily through the liver and gastrointestinal tract, with

Table 19-5 MEDICATIONS FOR PSYCHOSIS AND AGITATION

NAME	FDA APPROVED (AGE RANGE IN YEARS)	TARGET SYMPTOMS	USUAL DAILY DOSAGE	SUGGESTED TOP END OF DAILY DOSAGE
ATYPICAL ANTIPSYCHOTICS				
Aripiprazole (Abilify)	Bipolar disorder (10-17) Schizophrenia (13-17) Irritability in autism (6-17)	Psychosis Mania Aggression Agitation	2-30 mg	Child: 15 mg Teen: 30 mg
Ziprasidone (Geodon)	None	Psychosis Mania Aggression Agitation	20-160 mg	160 mg
Risperidone (Risperdal)	Bipolar disorder (10-17) Schizophrenia (13-17) Irritability in autism (5-16)	Psychosis Mania Aggression Agitation	Child: 0.25-3 mg Teen: 0.5-6 mg	Child: 3 mg Teen: 6 mg
Quetiapine (Seroquel)	Bipolar disorder (10-17) Schizophrenia (13-17)	Psychosis Mania Aggression Agitation	Child: 25-400 mg Teen: 50-800 mg	Child: 400 mg Teen: 800 mg
Olanzapine (Zyprexa)	Bipolar disorder (13-17) Schizophrenia (13-17)	Psychosis Mania Aggression Agitation	2.5-10 mg	20 mg
TYPICAL ANTIPSYCHOTICS				
Haloperidol (Haldol)	Psychosis (3-17) Tourette's (3-17) Severe behavioral disorders (3-17) Agitation (3-17)	Psychosis Mania Aggression Agitation	0.5-15 mg	100 mg (severe refractory)
ALPHA AGONISTS				
Clonidine (Catapres)	None	Agitation Sleep	60-90 lb: 0.05-0.2 mg >90 lb: 0.05-0.3 mg >100 lb: 0.05-0.4 mg	60-90 lb: 0.2 mg >90 lb: 0.3 mg >100 lb: 0.4 mg
Guanfacine (Tenex)	None	Agitation Sleep	60-90 lb: 0.5-2 mg >90 lb: 0.5-3 mg >100 lb: 0.5-4 mg	60-90 lb: 2 mg >90 lb: 3 mg >100 lb: 4 mg

Table 19-6 MEDICATIONS FOR MOOD INSTABILITY

	FDA APPROVED (AGE RANGE IN YEARS)	TARGET SYMPTOMS	USUAL DAILY DOSAGE	SUGGESTED TOP END OF DAILY DOSAGE
MOOD STABILIZERS				
Lithium carbonate (Eskalith, Eskalith CR, Lithobid)	Bipolar disorder (12-17)	Mania Depression	<50 lb: 600 mg 50-90 lb: 900 mg >90 lb: 1200 mg Blood lithium level 0.6-1.2 mmol/L	1800 mg Blood lithium level >1.2 mmol/L
Divalproex (Depakote, Depakote ER)	None	Mania	15-60 mg/kg/day Blood valproic acid level 50-100 μg/mL	Blood valproic acid level >125 μg/mL
Lamotrigine (Lamictal)	None	Depression in bipolar disorder	Teen: 25-200 mg	Teen: 200 mg
ATYPICAL ANTIPSYCHOTICS				
Aripiprazole (Abilify)	Bipolar disorder (10-17) Schizophrenia (13-17)	Psychosis Mania Aggression Agitation	2-30 mg	Child: 15 mg Teen: 30 mg
Risperidone (Risperdal)	Bipolar disorder (10-17) Schizophrenia (13-17) Aggression in autism (5-16)	Psychosis Mania Aggression Agitation	Child: 0.25-3 mg Teen: 0.5-6 mg	Child: 3 mg Teen: 6 mg

excretion via the kidney. Therefore, dosages may need to be adjusted in children with hepatic or renal impairment.

Hepatic Disease

It is often necessary to use lower doses of medications in patients with hepatic disease. Initial dosing of medications should be reduced and titration should proceed slowly. In steady-state situations, changes in protein binding can result in elevated unbound medication, resulting in increased drug action even in the presence of normal serum drug concentrations. Because it is often difficult to predict changes in protein binding, it is important to maintain attention to the clinical effects of psychotropic medications and not rely exclusively on serum drug concentrations.

In acute hepatitis, there is generally no need to modify dosing because metabolism is only minimally altered. In chronic hepatitis and cirrhosis, hepatocytes are destroyed and doses might need to be modified.

Medications with high baseline rates of liver clearance (e.g., haloperidol, sertraline, venlafaxine, and TCAs) are significantly affected by hepatic disease. For drugs that have significant hepatic metabolism, intravenous administration may be preferred because parenteral administration avoids first-pass liver metabolic effects and the dosing and action of parenteral medications are similar to those in patients with normal hepatic function. Valproic acid can impair the metabolism of the hepatocyte disproportionate to the degree of hepatocellular damage. In patients with valproate-induced liver injury, low albumin, high prothrombin, and high ammonia may be seen without significant elevation in liver transaminases.

Gastrointestinal Disease
Medications with anticholinergic side effects can slow gastrointestinal motility, affecting absorption and causing constipation. SSRIs increase gastric motility and can cause diarrhea. SSRIs have a potential to increase the risk of gastrointestinal bleeding, especially when they are co-administered with nonsteroidal antiinflammatory drugs. Extended-release or controlled-release preparations of medications can reduce gastrointestinal side effects, particularly where gastric distress is related to rapid increases in plasma drug concentrations.

Kidney Disease
With the exceptions of lithium and gabapentin, psychotropic medications do not generally require significant dosing adjustments in kidney failure. It is important to monitor serum concentrations in renal insufficiency, particularly for medications with a narrow therapeutic index; cyclosporine can elevate serum lithium levels by decreasing lithium excretion. Patients with kidney failure and those on dialysis appear to be more sensitive to TCA side effects, possibly because of the accumulation of hydroxylated tricyclic metabolites.

Because most psychotropic medications are highly protein-bound, they are not significantly cleared by dialysis. Lithium, gabapentin, and topiramate are essentially completely removed by dialysis, and the common practice is to administer these medications after dialysis. Patients on dialysis often have significant fluid shifts and are at risk for dehydration, with neuroleptic malignant syndrome being more likely in these situations.

Heart Disease
Cardiovascular effects of psychotropic medications can include orthostatic hypotension, conduction disturbances, and arrhythmias. Orthostatic hypotension is one of the most common cardiovascular side effects of TCAs. Trazodone can cause orthostatic hypotension and exacerbate myocardial instability; SSRIs and bupropion are preferred as antidepressant agents in patients with heart disease.

There is the potential for increased morbidity and mortality in patients with pre-existing cardiac conduction problems. Some of the calcium channel blocking agents (e.g., verapamil) can slow atrioventricular conduction and can theoretically interact with a TCA. Patients with Wolff-Parkinson-White syndrome who have a short PR interval (<0.12 sec) and widened QRS interval associated with paroxysmal tachycardia are at high risk for life-threatening ventricular tachycardia that may be exacerbated by the use of a TCA. Quinidine-like effects of TCAs and the antipsychotic agents can lead to prolongation of the QTc interval, with increased risk of ventricular tachycardia and ventricular fibrillation, particularly in patients with structural heart disease. Patients with a baseline QTc interval of >440 msec should be considered at particular risk. The range of normal QTc values in children is 400 msec ± 25-30 msec. A QTc value that exceeds 2 standard deviations (>450-460 msec) is considered too long and may be associated with increased mortality. An increase in the QTc from baseline of >60 msec is also associated with increased mortality.

Respiratory Disease
Anxiolytic agents can increase the risk of respiratory suppression in patients with pulmonary disease. SSRIs and buspirone are good alternative medications for treating anxiety. Consideration should be given to possible airway compromise due to acute laryngospasm when dopamine-blocking agents such as antipsychotic or antiemetic medications are used.

Neurological Disease
Psychotropic medications can be used safely with epilepsy following consideration of potential interactions between the psychotropic medication, the seizure disorder, and the anticonvulsant medication. Any behavioral toxicity of anticonvulsants used either alone or in combination should be considered before proceeding with psychotropic treatment. Simplification of combination anticonvulsant therapy or a change to another agent can result in a reduction of behavioral or emotional symptoms and obviate the need for psychotropic intervention. Clomipramine and bupropion possess significant seizure-inducing properties and should be avoided when the risk of seizures is present.

Neuroleptic Malignant Syndrome
Neuroleptic malignant syndrome (NMS) is a rare and potentially fatal reaction that can occur during treatment with antipsychotic agents (Chapter 169). The syndrome generally manifests with fever, muscle rigidity, autonomic instability, and delirium. It is associated with elevated serum creatine phosphokinase levels, a metabolic acidosis, and high end-tidal CO_2 excretion. It has been estimated to occur in 0.2-1% of patients treated with dopamine-blocking agents. Malnutrition and dehydration in the context of an organic brain syndrome and simultaneous treatment with lithium and antipsychotic agents can increase the risk. Mortality rates may be as high as 20-30% due to dehydration, aspiration, kidney failure, and respiratory collapse. Differential diagnosis of NMS includes heat stroke, malignant hyperthermia, lethal catatonia, serotonin syndrome, and anticholinergic toxicity

Serotonin Syndrome
Serotonin syndrome is characterized by a triad of mental status changes, autonomic hyperactivity, and neuromuscular abnormalities (Chapter 58). It is the result of an excess agonism of the central and peripheral nervous system serotoninergic receptors and can be caused by a range of drugs including SSRIs, valproate, and lithium. Drug-drug interactions that can cause serotonin syndrome include linezolid (an antibiotic that has MAOI properties) and anti-migraine preparations used with an SSRI, as well as combinations of SSRI, trazodone, buspirone, and venlafaxine. It is generally self-limited and can resolve spontaneously after the serotoninergic agents are discontinued. Severe cases require the control of agitation, autonomic instability, and hyperthermia as well as the administration of 5-HT_{2A} antagonists (e.g., cyproheptadine).

BIBLIOGRAPHY
Please visit the Nelson Textbook of Pediatrics *website at www.expertconsult.com for the complete bibliography.*

19.2 Psychotherapy

David R. DeMaso and Heather J. Walter

Psychotherapy in children may also be effective in reducing patient symptomatology. Effect sizes in research studies range from 0.71 to 0.84, which are as large as or larger than the effects of psychiatric medications or medicines for many physical illnesses. Despite benefit, only a minority of patients achieve the same level of functioning as average children, because in community settings the effect size of psychotherapy approaches zero. This poor response might reflect the fact that treatment in real-world community settings involves complex and co-occurring disorders, as opposed to the research or academic setting, where comorbid conditions are often excluded.

A variety of psychotherapeutic approaches exist with varying levels of evidence regarding their effectiveness. The following is a simplified rank ordering of the comparative effectiveness of the different therapeutic approaches: cognitive-behavioral therapy, which is considered to be the first-line treatment for anxiety and mild depressive disorders; family therapy; psychodynamic therapy; supportive therapy; and narrative therapy.

Differences between therapeutic approaches may be less pronounced in practice than in theory. The quality of the therapist-patient alliance consistently has been shown to be the strongest predictor of treatment outcome. A positive therapeutic relationship, expecting change to occur, facing problems assertively, increasing mastery, and attributing change to the participation in the therapy have all been connected to effective therapy.

The use of psychotherapy involves a series of interconnected steps including performing an assessment, deciding upon treatment and a monitoring plan, obtaining treatment assent or consent, and implementing treatment. Cognitive, emotional, and/or behavior symptoms are identified that become the targets for evidence-based psychotherapeutic interventions. Psychotherapists ideally develop a treatment plan by combining known evidence-based practices about specific interventions with their clinical judgment to arrive at a specific intervention plan for the individual patient. It is not unusual for the psychotherapist to use elements from more than one treatment approach, including psychopharmacology.

COGNITIVE-BEHAVIORAL THERAPY

Cognitive-behavioral therapy (CBT) is based on the theory that antecedent events stimulate thoughts and beliefs that in turn cause emotional consequences. CBT is problem-oriented treatment that seeks to identify and change cognitive distortions (e.g., learned helplessness or irrational fears), identify and avoid distressing situations, and identify and practice distress-reducing behavior. Self-monitoring (e.g., daily thought record), self-instruction (e.g., brief sentences asserting thoughts that are comforting and/or adaptive), and self-reinforcement (rewarding oneself) are internal analogues of the charts, prompts, and rewards that in behavior therapy are supplied by parents and/or significant others.

FAMILY THERAPY

The core idea in family therapy is that problems exist in families and not just in individuals. The cause of problems in individuals is thought to lie in patterns of family interaction, with other family members helping to maintain the problem. Family dysfunction can take a variety of forms, including enmeshment, disengagement, and maladaptive communication patterns (e.g., parent-child role reversal). Family therapy techniques involve helping family members communicate more effectively, reframing troublesome behavior, and giving directives to disrupt ingrained dysfunctional patterns. Family interventions that include behavioral therapy components are well-established treatments for ADHD and oppositional defiant disorder.

PSYCHODYNAMIC PSYCHOTHERAPY

At the core of psychodynamic psychotherapy lies a *dynamic* interaction between different parts or aspects of the mind. This approach is based on the belief that much of one's mental activity occurs outside one's awareness. The patient is often unaware of internal conflicts because threatening or painful emotions, impulses, and memories are repressed. Behavior is then controlled by what the patient does not know about himself or herself. Therapy objectives are to increase self-understanding, increase acceptance of feelings, shift to mature defense mechanisms, and develop realistic relationships between self and others. This therapy is nondirective to allow the patient's characteristic patterns to emerge so that self-understanding and a corrective emotional experience can then be fostered by the therapist.

SUPPORTIVE PSYCHOTHERAPY

Supportive psychotherapy aims to minimize levels of emotional distress. Treatment is focused on the here and now. The therapist is active and helpful in providing the patient with symptomatic relief by containing anxiety, sadness, and anger. The therapist provides education and encouragement to bolster a patient's existing coping mechanisms.

NARRATIVE THERAPY

Narrative therapy is based on the principle that self-stories organize, interpret, and assign meaning to events in a person's life. It emphasizes the construction of meaning by allowing patients to tell their personal story or narrative of the problem. Narratives typically center on 5 pervasive themes: *identity, cause, time-line, consequences,* and *cure* or *control*. The therapist helps the patient "make meaning" of his or her stories and correct misperceptions or misattributions. The therapist's role is to help the patient reframe negative narratives (re-storying) into ones that are more positive and progressive.

BIBLIOGRAPHY

Please visit the Nelson Textbook of Pediatrics *website at www.expertconsult.com for the complete bibliography.*

19.3 Psychiatric Hospitalization

David R. DeMaso and Heather J. Walter

Psychiatric hospital programs are meant to address the serious risks and severe impairments caused by the most acute and complex forms of psychiatric disorder that cannot be managed effectively at any other level of care. Their goal is to produce rapid clinical stabilization that allows an expeditious, safe, and appropriate treatment transition to a less-intensive level of mental health care outside of the hospital.

High levels of illness severity combined with significant functional impairment signal a need for hospitalization. Admission criteria must include significant signs and symptoms of active psychiatric disorder(s). Functional admission indicators generally include a significant risk of self-harm and/or harm to others, although in some cases the patient is unable to meet basic self-care or health care needs, jeopardizing well-being. Serious emotional disturbances that prevent participation in family, school, or community life can also rise to a level of global impairment that can only be addressed on an inpatient basis.

Discharge planning begins at the time of admission, when efforts are made to coordinate care with services and resources that are already in place for the child or adolescent in the community. Step-down care might be needed in partial hospital or residential settings if integrated services in a single location remain indicated after sufficient clinical stabilization has occurred in the hospital setting. Transition from the hospital entails active collaboration and communication with pediatric practitioners in the child's medical home.

BIBLIOGRAPHY

Please visit the Nelson Textbook of Pediatrics *website at www.expertconsult.com for the complete bibliography.*

Chapter 20
Psychosomatic Illness

Patricia Ibeziako, Richard J. Shaw, and David R. DeMaso

Psychosomatic medicine deals with the relation between physiologic and psychologic factors in the cause or maintenance of disease. Physical illnesses have accompanying emotional symptoms, and psychiatric illnesses commonly have associated somatic or physical symptoms. It is important for health care providers to avoid the dichotomy of approaching illness using a medical model in which diseases are considered either organic or psychologically based. A biobehavioral continuum of disease characterizes illness as occurring across a spectrum ranging from a biologic etiology on one end to predominantly a psychosocial etiology on the other (Fig. 20-1). Using the biopsychosocial approach, biologic, psychologic, social, and developmental realms are integrated into an understanding of an individual patient's presentation.

The interplay of physiologic and psychosocial factors is readily seen in children experiencing stressful life events. During periods of stress, neuroregulatory mechanisms undergo changes that render the body more vulnerable to infection and other disorders. The pathophysiologic basis of these changes can include immune activation with release of hormonal immune factors (cytokines) in response to acute stress as well as a decrease in the number and activity of natural killer cells in situations of more chronic stress. The hypothalamic-pituitary-adrenal axis may be affected, resulting in an excess secretion of cortisol, which can produce structural damage to various organ systems. Under acute stress, the sympathomimetic effects of catecholamines can cause elevated blood pressure and tachycardia.

In the *Diagnostic and Statistical Manual of Mental Disorders, Fourth Edition, Text Revision* (DSM-IV-TR), the diagnosis **psychological factors affecting general medical conditions** acknowledges the influence of emotional and behavioral factors on the onset and course of physical illness, including stress-related physiologic responses. This diagnosis requires physical findings of disease (e.g., asthma, diabetes, gastric ulcer, migraine headache, or ulcerative colitis) and evidence that psychologic factors are temporally related to the appearance, exacerbation, and/or maintenance of the physical symptoms.

The DSM-IV-TR defines the category of **Somatoform Disorders**, which are on the end of the continuum where predominantly psychologic factors contribute to the presentation of somatic symptoms. Somatization may be defined as the process whereby distress is experienced and/or expressed in physical modalities (recurrent abdominal pain, headache, and various neurologic symptoms). In children, recurrent poorly explained physical complaints generally fall into 4 distinct symptom clusters: cardiovascular, gastrointestinal, pain, and neurologic. In patients presenting with somatoform disorders, the physical findings are insufficient to explain the symptoms and/or the complaints are in excess of what would normally be expected based on the underlying physical illness.

The DSM-IV-TR category of somatoform disorders includes Somatization Disorder, Conversion Disorder, and Pain Disorders Associated with Both Psychological Factors and a General Medical Condition (Tables 20-1 to 20-4). Somatoform Disorder Not Otherwise Specified includes presentations with disabling somatic symptoms that do not meet the full DSM-IV-TR criteria for any of the aforementioned disorders. Hypochondriasis and Body Dysmorphic Disorder occur rarely in childhood.

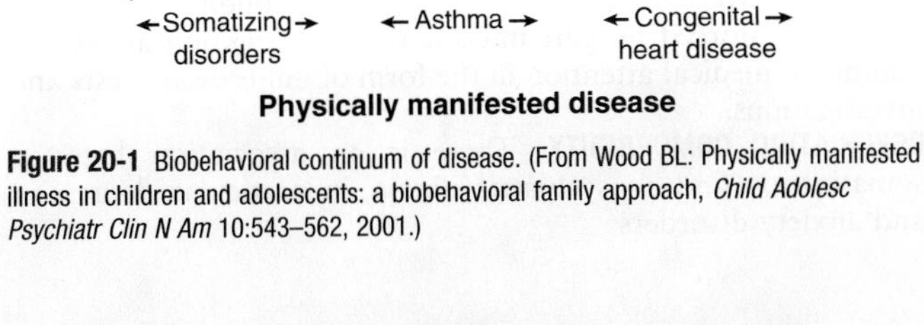

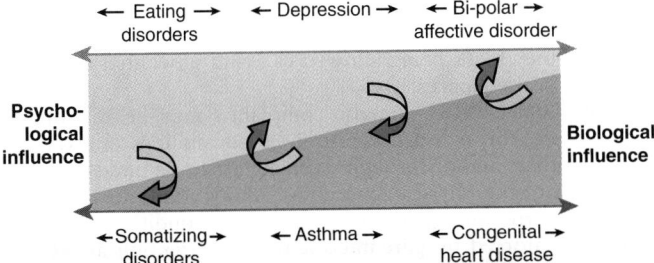

Figure 20-1 Biobehavioral continuum of disease. (From Wood BL: Physically manifested illness in children and adolescents: a biobehavioral family approach, *Child Adolesc Psychiatr Clin N Am* 10:543–562, 2001.)

EPIDEMIOLOGY

It is estimated that somatic complaints are seen in adolescents at a rate of 4.5-10% in boys and 10-15% in girls. Conversion Disorder has prevalence rates that vary between 0.5% and 10%. Headaches, recurrent abdominal pain, limb pain, and chest pain have been reported as having prevalence rates ranging from 7-30% in community and clinical samples.

RISK FACTORS

Family and Environmental

SOCIOCULTURAL Youngsters of lower socioeconomic status or those who live in rural areas have higher rates of somatoform disorders. Local cultural ideas about acceptable and credible ways to express psychologic distress might play a role in the expression of somatic symptoms. Conversion symptoms have also been reported more commonly in non-Western clinical settings.

Table 20-1 DSM-IV-TR DIAGNOSTIC CRITERIA FOR SOMATIZATION DISORDER

A. A history of many physical complaints beginning before age 30 years that occur over a period of several years and result in treatment being sought or significant impairment in social, occupational, or other important areas of functioning.
B. Each of the following criteria must have been met, with individual symptoms occurring at any time during the course of the disturbance:
   (1) *four pain symptoms:* a history of pain related to at least four different sites or functions (e.g., head, abdomen, back, joints, extremities, chest, rectum, during menstruation, during sexual intercourse, or during urination)
   (2) *two gastrointestinal symptoms:* a history of at least two gastrointestinal symptoms other than pain (e.g., nausea, bloating, vomiting other than during pregnancy, diarrhea, or intolerance of several different foods)
   (3) *one sexual symptom:* a history of at least one sexual or reproductive symptom other than pain (e.g., sexual indifference, erectile or ejaculatory dysfunction, irregular menses, excessive menstrual bleeding, vomiting throughout pregnancy)
   (4) *one pseudoneurological symptom:* a history of at least one symptom or deficit suggesting a neurological condition not limited to pain (conversion symptoms such as impaired coordination or balance, paralysis or localized weakness, difficulty swallowing or lump in throat, aphonia, urinary retention, hallucinations, loss of touch or pain sensation, double vision, blindness, deafness, seizures, dissociative symptoms such as amnesia; or loss of consciousness other than fainting)
C. Either (1) or (2):
   (1) after appropriate investigation, each of the symptoms in Criterion B cannot be fully explained by a known general medical condition or the direct effects of a substance (e.g., a drug of abuse, a medication)
   (2) when there is a related general medical condition, the physical complaints or resulting social or occupational impairment are in excess of what would be expected from the history, physical examination, or laboratory findings
D. The symptoms are not intentionally produced or feigned (as in Factitious Disorder or Malingering).

From American Psychiatric Association: *Diagnostic and statistical manual of mental disorders. fourth edition, text revision,* Washington, DC, 2000, American Psychiatric Association, p 490.

Table 20-2 DSM-IV-TR DIAGNOSTIC CRITERIA FOR UNDIFFERENTIATED SOMATOFORM DISORDER

A. One or more physical complaints (e.g., fatigue, loss of appetite, gastrointestinal or urinary complaints).
B. Either (1) or (2):
  1. After appropriate investigation, each of the symptoms in criterion B cannot be fully explained by a known general medical condition or the direct effects of a substance (e.g., a drug of abuse, a medication).
  2. When there is a related general medical condition, the physical complaints or resulting social or occupational impairment are in excess of what would be expected from the history, physical examination, or laboratory findings.
C. The symptoms cause clinically significant distress or impairment in social, occupational, or other important areas of functioning.
D. The duration of the disturbance is at least 6 months.
E. The disturbance is not better accounted for by another mental disorder (e.g., another somatoform disorder, sexual dysfunction, mood disorder, anxiety disorder, sleep disorder, or psychotic disorder).
F. The symptom is not intentionally produced or feigned (as in factitious disorder or malingering).

From American Psychiatric Association: *Diagnostic and statistical manual of mental disorders, fourth edition, text revision,* Washington, DC, 2000, American Psychiatric Association, p 492.

Table 20-3 DSM-IV-TR DIAGNOSTIC CRITERIA FOR CONVERSION DISORDER

A. One or more symptoms or deficits affecting voluntary motor or sensory function that suggest a neurological or other general medical condition.
B. Psychological factors are judged to be associated with the symptom or deficit because the initiation or exacerbation of the symptom or deficit is preceded by conflicts or other stressors.
C. The symptom or deficit is not intentionally produced or feigned (as in Factitious Disorder or Malingering).
D. The symptom or deficit cannot, after appropriate investigation, be fully explained by a general medical condition, or by the direct effects of a substance, or as a culturally sanctioned behavior or experience.
E. The symptom or deficit causes clinically significant distress or impairment in social, occupational, or other important areas of functioning or warrants medical evaluation.
F. The symptom or deficit is not limited to pain or sexual dysfunction, does not occur exclusively during the course of Somatization Disorder, and is not better accounted for by another mental disorder.

Specify type of symptom or deficit: With Motor Symptom or Deficit; With Sensory Symptom or Deficit; With Seizures of Convulsions; or With Mixed Presentation

From American Psychiatric Association: *Diagnostic and statistical manual of mental disorders, fourth edition, text revision,* Washington, DC, 2000, American Psychiatric Association, p 498.

GENETIC A possible genetic etiology in somatization disorders is suggested by findings of a 29% concordance rate in monozygotic twins and 10-20% of first-degree relatives of patients meeting criteria for this disorder. There is also a familial link between somatization disorders and other psychiatric disorders (e.g., higher rates of anxiety and depression in the family members).

SYMPTOM MODEL Children may be more prone to adopt somatic symptoms to express emotional distress if they observe their parents or other family members using similar strategies. Parental medical illness is associated with childhood somatization.

FAMILY FACTORS Parents of children with somatoform disorders might present with a persistent fear of disease and a conviction about its presence. Other common family factors include achievement-oriented families with high expectations for their children, psychologically inarticulate families, a pattern of overinvolved or enmeshed family interactions, and role reversal in which the child adopts a parental role.

STRESSFUL LIFE EVENTS Significant temporally related correlations are found between somatic symptoms and psychosocial stressors, including children subject to high academic expectations, social pressures, family conflict, physical injury, family illness, parental absence, and other significant losses.

Table 20-4 DSM-IV DIAGNOSTIC CRITERIA FOR PAIN DISORDER

A. Pain in one or more anatomical sites is the predominant focus of the clinical presentation and is of sufficient severity to warrant clinical attention.
B. The pain causes clinically significant distress or impairment in social, occupational, or other important areas of functioning.
C. Psychological factors are judged to have an important role in the onset, severity, exacerbation, or maintenance of the pain.
D. The symptom or deficit is not intentionally produced or feigned (as in Factitious Disorder or Malingering).
E. The pain is not better accounted for by a Mood, Anxiety, or Psychotic Disorder and does not meet criteria for Dyspareunia.

Code as Follows:
307.80 Pain Disorder Associated with Psychological Factors: psychological factors are judged to have the major role in the onset, severity, exacerbation, or maintenance of the pain. (If a general medical condition is present, it does not have a major role in the onset, severity, exacerbation, or maintenance of the pain.) This type of Pain Disorder is not diagnosed if criteria are also met for Somatization Disorder.

Specify If:
Acute: duration of less than 6 months
Chronic: duration of 6 months or longer
307.89 Pain Disorder Associated with Both Psychological Factors and a General Medical Condition: both psychological factors and a general medical condition are judged to have important roles in the onset, severity, exacerbation, or maintenance of the pain. The associated general medical condition or anatomical site of the pain (see below) is coded on Axis III.

Specify If:
Acute: duration of less than 6 months
Chronic: duration of 6 months or longer
Note: The following is not considered to be a mental disorder and is included here to facilitate differential diagnosis.
Pain Disorder Associated with a General Medical Condition: a general medical condition has a major role in the onset, severity, exacerbation, or maintenance of the pain. (If psychological factors are present, they are not judged to have a major role in the onset, severity, exacerbation, or maintenance of the pain.)

From American Psychiatric Association: *Diagnostic and statistical manual of mental disorders, fourth edition, text revision,* Washington, DC, 2000, American Psychiatric Association, p 503.

Individual

CHILDHOOD PHYSICAL ILLNESS There is a connection between childhood physical illness and the later development of somatization. Children who tend to somatize might have a tendency to experience normal somatic sensations as intense, noxious, and disturbing, referred to as *somatosensory amplification.* Children with somatoform disorders often have histories of disabling and poorly explained physical symptoms.

TEMPERAMENT AND COPING STYLES Somatic symptoms are more common in children who are conscientious, sensitive, insecure, and anxious and in those who strive for high academic achievement. Somatization can also occur in youngsters who are unable to verbalize emotional distress. Somatic symptoms are often seen as a form of psychologic defense against intrapsychic distress that allows the child to avoid confronting anxieties or conflicts, a process referred to as *primary gain.* Primary gain is obtained by keeping the conflict from consciousness and minimizing anxiety. The symptoms can also lead to secondary gain if the symptom results in the child's being allowed to avoid unwanted responsibilities or consequences.

LEARNED COMPLAINTS Somatic complaints may be reinforced, for example, through a decrease in responsibilities or expectations by others and/or through receiving attention and sympathy as a result of the physical symptoms. Many youngsters have an antecedent true underlying general medical condition that may then be reinforced by parental and/or peer attention as well as additional medical attention in the form of unnecessary tests and investigations.

PSYCHIATRIC COMORBIDITY There is an association between somatization and a psychiatric illness, in particular depressive and anxiety disorders.

ASSESSMENT

Medical

The medical evaluation of suspected psychosomatic illness should include an assessment of biologic, psychologic, social, and developmental realms both separately and in relation to each other. A comprehensive medical work-up to rule out serious physical illness must be carefully balanced with efforts to avoid unnecessary and potentially harmful tests and procedures. Although the likelihood of finding physical illness in patients with somatoform disorders at initial diagnosis is less than 10%, certain physical illnesses should be considered, such as Lyme disease (Chapter 214), systemic lupus erythematosus (Chapter 152), multiple sclerosis (Chapter 593), infectious mononucleosis (Chapter 246), irritable bowel syndrome (Chapter 334), migraine (Chapter 588.1), and seizure disorders (Chapter 586).

The presence of a physical illness does not exclude the possibility of somatization having an important role in the child's presentation. Somatic symptoms early in a disease course that can be directly attributed to a specific physical illness (e.g., acute respiratory illness) can evolve into psychologically based symptoms, particularly in situations in which the child experiences benefit from adopting the sick role. Somatic symptoms can also occur in excess of what would be expected of the symptoms experienced in true physical illness. Physical findings can occur secondary to the effects of a somatoform disorder (e.g., disuse atrophy).

Psychologic

Assessment of psychosomatic illness should consider inconsistent findings in the medical evaluation, the presence of psychosocial stressors, the presence of comorbid depressive or anxiety disorders, a past history of somatization in the child and/or family, a symptom model of illness behavior in the family, and the presence of secondary gain or reinforcement of physical illness. The presence of any one risk factor does not conclusively prove the presence of a somatoform disorder; psychiatric and social risk factors can increase the diagnostic likelihood.

If somatization is suspected, psychiatric consultation should be included early in the diagnostic workup. The reason for consultation should be carefully explained to the family to help avoid the parents' perception that their child's symptoms are not being taken seriously by the pediatric team (i.e., "it's in her head"). It should be explained that the goal of the psychiatric consultation is to understand the origins of the child's distress, why the child uses somatization as a way to express the distress, what perpetuates it, and which treatments are likely to be most effective.

Diagnosis and Differential Diagnosis

Conversion disorder denotes the loss or alteration of physical functioning without demonstrable organic pathology (see Table 20-3). It occurs in adolescence or adulthood, although numerous childhood cases have been reported. Conversion reactions usually start suddenly, can often be traced to a precipitating environmental event, and can end abruptly after a short duration. Voluntary musculature and organs of special sense are the most common target sites for expressions of conversion reactions. Such reactions can take the form of blindness, paralysis, diplopia, and postural or gait disturbances. Pseudoseizures are a common manifestation of a conversion disorder.

Physical examination often fails to reveal objective abnormalities. Histories might reveal a close relationship with someone who exhibited similar symptoms or had a recent episode of acute illness. Findings inconsistent with organic pathology are often seen. Deep tendon reflexes can be elicited in a paralyzed limb, or pupillary responses to light can be elicited in patients who report blindness. Video electroencephalography and postictal serum prolactin levels (elevated in true seizures) are useful in diagnosing pseudoseizures. Abasia-astasia is a conversion disorder manifest as an inability to stand or walk.

Table 20-5 CRITERIA FOR DIAGNOSIS OF FACTITIOUS DISORDER

A. Intentional production or feigning of physical or psychologic signs or symptoms B. The motivation for the behavior is to assume the sick role C. External incentives for the behavior (e.g., economic gain, avoiding legal responsibility, or improving physical well-being, as in malingering) are absent
CODE BASED ON TYPE
With predominantly psychological signs and symptoms: if psychologic signs and symptoms predominate in the clinical presentation **With predominantly physical signs and symptoms:** if physical signs and symptoms predominate in the clinical presentation **With combined psychological and physical signs and symptoms:** if psychologic and physical signs and symptoms are present, but neither predominates in the clinical persentation

From Kliegman RM, Marcdante KJ, Jenson HB, et al, editors: *Nelson essentials of pediatrics,* ed 5, Philadelphia, 2006, Elsevier/Saunders, p 84.

Vulnerability to conversion disorders is not clearly linked to any specific cause, although anxiety and family disturbance can be factors. Children with conversion disorders are highly *suggestible*, which often helps in treatment. Cultural background affects how illness and distress are expressed and should be considered before diagnosing conversion disorder. Follow-up studies indicate that about 30% of children with a diagnosis of conversion disorder are later found to have a medical disorder that can explain the original symptoms.

In **somatoform pain disorder,** pain is the primary physical symptom (see Table 20-4). These disorders are characterized by reoccurrence. Prevalence studies suggest that 11% of boys and 15% of girls have ongoing somatic symptoms. Recurrent abdominal pain accounts for 2-4% of all pediatric visits and headaches for an additional 1-2%. Most of these children do not have any positive clinical findings.

The primary differential diagnosis of psychosomatic illness is between that of somatoform disorder and a physical illness. Mood and anxiety disorders often include the presence of physical symptoms that tend to remit with treatment of the primary mood or anxiety symptoms and that appear distinct from physical complaints seen in somatoform disorders.

Additional diagnoses to consider include malingering and factitious disorders. **Malingering,** which is very rare in the pediatric setting, can be distinguished from somatoform disorders by looking at the motivation for the symptoms. Persons who are malingering will intentionally produce or exaggerate physical symptoms to receive some external reward. Persons with **factitious disorder** on the other hand are not motivated by external rewards but instead have an intrapsychic need to remain in the sick role (Table 20-5). Factitious disorders cause somatic and/or psychologic symptoms that are deliberately fabricated in the absence of any potential gain to the patient, other than the benefit of assuming the sick role (see Table 20-5). *Munchausen syndrome* is an example of a chronic factitious disorder typically seen in adults who persist in seeking medical treatments, including surgery, despite the lack of any real disease. *Factitious disorder by proxy* is a variant in which parents induce physical symptoms in their children in order to assume the sick role by proxy (Chapter 37.2). In such cases infants and young children can present with fractures, poisonings, persistent episodes of apnea, and other unusual ailments. It is considered a form of child abuse, which can be lethal, and must be reported to the appropriate authorities.

TREATMENT

It is generally believed that effective treatment needs to incorporate a number of different treatment modalities to target the

Table 20-6 STEPWISE APPROACH TO DEVELOPING AN INTEGRATED MEDICAL AND PSYCHIATRIC TREATMENT APPROACH TO SOMATOFORM DISORDERS

COMPLETE MEDICAL AND PSYCHIATRIC ASSESSMENTS
• Perform patient and family interviews • Obtain histories, examinations, and studies • Elicit risk factors for pediatric somatization • Remember somatoform illness is not a diagnosis by exclusion • Develop a developmental biopsychosocial formulation of the patient and family
CONVENE AN INFORMING CONFERENCE WITH THE FAMILY
• Convey integrated medical and psychiatric findings to family • Emphasize the positive nature of the medical findings • Acknowledge the patient's suffering and family's concerns and emphasize that the symptoms are not feigned or under voluntary control • Because the family has a medical model as their frame of reference, help reframe this understanding of symptoms into a developmental biopsychosocial formulation
IMPLEMENT TREATMENT INTERVENTIONS IN *BOTH* MEDICAL AND PSYCHIATRIC DOMAINS

• Consider the following medical interventions
  • Set up ongoing pediatric follow-up appointments
  • Physical therapy or other face-saving remedies may be added depending on symptoms
• Consider the following psychiatric interventions
  • Implement cognitive-behavioral intervention
  • Implement psychotherapy
  • Implement family therapy
  • Assess for the presence of target symptoms for psychotropic medications

Modified from DeMaso DR, Beasley PJ; The somatoform disorders. In Klykylo WM, Kay JL, Rube DM, editors: *Clinical child psychiatry*, ed 2, London, 2005, John Wiley & Sons, p 481, Table 26.3.

factors that are believed to be associated with the development of somatization. Given the "diagnostic uncertainty" in these disorders, a multidisciplinary approach is recommended, including a stepwise plan for developing an integrated medical and psychiatric treatment strategy to somatoform disorders (Table 20-6).

Education of the Patient and Family

With completion of the medical and psychologic assessments, it is crucial to present the findings to the patient and his or her family. The etiology of the child's symptoms should be reframed in a broader biopsychosocial understanding through an "informing conference" where the findings are conveyed to the family. It is critical to give both a physical and emotional interpretation of the child's symptoms in a supportive and nonjudgmental manner. It is important for the family to directly hear from the pediatric practitioner that the symptoms are not solely the result of a physical condition, thereby facilitating acceptance of the role of psychologic factors.

It is not unusual for parents to be doubtful or rejecting of the formulation and proposed treatment. In these instances it is helpful to gently explore the source of the parent's resistance. Common reasons include previous errors on the part of health care providers leading to lack of trust, the family's past experience of serious physical illness that can create a pattern of anxiety and hypervigilance, and concerns about the stigma of being labeled with a mental health illness. It is particularly important not to come across as dismissive of the family's concerns or the child's symptoms or suffering. It may be extremely beneficial to devote extra time to further discussion, clarification, education, and normalization of the child's presentation.

Regular team meetings should be encouraged to maintain close communication between health care providers and minimize inconsistencies and miscommunications that have the potential to increase the patient's and family's mistrust and frustration.

Implementing a Rehabilitation Model

A rehabilitation model approach provides a useful framework for the treatment that shifts the focus away from finding a cure for symptoms and instead emphasizes a return to normal adaptive functioning. This includes increased activities of daily living, improved nutrition, enhanced mobility, return to school, and socialization with peers. It is generally counterproductive to adopt a confrontational approach or try to talk patients into giving up their symptoms. Unlike malingering and factitious disorders, somatoform symptoms are not consciously produced and they are experienced as "real suffering" by the patient. Any implication that the symptoms are not real can lead to increased frustration and escalation of symptoms.

Treatment approaches include the use of intensive physical and occupational therapies that emphasize the recovery of function. Behavioral modification approaches include increasing attention and reward for adaptive functioning as well as reducing environmental reinforcers and unnecessary medical interventions to minimize the sick role. Relaxation strategies, biofeedback, hypnosis, and/or integrative therapies (e.g., acupuncture and massage therapy) are also useful.

Cognitive-behavioral therapy, individual psychotherapy, and/or family therapy can help a child adjust to the stress of the illness and to learn new coping strategies. Individual psychotherapy can play an important role in helping change a child's erroneous cognitions about his or her ability to resume functioning. Patients are encouraged to express their underlying emotions and to develop alternative ways to express their feelings of distress.

Psychotropic interventions may be beneficial if there is evidence of underlying or co-morbid depression or anxiety.

When the child is being managed as an outpatient, regularly scheduled visits to the pediatric practitioner can help alleviate anxiety and potentially reduce the frequency of unnecessary emergency department visits, diagnostic work-ups, and inpatient hospitalizations. It is also important to establish regular contact and liaison with key school personnel to provide guidance and education on how to address the child's physical symptoms and complaints in the school setting. Collaborative models of health care that integrate mental health consultation within the primary care setting may be especially helpful for this group of patients and families.

BIBLIOGRAPHY

Please visit the Nelson Textbook of Pediatrics *website at www.expertconsult.com for the complete bibliography.*

Chapter 21 Rumination, Pica, and Elimination (Enuresis, Encopresis) Disorders

21.1 Rumination Disorder

Emily R. Katz and David R. DeMaso

Rumination disorder is defined as the repeated regurgitation and rechewing of food for a period of at least 1 mo following a period of normal functioning. The rumination is not due to an associated gastrointestinal illness or other general medical condition (e.g., esophageal reflux). It does not occur exclusively during the course of anorexia nervosa or bulimia nervosa. Malnourishment with resultant weight loss or growth delay is a hallmark of this disorder. If the symptoms occur exclusively during the course of mental retardation or a pervasive developmental disorder, they must be sufficiently severe to warrant independent clinical attention.

EPIDEMIOLOGY

Rumination is a rare disorder that is potentially fatal, and some reports indicate that 5-10% of affected children die. In otherwise healthy children, this disorder typically appears in the 1st yr of life, generally between the ages of 3 and 6 mo. The disorder is more common in infants with severe mental retardation than in those with mild or moderate mental retardation.

ETIOLOGY AND DIFFERENTIAL DIAGNOSIS

Proposed causes of rumination disorder include a disturbed relationship with primary caregivers; lack of an appropriately stimulating environment; and learned behavior reinforced by pleasurable sensations, distraction from negative emotions, and/or inadvertent reinforcement (attention) from primary caregivers. The differential diagnosis includes congenital gastrointestinal system anomalies, pyloric stenosis, Sandifer's syndrome, increased intracranial pressure, diencephalic tumors, adrenal insufficiency, and inborn errors of metabolism.

TREATMENT

Treatment begins with a behavioral analysis to determine if the disorder serves as self-stimulation or is socially motivated. The behavior might begin as self-stimulation, but it subsequently becomes reinforced by the social attention given to the behavior. Treatment is generally directed at reinforcing correct eating behavior and minimizing attention to rumination. Aversive conditioning techniques (e.g., withdrawal of positive attention) are useful when a child's health is jeopardized. Successful treatment requires the child's primary caregivers to be involved in the intervention. The caretakers need counseling around responding adaptively to the child's behavior as well as altering any maladaptive responses. There is no current evidence supporting a psychopharmacologic response to these disorders.

BIBLIOGRAPHY

Please visit the Nelson Textbook of Pediatrics *website at www.expertconsult.com for the complete bibliography.*

21.2 Pica

Emily R. Katz and David R. DeMaso

Pica involves the persistent eating of nonnutritive substances (e.g., plaster, charcoal, clay, wool, ashes, paint, earth). The eating behavior is inappropriate to the developmental level (e.g., the normal mouthing and tasting of objects in infants and toddlers) and not part of a culturally sanctioned practice.

EPIDEMIOLOGY

Pica appears to be more common in children with mental retardation, pervasive developmental disorders, obsessive-compulsive disorders, and other neuropsychiatric disorders (e.g., Kleine-Levin syndrome, schizophrenia). It usually remits in childhood but can continue into adolescence and adulthood. Geophagia (eating earth) is associated with pregnancy and is not seen as abnormal in some cultures (e.g., rural or preindustrial societies in parts of Africa and India). Children with pica are at increased risk for lead poisoning (Chapter 702), iron-deficiency anemia (Chapter 449), obstruction, dental injury, and parasitic infections.

ETIOLOGY

Numerous etiologies have been proposed but not proved, ranging from psychosocial causes to physical ones. They include nutritional deficiencies (e.g., iron, zinc, and calcium), low socioeconomic factors (e.g., lead paint), child abuse and neglect, family disorganization (e.g., poor supervision), psychopathology, learned behavior, underlying (but undetermined) biochemical disorder, and cultural and familial factors.

TREATMENT

A combined medical and psychosocial approach is generally indicated for pica. The sequelae related to the ingested item can require specific treatment (e.g., lead toxicity, iron-deficiency anemia, parasitic infestation). Ingestion of hair can require medical or surgical intervention for a gastric bezoar (Chapter 326). Nutritional education, cultural factors, psychologic assessment, and behavior interventions are important in developing an intervention strategy for this disorder.

BIBLIOGRAPHY

Please visit the Nelson Textbook of Pediatrics *website at www.expertconsult.com for the complete bibliography.*

21.3 Enuresis (Bed-Wetting)

Emily R. Katz and David R. DeMaso

Enuresis is defined as the repeated voiding of urine into clothes or bed at least twice a week for at least 3 consecutive months in a child who is at least 5 yr of age. The behavior is not due exclusively to the direct physiologic effect of a substance (e.g., a diuretic) or a general medical condition (e.g., diabetes, spina bifida, a seizure disorder). *Diurnal enuresis* defines wetting while awake and *nocturnal enuresis* refers to voiding during sleep. *Primary enuresis* occurs in children who have never been consistently dry through the night, whereas *secondary enuresis* refers to the resumption of wetting after at least 6 months of dryness. *Monosymptomatic enuresis* has no associated daytime symptoms (urgency, frequency, daytime enuresis), and *nonmonosymptomatic enuresis*, which is more common, often has at least one subtle daytime symptom. Monosymptomatic enuresis is rarely associated with significant organic underlying abnormalities.

NORMAL VOIDING AND TOILET TRAINING

Urine storage consists of sympathetic and pudendal nerve–mediated inhibition of detrusor contractile activity accompanied by closure of the bladder neck and proximal urethra with increased activity of the external sphincter. The infant has coordinated reflex voiding as often as 15-20 times per day. Over time, bladder capacity increases. In children up to the age of 14 yr, the mean bladder capacity in ounces is equal to the age (in years) plus 2.

At 2-4 yr, the child is developmentally ready to begin toilet training. To achieve conscious bladder control, several conditions must be present: awareness of bladder filling, cortical inhibition (suprapontine modulation) of reflex (unstable) bladder contractions, ability to consciously tighten the external sphincter to prevent incontinence, normal bladder growth, and motivation by the child to stay dry. The transitional phase of voiding is the period when children are acquiring bladder control. Girls typically acquire bladder control before boys, and bowel control typically is achieved before bladder control.

EPIDEMIOLOGY

Prevalence estimates vary significantly. At age 5 yr, 7% of boys and 3% of girls have enuresis; by age 10 yr the percentages are 3% and 2%, respectively: by age 18 yr, 1% for men and less than 1% for women. Primary enuresis accounts for 85% of cases. Enuresis is more common in lower socioeconomic groups, in larger families, and in institutionalized children. There is an estimated spontaneous cure rate of 14-16% annually. Diurnal enuresis is more common in girls and rarely occurs after the age of 9 yr; overall, 25% of children have diurnal enuresis.

DIAGNOSIS AND DIFFERENTIAL DIAGNOSIS

Secondary etiologies of urinary incontinence include urinary tract infections (UTIs), chronic kidney disease, hypercalcemia, hypokalemia, chemical urethritis, constipation, diabetes mellitus or insipidus, sickle cell anemia, seizures, pinworm infection, spinal dysraphism, neurogenic bladder, hyperthyroidism, sleep-disordered breathing, drugs (selective serotonin reuptake inhibitor, valproic acid, clozapine) and giggle or stress incontinence. Children with combined nocturnal and diurnal enuresis are more likely to have abnormalities of the urinary tract, making ultrasonography or uroflowmetry indicated. Otherwise, anatomic abnormalities are rarely associated with either nocturnal or diurnal enuresis such that invasive studies are generally contraindicated. Urinalysis and urine culture will rule out infectious causes and the elevated urine osmolality associated with diabetes mellitus.

ETIOLOGY

The cause of enuresis likely involves biologic, emotional, and learning factors. Compared with a 15% incidence of enuresis in children from nonenuretic families, 44% and 77% of children were enuretic when one or both parents, respectively, were themselves enuretic. Twin studies show a marked familial pattern, with documented concordance rates of 68% in monozygotic twins and 36% in dizygotic twins. Linkage studies have implicated several chromosomes with varying patterns of transmission.

Children with nocturnal enuresis might hyposecrete arginine vasopressin (AVP) and may be less responsive to the lower urine osmolality associated with fluid loading. Many affected children also appear to have small functional bladder capacity. There is some support for a relationship among sleep architecture, diminished capacity to be aroused from sleep, and abnormal bladder function. A subgroup of patients with enuresis has been identified in whom there is no arousal to bladder distention and an unusual pattern of uninhibited bladder contractions before the enuretic episode. One specific sleep disorder, *sleep apnea*, has been associated with enuresis (Chapter 17). Although the mechanism is unknown, central nervous system immaturity with delays in motor and language milestones appears to be a relevant etiology of enuresis for some children.

Psychosocial stressors may be contributory. Children generally have *secondary enuresis* in the context of significant life stress or traumatic experiences (e.g., divorce, school trauma, physical or sexual abuse, hospitalization). Psychologic factors can be central in the rare instance in which family disorganization or neglect has resulted in there never having been a reasonable effort made at toilet training. Children with enuresis have a higher incidence of psychiatric disorders than those without enuresis, although no single disorder accounts for the difference. There is some support for enuresis being a cause of psychologic disturbance, rather than an effect of the disturbances, as emotional and behavioral functioning tends to improve significantly once enuresis resolves.

Children during their early years must master the learning task of controlling the reflexive behavior of urination. Children with enuresis have difficulty in learning this control.

Children with enuresis should be evaluated with a detailed history and physical exam, taking into consideration the underlying organic causes of secondary enuresis (see earlier). Particular attention should be paid to manifestations of UTIs; chronic kidney disease; spinal cord disorders; constipation; and the thirst, polyuria, and polydipsia associated with both type of diabetes. Laboratory evaluation should include a urinalysis to check for glycosuria or a low specific gravity; in children with daytime symptoms, bladder ultrasonography should be performed when the bladder is perceived to be full and after voiding.

TREATMENT

Given the steady progression in the spontaneous remission rate of enuresis each year, there is some question as to whether enuresis should be treated. Family conflict, parent-child antagonism, and/or peer teasing due to the enuresis are good reasons to institute treatment for enuresis with resultant beneficial effects on a child's well-being and self-esteem. Daytime wetting, abnormal voiding (unusual posturing, discomfort, straining, and/or a poor urine stream), a history of UTIs and/or evidence of infection on urinalysis or culture, and genital abnormalities are indications for urologic referral and treatment.

The treatment of monosymptomatic nocturnal enuresis should be marked by a conservative, gentle, and patient approach. Treatment can begin with parent-child education, charting with rewards for dry nights, voiding before bedtime, and night awakening 2-4 hr after bedtime, while at the same time making sure that parents do not punish the child for enuretic episodes (Table 21-1). In addition, the child should be encouraged to avoid holding urine and to void frequently during the day (to avoid day wetting). These children also need ready access to school toilets. Furthermore, if constipation and fecal impaction are problems (Chapter 22.4), children should be encouraged to have a daily bowel movement and taught optimal relaxation of pelvic floor muscles to improve bowel emptying.

If this approach fails, urine alarm treatment is recommended. Application of an alarm for a period of 8-12 wk can be expected to result in a 75-95% success in the arrest of bedwetting. The underlying conditioning principle likely lies in the alarm's being an annoying awakening stimulus that causes the child to awaken in time to go to the bathroom and/or retain urine in order to avoid the aversive stimulus. Urine alarm treatment has been shown to be of equal or superior effectiveness when compared to all other forms of treatment. Relapse rates are approximately 40%, with the simplest response being a second alarm course as well as considering the addition of intermittent schedules of reinforcement or the use of overlearning (drinking just before bedtime).

Pharmacotherapy for nocturnal enuresis is second-line treatment (Table 21-2). Desmopressin acetate (DDAVP) is a synthetic

Table 21-1 TREATMENT REGIMEN FOR MONOSYMPTOMATIC NOCTURNAL ENURESIS

- Limit fluids to 8 oz at supper 3 to 3.5 hours before bedtime; no fluids thereafter.
- Empty the bladder before sleeping.
- Make a bedtime "resolution" to stay dry.
- Discuss mode of action of drugs or moisture alarm and drug side effects; dispense drug or alarm.
- Advise that medication or alarm is the "coach" and the child is the "player."
- Advise that positive internal and external biofeedback signals help hasten central nervous system control of the bladder.
- Keep a calendar of dry and wet nights.
- Encourage the child's participation in cleaning up personal clothing and bedclothes.
- Schedule follow-up visits or phone calls at least every 2 wk, with positive reinforcement for dry nights and efforts.
- Continue use of alarm until 28 consecutive dry nights are achieved, then stop; use medications as directed.
- If bedwetting returns on tapering or discontinuation of medication or alarm, restart nightly medication or alarm.
- If the child is not dry every night, despite motivation and efforts, substitute or add another drug or alarm and rule out undisclosed diurnal voiding problems.

From Chandra MM: Enuresis and voiding dysfunction. In Burg FD, Ingelfinger JR, Polin RA, et al, editors: *Current pediatric therapy*, ed 18, Philadelphia, 2006, Elsevier/Saunders, p 591.

Table 21-2 MEDICATIONS FOR TREATMENT OF MONOSYMPTOMATIC NOCTURNAL ENURESIS

GENERIC NAME (TRADE NAME)	DOSAGE FORMULATION	DOSAGE REGIMEN	MECHANISM OF ACTION	COMMENTS
Desmopressin acetate (DDAVP)	Nasal spray pump: 10 µg/0.1 mL spray	1 spray (10 µg) per nostril qhs, increasing to 40 µg	Decreased urine volume, possible effect on sleep arousal through its action as a central nervous system neurotransmitter	Can cause nasal irritation; risk of water intoxication (headache, seizures); hence, restrict fluids 3 hr before the dose
	Tablets: 0.1 mg, 0.2 mg	0.2 mg PO qhs, increasing up to 0.6 mg		Risk of water intoxication
Imipramine hydrochloride (Tofranil)	Tablets: 10 mg, 25 mg, 50 mg; Tofranil PM capsule 75, 100, 125, 150 mg	1.5-2 mg/kg 2 hr before bedtime, not to exceed 2.5 mg/kg or 75 mg maximum	Anticholinergic effect on bladder, increased resistance of bladder outlet, possible central inhibition of micturition reflex, possible effect on sleep arousal by central noradrenergic facilitation	Can cause sleep disturbance, mood alteration, decreased appetite, risk of cardiac arrhythmia with overdose

From Chandra MM: Enuresis and voiding dysfunction. In Burg FD, Ingelfinger JR, Polin RA, et al, editors: *Current pediatric therapy*, ed 18, Philadelphia, 2006, Elsevier/Saunders, p 591.

analog of the antidiuretic hormone (ADH) vasopressin, which decreases nighttime urine production. The fast action of DDAVP suggests a role for special occasions (e.g., sleepovers), when rapid control of bedwetting is desired. Unfortunately, the relapse rate is high when DDAVP is discontinued. DDAVP is also associated with rare side effects of hyponatremia and water intoxication, with resulting seizures. Although imipramine has some usefulness, less than 50% of children respond, and most relapse when the medication is discontinued. Bothersome side effects and potential lethality in overdose also limit this medication's usefulness. Much less commonly used, oxybutynin and tolterodine are antimuscarinic drugs, which may be effective by reducing bladder spasm and increasing bladder capacity.

DIURNAL INCONTINENCE

Daytime incontinence not secondary to neurologic abnormalities is common in children. At age 5 yr, 95% have been dry during the day at some time and 92% are dry. At 7 yr, 96% are dry, although 15% have significant urgency at times. At 12 yr, 99% are dry during the day. The most common cause of daytime incontinence is a **pediatric unstable bladder** (also termed uninhibited or overactive bladder, bladder spasms).

Important points in the history include the pattern of incontinence, including the frequency, the volume of urine lost during incontinent episodes, whether the incontinence is associated with urgency or giggling, whether it occurs after voiding, and whether the incontinence is continuous. The frequency of voiding and whether there is nocturnal enuresis, a strong, continuous urinary stream, or sensation of incomplete bladder emptying should be assessed. A diary of when the child voids and whether he or she was wet or dry is helpful. Other urologic problems such as UTIs, reflux, neurologic disorders, or a family history of duplication anomalies should be assessed. Bowel habits also should be evaluated, because incontinence is common in children with constipation and/or encopresis. Diurnal incontinence can occur in girls with a history of sexual abuse.

Physical examination is directed at identifying signs of organic causes of incontinence: short stature, hypertension, enlarged kidneys and/or bladder, constipation, labial adhesion, ureteral ectopy, back or sacral spinal anomalies, and neurologic signs. A urinalysis and/or culture should be performed to check for infection. In some cases, assessing the postvoid residual urine volume or urinary flow rate is appropriate. Imaging is reserved for children who have significant physical findings, a family history of urinary tract anomalies, or UTIs, and for those who do not respond to therapy appropriately. A renal ultrasonogram with or without a voiding cystourethrogram is indicated. Urodynamics should be performed if there is evidence of neurologic disease and may be helpful if empiric therapy is ineffective.

21.4 Encopresis

Emily R. Katz and David R. DeMaso

The definition of encopresis requires the voluntary or involuntary passage of feces into inappropriate places at least once a month for 3 consecutive months once a chronologic or developmental age of 4 yr has been reached. Encopresis is not diagnosed when the behavior is due exclusively to the direct effects of a substance (e.g., laxatives) or a general medical condition (except through a mechanism involving constipation). Subtypes include **retentive encopresis** (with constipation and overflow incontinence) representing 65-95% of cases, and **nonretentive encopresis** (without constipation and overflow incontinence). Encopresis can persist from infancy onward (primary) or can appear after successful toilet training (secondary).

CLINICAL MANIFESTATIONS

Children with encopresis often present with reports of underwear soiling, and many parents initially presume that diarrhea, rather than constipation, is the cause. In retentive encopresis, associated complaints of difficulty with defecation, abdominal or rectal pain, impaired appetite with poor growth, and urinary (day and/or night) incontinence are common. Children often have large bowel movements that obstruct the toilet. There may also be retentive posturing or UTIs.

Nonretentive encopresis is more likely to occur as a solitary symptom and have associated primary underlying psychologic problems. Children with encopresis can present with poor school performance and attendance that is triggered by the scorn and derision from schoolmates because of the child's offensive odor.

EPIDEMIOLOGY

Functional encopresis does not begin before age 4 yr. The prevalence of encopresis is approximately 4% in 5-6 yr olds and 1.5% in 11-12 yr olds. Encopresis is 4-5 times more common in boys than in girls and tends to decrease with age.

DIAGNOSIS AND DIFFERENTIAL DIAGNOSIS

The first priority in evaluating a child with fecal incontinence is to rule out a general medical condition (e.g., tethered cord, Chapter 598.1) causing the problem. The presence of fecal retention should then be determined. A positive finding on rectal examination is sufficient to document fecal retention, but a

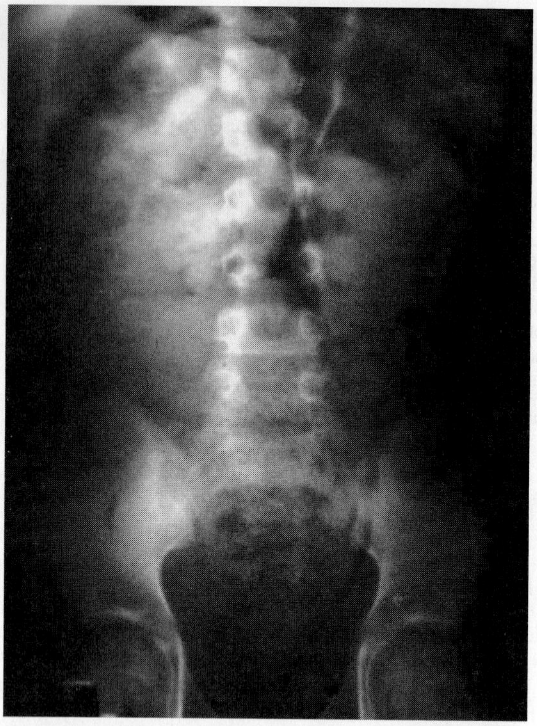

Figure 21-1 Radiograph revealing severe stool retention. (From Loening-Baucke V: Functional constipation with encopresis. In Wyllie R, Hyams JS, Kay M, editors: *Pediatric gastrointestinal and liver disease*, ed 3, Philadelphia, 2006, Elsevier/Saunders, p 182.)

negative finding requires plain abdominal films (Fig. 21-1). Additional diagnostic studies are rarely indicated.

ETIOLOGY

The etiology of encopresis lies in a combination of biologic, emotional, and learning factors. Although by definition encopresis is fecal incontinence based on a functional disorder, abnormal gastrointestinal mobility or sensation, hereditary predispositions, and developmental delays have been postulated as playing an etiologic role in encopresis. Although most children with encopresis do not have an emotional problem, a great deal of turmoil and conflict within the family is commonly found. Whether this turmoil is an effect or the cause is unclear; nevertheless, the common accompanying feelings of distress and low self-esteem improve with successful treatment.

Manipulative soiling appears to follow a reinforcement model. Complaints may lead to being excused from stressful circumstances. Stress and anxiety, along with an inherited tendency to react with intestinal distress, can lead to impaired bowel control and to loss of previously learned toileting behavior. Poor dietary choices and failure to establish good toilet habits can further contribute to the development of encopresis.

TREATMENT

The standard medical treatment of retentive encopresis involves the clearance of impacted fecal material followed by the short-term use of mineral oil or laxatives to prevent further constipation (Tables 21-3 and 21-4). There needs to be a focus on adherence with regular postprandial toilet sitting and adoption of a balanced diet. Once impacted stool is removed, the combination of constipation management and simple behavior therapy is successful in the majority of cases, although it is often a period of months before soiling stops completely. Compliance can wane, and failure of this standard treatment approach sometimes requires more intensive intervention, with a special emphasis on adherence to a high-fiber diet and family support for behavioral change. Keeping records of the child's progress is necessary. In cases where behavioral or psychiatric problems are evident, group or individual psychotherapy may be necessary.

From the outset, parents should be actively encouraged to reward the child for adherence to a healthy bowel regimen and to avoid power struggles. In addition, they should be instructed not to respond to soiling with retaliatory or punitive measures, because children are likely to become angry, ashamed, and resistant to intervention.

Whereas around 80% of children become continent on the above regimen, many relapse when removed from the protocol.

Table 21-3 SUGGESTED MEDICATIONS AND DOSAGES FOR DISIMPACTION

MEDICATION	AGE	DOSAGE
RAPID RECTAL DISIMPACTION		
Glycerin suppositories	Infants and toddlers	
Phosphate enema	<1 yr	60 mL
	>1 yr	6 mL/kg bodyweight, up to 135 mL twice
Milk of molasses enema	Older children	(1 : 1 milk : molasses) 200-600 mL
SLOW ORAL DISIMPACTION IN OLDER CHILDREN		
Over 2-3 Days		
Polyethylene glycol with electrolytes		25 mL/kg bodyweight/hr, up to 1000 mL/h until clear fluid comes from the anus
Over 5-7 Days		
Polyethylene without electrolytes		1.5 g/kg bodyweight per day for 3 days
Milk of magnesia		2 mL/kg bodyweight twice/day for 7 days
Mineral oil		3 mL/kg bodyweight twice/day for 7 days
Lactulose or sorbitol		2 mL/kg bodyweight twice/day for 7 days

From Loening-Baucke V: Functional constipation with encopresis. In Wyllie R, Hyams JS, Kay M, editors: *Pediatric gastrointestinal and liver disease*, ed 3, Philadelphia, 2006, Elsevier/Saunders, p 183.

Table 21-4 SUGGESTED MEDICATIONS AND DOSAGES FOR MAINTENANCE THERAPY OF CONSTIPATION

MEDICATION	AGE	DOSE
FOR LONG-TERM TREATMENT (YEARS):		
Milk of magnesia	>1 mo	1-3 mL/kg body weight/day, divide in 1-2 doses
Mineral oil	>12 mo	1-3 mL/kg body weight/day, divided in 1-2 doses
Lactulose or sorbitol	>1 mo	1-3 mL/kg body weight/day, divide in 1-2 doses
Polyethylene glycol 3350 (MiraLax)	>1 mo	0.7 g/kg body weight/day, divide in 1-2 doses
FOR SHORT-TERM TREATMENT (MONTHS):		
Senna (Senokot) syrup, tablets	1-5 yr	5 mL (1 tablet) with breakfast, max 15 mL daily
	5-15 yr	2 tablets with breakfast, maximum 3 tablets daily
Glycerin enemas	>10 yr	20-30 mL/day (1/2 glycerin and 1/2 normal saline)
Bisacodyl suppositories	>10 yr	10 mg daily

From Loening-Baucke V: Functional constipation with encopresis. In Wyllie R, Hyams JS, Kay M, editors: *Pediatric gastrointestinal and liver disease*, ed 3, Philadelphia, 2006, Elsevier/Saunders, p 185.

Children with behavioral problems are particularly prone to treatment failure, necessitating referral for psychologic intervention and behavioral management (e.g., behavior programs and/or biofeedback).

For children with chronic diarrhea and/or irritable bowel syndrome where stress and anxiety play a major role, stress reduction and learning effective coping strategies can play an important role in responding to the encopresis. Relaxation training, stress inoculation, assertiveness training, and/or general stress management procedures can be helpful.

In the infrequent case where the child is using soiling as a way of manipulating the environment, a combination of behavioral and family therapy is indicated. Reinforcement for soiling behavior needs to be identified and removed, and family counseling and intervention are required to do so.

BIBLIOGRAPHY

Please visit the Nelson Textbook of Pediatrics *website at www.expertconsult.com for the complete bibliography.*

Chapter 22
Habit and Tic Disorders

Colleen A. Ryan, Gary J. Gosselin, and David R. DeMaso

HABIT DISORDERS

Habits are common and can range from benign transient habits (e.g., skin picking) to significantly problematic repetitive behavior (e.g., bruxism). The *Diagnostic and Statistical Manual of Mental Disorders, Fourth Edition, Text Revision* (DSM-IV-TR) defines stereotypic movement disorders (habit disorders) as repetitive, seemingly driven, and nonfunctional motor behavior that markedly interferes with normal activities or results in self-inflicted bodily injury that requires medical treatment. The behavior persists for 4 wk or longer and is not better accounted for by a compulsion, a tic, a stereotypy that is part of a pervasive developmental disorder, or hair pulling (as in trichotillomania).

Clinical Manifestations

A child's presentation depends on the nature of the habit and level of the child's awareness of the behavior. Habit behaviors can be described as either automatic or focused, depending on the child's level of awareness. It has been suggested that a focused style (e.g., having awareness and receiving gratification from performing the behavior) is associated with higher levels of co-occurring habits. This style in hair pulling has been linked with increased depression, anxiety, and impairment in functioning, particularly during stressful events and onset of puberty.

Teeth grinding, or **bruxism**, is common, can begin in the first 5 yr of life, and may be associated with daytime anxiety. Untreated bruxism can cause problems with dental occlusion. Helping the child find ways to reduce anxiety might relieve the problem; bedtime can be made more relaxing by reading or talking with the child and allowing the child to discuss fears. Praise and other emotional support are useful. Persistent bruxism requires referral to a dentist and can manifest as muscular or temporomandibular joint pain.

Thumb sucking is normal in infancy and toddlerhood. Like other rhythmic patterns of behavior, thumb sucking is self-soothing. Basic behavioral management, including encouraging parents to ignore thumb sucking and instead focus on providing the child with praise for substitute behaviors, is often effective treatment. Simple reinforcers, such as giving the child a sticker for each block of time that he or she does not suck the thumb, can also be considered. Although some literature suggests that the use of noxious agents (bitter salves) may be effective in controlling thumb sucking, this approach should rarely be necessary.

Trichotillomania is the repetitive pulling of hair resulting in loss and strand breakage of hair (Chapter 654). The usual age of onset of trichotillomania is around 13 yr, although preschoolers have been described with this disorder. Children with trichotillomania have an increasing sense of tension immediately before pulling or when resisting the behavior, followed by pleasure or relief when pulling out the hair. The prevalence of trichotillomania in children is not well known but is believed to be 1-2% in college students. Although trichotillomania often remits spontaneously, treatment of those whose disorder has been present for >6 mo is unlikely to remit and requires behavioral treatment. Selective serotonin reuptake inhibitors (SSRIs) such as fluoxetine have some success as adjuncts.

Diagnosis and Differential Diagnosis

The child should be screened for current and past psychiatric symptoms (particularly anxiety, obsessions, compulsions, and depression) along with any accompanying functional limitations. The child should be examined for any significant physical injury from habit behaviors.

The differential diagnosis includes the stereotypic movements associated with mental retardation and pervasive developmental disorders. Compulsions with obsessive-compulsive disorder (OCD) and tic disorders as well as involuntary movements associated with neurologic conditions must be considered. Developmentally appropriate self-stimulatory behaviors in young children and in persons with sensory deficits (e.g., blindness) are other considerations.

Epidemiology

Prevalence rates remain unclear given the various different manifestations of habits. Thumb sucking is common in infancy and in as many as 25% of children age 2 yr and 15% in children age 5 yr. Nail biting has a reported child prevalence as high as 45-60%. Bruxism has been observed in 5-30% of children and breath-holding spells in up to 4-5% of children younger than 8 yr. The prevalence of self-injurious behaviors in the context of mental retardation varies from 2-3% in the community to 25% of institutionalized adults with severe mental retardation.

Certain habit disorders are more common in children with developmental delays, particularly those with pervasive developmental disorders. Self-injurious habits, such as self-biting or head banging, can occur in up to 25% of normally developing toddlers, but they are almost invariably associated with developmental delays in children older than 5 yr. Habit disorders in developmentally disabled children are more refractory to treatment than those in typically developing children, and referral to a developmental pediatrician or child psychiatrist for behavioral and/or psychopharmacologic management is often indicated. The pediatrician must also rule out severe neglect, which is associated with repetitive rocking, spinning, or other stereotypies. Institutionalized children have the highest rates of these kinds of stereotypies.

Etiology

Although habit disorders are limited and diverse, given the wider variety of habit behaviors (hand shaking, head banging, mouthing objects, body rocking, skin picking), the literature is suggestive of repetitive abnormal grooming-like behaviors with possibly evolutionary ties to early human experience with adversity. Brain regions implicated are those involved in navigating human experience through unpredictable, anxiety-provoked emotional states (e.g., amygdala and hippocampus) as well as regions related to pleasure and reward seeking (e.g., nucleus accumbens). The latter involves the hypothesis that individuals experience some level of gratification from performing the habit behavior.

Treatment

Often the initial approach to helping children with habit behaviors is for the parents to ignore the behavior and not convey worry to their children. Generally these behaviors disappear with time and elimination of attention. If distress in the child or family, social isolation, and/or physical injury is occurring, then treatment is indicated.

Behavior therapy is the mainstay of treatment using a variety of strategies including habit reversal, relaxation training, self-monitoring, reinforcement, competing responses, negative practice, and, rarely, the use of aversive-tasting substances (for thumb sucking or nail biting). SSRIs are helpful in reducing repetitive behaviors, and they might play a role in particularly disabling and problematic behaviors, particularly those co-occurring with anxiety and obsessive-compulsive behaviors.

TIC DISORDERS

In DSM-IV-TR, a tic is defined as a sudden, rapid, recurrent, nonrhythmic, stereotyped motor movement or vocalization that is experienced as irresistible, but can be suppressed for varying lengths of time. They are usually markedly diminished during sleep.

Tourette's disorder (TD) or syndrome (TS) is characterized by multiple motor and one or more vocal tics that have been present at some time in the illness, although not necessarily concurrently (Chapter 590.4). The tics occur many times a day nearly every day for more than 1 yr with no more than 3 consecutive tic-free months. Chronic motor or vocal tic disorder is similar, but each does not include both kinds of tics. Transient tic disorder involves motor and/or vocal tics that have been present for at least 4 wk, but less than 1 yr.

Clinical Manifestations

Motor tics generally involve muscles of the face, neck, shoulders, trunk, or hands. They can be divided into simple (eye blinking, neck jerking, shoulder shrugging, and cough) and complex (facial gestures and grooming behaviors). Vocal tics can also be simple (throat clearing, grunting, sniffing, barking) and complex (coprolalia [obscene words], palilalia [repetition of the patient's words], and echolalia [repetition of words said to the patient]).

Tic disorders can be associated with obsessions, compulsions, hyperactivity, distractibility, and impulsivity as well as social discomfort, anxiety, and depression. Although most children with TD have normal intelligence, learning difficulties are common.

Tics are differentiated from dyskinesias or dystonic movements because they can be consciously inhibited for brief periods, are not present continuously, are absent during sleep, and tend to be exacerbated by emotional stress or reduced during physical or mental activity. Tics are distinguished from absence seizures because the child with tics does not have loss of awareness of surroundings and/or amnesia.

Diagnosis and Differential Diagnosis

TD and associated tic disorders must be differentiated from abnormal movements that might accompany a general medical condition (e.g., head injury, Huntington's disease) or the direct effects of a substance (e.g., neuroleptic medication). They are different from the stereotyped movements seen in habit (or stereotypic movement) and pervasive developmental disorders. Tics must be differentiated from the compulsions seen in OCD (Chapter 23). Certain medications (e.g., stimulants) can exacerbate a pre-existing tic disorder.

Epidemiology

The onset of a tic disorder almost always occurs during childhood, developing in approximately 5-10% of early-school-aged children, with spontaneous disappearance in approximately 65% by the onset of adolescence. Multiple tics and complex vocal sounds can develop over time, peaking in severity by age 10-12 yr.

Etiology

Abnormalities in the dopamine, serotonin, and norepinephrine neurotransmitter systems have been identified in tic disorders as possible etiologic factors.

Autoimmune-mediated mechanisms continue to be investigated as having a potential etiologic role in movement disorders. **Pediatric autoimmune neuropsychiatric disorder associated with streptococcal infection** (PANDAS) is a condition in which antibodies to group A streptococcus (Chapter 176) cross-react with basal ganglia tissue and precipitate symptoms. Data supporting the pathophysiology of PANDAS include the ability to prevent tic relapses with antibiotic prophylaxis; high rates of cross-reactive antibodies for both group A streptococcus and basal ganglia proteins found in some samples from patients with tics compared with control subjects; and enlargement of the basal ganglia during acute exacerbations of neuropsychiatric symptoms in patients with PANDAS. Five clinical characteristics define the subgroup of patients with PANDAS: the presence of OCD and/or tic disorder; prepubertal age of onset; abrupt onset and relapsing-remitting course; association with neurologic abnormalities (chorea, hyperactivity, tics) during exacerbations; and temporal association between symptom exacerbations and group A streptococcal infection (a positive antistreptolysin O titer). Treatment of PANDAS includes acute antistreptococcal antibiotic therapy; prophylactic penicillin or azithromycin can decrease the number or episodes. The role of immunotherapy is controversial, with therapeutic plasma exchange indicated only for severely affected children.

Treatment

The treatment of tic disorder generally involves a multilevel approach including education, treating co-occurring conditions, and managing disabling tics. The child and family can be helped to understand the condition including what exacerbates and what reduces the tics. Supportive counselling can prove helpful for the child and/or the family.

Cognitive-behavioral therapy can be helpful in reducing impairing co-occurring anxiety and/or compulsive symptoms. Classroom level interventions might be needed when significant academic difficulties associated with co-occurring attention-deficit/hyperactivity disorder (ADHD) and/or learning disorders are present.

Medication for tic reduction is reserved for when the tics cause marked distress or significant impairments in psychosocial functioning. The α_2-adrenergic agonists (clonidine and guanfacine) are first-line agents in treating mild to moderate tic disorders. Sedation and low blood pressure are common side effects that require careful monitoring particularly when initiating treatment. The D_2 dopamine receptor-blocking medications (haloperidol and pimozide) are effective in reducing tics, but side effects including extrapyramidal symptoms have limited their use as first-line treatment. Risperidone, an atypical antipsychotic medication, has been shown to be equivalent to clonidine in reducing tics, though it too can have extrapyramidal as well as metabolic side effects (see Table 19-5).

Children with tic disorders might benefit from an SSRI for the treatment of comorbid OCD as well as anxiety and depressive disorders. Augmentation of the SSRI with an atypical antipsychotic medication is a consideration in patients with tic disorders and OCD who respond poorly to an SSRI alone. The presence of tics does not preclude the use of stimulants to address comorbid ADHD. However, close clinical monitoring is required for possible exacerbation of tics during stimulant treatment in an effort to strike a careful balance between reducing ADHD symptoms and controlling the tics.

TOURETTE'S SYNDROME

Clinical Manifestations

Tourette's syndrome (TS) is characterized by multiple motor and vocal tics (not necessarily present concurrently). TS occurs in approximately 4-5 persons per 10,000. It is 1.5-3 times more likely in boys than in girls. TS commonly manifests in childhood, beginning with simple motor tics, often before age 7 yr. In many cases, multiple tics and complex vocal sounds, such as barking and grunting, develop over time and peak in severity by age 10-12 yr. Shouting obscene words (**coprolalia**) is characteristic but is seen in only 10% of affected patients. The vocalizations can be suppressed temporarily but ultimately are uncontrollable and often jeopardize patients' social interaction with other children. Although TS is a lifelong condition, the ultimate prognosis can often be determined by the severity of the symptoms during adolescence. TS is more common in 1st-degree relatives of patients with TS than in the general population, and it affects boys 3-4 times more often than girls. In some, it is an autosomal dominant disorder with greater penetrance in males. Criteria for the diagnosis include multiple motor and vocal tics lasting >1 yr, with no tic-free interval lasting >3 mo, onset before age 18 yr, and no medical causes (drugs, central nervous system disease).

Children with TS often have behavioral, emotional, and academic problems. In particular, these children have higher rates of OCD (Chapter 23), ADHD (Chapter 30), and oppositional-defiant disorder (Chapter 27). The fact that TS is highly comorbid with these specific psychiatric disorders suggests dysfunction in particular regions of the brain. Neuroimaging studies suggest that there is a lack of normal asymmetry within the striatum and a decrease in the size of the cavum septum pellucidum. Single-photon emission computed tomography (SPECT) scan data implicate dysfunction in dopamine receptor binding in severely affected children. Studies have also implicated systemic and local cytokine responses in TS and in the exacerbation of symptoms.

Lyme disease rarely occurs with clinical manifestations of TS (Chapter 214). Many environmental factors are emotional stressors, which can also precipitate or increase tics. Laboratory studies are nonspecific; many patients with TS have nonspecific abnormal electroencephalographic findings.

Treatment

Treatment for TS should only occur after careful consideration of the functional limitations associated with the child's symptoms, any associated symptoms, and the risks and benefits of pharmacotherapy. In many cases, supportive management is all that is indicated. Many children with TS require medication for obsessive-compulsive symptoms or attention and impulsivity problems. There has been a concern that stimulants will unmask tics; studies have not consistently substantiated this concern. Tic disorders are not a contraindication to the judicious use of stimulants.

Pharmacotherapy, targeting the tics themselves, is indicated when tics interfere with social development or classroom function. For 1st-line treatment, haloperidol and pimozide reduce the severity of tics by 65%. Because potentially severe side effects are associated with traditional neuroleptics (cognitive impairment, lethargy, depression, dystonic reactions, parkinsonism, tardive dyskinesia), many clinicians recommend risperidone. Risperidone is equivalent to clonidine in reducing tics. Clonidine, an α_2-agonist, is effective; sedation and low blood pressure are common side effects of clonidine and require careful monitoring. The role of guanfacine (Tenex), which is a less sedating α_2-agonist, has not been firmly established (see Table 19-5).

Affected children and their families should be encouraged to be active participants in the management of TS. Support from organizations such as the Tourette Syndrome Association, which has a user-friendly website (*www.tsa-usa.org*), is often very beneficial to affected families. The natural course of TS includes a significant diminution or remission in symptoms in adolescence and early adulthood in approximately 65% of cases. It is difficult to predict which patients will experience fewer symptoms over time.

Obsessive-compulsive symptoms can persist into adulthood.

BIBLIOGRAPHY

Please visit the Nelson Textbook of Pediatrics *website at www.expertconsult.com for the complete bibliography.*

Chapter 23
Anxiety Disorders

David R. Rosenberg, Pankhuree Vandana, and Jennifer A. Chiriboga

Anxiety, defined as dread or apprehension, is a normal phenomenon. Anxiety by itself is not considered pathologic, is seen across the lifespan, and can be adaptive (e.g., the anxiety one might feel during an automobile crash). Anxiety has both a physiologic component, mediated by the autonomic nervous system, and a cognitive and behavioral component, expressed in worrying and wariness. Anxiety disorders are characterized by pathologic anxiety in which anxiety becomes disabling, interfering with social interactions, development, and achievement of goals or quality of life, and can lead to low self-esteem, social withdrawal, and academic underachievement. Diagnosis of a particular anxiety disorder in a child requires significant interference in the child's psychosocial and/or academic or occupational functioning, which can occur even with subthreshold symptoms that do not meet criteria in the *Diagnostic and Statistical Manual of Mental Disorders, Fourth Edition* (DSM-IV).

Separation anxiety disorder (**SAD**), childhood-onset social phobia or social anxiety disorder, generalized anxiety disorder (**GAD**), obsessive-compulsive disorder (**OCD**), phobias, post-traumatic stress disorder (**PTSD**), and panic disorder are all defined by the occurrence of either diffuse or specific anxiety, often related to predictable situations or cues. Anxiety disorders are the most common psychiatric disorders of childhood; they occur in 5-18% of all children and adolescents, prevalence rates comparable to physical disorders such as asthma and diabetes. Anxiety disorders are often comorbid with other psychiatric disorders (including a 2nd anxiety disorder); significant impairment in day-to-day functioning is common. High levels of fear in adolescence are also a significant risk factor for experiencing later episodes of major depression in adulthood. Anxiety and depressive disorder in adolescence predict increased risk of anxiety and depressive symptoms (including suicide attempts) in adulthood, underscoring the need to diagnose and treat these underreported, yet prevalent, conditions early.

Because anxiety is both a normal phenomenon and, when highly activated, strongly associated with impairment, the pediatrician must be able to differentiate normal anxiety from abnormal anxiety across development. Anxiety has an identifiable developmental progression for most children; most infants exhibit stranger wariness or anxiety beginning at 7-9 mo of age. Behavioral inhibition to the unfamiliar (withdrawal or fearfulness to novel stimuli associated with physiologic arousal) is evident in approximately 10-15% of the population at 12 mo of age and is moderately stable. Most children who show behavioral inhibition do not develop impairing levels of anxiety. A family history of anxiety disorders and maternal overinvolvement or enmeshment predicts later clinically significant anxiety in behaviorally inhibited infants. The infant who is excessively clingy and difficult to calm during pediatric visits should be followed for signs of increasing levels of anxiety.

Preschoolers typically have specific fears related to the dark, animals, and imaginary situations, in addition to normative separation anxiety. Preoccupation with orderliness and routines (*just right* phenomena) often takes on a quality of anxiety for preschool children. Parents' reassurance is usually sufficient to help the child through this period. Although most school-aged children abandon the imaginary fears of early childhood, some replace them with fears of bodily harm or other worries (Table 23-1). In adolescence, general worrying about school performance and worrying about social competence are common and remit as the teen matures.

Genetic or temperamental factors contribute more to the development of some anxiety disorders, whereas environmental factors are closely linked to the cause of others. Specifically, behavioral inhibition appears to be a heritable tendency and is linked with social phobia, generalized anxiety, and selective mutism. OCD and other disorders associated with OCD-like behaviors, such as Tourette syndrome and other tic disorders, tend to have high genetic risk as well (Chapter 590.4). Environmental factors, such as parent-infant attachment and exposure to trauma, contribute more to SAD and PTSD. Parental anxiety disorder is associated with an increased risk of anxiety disorder in offspring. Differences in the size of the amygdala and hippocampus are noted in patients with anxiety symptoms.

Separation anxiety disorder (SAD) is one of the most common childhood anxiety disorders with a prevalence of 3.5-5.4%. Approximately 30% of children presenting to an outpatient anxiety disorder clinic have SAD as a primary diagnosis. Separation anxiety is developmentally normal when it begins about 10 mo of age and tapers off by 18 mo. By 3 yr of age, most children can accept the temporary absence of their mother or primary caregiver.

Table 23-1 CRITERIA FOR DIAGNOSIS OF SPECIFIC PHOBIA

A. Marked and persistent fear that is excessive or unreasonable, cued by the presence or anticipation of a specific object or situation (e.g., flying, heights, animals, receiving an injection, seeing blood)
B. Exposure to the phobic stimulus almost invariably provokes an immediate anxiety response, which can take the form of a situationally bound or situationally predisposed panic attack. **Note:** In children, the anxiety may be expressed by crying, tantrums, freezing, or clinging
C. The person recognizes that the fear is excessive or unreasonable. **Note:** In children, this feature may be absent
D. The phobic situation is avoided or else is endured with intense anxiety or distress
E. The avoidance, anxious anticipation, or distress in the feared situation interferes significantly with the person's normal routine, occupational (or academic) functioning, or social activities or relationships, or there is marked distress about having the phobia
F. In children <18 yr, the duration is ≥6 mo
G. The anxiety, panic attacks, or phobic avoidance associated with the specific object or situation is not better accounted for by another mental disorder, such as obsessive-compulsive disorder (e.g., fear of dirt in someone with an obsession about contamination), post-traumatic stress disorder (e.g., avoidance of stimuli associated with a severe stressor), separation anxiety disorder (e.g., avoidance of school), social phobia (e.g., avoidance of social situations because of fear of embarrassment), panic disorder with agoraphobia, or agoraphobia without a history of panic disorder.
SPECIFY TYPE:
Animal type is fear elicited by animals or insects **Natural environment type** is elicited by, e.g., heights, storms, or water **Blood/injection/injury type** is fear related to seeing blood, injuries, or injections, or having an invasive medical procedure **Situational type** is fear caused by specific situations (e.g., airplanes, elevators, enclosed places) **Other types** include, e.g., fear of choking, vomiting, or contracting an illness; in children, fear of loud sounds or costumed characters

From Kliegman RM, Marcdante KJ, Jenson HB, et al, editors: *Nelson essentials of pediatrics,* ed 5, Philadelphia, 2006, Elsevier/Saunders, p 92.

SAD is more common in prepubertal children, with an average age of onset of 7.5 yr. Girls are more commonly affected than boys. SAD is characterized by unrealistic and persistent worries about separation from the home or a major attachment figure. Concerns include possible harm befalling the affected child or his or her primary caregivers, reluctance to go to school or to sleep without being near the parents, persistent avoidance of being alone, nightmares involving themes of separation, numerous somatic symptoms, and complaints of subjective distress. The 1st clinical sign might not appear until 3rd or 4th grade, typically after a holiday or a period where the child has been home because of illness, or when the stability of the family structure has been threatened by illness, divorce, or other psychosocial stressor.

Symptoms vary depending on the child's age: Children younger than 8 yr often have associated school refusal and excessive fear that harm will come to a parent; children 9-12 yr have excessive distress when separated from a parent; and those 13-16 yr often have school refusal and physical complaints. SAD may be more likely to develop in children with lower levels of psychosocial maturity. Parents are often unable to be assertive in returning the child to school. Mothers of children with SAD often have a history of an anxiety disorder. In these cases, the pediatrician should screen for parental depression or anxiety. Often referral for parental treatment or family therapy is necessary before SAD and concomitant school refusal can be successfully treated.

Comorbidity is common in SAD. In children with comorbid tic disorders and anxiety, SAD is especially associated with tic severity. SAD is a predictor for early onset of panic disorder. Children with SAD compared to those without SAD are 3 times more likely to develop panic disorder in adolescence.

When a child reports recurring acute severe anxiety, antidepressant or anxiolytic medication is often necessary. Controlled studies of tricyclic antidepressants (imipramine) and benzodiazepines (clonazepam) show that these agents are not generally effective. Data support the use of cognitive-behavioral therapy (CBT) and selective serotonin reuptake inhibitors (SSRIs) (see Table 19-4). One controlled trial of 488 children, 7-17 yr, which included children with a primary diagnosis of SAD, compared 12 wk of treatment with CBT, the SSRI, sertraline, their combination, and placebo. Nearly 81% of those treated with combination therapy improved, 55% for SSRI alone, 60% for CBT. All treatments were superior to placebo (24% response rate). The SSRI was well tolerated and had few side effects; adverse events, including suicidal and homicidal ideation, did not differ between the SSRI and placebo groups. There was no attempted suicide among the 488 children. CBT was associated with less insomnia, fatigue, sedation, and restlessness than SSRI. Combining SSRI with CBT may be the best approach to achieving a positive response; long-term SSRI treatment can provide additional benefit.

Childhood-onset social phobia (social anxiety disorder) is characterized by excessive anxiety in social settings (including the presence of unfamiliar peers, or unfamiliar adults) or performance situations, leading to social isolation (Table 23-2) and is associated with social scrutiny and fear of doing something embarrassing. Fear of social settings can also occur in other disorders, such as GAD. Avoidance or escape from the situation usually dissipates anxiety in **social phobia (SP)**, unlike GAD, where worry persists. Children and adolescents with SP often maintain the desire for involvement with family and familiar peers. When severe, the anxiety can manifest as a panic attack.

SP is associated with a decreased quality of life, with 38% of SP patients not graduating from high school. SP is associated with increased likelihood of having failed at least one grade. Its onset is typically during or before adolescence and is more common in girls. A family history of SP or extreme shyness is common. About 70-80% of patients with SP have at least one comorbid psychiatric disorder.

Table 23-2 CRITERIA FOR DIAGNOSIS OF SOCIAL PHOBIA

A. A marked and persistent fear of ≥1 social or performance situations in which the person is exposed to unfamiliar people or to possible scrutiny by others. The individual fears that he or she will act in a way (or show anxiety symptoms) that will be humiliating or embarrassing. **Note:** In children, there must be evidence of the capacity of age-appropriate social relationships with familiar people, and the anxiety must occur in peer settings, not just in interactions with adults
B. Exposure to the feared social situation almost invariably provokes anxiety, which may take the form of a situationally bound or situationally predisposed panic attack. **Note:** In children, the anxiety may be expressed by crying, tantrums, freezing, or shrinking from social situations or unfamiliar people
C. The person recognizes that the fear is excessive or unreasonable. **Note:** In children, this feature may be absent
D. The feared social or performance situations are avoided or else are endured with intense anxiety or distress
E. The avoidance, anxious anticipation, or distress in the feared social or performance situation interferes significantly with the person's normal routine, occupational (academic) functioning, or social activities or relationships, or there is marked distress about having the phobia
F. In children <18 yr, the duration is ≥6 mo
G. The fear or avoidance is not due to the direct physiologic effects of a drug of abuse, a medication, or a general medical condition and is not better accounted for by another mental disorder (e.g., panic disorder with or without agoraphobia, separation anxiety disorder, body dysmorphic disorder, pervasive developmental disorder, or schizoid personality disorder)
H. If a general medical condition or another mental disorder is present, the fear in criterion A is unrelated to it (e.g., the fear is not of stuttering, trembling in Parkinson's disease, or exhibiting abnormal eating behavior in anorexia nervosa or bulimia nervosa)

SPECIFY IF

Generalized: if the fears include most social situations (e.g., initiating or maintaining conversations, participating in small groups, dating, speaking to authority figures, attending parties). **Note:** Also consider the additional diagnosis of avoidant personality disorder

From Kliegman RM, Marcdante KJ, Jenson HB, et al, editors: *Nelson essentials of pediatrics,* ed 5, Philadelphia, 2006, Elsevier/Saunders, p 93.

Social effectiveness therapy for children (SET-C), alone or with SSRIs, is considered the treatment of choice for SP (see Table 19-4). SSRI and SET-C are superior to placebo in reducing social distress and behavioral avoidance and increasing general functioning. SET-C may be better than SSRI in reducing these symptoms. SET-C, but not SSRI, may be superior to placebo in improving social skills, decreasing anxiety in specific social interactions, and enhancing social competence. SSRIs have a maximum effect by 8 wk; SET-C provides continued improvement through 12 wk. A combination of SSRI and CBT is superior to either treatment alone in reducing severity of anxiety in children with SP and other anxiety disorders. β-Adrenergic blocking agents are used to treat SP, particularly the subtype with performance anxiety and stage fright. β-Blockers are not FDA approved for SP.

School refusal, which occurs in approximately 1-2% of children, is associated with anxiety in 40-50% of cases, depression in 50-60% of cases, and oppositional behavior in 50% of cases. Younger anxious children who refuse to attend school are more likely to have SAD, whereas older anxious children usually refuse to attend school because of SP. Somatic symptoms, especially abdominal pain and/or headaches, are common. There may be increasing tension in the parent-child relationship or other indicators of family disruption (domestic violence, divorce, or other major stressors) contributing to school refusal.

Management of school refusal typically requires parent management training and family therapy. Working with school personnel is always indicated; anxious children often require special attention from teachers, counselors, or school nurses. Parents who are coached to calmly send the child to school and to reward the child for each completed day of school are usually successful. In cases of ongoing school refusal, referral to a child psychiatrist and psychologist is indicated. SSRI treatment may be helpful.

Table 23-3 CRITERIA FOR DIAGNOSIS OF PANIC DISORDER

A. Both (1) and (2)
   1. Recurrent unexpected panic attacks
   2. At least 1 of the attacks has been followed by ≥1 mo of ≥1 of the following:
      a. Persistent concern about having additional attacks
      b. Worry about the implications of the attack or its consequences (e.g., losing control, having a heart attack, "going crazy")
      c. A significant change in behavior related to the attacks
B. The presence or absence of agoraphobia
C. The panic attacks are not due to the direct physiologic effects of a drug of abuse or a medication or a general medical condition (e.g., hyperthyroidism)
D. The panic attacks are not better accounted for by another mental disorder, such as social phobia (e.g., occurring on exposure to feared social situations), specific phobia (e.g., on exposure to a specific phobic situation), obsessive-compulsive disorder (e.g., on exposure to dirt in someone with an obsession about contamination), post-traumatic stress disorder (e.g., in response to stimuli associated with a severe stressor), or separation anxiety disorder (e.g., in response to being away from home or close relatives)

From Kliegman RM, Marcdante KJ, Jenson HB, et al, editors: *Nelson essentials of pediatrics,* ed 5, Philadelphia, 2006, Elsevier/Saunders, p 87.

Table 23-4 CRITERIA FOR DIAGNOSIS OF A PANIC ATTACK

A discrete period of intense fear or discomfort, in which ≥4 of the following symptoms developed abruptly and reached a peak within 10 min
- Palpitations, pounding heart, or accelerated heart rate
- Sweating
- Trembling or shaking
- Sensations of shortness of breath or being smothered
- Feeling of choking
- Chest pain or discomfort
- Nausea or abdominal distress
- Feeling dizzy, unsteady, light-headed, or faint
- Derealization (feelings of unreality) or depersonalization (being detached from oneself)
- Fear of losing control or going crazy
- Paresthesias (numbness or tingling sensations)
- Chills or hot flashes

From Kliegman RM, Marcdante KJ, Jenson HB, et al, editors: *Nelson essentials of pediatrics,* ed 5, Philadelphia, 2006, Elsevier/Saunders, p 87.

Young children with affective symptoms have a good prognosis, whereas adolescents with more insidious onset or with significant somatic complaints have a more guarded prognosis.

Selective mutism is conceptualized as a disorder that overlaps with SP. Children with selective mutism talk almost exclusively at home, although they are reticent in other settings, such as school, daycare, or even relatives' homes. Often, one or more stressors, such as a new classroom or conflicts with parents or siblings, drive an already shy child to become reluctant to speak. It may be helpful to obtain history of normal language use in at least one situation to rule out any communication disorder, neurologic disorder, or pervasive developmental disorder as a cause of mutism. Fluoxetine in combination with behavioral therapy is effective for children whose school performance is severely limited by their symptoms (Chapter 32).

Panic disorder is a syndrome of recurrent, discrete episodes of marked fear or discomfort in which patients experience abrupt onset of physical and psychologic symptoms called *panic attacks* (Tables 23-3 and 23-4). Physical symptoms can include palpitations, sweating, shaking, shortness of breath, dizziness, chest pain, and nausea. Children can present with acute respiratory distress but without fever, wheezing, or stridor, ruling out organic causes of the distress. The associated psychologic symptoms include fear of death, impending doom, loss of control, persistent concerns about having future attacks, and avoidance of settings where attacks have occurred (agoraphobia: Table 23-5).

Panic disorder is uncommon before adolescence, with the peak age of onset at 15-19 yr of age, occurring more often in girls.

Table 23-5 CRITERIA FOR DIAGNOSIS OF AGORAPHOBIA

Agoraphobia is anxiety about being in places or situations from which escape might be difficult (or embarrassing) or in which help might not be available in the event of having an unexpected or situationally predisposed panic attack or panic-like symptoms

Agoraphobic fears typically involve characteristic clusters of situations that include being outside the home alone; being in a crowd or standing in line; being on a bridge; and traveling in a bus, train, plane, or automobile

Note: Consider the diagnosis of specific phobia if the avoidance is limited to 1 or only a few specific situations or social phobia if the avoidance is limited to social situations in general

The anxiety or phobic avoidance is not better accounted for by another mental disorder, such as social phobia (e.g., avoidance limited to social situations because of fear of embarrassment), specific phobia (e.g., avoidance limited to a single situation, such as elevators), obsessive-compulsive disorder (e.g., avoidance of dirt in someone with an obsession about contamination), post-traumatic stress disorder (e.g., avoidance of stimuli associated with a severe stressor), or separation anxiety disorder (e.g., avoidance of leaving home or relatives)

From Kliegman RM, Marcdante KJ, Jenson HB, et al, editors: *Nelson essentials of pediatrics,* ed 5, Philadelphia, 2006, Elsevier/Saunders, p 88.

The postadolescence prevalence of panic disorder is 1-2%. Early-onset panic disorder and adult-onset panic disorder do not differ in symptom severity or social functioning. Early-onset panic disorder is associated with greater comorbidity, which can result from greater familial loading for anxiety disorders in the early-onset subtype. Children of parents with panic disorder are much more likely to develop panic disorder. A predisposition to react to autonomic arousal with anxiety may be a specific risk factor leading to panic disorder. Twin studies suggest that 30-40% of the variance is attributed to genetics. The increasing rates of panic attack are also directly related to earlier sexual maturity. Cued panic attacks can be present in other anxiety disorders and differ from the uncued "out of the blue" attacks in panic disorder.

SSRIs have shown effectiveness in the treatment of adolescents (see Table 19-4). CBT may also be helpful. The recovery rate is approximately 70%.

Generalized anxiety disorder (GAD) occurs in children who often experience unrealistic worries about different events or activities for at least 6 mo (Table 23-6) with at least one somatic complaint. The diffuse nature of the anxiety symptoms differentiates it from other anxiety disorders. Worries in children with GAD commonly center around concerns about competence and performance in school and athletics. GAD often manifests with somatic symptoms including restlessness, fatigue, problems concentrating, irritability, muscle tension, and sleep disturbance. Given the somatic symptoms characteristic of GAD, the differential diagnosis must consider other medical causes. Excessive use of caffeine or other stimulants in adolescence is common and should be determined with a careful history. When the history or physical exam is suggestive, the pediatrician should rule out hyperthyroidism, hypoglycemia, lupus, and pheochromocytoma.

Children with GAD are markedly self-conscious and perfectionistic and struggle with more intense distress than is evident to parents or others around them. They often have other anxiety disorders, such as simple phobia and panic disorder. Onset may be gradual or sudden, although GAD does not often become manifest until puberty. Boys and girls are equally affected before puberty, when GAD becomes more prevalent in girls. The prevalence of GAD ranges from 2.5% to 6% of children. Hypermetabolism in frontal precortical area and increased blood flow in right the dorsolateral prefrontal cortex may be present.

Children with GAD are good candidates for CBT, an SSRI, or their combination (see Table 19-4). Buspirone may be used as an adjunct to SSRI therapy. Combination of CBT and SSRI often results in a superior response in pediatric patients with anxiety disorders, including GAD. The recovery rate is approximately 80%.

Table 23-6 CRITERIA FOR DIAGNOSIS OF GENERALIZED ANXIETY DISORDER

A. Excessive anxiety and worry (apprehensive expectation), occurring more days than not for ≥6 mo, about numerous events or activities (e.g., work or school performance)
B. The person finds it difficult to control the worry
C. The anxiety and worry are associated with ≥3 of the following 6 symptoms (with at least some symptoms present for more days than not for the past 6 mo). **Note:** Only 1 symptom is required in children
   1. Restlessness or feeling keyed up or on edge
   2. Being easily fatigued
   3. Difficulty concentrating or mind going blank
   4. Irritability
   5. Muscle tension
   6. Sleep disturbance (difficulty falling or staying asleep or restless, unsatisfying sleep)
D. The focus of the anxiety and worry is not confined to features of a disorder (e.g., the anxiety or worry is not about having a panic attack, as in panic disorder; being embarrassed in public, as in social phobia; being contaminated, as in obsessive-compulsive disorder; being away from home or close relatives, as in separation anxiety disorder; gaining weight, as in anorexia nervosa; having multiple physical complaints, as in somatization disorder; or having a serious illness, as in hypochondriasis), and the anxiety and worry do not occur exclusively during post-traumatic stress disorder
E. The anxiety, worry, or physical symptoms cause clinically significant distress or impairment in social, occupational, or other important areas of functioning
F. The disturbance is not due to the direct physiologic effects of a drug (e.g., a drug of abuse or a medication) or a general medical condition (e.g., hyperthyroidism) and does not occur exclusively during a mood disorder, a psychotic disorder, or a pervasive developmental disorder

From Kliegman RM, Marcdante KJ, Jenson HB, et al, editors: *Nelson essentials of pediatrics,* ed 5, Philadelphia, 2006, Elsevier/Saunders, p 89.

It is important to distinguish children with GAD from those who present with specific repetitive thoughts that invade consciousness (**obsessions**) or repetitive rituals or movements that are driven by anxiety (**compulsions**). The most common obsessions are concerned with bodily wastes and secretions, the fear that something calamitous will happen, or the need for sameness. The most common compulsions are hand washing, continual checking of locks, and touching. At times of stress (bedtime, preparing for school), some children touch certain objects, say certain words, or wash their hands repeatedly. OCD is diagnosed when the thoughts or rituals cause distress, consume time, or interfere with occupational or social functioning (Table 23-7).

OCD is a chronically disabling illness characterized by repetitive, ritualistic behaviors over which the patient has little or no control. OCD has a lifetime prevalence of 1-3% worldwide, and as many as 80% of all cases have their onset in childhood and adolescence. Common obsessions include contamination (35%) and thoughts of harming loved ones or oneself (30%). Washing and cleaning compulsions are common in children (75%), as are checking (40%) and straightening (35%). Many children are observed to have visuospatial irregularities, memory problems, and attention deficits, causing academic problems not explained by OCD symptoms alone.

The Children's Yale-Brown Obsessive-Compulsive Scale (C-YBOCS) and the Anxiety Disorders Interview Schedule for Children (ADIS-C) are reliable and valid methods for identifying children with OCD. The C-YBOCS is helpful in following the progression of symptoms with treatment. The Leyton Obsessional Inventory (LOI) is a self-report measure of OCD symptoms that is quite sensitive. Patients with OCD have consistently identified abnormalities in the fronto-striatal-thalamic circuitry associated with severity of illness and treatment response. Comorbidity is common in OCD, with 30% of patients having comorbid tic disorders, 26% having comorbid major depression, and 24% having comorbid developmental disorders.

Consensus guidelines recommend that children and adolescents with OCD begin treatment with either CBT alone or CBT

Table 23-7 CRITERIA FOR DIAGNOSIS OF OBSESSIVE-COMPULSIVE DISORDER

A. Either obsessions or compulsions. Obsessions Are Defined by (1), (2), (3), and (4) 1. Recurrent and persistent thoughts, impulses, or images that are experienced, at some time during the disturbance, as intrusive and inappropriate and that cause marked anxiety or distress 2. The thoughts, impulses, or images are not simply excessive worries about real-life problems 3. The person attempts to ignore or suppress such thoughts, impulses, or images or to neutralize them with some other thought or action 4. The person recognizes that the obsessional thoughts, impulses, or images are a product of his or her own mind (not imposed from without, as in thought insertion) Compulsions Are Defined by (1) and (2) 1. Repetitive behaviors (e.g., handwashing, ordering, checking) or mental acts (e.g., praying, counting, repeating words silently) that the person feels driven to perform in response to an obsession or according to rules that must be applied rigidly 2. The behaviors or mental acts are aimed at preventing or reducing distress or preventing some dreaded event or situation; however, these behaviors or mental acts either are not connected in a realistic way with what they are designed to neutralize or prevent or are clearly excessive B. At some point during the course of the disorder, the person has recognized that the obsessions or compulsions are excessive or unreasonable. **Note:** This does not apply to children C. The obsessions or compulsions cause marked distress; are time-consuming (taking >1 hr/day); or significantly interfere with the person's normal routine, occupational (or academic) functioning, or usual social activities or relationships D. If another Axis I disorder is present, the content of the obsessions or compulsions is not restricted to it (e.g., preoccupation with food in the presence of an eating disorder, hair pulling in the presence of trichotillomania, concern with appearance in the presence of body dysmorphic disorder, preoccupation with drugs in the presence of a substance use disorder, preoccupation with having a serious illness in the presence of hypochondriasis, preoccupation with sexual urges or fantasies in the presence of a paraphilia, or guilty ruminations in the presence of major depressive disorder) E. The disturbance is not due to the direct physiologic effects of a drug of abuse, a medication, or a general medical condition
SPECIFY IF
With poor insight: if, for most of the time during the current episode, the person does not recognize that the obsessions and compulsions are excessive or unreasonable

From Kliegman RM, Marcdante KJ, Jenson HB, et al, editors: *Nelson essentials of pediatrics*, ed 5, Philadelphia, 2006, Elsevier/Saunders, p 98.

in combination with SSRI, when symptoms are moderate to severe (i.e., Y-BOCS >21). In OCD patients with comorbid tics, SSRI are no more effective than placebo, and combination of CBT and SSRI is superior to CBT; CBT alone is superior to placebo. Pediatric OCD patients with comorbid tics should begin treatment with CBT alone or the combination of CBT and SSRI.

There are four FDA-approved medications for pediatric OCD: fluoxetine, sertraline, fluvoxamine, and clomipramine. Clomipramine, a heterocylic antidepressant and nonselective serotonin and norepinephrine reuptake inhibitor, is only indicated when a patient has failed 2 or more SSRI trials. There may be a critical role for glutamate in the pathogenesis and treatment response of OCD. The glutamate inhibitor riluzole (Rilutek) is FDA-approved for amyotrophic lateral sclerosis (Chapter 604.3) and has a good safety record. The most common adverse event with riluzole is transient increase in liver transaminases. Riluzole in children with treatment-resistant OCD may be beneficial and is well tolerated. Referral of patients with OCD to a mental health professional is always indicated.

In 10% of children with OCD, symptoms are triggered or exacerbated by group A β-hemolytic streptococcal infection (GABHS) (Chapter 176). GABHS bacteria trigger antineuronal antibodies that cross react with basal ganglia neural tissue in genetically susceptible hosts, leading to swelling of this region and resultant obsessions and compulsions. This subtype of OCD, called **pediatric autoimmune neuropsychiatric disorders associated with streptococcal infection (PANDAS),** is characterized by sudden and dramatic onset or exacerbation of OCD or tic symptoms, associated neurologic findings, and a recent streptococcal infection. Increased antibody titers of antistreptolysin O and antideoxyribonuclease B correlates with increased basal ganglia volumes. Plasmapheresis is effective in reducing OCD symptoms in some patients with PANDAS and also decreasing enlarged basal ganglia volume. The pediatrician should be aware of the infectious cause of some cases of tic disorders, attention-deficit disorder, and OCD and follow management guidelines (Chapter 22).

Children with **phobias** avoid specific objects or situations that reliably trigger physiologic arousal (e.g., dogs or spiders) (see Table 23-1). The fear is excessive and unreasonable and can be cued by the presence or anticipation of the feared trigger, with anxiety symptoms occurring immediately. Neither obsessions nor compulsions are associated with the fear response; phobias only rarely interfere with social, educational, or interpersonal functioning. Assault by a relative and verbal aggression between parents can influence the onset of specific phobias. The parents of phobic children should remain calm in the face of the child's anxiety or panic. Parents who become anxious themselves may reinforce their children's anxiety, and the pediatrician can usefully interrupt this cycle by calmly noting that phobias are not unusual and rarely cause impairment. The prevalence of specific phobias in childhood is 0.5-2.0%.

Systematic desensitization is a form of behavior therapy that gradually exposes the patient to the fear-inducing situation or object, while simultaneously teaching relaxation techniques for anxiety management. Successful repeated exposure leads to extinguishing anxiety for that stimulus. When phobias are particularly severe, SSRIs can be used with behavioral intervention. Low-dose SSRI treatment may be especially effective for some children with severe, refractory choking phobia.

Post-traumatic stress disorder (PTSD; see Chapter 36) is typically precipitated by an extreme stressor. PTSD is an anxiety disorder resulting from the long- and short-term effects of trauma that cause behavioral and physiologic sequelae in toddlers, children, and adolescents (Table 23-8). Another diagnostic category, **acute stress disorder,** reflects the fact that traumatic events often cause acute symptoms that may or may not resolve. Previous trauma exposure, a history of other psychopathology, and symptoms of PTSD in parents predict childhood-onset PTSD. Many adolescent and adult psychopathologic conditions, such as conduct disorder, depression, and some personality disorders, might relate to previous trauma. PTSD is also linked to mood disorders and disruptive behavior. Separation anxiety is common in children with PTSD. The lifetime prevalence of PTSD by age 18 yr is approximately 6%. Up to 40% show symptoms, but do not fulfill the diagnostic criteria.

Life-threatening events that pose harm to the child or the caregiver and that produce considerable stress or fear are required to make the diagnosis of PTSD. Three clusters of symptoms are also essential for diagnosis: re-experiencing, avoidance, and hyperarousal. Persistent re-experiencing of the stressor through intrusive recollections, nightmares, and reenactment in play are typical responses in children. Persistent avoidance of reminders and numbing of emotional responsiveness, such as isolation, amnesia, and avoidance, constitute the 2nd cluster of behaviors. Symptoms of hyperarousal, such as hypervigilance, poor concentration, extreme startle responses, agitation, and sleep problems, complete the symptom profile of PTSD. Occasionally, children regress in some of their developmental milestones after a traumatic event. Avoidance symptoms are commonly observable in younger children, whereas older children may be more able to describe re-experiencing and hyperarousal symptoms. Repetitive

Table 23-8 CRITERIA FOR DIAGNOSIS OF POST-TRAUMATIC STRESS DISORDER

A. The person has been exposed to a traumatic event in which both of the following were present:
   1. The person experienced, witnessed, or was confronted with an event or events that involved actual or threatened death or serious injury or a threat to the physical integrity of self or others
   2. The person's response involved intense fear, helplessness, or horror. **Note:** In children, this may be expressed instead by disorganized or agitated behavior

B. The traumatic event is persistently re-experienced in ≥1 of the following ways:
   1. Recurrent and intrusive distressing recollections of the event, including images, thoughts, or perceptions. **Note:** In young children, repetitive play may occur in which themes or aspects of the trauma are expressed
   2. Recurrent distressing dreams of the event. **Note:** In children, there may be frightening dreams without recognizable content
   3. Acting or feeling as if the traumatic event were recurring (includes a sense of reliving the experience, illusions, hallucinations, and dissociative flashback episodes, including flashbacks that occur on awakening or when intoxicated). **Note:** In young children, trauma-specific reenactment may occur
   4. Intense psychologic distress on exposure to internal or external cues that symbolize or resemble an aspect of the traumatic event
   5. Physiologic reactivity on exposure to internal or external cues that symbolize or resemble an aspect of the traumatic event

C. Persistent avoidance of stimuli associated with the trauma and numbing of general responsiveness (not present before the trauma), as indicated by ≥3 of the following:
   1. Efforts to avoid thoughts, feelings, or conversations associated with the trauma
   2. Efforts to avoid activities, places, or people that arouse recollections of the trauma
   3. Inability to recall an important aspect of the trauma
   4. Markedly diminished interest or participation in significant activities
   5. Feeling of detachment or estrangement from others
   6. Restricted range of affect (e.g., unable to have loving feelings)
   7. Sense of a foreshortened future (e.g., does not expect to have a career, marriage, children, or a normal life span)

D. Persistent symptoms of increased arousal (not present before the trauma), as indicated by ≥2 of the following:
   1. Difficulty falling or staying asleep
   2. Irritability or outbursts of anger
   3. Difficulty concentrating
   4. Hypervigilance
   5. Exaggerated startle response

E. Duration of the disturbance (symptoms in criteria B, C, and D) is >1 mo

F. The disturbance causes clinically significant distress or impairment in social, occupational, or other important areas of functioning

SPECIFY IF

Acute: if duration of symptoms is <3 mo
Chronic: if duration of symptoms is ≥3 mo

SPECIFY IF

With delayed onset: if onset of symptoms is >6 mo after the stressor

From Kliegman RM, Marcdante KJ, Jenson HB, et al, editors: *Nelson essentials of pediatrics*, ed 5, Philadelphia, 2006, Elsevier/Saunders, p 90.

play involving the event, psychosomatic symptoms, and nightmares may also be observed.

Initial interventions after a trauma should focus on reunification with a parent and attending to the child's physical needs in a safe place. Aggressive treatment of pain might decrease the likelihood of PTSD, and facilitating a return to comforting routines, including regular sleep, is indicated. Long-term treatment may include individual, group, school-based, or family therapy, as well as pharmacotherapy, in selected cases. Individual treatment involves transforming the child's concept of himself or herself as victim to that of survivor and can occur through play therapy, psychodynamic therapy, or CBT. Group work is also helpful for identifying which children might need more intensive assistance. Goals of family work include helping the child establish a sense of security, validating his or her emotions, and anticipating situations when the child will need more support from the family. Clonidine or guanfacine may be helpful for sleep disturbance, persistent arousal, and exaggerated startle response. Comorbid depression and affective numbing might respond to an SSRI (see Table 19-4). As for many other anxiety disorders, CBT is the psychotherapeutic intervention with the most empiric support.

ANXIETY ASSOCIATED WITH MEDICAL CONDITIONS

It is prudent to rule out organic conditions such as hyperthyroidism, caffeinism (carbonated beverages), hypoglycemia, CNS disorders (delirium, brain tumors), migraine, asthma, lead poisoning, cardiac arrhythmias, and, rarely, pheochromocytoma, before making a diagnosis of an anxiety disorder. Some prescription drugs with side effects that can mimic anxiety include antiasthmatic agents, steroids, sympathomimetics, SSRIs (initiation), and antipsychotics. Nonprescription drugs causing anxiety include diet pills, antihistamines, and cold medicines.

SAFETY AND EFFICACY CONCERNS ABOUT SSRIS

No empiric evidence suggests the superiority of one SSRI over another. Data are limited as far as combining medications are concerned. SSRIs are usually well tolerated by most children and adolescents. The FDA issued a black box warning of increased agitation and suicidality among adolescents and children on these medications. This warning was based on review of studies in children and adolescents with major depression and not anxiety disorders. Close monitoring is always warranted.

BIBLIOGRAPHY

Please visit the Nelson Textbook of Pediatrics *website at www.expertconsult.com for the complete bibliography.*

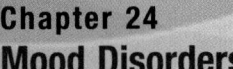

Chapter 24
Mood Disorders

Heather J. Walter and David R. DeMaso

The mood disorders have a disturbance in mood as the predominant feature, and are divided into the **depressive disorders**, in which the mood is depressed or irritable, and the **bipolar disorders**, in which the mood is elevated, expansive, or irritable. These mood disturbances exist on a dimensional spectrum ranging from sub-syndromal (i.e., some symptoms are present, but not enough to meet full diagnostic criteria) to syndromal (i.e., full diagnostic criteria are met). The syndromal disorders are themselves dimensional, ranging in severity from mild to severe.

24.1 Major Depression

Heather J. Walter and David R. DeMaso

DESCRIPTION

In the *Diagnostic and Statistical Manual of Mental Disorders, Fourth Edition, Text Revision* (DSM-IV-TR), major depressive disorder is characterized by a distinct period of at least 2 wk (an episode, Table 24-1) in which there is a depressed or irritable mood that is present for most of the day nearly every day, and/or loss of interest or pleasure in nearly all activities. There also are associated vegetative and cognitive symptoms, including disturbances in appetite, sleep, and energy; impaired concentration; and thoughts of worthlessness, guilt, and suicide. To meet the syndromal diagnosis, 5 or more symptoms (including depressed

Table 24-1 DSM-IV-TR DIAGNOSTIC CRITERIA FOR MAJOR DEPRESSIVE EPISODE

A. Five (or more) of the following symptoms have been present during the same 2-week period and represent a change from previous functioning; at least one of the symptoms is either (1) depressed mood or (2) loss of interest or pleasure.
1. Depressed most of the day, nearly every day, as indicated by either subjective report (e.g., feels sad or empty) or observation made by others (e.g., appears tearful). Note: In children and adolescents, can be irritable mood.
2. Markedly diminished interest or pleasure in all, or almost all, activities most of the day, nearly every day (as indicated by either subjective account or observation made by others).
3. Significant weight loss when not dieting or weight gain (e.g., a change of more than 5% of body weight in a month), or decrease or increase in appetite nearly every day. Note: In children, consider failure to make expected weight gains.
4. Insomnia or hypersomnia nearly every day.
5. Psychomotor agitation or retardation nearly every day (observable by others, not merely subjective feelings of restlessness or being slowed down).
6. Fatigue or loss of energy nearly every day.
7. Feelings of worthlessness or inappropriate guilt (which may be delusional) nearly every day (not merely self-reproach or guilt about being sick).
8. Diminished ability to think or concentrate, or indecisiveness, nearly every day (either by subjective account or as observed by others).
9. Recurrent thoughts of death (not just fear of dying), recurrent suicidal ideation without a specific plan, or a suicide attempt or a specific plan for committing suicide.

B. The symptoms do not meet criteria for a mixed episode.
C. The symptoms cause clinically significant distress or impairment in social, occupational, or other important areas of functioning.
D. The symptoms are not due to the direct physiological effects of a substance (e.g., a drug of abuse, a medication) or a general medical condition (e.g., hypothyroidism).
E. The symptoms are not better accounted for by bereavement, i.e., after the loss of a loved one, the symptoms persist for longer than 2 months or are characterized by marked functional impairment, morbid preoccupation with worthlessness, suicidal ideation, psychotic symptoms, or psychomotor retardation.

From American Psychiatric Association: *Diagnostic and statistical manual of mental disorders, fourth edition, text revision,* Washington, DC, 2000, American Psychiatric Association.

or irritable mood or loss of interest or pleasure) must be present and must represent a distinct change from previous functioning, cause clinically significant distress or impairment, not be better accounted for by bereavement or by other psychiatric disorders, and not be due to the direct physiologic effects of a substance or a general medical condition.

Major depressive disorder is categorized as **mild** if few symptoms in excess of those required to make the diagnosis are present and the symptoms result in only minor functional impairment, and it is categorized as **severe** if several symptoms in excess of those required are present and the symptoms markedly interfere with functioning. Severe major depression is subcategorized as occurring with or without psychotic features (hallucinations or delusions). Moderate major depression is intermediate between mild and severe.

Overall, the clinical presentation of major depressive disorder in children and adolescents is similar to that in adults. The prominence of the symptoms can change with age; somatic complaints, irritability, and social withdrawal may be more common in children (who are less able to verbalize their feeling states), and psychotic and melancholic symptoms or suicidal behavior may be more common in adolescents.

EPIDEMIOLOGY

The prevalence of major depressive disorder is estimated to be approximately 2% in children and 4-8% in adolescents, with a male-female ratio of 1:1 during childhood and 1:2 during adolescence. The risk of major depression increases by a factor of 2 to 4 after puberty, and the cumulative incidence by age 18 yr is approximately 20%.

DIFFERENTIAL DIAGNOSIS

A number of psychiatric disorders, general medical conditions, and medications can generate symptoms of depression and irritability and must be distinguished from the depressive disorders. The psychiatric disorders include anxiety (Chapter 23), attention-deficit/hyperactivity disorder (ADHD) (Chapter 30), disruptive behavior (Chapter 27), developmental disorders (Chapter 28), substance abuse (Chapter 108), and adjustment disorders. Medical conditions include neurologic disorders, endocrine disorders, infectious diseases, tumors, anemia, uremia, failure to thrive, chronic fatigue disorder, and pain disorder. Medications include narcotics, chemotherapy agents, cardiovascular medications, corticosteroids, and contraceptives. The diagnosis of a depressive disorder should be made after these other explanations for the observed symptoms have been ruled out.

COMORBIDITY

Major depressive and dysthymic disorders (Chapter 24.3) often co-occur with other psychiatric disorders, and both can occur concurrently (double depression). Depending on the setting and source of referral, 40-90% of youths with a depressive disorder have other psychiatric disorders, and up to 50% have 2 or more comorbid diagnoses. The most common comorbid diagnosis is an anxiety disorder, followed by disruptive behavior, ADHD, and substance use disorder.

CLINICAL COURSE

The median duration of a major depressive episode approximates 8 mo for clinically referred youths and 1 to 2 mo for community samples. Prepubertal depressive disorders can exhibit more heterotypic than homotypic continuity; thus, depressed children may be more likely to develop nondepressive psychiatric disorders in adulthood than depressive disorders. Adolescents might exhibit greater homotypic continuity, with the probability of recurrence of depression reaching 70% after 5 yr. Between 20% and 40% of these adolescents develop a bipolar disorder (Chapter 24.2), and the risk is higher among adolescents who have a high family loading for bipolar disorder, who have psychotic depression, or who have had pharmacologically induced mania.

SEQUELAE

Approximately 60% of youths with major depression report thinking about suicide, and 30% actually attempt suicide (Chapter 25). The risk of suicidal behavior increases if there is a history of suicide attempts, exposure to adverse psychosocial circumstances, a family history of suicidal behavior, or comorbid psychiatric disorders. Youths with depressive disorders are also at high risk of substance abuse, impaired academic performance, impaired family and peer relationships, and poor adjustment to life stressors, including physical illness.

ETIOLOGY AND RISK FACTORS

Major depression is a highly familial disorder, with both genetic and environmental influences. Environmental influences include parental psychopathology, impaired parenting, dysfunctional families, parent figure changes, loss of a parent, physical and sexual abuse, neglect, social isolation, lack of social supports, exposure to domestic and community violence, and other correlates of disadvantaged socioeconomic status. Longitudinal studies have suggested the greater importance of environmental influences in children who become depressed compared to adults who become depressed.

PREVENTION

Several experimental trials have demonstrated the effectiveness of cognitive-behavioral strategies in preventing the escalation of sub-syndromal to syndromal depression. These strategies include identifying negative mood states, linking mood states to environmental or cognitive precipitants, avoiding situations that are typically stressful, correcting automatic negative attributions, scheduling pleasurable activities, developing competencies to enhance self-esteem, and developing learning skills to deal with adversity. Other strategies that can prove helpful include lifestyle modification (e.g., regular and adequate sleep, exercise, and relaxation) and involvement with supportive mentors and peers.

EARLY IDENTIFICATION

Clinicians should screen all children and adolescents for the key depressive symptoms of sad mood, irritability, and anhedonia (Table 24-2). A diagnosis of a depressive disorder should be considered if these symptoms are present most of the time, affect the child's functioning, and are beyond what would be expected for the given circumstances. The use of standardized depression rating scales (Chapter 18) designed for self- or parent report can be helpful in the screening process. If the screening indicates clinically significant depressive symptoms, the clinician should refer to a specialist for a comprehensive diagnostic evaluation to determine the presence of depressive and other comorbid psychiatric and medical disorders. The evaluation must include assessment of the potential for harm to self or others.

Table 24-2 SCREENING AND TREATMENT FOR MAJOR DEPRESSIVE DISORDER IN YOUTHS

RECOMMENDATION	ADOLESCENTS (12-18 YR)	CHILDREN 7-11 YR)
Screening	Screen (when systems for diagnosis, treatment, and follow-up are in place) Grade B	No recommendations Grade I (insufficient evidence)
Risk assessment	Risk factors for major depressive disorder include parental depression, having comorbid mental health or chronic medical conditions, and having experience a major negative life event	
Screening tests	The following have been shown to do well in teens in primary care settings: Patient Health Questionnaire for Adolescents (PHQ-A) Beck Depression Inventory—Primary Care version (BDI-PC)	Screening instruments perform less well in younger children
Treatments	Among pharmacotherapies, fluoxetine, a selective serotonin reuptake inhibitor (SSRI) has been found efficacious. However, because of risk of suicidality, SSRIs should be considered only if clinical monitoring is possible. Various modes of psychotherapy, and pharmacotherapy combined with psychotherapy, have been found efficacious.	Evidence on the balance of benefits and harms of treatment of younger children is insufficient for a recommendation

For a summary of the evidence systematically reviewed in making these recommendations, the full recommendation statement, and supporting documents, please go to www.AHRQ.gov/clinic/USPSTF/USPSCHDEPR.htm.

TREATMENT

Treatment of the depressive disorders should begin with psychoeducation, family involvement, and school involvement. Psychoeducation refers to education of the family members and patient about the causes, symptoms, course, and different treatments for depression and the risks associated with each treatment and with no treatment. Written materials and reliable websites about depression can be helpful to the parents and patient. Because of the importance of environmental factors in the etiology of childhood depression, family involvement should focus on ameliorating these factors by strengthening the relationship between the identified patient and parent(s), providing parenting guidance, reducing family dysfunction, eliminating identified sources of stress, enhancing social supports, and facilitating treatment referral for parents as indicated.

With the patient's and parents' consent, school personnel should be informed about the need for accommodations until recovery has been achieved. Students with a depressive disorder may be eligible for an Individualized Education Program specifying school-based services and accommodations under the emotional disturbance disability category of the Individuals with Disabilities Education Act.

Because of the high rates of response to placebo and brief therapy in pediatric depression, it is reasonable in a patient with sub-syndromal (i.e., depressive disorder, not otherwise specified) or mild syndromal (i.e., dysthymic disorder or major depressive disorder) depression (Chapter 24.3), mild functional impairment, and absence of suicidality or psychosis to supplement the above-described interventions with 4 to 6 wk of weekly supportive therapy, focusing on enhancement of the youth's coping capabilities and amelioration of adverse environmental influences. In youths with moderate to severe syndromal depression, significant functional impairment, and suicidality or psychosis, specialized treatment with specific psychotherapies and/or with medication is indicated.

Moderate syndromal depression may respond to cognitive-behavioral or interpersonal therapy without medication. These types of therapy, typically administered in weekly doses over 8 to 12 wk, are more efficacious than supportive therapy alone when depression is more than mild. Severe syndromal depression requires treatment with antidepressants. In addition to level of severity, treatment decisions are influenced by treatment availability, comorbid disorders, and family preference.

Studies of the effectiveness of selective serotonin reuptake inhibitors (SSRIs) are mixed. Within the positive studies, approximately 50% of youths with depression respond to the medication, but only around 30% experience symptom remission. Studies of other classes of antidepressant medications have not demonstrated clear superiority over placebo.

The SSRIs and other antidepressants have been well tolerated by children and adolescents. The most common side effects include irritability, gastrointestinal symptoms, sleep disturbance, restlessness, diaphoresis, headaches, changes in appetite, and sexual dysfunction. Approximately 5% of youths, particularly children, develop increased impulsivity, agitation, and irritability (behavioral activation) on SSRIs, and the SSRI must be discontinued. More rarely, the use of antidepressants has been associated with serotonin syndrome, increased predisposition to bleeding, and increased suicidal thoughts. The excess risk for such thoughts appears to approximate 1.8 (relative risk) in youths with major depression.

Except for lower initial doses to avoid unwanted effects, the doses of antidepressants in youths are similar to those used for adult patients (Chapter 19 and Table 19-4). Some studies have reported that the half-lives of sertraline, citalopram, paroxetine, and bupropion SR are much shorter in children than in adults; therefore daily withdrawal side effects can be observed with these medications if they are administered once daily.

Patients should be treated with adequate and tolerable doses of medication for at least 4 wk. Clinical response, tolerability, and emergence of behavioral activation, mania, or suicidal thoughts should be assessed frequently (as often as weekly) for the first 4 wk. If the youth has safely tolerated the antidepressant, the dose may be increased at 4 wk if an adequate response (at least 50% reduction in symptom severity) has not been achieved. Patients can then be monitored slightly less frequently (as often as biweekly) until remission (no longer meets diagnostic criteria) has been achieved, and approximately monthly thereafter. Because of the high rate of relapse, successful treatment should continue for 6 to 12 mo. At the conclusion of treatment, all antidepressants (except fluoxetine) should be discontinued gradually to avoid withdrawal symptoms (tiredness, irritability, severe somatic symptoms).

Patients with recurrent (two or more), chronic, or severe major depression can require treatment beyond 12 mo. Patients who have shown minimal or no response to antidepressant medication at 8 wk, and patients who have not achieved remission by 12 wk, are likely to need referral for specialized treatment. Switching to another antidepressant combined with cognitive-behavioral therapy may be helpful in those who do not respond to the initial SSRI. Depressed patients with suicidality, psychosis, seasonal depression, or bipolar depression also should be referred for specialized treatment.

LEVEL OF CARE

Most children and adolescents with mild to moderate depressive disorders can be safely and effectively treated as outpatients, provided that a schedule of approximately weekly visits can be maintained through the acute phase of treatment. Youths who are suicidal, psychotic, or melancholic usually require inpatient care.

BIBLIOGRAPHY

Please visit the Nelson Textbook of Pediatrics *website at www.expertconsult.com for the complete bibliography.*

24.2 Bipolar Disorder

Heather J. Walter and David R. DeMaso

DESCRIPTION

In the DSM-IV-TR, bipolar I disorder is characterized by one or more episodes of mania, often alternating or concurrent with one or more episodes of major depression. Mania is characterized by a distinct period of at least 1 wk (an episode, Table 24-3) in which there is an unusually happy (elated), unusually enthusiastic (expansive), or unusually irritable mood. The mood represents a distinct change from previous functioning. There also are associated cognitive and behavioral symptoms, including unrealistically high self-esteem (grandiosity), needing little sleep (not being tired after sleeping very little), feeling the need to talk all the time, feeling that thoughts are racing, having difficulty concentrating, feeling agitated or engaging in a flurry of activity to accomplish tasks, and impulsively doing things that can be pleasurable but have the potential for harm in excess (e.g., shopping sprees, gambling). Psychotic symptoms can be an associated feature of the disorder.

To meet the syndromal diagnosis, 3 or more cognitive or behavioral symptoms in addition to elevated, expansive or irritable mood must be present, cause clinically significant impairment in multiple settings or require hospitalization to prevent harm to self or others, not be better accounted for by other psychiatric disorders, and not be due to the direct physiologic effects of a substance or a general medical condition.

Table 24-3 DSM-IV-TR DIAGNOSTIC CRITERIA FOR A MANIC EPISODE

A. A distinct period of abnormally and persistently elevated, expansive, or irritable mood, lasting at least 1 week (or any duration if hospitalization is necessary).
B. During the period of mood disturbance, three (or more) of the following symptoms have persisted (four if the mood is only irritable) and have been present to a significant degree:
1. Inflated self-esteem or grandiosity
2. Decreased need for sleep (e.g., feels rested after only 3 hours of sleep)
3. More talkative than usual or pressure to keep talking
4. Flight of ideas or subjective experience that thoughts are racing
5. Distractibility (i.e., attention too easily drawn to unimportant or irrelevant external stimuli)
6. Increase in goal-directed activity (either socially, at work or school, or sexually) or psychomotor agitation
7. Excessive involvement in pleasurable activities that have a high potential for painful consequences (e.g., engaging in unrestrained buying sprees, sexual indiscretions, or foolish business investments)
C. The symptoms do not meet criteria for a mixed episode.
D. The mood disturbance is sufficiently severe to cause marked impairment in occupational functioning or in usual social activities or relationships with others, or to necessitate hospitalization to prevent harm to self or others, or there are psychotic features.
E. The symptoms are not due to the direct physiological effects of a substance (e.g., a drug of abuse, a medication, or other treatment) or a general medical condition (e.g., hyperthyroidism).

From American Psychiatric Association: *Diagnostic and statistical manual of mental disorders, fourth edition, text revision,* Washington, DC, 2000, American Psychiatric Association.

Bipolar II disorder is characterized by 1 or more episodes of major depression alternating with 1 or more episodes of hypomania. **Hypomania** is similar to mania, but is briefer (at least 4 days) and less severe (causes less impairment in functioning, is not associated with psychosis, and would not require hospitalization). To meet the syndromal diagnosis, there must never have been a manic episode, and the symptoms must cause clinically significant distress or impairment and not be better accounted for by another psychiatric diagnosis.

Cyclothymic disorder is characterized by a period of at least 1 yr in which there are numerous episodes of hypomania and sub-syndromal depression. To meet the syndromal diagnosis, the symptoms must cause clinically significant distress or impairment, not be better accounted for by other psychiatric disorders, and not be due to the direct physiologic effects of a substance or a general medication condition.

Bipolar disorder, not otherwise specified (sub-syndromal bipolar disorder) is diagnosed when some symptoms of bipolar disorder are present but not enough to meet full diagnostic criteria for the bipolar or cyclothymic disorders. Although this diagnosis increasingly has been applied to children with severe and chronic mood and behavioral dysregulation who do not precisely fit other diagnostic categories, the empiric support for the validity of this practice is sparse.

In adolescents, the clinical manifestation of bipolar disorder is similar to that in adults. Psychosis (delusions, hallucinations) often is an associated symptom, and episodes often are mixed (concurrent mania and depression). There is controversy about the applicability of the bipolar diagnostic criteria to prepubertal children. It may be developmentally normal for children to be elated, expansive, or grandiose, reducing the specificity of these symptoms to psychiatric disorder. This makes the diagnosis of the bipolar disorders difficult in young children.

EPIDEMIOLOGY

The lifetime prevalence of each of the bipolar disorders and cyclothymic disorder is estimated to approximate 0.6%; the male-female ratio approximates 1. Offspring of parents with bipolar disorders are at high risk for early-onset bipolar disorders. Twin and adoption studies provide strong evidence of a genetic influence; first-degree relatives of patients with bipolar I have a 4- to 6-fold increased risk of bipolar and depressive disorders.

DIFFERENTIAL DIAGNOSIS

A number of psychiatric disorders, general medical conditions, and medications can generate symptoms of mania and must be distinguished from the bipolar disorders. The psychiatric disorders include ADHD, oppositional defiant, post-traumatic stress, substance abuse, pervasive developmental, communication, and borderline personality disorders. Medical conditions include neurologic disorders, endocrine disorders, infectious diseases, tumors, anemia, uremia, and vitamin deficiencies. Medications include androgens, bronchodilators, cardiovascular medications, corticosteroids, chemotherapy agents, thyroid preparations, and certain psychiatric medications (benzodiazepines, antidepressants, stimulants). The diagnosis of a bipolar disorder should be made after these other explanations for the observed symptoms have been ruled out. Some suggest that a diagnosis of bipolar disorder should not be given to youths in the absence of the cardinal symptoms of elation and grandiosity and an episodic course.

COMORBIDITY

The bipolar disorders can be comorbid with a number of other psychiatric disorders, including ADHD, anxiety, eating, and substance use disorders.

CLINICAL COURSE

Premorbid problems are common in bipolar disorder, especially difficulties with mood and behavioral regulation. Premorbid anxiety also is common. The bipolar disorders are highly recurrent, and more than 90% of bipolar I patients have additional episodes. Recurrent episodes can approximate 4 in 10 years, with the interepisode interval shortening as the patient ages. Although the majority of patients with bipolar I return to a fully functional level between episodes, approximately one third continue to be symptomatic and functionally impaired between episodes.

SEQUELAE

Completed suicide occurs in 10-15% of patients with bipolar I disorder. Youths with bipolar disorders are also at high risk for substance abuse, antisocial behavior, impaired academic performance, impaired family and peer relationships, and poor adjustment to life stressors. Cyclothymic disorder is thought to be a temperamental predisposition to bipolar disorder and as such may be an important target for treatment.

PREVENTION

Although empiric support is lacking, the course of cyclothymic disorder suggests that treatment with specific therapies that focus on regulation of mood and possibly the use of mood-stabilizing medication can prevent the evolution of cyclothymia into bipolar disorder.

EARLY IDENTIFICATION

Clinicians should screen all children and adolescents for the cardinal manic symptoms of elation and grandiosity. The diagnosis of bipolar disorder should be considered if the symptoms occur in the context of distinct episodes and do not represent developmentally normal emotional and behavioral expressions. If the screening indicates clinically significant bipolar symptoms, the clinician should refer to a specialist for a comprehensive diagnostic evaluation to determine the presence of bipolar and other comorbid psychiatric and medical disorders. The evaluation must include assessment of the potential for harm to self or others.

TREATMENT

Treatment of the bipolar disorders should begin with psychoeducation, family involvement, and school involvement. Family involvement should include the importance of treatment compliance and stable, positive family relationships with control of expressed emotion. Family-focused treatment is often beneficial. Students with a bipolar disorder may be eligible for an Individualized Educational Program specifying school-based services and accommodations under the emotional disturbance disability category of the Individuals with Disabilities Education Act (Chapter 15).

For **mania** in classically defined bipolar I disorder, medication is the primary treatment; medications used with adults may be less effective with youths (<50% response rate). Standard pharmacotherapy includes lithium, valproate, or atypical antipsychotics (aripiprazole, olanzapine, risperidone, quetiapine, ziprasidone) (Chapter 19 and Table 19-6). The choice of medication is based upon empiric support for safety and efficacy, medical considerations, adherence considerations, and a positive response of a family member.

Medication trials should be systematic, and the duration of trials should be sufficient (generally 6-8 wk) to determine the agent's effectiveness. Care should be taken to avoid unnecessary polypharmacy, in part by discontinuing agents that have not demonstrated significant benefit. Because all of these medications are associated with significant side effects, careful monitoring of baseline and follow-up indices is imperative. Side effects of lithium include cardiac, renal, thyroid, and hematologic effects; toxicity; and teratogenicity. Side effects of valproate include hematologic, hepatic, and ovarian effects and teratogenicity. Atypical antipsychotics cause weight gain, metabolic aberrations (diabetes, hyperlipidemia), and cardiac effects. Withdrawal of medication has been associated with increased risk of relapse.

The regimen needed to stabilize acute mania should be maintained for 12 to 24 mo. Maintenance therapy is often needed for youths with classic bipolar I disorder, and some patients need lifelong medication. Any attempts to discontinue prophylactic medication should be done gradually, while closely monitoring the patient for relapse.

For depression in **bipolar II disorder**, antidepressant medication may be used once a mood-stabilizing medication has been initiated. Lamotrigine as adjunctive or monotherapy also may be helpful for adolescents with bipolar depression. Comorbid ADHD can be treated with stimulant medication once a mood-stabilizing medication has been initiated.

Psychotherapy is a key adjunctive treatment for the bipolar disorders. The components deemed to be important in therapy include identification and management of unpleasant feeling states, mastering interpersonal skills, developing decision-making and problem-solving skills, and inculcating healthy lifestyle habits: getting regular sleep and exercise, reducing stress, stabilizing social relationships, and avoiding drugs, alcohol, and nonprescribed medications. Many of these components are present in dialectical behavioral therapy, which has emerging empiric support for the treatment of these disorders.

LEVEL OF CARE

Most youths with bipolar disorders can be safely and effectively treated as outpatients, provided that a schedule of frequent visits and laboratory tests can be maintained through the acute phase of treatment. Youths who are suicidal or psychotic usually require inpatient care.

Table 24-4 DSM-IV-TR DIAGNOSTIC CRITERIA FOR DYSTHYMIC DISORDER

A. Depressed mood for most of the day, for more days than not, as indicated either by subjective account or observation by others, for at least 2 years. Note: In children and adolescents, mood can be irritable and duration must be at least 1 year.
B. Presence, while depressed, of two (or more) of the following:
 1. Poor appetite or overeating
 2. Insomnia or hypersomnia
 3. Low energy or fatigue
 4. Low self-esteem
 5. Poor concentration or difficulty making decisions
 6. Feelings of hopelessness
C. During the 2-year period (1 year for children or adolescents) of the disturbance, the person has never been without the symptoms in Criteria A and B for more than 2 months at a time.
D. No major depressive episode has been present during the first 2 years of the disturbance (1 year for children and adolescents); i.e., the disturbance is not better accounted for by chronic major depressive episode or major depressive disorder, in partial remission. **Note:** There may have been a previous major depressive episode provided there was a full remission (no significant signs or symptoms for 2 months) before development of the dysthymic disorder. in addition, after the initial 2 years (1 year in children or adolescents) of dysthymic disorder, there may be superimposed episodes of major depressive disorder, in which case both diagnoses may be given when the criteria are met for a major depressive episode.
E. There has never been a manic episode, a mixed episode, or a hypomanic episode and criteria have never been met for cyclothymic disorder.
F. The disturbance does not occur exclusively during the course of a chronic psychotic disorder, such as schizophrenia or delusional disorder.
G. The symptoms are not due to the direct physiological effects of a substance (e.g., a drug of abuse, a medication) or a general medical condition (e.g., hypothyroidism).
H. The symptoms cause clinically significant distress or impairment in social, occupational, or other important areas of functioning.

From American Psychiatric Association: *Diagnostic and statistical manual of mental disorders, fourth edition, text revision,* Washington, DC, 2000, American Psychiatric Association.

BIBLIOGRAPHY

Please visit the Nelson Textbook of Pediatrics *website at* *www.expertconsult.com* *for the complete bibliography.*

24.3 Dysthymic Disorder

Heather J. Walter and David R. DeMaso

In the DSM-IV-TR, dysthymic disorder is characterized by a period of at least 1 yr in which there is a depressed or irritable mood for most of the day on more days than not (Table 24-4). There also are associated vegetative and cognitive symptoms, including disturbances in appetite, sleep, and energy and impaired concentration, low self-esteem, and thoughts of hopelessness. To meet the syndromal diagnosis, two or more symptoms in addition to depressed or irritable mood must be present and cause clinically significant distress or impairment, not be better accounted for by other psychiatric disorders, and not be due to the direct physiologic effects of a substance or a general medical condition.

Depressive disorder, not otherwise specified (sub-syndromal depression) is diagnosed when some symptoms of depressive disorders are present, but not enough to meet full diagnostic criteria for major depressive disorder or dysthymic disorder.

The prevalence of dysthymic disorder is estimated to approximate 1% in children and 5% in adolescents. Approximately 5-10% of children and adolescents are estimated to have sub-syndromal symptoms of depression (depressive disorder, not otherwise specified). The duration of a dysthymic episode approximates 3 to 4 years for both clinical and community samples. Both dysthymic disorder and sub-syndromal depression convey increased risk for the development of major depression and as such are important targets for treatment.

The Etiology, Prevention, Early Identification, and Treatment sections under Chapter 24.1 above are applicable to dysthymic disorder.

BIBLIOGRAPHY

Please visit the Nelson Textbook of Pediatrics *website at* *www.expertconsult.com* *for the complete bibliography.*

Chapter 25
Suicide and Attempted Suicide

Joanna C.M. Cole, Heather J. Walter, and David R. DeMaso

Youth suicide is a major and preventable public health problem. It ranks as the 3rd and 4th leading causes of death among young people ages 15-24 yr and 10-14 yr, respectively.

Each year, there are approximately 10 suicides for every 100,000 youngsters younger than 19 yr, an estimated 12 suicides every day. Morbidity from suicide attempts is high, with approximately 2 million young people attempting suicide each year and almost 700,000 receiving medical attention. There are a number of psychologic, social, cultural, and environmental risk factors for suicide, and knowledge of these risk factors can facilitate identification of youths at highest risk.

EPIDEMIOLOGY

Suicide Completions

Suicide is very rare before puberty. Rates of completed suicide increase steadily across the teen years and into young adulthood, peaking in the early 20s. Males complete suicide at a rate 4 times that of females and represent 79.4% of all suicides. Firearms remain the most commonly used method of completing suicide for males, whereas females are more likely to complete suicide by poisoning (Fig. 25-1). In the past 60 yr, the suicide rate has quadrupled among 15-24 yr old males and has doubled for females of the same age. The male:female ratio for completed suicide rises with age from 3:1 in young children to approximately 4:1 in 15-24 yr olds, and to greater than 6:1 among 20-24 yr olds.

The ethnic groups with the highest risk for completed suicide are American Indians and Alaska Natives. Within this population, suicide is the second leading cause of death, accounting for nearly 1 in 5 deaths among youth ages 15-24 yr. The ethnic groups with the lowest risk are African-Americans, Hispanics, Asians, and Pacific Islanders. The suicide rate among African-American, Hispanic, and other minority males has continued to increase, and the rate among white males has remained steady. Suicide risk also varies in different countries (Fig. 25-2).

Suicide Attempts

It is estimated that for every completed youth suicide, as many as 200 suicide attempts are made. Ingestion of medication is the most common method of attempted suicide. The 15 to 19 yr old age group is the most likely to intentionally harm themselves by ingestion, receive treatment in emergency departments, and survive. Attempts are more common in girls than boys (approximately 3:1), and in Hispanic girls than their non-Hispanic white or non-Hispanic African-American counterparts. Gay, lesbian, and bisexual youths are also at increased risk for suicide attempts. Suicide attempts among African-American adolescent males have more than doubled from 1991 to 2001. Attempters who have made prior suicide attempts, who used a method other than ingestion, and who still want to die are at increased risk for completed suicide.

Suicide Ideation

Based on the 2007 Youth Risk Behavior Survey, 14.5% of students in grades 9 through 12 reported that they had seriously considered attempting suicide in the 12 mo preceding the survey (18.7% of females and 10.3% of males). Nearly 7% of students reported that they had actually attempted suicide at least once during the same period.

RISK FACTORS

In addition to age, race and ethnicity, and a history of a previous suicide attempt, there are multiple risk factors that predispose youths to suicide.

Pre-existing Psychiatric Illness

The great majority (estimated at 90%) of youths who complete suicide have a pre-existing psychiatric illness, most commonly major depression (Chapter 24.1). Among girls, chronic anxiety, especially panic disorder, also is associated with suicide completion (Chapter 23). Among boys, conduct disorder and substance use convey increased risk. Comorbidity of a substance use disorder (Chapter 108), a mood disorder (Chapter 24), and conduct disorder (Chapter 27) has been linked to suicide by firearm.

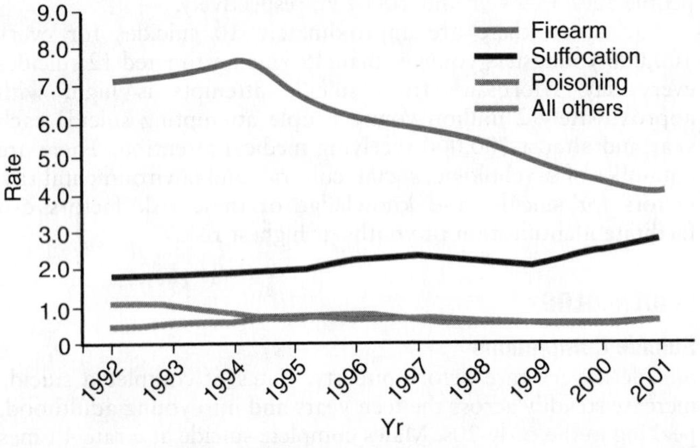

*Per 100,000 population.

Figure 25-1 Annual suicide rates among persons aged 15-19 yr, by year and method, United States, 1992-2001. (From Centers for Disease Control and Prevention: Methods of suicide among persons aged 10–19 years, United States, 1992–2001, *MMWR Morb Mortal Wkly Rep* 53:471–474, 2004.)

Cognitive Distortions

Negative self-attributions can contribute to the hopelessness that is commonly associated with suicidality; hopelessness may contribute to ~55% of the explained variance in continued suicidal ideation. Many suicidal youth hold negative views of their own competence, have poor self-esteem, and have difficulty identifying sources of support or reasons to live. Many youngsters lack the coping strategies necessary to manage strong emotions and instead tend to catastrophize and engage in all-or-nothing thinking.

Social, Cultural, and Environmental Factors

Of children and adolescents who attempt suicide, 65% can name a precipitating event for their action. Most adolescent suicide attempts are precipitated by stressful life events, such as academic or social problems, being bullied, trouble with the law, family instability, questioning one's sexual orientation, a newly diagnosed medical condition, or a recent or anticipated loss. Suicide may also be precipitated by exposure to news of another person's suicide or by reading about or viewing a suicide portrayed in a romantic light in the media.

For some recent immigrants, suicidal ideation is associated with high levels of acculturative stress, especially in the context of family separation and limited access to supportive resources. Physical and sexual abuse can also increase one's risk of suicide; 15-20% of female suicide attempters had a history of abuse. There is a more general association between family conflict and suicide attempts; this association is strongest in children and early adolescents. Family psychopathology and a family history of suicidal behavior convey excess risk. Supportive social relations with peers, parents, and school personnel have an interactive relationship in mitigating the risk of suicide among youth.

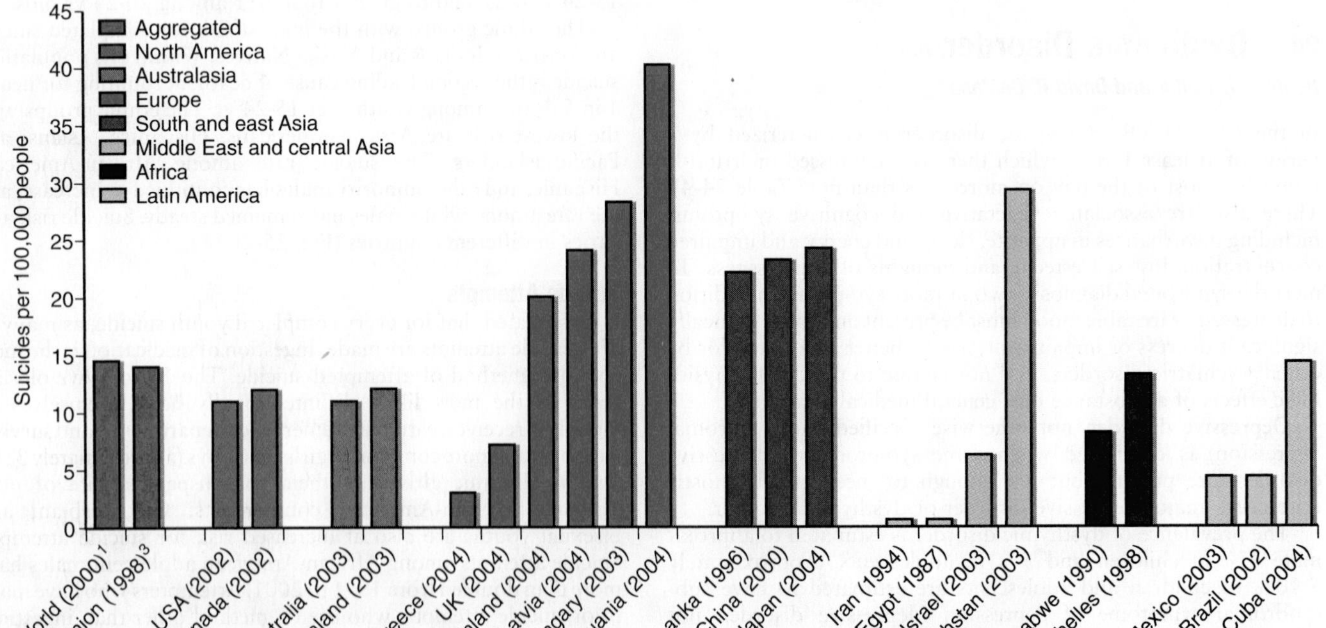

Figure 25-2 Suicide rates in selected regions and countries. (From Hawton K, van Heeringen K: Suicide. *Lancet* 373:1372–1380, 2009.)

ASSESSMENT AND INTERVENTION

Assessment of suicidal ideation should be a regular part of visits with young patients. Two thirds of youths who commit suicide visit a physician in the month before they kill themselves. When not specifically asked, youth are less likely to disclose depression, suicidal thoughts, and patterns of drug use. Distress is not always expressed in the same ways among persons from different cultural backgrounds.

Evaluating the presence and degree of suicidality and underlying risk factors is complex; clinical assessment is best conducted by a qualified mental health professional. All suicidal ideation and attempts should be taken seriously and require a thorough assessment to evaluate the youth's current state of mind, underlying psychiatric conditions, and ongoing risk of harm. Gathering information from multiple sources and by varied culturally and developmentally sensitive techniques are essential in evaluating suicidal risk indicators.

The reliability and validity of interview reporting of children and adolescents may be affected by their level of cognitive development and their understanding of the relationship between their emotions and behavior. Confirmation of the youth's suicidal behavior can be obtained from information gathered by interviewing others who know the child or adolescent. There is often a discrepancy between child and parent reports, with both children and adolescents being more likely to tell of suicidal ideation and suicidal actions than their parents.

Ideation can be assessed by the following series of questions: "Did you ever feel so upset that you wished you were not alive or wanted to die?" "Did you ever do something that you knew was so dangerous that you could get hurt or killed by doing it?" "Did you ever hurt yourself or try to hurt yourself?" "Did you ever try to kill yourself?"

The assessment of attempts should include a detailed exploration of the hours immediately preceding the attempt to identify precipitants, as well as the circumstances of the attempt itself to identify intent and potential lethality. Attempters at greatest risk for completed suicide are those who are male; have made a prior suicide attempt; have current ideation, intent, a written note, and a plan; have a mental status altered by depression, mania, anxiety, intoxication, psychosis, hopelessness, rage, humiliation, or impulsivity; and lack supportive family members who can provide supervision, safeguard the home (prevent access to firearms, medications, alcohol, drugs), and ensure adherence to treatment recommendations (Table 25-1).

Youth with these risk factors generally require inpatient level of care to ensure safety, clarify diagnosis, and comprehensively plan treatment. For those youth suitable for treatment in the outpatient setting, an appointment should be scheduled within a few days with a mental health professional. Ideally this appointment should be scheduled before leaving the assessment venue, because 50% of those who attempt suicide fail to complete the follow-up referral. A procedure should be in place to contact the family if the family fails to complete the referral. Therapies that have been found to be helpful with suicidal youth include cognitive-behavioral therapy, dialectical behavioral therapy, and interpersonal therapy. Psychotropic medications are used adjunctively to treat underlying psychiatric disorders.

Table 25-1 CHECKLISTS FOR ASSESSING CHILD OR ADOLESCENT SUICIDE ATTEMPTERS IN AN EMERGENCY DEPARTMENT OR CRISIS CENTER

ATTEMPTERS AT GREATER RISK FOR SUICIDE
Suicidal History
Still thinking of suicide Have made a prior suicide attempt
Demographics
Male Live alone
Mental State
Depressed, manic, hypomanic, severely anxious, or a mixture of these states Substance abuse alone or in association with a mood disorder Irritable, agitated, threatening violence to others, delusional, or hallucinating **Do not discharge such patients without a psychiatric evaluation.**
LOOK FOR SIGNS OF CLINICAL DEPRESSION:
Depressed mood most of the time Loss of interest or pleasure in usual activities Weight loss or gain Can't sleep or sleeps too much Restless or slowed down Fatigue, loss of energy Feelings of worthlessness or guilt Low self-esteem, disappointed with self Feelings of hopelessness about the future Can't concentrate, indecisive Recurring thoughts of death Irritable, upset by little things
LOOK FOR SIGNS OF MANIA OR HYPOMANIA:
Depressed mood most of the time Elated, expansive, or irritable mood Inflated self-esteem, grandiosity Decreased need for sleep More talkative than usual, pressured speech Racing thoughts Abrupt topic changes when talking Distractible Excessive participation in multiple activities Agitated or restless Hypersexual, spends foolishly, uninhibited remarks

From American Foundation for Suicide Prevention: *Today's suicide attempter could be tomorrow's suicide (poster),* New York, 1999, American Foundation for Suicide Prevention, 1-888-333-AFSP.

PREVENTION

At present there is insufficient evidence to either support or refute universal suicide prevention programs. Screening for suicidality is fraught with problems related to low specificity of the screening instrument, poor acceptability among school administrators, and paucity of referral sites. Gatekeeper (e.g., student support personnel) training is effective in improving skills among school personnel and is highly acceptable to administrators but has not been shown to prevent suicide. Peer helpers have not been shown to be efficacious.

One school-based prevention program (the Signs of Suicide program) has shown some preventive potential based on the results from a randomized trial among high school students. In this program, a curriculum to raise awareness of suicide is combined with a brief screening for depression and other risk factors associated with suicide. The curriculum promotes the concept that suicide is directly related to mental illness, typically depression, and is not a normal reaction to stress. Students are taught to recognize the signs of suicide and depression in themselves and others, and they are taught the specific action steps necessary for responding to these signs.

BIBLIOGRAPHY

Please visit the Nelson Textbook of Pediatrics *website at www.expertconsult.com for the complete bibliography.*

Chapter 26
Eating Disorders

Richard E. Kreipe

Eating disorders (EDs) are characterized by body dissatisfaction related to overvaluation of a thin body ideal associated with dysfunctional patterns of cognition and weight control behaviors that results in significant biologic, psychologic, and social complications. Although largely affecting white, adolescent girls, EDs also affect boys and cross all racial, ethnic, and cultural boundaries. Early intervention in EDs improves outcome.

DEFINITIONS

Anorexia nervosa (AN) involves significant overestimation of body size and shape, with a relentless pursuit of thinness that typically combines excessive dieting and compulsive exercising in the **restrictive** subtype; in the **binge-purge** subtype, patients might intermittently overeat and then attempt to rid themselves of calories by vomiting or taking laxatives, still with a strong drive for thinness (Table 26-1). **Bulimia nervosa** (BN) is characterized by episodes of eating large amounts of food in a brief period, followed by compensatory vomiting, laxative use, and exercise or fasting to rid the body of the effects of overeating in an effort to avoid obesity (Table 26-2).

The majority of children and adolescents with EDs do *not* fulfill all of the criteria for either of these syndromes in the *Diagnostic and Statistical Manual of Mental Disorders, Fourth Edition* (DSM-IV) classification system but fall instead into the category of **eating disorder, not otherwise specified (ED-NOS)** (Table 26-3). ED-NOS includes a wide variety of subthreshold clinical presentations. **Binge eating disorder** (BED), in which binge eating is not followed regularly by any compensatory behaviors, is included in ED-NOS in DSM-IV and shares many features with obesity (Chapter 44). ED-NOS, often called "disordered eating," can worsen into full syndrome EDs.

EPIDEMIOLOGY

The classic features of AN include a white, early to middle adolescent girl of above-average intelligence and socioeconomic status, who is a conflict-avoidant, risk-aversive, perfectionist struggling with disturbances of anxiety and/or mood. BN tends to emerge in later adolescence, sometimes evolving from AN, and is typified by impulsivity and features of borderline personality disorder that are associated with depression and mood swings. The 0.5-1% and 3-5% incidence rates among younger and older adolescent girls for AN and BN, respectively, probably reflect ascertainment bias in sampling and underdiagnosis in cases not fitting the typical profile. The same may be true of the significant gender disparity, in which female patients account for about 90% of patients with diagnosed EDs. Ten percent or more of some adolescent female populations have ED-NOS.

No single factor causes the development of an ED; sociocultural studies indicate a complex interplay of culture, ethnicity, gender, peers, and family. The gender dimorphism is presumably related to girls having a stronger relationship between body image and self-evaluation, as well as the influence of the Western culture's thin body ideal on the development of EDs. Race and ethnicity appear to moderate the association between risk factors and disordered eating, with African-American and Caribbean girls reporting lower body dissatisfaction and less dieting than Hispanic and non-Hispanic white girls. Because peer acceptance is central to healthy adolescent growth and development, especially in early adolescence when AN tends to have its initial

Table 26-1 DIAGNOSTIC CRITERIA FOR 307.1 ANOREXIA NERVOSA

A. Refusal to maintain body weight at or above a minimally normal weight for age and height (e.g., weight loss leading to maintenance of body weight less than 85% of that expected; or failure to make expected weight gain during period of growth, leading to body weight less than 85% of that expected).
B. Intense fear of gaining weight or becoming fat, even though underweight.
C. Disturbance in the way one's body weight or shape is experienced, undue influence of body weight or shape on self-evaluation, or denial of the seriousness of the current low body weight.
D. In post-menarcheal females, amenorrhea, i.e., the absence of at least three consecutive menstrual cycles. (A woman is considered to have amenorrhea if her periods occur only following hormone, e.g., estrogen, administration.)

Specify Type:

Restricting Type: during the current episode of anorexia nervosa, the person has not regularly engaged in binge-eating or purging behavior (i.e., self-induced vomiting or the misuse of laxatives, diuretics, or enemas)
Binge-Eating/Purging Type: during the current episode of anorexia nervosa, the person has regularly engaged in binge-eating or purging behavior (i.e., self-induced vomiting or the misuse of laxatives, diuretics, or enemas)

From American Psychiatric Association: *Diagnostic and statistical manual of mental disorders*, ed 4, Washington, DC, 1994, American Psychiatric Association.

Table 26-2 DIAGNOSTIC CRITERIA FOR 307.51 BULIMIA NERVOSA

A. Recurrent episodes of binge eating. An episode of binge eating is characterized by both of the following:
   1. Eating, in a discrete period of time (e.g., within any 2-hour period), an amount of food that is definitely larger than most people would eat during a similar period of time and under similar circumstances
   2. A sense of lack of control over eating during the episode (e.g., a feeling that one cannot stop eating or control what or how much one is eating)
B. Recurrent inappropriate compensatory behavior to prevent weight gain, such as self-induced vomiting; misuse of laxatives, diuretics, enemas, or other medications; fasting; or excessive exercise.
C. The binge eating and inappropriate compensatory behaviors both occur, on average, at least twice a week for 3 months.
D. Self-evaluation is unduly influenced by body shape and weight.
E. The disturbance does not occur exclusively during episodes of Anorexia Nervosa.

Specify Type:

Purging Type: during the current episode of Bulimia Nervosa, the person has regularly engaged in self-induced vomiting or the misuse of laxatives, diuretics, or enemas
Nonpurging Type: during the current episode of Bulimia Nervosa, the person has used other inappropriate compensatory behaviors, such as fasting or excessive exercise, but has not regularly engaged in self-induced vomiting or the misuse of laxatives, diuretics, or enemas

From American Psychiatric Association: *Diagnostic and statistical manual of mental disorders*, ed 4, Washington, DC, 1994, American Psychiatric Association.

Table 26-3 307.50 EATING DISORDER NOT OTHERWISE SPECIFIED

The Eating Disorder Not Otherwise Specified category is for disorders of eating that do not meet the criteria for any specific Eating Disorder. Examples include:
1. For females, all of the criteria for Anorexia Nervosa are met except that the individual has regular menses.
2. All of the criteria for Anorexia Nervosa are met except that, despite significant weight loss, the individual's current weight is in the normal range.
3. All of the criteria for Bulimia Nervosa are met except that the binge eating and inappropriate compensatory mechanisms occur at a frequency of less than twice a week or for a duration of less than 3 months.
4. The regular use of inappropriate compensatory behavior by an individual of normal body weight after eating small amounts of food (e.g., self-induced vomiting after the consumption of two cookies).
5. Repeatedly chewing and spitting out, but not swallowing, large amounts of food.
6. Binge-eating disorder: recurrent episodes of binge eating in the absence of the regular use of inappropriate compensatory behaviors characteristic of Bulimia Nervosa

From American Psychiatric Association: *Diagnostic and statistical manual of mental disorders*, ed 4, Washington, DC, 1994, American Psychiatric Association.

prevalence peak, the potential influence of peers on EDs is significant, as are the relationships among peers, body image, and eating. Teasing by peers or by family members (especially male) may be a contributing factor for overweight girls.

Family influence in the development of EDs is even more complex because of the interplay of environmental and genetic factors; shared elements of the family environment and immutable genetic factors account for significant (about equal) variance in disordered eating. There are associations between parents' and children's eating behaviors; dieting and physical activity levels suggest parental reinforcement of body-related societal messages. The influence of inherited genetic factors on the emergence of EDs during adolescence is also significant, but not in a direct fashion. Rather, the risk for developing an ED appears to be mediated through a genetic predisposition to anxiety (Chapter 23), depression (Chapter 24), or obsessive-compulsive traits that may be modulated through the internal milieu of puberty. There is little evidence that parents "cause" an ED in their child or adolescent; the importance of parents in treatment and recovery cannot be overestimated.

PATHOLOGY AND PATHOGENESIS

For the full continuation of this topic, please visit the Nelson Textbook of Pediatrics *website at www.expertconsult.com.*

CLINICAL MANIFESTATIONS

A central feature of EDs is the overestimation of body size, shape or parts (e.g., abdomen, thighs) leading to weight-control practices intended to reduce weight (AN) or prevent weight gain (BN). Associated practices include severe restriction of caloric intake and behaviors intended to reduce the effect of calories ingested, such as compulsive exercising or purging by inducing vomiting or taking laxatives. Eating and weight loss habits commonly found in EDs can result in a wide range of energy intake and output, the balance of which leads to a wide range in weight from extreme loss of weight in AN to fluctuation around a normal to moderately high weight in BN. Reported eating and weight-control habits (Table 26-4) thus inform the initial primary care approach.

Although weight-control patterns guide the initial pediatric approach, an assessment of commonly reported symptoms and findings on physical examination is essential to identify targets for intervention. When reported symptoms of excessive weight loss (feeling tired and cold; lacking energy; orthostasis; difficulty concentrating) are explicitly linked by the clinician to their associated physical signs (hypothermia with acrocyanosis and slow capillary refill, loss of muscle mass, bradycardia with orthostasis), it becomes more difficult for the patient to deny that a problem exists. Furthermore, awareness that bothersome symptoms can be eliminated by healthier eating and activity patterns can increase a patient's motivation to engage in treatment. Tables 26-5 and 26-6 detail common symptoms and signs that should be addressed in a pediatric assessment of a suspected ED.

DIFFERENTIAL DIAGNOSIS

In addition to identifying symptoms and signs that deserve targeted intervention for patients who have an ED or disordered eating, a comprehensive history and physical examination are required in the assessment of a suspected ED to rule out other conditions in the differential diagnosis. Weight loss can occur with any condition in which there is increased catabolism (e.g., malignancy or occult chronic infection) or malabsorption (e.g., inflammatory bowel disease or celiac disease), but these illnesses are generally associated with other findings and are not usually associated with decreased caloric intake. Patients with inflammatory bowel disease can reduce intake to minimize abdominal cramping; eating can cause abdominal discomfort and early satiety in AN because of gastric atony associated with significant weight loss, not malabsorption. Likewise, signs of weight loss in AN might include hypothermia, acrocyanosis with slow capillary refill, and neutropenia suggesting overwhelming sepsis, but the overall picture in EDs is one of relative cardiovascular stability compared to sepsis. Endocrinopathies are also in the differential of EDs. With BN, voracious appetite in the face of weight loss might suggest diabetes mellitus, but blood glucose levels are normal or low in EDs. Adrenal insufficiency mimics many physical symptoms and signs found in restrictive AN but is associated with elevated potassium levels and hyperpigmentation. Although thyroid disorders are often considered, due to changes in weight and other symptoms in AN, the overall presentation includes symptoms of both underactive and overactive thyroid, such as hypothermia, bradycardia, and constipation, as well as weight loss and excessive physical activity, respectively.

In the CNS, craniopharyngiomas and Rathke pouch tumors can mimic some of the findings of AN, such as weight loss and growth failure, and even some body image disturbances, but the latter are less fixed than in typical EDs and are associated with other findings, including evidence of increased intracranial pressure. Any patient with an atypical presentation of an ED, based on age, sex, or other factors not typical for AN or BN deserves a scrupulous search for an alternative explanation. Patients can have both an underlying illness and an ED. The core features of dysfunctional eating habits—body image disturbance and change in weight—can coexist with conditions such as diabetes mellitus, where patients might manipulate their insulin dosing to lose weight.

LABORATORY FINDINGS

Because the diagnosis of an ED is made clinically, there is no confirmatory laboratory test. Laboratory abnormalities, when found, are due to malnutrition, weight control habits used, or medical complications; studies should be chosen based on history and physical examination. A routine screening battery typically includes complete blood count, erythrocyte sedimentation rate (should be normal), and biochemical profile. Common abnormalities in ED include low white blood cell count with normal hemoglobin and differential; hypokalemic, hypochloremic metabolic alkalosis with severe vomiting; mildly elevated liver enzymes, cholesterol, and cortisol levels; low gonadotropins and blood glucose with marked weight loss; and generally normal total protein, albumin, and renal function. An electrocardiogram (ECG) may be useful when profound bradycardia or arrhythmia is detected; the ECG usually has low voltage, with nonspecific ST or T wave changes. Although prolonged QTc has been reported, prospective studies have not found an increased risk for this.

COMPLICATIONS

No organ is spared the harmful effects of dysfunctional weight control habits, but the most concerning targets of medical complications are the heart, brain, gonads, and bones. Some **heart** findings in EDs (e.g., sinus bradycardia and hypotension) are *physiologic* adaptations to starvation that conserve calories and reduce afterload. Cold, blue hands and feet with slow capillary refill that can result in tissue perfusion insufficient to meet demands also represent energy-conserving responses associated with inadequate intake. All of these acute changes are reversible with restoration of nutrition and weight. Significant orthostatic pulse changes, prolonged corrected QT interval, ventricular dysrhythmias, or reduced myocardial contractility reflect myocardial impairment that can be lethal. In addition, with extremely low weight, **refeeding syndrome** (due to rapid drop in serum phosphorous, magnesium, and potassium with excessive reintroduction of calories, especially carbohydrates), is associated with

Table 26-4 EATING AND WEIGHT CONTROL HABITS COMMONLY FOUND IN CHILDREN AND ADOLESCENTS WITH AN EATING DISORDER

HABIT	PROMINENT FEATURE		CLINICAL COMMENTS REGARDING EATING DISORDER HABITS	
	Anorexia Nervosa	Bulimia Nervosa	Anorexia Nervosa	Bulimia Nervosa
Overall intake	Inadequate energy (calories), although volume of food and beverages may be high due to very low caloric density of intake due to "diet" and nonfat choices	Variable, but calories normal to high; intake in binges often "forbidden" food or drink that differs from intake at meals.	Consistent inadequate caloric intake leading to wasting of the body is an essential feature of diagnosis	Inconsistent balance of intake, exercise and vomiting, but severe caloric restriction is short-lived
Food	Counts and limits calories, especially from fat; Emphasis on "healthy food choices" with reduced caloric density Monotonous, limited "good" food choices, often leading to vegetarian or vegan diet Strong feelings of guilt after eating more than planned leads to exercise and renewed dieting	Aware of calories and fat, but less regimented in avoidance than AN Frequent dieting interspersed with overeating, often triggered by depression, isolation, or anger	Obsessive-compulsive attention to nutritional data on food labels and may have "logical" reasons for food choices in highly regimented pattern, such as sports participation or family history of lipid disorder	Choices less structured, with more frequent diets
Beverages	Water or other low- or no-calorie drinks; nonfat milk	Variable, diet soda common; may drink alcohol to excess	Fluids often restricted to avoid weight gain	Fluids ingested to aid vomiting or replace losses
Meals	Consistent schedule and structure to meal plan Reduced or eliminated caloric content, often starting with breakfast, then lunch, then dinner Volume can increase with fresh fruits, vegetables, and salads as primary food sources	Meals less regimented and planned than in AN; more likely impulsive and unregulated, often eliminated following a binge-purge episode	Rigid adherence to "rules" governing eating leads to sense of control, confidence and mastery	Elimination of a meal following a binge-purge only reinforces the drive for binge later in the day
Snacks	Reduced or eliminated from meal plan	Often avoided in meal plans, but then impulsively eaten	Snack foods removed early because "unhealthy"	Snack "comfort foods" can trigger a binge
Dieting	Initial habit that becomes progressively restrictive, although often appearing superficially "healthy" Beliefs and "rules" about the patient's idiosyncratic nutritional requirements and response to foods are strongly held	Initial dieting gives way to chaotic eating, often interpreted by the patient as evidence of being "weak" or "lazy"	Distinguishing between healthy meal planning with reduced calories and dieting in ED may be difficult	Dieting tends to be impulsive and short-lived, with "diets" often resulting in unintended weight gain
Binge eating	None in restrictive subtype, but an essential feature in binge-purge subtype	Essential feature, often secretive Shame and guilt prominent afterward	Often "subjective" (more than planned but not large)	Relieves emotional distress, may be planned
Exercise	Characteristically obsessive-compulsive, ritualistic, and progressive May excel in dance, long-distance running	Less predictable May be athletic, or may avoid exercise entirely	May be difficult to distinguish active thin vs. ED	Males often use exercise as means of "purging"
Vomiting	Characteristic of binge-purge subtype May chew, then spit out, rather than swallow, food as a variant	Most common habit intended to reduce effects of overeating Can occur after meal as well as a binge	Physiologic and emotional instability prominent	Strongly "addictive" and self-punishing, but does not eliminate calories ingested—many still absorbed
Laxatives	If used, generally to relieve constipation in restrictive subtype, but as a cathartic in binge-purge subtype	Second most common habit used to reduce or avoid weight gain, often used in increasing doses for cathartic effect	Physiologic and emotional instability prominent	Strongly "addictive," self-punishing, but ineffective means to reduce weight (calories are absorbed in the small intestine, but laxatives work in the colon)
Diet pills	Very rare, if used; more common in binge-purge subtype	Used to either reduce appetite or increase metabolism	Use of diet pills implies inability to control eating	Control over eating may be sought by any means

AN, anorexia nervosa; BN, bulimia nervosa; ED, eating disorder.

acute heart failure and neurologic symptoms. With long-term malnutrition, the myocardium appears to be more prone to tachyarrhythmias, the second most common cause of death after suicide. In BN, dysrhythmias can also be related to electrolyte imbalance.

Clinically, the primary **brain** area affected acutely in EDs, especially with weight loss, is the hypothalamus. Hypothalamic dysfunction is reflected in problems with thermoregulation (warming and cooling), satiety, sleep, autonomic cardioregulatory imbalance (orthostasis) and endocrine function (reduced gonadal and excessive adrenal cortex stimulation), all of which are reversible. Anatomic studies of the brain in ED have focused on AN, with the most common finding being increased ventricular and sulcal volumes that normalize with weight restoration. Persistent gray-matter deficits following recovery, related to the degree of weight loss, have been reported. Elevated medial temporal lobe cerebral blood flow on positron emission tomography (PET) similar to that found in psychotic patients suggests that these changes may be related to body image distortion. Also, visualizing high-calorie foods is associated with exaggerated responses in the visual association cortex that are similar to those seen in patients with specific phobias. Patients with AN might have an imbalance between serotonin and dopamine pathways related to neurocircuits in which dietary restraint reduces anxiety.

Reduced **gonadal** function occurs in male and female patients; it is clinically manifested in AN as amenorrhea in female patients. It is related to understimulation from the hypothalamus as well as cortical suppression related to physical and emotional stress. Amenorrhea precedes significant dieting and weight loss in up to 30% of females with AN, and most adolescents with EDs perceive the absence of menses positively. The primary health concern is the negative effect of decreased ovarian function and estrogen on

Table 26-5 SYMPTOMS COMMONLY REPORTED BY PATIENTS WITH AN EATING DISORDER

SYMPTOMS	DIAGNOSIS: Anorexia Nervosa	DIAGNOSIS: Bulimia Nervosa	CLINICAL COMMENTS REGARDING ED SYMPTOMS
Body image	Feels fat, even with extreme emaciation, often with specific body distortions (e.g., stomach, thighs); Strong drive for thinness, with self-efficacy closely tied to appraisal of body shape, size, and/or weight	Variable body image distortion and dissatisfaction, but drive for thinness is less than the desire to avoid gaining weight	Challenging a patient's body image is both ineffective and countertherapeutic clinically Accepting the patient's expressed body image but noting its discrepancy with symptoms and signs reinforces concept that patient can "feel" fat but be also "be" too thin and unhealthy
Metabolism	Hypometabolic symptoms include feeling cold, tired, and weak and lacking energy May be both bothersome and reinforcing	Variable, depending on balance of intake and output and hydration	Symptoms are evidence of body's "shutting down" in an attempt to conserve calories with an inadequate diet Emphasizing reversibility of symptoms with healthy eating and weight gain can motivate patients to cooperate with treatment
Skin	Dry skin, delayed healing, easy bruising, goose flesh Orange-yellow skin on hands	No characteristic symptom, self-injurious behavior may be seen	Skin lacks good blood flow and the ability to heal in low weight Carotenemia with large intake of β-carotene foods; reversible
Hair	Lanugo-type hair growth on face and upper body Slow growth and increased loss of scalp hair	No characteristic symptom	Body hair growth conserves energy Scalp hair loss can worsen during refeeding "telogen effluvium" (resting hair is replaced by growing hair) Reversible with continued healthy eating
Eyes	No characteristic symptom	Subconjunctival hemorrhage	Caused by increased intrathoracic pressure during vomiting
Teeth	No characteristic symptom	Erosion of dental enamel erosion Decay, fracture, and loss of teeth	Intraoral stomach acid resulting from vomiting etches dental enamel, exposing softer dental elements
Salivary glands	No characteristic symptom	Enlargement (no to mild tenderness)	Caused by chronic binge eating and induced vomiting, with parotid enlargement more prominent than submandibular; reversible
Heart	Dizziness, fainting in restrictive subtype Palpitations more common in binge-purge subtype	Dizziness, fainting, palpitations	Dizziness and fainting due to postural orthostatic tachycardia and dysregulation at hypothalamic and cardiac level with weight loss, due to hypovolemia with binge-purge Palpitations and arrhythmias often caused by electrolyte disturbance Symptoms reverse with weight gain and/or cessation of binge-purge
Abdomen	Early fullness and discomfort with eating Constipation Perceives contour as "fat," often preferring well-defined abdominal musculature	Discomfort after a binge Cramps and diarrhea with laxative abuse	Weight loss is associated with reduced volume and tone of GI tract musculature, especially the stomach Laxatives may be used to relieve constipation or as a cathartic Symptom reduction with healthy eating can take weeks to occur
Extremities and musculoskeletal	Cold, blue hands and feet	No characteristic symptoms Self-cutting or burning on wrists or arms	Energy-conserving low body temperature with slow blood flow most notable peripherally Quickly reversed with healthy eating
Nervous system	No characteristic symptom	No characteristic symptom	Neurologic symptoms suggest a diagnosis other than an ED
Mental status	Depression, anxiety, obsessive-compulsive symptoms, alone or in combination	Depression; PTSD; borderline personality disorder traits	Underlying mood disturbances can worsen with dysfunctional weight control practices and can improve with healthy eating AN patients might report emotional "numbness" with starvation, preferable to emotionality associated with healthy eating

AN, anorexia nervosa; BN, bulimia nervosa; ED, eating disorder; GI, gastrointestinal; PTSD, post-traumatic stress disorder.

bones. Decreased bone mineral density (BMD) with osteopenia or the more severe osteoporosis is a significant complication of EDs (more pronounced in AN than BN). Data do not support the use of sex hormone replacement therapy because this alone does not improve other causes of low BMD (low body weight, lean body mass, and insulin-like growth factor [IGF]-1; high cortisol).

TREATMENT

Principles Guiding Primary Care Treatment

The approach in primary care should facilitate the acceptance by the patient (and parents) of the diagnosis and initial treatment recommendations. A **nurturant-authoritative** approach using the **biopsychosocial** model is useful. A pediatrician who explicitly acknowledges that the patient may disagree with the diagnosis and treatment recommendations and be ambivalent about changing eating habits, while also acknowledging that recovery requires strength, courage, will-power and determination, demonstrates *nurturance*. Parents also find it easier to be nurturant once they learn that the development of an ED is neither a willful decision by the patient nor a reflection of bad parenting. Framing the ED as a coping mechanism for a complex variety of issues with both positive and negative aspects avoids blame or guilt and can prepare the family for professional help that will focus on strengths and restoring health, rather than on the deficits in the adolescent or the family.

The **authoritative** aspect of a physician's role comes from expertise in health, growth, and physical development. A goal of primary care treatment should be attaining and maintaining health—not merely weight gain—although weight gain is a means to the goal of wellness. Providers who frame themselves as consultants to the patient with *authoritative* knowledge about health can avoid a countertherapeutic authoritarian stance. Primary care health-focused activities include monitoring the patient's physical status, setting limits on behaviors that threaten the patient's health, involving specialists with expertise in EDs on the treatment team, and continuing to provide primary care for health maintenance, acute illness, or injury.

Table 26-6 SIGNS COMMONLY FOUND IN PATIENTS WITH EATING DISORDERS RELATIVE TO PROMINENT FEATURE OF WEIGHT CONTROL

PHYSICAL SIGN	PROMINENT FEATURE Restrictive Intake	 Binge Eating/Purging	CLINICAL COMMENTS RELATED TO EATING DISORDER SIGNS
General appearance	Thin to cachetic, depending on balance of intake and output Might wear bulky clothing to hide thinness and ight resist being examined	Thin to overweight, depending on the balance of intake and output through various means	Examine in hospital gown Weight loss more rapid with reduced intake and excessive exercise Binge eating can result in large weight gain, regardless of purging behavior Appearance depends on balance of intake and output and overall weight control habits
Weight	Low and falling (if previously overweight may be normal or high); May be falsely elevated if patient drinks fluids or adds weights to body before being weighed	Highly variable, depending on balance of intake and output and state of hydration Falsification of weight is unusual	Weigh in hospital gown with no underwear, after voiding (measure urine SG) Remain in gown until physical exam completed to identify possible fluid loading (low urine SG, palpable bladder) or adding weights to body
Metabolism	Hypothermia: temp <35.5°C, pulse <60 Slowed psychomotor response with very low core temperature	Variable, but hypometabolic state is less common than in AN	Hypometabolism related to disruption of hypothalamic control mechanisms due to weight loss Signs of hypometabolism (cold skin, slow capillary refill, acryocyanosis) most evident in hands and feet, where energy conservation is most active.
Skin	Dry Increased prominence of hair follicles Orange or yellow hands	Calluses over proximal knuckle joints of hand (Russell's sign)	Carotenemia with large intake of β-carotene foods Russell's sign: maxillary incisors abrasion develops into callus with chronic digital pharyngeal stimulation, usually on dominant hand
Hair	Lanugo-type hair growth on face and upper body Scalp hair loss, especially prominent in parietal region	No characteristic sign	Body hair growth conserves energy Scalp hair loss "telogen effluvium" can worsen weeks after refeeding begins, as hair in resting phase is replaced by growing hair
Eyes	No characteristic sign	Subconjunctival hemorrhage	Increased intrathoracic pressure during vomiting.
Teeth	No characteristic sign	Eroded dental enamel and decayed, fractured, missing teeth	Perimolysis, worse on lingual surfaces of maxillary teeth, is intensified by brushing teeth without preceding water rinse
Salivary glands	No characteristic sign	Enlargement, relatively nontender	Parotid > submandibular involvement with frequent and chronic binge eating and induced vomiting
Throat	No characteristic sign	Absent gag reflex	Extinction of gag response with repeated pharyngeal stimulation
Heart	Bradycardia, hypotension, and orthostatic pulse differential >25 beats/min	Hypovolemia if dehydrated	Changes in AN due to central hypothalamic and intrinsic cardiac function Orthostatic changes less prominent if athletic, more prominent if associated with purging
Abdomen	Scaphoid, organs may be palpable but not enlarged, stool-filled left lower quadrant	Increased bowel sounds if recent laxative use	Presence of organomegaly requires investigation to determine cause Constipation prominent with weight loss
Extremities and musculoskeletal system	Cold, acrocyanosis, slow capillary refill Edema of feet Loss of muscle, subcutaneous, and fat tissue	No characteristic sign, but may have rebound edema after stopping chronic laxative use	Signs of hypometabolism (cold) and cardiovascular dysfunction (slow capillary refill and acryocyanosis) in hands and feet Edema, caused by capillary fragility more than hypoproteinemia in AN, can worsen in early phase of refeeding.
Nervous system	No characteristic sign	No characteristic sign	Water loading before weigh-ins can cause acute hyponatremia
Mental status	Anxiety about body image, irritability, depressed mood, oppositional to change	Depression, evidence of PTSD, more likely suicidal than AN	Mental status often improves with healthier eating and weight. SSRIs only shown to be effective for BN.

AN, anorexia nervosa; BN, bulimia nervosa; PTSD, post-traumatic stress disorder; SG, specific gravity; SSRI, selective serotonin reuptake inhibitor.

The **biopsychosocial** model uses a broad ecologic framework, starting with the biologic impairments of physical health related to dysfunctional weight control practices, evidenced by symptoms and signs. Explicitly linking ED behaviors to symptoms and signs can increase motivation to change. In addition, there are usually unresolved psychosocial conflicts in both the intrapersonal (self-esteem, self-efficacy) and interpersonal (family, peers, school) domains. Weight-control practices initiated as coping mechanisms become reinforced because of positive feedback. That is, external rewards (e.g., compliments about improved physical appearance) and internal rewards (e.g., perceived mastery over what is eaten or what is done to minimize the effects of overeating through exercise or purging) are more powerful to maintain behavior than negative feedback (e.g., conflict with parents, peers, and others about eating) is to change it. Thus, when definitive treatment is initiated, more productive alternative means of coping must be developed.

Nutrition and Physical Activity

The primary care provider generally begins the process of prescribing nutrition, although a dietitian should be involved eventually in the meal planning and nutritional education of patients with AN or BN. Framing food as fuel for the body and the source of energy for daily activities emphasizes the health goal of increasing the patient's energy level, endurance, and strength. For patients with AN and low weight, the nutrition prescription should work toward gradually increasing weight at the rate of about 0.5 to 1 lb/wk, by increasing energy intake at 100 to 200 kcal increments every few days toward a target of approximately 90% of average body weight for sex, height, and age.

Weight gain will not occur until intake exceeds output, and eventual intake for continued weight gain can exceed 3500 kcal/day, especially for patients who are anxious and have high levels of thermogenesis from non-exercise activity. Stabilizing intake is the goal for patients with BN, with a gradual introduction of forbidden foods while also limiting foods that might trigger a binge.

When initiating treatment of an ED in a primary care setting, the clinician should be aware of common cognitive patterns. Patients with AN typically have all-or-none thinking (related to perfectionism) with a tendency to over-generalize and jump to catastrophic conclusions, while assuming that their body is governed by rules that do not apply to others. These tendencies lead to the dichotomization of foods into good or bad categories, having a day ruined because of one unexpected event, or choosing foods based on rigid self-imposed restrictions. These thoughts may be related to neurocircuitry and neurotransmitter abnormalities related to executive function and rewards.

A standard nutritional balance of 15-20% calories from protein, 50-55% from carbohydrate, and 25-30% from fat is appropriate. The fat content may need to be lowered to 15-20% early in the treatment of AN because of continued fat phobia. With the risk of low BMD in patients with AN, calcium and vitamin D supplements are often needed to attain the recommended 1300 mg/day intake of calcium. Refeeding can be accomplished with frequent small meals and snacks consisting of a variety of foods and beverages (with minimal diet or fat-free products), rather than fewer high-volume high-calorie meals. Some patients find it easier to take in part of the additional nutrition as canned supplements (medicine) rather than food. Regardless of the source of energy intake, the risk for refeeding syndrome (acute tachycardia and heart failure with neurologic symptoms associated primarily with acute decline in serum phosphate and magnesium) increases with the degree of weight loss and the rapidity of caloric increases. Therefore, if the weight has fallen below 80% of expected weight for height, refeeding should proceed cautiously, possibly in the hospital (Table 26-7).

Patients with AN tend to have a highly structured day with restrictive intake, in contrast to BN, which is characterized by a lack of structure, resulting in chaotic eating patterns and binge-purge episodes. Patients with AN, BN, or ED-NOS all benefit from a daily structure for healthy eating that includes 3 meals and at least 1 snack a day, distributed evenly over the day, based on balanced meal planning. Breakfast deserves special emphasis because it is often the first meal eliminated in AN and is often avoided the morning after a binge-purge episode. In addition to structuring meals and snacks, patients should plan structure in their activities. Although overexercising is common in AN, completely prohibiting exercise can lead to further restriction of intake or to surreptitious exercise; inactivity should be limited to situations in which weight loss is dramatic or there is physiologic instability. Also, healthy exercise (once a day, for no more than 45 minutes, at no more than moderate intensity) can improve mood and make increasing calories more acceptable. Because patients with AN often are unaware of their level of activity and tend toward progressively increasing their output, exercising without either a partner or supervision is not recommended.

Table 26-7 INDICATIONS FOR IN-PATIENT MEDICAL HOSPITALIZATION OF PATIENTS WITH ANOREXIA NERVOSA

PHYSICAL AND LABORATORY
Heart rate <45 beats/min
Other cardiac rhythm disturbances
Blood pressure <80/50 mm Hg
Postural hypotension resulting in a >10 mm Hg drop or a >20 beats/min increase
Hypokalemia
Hypophosphatemia
Hypoglycemia
Dehydration
Body temperature <97°F
<80% healthy body weight
Hepatic, cardiac, or renal compromise
PSYCHIATRIC
Suicidal intent and plan
Very poor motivation to recover (in family and patient)
Preoccupation with ego-syntonic thoughts
Coexisting psychiatric disorders
MISCELLANEOUS
Requires supervision after meals and while using the restroom
Failed day treatment

Primary Care Treatment

Follow-up primary care visits are essential in the management of EDs; close monitoring of the response of the patient and the family to suggested interventions is required to determine which patients can remain in primary care treatment (patients with early, mildly disordered eating), which patients need to be referred to individual specialists for co-management (mildly progressive disordered eating), and which patients need to be referred for interdisciplinary team management (EDs). Between the initial and subsequent visits, the patient can record daily caloric intake (food, drink, amount, time, location), physical activity (type, duration, intensity), and emotional state (e.g., angry, sad, worried) in a journal that is reviewed jointly with the patient in follow-up. Focusing on the recorded data helps the clinician to identify dietary and activity deficiencies and excesses as well as behavioral and mental health patterns, and the patient to become objectively aware of the relevant issues to address in recovery.

Given the tendency of patients with AN to overestimate their caloric intake and underestimate their activity level, before reviewing the journal record it is important at each visit to measure weight, without underwear, in a hospital gown after voiding; urine specific gravity; temperature; and blood pressure and pulse in supine, sitting, and standing positions as objective data. In addition, a targeted physical examination focused on hypometabolism, cardiovascular stability, and mental status, as well as any related symptoms, should occur at each visit to monitor progress (or regression).

Referral to Mental Health Services

In addition to referral to a registered dietitian, mental health services are an important element of treatment of EDs. Depending on availability and experience, these services can be provided by a psychiatric social worker, psychologist, or psychiatrist, who should team with the primary care provider. Although patients with AN often are prescribed a selective serotonin reuptake inhibitor (SSRI) because of depressive symptoms, there is no evidence of efficacy for patients at low weight; food remains the initial treatment of choice to treat depression in AN. SSRIs, very effective in reducing binge-purge behaviors regardless of depression, are considered a standard element of therapy in BN. SSRI dosage in BN, however, may need to increase to an equivalent of more than 60 mg of fluoxetine to maintain effectiveness.

Cognitive-behavioral therapy (CBT), which focuses on restructuring "thinking errors" and establishing adaptive patterns of behavior, is more effective than interpersonal or psychoanalytic approaches. **Dialectical behavioral therapy** (DBT), in which distorted thoughts and emotional responses are challenged, analyzed, and replaced with healthier ones, with an emphasis on "mindfulness," requires adult thinking skills and is useful for older patients with BN. **Group therapy** can provide much needed support, but it requires a skilled clinician. Combining patients at various levels of recovery who experience variable reinforcement from dysfunctional coping behaviors can be challenging if group therapy patients compete with each other to be "thinner" or take up new behaviors such as vomiting.

The younger the patient, the more intimately the parents need to be involved in therapy. The only treatment approach with evidence-based effectiveness in the treatment of AN in children and adolescents is **family-based treatment**, exemplified by the Maudsley approach. This 3-phase intensive outpatient model helps parents play a positive role in restoring their child's eating and weight to normal, then returns control of eating to the child who has demonstrated the ability to maintain healthy weight, and then encourages healthy progression in the other domains of adolescent development. Features of effective family treatment include an agnostic approach in which the cause of the disease is unknown and irrelevant to weight gain, emphasizing that parents are *not* to blame for EDs; parents being actively nurturing and supportive of their child's healthy eating while reinforcing limits on dysfunctional habits, rather than an authoritarian food police or complete hands-off approach; and reinforcement of parents as the best resource for recovery for almost all patients, with professionals serving as consultants and advisors to help parents address challenges.

Referral to an Interdisciplinary Eating Disorder Team

The treatment of a child or adolescent diagnosed with an ED is ideally provided by an interdisciplinary team (physician, nurse, dietitian, mental health provider) with expertise treating pediatric patients. Because such teams, often led by specialists in adolescent medicine at medical centers, are not widely available, the primary care provider might need to convene such a team. Adolescent medicine–based programs report encouraging treatment outcomes, possibly related to patients entering earlier into care and the stigma that some patients and parents may associate with psychiatry-based programs. Specialty centers focused on treating EDs are generally based in psychiatry and often have separate tracks for younger and adult patients. The elements of treatment noted earlier (CBT, DBT, and family-based therapy), as well as individual and group treatment should all be available as part of interdisciplinary team treatment. Comprehensive services ideally include intensive outpatient and/or partial hospitalization as well as inpatient treatment. Regardless of the intensity, type, or location of the treatment services, the patient, parents, and primary care provider are essential members of the treatment team. A recurring theme in effective treatment is helping patients and families re-establish connections that are disrupted by the ED.

Inpatient medical treatment of EDs is generally limited to patients with AN, to stabilize and treat life-threatening starvation and to provide supportive mental health services. Inpatient medical care may be required to avoid refeeding syndrome in severely malnourished patients, provide nasogastric tube feeding for patients unable or unwilling to eat, or initiate mental health services, especially family-based treatment, if this has not occurred on an outpatient basis (see Table 26-7). Admission to a general pediatric or hospital unit is advised only for short-term stabilization in preparation for transfer to a medical unit with expertise in treating pediatric EDs. Inpatient psychiatric care of EDs should be provided on a unit with expertise in managing the often challenging behaviors (e.g., hiding or discarding food, vomiting, surreptitious exercise) and emotional problems (e.g., depression, anxiety). Suicidal risk is small, but patients with AN might threaten suicide if made to eat or gain weight in an effort to get their parents to back off.

An ED **partial hospital program** (PHP) offers outpatient services that are less intensive than round-the-clock inpatient care. Generally held 4 to 5 days a week for 6 to 9 hours each session, PHP services typically are group-based and include eating at least two meals as well as opportunities to address issues in a setting that more closely approximates "real life" than inpatient treatment. That is, patients sleep at home and are free-living on weekends, exposing them to challenges that can be processed during the 25 to 40 hours in program, also sharing group and family experiences.

Supportive Care

In relation to pediatric EDs, support groups are primarily designed for parents. Because their daughter or son with an ED often resists the diagnosis and treatment, parents often feel helpless and hopeless. Because of the historical precedent of blaming parents for causing EDs, parents often express feelings of shame and isolation (*www.maudsleyparents.org*). Support groups and multifamily therapy sessions bring parents together with other parents whose families are at various stages of recovery from an ED in ways that are educational and encouraging. Patients often benefit from support groups after intensive treatment or at the end of treatment because of residual body image or other issues after eating and weight have normalized.

PROGNOSIS

With early diagnosis and effective treatment, 80% or more of youth with AN recover: They develop normal eating and weight control habits, resume menses, maintain average weight for height, and function in school, work, and relationships, although some still have poor body image. With weight restored to normal, fertility returns as well, although the weight for resumption of menses (about 92% of average body weight for height) may be lower than the weight for ovulation. The prognosis for BN is less well established, but outcome improves with multidimensional treatment that includes SSRIs and attention to mood, past trauma, impulsivity, and any existing psychopathology. Even less is known about the prognosis for ED-NOS.

PREVENTION

Given the complexity of the pathogenesis of EDs, prevention is difficult. Targeted preventive interventions can reduce risk factors in older adolescents and college-age women. Universal prevention efforts to promote healthy weight regulation and discourage unhealthy dieting have not shown effectiveness in middle-school students. Programs that include recovered patients or focus on the problems associated with EDs can inadvertently normalize or even glamorize EDs and should be discouraged.

BIBLIOGRAPHY

Please visit the Nelson Textbook of Pediatrics *website at www.expertconsult.com for the complete bibliography.*

Chapter 27
Disruptive Behavioral Disorders

Heather J. Walter and David R. DeMaso

The disruptive behavior disorders are a group of mental health problems in children and adolescents characterized by out-of-control anger and/or behavior. These disturbances exist on a dimensional spectrum ranging from subsyndromal (i.e., some symptoms are present, but not enough to meet full diagnostic criteria) to syndromal (i.e., full diagnostic criteria are met).

DESCRIPTION

Oppositional defiant disorder is characterized by a persistent pattern of angry outbursts, arguing, vindictiveness, and disobedience, generally directed at authority figures (such as parents and teachers). To meet the diagnosis, ≥4 of these types of behavior must be more frequent and more severe than children of a given developmental stage normally exhibit (especially when tired, hungry, or under stress), must be present at least 6 mo, and must impair the youth's function at home, at school, or with peers (Table 27-1).

Table 27-1 DSM-IV-TR DIAGNOSTIC CRITERIA FOR OPPOSITIONAL DEFIANT DISORDER

A. A pattern of negativistic, hostile, and defiant behavior lasting at least 6 months, during which four (or more) of the following are present:
1. Often loses temper.
2. Often argues with adults.
3. Often actively defies or refuses to comply with adults' requests or rules.
4. Often deliberately annoys people.
5. Often blames others for his or her mistakes or misbehavior.
6. Is often touchy or easily annoyed by others.
7. Is often angry and resentful.
8. Is often spiteful or vindictive.

Note: Consider a criterion met only if the behavior occurs more frequently than is typically observed in individuals of comparable age and developmental level.

B. The disturbance in behavior causes clinically significant impairment in social, academic, or occupational functioning.

C. The behaviors do not occur exclusively during the course of a Psychotic or Mood Disorder.

D. Criteria are not met for Conduct Disorder, and, if the individual is age 18 years or older, criteria are not met for Antisocial Personality Disorder.

From American Psychiatric Association: *Diagnostic and statistical manual of mental disorders, fourth edition, text revision,* Washington, DC, 2000, American Psychiatric Association.

Conduct disorder is characterized by a persistent pattern of serious rule-violating behavior, including behaviors that harm (or have the potential to harm) others. The patient with conduct disorder typically shows little concern for the rights or needs of others. The symptoms of conduct disorder are divided into 4 major categories: physical aggression to people and animals including bullying, fighting, weapon carrying, cruelty to animals, and sexual aggression; destruction of property, including firesetting and breaking and entering; deceitfulness and theft; and serious rule violations, including running away from home, staying out late at night without permission, and truancy. To meet the diagnosis, ≥3 of these symptoms must be present at least 1 year (1 or more in the past 6 mo) and must impair the youth's function at home, at school, or with peers (Table 27-2).

Disruptive behavior disorder, not otherwise specified (subsyndromal disruptive behavior) is diagnosed when some symptoms of disruptive behavior disorders are present, but not enough to meet full diagnostic criteria for oppositional defiant disorder or conduct disorder.

EPIDEMIOLOGY

Estimates of the prevalence of the disruptive behavior disorders vary according to the methodologic characteristics of the study. Recent surveys using *Diagnostic and Statistical Manual of Mental Disorders, Fourth Edition* (DSM-IV) criteria suggests a point prevalence of oppositional defiant disorder and conduct disorder together of 5%. The male:female ratio is estimated at 3:1 to 5:1. Both disorders are believed to be more common in sociodemographically disadvantaged, urban populations.

DIFFERENTIAL DIAGNOSIS

Although oppositional defiant disorder and conduct disorder share a number of characteristics, oppositional defiant disorder can be distinguished from conduct disorder by the absence of physical aggression and other severe forms of antisocial behavior. When the youth's pattern of behavior meets the criteria for both oppositional defiant disorder and conduct disorder, the diagnosis of conduct disorder takes precedence. Other diagnoses to consider in the differential include attention-deficit/hyperactivity disorder (ADHD) (Chapter 30), bipolar disorder (Chapter 24), developmental disorders (Chapter 28), and communication disorders (Chapter 32), in which anger and disruptive behavior can be associated symptoms.

Table 27-2 DSM-IV-TR DIAGNOSTIC CRITERIA FOR CONDUCT DISORDER

A. A repetitive and persistent pattern of behavior in which the basic rights of others or major age-appropriate societal norms or rules are violated, as manifested by the presence of three (or more) of the following criteria in the past 12 months, with at least one criterion present in the past 6 months:

AGGRESSION TO PEOPLE AND ANIMALS
1. Often bullies, threatens, or intimidates others.
2. Often initiates physical fights.
3. Has used a weapon that can cause serious physical harm to others (e.g., a bat, brick, broken bottle, knife, gun).
4. Has been physically cruel to people.
5. Has been physically cruel to animals.
6. Has stolen while confronting a victim (e.g., mugging, purse snatching, extortion, armed robbery).
7. Has forced someone into sexual activity.

DESTRUCTION OF PROPERTY
8. Has deliberately engaged in fire setting with the intention of causing serious damage.
9. Has deliberately destroyed others' property (other than by fire setting).

DECEITFULNESS OR THEFT
10. Has broken into someone else's house, building, or car.
11. Often lies to obtain goods or favors or to avoid obligations (i.e., "cons" others).
12. Has stolen items of nontrivial value without confronting a victim (e.g., shoplifting, but without breaking and entering; forgery).

SERIOUS VIOLATION OF RULES
13. Often stays out at night despite parental prohibitions, beginning before age 13 years.
14. Has run away from home overnight at least twice while living in parental or parental surrogate home (or once without returning for a lengthy period).
15. Is often truant from school, beginning before age 13 years.

B. The disturbance in behavior causes clinically significant impairment in social, academic, or occupational functioning.

C. If the individual is 18 years or older, criteria are not met for Antisocial Personality Disorder.

Specify Type Based on Age at Onset:

Childhood-Onset Type: onset of at least one criterion characteristic of Conduct Disorder prior to age 10 years.

Adolescent-Onset Type: absence of any criteria characteristic of Conduct Disorder prior to age 10 years.

Specify Severity:

Mild: few if any conduct problems in excess of those required to make the diagnosis and conduct problems cause only mild harm to others.

Moderate: number of conduct problems and effect on others intermediate between "mild" and "severe."

Severe: many conduct problems in excess of those required to make the diagnosis or conduct problems cause considerable harm to others.

From American Psychiatric Association: *Diagnostic and statistical manual of mental disorders, fourth edition, text revision,* Washington, DC, 2000, American Psychiatric Association.

COMORBIDITY

ADHD, anxiety (Chapter 23), depression and bipolar disorders, post-traumatic stress disorder (Chapter 23), substance abuse (Chapter 108), and impulse control, learning, and communication disorders commonly co-occur with oppositional defiant disorder and conduct disorder. Treating comorbidities when they occur enhances the treatment of the disruptive behavior disorders.

CLINICAL COURSE

Oppositional behavior can occur in all children and adolescents from time to time, particularly during the toddler and early teenage periods when autonomy and independence are developmental tasks (see 27.1). Oppositional behavior becomes a concern when it is intense, persistent, and pervasive and when it affects the child's social, family, and academic life.

Some of the earliest manifestations of disruptive behavioral symptoms are stubbornness (3 yr), defiance and temper tantrums (4-5 yr), and argumentativeness (6 yr). Teachers' reports suggest that most disruptive symptoms peak between 8 and 11 years and then decline in frequency.

Approximately 65% of children with oppositional defiant disorder exit from the diagnosis after a 3-yr follow-up. Earlier age at onset of oppositional symptoms conveys a poorer prognosis; preschool children with oppositionality are at heightened risk for the development of other psychiatric disorders (most commonly, ADHD, mood disorders, and anxiety disorders) several years later. An estimated 30% of children with oppositional defiant disorder progress to conduct disorder; the risk of progression is higher with comorbid ADHD.

The onset of conduct disorder can occur in early childhood but usually occurs in late childhood or adolescence. In a majority of patients, the disorder remits by adulthood. A substantial fraction of patients develop antisocial personality disorder as adults. Early onset of conduct disorder, along with high frequency of diverse antisocial acts across multiple settings, predicts a worse prognosis and increased risk for antisocial personality disorder. Patients with conduct disorder also are at risk for the development of mood, anxiety, somatoform, and substance-use disorders as they move into adulthood.

SEQUELAE

The disruptive behavior disorders are associated with a wide range of psychiatric disorders in adulthood and with many other adverse outcomes such as suicidal behavior, delinquency, educational difficulties, unemployment, and teenage pregnancy. The disruptive behaviors often trigger a chain of adverse events (e.g., parental hostility, peer rejection) that heighten the risk for additional adverse events (e.g., conflict with authority, deviant peers) extending through adolescence into adulthood.

ETIOLOGY AND RISK FACTORS

Biologic, psychologic, and social factors all play a role in the etiology and/or course of the disruptive behavior disorders. Among the social risk factors, ineffective parenting strategies is one of the strongest. Ineffective parenting strategies include authoritarian parenting, in which the parent may be harsh and demanding, and inconsistent parenting, in which the parent may give in to the child when the child's demands become coercive. Other social risk factors include ecologic factors such as poverty, social disorganization, community violence, and exposure to stressful life events; peer factors such as association with antisocial friends; and parent/family factors such as parental antisocial behavior, substance use, or depression, lack of parental supervision and involvement, coercive family processes, problematic sibling relationships, marital conflict, family instability, inconsistent discipline, neglect, and outright abuse.

Among the biologic risk factors are a family history of disruptive behavior, ADHD, substance use, and mood, somatization, and personality disorders; prenatal, perinatal, and postnatal insults; cognitive and linguistic impairment (including impaired intellectual capacity, executive function, memory, judgment, and pragmatic language); difficult temperamental characteristics (e.g., inflexibility to change, low threshold for and low tolerance of frustration, a rigid cognitive style, relative imperviousness to rewards and consequences; mood lability, and sensitivities to hunger, fatigue, and sensory inputs): and certain personality characteristics (e.g., impulsivity, novelty seeking, reduced harm avoidance, reduced reward dependence). Neurochemical abnormalities in the serotoninergic, noradrenergic, and dopaminergic systems and low cortisol levels have also been implicated.

Among the psychologic risk factors are impaired attachment to the primary caregiver, impaired social information processing (i.e., habitually misattributing hostile intent), and impaired impulse control.

PREVENTION

A reliable sequence of events leads to the progression of subsyndromal disruptive behavior to oppositional defiant disorder to conduct disorder. This sequence often occurs in the context of a disadvantaged environment and begins with ineffective parenting strategies, followed by academic failure, parental hostility, and peer rejection, which leads to depressed mood, conflict with authority, and involvement in a deviant peer group. Children with difficult temperamental characteristics are more vulnerable to this sequence of events. Prevention efforts that intervene early in this sequence have the greatest chance of success.

In children predisposed to the development of disruptive behavioral disorders, repeated requests for compliance from authority figures often results in escalating anger and argumentativeness until the authority figure relents, thus inadvertently reinforcing the negative behavior. Parenting and teaching these children requires a high level of skill that can be enhanced by child development specialists who can teach parents and teachers effective behavior-management skills. Child-focused social-emotional skills training, which focuses on self-regulation, interpersonal regulation, problem-solving, and decision-making, also can be helpful and can be administered universally to at-risk populations such as disadvantaged preschoolers and students in inner city elementary schools.

EARLY IDENTIFICATION

All children should be screened for out-of-control behavior. A typical screening question would be "Does [name] have trouble controlling [his/her] anger or behavior?" If the question is answered affirmatively, a symptom-rating scale designed for parent report can be administered to standardize the assessment (Chapter 18). If the screening indicates clinically significant behavior symptoms, the pediatric practitioner should refer to a qualified mental health clinician for a comprehensive diagnostic evaluation to determine the presence of disruptive behavioral and other comorbid psychiatric and medical disorders. The evaluation must include assessment of the potential for harm to self or others.

TREATMENT

The treatment for oppositional defiant disorder with the strongest evidence base is parent management training directed at the child's caregivers. Parent management training includes understanding social learning principles, developing a warm, supportive relationship with the child, encouraging child-directed interaction and play, providing a predictable, structured household environment, setting clear and simple household rules, consistently praising and materially rewarding positive behavior, consistently ignoring annoying behavior (followed by praise when the annoying behavior ceases), and consistently giving consequences (such as time out or loss of privileges) for dangerous or destructive behavior. Other important targets for parenting training include understanding developmentally appropriate moods and behavior, managing difficult temperamental characteristics, and obtaining treatment and school-based remediation for comorbid disorders (especially ADHD and learning disorders).

Another treatment for oppositional defiant disorder that has some evidence supporting its effectiveness is social-emotional skills training directed at the child. Social-emotional skills training is targeted at modifiable cognitive, social, and emotional etiologic risk factors for disruptive behavior disorders. Training typically includes introducing a skill, verbally instructing the skill, modeling the skill for the child to observe, role-playing to practice the skill, coaching by the clinician during skill practice, summarizing the skill, and giving homework to practice the skill outside the training situation.

The primary evidence-based treatment for youths with conduct disorder is multisystemic therapy. Multisystemic therapy assumes that antisocial behavior becomes embedded in the life space of the patient; thus treatment involves extensive contact between the therapist and the multiple life contexts of the patient, especially the family, school, and peer group, with the goal of developing competencies and rewarding adaptive behavior. Interventions include social competence training, parent and family skills training, medications, academic engagement and skills building, school interventions and peer mediation, mentoring and after-school programs, and involvement of child-serving agencies.

The role of medication in the treatment of the disruptive behavior disorders primarily is limited to the treatment of comorbidities. There is an emerging evidence base for the utility of stimulants, selective serotonin reuptake inhibitors (SSRIs), valproate, and atypical antipsychotics for reactive, affective, defensive, and impulsive aggression. Because all of these medications are associated with significant side effects, careful monitoring of baseline and follow-up indices is imperative. Side effects include cardiac for stimulants; suicide, behavioral activation for SSRIs; hematologic, hepatic, ovarian, teratogenic for valproate; weight gain, metabolic aberrations (diabetes, hyperlipidemia), and cardiac for the atypical antipsychotics. The dosages for the stimulants, SSRIs, atypical antipsychotics, and valproate used in the treatment of aggression are similar to those used in the treatment of other psychiatric disorders in youths.

Most children and adolescents with a disruptive behavior disorder can be safely and effectively treated in the outpatient setting. Youths with intractable conduct disorder may benefit from residential or specialized foster care treatment.

BIBLIOGRAPHY

Please visit the Nelson Textbook of Pediatrics *website at www.expertconsult.com for the complete bibliography.*

27.1 Age-Specific Behavioral Disturbances

Heather J. Walter and David R. DeMaso

INFANCY AND TODDLERHOOD

Temper tantrums and *breath-holding spells* are common during the 1st yrs of life and are age-typical expressions of frustration or anger. Parents who respond to toddler defiance with punitive anger can reinforce oppositional behavior. Parents are best advised to attempt to avert defiance by giving the child choices; once the child has begun a tantrum, the child can be given a time-out. It is useful to advise parents to tell their child, once he or she is calm, that the reasons for frustration are understandable, but that defiance is not acceptable.

Parents are occasionally concerned about **breath-holding spells.** Although some children hold their breath until they lose consciousness, sometimes leading to a brief seizure, there is no increased risk of seizure disorders in children who have had a seizure during a breath-holding spell. Parents are best advised to ignore breath holding once it has started. Without sufficient reinforcement, breath holding generally disappears.

The first key to the office management of temper tantrums and breath-holding spells is to help parents to intercede before the child is highly distressed. The pediatrician should advise parents to intercede early in defiant behavior by calmly placing the child in time-out for 2-3 min. Iron supplements might reduce recurrent breath-holding spells if anemia is present. When breath holding does not respond to the parent's coaching or is accompanied by head banging or high levels of aggression, referral for a mental health evaluation is indicated.

If behavioral measures such as time-out fail, pediatricians must assess how the parents handle anger before making further recommendations about how to approach the child. Children can be frightened by the intensity of their own angry feelings and by angry feelings they arouse in their parents. Parents should model the anger control that they wish their children to exhibit. Some parents are unable to see that they lose control themselves; their own angry behavior does not help their children to internalize controls. Advising parents to calmly provide simple choices will help the child to feel more in control and to develop a sense of autonomy. Providing the child with options also typically helps reduce the child's feelings of anger and shame, which can later have adverse effects on social and emotional development.

Lying can be used by 2-4 yr olds as a method of playing with the language. By observing the reactions of parents, preschoolers learn about expectations for honesty in communication. Lying can also be a form of fantasy for children, who describe things as they wish them to be rather than as they are. To avoid an unpleasant confrontation, a child who has not done something that a parent wanted may say that it has been done. The child's sense of time and reason does not permit the realization that this only postpones a confrontation.

CHILDHOOD AND ADOLESCENCE

Lying

In **school-aged children,** lying is generally an effort to cover up something that the child does not want to accept in his or her own behavior. The lie is invented to achieve a temporary good feeling and to protect the child against a loss of self-esteem. Habitual lying also can be promoted by poor adult modeling. Many adolescents lie to avoid adults' disapproval; lying may be used as a method of rebellion. Chronic lying can occur in combination with several other antisocial behaviors and is a sign of underlying psychopathology or family dysfunction.

Regardless of age or developmental level, when lying becomes a common way of managing conflict, intervention is warranted. Initially, the parents should confront the child to give a clear message of what is acceptable. Sensitivity and support combined with limit-setting are necessary for a successful intervention. If this behavior cannot be resolved through the parents' understanding of the situation and the child's understanding that lying is not a reasonable alternative, a mental health evaluation is indicated.

Stealing

Many children **steal** something at some point in their lives. When preschoolers and school-aged children steal more than once or twice, the behavior may be a response to stressful environmental circumstances. Stealing can be an expression of anger or revenge for perceived frustrations with parents. In some instances, stealing becomes one way the child or adolescent can manipulate and attempt to control his world. Stealing also can be learned from adults.

It is important for parents to help the child undo the theft by returning the stolen articles or by rendering their equivalent either in money that the child can earn or in services. When stealing is part of a pattern of conduct problems, referral for a mental health evaluation is warranted.

Truancy and Running Away

Truancy and running away are never developmentally appropriate. Truancy may represent disorganization within the home, caretaking needs of younger siblings, developing conduct problems, or emotional problems including depression or anxiety. Whereas younger children may threaten to run away out of frustration or a desire to get back at parents, older children who run away are almost always expressing a serious underlying problem within themselves or their family, including violence, abuse, and neglect. Adolescent runaways are at high risk for substance abuse, unsafe sexual activity, and other risk-taking behaviors.

Fire Setting

Although interest in fire is common in early childhood, unsupervised **fire setting** is always inappropriate. Early school-aged children may set fires accidentally, or because of curiosity or latent hostility. These young children usually set fires by themselves within their homes. In adolescence, fire setting can be a sign of delinquency or a signal of traumatic experiences.

Fire setting always requires intervention by mental health clinicians. A thorough mental health evaluation is necessary to plan the components of a successful treatment program.

Aggression and Bullying (See Also Chapter 36.1)

Aggression and bullying are serious symptoms and are associated with significant morbidity and mortality. Children might not grow out of this behavior; early intervention is indicated for persistent aggressive behavior. Aggressive tendencies are heritable, although environmental factors can promote aggression in susceptible children. Both enduring and temporary stressors affecting a family can increase aggressive behavior in children. Aggression in childhood is correlated with family unemployment, discord, violence, criminality, and psychiatric disorders as well as births to teenage or unmarried mothers. Boys are almost universally reported to be more aggressive than girls. A difficult temperament and later aggressiveness are related, although there is evidence that these children elicit punitive caregiving within the family environment, setting up a cycle of increasing aggression. Aggressive children often misperceive social cues and react with inappropriate hostility toward peers and parents.

Clinically, it is important to differentiate the causes and motives for childhood aggression. Intentional aggression may be primarily instrumental, to achieve an end, or primarily hostile, to inflict physical or psychologic pain. Children who are callous and not empathetic and who are often aggressive require mental health intervention. These children are at high risk for suspension from school and eventual school failure. Learning disorders are common, and aggressive children should be screened. Other forms of psychopathology may be present; in particular, aggressive children with ADHD (Chapter 30) might have oppositional defiant disorder and/or conduct disorder. Some aggressive, impulsive children have bipolar disorder; a family history of bipolar disorder, grandiosity, elation, and cyclic mood disturbance may be evident in the history of these children.

Aggressive behavior in boys is relatively consistent from the preschool period through adolescence; a boy with a high level of aggressive behavior at 3-6 yr of age has a high probability of carrying this behavior into adolescence, especially without effective intervention. The developmental progression of aggression among girls is less well studied. There are fewer girls with physically aggressive behavior in early childhood; interpersonal coercive behavior, especially in peer relationships, is not uncommon among girls and may be related to the development of more physical aggression in adolescence (fighting, stealing).

Children exposed to aggressive models on television, in video games, or in play show more aggressive behavior compared with children not exposed to these models (Chapter 36). Parents' anger and aggressive or harsh punishment model behavior that children might imitate when they are physically or psychologically hurt. Parents' abuse may be transmitted to the next generation by several modes: children imitate aggression that they have witnessed, abuse can cause brain injury (which itself predisposes the child to violence), and internalized rage often results from abuse.

BIBLIOGRAPHY

Please visit the Nelson Textbook of Pediatrics *website at www.expertconsult.com for the complete bibliography.*

Chapter 28
Pervasive Developmental Disorders and Childhood Psychosis

Giuseppe Raviola, Gary J. Gosselin, Heather J. Walter, and David R. DeMaso

The pervasive developmental disorders (PDD) and childhood schizophrenia can be understood as disturbances of brain development with genetic underpinnings. PDD spectrum includes autistic, Asperger's, childhood disintegrative, Rett's, and PDD not otherwise specified (NOS) disorders. Children with these disorders all share the inability to attain expected social, communication, emotional, cognitive, and adaptive abilities (Table 28-1).

28.1 Autistic Disorder

Giuseppe Raviola, Gary J. Gosselin, Heather J. Walter, and David R. DeMaso

CLINICAL MANIFESTATIONS

The core features of autistic disorder (AD) include impairments in 3 symptom domains: social interaction; communication; and developmentally appropriate behavior, interests, or activities (Table 28-2). Stereotypical body movements, a marked need for sameness, and a very narrow range of interests are also common.

Aberrant development of social skills and impaired ability to engage in reciprocal social interactions are hallmark symptoms of AD. Early social skill deficits can include abnormal eye contact, failure to orient to name, failure to use gestures to point or show, lack of interactive play, failure to smile, lack of sharing, and lack of interest in other children. Some children with AD make no eye contact and seem totally aloof, whereas others show intermittent engagement with their environment and can make inconsistent eye contact, smile, or hug. Most children have some impairment in joint attention, which is the ability to use eye contact and pointing for the purposes of sharing experiences with others. These children show deficits in empathy for what another person might be feeling. They also demonstrate deficits in understanding what another person might be thinking, a lack of a theory of mind.

Children with AD vary in their verbal abilities. They can range from being nonverbal to having some speech (e.g., capable of imitating songs, rhymes, or television commercials). Speech might have an odd prosody or intonation and may be characterized by echolalia (imitative repetition of words), pronoun reversal, nonsense rhyming, and other idiosyncratic language forms. Early abnormal language concerns include absent babbling or gestures by 12 mo, absent single words by 16 mo, absent 2-word purposeful phrases by 24 mo, and any loss of language or social skills at any time.

Play skills in AD are typically aberrant, characterized by little symbolic play, ritualistic rigidity, and preoccupation with parts of objects. The child with AD is often withdrawn and spends hours in solitary play, often with restrictive or repetitive interests and behaviors. Ritualistic behavior prevails, reflecting the child's need to maintain a consistent, predictable environment. Tantrum-like rages can accompany disruptions of routine.

Intellectual functioning can vary from mental retardation to superior intellectual functioning in select areas (splinter skills, savant behavior). Some children show typical development in certain skills and can even show areas of strength in specific areas, such as puzzles, art, or music.

Visual scanning of hand and finger movements, mouthing of objects, and rubbing of surfaces can indicate a heightened awareness of and sensitivity to some stimuli, whereas diminished

Table 28-1 PERVASIVE DEVELOPMENTAL DISORDERS AND AUTISM SPECTRUM DISORDERS

AUTISM	ASPERGER'S SYNDROME	RETT'S SYNDROME	CHILDHOOD DISINTEGRATIVE DISORDER	PERVASIVE DEVELOPMENTAL DISORDER—NOT OTHERWISE SPECIFIED
Delayed and disordered communication Atypical social interaction Restricted range of interests Onset before 3 yr of age	Similar to autism except language skills relatively intact Usually not cognitively delayed	Almost always affects girls Regression in skills between 6 and 18 mo of age	Clinically significant regression in skills (language, social skills, bowel and bladder control, play motor skills) before 10 yr of age	Features of 1 of the other autism spectrum disorders, but insufficient for a specific diagnosis

From Manning-Courtney P, Brown J, Molloy CA, et al: Diagnosis and treatment of autism spectrum disorders, *Curr Probl Pediatr Adolesc Health Care* 33:283-312, 2003.

Table 28-2 DSM-IV-TR DIAGNOSTIC CRITERIA FOR AUTISTIC DISORDER

A. A total of six (or more) items from (1), (2), and (3), with at least two from (1), and one each from (2) and (3):
   1. Qualitative impairment in social interaction, as manifested by at least two of the following:
      a. Marked impairment in the use of multiple nonverbal behaviors such as eye-to-eye gaze, facial expression, body postures, and gestures to regulate social interaction
      b. Failure to develop peer relationships appropriate to developmental level
      c. A lack of spontaneous seeking to share enjoyment, interests, or achievements with other people (e.g., by a lack of showing, bringing, or pointing out objects of interest)
      d. Lack of social or emotional reciprocity
   2. Qualitative impairments in communication as manifested by at least one of the following:
      a. Delay in, or total lack of, the development of spoken language (not accompanied by an attempt to compensate through alternative modes of communication such as gesture or mime)
      b. In individuals with adequate speech, marked impairment in the ability to initiate or sustain a conversation with others
      c. Stereotyped and repetitive use of language or idiosyncratic language
      d. Lack of varied, spontaneous make-believe play or social imitative play appropriate to developmental level
   3. Restricted repetitive and stereotyped patterns of behavior, interests, and activities, as manifested by at least one of the following:
      a. Encompassing preoccupation with one or more stereotyped and restricted patterns of interest that is abnormal either in intensity or focus
      b. Apparently inflexible adherence to specific, nonfunctional routines or rituals
      c. Stereotyped and repetitive motor manners (e.g., hand or finger flapping or twisting, or complex whole-body movements)
      d. Persistent preoccupation with parts of objects

B. Delays or abnormal functioning in at least one of the following areas, with onset prior to age 3 years: (1) social interaction, (2) language as used in social communication, or (3) symbolic or imaginative play.

C. The disturbance is not better accounted for by Rett's Disorder or Childhood Disintegrative Disorder.

From American Psychiatric Association: *Diagnostic and statistical manual of mental disorders, fourth edition, text revision,* Washington, DC, 2000, American Psychiatric Association.

responses to pain and lack of startle responses to sudden loud noises reflect lowered sensitivity to other stimuli.

DIAGNOSIS

AD is diagnosed by the clinical examination. The gold standard diagnostic tools are the *Autism Diagnostic Interview—Revised* (ADI-R) and the *Autism Diagnostic Observation Schedule* (ADOS), which require referral to a trained professional for administration.

Neuropsychologic and achievement assessment should include intelligence testing to establish overall cognitive function and eligibility for services. Intelligence, as measured by conventional psychologic testing, falls in the functionally retarded range in 30-60% of children with AD. Deficits in language and socialization often make it difficult to obtain an accurate estimate of a child's intellectual potential. Some children with AD perform adequately in nonverbal tests, and those with developed speech can show adequate intellectual capacity. Separate estimates of verbal and nonverbal (performance) intelligence quotient (IQ) should be obtained. A measure of adaptive functioning such as the *Vineland Adaptive Behavior Scales* is essential to establish priorities for treatment planning.

Critical elements of the evaluation should include a detailed developmental history with a review of communicative and motor milestones, a medical history including discussion of possible seizures, sensory deficits such as hearing or visual impairment, or other medical conditions associated with AD including fragile-X, Prader-Willi, Smith-Lemli-Opitz, Rett's, and Angelman's syndromes, fetal alcohol syndrome, tuberous sclerosis, neurofibromatosis, congenital rubella, or untreated phenylketonuria. The family history should be reviewed for the presence of other developmental disorders. A review of current and past psychotropic medications should include a review of medication dosages and behavioral response, along with adverse effects. The impact of other medications on behavioral status should also be reviewed.

The medical and genetic evaluation of children with PDD must consider a broad range of disorders (Table 28-3). Approximately 20% of children with AD have macrocephaly, but enlarged head size might not be apparent until after the 2nd yr of life. In the absence of dysmorphic features or focal neurologic signs, additional neuroimaging for investigation of macrocephaly is not usually indicated. Multidisciplinary assessment of AD is optimal in facilitating early diagnosis, treatment, and coordinated multiagency collaboration. Evaluations from various other professionals, including a developmental pediatrician or pediatric neurologist, medical geneticist, child and adolescent psychiatrist, speech-language pathologist, occupational or physical therapist, or medical social worker may be indicated.

DIFFERENTIAL DIAGNOSIS

The differential diagnosis includes consideration of the various PDD, mental retardation not associated with PDD (Chapter 33), specific developmental disorders (e.g., of language), early onset psychosis (e.g., schizophrenia), selective mutism, social anxiety (Chapter 23), obsessive-compulsive disorder, stereotypic movement disorder, inhibited-type reactive attachment disorder, and rarely, childhood-onset dementia.

EPIDEMIOLOGY

The incidence of AD has increased steadily over the past 15 yr. There is evidence that the increase in the number of children identified with AD is likely related to changes in the definition of and diagnostic criteria for AD, as well as improvements in the recognition of AD at younger ages. Current estimates of the prevalence rate of all PDD (63.7/10,000) are approximately 1 in 150-160. Disorder-specific prevalence rate estimates includes AD (20.6/10,000), Asperger's disorder (6/10,000), PDD-NOS

Table 28-3 MEDICAL AND GENETIC EVALUATION OF CHILDREN WITH PERVASIVE DEVELOPMENTAL DISORDERS

REQUIRED EVALUATIONS
Careful physical examination to identify dysmorphic physical features
Macrocephaly
Wood's lamp examination for tuberous sclerosis
Formal audiologic evaluation
Lead test; repeat periodically in children with pica
High-resolution karyotype
Molecular DNA testing for fragile X syndrome
CONSIDER IF RESULTS OF ABOVE EVALUATIONS ARE NORMAL, AND IN CHILDREN WITH COMORBID MENTAL RETARDATION
FISH test for region 15q11q13 to rule out duplications in Prader-Willi / Angelman's syndrome region
FISH test for telomeric abnormalities
Test for mutations in *MECP2* gene (Rett's syndrome)
DNA testing for fragile X syndrome
METABOLIC TESTING TO CONSIDER BASED ON OTHER CLINICAL FEATURES
Fasting blood glucose
Plasma amino acids
Ammonia and lactate
Fatty acid profile, paroxysmal
Carnitine
Acylcarnitine, quantitative
Homocysteine
Plasma 7-dehydrocholesterol (Smith-Lemli-Opitz disease screening)
Urine amino acids
Urine organic acids
Urine testing for purines and pyrimidines
Urine acylglycine, random
OTHER TESTING TO CONSIDER BASED ON CLINICAL FEATURES
Liver enzymes
Thyroxine, thyroid-stimulating hormone
Biotinidase
Complete blood cell count
Ceruloplasmin and serum copper
ELECTROENCEPHALOGRAPHY IF THE FOLLOWING CLINICAL FEATURES ARE NOTED
Clinically observable seizures
History of significant regression in social or communication functioning
FISH, fluorescence in situ hybridization.

From Barbaresi WJ, Katusic SK, Voigt R: Autism: a review of the state of the science for pediatric primary care clinicians, *Arch Pediatr Adolesc Med* 160:1169, 2006.

(37.1/10,000), Rett's disorder (0.5-1/10,000 females), and childhood disintegrative disorder (2/100,000). The male : female ratios are estimated to be 4 : 1 for AD and 5 : 1 for Asperger's disorder.

PATHOLOGY

Retrospective analysis of head circumference, in conjunction with MRI studies, has shown differences in the brain structure of children with AD. The head circumference in AD is normal or slightly smaller than normal at birth until 2 mo of age. Afterward children with AD show an abnormally rapid increase in head circumference from 6-14 mo of age, increased brain volume in 2-4 yr olds, increased volume of the cerebellum, cerebrum, and amygdala, and marked abnormal growth in the frontal, temporal, cerebellar, and limbic regions of the brain. Early, accelerated brain growth during the 1st several years of life is followed by abnormally slow or arrested growth, resulting in areas of underdeveloped and abnormal circuitry in parts of the brain. Areas of the brain responsible for higher-order cognitive, language, emotional, and social functions are most affected.

ETIOLOGY

The basis for AD is diverse and complex. Multiple genetic regions (chromosomes 16p11.2, 15q24, 11p12-p13) and gene variants (copy number variation, deletions, microdeletions, duplications, inversions, translocations) potentially contribute to abnormal neuronal and axonal growth, synapse formation, and myelination via gene-gene and gene-environment interactions over the course of prenatal and postnatal development. Inheritance patterns of AD demonstrate a 60% concordance rate for monozygotic twins and no concordance in dizygotic twins. A 4 : 1 male : female AD prevalence ratio suggests a sex-linked mechanism in a significant number of cases. An emerging etiologic hypothesis of AD describes spontaneous paternal or maternal genetic mutations that delete or inactivate areas of the genome affecting early brain development.

In utero toxic insults are also thought to carry the potential to produce disruptions in CNS development that can manifest as mental retardation and autistic symptoms. There is no scientifically substantiated association between the administration of the measles-mumps-rubella vaccine and the development of AD. As yet undiscovered environmental factors cannot be ruled out. There may be genetic associations between AD and premature birth as well as childhood-onset schizophrenia, suggesting possible common core neurobiologic processes for subsets of these two heterogeneous clinical groups.

EARLY IDENTIFICATION

Early identification and intervention of PDD are associated with better outcomes. Several instruments have been developed for screening of PDD in primary care settings including the Checklist for Autism in Toddlers (CHAT), the Modified Checklist for Autism in Toddlers (M-CHAT), and the Pervasive Developmental Disorders Screening Test (PDDST) (Chapter 18) (Fig. 28-1). Failures to meet age-expected language or social milestones are important early red flags for PDD and should prompt an immediate evaluation. Early signs include unusual use of language or loss of language skills, nonfunctional rituals, inability to adapt to new settings, lack of imitation, and absence of imaginary play. Deviations in social and emotional development (such as decreased eye contact, failure to orient to name, and lack of joint attention) can often be detected by 1 yr of age. The absence of expected social, communication, and play behavior often precedes the emergence of odd or stereotypical behaviors or the unusual language usage that is seen in AD in the later years.

TREATMENT

The primary goals of treatment are to maximize the child's ultimate functional independence and quality of life by minimizing the core features of the disorder, facilitating development and learning, promoting socialization, reducing maladaptive behaviors, and educating and supporting families. Educational interventions, including behavioral and habilitative (speech, occupational, and physical) therapies, are the cornerstones of treatment for the PDDs. These interventions address communication, social skills, daily-living skills, play and leisure skills, academic achievement, and maladaptive behaviors.

Model early childhood educational programs for children with PDD can be categorized as behavior analytic, developmental, or structured teaching on the basis of the underlying theoretical orientation. Although programs differ in relative emphasis, they share many common goals, including beginning intervention as early as possible; providing intensive intervention (at least 25 hr/wk, 12 mo/yr) in systematically planned educational activities; providing a low student-to-teacher ratio; including parent training; promoting opportunities for interaction with typically developing peers incorporating a high degree of structure through elements such as a predictable routine, visual activity schedules, and clear physical boundaries; implementing strategies to apply learned skills to new environments and situations; and using curricula that address functional spontaneous communication,

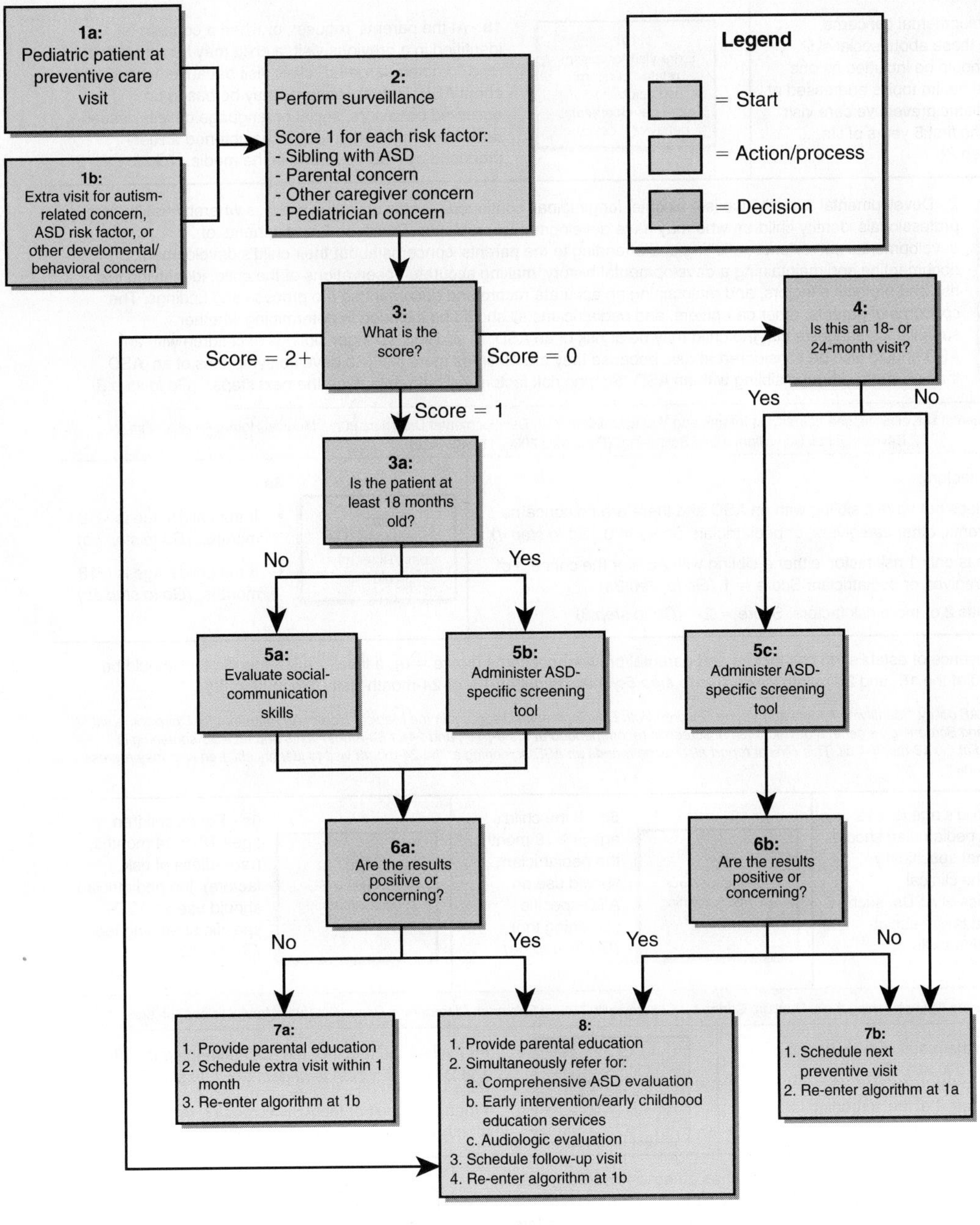

Figure 28-1 Surveillance and screening algorithm: autism spectrum disorders (ASDs). (From Plauche Johnson C, Myers SM, Council on Children with Disabilities: Identification and evaluation of children with autism spectrum disorders, *Pediatrics* 120:1183–1215, 2007.)

Continued

social skills, functional adaptive skills, reduction of maladaptive behaviors, cognitive skills, and traditional academic skills. Some well-regarded programs that address at least some of these skills include Applied Behavioral Analysis (ABA), Discrete Trial Training (DTT), and Treatment and Education of Autistic and related Communication-handicapped Children (TEACCH). Most educational programs available to young children with PDDs are based in communities in the context of an Individualized Education Program (Chapter 15), and offer an eclectic treatment approach, which may be less effective than standardized protocols.

Parent training and family involvement includes educating parents about PDDs, providing access to needed ongoing supports and services, training and involving them as co-therapists, assisting them in advocating for their child's needs, and providing emotional support.

Older children and adolescents with relatively higher intelligence, but with poor social skills and psychiatric symptoms, can benefit from more-intensive behavioral or cognitive-behavioral therapy (CBT) and/or supportive psychotherapy. The focus on achieving social communication competence, emotional and behavioral regulation, and functional adaptive skills necessary for independence continues. Every adolescent should be provided with a school-based individualized transition plan, where the focus may shift from academic to vocational services and from remediating deficits to fostering abilities. A vocational assessment can be helpful in this regard.

Pharmacotherapy can increase the ability of persons with AD to benefit from educational and other interventions and to remain in less-restrictive environments (Table 28-4). Common targets for pharmacological intervention include associated comorbid conditions and problematic behaviors such as aggression, self-injurious behavior, hyperactivity, inattention, anxiety, mood lability, irritability, compulsive-like behaviors, stereotypic behaviors, and sleep disturbances. After treatable medical causes and modifiable environmental factors have been ruled out, a trial of medication may be considered if the behavioral symptoms cause significant impairment in functioning. Prescribing is best approached with

1a:
Pediatric patient at preventive care visit

1a - Developmental concerns, including those about social skill deficits should be included as one of several health topics addressed at each pediatric preventive care visit through the first 5 years of life. *(Go to step 2)*

1b:
Extra visit for autism-related concern, asd risk factor, or other developmental/behavioral concern

1b - At the parents' request, or when a concern is identified in a previous visit, a child may be scheduled for a "problem-targeted" clinic visit because of concerns about ASD. Parent concerns may be based on observed behaviors, social or language deficits, issues raised by other caregivers, or heightened anxiety produced by ASD coverage in the media. *(Go to step 2)*

2:
Perform surveillance

Score 1 for each risk factor:
- Sibling with ASD
- Parental concern
- Other caregiver concern
- Pediatrician concern

2 - Developmental surveillance is a flexible, longitudinal, continuous, and cumulative process whereby health care professionals identify children who may have developmental problems. There are 5 components of developmental surveillance: eliciting and attending to the parents' concerns about their child's development, documenting and maintaining a developmental history, making accurate observations of the child, identifying the risk and protective factors, and maintaining an accurate record and documenting the process and findings. The concerns of parents, other caregivers, and pediatricians all should be included in determining whether surveillance suggests that the child may be at risk of an ASD. In addition, younger siblings of children with an ASD should also be considered at risk, because they are 10 times more likely to develop symptoms of an ASD than children without a sibling with an ASD. Scoring risk factors will help determine the next steps, *(Go to step 3)*

For more information on developmental surveillance, see "Identifying Infants and Young Children With Developmental Disorders in the Medical Home: An Algorithm for Developmental Surveillance and Screening" (Pediatrics 2006; 118:405-420).

3:
What is the score?

3 - Scoring risk factors:
- If the child does not have a sibling with an ASD and there are no concerns from the parents, other caregivers, or pediatrician: Score = 0 *(Go to step 4)*
- If the child has only 1 risk factor, either a sibling with ASD or the concern of a parent, caregiver, or pediatrician: Score = 1 *(Go to step 3a)*
- If the child has 2 or more risk factors: Score = 2+ *(Go to step 8)*

3a:
Is the patient at least 18 months old?

3a -
- If the child's age is <18 months, *(Go to step 5a)*
- If the child's age is ≥18 months, *(Go to step 5b)*

4:
Is this an 18-or 24-month visit?

4 - In the absence of established risk factors and parental/provider concerns (score = 0), a level-1 ASD-specific tool should be administered at the 18- and 24-month visits. *(Go to step 5c)* If this is not an 18- or 24-month visit, *(Go to step 7b).*

Note: In the AAP policy, "Identifying Infants and Young Children With Developmental Disorders in the Medical Home: An Algorithm for Developmental Surveillance and Screening", a general developmental screen is recommended at the 9-, 18-, and 24-or 30-month visits and an ASD screening is recommended at the 18-month visit. This clinical report also recommends an ASD screening at the 24-month visit to identify children who may regress after 18 months of age.

5a:
Evaluate social-communication skills

5a - If the child's age is <18 months, the pediatrician should use a tool that specifically addresses the clinical characteristics of ASDs, such as those that target social-communication skills. *(Go to step 6a)*

5b:
Administer ASD-specific screening tool

5b - If the child's age is ≥18 months, the pediatrician should use an ASD-specific screening tool. *(Go to step 6a)*

5c:
Administer ASD-specific screening tool

5c - For all children ages 18 or 24 months, (regardless of risk factors), the pediatrician should use an ASD-specific screening tool. *(Go to step 6b)*

AAP-recommended strategies for using ASD screening tools: "Autism: Caring for Children with Autism Spectrum Disorders: A Resource Toolkit for Clinicians" (in press)*

6a:
Are the results positive or concerning?

6a - When the result of the screening is *negative*, Go to step 7a

When the result of the screening is *positive*, Go to step 8

6b:
Are the results positive or concerning?

6b - When the result of the ASD screening (at 18- and 24-month visits) is *negative*, Go to step 7b

When the result of the ASD screening (at 18- and 24-month visits) is *positive*, Go to step 8

7a:
1. Provide parental education
2. Schedule extra visit within 1 month
3. Re-enter algorithm at 1b

7a - If the child demonstrates risk but has a negative screening result, information about ASDs should be provided to parents. The pediatrician should schedule an extra visit within 1 month to address any residual ASD concerns or additional developmental/behavioral concerns after a negative screening result. The child will then re-enter the algorithm at 1b. A "wait-and-see" approach is discouraged. If the only risk factor is a sibling with an ASD, the pediatrician should maintain a higher index of suspicion and address ASD symptoms at each preventive care visit, but an early follow-up within 1 month is not necessary unless a parental concern subsequently arises.

7b:
1. Schedule next preventive visit
2. Re-enter algorithm at 1a

7b - If this is not an 18- or 24-month visit, or when the result of the ASD screening is *negative*, the pediatrician can inform the parents and schedule the next routine preventive visit. The child will then re-enter the algorithm at 1a.

8:
1. Provide parental education
2. Simultaneously refer for:
   a. Comprehensive ASD evaluation
   b. Early intervention/early childhood education services
   c. Audiologic evaluation
3. Schedule follow-up visit
4. Re-enter algorithm at 1b

8 - If the screening result is *positive* for possible ASD in step 6a or 6b, the pediatrician should provide peer reviewed and/or consensus-developed ASD materials. Because a positive screening result does not determine a diagnosis of ASD, the child should be referred for a comprehensive ASD evaluation, to early intervention/early childhood education services (depending on child's age), and an audiologic evaluation. A categorical diagnosis is not needed to access intervention services. These programs often provide evaluations and other services even before a medical evaluation is complete. A referral to intervention services or school also is indicated when other developmental/behavioral concerns exist, even though the ASD screening result is negative. The child should be scheduled for a follow-up visit and will then re-enter the algorithm at 1b. All communication between the referral sources and the pediatrician should be coordinated.

AAP information for parents about ASDs includes: "*Is Your One-Year-Old Communicating with You?*"* and "*Understanding Autism Spectrum Disorders.*"*

*Available at www.aap.org

Figure 28-1, cont'd Surveillance and screening algorithm: autism spectrum disorders (ASDs). (From Plauche Johnson C, Myers SM, Council on Children with Disabilities: Identification and evaluation of children with autism spectrum disorders, *Pediatrics* 120:1183–1215, 2007.)

Table 28-4 SELECTED POTENTIAL MEDICATION OPTIONS FOR COMMON TARGET SYMPTOMS OR COEXISTING DIAGNOSIS IN CHILDREN WITH AUTISM SPECTRUM DISORDERS

TARGET SYMPTOM CLUSTERS	POTENTIAL COEXISTING DIAGNOSES	SELECTED MEDICATION CONSIDERATIONS
Repetitive behavior, behavioral rigidity, obsessive-compulsive symptoms	Obsessive-compulsive disorder, stereotypic movement disorder	SSRIs: fluoxetine, fluvoxamine, citalopram, escitalopram, paroxetine, sertraline
Hyperactivity, impulsivity, inattention	Attention-deficit/hyperactivity disorder	Stimulants: methylphenidate, dextroamphetamine, mixed amphetamine salts Atomoxetine Atypical antipsychotic agents: risperidone, aripiprazole, olanzapine, quetiapine, ziprasidone α_2-Agonists: clonidine, guanfacine Mood stabilizers (levetiracetam, topiramate, valproic acid) SSRIs (fluoxetine, fluvoxamine, citalopram, escitalopram, paroxetine, sertraline) β-blockers (propranolol, nadolol, metoprolol, pindolol)
Sleep dysfunction	Circadian rhythm sleep disorder, dyssomnia–not otherwise specified	Melatonin Ramelteon Antihistamines (diphenhydramine, hydroxyzine) α_2-Agonists: clonidine, guanfacine Mirtazapine
Anxiety	Generalized anxiety disorder, anxiety disorder–not otherwise specified	SSRIs (fluoxetine, fluvoxamine, citalopram, escitalopram, paroxetine, sertraline) Buspirone Mirtazapine
Depressive phenotype (marked change from baseline including symptoms such as social withdrawal, irritability, sadness or crying spells, decreased energy, anorexia, weight loss, sleep dysfunction)	Major depressive disorder, depressive disorder–not otherwise specified	SSRIs (fluoxetine, fluvoxamine, citalopram, escitalopram, paroxetine, sertraline) Mirtazapine
Bipolar phenotype (behavioral cycling with rages and euphoria, decreased need for sleep, manic-like hyperactivity, irritability, aggression, self-injury, sexual behaviors)	Bipolar I disorder, bipolar disorder–not otherwise specified	Anticonvulsant mood stabilizers (carbamazepine, gabapentin, lamotrigine, oxcarbazepine, topiramate, valproic acid) Atypical antipsychotic agents (risperidone, aripiprazole, olanzapine, quetiapine, ziprasidone) Lithium

SSRI, selective serotonin reuptake inhibitor.
Modified from Myers SM, Plauche Johnson C, Council on Children with Disabilities: Management of children with autism spectrum disorders, *Pediatrics* 120:1162-1182, 2007.

consultation from a practitioner with background and training in developmental disabilities.

Selective serotonin reuptake inhibitors appear to have efficacy for the treatment of co-occurring mood and anxiety symptoms and compulsive-like behaviors among persons with AD. Of the typical antipsychotics, haloperidol has evidence supporting a role in reducing stereotypy and facilitating learning. There has been concern about its use given the high rates of dyskinesias that are incurred. Given a more favorable side-effect profile in this population, atypical neuroleptics have been increasingly used with demonstrated efficacy on the symptoms of agitation, irritability, aggression, self-injury, and severe temper outbursts (Table 28-5; Chapter 19). Risperidone and aripiprazole have been approved by the U.S. Food and Drug Administration (FDA) for treating irritability associated with autism. In moderate doses, stimulants can benefit children with hyperactivity and impulsivity. α-Adrenergic agonists can reduce hyperarousal symptoms including hyperactivity, irritability, impulsivity, and repetitive behavior. The evidence for mood stabilizers in AD is limited.

PROGNOSIS

Most persons with PDD remain within the spectrum as adults, and regardless of their intellectual functioning, they continue to experience problems with independent living, employment, social relationships, and mental health. Some children, especially those with communication abilities, can grow up to live self-sufficient lives in the community with employment. Others remain dependent on their family or require placement in facilities outside the home. Because early, intensive therapy can improve language and social function, delayed diagnosis can lead to a poorer outcome. A better prognosis is associated with higher intelligence, functional speech,

Table 28-5 DSM-IV-TR DIAGNOSTIC CRITERIA FOR ASPERGER'S DISORDER

A. Qualitative impairment in social interaction, as manifested by at least two of the following:
   1. Marked impairment in the use of multiple nonverbal behaviors such as eye-to-eye gaze, facial expression, body postures, and gestures to regulate social interaction
   2. Failure to develop peer relationships appropriate to developmental level
   3. A lack of spontaneous seeking to share enjoyment, interests, or achievements with other people (e.g., by a lack of showing, bringing, or pointing out objects of interest to other people)
   4. Lack of social or emotional reciprocity
B. Restricted repetitive and stereotyped patterns of behavior, interests, and activities, as manifested by at least one of the following:
   1. Encompassing preoccupation with one or more stereotyped and restricted patterns of interest that is abnormal either in intensity or focus
   2. Apparently inflexible adherence to specific, nonfunctional routines or rituals
   3. Stereotyped and repetitive motor mannerisms (e.g., hand or finger flapping or twisting, or complex whole-body movements)
   4. Persistent preoccupation with parts of objects
C. The disturbance causes clinically significant impairment in social, occupational, or other important areas of functioning.
D. There is no clinically significant general delay in language (e.g., single words used by age 2 years, communicative phrases used by age 3 years).
E. There is no clinically significant delay in cognitive development or in the development of age-appropriate self-help skills, adaptive behavior (other than in social interaction), and curiosity about the environment in childhood.
F. Criteria are not met for another specific Pervasive Developmental Disorder or Schizophrenia.

From American Psychiatric Association: *Diagnostic and statistical manual of mental disorders, fourth edition, text revision,* Washington, DC, 2000, American Psychiatric Association.

and less-bizarre symptoms and behavior. The symptom profile for some children might change as they grow older, and risk of seizures or self-injurious behavior becomes more common.

BIBLIOGRAPHY

Please visit the Nelson Textbook of Pediatrics *website at www.expertconsult.com for the complete bibliography.*

28.2 Asperger's Disorder

Giuseppe Raviola, Gary J. Gosselin, Heather J. Walter, and David R. DeMaso

Children with Asperger's disorder have a qualitative impairment in the development of reciprocal social interaction. They often show repetitive behaviors with restricted, obsessional, and idiosyncratic interests. To meet the DSM-IV-TR diagnostic criteria for Asperger's disorder, a child must manifest impairments in social interactions and show restrictive, repetitive patterns of behavior, interests, or achievements with other people. These disturbances must cause significant impairments in social or occupational functioning (see Table 28-5).

Unlike children with AD, those with Asperger's disorder have a history of normal language milestones with single words used by age 2 yr and communicative phrases used by age 3 yr. They have deficits in nonverbal and pragmatic aspects of communication (facial expressions, gestures) but do not have the severe language delays and impairments that characterize AD. Neuropsychologic testing can reveal a pattern consistent with nonverbal learning disability.

Although they are somewhat socially aware, these children appear to others to be peculiar or eccentric. They can be awkward and clumsy and have unusual postures and gait. There are often similar traits in family members. This disorder might represent a form of high-functioning AD (children with autism without cognitive impairment), although this distinction remains controversial. Group social skills training is an effective intervention. CBT has been useful in patients with associated anxiety, and risperidone can improve negative symptoms similar to those seen in schizophrenia. Because children with Asperger's disorder are at high risk for other psychiatric disorders, particularly mood (Chapter 24) and anxiety disorders (Chapter 23) screening for such problems is an important part of the evaluation.

Children with Asperger's disorder tend to improve symptomatically and functionally as they mature, with superior IQ conveying an improved prognosis. Thirty percent of children with this disorder develop comorbid psychiatric disorders.

A child who has some symptoms but who does not meet full criteria for AD or Asperger's disorder is diagnosed as **PDD Not Otherwise Specified**. This "atypical autism" has a lifelong course with variable outcome and is often associated with comorbid psychiatric disorders.

BIBLIOGRAPHY

Please visit the Nelson Textbook of Pediatrics *website at www.expertconsult.com for the complete bibliography.*

28.3 Childhood Disintegrative Disorder

Giuseppe Raviola, Gary J. Gosselin, Heather J. Walter, and David R. DeMaso

The essential feature of childhood disintegrative disorder (also termed Heller's syndrome, dementia infantilis, or disintegrative psychosis) is a marked regression in multiple areas of functioning following a period of at least 2 yr of apparently normal development.

For the full continuation of this chapter, please visit the Nelson Textbook of Pediatrics *website at www.expertconsult.com.*

28.4 Childhood Schizophrenia

Giuseppe Raviola, Gary J. Gosselin, Heather J. Walter, and David R. DeMaso

The signs and symptoms of schizophrenia in children are classified in the DSM-IV-TR into 2 broad domains of positive and negative symptoms (see Table 28-6 on the *Nelson Textbook of Pediatrics* website at www.expertconsult.com). **Positive symptoms** include hallucinations, delusions, disorganized speech, and/or disorganized or catatonic behavior. **Negative symptoms** include flattening of affect, social withdrawal, loss of motivation, and cognitive impairments. These latter symptoms are related to poorer premorbid functioning and an increased familial risk of schizophrenia. Children with schizophrenia have more-severe premorbid neurodevelopmental abnormalities, increased cytogenetic anomalies, and stronger family histories of psychotic disorders in comparison to their adult counterparts.

For the full continuation of this chapter, please visit the Nelson Textbook of Pediatrics *website at www.expertconsult.com.*

28.5 Psychosis Associated with Epilepsy

Robert M. Kliegman

Psychosis associated with epilepsy has been reported in children and adults and may be more common than expected. Also called schizophrenic-like psychosis of epilepsy, the disorder can manifest delusions, hallucinations, and poor insight. The characterization is complicated by the facts that anticonvulsant drugs can precipitate psychosis and antipsychotic drugs can lower the seizure threshold, producing seizures. In addition, epilepsy may be a risk factor for schizophrenia.

For the full continuation of this chapter, please visit the Nelson Textbook of Pediatrics *website at www.expertconsult.com.*

28.6 Acute Phobic Hallucinations of Childhood

Giuseppe Raviola, Gary J. Gosselin, Heather J. Walter, and David R. DeMaso

Among adults, hallucinations are viewed as synonymous with psychosis and as harbingers of serious psychopathology. In children, hallucinations can be part of normal development or can be associated with nonpsychotic psychopathology, psychosocial stressors, drug intoxication, or physical illness. The first clinical task in evaluating children and adolescents who report hallucinations is to sort out those that are associated with severe mental illness from those that derive from other causes (Fig. 28-2).

CLINICAL MANIFESTATIONS

Hallucinations are perceptions (typically auditory, visual, tactile, or olfactory) that occur in the absence of identifiable external stimuli. Hallucinations can be further categorized as nondiagnostic (such as hearing footsteps, knocking, or one's name) and diagnostic (such as hearing one or more voices saying words other than one's own name).

In children with nonpsychotic hallucinations, the symptoms of psychosis are absent. Nonpsychotic hallucinations commonly occur in the context of severe traumatic stress, developmental difficulties, social and emotional deprivation, parents whose own psychopathology promotes a breakdown in the child's sense of reality, cultural beliefs in mysticism, and unresolved mourning.

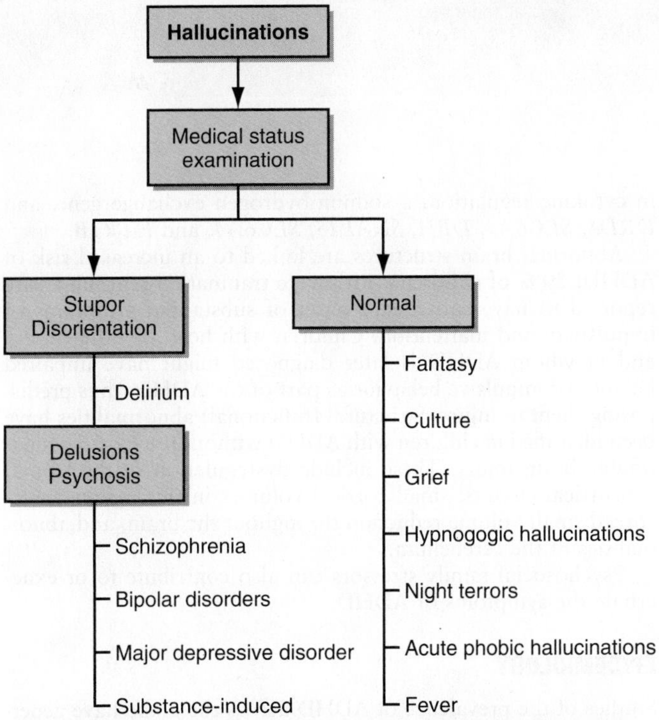

Figure 28-2 Evaluation of hallucinations. (From Kliegman RM, Greenbaum LA, Lye PS: *Practical strategies in pediatric diagnosis and therapy,* ed 2, Philadelphia, 2004, Elsevier/Saunders, p 601.)

Auditory hallucinations of voices telling the child to do bad things may be more often associated with disruptive behavior disorders than with psychotic diagnoses. Hearing a voice invoking suicide is often associated with depression. Trauma-related auditory hallucinations are commonly associated with post-traumatic stress disorder or a brief psychotic disorder with marked stressors. Thus, the content of the hallucinations may be relevant in understanding the underlying psychopathology and/or developmental issues.

DIAGNOSIS AND DIFFERENTIAL DIAGNOSIS

The differential diagnosis of hallucinations comprises a broad range of psychiatric disorders, including diagnoses in which hallucinations are not the hallmark feature, but may be viewed as associated symptoms (e.g., post-traumatic stress disorder, nonpsychotic mood disorders, and disruptive behavior disorders); diagnoses that are defined by psychotic features (e.g., brief psychotic disorder, schizophrenia, major depression with psychotic features, bipolar disorder with psychotic features); and at-risk clinical states (poor reality testing). In addition, nonpsychiatric disorders can manifest with hallucinations, including drug intoxications (cannabis, LSD, cocaine, amphetamines, barbiturates), medication side effects (steroids, anticholinergic medications, stimulant medications), and physical illnesses (thyroid, parathyroid, adrenal, and Wilson's disease; electrolyte imbalance; infections; migraines; seizures; and brain tumors).

Acute phobic hallucinations are benign and common and occur in previously healthy preschool children. The hallucinations are often visual or tactile, last 10-60 min, and occur at any time but most often at night. The child is quite frightened and might complain that bugs or snakes are crawling over him or her and attempt to remove them. The cause is unknown. The differential diagnosis includes drug overdose or poisoning, high fever, encephalitis, and psychosis. The child's fear is not alleviated by reassurance by the parents or physician, and the child is not amenable to reason. Findings on physical and mental status examinations are otherwise normal. Symptoms can persist for 1-3 days, slowly abating over 1-2 wk. Treatment with benzodiazepines may be beneficial.

TREATMENT

The evaluation of the underlying condition directs the type of treatment needed. Nonpsychotic hallucinations suggest the need for disorder-specific psychotherapy (e.g., trauma-focused CBT for post-traumatic stress disorder) and perhaps adjunctive medication (e.g., an antidepressant for depression or anxiety, or a brief trial of antipsychotic medication). CBT focused on helping the youth understand the origin of the hallucinations and develop coping strategies for stressful situations also may be helpful for older children and adolescents. Psychotic hallucinations suggest the need for antipsychotic medication.

BIBLIOGRAPHY

Please visit the Nelson Textbook of Pediatrics *website at www.expertconsult.com for the complete bibliography.*

PART IV Learning Disorders

Chapter 29
Neurodevelopmental Function and Dysfunction in the School-Aged Child

Desmond P. Kelly and Mindo J. Natale

A **neurodevelopmental function** is a basic brain process needed for learning and productivity. **Neurodevelopmental variation** refers to differences in neurodevelopmental functioning. Wide variations in these functions exist within and between individuals. These differences can change over time and need not represent pathology or abnormality. **Neurodevelopmental dysfunctions** reflect disruptions of neuroanatomic structure or psychophysiologic function that may be associated with problems related to cognition, academics, and/or behavioral, emotional, social, and adaptive functioning.

For the full continuation of this chapter, please visit the Nelson Textbook of Pediatrics *website at www.expertconsult.com.*

Chapter 30
Attention-Deficit/Hyperactivity Disorder

Natoshia Raishevich Cunningham and Peter Jensen

Attention-deficit/hyperactivity disorder (ADHD) is the most common neurobehavioral disorder of childhood, among the most prevalent chronic health conditions affecting school-aged children, and the most extensively studied mental disorder of childhood. ADHD is characterized by inattention, including increased distractibility and difficulty sustaining attention; poor impulse control and decreased self-inhibitory capacity; and motor overactivity and motor restlessness (Table 30-1). Definitions vary in different countries (Table 30-2). Affected children commonly experience academic underachievement, problems with interpersonal relationships with family members and peers, and low self-esteem. ADHD often co-occurs with other emotional, behavioral, language, and learning disorders (Table 30-3).

ETIOLOGY

No single factor determines the expression of ADHD; ADHD may be a final common pathway for a variety of complex brain developmental processes. Mothers of children with ADHD are more likely to experience birth complications, such as toxemia, lengthy labor, and complicated delivery. Maternal drug use has also been identified as a risk factor in the development of ADHD. Maternal smoking and alcohol use during pregnancy and prenatal or postnatal exposure to lead are commonly linked to attentional difficulties associated with the development of ADHD. Food colorings and preservatives have inconsistently been associated with hyperactivity in previously hyperactive children.

There is a strong genetic component to ADHD. Genetic studies have primarily implicated 2 candidate genes, the dopamine transporter gene *(DAT1)* and a particular form of the dopamine 4 receptor gene *(DRD4)*, in the development of ADHD. Additional genes that might contribute to ADHD include *DOCK2* associated with a pericentric inversion 46N inv(3)(p14:q21) involved in cytokine regulation, a sodium-hydrogen exchange gene, and *DRD5, SLC6A3, DBH, SNAP25, SLC6A4,* and *HTR1B.*

Abnormal brain structures are linked to an increased risk of ADHD; 20% of children with severe traumatic brain injury are reported to have subsequent onset of substantial symptoms of impulsivity and inattention. Children with head or other injury and in whom ADHD is later diagnosed might have impaired balance or impulsive behavior as part of the ADHD, thus predisposing them to injury. Structural (functional) abnormalities have been identified in children with ADHD without pre-existing identifiable brain injury. These include dysregulation of the frontal subcortical circuits, small cortical volumes in this region, widespread small-volume reduction throughout the brain, and abnormalities of the cerebellum.

Psychosocial family stressors can also contribute to or exacerbate the symptoms of ADHD.

EPIDEMIOLOGY

Studies of the prevalence of ADHD across the globe have generally reported that 5-10% of school-aged children are affected, although rates vary considerably by country, perhaps in part due to differing sampling and testing techniques. Rates may be higher if symptoms (inattention, impulsivity, hyperactivity) are considered in the absence of functional impairment. The prevalence rate in adolescent samples is 2-6%. Approximately 2% of adults have ADHD. ADHD is often underdiagnosed in children and adolescents. Youth with ADHD are often undertreated with respect to what is known about the needed and appropriate doses of medications. Many children with ADHD also present with comorbid psychiatric diagnoses, including opposition defiant disorder, conduct disorder, learning disabilities, and anxiety disorders (see Table 30-3).

PATHOGENESIS

For the full continuation of this topic, please visit the Nelson Textbook of Pediatrics *website at www.expertconsult.com.*

CLINICAL MANIFESTATIONS

Development of the *Diagnostic and Statistical Manual of Mental Disorders*, 4th edition (DSM-IV) criteria leading to the diagnosis of ADHD has occurred mainly in field trials with children 5-12 yr of age (see Table 30-1). The current DSM-IV criteria state that the behavior must be developmentally inappropriate (substantially different from that of other children of the same age and developmental level), must begin before age 7 yr, must be present for at least 6 mo, must be present in 2 or more settings, and must not be secondary to another disorder. DSM-IV identifies 3 subtypes of ADHD. The 1st subtype, *attention-deficit/hyperactivity disorder, predominantly inattentive type,* often includes cognitive impairment and is more common in females. The other 2 subtypes, *attention-deficit/hyperactivity disorder, predominantly hyperactive-impulsive type,* and *attention deficit/hyperactivity disorder, combined type,* are more commonly diagnosed in males. Clinical manifestations of ADHD may change with age. The symptoms may vary from motor restlessness and aggressive and disruptive behavior, which are common in preschool children, to disorganized, distractible, and inattentive symptoms, which are more typical in older adolescents and adults. ADHD is often difficult to diagnose in preschoolers because distractibility and

Table 30-1 DSM-IV DIAGNOSTIC CRITERIA FOR ATTENTION-DEFICIT/HYPERACTIVITY DISORDER

A. **Either 1 or 2** 1. Six (or more) of the following symptoms of inattention have persisted for ≥6 mo to a degree that is maladaptive and inconsistent with development level: Inattention a. Often fails to give close attention to details or makes careless mistakes in schoolwork, work, or other activities b. Often has difficulty sustaining attention in tasks or play activities c. Often does not seem to listen when spoken to directly d. Often does not follow through on instructions and fails to finish schoolwork, chores, or duties in the workplace (not due to oppositional behavior or failure to understand instructions) e. Often has difficulty organizing tasks and activities f. Often avoids, dislikes, or is reluctant to engage in tasks that require sustained mental effort (such as schoolwork or homework) g. Often loses things necessary for tasks or activities (e.g., toys, school assignments, pencils, books, tools) h. Is often easily distracted by extraneous stimuli i. Is often forgetful in daily activities 2. Six (or more) of the following symptoms of hyperactivity-impulsivity have persisted for ≥6 mo to a degree that is maladaptive and inconsistent with developmental level: Hyperactivity a. Often fidgets with hands or feet or squirms in seat b. Often leaves seat in classroom or in other situations in which remaining seated is expected c. Often runs about or climbs excessively in situations in which it is inappropriate (in adolescents or adults, may be limited to subjective feelings of restlessness) d. Often has difficulty playing or engaging in leisure activities quietly e. Is often "on the go" or often acts as if "driven by a motor" f. Often talks excessively Impulsivity g. Often blurts out answers before questions have been completed h. Often has difficulty awaiting turn i. Often interrupts or intrudes on others (e.g., butts into conversations or games) B. Some hyperactive-impulsive or inattentive symptoms that caused impairment were present before 7 yr of age C. Some impairment from the symptoms is present in 2 or more settings (e.g., at school [or work] or at home) D. There must be clear evidence of clinically significant impairment in social, academic, or occupational functioning E. Symptoms do not occur exclusively during the course of a pervasive developmental disorder, schizophrenia, or other psychotic disorder, and are not better accounted for by another mental disorder (e.g., mood disorder, anxiety disorder, dissociative disorder, personality disorder)
CODE BASED ON TYPE
314.01 Attention-deficit/hyperactivity disorder, combined type: if both criteria A1 and A2 are met for the past 6 mo 314.00 Attention-deficit/hyperactivity disorder, predominantly inattentive type: if criterion A1 is met but criterion A2 is not met for the past 6 mo 314.01 Attention-deficit/hyperactivity disorder, predominantly hyperactive-impulsive type: if criterion A2 is met but criterion A1 is not met for the past 6 mo

Reprinted with permission from American Psychiatric Association: *Diagnostic and statistical manual of mental disorders, fourth edition, text revision,* Washington, DC, 2000, American Psychiatric Association. Copyright 2000 American Psychiatric Association.

inattention are often considered developmental norms during this period.

DIAGNOSIS AND DIFFERENTIAL DIAGNOSIS

A diagnosis of ADHD is made primarily in clinical settings after a thorough evaluation, including a careful history and clinical interview to rule in or to identify other causes or contributing factors; completion of behavior rating scales; a physical examination; and any necessary or indicated laboratory tests. It is important to systematically gather and evaluate information from a variety of sources, including the child, parents, teachers, physicians, and, when appropriate, other caretakers.

Table 30-2 DIFFERENCES BETWEEN U.S. AND EUROPEAN CRITERIA FOR ADHD OR HKD

DSM-IV ADHD	ICD-10 HKD
SYMPTOMS	
Either or both of following: At least 6 of 9 inattentive symptoms At least 6 of 9 hyperactive or impulsive symptoms	All of following: At least 6 of 8 inattentive symptoms At least 3 of 5 hyperactive symptoms At least 1 of 4 impulsive symptoms
PERVASIVENESS	
Some impairment from symptoms is present in >1 setting	Criteria are met for >1 setting

ADHD, attention-deficit/hyperactivity disorder; DSM-IV, *Diagnostic and Statistical Manual of Mental Disorders,* 4th edition; HKD, hyperkinetic disorder; ICD-10, *International Classification of Diseases,* 10th edition.
From Biederman J, Faraone S: Attention-deficit hyperactivity disorder, *Lancet* 366:237–248, 2005.

Table 30-3 DIFFERENTIAL DIAGNOSIS OF ATTENTION-DEFICIT/HYPERACTIVITY DISORDER

PSYCHOSOCIAL FACTORS
Response to physical or sexual abuse Response to inappropriate parenting practices Response to parental psychopathology Response to acculturation Response to inappropriate classroom setting
DIAGNOSES ASSOCIATED WITH ADHD BEHAVIORS
Fragile X syndrome Fetal alcohol syndrome Pervasive developmental disorders Obsessive-compulsive disorder Tourette's syndrome Attachment disorder with mixed emotions and conduct
MEDICAL AND NEUROLOGIC CONDITIONS
Thyroid disorders (including general resistance to thyroid hormone) Heavy metal poisoning (including lead) Adverse effects of medications Effects of abused substances Sensory deficits (hearing and vision) Auditory and visual processing disorders Neurodegenerative disorder Post-traumatic head injury Post-encephalitic disorder

Note: Coexisting conditions with possible ADHD presentation include oppositional defiant disorder, anxiety disorders, conduct disorder, depressive disorders, learning disorders, and language disorders. Presence of one or more of the symptoms of these disorders can fall within the spectrum of normal behavior, whereas a range of these symptoms may be problematic but fall short of meeting the full criteria for the disorder.
From Reiff MI, Stein MT: Attention-deficit/hyperactivity disorder evaluation and diagnosis: a practical approach in office practice, *Pediatr Clin North Am* 50:1019–1048, 2003. Adapted from Reiff MI: Attention-deficit/hyperactivity disorders. In Bergman AB, editor: *20 Common problems in pediatrics,* New York, 2001, McGraw-Hill, p 273.

Clinical Interview and History

The clinical interview allows a comprehensive understanding of whether the symptoms meet the diagnostic criteria for ADHD. During the interview, the clinician should gather information pertaining to the history of the presenting problems, the child's overall health and development, and the social and family history. The interview should emphasize factors that might affect the development or integrity of the central nervous system or reveal chronic illness, sensory impairments, or medication use that might affect the child's functioning. Disruptive social factors, such as family discord, situational stress, and abuse or neglect, can result in hyperactive or anxious behaviors. A family history of 1st-degree relatives with ADHD, mood or anxiety disorders, learning disability, antisocial disorder, or alcohol or substance abuse might indicate an increased risk of ADHD and/or comorbid conditions.

Behavior Rating Scales

Behavior rating scales are useful in establishing the magnitude and pervasiveness of the symptoms, but are not sufficient alone to make a diagnosis of ADHD. There are a variety of well-established behavior rating scales that have obtained good results in discriminating between children with ADHD and control subjects. These measures include, but are not limited to, the Vanderbilt ADHD Diagnostic Rating Scale, the Conner Rating Scales (parent and teacher); the ADHD Index; the Swanson, Nolan, and Pelham Checklist (SNAP); and the ADD-H: Comprehensive Teacher Rating Scale (ACTeRS). Other broadband checklists, such as the Achenbach Child Behavior Checklist (CBCL), are useful, particularly in instances where the child may be experiencing co-occurring problems in other areas (anxiety, depression, conduct problems).

Physical Examination and Laboratory Findings

There are no laboratory tests available to identify ADHD in children. The presence of hypertension, ataxia, or a thyroid disorder should prompt further diagnostic evaluation. Impaired fine motor movement and poor coordination and other **soft signs** (finger tapping, alternating movements, finger-to-nose, skipping, tracing a maze, cutting paper) are common, but they are not sufficiently specific to contribute to a diagnosis of ADHD. The clinician should also identify any possible vision or hearing problems. The clinician should consider testing for elevated lead levels in children who present with some or all of the diagnostic criteria, if these children are exposed to environmental factors that might put them at risk (substandard housing, old paint). Behavior in the structured laboratory setting might not reflect the child's typical behavior in the home or school environment. Therefore, reliance on observed behavior in a physician's office can result in an incorrect diagnosis. Computerized attentional tasks and electroencephalographic assessments are not needed to make the diagnosis, and compared to the clinical gold standard they are subject to false-positive and false-negative errors.

Differential Diagnosis

Chronic illnesses, such as migraine headaches, absence seizures, asthma and allergies, hematologic disorders, diabetes, childhood cancer, affect up to 20% of children in the U.S. and can impair children's attention and school performance, either because of the disease itself or because of the medications used to treat or control the underlying illness (medications for asthma, steroids, anticonvulsants, antihistamines) (see Table 30-3). In older children and adolescents, **substance abuse** (Chapter 108) can result in declining school performance and inattentive behavior.

Sleep disorders, including those secondary to chronic upper airway obstruction from enlarged tonsils and adenoids, often result in behavioral and emotional symptoms, although such problems are not likely to be principal contributing causes of ADHD (Chapter 17). Behavioral and emotional disorders can cause disrupted sleep patterns.

Depression and anxiety disorders (Chapters 23 and 24) can cause many of the same symptoms as ADHD (inattention, restlessness, inability to focus and concentrate on work, poor organization, forgetfulness), but can also be comorbid conditions. Obsessive-compulsive disorder can mimic ADHD, particularly when recurrent and persistent thoughts, impulses, or images are intrusive and interfere with normal daily activities. Adjustment disorders secondary to major life stresses (death of a close family member, parents' divorce, family violence, parents' substance abuse, a move) or parent-child relationship disorders involving conflicts over discipline, overt child abuse and/or neglect, or overprotection can result in symptoms similar to those of ADHD.

Although ADHD is believed to result from primary impairment of attention, impulse control, and motor activity, there is a high prevalence of comorbidity with other psychiatric disorders (see Table 30-3). Of children with ADHD, 15-25% have learning disabilities, 30-35% have language disorders, 15-20% have diagnosed mood disorders, and 20-25% have coexisting anxiety disorders. Children with ADHD can also have co-occurring diagnoses of sleep disorders, memory impairment, and decreased motor skills.

TREATMENT

Psychosocial Treatments

Once the diagnosis of ADHD has been established, the parents and child should be educated with regard to the ways ADHD can affect learning, behavior, self-esteem, social skills, and family function. The clinician should set goals for the family to improve the child's interpersonal relationships, develop study skills, and decrease disruptive behaviors.

Behaviorally Oriented Treatments

Treatments geared toward behavioral management often occur in the time frame of 8-12 sessions. The goal of such treatment is for the clinician to identify targeted behaviors that cause impairment in the child's life (disruptive behavior, difficulty in completing homework, failure to obey home or school rules) and for the child to work on progressively improving his or her skill in these areas. The clinician should guide the parents and teachers in implementing rules, consequences, and rewards to encourage desired behaviors. In short-term comparison trials, stimulants have been more effective than behavioral treatments used alone; behavioral interventions are only modestly successful at improving behavior, but they may be particularly useful for children with complex comorbidities and family stressors, when combined with medication.

Medications

The most widely used medications for the treatment of ADHD are the psychostimulant medications, including methylphenidate (Ritalin, Concerta, Metadate, Focalin, Daytrana), amphetamine, and/or various amphetamine and dextroamphetamine preparations (Dexedrine, Adderall, Vyvanse) (Table 30-4). Longer-acting, once-daily forms of each of the major types of stimulant medications are available and facilitate compliance with treatment. The clinician should prescribe a stimulant treatment, either methylphenidate or an amphetamine compound. If a full range of methylphenidate dosages is used, approximately 25% of patients have an optimal response on a low (<20 mg/day), medium (20-50 mg/day), or high (>50 mg/day) daily dosage; another 25% will be unresponsive or will have side effects, making that drug particularly unpalatable for the family.

Over the first 4 wk, the physician should increase the medication dose as tolerated (keeping side effects minimal to absent) to achieve maximum benefit. If this strategy does not yield satisfactory results, or if side effects prevent further dose adjustment in the presence of persisting symptoms, the clinician should use an alternative class of stimulants that was not used previously. If a methylphenidate compound is unsuccessful, the clinician should switch to an amphetamine product. If satisfactory treatment results are not obtained with the 2nd stimulant, clinicians may choose to prescribe atomoxetine, a noradrenergic reuptake inhibitor that is superior to placebo in the treatment of ADHD in children, adolescents, and adults and that has been approved by the U.S Food and Drug Administration (FDA) for this indication. Atomoxetine should be initiated at a dose of 0.3 mg/kg/day and titrated over 1-3 wk to a maximum dosage of 1.2-1.8 mg/kg/day. Guanfacine, an antihypertension agent, is also FDA approved for the treatment of ADHD.

Table 30-4 MEDICATIONS USED IN THE TREATMENT OF ATTENTION-DEFICIT/HYPERACTIVITY DISORDER

GENERIC NAME	BRAND NAME	DURATION	DOSAGE RANGE	SIDE EFFECTS
METHYLPHENIDATE				
Immediate-release	Ritalin, Methylin	3-4 hr	5, 10, 20 mg tabs	Moderate appetite suppression, mild sleep disturbances, transient weight loss, irritability, emergence of tics
Extended-release	Metadate ER, Methylin ER,	4-6 hr	10, 20 mg extended-release tabs	Moderate appetite suppression, mild sleep disturbances, transient weight loss, irritability, emergence of tics
	Metadate-CD	8-10 hr	10, 20, 30 mg extended-release caps	
	Ritalin LA	8-10 hr	20, 30, 40 mg caps	
	Concerta	10-12 hr	18, 27, 36, 54 mg caps	Moderate appetite suppression, mild sleep disturbances, transient weight loss, irritability, emergence of tics
Sustained-release	Ritalin SR, Methylphenidate SR	4-6 hr	20 mg sustained release tabs	Moderate appetite suppression, mild sleep disturbances, transient weight loss, irritability, emergence of tics
Transdermal system	Daytrana	≥12 hr	patch	Moderate appetite suppression, mild sleep disturbances, transient weight loss, irritability, emergence of tics
DEXMETHYLPHENIDATE				
	Focalin	4-6 hr	2.5, 5, and 10 mg tabs	Moderate appetite suppression, mild sleep disturbances, transient weight loss, irritability, emergence of tics
Extended-release	Focalin XR	6-8 hr		Moderate appetite suppression, mild sleep disturbances, transient weight loss, irritability, emergence of tics
DEXTROAMPHETAMINE				
Short-acting	Dexedrine, DextroStat	4-6 hr	5, 10, and 15 mg tabs	Moderate appetite suppression, mild sleep disturbances, transient weight loss, irritability, emergence of tics
Intermediate-acting	Dexedrine Spansule	6-8 hr	5, 10, and 20 mg tabs	Moderate appetite suppression, mild sleep disturbances, transient weight loss, irritability, emergence of tics
Lisdexamfetamine	Vyvanse	≤12 hr	30 mg, 50 mg and 70 mg tablets	Moderate appetite suppression, mild sleep disturbances, transient weight loss, irritability, emergence of tics
MIXED AMPHETAMINE SALTS				
Intermediate-acting	Adderall	4-6 hr	5, 10, 20 mg tabs	Moderate appetite suppression, mild sleep disturbances, transient weight loss, irritability, emergence of tics
Extended-release	Adderall XR	8-12 hr	5, 10, 15, 20, 25, 30 mg caps	Moderate appetite suppression, mild sleep disturbances, transient weight loss, irritability, emergence of tics
ATOMOXETINE				
Extended-release	Strattera	12 hr	10, 18, 25, 40, 60 mg caps	Nervousness, sleep problems, fatigue, stomach upset, dizziness, dry mouth Can lead in rare cases to severe liver injury or to suicidal ideation
Bupropion	Wellbutri	4-5 hr	100 150 mg tabs	Difficulty sleeping, headache, seizures
Bupropion	Wellbutrin SR, Wellbutrin XL		100, 150, 200 mg tabs	
TRICYCLIC ANTIDEPRESSANTS				
Imipramine	Tofranil	Variable	See Table 19-4	Nervousness, sleep problems, fatigue, stomach upset, dizziness, dry mouth, accelerated heart rate
Desipramine*	Norpramin			
Nortriptyline	Aventyl, Pamelor			
α-AGONISTS				
Clonidine		6-12 hr	3-10 μg/kg/day bid-qid	Sedation, depression, dry mouth, rebound hypertension on discontinuing, confusion
Guanfacine	Tenex, Intuniv	6-12 hr	1, 2, 3 mg tabs	Hypotension, lightheadedness

*Has been associated with deaths due to cardiac problems. Not recommended for children.
cap, capsule; tab, tablet.

The clinician should consider careful monitoring of medication a necessary component of treatment in children with ADHD. When physicians prescribe medications for the treatment of ADHD, they tend to use lower than optimal doses. Optimal treatment usually requires somewhat higher doses than tend to be found in routine practice settings. All-day preparations are also useful to maximize positive effects and minimize side effects, and regular medication follow-up visits should be offered (4 or more times/yr) vs the twice-yearly medication visits often used in standard community-care settings.

Medication alone is not always sufficient to treat ADHD in children, particularly in instances where children have multiple psychiatric disorders or stressed home environments. When children do not respond to medication, it may be appropriate to refer them to a mental health specialist. Consultation with a child psychiatrist or psychologist can also be beneficial to determine the next steps for treatment, including adding other components and supports to the overall treatment program. Evidence suggests that children who receive careful medication management, accompanied by frequent treatment follow-up, all within the context of an educative, supportive relationship with the primary care provider, are likely to experience behavioral gains for up to 24 mo.

Stimulant drugs used to treat ADHD may be associated with an increased risk of adverse cardiovascular events, including sudden cardiac death, myocardial infarction, and stroke in young adults and rarely in children. In some of the reported cases, the patient had an underlying disorder, such as hypertrophic obstructive cardiomyopathy, which is made worse by sympathomimetic agents. These events are rare, but they nonetheless warrant

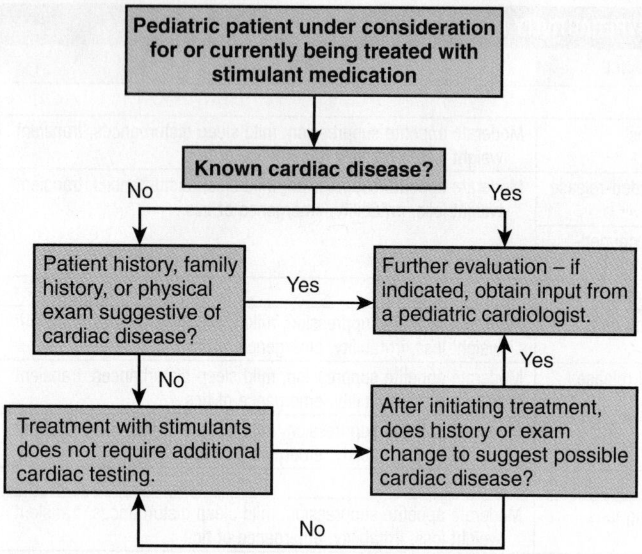
Pediatric patient under consideration for or currently being treated with stimulant medication
Known cardiac disease?
No
Yes
Patient history, family history, or physical exam suggestive of cardiac disease?
Yes
Further evaluation – if indicated, obtain input from a pediatric cardiologist.
Yes
No
Treatment with stimulants does not require additional cardiac testing.
After initiating treatment, does history or exam change to suggest possible cardiac disease?
No

Figure 30-1 Cardiac evaluation of children and adolescents receiving or being considered for stimulant medications. (From Perrin JM, Friedman RA, Knilans TK: Cardiovascular monitoring and stimulant drugs for attention-deficit/hyperactivity disorder, *Pediatrics* 122:451-453, 2008.)

consideration before initiating treatment and during monitoring of treatment with stimulant medications. Children with a positive or personal family history of cardiomyopathy, or arrhythmias, or syncope will require an electrocardiogram and possible cardiology consultation before a stimulant is prescribed (Fig. 30-1).

PROGNOSIS

A childhood diagnosis of ADHD often leads to persistent ADHD throughout the life span. From 60-80% of children with ADHD continue to experience symptoms in adolescence, and up to 40-60% of adolescents exhibit ADHD symptoms into adulthood. In children with ADHD, a reduction in hyperactive behavior often occurs with age. Other symptoms associated with ADHD can become more prominent with age, such as inattention, impulsivity, and disorganization, and these exact a heavy toll on young adult functioning. A variety of risk factors can affect children with untreated ADHD as they become adults. These risk factors include engaging in risk-taking behaviors (sexual activity, delinquent behaviors, substance use), educational underachievement or employment difficulties, and relationship difficulties. With proper treatment, the risks associated with the disorder can be significantly reduced.

PREVENTION

Parent training can lead to significant improvements in preschool children with ADHD symptoms, and parent training for preschool youth with ADHD can reduce oppositional behavior. To the extent that parents, teachers, physicians, and policymakers support efforts for earlier detection, diagnosis, and treatment, prevention of long-term adverse effects of ADHD on affected children's lives should be reconsidered within the lens of prevention. Given the effective treatments for ADHD now available, and the well-documented evidence about the long-term effects of untreated or ineffectively treated ADHD on children and youth, prevention of these consequences should be within the grasp of physicians and the children and families with ADHD for whom we are responsible.

BIBLIOGRAPHY

Please visit the Nelson Textbook of Pediatrics *website at* *www.expertconsult.com* *for the complete bibliography.*

Chapter 31
Dyslexia

G. Reid Lyon, Sally E. Shaywitz, and Bennett A. Shaywitz

Dyslexia is characterized by an unexpected difficulty in reading in persons who otherwise possess the necessary intelligence and motivation that should permit accurate and fluent reading. Dyslexia is the most common of the **learning disabilities**, affecting at least 80% of children identified as manifesting learning disabilities. In attempting to read aloud, most children and adults with dyslexia display an effortful approach to decoding and recognizing single words, an approach in children characterized by hesitations, mispronunciations, and repeated attempts to sound out unfamiliar words. In contrast to the difficulties they experience in decoding single words, persons with dyslexia typically possess the vocabulary, syntax, and other higher-level abilities involved in comprehension.

ETIOLOGY

There are numerous theories regarding the etiology of dyslexia, including those implicating deficits in the temporal processing of auditory and visual stimuli and those that hypothesize language-specific impairments. The latter category posits that at a cognitive-linguistic level, dyslexia reflects deficits within a specific component of the language system, the phonologic module, which is engaged in processing the sounds of speech. As predicted by this model, dyslexic persons have difficulty developing an awareness that words, both spoken and written, can be segmented into smaller elemental units of sound (**phonemes**)—an essential ability given that reading an alphabetic language (English) requires that the reader map or link printed symbols to sound. The linguistic abilities related to learning to read involve phonology, and deficits in phonologic awareness are a strong predictor of dyslexia. There is some evidence that other cognitive processes are involved in reading, including attentional mechanisms, the disruption of which can play a causal role in reading difficulties.

Dyslexia is both familial and heritable. Family history is one of the most important risk factors; approximately 50% of children who have a parent with dyslexia, 50% of the siblings of dyslexic persons, and 50% of the parents of dyslexics may have the disorder. Dyslexia reflects a multifactorial model of the interaction between genetic and environmental factors. Multiple genes can influence the disorder, with each gene individually contributing a small amount of variance and with a single etiologic factor insufficient to cause or explain dyslexia. The neural systems are the final common pathway for multiple influences, and it is unlikely that a single gene or even several genes cause or explain dyslexia.

EPIDEMIOLOGY

Dyslexia may be the most common neurobehavioral disorder affecting children, with prevalence rates ranging from 5-10% in clinic- and school-identified samples to 17.5% in unselected population-based samples in the U.S. and other countries. Dyslexia fits a dimensional model in which reading ability and disability occur along a continuum, with dyslexia representing the lower tail of a normal distribution of reading ability. Dyslexia affects both boys and girls; epidemiologic samples indicate slightly more boys. Dyslexia is a persistent, chronic condition rather than a transient developmental lag. Although dyslexic and poor readers maintain their relative positions along the distribution of reading ability, approaches using focused, early, and intensive intervention provide indications that these trends possibly can be modified. There are no reports of closure of the gap in reading fluency between typical and dyslexic readers, and this goal appears elusive at this time. Furthermore, longitudinal data indicate that in typical readers, intelligence and reading track together and are dynamically linked. In contrast, in dyslexic readers, intelligence and reading are quite separate and are not dynamically linked, providing empirical evidence for the "unexpected" nature of the reading difficulty in dyslexia.

PATHOGENESIS

A range of neurobiologic investigations using primarily functional brain imaging suggest that there are differences in the *left temporo-parieto-occipital brain regions* between dyslexic and nonimpaired readers. Functional brain imaging in both children with dyslexia and adult dyslexic readers demonstrates a failure of the left hemisphere posterior brain systems to function properly during reading, with increased activation in the frontal regions, a pattern referred to as the *neural signature of dyslexia.* Thus, functional brain imaging has for the first time made visible what has always been a hidden disability. These data suggest that rather than the smoothly functioning and integrated reading systems observed in nonimpaired children (Fig. 31-1), inefficient functioning of the posterior reading systems results in dyslexic children's attempting to compensate by shifting to other, ancillary systems, for example, anterior sites, such as the inferior frontal gyrus. In dyslexic readers, inefficient functioning of the posterior reading systems underlies the failure of skilled reading to develop, whereas a shift to ancillary systems supports accurate, but *not* automatic word reading.

CLINICAL MANIFESTATIONS

Reflecting the underlying phonologic weakness, dyslexics manifest problems in both spoken and written language. Spoken language difficulties are typically manifest by mispronunciations, lack of glibness, speech that lacks fluency with many pauses or hesitations and "ums" heard, word-finding difficulties with the need for time to summon an oral response and the inability to come up with a verbal response quickly when questioned; these reflect sound-based, and not semantic or knowledge-based difficulties.

Struggles in decoding and word recognition can vary according to age and developmental level. The cardinal signs of dyslexia observed in school-aged children and adults are a labored, effortful approach to decoding, word recognition, and text reading. Listening comprehension is typically robust. Older children have been found to improve reading accuracy over time, albeit without commensurate gains in reading fluency; they remain slow readers. Difficulties in spelling typically reflect the phonologically based difficulties observed in oral reading. Handwriting is often affected as well.

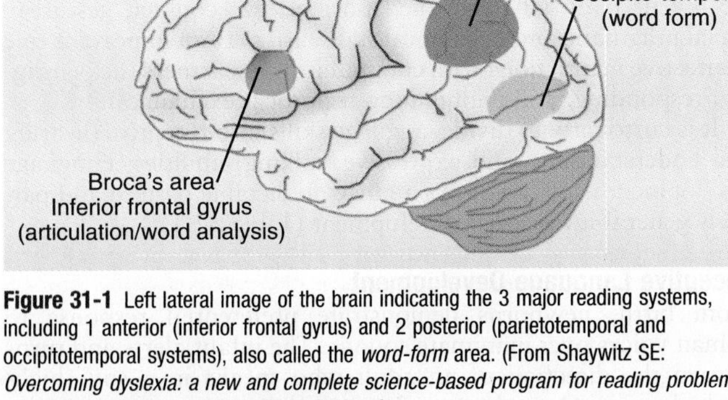

Figure 31-1 Left lateral image of the brain indicating the 3 major reading systems, including 1 anterior (inferior frontal gyrus) and 2 posterior (parietotemporal and occipitotemporal systems), also called the *word-form* area. (From Shaywitz SE: *Overcoming dyslexia: a new and complete science-based program for reading problems at any level,* New York, 2003, Alfred A. Knopf.)

A parental history often identifies early subtle language difficulties in dyslexic children. During the preschool and kindergarten years, at-risk children display difficulties playing rhyming games and learning the names for letters and numbers. Kindergarten assessments of these language skills can help identify children at risk for dyslexia. Although a dyslexic child enjoys and benefits from being read to, he or she might avoid reading aloud to the parent or reading independently.

Anxiety is often present and increases over time. Dyslexia may co-occur with attention-deficit/hyperactivity disorder (Chapter 30); this comorbidity has been documented in both referred samples (40% comorbidity) and nonreferred samples (15% comorbidity).

DIAGNOSIS

Dyslexia is a clinical diagnosis, and history is especially critical. The clinician seeks to determine through history, observation, and psychometric assessment, if there are unexpected difficulties in reading (based on the person's cognitive capacity as shown by age, intelligence, or level of education or professional status) and associated linguistic problems at the level of phonologic processing. There is no single test score that is pathognomonic of dyslexia. The diagnosis of dyslexia should reflect a thoughtful synthesis of all clinical data available.

Dyslexia is distinguished from other disorders that can prominently feature reading difficulties by the unique, circumscribed nature of the phonologic deficit, one that does not intrude into other linguistic or cognitive domains. Family history, teacher and classroom observation, and tests of language (particularly phonology), reading including fluency, and spelling represent a core assessment for the diagnosis of dyslexia in children; additional tests of intellectual ability, attention, memory, general language skills, and mathematics may be administered as part of a more comprehensive evaluation of cognitive, linguistic, and academic function. Once a diagnosis has been made, dyslexia is a permanent diagnosis and need not be reconfirmed by new assessments.

For informal screening, in addition to a careful history, the primary care physician in an office setting can listen to the child read aloud from his or her own grade-level reader. Keeping a set of graded readers available in the office serves the same purpose and eliminates the need for the child to bring in schoolbooks. Oral reading is a sensitive measure of reading accuracy and fluency. The most consistent and telling sign of a reading disability in an accomplished young adult is slow and laborious reading and writing.

It must be emphasized that the failure either to recognize or to measure the lack of fluency in reading is perhaps the most common error in the diagnosis of dyslexia in older children and accomplished young adults. Simple word identification tasks will not detect dyslexia in a person who is accomplished enough to be in honors high school classes or to graduate from college or obtain a graduate degree. Tests relying on the accuracy of word identification alone are inappropriate to use to diagnose dyslexia because they show little to nothing of the struggle to read. It is important to recognize that because they assess reading accuracy but not automaticity (speed), the kinds of reading tests commonly used for school-aged children might provide misleading data on bright adolescents and young adults. The most critical tests are those that are timed; they are the most sensitive in detecting dyslexia in a bright adult. There are few standardized tests for young adult readers that are administered under timed and untimed conditions; the Nelson-Denny Reading Test is an exception. The helpful Test of Word Reading Efficiency (TOWRE) examines simple word reading under timed conditions. Any scores obtained on testing must be considered relative to peers with the same degree of education or professional training.

MANAGEMENT

The management of dyslexia demands a life-span perspective. Early on, the focus is on remediation of the reading problem. Application of knowledge of the importance of early language and phonologic skills leads to significant improvements in children's reading accuracy, even in predisposed children. As a child matures and enters the more time-demanding setting of secondary school, the emphasis shifts to the important role of providing accommodations. Based on the work of the National Reading Panel, evidence-based reading intervention methods and programs are identified. Effective intervention programs provide systematic instruction in 5 key areas: phonemic awareness, phonics, fluency, vocabulary, and comprehension strategies. These programs also provide ample opportunities for writing, reading, and discussing literature.

Taking each component of the reading process in turn, effective interventions improve **phonemic awareness:** the ability to focus on and manipulate phonemes (speech sounds) in **spoken** syllables and words. The elements found to be most effective in enhancing phonemic awareness, reading, and spelling skills include teaching children to manipulate phonemes with letters; focusing the instruction on 1 or 2 types of phoneme manipulations rather than multiple types; and teaching children in small groups. Providing instruction in phonemic awareness is necessary but not sufficient to teach children to read. Effective intervention programs include teaching **phonics,** or making sure that the beginning reader understands how letters are linked to sounds (phonemes) to form letter-sound correspondences and spelling patterns. The instruction should be explicit and systematic; phonics instruction enhances children's success in learning to read, and systematic phonics instruction is more effective than instruction that teaches little or no phonics or teaches phonics casually or haphazardly.

Fluency is of critical importance because it allows the automatic, rapid recognition of words. Although it is generally recognized that fluency is an important component of skilled reading, it is often neglected in the classroom. The most effective method to build reading fluency is a procedure referred to as **guided repeated oral reading:** the teacher models reading a passage aloud, and the student rereads the passage repeatedly to the teacher, another adult, or a peer, receiving feedback until he or she is able to read the passage correctly. Evidence indicates that guided repeated oral reading has some positive effect on word recognition, fluency, and comprehension at a variety of grade levels. The evidence is less clear for programs for struggling readers that encourage large amounts of independent reading, that is, silent reading without any feedback to the student. Thus, even though independent silent reading is intuitively appealing, at this time, the evidence is insufficient to support the notion that in struggling readers, reading fluency improves. In contrast to teaching phonemic awareness, phonics, and fluency, interventions for **vocabulary development and reading comprehension** are not as well established. The most effective methods to teach reading comprehension involve teaching vocabulary and strategies that encourage active interaction between the reader and the text.

For those in high school, college, and graduate school, provision of accommodation rather than remediation most often represents the most effective approach to dyslexia. Imaging studies now provide neurobiologic evidence for the need for extra time for dyslexic students; accordingly, college students with a childhood history of dyslexia require extra time in reading and writing assignments as well as examinations. Many adolescent and adult students have been able to improve their reading accuracy but without commensurate gains in reading speed. Other helpful accommodations include the use of laptop computers with spelling checkers, use of recorded books, access to lecture notes, tutorial services, alternatives to multiple-choice tests, and a separate quiet room for taking tests. In addition, the impact of the primary phonologic weakness mandates special consideration during oral examinations so that students are not graded on their lack of glibness or speech hesitancies but on their content knowledge. Unfortunately, often speech hesitancies or difficulties in word retrieval are wrongly confused with insecure content knowledge. Thus, such "performance" tests are inappropriate for children and adults who are dyslexic.

PROGNOSIS

Application of evidence-based methods to young children (kindergarten to grade 3), provided with sufficient intensity and duration, can result in improvements in reading accuracy and, to a much lesser extent, fluency. In older children and adults, interventions result in improved accuracy but not fluency. Accommodations are critical in allowing the dyslexic child to demonstrate his or her knowledge. Parents should be informed that with proper support, dyslexic children can succeed in a range of future occupations that might seem out of the reach of dyslexic children including medicine, law, journalism, and writing.

BIBLIOGRAPHY

Please visit the Nelson Textbook of Pediatrics *website at www.expertconsult.com for the complete bibliography.*

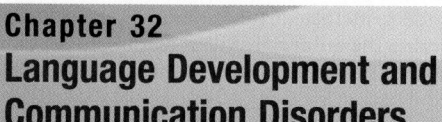

Chapter 32
Language Development and Communication Disorders

Mark D. Simms and Robert L. Schum

For most children, learning to communicate in their native language is a naturally acquired skill whose potential is present at birth. No specific instruction is required, although children must be exposed to a language-rich environment. Normal development of speech and language is predicated on the infant's ability to hear, see, comprehend, and remember. Equally important are sufficient motor skills to imitate oral motor movements, and the social ability to interact with others.

NORMAL LANGUAGE DEVELOPMENT

For the purposes of analysis, language is subdivided into several essential components. **Communication** consists of a wide range of behaviors and skills. At the level of basic verbal ability, **phonology** refers the correct use of speech sounds to form words, **semantics** refers to the correct use of words, and **syntax** refers to the appropriate use of grammar to make sentences. At a more abstract level, verbal skills include the ability to link thoughts together in a coherent fashion and to maintain a topic of conversation. **Pragmatic** abilities include verbal and nonverbal skills that facilitate the exchange of ideas, including the appropriate choice of language for the situation and circumstance and the appropriate use of body language (i.e., posture, eye contact, gestures). Social pragmatic and behavioral skills also play an important role in effective interactions with communication partners (i.e., engaging, responding, and maintaining reciprocal exchanges).

It is customary to divide language skills into receptive (hearing and understanding) and expressive (talking) abilities. Language development usually follows a fairly predictable pattern and parallels general intellectual development (Table 32-1).

Receptive Language Development

From birth, newborns demonstrate preferential response to human voices over inanimate sounds. The infant alerts and turns toward the direction of an adult who speaks in a soft, high-pitched voice. Over the first 3 mo, infants appear to recognize

Table 32-1 NORMAL LANGUAGE MILESTONES

HEARING AND UNDERSTANDING	TALKING
BIRTH TO 3 MONTHS	
Startles to loud sounds Quiets or smiles when spoken to Seems to recognize your voice and quiets if crying Increases or decreases sucking behavior in response to sound	Makes pleasure sounds (cooing, gooing) Cries differently for different needs Smiles when sees you
4 TO 6 MONTHS	
Moves eyes in direction of sounds Responds to changes in tone of your voice Notices toys that make sounds Pays attention to music	Babbling sounds more speech-like, with many different sounds, including *p, b,* and *m* Vocalizes excitement and displeasure Makes gurgling sounds when left alone and when playing with you
7 MONTHS TO 1 YEAR	
Enjoys games such as peekaboo and pat-a-cake Turns and looks in direction of sounds Listens when spoken to Recognizes words for common items, such as *cup, shoe,* and *juice* Begins to respond to requests (*Come here. Want more?*)	Babbling has both long and short groups of sounds, such as *tata upup bibibibi.* Uses speech or noncrying sounds to get and keep attention Imitates different speech sounds Has 1 or 2 words (*bye-bye, Dada, Mama*), although they might not be clear
1 TO 2 YEARS	
Points to a few body parts when asked Follows simple commands and understands simple questions (*Roll the ball. Kiss the baby. Where's your shoe?*) Listens to simple stories, songs, and rhymes Points to pictures in a book when named	Says more words every month Uses some 1-2 word questions (*Where kitty? Go bye-bye? What's that?*) Puts 2 words together (*more cookie, no juice, mommy book*) Uses many different consonant sounds at the beginning of words
2 TO 3 YEARS	
Understands differences in meaning (e.g., go-stop, in-on, big-little, up-down) Follows 2-step requests (*Get the book and put it on the table.*)	Has a word for almost everything Uses 2-3 word "sentences" to talk about and ask for things Speech is understood by familiar listeners most of the time Often asks for or directs attention to objects by naming them
3 TO 4 YEARS	
Hears you when you call from another room Hears television or radio at the same loudness level as other family members Understands simple *who, what, where, why* questions	Talks about activities at school or at friends' homes Usually understood by people outside the family Uses a lot of sentences that have ≥4 words Usually talks easily without repeating syllables or words
4 TO 5 YEARS	
Pays attention to a short story and answers simple questions about it Hears and understands most of what is said at home and in school	Voice sounds as clear as other children's Uses sentences that include details (*I like to read my books.*) Tells stories that stick to a topic Communicates easily with other children and adults Says most sounds correctly except a few, such as *l, s, r, v, z, ch, sh,* and *th* Uses the same grammar as the rest of the family

From American Speech-Language-Hearing Association, 2005. http://professional.asha.org.

their parent's voice and quiet if crying. Between 4 and 6 mo, infants visually search for the source of sounds, again showing a preference for the human voice over other environmental sounds. By 5 mo, infants can passively follow the adult's line of visual regard, resulting in a "joint reference" to the same objects and events in the environment. The ability to share the same experience is critical to the development of further language, social, and cognitive skills. By 8 mo, the infant can actively show, give, and point to objects. Comprehension of words often becomes apparent by 9 mo, when the infant selectively responds to his or her name and appears to comprehend the word "no." Social games, such as "peek-a-boo," "so big," and waving "bye-bye" can be elicited by simply mentioning the words. At 12 mo, many children can follow a simple, one-step request without a gesture (e.g., "Give it to me!").

Between 1 and 2 yr, comprehension of language accelerates rapidly. Toddlers can point to body parts on command, identify pictures in books when named, and respond to simple questions (e.g., "Where's your shoe?"). The 2 yr old is able to follow a 2-step command, employing unrelated tasks (e.g., "Take off your shoes, then go sit at the table"), and can point to objects described by their use (e.g., "Give me the one we drink from"). By 3 yr, children typically understand simple "wh-" question forms (e.g., who, what, where, why). By 4 yr, most children can follow adult conversation. They can listen to a short story and answer simple questions about it. Five yr olds typically have a receptive vocabulary of over 2000 words and can follow 3- and 4-step commands.

Expressive Language Development

Cooing noises are established by 4 to 6 wk of age. Over the first 3 mo of life, parents may distinguish their infant's different vocal sounds for pleasure, pain, fussing, tiredness, etc. Many 3 mo old infants vocalize in a reciprocal fashion with an adult to maintain a social interaction ("vocal tennis"). By 4 mo, infants begin to make bilabial ("raspberry") sounds, and by 5 mo monosyllables and laughing are noticeable. Between 6 and 8 mo, polysyllabic babbling ("lalala" or "mamama") is heard and the infant might begin to communicate with gestures. Between 8 and 10 mo, babbling makes a phonologic shift toward the particular sound patterns of the child's native language (i.e., they produce more native sounds than nonnative sounds). At 9 to 10 mo, babbling becomes truncated into specific words (e.g., "mama," or "dada") for their parents.

Over the next several mo, infants learn 1 or 2 words for common objects and begin to imitate words presented by an adult. These words might appear to come and go from the child's repertoire until a stable group of 10 or more words is established.

The rate of acquisition of new words is approximately 1 new word per wk at 12 mo, but it accelerates to approximately 1 new word per day by 2 yr. The first words to appear are used primarily to label objects (nouns) or to ask for objects and people (requests). By 18 to 20 mo, toddlers should use a minimum of 20 words and produce jargon (strings of word-like sounds) with language-like inflection patterns (rising and falling speech patterns). This jargon usually contains some embedded true words. Spontaneous 2-word phrases (pivotal speech), consisting of the flexible juxtaposition of words with clear intention (e.g., "Want juice!" or "Me down!"), is characteristic of 2 yr olds and reflects the emergence of grammatical ability (syntax).

Two-word, combinational phrases do not usually emerge until the child has acquired 50-100 words in their lexicon. Thereafter, the acquisition of new words accelerates rapidly. As knowledge of grammar increases, there is a proportional increase in verbs, adjectives, and other words that serve to define the relation between objects and people (predicates). By 3 yr, sentence length increases and the child uses pronouns and simple present tense verb forms. These 3-5 word sentences typically have a subject and verb but lack conjunctions, articles, and complex verb forms. The Sesame Street character Cookie Monster ("Me want cookie!") typifies the "telegraphic" nature of the 3 yr old's sentences. By 4-5 yr, children should be able to carry on conversations using adult-like grammatical forms and use sentences that provide details (e.g., "I like to read my books").

Variations of Normal

Language milestones have been found to be largely universal across languages and cultures, with some variations depending on the complexity of the grammatical structure of individual languages. In Italian (where verbs often occupy a prominent position at the beginning or end of sentences), 14 mo olds produce a greater proportion of verbs compared with English speaking infants. Within a given language, development usually follows a fairly predictable pattern, paralleling general cognitive development. Although the sequences are predictable, the exact timing of achievement is not. There are marked variations among normal children in the rate of development of babbling, comprehension of words, production of single words, and use of combinational forms within the first 2-3 yr of life.

Two basic patterns of language learning have been identified: "analytic" and "holistic." The analytic pattern is the most common and reflects the mastery of increasingly larger units of language form. As reflected in the previous discussion of milestones, the child's analytic skills proceed from simple to more complex and lengthy forms. Children who follow a holistic or gestalt learning pattern might start by using relatively large chunks of speech in familiar contexts. They might memorize familiar phrases or dialogs from movies or stories and repeat them in an over-generalized fashion. Their sentences often have a formulaic pattern, reflecting inadequate mastery of the use of grammar to flexibly and spontaneously combine words appropriately in the child's own unique utterance. Over time, these children gradually break down the meanings of phrases and sentences into their component parts, and they learn to analyze the linguistic units of these memorized forms. As this occurs, more original speech productions emerge and the child is able to assemble thoughts in a more flexible manner. Both analytic and holistic learning processes are necessary for normal language development to occur.

LANGUAGE AND COMMUNICATION DISORDERS

Epidemiology

Disorders of speech and language affect up to 8% of preschool-aged children. Nearly 20% of 2 yr olds are thought to have delayed onset of speech. By age 5 yr, 19% of children are identified as having a speech and language disorder (6.4% speech impairment, 4.6% both speech and language impairment, and 8% language impairment). Boys are nearly twice as likely to have an identified speech or language impairment as girls.

Etiology

Normal language ability is a complex function that is widely distributed across the brain through interconnected neural networks that are synchronized for specific activities. Early researchers in language disorders, noting what appeared to be clinical parallels between acquired aphasia in adults and childhood language disorders, expected to find similar lesions in the brains of affected children. For the most part, unilateral, focal lesions acquired in early life do not seem to have the same effects in children as in adults. Furthermore, risk factors for neurologic injury are absent in the vast majority of children with language impairment.

Genetic factors appear to play a major role in influencing how children learn to talk. Language disorders appear to cluster in families. A careful family history may identify current or past speech or language problems in up to 30% of 1st-degree relatives of proband children. Although children who are exposed to parents with language difficulty might be expected to experience poor language stimulation and inappropriate language modeling, studies of twins have shown the concordance rate for low language test score and/or a history of speech therapy to be approximately 50% in dizygotic pairs, rising to over 90% in monozygotic pairs. A number of potential gene loci have been identified, but no consistent genetic markers have been established.

The most plausible genetic mechanism involves a disruption in the timing of early prenatal neurodevelopmental events affecting migration of nerve cells from the germinal matrix to the cerebral cortex. Chromosomal lesions and point mutations of the *FOXP2* gene and polymorphisms of the *CNTNAP2* gene are associated with an uncommon but distinct speech and language disorder characterized by difficulties in learning and producing oral movement sequences (**developmental verbal dyspraxia**, childhood apraxia of speech). Affected children have a spectrum of impairment in expressive and receptive language as well as problems understanding grammar.

Pathogenesis

Language disorders are associated with a fundamental deficit in the brain's capacity to process complex information rapidly. Simultaneous evaluation of words (semantics), sentences (syntax), prosody (tone of voice), and social cues can overtax the child's ability to comprehend and respond appropriately in a verbal setting. Limitations in the amount of information that can be stored in verbal working memory can further limit the rate at which language information is processed. Electrophysiologic studies have shown abnormal latency in the early phase of auditory processing in children with language disorders. Neuroimaging studies have identified an array of anatomic abnormalities in regions of the brain that are central to language processing. MRI scans in children with **specific language impairment (SLI)** can reveal white matter lesions, white matter volume loss, ventricular enlargement, focal gray matter heterotopia within the right and left parietotemporal white matter, abnormal morphology of the inferior frontal gyrus, atypical patterns of asymmetry of language cortex, or increased thickness of the corpus callosum. Postmortem studies of children with language disorders have found evidence of atypical symmetry in the plana temporale and cortical dysplasia in the region of the sylvian fissure. Additionally, some researchers have identified a high incidence of paroxysmal EEG anomalies during sleep in children with SLI. Although these findings might represent a mild variant of the Landau-Kleffner syndrome (acquired verbal auditory agnosia), they likely represent an epiphenomenon in which paroxysmal activity is related to architectural dysplasia. In support of a genetic mechanism affecting cerebral development, a high rate of atypical perisylvian asymmetries has also been documented in the parents of children with SLI.

Clinical Manifestations

Primary disorders of speech and language development are often found in the absence of broader cognitive or motor dysfunction. Disorders of communication are the most common comorbid condition in persons with generalized cognitive disorders (intellectual disability or autism), structural anomalies of the organs of speech (velopharyngeal insufficiency from cleft palate), and neuromotor conditions affecting oral motor coordination (dysarthria from cerebral palsy or other neuromuscular disorders).

Classification

Each professional discipline has adopted a somewhat different classification system, based on cluster patterns of symptoms. One of the simplest classifications is the American Psychiatric Association's *Diagnostic and Statistical Manual of Mental Disorders* (DSM-IV) (Table 32-2). This system recognizes 4 types of communication disorders: expressive language disorder, mixed receptive-expressive language disorder, phonological disorder, and stuttering. In clinical practice, childhood speech and language disorders occur as a number of distinct entities.

Specific Language Impairment

Also referred to as **developmental dysphasia**, or developmental language disorder, SLI is characterized by a significant discrepancy between the child's overall cognitive level (typically nonverbal measures of intelligence) and functional language level. In addition, these children follow an atypical pattern of language acquisition and use. Closer examination of the child's skills might reveal deficits in understanding and use of word meaning (semantics) and grammar (syntax). Often, children with SLI are delayed in starting to talk. Most significantly, they usually have difficulty understanding spoken language. The problem may stem from insufficient understanding of single words or from the inability to deconstruct and analyze the meaning of sentences. Many affected children show a holistic pattern of language development, repeating memorized phrases or dialog from movies or stories (echolalia). In contrast to their difficulty with spoken language, children with SLI appear to learn visually and demonstrate their ability on nonverbal tests of intelligence.

Although they have difficulty interacting with peers who are more verbally adept, many children with SLI play appropriately with younger or older children. Despite their communication impairment, they engage in pretend play, show imagination, share emotions (affective reciprocity), and demonstrate joint referencing behaviors appropriate to their age. Of note is the high incidence of fine-motor coordination difficulty found in these children. A combination of increased joint mobility and mild muscular hypotonia often results in motor clumsiness.

Over time, children with SLI respond to therapeutic/educational interventions and show a trend toward improvement of communication skills. Adults with a history of childhood language disorder continue to show evidence of impaired language ability, even when surface features of the communication difficulty have improved considerably. This suggests that many persons find successful ways of adapting to their impairment.

Many children with SLI show difficulties with social interaction, particularly with same-aged peers. Social interaction is mediated by oral communication, and a child deficient in communication is at a distinct disadvantage in the social arena. Children with SLI tend to be more dependent on older children or adults, who can adapt their communication to match the child's level of function. They might gravitate toward younger children who communicate at a level they can comprehend. Generally, social interaction skills are more closely correlated with language level than with nonverbal cognitive level. Using this as a guide, one usually sees a developmental progression of increasingly

Table 32-2 DSM-IV DIAGNOSTIC CRITERIA FOR COMMUNICATION DISORDERS

EXPRESSIVE LANGUAGE DISORDER
A. The scores obtained from standardized individually administered measures of expressive language development are substantially below those obtained from standardized measures of both nonverbal intellectual capacity and receptive language development. The disturbance may be manifest clinically by symptoms that include having a markedly limited vocabulary, making errors in tense, or having difficulty recalling words or producing sentences with developmentally appropriate length or complexity B. The difficulties with expressive language interfere with academic or occupational achievement or with social communication C. Criteria are not met for mixed receptive-expressive language disorder or a pervasive developmental disorder D. If mental retardation, a speech-motor or sensory deficit, or environmental deprivation is present, the language difficulties are in excess of those usually associated with these problems
Coding note: If a speech-motor or sensory deficit or a neurologic condition is present, code the condition on Axis III
MIXED RECEPTIVE-EXPRESSIVE LANGUAGE DISORDER
A. The scores obtained from a battery of standardized individually administered measures of both receptive and expressive language development are substantially below those obtained from standardized measures of nonverbal intellectual capacity. Symptoms include those for expressive language disorder as well as difficulty understanding words, sentences, or specific types of words, such as spatial terms B. The difficulties with receptive and expressive language significantly interfere with academic or occupational achievement or with social communication C. Criteria are not met for a pervasive developmental disorder D. If mental retardation, a speech-motor or sensory deficit, or environmental deprivation is present, the language difficulties are in excess of those usually associated with these problems
Coding note: If a speech-motor or sensory deficit or a neurologic condition is present, code the condition on Axis III
PHONOLOGICAL DISORDER
A. Failure to use developmentally expected speech sounds that are appropriate for age and dialect (e.g., errors in sound production, use, representation, or organization such as, but not limited to, substitutions of 1 sound for another [use of /t/ for target /k/ sound] or omissions of sounds such as final consonants) B. The difficulties in speech sound production interfere with academic or occupational achievement or with social communication C. If mental retardation, a speech-motor or sensory deficit, or environmental deprivation is present, the speech difficulties are in excess of those usually associated with these problems
Coding note: If a speech-motor a sensory deficit or a neurologic condition is present, code the condition on Axis III
STUTTERING
A. Disturbance in the normal fluency and time patterning of speech (inappropriate for the individual's age), characterized by frequent occurrences of ≥1 of the following: 1. Sound and syllable repetitions 2. Sound prolongations 3. Interjections 4. Broken words (e.g., pauses within a word) 5. Audible or silent blocking (filled or unfilled pauses in speech) 6. Circumlocutions (word substitutions to avoid problematic words) 7. Words produced with an excess of physical tension 8. Monosyllabic whole-word repetitions (e.g., *I-I-I-I see him*) B. The disturbance in fluency interferes with academic or occupational achievement or with social communication C. If a speech-motor or sensory deficit is present, the speech difficulties are in excess of those usually associated with these problems
Coding note: If a speech-motor or sensory deficit or a neurologic condition is present, code the condition on Axis III
COMMUNICATION DISORDER NOT OTHERWISE SPECIFIED
This category is for disorders in communication that do not meet the criteria for any specific communication disorder; for example, a voice disorder (i.e., an abnormality of vocal pitch, loudness, quality, tone, or resonance)

Reprinted with permission from the *Diagnostic and statistical manual of mental disorders,* ed 4, Washington, DC, 1994, American Psychiatric Association, pp 58, 60–61, 63, 65.

more sophisticated social interaction as the child's language abilities improve. In this context, social ineptitude is not necessarily a sign of asocial distancing (e.g., autism) but rather a delay in the ability to negotiate social interactions.

Pragmatic Language Disorder

The ability to communicate effectively with others depends on mastery of a range of skills that go beyond basic understanding of words and rules of grammar. These higher-order abilities include knowledge of the conversational partner, knowledge of the social context in which the conversation is taking place, and general knowledge of the world. Social and linguistic aspects of communication are often difficult to tease apart, and persons who have trouble interpreting these relatively abstract aspects of communication typically experience difficulty forming and maintaining relationships. Symptoms of pragmatic difficulty include extreme literalness and inappropriate verbal and social interactions. Proper use and understanding of humor, slang, and sarcasm depend on correct interpretation of the meaning and the context of language and the ability to draw proper inferences. Failure to provide a sufficient referential base to one's conversational partner—to take the perspective of another person—results in the appearance of talking or behaving randomly or incoherently. Pragmatic language impairment often occurs in the context of SLI, but it has been recognized as a symptom of a wide range of disorders, including right-hemisphere damage to the brain, autism, Asperger's syndrome, Williams syndrome, and nonverbal learning disabilities.

Mental Retardation

Most children with a mild degree of mental retardation learn to talk at a slower than normal rate; they follow a normal sequence of language acquisition and eventually master basic communication skills. Difficulties may be encountered with higher-level language concepts and use. Persons with moderate to severe degrees of cognitive retardation can have great difficulty in acquiring basic communication skills. About half of persons with IQ <50 are able to communicate using single words or simple phrases; the rest are typically nonverbal.

Autism and Pervasive Developmental Disorders

A disordered pattern of language development is one of the core features of autism and other pervasive developmental disorders (Chapter 28). In fact, the language profile of children with autism is indistinguishable from that in children with SLIs. The key points of distinction between these conditions are the lack of reciprocal social relationships that characterizes children with autism, limitation in the ability to develop functional, symbolic, or pretend play, and an obsessive need for sameness and resistance to change. Approximately 75-80% of children with autism are also mentally retarded, and this can limit their ability to develop functional communication skills. Language abilities can range from absent to grammatically intact, but with limited pragmatic features and/or odd prosody patterns. Some autistic persons have highly specialized, but isolated, "savant" skills, such as calendar calculations and hyperlexia (the precocious ability to recognize written words beyond expectation based on general intellectual ability). Regression in language and social skills (**autistic regression**) occurs in approximately one third of children with autism, usually before 2 yr of age. No explanation for this phenomenon has been identified. Once the regression has "stabilized," recovery of function does not usually occur (Fig. 32-1).

Asperger's Syndrome (Chapter 28.2)

Although sharing many characteristics of autism (deficits in social relatedness and restricted range of interests), individuals with Asperger syndrome typically show normal early language development (syntax and semantics). As they mature, higher-order social and language pragmatic impairments become prominent

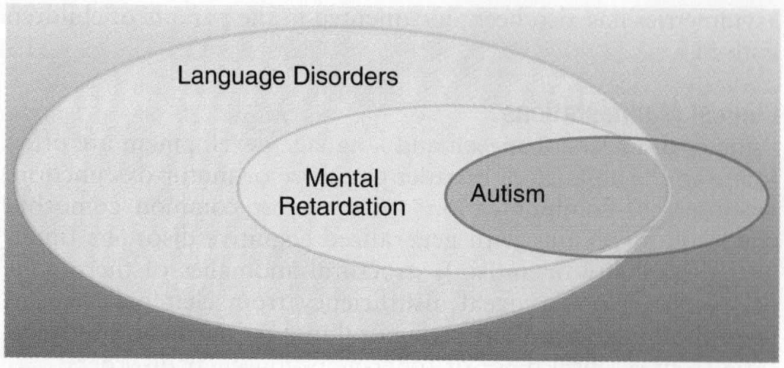

Figure 32-1 Relationship of autism, language disorders, and mental retardation. (From Simms MD, Schum RL: Preschool children who have atypical patterns of development, *Pediatr Rev* 21:147–158, 2000.)

features of this disorder. Affected children have an unusually circumscribed range of interests, which are all-absorbing and interfere with learning of other skills and with social adaptation. These children may engage in long-winded, verbose monologues about their topics of special interest, with little regard to the reaction of others. Their inflection pattern (prosody) may be inappropriate to the content of their conversation, and they might not adjust their rate of speech or vocal volume to the setting.

Selective Mutism

Selective mutism is defined as a failure to speak in specific social situations despite speaking in other situations, and it is typically a symptom of an underlying anxiety disorder. Children with selective mutism can speak normally in certain settings, such as within their home or when they are alone with their parents. They fail to speak in other social settings, such as at school or at other places outside their home. Other symptoms associated with selective mutism can include excessive shyness, withdrawal, dependency on parents, and oppositional behavior. Most cases of selective mutism are not the result of a single traumatic event, but rather are the manifestation of a chronic pattern of anxiety. Mutism is not passive-aggressive behavior. Mute children report that they want to speak in social settings but are afraid to do so. It is important to emphasize that the underlying anxiety disorder is the likely origin of selective mutism. Often, one or both parents of a child with selective mutism has a history of anxiety symptoms, including childhood shyness, social anxiety, or panic attacks. This suggests that the child's anxiety represents a familial trait. For some unknown reason, the child converts the anxiety into the mute symptom. The mutism is highly functional for the child in that it reduces anxiety and protects the child from the perceived challenge of social interaction. Treatment of selective mutism should focus on reducing the general anxiety, rather than focusing only on the mute behaviors (Chapter 23). Selective mutism reflects a difficulty of social interaction and not a disorder of language processing.

Isolated Expressive Language Disorder

More commonly seen in boys than girls, isolated expressive language disorder (late talker syndrome) is a diagnosis best made in retrospect. These children have age-appropriate receptive language and social ability. Once they start talking, their speech is clear. There is no increased risk for language or learning disability as they progress through school. A family history of other males with a similar developmental pattern is often reported. This pattern of language development likely reflects a variation of normal.

MOTOR SPEECH DISORDERS

Dysarthria

Motor speech disorders can originate from neuromotor disorders such as cerebral palsy, muscular dystrophy, myopathy, facial palsy. The resulting dysarthria affects both speech and nonspeech functions (smiling and chewing). Lack of strength and muscular control manifests as slurring of words and distorting of vowels. Speech patterns are often slow and labored. Poor velopharyngeal function can result in mixed nasal resonance (hyper- or hyponasal speech). In many cases, feeding difficulty, drooling, open mouth posture, and a protruding tongue accompany the dysarthric speech.

Verbal Apraxia

Difficulty in planning and coordinating movements for speech production can result in inconsistent distortion of speech sounds. The same word may be pronounced differently each time. Intelligibility tends to decline as the length and complexity of the child's speech increases. Consonants may be deleted and sounds transposed. As they try to talk spontaneously, or imitate other's speech, children with verbal apraxia may display oral groping or struggling behaviors. Often, children with verbal apraxia have a history of early feeding difficulty, limited sound production as infants, and delayed onset of spoken words. They may point, grunt, or develop an elaborate gestural communication system in an attempt to overcome their verbal difficulty. Apraxia may be limited to oral-motor function, or it may be a more generalized problem affecting fine and/or gross motor coordination.

Phonologic Disorder

Children with phonologic speech disorder are often unintelligible, even to their parents. Articulation errors are not the result of neuromotor impairment but seem to reflect an inability to correctly process the words they hear. As a result, they lack understanding of how to fit sounds together properly to create words. In contrast to children with apraxia, those with phonologic disorder are fluent—although unintelligible—and produce a consistent, highly predictable pattern of articulation errors. Children with phonologic speech disorder are at high risk for later reading and learning disability.

Hearing Impairment

Hearing loss can be a major cause of delayed or disordered language development (Chapter 629). Approximately 16-30 per 1,000 children have mild to severe hearing loss, significant enough to affect educational progress. In addition to these "hard of hearing" children, approximately another 1 per 1,000 are deaf (profound bilateral hearing loss). Hearing loss can be present at birth or acquired postnatally. Newborn screening programs can identify many forms of congenital hearing loss, but children can develop progressive hearing loss or acquire deafness after birth.

The most common types of hearing loss are due to conductive (middle ear) or sensorineural deficit. Although it is not possible to accurately predict the impact of hearing loss on a child's language development, the type and degree of hearing loss, the age of onset, and the duration of the auditory impairment clearly play important roles. Children with significant hearing impairment often have problems developing facility with language and often have related academic difficulties. Presumably, the language impairment is caused by lack of exposure to fluent language models starting in infancy.

Approximately 30% of hearing-impaired children have at least one other disability that affects development of speech and language (e.g., mental retardation, cerebral palsy, craniofacial anomalies). Any child who shows developmental warning signs of a speech or language problem should have a hearing assessment by an audiologist and an examination by a geneticist as part of a comprehensive evaluation.

Hydrocephalus

Children with hydrocephalus are described as having "cocktail-party syndrome." Although they may use sophisticated words, their comprehension of abstract concepts is limited, and their pragmatic conversational skills are weak. As a result, they speak superficially about topics and appear to be carrying on a monologue (Chapter 585.11).

RARE CAUSES OF LANGUAGE IMPAIRMENT

Hyperlexia

Hyperlexia is the precocious development of reading single words that spontaneously occurs in some young children (2-5 yr) without specific instruction. It is typically associated with children who have a pervasive developmental disorder (PDD) or SLI. It stands in contrast to precocious reading development in young children who do not have any other developmental disorders. Hyperlexia is a variation seen in young children with disordered language who do not have the social deficits or restricted or repetitive behaviors associated with autism. A typical manifestation is for a child with SLI to orally read single words, or match pictures with single words. Although hyperlexic children show early and well-developed word-decoding skills, they usually have no precocious ability for comprehension of text. Rather, text comprehension is closely intertwined with oral comprehension, and children who have difficulty decoding the syntax of language are also at risk for having reading comprehension problems.

Landau-Kleffner Syndrome (Verbal Auditory Agnosia)

Children with Landau-Kleffner syndrome have a history of normal language development until they experience a regression in their ability to comprehend spoken language (verbal auditory agnosia). The regression may be sudden or gradual, and it usually occurs between 3 and 7 yr of age. Expressive language skills typically deteriorate, and some children may become mute. Despite their language regression, these children typically retain appropriate play patterns and the ability to interact in a socially appropriate manner. An EEG might show a distinct pattern of status epilepticus in sleep (continuous spike-wave in slow-wave sleep), and up to 80% of children with this condition eventually exhibit clinical seizures. A number of treatment approaches have been reported, including antiepileptic medication, steroids, and intravenous gamma globulin, with varying results. The prognosis for return of normal language ability is uncertain, even with resolution of the EEG abnormality, which can represent an epiphenomenon of an underlying brain abnormality.

Metabolic and Neurodegenerative Disorders (See Also Part XI)

Regression of language development may accompany loss of neuromotor function at the outset of a number of metabolic diseases including lysosomal storage disorders (metachromatic leukodystrophy), peroxisomal disorders (adrenal leukodystrophy), ceroid lipofuscinosis (Batten's disease), and mucopolysaccharidosis (Hunter's disease, Hurler's disease). Recently, creatine transporter deficiency was identified as an X-linked disorder that manifests with language delay in boys and mild learning disability in female carriers.

SCREENING

At each well child visit, developmental surveillance should include specific questions about normal language developmental milestones and observations of the child's behavior. Clinical judgment, defined as eliciting and responding to parents' concerns, can detect the majority of children with speech and language problems. Many clinicians employ standardized developmental screening questionnaires and observation checklists designed for use in a pediatrics office (Chapter 14).

The U.S. Preventive Services Task Force reviewed screening instruments for speech and language delays in young children that can be used in primary care settings. The Task Force focused

Table 32-3 SPEECH AND LANGUAGE SCREENING

REFER FOR SPEECH-LANGUAGE EVALUATION IF:

AT AGE	RECEPTIVE	EXPRESSIVE
15 mo	Does not look/point at 5-10 objects	Is not using 3 words
18 mo	Does not follow simple directions ("get your shoes")	Is not using Mama, Dad, or other names
24 mo	Does not point to pictures or body parts when they are named	Is not using 25 words
30 mo	Does not verbally respond or nod/shake head to questions	Is not using unique 2-word phrases, including noun-verb combinations
36 mo	Does not understand prepositions or action words; does not follow 2-step directions	Has a vocabulary <200 words; does not ask for things; echolalia to questions; language regression after attaining 2-word phrases

on brief measures that require <10 minutes to complete. There was insufficient evidence that screening instruments are more effective than using physician's clinical observations and parents' concerns to identify children who require further evaluation. The Task Force noted that there is no single gold standard for screening, owing to inconsistent measures and terminology, and did not recommend the use of screening instruments. Furthermore, the Task Force determined that the use of formal measures was not time or cost efficient and deferred to pediatrician's and parents' concerns as indicators of potential problems. Table 32-3 offers guidelines for raising concerns and referring a child for specialized speech and language evaluation. Because of the high prevalence of speech and language disorders in the general population, referral to a speech-language pathologist for further evaluation should be made whenever there is a suspicion of delay.

NON-CAUSES OF LANGUAGE DELAY

Twinning, birth order, "laziness," exposure to multiple languages (bilingualism), tongue-tie, or otitis media are not adequate explanations for significant language delay. Normal twins learn to talk at the same age as normal single-born children, and birth order effects on language development have not been consistently found. The drive to communicate and the rewards for successful verbal interaction are so strong that children who let others talk for them usually can't talk for themselves and are not "lazy." Toddlers exposed to more than one language can show a mild delay in starting to talk, and they can initially mix elements (vocabulary and syntax) of the different languages they are learning (code switching). However, they learn to segregate each language by 24-30 mo and are equal to their monolingual peers by 3 yr of age. An extremely tight lingual frenulum (tongue-tie) can affect feeding and speech articulation but does not prevent the acquisition of language abilities. Finally, prospective studies have shown that frequent ear infections and/or serous otitis media in early childhood do not result in language disorder.

DIAGNOSTIC EVALUATION

It is important to distinguish developmental delay (abnormal timing) from developmental disorder (abnormal patterns or sequences). A child's language and communication skills must also be interpreted within the context of his or her overall cognitive and physical abilities. Finally, it is important to evaluate the child's use of language to communicate with others in the broadest sense (communicative intent). Thus, a multidisciplinary evaluation is often warranted. At a minimum this should include psychologic evaluation, neurologic assessment, and speech and language examination.

Psychologic Evaluation

There are two main goals for the psychologic evaluation of a young child with a communication disorder. Nonverbal cognitive ability must be assessed to determine if the child is mentally retarded, and the child's social behaviors must be assessed to determine whether autism or a form of PDD is present. Additional diagnostic considerations may include emotional disorders such as anxiety, depression, mood disorder, obsessive-compulsive disorder, academic learning disorders, and attention-deficit/hyperactivity disorder (ADHD).

COGNITIVE ASSESSMENT Mental retardation (intellectual disability) is defined as retardation in development of cognitive abilities and adaptive behaviors. In this context, children with mental retardation show delayed development of communication skills; however, delayed communication does not necessarily signal mental retardation. Therefore, a broad-based cognitive assessment is an important component to the evaluation of children with language delays, including evaluation of both verbal and nonverbal skills. If a child has mental retardation, both verbal and nonverbal scores will be low compared to norms (≤2nd percentile). In contrast, a typical cognitive profile for a child with SLI includes a significant difference between nonverbal and verbal abilities, with nonverbal IQ > verbal IQ and the nonverbal score within an average range.

EVALUATION OF SOCIAL BEHAVIORS Social interest is the key difference between children with a primary language disorder (SLI) and those with a communication disorder secondary to autism or PDD. Children with SLI have an interest in social interaction, but they may have difficulty enacting their interest because of their limitations to communication. In contrast, autistic children show little social interest. Four key nonverbal behaviors that are often shown by children with SLI—but not autistic children (especially toddlers and preschoolers)—are joint attention, affective reciprocity, pretend play, and direct imitation.

RELATIONSHIP OF LANGUAGE AND SOCIAL BEHAVIORS TO MENTAL AGE Cognitive assessment provides a mental age for the child, and the child's behavior must be evaluated in that context. Most 4 yr old children typically engage peers in interactive play, but most 2 yr olds are playful but primarily focused on interactions with adult caretakers. A 4 yr old with mild to moderate mental retardation and a mental age of 2 yr might not play with peers yet because of cognitive limitation, not a lack of desire for social interaction.

Speech and Language Evaluation

A certified speech-language pathologist should perform a speech and language evaluation. A typical evaluation includes assessment of language, speech, and the physical mechanisms associated with speech production. Both expressive and receptive language is assessed by a combination of standardized measures and informal interactions and observations. All components of language are assessed, including syntax, semantics, pragmatics, and fluency. Speech assessment similarly uses a combination of standardized measures and informal observations. Assessment of physical structures includes oral structures and function, respiratory function, and vocal quality. In many settings, a speech-language pathologist works in conjunction with an audiologist, who can do appropriate hearing evaluation of the child. If an audiologist is not available in that setting, then a separate referral should be made. No child is too young for a speech and language or hearing evaluation. A referral for evaluation is appropriate whenever there is suspicion of language impairment.

Medical Evaluation

As in any developmental disorder, careful history and physical examination should focus on the identification of potential contributors to the child's language and communication difficulties. A family history of delay in talking, need for speech and language therapy, or academic difficulty can suggest a genetic predisposition to language disorders. Pregnancy history might reveal risk factors for prenatal developmental anomalies, such as polyhydramnios or decreased fetal movement patterns. Small size for gestational age at birth, symptoms of neonatal encephalopathy, or early and persistent oral-motor feeding difficulty may presage speech and language difficulty. Developmental history should focus on the age at which various language skills were mastered and the sequences and patterns of milestone acquisition. Regression or loss of acquired skills should raise immediate concern.

Physical examination should include measurement of height (length), weight, and head circumference. The skin should be examined for lesions consistent with phakomatosis (e.g., tuberous sclerosis, neurofibromatosis, Sturge-Weber syndrome) and other disruptions of pigment (hypomelanosis of Ito). Anomalies of the head and neck, such as white forelock and hypertelorism (Waardenberg syndrome), ear malformations (Goldenhar syndrome), facial and cardiac anomalies (Williams syndrome, velocardiofacial syndrome), retrognathism of the chin (Pierre-Robin anomaly), or cleft lip and/or palate, are associated with hearing and speech abnormalities. Neurologic examination might reveal muscular hypertonia or hypotonia, both of which can affect neuromuscular control of speech. Generalized muscular hypotonia, with increased range of motion of the joints, is commonly seen in children with SLI. The reason for this association is not clear but it might account for the fine and gross motor clumsiness often seen in these children. However, mild hypotonia is not a sufficient explanation for the impairments of expressive and receptive language.

No routine diagnostic studies are indicated for SLI or isolated language disorders. When language delay is a part of a generalized cognitive or physical disorder, referral for further genetic evaluation, chromosome testing (including high resolution banding karyotype, fragile X testing, and microarray comparative genomic hybridization), neuroimaging studies, and EEG may be considered, if clinically indicated.

TREATMENT

The federal IDEA laws (Individuals with Disabilities Education Act) require that schools provide special education services to children who have learning difficulties. This includes children with speech and language disorders. Services are provided to children from birth through 21 yr of age. Each state has various methods for providing services, and for young children these can include Birth-to-Three, Early Childhood, and Early Learning programs. These programs provide speech-language therapy as part of public education, in conjunction with other special education resources. Children can also receive therapy from nonprofit service agencies, hospital and rehabilitation centers, and speech pathologists in private practice.

Speech-language therapy includes a variety of goals. Sometimes both speech and language activities are incorporated in therapy. The speech goals focus on development of more intelligible speech. Language goals can focus on expanding vocabulary (lexicon) and understanding of the meaning of words (semantics), improving syntax by using proper forms or learning to expand single words into sentences, and social use of language (pragmatics). Therapy can include individual sessions, group sessions, and mainstream classroom integration. Individual sessions may use drill activities for older children or play activities for younger children to target specific goals. Group sessions can include several children with similar language goals to help them practice peer communication activities and to help them bridge the gap into more naturalistic communication situations. Classroom integration might include the therapist team-teaching or consulting with the teacher to facilitate the child's use of language in common academic situations.

For children with severe language impairment, alternative methods of communication are often included in therapy. These may include use of manual sign language, use of pictures (e.g., Picture Exchange Communication System—PECS), and computerized devices for speech output. Often the ultimate goal is to achieve better spoken language. Early use of signs or pictures can help the child to establish better functional communication and help the child to understand the symbolic nature of words to facilitate the language process. There is no evidence that use of signs or pictures interferes with development of oral language if the child has the capacity to speak. Many clinicians believe that these alternative methods accelerate the learning of language. They also reduce frustration of parents and children who cannot communicate for basic needs.

Parents can consult with their child's speech-language therapist about home activities to enhance language development and extend therapy activities through appropriate language-stimulating activities and recreational reading. Parents' language activities should focus on emerging communication skills that are within the child's repertoire, rather than teaching the child new skills. The speech pathologist can guide parents on effective modeling and eliciting communication from their child.

Recreational reading focuses on expanding the child's comprehension of language. Sometimes the child's avoidance of reading is a sign that the parent is presenting material that is too complex for the child. The speech-language therapist can guide the parent in selecting an appropriate level of reading material.

PROGNOSIS

Although the majority of children improve their communication ability with time, 50-80% of preschoolers with language delay and normal nonverbal intelligence continue to show language difficulties up to 20 yr beyond the initial diagnosis. Early language difficulty is strongly related to later reading disorder. Approximately 50% of children with early language difficulty develop reading disorder, and 55% of children with reading disorder have a history of impaired early oral language development. Studies have shown that children who eventually manifest a specific reading disorder produce fewer words per utterance, express less-complicated sentences, and show more pronunciation difficulties at 2-3 yr of age compared with peers who do not have reading disorders. By 5 yr of age, verbal sentence complexity had little predictive power, but expressive vocabulary and phonologic awareness of words (the ability to manipulate the component sounds of words) were highly correlated with later reading achievement.

COMORBID PSYCHIATRIC DISORDERS

Early language disorder, particularly difficulty with auditory comprehension, appears to be a specific risk factor for later emotional dysfunction. Boys and girls with language disorder have a higher than expected rate of anxiety disorder (principally social phobia). Boys with language disorder are more likely to develop symptoms of ADHD, conduct disorder, and antisocial personality disorder compared with normally developing peers. Language disorders are common in children referred for psychiatric services, but they are often underdiagnosed, and their impact on children's behavior and emotional development is often overlooked.

Preschoolers with language difficulty commonly express their frustration through anxious, socially withdrawn, or aggressive behavior. As their ability to communicate improves, parallel improvements are usually noted in their behavior, suggesting a cause-and-effect relationship between language and behavior. However, the persistence of emotional and behavioral problems over the lifespan of persons with early language disability suggests a strong biologic or genetic connection between language development and subsequent emotional disorders.

BIBLIOGRAPHY

Please visit the Nelson Textbook of Pediatrics *website at www.expertconsult.com for the complete bibliography.*

32.1 Dysfluency (Stuttering, Stammering)

Robert M. Kliegman

Fluent speech requires timely synchronization of phonatory and articulatory muscle groups. There is also an important interaction between speech and language skills. Stuttering involves involuntary frequent repetitions, lengthenings (prolongations) or arrests (blocks, pauses) of syllables, or sounds that are exacerbated by emotionally or syntactically demanding speech. The World Health Organization's definition of *stuttering* is a disorder in the rhythm of speech in which the person knows precisely what he or she wishes to say but at the same time may have difficulty saying it because of an involuntary repetition, prolongation, or cessation of sound. Stuttering often leads to frustration and avoidance of speaking situations. Stuttering can lead to being bullied or teased and to speech-related anxiety and social phobia.

EPIDEMIOLOGY AND ETIOLOGY

Stuttering usually begins at 2-4 yr of age and is seen more often in boys (4:1). Approximately 3-5% of preschool children stutter to some degree; only 0.7-1% of young adults stutter. Stuttering is common in families. Stuttering may occur suddenly and often begins when word combinations are involved. Higher vocabulary at age 2 yr and higher material education may also be associated with stuttering. Girls and those with a family history of recovery are most likely to have spontaneous recovery by adolescence. This recovery is not related to the severity of the stuttering. About 75% stop stuttering by adolescence, ~ 90% for girls.

Stuttering may be due to impaired timing between areas of the brain involved in language preparation and execution. Adults who stutter and those with fluent speech activate similar areas of the brain. In addition, adults who stutter overactivate parts of the motor cortex and cerebellar vermis, show right-sided laterality, and have no auditory activation on hearing their own speech.

DIAGNOSIS

Stuttering must be differentiated from the normal developmental dysfluency of preschool children (Tables 32-4 and 32-5). Developmental dysfluency is characterized by brief periods of stuttering that resolve by school age, and it usually involves whole words, with <10 dysfluencies per 100 words. The DSM-IV diagnostic criteria for stuttering are noted in Table 32-2. Stuttering that persists and is associated with tics may be a manifestation of **Tourette's syndrome** (Chapters 23 and 590).

TREATMENT

Preschool children with developmental dysfluency (see Table 32-5) can be observed with parental education and reassurance. Parents should not reprimand the child or create undue anxiety. Preschool or older children with stuttering should be referred to a speech pathologist. Therapy is most effective if started during the preschool period. In addition to the risks noted in Table 32-3, indications for referral include 3 or more dysfluencies per 100 syllables (*b-b-but; th-th-the; you, you, you*), avoidances or escapes (pauses, head nod, blinking), discomfort or anxiety while speaking, and suspicion of an associated neurologic or psychotic disorder.

Most preschool children respond to interventions taught by speech pathologists and to behavioral feedback by parents. Parents should not yell at the child, but should calmly praise periods of fluency ("That was smooth") or nonjudgmentally note episodes of stuttering ("That was a bit bumpy"). The child can be involved with self-correction and respond to requests ("Can you say that again?") made by a calm parent.

Table 32-4 DIFFERENCES BETWEEN STUTTERING AND DEVELOPMENTAL DYSFLUENCY

BEHAVIOR	STUTTERING	DEVELOPMENTAL DYSFLUENCY
Frequency of syllable repetition per word	≥2	≤1
Tempo	Faster than normal	Normal
Airflow	Often interrupted	Rarely interrupted
Vocal tension	Often apparent	Absent
Frequency of prolongations per 100 words	≥2	≤1
Duration of prolongation	≥2 sec	≤1 sec
Tension	Often present	Absent
Silent pauses within a word	May be present	Absent
Silent pauses before a speech attempt	Unusually long	Not marked
Silent pauses after the dysfluency	May be present	Absent
Articulating postures	May be inappropriate	Appropriate
Reaction to stress	More broken words	No change in dysfluency
Frustration	May be present	Absent
Eye contact	May waver	Normal

Adapted with permission from Van Riper C: *The nature of stuttering,* Englewood Cliffs, NJ, Prentice-Hall, 1971, p 28. From Lawrence M, Barclay DM III: Stuttering: a brief review, *Am Fam Physician* 57:2175-2178, 1998.

Table 32-5 EXAMPLES OF NORMAL DYSFLUENCY IN PRESCHOOLERS

TYPE OF DYSFLUENCY	EXAMPLES
Voiced repetitions	Occasionally 2 word parts (*mi … milk*) Single-syllable words (*I … I see you*) Multisyllabic words (*Barney … Barney is coming!*) Phrases (*I want … I want Elmo.*)
Interjections	*We went to the … uh … cottage.*
Revisions: incomplete phrases	*I lost my. … Where is Daddy going?*
Prologations	*I am Tooоommy Baker.*
Tense pauses	Lips together, no sound produced

From Costa D, Kroll R: Stuttering: an update for physicians, *CMAJ* 162:1849–1855, 2000.

Older children, adolescents, and adults have also been treated with risperidone or olanzapine with varying but usually positive results if behavioral speech therapy is unsuccessful.

BIBLIOGRAPHY

Please visit the Nelson Textbook of Pediatrics *website at www.expertconsult.com for the complete bibliography.*

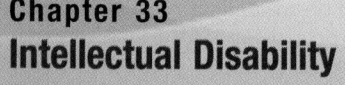

Chapter 33
Intellectual Disability

Bruce K. Shapiro and Mark L. Batshaw

Intellectual disability (formerly called mental retardation) refers to a group of disorders that have in common deficits of adaptive and intellectual function and an age of onset before maturity is reached.

DEFINITION

Three criteria must be met to establish the diagnosis of intellectual disability: significantly subaverage intellectual function, significant impairments in adaptive function, and onset before

Table 33-1 DIAGNOSTIC CRITERIA FOR INTELLECTUAL DISABILITY

A. Significantly subaverage intellectual functioning: an IQ score of 70 or below on an individually administered IQ test (for infants, a clinical judgment of significantly subaverage intellectual functioning).
B. Concurrent deficits or impairments in present adaptive functioning (i.e., the person's effectiveness in meeting the standards expected for his or her age by his or her cultural group) in at least two of the following areas: communication, self-care, home living, social and interpersonal skills, use of community resources, self-direction, functional academic skills, work, leisure, health, and safety.
C. The onset is before age 18 years.

Code based on degree of severity reflecting level of intellectual impairment:

317: Mild Intellectual disability, IQ level 50-55 to ≈70
318.0: Moderate Intellectual disability, IQ level 35-40 to 50-55
318.1: Severe Intellectual disability, IQ level 20-25 to 35-40
318.2: Profound Intellectual disability, IQ level below 20-25
319: Intellectual disability, Severity Unspecified, when there is a strong presumption of intellectual disability but the person's intelligence is untestable by standard tests

From American Psychiatric Association: *Diagnostic and statistical manual of mental disorders, fourth edition, text revision,* Washington, DC, 2000, American Psychiatric Association, p 49, reprinted by permission.

Table 33-2 IDENTIFICATION OF CAUSE IN CHILDREN WITH SEVERE INTELLECTUAL DISABILITY

CAUSE	EXAMPLES	PERCENT OF TOTAL
Chromosomal disorder	Trisomies 21, 18, 13, Deletion 1p36 Klinefelter's syndrome Wolf Hirschhorn syndrome	~20
Genetic syndrome	Fragile X syndrome Prader-Willi syndrome Rett syndrome	~20
Nonsyndromic autosomal mutations	Variations in copy number, Mutations in *SYNGAP1, GRIK2, TUSC3* and oligosaccharyl transferase	~10
Developmental brain abnormality	Hydrocephalus ± meningomyelocele, lissencephaly	~8
Inborn errors of metabolism or neurodegenerative disorder	PKU, Tay-Sachs, various storage diseases	~7
Congenital infections	HIV, toxoplasmosis, rubella, CMV, syphilis, herpes simplex	~3
Familial intellectual disability	Environment, syndromic, or genetic	~5
Perinatal causes	HIE, meningitis, IVH, PVL, fetal alcohol syndrome	4
Postnatal causes	Trauma (abuse), meningitis, hypothyroidism	~4
Unknown	Cerebral palsy	20

CMV, cytomegalovirus; HIE, hypoxic ischemic encephalopathy; HIV, human immunodeficiency virus; IVH, intraventricular hemorrhage; PKU, phenylketonuria; PVL, periventricular leukomalacia. Modified from Stromme P, Hayberg G: Aetiology in severe and mild mental retardation: a population based study of Norwegian children, *Dev Med Child Neurol* 42:76–86, 2000.

18 years of age. The three diagnostic formulations—*Diagnostic and Statistical Manual of Mental Disorders, Fourth Edition, Text Revision* (DSM-IV-TR), American Association on Intellectual and Developmental Disabilities (AAIDD), and Individuals with Disabilities Education Act (IDEA)—agree on the 3 criteria but define them differently.

Significantly subaverage general intellectual function refers to performance on an individually administered test of intelligence that is approximately two standard deviations (SD) below the mean. For a test that has a mean of 100 and SD of 15, IQ scores below 70 would meet these criteria. If the standard error of measurement is considered, the upper limits of subaverage intellectual function may extend to an IQ of 75. Using a score of 75 to delineate intellectual disability might double the number of children with intellectual disability, but the requirement for impairment of adaptive skills limits the false positives. Children with intellectual disability often show a variable pattern of strengths and weaknesses. Not all of their partial scores on IQ tests fall into the significantly subaverage range.

Significant impairment in adaptive behavior reflects the degree that the cognitive dysfunction impairs daily function. Adaptive behavior refers to the skills that are required for people to function in their everyday lives. Adaptive behavior may be assessed by three different constructs: the classification of DSM-IV-TR, the classification of AAIDD, and the IDEA.

The **DSM-IV-TR** classification of adaptive behavior addresses 10 domains: communication, self-care, home living, social and interpersonal skills, use of community resources, self-direction, functional academics, work, leisure, and health and safety. For a deficit in adaptive behavior to be present, a significant delay in 2 of the 10 areas must be present.

The **AAIDD** classification of adaptive behavior addresses 3 broad sets of skills: conceptual, social, and practical. Conceptual skills include language, reading and writing, money concepts, and self-direction. Social skills include interpersonal skills, personal responsibility, self-esteem, gullibility, naiveté, and ability to follow rules, obey laws, and avoid victimization. Representative practical skills are performance of activities of daily living (dressing, feeding, toileting and bathing, mobility), instrumental activities of daily living (housework, managing money, taking medication, shopping, preparing meals, using the telephone, etc) occupational skills, and the maintenance of a safe environment. For a deficit in adaptive behavior to be present, a significant delay in 1 of the 3 areas must be present. The rationale for requiring only 1 of the 3 areas is the empirically derived finding that people with intellectual disability can have varying patterns of ability and may not have deficits in all 3 areas.

The **IDEA** requires that the cognitive dysfunction affect school performance.

The requirement for adaptive behavior deficits is the most controversial aspect of the diagnostic formulation. The controversy centers on 2 broad areas: whether impairments in adaptive behavior are necessary for the construct of intellectual disability and what to measure. The adaptive behavior criterion may be irrelevant for many children; adaptive behavior is impaired in virtually all children who have IQ scores <50. The major utility of the adaptive behavior criterion is to confirm intellectual disability in children with IQ scores in the 65-75 range. It should be noted that deficits in adaptive behavior are often found in disorders such as Asperger syndrome (Chapter 28) and ADHD (Chapter 30) in the presence of typical intellectual function.

The issues of measurement are important as well. The independence of the 3 domains of the AAIDD and the 10 domains of the DSM-IV-TR has not been validated with research. The relationship between adaptive behavior and IQ performance is insufficiently explored. Most adults with mild intellectual disability do not have significant impairments in practical skills. It should be noted that adaptive behavior deficits must be distinguished from maladaptive behavior (e.g., aggression, inappropriate sexual contact).

Onset before age 18 yr distinguishes dysfunctions that originate during the developmental period. The diagnosis of intellectual disability may be made after 18 years of age, but the cognitive and adaptive dysfunction must have been manifested before age 18. The IDEA, because of its focus on school-aged children, does not require a limit of 18 years but refers to the "developmental period."

The most commonly used medical diagnostic criteria for intellectual disability are those contained in the DSM-IV-TR (Table 33-1). The classification of intellectual disability that results from these definitions has been criticized for depending on IQ test performance rather than adaptive behavior, not taking the standard error of measurement into account, and not being predictive of outcomes for individuals. A new edition is currently being prepared that might address these issues. The AAIDD has proposed a different classification system. Instead of defining degrees of deficit (mild to profound), the AAIDD definition substitutes levels of support required in areas of adaptive function (intermittent, limited, extensive, or pervasive). The reliability of this approach has been challenged, and it blurs the distinction between intellectual and other developmental disabilities (communication disorder, autism, specific learning disabilities).

The term **mental retardation** should be cast aside because it is stigmatizing, has been used to limit the achievements of the individual, and has not met its initial objective of providing assistance to people with the disorder. The term **intellectual disability** is increasingly used in its place but has not been adopted universally; existing laws and their attendant entitlements still use the term mental retardation. In Europe, the term **learning disability** is often used to describe intellectual disability. **Global developmental delay** is a term often used to describe young children whose limitations have not yet resulted in a formal diagnosis of intellectual disability; it is often inappropriately used beyond the point when it is clear the child has intellectual disability, usually age 3 years.

ETIOLOGY

There appear to be 2 overlapping populations of children with intellectual disability: mild (IQ >50-70), which is more associated with environmental influences, and severe (IQ < 50), which is more frequently linked to biologic causes. Mild intellectual disability is 4 times more likely to be found in the offspring of women who have not completed high school than in women who have graduated. This is presumably a consequence of both genetic (children can inherit an intellectual impairment) and socioeconomic (poverty, malnutrition) factors. The specific causes of mild intellectual disability are identifiable in <50% of affected individuals. The most common biologic causes of mild intellectual disability include genetic or chromosomal syndromes with multiple, major, or minor congenital anomalies (velocardiofacial syndrome, Williams syndrome, Noonan's syndrome), intrauterine growth restriction, prematurity, perinatal insults, intrauterine exposure to drugs of abuse (including alcohol), and sex chromosomal abnormalities. Familial clustering is common.

In children with severe intellectual disability, a biologic cause (most commonly prenatal) can be identified in >75% of cases. Causes include chromosomal (e.g., Down syndrome Wolf-Hirschhorn syndrome, deletion 1p36 syndrome) and other genetic and epigenetic disorders (e.g., fragile X syndrome, Rett syndrome, Angelman and Prader-Willi syndromes), abnormalities of brain development (e.g., lissencephaly), and inborn errors of metabolism or neurodegenerative disorders (e.g, mucopolysaccharidoses) (Table 33-2). Consistent with the finding that disorders that alter early embryogenesis are the most common and severe, the earlier the problem occurs in development, the more severe its consequences tend to be.

EPIDEMIOLOGY

The prevalence of intellectual disability depends on the definition, the method of ascertainment, and the population. According to statistics (based on the DSM-IV-TR definition), 2.5% of the population should have intellectual disability, and 85% of these individuals should fall into the mild range. In 2005-2006, ~556,000 or only 1.1% of school-aged children received services for intellectual disability in federally supported school programs in the US. For several reasons, fewer children than predicted are identified as having mild intellectual disability. Because it is more difficult to diagnose mild intellectual disability than the more severe forms, professionals might defer the diagnosis and give the benefit of the doubt to the child. Other reasons that contribute to the discrepancy are use of instruments that underidentify young children with mild intellectual disability, some children being diagnosed as having autism spectrum disorders and their intellectual disability not addressed, and a disinclination to make the diagnosis in poor or minority students because of previous overdiagnosis.

Young children might show cognitive limitations without significant delays in adaptive behavior. As a result, new cases of mild intellectual disability continue to be diagnosed among children up to 9 yr of age. Children with intellectual disability also may be incorporated into another diagnosis (e.g., autism, cerebral palsy). Furthermore, it is possible that the number of children with mild intellectual disability is actually decreasing as a result of public health and education measures to prevent prematurity and provide early intervention and head start programs. In fact, the number of school children who receive services for intellectual disability has not changed appreciably since 1997.

Unlike mild intellectual disability, where the prevalence may be decreasing, the occurrence of severe intellectual disability has not changed appreciably since the 1940s and is 0.3-0.5% of the population. Many of the causes of severe intellectual disability involve genetic or congenital brain malformations that can neither be anticipated nor treated at present. In addition, new populations with severe intellectual disability have offset the decreases in the prevalence of severe intellectual disability that have resulted from improved health care. Although prenatal diagnosis and subsequent pregnancy terminations have resulted in a decreased prevalence of Down syndrome (Chapter 76), and newborn screening with early treatment has virtually eliminated intellectual disability caused by phenylketonuria and congenital hypothyroidism, an increased prevalence of maternal prenatal drug use (Chapter 90.4) and improved survival of very low birthweight premature infants has counterbalanced this effect.

Overall, intellectual disability occurs more in boys than in girls: 2:1 in mild intellectual disability and 1.5:1 in severe intellectual disability. In part this may be a consequence of the many X-linked disorders associated with intellectual disability, the most prominent being fragile X syndrome.

PATHOLOGY AND PATHOGENESIS

For the full continuation of this topic, please visit the Nelson Textbook of Pediatrics *website at* *www.expertconsult.com.*

CLINICAL MANIFESTATIONS

Early diagnosis of intellectual disability facilitates earlier intervention, identification of abilities, realistic goal setting, easing of parental anxiety, and greater acceptance of the child in the community. Most children with intellectual disability first come to the pediatrician's attention in infancy because of dysmorphisms, associated developmental disabilities, or failure to meet age-appropriate developmental milestones. There are no specific physical characteristics of intellectual disability, but dysmorphisms may be the earliest signs that bring children to the attention of the pediatrician. They might fall within a genetic syndrome such as Down syndrome or be isolated, as in microcephaly or failure to thrive. Associated developmental disabilities include seizure disorders, cerebral palsy, hypotonia, and autism; these conditions are seen more commonly in conjunction with intellectual disability than in the general population.

Most children with intellectual disability do not keep up with their peers and fail to meet age-expected norms. In early infancy,

Table 33-3 COMMON PRESENTATIONS OF INTELLECTUAL DISABILITY BY AGE

AGE	AREA OF CONCERN
Newborn	Dysmorphic syndromes, (multiple congenital anomalies), microcephaly Major organ system dysfunction (e.g., feeding and breathing)
Early infancy (2-4 mo)	Failure to interact with the environment Concerns about vision and hearing impairments
Later infancy (6-18 mo)	Gross motor delay
Toddlers (2-3 yr)	Language delays or difficulties
Preschool (3-5 yr)	Language difficulties or delays Behavior difficulties, including play Delays in fine motor skills: cutting, coloring, drawing
School age (>5 yr)	Academic underachievement Behavior difficulties (attention, anxiety, mood, conduct, etc.)

failure to meet age-appropriate expectations can include a lack of visual or auditory responsiveness, unusual muscle tone (hypo- or hypertonia) or posture, and feeding difficulties. Between 6 and 18 mo of age, gross motor delay (lack of sitting, crawling, walking) is the most common complaint. Language delay and behavior problems are common concerns after 18 mo (Table 33-3). Earlier identification of atypical development is likely to occur with more severe impairments; and intellectual disability is usually identifiable by age 3 yr.

For some children with mild intellectual disability the diagnosis remains uncertain during the early school years. It is only after the demands of the school setting increase over the years, changing from "learning to read" to "reading to learn," that the child's limitations are clarified.

Adolescents with mild intellectual disability can present a diagnostic challenge. Adolescents with mild intellectual disability "talk the talk" but do not "walk the walk." Typically they are up to date on current trends and are conversant as to who, what, and where. It isn't until the "why" and "how" questions are asked that their limitations become apparent. If allowed to interact at a superficial level, their mild intellectual disability might not be appreciated, even by professionals who may be their special education teachers or health care providers. Because of the stigma associated with intellectual disability, they may use euphemisms to avoid being thought of as "stupid" or "retarded" and refer to themselves as learning disabled, dyslexic, language disordered, or slow learners. Some people with intellectual disability emulate their social milieu to be accepted. They may be social chameleons and assume the morals of the group to which they are attached. Some would rather be thought "bad" than "incompetent."

LABORATORY FINDINGS

The most commonly used medical diagnostic testing for children with intellectual disability include neuroimaging; metabolic, genetic, and chromosomal testing; microarray analysis; and electroencephalography (EEG). These tests should not be used as screening tools for all children with an intellectual disability. In some children, there is a reasonable yield for testing, whereas in others the yield of <1% does not support its use. Decisions on diagnostic testing should be based on the medical and family history, physical examination, testing by other disciplines, and the family's wishes (Fig. 33-1). Table 33-4 summarizes clinical practice guidelines that have been published to assist in evaluating the child with global developmental delay or intellectual disability. Karyotyping, particularly focusing on the number of chromosomes, duplications, deletions, or chromosomal translocations and the **subtelomeric region** (a hot spot), is indicated in children with multiple anomalies or a positive family history. Microarray analysis for copy number variation detects deletions and duplications when traditional chromosome banding techniques are normal and should be performed if a normal karyotype is reported and other tests are unrevealing. Deletion 1p36 syndrome, the most common subtelomeric microdeletion syndrome (1:5,000 births), accounts for ~1% of children with developmental disabilities and is characterized by failure to thrive, microcephaly, deep-set eyes, midface hypoplasia, broad nasal bridge, heart deficits, and CNS anomalies. Noncompaction cardiomyopathy and seizures are also noted. The diagnosis is made by standard chromosomes in only ~20% and requires fluorescent in situ hybridization (FISH) or microarray comparative genomic hybridization methods for remaining patients.

Molecular genetic testing for fragile X syndrome is appropriate for a boy with moderate intellectual disability, unusual physical features, and/or a family history of intellectual disability or for a girl with more subtle cognitive deficits associated with severe shyness and a relevant family history. A child with a progressive neurologic disorder or acute behavioral changes needs metabolic investigation (urinary organic acids, plasma amino acids, blood lactate, lysosomal enzymes in lymphocytes); a child with seizure-like episodes should have an EEG performed. Children with micro- or macrocephaly or changes in head growth trajectory or asymmetric head shapes, as well as those with new or focal neurologic findings, including seizures, should have a neuroimaging procedure.

Some children with more subtle physical or neurologic findings can also have determinable biologic causes of their intellectual disability. About 6% of unexplained intellectual disability can be accounted for by micro chromosomal abnormalities that can be identified by high-resolution chromosomal banding, FISH, or chromosome painting for subtelomeric rearrangements. Microarray genome analysis with gene chip technology is replacing subtelomeric FISH probes; it can identify variants of unknown significance or benign variants, and therefore it should be used in conjunction with a genetic consultation. Magnetic resonance imaging scans identify a significant number of subtle markers of cerebral dysgenesis in children with intellectual disability. Formes frustes of amino acid and organic acid disorders are associated with intellectual disability in the absence of the more commonly associated manifestations of behavior change, lethargy, and coma.

How intensively one investigates the cause of a child's intellectual disability is based on a number of factors:

What is the degree of intellectual disability? One is less likely to find a biologic cause in a child with mild intellectual disability than in a child with a severe intellectual disability.

Is there a specific diagnostic path to follow? If there is a medical history or a family history, or if physical findings pointing to a specific disorder, a diagnosis is more likely to be made. In the absence of these indicators, it is difficult to choose specific tests to perform.

Are the parents planning on having additional children? If so, one would be more likely to intensively seek disorders for which prenatal diagnosis or a specific early treatment option is available.

What are the parents' wishes? Some parents have little interest in searching for the cause of the intellectual disability and focus exclusively on treatment. Others are so focused on obtaining a diagnosis that they have difficulty following through on interventions until a cause has been found. The entire spectrum of responses must be respected, and supportive guidance should be provided in the context of the parents' education.

DIFFERENTIAL DIAGNOSIS

One of the important roles of pediatricians is the early recognition and diagnosis of cognitive deficits. The developmental

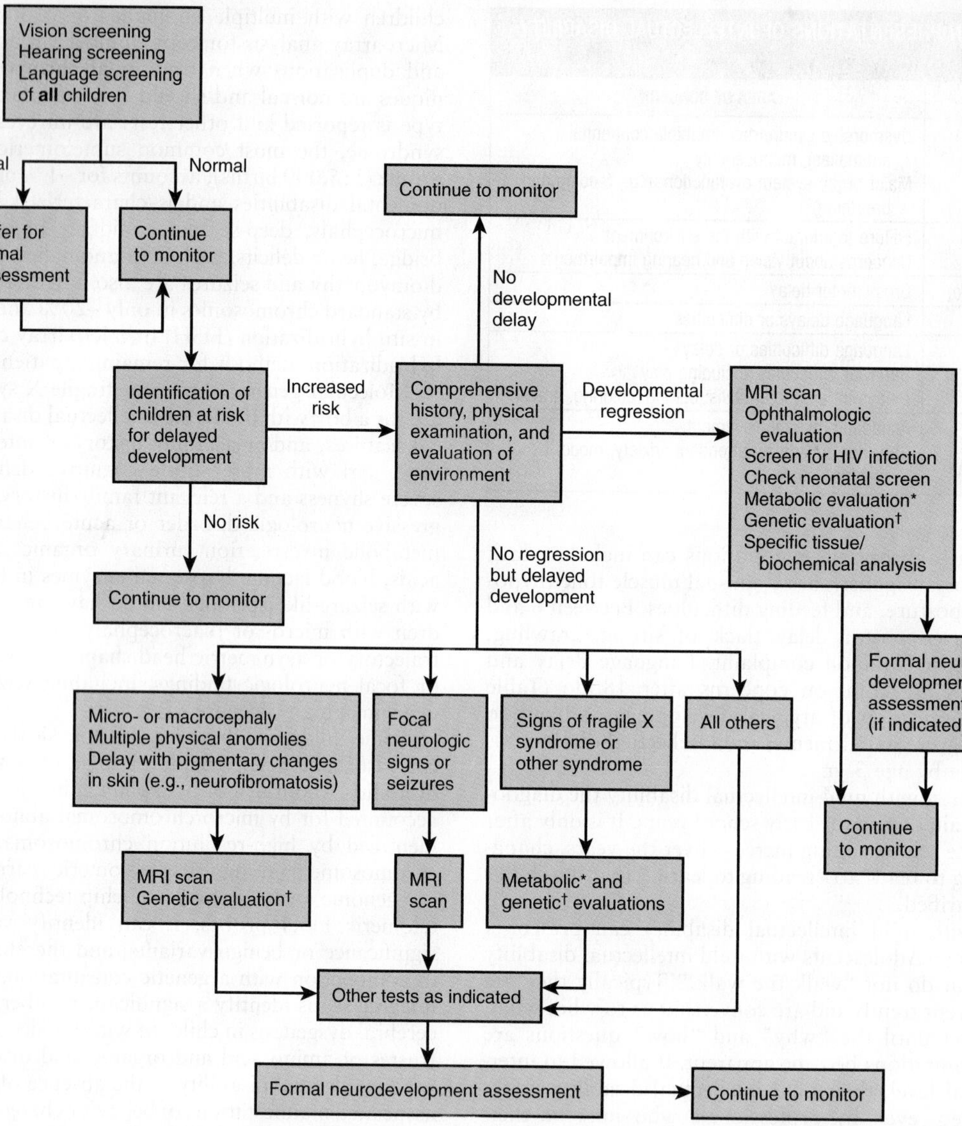

Figure 33-1 Diagnostic strategy for identifying and assessing children with developmental delay. *Metabolic evaluation includes serum amino acids, serum and urine organic acids, serum lactate, and ammonia. †Genetic evaluation includes karyotype, microarray analysis, and dysmorphology consultation if indicated. (From Kliegman RM, Greenbaum LA, Lye PS: *Practical strategies in pediatric diagnosis and therapy,* ed 2, Philadelphia, 2004, Elsevier/Saunders, p 553.)

surveillance approach to early diagnosis of intellectual disability should be multifaceted. Parents' concerns and observations about their child's development should be listened to carefully, because their observations have been found to be as accurate as developmental screening tests. Medical, genetic, and environmental risk factors should be recognized. Infants at high risk (prematurity, maternal substance abuse, perinatal insult) should be registered in newborn follow-up programs in which they are evaluated periodically for developmental lags in the first 2 yr of life; they should be referred to early intervention (Child Find) programs as appropriate. Developmental milestones should be recorded routinely during health care maintenance visits. The American Academy of Pediatrics (AAP) has formulated a schema for developmental surveillance and screening. Whether developmental surveillance is a more effective technique for identifying than recognizing failure to meet age-appropriate milestones has not been clearly established.

Before making the diagnosis of intellectual disability, other disorders that affect cognitive abilities and adaptive behavior should be considered. These include conditions that mimic intellectual disability and others that involve intellectual disability as an associated impairment. Sensory deficits (severe hearing and vision loss), communication disorders, and poorly controlled seizure disorders can mimic intellectual disability; certain progressive neurologic disorders can appear as intellectual disability before regression is appreciated. More than half of children with cerebral palsy (Chapter 591.1) or autism spectrum disorders (Chapter 28) also have intellectual disability as an associated deficit. Differentiation of isolated **cerebral palsy** from intellectual disability relies on motor skills being more affected than cognitive skills and on the presence of pathologic reflexes and tone changes. In **autism spectrum disorders,** language and social adaptive skills are more affected than nonverbal reasoning skills, whereas in intellectual disability there are usually more equivalent deficits in social, motor, adaptive, and cognitive skills.

DIAGNOSTIC PSYCHOLOGIC TESTING

The formal diagnosis of intellectual disability requires the administration of individual tests of intelligence and adaptive functioning.

The **Bayley Scales of Infant Development (BSID-II),** the most commonly used infant intelligence scale, assesses language, visual

Table 33-4 SUGGESTED EVALUATION OF THE CHILD WITH INTELLECTUAL DISABILITY/GLOBAL DEVELOPMENTAL DELAY

TEST	COMMENT
In-depth history	Includes pre-, peri- and postnatal events (including seizures); developmental attainments; and 3-generation pedigree in family history
Physical examination	Particular attention to minor or subtle abnormalities; neurologic examination for focality and skull abnormalities Behavioral phenotype
Vision and hearing evaluation	Essential to detect and treat; can mask as developmental delay
Karyotype	Must include microarray copy number variation determinates if karyotype and chromosome banding are normal
Fragile X screen	Preselection on clinical grounds can increase yield to 7.6%
Neuroimaging	MRI preferred. Positives increased by abnormalities of skull contour or microcephaly and macrocephaly, or focal neurologic examination. Overall has a higher yield. Identification of specific etiologies is rare. Most conditions that are found do not alter the treatment plan. Need to weigh risk of sedation against possible yield.
Thyroid (T_4, TSH)	Near 0% in settings with universal newborn screening program
Serum lead	If there are identifiable risk factors for excessive environmental lead exposure
Metabolic testing	Urine organic acids, plasma amino acids, ammonia, lactate, and a capillary blood gas. Focused testing based on clinical findings is warranted.
Subtelomeric deletion replaced by CGH	Obtain in the presence of dysmorphisms but with a normal karyotype and fragile X DNA study. Higher in severe intellectual disability.
MECP2 for Rett syndrome	Females with severe intellectual disability
EEG	May be deferred in absence of history of seizures
Repeated history and physical examination	Can give time for maturation of physical and behavioral phenotype. New technology may be available for evaluation.

CGH, comparative genomic hybridization; EEG, electroencephalogram; T_4, thyroxine; TSH, thyroid-stimulating hormone.
Based on Curry et al, 1997; Shapiro BK, Batshaw ML: Mental retardation. In Burg FD, Ingelfinger JR, Polin RA, et al: *Gellis and Kagan's current pediatric therapy*, ed 18, Philadelphia, 2005, WB Saunders, used with permission; and Shevell M, Ashwal S, Donley D, et al: Practice parameter: evaluation of the child with global developmental delay, *Neurology* 60:367–380, 2003.

problem-solving skills, behavior, fine motor skills, and gross motor skills in children between 1 mo and 3 yr of age. A Mental Developmental Index (MDI) and a Psychomotor Development Index score (PDI, a measure of motor competence) are derived from the results. This test permits the differentiation of infants with severe intellectual disability from typically developing infants, but it is less helpful in distinguishing between a typical child and one with mild intellectual disability.

The most commonly used psychologic tests for children >3 yr of age are the **Wechsler Scales**. The Wechsler Preschool and Primary Scale of Intelligence, 3rd edition (WPPSI-III) is used for children with mental ages of 2.5-7.3 yr. The Wechsler Intelligence Scale for Children, 4th edition (WISC-IV), is used for children who function above a 6 yr mental age. Both scales contain a number of subtests in the areas of verbal and performance skills. Although children with intellectual disability usually score below average on all subscale scores, they occasionally score in the average range in one or more performance areas.

The most commonly used test of adaptive behavior is the **Vineland Adaptive Behavior Scale** (VABS), which involves semi-structured interviews with parents and/or caregivers and teachers that assess adaptive behavior in four domains: communication, daily living skills, socialization, and motor skills. Other tests of adaptive behavior include the Woodcock-Johnson Scales of Independent Behavior—Revised, the American Association on Intellectual and Developmental Disability Adaptive Behavior Scale (ABS-2nd edition) and the Adaptive Behavior Assessment System (ABAS-2nd edition). There is usually (but not always) a good correlation between scores on the intelligence and adaptive scales. Basic adaptive abilities (feeding, dressing, hygiene) are more responsive to remedial efforts than is the IQ score. Adaptive abilities are also more variable, which can relate to the underlying condition and to environmental expectations. Although persons with Prader-Willi syndrome (Chapter 76) have stability of adaptive skills through adulthood, those with fragile X syndrome (Chapter 76) may have increasing deficits over time.

COMPLICATIONS

Children with intellectual disability have higher rates of vision, hearing, neurologic, orthopedic, and behavioral or emotional disorders than do typically developing children. These other problems are often detected later in children with intellectual disability. If untreated, the associated impairments can potentially adversely affect the individual's outcome more than the intellectual disability itself.

The most common associated deficits are motor impairments, behavioral and emotional disorders, medical complications, and seizures. The more severe the intellectual disability, the greater are the number and severity of associated impairments. Knowing the cause of the intellectual disability can help predict which associated impairments are most likely to occur. Fragile X syndrome and fetal alcohol syndrome (Chapter 100.2) are associated with a high rate of behavioral disorders; Down syndrome has many medical complications (hypothyroidism, celiac disease, congenital heart disease, atlantoaxial subluxation). Associated impairments can require ongoing physical therapy, occupational therapy, speech-language therapy, adaptive equipment, glasses, hearing aids, and medication. Failure to identify and treat these impairments adequately can hinder successful habilitation and result in difficulties in the school, home, and/or neighborhood environment.

PREVENTION

Examples of primary programs to prevent intellectual disability include:

Increasing the public's awareness of the adverse effects of alcohol and other drugs of abuse on the fetus
Preventing teen pregnancy and promoting early prenatal care
Preventing traumatic injury: Encouraging the use of guards and railings to prevent falls and other avoidable injuries in the home; using appropriate seat restraints when driving and wearing a safety helmet when biking or skateboarding; teaching firearms safety
Preventing poisonings: Teaching parents about locking up medications and potential poisons
Encouraging safe sexual practices to prevent the transmission of diseases, most prominently HIV
Implementing immunization programs to reduce the risk of intellectual disability due to encephalitis, meningitis, and congenital infection

Presymptomatic detection of certain disorders can result in treatment that prevents adverse consequences. State newborn screening by tandem mass spectrometry (now including >50 rare genetic disorders in most states), newborn hearing screening, and preschool lead poisoning prevention programs are examples. Radiologic screening for atlantoaxial subluxation in a child with Down syndrome is an example of presymptomatic testing in a disorder associated with intellectual disability.

TREATMENT

Although intellectual disability is not treatable, many associated impairments are amenable to intervention and therefore benefit from early identification. Most children with an intellectual disability do not have a behavioral or emotional disorder as an associated impairment, but challenging behaviors (aggression, self-injury, oppositional defiant behavior) and mental illness (mood and anxiety disorders) occur with greater frequency in this population than among children with typical intelligence. These behavioral and emotional disorders are the primary cause for out-of-home placements, reduced employment prospects, and decreased opportunities for social integration. Some behavioral and emotional disorders are difficult to diagnose in children with more severe intellectual disability because of the child's limited abilities to understand, communicate, interpret, or generalize. Other disorders are masked by the intellectual disability. The detection of ADHD (Chapter 30) in the presence of moderate to severe intellectual disability may be difficult, as may be discerning a thought disorder (psychosis) in someone with autism and intellectual disability.

Although mental illness is generally of biologic origin and responds to medication, behavioral disorders can result from a mismatch between the child's abilities and the demands of the situation, organic problems, and/or family difficulties. They may represent attempts by the child to communicate, gain attention, or avoid frustration. In assessing the challenging behavior, one must also consider whether it is inappropriate for the child's *mental age,* rather than the *chronological age.* When intervention is needed, an environmental change, such as a more appropriate classroom setting, may improve certain behavior problems. Behavior management techniques are useful; psychopharmacologic agents may be appropriate in certain situations.

Medication is not useful in treating the core symptoms of intellectual disability; no agent has been found to improve intellectual function. Medication may be helpful in treating associated behavioral and psychiatric disorders. Psychopharmacology is generally directed at specific symptom complexes including ADHD (stimulant medication), self-injurious behavior and aggression (neuroleptics), and anxiety obsessive-compulsive disorder, and depression (selective serotonin reuptake inhibitors). Before long-term therapy with any psychopharmacologic agent is initiated, a short trial should be conducted. Even if a medication proves successful, its use should be re-evaluated at least yearly to assess the need for continued treatment.

SUPPORTIVE CARE AND MANAGEMENT

Each child with intellectual disability needs a medical home with a pediatrician who is readily accessible to the family to answer questions, help coordinate care, and discuss concerns. Pediatricians can have effects on patients and their families that are still felt decades later. The role of the pediatrician includes involvement in prevention efforts, early diagnosis, identification of associated deficits, referral for appropriate diagnostic and therapeutic services, interdisciplinary management, provision of primary care, and advocacy for the child and family. The management strategies for children with an intellectual disability should be multimodal, with efforts directed at all aspects of the child's life: health, education, social and recreational activities, behavior problems, and associated impairments. Support for parents and siblings should also be provided.

Primary Care

For children with an intellectual disability, primary care has a number of important components:

Provision of the same primary care received by all other children of similar chronological age (Chapter 5)

Anticipatory guidance relevant to the child's level of function: feeding, toileting, school, accident prevention, sexuality education

Assessment of issues that are relevant to that child's disorder: e.g., examination of the teeth in children who exhibit bruxism, thyroid function in children with Down syndrome, cardiac function in Williams syndrome (Chapter 102)

The AAP has published a series of guidelines for children with specific genetic disorders associated with intellectual disability (Down syndrome, fragile X syndrome, and Williams syndrome). Goals should be considered and programs adjusted as needed during the primary care visit. Decisions should also be made about what additional information is required for future planning or to explain why the child is not meeting expectations. Other evaluations, such as formal psychologic or educational testing, may need to be scheduled.

Interdisciplinary Management

The pediatrician has the responsibility for consulting with other disciplines to make the diagnosis of intellectual disability and coordinate treatment services. Consultant services may include psychology, speech-language pathology, physical therapy, occupational therapy, audiology, nutrition, nursing, and/or social work, as well as medical specialties such as neurodevelopmental disabilities, neurology, genetics, psychiatry, and/or surgical specialties. Contact with early intervention and school personnel is equally important to help prepare the child's Individual Family Service Plan (IFSP). The family should be an integral part of the planning and direction of this process. Care should be family centered and culturally sensitive; for older children, their participation in planning and decision-making should be promoted to whatever extent possible.

Periodic Re-evaluation

The child's abilities and the family's needs change over time. As the child grows, more information must be provided to the child and family, goals must be reassessed, and programming needs should be adjusted. A periodic review should include information about the child's health status as well as his or her functioning at home, at school, and in other community settings. Other information, such as formal psychologic or educational testing, may be helpful. Re-evaluation should be undertaken at routine intervals (6-12 mo during early childhood), at any time the child is not meeting expectations, or when he or she is moving from one service delivery system to another. This is especially true during the transition to adulthood, beginning at age 14 yr as mandated by the IDEA Amendments of 2004. This transitioning should include the transfer of care to the adult health care system by age 21 yr.

Educational Services

Education is the single most important discipline involved in the treatment of children with an intellectual disability. The educational program must be relevant to the child's needs and address the child's individual strengths and weaknesses. The child's developmental level, his or her requirements for support, and goals for independence provide a basis for establishing an Individualized Education Program (IEP) for school-aged children, as mandated by federal legislation.

Leisure and Recreational Activities

The child's social and recreational needs should be addressed. Although young children with intellectual disability are generally included in play activities with children who have typical development, adolescents with intellectual disability often do not have opportunities for appropriate social interactions. Participation in sports should be encouraged, even if the child is not competitive, because it offers many benefits, including weight management, development of physical coordination, maintenance of cardiovascular fitness, and improvement of self-image. Social activities are equally important, including dances, trips, dating, and other typical social and recreational events.

Family Counseling

Many families adapt well to having a child with intellectual disability, but some have emotional or social difficulties. The risks of parents' depression and child abuse and neglect are higher in this group of children than in the general population. Among the factors that have been associated with good family coping and parenting skills are stability of the marriage, good parental self-esteem, limited number of siblings, higher socioeconomic status, lower degree of disability or associated impairments, parents' appropriate expectations and acceptance of the diagnosis, supportive extended family members, and availability of community programs and respite care services. In families in which the emotional burden of having a child with intellectual disability is great, family counseling, parent support groups, respite care, and home health services should be an integral part of the treatment plan.

Advocacy

The pediatrician can play a number of advocacy roles: maintaining close contact with the department of health or local school district to advocate for an appropriate IFSP/IEP; identifying eligibility for financial supports via Supplemental Security Income (SSI) through the Social Security Administration; assessing the impact of the Americans with Disabilities Act (ADA) on the adolescent's access to jobs and community activities; referring families to appropriate parental support groups or websites for their specific disorder or syndrome; ensuring adequate respite care services for the family; becoming involved in the community to help develop educational, recreational, and leisure programs for children with disabilities; and advocating for improved health care coverage by private and government insurers.

PROGNOSIS

In children with severe intellectual disability, the prognosis is often evident by early childhood. Mild intellectual disability might not always be a lifelong disorder. Children might meet criteria for intellectual disability at an early age, but later the disability can evolve into a more specific developmental disorder (communication disorder, autism, slow learner, or borderline normal intelligence). Others with a diagnosis of mild intellectual disability during their school years develop sufficient adaptive behavior skills so that they no longer fit the diagnosis as adolescents, or the effects of maturation and plasticity can result in children moving from one diagnostic category to another (from moderate to mild retardation). Some children who have a diagnosis of a specific learning disability or communication disorder might not maintain their rate of cognitive growth and fall into the range of intellectual disability over time. By adolescence, the diagnosis has generally stabilized.

The long-term outcome of persons with intellectual disability depends on the underlying cause, the degree of cognitive and adaptive deficits, the presence of associated medical and developmental impairments, the capabilities of the families, and the school and community supports, services, and training provided to the child and family (Table 33-5). As adults, many persons with mild intellectual disability are capable of gaining economic and social independence with functional literacy. They might need periodic supervision, especially when under social or economic stress. Most live successfully in the community, either independently or in supervised settings. Life expectancy is not adversely affected by intellectual disability itself.

Table 33-5 SEVERITY OF INTELLECTUAL DISABILITY AND ADULT AGE FUNCTIONING

LEVEL	MENTAL AGE AS ADULT*	ADULT ADAPTATION
Mild	9-11 yr	Reads at 4th-5th grade level; simple multiplication and division; writes simple letter, lists; completes job application; basic independent job skills (arrive on time, stay at task, interact with coworkers); uses public transportation, might qualify for driver's license; keeps house, cooks using recipes
Moderate	6-8 yr	Sight-word reading; copies information, e.g., address from card to job application; matches written number to number of items; recognizes time on clock; communicates; some independence in self-care; housekeeping with supervision or cue cards; meal preparation, can follow picture recipe cards; job skills learned with much repetition; uses public transportation with some supervision
Severe	3-5 yr	Needs continuous support and supervision; might communicate wants and needs, sometimes with augmentative communication techniques
Profound	<3 yr	Limitations of self-care, continence, communication, and mobility; might need complete custodial or nursing care

**International Statistical Classification of Diseases and Related Health Problems*, 10th edition (World Health Organization).
From Dr. Robert L. Schum, Grand Rounds Presentation at Children's Hospital of Wisconsin, 2003.

For persons with moderate intellectual disability, the goals of education are to enhance adaptive abilities and "survival" academic and vocational skills so they are better able to live in the adult world (see Table 33-5). The concept of supported employment has been very beneficial to these individuals; the person is trained by a coach to do a specific job in the setting in which the person is to work. This bypasses the need for a sheltered workshop experience and has resulted in successful work adaptation in the community for many people with an intellectual disability. These persons generally live at home or in a supervised setting in the community.

As adults, people with severe to profound intellectual disability usually require extensive to pervasive supports (see Table 33-5). These individuals may have associated impairments, such as cerebral palsy, behavioral disorders, epilepsy, or sensory impairments, that further limit their adaptive functioning. They can perform simple tasks in supervised settings. Most people with this level of intellectual disability are able to live in the community with appropriate supports.

BIBLIOGRAPHY

Please visit the Nelson Textbook of Pediatrics *website at www.expertconsult.com for the complete bibliography.*

PART V Children with Special Needs

Chapter 34
Adoption

Mark D. Simms and Samantha L. Wilson

Adoption is a social, emotional, and legal process that provides a new family for a child when the birth family is unable or unwilling to parent. In the USA, about 1 million children are adopted; 2-4% of all American families have adopted. In 2007, approximately 135,000 children were adopted. Of these, approximately 40% were stepparent or relative adoptions. Of nonstepparent adoptions, approximately 60% were from the child welfare system, 25% were international, and 15% were voluntarily adoption-placed domestic infants. Private agencies or independent practitioners, such as lawyers, handle approximately one third of adoptions.

The Adoption and Safe Families Act (P.L. 105-89) requires that children in foster care who cannot be safely returned to their families within a reasonable period of time should be placed with adoptive families. As a result, adoptions of children in foster care increased from about 18,000 per yr to a peak of 53,000 in 2002. Nonetheless, approximately 130,000 children are "waiting to be adopted" from foster care, a number that has remained stable since 2003. Many children awaiting adoption have "special needs" because they are of school age, part of a sibling group, members of ethnic or racial minority groups, or because they have physical, emotional, or developmental needs. Federal adoption subsidies, tax credits, special minority recruitment efforts, increased preplacement services, and approval of adoptions by "nontraditional" families (particularly single adults and older couples) are aimed at increasing the adoption opportunities for these children.

Over the past quarter century, the number of families wanting to adopt children from other countries has grown dramatically. Between the late 1960s and the early 2000s, Sweden received well over 40,000 foreign children. In France, 3 out of 4 children adopted are foreign, from over 75 countries. The number of children adopted into the USA from other countries varies each year as a result of political and social changes across the globe. In 2008, U.S. families adopted 17,438 children from other countries (compared with 7,093 in 1990). In 2008, Guatemala, China, Russia, Ethiopia, and South Korea were the 5 primary sending countries for children to the USA. Most children placed for international adoption have histories of poverty and social hardship in their home countries, and approximately 65% are adopted from orphanage/institutional settings. Although many young infants are abandoned shortly after birth, some older children have experienced family disruption resulting from parental illness, war, or natural disasters. The effects of institutionalization and other life stresses impact all areas of early development, creating distinctive risk factors for these children.

Worldwide, according to UNICEF, there are 50 prospective adopters for every available child. There is concern that in some countries of origin the demand for adoptive children from other countries outstrips regulation and oversight to protect these children. Opportunities for financial gain have lead to abuses including the sale and abduction of children, bribery, and financial coercion of families.

ROLE OF PEDIATRICIANS

Preadoption Medical Record Reviews

Adoption agencies are making increased efforts to obtain biological family health information and genetic histories to share with adoptive families prior to adoption. Pediatricians can help prospective adoptive parents evaluate the health and developmental history of a child and available background information from birth families in order to assess actual and potential problems or risks that children may have. Under the Hague Convention on Protection of Children and Co-operation in Respect of Intercountry Adoption (implemented in the USA on April 1, 2008), agencies in the USA that arrange international adoptions must make efforts to obtain accurate and complete health histories on children awaiting adoption.

The nature and quality of preadoption medical records of children living outside of the USA vary widely. Poor translation and use of medical terminology and medications that are unfamiliar to U.S. trained physicians are quite common. Results of specific diagnostic studies and laboratory tests performed in the child's home country should not be relied on and **should be repeated** once the child arrives in the USA. Paradoxically, review of the child's medical records may raise more questions than provide answers. Each medical diagnosis should be considered carefully before being rejected or accepted. Country-specific growth curves should be avoided as they may be inaccurate or reflect a general level of poor health and nutrition in the country of origin. Instead, serial growth data should be plotted on U.S. standard growth curves; they may reveal a pattern of poor growth due to malnutrition or other chronic illness. Photographs or videotapes/DVDs may provide the only objective data regarding a child's health status. The quality of this information, however, is often of questionable value. Nonetheless, full-face photographs may reveal dysmorphic features consistent with fetal alcohol syndrome (Chapter 100.2) or findings suggestive of other congenital disorders.

Frank interpretations of available information should be shared with the prospective adoptive parents. As noted by the American Academy of Pediatrics Committee on Early Childhood, Adoption and Dependent Care (1991), "It is not the pediatrician's role to judge the advisability of a proposed adoption, but it is appropriate and necessary that the prospective parents and any involved agency be apprised clearly and honestly of any special health needs detected now or anticipated in the future."

Postadoption Care

ARRIVAL VISIT After the child is settled in the new home, pediatricians should encourage adoptive parents to seek a comprehensive assessment of the child's health and development. The unique medical and developmental needs of internationally adopted children have led to the creation of specialty clinics throughout the USA. A significant number of internationally adopted children have acute or chronic medical problems, including growth deficiencies, anemia, elevated blood lead, dental decay, strabismus, birth defects, developmental delay, feeding and sensory difficulty, and social-emotional concerns (Chapter 34.1). All children with symptoms of an acute illness should receive immediate medical care. The American Academy of Pediatrics recommends that all children who are adopted from other countries undergo routine screening for infectious diseases and disorders of growth,

Table 34-1 RECOMMENDED SCREENING TESTS FOR NEWLY ARRIVING ADOPTEES

Screening tests
- Complete blood cell count
- Hemoglobin identification
- Blood lead level
- Urinalysis
- Newborn screening (children <12 mo)
- Vision and hearing screening
- Developmental testing

Other screening tests to consider based on clinical findings and age of the child
- Detection of *Helicobacter pylori* antibody or ^{13}C-urea breath test
- Stool cultures for bacterial pathogens
- Glucose-6-phosphate dehydrogenase deficiency screening
- Sickle cell
- Urine pregnancy test

Infectious disease screening (see Table 34-2)

Table 34-2 SCREENING TESTS FOR INFECTIOUS DISEASES IN IMMIGRANT CHILDREN

RECOMMENDED TESTS
Hepatitis B virus serologic testing*
• Hepatitis B surface antigen (HBsAg)
• Antibody to hepatitis B surface antigen (anti-HBs)
Hepatitis C virus serologic testing*†
Hepatitis A virus serologic testing†
Varicella virus serologic testing†
Syphilis serologic testing
• Nontreponemal test (RPR, VDRL, or ART)
• Treponemal test (MHA-TP or FTA-ABS)
Human immunodeficiency virus 1 and 2 testing (ELISA if >18 mo, PCR if <18 mo)*
Complete blood cell count with red blood cell indices and differential (if eosinophilia, see text)
Stool examination for ova and parasites (2-3 specimens)†
Stool examination for *Giardia lamblia* and *Cryptosporidium* antigen (1 specimen)†
Tuberculin skin test (with CXR if >5 mm induration)*†
OPTIONAL TESTS (FOR SPECIAL POPULATIONS OR CIRCUMSTANCES)
GC/Chlamydia
Malaria thick and thin smears
Urine for O&P for schistosomiasis, if hematuria present

*Repeat 3-6 mo after arrival.
†See text.
ART, automated reagin test; FTA-ABS, fluorescent treponemal antibody absorption; MHA-TP, microhemagglutination test for *Treponema pallidum*; RPR, rapid plasma reagin; VDRL, Venereal Disease Research Laboratories.

development, vision, and hearing (Tables 34-1 and 34-2). Additional tests (e.g., malaria) should be ordered depending on the prevalence of disease in the child's country of origin. If the child's PPD is negative, a repeat skin test should be performed in 4-6 mo, since children may have false negative tests due to poor nutrition. A positive PPD should be followed by a QuantiFERON-TB Gold test to determine if the response is the result of prior BCG vaccination (Chapter 207). If they have not received hepatitis A vaccine prior to leaving the USA, parents and other household contacts (siblings, grandparents, etc.) should also be immunized. In 1 survey, 65% of internationally adopted children had no written records of overseas immunizations; however, those with records appeared to have valid records, although doses were not necessarily acceptable according to the U.S. schedule (Chapter 165).

DEVELOPMENTAL DELAYS At the time of international adoption, many children exhibit delays in at least 1 area of development, but most exhibit significant gains within the 1st 12 mo after adoption. Those adopted before 6 mo of age usually demonstrate typical development, whereas those adopted at older ages have more variable outcomes.

GROWTH DELAYS Physical growth delays are common among internationally adopted children and may represent the combined result of many factors, including unknown/untreated medical conditions, malnutrition, and psychological deprivation. Weight and height at the time of adoption have been negatively correlated with the amount of time spent in institutional settings. Though most children experience a significant catch-up in physical growth following adoption, many remain shorter than their U.S. peers.

LANGUAGE DEVELOPMENT The majority of internationally adopted children have had little exposure to English. Within 24 mo postadoption, most preschool-age children attain English language skills equal to those of born in the USA. In older children, delays in native language skills often predict delays in English acquisition.

EATING CONCERNS Initial concerns about eating, sleep regulation, and repetitive (e.g., self-stimulating or self-soothing) behaviors are common, especially among children adopted from institutional settings. Feeding concerns are often linked to limited exposure to textured or solid foods. Also, children may not have developed an awareness of satiation cues, leading to hoarding or frequent vomiting. Feeding concerns often subside gradually with introduction of age-appropriate foods and parental limits to portion sizes. Occasionally, additional support from a speech pathologist or feeding specialist is warranted to address possible physical concerns that could impede proper feeding.

SLEEP CONCERNS Sleep is often disrupted as the child reacts to changes in routines and environments. Efforts to create continuity between the preadoption and postadoption environment can be helpful. Within the first few months, as the child's emotional self-regulation improves, many sleep concerns subside. Similarly, stereotypic behaviors, such as rocking or head banging, often diminish within the first few months following adoption.

SOCIAL AND EMOTIONAL DEVELOPMENT Through the attentive presence of a consistent caregiver, the infant's developing brain becomes more adept at regulating high arousal and emotional reactions. These dyadic interactions between child and caretaker are a critical component to later regulatory functioning and social-emotional development. The amount and quality of individualized caretaking children have received prior to their adoption is usually unknown. In many instances, entry into a secure, stable home setting with consistent caregivers is sufficient to support the child's emerging social-emotional development. At times, the child's prior experiences or biological disposition may result in behavior that is confusing to the adoptive parents. As such, the child's reactions may be subtle or difficult to interpret, interfering with the parents' ability to respond in a sensitive manner. In these circumstances, additional support may be helpful to foster the emerging relationships and behavioral regulation in the newly formed family.

FAMILY CONCERNS There are unique aspects to adoptive family formation that can create familial stress and impact child and family functioning. Specifically, some adoptive families may have to address infertility, creation of a multiracial family, disclosure of adoptive status, concerns and questions the child may have about their biological origins, and ongoing scrutiny by adoption agencies. Although most families acclimate well to the transition following adoption, some parents experience postadoption depression and may benefit from additional support to ease the family transition.

Families should be encouraged to speak openly and repeatedly about adoption with the child, beginning in the toddler years and continuing through adolescence. A child's understanding of adoption is related to overall cognitive development. It is common, and normal, for children to have questions about their adoption, typically between the ages of 7 and 10 yr. Pediatricians may need to respond to a number of concerns and questions on the part of adoptive parents or adopted adolescents when the adoptee's health and genetic history is incomplete or unknown. At any time, concerns about development, behavior and emotional functioning may or may not be related to the child's adoption history.

Most adopted children and families adjust well and lead healthy, productive lives. It is not common that adoptions disrupt; disruption rates are higher among children adopted from foster care, which the research associates with their older ages at time of adoption and their histories of multiple placements prior to adoption. As a result of a greater understanding of the needs of families who adopt children from foster care, agencies are placing greater emphasis on the preparation of adoptive parents and ensuring the availability of a full range of postadoption services, including physical health, mental health, and developmental services for their adopted children.

BIBLIOGRAPHY

Please visit the Nelson Textbook of Pediatrics *website at www.expertconsult.com for the complete bibliography.*

34.1 Medical Evaluation of Immigrant (Foreign-Born) Children for Infectious Diseases

Stacene R. Maroushek

Annually, more than 210,000 foreign-born children (≤16 yr old) enter the USA as asylees, refugees, and immigrants including international adoptees. This does not include undocumented children living and working in the USA, the U.S.-born children of foreign-born parents, or the ~2.7 million nonimmigrant visitors ≤16 yr old that legally enter the USA annually with temporary visas. It is estimated that 20% of children living in the USA are either immigrants or members of an immigrant family. With the exception of internationally adopted children, pediatric guidelines for screening these newly arrived children are sparse. The diverse countries of origin and patterns of infectious disease, the possibility of previous high-risk living circumstances (e.g., refugee camps, orphanages, foster care, rural/urban poor), the limited availability of reliable health care in many economically developing countries, the generally unknown past medical histories, and interactions with parents that may have limited English proficiency, varied educational, or economic experiences, make the medical evaluation of immigrant children a challenging but important task.

Before admission to the USA, all immigrant children are required to have a medical examination performed by a physician designated by the U.S. Department of State in their country of origin. This examination is limited to completing legal requirements for screening for certain communicable diseases and examination for serious physical or mental defects that would prevent the issue of a permanent residency visa. This evaluation is not a comprehensive assessment of the child's health and, except in limited circumstances, laboratory or radiographic screening for infectious diseases **is not required** for children <15 yr old. After entry into the USA, health screenings of refugees, but not other immigrants, are recommended to be done by the resettlement state. These postarrival assessments are not legally required, and there is little tracking of refugees as they move to different cities or states. Thus, many foreign-born children have had minimal prearrival or postarrival screening for infectious diseases or other health issues.

Immunization requirements and records are also varied depending on entry status. Internationally adopted children who are younger than 10 yr are exempt from Immigration and Nationality Act (INA) regulations pertaining to immunization of immigrants before arrival in the USA. Adoptive parents are required to sign a waiver indicating their intention to comply with U.S.-recommended immunizations, whereas other immigrants need only show evidence of up-to-date, not necessarily complete, immunizations before application for permanent resident (green card) status after arrival in the USA.

Immigrants having arrived in the USA years to decades ago likely have had more limited screening than those recently arrived immigrants. If adequate records of previous screenings cannot be obtained, full to limited re-screen, especially in an ill or failing to thrive child or youth should be considered.

Infectious diseases are among the most common medical diagnoses identified in immigrant children after arrival in the USA. Children may be asymptomatic; therefore, diagnoses must be made by screening tests in addition to history and physical examination. Because of inconsistent perinatal screening for hepatitis B and hepatitis C viruses, syphilis, and HIV and the high prevalence of certain intestinal parasites and tuberculosis, all foreign-born children should be screened for these infections on arrival in the USA. Suggested screening tests for infectious diseases are listed in Table 34-2. In addition to these infections, other medical and developmental issues, including hearing, vision, dental, and mental health assessments; evaluation of growth and development; nutritional assessment; lead exposure risk; complete blood cell count with red blood cell indices; microscopic urinalysis; newborn screening (this could be done in non-neonates, too) and/or measurement of thyroid-stimulating hormone concentration; and examination for congenital anomalies (including fetal alcohol syndrome) should be considered as part of the initial evaluation of any immigrant child.

Children should be examined within 1 mo of arrival in the USA or earlier if there are immediate health concerns, but foreign-born parents may not access the health care system with their children unless prompted by illness, school vaccination, or other legal requirements. **Thus, it is important to assess the completeness of previous medical screenings at any first visit with a foreign-born child.**

COMMONLY ENCOUNTERED INFECTIONS

Hepatitis B (Chapter 350)

The prevalence of hepatitis B surface antigen (HBsAg) in international adoptees and refugee children ranges from 1-5% and 4-14%, respectively, depending on the country of origin, age, and year studied. Prevalence of markers of past hepatitis B virus (HBV) infection is higher. Hepatitis B virus infection is most prevalent in immigrants from Asia, Africa, and some countries in Central and Eastern Europe and former Soviet Union (e.g., Bulgaria, Romania, Russia, and Ukraine) but also occurs in immigrants born in other countries. All immigrant children, even if previously vaccinated, coming from high-risk countries (HBsAg seropositivity >2%) should undergo serologic testing for HBV infection, including both HBsAg and antibody to HBsAg (anti-HBs), to identify current or chronic infection, past resolved infection, or evidence of previous immunization. Because HBV has a long incubation period (6 wk to 6 mo), the child may have become infected at or near the time of migration and initial testing might be falsely negative. Therefore, strong consideration should be given to a repeated evaluation 6 mo after arrival for all children, especially those from highly endemic countries. Chronic HBV infection is indicated by persistence of HBsAg for more than 6 mo. Children with HBsAg-positive test results should be evaluated to identify the presence of chronic HBV infection because chronic hepatitis B infection occurs in >90% of infants infected at birth or in the 1st year of life, and in 30% of children exposed at ages 1-5 yr. Once identified as being infected, additional testing to assess for biochemical evidence of severe or chronic liver disease or liver cancer should take place.

All exposed household or sexual contacts of a child or youth found to be HBsAg positive should be tested or have documentation of HBV immunization reviewed. Those found to be susceptible should have the series initiated. Immigrant children who test negative for HBV should receive immunization for HBV as soon as possible according to the recommended childhood and adolescent immunization schedule. Children who test positive for

HBsAg are infected with HBV acutely or chronically and do not need to be immunized, but should be educated about hepatitis B disease, transmission, monitoring, and treatment.

Hepatitis A (Chapter 350)

Many immigrant children have acquired hepatitis A virus (HAV) infection early in life and are, therefore, protected. Routine serologic screening for HAV antibody generally is not indicated to detect susceptible children. However, because routine childhood immunization against HAV is recommended in the USA beginning at 1-2 yr (12-35 mo) of age, antibody testing for HAV may be considered reasonable to determine whether these children have evidence of previous infection. If a child has no evidence of previous infection, the child should be immunized against HAV as recommended.

Hepatitis C (Chapter 350)

Children from Eastern Mediterranean and Western Pacific countries, Africa, China, and Southeast Asia should be considered for hepatitis C infection screening. The decision to screen children should depend on history (e.g., receipt of blood products; traditional percutaneous procedures such as tattooing, body piercing, circumcisions, or other exposures to reused, unsterile medical devices) and the prevalence of infection in the child's country of origin. All children coming from Egypt, which has the highest known seroprevalence (12% nationally and 40% in some villages), should be tested for hepatitis C. To distinguish chronic HCV from past/resolved HCV infection, complete testing must include serologic antibody screening (anti-HCV), followed by confirmatory HCV test (HCV RIBA or a nucleic acid test for HCV RNA).

Intestinal Pathogens

Fecal examinations for ova and parasites by an experienced laboratory will identify a pathogen in 15-35% of internationally adopted children; prevalence rates in immigrants and refugees range from 8-86%. The prevalence of intestinal parasites varies by country of origin, time period when studied, previous living conditions (including water quality, sanitation, and access to footwear) and the age of the child, with toddler/young school-aged children being most affected.

The most common pathogens identified are *Giardia lamblia* (Chapter 274), *Trichuris trichiura* (Chapter 285), *Hymenolepis* species (Chapter 294), *Entamoeba histolytica/dispar* (Chapter 273), *Schistosoma* species (Chapter 292), *Strongyloides stercoralis* (Chapter 287), *Ascaris lumbricoides* (Chapter 283), and hookworm (Chapter 284). All nonpregnant refugees over 2 yr of age coming from sub-Saharan Africa and Southeast Asia should be presumptively treated with predeparture albendazole. Rates of intestinal helminth infections susceptible to albendazole (*Ascaris*, *Trichuris*, or hookworm) from these areas have decreased. Nonrefugee immigrants do not receive predeparture treatment.

If documented predeparture treatment was given, an eosinophil count should be performed. An absolute eosinophil count of >400 cells/μL, if persistently elevated for 3-6 mo after arrival, should prompt further investigation for tissue-invasive parasites such as *Strongyloides* and *Schistosoma* species. If no documented predeparture treatment was given, 2 stool ova and parasite specimens obtained from separate morning stools should be examined by the concentration method, and an eosinophil count should be performed. If the child is symptomatic, including evidence of poor physical growth, but no eosinophilia is present, a single stool specimen should also be sent for *G. lamblia* and *Cryptosporidium parvum* antigen detection. All potentially pathogenic parasites found should be treated appropriately.

Therapy for intestinal parasites will be successful, but complete eradication may not occur always. Therefore, repeat ova and parasite testing after treatment in children who remain symptomatic is important to ensure successful elimination of all parasites. A follow-up eosinophil count is also recommended 3-6 mo later, and if still elevated, further evaluation is warranted. In addition, testing stool specimens for *Salmonella* species (Chapter 190), *Shigella* species (Chapter 191), *Campylobacter* species (Chapter 194), and *Escherichia coli* O157:H7 (Chapter 192) should be considered in children with diarrhea, especially if stools are bloody.

Tuberculosis (Chapter 207)

Tuberculosis (TB) commonly is encountered in immigrants from all countries because *Mycobacterium tuberculosis* infects ~30% of the world's population. Latent tuberculosis infection rates range from 0.6-30% in adoptees and up to 60% in some refugee children from North Africa and the Middle East. Prior to 2007, chest radiographs or tuberculin skin tests (TST) were generally not administered in children less than 15 yr of age and reports indicate that 1-2% of these unscreened children may enter the USA with undiagnosed active TB disease.

Since 2007, TB Technical Instructions for Medical Evaluation of Aliens have required that children aged 2-14 yr undergo a TB skin test if they are medically screened in countries where the TB rate is 20 cases or more per 100,000 population. If the skin test is positive, a chest x-ray is required. If the chest x-ray suggests TB, cultures and three sputum smears are required, all before arrival in the USA. This requirement is being phased in over a number of years, and some countries with a case rate of 20 per 100,000 may not currently be screening children. Check with the Centers for Disease Control and Prevention, Division of Global Migration and Quarantine for latest information (*www.cdc.gov/ncidod/dq/technica.htm*).

Because active tuberculosis disease may be more severe in young children, and latent TB infection may reactivate in later years, screening with the TST is highly important in this high-risk population. Serologic-based interferon gamma release assays such as QuantiFERON-TB Gold or T-SPOT. TB tests, although being used more frequently in adults, have not been extensively studied in children. Several studies indicate they may be unreliable in toddlers and infants.

Routine chest radiography is not indicated in asymptomatic children with negative TST results. However, some immigrants may be anergic because of malnutrition or underlying HIV infection. If malnutrition is suspected, the TST should be repeated once the child is better nourished. Receipt of bacille Calmette-Guérin (BCG) vaccine is not a contraindication to a TST, and a positive TST result should not routinely be attributed to BCG vaccine. In these children, further investigation is necessary to determine whether latent tuberculosis infection or active disease is present and therapy is needed. Empirical therapy should be considered for any child younger than 4 yr with a known recent exposure to sputum positive TB disease. Some experts repeat TST 3-6 mo after a child has left an area with high prevalence of tuberculosis. When tuberculosis is suspected in an immigrant child, serious efforts to isolate and test the organism for drug susceptibilities are imperative because of the high prevalence of drug resistance in many countries.

Syphilis (Chapter 210)

Congenital syphilis, especially with involvement of the central nervous system, may not have been diagnosed or may have been treated inadequately in immigrants from some developing countries. Each immigrant child should be screened for syphilis by reliable nontreponemal and treponemal serologic tests, regardless of history or a report of treatment. Children with positive treponemal serologic test results should be evaluated by an individual with special expertise to assess the differential diagnosis of pinta, yaws, syphilis, or other noninfectious causes of false-positive tests, and to determine the extent of the infection so appropriate treatment can be administered.

HIV Infection (Chapter 268)

The risk of HIV infection in immigrant children depends on the country of origin and individual risk factors. Because of the rapidly changing epidemiology of HIV infection, because immigrants may come from populations at high risk of infection, and because those less than 15 yr of age are not required to be tested prior to arrival, screening for HIV should be performed on all immigrant children. Although many adoptee children will have HIV test results documented in their referral information, test results from the child's country of origin may not be reliable. Conversely, refugee testing, if performed on children, is generally done in a highly regulated International Organization for Migration laboratory. Transplacentally acquired maternal antibody in the absence of infection can be detected in a child younger than 18 mo, thus HIV antibody tests should only be used in children >18 mo of age. PCR tests for HIV RNA or DNA should be used in those less than 18 mo old. Positive HIV antibody or PCR test results in any child or youth requires immediate clinical and laboratory evaluation as well as specialist counseling.

Other Infectious Diseases

Skin infections that occur commonly in immigrant children include bacterial (e.g., impetigo), fungal (e.g., candidiasis, tinea), and ectoparasitic (e.g., scabies, pediculosis) infections. Diseases such as typhoid fever, malaria, leprosy, or melioidosis are encountered sporadically in immigrant children. Although routine screening for these diseases is not recommended, findings of fever, splenomegaly, respiratory tract infection, anemia, or eosinophilia should prompt an appropriate evaluation on the basis of the epidemiology of infectious diseases that occur in the child's country of origin. If the child arrived within the previous year from a country where malaria is endemic, malaria should be considered in the differential diagnosis of any febrile illness, especially if no predeparture antimalarial treatment was given.

In the USA, multiple outbreaks of measles have been reported in immigrant children, including those adopted from China, and in their U.S. contacts. Prospective parents traveling internationally to adopt children, as well as their household contacts, should ensure that they have a history of natural disease or have been adequately immunized for measles according to U.S. guidelines. All people born after 1957 should receive 2 doses of measles-containing vaccine in the absence of documented measles infection or contraindication to the vaccine. Susceptible immigrant children and their families should be immunized as soon as possible after arrival according to recommended childhood, adolescent, and adult immunization schedules (Chapter 238).

Clinicians should be aware of potential diseases in high-risk immigrant children and their clinical manifestations. Some diseases, such as central nervous system cysticercosis, may have incubation periods as long as several years, and thus may not be detected during initial screening. On the basis of findings at the initial evaluation, consideration should be given to a repeat evaluation 6 mo after arrival. In most cases, the longer the interval from arrival to development of a clinical syndrome, the less likely the syndrome can be attributed to a pathogen acquired in the country of origin.

Immunizations

Some immigrants will have written documentation of immunizations received in their birth or home country. Although immunizations such as BCG, diphtheria and tetanus toxoids, and pertussis (DTP), poliovirus, measles, and hepatitis B virus vaccines often are documented, other immunizations, such as *Haemophilus influenzae* type b, mumps, and rubella vaccines, are given less frequently; and *Streptococcus pneumoniae*, human papillomavirus, meningococcal, and varicella vaccines are given rarely. Immigrant children and adolescents should receive immunizations according to the recommended schedules in the USA for healthy children and adolescents (Chapter 165). Although some vaccines with inadequate potency are used in other countries, most vaccines available worldwide are produced with adequate quality control standards and are reliable. Written documentation of immunizations can usually be accepted as evidence of adequacy of previous immunization if the vaccines, dates of administration, number of doses, intervals between doses, and age of the child at the time of immunization are consistent internally and comparable to current U.S. or World Health Organization schedules. Given the limited data available regarding verification of immunization records from other countries, measurements of serum antibodies to vaccine antigens is an option to ensure that vaccines were given and were immunogenic. *An equally acceptable alternative when doubt exists is to reimmunize the child.* Because the rate of more serious local reactions after diphtheria and tetanus toxoids and acellular pertussis (DTaP) vaccine increases with the number of doses administered, serologic testing for antibody to tetanus and diphtheria toxins before reimmunizing or if a serious reaction occurs can decrease risk.

In children older than 6 mo with or without written documentation of immunization, testing for antibodies to diphtheria and tetanus toxoids and poliovirus may be considered to determine whether the child has protective antibody concentrations. If the child has protective concentrations, then the immunization series should be completed as appropriate for that child's age. In children older than 12 mo, measles, mumps, rubella, and varicella antibody concentrations may be measured to determine whether the child is immune; these antibody tests should not be performed in children younger than 12 mo because of the potential presence of maternal antibody. Many immigrant children will need a dose of mumps and rubella vaccines, because these vaccines are administered infrequently in developing countries. Measles-mumps-rubella (MMR) vaccine should be administered for mumps and rubella coverage, even if measles antibodies are present. At this time, no antibody testing is reliable or available routinely to assess immunity to pertussis. As discussed previously, serologic testing for hepatitis B should be performed for all children to determine their hepatitis B immunity status. If serologic testing is not available and receipt of immunogenic vaccines cannot be ensured, the prudent course is to provide the series.

BIBLIOGRAPHY

Please visit the Nelson Textbook of Pediatrics *website at www.expertconsult.com for the complete bibliography.*

Chapter 35
Foster and Kinship Care

Moira Szilagyi and Sara B. Eleoff

The mission of foster care is to provide for the health, safety, and well-being of children while assisting their families with services to promote reunification. The placement of children in another family has served the needs of children in many societies worldwide throughout history. The institution of foster care was developed in the USA as a temporary resource for children during times of family crisis and is rooted in the principle that children fare best when raised in family settings. The 1989 United Nations Convention on the Rights of the Child, a legally binding international instrument, addresses the need for such care for all children worldwide.

For the full continuation of this chapter, please visit the Nelson Textbook of Pediatrics *website at www.expertconsult.com.*

Chapter 36
Impact of Violence on Children

Marilyn Augustyn and Barry Zuckerman

Violence, whether as the victim, perpetrator, or witness, whether in person or through the media, is a major public health problem throughout the world (Chapter 1). The focus of pediatrics should not be limited to the traditional care of violence-related injury. Exposure to violence disrupts the healthy development of children; pediatricians need to be aware of this risk factor. Pediatric providers also have a wider responsibility to advocate on local, state, national, and international levels for safer environments in which all children can grow and thrive.

For the full continuation of this chapter, please visit the Nelson Textbook of Pediatrics *website at www.expertconsult.com.*

36.1 Bullying and School Violence

Douglas Vanderbilt and Marilyn Augustyn

BULLYING

Definition

Bullying is the assertion of power through aggression that involves a bully repeatedly and intentionally targeting a weaker victim through social, emotional, or physical means. Bullying affects a large number of children and lays the groundwork for long-term depression, suicidality, psychotic symptoms, conduct problems, and psychosomatic concerns seen in children. Children can move between being a bully, victim, bully-victim (both a bully and a victim at different times), or bystander. Bullying can be **direct,** involving physical aggression such as hitting, stealing, and threatening with a weapon or verbal aggression such as name-calling, public humiliation, and intimidation, or it can be **indirect,** involving relational aggression such as spreading rumors, social rejection, exclusion from peer groups, and ignoring. Bullying occurs most frequently at school when there is minimal supervision during breaks, recess, and lunch at playgrounds, in hallways, and en route to and from school. Technology creates unique venues for this behavior through text messaging, mass emailing, and Internet chat rooms and message boards.

For the full continuation of this chapter, please visit the Nelson Textbook of Pediatrics *website at www.expertconsult.com.*

36.2 Effects of War on Children

Isaiah D. Wexler and Eitan Kerem

The impact of war on children is devastating, and its effects can last for decades after hostilities have ceased. In collected health surveys it was found that for 13 war-prone countries, 7.5% of the victims were children aged <15 yr. Based on statistics accrued by the United Nations Children's Fund (UNICEF), of the 3.6 million people killed as a result of military conflict between the years 1990 and 2003, 90% were civilian and 50% were children. During the past decade, the effects of war on children has not abated, and children continue to be the victims of warfare taking place on the Asian subcontinent, sub-Saharan Africa, and the Middle East.

For the full continuation of this chapter, please visit the Nelson Textbook of Pediatrics *website at www.expertconsult.com.*

Chapter 37
Abused and Neglected Children

Howard Dubowitz and Wendy G. Lane

The abuse and neglect (maltreatment) of children are pervasive problems worldwide, with short- and long-term physical and mental health and social consequences. Child health care professionals have an important role in helping address this problem. In addition to their responsibility to identify maltreated children and help ensure their protection and health, child health care professionals can also play vital roles related to prevention, treatment, and advocacy. Rates and policies vary greatly between nations and often within nations. Rates of maltreatment and provision of services are affected by the overall policies of the country, province, or state governing recognition and response to child abuse and neglect. Two broad approaches have been identified: a child and family welfare approach and a child safety approach. Though overlapping, the focus in the former is the family as a whole, and in the latter, on the child perceived to be at risk. The USA has a child safety approach.

DEFINITIONS

Abuse is defined as acts of commission and **neglect** as acts of omission. The U.S. government defines child abuse as "any recent act or failure to act on the part of a parent or caretaker, which results in death, serious physical or emotional harm, sexual abuse or exploitation, or an act or failure to act which presents an imminent risk of serious harm." Some states in the USA also include other household members. Children may be found in situations in which no actual harm has occurred and no imminent risk of serious harm is evident, but potential harm may be a concern. Many states include potential harm in their child abuse laws. Consideration of potential harm enables preventive intervention, although predicting potential harm is inherently difficult. Two aspects should be considered. One is the likelihood of harm; the other is the severity.

Physical abuse includes beating, shaking, burning, and biting. Corporal punishment is widely accepted in many countries: the World Health Organization (WHO) reported in 2006 that 106 countries do not prohibit the use of corporal punishment in schools, 147 do not prohibit it within alternative care settings, and only 16 prohibit its use in the home. Within the USA, the threshold for defining corporal punishment as abuse is unclear. One can consider any injury beyond transient redness as abuse. If parents spank a child, it should be limited to the buttocks, should occur over clothing, and should never involve the head and neck. When parents use objects other than a hand, the potential for serious harm increases. Acts of serious violence (e.g., throwing a hard object, slapping an infant's face) should be seen as abusive even if no injury ensues; significant risk of harm exists. While some child health care professionals think that hitting is acceptable under limited conditions, almost all believe that more constructive approaches to discipline are preferable. Although many think that hitting a child should never be accepted, and several studies have documented the potential harm, there remains a reluctance to label hitting as abuse unless there is an injury. It is clear that the emotional impact of being hit may leave the most worrisome scar, long after the bruises fade and the fracture heals.

Sexual abuse has been defined as "the involvement of dependent, developmentally immature children and adolescents in sexual activities which they do not fully comprehend, to which they are unable to give consent, or that violate the social taboos of family roles." Sexual abuse includes exposure to sexually explicit materials, oral-genital contact, genital-to-genital contact, genital fondling, and genital-to-anal contact. Any touching of private areas by parents or caregivers in a context other than necessary care is inappropriate.

Neglect refers to omissions in care, resulting in actual or potential harm. Omissions may include inadequate health care, education, supervision, protection from hazards in the environment, physical needs (e.g., clothing, food), and/or emotional support. A preferable alternative to focusing on caregiver omissions is to instead consider the basic needs (or rights) of children (e.g., adequate food, clothing, shelter, health care, education, nurturance); neglect occurs when a need is not adequately met, whatever the reasons. A child whose health is jeopardized or harmed by not receiving necessary care experiences medical neglect. Not all such situations necessarily require a report to child protective services (CPS); less intrusive initial efforts may be appropriate.

Psychological abuse includes verbal abuse and humiliation and acts that scare or terrorize a child. Although this form of abuse may be extremely harmful to children, resulting in depression, anxiety, estrangement, poor self-esteem, or lack of empathy, CPS seldom becomes involved because of the difficulty in proving such allegations. Child health care professionals should still carefully consider this form of maltreatment, even if the concern fails to reach a legal or agency threshold for reporting. These children and families can benefit from counseling and referrals to social support, as well as behavioral, educational, and mental health services. Many children experience more than one form of maltreatment; CPS may address psychologic abuse in the context of investigating other forms of maltreatment.

Internationally, problems of **trafficking** in children, for purposes of cheap labor and/or sexual exploitation, expose children to all of the forms of abuse just noted.

INCIDENCE AND PREVALENCE

Global Situation

Child abuse and neglect are not rare and occur worldwide. WHO has estimated that 40 million children under the age of 15 yr suffer from abuse and neglect; it has been estimated that over 1 million children have been trafficked. Studies from many countries across the globe indicate that more than 80% of children suffer physical punishment in their homes, with over 30% experiencing severe physical punishment. Surveys reported by UNICEF confirm these reports; 1 survey conducted in the Middle East reported that 30% of children had been beaten or tied up by parents, and in a 2nd survey in a Southeast Asian country, 30% of mothers reported having hit their child with an object in the past 6 mo.

United States Situation

In the USA, abuse and neglect mostly occur behind closed doors and often are a well kept secret. Nevertheless, there were over 3 million reports to CPS involving over 6 million children in the USA in 2008—a rate of 49.4 per 1000 children. Of the 772,000 substantiated reports, 71% were for neglect, 2.2% for medical neglect, 16% for physical abuse, 9% for sexual abuse, and 7.3% for psychologic maltreatment. This translates to a rate of 8 per 1000 children identified as neglected, a rate that has been steady since the early 1990s; this is in contrast to declining rates of sexual abuse (down 53%) and physical abuse (down 48%) between 1992 and 2006. Medical personnel make about 12% of all reports.

The highest rate of maltreatment, 16.4 per 1000, was for children 0 to 3 yr old. The rate for black children was almost twice that of white children (20.4 vs 11.0 per 1000). This rate is likely due, in part, to professional bias in identifying, reporting, and investigating low-income and minority families for maltreatment. Sources independent from the official CPS statistics cited above confirm the prevalence of child maltreatment. In a community survey, 3% of parents reported using very severe violence (e.g., hitting with fist, burning, using gun or knife) against their child in the prior year. Considering a natural disinclination to disclose socially undesirable information, such rates are both conservative and alarming.

Etiology

Child maltreatment seldom has a single cause; rather, multiple and interacting biopsychosocial **risk factors** at 4 levels usually exist. At the *individual level*, a child's disability or a parent's depression or substance abuse predispose a child to maltreatment. At the *familial level*, intimate partner (or domestic) violence presents risks for children. Influential *community factors* include stressors such as dangerous neighborhoods or a lack of recreational facilities. Professional inaction may contribute to neglect, such as when the treatment plan is not clearly communicated. Broad *societal factors*, such as poverty and its associated burdens, also contribute to maltreatment. WHO estimates the rate of homicide of children is approximately twofold higher in low-income compared to high-income countries (2.58 vs 1.21 per 100,000 population), but clearly homicide occurs in high-income countries (Table 37-1). Children in all social classes can be maltreated, and child health care professionals need to guard against biases concerning low-income families.

In contrast, **protective factors**, such as family supports, or a mother's concern for her child, may buffer risk factors and protect children from maltreatment. Identifying and building on protective factors can be vital to intervening effectively. One can say to a parent, for example, "I can see how much you love ____. What can we do to keep her out of the hospital?" Child maltreatment results from a complex interplay among risk and protective

Table 37-1 CHILD MALTREATMENT DEATHS BY NATION

COUNTRY	DEATHS PER 100,000 CHILDREN*
Spain	0.1
Greece	0.2
Italy	0.2
Ireland	0.3
Norway	0.3
Netherlands	0.6
Sweden	0.6
Korea	0.8
Australia	0.8
Germany	0.8
Denmark	0.8
Finland	0.8
Poland	0.9
UK	0.9
Switzerland	0.9
Canada	1.0
Austria	1.0
Japan	1.0
Slovak Republic	1.0
Belgium	1.1
Czech Republic	1.2
New Zealand	1.3
Hungary	1.3
France	1.4
USA	2.4
Mexico	3.0
Portugal	3.7

*Deaths include obvious maltreatment and those of undetermined intent.

From UNICEF: A league table of child maltreatment deaths in rich nations. In *Inocenti Report Card No 5*, Florence, September 2003, UNICEF Innocenti Research Centre, Figure 1b, p 4.

factors. A single mother who has a colicky baby and who recently lost her job is at risk for maltreatment, but a loving grandmother may be protective. A good understanding of factors that contribute to maltreatment, as well as those that are protective, should guide an appropriate response.

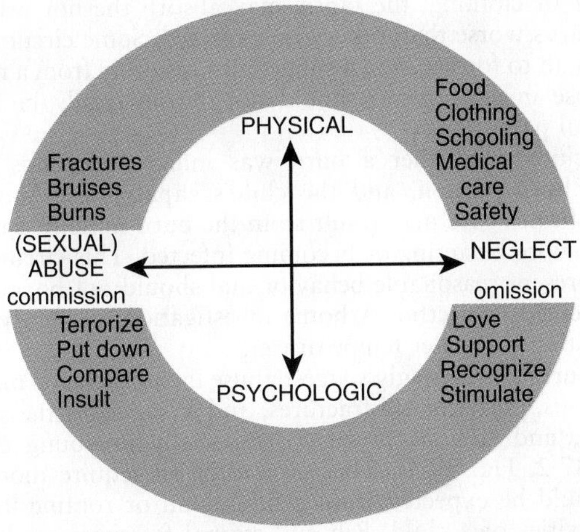

Figure 37-1 The spectrum of child maltreatment. Child maltreatment encompasses acts of commission, abuse, and acts of omission or neglect by a caretaker that adversely affect children. The act can be physical or psychologic. The boundaries between these areas are indistinct and psychologic; physical abuse and neglect overlap and may exist at the same time or various times in a child's life. Sexual abuse may be considered a specific type of physical abuse that has strong emotional components. Physical abuse and neglect invariably have short- and long-term psychologic consequences. Psychologic consequences may persist long after the physical wounds heal.

Clinical Manifestations

Child abuse and neglect can manifest in many different ways (Fig. 37-1). With regard to physical abuse, a critical element is the lack of a plausible history other than inflicted trauma. As with any medical condition, the onus is on the clinician to carefully consider the differential diagnosis and not jump to conclusions.

Bruises are the most common manifestation of physical abuse. Features suggestive of inflicted bruises include (1) bruising in a preambulatory infant (occurring in just 2% of infants), (2) bruising of padded and less exposed areas (buttocks, cheeks, under the chin, genitalia), (3) patterned bruising or burns conforming to shape of an object or ligatures around the wrists (Figs. 37-2 and 37-3), and (4) multiple bruises, especially if clearly of different ages. Estimating the age of bruises needs to be done cautiously. Red suggests less than a week, yellow suggests more than 1-2 days. It is very difficult to precisely determine the ages of bruises.

Other conditions such as birthmarks and Mongolian spots can be confused with bruises and abuse. These skin markings are not tender and do not rapidly change color or size. An underlying medical explanation for bruises may exist, such as blood dyscrasias or connective tissue disorders (hemophilia, Ehlers-Danlos). The history or examination usually provides clues to these conditions. Henoch-Schönlein purpura, the most common vasculitis in young children, may be confused with abuse. The pattern and location of bruises caused by abuse are usually different from those due to a coagulopathy. Noninflicted bruises are characteristically anterior and over bony prominences, such as shins and forehead. The presence of a medical disorder does not preclude abuse.

Cultural practices can cause bruising. Cao gio, or *coining*, is a Southeast Asian folkloric therapy. A hard object is vigorously

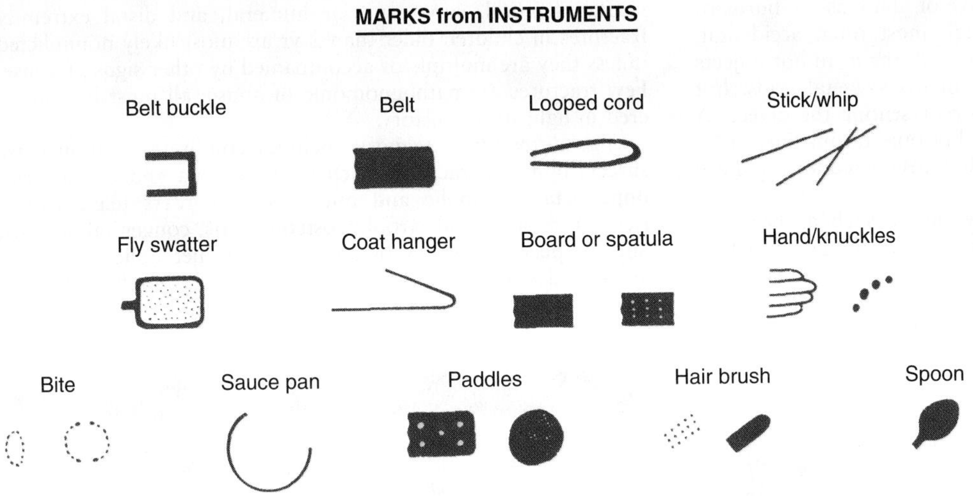

Figure 37-2 A variety of instruments may be used to inflict injury on a child. Often the choice of an instrument is a matter of convenience. Marks tend to silhouette or outline the shape of the instrument. The possibility of intentional trauma should prompt a high degree of suspicion when injuries to a child are geometric, paired, mirrored, of various ages or types, or on relatively protected parts of the body. Early recognition of intentional trauma is important to provide therapy and prevent escalation to more serious injury.

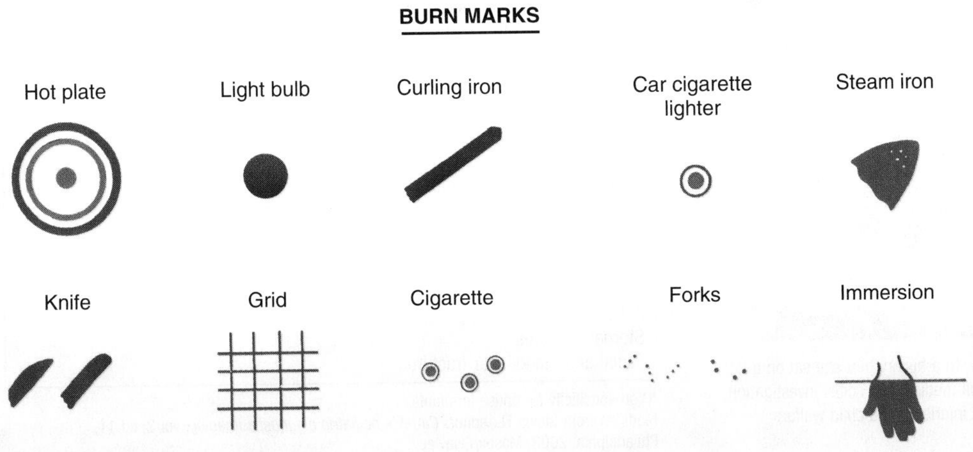

Figure 37-3 Marks from heated objects cause burns in a pattern that duplicates that of the object. Familiarity with the common heated objects that are used to traumatize children facilitates recognition of possible intentional injuries. The location of the burn is important in determining its cause. Children tend to explore surfaces with the palmar surface of the hand and rarely touch a heated object repeatedly or for a long time.

rubbed on the skin, causing petechiae or purpura. Cupping is another approach, popular in the Middle East. A heated glass is applied to the skin, often on the back. As it cools, a vacuum results, leading to perfectly circular bruises. The context here is important, and such circumstances should not be considered abusive.

A careful history of bleeding problems in the patient and first degree relatives is needed. If a bleeding disorder is suspected, a platelet count, prothrombin time, international normalized ratio (the ratio of the prothrombin time to a control sample, raised to the power of the International Sensitivity Index), and partial thromboplastin time should be obtained (Chapter 469). More extensive testing should be considered in consultation with a hematologist.

Bites have a characteristic pattern of 1 or 2 opposing arches with multiple bruises (see Fig. 37-2). They can be inflicted by an adult, another child, an animal, or the patient. Bites by a child (younger than approximately 8 yr with primary teeth) typically have a distance of less than 2.5 cm between the canines—often the most prominent bruises. The appearance of animal bites is variable (Chapter 705); they usually have narrower arches than human bites and are often deep. Self-inflicted bites are on accessible areas, particularly the hands. Adult bites raise concern for abuse. Multiple bites by another child suggest inadequate supervision and neglect.

Burns may be inflicted or due to inadequate supervision. Scalding burns may result from immersion or splash (Fig. 37-4; also see Fig. 37-3). Immersion burns, when a child is forcibly held in hot water, show clear delineation between the burned and healthy skin and uniform depth (see Fig. 37-4). They may have a sock or glove distribution. Splash marks are usually absent, unlike when a child inadvertently encounters hot water. Symmetrical burns are especially suggestive of abuse as are burns of the buttocks and perineum. Although most often accidental, splash burn may also result from abuse. Burns from hot objects such as curling irons, radiators, steam irons, metal grids, hot knives, and cigarettes leave patterns representing the object. A child is likely to try to escape from a hot object; thus burns that are extensive and deep reflect more than fleeting contact and are suggestive of abuse.

Several conditions mimic abusive burns, such as brushing against a hot radiator, car seat burns, hemangiomas, and folk remedies such as moxibustion. Impetigo may resemble cigarette burns. Cigarette burns are usually 7-10 mm across, whereas impetigo has lesions of varying size. Noninflicted cigarette burns are usually oval and superficial.

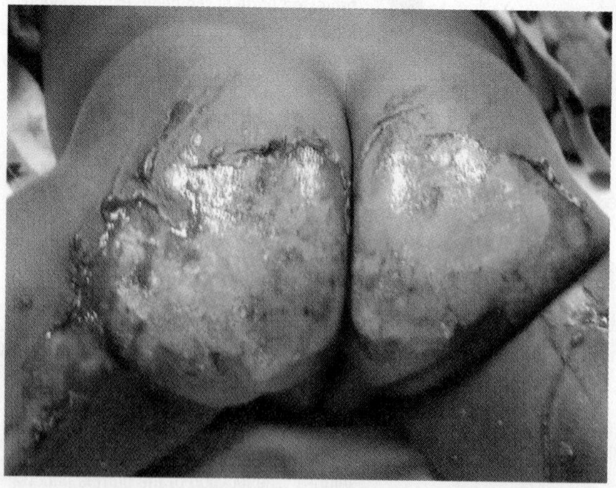

Figure 37-4 A 1 yr old child brought to a hospital with a history that she sat on a hot radiator. Suspicious injuries such as this require a full medical and social investigation including a skeletal survey to look for occult skeletal injuries and a child welfare evaluation.

Neglect frequently contributes to childhood burns (Chapter 68). Children, home alone, may be burned in house fires. A parent taking drugs may cause a fire and may be unable to protect a child. Exploring children may pull hot liquids left unattended onto themselves. Liquids cool as they flow downward so that the burn is most severe and broad proximally. If the child is wearing a diaper or clothing, the fabric may absorb the hot water and cause burns worse than otherwise expected. Some circumstances are difficult to foresee, and a single burn resulting from a momentary lapse in supervision should not automatically be seen as neglectful parenting.

Concluding whether a burn was inflicted depends on the history, burn pattern, and the child's capabilities. A delay in seeking health care may result from the burn initially appearing minor, before blistering or becoming infected. This circumstance may represent reasonable behavior and should not be automatically deemed neglectful. A home investigation is often valuable (e.g., testing the water temperature).

Fractures that strongly suggest abuse include: classic metaphyseal lesions, posterior rib fractures, and fractures of the scapula, sternum, and spinous processes, especially in young children (Table 37-2, Fig. 37-5). These fractures all require more force than would be expected from a minor fall or routine handling and activities of a child. Rib and sternal fractures rarely result from cardiopulmonary resuscitation, even when performed by untrained adults. In abused infants, rib, metaphyseal, and skull fractures are most common. Femoral and humeral fractures in nonambulatory infants are also very worrisome for abuse. With increasing mobility and running, toddlers can fall with enough rotational force to cause a spiral, femoral fracture. Multiple fractures in various stages of healing are suggestive of abuse; nevertheless, underlying conditions need to be considered. Clavicular, femoral, supracondylar humeral, and distal extremity fractures in children older than 2 yr are most likely noninflicted unless they are multiple or accompanied by other signs of abuse. Few fractures are pathognomonic of abuse; all must be considered in light of the history.

The *differential diagnosis* includes conditions that increase susceptibility to fractures, such as osteopenia and osteogenesis imperfecta, metabolic and nutritional disorders (e.g., scurvy, rickets), renal osteodystrophy, osteomyelitis, congenital syphilis, and neoplasia. Features of congenital or metabolic conditions associated with nonabusive fractures include family history of recurrent fractures after minor trauma, abnormally shaped

Table 37-2 SKELETAL INJURIES FROM ABUSE

COMMON
*Multiple fractures (unsuspected and/or varying in age especially if bilateral)**
*Classic metaphyseal lesions**
*Multiple rib fractures (especially posterior)**
Diaphyseal fractures (nonambulatory infant/child)
Skull fractures (often complex)
Subperiosteal new bone formation
LESS COMMON
Spinous process, vertebral body
Small bones of hands and feet
Clavicular fractures (usually low risk for abuse)
Femoral fracture in nonambulatory children
Humeral fractures (especially mid shaft) in children under 3 yr
Dislocations and epiphyseal separations
UNCOMMON
*Scapular fractures**
Pelvic fractures
Sternal fractures
Facial and mandibular fractures

*High specificity for abuse in infants.
Modified from Slovis TL, editor: *Caffey's pediatric diagnostic imaging*, vol 2, ed 11, Philadelphia, 2008, Mosby/Elsevier.

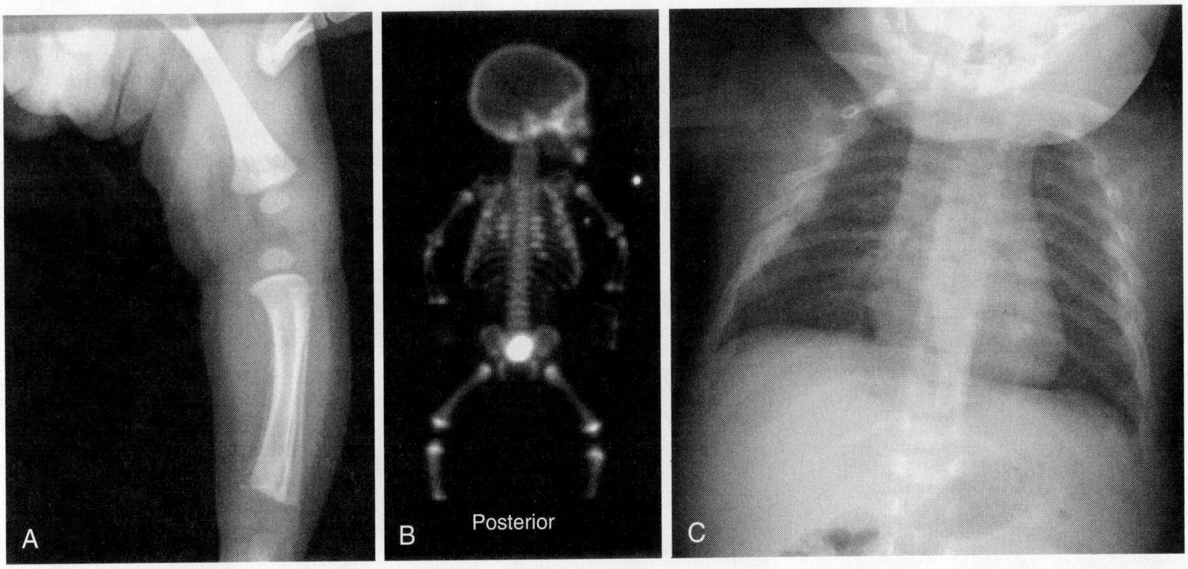

Figure 37-5 *A,* Metaphyseal fracture of the distal tibia in a 3 mo old infant admitted to the hospital with severe head injury. There is also periosteal new bone formation of the tibia, perhaps from previous injury. *B,* Bone scan of same infant. Initial chest x-ray showed a single fracture of the right posterior 4th rib. A radionuclide bone scan performed 2 days later revealed multiple previously unrecognized fractures of the posterior and lateral ribs. *C,* Follow-up radiographs 2 wk later showed multiple healing rib fractures. This pattern of fracture is highly specific for child abuse. The mechanism of these injuries is usually violent squeezing of the chest.

cranium, dentinogenesis imperfecta, blue sclera, craniotabes, ligamentous laxity, bowed legs, hernia, and translucent skin. Subperiosteal new bone formation is a nonspecific finding seen in infectious, traumatic, and metabolic disorders. In young infants, new bone formation may be a normal physiologic finding, usually bilateral, symmetric, and less than 2 mm in depth.

The evaluation of a fracture should include a skeletal survey in children less than 2 yr of age when abuse seems possible. Multiple films with different views are needed; "babygrams" (1 or 2 films of the entire body) should be avoided. If the survey is normal, but concern for an occult injury remains, a radionucleotide bone scan should be performed to detect a possible acute injury (see Fig. 37-5). Follow-up films after 2 wk may also reveal fractures not apparent initially (see Fig 37-5).

In corroborating the history and the injury, the age of a fracture can only be crudely estimated (Table 37-3). Soft-tissue swelling subsides in 2-21 days. Periosteal new bone is visible within 4-21 days. Loss of definition of the fracture line occurs between 10-21 days. Soft callus can be visible after 10 days and hard callus between 14-90 days. These time frames are shorter in infancy and longer in children with poor nutritional status or a chronic underlying disease. Fractures of flat bones such as the skull do not form callus and cannot be aged.

Abusive head trauma (AHT) results in the most significant morbidity and mortality. Abusive injury may be caused by direct impact, asphyxia, or shaking. Subdural hematomas (Fig. 37-6), retinal hemorrhages (especially when extensive and involving multiple layers) (Fig. 37-7), and diffuse axonal injury strongly suggest AHT, especially when they co-occur (Chapter 63). The poor neck muscle tone and relatively large heads of infants make them vulnerable to acceleration-deceleration forces associated with shaking, leading to AHT. Children may lack external signs of injury, even with serious intracranial trauma. Signs and symptoms may be nonspecific, ranging from lethargy, vomiting (without diarrhea), changing neurologic status or seizures, and coma. In all preverbal children, an index of suspicion for AHT should exist when children present with these signs and symptoms.

Acute intracranial trauma is best evaluated via initial and follow-up CT. MRIs are helpful in differentiating extra axial fluid, determining timing of injuries, assessing parenchymal injury, and identifying vascular anomalies. MRIs are best obtained

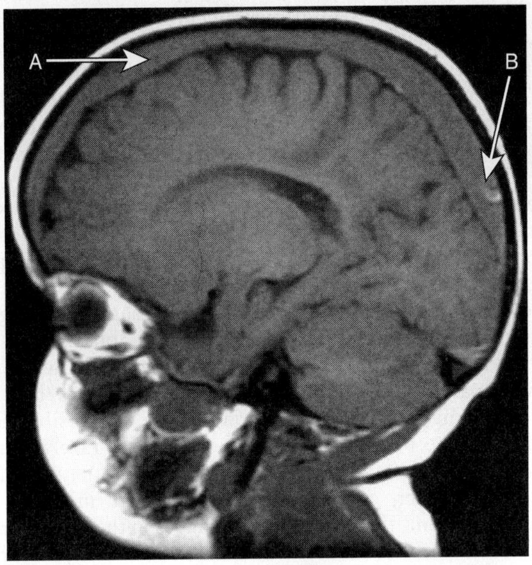

Figure 37-6 CT scan indicating intracranial bleeding. *A,* Older blood. *B,* New blood.

Table 37-3 TIMETABLE OF RADIOLOGIC CHANGES IN CHILDREN'S FRACTURES*

CATEGORY	EARLY	PEAK	LATE
1) Resolution of soft-tissue swelling	2-5 days	4-10 days	10-21 days
2) SPNBF	4-10 days	10-14 days	14-21 day
3) Loss of fracture line definition, days		10-14 days	14-21 days
4) Soft callus		10-14 days	14-21 days
5) Hard callus	14-21 days	21-42 days	42-90 days
6) Remodeling of fracture	3 mo	1 yr	2 yr to physeal closure

*Repetitive injuries may prolong categories 1, 2, 5, and 6.
SPNBF, subperiosteal new bone formation.
From Kleinman PK: *Diagnostic imaging of child abuse,* ed 2, St Louis, 1998, Mosby, p 176.

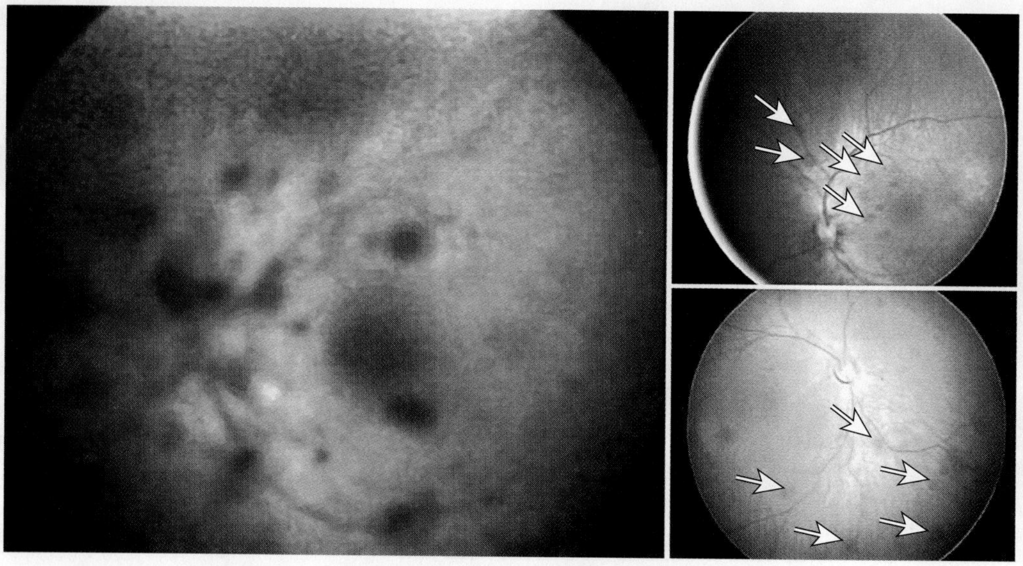

Figure 37-7 Retinal hemorrhages. Lines point to hemorrhages of various sizes.

5-7 days after an acute injury. Glutaric aciduria type 1 can present with intracranial bleeding and should be considered. Other causes of subdural hemorrhage in infants include arteriovenous malformations, coagulopathies, birth trauma, tumor, or infections. When AHT is suspected, injuries elsewhere—skeletal and abdominal—should be ruled out.

Retinal hemorrhages are an important marker of AHT (see Fig. 37-7). Whenever AHT is being considered, a dilated indirect ophthalmologic examination by a pediatric ophthalmologist should be performed. Although retinal hemorrhages can be found in other conditions, hemorrhages that are multiple, involve more than one layer of the retina, and extend to the periphery are very suspicious for abuse. The mechanism is likely repeated acceleration-deceleration due to shaking. Traumatic retinoschisis points strongly to abuse.

There are other causes of retinal hemorrhages, although the pattern is usually different than seen in child abuse. After birth, many newborns have them, but they disappear in 2-6 wk. Coagulopathies (particularly leukemia), retinal diseases, carbon monoxide poisoning, or glutaric aciduria may be responsible. Severe noninflicted direct crush injury to the head can rarely cause an extensive hemorrhagic retinopathy. Cardiopulmonary resuscitation rarely, if ever, causes retinal hemorrhage in infants and children; if present, there a few hemorrhages in the posterior pole. Hemoglobinopathies, diabetes mellitus, routine play, minor noninflicted head trauma, and vaccinations do not appear to cause retinal hemorrhage. Severe coughing or seizures rarely cause retinal hemorrhages that could be confused with AHT.

The dilemma frequently posed is whether minor, "everyday" forces can explain the findings seen in AHT. Simple linear skull fractures in the absence of other suggestive evidence can be explained by a short fall, although even that is rare (1-2%), and underlying brain injury from short falls is exceedingly rare. Timing of brain injuries in cases of abuse is not precise. In fatal cases, the trauma most likely occurred very soon before the child became symptomatic.

Other manifestations of abusive head trauma may be seen. "Raccoon" eyes occur in association with subgaleal hematomas after traction on the anterior hair and scalp, or after a blow to the forehead. Neuroblastoma can present similarly, and should be considered (Chapter 492). Bruises from attempted strangulation may be visible on the neck. Choking or suffocation can cause hypoxic brain injury, often with no external signs.

Abdominal trauma accounts for significant morbidity and mortality in abused children (Chapter 66). Young children are especially vulnerable because of their relatively large abdomens and lax abdominal musculature. A forceful blow or kick can cause hematomas of solid organs (liver, spleen, kidney) from compression against the spine, as well as hematoma (duodenal) or rupture (stomach) of hollow organs. Intra-abdominal bleeding may result from trauma to an organ or from shearing of a vessel. More than one organ may be affected. Children may present with cardiovascular failure or an acute condition of the abdomen, often after a delay in care. Bilious vomiting without fever or peritoneal irritation suggests a duodenal hematoma, often due to abuse.

The manifestations of abdominal trauma are often subtle, even with severe injuries. Bruising of the abdominal wall is unusual, and symptoms may evolve slowly. Delayed perforation may occur days after the injury; bowel strictures or a pancreatic pseudocyst may occur weeks or months later. Child health care professionals should consider screening for occult abdominal trauma when other evidence of physical abuse exists. Screening should include liver and pancreatic enzyme levels, and testing urine and stool for blood. Children with lab results indicating possible injury should have abdominal CT performed. CT or ultrasound should also be performed if there is concern about possible splenic, adrenal, or reproductive organ injury.

Neglect is the most prevalent form of child maltreatment, with potentially severe and lasting sequelae. It may manifest in many ways, depending on which needs are not adequately met. Nonadherence to medical treatment may aggravate the condition as may a delay in seeking care. Inadequate food may manifest as impaired growth; inattention to obesity may compound that problem. Poor hygiene may contribute to infected cuts or lesions. Inadequate supervision contributes to injuries and ingestions. Children's needs for mental health care, dental care, and other health-related needs may be unmet, manifesting as problems in those areas. Educational needs, particularly for children with learning disabilities, are often not met.

The evaluation of possible neglect requires addressing several critical questions. "Is this neglect?" "Have the circumstances harmed the child, or jeopardized the child's health and safety?" For example, suboptimal treatment adherence may lead to few or no clear consequences. Inadequacies in the care children receive naturally fall along a continuum, requiring a range of responses tailored to the individual situation. Legal considerations or CPS policies may discourage physicians from labeling many circumstances as neglect. Even if neglect does not meet a threshold for reporting to CPS, child health care professionals can still help ensure children's needs are adequately met.

GENERAL PRINCIPLES FOR ASSESSING POSSIBLE ABUSE AND NEGLECT

The heterogeneity of circumstances in situations of child maltreatment precludes specific details. The following are general principles.

- Given the complexity and possible ramifications of determining child maltreatment, an interdisciplinary assessment is optimal, with input from all involved professionals. Consultation with a physician expert in child maltreatment is recommended.
- A thorough history should be obtained from the parent(s) optimally via separate interviews.
- Verbal children should be interviewed separately, in a developmentally appropriate manner. Open-ended questions (e.g., "Tell me what happened") are best. Many need more directed questioning (e.g., "How did you get that bruise?"); some need multiple choice questions. Leading questions must be avoided (e.g., "Did your daddy hit you?").
- A thorough physical examination is necessary.
- Careful documentation of the history and physical is essential. Verbatim quotes are valuable, including the question that prompted the response. Photographs are helpful.
- For abuse: What is the evidence for concluding abuse? Have other diagnoses been ruled out? What is the likely mechanism of the injury? When did the injury likely occur?
- For neglect: Do the circumstances indicate that the child's needs have not been adequately met? Is there evidence of actual harm? Is there evidence of potential harm and on what basis? What is the nature of the neglect? Is there a pattern of neglect?
- Are there indications of other forms of maltreatment? Has there been prior CPS involvement?
- A child's safety is a paramount concern. What is the risk of imminent harm, and of what severity?
- What is contributing to the maltreatment? Consider the factors listed under the section on etiology.
- What strengths/resources are there? This is as important as identifying problems.
- What interventions have been tried, with what results? Knowing the nature of these interventions can be useful, including from the parent's perspective.
- What is the prognosis? Is the family motivated to improve the circumstances and accept help, or resistant? Are suitable resources, formal and informal, available?
- Are there other children in the household who should be assessed for maltreatment?

GENERAL PRINCIPLES FOR ADDRESSING CHILD MALTREATMENT

The heterogeneity of circumstances precludes specific details. The following are general principles.

- Treat any medical problems.
- Help ensure the child's safety, often in conjunction with CPS; this is a priority.
- Convey concerns of maltreatment to parents, kindly but forthrightly. Avoid blaming. It is natural to feel anger or pain towards parents of maltreated children, but they need support and deserve respect.
- Have a means of addressing the difficult emotions child maltreatment can evoke in us.
- Be empathic and state interest in helping, or suggest another pediatrician.
- Know your national and state laws and/or local CPS policies on reporting child maltreatment. In the USA, the legal threshold for reporting is typically "reason to believe"; one does not need to be certain. Physical abuse and moderate to severe neglect warrant a report. In less severe neglect, less intrusive interventions may be an appropriate initial response. For example, if an infant's mild failure to thrive is due to an error in mixing the formula, parent education and perhaps a visiting nurse should be tried. In contrast, severe failure to thrive may require hospitalization, and, if the contributing factors are particularly serious (e.g., a psychotic mother), out-of-home placement may be needed. CPS can assess the home environment, providing valuable insights.
- Remember that reporting child maltreatment is never easy. Parental inadequacy or culpability is at least implicit, and parents may express considerable anger. Child health care professionals should supportively inform families directly of the report; it can be explained as an effort to clarify the situation and provide help, as well as a professional (and legal) responsibility. Explaining what the ensuing process is likely to entail (e.g., a visit from a CPS worker and sometimes a police officer) may ease a parent's anxiety. Parents are frequently concerned that they might lose their child. Child health care professionals can cautiously reassure parents that CPS is responsible for helping children and families and that, in most instances, children remain with their parents. Even when CPS does not accept a report or when a report is not substantiated, they may offer voluntary supportive services such as food, shelter, homemaker services, and child care. Child health care professionals can be a useful liaison between the family and the public agencies, and should try to remain involved after reporting to CPS.
- Help address contributory factors, prioritizing those most important and amenable to being remedied. Concrete needs should not be overlooked; accessing nutrition programs, obtaining health insurance, enrolling children in preschool programs, and help finding safe housing can make a valuable difference. Parents may need their own problems addressed before they can adequately care for their children.
- Establish specific objectives (e.g., no hitting, diabetes will be adequately controlled), with measurable outcomes (e.g., urine dipsticks, hemoglobin A1c). Similarly, advice should be specific and limited to a few reasonable steps. A written contract can be very helpful.
- Engage the family in developing the plan, solicit their input and agreement.
- Build on strengths; there are always some. These provide a valuable way to engage parents.
- Encourage informal supports (e.g., family, friends; invite fathers to office visits). This is where most people get their support, not from professionals. Consider support available through a family's religious affiliation.
- Consider children's specific needs. Too often, maltreated children do not receive direct services.
- Be knowledgeable about community resources, and facilitate appropriate referrals.
- Provide support, follow-up, review of progress, and adjust the plan if needed.
- Recognize that maltreatment often requires long-term intervention with ongoing support and monitoring.

OUTCOMES OF CHILD MALTREATMENT

Child maltreatment often has significant short- and long-term medical, mental health, and social sequelae. Physically abused children are at risk for behavioral and functional problems, including conduct disorders, aggressive behavior, decreased cognitive functioning, and poor academic performance. Neglect is similarly associated with many potential problems. Even if a maltreated child appears to be functioning well, health care professionals and parents need to be sensitive to the possibility of later problems. Maltreatment is associated with increased risk in adulthood for several health risk behaviors and physical and mental health problems. Maltreated children are at risk for becoming abusive parents. The neurobiologic effects of child abuse and neglect on the developing brain may partly explain some of these sequelae.

Some children appear to be resilient and may not exhibit sequelae of maltreatment, perhaps owing to protective factors or interventions. The benefits of intervention have been found in even the most severely neglected children, such as those from Romanian orphanages, who were adopted—the earlier the better.

PREVENTION OF CHILD ABUSE AND NEGLECT

An important aspect of prevention is that many of the efforts to strengthen families and support parents should enhance children's health, development, and safety, as well as prevent child abuse and neglect. Medical responses to child maltreatment have typically occurred after the fact; preventing the problem is preferable. Child health care professionals can help in several ways. An ongoing relationship offers opportunities to develop trust and knowledge of a family's circumstances. Astute observation of parent-child interactions can reveal useful information.

Parent and child education regarding medical conditions helps to ensure implementation of the treatment plan and to prevent neglect. Possible barriers to treatment should be addressed. Practical strategies such as writing down the plan can help. In addition, anticipatory guidance may help with child rearing, diminishing the risk of maltreatment. Hospital-based programs that educate parents about infant crying and the risks of shaking the infant may help prevent abusive head trauma.

Screening for major psychosocial risk factors for maltreatment (depression, substance abuse, intimate partner violence, major stress), and helping address identified problems, often via referrals, may help prevent maltreatment. The primary care focus on prevention offers excellent opportunities to screen briefly for psychosocial problems. The traditional organ system–focused review of systems can be expanded to probe areas such as feelings about the child, the parent's own functioning, possible depression, substance abuse, intimate partner violence, disciplinary approaches, stressors, and supports. Obtaining information directly from children or youth is also important, especially given that separate interviews with teens have become the norm. Any concerns identified on such screens require at least brief assessment and initial management, which may lead to a referral for further evaluation and treatment. More frequent office visits can be scheduled for support and counseling while monitoring the situation. Other key family members (e.g., fathers) might be invited to participate, thereby encouraging informal support. Practices might arrange parent groups through which problems and solutions are shared.

Child health care professionals also need to recognize their limitations, providing referral to other community resources when indicated. Finally, the problems underpinning child maltreatment, such as poverty, parental stress, substance abuse, and limited child-rearing resources require policies and programs that enhance families' abilities to care for their children adequately. Child health care professionals can help advocate for such policies and programs.

Advocacy

Child health care professionals can assist in understanding what contributed to the child's maltreatment. When advocating for the best interest of the child and family, addressing risk factors at the individual, family, and community levels is optimal. At the individual level, an example of advocating on behalf of a child is explaining to a parent that an active toddler is behaving normally and not intentionally challenging the parent. Encouraging a mother to seek help dealing with a violent spouse, saying, "You and your life are very important," asking about substance abuse and helping parents obtain health insurance for their children are all forms of advocacy.

Efforts to improve family functioning, such as encouraging fathers' involvement in child care are also examples of advocacy. Remaining involved after a report to CPS and helping ensure appropriate services are provided is advocacy as well. In the community, child health care professionals can be influential advocates for maximizing resources devoted to children and families. These include parenting programs, services for abused women and children, and recreational facilities. Finally, child health care professionals can play an important role in advocating for policies and programs at the local, state, and national levels to benefit children and families. Child maltreatment is a complex problem that has no easy solutions. Through partnerships with colleagues in child protection, mental health, education, and law enforcement, child health care professionals can make a valuable difference in the lives of many children and families.

BIBLIOGRAPHY

Please visit the Nelson Textbook of Pediatrics *website at www.expertconsult.com for the complete bibliography.*

37.1 Sexual Abuse

(See Also Adolescent Rape, Chapter 113)

Howard Dubowitz and Wendy G. Lane

Approximately 25% of girls and 10% of boys in the USA will be sexually abused at some point during their childhood. Whether children and families share this information with their pediatrician will depend, in large part, on the pediatrician's comfort with and openness to discussing possible sexual abuse with families.

Pediatricians may play a number of different roles in addressing sexual abuse, including identification, reporting to CPS, testing for and treating sexually transmitted infections, and providing support and reassurance to children and families. Pediatricians may also play a role in the prevention of sexual abuse by advising parents and children about ways to help keep safe from sexual abuse. In many jurisdictions throughout the USA, general pediatricians will play a triage role, with the definitive medical evaluation conducted by a child abuse specialist.

DEFINITION

Sexual abuse may be defined as any sexual behavior or action toward a child that is unwanted or exploitative. Some legal definitions distinguish sexual abuse from sexual assault; the former being committed by a caregiver or household member, and the latter being committed by someone with a noncustodial relationship or no relationship with the child. For this chapter, the term sexual abuse will encompass both abuse and assault. It is important to note that sexual abuse does not have to involve direct touching or contact by the perpetrator. Showing pornography to a child, filming or photographing a child in sexually explicit poses, and encouraging or forcing one child to perform sex acts on another also constitute sexual abuse.

PRESENTATION OF SEXUAL ABUSE

Caregivers may readily entertain the possibility of sexual abuse when children exhibit sexually explicit behavior. This behavior includes that which is outside the norm for a child's age and developmental level. For preschool and school-aged children, sexually explicit behavior may include compulsive masturbation, attempting to perform sex acts on adults or other children, or asking adults or children to perform sex acts on them. Teenagers may become sexually promiscuous and even engage in prostitution. Older children and teenagers may respond by sexually abusing younger children. It is important to recognize that this behavior could also result from accidental exposure (e.g., the child who enters his parent's bedroom at night to find his parents having sex), or from neglect (e.g., watching pornographic movies where a child can see them).

Children who have been sexually abused sometimes provide a clear, spontaneous disclosure to a trusted adult. Often the signs of sexual abuse are much more subtle. For some children, behavioral changes are the first indication that something is amiss. Nonspecific behavior changes such as social withdrawal, acting out, increased clinginess or fearfulness, distractibility, and learning difficulties may be attributed to a variety of life changes or stressors. Regression in developmental milestones, including new-onset bed-wetting or encopresis (Chapter 21), is another behavior that caregivers may overlook as an indicator of sexual abuse. Teenagers may respond by becoming depressed, experimenting with drugs or alcohol, or running away from home. Because nonspecific symptoms are very common among children who have been sexually abused, it should nearly always be included in one's differential diagnosis of child behavior changes.

Some children may not exhibit behavioral changes or provide any other indication that something is wrong. For these children, sexual abuse may be discovered when another person witnesses the abuse or discovers evidence such as sexually explicit photographs or videos. Pregnancy may be another way that sexual abuse is identified. There are also children, some with and others without symptoms, that will not be identified at any point during their childhood.

THE ROLE OF THE GENERAL PEDIATRICIAN IN THE ASSESSMENT AND MANAGEMENT OF POSSIBLE SEXUAL ABUSE

Before determining where and how a child with suspected sexual abuse is evaluated, it is important to assess for and rule out any medical problems that can be confused with abuse. A number of genital findings may raise concern about abuse but often have nonabusive explanations. For example, genital redness in a prepubertal child is more often caused by nonspecific vulvovaginitis, eczema, or infection with staphylococcus, group A streptococcus, *Haemophilus*, *Neisseria*, or yeast. Lichen sclerosis is a less common cause of redness. Vaginal discharge can be caused by sexually transmitted infections, but also by vaginal foreign body, onset of puberty, or infection with *Salmonella*, *Shigella*, or *Yersinia*. Genital ulcers can be caused by herpes simplex virus (HSV) and syphilis, but also by Epstein-Barr virus, varicella-zoster, Crohn's disease, and Behçet's disease. Vaginal bleeding can be caused by urethral prolapse, vaginal foreign body, accidental trauma, and vaginal tumor.

When other medical conditions are not under consideration, have been ruled out, or are less likely than abuse, the triage process for suspected sexual abuse should be activated (Fig. 37-8). Where and how a child with suspected sexual abuse is evaluated should be determined by how long ago the last incident of abuse likely occurred, and whether the child is prepubertal or postpubertal. For the prepubertal child, if abuse has occurred in the previous 72 hr, forensic evidence collection (e.g., external genital, vaginal, anal, and oral swabs, sometimes referred to as a "rape kit") is often indicated, and the child should be referred to a site equipped to collect forensic evidence. Depending on the jurisdiction, this site may be an emergency department, a child advocacy center, or an outpatient clinic. If the last incident of abuse occurred more than 72 hours prior, the likelihood of recovering forensic evidence is extremely low, and forensic evidence collection is not necessary. For postpubertal females, many experts recommend forensic evidence collection up to 120 hr following the abuse—the same time limit as for adult women. The extended time frame is justified because some studies have demonstrated that semen can remain in the postpubertal vaginal vault for more than 72 hr.

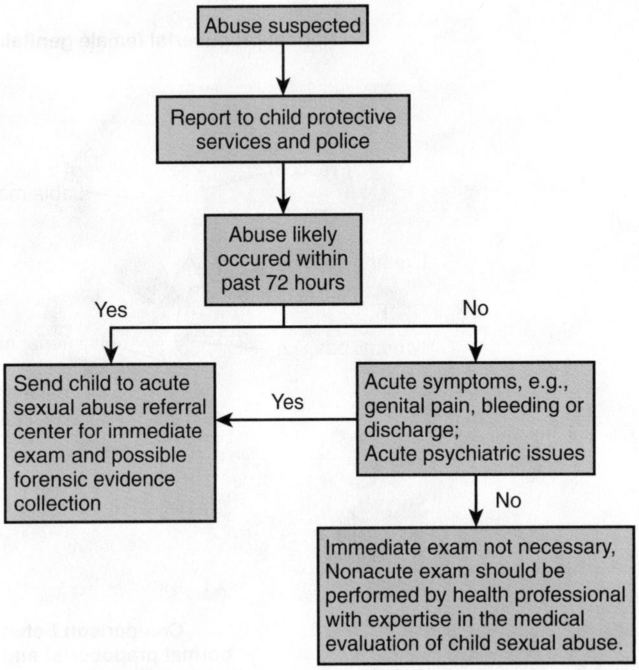

Figure 37-8 Triage protocol for children with suspected sexual abuse.

The referral site may be different when the child does not present until after the cutoff for an acute exam. Because emergency departments may not have a child abuse expert, and can be busy, noisy, and lacking in privacy, examination at an alternate location such as a child advocacy center or outpatient clinic is recommended. If the exam is not urgent, waiting until the next morning is recommended because it is easier to interview and examine a child who is not tired and cranky. Referring physicians should be familiar with the triage procedures in their communities, including the referral sites for both acute and chronic exams, and whether there are separate referral sites for prepubertal and postpubertal children.

Children with suspected sexual abuse may present to the pediatrician's office with a clear disclosure of abuse or more subtle indicators. In this situation, a private conversation between pediatrician and child can provide an opportunity for the child to speak in his or her own words without the parent speaking for him or her. Doing this may be especially important when the caregiver does not believe the child, or is unwilling or unable to offer emotional support and protection. Telling caregivers that a private conversation is part of the routine assessment for the child's concerns can help comfort a hesitant parent.

When speaking with the child, experts recommend establishing rapport by starting with general and open-ended questions; for example: "Who lives at home?" and "What are your favorite things to do?" Questions about sexual abuse should be nonleading. A pediatrician should explain that sometimes children are hurt or bothered by others, and that he or she wonders whether that might have happened to the child. Open-ended questions, such as "Can you tell me more about that?" allow the child to provide additional information and clarification in his or her own words. It is not necessary to obtain extensive information about what happened because the child will usually have a forensic interview once a report is made to CPS and an investigation begins. Very young children and those with developmental delay may lack the verbal skills to describe what happened. In this situation, the caregiver's history may provide enough information to warrant a report to CPS without interviewing the child.

All 50 U.S. states mandate that professionals report suspected maltreatment to child protective services. The specific criteria for "reason to suspect" are generally not defined by state law. It is

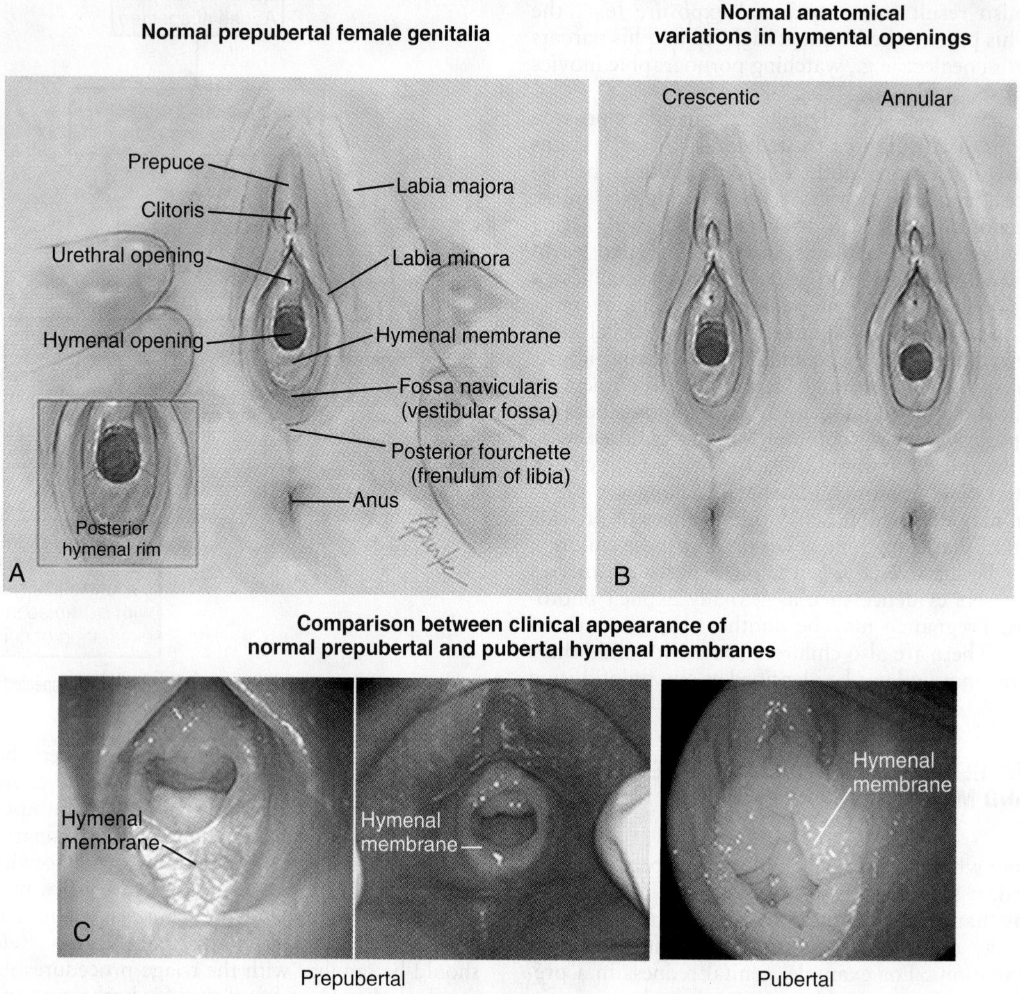

Figure 37-9 Female prepubertal genital anatomy. *A,* Inset shows the region defined as the posterior hymenal rim, between the 4 and 8 o'clock positions, shaded blue. *B,* There is a range of normal anatomic variations in hymenal openings. Crescentic and annular are 2 of the most common shapes. *C,* The photographs illustrate the range of normal prepubertal hymenal membranes. In most children, the hymen becomes thicker and more redundant during puberty. (From Berkoff MC, Zolotor AJ, Makoroff KL, et al: Has this prepubertal girl been sexually abused? *JAMA* 300:2779–2792, 2008.)

clear that reporting does not require certainty that abuse has occurred. Therefore, it may be appropriate to report a child with sexual behavior concerns when no accidental sexual exposure can be identified and the child does not clearly confirm or deny abuse during your conversation with her.

PHYSICAL EXAMINATION OF THE CHILD WITH SUSPECTED SEXUAL ABUSE

Unfortunately, many physicians are unfamiliar with genital anatomy and examination, particularly in the prepubertal child (Figs. 37-9 and 37-10). Because about 95% of children who undergo a medical evaluation following sexual abuse have normal exams, the role of the primary care provider is often simply to be able to distinguish a normal exam from findings indicative of common medical concerns or trauma. The absence of physical findings can often be explained by the type of sexual contact that has occurred. Abusive acts such as fondling or even digital penetration can occur without causing injury. In addition, many children do not disclose abuse until days, weeks, months, or even years after the abuse has occurred. Because genital injuries can heal rapidly, injuries are often completely healed by the time a child presents for medical evaluation. A normal genital exam does not rule out the possibility of abuse, and should not influence the decision to report to CPS.

Even with the high proportion of normal genital exams, there is value in conducting a thorough physical exam. Unsuspected injuries or medical problems such as labial adhesions, imperforate hymen, or a small urethral prolapse may be identified. In addition, reassurance about the child's physical health may allay fears and reduce anxiety for the child and family.

Few findings on the genital examination are diagnostic for physical abuse. In the acute time frame, lacerations or bruising of the labia, penis, scrotum, perianal tissues, or perineum are indicative of trauma. Likewise, hymenal bruising and lacerations, and perianal lacerations extending deep to the external anal sphincter indicate penetrating trauma. Several nonacute findings are also concerning for sexual abuse. A complete transection of the hymen to the base between the 4 and 8 o'clock positions (i.e., absence of hymenal tissue in the posterior rim) is considered diagnostic for trauma (see Fig. 37-10). For all of these findings, the cause of injury must be elucidated through the child and caregiver history. If there is any concern that the finding may be the result of sexual abuse, CPS should be notified and a medical evaluation should be performed by an experienced child abuse pediatrician.

Testing for sexually transmitted infections is not indicated for all children, but is warranted in the situations described in Table 37-4. Culture is still considered the gold standard for the diagnosis of gonorrhea (Chapter 185) and chlamydia (Chapter 218)

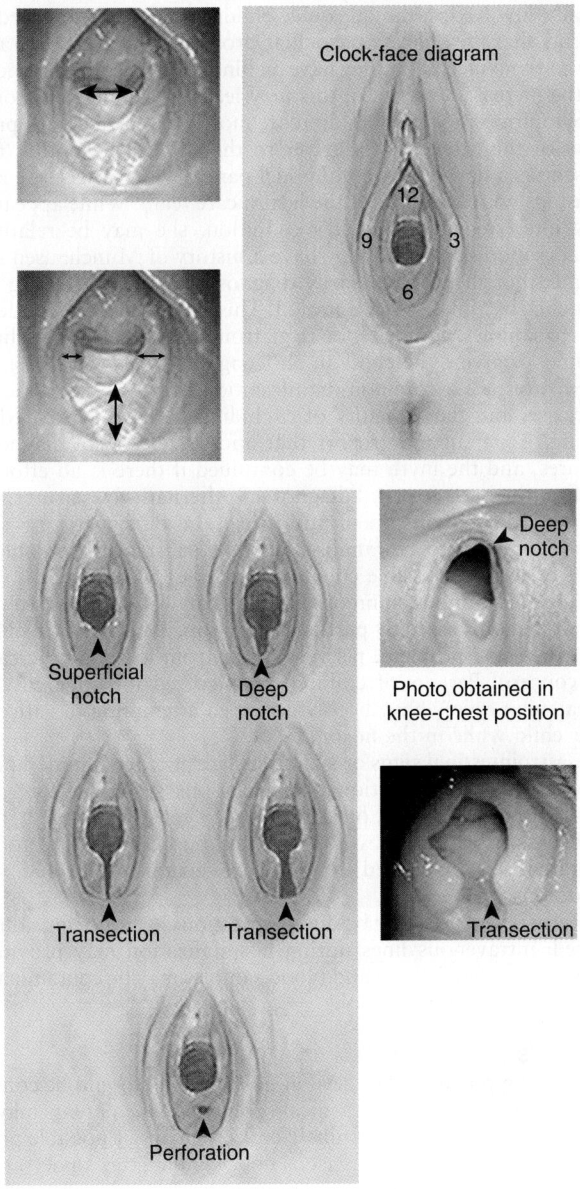

Figure 37-10 Hymenal membrane characteristics. When considering the possibility of sexual abuse during an examination, the examiner should document pertinent positive and negative findings. In addition to the clinical signs depicted in the figure, other possible findings include prominent hymenal vessels, bumps, tags, longitudinal intravaginal ridge, external ridge, periurethral bands, or vestibular bands. Perforation of the hymen is not a finding commonly discussed in the literature. (From Berkoff MC, Zolotor AJ, Makoroff KL, et al: Has this prepubertal girl been sexually abused? *JAMA* 300:2779–2792, 2008.)

in children. Because obtaining vaginal swabs can be uncomfortable for prepubertal children, a urine specimen for nucleic acid amplification testing (NAAT) can be collected as a screening test. However, if only NAAT testing is done, the child should NOT receive presumptive treatment at the time of testing. Instead, a positive NAAT test should be confirmed by culture prior to treatment. Because gonorrhea and chlamydia in prepubertal children do not typically cause ascending infection, waiting for a definitive diagnosis before treatment will not increase the risk for pelvic inflammatory disease.

A number of sexually transmitted infections should raise concern for abuse (Table 37-5). In a prepubertal child, a positive culture for gonorrhea beyond the neonatal period, trichomonas beyond 1 yr of age, or chlamydia beyond 3 yr of age indicates that the child has had some contact with infected genital secretions, almost always as a result of sexual abuse. Syphilis (Chapter 210) and HIV are diagnostic for sexual abuse if other means of transmission have been excluded. Because of the potential for transmission either perinatally or through nonsexual contact, the presence of genital warts has a low specificity for sexual abuse. The possibility of sexual abuse should be considered and addressed with the family, especially in children whose warts first appear beyond 3 yr of age. Type 1 or 2 genital herpes is concerning for sexual abuse, but not diagnostic given other possible routes of transmission. For both human papillomavirus and HSV, the American Academy of Pediatrics recommends reporting to child protective services unless perinatal or horizontal transmission is considered likely.

Table 37-4 SITUATIONS INVOLVING A HIGH RISK FOR TRANSMISSION OF SEXUALLY TRANSMITTED INFECTIONS

1. Child has signs or symptoms of STI, including vaginal discharge or pain, genital itching or odor, urinary symptoms, and genital ulcers or lesions.
2. The suspected perpetrator is known to have an STI, or is at high risk for having an STI because of multiple partners, substance abuse, or other reasons.
3. Any other person living in the child's household has an STI.
4. There is a high prevalence of STIs in the child's community.
5. There is evidence of genital, oral, or anal penetration or ejaculation.
6. The patient or parent requests testing.

STI, sexually transmitted infection.
From Centers for Disease Control and Prevention, Workowski KA, Berman SM: Sexually transmitted diseases treatment guidelines, 2006, *MMWR Recomm Rep* 55(RR-11):1-94, 2006.

Table 37-5 IMPLICATIONS OF COMMONLY ENCOUNTERED SEXUALLY TRANSMITTED (ST) OR SEXUALLY ASSOCIATED (SA) INFECTIONS FOR DIAGNOSIS AND REPORTING OF SEXUAL ABUSE AMONG INFANTS AND PREPUBERTAL CHILDREN

ST/SA CONFIRMED	EVIDENCE FOR SEXUAL ABUSE	SUGGESTED ACTION
Gonorrhea*	Diagnostic†	Report‡
Syphilis*	Diagnostic	Report‡
HIV§	Diagnostic	Report‡
*Chlamydia trachomatis**	Diagnostic†	Report‡
Trichomonas vaginalis	Highly suspicious	Report‡
Condylomata acuminate (anogenital warts)	Suspicious	Report‡
Genital herpes*	Suspicious	Report‡¶
Bacterial vaginosis	Inconclusive	Medical follow-up

*Report if not likely to be perinatally acquired and rare nonsexual vertical transmission is excluded.
†Although culture is the gold standard, current studies are investigating the use of nucleic acid amplification tests as an alternative diagnostic method.
‡Report to the agency mandated to receive reports of suspected child abuse.
§Report if not likely to be acquired perinatally or through transfusion.
¶Report unless a clear history of autoinoculation is evident.
From MMWR 2006 STD guidelines. Adapted from Kellogg N, American Academy of Pediatrics Committee on Child Abuse and Neglect: The evaluation of sexual abuse in children, *Pediatrics* 116:506–512, 2005.

SEXUAL ABUSE PREVENTION

Pediatricians can play a role in the prevention of sexual abuse by educating parents and children about sexual safety at well child visits. During the genital exam the pediatrician can inform the child that only the doctor and select adult caregivers should be permitted to see their "private parts," and that a trusted adult should be told if anyone else attempts to do so. Pediatricians can raise parental awareness that sometimes older kids or adults may try engage in sexual behavior with children. The pediatrician can teach parents how to minimize the opportunity for perpetrators to access children, for example, by limiting one-adult/one-child situations and being sensitive to any adult's unusual interest in young children. In addition, pediatricians can help parents talk to children about what to do if confronted with a potentially abusive situation. Some examples include telling children to say "no," to leave, and to tell a parent and/or another adult. If abuse does occur, the pediatrician can tell parents how to recognize possible signs and symptoms, and how to reassure the child that she or he was not at fault. Finally, pediatricians can provide parents with suggestions about how to maintain open communication with their children so that these conversations can occur with minimal parent and child discomfort.

BIBLIOGRAPHY

Please visit the Nelson Textbook of Pediatrics *website at www.expertconsult.com for the complete bibliography.*

37.2 Factitious Disorder by Proxy (Munchausen Syndrome by Proxy)

Howard Dubowitz and Wendy G. Lane

The term *Munchausen syndrome* is used to describe situations in which adults falsify their own symptoms. In *Munchausen syndrome by proxy*, a parent, typically a mother, simulates or causes disease in her child. Several terms have been suggested to describe this phenomenon: factitious disorder by proxy, pediatric condition falsification, and medical child abuse. **Factitious disorder by proxy** (FDP) appears relatively straightforward and optimal. In some instances, such as partial suffocation, "child abuse" may be most appropriate. Factitious is defined as "produced by humans, rather than by natural forces."

The core dynamic is that a parent falsely presents a child for medical attention. This may be via fabricating a history, such as reporting seizures that never occurred. A parent may directly cause a child's illness, for example by exposing a child to a toxin, medication, or infectious agent (e.g., injecting stool into an intravenous line). Signs or symptoms may also be manufactured, such as when a parent smothers a child, or alters laboratory samples or temperature measurements. Each of these actions may lead to unnecessary medical care, sometimes including intrusive tests and surgeries. The "problems" often recur repeatedly over several years. In addition to the physical concomitants of testing and treatment, there are potentially serious and lasting social and psychologic sequelae.

Child health care professionals are typically misled into thinking that the child really has a medical problem. Parents, sometimes working in a medical field, may be adept at constructing somewhat plausible presentations; a convincing seizure history may be offered, and a normal electroencephalogram (EEG) cannot fully rule out the possibility of a seizure disorder. Even after extensive testing fails to lead to a diagnosis or treatment proves ineffective, child health care professionals may think they are confronting a "new or rare disease." Unwittingly, this can lead to continued testing (leaving no stone unturned) and interventions, thus perpetuating the FDP. Pediatricians generally rely on and trust parents to provide an accurate history. As with other forms of child maltreatment, accurate diagnosis of FDP requires that the pediatrician maintain a healthy skepticism under certain circumstances.

Clinical Manifestations

As with other forms of child abuse, the presentation of FDP may vary in nature and severity. Consideration of FDP should be triggered when the reported symptoms are repeatedly noted by only one parent, appropriate testing fails to confirm a diagnosis, and seemingly appropriate treatment is ineffective. At times, the child's symptoms, their course, or the response to treatment may be incompatible with any recognized disease. Preverbal children are usually involved, although older children may be convinced by parents that they have a particular problem. Older children may become convinced that they have an illness and become dependent on the increased attention; this may lead to feigning symptoms.

Symptoms in young children are mostly associated with proximity of the offending caregiver to the child. The mother may present as a devoted or even model parent who forms close relationships with members of the health care team. While appearing very interested in her child's condition, she may be relatively distant emotionally. She may have a history of Munchausen syndrome, though not necessarily diagnosed as such. **Bleeding** is a particularly common presentation. This may be caused by adding dyes to samples, adding blood (e.g., from the mother) to the child's sample, or giving the child an anticoagulant (e.g., warfarin).

Seizures are a common manifestation, with a history easy to fabricate, and the difficulty of excluding the problem based on testing. A parent may report that another physician diagnosed seizures, and the myth may be continued if there is no effort to confirm the basis for the "diagnosis." Alternatively, seizures may be induced by toxins, medications (e.g., insulin), water, or salts. Physicians need to be familiar with the substances available to families and the possible consequences of exposure.

Apnea is another common presentation. The observation may be falsified or created by partial suffocation. A history of a sibling with the same problem, perhaps dying from it, should be cause for concern. Parents of children hospitalized for apparent life-threatening events have been videotaped attempting to suffocate their child while in the hospital.

Gastrointestinal signs or symptoms are another common manifestation. Forced ingestion of medications such as ipecac may cause chronic vomiting, or laxatives may cause diarrhea.

The **skin**, easily accessible, may be burned, dyed, tattooed, lacerated, or punctured to simulate acute or chronic skin conditions.

Recurrent sepsis may be due to infectious agents being administered; intravenous lines during hospitalization may provide a convenient portal. Urine and blood samples may be contaminated with foreign blood or stool.

Diagnosis

In assessing possible FDP, several explanations should be considered in addition to a true medical problem. Some parents may be extremely anxious and genuinely concerned about possible problems. There may be many reasons underpinning this anxiety, such as a personality trait, the death of neighbor's child, or something read on the Internet. Alternatively, parents may believe something told to them by a trusted physician despite subsequent evidence to the contrary and efforts to correct the earlier misdiagnosis. Physicians may unwittingly contribute to a parent's belief that a real problem exists by, perhaps reasonably, persistently pursuing a medical diagnosis. There is a need to discern commonly used hyperbole (e.g., exaggerating the height of the fever) in order to evoke concern and perhaps justify a visit to an emergency department. In the end, a diagnosis of FDP rests on clear evidence of a child repeatedly being subjected to unnecessary medical tests and treatment, primarily stemming from a parent's actions. Determining the parent's underlying psychopathology is the responsibility of mental health professionals.

Once FDP is suspected, gathering and reviewing **all** the child's medical records is an onerous but critical first step. It is often important to confer with other treating physicians about what specifically was conveyed to the family. A mother may report that the child's physician insisted that a certain test be done when it may be the mother instead who demanded the test. It is also necessary to confirm the basis for a given diagnosis, rather than simply accepting a parent's account.

Pediatricians may face the dilemma of when to accept that all plausible diagnoses have been reasonably ruled out, the circumstances fit FDP, and further testing and treatment should cease. The likelihood of FDP must be balanced with concerns about possibly missing an important diagnosis. Consultation with a pediatrician expert in child abuse is recommended. In evaluating possible FDP, specimens should be carefully collected, with no opportunity for tampering with them. Similarly, temperature measurements should be closely observed.

Depending on the severity and complexity, hospitalization may be needed for careful observation to help make the diagnosis. In some instances, such as repeated apparent life-threatening events, covert video surveillance accompanied by close monitoring (to rapidly intervene in case a parent attempts to suffocate a child) can be valuable. It is important that there be close coordination among hospital staff, especially as some may side with the mother and resent even the possibility of FDP being raised. Parents should not be informed of the evaluation for FDP until the diagnosis is made. Doing so could naturally influence their behavior and jeopardize establishing the diagnosis. All steps in making the diagnosis and all pertinent information should be very carefully documented, perhaps using a "shadow" chart that the parent does not have access to.

Treatment

Once the diagnosis is established, the treatment plan should be worked out by the medical team and CPS; it may require out-of-home placement and should include mental health care for the offending parent as well as for older affected children. Further medical care should be carefully organized and coordinated by 1 primary care provider. CPS should be encouraged to meet with the family only after the medical team has informed the offending parent of the diagnosis; their earlier involvement may hamper the evaluation. Parents often respond with resistance, denial, and threats. It may be prudent to have hospital security in the vicinity.

BIBLIOGRAPHY

Please visit the Nelson Textbook of Pediatrics *website at www.expertconsult.com for the complete bibliography.*

Chapter 38
Failure to Thrive

Heather S. McLean and David T. Price

Failure to thrive (FTT) is the result of inadequate usable calories necessary for a child's metabolic and growth demands, and it manifests as physical growth that is significantly less than that of peers. No one set of growth parameters provides the criteria for a universal definition of FTT, although the pattern may be helpful (Fig. 38-1). FTT has classically been grouped into organic and nonorganic causes, but FTT is better defined as the end result of inadequate usable calories with contributing risk factors from multiple categories.

EPIDEMIOLOGY

The prevalence of FTT depends on the risks within populations. In developing countries or countries torn by conflict, infectious diseases, and inadequate nutrition are the primary risks. In developed countries, the primary risks are preterm birth and family dysfunction. In all settings there are a myriad of other causes (Table 38-1).

CLINICAL MANIFESTATIONS

The most common clinical presentation of FTT is poor growth, which is depicted using standardized growth charts. Poor growth may be accompanied by physical signs such as alopecia, reduced

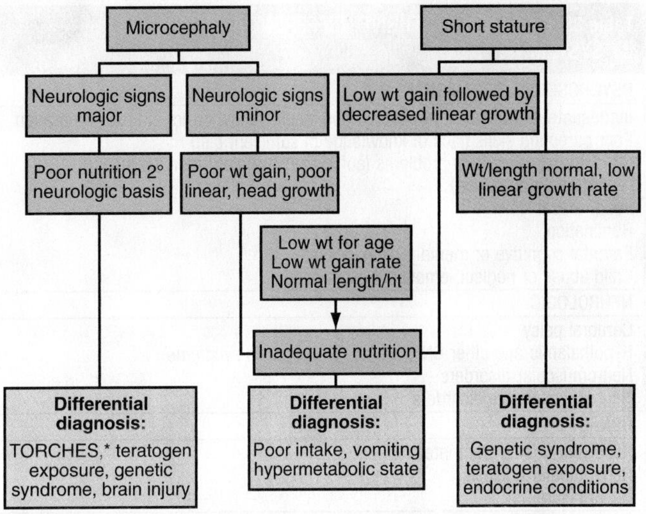

Figure 38-1 Approach to the differential diagnosis of failure to thrive. *See key to Table 38-1. (Derived from Gahagan S: Failure to thrive: a consequence of undernutrition, *Pediatr Rev* 27:e1–e11, 2006.)

subcutaneous fat or muscle mass, and dermatitis. Syndromes of marasmus or kwashiorkor are more common in developing countries (Chapter 43).

Weight for corrected age, weight for height, body mass index, and failure to gain adequate weight over a period of time help define FTT (Chapter 13). Growth parameters should be measured serially and plotted on growth charts appropriate for the child's sex, age, and, if preterm, postconceptual age. Growth charts are also available for some known chromosomal abnormalities, such as Down syndrome or Turner syndrome.

ETIOLOGY AND DIAGNOSIS

The causes of insufficient growth include (1) failure of a caregiver to offer adequate calories, (2) failure of the child to take in sufficient calories, (3) failure of the child to retain and use sufficient calories, and (4) increased metabolic demands. History, physical examination, and observation of the parent-child interaction in the clinical or home environment usually suggest the most likely etiologies and thus direct appropriate workup and management (see Fig. 38-1). A complete history should include a detailed nutritional, family, and prenatal history; documentation of who feeds and cares for the child; further information regarding the timing of the growth failure; and a thorough review of systems. In young infants it is important to obtain a detailed dietary history, including quantity, quality, and frequency of meals, in addition to information about the caregiver's response to excessive crying or sleeping.

The causes of FTT are numerous, involving every organ system (see Table 38-1). The clinician may approach the diagnosis in terms of age (Table 38-2) or signs and symptoms (Table 38-3). The timing of the growth deficiency can indicate a cause, such as the introduction of gluten into the diet of a child with celiac disease or a coincidental psychosocial event. Regardless of gestational age, a chromosomal abnormality, intrauterine infection, or teratogen exposure should be considered in a child with symmetric growth failure since birth.

The physical examination should focus on identifying chronic illnesses, recognizing syndromes that may alter growth, and documenting the effects of malnutrition (Table 38-4).

The laboratory evaluation of children with FTT should be judicious and based on findings from the history and physical (see Fig. 38-1). Obtaining the state's newborn screening results, a complete blood count, and urinalysis represent a reasonable initial screen.

Table 38-1 FAILURE TO THRIVE: DIFFERENTIAL DIAGNOSIS BY SYSTEM

PSYCHOSOCIAL/BEHAVIORAL
Inadequate diet because of poverty/food insufficiency, errors in food preparation Poor parenting skills (lack of knowledge of sufficient diet) Child/parent interaction problems (autonomy struggles, coercive feeding, maternal depression) Food refusal Rumination Parental cognitive or mental health problems Child abuse or neglect; emotional deprivation
NEUROLOGIC
Cerebral palsy Hypothalamic and other CNS tumors (diencephalic syndrome) Neuromuscular disorders Neurodegenerative disorders
RENAL
Recurrent urinary tract infection Renal tubular acidosis Renal failure
ENDOCRINE
Diabetes mellitus Diabetes insipidus Hypothyroidism/hyperthyroidism Growth hormone deficiency Adrenal insufficiency
GENETIC/METABOLIC/CONGENITAL
Sickle cell disease Inborn errors of metabolism (organic acidosis, hyperammonemia, storage disease) Fetal alcohol syndrome Skeletal dysplasias Chromosomal disorders Multiple congenital anomaly syndromes (VATER, CHARGE)*
GASTROINTESTINAL
Pyloric stenosis Gastroesophageal reflux Repair of tracheoesophageal fistula Malrotation Malabsorption syndromes Celiac disease Milk intolerance: lactose, protein Pancreatic insufficiency syndromes (cystic fibrosis) Chronic cholestasis Inflammatory bowel disease Chronic congenital diarrhea states Short bowel syndrome Pseudo-obstruction Hirschsprung disease Food allergy
CARDIAC
Cyanotic heart lesions Congestive heart failure Vascular rings
PULMONARY/RESPIRATORY
Severe asthma Cystic fibrosis; bronchiectasis Chronic respiratory failure Bronchopulmonary dysplasia Adenoid/tonsillar hypertrophy Obstructive sleep apnea
MISCELLANEOUS
Collagen-vascular disease Malignancy Primary immunodeficiency Transplantation
INFECTIONS
Perinatal infection (TORCHES)* Occult/chronic infections Parasitic infestation Tuberculosis HIV

*CHARGE, coloboma, heart disease, atresia choanae, retarded growth and retarded development and/or central nervous system anomalies, genital hypoplasia, and ear anomalies and/or deafness; TORCHES, toxoplasma, other, rubella, cytomegalovirus, herpes simplex; VATER, vertebral defects, imperforate anus, tracheoesophageal fistula, and radial and renal dysplasia.

Table 38-2 COMMON CAUSES OF MALNUTRITION IN EARLY LIFE

0-6 MO
Breastfeeding difficulties Improper formula preparation Impaired parent/child interaction Congenital syndromes Prenatal infections or teratogenic exposures Poor feeding (sucking, swallowing) or feeding refusal (aversion) Maternal psychological disorder (depression or attachment disorder) Congenital heart disease Cystic fibrosis Neurologic abnormalities Child neglect Recurrent infections
6-12 MO
Celiac disease Food intolerance Child neglect Delayed introduction of age-appropriate foods or poor transition to food Recurrent infections Food allergy
AFTER INFANCY
Acquired chronic diseases Highly distractible child Inappropriate mealtime environment Inappropriate diet (e.g., excessive juice consumption, avoidance of high-calorie foods) Recurrent infections

Table 38-3 APPROACH OF FAILURE TO THRIVE BASED ON SIGNS AND SYMPTOMS

HISTORY/PHYSICAL EXAMINATION	DIAGNOSTIC CONSIDERATION
Spitting, vomiting, food refusal	Gastroesophageal reflux, chronic tonsillitis, food allergies
Diarrhea, fatty stools	Malabsorption, intestinal parasites, milk protein intolerance
Snoring, mouth breathing, enlarged tonsils	Adenoid hypertrophy, obstructive sleep apnea
Recurrent wheezing, pulmonary infections	Asthma, aspiration, food allergy
Recurrent infections	HIV or congenital immunodeficiency diseases
Travel to/from developing countries	Parasitic or bacterial infections of the gastrointestinal tract

A minority of children with FTT will be solely categorized as child neglect (Chapter 37). Risk factors for neglect are often shared by those with FTT, such as poverty, social isolation, and caregiver mental health issues.

TREATMENT

Treatment requires a multidisciplinary approach, understanding all the elements that contribute to a child's growth: a child's health and nutritional status, family issues, and the parent-child interaction. An appropriate feeding atmosphere at home is important for all children with FTT.

Indications for hospitalization include severe malnutrition or failure of outpatient management. If a child without other conditions requiring hospitalization has not responded after 2-3 mo of outpatient management, then a specialized, multidisciplinary inpatient assessment should be considered. Inpatient care may include further diagnostic and laboratory evaluation, an assessment and implementation of adequate nutrition, and further evaluation of the parent-child feeding interaction.

Table 38-4 APPROACH TO PHYSICAL EXAMINATION

Vital signs	Blood pressure, temperature, pulse respirations, anthropometry
General appearance	Activity, affect, posture
Skin	Hygiene, rashes, neurocutaneous markings, signs of trauma (bruises, burns, scars)
Head	Hair whorls, quality of hair, alopecia, fontanel size, frontal bossing, sutures, shape, dysmorphisms, philtrum
Eyes	Ptosis, strabismus, palpebral fissures, conjunctival pallor, fundoscopic exam
Ears	External form, rotation, tympanic membranes
Mouth, nose, throat	Thinness of lip, hydration, dental health, glossitis, cheilosis, gum bleeding
Neck	Hairline, masses, lymphadenopathy
Abdomen	Protuberance, hepatosplenomegaly, masses
Genitalia	Malformations, hygiene, trauma
Rectum	Fissures, trauma, hemorrhoids
Extremities	Edema, dysmorphisms, rachitic changes, nails
Neurologic	Cranial nerves, reflexes, tone, retention of primitive reflexes, voluntary movement

Adapted from American Academy of Pediatrics: Failure to thrive. In Kleinman RE, editor: *Pediatric nutrition handbook*, ed 6, Elk Grove Village, IL, 2009, American Academy of Pediatrics, pp 601–636.

Children with severe malnutrition must be re-fed carefully with an incremental increase in calories to avoid re-feeding syndrome (Chapter 43). The type of caloric supplementation is based on the severity of FTT and the underlying medical condition. The response to feeding depends on the specific diagnosis, medical treatment, and severity of FTT. Minimal catch-up growth should generally be 2-3 times the average weight gain for corrected age. Multivitamin supplementation should be given to all children with FTT to meet the recommended dietary allowance, because these children commonly have iron, zinc, and vitamin D deficiencies, as well as increased micronutrient demands with catch-up growth.

PROGNOSIS

FTT in the first year of life, regardless of cause, is particularly ominous. Maximal postnatal brain growth occurs in the first 6 mo of life. The prognosis for children with FTT is variable, depending on the specific diagnosis and severity of FTT. Children with early FTT are at higher risk for short stature, and behavioral and academic difficulties. Community-based studies of children with a history of FTT have found IQ scores to be about 4 points lower than children with a history of adequate growth. Appropriate assessment and intervention of cognitive and emotional development is necessary for all children with FTT. Referrals to early intervention, Head Start, or Supplemental Security Income (SSI) may be beneficial. Home intervention may attenuate some of these negative effects of early failure to thrive.

BIBLIOGRAPHY

Please visit the Nelson Textbook of Pediatrics *website at* *www.expertconsult.com* *for the complete bibliography.*

Chapter 39
Chronic Illness in Childhood

Lisa J. Chamberlain and Paul H. Wise

EPIDEMIOLOGY

Patterns of chronic illness in childhood are both complex and dynamic. Compared to chronic disease in adults, serious chronic illness in children is less common and widely heterogeneous. This has profound implications for the organization of children's health services, as pediatricians have the difficult task of identifying and caring for children with unusual and varied conditions. Accordingly, child health services have become far more reliant on standardized screening programs and formal systems of referral to regional specialty care programs than are health care systems for adults. Pediatrics has been characterized by rapid progress in preventing serious acute illnesses and in extending the lives of children who previously would have succumbed to their illness early in life. These factors have made the epidemiology of childhood far more dynamic than that of the adult world.

For the full continuation of this chapter, please visit the Nelson Textbook of Pediatrics *website at* *www.expertconsult.com*.

Chapter 40
Pediatric Palliative Care

Christina Ullrich, Janet Duncan, Marsha Joselow, and Joanne Wolfe

According to the World Health Organization, "Palliative care for children is the active total care of the child's body, mind and spirit, and also involves giving support to the family...Optimally, this care begins when a life-threatening illness or condition is diagnosed and continues regardless of whether or not a child receives treatment directed at the underlying illness." Provision of palliative care applies not only to children with cancer or cystic fibrosis but also those with diagnoses such as complex or severe cardiac disease, neurodegenerative diseases, or trauma with life-threatening sequelae (Table 40-1). While palliative care is often mistakenly understood as equivalent to end-of-life care, its scope and potential benefit extend before and well after end-of-life care and is applicable throughout the illness trajectory. Palliative care emphasizes optimization of quality of life, communication, and

Table 40-1 CONDITIONS APPROPRIATE FOR PEDIATRIC PALLIATIVE CARE

CONDITIONS FOR WHICH CURATIVE TREATMENT IS POSSIBLE BUT MAY FAIL
Advanced or progressive cancer or cancer with a poor prognosis Complex and severe congenital or acquired heart disease
CONDITIONS REQUIRING INTENSIVE LONG-TERM TREATMENT AIMED AT MAINTAINING THE QUALITY OF LIFE
Human immunodeficiency virus infection Cystic fibrosis Severe gastrointestinal disorders or malformations such as gastroschisis Severe epidermolysis bullosa Severe immunodeficiencies High-risk solid organ transplant candidates and/or recipients such as lung or multivisceral Chronic or severe respiratory failure Muscular dystrophy
PROGRESSIVE CONDITIONS IN WHICH TREATMENT IS ALMOST EXCLUSIVELY PALLIATIVE AFTER DIAGNOSIS
Progressive metabolic disorders Certain chromosomal abnormalities such as trisomy 13 or trisomy 18 Severe forms of osteogenesis imperfecta
CONDITIONS INVOLVING SEVERE, NONPROGRESSIVE DISABILITY, CAUSING EXTREME VULNERABILITY TO HEALTH COMPLICATIONS
Severe cerebral palsy with recurrent infection or difficult-to-control symptoms Extreme prematurity Severe neurologic sequelae of infectious disease Hypoxic or anoxic brain injury Holoprosencephaly or other severe brain malformations

Adapted from Himelstein BP, Hilden JM, Boldt AM, et al: Pediatric palliative care, *N Engl J Med* 350:1752–1762, 2004.

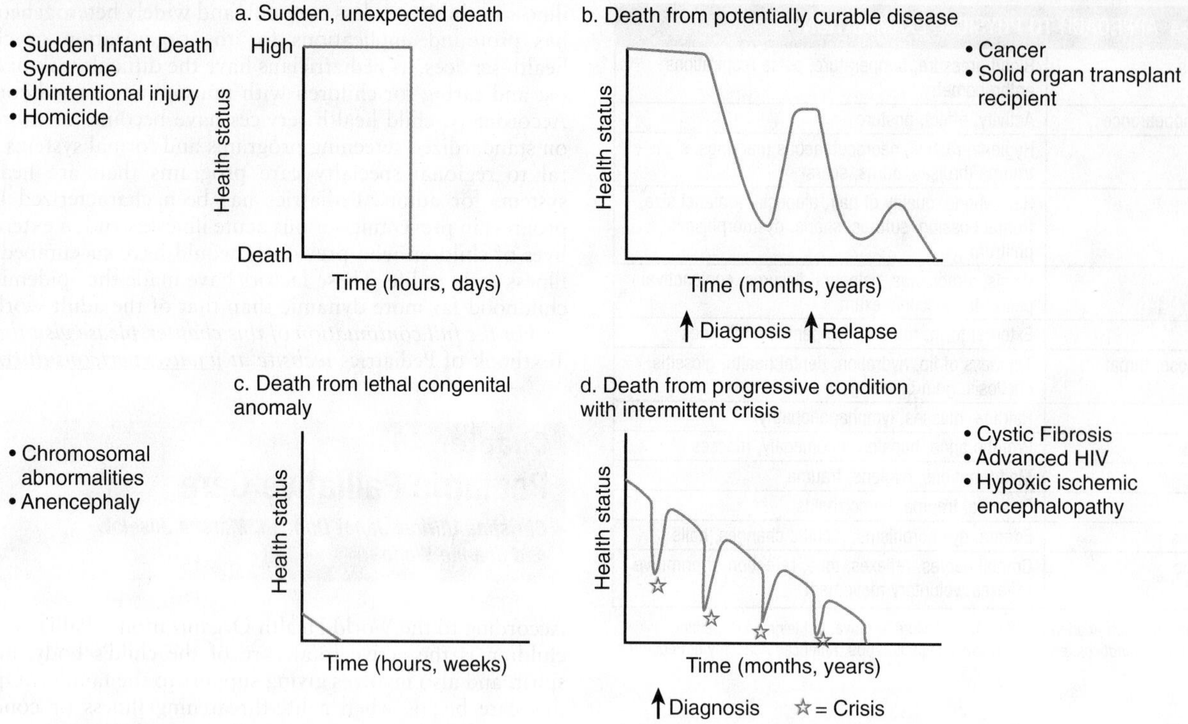

Figure 40-1 Typical illness trajectories for children with life-threatening illness. (From Field M, Behrman R, editors: *When children die: improving palliative and end-of-life care for children and their families*, Washington, DC, 2003, National Academies Press, p 74.)

symptom control, aims that may be congruent with maximal treatment aimed at sustaining life.

Such comprehensive physical, psychologic, social, and spiritual care requires an interdisciplinary approach. Worldwide this is possible with creative use of professional and community providers. Organizations such as the Children's International Project on Palliative/Hospice Services share existing clinical and scientific knowledge in an attempt to establish international standards for palliative care. In the USA, the American Academy of Pediatrics has delineated essential elements of pediatric palliative care. The National Consensus Project released its second edition of *Clinical Practice Guidelines for Quality Palliative Care*, endorsed by 39 medical, nursing, and social work organizations as well as the International Association for Hospice and Palliative Care.

Approximately 54,000 children (birth to 19 yr) died in 2005 in the USA. This number has remained relatively unchanged over the past several years, and half of the deaths occur in acute-care hospitals. Among children who die from cancer, about 50% die in the hospital and 50% at home. Approximately 65% of childhood AIDS deaths occur in the hospital. In many developing countries, the majority of pediatric deaths occur at home, with or without palliative care.

Pediatric palliative care should be provided across settings, including the hospital, outpatient settings, the home, and sometimes in hospice programs. In the USA, the insurance structure and frequent use of medical technology (e.g., home ventilatory support) precludes formal enrollment of a child on the hospice benefit. A growing number of home care agencies offer palliative care programs that serve as a bridge to hospice services. Some freestanding hospice houses will accept children, although many families and children prefer to be at home, if at all possible, through the end of life. Despite establishment of such programs, provision of palliative care for children is often limited by the availability of clinicians who have training or experience in caring for seriously ill children.

The mandate of the pediatrician and other health care providers to oversee children's physical, mental, and emotional health and development includes the practice of palliative care for those children who live with a significant possibility of death before adulthood (Fig. 40-1). Many pediatric subspecialists care for children with life-threatening illnesses.

Compared with adult palliative care, pediatric palliative care has:

- Smaller numbers of children who die. Professionals specializing in the care of children may only rarely encounter the death of a child.
- A broad spectrum of illnesses, including many rare diseases. In pediatrics, the wide range of often poorly understood disorders limits generalization from one disease-specific research study to another.
- Unpredictable illness trajectories with significant prognostic uncertainty. It is difficult to predict accurately the progression of illness for many life-threatening illnesses in pediatrics. Such uncertainty may compound child and family distress. Unpredictable trajectories may require palliative care services for months or years, which may not be easily sustained by some programs.
- More confusion about the integration of palliative care with life-prolonging care. Parents and professionals who care for children often consider interventions that are accepted as life-extending, but may also be palliative, such as noninvasive respiratory ventilation, blood transfusions, or parenteral nutrition.
- Parents are most often the decision-makers, but involving the child/adolescent in a manner consistent with the family communication style is also important. This triad (parent–child–interdisciplinary providers) of decision-makers also complicates the process of assessing symptoms, choosing therapies, and evaluating outcomes.
- The added emotional burden of child death. For a parent, this is unnatural and out of order and considered to be among life's most significant tragedies. The cumulative emotional impact on pediatric clinicians is also substantial.

Medical and technological advances have resulted in an increase in the number of children who live longer, often with significant dependence on new and expensive technologies. These children have complex chronic conditions across the spectrum of congenital and acquired life-threatening disorders (Chapter 39). Children with complex chronic conditions may benefit from simultaneous palliative and curative therapies. These children, who often survive near-death crises followed by the renewed need for rehabilitative and life-prolonging treatments, are best served by a system that is flexible and responsive to changing needs.

CARE SETTINGS

Home care for the child with a life-threatening illness requires 24 hr per day accessibility to experts in pediatric palliative care, a team approach, and an identified coordinator who serves as a link between hospitals, the community, and specialists and who may assist in preventing and/or arranging for hospital admissions, respite care, and increased home care support as needed. Adequate home care support and respite care, though sorely needed, is often not readily available. Furthermore, families may feel using respite care is a personal failure, or they may worry that others cannot adequately care for their child's special needs.

At the end of life, children and families may need intensive support. This may be provided in the home, hospital, or hospice house. Families need to feel safe and well cared for and given permission, if possible, to choose location of care. In tertiary care hospitals, most children die in the neonatal and pediatric intensive care units (ICUs). The philosophy of palliative care can be successfully integrated into a hospital setting, including the ICU, when the focus of care also includes the prevention or amelioration of suffering and improving comfort and quality of life. All interventions that affect the child and family need to be assessed in relationship to these goals. This proactive approach asks the question "What can we offer that will improve the quality of this child's life?" instead of "What therapies are we no longer going to offer this patient?" Staff need education, support, and guidance since pediatric palliative care, like other types of intensive care, is an area of specialty. Comprehensive palliative care also requires an interdisciplinary approach that may include nurses, physicians, psychologists, psychiatrists, social workers, religious counselors, child-life specialists, and trained volunteers.

COMMUNICATION, ADVANCE CARE PLANNING, AND ANTICIPATORY GUIDANCE

Although accurate prognostication is a particular challenge in pediatrics, the medical team often recognizes a terminal prognosis before the prognosis is understood by parents. This time delay may impede informed decision-making about how the child lives at the end of life. Given the inherent prognostic uncertainty of a life-limiting diagnosis, discussions concerning resuscitation, symptom control, and end-of-life care planning should be initiated when the physician recognizes that a significant possibility of patient mortality exists. These conversations should not happen during a crisis, but should occur well in advance of the crisis or when the patient has recovered from a crisis, but is at high risk for others. Patients and families are most comfortable being cared for by physicians and other care providers with whom they have an established relationship; these individuals may not have had the benefit of palliative care training. The services of a palliative care team or hospice program can be consultative to the primary or subspecialty care team and/or the patient and family, and help alleviate physician discomfort in discussions regarding advanced care planning. A consultative palliative care team provides the family with an opportunity to engage in sensitive conversations that they may feel less comfortable having with their primary team, at least initially. Perhaps resulting from long-standing and highly connected relationships, primary providers and families can be mutually protective of one another, and may not engage in conversations that are perceived as promoting hopelessness. The palliative care team can help to begin conversations about difficult and emotional topics in a manner that concurrently promotes **hopefulness.**

The population of children who die before reaching adulthood includes a disproportionate number of nonverbal and preverbal children who are developmentally unable to make autonomous care decisions. Although parents are legally the primary decision-maker in most situations in the USA, children should be as fully involved in discussions and decisions about their care as appropriate for their developmental status. Utilizing communication experts, child life therapists, chaplains, social workers, psychologists, or psychiatrist to allow children to express themselves through art, play, music, talk, and writing will enhance the provider's knowledge of the child's understanding and hopes. Tools such as "Five Wishes" and "My Wishes" have proven to be useful in helping to gently introduce advance care planning to children, adolescents, and their families (*www.agingwithdignity.org/index.php*).

The Parents

For parents, compassionate communication with medical providers who understand their child's illness, treatment options, and family preferences and goals is the cornerstone of caring for children with life threatening illness. During this period of time, one of the most significant relationships is that with the child's pediatrician, who often has an enduring relationship with the child and family, including healthy siblings. Parents need to know that their child's pediatrician will not abandon them as the goals of care shift to include palliative care. A family's goals may shift and change with the child's evolving clinical condition and other variable factors. A flexible approach rooted in ongoing communication and guidance that incorporates understanding of the family's values, goals, and religious, cultural, spiritual, and personal beliefs is of paramount importance.

Pediatricians should recognize the important role they have in continuing to care for the child and family as the primary goal of treatment simultaneously may be prolongation of life and comfort, relief of suffering and promoting quality of life. Regular meetings between caregivers and the family are essential in order to reassess and manage symptoms, explore the impact of illness on immediate family members, and provide anticipatory guidance. At these meetings, important issues with lifelong implications for parents and their child may be discussed. Such discussions should be planned with care, ensuring that adequate time for in-depth conversation is allotted; a private, physical setting is arranged; and that both parents and/or others who might be identified by the family as primary supports are present. These meetings should first and foremost elicit what parents are thinking or worried about. Included is a review of what was previously discussed, listening to other concerns and issues as they are revealed, having parents repeat back what was said to ensure clarity, and responding with honest, factual answers in areas of uncertainty. By offering medical recommendations based on family goals and the clinical reality, the team can decrease the burden of responsibility for decision-making that parents carry.

Families may look to their pediatrician for assurance that all treatment options have been explored. Assisting a patient's family to arrange a second opinion may be helpful. Listening to families and children speak about the future even in the face of poor prognosis may help keep the focus on living even while the child may be dying. Hoping for a miracle can coexist for parents even as they are facing and accepting the more likely reality of death.

Parents also need to know about the availability of home care, respite services, web-based support and information, educational books and videotapes, and support groups. Responding to parent requests or need for counseling referrals for themselves, other children, or family is essential.

While broaching the topic may seem daunting, exploration of how parents envision their child's death, addressing their previous loss experiences (most often with death of an adult relative) and any misconceptions they may have, is often a great relief to parents. Learning about cultural, spiritual, and family values regarding pain management, suffering, and the preferred place of end-of-life care is essential before death. Even raising the thoughts about funeral arrangements, the possibility of autopsy, and tissue donation can be helpful to give parents choices and know that these things can be discussed without fear. A major worry of many parents is in how to involve and communicate with siblings as well as the child about the fact that most likely death is going to occur.

Ratings of high satisfaction with physician care have been directly correlated with receiving clear communication around end-of-life issues, delivered with sensitivity and caring; such communication included speaking directly to the child when appropriate. Communication is complicated by an assumed need for mutual protection in which the child wants to protect his or her parents and likewise the parents want to protect their child from painful information or sadness. Honoring the family's communication style, values, spirituality, and culture, which may be impacted by the child's personality style, is critical in these highly sensitive conversations. Evidence shows that parents who have open conversations with their child about death and dying do not regret having done so.

In communications with the child and family, the physician should avoid giving estimates of survival length, even when the child or family explicitly asks for them. These predictions are invariably inaccurate because population-based statistics do not predict the course for individual patients. A more honest approach may be to explore ranges of time in general terms ("weeks to months," "months to years"). The physician can also ask parents what they might do differently if they knew how long their child would live and then assist them in thinking through the options relating to their specific concerns (suggest celebrating upcoming holidays/important events earlier in order to take advantage of times when the child may be feeling better). It is generally wise to suggest that relatives who wish to visit might do so earlier rather than later, given the unpredictability of the time course of many illnesses.

For the child and family, the integration of bad news is a process, not an event, and when done sensitively does not take away hope or alter the relationship between the family and physician. The physician should expect that some issues previously discussed may not be fully resolved for the child and parents (do-not-resuscitate [DNR] orders, artificial nutrition or hydration) and may need to be revisited over time. Parents of a child with chronic illness may reject the reality of an impending death because past predictions may not have been accurate. Whether they are parents of a child with a chronic illness or of a child whose death is the result of accident or sudden catastrophic illness, they may experience great anxiety, guilt, or despair.

The Child

Truthful communication that takes into account the child's developmental stage and unique lived experience can help to address the fear and anxiety commonly experienced among children with life-threatening illness. Responding in a developmentally appropriate fashion (Table 40-2) to a child's questions about death, such as "What's happening to me?" or "Am I dying?" requires a careful exploration of what is already known by the child, what is really being asked (the question behind the question), and why the question is being asked at this particular time and in this setting. It may signal a need to be with someone who is comfortable listening to such unanswerable questions. Many children find nonverbal expression much easier than talking; art, play therapy, and storytelling may be more helpful than direct conversation.

A child's perception of death depends on his or her conceptual understanding of *universality* (that all things inevitably die), *irreversibility* (that dead people cannot come back to life), *nonfunctionality* (that being dead means that all biologic functions cease), and *causality* (that there are objective causes of death).

Very young children may struggle with the concepts of irreversibility and nonfunctionality. For young school-aged children, who are beginning to understanding the finality of death, worries may include magical thinking in which their thoughts, wishes, or bad behavior might be the underlying cause for their illness. Older children seek more factual information to gain some control over the situation.

Children's fears of death are often centered on the concrete fear of being separated from parents and other loved ones and what will happen to their parents rather than themselves. This can be true for teens and young adults as well. This fear may be responded to in different ways: some families may give reassurance that loving relatives will be waiting, while others use religious figures to refer to an eternal spiritual connection.

While adolescents may have a conceptual understanding of death similar to that of adults, working with the adolescent with life-threatening illness presents unique concerns and issues. The developmental work of adolescence includes separating from their parents, developing strong peer relationships, and moving towards independent adulthood. For this particular population, the teenager's developmental need to separate is complicated by the often increasing dependence both physically and emotionally on their parents. At the same time, adolescents are often asked to be part of the decision-making process without always having the emotional experience to fully understand the impact.

In addition to developmental considerations, understanding related to the child's life experiences, the length of the child's illness, the understanding of the nature and prognosis of the illness, the child's role in the family (peacemaker, clown, troublemaker, the "good" child) should be considered in communication with children.

Parents have an instinctive and strong desire to protect their children from harm. When facing the death of their child, many parents attempt to keep the reality of impending death hidden from their child with the hope that the child can be "protected" from the harsh reality. Although it is important to respect parental wishes, it is also true that most children already have a sense of what is happening to their bodies even when it has been purposely left unspoken. Children may blame themselves for their illness and the hardships that it causes for their loved ones. Perpetuating the myth that "everything is going to be all right" takes away the chance to explore fears and provide reassurance. Honest communication also allows opportunities for memory and legacy making and saying goodbye.

School is the "work" of childhood and is important in optimizing quality of life for a child seeking "normalcy" in the face of illness. Finding ways to help children and their families to maintain these connections through modification of the school day and exploring options to promote educational and social connections into the home or into the hospital room can be meaningful in the event that a child is not well enough to attend school.

As with the younger child, finding ways to help the adolescent maintain peer relationships and school based programming can be important in maximizing quality of life.

The Siblings

Brothers and sisters are at special risk both during their sibling's illness and after the death. Because of the extraordinary demands placed on parents to meet the needs of their ill child, healthy siblings may feel that their own needs are not being acknowledged or fulfilled. These feelings of neglect may then trigger guilt about their own good health and resentment toward their parents and ill sibling. Younger siblings may react to the stress by becoming seemingly oblivious to the turmoil around them. Some

Table 40-2 DEVELOPMENTAL QUESTIONS, THOUGHTS, AND CONCEPTS OF DYING AND WITH RESPONSIVE STRATEGIES

TYPICAL QUESTIONS AND STATEMENTS ABOUT DYING	THOUGHTS THAT GUIDE BEHAVIOR	DEVELOPMENTAL UNDERSTANDING OF DEATH	STRATEGIES AND RESPONSES
MOs-3 YR			
"Mommy, don't cry" *"Daddy, will you still tickle me when I'm dead?"*	Limited understanding of events, future and past, and of the difference between living and nonliving.	May have "sense" that something is wrong. Death is often viewed as continuous with life. Like being awake and being asleep.	Optimize comfort, and consistency; familiar persons, objects, routines. Use soothing songs, words, and touch. *"I will always love you."* *"I will always take care of you."* *"I will tickle you forever."*
3-5 YR			
"I did something bad and so I will die." *"Can I eat anything I want in heaven?"*	Concepts are simple and reversible. Variations between reality and fantasy.	The child may see death as temporary and reversible, and not universal. May feel responsible for illness. Death may be perceived as an external force that can get you.	Assure child that illness not his/her fault. Provide consistent caregivers. Promote honest simple language. Use books to explain the life cycle and promote questions and answers. *"You did not do anything to cause this."* *"You are so special to us and we will always love you."* *"We know (God, Jesus, Grandma, Grandpa) are waiting to see you."*
5-10 YR			
"How will I die?" *"Will it hurt?"* *"Is dying scary?"*	The child begins to demonstrate organized, logical thought. Thinking becomes less esoteric. The child begins to problem solve concretely, reason logically, and organize thoughts coherently. However, he or she has limited abstract reasoning.	The child begins to understand death as real and permanent. Death means that your heart stops, your blood does not circulate, and you do not breathe. It may be viewed as a violent event. The child may not accept death could happen to himself or herself or anyone he or she knows but starts to realize that people he or she knows will die.	Be honest and provide specific details if they are requested. Help and support the child's need for control. Permit and encourage the child's participation in decision making. *"We will work together to help you feel comfortable. It is very important that you let us know how you are feeling and what you need. We will always be with you so that you do not need to be afraid."*
10-18 YR			
"I'm afraid if I die my mom will just break down." *"I'm too young to die. I want to get married and have children."* *"Why is God letting this happen?"*	Abstract thoughts and logic possible. Body image is important. Need peer relationships for support and for validation. Altruistic values — staying alive for family — parents, siblings — donating organs/tissue Disbelief that he/she is dying.	Understand death as irreversible, inevitable and universal. Needs reassurance of continued care and love. Search for meaning and purpose of life.	Reinforce child/adolescent's self-esteem, sense of worth, and self-respect. Allow need for privacy, independence, access to friends and peers. Tolerate expression of strong emotions and permit participation in decision-making. *"I can't imagine how you must be feeling. Despite it all, you are doing an incredible job. I wonder how I can help?"* *"What's most important to you now?"* *"What are your hopes…your worries?"* *"You have taught me so much, I will always remember you."*

Adapted from Hurwitz C, Duncan J, Wolfe J: Caring for the child with cancer at the close of life, *JAMA* 292:2141–2149, 2003.

younger siblings may feel guilty as a result of "wishing" the affected child would die so they could get their parents back ("magical thinking"). Parents need to know that these are normal responses, and siblings should be encouraged to maintain the typical routines of daily living. Siblings who are most involved with their sick brothers or sisters before death usually adjust better both at the time of and after the death. Acknowledging and validating sibling feelings, being honest and open, and appropriately involving them in the life of their sick sibling provide a good foundation for the grief process.

The Staff

Inadequate support for the staff providing palliative care can result in depression, emotional withdrawal, and other symptoms. Offering educational opportunities and emotional support for staff at various stages of caring for a child with life-threatening illness can be helpful in bettering patient/family care and preventing staff from experiencing long-term repercussions, including the possibility of leaving the field.

Decision-Making

In the course of a child's life-limiting illness, a series of difficult decisions need to be made in relation to location of care, medications with risks and benefits, withholding and or withdrawing life-prolonging treatments, experimental treatments in research protocols, and the use of complementary therapies (Chapter 3). Such family decisions are greatly facilitated by opportunities for in-depth and guided discussions around **goals of care** for their child. This is often accomplished by asking open-ended questions that explore the parent's and child's hopes, worries, and family values. Goals of care conversations include what is most important for them as a family, considerations of their child's clinical condition, and their values and beliefs, including cultural, religious, and spiritual considerations.

Decision-making should be focused on the goals of care, as opposed to limitations of care; "This is what we can offer" instead of "This is what we can no longer do." Instead of meeting specifically to discuss "withdrawing support" or a DNR order, a more general discussion centered on the goals of care will naturally lead to considering which interventions are in the **child's best interests.**

Resuscitation Status

Many parents do not understand the legal mandate requiring attempted resuscitation for cardiorespiratory arrest unless a written DNR order is in place. In broaching this topic, rather than asking parents if they want to forgo cardiopulmonary resuscitation for their child (and placing the full burden of decision-making on them), it is preferable to discuss whether or not resuscitative interventions are likely to benefit the child. It is important to make recommendations based on overall goals of care and medical knowledge of potential benefit and/or harm of these interventions. Once the goals of therapy are agreed upon, the physician is required to write a formal order; it is also extremely beneficial to write a letter delineating decisions regarding resuscitation interventions and supportive care measures to be undertaken for the child. The letter should be as detailed as possible, including recommendations for comfort medications and contact information for caregivers best known to the patient. Such a letter, given to the parents, with copies to involved caregivers and institutions, can be a useful communication aid, especially in times of crisis. Many states have out of hospital DNR verification forms, which if completed on behalf of the child, affirm that rather than initiating resuscitative efforts, emergency response teams are obligated to provide comfort measures when called to the scene.

Conflicts in decision-making can occur within families, within health care teams, between the child and family, and between the family and professional caregivers (Chapter 3). For children who are developmentally unable to provide guidance in decision-making (neonates, very young children, or children with cognitive impairment), parents and health care professionals may come to different conclusions as to what is in the child's best interests. Decision-making around the care of adolescents presents specific challenges, given the shifting boundary that separates childhood from adulthood. In some families and cultures, truth telling and autonomy are much less valued compared with family integrity (Chapter 4). Although frequently encountered, differences in opinion are often manageable for all involved when lines of communication are kept open, team and family meetings are held, and the goals of care are clear (Chapters 3, 12, and 106).

Symptom Management

Intensive symptom control is another cornerstone of pediatric palliative care. Alleviation of symptoms reduces suffering of the child and family, and allows them to focus on other concerns and participate in meaningful experiences. Despite increasing attention to symptoms, and pharmacologic and technical advances in medicine, children often suffer from multiple symptoms. Key elements and general approaches to managing symptoms are provided in Table 40-3.

Pain is a complex sensation triggered by actual or potential tissue damage and influenced by cognitive, behavioral, emotional, social, and cultural factors. Effective pain relief is essential to prevent central desensitization, a central hyperexcitation response that may lead to escalating pain, and to diminish a stress response that may have a variety of physiologic effects. Assessment tools include self-report tools for children who are able to communicate their pain verbally, as well as tools based on behavioral cues for children who are unable to do so because of developmental or cognitive limitations. Management of pain is addressed in Tables 40-4 and 40-5 (Chapter 71). Many children with life-threatening illness require opioids for pain at some point in their illness trajectory. Though a stepwise approach to pain is recommended, the step consisting of "weak opioids" is often skipped. The primary opioid in this category, codeine, should generally be avoided because of its side effect profile and lack of superiority over nonopioid analgesics. Furthermore, relatively common genetic polymorphisms in the CYP2D6 gene lead to wide variation in codeine metabolism. Specifically, 10-40% of individuals carry polymorphisms causing them to be "poor metabolizers" who cannot convert codeine to its active form, morphine, and therefore are at risk for inadequate pain control; others are "ultra metabolizers" who may even experience respiratory depression from rapid generation of morphine from codeine. It is therefore

Table 40-3 KEY ELEMENTS OF EFFECTIVE SYMPTOM MANAGEMENT

Establish and periodically revisit goals of care. Communicate goals to care team.
Anticipate and plan for symptoms before they occur.
Assess the child for symptoms regularly, using consistent and developmentally appropriate assessment tools.
- Utilize self report, if the child is able to reliably report symptoms.
- Evaluate all aspects of the symptom, including quality, frequency, duration, and intensity.

Consider the holistic nature of symptoms.
- Explore the meaning that symptoms may have for families in cultural, religious context.
- Assess distress caused by the symptom.
- Evaluate the degree of functional impairment from the symptom.

Understand the pathophysiology of the symptom and establish a complete differential diagnosis.
Treat the underlying cause if possible, weighing benefits and risks, in the context of goals of care.
Choose the least invasive route for medications—by mouth whenever possible.
Prescribe regular medications for constant symptoms, and consider prn doses for breakthrough or uncontrolled symptoms.
Consider both pharmacologic and nonpharmacologic approaches.
Reassess the symptom and response to interventions regularly.
- For refractory symptoms, revisit the differential diagnosis and review potentially contributing factors.
- Effective interventions relieve the symptom and reduce distress and functional impairment.

Partner with families to identify and address any barriers to optimal control of symptoms.
Address spiritual, emotional, and existential suffering in addition to physical suffering since these are often inter-related.

Table 40-4 GUIDELINES FOR PAIN MANAGEMENT

Utilize nonopioid analgesics as monotherapy for mild pain and together with opioids for more severe pain.
- Nonopioid analgesics include acetaminophen, nonsteroidal antiinflammatory drugs (NSAIDs), salicylates, and selective cyclo-oxygenase (COX-2) inhibitors.

For moderate or severe pain, start with a short-acting opioid at regular intervals.
- When dose requirements have stabilized, consider converting opioid to a long-acting formulation with doses available for breakthrough or uncontrolled pain, as needed.
- Avoid codeine and opioids with mixed agonist activity (e.g., butorphanol, pentazocine)

Administer medications via the simplest, most effective, and least distressing route.
Dispel the myth that strong medications should be saved for extreme situations or the very end of life.
- Opioids do not have a "ceiling effect," and escalating symptoms may be treated with an increase in dose.

Clarify for families the differences between tolerance, physical dependence, and addiction.
Anticipate and treat/prevent common analgesic side effects (gastritis with NSAIDs; constipation, pruritus, nausea, sedation with opioids).
- Always initiate a bowel regimen to prevent constipation when starting opioids.
- Consider stimulants for opioid-induced somnolence.
- Pruritus rarely indicates a true allergy. If not responsive to an antihistamine, consider low-dose naloxone or switching opioids.

Consider switching to a different opioid for intolerable side effects or neurotoxicity (e.g., myoclonus).
- Use an equianalgesic conversion table when switching opioids, and account for incomplete cross-tolerance.

Consider the use of adjuvant drugs for specific pain syndromes, and for their opioid-sparing effect:
- Antidepressants (e.g., amitriptyline, nortriptyline) and anticonvulsants (e.g., gabapentin, carbamazepine, topiramate) for neuropathic pain
- Steroids or NSAIDs for bone pain
- Sedatives and hypnotics for anxiety and muscle spasm
- Use topical local anesthetics when possible
- To enhance analgesia from opioids, consider clonidine or ketamine
- Local anesthetics (lidocaine, prilocaine, bupivacaine)

Consider anesthetic blocks for regional pain.
Consider palliative radiation therapy.
Consider psychologic approaches (e.g., cognitive or behavioral therapy) and complementary therapies (e.g., acupuncture, massage).

Table 40-5 PHARMACOLOGIC APPROACH TO SYMPTOMS COMMONLY EXPERIENCED BY CHILDREN WITH LIFE-THREATENING ILLNESS

SYMPTOM	MEDICATION	STARTING DOSE	COMMENTS
Pain—mild	Acetaminophen	15 mg/kg po Q 4 hr, max of 4 g/day	Available po (including liquid), pr
	Ibuprofen	10 mg/kg po Q 6 hr	PO (including liquid) only; avoid if risk of bleeding; use only in infants ≥6 months. Use with caution in congestive heart failure. Chewable tablets contain phenylalanine.
	Trilisate	10-15 mg/kg po tid	Trilisate may have less anti-platelet activity and therefore pose less risk for bleeding than other salicylates. Salicylates, however, have been associated with Reye Syndrome in children under 2 yr.
Pain—moderate/ severe	Morphine immediate release (i.e., MSIR)	0.3 mg/kg po Q 4 hr if <50 kg; 5-10 mg po Q 4 hr*†	Also available in IV/SQ formulation.‡§
	Oxycodone	0.1 mg/kg po Q 4 hr if <50 kg; 5-10 mg po Q 4 hr if >50 kg*†	No injectable formulation.‡§
	Hydromorphone	0.05 mg/kg po Q 4 hr if <50 kg; 1-2 mg po Q 4 hr if >50 kg*†	Also available in IV/SQ formulation. Injectable form very concentrated, facilitating subcutaneous delivery.‡§
	Fentanyl	0.5-1.5 μg/kg IV/SQ Q 30 min*†	Rapid infusion may cause chest wall rigidity.‡§
	Methadone	Starting dose 0.1-0.2 mg/kg po bid. May give tid if needed. Recommend consultation with experienced clinician for equivalence dosing from other opioids.*†	Only opioid with immediate and prolonged effect available as a liquid; do not adjust dose more often than every 72 hours as prolonged biologic half-life > than therapeutic half-life. Knowledge of the pharmacokinetics of methadone is needed for converting to and from doses of other opioids. Also available IV/SQ. May cause QT interval prolongation, especially in adults on >200 mg/day or in those at risk for QT prolongation. Interacts with several antiretrovirals.§
Pain—sustained release	MS Contin Kadian (contains sustained release pellets), Avinza (contains immediate and extended release beads) Oramorph	Total daily dose of MSIR divided bid-tid	Do not crush MS Contin. For those unable to swallow pills, Kadian and Avinza capsules may be opened and contents mixed with food but *cannot be chewed.* Kadian contents may be mixed in 10 mL water and given via 16-French G-tube. Avoid alcohol with Avinza. Larger dose formulation may not be suitable for small children.§
	Oxycontin	Total daily dose of oxycodone divided bid-tid	Do not crush.§
	Transdermal fentanyl patch	Divide 24-hr po morphine dose by 2 to determine starting dose of transdermal fentanyl. There is no data on the equianalgesic conversion from transdermal fentanyl to any oral opioid.	Smallest patch size may be too high for small children. For children >2 yr. Apply to upper back in young children. Patch may not be cut. Typically for patients on at least 60 mg morphine/day or its equivalent. Not appropriate when dosage changes are frequent or for opioid-naïve patients. Fever >40°C results in higher serum concentrations.§
Pain—neuropathic	Nortriptyline	0.5 mg/kg po at bedtime to maximum of 150 mg/day	Fewer anticholinergic side effects than amitriptyline. May cause constipation, postural hypotension, dry mouth
	Gabapentin	Start at 5 mg/kg/day daily and gradually increase to 10-15 mg/kg/day divided tid; titrate as needed but not to exceed 3600 mg/day	May cause neuropsychiatric events in children (aggression, emotional lability, hyperkinesia), usually mild but may require discontinuation of gabapentin. May cause dizziness or drowsiness.
	Methadone	See previous listing	See previous listing
Dyspnea	Morphine, immediate release (i.e., MSIR)	0.1 mg/kg po Q 4 hr prn*†	All opioids may relieve dyspnea. For dyspnea, the starting dose is 30% of the dose that would be administered for pain.§
	Lorazepam	0.025-0.05 mg/kg iv/po Q 6 hr, up to 2 mg/dose	See previous listing
Respiratory secretions	Scopolamine patch	1.5 mg patch, change Q 72 hrs	Excessive drying of secretions can cause mucus plugging of airways. Good for motion-induced nausea and vomiting. Handling patch and contacting eye may cause anisocoria and blurry vision. May fold patches but do not cut them. Anticholinergic side effects possible.
	Glycopyrrolate	0.04-0.1 mg/kg po Q 4-8 hr	Excessive drying of secretions can cause mucus plugging of airways. Anticholinergic side effects possible.
	Hyoscyamine sulfate	4 gtt po Q 4 hr prn if <2 yrs; 8 gtt po Q 4 hr prn if 2-12 yr; do not exceed 24 gtt/24 hr	Anticholinergic side effects possible.
Nausea	Metoclopramide	0.1-0.2 mg/kg/dose Q 6 hrs, up to 10 mg/dose (prokinetic and mild nausea dosing). For chemotherapy-associated nausea 0.5-1 mg/kg Q 6 hr prn po/IV/SC, give with diphenhydramine	Helpful when dysmotility is an issue; may cause extrapyramidal reactions, particularly in children following IV administration of high doses. Contraindicated in complete bowel obstruction or pheochromocytoma.
	Ondansetron	0.15 mg/kg dose Q 8 hr to max of 8 mg/dose. Some institutions also use daily dosing for chemotherapy.	Significant experience in pediatrics. Good empiric therapy for nausea in palliative care population. Higher doses used with chemotherapy. Oral dissolving tablet contains phenylalanine.
	Dexamethasone	0.1 mg/kg/dose tid po/IV; max dose 10 mg/day	Also helpful with hepatic capsular distension, bowel wall edema, anorexia, increased ICP. May cause mood swings or psychosis.

Continued

Table 40-5 PHARMACOLOGIC APPROACH TO SYMPTOMS COMMONLY EXPERIENCED BY CHILDREN WITH LIFE-THREATENING ILLNESS—cont'd

SYMPTOM	MEDICATION	STARTING DOSE	COMMENTS
	Lorazepam	See previous listing	See previous listing
	Dronabinol	2.5-5 mg/m^2/dose Q 3-4 hrs	Available in 2.5- and 5-mg capsules. May remove liquid contents from capsules for children who cannot swallow capsules. Avoid in patients with sesame oil hypersensitivity or history of schizophrenia. May cause euphoria, dysphoria or other mood changes. Tolerance to CNS side effects usually develops in 1-3 days of continuous use. Avoid in patients with depression or mania.
	Scopolamine patch	See previous listing	See previous listing
Anxiety	Lorazepam	See previous listing	See previous listing
Agitation	Haloperidol	0.01 mg/kg po tid prn for acute onset: 0.025-0.050 mg/kg po, may repeat 0.025 mg/kg in 1 hr prn	May cause extrapyramidal reactions, which can be reversed with diphenhydramine or Cogentin. Safety not established in children <3 yr.
Sleep disturbance/ insomnia	Lorazepam	See previous listing	See previous listing
	Trazodone	Children 6-18 yr: 0.75-1 mg/kg/dose, given bid-tid if needed If >18 yr, start at 25-50 mg/dose, given bid-tid if needed	Potentially arrhythmogenic
Fatigue	Methylphenidate	0.3 mg/kg/dose titrated as needed, up to 60 mg/day	Rapid antidepressant effect; also improves cognition. Take before meals to avoid appetite suppression. Use with caution in children at risk for cardiac arrhythmia. Available as liquid and chewable tablet.
Pruritus	Diphenhydramine	0.5-1 mg/kg Q 6 hr IV/po (100 mg max per day)	May reverse phenothiazine-induced dystonic reactions. Topical formulation on large areas of the skin or open area may cause toxic reactions. May cause paradoxical reaction in young children.
	Hydroxyzine	0.5-1 mg/kg Q 6 hr IV/po (600 mg maximum per day)	
Constipation	Docusate	40-150 mg/day po in 1-4 divided doses	Stool softener available as liquid or capsule
	Miralax	<5 years: ½ scoop (8.5 g) in 4 oz of water daily >5 years: 1 scoop (17 g) in 8 oz of water daily	Tasteless powder may be mixed in beverage of choice. Now available over the counter.
	Lactulose	5-10 mL po up to Q 2 hr until BM	Bowel stimulant; dosing Q 2 hr may cause cramping
	Senna	2.5 mL po daily (for children >27 kg)	Bowel stimulant; available as granules
	Dulcolax	3-12 yr: 5-10 mg po daily >12 yr 5-15 mg po daily	Available in oral or rectal formulation
	Pediatric Fleets Enema	2.5 oz pediatric enema for children 2-11 yr; adult enema for children ≥12 yr	May repeat ×1 if needed. Do not use in neutropenic patients.
Muscle spasm	Diazepam	0.5 mg/kg/dose IV/po Q 6 hr prn; initial dose for children <5 yr is 5 mg dose; for children ≥5 yr dose is 10 mg/dose	May be irritating if given by peripheral IV
	Baclofen	5 mg po tid, increase by 5 mg/dose as needed	Helpful with neuropathic pain and spasticity; abrupt withdrawal may result in hallucinations and seizures; not for children <10 yr
Seizures	Lorazepam	0.1 mg/kg IV/po/SL/PR; repeat Q 10 min ×2	
	Diazepam	0.1 mg/kg Q 6 hr (max 5 mg/dose if <5 yr; max 10 mg/dose if >5 yr)	May be given PR as Diastat (0.2 mg/kg/dose Q 15 minutes ×3 doses)
Neuroirritability	Gabapentin	See previous listing	
	Clonidine	Starting dose: 0.05 mg/day. May increase every 3-5 days by 0.05 mg/day to 3-5 μg/kg/day given in divided doses 3-4 times/day; maximum dose is 0.3 mg/day. May switch from oral to transdermal route once optimal oral dose is established; Transdermal dose is equivalent to the total oral daily dose (e.g., if total oral dose is 0.1 mg/day, apply one patch (delivers 0.1 mg/day). Change patch every 7 days.	Transdermal patch may contain metal (e.g., aluminum) that may cause burns if worn during MRI scan. Remove patch prior to MRI. Patch may be cut into ¼ or ½ fractions based on dose needed.
	Clonazepam	<10 yr or <30 kg Initial dose: 0.01-0.03 mg/kg/day divided tid; ≥10 yr (≥30 kg) Initial dose: up to 0.25 mg po tid; may increase by 0.5-1 mg/day every 3 days Maintenance dose: 0.05-0.2 mg/kg/day up to 20 mg/day	
Anorexia	Megestrol acetate	10 mg/kg/day in 1-4 divided doses, may titrate up to 15 mg/kg/day or 800 mg/day	For children >10 yr. Acute adrenal insufficiency may occur with abrupt withdrawal after long-term use. Use with caution in patients with diabetes mellitus or history of thromboembolism. May cause photosensitivity.
	Dronabinol	See previous listing	See previous listing

*Infants <6 mo should receive 25-30% of the usual opioid starting dose.
†Although the usual opioid starting dose is presented, dose may be titrated as needed. There is no ceiling/maximum dose for opioids.
‡Breakthrough dose is 10% of 24 hr dose. See Chapter 71 for information regarding titration of opioids.
§Side effects from opioids include constipation, respiratory depression, pruritus, nausea, urinary retention, physical dependence.
hr, hour; IV, intravenously; po, by mouth; pr, rectally; prn, as needed; SC, subcutaneously.
Adapted from Ullrich C, Wolfe J: Pediatric pain and symptom control. In Walsh TD, Caraceni AT, Fainsinger R, et al: *Palliative medicine*, Philadelphia, 2008, Saunders.

preferable to use a known amount of the active agent, morphine.

It is important to explore with families, as well as members of the care team, misconceptions that they may have regarding addiction, dependence, the symbolic meaning of starting morphine and/or a morphine drip, and the potential for opioids to hasten death. There is no association between administration or escalation of opioids and length of survival. Evidence supports longer survival in individuals with symptoms that are well controlled.

Children also often experience a multitude of **nonpain symptoms.** A combination of both pharmacologic (see Table 40-5) and nonpharmacologic approaches (Table 40-6) is often optimal. **Fatigue** is one of the most common symptoms in children with advanced illness. Children may experience fatigue as a physical symptom (e.g., weakness or somnolence), a decline in cognition (e.g., diminished attention or concentration), and/or impaired emotional function (e.g., depressed mood or decreased motivation). Because of its multidimensional and incapacitating nature, fatigue can prevent children from participating in meaningful or pleasurable activities, thereby impairing quality of life. Fatigue is usually multifactorial in etiology. A careful history may reveal contributing physical factors (uncontrolled symptoms, medication side effects), psychologic factors (anxiety, depression), spiritual distress, or sleep disturbance. Interventions to reduce fatigue include treatment of contributing factors, exercise, pharmacologic agents, and behavior modification strategies. Challenges to effectively addressing fatigue include the common belief that fatigue is inevitable, lack of communication between families and care teams about it, and limited awareness of potential interventions for fatigue.

Dyspnea (the subjective sensation of shortness of breath) is due to a mismatch between afferent sensory input to the brain and the outgoing motor signal from the brain. It may stem from respiratory causes (e.g., airway secretions, obstruction, infection) or other factors (e.g., cardiac), and may also be influenced by psychologic factors (e.g., anxiety). Respiratory parameters such as respiratory rate and oxygen saturation correlate unreliably with the degree of dyspnea present. Therefore, giving oxygen to a cyanotic or hypoxic child who is otherwise quiet and relaxed may relieve staff discomfort while having no impact on patient distress. Dyspnea can be relieved with the use of regularly scheduled plus as-needed doses of opioids. Opioids work *directly* on the brainstem to reduce the sensation of respiratory distress, as opposed to relieving dyspnea via sedation. The dose of opioid needed to reduce dyspnea is as little as 25% of the amount that would be given for analgesia. Nonpharmacologic interventions, including guided imagery or hypnosis to reduce anxiety, or cool, flowing air, aimed toward the face, are also frequently helpful in alleviating dyspnea. While oxygen may relieve hypoxemia-related headaches, it is no more effective than blowing room air in reducing the distressing sensation of shortness of breath.

As death approaches, a buildup of secretions may result in noisy respiration sometimes referred to as a "death rattle." Patients at this stage are usually unconscious, and noisy respirations are often more distressing for others than for the child. It is often helpful to discuss this anticipated phenomenon with families in advance, and if it occurs, to point out the child's lack of distress from it. If treatment is needed, an anticholinergic medication, such as hyoscine, may reduce secretions.

Neurologic symptoms include **seizures** that are often part of the antecedent illness but may increase in frequency and severity toward the end of life. A plan for managing seizures should be made in advance and anticonvulsants should be readily available in the event of seizure. Parents can be taught to use rectal diazepam at home. Increased **neuroirritability** accompanies some neurodegenerative disorders; it may be particularly disruptive because of the resultant break in normal sleep-wake patterns and the difficulty in finding respite facilities for children who have prolonged crying. Such neuroirritability may respond to gabapentin. Judicious use of sedatives, benzodiazepines, clonidine, or methadone may also reduce irritability without inducing excessive sedation; this combination can dramatically improve the quality of life for both child and caregivers. **Increased intracranial pressure** and **spinal cord compression** are most often encountered in children with brain tumors or metastatic and solid tumors. Depending on the clinical situation and the goals of care,

Table 40-6 NONPHARMACOLOGIC APPROACH TO SYMPTOMS COMMONLY EXPERIENCED BY CHILDREN WITH LIFE-THREATENING ILLNESS

SYMPTOM	APPROACH TO MANAGEMENT
Pain	Prevent pain when possible by limiting unnecessary painful procedures, providing sedation, and giving pre-emptive analgesia prior to a procedure (e.g., including sucrose for procedures in neonates)
	Address coincident depression, anxiety, sense of fear or lack of control
	Consider guided imagery, relaxation, hypnosis, art/pet/play therapy, acupuncture/acupressure, biofeedback, massage, heat/cold, yoga, transcutaneous electric nerve stimulation, distraction
Dyspnea or air hunger	Suction secretions if present, positioning, comfortable loose clothing, fan to provide cool, blowing air
	Limit volume of IV fluids, consider diuretics if fluid overload/ pulmonary edema present
	Behavioral strategies including breathing exercises, guided imagery, relaxation, music
Fatigue	Sleep hygiene
	Gentle exercise
	Address potentially contributing factors (e.g., anemia, depression, side effects of medications)
Nausea/vomiting	Consider dietary modifications (bland, soft, adjust timing/ volume of foods or feeds)
	Aromatherapy: peppermint, lavender; acupuncture/ acupressure
Constipation	Increase fiber in diet, encourage fluids
Oral lesions/ dysphagia	Oral hygiene and appropriate liquid, solid and oral medication formulation (texture, taste, fluidity). Treat infections, complications (mucositis, pharyngitis, dental abscess, esophagitis).
	Orophayngeal motility study and speech (feeding team) consultation.
Anorexia/ cachexia	Manage treatable lesions causing oral pain, dysphagia, anorexia. Support caloric intake during phase of illness when anorexia is reversible. Acknowledge that anorexia/ cachexia is intrinsic to the dying process and may not be reversible.
	Prevent/treat coexisting constipation
Pruritus	Moisturize skin
	Trim child's nails to prevent excoriation
	Try specialized anti-itch lotions
	Apply cold packs
	Counterstimulation, distraction, relaxation
Diarrhea	Evaluate/treat if obstipation
	Assess and treat infection
	Dietary modification
Depression	Psychotherapy, behavioral techniques
Anxiety	Psychotherapy (individual and family), behavioral techniques
Agitation/terminal restlessness	Evaluate for organic or drug causes
	Educate family
	Orient and reassure child; provide calm, nonstimulating environment

From Sourkes B, Frankel L, Brown M, et al: Food, toys, and love: pediatric palliative care, *Curr Probl Pediatr Adolesc Health Care* 35:345–392, 2005.

radiation therapy, surgical interventions, and steroids are potential therapeutic options.

Feeding and hydration issues can raise ethical questions that evoke intense emotions in families and medical caregivers alike. Options that may be considered to artificially support nutrition and hydration in a child who can no longer feed by mouth include nasogastric and gastrostomy feedings or intravenous nutrition or hydration (Chapter 3). These complex decisions require evaluating the risks and benefits of artificial feedings and taking into consideration the child's functional level and prognosis. At times, it may be appropriate to initiate a trial of tube feedings with the understanding that they may be discontinued at a later stage of the illness. A commonly held but unsubstantiated belief is that artificial nutrition and hydration are "comfort measures," without which a child may suffer from starvation or thirst. This may result in well-meaning but disruptive and invasive attempts to administer nutrition or fluids to a dying child. In dying adults, the sensation of thirst may be alleviated by careful efforts to keep the mouth moist and clean. There may also be deleterious side effects to artificial hydration in the form of increased secretions, need for frequent urination, and exacerbation of dyspnea. For these reasons, it is important to educate families about anticipated decreases in appetite/thirst and therefore little need for nutrition and hydration as the child approaches death. In addition, exploring the meaning that provision of nutrition and hydration may hold for families, as well alternative ways that they may love and nurture their child, may be a helpful way to approach this issue.

Nausea and vomiting may be due to a variety of causes, including medications/toxins, irritation to or obstruction of the gastrointestinal tract, motion, and emotions. Drugs such as metoclopramide, 5-hydroxytryptamine antagonists, steroids, and aprepitant may be used, and should be chosen depending on the underlying pathophysiology and neurotransmitters involved. Vomiting may accompany nausea but may also occur without nausea, such as in the instance of increased intracranial pressure. **Constipation** is commonly encountered in children with neurologic impairment or children receiving medications that impair gastrointestinal motility (most notably, opioids). Stool frequency and quantity should be evaluated in the context of the child's diet and usual bowel pattern. Children on regular opioids should routinely be placed on stool softeners (docusate) in addition to a laxative agent (e.g., senna). **Diarrhea** may be particularly difficult for the child and family and may be treated with loperamide and opioids. Paradoxical diarrhea, a result of overflow resulting from constipation, must also be considered.

Hematologic issues include consideration of anemia and thrombocytopenia or bleeding. If the child has symptomatic anemia (weakness, dizziness, shortness of breath, tachycardia), red blood cell transfusions may be considered. Platelet transfusions may be an option if the child has symptoms of bleeding. Life-ending hemorrhage is disturbing for all concerned, and a plan involving the use of fast-acting sedatives should be prepared in advance if such an event is a possibility.

Skin care issues include primary prevention of problems by frequent turning and repositioning and alleviating pressure wherever possible (e.g., elevating heels with pillows). Pruritus may be secondary to systemic disorders or drug therapy. Treatment includes avoiding excessive use of drying soaps, using moisturizers, trimming fingernails, and wearing loose-fitting clothing, in addition to administering topical or systemic steroids. Oral antihistamines and other specific therapies may also be indicated (e.g., cholestyramine in biliary disease). While opioids can cause histamine release from mast cells, this does not account for most of the pruritus caused by opioids. A trial of diphenhydramine may provide relief; alternatively, switching opioids or instituting a low dose of opioid antagonist may be needed for refractory pruritus.

Children with life-threatening illness may experience psychologic symptoms such as **anxiety** and **depression.** Such symptoms are frequently multifactorial, and sometimes interrelated with uncontrolled symptoms such as pain and fatigue. Diagnosing depression in the context of serious illness may pose challenges since neurovegetative symptoms may not be reliable indicators. Instead, expressions of hopelessness, helplessness, worthlessness, and guilt may be more useful. While psychopharmacologic agents may improve psychologic symptoms, psychologic interventions and opportunities for children to explore worries, hopes, and concerns in an open, supportive, and nonjudgmental setting are equally if not more important. Skilled members from a variety of disciplines, including psychology, social work, chaplaincy, child life, expressive therapy, among others, may help children and their families in this regard. Such opportunities may in fact create positive moments in which meaning, connection, and new definitions of hope are found.

When discussing possible therapies or interventions with adolescent patients or with the parents of any ill child, it is important to raise the issue of **complementary or alternative medicine.** Many families use some form of alternative medicine therapy but do not bring it up with their physician unless explicitly asked (Chapter 59). Although largely unproven, some therapies are inexpensive and provide relief to individual patients. Other therapies may be expensive, painful, intrusive, and even toxic. By initiating conversation and inviting discussion in a nonjudgmental way, the physician can offer advice on the safety of different therapies and may help avoid expensive, dangerous, or burdensome interventions.

Intensive Symptom Management

When intensive efforts to relieve the symptom have been exhausted, or when efforts to address suffering are incapable of providing relief with acceptable toxicity/morbidity or in an acceptable time frame, **palliative sedation** may be considered. Palliative sedation may relieve suffering from refractory symptoms by reducing a child's level of consciousness. It is most often used for intractable pain, dyspnea, or agitation, but is not limited to these distressing indications.

The *principle of double effect* is often invoked to justify escalation of symptom-relieving medications or palliative sedation for uncontrolled symptoms at the end of life. Use of this principle emphasizes the risk of hastening death posed by escalating opioids or sedation, which is theoretical and unproven. There is mounting evidence that patients with well-controlled symptoms live longer.

The Terminal Phase

As death seems imminent, the major task of the physician and team are to help the child have as many good days as possible and not suffer. Gently preparing the family for what to expect and offering choices, when possible, will allow them a sense of control in the midst of tragic circumstances. Before death, it can be very helpful to discuss:

- Support of siblings or other family members
- Resuscitation status
- Limiting technology when no longer beneficial to the child
- Cultural, spiritual, or religious needs
- Location of death
  - Who will pronounce if death occurs at home
- Funeral arrangements
  - Offering siblings choice and appropriate support to attend
- Autopsy and/or tissue or organ donation
  - Legacy building, benefits others, informs science and family

Families will inform the provider of what they can tolerate thinking about. It may help to let the family know this is not about *whether* the child will die but *how* the child may die.

Families gain tremendous support from having a physician who will continue to stay involved in the child's care. If the child is at home or hospitalized, regular phone calls or visits, assisting with symptom management, and offering emotional support is invaluable for families.

In an intensive care setting, where technology can be overwhelming and put distance between the child and parent, the physician can offer discontinuation of that which is not benefiting the child or adding to quality of life. Parents may be afraid to ask about holding or sleeping next to their child. They may need reassurance and assistance in holding, touching, and speaking with their child, despite tubes and technology, even if the child appears unresponsive.

It is believed that hearing and the ability to sense touch is often present until death; all family members should be encouraged to continue interacting with their loved one through the dying process. Parents may be afraid to leave the bedside so that their child will not die alone. In most instances the moment of death cannot be predicted. Some propose that children wait to die until parents are "ready," an important event has passed, or until they are given permission. Caregivers need not dispute this, nor the hope for a miracle often held by families until the child takes the very last breath.

For the family, the moment of death is an event that is recalled in detail for years to come, and so enhancing opportunity for dignity and limited suffering is essential. Families may find solace in having a clinician present. After death, they should be given the option of remaining with their child for as long as they would like. During this time, physicians and other professionals may ask permission to "say goodbye." The family may be invited to bathe and dress the body as a final act of caring for the child.

The physician's decision to attend the funeral is a personal one. Participation may serve the dual purpose of showing respect as well as helping the clinician cope with a personal sense of loss. If unable to attend services, families report highly valuing the importance of receiving a card or note from the physician. To know that their child made a difference and will not be forgotten is incredibly important to families in their bereavement.

The Pediatrician

While optimal palliative care for children entails caregivers from a variety of disciplines, pediatricians are well-positioned to support children and their families, particularly if they have a long-standing relationship with multiple family members. A pediatrician who has cared for a family over time may already know and care for other family members, understand pre-existing stressors for the family, and may be familiar with coping strategies used by family members. Pediatricians are familiar with the process of eliciting concerns and providing anticipatory guidance for parents, as well as developmentally appropriate explanations for children.

BIBLIOGRAPHY

Please visit the Nelson Textbook of Pediatrics *website at* *www.expertconsult.com* *for the complete bibliography.*

PART VI Nutrition

Chapter 41
Nutritional Requirements

Asim Maqbool, Nicolas Stettler, and Virginia A. Stallings

Nutritional intakes for infants, children, and adolescents should provide for maintenance of current weight and support normal growth and development. The infancy growth period is rapid, is critical for neurocognitive development, and bears higher metabolic rate and nutrient requirements, relative to body size, than other periods of growth. It is followed by the childhood period of growth, during which 60% of total growth occurs, and then by the puberty phase. Nutrition and growth during the first 3 yr of life predict adult stature and some health outcomes. The major risk period for growth stunting (impaired linear growth) is between 4 mo and 2 yr of age, and it may be followed by a delay in the childhood phase of growth. It is critical to identify nutrient deficiencies promptly and to address them aggressively early in life, because they can impart lasting effects on growth and development.

For the full continuation of this chapter, please visit the Nelson Textbook of Pediatrics *website at www.expertconsult.com.*

Chapter 42
Feeding Healthy Infants, Children, and Adolescents

Nicolas Stettler, Jatinder Bhatia, Anjali Parish, and Virginia A. Stallings

Early feeding and nutrition play important roles in the origin of adult diseases such as type 2 diabetes, hypertension, obesity, and the metabolic syndrome; therefore, appropriate feeding practices should be established in the neonatal period and carried out as a continuum from childhood and adolescence to adulthood. Optimal neonatal feeding practices require a multidisciplinary approach among health care providers, including physicians, nursing staff, nutritionists, and lactation consultants. Whether by breast or by bottle, successful infant feeding requires education and a supportive environment conducive to successful transition from fetal to neonatal life.

FEEDING DURING THE FIRST YEAR OF LIFE

Breast-feeding

Feedings should be initiated soon after birth unless medical conditions preclude them. The American Academy of Pediatrics (AAP) and World Health Organization (WHO) strongly advocate breast-feeding as the preferred feeding for all infants. The success of breast-feeding initiation and continuation depends on multiple factors, such as education about breast-feeding, hospital breast-feeding practices and policies, routine and timely follow-up care, and family and societal support (Table 42-1). The AAP recommends exclusive breast-feeding for a minimum of 4 mo and preferably for 6 mo. The advantages of breast-feeding are well documented (Tables 42-2 and 42-3), and contraindications are rare (Table 42-4).

Mothers should be encouraged to nurse at each breast at each feeding starting with the breast offered 2nd at the last feeding. It is not unusual for an infant to fall asleep after the 1st breast and refuse the 2nd. It is preferable to empty the 1st breast before offering the 2nd in order to allow complete emptying and therefore better milk production. Table 42-5 summarizes patterns of milk supply in the 1st week.

New mothers should be instructed about infant hunger cues, correct nipple latch, positioning of the infant on the breast, and feeding frequency. It is also suggested that a physician or a lactation expert observe a feeding to evaluate positioning, latch, milk transfer and maternal responses, and infant satiety. Attention to these issues during the birth hospitalization allows dialogue with the mother and family and can prevent problems that could occur with improper technique or knowledge of breast-feeding. As part of the discharge teaching process, issues surrounding infant feeding, elimination patterns, breast engorgement, basic breast care, and maternal nutrition should be discussed. A follow-up appointment is recommended within 24-48 hr after hospital discharge.

Nipple Pain

Nipple pain is one of the most common complaints of breast-feeding mothers in the immediate postpartum period. Poor infant positioning and improper latch are the most common reasons for nipple pain beyond the mild discomfort felt early in breast-feeding. If the problem persists and the infant refuses to feed, consideration needs to be given to nipple candidiasis, and both mother and baby should be treated if candidiasis is found. In some cases, especially if accompanied by engorgement, it may be necessary to express milk manually until healing has occurred.

Engorgement

In the 2nd stage of lactogenesis, physiologic fullness of the breast occurs. If the breasts are firm, overfilled, and painful, the cause may be incomplete removal of milk due to poor breast-feeding technique or other reasons such as infant illness. Frequent breast-feeding or, in some cases, manual milk expression before breast-feeding may be required.

Mastitis

Mastitis occurs in 2-3% of lactating women and is usually unilateral, manifesting with localized warmth, tenderness, edema, and erythema after the 2nd postdelivery week. Sudden onset of breast pain, myalgia, and fever with fatigue, nausea, vomiting, and headache can also occur. Organisms implicated in mastitis include *Staphylococcus aureus*, *Escherichia coli*, group A streptococcus, *Haemophilus influenzae*, *Klebsiella pneumoniae*, and *Bacteroides* spp. Diagnosis is confirmed by physical examination. Oral antibiotics and analgesics, while promoting breast-feeding or emptying of the affected breast, usually resolve the infection. A breast abscess is a less-common complication of mastitis, but it is a more serious infection that requires intravenous antibiotics as well as incision and drainage, along with temporary cessation of feeding from that breast.

Milk Leakage

Milk leakage is a common event in which milk is involuntarily lost from the breast either in response to breast-feeding on the opposite side or as a reflex in response to other stimuli, such as an infant's cry. Milk leakage usually resolves spontaneously as lactation proceeds.

Table 42-1 STEPS TO ENCOURAGE BREAST-FEEDING IN THE HOSPITAL: UNICEF/WHO BABY-FRIENDLY

HOSPITAL INITIATIVES
Provide all pregnant women with information and counseling Document the desire to breast-feed in the medical record Document the method of feeding in the infant's record Place the newborn and mother skin-to-skin, and initiate breast-feeding within 1 hr of birth Continue skin-to-skin contact at other times and encourage rooming in Assess breast-feeding and continue encouragement and teaching on each shift
MOTHERS TO LEARN
Proper position and latch on Nutritive sucking and swallowing Milk production and release Frequency and feeding cues Expression of milk if needed Assessment of the infant's nutritional status When to contact the clinician
ADDITIONAL INSTRUCTIONS
Refer to lactation consultation if any concerns arise Infants should go to the breast at least 8-12 times/24 hr day and night Avoid time limits on the breasts; offer both breasts at each feeding Do not give sterile water, glucose, or formula unless indicated If supplements are given, use cup feeding, a Haberman feeder, fingers, or syringe feedings Avoid pacifiers in the newborn nursery except during painful procedures Avoid antilactation drugs

UNICEF, United Nations Children's Fund; WHO, World Health Organization.

Table 42-2 SELECTED BENEFICIAL PROPERTIES OF HUMAN MILK COMPARED TO INFANT FORMULA

Secretory IgA	Specific antigen-targeted anti-infective action
Lactoferrin	Immunomodulation, iron chelation, antimicrobial action, antiadhesive, trophic for intestinal growth
κ-casein	Antiadhesive, bacterial flora
Oligosaccharides	Prevention of bacterial attachment
Cytokines	Anti-inflammatory, epithelial barrier function
Growth factors	
Epidermal growth factor	Luminal surveillance, repair of intestine
Transforming growth factor (TGF)	Promotes epithelial cell growth (TGF-β) Suppresses lymphocyte function (TGF-β)
Nerve growth factor	Promotes neural growth
Enzymes	
Platelet-activating factor-acetylhydrolase	Blocks action of platelet activating factor
Glutathione peroxidase	Prevents lipid oxidation
Nucleotides	Enhance antibody responses, bacterial flora

Table 42-3 CONDITIONS FOR WHICH HUMAN MILK HAS BEEN SUGGESTED TO HAVE A PROTECTIVE EFFECT

- Acute disorders
  - Diarrhea
  - Otitis media
  - Urinary tract infection
  - Necrotizing enterocolitis
  - Septicemia
  - Infant botulism
- Chronic disorders
  - Insulin-dependent diabetes mellitus
  - Celiac disease
  - Crohn's disease
  - Childhood cancer
    - Lymphoma
    - Leukemia
  - Recurrent otitis media
  - Allergy
- Obesity and overweight
- Hospitalizations
- Infant mortality

Adapted from the Schanler RJ, Dooley S: *Breastfeeding handbook for physicians*, Elk Grove Village, IL, 2006, American Academy of Pediatrics.

Table 42-4 ABSOLUTE AND RELATIVE CONTRAINDICATIONS TO BREAST-FEEDING DUE TO MATERNAL HEALTH CONDITIONS

MATERNAL HEALTH CONDITIONS	DEGREE OF RISK
HIV and HTLV infection	In the USA, breast-feeding is contraindicated In other settings, health risks of not breast-feeding must be weighed against the risk of transmitting virus to the infant
Tuberculosis infection	Breast-feeding is contraindicated until completion of approximately 2 wk of appropriate maternal therapy
Varicella-zoster infection	Infant should not have direct contact to active lesions Infant should receive immune globulin
Herpes simplex infection	Breast-feeding is contraindicated with active herpetic lesions of the breast
CMV infection	May be found in milk of mothers who are CMV seropositive Transmission through human milk Causing symptomatic illness in term infants is uncommon.
Hepatitis B infection	Infants routinely receive hepatitis B immune globulin and hepatitis B vaccine if mother is HbsAg positive No delay in initiation of breast-feeding is required
Hepatitis C infection	Breast-feeding is not contraindicated
Alcohol intake	Limit maternal alcohol intake to <0.5 g/kg/day (for a woman of average weight, this is the equivalent of 2 cans of beer, 2 glasses of wine, or 2 oz of liquor)
Cigarette smoking	Discourage cigarette smoking, but smoking is not a contraindication to breast-feeding
Chemotherapy, radiopharmaceuticals	Breast-feeding is generally contraindicated

CMV, cytomegalovirus; HbsAg, hepatitis B surface antigen; HIV, human immunodeficiency virus; HTLV, human T-lymphotropic virus.

Inadequate Milk Intake

Insufficient milk intake, dehydration, and jaundice in the infant can surface after the first 48 hr of life. The infant might cry or be lethargic and have delayed stooling, decreased urine output, weight loss >7% of birth weight, hypernatremic dehydration, and increased hunger. Insufficient milk intake may be due to insufficient milk production or failure of established breast-feeding, but it can also result from health conditions in the infant that prevent proper breast stimulation. Parents should be counseled that breast-fed neonates must feed a minimum of 8 times per day. Careful attention to prenatal history can identify maternal factors that may be associated with this problem, for example, failure of breasts to enlarge during pregnancy or within the first few days after delivery. Direct observation of breast-feeding can help identify improper technique. If a large volume of milk is expressed manually after breast-feeding, then the infant might not be extracting enough milk, eventually leading to decreased milk output. Late preterm infants (34-36 wk) are at risk for insufficient milk syndrome because of poor suck and swallow patterns or medical issues.

Jaundice

Breast-feeding jaundice is a common reason for hospital readmission of healthy breast-fed infants and is largely related to insufficient fluid intake (Chapter 96.3). It may also be associated with dehydration and hypernatremia. Breast milk jaundice causes persistently high serum indirect bilirubin in a thriving healthy baby. Jaundice generally declines in the 2nd wk of life. Infants with severe or persistent jaundice should be evaluated for problems such as galactosemia, hypothyroidism, urinary tract infection, and hemolysis before ascribing the jaundice to breast milk that might contain inhibitors of glucuronyl transferase or enhanced absorption of bilirubin from the gut. Persistently high bilirubin can require changing from breast milk to infant formula for 24-48 hr and/or phototherapy without cessation of breast-feeding. Breast-feeding should resume after the decline in serum bilirubin. Parents should be reassured and encouraged to continue collecting breast milk during the period when the infant is taking formula.

Collecting Breast Milk

The pumping of breast milk is a common practice when the mother and baby are separated, such as when the mother returns to work or when there is an illness or hospitalization of the mother or infant that precludes breast-feeding. Good handwashing and hygiene should be emphasized. Electric breast pumps are more efficient and better tolerated by mothers than mechanical pumps or manual expression. Collection kits should be rinsed, cleaned with hot soapy water, and air dried after every use. Glass or plastic containers should be used to collect the milk, and milk should be refrigerated and then used within 48 hr. Expressed breast milk can be frozen and used for up to 6 mo. Milk should be thawed rapidly by holding under running tepid water and used completely within 24 hr after thawing. Milk should not be microwaved.

Table 42-5 PATTERNS OF MILK SUPPLY

DAY OF LIFE	MILK SUPPLY
Day 1	Some milk (~5 mL) may be expressed
Days 2-4	Lactogenesis, milk production increases
Day 5	Milk present, fullness, leaking felt
Day 6 onward	Breasts should feel "empty" after feeding

Adapted from Neifert MR: Clinical aspects of lactation: promoting breastfeeding success, *Clin Perinatol* 26:281–306, 1999.

Growth of the Breast-fed Infant

The rate of weight gain of the breast-fed infant differs from that of the formula-fed infant, and the infant's risk for excess weight gain during late infancy may be associated with bottle feeding. Some of the differences in weight gain are explained by the use of growth charts derived from predominantly formula-fed children, and several studies suggest that the growth pattern of the population of breast-fed infants should be considered the norm. The WHO, has published a growth reference based on the growth of healthy breast-fed infants through the 1st yr of life. The new standards (*http://www.who.int/childgrowth*) are the result of a study in which >8,000 children were selected from 6 countries. The infants were selected based on healthy feeding practices (breast-feeding), good health care, high socioeconomic status, and nonsmoking mothers, so that they reflect the growth of breast-fed infants in the optimal conditions and can be used as prescriptive rather than normative curves. Charts are available for growth monitoring from birth to age 6 yr. The Centers for Disease Control and Prevention now recommends use of these charts for infants 0 to 23 months of age.

Formula Feeding (Fig. 42-1)

Most women make their feeding choices for their infant early in pregnancy. In a U.S. survey, although 83% of respondents initiated breast-feeding, the percentage who continued to breast-feed declined to 50% at 6 mo. Fifty-two percent of infants received formula while in the hospital and by 4 mo 40% had

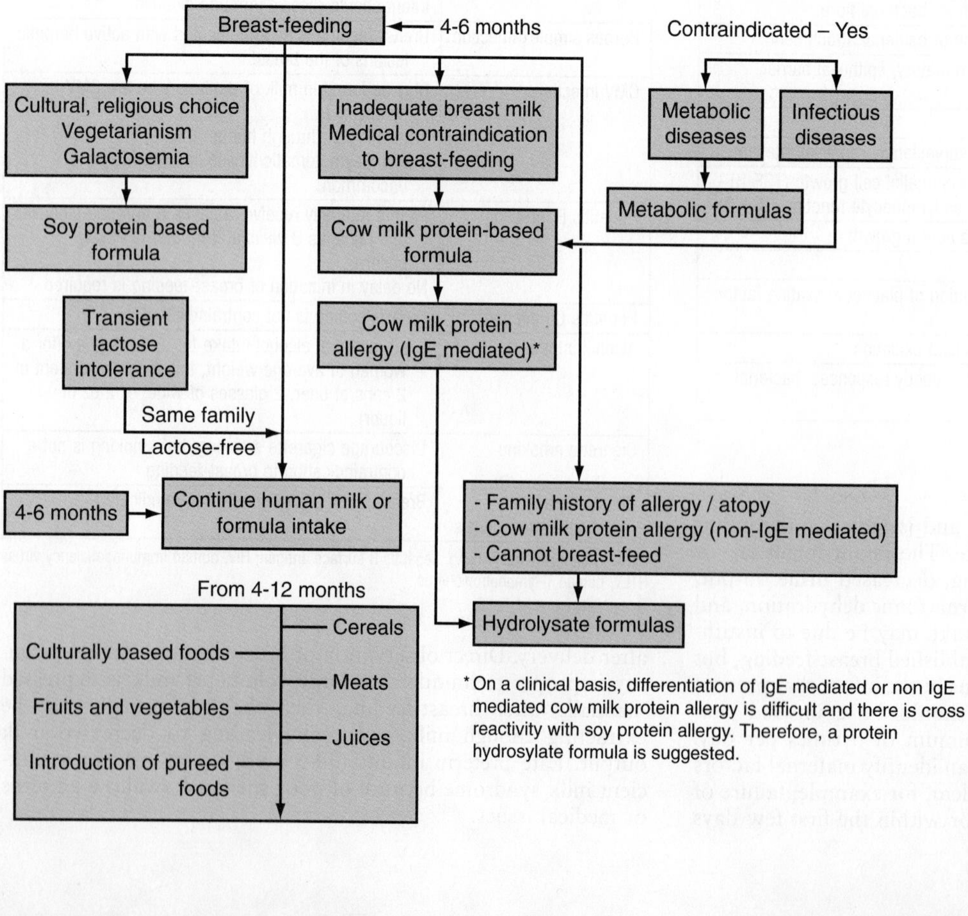

Figure 42-1 Feeding algorithm for term infants. (From Gamble Y, Bunyapen C, Bhatia J: Feeding the term infant. In Berdanier CD, Dwyer J, Feldman EB, editors: *Handbook of nutrition and food,* Boca Raton, FL, 2008, CRC Press, Taylor and Francis Group, pp 271–284, Fig. 15-3.)

consumed other foods as well. Despite efforts to promote breast-feeding and discourage complementary foods before 4 mo of age, supplementing breast-feeding with infant formula and early introduction of complementary foods remain common in the USA. Indications for the use of infant formula are as a substitute or a supplement for breast milk or as a substitute for breast milk when breast milk is medically contraindicated by maternal (see Table 42-4) or infant factors.

Infant formulas marketed in the USA are safe and nutritionally adequate as the sole source of nutrition for healthy infants for the first 4-6 mo of life. Infant formulas are available in ready-to-feed, concentrated liquid or powder forms. Ready-to-feed products generally provide 20 kcal/30 mL (1 oz) and approximately 67 kcal/dL. Concentrated liquid products when diluted according to instructions provide a preparation with the same concentration. Powder formulas come in single or multiple servings and when mixed according to instructions will result in similar caloric density.

Although infant formulas are manufactured in adherence to good manufacturing practices and are inspected by the U.S. Food and Drug Administration (FDA), there are potential issues. Powder preparations are not sterile, and although the number of bacterial colony-forming units per gram of formula is generally lower than allowable limits, outbreaks of infections with *Enterobacter sakazakii* have been documented, especially in premature infants. The powder preparations can contain other coliform bacteria but have not been linked to disease in healthy term infants. Care also needs to be taken in following the mixing instructions to avoid over or under dilution, using water either boiled or sterilized, and using the specific scoops provided by the manufacturer, because scoop sizes vary. Well water needs to be tested regularly for bacteria and toxin contamination. Municipal water can contain variable concentrations of fluoride, and if the concentrations are high, bottled water that is defluoridated should be used to avoid toxicity.

Parents should be instructed to use proper handwashing techniques when preparing formula or feeding the infant. Guidance to follow written instructions for storage should also be given. Once opened, ready-to-feed and concentrated liquid containers can be covered with aluminum foil or plastic wrap and stored in the refrigerator for no longer than 48 hr. Powder formula should be stored in a cool, dry place; once opened, cans should be covered with the original plastic cap or aluminum foil, and the powdered product can be used for up to 4 wk. Prepared formula stored in the refrigerator should be warmed by placing the container in warm water for ~5 min; similar to breast milk, formula should not be heated in a microwave, because the formula can be heated unevenly and result in burns despite appearing to be at the right temperature when the surface is tested.

Formula feedings should be ad libitum, with the goal of achieving growth and development to the child's genetic potential. The usual intake to allow a weight gain of 25-30 g/day will be 140-200 mL/kg/day in the first 3 mo of life. Between 3 and 6 mo of age and between 6 and 12 mo of age, the rate of weight gain declines. The protein and energy content of infant formulas in the USA for term infants is ~2.1 g/100 kcal and 67 kcal/dL. No recommendations have been made for follow-up or weaning formulas, although these are available and marketed.

If feedings are adequate and weight, length, and head circumference trajectories are appropriate, then infants do not need additional water, unless dictated by high environmental temperature. Vomiting and spitting up are common, and when weight gain and general well-being are noted, no change in formula is necessary. Most infants thrive on cow's milk protein–based formulas, although some infants exhibit intolerance or allergy to cow's milk protein.

In addition to complementary foods introduced between 4 and 6 mo of age, continued breast-feeding or the use of infant formula for the entire 1st year of life should be encouraged. Whole cow's milk should not be introduced until 12 mo of age. In children between 12 and 24 mo of age for whom overweight or obesity is a concern or who have a family history of obesity, dyslipidemia, or cardiovascular disease, the use of reduced-fat milk would be appropriate.

COW'S MILK PROTEIN–BASED FORMULAS Intact cow's milk–based formulas in the USA contain a protein concentration varying from 1.45 to 1.6 g/dL, considerably higher than in mature breast milk (~1 g/dL). The whey:casein ratio varies from 18:82 to 60:40; one manufacturer markets a formula that is 100% whey. The predominant whey protein is β-globulin in bovine milk and α-lactalbumin in human milk. This and other differences between human milk and bovine milk–based formulas result in different plasma amino acid profiles in infants on different feeding patterns, but a clinical significance of these differences has not been demonstrated.

Plant or a mixture of plant and animal oils are the source of fat in infant formulas, and fat provides 40-50% of the energy in cow's milk–based formulas. Fat blends are better absorbed than dairy fat and provide saturated, monounsaturated, and polyunsaturated fatty acids (PUFAs). All infant formulas are supplemented with long-chain PUFAs, docosahexaenoic acid (DHA), and arachidonic acid (ARA) at varying concentrations. ARA and DHA are found at varying concentrations in human milk and vary by geographic region and maternal diet. No studies in term infants have found a negative effect of DHA and ARA supplementation, but some studies have demonstrated positive effects on visual acuity and neurocognitive development. A critical review concluded that there are no consistent effects of long-chain PUFAs (LCPUFAs) on visual acuity in term infants. A Cochrane review concluded that routine supplementation of milk formula with LCPUFAs to improve the physical, neurodevelopmental, or visual outcomes of infants born at term cannot be recommended based on the current evidence. DHA and ARA derived from single-cell microfungi and microalgae are classified as generally recognized as safe for use in infant formulas at approved concentrations and ratios.

Lactose is the major carbohydrate in mother's milk and in standard cow's milk–based infant formulas for term infants. Formulas for older infants might also contain modified starch or other complex carbohydrates.

SOY FORMULAS Soy protein–based formulas on the market are all free of cow's milk protein and lactose and provide 67 kcal/dL. They meet the vitamin, mineral, and electrolyte guidelines from the AAP and the FDA for feeding term infants. The protein is a soy isolate supplemented with L-methionine, L-carnitine, and taurine to provide a protein content of 2.45-2.8 g per 100 kcal or 1.65-1.9 g/dL.

The quantity of specific fats varies by manufacturer and is usually similar to the manufacturer's corresponding cow's milk–based formula. The fat content is 5.0-5.5 g per 100 kcal or 3.4-3.6 g/dL. The oils used include soy, palm, sunflower, olein, safflower, and coconut. DHA and ARA are now added routinely.

In term infants, although soy protein–based formulas have been used to provide nutrition resulting in normal growth patterns, there are few indications for use in place of cow's milk–based formula. These indications include galactosemia and hereditary lactase deficiency, because soy-based formulas are lactose-free; and situations in which a vegetarian diet is preferred. Most previously well infants with acute gastroenteritis can be managed after rehydration with continued use of mother's milk or cow's milk–based formulas and do not require lactose-free formula, such as soy-based formula. However, soy protein–based formulas may be indicated when documented secondary lactose intolerance occurs. Soy protein–based formulas have no advantage over cow's milk protein–based formulas as a supplement for the breast-fed infant, unless the infant has one of the indications noted previously. The routine use of soy protein–based formula has no proven value in the prevention or management of infantile colic, fussiness, or atopic disease. Infants with documented cow's milk protein–induced enteropathy or enterocolitis often are also sensitive to soy protein and should not be given isolated soy protein–based formula. They should be provided formula derived from extensively hydrolyzed protein or synthetic amino acids. Soy formulas can contain phytoestrogens, which have increased caution for their use in infants.

PROTEIN HYDROLYSATE FORMULA Protein hydrolysate formulas may be partially hydrolyzed, containing oligopeptides with a molecular weight of <5000 d, or extensively hydrolyzed, containing peptides with a molecular weight <3000 d. Partially hydrolyzed proteins have fat blends similar to cow's milk–based formulas, and carbohydrates are supplied by corn maltodextrin or corn syrup solids. Because the protein is not extensively hydrolyzed, these formulas should not be fed to infants who are allergic to cow's milk protein. In studies of infants who are at high risk of developing atopic disease and who are not breast-fed exclusively for 4-6 mo, there is modest evidence that atopic dermatitis may be delayed or prevented in early childhood by the use of extensively or partially hydrolyzed formulas, compared with cow's milk formula. Comparative studies of the various hydrolyzed formulas have also indicated that not all formulas have the same protective benefit. Extensively hydrolyzed formulas may be more effective than partially hydrolyzed in preventing atopic disease. Extensively hydrolyzed formulas are the preferred formulas for infants intolerant to cow's milk or soy proteins. These formulas are lactose free and can include medium-chain triglycerides, making them useful in infants with gastrointestinal malabsorption due to cystic fibrosis, short gut syndrome, and prolonged diarrhea.

AMINO ACID FORMULAS Amino acid formulas are peptide-free formulas that contain mixtures of essential and nonessential amino acids. They are specifically designed for infants with dairy protein allergy who failed to thrive on extensively hydrolyzed protein formulas. The use of amino acid formulas to prevent atopic disease has not been studied.

Complementary Feeding

The timely introduction of complementary foods (all solid foods and liquid foods other than breast milk or formula, also called weaning foods or beikost) during infancy is necessary to enable transition from milk feedings to other foods and is important for nutritional and developmental reasons (Table 42-6). The dilemmas of the weaning period are different in different societies. The ability of exclusive breast-feeding to meet macronutrient and micronutrient requirements becomes limiting with increasing age of the infant. Current WHO recommendations on the age at which complementary food should be introduced are based on the optimal duration of exclusive breast-feeding. A WHO-commissioned systematic review of the optimal duration of exclusive breast-feeding compared outcomes with exclusive breast-feeding for 6 vs 3-4 mo. The review concluded that there were no differences in growth between the 2 durations of exclusive breast-feeding. Another systematic review concluded that there was no compelling evidence to change the recommendations for starting complementary foods at 4-6 mo. The AAP Pediatric Nutrition Handbook also states that there is no significant harm associated with introduction of complementary foods at 4 mo of age and no significant benefit from exclusive breast-feeding for 6 mo in terms of growth, zinc and iron nutriture, allergy, or infections. The European Society for Pediatric Gastroenterology, Hepatology, and Nutrition Committee on Nutrition considers that exclusive breast-feeding for ~6 mo is desirable, but that the introduction of complementary foods should not occur before 17 weeks (~4 mo) and should not be delayed beyond 26 weeks (~6 mo).

Evidence for the optimal timing for introducing specific complementary foods is lacking and is largely based on consensus and traditions. Practices vary widely among regions and cultures. Ideally, complementary foods are combined with human milk or formula to provide the nutrients required for appropriate growth. Current complementary feeding practices largely meet infants' energy and nutrient needs. Because some complementary foods are more nutritionally appropriate than others to complement breast milk or infant formula, improved evidence-based guidelines about types, quantities, and timing of introducing complementary foods would be desirable. For example, the Feeding and Toddlers Study collected data on the food consumption patterns of U.S. infants and toddlers and showed that nearly all infants ≤12 mo consumed some form of milk every day; more infants >4 mo consumed more formula than human milk, and by 9-11 mo of age 20% consumed whole cow's milk and 25% consumed nonfat or reduced-fat milk. These patterns are somewhat similar to patterns in Denmark, Sweden, and Canada, where whole cow's milk can be introduced between 9 and 10 mo of age.

The most commonly fed complementary foods between 4 and 11 mo are infant cereals. Nearly 45% of infants between 9 and 11 mo consume noninfant cereals. Infant eating patterns also varied, with up to 61% of infants 4-11 mo of age consuming no vegetables. Among those who consumed vegetables, French fries were one of the common foods fed as vegetables.

The AAP provides the following recommendations for initiating complementary foods (*Pediatric Nutrition Handbook*, 6th edition):

- Introduce 1 single nutrient ingredient food at a time, and do not introduce other new foods for 3-5 days to observe for tolerance. Although iron-fortified rice cereal is most commonly introduced, ethnic and cultural variations should be respected and understood. There is no good evidence that delaying the introduction of other foods such as wheat, fish, and shellfish affects the overall incidence of atopic disease in infants and children.
- Choose foods that provide key nutrients and help meet energy needs: iron-fortified cereals or pureed meats that are rich in protein, iron, and zinc.
- Introduce a variety of foods by the end of the 1st yr, helping to establish healthy eating habits. When offering a new food, 8-10 attempts to offer might need to be made before the infant accepts the new food.
- Withhold cow's milk and other milks not formulated for infants during the 1st yr of life.
- Ensure adequate calcium intake while transitioning to complementary foods.
- Do not give fruit juices during the first 6 mo of life and limited amounts of 100% juices thereafter (4-6 oz/day for ages 1-6 yr, and 8-12 oz per day for ages 7-18 yr).
- Ensure safe ingestion to decrease choking hazard and adequate nutrition when choosing and preparing homemade foods: mash or puree solid foods; avoid hot dogs, nuts, grapes, and popcorn in the first 3-4 yr of life; avoid adding salt or sugar; and ensure nutrient and energy sufficiency

Table 42-6 IMPORTANT PRINCIPLES FOR WEANING

Begin at 4-6 mo of age
At the proper age, encourage a cup rather than a bottle
Introduce 1 food at a time
Energy density should exceed that of breast milk
Iron-containing foods (meat, iron-supplemented cereals) are required
Zinc intake should be encouraged with foods such as meat, dairy products, wheat, and rice
Phytate intake should be low to enhance mineral absorption
Breast milk should continue to 12 mo, formula or cow's milk is then substituted.
• **Give no more than 24 oz/day of cow's milk**
Fluids other than breast milk, formula, and water should be discouraged.
• **Give no more than 4-6 oz/day of fruit juices. No soda.**

The period of introducing increasingly diverse complementary foods gives the opportunity to provide adequate nutrition or to increase the risk of over- or underfeeding. Overconsumption of energy-dense complementary foods can support excessive weight gain in infancy, resulting in an increased risk of obesity in childhood.

FEEDING TODDLERS AND PRESCHOOL-AGE CHILDREN

The 2nd yr of life is a period when eating behavior and healthful habits can be established and is often a confusing and anxiety-generating period for parents. Growth after the 1st yr slows down, motor activity increases, and appetites decrease. Birth weight triples during the 1st yr of life and quadruples by 2 yr of age, reflecting this slowing in growth velocity. Birth length increases during the 1st yr of life and doubles by 4 yr of age. Eating behavior is erratic, and the child appears distracted as he or she explores the environment. Children consume a limited variety of foods and often only "like" a particular food for a period of time and then reject the favored food. These concerns need to be addressed in the context of growth and development and with appropriate nutritional counseling. Demonstrating adequate growth and providing guidance about behavior and eating habits will go a long way in allaying concerns of parents and other caregivers. Important goals of early childhood nutrition are to foster healthful eating habits and to offer foods that are developmentally appropriate, while not always giving in to every child's requests, such as for sweets or French fries.

Feeding Practices

The period starting after 6 mo until 15 mo is characterized by the acquisition of self-feeding skills because the infant can grasp finger foods, learn to use a spoon, and eat soft foods (Table 42-7).

Table 42-7 FEEDING SKILLS BIRTH TO 36 MONTHS

AGE (mo)	FEEDING/ORAL SENSORIMOTOR
Birth to 4-6	Nipple feeding, breast, or bottle Hand on bottle during feeding (2-4 mo) Maintains semiflexed posture during feeding Promotion of infant-parent interaction
6-9 (transition feeding)	Feeding more in upright position Spoon feeding thin, pureed foods Suckle pattern initially suckle → suck Both hands to hold bottle Finger feeding introduced Vertical munching of easily dissolvable solids Preference for parents to feed
9-12	Cup drinking Eats lumpy, mashed food Finger feeding for easily dissolvable solids Chewing includes rotary jaw action
12-18	Self-feeding; grasps spoon with whole hand Holds cup with 2 hands Drinking with 4-5 consecutive swallows Holding and tipping bottle
>18-24	Swallowing with lip closure Self-feeding predominates Chewing broad range food Up-down tongue movements precise
24-26	Circulatory jaw rotations Chewing with lips closed One-handed cup holding and open cup drinking with no spilling Using fingers to fill spoon Eating wide range of solid food Total self-feeding, using fork

Modified from Udall Jr JN: Infant feeding: initiation, problems, approaches, *Curr Prob Pediatr Adolesc Health Care* 37:369–408, 2007.

Around 15 mo, the child learns to feed himself or herself and to drink from a cup, messy as that may be. Infants may still breast-feed or desire formula bottle feeding, but bedtime bottles should be discouraged because of the association with dental caries. Even breast-fed babies can develop caries; therefore, drinking juices and other sugared drinks from a bottle should be discouraged in all infants at all times. In the 2nd yr of life, self-feeding becomes a norm and provides the opportunity for the family to eat together with less stress. Self-feeding allows the child to limit his or her intake while also observing parental reactions to the child's eating behavior. Encouraging positive eating behaviors and ignoring negative ones unless they jeopardize the health and safety of the infant should be the family's goal.

The child should progress from soft, nonsticky foods or foods with small particle size (to avoid choking and gagging) to prepared table foods with the same precautions. At this stage, the child is not capable of completely chewing and swallowing foods, and foods with a choking risk, such as hard candies and peanuts, should be avoided. Caregivers should always be vigilant and present during feeding, and the child should be placed in a high chair. The AAP and other organizations discourage eating in the presence of distractions such as television or eating in a car where an adult cannot adequately supervise or observe the child.

A newborn infant can already discriminate between sweet and sour. This same phenomenon is observed in infancy and early childhood as a preference for sweetened foods and beverages. A new food has to be offered multiple times before being considered rejected by the child. This, as well as reluctance to accept new foods, is a common developmental phase, and persistence and patience are the keys to successful feeding.

Toddlers eat or need to eat 5-7 times a day, and parents need to capitalize on these habits by offering tasty and healthful snacks. Milk continues to be an important source of nutrition, because it includes important nutrients such as vitamin D. Guidelines for vitamin D supplementation recommend a daily vitamin D intake of 400 IU/day for all infants beginning in the first few days of life, children, and adolescents who are ingesting <1000 mL/day of vitamin D-fortified milk or formula. About 2/3 of toddlers consume fruits and vegetables, and more than 75% consume a serving of vegetables on any given day, with French fries being the most commonly consumed vegetable. Preschool children also lag behind current recommendations for the number of servings of fruits, vegetables, and fiber, whereas intakes of food with fat and added sugar are high.

Feeding infants and children is a challenge, and there is no one right way to nurture a child. It takes education, encouragement, and patience to go through this period, and the medical home for the child plays a very important role in supporting the family-infant dyad.

Eating in the Daycare Setting

Many U.S. toddlers and preschool children attend daycare and receive meals and snacks in this setting. There is a wide variation in the quality of the food offered and the level of supervision during meals. Parents are encouraged to assess the quality of the food served at daycare by asking questions, visiting the center, and taking part in parents' committees. Pediatricians should also become familiar with the quality of daycare centers in their regions. Free or reduced-price snacks and meals are provided in daycare centers of low- and medium-income communities through the U.S. Department of Agriculture (USDA) Child and Adult Care Food Program. Participating programs are required to provide meals and snacks that meet the dietary guidelines, also set by the USDA, and therefore guarantee a level of food quality. Because the reimbursement is typically low, many daycare centers still struggle in providing high-quality meals and snacks through the day.

FEEDING SCHOOL-AGE CHILDREN AND ADOLESCENTS

MyPyramid

Most U.S. professional organizations and governmental agencies recommend the use of the USDA MyPyramid (*www.mypyramid.gov*) as a basis for building an optimal diet for children and adolescents. MyPyramid is based on the Dietary Guidelines for Americans. A personalized eating plan based on these guidelines provide, on average over a few days, all the essential nutrients necessary for health and growth, while limiting nutrients associated with chronic disease development. MyPyramid is aimed at the general public and differs from previous versions of the food pyramid in many ways. The intent is to primarily use MyPyramid as an Internet interactive tool that allows customization of recommendations, based on age, sex, physical activity, and, for some populations, weight and height. Print material is also available for families without Internet access.

Recommendations based on MyPyramid are given within 5 food groups (grains, vegetables, fruits, milk, and meat and beans) plus oils, with the general recommendations to eat, over time, a variety of foods within each food group. The graphic representation (Fig. 42-2) of slices symbolizes the average number of servings that should be consumed daily from each food group. In addition to these food groups, MyPyramid offers recommendations for physical activity to achieve a healthful energy balance. MyPyramid also provides information on discretionary calories, which are the foods that are not included in MyPyramid guidelines because of their low nutritional value, such as sweetened beverages, sweetened bakery products, or higher-fat meats. It should be noted that a diet based on MyPyramid, in order to provide all the necessary nutrients, allows a very small amount of discretionary calories available each day.

In the USA and in an increasing number of other countries the vast majority of children and adolescents do not consume a diet that follows the recommendations of MyPyramid. In general, intake of discretionary calories is much higher than recommended, with frequent consumption of sweetened beverages (soda, juice drinks, iced tea, sport drinks), snack foods, high-fat meat (bacon, sausage), and high-fat dairy products (cheese, ice cream). Intake of dark green and orange vegetables (as opposed to fried white potatoes), whole fruits, reduced-fat dairy products, and whole grain is typically lower than recommended. Furthermore, unhealthful eating habits—such as larger-than-recommended portion sizes; food preparation that adds fat, sugar, or salt; skipping breakfast and/or lunch; grazing; or following fad diets—is prevalent and associated with a poorer diet quality. Therefore, MyPyramid offers a helpful and customer-friendly tool to assist pediatricians counseling families on optimal eating plans for short- and long-term health.

Eating at Home

At home, much of what children and adolescents eat is under the control of their parents. Typically, parents shop for groceries and they control, to some extent, what food is available in the house. It has been demonstrated that modeling of healthful eating behavior by parents is a critical determinant of the food choices of children and adolescents (Table 42-8). Therefore, pediatric counseling to improve diet should include guiding parents in using their influence to make healthier food choices available and attractive at home.

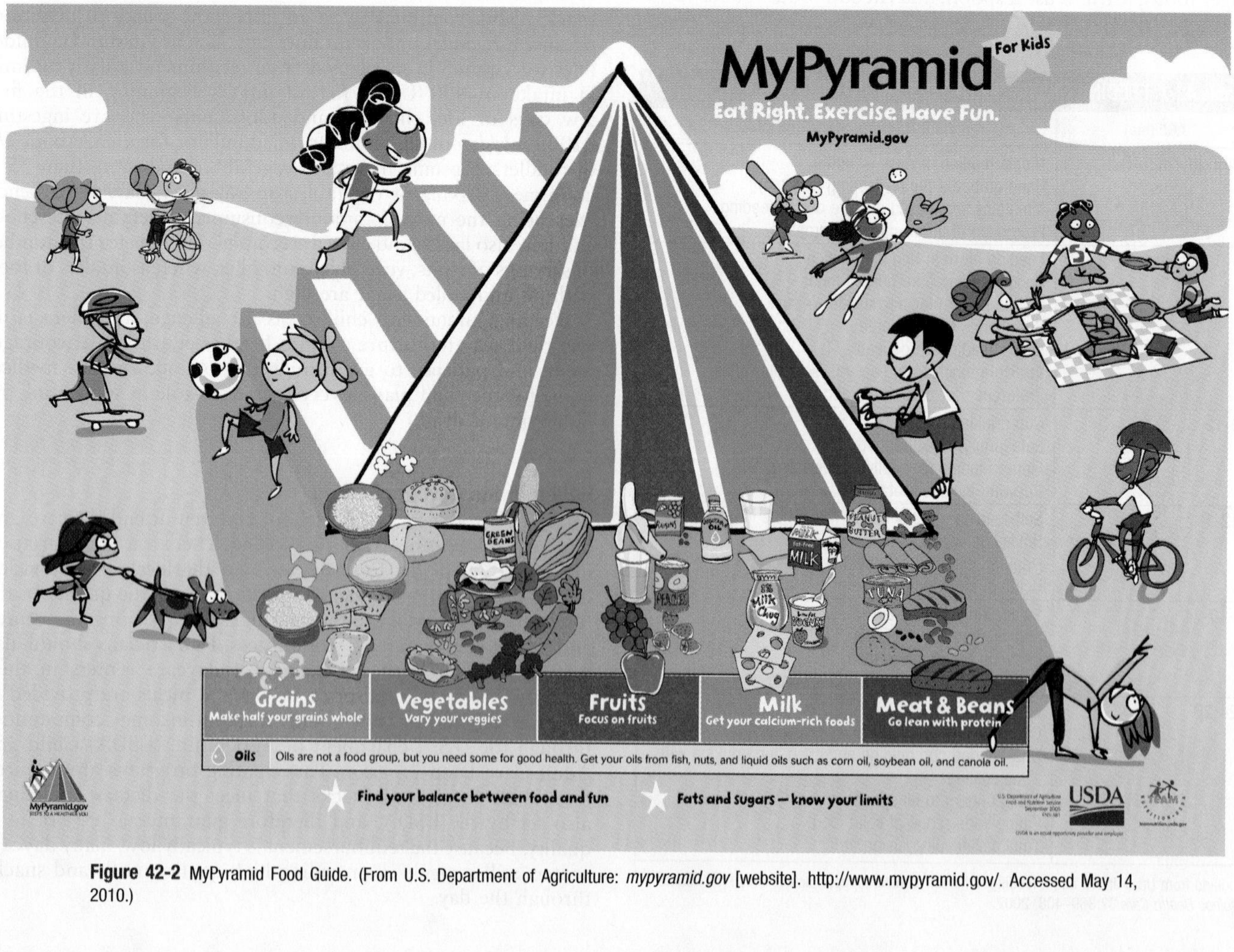

Figure 42-2 MyPyramid Food Guide. (From U.S. Department of Agriculture: *mypyramid.gov* [website]. http://www.mypyramid.gov/. Accessed May 14, 2010.)

Table 42-8 FEEDING GUIDELINES FOR PARENTS

Parents' responsibilities include:
- Choosing food
- Setting routine
- Creating a positive, nonstressful mealtime environment
- Being a role model for their child
- Regarding mealtime as a family time

Parents need to:
- Offer new foods repeatedly (8-10 times) to establish acceptance or rejection of that food
- Offer 3 meals and 2 healthful snacks per day
- Teach skills such as handling of spoons and drinking from a cup to encourage self-feeding

Adapted from Kleinman RE and the AAP Committee on Nutrition: *Pediatric nutrition handbook*, ed 6, Elk Grove Village, IL, 2009, American Academy of Pediatrics.

Regular family meals sitting at a table, as opposed to eating alone, in the living room, or watching television, have been associated with improved diet quality, perhaps because of increased opportunities for positive parenting during meals. Such an ideal situation is recommended but a challenge for many families who, with busy schedules and other stressors, are unable to provide such a setting. Pediatricians should work with families to set realistic goals around these eating issues. Another parenting challenge is to control the excess appetite of some children and adolescents. Useful strategies, when the child is still hungry after a meal, include a 15- to 20-min pause before a 2nd serving or offering foods that are insufficiently consumed, such as vegetables, whole grains, or fruits.

Eating at School

Food quality and availability of healthy options vary greatly among U.S. schools. Schools that participate in federally reimbursed lunch or breakfast programs are required to comply with minimum standards for those meals, but regulation of other foods and beverages available in the school are less consistent. These competitive foods, often sold through vending machines, are available through exclusivity contracts with food and beverage companies that represent significant sources of revenue for many schools for funding important programs. Low reimbursement levels from federal programs, unavailable or inadequate cooking facilities, insufficient training of school cafeteria staff, and competing academic requirements are additional barriers to offering healthy nutrition in schools. This is an important issue, because most U.S. children take 1 or 2 meals a day in school. Pediatricians and parents should therefore keep themselves informed of the school's nutrition policies and menus in their districts and advocate for improved standards. Where the quality of school nutrition is problematic, a practical alternative is to suggest that children pack their own lunch from home.

Eating Out

The number of meals eaten outside the home or brought home from take-out restaurants has increased in all age groups of the U.S. population. The increased convenience of this meal pattern is undermined by the generally lower nutritional value of the meals, compared to home-cooked meals. Typically, meals consumed or purchased in fast-food or casual restaurants are of large portion size, are dense in calories, and contain large amounts of saturated and *trans* fats, salt, and sugar and low amounts of whole grains, fruits, and vegetables. Although an increasing number of restaurants offer healthier alternatives, the vast majority of what is consumed at restaurants does not fit MyPyramid. Parents can use these opportunities to teach and model healthful choices within the choices offered.

With increasing age, an increasing number of meals and snacks are also consumed during peer social gatherings at friends' houses and parties. When a large part of a child's or adolescent's diet is consumed on these occasions, the diet quality can suffer, because food offerings are typically of low nutritional value. Parents and pediatricians need to guide teens in navigating these occasions while maintaining a healthful diet and enjoying meaningful social interactions. These occasions often are also opportunities for teens to consume alcohol; therefore, adult supervision is important.

NUTRITION ISSUES OF IMPORTANCE ACROSS PEDIATRIC AGES

Food Environment

Most families have some knowledge of how to optimize nutrition and intend to provide their children with a healthful diet. The discrepancy between this fact and the actual quality of the diet consumed by U.S. children is often explained by difficulties and barriers for families to make healthful food choices. Because the final food choice is made by individual children or their parents, interventions to improve diet have focused on individual knowledge and behavior changes, but these have had limited success. One of the main determinants of food choice is taste, but other factors also influence these choices. One of the most useful conceptual frameworks to understand the child's food environment in the context of obesity illustrates the variety and levels of the determinants of individual food and physical activity choices. Many of these determinants are not under the direct control of individual children or parents (Fig. 42-3). Understanding the context of food and lifestyle choices helps in understanding lack of changes or "poor compliance" and can decrease the frustration often experienced by the pediatricians who might "blame the victim" for behavior that is not entirely under their control.

Marketing and advertising of food to children is a particularly illustrative aspect of the food environment. Marketing includes strategies as diverse as shelf placements, association of cartoon characters with food products, coupons, and special offers or pricing, all of which influence food choices. Television advertising is an important part of how children and adolescents hear about food, with an estimated 40,000 TV commercials seen by the average U.S. child, many of which are for food, as compared to the few hours of nutrition education they receive in school. Additional food advertisement increasingly occurs as brand placement in movies and TV shows, on websites, and even video games.

Using Food as Reward

It is a prevalent habit to use food as a reward or sometimes withdraw food as punishment at various ages and in various settings. Most parents use this practice occasionally, and some use it almost systematically, starting at a young age. The practice is also commonly used in other settings where children spend time, such as daycare, school, or even athletic settings. Although it might be a good idea to limit some unhealthy but desirable food categories to special occasions, using food as a reward is problematic. Limiting access to some foods and making its access contingent on a particular accomplishment increases the desirability of that type of food. Conversely, encouraging the consumption of some foods renders them less desirable. Therefore, phrases such as "finish your vegetables, and you will get ice cream for dessert" can result in establishing unhealthy eating habits once the child has more autonomy in food choices. Parents should be counseled on such issues and encouraged to choose items other than food as reward, such as toys or sporting equipment, special family events, or collectable items. Daycare and school teachers should also be discouraged from using food as a reward or to withhold food as punishment.

Cultural Considerations in Nutrition and Feeding

Food choices, food preparation, eating patterns, and infant feeding practices all have very deep cultural roots. In fact, beliefs,

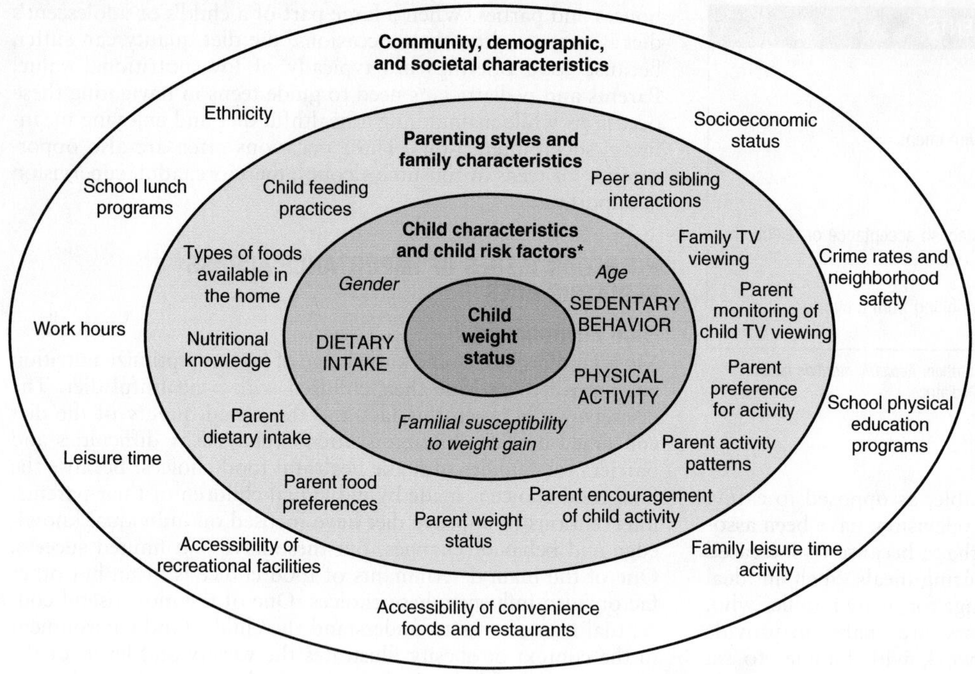

Figure 42-3 A conceptual framework of the context of food and lifestyle choices. *Child risk factors (shown in upper case lettering) refer to child behaviors associated with the development of overweight. Characteristics of the child (shown in italic lettering) interact with child risk factors and contextual factors to influence the development of overweight (i.e., moderator variables). (From Davison KK, Birch LL: Childhood overweight: a contextual model and recommendations for future research, *Obes Rev* 2:159–171, 2001. © 2001 The International Association for the Study of Obesity.)

attitudes, and practices surrounding food and eating are some of the most important components of cultural identity. Therefore, it is not surprising that in multicultural societies, great variability exists in the cultural characteristics of the diet. Even in a world where global marketing forces tend to reduce geographic differences in the types of food, or even brands, that are available, most families, especially during family meals at home, are still much influenced by their cultural background. Therefore, pediatricians should become familiar with the dietary characteristics of various cultures in their community, so that they can identify and address, in a nonjudgmental way and avoiding stereotypes, the likely nutritional issues related to the diet of their patients.

Many differences exist in infant-feeding practices as well. Even if many of these practices do not follow the usual recommendations, often based themselves more on tradition than science, they are compatible with healthy growth and should only be challenged when clear evidence of their negative effects is available.

Vegetarianism

Vegetarianism is the practice of following a diet that excludes meat (including game and slaughter by-products; fish, shellfish, and other sea animals; and poultry). There are several variants of the diet, some of which also exclude eggs and/or some products produced from animal labor, such as dairy products and honey. There are many different variations in vegetarianism:

- Veganism: excludes all animal products. It may be part of a larger practice of abstaining from the use of animals for any purpose.
- Ovovegetarianism: includes eggs but not dairy
- Lactovegetarianism: includes dairy products but excludes eggs
- Lactoovovegetarianism: includes eggs and dairy

A generic expression often used for vegetarianism and veganism is "plant-based diets." Other dietary practices commonly associated with vegetarianism include fruitarian diet (fruits, nuts, seeds, and other plant matter gathered without harm to the plant); su vegetarian diet (a diet that excludes all animal products as well as onion, garlic, scallions, leeks, or shallots); a macrobiotic diet (whole grains and beans and in some cases fish); and raw vegan diet (fresh and uncooked fruits, nuts, seeds, and vegetables).

Vegetarianism is considered a healthful and viable diet, and both the American Dietetic Association and the Dietitians of Canada have found that a properly planned vegetarian diet can satisfy the nutritional goals for all stages of life. Various reports find lower risks of cancer and ischemic heart disease. These authoritative bodies have stated that "Vegetarian diets offer a number of nutritional benefits, including lower levels of saturated fat, cholesterol, and animal protein, as well as higher levels of carbohydrates, fiber, magnesium, potassium, folate, and antioxidants such as vitamins C and E and phytochemicals." Vegetarians also tend to have lower body mass index, lower cholesterol, and lower blood pressure than nonvegetarians.

Specific nutrients of concern in vegetarian diets include:

- **Iron:** Vegetarian diets have similar levels of iron compared to nonvegetarian diets, but the iron may have lower bioavailability than iron from meat sources, and iron absorption may be inhibited by other dietary constituents. Foods rich in iron include black beans, cashews, kidney beans, lentils, oatmeal, raisins, black-eyed peas, soybeans, sunflower seeds, chickpeas, molasses, and tempeh. Vegan diets are low in iron; iron stores are lower in vegetarians than nonvegetarians; and iron deficiency is more common in vegetarian and vegan women and children.
- **Vitamin B_{12}:** Plants are not generally a good source of B_{12}. Additional vitamin B_{12} can be obtained through dairy products and eggs, and vegans typically need fortified foods or supplements. Breast-feeding by vegan mothers can place an infant at risk for vitamin B_{12} deficiency.
- **Fatty acids:** Vegetarians and vegans are at risk for low levels of eicosapentaenoic acid (EPA) and DHA.
- **Calcium:** Vegans are at risk for impaired bone mineralization unless they consume enough leafy greens, a good source of calcium, to meet the age and gender recommendations.
- **Zinc:** Foods such as red meat contain large amounts of zinc and protein. Human milk contains zinc, but does not satisfy zinc needs after 6 mo of age, resulting in the recommendation that zinc-containing foods be consumed at that age in this population. Bioavailability of zinc in plant sources tends to be low due to the concomitant presence of inhibitors of zinc absorption such as phytate and fiber.

Organic Foods

The increasing interest in using organic foods, especially to feed children, results in frequent questions to pediatricians. Unfortunately, the scientific basis available to answer these questions is slim, and no clear benefit or harm associated with organic food consumption has been clearly demonstrated. Children consuming organic foods have lower or no detectable levels of pesticides in their urine compared to those consuming nonorganic foods. Some families also choose organic foods for their perceived environmental benefit more than for the human health reasons. As the cost of these foods is generally higher than the cost of other food, a prudent approach is to explain to families that the scientific basis for choosing organic foods is limited, but if it is their preference and they can afford the added cost, there is no reason not to eat organic foods.

Nutrition as Part of Complementary and Alternative Medicine, Functional Foods, Dietary Supplements, Vitamin Supplements, and Botanical and Herbal Products

The use of nutrition or nutritional supplements as complementary or alternative medicine is increasing, despite very limited data on safety and efficacy, especially in children. Many parents assume that if a food or supplement is natural or organic, then there is no potential for risk and that there might be some potential for benefits. We know, of course, that this is not the case, and the adverse effects of some dietary supplements have come to light, including evidence of severe adverse effects. However, it is difficult for pediatricians using evidence-based messages to compete against the aggressive marketing of food supplements to families of healthy and chronically ill children; through the Internet, television shows, and magazines; or simply against the word-of-mouth or advice from people without a scientific background or with significant conflicts of interest. One reason to recommend caution to parents when it comes to dietary supplements, including botanical and herbal products, is that in the USA, unlike medications, these products are not evaluated for safety and efficacy before marketing and do not undergo the same level of quality control as medications. The potential for adverse effects or simply for inefficacy is therefore high.

Some dietary components, either available as supplements or within so-called functional foods, have been more carefully evaluated. These include emerging evidence for safety and efficacy of using pre- and probiotics for various gastrointestinal conditions, plant sterols for dyslipidemia, fish oils for elevated triglycerides, or an elemental diet for inflammatory bowel disease.

Pediatricians are often asked by parents if their children need to receive a daily multivitamin. Unless the child follows a particular diet that may be poor in one or more nutrients for health, cultural, or religious reasons, or if the child has a chronic health condition that puts him or her at risk for deficiency in one or more nutrients, multivitamins are not indicated. A diet that follows the guidelines of MyPyramid contains sufficient nutrients to support healthy growth. Of course, many children do not follow all the guidelines of MyPyramid, and parents and pediatricians may be tempted to use multivitamin supplements just to make sure that nutrient deficiencies are avoided. The problem with this approach is that multivitamin supplements do not provide all the nutrients that are necessary for good health, such as fiber or some of the antioxidants contained in food. Use of a daily multivitamin supplement can result in a false impression that the child's diet is complete and in decreased efforts to meet dietary recommendations with food rather than the intake of supplements. As discussed in Chapter 41, the average U.S. diet provides more than a sufficient amount of most nutrients, including most vitamins. Therefore, multivitamins should not be routinely recommended.

The AAP recommends daily supplementation of 400 IU of vitamin D per day in all children who drink less than 1,000 mL/day of vitamin D–fortified milk, representing the majority of U.S. children and adolescents. In some specific populations of children at risk for deficiency, supplements of vitamin B_{12}, iron, fat-soluble vitamins, or zinc may be considered.

Food Safety

Constantly keeping food safety issues in mind is an important aspect of feeding infants, children, and adolescents. In addition to choking hazards and food allergies, pediatricians and parents should be aware of food safety issues related to infectious agents and environmental contaminants. Food poisoning with infectious agents, either live bacteria or viruses or chemicals produced by these infectious agents, are most common with food consumed raw or undercooked, such as oysters, beef, eggs, and tomatoes, or cooked foods that have not been handled or stored properly. The specific infectious agents involved in food poisoning are described in Chapter 332. A good source of information for patients and parents can be found at *www.foodsafety.gov*.

Many chemical contaminants, such as heavy metals, pesticides, and organic compounds, are present in various foods, usually in small amounts. Because of concerns regarding their child's neurologic development and cancer risk, many questions arise from parents, especially after media coverage of specific isolated incidents. Pediatricians therefore need to become familiar with reliable sources of information, such as the websites of the U.S. Environmental Protection Agency (EPA), the FDA, or the Centers for Disease Control and Prevention (CDC). For example, a recurrent debate is the balance between the benefits of seafood for the growing brain and cardiovascular health and the risk of mercury contamination from consuming large predatory fish species.

Nutritional Programming

Emerging epidemiologic evidence suggests that early nutrition can have a long-term impact on adult health. It is well established that undernutrition in early life can exert a long-term impact in terms of reduced adult height and academic achievements, but other data suggest that intrauterine growth restriction (IUGR) is associated with adult cardiovascular risk factors and disease. Rapid weight gain in infancy, either following IUGR or a period of malnutrition, is associated with an increased risk for later obesity.

Preventive Nutrition Counseling in Pediatric Primary Care

An important part of the primary care well child visit focuses on nutrition and growth, because most families turn to pediatricians for guidance on child nutrition. Preventive nutrition is one of the cornerstones of preventive pediatrics and a critical aspect of anticipatory guidance. The first steps of nutrition counseling are nutritional status assessments, primarily done through growth monitoring and dietary intake assessment. Although dietary assessment is somewhat simple in infants who have a relatively monotonous diet, it is more challenging at older ages. Even the most sophisticated and time-consuming research tools of dietary assessments are imprecise. Therefore, the goals of dietary assessment in the primary care setting need to remain modest, including simply getting an idea of the eating patterns (time, location, environment) and usual diet by asking the parent to describe the child's dietary intake on a typical day or in the last 24 hr. For more ambitious goals of dietary assessment, referral to a registered dietician with pediatric experience is recommended.

Once some understanding of the child's usual diet has been acquired, existing or anticipated nutritional problems should be addressed, such as diet quality, dietary habits, or portion size. For a few nutritional problems, a lack of knowledge can be addressed with nutrition education, but most pediatric preventive nutritional issues, such as overeating or poor food choices, are not the result of lack of parents' knowledge. Therefore, nutrition education alone is insufficient in these situations, and pediatricians need to acquire training in behavior-modification techniques or refer to specialists to assist their patients in making healthy choices more often. The physical, cultural, and family environments in which the child lives should be kept in mind at all times, so that nutrition counseling is relevant and changes are feasible.

One important aspect of nutrition counseling is providing families with sources of additional information and behavioral change tools. Although some handouts are available from government agencies, the AAP, and other professional organizations for families without Internet access, an increasing number of families rely on the Internet to find nutrition information. Therefore, pediatricians need to become familiar with commonly used websites so that they can point families to reliable and unbiased sources of information. Perhaps the most useful websites for reliable and unbiased nutrition information for children are the USDA MyPyramid website, the sites of the CDC, FDA, National Institutes of Health (NIH), and Institute of Medicine Food and Nutrition Board for government sources and the AAP, American Heart Association, and American Dietetic Association for professional organization resources. Pediatricians should also be aware of sites that provide biased or even dangerous information, so that they can warn families accordingly. Examples include dieting sites, sites that openly promote dietary supplements or other food products, and the sites of "nonprofit" organizations that are mainly sponsored by food companies or that have other social or political agendas.

Food Assistance Programs in the USA

Several programs exist in the USA to ensure sufficient and high-quality nutrition for children of families who cannot always afford optimal nutrition. One of the most popular federal programs is the Special Supplemental Nutrition Program for Women, Infants, and Children (WIC). This program provides nutrition supplements to a large proportion of pregnant women, postpartum women, and children up to their 5th birthday. One of its strengths is that in order to qualify, families need to regularly visit a WIC nutritionist, who can be a useful resource for nutritional counseling. Other popular programs include school lunches, breakfasts, and after-school meals, as well as daycare and summer nutrition programs. Lower-income families are also eligible for the Supplemental Nutrition Assistance Program, formerly known as the Food Stamp Program. This program provides funds directly to families to purchase various food items in regular food stores.

BIBLIOGRAPHY

Please visit the Nelson Textbook of Pediatrics *website at www.expertconsult.com for the complete bibliography.*

Chapter 43
Nutrition, Food Security, and Health

Harold Alderman and Meera Shekar

MALNUTRITION AS THE INTERSECTION OF FOOD SECURITY AND HEALTH SECURITY

Undernutrition is usually an outcome of 3 factors: household level food security, access to health and sanitation services, and child caring practices. A mother with few economic resources who knows how to care for her children and is enabled to do so can often use available food and health services to produce well-nourished children. If food resources and health services are available in a community, but the mother does not access immunizations or does not know how or when to properly add complementary foods to her child's diet, that child might become malnourished (Table 43-1).

Undernutrition is not simply a result of food insecurity, although food security is often a necessary but insufficient condition for nutrition security. Many children in food-secure environments and from better-off families are underweight or stunted because of inappropriate infant feeding and child care practices, poor access to health services, or poor sanitation. In many countries where malnutrition is widespread, food production or even access to food might not be the most limiting factor. The most important causes of undernutrition are often inadequate knowledge about the benefits of exclusive breast-feeding and complementary feeding practices, the role of micronutrients, and the lack of time women have available for appropriate infant care practices and their own care during pregnancy. The situation is different in famine and emergency settings, where food insecurity is often among the most important factors.

Table 43-1 THREE MYTHS ABOUT NUTRITION

Myth 1: *Malnutrition is primarily a matter of inadequate food intake.* Not so. Food is of course important. But most serious malnutrition is caused by bad sanitation and disease, leading to diarrhea, especially among young children. Women's status and women's education play big parts in improving nutrition. Improving care of young children is vital.
Myth 2: *Improved nutrition is a by-product of other measures of poverty reduction and economic advance. It is not possible to jump-start the process.* Again, untrue. Improving nutrition requires focused action by parents and communities, backed by local and national action in health and public services, especially water and sanitation. Thailand has shown that moderate and severe malnutrition can be reduced by 75% or more in a decade by such means.
Myth 3: *Given scarce resources, broad-based action on nutrition is hardly feasible on a mass scale, especially in poor countries.* Wrong again. In spite of severe economic setbacks, many developing countries have made impressive progress. More than two thirds of the people in developing countries now eat iodized salt, combating the iodine deficiency and anemia that affect about 3.5 billion people, especially women and children in some 100 nations. About 450 million children a year now receive vitamin A capsules, tackling the deficiency that causes blindness and increases child mortality. New ways have been found to promote and support breast-feeding, and breast-feeding rates are being maintained in many countries and increased in some. Mass immunization and promotion of oral rehydration to reduce deaths from diarrhea have also done much to improve nutrition.

From World Bank: *Repositioning nutrition as central to development, 2006* (PDF). http://web.worldbank.org/WBSITE/EXTERNAL/TOPICS/EXTHEALTHNUTRITIONANDPOPULATION/EXTNUTRITION/0,,contentMDK:20787550~menuPK:282580~pagePK:64020865~piPK:149114~theSitePK:282575,00.html. Accessed May 23, 2010.

Economic growth and food production as well as birth spacing and women's education are also important but less-direct routes to improving nutrition outcomes in developing countries. Shorter routes to nutrition improvements often come through the provision of health, sanitation, and nutrition education and counseling services, including the promotion of exclusive breast-feeding and appropriate and timely complementary feeding, coupled with prenatal care and basic maternal and child health services. In many contexts, micronutrient supplementation and fortification are also key elements of a public health strategy aimed at addressing undernutrition.

FOOD INSECURITY

Governments seek to promote the food security of their population both for its intrinsic value and for its instrumental value as well. The former refers to the fact that individuals value food security in its own right, whereas the latter acknowledges the contribution that food security makes toward improved nutrition. But what is food security? One prevalent definition of food security views it as *access* by all people at all times to *sufficient* food in terms of quality, quantity, and diversity for an active and *healthy life* without risk of loss of such access. To achieve food security, it is necessary to look at 3 dimensions of food security: **availability, access,** and **utilization.** *Availability* refers to the supply of food (generally grain in the market, reflecting economic conditions of production and trade), whereas *access* is at the household level, reflecting purchasing power as well as transfer programs. Access also has an intrahousehold dimension, because food is not necessarily shared equitably within a household. The *utilization* pillar reflects the fact that even when a household has access to food, it does not necessarily achieve nutritional security.

Measurement of Food Insecurity

The most commonly used measurement of food insecurity is the Food and Agriculture Organization's (FAO's) measure of undernourishment, expressed in terms of the number of persons who are assumed to be unable to meet daily calorie requirements necessary for light activities. In the period 2003-2005, the FAO estimated that 848 million individuals were hungry or undernourished, and 97% of these individuals were in developing countries, an increase of 20 million undernourished individuals in *developing* countries compared to 1995-1997.

This estimate of undernourished individuals is based on country-level annual food balance sheets that take into account food production plus net imports minus net trade. This gross availability is also adjusted for seeds used for replanting as well as grain fed to animals and an allowance for waste. The estimates also acknowledge that the average national food availability is not uniformly distributed, and they thus make adjustments for an assumed inequality of access based on historical patterns.

This estimate is, therefore, not based on direct measurement of household or individual consumption. However, it has the advantage of being available on an annual basis for virtually all countries. Therefore, it assists in monitoring global trends. Reductions in the number of undernourished individuals as calculated using this indicator of food access have been used as a measure of progress in reducing poverty, albeit other indicators (percent underweight or stunted children) are better indicators for tracking changes at household and national levels.

The undernourishment measure being based on national food balance sheets cannot be disaggregated by regions or by income or other household characteristics and is therefore not a very useful measure, especially at household or individual levels. There are often differences with estimated levels of hunger using this indirect approach and levels derived based on surveys of consumption or expenditure recorded at the household level. Such surveys are commonly undertaken in most countries, often with samples that are representative at regional or subregional levels and that permit analysis of correlates of food insecurity. The surveys often are collected over rounds, and they thus allow an understanding of seasonal food insecurity. Consumption may be based on recall or on a diary of expenditures and home consumption. There is no consensus on the relative advantages of diary approaches compared with interviews given the level of education in food-insecure regions of the world, and there is not full agreement on the period of recall that provides the greatest accuracy of reporting. Nevertheless, with the widespread availability and range of data contained in these surveys, they provide the basis for substantial analysis on the determinants of household food insecurity.

Individual food insecurity is better understood using 24-hr food recall data. Such methods, preferably repeated over a period of days within a week, allow a measure of individual intake and of intrahousehold variation of food consumption. Although these data are harder to collect and less available, they are a better source of information on diet diversity than household or national indicators. Diet diversity is a strong predictor of child growth and a valuable tool for understanding micronutrient intakes, a dimension of nutritional security that is generally not emphasized in data on food security based on food balance sheets.

UNDERNUTRITION

The greatest risk of undernutrition occurs during pregnancy and in the first 2 years of life (Fig. 43-1); the effects of this early damage on health, brain development, intelligence, educability, and productivity are potentially irreversible (Table 43-2). Governments with limited resources are therefore best advised to focus publicly funded actions on this critical window of opportunity, between preconception and 24 mo of age. Folate deficiency also increases the risk of birth defects; this particular window of opportunity is before conception, as it is with iodine. Iron deficiency anemia is another dimension of undernutrition that has measurable risks that extend outside of the early years of life, with particular risks to the health of a mother as well as for the birth weight of her child. Anemia can also reduce physical and cognitive function and economic productivity of adults of both sexes.

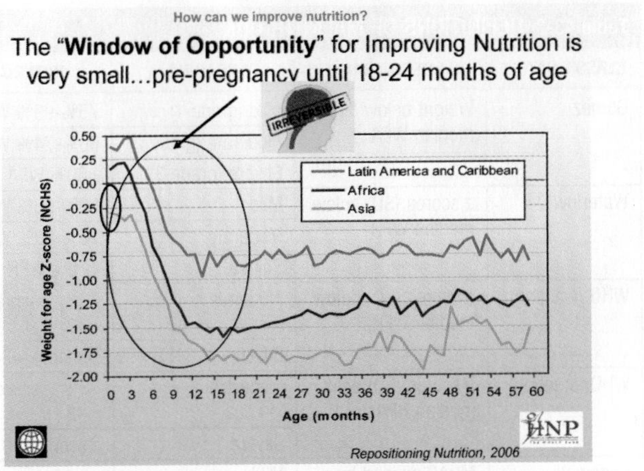

Figure 43-1 The window of opportunity for improving nutrition is very small: prepregnancy until 18-24 mo of age. (From The World Bank's Human Development Network: *Better nutrition = less poverty: repositioning nutrition as central to development: a strategy for large scale action, 2006* [PDF]. http://siteresources.worldbank.org/NUTRITION/Resources/281846-1114108837888/RepositioningNutritionLaunchJan30Final.pdf. Accessed May 23, 2010.)

Table 43-2 WHY MALNUTRITION PERSISTS IN MANY FOOD-SECURE HOUSEHOLDS

- Pregnant and nursing women eat too few calories and too little protein, have untreated infections, such as sexually transmitted diseases that lead to low birthweight, or do not get enough rest.
- Mothers have too little time to take care of their young children or themselves during pregnancy.
- Mothers of newborns discard colostrum, the first milk, which strengthens the child's immune system.
- Mothers often feed children <6 mo of age foods other than breast milk even though exclusive breast-feeding is the best source of nutrients and the best protection against many infectious and chronic diseases.
- Caregivers start introducing complementary solid foods too late.
- Caregivers feed children <2 yr of age too little food or foods that are not energy dense.
- Though food is available, because of inappropriate household food allocation, women and young children's needs are not met and their diets often do not contain enough of the right micronutrients or protein.
- Caregivers do not know how to feed children during and following diarrhea or fever.
- Caregivers' poor hygiene contaminates food with bacteria or parasites.

From World Bank: *Repositioning nutrition as central to development, 2006* (PDF). http://web.worldbank.org/WBSITE/EXTERNAL/TOPICS/EXTHEALTHNUTRITIONANDPOPULATION/EXTNUTRITION/0,,contentMDK:20787550~menuPK:282580~pagePK:64020865~piPK:149114~theSitePK:282575,00.html. Accessed May 23, 2010.

Measurement of Undernutrition

The term *malnutrition* encompasses both ends of the nutrition spectrum, from undernutrition (underweight, stunting, wasting, and micronutrient deficiencies) to overweight. Many poor nutritional outcomes begin in utero and are manifest as low birth-

Table 43-3 DEFINITIONS OF MALNUTRITION

CLASSIFICATION	DEFINITION	GRADING	CRITERIA
Gomez	Weight below % median WFA	Mild (grade 1)	75%-90% WFA
		Moderate (grade 2)	60%-74% WFA
		Severe (grade 3)	<60% WFA
Waterlow	*z* scores (SD) below median WFH	Mild	80%-90% WFH
		Moderate	70%-80% WFH
		Severe	<70% WFH
WHO (wasting)	*z* scores (SD) below median WFH	Moderate	$-3 \leq z$ score <-2
		Severe	*z* score <–3
WHO (stunting)	*z* scores (SD) below median HFA	Moderate	$-3 \leq z$ score <-2
		Severe	*z* score <–3
Kanawati	MUAC divided by occipitofrontal head circumference	Mild	<0.31
		Moderate	<0.28
		Severe	<0.25
Cole	*z* scores of BMI for age	Grade 1	*z* score <–1
		Grade 2	*z* score <–2
		Grade 3	*z* score <–3

BMI, body mass index; HFA, height for age; MUAC, mid-upper arm circumference; NCHS, U.S. National Center for Health Statistics; SD, standard deviation; WFA, weight for age; WFH, weight for height; WHO, World Health Organization.
From Grover Z, Ee LC: Protein energy malnutrition, *Pediatr Clin N Am* 56:1055–1068, 2009.

weight (LBW). Prematurity and intrauterine growth restriction (IUGR) are the two main causes of LBW, with prematurity relatively more important in developed countries and IUGR relatively more important in developing countries (Chapter 90).

In preschool- and school-aged children, nutritional status is often assessed in terms of anthropometry. International references have been established that allow normalization of anthropometric measures in terms of *z* scores defined as the child's height (weight) minus the median height (weight) for the age and sex of the child divided by the relevant standard deviation (Table 43-3). The World Health Organization (WHO) recently revised the child growth references based on data from healthy children in 5 countries. Comparisons of malnutrition rates across countries are meaningful, and these growth references are applicable to all children across the globe.

Height for age is useful for assessing the nutritional status of populations, because this measure of skeletal growth reflects the cumulative impact of events affecting nutritional status that result in *stunting* and is also referred to as **chronic malnutrition.** This measure contrasts with **weight for height**, or *wasting*, which is a measure of **acute malnutrition. Weight for age** is an additional commonly used measurement of nutritional status. Although it has less clinical significance because it combines stature with current health conditions, it has the advantage of being somewhat easier to measure: Current weighing scales allow a child to be weighed in a caregiver's arms, but weight for height requires 2 different instruments for measurement. Height for age is particularly difficult to measure for the most vulnerable children <2 yr of age for whom recumbent length is the preferred indicator for height. In emergencies and in some field settings, **mid-upper arm circumference** (**MUAC**) is often used for screening in lieu of weight for height (see Table 43-3).

Obesity as well as energy deficiency among adults is often reported in terms of the Body Mass Index (BMI). BMI is calculated by dividing weight in kilograms by the square of height in meters. Individuals are considered to be chronically energy deficient if they have a BMI below 18.5, overweight if they have a BMI greater than 25, and obese if they have a BMI greater than 30.

Another dimension of malnutrition is micronutrient deficiencies. The micronutrients of particular public-health significance are iodine, vitamin A, iron, folic acid, and zinc. Iodine deficiency and its sequelae (goiter, hypothyroidism, and developmental disabilities including severe mental retardation) are assessed by clinical inspection of enlarged thyroids (goiter) or by iodine concentrations in urine (µg/L). Even mild forms of iodine deficiency during pregnancy have been implicated in poor mental and physical development among children as well as fetal losses. The public-health benchmark for eliminating iodine deficiency in a population is <20% of the population with urinary iodine levels <50 µg/L (Chapter 51).

Vitamin A deficiency is caused by low intake of retinol or its precursor, beta-carotene. Absorption can be inhibited by a lack of fats in the diet or by parasite infestations. Clinical deficiency is estimated by combining night blindness and eye changes—principally Bitot spots and total xerophthalmia prevalence. Subclinical deficiency is assessed as prevalence of serum retinal concentrations <0.70 µmol/L (Chapter 45). The greatest public-health significance of vitamin A deficiency is its association with a higher mortality among young children. Prophylactic supplementation of vitamin A among deficient populations for children <5 yr of age can reduce child mortality by as much as 23%.

Children commonly suffer from anemia, either as a result of low iron intakes or poor absorption or as a result of illness or parasite infestation, although severe protein-energy malnutrition and vitamin B_{12} or folate deficiency can also lead to anemia. Women also have relatively high rates of anemia as a result of low iron intakes, poor absorption, illness, or excessive losses of blood. Severe protein-energy malnutrition and vitamin B_{12} or folate deficiency can also lead to anemia. Anemia is most commonly measured as grams of hemoglobin per liter of blood. Cutoffs to define anemia are 11 g/dL for children 6-59 mo, 11.5 g/dL for children 5-11 yr, and 12 g/dL for children 12-14 yr. Cutoffs to define anemia are 12 g/dL for nonpregnant women, 11 g/dL for pregnant women, and 13 g/dL for men.

Zinc supplementation can reduce child mortality, especially when combined with oral rehydration therapy for diarrheal disease. Plasma concentrations respond in a dose-dependent manner to dietary changes, and urinary excretion correlates with zinc status overall, but there is not yet a biomarker standard that is widely used as a cutoff to define a public health concern.

Prevalence of Undernutrition

Maternal and child undernutrition is prevalent in many developing countries and in some middle-income countries. It is estimated that about 16% of children across developing countries are born with low birthweight (LBW). LBW rates are highest in the south-central Asia region (27%) and lowest in South America. In 2005, 20% of children <5 years of age in low- and middle-income countries were underweight (weight-for-age <–2 standard deviations [SD]), and 32% were stunted (height-for-age <–2 SD). Somewhat surprisingly, underweight rates in many south Asian countries (India, Bangladesh, Nepal, and Pakistan) are much higher than, and often nearly double, the rates in many sub-Saharan African countries. The combination of the high prevalence rates and the large population sizes in Asia mean that this region carries the highest burden of underweight children. Even though underweight and stunting are more prevalent among the poor, the prevalence rates among the highest income quintiles are also high, thereby reiterating the fact that undernutrition is not just a result of food insecurity.

About 42% of pregnant women and 47% of children <5 yr of age in developing countries are anemic. Zinc deficiency is harder to measure and is assessed on the basis of indirect indicators such as stunting; it is estimated to be high in south Asia, sub-Saharan Africa, and some countries in Central and South America. Vitamin A deficiency rates have improved significantly in most developing countries, primarily owing to high coverage with high-dose vitamin A supplements given twice a year to every child <5 yr of age as part of public-health programs. Nevertheless, 100-140 million people are considered deficient in vitamin A, with deficient populations found in Brazil and Andean South America as well as much of sub-Saharan Africa and South Asia. Large-scale availability of iodized salt has reduced the rates of iodine deficiency; nonetheless, approximately 1 billion people do not have regular access to iodized salt, including in large areas of Africa and the former Soviet Union.

Consequences of Undernutrition

The most immediate consequence of undernutrition is premature death. The global estimates conclude that stunting, severe wasting, and IUGR jointly contributes to 2.2 million deaths of children <5 yr of age. This accounts for 35% of all child mortality globally, even though this estimate is lower than those previously reported. The earlier and widely cited estimate had suggested that undernutrition was associated with nearly 53% of all child deaths. The risk of death increases even with mild undernutrition, and as the severity of undernutrition increases, the risk increases exponentially; the probability of mortality for a child <5 yr of age with a *z* score of weight for age below −3 is nearly 4 times the elevated risk for a child with a *z* score between −3 and −2. Because there are more children with less-severe malnutrition, it is this category that contributes the greater share of the global burden of malnutrition. After controlling for the occurrence of multiple nutritional deficits, deficiencies of vitamin A and zinc are estimated to be responsible for an additional 0.6 million and 0.4 million child deaths, respectively. More than 3.5 million mothers and children under 5 years die every year due to undernutrition-related causes, and many millions more are disabled or stunted for life. By the time children reach their first birthday, if undernourished, they could suffer irreversible physical and cognitive damage, thereby impacting their future health, welfare, and economic well being. These consequences continue into adulthood, and the cycle of undernutrition is passed on to the next generation when undernourished women give birth to low birth weight babies.

Hunger and undernutrition have substantial consequences for survivors and their families by requiring them to spend additional resources on health care and by affecting the productivity of malnourished persons. There is substantial evidence that early child malnutrition is detrimental to productivity in adulthood. The consequences of malnutrition can be identified and quantified in 5 categories: excess costs of health care, either neonatal care for LBW babies or excess costs of infant and child illness for malnourished children; productivity losses associated with stunting; productivity losses from reduced cognitive ability and achievement; increased costs of chronic diseases associated with fetal and early child malnutrition; and consequences of impaired maternal nutrition on future generations.

There is a 2-way causality from malnutrition to infections and vice versa. Deficiencies of both macro- and micronutrients impair the immune system, with well-documented consequences. Conversely, helminthic and other infections lead to reduced nutrient absorption, and fevers lead to catabolism and anorexia and thus contribute to malnutrition. Additionally, caregivers might respond to episodes of diarrhea by withholding food.

In many low-income settings, the consequence of malnutrition leads to reduced lifetime earnings. These effects can come about through impaired cognitive development, late school entrance leading to delayed entry into the labor force, fewer completed years of schooling, less learning per year of schooling, or a combination of these.

The evidence base for the impact of nutrition on earnings is substantial and growing. While separating the factors that lead to undernutrition from the constraints of poverty that will independently affect cognitive ability and limit schooling regardless of nutritional status can be problematic, studies confirm that the impact of improved nutrition is distinct from the contribution of poverty reduction. One study assessed the earnings of adults in Guatemala up to 42 years of age who received nutritional supplements as children or whose mothers received them during their pregnancy. The men who received nutritional supplements before reaching age 3 earned wages that were 46% higher than the wages earned by men who were not supplemented. Evidence from Africa confirms that children who are under 2 years old when a drought hits their community in Africa are likely to be shorter and to complete fewer years of school than their siblings or in contrast to children in different age cohorts in the village. Elsewhere, spikes in the price of food during these critical years lead both to stunting and to diminished schooling.

In addition to the association of stunting and cognitive impairment, some micronutrient deficiencies lead to loss of cognitive potential. Individuals with an iodine deficiency have, on average, 13.5 points lower IQs than comparison groups. Interventions have shown that provision of iodine to pregnant women can reduce this gap. In the case of iron deficiencies, anemia is regularly associated with impaired cognitive development. Moreover, supplementation trials for school-age children confirm this conclusion because they regularly indicate improved cognition, although this is less regularly observed with interventions aimed at deficient younger children.

Tracking the consequences of fetal or childhood deprivation for adult chronic illness imposes additional challenges given the long latency. The hypothesis that early nutritional challenges are part of the etiology of diabetes and cardiovascular disease has first proposed on the basis of epidemiological evidence, including tracking cohorts that suffered from famines in Holland and China. This hypothesis has been bolstered by studies with animal models that help define a mechanism of embryonic development that provides a conceptual basis for the epidemiological evidence. The increased risk of adult chronic disease from this malnutrition in early life is estimated to be a particular challenge to low-income countries with rapid economic growth such as China and India, leading to premature death as well as substantial economic costs from medical expenses and lost productivity.

Quantifying the magnitude of such losses of potential for malnourished children who survive is, of course, context specific, but various studies have shown that investments in nutrition—that is, preventing these losses—can yield considerable economic returns. These preventive investments cover a broad range, including nutrition as well as a diverse set of interventions in education, water and sanitation, trade reform, and private sector deregulation. Addressing micronutrient deficiencies has the highest rate of economic return. For example, every $1 of expenditures on vitamin A supplementation is likely to produce $100 of benefits. To be fair, such estimates are based on a variety of assumptions, such as the value of future benefits compared to current benefits; economists generally view a dollar today as worth more than a dollar sometime in the future.

NUTRITION, FOOD SECURITY, AND POVERTY Household food security tracks income closely. This is not the case for malnutrition, which is often observed even within better-off households in Asia and Africa. Data from household surveys as well as from cross-country comparisons confirm that income growth, even when evenly distributed over a population, has a modest impact on malnutrition rates, even though this impact is statistically significant and positive. On a global average, a 10% increase of national income per capita would lead to a 10% decline in the poverty rate in the country but only a 5% decline in the rate of malnutrition as measured by low weights for age. Global evidence indicates that such a rate of income growth would lead to only a 2.5% decline in anemia.

The international development community has collectively agreed upon 8 Millennium Development Goals (MDGs). The first of these 8 goals refers to poverty and hunger. The recognition of the close relation of food insecurity and poverty is evident in the definition of this first MDG, which aims to eradicate extreme poverty and hunger. The two targets originally proposed (a third on employment was added later) are to halve, between 1990 and 2015:

The proportion of people whose income is less than $1 a day
The proportion of people who suffer from hunger

Two measureable indicators of progress are used for the second target, the percentage of individuals who cannot meet their calorie requirements as measured by the estimate of undernourishment and by the percentage of children under 5 who are underweight as measured in nationally representative household surveys.

While prior to the global financial crisis, the prognosis in general had been that most countries were on track for achieving the poverty goal. But of 143 countries, only 34 (24%) were on track to achieve the nutrition MDG goal. No country in South Asia, where undernutrition rates are the highest, is likely to achieve this MDG—although Bangladesh was most likely to come close to achieving it, and Asia as a whole was likely to achieve it because of the improvements in China. Nutrition status was actually deteriorating in 26 countries, many of them in Africa, where the nexus between HIV and undernutrition is particularly strong and mutually reinforcing. And in 57 countries, no trend data were available to tell whether progress is being made. A renewed focus on this non-income poverty target is clearly central to any poverty reduction efforts.

KEY INTERVENTIONS There is substantial consensus regarding which interventions work to address child undernutrition based on accumulated field evidence (Fig. 43-2). Many of these interventions lie within the responsibility of the health sector, albeit investments in other sectors may be necessary to sustain the benefits from the health sector interventions. Key interventions that have been proved to be cost effective in reducing infant and child mortality, improving underweight rates, and reversing micronutrient deficiencies include:

Interventions with sufficient evidence to implement in all countries

Maternal and birth outcomes	Newborn babies	Infants and children
• Iron folate supplementation • Maternal supplements of multiple micronutrients • Maternal iodine through iodization of salt • Maternal calcium supplementation • Interventions to reduce tobacco consumption or indoor air pollution	• Promotion of breastfeeding (individual and group counseling)	• Promotion of breastfeeding (individual and group counseling) • Behavior change communication for improved complementary feeding • Zinc supplementation • Zinc in management of diarrhea • Vitamin A fortification or supplementation • Universal salt iodization • Handwashing or hygiene interventions • Treatment of SAM

Interventions with sufficient evidence to implement in specific situational contexts

Maternal and birth outcomes	Newborn babies	Infants and children
• Maternal supplementation of balanced energy and protein • Maternal iodine supplements • Maternal deworming in pregnancy • Intermittent preventative treatment for malaria • Insecticide-treated bednets	• Neonatal vitamin A supplementation • Delayed cord clamping	• Conditional cash tranfer programs (with nutrition education) • Deworming • Iron fortification and supplementation programs • Insecticide-treated bednets

Figure 43-2 Key interventions. SAM, severe acute malnutrition. (From World Health Organization and Lancet Global Nutrition Series. www.who.int/nutrition/topics/lancetseries_maternal_and_childundernutrition/en/index.htm.)

- Promoting exclusive breast-feeding
- Promoting adequate and timely complementary feeding (at ~6 mo of age)
- Promoting key hygiene behavior (e.g., hand-washing with soap)
- Providing micronutrient interventions such as vitamin A and iron supplements for pregnant and lactating women and young children
- Presumptive treatment for malaria for pregnant women in endemic malarial regions and promoting long-lasting insecticide treated bednets
- Deworming in endemic parasitic areas and oral rehydration in high-diarrhea regions
- Fortifying commonly eaten foods with micronutrients (such as salt fortified with iodine) and staple foods like wheat, oil, and sugar with iron, vitamin A, and zinc

Birth-spacing and family planning interventions, as well as strategies to address women's empowerment and gender, also have strong impacts on nutrition and child health outcomes. Additionally, community growth promotion programs can provide an opportunity to impart knowledge on a face-to-face basis—hence the stress on community mobilization in many programs. Many growth promotion programs also facilitate the provision of immunizations, vitamin supplements, and deworming medicine as well as being a platform to promote behavioral change.

The emergence of HIV/AIDS as a public health concern has introduced new issues for public health nutrition. One issue is the increased requirements for both macro- and micro-nutrients of individuals with HIV/AIDS, especially those who are able to access anti-retroviral treatment (ART). In addition, there is a particular concern for the prevention of maternal child transmission from HIV-positive mothers. In 2007, an estimated 1.5 million pregnant women in low- and middle-income countries were living with HIV. Seventy-five percent of these were concentrated in 12 countries, which include South Africa, Nigeria, United Republic of Tanzania, and Mozambique.

Even if the mother is able to receive nevirapine or other ART during pregnancy and delivery, she faces a dilemma regarding breastfeeding. The overall risk of mother-to-child HIV transmission by a non-breastfeeding mother is 15-25% (without interventions to reduce transmission) and of a breastfeeding mother is 20-45%. However, the risk is less when the mother is exclusively breastfeeding and increases with duration; the majority of the transmission after delivery occurs after 6 months of breastfeeding. Breast milk substitutes are costly and risky in low-income settings; an outbreak of diarrheal disease linked to formula feeding in Botswana where substitutes are provided free by the government proved fatal to more than 30 children in 2007. Thus, in most low-income settings, HIV-positive mothers are advised to continue with exclusive breastfeeding for 6 months and to wean more abruptly than is otherwise recommended.

Clinical Manifestations and Treatment of Undernutrition

Treatment of vitamin and mineral deficiencies is discussed in Chapters 45-51.

SEVERE ACUTE MALNUTRITION (PROTEIN-ENERGY MALNUTRITION)

Deficiency of a single nutrient is an example of undernutrition or malnutrition, but deficiency of a single nutrient usually is accompanied by a deficiency of several other nutrients. Protein-energy malnutrition (PEM) is manifested primarily by inadequate dietary intakes of protein and energy, either because the dietary intakes of these 2 nutrients are less than required for normal growth or because the needs for growth are greater than can be supplied by what otherwise would be adequate intakes. PEM is almost always accompanied by deficiencies of other nutrients.

Historically, the most severe forms of malnutrition, **marasmus** (nonedematous malnutrition with severe wasting) and **kwashiorkor** (edematous malnutrition), were considered distinct disorders. Nonedematous malnutrition was believed to result primarily from inadequate energy intake or inadequate intakes of both energy and protein, whereas edematous malnutrition was believed to result primarily from inadequate protein intake. A third disorder, **marasmic kwashiorkor,** has features of both disorders (wasting and edema). The 3 conditions have distinct clinical and metabolic features, but they also have a number of overlapping features. A low plasma albumin concentration, often believed to be a manifestation of edematous malnutrition, is common in children with both edematous and nonedematous malnutrition.

In the USA, severe malnutrition has been reported in families who use unusual and inadequate foods to feed infants whom the parents believe to be at risk for milk allergies and also in families who believe in fad diets. Many cases are associated with rice milk diets, a product that is very low in protein content. In addition, protein-calorie malnutrition has been noted in chronically ill patients in neonatal or pediatric intensive care units as well as among patients with burns, HIV, cystic fibrosis, failure to thrive, chronic diarrhea syndromes, malignancies, bone marrow transplantation, and inborn errors of metabolism.

Clinical Manifestations of Severe Protein Calorie Malnutrition

Nonedematous malnutrition (marasmus) is characterized by failure to gain weight and irritability, followed by weight loss and listlessness until emaciation results. The skin loses turgor and becomes wrinkled and loose as subcutaneous fat disappears. Loss of fat from the sucking pads of the cheeks often occurs late in the course of the disease; thus, the infant's face may retain a relatively normal appearance compared with the rest of the body, but this, too, eventually becomes shrunken and wizened. Infants are often constipated, but they can have starvation diarrhea, with frequent small stools containing mucus. The abdomen may be distended or flat, with the intestinal pattern readily visible. There is muscle atrophy and resultant hypotonia. As the condition progresses, the temperature usually becomes subnormal and the pulse slows (Table 43-4).

Edematous malnutrition (kwashiorkor) can occur initially as vague manifestations that include lethargy, apathy, and/or irritability. When kwashiorkor is advanced, there is lack of growth, lack of stamina, loss of muscle tissue, increased susceptibility to infections, vomiting, diarrhea, anorexia, flabby subcutaneous tissues, and edema. The edema usually develops early and can mask the failure to gain weight. It is often present in internal organs before it is recognized in the face and limbs. Liver enlargement can occur early or late in the course of disease. Dermatitis is common, with darkening of the skin in irritated areas, but in contrast to pellagra (Chapter 46) not in areas exposed to sunlight. Depigmentation can occur after desquamation in these areas, or it may be generalized (Figs. 43-3, 43-4, 43-5). The hair is sparse and thin, and in dark-haired children, it can become streaky red or gray. Eventually, there is stupor, coma, and death (see Table 43-4).

Noma is a chronic necrotizing ulceration of the gingiva and the cheek (Fig. 43-6). It is associated with malnutrition and is often preceded by a debilitating illness (measles, malaria, tuberculosis, diarrhea, ulcerative gingivitis) in a nutritionally compromised host. Noma manifests with fever, malodorous breath, anemia, leukocytosis, and signs of malnutrition. Untreated, it produces sever disfiguration. Polymicrobial infection with *Fusobacterium necrophorum* and *Prevotella intermedia* may be inciting agents.

Treatment of noma includes local wound care, penicillin, and metronidazole as well as therapy for the underlying predisposing condition.

Pathophysiology of Severe Protein-Calorie Malnutrition

Why edematous malnutrition develops in some children and nonedematous malnutrition develops in others is unknown. One factor may be the variability among infants in nutrient requirements and in body composition at the time the dietary deficit is incurred. It also has been proposed that giving excess carbohydrate to a child with nonedematous malnutrition reverses the adaptive responses to low protein intake, resulting in mobilization of body protein stores. Eventually, albumin synthesis

Table 43-4 CLINICAL SIGNS OF MALNUTRITION

SITE	SIGNS
Face	Moon face (kwashiorkor), simian facies (marasmus)
Eye	Dry eyes, pale conjunctiva, Bitot spots (vitamin A), periorbital edema
Mouth	Angular stomatitis, cheilitis, glossitis, spongy bleeding gums (vitamin C), parotid enlargement
Teeth	Enamel mottling, delayed eruption
Hair	Dull, sparse, brittle hair, hypopigmentation, flag sign (alternating bands of light and normal color), broomstick eyelashes, alopecia
Skin	Loose and wrinkled (marasmus), shiny and edematous (kwashiorkor), dry, follicular hyperkeratosis, patchy hyper- and hypopigmentation (crazy paving or flaky paint dermatoses), erosions, poor wound healing
Nails	Koilonychia, thin and soft nail plates, fissures or ridges
Musculature	Muscle wasting, particularly buttocks and thighs; Chvostek or Trousseau signs (hypocalcemia)
Skeletal	Deformities, usually as a result of calcium, vitamin D, or vitamin C deficiencies
Abdomen	Distended: hepatomegaly with fatty liver; ascites may be present
Cardiovascular	Bradycardia, hypotension, reduced cardiac output, small vessel vasculopathy
Neurologic	Global developmental delay, loss of knee and ankle reflexes, impaired memory
Hematologic	Pallor, petechiae, bleeding diathesis
Behavior	Lethargic, apathetic, irritable on handling

From Grover Z, Ee LC: Protein energy malnutrition, *Pediatr Clin N Am* 56:1055–1068, 2009.

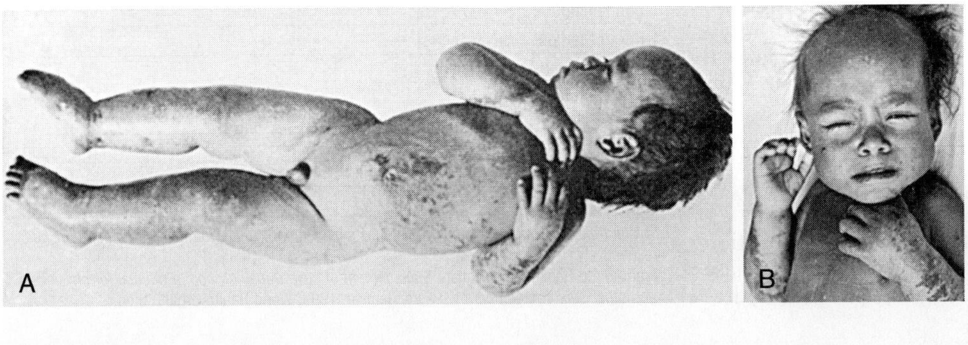

Figure 43-3 *A,* Kwashiorkor in a 2 yr old boy. Note the generalized edema, the typical skin lesions, and the state of prostration. *B,* Close-up view of the same child showing the hair changes and psychic alterations (apathy and misery); the edema of the face and skin lesions can be seen more clearly. (Photographs made available by the Institute of Nutrition of Central Panama, Guatemala, courtesy of Moises Behar, MD.)

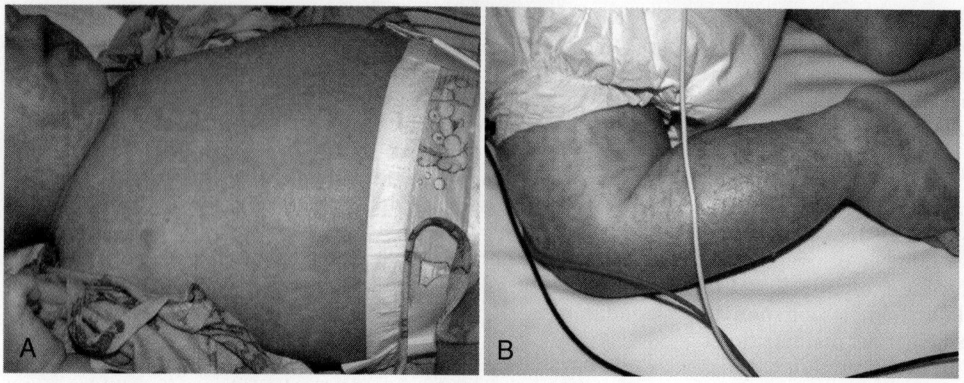

Figure 43-4 *A* and *B,* A 7 mo old boy with diffuse erythematous papules and plaques, some scaly, and edema of the extremities. (From Katz KA, Mahlberg MH, Honig PJ, et al: Rice nightmare: kwashiorkor in 2 Philadelphia-area infants fed Rice Dream beverage, *J Am Acad Dermatol* 52[5 Suppl 1]:S69–S72, 2005.)

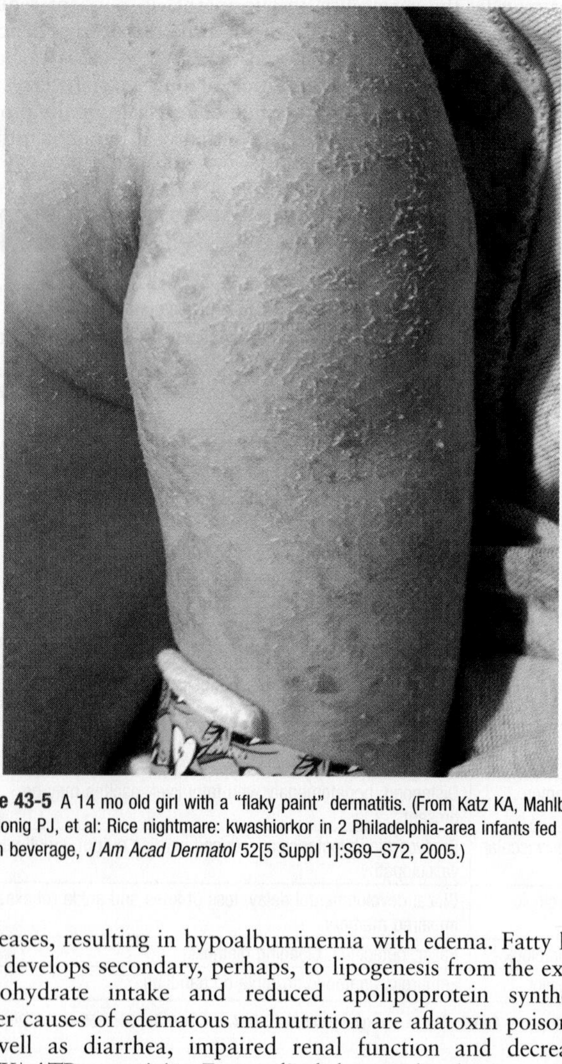

Figure 43-5 A 14 mo old girl with a "flaky paint" dermatitis. (From Katz KA, Mahlberg MH, Honig PJ, et al: Rice nightmare: kwashiorkor in 2 Philadelphia-area infants fed Rice Dream beverage, *J Am Acad Dermatol* 52[5 Suppl 1]:S69–S72, 2005.)

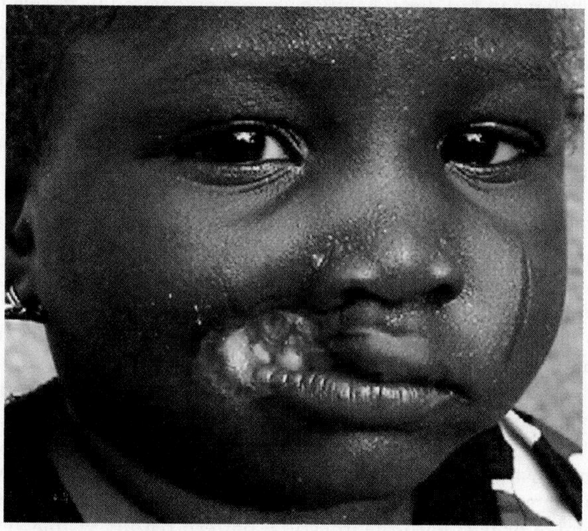

Figure 43-6 Noma lesion. (From Baratti-Mayer D, Pittet B, Montandon D, et al for the Geneva Study Group on Noma [GESNOMA]: Noma: an infectious disease of unknown aetiology, *Lancet Infect Dis* 3:419–431, 2003.)

decreases, resulting in hypoalbuminemia with edema. Fatty liver also develops secondary, perhaps, to lipogenesis from the excess carbohydrate intake and reduced apolipoprotein synthesis. Other causes of edematous malnutrition are aflatoxin poisoning as well as diarrhea, impaired renal function and decreased Na^+/K^+-ATPase activity. Free radical damage has been proposed as an important factor in the development of edematous malnutrition. This proposal is supported by low plasma concentrations of methionine, a dietary precursor of cysteine, which is needed for synthesis of the major antioxidant factor, glutathione. This possibility also is supported by lower rates of glutathione synthesis in children with edematous compared with nonedematous malnutrition.

Treatment

The usual approach to the treatment of severe acute malnutrition includes 3 phases (Table 43-5 and Fig. 43-7). The initial phase (1-7 days) is a stabilization phase. During this phase, dehydra-

Table 43-5 TIME FRAME FOR THE MANAGEMENT OF A CHILD WITH SEVERE MALNUTRITION*

ACTIVITY	INITIAL TREATMENT Days 1-2	Days 3-7	REHABILITATION Weeks 2-6	FOLLOW-UP Weeks 7-26
Treat or prevent				
Hypoglycemia	------->			
Hypothermia	------->			
Dehydration	------->			
Correct electrolyte imbalance	------------	------------	------------>	
Treat infection	------------	------>		
Correct micronutrient deficiencies	<--without iron--	-->	<--with iron-->	
Begin feeding	------------	------>		
Increase feeding to recover lost weight ("catch-up growth")			------------	------------>
Stimulate emotional and sensorial development	------------	------------	------------	------------>
Prepare for discharge			------------>	

**Malnutrition* and *malnourished* are used as synonyms for *undernutrition* and *undernourished*, respectively.

From World Health Organization: *Management of severe malnutrition: a manual for physicians and other senior health care workers*, Geneva, 1999, World Health Organization.

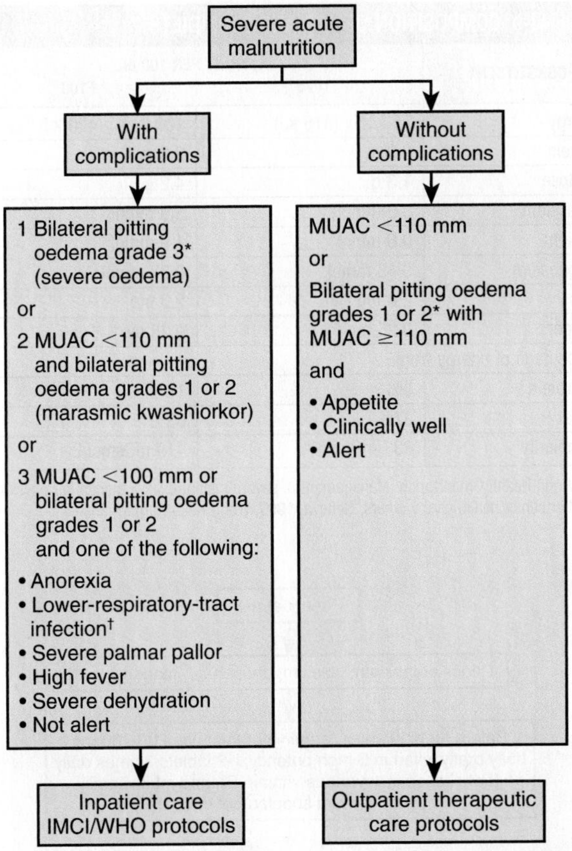

Figure 43-7 Classification of severe acute malnutrition used in community-based therapeutic care. ICMI, integrated management of childhood illness; MUAC, mid-upper arm circumference; WHO, Word Health Organization. *Grade 1, mild edema on both feet or ankles; grade 2, moderate edema on both feet, plus lower legs, hands, or lower arms; grade 3, severe generalized edema affecting both feet, legs, hands, arms, and face. †IMCI criteria[39]: 60 respirations/min children age <2 mo; 50 respirations/min for age 2-12 mo; 40 respirations/min for ages 1-5 yr; 30 respirations for age >5 yr. (From Collins S, Dent N, Binns P, et al: Management of severe acute malnutrition in children, *Lancet* 368:1992–2000, 2006.)

tion, if present, is corrected and antibiotic therapy is initiated to control bacterial or parasitic infection. Because of the difficulty of estimating hydration, **oral rehydration** therapy is preferred (Chapters 55 and 332). If intravenous therapy is necessary, estimates of dehydration should be reconsidered frequently, particularly during the first 24 hr of therapy. Oral feedings are also started with specialized high-calorie formula (see Fig. 43-7 and Table 43-6), proposed by the World Health Organization, that can be made with simple ingredients. The initial phase of oral treatment is with the F75 diet (75 kcal or 315 kJ/100 mL). The rehabilitation diet is with the F100 diet (100 kcal or 420 kJ/100 mL). Feedings are initiated with higher frequency and smaller volumes; over time, the frequency is reduced from 12 to 8 to 6 feedings per 24 hr. The initial caloric intake is estimated at 80-100 kcal/kg/day. In developed countries, 24-27 calorie/oz infant formulas may be initiated with the same daily caloric goals. If diarrhea starts or fails to resolve and lactose intolerance is suspected, a non–lactose-containing formula should be substituted. If milk protein intolerance is suspected, a soy protein hydrolysate formula may be used.

Another approach is the use of **ready to use therapeutic foods** (RUTFs) (Fig. 43-8). RUTFs reduce mortality in a cost-effective manner, in part because they are less susceptible to spoilage than powdered milk–based supplementary foods. F100 is water based and subject to bacterial contamination, whereas RUTF is an oil-based paste that has little water content and a similar nutrient profile but a higher calorie density and is equally palatable to

SAM management

Independent additional criteria	• No appetite • Medical complications		• Appetite • No medical complications
	↓		↓
Type of therapeutic feeding	**Facility-based**	→	**Community-based**
Intervention	F75→ F100/RUTF and 24 hour medical care		RUTF, basic medical care
Discharge criteria (transition criteria from facility to community-based care)	Reduced oedema Good appetite (with acceptable[a] intake of RUTF)		15 to 20% weight gain

[a] Child eats at least 75% of his/her calculated RUTF ration for the day

Figure 43-8 Severe acute malnutrition (SAM) management. RUTF, ready to use therapeutic foods. (From World Health Organization and the United Nations Children's Fund: *WHO child growth standards and the identification of severe acute malnutrition in infants and children, 2009* (PDF). www.who.int/nutrition/publications/severemalnutrition/9789241598163/en/index.html. Accessed May 23, 2010.)

Table 43-6 PREPARATION OF F75 AND F100 DIETS

INGREDIENT	AMOUNT F75*	AMOUNT F100†
Dried skim milk	25 g	80 g
Sugar	70 g	50 g
Cereal flour	35 g	
Vegetable oil	27 g	60 g
Mineral mix‡	20 mL	20 mL
Vitamin mix‡	140 mg	140 mg
Water to make	1,000 mL	1,000 mL

*To prepare the F75 diet, add the dried skim milk, sugar, cereal flour, and oil to some water and mix. Boil for 5-7 min. Allow to cool, then add the mineral mix and vitamin mix, and mix again. Make up the volume to 1,000 mL with water.

†To prepare the F100 diet, add the dried skim milk, sugar, and oil to some warm boiled water and mix. Add the mineral mix and vitamin mix, and mix again. Make up the volume to 1,000 mL with water.

‡If only small amounts of feed are being prepared, it is not feasible to prepare the vitamin mix because of the small amounts involved. In this case, give a proprietary multivitamin supplement. Alternatively, a combined mineral and vitamin mix for malnourished children is available commercially and may be used in these diets. A comparable formula can be made from 35 g whole dried milk, 70 g sugar, 35 g cereal flour, 17 g oil, 20 mL mineral mix, 140 mg vitamin mix, and water to make 1,000 mL. Alternatively, use 300 mL fresh cow's milk, 70 g sugar, 35 g cereal flour, 17 g oil, 20 mL mineral mix, 140 mg vitamin mix, and water to make 1,000 mL. Isotonic versions of F75 (280 mOsmol/L), which contain maltodextrins instead of cereal flour and some of the sugar and which include all the necessary micronutrients, are available commercially. If cereal flour is not available or there are no cooking facilities, a comparable formula can be made from 25 g dried skim milk, 100 g sugar, 27 g oil, 20 mL mineral mix, 140 mg vitamin mix, and water to make 1,000 mL. However, this formula has a high osmolarity (415 mOsmol/L) and might not be well tolerated by all children, especially those with diarrhea. A comparable formula can be made from 110 g whole dried milk, 50 g sugar, 30 g oil, 20 mL mineral mix, 140 mg vitamin mix, and water to make 1,000 mL. Alternatively, use 880 mL fresh cow's milk, 75 g sugar, 20 g oil, 20 mL mineral mix, 140 mg vitamin mix, and water to make 1,000 mL.

From World Health Organization: *Management of severe malnutrition: a manual for physicians and other senior health care workers,* Geneva, 1999, World Health Organization.

F100. RUTF is a mixture of powdered milk, peanuts, sugar, vitamins, and minerals.

One advantage of RUTFs is that in many cases it can be used in community settings rather than in rehabilitation centers where there is a high risk of infection. Indeed, it may be hard to separate out the intrinsic advantage of the RUTF products from the advantages of the community-based management of care.

Laboratory evaluation (Table 43-7) and ongoing monitoring (Table 43-8), when available, help guide therapy and prevent complications. Fluid status must be monitored very carefully in

Table 43-7 LABORATORY FEATURES OF SEVERE MALNUTRITION

BLOOD OR PLASMA VARIABLES	INFORMATION DERIVED
Hemoglobin, hematocrit, erythrocyte count, mean corpuscular volume	Degree of dehydration and anemia; type of anemia (iron/folate and vitamin B_{12} deficiency, hemolysis, malaria)
Glucose	Hypoglycemia
Electrolytes and alkalinity	
• Sodium	Hyponatremia, type of dehydration
• Potassium	Hypokalemia
• Chloride, pH, bicarbonate	Metabolic alkalosis or acidosis
Total protein, transferrin, (pre)albumin	Degree of protein deficiency
Creatinine	Renal function
C-reactive protein, lymphocyte count, serology, thick and thin blood films	Presence of bacterial or viral infection or malaria
Stool examination	Presence of parasites

From Müller O, Krawinkel M: Malnutrition and health in developing countries, *CMAJ* 173(3):279–286, 2006. © 2005 Canadian Medical Association. Reprinted with permission of the publisher.

Table 43-8 ELEMENTS IN THE MANAGEMENT OF SEVERE PROTEIN-ENERGY MALNUTRITION

PROBLEM	MANAGEMENT
Hypothermia	Warm patient up; maintain and monitor body temperature
Hypoglycemia	Monitor blood glucose; provide oral (or intravenous) glucose
Dehydration	Rehydrate carefully with oral solution containing less sodium and more potassium than standard mix
Micronutrients	Provide copper, zinc, iron, folate, multivitamins
Infections	Administer antibiotic and antimalarial therapy, even in the absence of typical symptoms
Electrolytes	Supply plenty of potassium and magnesium
Starter nutrition	Keep protein and volume load low
Tissue-building nutrition	Furnish a rich diet dense in energy, protein, and all essential nutrients that is easy to swallow and digest
Stimulation	Prevent permanent psychosocial effects of starvation with psychomotor stimulation
Prevention of relapse	Start early to identify causes of protein-energy malnutrition in each case; involve the family and the community in prevention

From Müller O, Krawinkel M: Malnutrition and health in developing countries, *CMAJ* 173(3):279–286, 2006. © 2005 Canadian Medical Association. Reprinted with permission of the publisher.

anemic patients, who might require a packed red blood cell transfusion.

The second rehabilitation phase (wk 2-6) may include continued antibiotic therapy with appropriate changes, if the initial combination was not effective, and introduction of the F100 or RUTF diet (Tables 43-6 and 43-9) with a goal of at least 100 kcal/kg/day. This phase usually lasts an additional 4 wk. At any time, if the infant is unable to take the feedings from a cup, syringe, or dropper, administration by a nasogastric tube rather than by the parenteral route is preferred. Bottles may be contaminated in certain locales, and their use is discouraged unless cleanliness is assured. Once ad libitum feedings are allowed, intakes of both energy and protein are often substantial. Iron therapy usually is not started until this phase of treatment; iron can interfere with the protein's host defense mechanisms. There also is concern that free iron during the early phase of treatment might exacerbate oxidant damage, precipitating infections (malaria), clinical kwashiorkor, or marasmic kwashiorkor in a child with clinical marasmus. Some recommend treatment with antioxidants.

Table 43-9 COMPOSITION OF F75 AND F100 DIETS

CONSTITUENT	AMOUNT PER 100 mL F75	F100
Energy	75 $kcal_{th}$ (315 kJ)	100 $kcal_{th}$ (420 kJ)
Protein	0.9 g	2.9 g
Lactose	1.3 g	4.2 g
Potassium	3.6 mmol	5.9 mmol
Sodium	0.6 mmol	1.9 mmol
Magnesium	0.43 mmol	0.73 mmol
Zinc	2.0 mg	2.3 mg
Copper	0.25 mg	0.25 mg
Percentage of energy from:		
Protein	5%	12%
Fat	32%	53%
Osmolarity	333 mOsmol/L	419 mOsmol/L

From World Health Organization: Management of severe malnutrition: a manual for physicians and other senior health care workers, Geneva, 1999, World Health Organization.

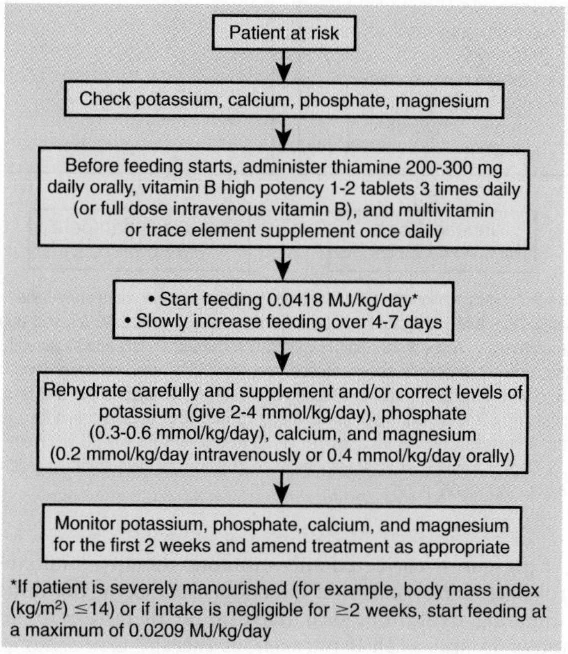

Figure 43-9 Guidelines for management. (From Mehanna HM, Moledina J, Travis J: Refeeding syndrome: what it is, and how to prevent and treat it. *BMJ* 336:1495–1498, 2008.)

By the end of the 2nd phase, any edema that was present has usually been mobilized, infections are under control, the child is becoming more interested in his or her surroundings, and his or her appetite is returning. The child is then ready for the final follow-up phase, which consists of feeding to cover catch-up growth as well as providing emotional and sensory stimulation. The child should be fed ad libitum.

In developing countries, this final phase is often carried out at home. In all phases, parental education is crucial for continued effective treatment as well as preventing additional episodes.

Refeeding syndrome can complicate the acute nutritional rehabilitation of children who are undernourished from any cause (Fig. 43-9, Table 43-10). The hallmark of refeeding syndrome is the development of severe hypophosphatemia after the cellular uptake of phosphate during the 1st week of starting to refeed. Serum phosphate levels of ≤0.5 mmol/L can produce weakness, rhabdomyolysis, neutrophil dysfunction, cardiorespiratory failure, arrhythmias, seizures, altered level of conscious-

Table 43-10 CLINICAL SIGNS AND SYMPTOMS OF REFEEDING SYNDROME

HYPOPHOSPHATEMIA	HYPOKALEMIA	HYPOMAGNESEMIA	VITAMIN/THIAMINE DEFICIENCY	SODIUM RETENTION	HYPERGLYCEMIA
Cardiac Hypotension Decreased stroke volume **Respiratory** Impaired diaphragm contractility Dyspnea Respiratory failure **Neurologic** Paresthesia Weakness Confusion Disorientation Lethargy Areflexic paralysis Seizures Coma **Hematologic** Leukocyte dysfunction Hemolysis Thrombocytopenia **Other** Death	**Cardiac** Arrhythmias **Respiratory** Failure **Neurologic** Weakness Paralysis **Gastrointestinal** Nausea Vomiting Constipation **Muscular** Rhabdomyolysis Muscle necrosis **Other** Death	**Cardiac** Arrhythmias **Neurologic** Weakness Tremor Tetany Seizures Altered mental status Coma **Gastrointestinal** Nausea Vomiting Diarrhea **Other** Refractory hypokalemia and hypocalcemia Death	Encephalopathy Lactic acidosis Death	Fluid overload Pulmonary edema Cardiac compromise	**Cardiac** Hypotension **Respiratory** Hypercapnea Failure **Other** Ketoacidosis Coma Dehydration Impaired immune function

Data from Kraft MD, Btaiche IF, Sacks GS: Review of RFS, *Nutr Clin Pract* 20:625–633, 2005. From Fuentebella J, Kerner JA: Refeeding syndrome, *Pediatr Clin N Am* 56:1201–1210, 2009.

ness, or sudden death. Phosphate levels should be monitored during refeeding, and if they are low, phosphate should be administered during refeeding to treat severe hypophosphatemia (Chapter 52.6).

BIBLIOGRAPHY

Please visit the Nelson Textbook of Pediatrics *website at www.expertconsult.com for the complete bibliography.*

Chapter 44
Overweight and Obesity
Sheila Gahagan

Obesity is an important pediatric public health problem associated with risk of complications in childhood and increased morbidity and mortality throughout adult life. The prevalence of childhood obesity has increased, and the prevention and treatment of obesity has emerged as an important focus of pediatric research and clinical care.

EPIDEMIOLOGY

Obesity is a global public health problem, sparing only dramatically poor regions with chronic food scarcity such as sub-Saharan Africa and Haiti. As of 2005, more than 1.6 billion persons ≥15 yr old are overweight or obese (WHO).

In the USA, 30% of adults are obese, and an additional 35% of adults are overweight. In children, the prevalence of obesity increased 300% over approximately 40 years. The National Health and Nutrition Examination Survey (NHANES) IV, 1999-2002, found 31% of children older than 2 yr to be overweight or obese, and 16% of children and adolescents 6-19 years were in the obese range. Children's risk varies by socioeconomic status, race, maternal education level, and gender. African-American adolescent girls and Mexican-American 6-12 yr old boys have higher rates of obesity compared to other groups. Childhood obesity is also increasingly common in some Native American groups. Across all racial groups, higher maternal education confers protection against childhood obesity.

Parental obesity correlates with a higher risk for obesity in their children. Prenatal factors including weight gain during pregnancy, high birth weight, and gestational diabetes are associated with increased risk for later obesity. Paradoxically, intrauterine growth restriction with early infant catch-up growth is associated with the development of central adiposity and cardiovascular risk.

BODY MASS INDEX

Health care professionals define obesity or increased adiposity using the body mass index (BMI), which is an excellent proxy for more direct measurement of body fat. BMI = weight in kg/(height in meters)^2. Adults with a BMI ≥30 meet the criterion for obesity, and those with a BMI 25-30 fall in the overweight range. During childhood, levels of body fat change beginning with high adiposity during infancy. Body fat levels decrease for approximately 5.5 yr until the period called *adiposity rebound,* when body fat is typically at the lowest level. Adiposity then increases until early adulthood (Fig. 44-1). Consequently, obesity and overweight are defined using BMI percentiles; children >2 yr old with a BMI ≥95th percentile meet the criterion for obesity, and those with a BMI between the 85th and 95th percentiles fall in the overweight range. The terminology used for pediatric obesity previously was "overweight" and "risk for overweight." This terminology has changed to improve consistency with the adult criteria and international definitions of pediatric obesity.

ETIOLOGY

Humans have the capacity to store energy in adipose tissue, allowing improved survival in times of famine. Simplistically, obesity results from an imbalance of caloric intake and energy expenditure. Even incremental but sustained caloric excess results in excess adiposity. Individual adiposity is the result of a complex interplay among genetically determined body habitus, appetite, nutritional intake, physical activity, and energy expenditure. Environmental factors determine levels of available food, preferences for types of foods, levels of physical activity, and preferences for types of activities.

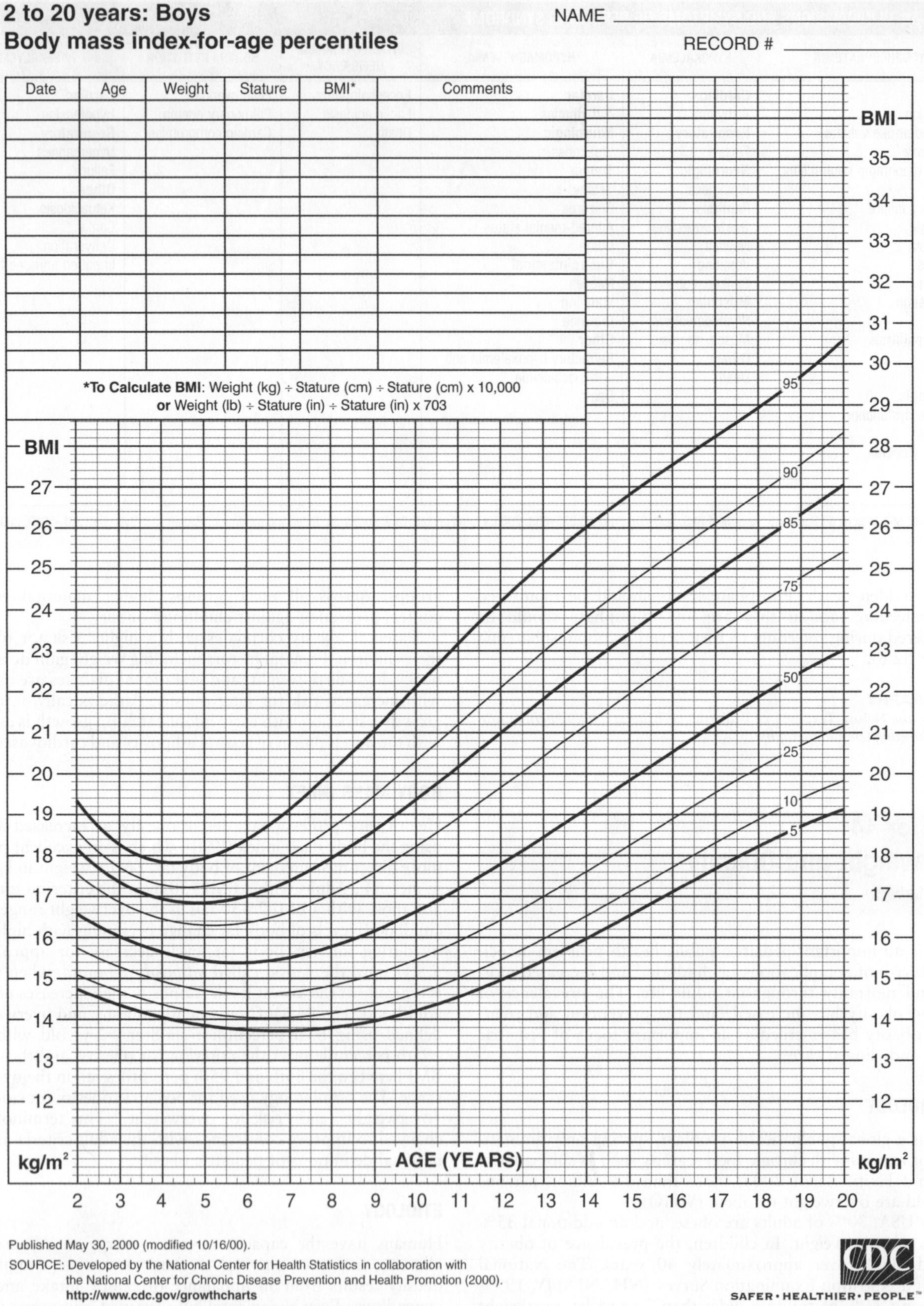

A

Figure 44-1 Body mass index (BMI)-for-age profiles for boys and men *(A)* and girls and women *(B)*.

2 to 20 years: Girls
Body mass index-for-age percentiles

NAME
RECORD #

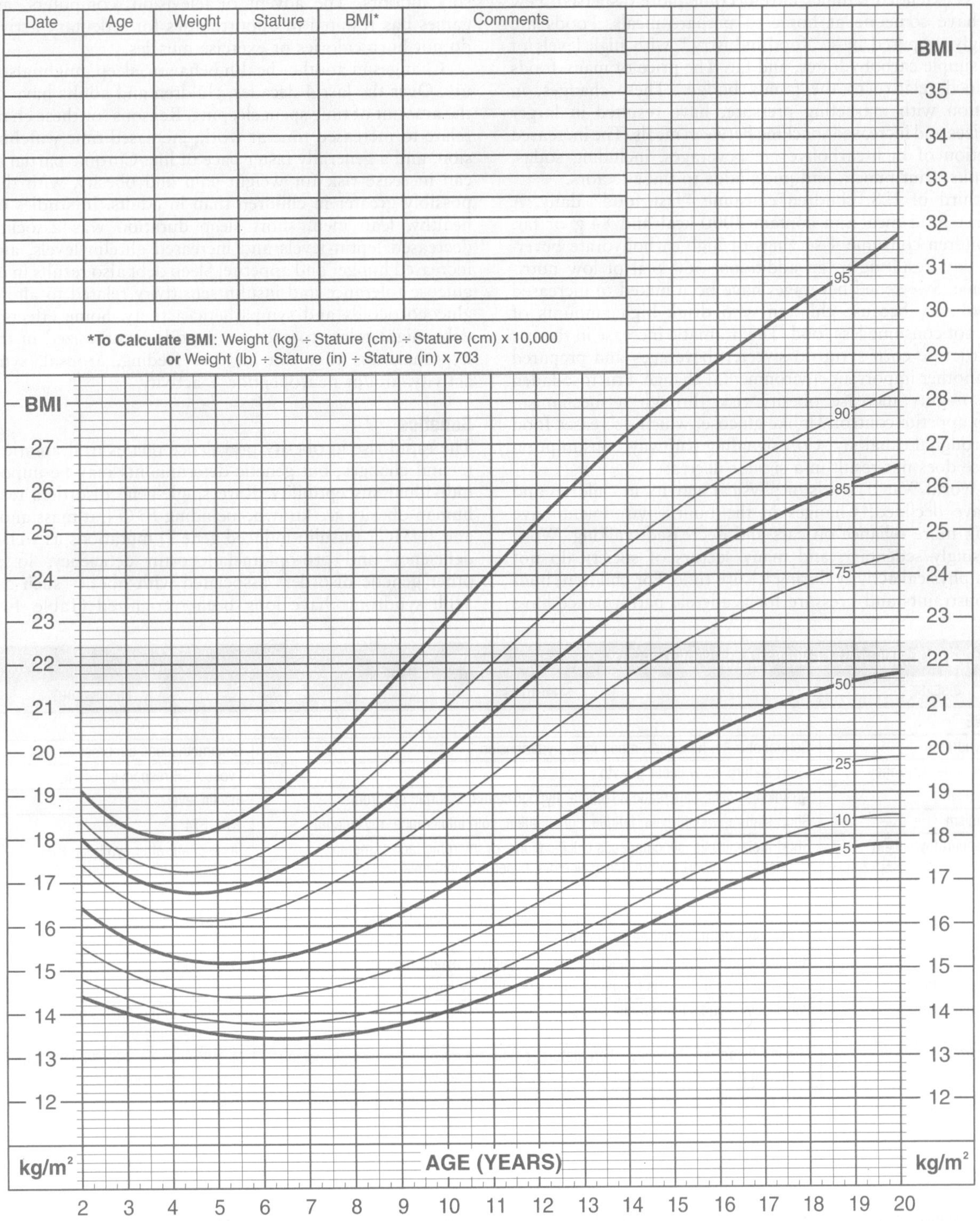

Published May 30, 2000 (modified 10/16/00).
SOURCE: Developed by the National Center for Health Statistics in collaboration with the National Center for Chronic Disease Prevention and Health Promotion (2000).
http://www.cdc.gov/growthcharts

CDC
SAFER • HEALTHIER • PEOPLE™

B

Figure 44-1, cont'd For legend see facing page.

Environmental Changes

Over the last 4 decades, the food environment has changed dramatically. Changes in the food industry relate in part to social changes, as extended families have become more dispersed. Few families have someone at home to prepare meals. Foods are increasingly prepared by a "food industry," with high levels of calories, simple carbohydrates, and fat. The price of many foods has declined relative to the family budget. These changes, in combination with marketing pressure, have resulted in larger portion sizes and increased snacking between meals. The increased consumption of high-carbohydrate beverages, including sodas, sport drinks, fruit punch, and juice, adds to these factors.

One third of U.S. children consume "fast food" daily. A typical fast food meal can contain 2000 kcal and 84 g of fat. Many children consume 4 servings of high-carbohydrate beverages per day, resulting in an additional 560 kcal of low nutritional value. Sweetened beverages have been linked to increased risk for obesity because children who drink high amounts of sugar do not consume less food. The dramatic increase in the use of high-fructose corn syrup to sweeten beverages and prepared foods is another important environmental change. Fructose-laden products mighty increase obesity risk through a mechanism related to appetite control. Unlike glucose, which decreases food intake through the malonyl-CoA signaling pathway, consumption of fructose does not result in a similar decrease.

Since World War II, levels of physical activity in children and adults have declined. Changes in the built environment have resulted in more reliance on cars and decreased walking. Work is increasingly sedentary, and many sectors of society do not engage in physical activity during leisure time. For children, budgetary constraints and pressure for academic performance have led to less time devoted to physical education in schools. Perception of poor neighborhood safety is another factor that can lead to lower levels of physical activity when children are required to stay indoors. The advent of television, computers, and video games has resulted in opportunities for sedentary activities that do not burn calories or exercise muscles.

Changes in another health behavior, sleep, might also contribute. Over the last 4 decades, children and adults have decreased the amount of time spent sleeping. Reasons for these changes may relate to increased time at work, increased time watching television, and a generally faster pace of life. Chronic partial sleep loss can increase risk for weight gain and obesity, with the impact possibly greater in children than in adults. In studies of young, healthy, lean men, short sleep duration was associated with decreased leptin levels and increased ghrelin levels, along with increased hunger and appetite. Sleep debt also results in decreased glucose tolerance and insulin sensitivity related to alterations in glucocorticoids and sympathetic activity. Some effects of sleep debt might relate to orexins, peptides synthesized in the lateral hypothalamus that can increase feeding, arousal, sympathetic activity, and/or neuropeptide Y activity.

Genetics

The rapid rise in obesity prevalence relates to dramatic environmental changes, but genetic determinants may be important for individual susceptibility. Rare single-gene disorders resulting in human obesity are known, including *FTO* (fat mass and obesity) and *INSIG2* (insulin-induced gene 2) mutations as well as leptin deficiency and pro-opiomelanocortin deficiency. In addition, other genetic disorders associated with obesity such as Prader-Willi syndrome have long been recognized (Table 44-1). It is

Table 44-1 ENDOCRINE AND GENETIC CAUSES OF OBESITY

DISEASE	SYMPTOMS	LABORATORY
ENDOCRINE		
Cushing syndrome	Central obesity, hirsutism, moon face, hypertension	Dexamethasone suppression test
Growth hormone deficiency	Short stature, slow linear growth	Evoked GH response, IGF-1
Hyperinsulinism	Nesidioblastosis, pancreatic adenoma, hypoglycemia, Mauriac syndrome	Insulin level
Hypothyroidism	Short stature, weight gain, fatigue, constipation, cold intolerance, myxedema	TSH, FT4
Pseudohypoparathyroidism	Short metacarpals, subcutaneous calcifications, dysmorphic facies, mental retardation, short stature, hypocalcemia, hyperphosphatemia	Urine cAMP after synthetic PTH infusion
GENETIC		
Alstrom syndrome	Cognitive impairment, retinitis pigmentosa, diabetes mellitus, hearing loss, hypogonadism, retinal degeneration	*ALMS1* gene
Bardet-Biedl syndrome	Retinitis pigmentosa, renal abnormalities, polydactyly, hypogonadism	*BBS1* gene
Biemond syndrome	Cognitive impairment, iris coloboma, hypogonadism, polydactyly	
Carpenter syndrome	Polydactyly, syndactyly, cranial synostosis, mental retardation	Mutations in the *RAB23* gene, located on chromosome 6 in humans
Cohen syndrome	Mid-childhood-onset obesity, short stature, prominent maxillary incisors, hypotonia, mental retardation, microcephaly, decreased visual activity	Mutations in the *VPS13B* gene (often called the *COH1* gene) at locus 8q22
Deletion 9q34	Early-onset obesity, mental retardation, brachycephaly, synophrys, prognathism, behavior and sleep disturbances	Deletion 9q34
Down syndrome	Short stature, dysmorphic facies, mental retardation	Trisomy 21
ENPP1 gene mutations	Insulin resistance, childhood obesity	Gene mutation on chromosome 6q
Frohlich syndrome	Hypothalamic tumor	
Leptin or leptin receptor gene deficiency	Early-onset severe obesity, infertility (hypogonadotropic hypogonadism)	Leptin
Melanocortin 4 receptor gene mutation	Early-onset severe obesity, increased linear growth, hyperphagia, hyperinsulinemia Most common known genetic cause of obesity Homozygous worse than heterozygous	*MC4R* mutation
Prader-Willi Syndrome	Neonatal hypotonia, slow infant growth, small hands and feet, mental retardation, hypogonadism, hyperphagia leading to severe obesity, paradoxically elevated ghrelin	Partial deletion of chromosome 15 or loss of paternally expressed genes
Pro-opiomelanocortin deficiency	Obesity, red hair, adrenal insufficiency, hyperproinsulinemia	Loss-of-function mutations of the POMC gene
Turner syndrome	Ovarian dysgenesis, lymphedema, web neck, short stature, cognitive impairment	XO chromosome

cAMP, cyclic adenosine monophosphate; FT4, free throxine; GH, growth hormone; IGF, insulin-like growth factor; PTH, parathyroid hormone; TSH, thyroid-stimulating hormone.

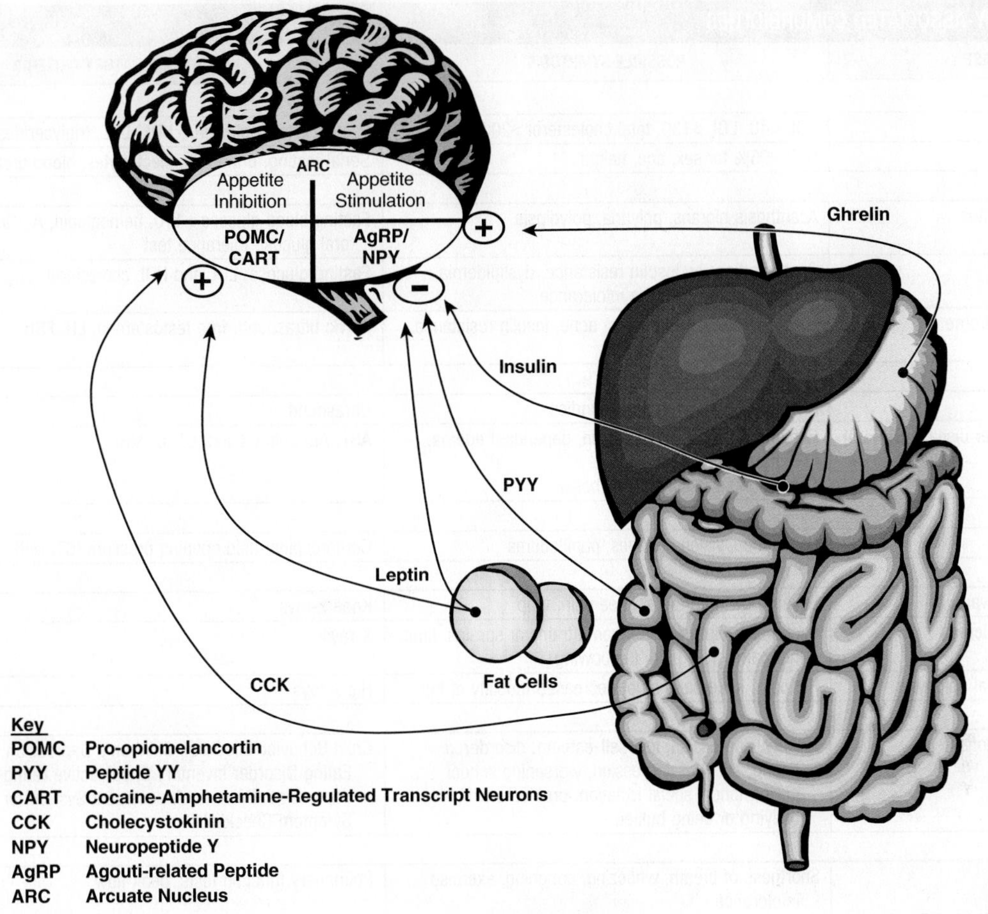

Figure 44-2 Control of appetite.

likely that genes are involved in behavioral phenotypes related to appetite regulation and preference for physical activity. More than 600 genes, markers, and chromosomal regions have been associated with human obesity.

Endocrine and Neural Physiology

Monitoring of "stored fuels" and short-term control of food intake (appetite and satiety) occurs through neuroendocrine feedback loops linking adipose tissue, the gastrointestinal (GI) tract, and the central nervous system (Fig. 44-2). GI hormones, including cholecystokinin, glucagon-like peptide-1, peptide YY, and vagal neuronal feedback promote satiety. Ghrelin stimulates appetite. Adipose tissue provides feedback regarding energy storage levels to the brain through hormonal release of adiponectin and leptin. These hormones act on the arcuate nucleus in the hypothalamus and on the solitary tract nucleus in the brainstem and in turn activate distinct neuronal networks. Adipocytes secrete adiponectin into the blood, with reduced levels in response to obesity and increased levels in response to fasting. Reduced adiponectin levels are associated with lower insulin sensitivity and adverse cardiovascular outcomes. Leptin is directly involved in satiety, as low leptin levels stimulate food intake and high leptin levels inhibit hunger in animal models and in healthy human volunteers. Adiposity correlates to serum leptin levels among children and adults, with the direction of effect remaining unclear.

Numerous neuropeptides in the brain, including neuropeptide Y, agouti-related peptide, and orexin, appear to affect appetite stimulation, whereas melanocortins and α-melanocortin-stimulating hormone are involved in satiety. The neuroendocrine control of appetite and weight involves a negative-feedback system, balanced between short-term control of appetite (including ghrelin, PPY) and long-term control of adiposity (including leptin).

COMORBIDITIES

Complications of pediatric obesity occur during childhood and adolescence and persist into adulthood. An important reason to prevent and treat pediatric obesity is the increased risk for morbidity and mortality later in life. The Harvard Growth Study found that boys who were overweight during adolescence were twice as likely to die from cardiovascular disease as those who had normal weight. More immediate comorbidities include type 2 diabetes, hypertension, hyperlipidemia, and nonalcoholic fatty liver disease (Table 44-2). Insulin resistance increases with increasing adiposity and independently affects lipid metabolism and cardiovascular health. Nonalcoholic fatty liver disease occurs in 10-25% of obese adolescents and can progress to cirrhosis.

In adults, the combination of central obesity, hypertension, glucose intolerance, and hyperlipidemia is the metabolic syndrome. Persons with the metabolic syndrome are at increased risk for cardiovascular morbidity and mortality. Experts do not uniformly agree that this symptom cluster in the pediatric age group has prognostic significance.

There is increasing evidence that obesity may be associated with chronic inflammation. Adiponectin, a peptide with anti-inflammatory properties, occurs in reduced levels in obese patients as compared to insulin-sensitive, lean persons. Low adiponectin levels correlate with elevated levels of free fatty acids and plasma triglycerides as well as a high BMI, and high adiponectin levels correlate with peripheral insulin sensitivity. Adipocytes secrete peptides and cytokines into the circulation, and pro-inflammatory peptides such interleukin (IL)-6 and tumor necrosis

Table 44-2 OBESITY-ASSOCIATED COMORBIDITIES

DISEASE	POSSIBLE SYMPTOMS	LABORATORY CRITERIA
CARDIOVASCULAR		
Dyslipidemia	HDL <40, LDL >130, total cholesterol >200	Fasting total cholesterol, HDL, LDL, triglycerides
Hypertension	SBP >95% for sex, age, height	Serial testing, urinalysis, electrolytes, blood urea nitrogen, creatinine
ENDOCRINE		
Type 2 diabetes mellitus	Acanthosis nigrans, polyuria, polydipsia	Fasting blood glucose >110, hemoglobin, A_{1c}, insulin level, C-peptide, oral glucose tolerance test
Metabolic syndrome	Central adiposity, insulin resistance, dyslipidemia, hypertension, glucose intolerance	Fasting glucose, LDL and HDL cholesterol
Polycystic ovary syndrome	Irregular menses, hirsutism, acne, insulin resistance, hyperandrogenemia	Pelvic ultrasound, free testosterone, LH, FSH
GASTROINTESTINAL		
Gallbladder disease	Abdominal pain, vomiting, jaundice	Ultrasound
Nonalcoholic fatty liver disease (NAFLD)	Hepatomegaly, abdominal pain, dependent edema, ↑ transaminases Can progress to fibrosis, cirrhosis	AST, ALT, ultrasound, CT, or MRI
NEUROLOGIC		
Pseudotumor cerebri	Headaches, vision changes, papilledema	Cerebrospinal fluid opening pressure, CT, MRI
ORTHOPEDIC		
Blount disease (tibia vara)	Severe bowing of tibia, knee pain, limp	Knee x-rays
Musculoskeletal problems	Back pain, joint pain, frequent strains or sprains, limp, hip pain, groin pain, leg bowing	X-rays
Slipped capital femoral epiphysis	Hip pain, knee pain, limp, decreased mobility of hip	Hip x-rays
PSYCHOLOGICAL		
Behavioral complications	Anxiety, depression, low self-esteem, disordered eating, signs of depression, worsening school performance, social isolation, problems with bullying or being bullied	Child Behavior Checklist, Children's Depression Inventory, Peds QL, Eating Disorder Inventory 2, subjective ratings of stress and depression, Behavior Assessment System for Children, Pediatric Symptom Checklist
PULMONARY		
Asthma	Shortness of breath, wheezing, coughing, exercise intolerance	Pulmonary function tests, peak flow
Obstructive sleep apnea	Snoring, apnea, restless sleep, behavioral problems	Polysomnography, hypoxia, electrolytes (respiratory acidosis with metabolic alkalosis)

ALT, alanine aminotransferase; AST, aspartate aminotransferase; CT, computed tomography; FSH, follicle-stimulating hormone; HDL, high-density lipoprotein; LDL, low-density lipoprotein; LH, luteinizing hormone; MRI, magnetic resonance imaging; Peds QL, Pediatric Quality of Life Inventory.

factor-α (TNF-α) occur in higher levels in obese patients. Specifically, IL-6 stimulates production of C-reactive protein (CRP) in the liver. CRP is a marker of inflammation and might link obesity, coronary disease, and subclinical inflammation.

Some complications of obesity are mechanical, including obstructive sleep apnea and orthopedic complications. Orthopedic complications include Blount disease and slipped femoral capital epiphysis (Chapters 669, 670.4).

Mental health problems can coexist with obesity, with the possibility of bidirectional effects. These associations are modified by gender, ethnicity, and socioeconomic status. Self-esteem may be lower in obese adolescent girls compared to nonobese peers. Some studies have found an association between obesity and adolescent depression. There is considerable interest in the co-occurrence of eating disorders and obesity.

IDENTIFICATION

Overweight and obese children are often identified as part of routine medical care, and the child and family may be unaware that the child has increased adiposity. They may be unhappy with the medical provider for raising this issue and respond with denial or apparent lack of concern. It is often necessary to begin by helping the family understand the importance of healthy weight for current and future health, especially because intervention requires considerable effort by the child and the family. Forging a good therapeutic relationship is important, because obesity intervention requires a chronic disease management approach. Successful resolution of this problem necessitates considerable family and child effort over an extended period in order to change eating and activity behaviors.

EVALUATION

The evaluation of the overweight or obese child begins with examination of the growth chart for weight, height, and BMI trajectories; consideration of possible medical causes of obesity; and detailed exploration of family eating, nutritional, and activity patterns. A complete pediatric history is used to uncover comorbid disorders. The family history focuses on the adiposity of other family members and the family history of obesity-associated disorders. The physical examination adds data that can lead to important diagnoses. Laboratory testing is guided by the need to identify comorbid conditions.

Examination of the growth chart reveals the severity, duration, and timing of obesity onset. Children who are overweight (BMI in the 85th-95th percentile) are less likely to have developed comorbid conditions than those who are obese (BMI ≥95th percentile). Those with a BMI ≥99th percentile are even more likely to have coexisting medical problems. Once obesity severity is determined, the BMI trajectory is examined to elucidate when the child became obese. Several periods during childhood are considered sensitive periods or times of increased risk for developing obesity, including infancy, adiposity rebound (when body fat is lowest at approximately age 5.5 years), and adolescence. Severe obesity and obesity of long duration can require more intensive family intervention unless the family is highly motivated to make dietary and activity changes. An abrupt change in BMI might signal the onset of a medical problem or a period of family or personal stress for the child. Examination of the weight trajectory can further expand understanding of how the problem developed. A young child might exhibit high weight and high height, because linear growth can increase early in childhood if a child consumes excess energy. At some point, the weight percentile exceeds the height percentile and the child's BMI climbs into the obese range. Another example is a child whose weight rapidly increases when she reduces her activity level and consumes more meals away from home. Examination of the height trajectory can reveal endocrine problems, which often occur with slowing of linear growth.

Consideration of possible medical causes of obesity is essential, even though endocrine and genetic causes are rare (see Table 44-1). Growth hormone deficiency, hypothyroidism, and Cushing syndrome are examples of endocrine disorders that can lead to obesity. In general, these disorders manifest with slow linear growth. Because children who consume excessive amounts of calories tend to experience accelerated linear growth, short stature warrants further evaluation. Genetic disorders associated with obesity can have coexisting dysmorphic features, cognitive impairment, vision and hearing abnormalities, or short stature. In some children with congenital disorders such as myelodysplasia or muscular dystrophy, lower levels of physical activity can lead to secondary obesity. Some medications can cause excessive appetite and hyperphagia, resulting in obesity. Atypical antipsychotic medications most commonly have this dramatic side effect. Rapid weight gain in a child or adolescent taking one of these medications might require a discontinuation of that medication. Poor linear growth and rapid changes in weight gain are indications for evaluation of possible medical causes.

Exploration of family eating and nutritional and activity patterns begins with a description of regular meal and snack times and family habits for walking, bicycle riding, active recreation, television, computer, and video-game time. It is useful to request a 24-hour dietary recall with special attention to intake of fruits, vegetables, and water, as well as high-calorie foods and high-carbohydrate beverages. When possible, evaluation by a nutritionist is extremely helpful. This information will form the basis for incremental changes in eating behavior, caloric intake, and physical activity during the intervention.

Initial assessment of the overweight or obese child includes a complete review of bodily systems focusing on the possibility of comorbid conditions (see Table 44-2). Developmental delay and visual and hearing impairment can be associated with genetic disorders. Difficulty sleeping, snoring, or daytime sleepiness suggests the possibility of sleep apnea. Abdominal pain might suggest nonalcoholic fatty liver disease. Symptoms of polyuria, nocturia, or polydipsia may be the result of type 2 diabetes. Hip or knee pain can be caused by secondary orthopedic problems, including Blount disease and slipped capital femoral epiphysis. Irregular menses may be associated with polycystic ovary syndrome. Acanthosis nigricans can suggest insulin resistance and type 2 diabetes (Fig. 44-3).

The family history begins with identifying other obese family members. Parental obesity is an important risk for child obesity. If all family members are obese, focusing the intervention on the entire family is reasonable. The child may be at increased risk for developing type 2 diabetes if a family history exists. Patients of African-American, Hispanic, or Native American heritage are also at increased risk for developing type 2 diabetes. Identification of a family history of hypertension, cardiovascular disease, or metabolic syndrome indicates increased risk for developing these obesity-associated conditions. If one helps the family to understand that childhood obesity increases risk for developing these chronic diseases, this educational intervention might serve as motivation to improve their nutrition and physical activity.

Physical examination should be thorough, focusing on possible comorbid conditions (see Table 44-2). Careful screening for hypertension using an appropriately sized blood pressure cuff is important. Systematic examination of the skin can reveal acanthosis nigricans, suggesting insulin resistance, or hirsutism, suggesting polycystic ovary syndrome. Tanner staging can reveal premature adrenarche secondary to advanced sexual maturation in overweight and obese girls.

Laboratory testing for fasting plasma glucose, triglycerides, low-density lipoprotein (LDL) and high-density lipoprotein (HDL) cholesterol, and liver function tests are recommended as part of the initial evaluation for newly identified pediatric obesity (Table 44-3). Overweight children (BMI 85th-95th percentile) who have a family history of diabetes mellitus or signs of insulin resistance should also be evaluated with a fasting plasma glucose test. Other laboratory testing should be guided by history or physical examination findings.

INTERVENTION

Successful intervention for obesity is challenging and is best accomplished using multimodal approaches to accomplish substantial lifestyle change. In adults, long-term weight loss is uncommon despite the availability of a wide variety of diet plans, commercial products, and medications. Cognitive-behavioral therapy approaches to improve motivation have been promising.

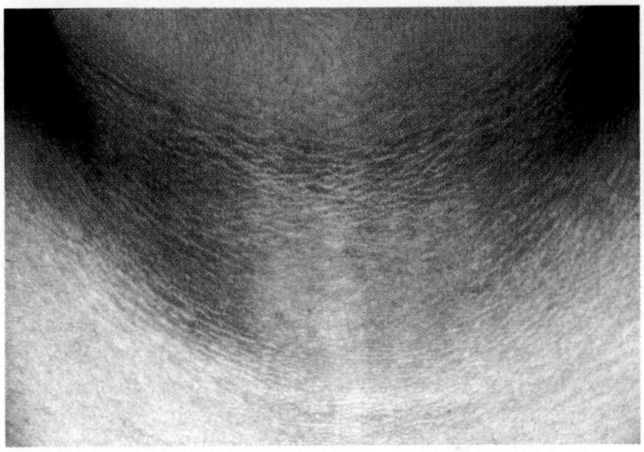

Figure 44-3 Acanthosis nigricans. (From Gahagan S: Child and adolescent obesity, *Curr Probl Pediatr Adolesc Health Care* 34:6–43, 2004.)

Table 44-3 NORMAL LABORATORY VALUES FOR RECOMMENDED TESTS

LABORATORY TEST	NORMAL VALUE
Glucose	<110 mg/dL
Insulin	<15 mU/L
Hemoglobin A_{1c}	<5.7%
AST 2-8 yr	<58 U/L
AST 9-15 yr	<46 U/L
AST 15-18 yr	<35 U/L
ALT	<35 U/L
Total cholesterol	<170 mg/dL
LDL	<110 mg/dL
HDL	<35 mg/dL
Triglycerides 2-15 yr	<100 mg/dL
Triglycerides 15-19 yr	<125 mg/dL

AST, aspartate aminotransferase; ALT, alanine aminotransferase; LDL, low-density lipoprotein; HDL, high-density lipoprotein.

From Children's Hospital of Wisconsin: *The NEW (nutrition, exercise and weight management) kids program* (PDF file). www.chw.org/display/displayFile.asp?docid=33670&filename=/Groups/NEWKids/08_Referral_Form.pdf. Accessed February 2, 2011.

A combination of nutritional advice, exercise, and cognitive behavioral approaches usually work best. Bariatric surgery can accomplish considerable weight loss in adolescents. It is not yet clear whether these patients will maintain a healthy weight permanently, and long-term safety has yet to be established.

It is important to begin with clear recommendations about appropriate caloric intake for the obese child (Table 44-4). Working with a dietitian is very helpful. Meals should be based on fruits, vegetables, whole grains, lean meat, fish, and poultry. Prepared foods should be chosen for their nutritional value, with attention to calories and fat. Foods that provide excessive calories and low nutritional value should be reserved for infrequent treats. Because many obese children are consuming calories greatly in excess of their needs, it is often impossible to achieve an immediate reduction to the recommended daily calorie level. Instead, a gradual approach is recommended. A 10 yr old child who requires 2000 kcal/day and consumes 3500 kcal/day could reduce his typical daily intake by 280 kcal by forgoing two cans of high-carbohydrate beverage and drinking water instead. Although this dietary change will not result in weight loss, it will probably result in slightly slower weight gain. Once this change has been successfully incorporated, the child could make another change such as cutting out a snack, thereby eliminating an additional 300 kcal.

Weight-reduction diets in adults generally do not lead to sustained weight loss. Therefore, the focus should be on changes that can be maintained for life. Attention to eating patterns is helpful. Families should be encouraged to plan family meals, including breakfast. It is almost impossible for a child to make changes in nutritional intake and eating patterns if other family members do not make the same changes. Dietary needs also change developmentally, as adolescents require greatly increased calories during their growth spurts, and adults who lead inactive lives need fewer calories than active and growing children.

Psychological strategies are helpful. The "traffic light" diet groups foods into those that can be consumed without any limitations (green), in moderation (yellow), or reserved for infrequent treats (red) (Table 44-5). The concrete categories are very helpful to children and families. This approach can be adapted to any ethnic group or regional cuisine. Motivational interviewing, a strategy with proven efficacy for decreasing tobacco and substance use, shows promise for assisting patients in changing their nutritional patterns. This approach begins with assessing how ready the patient is to make important behavioral changes. The professional then engages the patient in developing a strategy to take the next step toward the ultimate goal of healthy nutritional intake. This method allows the professional to take the role of a coach, helping the child and family reach their goals. Other behavioral approaches include family rules about where food may be consumed—for example, "not in the bedroom." Evidence-based strategies can be used to tailor interventions, given individual and environmental differences.

It is very difficult to achieve weight loss by increasing physical activity alone. Nonetheless, increasing fitness improves cardiovascular health even without weight loss. Therefore, increasing physical activity can decrease risk for cardiovascular disease, improve well-being, and contribute to weight loss. Increased physical activity can be accomplished by walking to school, engaging in physical activity during leisure time with family and friends, or enrolling in organized sports. Children are more likely to be active if their parents are active. Just as family meals are recommended, family physical activity is recommended.

Active pursuits can replace more sedentary activities. The American Academy of Pediatrics recommends that screen time be restricted to no more than 2 hr/day for children >2 yr old and that children <2 yr old not watch television. Television watching is often associated with eating, and many highly caloric food products are marketed directly to children during child-oriented television programs.

Pediatric providers should assist families to develop goals to change nutritional intake and physical activity. They can also provide the child and family with needed information. The family should not expect immediate lowering of BMI percentile related to behavioral changes but can instead count on a gradual decrease in the rate of BMI percentile increase until it stabilizes, followed by a gradual decrease in BMI percentile. Referral to multidisciplinary, comprehensive pediatric weight-management programs is ideal for obese children whenever possible. As part of a comprehensive program, adolescents may receive adjunctive pharmacologic therapy. In adults, the addition of antiobesity drugs to comprehensive lifestyle modification can produce more weight loss than lifestyle modification alone, with a BMI-lowering effect of 4%. Sibutramine, a norepinephrine and serotonin reuptake inhibitor, and Orlistat, an intestinal lipase inhibitor, is as effective as adjunctive therapy to behavior modification for weight loss in overweight adolescents (Table 44-6). The effect on long-term weight maintenance is not yet known. The pediatric provider also makes referrals to specialists to treat comorbid conditions, including type 2 diabetes, hypertension, nonalcoholic fatty liver disease, and orthopedic disorders.

In some cases, it is reasonable to refer adolescents for evaluation for bariatric surgery. The American Pediatric Surgical Association Guidelines recommends that surgery be considered only in children with complete or near-complete skeletal maturity, a BMI ≥40, and a medical complication resulting from obesity, *after* they have failed 6 mo of a multidisciplinary weight management program. Current surgical approaches include the Roux-en-Y and the adjustable gastric band.

PREVENTION

Prevention of child and adolescent obesity is essential for public health in the USA and most other countries (Tables 44-7 and 44-8). Efforts by pediatric providers can supplement national- and community-level public health programs. The National

Table 44-4 RECOMMENDED CALORIC INTAKE DESIGNATED BY AGE AND GENDER

LIFE STAGE GROUP	AGE (yr)	RELATIVELY SEDENTARY LEVEL OF ACTIVITY (kcal)	MODERATE LEVEL OF ACTIVITY (kcal)	ACTIVE (kcal)
Child	2-3	1,000	1,000-1,400	1,000-1,400
Female	4-8	1,200	1,400-1,600	1,400-1,800
	9-13	1,600	1,600-2,000	1,800-2,200
	14-18	1,800	2,000	2,400
Male	4-8	1,400	1,400-1,600	1,600-2,000
	9-13	1,800	1,800-2,200	2,000-2,600
	14-18	2,200	2,400-2,800	2,800-3,200

Adapted from U.S. Department of Agriculture: *Dietary guidelines for Americans, 2005* (website). www.health.gov/DIETARYGUIDELINES/dga2005/document/html/chapter2.htm. Accessed May 23, 2010.

Table 44-5 TRAFFIC LIGHT DIET PLAN

FEATURE	GREEN LIGHT FOOD	YELLOW LIGHT FOODS	RED LIGHT FOODS
Quality	Low-calorie, high-fiber, low-fat, nutrient-dense	Nutrient-dense, but higher in calories and fat	High in calories, sugar, and fat
Types of food	Fruits, vegetables	Lean meats, dairy, starches, grains	Fatty meats, sugar, fried foods
Quantity	Unlimited	Limited	Infrequent or avoided

Table 44-6 MEDICATIONS USED FOR WEIGHT LOSS IN ADULTS

DRUG	MECHANISM OF ACTION	SIDE EFFECTS
Sibutramine*†	Appetite suppressant: combined norepinephrine and serotonin reuptake inhibitor	Modest increases in heart rate and blood pressure, nervousness, insomnia
Phentermine*†	Appetite suppressant: sympathomimetic amine	Cardiovascular, gastrointestinal
Diethylpropion*†	Appetite suppressant: sympathomimetic amine	Palpitations, tachycardia, insomnia, gastrointestinal
Orlistat*	Lipase inhibitor: decreased absorption of fat	Diarrhea, flatulence, bloating, abdominal pain, dyspepsia
Bupropion	Appetite suppressant: mechanism unknown	Paresthesia, insomnia, central nervous system effects
Fluoxetine	Appetite suppressant: selective serotonin reuptake inhibitor	Agitation, nervousness, gastrointestinal
Sertraline	Appetite suppressant: selective serotonin reuptake inhibitor	Agitation, nervousness, gastrointestinal
Topiramate	Mechanism unknown	Paresthesia, changes in taste
Zonisamide	Mechanism unknown	Somnolence, dizziness, nausea

*Approved by the U.S. Food and Drug Administration for weight loss.
†Drug Enforcement Administration schedule IV.
From Snow V, Barry P, Fitterman N, et al: Pharmacologic and surgical management of obesity in primary care: a clinical practice guideline from the American College of Physicians, *Ann Intern Med* 142:525–531, 2005.

Institutes of Health (NIH) and Centers for Disease Control and Prevention (CDC) recommend a variety of initiatives to combat the current obesigenic environment, including promotion of breast-feeding, access to fruits and vegetables, walkable communities, and 60 min/day of activity for children. The USDA sponsors programs promoting 5.5 cups of fruits and vegetables per day. Incentives for the food industry to promote consumption of healthier foods should be considered. Marketing of unhealthy foods to children has begun to be regulated. We expect to see changes in federal food programs including commodity foods, the Women, Infant, and Children Supplemental Food Program (WIC), and school-lunch programs to meet the needs of today's children.

The Ways to Enhance Children's Activity and Nutrition (WE CAN) program is an example of a community-based child obesity prevention effort aimed at 8- to 12-year old children. This national program, designed for families and communities, focuses on three important behaviors: *improved* food choices, *increased* physical activity, and *reduced* screen time. Child health professionals can serve as leaders and topic experts for community programs. Speeches at schools, at community centers, and on local radio and television programs emphasize the importance of nutrition and physical activity for health.

Pediatric prevention efforts begin with careful monitoring of weight and BMI percentiles at health care maintenance visits. Attention to changes in BMI percentiles can alert the pediatric provider to increasing adiposity before the child becomes overweight or obese. All families should be counseled about healthy nutrition for their children because the current prevalence of overweight and obesity in adults is 65%. Therefore, approximately 2/3 of all children can be considered at risk for becoming overweight or obese at some time in their lives. Those who have an obese parent are at increased risk. Prevention efforts begin with promotion of exclusive breast-feeding for 6 mo and total breast-feeding for 12 mo. Introduction of infant foods at 6 months should focus on cereals, fruits, and vegetables. Lean meats, poultry, and fish may be introduced later in the 1st year of life. Parents should be specifically counseled to avoid

Table 44-7 PROPOSED SUGGESTIONS FOR PREVENTING OBESITY

PREGNANCY
Normalize body mass index before pregnancy. Do not smoke. Maintain moderate exercise as tolerated. In gestational diabetics, provide meticulous glucose control.
POSTPARTUM AND INFANCY
Breast-feeding is preferred for a minimum of 3 mo. Postpone the introduction of solid foods and sweet liquids.
FAMILIES
Eat meals as a family in a fixed place and time. Do not skip meals, especially breakfast. No television during meals. Use small plates, and keep serving dishes away from the table. Avoid unnecessary sweet or fatty foods and soft drinks. Remove televisions from children's bedrooms; restrict times for television viewing and video games.
SCHOOLS
Eliminate fundraisers with candy and cookie sales. Review the contents of vending machines and replace with healthier choices. Install water fountains. Educate teachers, especially physical education and science faculty, about basic nutrition and the benefits of physical activity. Educate children from preschool through high school on appropriate diet and lifestyle. Mandate minimum standards for physical education, including 30-45 min of strenuous exercise 2-3 times weekly. Encourage "the walking schoolbus": Groups of children walking to school with an adult.
COMMUNITIES
Increase family-friendly exercise and play facilities for children of all ages. Discourage the use of elevators and moving walkways. Provide information on how to shop and prepare healthier versions of culture-specific foods.
HEALTH CARE PROVIDERS
Explain the biologic and genetic contributions to obesity. Give age-appropriate expectations for body weight in children. Work toward classifying obesity as a disease to promote recognition, reimbursement for care, and willingness and ability to provide treatment.
INDUSTRY
Mandate age-appropriate nutrition labeling for products aimed at children (e.g., red light/green light foods, with portion sizes). Encourage marketing of interactive video games in which children must exercise in order to play. Use celebrity advertising directed at children for healthful foods to promote breakfast and regular meals.
GOVERNMENT AND REGULATORY AGENCIES
Classify obesity as a legitimate disease. Find novel ways to fund healthy lifestyle programs, (e.g., with revenues from food and drink taxes). Subsidize government-sponsored programs to promote the consumption of fresh fruits and vegetables. Provide financial incentives to industry to develop more healthful products and to educate the consumer on product content. Provide financial incentives to schools that initiate innovative physical activity and nutrition programs. Allow tax deductions for the cost of weight loss and exercise programs. Provide urban planners with funding to establish bicycle, jogging, and walking paths. Ban advertising of fast foods directed at preschool children, and restrict advertising to school-aged children.

From Speiser PW, Rudolf MCJ, Anhalt H, et al: Consensus statement: childhood obesity, *J Clin Endocrinol Metabol* 90:1871–1887, 2005.

introducing highly sugared beverages and foods in the 1st year of life. Instead, they should expose their infants and young children to a rich variety of fruits, vegetables, grains, lean meats, poultry, and fish to facilitate acceptance of a diverse and healthy diet. Parenting matters, and authoritative parents are more likely to have children with a healthy weight than those who are

Table 44-8 ANTICIPATORY GUIDANCE: ESTABLISHING HEALTHY EATING HABITS IN CHILDREN

Do not punish a child during mealtimes with regard to eating. The emotional atmosphere of a meal is very important. Interactions during meals should be pleasant and happy.
Do not use foods as rewards.
Parents, siblings, and peers should model healthy eating, tasting new foods, and eating a well-balanced meal.
Children should be exposed to a wide range of foods, tastes, and textures.
Foods should be offered multiple times. Repeated exposure to initially disliked foods will break down resistance.
Offering a range of foods with low energy density helps children balance energy intake.
Restricting access to foods will increase rather than decrease a child's preference for that food.
Forcing a child to eat a certain food will decrease his or her preference for that food. Children's wariness of new foods is normal and should be expected.
Children tend to be more aware of satiety than adults, so allow children to respond to satiety, and let that dictate servings. Do not force children to "clean their plate."

Adapted from Benton D: Role of parents in the determination of food preferences of children and the development of obesity, *Int J Obes Relat Metab Disord* 28:858–869, 2004. Copyright 2004. Reprinted by permission from Macmillan Publishers Ltd.

authoritarian or permissive. Families who eat regularly scheduled meals together are less likely to have overweight or obese children. Child health professionals are able to address a child's nutritional status and to provide expertise in child growth and development.

Child health professionals can also promote physical activity during regular health care maintenance visits. Parents who spend some of their leisure time in physical activity promote healthy weight in their children. Beginning in infancy, parents should be cognizant of their child's developmental capability and need for physical activity. Because television, computer, and video-game time can replace health-promoting physical activity, physicians should counsel parents to limit screen time for their children. Snacking during television watching should be discouraged. Parents can help their children to understand that television commercials intend to sell a product. Children can learn that their parents will help them by responsibly choosing healthy foods.

BIBLIOGRAPHY

Please visit the Nelson Textbook of Pediatrics *website at www.expertconsult.com for the complete bibliography.*

Chapter 45 Vitamin A Deficiencies and Excess

Maija H. Zile

OVERVIEW OF VITAMINS

Vitamins are essential organic compounds that are required in very small amounts (micronutrients) and are involved in fundamental functions in the body, such as growth, maintenance of health, and metabolism. A vitamin can have several functions. Because our bodies cannot biosynthesize vitamins, vitamins must be supplied by the diet or as supplements. The dietary reference intakes (DRIs) for infants and children are summarized in Table 41-5. Vitamins are not chemically similar. Based on their chemical properties, they are classified as either water-soluble or fat-soluble; these 2 groups are handled differently by the body. The water-soluble vitamins (except vitamin C) are members of the B complex.

Deficiency states in developed countries are rare, except in some impoverished populations (Chapter 43) or after mistakes in food preparation or with fad diets, but they are common in many developing countries and are often associated with global malnutrition (Chapter 43). In the clinical setting, vitamin deficiencies can also occur as complications in children with various chronic disorders or diseases. Information obtained in the medical history related to dietary habits can be important in identifying the possibility of such nutritional problems. Except for vitamin A, toxicity from excess intake of vitamins is rare. The food sources, functions, and deficiency and excess symptoms of the vitamins are summarized in Tables 45-1 and 48-1.

VITAMIN A

Vitamin A is an essential micronutrient because it cannot be biogenerated de novo by animals. It must be obtained from plants in the form of provitamin-A carotenoids: α-, β-, and γ-carotenes and β-cryptoxanthin. These substances can be converted to vitamin A compounds in the body.

The term *vitamin A* refers to all-*trans*-retinol, the alcohol form of the vitamin. The storage form of vitamin A is retinyl palmitate. The aldehyde form of vitamin A is retinal and functions in vision. The physiologically most important vitamin A metabolite is the acid derivative, retinoic acid. Retinoic acid functions at the gene level as a ligand for specific nuclear transcription factors that regulate many genes involved in fundamental biologic activities of the cell. The term *retinoids* includes both natural and synthetic compounds with vitamin A activity and is most often used in the context of vitamin A action at the gene level.

Absorption, Transport, Metabolism, Storage

The body acquires vitamin A either as preformed vitamin A (usually as esters) or as provitamin-A carotenoids. In the USA, grains and vegetables supply approximately 55% and dairy and meat products supply approximately 30% of vitamin A intake from food. Vitamin A and the provitamins-A are fat-soluble, and their absorption depends on the presence of adequate lipid and protein within the meal. Chronic intestinal disorders or lipid malabsorption syndromes can result in vitamin A deficiency. Ingested and absorbed provitamins-A are bioconverted to vitamin A molecules in the small intestine by the carotene cleavage enzyme dioxygenase; β-carotene provides twice the vitamin A activity of the other provitamins-A. Further processing in the enterocyte involves the esterification of vitamin A to retinyl palmitate for incorporation into chylomicrons, which are released into lymph and transported via the circulation to the liver for storage or to other tissues. The vitamin A content in the liver is low at birth, but it increases 60-fold during the first 6 mo of life. If the growing child has a well-balanced diet and obtains vitamin A from foods that are rich in vitamin A or provitamin-A (see Table 45-1), the risk of vitamin A deficiency is small. However, even subclinical vitamin A deficiency can have serious consequences.

Stored vitamin A is released from the liver into the circulation as retinol bound to its specific transport protein, retinol-binding protein (RBP), which binds to the thyroid hormone transport protein, transthyretin; this complex delivers retinol (as well as the thyroid hormone) to tissues. Normal plasma levels of retinol are 20-50 μg/dL in infants and 30-225 μg/dL in older children and adults. Uncleaved provitamin-A carotenoids in the intestine are also incorporated into chylomicrons and delivered to various tissues. Malnutrition, particularly protein deficiency, can cause vitamin A deficiency by the impaired synthesis of retinol transport protein. However, if dietary vitamin A is provided in the absence of RBP, vitamin A is transported to the tissues via chylomicrons and almost completely alleviates the symptoms of vitamin A deficiency. In developing countries, subclinical or clinical zinc deficiency can increase the risk of vitamin A deficiency. There is also some evidence of marginal zinc intakes in children in the USA.

Table 45-1 VITAMIN A

NAMES AND SYNONYMS	CHARACTERISTICS	BIOCHEMICAL ACTION	EFFECTS OF DEFICIENCY	EFFECTS OF EXCESS	SOURCES
Retinol (vitamin A_1); 1 μg retinol = 3.3 IU vitamin A = 1 RAE Provitamins A: the plant pigments α-, β-, and γ-carotenes and cryptoxanthin have partial retinol activity: 12 μg β-carotene, or 24 μg other provitamin A carotenoids = 1 μg retinol	Fat-soluble; heat-stable; destroyed by oxidation, drying Bile necessary for absorption Stored in liver Protected by vitamin E	In vision, as retinal, for synthesis of the visual pigments rhodopsin and iodopsin In growth, reproduction, embryonic and fetal development, bone growth, immune and epithelial functions, via retinoic acid as a ligand for specific nuclear transcription factors, regulating genes involved in many fundamental cellular processes	Nyctalopia Photophobia, xerophthalmia, Bitot spots, conjunctivitis, keratomalacia leading to blindness Faulty epiphyseal bone formation Defective tooth enamel Keratinization of mucous membranes and skin Retarded growth Impaired resistance to infection, anemia, reproductive failure, fetal abnormalities	Anorexia, slow growth, drying and cracking of skin, enlargement of liver and spleen, swelling and pain of long bones, bone fragility, increased intracranial pressure, alopecia, carotenemia Fetal abnormalities	Liver, fish liver oils Dairy products, except skim milk Egg yolk, fortified margarine, fortified skim milk Carotenoids from plants: green vegetables, yellow fruits and vegetables

RAE, retinol activity equivalent.

Function and Mechanism of Action

Vitamin A is required throughout the life cycle, beginning with embryogenesis. Except for its role in vision, the pleiotropic actions of this micronutrient include many systemic functions that are mediated at the gene level by all-*trans*-retinoic acid (RA), which is a ligand for specific nuclear transcription factors, the retinoid receptors: RARs and RXRs. When an RAR is activated by the presence of RA, it combines with an RXR, and the resulting heterodimer binds to target genes that have specific recognition sites. Thus, vitamin A, via its active form, retinoic acid, regulates many genes that are involved in the fundamental biologic activities of cells, such as cell division, cell death, and cell differentiation.

Retinoic acid is among the most important signaling molecules in vertebrate ontogenesis. It affects many physiologic processes, including reproduction, growth, embryonic and fetal development, and bone development, in addition to respiratory, gastrointestinal, hematopoietic, and immune functions. The role of vitamin A in immune function and host defense is particularly important in developing countries, where vitamin A supplementation or therapy reduces the morbidity and mortality rates of various diseases, such as measles (Chapter 238).

The best understood function of vitamin A is its nongenomic role in vision. The human retina has two distinct photoreceptor systems: the rods, containing rhodopsin, which can detect low-intensity light, and the cones, containing iodopsin, which can detect different colors. The aldehyde form of vitamin A, retinal, is the prosthetic group on both visual proteins. The mechanism of vitamin A action in vision is based on the ability of the vitamin A molecule to photoisomerize (change shape when exposed to light). Thus, in the dark, low-intensity light isomerizes the rhodopsin prosthetic group, 11-*cis* retinal, to all-*trans*-retinal, generating an electrical signal that is transmitted via the optic nerve to the brain and results in visual sensation.

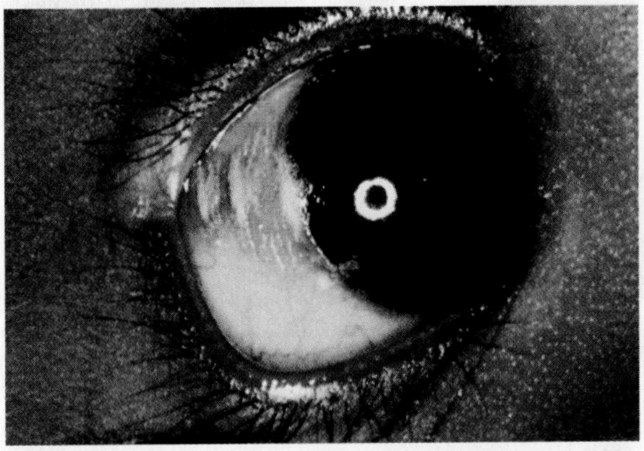

Figure 45-1 Bitot spots with hyperpigmentation seen in a 10 mo old Indonesian boy. (From Oomen HAPC: Vitamin A deficiency, xerophthalmia and blindness, *Nutr Rev* 6:161–166, 1974.)

VITAMIN A DEFICIENCY

Clinical Manifestations

The most obvious symptoms of vitamin A deficiency are associated with the requirement of this vitamin for the maintenance of epithelial functions. In the intestines, a normal mucus-secreting epithelium is an effective barrier against a pathogenic attack that can cause diarrhea. Similarly, in the respiratory tract, a mucus-secreting epithelium is essential for the disposal of inhaled pathogens and toxicants. Epithelial changes in the respiratory system can result in bronchial obstruction. Characteristic changes due to vitamin A deficiency in the epithelia include a proliferation of basal cells, hyperkeratosis, and formation of stratified cornified squamous epithelium. Squamous metaplasia of the renal pelves, ureters, vaginal epithelium, and the pancreatic and salivary ducts can lead to increased infections in these areas. In the urinary bladder, loss of epithelial integrity can result in pyuria and hematuria. Epithelial changes in the skin due to vitamin A deficiency are manifested as dry, scaly, hyperkeratotic patches, commonly on the arms, legs, shoulders, and buttocks. The combination of defective epithelial barriers to infection, low immune response, and lowered response to inflammatory stress, all due to insufficient vitamin A, can cause poor growth and serious health problems in children.

The most characteristic and specific signs of vitamin A deficiency are eye lesions. Lesions due to vitamin A deficiency develop insidiously and rarely occur before 2 yr of age. An early symptom is delayed adaptation to the dark; later when vitamin A deficiency is more advanced, it leads to **night blindness** due to the absence of retinal in the visual pigment, rhodopsin, of the retina. Photophobia is a common symptom. As vitamin A deficiency progresses, the epithelial tissues of the eye become severely altered.

The cornea protects the eye from the environment and is also important in light refraction. In early vitamin A deficiency, the cornea keratinizes, becomes opaque, is susceptible to infection, and forms dry, scaly layers of cells (**xerophthalmia**). In later stages, infection occurs, lymphocytes infiltrate, and the cornea becomes wrinkled; it degenerates irreversibly (keratomalacia), resulting in blindness. The conjunctiva keratinizes and develops plaques (**Bitot spots** [Fig. 45-1]). The pigment epithelium is the structural element of the retina and keratinizes. When the pigment

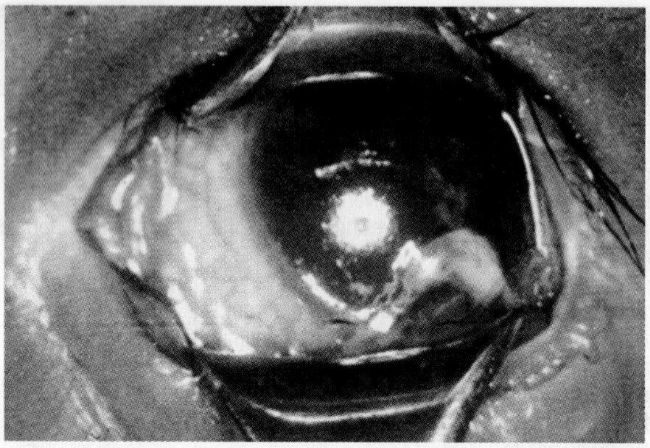

Figure 45-2 Advanced xerophthalmia with an opaque, dull cornea and some damage to the iris in a 1 yr old boy. (From Oomen HAPC: Vitamin A deficiency, xerophthalmia and blindness, *Nutr Rev* 6:161–166, 1974.)

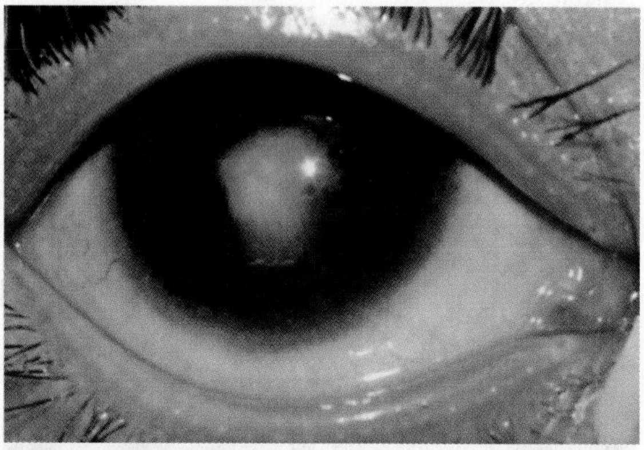

Figure 45-3 Recovery from xerophthalmia, showing a permanent eye lesion. (From Bloch CE: Blindness and other disease arising from deficient nutrition [lack of fat soluble A factor], *Am J Dis Child* 27:139, 1924.)

epithelium degenerates, the rods and cones have no support and eventually break down, resulting in blindness. Advanced xerophthalmia is shown in Figure 45-2, and xerophthalmia with permanent damage to the eye is shown in Figure 45-3. These eye lesions are primarily diseases of the young and are a major cause of blindness in developing countries.

Other clinical signs of vitamin A deficiency include poor overall growth, diarrhea, susceptibility to infections, anemia, apathy, mental retardation, and increased intracranial pressure, with wide separation of the cranial bones at the sutures. There may be vision problems due to bone overgrowth causing pressure on the optic nerve.

Diagnosis

Dark adaptation tests can be used to assess early-stage vitamin A deficiency. Although Bitot spots develop early, those related to active vitamin A deficiency are usually confined to preschool-aged children. Xerophthalmia is a very characteristic lesion of vitamin A deficiency. Caution must be exercised to exclude other, similar eye abnormalities from those associated with vitamin A deficiency. To detect marginal vitamin A status, there are 3 useful indicators: conjunctival impression cytology, relative dose response, and modified relative dose response. There is a relatively high prevalence of marginal vitamin A state among pregnant and lactating women. The plasma retinol level is not an accurate indicator of vitamin A status unless the deficiency is severe and liver stores are depleted. The range of normal vitamin A levels is 20-60 μg/dL; a level <20 μg/dL occurs in deficiency.

Prevention

The daily recommended dietary allowance (RDA) is expressed as retinol activity equivalents (RAEs; 1 RAE = 1 μg all-*trans*-retinol; equivalents for provitamin-A in foods = 12 μg β-carotene, 24 μg α-carotene, or 24 μg β-cryptoxanthin). The RAE for infants 0-1 yr of age is 400-500 μg; for children 3 yr of age is 300 μg; for children 4-8 yr of age is 400 μg; for children 9-13 yr of age is 600 μg; for boys 14-18 yr of age and men is 900 μg; and for girls 14-18 of age and women is 700 μg (also see Table 41-8). During pregnancy, the RDA is 750-770 μg, and during lactation, the RDA is increased to 1,200-1,300 μg to ensure sufficient vitamin A content during breast-feeding. A daily tolerable upper level of vitamin A for adults is 3,000 μg of preformed vitamin A. Approximately 80% of dietary vitamin A is absorbed as long as the meal contains some fat (>10 g). Low-fat diets may need to be supplemented with vitamin A. In disorders with poor fat absorption or increased excretion of vitamin A, water-miscible preparations should be administered in amounts higher than the RDAs. Premature infants have poor lipid absorption and thus should receive water-miscible vitamin A and be monitored closely.

Epidemiology and Public Health Issues

Vitamin A deficiency and xerophthalmia occur throughout much of the developing world and are linked to undernourishment and complicated by illness. More than 350,000 cases of childhood blindness are reported annually due to severe vitamin A deficiency. Because maternal vitamin A status is reflected in the vitamin A content of breast milk, intervention trials are ongoing with mothers of breast-fed infants living in regions where vitamin A deficiency is common. In these trials, 2 doses of 200,000 IU (60 mg) each of vitamin A are given to the mother immediately after delivery, and the infant is given 3 doses of 25,000 IU (7.5 mg) each of vitamin A at 1-3 mo of age (1 IU = 0.3 μg retinol).

Treatment

The safety and efficacy of vitamin A supplementation depend on the patient's state of health and the regimens of other treatments. A daily supplement of 1,500 μg of vitamin A is sufficient for treating latent vitamin A deficiency. In children without overt vitamin A deficiency, morbidity and mortality rates from viral infections such as measles can be lowered by daily administration of 1,500-3,000 μg of vitamin A, under careful monitoring to avoid toxicity associated with excess vitamin A. Xerophthalmia is treated by giving 1,500 μg/kg body weight orally for 5 days followed by intramuscular injection of 7,500 μg of vitamin A in oil, until recovery.

HYPERVITAMINOSIS A

Chronic hypervitaminosis A results from excessive ingestion of vitamin A for several weeks or months. Toxicity can be induced in adults and children with chronic daily intakes of 15,000 μg and 6,000 μg, respectively. Symptoms subside rapidly on withdrawal of the vitamin. Signs of subacute or chronic toxicity can include headache; vomiting; anorexia; dry, itchy desquamating skin; seborrheic cutaneous lesions; fissuring at the corners of the mouth; alopecia and/or coarsening of the hair; bone abnormalities; swelling of the bones; enlargement of the liver and spleen; diplopia; increased intracranial pressure; irritability; stupor; limited motion; and dryness of the mucous membranes. In addition, desquamation of the palms and the soles of the feet is common. Radiographs show **hyperostosis** affecting several long bones, especially in the middle of the shafts (Fig. 45-4). Serum levels of vitamin A are elevated. Hypercalcemia and/or liver cirrhosis may be present. Hypervitaminosis A is distinct from cortical hyperostosis (Chapter 691).

In young children, toxicity is associated with vomiting and bulging fontanels. An affected child has anorexia, pruritus, and a lack of weight gain. Acute hypervitaminosis A toxicity has

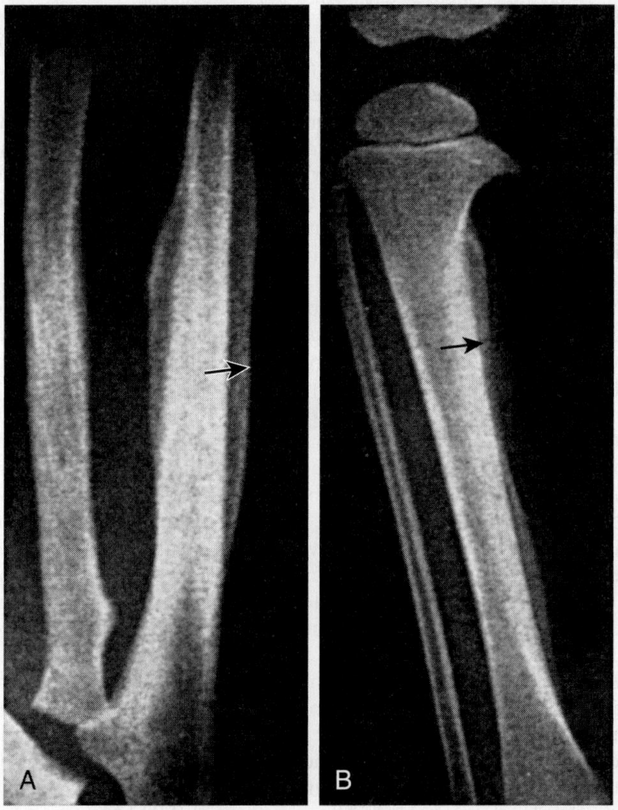

Figure 45-4 Hyperostosis of the ulna and tibia in an infant 21 mo of age, resulting from vitamin A positioning. *A,* Long, wavy cortical hyperostosis of the ulna *(arrow). B,* Long, wavy cortical hyperostosis of the right tibia *(arrow),* with a striking absence of metaphyseal changes. (From Caffey J: *Pediatric x-ray diagnosis,* ed 5, Chicago, 1967, Year Book, p 994.)

occurred in infants in developing countries after ingestion of very large amounts of vitamin A during vaccine administration. Symptoms include nausea, vomiting, and drowsiness; less-common symptoms include diplopia, papilledema, cranial nerve palsies, and other symptoms suggesting **pseudotumor cerebri.** Severe congenital malformations occur in infants of mothers who consumed therapeutic doses (0.5-1.5 mg/kg) of oral 13-*cis*-retinoic acid during the 1st trimester of pregnancy for treatment of acne or cancer. These malformations result in a high incidence (>20%) of spontaneous abortions and birth defects.

Excessive intake of carotenoids is not associated with toxicity but can cause yellow coloration of the skin that disappears when intake is reduced; this disorder (carotenemia) is especially likely to occur in children with liver disease, diabetes mellitus, or hypothyroidism and in those who do not have enzymes that metabolize carotenoids.

BIBLIOGRAPHY

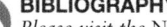

Please visit the Nelson Textbook of Pediatrics *website at www.expertconsult.com for the complete bibliography.*

Chapter 46
Vitamin B Complex Deficiency and Excess

H.P.S. Sachdev and Dheeraj Shah

Vitamin B complex includes a number of water soluble nutrients, including thiamine (B_1), riboflavin (B_2), niacin (B_3), pyridoxine (B_6), folate, cobalamin (B_{12}), biotin, and pantothenic acid. Choline and inositol are also considered part of the B complex and are important for normal body functions, but specific deficiency syndromes have not been attributed to a lack of these factors in the diet.

B-complex vitamins serve as coenzymes in many metabolic pathways that are functionally closely related. Consequently, a lack of one of the vitamins has the potential to interrupt a chain of chemical processes, including reactions that are dependent on other vitamins, and ultimately can produce diverse clinical manifestations. Because diets deficient in any one of the B-complex vitamins are often poor sources of other B vitamins, manifestations of several vitamin B deficiencies usually can be observed in the same person. It is therefore a general practice in a patient who has evidence of deficiency of a specific B vitamin to treat with the entire B-complex group of vitamins.

46.1 Thiamine (Vitamin B_1)

H.P.S. Sachdev and Dheeraj Shah

Thiamine (vitamin B_1) consists of thiazole and pyrimidine rings joined by a methylene bridge. Thiamine diphosphate, the active form of thiamine, serves as a cofactor for several enzymes involved in carbohydrate catabolism such as pyruvate dehydrogenase, transketolase, and α-ketoglutarate. These enzymes also play a role in the hexose monophosphate shunt that generates nicotinamide adenine dinucleotide phosphate (NADP) and pentose for nucleic acid synthesis. Thiamine is also required for the synthesis of acetylcholine and gamma-aminobutyric acid (GABA), which have important roles in nerve conduction. Thiamine is absorbed efficiently in the gastrointestinal (GI) tract, and may be deficient in persons with GI or liver disease. The requirement of thiamine is increased when carbohydrates are taken in large amounts and during periods of increased metabolism, for example, fever, muscular activity, hyperthyroidism, and pregnancy and lactation. Alcohol affects various aspects of thiamine transport and uptake, contributing to the deficiency in alcoholics.

Pork (especially lean), fish, and poultry are good nonvegetarian **dietary sources** of thiamine. Main sources of thiamine for vegetarians are rice, oat, wheat, and legumes. Most ready-to-eat breakfast cereals are enriched with thiamine. Thiamine is water soluble and heat-labile; most of the vitamin is lost when the rice is repeatedly washed and the cooking water is discarded. The breast milk of a well-nourished mother provides adequate thiamine; breast-fed infants of thiamine-deficient mothers are at risk for deficiency. Most infants and older children consuming a balanced diet obtain an adequate intake of thiamine from food and do not require supplements.

DEFICIENCY

Deficiency of thiamine is associated with severely malnourished states, including malignancy and following surgery. The disorder (or spectrum of disorders) is classically associated with a diet consisting largely of polished rice (oriental beriberi), it can also arise if highly refined wheat flour forms a major part of the diet, in alcoholics, and in food faddists (occidental beriberi). Thiamine deficiency has often been reported from inhabitants of refugee camps consuming the polished rice–based monotonous diets. **Thiamine-responsive megaloblastic anemia (TRMA) syndrome** is a rare autosomal recessive disorder characterized by megaloblastic anemia, diabetes mellitus, and sensorineural deafness, responding in varying degrees to thiamine treatment. The syndrome occurs because of mutations in the *SLC19A2* gene, encoding a thiamine transporter protein, leading to abnormal thiamine transportation and vitamin deficiency in the cells. Thiamine and related vitamins can improve the outcome in children with Leigh encephalomyelopathy and type 1 diabetes mellitus.

Clinical Manifestations

Thiamine deficiency can develop within 2-3 mo of a deficient intake. Early symptoms of thiamine deficiency are nonspecific such as fatigue, apathy, irritability, depression, drowsiness, poor mental concentration, anorexia, nausea, and abdominal discomfort. As the condition progresses, more-specific manifestations of **beriberi** such as peripheral neuritis (manifesting as tingling, burning, paresthesias of the toes and feet), decreased deep tendon reflexes, loss of vibration sense, tenderness and cramping of the leg muscles, congestive heart failure, and psychic disturbances develop. Patients can have ptosis of the eyelids and atrophy of the optic nerve. Hoarseness or aphonia caused by paralysis of the laryngeal nerve is a characteristic sign. Muscle atrophy and tenderness of the nerve trunks are followed by ataxia, loss of coordination, and loss of deep sensation. Later signs include increased intracranial pressure, meningismus, and coma. The clinical picture of thiamine deficiency is usually divided into a **dry (neuritic) type** and a **wet (cardiac) type**. The disease is wet or dry depending on the amount of fluid that accumulates in the body due to factors such as cardiac and renal dysfunction, even though the exact cause for this edema has not been explained. Many cases of thiamine deficiency show a mixture of the 2 main features and are more properly termed *thiamine deficiency with cardiopathy* and *peripheral neuropathy*.

The classic clinical triad of **Wernicke encephalopathy** (mental status changes, ocular signs, ataxia) is rarely reported in infants and young children with severe deficiency secondary to malignancies or feeding of defective formula. An epidemic of life-threatening thiamine deficiency was seen in infants fed a defective soy-based formula that had undetectable thiamine levels. Manifestations included emesis, lethargy, restlessness, ophthalmoplegia, abdominal distention, developmental delay, failure to thrive, lactic acidosis, nystagmus, diarrhea, apnea, and seizures. Intercurrent illnesses that resembled Wernicke encephalopathy often precipitated the symptoms.

Death from thiamine deficiency usually is secondary to cardiac involvement. The initial signs are slight cyanosis and dyspnea, but tachycardia, enlargement of the liver, loss of consciousness, and convulsions can develop rapidly. The heart, especially the right side, is enlarged. The electrocardiogram shows an increased Q-T interval, inverted T waves, and low voltage. These changes as well as the cardiomegaly rapidly revert to normal with treatment, but without prompt treatment, cardiac failure can develop rapidly and result in death. In fatal cases of beriberi, lesions are located principally in the heart, peripheral nerves, subcutaneous tissue, and serous cavities. The heart is dilated, and fatty degeneration of the myocardium is common. Generalized edema or edema of the legs, serous effusions, and venous engorgement are often present. Degeneration of myelin and axon cylinders of the peripheral nerves, with wallerian degeneration beginning in the distal locations, also is common, particularly in the lower extremities. Lesions in the brain include vascular dilation and hemorrhage.

Diagnosis

The diagnosis is often suspected on the basis of clinical setting and compatible symptoms. Objective biochemical tests of thiamine status include measurement of erythrocyte transketolase activity (ETKA) and the thiamine pyrophosphate effect (TPPE). The biochemical diagnostic criteria of thiamine deficiency consist of low ETKA and high TPPE (normal range, 0-14%). Urinary excretion of thiamine or its metabolites (thiazole or pyrimidine) after an oral loading dose of thiamine may also be measured to help identify the deficiency state. MRI changes of thiamine deficiency in infants are characterized by bilateral symmetric hyperintensities of the frontal lobes and basal ganglia, in addition to the lesions in the periaqueductal region, thalami, and the mammillary bodies described in adults.

Prevention

A maternal diet containing sufficient amounts of thiamine prevents thiamine deficiency in breast-fed infants, and infant formulas marketed in all developed countries provide recommended levels of intake. During complementary feeding, adequate thiamine intake can be achieved with a varied diet that includes meat and enriched or whole-grain cereals. When the staple cereal is polished rice, special efforts need to be made to include legumes and/or nuts in the ration. Thiamine and other vitamins can be retained in rice by parboiling, a process of steaming the rice in the husk before milling. Improvement in cooking techniques, such as not discarding the water used for cooking, minimal washing of grains, and reduction of cooking time help to minimize the thiamine losses during the preparation of food.

Treatment

In the absence of GI disturbances, oral administration of thiamine is effective. Children with cardiac failure, convulsions, or coma should be given 10 mg of thiamine intramuscularly or intravenously daily for the 1st week. This treatment should then be followed by 3-5 mg of thiamine per day orally for at least 6 wk. The response is dramatic in infants and in those having predominantly cardiovascular manifestations, whereas the neurologic response is slow and often incomplete. Patients with beriberi often have other B-complex vitamin deficiencies; therefore, all other B-complex vitamins should also be administered. Treatment of TRMA and other dependency states require higher dosages (100-200 mg/day). The anemia responds well to thiamine administration, and insulin for associated diabetes mellitus can also be discontinued in many cases of TRMA.

TOXICITY

There are no reports of adverse effects from consumption of excess thiamine by ingestion of food or supplements. A few isolated cases of pruritus and anaphylaxis have been reported in patients after parenteral administration of the vitamin.

BIBLIOGRAPHY

Please visit the Nelson Textbook of Pediatrics *website at www.expertconsult.com for the complete bibliography.*

46.2 Riboflavin (Vitamin B_2)

H.P.S. Sachdev and Dheeraj Shah

Riboflavin is part of the structure of the coenzymes flavin adenine dinucleotide (FAD) and flavin mononucleotide, which participate in oxidation-reduction reactions in numerous metabolic pathways and in energy production via the mitochondrial respiratory chain. Riboflavin is stable to heat but is destroyed by light.

Milk, eggs, organ meats, legumes, and mushrooms are rich **dietary sources** of riboflavin. Most commercial cereals, flours, and breads are enriched with riboflavin.

DEFICIENCY

The causes of riboflavin deficiency are mainly related to malnourished and malabsorptive states, including GI infections. Treatment with some drugs, such as probenecid, phenothiazine, or oral contraceptives, can also cause the deficiency. The side chain of the vitamin is photochemically destroyed during phototherapy for hyperbilirubinemia, as it is involved in the photosensitized oxidation of bilirubin to more polar excretable compounds. Isolated **complex II deficiency**, a rare mitochondrial disease manifesting in infancy and childhood, responds favorably to riboflavin supplementation and thus can be termed a dependency state.

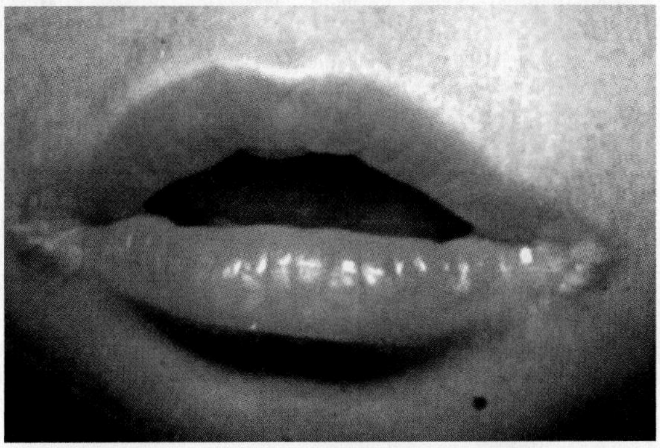

Figure 46-1 Angular cheilosis with ulceration and crusting. (Courtesy of National Institute of Nutrition, Indian Council of Medical Research, Hyderabad, India.)

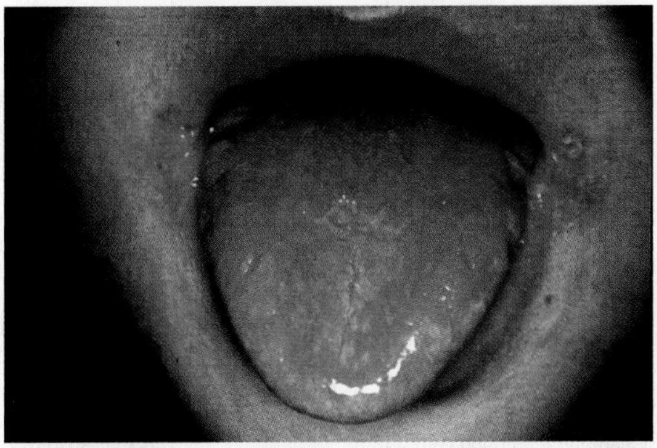

Figure 46-2 Glossitis as seen in riboflavin deficiency. (From Zappe HA, Nuss S, Becker K, et al: *Riboflavin deficiency in baltistan* (website). www.rzuser.uni-heidelberg.de/%7Ecn6/baltista/ribofl_e.htm. Accessed May 23, 2010.)

Clinical Manifestations

Clinical features of riboflavin deficiency include cheilosis, glossitis, keratitis, conjunctivitis, photophobia, lacrimation, corneal vascularization, and seborrheic dermatitis. Cheilosis begins with pallor at the angles of the mouth and progresses to thinning and maceration of the epithelium, leading to fissures extending radially into the skin (Fig. 46-1). In glossitis, the tongue becomes smooth, with loss of papillary structure (Fig. 46-2). Normochromic, normocytic anemia may also be seen because of the impaired erythropoiesis. A low riboflavin content of the maternal diet has been linked to congenital heart defects, but the evidence is weak.

Diagnosis

Most often, the diagnosis is based on the clinical features of angular cheilosis in a malnourished child, which responds promptly to riboflavin supplementation. A functional test of riboflavin status is done by measuring the activity of erythrocyte glutathione reductase (EGR), with and without the addition of FAD. An EGR activity coefficient (ratio of EGR activity with added FAD to EGR activity without FAD) of >1.4 is used as an indicator of deficiency. Urinary excretion of riboflavin <30 μg/24 hr also suggests low intakes.

Prevention

The recommended daily allowance (RDA) of riboflavin for infants, children and adolescents is presented in Table 46-1. Adequate consumption of milk, milk products, and eggs prevents riboflavin deficiency. Fortification of cereal products is helpful for those who follow vegan diets or are consuming inadequate amounts of milk products because of other reasons.

Treatment

Treatment includes oral administration of 3-10 mg/day of riboflavin, often as an ingredient of a vitamin B-complex mix. The child should also be given a well-balanced diet, including milk and milk products.

TOXICITY

No adverse effects associated with riboflavin intakes from food or supplements have been reported, and the upper safe limit for consumption has not been established. Though the photosensitizing property of this vitamin raises the possibility for some potential risks, limited absorption in high-intake situations precludes such concerns.

BIBLIOGRAPHY

Please visit the Nelson Textbook of Pediatrics *website at www.expertconsult.com for the complete bibliography.*

46.3 Niacin (Vitamin B_3)

H.P.S. Sachdev and Dheeraj Shah

Niacin (nicotinamide or nicotinic acid) forms part of 2 cofactors, nicotinamide adenine dinucleotide (NAD) and NADP, which are important in several biologic reactions, including the respiratory chain, fatty acid and steroid synthesis, cell differentiation, and DNA processing. Niacin is rapidly absorbed from the stomach and the intestines and can also be synthesized from tryptophan in the diet.

Major **dietary sources** of niacin are meat, fish, and poultry for nonvegetarians and cereals, legumes, and green leafy vegetables for vegetarians. Enriched and fortified cereal products and legumes also are major contributors to niacin intake. Milk and eggs contain little niacin but are good sources of tryptophan, which can be converted to NAD (60 mg tryptophan = 1 mg niacin).

DEFICIENCY

Pellagra, the classic niacin deficiency disease, occurs chiefly in populations where corn (maize), a poor source of tryptophan, is the major foodstuff. A severe dietary imbalance such as in anorexia nervosa and in war or famine conditions also can cause pellagra. Pellagra can also develop in conditions associated with disturbed tryptophan metabolism such as carcinoid syndrome and Hartnup's disease.

Clinical Manifestations

The early symptoms of pellagra are vague: anorexia, lassitude, weakness, burning sensations, numbness, and dizziness. After a long period of deficiency, the classic triad of dermatitis, diarrhea, and dementia appears. **Dermatitis,** the most characteristic manifestation of pellagra, can develop suddenly or insidiously and may be initiated by irritants, including intense sunlight. The lesions first appear as symmetric areas of erythema on exposed surfaces, resembling sunburn, and might go unrecognized. The lesions are usually sharply demarcated from the surrounding healthy skin, and their distribution can change frequently. The lesions on the hands and feet often have the appearance of a glove or stocking (Fig. 46-3). Similar demarcations can also occur around the neck (Casal necklace) (see Fig. 46-3). In some cases, vesicles and bullae develop (wet type). In others, there may be suppuration beneath the scaly, crusted epidermis, and in still others, the swelling can disappear after a short time, followed by desquamation (Fig. 46-4). The healed parts of the skin might remain pigmented. The cutaneous lesions may be preceded by or accompanied by stomatitis, glossitis, vomiting, and/or diarrhea. Swelling and redness of the tip of the tongue and its lateral margins is often followed by intense redness, even ulceration, of

Table 46-1 WATER-SOLUBLE VITAMINS

NAMES AND SYNONYMS	BIOCHEMICAL ACTION	EFFECTS OF DEFICIENCY	TREATMENT OF DEFICIENCY	CAUSES OF DEFICIENCY	DIETARY SOURCES	RDA*
Thiamine (vitamin B_1)	Coenzyme in carbohydrate metabolism Nucleic acid synthesis Neurotransmitter synthesis	Neurologic (dry beriberi): Irritability, peripheral neuritis, muscle tenderness, ataxia Cardiac (wet beriberi): tachycardia, edema, cardiomegaly, cardiac failure	3-5 mg/day PO thiamine for 6 wk	Polished rice–based diets Malabsorptve states Severe malnutrition Malignancies Alcoholism	Meat, especially pork; fish; liver Rice (unmilled), wheat germ; enriched cereals; legumes	0-6 mo: 0.2 mg/day 7-12 mo: 0.3 mg/day 1-3 yr: 0.5 mg/day 4-8 yr: 0.6 mg/day 9-13 yr: 0.9 mg/day 14-18 yr: Girls: 1.0 mg/day Boys: 1.2 mg/day
Riboflavin (vitamin B_2)	Constituent of flavoprotein enzymes important in oxidation-reduction reactions: amino acid, fatty acid, and carbohydrate metabolism and cellular respiration	Glossitis, photophobia, lacrimation, corneal vascularization, poor growth, cheilosis	3-10 mg/day PO riboflavin	Severe malnutrition Malabsorptive states Prolonged treatment with phenothiazines, probenecid, or OCPs	Milk, milk products, eggs, fortified cereals, green vegetables	0-6 mo: 0.3 mg/day 7-12 mo: 0.4 mg/day 1-3 yr: 0.5 mg/day 4-8 yr: 0.6 mg/day 9-13 yr: 0.9 mg/day 14-18 yr: Girls: 1.0 mg/day Boys: 1.3 mg/day
Niacin (vitamin B_3)	Constituent of NAD and NADP, important in respiratory chain, fatty acid synthesis, cell differentiation, and DNA processing	Pellagra manifesting as diarrhea, symmetric scaly dermatitis in sun-exposed areas, and neurologic symptoms of disorientation and delirium	50-300 mg/day PO niacin	Predominantly maize-based diets Anorexia nervosa Carcinoid syndrome	Meat, fish, poultry Cereals, legumes, green vegetables	0-6 mo: 2 mg/day 7-12 mo: 4 mg/day 1-3 yr: 6 mg/day 4-8 yr: 8 mg/day 9-13 yr: 12 mg/day 14-18 yr: Girls: 14 mg/day Boys: 16 mg/day
Pyridoxine (vitamin B_6)	Constituent of coenzymes for amino acid and glycogen metabolism, heme synthesis, steroid action, neurotransmitter synthesis	Irritability, convulsions, hypochromic anemia Failure to thrive Oxaluria	5-25 mg/day PO for deficiency states 100 mg IM or IV for pyridoxine-dependent seizures	Prolonged treatment with INH, penicillamine, OCPs	Fortified ready-to-eat cereals, meat, fish, poultry, liver, bananas, rice. potatoes	0-6 mo: 0.1 mg/day 7-12 mo: 0.3 mg/day 1-3 yr: 0.5 mg/day 4-8 yr: 0.6 mg/day 9-13 yr: 1.0 mg/day 14-18 yr: Girls: 1.2 mg/day Boys: 1.3 mg/day
Biotin	Cofactor for carboxylases, important in gluconeogenesis, fatty acid and amino acid metabolism	Scaly periorificial dermatitis, conjunctivitis, alopecia, lethargy, hypotonia and withdrawn behavior	1-10 mg/day PO biotin	Consumption of raw eggs for prolonged periods Parenteral nutrition with infusates lacking biotin Valproate therapy	Liver, organ meats, fruits	0-6 mo: 5 µg/day 7-12 mo: 6 µg/day 1-3 yr: 8 µg/day 4-8 yr: 12 µg/day 9-13 yr: 20 µg/day 14-18 yr: 25 µg/day
Pantothenic acid (vitamin B_5)	Component of coenzyme A and acyl carrier protein involved in fatty acid metabolism	Experimentally produced deficiency in humans: irritability, fatigue, numbness, paresthesias (burning feet syndrome), muscle cramps		Isolated deficiency extremely rare in humans	Beef, organ meats, poultry, seafood, egg yolk Yeast, soybeans, mushrooms	0-6 mo: 1.7 mg/day 7-12 mo: 1.8 mg/day 1-3 yr: 2 mg/day 4-8 yr: 3 mg/day 9-13 yr: 4 mg/day 14-18 yr: 5 mg/day
Folic acid	Coenzymes in amino acid and nucleotide metabolism as an acceptor and donor of one-carbon units	Megaloblastic anemia Growth retardation, glossitis Neural tube defects in progeny	0.5-1 mg/day PO folic acid	Malnutrition Malabsorptive states Malignancies Hemolytic anemias Anticonvulsant therapy	Enriched cereals, beans, leafy vegetables, citrus fruits, papaya	0-6 mo: 65 µg/day 7-12 mo: 80 µg/day 1-3 yr: 150 µg/day 4-8 yr: 200 µg/day 9-13 yr: 300 µg/day 14-18 yr: 400 µg/day
Cobalamin (vitamin B_{12})	As deoxy-adenosylcobalamin, acts as cofactor for lipid and carbohydrate metabolism As methycobalamin, important for conversion of homocysteine to methionine and folic acid metabolism	Megaloblastic anemia, irritability, developmental delay, developmental regression, involuntary movements, hyperpigmentation	1,000 µg IM vitamin B_{12}	Vegan diets Malabsorptive states Crohn disease Intrinsic factor deficiency (pernicious anemia)	Organ meats, sea foods poultry, egg yolk, milk, fortified ready-to-eat cereals	0-6 mo: 0.4 µg/d 7-12 mo: 0.5 µg/d 1-3 yr: 0.9 µg/d 4-8 yr: 1.2 µg/d 9-13 yr: 1.8 µg/d 14-18 yr: 2.4 µg/d
Ascorbic acid (vitamin C)	Important for collagen synthesis, metabolism of cholesterol and neurotransmitters Antioxidant functions and nonheme iron absorption	Scurvy manifesting as irritability, tenderness and swelling of legs, bleeding gums, petechiae, ecchymoses, follicular hyperkeratosis, and poor wound healing	100-200 mg/day PO ascorbic acid for up to 3 mo	Predominantly milk-based (non–human milk) diets Severe malnutrition	Citrus fruits and fruit juices, peppers, berries, melons, tomatoes, cauliflower, leafy green vegetables	0-6 mo: 40 mg/day 7-12 mo: 50 mg/day 1-3 yr: 15 mg/day 4-8 yr: 25 mg/day 9-13 yr: 45 mg/day 14-18 yr: Girls: 65 mg/day Boys: 75 mg/day

*For healthy breast-fed infants, the values represent adequate intakes (AI), i.e., the mean intake of apparently "normal" infants.
INH, isoniazid; NAD, nicotinamide adenine dinucleotide ; NADP, nicotinamide adenine dinucleotide phosphate; OCP, oral contraceptive pill; RDA, recommended dietary allowance.

the entire tongue and the papillae. Nervous symptoms include depression, disorientation, insomnia, and delirium.

The classic symptoms of pellagra usually are not well developed in infants and young children, but anorexia, irritability, anxiety, and apathy are common. Young patients might also have sore tongues and lips and usually have dry and scaly skin. Diarrhea and constipation can alternate, and anemia can occur. Children who have pellagra often have evidence of other nutritional deficiency diseases.

Diagnosis

Because of lack of a good functional test to evaluate niacin status, the diagnosis of deficiency is usually made from the physical signs of glossitis, GI symptoms, and a symmetric dermatitis. Rapid clinical response to niacin is an important confirmatory test. A decrease in the concentration and/or a change in the proportion of the niacin metabolites N^1-methyl-nicotinamide (1-mn) and 2-pyridone (2-pyr) in the urine provide biochemical evidence of deficiency and can be seen before the appearance of overt signs of deficiency. Serum levels of NAD and NADP do not correlate well with clinical deficiency.

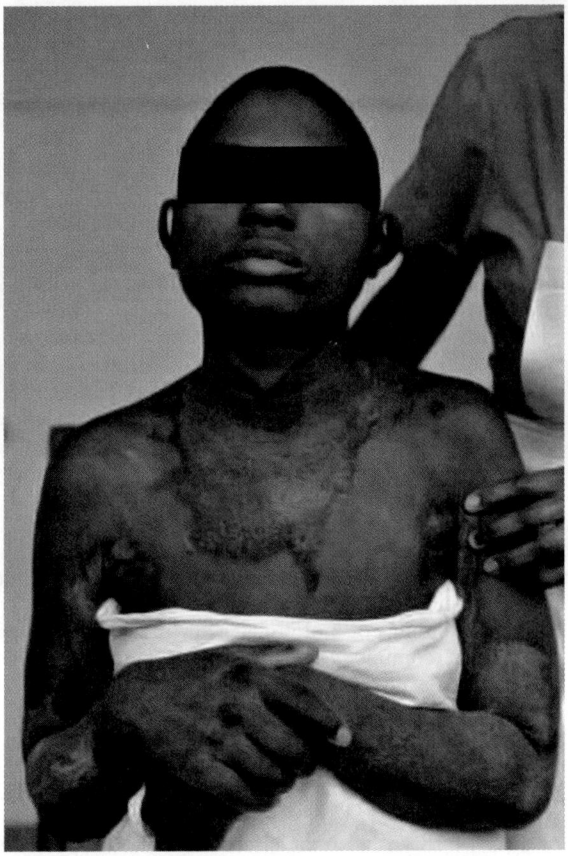

Figure 46-3 Characteristic skin lesions of pellagra on hands and lesions on the neck (Casal necklace). (Courtesy of Dr. J.D. MacLean, McGill Centre for Tropical Diseases, Montreal, Canada.)

Prevention

Adequate intakes of niacin are easily met by consumption of a diet that consists of a variety of foods and includes meat, eggs, milk, and enriched or fortified cereal products. The dietary reference intake (DRI) is expressed in mg niacin equivalents (NE) in which 1 mg NE = 1 mg niacin or 60 mg tryptophan. An intake of 2 mg of niacin is considered adequate for infants 0-6 mo of age; and 4 mg is adequate for infants 7-12 mo of age. For older children, the recommended intakes are 6 mg for 1-3 yr of age, 8 mg for 4-8 yr of age, 12 mg for 9-13 yr of age, and 14-16 mg for 14-18 yr of age.

Treatment

Children usually respond rapidly to treatment. A liberal and varied diet should be supplemented with 50-300 mg/day of niacin; in severe cases or in patients with poor intestinal absorption, 100 mg may be given intravenously. The diet should also be supplemented with other vitamins, especially other B-complex vitamins. Sun exposure should be avoided during the active phase of pellagra, and the skin lesions may be covered with soothing applications. Other coexisting nutrient deficiencies such as iron deficiency anemia should be treated. Even after successful treatment, the diet should continue to be monitored to prevent recurrence.

TOXICITY

There are no toxic effects associated with the intake of naturally occurring niacin in foods. Shortly after the ingestion of large doses of nicotinic acid taken as a supplement or a pharmacologic agent, a person often experiences a burning, tingling, and itching sensation as well as flushing on the face, arms, and chest. Large doses of niacin also can have nonspecific GI effects and can cause cholestatic jaundice or hepatotoxicity. Tolerable upper intake levels for children are approximately double the recommended dietary allowance.

BIBLIOGRAPHY

Please visit the Nelson Textbook of Pediatrics *website at www.expertconsult.com for the complete bibliography.*

46.4 Vitamin B_6 (Pyridoxine)

H.P.S. Sachdev and Dheeraj Shah

Vitamin B_6 includes a group of closely related compounds: pyridoxine, pyridoxal, pyridoxamine, and their phosphorylated derivatives. Pyridoxal 5′-phosphate (PLP) and, to a lesser extent, pyridoxamine phosphate function as coenzymes for many enzymes involved in amino acid metabolism, neurotransmitter

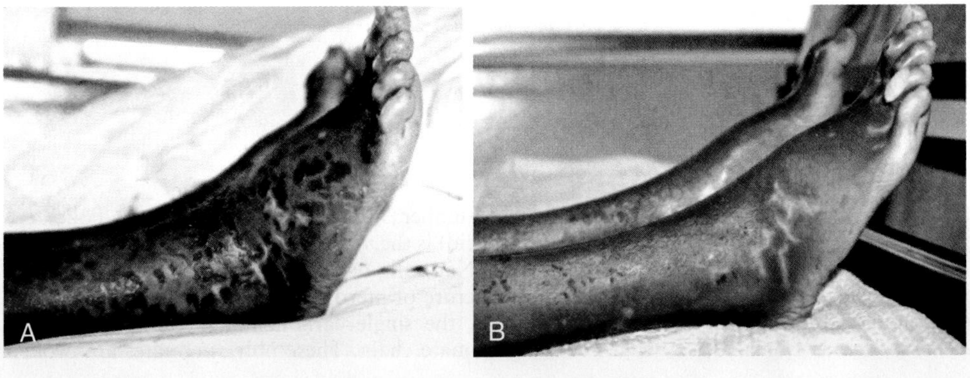

Figure 46-4 Clinical manifestations of niacin deficiency before *(A)* and after *(B)* therapy. (From Weinsier RL, Morgan SL: *Fundamentals of clinical nutrition*, St Louis, 1993, Mosby, p 99.)

synthesis, glycogen metabolism, and steroid action. If vitamin B_6 is lacking, glycine metabolism can lead to oxaluria. The major excretory product in the urine is 4-pyridoxic acid.

The vitamin B_6 content of human milk and infant formulas is adequate. Good **food sources** of the vitamin include fortified ready-to-eat cereals, meat, fish, poultry, liver, bananas, rice, and certain vegetables. Large losses of the vitamin can occur during high-temperature processing of foods or milling of cereals, whereas parboiling of rice prevents its loss.

DEFICIENCY

Because of the importance of vitamin B_6 in amino acid metabolism, high protein intakes can increase the requirement for the vitamin; the RDAs are sufficient to cover the expected range of protein intake in the population. The risk of deficiency is increased in persons taking medications that inhibit the activity of vitamin B_6 (isoniazid, penicillamine, corticosteroids, anticonvulsants), in young women taking oral progesterone-estrogen contraceptives, and in patients receiving maintenance dialysis.

Clinical Manifestations

The deficiency symptoms seen in infants are listlessness, irritability, seizures, vomiting, and failure to thrive. Peripheral neuritis is a feature of deficiency in adults but is not usually seen in children. Electroencephalogram (EEG) abnormalities have been reported in infants as well as in young adult subjects in controlled depletion studies. Skin lesions include cheilosis, glossitis, and seborrheic dermatitis around the eyes, nose, and mouth. Microcytic anemia can occur in infants but is not common. Oxaluria, oxalic acid bladder stones, hyperglycinemia, lymphopenia, decreased antibody formation, and infections also have been associated with vitamin B_6 deficiency.

Several types of vitamin B_6 **dependence syndromes,** presumably due to errors in enzyme structure or function, respond to very large amounts of pyridoxine (see Table 46-1). These syndromes include pyridoxine-dependent seizures, a vitamin B_6–responsive anemia, xanthurenic aciduria, cystathioninuria, and homocystinuria (Chapters 79, 448, and 586).

Diagnosis

The activity of the erythrocyte transaminases glutamic oxaloacetic transaminase and glutamic pyruvic transaminase is low in vitamin B_6 deficiency; tests measuring the activity of these enzymes before and after the addition of PLP may be useful as indicators of vitamin B_6 status. Abnormally high xanthurenic acid excretion after tryptophan ingestion also provides evidence of deficiency. Plasma PLP assays are being used more often, but factors other than deficiency can influence the results. Vitamin B_6 deficiency or dependence should be suspected in all infants with seizures. If more common causes of infantile seizures have been eliminated, 100 mg of pyridoxine can be injected, with EEG monitoring if possible. If the seizure stops, vitamin B_6 deficiency should be suspected. In older children, 100 mg of pyridoxine may be injected intramuscularly while the EEG is being recorded; a favorable response of the EEG suggests pyridoxine deficiency.

Prevention

Deficiency is unlikely in children consuming diets that meet their energy needs and contain a variety of foods. Parboiling of rice prevents the loss of vitamin B_6 from the grains. The DRIs for vitamin B_6 are 0.1 mg/day for infants up to 6 mo of age; 0.3 mg/day for ages 6 mo to 1 yr; 0.5 mg/day for ages 1-3 yr; 0.6 mg/day for ages 4-8 yr; 1.0 mg/day for ages 9-13 yr; and 1.2-1.3 mg/day for ages 14-18 yr. Infants whose mothers have received large doses of pyridoxine during pregnancy are at increased risk for seizures from pyridoxine dependence, and supplements during the 1st few weeks of life should be considered. Any child receiving a pyridoxine antagonist, such as isoniazid, should be carefully observed for neurologic manifestations; if these develop, vitamin B_6 should be administered or the dose of the antagonist should be decreased.

Treatment

Intramuscular or intravenous administration of 100 mg of pyridoxine is used to treat convulsions due to vitamin B_6 deficiency. One dose should be sufficient if adequate dietary intake follows. For pyridoxine-dependent children, daily doses of 2-10 mg intramuscularly or 10-100 mg orally may be necessary. Occasionally vitamin B_6 has been used in large doses along with magnesium in children said to have "autism"; the functional benefit of such intervention is minimal.

TOXICITY

Adverse effects have not been associated with high intakes of vitamin B_6 from food sources. However, ataxia and sensory neuropathy have been reported with dosages as low as 100 mg/day in adults taking vitamin B_6 supplements for several months.

BIBLIOGRAPHY

Please visit the Nelson Textbook of Pediatrics *website at www.expertconsult.com for the complete bibliography.*

46.5 Biotin

H.P.S. Sachdev and Dheeraj Shah

Biotin functions as a cofactor for enzymes involved in carboxylation reactions within and outside mitochondria. These biotin-dependent carboxylases catalyze key reactions in gluconeogenesis, fatty acid metabolism, and amino acid catabolism.

There is limited information on the biotin content of foods; it is believed to be widely distributed, thus making a deficiency unlikely. Avidin found in raw egg whites acts as a biotin antagonist. Signs of biotin deficiency have been demonstrated in persons who consume large amounts of raw egg whites over long periods. Deficiency also has been described in infants and children receiving enteral and parenteral nutrition infusates that lack biotin. Treatment with valproic acid may result in a low biotinidase activity and/or biotin deficiency.

The clinical findings of biotin deficiency include scaly periorificial dermatitis, conjunctivitis, thinning of hair, and alopecia. Central nervous system abnormalities seen with biotin deficiency are lethargy, hypotonia, and withdrawn behavior. Biotin deficiency can be successfully treated using 1-10 mg of biotin orally daily. The adequate dietary intake values for biotin are 5 μg/day for 0-6 mo, 6 μg/day for 7-12 mo, 8 μg/day for ages 1-3 yr, 12 μg/day for ages 4-8 yr, 20 μg/day for ages 9-13 yr, and 25 μg/day for ages 14-18 yr. No toxic effects have been reported with very high doses. Conditions involving deficiencies in the enzymes holocarboxylase synthetase and biotinidase that respond to treatment with biotin are described in Chapter 79.6.

BIBLIOGRAPHY

Please visit the Nelson Textbook of Pediatrics *website at www.expertconsult.com for the complete bibliography.*

46.6 Folate

H.P.S. Sachdev and Dheeraj Shah

Folate exists in a number of different chemical forms. Folic acid (pteroylglutamic acid) is the synthetic form used in fortified foods and supplements. Naturally occurring folates in foods retain the core chemical structure of pteroylglutamic acid but vary in their state of reduction, the single carbon moiety they bear, or the length of the glutamate chain. These polyglutamates are broken down and reduced in the small intestine to dihydro- and tetrahydrofolates, which are involved as coenzymes in amino acid and nucleotide metabolism as acceptors and donors of 1-carbon units.

Rice and cereals are rich **dietary sources** of folate, especially if enriched. Beans, leafy vegetables, and fruits such as oranges and papaya are good sources, too. The vitamin is readily absorbed from the small intestine and is broken down to monoglutamate derivatives by mucosal polyglutamate hydrolases. A high-affinity proton-coupled folate transporter (PCFT) seems to be essential for absorption of folate in intestine and in various cell types at low pH. The vitamin is also synthesized by the colonic bacteria, and the half-life of the vitamin is prolonged by enterohepatic recirculation.

DEFICIENCY

Because of its role in protein, DNA, and RNA synthesis, the risk of deficiency is increased during periods of rapid growth or increased cellular metabolism. Folate deficiency can result from poor nutrient content in diet, inadequate absorption (celiac disease, inflammatory bowel disease), increased requirement (sickle cell anemia, psoriasis, malignancies, periods of rapid growth as in infancy and adolescence), or inadequate utilization (long-term treatment with high-dose nonsteroidal anti-inflammatory drugs, anticonvulsants such as phenytoin and phenobarbital, and methotrexate). Rare causes of deficiency are hereditary folate malabsorption, inborn errors of folate metabolism (methylene tetrahydrofolate reductase, methionine synthase reductase, and glutamate formiminotransferase deficiencies), and cerebral folate deficiency. A loss-of-function mutation in the gene coding for proton-coupled folate transporter (PCFT) is the molecular basis for hereditary folate malabsorption. A high-affinity blocking autoantibody against the membrane-bound folate receptor in the choroid plexus preventing its transport across the blood-brain barrier is the likely cause of the infantile cerebral folate deficiency.

Clinical Manifestations

Folic acid deficiency results in megaloblastic anemia and hypersegmentation of neutrophils. Nonhematologic manifestations include glossitis, listlessness, and growth retardation not related to anemia. There is an association between low maternal folic acid status and neural tube defects, primarily spina bifida and anencephaly, and the role of periconceptional folic acid in their prevention is well established.

Hereditary folate malabsorption manifests at 1-3 mo of age with recurrent or chronic diarrhea, failure to thrive, oral ulcerations, neurologic deterioration, megaloblastic anemia, and opportunistic infections. Cerebral folate deficiency manifests at 4-6 mo of age with irritability, microcephaly, developmental delay, cerebellar ataxia, pyramidal tract signs, choreoathetosis, ballismus, seizures, and blindness due to optic atrophy. 5-Methyltetrahydrofolate levels are normal in serum and red blood cells (RBCs) but are markedly depressed in the cerebrospinal fluid (CSF).

Diagnosis

The diagnosis of folic acid deficiency anemia is made in the presence of macrocytosis along with low folate levels in serum and/or RBCs. Normal serum folic acid levels are 5-20 ng/mL; with deficiency, serum folic acid levels are <3 ng/mL. Levels of RBC folate are a better indicator of chronic deficiency. The normal RBC folate level is 150-600 ng/mL of packed cells. The bone marrow is hypercellular because of erythroid hyperplasia, and megaloblastic changes are prominent. Large, abnormal neutrophilic forms (giant metamyelocytes) with cytoplasmic vacuolation also are seen.

Cerebral folate deficiency is associated with low levels of 5-methyltetrahydrofolate in the CSF and normal folate levels in the plasma and red blood cells. Mutations in the PCFT gene are demonstrated in the hereditary folate malabsorption.

Prevention

Breast-fed infants have better folate nutriture than non–breast-fed infants throughout infancy. Consumption of folate-rich foods and food-fortification programs are important to ensure adequate intake in children and in women of childbearing age. The DRIs for folate are 65 µg of dietary folate equivalent (DFE) for infants 0-6 mo and 80 µg of DFE for infants aged between 6 and 12 mo. (1 DFE = 1 µg food folate = 0.6 µg of folate from fortified food or as a supplement consumed with food = 0.5 µg of a supplement taken on an empty stomach.) For older children, the DRIs are 150 µg of DFE for ages 1-3 yr; 200 µg of DFE for ages 4-8 yr; 300 µg of DFE for ages 9-13 yr; and 400 µg of DFE for ages 14-18 yr. Providing iron and folic acid tablets for prevention of anemia in children and pregnant women is a routine strategy in at-risk populations. Health-education programs increase women's knowledge and use of folate supplements to prevent birth defects.

Treatment

When the diagnosis of folate deficiency is established, folic acid may be administered orally or parenterally at 0.5-1.0 mg/day. Folic acid therapy should be continued for 3-4 wk or until a definite hematologic response has occurred. Maintenance therapy with 0.2 mg of folate is adequate. Prolonged treatment with oral folinic acid is required in cerebral folate deficiency, and the response may be incomplete. Treatment of hereditary folate malabsorption may be possible with intramuscular folinic acid; some patients may respond to high-dose oral folinic acid therapy.

TOXICITY

No adverse effects have been associated with consumption of the amounts of folate normally found in fortified foods. Excessive intake of folate supplements might obscure and potentially delay the diagnosis of vitamin B_{12} deficiency. Massive doses given by injection have the potential to cause neurotoxicity.

BIBLIOGRAPHY

Please visit the Nelson Textbook of Pediatrics *website at www.expertconsult.com for the complete bibliography.*

46.7 Vitamin B_{12} (Cobalamin)

H.P.S. Sachdev and Dheeraj Shah

Vitamin B_{12} in the form of deoxyadenosylcobalamin functions as a cofactor for isomerization of methylmalonyl-CoA to succinyl-CoA, an essential reaction in lipid and carbohydrate metabolism. Methylcobalamin is another circulating form of vitamin B_{12} and is essential for methyl group transfer during the conversion of homocysteine to methionine. This reaction also requires a folic acid cofactor and is important for protein and nucleic acid biosynthesis.

Dietary sources of vitamin B_{12} are almost exclusively from animal foods. Organ meats, muscle meats, sea foods (mollusks, oysters, fish), poultry, and egg yolk are rich sources. Fortified ready-to-eat cereals and milk and their products are the important sources of the vitamin for vegetarians. Human milk is an adequate source for breast-feeding infants if the maternal serum B_{12} levels are adequate. The vitamin is absorbed from ileum at alkaline pH after binding with intrinsic factor. Enterohepatic circulation, direct absorption, and synthesis by intestinal bacteria are additional mechanisms helping to maintain the vitamin B_{12} nutriture.

DEFICIENCY

Vitamin B_{12} deficiency due to inadequate dietary intake occurs primarily in persons consuming strict vegetarian or vegan diets. Prevalence of vitamin B_{12} deficiency is high in predominantly vegetarian or lacto-vegetarian populations. Malabsorption of B_{12}

occurs in pernicious anemia due to intrinsic factor deficiency, and in ileal resections and Crohn disease. Breast-feeding infants of B_{12}-deficient mothers are also at risk for significant deficiency. Newborn metabolic screening can detect high levels of methylmalonic acid in the neonate's blood spot, which suggests maternal and neonatal B_{12} deficiencies.

Clinical Manifestations

The hematologic manifestations of vitamin B_{12} deficiency are similar to manifestations of folate deficiency and are discussed in Chapter 448.2. Irritability, hypotonia, developmental delay, developmental regression, and involuntary movements are the common neurologic symptoms in infants and children, whereas sensory deficits, paresthesias, and peripheral neuritis are seen in adults. Hyperpigmentation of the knuckles and palms is another common observation with B_{12} deficiency in children.

Diagnosis

See Chapter 448.2.

Treatment

The hematologic symptoms respond promptly to parenteral administration of 1,000 µg vitamin B_{12}. Oral administration has also been found to be equally effective in achieving hematologic and neurologic responses in adults, but the data are inadequate in children.

Prevention

The DRIs are 0.4 µg/day at age 0-6 mo, 0.5 µg/day at age 6-12 mo, 0.9 µg/day at age 1-3 yr, 1.2 µg/day at age 4-8 yr, 1.8 µg/day at age 9-13 yr, 2.4 µg/day at age 14-18 yr and in adults, 2.6 µg/day in pregnancy, and 2.8 µg/day in lactation. Pregnant and breastfeeding women should ensure an adequate consumption of animal products to prevent the deficiency in infants. Food fortification with the vitamin helps to prevent deficiency in predominantly vegetarian populations.

BIBLIOGRAPHY

Please visit the Nelson Textbook of Pediatrics *website at www.expertconsult.com for the complete bibliography.*

Chapter 47
Vitamin C (Ascorbic Acid)

Dheeraj Shah and H.P.S. Sachdev

Vitamin C is important for synthesis of collagen at the level of hydroxylation of lysine and proline in precollagen. It is also involved in neurotransmitter metabolism (conversion of dopamine to norepinephrine and tryptophan to serotonin), cholesterol metabolism (conversion of cholesterol to steroid hormones and bile acids), and the biosynthesis of carnitine. In these reactions, vitamin C functions to maintain the iron and copper atoms, cofactors of the metalloenzymes, in a reduced (active) state. Vitamin C is an important antioxidant (electron donor) in the aqueous milieu of the body. This function of ascorbic acid may be important in preventing degenerative diseases, cardiovascular diseases, and some cancers. Vitamin C enhances nonheme iron absorption, the transfer of iron from transferrin to ferritin, and the formation of tetrahydrofolic acid and thus can affect the cellular and immunologic functions of the hematopoietic system.

DIETARY NEEDS AND SOURCES

Humans depend on dietary sources for vitamin C. An adequate intake is 40 mg for age 0-6 mo and 50 mg for age 6-12 mo. For older children, the RDA is 15 mg for age 1-3 yr, 25 mg for age 4-8 yr, 45 mg for age 9-13 yr, and 65-75 mg for age 14-18 yr. The RDAs during pregnancy and lactation are 85 mg/day and 120 mg/day, respectively. The requirement for vitamin C is increased during infectious and diarrheal diseases. Children exposed to smoking or environmental tobacco smoke also require increased amounts of foods rich in vitamin C. The best food sources of vitamin C are citrus fruits and fruit juices, peppers, berries, melons, tomatoes, cauliflower, and green leafy vegetables. Vitamin C is easily destroyed by prolonged storage, overcooking, and processing of foods.

Absorption of vitamin C occurs in the upper small intestine by an active process or by simple diffusion when large amounts are ingested. Vitamin C is not stored in the body but is taken up by all tissues; the highest levels are found in the pituitary and adrenal glands. The brain ascorbate content in the fetus and neonate is many-fold higher than the content in the adult brain, a finding probably related to its function in neurotransmitter synthesis.

When a mother's intake of vitamin C during pregnancy and lactation is adequate, the newborn will have adequate tissue levels of vitamin C related to active placental transfer, subsequently maintained by the vitamin C in breast milk or commercial infant formulas. Breast milk contains sufficient vitamin C to prevent deficiency throughout infancy. Infants consuming pasteurized or boiled animal milk are at significant risk of developing deficiency if the other sources of vitamin C are also lacking in the diet. Neonates whose feeding has been delayed because of clinical condition can also suffer from ascorbic acid deficiency. For patients on total parenteral nutrition (TPN), a parenteral dose of 80 mg/day is recommended for full-term infants and a parenteral dose of 25 mg/kg/day is recommended for preterm infants.

DEFICIENCY

A deficiency of vitamin C results in the clinical presentation of **scurvy**, the oldest nutritional deficiency disease to be recognized. Children fed predominantly heat-treated (ultra-high-temperature or pasteurized) milk or unfortified formulas and not receiving fruits and fruit juices are at significant risk for symptomatic disease. In scurvy, there is defective formation of connective tissues and collagen in skin, cartilage, dentine, bone, and blood vessels, leading to their fragility. In the long bones, osteoid is not deposited by osteoblasts, cortex is thin, and the trabeculae become brittle and fracture easily.

Clinical Features

The early manifestations are irritability, loss of appetite, low-grade fever, and tenderness in the legs. These signs and symptoms are followed by leg swelling—most marked at the knees and the ankles—and pseudoparalysis. The infant might lie in the "pithed frog" position, with the hips and knees semiflexed and the feet rotated outward. Subperiosteal hemorrhages in the lower limb bones sometimes acutely increase the swelling and pain, and the condition might mimic acute osteomyelitis or arthritis. A "rosary" at the costochondral junctions and depression of the sternum are other typical features (Fig. 47-1). The angulation of scorbutic beads is usually sharper than the angulation of a rachitic rosary. Gum changes are seen in older children after teeth have erupted and are manifested as bluish purple, spongy swellings of the mucous membrane, especially over the upper incisors (Fig. 47-2). Anemia, a common finding in infants and young children with scurvy, is related to impaired iron absorption and coexistent hematopoietic nutrient deficiencies including iron, vitamin B_{12}, and folate. Hemorrhagic manifestations of scurvy include petechiae, purpura, and ecchymoses at pressure points; epistaxis; gum bleeding; and the characteristic perifollicular hemorrhages (Fig. 47-3). Other manifestations are poor wound and fracture

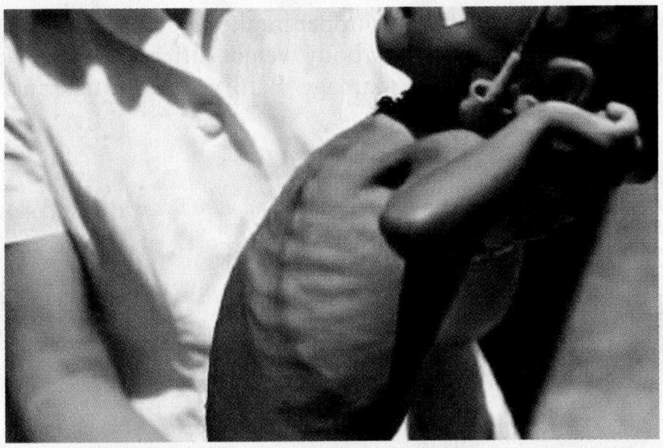

Figure 47-1 Scorbutic rosary. (Courtesy of Dr J.D. MacLean, McGill Centre for Tropical Diseases, Montreal.)

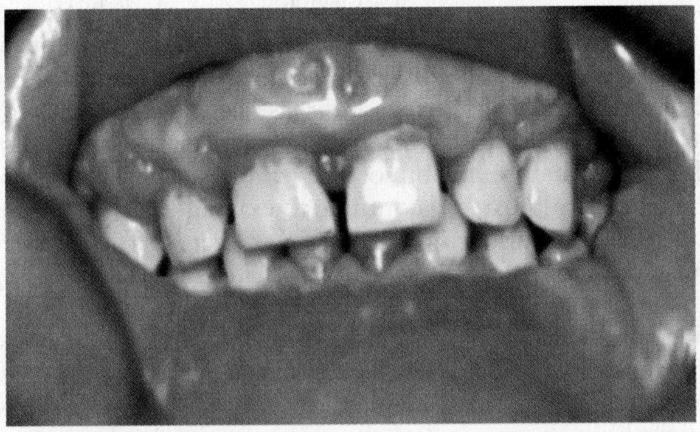

Figure 47-2 Gingival lesions in advanced scurvy. (From *Nutrition,* ed 4, Kalamazoo, MI, 1980, The Upjohn Company, p 80. Used with permission of Pfizer, Inc.)

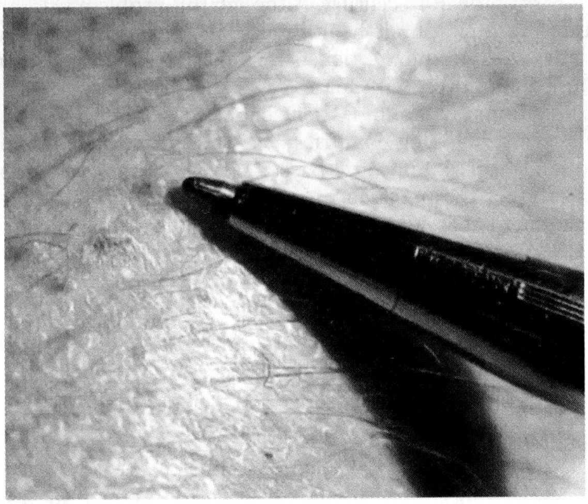

Figure 47-3 Perifollicular petechiae in scurvy. (From Weinsier RL, Morgan SL: *Fundamentals of clinical nutrition,* St Louis, 1993, Mosby, p 85.)

healing, hyperkeratosis of hair follicles, arthralgia, and muscle weakness.

Laboratory Findings and Diagnosis

The diagnosis of vitamin C deficiency is usually based on the characteristic clinical picture, the radiographic appearance of the long bones, and a history of poor vitamin C intake. The typical **radiographic changes** occur at the distal ends of the long bones and are particularly common at the knees. The shafts of the long bones have a ground-glass appearance due to trabecular atrophy. The cortex is thin and dense, giving the appearance of *pencil outlining* of the diaphysis and epiphysis. The *white line of Fränkel,* an irregular but thickened white line at the metaphysis, represents the zone of well-calcified cartilage. The epiphyseal centers of ossification also have a ground-glass appearance and are surrounded by a sclerotic ring (Fig. 47-4). The more specific but late radiologic feature of scurvy is a zone of rarefaction under the white line at the metaphysis. This zone of rarefaction *(Trumerfeld zone),* a linear break in the bone that is proximal and parallel to the white line, represents area of debris of broken-down bone trabeculae and connective tissue. A *Pelkan spur* is a lateral prolongation of the white line and may be present at cortical ends. Epiphyseal separation can occur along the line of destruction, with either linear displacement or compression of the epiphysis against the shaft. Subperiosteal hemorrhages are not visible using plain radiographs during the active phase of scurvy. However, during healing the elevated periosteum becomes calcified and radiopaque, giving a dumbbell or club shape to the affected bone (Fig. 47-5). MRI can demonstrate acute as well as healing subperiosteal hematomas along with periostitis, metaphyseal changes, and heterogeneous bone marrow signal intensity.

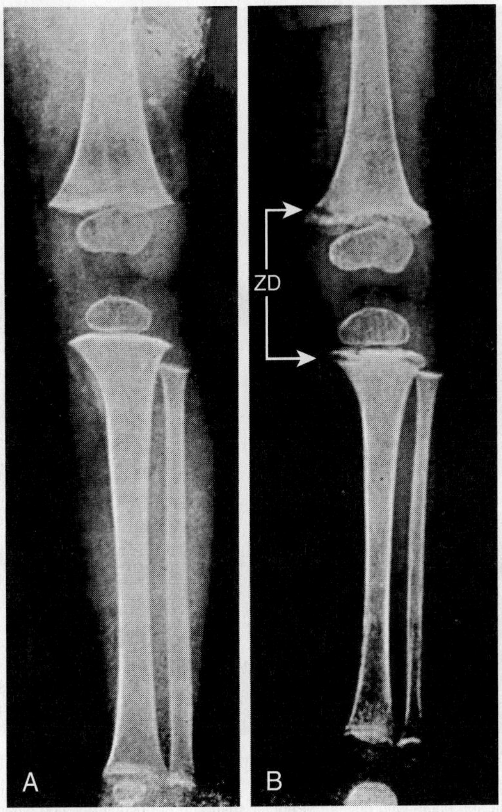

Figure 47-4 Radiographs of a leg. *A,* An early scurvy "white line" is visible on the ends of the shafts of the tibia and fibula; sclerotic rings (Wimberger sign) are shown around the epiphyses of the femur and tibia. *B,* More advanced scorbutic changes; zones of destruction (ZD) are evident in the femur and tibia. Pelkan spur is also seen at the cortical end.

Biochemical tests are not very useful in the diagnosis of scurvy, because they do not reflect the tissue status. A plasma ascorbate concentration of <0.2 mg/dL usually is considered deficient. Leukocyte concentration of vitamin C is a better indicator of body stores, but this measurement is technically more difficult to perform. Leukocyte concentrations of ≤10 μg/10^8 white blood cells (WBCs) are considered deficient and indicate latent scurvy, even in the absence of clinical signs of deficiency. Saturation of the tissues with vitamin C can be estimated from the urinary excretion of the vitamin after a test dose of ascorbic acid. In healthy children, 80% of the test dose appears in the urine within 3-5 hr after parenteral administration. Generalized nonspecific

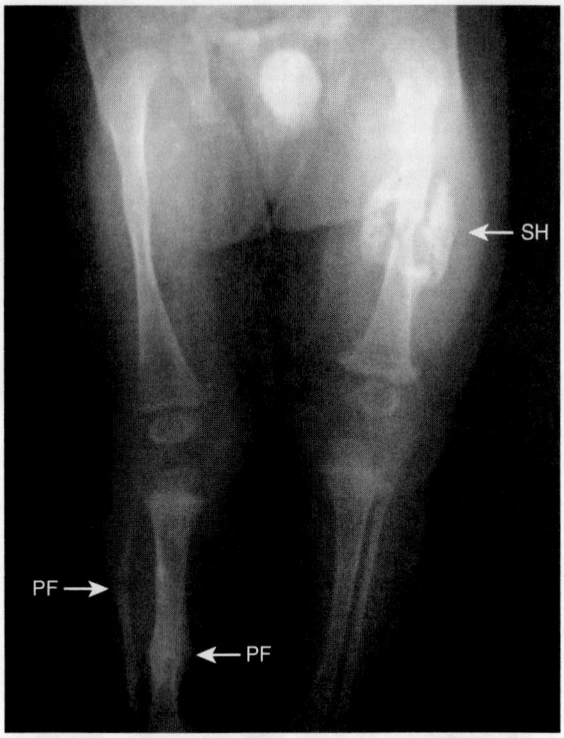

Figure 47-5 Calcified subperiosteal hematoma (SH) is seen along the midshaft of left femur of an infant with advanced scurvy; pathologic fractures (PF) are seen in the shafts of right tibia and fibula with bowing of fibular shaft and periosteal reaction along the tibia. (Courtesy of Prof. Anita Khalil.)

aminoaciduria is common in scurvy, whereas plasma amino acid levels remain normal.

Differential Diagnosis

Scurvy is often misdiagnosed as arthritis, osteomyelitis, battered child syndrome, or acrodynia. The early irritability and bone pain are sometimes attributed to nonspecific pains or other nutritional deficiencies. Copper deficiency results in a radiographic picture very similar to that of scurvy. Henoch-Schönlein purpura, thrombocytopenic purpura, or leukemia is sometimes suspected in children presenting with hemorrhagic manifestations.

Treatment

Vitamin C supplements of 100-200 mg/day orally or parenterally ensure rapid and complete cure. The clinical improvement is seen within a week in most cases, but the treatment should be continued for up to 3 months for complete recovery.

Prevention

Breast-feeding protects against vitamin C deficiency throughout infancy. In children consuming milk formula, fortification with vitamin C must be ensured. Children consuming heat-treated milk should consume adequate vitamin C–rich foods in infancy. Dietary or medicinal supplements are required in severely malnourished children.

TOXICITY

Daily intake of <2 g of vitamin C is generally without adverse effects in adults. Larger doses can cause gastrointestinal problems, such as abdominal pain and osmotic diarrhea. In general, megadoses of vitamin C should be avoided in patients with a history of urolithiasis or conditions related to excessive iron accumulation such as thalassemia and hemochromatosis. There is a paucity of data regarding vitamin C toxicity in children. The following values for tolerable upper intake levels are extrapolated from data for adults based on body weight differences: age 1-3 yr, 400 mg; age 4-8 yr, 650 mg; age 9-13 yr, 1200 mg; and age 14-18 yr, 1800 mg.

BIBLIOGRAPHY

Please visit the Nelson Textbook of Pediatrics *website at www.expertconsult.com for the complete bibliography.*

Chapter 48
Rickets and Hypervitaminosis D

Larry A. Greenbaum

RICKETS

Bone consists of a protein matrix called *osteoid* and a mineral phase, principally composed of calcium and phosphate, mostly in the form of hydroxyapatite. Osteomalacia is present when there is inadequate mineralization of bone osteoid and occurs in children and adults. Rickets is a disease of growing bone that is due to unmineralized matrix at the growth plates and occurs in children only before fusion of the epiphyses. Because growth plate cartilage and osteoid continue to expand but mineralization is inadequate, the growth plate thickens. There is also an increase in the circumference of the growth plate and the metaphysis, increasing bone width at the location of the growth plates and causing some of the classic clinical manifestations, such as widening of the wrists and ankles. There is a general softening of the bones that causes them to bend easily when subject to forces such as weight bearing or muscle pull. This softening leads to a variety of bone deformities.

Rickets is principally due to vitamin D deficiency (Table 48-1) and was rampant in northern Europe and the USA during the early years of the 20th century. Although this problem was largely corrected through public health measures that provided children with adequate vitamin D, rickets remains a persistent problem in developed countries, with many cases still secondary to preventable nutritional vitamin D deficiency It remains a significant problem in developing countries as well, with some community-based and general hospital-based surveys among children in Africa finding the prevalence of rickets exceeds 10%. UNICEF has estimated that up to 25% of children in China have some evidence of rickets.

Etiology

There are many causes of rickets (Table 48-2), including vitamin D disorders, calcium deficiency, phosphorous deficiency, and distal renal tubular acidosis.

Clinical Manifestations

Most manifestations of rickets are due to skeletal changes (Table 48-3). **Craniotabes** is a softening of the cranial bones and can be detected by applying pressure at the occiput or over the parietal bones. The sensation is similar to the feel of pressing into a Ping-Pong ball and then releasing. Craniotabes may also be secondary to osteogenesis imperfecta, hydrocephalus, and syphilis. It is a normal finding in many newborns, especially near the suture lines, but it typically disappears within a few months of birth. Widening of the costochondral junctions results in a **rachitic rosary**, which feels like the beads of a rosary as the examiner's fingers move along the costochondral junctions from rib to rib (Fig. 48-1). **Growth plate** widening is also responsible for the enlargement at the wrists and ankles. The horizontal depression along the lower anterior chest known as **Harrison groove** occurs from pulling of the softened ribs by the diaphragm during inspiration (Fig. 48-2). Softening of the ribs also impairs air movement and predisposes patients to atelectasis and pneumonia.

Table 48-1 PHYSICAL AND METABOLIC PROPERTIES AND FOOD SOURCES OF THE VITAMINS (D, E, AND K)

NAMES AND SYNONYMS	CHARACTERISTICS	BIOCHEMICAL ACTION	EFFECTS OF DEFICIENCY	EFFECTS OF EXCESS	SOURCES
VITAMIN D					
Vitamin D_3 (3-cholecalciferol), which is synthesized in the skin, and vitamin D_2 (from plants or yeast) are biologically equivalent; 1 μg = 40 IU vitamin D	Fat-soluble, stable to heat, acid alkali, and oxidation; bile necessary for absorption; hydroxylation in the liver and kidney necessary for biologic activity	Necessary for GI absorption of calcium; also increases absorption of phosphate; direct actions on bone, including mediating resorption	Rickets in growing children; osteomalacia; hypocalcemia can cause tetany and seizures	Hypercalcemia, which can cause emesis, anorexia, pancreatitis, hypertension, arrhythmias, CNS effects, polyuria, nephrolithiasis, renal failure	Exposure to sunlight (UV light); fish oils, fatty fish, egg yolks, and vitamin D–fortified formula, milk, cereals, bread
VITAMIN E					
Group of related compounds with similar biologic activities; α-tocopherol is the most potent and the most common form	Fat-soluble; readily oxidized by oxygen, iron, rancid fats; bile acids necessary for absorption	Antioxidant; protection of cell membranes from lipid peroxidation and formation of free radicals	Red cell hemolysis in premature infants; posterior column and cerebellar dysfunction; pigmentary retinopathy	Unknown	Vegetable oils, seeds, nuts, green leafy vegetables, margarine
VITAMIN K					
Group of naphthoquinones with similar biologic activities; K_1 (phylloquinone) from diet; K_2 (menaquinones) from intestinal bacteria	Natural compounds are fat-soluble; stable to heat and reducing agents; labile to oxidizing agent, strong acids, alkali, light; bile salts necessary for intestinal absorption	Vitamin K–dependent proteins include coagulation factors II, VII, IX, and X; proteins C, S, Z; matrix gla protein, osteocalcin	Hemorrhagic manifestations; long-term bone and vascular health	Not established; analogs (no longer used) caused hemolytic anemia, jaundice, kernicterus, death	Green leafy vegetables, liver, certain legumes and plant oils; widely distributed

CNS, central nervous system; GI, gastrointestinal; UV, ultraviolet.

Table 48-2 CAUSES OF RICKETS

VITAMIN D DISORDERS
Nutritional vitamin D deficiency
Congenital vitamin D deficiency
Secondary vitamin D deficiency
Malabsorption
Increased degradation
Decreased liver 25-hydroxylase
Vitamin D–dependent rickets type 1
Vitamin D–dependent rickets type 2
Chronic renal failure
CALCIUM DEFICIENCY
Low intake
Diet
Premature infants (rickets of prematurity)
Malabsorption
Primary disease
Dietary inhibitors of calcium absorption
PHOSPHORUS DEFICIENCY
Inadequate intake
Premature infants (rickets of prematurity)
Aluminum-containing antacids
RENAL LOSSES
X-linked hypophosphatemic rickets*
Autosomal dominant hypophosphatemic rickets*
Autosomal recessive hypophosphatemic rickets*
Hereditary hypophosphatemic rickets with hypercalciuria
Overproduction of phosphatonin
Tumor-induced rickets*
McCune-Albright syndrome*
Epidermal nevus syndrome*
Neurofibromatosis*
Fanconi syndrome
Dent disease
Distal renal tubular acidosis

*Disorders secondary to excess phosphatonin.

Table 48-3 CLINICAL FEATURES OF RICKETS

GENERAL
Failure to thrive
Listlessness
Protruding abdomen
Muscle weakness (especially proximal)
Fractures
HEAD
Craniotabes
Frontal bossing
Delayed fontanel closure
Delayed dentition; caries
Craniosynostosis
CHEST
Rachitic rosary
Harrison groove
Respiratory infections and atelectasis*
BACK
Scoliosis
Kyphosis
Lordosis
EXTREMITIES
Enlargement of wrists and ankles
Valgus or varus deformities
Windswept deformity (combination of valgus deformity of 1 leg with varus deformity of the other leg)
Anterior bowing of the tibia and femur
Coxa vara
Leg pain
HYPOCALCEMIC SYMPTOMS†
Tetany
Seizures
Stridor due to laryngeal spasm

*These features are most commonly associated with the vitamin D deficiency disorders.
†These symptoms develop only in children with disorders that produce hypocalcemia (see Table 48-4).

There is some variation in the clinical presentation of rickets based on the etiology. Changes in the lower extremities tend to be the dominant feature in X-linked hypophosphatemic rickets. Symptoms secondary to hypocalcemia occur only in those forms of rickets associated with decreased serum calcium (Table 48-4).

The chief complaint in a child with rickets is quite variable. Many children present because of skeletal deformities, whereas others have difficulty walking owing to a combination of deformity and weakness. Other common presenting complaints include failure to thrive and symptomatic hypocalcemia (Chapter 565).

Radiology

Rachitic changes are most easily visualized on posteroanterior radiographs of the wrist, although characteristic rachitic changes can be seen at other growth plates (Figs. 48-3 and 48-4). Decreased calcification leads to thickening of the growth plate. The edge of the metaphysis loses its sharp border, which is described as *fraying*. The edge of the metaphysis changes from a convex or flat surface to a more concave surface. This change to a concave surface is termed *cupping* and is most easily seen at the distal ends of the radius, ulna, and fibula. There is widening of the distal end of the metaphysis, corresponding to the clinical observation of thickened wrists and ankles as well as the rachitic rosary. Other radiologic features include coarse trabeculation of the diaphysis and generalized rarefaction.

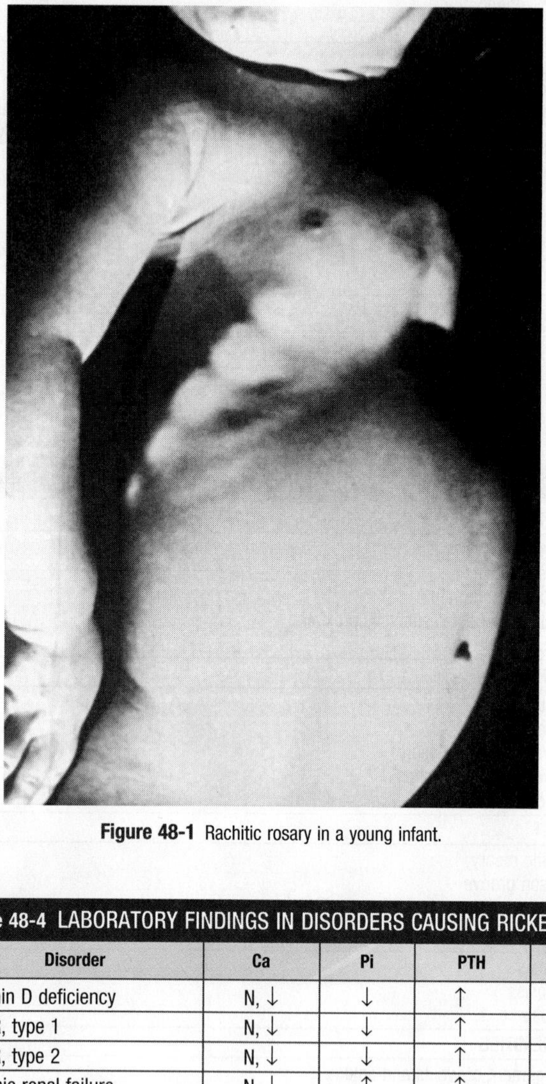

Figure 48-1 Rachitic rosary in a young infant.

Diagnosis

Most cases of rickets are diagnosed based on the presence of classic radiographic abnormalities. The diagnosis is supported by physical examination findings (see Table 48-3) and a history and laboratory test results that are consistent with a specific etiology.

Clinical Evaluation

Because the majority of children with rickets have a nutritional deficiency, the initial evaluation should focus on a dietary history, emphasizing intake of vitamin D and calcium. Most children in industrialized nations receive vitamin D from formula, fortified milk, or vitamin supplements. Along with the amount, the exact composition of the formula or milk is pertinent, because rickets has occurred in children given products that are called *milk* (soy milk) but are deficient in vitamin D and/or minerals.

Cutaneous synthesis mediated by sunlight exposure is an important source of vitamin D. It is important to ask about time

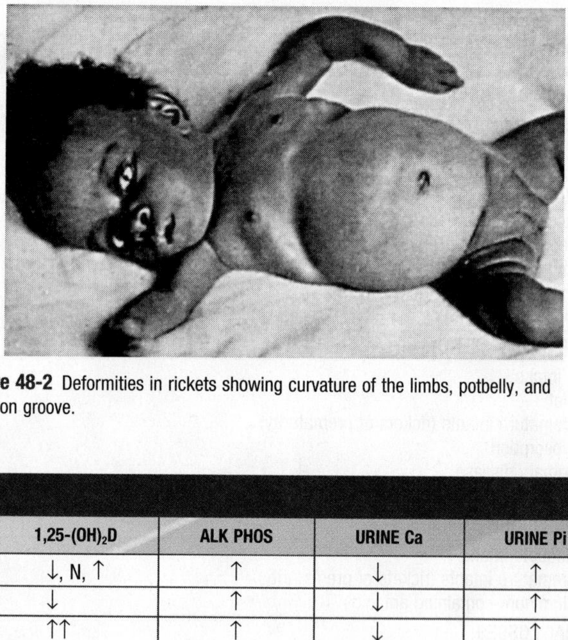

Figure 48-2 Deformities in rickets showing curvature of the limbs, potbelly, and Harrison groove.

Table 48-4 LABORATORY FINDINGS IN DISORDERS CAUSING RICKETS

Disorder	Ca	Pi	PTH	25-(OH)D	1,25-$(OH)_2D$	ALK PHOS	URINE Ca	URINE Pi
Vitamin D deficiency	N, ↓	↓	↑	↓	↓, N, ↑	↑	↓	↑
VDDR, type 1	N, ↓	↓	↑	N	↓	↑	↓	↑
VDDR, type 2	N, ↓	↓	↑	N	↑↑	↑	↓	↑
Chronic renal failure	N, ↓	↑	↑	N	↓	↑	N, ↓	↓
Dietary Pi deficiency	N	↓	N, ↓	N	↑	↑	↑	↓
XLH	N	↓	N	N	RD	↑	↓	↑
ADHR	N	↓	N	N	RD	↑	↓	↑
HHRH	N	↓	N, ↓	N	RD	↑	↑	↑
ARHR	N	↓	N	N	RD	↑	↓	↑
Tumor-induced rickets	N	↓	N	N	RD	↑	↓	↑
Fanconi syndrome	N	↓	N	N	RD or ↑	↑	↓ or ↑	↑
Dietary Ca deficiency	N, ↓	↓	↑	N	↑	↑	↓	↑

ADHR, autosomal dominant hypophosphatemic rickets; Alk Phos, alkaline phosphatase; ARHR, autosomal recessive hypophosphatemic rickets; Ca, calcium; HHRH, hereditary hypophosphatemic rickets with hypercalciuria; N, normal; Pi, inorganic phosphorus; PTH, parathyroid hormone; RD, relatively decreased (because it should be increased given the concurrent hypophosphatemia); VDDR, vitamin D–dependent rickets; XLH, X-linked hypophosphatemic rickets; 1,25-$(OH)_2D$, 1,25-dihydroxyvitamin D; 25-OHD, 25-hydroxyvitamin D; ↓, decreased; ↑, increased; ↑↑, extremely increased.

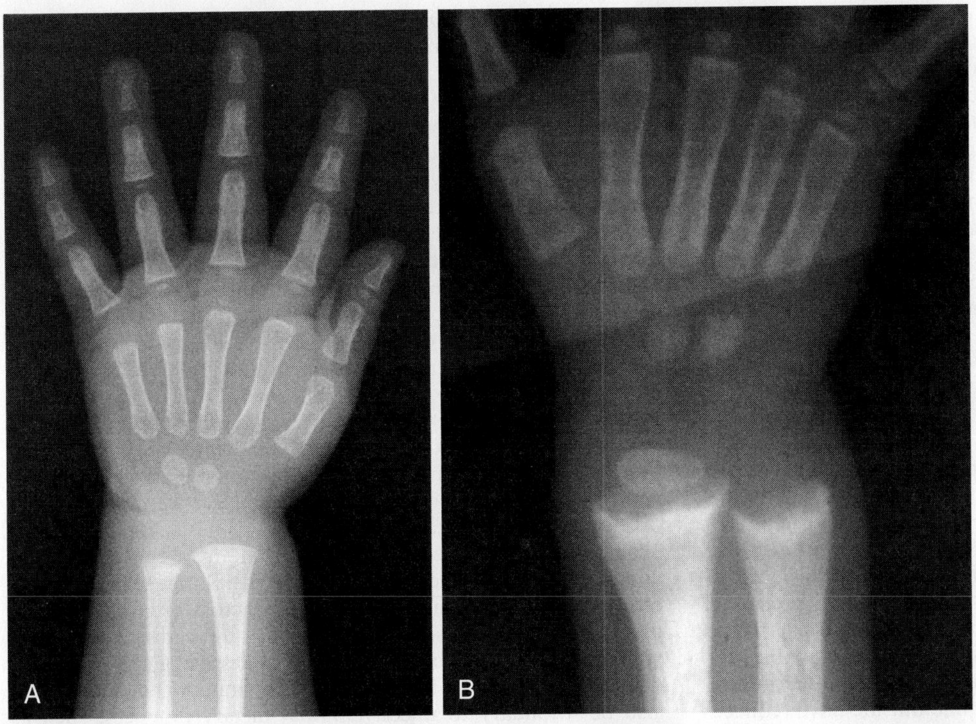

Figure 48-3 Wrist x-rays in a normal child *(A)* and a child with rickets *(B)*. The child with rickets has metaphyseal fraying and cupping of the distal radius and ulna.

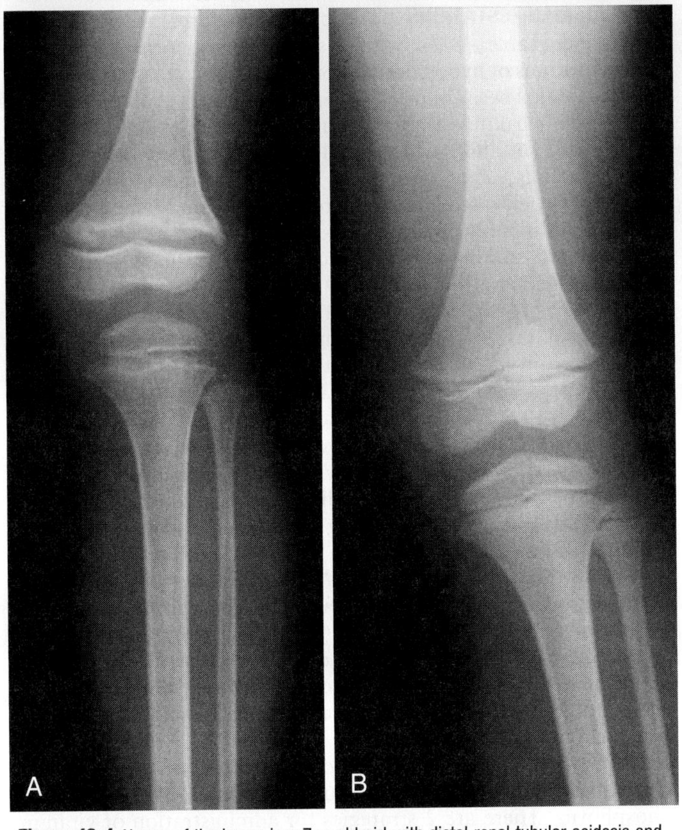

Figure 48-4 X-rays of the knees in a 7 yr old girl with distal renal tubular acidosis and rickets. *A*, At initial presentation, there is widening of the growth plate and metaphysical fraying. *B*, Dramatic improvement after 4 mo of therapy with alkali.

spent outside, sunscreen use, and clothing, especially if there may be a cultural reason for increased covering of the skin. Because winter sunlight is ineffective at stimulating cutaneous synthesis of vitamin D, the season is an additional consideration. Children with increased skin pigmentation are at increased risk for vitamin D deficiency because of decreased cutaneous synthesis.

The presence of **maternal risk** factors for nutritional vitamin D deficiency, including diet and sun exposure, is an important consideration when a neonate or young infant has rachitic findings, especially if the infant is breast-fed. Determining a child's intake of dairy products, the main dietary source of calcium, provides a general sense of calcium intake. High dietary fiber can interfere with calcium absorption.

The child's **medication** use is relevant, because certain medications such as the anticonvulsants phenobarbital and phenytoin increase degradation of vitamin D, and aluminum-containing antacids interfere with the absorption of phosphate.

Malabsorption of vitamin D is suggested by a history of liver or intestinal disease. Undiagnosed liver or intestinal disease should be suspected if the child has gastrointestinal (GI) symptoms, although occasionally rickets is the presenting complaint. Fat malabsorption is often associated with diarrhea or oily stools, and there may be signs or symptoms suggesting deficiencies of other fat-soluble vitamins (A, E, and K; Chapters 45, 49, and 50).

A history of **renal disease** (proteinuria, hematuria, urinary tract infections) is an additional significant consideration, given the importance of chronic renal failure as a cause of rickets. Polyuria can occur in children with chronic renal failure or Fanconi syndrome.

Children with rickets might have a history of dental caries, poor growth, delayed walking, waddling gait, pneumonia, and hypocalcemic symptoms.

The family history is critical, given the large number of **genetic causes** of rickets, although most of these causes are rare. Along with bone disease, it is important to inquire about leg deformities, difficulties with walking, or unexplained short stature, because some parents may be unaware of their diagnosis. Undiagnosed disease in the mother is not unusual in X-linked hypophosphatemia. A history of a unexplained sibling death during infancy may be present in the child with cystinosis, the most common cause of Fanconi syndrome in children.

The physical examination focuses on detecting manifestations of rickets (see Table 48-3). It is important to observe the child's gait, auscultate the lungs to detect atelectasis or pneumonia, and plot the patient's growth. Alopecia suggests vitamin D-dependent rickets type 2.

The **initial laboratory** tests in a child with rickets should include serum calcium, phosphorus, alkaline phosphatase, parathyroid hormone (PTH), 25-hydroxyvitamin D, 1,25-dihydroxyvitamin D_3, creatinine, and electrolytes (see Table 48-4 for interpretation). Urinalysis is useful for detecting the glycosuria and aminoaciduria (positive dipstick for protein) seen with Fanconi syndrome. Evaluation of urinary excretion of calcium (24 hr collection for calcium or calcium:creatinine ratio) is helpful if hereditary hypophosphatemic rickets with hypercalciuria or Fanconi syndrome is suspected. Direct measurement of other fat-soluble vitamins (A, E, and K) or indirect assessment of deficiency (prothrombin time for vitamin K deficiency) is appropriate if malabsorption is a consideration.

VITAMIN D DISORDERS

Vitamin D Physiology

Vitamin D can be synthesized in skin epithelial cells and therefore technically is not a vitamin. Cutaneous synthesis is normally the most important source of vitamin D and depends on the conversion of 7-dehydrochlesterol to vitamin D_3 (3-cholecalciferol) by ultraviolet B radiation from the sun. The efficiency of this process is decreased by melanin; hence, more sun exposure is necessary for vitamin D synthesis in people with increased skin pigmentation. Measures to decrease sun exposure, such as covering the skin with clothing or applying sunscreen, also decrease vitamin D synthesis. Children who spend less time outside have reduced vitamin D synthesis. The winter sun away from the equator is ineffective at mediating vitamin D synthesis.

There are few natural dietary sources of vitamin D. Fish liver oils have a high vitamin D content. Other good dietary sources include fatty fish and egg yolks. Most children in industrialized countries receive vitamin D via fortified foods, especially formula and milk (both of which contain 400 IU/L) and some breakfast cereals and breads. Supplemental vitamin D may be vitamin D_2 (which comes from plants or yeast) or vitamin D. Breast milk has a low vitamin D content, approximately 12-60 IU/L.

Vitamin D is transported bound to vitamin D–binding protein to the liver, where 25-hydroxlase converts vitamin D into 25-hydroxyvitamin D (25-D), the most abundant circulating form of vitamin D. Because there is little regulation of this liver hydroxylation step, measurement of 25-D is the standard method for determining a patient's vitamin D status. The final step in activation occurs in the kidney, where 1α-hydroxylase adds a second hydroxyl group, resulting in 1,25-dihydroxyvitamin D (1,25-D). The 1α-hydroxylase is upregulated by PTH and hypophosphatemia; hyperphosphatemia and 1,25-D inhibit this enzyme. Most 1,25-D circulates bound to vitamin D–binding protein.

1,25-D acts by binding to an intracellular receptor, and the complex affects gene expression by interacting with vitamin D–response elements. In the intestine, this binding results in a marked increase in calcium absorption, which is highly dependent on 1,25-D. There is also an increase in phosphorus absorption, but this effect is less significant because most dietary phosphorus absorption is vitamin D independent. 1,25-D also has direct effects on bone, including mediating resorption. 1,25-D directly suppresses PTH secretion by the parathyroid gland, thus completing a negative feedback loop. PTH secretion is also suppressed by the increase in serum calcium mediated by 1,25-D. 1,25-D inhibits its own synthesis in the kidney and increases the synthesis of inactive metabolites.

Nutritional Vitamin D Deficiency

Vitamin D deficiency remains the most common cause of rickets globally and is prevalent, even in industrialized countries. Because vitamin D can be obtained from dietary sources or from cutaneous synthesis, most patients in industrialized countries have a combination of risk factors that lead to vitamin D deficiency.

ETIOLOGY Vitamin D deficiency most commonly occurs in infancy due to a combination of poor intake and inadequate cutaneous synthesis. Transplacental transport of vitamin D, mostly 25-D, typically provides enough vitamin D for the 1st 2 mo of life unless there is severe maternal vitamin D deficiency. Infants who receive formula receive adequate vitamin D, even without cutaneous synthesis. Because of the low vitamin D content of breast milk, breast-fed infants rely on cutaneous synthesis or vitamin supplements. Cutaneous synthesis can be limited due to the ineffectiveness of the winter sun in stimulating vitamin D synthesis; avoidance of sunlight due to concerns about cancer, neighborhood safety, or cultural practices; and decreased cutaneous synthesis because of increased skin pigmentation.

The effect of skin pigmentation explains why most cases of nutritional rickets in the USA and northern Europe occur in breast-fed children of African descent or other dark-pigmented populations. The additional impact of the winter sun is supported by the fact that such infants more commonly present in the late winter or spring. In some groups, complete covering of infants or the practice of not taking infants outside has a significant role, explaining the occurrence of rickets in infants living in areas of abundant sunshine, such as the Middle East. Because the mothers of some infants can have the same risk factors, decreased maternal vitamin D can also contribute, both by leading to reduced vitamin D content in breast milk and by lessening transplacental delivery of vitamin D. Rickets caused by vitamin D deficiency can also be secondary to unconventional dietary practices, such as vegan diets that use unfortified soy milk or rice milk.

CLINICAL MANIFESTATIONS The clinical features are typical of rickets (see Table 48-3), with a significant minority presenting with symptoms of hypocalcemia; prolonged laryngospasm is occasionally fatal. These children have an increased risk of pneumonia and muscle weakness leading to a delay in motor development.

LABORATORY FINDINGS Table 48-4 summarizes the principal laboratory findings. Hypocalcemia is a variable finding due to the actions of the elevated PTH to increase the serum calcium concentration. The hypophosphatemia is due to PTH-induced renal losses of phosphate, combined with a decrease in intestinal absorption.

The wide variation in 1,25-D levels (low, normal, or high) is secondary to the upregulation of renal 1α-hydroxylase due to concomitant hypophosphatemia and hyperparathyroidism. Because serum levels of 1,25-D are much lower than the levels of 25-D, even with low levels of 25-D there is still often enough 25-D present to act as a precursor for 1,25-D synthesis in the presence of an upregulated 1α-hydroxylase. The level of 1,25-D is only low when there is severe vitamin D deficiency.

Some patients have a metabolic acidosis secondary to PTH-induced renal bicarbonate wasting. There may also be generalized aminoaciduria.

DIAGNOSIS AND DIFFERENTIAL DIAGNOSIS The diagnosis of nutritional vitamin D deficiency is based on the combination of a history of poor vitamin D intake and risk factors for decreased cutaneous synthesis, radiographic changes consistent with rickets, and typical laboratory findings (see Table 48-4). A normal PTH level almost never occurs with vitamin D deficiency and suggests a primary phosphate disorder.

TREATMENT Children with nutritional vitamin D deficiency should receive vitamin D and adequate nutritional intake of calcium and phosphorus. There are 2 strategies for administration of vitamin D. With stoss therapy, 300,000-600,000 IU of vitamin D are administered orally or intramuscularly as 2-4 doses over 1 day. Because the doses are observed, stoss therapy is ideal in situations where adherence to therapy is questionable. The alternative is daily, high-dose vitamin D, with doses ranging from 2,000-5,000 IU/day over 4-6 wk. Either strategy should be followed by daily vitamin D intake of 400 IU/day if <1 yr old or 600 IU/day if >1 yr, typically given as a multivitamin. It is important to ensure that children receive adequate dietary calcium and phosphorus; this dietary intake is usually provided by milk, formula, and other dairy products.

Children who have symptomatic hypocalcemia might need intravenous calcium acutely, followed by oral calcium supplements, which typically can be tapered over 2-6 wk in children who receive adequate dietary calcium. Transient use of intravenous or oral 1,25-D (calcitriol) is often helpful in reversing hypocalcemia in the acute phase by providing active vitamin D during the delay as supplemental vitamin D is converted to active vitamin D. Calcitriol doses are typically 0.05 µg/kg/day. Intravenous calcium is initially given as an acute bolus for symptomatic hypocalcemia (20 mg/kg of calcium chloride or 100 mg/kg of calcium gluconate). Some patients require a continuous intravenous calcium drip, titrated to maintain the desired serum calcium level. These patients should transition to enteral calcium, and most infants require approximately 1,000 mg of elemental calcium.

PROGNOSIS Most children have an excellent response to treatment, with radiologic healing occurring within a few months. Laboratory test results should also normalize rapidly. Many of the bone malformations improve dramatically, but children with severe disease can have permanent deformities and short stature. Rarely, patients benefit from orthopedic intervention for leg deformities, although this is generally not done until the metabolic bone disease has healed, there is clear evidence that the deformity will not self-resolve, and the deformity is causing functional problems.

PREVENTION Most cases of nutritional rickets can be prevented by universal administration of a daily multivitamin containing 400 IU of vitamin D to infants who are breast-fed. Older children should receive 600 IU/day.

Congenital Vitamin D Deficiency

Congenital rickets is quite rare in industrialized countries and occurs when there is severe maternal vitamin D deficiency during pregnancy. Maternal risk factors include poor dietary intake of vitamin D, lack of adequate sun exposure, and closely spaced pregnancies. These newborns can have symptomatic hypocalcemia, intrauterine growth retardation, and decreased bone ossification, along with classic rachitic changes. More subtle maternal vitamin D deficiency can have an adverse effect on neonatal bone density and birthweight, cause a defect in dental enamel, and predispose infants to neonatal hypocalcemic tetany. Treatment of congenital rickets includes vitamin D supplementation and adequate intake of calcium and phosphorus. Use of prenatal vitamins containing vitamin D prevents this entity.

Secondary Vitamin D Deficiency

ETIOLOGY Along with inadequate intake, vitamin D deficiency can develop due to inadequate absorption, decreased hydroxylation in the liver, and increased degradation. Because vitamin D is fat-soluble, its absorption may be decreased in patients with a variety of liver and GI diseases, including cholestatic liver disease, defects in bile acid metabolism, cystic fibrosis and other causes of pancreatic dysfunction, celiac disease, and Crohn disease. Malabsorption of vitamin D can also occur with intestinal lymphangiectasia and after intestinal resection.

Severe liver disease, which is usually also associated with malabsorption, can cause a decrease in 25-D formation due to insufficient enzyme activity. Because of the large reserve of 25-hydroxlase activity in the liver, vitamin D deficiency due to liver disease usually requires a loss of >90% of liver function. A variety of medications increase the degradation of vitamin D by inducing the cytochrome P450 (CYP) system. Rickets due to vitamin D deficiency can develop in children receiving anticonvulsants such as phenobarbital or phenytoin or antituberculosis medications such as isoniazid or rifampin.

TREATMENT Treatment of vitamin D deficiency due to malabsorption requires high doses of vitamin D. Because of its better absorption, 25-D (25-50 µg/day or 5-7 µg/kg/day) is superior to vitamin D_3. The dose is adjusted based on monitoring of serum levels of 25-D. Alternatively, patients may be treated with 1,25-D, which also is better absorbed in the presence of fat malabsorption, or with parenteral vitamin D. Children with rickets due to increased degradation of vitamin D by the CYP system require the same acute therapy as indicated for nutritional deficiency (discussed earlier), followed by long-term administration of high doses of vitamin D (e.g., 1,000 IU/day), with dosing titrated based on serum levels of 25-D. Some patients require as much as 4,000 IU/day.

Vitamin D–Dependent Rickets, Type 1

Children with vitamin D–dependent rickets type 1, an autosomal recessive disorder, have mutations in the gene encoding renal 1α-hydroxylase, preventing conversion of 25-D into 1,25-D. These patients normally present during the 1st 2 yr of life and can have any of the classic features of rickets (see Table 48-3), including symptomatic hypocalcemia. They have normal levels of 25-D but low levels of 1,25-D (see Table 48-4). Occasionally, 1,25-D levels are at the lower limit of normal, inappropriately low given the high PTH and low serum phosphorus levels, both of which should increase the activity of renal 1α-hydroxylase and cause elevated levels of 1,25-D. As in nutritional vitamin D deficiency, renal tubular dysfunction can cause a metabolic acidosis and generalized aminoaciduria.

TREATMENT These patients respond to long-term treatment with 1,25-D (calcitriol). Initial doses are 0.25-2 µg/day, and lower doses are used once the rickets has healed. Especially during initial therapy, it is important to ensure adequate intake of calcium. The dose of calcitriol is adjusted to maintain a low-normal serum calcium level, a normal serum phosphorus level, and a high-normal serum PTH level. Targeting a low-normal calcium concentration and a high-normal PTH level avoids excessive dosing of calcitriol, which can cause hypercalciuria and nephrocalcinosis. Hence, patient monitoring includes periodic assessment of urinary calcium excretion, with a target of <4 mg/kg/day.

Vitamin D–Dependent Rickets, Type 2

Patients with vitamin D–dependent rickets type 2 have mutations in the gene encoding the vitamin D receptor, preventing a normal physiologic response to 1,25-D. Levels of 1,25-D are extremely elevated in this autosomal recessive disorder (see Table 48-4). Most patients present during infancy, although rickets in less severely affected patients might not be diagnosed until adulthood. Less-severe disease is associated with a partially functional vitamin D receptor. Approximately 50-70% of children have **alopecia**, which tends to be associated with a more severe form of the disease and can range from alopecia areata to alopecia totalis. Epidermal cysts are a less common manifestation.

TREATMENT Some patients respond to extremely high doses of vitamin D_2, 25-D or 1,25-D, especially patients without alopecia. This response is due to a partially functional vitamin D receptor. All patients with this disorder should be given a 3-6 mo trial of high-dose vitamin D and oral calcium. The initial dose of 1,25-D should be 2 µg/day, but some patients require doses as high as 50-60 µg/day. Calcium doses are 1,000-3,000 mg/day. Patients who do not respond to high-dose vitamin D may be treated with long-term intravenous calcium, with possible transition to very high dose oral calcium supplements. Treatment of patients who do not respond to vitamin D is difficult.

Chronic Renal Failure (Chapter 529.2)

With chronic renal failure, there is decreased activity of 1α-hydroxylase in the kidney, leading to diminished production of 1,25-D. In chronic renal failure, unlike the other causes of vitamin D deficiency, patients have hyperphosphatemia as a result of decreased renal excretion (see Table 48-4).

TREATMENT Therapy requires the use of a form of vitamin D that can act without 1-hydroxylation by the kidney (calcitriol), which both permits adequate absorption of calcium and directly suppresses the parathyroid gland. Because hyperphosphatemia is a stimulus for PTH secretion, normalization of the serum phosphorus level via a combination of dietary phosphorus restriction and the use of oral phosphate binders is as important as the use of activated vitamin D.

CALCIUM DEFICIENCY

Pathophysiology

Rickets secondary to inadequate dietary calcium is a significant problem in some countries in Africa, although there are cases in other regions of the world, including industrialized countries. Because breast milk and formula are excellent sources of calcium, this form of rickets develops after children have been weaned from breast milk or formula and is more likely to occur in children who are weaned early. Rickets develops because the diet has low calcium content, typically <200 mg/day. There is little intake of dairy products or other sources of calcium. In addition, because of reliance on grains and green leafy vegetables, the diet may be high in phytate, oxalate, and phosphate, which decrease absorption of dietary calcium. In industrialized countries, rickets due to calcium deficiency can occur in children who consume an unconventional diet. Examples include children with milk allergy who have low dietary calcium and children who transition from formula or breast milk to juice, soda, or a calcium-poor soy drink, without an alternative source of dietary calcium.

This type of rickets can develop in children who receive intravenous nutrition without adequate calcium. Malabsorption of calcium can occur in celiac disease, intestinal abetalipoproteinemia, and after small bowel resection. There may be concurrent malabsorption of vitamin D.

Clinical Manifestations

Children have the classic signs and symptoms of rickets (see Table 48-3). Presentation can occur during infancy or early childhood, although some cases are diagnosed in teenagers. Because calcium deficiency occurs after the cessation of breast-feeding, it tends to occur later than the nutritional vitamin D deficiency that is associated with breast-feeding. In Nigeria, nutritional vitamin D deficiency is most common at 4-15 mo of age, whereas calcium-deficiency rickets typically occurs at 15-25 mo of age.

Diagnosis

Laboratory findings include increased levels of alkaline phosphatase, PTH, and 1,25-D (see Table 48-4). Calcium levels may be normal or low, although symptomatic hypocalcemia is uncommon. There is decreased urinary excretion of calcium, and serum phosphorus levels may be low due to renal wasting of phosphate from secondary hyperparathyroidism, which can also cause aminoaciduria. In some children, there is coexisting nutritional vitamin D deficiency, with low 25-D levels.

Treatment

Treatment focuses on providing adequate calcium, typically as a dietary supplement (doses of 700 [1-3 yr age], 1,000 [4-8 yr age], 1,300 [9-18 yr age] mg/day of elemental calcium are effective). Vitamin D supplementation is necessary if there is concurrent vitamin D deficiency (discussed earlier). Prevention strategies include discouraging early cessation of breast-feeding and increasing dietary sources of calcium. In countries such as Kenya, where many children have diets high in cereal with negligible intake of cow's milk, school-based milk programs have been effective in reducing the prevalence of rickets.

PHOSPHOROUS DEFICIENCY

Inadequate Intake

With the exception of starvation or severe anorexia, it is almost impossible to have a diet that is deficient in phosphorus, because phosphorus is present in most foods. Decreased phosphorus absorption can occur in diseases associated with malabsorption (celiac disease, cystic fibrosis, cholestatic liver disease), but if rickets develops, the primary problem is usually malabsorption of vitamin D and/or calcium.

Isolated malabsorption of phosphorus occurs in patients with long-term use of aluminum-containing antacids. These compounds are very effective at chelating phosphate in the GI tract, leading to decreased absorption. This decreased absorption results in hypophosphatemia with secondary osteomalacia in adults and rickets in children. This entity responds to discontinuation of the antacid and short-term phosphorus supplementation.

Phosphatonin

Phosphatonin is a humoral mediator that decreases renal tubular reabsorption of phosphate and therefore decreases serum phosphorus. Phosphatonin also decreases the activity of renal 1α-hydroxylase, resulting in a decrease in the production of 1,25-D. Fibroblast growth factor–23 (FGF-23) is the most well characterized phosphatonin, but there are a number of other putative phosphatonins (discussed later). Increased levels of phosphatonin cause many of the phosphate-wasting diseases (see Table 48-2).

X-Linked Hypophosphatemic Rickets

Among the genetic disorders causing rickets due to hypophosphatemia, X-linked hypophosphatemic rickets (XLH) is the most common, with a prevalence of 1/20,000. The defective gene is on the X chromosome, but female carriers are affected, so it is an X-linked dominant disorder.

PATHOPHYSIOLOGY The defective gene is called *PHEX* because it is a PHosphate-regulating gene with homology to Endopeptidases on the X chromosome. The product of this gene appears to have an indirect role in inactivating the phosphatonin FGF-23. Mutations in the *PHEX* gene lead to increased levels of FGF-23. Because the actions of FGF-23 include inhibition of phosphate reabsorption in the proximal tubule, phosphate excretion is increased. FGF-23 also inhibits renal 1α-hydroxylase, leading to decreased production of 1,25-D.

CLINICAL MANIFESTATIONS These patients have rickets, but abnormalities of the lower extremities and poor growth are the dominant features. Delayed dentition and tooth abscesses are also common. Some patients have hypophosphatemia and short stature without clinically evident bone disease.

LABORATORY FINDINGS Patients have high renal excretion of phosphate, hypophosphatemia, and increased alkaline phosphatase; PTH and serum calcium levels are normal (see Table 48-4). Hypophosphatemia normally upregulates renal 1α-hydroxylase and should lead to an increase in 1,25-D, but these patients have low or inappropriately normal levels of 1,25-D.

TREATMENT Patients respond well to a combination of oral phosphorus and 1,25-D (calcitriol). The daily need for phosphorus supplementation is 1-3 g of elemental phosphorus divided into 4-5 doses. Frequent dosing helps to prevent prolonged decrements in serum phosphorus because there is a rapid decline after each dose. In addition, frequent dosing decreases diarrhea, a complication of high-dose oral phosphorus. Calcitrol is administered 30-70 ng/kg/day divided into 2 doses.

Complications of treatment occur when there is not an adequate balance between phosphorus supplementation and calcitriol. Excess phosphorus, by decreasing enteral calcium absorption, leads to secondary hyperparathyroidism, with worsening of the bone lesions. In contrast, excess calcitriol causes hypercalciuria and nephrocalcinosis and can even cause hypercalcemia. Hence, laboratory monitoring of treatment includes serum calcium, phosphorus, alkaline phosphatase, PTH, and urinary calcium, as well as periodic renal ultrasounds to evaluate patients for nephrocalcinosis. Because of variation in the serum phosphorus level and the importance of avoiding excessive phosphorus dosing, normalization of alkaline phosphatase levels is a more useful method of assessing the therapeutic response than measuring serum phosphorus. For children with significant short stature, growth hormone is an effective option. Children with severe deformities might need osteotomies, but these procedures should be done only when treatment has led to resolution of the bone disease.

PROGNOSIS The response to therapy is usually good, although frequent dosing can lead to problems with compliance. Girls generally have less severe disease than boys, probably due to the X-linked inheritance. Short stature can persist despite healing of the rickets. Adults generally do well with less aggressive treatment, and some receive calcitriol alone. Adults with bone pain or other symptoms improve with oral phosphorus supplementation and calcitriol.

Autosomal Dominant Hypophosphatemic Rickets

Autosomal dominant hypophosphatemic rickets (ADHR) is much less common than XLH. There is incomplete penetrance and variable age of onset. Patients with ADHR have a mutation in the gene encoding FGF-23. The mutation prevents degradation of FGF-23 by proteases, leading to increased levels of this phosphatonin. The actions of FGF-23 include decreased reabsorption of phosphate in the renal proximal tubule, which results in hypophosphatemia, and inhibition of the 1α-hydroxylase in the kidney, causing a decrease in 1,25-D synthesis.

In ADHR, as in XLH, abnormal laboratory findings are hypophosphatemia, an elevated alkaline phosphatase level, and a low or inappropriately normal 1,25-D level (see Table 48-4). Treatment is similar to the approach used in XLH.

Autosomal Recessive Hypophosphatemic Rickets

Autosomal recessive hypophosphatemic rickets is an extremely rare disorder due to mutations in the gene encoding dentin matrix protein 1, which results in elevated levels of FGF-23, leading to renal phosphate wasting, hypophosphatemia, and low or inappropriately normal levels of 1.,25-D. Treatment is similar to the approach used in XLH.

Hereditary Hypophosphatemic Rickets with Hypercalciuria

Hereditary hypophosphatemic rickets with hypercalciuria (HHRH) is a rare disorder that is mainly described in the Middle East.

PATHOPHYSIOLOGY This autosomal recessive disorder is due to mutations in the gene for a sodium-phosphate cotransporter in the proximal tubule. The renal phosphate leak causes hypophosphatemia, which then stimulates production of 1,25-D. The high level of 1,25-D increases intestinal absorption of calcium, suppressing PTH. Hypercalciuria ensues due to the high absorption of calcium and the low level of PTH, which normally decreases renal excretion of calcium.

CLINICAL MANIFESTATIONS The dominant symptoms are rachitic leg abnormalities (see Table 48-3), muscle weakness, and bone pain. Patients can have short stature, with a disproportionate decrease in the length of the lower extremities. The severity of the disease varies, and some family members have no evidence of rickets but have kidney stones secondary to hypercalciuria.

LABORATORY FINDINGS Laboratory findings include hypophosphatemia, renal phosphate wasting, elevated serum alkaline phosphatase levels, and elevated 1,25-D levels. PTH levels are low (see Table 48-4).

TREATMENT Therapy relies on oral phosphorus replacement (1-2.5 g/day of elemental phosphorus in 5 divided oral doses). Treatment of the hypophosphatemia decreases serum levels of 1,25-D and corrects the hypercalciuria. The response to therapy is usually excellent, with resolution of pain, weakness, and radiographic evidence of rickets.

Overproduction of Phosphatonin

Tumor-induced osteomalacia is more common in adults than in children, where it can produce classic rachitic findings. Most tumors are mesenchymal in origin and are usually benign, small, and located in bone. These tumors secrete a number of different putative phosphatonins (FGF-23, frizzled-related protein 4, and matrix extracellular phosphoglycoprotein); different tumors secrete different phosphatonins or combinations of phosphatonins. These phosphatonins produce a biochemical phenotype that is similar to XLH, including urinary phosphate wasting, hypophosphatemia, elevated alkaline phosphatase levels, and low or inappropriately normal 1,25-D levels (see Table 48-4). Curative treatment is excision of the tumor. If the tumor cannot be removed, treatment is identical to that used for XLH.

Renal phosphate wasting leading to hypophosphatemia and rickets (or osteomalacia in adults) is a potential complication in **McCune-Albright syndrome,** an entity that includes the triad of polyostotic fibrous dysplasia, hyperpigmented macules, and polyendocrinopathy (Chapter 556.6). Affected patients have inappropriately low levels of 1,25-D and elevated levels of alkaline phosphatase. The renal phosphate wasting and inhibition of 1,25-D synthesis are related to the polyostotic fibrous dysplasia. Patients have elevated levels of the phosphatonin FGF-23, presumably produced by the dysplastic bone. Hypophosphatemic rickets can also occur in children with isolated polyostotic fibrous dysplasia. Although it is rarely possible, removal of the abnormal bone can cure this disorder in children with McCune-Albright syndrome. Most patients receive the same treatment as children with XLH. Bisphosphonate treatment decreases the pain and fracture risk associated with the bone lesions.

Rickets is an unusual complication of **epidermal nevus syndrome** (Chapter 643). Patients have hypophosphatemic rickets due to renal phosphate wasting and also have an inappropriately normal or low level of 1,25-D due to excessive production of FGF-23. The timing of presentation with rickets varies from infancy to early adolescence. Resolution of hypophosphatemia and rickets has occurred after excision of the epidermal nevi in some patients but not in others. In most cases, the skin lesions are too extensive to be removed, necessitating treatment with phosphorus supplementation and 1,25-D. Rickets due to phosphate wasting is an extremely rare complication in children with **neurofibromatosis** (Chapter 589.1), again presumably due to the production of a phosphatonin.

Fanconi Syndrome

Fanconi syndrome is secondary to generalized dysfunction of the renal proximal tubule (Chapter 523.1). There are renal losses of phosphate, amino acids, bicarbonate, glucose, urate, and other molecules that are normally reabsorbed in the proximal tubule. Some patients have partial dysfunction, with less generalized losses. The most clinically relevant consequences are hypophosphatemia due to phosphate losses and proximal renal tubular acidosis due to bicarbonate losses. Patients have rickets as a result of hypophosphatemia, with exacerbation from the chronic metabolic acidosis, which causes bone dissolution. Failure to thrive is a consequence of both rickets and renal tubular acidosis. Treatment is dictated by the etiology (Chapters 523.1 and 523.4).

Dent Disease (Chapter 525.3)

Dent disease is an X-linked disorder usually caused by mutations in the gene encoding a chloride channel that is expressed in the kidney. Some patients have mutations in the *OCRL 1* gene, which can also cause Lowe syndrome (Chapter 523.1). Affected males have variable manifestations, including hematuria, nephrolithiasis, nephrocalcinosis, rickets, and chronic renal failure. Almost all patients have low molecular weight proteinuria and hypercalciuria. Other, less universal abnormalities are aminoaciduria, glycosuria, hypophosphatemia, and hypokalemia. Rickets occurs in approximately 25% of patients, and it responds to oral phosphorus supplements. Some patients also need 1,25-D, but this treatment should be used cautiously because it can worsen the hypercalciuria.

RICKETS OF PREMATURITY (CHAPTER 100)

Rickets in very low birthweight infants has become a significant problem, as the survival rate for this group of infants has increased.

Pathogenesis

The transfer of calcium and phosphorus from mother to fetus occurs throughout pregnancy, but 80% occurs during the 3rd trimester. Premature birth interrupts this process, with rickets developing when the premature infant does not have an adequate supply of calcium and phosphorus to support mineralization of the growing skeleton.

Most cases of rickets of prematurity occur in infants with a birthweight <1,000 g. It is more likely to develop in infants with lower birthweight and younger gestational age. Rickets occurs because unsupplemented breast milk and standard infant formula do not contain enough calcium and phosphorus to supply the needs of the premature infant. Other risk factors include cholestatic jaundice, a complicated neonatal course, prolonged use of parenteral nutrition, the use of soy formula, and medications such as diuretics and corticosteroids.

Clinical Manifestations

Rickets of prematurity occurs 1-4 mo after birth. Infants can have nontraumatic fractures, especially of the legs, arms, and ribs. Most fractures are not suspected clinically. Because fractures and softening of the ribs lead to decreased chest compliance, some infants have respiratory distress due to atelectasis and poor ventilation. This rachitic respiratory distress usually develops >5 wk after birth, distinguishing it from the early-onset respiratory disease of premature infants. These infants have poor linear growth, with negative effects on growth persisting beyond 1 yr of age. An additional long-term effect is enamel hypoplasia. Poor bone mineralization can contribute to dolichocephaly. There may be classic rachitic findings, such as frontal bossing, rachitic rosary, craniotabes, and widened wrists and ankles (see Table 48-3). Most infants with rickets of prematurity have no clinical manifestations, and the diagnosis is based on radiographic and laboratory findings.

Laboratory Findings

Due to inadequate intake, the serum phosphorus level is low or low-normal in rickets of prematurity. The renal response is appropriate, with conservation of phosphate leading to a low urine phosphate level; the tubular reabsorption of phosphate is >95%. Most patients have normal levels of 25-D, unless there has been inadequate intake or poor absorption (discussed earlier). The hypophosphatemia stimulates renal 1α-hydroxylase, so levels of 1,25-D are high or high-normal. These high levels can contribute to bone demineralization, because 1,25-D stimulates bone resorption. Serum levels of calcium are low, normal, or high, and patients often have hypercalciuria. Elevated serum calcium levels and hypercalciuria are secondary to increased intestinal absorption and bone dissolution due to elevation of 1,25-D levels and the inability to deposit calcium in bone because of an inadequate phosphorus supply. The hypercalciuria indicates that phosphorus is the limiting nutrient for bone mineralization, although increased provision of phosphorus alone often cannot correct the mineralization defect; increased calcium is also necessary. Hence, there is an inadequate supply of calcium and phosphorus, but the deficiency in phosphorus is greater.

Alkaline phosphatase levels are often elevated, but some affected infants have normal levels. In some instances, normal alkaline phosphatase levels may be secondary to resolution of the bone demineralization because of an adequate mineral supply despite the continued presence of radiologic changes, which take longer to resolve. However, alkaline phosphatase levels may be normal despite active disease. No single blood test is 100% sensitive for the diagnosis of rickets. The diagnosis should be suspected in infants with an alkaline phosphatase level that is >5-6 times the upper limit of normal for adults (unless there is concomitant liver disease) or a phosphorus level <5.6 mg/dL. The diagnosis is confirmed by radiologic evidence of rickets, which is best seen on films of the wrists and ankles. Films of the arms and legs might reveal fractures. The rachitic rosary may be visible on chest x-ray. Unfortunately, x-rays cannot show early demineralization of bone because changes are not evident until there is >20-30% reduction in the bone mineral content.

Diagnosis

Because many premature infants have no overt clinical manifestations of rickets, screening tests are recommended. These tests should include weekly measurements of calcium, phosphorus, and alkaline phosphatase. Periodic measurement of the serum bicarbonate concentration is also important, because metabolic acidosis causes dissolution of bone. At least 1 screening x-ray for rickets at 6-8 wk of age is appropriate in infants who are at high risk for rickets; additional films may be indicated in very high risk infants.

Prevention

Provision of adequate amounts of calcium, phosphorus, and vitamin D significantly decreases the risk of rickets of prematurity. Parenteral nutrition is often necessary initially in very premature infants. In the past, adequate parenteral calcium and phosphorus delivery was difficult because of limits secondary to insolubility of these ions when their concentrations were increased. Current amino acid preparations allow higher concentrations of calcium and phosphate, decreasing the risk of rickets. Early transition to enteral feedings is also helpful. These infants should receive either human milk fortified with calcium and phosphorus or preterm infant formula, which has higher concentrations of calcium and phosphorus than standard formula. Soy formula should be avoided because there is decreased bioavailability of calcium and phosphorus. Increased mineral feedings should continue until the infant weighs 3-3.5 kg. These infants should also receive approximately 400 IU/day of vitamin D via formula and vitamin supplements.

Treatment

Therapy for rickets of prematurity focuses on ensuring adequate delivery of calcium, phosphorus, and vitamin D. If mineral delivery has been good and there is no evidence of healing, then it is important to screen for vitamin D deficiency by measuring serum 25-D. Measurement of PTH, 1,25-D, and urinary calcium and phosphorus may be helpful in some cases.

DISTAL RENAL TUBULAR ACIDOSIS (CHAPTER 523)

Distal renal tubular acidosis usually manifests with failure to thrive. Patients have a metabolic acidosis with an inability to acidify the urine appropriately. Hypercalciuria and nephrocalcinosis are typically present. There are many possible etiologies, including autosomal recessive and autosomal dominant forms. Rickets is variable, and it responds to alkali therapy (see Fig. 48-4).

HYPERVITAMINOSIS D

Etiology

Hypervitaminosis D is secondary to excessive intake of vitamin D. It can occur with long-term high intake or with a substantial, acute ingestion (see Table 48-1). Most cases are secondary to misuse of prescribed or over-the-counter vitamin D supplements, but other cases have been secondary to accidental overfortification of milk, contamination of table sugar, and inadvertent use of vitamin D supplements as cooking oil. The recommended upper limits for long-term vitamin D intake are 1,000 IU for children <1 year old and 2,000 IU for older children and adults. Hypervitaminosis D can also result from excessive intake of synthetic vitamin D analogs (25-D, 1,25-D). Vitamin D intoxication is never secondary to excessive exposure to sunlight, probably because ultraviolet irradiation can transform vitamin D_3 and its precursor into inactive metabolites.

Pathogenesis
Although vitamin D increases intestinal absorption of calcium, the dominant mechanism of the hypercalcemia is excessive bone resorption.

Clinical Manifestations
The signs and symptoms of vitamin D intoxication are secondary to hypercalcemia. GI manifestations include nausea, vomiting, poor feeding, constipation, abdominal pain, and pancreatitis. Possible cardiac findings are hypertension, decreased Q-T interval, and arrhythmias. The central nervous system effects of hypercalcemia include lethargy, hypotonia, confusion, disorientation, depression, psychosis, hallucinations, and coma. Hypercalcemia impairs renal concentrating mechanisms, which can lead to polyuria, dehydration, and hypernatremia. Hypercalcemia can also lead to acute renal failure, nephrolithiasis, and nephrocalcinosis, which can result in chronic renal insufficiency. Deaths are usually associated with arrhythmias or dehydration.

Laboratory Findings
The classic findings in vitamin D intoxication are hypercalcemia and extremely elevated levels of 25-D (>150 ng/mL). Hyperphosphatemia is also common. PTH levels are appropriately decreased owing to hypercalcemia. Hypercalciuria is universally present and can lead to nephrocalcinosis, which is visible on renal ultrasound. Hypercalcemia and nephrocalcinosis can lead to renal insufficiency.

Surprisingly, levels of 1,25-D are usually normal. This may be due to downregulation of renal 1α-hydroxylase by the combination of low PTH, hyperphosphatemia, and a direct effect of 1,25-D. There is evidence indicating that the level of free 1,25-D may be high, owing to displacement from vitamin D–binding proteins by 25-D. Nephrocalcinosis is often visible on ultrasound or CT scan. Anemia is sometimes present; the mechanism is unknown.

Diagnosis and Differential Diagnosis
The diagnosis is based on the presence of hypercalcemia and an elevated serum 25-D level, although children with excess intake of 1,25-D or another synthetic vitamin D preparation have normal levels of 25-D. With careful sleuthing, there is usually a history of excess intake of vitamin D, although in some situations (overfortification of milk by a dairy) the patient and family may be unaware.

The **differential diagnosis** of vitamin D intoxication focuses on other causes of hypercalcemia. **Hyperparathyroidism** produces hypophosphatemia, whereas vitamin D intoxication usually causes hyperphosphatemia. **Williams syndrome** is often suggested by phenotypic features and accompanying cardiac disease. **Subcutaneous fat necrosis** is a common cause of hypercalcemia in young infants; skin findings are usually present. The hypercalcemia of **familial benign hypocalciuric hypercalcemia** is mild, asymptomatic, and associated with hypocalciuria. Hypercalcemia of **malignancy** is an important consideration. High intake of calcium can also cause hypercalcemia, especially in the presence of renal insufficiency. Questioning about calcium intake should be part of the history in a patient with hypercalcemia. Occasionally, patients are intentionally taking high doses of calcium and vitamin D.

Treatment
The treatment of vitamin D intoxication focuses on control of hypercalcemia. Many patients with hypercalcemia are dehydrated as a result of polyuria from nephrogenic diabetes insipidus, poor oral intake, and vomiting. Rehydration lowers the serum calcium level via dilution and corrects prerenal azotemia. The resultant increased urine output increases urinary calcium excretion. Urinary calcium excretion is also increased by high urinary sodium excretion. The mainstay of the initial treatment is aggressive therapy with normal saline, often in conjunction with a loop diuretic to further increase calcium excretion.

Normal saline, with or without a loop diuretic, is often adequate for treating mild or moderate hypercalcemia. More significant hypercalcemia usually requires other therapies. Glucocorticoids decrease intestinal absorption of calcium by blocking the action of 1,25-D. There is also a decrease in the levels of 25-D and 1,25-D. The usual dosage of prednisone is 1-2 mg/kg/24 hr.

Calcitonin, which lowers calcium by inhibiting bone resorption, is a useful adjunct, but its effect is usually not dramatic. There is an excellent response to intravenous or oral bisphosphonates in vitamin D intoxication. Bisphosphonates inhibit bone resorption through their effects on osteoclasts. Hemodialysis using a low or 0 dialysate calcium can rapidly lower serum calcium in patients with severe hypercalcemia that is refractory to other measures.

Along with controlling hypercalcemia, it is imperative to eliminate the source of excess vitamin D. Additional sources of vitamin D such as multivitamins and fortified foods should be eliminated or reduced. Avoidance of sun exposure, including the use of sunscreen, is prudent. The patient should also restrict calcium intake.

Prognosis
Most children make a full recovery, but hypervitaminosis D may be fatal or can lead to chronic renal failure. Because vitamin D is stored in fat, levels can remain elevated for months, necessitating regular monitoring of 25-D, serum calcium, and urine calcium.

BIBLIOGRAPHY
Please visit the Nelson Textbook of Pediatrics *website at www.expertconsult.com for the complete bibliography.*

Chapter 49
Vitamin E Deficiency
Larry A. Greenbaum

Vitamin E is a fat-soluble vitamin and functions as an antioxidant, but its precise biochemical functions are not known. Vitamin E deficiency can cause hemolysis or neurologic manifestations and occurs in premature infants, in patients with malabsorption, and in an autosomal recessive disorder affecting vitamin E transport. Because of its role as an antioxidant, there is considerable research on the potential role of vitamin E supplementation in chronic illnesses.

For the full continuation of this chapter, please visit the Nelson Textbook of Pediatrics *website at www.expertconsult.com.*

Chapter 50
Vitamin K Deficiency
Larry A. Greenbaum

Vitamin K is necessary for the synthesis of clotting factors II, VII, IX, and X, and deficiency of vitamin K can result in clinically significant bleeding. Vitamin K deficiency typically affects infants, who experience a transient deficiency related to inadequate intake, or patients of any age who have decreased vitamin K absorption. Mild vitamin K deficiency can affect long-term bone and vascular health (Chapters 97.4 and 474).

PATHOGENESIS

Vitamin K is a group of compounds that have a common naphthoquinone ring structure. Phylloquinone, called *vitamin K_1*, is present in a variety of dietary sources, with green leafy vegetables, liver, and certain legumes and plant oils having the highest content. Vitamin K_1 is the form used to fortify foods and as a medication in the USA. Vitamin K_2 is a group of compounds called *menaquinones,* which are produced by intestinal bacteria. There is uncertainty regarding the relative importance of intestinally produced vitamin K_2. Menaquinones are also present in meat, especially liver, and cheese. A menaquinone is used pharmacologically in some countries.

Vitamin K is a cofactor for γ-glutamyl carboxylase, an enzyme that performs post-translational carboxylation, converting glutamate residues in proteins to γ-carboxyglutamate (Gla). The Gla residues, by facilitating calcium binding, are necessary for protein function.

The classic Gla-containing proteins involved in blood coagulation that are decreased in vitamin K deficiency are factors II (prothrombin), VII, IX, and X. Vitamin K deficiency causes a decrease in proteins C and S, which inhibit blood coagulation, and protein Z, which also has a role in coagulation. All of these proteins are made only in the liver, except for protein S, a product of various tissues.

Gla-containing proteins are also involved in bone biology (e.g., osteocalcin and protein S) and vascular biology (matrix Gla protein and protein S). Based on the presence of reduced levels of Gla, these proteins appear more sensitive than the coagulation proteins to subtle vitamin K deficiency. There is evidence suggesting that mild vitamin K deficiency might have a deleterious effect on long-term bone strength and vascular health.

Because it is fat-soluble, vitamin K requires the presence of bile salts for its absorption. Unlike other fat-soluble vitamins, there are limited body stores of vitamin K. In addition, there is high turnover of vitamin K, and the vitamin K–dependent clotting factors have a short half-life. Hence, symptomatic vitamin K deficiency can develop within weeks when there is inadequate supply due to low intake or malabsorption.

There are 3 forms of **vitamin K–deficiency bleeding (VKDB)** of the newborn (Chapter 97.4). Early VKDB was formerly called *classic hemorrhagic disease of the newborn* and occurs at 1-14 days of age. Early VKDB is secondary to low stores of vitamin K at birth due to the poor transfer of vitamin K across the placenta and inadequate intake during the 1st few days of life. In addition, there is no intestinal synthesis of vitamin K_2 because the newborn gut is sterile. Early VKDB occurs mostly in breast-fed infants due to the low vitamin K content of breast milk (formula is fortified). Delayed feeding is an additional risk factor.

Late VKDB most commonly occurs at 2-12 wk of age, although cases can occur up to 6 mo after birth. Almost all cases are in breast-fed infants due to the low vitamin K content of breast milk. An additional risk factor is occult malabsorption of vitamin K, as occurs in children with undiagnosed cystic fibrosis or cholestatic liver disease (e.g., biliary atresia, α_1-antitrypsin deficiency). Without vitamin K prophylaxis, the incidence is 4-10/100,000 newborns.

The 3rd form of VKDB of the newborn occurs at birth or shortly thereafter. It is secondary to maternal intake of medications (warfarin, phenobarbital, phenytoin) that cross the placenta and interfere with vitamin K function.

Vitamin K–deficiency bleeding due to fat malabsorption can occur in children of any age. Potential etiologies include cholestatic liver disease, pancreatic disease, and intestinal disorders (celiac sprue, inflammatory bowel disease, short-bowel syndrome). Prolonged diarrhea can cause vitamin K deficiency, especially in breast-fed infants. Children with cystic fibrosis are most likely to have vitamin K deficiency if they have pancreatic insufficiency and liver disease.

Beyond infancy, low dietary intake by itself never causes vitamin K deficiency. However, the combination of poor intake and the use of broad-spectrum antibiotics that eliminate the intestine's vitamin K_2-producing bacteria can cause vitamin K deficiency. This scenario is especially common in the intensive care unit. Vitamin K deficiency can also occur in patients who receive total parenteral nutrition without vitamin K supplementation.

CLINICAL MANIFESTATIONS

In early VKDB, the most common sites of bleeding are the gastrointestinal (GI) tract, mucosal and cutaneous tissue, the umbilical stump, and the post-circumcision site; intracranial bleeding is less common. Gastrointestinal blood loss can be severe enough to require a transfusion. In contrast, the most common site of bleeding in late VKDB is intracranial, although cutaneous and GI bleeding may be the initial manifestation. Intracranial bleeding can cause convulsions, permanent neurologic sequelae, or death. In some cases of late VKDB, the presence of an underlying disorder may be suggested by jaundice or failure to thrive. Older children with vitamin K deficiency can present with bruising, mucocutaneous bleeding, or more serious bleeding.

LABORATORY FINDINGS

In patients with bleeding due to vitamin K deficiency, the prothrombin time (PT) is prolonged. The PT must be interpreted based on the patient's age, because it is normally prolonged in newborns (Chapter 469). The partial thromboplastin time (PTT) is usually prolonged, but it may be normal in early deficiency; factor VII has the shortest half-life of the coagulation factors and is the first to be affected by vitamin K deficiency, but isolated factor VII deficiency does not affect the PTT. The platelet count and fibrinogen level are normal.

When there is mild vitamin K deficiency, the PT is normal, but there are elevated levels of the undercarboxylated forms of the proteins that are normally carboxylated in the presence of vitamin K. These undercarboxylated proteins are called *proteins induced by vitamin K absence* (PIVKA). Measurement of undercarboxylated factor II (PIVKA-II) can be used to detect mild vitamin K deficiency. Determination of blood vitamin K levels is less useful because of significant variation based on recent dietary intake; levels do not always reflect tissue stores.

DIAGNOSIS AND DIFFERENTIAL DIAGNOSIS

The diagnosis is established by the presence of a prolonged PT that corrects rapidly after administration of vitamin K, which stops the active bleeding. Other possible causes of bleeding and a prolonged PT include **disseminated intravascular coagulation** (DIC), liver failure, and rare hereditary deficiencies of clotting factors. DIC, which is most commonly secondary to sepsis, is associated with thrombocytopenia, low fibrinogen, and elevated D-dimers. Most patients with DIC have hemodynamic instability that does not correct with restoration of blood volume. Severe liver disease results in decreased production of clotting factors; the PT does not fully correct with administration of vitamin K. Children with a hereditary disorder have a deficiency in a specific clotting factor (I, II, V, VII, X).

Coumarin derivatives inhibit the action of vitamin K by preventing its recycling to an active form after it functions as a cofactor for γ-glutamyl carboxylase. Bleeding can occur with overdosage of the commonly used anticoagulant warfarin or with ingestion of rodent poison, which contains a coumarin derivative.

High doses of salicylates also inhibit vitamin K regeneration, potentially leading to a prolonged PT and clinical bleeding.

TREATMENT

Infants with VKDB should receive 1 mg of parenteral vitamin K. The PT should decrease within 6 hr and normalize within 24 hr. For rapid correction in adolescents, the parenteral dose is 2.5-10 mg. In addition to vitamin K, a patient with severe, life-threatening bleeding should receive an infusion of fresh frozen plasma, which corrects the coagulopathy rapidly. Children with vitamin K deficiency due to malabsorption require chronic administration of high doses of oral vitamin K (2.5 mg twice/wk to 5 mg/day). Parenteral vitamin K may be necessary if oral vitamin K is ineffective.

PREVENTION

Administration of either oral or parenteral vitamin K soon after birth prevents early VKDB of the newborn. In contrast, a single dose of oral vitamin K does not prevent a substantial number of cases of late VKDB. However, a single intramuscular injection of vitamin K (1 mg), the current practice in the USA, is almost universally effective, except in children with severe malabsorption. This increased efficacy of the intramuscular form is believed to be due to a depot effect. Concerns about an association between parenteral vitamin K at birth and the later development of malignancy are unsubstantiated.

Discontinuing the offending medications before delivery can prevent VKDB due to maternal medications. If this is not possible, administration of vitamin K to the mother may be helpful. In addition, the neonate should receive parenteral vitamin K immediately after birth. If parenteral vitamin K does not correct the coagulopathy rapidly, then the child should receive fresh frozen plasma.

Children at high risk for malabsorption of vitamin K should receive supplemental vitamin K and periodic measurement of the PT.

BIBLIOGRAPHY

Please visit the Nelson Textbook of Pediatrics *website at www.expertconsult.com for the complete bibliography.*

Chapter 51
Micronutrient Mineral Deficiencies

Larry A. Greenbaum

Micronutrients include vitamins (Chapters 45-50) and trace elements. By definition, a trace element is <0.01% of the body weight. Trace elements have a variety of essential functions (see Table 51-1 on the *Nelson Textbook of Pediatrics* website at www.expertconsult.com). With the exception of iron deficiency, trace element deficiency (see Table 51-1) is uncommon in developed countries, but some deficiencies (iodine, zinc, selenium) are important public health problems in a number of developing countries. Because of low nutritional requirements and plentiful supply, deficiencies of some of the trace elements are extremely rare in humans and typically occur in patients receiving unusual diets or prolonged total parenteral nutrition without adequate delivery of a specific trace element. They can also occur in children with short bowel or malabsorption. Excess intake of trace elements (see Table 51-1) is uncommon, but it can result from environmental exposure or overuse of supplements.

For the full continuation of this chapter, please visit the Nelson Textbook of Pediatrics *website at www.expertconsult.com.*

PART VII Pathophysiology of Body Fluids and Fluid Therapy

Chapter 52 Electrolyte and Acid-Base Disorders

Larry A. Greenbaum

52.1 Composition of Body Fluids

Larry A. Greenbaum

TOTAL BODY WATER

Water is the most plentiful constituent of the human body. Total body water (TBW) as a percentage of body weight varies with age (Web Fig. 52-1). The fetus has very high TBW, which gradually decreases to approximately 75% of birthweight for a term infant. Premature infants have higher TBW than term infants. During the 1st yr of life, TBW decreases to approximately 60% of body weight and basically remains at this level until puberty. At puberty, the fat content of females increases more than that of males, who acquire more muscle mass than females. Because fat has very low water content and muscle has high water content, by the end of puberty TBW in males remains at 60%, but TBW in females decreases to approximately 50% of body weight. The high fat content in overweight children causes a decrease in TBW as a percentage of body weight. During dehydration, TBW decreases and, thus, is a smaller percentage of body weight.

For the full continuation of this chapter, please visit the Nelson Textbook of Pediatrics *website at* *www.expertconsult.com*.

52.2 Regulation of Osmolality and Volume

Larry A. Greenbaum

The regulation of plasma osmolality and the intravascular volume are controlled by independent systems for water balance, which determines osmolality, and sodium balance, which determines volume status. Maintenance of normal osmolality depends on control of water balance. Control of volume status depends on regulation of sodium balance. When volume depletion is present, it takes precedence over regulation of osmolality, and retention of water contributes to the maintenance of intravascular volume.

For the full continuation of this chapter, please visit the Nelson Textbook of Pediatrics *website at* *www.expertconsult.com*.

52.3 Sodium

Larry A. Greenbaum

SODIUM METABOLISM

Body Content and Physiologic Function

Sodium is the dominant cation of the ECF (see Web Fig. 52-3), and it is the principal determinant of extracellular osmolality. Sodium is therefore necessary for the maintenance of intravascular volume. Less than 3% of sodium is intracellular. More than 40% of total body sodium is in bone; the remainder is in the interstitial and intravascular spaces. The low intracellular sodium concentration, approximately 10 mEq/L, is maintained by Na^+,K^+-ATPase, which exchanges intracellular sodium for extracellular potassium.

Intake

A child's diet determines the amount of sodium ingested—a predominantly cultural determination in older children. An occasional child has salt craving because of an underlying salt-wasting renal disease or adrenal insufficiency. Children in the USA tend to have very high sodium intakes because their diets include a large amount of "junk" food or fast food. Infants receive sodium from breast milk (≈7 mEq/L) and formula (7-13 mEq/L, for 20 calorie/oz formula). Lower recommended sodium intake limits for adults and children are being considered by the U.S. Department of Health and Human Services. In 2005-2006, the average daily sodium intake in those aged ≥2 yr was 3436 mg/day. Sodium intake is now recommended not to exceed 2500 mg/day.

Sodium is readily absorbed throughout the gastrointestinal tract. Mineralocorticoids increase sodium transport into the body, although this effect has limited clinical significance. The presence of glucose enhances sodium absorption owing to the presence of a cotransport system. This is the rationale for including sodium and glucose in oral rehydration solutions (Chapter 332).

Excretion

Sodium excretion occurs in stool and sweat, but the kidney regulates sodium balance and is the principal site of sodium excretion. There is some sodium loss in stool, but it is minimal unless diarrhea is present. Normally, sweat has 5-40 mEq/L of sodium. Sweat sodium concentration is increased in children with cystic fibrosis, aldosterone deficiency, or pseudohypoaldosteronism. The higher sweat losses in these conditions may cause or contribute to sodium depletion.

Sodium is unique among electrolytes because water balance, not sodium balance, usually determines its concentration. When the sodium concentration increases, the resultant higher plasma osmolality causes increased thirst and increased secretion of ADH, which leads to renal conservation of water. Both of these mechanisms increase the water content of the body, and the sodium concentration returns to normal. During hyponatremia, the decrease in plasma osmolality stops ADH secretion, and consequent renal water excretion leads to an increase in the sodium concentration. Even though water balance is usually regulated by osmolality, volume depletion does stimulate thirst, ADH secretion, and renal conservation of water. Volume depletion takes precedence over osmolality; volume depletion stimulates ADH secretion, even if a patient has hyponatremia.

The excretion of sodium by the kidney is *not* regulated by the plasma osmolality. The patient's effective plasma volume determines the amount of sodium in the urine. This is mediated by a variety of regulatory systems, including the renin-angiotensin-aldosterone system and intrarenal mechanisms. In hyponatremia or hypernatremia, the underlying pathophysiology determines the amount of urinary sodium, not the serum sodium concentration.

HYPERNATREMIA

Hypernatremia is a sodium concentration >145 mEq/L, although it is sometimes defined as >150 mEq/L. Mild hypernatremia is fairly common in children, especially among infants with gastroenteritis. Hypernatremia in hospitalized patients may be iatrogenic—caused by inadequate water administration or, less often, by excessive sodium administration. Moderate or severe hypernatremia has significant morbidity, including the result of underlying disease, the effects of hypernatremia on the brain, and the risks of overly rapid correction.

Etiology and Pathophysiology

There are 3 basic mechanisms of hypernatremia (Table 52-1). Sodium intoxication is frequently iatrogenic in a hospital setting as a result of correction of metabolic acidosis with sodium bicarbonate. Baking soda, a putative home remedy for upset stomach, is another source of sodium bicarbonate; the hypernatremia is accompanied by a profound metabolic alkalosis. In hyperaldosteronism, there is renal retention of sodium and resultant hypertension; the hypernatremia is usually mild.

The classic causes of hypernatremia from a water deficit are **nephrogenic** and **central diabetes insipidus** (Chapters 524 and 552). Hypernatremia develops in diabetes insipidus only if the patient does not have access to water or cannot drink adequately because of immaturity, neurologic impairment, emesis, or anorexia. Infants are at high risk because of their inability to control their own water intake. Central diabetes insipidus and the genetic forms of nephrogenic diabetes insipidus typically cause massive urinary water losses and very dilute urine. The water losses are less dramatic, and the urine often has the same osmolality as plasma when nephrogenic diabetes insipidus is secondary to disease (obstructive uropathy, renal dysplasia, sickle cell disease).

The other causes of a water deficit are also secondary to an imbalance between losses and intake. Newborns, especially if premature, have high insensible water losses. Losses are further increased if the infant is placed under a radiant warmer or with the use of phototherapy for hyperbilirubinemia. The renal concentrating mechanisms are not optimal at birth, providing an additional source of water loss. Ineffective breast-feeding, often in a primiparous mother, can cause severe hypernatremic dehydration. Adipsia, the absence of thirst, is usually secondary to damage to the hypothalamus, such as from trauma, tumor, hydrocephalus, or histiocytosis. Primary adipsia is rare.

When hypernatremia occurs in conditions with deficits of sodium and water, the water deficit exceeds the sodium deficit. This occurs only if the patient is unable to ingest adequate water. Diarrhea results in depletion of both sodium and water. Because diarrhea is hypotonic—typical sodium concentration of 35-65 mEq/L—water losses exceed sodium losses, potentially leading to hypernatremia. Most children with gastroenteritis do not have hypernatremia because they drink enough hypotonic fluid to compensate for stool water losses (Chapter 332). Fluids such as water, juice, and formula are more hypotonic than the stool losses, allowing correction of the water deficit and potentially even causing hyponatremia. Hypernatremia is most likely to occur in the child with diarrhea who has inadequate intake because of emesis, lack of access to water, or anorexia.

Osmotic agents, including mannitol, and glucose in diabetes mellitus, cause excessive renal losses of water and sodium. Because the urine is hypotonic—sodium concentration of approximately 50 mEq/L—during an osmotic diuresis, water loss exceeds sodium loss, and hypernatremia may occur if water intake is inadequate. Certain chronic kidney diseases, such as renal dysplasia and obstructive uropathy, are associated with tubular dysfunction, leading to excessive losses of water and sodium. Many children with such diseases have disproportionate water loss and are at risk for hypernatremic dehydration, especially if gastroenteritis supervenes. Similar mechanisms occur during the polyuric phase of acute tubular necrosis and after relief of urinary obstruction (postobstructive diuresis). Patients with either condition may have an osmotic diuresis from urinary losses of urea and an inability to conserve water because of tubular dysfunction.

Table 52-1 CAUSES OF HYPERNATREMIA

EXCESSIVE SODIUM
Improperly mixed formula
Excess sodium bicarbonate
Ingestion of seawater or sodium chloride
Intentional salt poisoning (child abuse or Munchausen syndrome by proxy)
Intravenous hypertonic saline
Hyperaldosteronism
WATER DEFICIT
Nephrogenic diabetes insipidus:
Acquired
X-linked (MIM 304800)
Autosomal recessive (MIM 222000)
Autosomal dominant (MIM 125800)
Central diabetes insipidus:
Acquired
Autosomal recessive (MIM 125700)
Autosomal dominant (MIM 125700)
Wolfram syndrome (MIM 222300/598500)
Increased insensible losses:
Premature infants
Radiant warmers
Phototherapy
Inadequate intake:
Ineffective breast-feeding
Child neglect or abuse
Adipsia (lack of thirst)
WATER AND SODIUM DEFICITS
Gastrointestinal losses:
Diarrhea
Emesis/nasogastric suction
Osmotic cathartics (lactulose)
Cutaneous losses:
Burns
Excessive sweating
Renal losses:
Osmotic diuretics (mannitol)
Diabetes mellitus
Chronic kidney disease (dysplasia and obstructive uropathy)
Polyuric phase of acute tubular necrosis
Postobstructive diuresis

MIM, database number from the Mendelian Inheritance in Man (*http://www3.ncbi.nlm.nih.gov/Omim/*).

Clinical Manifestations

Most children with hypernatremia are dehydrated and show the typical clinical signs and symptoms (Chapter 54). Children with hypernatremic dehydration tend to have better preservation of intravascular volume because of the shift of water from the intracellular space to the extracellular space. This shift maintains blood pressure and urine output and allows hypernatremic infants to be less symptomatic initially and potentially to become more dehydrated before medical attention is sought. Breast-fed infants with hypernatremia are often profoundly dehydrated, with failure to thrive. Probably because of intracellular water loss, the pinched abdominal skin of a dehydrated, hypernatremic infant has a "doughy" feel.

Hypernatremia, even without dehydration, causes central nervous system (CNS) symptoms that tend to parallel the degree of sodium elevation and the acuity of the increase. Patients are irritable, restless, weak, and lethargic. Some infants have a high-pitched cry and hyperpnea. Alert patients are very thirsty, even though nausea may be present. Hypernatremia may cause fever, although many patients have an underlying process that contributes to the fever. Hypernatremia is associated with hyperglycemia and mild hypocalcemia; the mechanisms are unknown. Beyond the sequelae of dehydration, there is no clear direct effect of hypernatremia on other organs or tissues, except the brain.

Brain hemorrhage is the most devastating consequence of hypernatremia. As the extracellular osmolality increases, water moves out of brain cells, leading to a decrease in brain volume. This decrease can result in tearing of intracerebral veins and bridging blood vessels as the brain moves away from the skull and the meninges. Patients may have subarachnoid, subdural, and parenchymal hemorrhages. Seizures and coma are possible sequelae of the hemorrhage, although seizures are more common during correction of hypernatremia. The cerebrospinal fluid (CSF) protein is often elevated in infants with significant hypernatremia, probably owing to leakage from damaged blood vessels. Neonates, especially if premature, seem especially vulnerable to hypernatremia and excessive sodium intake. There is an association between rapid or hyperosmolar sodium bicarbonate administration and the development of intraventricular hemorrhages in neonates. Even though central pontine myelinolysis (CPM) is classically associated with overly rapid correction of hyponatremia, both CPM and extrapontine myelinolysis can occur in children with hypernatremia. Thrombotic complications occur in severe hypernatremic dehydration; they include stroke, dural sinus thrombosis, peripheral thrombosis, and renal vein thrombosis. This is secondary to dehydration and possibly hypercoagulability associated with hypernatremia.

Diagnosis

The etiology of hypernatremia is usually apparent from the history. Hypernatremia resulting from water loss occurs only if the patient does not have access to water or is unable to drink. In the absence of dehydration, it is important to ask about sodium intake. Children with excess sodium intake do not have signs of dehydration, unless another process is present. Severe sodium intoxication causes signs of volume overload, such as pulmonary edema and weight gain. **Salt poisoning** is associated with an elevated fractional excretion of sodium, whereas hypernatremic dehydration causes a low fractional excretion of sodium. In hyperaldosteronism, hypernatremia is usually mild or absent and is associated with edema, hypertension, hypokalemia, and metabolic alkalosis.

When there is isolated water loss, the signs of volume depletion are usually less severe initially because much of the loss is from the intracellular space. When pure water loss causes signs of dehydration, the hypernatremia and water deficit are usually severe. In the child with renal water loss, either central or nephrogenic diabetes insipidus, the urine is inappropriately dilute and urine volume is not low. The urine is maximally concentrated and urine volume is low if the losses are extrarenal or due to inadequate intake. With extrarenal causes of loss of water, the urine osmolality should be >1,000 mOsm/kg. When diabetes insipidus is suspected, the evaluation may include measurement of ADH and a water deprivation test, including a trial of desmopressin acetate (synthetic ADH analog) to differentiate between nephrogenic diabetes insipidus and central diabetes insipidus (Chapter 552.1). A water deprivation test is unnecessary if the patient has simultaneous documentation of hypernatremia and poorly concentrated urine (osmolality lower than that of plasma). In children with central diabetes insipidus, administration of desmopressin acetate increases the urine osmolality above the plasma osmolality, although maximum osmolality does not occur immediately because of the decreased osmolality of the renal medulla due to the chronic lack of ADH. In children with nephrogenic diabetes insipidus, there is no response to desmopressin acetate.

With combined sodium and water deficits, analysis of the urine differentiates between renal and nonrenal etiologies. When the losses are extrarenal, the kidney responds to volume depletion with low urine volume, concentrated urine, and sodium retention (urine sodium <20 mEq/L, fractional excretion of sodium <1%). With renal causes, the urine volume is not appropriately low, the urine is not maximally concentrated, and the urine sodium may be inappropriately elevated.

Treatment

As hypernatremia develops, the brain generates **idiogenic osmoles** to increase the intracellular osmolality and prevent the loss of brain water. This mechanism is not instantaneous and is most prominent when hypernatremia has developed gradually. If the serum sodium concentration is lowered rapidly, there is movement of water from the serum into the brain cells to equalize the osmolality in the 2 compartments (Fig. 52-1). The resultant brain swelling manifests as seizures or coma.

Because of the associated dangers, hypernatremia should not be corrected rapidly. The goal is to decrease the serum sodium by <12 mEq/L every 24 hr, a rate of 0.5 mEq/L/hr. The most important component of correcting moderate or severe hypernatremia is frequent monitoring of the serum sodium value so that fluid therapy can be adjusted to provide adequate correction, neither too slow nor too fast. If a child has seizures as a result of brain edema secondary to rapid correction, administration of hypotonic fluid should be stopped. An infusion of 3% saline can acutely increase the serum sodium, reversing the cerebral edema.

In the child with hypernatremic dehydration, as in any child with dehydration, the **first priority is restoration of intravascular volume** with isotonic fluid (Chapter 54). Normal saline is preferable to lactated Ringer solution because the lower sodium concentration of the latter can cause the serum sodium to decrease too rapidly, especially if multiple fluid boluses are given. Repeated boluses of normal saline (10-20 mL/kg) may be required to treat hypotension, tachycardia, and signs of poor perfusion (peripheral pulses, capillary refill time) (Chapters 54 and 64).

The sodium concentration of the deficit replacement fluid, the rate of fluid administration, and the presence of continued water losses determine the rate of decrease of the sodium concentration. The following formula is often cited for calculating the water deficit:

$$\text{Water deficit} = \text{Body weight} \times 0.6\ (1\text{-}145/[\text{current sodium}])$$

This calculation is equivalent to 3-4 mL of water per kg for each 1 mEq that the current sodium level exceeds 145 mEq. The utility of such formulas has never been proven in clinical practice. Most patients with hypernatremic dehydration do well with a fluid sodium concentration of approximately half-normal saline, but with a fluid rate that is only 20-30% greater than maintenance fluid. Use of this concentration prevents excessive delivery of free water and too rapid a decrease in the serum sodium level. Patients with pure water loss may require a more hypotonic fluid (0.2 normal saline). Excessive water and sodium losses may also need to be replaced. If signs or symptoms of volume depletion

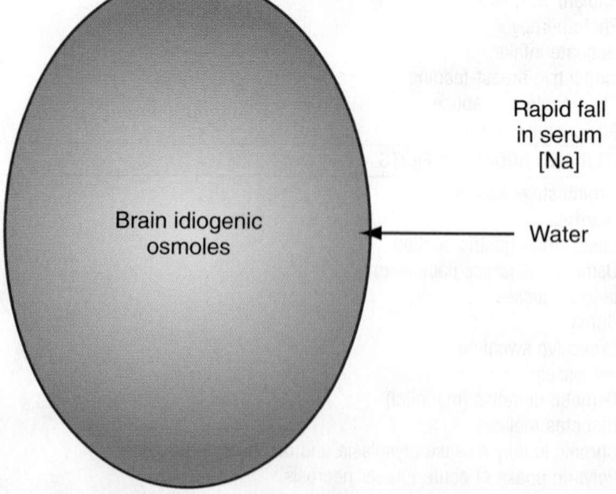

Figure 52-1 Mechanism of brain edema during correction of hypernatremia. A rapid decrease of the serum concentration during treatment of hypernatremia causes movement of water into brain cells, leading to cerebral edema. The presence of idiogenic osmoles in brain cells is responsible for the osmotic gradient.

develop, the patient receives additional boluses of isotonic saline. Monitoring of the rate of decrease of the serum sodium concentration permits adjustment in the rate and sodium concentration of the fluid that the patient is receiving, avoiding overly rapid correction of the hypernatremia. Many patients with mild to moderate hypernatremic dehydration due to gastroenteritis can be managed with oral rehydration (Chapter 332).

Acute, severe hypernatremia, usually secondary to sodium administration, can be corrected more rapidly because idiogenic osmoles have not had time to accumulate. This fact balances the high morbidity and mortality rates associated with hypernatremia with the dangers of overly rapid correction. When hypernatremia is severe and is due to sodium intoxication, it may be impossible to administer enough water to correct the hypernatremia rapidly without worsening the volume overload. In this situation, peritoneal dialysis allows for removal of the excess sodium. This requires dialysis fluid with a high glucose concentration and a low sodium concentration. In less severe cases, the addition of a loop diuretic increases the removal of excess sodium and water, decreasing the risk of volume overload. With sodium overload, hypernatremia is corrected with sodium-free intravenous fluid (5% dextrose in water [D5W]).

Hyperglycemia from hypernatremia is not usually a problem and is not treated with insulin because the acute decrease in glucose may precipitate cerebral edema by lowering plasma osmolality. Rarely, the glucose concentration of intravenous fluids must be reduced (from D5W to D2.5W). The secondary hypocalcemia is treated as needed.

It is important to address the underlying cause of the hypernatremia, if possible. The child with central diabetes insipidus should receive desmopressin acetate. Because this treatment reduces renal excretion of water, excessive intake of water must consequently be avoided to prevent both overly rapid correction of the hypernatremia and the development of hyponatremia. Over the long term, reduced sodium intake and the use of medications can somewhat ameliorate the water losses in nephrogenic diabetes insipidus (Chapter 524). The daily water intake of a child who is receiving tube feeding may need to be increased to compensate for high losses. The patient with significant ongoing losses, such as through diarrhea, may need supplemental water and electrolytes (Chapter 53). Sodium intake is reduced if it contributed to the hypernatremia.

HYPONATREMIA

Hyponatremia, a very common electrolyte abnormality in hospitalized patients, is a serum sodium level <135 mEq/L. Both total body sodium and TBW determine the serum sodium concentration. Hyponatremia exists when the ratio of water to sodium is increased. *This condition can occur with low, normal, or high levels of body sodium.* Similarly, body water can be low, normal, or high.

Etiology and Pathophysiology

The causes of hyponatremia are listed in Table 52-2. Pseudohyponatremia is a laboratory artifact that is present when the plasma contains very high concentrations of protein (multiple myeloma, intravenous immunoglobulin infusion) or lipid (hypertriglyceridemia, hypercholesterolemia). It does not occur when a direct ion-selective electrode determines the sodium concentration in undiluted plasma, a technique that is used by the instruments used for measuring arterial blood gases. In true hyponatremia, the measured osmolality is low, whereas it is normal in pseudohyponatremia. Hyperosmolality, as may occur with hyperglycemia, causes a low serum sodium concentration because water moves down its osmotic gradient from the intracellular space into the extracellular space, diluting the sodium concentration. However, because the manifestations of hyponatremia are due to the low plasma osmolality, patients with hyponatremia resulting from hyperosmolality do not have symptoms of hyponatremia.

Table 52-2 CAUSES OF HYPONATREMIA

PSEUDOHYPONATREMIA
Hyperosmolality:
Hyperglycemia
Iatrogenic (mannitol, sucrose)
Hypovolemic hyponatremia
EXTRARENAL LOSSES
Gastrointestinal (emesis, diarrhea)
Skin (sweating or burns)
(Third space losses)
RENAL LOSSES
Thiazide or loop diuretics
Osmotic diuresis
Postobstructive diuresis
Polyuric phase of acute tubular necrosis
Juvenile nephronophthisis (MIM 256100/606966/602088/604387/611498)
Autosomal recessive polycystic kidney disease (MIM 263200)
Tubulointerstitial nephritis
Obstructive uropathy
Cerebral salt wasting
Proximal (type II) renal tubular acidosis (MIM 604278)*
Lack of aldosterone effect (high serum potassium):
Absence of aldosterone (e.g., 21-hydroxylase deficiency [MIM 201910])
Pseudohypoaldosteronism type I (MIM 264350 and 177735)
Urinary tract obstruction and/or infection
EUVOLEMIC HYPONATREMIA
Syndrome of inappropriate antidiuretic hormone secretion
Nephrogenic syndrome of inappropriate antidiuresis (MIM 304800)
Desmopressin acetate
Glucocorticoid deficiency
Hypothyroidism
Water intoxication:
Iatrogenic (excess hypotonic intravenous fluids)
Feeding infants excessive water products
Swimming lessons
Tap water enema
Child abuse
Psychogenic polydipsia
Diluted formula
Marathon running with excessive water intake
Beer potomania
HYPERVOLEMIC HYPONATREMIA
Congestive heart failure
Cirrhosis
Nephrotic syndrome
Renal failure
Capillary leak due to sepsis
Hypoalbuminemia due to gastrointestinal disease (protein-losing enteropathy)

*Most cases of proximal renal tubular acidosis are not due to this primary genetic disorder. Proximal renal tubular acidosis is usually part of Fanconi syndrome, which has multiple etiologies.

MIM, database number from the Mendelian Inheritance in Man (*http://www3.ncbi.nlm.nih.gov/Omim/*).

When the etiology of the hyperosmolality resolves, such as hyperglycemia in diabetes mellitus, water moves back into the cells and the sodium concentration rises to its "true" value. Mannitol or sucrose, a component of intravenous immunoglobulin preparations, may cause hyponatremia due to hyperosmolality.

Classification of hyponatremia is based on the patient's volume status. In **hypovolemic hyponatremia,** the child has lost sodium from the body. The water balance may be positive or negative, but sodium loss has been higher than water loss. The pathogenesis of the hyponatremia is usually a combination of sodium loss and water retention to compensate for the volume depletion. The patient has a pathologic increase in fluid loss, and this fluid contains sodium. Most fluid that is lost has a lower sodium concentration than that of plasma. Viral diarrhea fluid has, on average, a sodium concentration of 50 mEq/L. Replacing diarrhea fluid, which has a sodium concentration of 50 mEq/L, with formula, which has only approximately 10 mEq/L of sodium, reduces the sodium concentration. Intravascular volume depletion interferes with renal water excretion, the body's usual mechanism for preventing hyponatremia. The volume depletion stimulates ADH synthesis, resulting in renal water retention. Volume depletion also decreases the GFR and enhances water resorption in the proximal tubule, thereby reducing water delivery to the collecting duct.

Diarrhea due to gastroenteritis is the most common cause of **hypovolemic hyponatremia** in children. Emesis causes hyponatremia if the patient takes in hypotonic fluid, either intravenously or enterally, despite the emesis. Most patients with emesis have either a normal sodium concentration or hypernatremia. Burns may cause massive losses of isotonic fluid and resultant volume depletion. Hyponatremia develops if the patient receives hypotonic fluid. Losses of sodium from sweat are especially high in children with cystic fibrosis, aldosterone deficiency, or pseudohypoaldosteronism, although high losses can occur simply in a hot climate. Third space losses are isotonic and can cause significant volume depletion, leading to ADH production and water retention, which can cause hyponatremia if the patient receives hypotonic fluid. In diseases that cause volume depletion through extrarenal sodium loss, the urine sodium level should be low (<10 mEq/L) as part of the renal response to maintain the intravascular volume. The only exceptions are diseases that cause both extrarenal and renal sodium losses: adrenal insufficiency and pseudohypoaldosteronism.

Renal sodium loss may occur in a variety of situations. In some situations, the urine sodium concentration is >140 mEq/L; thus, hyponatremia may occur without any fluid intake. In many cases, the urine sodium level is less than the serum concentration; thus, the intake of hypotonic fluid is necessary for hyponatremia to develop. In diseases associated with urinary sodium loss, the urine sodium level is >20 mEq/L despite volume depletion. This may not be true if the urinary sodium loss is no longer occurring, as is frequently the case if diuretics are discontinued. Because loop diuretics prevent generation of a maximally hypertonic renal medulla, the patient can neither maximally dilute nor concentrate the urine. The inability to maximally retain water provides some protection against severe hyponatremia. The patient receiving thiazide diuretics can concentrate the urine and is at higher risk for severe hyponatremia. Osmotic agents, such as glucose during diabetic ketoacidosis, cause loss of both water and sodium. Urea accumulates during renal failure and then acts as an osmotic diuretic after relief of urinary tract obstruction and during the polyuric phase of acute tubular necrosis. Transient tubular damage in these conditions further impairs sodium conservation. The serum sodium concentration in these conditions depends on the sodium concentration of the fluid used to replace the losses. Hyponatremia develops when the fluid is hypotonic relative to the urinary losses.

Renal salt wasting occurs in hereditary kidney diseases, such as juvenile nephronophthisis and autosomal recessive polycystic kidney disease. Obstructive uropathy, most commonly a consequence of posterior urethral valves, produces salt wasting, but patients with the disease may also have hypernatremia as a result of impaired ability to concentrate urine and high water loss. Acquired tubulointerstitial nephritis, usually secondary to either medications or infections, may cause salt wasting, along with other evidence of tubular dysfunction. CNS injury may produce cerebral salt wasting, which is theoretically due to the production of a natriuretic peptide that causes renal salt wasting. In type II renal tubular acidosis (RTA), usually associated with Fanconi syndrome (Chapter 523), there is increased excretion of sodium and bicarbonate in the urine. Patients with Fanconi syndrome also have glycosuria, aminoaciduria, and hypophosphatemia due to renal phosphate wasting.

Aldosterone is necessary for renal sodium retention and for the excretion of potassium and acid. In congenital adrenal hyperplasia due to 21-hydroxylase deficiency, the absence of aldosterone produces hyponatremia, hyperkalemia, and metabolic acidosis. In pseudohypoaldosteronism, aldosterone levels are elevated, but there is no response because of either a defective sodium channel or a lack of aldosterone receptors. A lack of tubular response to aldosterone may occur in children with urinary tract obstruction, especially during an acute urinary tract infection.

In **hypervolemic hyponatremia,** there is an excess of TBW and sodium, although the increase in water is greater than the increase in sodium. In most of the conditions that cause hypervolemic hyponatremia, there is a decrease in the effective blood volume, due to third space fluid loss, vasodilation, or poor cardiac output. The regulatory systems sense a decrease in effective blood volume and attempt to retain water and sodium to correct the problem. ADH causes renal water retention, and the kidney, under the influence of aldosterone and other intrarenal mechanisms, retains sodium. The patient's sodium concentration decreases because water intake exceeds sodium intake and ADH prevents the normal loss of excess water.

In these disorders, there is a low urine sodium concentration (<10 mEq/L) and an excess of both TBW and sodium. The only exception is in patients with renal failure and hyponatremia. These patients have an expanded intravascular volume, and hyponatremia can therefore appropriately suppress ADH production. Water cannot be excreted because very little urine is being made. Serum sodium is diluted through ingestion of water. Because of renal dysfunction, the urine sodium concentration may be elevated, but urine volume is so low that urine sodium excretion has not kept up with sodium intake, leading to sodium overload. The urine sodium concentration in renal failure varies. In patients with acute glomerulonephritis, because it does not affect the tubules, the urine sodium level is usually low, whereas in patients with acute tubular necrosis, it is elevated because of tubular dysfunction.

Patients with hyponatremia and no evidence of volume overload or volume depletion have **euvolemic hyponatremia.** These patients typically have an excess of TBW and a slight decrease in total body sodium. Some of these patients have an increase in weight, implying that they are volume-overloaded. Nevertheless, from a clinical standpoint, they usually appear normal or have subtle signs of fluid overload.

In SIADH, the secretion of ADH is not inhibited by either low serum osmolality or expanded intravascular volume (Chapter 553). The result is that the child with SIADH is unable to excrete water. This results in dilution of the serum sodium and hyponatremia. The expansion of the extracellular volume due to the retained water causes a mild increase in intravascular volume. The kidney increases sodium excretion in an effort to decrease intravascular volume to normal; thus, the patients has a mild decrease in body sodium. SIADH most commonly occurs with disorders of the CNS (infection, hemorrhage, trauma, tumor, thrombosis), but lung disease (infection, asthma, positive pressure ventilation) and malignant tumors (producing ADH) are other potential causes. A variety of medications may cause SIADH, including recreational use of 3,4-methylenedioxymethylamphetamine (MDMA, or "Ecstasy"), opiates, antiepileptic drugs (carbamazepine, oxcarbamazepine, valproate), tricyclic antidepressants, vincristine, cytoxan, and selective serotonin reuptake inhibitors. The diagnosis of SIADH is one of exclusion, because other causes of hyponatremia must be eliminated (Table 52-3). Because SIADH is a state of intravascular volume expansion, low serum uric acid and BUN levels are supportive of the diagnosis.

A rare gain-of-function mutation in the renal ADH receptor causes **nephrogenic syndrome of inappropriate antidiuresis.** Patients with this X-linked disorder appear to have SIADH but have undetectable levels of ADH.

Table 52-3 DIAGNOSTIC CRITERIA FOR SYNDROME OF INAPPROPRIATE ANTIDIURETIC HORMONE SECRETION

Absence of:
Renal, adrenal, or thyroid insufficiency
Heart failure, nephrotic syndrome, or cirrhosis
Diuretic ingestion
Dehydration
Urine osmolality > 100 mOsm/kg (usually > plasma)
Serum osmolality < 280 mOsm/kg and serum sodium < 135 mEq/L
Urine sodium > 30 mEq/L
Reversal of "sodium wasting" and correction of hyponatremia with water restriction

Hyponatremia in hospitalized patients is frequently due to inappropriate production of ADH and administration of hypotonic intravenous fluids. Causes of inappropriate ADH production include stress, medications such as narcotics or anesthetics, nausea, and respiratory illness. The synthetic analog of ADH, desmopressin acetate, causes water retention and may cause hyponatremia if fluid intake is not appropriately limited. The main uses of desmopressin acetate in children are for the management of central diabetes insipidus and of nocturnal enuresis.

Excess water ingestion can produce hyponatremia. In these cases, the sodium concentration decreases as a result of dilution. This decrease suppresses ADH secretion, and there is a marked water diuresis by the kidney. Hyponatremia develops only because the intake of water exceeds the kidney's ability to eliminate water. This condition is more likely to occur in infants because their lower GFR limits their ability to excrete water. In some situations, the water intoxication causes acute hyponatremia and is due to a massive acute water load. Examples of causes of this water load include infant swimming lessons, inappropriate use of hypotonic intravenous fluids, water enemas, and forced water intake as a form of child abuse. Chronic hyponatremia occurs in children who receive water, but limited sodium and protein. The minimum urine osmolality is approximately 50 mOsm/kg, so the kidney can excrete 1 L of water only if there is enough solute ingested to produce 50 mOsm for urinary excretion. Because sodium and urea (a breakdown product of protein) are the principal urinary solutes, a lack of intake of sodium and protein prevents adequate water excretion. This occurs with the use of diluted formula or other inappropriate diets. Subsistence on beer, a poor source of sodium and protein, causes hyponatremia due to the inability to excrete the high water load ("beer potomania").

The pathogenesis of the hyponatremia in glucocorticoid deficiency or hypothyroidism is incompletely understood. There is an inappropriate retention of water by the kidney, but the precise mechanisms are not clearly elucidated.

Clinical Manifestations

Hyponatremia causes a decrease in the osmolality of the extracellular space. Because the intracellular space then has a higher osmolality, water moves from the extracellular space to the intracellular space to maintain osmotic equilibrium. The increase in intracellular water causes cells to swell. Although cell swelling is not problematic in most tissues, it is dangerous for the brain, which is confined by the skull. As brain cells swell, there is an increase in intracranial pressure, which impairs cerebral blood flow. Acute, severe hyponatremia can cause brainstem herniation and apnea; respiratory support is often necessary. Brain cell swelling is responsible for most of the symptoms of hyponatremia. Neurologic symptoms of hyponatremia include anorexia, nausea, emesis, malaise, lethargy, confusion, agitation, headache, seizures, coma, and decreased reflexes. Patients may have hypothermia and Cheyne-Stokes respirations. Hyponatremia can cause muscle cramps and weakness; rhabdomyolysis can occur with water intoxication.

The symptoms of hyponatremia are mostly due to the decrease in extracellular osmolality and the resulting movement of water down its osmotic gradient into the intracellular space. Brain swelling can be significantly obviated if the hyponatremia develops gradually, because brain cells adapt to the decreased extracellular osmolality by reducing intracellular osmolality. This reduction is achieved by extrusion of the main intracellular ions (potassium and chloride) and a variety of small organic molecules. This process explains why the range of symptoms in hyponatremia is related to both the serum sodium level and its rate of decrease. A patient with chronic hyponatremia may have only subtle neurologic abnormalities with a serum sodium level of 110 mEq/L, but another patient may have seizures because of an acute decline in serum sodium level from 140 to 125 mEq/L.

Diagnosis

The history usually points to a likely etiology of the hyponatremia. Most patients with hyponatremia have a history of volume depletion. Diarrhea and diuretic use are very common causes of hyponatremia in children. A history of polyuria, perhaps with enuresis, and/or salt craving is present in children with primary kidney diseases or absence of aldosterone effect. Children may have signs or symptoms suggesting a diagnosis of hypothyroidism or adrenal insufficiency (Chapters 559 and 569). Brain injury raises the possibility of SIADH or cerebral salt wasting, with the caveat that SIADH is much more likely. Liver disease, nephrotic syndrome, renal failure, or congestive heart failure may be acute or chronic. The history should include a review of the patient's intake, both intravenous and enteral, with careful attention to the amounts of water, sodium, and protein.

The traditional 1st step in the diagnostic process is determination of the plasma osmolality. This is done because some patients with a low serum sodium value do not have low osmolality. The clinical effects of hyponatremia are secondary to the associated low osmolality. Without a low osmolality, there is no movement of water into the intracellular space.

A patient with hyponatremia can have a low, normal, or high osmolality. A normal osmolality in combination with hyponatremia occurs in pseudohyponatremia. Children with elevation of serum glucose concentration or of another effective osmole (mannitol) have a high plasma osmolality and hyponatremia. The presence of a low osmolality indicates "true" hyponatremia. Patients with low osmolality are at risk for neurologic symptoms and require further evaluation to determine the etiology of the hyponatremia.

In some situations, true hyponatremia is present despite a normal or elevated plasma osmolality. The presence of an ineffective osmole, most commonly urea, increases the plasma osmolality, but because the osmole has the same concentration in the intracellular space, it does not cause fluid to move into the extracellular space. There is no dilution of the serum sodium by water, and the sodium concentration remains unchanged if the ineffective osmole is eliminated. Most importantly, the ineffective osmole does not protect the brain from edema due to hyponatremia. Hence, a patient may have symptoms of hyponatremia despite having a normal or increased osmolality because of uremia.

In patients with true hyponatremia, the next step in the diagnostic process is to clinically evaluate the volume status. Patients with hyponatremia can be hypovolemic, hypervolemic, or euvolemic. The diagnosis of volume depletion relies on the usual findings with dehydration (Chapter 54), although subtle volume depletion may not be clinically apparent. In a patient with subtle volume depletion, a fluid bolus results in a decrease in the urine osmolality and an increase in the serum sodium concentration. Children with hypervolemia are **edematous** on physical examination. They may have ascites, pulmonary edema, pleural effusion, or hypertension.

Hypovolemic hyponatremia can have renal or nonrenal causes. The urine sodium concentration is very useful in differentiating between renal and nonrenal causes. When the losses are nonrenal and the kidney is working properly, there is renal retention of sodium, a normal homeostatic response to volume depletion. Thus, the urinary sodium concentration is low, typically <10 mEq/L, although sodium conservation in neonates is less avid. When the kidney is the cause of the sodium loss, the urine sodium concentration is >20 mEq/L, reflecting the defect in renal sodium retention. The interpretation of the urine sodium level is challenging with diuretic therapy because it is high when diuretics are being used but low after the diuretic effect is gone. This becomes an issue only when diuretic use is surreptitious. The urine sodium concentration is not useful if a metabolic alkalosis is present; the urine chloride concentration must be used instead (Chapter 52.7).

Differentiating among the nonrenal causes of hypovolemic hyponatremia is usually facilitated by the history. Although the renal causes are more challenging to distinguish, a high serum potassium concentration is associated with disorders in which the sodium wasting is due to absence of or ineffective aldosterone.

In the patient with hypervolemic hyponatremia, the urine sodium concentration is a helpful parameter. It is usually <10 mEq/L, except in the patient with renal failure.

Treatment

The management of hyponatremia is based on the pathophysiology of the specific etiology. The management of all causes requires judicious monitoring and avoidance of an overly quick normalization of the serum sodium concentration. A patient with severe symptoms (seizures), no matter the etiology, should be given a bolus of hypertonic saline to produce a small, rapid increase in serum sodium. Hypoxia worsens cerebral edema, and hyponatremia may cause hypoxia. Hence, pulse oximetry should be monitored, and hypoxia aggressively corrected.

With all causes of hyponatremia, it is important to avoid "overly rapid" correction. The reason is that rapid correction of hyponatremia may cause **central pontine myelinolysis** (CPM). This syndrome, which occurs within several days of rapid correction of hyponatremia, produces neurologic symptoms, including confusion, agitation, flaccid or spastic quadriparesis, and death. There are usually characteristic pathologic and radiologic changes in the brain, especially in the pons.

CPM is more common in patients who are treated for chronic hyponatremia than in those treated for acute hyponatremia. Presumably, this difference is based on the adaptation of brain cells to the hyponatremia. The reduced intracellular osmolality that is an adaptive mechanism for chronic hyponatremia makes brain cells susceptible to dehydration during rapid correction of the hyponatremia, and this may be the mechanism of CPM. Even though CPM is rare in pediatric patients, it is advisable to avoid correcting the serum sodium concentration by >12 mEq/L/24 hr or > 18 mEq/L/48 hr. Desmopressin is a potential option if the serum sodium level is increasing too rapidly. This guideline does not apply to acute hyponatremia, as may occur with water intoxication, because the hyponatremia is more often symptomatic and there has not been time for the adaptive decrease in brain osmolality to occur. The consequences of brain edema in acute hyponatremia exceed the small risk of CPM.

Patients with hyponatremia can have severe neurologic symptoms, such as seizures and coma. The seizures associated with hyponatremia generally are poorly responsive to anticonvulsants. The child with hyponatremia and severe symptoms needs to receive treatment that will quickly reduce cerebral edema. This goal is best accomplished by increasing the extracellular osmolality so that water moves down its osmolar gradient from the intracellular space to the extracellular space.

Intravenous hypertonic saline rapidly increases serum sodium, and the effect on serum osmolality leads to a decrease in brain edema. Each mL/kg of 3% sodium chloride increases the serum sodium by approximately 1 mEq/L. A child with active symptoms often improves after receiving 4-6 mL/kg of 3% sodium chloride.

The child with **hypovolemic hyponatremia** has a deficiency in sodium and may have a deficiency in water. The cornerstone of therapy is to replace the sodium deficit and any water deficit that is present. The 1st step in treating any dehydrated patient is to restore the intravascular volume with isotonic saline. Ultimately, complete restoration of intravascular volume suppresses ADH production, thereby permitting excretion of the excess water. Chapter 54 discusses the management of hyponatremic dehydration.

The management of **hypervolemic hyponatremia** is difficult. Patients with this disorder have an excess of both water and sodium. Administration of sodium leads to worsening volume overload and edema. In addition, the patients are retaining water and sodium because of their ineffective intravascular volume or renal insufficiency. The cornerstone of therapy is water and sodium restriction, because the patients have volume overload. Diuretics may help by causing excretion of both sodium and water. Vasopressin antagonists (tolvaptan), by blocking the action of ADH and causing a water diuresis, are effective in correcting the hypervolemic hyponatremia due to heart failure or cirrhosis.

Some patients with low albumin due to nephrotic syndrome have a better response to diuretics after an infusion of 25% albumin; the sodium concentration often normalizes as a result of expansion of the intravascular volume. A child with congestive heart failure may have an increase in renal water and sodium excretion if there is an improvement in cardiac output. This improvement will "turn off" the regulatory hormones that are causing renal water (ADH) and sodium (aldosterone) retention. The patient with renal failure cannot respond to any of these therapies except fluid restriction. Insensible fluid losses eventually result in an increase in the sodium concentration as long as insensible and urinary losses are greater than intake. A more definitive approach in children with renal failure is to perform dialysis, which removes water and sodium.

In **isovolumic hyponatremia,** there is usually an excess of water and a mild sodium deficit. Therapy is directed at eliminating the excess water. The child with acute excessive water intake loses water in the urine because ADH production is turned off as a result of the low plasma osmolality. Children may correct their hyponatremia spontaneously over 3-6 hr. For acute, symptomatic hyponatremia due to water intoxication, hypertonic saline may be needed to reverse cerebral edema. For chronic hyponatremia due to poor solute intake, the child needs to receive an appropriate formula, and excess water intake should be eliminated.

Children with iatrogenic hyponatremia due to the administration of hypotonic intravenous fluids should receive 3% saline if they are symptomatic. Subsequent management is dictated by the patient's volume status. The hypovolemic child should receive isotonic intravenous fluids. The child with nonphysiologic stimuli for ADH production should undergo fluid restriction. Prevention of this iatrogenic complication requires judicious use of intravenous fluids (Chapter 53).

Specific hormone replacement is the cornerstone of therapy for the hyponatremia of hypothyroidism or cortisol deficiency. Correction of the underlying defect permits appropriate elimination of the excess water.

SIADH is a condition of excess water, with limited ability of the kidney to excrete water. The mainstay of its therapy is fluid restriction. Furosemide is effective in the patient with SIADH and severe hyponatremia. Even in a patient with SIADH, furosemide causes an increase in water and sodium excretion. The loss of sodium is somewhat counterproductive, but this sodium can be replaced with hypertonic saline. Because the patient has a net loss of water and the urinary losses of sodium have been replaced, there is an increase in the sodium concentration, but no significant increase in blood pressure. Vasopressin antagonists (conivaptan, tolvaptan), which block the action of ADH and cause a water diuresis, are effective at correcting euvolemic hyponatremia, but overly rapid correction is a potential complication.

Treatment of chronic SIADH is challenging. Fluid restriction in children is difficult for nutritional and behavioral reasons. Other options are long-term furosemide therapy with sodium supplementation, an oral vasopressin antagonist (tolvaptan), or oral urea.

BIBLIOGRAPHY

Please visit the Nelson Textbook of Pediatrics *website at* *www.expertconsult.com* *for the complete bibliography.*

52.4 Potassium

Larry A. Greenbaum

POTASSIUM METABOLISM

Body Content and Physiologic Function

The intracellular concentration of potassium, approximately 150 mEq/L, is much higher than the plasma concentration (see Web Fig. 52-3). The majority of body potassium is contained in muscle. As muscle mass increases, there is an increase in body potassium. There is thus an increase in body potassium during puberty, and it is more significant in males. The majority of extracellular potassium is in bone; <1% of total body potassium is in plasma.

Because most potassium is intracellular, the plasma concentration does not always reflect the total body potassium content. A variety of conditions alter the distribution of potassium between the intracellular and extracellular compartments. The Na^+,K^+-ATPase maintains the high intracellular potassium concentration by pumping sodium out of the cell and potassium into the cell. This activity balances the normal leak of potassium out of cells via potassium channels that is driven by the favorable chemical gradient. Insulin increases potassium movement into cells by activating the Na^+,K^+-ATPase. Hyperkalemia stimulates insulin secretion, which helps mitigate the hyperkalemia. Acid-base status affects potassium distribution, probably via potassium channels and the Na^+,K^+-ATPase. A decrease in pH drives potassium extracellularly; an increase in pH has the opposite effect. β-Adrenergic agonists stimulate the Na^+,K^+-ATPase, increasing cellular uptake of potassium. This increase is protective, in that hyperkalemia stimulates adrenal release of catecholamines. α-Adrenergic agonists and exercise cause a net movement of potassium out of the intracellular space. An increase in plasma osmolality, as with mannitol infusion, leads to water movement out of the cells, and potassium follows as a result of solvent drag. The serum potassium concentration increases by approximately 0.6 mEq/L with each 10-mOsm rise in plasma osmolality.

The high intracellular concentration of potassium, the principal intracellular cation, is maintained via the Na^+,K^+-ATPase. The resulting chemical gradient is used to produce the resting membrane potential of cells. Potassium is necessary for the electrical responsiveness of nerve and muscle cells and for the contractility of cardiac, skeletal, and smooth muscle. The changes in membrane polarization that occur during muscle contraction or nerve conduction make these cells susceptible to changes in serum potassium levels. The ratio of intracellular to extracellular potassium determines the threshold for a cell to generate an action potential and the rate of cellular repolarization. The intracellular potassium concentration affects cellular enzymes. Potassium is necessary for maintaining cell volume because of its important contribution to intracellular osmolality.

Intake

Potassium is plentiful in food. Dietary consumption varies considerably, even though 1-2 mEq/kg is the recommended intake. The intestines normally absorb approximately 90% of ingested potassium. Most absorption occurs in the small intestine, whereas the colon exchanges body potassium for luminal sodium. Regulation of intestinal losses normally has a minimal role in maintaining potassium homeostasis, although renal failure, aldosterone, and glucocorticoids increase colonic secretion of potassium. The increase in intestinal losses in the setting of renal failure and hyperkalemia, which stimulates aldosterone production, is clinically significant, helping to protect against hyperkalemia.

Excretion

There is some loss of potassium in sweat, but it is normally minimal. The colon has the ability to eliminate some potassium. In addition, after an acute potassium load, much of the potassium, >40%, moves intracellularly, through the actions of epinephrine and insulin, which are produced in response to hyperkalemia. This process provides transient protection from hyperkalemia, but most ingested potassium is eventually excreted in the urine. The kidneys principally regulate long-term potassium balance, and they alter excretion in response to a variety of signals. Potassium is freely filtered at the glomerulus, but 90% is resorbed before the distal tubule and collecting duct, the principal sites of potassium regulation. The distal tubule and the collecting duct have the ability to absorb and secrete potassium. It is the amount of tubular secretion that regulates the amount of potassium that appears in the urine. The plasma potassium concentration directly influences secretion in the distal nephron. As the potassium concentration increases, secretion increases.

The principal hormone regulating potassium secretion is aldosterone, which is released by the adrenal cortex in response to increased plasma potassium. Its main site of action is the cortical collecting duct, where aldosterone stimulates sodium movement from the tubule into the cells. This movement creates a negative charge in the tubular lumen, facilitating potassium excretion. In addition, the increased intracellular sodium stimulates the basolateral Na^+,K^+-ATPase, causing more potassium to move into the cells lining the cortical collecting duct. Glucocorticoids, ADH, a high urinary flow rate, and high sodium delivery to the distal nephron also increase urinary potassium excretion. Potassium excretion is decreased by insulin, catecholamines, and urinary ammonia. Whereas ADH increases potassium secretion, it also causes water resorption, decreasing urinary flow. The net effect is that ADH has little overall impact on potassium balance. Alkalosis causes potassium to move into cells, including the cells lining the collecting duct. This movement increases potassium secretion, and because acidosis has the opposite effect, it decreases potassium secretion.

The kidney can dramatically vary potassium excretion in response to changes in intake. Normally, approximately 10-15% of the filtered load is excreted. In an adult, excretion of potassium can vary from 5-1,000 mEq/day.

HYPERKALEMIA

Hyperkalemia—because of the potential for lethal arrhythmias—is one of the most alarming electrolyte abnormalities.

Etiology and Pathophysiology

Three basic mechanisms cause hyperkalemia (Table 52-4). In the individual patient, the etiology is sometimes multifactorial.

Fictitious or spurious hyperkalemia is very common in children because of the difficulties in obtaining blood specimens. This laboratory result is usually due to hemolysis during a heelstick or phlebotomy, but it can be the result of prolonged tourniquet application or fist clenching, either of which causes local potassium release from muscle.

Table 52-4 CAUSES OF HYPERKALEMIA
SPURIOUS LABORATORY VALUE
Hemolysis
Tissue ischemia during blood drawing
Thrombocytosis
Leukocytosis
INCREASED INTAKE
Intravenous or oral
Blood transfusions
TRANSCELLULAR SHIFTS
Acidosis
Rhabdomyolysis
Tumor lysis syndrome
Tissue necrosis
Hemolysis/hematomas/gastrointestinal bleeding
Succinylcholine
Digitalis intoxication
Fluoride intoxication
β-Adrenergic blockers
Exercise
Hyperosmolality
Insulin deficiency
Malignant hyperthermia (MIM 145600/601887)
Hyperkalemic periodic paralysis (MIM 170500)
DECREASED EXCRETION
Renal failure
Primary adrenal disease:
Acquired Addison disease
21-Hydroxylase deficiency (MIM 201910)
3β-Hydroxysteroid dehydrogenase deficiency (MIM 201810)
Lipoid congenital adrenal hyperplasia (MIM 201710)
Adrenal hypoplasia congenita (MIM 300200)
Aldosterone synthase deficiency (MIM 203400/610600)
Adrenoleukodystrophy (MIM 300100)
Hyporeninemic hypoaldosteronism:
Urinary tract obstruction
Sickle cell disease (MIM 603903)
Kidney transplant
Lupus nephritis
Renal tubular disease:
Pseudohypoaldosteronism type I (MIM 264350 and 177735)
Pseudohypoaldosteronism type II (MIM 145260)
Bartter syndrome, type 2 (MIM 241200)
Urinary tract obstruction
Sickle cell disease
Kidney transplant
Medications:
Angiotensin-converting enzyme inhibitors
Angiotensin II blockers
Potassium-sparing diuretics
Calcineurin inhibitors
Nonsteroidal anti-inflammatory drugs
Trimethoprim
Heparin
Yasmin-28 (oral contraceptive)

MIM, database number from the Mendelian Inheritance in Man (*http://www3.ncbi.nlm.nih.gov/Omim/*).

The serum potassium level is normally 0.4 mEq/L higher than the plasma value, secondary to potassium release from cells during clot formation. This phenomenon is exaggerated with thrombocytosis because of potassium release from platelets. For every 100,000/m^3 increase in the platelet count, the serum potassium level rises by approximately 0.15 mEq/L. This phenomenon also occurs with the marked white blood cell count elevations sometimes seen with leukemia. Elevated white blood cell counts, typically >200,000/m^3, can cause a dramatic elevation in the serum potassium concentration. Analysis of a plasma sample usually provides an accurate result. It is important to analyze the sample promptly to avoid potassium release from cells, which occurs if the sample is stored in the cold, or cellular uptake of potassium and spurious hypokalemia, which occurs with storage of the sample at room temperature.

Because of the kidney's ability to excrete potassium, it is unusual for excessive intake, by itself, to cause hyperkalemia. This condition can occur in a patient who is receiving large quantities of intravenous or oral potassium for excessive losses that are no longer present. Frequent or rapid blood transfusions can acutely increase the potassium level because of the potassium content of blood, which is variably elevated. Increased intake may precipitate hyperkalemia if there is an underlying defect in potassium excretion.

The intracellular space has a very high potassium concentration, so a shift of potassium from the intracellular space to the extracellular space can have a significant effect on the plasma potassium level. This shift occurs with metabolic acidosis, but the effect is minimal with an organic acid (lactic acidosis, ketoacidosis). A respiratory acidosis has less impact than a metabolic acidosis. Cell destruction, as seen with rhabdomyolysis, tumor lysis syndrome, tissue necrosis, or hemolysis, releases potassium into the extracellular milieu. The potassium released from red blood cells in internal bleeding, such as hematomas, is resorbed and enters the extracellular space.

Normal doses of succinylcholine or β-blockers and fluoride or digitalis intoxication all cause a shift of potassium out of the intracellular compartment. Succinylcholine should not be used during anesthesia in patients at risk for hyperkalemia. β-Blockers prevent the normal cellular uptake of potassium mediated by binding of β-agonists to the β_2-adrenergic receptors. Potassium release from muscle cells occurs during exercise, and levels can increase by 1-2 mEq/L with high activity. With an increased plasma osmolality, water moves from the intracellular space and potassium follows. This process occurs with hyperglycemia, although in nondiabetic patients, the resultant increase in insulin causes potassium to move intracellularly. In diabetic ketoacidosis, the absence of insulin causes potassium to leave the intracellular space, and the problem is compounded by the hyperosmolality. The effect of hyperosmolality causes a transcellular shift of potassium into the extracellular space after mannitol or hypertonic saline infusions. **Malignant hyperthermia,** which is triggered by some inhaled anesthetics, causes muscle release of potassium (Chapter 603.2). **Hyperkalemic periodic paralysis** is an autosomal dominant disorder caused by a mutated sodium channel. It results in episodic cellular release of potassium and attacks of paralysis (Chapter 603.1).

The kidneys excrete most of the daily potassium intake, so a decrease in kidney function can cause hyperkalemia. Newborn infants in general, and especially premature infants, have decreased kidney function at birth and thus are at increased risk for hyperkalemia despite an absence of intrinsic renal disease. Neonates also have decreased expression of potassium channels, further limiting potassium excretion.

A wide range of primary **adrenal disorders,** both hereditary and acquired, can cause decreased production of aldosterone, with secondary hyperkalemia (Chapters 569 and 570). Patients with these disorders typically have metabolic acidosis and salt wasting with hyponatremia. Children with more subtle adrenal insufficiency may have electrolyte problems only during acute illnesses. The most common form of **congenital adrenal hyperplasia,** 21-hydroxylase deficiency, typically manifests in male infants as hyperkalemia, metabolic acidosis, hyponatremia, and volume depletion. Females with this disorder usually are diagnosed as newborns because of their ambiguous genitalia; treatment prevents the development of electrolyte problems.

Renin, via angiotensin II, stimulates aldosterone production. A deficiency in renin, a result of kidney damage, can lead to decreased aldosterone production. Hyporeninemia occurs in many kidney diseases, with some of the more common pediatric causes listed in Table 52-4. These patients typically have hyperkalemia and a metabolic acidosis, without hyponatremia. Some of these patients have impaired renal function, partially accounting for the hyperkalemia, but the impairment in potassium excretion is more extreme than expected for the degree of renal insufficiency.

A variety of **renal tubular disorders** impair renal excretion of potassium. Children with **pseudohypoaldosteronism type 1** have hyperkalemia, metabolic acidosis, and salt wasting leading to hyponatremia and volume depletion; aldosterone values are elevated. In the autosomal recessive variant, there is a defect in the renal sodium channel that is normally activated by aldosterone. Patients with this variant have severe symptoms, beginning in infancy. Patients with the autosomal dominant form have a defect in the aldosterone receptor, and the disease is milder, often remitting in adulthood. **Pseudohypoaldosteronism type 2,** also called **Gordon syndrome,** is an autosomal dominant disorder characterized by hypertension due to salt retention and impaired excretion of potassium and acid, leading to hyperkalemia and metabolic acidosis. Activating mutations in either WNK1 or WNK4, both serine-threonine kinases located in the distal nephron, cause Gordon syndrome. In **Bartter syndrome** due to mutations in the potassium channel ROMK (type 2 Bartter syndrome), there can be transient hyperkalemia in neonates, but hypokalemia subsequently develops (Chapter 525).

Acquired renal tubular dysfunction, with an impaired ability to excrete potassium, occurs in a number of conditions. These disorders, all characterized by tubulointerstitial disease, are often associated with impaired acid secretion and a secondary metabolic acidosis. In some affected children, the metabolic acidosis is the dominant feature, although a high potassium intake may unmask the defect in potassium handling. The tubular dysfunction can cause renal salt wasting, potentially leading to hyponatremia. Because of the tubulointerstitial damage, these conditions may also cause hyperkalemia as a result of hyporeninemic hypoaldosteronism.

The risk of hyperkalemia resulting from medications is greatest in patients with underlying renal insufficiency. The predominant mechanism of medication-induced hyperkalemia is impaired renal excretion, although ACE inhibitors may worsen hyperkalemia in anuric patients, probably by inhibiting gastrointestinal potassium loss, which is normally upregulated in renal insufficiency. The hyperkalemia caused by trimethoprim generally occurs only at the very high doses used to treat *Pneumocystis jiroveci* pneumonia in patients with AIDS. Potassium-sparing diuretics may easily cause hyperkalemia, especially because they are often used in patients who are receiving oral potassium supplements. The oral contraceptive Yasmin-28 contains drospirenone, which blocks the action of aldosterone.

Clinical Manifestations

The most important effects of hyperkalemia are due to the role of potassium in membrane polarization. The cardiac conduction system is usually the dominant concern. Changes in the electrocardiogram (ECG) begin with peaking of the T waves. This is followed, as the potassium level increases, by ST-segment depression, an increased PR interval, flattening of the P wave, and widening of the QRS complex. This process can eventually progress to ventricular fibrillation. Asystole may also occur. Some patients have paresthesias, fasciculations, weakness, and even an ascending paralysis, but cardiac toxicity usually precedes these clinical symptoms, emphasizing the danger of assuming that an absence of symptoms implies an absence of danger. Chronic hyperkalemia is generally better tolerated than acute hyperkalemia.

Diagnosis

The etiology of hyperkalemia is often readily apparent. Spurious hyperkalemia is very common in children, so obtaining a second potassium measurement is often appropriate. If there is a significant elevation of the white blood cell or platelet count, the second measurement should be performed on a plasma sample that is evaluated promptly. The history should initially focus on potassium intake, risk factors for transcellular shifts of potassium, medications that cause hyperkalemia, and the presence of signs of renal insufficiency, such as oliguria and edema. Initial **laboratory evaluation** should include creatinine, BUN, and assessment of the acid-base status. Many etiologies of hyperkalemia cause a metabolic acidosis; a metabolic acidosis worsens hyperkalemia through the transcellular shift of potassium out of cells. Renal insufficiency is a common cause of the combination of metabolic acidosis and hyperkalemia. This association is also seen in diseases associated with aldosterone insufficiency or aldosterone resistance. Children with absence of or ineffective aldosterone often have hyponatremia and volume depletion because of salt wasting. Genetic diseases, such as congenital adrenal hyperplasia and pseudohypoaldosteronism, usually manifest in infancy and should be strongly considered in the infant with hyperkalemia and metabolic acidosis, especially if hyponatremia is present. It is important to consider the various etiologies of a transcellular shift of potassium. In some of these disorders, the potassium level continues to increase, despite the elimination of all potassium intake, especially when there is concurrent renal insufficiency. This increase is potentially seen in tumor lysis syndrome, hemolysis, rhabdomyolysis, and other causes of cell death. All of these entities can cause concomitant hyperphosphatemia and hyperuricemia. Rhabdomyolysis produces an elevated creatinine phosphokinase (CPK) value and hypocalcemia, whereas children with hemolysis have hemoglobinuria and a decreasing hematocrit. For the child with diabetes, an elevated blood glucose value suggests a transcellular shift of potassium.

When there is no clear etiology of hyperkalemia, the diagnostic approach should focus on differentiating decreased potassium excretion from the other etiologies. Measuring urinary potassium assesses renal excretion of potassium. The transtubular potassium gradient (TTKG) is a useful method to evaluate the renal response to hyperkalemia, as follows:

$$\text{TTKG} = [\text{K}]_{\text{urine}}/[\text{K}]_{\text{plasma}} \times (\text{plasma osmolality}/\text{urine osmolality})$$

where $[K]_{urine}$ is urine potassium concentration and $[K]_{plasma}$ is plasma potassium concentration. For the result to be valid, the urine osmolality must be greater than the serum osmolality. The TTKG normally varies widely, ranging from 5-15. The TTKG should be >10 in the setting of hyperkalemia, assuming normal renal excretion of potassium. A TTKG <8 during hyperkalemia suggests a defect in renal potassium excretion, which is usually due to lack of aldosterone or an inability to respond to aldosterone. Measurement of aldosterone is useful for differentiating these possible mechanisms. Patients with a lack of aldosterone respond to fludrocortisone, an oral mineralocorticoid, by increasing urinary potassium and decreasing serum potassium. An appropriate TTKG with normal kidney function argues for a nonrenal cause of hyperkalemia.

Treatment

The plasma potassium level, the ECG, and the risk of the problem worsening determine the aggressiveness of the therapeutic approach. High serum potassium levels and the presence of ECG changes require vigorous treatment. An additional source of concern is the patient in whom plasma potassium levels are rising despite minimal intake. This situation can happen if there is cellular release of potassium (tumor lysis syndrome), especially in the setting of diminished excretion (renal failure).

The 1st action in a child with a concerning elevation of plasma potassium is to stop all sources of additional potassium (oral, intravenous) (Chapter 529). Washed red blood cells can be used for patients who require blood transfusions. If the potassium level is >6.0-6.5 mEq/L, an ECG should be obtained to help assess the urgency of the situation. Peak T waves are the first sign of hyperkalemia followed by a prolonged PR interval and, when most severe, a prolonged QRS complex. Life-threatening ventricular arrhythmias may also develop. The treatment of hyperkalemia has 2 basic goals: (1) to stabilize the heart to prevent life-threatening arrhythmias and (2) to remove potassium from the body. The treatments that acutely prevent arrhythmias all have the advantage of working quickly (within minutes) but do not remove potassium from the body. Calcium stabilizes the cell membrane of heart cells, preventing arrhythmias. It is given intravenously over a few minutes, and its action is almost immediate. Calcium should be given over 30 min in a patient receiving digitalis, because otherwise the calcium may cause arrhythmias. Bicarbonate causes potassium to move intracellularly, lowering the plasma potassium level. It is most efficacious in a patient with a metabolic acidosis. Insulin causes potassium to move intracellularly but must be given with glucose to avoid hypoglycemia. The combination of insulin and glucose works within 30 min. Nebulized albuterol, by stimulation of β_1-receptors, leads to rapid intracellular movement of potassium. This has the advantage of not requiring an intravenous route of administration, allowing it to be given concurrently with the other measures.

It is critical to begin measures that remove potassium from the body. In patients who are not anuric, a loop diuretic increases renal excretion of potassium. A high dose may be required in a patient with significant renal insufficiency. Sodium polystyrene sulfonate (Kayexalate) is an exchange resin that is given either rectally or orally. Sodium in the resin is exchanged for body potassium, and the potassium-containing resin is then excreted from the body. Some patients require dialysis for acute potassium removal. Dialysis is often necessary if the patient has either severe renal failure or an especially high rate of endogenous potassium release, as is sometimes present with tumor lysis syndrome or rhabdomyolysis. Hemodialysis rapidly lowers plasma potassium levels. Peritoneal dialysis is not nearly as quick or reliable, but it is usually adequate as long as the acute problem can be managed with medications and the endogenous release of potassium is not high.

Long-term management of hyperkalemia includes reducing intake via dietary changes and eliminating or reducing medications that cause hyperkalemia (Chapter 529). Some patients require medications to increase potassium excretion, such as sodium polystyrene sulfonate and loop or thiazide diuretics. Some infants with chronic renal failure may need to start dialysis to allow adequate caloric intake without hyperkalemia. It is unusual for an older child to require dialysis principally to control chronic hyperkalemia. The disorders that are due to a deficiency in aldosterone respond to replacement therapy with fludrocortisone.

HYPOKALEMIA

Hypokalemia is common in children, with most cases related to gastroenteritis.

Etiology and Pathophysiology

There are 4 basic mechanisms of hypokalemia (Table 52-5). Spurious hypokalemia occurs in patients with leukemia and very elevated white blood cell counts if plasma for analysis is left at room temperature, permitting the white blood cells to take up potassium from the plasma. With a transcellular shift, there is no change in total body potassium, although there may be concomitant potassium depletion resulting from other factors. Decreased intake, extrarenal losses, and renal losses are all associated with total body potassium depletion.

Because the intracellular potassium concentration is much higher than the plasma level, a significant amount of potassium can move into cells without markedly changing the intracellular potassium concentration. Alkalemia is one of the more common causes of a transcellular shift. The effect is much greater with a metabolic alkalosis than with a respiratory alkalosis. The impact of exogenous insulin on potassium movement into the cells is substantial in patients with diabetic ketoacidosis. Endogenous insulin may be the cause when a patient is given a bolus of glucose. Both endogenous (epinephrine in stress) and exogenous (albuterol) β-adrenergic agonists stimulate cellular uptake of potassium. Theophylline overdose, barium intoxication, administration of cesium chloride (a homeopathic cancer remedy), and toluene intoxication from paint or glue sniffing can cause a transcellular shift hypokalemia, often with severe clinical manifestations. Children with **hypokalemic periodic paralysis**, a rare autosomal dominant disorder, have acute cellular uptake of

Table 52-5 CAUSES OF HYPOKALEMIA

SPURIOUS
High white blood cell count
TRANSCELLULAR SHIFTS
Alkalemia
Insulin
α-Adrenergic agonists
Drugs/toxins (theophylline, barium, toluene, cesium chloride, hydroxychloroquine)
Hypokalemic periodic paralysis (MIM 170400)
Thyrotoxic period paralysis
Refeeding syndrome
DECREASED INTAKE
Anorexia nervosa
EXTRARENAL LOSSES
Diarrhea
Laxative abuse
Sweating
Sodium polystyrene sulfonate (Kayexalate) or clay ingestion
RENAL LOSSES
With metabolic acidosis:
Distal rental tubular acidosis (MIM 179800/602722/267300)
Proximal renal tubular acidosis (MIM 604278)*
Ureterosigmoidostomy
Diabetic ketoacidosis
Without specific acid-base disturbance:
Tubular toxins: amphotericin, cisplatin, aminoglycosides
Interstitial nephritis
Diuretic phase of acute tubular necrosis
Postobstructive diuresis
Hypomagnesemia
High urine anions (e.g., penicillin or penicillin derivatives)
With metabolic alkalosis:
Low urine chloride:
Emesis or nasogastric suction
Chloride-losing diarrhea (MIM 214700)
Cystic fibrosis (MIM 219700)
Low-chloride formula
Post-hypercapnia
Previous loop or thiazide diuretic use
High urine chloride and normal blood pressure:
Gitelman syndrome (MIM 263800)
Bartter syndrome (MIM 607364/602522/241200/601678)
Autosomal dominant hypoparathyroidism (MIM 146200)
EAST syndrome (MIM 612780)
Loop and thiazide diuretics
High urine chloride and high blood pressure:
Adrenal adenoma or hyperplasia
Glucocorticoid-remediable aldosteronism (MIM 103900)
Renovascular disease
Renin-secreting tumor
17β-Hydroxylase deficiency (MIM 202110)
11β-Hydroxylase deficiency (MIM 202010)
Cushing syndrome
11β-Hydroxysteroid dehydrogenase deficiency (MIM 218030)
Licorice ingestion
Liddle syndrome (MIM 177200)

*Most cases of proximal renal tubular acidosis are not due to this primary genetic disorder. Proximal renal tubular acidosis is usually part of Fanconi syndrome, which has multiple etiologies.

EAST, epilepsy, ataxia, sensorineural hearing loss, and tubulopathy; MIM, database number from the Mendelian Inheritance in Man *(http://www3.ncbi.nlm.nih.gov/Omim/)*.

potassium (Chapter 603). **Thyrotoxic periodic paralysis,** which is more common in Asians, is an unusual initial manifestation of hyperthyroidism. Affected patients have dramatic hypokalemia as a result of a transcellular shift of potassium. Hypokalemia can occur during refeeding syndrome (Chapter 330.08).

Inadequate potassium intake occurs in **anorexia nervosa;** accompanying bulimia and laxative or diuretic abuse exacerbates the potassium deficiency. Sweat losses of potassium can be significant during vigorous exercise in a hot climate. Associated volume depletion and hyperaldosteronism increase renal losses of potassium (discussed later). Diarrheal fluid has a high concentration of potassium, and hypokalemia due to diarrhea is usually associated with a metabolic acidosis resulting from stool losses of bicarbonate. In contrast, a normal acid-base balance or a mild metabolic alkalosis is seen with laxative abuse. Intake of sodium polystyrene sulfonate or ingestion of clay due to pica increases stool losses of potassium.

Urinary potassium wasting may be accompanied by a metabolic acidosis (proximal or distal RTA). In diabetic ketoacidosis, although it is often associated with normal plasma potassium caused by transcellular shifts, there is significant total body potassium depletion from urinary losses due to the osmotic diuresis, and the potassium level may decrease dramatically with insulin therapy (Chapter 583). Both the polyuric phase of acute tubular necrosis and postobstructive diuresis cause transient, highly variable potassium wasting and may be associated with a metabolic acidosis. Tubular damage, which occurs either directly from medications or secondary to interstitial nephritis, is often accompanied by other tubular losses of nutrients, including magnesium, sodium, and water. Such tubular damage may cause a secondary RTA with a metabolic acidosis. Isolated magnesium deficiency causes renal potassium wasting. Penicillin is an anion that is excreted in the urine, resulting in increased potassium excretion because the penicillin anion must be accompanied by a cation. Hypokalemia from penicillin therapy occurs only with the sodium salt of penicillin, not with the potassium salt.

Urinary potassium wasting is often accompanied by a metabolic alkalosis. This condition is usually associated with increased aldosterone, which increases urinary potassium and acid losses, contributing to the hypokalemia and the metabolic alkalosis. Other mechanisms often contribute to both the potassium losses and the metabolic alkalosis. With emesis or nasogastric suction, there is gastric loss of potassium, but this is fairly minimal, given the low potassium content of gastric fluid (≈10 mEq/L). More important is the gastric loss of hydrochloric acid (HCl), leading to a metabolic alkalosis and a state of volume depletion. The kidney compensates for the metabolic alkalosis by excreting bicarbonate in the urine, but there is obligate loss of potassium and sodium with the bicarbonate. The volume depletion raises aldosterone levels, further increasing urinary potassium losses and preventing correction of the metabolic alkalosis and hypokalemia until the volume depletion is corrected. Urinary chloride is low as a response to the volume depletion. Because the volume depletion is secondary to chloride loss, this is a state of chloride deficiency. There were cases of chloride deficiency resulting from infant formula deficient in chloride, which caused a metabolic alkalosis with hypokalemia and low urine chloride levels. Current infant formula is not deficient in chloride. A similar mechanism occurs in cystic fibrosis because of chloride loss in sweat. In **congenital chloride-losing diarrhea**, an autosomal recessive disorder, there is high stool loss of chloride, leading to metabolic alkalosis, an unusual sequela of diarrhea. Because of stool potassium losses, chloride deficiency, and metabolic alkalosis, patients with this disorder have hypokalemia. During respiratory acidosis, there is renal compensation, with retention of bicarbonate and excretion of chloride. After the respiratory acidosis is corrected, the patients have chloride deficiency and post-hypercapnic alkalosis with secondary hypokalemia. Patients with chloride deficiency, metabolic alkalosis, and hypokalemia have a urinary chloride level of <10 mEq/L. Loop and thiazide diuretics lead to hypokalemia, metabolic alkalosis, and chloride deficiency. During treatment, these patients have high urine chloride levels resulting from the effect of the diuretic. However, after the diuretics are discontinued, there is residual chloride deficiency, the urinary chloride level is appropriately low, and neither the hypokalemia nor the alkalosis resolves until the chloride deficiency is corrected.

The combination of metabolic alkalosis, hypokalemia, a high urine chloride level, and normal blood pressure is characteristic of **Bartter syndrome, Gitelman syndrome,** and **current diuretic use.** Patients with any of these conditions have high urinary losses of potassium and chloride, despite a state of relative volume depletion with secondary hyperaldosteronism. Bartter and Gitelman syndromes are autosomal recessive disorders caused by defects in tubular transporters (Chapter 525). Bartter syndrome is usually associated with hypercalciuria, and often with nephrocalcinosis, whereas children with Gitelman syndrome have low urinary calcium losses but hypomagnesemia due to urinary magnesium losses. Some patients with Bartter syndrome have hypomagnesemia.

Some patients with hypoparathyroidism and hypocalcemia due to an activating mutation of the calcium-sensing receptor (autosomal dominant hypoparathyroidism) have hypokalemia, hypomagnesemia, and metabolic alkalosis. The reason is that activation of the calcium-sensing receptor in the loop of Henle impairs tubular resorption of sodium and chloride, causing volume depletion and secondary hyperaldosteronism **EAST syndrome,** an autosomal recessive disorder due to mutations in the gene for a potassium channel present in the kidney, inner ear and brain, consists of *e*pilepsy, *a*taxia, *s*ensorineural hearing loss, and *t*ubulopathy (hypokalemia, metabolic alkalosis, hypomagnesemia, and hypocalciuria).

In the presence of high aldosterone levels, there is urinary loss of potassium, hypokalemia, metabolic alkalosis, and an elevated urinary chloride level. Also ,renal retention of sodium leads to hypertension. Primary hyperaldosteronism caused by adenoma or hyperplasia is much less common in children than in adults (Chapter 572). Glucocorticoid-remediable aldosteronism, an autosomal dominant disorder that leads to high levels of aldosterone, is often diagnosed in childhood, although hypokalemia is not always present.

Increased aldosterone levels may be secondary to increased renin production. Renal artery stenosis leads to hypertension from increased renin and secondary hyperaldosteronism. The increased aldosterone can cause hypokalemia and metabolic alkalosis, although most patients have normal electrolyte levels. Renin-producing tumors, which are extremely rare, can cause hypokalemia.

A variety of disorders causes hypertension and hypokalemia without increased aldosterone levels. Some are due to increased levels of mineralocorticoids other than aldosterone. Such increases occur in 2 forms of **congenital adrenal hyperplasia** (Chapter 570). In 11β-hydroxylase deficiency, which is associated with virilization, the value of 11-deoxycorticosterone (DOC) is elevated, causing variable hypertension and hypokalemia. A similar mechanism, increased DOC, occurs in 17α-hydroxylase deficiency, but patients with this disorder are more uniformly hypertensive and hypokalemic, and they have a defect in sex hormone production. Cushing syndrome, frequently associated with hypertension, less commonly causes metabolic alkalosis and hypokalemia. This is secondary to the mineralocorticoid activity of cortisol. In 11β-hydroxysteroid dehydrogenase deficiency, an autosomal recessive disorder, the enzymatic defect prevents the conversion of cortisol to cortisone in the kidney. Because cortisol binds to and activates the aldosterone receptor, children with this deficiency have all the features of excessive mineralocorticoids, including hypertension, hypokalemia, and metabolic alkalosis. Patients with this disorder, which is also called *apparent mineralocorticoid excess,* respond to spironolactone therapy, which blocks the mineralocorticoid receptor. An acquired form of 11β-hydroxysteroid dehydrogenase deficiency occurs from the ingestion of substances that inhibit this enzyme. A classic example is glycyrrhizic acid, which is found in natural licorice. **Liddle syndrome** is an autosomal dominant disorder that results from an activating mutation of the distal nephron sodium channel that is normally upregulated by aldosterone. Patients have the characteristics of hyperaldosteronism—hypertension, hypokalemia, and alkalosis—but low serum aldosterone levels. These patients respond to the potassium-sparing diuretics (triamterene and amiloride) that inhibit this sodium channel (Chapter 525.3).

Clinical Manifestations
The heart and skeletal muscle are especially vulnerable to hypokalemia. ECG changes include a flattened T wave, a depressed ST segment, and the appearance of a U wave, which is located between the T wave (if still visible) and the P wave. Ventricular fibrillation and torsades de pointes may occur, although usually only in the context of underlying heart disease. Hypokalemia makes the heart especially susceptible to digitalis-induced arrhythmias, such as supraventricular tachycardia, ventricular tachycardia, and heart block (Chapter 429).

The clinical consequences of hypokalemia in skeletal muscle include muscle weakness and cramps. Paralysis is a possible complication, generally only at potassium levels <2.5 mEq/L. It usually starts in the legs and moves to the arms. Respiratory paralysis may require mechanical ventilation. Some patients have rhabdomyolysis; the risk increases with exercise. Hypokalemia slows gastrointestinal motility. This effect manifests as constipation; with potassium levels <2.5 mEq/L, an ileus may occur. Hypokalemia impairs bladder function, potentially leading to urinary retention.

Hypokalemia causes **polyuria** and **polydipsia** by 2 mechanisms, primary polydipsia and impairment of urinary concentrating ability, which produces nephrogenic diabetes insipidus. Hypokalemia stimulates renal ammonia production, an effect that is clinically significant if hepatic failure is present, because the liver cannot metabolize the ammonia. Hypokalemia may therefore worsen hepatic encephalopathy.

Chronic hypokalemia may cause kidney damage, including interstitial nephritis and renal cysts. In children, chronic hypokalemia, like Bartter syndrome, leads to poor linear growth.

Diagnosis
Most causes of hypokalemia are readily apparent from the history. It is important to review the child's diet, gastrointestinal losses, and medications. Both emesis and diuretic use can be surreptitious. The presence of hypertension suggests excess mineralocorticoids. Concomitant electrolyte abnormalities are useful clues. The combination of hypokalemia and metabolic acidosis is characteristic of diarrhea and of distal and proximal RTA. A concurrent metabolic alkalosis is characteristic of emesis or nasogastric losses, aldosterone excess, use of diuretics, and Bartter and Gitelman syndromes. An approach to persistent hypokalemia is shown in Figure 52-2.

If a clear etiology is not apparent, the measurement of urinary potassium distinguishes between renal and extrarenal losses. The kidneys should conserve potassium in the presence of extrarenal losses. Urinary potassium losses can be assessed with a 24-hr urine collection, a spot potassium-creatinine ratio, a fractional excretion of potassium, or calculation of the TTKG, which is the most widely used approach in children:

$$\text{TTKG} = [\text{K}]_{urine}/[\text{K}]_{plasma} \times (\text{plasma osmolality}/\text{urine osmolality})$$

where $[K]_{urine}$ = urine potassium concentration and $[K]_{plasma}$ = plasma potassium concentration.

The urine osmolality must be greater than the serum osmolality for the result of this calculation to be valid. A TTKG >4 in the presence of hypokalemia suggests excessive urinary losses of potassium. The urinary potassium excretion value can be misleading if the stimulus for renal loss, such as a diuretic, is no longer present.

Treatment
Factors that influence the treatment of hypokalemia include the potassium level, clinical symptoms, renal function, the presence of transcellular shifts of potassium, ongoing losses, and the patient's ability to tolerate oral potassium. Severe, symptomatic hypokalemia requires aggressive treatment. Supplementation is more cautious if renal function is decreased because of the kidney's limited ability to excrete excessive potassium. The plasma potassium level does not always provide an accurate estimation of the total body potassium deficit because there may be shifts of potassium from the intracellular space to the plasma. Clinically, such shifts occur most commonly with metabolic acidosis and the insulin deficiency of diabetic ketoacidosis; the plasma potassium measurement underestimates the degree of total body potassium depletion. When these problems are corrected, potassium moves into the intracellular space, so more potassium supplementation is required to correct the hypokalemia. Likewise, the presence of a transcellular shift of potassium into the cells indicates that the total body potassium depletion is less severe. In an isolated transcellular shift, as occurs in hypokalemic periodic paralysis, potassium supplementation should be used cautiously, given the risk of hyperkalemia when the transcellular shift resolves. This caution is especially required in thyrotoxic periodic paralysis, which responds dramatically to propranolol, with correction of weakness and hypokalemia. Patients who have ongoing losses of potassium need correction of the deficit and replacement of the ongoing losses.

Because of the risk of hyperkalemia, intravenous potassium should be used very cautiously. Oral potassium is safer, albeit not as rapid in urgent situations. Liquid preparations are bitter tasting; microencapsulated or wax matrix formulations are less irritating than tablets to the gastric mucosa (oral dose: 2-4 mEq/kg/day with a maximum of 120-240 mEq/day in divided doses). The dose of intravenous potassium is 0.5-1 mEq/kg, usually given over 1 hr. The adult maximum dose is 40 mEq. Conservative dosing is generally preferred. Potassium chloride is the usual choice for supplementation, although the presence of concurrent electrolyte abnormalities may dictate other options. Patients with acidosis and hypokalemia can receive potassium acetate or potassium citrate. If hypophosphatemia is present, then some of the potassium deficit can be replaced with potassium phosphate. It is sometimes possible to decrease ongoing losses of potassium. For patients with excessive urinary losses, potassium-sparing diuretics are effective, but they need to be used cautiously in patients with renal insufficiency. If hypokalemia, metabolic alkalosis, and volume depletion are present (with gastric losses), then restoration of intravascular volume with adequate sodium chloride will decrease urinary potassium losses. Correction of concurrent hypomagnesemia is important because hypomagnesemia may cause hypokalemia. Disease-specific therapy is effective in many of the genetic tubular disorders.

BIBLIOGRAPHY

Please visit the Nelson Textbook of Pediatrics *website at www.expertconsult.com for the complete bibliography.*

52.5 Magnesium

Larry A. Greenbaum

MAGNESIUM METABOLISM

Body Content and Physiologic Function
Magnesium is the 4th most common cation in the body and the 3rd most common intracellular cation (see Web Fig. 52-3).

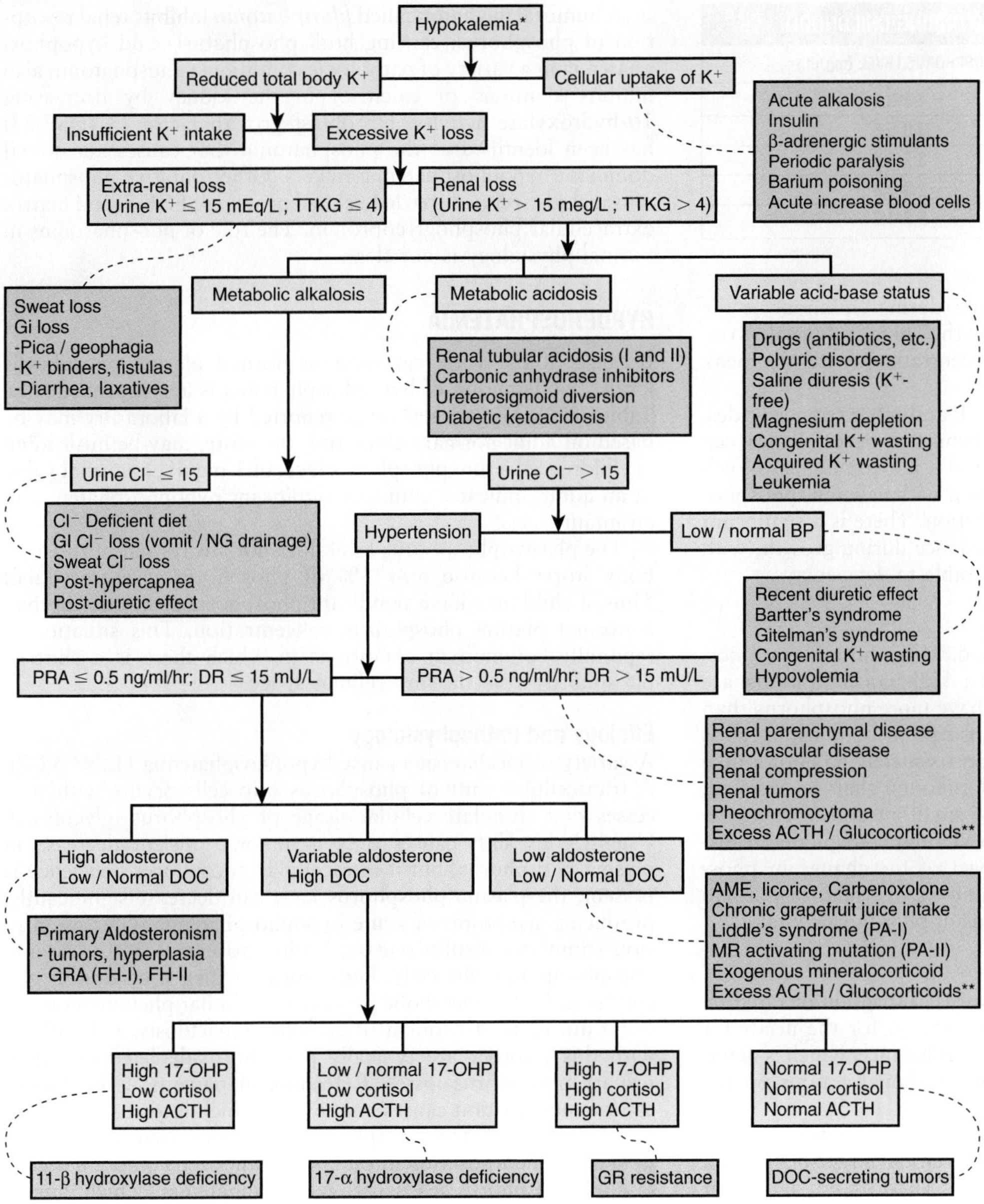

Figure 52-2 Diagnostic algorithm to evaluate persistent hypokalemia. *Spurious hypokalemia must be excluded. **Hypokalemia is uncommon in uncomplicated edematous disorders and in conditions associated with excessive glucocorticosteroids. Conditions associated with high circulating levels of glucocorticosteroids often have normal renin activity. 17-OHP, 17-hydroxyprogesterone; ACTH, adrenocorticotropic hormone; AME, apparent mineralocorticoid excess; BP, blood pressure; Cl^-, chloride; DOC, 11-deoxycorticosterone; DR, direct renin assay; GI, gastrointestinal; FH-II, familial hyperaldosteronism type II; GR, glucocorticoid receptor; GRA (FH-I), glucocorticoid remediable aldosteronism (familial hyperaldosteronism type I); K^+, potassium; MR, mineralocorticoid receptor; PA-I, pseudoaldosteronism type I; PA-II, pseudoaldosteronism type II; PRA, plasma renin activity; TTKG, transtubular potassium gradient. (From Shoemaker LR, Eaton BV, Buchino JJ: A three-year-old with persistent hypokalemia, *J Pediatr* 151:696–699, 2007.)

Between 50% and 60% of body magnesium is in bone, where it serves as a reservoir because 30% is exchangeable, allowing movement to the extracellular space. Most intracellular magnesium is bound to proteins; only approximately 25% is exchangeable. Because cells with higher metabolic rates have higher magnesium concentrations, most intracellular magnesium is present in muscle and liver.

For the full continuation of this chapter, please visit the Nelson Textbook of Pediatrics *website at* *www.expertconsult.com*.

52.6 Phosphorus

Larry A. Greenbaum

Approximately 65% of plasma phosphorus is in phospholipids, but these compounds are insoluble in acid and are not measured by clinical laboratories. It is the phosphorus content of plasma phosphate that is determined. The result is reported as either phosphate or phosphorus, although even when the term *phosphate* is used, it is actually the phosphorus concentration that is measured and reported. The result is that the terms *phosphate* and *phosphorus* are often used interchangeably. The term *phosphorus* is preferred when one is referring to the plasma concentration. Conversion from the units used in the USA (mg/dL) to mmol/L is straightforward (see Web Table 52-1).

PHOSPHORUS METABOLISM

Body Content and Physiologic Function

Most phosphorus is in bone or is intracellular, with <1% in plasma. At a physiologic pH, there are monovalent and divalent forms of phosphate because the pK of these forms is 6.8. Approximately 80% is divalent, and the remainder is monovalent at a pH of 7.4. A small percentage of plasma phosphate, approximately 15%, is protein bound. The remainder can be filtered by the glomerulus, with most existing as free phosphate and a small percentage complexed with calcium, magnesium, or sodium. Phosphate is the most plentiful intracellular anion, although the majority is part of a larger compound (ATP).

More than that of any other electrolyte, the phosphorus concentration varies with age (Table 52-6). The teleologic

Table 52-6 SERUM PHOSPHORUS LEVELS DURING CHILDHOOD

AGE	PHOSPHORUS LEVEL (mg/dL)
0-5 day	4.8-8.2
1-3 yr	3.8-6.5
4-11 yr	3.7-5.6
12-15 yr	2.9-5.4
16-19 yr	2.7-4.7

explanation for the high concentration during childhood is the need for phosphorus to facilitate growth. There is diurnal variation in the plasma phosphorus concentration, with the peak during sleep.

Phosphorus, as a component of ATP and other trinucleotides, is critical for cellular energy metabolism. It is necessary for cell signaling and nucleic acid synthesis, and it is a component of cell membranes and other structures. Along with calcium, phosphorus is necessary for skeletal mineralization. There is a significant need for a net positive phosphorus balance during growth, with the growing skeleton especially vulnerable to deficiency.

Intake

Phosphorus is readily available in food. Milk and milk products are the best sources of phosphorus; high concentrations are present in meat and fish. Vegetables have more phosphorus than fruits and grains. Gastrointestinal absorption of phosphorus is fairly proportional to intake, with approximately 65% of intake being absorbed, including a small amount that is secreted. Absorption, almost exclusively in the small intestine, occurs via a paracellular diffusive process and a vitamin D–regulated transcellular pathway. However, the impact of the change in phosphorus absorption caused by vitamin D is relatively small compared with the effect of variations in phosphorus intake.

Excretion

Despite the wide variation in phosphorus absorption dictated by oral intake, excretion matches intake, except for the needs for growth. The kidney regulates phosphorus balance, which is determined by intrarenal mechanisms and hormonal actions on the nephron.

Approximately 90% of plasma phosphate is filtered at the glomerulus, although there is some variation based on plasma phosphate and calcium concentrations. There is no significant secretion of phosphate along the nephron. Resorption of phosphate occurs mostly in the proximal tubule, although a small amount can be resorbed in the distal tubule. Normally, approximately 85% of the filtered load is resorbed. A sodium-phosphate cotransporter mediates the uptake of phosphate into the cells of the proximal tubule.

The dietary phosphorus determines the amount of phosphate resorbed by the nephron. There are both acute and chronic changes in phosphate resorption that are based on intake. Many of these changes appear to be mediated by intrarenal mechanisms that are independent of regulatory hormones. PTH, which is secreted in response to a low plasma calcium level, decreases resorption of phosphate, increasing the urinary phosphate level. This process appears to have a minimal effect during normal physiologic variation in PTH levels. However, it does have an impact in the setting of pathologic changes in PTH synthesis.

Low plasma phosphorus stimulates the 1α-hydroxylase in the kidney that converts 25-hydroxyvitamin D to 1,25-dihydroxyvitamin D (calcitriol). Calcitriol increases intestinal absorption of phosphorus and is necessary for maximal renal resorption of phosphate. The effect of a change in calcitriol on urinary phosphate is significant only when the level of calcitriol was initially low, arguing against a role for calcitriol in nonpathologic conditions.

A humoral mediator called *phosphatonin* inhibits renal resorption of phosphorus, causing both phosphaturia and hypophosphatemia in a variety of pathologic conditions. Phosphatonin also inhibits synthesis of calcitriol in the kidney by decreasing 1α-hydroxylase activity. Fibroblast growth factor-23 (FGF-23) has been identified as the phosphatonin that causes autosomal dominant hypophosphatemic rickets. Other putative phosphatonins include secreted frizzled-related protein 4, FGF-7, and matrix extracellular phosphoglycoprotein. The role of phosphatonins in normal physiology is not clear.

HYPOPHOSPHATEMIA

Because of the wide variation in normal plasma phosphorus levels, the definition of hypophosphatemia is age-dependent (see Table 52-6). The normal range reported by a laboratory may be based on adult normal values and, therefore, may be misleading in children. A serum phosphorus level of 3 mg/dL, a normal value in an adult, indicates clinically significant hypophosphatemia in an infant.

The plasma phosphorus level does not always reflect the total body stores because only 1% of phosphorus is extracellular. Thus, a child may have significant phosphorus deficiency despite a normal plasma phosphorus concentration. This situation is especially common in conditions in which there is a shift of phosphorus from the intracellular space.

Etiology and Pathophysiology

A variety of mechanisms cause hypophosphatemia (Table 52-7). A transcellular shift of phosphorus into cells occurs with processes that stimulate cellular usage of phosphorus (glycolysis). Usually, this shift causes only a minor, transient decrease in plasma phosphorus, but if intracellular phosphorus deficiency is present, the plasma phosphorus level can decrease significantly, producing symptoms of acute hypophosphatemia. Glucose infusion stimulates insulin release, leading to entry of glucose and phosphorus into the cells. Phosphorus is then used during glycolysis and other metabolic processes. A similar phenomenon can occur during the treatment of diabetic ketoacidosis, and patients with this disorder are typically phosphorus-depleted owing to urinary phosphorus losses. **Refeeding** of patients with protein-calorie malnutrition causes anabolism, which leads to significant cellular demand for phosphorus. The increased phosphorus uptake for incorporation into newly synthesized compounds containing phosphorus leads to hypophosphatemia, which can be severe and symptomatic. Refeeding hypophosphatemia occurs frequently during treatment of severe anorexia nervosa. It can occur during treatment of children with malnutrition due to any cause, such as cystic fibrosis, Crohn disease, burns, neglect, chronic infection, or famine. Hypophosphatemia usually occurs within the 1st 5 days of refeeding and is prevented by a gradual increase in nutrition with appropriate phosphorus supplementation (Chapter 43). Total parenteral nutrition without adequate phosphorus can cause hypophosphatemia.

Phosphorus moves into the intracellular space during a respiratory alkalosis and during recovery from a respiratory acidosis. An acute decrease in the carbon dioxide concentration, by raising the intracellular pH, stimulates glycolysis, leading to intracellular use of phosphorus and hypophosphatemia. Because a metabolic alkalosis has less effect on the intracellular pH (carbon dioxide diffuses across cell membranes much faster than bicarbonate), there is minimal transcellular phosphorus movement with a metabolic alkalosis.

Tumors that grow rapidly, such as leukemia and lymphoma, may use large amounts of phosphorus, leading to hypophosphatemia. A similar phenomenon may occur during the hematopoietic reconstitution that follows bone marrow transplantation. In **hungry bone syndrome,** there is avid bone uptake of phosphorus, along with calcium and magnesium, which can produce plasma

Table 52-7 CAUSES OF HYPOPHOSPHATEMIA

TRANSCELLULAR SHIFTS
Glucose infusion
Insulin
Refeeding
Total parenteral nutrition
Respiratory alkalosis
Tumor growth
Bone marrow transplantation
Hungry bone syndrome
DECREASED INTAKE
Nutritional
Premature infants
Low phosphorus formula
Antacids and other phosphate binders
RENAL LOSSES
Hyperparathyroidism
Parathyroid hormone–related peptide
X-linked hypophosphatemic rickets (MIM 307800)
Tumor-induced osteomalacia
Autosomal dominant hypophosphatemic rickets (MIM 193100)
Autosomal recessive hypophosphatemic rickets (MIM 241520)
Fanconi syndrome
Dent disease (MIM 300009/300555)
Hypophosphatemic rickets with hypercalciuria (MIM 241530)
Hypophosphatemic nephrolithiasis/osteoporosis type 1 (MIM 612286)
Hypophosphatemic nephrolithiasis/osteoporosis type 2 (MIM 612287)
Volume expansion and intravenous fluids
Metabolic acidosis
Diuretics
Glycosuria
Glucocorticoids
Kidney transplantation
MULTIFACTORIAL
Vitamin D deficiency
Vitamin D–dependent rickets type 1 (MIM 264700)
Vitamin D–dependent rickets type 2 (MIM 277440)
Alcoholism
Sepsis
Dialysis

MIM, database number from the Mendelian Inheritance in Man (*http://www3.ncbi.nlm.nih.gov/Omim/*).

deficiency of all 3 ions. Hungry bone syndrome is most common after parathyroidectomy for hyperparathyroidism because the stimulus for bone dissolution is acutely removed, but bone synthesis continues.

Nutritional phosphorus deficiency is unusual because most foods contain phosphorus. However, infants are especially susceptible because of their high demand for phosphorus to support growth, especially of the skeleton. Very low birthweight infants have particularly rapid skeletal growth, and phosphorus deficiency and rickets may develop if they are fed human milk or formula for term infants. There is also a relative deficiency of calcium. The provision of additional calcium and phosphorus, using breast milk fortifier or special premature infant formula, prevents this complication. Phosphorus deficiency, sometimes with concomitant calcium and vitamin D deficiencies, occurs in infants who are not given enough milk or who receive a milk substitute that is nutritionally inadequate.

Antacids containing aluminum hydroxide, such as Maalox and Mylanta, bind dietary phosphorus and secreted phosphorus, preventing absorption. This process can cause phosphorus deficiency and rickets in growing children. A similar mechanism causes hypophosphatemia in patients who are overtreated for hyperphosphatemia with phosphorus binders. In children with kidney failure, the addition of dialysis to phosphorus binders increases the risk of iatrogenic hypophosphatemia in these normally hyperphosphatemic patients. This complication, which is more common in infants, can worsen renal osteodystrophy.

Excessive renal losses of phosphorus occur in a variety of inherited and acquired disorders. Because PTH inhibits the resorption of phosphorus in the proximal tubule, **hyperparathyroidism** causes hypophosphatemia (Chapter 567). The dominant clinical manifestation, however, is hypercalcemia, and the hypophosphatemia is usually asymptomatic. The phosphorus level in hyperparathyroidism is not extremely low, and there is no continued loss of phosphorus because a new steady state is achieved at the lower plasma phosphorus level. Renal excretion, therefore, does not exceed intake over the long term. There are occasional malignancies that produce PTH-related peptide, which has the same actions as PTH and causes hypophosphatemia and hypercalcemia.

A variety of diseases cause renal phosphate wasting, hypophosphatemia, and rickets due to excess phosphatonin (Chapter 48). These disorders include **X-linked hypophosphatemic rickets, tumor-induced osteomalacia, autosomal dominant hypophosphatemic rickets,** and **autosomal recessive hypophosphatemic rickets.** Heterozygous mutations in a phosphate transporter or a regulator of proximal tubule phosphate transport cause hypophosphatemia, osteoporosis and nephrolithiasis (**hypophosphatemic nephrolithiasis/osteoporosis type 1 or 2**).

Fanconi syndrome is a generalized defect in the proximal tubule leading to urinary wasting of bicarbonate, phosphorus, amino acids, uric acid, and glucose (Chapter 523). The clinical sequelae are due to the metabolic acidosis and hypophosphatemia. In children, an underlying genetic disease, most commonly cystinosis, often causes Fanconi syndrome, but it can be secondary to a variety of toxins and acquired diseases. Some patients have incomplete Fanconi syndrome, and phosphorus wasting may be one of the manifestations.

Dent disease, an X-linked disorder, can cause renal phosphorus wasting and hypophosphatemia, although the latter is not present in most cases. Other possible manifestations of Dent disease include tubular proteinuria, hypercalciuria, nephrolithiasis, rickets, and chronic renal failure. Dent disease may be secondary to mutations in a gene that encodes a chloride channel or the *OCRL1* gene, which may also cause Lowe syndrome (Chapter 523.1). **Hypophosphatemic rickets with hypercalciuria** is a rare disorder, principally described in kindreds from the Middle East. Mutations in a sodium-phosphate cotransporter cause hypophosphatemia in this disorder, and complications may include nephrolithiasis and osteoporosis; the disorder is autosomal dominant.

Metabolic acidosis inhibits resorption of phosphorus in the proximal tubule. In addition, metabolic acidosis causes a transcellular shift of phosphorus out of cells because of intracellular catabolism. This released phosphorus is subsequently lost in the urine, leading to significant phosphorus depletion, even though the plasma phosphorus level may be normal. This classically occurs in diabetic ketoacidosis in which renal phosphorus loss is further increased by the osmotic diuresis. With correction of the metabolic acidosis and the administration of insulin, both of which cause a transcellular movement of phosphorus into the cells, there is a marked decrease in the plasma phosphorus level.

Volume expansion from any cause, such as hyperaldosteronism or SIADH, inhibits resorption of phosphorus in the proximal tubule. This effect also occurs with high rates of intravenous fluids. Thiazide and loop diuretics can increase renal phosphorus excretion, but the increase is seldom clinically significant. Glycosuria and glucocorticoids inhibit renal conservation of phosphorus. Hypophosphatemia is common after kidney transplantation as a result of urinary phosphorus losses. Possible explanations include pre-existing secondary hyperparathyroidism from chronic renal failure, glucocorticoid therapy, and upregulation of phosphatonins before transplantation. The hypophosphatemia usually resolves in a few months.

Both acquired and genetic causes of **vitamin D deficiency** are associated with hypophosphatemia (Chapter 48). The pathogenesis is multifactorial. Vitamin D deficiency, by impairing intestinal calcium absorption, causes secondary hyperparathyroidism that leads to increased urinary phosphorus wasting. An absence of vitamin D decreases intestinal absorption of phosphorus and directly decreases renal resorption of phosphorus. The dominant clinical manifestation is rickets, although some patients have muscle weakness that may be related to phosphorus deficiency.

Alcoholism is the most common cause of severe hypophosphatemia in adults. Fortunately, many of the risk factors that predispose adult alcoholics to hypophosphatemia are not usually present in adolescents (malnutrition, antacid abuse, recurrent episodes of diabetic ketoacidosis). Hypophosphatemia often occurs in sepsis, but the mechanism is not clear. Aggressive, protracted hemodialysis, as might be used for the treatment of methanol or ethylene glycol ingestion, can cause hypophosphatemia.

Clinical Manifestations

There are acute and chronic manifestations of hypophosphatemia. Rickets occurs in children with long-term phosphorus deficiency. The clinical features of rickets are described in Chapter 48.

Severe hypophosphatemia, typically at levels <1-1.5 mg/dL, may affect every organ in the body because phosphorus has a critical role in maintaining adequate cellular energy. Phosphorus is a component of ATP and is necessary for glycolysis. With inadequate phosphorus, red blood cell 2,3-diphosphoglycerate levels decrease, impairing release of oxygen to the tissues. Severe hypophosphatemia can cause hemolysis and dysfunction of white blood cells. Chronic hypophosphatemia causes proximal muscle weakness and atrophy. In the intensive care unit, phosphorus deficiency may slow weaning from mechanical ventilation or cause acute respiratory failure. **Rhabdomyolysis** is the most common complication of acute hypophosphatemia, usually in the setting of an acute transcellular shift of phosphorus into cells in a child with chronic phosphorus depletion (anorexia nervosa). The rhabdomyolysis is actually somewhat protective, in that there is cellular release of phosphorus. Other manifestations of severe hypophosphatemia include cardiac dysfunction and neurologic symptoms, such as tremor, paresthesia, ataxia, seizures, delirium, and coma.

Diagnosis

The history and basic laboratory evaluation often suggest the etiology of hypophosphatemia. The history should investigate nutrition, medications, and familial disease. Hypophosphatemia and rickets in an otherwise healthy young child suggests a genetic defect in renal phosphorus conservation, Fanconi syndrome, inappropriate use of antacids, poor nutrition, vitamin D deficiency, or a genetic defect in vitamin D metabolism. The patient with Fanconi syndrome usually has metabolic acidosis, glycosuria, aminoaciduria, and a low plasma uric acid level. Measurement of 25-hydroxyvitamin D and 1,25-dihydroxyvitamin D, calcium, and PTH differentiates among the various vitamin D deficiency disorders and primary renal phosphate wasting (Chapter 48). Hyperparathyroidism is easily distinguished by the presence of elevated plasma PTH and calcium values.

Treatment

The plasma phosphorus level, the presence of symptoms, the likelihood of chronic depletion, and the presence of ongoing losses dictate the approach to therapy. Mild hypophosphatemia does not require treatment unless the clinical situation suggests that chronic phosphorus depletion is present or that losses are ongoing. Oral phosphorus can cause diarrhea, so the doses should be divided. Intravenous therapy is effective in patients who have severe deficiency or who cannot tolerate oral medications. Intravenous phosphorus is available as either sodium phosphate or potassium phosphate, with the choice usually based on the patient's plasma potassium level. Starting doses are 0.08-0.16 mmol/kg over 6 hr. The oral preparations of phosphorus are available with various ratios of sodium and potassium. This is an important consideration because some patients may not tolerate the potassium load, whereas supplemental potassium may be helpful in some diseases, such as Fanconi syndrome and malnutrition. Oral maintenance dosages are 2-3 mmol/kg/day in divided doses.

Increasing dietary phosphorus is the only intervention needed in infants with inadequate intake. Other patients may also benefit from increased dietary phosphorus, usually from dairy products. Phosphorus-binding antacids should be discontinued in patients with hypophosphatemia. Certain diseases require specific therapy (Chapter 48).

HYPERPHOSPHATEMIA

Etiology and Pathophysiology

Renal insufficiency is the most common cause of hyperphosphatemia, with the severity proportional to the degree of kidney impairment (Chapter 529). This occurs because gastrointestinal absorption of the large dietary intake of phosphorus is unregulated, and the kidneys normally excrete this phosphorus. As renal function deteriorates, increased excretion of phosphorus is able to compensate. When kidney function is <30% of normal, hyperphosphatemia usually develops, although the time of its development may vary considerably according to dietary phosphorus absorption. Many of the other causes of hyperphosphatemia are more likely to develop in the setting of renal insufficiency (Table 52-8).

Cellular content of phosphorus is high relative to plasma phosphorus, and cell lysis can release substantial phosphorus. This is the etiology of hyperphosphatemia in **tumor lysis syndrome, rhabdomyolysis,** and **acute hemolysis.** These disorders cause concomitant potassium release and the risk of hyperkalemia. Additional features of tumor lysis and rhabdomyolysis are hyperuricemia and hypocalcemia, whereas indirect hyperbilirubinemia and elevated lactate dehydrogenase values are often present with hemolysis. An elevated CPK level is suggestive of rhabdomyolysis. During lactic acidosis or diabetic ketoacidosis, usage of phosphorus by cells decreases, and phosphorus shifts into the extracellular space. This problem reverses when the underlying problem is corrected, and especially with diabetic ketoacidosis, patients subsequently become hypophosphatemic as a result of previous renal phosphorus loss.

Excessive intake of phosphorus is especially dangerous in children with renal insufficiency. Neonates are at risk because renal function is normally reduced during the 1st few months of life.

Table 52-8 CAUSES OF HYPERPHOSPHATEMIA

TRANSCELLULAR SHIFTS
Tumor lysis syndrome
Rhabdomyolysis
Acute hemolysis
Diabetic ketoacidosis and lactic acidosis
INCREASED INTAKE
Enemas and laxatives
Cow's milk in infants
Treatment of hypophosphatemia
Vitamin D intoxication
DECREASED EXCRETION
Renal failure
Hypoparathyroidism or pseudohypoparathyroidism (MIM 146200/603233/103580 /241410/203330)
Acromegaly
Hyperthyroidism
Tumoral calcinosis with hyperphosphatemia (MIM 211900)

MIM, database number from the Mendelian Inheritance in Man (*http://www3.ncbi.nlm.nih.gov/Omim/*).

In addition, they may erroneously be given doses of phosphorus that are meant for an older child or adult. In infants fed cow's milk, which has higher phosphorus content than breast milk or formula, hyperphosphatemia may develop. **Fleet Enema** has a high amount of phosphorus that can be absorbed, especially in the patient with an ileus. Infants and children with Hirschsprung disease are especially vulnerable. There is often associated hypernatremia owing to sodium absorption and water loss from diarrhea. Sodium phosphorus laxatives may cause hyperphosphatemia if the dose is excessive or if renal insufficiency is present. Hyperphosphatemia occurs in children who receive overly aggressive treatment for hypophosphatemia. Vitamin D intoxication causes excessive gastrointestinal absorption of both calcium and phosphorus, and the suppression of PTH by hypercalcemia decreases renal phosphorus excretion.

The absence of PTH in **hypoparathyroidism** or PTH responsiveness in **pseudohypoparathyroidism** causes hyperphosphatemia because of increased resorption of phosphorus in the proximal tubule of the kidney (Chapters 565 and 566). The associated hypocalcemia is responsible for the clinical symptoms. The hyperphosphatemia in hyperthyroidism or acromegaly is usually minor. It is secondary to increased resorption of phosphorus in the proximal tubule due to the actions of thyroxine or growth hormone. Excessive thyroxine can also cause bone resorption, which may contribute to the hyperphosphatemia and cause hypercalcemia. Patients with **familial tumoral calcinosis,** a rare autosomal recessive disorder, have hyperphosphatemia due to decreased renal phosphate excretion and heterotopic calcifications. The disease may be secondary to mutations in the genes for a glycosyltransferase, the phosphatonin FGF-23, or the gene for Klotho, which encodes the co-receptor for FGF-23.

Clinical Manifestations

The principal clinical consequences of hyperphosphatemia are hypocalcemia and systemic calcification. The hypocalcemia is probably due to tissue deposition of calcium-phosphorus salt, inhibition of 1,25-dihydroxyvitamin D production, and decreased bone resorption. Symptomatic hypocalcemia is most likely to occur when the phosphorus level increases rapidly or when diseases predisposing to hypocalcemia are present (chronic renal failure, rhabdomyolysis). Systemic calcification occurs because the solubility of phosphorus and calcium in the plasma is exceeded. This is believed to happen when plasma calcium × plasma phosphorus, both measured in mg/dL, is more than 70. Clinically, this condition is often apparent in the conjunctiva, where it manifests as a foreign body feeling, erythema, and injection. More ominous manifestations are hypoxia from pulmonary calcification and renal failure from nephrocalcinosis.

Diagnosis

Plasma creatinine and BUN levels should be assessed in any patient with hyperphosphatemia. The history should focus on intake of phosphorus and the presence of chronic diseases that may cause hyperphosphatemia. Measurement of potassium, uric acid, calcium, lactate dehydrogenase, bilirubin, and CPK may be indicated if rhabdomyolysis, tumor lysis, or hemolysis is suspected. With mild hyperphosphatemia and significant hypocalcemia, measurement of the serum PTH level distinguishes between hypoparathyroidism and pseudohypoparathyroidism.

Treatment

The treatment of acute hyperphosphatemia depends on its severity and etiology. Mild hyperphosphatemia in a patient with reasonable renal function spontaneously resolves; the resolution can be accelerated by dietary phosphorus restriction. If kidney function is not impaired, then intravenous fluids can enhance renal phosphorus excretion. For more significant hyperphosphatemia or a situation such as tumor lysis or rhabdomyolysis, in which endogenous phosphorus generation is likely to continue, addition of an oral phosphorus binder prevents absorption of dietary phosphorus and can remove phosphorus from the body by binding what is normally secreted and absorbed by the gastrointestinal tract. Phosphorus binders are most effective when given with food. Binders containing aluminum hydroxide are especially efficient, but calcium carbonate is an effective alternative and may be preferred if there is a need to treat concomitant hypocalcemia. Preservation of renal function, for example with high urine flow in rhabdomyolysis or tumor lysis, is an important adjunct because it will permit continued excretion of phosphorus. If the hyperphosphatemia is not responding to conservative management, especially if renal insufficiency is supervening, then dialysis may be necessary to increase phosphorus removal.

Dietary phosphorus restriction is necessary for diseases causing chronic hyperphosphatemia. However, such diets are often difficult to follow, given the abundance of phosphorus in a variety of foods. Dietary restriction is often sufficient in conditions such as hypoparathyroidism and mild renal insufficiency. For more problematic hyperphosphatemia, such as with moderate renal insufficiency and end-stage renal disease, phosphorus binders are usually necessary. They include calcium carbonate, calcium acetate, and sevelamer hydrochloride. Aluminum-containing phosphorus binders are no longer used in chronic renal insufficiency because of the risk of aluminum toxicity. Dialysis directly removes phosphorus from the blood in patients with end-stage renal disease, but it is only an adjunct to dietary restriction and phosphorus binders, in that elimination of phosphorus by dialysis is not efficient enough to keep up with normal dietary intake.

BIBLIOGRAPHY

Please visit the Nelson Textbook of Pediatrics *website at www.expertconsult.com for the complete bibliography.*

52.7 Acid-Base Balance

Larry A. Greenbaum

ACID-BASE PHYSIOLOGY

Introduction and Terminology

Close regulation of pH is necessary for cellular enzymes and other metabolic processes, which function optimally at normal pH. Chronic, mild derangements in acid-base status may interfere with normal growth and development, whereas acute, severe changes in pH can be fatal. Control of acid-base balance depends on the kidneys, the lungs, and intracellular and extracellular buffers.

For the full continuation of this chapter, please visit the Nelson Textbook of Pediatrics *website at www.expertconsult.com.*

CLINICAL ASSESSMENT OF ACID-BASE DISORDERS

The following equation, a rearrangement of the Henderson-Hasselbalch equation, emphasizes the relationship among the P_{CO_2}, the bicarbonate concentration, and the hydrogen ion concentration:

$$[H^+] = 24 \times P_{CO_2}/[HCO_3^-]$$

An increase in the P_{CO_2} or a decrease in the bicarbonate concentration increases the hydrogen ion concentration; the pH decreases. A decrease in the P_{CO_2} or an increase in the bicarbonate concentration decreases the hydrogen ion concentration; the pH increases.

Terminology

Acidemia is a pH below normal (<7.35), and **alkalemia** is a pH above normal (>7.45). An *acidosis* is a pathologic process that causes an increase in the hydrogen ion concentration, and an *alkalosis* is a pathologic process that causes a decrease in the hydrogen ion concentration. Whereas acidemia is always accompanied by an acidosis, a patient can have an acidosis and a low, normal, or high pH. For example, a patient may have a mild metabolic acidosis but a simultaneous, severe respiratory alkalosis; the net result may be alkalemia. Acidemia and alkalemia indicate the pH abnormality; acidosis and alkalosis indicate the pathologic process that is taking place.

A **simple acid-base disorder** is a single primary disturbance. During a simple metabolic disorder, there is respiratory compensation. With a metabolic acidosis, the decrease in the pH increases the ventilatory drive, causing a decrease in the P_{CO_2}. The decrease in the carbon dioxide concentration leads to an increase in the pH. This appropriate respiratory compensation is expected with a primary metabolic acidosis. Despite the decrease in the carbon dioxide concentration, appropriate respiratory compensation is not a respiratory alkalosis, even though it is sometimes erroneously called a *compensatory respiratory alkalosis.* A low P_{CO_2} can be due either to a primary respiratory alkalosis or to appropriate respiratory compensation for a metabolic acidosis. Appropriate respiratory compensation also occurs with a primary metabolic alkalosis, although in this case the carbon dioxide concentration increases to attenuate the increase in the pH. The respiratory compensation for a metabolic process happens quickly and is complete within 12-24 hr; it cannot overcompensate for or normalize the pH.

During a primary respiratory process, there is metabolic compensation, mediated by the kidneys. The kidneys respond to a respiratory acidosis by increasing hydrogen ion excretion, thereby increasing bicarbonate generation and raising the serum bicarbonate concentration. The kidneys increase bicarbonate excretion to compensate for a respiratory alkalosis; the serum bicarbonate concentration decreases. Unlike respiratory compensation, which occurs rapidly, it takes 3-4 days for the kidneys to complete appropriate metabolic compensation. There is, however, a small and rapid compensatory change in the bicarbonate concentration during a primary respiratory process. The expected appropriate metabolic compensation for a respiratory disorder depends on whether the process is acute or chronic.

A **mixed acid-base disorder** is present when there is more than 1 primary acid-base disturbance. An infant with bronchopulmonary dysplasia may have a respiratory acidosis from chronic lung disease and a metabolic alkalosis from the furosemide used to treat the chronic lung disease. More dramatically, a child with pneumonia and sepsis may have severe acidemia due to a combined metabolic acidosis caused by lactic acid and respiratory acidosis caused by ventilatory failure.

There are formulas for calculating the appropriate metabolic or respiratory compensation for the 6 primary simple acid-base disorders (Table 52-9). The appropriate compensation is expected in a simple disorder; it is not optional. If a patient does not have the appropriate compensation, then a mixed acid-base disorder is present. A patient has a primary metabolic acidosis with a serum bicarbonate concentration of 10m Eq/L. The expected respiratory compensation is a carbon dioxide concentration of 23 mm Hg ± 2 ($1.5 \times 10 + 8 \pm 2 = 23 \pm 2$; see Table 52-9). If the patient's carbon dioxide concentration is >25 mm Hg, a concurrent respiratory acidosis is present; the carbon dioxide concentration is higher than expected. A patient may have a respiratory acidosis despite a carbon dioxide level below the "normal" value of 35-45 mm Hg. In this example, a carbon dioxide concentration <21 mm Hg indicates a concurrent respiratory alkalosis; the carbon dioxide concentration is lower than expected.

Table 52-9 APPROPRIATE COMPENSATION DURING SIMPLE ACID-BASE DISORDERS

DISORDER	EXPECTED COMPENSATION
Metabolic acidosis	$P_{CO_2} = 1.5 \times [HCO_3^-] + 8 \pm 2$
Metabolic alkalosis	P_{CO_2} increases by 7 mm Hg for each 10-mEq/L increase in serum $[HCO_3^-]$
Respiratory acidosis	
Acute	$[HCO_3^-]$ increases by 1 for each 10–mm Hg increase in P_{CO_2}
Chronic	$[HCO_3^-]$ increases by 3.5 for each 10–mm Hg increase in P_{CO_2}
Respiratory alkalosis	
Acute	$[HCO_3^-]$ falls by 2 for each 10–mm Hg decrease in P_{CO_2}
Chronic	$[HCO_3^-]$ falls by 4 for each 10–mm Hg decrease in P_{CO_2}

Table 52-10 NORMAL VALUES OF ARTERIAL BLOOD GASES

pH	7.35-7.45
$[HCO_3^-]$	20-28 mEq/L
P_{CO_2}	35-45 mm Hg

Diagnosis

A systematic evaluation of an arterial blood gas sample, combined with the clinical history, can usually explain the patient's acid-base disturbance. Assessment of an arterial blood gas sample requires knowledge of normal values (Table 52-10). In most cases, this is accomplished via a 3-step process (Fig. 52-3):

- Determine whether acidemia or alkalemia is present.
- Determine a cause of the acidemia or alkalemia.
- Determine whether a mixed disorder is present.

Most patients with an acid-base disturbance have an abnormal pH, although there are 2 exceptions. The 1st exception is in the patient with a mixed disorder, wherein the 2 processes have opposite effects on pH (a metabolic acidosis and a respiratory alkalosis) and cause changes in the hydrogen ion concentration that are comparable in magnitude, albeit opposite. The 2nd exception is in the patient with a simple chronic respiratory alkalosis; in some instances, the appropriate metabolic compensation is enough to normalize the pH. In both of these situations, the presence of an acid-base disturbance is deduced because of the abnormal carbon dioxide and/or bicarbonate levels. Determining the acid-base disturbance in these situations requires proceeding to the 3rd step of this process.

The 2nd step requires inspection of the serum bicarbonate and carbon dioxide concentrations to determine a cause of the abnormal pH (see Fig. 52-3). In most cases, there is only 1 obvious explanation for the abnormal pH. In some mixed disorders, however, there may be 2 possibilities (a high P_{CO_2} and a low $[HCO_3^-]$ in a patient with acidemia). In such cases, the patient has 2 causes for abnormal pH (a metabolic acidosis and a respiratory acidosis, in this instance), and it is unnecessary to proceed to the 3rd step.

The 3rd step requires determining whether the patient's compensation is appropriate. It is assumed that the primary disorder was diagnosed in the 2nd step, and the expected compensation is calculated (see Table 52-9). If the compensation is appropriate, then a simple acid-base disorder is present. If the compensation is not appropriate, then a mixed disorder is present. The identity of the 2nd disorder is determined by deciding whether the compensation is too little or too much compared with what was expected (see Fig. 52-3).

The history is always useful in evaluating and diagnosing patients with acid-base disturbances. It is especially helpful in a respiratory process. The expected metabolic compensation for a respiratory process changes according to whether the process is acute or chronic, which can be deduced only from the history. The metabolic compensation for an acute respiratory acidosis is less

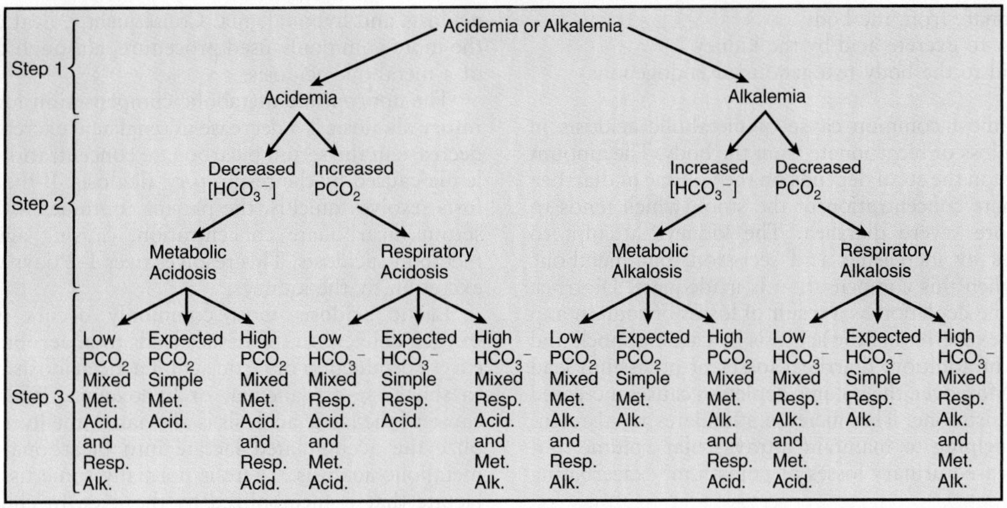

Figure 52-3 Three-step process for interpreting acid-base disturbances. In step 1, determine whether the pH is low (acidemia) or high (alkalemia). In step 2, establish an explanation for the acidemia or alkalemia. In step 3, calculate the expected compensation (see Table 52-9) and determine whether a mixed disturbance is present. Met. alk., metabolic alkalosis; Met. Acid., metabolic acidosis; Resp. Alk., respiratory alkalosis; Resp. Acid., respiratory acidosis.

than that for a chronic respiratory acidosis. In a patient with a respiratory acidosis, a small increase in the bicarbonate concentration would be consistent with a simple acute respiratory acidosis or a mixed disorder (a chronic respiratory acidosis and a metabolic acidosis). Only the history can differentiate among the possibilities. Knowledge of the length of the respiratory process and the presence or absence of a risk factor for a metabolic acidosis (diarrhea) allows the correct conclusion to be reached.

METABOLIC ACIDOSIS

Metabolic acidosis occurs frequently in hospitalized children; diarrhea is the most common etiology. For a patient with an unknown medical problem, the presence of a metabolic acidosis is often helpful diagnostically, because it suggests a relatively narrow differential diagnosis.

Patients with a metabolic acidosis have a low serum bicarbonate concentration, although not every patient with a low serum bicarbonate concentration has a metabolic acidosis. The exception is the patient with a respiratory alkalosis, which causes a decrease in the serum bicarbonate concentration as part of appropriate renal compensation. In a patient with an isolated metabolic acidosis, there is a predictable decrease in the blood carbon dioxide concentration, as follows:

$$P_{CO_2} = 1.5 \times [HCO_3^-] + 8 \pm 2$$

A mixed acid-base disturbance is present if the respiratory compensation is not appropriate. If the P_{CO_2} is greater than predicted, then the patient has a concurrent respiratory acidosis. A lower P_{CO_2} than predicted indicates a concurrent respiratory alkalosis or, less commonly, an isolated respiratory alkalosis. Because the appropriate respiratory compensation for a metabolic acidosis **never normalizes** the patient's pH, the presence of a normal pH and a low bicarbonate concentration occurs only if some degree of respiratory alkalosis is present. In this situation, distinguishing an isolated chronic respiratory alkalosis from a mixed metabolic acidosis and acute respiratory alkalosis may be possible only clinically. In contrast, the combination of a low serum pH and a low bicarbonate concentration occurs only if a metabolic acidosis is present.

Etiology and Pathophysiology

There are many causes of a metabolic acidosis (Table 52-11), which occur via 3 basic mechanisms:

Table 52-11 CAUSES OF METABOLIC ACIDOSIS

NORMAL ANION GAP
Diarrhea
Renal tubular acidosis (RTA):
Distal (type I) RTA (MIM 179800/602722/267300)[*]
Proximal (type II) RTA (MIM 604278)[†]
Hyperkalemic (type IV) RTA (MIM 201910/264350/177735/145260)[‡]
Urinary tract diversions
Post-hypocapnia
Ammonium chloride intake
INCREASED ANION GAP
Lactic acidosis:
Tissue hypoxia:
Shock
Hypoxemia
Severe anemia
Liver failure
Malignancy
Intestinal bacterial overgrowth
Inborn errors of metabolism
Medications:
Nucleoside reverse transcriptase inhibitors
Metformin
Propofol
Ketoacidosis:
Diabetic ketoacidosis
Starvation ketoacidosis
Alcoholic ketoacidosis
Kidney failure
Poisoning:
Ethylene glycol
Methanol
Salicylate
Toluene
Paraldehyde
Inborn errors of metabolism

*Along with these genetic disorders, distal renal tubular acidosis may be secondary to renal disease or medications.

†Most cases of proximal RTA are not due to this primary genetic disorder. Proximal RTA is usually part of Fanconi syndrome, which has multiple etiologies.

‡Hyperkalemic RTA can be secondary to a genetic disorder (some of the more common are listed) or other etiologies.

MIM, database number from the Mendelian Inheritance in Man (*http://www3.ncbi.nlm.nih.gov/Omim/*).

- Loss of bicarbonate from the body
- Impaired ability to excrete acid by the kidney
- Addition of acid to the body (exogenous or endogenous)

Diarrhea, the most common cause of metabolic acidosis in children, causes a loss of bicarbonate from the body. The amount of bicarbonate lost in the stool depends on the volume of diarrhea and the bicarbonate concentration of the stool, which tends to increase with more severe diarrhea. The kidneys attempt to balance the losses by increasing acid secretion, but metabolic acidosis occurs when this compensation is inadequate. Diarrhea often causes volume depletion as a result of losses of sodium and water, potentially exacerbating the acidosis by causing shock and a lactic acidosis. In addition, diarrheal losses of potassium lead to hypokalemia. Moreover, the volume depletion causes increased production of aldosterone. This increase stimulates renal retention of sodium, helping to maintain intravascular volume, but also leads to increased urinary losses of potassium, exacerbating the hypokalemia.

There are 3 forms of **renal tubular acidosis** (RTA): distal (type I), proximal (type II), and hyperkalemic (type IV) [Chapter 523]. In distal RTA, children may have accompanying hypokalemia, hypercalciuria, nephrolithiasis, and nephrocalcinosis. Failure to thrive due to chronic metabolic acidosis is the most common presenting complaint. Patients with distal RTA cannot acidify their urine and, thus, have a urine pH >5.5 despite a metabolic acidosis.

Proximal RTA is rarely present in isolation. In most patients, proximal RTA is part of Fanconi syndrome, a generalized dysfunction of the proximal tubule. The dysfunction leads to glycosuria, aminoaciduria, and excessive urinary losses of phosphate and uric acid. The presence of a low serum uric acid level, glycosuria, and aminoaciduria is helpful diagnostically. Chronic hypophosphatemia leads to rickets in children (Chapter 48). Rickets and/or failure to thrive may be the presenting complaint. The ability to acidify the urine is intact in proximal RTA; thus, untreated patients have a urine pH <5.5. However, bicarbonate therapy increases bicarbonate losses in the urine, and the urine pH increases.

In hyperkalemic RTA, renal excretion of acid and potassium is impaired. Hyperkalemic RTA is due to either an absence of aldosterone or an inability of the kidney to respond to aldosterone. In severe aldosterone deficiency, as occurs with congenital adrenal hyperplasia due to 21α-hydroxylase deficiency, the hyperkalemia and metabolic acidosis are accompanied by hyponatremia and volume depletion from renal salt wasting. Incomplete aldosterone deficiency causes less severe electrolyte disturbances; children may have isolated hyperkalemic RTA, hyperkalemia without acidosis, or isolated hyponatremia. Patients may have aldosterone deficiency due to decreased renin production by the kidney; renin normally stimulates aldosterone synthesis. Children with hyporeninemic hypoaldosteronism usually have either isolated hyperkalemia or hyperkalemic RTA. The manifestations of aldosterone resistance depend on the severity of the resistance. In the autosomal recessive form of pseudohypoaldosteronism type I, which is due to an absence of the sodium channel that normally responds to aldosterone, there is often severe salt wasting and hyponatremia. In contrast, the aldosterone resistance in kidney transplant recipients usually produces either isolated hyperkalemia or hyperkalemic RTA; hyponatremia is unusual. Similarly, the medications that cause hyperkalemic RTA do not cause hyponatremia. Pseudohypoaldosteronism type II, an autosomal recessive disorder also known as **Gordon syndrome,** is a unique cause of hyperkalemic RTA because the genetic defect causes volume expansion and hypertension.

Children with **abnormal urinary tracts,** usually secondary to congenital malformations, may require diversion of urine through intestinal segments. Ureterosigmoidostomy, anastomosis of a ureter to the sigmoid colon, almost always produces a metabolic acidosis and hypokalemia. Consequently, ileal conduits are now the more commonly used procedure, although there is still a risk of a metabolic acidosis.

The **appropriate metabolic compensation for a chronic respiratory alkalosis** is a decrease in renal acid excretion. The resultant decrease in the serum bicarbonate concentration lessens the alkalemia caused by the respiratory alkalosis. If the respiratory alkalosis resolves quickly, the patient continues to have a decreased serum bicarbonate concentration, causing acidemia due to a metabolic acidosis. This resolves over 1-2 days via increased acid excretion by the kidneys.

Lactic acidosis most commonly occurs when inadequate oxygen delivery to the tissues leads to anaerobic metabolism and excess production of lactic acid. Lactic acidosis may be secondary to shock, severe anemia, or hypoxemia. When the underlying cause of the lactic acidosis is alleviated, the liver is able to metabolize the accumulated lactate into bicarbonate, correcting the metabolic acidosis. There is normally some tissue production of lactate that is metabolized by the liver. In children with severe liver dysfunction, impairment of lactate metabolism may produce a lactic acidosis. Rarely, a metabolically active malignancy grows so fast that its blood supply becomes inadequate, with resultant anaerobic metabolism and lactic acidosis. Patients who have short bowel syndrome due to small bowel resection can have bacterial overgrowth. In these patients, excessive bacterial metabolism of glucose into D-lactic acid can cause a lactic acidosis. Lactic acidosis occurs in a variety of inborn errors of metabolism, especially those affecting mitochondrial oxidation (Chapter 81.4). Finally, medications can cause lactic acidosis. Nucleoside reverse transcriptase inhibitors that are used to treat HIV infection inhibit mitochondrial replication; lactic acidosis is a rare complication, although elevated serum lactate concentrations without acidosis are quite common. Metformin, commonly used for treating type 2 diabetes mellitus, is most likely to cause a lactic acidosis in patients with renal insufficiency. High dosages and prolonged use of propofol can cause lactic acidosis.

In **insulin-dependent diabetes mellitus,** inadequate insulin leads to hyperglycemia and diabetic ketoacidosis (Chapter 583). Production of acetoacetic acid and β-hydroxybutyric acid causes the metabolic acidosis. Administration of insulin corrects the underlying metabolic problem and permits conversion of acetoacetate and β-hydroxybutyrate into bicarbonate, which helps correct the metabolic acidosis. However, in some patients, urinary losses of acetoacetate and β-hydroxybutyrate may be substantial, preventing rapid regeneration of bicarbonate. In these patients, full correction of the metabolic acidosis requires renal regeneration of bicarbonate, a slower process. The hyperglycemia causes an osmotic diuresis, usually producing volume depletion, along with substantial losses of potassium, sodium, and phosphate.

In **starvation ketoacidosis,** the lack of glucose leads to keto acid production, which in turn can produce a metabolic acidosis, although it is usually mild as a result of increased acid secretion by the kidney. In alcoholic ketoacidosis, which is much less common in children than in adults, the acidosis usually follows a combination of an alcoholic binge with vomiting and poor intake of food. The acidosis is potentially more severe than with isolated starvation, and the blood glucose level may be low, normal, or high. Hypoglycemia and acidosis also suggest an inborn error of metabolism.

Renal failure causes a metabolic acidosis because of the need for the kidneys to excrete the acid produced by normal metabolism. With mild or moderate renal insufficiency, the remaining nephrons are usually able to compensate by increasing acid excretion. When the GFR is <20-30% of normal, the compensation is inadequate and a metabolic acidosis develops. In some children, especially those with chronic renal failure due to tubular damage, the acidosis develops at a higher GFR because of a concurrent defect in acid secretion by the distal tubule (a distal RTA).

A variety of **toxic ingestions** (Chapter 58) can cause a metabolic acidosis. **Salicylate** intoxication is now much less common because aspirin is no longer recommended for fever control in children. Acute salicylate intoxication occurs after a large overdose. Chronic salicylate intoxication is possible with gradual buildup of the drug. Especially in adults, respiratory alkalosis may be the dominant acid-base disturbance. In children, the metabolic acidosis is usually the more significant finding. Other symptoms of salicylate intoxication are fever, seizures, lethargy, and coma. Hyperventilation may be particularly marked. Tinnitus, vertigo, and hearing impairment are more likely with chronic salicylate intoxication.

Ethylene glycol, a component of antifreeze, is converted in the liver to glyoxylic and oxalic acids, causing a severe metabolic acidosis. Excessive oxalate excretion causes calcium oxalate crystals to appear in the urine, and calcium oxalate precipitation in the kidney tubules can cause renal failure. The toxicity of methanol ingestion also depends on liver metabolism; formic acid is the toxic end product that causes the metabolic acidosis and other sequelae, which include damage to the optic nerve and CNS. Symptoms may include nausea, emesis, visual impairment, and altered mental status. Toluene inhalation and paraldehyde ingestion are other potential causes of a metabolic acidosis.

Many **inborn errors of metabolism** cause a metabolic acidosis (Chapters 78-81). The metabolic acidosis may be due to excessive production of keto acids, lactic acid, and/or other organic anions. Some patients have accompanying hypoglycemia or hyperammonemia. In most patients, the acidosis occurs episodically, only during acute decompensations, which may be precipitated by ingestion of specific dietary substrates, the stress of a mild illness, or poor compliance with dietary or medical therapy. In a few inborn errors of metabolism, patients have a chronic metabolic acidosis.

Clinical Manifestations

The underlying disorder usually produces most of the signs and symptoms in children with a mild or moderate metabolic acidosis. The clinical manifestations of the acidosis are related to the degree of acidemia; patients with appropriate respiratory compensation and less severe acidemia have fewer manifestations than those with a concomitant respiratory acidosis. At a serum pH <7.20, there may be impaired cardiac contractility and an increased risk of arrhythmias, especially if underlying heart disease or other predisposing electrolyte disorders are present. With acidemia, there may be a decrease in the cardiovascular response to catecholamines, potentially exacerbating hypotension in children with volume depletion or shock. Acidemia causes vasoconstriction of the pulmonary vasculature, which is especially problematic in newborn infants with persistent pulmonary hypertension (Chapter 95.7).

The normal respiratory response to metabolic acidosis—compensatory hyperventilation—may be subtle with mild metabolic acidosis, but it causes discernible increased respiratory effort with worsening acidemia. The acute metabolic effects of acidemia include insulin resistance, increased protein degradation, and reduced ATP synthesis. Chronic metabolic acidosis causes failure to thrive in children. Acidemia causes potassium to move from the intracellular space to the extracellular space, thereby increasing the serum potassium concentration. Severe acidemia impairs brain metabolism, eventually resulting in lethargy and coma.

Diagnosis

The etiology of a metabolic acidosis is often apparent from the history and physical examination. Acutely, diarrhea and shock are common causes of a metabolic acidosis. Shock, which causes a lactic acidosis, is usually apparent on physical examination and can be secondary to dehydration, acute blood loss, sepsis, or heart disease. Failure to thrive suggests a chronic metabolic acidosis, as happens with renal insufficiency or RTA. New onset of polyuria occurs in children with undiagnosed diabetes mellitus and diabetic ketoacidosis. Metabolic acidosis with seizures and/or a depressed sensorium, especially in an infant, warrants consideration of an inborn error of metabolism. Meningitis and sepsis with lactic acidosis are more common explanations for metabolic acidosis with neurologic signs and symptoms. Identification of a toxic ingestion, such as of ethylene glycol or methanol, is especially important because of the potentially excellent response to specific therapy. A variety of medications can cause a metabolic acidosis; they may be prescribed or accidentally ingested. Hepatomegaly and metabolic acidosis may occur in children with sepsis, congenital or acquired heart disease, hepatic failure, or inborn errors of metabolism.

Basic laboratory tests in a child with a metabolic acidosis should include measurements of BUN, serum creatinine, serum glucose, urinalysis, and serum electrolytes. Elevated BUN and creatinine values are present in renal insufficiency, whereas an elevated BUN:creatinine ratio (>20:1) supports a diagnosis of prerenal azotemia and the possibility of poor perfusion with lactic acidosis. Metabolic acidosis, hyperglycemia, glycosuria, and ketonuria support a diagnosis of diabetic ketoacidosis. Starvation causes ketosis, but the metabolic acidosis, if present, is usually mild (HCO_3^- >18). In most children with ketosis due to poor intake and metabolic acidosis, there is a concomitant disorder, such as gastroenteritis with diarrhea, that explains the metabolic acidosis. Alternatively, metabolic acidosis with or without ketosis occurs in inborn errors of metabolism; patients with these disorders may have hyperglycemia, normoglycemia, or hypoglycemia. Adrenal insufficiency may cause metabolic acidosis and hypoglycemia. Metabolic acidosis with hypoglycemia also occurs with liver failure. Metabolic acidosis, normoglycemia, and glycosuria occur in children when type II RTA is part of Fanconi syndrome; the defect in resorption of glucose by the proximal tubule of the kidney causes the glycosuria.

The serum potassium level is often abnormal in children with a metabolic acidosis. Even though a metabolic acidosis causes potassium to move from the intracellular space to the extracellular space, many patients with a metabolic acidosis have a low serum potassium level owing to excessive body losses of potassium. With diarrhea, there are high stool losses of potassium and often secondary renal losses of potassium, whereas in type I or type II RTA, there are increased urinary losses of potassium. In diabetic ketoacidosis, urinary losses of potassium are high, but the shift of potassium out of cells due to lack of insulin and metabolic acidosis is especially significant. Consequently, the initial serum potassium level can be low, normal, or high, even though total body potassium is almost always decreased. The serum potassium level is usually increased in patients with acidosis due to renal insufficiency; urinary potassium excretion is impaired. The combination of metabolic acidosis, hyperkalemia, and hyponatremia occurs in patients with severe aldosterone deficiency (adrenogenital syndrome) or aldosterone resistance. Patients with less severe, type IV RTA often have only hyperkalemia and metabolic acidosis. Very ill children with metabolic acidosis may have an elevated serum potassium value as a result of a combination of renal insufficiency, tissue breakdown, and a shift of potassium from the intracellular space to the extracellular space secondary to the metabolic acidosis.

The **plasma anion gap** is useful for evaluating patients with a metabolic acidosis. It divides patients into 2 diagnostic groups, those with normal anion gap and those with increased anion gap. The following formula determines the anion gap:

$$\text{Anion gap} = [Na^+] - [Cl^-] - [HCO_3^-]$$

A normal anion gap is 4-11, although there is variation among laboratories. The number of serum anions must equal the number of serum cations to maintain electrical neutrality (Fig. 52-4). The anion gap is the difference between the measured cation (sodium)

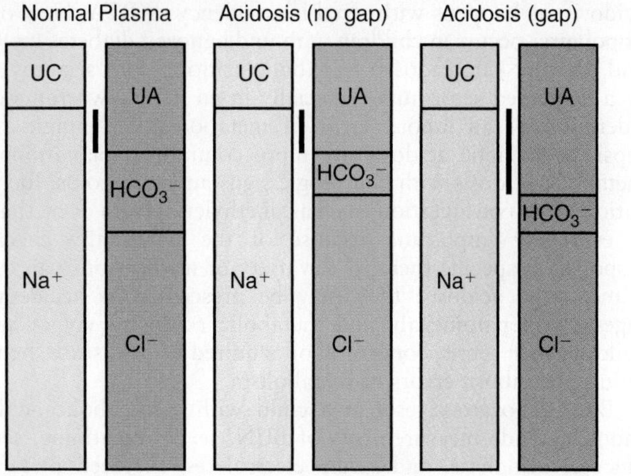

Figure 52-4 The anion gap, which is the difference between the sodium concentration and the combined concentrations of chloride and bicarbonate *(vertical line).* In both a gap and a non-gap metabolic acidosis, there is a decrease in the bicarbonate concentration. There is an increase in unmeasured anions (UA) in patients with a gap metabolic acidosis. In a non-gap metabolic acidosis, there is an increase in the serum chloride concentration. UC, unmeasured cations.

and the measured anions (chloride + bicarbonate). The anion gap is also the difference between the unmeasured cations (potassium, magnesium, calcium) and the unmeasured anions (albumin, phosphate, urate, sulfate). An increased anion gap occurs when there is an increase in unmeasured anions. With a lactic acidosis, there is endogenous production of lactic acid, which is composed of positively charged hydrogen ions and negatively charged lactate anions. The hydrogen ions are largely buffered by serum bicarbonate, resulting in a decrease in the bicarbonate concentration. The hydrogen ions that are not buffered by bicarbonate cause the serum pH to decrease. The lactate anions remain, causing the increase in the anion gap.

An increase in unmeasured anions, along with hydrogen ion generation, is present in all causes of an increased gap metabolic acidosis (see Table 52-11). In diabetic ketoacidosis, the keto acids β-hydroxybutyrate and acetoacetate are the unmeasured anions. In renal failure, there is retention of unmeasured anions, including phosphate, urate, and sulfate. The increase in unmeasured anions in renal failure is usually less than the decrease in the bicarbonate concentration. Renal failure is thus a mix of an increased gap and a normal gap metabolic acidosis. The normal gap metabolic acidosis is especially prominent in children with renal failure due to tubular damage, as occurs with renal dysplasia or obstructive uropathy, because these patients have a concurrent RTA. The unmeasured anions in toxic ingestions vary: formate in methanol intoxication, glycolate in ethylene glycol intoxication, and lactate and keto acids in salicylate intoxication. In inborn errors of metabolism, the unmeasured anions depend on the specific etiology and may include keto acids, lactate, and other organic anions. In a few inborn errors of metabolism, the acidosis occurs without generation of unmeasured anions; thus, the anion gap is normal.

A **normal anion gap** metabolic acidosis occurs when there is a decrease in the bicarbonate concentration without an increase in the unmeasured anions. With diarrhea, there is a loss of bicarbonate in the stool, causing a decrease in the serum pH and bicarbonate concentration; the serum chloride concentration increases to maintain electrical neutrality (see Fig. 52-4). Hyperchloremic metabolic acidosis is an alternative term for a normal anion gap metabolic acidosis. Calculation of the anion gap is more precise than using the chloride concentration to differentiate between a normal and an increased gap metabolic acidosis, in that the anion gap directly determines the presence of unmeasured anions. Electrical neutrality dictates that the chloride concentration increases or decreases according to the serum sodium concentration, making the chloride concentration a less reliable predictor of unmeasured anions than the more direct measure, calculation of the anion gap.

Approximately 11 mEq of the anion gap is normally secondary to albumin. A 1-g/dL decrease in the albumin concentration decreases the anion gap by roughly 2.5 mEq/L. Similarly, an increase in unmeasured cations, such as calcium, potassium, and magnesium, decreases the anion gap. Conversely, a decrease in unmeasured cations is a very unusual cause of an increased anion gap. Because of these variables, the broad range of a normal anion gap, and other variables, the presence of a normal or an increased anion gap is not always reliable in differentiating among the causes of a metabolic acidosis, especially when the metabolic acidosis is mild. In some patients there is more than one explanation for the metabolic acidosis, such as the child with diarrhea and lactic acidosis due to poor perfusion. The anion gap should not be interpreted in dogmatic isolation; consideration of other laboratory abnormalities and the clinical history improves its diagnostic utility.

Treatment

The most effective therapeutic approach for patients with a metabolic acidosis is repair of the underlying disorder, if possible. The administration of insulin in diabetic ketoacidosis and the restoration of adequate perfusion with intravenous fluids in lactic acidosis due to hypovolemia or shock eventually result in normalization of the acid-base balance. In other diseases, the use of bicarbonate therapy is indicated because the underlying disorder is irreparable. Children with metabolic acidosis due to RTA or chronic renal failure require long-term base therapy. Patients with acute renal failure and metabolic acidosis need base therapy until their kidneys' ability to excrete hydrogen normalizes. In other disorders, the cause of the metabolic acidosis eventually resolves, but base therapy is necessary during the acute illness. In salicylate poisoning, alkali administration increases renal clearance of salicylate and decreases the amount of salicylate in brain cells. Short-term base therapy is often necessary in other poisonings (ethylene glycol, methanol) and inborn errors of metabolism (pyruvate carboxylase deficiency, propionic acidemia). Some inborn errors of metabolism require long-term base therapy.

The use of base therapy in diabetic ketoacidosis and lactic acidosis is controversial; there is little evidence that it improves patient outcome, and it has a variety of potential side effects. The risks of giving sodium bicarbonate include the possibility of causing hypernatremia or volume overload. Furthermore, the patient may have overcorrection of the metabolic acidosis once the underlying disorder resolves, because metabolism of lactate or keto acids generates bicarbonate. The rapid change from acidemia to alkalemia can cause a variety of problems, including hypokalemia and hypophosphatemia. Bicarbonate therapy increases the generation of carbon dioxide, which can accumulate in patients with respiratory failure. Because carbon dioxide readily diffuses into cells, the administration of bicarbonate can lower the intracellular pH, potentially worsening cell function. Base therapy is usually reserved for children with severe acute lactic acidosis and severe diabetic ketoacidosis.

Oral base therapy is given to children with chronic metabolic acidosis. Sodium bicarbonate tablets are available for older children. Younger children generally take citrate solutions; the liver generates bicarbonate from citrate. Citrate solutions are available as sodium citrate, potassium citrate, and a 1 : 1 mix of sodium citrate and potassium citrate. The patient's potassium needs dictate the choice. Children with type I or type II RTA may have hypokalemia and may benefit from potassium supplements, whereas most children with chronic renal failure cannot tolerate additional potassium.

Oral or intravenous base can be used in acute metabolic acidosis; intravenous therapy is generally used when a rapid response is necessary. Sodium bicarbonate may be given as a bolus, usually at a dose of 1 mEq/kg, in an emergency situation. Another approach is to add sodium bicarbonate or sodium acetate to the patient's intravenous fluids, remembering to remove an equal amount of sodium chloride from the solution to avoid giving an excessive sodium load. Careful monitoring is mandatory so that the dose of base can be titrated appropriately. Tris-hydroxymethyl aminomethane (THAM) is an option in patients with a metabolic acidosis and a respiratory acidosis, because it neutralizes acids without releasing CO_2. THAM also diffuses into cells and therefore provides intracellular buffering.

Hemodialysis is another option for correcting a metabolic acidosis, and it is an appropriate choice in patients with renal insufficiency, especially if significant uremia or hyperkalemia is also present. Hemodialysis is advantageous for correcting the metabolic acidosis due to methanol or ethylene glycol intoxication, because hemodialysis removes the offending toxin. In addition, these patients often have a severe metabolic acidosis that does not respond easily to intravenous bicarbonate therapy. Peritoneal dialysis is another option for correcting the metabolic acidosis due to renal insufficiency, although, because it relies on lactate as the source of base, it may not correct the metabolic acidosis in patients with concomitant renal failure and lactic acidosis.

Many causes of metabolic acidosis require specific therapy. Administration of a glucocorticoid and a mineralocorticoid is necessary in patients with adrenal insufficiency. Patients with diabetic ketoacidosis require insulin therapy, whereas patients with lactic acidosis respond to measures that alleviate tissue hypoxia. Along with correction of acidosis, patients with methanol or ethylene glycol ingestion should receive an agent that prevents the breakdown of the toxic substance to its toxic metabolites. Fomepizole has supplanted ethanol as the treatment of choice. These agents work by inhibiting alcohol dehydrogenase, the enzyme that performs the 1st step in the metabolism of ethylene glycol or methanol. There are a variety of disease-specific therapies for patients with a metabolic acidosis due to an inborn error of metabolism.

METABOLIC ALKALOSIS

Metabolic alkalosis in children is most commonly secondary to emesis or diuretic use. The serum bicarbonate concentration is increased with a metabolic alkalosis, although a respiratory acidosis also leads to a compensatory elevation of the serum bicarbonate concentration. With a simple metabolic alkalosis, however, the pH is elevated; alkalemia is present. Patients with a respiratory acidosis are acidemic. A metabolic alkalosis, by decreasing ventilation, causes appropriate respiratory compensation. Pco_2 increases by 7 mm Hg for each 10-mEq/L increase in the serum bicarbonate concentration. Appropriate respiratory compensation never exceeds a Pco_2 of 55-60 mm Hg. The patient has a concurrent respiratory alkalosis if the Pco_2 is lower than the expected compensation. A greater than expected Pco_2 occurs with a concurrent respiratory acidosis.

Etiology and Pathophysiology

The kidneys normally respond promptly to a metabolic alkalosis by increasing base excretion. Two processes are therefore usually present to produce a metabolic alkalosis. The 1st process is the generation of the metabolic alkalosis, which requires the addition of base to the body. The 2nd process is the maintenance of the metabolic alkalosis, which requires impairment in the kidney's ability to excrete base.

The etiologies of a metabolic alkalosis are divided into 2 categories on the basis of urinary chloride level (Table 52-12). The alkalosis in patients with a **low urinary chloride** level is maintained by **volume depletion;** thus, volume repletion is necessary for correction of the alkalosis. The volume depletion in these patients is due to losses of sodium and potassium, but the loss of chloride is usually greater than the losses of sodium and potassium combined. Because chloride losses are the dominant cause of the volume depletion, these patients require chloride to correct the volume depletion and metabolic alkalosis; they are said to have **chloride-responsive metabolic alkalosis.** In contrast, the alkalosis in a patient with an elevated urinary chloride concentration does not respond to volume repletion and so is termed **chloride-resistant metabolic alkalosis.**

Table 52-12 CAUSES OF METABOLIC ALKALOSIS

CHLORIDE-RESPONSIVE (URINARY CHLORIDE < 15 mEq/L)
Gastric losses:
Emesis
Nasogastric suction
Diuretics (loop or thiazide)
Chloride-losing diarrhea (MIM 214700)
Chloride-deficient formula
Cystic fibrosis (MIM 219700)
Post-hypercapnia
CHLORIDE-RESISTANT (URINARY CHLORIDE > 20 mEq/L)
High blood pressure:
Adrenal adenoma or hyperplasia
Glucocorticoid-remediable aldosteronism (MIM 103900)
Renovascular disease
Renin-secreting tumor
17β-Hydroxylase deficiency (MIM 202110)
11β-Hydroxylase deficiency (MIM 202010)
Cushing syndrome
11β-Hydroxysteroid dehydrogenase deficiency (MIM 218030)
Licorice ingestion
Liddle syndrome (MIM 177200)
Normal blood pressure:
Gitelman syndrome (MIM 263800)
Bartter syndrome (MIM 607364/602522/241200/601678)
Autosomal dominant hypoparathyroidism (MIM 146200)
EAST syndrome (MIM 612780)
Base administration

EAST, epilepsy, ataxia, sensorineural hearing loss, and tubulopathy; MIM, database number from the Mendelian Inheritance in Man (*http://www3.ncbi.nlm.nih.gov/Omim/*).

Emesis or nasogastric suction results in **loss of gastric fluid,** which has a high content of HCl. Generation of hydrogen ions by the gastric mucosa causes simultaneous release of bicarbonate into the bloodstream. Normally, the hydrogen ions in gastric fluid are reclaimed in the small intestine (by neutralizing secreted bicarbonate). Thus, there is no net loss of acid. With loss of gastric fluid, this does not occur, and a metabolic alkalosis develops. This period is the generation phase of the metabolic alkalosis.

The maintenance phase of the metabolic alkalosis from gastric losses is due to the volume depletion ("chloride depletion" from gastric loss of HCl). Volume depletion interferes with urinary loss of bicarbonate, the normal renal response to a metabolic alkalosis. During volume depletion, several mechanisms prevent renal bicarbonate loss. First, there is a reduction in the GFR, so less bicarbonate is filtered. Second, volume depletion increases resorption of sodium and bicarbonate in the proximal tubule, limiting the amount of bicarbonate that can be excreted in the urine. This effect is mediated by angiotensin II and by adrenergic stimulation of the kidney, which are both increased in response to volume depletion. Third, the increase in aldosterone during volume depletion increases bicarbonate resorption and hydrogen ion secretion in the collecting duct.

In addition to volume depletion, gastric losses are usually associated with hypokalemia as a result of both gastric loss of potassium and, most importantly, increased urinary potassium losses. The increased urinary losses of potassium are mediated by aldosterone, through volume depletion, and by the increase in intracellular potassium secondary to the metabolic alkalosis, which causes potassium to move into the cells of the kidney, causing increased potassium excretion. Hypokalemia contributes to the maintenance of the metabolic alkalosis by decreasing bicarbonate loss. Hypokalemia increases hydrogen ion secretion in the distal nephron and stimulates ammonia production in the proximal tubule. Ammonia production enhances renal excretion of hydrogen ions.

A metabolic alkalosis can develop in patients receiving **loop** or **thiazide diuretics.** Diuretic use leads to volume depletion, which increases angiotensin II, aldosterone, and adrenergic stimulation of the kidney. Diuretics increase the delivery of sodium to the distal nephron, further enhancing acid excretion. Moreover, these diuretics cause hypokalemia, which increases acid excretion by the kidney. The increase in renal acid excretion generates the metabolic alkalosis, and the decrease in bicarbonate loss maintains it. In addition, patients who are receiving diuretics have a "contraction alkalosis." Diuretic use causes fluid loss without bicarbonate; thus, the remaining body bicarbonate is contained in a smaller total body fluid compartment. The bicarbonate concentration increases, helping to generate the metabolic alkalosis.

Diuretics are often used in patients with edema, such as those with nephrotic syndrome, heart failure, or liver failure. In many of these patients, metabolic alkalosis resulting from diuretic use develops despite the continued presence of edema. This is because the effective intravascular volume is low, and it is the effective intravascular volume that stimulates the compensatory mechanisms that cause and maintain a metabolic alkalosis. Many of these patients have a decreased effective intravascular volume before they begin diuretic therapy, increasing the likelihood of diuretic-induced metabolic alkalosis.

Diuretic use increases chloride excretion in the urine. Consequently, while a patient is receiving diuretics, the urine chloride level is typically high (>20 mEq/L). After the diuretic effect has worn off, the urinary chloride level is low (<15 mEq/L) owing to appropriate renal chloride retention in response to volume depletion. Thus, categorization of diuretics on the basis of urinary chloride level depends on the timing of the measurement. However, the metabolic alkalosis from diuretics is clearly chloride responsive; it is corrected after adequate volume repletion. This is the rationale for including this process among the chloride-responsive causes of a metabolic alkalosis.

Most patients with diarrhea have a metabolic acidosis due to stool losses of bicarbonate. In **chloride-losing diarrhea,** an autosomal recessive disorder, there is a defect in the normal intestinal exchange of bicarbonate for chloride, causing excessive stool losses of chloride (Chapter 330). In addition, stool losses of hydrogen ions and potassium cause metabolic alkalosis and hypokalemia, both of which are exacerbated by increased renal hydrogen and potassium losses due to volume depletion. Treatment is with oral supplements of potassium and sodium chloride. Use of a gastric proton pump inhibitor, by decreasing gastric HCl production, reduces both the volume of diarrhea and the need for electrolyte supplementation.

An infant formula with extremely low chloride content has led to chloride deficiency and volume depletion. The infants fed this formula, which is no longer available, had a metabolic alkalosis and hypokalemia. **Cystic fibrosis** can rarely cause metabolic alkalosis, hypokalemia, and hyponatremia due to excessive losses of sodium chloride in sweat (Chapter 395). The volume depletion causes the metabolic alkalosis and hypokalemia through increased urinary losses, whereas the hyponatremia, a less common finding, is secondary to sodium loss combined with renal water conservation in an effort to protect the intravascular volume ("appropriate" ADH production).

A **post-hypercapnic metabolic alkalosis** occurs after the correction of a chronic respiratory acidosis. This is typically seen in patients with chronic lung disease who are started on mechanical ventilation. During chronic respiratory acidosis, appropriate renal compensation leads to an increase in the serum bicarbonate concentration. This elevated bicarbonate concentration, because it is still present after acute correction of the respiratory acidosis, causes a metabolic alkalosis. The metabolic alkalosis persists because the patient with a chronic respiratory acidosis is intravascularly depleted because of the chloride loss that occurred during the initial metabolic compensation for the primary respiratory acidosis. In addition, many children with a chronic respiratory acidosis receive diuretics, which further decrease the intravascular volume. The metabolic alkalosis responds to correction of the intravascular volume deficit.

The **chloride-resistant** causes of metabolic alkalosis can be subdivided according to blood pressure status. Patients with **hypertension** either have increased aldosterone levels or act as if they do. Aldosterone levels are elevated in children with adrenal adenomas or hyperplasia. Aldosterone causes renal retention of sodium, with resultant hypertension. Metabolic alkalosis and hypokalemia result from aldosterone-mediated renal excretion of hydrogen ions and potassium. The urinary chloride level is not low because these patients are volume-overloaded, not volume-depleted. The volume expansion and hypertension allow normal excretion of sodium and chloride despite the presence of aldosterone. This is known as the *mineralocorticoid escape phenomenon.*

In **glucocorticoid-remediable aldosteronism,** an autosomal dominant disorder, there is excess production of aldosterone owing to the presence of an aldosterone synthase gene that is regulated by adrenocorticotropic hormone (ACTH) (Chapter 570.8). Glucocorticoids effectively treat this disorder by inhibiting ACTH production by the pituitary, downregulating the inappropriate aldosterone production. Renovascular disease and renin-secreting tumors both cause excessive renin, leading to an increase in aldosterone, although hypokalemia and metabolic alkalosis are less common findings than hypertension. In 2 forms of **congenital adrenal hyperplasia,** 11β-hydroxylase deficiency and 17α-hydroxylase deficiency, there is excessive production of the mineralocorticoid 11-deoxycorticosterone (Chapters 570.2 and 570.4). Hypertension, hypokalemia, and metabolic alkalosis are more likely in 17α-hydroxylase deficiency than in 11β-hydroxylase deficiency. These disorders respond to glucocorticoids because the excess production of 11-deoxycorticosterone is under the control of ACTH.

Cushing syndrome frequently causes hypertension. Cortisol has some mineralocorticoid activity, and high levels can produce hypokalemia and metabolic alkalosis in patients with Cushing syndrome.

Cortisol can bind to the mineralocorticoid receptors in the kidney and function as a mineralocorticoid. This binding normally does not occur because 11β-hydroxysteroid dehydrogenase in the kidney converts cortisol to cortisone, which does not bind to the mineralocorticoid receptor. In 11β-hydroxysteroid dehydrogenase deficiency, also called **apparent mineralocorticoid excess,** however, cortisol is not converted in the kidney to cortisone. Cortisol is therefore available to bind to the mineralocorticoid receptor in the kidney and act as a mineralocorticoid. Patients with this deficiency, despite low levels of aldosterone, are hypertensive and hypokalemic, and they have a metabolic alkalosis. The same phenomenon can occur with excessive intake of natural licorice, a component of which, glycyrrhizic acid, inhibits 11β-hydroxysteroid dehydrogenase. The autosomal dominant disorder **Liddle syndrome** is secondary to an activating mutation of the sodium channel in the distal nephron (Chapter 525.3). Upregulation of this sodium channel is 1 of the principal actions of aldosterone. Because this sodium channel is continuously open, children with Liddle syndrome have the features of hyperaldosteronism, including hypertension, hypokalemia, and metabolic alkalosis, but low serum levels of aldosterone.

Bartter syndrome and **Gitelman syndrome** are autosomal recessive disorders associated with **normal blood pressure,** elevations of urinary chloride, metabolic alkalosis, and hypokalemia

(Chapter 525). In Bartter syndrome, patients have a defect in sodium and chloride resorption in the loop of Henle. This leads to excessive urinary losses of sodium and chloride, and as in patients receiving loop diuretics, volume depletion and secondary hyperaldosteronism occur, causing hypokalemia and metabolic alkalosis. Gitelman syndrome is usually milder than Bartter syndrome. Patients have renal sodium and chloride wasting with volume depletion due mutations in the gene encoding the thiazide-sensitive sodium-chloride transporter in the distal tubule. As in patients receiving a thiazide diuretic, affected patients have volume depletion and secondary hyperaldosteronism with hypokalemia and metabolic alkalosis. Children with Gitelman syndrome have hypocalciuria and hypomagnesemia. Some patients with autosomal dominant hypoparathyroidism have hypokalemia and metabolic alkalosis due to impaired sodium and chloride resorption in the loop of Henle. **EAST syndrome** (epilepsy, ataxia, sensorineural deafness and tubulopathy) causes hypokalemia, metabolic alkalosis and hypokalemia.

Excessive base intake can cause a metabolic alkalosis. Affected patients do not have a low urine chloride level, unless there is associated volume depletion. In the absence of volume depletion, excess base is rapidly corrected via renal excretion of bicarbonate. Rarely, massive base intake can cause a metabolic alkalosis by overwhelming the kidney's ability to excrete bicarbonate. This may occur in infants who are given baking soda as a "home remedy" for colic or stomach upset. Each teaspoon of baking soda has 42 mEq of sodium bicarbonate. Infants have increased vulnerability because of a lower GFR, limiting the rate of compensatory renal bicarbonate excretion. A metabolic alkalosis may also occur in patients who receive a large amount of sodium bicarbonate during cardiopulmonary resuscitation. Blood products are anticoagulated with citrate, which is converted into bicarbonate by the liver. Patients who receive large amounts of blood products may have a metabolic alkalosis. Iatrogenic metabolic alkalosis can occur as a result of acetate in total parenteral nutrition. Aggressive use of bicarbonate therapy in a child with a lactic acidosis or diabetic ketoacidosis may cause a metabolic alkalosis. This event is especially likely in a patient in whom the underlying cause of the lactic acidosis is successfully corrected (restoration of intravascular volume in a patient with severe dehydration). Once the cause of the lactic acidosis resolves, lactate can be converted by the liver into bicarbonate, which when combined with infused bicarbonate can create a metabolic alkalosis. A similar phenomenon can occur in a child with diabetic ketoacidosis because the administration of insulin allows keto acids to be metabolized, producing bicarbonate. However, this phenomenon rarely occurs because of judicious use of bicarbonate therapy in diabetic ketoacidosis and because there are usually significant pretreatment losses of keto acids in the urine, preventing massive regeneration of bicarbonate. Base administration is most likely to cause a metabolic alkalosis in patients who have an impaired ability to excrete bicarbonate in the urine. This impairment occurs in patients with concurrent volume depletion or renal insufficiency.

Clinical Manifestations

The symptoms in patients with a metabolic alkalosis are often related to the underlying disease and associated electrolyte disturbances. Children with chloride-responsive causes of metabolic alkalosis often have symptoms related to volume depletion, such as thirst and lethargy. In contrast, children with chloride-unresponsive causes may have symptoms related to hypertension.

Alkalemia causes potassium to shift into the intracellular space, producing a decrease in the extracellular potassium concentration. Alkalemia leads to increased urinary losses of potassium. Increased potassium losses are present in many of the conditions that cause a metabolic alkalosis. Therefore, most patients with a metabolic alkalosis have hypokalemia, and their symptoms may be related to the hypokalemia (Chapter 52.4).

The symptoms of a metabolic alkalosis are due to the associated alkalemia. The magnitude of the alkalemia is related to the severity of the metabolic alkalosis and the presence of concurrent respiratory acid-base disturbances. During alkalemia, the ionized calcium concentration decreases as a result of increased binding of calcium to albumin. The decrease in the ionized calcium concentration may cause symptoms of **tetany** (carpopedal spasm).

Arrhythmias are a potential complication of a metabolic alkalosis, and the risk for arrhythmia increases if there is concomitant hypokalemia. Alkalemia increases the risk of digoxin toxicity, and antiarrhythmic medications are less effective in the presence of alkalemia. In addition, alkalemia may decrease cardiac output. A metabolic alkalosis causes a compensatory increase in the P_{CO_2} by decreasing ventilation. In patients with underlying lung disease, the decrease in ventilatory drive can cause hypoxia. In patients with normal lungs, the hypoventilation seen in severe metabolic alkalosis can cause hypoxia.

Diagnosis

Measurement of the urinary chloride concentration is the most helpful test in differentiating among the causes of a metabolic alkalosis. The urine chloride level is low in patients with a metabolic alkalosis resulting from volume depletion, unless there is a defect in renal handling of chloride. The urine chloride level is superior to the urine sodium level in assessment of volume status in patients with a metabolic alkalosis, because the normal renal response to a metabolic alkalosis is to excrete bicarbonate. Because bicarbonate is negatively charged, it can be excreted only with a cation, usually sodium and potassium. Hence, a patient with a metabolic alkalosis may excrete sodium in the urine despite the presence of volume depletion, which normally causes avid sodium retention. The urine chloride level is usually a good indicator of volume status, and it differentiates among the chloride-resistant and chloride-responsive causes of a metabolic alkalosis.

Diuretics and gastric losses are the most common causes of metabolic alkalosis and are usually readily apparent from the patient history. Occasionally, metabolic alkalosis, usually with hypokalemia, may be a clue to the presence of bulimia or surreptitious diuretic use (Chapter 26). Patients with bulimia have a low urine chloride level, indicating that they have volume depletion as a result of an extrarenal etiology, but there is no alternative explanation for their volume depletion. Surreptitious diuretic use may be diagnosed by obtaining a urine toxicology screen for diuretics. The urine chloride level is increased while a patient is using diuretics but is low when the patient stops taking them. Rarely, children with mild Bartter syndrome or Gitelman syndrome are misdiagnosed as having bulimia or abusing diuretics. The urine chloride value is always elevated in Bartter syndrome and Gitelman syndrome, and the urine toxicology screen for diuretics has a negative result. Metabolic alkalosis with hypokalemia is occasionally the initial manifestation of cystic fibrosis. An elevated sweat chloride finding is diagnostic.

Patients with a metabolic alkalosis and a high urinary chloride level are subdivided according to blood pressure status. Children with normal blood pressure may have Bartter syndrome or Gitelman syndrome. Excess base administration is another diagnostic possibility, but it is usually apparent from the history. In patients with sodium bicarbonate ingestion (baking soda), which may be unreported by the parent, the metabolic alkalosis usually occurs with significant hypernatremia. In addition, unless volume depletion is superimposed, the metabolic alkalosis from base ingestion resolves itself once the source of base is eliminated.

Measuring serum concentrations of renin and aldosterone differentiates children with a metabolic alkalosis, a high urinary chloride level, and elevated blood pressure. Both renin and aldosterone are elevated in children with either renovascular disease or a renin-secreting tumor. Aldosterone is high and renin is low in patients with adrenal adenomas or hyperplasia and glucocorticoid-remediable aldosteronism. Renin and aldosterone are low in children with Cushing syndrome, Liddle syndrome, licorice ingestion, 17α-hydroxylase deficiency, 11β-hydroxylase deficiency, and 11β-hydroxysteroid dehydrogenase deficiency. An elevated 24-hr urine cortisol value is diagnostic of Cushing syndrome, which is suspected from the presence of the other classic features of this disease (Chapter 571). Elevations of 11-Deoxycorticosterone values are seen in 17α-hydroxylase deficiency and 11β-hydroxylase deficiency.

Treatment

The approach to treatment of metabolic alkalosis depends on the severity of the alkalosis and the underlying etiology. In children with a mild metabolic alkalosis ($[HCO_3^-]$ <32), intervention is often unnecessary, although this depends on the specific circumstances. In a child with congenital heart disease who is receiving a stable dose of a loop diuretic, a mild alkalosis does not require treatment. In contrast, intervention may be appropriate in a child with a worsening mild metabolic alkalosis due to nasogastric suction. The presence of a concurrent respiratory acid-base disturbance also influences therapeutic decision-making. A patient with a concurrent respiratory acidosis should have some increase in bicarbonate owing to metabolic compensation; thus, the severity of the pH elevation is more important than the bicarbonate concentration. In contrast, a patient with a respiratory alkalosis and a metabolic alkalosis is at risk for severe alkalemia; treatment may be indicated, even if the increase in bicarbonate value is only mild.

Intervention is usually necessary in children with moderate or severe metabolic alkalosis. The most effective approach is to address the underlying etiology. In some children, nasogastric suction may be decreased or discontinued. Alternatively, the addition of a gastric proton pump inhibitor reduces gastric secretion and losses of HCl. Diuretics are an important cause of metabolic alkalosis, and if a change is tolerated, they should be eliminated or the dose reduced. Adequate potassium supplementation or the addition of a potassium-sparing diuretic is also helpful in a child with a metabolic alkalosis due to diuretics. Potassium-sparing diuretics not only decrease renal potassium losses but, by blocking the action of aldosterone, also decrease hydrogen ion secretion in the distal nephron, increasing urinary bicarbonate excretion. Many children cannot tolerate discontinuation of diuretic therapy; thus, potassium supplementation and potassium-sparing diuretics are the principal therapeutic approach. Arginine HCl may also be used to treat chloride-responsive metabolic acidosis if sodium or potassium salts are not appropriate. Arginine HCl may raise the serum potassium levels during administration. Rarely, in cases of severe metabolic alkalosis, acetazolamide is an option. A carbonic anhydrase inhibitor, acetazolamide decreases resorption of bicarbonate in the proximal tubule, causing significant bicarbonate loss in the urine. The patient receiving this drug must be monitored closely, because acetazolamide produces major losses of potassium in the urine and increases fluid losses, potentially necessitating a reduction in dosage of other diuretics.

Most children with a metabolic alkalosis have one of the chloride-responsive etiologies. In these situations, administration of sufficient sodium chloride and potassium chloride to correct the volume deficit and the potassium deficit is necessary to correct the metabolic alkalosis. This approach may not be an option in the child who has volume depletion due to diuretics, because volume repletion may be contraindicated. Adequate replacement of gastric losses of sodium and potassium in a child with a nasogastric tube can minimize or prevent the development of the metabolic alkalosis. With adequate intravascular volume and a normal serum potassium concentration, the kidney is able to excrete the excess bicarbonate within a couple of days.

In children with the chloride-resistant causes of a metabolic alkalosis that are associated with hypertension, volume repletion is contraindicated because it would exacerbate the hypertension and would not repair the metabolic alkalosis. Ideally, treatment focuses on eliminating the excess aldosterone effect. Adrenal adenomas can be resected, licorice intake can be eliminated, and renovascular disease can be repaired. Glucocorticoid-remediable aldosteronism, 17α-hydroxylase deficiency, and 11β-hydroxylase deficiency respond to the administration of glucocorticoids. The mineralocorticoid effect of cortisol in 11β-hydroxysteroid dehydrogenase deficiency can be decreased with the use of spironolactone, which blocks the mineralocorticoid receptor. In contrast, the metabolic alkalosis in children with Liddle syndrome does not respond to spironolactone; however, either triamterene or amiloride is effective therapy because both agents block the sodium channel that is constitutively active in Liddle syndrome.

In children with Bartter syndrome and Gitelman syndrome, therapy includes oral potassium supplementation and potassium-sparing diuretics. Children with Gitelman syndrome often require magnesium supplementation, whereas children with severe Bartter syndrome often benefit from indomethacin.

RESPIRATORY ACIDOSIS

A respiratory acidosis is an inappropriate increase in blood carbon dioxide (Pco_2). Carbon dioxide is a byproduct of metabolism, and it is removed from the body by the lungs. During a respiratory acidosis, there is a decrease in the effectiveness of carbon dioxide removal by the lungs. A respiratory acidosis is secondary to either pulmonary disease, such as severe bronchiolitis, or nonpulmonary disease, such as a narcotic overdose. Even though body production of carbon dioxide can vary, normal lungs are able to accommodate this variation; excess production of carbon dioxide is not an isolated cause of a respiratory acidosis. With impairment of alveolar ventilation, the rate of body production of carbon dioxide may affect the severity of the respiratory acidosis, but this is usually not a significant factor.

A respiratory acidosis causes a decrease in the blood pH, but there is normally a metabolic response that partially compensates, minimizing the severity of the acidemia. The acute metabolic response to a respiratory alkalosis occurs within minutes. The metabolic compensation for an acute respiratory acidosis is secondary to titration of acid by nonbicarbonate buffers. This buffering of hydrogen ions causes a predictable increase in the serum bicarbonate concentration: Plasma bicarbonate increases by 1 for each 10–mm Hg increase in the Pco_2 (acute compensation).

With a chronic respiratory acidosis, there is more significant metabolic compensation and, thus, less severe acidemia than in an acute respiratory acidosis with the same increase in Pco_2. During a chronic respiratory acidosis, the kidneys increase acid excretion. This response occurs over 3-4 days and causes a predictable increase in the serum bicarbonate concentration: Plasma bicarbonate increases by 3.5 for each 10–mm Hg increase in the Pco_2 (chronic compensation).

The increase of serum bicarbonate concentration during a chronic respiratory acidosis is associated with a decrease in body chloride. After acute correction of a chronic respiratory acidosis, the plasma bicarbonate continues to be increased, and the patient has a metabolic alkalosis. Because of the chloride deficit, this is a chloride-responsive metabolic alkalosis; it corrects once the patient's chloride deficit is replaced.

A mixed disorder is present if the metabolic compensation is inappropriate. A higher than expected bicarbonate value occurs in the setting of a concurrent metabolic alkalosis, and a lower than expected bicarbonate value occurs in the setting of a concurrent metabolic acidosis. Evaluating whether compensation is appropriate during a respiratory acidosis requires clinical knowledge of the acuity of the process, because the expected compensation is different, depending on whether the process is acute or chronic.

The Pco_2 cannot be interpreted in isolation to determine whether a patient has a respiratory acidosis. A respiratory acidosis is always present if a patient has acidemia and an elevated PCO_2. However, an elevated PCO_2 also occurs as appropriate respiratory compensation for a simple metabolic alkalosis. The patient is alkalemic; this is not a respiratory acidosis. During a mixed disturbance, a patient can have a respiratory acidosis and a normal or even low PCO_2. This condition may occur in a patient with a metabolic acidosis; a respiratory acidosis is present if the patient does not have appropriate respiratory compensation (the PCO_2 is higher than expected from the severity of the metabolic acidosis).

Etiology and Pathophysiology

The causes of a respiratory acidosis are either pulmonary or nonpulmonary (Table 52-13). CNS disorders can decrease the activity of the central respiratory center, reducing ventilatory drive. A variety of medications and illicit drugs suppress the respiratory center. The signals from the respiratory center need to be transmitted to the respiratory muscles via the nervous system. Respiratory muscle failure can be secondary to disruption of the signal from the CNS in the spinal cord, the phrenic nerve, or the neuromuscular junction. Disorders directly affecting the muscles of respiration can prevent adequate ventilation, causing a respiratory acidosis.

Mild or moderate lung disease often causes a respiratory alkalosis as a result of hyperventilation secondary to hypoxia or stimulation of lung mechanoreceptors or chemoreceptors. Only more severe lung disease causes a respiratory acidosis. Upper airway diseases, by impairing air entry into the lungs, may decrease ventilation, producing a respiratory acidosis.

Increased production of carbon dioxide is never the sole cause of a respiratory acidosis, but it can increase the severity of the disease in a patient with decreased ventilation of carbon dioxide. Increased production of carbon dioxide occurs in patients with fever, hyperthyroidism, excess caloric intake, and high levels of physical activity. Increased respiratory muscle work also increases carbon dioxide production.

Clinical Manifestations

Patients with a respiratory acidosis are often tachypneic in an effort to correct the inadequate ventilation. Exceptions include patients with a respiratory acidosis resulting from CNS depression and patients who are on the verge of complete respiratory failure secondary to fatigue of the respiratory muscles.

The symptoms of respiratory acidosis are related to the severity of the hypercarbia. Acute respiratory acidosis is usually more symptomatic than chronic respiratory acidosis. Symptoms are also increased by concurrent hypoxia or metabolic acidosis. In a patient breathing room air, hypoxia is always present if a respiratory acidosis is present. The potential CNS manifestations of respiratory acidosis include anxiety, dizziness, headache, confusion, asterixis, myoclonic jerks, hallucinations, psychosis, coma, and seizures.

Acidemia, no matter the etiology, affects the cardiovascular system. An arterial pH <7.20 impairs cardiac contractility and the normal response to catecholamines, in both the heart and the peripheral vasculature. Hypercapnia causes vasodilation, most dramatically in the cerebral vasculature, but hypercapnia produces vasoconstriction of the pulmonary circulation. Respiratory acidosis increases the risk of cardiac arrhythmias, especially in a child with underlying cardiac disease.

Diagnosis

The history and physical findings often point to a clear etiology. For the obtunded patient with poor respiratory effort, evaluation of the CNS is often indicated. This may include imaging studies (CT or MRI) and, potentially, a lumbar puncture for CSF analysis. A toxicology screen for illicit drugs may also be appropriate. A response to naloxone is both diagnostic and therapeutic. In many of the diseases affecting the respiratory muscles, there is evidence

Table 52-13 CAUSES OF RESPIRATORY ACIDOSIS

CENTRAL NERVOUS SYSTEM DEPRESSION
Encephalitis
Head trauma
Brain tumor
Central sleep apnea
Primary pulmonary hypoventilation (Ondine curse)
Stroke
Hypoxic brain damage
Obesity-hypoventilation (Pickwickian syndrome)
Increased intracranial pressure
Medications:
Narcotics
Barbiturates
Anesthesia
Benzodiazepines
Propofol
Alcohols
DISORDERS OF THE SPINAL CORD, PERIPHERAL NERVES, OR NEUROMUSCULAR JUNCTION
Diaphragmatic paralysis
Guillain-Barré syndrome
Poliomyelitis
Spinal muscular atrophies
Tick paralysis
Botulism
Myasthenia
Multiple sclerosis
Spinal cord injury
Medications:
Vecuronium
Aminoglycosides
Organophosphates (pesticides)
RESPIRATORY MUSCLE WEAKNESS
Muscular dystrophy
Hypothyroidism
Malnutrition
Hypokalemia
Hypophosphatemia
Medications:
Succinylcholine
Corticosteroids
PULMONARY DISEASE
Pneumonia
Pneumothorax
Asthma
Bronchiolitis
Pulmonary edema
Pulmonary hemorrhage
Adult respiratory distress syndrome
Neonatal respiratory distress syndrome
Cystic fibrosis
Bronchopulmonary dysplasia
Hypoplastic lungs
Meconium aspiration
Pulmonary thromboembolus
Interstitial fibrosis
UPPER AIRWAY DISEASE
Aspiration
Laryngospasm
Angioedema
Obstructive sleep apnea
Tonsillar hypertrophy
Vocal cord paralysis
Extrinsic tumor
Extrinsic or intrinsic hemangioma
MISCELLANEOUS
Flail chest
Cardiac arrest
Kyphoscoliosis
Decreased diaphragmatic movement due to ascites or peritoneal dialysis

of weakness in other muscles. Stridor is a clue that the child may have upper airway disease. Along with a physical examination, a chest radiograph is often helpful in diagnosing pulmonary disease.

In many patients, respiratory acidosis may be multifactorial. A child with bronchopulmonary dysplasia, an intrinsic lung disease, may worsen because of respiratory muscle dysfunction due to severe hypokalemia resulting from long-term diuretic therapy. Conversely, a child with muscular dystrophy, a muscle disease, may worsen because of aspiration pneumonia.

For a patient with respiratory acidosis, calculation of the gradient between the alveolar oxygen concentration and the arterial oxygen concentration, the A-aO2 gradient, is useful for distinguishing between poor respiratory effort and intrinsic lung disease. The A-aO2 gradient is increased if the hypoxemia is due to intrinsic lung disease (Chapter 365).

Treatment

Respiratory acidosis is best managed by treatment of the underlying etiology. In some instances, the response is very rapid, such as after the administration of naloxone to a patient with a narcotic overdose. In contrast, in the child with pneumonia, a number of days of antibiotic therapy may be required before the respiratory status improves. In many children with a chronic respiratory acidosis, there is no curative therapy, although an acute respiratory illness superimposed on a chronic respiratory condition is usually reversible.

All patients with an acute respiratory acidosis are hypoxic and therefore need to receive supplemental oxygen. Mechanical ventilation is necessary in some children with a respiratory acidosis. Children with a significant respiratory acidosis due to a CNS disease usually require mechanical ventilation because such a disorder is unlikely to respond quickly to therapy. In addition, hypercarbia causes cerebral vasodilation, and the increase in intracranial pressure can be dangerous in a child with an underlying CNS disease. Readily reversible CNS depression, such as from a narcotic overdose, may not require mechanical ventilation. Decisions on mechanical ventilation for other patients depend on a number of factors. Patients with severe hypercarbia—P_{CO_2} > 75 mm Hg—usually require mechanical ventilation (Chapters 65 and 366). The threshold for intubation is lower if there is concomitant metabolic acidosis, a slowly responsive underlying disease, or hypoxia that responds poorly to oxygen, or if the patient appears to be tiring and respiratory arrest seems likely.

In patients with a chronic respiratory acidosis, the respiratory drive is often less responsive to hypercarbia and more responsive to hypoxia. Hence, with chronic respiratory acidosis, excessive use of oxygen can blunt the respiratory drive and therefore increase the P_{CO_2}. In these patients, oxygen must be used cautiously.

When possible, it is best to avoid mechanical ventilation in a patient with a chronic respiratory acidosis because extubation is often difficult. However, an acute illness may necessitate mechanical ventilation in a child with a chronic respiratory acidosis. When intubation is necessary, the P_{CO_2} should be lowered only to the patient's normal baseline, and this should be done gradually. These patients normally have an elevated serum bicarbonate concentration as a result of metabolic compensation for their respiratory acidosis. A rapid lowering of the P_{CO_2} can cause a severe metabolic alkalosis, potentially leading to complications, including cardiac arrhythmias, decreased cardiac output, and decreased cerebral blood flow. In addition, prolonged mechanical ventilation at a normal P_{CO_2} causes the metabolic compensation to resolve. When the patient is subsequently extubated, the patient will no longer benefit from metabolic compensation, causing a more severe acidemia because of the respiratory acidosis.

RESPIRATORY ALKALOSIS

A respiratory alkalosis is an inappropriate reduction in the blood carbon dioxide concentration. This is usually secondary to hyperventilation, initially causing removal of carbon dioxide to surpass production. Eventually, a new steady state is achieved, with removal equaling production, albeit at a lower carbon dioxide tension (P_{CO_2}). A respiratory alkalosis that is not due to hyperventilation may occur in children receiving extracorporeal membrane oxygenation or hemodialysis, with carbon dioxide lost directly from the blood in the extracorporeal circuit.

With a simple respiratory alkalosis, the pH increases but there is a normal metabolic response that attenuates some of the change in the blood pH. A metabolic response to an acute respiratory alkalosis occurs within minutes, mediated by hydrogen ion release from nonbicarbonate buffers. The metabolic response to an acute respiratory alkalosis is predictable: Plasma bicarbonate falls by 2 for each 10– mm Hg decrease in the P_{CO_2} (acute compensation).

A chronic respiratory alkalosis leads to more significant metabolic compensation because of the actions of the kidneys, which decrease acid secretion, producing a decrease in the serum bicarbonate concentration. Both the proximal and distal tubules decrease acid secretion. Metabolic compensation for a respiratory alkalosis develops gradually and takes 2-3 days to produce the full effect: Plasma bicarbonate falls by 4 for each 10-mm Hg decrease in the P_{CO_2} (chronic compensation).

A chronic respiratory alkalosis is the only acid-base disturbance wherein appropriate compensation may normalize the pH, albeit >7.40.

A mixed disorder is present if the metabolic compensation is inappropriate. A higher than expected bicarbonate level occurs in the setting of a concurrent metabolic alkalosis, and a lower than expected bicarbonate level occurs in the setting of a concurrent metabolic acidosis. Evaluating whether compensation is appropriate during a respiratory alkalosis requires clinical knowledge of the acuity of the process, because the expected compensation differs according to whether the process is acute or chronic.

A low P_{CO_2} value does not always indicate a respiratory alkalosis. The P_{CO_2} also decreases as part of the appropriate respiratory compensation for a metabolic acidosis; this is not a respiratory alkalosis. A metabolic acidosis is the dominant acid-base disturbance in a patient with acidemia and a low P_{CO_2}, even though there could still be a concurrent respiratory alkalosis. In contrast, a respiratory alkalosis is always present in a patient with alkalemia and a low P_{CO_2}. Even a normal P_{CO_2} value may be consistent with a respiratory alkalosis in a patient with a metabolic alkalosis because an elevated P_{CO_2} is expected as part of appropriate respiratory compensation for the metabolic alkalosis.

Etiology and Pathophysiology

A variety of stimuli can increase the ventilatory drive and cause a respiratory alkalosis (Table 52-14). Arterial hypoxemia or tissue hypoxia stimulates peripheral chemoreceptors to signal the central respiratory center in the medulla to increase ventilation. The resultant greater respiratory effort increases the oxygen content of the blood but depresses the P_{CO_2}. The effect of hypoxemia on ventilation begins when the oxygen saturation decreases to approximately 90% (P_{O_2} = 60 mm Hg), and hyperventilation increases as hypoxemia worsens. Acute hypoxia is a more potent stimulus for hyperventilation than chronic hypoxia; thus, chronic hypoxia, as occurs in cyanotic heart disease, causes a much less severe respiratory alkalosis than an equivalent degree of acute hypoxia. There are many causes of hypoxemia or tissue hypoxia, including primary lung disease, severe anemia, and carbon monoxide poisoning.

The lungs contain chemoreceptors and mechanoreceptors that respond to irritants and stretching and send signals to the respiratory center to increase ventilation. Aspiration or pneumonia may stimulate the chemoreceptors, whereas pulmonary edema may stimulate the mechanoreceptors. Most of the diseases that activate these receptors may also cause hypoxemia and can, therefore, potentially lead to hyperventilation via 2 mechanisms.

Table 52-14 CAUSES OF RESPIRATORY ALKALOSIS

HYPOXEMIA OR TISSUE HYPOXIA
Pneumonia
Pulmonary edema
Cyanotic heart disease
Congestive heart failure
Asthma
Severe anemia
High altitude
Laryngospasm
Aspiration
Carbon monoxide poisoning
Pulmonary embolism
Interstitial lung disease
Hypotension
LUNG RECEPTOR STIMULATION
Pneumonia
Pulmonary edema
Asthma
Pulmonary embolism
Hemothorax
Pneumothorax
Respiratory distress syndrome (adult or infant)
CENTRAL STIMULATION
Central nervous system disease:
Subarachnoid hemorrhage
Encephalitis or meningitis
Trauma
Brain tumor
Stroke
Fever
Pain
Anxiety (panic attack)
Psychogenic hyperventilation or anxiety
Liver failure
Sepsis
Pregnancy
Medications:
Salicylate intoxication
Theophylline
Progesterone
Exogenous catecholamines
Caffeine
Mechanical ventilation
Hyperammonemia
Extracorporeal membrane oxygenation or hemodialysis

Patients with primary lung disease may initially have a respiratory alkalosis, but worsening of the disease, combined with respiratory muscle fatigue, often causes respiratory failure and the development of a respiratory acidosis.

Hyperventilation in the absence of lung disease occurs with direct stimulation of the central respiratory center. This occurs with CNS diseases, such as meningitis, hemorrhage, and trauma. Central hyperventilation due to lesions, such as infarcts or tumors near the central respiratory center in the midbrain, increases the rate and depth of the respiratory effort. This respiratory pattern portends a poor prognosis because these midbrain lesions are frequently fatal. Systemic processes may cause centrally mediated hyperventilation. Although the exact mechanisms are not clear, liver disease causes a respiratory alkalosis that is usually proportional to the degree of liver failure. Pregnancy causes a chronic respiratory alkalosis, probably mediated by progesterone acting on the respiratory centers. Salicylates, although often causing a concurrent metabolic acidosis, directly stimulate the respiratory center to produce a respiratory alkalosis. The respiratory alkalosis during sepsis is probably due to cytokine release.

Hyperventilation may be secondary to an underlying disease that causes pain, stress, or anxiety. In psychogenic hyperventilation, there is no disease process accounting for the hyperventilation. This disorder may occur in a child who has had an emotionally stressful experience. Alternatively, it may be part of a panic disorder, especially if there are repeated episodes of hyperventilation. In such a patient, the symptoms of acute alkalemia increase anxiety, potentially perpetuating the hyperventilation.

A respiratory alkalosis is quite common in children receiving mechanical ventilation because the respiratory center is not controlling ventilation. In addition, these children may have a decreased metabolic rate and hence less carbon dioxide production because of sedation and paralytic medications. Normally, decreased carbon dioxide production and the resultant hypocapnia decrease ventilation, but this physiologic response cannot occur in a child who cannot reduce the ventilatory effort.

Clinical Manifestations

The disease process that is causing the respiratory alkalosis is usually more concerning than the clinical manifestations of the respiratory alkalosis. Chronic respiratory alkalosis is usually asymptomatic because metabolic compensation decreases the magnitude of the alkalemia.

Acute respiratory alkalosis may cause chest tightness, palpitations, lightheadedness, circumoral numbness, and paresthesias of the extremities. Less common manifestations include tetany, seizures, muscle cramps, and syncope. The lightheadedness and syncope are probably due to the reduction in cerebral blood flow that is caused by hypocapnia. The reduction in cerebral blood flow is the rationale for using hyperventilation to treat children with increased intracranial pressure. The paresthesias, tetany, and seizures may be partially related to the reduction in ionized calcium that occurs because alkalemia causes more calcium to bind to albumin. A respiratory alkalosis also causes a mild reduction in the serum potassium level. Patients with psychogenic hyperventilation tend to be most symptomatic as a result of the respiratory alkalosis, and these symptoms, along with a sensation of breathlessness, exacerbate the hyperventilation.

Diagnosis

In many patients, hyperventilation producing a respiratory alkalosis is not clinically detectable, even with careful observation of the patient's respiratory effort. Metabolic compensation for a respiratory alkalosis causes a low serum bicarbonate concentration. When hyperventilation is not appreciated and only serum electrolytes are evaluated, there is often a presumptive diagnosis of a metabolic acidosis. If a respiratory alkalosis is suspected, only a blood gas determination can make the diagnosis.

Hyperventilation does not always indicate a primary respiratory disorder. In some patients, the hyperventilation is appropriate respiratory compensation for a metabolic acidosis. With a primary metabolic acidosis, acidemia is present and the serum bicarbonate level is usually quite low if there is clinically detectable hyperventilation. In contrast, the serum bicarbonate level never goes below 17 mEq/L as part of the metabolic compensation for acute respiratory alkalosis, and simple acute respiratory alkalosis causes alkalemia.

The etiology of a respiratory alkalosis is often apparent from the physical examination or history, and it may consist of lung disease, neurologic disease, or cyanotic heart disease. Hypoxemia is a common cause of hyperventilation, and it is important to diagnose because it suggests a significant underlying disease that requires expeditious treatment. Hypoxemia may be detected on physical examination (cyanosis) or by pulse oximetry. However, normal pulse oximetry values do not completely eliminate hypoxemia as the etiology of the hyperventilation. There are 2 reasons why pulse oximetry is not adequate for eliminating hypoxemia as a cause of a respiratory alkalosis. First, pulse oximetry is not very sensitive at detecting a mildly low pO_2. Second, the hyperventilation during a respiratory alkalosis causes the pO_2 to increase, possibly to a level that is not identified as abnormal by pulse oximetry. Only an arterial blood gas measurement can completely eliminate hypoxia as an explanation for a respiratory alkalosis. Along with hypoxemia, it is important to consider processes that cause tissue hypoxia without necessarily causing hypoxemia. Examples are carbon monoxide poisoning, severe anemia, and congestive heart failure.

Lung disease without hypoxemia may cause hyperventilation. Although lung disease is often apparent by history or physical examination, a chest radiograph may detect more subtle disease. The patient with a pulmonary embolism may have benign chest radiograph findings, normal pO_2, and isolated respiratory alkalosis, although hypoxia may eventually occur. Diagnosis of a pulmonary embolism requires a high index of suspicion and should be considered in children without another explanation for respiratory alkalosis, especially if risk factors are present, such as prolonged bed rest and a hypercoagulable state (e.g., nephrotic syndrome or lupus anticoagulant).

Treatment

There is seldom a need for specific treatment of respiratory alkalosis. Rather, treatment focuses on the underlying disease. Mechanical ventilator settings are adjusted to correct iatrogenic respiratory alkalosis, unless the hyperventilation has a therapeutic purpose (e.g., treatment of increased intracranial pressure).

For the patient with hyperventilation secondary to anxiety, efforts should be undertaken to reassure the child, usually enlisting the parents. Along with reassurance, patients with psychogenic hyperventilation may benefit from benzodiazepines. During an acute episode of psychogenic hyperventilation, rebreathing into a paper bag increases the patient's Pco_2. Using a paper bag, instead of a plastic bag, allows adequate oxygenation but permits the carbon dioxide concentration in the bag to increase. The resultant increase in the patient's Pco_2 decreases the symptoms of the respiratory alkalosis that tend to perpetuate the hyperventilation. Rebreathing should be performed only once other causes of hyperventilation have been eliminated; pulse oximetry during the rebreathing is prudent.

BIBLIOGRAPHY

Please visit the Nelson Textbook of Pediatrics *website at www.expertconsult.com for the complete bibliography.*

Chapter 53
Maintenance and Replacement Therapy

Larry A. Greenbaum

Maintenance intravenous fluids are used in a child who cannot be fed enterally. Along with maintenance fluids, children may require concurrent **replacement fluids** if they have continued excessive losses, such as may occur with drainage from a nasogastric (NG) tube or with high urine output due to nephrogenic diabetes insipidus. If dehydration is present, the patient also needs to receive **deficit** replacement (Chapter 54). A child awaiting surgery may need only maintenance fluids, whereas a child with diarrheal dehydration needs maintenance and deficit therapy and also may require replacement fluids if significant diarrhea continues.

MAINTENANCE THERAPY

Children normally have large variations in their daily intake of water and electrolytes. The only exceptions are patients who receive fixed dietary regimens orally, via a gastric tube, or as intravenous total parenteral nutrition. Healthy children can tolerate significant variations in intake because of the many homeostatic mechanisms that can adjust absorption and excretion of water and electrolytes (Chapter 52). The calculated water and electrolyte needs that form the basis of maintenance therapy are not absolute requirements. Rather, these calculations provide reasonable guidelines for a starting point to estimate intravenous therapy. Children do not need to be started on intravenous fluids simply because their intake is being monitored in a hospital and they are not taking "maintenance fluids" orally, unless there is a pathologic process present that necessitates high fluid intake.

Maintenance fluids are most commonly necessary in preoperative and postoperative surgical patients; many nonsurgical patients also require maintenance fluids. It is important to recognize when it is necessary to begin maintenance fluids. A normal teenager who is given nothing by mouth (NPO) overnight for a morning procedure does not require maintenance fluids because a healthy adolescent can easily tolerate 12 or 18 hr without oral intake. In contrast, a 6 mo old child waiting for surgery should begin receiving intravenous fluids within 8 hr of the last feeding. Infants become dehydrated more quickly than older patients. A child with obligatory high urine output from nephrogenic diabetes insipidus should begin receiving intravenous fluids soon after being classified as NPO.

Maintenance fluids are composed of a solution of water, glucose, sodium, and potassium. This solution has the advantages of simplicity, long shelf life, low cost, and compatibility with peripheral intravenous administration. Such a solution accomplishes the major objectives of maintenance fluids (Table 53-1). Patients lose water, sodium, and potassium in their urine and stool; water is also lost from the skin and lungs. Maintenance fluids replace these losses and therefore avoid the development of dehydration and deficiency of sodium or potassium.

The glucose in maintenance fluids provides approximately 20% of the normal caloric needs of the patient, prevents the development of starvation ketoacidosis, and diminishes the protein degradation that would occur if the patient received no calories. Glucose also provides added osmoles, thus avoiding the administration of hypotonic fluids that may cause hemolysis.

Maintenance fluids do not provide adequate calories, protein, fat, minerals, or vitamins. This fact is typically not problematic for a patient receiving intravenous fluids for a few days. A patient receiving maintenance intravenous fluids is receiving inadequate calories and will lose 0.5-1% of weight each day. It is imperative that patients not remain on maintenance therapy indefinitely; total parental nutrition should be used for children who cannot be fed enterally for more than a few days, especially patients with underlying malnutrition.

Prototypical maintenance fluid therapy does not provide electrolytes such as calcium, phosphorus, magnesium, and bicarbonate. For most patients, this lack is not problematic for a few days, although there are patients who will not tolerate this omission, usually because of excessive losses. A child with renal tubular acidosis wastes bicarbonate in urine. Such a patient will rapidly become acidemic unless bicarbonate (or acetate) is added to the maintenance fluids. It is important to remember the limitations of maintenance fluid therapy.

MAINTENANCE WATER

Water is a crucial component of maintenance fluid therapy because of the obligatory daily water losses. These losses are both measurable (urine, stool) and not measurable (insensible losses from the

Table 53-1 GOALS OF MAINTENANCE FLUIDS
Prevent dehydration
Prevent electrolyte disorders
Prevent ketoacidosis
Prevent protein degradation

skin and lungs). Failure to replace these losses leads to a child who is thirsty, uncomfortable, and, ultimately, dehydrated.

The goal of maintenance water is to provide enough water to replace these losses. Although urinary losses are approximately 60% of the total, the normal kidney has the ability to markedly modify water losses, with daily urine volume potentially varying by more than a factor of 20. Maintenance water is designed to provide enough water so that the kidney does not need to significantly dilute or concentrate the urine. It also provides a margin of safety, so that normal homeostatic mechanisms can adjust urinary water losses to prevent overhydration and dehydration. This adaptability obviates the need for absolute precision in determining water requirements. This fact is important, given the absence of absolute accuracy in the formulas for calculation of water needs. Table 53-2 provides a system for calculating maintenance water on the basis of the patient's weight and emphasizes the high water needs of smaller, less mature patients. This approach is reliable, although calculations based on weight do overestimate the water needs of an overweight child, in whom it is better to base the calculations on the lean body weight, which can be estimated by using the 50th percentile of body weight for the child's height. It is also important to remember that there is an upper limit of 2.4 L/24 hr in adult-sized patients. Intravenous fluids are written as an hourly rate. The formulas in Table 53-3 enable rapid calculation of the rate of maintenance fluids.

INTRAVENOUS SOLUTIONS

The components of the commonly available solutions are shown in Table 53-4. Normal saline (NS) and Ringer lactate (LR) are isotonic solutions; they have approximately the same tonicity as plasma. Isotonic fluids are generally used for the acute correction of intravascular volume depletion (Chapter 54). The usual choices for maintenance fluid therapy in children are half-normal saline (½NS) and 0.2NS. These solutions are available with 5% dextrose (D5). In addition, they are available with 20 mEq/L of potassium chloride, 10 mEq/L of potassium chloride, or no potassium. A hospital pharmacy can also prepare custom-made solutions with different concentrations of glucose, sodium, or potassium. In addition, other electrolytes, such as calcium, magnesium, phosphate, acetate, and bicarbonate, can be added to intravenous solutions. Custom-made solutions take time to prepare and are much more expensive than commercial solutions. The use of custom-made solutions is necessary only for patients who have underlying disorders that cause significant electrolyte imbalances. The use of commercial solutions saves both time and expense.

A normal plasma osmolality is 285-295 mOsm/kg. Infusing an intravenous solution peripherally with a much lower osmolality can cause water to move into red blood cells, leading to hemolysis. Thus, intravenous fluids are generally designed to have an osmolality that is either close to 285 or greater (fluids with moderately higher osmolality do not cause problems). Thus, 0.2NS (osmolality = 68) should not be administered peripherally, but D5 0.2NS (osmolality = 346) or D5 ½NS + 20 mEq/L KCl (osmolality = 472) can be administered.

There is controversy about the appropriate sodium content of maintenance fluids, considering the suggestion that excessive amounts of hypotonic fluids may cause hyponatremia, which at times may have serious sequelae. One approach to avoid water intoxication is to reduce the rate of infusion of fluids containing 0.2NS or ½NS. The other recommends that normal saline be used as the maintenance fluid; most centers have not adopted the routine use of NS as the initiating maintenance solution.

Table 53-2 BODY WEIGHT METHOD FOR CALCULATING DAILY MAINTENANCE FLUID VOLUME

BODY WEIGHT	FLUID PER DAY
0-10 kg	100 mL/kg
11-20 kg	1,000 mL + 50 mL/kg for each kg >10 kg
>20 kg	1,500 mL + 20 mL/kg for each kg >20 kg*

*The maximum total fluid per day is normally 2,400 mL.

Table 53-3 HOURLY MAINTENANCE WATER RATE

For body weight of 0-10 kg: 4 mL/kg/hr
For body weight of 10-20 kg: 40 mL/hr + 2 mL/kg/hr × (wt − 10 kg)
For body weight of >20 kg: 60 mL/hr + 1 mL/kg/hr × (wt − 20 kg)*

*The maximum fluid rate is normally 100 mL/hr.

Table 53-4 COMPOSITION OF INTRAVENOUS SOLUTIONS

FLUID	[Na]	[Cl⁻]	[K⁺]	[Ca²⁺]	[LACTATE⁻]
Normal saline (0.9% NaCl)	154	154	—	—	—
Half-normal saline (0.45% NaCl)	77	77	—	—	—
0.2 normal saline (0.2% NaCl)	34	34	—	—	—
Ringer lactate	130	109	4	3	28

GLUCOSE

Maintenance fluids usually contain D5, which provides 17 calories/100 mL and nearly 20% of the daily caloric needs. This level is enough to prevent ketone production and helps minimize protein degradation, but the child will lose weight on this regimen. The weight loss is the principal reason why a patient needs to be started on total parental nutrition after a few days of maintenance fluids if enteral feedings are still not possible. Maintenance fluids are also lacking in such crucial nutrients as protein, fat, vitamins, and minerals.

SELECTION OF MAINTENANCE FLUIDS

After calculation of water and electrolyte needs, children typically receive either D5 ½NS + 20 mEq/L KCl or D5 0.2NS + 20 mEq/L KCl. Children weighing less than approximately 10 kg do best with the solution containing 0.2NS because of their high water needs per kilogram. Larger children and adults may receive the solution with ½NS. These guidelines assume that there is no disease process present that would require an adjustment in either the volume or the electrolyte composition of maintenance fluids (children with renal insufficiency may be hyperkalemic or unable to excrete potassium and may not tolerate 20 mEq/L of potassium). These solutions work well in children who have normal homeostatic mechanisms for adjusting urinary excretion of water, sodium, and potassium. In children with complicated pathophysiologic derangements, it may be necessary to empirically adjust the electrolyte composition and rate of maintenance fluids on the basis of electrolyte measurements and assessment of fluid balance. **In all children, it is critical to carefully monitor weight, urine output, and electrolytes to identify overhydration or underhydration, hyponatremia, and other electrolyte disturbances, and to then adjust the rate or composition of the intravenous solution accordingly.**

MAINTENANCE FLUIDS AND HYPONATREMIA

Patients who are producing antidiuretic hormone (ADH) may retain water, creating a risk of hyponatremia due to water intoxication. Patients who may be producing ADH owing to subtle volume depletion or other mechanisms (respiratory disease, stress, pain, nausea, medications such as narcotics) may be more safely treated with fluids that have a higher sodium concentration, with a decrease in fluid rate, or with a combination of these strategies. Patients with persistent ADH production due to an underlying disease process (syndrome of inappropriate ADH secretion [SIADH], congestive heart failure, nephrotic syndrome, liver disease) should receive less than maintenance fluids. Treatment is individualized, and careful monitoring is critical. Special caution is needed in patients who are known to have low-normal serum sodium concentrations or hyponatremia.

Hyponatremia as a complication of intravenous fluids is particularly a concern in the postoperative patient who is intravascularly volume-depleted from surgical losses, third space losses (discussed later), and venous pooling (due to lying supine and the effects of anesthesia and sedation). Surgical patients typically receive isotonic fluids (NS, LR) during surgery and in the recovery room for 6-8 hr postoperatively; the rate is typically approximately ⅔ of the calculated maintenance rate. Subsequent maintenance fluids should contain ½NS, even in smaller patients, unless there is a specific indication to use 0.2NS. Electrolytes should be measured at least daily.

Patients with other potential causes of ADH production must have careful monitoring of their electrolytes and fluid input and output. Patients with possible subtle volume depletion (Chapter 54) should receive 20 mL/kg (maximum of 1 L) of isotonic fluid (NS, LR) over 1-2 hr to restore their intravascular volume before maintenance fluids are initiated. The patient can then be switched to D5 ½NS + 20 mEq/L KCl at a standard maintenance rate. Patients of any weight with possible volume depletion should not routinely receive fluids with 0.2NS, unless there is a specific indication. Patients who are at risk for producing ADH owing to etiologies other than volume depletion may need to receive less than maintenance fluids to avoid hyponatremia.

VARIATIONS IN MAINTENANCE WATER AND ELECTROLYTES

The calculation of maintenance water is based on standard assumptions regarding water losses. There are patients, however, in whom these assumptions are incorrect. To identify such situations, it is helpful to understand the source and magnitude of normal water losses. Table 53-5 lists the 3 sources of normal water loss.

Urine is the most important contributor to normal water loss. Insensible losses represent approximately ⅓ of total maintenance water (40% in infants and closer to 25% in adolescents and adults). Insensible losses are composed of evaporative losses from the skin and lungs that cannot be quantitated. The evaporative losses from the skin do not include sweat, which would be considered an additional (sensible) source of water loss. Stool normally represents a minor source of water loss.

Maintenance water and electrolyte needs may be increased or decreased, depending on the clinical situation. This may be obvious, in the case of the infant with profuse diarrhea, or subtle, in the case of the patient who has decreased insensible losses while receiving mechanical ventilation. It is helpful to consider the sources of normal water and electrolyte losses and to determine whether any of these sources is being modified in a specific patient. It is then necessary to adjust maintenance water and electrolyte calculations.

Table 53-6 lists a variety of clinical situations that modify normal water and electrolyte losses. The skin can be a source of very significant water loss, particularly in neonates, especially premature infants, who are under radiant warmers or are receiving phototherapy. Very low birthweight infants can have insensible losses of 100-200 mL/kg/24 hr. Burns can result in massive losses of water and electrolytes, and there are specific guidelines for fluid management in children with burns (Chapter 68). Sweat losses of water and electrolytes, especially in a warm climate, can also be significant. Children with cystic fibrosis have increased sodium losses from the skin. Some children with pseudohypoaldosteronism also have increased cutaneous salt losses.

Fever increases evaporative losses from the skin. These losses are somewhat predictable, leading to a 10-15% increase in maintenance water needs for each 1°C increase in temperature above 38°C. These guidelines are for a patient with a persistent fever; a 1-hr fever spike does not cause an appreciable increase in water needs.

Tachypnea or a tracheostomy increases evaporative losses from the lungs. A humidified ventilator causes a decrease in insensible losses from the lungs and can even lead to water absorption via the lungs; a ventilated patient has a decrease in maintenance water requirements. It may be difficult to quantify the changes that take place in the individual patient in these situations.

REPLACEMENT FLUIDS

The gastrointestinal (GI) tract is potentially a source of considerable water loss. GI water losses are accompanied by electrolytes and thus may cause disturbances in intravascular volume and electrolyte concentrations. GI losses are often associated with loss of potassium, leading to hypokalemia. Because of the high bicarbonate concentration in stool, children with diarrhea usually have a metabolic acidosis, which may be accentuated if volume depletion causes hypoperfusion and a concurrent lactic acidosis. Emesis or losses from an NG tube can cause a metabolic alkalosis (Chapter 52).

In the absence of vomiting, diarrhea, or NG drainage, GI losses of water and electrolytes are usually quite small. All GI losses are considered excessive, and the increase in the water requirement is equal to the volume of fluid losses. Because GI water and electrolyte losses can be precisely measured, it is possible to use an appropriate replacement solution.

It is impossible to predict the losses for the next 24 hr; it is better to replace excessive GI losses as they occur. The child should receive an appropriate maintenance fluid that does not consider the GI losses. The losses should then be replaced after they occur, with use of a solution with the same approximate electrolyte concentration as the GI fluid. The losses are usually replaced every 1-6 hr, depending on the rate of loss, with very rapid losses being replaced more frequently.

Diarrhea is a common cause of fluid loss in children. It can cause dehydration and electrolyte disorders. In the unusual

Table 53-5 SOURCES OF WATER LOSS

Urine: 60%
Insensible losses: ≈35% (skin and lungs)
Stool: 5%

Table 53-6 ADJUSTMENTS IN MAINTENANCE WATER

SOURCE	CAUSES OF INCREASED WATER NEEDS	CAUSES OF DECREASED WATER NEEDS
Skin	Radiant warmer	Incubator (premature infant)
	Phototherapy	
	Fever	
	Sweat	
	Burns	
Lungs	Tachypnea	Humidified ventilator
	Tracheostomy	
Gastrointestinal tract	Diarrhea	—
	Emesis	
	Nasogastric suction	
Renal	Polyuria	Oliguria/anuria
Miscellaneous	Surgical drain	Hypothyroidism
	Third spacing	

Table 53-7 REPLACEMENT FLUID FOR DIARRHEA

AVERAGE COMPOSITION OF DIARRHEA
Sodium: 55 mEq/L Potassium: 25 mEq/L Bicarbonate: 15 mEq/L
APPROACH TO REPLACEMENT OF ONGOING LOSSES
Solution: D5 0.2 normal saline + 20 mEq/L sodium bicarbonate + 20 mEq/L KCl Replace stool mL/mL every 1-6 hr

Table 53-8 REPLACEMENT FLUID FOR EMESIS OR NASOGASTRIC LOSSES

AVERAGE COMPOSITION OF GASTRIC FLUID
Sodium: 60 mEq/L Potassium: 10 mEq/L Chloride: 90 mEq/L
APPROACH TO REPLACEMENT OF ONGOING LOSSES
Solution: normal saline + 10 mEq/L KCl Replace output mL/mL every 1-6 hr

patient with significant diarrhea and a limited ability to take oral fluid, it is important to have a plan for replacing excessive stool losses. The volume of stool should be measured, and an equal volume of replacement solution should be given. Data are available on the average electrolyte composition of diarrhea in children (Table 53-7). With use of this information, it is possible to design an appropriate replacement solution. The solution shown in Table 53-7 replaces stool losses of sodium, potassium, chloride, and bicarbonate. Each 1 mL of stool should be replaced by 1 mL of this solution. The average electrolyte composition of diarrhea is just an average, and there may be considerable variation. It is therefore advisable to consider measuring the electrolyte composition of a patient's diarrhea if the amount is especially excessive or if the patient's serum electrolyte levels are problematic.

Loss of gastric fluid, via either emesis or NG suction, is also likely to cause dehydration, in that most patients with either condition have impaired oral intake of fluids. Electrolyte disturbances, particularly hypokalemia and metabolic alkalosis, are also common. These complications can be avoided by judicious use of a replacement solution. The composition of gastric fluid shown in Table 53-8 is the basis for designing a replacement solution.

Patients with gastric losses frequently have hypokalemia, although the potassium concentration of gastric fluid is relatively low. The associated urinary loss of potassium is an important cause of hypokalemia in this situation (Chapter 52). These patients may need additional potassium either in their maintenance fluids or in their replacement fluids to compensate for prior or ongoing urinary losses. Restoration of the patient's intravascular volume, by decreasing aldosterone synthesis, lessens the urinary potassium losses.

Urine output is normally the largest cause of water loss. Diseases such as renal failure and SIADH can lead to a decrease in urine volume. The patient with oliguria or anuria has a decreased need for water and electrolytes; continuation of maintenance fluids produces fluid overload. In contrast, postobstructive diuresis, the polyuric phase of acute tubular necrosis, diabetes mellitus, and diabetes insipidus increase urine production. To prevent dehydration, the patient must receive more than standard maintenance fluids when urine output is excessive. The electrolyte losses in patients with polyuria are variable. In diabetes insipidus, the urine electrolyte concentration is usually low, whereas children with diseases such as juvenile nephronophthisis and obstructive uropathy usually have increased losses of both water and sodium.

The approach to decreased or increased urine output is similar (Table 53-9). The patient receives fluids at a rate to replace insensible losses. This is accomplished by a rate of fluid administration that is 25-40% of the normal maintenance rate, depending on the patient's age. Replacing insensible losses in the anuric child will theoretically maintain an even fluid balance, with the caveat that 25-40% of the normal maintenance rate is only an estimate of insensible losses. In the individual patient, this rate is adjusted on the basis of monitoring of the patient's weight and volume status. Most children with renal insufficiency receive little or no potassium because the kidney is the principal site of potassium excretion.

Table 53-9 ADJUSTING FLUID THERAPY FOR ALTERED RENAL OUTPUT

OLIGURIA/ANURIA
Start patient on replacement of insensible fluid losses (25-40% of maintenance) Replace urine output mL/mL with half-normal saline
POLYURIA
Start patient on replacement of insensible fluid losses (25-40% of maintenance) Measure urine electrolytes Replace urine output mL/mL with solution based on measured urine electrolytes

For the oliguric child, it is important to add a urine replacement solution to prevent dehydration. This issue is especially important in the patient with acute renal failure, in whom output may increase slowly, potentially leading to volume depletion and worsening of renal failure if the patient remains on only insensible fluids. A replacement solution of D5 ½NS is usually appropriate initially, although its composition may have to be adjusted if urine output increases significantly.

Most children with polyuria (except in diabetes mellitus; Chapter 583) should be started on replacement of insensible fluid plus urine losses. This approach avoids the need to attempt to calculate the volume of urine output that is "normal" so that the patient can be given replacement fluid for the excess. In these patients, urine output is, by definition, excessive, and it is important to measure the sodium and potassium concentrations of the urine to help in formulating the urine replacement solution.

Surgical drains and chest tubes can produce measurable fluid output. These fluid losses should be replaced when they are significant. They can be measured and replaced with an appropriate replacement solution. Third space losses, which manifest as edema and ascites, are due to a shift of fluid from the intravascular space into the interstitial space. Although these losses cannot be quantitated easily, third space losses can be large and may lead to intravascular volume depletion, despite the patient's weight gain. Replacement of third space fluid is empirical but should be anticipated in patients who are at risk, such as children who have burns or abdominal surgery. Third space losses and chest tube output are isotonic; thus, they usually require replacement with an isotonic fluid, such as NS or LR. Adjustments in the amount of replacement fluid for third space losses are based on continuing assessment of the patient's intravascular volume status. Protein losses from chest tube drainage can be significant, occasionally necessitating that 5% albumin be used as a replacement solution.

BIBLIOGRAPHY

Please visit the Nelson Textbook of Pediatrics *website at www.expertconsult.com for the complete bibliography.*

Chapter 54
Deficit Therapy

Larry A. Greenbaum

Dehydration, most often due to gastroenteritis, is a common problem in children. Most cases can be managed with oral rehydration (Chapter 332). **Even children with mild to moderate**

Table 54-1 CLINICAL EVALUATION OF DEHYDRATION

Mild dehydration (<5% in an infant; <3% in an older child or adult): Normal or increased pulse; decreased urine output; thirsty; normal physical findings
Moderate dehydration (5-10% in an infant; 3-6% in an older child or adult): Tachycardia; little or no urine output; irritable/lethargic; sunken eyes and fontanel; decreased tears; dry mucous membranes; mild delay in elasticity (skin turgor); delayed capillary refill (>1.5 sec); cool and pale
Severe dehydration (>10% in an infant; >6% in an older child or adult): Peripheral pulses either rapid and weak or absent; decreased blood pressure; no urine output; very sunken eyes and fontanel; no tears; parched mucous membranes; delayed elasticity (poor skin turgor); very delayed capillary refill (>3 sec); cold and mottled; limp, depressed consciousness

hyponatremic or hypernatremic dehydration can be managed with oral rehydration. This chapter focuses on the child who requires intravenous therapy, although many of the same principles are used in oral rehydration.

CLINICAL MANIFESTATIONS

The first step in caring for the child with dehydration is to assess the degree of dehydration (Table 54-1), which dictates both the urgency of the situation and the volume of fluid needed for rehydration. The infant with mild dehydration (3-5% of body weight dehydrated) has few clinical signs or symptoms. The infant may be thirsty; the alert parent may notice a decline in urine output. The history is most helpful. The infant with moderate dehydration has clear physical signs and symptoms. Intravascular space depletion is evident from an increased heart rate and reduced urine output. This patient needs fairly prompt intervention. The infant with severe dehydration is gravely ill. The decrease in blood pressure indicates that vital organs may be receiving inadequate perfusion. Immediate and aggressive intervention is necessary. If possible, the child with severe dehydration should initially receive intravenous therapy. For older children and adults, mild, moderate, or severe dehydration represents a lower percentage of body weight lost. This difference occurs because water accounts for a higher percentage of body weight in infants (Chapter 52).

Clinical assessment of dehydration is only an estimate; thus, the patient must be continually reevaluated during therapy. The degree of dehydration is underestimated in hypernatremic dehydration because the movement of water from the intracellular space to the extracellular space helps preserve the intravascular volume.

The history usually suggests the etiology of the dehydration and may predict whether the patient will have a normal sodium concentration (isotonic dehydration), hyponatremic dehydration, or hypernatremic dehydration. The neonate with dehydration due to poor intake of breast milk often has hypernatremic dehydration. Hypernatremic dehydration is likely in any child with losses of hypotonic fluid and poor water intake, such as may occur with diarrhea, and poor oral intake due to anorexia or emesis. Hyponatremic dehydration occurs in the child with diarrhea who is taking in large quantities of low-salt fluid, such as water or diluted formula.

Some children with dehydration are appropriately thirsty, but in others, the lack of intake is part of the pathophysiology of the dehydration. Even though decreased urine output is present in most children with dehydration, good urine output may be deceptively present if a child has an underlying renal defect, such as diabetes insipidus or a salt-wasting nephropathy, or in infants with hypernatremic dehydration.

Physical examination findings are usually proportional to the degree of dehydration. Parents may be helpful in assessment of the child for the presence of sunken eyes, because this finding may be subtle. Pinching and gently twisting the skin of the abdominal or thoracic wall detects tenting of the skin (turgor, elasticity). Tented skin remains in a pinched position rather than springing quickly back to normal. It is difficult to properly assess tenting of the skin in premature infants or severely malnourished children. Activation of the sympathetic nervous system causes tachycardia in children with intravascular volume depletion; diaphoresis may also be present. Postural changes in blood pressure are often helpful for evaluating and assessing the response to therapy in children with dehydration. Tachypnea in children with dehydration may be present secondary to a metabolic acidosis from stool losses of bicarbonate or due to lactic acidosis from shock (Chapter 64).

LABORATORY FINDINGS

Several laboratory findings are useful for evaluating the child with dehydration. The serum sodium concentration determines the type of dehydration. Metabolic acidosis may be due to stool bicarbonate losses in children with diarrhea, secondary renal insufficiency, or lactic acidosis from shock. The anion gap is useful for differentiating among the various causes of a metabolic acidosis (Chapter 52). Emesis or nasogastric losses usually cause a metabolic alkalosis. The serum potassium concentration may be low as a result of diarrheal losses. In children with dehydration due to emesis, gastric potassium losses, metabolic alkalosis, and urinary potassium losses all contribute to hypokalemia. Metabolic acidosis, which causes a shift of potassium out of cells, and renal insufficiency may lead to hyperkalemia. A combination of mechanisms may be present; thus, it may be difficult to predict the child's acid-base status or serum potassium level from the history alone.

The blood urea nitrogen (BUN) value and serum creatinine concentration are useful in assessing the child with dehydration. Volume depletion without parenchymal renal injury may cause a disproportionate increase in the BUN with little or no change in the creatinine concentration. This condition is secondary to increased passive resorption of urea in the proximal tubule due to appropriate renal conservation of sodium and water. The increase in the BUN with moderate or severe dehydration may be absent or blunted in the child with poor protein intake, because urea production depends on protein degradation. The BUN may be disproportionately increased in the child with increased urea production, as occurs with a gastrointestinal bleed or with the use of glucocorticoids, which increase catabolism. A significant elevation of the creatinine concentration suggests renal insufficiency, although a small, transient increase can occur with dehydration. **Acute tubular necrosis** (Chapter 529) due to volume depletion is the most common etiology of renal insufficiency in a child with volume depletion, but occasionally the child may have previously undetected chronic renal insufficiency or an alternative explanation for the acute renal failure. Renal vein thrombosis is a well-described sequela of severe dehydration in infants; possible findings include thrombocytopenia and hematuria (Chapter 513.7).

Hemoconcentration due to dehydration causes increases in hematocrit, hemoglobin, and serum proteins. These values normalize with rehydration. A normal hemoglobin concentration during acute dehydration may mask an underlying anemia. A decreased albumin level in a dehydrated patient suggests a chronic disease, such as malnutrition, nephrotic syndrome, or liver disease, or an acute process, such as capillary leak. An acute or chronic protein-losing enteropathy may also cause a low serum albumin concentration.

CALCULATION OF THE FLUID DEFICIT

Determining the fluid deficit necessitates clinical determination of the percentage of dehydration and multiplication of this percentage by the patient's weight; a child who weighs 10 kg and is 10% dehydrated has a fluid deficit of 1 L.

APPROACH TO DEHYDRATION

The child with dehydration needs acute intervention to ensure that there is adequate tissue perfusion. This resuscitation phase requires rapid restoration of the circulating intravascular volume and treatment of shock with an isotonic solution, such as normal saline (NS) or Ringer lactate (LR) (Chapter 64). The child is given a fluid bolus, usually 20 mL/kg of the isotonic fluid, over approximately 20 min. The child with severe dehydration may require multiple fluid boluses and may need to receive the boluses as fast as possible. In a child with a known or probable metabolic alkalosis (the child with isolated vomiting), LR should not be used because the lactate would worsen the alkalosis.

Colloids, such as blood, 5% albumin, and plasma, are rarely needed for fluid boluses. A crystalloid solution (NS or LR) is satisfactory, with both less infectious risk and lower cost. Blood is obviously indicated in the child with significant anemia or acute blood loss. Plasma is useful for children with a coagulopathy. The child with hypoalbuminemia may benefit from 5% albumin, although there is evidence that albumin infusions increase mortality in adults. The volume and the infusion rate for colloids are generally modified compared with crystalloids (Chapters 464 and 467).

The initial resuscitation and rehydration phase is complete when the child has an adequate intravascular volume. Typically, the child shows clinical improvement, including a lower heart rate, normalization of blood pressure, improved perfusion, better urine output, and a more alert affect.

With adequate intravascular volume, it is appropriate to plan the fluid therapy for the next 24 hr. A general approach is outlined in Table 54-2, with the caveat that there are many different approaches to correcting dehydration. In isonatremic or hyponatremic dehydration, the entire fluid deficit is corrected over 24 hr; a slower approach is used for hypernatremic dehydration (discussed later). To assure that the intravascular volume is restored, the patient receives an additional 20-mL/kg bolus of an isotonic fluid over 2 hr. The child's total fluid needs are added together (maintenance + deficit). The volume of isotonic fluids that the patient has received is subtracted from this total. The remaining fluid volume is then administered over 24 hr. The potassium concentration may need to be decreased or, less commonly, increased, depending on the clinical situation. Potassium is not usually included in the intravenous fluids until the patient voids. Children with significant ongoing losses need to receive an appropriate replacement solution (Chapter 53).

MONITORING AND ADJUSTING THERAPY

The formulation of a plan for correcting a child's dehydration is only the beginning of management. **All calculations in fluid therapy are only approximations.** This statement is especially true for the assessment of percentage dehydration. It is equally important to monitor the patient during treatment and to modify therapy on the basis of the clinical situation. The cornerstones of patient monitoring are listed in Table 54-3. The patient's vital signs are useful indicators of intravascular volume status. The child with decreased blood pressure and an increased heart rate will probably benefit from a fluid bolus. Central venous pressure is an excellent indicator of fluid status in the critically ill child with shock.

The patient's intake and output are critically important in the dehydrated child. The child who, after 8 hr of therapy, has more output than input because of continuing diarrhea needs to be started on a replacement solution. See the guidelines in Chapter 53 for selecting an appropriate replacement solution. Urine output is useful for evaluating the success of therapy. Good urine output indicates that rehydration has been successful.

Signs of dehydration on physical examination suggest the need for continued rehydration. Signs of fluid overload, such as edema and pulmonary congestion, are present in the child who is overhydrated. An accurate daily weight measurement is critical for the management of the dehydrated child. There should be a gain in weight during successful therapy.

Measurement of serum electrolyte levels at least daily is appropriate for any child who is receiving intravenous rehydration. Such a child is at risk for sodium, potassium, and acid-base disorders. It is always important to look at trends. For instance, a sodium value of 144 mEq/L is normal; but if the sodium concentration was 136 mEq/L 12 hr earlier, then there is a distinct risk that the child will be hypernatremic in 12 or 24 hr. It is advisable to be proactive in adjusting fluid therapy.

Both hypokalemia and hyperkalemia are potentially serious (Chapter 52). Because dehydration can be associated with acute renal failure and hyperkalemia, potassium is withheld from intravenous fluids until the patient has voided. The potassium concentration in the patient's intravenous fluids is not rigidly prescribed. Rather, the patient's serum potassium level and underlying renal function are used to modify potassium delivery. The patient with an elevated creatinine value and a potassium level of 5 mEq/L does not receive any potassium until the serum potassium level decreases. Conversely, the patient with a potassium level of 2.5 mEq/L may require additional potassium.

Metabolic acidosis can be quite severe in dehydrated children. Although normal kidneys eventually correct this problem, a child with renal dysfunction may be unable to correct a metabolic acidosis, and a portion of the patient's intravenous sodium chloride may have to be replaced with sodium bicarbonate or sodium acetate.

The serum potassium level is modified by the patient's acid-base status. Acidosis increases serum potassium by causing intracellular potassium to move into the extracellular space. Thus, as acidosis is corrected, the potassium concentration decreases. Again, it is best to anticipate this problem and to monitor the serum potassium concentration and adjust potassium administration appropriately.

HYPONATREMIC DEHYDRATION

The pathogenesis of hyponatremic dehydration usually involves a combination of sodium and water loss and water retention to compensate for the volume depletion. The patient has a pathologic increase in fluid loss, and the lost fluid contains sodium.

Table 54-2 FLUID MANAGEMENT OF DEHYDRATION

Restore intravascular volume:
Normal saline: 20 mL/kg over 20 min
Repeat as needed
Rapid volume repletion: 20 mL/kg normal saline or Ringer lactate (maximum = 1 L) over 2 hr
Calculate 24-hr fluid needs: maintenance + deficit volume
Subtract isotonic fluid already administered from 24-hr fluid needs
Administer remaining volume over 24 hr using D5 half-normal saline + 20 mEq/L KCl
Replace ongoing losses as they occur

Table 54-3 MONITORING THERAPY

Vital signs:
Pulse
Blood pressure
Intake and output:
Fluid balance
Urine output
Physical examination:
Weight
Clinical signs of depletion or overload
Electrolytes

Most fluid that is lost has a lower sodium concentration, so patients with only fluid loss would have hypernatremia. Diarrhea has, on average, a sodium concentration of 50 mEq/L. Replacing diarrheal fluid with water, which has almost no sodium, causes a reduction in the serum sodium concentration. The volume depletion stimulates synthesis of antidiuretic hormone, resulting in reduced renal water excretion. Hence, the body's usual mechanism for preventing hyponatremia, renal water excretion, is blocked. The risk of hyponatremia is further increased if the volume depletion is due to loss of fluid with a higher sodium concentration, as may occur with renal salt wasting, third space losses, or diarrhea with high sodium content (cholera).

The initial goal in treating hyponatremia is correction of intravascular volume depletion with isotonic fluid (NS or LR). An overly rapid (>12 mEq/L over the first 24 hr) or overcorrection in the serum sodium concentration (>135 mEq/L) is associated with an increased risk of **central pontine myelinolysis** (Chapter 52). Most patients with hyponatremic dehydration do well with the same basic strategy that is outlined in Table 54-2. Again, potassium delivery is adjusted according to the initial serum potassium level and the patient's renal function. Potassium is not given until the patient voids.

The patient's sodium concentration is monitored closely to ensure appropriate correction, and the sodium concentration of the fluid is adjusted accordingly. Patients with ongoing losses require an appropriate replacement solution (Chapter 53). Patients with neurologic symptoms (seizures) as a result of hyponatremia need to receive an acute infusion of hypertonic (3%) saline to increase the serum sodium concentration rapidly (Chapter 52).

HYPERNATREMIC DEHYDRATION

Hypernatremic dehydration is the most dangerous form of dehydration due to complications of hypernatremia and of therapy. Hypernatremia can cause serious neurologic damage, including central nervous system hemorrhages and thrombosis. This damage appears to be secondary to the movement of water from the brain cells into the hypertonic extracellular fluid, causing brain cell shrinkage and tearing blood vessels within the brain (Chapter 52).

The movement of water from the intracellular space to the extracellular space during hypernatremic dehydration partially protects the intravascular volume. Unfortunately, because the initial manifestations are milder, children with hypernatremic dehydration are often brought for medical attention with more profound dehydration.

Children with hypernatremic dehydration are often lethargic, and they may be irritable when touched. Hypernatremia may cause fever, hypertonicity, and hyperreflexia. More severe neurologic symptoms may develop if cerebral bleeding or thrombosis occurs.

Overly rapid treatment of hypernatremic dehydration may cause significant morbidity and mortality. Idiogenic osmoles are generated within the brain during the development of hypernatremia. These idiogenic osmoles increase the osmolality within the cells of the brain, providing protection against brain cell shrinkage caused by movement of water out of the cells and into the hypertonic extracellular fluid. They dissipate slowly during the correction of hypernatremia. With overly rapid lowering of the extracellular osmolality during the correction of hypernatremia, an osmotic gradient may be created that causes water movement from the extracellular space into the cells of the brain, producing cerebral edema. Symptoms of the resultant cerebral edema can range from seizures to brain herniation and death.

To minimize the risk of cerebral edema during the correction of hypernatremic dehydration, the serum sodium concentration should not decrease by >12 mEq/L every 24 hr. The deficits in severe hypernatremic dehydration may need to be corrected over 2-4 days (Table 54-4).

Table 54-4 TREATMENT OF HYPERNATREMIC DEHYDRATION

Restore intravascular volume:
- Normal saline: 20 mL/kg over 20 min (repeat until intravascular volume restored)
- Determine time for correction on basis of initial sodium concentration:
  - [Na] 145-157 mEq/L: 24 hr
  - [Na] 158-170 mEq/L: 48 hr
  - [Na] 171-183 mEq/L: 72 hr
  - [Na] 184-196 mEq/L: 84 hr

Administer fluid at constant rate over time for correction:
- Typical fluid: D5 half-normal saline (with 20 mEq/L KCl unless contraindicated)
- Typical rate: 1.25-1.5 times maintenance

Follow serum sodium concentration

Adjust fluid on basis of clinical status and serum sodium concentration:
- Signs of volume depletion: administer normal saline (20 mL/kg)
- Sodium decreases too rapidly; either:
  - Increase sodium concentration of intravenous fluid
  - Decrease rate of intravenous fluid
- Sodium decreases too slowly; either:
  - Decrease sodium concentration of intravenous fluid
  - Increase rate of intravenous fluid

Replace ongoing losses as they occur

The initial resuscitation of hypernatremic dehydration requires restoration of the intravascular volume with NS. LR should not be used because it is more hypotonic than NS and may cause too rapid a decrease in the serum sodium concentration, especially if multiple fluid boluses are necessary.

To avoid cerebral edema during correction of hypernatremic dehydration, the fluid deficit is corrected slowly. The rate of correction depends on the initial sodium concentration (see Table 54-4). There is no general agreement on the choice or the rate of fluid for correcting hypernatremic dehydration. The choice and the rate of fluid administration are not nearly as important as vigilant monitoring of the serum sodium concentration and adjustment of the therapy according to the result (see Table 54-4). The rate of decrease of the serum sodium concentration is roughly related to the "free water" delivery, although there is considerable variation between patients. Free water is water without sodium. NS contains no free water, half-normal saline (½NS) is 50% free water, and water is 100% free water. Smaller patients, to achieve the same decrease in the sodium concentration, tend to need higher amounts of free water delivery per kilogram because of higher insensible fluid losses. Five percent dextrose (D5) with ½NS is usually an appropriate starting solution for a patient with hypernatremic dehydration. Some patients, especially infants with ongoing high insensible water losses, may need to receive D5 0.2NS. Others require a higher sodium concentration than is present in D5 ½NS. A child with dehydration due to pure free water loss, as usually occurs with diabetes insipidus, usually needs a more hypotonic fluid than a child with depletion of both sodium and water due to diarrhea.

Adjustment in the sodium concentration of the intravenous fluid is the most common approach to modifying the rate of decrease in the serum concentration (see Table 54-4). For difficult patients with severe hypernatremia, having 2 intravenous solutions (D5 ¼NS and D5 NS, both with the same concentration of potassium) at the bedside can facilitate this approach by allowing for rapid adjustments of the rates of the 2 fluids. If the serum sodium concentration decreases too rapidly, the rate of D5 NS can be increased and the rate of D5 ½NS can be decreased by the same amount. Adjustment in the total rate of fluid delivery is another approach to modifying free water delivery. For example, if the serum sodium concentration is decreasing too slowly, the rate of the intravenous fluid can be increased, thereby increasing the delivery of free water. There is limited flexibility in modifying the rate of the intravenous fluid because patients generally should receive 1.25-1.5 times the normal maintenance fluid rate. Nevertheless, in some situations, it can be a helpful adjustment.

Because increasing the rate of the intravenous fluid increases the rate of decline of the sodium concentration, signs of volume depletion are treated with additional isotonic fluid boluses. The serum potassium concentration and the level of renal function dictate the potassium concentration of the intravenous fluid; potassium is withheld until the patient voids. Patients with hypernatremic dehydration need an appropriate replacement solution if they have ongoing, excessive losses (Chapter 53).

Seizures are the most common manifestation of **cerebral edema** from an overly rapid decrease of the serum sodium concentration during correction of hypernatremic dehydration. Acutely, increasing the serum concentration via an infusion of 3% sodium chloride can reverse the cerebral edema. Each 1-mL/kg of 3% sodium chloride increases the serum sodium concentration by approximately 1 mEq/L. An infusion of 4 mL/kg often results in resolution of the symptoms. This strategy is similar to that used for treating symptomatic hyponatremia (Chapter 52).

In patients with severe hypernatremia, oral fluids must be used cautiously. Infant formula, because of its low sodium concentration, has a high free water content, and especially if added to intravenous therapy, it may contribute to a rapid decrease in the serum sodium concentration. Less hypotonic fluid, such as an oral rehydration solution, may be more appropriate initially (Chapter 332). If oral intake is allowed, its contribution to free water delivery must be taken into account, and adjustment in the intravenous fluid is usually appropriate. Judicious monitoring of the serum sodium concentration is critical.

BIBLIOGRAPHY

Please visit the Nelson Textbook of Pediatrics *website at www.expertconsult.com for the complete bibliography.*

Chapter 55
Fluid and Electrolyte Treatment of Specific Disorders

ACUTE DIARRHEA

See Chapter 332.

PYLORIC STENOSIS

See Chapter 321.1.

PERIOPERATIVE FLUIDS

See Chapter 70.

PART VIII Pediatric Drug Therapy

Chapter 56
Pediatric Pharmacogenetics, Pharmacogenomics, and Pharmacoproteomics

Kathleen A. Neville and J. Steven Leeder

Interindividual variability in the response to similar doses of a given medication is an inherent characteristic of adult and pediatric populations. The role of genetic factors in drug disposition and response, **pharmacogenetics**, has resulted in many examples of how variations in human genes can lead to interindividual differences in pharmacokinetics and drug response at the level of individual patients. Just as in adults, pharmacogenetic variability contributes to the broad range of drug responses observed in children at any given age or developmental stage. Therefore, it is expected that children will benefit from the promise of **personalized medicine**: identifying the right drug for the right patient at the right time (see Fig. 56-1 on the *Nelson Textbook of Pediatrics* website at www.expertconsult.com). However, pediatricians are keenly aware that children are not merely small adults. Numerous maturational processes occur from birth through adolescence, and using information resulting from the Human Gene Project and related initiatives must take into account the changing patterns of gene expression that occur over development to improve pharmacotherapeutics in children.

For the full continuation of this chapter, please visit the Nelson Textbook of Pediatrics *website at www.expertconsult.com.*

Chapter 57
Principles of Drug Therapy

Jennifer A. Lowry, Bridgette L. Jones, Tracy Sandritter, Susanne Liewer, and Gregory L. Kearns

Regulatory mandates and economic opportunities have positioned pediatric patients for inclusion as subjects in pediatric clinical drug trials, but the majority of drugs used to treat sick infants and children do not have complete, approved product labeling sufficient to guide their use. Thus, off-label (or off-license) use of drugs in pediatrics continues to be the rule as opposed to the exception. Nonetheless, any important therapeutic advances have been made in pediatrics because physicians most often do not prescribe drugs from an "off-knowledge" basis. Rather, scientific and technical information published in the peer-reviewed medical literature and distilled into compendia for pediatric therapeutics have been used to support prudent, safe, and effective drug prescribing. Much of this information has resulted from investigations in the field of pediatric clinical pharmacology, which have explored the association with development (most often represented by the surrogate of age) of both drug disposition and action.

For the full continuation of this chapter, please visit the Nelson Textbook of Pediatrics *website at www.expertconsult.com.*

Chapter 58
Poisonings

Katherine A. O'Donnell and Michele Burns Ewald

Of the more than 2 million human poisoning exposures reported annually to the National Poison Data Systems of the American Association of Poison Control Centers (AAPCC), more than 50% occur in children <6 yr old. Almost all of these exposures are unintentional and reflect the propensity for young children to put virtually anything in their mouths.

More than 90% of toxic exposures in children occur in the home, and most involve only a single substance. Ingestion accounts for the vast majority of exposures, with a minority occurring via the dermal, inhalational, and ophthalmic routes. Approximately 50% of cases involve nondrug substances, such as cosmetics, personal care items, cleaning solutions, plants, and foreign bodies. Pharmaceutical preparations account for the remainder of exposures, and analgesics, topical preparations, cough and cold products, and vitamins are the most commonly reported categories.

The majority of poisoning exposures in children <6 yr can be managed without direct medical intervention, either because the product involved is not inherently toxic or the quantity of the material involved is not sufficient to produce clinically relevant toxic effects (Table 58-1). However, a number of substances are potentially highly toxic to toddlers in small doses (Table 58-2). In recent years, carbon monoxide, prescription opioids, antidepressants, and cardiovascular drugs have been the leading causes of poison-related fatalities in young children. Although the majority of exposures are in children <6 yr, only 2% of the reported deaths occur in this age group. In addition to the exploratory nature of ingestions in young children, product safety measures, poison prevention education, early recognition of exposures, and around-the-clock access to regionally based poison control centers all contribute to the favorable outcomes in this age group.

Poison prevention education should be an integral part of all well child visits, starting at the 6-mo visit. Counseling parents and other caregivers about potential poisoning risks, how to poison-proof a child's environment, and what to do if an ingestion or exposure occurs diminishes the likelihood of serious morbidity or mortality. Poison prevention education materials are available from the American Academy of Pediatrics and regional poison control centers. A network of poison control centers exists in the U.S., and anyone at any time can contact a regional poison center by calling a toll-free number: **1-800-222-1222.** Parents should be encouraged to share this number with grandparents, relatives, and any other caregivers.

Poisoning exposures in children 6-12 yr old are much less common, involving only ~ 6% of all reported pediatric exposures. A second peak in pediatric exposures occurs in adolescence. Exposures in the adolescent age group are primarily intentional (suicide or abuse or misuse of substances) and thus often result in more severe toxicity (Chapter 108). Families should be informed and given anticipatory guidance that over-the-counter (OTC) and prescription medications and even household products (e.g., inhalants) are common sources of adolescent exposures. Adolescents (ages 13-19 yr) accounted for 74 of the 108 poison-related pediatric deaths in 2008 reported to the National Poison Data System. Pediatricians should be aware of the signs of drug abuse or suicidal ideation in this population and should aggressively intervene (Chapter 108).

Table 58-1 COMMON NONTOXIC AND MINIMALLY TOXIC* PRODUCTS

Abrasives
Antacids, non-salicylate-containing
Antibiotics, topical
Antifungals, topical
Ballpoint pen ink
Bathtub floating toys
Bath oil (unless aspirated)
Body conditioners
Bubble bath soap
Calamine lotion
Candles (beeswax or paraffin)
Caps (toy pistols, potassium chlorate)
Chalk (calcium carbonate)
Children's toy cosmetics
Clay (modeling)
Contraceptives (oral) without iron
Corticosteroids, topical
Cosmetics
Crayons
Dehumidifying packets (e.g., silica)
Deodorants, underarm
Fabric softeners
Fertilizers (no insecticides or herbicides)
Detergents: hand, liquid dishwashing
Diaper rash creams and ointments
Fishbowl additives
Glow products (glowsticks)
Glues and paste
Golf ball (core can cause mechanical injury)
Grease
Hand lotions and creams
Hydrogen peroxide (medicinal 3%)
Incense
Indelible markers
Ink (black or blue, nonpermanent)
Iodophil disinfectants (unless the person is allergic)
Laxatives
Lipstick
Lozenges (without anesthetics)
Lubricating oils (unless aspirated)
Magazines
Markers, porous tip
Makeup
Matches
Mineral oil (unless aspirated)
Modeling compound (Play-Doh)
Newspaper (chronic ingestion can result in lead poisoning)
Paint, indoor latex, water-based
Paints, watercolor
Pencil lead (graphite, coloring)
Petroleum jelly (Vaseline)
Plant food (no insecticides or herbicides)
Polaroid picture coating fluid
Putty
Rubber cement
Shampoo
Shaving creams and lotions
Silica gel
Soap and soap products (noncaustic)
Spackle
Starch
Sunscreen
Sweetening agents (saccharin, aspartame)
Toothpaste (with and without fluoride)
Warfarin rodenticides (<0.5%)
Watercolor paints
Zinc oxide

*The potential for toxicity depends on the magnitude and amount of exposure. These agents are considered nontoxic or minimally toxic for mild to moderate exposure. The potential for toxicity increases with increased amount of exposure.

Table 58-2 MEDICATIONS POTENTIALLY TOXIC TO YOUNG CHILDREN IN SMALL DOSES*

SUBSTANCE	TOXICITY
Antimalarials (chloroquine, quinine)	Seizures, cardiac arrhythmias
Benzocaine	Methemoglobinemia
β-Blockers (lipid-soluble β-blockers [e.g., propranolol] are more toxic than water-soluble β-blockers [e.g., atenolol])	Bradycardia, hypotension, hypoglycemia
Calcium channel blockers	Bradycardia, hypotension, hyperglycemia
Camphor	Seizures
Clonidine	Lethargy, bradycardia, hypotension
Diphenoxylate and atropine (Lomotil)	CNS depression, respiratory depression
Hypoglycemics, oral (sulfonylureas and meglitinides)	Hypoglycemia, seizures
Lindane	Seizures
Monoamine oxidase Inhibitors	Hypertension followed by delayed cardiovascular collapse
Methyl salicylates	Tachypnea, metabolic acidosis, seizures
Opioids (especially methadone, lomotil and suboxone)	CNS depression, respiratory depression
Phenothiazines (chlorpromazine, thioridazine)	Seizures, cardiac arrhythmias
Theophylline	Seizures, cardiac arrhythmias
Tricyclic antidepressants	CNS depression, seizures, cardiac arrhythmias, hypotension

*"Small dose" typically implies 1 or 2 pills or 5 mL.
CNS, central nervous system.

APPROACH TO THE POISONED PATIENT

The initial approach to the patient with a witnessed or suspected poisoning should be no different than that in any other sick child, starting with stabilization and rapid assessment of the airway, breathing, circulation, and mental status (Chapter 62). A serum dextrose concentration should be obtained early in the evaluation of any patient with altered mental status. A targeted history and physical examination serves as the foundation for a thoughtful differential diagnosis, which can then be further refined through laboratory testing and other diagnostic studies.

INITIAL EVALUATION

History

Obtaining an accurate problem-oriented history is of paramount importance. Intentional poisonings (suicide attempts; abuse or misuse) are typically more severe than unintentional, exploratory ingestions. In patients without a witnessed exposure, historical features such as age of the child (toddler or adolescent), acute onset of symptoms without prodrome, sudden alteration of mental status, multiple system organ dysfunction, or highs levels of household stress should suggest a possible diagnosis of poisoning.

DESCRIPTION OF THE EXPOSURE For household and workplace products, names (brand, generic, chemical) and specific ingredients, along with their concentrations, can often be obtained from the labels. Poison control center specialists can also help to identify possible ingredients and review the potential toxicities of each component. In cases of suspected ingestion, poison center specialists can help identify pills based on markings, shape, and color. If referred to the hospital for evaluation, parents should be instructed to bring the products, pills, and/or containers with them to assist with identifying and quantifying the exposure. If a child is found with an unknown pill in his or her mouth, the history must include a list of all medications in the child's environment (including medications that grandparents, caregivers, or other visitors might have brought into the house). In the case of an unknown exposure, clarifying where the child was found (e.g., garage, kitchen, laundry room, bathroom, backyard, workplace) can help to generate a list of potential toxins.

Next, it is important to clarify the timing of the ingestion and to obtain some estimate of how much of the substance was ingested. In general, it is better to overestimate the amount ingested in order to prepare for the worst-case scenario. Counting pills or measuring the remaining volume of a liquid ingested can sometimes be useful in generating estimates.

For inhalational, ocular, or dermal exposures, the concentration of the agent and the length of contact time with the material should be determined if possible.

SYMPTOMS Obtaining a description of symptoms experienced after ingestion, including their timing of onset relative to the time of ingestion and their progression, can help to generate a list of potential toxins and to predict the severity of the ingestion. Coupled with physical exam findings, reported symptoms assist practitioners in identifying **toxidromes** or recognized poisoning syndromes suggestive of poisoning from specific substances or classes of substances (Tables 58-3 and 58-4).

PAST MEDICAL HISTORY Underlying diseases can make a child more susceptible to the effects of a toxin. Concurrent drug therapy can also increase susceptibility because certain drugs may interact with the toxin. Pregnancy is a common precipitating factor in adolescents' suicide attempts and can influence both evaluation of the patient and subsequent treatment. A history of

Table 58-3 HISTORICAL AND PHYSICAL FINDINGS IN POISONING

SIGN	TOXIN
ODOR	
Bitter almonds	Cyanide
Acetone	Isopropyl alcohol, methanol, paraldehyde, salicylates
Alcohol	Ethanol
Wintergreen	Methyl salicylate
Garlic	Arsenic, thallium, organophosphates, selenium
OCULAR SIGNS	
Miosis	Opioids (except propoxyphene, meperidine, and pentazocine), organophosphates and other cholinergics, clonidine, phenothiazines, sedative-hypnotics, olanzapine
Mydriasis	Atropine, cocaine, amphetamines, antihistamines, TCAs, carbamazepine, serotonin syndrome, PCP, LSD, post-anoxic encephalopathy
Nystagmus	Phenytoin, barbiturates, sedative-hypnotics, alcohols, carbamazepine, PCP, ketamine, dextromethorphan
Lacrimation	Organophosphates, irritant gas or vapors
Retinal hyperemia	Methanol
CUTANEOUS SIGNS	
Diaphoresis	Organophosphates, salicylates, cocaine and other sympathomimetics, serotonin syndrome, withdrawal syndromes
Alopecia	Thallium, arsenic
Erythema	Boric acid, elemental mercury, cyanide, carbon monoxide, disulfuram, scombroid, anticholinergics
Cyanosis (unresponsive to oxygen)	Methemoglobinemia (e.g., benzocaine, dapsone, nitrites, phenazopyridine), amiodarone, silver
ORAL SIGNS	
Salivation	Organophosphates, salicylates, corrosives, ketamine, PCP, strychnine
Oral Burns	Corrosives, oxalate-containing plants
Gum lines	Lead, mercury, arsenic, bismuth
GASTROINTESTINAL SIGNS	
Diarrhea	Antimicrobials, arsenic, iron, boric acid, cholinergics, colchicine, withdrawal
Hematemesis	Arsenic, iron, caustics, NSAIDs, salicylates
CARDIAC SIGNS	
Tachycardia	Sympathomimetics (e.g., amphetamines, cocaine), anticholinergics, antidepressants, theophylline, caffeine, antipsychotics, atropine, salicylates, cellular asphyxiants (cyanide, carbon monoxide, hydrogen sulfide), withdrawal
Bradycardia	β-Blockers, calcium channel blockers, digoxin, clonidine and other central α_2 agonists, organophosphates, opioids, sedative-hypnotics
Hypertension	Sympathomimetics (amphetamines, cocaine, LSD), anticholinergics, clonidine (early), monoamine oxidase inhibitors
Hypotension	β blockers, calcium channel blockers, cyclic antidepressants, iron, phenothiazines, barbiturates, clonidine, theophylline, opioids, arsenic, amatoxin mushrooms, cellular asphyxiants (cyanide, carbon monoxide, hydrogen sulfide), snake envenomation
RESPIRATORY SIGNS	
Depressed respirations	Opioids, sedative-hypnotics, alcohol, clonidine, barbiturates
Tachypnea	Salicylates, amphetamines, caffeine, metabolic acidosis (ethylene glycol, methanol, cyanide), carbon monoxide, hydrocarbons
CENTRAL NERVOUS SYSTEM SIGNS	
Ataxia	Alcohol, anticonvulsants, benzodiazepines, barbiturates, lithium, dextromethorphan, carbon monoxide, inhalants
Coma	Opioids, sedative-hypnotics, anticonvulsants, cyclic antidepressants, antipsychotics, ethanol, anticholinergics, clonidine, GHB, alcohols, salicylates, barbiturates
Seizures	Sympathomimetics, anticholinergics, antidepressants (especially TCAs, bupropion, venlafaxine), isoniazid, camphor, lindane, salicylates, lead, organophosphates, carbamazepine, tramadol, lithium, ginkgo seeds, water hemlock, withdrawal
Delirium/psychosis	Sympathomimetics, anticholinergics, LSD, PCP, hallucinogens, lithium, dextromethorphan, steroids, withdrawal
Peripheral neuropathy	Lead, arsenic, mercury, organophosphates

PCP, phencyclidine; LSD, lysergic acid diethylamide; TCA, tricylic antidepressants; NSAID, nonsteroidal anti-inflammatory drug; GHB, gamma hydroxybutyrate.

Table 58-4 RECOGNIZABLE POISON SYNDROMES

POISON SYNDROME	SIGNS: Vital	Mental Status	Pupils	Skin	Bowel Sounds	Other	POSSIBLE TOXINS
Sympathomimetic	Hypertension, tachycardia, hyperthermia	Agitated, psychosis, delirium	Dilated	Diaphoretic	Normal to increased		Amphetamines, cocaine, ecstasy, pseudoephedrine, caffeine, theophylline
Anticholinergic	Hypertension, tachycardia, hyperthermia	Agitation, delirium, mumbling speech	Dilated	Dry	Decreased		Antihistamines, tricyclic antidepressants, atropine, jimson weed, phenothiazines
Cholinergic	Bradycardia (though may show tachycardia), BP and temp typically normal	Confusion, coma, fasciculations	Small	Diaphoretic	Hyperactive	Diarrhea, urination, bronchorrhea, bronchospasm, emesis, lacrimation, salivation	Organophosphates, nerve gases, Alzheimer medications
Opioids	Vitals: Respiratory depression (hallmark of toxicity), bradycardia, hypotension, hypothermia	Depression, coma	Pinpoint	Normal	Normal to decreased		Methadone, suboxone, morphine, oxycodone, heroin, etc.
Sedative-Hypnotics	Respiratory depression, HR normal to decreased, BP normal to decreased, temp normal to decreased	Somnolence, coma	Small	Normal	Normal		Barbiturates, benzodiazepines, ethanol
Serotonin syndrome	Hyperthermia, tachycardia, hypertension or hypotension (autonomic instability)	Agitation, confusion, coma	Dilated	Diaphoretic	Increased	Neuromuscular hyperexcitability: clonus, hyperreflexia (lower extremities > upper extremities)	SSRIs, lithium, MAOIs, linezolid, tramadol, meperidine, dextromethorphan
Salicylates	Tachypnea, hyperpnea, tachycardia, hyperthermia	Agitation, confusion, coma	Normal	Diaphoretic	Normal	Nausea, vomiting, tinnitus, ABG with primary respiratory alkalosis and primary metabolic acidosis	Aspirin, bismuth subsalicylate (Pepto-Bismol), methyl salicylates
Withdrawal	Tachycardia, tachypnea, hyperthermia	Lethargy, confusion, delirium	Dilated	Diaphoretic	Increased		Withdrawal from opioids, sedative-hypnotics, ethanol

HR, heart rate; BP, blood pressure; temp, temperature; SSRI, selective serotonin reuptake inhibitor; MAOI, monoamine oxidase inhibitor; ABG, arterial blood gas.

psychiatric illness can make patients more prone to substance abuse, misuse, or intentional ingestions. A developmental history is important to ensure that the history provided is appropriate for the child's developmental stage (e.g., a report of a 6 mo old picking up a large container of laundry detergent and drinking it should raise a red flag).

SOCIAL HISTORY Understanding the child's social environment helps to identify potential sources of exposures (caregivers, visitors, grandparents, recent parties or social gatherings) and environmental stressors (new baby, parent's illness, financial stress) that might have contributed to the ingestion. Unfortunately, some poisonings occur in the setting of serious neglect or intentional abuse.

Physical Examination

A targeted physical exam is important to identifying the toxin and assessing the severity of the exposure. Initial efforts should be directed toward assessing and stabilizing the airway, breathing, circulation, and mental status. Once one has ensured that the airway is secure and the patient is stable from a cardiopulmonary standpoint, a more extensive physical exam can help to identify characteristics of specific toxins or classes of toxins.

In the poisoned patient, the key features of the physical exam are the vital signs, mental status, pupils (size, reactivity, nystagmus), skin, bowel sounds, and odors. Together, these findings might suggest a toxidrome (see Tables 58-3 and 58-4) that can guide the differential diagnosis and initial management.

Laboratory Evaluation

For select intoxications (salicylates, some anticonvulsants, acetaminophen, iron, digoxin, methanol, lithium, theophylline, ethylene glycol, carbon monoxide), quantitative blood concentrations are integral to confirming the diagnosis and formulating a treatment plan. For most exposures, quantitative measurement is not readily available and is not likely to alter management. Comprehensive drug screens vary widely in their ability to detect toxins and generally add little information to the clinical assessment, particularly if the agent is known and the patient's symptoms are consistent with that agent. If a drug screen is ordered, it is important to know that the components screened for in a toxicology screen, and the lower limits of detection, vary from hospital to hospital. In addition, the interpretation of most drug screens is hampered by false-positive and false-negative results. Most standard urine opiate screens won't be positive after ingestion of a synthetic opioid (e.g., methadone, suboxone). Although the presence of some drugs (e.g., marijuana) might not be clinically useful, it can identify use of "gateway drugs" and an adolescent at risk for substance abuse. Consultation with a medical toxicologist can be helpful in interpreting drug screens and ordering specific drug levels or metabolites that can aid in patient management.

Toxicology screens may be indicated in the assessment of the neglected or allegedly abused child, because a positive toxicology screen can add substantial weight to a claim of abuse or neglect. In these cases and any case with medicolegal implications, any positive screen *must* be confirmed with gas chromatography/mass spectroscopy (GC/MS), which is considered the gold standard measurement for legal purposes.

Acetaminophen is a widely available medication and a commonly detected co-ingestant with the potential for severe toxicity. Given that patients might initially be asymptomatic and might not report acetaminophen as a co-ingestant, an acetaminophen

Table 58-5 SCREENING LABORATORY CLUES IN TOXICOLOGIC DIAGNOSIS

ANION GAP METABOLIC ACIDOSIS (MNEMONIC = MUDPILES)
Methanol, metformin **U**remia **D**iabetic ketoacidosis **P**araldehyde, phenformin **I**soniazid, iron, massive ibuprofen **E**thylene glycol, ethanol **L**actic Acidosis (i.e. cyanide, carbon monoxide) **S**alicylates
ELEVATED OSMOLAR GAP
Alcohols: ethanol, isopropyl, methanol, ethylene glycol
HYPOGLYCEMIA (MNEMONIC = HOBBIES)
Hypoglycemics, oral: sulfonylureas, meglitinides **O**ther: quinine, unripe ackee fruit **B**eta-**B**lockers **I**nsulin **E**thanol **S**alicylates (late)
HYPERGLYCEMIA
Salicylates (early) Calcium channel blockers Caffeine
HYPOCALCEMIA
Ethylene glycol Fluoride
RHABDOMYOLYSIS
Diphenhydramine, doxylamine Neuroleptic malignant syndrome Statins Mushrooms (*tricholoma equestre*) Any toxin causing prolonged immobilization (e.g., opioids) or excessive muscle activity or seizures (e.g., sympathomimetics)
RADIOPAQUE SUBSTANCE ON KUB (MNEMONIC = CHIPPED)
Chloral hydrate, calcium carbonate **H**eavy metals (lead, zinc, barium, arsenic, lithium, bismuth, as in Pepto-Bismol) **I**ron **P**henothiazines **P**lay-Doh, potassium chloride **E**nteric-coated pills **D**ental amalgam

KUB, kidney-ureter-bladder radiograph.

Table 58-6 ELECTROCARDIOGRAPHIC FINDINGS IN POISONING

PR INTERVAL PROLONGATION
Digoxin Lithium
QRS PROLONGATION
Tricyclic antidepressants Diphenhydramine Carbamazepine Cardiac glycosides Chloroquine, hydoxychloroquine Cocaine Lamotrigine Quindine, quinine, procainamide, disopyramide Phenothiazines Propoxyphene Propranolol Bupropion, venlafaxine (rare)
QTc PROLONGATION*
Amiodarone Antipsychotics (typical and atypical) Arsenic Cisapride Citalopram and other SSRIs Clarithromycin, Erythromycin Disopyramide, Dofetilide, Ibutilide Fluconazole, ketoconazole, itraconazole Methadone Pentamadine Phenothiazines Sotalol

*This is a select list of important toxins, but other medications are also associated with QTc prolongation.
SSRI, selective serotonin reuptake inhibitor.

level should be checked in all patients who present after an intentional exposure or ingestion. Furthermore, in *any* clinical situation with potential medicolegal implications, any positive drug screen should be confirmed by a more sensitive and specific method (typically GC/MS).

Based on the clinical presentation, additional labs tests that may be helpful include electrolytes and renal function (an elevated anion gap suggests a number of ingestions), serum osmolarity (toxic alcohols), complete blood count, liver function tests, urinalysis (crystals), co-oximetry, and a serum creatine kinase level (Table 58-5).

Additional Diagnostic Testing

An electrocardiogram (ECG) is a quick and noninvasive bedside test that can yield important clues to diagnosis and prognosis. Toxicologists pay particular attention to the ECG intervals (Table 58-6). A widened QRS interval suggests blockade of fast sodium channels, as may be seen after ingestion of tricyclic antidepressants, diphenhydramine, cocaine, propoxyphene, and carbamazepine, among others. A widened QTc interval suggests effects at the potassium rectifier channels and portends a risk of torsades de pointes.

Chest x-ray may reveal signs of pneumonitis (e.g., hydrocarbon ingestion), pulmonary edema (e.g., salicylate toxicity), or a foreign body. Abdominal x-ray can suggest the presence of a bezoar, demonstrate radiopaque tablets, or reveal drug packets in a body packer. Endoscopy may be useful after significant caustic ingestions. Further diagnostic testing is based on the differential diagnosis and pattern of presentation (Table 58-7).

PRINCIPLES OF MANAGEMENT

The four principles of management of the poisoned patient are decontamination, enhanced elimination, antidotes, and supportive care. Few patients meet criteria for all of these interventions, though clinicians should consider each option in every poisoned patient so as not to miss a potentially lifesaving therapy. Antidotes are available for relatively few poisons (Table 58-8), thus emphasizing the importance of meticulous supportive care and close clinical monitoring.

Poison control centers are staffed by nurses, pharmacists, and physicians specifically trained to provide expertise in the management of poisoning exposures. Parents should be instructed to call the poison control center (**1-800-222-1222**) for any concerning exposure. Poison specialists can assist parents in assessing the potential toxicity and severity of the exposure. In doing so, they can further determine which children can be safely monitored at home and which children should be referred to the emergency department (ED) for further evaluation and care. The American Academy of Clinical Toxicology has generated consensus statements for out-of-hospital management of common ingestions (e.g., acetaminophen, iron, selective serotonin reuptake inhibitors) that serve to guide poison center recommendations.

Decontamination

The majority of poisonings in children are due to ingestion, though exposures can also occur via inhalational, dermal, and ocular routes. The goal of decontamination is to prevent absorption of the toxic substance. The specific method employed

Table 58-7 DRUGS ASSOCIATED WITH MAJOR MODES OF PRESENTATION

COMMON TOXIC CAUSES OF CARDIAC ARRHYTHMIA
Amphetamine Antiarrhythmics Anticholinergics Antihistamines Arsenic Carbon monoxide Chloral hydrate Cocaine Cyanide Cyclic antidepressants Digitalis Freon Phenothiazines Physostigmine Propranolol Quinine, quinidine Theophylline
CAUSES OF COMA
Alcohol Anticholinergics Antihistamines Barbiturates Carbon monoxide Clonidine Cyanide Cyclic antidepressants Hypoglycemic agents Lead Lithium Methemoglobinemia* Methyldopa Narcotics Phencyclidine Phenothiazines Salicylates
COMMON AGENTS CAUSING SEIZURES (MNEMONIC = CAPS)
Camphor, carbamazepine, carbon monoxide, cocaine, cyanide **A**minophylline, amphetamine, anticholinergics, antidepressants (cyclic) **P**b (lead) [also lithium], pesticide (organophosphate), phencyclidine, phenol, phenothiazines, propoxyphene **S**alicylates, strychnine

*Causes of methemoglobinemia: amyl nitrite, aniline dyes, benzocaine, bismuth subnitrate, dapsone, primaquone, quinones, spinach, sulfonamides.
From Kliegman RM, Mascdante KJ, Jenson HB, editors: *Nelson essentials of pediatrics*, ed 5, Philadelphia, 2006, Elsevier, p 208.

depends on the properties of the toxin itself and the route of exposure. Regardless of the decontamination method used, the efficacy of the intervention decreases with increasing time since exposure. **Thus, decontamination should not be routinely employed for every poisoned patient.** Instead, careful decisions regarding the utility of decontamination should be made for each patient and should include consideration of the toxicity and pharmacologic properties of the exposure, the route of the exposure, the time since the exposure, and the risks versus the benefits of the decontamination method.

Dermal and ocular decontamination begin with removal of any contaminated clothing and particulate matter, followed by flushing of the affected area with tepid water or normal saline. Treating clinicians should wear proper protective gear when performing irrigation. Flushing for a minimum of 10 to 20 minutes is recommended for most exposures, although some chemicals (e.g., alkaline corrosives) require much longer periods of flushing. Dermal decontamination, especially after exposure to adherent or lipophilic (e.g., organophosphates) agents, should include thorough cleansing with soap and water. Water should *not* be used for decontamination after exposure to highly reactive agents, such as elemental sodium, phosphorus, calcium oxide, and titanium tetrachloride. After an inhalational exposure, decontamination involves moving the patient to fresh air and administering supplemental oxygen if indicated.

Gastrointestinal (GI) decontamination is a controversial topic among medical toxicologists, with numerous studies documenting marked variability in recommendations. *In general, GI decontamination strategies are most likely to be effective in the first hour after an acute ingestion.* GI absorption may be delayed after ingestion of agents that slow GI motility (anticholinergic medications, opioids), massive pill ingestions, sustained-release preparations, and ingestions of agents that can form pharmacologic bezoars (e.g., enteric-coated salicylates). Thus, GI decontamination at >1 hr after ingestion may be considered in patients who ingest toxic substances with these properties. Described methods of GI decontamination include induced emesis with ipecac, gastric lavage, cathartics, activated charcoal, and whole-bowel irrigation (WBI). Of these, only activated charcoal and WBI are likely to have significant clinical benefit in management of the poisoned patient.

SYRUP OF IPECAC Syrup of ipecac contains 2 emetic alkaloids that work in both the central nervous system (CNS) and locally in the GI tract to produce vomiting. In the 1960s, the American Academy of Pediatrics (AAP) lobbied for OTC availability of ipecac and in the 1980s recommended that ipecac be given to parents at the 6-month well child check, coupled with a discussion about poison prevention strategies. Since that time, studies have failed to document a significant clinical impact from the use of ipecac and have documented multiple adverse events from its use. Ipecac-induced emesis is especially contraindicated after the ingestion of caustics (acids and bases), hydrocarbons, and agents likely to cause rapid onset of CNS or cardiovascular symptoms. Ipecac abuse and cardiac toxicity is described in some adolescents with bulimia, and syrup of ipecac has been used in reported cases of factitious disorder by proxy.

After a review of the evidence and assessment of the risks and benefits of ipecac use, the American Academy of Pediatrics no longer recommends the use of syrup of ipecac. The 2004 American Academy of Clinical Toxicology (AACT)/European Association of Poison Control Centers and Clinical Toxicology (EAPCCT) position paper suggests that the use of ipecac in the ED be abandoned. A further review by the American Association of Poison Control Centers in 2005 suggests that out-of-hospital ipecac use *only be considered in consultation with a medical toxicologist or poison control center if all of the following characteristics are met:*

- There will be a delay of 1 hr before the child will reach an emergency medical facility and the ipecac can be administered within 30-90 min of the ingestion.
- There is a substantial risk of serious toxicity to the patient.
- There are no contraindications to the use of ipecac (see above).
- There is no alternative therapy available to decrease GI absorption.
- The use of ipecac will not adversely affect more definitive therapy that may be provided at the hospital.

GASTRIC LAVAGE Gastric lavage involves placing a tube into the stomach to aspirate contents, followed by flushing with aliquots of fluid, usually normal saline. Although gastric lavage was used routinely for many years, objective data do not document or support clinically relevant efficacy. This is particularly true in children, in whom only small-bore tubes can be used. Lavage is time-consuming, can induce bradycardia via a vagal response to tube placement, can delay administration of more definitive treatment (activated charcoal), and under the best circumstances only removes a fraction of gastric contents. **Thus, in most clinical scenarios, the use of gastric lavage is no longer recommended.**

In consultation with a poison control center or toxicologist, lavage *may* be considered in the extremely rare instance of a child who presents very soon (30-60 min) after an ingestion of a highly toxic agent for which antidotal therapy or supportive care is

Table 58-8 COMMON ANTIDOTES FOR POISONING

POISON	ANTIDOTE	DOSAGE	ROUTE	ADVERSE EFFECTS, WARNINGS, COMMENTS
Acetaminophen	*N*-Acetylcysteine (Mucomyst)	140 mg/kg loading, followed by 70 mg/kg q4h for 17 doses*	PO	Nausea, vomiting *Consider shorter patient-tailored regimens (see text) Most effective if given within 8 hr of ingestion
	N-Acetylcysteine (Acetadote)	150 mg/kg over 1hr, followed by 50 mg/kg over 4 hr, followed by 100 mg/kg over 16 hr	IV	Anaphylactoid reactions (most commonly seen with loading dose)
Anticholinergics	Physostigmine	0.02 mg/kg over 5 min; may repeat q5-10min to 2 mg max	IV/IM	Bradycardia, asystole, seizures, bronchospasm, vomiting, headache *Note*: Do not use if conduction delays on ECG
Benzodiazepines	Flumazenil	0.2 mg over 30 sec; if response is inadequate, repeat q1min to 1 mg max	IV	Nausea, vomiting, facial flushing, agitation, headache, dizziness, seizures; **do not use for unknown or antidepressant ingestions**
β-Blockers	Glucagon	0.15 mg/kg bolus followed by infusion of 0.05-0.15 mg/kg/hr	IV	Hyperglycemia, nausea, vomiting
Calcium channel blockers	Insulin	1 U/kg bolus followed by infusion of 0.5-1 U/kg/hr	IV	Hypoglycemia Follow serum potassium and glucose closely
	Calcium salts	Dose depends on the specific calcium salt	IV	
Carbon monoxide	Oxygen	100% FiO_2 via non-rebreather mask (or ET if intubated)	Inhalational	Some patients may benefit from hyperbaric oxygen (see text)
Cyanide	Cyanide kit			
	1. Amyl nitrate	1 crushable ampule; inhale 30 sec of each min	Inhalation	Methemoglobinemia
	2. Sodium nitrate	0.33 mL/kg of 3% solution if hemoglobin level is not known; otherwise, based on tables with product	IV	Methemoglobinemia Hypotension
	3. Sodium thoisulfate	1.6 mL/kg of 25% solution; may be repeated q30-60min to max of 50 mL	IV	If inducing methemoglobinemia is contraindicated; consider only using the thiosulfate component of the kit
	Hydoxocobalamin (Cyanokit)	70 mg/kg (Adults: 5 g) given over 15 min	IV	Flushing/erythema, nausea, rash, chromaturia, hypertension, headache
Digitalis	Digoxin-specific Fab antibodies (Digibind; DigiFab)	1 vial binds 0.6 mg of digitalis glycoside; ingested dose may be estimated from the serum level (see table with product)	IV	Allergic reactions (rare), return of condition being treated with digitalis glycoside
Ethylene glycol Methanol	Fomepizole	15 mg/kg load; 10 mg/kg q12h × 4 doses; 15 mg/kg q12h until EG level is <20 mg/dL	IV	Infuse slowly over 30 min; increase doses to q4h if being dialyzed If Fomepizole is not available, treat with an ethanol infusion
Iron	Deferoxamine	Infusion of 5-15 mg/kg/hr (max, 6 g/24 hr)	IV	Hypotension (minimized by avoiding rapid infusion rates)
Isoniazid (INH)	Pyridoxine	Empirical dosing: 70 mg/kg (max dose = 5 g) If ingested dose is known: 1 g per gram of INH	IV	May also be used for *Gyromitra* mushroom ingestions
Lead and other heavy metals (e.g., arsenic, inorganic mercury)	BAL (dimercaprol)	3-5 mg/kg/dose q4hr, for the 1st day; subsequent dosing depends on the toxin	Deep IM	Local injection site pain and sterile abscess, nausea, vomiting, fever, salivation, nephrotoxicity *Caution:* Prepared in peanut oil; contraindicated in patients with peanut allergy
	Calcium disodium EDTA	35-50 mg/kg/day × 5 days; may be given as a continuous infusion or 2 divided doses/day	IV IM	Nausea, vomiting, fever, hypertension, arthralgias, allergic reactions, local inflammation, nephrotoxicity (maintain adequate hydration, follow UA and renal function) IV preferred, IM injections very painful
	Dimercaptosuccinic acid (succimer, DMSA, Chemet)	10 mg/kg/dose q8h × 5 days, then 10 mg/kg q12h × 14 days	PO	Nausea and vomiting, neutropenia, transaminitis, rash; repeated courses may be needed
Methemoglobinemia	Methylene blue, 1% solution	0.1-0.2 mL/kg (1-2 mg/kg) over 5-10 min; may be repeated q30-60 min	IV	Nausea, vomiting, headache, dizziness
Opioids	Naloxone	0.01-0.1 mg/kg; Adults: 0.4-2 mg, may be repeated as needed; may give continuous infusion	IV	Acute withdrawal symptoms if given to addicted patients May also be useful for clonidine ingestions (inconsistent response)
Organophosphates	Atropine	0.05-0.1 mg/kg repeated q5-10min as needed	IV/ET	Tachycardia, dry mouth, blurred vision, urinary retention
	Pralidoxime (2PAM)	25-50 mg/kg over 5-10 min (max, 200 mg/min); can be repeated after 1-2 hr, then q10-12hr as needed	IV/IM	Nausea, dizziness, headache, tachycardia, muscle rigidity, bronchospasm (rapid administration)

Table 58-8 COMMON ANTIDOTES FOR POISONING—cont'd

POISON	ANTIDOTE	DOSAGE	ROUTE	ADVERSE EFFECTS, WARNINGS, COMMENTS
Salicylates	Sodium bicarbonate	Bolus 1-2 mEq/kg followed by a continuous infusion	IV	Follow potassium closely and replete as necessary Avoid severe alkalosis (serum pH >7.55)
Sulfonylureas	Octreotide	1-2 µg/kg/dose (adults 50-100 µg) q6-8 hr.	IV/SC	
Tricyclic antidepressants	Sodium bicarbonate	Bolus 1-2 mEq/kg followed by continuous infusion	IV	Indications: QRS widening (>100 ms), hemodynamic instability Avoid severe alkalosis (serum pH >7.55) Follow potassium

max, maximum; ECG, electrocardiogram; ET, endotracheal; EG, ethylene glycol; BAL, British antilewisite; EDTA, ethylenediaminetetraacetic acid; UA, urinalysis; DMSA, dimercaptosuccinic acid.

unlikely to be of substantial benefit. If the treating clinician does decide to pursue lavage, careful attention should be paid to protecting the airway and to performing lavage with proper technique.

SINGLE-DOSE ACTIVATED CHARCOAL Of all the described modalities of gastric decontamination, activated charcoal is thought to potentially be the most useful, though clinical data to support this claim is somewhat limited. Charcoal is "activated" via heating to extreme temperatures, creating an extensive network of pores that provides a very large adsorptive surface area. Many, but not all, toxins are adsorbed onto its surface, thus preventing absorption from the GI tract. **Charcoal is most likely to be effective when given within 1 hr of ingestion.** Some toxins, including heavy metals, iron, lithium, hydrocarbons, cyanide, and low-molecular-weight alcohols, are not significantly bound to charcoal (Table 58-9). Charcoal administration should also be avoided after ingestion of a caustic substance, because the presence of charcoal can impede subsequent endoscopic evaluation.

The dose of activated charcoal is 1 g/kg in children or 50-100 g in adolescents and adults. Before administering charcoal, one *must* ensure that the patient's airway is intact or protected and that he or she has a benign abdominal exam. Approximately 20% of children vomit after receiving a dose of charcoal, emphasizing the importance of an intact airway and avoiding administration of charcoal after ingestion of substances that are particularly toxic when aspirated (e.g., hydrocarbons). If charcoal is given through a gastric tube, placement of the tube should be carefully confirmed before activated charcoal is given because instillation of charcoal directly into the lungs has disastrous effects. Constipation is another common side effect of activated charcoal, and in extreme cases, bowel perforation has been reported.

In young children, practitioners may attempt to improve palatability by adding flavorings (chocolate or cherry syrup) or giving the mixture over ice cream. Cathartics (sorbitol, magnesium sulfate, magnesium citrate) have been used in conjunction with activated charcoal to prevent constipation and accelerate evacuation of the charcoal-toxin complex. There is no evidence demonstrating their value and there are numerous reports of adverse effects from cathartics. Cathartics should be used with care in young children and should never be used in multiple doses because of the risk of dehydration and electrolyte imbalance.

WHOLE-BOWEL IRRIGATION WBI involves instilling large volumes (35 mL/kg/hr in children or 1-2 L/hr in adolescents) of a polyethylene glycol electrolyte solution (e.g., GoLYTELY) to "cleanse" the entire GI tract. This technique may have some success after the ingestion of slowly absorbed substances (sustained-release preparations), substances not well adsorbed by charcoal (e.g., lithium, iron), transdermal patches, and drug packets. WBI can be combined with the use of activated charcoal, if appropriate (cocaine or heroin body packers).

Careful attention should be paid to assessment of the airway and abdominal exam before initiating WBI. Given the rate of administration and volume needed to flush the system, WBI is typically administered via a nasogastric tube. WBI is continued until the rectal effluent is clear. Complications of WBI include vomiting, abdominal pain, and abdominal distention. Bezoar formation might respond to WBI but may require endoscopy or surgery (Table 58-10).

Table 58-9 SUBSTANCES POORLY ADSORBED BY ACTIVATED CHARCOAL

Alcohols Caustics: alkalis and acids Cyanide Heavy metals (e.g., lead) Hydrocarbons Iron Lithium

Table 58-10 COMMON MEDICATIONS IMPLICATED IN BEZOAR FORMATION

ANTACIDS
Aluminum hydroxide
BULK-FORMING LAXATIVES
Combination laxatives (e.g., Perdiem) Psyllium
EXTENDED-RELEASE PRODUCTS
Nifedipine Procainamide Verapamil
ION-EXCHANGE RESINS
Sodium polystyrene sulfonate Calcium polystyrene sulfonate
VITAMIN AND NATURAL PRODUCTS
Ascorbic acid Ferrous sulfate Lecithin
OTHER MEDICATIONS
Carbamazepine Cholestyramine Enteric-coated aspirin Lithium Salicylic acid Sucralfate

Enhanced Elimination

Enhancing excretion is only useful for a few toxins; in these cases, enhancing elimination is a potentially lifesaving intervention (e.g., hemodialysis for methanol toxicity).

MULTIPLE-DOSE ACTIVATED CHARCOAL Whereas single-dose activated charcoal is used as a method of decontamination, multiple doses of charcoal (MDAC) can help to enhance the elimination of some toxins. MDAC is typically given as 0.5 g/kg every 4-6 hr (for ≤24 hr) and continued until there is significant clinical improvement, including satisfactory decline of serum drug concentrations. Multiple doses of charcoal enhance elimination via two proposed mechanisms: interruption of enterohepatic recirculation and "GI dialysis," which uses the intestinal mucosa as the dialysis membrane and pulls toxins from the bloodstream back into the intraluminal space, where they are adsorbed to the charcoal. The AACT/EAPCCT position statement recommends MDAC in managing significant ingestions of carbamazepine, dapsone, phenobarbital, quinine, and theophylline. Many toxicologists consider using MDAC to manage salicylate toxicity that has persistently rising or inadequately falling salicylate levels (suggesting the presence of a pharmacobezoar).

As with single-dose activated charcoal, contraindications to use of MDAC include an unprotected airway and a concerning abdominal exam (e.g., ileus, distention, peritoneal signs); thus the airway and abdominal exam *should be assessed before each dose.* A cathartic (e.g., sorbitol) may be given with the first dose, but it should not be used with subsequent doses owing to the risk of dehydration and electrolyte derangements.

URINARY ALKALINIZATION Alkalinizing the urine enhances the elimination of some drugs that are weak acids by forming charged particles that are "trapped" within the renal tubules and thus excreted. Urinary alkalinization is accomplished with a continuous infusion of sodium bicarbonate–containing intravenous fluids, with a goal urine pH of 7.5-8. Alkalinization of the urine is most useful in managing salicylate and methotrexate toxicity. Alkalinization may also be beneficial in managing phenobarbital toxicity, though MDAC is thought to be a superior method of enhancing elimination of phenobarbital.

Serum pH should be closely monitored because a serum pH of >7.55 is potentially dangerous to cellular functions. Other complications of urinary alkalinization include electrolyte derangements, such as hypokalemia and hypocalcemia. This method of enhanced elimination is contraindicated in patients who are unable to tolerate the large volumes of fluid needed to achieve alkalinization, including patients with heart failure, kidney failure, pulmonary edema, or cerebral edema.

DIALYSIS Few drugs or toxins are removed by dialysis in amounts sufficient to justify the risks and difficulty of dialysis. Toxins that are amenable to dialysis have the following properties: low volume of distribution (<1 L/kg), low molecular weight, low degree of protein binding, and high degree of water solubility. Examples of toxins for which dialysis may be useful include methanol and ethylene glycol, as well as large symptomatic ingestions of salicylates, theophylline, bromide, or lithium. In addition to enhancing the elimination of the toxin itself, hemodialysis can also be useful to correct severe electrolyte disturbances and acid-base derangements resulting from the ingestion (e.g., metformin-associated lactic acidosis).

Antidotes

Antidotes are available for relatively few toxins (Table 58-11, and see Table 58-8), but early and appropriate use of an antidote is a key element in managing the poisoned patient. Consensus guidelines indicate the important antidotes to stock in facilities that provide emergency care.

SUPPORTIVE CARE

Many poisoned patients arrive to medical care too late for decontamination, having ingested a substance that is neither amenable to enhancing elimination nor a candidate for antidotal therapy. Particularly in these patients, but truly in any poisoned patient, excellent supportive care and frequent clinical assessments are the keys to effective management and improved outcomes. Supportive care entails careful attention to airway support, ventilator management, blood pressure support, and appropriate and timely management of seizures, dysrhythmias, conduction delays, and electrolyte and metabolic derangements. The goal is to support the vital functions of the patient until the patient can eliminate the toxin from the system.

Table 58-11 ADDITIONAL ANTIDOTES

ANTIDOTES	TOXIN OR POISON
Latrodectus antivenin	Black widow spider
Botulin antitoxin	Botulinum toxin
Insulin and glucose	Calcium channel antagonists
Diphenhydramine and/or benztropine	Dystonic reactions
Calcium salts	Fluoride, calcium channel blockers
Protamine	Heparin
Folinic acid	Methotrexate, trimethoprim, pyrimethamine
Crotalidae-specific Fab antibodies	Rattlesnake envenomation
Sodium bicarbonate	Sodium channel blockade (tricyclic antidepressants, type 1 antiarrhythmics)

SELECTED COMPOUNDS COMMONLY INVOLVED IN PEDIATRIC POISONINGS

Herbal medicines (Chapter 59), drugs of abuse (Chapter 108), and environmental health hazards (Chapters 699-706) are covered elsewhere.

Pharmaceuticals

ANALGESICS

Acetaminophen Acetaminophen is the most widely used analgesic and antipyretic in pediatrics, available in multiple formulations, strengths, and combinations. Consequently, acetaminophen is commonly available in the home, where it can be unintentionally ingested by young children, taken in an intentional overdose by adolescents and adults, or inappropriately dosed in all ages. Acetaminophen toxicity remains the most common cause of acute liver failure in the United States.

PATHOPHYSIOLOGY Acetaminophen toxicity results from the formation of a highly reactive intermediate metabolite, *N*-acetyl-*p*-benzoquinone imine (NAPQI). In therapeutic use, only a small percentage of a dose (approximately 5%) is metabolized by the hepatic cytochrome P450 enzyme CYP2E1 to NAPQI, which is then immediately conjugated with glutathione to form a nontoxic mercapturic acid conjugate. In overdose, glutathione stores are overwhelmed, and free NAPQI is able to combine with hepatic macromolecules to produce hepatocellular damage. The single acute toxic dose of acetaminophen is generally considered to be >200 mg/kg in children and >7.5-10 g in adolescents and adults. Repeated administration of acetaminophen at supratherapeutic doses (>75 mg/kg/day for consecutive days) can lead to hepatic injury or failure in some children, especially in the setting of fever, dehydration, poor nutrition, and other conditions that serve to reduce glutathione stores.

Any child with a history of acute ingestion of >200 mg/kg (unusual in children <6 yr old) or with an acute intentional ingestion of any amount should be referred to a health care facility for clinical assessment and measurement of a serum acetaminophen level.

CLINICAL AND LABORATORY MANIFESTATIONS Classically, four stages of acetaminophen toxicity have been described (Table 58-12). The initial signs of acetaminophen toxicity are nonspecific, including nausea and vomiting, and are often followed by an asymptomatic period. Thus, the diagnosis of acetaminophen toxicity cannot be based on clinical symptoms alone, but instead requires consideration of the combination of the patient's history, symptoms, and laboratory findings.

Table 58-12 CLASSIC STAGES IN THE CLINICAL COURSE OF ACETAMINOPHEN TOXICITY

STAGE	TIME AFTER INGESTION	CHARACTERISTICS
I	0.5-24 hr	Anorexia, nausea, vomiting, malaise, pallor, diaphoresis Labs typically normal, except for acetaminophen level
II	24-48 hr	Resolution of earlier symptoms; right upper quadrant abdominal pain and tenderness; elevated bilirubin, prothrombin time, and hepatic enzymes; oliguria
III	72-96 hr	Peak liver function abnormalities; fulminant hepatic failure; multisystem organ failure and potential death
IV	4 days-2 wk	Resolution of liver function abnormalities Clinical recovery precedes histologic recovery

If a toxic ingestion is suspected, a serum acetaminophen level should be measured 4 hr after the reported time of ingestion. For patients who present to medical care >4 hr after ingestion, a stat acetaminophen level should be obtained. **Acetaminophen levels obtained <4 hr after ingestion are difficult to interpret and cannot be used to estimate the potential for toxicity.** Other important baseline labs include hepatic transaminases, renal function tests, and coagulation parameters.

Any patient with a serum acetaminophen level in the possible or probable hepatotoxicity range per the Rumack-Matthew nomogram (see Fig. 58-1) should be treated with *N*-acetylcysteine (NAC). **This nomogram is only intended for use in patients who present within 24 hr of a single acute acetaminophen ingestion with a known time of ingestion.** Patients who have an initially nontoxic level and have ingested combination products or co-ingestants that can slow GI motility (e.g., diphenhydramine, opioids) should have a second acetaminophen level drawn 6-8 hr after ingestion to ensure that ongoing absorption in the setting of poor motility has not caused the acetaminophen level to cross the line into the possible or probable hepatotoxicity range.

Assessment of the patient who presents with an unknown time of ingestion or a history of chronic supratherapeutic ingestion is more complicated. One approach is to check an acetaminophen level, hepatic transaminases, and coagulation parameters. If the acetaminophen level is >10 µg/mL, even with normal liver function tests, this patient is a candidate to be treated with NAC. This practice serves to catch patients in the asymptomatic phase of toxicity, before hepatotoxicity develops, because a level of 10 µg/mL is potentially toxic at ≥20 hr after ingestion. Patients who have any signs of hepatotoxicity (elevated transaminases and international normalized ratio [INR]), even with a low or nondetectable acetaminophen level, are also candidates for antidotal therapy. However, patients who have an acetaminophen level <10 µg/mL and normal transaminases are unlikely to develop significant toxicity. Although this is a conservative approach, the benefits of treating with NAC likely outweigh the risks of treatment or missing potential hepatotoxicity in most of these cases. Consultation with the poison control center (**1-800-222-1222**) or a medical toxicologist is recommended in these difficult cases.

TREATMENT Initial treatment should focus on the ABCs and consideration of decontamination with activated charcoal in patients who present within 1-2 hr of ingestion. The antidote for acetaminophen poisoning is NAC, which works primarily via replenishing hepatic glutathione stores. NAC therapy is most effective when initiated within 8 hr of ingestion, though it has been shown to have benefit even in patients who present in fulminant hepatic failure, likely due to its antioxidant properties. There is no demonstrated benefit to giving NAC before the 4 hr postingestion mark. Thus, patients who present early after ingestion should have a 4 hr level drawn, and decision to initiate NAC should be based on this level. Patients with a history of a potentially toxic ingestion who present >8 hr after ingestion should be given the loading dose of NAC, and decision to continue treatment should be based on the stat acetaminophen level and/or other lab parameters as noted earlier.

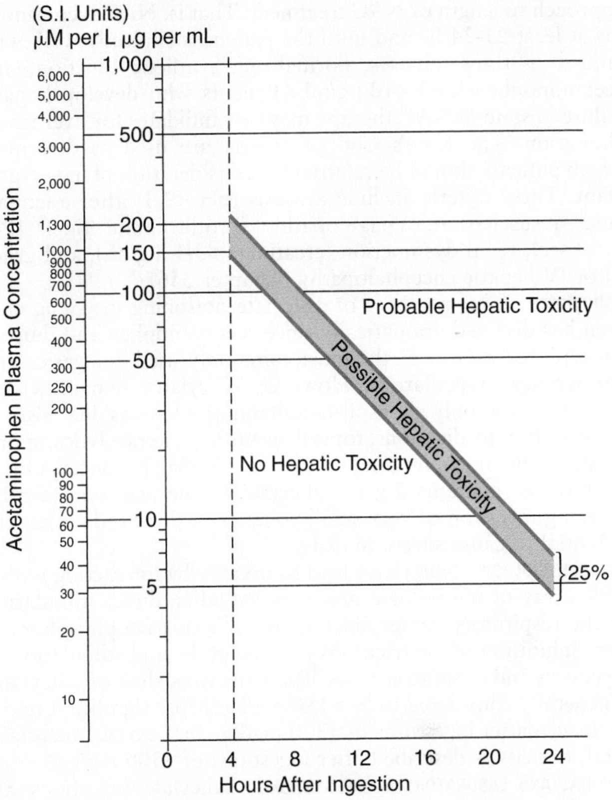

Figure 58-1 Rumack-Matthew nomogram for acetaminophen poisoning, a semilogarithmic plot of plasma acetaminophen concentrations vs time. Cautions for the use of this chart: The time coordinates refer to time after ingestion, serum concentrations obtained before 4 hr are not interpretable, and the graph should be used only in relation to a single acute ingestion with a known time of ingestion. This nomogram is not useful for chronic exposures or unknown time of ingestion and should be used with caution in the setting of co-ingestants that that slow gastrointestinal motility. The *lower solid line* is typically used in the United States to define toxicity and direct treatment, whereas the *upper line* is generally used in Europe. (From Rumack BH, Hess AJ, editors: *Poisindex*, Denver, 1995, Micromedix. Adapted from Rumack BH, Matthew H: Acetaminophen poisoning and toxicity, *Pediatrics* 55:871–876, 1975.)

NAC is available in oral and intravenous forms, and both forms are equally efficacious (see Table 58-8 for the dosing regimens of the oral vs. IV form). The intravenous form is generally preferred, especially in patients with intractable vomiting, those with evidence of hepatic failure, and pregnant patients. NAC has an unpleasant taste and smell, and it should be mixed in soft drink or fruit juice or given via nasogastric tube to improve tolerability of the oral regimen. Administration of IV NAC (as a standard 3% solution to avoid administering excess free water, typically in 5% dextrose), especially the initial loading dose, is associated in some patients with the development of anaphylactoid reactions (non–immunoglobulin E [IgE] mediated). These reactions are typically managed by stopping the infusion; treating with diphenhydramine, albuterol, and/or epinephrine as indicated; and restarting the infusion at a slower rate once symptoms have resolved. IV NAC is also associated with mild elevation in measured INR (1.2-1.5 range).

Transaminases, synthetic function, and renal function should be followed daily while the patient is being treated with NAC. Patients with worsening hepatic function or clinical status might benefit from more frequent lab monitoring. Instead of a standard time course of therapy for all patients with acetaminophen poisoning, current literature suggests a more patient-tailored approach to length of NAC treatment. That is, NAC is continued for at least 21-24 hr and until the patient is clinically well, with improving transaminases, normalizing synthetic function, and acetaminophen level <10 µg/mL. Patients who develop hepatic failure in spite of NAC therapy may be candidates for liver transplantation. The King's College criteria are used to determine which patients should be referred for consideration of liver transplant. These criteria include acidosis (pH <7.3) after adequate fluid resuscitation, coagulopathy (prothrombin time [PT] >100 sec), renal dysfunction (creatinine >3.4 mg/dL), and grade III or IV hepatic encephalopathy (Chapter 356).

Salicylates The incidence of salicylate poisoning in young children has declined dramatically since acetaminophen and ibuprofen replaced aspirin as the most commonly used analgesics and antipyretics in pediatrics. However, salicylates remain widely available, not only in aspirin-containing products but also in antidiarrheal medications, topical agents (e.g., keratolytics, sports creams), oil of wintergreen, and some herbal products. Oil of wintergreen contains 5 g of salicylate in one teaspoon (5 mL), meaning ingestion of very small volumes of this product has the potential to cause severe toxicity.

PATHOPHYSIOLOGY Salicylates lead to toxicity by interacting with a wide array of physiologic processes including direct stimulation of the respiratory center, uncoupling of oxidative phosphorylation, inhibition of the tricarboxylic acid cycle, and stimulation of glycolysis and gluconeogenesis. The acute toxic dose of salicylates is generally considered to be >150 mg/kg. More significant toxicity is seen after ingestions of >300 mg/kg, and severe, potentially fatal, toxicity is described after ingestions of >500 mg/kg.

CLINICAL AND LABORATORY MANIFESTATIONS Salicylate ingestions are classified as acute or chronic, and acute toxicity is far more common in pediatric patients. Early signs of acute salicylism include nausea, vomiting, diaphoresis, and tinnitus. Moderate salicylate toxicity can manifest as tachypnea and hyperpnea, tachycardia, and altered mental status. The tachycardia results in large part from marked insensible losses from vomiting, tachypnea, diaphoresis, and uncoupling of oxidative phosphorylation. Thus, careful attention should be paid to volume status and early volume resuscitation in the significantly poisoned patient. Signs of severe salicylate toxicity include hyperthermia, coma, and seizures. Chronic salicylism can have a more insidious presentation, and patients can show marked toxicity at significantly lower salicylate levels than in acute toxicity.

The classic blood gas of salicylate toxicity reveals a primary respiratory alkalosis and a primary, anion gap, metabolic acidosis. Hyperglycemia (early) and hypoglycemia (late) have been described. Abnormal coagulation studies, clinically manifested as bleeding and easy bruising, may also be seen.

Serial serum salicylate levels should be closely monitored (every 2 hr initially) until they are consistently down trending. **Salicylate absorption in overdose is often unpredictable and erratic, and levels can rapidly increase into the highly toxic range.** The Done nomogram is of poor value and should not be used. Serum and urine pH and electrolytes should be followed closely. An acetaminophen level should be checked in any patient who intentionally overdoses on salicylates, because acetaminophen is a common co-ingestant and because people often confuse or combine their OTC analgesic medications. Salicylate toxicity can cause a noncardiogenic pulmonary edema, especially in chronic overdose; thus a chest x-ray is recommended in any patient with signs and symptoms of pulmonary edema.

TREATMENT For the patient who presents soon after an acute ingestion, initial treatment should include gastric decontamination with activated charcoal. Salicylate pills occasionally form concretions called *bezoars,* which should be suspected if serum salicylate concentrations continue to rise many hours after ingestion or are persistently elevated in spite of appropriate management. Gastric decontamination is typically not useful after chronic exposure.

Initial therapy focuses on aggressive volume resuscitation and prompt initiation of sodium bicarbonate therapy in the symptomatic patient, even before obtaining serum salicylate levels. Therapeutic salicylate levels are 10-20 mg/dL, and levels >30 mg/dL warrant treatment.

The primary mode of therapy for salicylate toxicity is urinary alkalinization. Urinary alkalinization enhances the elimination of salicylates by converting salicylate to its ionized form, "trapping" it in the renal tubules, and thus enhancing elimination. In addition, maintaining an alkalemic serum pH decreases CNS penetration of salicylates because charged particles are less able to cross the blood-brain barrier. Alkalinization is achieved by administration of a sodium bicarbonate infusion at approximately 1.5 times maintenance fluid rates. **The goals of therapy include a urine pH of 7.5-8, a serum pH of 7.45-7.55, and decreasing serum salicylate levels.** Careful attention should be paid to serial potassium levels, because hypokalemia impairs alkalinization of the urine. Multiple doses of charcoal may be beneficial if a salicylate bezoar is suspected.

In cases of severe toxicity, dialysis may be required. Indications for dialysis include serum salicylate concentrations of >90-100 mg/dL in acute ingestions and >60 mg/dL in chronic ingestions, altered mental status, seizures, pulmonary edema, cerebral edema, renal failure, and worsening clinical status in spite of appropriate alkalinization.

Ibuprofen and Other Nonsteroidal Anti-inflammatory Drugs Ibuprofen and other nonsteroidal anti-inflammatory drugs (NSAIDs) are often involved in unintentional and intentional overdoses owing their widespread availability and common use as analgesics and antipyretics. Fortunately, serious effects after NSAID overdose are rare owing to their wide therapeutic index.

PATHOPHYSIOLOGY NSAIDs inhibit prostaglandin synthesis by reversibly inhibiting the activity of cyclo-oxygenase (COX), the primary enzyme responsible for the biosynthesis of prostaglandins. In therapeutic use, side effects include GI irritation, reduced renal blood flow, and platelet dysfunction. In an attempt to minimize these side effects, NSAID analogs have been developed that are more specific for the inducible form of COX (the COX-2 isoform) than the constitutive form, COX-1. However, overdose of the more selective COX-2 inhibitors (e.g., celecoxib [Celebrex]) is treated the same as overdose of nonspecific COX inhibitors (e.g., ibuprofen) because at higher doses, COX-2–selective agents lose their COX inhibitory selectivity.

Ibuprofen, the primary NSAID used in pediatrics, is well tolerated, even in overdose. In children, acute doses of <200 mg/kg rarely cause toxicity, but ingestions of >400 mg/kg can produce more serious effects, including altered mental status and metabolic acidosis.

CLINICAL AND LABORATORY MANIFESTATIONS Symptoms usually develop within 4-6 hr of ingestion and resolve within 24 hr. If toxicity does develop, it is typically manifested as nausea, vomiting, and abdominal pain. Though GI bleeding and ulcers have been described with chronic use, they are rare in the setting of acute ingestion. After massive ingestions, patients can develop marked CNS depression, anion gap metabolic acidosis, renal insufficiency, and (rarely) respiratory depression. Seizures have also been described, especially after overdose of mefenamic acid. Specific drug levels are not readily available nor do they inform management decisions. Renal function studies, acid-base balance, complete blood count, and coagulation parameters should be monitored after very large ingestions. Co-ingestants, especially acetaminophen, should be ruled out after any intentional ingestion.

TREATMENT Meticulous supportive care, including use of antiemetics and acid blockade as indicated, is the primary therapy for NSAID toxicity. Decontamination with activated charcoal should be considered if a patient presents within 1-2 hr of a potentially toxic ingestion. There is no specific antidote for this class of drugs. Given the high degree of protein binding and excretion pattern of NSAIDs, none of the modalities used to enhance elimination are particularly useful in managing these overdoses. Unlike in patients with salicylate toxicity, urinary alkalinization is not helpful for NSAID toxicity. Patients who develop significant clinical signs of toxicity should be admitted to the hospital for ongoing supportive care and monitoring. Patients who remain asymptomatic for 4-6 hr after ingestion may be considered medically cleared.

Oral Opioids Opioids are a commonly abused class of medications (Chapter 108), both in their IV and oral forms. Two specific oral opioids, suboxone and methadone, merit particular mention given their potential for life-threatening toxicity in toddlers with ingestion of even 1 pill. Suboxone, a combination of buprenorphine and naloxone, and methadone are primarily used in managing opioid dependence. However, methadone is also used in the treatment of chronic pain, and both drugs are readily available for illicit purchase and potential abuse. In contrast to methadone in most dependence-treatment programs, suboxone is prescribed in a multiday supply, meaning it is available in homes and particularly susceptible to unintentional ingestion by toddlers.

PATHOPHYSIOLOGY Methadone is a lipophilic synthetic opioid with potent agonist effects at μ-opioid receptors, leading to both its desired analgesic effects and undesired side effects including sedation, respiratory depression, and impaired GI motility. Methadone is thought to cause QTc interval prolongation via interactions with the human ether-a-go-go–related gene (hERG)-encoded potassium rectifier channel. Methadone has an average half-life of >25 hr, which may be extended to >50 hr in overdose.

Suboxone is a combination of buprenorphine, a potent opioid with partial agonism at μ-opioid receptors and weak antagonism at κ-opioid receptors, and naloxone. Naloxone has poor oral bioavailability but is included in the formulation to discourage diversion for intravenous use, during which it precipitates withdrawal. Suboxone is formulated for buccal or sublingual administration; consequently, toddlers can absorb significant amounts of drug even by sucking on a tablet. Buprenorphine has an average half-life of 37 hr.

CLINICAL AND LABORATORY MANIFESTATIONS In children, methadone and suboxone ingestions can manifest with the classic opioid toxidrome of respiratory depression, sedation, and miosis. Signs of more-severe toxicity can include bradycardia, hypotension, and hypothermia. Even in therapeutic use, methadone has been associated with a prolonged QTc interval and risk of torsades de pointes. Accordingly, an ECG should be part of the initial evaluation after ingestion of methadone or any unknown opioid. Neither drug is detected on routine urine opiate screens, though some centers have added a separate urine methadone screen. Levels of both drugs can be measured, though this is rarely done clinically and is seldom helpful in the acute setting. An exception may be in the cases involving concerns about neglect or abuse, at which point urine for gas chromatography/mass spectroscopy (GC/MS), the legal gold standard, should be sent to confirm and document the presence of the drug.

TREATMENT Patients with significant respiratory depression or CNS depression should be treated with the opioid antidote, naloxone (see Table 58-8). In pediatric patients who are not chronically on opioids, the full reversal dose of 0.1 mg/kg (max, 2 mg/dose) should be used. In contrast, opioid-dependent patients should be treated with smaller initial doses (0.01 mg/kg), which can then be repeated as needed to achieve the desired clinical response, hopefully avoiding abrupt induction of withdrawal. Because the half-lives of methadone and suboxone are far longer than that of naloxone, patients can require multiple doses of naloxone. These patients may benefit from a continuous infusion of naloxone, typically started at 2/3 of the reversal dose/hr and titrated to maintain an adequate respiratory rate and level of consciousness. Patients who have ingested methadone should be placed on a cardiac monitor and have serial ECGs to monitor for the development of a prolonged QTc interval. If a patient does develop a prolonged QTc, management includes close cardiac monitoring, repletion of electrolytes (potassium, calcium, and magnesium), and having magnesium readily available should the patient develop torsades de pointes.

Given the potential for clinically significant and prolonged toxicity, any toddler who has ingested methadone, even if asymptomatic, should be admitted to the hospital for at least 24 hr of monitoring. Some experts advocate a similar approach to management of suboxone ingestions, even in the asymptomatic patient. As we gain more experience with pediatric suboxone exposures, some patients who remain absolutely asymptomatic for 6-8 hr after ingestion and *have a stable social setting* may be candidates for earlier discharge. In the meantime, these cases should be discussed with a poison control center or medical toxicologist before determining disposition.

CARDIOVASCULAR MEDICATIONS

β-Adrenergic Receptor Blockers β-Blockers competitively inhibit the action of catecholamines at the β receptor. Therapeutically, β-blockers are used for a variety of conditions, including hypertension, coronary artery disease, tachydysrhythmias, anxiety disorders, migraines, essential tremor, and hyperthyroidism. Because of its lipophilicity and blockade of fast sodium channels, propranolol is considered to be the most toxic member of the β-blocker class. Overdoses of water-soluble β-blockers (e.g., atenolol) are associated with milder symptoms.

PATHOPHYSIOLOGY In overdose, β-blockers decrease chronotropy and inotropy in addition to slowing conduction through AV nodal tissue. Clinically, these effects are manifested as bradycardia, hypotension, and heart block. Patients with reactive airways disease can experience bronchospasm due to blockade of β_2-mediated bronchodilation. β_2-Blockers interfere with glycogenolysis and gluconeogenesis, which can lead to hypoglycemia, especially in patients with poor glycogen stores (e.g., toddlers).

CLINICAL AND LABORATORY MANIFESTATIONS Toxicity typically develops within 6 hr of ingestion, though it may be delayed after ingestion of sotalol or sustained-release preparations. The most common features of severe poisoning are bradycardia and hypotension. Lipophilic agents, including propranolol, can enter the CNS and cause altered mental status, coma, and seizures. Overdose of β-blockers with membrane-stabilizing properties (e.g., propranolol) can cause QRS interval widening and ventricular dysrhythmias.

Evaluation after β-blocker overdose should include an ECG and frequent reassessments of hemodynamic status. Hypoglycemia may be seen, especially in children, and blood glucose should be measured in all patients. Serum levels of β-blockers are not readily available for routine clinical use and are not useful in management of the poisoned patient.

TREATMENT In addition to supportive care and GI decontamination as indicated, glucagon is the antidote of choice for β-blocker toxicity (see Table 58-8). Glucagon stimulates adenyl cyclase and increases levels of cyclic AMP independent of the β receptor. Glucagon is typically given as a bolus and, if this is effective, followed by a continuous infusion. Other potentially useful interventions include atropine, calcium, vasopressors, and high-dose insulin. Seizures are managed with benzodiazepines, and QRS widening should be treated with sodium bicarbonate. Children who ingest 1 or 2 water-soluble β-blockers are unlikely to develop toxicity and can typically be discharged to home if they remain asymptomatic over a 6-hr observation period. Children who ingest sustained-release products, highly lipid soluble agents, and sotalol can require longer periods of observation before safe discharge. Any symptomatic child should be admitted for ongoing monitoring and directed therapy.

Calcium Channel Blockers Calcium channel blockers (CCBs) are used for a variety of therapeutic indications and have the potential to cause severe toxicity, even after exploratory ingestions. Specific agents include nifedipine, diltiazem, verapamil, amlodipine, and felodipine. Of these, diltiazem and verapamil are the most dangerous in overdose.

PATHOPHYSIOLOGY CCBs antagonize L-type calcium channels, inhibiting calcium influx into myocardial and vascular smooth muscle cells. This results in depressed myocardial contractility and conduction as well as peripheral vasodilation, with subsequent development of hypotension and bradydysrhythmias. Though receptor selectivity is often lost in overdose, ingestion of certain CCBs with more peripheral activity (e.g., nifedipine) can result in an initial reflex tachycardia or normal heart rate. Metabolic acidosis develops in the setting of poor perfusion.

CLINICAL AND LABORATORY MANIFESTATIONS The onset of symptoms typically is soon after ingestion, though it may be delayed with ingestions of sustained-release products. Overdoses of CCBs lead to hypotension, accompanied by bradycardia, normal heart rate, or even tachycardia, depending on the agent. One unique characteristic of CCB overdose is that patients can exhibit profound hypotension with preserved consciousness.

Initial evaluation should include an ECG, continuous and careful hemodynamic monitoring, and rapid measurement of serum glucose levels. Both the absolute degree of hyperglycemia and the percentage increase in serum glucose have been correlated with the severity of CCB toxicity in adults. The development of hyperglycemia can even precede the development of hemodynamic instability. Blood levels of CCBs are not readily available and are not useful in guiding therapy.

TREATMENT Once initial supportive care has been instituted, GI decontamination should begin with activated charcoal as appropriate. WBI may be beneficial after ingestion of a sustained-release product. Calcium channel blockade in the smooth muscles of the GI tract can lead to greatly diminished motility; thus, any form of GI decontamination should be undertaken with careful attention to serial abdominal exams. **High-dose insulin therapy is considered the antidote of choice for CCB toxicity.** An initial bolus of 1 U/kg of regular insulin is followed by an infusion at 0.5-1 U/kg/hr (see Table 58-8). Blood glucose levels should be closely monitored, and supplemental glucose may be given to maintain euglycemia, though this is rarely necessary in the severely poisoned patient. Calcium salts are typically administered in an overdose setting, although they might not provide substantial clinical benefit. Additional therapies include IV fluid boluses, vasopressors, and cardiac pacing. In extreme cases, extracorporeal membrane oxygenation (ECMO), cardiac assist devices, and lipid emulsion therapy may be lifesaving. Given the potential for profound and sometimes delayed toxicity in toddlers after ingestion of 1 or 2 CCB tablets, hospital admission and 24 hr of monitoring for all of these patients is strongly recommended.

Clonidine Though originally intended for use as an antihypertensive, clonidine prescriptions in the pediatric population have increased markedly, owing to its reported efficacy in the management of attention-deficit/hyperactivity disorder (ADHD), tic disorders, and other behavioral disorders. With this increased use has come a significant increase in pediatric ingestions and therapeutic misadventures. Clonidine is available in pill and transdermal patch forms.

PATHOPHYSIOLOGY Clonidine is a centrally acting α_2 agonist with a very narrow therapeutic index. Agonism at central α_2 receptors decreases sympathetic outflow, producing lethargy, bradycardia, and hypotension. Toxicity can develop after ingestion of as little as 1 pill or after sucking on or swallowing a discarded transdermal patch.

CLINICAL AND LABORATORY MANIFESTATIONS The most common clinical manifestations of clonidine toxicity include lethargy, miosis, and bradycardia. Hypotension, respiratory depression, and apnea may be seen in severe cases. Very early after ingestion, patients may be hypertensive in the setting of agonism at peripheral α receptors and resulting vasoconstriction. Symptoms develop relatively soon after ingestion and typically resolve within 24 hr. Serum clonidine concentrations are not readily available and are of no clinical value in the acute setting. Though signs of clinical toxicity are common after clonidine overdose, death from clonidine alone is extremely unusual.

TREATMENT Given the potential for significant toxicity, most young children warrant referral to a health care facility for evaluation after unintentional ingestions of clonidine. Gastric decontamination is usually of little value, owing to the small quantities ingested and the rapid onset of serious symptoms. Aggressive supportive care is imperative and is the cornerstone of management. Naloxone, often in high doses, has shown variable efficacy in treating clonidine toxicity. Other potentially useful therapies include atropine, IV fluid boluses, and vasopressors. Symptomatic children should be admitted to the hospital for close cardiovascular and neurologic monitoring.

Digoxin Digoxin is a cardiac glycoside extracted from the leaves of *Digitalis lanata*. Other natural sources of cardiac glycosides include *Digitalis purpura* (foxglove), *Nerium oleander* (oleander), *Convallaria majalis* (lily of the valley), Siberian ginseng, and the *Bufo marinus* toad. Therapeutically, digoxin is used in the management of heart failure and some supraventricular tachydysrhythmias. Acute overdose can occur in the setting of dosing errors (especially in younger children), unintentional or intentional medication ingestion, or exposure to plant material containing digitalis glycosides. Chronic toxicity can result from alteration of the digoxin dose, alteration in digoxin clearance due to renal impairment, or drug interactions.

PATHOPHYSIOLOGY Digoxin blocks the Na^+, K^+-ATPase pump, leading to intracellular loss of K^+ and gain of Na^+ and Ca^{2+}. This resulting rise in Ca^{2+} available to the contractile myocardium improves inotropy. An increase in myocardial automaticity leads to subsequent atrial, nodal, and ventricular ectopy. Digoxin also affects nodal conduction, leading to a prolonged refractory period, decreased sinus node firing, and slowed conduction through the AV node. Impaired Na-K exchange results in dangerously high levels of serum potassium. Overall, digoxin overdose manifests as a combination of slowed or blocked conduction and increased ectopy.

Digoxin has a very narrow therapeutic index. Therapeutic plasma digoxin concentrations are 0.5-2.0 ng/mL; a level of >2 ng/mL is considered toxic and a level of >6 ng/mL is considered potentially fatal. Numerous drug interactions have been shown to affect plasma digoxin concentrations. Medications known to increase serum digoxin concentrations include the macrolides, erythromycin and clarithromycin, spironolactone, verapamil, amidarone, and itraconazole.

CLINICAL AND LABORATORY MANIFESTATIONS Nausea and vomiting are common initial symptoms of acute digoxin toxicity, manifesting within 6 hr of overdose. Cardiovascular manifestations include bradycardia, heart block, and a wide variety of dysrhythmias. CNS manifestations consist of lethargy, confusion, and weakness. Chronic toxicity is more insidious and manifests with GI symptoms, altered mental status, and visual disturbances.

Initial assessment should include an ECG, serum digoxin level, serum potassium, and kidney function tests. The serum digoxin level should be assessed at least 6 hr after ingestion and carefully interpreted in the setting of clinical symptoms because the digoxin level alone does not entirely reflect the severity of intoxication. In acute ingestions, serum potassium is an independent marker of morbidity and mortality, with levels >5.5 mEq/L predicting poor outcomes. In chronic toxicity, serum potassium is less useful as a prognostic marker and may be altered due to concomitant use of diuretics.

TREATMENT Initial treatment includes good general supportive care and gastric decontamination with activated charcoal if the ingestion was recent. An antidote for digoxin, digoxin-specific Fab antibody fragments (Digibind or DigiFab) is available (see Table 58-8). Fab fragments bind free digoxin in both the intravascular and the interstitial spaces to form a pharmacologically inactive complex that is subsequently renally eliminated. Indications for Fab fragments include life-threatening dysrhythmias, K^+ value of >5-5.5 mEq/L in the setting of acute overdose, serum digoxin level of >15 ng/mL at any time or >10 ng/mL 6 hr after ingestion, and ingestion of >4 mg in children or >10 mg in adults. If Digibind or DigiFab are not readily available, phenytoin or lidocaine may be beneficial in managing ventricular irritability. Atropine is potentially useful in managing symptomatic bradycardia. Consultation with a cardiologist is recommended in the management of patients chronically on digoxin, because administration of Fab fragments can lead to recurrence of the patient's underlying dysrhythmias or dysfunction.

IRON Historically, iron was a common cause of childhood poisoning deaths. However, preventive measures such as childproof packaging have significantly decreased the rates of serious iron toxicity in young children. Iron-containing products remain widely available, with the most potentially toxic being adult iron preparations and prenatal vitamins. The severity of an exposure is related to the amount of *elemental iron* ingested. Ferrous sulfate contains 20% elemental iron, ferrous gluconate 12%, and ferrous fumarate 33%. Multivitamin preparations and children's vitamins rarely contain enough elemental iron to cause significant toxicity.

Pathophysiology Iron is directly corrosive to the GI mucosa, leading to hematemesis, melena, ulceration, infarction, and potential perforation. Early iron-induced hypotension is due to massive volume losses, increased permeability of capillary membranes, and venodilation mediated by free iron. Iron accumulates in tissues, including the Kupffer cells of the liver and myocardial cells, leading to hepatotoxicity, coagulopathy, and cardiac dysfunction. Metabolic acidosis develops in the setting of hypotension, hypovolemia, and iron's direct interference with oxidative phosphorylation and the Krebs cycle. Pediatric patients who ingest >40 mg/kg of elemental iron should be referred to medical care for evaluation, though moderate to severe toxicity is typically seen with ingestions of >60 mg/kg.

Clinical and Laboratory Manifestations Iron toxicity is classically described in 4, often overlapping, stages. The initial stage, 30 min to 6 hr after ingestion, consists of profuse vomiting and diarrhea (often bloody), abdominal pain, and significant volume losses leading to potential hypovolemic shock. Patients who do not develop GI symptoms within 6 hr of ingestion are unlikely to develop serious toxicity. The second stage, 6 to 24 hr after ingestion, is the quiescent phase, as GI symptoms typically resolve. However, careful clinical exam can reveal subtle signs of hypoperfusion, including tachycardia, pallor, and fatigue. During the third stage, occurring 12 to 24 hr after ingestion, patients develop multisystem organ failure, shock, hepatic and cardiac dysfunction, acute lung injury or ARDS, and profound metabolic acidosis. Death occurs most commonly during this stage. In patients who survive, the fourth stage (4 to 6 wk after ingestion) is marked by formation of strictures and signs of GI obstruction.

Symptomatic patients and patients with a large exposure by history should have serum iron levels drawn 4-6 hr after ingestion. Serum iron concentrations of <500 µg/dL 4-8 hr after ingestion suggest a low risk of significant toxicity, whereas concentrations of >500 µg/dL indicate that significant toxicity is likely. Additional lab evaluation in the ill patient should include arterial blood gas, complete blood count, serum glucose level, liver function tests, and coagulation parameters. Careful attention should be paid to ongoing monitoring of the patient's hemodynamic status. An abdominal x-ray might reveal the presence of iron tablets, though not all formulations of iron are radiopaque.

Treatment Close clinical monitoring, combined with aggressive supportive and symptomatic care, is essential to the management of iron poisoning. Activated charcoal does not adsorb iron, and WBI remains the decontamination strategy of choice. Deferoxamine, a specific chelator of iron, is the antidote for moderate to severe iron intoxication (see Table 58-8). Indications for deferoxamine treatment include a serum iron concentration of >500 mg/dL or moderate to severe symptoms of toxicity, regardless of serum iron concentration. Deferoxamine is preferably given via continuous IV infusion at a rate of 15 mg/kg/hr. Hypotension is a common side effect of deferoxamine infusion and is managed by slowing the rate of the infusion and administering fluids and/or vasopressors as needed. Prolonged deferoxamine infusion (>24 hr) has been associated with pulmonary toxicity (acute respiratory distress syndrome) and *Yersinia* sepsis. The deferoxamine-iron complex can color the urine reddish ("vin rosé"), though this is an unreliable indicator of iron excretion. Clear endpoints for deferoxamine chelation are not well defined, but therapy is typically continued until clinical symptoms resolve. Consultation with a poison control center or medical toxicologist can yield guidelines for discontinuing deferoxamine.

ORAL HYPOGLYCEMICS Oral medications used in the management of type 2 diabetes include sulfonylureas, biguanides (e.g., metformin), thiazolidinediones, and meglitinides. Of these, only the sulfonylureas and meglitinides have the potential to cause profound hypoglycemia in both diabetic and nondiabetic patients. These classes of medications are widely prescribed and thus readily available for both unintentional and intentional exposures. In toddlers, ingestion of a single sulfonylurea tablet can lead to significant toxicity.

Pathophysiology Sulfonylureas work primarily by enhancing endogenous insulin secretion. In binding to the sulfonylurea receptor, these drugs induce closure of potassium channels, leading to membrane depolarization, opening of calcium channels, and stimulation of calcium-mediated insulin release. Even in therapeutic use, the duration of hypoglycemic action can last up to 24 hr.

Clinical and Laboratory Manifestations Hypoglycemia and symptoms associated with hypoglycemia are the primary clinical manifestations of sulfonylurea toxicity. These signs and symptoms can include diaphoresis, tachycardia, lethargy, irritability, coma, seizures, and even focal neurologic findings. As with other hyperinsulinemic states, sulfonylurea overdoses are associated with a nonketotic hypoglycemia. In the majority of cases, hypoglycemia develops within 6 hr of ingestion but can be delayed up to 16-18 hr after ingestion. Toddlers are particularly susceptible to hypoglycemia during an overnight fast.

Treatment Patients with symptomatic hypoglycemia should be promptly treated with dextrose. In patients with mild symptoms, oral dextrose may be sufficient. However, patients with severe symptoms or profound hypoglycemia should be treated with a bolus of IV dextrose. Continuous dextrose infusions and repeated IV dextrose boluses should be avoided if possible, because this can stimulate further insulin release and lead to recurrent and prolonged hypoglycemia. Instead, the preferred antidote for symptomatic sulfonylurea toxicity is octreotide (see Table 58-8). Octreotide is a somatostain analogue that works via inhibiting insulin release. Octreotide is given IV or SC, typically in doses of 1-2 µg/kg (50-100 µg in adults) every 6-8 hr.

Given the potential for significant hypoglycemia, toddlers with witnessed or suspected sulfonylurea ingestions should be admitted to the hospital for monitoring and serial glucose measurements, at least through an overnight fast. Patients of any age who develop hypoglycemia are also candidates for admission given the prolonged duration of hypoglycemic activity. Prophylactic IV dextrose infusions are not recommended because they can mask the symptoms of toxicity and stimulate further insulin secretion. Patients who require IV dextrose and/or octreotide should be monitored until they can demonstrate euglycemia for at least 8-12 hr off of all therapy.

PSYCHIATRIC MEDICATIONS: ANTIDEPRESSANTS Selective serotonin reuptake inhibitors (SSRIs; e.g., fluoxetine, sertraline, paroxetine, citalopram) are the most commonly prescribed class of antidepressants. This trend results in large part from their wide therapeutic index and more favorable side-effect profile when compared to older agents such as tricylic antidepressants (TCAs; amitriptyline, clomipramine, desipramine, doxepin, nortriptyline, imipramine) and monoamine oxidase inhibitors (MAOIs). Newer agents include the serotonin and norepinephine reuptake inhibitors (SNRIs; e.g., venlafaxine) and other atypical antidepressants (e.g., bupropion).

Tricyclic Antidepressants Though TCAs are now prescribed less commonly for depression, they remain in use for a variety of other conditions, including chronic pain syndromes, enuresis, ADHD, and obsessive compulsive disorder. TCAs can cause significant toxicity in children, even with ingestion of 1 or 2 pills (10-20 mg/kg).

PATHOPHYSIOLOGY TCAs achieve their desired antidepressant effects primarily via blockade of norepinephrine and serotonin reuptake. TCAs have complex interactions with other receptor types. Antagonism at muscarinic acetylcholine receptors leads to clinical features of the anticholinergic toxidrome. Antagonism at peripheral α-receptors leads to hypotension and syncope. Key to the toxicity of TCAs is their ability to block fast sodium channels, leading to impaired cardiac conduction and arrhythmias.

CLINICAL AND LABORATORY MANIFESTATIONS Cardiovascular and CNS symptoms dominate the clinical presentation of TCA toxicity. Symptoms typically develop within 1-2 hr of ingestion, and serious toxicity usually manifests within 6 hr of ingestion. Patients can have an extremely rapid progression from mild symptoms to life-threatening arrhythmias. Patients often develop features of the anticholinergic toxidrome, including delirium, mydriasis, dry mucous membranes, tachycardia, hyperthermia, mild hypertension, urinary retention, and slow GI motility. CNS toxicity can include lethargy, coma, myoclonic jerks, and seizures. Sinus tachycardia is the most common cardiovascular manifestation of toxicity; however, patients can develop widening of the QRS complex, premature ventricular contractions, and ventricular arrhythmias. Refractory hypotension is a poor prognostic indicator and is the most common cause of death in TCA overdose.

An ECG is a readily available bedside test that can help determine the diagnosis and prognosis of the TCA-poisoned patient (see Fig. 58-2). A QRS duration of >100 ms identifies patients who are at risk for seizures and cardiac arrhythmias. An R wave in lead aVR of >3 mm is also an independent predictor of toxicity. Both of these ECG parameters are superior to measured serum TCA concentrations in identifying patients at risk for serious toxicity, and obtaining levels is rarely helpful in management of the acutely ill patient.

TREATMENT Initial attention should be directed to supporting vital functions, including airway and ventilation support as needed. Gastric decontamination can be accomplished with activated charcoal in appropriate patients. Because mental status can deteriorate rapidly, airway protective reflexes must be carefully assessed and the airway must be protected, if necessary, before decontamination. Treating clinicians should obtain an ECG as soon as possible and follow serial ECGs to monitor for progression of toxicity.

Sodium bicarbonate is the antidote of choice for TCA toxicity and works via overcoming the sodium channel blockade by providing a sodium load and via inducing an alkalosis to decrease drug binding to sodium channels. **Indications for sodium bicarbonate include a QRS duration >100 ms, ventricular dysrhythmias, and hypotension.** An initial bolus of 1-2 mEq/kg of sodium bicarbonate is given followed by initiation of a continuous infusion. Additional boluses may be given if the QRS duration continues to widen, with the goals of therapy being a serum pH of 7.45-7.55, improved hemodynamic stability, and narrowing of the QRS complex. Hypertonic (3%) saline, lidocaine, or lipid emulsion therapy may be beneficial in the setting of refractory arrhythmias. Consultation with a poison control center or medical toxicologist is suggested in these cases. Sodium bicarbonate therapy should be continued for at least 12-24 hr after the patient is stabilized because TCAs have the propensity to redistribute from the tissues back into the serum.

Hypotension can require vasopressor therapy, with direct-acting agents such as norepinephrine being the preferred pressors. Physostigmine, once promoted as an "antidote" for TCA toxicity, can cause seizures or dysrhythmias, especially in the setting of impaired cardiac conduction. Thus, physostigmine is currently considered relatively contraindicated in management of TCA ingestions. In the few patients who demonstrate prominent anticholinergic signs without *any* evidence of cardiac conduction abnormalities or seizures, use of physostigmine may be considered in consultation with a medical toxicologist. Seizures are typically brief and can be managed with benzodiazepines.

Asymptomatic children should be observed with continuous cardiac monitoring and serial ECGs for at least 6 hr. If any manifestations of toxicity develop, the child should be admitted to a monitored setting. Children who remain completely asymptomatic with normal serial ECGs may be candidates for discharge after 6 hr of close observation.

Selective Serotonin Reuptake Inhibitors In overdose, SSRIs are considerably less toxic than TCAs. SSRIs are unlikely to cause significant toxicity in exploratory ingestions. Some data suggest that initiating SSRI therapy is associated with an increased risk of suicidal ideation and behavior (Chapter 19).

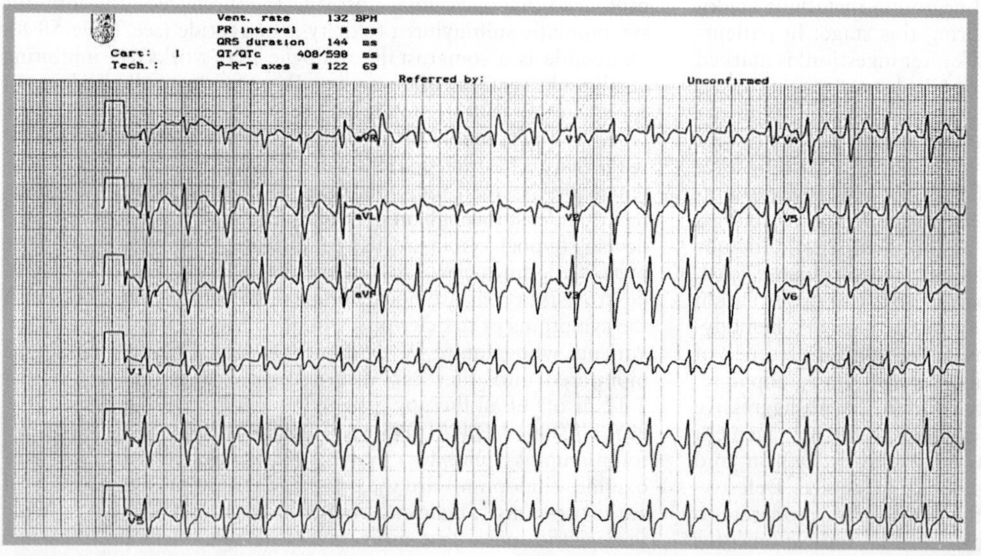

Figure 58-2 Electrocardiographic findings in tricylic antidepressant toxicity. Note the tachycardia, widened QRS interval (144 ms), and prominent R wave in lead aVR. These findings are consistent with blockade of fast sodium channels.

PATHOPHYSIOLOGY SSRIs selectively block the reuptake of serotonin in the CNS. In contrast to TCAs and atypical antidepressants, SSRIs do not directly interact with other receptor types.

CLINICAL AND LABORATORY MANIFESTATIONS In overdose, the principal manifestations of toxicity are sedation and tachycardia. Cardiac conduction abnormalities (primarily QTc prolongation) and seizures have been described in significant overdoses, especially after ingestions of citalopram. An ECG should be part of the initial assessment after SSRI ingestion.

Though development of the serotonin syndrome is seen more often after therapeutic use or overdose of several serotoninergic agents in combination, it has also been described in ingestions of SSRIs alone (Table 58-13). **Clinically, serotonin syndrome is a triad of altered mental status, autonomic instability, and neuromuscular hyperactivity (hyperreflexia, tremors, clonus in the lower extremities more than the upper extremities)** (see Figure 58-3).

Table 58-13 DRUGS ASSOCIATED WITH THE SEROTONIN SYNDROME

DRUG TYPE	DRUGS
Selective serotonin reuptake inhibitors	Sertraline, fluoxetine, fluvoxamine, paroxetine, citalopram
Antidepressant drugs	Trazodone, nefazodone, buspirone, clomipramine, venlafaxine
Monoamine oxidase inhibitors	Phenelzine, moclobemide, clorgyline, isocarboxazid
Anticonvulsants	Valproate
Analgesics	Meperidine, fentanyl, tramadol, pentazocine
Antiemetic agents	Ondansetron, granisetron, metoclopramide
Antimigraine drugs	Sumatriptan
Bariatric medications	Sibutramine
Antibiotics	Linezolid (a monoamine oxidase inhibitor), ritonavir (through inhibition of cytochrome P450 enzyme isoform 3A4)
Over-the-counter cough and cold remedies	Dextromethorphan
Drugs of abuse	Methylenedioxymethamphetamine (MDMA, or "ecstasy"), lysergic acid diethylamide (LSD), 5-methoxydiisopropyltryptamine ("foxy methoxy"), Syrian rue (contains harmine and harmaline, both monoamine oxidase inhibitors)
Dietary supplements and herbal products	Tryptophan, *Hypericum perforatum* (St. John's wort), *Panax ginseng* (ginseng)
Other	Lithium

From Boyer EW, Shannon M: The serotonin syndrome, *N Engl J Med* 352:1112–1120, 2005.

TREATMENT Initial management includes a careful assessment for signs and symptoms of serotonin syndrome and an ECG. Most patients simply require supportive care and observation until their mental status improves and tachycardia, if present, resolves. Management of serotonin syndrome is directed by the severity of symptoms; possible therapeutic interventions include benzodiazepines in mild cases and intubation, sedation, and paralysis in patients with severe manifestations (e.g., significant hyperthermia). Because agonism at the 5-HT_{2A} serotonin receptor is thought to be primarily responsible for the development of serotonin syndrome, use of the $5HT_{2A}$ receptor antagonist cyproheptadine has also been shown to be beneficial. Cyproheptadine is only available in an oral form.

Atypical Antidepressants The class known as atypical antidepressants includes agents such as venlafaxine and duloxetine (SNRIs), bupropion (dopamine, norepinephrine, and some serotonin reuptake blockade), and trazodone (serotonin reuptake blockade and peripheral α-receptor antagonism). The variable receptor affinities of these agents lead to some distinctions in their clinical manifestations and management.

CLINICAL AND LABORATORY MANIFESTATIONS In overdose, venlafaxine and other SNRIs have been associated with cardiac conduction defects, including QRS and QTc prolongation, and seizures. Bupropion is one of the most common etiologies of toxicant-induced seizures in the United States. After ingestion of sustained or extended-release preparations, seizures can occur as late as 18-20 hr after ingestion. In addition, bupropion can cause tachycardia, agitation, and QRS and QTc prolongation. The structure of bupropion contains an amphetamine moiety, which can cause a false-positive result on the urine amphetamine screen. In addition to sedation and signs of serotonin excess, trazodone overdose may be associated with hypotension due to blockade of peripheral α-receptors.

TREATMENT Management is directed to clinical signs and symptoms. QRS interval prolongation may be treated with IV sodium bicarbonate as described in detail earlier. Seizures are often brief and self-limited, but they can be treated with benzodiazepines if necessary. Trazodone-associated hypotension typically responds to fluids, though it can require vasopressors in extreme cases. Because of the potential for delayed seizures, patients who ingest a sustained-release preparation of bupropion should be admitted to a monitored setting for at least 20-24 hr of observation.

Monoamine Oxidase Inhibitors Monoamine oxidase inhibitors are now rarely used therapeutically; however, they remain important

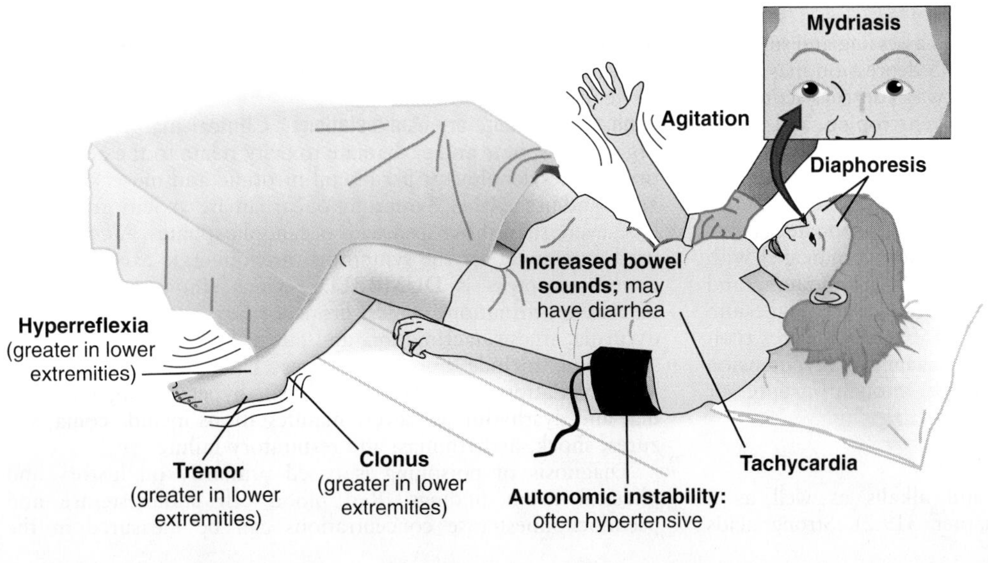

Figure 58-3 Findings in a patient with moderately severe serotonin syndrome. Hyperkinetic neuromuscular findings of tremor or clonus and hyperreflexia should lead the clinician to consider the diagnosis of the serotonin syndrome. (From Boyer EW, Shannon M: The serotonin syndrome, *N Engl J Med* 352:1112–1120, 2005.)

agents to know about given their potential for serious and delayed toxicity. Ingestions of as little as 1 or 2 pills (6 mg/kg) have been associated with toxicity in children. Clinical manifestations initially include hypertension, hyperthermia, tachycardia, muscle rigidity, and seizures followed up to 24 hr later by hemodynamic instability and cardiovascular collapse. **Any child who ingests an MAOI should be admitted to a monitored setting for at least 24 hr, regardless of symptoms.** Management includes blood pressure control, cooling and benzodiazepines for hyperthermia, serial monitoring of creatine kinase and renal function, and fluid and vasopressor therapy for hemodynamic instability.

PSYCHIATRIC MEDICATIONS: ANTIPSYCHOTICS Clinicians are increasingly prescribing antipsychotic medications in the pediatric population. Antipsychotic medications are commonly classified as either typical or atypical. In general, typical agents are associated with more side effects and toxicity than the atypical agents.

Pathophysiology Typical or traditional antipsychotics (i.e. haloperidol, thioridazine, chlorpromazine, and fluphenazine) are characterized by their antagonism at D_2 dopamine receptors. In therapeutic use, these agents are associated with extrapyramidal symptoms, tardive dyskinesia, and development of the neuroleptic malignant syndrome (NMS). The atypical agents (i.e. aripiprazole, clozapine, quetiapine, risperidone, ziprasidone) were developed with less dopamine (D_2-receptor) antagonism in efforts to avoid these side effects and improve their efficacy in managing the "negative" symptoms of schizophrenia. Instead, these agents have complex and varied interactions with multiple receptor types, including α-receptors, serotonin receptors, muscarinic acetylcholine receptors, and histamine receptors.

Clinical and Laboratory Manifestations Typical antipsychotic toxicity commonly includes sedation, tachycardia, and prolongation of the QTc interval. Patients can present with acute dystonia, akathisia, and NMS, though these are seen less commonly in acute overdoses than in therapeutic use. The phenothiazines (e.g., thioridazine) can cause widening of the QRS interval owing to blockade of fast sodium channels.

Though the presentation of atypical antipsychotic toxicity can vary based on the receptor affinities of the specific agent, sedation, tachycardia, and QTc prolongation are common. Overdose of agents with muscarinic receptor activity leads to features of the anticholinergic toxidrome (see Table 58-4). Peripheral α-receptor blockade (e.g., with quetiapine) is associated with hypotension. In therapeutic use, clozapine is associated with agraulocytosis.

Diagnostic testing should include an ECG. Patients with hyperthermia or muscle rigidity should have a serum creatine kinase level sent to monitor for possible rhabodomyolysis. Antipsychotic levels are not readily available and are not helpful in managing acute poisoning.

Management Initial management involves assessing and supporting vital functions. In some patients, CNS depression may be so profound as to require intubation for airway control. Acute dystonia is treated with diphenhydramine, benztropine, and sometimes benzodiazepines. Management of NMS includes conscientious supportive care, IV fluids, cooling, benzodiazepines, and bromocriptine or dantrolene in severe cases. QRS prolongation is managed with IV sodium bicarbonate as discussed in the TCA section. QTc prolongation is managed with repletion of electrolytes (especially calcium, magnesium, and potassium), continuous cardiac monitoring, and IV magnesium sulfate if the patient develops torsades de pointes. Seizures typically are well controlled with benzodiazepines. Hypotension usually responds to boluses of IV fluids, though vasopressor therapy is necessary in some cases.

Household Products

CAUSTICS Caustics include acids and alkalis as well as a few common oxidizing agents (Chapter 319.2). Strong acids and alkalis can produce severe injury even in small-volume ingestions.

Pathophysiology Alkalis produce a liquefaction necrosis, allowing further tissue penetration of the toxin and setting the stage for possible perforation. Acids produce a coagulative necrosis, which limits further tissue penetration, though perforation can still occur. The severity of the corrosive injury depends on the pH and concentration of the product as well as the length of contact time with the product. Agents with a pH of <2 or >12 are most likely to produce significant injury.

Clinical Manifestations Ingestion of caustic materials can produce injury to the oral mucosa, esophagus, and stomach. Patients can have significant esophageal injury even in the absence of visible oral burns. Symptoms include pain, drooling, vomiting, abdominal pain, and difficulty swallowing or refusal to swallow. Laryngeal injury can manifest as stridor and respiratory distress, necessitating intubation. In the most severe cases, patients can present in shock after perforation of a hollow viscus. Circumferential burns of the esophagus are likely to cause strictures when they heal, which can require repeated dilation or surgical correction and long-term follow-up for neoplastic changes in adulthood (Chapter 319.2). Caustics on the skin or in the eye can cause significant tissue damage.

Treatment Initial treatment of caustic exposures includes thorough removal of the product from the skin or eye by flushing with water. Emesis and lavage are contraindicated. Activated charcoal should not be used because it does not bind these agents and can predispose the patient to vomiting and subsequent aspiration. Endoscopy should be performed within 12-24 hr of ingestion in symptomatic patients or those in whom injury is suspected on the basis of history and known characteristics of the ingested product. The use of corticosteroids is not beneficial in managing grade I and grade III injuries, and it is controversial in the management of grade II injuries. Prophylactic antibiotics do not improve outcomes.

CHOLINESTERASE-INHIBITING INSECTICIDES The most commonly used insecticides are organophosphates and carbamates; both are inhibitors of cholinesterase enzymes (acetylcholinesterase, pseudocholinesterase, and erythrocyte acetylcholinesterase). Most pediatric poisonings occur as the result of unintentional exposure to insecticides in and around the home or farm.

Pathophysiology Organophosphates and carbamates produce toxicity by binding to and inhibiting acetylcholinesterase, preventing the degradation of acetylcholine and resulting in its accumulation at nerve synapses. If left untreated, organophosphates form an irreversible bond to acetylcholinesterase, permanently inactivating the enzyme. This process, called *aging*, occurs over a variable time period depending on the characteristics of the specific organophosphate. Afterwards, a period of weeks to months is required to regenerate inactivated enzymes. In contrast, carbamates form a temporary bond to the enzymes, typically allowing reactivation of acetylcholinesterase within 24 hr.

Clinical and Laboratory Manifestations Clinical manifestations of organophosphate and carbamate toxicity relate to the accumulation of acetylcholine at peripheral nicotinic and muscarinic synapses and in the CNS. Symptoms of carbamate toxicity are usually less severe than those seen with organophosphates. A commonly used mnemonic for the symptoms of cholinergic excess at muscarinic receptors is **DUMBBELS**, which stands for *d*iarrhea/defecation, *u*rination, *m*iosis, *b*ronchorrhea/*b*ronchospasm, *b*radycardia, *e*mesis, *l*acrimation, and *s*alivation. Nicotinic signs and symptoms include muscle weakness, fasciculations, tremors, hypoventilation (diaphragm paralysis), hypertension, tachycardia, and dysrhythmias. Severe manifestations include coma, seizures, shock, arrhythmias, and respiratory failure.

Diagnosis of poisoning is based primarily on history and physical exam findings. Red blood cell cholinesterase and pseudocholinesterase concentrations can be measured in the laboratory. These may be useful in documenting an exposure, but they are not reported in time to direct management and they do not correlate well with the magnitude of acute exposure or symptoms.

Treatment Basic decontamination should be performed, including washing all exposed skin with soap and water and immediately removing all exposed clothing. Administering activated charcoal after ingestion of insecticides is controversial, with recent literature suggesting its value is limited, at least in rural Asian-Pacific settings. Basic supportive care should be provided, including fluid and electrolyte replacement and intubation and ventilation if necessary.

Two antidotes are useful in treating cholinesterase inhibitor poisoning: atropine and pralidoxime (see Table 58-8). Atropine, which antagonizes the muscarinic acetylcholine receptor, is useful for both organophosphate and carbamate intoxication. Often, large doses of atropine must be administered by intermittent bolus or via continuous infusion to control symptoms. Atropine dosing is primarily targeted to resolving respiratory secretions and bronchospasm. Heart rate is not an appropriate endpoint because tachycardia can result from nicotinic effects. Pralidoxime breaks the bond between the organophosphate and the enzyme, reactivating acetylcholinesterase. Pralidoxime is only effective if it is used before the bond ages and becomes permanent. Pralidoxime is not necessary for carbamate poisonings because the bond between the insecticide and the enzyme degrades spontaneously.

Without treatment, symptoms of organophosphate poisoning can persist for weeks, requiring continuous supportive care. Even with treatment, some patients develop a delayed polyneuropathy and a range of chronic neuropsychiatric symptoms.

HYDROCARBONS Hydrocarbons include a wide array of chemical substances found in thousands of commercial products. Specific characteristics of each product determine whether exposure will produce systemic toxicity, local toxicity, both, or neither. Nevertheless, aspiration of even small amounts of certain hydrocarbons can lead to serious, potentially life-threatening toxicity.

Pathophysiology The most important manifestation of hydrocarbon toxicity is aspiration pneumonitis via inactivation of the type II pneumocytes and resulting surfactant deficiency (Chapter 389). Aspiration usually occurs during coughing and gagging at the time of ingestion or vomiting after the ingestion. The propensity of a hydrocarbon to cause aspiration pneumonitis is inversely proportional to its viscosity. Compounds with low viscosity, such as mineral spirits, naphtha, kerosene, gasoline, and lamp oil, spread rapidly across surfaces and cover large areas of the lungs when aspirated. Only small quantities (<1 mL) of low-viscosity hydrocarbons need be aspirated to produce significant injury. Pneumonitis does not result from dermal absorption of hydrocarbons or from ingestion in the absence of aspiration. Gasoline and kerosene are poorly absorbed, but they often cause considerable irritation of the GI mucosa as they pass through the intestines.

Certain hydrocarbons have unique toxicities and can cause symptoms after ingestion, inhalation, or dermal exposures. Several chlorinated solvents, most notably **carbon tetrachloride**, can produce hepatic toxicity. **Methylene chloride**, found in some paint removers, is metabolized to carbon monoxide. Benzene is known to cause cancer, most commonly acute myelogenous leukemia, after long-term exposure. Nitrobenzene, aniline, and related compounds can produce methemoglobinemia. Methemoglobinemia is suggested by the classic "chocolate brown" blood and confirmed via co-oximetry. Methemoglobinemia is treated with methylene blue (see Table 58-8).

A number of volatile hydrocarbons, including toluene, propellants, refrigerants, and volatile nitrites, are commonly **abused** by inhalation. Some of these substances, principally the halogenated hydrocarbons (which contain a chlorine, bromine, or fluorine), can sensitize the myocardium to the effects of endogenous catecholamines. This can result in dysrhythmias and "sudden sniffing death." Chronic abuse of these agents can lead to cerebral atrophy, neuropsychological changes, peripheral neuropathy, and kidney disease (Chapter 108.4).

Clinical and Laboratory Manifestations Transient, mild CNS depression is common after hydrocarbon ingestion or inhalation. Aspiration is characterized by coughing, which usually is the first clinical finding. Chest radiographs may initially be normal, but they often show abnormalities within 6 hr of exposure in patients who have aspirated. Respiratory symptoms can remain mild or progress rapidly to the acute respiratory distress syndrome (ARDS) and respiratory failure. Fever and leukocytosis are common accompanying signs in patients with pneumonitis and don't necessarily imply bacterial superinfection. Chest radiographs can remain abnormal long after the patient is clinically normal. Pneumatoceles can appear on the chest radiograph 2-3 wk after exposure.

After inhalational exposures to halogenated hydrocarbons, patients can present with ventricular dysrhythmias, often refractory to conventional management.

Treatment Emesis and lavage are contraindicated given the risk of aspiration. Activated charcoal is not useful because it does not bind the common hydrocarbons and can also induce vomiting. If hydrocarbon-induced pneumonitis develops, respiratory treatment is supportive (Chapter 389). Neither corticosteroids nor prophylactic antibiotics have shown any clear benefit. Standard mechanical ventilation, high-frequency ventilation, and ECMO have all been used to manage the respiratory failure and ARDS associated with severe hydrocarbon-induced pneumonitis.

Patients with dysrhythmias in the setting of halogenated hydrocarbon inhalation should be treated with β-blockers (usually esmolol) to block the effects of endogenous catecholamines on the sensitized myocardium.

TOXIC ALCOHOLS **Methanol** is commonly found in windshield washer fluids, de-icers, paint removers, fuel additives, liquid fuel canisters, and industrial solvents. **Ethylene glycol** is commonly found in antifreeze. Unintentional ingestion is the most common exposure in children, and small-volume ingestions of concentrated products have the potential for severe toxicity. The pathophysiology, acid-base derangements, and treatment of both chemicals are similar, though they differ in their primary end-organ toxicity. In both cases, the metabolites of the parent compounds are responsible for the serious clinical effects that can follow exposure.

Isopropyl alcohol (rubbing alcohol, hand sanitizers) causes intoxication similar to that associated with ethanol but can also cause a hemorrhagic gastritis and myocardial depression in massive ingestions. Unlike ethylene glycol and methanol, isopropyl alcohol is metabolized to a ketone and does not cause a metabolic acidosis. Management is similar to that of ethanol ingestions (Chapter 108.1) and is not further discussed here.

Methanol

PATHOPHYSIOLOGY Methanol is metabolized in the liver by alcohol dehydrogenase to formaldehyde, which is further metabolized to formic acid by aldehyde dehydrogenase. Toxicity is caused primarily by formic acid, which inhibits mitochondrial respiration.

CLINICAL AND LABORATORY MANIFESTATIONS Drowsiness, mild inebriation, nausea, and vomiting develop early after ingestion. The onset of serious effects, including profound metabolic acidosis and visual disturbances, is often delayed for up to 12-24 hr as the parent methanol is undergoing metabolism to its toxic metabolites. Visual disturbances include blurred or cloudy vision, constricted visual fields, decreased acuity, and the "feeling of being in a snowstorm." These visual defects may be reversible if treated early, but untreated they can lead to permanent blindness. On exam, dilated pupils, retinal edema, and optic disc hyperemia may be noted. Initially, patients have an elevated osmolar gap and then develop an anion gap metabolic acidosis as the parent compound is metabolized to formic acid.

In young children, determining if a significant exposure has occurred is usually difficult based on history. Methanol blood levels are available at some laboratories and should be sent after a concerning exposure. If methanol blood levels are not readily available, estimation of an osmolar gap may be used as a surrogate marker. Serum osmolarity is measured by the freezing point depression method and compared with a calculated serum osmolarity. The osmolar gap can be used to estimate the serum methanol concentration using the following formula:

$$\text{Osmolar gap} \times 3.2 = \text{estimated methanol blood concentration (mg/dL)}$$

TREATMENT Treatment is as discussed ethylene glycol toxicity.

Ethylene Glycol

PATHOPHYSIOLOGY Ethylene glycol is metabolized by alcohol dehydrogenase in the liver to glycoaldehyde, which is further converted to glycolic acid by aldehyde dehydrogenase. Glycolic acid is metabolized to glyoxylic acid and oxalic acid, which are responsible for most of the observed toxicity. Oxalic acid combines with serum and tissue calcium, causing hypocalcemia and the formation of calcium oxalate crystals.

CLINICAL AND LABORATORY MANIFESTATIONS Early symptoms include nausea, vomiting, CNS depression, and inebriation. Delayed manifestations include an anion gap metabolic acidosis, hypocalcemia, and kidney failure (secondary to deposition of calcium oxalate crystals in the renal tubules). Even later, patients can develop cranial nerve palsies.

Ethylene glycol blood concentrations are available at some laboratories. In the absence of readily available ethylene glycol concentrations, calculation of the osmolar gap may be used as a surrogate marker. Serum osmolarity is measured by the freezing point depression method and compared with a calculated serum osmolarity. The osmolar gap can be used to estimate the serum ethylene glycol concentration using the following formula:

$$\text{Osmolar gap} \times 6.2 = \text{estimated ethylene glycol concentration (mg/dL)}$$

Examination of the urine with a Wood lamp is neither sensitive nor specific for ethylene glycol ingestion. Calcium oxalate crystals can be seen on urine microscopy but might not be evident early after exposure. Electrolytes (including calcium), acid-base status, kidney function, and ECG should be closely monitored in poisoned patients.

TREATMENT Because methanol and ethylene glycol are rapidly absorbed, gastric decontamination is generally not of value. The classic antidote for methanol and ethylene glycol poisoning was ethanol, a preferential substrate for alcohol dehydrogenase, thus preventing the metabolism of parent compounds to toxic metabolites. **Fomepizole** (see Table 58-8), a potent competitive inhibitor of alcohol dehydrogenase, has almost entirely replaced the use of ethanol owing to its ease of administration, lack of CNS and metabolic effects, and overall excellent patient tolerability profile. Indications for fomepizole include ethylene glycol or methanol level >20 mg/dL, history of potentially toxic ingestion and an elevated osmolar gap, or history of ingestion with evidence of acidosis. There are few disadvantages to giving the initial dose of fomepizole to patients with a concerning history of ingestion or lab findings, and given the dosing schedule of fomepizole (every 12 hr), this strategy buys the clinician time to confirm or exclude the diagnosis before giving a second dose. Adjunctive therapy includes folate (methanol toxicity) and pyridoxine (ethylene glycol toxicity).

Hemodialysis effectively removes ethylene glycol, methanol, and their metabolites and corrects acid-base and electrolyte disturbances. Dialysis also removes fomepizole, so dosing should be changed to every 4 hr during dialysis. Indications for dialysis include a methanol level of >50 mg/dL, acidosis, severe electrolyte disturbances, and renal failure. However, in the absence of acidosis and kidney failure, even massive ethylene glycol ingestions have been managed without dialysis. Methanol is another story, because its elimination in the setting of alcohol dehydrogenase inhibition is very prolonged, thus often warranting dialysis to remove the parent compound. Therapy (fomepizole and/or dialysis) should be continued until ethylene glycol and methanol levels are <20 mg/dL. Consultation with a poison control center, medical toxicologist, and nephrologist may be helpful in managing toxic alcohol ingestions.

Plants

Exposure to plants, both inside the home and outside in backyards and fields, is one of the most common causes of unintentional poisoning in children. Fortunately, the majority of ingestions of plant parts (leaves, seeds, flowers) result in either no toxicity or mild, self-limiting effects (Table 58-14). However, ingestion of certain plants (Table 58-15) outlines some of the most toxic plants) can lead to serious toxicity.

The potential toxicity of a particular plant is highly variable, depending on the part of the plant involved (flowers are generally less toxic than the root or seed), the time of year, growing conditions, and the route of exposure. Assessment of the potential severity after an exposure is also complicated by the difficulty in properly identifying the plant. Many plants are known by several common names, which can vary among communities. Poison control centers have access to professionals who can assist in properly identifying plants. They also are well versed in the

Table 58-14 NONTOXIC AND MINIMALLY TOXIC PLANTS*
African violet
Aluminum plant
Aralia, false
Aster
Begonia species
Boston fern
Carnation
Chinese evergreen
Christmas cactus
Coleus
Corn plant
Dandelion
Daylily
Dogwood
Dracaena
Fern species (not asparagus fern)
Fig
Gardenia
Geranium
Hen and chicks
Honeysuckle
Impatiens
Jade plant
Kalanchoe
Magnolia
Marigold
Nasturtium
Norfolk Island pine
Palm
Peperomia
Petunia
Poinsettia
Pyracantha
Rose
Rubber plant
Schefflera
Snake plant
Spider plant
Violet
Wandering Jew
Yucca

*The potential for toxicity depends on the magnitude and amount of exposure. These agents are considered nontoxic or minimally toxic for mild to moderate exposure. The potential for toxicity increases with increased amount of exposure. Many plants contain substances that can be irritating to the mucosa (dermal/oroesophageal) and/or can precipitate allergic responses.

Table 58-15 COMMONLY INGESTED PLANTS WITH SIGNIFICANT TOXIC POTENTIAL

PLANT	SYMPTOMS	MANAGEMENT
Autumn crocus *(Colchicum autumnlae)*	Vomiting Diarrhea Initial leukocytosis followed by bone marrow failure Multisystem organ failure	Activated charcoal decontamination Aggressive fluid resuscitation and supportive care
Belladonna alkaloids: jimson weed *(Datura stramonium)* Belladonna ("deadly nightshade"; *Atropa belladonna*)	Anticholinergic toxidrome Seizures	Supportive care, benzodiazepines Consider physostigmine if pt is a threat to self or others; only use if no conduction delays on ECG
Cardiac glycoside–containing plants (foxglove, lily of the valley, oleander, yellow oleander, etc)	Nausea Vomiting Bradycardia Dysrhythmias (AV block, ventricular ectopy) Hyperkalemia	Digoxin-specific Fab fragments
Jequirity bean and other abrin-containing species (e.g., rosary pea, precatory bean)	Oral pain Vomiting Diarrhea Shock Hemolysis Renal failure	Supportive care, including aggressive volume resuscitation and correction of electrolyte abnormalities
Monkshood (*Aconitum* species)	Numbness and tingling of lips/tongue Vomiting Bradycardia	Atropine for bradycardia Supportive care
Oxalate-containing plants: *Philodendron, Diffenbachia, Colocasia* ("elephant ear")	Local tissue injury Oral pain Vomiting	Supportive care, pain control
Poison hemlock *(Conium maculatum)*	Vomiting Agitation followed by CNS depression Paralysis Respiratory failure	Supportive care
Pokeweed	Hemorrhagic gastroenteritis Burning of mouth and throat	Supportive care
Rhododendron	Vomiting Diarrhea Bradycardia	Atropine for symptomatic bradycardia Supportive care
Tobacco	Vomiting Agitation Diaphoresis Fasciculations Seizures	Supportive care
Water hemlock (*Cicuta* species)	Abdominal pain Vomiting Delirium Seizures	Supportive care, including benzodiazepines for seizures
Yew (*Taxus*` species)	GI symptoms QRS widening Hypotension CV collapse	Supportive care Atropine for bradycardia Sodium bicarbonate does not appear to be effective

pt, patient; ECG, electrocardiogram; AV, atrioventricular; Fab, fragment, antigen binding; CNS, central nervous system; GI, gastrointestinal; CV, cardiovascular.

common poisonous plants in their service area and the seasons when they are more abundant. For these reasons, consultation with the local poison control center may be very helpful in the management of these ingestions.

For potentially toxic plant ingestions, consider decontamination with activated charcoal in patients who present within 1-2 hr of ingestion; otherwise, treatment is primarily supportive and symptomatic. The most common manifestation of toxicity after plant ingestion is GI upset, which can be managed with antiemetics and fluid and electrolyte support. Management strategies for a few specific toxicities are outlined in Table 58-15.

Toxic Gases

CARBON MONOXIDE Although many industrial and naturally occurring gases pose a health risk by inhalation, the most common gas involved in pediatric exposures is carbon monoxide (CO). In recent years, CO released from malfunctioning and improperly used portable generators has been implicated in hurricane-related visits to hospitals and emergency facilities, hospitalizations, and deaths, many of them involving children. CO is a colorless, odorless gas produced during the combustion of any carbon-containing fuel. The less efficient the combustion, the greater the amount of CO produced. Wood-burning stoves, old furnaces, and automobiles are a few of the potential sources of CO.

Pathophysiology CO binds to hemoglobin with an affinity >200 times that of oxygen, forming carboxyhemoglobin (COHb). In doing so, CO displaces oxygen and creates a conformational change in hemoglobin that impairs the delivery of oxygen to the tissues, leading to tissue hypoxia. COHb levels are not well correlated with clinical signs of toxicity, likely because CO interacts with multiple proteins in addition to hemoglobin. CO binds to cytochrome oxidase, disrupting cellular respiration. CO displaces nitric oxide (NO) from proteins, allowing NO to bind with free radicals to form the toxic metabolite peroxynitrate. NO is also a potent vasodilator, in part responsible for clinical symptoms including headache, syncope, and hypotension.

Clinical and Laboratory Manifestations Early symptoms are nonspecific and include headache, malaise, nausea, and vomiting. These symptoms are often misdiagnosed as indicating flu or food poisoning. At higher exposure levels, patients can develop mental status changes, confusion, ataxia, syncope, tachycardia, and tachypnea. Severe poisoning is manifested by coma, seizures, myocardial ischemia, acidosis, cardiovascular collapse, and potentially death. On exam, patients might have cherry-red skin. ED evaluation should include a COHb level in all symptomatic patients, arterial blood gas and creatine kinase in severely poisoned patients, and an ECG in any patient with cardiac symptoms.

Treatment In addition to general supportive care, treatment requires the administration of 100% oxygen to enhance elimination of CO. In ambient air, the average half-life of COHb is 4-6 hr. This is dramatically reduced to 60-90 min by providing 100% oxygen at normal atmospheric pressures via a nonrebreather facemask. Severely poisoned patients might benefit from **hyperbaric oxygen (HBO)**, which decreases the half-life of COHb to 20-30 minutes. Though the clinical benefits and referral guidelines for HBO therapy remain controversial, commonly cited indications include syncope, coma, seizure, altered mental status, COHb level >25%, abnormal cerebellar examination, and pregnancy. Consultation with a poison control center, medical toxicologist, or hyperbaric oxygen facility can assist clinicians in determining which patients could benefit from HBO therapy. Sequelae of CO poisoning include persistent and delayed cognitive effects. Prevention of CO poisoning should involve educational initiatives and the use of home CO detectors.

HYDROGEN CYANIDE

Pathophysiology Cyanide inhibits cytochrome oxidase, part of the electron transport chain, interrupting cellular respiration and leading to profound tissue hypoxia. Patients may be exposed to hydrogen cyanide gas in the workplace (manufacturing of synthetic fibers, nitriles, and plastics) or via smoke inhalation in a fire.

Clinical and Laboratory Manifestations Onset of symptoms is rapid after a significant exposure. Clinical manifestations of toxicity include headache, agitation and confusion, sudden loss of consciousness or "knock-down," tachycardia, cardiac dysrhythmias, and metabolic acidosis. Cyanide levels can be measured in whole blood, but they are not readily available at most institutions and thus are not useful in emergent management of the poisoned patient. A severe lactic acidosis (lactate >10 mmol/L) in fire victims suggests cyanide toxicity. Impaired oxygen extraction by tissues is implied by elevated mixed venous oxygen saturation, another laboratory finding suggesting cyanide toxicity.

Treatment Treatment includes removal from the source of exposure, rapid administration of high concentrations of oxygen, and antidotal therapy. The cyanide antidote kit includes nitrites (amyl nitrite and sodium nitrite) used to produce methemoglobin, which then reacts with cyanide to form cyanmethemoglobin (see Table 58-8). The third part of the kit is sodium thiosulfate, given to hasten the metabolism of cyanmethemoglobin to hemoglobin and the less-toxic thiocyanate. In patients for whom induction of methemoglobinemia could produce more risk than benefit, the sodium thiosulfate component of the kit may be given alone. **In 2006, the FDA approved hydroxocobalamin (a form of vitamin B_{12}) for use in known or suspected cyanide poisoning.** This antidote, used for many years in Europe, reacts with cyanide to form the nontoxic cyanocobalamin, which is then excreted in urine. Side effects of hydroxocobalamin include red discoloration of the skin and urine, transient hypertension, and interference with colorimetric lab assays. *Overall, the safety profile of hydoxocobalamin appears superior to that of the cyanide antidote kit; thus this is becoming the preferred antidote for cyanide poisoning.*

BIBLIOGRAPHY

Please visit the Nelson Textbook of Pediatrics *website at www.expertconsult.com for the complete bibliography.*

Chapter 59
Herbs, Complementary Therapies, and Integrative Medicine

Paula Gardiner and Kathi J. Kemper

Integrative medicine focuses on promoting health to achieve physical, mental, emotional, spiritual, and social well-being in the context of a medical home in a healthy community. The foundations of integrative medicine are health-promoting practices including optimal nutrition, dietary supplements to avoid deficiencies, physical activity, adequate sleep, a healthy environment, stress management, and supportive social relationships. Other complementary therapies recommended by some integrative practitioners include herbal remedies, massage and other forms of bodywork, and acupuncture. Although prayer, healing touch, and healing rituals are sometimes included under the rubric of complementary and integrative therapies, they are not covered in this chapter.

DIETARY SUPPLEMENTS

Herbs and other dietary supplements are the most commonly used complementary therapies for children and adolescents. The U.S. Food and Drug Administration (FDA) defines dietary supplements as oral preparations that may include vitamins, minerals, single or multiple herbal ingredients, amino acids, essential fatty acids, hormones (such as melatonin and DHEA), and probiotics. More than $4 billion are spent on these products each year in the USA. Some uses are common and recommended, such as vitamin D supplements for breast-fed infants, whereas other uses are more controversial, such as using echinacea to treat upper respiratory infections. Use of dietary supplements is most common among children whose families have higher income and education and whose parents use them, and among older children and those suffering from chronic, incurable, or recurrent conditions. Less than 50% of patients who use supplements talk with their physician about their use. Even when asked directly, some patients deny using herbs (such as coffee, cranberry, protein powders, probiotics, or fish oil) because they do not consider their use to be medicinal and they consider them to be safe because they are "natural." To elicit a complete history, clinicians need to ask patients routinely about and provide examples of dietary supplements.

Although they are generally safe, natural products can cause serious toxicity (Tables 59-1 to 59-5). For example, acute hepatic toxicity and death can result from ingestion of even small amounts of *Amanita* mushrooms. Ephedra, also known as ma huang, is banned as a weight loss or sports supplement in the United States because of its toxicity. Even when a product is safe when used correctly, it can cause mild or severe toxicity when used incorrectly. For example, although peppermint is a commonly used and usually benign gastrointestinal spasmolytic included in after-dinner mints, it can exacerbate gastroesophageal reflux. Probiotics are generally safe when taken orally, but in an immune-compromised patient in an ICU setting, they can cause sepsis. Excessive vitamin C or magnesium can cause diarrhea.

Product labels might not accurately reflect the contents or the concentrations of ingredients. Because of natural variability, variations of 10- to 1,000-fold have been reported for several popular herbs, even across lots produced by the same manufacturer. Herbal products may be unintentionally contaminated with pesticides, animal wastes, or the wrong herb that was misidentified during harvesting. Some DHEA supplements have been found to contain banned stimulants and steroids. Products from developing countries (e.g., ayurvedic products from South

Table 59-1 POSSIBLE HERBS FOR ASTHMA

HERB OR COMBINATION	RCTs	DEMONSTRATED BENEFIT	ADVERSE EFFECTS AND DRUG INTERACTIONS	PURPORTED MECHANISM
Coffee, tea	None recently in children	Epidemiologic data suggest fewer symptoms in coffee drinkers	Tachycardia, insomnia, jitteriness, decreased appetite; potential interaction with β-agonists	Methylxanthines Increased intracellular cAMP Bronchodilator
Shinpi-to	None in children	Yes, in historical data	Unknown; potential interaction with leukotriene blockers	Blocks 5-lipo- oxygenase and phospholipase A_2
Saiboku-to	Yes, in adults	Yes, corticosteroid-sparing effects in adults	Unknown; potential increase in corticosteroid adverse effects	Inhibits 11 β-hydroxylase (blocks steroid breakdown) Blocks 5-lipo-oxygenase Inhibits platelet-activating factor
Ma huang *(Ephedra sinica)*	Yes	Yes	Cardiovascular and CNS toxicity, deaths reported, potential interaction with β-agonists	β-Agonist Bronchodilator
Licorice *(Glycyrrhize glabra)*	No	Case series suggest corticosteroid-sparing effects	Pseudohyperaldosteronism, hypertension, peripheral edema, potential increase in corticosteroid adverse effects	Inhibits 11 β-hydroxylase and cortisol breakdown
Coleus forskohlii	No	Case series in adults	Unknown	Decreased cAMP metabolism Bronchodilator
Tylophora indica	Yes, in adults	Yes	Unknown	Unknown
Ginkgo biloba	No	Yes, in a pilot study	Unknown	Platelet-activating factor antagonist
Onions *(Allium cepa)*	No	In vitro and animal data support use	Hypersensitivity is rare	Antioxidant Blocks leukotriene synthesis
Bee pollen	No	No	Anaphylaxis	Unknown

RCTs, randomized controlled trials; CNS, central nervous system; cAMP, cyclic adenosine monophosphate.
From Kemper KJ, Lester MR: Alternative asthma therapies: an evidence-based review, *Contemp Pediatr* 16:162–195, 1999.

Table 59-2 COMMONLY USED SEDATIVE HERBS

ADVERSE EFFECTS OR INTERACTIONS	SCIENTIFIC STUDIES	POTENTIAL ADVERSE EFFECTS OR INTERACTIONS			ADULT DOSE
		Adverse Effects	Pregnancy and Lactation	Drug Interactions	
German chamomile	In controlled trials, chamomile and its constituents have positive effects as a mild sedative	Allergic reactions	No known adverse effects in pregnancy, lactation, and childhood	None known	**Tea:** 150 mL boiling water over 3 g fresh flower heads, steep for 5-10 min; tid
Hops *(Humulus lupulus)*	Historical and anecdotal use Controlled trials have used hops/valerian combinations; these show improvements in sleep with the combination	Allergic reactions, skin irritation	No data available	Sedative activity increases the sleeping time induced by pentobarbital	**Tea:** 0.5-1.0 g dried hops before bed, typically in combination with valerian
Kava kava *(Piper methysticum)*	Randomized, controlled trials in adults show anxiolytic effects	Drowsiness, lethargy; slowed reaction time; withdrawal syndrome; chronic use can lead to yellow, dry skin and red eyes	Insufficient information available	Can potentiate sedative and anxiolytic effects of other herbs and medications	**Capsules:** 60-120 mg kava lactones, up to 300 mg of kava lactones daily to dried root/rhizome; 1.5-3.0 g/day in divided doses
Lavender *(Lavandula)*	Animal data, adult case series, and controlled trials suggest anticonvulsant and sedative effects	Allergies with topical use; toxic if large doses are taken internally	Historically contraindicated during pregnancy owing to possible emmenagogic effects; no documented adverse effects	Can potentiate sedative and anticonvulsant effects of other drugs	**Massage aromatherapy:** 1-10 mL of the essential oil can be added to 25 mL of a carrier oil **Bath soak:** add ¼-½ cup of dried lavender flowers to hot bath water
Lemon balm *(Melissa officinalis)*	Animal data suggest sedative-hypnotic effects All RCTs have examined lemon balm/valerian combinations; most show enhanced sleep quality	Allergic reactions are possible	Insufficient data; generally recognized as safe	None known	**Tea:** 2-3 g of dried herb, steeped in water; usually combined with valerian or lavender
Passionflower *(Passiflora alata)*	Case reports and historical use; most often combined with other herbs, such as valerian	Allergic reactions are possible	Insufficient data	None known	**Tea:** 0.25-1 g (about 1 tsp of crushed dried flowers/ cup of water) **Solid extract:** 150-300 mg (sold in capsules) daily
Valerian *(Valeriana officinalis)*	Randomized, double-blind, placebo-controlled studies in adults show decreased sleep latency and improved sleep quality	Headaches, insomnia	Insufficient data	Sedative activity increases the sleeping time induced by pentobarbital	**Tea:** 2-3 g of fresh or dried root/cup; 1-3× a day **Capsules:** 400 mg before bed

From Gardiner P, Kemper KJ: Herbs for sleep problems, *Contemp Pediatr* 19(2):69–87, 2002; and Gardiner P, Kemper KJ: Herbs in pediatric and adolescent medicine, *Pediatr Rev* 21:44–57, 2000.

Table 59-3 HERBS FOR SKIN CONDITIONS

ACTION	HERB OR SUPPLEMENT FOR TOPICAL USE
Soothing, emollient	Aloe, calendula
Anti-inflammatory	Aloe, chamomile, evening primrose oil, lemon balm
Antiviral	Aloe vera, calendula, chamomile, lemon balm
Antibacterial	Aloe vera, calendula, chamomile, lavender, lemon balm, tea tree oil
Antifungal	Lavender, tea tree oil

From Gardiner P, Coles D, Kemper KJ: The skinny on herbal remedies for dermatologic disorders, *Contemp Pediatr* 18:103–104, 107–110, 112–114, 2001.

Asia) might contain toxic levels of mercury, cadmium, arsenic, or lead, either from unintentional contamination during manufacturing or from intentional additions by producers who believe that these metals have therapeutic value. Approximately 30-40% of Asian patent medicines include potent pharmaceuticals, such as analgesics, antibiotics, hypoglycemic agents, or corticosteroids; typically, the labels for these products are not written in English and do not note the inclusion of pharmaceutical agents. Even mineral supplements, such as calcium, have been contaminated with lead or had significant problems with product variability.

Table 59-4 POTENTIALLY TOXIC HERBS

HERB	TOXIC CONSTITUENTS	TYPICAL USES	POTENTIAL ACUTE ADVERSE EFFECTS	HOW TO TREAT OVERDOSE
Aconitum (monkshood, wolfsbane)	**Diester alkaloids:** Hypaconitine and aconitine (aconitine increases permeability for sodium ions and slows down repolarization, leading to paralysis of the nerve)	Facial neuralgia and sciatica Headache and migraines Rheumatic pain, arthritis, gout Pericarditis sicca	Nausea, vomiting, hypersalivation **CNS:** Paresthesias, muscular weakness, dizziness, ataxia, seizures, coma **Cardiac:** Bradycardia, hypotension, rhythm disorders	Supportive care Dioxin-specific antibodies, unless history excludes cardiac glycosides Do not give ipecac Activated charcoal and gastric emptying might help Avoid type 1 antiarrhythmics
Artemisia absinthium (wormwood)	**Thujone and isothujone:** Neurotoxins	Anorexia Dyspeptic conditions Liver and gallbladder disorders	**Mental status changes:** Restlessness, vertigo, tremors, agitation, seizures, headache Vomiting; stomach and intestinal cramps Rhabdomyolysis and renal failure	Supportive care Benzodiazepines
Atropa belladonna (deadly nightshade) of atropline)	**Alkaloids:** Hyoscyamine (the L-isomer)	Gastrointestinal symptoms Cardiac insufficiency and arrhythmia Asthma	**Anticholinergic reaction:** Tachycardia, hyperthermia, mydriasis, urine and feces retention, restlessness Nervous system and respiratory depression	Gastric lavage Physostigmine given in consultation with a poison specialist External cooling if temperature is >102°F Benzodiazepines Hydration
Ayurvedic herbal remedies	Contaminated with lead, mercury, or arsenic	Traditional medicine from India; many purposes	Acute or chronic heavy metal toxicity	Depends on heavy metal
Digitalis purpurea (foxglove)	**Cardioactive glycosides:** Purpurea glycoside, digitoxin	Ulcers, boils, headaches, abscesses, paralysis, cardiac insufficiency	Nausea and vomiting, headache, loss of appetite Cardiac rhythm disorders **CNS:** Stupor, confusion, visual disorders, depression, psychosis, hallucinations	Supportive care Gastric lavage Activated charcoal Treatment of symptoms
Ephedra sinica (ma huang) Common names: Miner's tea, Mexican tea, Desert herb	**Alkaloids:** Ephedrine, pseudoephedrine (stimulates sympathomimetic receptors and the CNS)	Decongestant for upper respiratory infection Asthma Weight loss Stimulant	**Cardiac:** Hypertension, cardiomyopathy, myocardial infarction, arrhythmias **CNS:** Dizziness, restlessness, headaches, anxiety, hallucinations, tremors, seizures, psychosis, strokes Nausea and vomiting Contraindicated in diabetes or hypertension, angle-closure glaucoma, anxiety, prostate adenoma, thyroid disease, pheochromocytoma	Activated charcoal Benzodiazepine for seizures and sedation Vasodilators for hypertension Lidocaine and β-blockers for arrhythmias External cooling if temperature is >102°F Hydration therapy
Illicium anisatum (Japanese star anise tea)	Anisatins; block γ-aminobutyric acid	Colic in Latino and Caribbean populations	Seizures, tonic postures, myoclonus, hyperexcitability, irritability	Recovery with supportive care within 48 hr
Lobelia inflata (lobelia)	**Piperidine alkaloid:** L-Lobeline (stimulates nicotinic receptors)	Expectorant Asthma Spasmolytic Emetic To induce mental clarity and a feeling of well-being	**Gastrointestinal:** Nausea and vomiting, abdominal pain, diarrhea **CNS:** Anxiety, headache, dizziness, tremors, seizures, paresthesias, euphoria **Cardiac:** Arrhythmias, bradycardia, transient increase in blood pressure, decreased respiratory rate In overdose, lobeline can cause hypotension. Diaphoresis, muscle fasciculations and weakness, tremors, respiratory depression Dermatitis	Supportive care Gastric emptying Activated charcoal Benzodiazepines
Longdan xieganwan	Aristolochic acid	Enhance health	Renal interstitial fibrosis End-stage renal failure Renal cell carcinoma	Supportive care

Table 59-4 POTENTIALLY TOXIC HERBS—cont'd

HERB	TOXIC CONSTITUENTS	TYPICAL USES	POTENTIAL ACUTE ADVERSE EFFECTS	HOW TO TREAT OVERDOSE
Mentha pulegium (pennyroyal)	Pennyroyal oil has a hepatotoxic effect Acute poisoning is not found with proper administration of the designated therapeutic use of pennyroyal leaf; however, the drug is not recommended owing to hepatotoxicity	Insect repellent Respiratory illness Digestive disorders Emmenagogue Abortifacient Wound treatment Gout	Uterine contractions **Gastrointestinal:** Nausea, vomiting, abdominal pain, hepatitis **Neurotoxin:** Delirium, dizziness, convulsions, seizures, paralysis, encephalopathy, coma Renal failure and hypertension Shock and disseminated Intravascular coagulation Contraindicated in pregnancy	Supportive care N-Acetylcysteine
Pausinystalia yohimbe (yohimbe)	Indole alkaloids **Yohimbe:** α_2-Adrenoreceptor antagonist	Sexual disorders Exhaustion Improve muscle function	**Adverse reactions:** Dizziness, headache, anxiety, hypertension, indigestion, rash, insomnia, tachycardia, tremor, vomiting, hallucinations, nervousness, paresthesias, hypothermia, salivation, mydriasis, diarrhea, palpations, tachycardia Contraindicated in kidney and liver disease	Gastric emptying Activated charcoal Antiarrhythmics Hydration
Phytolacca americana (pokeweed, American nightshade)	Triterpene saponins (irritate mucous membranes) Lectins (toxic)	Anti-inflammatory Arthritis Cancer Emetic and cathartic Rheumatism	Dizziness, somnolence, nausea, vomiting, diarrhea, tachycardia, hemorrhagic gastritis, hypotension, lymphocytosis, headache, respiratory depression, seizures	Hydration therapy, electrolyte correction, gastric emptying Activated charcoal Electrolyte replacement Emesis should not be induced if patient is experiencing symptoms of overdose
Stramonium folium (jimsonweed)	**Alkaloids:** Hyoscyamine (the L-isomer of atropine)	Asthma and cough Diseases of the autonomic nervous system	In high doses, leads to restlessness, mania, hallucinations, delirium **Overdose:** Tachycardia, mydriasis, flushing, dry mouth, decreased sweating, miction, constipation	Supportive care Gastric lavage Decreasing temperature Physostigmine Benzodiazepines
Viscum album (mistletoe)	Alkaloids Viscotoxins *(Viscum album)* cause hypotension, bradycardia, and arterial vasoconstriction Lectins	Antineoplastic adjuvant Antihypertensive Nervous disorders: calmative agent Rheumatism Antispasmodic	Fever, headaches, nausea, vomiting, diarrhea, bradycardia, angina, change in blood pressure, seizures, confusion, hallucination, allergic reactions, miosis, mydriasis, chills, coma 2 reported deaths in the last 35 yr; most ingestions lead to mild reactions	Supportive therapy Data inconclusive for inducing emesis Activated charcoal

CNS, central nervous system.

From Gardiner P, Kemper KJ: Herbs for sleep problems, *Contemp Pediatr* 2:69–87, 2007; and Gardiner P, Kemper KJ: Herbs in pediatric and adolescent medicine, *Pediatr Rev* 21:44–57, 2000.

Many families use supplements concurrently with medications, posing hazards of interactions. For example, St. John's wort induces CYP3A4 activity of the P450 enzyme system and thus can enhance elimination of digoxin, cyclosporine, protease inhibitors, oral contraceptives, and numerous antibiotics, leading to subtherapeutic serum levels. It can also increase the risk of serotonin syndrome in patients taking antidepressant medications.

In the USA, dietary supplements do not undergo the same stringent evidence-based evaluation and post-marketing surveillance as prescription medications. Although they may not claim to prevent or treat specific medical conditions, product labels may make "structure-function" claims. A label may claim that a product "promotes a healthy immune system," but it may not claim to cure the common cold. The FDA can only restrict sales of certain products after receiving reports of adverse effects. Adverse reactions should be reported to the FDA's MedWatch program; failure to do so limits the FDA's ability to monitor and manage the clinical and public health risks of these products.

Evidence about the effectiveness of dietary supplements to prevent or treat pediatric problems is mixed, depending on the product used and condition treated; research in this area is growing rapidly. Some herbal products may be helpful adjunctive treatments for common childhood problems. For example, some herbs have proved helpful for colic (fennel and the combination of chamomile, fennel, vervain, licorice, balm mint), nausea (ginger), irritable bowel syndrome (peppermint), and diarrhea (probiotics) (Chapter 332).

MASSAGE AND OTHER BODYWORK THERAPIES

Massage is commonly provided at home by parents and by licensed massage therapists and nurses in clinical settings. Infant massage is routinely provided in many neonatal intensive care units to promote growth and development in preterm infants. Massage also has been demonstrated to be beneficial for pediatric patients suffering from asthma, insomnia, colic, cystic fibrosis, and juvenile rheumatoid arthritis. Massage therapy is generally safe.

Chiropractic is one of the most common professionally provided complementary practices. More than 50,000 chiropractors are licensed in the United States, and up to 14% of all chiropractic visits are for pediatric patients. Few randomized, controlled trials have demonstrated significant clinical benefits of chiropractic for pediatric patients; parents need to be cautioned not to rely on chiropractic as the primary treatment for serious conditions, such as cancer. Although anecdotal data suggest that severe complications are possible with chiropractic treatment of infants and children, such adverse effects appear to be rare. Further controlled trials are needed to determine the costs, benefits, and safety of chiropractic.

ACUPUNCTURE

Modern acupuncture incorporates treatment traditions from China, Japan, Korea, France, and other countries. The technique that has undergone most scientific study involves penetrating the skin with thin, solid, metallic needles that are manipulated by

Table 59-5 SPANISH-ENGLISH BOTANICAL NAME TRANSLATION CHART*

SPANISH NAME	ENGLISH NAME	BOTANICAL NAME
Ajo	Garlic	*Allium sativum*
Azarcon	Lead tetraoxide	Not a plant
Azogue	Mercury	Not a plant
Cebolla	Onion	*Allium cepa*
Cenela	Cinnamon	*Cinnamomum aromaticum*
Clavo	Cloves	*Eugenia aromatica*
Comino	Cumin	*Cuminum cyminum*
Epasote or herba Sancti Mariae	Wormseed	*Chenopodium anthelminticum*
Estafiate	Wormwood	*Artemisia absinthium*
Eucalipto	Eucalyptus	*Eucalyptus globulus*
Granada	Pomegranate	*Punica granatum*
Jengibre	Ginger	*Zingiber officinale*
Limon	Lemon	*Citrus limon*
Manzanilla	Chamomile	*Anthemis nobilis* or *Chamomilla recutita* or *Matricaria chamomilla*
Oregano	Oregano	*Origanum vulgare*
Pelos de elote	Corn silk	*Zea mays*
Savila	Aloe vera	*Aloe vera*
Siete jarabes	Mixture of syrup of sweet almond, castor oil, balsam resin, wild cherry, licorice, cocillana bark, honey	
Tomillo	Thyme	*Thymus vulgaris*
Una de gato	Cat's claw	*Uncaria tomentosa*
Valeriana	Valerian	*Valeriana officinalis*
Yerba buena	Spearmint	*Mentha spicata*

*Prepared with assistance of Laura Howell, MD.

hand or by electrical stimulation. Variants of needle therapy include stimulation of acupuncture points by rubbing (shiatsu), heat (moxibustion), lasers, magnets, pressure (acupressure), or electrical currents.

Acupuncture is used by an increasing number of pediatric patients. Although most pediatric patients are averse to needles, patients who suffer from severe chronic pain may be amenable to trying acupuncture and often report that it is helpful. Acupuncture services are offered by more than ⅓ of North American academic pediatric pain treatment programs. Although additional studies are needed in children, research in adults suggests that acupuncture can offer significant benefits in the treatment of recurrent headache, depression, and nausea. As with any therapy involving needles, infections and bleeding are expected, but uncommon complications and more serious complications, such as pneumothorax, occur in <1 in 30,000 treatments.

BIBLIOGRAPHY

Please visit the Nelson Textbook of Pediatrics *website at* *www.expertconsult.com* *for the complete bibliography.*

PART IX The Acutely Ill Child

Chapter 60
Evaluation of the Sick Child in the Office and Clinic

Mary Saunders and Marc H. Gorelick

Acutely ill children pose a challenge to a busy pediatrician's office. Illnesses can span the spectrum from simple viral infections to life-threatening emergencies. Pediatricians need to distinguish between patients who can be managed with close follow-up and those that need to be stabilized and transported to a higher level of care. Although patients of all ages can present with similar symptoms, the etiology of the illness can be age-dependent. The initial approach must focus on the general evaluation and stabilization of the acutely ill infant and child.

HISTORY

A thorough history is paramount to arriving at the correct diagnosis. In younger patients, parents must interpret how their child is "feeling." Older children may not be able to completely define or localize their symptoms. On the basis of the chief complaint, the pediatrician must ask questions that help distinguish between common and potentially life-threatening entities. Common complaints leading to acute care visits include altered mental status, vomiting, respiratory distress, fever, and abdominal pain.

For patients presenting with **altered mental status**, the pediatrician should inquire about the presence of other symptoms such as fever or headache. Screening questions regarding feeding changes, medications in the household, or the possibility of trauma should be asked. Parents will often describe a febrile child as "lethargic," but further questioning will reveal a tired appearing child who interacts appropriately when he or she has defervesced. Febrile patients need to be differentiated from the lethargic child who presents with sepsis or meningitis. Infants with meningitis or sepsis may have a history of irritability and/or inconsolability, not waking up for feedings, poor feeding, grunting respirations, seizures, and decreased urine output. Patients with poisonings or inborn errors of metabolism can also present with lethargy, poor feeding, seizures, and vomiting. Nonaccidental trauma should always be considered in a lethargic infant. Older children may present with altered mental status due to meningitis/encephalitis, trauma, or ingestions. Children with meningitis may have a history of fever and complaints of neck pain; other associated symptoms can include photophobia and vomiting. Children with ingestions can present with other abnormal neurologic symptoms such as ataxia, slurred speech, seizures, or characteristic constellations of vital sign changes and other physical findings (toxidromes).

Vomiting is a very common complaint of intestinal, abdominal (pancreas, liver) or non-gastrointestinal (hyperammonemia, increased intracranial pressure) origin. Care should be taken to determine whether the emesis is bilious, which is suggestive of intestinal obstruction. Other historical data to be gathered include the presence of abdominal distention, weight changes, presence of diarrhea, obstipation or hematochezia, history of trauma, and presence of headache. Although common causes of vomiting are gastroesophageal reflux and viral gastroenteritis, the pediatrician needs to be aware of other serious causes. In the infant, bilious emesis and abdominal distention and/or pain are worrisome for obstruction, as may be seen with malrotation with midgut volvulus or Hirschsprung disease. It is important to consider extra-abdominal causes of vomiting in the neonate, including hydrocephalus, incarcerated hernia, inborn errors of metabolism, and nonaccidental trauma. Markedly increasing head circumference or a bulging fontanel can be the result of congenital hydrocephalus or can signal the presence of subdural hematomas from nonaccidental trauma. In an older child, the differential diagnosis includes intussusception, incarcerated hernia, diabetic ketoacidosis, appendicitis, poisonings, and trauma. Patients with intussusception may present with vomiting and colicky abdominal pain. A history of increased urination in the presence of vomiting may herald the diagnosis of diabetes mellitus. Patients with headache and vomiting raise a concern for increased intracranial pressure and should be questioned about neurologic changes, meningismus, and fever. Vomiting may be also a nonspecific symptom of a systemic illness (otitis media, sinusitis).

Parents can interpret different symptoms as **respiratory distress**. Tachypnea secondary to fever is quite concerning. Parents of newborn infants are sometimes alarmed by the presence of periodic breathing. Normal variations in respiratory patterns must be distinguished from true respiratory distress. Parents need to be questioned regarding associated symptoms such as fever, limitation of neck movement, drooling, choking, and the presence of stridor or wheezing. A history of apnea or cyanosis warrants further investigation. Although wheezing is often secondary to bronchospasm, it can also be caused by cardiac disease or congenital anomalies such as vascular rings. Infants with congenital heart defects may be tachypneic but may lack any signs of respiratory distress as a compensatory mechanism for shock or metabolic acidosis. Older children who present with wheezing after a coughing or choking episode should be evaluated for a foreign body aspiration. Stridor is most commonly due to croup. However, anatomic abnormalities such as laryngeal webs, laryngomalacia, subglottic stenosis, and paralyzed vocal cords also cause stridor. In toxic-appearing children with respiratory distress, the pediatrician should entertain the possibilities of epiglottitis, bacterial tracheitis, or a rapidly expanding retropharyngeal abscess. The incidence of epiglottitis has markedly declined with the advent of the *Haemophilus influenzae type b* (Hib) vaccine, but remains a possibility in the unimmunized or partially immunized patient. Children with retropharyngeal abscesses may present with drooling and limitation of neck movement, especially hyperextension.

Fever is the most common reason for a sick child visit. Most fevers are the result of self-limited viral infections. However, pediatricians need to be aware of the age-dependent potential for serious bacterial infections (urinary tract infections, sepsis, meningitis, dysentery, osteoarticular infection). During the first 3 mo of life, the neonate is at risk for sepsis due to pathogens that are uncommon in older children. These organisms include group B streptococcus, *Escherichia coli, Listeria monocytogenes,* and herpes simplex virus. In neonates, the history must include maternal obstetric information and the patient's birth history. Risk factors for sepsis include maternal group B streptococcus colonization, prematurity, chorioamnionitis, and prolonged rupture of membranes. If there is a maternal history of sexually transmitted infections during the pregnancy, the differential diagnosis must be expanded to include those pathogens. Septic infants can present with lethargy, poor feeding, grunting respirations, and impaired perfusion, in addition to fever. Infants with fever, irritability, and a bulging fontanel should be evaluated for meningitis. As the infant matures beyond 3 mo of age, the bacterial pathogens that usually cause bacteremia, sepsis, and meningitis are *Streptococcus pneumoniae, H. influenzae* type b (if the child is unimmunized or only partially immunized), and *Neisseria meningitidis*. Immunization against some serotypes of *S. pneumoniae* appears to be reducing the occurrence of occult bacteremia and serious infections caused by that organism, as has immunization against *H. influenzae* type b. Other ailments that manifest with fever include septic arthritis and osteomyelitis, juvenile rheumatoid arthritis, and Kawasaki disease. Children with a septic joint generally present with only one joint that is painful and often have pseudoparalysis of that joint. In contrast, patients with juvenile rheumatoid arthritis may present with pain, stiffness, swelling, and warmth of several joints. The diagnosis of Kawasaki disease should be considered if the patient meets the diagnostic criteria for this illness (Chapter 160).

Abdominal pain is another frequent complaint. Often this symptom is due to a minor illness such as constipation, functional abdominal pain, urinary tract infection, or gastroenteritis. Parents should be questioned about associated symptoms including stooling patterns, abdominal distention, fever, urinary symptoms, and vomiting. In neonates, a tender abdomen is concerning for the presence of a small bowel obstruction; these infants tend to appear ill. There may be a history of vomiting and decreased or no stooling. Pediatricians also need to be wary of neonates with abdominal tenderness and bloody stools, as 10% of cases of necrotizing enterocolitis occur in term infants. Infants with milk protein intolerance can also present with bloody stools, but these infants are well appearing and do not have abdominal tenderness. In older patients, the differential diagnosis for abdominal pain expands to include intussusceptions and appendicitis. Patients with intussusception can present in a variety of ways, ranging from having episodes of colicky abdominal pain, but otherwise well in between episodes, to being in a shock-like state. The diagnosis of appendicitis in the child younger than 3 yr is extremely difficult because children in this age group do not localize their pain well. Often the diagnosis is made after the appendix has ruptured.

The child's **past medical history** also needs to be obtained. It is important to be aware of any underlying chronic problems that might predispose the child to recurring infections or a serious acute illness. The child with sickle cell anemia is at increased risk for bacteremia as well as painful vasoocclusive crisis. A careful review of systems can help in identifying the nature of the acute illness, as well as any complications needing intervention, such as dehydration accompanying an otherwise minor viral illness.

PHYSICAL EXAM

Observation is important in the evaluation of the acutely ill child. Most observational data that the pediatrician gathers during an acute illness should focus on assessing the child's response to stimuli. How does the crying child respond to the parents' comforting? How quickly does the sleeping child awaken with a stimulus? Does the child smile when the examiner interacts with him or her? Assessing responses to stimuli requires knowledge of normal responses for different age groups, the manner in which those normal responses are elicited, and to what degree a response might be impaired. Thus, the pediatrician must be both clinically and developmentally oriented.

During the **physical examination**, the pediatrician seeks evidence of illness. The portions of the physical examination that require the child to be optimally cooperative are completed first. Initially, it is best to seat the child on the parent's lap; the older child may be seated on the examination table. Vital signs are often overlooked but are valuable in assessing ill children. The degree of fever, the presence of tachycardia out of proportion to the fever, and the presence of tachypnea and hypotension all suggest a serious infection. The respiratory evaluation includes determining respiratory rate and noting any evidence of inspiratory stridor, expiratory wheezing, grunting, or coughing. Evidence of increased work of breathing—retraction, nasal flaring, and the use of abdominal musculature—is sought. Because acute infections in children are most often caused by viral infections, the presence of nasal discharge may be noted. It is possible at this time to assess the skin for rashes. Frequently, viral infections cause an exanthematous eruption, and many of these eruptions are diagnostic (the reticulated rash and "slapped-cheek" appearance caused by parvovirus infections or the typical appearance of hand-foot-and-mouth disease caused by coxsackieviruses). The skin examination may also yield evidence of more serious infections (bacterial cellulitis or petechiae and purpura associated with bacteremia). Cutaneous perfusion should be assessed by warmth and capillary refill time. When the child is seated and is least perturbed, an assessment of the fontanel can be completed; the examiner can determine whether the fontanel is depressed, flat, or bulging. It is also important to assess the child's willingness to move and ease of movement. It is reassuring to see the child moving about on the parent's lap with ease and without discomfort.

During this initial portion of the physical examination, when the child is most comfortable, the heart and lungs are auscultated. In the acutely febrile child, because of the relatively frequent occurrence of respiratory illnesses, it is important to assess adequacy of air entry into the lungs, equality of breath sounds, and evidence of adventitial breath sounds, especially wheezes, rales, and rhonchi. The coarse sound of air moving through a congested nasal passage is frequently transmitted to the lungs. The examiner can become attuned to these coarse sounds by placing the stethoscope near the child's nose and then compensating for this sound as the chest is auscultated. The cardiac examination is next; findings such as pericardial friction rub, loud murmurs, and distant heart sounds may indicate an infectious process involving the heart. The eyes are examined to identify features that might indicate an infectious process. Often, viral infections result in a watery discharge or redness of the bulbar conjunctivae. Bacterial infection, if superficial, results in purulent drainage; if the infection is more deep-seated, tenderness, swelling, and redness of the tissues surrounding the eye are present, as well as proptosis, reduced visual acuity, and altered extraocular movement. The extremities may then be evaluated not only for ease of movement but also for the possibility of swelling, heat, or tenderness; such abnormalities may indicate focal infections.

The components of the physical examination that are more bothersome to the child are completed last. This is best done with the patient on the examination table. Initially, the neck is examined to assess for areas of swelling, redness, or tenderness, as may be seen in cervical adenitis. The neck is then flexed to evaluate suppleness; resistance to flexion is indicative of meningeal irritation. The Kernig and Brudzinski signs may be sought at this time. In children younger than 18 mo, meningeal signs may not always be present with meningitis; if they are present, the diagnostic implications are the same as for the older child. During examination of the abdomen, the diaper is removed. The abdomen is inspected for distention. Auscultation is performed to assess adequacy of bowel sounds, followed by palpation. The child often fusses as the abdomen is auscultated and palpated. Every attempt should be made to quiet the child; if this is not possible, increased fussing as the abdomen is palpated may indicate tenderness, especially if this finding is reproducible. In addition to focal tenderness, palpation may elicit involuntary guarding or rebound tenderness (including tenderness to percussion); these findings indicate peritoneal irritation, as is seen in appendicitis. The inguinal area and genitals are then sequentially examined. The child is then placed in the prone position, and abnormalities of the back are sought. The spine and costovertebral angle areas are percussed to elicit any tenderness; such a finding may be indicative of vertebral osteomyelitis or diskitis and pyelonephritis, respectively.

Examining the ears and throat completes the physical examination. These are usually the most bothersome parts of the examination for the child, and parents frequently can be helpful in minimizing head movement. During the oropharyngeal examination, it is important to document the presence of enanthemas; these may be seen in many infectious processes, such as hand-foot-and-mouth disease caused by coxsackievirus. This portion of the examination is also important in documenting inflammation or exudates on the tonsils, which may be viral or bacterial.

Repeating portions of the assessment may be indicated. If the child cried continuously during the initial clinical evaluation, the examiner may not be certain whether the crying was caused by the high fever, stranger anxiety, or pain, or is indicative of a serious illness. Constant crying also makes portions of the physical examination, such as auscultation of the chest, more difficult. Before a repeat assessment is performed, efforts to make the child as comfortable as possible are indicated.

Febrile children can appear very ill. The elevated temperature is often accompanied by listlessness, tachycardia, and tachypnea. These patients should receive antipyretic medications and be reassessed once they have defervesced. In the majority of children with uncomplicated viral illnesses, the vital signs normalize. Persistence of abnormal vital signs should prompt the clinician to further investigate the source of fever. Continued tachycardia and poor perfusion may be secondary to myocarditis. Tachypnea may be the sole symptom in patients with pneumonia, especially in children whose chief complaint is abdominal pain due to lower lobe pneumonia. Persistent irritability suggests meningitis.

RISK FACTORS

The sensitivity of the carefully performed clinical assessment, observation, history, and physical examination for the presence of serious illness is approximately 90%. Careful data gathering is necessary in the observation, history, and physical examination, because each component of the evaluation is as effective as the others in identifying serious illness. Other data should be sought to improve this sensitivity level. In the child with an acute febrile illness, important supplemental data are age, body temperature, and the results of screening laboratory tests. Febrile children in the first 3 mo of life have yet to achieve immunologic maturity and therefore are more susceptible to severe infections. Thus, the febrile infant is at greater risk for serious bacterial infection than the child beyond 3 mo of age. In febrile children, the higher the fever is, the greater the risk of serious illness. The risk of bacteremia in infants increases as the magnitude of fever increases.

Screening laboratory tests may be helpful in identifying the febrile child at increased risk for selected serious illnesses. *S. pneumoniae* is a cause of occult bacteremia not associated with a focal soft tissue infection. A total white blood cell count of ≥15,000/mm^3 and/or an absolute neutrophil count of ≥10,000/mm^3, in addition to age 3-36 mo, higher grades of fever, and a more ill appearance, are indicators of increased risk for occult bacteremia caused by *S. pneumoniae.* The incidence of occult pneumococcal bacteremia in febrile children is declining because of the introduction of conjugated pneumococcal vaccine. Urinalysis and urine culture must always be considered when the source of fever is not apparent, especially in the highest-risk groups: females and uncircumcised males younger than 2 yr and all boys younger than 1 yr. The presence of leukocyte esterase, >5 white blood cells/high-power field on a spun urine specimen, or bacteria detected by Gram stain on an unspun urine specimen suggests urinary tract infection, but the sensitivity of these indicators is, on average, only 75-85% and urine culture is the definitive test. An elevated C-reactive protein value may also distinguish bacterial from viral infection.

MANAGEMENT

Most patients who present to the pediatrician's office with an acute illness will not require resuscitation. The pediatrician needs to be prepared to evaluate and begin resuscitation for the seriously ill or unstable child. The pediatrician's office should be stocked with appropriate equipment necessary to stabilize an acutely ill child. Maintenance of that equipment and ongoing training of the office staff in use of the equipment and procedures is required (Chapter 61). The evaluation must begin with assessment of the ABCs—airway, breathing, and circulation. When assessing the airway, chest rise should be evaluated, and evidence of increased work of breathing sought. The examiner should ensure that the trachea is midline. If the airway is patent and no signs of airway obstruction are present, the patient is allowed to assume a position of comfort. If the child shows signs of airway obstruction, repositioning of the head with the chin lift maneuver may alleviate the obstruction. An oral or nasal airway may be necessary in patients in whom airway patency cannot be maintained. These devices are not well tolerated in conscious patients and may induce gagging or vomiting. Once airway patency has been established, the adequacy of breathing should be evaluated. Auscultation of the lung fields should assess for air entry, symmetry of breath sounds, and presence of adventitious breath sounds such as crackles or wheezes. Pulse oximetry can be used to evaluate oxygenation. Bronchodilator therapy can be initiated to alleviate bronchospasm. Oxygen should be administered to all seriously ill children via nasal cannula or face mask. Cyanosis or slow respiratory rates may signal respiratory failure. If the airway is patent but the child's respiratory effort is deemed inadequate, positive pressure ventilation via a bag-valve-mask device should be initiated. Once airway and breathing have been addressed, circulation must be evaluated. This involves assessment of cardiac output. Symptoms of shock include tachycardia, cool extremities, delayed capillary refill time, mottled or pale skin, and effortless tachypnea. Hypotension is a late finding in shock. Vascular access is necessary for volume resuscitation in patients with impaired circulation. Once an intervention is performed, the clinician must reassess the patient.

If the febrile child is older than 3 mo and appears well, if the history or physical examination does not suggest a serious illness, and if no age or temperature risk factors are present, the child may be followed expectantly. If otitis media is present, it should be treated. This profile applies to most children with acute febrile illnesses. If, on the other hand, the child appears ill or the history or physical examination suggests a serious infection, definitive laboratory tests appropriate for those findings are indicated (e.g., chest radiograph for a child with grunting). The area of greatest controversy is whether laboratory studies are needed in a febrile child who appears well and has no abnormalities on history and physical examination, but who is younger than 3 mo or whose temperature is high. Many would agree that a sepsis work-up is indicated in the febrile child younger than 1 mo and possibly younger than 3 mo. Obtaining blood and urine cultures in children older than 3 mo with higher grades of fever without a focus has also gained increased acceptance.

DISPOSITION

The majority of children evaluated in the office for an acute illness can be managed on an outpatient basis. These patients should have reassuring physical examinations, stable vital signs, and adequate follow-up. A mildly dehydrated patient can be discharged to home for a trial of oral rehydration. Patients with a respiratory illness who are exhibiting signs of mild respiratory distress may be monitored at home with a repeat examination scheduled for the next day. Depending on the child's status, the comfort of the parents, and the relationship of the family with the physician, telephone follow-up may be all that is necessary.

If the physician feels comfortable in following as an outpatient the child in whom no specific diagnosis has been established, a follow-up examination may yield the diagnosis. During the initial visit, or from one visit to the next during the acute illness, the change in symptoms or in the findings on physical examination over time may provide important diagnostic clues. For the child in whom a diagnosis has already been established and who does not require hospitalization, follow-up by telephone or an office visit should be used to monitor the course of the illness and to further educate and support the parents.

However, if it is deemed that the child needs a higher level of care, it is the pediatrician's responsibility to decide what method of transfer is appropriate. Physicians may be reluctant to call for help because of a misperception that 911 services should be activated only for full-blown resuscitations. Emergency Medical Services (EMS) transport should be initiated for any child who is physiologically unstable (i.e., with severe respiratory distress, cyanosis, signs of shock, or altered mental status). If the family's ability to comply promptly with recommendation for emergency department evaluation is in question, that patient should also be transported by EMS. Some physicians and families may defer calling EMS because of the perception that a parent can get to the hospital faster by private car. Although rapidity of transport should be considered, the need for further interventions during transport and the risk of clinical decompensation are other important factors in the decision to activate EMS. Ultimately, the legal responsibility for a patient lies with the referring physician, until responsibility of care is officially transferred to another medical provider.

BIBLIOGRAPHY

Please visit the Nelson Textbook of Pediatrics *website at www.expertconsult.com for the complete bibliography.*

Chapter 61
Emergency Medical Services for Children

Joseph L. Wright and Steven E. Krug

The overwhelming majority of the 30 million children who present annually for emergency care in the USA are seen at community hospital emergency departments (EDs). Visits to children's hospital EDs account for just 11% of initial emergency care encounters. This distribution suggests that the greatest opportunity to optimize care for acutely ill or injured pediatric patients, on a population basis, occurs broadly as part of a systems-based approach to emergency services, an approach that incorporates the unique needs of children at every level. Conceptually, emergency medical services for children (EMSC) are characterized by an integrated, continuum of care model (see Fig. 61-1 on the *Nelson Textbook of Pediatrics* website at www.expertconsult.com). The model is designed such that patient care flows seamlessly from the primary care medical home through transport and on to hospital-based definitive care. It includes the following 5 principal domains of activity:

1. Prevention, primary and secondary
2. Out-of-hospital care, both emergency response and prehospital transport
3. Hospital-based care: emergency department and inpatient
4. Interfacility transport, as necessary, for definitive or subspecialty care (Chapter 61.1)
5. Rehabilitation.

For the full continuation of this chapter, please visit the Nelson Textbook of Pediatrics *website at www.expertconsult.com.*

61.1 Interfacility Transport of the Seriously Ill or Injured Pediatric Patient*

Elizabeth A. Edgerton and Bruce L. Klein

Patients often seek treatment at facilities that lack sufficient expertise to treat their conditions, necessitating transfer to more appropriate specialty centers. This is especially pronounced in pediatrics. EMS providers or parents usually take children to local EDs first, where their conditions and physiologic stabilities are assessed. Although bringing a child directly to the local ED may be proper logistically, local EDs can be less than ideal for pediatric emergencies. Children account for 27% of all ED visits but only 6% of EDs have all the necessary supplies for pediatric emergencies. Also, general EDs are less likely to have pediatric expertise or policies in place for the care of children. Outcomes for critically ill children treated in pediatric intensive care units (PICUs) are better than for those treated in adult ICUs. When pediatric critical care is required, transport to a regional PICU is indicated. In addition, often the type of subspecialty care needed (e.g., pediatric orthopedics) is available only at the pediatric center.

For the full continuation of this chapter, please visit the Nelson Textbook of Pediatrics *website at www.expertconsult.com.*

61.2 Outcomes and Risk Adjustment

Evaline A. Alessandrini

The publication of the IOM reports *To Err is Human: Building a Safer Health System* and *Crossing the Quality Chasm: A New Health System for the 21st Century* marked the beginning of a heightened public and professional urgency to improve the quality of health care. Health services research has documented wide variation in the likelihood that patients receive quality, evidence-based health care, and this can negatively impact the health of children and youth. The complexities of delivering high-quality health care are magnified in the ED. Patients are in crisis, EDs are often overcrowded, patient-physician relationships are based on brief interactions, and the variety of complaints and diagnoses is immense. Furthermore, in this complex era, health care professionals, patients, purchasers, and policy makers are demanding more transparency and accountability from health care providers.

For the full continuation of this chapter, please visit the Nelson Textbook of Pediatrics *website at www.expertconsult.com.*

61.3 Principles Applicable to the Developing World

Jennifer I. Chapman and David M. Walker

International pediatric emergency medicine, or IPEM, is an emerging academic field whose practitioners are committed to international collaboration aimed at improving the quality of care for children outside their national borders (see Tables 61-5 and 61-6 on the *Nelson Textbook of Pediatrics* website at www.expertconsult.com).

For the full continuation of this chapter, please visit the Nelson Textbook of Pediatrics *website at www.expertconsult.com.*

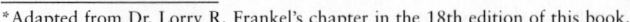

*Adapted from Dr. Lorry R. Frankel's chapter in the 18th edition of this book.

Chapter 62
Pediatric Emergencies and Resuscitation

Mary E. Hartman and Ira M. Cheifetz

Injuries are the leading cause of death in American children and young adults and are responsible for more childhood deaths than all other causes combined (Chapter 5.1). Children are particularly vulnerable to injury for a number of reasons, including their small size, relative physical uncoordination, and limited ability to predict or understand danger. In addition, the immaturity of their developing bones, ligaments, and muscles; their thin body walls; and their relatively large heads, compared with total body surface area, make young children susceptible to serious or fatal injury from falls and collisions.

Most injuries in childhood are unintentional, and many are preventable. Motor vehicle–related injuries account for nearly half of all pediatric deaths in the USA every year, many of which are related to speeding, aggressive driving, failure to use proper passenger restraints, and/or alcohol. Consistent use of bicycle helmets could reduce the severity of head injuries, the leading cause of death when a bicyclist is struck by a car, by more than 80%. Four-sided fencing around swimming pools and use of flotation devices for every passenger in a boat could greatly reduce the risk of drowning, the second leading cause of accidental death in children younger than 5 yr and the third major cause of death in adolescents.

Serious injuries can become fatal when appropriate medical care is delayed.

Rapid, effective bystander cardiopulmonary resuscitation (CPR) for children is associated with survival rates as high as 70%, with good neurologic outcome. However, bystander CPR is still provided for less than 50% of children who experience cardiac arrest outside medical settings. This has lead to long-term survival rates of <20%, with most survivors suffering a poor neurologic outcome.

APPROACH TO THE EMERGENCY EVALUATION OF A CHILD

The first response to a pediatric emergency of any cause is a systematic, rapid **general assessment** of the scene and the child to identify immediate threats to the child, care providers, or others. If an emergency is identified, the emergency response system (emergency medical services [EMS]) should be activated immediately. Care providers should then proceed through **primary**, **secondary**, and **tertiary assessments** as allowed by the child's condition, safety of the scene, and resources available. This standardized approach provides organization to what might otherwise be a confusing or chaotic situation and reinforces an organized thought process for care providers. If, at any point in these assessments, the caregiver identifies a life-threatening problem, the assessment is halted and lifesaving interventions are begun. Further assessment and intervention should be delayed until other caregivers arrive or the condition is successfully treated.

General Assessment

Upon arrival at the scene of a compromised child, a caregiver's first task is a quick survey of the scene itself. Is the rescuer or child in imminent danger because of circumstances at the scene (fire, high-voltage electricity)? If so, can the child be safely extricated to a safe location for assessment and treatment? Can the child be safely moved with the appropriate precautions (i.e., cervical spine protection), if indicated? A rescuer is expected to proceed only if these safety conditions have been met.

Once the caregiver and patient's safety has been ensured, the caregiver performs **a rapid visual survey** of the child, assessing the child's **general appearance and cardiopulmonary function**. This action should be very quick (only a few seconds) and should include assessment of (1) general appearance (determining color, tone, alertness, and responsiveness); (2) adequacy of breathing (distinguishing between normal, comfortable respirations and respiratory distress or apnea); and (3) adequacy of circulation (identifying cyanosis, pallor, or mottling). A child found unresponsive from an *unwitnessed* collapse should be approached with a gentle touch and the verbal question, "Are you OK?" If there is no response, the caregiver should immediately shout for help and send someone to both activate the emergency response system (EMS) and locate an automated external defibrillator (AED) (Fig. 62-1). The provider should then determine whether the child is breathing and, if not, provide 2 rescue breaths as described later under Recognition and Treatment of Respiratory Distress and Failure. If the child is adequately breathing, then the circulation is quickly assessed. Any child with a heart rate below 60 beats/min or without a pulse requires immediate CPR, as described under Cardiac Arrest. If the caregiver *witnesses* the sudden collapse of a child, the caregiver should have a higher suspicion for a sudden cardiac event. In this case, rapid deployment of an AED is of paramount importance. The provider should very briefly delay care of the child to activate EMS and locate the nearest AED.

Primary Assessment

Once the emergency response system has been activated and the child is determined not to need CPR, the caregiver should proceed with a primary assessment that includes a **brief, hands-on assessment of cardiopulmonary and neurologic function and stability**. This assessment includes a limited physical exam, evaluation of vital signs, and measurement of pulse oximetry if possible. Again, a standardized approach is best. The American Heart Association, in its pediatric advanced life support (PALS) curriculum, supports the structured format of **Airway, Breathing, Circulation, Disability, Exposure (ABCDE)**. The goal of the primary assessment is to obtain a focused, systems-based assessment of the child's injuries or abnormalities, so that resuscitative efforts can be directed to these areas; if the caregiver identifies a life-threatening abnormality, further evaluation is postponed until appropriate corrective action has been taken.

The exam and vital sign data can be interpreted only if the caregiver has a thorough understanding of normal values. In pediatrics, normal respiratory rate, heart rate, and blood pressure have age-specific norms (Table 62-1). These ranges can be difficult to remember, especially if used infrequently. However, several standard principals apply: (1) no child's respiratory rate should be >60 breaths/min for a sustained period; (2) normal heart rate is roughly 2-3 times normal respiratory rate for age; and (3) a simple guide for pediatric blood pressure (BP) is that the lower limit of systolic BP should be <60 mm Hg for neonates; <70 mm Hg for 1 mo–1 yr olds; <70 mm Hg + (2 × age) for 1-10 yr olds; and <90 mm Hg for any child older than 10 yr.

AIRWAY AND BREATHING The most common precipitating event for cardiac instability in infants and children is respiratory insufficiency. Therefore, rapid assessment of respiratory failure and immediate restoration of adequate ventilation and oxygenation remain the first priority in the resuscitation of a child. Using a systematic approach, the caregiver should first assess whether the child's airway is patent and maintainable. A healthy, patent airway is open and unobstructed, allowing normal respiration without noise or effort. A maintainable airway is one that is either already patent or can be made patent with a simple maneuver. To assess airway patency, the provider should look for breathing movements in the child's chest and abdomen, listen for breath sounds, and feel the movement of air at the child's mouth and nose. Abnormal breathing sounds (i.e., snoring or stridor), increased work of breathing, and apnea are all findings potentially consistent with airway obstruction. If there is evidence of

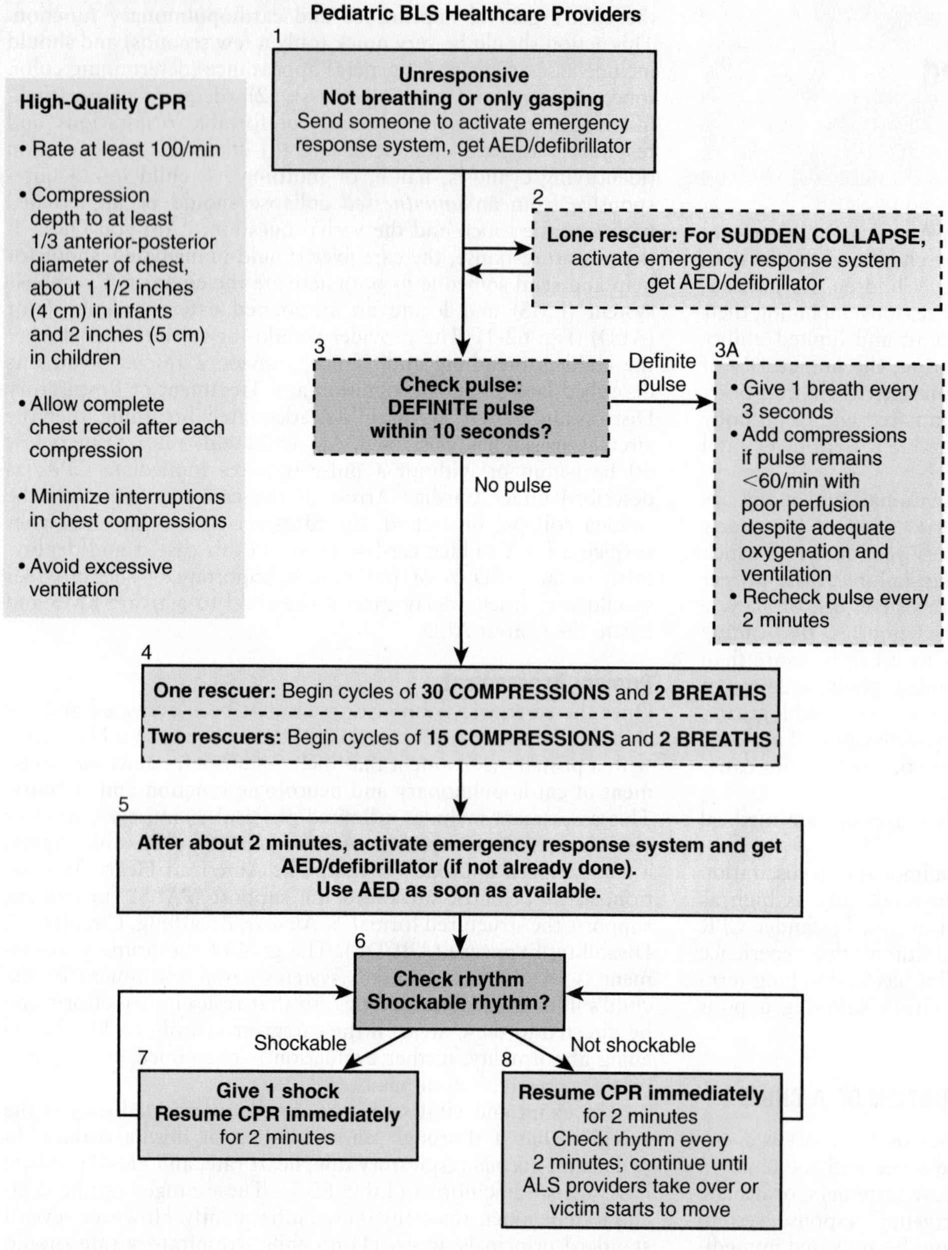
Pediatric BLS Healthcare Providers
High-Quality CPR
• Rate at least 100/min
• Compression depth to at least 1/3 anterior-posterior diameter of chest, about 1 1/2 inches (4 cm) in infants and 2 inches (5 cm) in children
• Allow complete chest recoil after each compression
• Minimize interruptions in chest compressions
• Avoid excessive ventilation
1
Unresponsive
Not breathing or only gasping
Send someone to activate emergency response system, get AED/defibrillator
2
Lone rescuer: For SUDDEN COLLAPSE, activate emergency response system get AED/defibrillator
3
Check pulse: DEFINITE pulse within 10 seconds?
Definite pulse
3A
• Give 1 breath every 3 seconds
• Add compressions if pulse remains <60/min with poor perfusion despite adequate oxygenation and ventilation
• Recheck pulse every 2 minutes
No pulse
4
One rescuer: Begin cycles of 30 COMPRESSIONS and 2 BREATHS
Two rescuers: Begin cycles of 15 COMPRESSIONS and 2 BREATHS
5
After about 2 minutes, activate emergency response system and get AED/defibrillator (if not already done). Use AED as soon as available.
6
Check rhythm
Shockable rhythm?
Shockable
Not shockable
7
Give 1 shock
Resume CPR immediately
for 2 minutes
8
Resume CPR immediately
for 2 minutes
Check rhythm every 2 minutes; continue until ALS providers take over or victim starts to move

Note: The boxes bordered with dashed lines are performed by healthcare providers and not by rescuers

Figure 62-1 Pediatric basic life support algorithm. AED, automated external defibrillator; ALS, advanced life support; CPR, cardiopulmonary resuscitation. (From Berg MD, Schexnayder SM, Chameides L, et al: 2010 American Heart Association guidelines for cardiopulmonary resuscitation and emergency cardiovascular care, part 13, *Circulation* 122[suppl 3]: S862–S875, 2010, Fig 3, p S866.)

Table 62-1 NORMAL VITAL SIGNS ACCORDING TO AGE

AGE	HEART RATE (beats/min)	BLOOD PRESSURE (mm Hg)	RESPIRATORY RATE (breaths/min)
Premature	120-170*	55-75/35-45†	40-70‡
0-3 mo	100-150*	65-85/45-55	35-55
3-6 mo	90-120	70-90/50-65	30-45
6-12 mo	80-120	80-100/55-65	25-40
1-3 yr	70-110	90-105/55-70	20-30
3-6 yr	65-110	95-110/60-75	20-25
6-12 yr	60-95	100-120/60-75	14-22
12+yr	55-85	110-135/65-85	12-18

*In sleep, infant heart rates may drop significantly lower, but if perfusion is maintained, no intervention is required.
†A blood pressure cuff should cover approximately ⅔ of the arm; too small a cuff yields spuriously high pressure readings, and too large a cuff yields spuriously low pressure readings.
‡Many premature infants require mechanical ventilatory support, making their spontaneous respiratory rate less relevant.

airway obstruction, then maneuvers to relieve the obstruction should be instituted before the caregiver proceeds to evaluate the child's breathing (see under Recognition and Treatment of Respiratory Distress and Failure, Initial Management).

Assessment of breathing includes evaluation of the child's respiratory rate, respiratory effort, abnormal sounds, and pulse oximetry. Normal breathing appears comfortable, is quiet, and occurs at an age-appropriate rate. Abnormal respiratory rates include apnea and rates that are either too slow (bradypnea) or too fast (tachypnea). **Bradypnea and irregular respiratory patterns require urgent attention, as they are often signs of impending respiratory failure and apnea.** Signs of increased respiratory effort include nasal flaring, grunting, chest or neck muscle retractions, head bobbing, and "seesaw" respirations. Hemoglobin oxygen desaturation, as measured by pulse oximetry, often accompanies parenchymal lung disease apnea or airway obstruction. However, providers should keep in mind that adequate perfusion is required to produce a reliable oxygen saturation measurement. A child with low oxygen saturation is a child in distress. Central cyanosis is a sign of severe hypoxia and indicates an emergency need for oxygen and respiratory support.

CIRCULATION Cardiovascular function is assessed by evaluation of skin color and temperature, heart rate, heart rhythm, pulses, capillary refill time, and blood pressure. In nonhospital settings, much of the important information can be obtained without measuring the blood pressure; lack of blood pressure data should not prevent the provider for determining adequacy of circulation or implementing a lifesaving response. Mottling, pallor, delayed capillary refill, cyanosis, poor pulses, and cool extremities are all signs of diminished perfusion and compromised cardiac output. Tachycardia is the earliest and most reliable sign of shock, but is itself fairly nonspecific and should be correlated with other components of the exam, such as weakness, threadiness, and absence of pulses. An age-specific approach to pulse assessment will yield best results.

DISABILITY In the setting of a pediatric emergency, *disability* refers to a child's neurologic function in terms of the level of consciousness and cortical function. Standard evaluation of a child's neurologic condition can be done quickly with an assessment of pupillary response to light (if one is available) and use of either of the standard scores used in pediatrics: the Alert, Verbal, Pain, Unresponsive (AVPU) Pediatric Response Scale and the Glasgow Coma Scale (GCS) (Tables 62-2 and 62-3). The causes of decreased level of consciousness in children are numerous and include conditions as diverse as respiratory failure with hypoxia or hypercarbia, hypoglycemia, poisonings or drug overdose, trauma, seizures, infection, and shock. **Most commonly, an ill or injured child has an altered level of consciousness because of respiratory compromise, circulatory compromise, or both.** Any child with a depressed level of consciousness should be immediately assessed for abnormalities in cardiorespiratory status.

The Alert, Verbal, Pain, Unresponsive Pediatric Response Scale The AVPU scoring system is used to determine both a child's level of consciousness and cerebral cortex function. Unlike the GCS (see later), the AVPU scale is not developmentally dependent—a child does not have to understand spoken language or follow commands, merely respond to a stimulus. The child is scored according to the amount of stimulus required to get a response, from alert (no stimulus, the child is already awake and interactive) to unresponsive (child does not respond to any stimulus) (see Table 62-2).

The Glasgow Coma Scale Although the GCS has not been validated as a prognostic scoring system for infants and young children as it has been in adults, it is commonly used in the assessment of pediatric patients with an altered level of consciousness. The GCS is the most widely used method of evaluating a child's neurologic function and has 3 components. Individual scores for eye opening, verbal response, and motor response are added together, with a maximum of 15 points (see Table 62-3). Patients with a GCS score ≤8 require aggressive management, including stabilization of the airway and breathing with endotracheal intubation and mechanical ventilation, respectively, and, if indicated, placement of an intracranial pressure monitoring device.

EXPOSURE Exposure is the final component of the pediatric primary assessment. This component of the exam is reached only after the child's airway, breathing, and circulation have been assessed and determined to be stable or have been stabilized through simple interventions. In this setting, *exposure* stands for the dual responsibility of the provider to both expose the child to assess for previously unidentified injures and consider prolonged exposure in a cold environment as a possible cause of hypothermia and cardiopulmonary instability. The provider should undress the child (as is feasible and reasonable) to perform a focused physical exam, assessing for burns, bruising, bleeding, joint laxity, and fractures. If possible, the provider should assess the child's temperature. All maneuvers should be performed with careful maintenance of cervical spine precautions.

Table 62-2 AVPU NEUROLOGIC ASSESSMENT

A	The child is awake, alert, and interactive with parents and care providers
V	The child responds only if the care provider or parents call the child's name or speak loudly
P	The child responds only to painful stimuli, such as pinching the nail bed of a toe or finger
U	The child is unresponsive to all stimuli

From Ralston M, Hazinski MF, Zaritsky AL, et al, editors: *Pediatric advanced life support course guide and PALS provider manual: provider manual*, Dallas, 2007, American Heart Association.

Table 62-3 GLASGOW COMA SCALE

EYE OPENING (TOTAL POSSIBLE POINTS 4)			
Spontaneous	4		
To voice	3		
To pain	2		
None	1		
VERBAL RESPONSE (TOTAL POSSIBLE POINTS 5)			
OLDER CHILDREN		**INFANTS AND YOUNG CHILDREN**	
Oriented	5	Appropriate words; smiles, fixes, and follows	5
Confused	4	Consolable crying	4
Inappropriate	3	Persistently irritable	3
Incomprehensible	2	Restless, agitated	2
None	1	None	1
MOTOR RESPONSE (TOTAL POSSIBLE POINTS 6)			
Obeys	6		
Localizes pain	5		
Withdraws	4		
Flexion	3		
Extension	2		
None	1		

Adapted and modified from Teasdale G, Jennett B: Assessment of coma and impaired consciousness: a practical scale, *Lancet* 2:81–84, 1974.

Secondary Assessment

For care providers in community or outpatient settings, transfer of care of a child to emergency or hospital personnel may occur before a full secondary assessment is possible. However, before the child is removed from the scene and separated from witnesses or family, a brief history should be obtained for medical providers at the accepting facility. **The components of a secondary assessment include a focused history and focused physical exam.**

The history should be targeted to information that could explain cardiorespiratory or neurologic dysfunction and should take the form of a **SAMPLE history (Signs/symptoms, Allergies, Medications, Past medical history, timing of Last meal, and Events leading to this situation)**. Medical personnel not engaged in resuscitative efforts can be dispatched to elicit history from witnesses or relatives. The physical exam during the secondary assessment is a thorough head-to-toe exam, although the severity of the child's illness or injury could necessitate curtailing portions of the exam or postponing nonessential elements until a later time.

Tertiary Assessment

The tertiary assessment occurs in a hospital setting, where ancillary laboratory and radiographic assessments contribute to a thorough understanding of the child's condition. A basic blood chemistry profile, complete blood count, liver function tests, coagulation studies, and arterial blood gas analyses give fairly broad (but somewhat nonspecific) estimates of renal function, acid-base balance, cardiorespiratory function, and presence or absence of shock. Chest radiographs can be useful to evaluate both the heart and lungs, although more detailed estimates of heart function and cardiac output can be made with echocardiography. Arterial and central venous catheters can be placed to monitor arterial and central venous pressure (see under Vascular Access).

RECOGNITION AND TREATMENT OF RESPIRATORY DISTRESS AND FAILURE

The goals of initial management of respiratory distress or failure are to rapidly stabilize the child's airway and breathing and to identify the cause of the problem so that further therapeutic efforts can be appropriately directed.

Airway Obstruction

Children <5 yr old are particularly susceptible to foreign body aspiration and choking. Liquids are the most common cause of choking in infants, whereas small objects and food (e.g., grapes, nuts, hot dogs, candies) are the most common source of foreign bodies in the airways of toddlers and older children. A history consistent with foreign body aspiration is considered diagnostic. Any child in the proper setting with the sudden onset of choking, stridor, or wheezing has foreign body aspiration until proven otherwise.

Airway obstruction is treated with a sequential approach, starting with the head-tilt/chin-lift maneuver to open and support the airway, followed by inspection for a foreign body, and finger-sweep clearance or suctioning if one is visualized (Fig. 62-2). Blind suctioning or finger sweeps of the mouth **are not recommended.** A nasopharyngeal airway (NPA) or oropharyngeal airway (OPA) can be inserted for airway support, if indicated. A conscious child suspected of having a partial foreign body obstruction should be permitted to cough spontaneously until coughing is no longer effective, respiratory distress and stridor increase, or the child becomes unconscious.

If the child becomes unconscious, the child should be gently placed on the ground, supine. The provider should then open the airway with the head-tilt/chin-lift maneuver and attempt mouth-to-mouth ventilation (Figs. 62-3 and 62-4). If ventilation is unsuccessful, the airway is repositioned, and ventilation attempted again. If there is still no chest rise, attempts to remove a foreign body are indicated. In an infant <1 yr old, a combination of 5 back blows and 5 chest thrusts is administered (Fig. 62-5). After each cycle of back blows and chest thrusts, the child's mouth should be visually inspected for the presence of the foreign body. If identified within finger's reach, it should be removed with a gentle finger sweep. If no foreign body is visualized, ventilation is again attempted. If this is unsuccessful, the head is repositioned, and ventilation attempted again. If there is no chest rise, the series of back blows and chest thrusts is repeated.

For a conscious child >1 yr old, providers should give a series of 5 abdominal thrusts (Heimlich maneuver) with the child standing or sitting (Fig. 62-6); this should occur with the child lying down if unconscious (Fig. 62-7). After the abdominal thrusts, the airway is examined for a foreign body, which should be removed

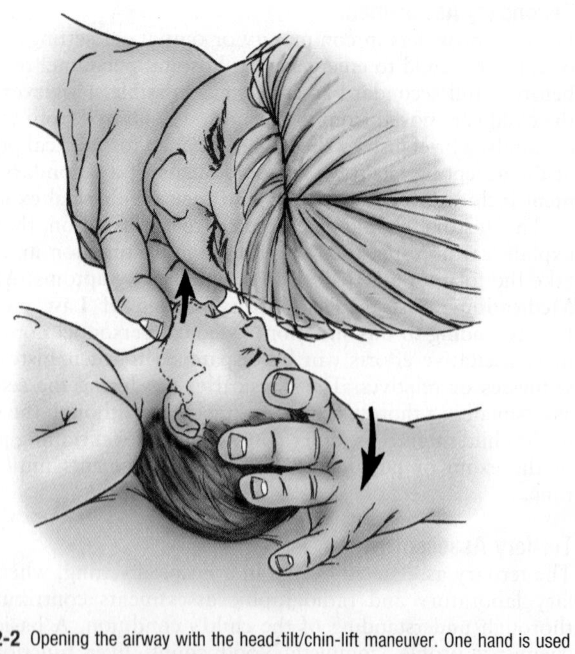

Figure 62-2 Opening the airway with the head-tilt/chin-lift maneuver. One hand is used to tilt the head, extending the neck. The index finger of the rescuer's other hand lifts the mandible outward by lifting the chin. Head-tilt should not be performed if a cervical spine injury is suspected. (From Guidelines for cardiopulmonary resuscitation and emergency cardiac care. Emergency Cardiac Care Committee and Subcommittees, American Heart Association. Part V. Pediatric basic life support, *JAMA* 268:2251–2261, 1992.)

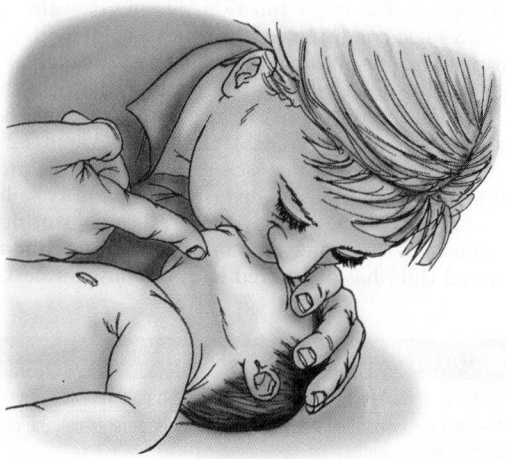

Figure 62-3 Rescue breathing in an infant. The rescuer's mouth covers the infant's nose and mouth, creating a seal. One hand performs the head-tilt while the other hand lifts the infant's jaw. Avoid head-tilt if the infant has sustained head or neck trauma. (From Guidelines for cardiopulmonary resuscitation and emergency cardiac care. Emergency Cardiac Care Committee and Subcommittees, American Heart Association. Part V. Pediatric basic life support, *JAMA* 268:2251–2261, 1992.)

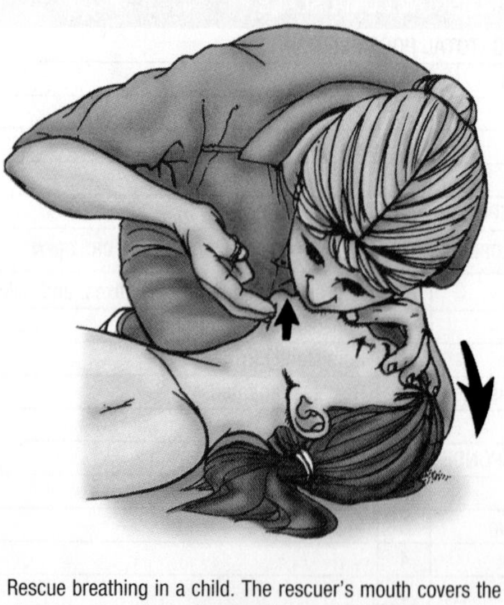

Figure 62-4 Rescue breathing in a child. The rescuer's mouth covers the child's mouth, creating a mouth-to-mouth seal. One hand maintains the head-tilt; the thumb and forefinger of the same hand are used to pinch the child's nose. (From Guidelines for cardiopulmonary resuscitation and emergency cardiac care. Emergency Cardiac Care Committee and Subcommittees, American Heart Association. Part V. Pediatric basic life support, *JAMA* 268:2251–2261, 1992.)

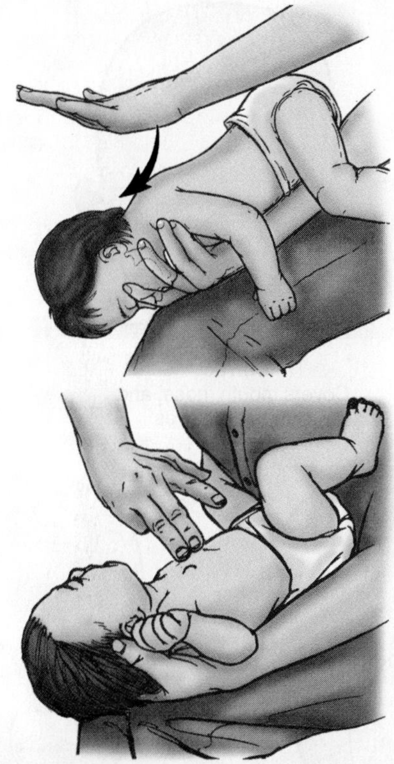

Figure 62-5 Back blows *(top)* and chest thrusts *(bottom)* to relieve foreign body airway obstruction in the infant. (From Guidelines for cardiopulmonary resuscitation and emergency cardiac care. Emergency Cardiac Care Committee and Subcommittees, American Heart Association. Part V. Pediatric basic life support, *JAMA* 268:2251–2261, 1992.)

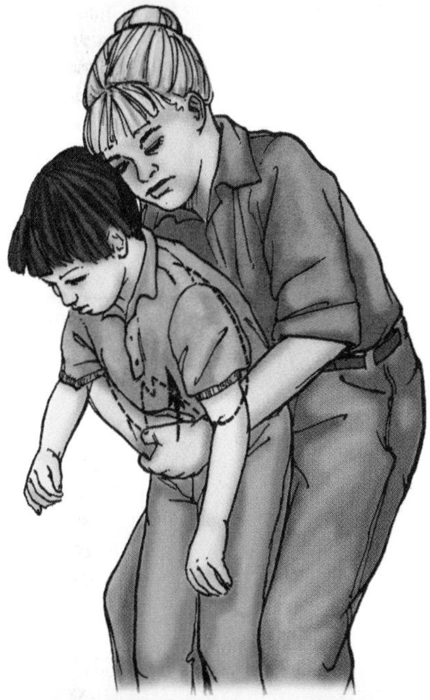

Figure 62-6 Abdominal thrusts with the victim standing or sitting (conscious). (From Guidelines for cardiopulmonary resuscitation and emergency cardiac care. Emergency Cardiac Care Committee and Subcommittees, American Heart Association. Part V. Pediatric basic life support, *JAMA* 268:2251–2261, 1992.)

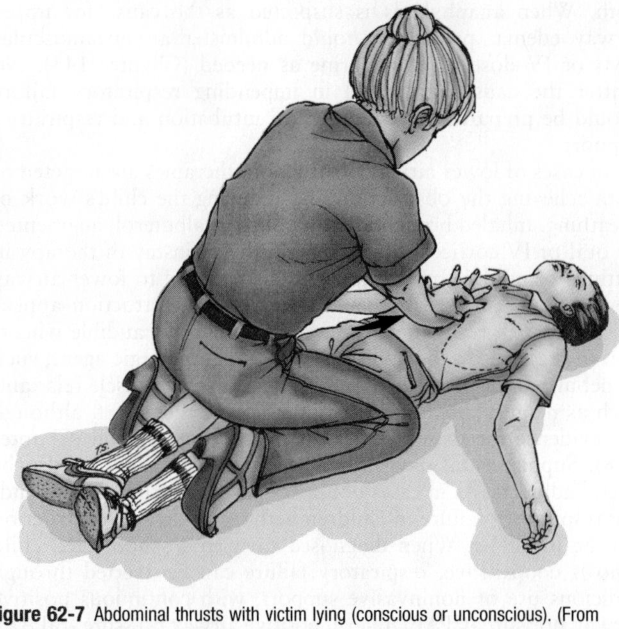

Figure 62-7 Abdominal thrusts with victim lying (conscious or unconscious). (From Guidelines for cardiopulmonary resuscitation and emergency cardiac care. Emergency Cardiac Care Committee and Subcommittees, American Heart Association. Part V. Pediatric basic life support, *JAMA* 268:2251–2261, 1992.)

if visualized. If no foreign body is seen, the head is repositioned, and ventilation attempted. If it is unsuccessful, the head is repositioned and ventilation is attempted again. If these efforts are unsuccessful, the Heimlich sequence is repeated.

Airway Narrowing

Airway obstruction can also be caused by airway narrowing, in both the upper and lower airways. *Upper airway obstruction* refers to narrowing of the extrathoracic portion of the airway, including the oropharynx, larynx, and trachea. In the upper airways, narrowing is most often caused by airway edema (croup or anaphylaxis). Lower airway disease affects all intrathoracic airways, notably the bronchi and bronchioles. In the lower airways, bronchiolitis and acute asthma exacerbations are the major contributors to intrathoracic airway obstruction in children, causing airway narrowing through a combination of airway swelling, mucus production, and circumferential smooth muscle constriction of smaller airways.

Airway support for these processes is dictated by both the underlying condition and the clinical severity of the problem. In cases of mild upper airway obstruction, the child has minimally elevated work of breathing (evidenced by tachypnea and few to mild retractions). Stridor, if present at all, should be audible with only coughing or activity. Children with these findings can be supported with nebulized cool mist and supplemental oxygen as needed. In cases with moderate obstruction, in which the child has a higher work of breathing and more pronounced stridor, nebulized racemic epinephrine and oral or intravenous (IV) dexamethasone can be added. Children with severe upper airway obstruction have marked retractions, prominent stridor, and decreased air entry on auscultation of the lung fields. Most children with significant airway obstruction are also hypoxic, and many appear dyspneic and agitated. A child in severe distress needs to be closely observed, as the signs of impending respiratory failure may be initially confused with improvement. Stridor becomes quieter and retractions less prominent when a child's respiratory effort begins to diminish. The child in respiratory failure can be distinguished from one who is improving by evidence of poor air movement on auscultation and lethargy or decreased level of consciousness from hypercarbia, hypoxia, or both. When anaphylaxis is suspected as the cause for upper airway edema, providers should administer an intramuscular (IM) or IV dose of epinephrine as needed (Chapter 143). No matter the cause, any child in impending respiratory failure should be prepared for endotracheal intubation and respiratory support.

In cases of lower airway obstruction, therapies are targeted to both relieving the obstruction and reducing the child's work of breathing. Inhaled bronchodilators, such as albuterol, augmented by oral or IV corticosteroids, remain the mainstay of therapy in settings of mild to moderate acute distress due to lower airway obstruction. Children with more significant obstruction appear dyspneic, with tachypnea, retractions, and easily audible wheezing. In these cases, the addition of an anticholinergic agent, such as nebulized ipratropium bromide, or a smooth muscle relaxant, such as magnesium sulfate, may provide further relief, although the evidence for these measures remains controversial (Chapter 138). Supplemental oxygen and IV fluid hydration can also be useful adjuncts. As in cases of upper airway obstruction, impending respiratory failure in children with lower airway obstruction can be insidious. When diagnosed early in a school-aged child who is cooperative, respiratory failure can be averted through judicious use of noninvasive support, with continuous positive airway pressure (CPAP), bilevel positive airway pressure (BiPAP), or heliox (combined helium-oxygen therapy). Endotracheal intubation should be performed only by skilled providers, preferably in a hospital setting, because there is a high risk of respiratory and circulatory compromise in patients with lower airway obstruction during the procedure.

Parenchymal Lung Disease

Parenchymal lung disease includes a heterogeneous list of conditions, such as pneumonia, acute respiratory distress syndrome, pneumonitis, bronchopulmonary dysplasia, cystic fibrosis, and pulmonary edema. The commonalities of these conditions are their effects on the alveoli, including inflammation and exudation leading to consolidation of lung tissue, decreased gas exchange, and increased work of breathing. Clinical management of these conditions includes specific treatment as indicated (i.e., antibiotics for bacterial pneumonia) and supportive care in the form of supplemental oxygen, noninvasive respiratory support (with CPAP or BiPAP), or invasive mechanical ventilation.

Advanced Airway Management Techniques

BAG-VALVE-MASK POSITIVE PRESSURE VENTILATION Rescue breathing with a bag-valve-mask apparatus can be as effective as endotracheal intubation and safer when the provider is inexperienced with intubation. Bag-valve-mask ventilation itself requires training to ensure that the provider is competent to select the correct mask size, open the child's airway, form a tight seal between the mask and the child's face, deliver effective ventilation, and assess the effectiveness of the ventilation. An appropriately sized mask is one that fits over the child's mouth and nose but does not extend below the chin or over the eyes (Fig. 62-8). An adequate seal is best achieved via a combination "C–E" grip on the mask, in which the thumb and index finger form the letter "C" on top of the mask, pressing the mask downward onto the child's face, and the remaining three fingers form an "E" grip under the child's mandible, holding the jaw forward and extending the head up toward the mask. Using this method, the care provider can secure the mask to the child's face with one hand and use the other hand to compress the ventilation bag (Fig. 62-9).

The provider may have to move the head and neck through a range of positions to find the one that best maintains airway patency and allows maximal ventilation. In infants and young children, optimal ventilation is often provided when the child's head is in the neutral "sniffing" position without hyperextension of the head (Fig. 62-10). Poor chest rise and persistently low

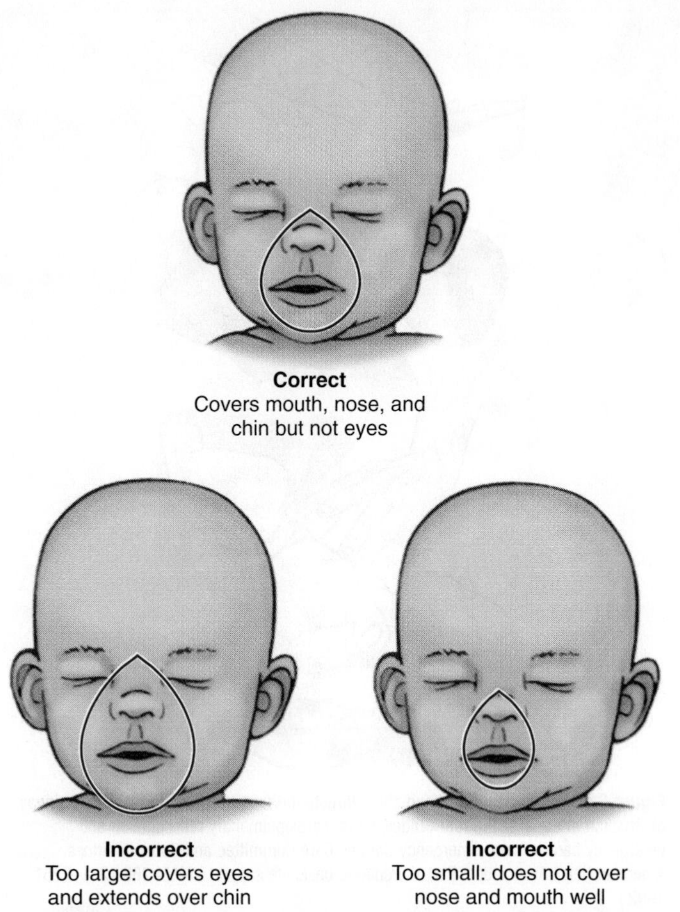

Figure 62-8 Appropriate sizing technique for pediatric bag-valve-mask apparatus. (From American Academy of Pediatrics and the American Heart Association; Short J, editor: *Textbook of neonatal resuscitation,* ed 5, Elk Grove, IL, American Academy of Pediatrics, 2006, pp 3–16.)

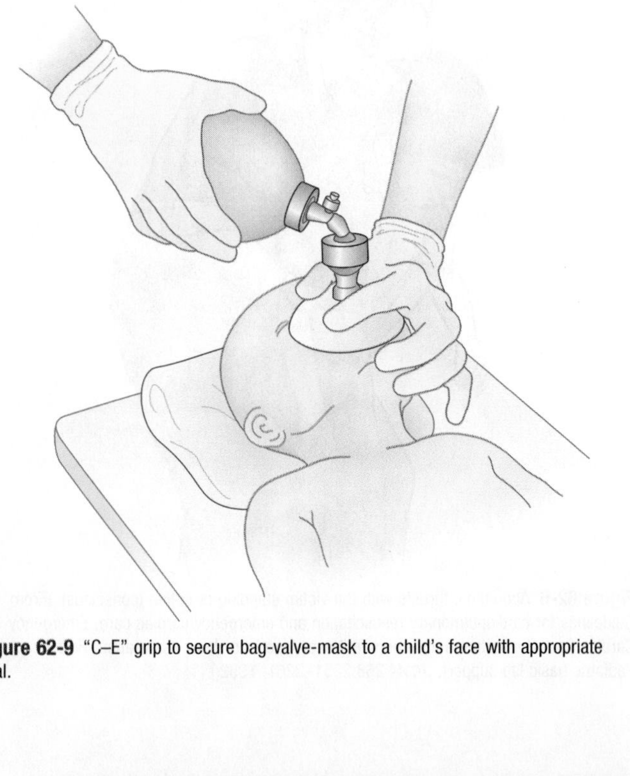

Figure 62-9 "C–E" grip to secure bag-valve-mask to a child's face with appropriate seal.

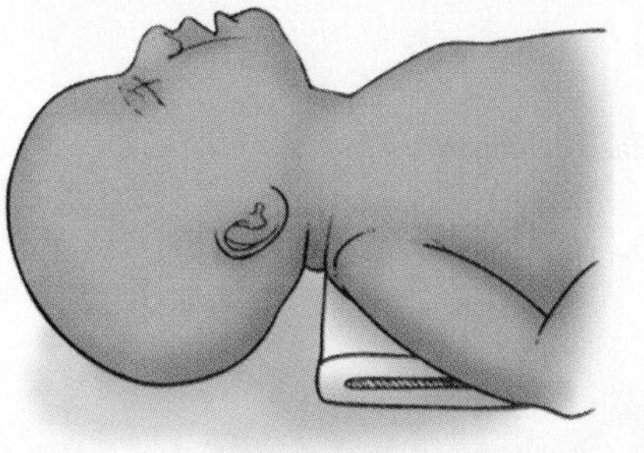

Figure 62-10 Appropriate head position for bag-valve-mask ventilation. (From American Academy of Pediatrics and the American Heart Association; Short J, editor: *Textbook of neonatal resuscitation*, ed 5, Elk Grove, IL, 2006, American Academy of Pediatrics, pp 3–18.)

oxygen saturation values indicate inadequate ventilation. In this setting, the care provider should recheck the mask's seal on the child's face, reposition the child's head, and consider suctioning the airway if indicated. If these maneuvers do not restore ventilation, then the provider should consider endotracheal intubation.

ENDOTRACHEAL INTUBATION A child requires intubation when at least one of these conditions exists: (1) the child is unable to maintain airway patency or protect the airway against aspiration (as occurs in settings of neurologic compromise), (2) the child is failing to maintain adequate oxygenation, (3) the child is failing to control blood carbon dioxide levels and maintain safe acid-base balance, (4) sedation and/or paralysis is required for a procedure, and (5) care providers anticipate a deteriorating course that will eventually lead to the first 4 conditions. There are few *absolute contraindications* to tracheal intubation, but experts generally agree that in settings of known complete airway obstruction, endotracheal intubation should be avoided, and emergency cricothyroidotomy performed instead. Another important consideration is to ensure that caregivers provide appropriate cervical spine protection during the intubation procedure when neck or spinal cord injury is suspected.

The most important phase of the intubation procedure is the preprocedure preparation, when the provider ensures all the equipment and staff needed for safe intubation are present and functioning. An easy pneumonic for this is **SOAP MM**: suction (Yankauer suction catheter attached to wall suction); oxygen (both preoxygenation of the patient and devices needed to deliver oxygen, such as a bag-valve-mask device); airway (appropriately sized endotracheal tube and laryngoscope); people (all those needed during and immediately after the procedure, such as respiratory therapists and nurses); monitor (to monitor the child's oxygen saturation, heart rate, and blood pressure); and medications (to sedate the child and allow the provider to control the airway). A simple formula for selecting the appropriately sized ET tube is as follows:

$$\text{Uncuffed ET size (in mm)} = \left(\frac{\text{age in years}}{4}\right) + 4$$

Analgesia is recommended to reduce metabolic stress, discomfort, and anxiety during intubation. Pretreatment with a sedative, an analgesic, and possibly a muscle relaxant is recommended unless the situation is an emergency (i.e., apnea, asystole, unresponsiveness) and the administration of drugs would cause an unacceptable delay.

Because many intubations in critically ill children are emergency procedures, caregivers should be prepared for rapid sequence intubation (RSI) (Fig. 62-11; Table 62-4). The goals of RSI are to induce anesthesia and paralysis and to complete intubation quickly. This approach minimizes elevations of intracranial pressure and blood pressure that may accompany intubation in awake or lightly sedated patients. Because the stomach generally cannot be emptied before RSI, the Sellick maneuver (downward pressure on the cricoid cartilage to compress the esophagus against the vertebral column) should be used to prevent aspiration of gastric contents.

Once the patient is intubated, proper tube placement should be assessed by auscultation of breath sounds, evidence of symmetric chest rise, and analysis of exhaled carbon dioxide (CO_2) by a colorimetric device placed within the respiratory tubing near the endotracheal tube or a device that directly measures carbon dioxide elimination (i.e., capnogram or capnograph). Chest radiography is necessary to confirm appropriate tube position.

RECOGNITION AND MANAGEMENT OF SHOCK

In simple terms, shock occurs when oxygen and nutrient delivery to the tissues is inadequate to meet metabolic demands (Chapter 64). The definition of shock does not include hypotension, and it is important for care providers to understand that **shock does not begin when blood pressure drops but merely worsens and becomes more difficult to treat once blood pressure is abnormal.**

Early *compensated* shock, whereby oxygen delivery is mostly preserved through compensatory mechanisms, is defined by the presence of normal blood pressure. When compensatory mechanisms fail, the shock progresses to *decompensated* shock, which is defined by hypotension and organ dysfunction. In *irreversible* shock, organ failure progresses and death ensues.

Shock is also often described according to the underlying pathophysiology, which dictates the appropriate therapeutic response. *Hypovolemic shock* is the most common type of shock in children worldwide, usually related to fluid losses from severe diarrhea. Hemorrhage is a cause of hypovolemic shock after trauma or intestinal hemorrhage. When hypovolemia occurs as a result of third spacing of intravascular fluids into the extravascular compartment, the shock is described as *distributive shock*. The most common causes of distributive shock are sepsis and burn injuries, in which release of inflammatory cytokines causes massive capillary leak of fluid and proteins, leading to low oncotic pressure and intravascular volume. In settings of profound myocardial dysfunction, a child has tissue hypoperfusion from *cardiogenic shock*. The most common causes of cardiogenic shock are congenital heart disease, myocarditis, and cardiomyopathies. *Obstructive shock* occurs when cardiac output is lowered by obstruction of blood flow to the body, as occurs when a ductus arteriosus closes in a child with ductus-dependent systemic blood flow in pericardial tamponade, tension pneumothorax, or massive pulmonary embolism.

The evaluation of a child in shock should proceed as described in the preceding sections on primary, secondary, and tertiary assessments. If the child presents in a hospital setting, providers should obtain central venous and arterial access to permit a more thorough laboratory assessment of all organ systems, including studies of renal and liver function, acid-base balance and presence of lactic acidosis, hypoxemia and/or hypercapnia, and evidence of coagulopathy or disseminated intravascular coagulation (DIC). Chest radiography and more sophisticated assessments, such as echocardiography, may also be useful. Respiratory and cardiovascular support should be provided as indicated.

The treatment of shock focuses on the modifiable determinants of oxygen delivery while reducing the imbalance between oxygen demand and supply. A multipronged approach is recommended; it consists of optimizing the oxygen content of the blood, improving the volume and distribution of cardiac output, correcting metabolic derangements, and reducing oxygen demand. Blood oxygen content is maximized when hemoglobin values are normal and 100% of available hemoglobin is saturated with oxygen. Transfusion should be considered in the presence of hemorrhagic or distributive shock, in which crystalloid volume resuscitation has led to hemodilution and anemia. High oxygen

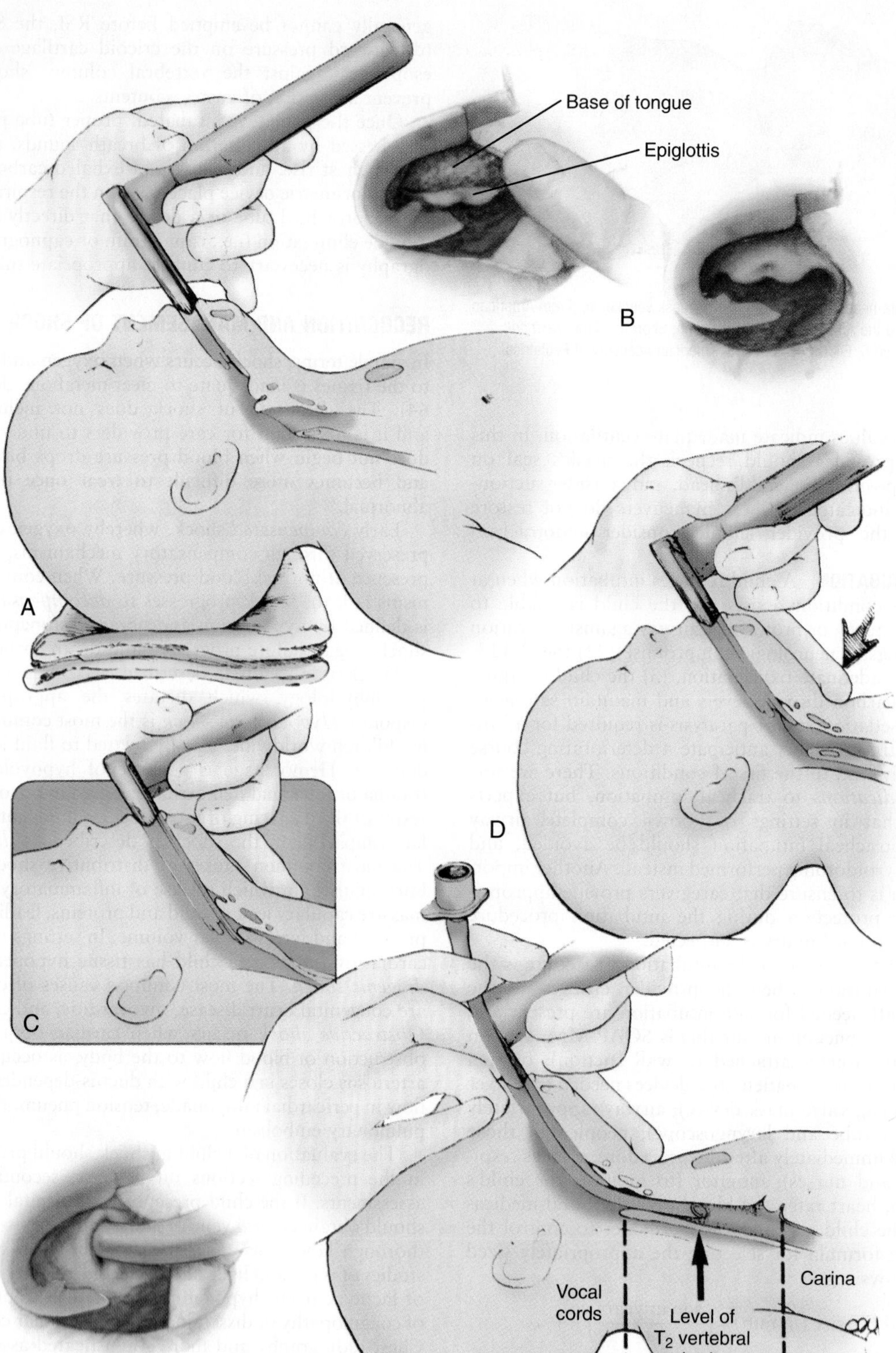

Figure 62-11 *A-E,* Intubation technique. (From Fleisher G, Ludwig S: *Textbook of pediatric emergency medicine.* Baltimore, 1983, Williams & Wilkins, p 1250.)

saturations may be achieved by simple maneuvers such as oxygen administration via nasal cannula or face mask, but supportive measures that provide positive pressure, such as CPAP, BiPAP, or even mechanical ventilation, may be necessary. Therapies to increase cardiac output should be selected on the basis of underlying pathophysiology. For hypovolemic and distributive shock, aggressive volume resuscitation, guided by arterial and central venous pressures, is the mainstay of therapy. In obstructive shock, relief of the obstruction is critical. The ductus arteriosus can often be reopened with prostaglandin administration, and tamponade physiology can be relieved with appropriate drain placement, as described under Nonvascular Emergency Procedures.

Table 62-4 RAPID SEQUENCE INTUBATION

STEP	PROCEDURE	COMMENT/EXPLANATION
1	Obtain a brief history and perform an assessment	Rule out drug allergies; examine the airway anatomy (e.g., micrognathia, cleft palate)
2	Assemble equipment, medications, etc.	See lists below
3	Preoxygenate the patient	With bag/mask, nasal cannula, hood or blow-by
4	Premedicate the patient with lidocaine, atropine	Lidocaine minimizes the ICP rise with intubation and can be applied topically to the airway mucosa for local anesthesia
		Atropine helps blunt the bradycardia associated with upper airway manipulation and reduces airway secretions
5	Induce sedation and analgesia	Sedatives:
		Thiopental (2-5 mg/kg): Very rapid onset; can cause hypotension.
		Diazepam (0.1 mg/kg): Onset 2-5 min; elimination in 30-60 min or more.
		Ketamine (2 mg/kg): Onset 1-2 min; elimination in 30-40 min. May cause hallucinations if used alone; causes higher ICP, mucous secretions, increased vital signs, and bronchodilation.
		Analgesics:
		Fentanyl (3-10 µg/kg, may repeat 3-4×): Rapid administration risks "tight chest" response, with no effective ventilation. Effects wear off in 20-30 min.
		Morphine (0.05-0.1 mg/kg dose): May last 30-60 min; may lead to hypotension in hypovolemic patients.
6	Pretreat with nondepolarizing paralytic agent	Small dose of a nondepolarizing paralytic agent (see below), with intent of diminishing the depolarizing effect of succinylcholine, which is administered next
7	Administer muscle relaxants	Succinylcholine dose is 1-2 mg/kg; causes initial contraction of muscles, then relaxation. This depolarization can, however, raise ICP and blood pressure. Onset of paralysis in 30-40 sec; duration is 5-10 min.
		Increased use of pretreatment with a nondepolarizing muscle relaxant, especially rocuronium (1 mg/kg), which has a very rapid onset and short duration. Other nondepolarizing agents include vecuronium and pancuronium, both dosed at 0.1 mg/kg.
8	Perform a Sellick maneuver	Pressure on the cricoid cartilage, to occlude the esophagus and prevent regurgitation or aspiration
9	Perform endotracheal intubation	ET: Select the proper size for the age and weight of the child
		Laryngoscope blades: A variety of Miller and the Macintosh blades
		Patient supine; the neck is extended moderately to the "sniffing" position
10	Secure the tube and verify the position with a roentgenogram	ET secured with tape to the cheeks and upper lip or to an adhesive patch applied to the skin near the mouth.
11	Begin mechanical ventilation	Verify tube placement before ventilating with positive pressure; if an ET tube is in one bronchus, barotraumas may occur

ET, endotracheal tube; ICP, intracranial pressure.

RECOGNITION OF BRADYARRHYTHMIAS AND TACHYARRHYTHMIAS

In the advanced life support setting, arrhythmias are most usefully classified according to the observed heart rate (slow or fast) and its effect on perfusion (adequate or poor). If, in the primary survey, a caregiver finds a child with an abnormal heart rate plus poor perfusion and/or altered mental status, then the rhythm is inadequate no matter its rate. In those settings, the child is diagnosed with shock, and further evaluation is halted until appropriate resuscitation has been initiated.

Bradyarrhythmias

By definition, a child is *bradycardic* when the heart rate is slower than the normal range for age (see Table 62-1). Sinus bradycardia can be a harmless incidental finding in an otherwise healthy person and is not commonly associated with cardiac compromise. A relative bradycardia occurs when the heart rate is too slow for a child's activity level or metabolic needs. A clinically significant bradycardia occurs when the heart rate is slow and there are signs of systemic hypoperfusion (i.e., pallor, altered mental status, hypotension, acidosis). Symptomatic bradycardia occurs most often in the setting of hypoxia but can also be caused by hypoglycemia, hypocalcemia, other electrolyte abnormalities, and intracranial hypertension. Bradyarrhythmias are often the most common pre-arrest rhythms in young children.

Initial management of symptomatic bradycardia includes support or opening of the airway and confirming or establishing adequate oxygenation and ventilation (Fig. 62-12). After the child's breathing has been secured, the child should be reassessed for continued bradycardia and poor perfusion—if cardiac compromise was solely the result of respiratory insufficiency, support of the child's airway and breathing may have been sufficient to restore normal hemodynamics. If respiratory support does not correct the perfusion abnormalities, then further care is based on the quality of perfusion and the degree of bradycardia. **A heart rate less than 60 beats/min with poor perfusion is an indication to begin chest compressions.** If the child's heart rate is above 60 beats/min, vascular access should be obtained; resuscitative epinephrine should be administered, and it should be repeated every 3-5 min for persistent symptomatic bradycardia. If increased vagal tone (e.g., in the setting of head injury with raised intracranial pressure) or primary atrioventricular block is suspected, atropine can also be given. For cases of refractory bradycardia, cardiac pacing should be considered. During the resuscitation of a child with bradycardia, providers should assess and treat factors known to cause bradycardia, referred to collectively as the **6 Hs** (hypoxia, hypovolemia, hydrogen ions [acidosis], hypokalemia or hyperkalemia, hypoglycemia, hypothermia), and **4 Ts** (toxins, tamponade, tension pneumothorax, and trauma [causing hypovolemia, intracranial hypertension, cardiac compromise or tamponade]) (Table 62-5).

Tachyarrhythmias

Tachyarrhythmias represent a variety of rhythm disturbances of both atrial and ventricular origin. Sinus tachycardia is a normal physiologic response to the body's need for increased cardiac output or oxygen delivery, as occurs with fever, exercise, or stress. It can also occur in more pathologic states, such as hypovolemia, anemia, pain, anxiety, and metabolic stress. Tachyarrhythmias

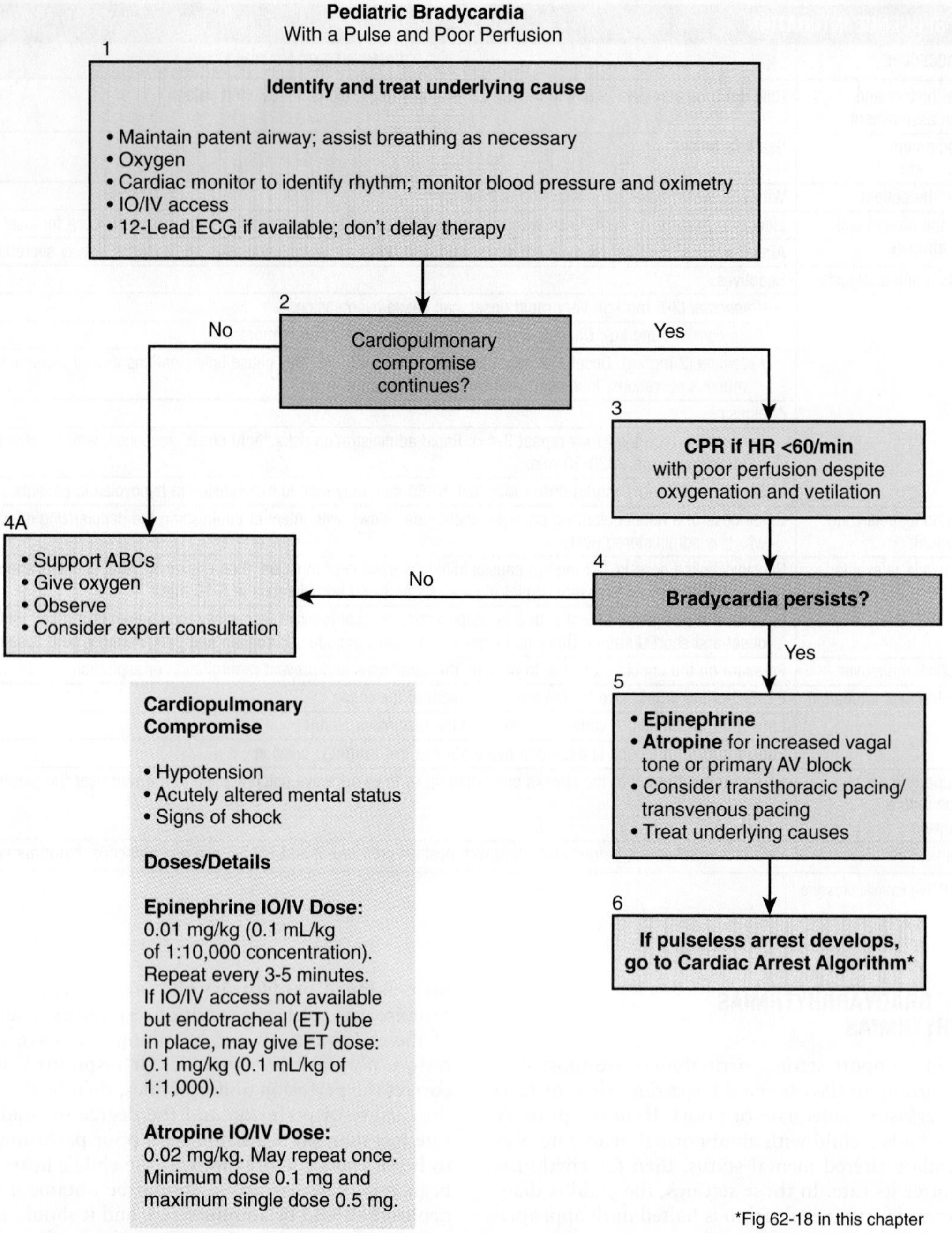
Pediatric Bradycardia
With a Pulse and Poor Perfusion
1
Identify and treat underlying cause
• Maintain patent airway; assist breathing as necessary
• Oxygen
• Cardiac monitor to identify rhythm; monitor blood pressure and oximetry
• IO/IV access
• 12-Lead ECG if available; don't delay therapy
2
Cardiopulmonary compromise continues?
No
Yes
3
CPR if HR <60/min
with poor perfusion despite oxygenation and vetilation
4A
• Support ABCs
• Give oxygen
• Observe
• Consider expert consultation
4
Bradycardia persists?
No
Yes
5
• Epinephrine
• Atropine for increased vagal tone or primary AV block
• Consider transthoracic pacing/ transvenous pacing
• Treat underlying causes
6
If pulseless arrest develops, go to Cardiac Arrest Algorithm*
Cardiopulmonary Compromise
• Hypotension
• Acutely altered mental status
• Signs of shock
Doses/Details
Epinephrine IO/IV Dose:
0.01 mg/kg (0.1 mL/kg of 1:10,000 concentration). Repeat every 3-5 minutes. If IO/IV access not available but endotracheal (ET) tube in place, may give ET dose: 0.1 mg/kg (0.1 mL/kg of 1:1,000).
Atropine IO/IV Dose:
0.02 mg/kg. May repeat once. Minimum dose 0.1 mg and maximum single dose 0.5 mg.
*Fig 62-18 in this chapter

Figure 62-12 Pediatric advanced life support bradycardia algorithm. ABCs, airway, breathing, and circulation; AV, atrioventricular (conductor); ECG, electrocardiogram; HR, heart rate. (From Kleinman ME, Chameides L, Schexnayder SM, et al: 2010 American Heart Association guidelines for cardiopulmonary resuscitation and emergency cardiovascular care, part 14, *Circulation* 122 [suppl 3]:S876–S908, 2010, Fig 2, p S887.)

that do not originate in the sinus node are often categorized as narrow complex rhythms (those originating in the atrium, such as atrial flutter or supraventricular tachycardia [SVT]) and wide complex rhythms (those rhythms of ventricular origin, such as ventricular tachycardia).

As in the bradycardia algorithm, the initial management of tachycardia includes confirmation that the child has an adequate airway and life-sustaining breathing and circulation (Fig. 62-13). For children with persistent symptoms, further treatment is based on whether the QRS complex of the electrocardiogram (ECG) is narrow (≤0.08 sec) or wide (>0.08 sec). For narrow complex tachycardia, providers must distinguish between sinus tachycardia and SVT. In sinus tachycardia, (1) the history and onset are consistent with a known cause of tachycardia, such as fever or dehydration and (2) P waves are consistently present, are of normal morphology, and occur at a rate that varies somewhat. In SVT, (1) onset is often abrupt without prodrome and (2) P waves are absent or polymorphic, and when present, their rate is often fairly steady at or above 220 beats/min. For children with SVT and good perfusion, vagal maneuvers can be attempted. In cases in which SVT is associated with poor perfusion, providers should rapidly move to convert the child's heart rhythm back to sinus rhythm. If the child already has IV access, then adenosine can be given via IV with rapid "push." Adenosine has an extremely short half-life, so a proximal IV is best, and the adenosine should be set up with a three-way stopcock so it can be given and immediately flushed into the circulation. If the child does not have IV access, or adenosine does not successfully convert the

Table 62-5 POTENTIALLY TREATABLE CONDITIONS ASSOCIATED WITH CARDIAC ARREST

CONDITION	COMMON CLINICAL SETTINGS	CORRECTIVE ACTIONS
Acidosis	Pre-existing acidosis, diabetes, diarrhea, drugs and toxins, prolonged resuscitation, renal disease, and shock	Reassess the adequacy of cardiopulmonary resuscitation, oxygenation, and ventilation; reconfirm endotracheal tube placement Hyperventilate Consider intravenous bicarbonate if pH <7.20 after above actions have been taken
Cardiac tamponade	Hemorrhagic diathesis, cancer, pericarditis, trauma, after cardiac surgery, and after myocardial infarction	Administer fluids; obtain bedside echocardiogram, if available Perform pericardiocentesis; immediate surgical intervention is appropriate if pericardiocentesis is unhelpful but cardiac tamponade is known or highly suspected
Hypothermia	Alcohol abuse, burns, central nervous system disease, debilitated patient, drowning, drugs and toxins, endocrine disease, history of exposure, homelessness, extensive skin disease, spinal cord disease, and trauma	If hypothermia is severe (temperature <30°C), limit initial shocks for ventricular fibrillation or pulseless ventricular tachycardia to 3; initiate active internal rewarming and cardiopulmonary support; hold further resuscitation medications or shocks until core temperature is >30°C If hypothermia is moderate (temperature 30-34°C), proceed with resuscitation (space medications at longer intervals than usual), passively rewarm child, and actively rewarm truncal body areas
Hypovolemia, hemorrhage, anemia	Major burns, diabetes, gastrointestinal losses, hemorrhage, hemorrhagic diathesis, cancer, pregnancy, shock, and trauma	Administer fluids Transfuse packed red blood cells if hemorrhage or profound anemia is present Thoracotomy is appropriate when a patient has cardiac arrest from penetrating trauma and a cardiac rhythm and the duration of cardiopulmonary resuscitation before thoracotomy is <10 min
Hypoxia	Consider in all patients with cardiac arrest	Reassess the technical quality of cardiopulmonary resuscitation, oxygenation, and ventilation; reconfirm endotracheal tube placement
Hypomagnesemia	Alcohol abuse, burns, diabetic ketoacidosis, severe diarrhea, diuretics, and drugs (e.g., cisplatin, cyclosporine, pentamidine)	Administer 1-2 g magnesium sulfate IV over 2 min
Poisoning	Alcohol abuse, bizarre or puzzling behavioral or metabolic presentation, classic toxicologic syndrome, occupational or industrial exposure, and psychiatric disease	Consult a toxicologist for emergency advice on resuscitation and definitive care, including an appropriate antidote Prolonged resuscitation efforts may be appropriate; immediate cardiopulmonary bypass should be considered, if available
Hyperkalemia	Metabolic acidosis, excessive administration of potassium, drugs and toxins, vigorous exercise, hemolysis, renal disease, rhabdomyolysis, tumor lysis syndrome, and clinically significant tissue injury	If hyperkalemia is identified or strongly suspected, treat* with all of the following: 10% calcium chloride (5-10 mL by slow IV push; do not use if hyperkalemia is secondary to digitalis poisoning), glucose and insulin (50 mL of 50% dextrose in water and 10 units of regular insulin IV), sodium bicarbonate (50 mmol IV; most effective if concomitant metabolic acidosis is present), and albuterol (15-20 mg nebulized or 0.5 mg by IV infusion)
Hypokalemia	Alcohol abuse, diabetes, use of diuretics, drugs and toxins, profound gastrointestinal losses, hypomagnesemia	If profound hypokalemia (<2-2.5 mmol of potassium V) is accompanied by cardiac arrest, initiate urgent IV replacement (2 mmol/min IV for 10-15 mmol)*; then reassess
Pulmonary embolism	Hospitalized patient, recent surgical procedure, peripartum, known risk factors for venous thromboembolism, history of venous thromboembolism, or pre-arrest presentation consistent with a diagnosis of acute pulmonary embolism	Administer fluids; augment with vasopressors as necessary Confirm the diagnosis, if possible; consider immediate cardiopulmonary bypass to maintain patient's viability Consider definitive care (e.g., thrombolytic therapy, embolectomy by interventional radiology or surgery)
Tension pneumothorax	Placement of a central catheter, mechanical ventilation, pulmonary disease (including asthma, chronic obstructive pulmonary disease, and necrotizing pneumonia), thoracentesis, and trauma	Needle decompression, followed by chest tube insertion

*Adult dose. Adjust for size of child. See Table 62-6.
IV, intravenously.
From Eisenbery MS, Mengert TJ: Cardiac resuscitation, *N Engl J Med* 344:1304–1313, 2001.

heart rhythm back to sinus rhythm, then **synchronized cardioversion**, using 0.5-1 joule/kg, should be performed. In cases of wide complex tachycardia, providers should move immediately to cardioversion and increase the dose to 2 joules/kg if 1 joule/kg is not effective. As with cases of bradycardia, providers should review the 6 Hs and 4 Ts to identify factors that might be contributing to the tachycardia (see Table 62-5).

RECOGNITION AND MANAGEMENT OF CARDIAC ARREST

Cardiac arrest occurs when the heart fails as an effective pump and blood flow ceases. Outwardly, the patient in cardiac arrest presents as unresponsive and apneic with no palpable pulse. Internally, the cessation of nutrient flow causes progressive tissue ischemia and organ dysfunction. If not rapidly reversed, cardiac arrest leads to progressive deterioration in brain and heart function such that resuscitation and recovery are no longer possible.

Pediatric cardiac arrest is rarely the cause of a sudden coronary event or arrhythmia. Instead, cardiac arrest in children is most often the end result of progressive asphyxia, caused by tissue hypoxia, acidosis, and nutrient depletion at the end stages of respiratory deterioration, shock, or heart failure. Therefore, **the most important treatment of cardiac arrest is anticipation and preventive: Intervening when a child manifests respiratory distress or early stages of shock can prevent deterioration to full-blown arrest.** When sudden cardiac arrest does occur, it is most often associated with an arrhythmia, specifically ventricular fibrillation (VF) or pulseless ventricular tachycardia (VT). In sudden events such as these, the key to successful resuscitation is early recognition of the arrhythmia and prompt treatment with high-quality CPR and defibrillation.

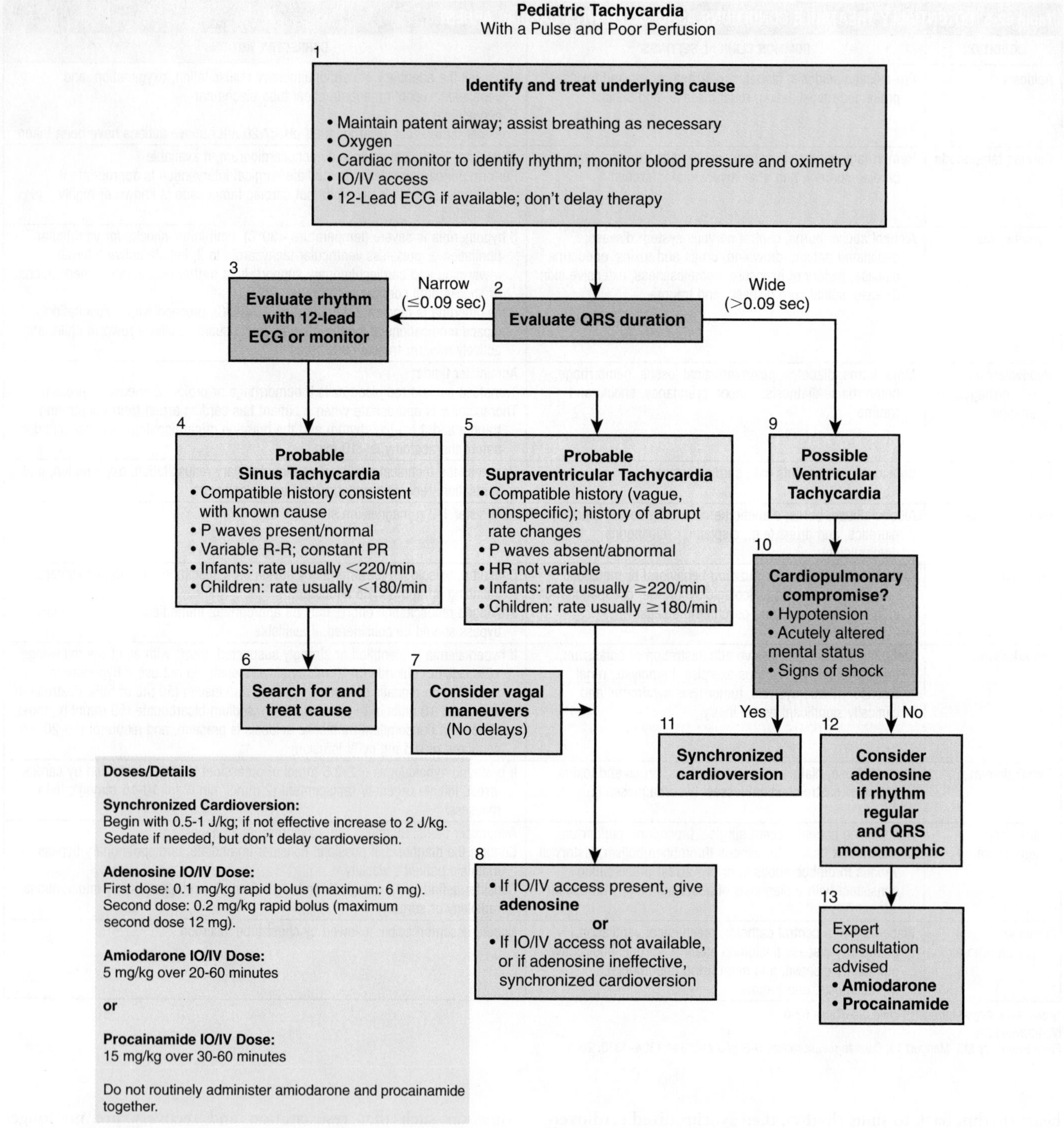

Figure 62-13 Pediatric advanced life support tachycardia algorithm. AV, atrioventricular (conductor); ECG, electrocardiogram; HR, heart rate. (From Kleinman ME, Chameides L, Schexnayder SM, et al: 2010 American Heart Association guidelines for cardiopulmonary resuscitation and emergency cardiovascular care, part 14, *Circulation* 122 [suppl 3]:S876–S908, 2010, Fig 3, p S888.)

The principle behind high-quality CPR is that adequate chest compressions—those that circulate blood around the body with a good pulse pressure—are the most important component of CPR. The caregiver providing chest compressions should push hard, push fast, allow for complete chest recoil, and minimize interruptions. Ideally, chest compressions should be interrupted only for ventilation, a rhythm check, or delivery of a defibrillating shock.

Cardiac arrest is recognized from general and primary survey findings consistent with a pale or cyanotic child who is unresponsive, apneic, and pulseless. Even experienced providers have a relatively high error rate when asked to determine presence or absence of pulse in a child. Therefore, any child found unresponsive and apneic can be presumed to be in cardiac arrest, and a rescuer should respond accordingly. **A lone rescuer for an unwitnessed pediatric cardiac arrest in an outpatient setting should treat the arrest as asphyxial in nature and should immediately initiate CPR.** The rescuer should perform initial rescue breaths and 2 min of chest compressions and ventilations before leaving the child to activate the emergency response system. For

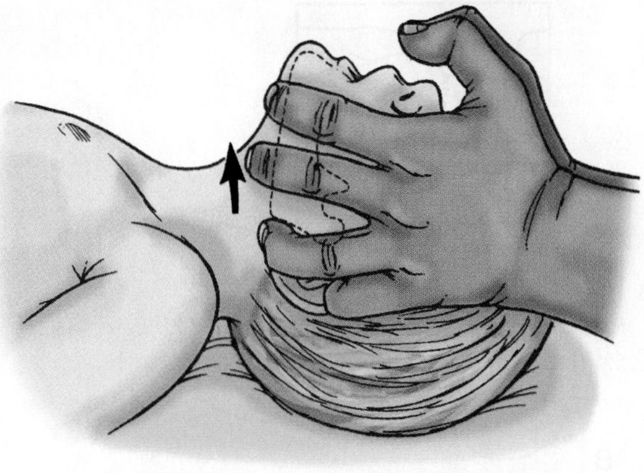

Figure 62-14 Combined jaw-thrust/spine stabilization maneuver for the pediatric trauma victim. (From Guidelines for cardiopulmonary resuscitation and emergency cardiac care. Emergency Cardiac Care Committee and Subcommittees, American Heart Association. Part V. Pediatric basic life support, *JAMA* 268:2251–2261, 1992.)

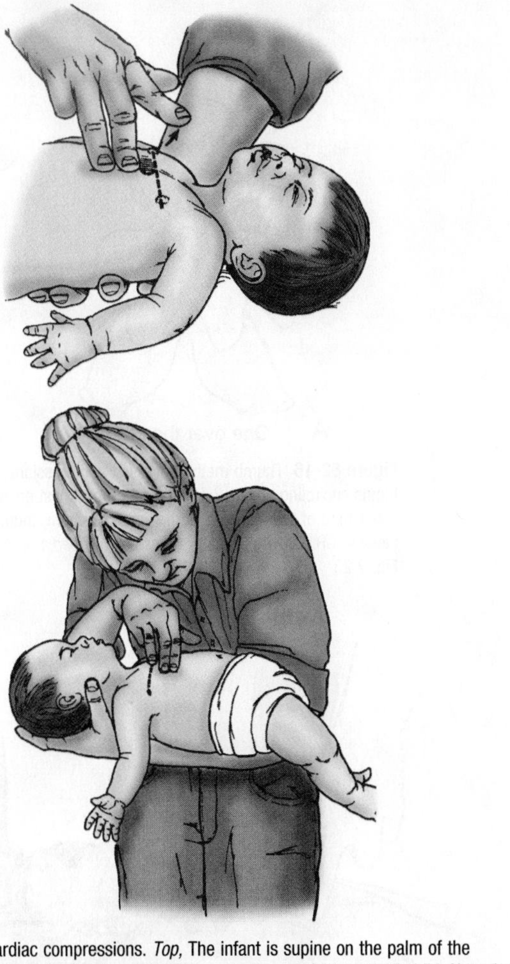

Figure 62-15 Cardiac compressions. *Top,* The infant is supine on the palm of the rescuer's hand. *Bottom,* Performing CPR while carrying an infant or small child. Note that the head is kept level with the torso. (From Guidelines for cardiopulmonary resuscitation and emergency cardiac care. Emergency Cardiac Care Committee and Subcommittees, American Heart Association. Part V. Pediatric basic life support, *JAMA* 268:2251–2261, 1992.)

an in-hospital arrest, the provider should call for help and send someone else to activate the emergency response system while beginning CPR. **A lone rescuer in an outpatient setting who witnesses a child suddenly collapse should treat the arrest as a primary arrhythmia, should immediately activate the EMS system, and should obtain an AED.** Upon returning to the child, the rescuer should confirm pulselessness, turn on the AED, place the leads on the child's chest, and follow the defibrillator's voice commands.

The initial step in CPR for a child of any age is to restore ventilation and oxygenation as quickly as possible. Upon confirmation of unresponsiveness, apnea, and pulselessness, the provider should open the airway with a head-tilt/chin-lift maneuver (or jaw-thrust if cervical spine trauma is suspected) and provide 2 initial rescue breaths (Fig. 62-14). These breaths are deep and slow, lasting approximately 1 sec per breath. The breaths are adequate if they cause the chest to rise and fall and improve the child's color. If the breaths appear inadequate, the child should be repositioned, and the breaths delivered again. If the breaths remain ineffective, the provider should assess the child for foreign body aspiration. After 2 effective rescue breaths, the child's pulse should be assessed. If the child has a pulse but remains apneic (or with ineffective breathing), then the rescuer should continue to provide assisted ventilation at an age-appropriate rate. Infants and children ≤8 yr old should receive rescue breathing at a rate of roughly 15-20 breaths/min, or roughly 1 breath every 3-5 sec. Children >8 yr old should receive 10-12 breaths/min, or 1 breath every 5-6 sec.

If the child remains pulseless, chest compressions should be initiated. Chest compressions in infants <1 yr old may be performed by placing 2 thumbs on the midsternum with the hands encircling the thorax or by placing 2 fingers over the midsternum and compressing (Figs. 62-15 and 62-16). For children >1 yr old, the care provider should perform chest compressions over the lower half of the sternum with the heel of 1 hand, or with 2 hands as used for adult resuscitation (Fig. 62-17). In all cases, care should be taken to avoid compression of the xiphoid and the ribs. When feasible, a cardiac resuscitation board should be placed under the child's back to maximize the efficiency of compressions. When a lone rescuer provides CPR, the universal ratio of 30 compressions to 2 ventilations is used. Pediatric patients in cardiac arrest are thought to have the best chance of survival if more frequent ventilation is offered. Therefore, the ratio should be lowered to 15 compressions to 2 ventilations for children ≤8 yr old as soon as a second care provider is available. In the outpatient setting, resuscitation effort should pause periodically to allow the provider to make an assessment of the possible return of spontaneous heart rate, pulse, and respirations. The goal of CPR is to re-establish spontaneous circulation at a level that is compatible with survival. If resuscitative efforts do not succeed in re-establishing life-sustaining breathing and circulation, the medical team must decide whether continued efforts are warranted or whether the resuscitation should be stopped. If EMS care is en route, bringing the potential for further escalation in care such as endotracheal intubation, vascular access, and medications, CPR should be continued as long as possible or deemed reasonable by the rescuers.

In the in-hospital setting, the ECG should dictate further resuscitative efforts. For children without a pulse and in asystole or electromechanical dissociation (pulseless electrical activity [PEA]), providers should continue rescue breathing and CPR, obtain vascular access, and give emergency IV epinephrine (Fig. 62-18). For continued asystole or PEA, epinephrine can be repeated every 3-5 min. Patient history, physical exam findings, and laboratory evaluation should be used to elicit correctable causes of arrest (such as the 6 Hs and 4 Ts) (see Table 62-5). CPR should be continued after epinephrine administration, to circulate the drug through the body. After 5 cycles of CPR, providers should reassess the child for the presence of a pulse or a change in the ECG rhythm that would necessitate a different response.

For those children with pulseless VT or VF, emergency defibrillation is indicated (see Fig. 62-18). Providers should apply the pads to the child's bare chest and back and follow the verbal instructions given by the AED. For younger children, a

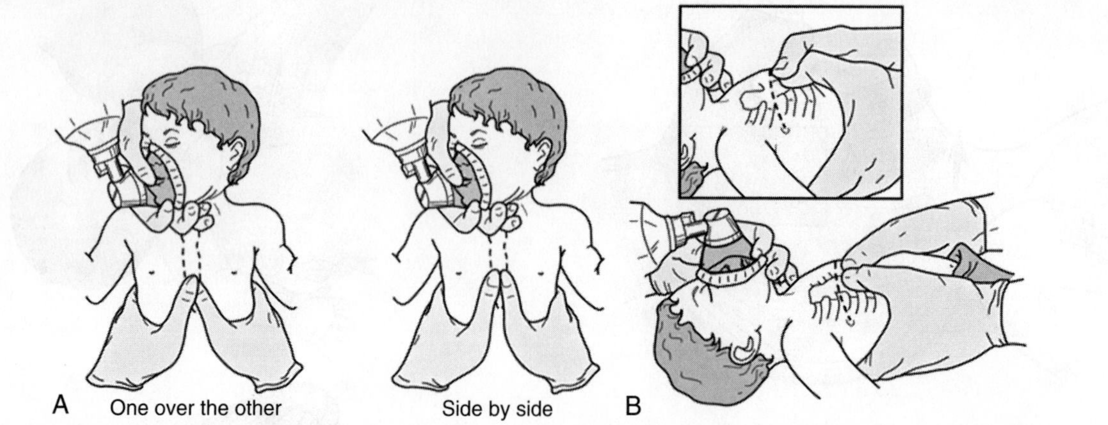

Figure 62-16 Thumb method of chest compressions. *A,* Infant receiving chest compressions with thumb 1 fingerbreadth below the nipple line and hands encircling chest. *B,* Hand position for chest encirclement technique for external chest compressions in neonates. Thumbs are side by side over the lower third of the sternum. In the small newborn, thumbs may need to be superimposed (*inset*). Gloves should be worn during resuscitation. (From Fleisher GR, Ludwig S, editors: *Textbook of pediatric emergency medicine,* Philadelphia, 2010, Wolters Kluwer/Lippincott Williams & Wilkins Health, Fig. 2.2.)

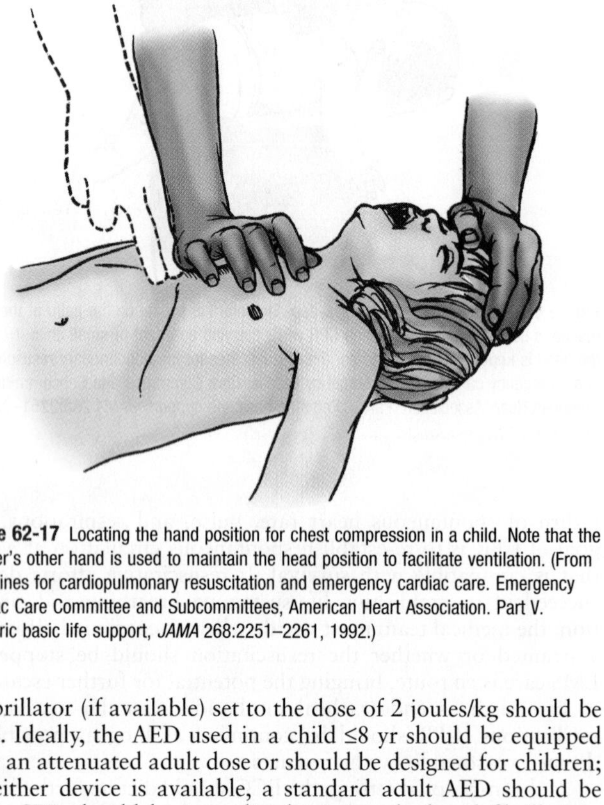

Figure 62-17 Locating the hand position for chest compression in a child. Note that the rescuer's other hand is used to maintain the head position to facilitate ventilation. (From Guidelines for cardiopulmonary resuscitation and emergency cardiac care. Emergency Cardiac Care Committee and Subcommittees, American Heart Association. Part V. Pediatric basic life support, *JAMA* 268:2251–2261, 1992.)

defibrillator (if available) set to the dose of 2 joules/kg should be used. Ideally, the AED used in a child ≤8 yr should be equipped with an attenuated adult dose or should be designed for children; if neither device is available, a standard adult AED should be used. CPR should be immediately restarted after defibrillation. Emergency dose epinephrine can also be administered with another 5 cycles of CPR to ensure its circulation throughout the child's body. If the ECG rhythm continues to show VF or VT, defibrillation can be alternated with epinephrine. For refractory VF or VT, an IV antiarrhythmic, such as amiodarone or lidocaine, can be given (Tables 62-6 and 62-7).

VASCULAR ACCESS

Venous Access

Veins suitable for cannulation are numerous, but there is considerable anatomic variation from patient to patient. In the upper extremities, the median antecubital vein, located in the antecubital fossa, is often the largest and easiest to access (Fig. 62-19). Many veins on the dorsum of the hand are also suitable for cannulation because they are often large and easily located on the flat surface of the dorsum of the hand, and their cannulation is well tolerated. The cephalic vein is usually cannulated at the wrist, along the forearm, or at the elbow. The median vein of the forearm is also suitable because it lies along a flat surface of the forearm. In the lower extremity, the great saphenous vein, located just anterior to the medial malleolus, is accessible in most patients. The dorsum of the foot usually has a large vein in the midline, passing across the ankle joint, but catheters are difficult to maintain in this vein because dorsiflexion tends to dislodge them. A second large vein on the lateral side of the foot, running in the horizontal plane, usually 1-2 cm dorsal to the lower margin of the foot, is preferable (Fig. 62-20). The most notable scalp veins are the superficial temporal (just anterior to the ear) and posterior auricular (just behind the ear).

Deeper and larger central veins can provide more reliable, larger-bore access for medications, nutritive solutions, and blood sampling than peripheral venous lines. They may be reached by percutaneous cannulation or surgical exposure. In infants and young children, the femoral vein is often the easiest to access and cannulate, but the internal jugular and subclavian veins may also be used (Figs. 62-21 and 62-22). Because of its proximity to the median nerve, the brachial vein is not often recommended for cannulation.

Intraosseous Access

Intraosseous (IO) needles are special rigid, large-bore needles that resemble those used for bone marrow aspiration. IO cannulation is recommended for patients for whom IV access proves difficult or unattainable, even in older children. If venous access is not available within 1 min in a child with cardiopulmonary arrest, an IO needle should be placed in the anterior tibia (with care taken to avoid traversing the epiphyseal plate). The needle should penetrate the anterior layer of compact bone, and its tip advanced into the spongy interior of the bone (Fig. 62-23). Any and all medications, blood products, and fluids may be administered through this route, including those involved in emergency resuscitations.

Arterial Access

Arterial access is indicated when care providers need frequent blood sampling, particularly to assess adequacy of oxygenation, ventilation, or acid-base balance, and/or continuous blood pressure monitoring. The radial artery, the most commonly cannulated artery, lies on the lateral side of the anterior wrist, just medial to the styloid process of the radius (Fig. 62-24). The ulnar

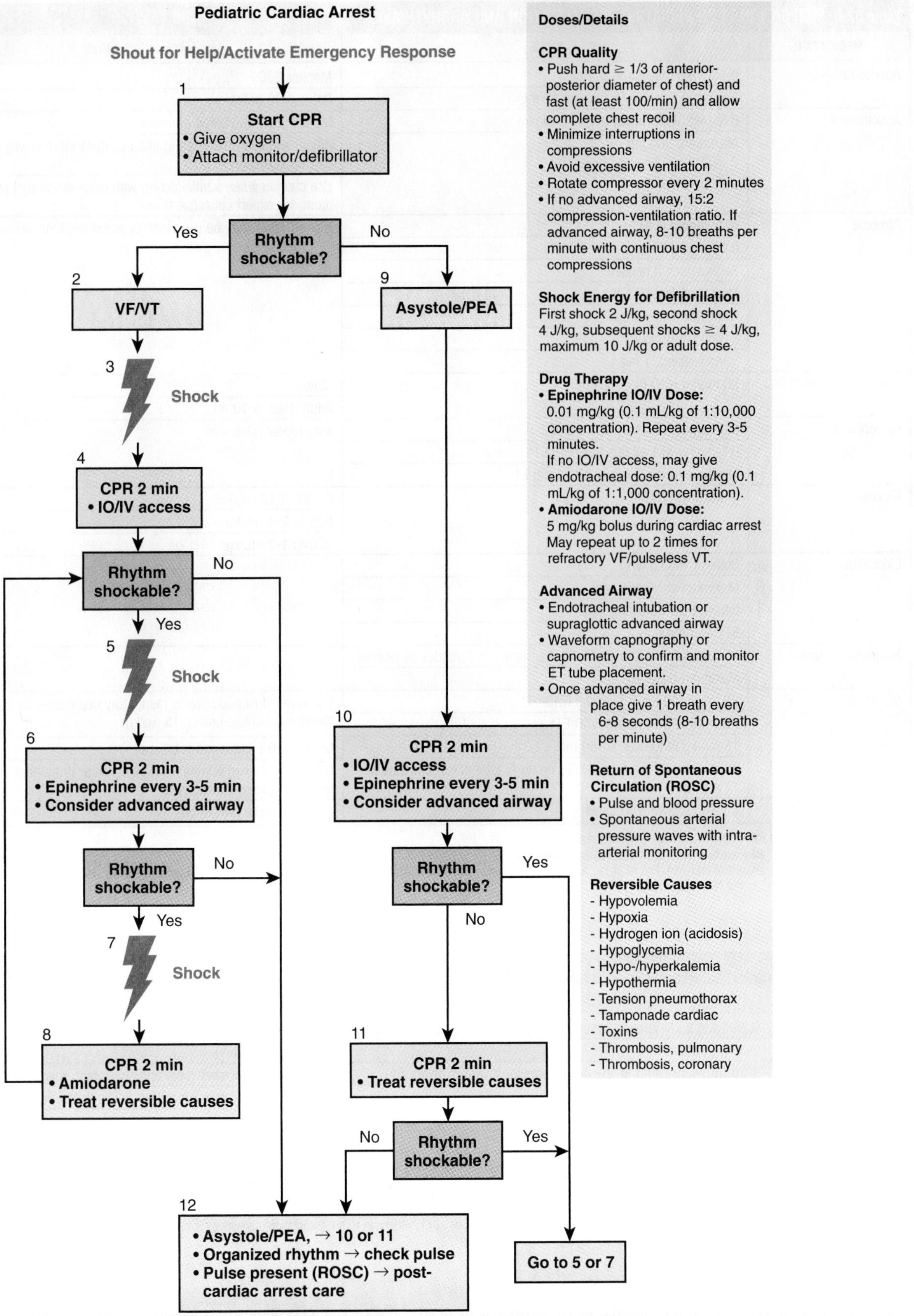

Figure 62-18 Pediatric advanced life support pulseless arrest algorithm. (From Kleinman ME, Chameides L, Schexnayder SM, et al: 2010 American Heart Association guidelines for cardiopulmonary resuscitation and emergency cardiovascular care, part 14, *Circulation* 122 [suppl 3]:S876–S908, 2010, Fig 1, p S885.)

Table 62-6 MEDICATIONS FOR PEDIATRIC RESUSCITATION AND ARRHYTHMIAS

MEDICATION	DOSE	REMARKS
Adenosine	0.1 mg/kg (maximum 6 mg)	Monitor ECG
	Repeat: 0.2 mg/kg (maximum 12 mg)	Rapid IV/IO bolus
Amiodarone	5 mg/kg IV/IO; repeat up to 15 mg/kg	Monitor ECG and blood pressure
	Maximum: 300 mg	Adjust administration rate to urgency (give more slowly when perfusing rhythm is present)
		Use caution when administering with other drugs that prolong QT interval (consider expert consultation)
Atropine	0.02 mg/kg IV/IO	Higher doses may be used with organophosphate poisoning
	0.03 mg/kg ET*	
	Repeat once if needed	
	Minimum dose: 0.1 mg	
	Minimum single dose:	
	Child, 0.5 mg	
	Adolescent, 1 mg	
Calcium chloride (10%)	20 mg/kg IV/IO (0.2 mL/kg)	Slowly
		Adult dose: 5-10 mL
Epinephrine	0.01 mg/kg (0.1 mL/kg 1:10,000) IV/IO	May repeat q3-5 min
	0.1 mg/kg (0.1 mL/kg 1:1,000) ET*	
	Maximum dose: 1 mg IV/IO; 10 mg ET	
Glucose	0.5-1 g/kg IV/IO	D10W: 5-10 mL/kg
		D25W: 2-4 mL/kg
		D50W: 1-2 mL/kg
Lidocaine	Bolus: 1 mg/kg IV/IO	
	Maximum dose: 100 mg	
	Infusion: 20-50 μg/kg/min	
	ET*: 2-3 mg	
Magnesium sulfate	25-50 mg/kg IV/IO over 10-20 min; faster in Torsades de pointes	
	Maximum dose: 2g	
Naloxone	<5 yr or ≤20 kg: 0.1 mg/kg IV/IO/ET*	Use lower doses to reverse respiratory depression associated with therapeutic opioid use (1-15 μg/kg)
	≥5 yr or >20 kg: 2 mg IV/IO/ET*	
Procainamide	15 mg/kg IV/IO over 30-60 min	Monitor EGG and blood pressure
	Adult dose: 20 mg/min IV infusion up to total maximum dose of 17 mg/kg	Use caution when administering with other drugs that prolong QT interval (consider expert consultation)
Sodium bicarbonate	1 mEq/kg/dose IV/IO slowly	After adequate ventilation

*Flush with 5 mL of normal saline and follow with 5 ventilations.
ECG, electrocardiogram; ET, endotracheal tube; IO, intraosseous; IV, intravenous.
From ECC Committee, Subcommittees and Task Forces of the American Heart Association: 2005 American Heart Association guidelines for cardiopulmonary resuscitation and emergency cardiovascular care, *Circulation* 112:IV1–203, 2005.

Table 62-7 MEDICATIONS TO MAINTAIN CARDIAC OUTPUT AND FOR POST-RESUSCITATION STABILIZATION*

MEDICATION	DOSE RANGE	COMMENT
Inamrinone	0.75-1 mg/kg IV/IO over 5 min; may repeat 2×; then: 2-20 μg/kg/min	Inodilator
Dobutamine	2-20 μg/kg/min IV/IO	Inotrope; vasodilator
Dopamine	2-20 μg/kg/min IV/IO in low doses; pressor in higher doses	Inotrope; chronotrope; renal and splanchnic vasodilator
Epinephrine	0.1-1 μg/kg/min IV/IO	Inotrope; chronotrope; vasodilator in low doses; vasopressor in higher doses
Milrinone	50-75 μg/kg IV/IO over 10-60 min then 0.5-0.75 μg/kg/min	Inodilator
Norepinephrine	0.1-2 μg/kg/min	Inotrope; vasopressor
Sodium nitroprusside	1-8 μg/kg/min	Vasodilator; prepare only in D5W

*Alternative formula for calculating an infusion: Infusion rate (mL/hr) = [weight (kg) × dose (μg/kg/min) × 60 (min/hr)]/concentration μg/mL).
IO, intraosseous; IV, intravenous.
From ECC Committee, Subcommittees and Task Forces of the American Heart Association: 2005 American Heart Association guidelines for cardiopulmonary resuscitation and emergency cardiovascular care, *Circulation* 112:IV1–203, 2005.

artery, just lateral to the tendon of the flexor carpi ulnaris, is used less often because of its proximity to the ulnar nerve. Useful sites in the lower extremity, particularly in neonates and infants, are the dorsalis pedis artery, on the dorsum of the foot between the tendons of the tibialis anterior and the extensor hallucis longus, and the posterior tibial artery, posterior to the medial malleolus. Arterial catheters require special care for insertion and subsequent management because the blood flow to tissue can be compromised and considerable hemorrhage can occur if an arterial catheter is dislodged.

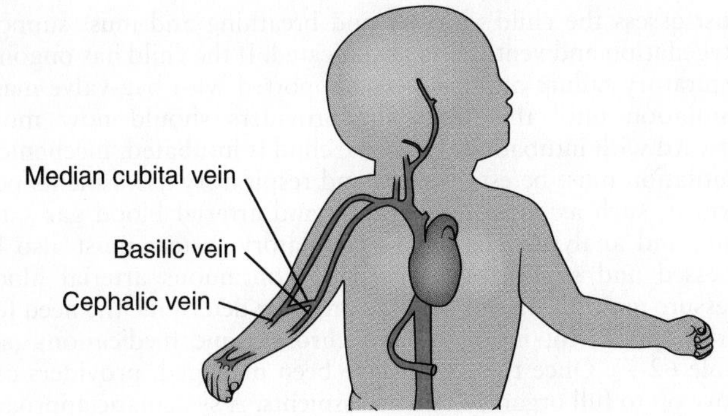

Figure 62-19 Veins of the upper extremity. (From Roberts JR, Hedges JR, editors: *Clinical procedures in emergency medicine,* ed 4, Philadelphia, 2004, Saunders.)

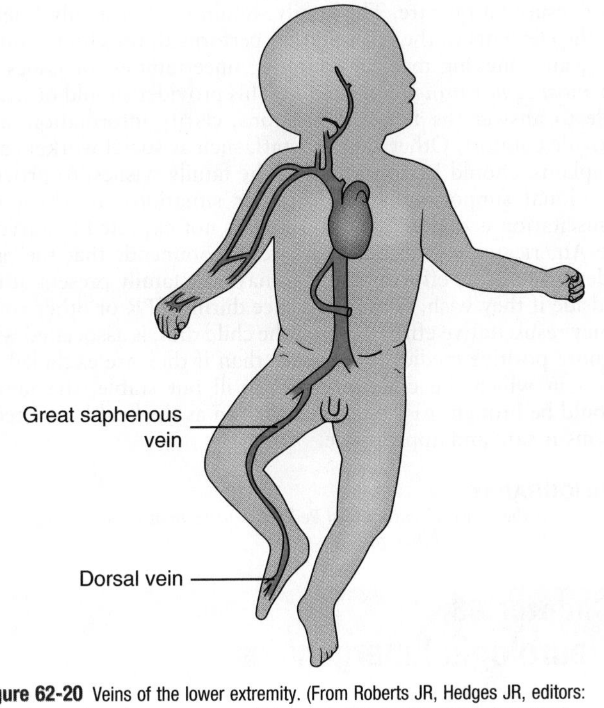

Figure 62-20 Veins of the lower extremity. (From Roberts JR, Hedges JR, editors: *Clinical procedures in emergency medicine,* ed 4, Philadelphia, 2004, Saunders.)

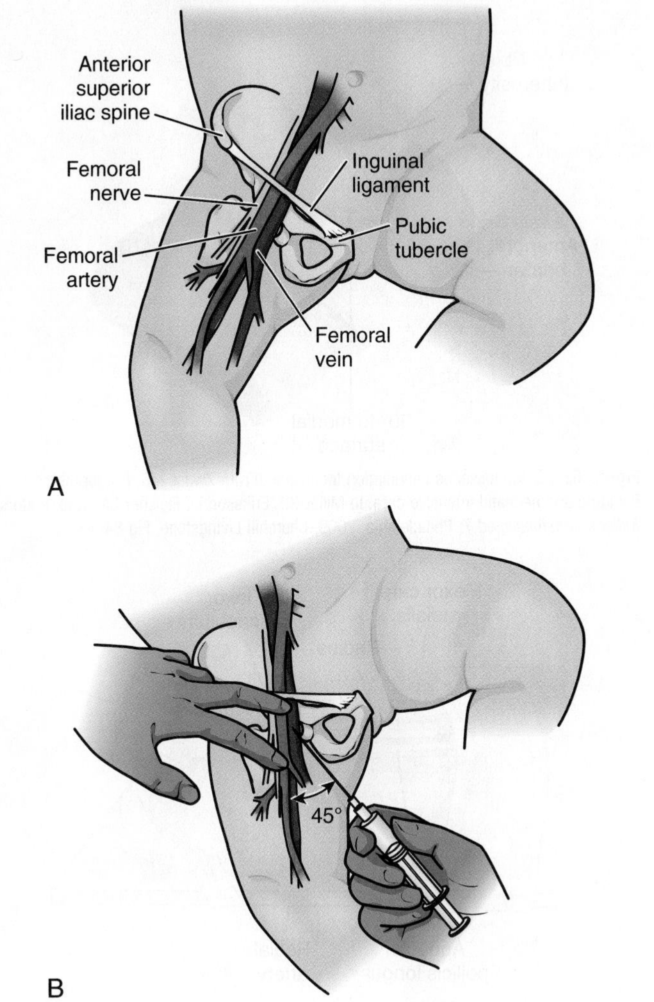

Figure 62-21 Femoral vein approach. Remember the mnemonic NAVEL for nerve, artery, vein, empty space, and lymphatics. (From Putigna F, Solenberger R: *Central venous access* [website]. http://emedicine.medscape.com/article/940865-overview. Accessed February 7, 2011.)

NONVASCULAR EMERGENCY PROCEDURES

Thoracentesis and Chest Tube Placement

Thoracentesis is the placement of a needle or catheter into the pleural space to evacuate fluid, blood, or air. Most insertions are performed in one of the intercostal spaces between the 4th and 9th ribs in the plane of the midaxillary line. After appropriate systemic and local anesthesia/sedation is performed as clinically indicated, a skin incision is made, and dissection through the chest wall is accomplished in layers with use of blunt dissection techniques. The needle (and later, the chest tube) that enters the pleural space should penetrate the intercostal space by passing over the superior edge of the lower rib, because there are larger vessels along the inferior edge of the rib. Ideally, the chest tube should lie anterior in the pleural space for air accumulation, and posterior for fluid accumulation. A radiograph must be obtained to verify chest tube placement and evacuation of the pleural space.

Pericardiocentesis

When fluid, blood, or gas accumulates in the pericardial sac, a danger is that the heart will be compressed and will not be able to fill and empty with normal volumes of blood, leading to

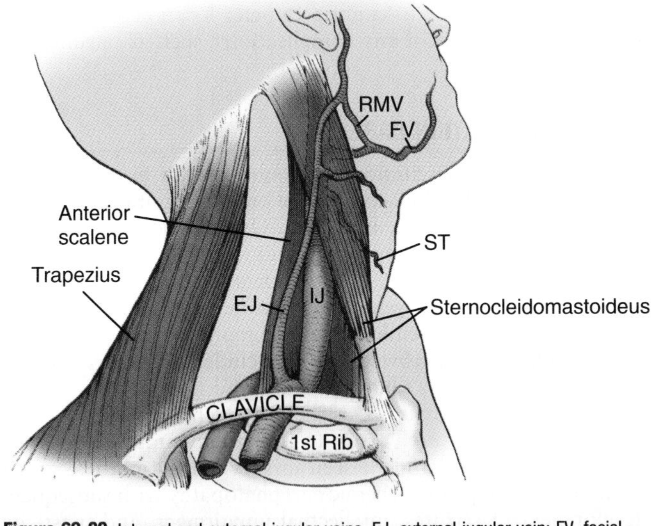

Figure 62-22 Internal and external jugular veins. EJ, external jugular vein; FV, facial vein; IJ, internal jugular vein; RMV, retromandibular vein; ST, superior thyroid vein. The 2 heads of the sternocleidomastoideus are indicated by the *lines.* (From Mathers LW, Smith DW, Frankel L: Anatomic considerations in placement of central venous catheters, *Clin Anat* 5:89, 1992. Reprinted by permission of Wiley-Liss.)

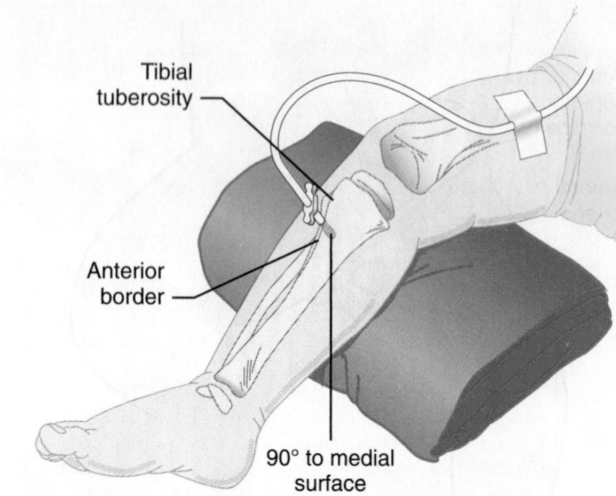

Figure 62-23 Intraosseous cannulation technique. (From Zwass MS, Gregory GA: Pediatric and neonatal intensive care. In Miller RD, Eriksson LI, Fleisher LA, et al, editors: *Miller's anesthesia,* ed 7, Philadelphia, 2009, Churchill Livingstone, Fig 84-1.)

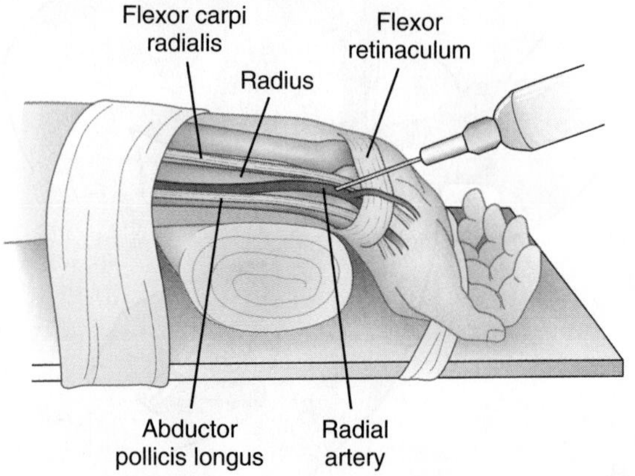

Figure 62-24 Radial artery anatomy and cannulation.

diminished cardiac output. The cardinal signs of such a restrictive pericardial effusion are tachycardia, hypotension, and decreasing oxygen saturation. Pericardiocentesis includes needle aspiration of the pericardial sac, often followed by the placement of a catheter for continuous drainage. As for thoracentesis, chest radiography should be done to confirm catheter location as well as to evaluate for presence of any complications, such as pneumothorax or hemothorax.

POST-RESUSCITATION CARE

After successful resuscitation, close observation in an intensive care unit, where the child can receive ongoing multiorgan system assessments and support, is critical. Optimal post-resuscitation care includes ongoing support of cardiovascular and respiratory system function as needed and the identification and treatment of other organ system dysfunction that may have contributed to (or resulted from) the child's cardiopulmonary instability. Good post-resuscitation intensive care also includes supportive services for the child's parents, siblings, family, and friends.

Induced hypothermia (32-33°C for ≈ 24 hr) has been used in adult and pediatric survivors of CPR in an attempt to reduce the high neurologic impairment seen in survivors of cardiac arrest (Chapter 63). Hypoxic-ischemic encephalopathy with subsequent development of seizures, intellectual impairment, and spasticity is a serious and common complication of cardiac arrest. In addition hyperglycemia and hypoglycemia should be avoided.

Post-resuscitation management generally has two phases, similar to earlier, emergency resuscitative care. First, the providers must assess the child's airway and breathing and must support oxygenation and ventilation as indicated. If the child has ongoing respiratory failure and has been supported with bag-valve-mask ventilation until this time, the providers should now move forward with intubation. Once the child is intubated, mechanical ventilation must be established, and respiratory assessments performed, such as chest radiography and arterial blood gas sampling and analysis. The child's circulatory system must also be assessed and supported as needed. Continuous arterial blood pressure monitoring can help the provider determine the need for, and response to, inotropic and chronotropic medications (see Table 62-7). Once the ABCs have been managed, providers can move on to full organ system assessments. A systematic approach that employs a full physical exam and laboratory evaluation to reveal the child's respiratory, cardiovascular, neurologic, gastrointestinal, renal, and hematologic system function should be used.

Communication with the family is an essential element of post-resuscitation care. The family should be thoroughly briefed on the elements of the resuscitation performed, the child's condition, and ongoing medical concerns, uncertainties, or issues by the *most senior provider available*. This provider should be available to answer the family's questions, clarify information, and provide comfort. Other support staff, such as social workers and chaplains, should be contacted, as the family wishes, to provide additional support and comfort. For situations in which the resuscitation is ongoing and the child is not expected to survive, the American Academy of Pediatrics recommends that the provider make every effort possible to have the family present at the bedside if they wish. Family presence during CPR or other emergency resuscitative efforts, even if the child dies, is associated with a more positive medical experience than if they are excluded. In cases in which the child is critically ill but stable, the family should be brought to the bedside as soon as the health care team deems it safe and appropriate.

BIBLIOGRAPHY

Please visit the Nelson Textbook of Pediatrics *website at* www.expertconsult.com *for the complete bibliography.*

Chapter 63
Neurologic Emergencies and Stabilization

Patrick M. Kochanek and Michael J. Bell

The care of critically ill children has advanced greatly over the past decades, and mortality rates have fallen. A remaining challenge is optimizing recovery after critical neurologic insults.

NEUROCRITICAL CARE PRINCIPLES

The brain has high metabolic demands, which are further increased during growth and development. Preservation of nutrient supply to the brain is the mainstay of care for children with evolving brain injuries. *Intracranial dynamics* describes the physics of the interactions of the contents—brain parenchyma, blood (arterial, venous, capillary) and cerebrospinal fluid (CSF)—within the cranium. Normally, brain parenchyma accounts for up to 85% of the contents of the cranial vault, and the remaining portion is divided between CSF and blood. The brain resides in a relatively rigid cranial vault, and cranial compliance decreases with age as the skull ossification centers gradually replace cartilage with bone. The **intracranial pressure (ICP)** is derived from the volume of its components and the bony compliance. The **perfusion pressure** of the brain (cerebral perfusion pressure [CPP]) is equal to the pressure of blood entering the cranium (mean arterial pressure [MAP]) minus the ICP, in most cases.

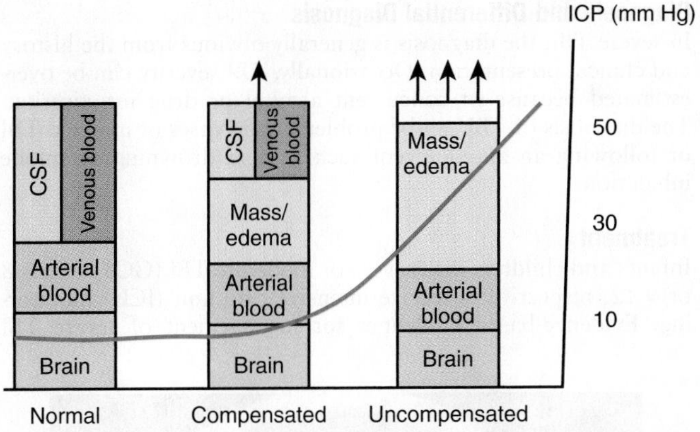

Figure 63-1 The Munro-Kellie doctrine describes intracranial dynamics in the setting of an expanding mass lesion (i.e., hemorrhage, tumor) or brain edema. In the normal state, the brain parenchyma, arterial blood, cerebrospinal fluid (CSF), and venous blood occupy the cranial vault at a low pressure, generally <10 mm Hg. With an expanding mass lesion or brain edema, initially there is a compensated state as a result of reduced CSF and venous blood volumes, and intracranial pressure (ICP) remains low. Further expansion of the lesion, however, leads to an uncompensated state when compensatory mechanisms are exhausted and intracranial hypertension results. See text for details.

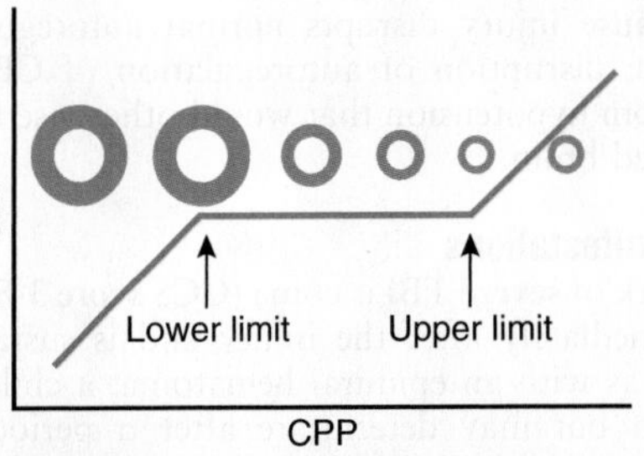

Figure 63-2 Schematic of the relationship between cerebral blood flow (CBF) and cerebral perfusion pressure (CPP). The diameter of a representative cerebral arteriole is also shown across the center of the y axis to facilitate understanding of the vascular response across CPP that underlies blood pressure autoregulation of CBF. CPP is generally defined as the mean arterial pressure (MAP) minus the intracranial pressure (ICP). At normal values for ICP, this generally represents MAP. Thus, normally, CBF is kept constant between the lower limit and upper limit of autoregulation; in normal adults, these values are ≈50 mm Hg and 150 mm Hg, respectively. In children, the upper limit of autoregulation is likely proportionally lower than the adult value relative to normal MAP for age. However, according to the work of Vavilala et al (2003), lower limit values are surprisingly similar in infants and older children. Thus, infants and young children may have less reserve for adequate CPP. See text for details.

Increases in intracranial volume can result from swelling, masses, or increases in blood and CSF volumes. As these volumes increase, compensatory mechanisms decrease ICP by (1) decreasing CSF volume (CSF is displaced into the spinal canal or absorbed by arachnoid villi), (2) decreasing cerebral blood volume (venous blood return to the thorax is augmented), and/or (3) increasing cranial volume (sutures pathologically expand or bone is remodeled). Once compensatory mechanisms are exhausted (the increase in cranial volume is too large), small increases in volume lead to large increases in ICP or intracranial hypertension (Fig. 63-1). As ICP continues to increase, brain ischemia can occur as CPP falls. Further increases in ICP can ultimately displace the brain downward into the foramen magnum—a process called **cerebral herniation,** which can become irreversible in minutes and may lead to severe disability or death.

Oxygen and glucose are required by brain cells for normal functioning, and these nutrients must be constantly supplied by cerebral blood flow (CBF). Normally, CBF is constant over a wide range of blood pressures (blood pressure autoregulation of CBF) via actions mainly within the cerebral arterioles. Cerebral arterioles are maximally dilated at lower blood pressures and maximally constricted at higher pressures so that CBF does not vary during normal fluctuations (Fig. 63-2). Acid-base balance of the CSF (often reflected by acute changes in $Paco_2$), body/brain temperature, glucose utilization, and other vasoactive mediators (i.e., adenosine, nitric oxide) can also affect the cerebral vasculature.

Knowledge of these concepts is instrumental to preventing secondary brain injury. Increases in CSF pH that occur because of inadvertent hyperventilation (decreased $Paco_2$) can produce cerebral ischemia. Hyperthermia-mediated increases in cerebral metabolic demands may damage vulnerable brain regions after injury. Hypoglycemia can produce neuronal death when CBF fails to compensate. Prolonged seizures can lead to permanent injuries if hypoxemia occurs from loss of airway control.

Attention to detail and constant reassessment are paramount in managing children with critical neurologic insults. Among the most valuable tools for serial, objective assessments of neurologic condition is the Glasgow Coma Scale (GCS) (see Table 62-3). Originally developed to assess level of consciousness after traumatic brain injury (TBI) in adults, the GCS is also valuable in pediatrics. Modifications to the GCS have been made for nonverbal children and are available for infants and toddlers (see Table 62-3). Serial assessments of the GCS score along with a focused neurologic examination are invaluable to detection of injuries before permanent damage occurs in the vulnerable brain.

The best-studied monitoring device in clinical practice is the **ICP monitor.** Monitoring is accomplished by a catheter inserted either into the cerebral ventricle (externalized ventricular drain) or into brain parenchyma (parenchymal transducer). ICP-directed therapies are standard of care in TBI and are used in other conditions such as intracranial hemorrhage, Reye syndrome, and some cases of encephalopathy, meningitis, and encephalitis. Other devices being studied include catheters that measure brain tissue oxygen concentration ($Pbto_2$), external probes that noninvasively assess brain oxygenation by absorbance of near-infrared light (near-infrared spectroscopy [NIRS]), monitors of brain electrical activity (continuous electroencephalography [EEG] or somatosensory, visual, or auditory evoked potentials), and CBF monitors (transcranial Doppler, xenon CT, perfusion MRI, or tissue probes).

TRAUMATIC BRAIN INJURY

Etiology

Mechanisms of TBI include motor vehicle crashes, falls, assaults, and abusive head trauma. Most TBIs in children are from closed-head injury.

Epidemiology

TBI is one of the most important pediatric public health problems, resulting in the death of about 7,000 children annually in the USA.

Pathology

Epidural, subdural, and parenchymal intracranial hemorrhages can result. Injury to gray or white matter is also commonly seen and includes focal cerebral contusions, diffuse cerebral swelling, axonal injury, and injury to the cerebellum or brainstem. Patients with severe TBI often have multiple findings; diffuse and potentially delayed cerebral swelling is common.

Pathogenesis

TBI results in primary and secondary injury. Primary injury from the impact produces irreversible tissue disruption. In contrast, 2 types of secondary injury are targets of neurointensive care. First, some of the ultimate damage seen in the injured brain evolves over hours or days, and the underlying mechanisms involved (edema, apoptosis, and secondary axotomy) are therapeutic targets. Second, the injured brain is vulnerable to additional insults because injury disrupts normal autoregulatory defense mechanisms; disruption of autoregulation of CBF can lead to ischemia from hypotension that would otherwise be tolerated by the uninjured brain.

Clinical Manifestations

The hallmark of **severe TBI** is coma (**GCS score** 3-8). Often, coma is seen immediately after the injury and is sustained. In some cases, such as with an epidural hematoma, a child may be alert presentation but may deteriorate after a period of hours. A similar picture can be seen in children with diffuse swelling, in whom a *talk and die* scenario has been described. Clinicians should also not be lulled into underappreciating the potential for deterioration of a child with **moderate TBI** (**GCS score 9-12**) with a significant contusion, because progressive swelling can potentially lead to devastating complications. In the comatose child with severe TBI, the second key clinical manifestation is the development of intracranial hypertension. The development of increased ICP with impending herniation may be heralded by new-onset or worsening headache, depressed level of consciousness, vital sign changes (hypertension, bradycardia, irregular respirations), and signs of 6th (lateral rectus palsy) or 3rd (anisocoria [dilated pupil], ptosis, down-and-out position of globe due to rectus muscle palsies) cranial nerve compression. Increased ICP can be appropriately managed only with continuous ICP monitoring. The development of brain swelling is progressive. Significantly raised ICP (>20 mm Hg) can occur early after severe TBI, but peak ICP generally is seen at 48-72 hr. Need for ICP-directed therapy may persist for longer than a week. A few children have coma without increased ICP, resulting from axonal injury or brainstem injury.

Laboratory Findings

Cranial CT should be obtained immediately after stabilization (Figs. 63-3 to 63-11). Generally, other laboratory findings are normal in isolated TBI, although occasionally coagulopathy or the development of the syndrome of inappropriate antidiuretic hormone secretion (SIADH) or, rarely, cerebral salt wasting is seen. In the setting of TBI with polytrauma, other injuries can result in laboratory abnormalities, and a full trauma survey is important in all patients with severe TBI (Chapter 66).

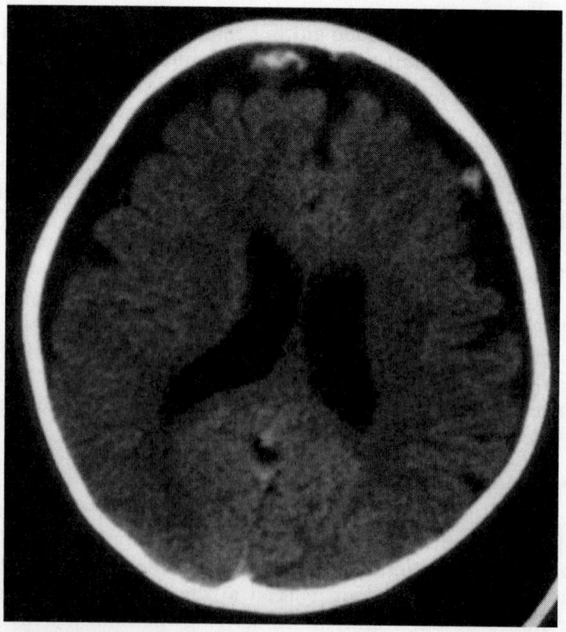

Figure 63-3 Abusive head trauma in an infant. Note the subdural fluid collections, dilated ventricles, and blood.

Diagnosis and Differential Diagnosis

In severe TBI, the diagnosis is generally obvious from the history and clinical presentation. Occasionally, TBI severity can be overestimated because of concurrent alcohol or drug intoxication. The diagnosis of TBI can be problematic in cases of inflicted TBI or following an anoxic event such as near drowning or smoke inhalation.

Treatment

Infants and children with severe or moderate TBI (GCS score 3-8 or 9-12, respectively) receive intensive care unit (ICU) monitoring. Evidence-based guidelines for management of severe TBI

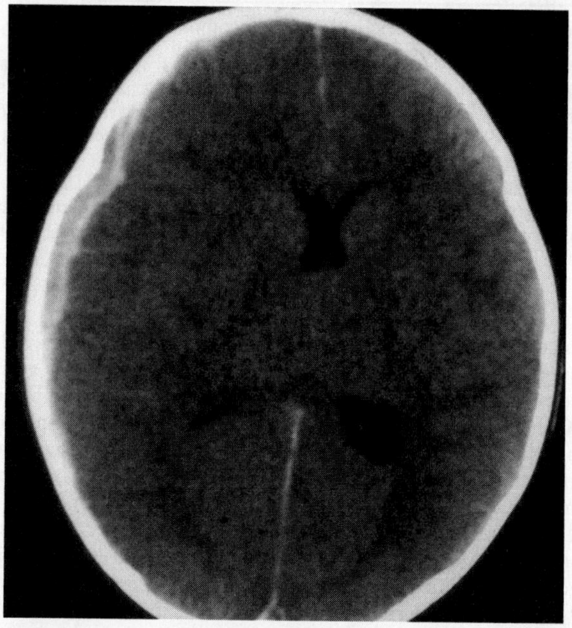

Figure 63-4 Abusive head trauma with a subdural collection of fluid and a midline shift.

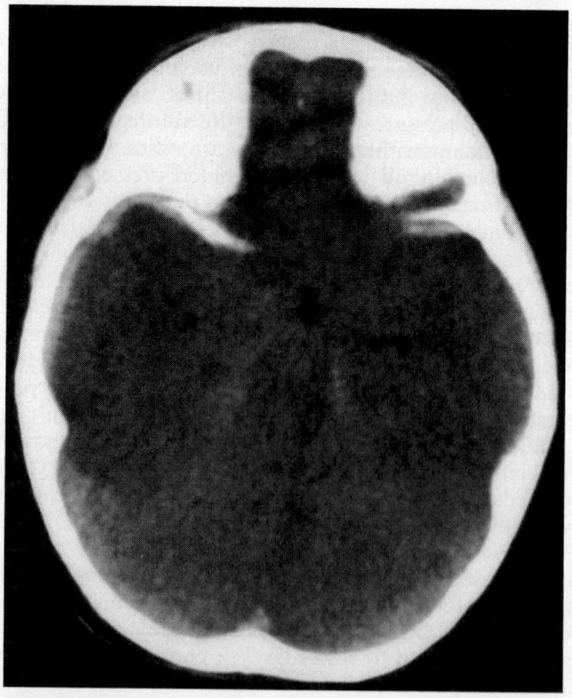

Figure 63-5 Abusive head trauma with massive cerebral edema, with loss of gray matter–white matter differentiation, loss of the ventricular system, and probable herniation of the brainstem.

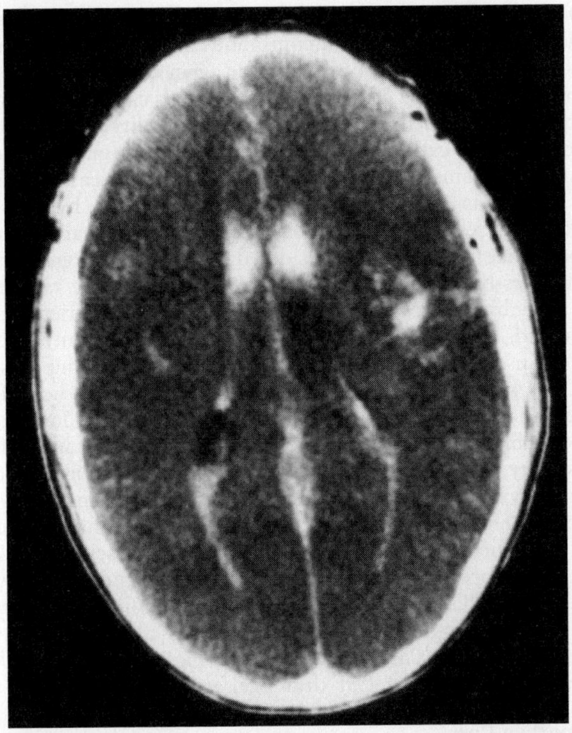

Figure 63-6 Abusive head trauma with significant intraventricular, intracerebral, and subdural hematomas, with loss of gray matter–white matter differentiation, suggestive of massive cerebral edema.

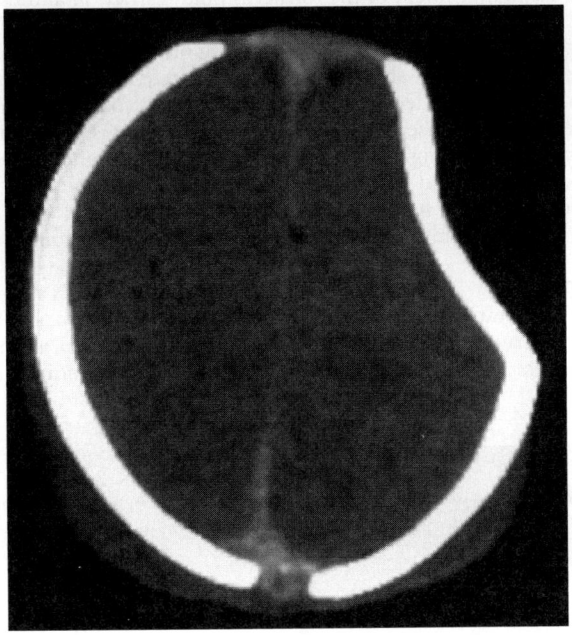

Figure 63-7 A depressed skull fracture due to traumatic delivery with forceps. Brain swelling can be seen.

have been published (Fig. 63-12). This approach to ICP-directed therapy is also reasonable for other conditions in which ICP is monitored. Care involves a multidisciplinary team comprising pediatric caregivers from neurologic surgery, critical care medicine, surgery, and rehabilitation, and is directed at preventing secondary insults and managing raised ICP. Initial stabilization of infants and children with severe TBI includes rapid sequence tracheal intubation with spine precautions along with maintenance of normal extracerebral hemodynamics, including blood gas values (Pa_{O_2}, Pa_{CO_2}), MAP, and temperature. Intravenous

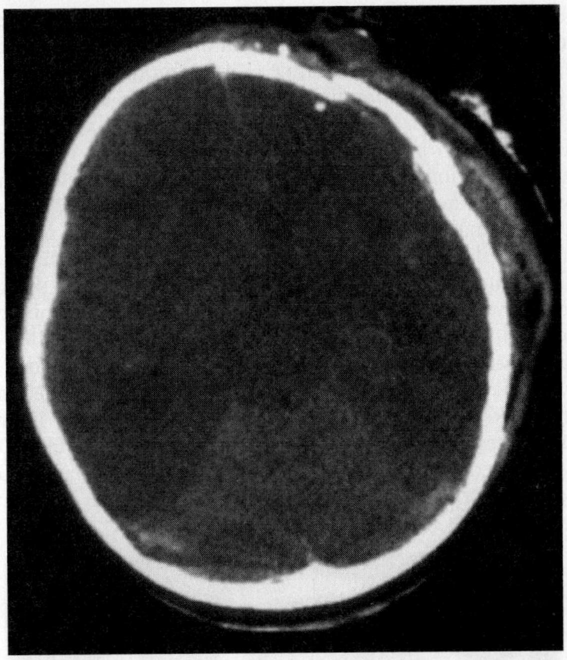

Figure 63-8 Malignant brain edema. A common pattern in severe head injury that is associated with significant secondary brain injury and a very high mortality rate. Cisterns are absent on the CT scan. This type of injury is associated with hypoxia and hypoxemia and hypotension.

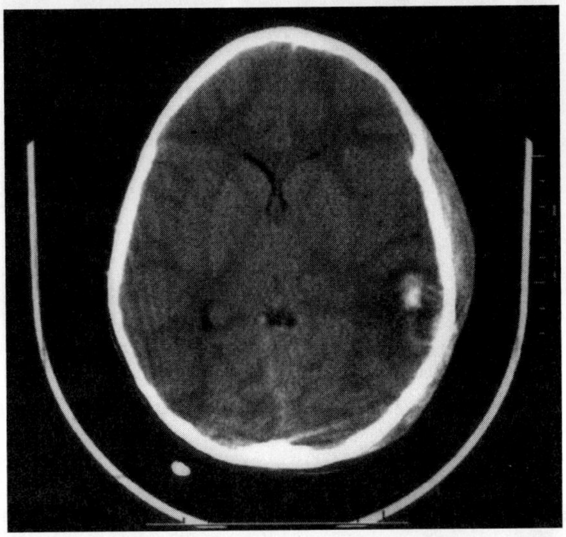

Figure 63-9 Significant closed-head injury with subgaleal hematoma, intracerebral hemorrhage, and loss of gray matter–white matter differentiation.

fluid boluses may be required to treat hypotension. Euvolemia is the target, and hypotonic fluids should be rigorously avoided; normal saline is the fluid of choice. Pressors may be needed as guided by monitoring of central venous pressure (CVP), with avoidance of both fluid overload and exacerbation of brain edema. A trauma survey should be performed. Once stabilized, the patient should be taken for CT scanning to rule out the need for emergency neurosurgical intervention. If surgery is not required, an ICP monitor should be inserted to guide the treatment of intracranial hypertension.

During stabilization or at any time during the treatment course, patients can present with signs and symptoms of cerebral **herniation** (pupillary dilatation, systemic hypertension, bradycardia, extensor posturing). Because herniation and its devastating consequences can sometimes be reversed if promptly addressed, it should be treated as a medical emergency, with use of hyperventilation with an FIO_2 of 1.0, and intubating doses of either thiopental or pentobarbital and either mannitol (0.25-1.0 g/kg, IV) or hypertonic saline (3% solution, 5-10 mL/kg IV).

ICP should be maintained <20 mm Hg; age-dependent CPP targets are ≈50 mm Hg for children 2-6 yr; 55 mm Hg for those 7-10 yr; and 65 mm Hg for those 11-16 yr. First-tier therapy includes elevation of the head of the bed, ensuring midline positioning of the head, controlled mechanical ventilation, and sedation and analgesia (i.e., benzodiazepines and narcotics). If neuromuscular blockade is needed, it may be desirable to monitor EEG continuously because *status epilepticus* can occur; this complication will not be recognized in a paralyzed patient and is associated with raised ICP and unfavorable outcome. If a ventricular rather than parenchymal catheter is used to monitor ICP, therapeutic CSF drainage is available and can be provided either continuously (often targeting an ICP > 5 mm Hg) or intermittently in response to ICP spikes, generally 20 mm Hg. Other first-tier therapies include the osmolar agents mannitol (0.25-1.0 g/kg IV over 20 min), given in response to ICP spikes >20 mm Hg or with a fixed (q4-6h) dosing interval, and hypertonic saline (often given as a continuous infusion of 3% saline at 0.1-1.0 mL/kg/hr). Choice of osmolar agent depends on the preference of the treating center. These two agents can be used concurrently. It is recommended to avoid serum osmolality >320 mOsm/L. A Foley urinary catheter should be placed to monitor urine output.

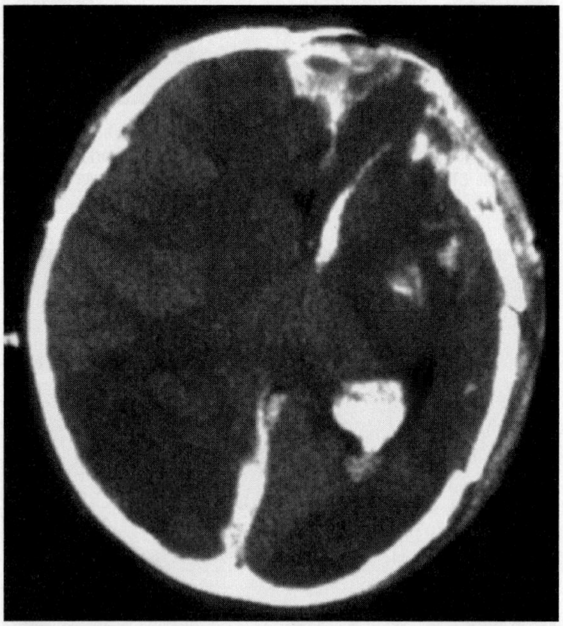

Figure 63-10 Severe traumatic brain injury with multiple depressed skull fractures and intraparenchymal hemorrhage.

If ICP remains refractory to treatment, careful reassessment of the patient is needed to rule out unrecognized hypercarbia, hypoxemia, fever, hypotension, hypoglycemia, pain, and seizures. Repeat imaging should be considered to rule out a surgical lesion. Guidelines-based second-tier therapies for refractory raised ICP are available, but evidence favoring a given second-tier therapy is limited. In some centers, decompressive craniectomy is used. Others use a pentobarbital infusion, with a loading dose of 5-10 mg/kg over 30 min followed by 5 mg/kg every hour for 3 doses and then maintenance with an infusion of 1 mg/kg/hr. Careful blood pressure monitoring is required because of the possibility of drug-induced hypotension and the frequent need for support with fluids and/or pressors. Mild hypothermia (32-34°C) to control refractory ICP can be induced and maintained by means of surface cooling. Sedation and neuromuscular blockade are used to prevent shivering, and rewarming should be slow, no faster than 1°C every 4-6 hr. Hypotension should be prevented during rewarming. Refractory raised ICP can also be treated with hyperventilation ($PaCO_2$ = 25-30 mm Hg). Other second-tier therapies (e.g., lumbar CSF drainage) are options.

Supportive Care

Euvolemia should be maintained, and isotonic fluids are recommended until resolution of intracranial hypertension. SIADH and salt wasting can develop and are important to differentiate, because management of the former is fluid restriction and that of the latter is sodium replacement. Severe hyperglycemia (blood glucose level >200 mg/dL) should be avoided and treated. The blood glucose level should be monitored frequently. Early nutrition with enteral feedings is advocated. Corticosteroids should generally not be used unless adrenal insufficiency is documented. Tracheal suctioning can exacerbate raised ICP. Timing of the use of sedation around suctioning events and/or use of tracheal or IV lidocaine can be helpful. Anticonvulsant prophylaxis with phenytoin or carbamazepine is a common treatment option.

Prognosis

Mortality rates for children with severe TBI who reach the PICU range between 10% and 30%. Ability to control ICP is related to patient survival, and the extent of cranial and systemic injuries

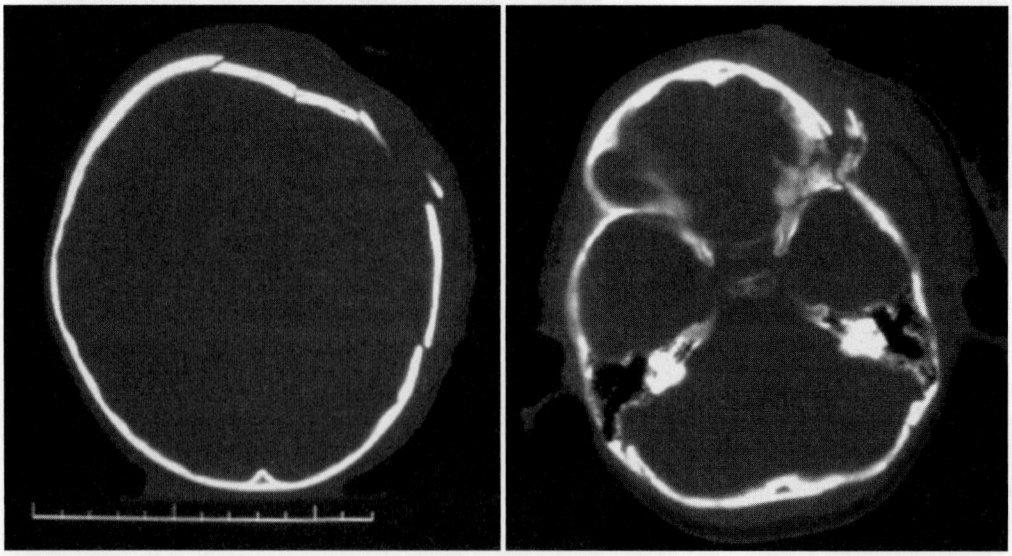

Figure 63-11 Bone widows associated with severe traumatic brain injury, showing multiple skull fractures.

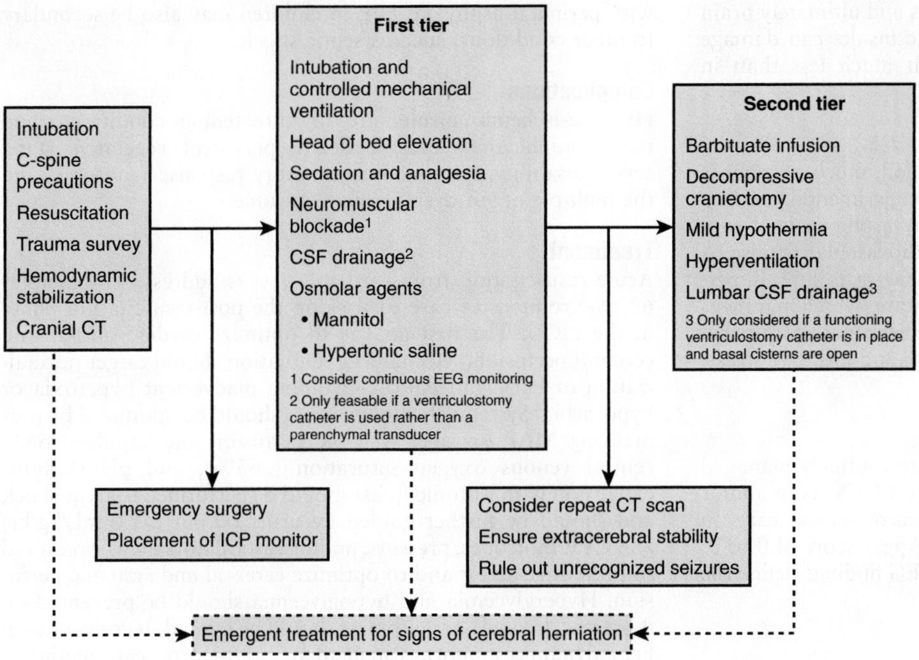

Figure 63-12 Schematic outlining the approach to management of a child with severe traumatic brain injury (TBI). It is based on the 2003 guidelines for the management of severe TBI, along with minor modifications from later literature. The intracranial pressure (ICP) and cerebral perfusion pressure (CPP) targets are discussed in the text. This schematic is specifically presented for severe TBI, for which the experience with ICP-directed therapy is greatest. Nevertheless, the general approach provided here is relevant to the management of intracranial hypertension in other conditions for which evidence-based data on ICP monitoring and ICP-directed therapy are lacking. Please see text for details.

correlates with quality of life. Motor and cognitive sequelae resulting from severe TBI generally benefit from rehabilitation to minimize long-term disabilities. Recovery from TBI may take months to achieve. Physical therapy, and in some centers methylphenidate, helps with motor and behavioral recovery.

MILD TRAUMATIC BRAIN INJURY

The majority (>90%) of children with blunt, closed-head trauma do not experience severe life- or brain-threatening complications. Children with mild TBI are defined as having a GCS score between 13 and 15 upon arrival at the hospital with or without the following acute symptoms: a history of loss of consciousness and antegrade or retrograde amnesia, as well as headache, vomiting, nausea, dizziness, or disorientation.

Cranial CT scanning is often considered in the evaluation of children with mild TBI, and findings are often negative. Nonetheless, the concern that the patient may have an acute intracranial hematoma that will necessitate immediate neurosurgical evacuation has resulted in identifying high-risk criteria to help determine whether the patient needs CT scanning. Although not all studies agree on all the criteria, the following are reasonable indications for CT imaging: loss of consciousness or amnesia >5 min; persistent dizziness; mental status changes; seizures; focal neurologic defects; a depressed skull fracture; signs of a basilar skull fracture; drug or alcohol use; and age <2 yr. The mechanisms of the injury are also important; they include: suspected child abuse; falls from >3 m; and high-speed injuries from projectiles, automobile, bicycle, or pedestrian-automobile crashes.

The **postconcussive syndrome** is an important sequela of an acute mild TBI. It often includes subjective complaints related to somatic, cognitive, or emotional symptoms. These include tiredness, headache, memory loss, dizziness, irritability, poor attention, depression, difficulty thinking (concentration), sleep problems, and personality changes. Postconcussive symptoms are more common after high-risk complications of mild TBI. The postconcussive syndrome usually resolves in 2-3 months, but subtle symptoms may last longer. Management includes avoiding excessive "brain activity" (TV, computer games, home or school work) and permitting the child to rest or sleep. In some high-risk children, symptoms may persist longer than a year after the acute injury. Children may need support in school with individualized learning programs. Parents need to know the spectrum of the postconcussive syndrome and to be assured that their children are not malingering or seeking attention.

ABUSIVE HEAD TRAUMA

Abusive head trauma is the most common cause of death from TBI in infants (Chapter 37) (see Figs. 63-3 to 63-6). Most cases occur in the initial 2 years of life. Affected infants can be initially misdiagnosed; severe inflicted TBI can be complicated by repeated injury and/or extracerebral injuries. Delayed deterioration despite normal initial GCS score can be seen. MRI findings and serum biomarker test results indicate that these patients often exhibit more evidence of hypoxic-ischemic brain injury than is seen in non-inflicted TBI. This may result from delay in presentation, seizures, apnea, or other factors; the history is often conflicting, and time of injury may be unclear. The patients are often managed with an approach similar to that outlined previously for non-inflicted TBI, including ICP-directed therapy. Severe TBI secondary to abuse often has a poor prognosis.

GLOBAL HYPOXIC-ISCHEMIC INSULTS AND HYPOXIC-ISCHEMIC ENCEPHALOPATHY

Etiology

The leading cause of global hypoxic-ischemic insults resulting in hypoxic-ischemic encephalopathy (HIE) in infants and children is asphyxial arrest. This event can result from a variety of conditions, such as drowning, airway obstruction, trauma, hanging, infections, and perinatal asphyxia.

Epidemiology

Cardiac arrest is seen in about 8-20/100,000 children in the USA (Chapter 62). The incidence of perinatal HIE is between 1and 6/1,000 live full-term births.

Pathology

Global hypoxic-ischemic insults damage selectively vulnerable brain regions such as the hippocampus, Purkinje neurons in the cerebellum, the basal ganglia, and brainstem. Longer durations of arrest produce infarcts in watershed areas and ultimately brain death. In term newborns, hypoxic-ischemic insults can damage periventricular white matter tracks—albeit much less than in preterm babies (Chapter 93).

Pathogenesis

The pathogenesis of HIE is poorly understood; much of what is believed to occur is based on studies in experimental models. Threshold insults to the brain produced by asphyxia lead to a period of anoxic perfusion followed by cardiovascular demise. A period of "no flow" follows, with cerebral energy failure. Reperfusion may trigger secondary injury in the brain, which manifests as excitotoxicity and seizures, activation of neuronal death pathways (i.e., apoptosis and necrosis), oxidative and nitrative stress, mitochondrial damage, and inflammation.

Clinical Manifestations

After cardiac arrest, infants and children are routinely managed in the ICU, and coma or acute HIE based on GCS score and/or seizures are generally the indications for neurointensive care. In perinatal asphyxia, fetal acidosis, a 5-min Apgar score of 0 to 3, neurologic dysfunction, and/or abnormal EEG findings define the need for neuroprotective interventions.

Laboratory Findings

In the ICU, blood gas, lactate, or electrolyte abnormalities may be seen and should be serially followed. Evidence of multiorgan injury or failure, including markers of myocardial, renal, and hepatic injury/function, can be seen and should be serially evaluated. Acute echocardiographic assessment and cranial CT should be strongly considered. EEG can identify encephalopathy, seizures, and subclinical electrical status epilepticus, particularly in the child with post-resuscitation coma. If neuromuscular blockade is required, continuous EEG should be considered. MRI is useful in the subacute period to define the extent of brain injury (Fig. 63-13).

Diagnosis and Differential Diagnosis

The history is often clear with regard to the etiology of the hypoxic-ischemic insult, but if it is not, the cause of the arrest should be determined. In children, poisoning, hyperkalemia, unrecognized trauma, child abuse, myocarditis, cardiomyopathy, and prolonged QT syndrome should be considered (Chapter 430). Pertinent obstetric history should be sought in a newborn with perinatal asphyxia. HIE in children may also be secondary to other conditions, such as septic shock.

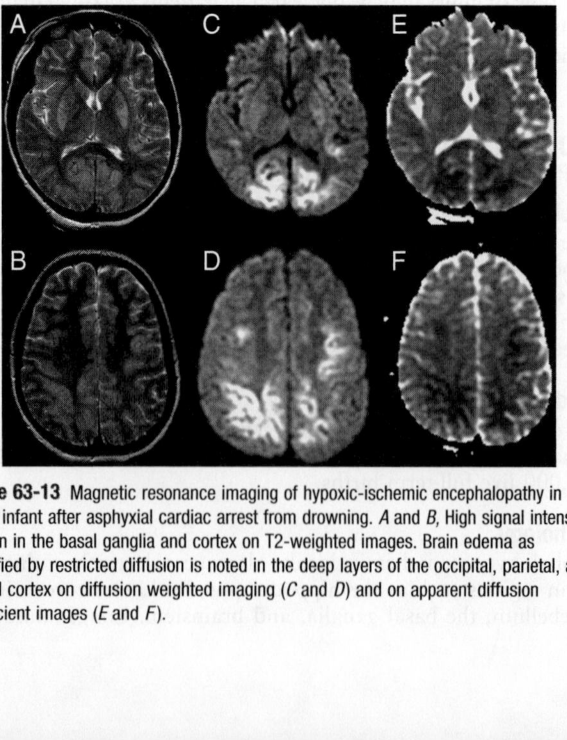

Figure 63-13 Magnetic resonance imaging of hypoxic-ischemic encephalopathy in a 1 yr old infant after asphyxial cardiac arrest from drowning. *A* and *B*, High signal intensity is seen in the basal ganglia and cortex on T2-weighted images. Brain edema as identified by restricted diffusion is noted in the deep layers of the occipital, parietal, and frontal cortex on diffusion weighted imaging (*C* and *D*) and on apparent diffusion coefficient images (*E* and *F*).

Complications

Hypoxic-ischemic insults are life-threatening conditions, and their complications include death, persistent vegetative state, severe disability, systemic inflammatory response syndrome, and the multiple organ dysfunction syndrome.

Treatment

Acute resuscitation from cardiac arrest is addressed in Chapter 62. Neurointensive care focuses on the post-resuscitation phase in the PICU. The first goal is to optimize cardiac output and cerebral perfusion. Mechanical ventilation should target normalization of Pa_{O_2} and Pa_{CO_2}—avoiding inadvertent hyperoxia or hypocarbia. Systemic hemodynamics should be optimized by normalizing MAP for age; systemic perfusion and capillary refill; central venous oxygen saturation (>65%); and pH. Volume expansion with isotonic fluids should be performed to treat shock and should be further guided by urine output (>1.0 mL/kg/hr) and CVP. Inotropes, pressors, and/or vasodilators may be required to prevent re-arrest and to optimize cerebral and systemic perfusion. Hyperglycemia and hypoglycemia should be prevented or, if present, treated. Arrhythmias should be treated. If conventional hemodynamic support is inadequate, extracorporeal membrane oxygenation (ECMO) should be considered.

Mild hypothermia should be considered as a treatment option in comatose children after cardiac arrest when restoration of spontaneous circulation (ROSC) with hemodynamic stability has been achieved. Similarly, in perinatal asphyxia, fetal acidosis, an Apgar score of 0 to 3 after 5 min, neurologic dysfunction, and/or abnormal EEG findings are criteria for use of this therapy in term neonates. Exclusion criteria have included coagulopathy, bleeding, and hemodynamic instability. According to the American Heart Association (AHA) guidelines (predominantly for adults after a cardiac arrest when the initial event was associated with ventricular fibrillation), cooling should be initiated as soon as possible after ROSC but may be beneficial even if delayed (4-6 hr); it should be induced by means of surface cooling with cooling blankets, application of ice packs to the groin, axillae, and neck, use of wet towels, and fanning. Infusion of 20 mL/kg IV of ice-cold saline over 30 min can be considered in children and may reduce core temperature by ≈2°C. If hypothermia is used in children, a temperature of 32-34°C should be use for 12-72 hr, according to physician preference. The rewarming rate should be no greater than 1°C every 4-6 hr. In perinatal asphyxia, cooling should be maintained for 72 hr. Shivering should be prevented with sedation and neuromuscular blockade. Temperature should be continuously monitored. Hypothermia in children has been associated with an increased risk for neutropenia, sepsis, and, in some studies (traumatic injury), no improvement in neurologic sequelae.

Supportive Care

Optimal supportive care includes maintenance of euvolemia with isotonic fluids. Hyperglycemia, hypoglycemia, hyponatremia, hyperosmolality, and metabolic acidosis should be prevented. If hypothermia is not used, careful attention should be paid to preventing fever in the initial 72 hr. Therapies needed to treat underlying conditions should be included in the post-resuscitation treatment plan when appropriate.

Prognosis

Outcome from HIE in children depends on the location of the insult. In out-of-hospital cardiac arrest, survival to discharge is only ≈10%, and < 50% of survivors have favorable neurologic outcome. In-hospital cardiac arrests survival is ≈30%, with favorable outcome in most survivors. In perinatal asphyxia, moderate encephalopathy is associated with 10% and 30% risks of mortality and disability, respectively; severe encephalopathy is associated with 60% mortality and nearly 100% disability.

Therapeutic Directives

AHA guidelines for the management of pediatric victims of cardiac arrest have been published and are the basis for the treatment recommendations for HIE.

STATUS EPILEPTICUS

Etiology

Status epilepticus is defined as a seizure of sufficient duration to provide an enduring epileptic focus. In more practical terms, persistent, disorganized, involuntary brain activity lasting for more than a proscribed amount of time (varying from 1 min to 30 min; usually 15-30 min) is characteristic of status epilepticus. The causes are myriad; epilepsy, abrupt discontinuation of anticonvulsive medications, febrile seizures, TBI, and encephalitis and other central nervous system infections are the leading causes in children (Chapter 586.8).

Epidemiology

The incidence of status epilepticus ranges between 10 and 60/100,000 population in various studies. Status epilepticus is most common in children <5 yr of age, with incidence in this age group >100/100,000.

Pathology and Pathogenesis

Status epilepticus can cause injury to the brain. It increases cerebral oxygen and glucose consumption markedly. In self-limited seizures, a concomitant increase in CBF to prevent energy failure is seen. As seizures persist, compensatory mechanisms fail, and relative cerebral ischemia can occur. Status epilepticus is associated with increases in brain levels of excitatory amino acids (glutamate), which bind to specific receptors (*N*-methyl-D-aspartate), causing greater neuronal activity and activation of intracellular pathways leading to cell death.

Clinical Manifestations

In the ICU, presentations of status epilepticus vary between easily recognizable signs and symptoms, such as tonic-clonic movements of all extremities, to a lack of physical findings in a comatose child in whom subclinical (or nonconvulsive) electrical status epilepticus is manifest only on EEG.

Laboratory Findings

Status epilepticus is not associated with significant laboratory abnormalities. Electrolyte abnormalities (i.e., hyponatremia, hypocalcemia, hypoglycemia) should be ruled out. Examination of CSF is warranted when infections are suspected. Determination of serum concentrations of chronically administered antiepileptic drugs is important to define potential etiology, adjust dosages, and ensure future compliance in these refractory cases. The definitive diagnosis of status epilepticus is made from EEG findings.

Diagnosis and Differential Diagnosis

Diagnosis is made with EEG, which shows disorganized, abnormal seizure activity during an event. The differential diagnosis for convulsive status epilepticus includes movement disorders (chorea, tics), rigors, clonus with stimulation, and decerebrate/decorticate posturing. For nonconvulsive status epilepticus, other causes of coma must be considered and eliminated by thorough testing.

Complications

Untreated status epilepticus can lead to relative cerebral ischemia and permanent brain injury. Physical injuries can occur from convulsions and should be prevented through control of the child's environment during this critical period.

Treatment

Several antiepileptic drugs have been advocated as first-line therapies for status epilepticus, including benzodiazepines (rectal valium, IV midazolam or lorazepam), phenytoin (or fosphenytoin), and barbiturates (phenobarbital). Therapy is adjusted for both symptoms and EEG evidence of seizures. In the PICU, for refractory cases, a continuous infusion of barbiturates and/or benzodiazepines may be necessary. Specifically, continuous IV infusions of midazolam (starting at 0.1 mg/kg/hr) or pentobarbital (loading dose of 2-10 mg/kg and a continuous infusion starting at 1 mg/kg/hr) should be considered. Bolus doses in the lower portion of this range may minimize untoward cardiovascular side effects. For refractory cases that progress to this level of therapeutic intensity, respiratory support and hemodynamic monitoring and/or support should already be in place. As therapy escalates, continuous EEG monitoring should be considered to help titrate therapy. For refractory status epilepticus, newer therapies include mapping of the seizure focus followed by neurosurgical resection, IV lidocaine, or levetiracetam.

Supportive Care

Effective cardiopulmonary resuscitation is critical to maximize outcome, because airway compromise can be common during the ictal event or may result from the drugs used to treat the seizure. Tracheal intubation should be strongly considered if the child becomes obtunded, loses airway reflexes, or has respiratory insufficiency. Neuromuscular blockade to facilitate intubation will mask epileptic movements but not the abnormal brain activity, and thus, treatment for the underlying ictus should be continued. Hypotension and decreased cardiac output may also be seen in severe cases or with high-dose anticonvulsant drug therapy; administration of fluids or inotropic drugs or use of hemodynamic monitoring may be indicated. In cases of prolonged refractory status epilepticus, meticulous ICU care, including pulmonary toilet, optimal nutrition, and infection surveillance and treatment, is needed to minimize morbidity.

Prognosis

Case fatality rates for children with status epilepticus range between 2-3%. Development of epilepsy after status epilepticus occurs in up to 30% of children (excluding children with febrile seizures, in whom the incidence is 1-2%).

STROKE AND INTRACEREBRAL HEMMORRHAGE

Etiology

The predominant causes of ischemic stroke in children are sickle cell disease and heart disease (either acquired or congenital), which are responsible for ≈50% of strokes after the neonatal period (Chapter 594). A variety of other conditions, including carotid or vertebral arterial dissection, infectious (meningitis, sinusitis), hematologic (prothrombotic states, polycythemia, chronic anemias), traumatic, and autoimmune (systemic lupus erythematosus, inflammatory bowel) disorders, and vasculitis, are risk factors. Intracerebral hemorrhage results from abnormal vascular development and subsequent rupture of cerebral vessels, with arteriovenous malformations, hemangiomas, or aneurysms. Cerebral venous sinus thrombosis is often caused by severe dehydration and hypercoagulable states.

Epidemiology

In the USA, there is an overall incidence of 2.3/100,000 (1.2/100,000 for ischemic stroke and 1.1/100,000 for intracerebral hemorrhage) in children.

Pathology and Pathogenesis

Ischemic strokes in children are generally not the result of atherosclerotic plaque migration, as they are in adults. Instead, damage to the intima of cerebral arteries can form a thrombotic nidus. In sickle cell disease, chronic turbulent blood flow likely leads to vascular damage. In intracerebral hemorrhage, blood vessel wall integrity is compromised, leading to extravasation of blood into the parenchyma or dural spaces. The usual pathology in children with heart disease is embolism from diseased valves (or intracardiac devices) and right-to-left shunts that leads to cerebrovascular occlusion.

Clinical Manifestations
The predominant presentation of children with stroke consists of the abrupt onset of focal neurologic deficits, and that of children with intracerebral hemorrhage is coma (if large portions of the cortex or brainstem are involved). In sickle cell disease, strokes are often unrecognized until imaging studies are obtained.

Laboratory Findings
In large hemorrhagic infarctions, release of tissue factor from the brain can lead to a prolonged prothrombin time (PT), which can exacerbate the injury. Conversely, in children with hypercoagulable phenotypes, abnormalities in factor V Leiden, protein S, protein C, or other factors may be present. Homocystinuria is another cause of hypercoagulable state in children.

Diagnosis and Differential
Detailed history and physical examination can often localize the location of lesions. However, CT or MRI studies of the brain are required. Differential diagnoses can include complex migraines, seizures, and other organic brain syndromes.

Complications
The major complications of stroke are hemorrhagic transformation of thrombotic lesions and vasospasm after aneurysmal subarachnoid hemorrhage (SAH). The incidence of hemorrhagic transformation in children has not been defined, but the incidence in adults is ≈3%. The incidence of vasospasm in children is unclear; case reports suggest that vasospasm can occur for up to 14 days after SAH.

Treatment
Close monitoring in a PICU or intermediate care unit is appropriate for most acute cases of stroke or intracerebral hemorrhage. The child with an evolving stroke may have progressive neurologic deterioration, particularly if the stroke affects motor control of the airway or is associated with cerebral edema. The only approved acute therapy for ischemic stroke is recombinant tissue plasminogen activator (rTPA) in adults with known thrombosis of a major cerebral artery by imaging—with the limitation that therapy be initiated within 3 hr if rTPA is given IV or within 6 hr if it is given intra-arterially into the occlusion. Recombinant TPA has been reported as effective in individual cases or small series in children, but dosing of this potentially dangerous agent has not been studied. Moreover, risk factors for hemorrhagic transformation in adults (extent of parenchymal hypoattenuation on baseline CT scan, a history of heart failure, increasing age, and baseline systolic blood pressure) may not be applicable to children. A focus at this time is determining which children would benefit from anticoagulation therapy (standard heparin, low-molecular-weight heparin, warfarin, aspirin) after stroke. Pediatric guidelines-based recommendations germane to the neurocritical care aspects of stroke include (1) consideration of ICP monitoring for spontaneous intracerebral hemorrhage (classification of recommendation: I, level of evidence: C), (2) providing red blood cell exchange/transfusion therapy for children with sickle cell disease and acute stroke (class IIa, level C), (3) anticoagulation and/or thrombolytics in the acute period if ICP management is not warranted (class IIa, level C and class IIb, level C, respectively), continuous EEG monitoring for children with tracheal intubation (class IIb, level C), and consideration of thrombolytics for children with cerebral sinus venous thrombosis (class IIb, level C).

In SAH, there are no pediatric guidelines. Adult guidelines recommend surgical clipping or endovascular coiling, along with medical management of vasospasm that includes induced hypertension and hypervolemic therapy, administration of calcium channel blockers, particularly nimodipine, and ICP monitoring in some cases. Collaboration between pediatric neurosurgery and ICU teams is essential.

Supportive Care
Controlling airway and respiration and avoiding secondary injury are essential. Hypotension should be treated. Hypertension, however, is a more difficult problem. Adult guidelines for acute ischemic stroke recommend antihypertensive therapies only if thrombolytic treatments are used, because a 25% risk of hemorrhagic transformation has been reported in adults with systolic blood pressure >165 mm Hg with use of rTPA. The conundrum faced by the clinician is whether the cause of the hypertension is related to a Cushing response due to raised ICP or is independent of ICP. Treatment of the former should target a reduction in ICP, whereas that of the latter should target a safe reduction in MAP—maintaining adequate CPP in the injured brain while preventing cerebral edema formation if blood pressure has exceeded the upper limit of the autoregulation. This problem is compounded in children by the fact that the upper limit of blood pressure autoregulation has not been defined. It is probably less than the adult value of MAP, 150 mm Hg, and is age-dependent. When this upper limit is exceeded, CBF rises proportionately with increases in MAP, leading to the propensity for cerebral edema formation. In intracerebral hemorrhage, the 2007 AHA Guidelines recommend aggressive reduction of blood pressure in patients with systolic blood pressure >200 mm Hg. What that threshold represents in children across the age spectrum is unclear. If a reduction of MAP is desired in a child with brain injury, it is best accomplished by means of continuous infusions of medications that have minimal effects on cerebral vasomotor tone (i.e., β-blockers such as esmolol or mixed α/β-blockers such as labetalol). These agents minimize the vasodilation and increases in cerebral blood volume that may exacerbate ICP. If such agents are contraindicated (i.e., by bradycardia or reactive airway disease), continuous infusion of a calcium channel blocker (nicardipine or diltiazem) can be effective.

Prognosis
Data are limited, but in general, larger strokes, especially during the newborn period, are associated with developmental delay and development of epilepsy.

Therapeutic Directives
Guidelines for management of stroke and cerebral hemorrhage have been published, and the recommendations relevant to ICU care can be found under Treatment.

BIBLIOGRAPHY
Please visit the Nelson Textbook of Pediatrics *website at www.expertconsult.com for the complete bibliography.*

63.1 Brain Death

K. Jane Lee

Brain death is the irreversible cessation of all functions of the entire brain, including the brainstem. It is also known as the determination of death using neurologic criteria. Although brain death is legally accepted in the USA as the equivalent of death due to the irreversible cessation of circulatory and respiratory functions, it remains a concept that is sometimes difficult to understand and is not universally accepted.

For the full continuation of this chapter, please visit the Nelson Textbook of Pediatrics *website at www.expertconsult.com.*

Chapter 64
Shock

David A. Turner and Ira M. Cheifetz

Shock is an acute syndrome characterized by the body's inability to deliver adequate oxygen to meet the metabolic demands of vital organs and tissues. Patients in shock have insufficient oxygen at the tissue level to support normal aerobic cellular metabolism, resulting in a shift to less efficient anaerobic metabolism. Increases in tissue oxygen extraction are unable to compensate for this deficiency in oxygen delivery, leading to progressive lactic acidosis and possible clinical deterioration. If inadequate tissue perfusion persists, adverse vascular, inflammatory, metabolic, cellular, endocrine, and systemic responses worsen the physiologic instability.

Compensation for inadequate oxygen delivery involves a complex set of responses that attempt to preserve oxygenation of the vital organs (i.e., brain, heart, kidneys, liver) at the expense of other organs (i.e., skin, gastrointestinal tract, muscles). Of importance, the brain is especially sensitive to periods of poor oxygen supply, given its lack of capacity for anaerobic metabolism. Initially, shock may be well compensated, but it may rapidly progress to an uncompensated state requiring more aggressive therapies to achieve clinical recovery or improvement. The combination of a continued presence of an inciting trigger and a body's exaggerated and potentially harmful neurohumoral, inflammatory, and cellular responses leads to the progression of shock. Untreated shock causes irreversible tissue and organ injury (i.e., irreversible shock) and, ultimately, death. Irrespective of the underlying cause of shock, the specific pattern of response, pathophysiology, clinical manifestations, and treatments may vary significantly, depending on the specific etiology (which may be unknown), the clinical circumstances, and an individual patient's biologic response to the shock state.

EPIDEMIOLOGY

Shock occurs in approximately 2% of all hospitalized infants, children, and adults in the USA (≈400,000 cases/yr), and the mortality rate varies according to the clinical circumstances. Most patients who die do so not in the acute hypotensive phase of shock, but rather as a result of associated complications. **Multiple organ dysfunction syndrome (MODS)** is defined as any alteration of organ function that requires medical support for maintenance, and the presence of MODS in patients with shock substantially increases the probability of death. In pediatrics, the mortality rate for shock is decreasing as a consequence of educational efforts and the utilization of standardized management guidelines, which emphasize early recognition and intervention along with the rapid transfer of critically ill patients to a pediatric intensive care unit (Fig. 64-1).

DEFINITION

Shock classification systems generally define 5 major types of shock: hypovolemic, cardiogenic, distributive, obstructive, and septic (Table 64-1). **Hypovolemic shock,** the most common cause of shock in children worldwide, is most frequently caused by diarrhea, vomiting, or hemorrhage. **Cardiogenic shock** is seen in patients with congenital heart disease (before or after surgery, including heart transplantation) or with congenital or acquired cardiomyopathies, including acute myocarditis. **Obstructive shock** stems from any lesion that creates a mechanical barrier that impedes adequate cardiac output; examples of this obstructive process are pericardial tamponade, tension pneumothorax, pulmonary embolism, and ductus-dependent congenital heart lesions when systemic blood flow decreases as the ductus arteriosus closes. **Distributive shock** is caused by inadequate vasomotor tone, which leads to capillary leak and maldistribution of fluid into the interstitium. **Septic shock** is often discussed synonymously with distributive shock, but the septic process usually involves a more complex interaction of distributive, hypovolemic, and cardiogenic shock.

PATHOPHYSIOLOGY

An initial insult triggers shock, leading to inadequate oxygen delivery to organs and tissues. Compensatory mechanisms attempt to maintain blood pressure by increasing cardiac output and systemic vascular resistance. The body also attempts to optimize oxygen delivery to the tissues by increasing oxygen extraction and redistributing blood flow to the brain, heart, and kidneys (at the expense of the skin and gastrointestinal tract). These responses lead to an initial state of **compensated shock,** in which blood pressure is maintained. If treatment is not initiated or is inadequate during this period, **decompensated shock** develops, with hypotension and tissue damage that may lead to multisystem organ dysfunction and ultimately to death (Fig. 64-2, Tables 64-2 and 64-3).

In the early phases of shock, multiple compensatory physiologic mechanisms act to maintain blood pressure and preserve tissue perfusion and oxygen delivery. These responses include increases in heart rate, stroke volume, and vascular smooth muscle tone, which are regulated through sympathetic nervous system activation and neurohormonal responses. Increased respiratory rate with greater CO_2 elimination is a compensatory response to the metabolic acidosis and increased CO_2 production from poor tissue perfusion. Renal excretion of hydrogen ions and retention of bicarbonate also increase in an effort to maintain normal body pH (Chapter 52.7). Maintenance of intravascular volume is facilitated via sodium regulation through the renin-angiotensin-aldosterone and atrial natriuretic factor axes, cortisol and catecholamine synthesis and release, and antidiuretic hormone secretion. Despite these compensatory mechanisms, the underlying shock and host response lead to vascular endothelial cell injury and significant leakage of intravascular fluids into the interstitial extracellular space.

All forms of shock affect cardiac output via several mechanisms. Changes in heart rate, preload, afterload, and myocardial contractility may occur separately or in combination (Table 64-4). **Hypovolemic shock** is characterized primarily by fluid loss and decreased preload. Tachycardia and an increase in systemic vascular resistance are the initial compensatory responses to maintain cardiac output and systemic blood pressure. Without adequate volume replacement, hypotension develops, followed by tissue ischemia and further clinical deterioration. When there is pre-existing low plasma oncotic pressure (due to nephrotic syndrome, malnutrition, hepatic dysfunction, acute severe burns, etc.), even further volume loss and exacerbation of shock may occur because of endothelial breakdown and worsening capillary leak.

In contrast, the underlying pathophysiologic mechanism leading to **distributive shock** is a state of abnormal vasodilation. Sepsis, hypoxia, poisonings, anaphylaxis, spinal cord injury, or mitochondrial dysfunction can cause vasodilatory shock (Fig. 64-3). The lowering of systemic vascular resistance (SVR) is accompanied initially by a maldistribution of blood flow away from vital organs and a compensatory increase in cardiac output. This process leads to significant decreases in both preload and afterload. Therapies for distributive shock must address both of these problems simultaneously.

Cardiogenic shock may be seen in patients with myocarditis, cardiomyopathy, congenital heart disease, or arrhythmias, or following cardiac surgery (Chapter 433). In these instances, myocardial contractility is affected, leading to systolic and/or diastolic dysfunction. The later phases of all forms of shock frequently

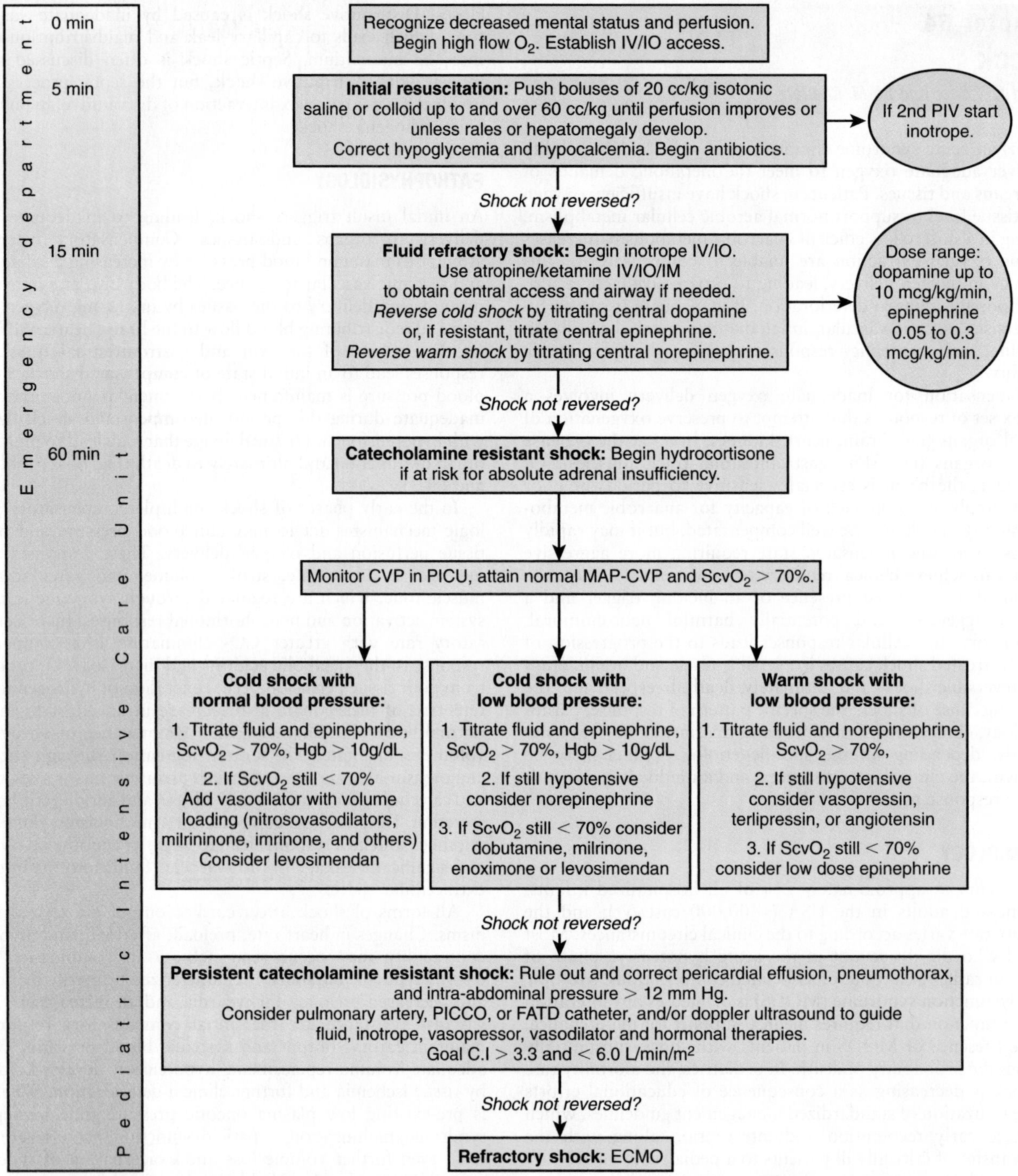

Figure 64-1 Algorithm for time-sensitive, goal-directed, stepwise management of hemodynamic support in infants and children. CI, cardiac index; CRRT, continuous renal replacement therapy; CVP, central venous pressure; ECMO, extracorporeal membrane oxygenation; FATD, femoral arterial thermodilution; Hgb, hemoglobin; IM, intramuscular; IO, intraosseous; IV, intravenous; MAP, mean arterial pressure; PICCO, pulse contour cardiac output. (From Brierly J, Carcillo JA, Choong K, et al: Clinical practice parameters for hemodynamic support of pediatric and neonatal septic shock: 2007 update from the American College of Critical Care Medicine, *Crit Care Med* 37:666–688, 2009. Copyright 2009, Society of Critical Care Medicine and Lippincott Williams & Wilkins.)

have a negative impact on the myocardium, leading to development of a cardiogenic component to the shock state.

Septic shock is often a unique combination of distributive, hypovolemic, and cardiogenic shock. Hypovolemia from intravascular fluid losses occurs through capillary leak. Cardiogenic shock results from the myocardium-depressant effects of sepsis, and distributive shock is the result of decreased systemic vascular resistance. The degree to which a patient exhibits each of these responses varies, but there are frequently alterations in preload, afterload, and myocardial contractility.

In septic shock, it is important to distinguish between the inciting infection and the host inflammatory response. Normally, host immunity prevents the development of sepsis via activation of the reticular endothelial system along with the cellular and humoral immune systems. This host immune response produces an inflammatory cascade of toxic mediators, including hormones,

Table 64-1 TYPES OF SHOCK

HYPOVOLEMIC	CARDIOGENIC	DISTRIBUTIVE	SEPTIC	OBSTRUCTIVE
Decreased preload secondary to internal or external losses	Cardiac pump failure secondary to poor myocardial function	Abnormalities of vasomotor tone due to loss of venous and arterial capacitance	Encompasses multiple forms of shock Hypovolemic: third spacing of fluids into the extracellular, interstitial space Distributive: early shock with decreased afterload Cardiogenic: depression of myocardial function by endotoxins	Decreased cardiac output secondary to direct impediment to right or left heart outflow or restriction of all cardiac chambers
POTENTIAL ETIOLOGIES				
Blood loss: hemorrhage; Plasma loss: burns, nephrotic syndrome; Water/electrolyte loss: vomiting, diarrhea	Congenital heart disease Cardiomyopathies: infectious or acquired, dilated or restrictive Ischemia Arrhythmias	Anaphylaxis Neurologic: loss of sympathetic vascular tone secondary to spinal cord or brainstem injury Drugs	Bacterial Viral Fungal (immunocompromised patients are at increased risk)	Tension pneumothorax Pericardial tamponade Pulmonary embolism Anterior mediastinal masses Critical coarctation of the aorta

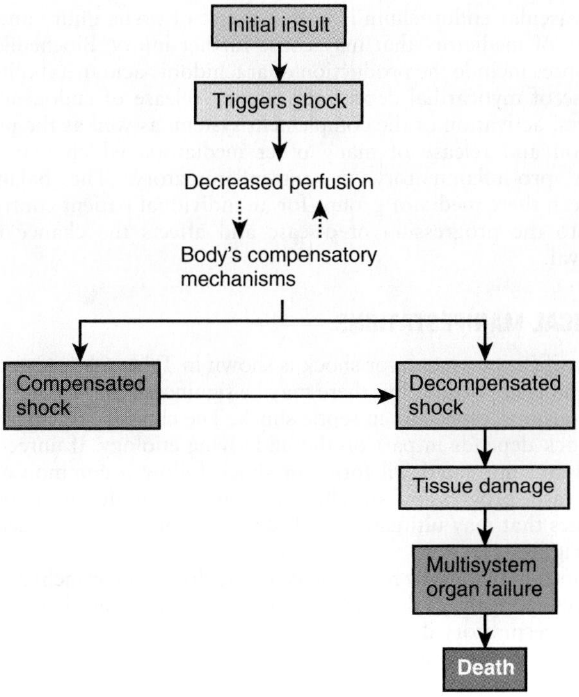

Figure 64-2 Algorithm for decompensated shock.

cytokines, and enzymes. If this inflammatory cascade is uncontrolled, derangement of the microcirculatory system leads to subsequent organ and cellular dysfunction.

The **systemic inflammatory response syndrome (SIRS)** is an inflammatory cascade that is initiated by the host response to an infectious or noninfectious trigger (Table 64-5). This inflammatory cascade is triggered when the host defense system does not adequately recognize and/or clear the triggering event. The inflammatory cascade initiated by shock can lead to hypovolemia, cardiac and vascular failure, acute respiratory distress syndrome (ARDS), insulin resistance, decreased cytochrome P450 (CYP450) activity (decreased steroid synthesis), coagulopathy, and unresolved or secondary infection. Tumor necrosis factor (TNF) and other inflammatory mediators increase vascular permeability, causing diffuse capillary leak, decreased vascular tone, and an imbalance between perfusion and metabolic demands of the tissues. TNF and interleukin-1 (IL-1) stimulate the release of proinflammatory and anti-inflammatory mediators, causing fever and vasodilatation. Arachidonic acid metabolites lead to the development of fever, tachypnea, ventilation-perfusion abnormalities, and lactic acidosis. Nitric oxide, released from the endothelium or inflammatory cells, is a major contributor to hypotension. Myocardial depression is caused by myocardium-depressant factors, TNF, and some interleukins through direct myocardial injury, depleted catecholamines, increased β-endorphin, and production of myocardial nitric oxide.

Table 64-2 CRITERIA FOR ORGAN DYSFUNCTION

ORGAN SYSTEM	CRITERIA FOR DYSFUNCTION
Cardiovascular	Despite administration of isotonic intravenous fluid bolus ≥60 mL/kg in 1 hour: Decrease in BP (hypotension) <5th percentile for age or systolic BP <2 SD below normal for age *OR* Need for vasoactive drug to maintain BP in normal range (dopamine >5 μg/kg/min or dobutamine, epinephrine, or norepinephrine at any dose) *OR* Two of the following: Unexplained metabolic acidosis: base deficit > 5.0 mEq/L Increased arterial lactate: >2× upper limit of normal Oliguria: urine output <0.5 mL/kg/hr Prolonged capillary refill: >5 sec Core to peripheral temperature gap >3°C
Respiratory	PaO_2/FIO_2 ratio <300 in absence of cyanotic heart disease or pre-existing lung disease *OR* $PaCO_2$ >65 torr or 20 mm Hg over baseline $PaCO_2$ *OR* Proven need for >50% FIO_2 to maintain saturation ≥92% *OR* Need for nonelective invasive or noninvasive mechanical ventilation
Neurologic	GCS score ≤11 *OR* Acute change in mental status with a decrease in GCS score ≥3 points from abnormal baseline
Hematologic	Platelet count <80,000/mm^3 or a decline of 50% in the platelet count from the highest value recorded over the last 3 days (for patients with chronic hematologic or oncologic disorders) *OR* INR >2
Renal	Serum creatinine ≥2× upper limit of normal for age or 2-fold increase in baseline creatinine value
Hepatic	Total bilirubin ≥4 mg/dL (not applicable for newborn) Alanine transaminase level 2× upper limit of normal for age

BP, blood pressure; GCS, Glasgow Coma Scale; INR, International Normalized Ratio; SD, standard deviation.

Table 64-3 SIGNS OF DECREASED PERFUSION

ORGAN SYSTEM	↓ PERFUSION	↓↓ PERFUSION	↓↓↓ PERFUSION
Central nervous system	—	Restless, apathetic, anxious	Agitated/confused, stuporous, coma
Respiration	—	↑ Ventilation	↑↑ Ventilation
Metabolism	—	Compensated metabolic acidemia	Uncompensated metabolic acidemia
Gut	—	↓ Motility	Ileus
Kidney	↓ Urine volume ↑ Urinary specific gravity	Oliguria (<0.5 mL/kg/hr)	Oliguria/anuria
Skin	Delayed capillary refill	Cool extremities	Mottled, cyanotic, cold extremities
Cardiovascular system	↑ Heart rate	↑↑ Heart rate ↓ Peripheral pulses	↑↑ Heart rate ↓ Blood pressure, central pulses only

Table 64-4 PATHOPHYSIOLOGY OF SHOCK

EXTRACORPOREAL FLUID LOSS
Hypovolemic shock may be due to direct blood loss through hemorrhage or abnormal loss of body fluids (diarrhea, vomiting, burns, diabetes mellitus or insipidus, nephrosis)
LOWERING PLASMA ONCOTIC FORCES
Hypovolemic shock may also result from hypoproteinemia (liver injury, or as a progressive complication of increased capillary permeability)
ABNORMAL VASODILATION
Distributive shock (neurogenic, anaphylaxis, or septic shock) occurs when there is loss of vascular tone—venous, arterial, or both (sympathetic blockade, local substances affecting permeability, acidosis, drug effects, spinal cord transection)
INCREASED VASCULAR PERMEABILITY
Sepsis may change the capillary permeability in the absence of any change in capillary hydrostatic pressure (endotoxins from sepsis, excess histamine release in anaphylaxis)
CARDIAC DYSFUNCTION
Peripheral hypoperfusion may result from any condition that affects the heart's ability to pump blood efficiently (ischemia, acidosis, drugs, constrictive pericarditis, pancreatitis, sepsis)

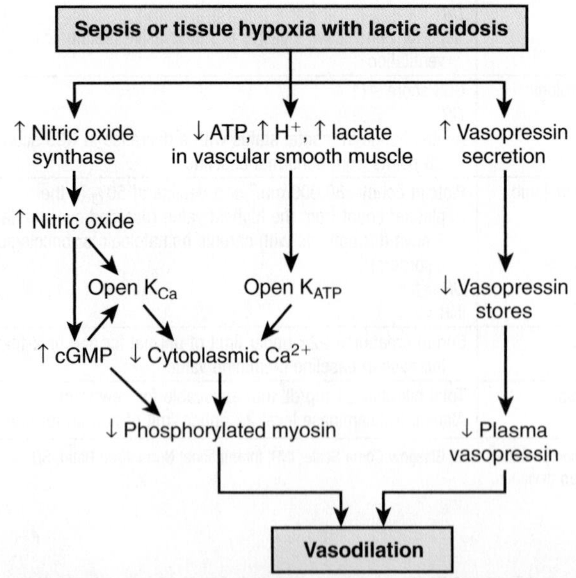

Figure 64-3 Mechanisms of vasodilatory shock. Septic shock and states of prolonged shock causing tissue hypoxia with lactic acidosis increase nitric oxide synthesis, activate the adenosine triphosphate (ATP)–sensitive and calcium-regulated potassium channels (K_{ATP} and K_{Ca}, respectively) in vascular smooth muscle, and lead to depletion of vasopressin. cGMP, cyclic guanosine monophosphate. (From Landry DW, Oliver JA: The pathogenesis of vasodilatory shock, *N Engl J Med* 345:588–595, 2001.)

The inflammatory cascade (Fig. 64-4) is initiated by toxins or superantigens via macrophage binding or lymphocyte activation. The vascular endothelium is both a target of tissue injury and a source of mediators that may cause further injury. Biochemical responses include the production of arachidonic acid metabolites, release of myocardial depressant factors, release of endogenous opiates, activation of the complement system, as well as the production and release of many other mediators, which may be either pro-inflammatory or anti-inflammatory. The balance between these mediator groups for an individual patient contributes to the progression of disease and affects the chance for survival.

CLINICAL MANIFESTATIONS

A classification system for shock is shown in Table 64-1. Categorization is important, but there may be significant overlap among these groups, especially in septic shock. The clinical presentation of shock depends in part on the underlying etiology. If unrecognized and untreated, all forms of shock follow a common and untoward progression of clinical signs and pathophysiologic changes that may ultimately lead to irreversible shock and death (see Fig. 64-2).

Shock may initially manifest as only tachycardia or tachypnea. Progression leads to decreased urine output, poor peripheral perfusion, respiratory distress or failure, alteration of mental status, and low blood pressure (see Table 64-3). A significant misconception is that shock occurs only with low blood pressure. Because of compensatory mechanisms, hypotension is often a late finding and is not a criterion for the diagnosis of shock. Tachycardia, with or without tachypnea, may be the first or only sign of early compensated shock. Hypotension reflects an advanced state of decompensated shock and is associated with increased mortality.

Hypovolemic shock often manifests initially as orthostatic hypotension and is associated with dry mucous membranes, dry axillae, poor skin turgor, and decreased urine output. Depending on the degree of dehydration, the patient with hypovolemic shock may present with either normal or slightly cool distal extremities, and peripheral or even central (femoral) pulses may be normal, decreased, or absent. Because of decreased cardiac output and compensatory peripheral vasoconstriction, the presenting signs of **cardiogenic shock** are tachypnea, cool extremities, delayed capillary filling time, poor peripheral and/or central pulses, declining mental status, and decreased urine output (Chapter 436.1). **Obstructive shock** often also manifests as inadequate cardiac output due to a physical restriction of forward blood flow; the acute presentation may quickly progress to cardiac arrest. **Distributive shock** manifests initially as peripheral vasodilation and increased but inadequate cardiac output.

Regardless of etiology, uncompensated shock, with hypotension, high systemic vascular resistance, decreased cardiac output,

Table 64-5 DIFFERENTIAL DIAGNOSIS OF SYSTEMIC INFLAMMATORY RESPONSE SYNDROME

INFECTION
Bacteremia or meningitis (*Streptococcus pneumoniae, Haemophilus influenzae* type b, *Neisseria meningitidis,* group A *streptococcus, S. aureus*)
Viral illness (influenza, enteroviruses, hemorrhagic fever group, herpes simple virus, respiratory syncytial virus, cytomegalovirus, Epstein-Barr virus)
Encephalitis (arboviruses, enteroviruses, herpes simplex virus)
Rickettsiae (Rocky Mountain spotted fever, *Ehrlichia,* Q fever)
Syphilis
Vaccine reaction (pertussis, influenza, measles)
Toxin-mediated reaction (toxic shock, staphylococcal scalded skin syndrome)
CARDIOPULMONARY
Pneumonia (bacteria, virus, mycobacteria, fungi, allergic reaction)
Pulmonary emboli
Heart failure
Arrhythmia
Pericarditis
Myocarditis
METABOLIC-ENDOCRINE
Adrenal insufficiency (adrenogenital syndrome, corticosteroid withdrawal)
Electrolyte disturbances (hyponatremia or hypernatremia; hypocalcemia or hypercalcemia)
Diabetes insipidus
Diabetes mellitus
Inborn errors of metabolism (organic acidosis, urea cycle, carnitine deficiency, mitochondrial disorders)
Hypoglycemia
Reye syndrome
GASTROINTESTINAL
Gastroenteritis with dehydration
Volvulus
Intussusception
Appendicitis
Peritonitis (spontaneous, associated with perforation or peritoneal dialysis)
Necrotizing enterocolitis
Hepatitis
Hemorrhage
Pancreatitis
HEMATOLOGIC
Anemia (sickle cell disease, blood loss, nutritional)
Methemoglobinemia
Splenic sequestration crisis
Leukemia or lymphoma
Hemophagocytic syndromes
NEUROLOGIC
Intoxication (drugs, carbon monoxide, intentional or accidental overdose)
Intracranial hemorrhage
Infant botulism
Trauma (child abuse, accidental)
Guillain-Barré syndrome
Myasthenia gravis
OTHER
Anaphylaxis (food, drug, insect sting)
Hemolytic-uremic syndrome
Kawasaki disease
Erythema multiforme
Hemorrhagic shock–encephalopathy syndrome
Poisoning
Toxic envenomation
Macrophage activation syndrome

respiratory failure, obtundation, and oliguria, occurs late in the progression of disease. Hemodynamic findings in various shock states are listed in Table 64-6. Additional clinical findings in shock include cutaneous lesions such as petechiae, diffuse erythema, ecchymoses, ecthyma gangrenosum, and peripheral gangrene. Jaundice can be present either as a sign of infection or as a result of **MODS**.

Sepsis is defined as **SIRS** resulting from a suspected or proven infectious etiology. The clinical spectrum of sepsis begins when a systemic (e.g., bacteremia, rickettsial disease, fungemia, viremia) or localized (e.g., meningitis, pneumonia, pyelonephritis) infection progresses from sepsis to **severe sepsis** (the presence of sepsis combined with organ dysfunction). Further deterioration leads to **septic shock** (severe sepsis plus the persistence of hypoperfusion or hypotension despite adequate fluid resuscitation or a requirement for vasoactive agents), **MODS**, and possibly death (Table 64-7). This is a complex spectrum of clinical problems that is a leading cause of mortality in children worldwide. Outcomes improve with early recognition and treatment.

Although **septic shock** is primarily distributive in nature, other and multiple elements of pathophysiology are represented in this disease process. The initial signs and symptoms of sepsis include alterations in temperature regulation (hyperthermia or hypothermia), tachycardia, and tachypnea. In the early stages (hyperdynamic phase or "warm" shock), the cardiac output increases in an attempt to maintain adequate oxygen delivery and meet the greater metabolic demands of the organs and tissues. As septic shock progresses, cardiac output falls in response to the effects of numerous inflammatory mediators, leading to a compensatory elevation in systemic vascular resistance and the development of "cold" shock.

DIAGNOSIS

Shock is diagnosed clinically on the basis of a thorough history and physical exam (see Tables 64-2 and 64-3). Of note, septic shock has a specific consensus conference definition (see Table 64-7). In cases of suspected septic shock, an infectious etiology should be sought through culture of clinically appropriate specimens and prompt initiation of empiric antimicrobial therapy based on patient age, underlying disease, and geographic location. Cultures take time for incubation and their results may not always be positive. Additional evidence for identifying an infectious etiology as the cause of SIRS includes physical examination findings, imaging findings, presence of white blood cells in normally sterile body fluids, and suggestive rashes such as petechiae and purpura. Affected children should be admitted to an intensive care unit or other highly monitored environment, as indicated by clinical status and the resources of the medical facility, where continuous, close invasive monitoring can be performed, including central venous pressure and arterial blood pressure monitoring as clinically indicated.

LABORATORY FINDINGS

Laboratory findings often include evidence of hematologic abnormalities and electrolyte disturbances. Hematologic abnormalities may include thrombocytopenia, prolonged prothrombin and partial thromboplastin times, reduced serum fibrinogen level, elevations of fibrin split products, and anemia. Elevated neutrophil counts and increased immature forms (i.e., bands, myelocytes, promyelocytes), vacuolation of neutrophils, toxic granulations, and Döhle bodies can be seen with infection. Neutropenia or leukopenia may be an ominous sign of overwhelming sepsis.

Glucose dysregulation, a common stress response, may manifest as hyperglycemia or hypoglycemia. Other electrolyte abnormalities are hypocalcemia, hypoalbuminemia, and metabolic acidosis. Renal and/or hepatic function may also be abnormal. Patients with ARDS or pneumonia have impairment of oxygenation (decreased PaO_2) as well as of ventilation (increased $PaCO_2$) in the later stages of lung injury (Chapter 65).

The hallmark of uncompensated shock is an imbalance between oxygen delivery (DO_2) and oxygen consumption ($\dot{V}O_2$).

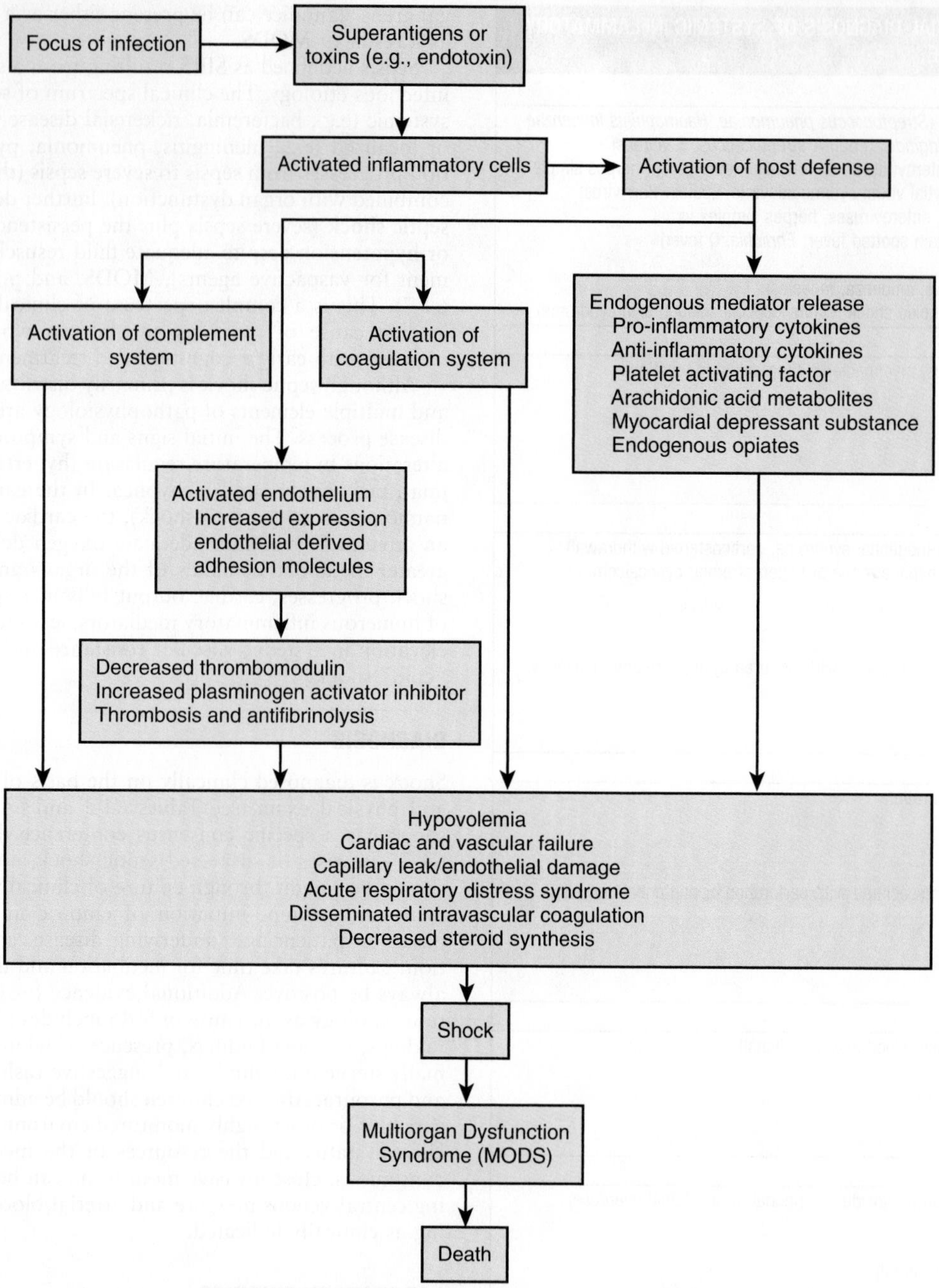

Figure 64-4 Hypothetical pathophysiology of the septic process.

This state is manifested clinically by increased lactic acid production (high anion gap, metabolic acidosis) due to anaerobic metabolism and a low **mixed venous oxygen saturation** ($S\dot{v}O_2$) due to the compensatory increase in tissue oxygen extraction. The gold standard measurement of $S\dot{v}O_2$ is from a pulmonary arterial catheter measurements from this location are often not clinically feasible. Sites such as the right ventricle, right atrium, superior vena cava ($ScvO_2$), or inferior vena cava are often used as for surrogate measures of mixed venous blood.

Oxygen delivery normally exceeds oxygen consumption by threefold. The oxygen extraction ratio is approximately 25%, thus producing a normal $S\dot{v}O_2$ of 75-80%. A falling $S\dot{v}O_2$ value, as measured by co-oximetry, reflects an increasing oxygen extraction ratio and documents a decrease in oxygen delivery relative to consumption. This increase in oxygen extraction by the end-organs is an attempt to maintain adequate oxygen delivery at the cellular level. Along with $S\dot{v}O_2$, serum lactate measurements may be used as a marker for the adequacy of oxygen delivery and the effectiveness of therapeutic interventions.

TREATMENT

Initial Management

Early recognition and prompt intervention are extremely important in the management of all forms of shock (Table 64-8). Baseline mortality is much lower in pediatric shock than in adult shock, and further improvements in mortality may occur with early interventions (see Fig. 64-1). The initial assessment and treatment of the pediatric shock patient should include stabilization of airway, breathing, and circulation (the ABCs) as established by the American Heart Association's pediatric advanced life support (PALS) and neonatal advanced life support (NALS) guidelines (Chapter 62). Depending on the severity of shock, further airway intervention, including intubation and mechanical

Table 64-6 HEMODYNAMIC VARIABLES IN DIFFERENT SHOCK STATES

TYPE OF SHOCK	CARDIAC OUTPUT	SYSTEMIC VASCULAR RESISTANCE	MEAN ARTERIAL PRESSURE	CAPILLARY WEDGE PRESSURE	CENTRAL VENOUS PRESSURE
Hypovolemic	↓	↑	↔ or ↓	↓↓↓	↓↓↓
Cardiogenic*:					
Systolic	↓↓	↑↑↑	↔ or ↓	↑↑	↑↑
Diastolic	↔	↑↑	↔	↑↑	↑
Obstructive	↓	↑	↔ or ↓	↑↑[†]	↑↑[†]
Distributive	↑↑	↓↓↓	↔ or ↓	↔ or ↓	↔ or ↓
Septic:					
Early	↑↑↑	↓↓↓	↔ or ↓[‡]	↓	↓
Late	↓↓	↓↓	↓↓	↑	↑ or ↔

*Systolic or diastolic dysfunction.
[†]Wedge pressure, central venous pressure, and pulmonary artery diastolic pressures are equal.
[‡]Wide pulse pressure.

Table 64-7 INTERNATIONAL CONSENSUS DEFINITIONS FOR PEDIATRIC SEPSIS

Infection	Suspected or proven infection or a clinical syndrome associated with high probability of infection
Systemic inflammatory response syndrome (SIRS)	2 out of 4 criteria, 1 of which must be abnormal temperature or abnormal leukocyte count: 1. Core temperature >38.5°C or <36°C (rectal, bladder, oral, or central catheter) 2. Tachycardia: Mean heart rate >2 SD above normal for age in absence of external stimuli, chronic drugs or painful stimuli *OR* Unexplained persistent elevation over 0.5-4 hr *OR* In children <1 year old, persistent bradycardia over 0.5 hour (mean heart rate <10th percentile for age in absence of vagal stimuli, β-blocker drugs, or congenital heart disease) 3. Respiratory rate >2 SD above normal for age or acute need for mechanical ventilation not related to neuromuscular disease or general anesthesia 4. Leukocyte count elevated or depressed for age (not secondary to chemotherapy) or >10% immature neutrophils
Sepsis	SIRS plus a suspected or proven infection
Severe sepsis	Sepsis plus 1 of the following: 1. Cardiovascular organ dysfunction, defined as: • Despite >40 mL/kg of isotonic intravenous fluid in 1 hour: • Hypotension <5th percentile for age or systolic blood pressure <2 SD below normal for age *OR* • Need for vasoactive drug to maintain blood pressure *OR* • 2 of the following: • Unexplained metabolic acidosis: base deficit > 5 mEq/L • Increased arterial lactate: >2 times upper limit of normal • Oliguria: urine output <0.5 mL/kg/hr • Prolonged capillary refill: >5 sec • Core to peripheral temperature gap >3°C 2. Acute respiratory distress syndrome (ARDS) as defined by the presence of a PaO_2/FIO_2 ratio ≤300 mm Hg, bilateral infiltrates on chest radiograph, and no evidence of left heart failure *OR* Sepsis plus 2 or more organ dysfunctions (respiratory, renal, neurologic, hematologic, or hepatic)
Septic shock	Sepsis plus cardiovascular organ dysfunction as defined above
Multiple organ dysfunction syndrome (MODS)	Presence of altered organ function such that homeostasis cannot be maintained without medical intervention

SD, standard deviation.

ventilation, may be necessary to lessen the workload of breathing and decrease the body's overall metabolic demands. Neonates and infants in particular may have profound glucose dysregulation in association with shock. Glucose levels should be checked routinely and treated appropriately, especially early in the course of illness.

Given the predominance of sepsis and hypovolemia as the most common causes of shock in the pediatric population, most therapeutic regimens are based on guidelines established in these settings. Immediately following establishment of intravenous (IV) or intraosseous (IO) access, aggressive, early goal-directed therapy (EGDT) should be initiated unless there are significant concerns for cardiogenic shock as an underlying pathophysiology. Rapid IV administration of 20 mL/kg isotonic saline or, less often, colloid should be initiated in an attempt to reverse the shock state. This bolus should be repeated quickly up to 60-80 mL/kg; it is not unusual for severely affected patients to require this volume within the first hour.

If shock remains refractory following 60-80 mL/kg of volume resuscitation, inotropic therapy (dopamine, norepinephrine, or epinephrine) should be instituted while additional fluids are administered. Current guidelines recommend administration of these inotropic agents via peripheral intravenous (PIV) lines, with very close monitoring of the PIV sites while central venous access is being obtained, because a delay in the initiation of inotropes in shock has been associated with increased mortality.

Rapid fluid resuscitation using 60-80 mL/kg or more is associated with improved survival without an increased incidence of

Table 64-8 GOAL-DIRECTED THERAPY OF ORGAN SYSTEM DYSFUNCTION IN SHOCK

SYSTEM	DISORDERS	GOALS	THERAPIES
Respiratory	Acute respiratory distress syndrome	Prevent/treat: hypoxia and respiratory acidosis	Oxygen
	Respiratory muscle fatigue	Prevent barotrauma	Early endotracheal intubation and mechanical ventilation
	Central apnea	Decrease work of breathing	Positive end-expiratory pressure (PEEP) Permissive hypercapnia High-frequency ventilation Extracorporeal membrane oxygenation (ECMO)
Renal	Prerenal failure Renal failure	Prevent/treat: hypovolemia, hypervolemia, hyperkalemia, metabolic acidosis, hypernatremia/hyponatremia, and hypertension Monitor serum electrolytes	Judicious fluid resuscitation Low-dose dopamine Establishment of normal urine output and blood pressure for age Furosemide (Lasix) Dialysis, ultrafiltration, hemofiltration
Hematologic	Coagulopathy (disseminated intravascular coagulation)	Prevent/treat: bleeding	Vitamin K Fresh frozen plasma Platelets
	Thrombosis	Prevent/treat: abnormal clotting	Heparinization Activated protein C
Gastrointestinal	Stress ulcers	Prevent/treat: gastric bleeding Avoid aspiration, abdominal distention	Histamine H_2 receptor–blocking agents or proton pump inhibitors Nasogastric tube
	Ileus Bacterial translocation	Avoid mucosal atrophy	Early enteral feedings
Endocrine	Adrenal insufficiency, primary or secondary to chronic steroid therapy	Prevent/treat: adrenal crisis	Stress-dose steroids in patients previously given steroids Physiologic dose for presumed primary insufficiency in sepsis
Metabolic	Metabolic acidosis	Correct etiology Normalize pH	Treatment of hypovolemia (fluids), poor cardiac function (fluids, inotropic agents) Improvement of renal acid excretion Low-dose (0.5-2 mEq/kg) sodium bicarbonate if the patient is not showing response, pH < 7.1, and ventilation (CO_2 elimination) is adequate

pulmonary edema. Fluid resuscitation in increments of 20 mL/kg should be titrated to normalize heart rate (according to age-based heart rates), urine output (to 1 mL/kg/hr), capillary refill time (to <2 sec), and mental status. Fluid resuscitation may sometimes require as much as 200 mL/kg. It must be stressed that hypotension is often a late and ominous finding, and normalization of blood pressure alone is not a reliable endpoint for assessing the effectiveness of resuscitation. Although the type of fluid (crystalloid vs colloid) is an area of ongoing debate, fluid resuscitation in the first hour is unquestionably essential to survival in septic shock, regardless of the fluid type administered.

Additional Early Considerations

In **septic shock** specifically, early administration of broad-spectrum antimicrobial agents is associated with a reduction in mortality. The choice of antimicrobial agents depends on the predisposing risk factors and the clinical situation. Bacterial resistance patterns in the community and/or hospital should be considered in the selection of optimal antimicrobial therapy. Neonates should be treated with ampicillin plus cefotaxime and/or gentamicin. Acyclovir should be added if herpes simplex virus is suspected clinically. In infants and children, community-acquired infections with *Neisseria meningitidis* can be treated empirically with a 3rd-generation cephalosporin (ceftriaxone or cefotaxime) or high-dose penicillin. *Haemophilus influenzae* infections can be treated empirically with a 3rd-generation cephalosporin (ceftriaxone or cefotaxime). The prevalence of resistant *Streptococcus pneumoniae* often requires the addition of vancomycin, depending on the specific clinical scenario. Suspicion of community- or hospital-acquired, methicillin-resistant *Staphylococcus aureus* infection warrants coverage with vancomycin, depending on local resistance patterns. If an intra-abdominal process is suspected, anaerobic coverage should be included with an agent such as metronidazole, clindamycin, or piperacillin-tazobactam.

Nosocomial sepsis should generally be treated with at least a 3rd- or 4th-generation cephalosporin or a penicillin with an extended gram-negative spectrum (e.g., piperacillin-tazobactam). An aminoglycoside should be added as the clinical situation warrants. Vancomycin should be added to the regimen if the patient has an indwelling medical device (Chapter 172), gram-positive cocci are isolated from the blood, or methicillin-resistant *S. aureus* infection is suspected, or as empiric coverage for *S. pneumoniae* in a patient with meningitis. Empirical coverage for fungal infections should be considered for selected immunocompromised patients (Chapter 171). It should be noted that these are broad, generalized recommendations that must be tailored to the individual clinical scenario and to the local resistance patterns of the community and/or hospital.

Distributive shock that is not secondary to sepsis is caused by a primary abnormality in vascular tone. Cardiac output in affected patients is usually maintained and may initially be supranormal. These patients may benefit temporarily from volume resuscitation, but the early initiation of a vasoconstrictive agent to increase SVR is an important element of clinical care. Patients with spinal cord injury and spinal shock may benefit from either phenylephrine or vasopressin to increase SVR. Epinephrine is the treatment of choice for patients with anaphylaxis (Table 64-9). This agent has peripheral α-adrenergic as well as inotropic effects that may improve the myocardial depression seen with anaphylaxis and its associated inflammatory response (Chapter 143).

Patients with **cardiogenic shock** have poor cardiac output secondary to systolic and/or diastolic myocardial depression, often with a compensatory elevation in SVR. These patients may show poor response to aggressive fluid resuscitation and, in fact, may demonstrate decompensation quickly when fluids are administered. Smaller boluses of fluid (5-10 mL/kg) should be given in cardiogenic shock. In any patient with shock whose clinical status deteriorates with fluid resuscitation, a cardiogenic etiology should

Table 64-9 CARDIOVASCULAR DRUG TREATMENT OF SHOCK

DRUG	EFFECT(S)	DOSING RANGE	COMMENT(S)
Dopamine	↑ Cardiac contractility	3-20 μg/kg/min	↑ Risk of arrhythmias at high doses
	Significant peripheral vasoconstriction at >10 μg/kg/min		
Epinephrine	↑ Heart rate and ↑ cardiac contractility	0.05-3.0 μg/kg/min	May ↓ renal perfusion at high doses
	Potent vasoconstrictor		↑ Myocardial O_2 consumption
			Risk of arrhythmia at high doses
Dobutamine	↑ Cardiac contractility	1-10 μg/kg/min	—
	Peripheral vasodilator		
Norepinephrine	Potent vasoconstriction	0.05-1.5 μg/kg/min	↑ Blood pressure secondary to ↑ systemic vascular resistance
	No significant effect on cardiac contractility		↑ Left ventricular afterload
Phenylephrine	Potent vasoconstriction	0.5-2.0 μg/kg/min	Can cause sudden hypertension
			↑ O_2 consumption

Table 64-10 VASODILATORS/AFTERLOAD REDUCERS

DRUG	EFFECT(S)	DOSING RANGE	COMMENT(S)
Nitroprusside	Vasodilator (mainly arterial)	0.5-4.0 μg/kg/min	Rapid effect
			Risk of cyanide toxicity with prolonged use (>96 hours)
Nitroglycerin	Vasodilator (mainly venous)	1.0-20 μg/kg/min	Rapid effect
			Risk of increased intracranial pressure
Prostaglandin E_1	Vasodilator	0.01-0.2 μg/kg/min	Can lead to hypotension
	Maintains an open ductus arteriosus in the newborn with ductal-dependent congenital heart disease		Risk of apnea
Milrinone	Increased cardiac contractility	Load 50 μg/kg over 15 min	Phosphodiesterase inhibitor—slows cyclic adenosine monophosphate breakdown
	Improves cardiac diastolic function	0.5-1 μg/kg/min	
	Peripheral vasodilation		

be considered, and further administration of intravenous fluids should be performed cautiously. Early initiation of myocardial support with dopamine or epinephrine to improve cardiac output is important in this context. Consideration should be given to administering an inodilator, such as milrinone, early in the process.

Despite adequate cardiac output with the support of inotropic agents, a high SVR with poor peripheral perfusion and acidosis may persist in cardiogenic shock. Therefore, if not already started, milrinone therapy may improve systolic function and decrease SVR without causing a significant increase in heart rate. Furthermore, this agent has the added benefit of enhancing diastolic relaxation. Dobutamine or other vasodilating agents, such as nitroprusside, may also be considered in this setting (Table 64-10). Dosage titration of these agents should target clinical endpoints, including increased urine output, improved peripheral perfusion, resolution of acidosis, and normalization of mental status. Agents that improve blood pressure by increasing SVR, such as norepinephrine and vasopressin, should generally be avoided in patients with cardiogenic shock (although they may be helpful for other causes of shock). These agents may cause further decompensation and potentially precipitate cardiac arrest as a result of the increased afterload and additional work imposed on the myocardium. The combination of inotropic and vasoactive agents administered must be tailored to the pathophysiology of the individual patient. Close and frequent reassessment of the patient's cardiovascular status is essential.

For patients with **obstructive shock**, fluid resuscitation may be briefly temporizing in maintaining cardiac output, but the primary insult must be immediately addressed. Examples of lifesaving therapeutic interventions for such patients are pericardiocentesis for pericardial effusion, pleurocentesis or chest tube placement for pneumothorax, thrombectomy/thrombolysis for pulmonary embolism, and the initiation of a prostaglandin infusion for ductus-dependent cardiac lesions. There is often a "last drop" or "last straw" phenomenon associated with some obstructive lesions, in that further small amounts of intravascular volume depletion may lead to a rapid deterioration, including cardiac arrest, if the obstructive lesion is not corrected.

Regardless of the etiology of shock, metabolic status should be meticulously maintained (see Table 64-8). Electrolyte levels should be monitored closely and corrected as needed. Hypoglycemia is common and should be promptly treated. Hypocalcemia, which may contribute to myocardial dysfunction, should be treated with a goal of normalizing the ionized calcium concentration. There is no evidence that supranormal calcium levels benefit the myocardium, and hypercalcemia may actually be associated with increased myocardial toxicity.

Hydrocortisone replacement may be beneficial in pediatric shock. Up to 50% of critically ill patients may have absolute or relative adrenal insufficiency. Patients at risk for adrenal insufficiency include those with congenial adrenal hypoplasia, abnormalities of the hypothalamic-pituitary axis, and recent therapy with corticosteroids (including patients with asthma, rheumatic diseases, malignancies, and inflammatory bowel disease). These patients are at high risk for adrenal dysfunction and should receive stress doses of hydrocortisone. Steroids may also be considered in patients with shock that is unresponsive to fluid resuscitation and catecholamines. Determination of baseline cortisol levels prior to steroid administration may be beneficial in guiding therapy, although this idea remains controversial.

Considerations for Continued Therapy

After the first hour of therapy and attempts at early reversal of shock, focusing of therapies on goal-directed endpoints should continue in an intensive care setting (see Fig. 64-1 and Table 64-8). These clinical endpoints serve as global markers for organ perfusion and oxygenation. Laboratory parameters such as $S\bar{v}O_2$ (or $ScvO_2$), serum lactate concentration, cardiac index, and hemoglobin level serve as adjunctive measures of tissue oxygen delivery. On the basis of guidelines published in 2009, hemoglobin should be maintained >10 g/dL, $S\dot{v}O_2$ (or $ScvO_2$) >70%, and cardiac index at 3.3-6 L/min/m^2 to optimize oxygen delivery in the acute phase of shock (although it should be noted that cardiac index is rarely monitored in the clinical setting owing to the limited use of pulmonary artery catheters and the lack of accurate noninvasive cardiac output monitors for infants and children). Blood lactate levels and calculation of base deficit from arterial blood gas values are very useful markers for the adequacy of oxygen delivery. It is important to note that these parameters are all indicators of global oxygen delivery and utilization, but there are no currently available clear indicators for adequate measurement of local tissue oxygenation.

Respiratory support should be used as clinically appropriate. When shock leads to ARDS or acute lung injury (ALI) requiring mechanical ventilation, lung-protective strategies to keep plateau pressure below 30 cm H_2O and maintain tidal volume at 6 mL/kg have been shown to improve mortality in adult patients (Chapter 65). These data are extrapolated to pediatric patients because of the lack of definitive pediatric studies in this area. Additionally, after the initial shock state has been reversed, renal replacement therapy and fluid removal may also be useful in children with anuria or oliguria and resultant severe fluid overload (Chapter 529). Intravenous immunoglobulin infusion or plasmapheresis may also be considered in certain circumstances as therapeutic adjuncts for shock. Other interventions include correction of coagulopathy with fresh frozen plasma or cryoprecipitate and platelet transfusions as necessary, especially in the presence of active bleeding.

In addition to symptomatic care and treatment of any underlying infectious causes, therapies to augment host defense, block trigger events, prevent leukocyte-endothelium interaction, and inhibit vasoactive substances, cytokines, or lipid mediators are being investigated. To date, the results of clinical trials investigating drugs targeting the mediators of SIRS have been disappointing. Trials have been conducted with anti-endotoxin antibodies, antioxidant compounds, an IL-1 receptor antagonist, IL-1 antibodies, bradykinin receptor antibodies, cyclooxygenase inhibitors, thromboxane antagonists, platelet-activating factor (PAF) antagonists, inhibitors of leukocyte adhesion molecules, nitric oxide antagonists, anti-TNF antibody, bactericidal permeability–increasing protein, and recombinant human activated protein C (drotrecogin-α). Studies of drotrecogin-α have shown improvement in the 28-day survival rate in adults, but enrollment in the pediatric trial was closed early because of an increased risk of intracranial bleeding and an unfavorable risk : benefit ratio, particularly in neonates. The best treatment for shock consists of early recognition, early antimicrobial therapy (for suspected septic shock), aggressive fluid resuscitation (except in cardiogenic shock), and early goal-directed therapy.

If shock remains refractory despite maximal therapeutic interventions, mechanical support with **extracorporeal membrane oxygenation (ECMO)** or a **ventricular assist device (VAD)** may be indicated. ECMO may be lifesaving in cases of refractory shock regardless of underlying etiology. Similarly, a VAD may be indicated for refractory cardiogenic shock in the setting of cardiomyopathy or recent cardiac surgery. Systemic anticoagulation, which is required while patients are receiving mechanical support, may be difficult, given the significant coagulopathy often encountered in refractory shock, especially when the underlying etiology is sepsis. Mechanical support in refractory shock poses substantial risks but can improve survival in specific populations of patients.

PROGNOSIS

In septic shock, mortality rates are as low as 3% in previously healthy children and 6-9% in children with chronic illness (compared with 25-30% in adults). With early recognition and therapy, the mortality rate for pediatric shock continues to improve, but shock and MODS remain one of the leading causes of death in infants and children. The risk of death involves a complex interaction of factors, including the underlying etiology, presence of chronic illness, host immune response, and timing of recognition and therapy.

BIBLIOGRAPHY

Please visit the Nelson Textbook of Pediatrics *website at* *www.expertconsult.com* *for the complete bibliography.*

Chapter 65
Respiratory Distress and Failure

Ashok P. Sarnaik and Jeff A. Clark

The term **respiratory distress** is often used to indicate signs and symptoms of abnormal respiratory pattern. A child with nasal flaring, tachypnea, chest wall retractions, stridor, grunting, dyspnea, and wheezing is often judged as having respiratory distress. The magnitude of these findings is used to judge the clinical severity of respiratory distress. Although nasal flaring is a nonspecific sign, the other signs may be useful in localizing the site of pathology (Chapter 365). Respiratory failure is defined as inability of the lungs to provide sufficient oxygen (hypoxic respiratory failure) or remove carbon dioxide (ventilatory failure) to meet metabolic demands. Whereas respiratory distress is a clinical impression, the diagnosis of **respiratory failure** indicates inadequacy of oxygenation or ventilation or both. Respiratory distress can occur in patients without respiratory disease, and respiratory failure can occur in patients without respiratory distress.

RESPIRATORY DISTRESS

Nasal flaring is an extremely important sign of distress, especially in infants. It is indicative of discomfort, pain, fatigue, or breathing difficulty. The state of responsiveness is another crucial sign. Lethargy, disinterest in surroundings, and poor cry are suggestive of exhaustion, hypercarbia, and impending respiratory failure. Abnormalities of the rate and depth of respirations can occur with both pulmonary and nonpulmonary causes of respiratory distress. In diseases of decreased lung compliance, such as pneumonia and pulmonary edema, respirations are characteristically rapid and shallow (decreased tidal volume). In obstructive airway diseases, such as asthma and laryngotracheitis, respirations are deep (increased tidal volume) but less rapid. Rapid and deep respirations without other respiratory signs should alert the physician to the possibility of nonrespiratory causes of respiratory distress, such as response to metabolic acidosis (diabetic ketoacidosis, renal tubular acidosis) or stimulation of the respiratory center (encephalitis, ingestion of central nervous system [CNS] stimulants). Chest wall, suprasternal, and subcostal retractions are manifestations of increased inspiratory effort, weak chest wall, or both. Inspiratory stridor indicates airway obstruction above the thoracic inlet, whereas expiratory wheezing results from airway obstruction below the thoracic inlet. Grunting is most commonly heard in diseases with decreased functional residual capacity (e.g., pneumonia, pulmonary edema) and peripheral airway obstruction (e.g., bronchiolitis).

Respiratory Disease Manifesting as Respiratory Distress

Clinical examination is important in localizing the site of pathology (Chapter 365). Extrathoracic airway obstruction occurs anywhere above the thoracic inlet. Inspiratory stridor, suprasternal, chest wall, and subcostal retractions, and prolongation of inspiration are hallmarks of extrathoracic airway obstruction. By

Table 65-1 TYPICAL LOCALIZING SIGNS FOR PULMONARY PATHOLOGY

SITE OF PATHOLOGY	RESPIRATORY RATE	RETRACTIONS	AUDIBLE SOUNDS
Extrathoracic airway	↑	↑↑↑↑	Stridor
Intrathoracic extra-pulmonary	↑	↑↑	Wheezing
Intrathoracic intrapulmonary	↑↑	↑↑	Wheezing
Alveolar interstitial	↑↑↑	↑↑↑	Grunting

Table 65-2 EXAMPLES OF ANATOMIC SITES OF LESIONS CAUSING RESPIRATORY FAILURE

LUNG	RESPIRATORY PUMP
CENTRAL AIRWAY OBSTRUCTION	**THORACIC CAGE**
Choanal atresia Tonsillo-adenoidal hypertrophy Retropharyngeal/peritonsillar abscess Laryngomalacia Epiglottitis Vocal cord paralysis Laryngotracheitis Subglottic stenosis Vascular ring/pulmonary sling Mediastinal mass Foreign body aspiration Obstructive sleep apnea	Kyphoscoliosis Diaphragmatic hernia Flail chest Eventration of diaphragm Asphyxiating thoracic dystrophy Prune-belly syndrome Dermatomyositis Abdominal distention
PERIPHERAL AIRWAY OBSTRUCTION	**BRAINSTEM**
Asthma Bronchiolitis Foreign body aspiration Aspiration pneumonia Cystic fibrosis α-1-antitrypsin deficiency	Arnold Chiari malformation Central hypoventilation syndrome CNS depressants Trauma Increased intracranial pressure CNS infections
ALVEOLAR-INTERSTITIAL DISEASE	**SPINAL CORD**
Lobar pneumonia ARDS/hyaline membrane disease Interstitial pneumonia Hydrocarbon pneumonia Pulmonary hemorrhage/hemosiderosis	Trauma Transverse myelitis Spinal muscular atrophy Poliomyelitis Tumor/abscess
	NEUROMUSCULAR
	Phrenic nerve injury Birth trauma Infant botulism Guillain-Barré syndrome Muscular dystrophy Myasthenia gravis Organophosphate poisoning

ARDS, acute respiratory distress syndrome; CNS, central nervous system.

comparison, features of intrathoracic airway obstruction are prolongation of expiration and expiratory wheezing. Typical manifestations of alveolar interstitial pathology are rapid, shallow respirations, chest wall retractions, and grunting. The site of pathology can be localized and the differential diagnosis established on the basis of the clinical signs and symptoms (Tables 65-1 and 65-2).

Respiratory Distress without Respiratory Disease

Although respiratory distress most commonly results from diseases of lungs, airways, and chest wall, pathology in other organ systems can manifest as "respiratory distress" and lead to misdiagnosis and inappropriate management (Table 65-3). Respiratory distress resulting from heart failure or diabetic ketoacidosis may be misdiagnosed as asthma and improperly treated with albuterol, resulting in worsened hemodynamic state or ketoacidosis.

Table 65-3 NONPULMONARY CAUSES OF RESPIRATORY DISTRESS

	EXAMPLE(S)	MECHANISM(S)
Cardiovascular	Left-to-right shunt Congestive heart failure Cardiogenic shock	↑ Pulmonary blood/water content Metabolic acidosis Baroreceptor stimulation
Central nervous system	Increased intracranial pressure Encephalitis Neurogenic pulmonary edema Toxic encephalopathy	Stimulation of brainstem respiratory centers
Metabolic	Diabetic ketoacidosis Organic acidemia Hyperammonemia	Stimulation of central and peripheral chemoreceptors
Renal	Renal tubular acidosis	Stimulation of central and peripheral chemoreceptors
	Hypertension	Left ventricular dysfunction → increased pulmonary blood/water content
Sepsis	Toxic shock syndrome Meningococcemia	Cytokine stimulation of respiratory centers Baroreceptor stimulation from shock Metabolic acidosis

Table 65-4 CARDIOVASCULAR PATHOLOGY MANIFESTING AS RESPIRATORY DISTRESS

I. DECREASED LUNG COMPLIANCE
- A. Left-to-Right Shunts
  - 1. Ventricular septal defect, atrial septal defect, patent ductus arteriosus, atrioventricular canal, truncus arteriosus
  - 2. Cerebral or hepatic arteriovenous fistula
- B. Ventricular Failure
  - 1. Left-heart obstructive lesions
    - a) aortic stenosis
    - b) coarctation of the aorta
    - c) mitral stenosis
    - d) Interrupted aortic arch
    - e) hypoplastic left heart syndrome
  - 2. Myocardial infarction
    - a) anomalous left coronary artery arising from the pulmonary artery
  - 3. Hypertension
    - a) acute glomerulonephritis
  - 4. Inflammatory/Infectious
    - a) myocarditis
    - b) pericardial effusion
  - 5. Idiopathic
    - a) dilated cardiomyopathy
    - b) hypertophic obstructive cardiomyopathy
- C. Pulmonary Venous Obstruction
  - 1. Total anomalous pulmonary venous return with obstruction
  - 2. Cor triatriatum

II. SHOCK RESULTING IN METABOLIC ACIDOSIS
- A. Left-Heart Obstructive Lesions
- B. Acute Ventricular Failure
  - 1. Myocarditis, myocardial infarction

CARDIOVASCULAR DISEASE MANIFESTING AS RESPIRATORY DISTRESS

A child with cardiovascular pathology may present with respiratory distress caused by 2 mechanisms: (1) decreased lung compliance and (2) cardiogenic shock (Table 65-4). Diseases that result in an increased pulmonary arterial blood flow (e.g., left-to-right shunts) or increased pulmonary venous pressure (e.g., left ventricular dysfunction from hypertension or myocarditis, obstructed total anomalous pulmonary venous return) cause an increase in pulmonary capillary pressure and transudation of fluid into the pulmonary interstitium and alveoli. The increased pulmonary blood and water content leads to decreased lung compliance and results in rapid shallow respirations.

Interstitial edema often results in small airway obstruction, manifesting as expiratory wheezing. Patients with cardiac lesions that result in a low cardiac output state, such as obstructive lesions of left side of the heart and acquired or congenital cardiomyopathy, often present in a state of shock with decreased tissue perfusion and metabolic acidosis. Such children demonstrate respiratory distress because of stimulation of chemoreceptors by metabolic acidosis and stimulation of baroreceptors by decreased blood pressure.

NEUROLOGIC DISEASE MANIFESTING AS RESPIRATORY DISTRESS CNS dysfunction can lead to alterations in respiratory patterns. Increased intracranial pressure (ICP) may manifest as respiratory distress. Early rise in ICP results in stimulation of respiratory centers, leading to increases in the rate (tachypnea) and depth (hyperpnea) of respiration. The resultant decrease in $Paco_2$ and elevation of cerebrospinal fluid pH lead to cerebral vasoconstriction and amelioration of intracranial hypertension. Cerebral hemispheric and midbrain lesions often result in hyperpnea as well as tachypnea. In such situations, blood gas measurements typically show respiratory alkalosis without hypoxemia. Pathology affecting the pons and medulla manifests as irregular breathing patterns such as apneustic breathing (prolonged inspiration with brief expiratory periods), Cheyne-Stokes breathing (alternate periods of rapid and slow breathing), and irregular, ineffective breathing or apnea. Level of consciousness is most often impaired when abnormal breathing pattern from a brainstem disorder is present. Along with respiratory changes, other manifestations of CNS dysfunction and increased ICP may be present, such as focal neurologic signs, pupillary changes, hypertension, and bradycardia (Chapter 63). Occasionally, severe CNS dysfunction can result in **neurogenic pulmonary edema** (NPE) and respiratory distress, which may be due to excessive sympathetic discharge resulting in increased pulmonary venous hydrostatic pressure as well as increased pulmonary capillary permeability. **Central neurogenic hyperventilation** is characteristically observed in CNS involvement by illnesses such as Reye syndrome and encephalitis. **Bradycardia and apnea** may be due to CNS-depressant medications, poisoning, prolonged hypoxia, trauma, or infection (see Table 65-2).

TOXIC-METABOLIC STATES MANIFESTING AS RESPIRATORY DISTRESS Direct stimulation of respiratory centers resulting in respiratory alkalosis is encountered in certain intoxications, such as those involving salicylates and theophylline. Similarly, intoxication with general CNS stimulants such as cocaine and amphetamines may manifest as increased respirations. Presence of endogenous and exogenous toxins, such as organic acidemias, ingestion of methanol and ethylene glycol, and late stages of salicylism, cause metabolic acidosis and compensatory hyperventilation, which can manifest as respiratory distress. Blood gas measurements show decreased pH and compensatory hypocarbia with normal oxygenation. Metabolic disorders causing hyperammonemia, on the other hand, cause respiratory alkalosis (decreased $Paco_2$ with increased pH) because ammonia is a stimulant of respiratory centers.

OTHER NONPULMONARY ENTITIES MANIFESTING AS RESPIRATORY DISTRESS Sepsis and septic shock may manifest as respiratory distress by causing acute respiratory distress syndrome [ARDS], hypovolemic stimulation of baroreceptors, stimulation of respiratory centers by cytokines, and lactic acidosis. Similarly, renal disease may manifest as respiratory distress by causing metabolic acidosis (e.g., renal tubular acidosis or renal failure) or hypertensive left ventricular failure and fluid overload.

RESPIRATORY FAILURE

Respiratory failure occurs when oxygenation and ventilation are insufficient to meet the metabolic demands of the body. Respiratory failure may result from an abnormality in (1) lung and airways, (2) chest wall and muscles of respiration, or (3) central and peripheral chemoreceptors (Fig. 65-1). Clinical manifestations depend largely on the site of pathology. Although respiratory failure is traditionally defined as respiratory dysfunction resulting in $Pao_2 < 60$ torr with breathing of room air and $Paco_2 > 50$ torr resulting in acidosis, the patient's general state, respiratory effort, and potential for impending exhaustion are more important indicators than blood gas values.

Acute lung injury due to pneumonia, sepsis, aspiration, drowning, embolism, trauma, smoke inhalation, or drug overdose often leads to the **acute respiratory distress syndrome** (Table 65-5; Fig. 65-2).

Pathophysiology of Respiratory Failure

Respiratory failure can be classified into 2 categories: (1) hypoxic respiratory failure (failure of oxygenation) and (2) hypercarbic respiratory failure (failure of ventilation). The two entities may coexist as a combined failure of oxygenation and ventilation. The main function of the respiratory system is to move atmospheric gases into the alveolar capillary units of the lung and to move alveolar gas back out into the atmosphere. Systemic venous (pulmonary arterial) blood is arterialized after mixing with the alveolar gas and being carried back to the heart by pulmonary veins. The arterial gas composition depends on the gas composition of the atmosphere and the effectiveness of alveolar ventilation, pulmonary capillary perfusion, and diffusion across the alveolar capillary membrane. Abnormality at any of these steps can result in respiratory failure.

INSPIRED GAS COMPOSITION Unless modified by the caretaker, inspired gas consists mainly of oxygen and nitrogen. The atmospheric pressure of inspired air depends on altitude. At sea level, it is 760 torr (mm Hg). At higher altitude, atmospheric pressure is lower; in Denver, for instance, the barometric pressure is around 630 torr. When the atmospheric gas reaches alveoli, it is 100% humidified. At 100% humidity and a temperature of 37°C, the water vapor pressure is 47 torr regardless of altitude. Therefore, pressure of inspired gases is calculated as barometric pressure minus 47 torr. Because the fraction of inspired oxygen (Fio_2) is 0.2093 (close to 0.21) throughout our atmosphere, the Po_2 of inspired gas (Pio_2) is $(760 - 47) \times 0.21 = 150$ torr in San Diego (sea level) and $(630 - 47) \times 0.21 = 122$ torr in Denver. Lower Pio_2 value at a higher altitude has a potentially adverse effect on oxygenation in respiratory disease. Pio_2 can be increased by either an increase in Fio_2 or administration of oxygen at greater than atmospheric pressure, such as in a hyperbaric chamber. For a person breathing 40% oxygen, the Pio_2 would be 285 torr in San Diego and 234 torr in Denver.

ALVEOLAR GAS COMPOSITION When atmospheric gas enters alveoli, oxygen is exchanged for carbon dioxide. This exchange is not equimolar because the body's average oxygen consumption is greater than carbon dioxide production, as represented by the respiratory quotient (R), which is CO_2 production ÷ O_2 consumption. Alveolar gas composition is roughly estimated by the following equation:

$$P_AO_2 = Pio_2 - (Paco_2 \div R)$$

where P_AO_2 is the expected partial pressure of oxygen in alveoli. Under normal metabolic conditions, R is assumed to be 0.8. P_AO_2 is traditionally compared with Pao_2 to determine the extent of oxygenation abnormality; this comparison is referred to as the alveolar-arterial oxygen gradient (A-ao_2).

ALVEOLAR VENTILATION AND DEAD SPACE VENTILATION The amount of air breathed in a minute is termed *minute volume*, which is a product of tidal volume (V_T) and respiratory rate. Part of the V_T occupies conducting airways (*anatomic dead space*) and does not participate in gas exchange. Additionally, air that enters alveoli that are not perfused (e.g., from pulmonary embolism) or poorly perfused (e.g., because of decreased cardiac output) also does not contribute to gas exchange (*physiologic dead space*). *Total dead space* (V_D) is a sum of anatomic and

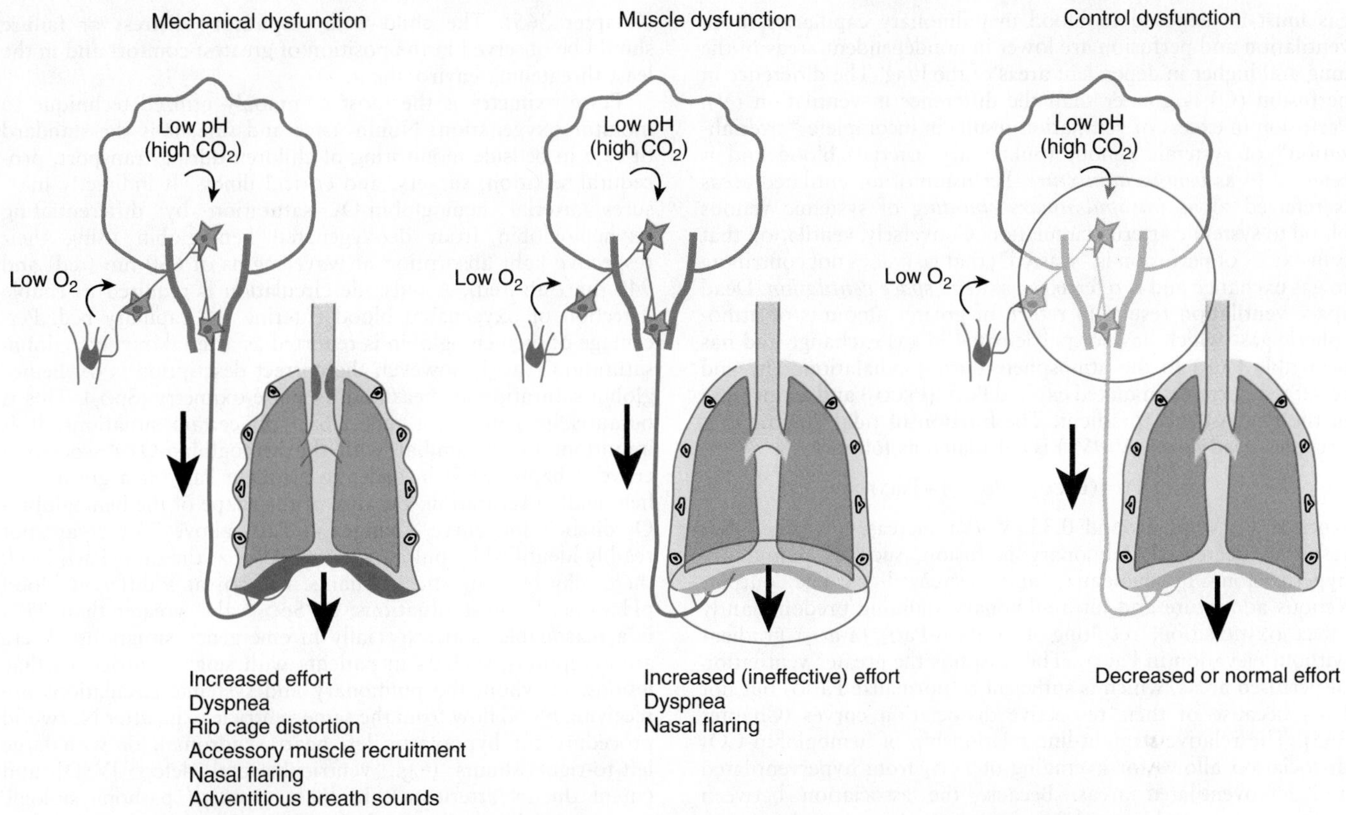

Figure 65-1 Presentation profiles of respiratory failure in childhood. When a mechanical dysfunction is present (by far, the most common circumstance), arterial hypoxemia and hypercapnia (and hence pH) are sensed by peripheral (carotid bodies) and central (medullary) chemoreceptors. After the information is integrated with other sensory information from the lungs and chest wall, chemoreceptor activation triggers an increase in the neural output to the respiratory muscles *(vertical arrows),* which results in the physical signs that characterize respiratory distress. When the problem resides with the respiratory muscles (or their innervation), the same increase in neural output occurs *(arrow),* but the respiratory muscles cannot increase their effort as demanded; therefore, the physical signs of distress are more subtle. Finally, when the control of breathing is itself affected by disease, the neural response to hypoxemia and hypercapnia is absent or blunted, and the gas exchange abnormalities are not accompanied by respiratory distress.

Table 65-5 SIMPLIFIED CONSENSUS DEFINITION OF ACUTE LUNG INJURY

- Acute onset (<7 days)
- Severe hypoxemia (Pa_{O_2}/F_{IO_2} < 300 for acute lung injury, or <200 for acute respiratory distress syndrome)
- Diffuse bilateral pulmonary infiltrates on frontal radiograph consistent with pulmonary edema (these can be patchy and asymmetric, and pleural effusions can be present)
- Absence of left atrial hypertension (pulmonary artery wedge pressure <18 mm Hg if measured)

From Wheeler AP, Bernard GR: Acute lung injury and the acute respiratory distress syndrome: a clinical review, *Lancet* 369:1553–1564, 2007.

physiologic dead spaces. Alveolar ventilation (VA) therefore is calculated as follows:

$$V_A = (V_T - V_D) \times \text{respiratory rate}$$

At a constant level of CO_2 production, Pa_{CO_2} is inversely proportional to alveolar ventilation. An increase in Pa_{CO_2} from 40 torr to 80 torr is indicative of a 50% decrease in VA, and a decrease in Pa_{CO_2} from 40 torr to 20 torr reflects doubling of VA. An elevated Pa_{CO_2}, which is indicative of alveolar hypoventilation, can occur from airway obstruction, weakness of respiratory muscles, or CNS dysfunction (hypoventilation).

VENTILATION-PERFUSION MISMATCH, VENOUS ADMIXTURE, INTRAPULMONARY SHUNT For exchange of O_2 and CO_2 to occur, alveolar

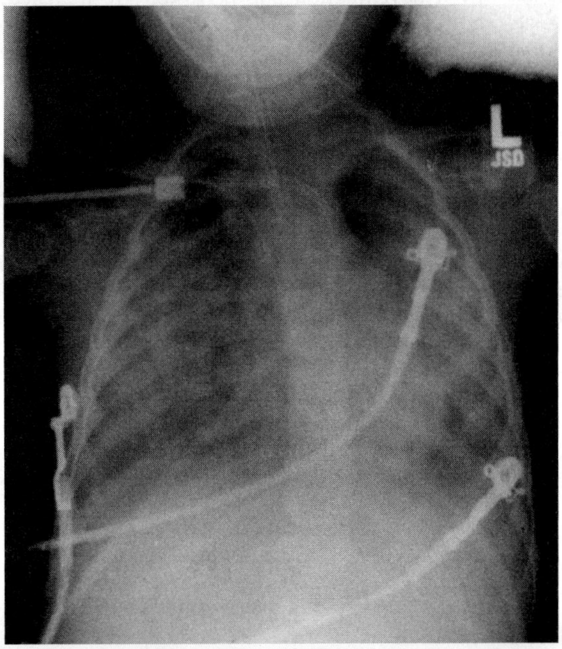

Figure 65-2 Frontal portal chest radiograph showing diffuse bilateral infiltrates consistent with acute lung injury. (From Wheeler AP, Bernard GR: Acute lung injury and the acute respiratory distress syndrome: a clinical review, *Lancet* 369:1553–1564, 2007.)

gas must be exposed to blood in pulmonary capillaries. Both ventilation and perfusion are lower in nondependent areas of the lung and higher in dependent areas of the lung. The difference in perfusion ($\dot{Q}$) is greater than the difference in ventilation ($\dot{V}$). Perfusion in excess of ventilation results in incomplete "arterialization" of systemic venous (pulmonary arterial) blood and is referred to as *venous admixture*. Perfusion of unventilated areas is referred to as *intrapulmonary shunting* of systemic venous blood to systemic arterial circulation. Conversely, ventilation that is in excess of perfusion is "wasted"; that is, it does not contribute to gas exchange and is referred to as *dead space ventilation*. Dead space ventilation results in return of greater amounts of atmospheric gas (which has not participated in gas exchange and has negligible CO_2) to the atmosphere during exhalation. The end result is a decrease in mixed expired PCO_2 (P_ECO_2) and an increase in the $Paco_2$-P_ECO_2 gradient. The fraction of tidal volume that occupies dead space (V_D/V_T) is calculated as follows:

$$V_D/V_T = (Paco_2 - P_ECO_2) \div Paco_2$$

Normal V_D/V_T is around 0.33. V_D/V_T increases in states that result in decreased pulmonary perfusion, such as pulmonary hypertension, hypovolemia, and decreased cardiac output. Venous admixture and intrapulmonary shunting predominantly affect oxygenation, resulting in a P_AO_2-Pao_2 (A-ao_2) gradient without elevation in $Paco_2$. The reason is the greater ventilation of perfused areas, which is sufficient to normalize $Paco_2$ but not Pao_2 because of their respective dissociation curves (Chapter 365). The relative straight-line relationship of hemoglobin-CO_2 dissociation allows for averaging of PCO_2 from hyperventilated and hypoventilated areas. Because the association between oxygen tension and hemoglobin saturation plateaus with increasing Pao_2, the decreased hemoglobin-O_2 saturation in poorly ventilated areas cannot be compensated for by well-ventilated areas where hemoglobin-O_2 saturation has already reached near-maximum. This results in decreased Sao_2 and Pao_2. Elevation of $Paco_2$ in such situations is indicative of attendant alveolar hypoventilation. Examples of diseases leading to venous admixture include asthma and aspiration pneumonia, and those of intrapulmonary shunt include lobar pneumonia and acute respiratory distress syndrome.

DIFFUSION Even if ventilation and perfusion are matched, gas exchange requires diffusion across the interstitial space between alveoli and pulmonary capillaries. Under normal conditions, there is sufficient time for the pulmonary capillary blood to equilibrate with alveolar gas across the interstitial space. When the interstitial space is filled with inflammatory cells or fluid, diffusion is impaired. Because the diffusion capacity of CO_2 is 20 times greater than that of O_2, diffusion defects manifest as hypoxemia rather than hypercarbia. Even with the administration of 100% oxygen, P_AO_2 increases to around 660 torr from 100 torr at sea level, and the concentration gradient for diffusion of O_2 is increased by only 6.6 times. Therefore, with diffusion defects, lethal hypoxemia will set in before clinically significant CO_2 retention results. In fact, in such situations PCO_2 is often decreased because of the hyperventilation that accompanies hypoxemia. Presence of hypercarbia in diseases that impair diffusion is indicative of alveolar hypoventilation from coexisting airway obstruction, exhaustion, or CNS depression. Examples of disease that impair diffusion are interstitial pneumonia, ARDS, scleroderma, and pulmonary lymphangiectasia.

MONITORING A CHILD IN RESPIRATORY DISTRESS AND RESPIRATORY FAILURE

Clinical Examination

Clinical observation is the most important component of monitoring. The presence and magnitude of abnormal clinical findings, their progression with time, and their temporal relation to therapeutic interventions serve as guides to diagnosis and management (Chapter 365). The child with respiratory distress or failure should be observed in the position of greatest comfort and in the least threatening environment.

Pulse oximetry is the most commonly utilized technique to monitor oxygenation. Noninvasive and safe, it is the standard of care in bedside monitoring of children during transport, procedural sedation, surgery, and critical illness. It indirectly measures arterial hemoglobin-O_2 saturation by differentiating oxyhemoglobin from deoxygenated hemoglobin using their respective light absorption at wavelengths of 660 nm (red) and 940 nm (infrared). A pulsatile circulation is required to enable detection of oxygenated blood entering the capillary bed. Percentage of oxyhemoglobin is reported as arterial oxyhemoglobin saturation (Sao_2); however, the correct description is oxyhemoglobin saturation as measured by pulse oximetry (Spo_2). This is because Spo_2 may not reflect Sao_2 in certain situations. It is important to be familiar with the hemoglobin-O_2 dissociation curve (Chapter 365) in order to estimate Pao_2 at a given oxyhemoglobin saturation. Because of the shape of the hemoglobin-O_2 dissociation curve, changes in Pao_2 above 70 torr are not readily identified by pulse oximetry. Also, at the same Pao_2 level, there may be a significant change in Spo_2 at a different blood pH value. In most situations, an Spo_2 value greater than 95% is a reasonable goal, especially in emergency situations. There are exceptions, such as in patients with single ventricle cardiac lesions, in whom the pulmonary and systemic circulations are receiving blood flow from the same ventricle (e.g., after Norwood procedure for hypoplastic left heart syndrome), or with large left-to-right shunts (e.g., ventriculoseptal defect [VSD] and patent ductus arteriosus). In these types of pathophysiologic situations, a lower Spo_2 is desired to avoid excessive blood flow to the lungs and pulmonary edema from the pulmonary vasodilatory effects of oxygen, and, in the patient with a single ventricle, diverting blood flow away from the systemic circulation. Because pulse oximetry recognizes all types of hemoglobin as either oxyhemoglobin or deoxygenated hemoglobin, it provides inaccurate information in the presence of carboxyhemoglobin and methemoglobin. Percentage of oxyhemoglobin is overestimated in carbon monoxide poisoning and methemoglobinemia. It should be recognized that dangerous levels of hypercarbia may exist in patients with ventilatory failure, who have satisfactory Spo_2 if they are receiving supplemental oxygen. Pulse oximetry should not be the only monitoring method in patients with primary ventilatory failure, such as neuromuscular weakness and CNS depression. It is also unreliable in patients with poor perfusion and poor pulsatile flow to the extremities. Despite these limitations, pulse oximetry is a noninvasive, easily applicable, and effective means of evaluating the percentage of oxyhemoglobin in most patients.

Capnography (end-tidal CO_2 measurement) is helpful in determining the effectiveness of ventilation and pulmonary circulation. This method is especially useful for monitoring the level of ventilation in intubated patients. It should be kept in mind that diseases that increase dead space or decrease pulmonary blood flow lead to decreases in end-tidal CO_2 and an overestimation of the adequacy of ventilation.

Blood Gas Abnormalities in Respiratory Distress and Respiratory Failure

(See Chapters 52.7 and 365.)

Assessment of Oxygenation and Ventilation Deficits

Indicators for following clinical progress and for determining the prognosis in patients with defects in oxygenation or ventilation include:

A-ao_2 gradient: Calculated by subtracting arterial Po_2 from alveolar Po_2 ($P_AO_2 - Pao_2$). For the comparison to be valid, it must be at the same FIO_2.

Pa_{O_2}/F_{IO_2} is calculated by dividing arterial P_{O_2} by F_{IO_2}. In hypoxic respiratory failure, a Pa_{O_2}/F_{IO_2} value <300 is consistent with acute lung injury, and a value <200 is consistent with acute respiratory distress syndrome. Although the intent is to measure $\dot{V}/\dot{Q}$ mismatch, intrapulmonary shunt, and diffusion defect, the status of alveolar hypoventilation could have a significant impact on Pa_{O_2}/F_{IO_2}.

Pa_{O_2}/PA_{O_2} is determined by dividing arterial P_{O_2} by alveolar P_{O_2}. The level of alveolar ventilation is accounted for in the calculation of PA_{O_2}. Therefore, Pa_{O_2}/PA_{O_2} is more indicative of $\dot{V}/\dot{Q}$ mismatch and alveolar capillary integrity.

Oxygenation index (OI) is aimed at standardizing oxygenation to the level of therapeutic interventions such as mean airway pressure (MAP) and F_{IO_2}, which are directed toward improving oxygenation. None of the previously mentioned indicators of oxygenation account for the degree of positive pressure respiratory support. OI is calculated as follows:

$$OI = [(MAP \times F_{IO_2}) \div Pa_{O_2}] \times 100$$

The limitation of OI is that level of ventilation is not accounted for in the assessment.

Ventilation index (VI) is aimed at standardizing alveolar ventilation to the level of therapeutic interventions (such as peak inspiratory pressure [PIP] and ventilator rate) directed toward lowering Pa_{CO_2}. VI is calculated as follows:

$$VI = (PIP \times \text{ventilator rate/min} \times Pa_{CO_2}) \div 1000$$

MANAGEMENT

The goal of management for respiratory distress and respiratory failure is to ensure a patent airway and provide necessary support for adequate oxygenation of the blood and removal of CO_2. Compared with hypercapnia, hypoxemia is a life-threatening condition, initial therapy for which should be aimed at ensuring adequate oxygenation.

Oxygen Administration

Supplemental oxygen administration is the least invasive and most easily tolerated therapy for hypoxemic respiratory failure. *Nasal cannula* oxygen provides low levels of oxygen supplementation and is easy to administer. Oxygen is humidified in a bubble humidifier and delivered via nasal prongs inserted in to the nares. In children, a flow rate <5 L/min is most often used because of increasing nasal irritation with higher rates. A common formula for an estimation of the F_{IO_2} during use of a nasal cannula in older children and adults is as follows:

$$F_{IO_2} = 21\% + (\text{nasal cannula flow (L/min)} \times 3)$$

The typical F_{IO_2} value using this method is between 23 and 40%, although the fraction of inspired oxygen varies according to the size of the child, the respiratory rate, and the volume of air moved with each breath. In a young child, because typical nasal cannula flows are a greater percentage of total minute ventilation, significantly higher F_{IO_2} may be provided. Alternately, a *simple mask* may be employed, which consists of a mask with open side ports and a valveless oxygen source. Variable amounts of room air are entrained through the ports and around the side of the mask, depending on the fit, size, and minute volume of the child. Oxygen flow rates vary from 5 to 10 L/min, yielding typical F_{IO_2} values between 0.30 and 0.65. If more precise delivery of oxygen is desired, other mask devices should be used.

A *Venturi mask* delivers preset fractions of oxygen through a mask and reservoir system by entraining precise amounts of room air into the reservoir with high-flow oxygen. The amount of room air entrainment and subsequent F_{IO_2} are determined by the adapter at the end of each mask reservoir. The adapter can be chosen to provide between 30 and 50% oxygen concentrations. Oxygen flow rates of 5-10 L/min are recommended to achieve desired F_{IO_2} and to prevent rebreathing. *Partial rebreather* and *nonrebreather* masks utilize a reservoir bag attached to a mask to provide higher fractions of oxygen. Partial rebreather masks have two open exhalation ports and contain a valveless oxygen reservoir bag. Some exhaled gas can mix with reservoir gas during exhalation, although most exits the mask via the exhalation ports. Through these ports, room air is also entrained during inspiration. A partial rebreather mask can provide up to 0.6 F_{IO_2} as long as oxygen flow is adequate to keep the bag from collapsing (typically 10-15 L/min). As with nasal cannulas, smaller children with smaller tidal volumes entrain less room air, and their F_{IO_2} values will be higher. Nonrebreather masks include two one-way valves, one between the oxygen reservoir bag and the mask and one on one of the two exhalation ports. This arrangement minimizes mixing of exhaled and fresh gas and entrainment of room air during inspiration. The second exhalation port has no valve, a safeguard to allow some room air to enter the mask in the event of disconnection from the oxygen source. A nonrebreather mask can provide up to 0.95 F_{IO_2}. The use of a nonrebreather mask in conjunction with an oxygen blender allows delivery of fractions of oxygen between 0.50 and 0.95. When supplemental oxygen alone is inadequate to improve oxygenation, or when ventilation problems coexist, additional therapies may be necessary.

Airway Adjuncts

Maintenance of a patent airway is a critical step in maintaining adequate oxygenation and ventilation. Artificial pharyngeal airways may be useful in patients with oropharyngeal or nasopharyngeal airway obstruction and in those with neuromuscular weakness in whom native extrathoracic airway resistance contributes to respiratory compromise. An *oropharyngeal airway* is a stiff plastic spacer with grooves along each side that can be placed in the mouth to run from the teeth along the tongue to its base just above the vallecula. The spacer prevents the tongue from opposing the posterior pharynx and occluding the airway. Because the tip sits at the base of the tongue, it is usually not tolerated by patients who are awake or whose gag reflex is strong. The *nasopharyngeal airway*, or nasal trumpet, is a flexible tube that can be inserted into the nose to run from the nasal opening along the top of the hard and soft palate with the tip ending in the hypopharynx. It is useful in bypassing obstruction from enlarged adenoids or from contact of the soft palate with the posterior nasopharynx. Because it is inserted past the adenoids, a nasopharyngeal airway should be used with caution in patients with bleeding tendencies.

Inhaled Gases

Helium-oxygen mixture (heliox) is useful in overcoming airway obstruction and improving ventilation. Helium is much less dense and slightly more viscous than nitrogen. When substituted for nitrogen, helium helps maintain laminar flow across an obstructed airway, decreases airway resistance, and improves ventilation. It is especially helpful in diseases of large airway obstruction in which turbulent airflow is more common, such as acute laryngotracheobronchitis, subglottic stenosis, and vascular ring. It is also used in patients with severe status asthmaticus. To be effective, helium should be administered in concentrations of at least 60%, so associated hypoxemia may limit its use in patients requiring more than 40% oxygen. *Nitric oxide (NO)* is a powerful inhaled pulmonary vasodilator. Its use may improve pulmonary blood flow and $\dot{V}/\dot{Q}$ mismatch in patients with diseases that elevate pulmonary vascular resistance, such as persistent pulmonary hypertension of the newborn (PPHN), primary pulmonary hypertension, and secondary pulmonary hypertension due to chronic excess pulmonary blood flow (e.g., VSD) or collagen vascular diseases. NO is administered in doses ranging from 5 to 20 parts per million (ppm). Although administration of NO to unintubated patients is possible, it is usually administered to patients receiving mechanical ventilation through endotracheal tubes, because of the need for precision in NO dosing.

Positive Pressure Respiratory Support

Noninvasive positive pressure respiratory support is useful in treating both hypoxemic and hypoventilatory respiratory failure. Positive airway pressure helps aerate partially atelectatic or filled alveoli, prevent alveolar collapse at end exhalation, and increase functional residual capacity (FRC). This improves pulmonary compliance and hypoxemia and decreases intrapulmonary shunt. In addition, positive pressure ventilation is useful in preventing collapse of extrathoracic airways by maintaining positive airway pressure during inspiration. Improving compliance and overcoming airway resistance also improves tidal volume and therefore ventilation. A *high-flow nasal cannula* delivers gas flow at 4-16 L/min, providing significant continuous positive airway pressure (CPAP). The amount of CPAP provided is not quantifiable and varies with each patient, depending on the percentage of total inspiratory flow that is delivered from the cannula, airway anatomy, and degree of mouth breathing. In small children, the relative amount of CPAP for a given flow is usually greater than in older children and may provide significant positive pressure. The FIO_2 can be adjusted by provision of gas flow through an oxygen blender. For delivery of high-flow air or oxygen, adequate humidification is essential and is achieved with use of a separate heated humidification chamber. CPAP can also be provided through snugly fitting nasal prongs or a tight-fitting facial mask attached to a ventilator or other positive pressure device. Noninvasive CPAP is most useful in diseases of mildly decreased lung compliance and low FRC, such as atelectasis and pneumonia. Diseases of extrathoracic airway obstruction in which extrathoracic negative airway pressures during inspiration lead to airway narrowing (e.g., laryngotracheitis, obstructive sleep apnea, postextubation airway edema) may also benefit from CPAP.

Bilevel positive airway pressure (BiPAP) machines provide positive airway pressure during exhalation and additional positive pressure during inspiration. A BiPAP device allows one to set an expiratory positive pressure (EPAP) and an inspiratory positive pressure (IPAP). The additional positive pressure during inspiration helps augment tidal volume and improve alveolar ventilation in low compliance and obstructive lung disease. The inspiratory and expiratory pressures can be adjusted independently to suit individual needs and comfort. Because of the additional support during inspiration, patients with neuromuscular weakness in particular tend to benefit from BiPAP support.

Endotracheal Intubation and Mechanical Ventilation

When hypoxemia or significant hypoventilation persists despite the interventions already described, tracheal intubation and mechanical ventilation are indicated. Additional indications for intubation include maintaining airway patency in patients who have the potential for airway compromise, such as those with actual or potential neurologic deterioration, and in patients with hemodynamic instability.

Proper monitoring is essential to ensuring a safe and successful tracheal intubation. Pulse oximetry, heart rate, and blood pressure monitoring are mandatory and should be forgone only in situations calling for emergency intubation. All necessary equipment, including bag-mask ventilation device, laryngoscope, tracheal tube with stylet, and suction equipment, must be available and working properly prior to initiation of intubation. The proper internal diameter (ID) for the tracheal tube can be estimated using the following formula:

$$ID = (\text{Age (yr)}/4) + 4$$

Average values for age, size, and depth of insertion for tracheal tubes are given in Table 65-6. Preoxygenation of the patient with high fractions of inspired oxygen is essential and will allow maximum procedure time prior to the onset of hypoxemia.

Table 65-6 AVERAGE SIZE AND DEPTH DIMENSIONS FOR TRACHEAL TUBES

PATIENT AGE	INTERNAL DIAMETER (mm)	OROTRACHEAL DEPTH (cm)	NASOTRACHEAL DEPTH (cm)
Premature	2.0-3.0	8-9	9-10
Full-term neonate	3.0-3.5	10	11
6 mo	4.0	11	13
12-24 mo	4.5	13-14	16-17
4 yr	5.0	15	17-18
6 yr	5.5	17	19-20
8 yr	6.0	19	21-22
10 yr	6.5	20	22-23
12 yr	7.0	21	23-24
14 yr	7.5	22	24-25
Adult	8.0-9.0	23-25	25-28

Although intubation can be accomplished without sedation and pharmacologic paralysis in selected patients, the physiologic benefits of these measures to the patient as well as to the facilitation of the intubation usually far outweigh the risks; sedation and paralysis should be considered standard unless contraindicated. Administration of a sedative and analgesic followed by a paralytic agent is a common pharmacologic regimen for facilitating intubation. The particular type and dose of each agent often depends on the underlying disease and clinician preference. Commonly used agents are listed in Table 65-7. An alternative to this pharmacologic approach, especially when intubation is urgent or the patient is suspected of having a full stomach, increasing the risk of aspiration, is rapid sequence intubation (Chapter 62).

Once adequate sedation and/or paralysis has been achieved, ventilation should be assisted with a bag-mask device. After optimal preoxygenation, intubation can be performed. The clinician uses his/her dominant hand to open the patient's mouth and inserts the laryngoscope blade gently along the tongue to its base. The airway opening can be visualized by applying lift up and away from the clinician, along the axis of the laryngoscope handle. If a straight (Miller) laryngoscope blade is used, the epiglottis is lifted anteriorly by the tip of the blade to visualize the glottis. If a curved (Macintosh) blade is used, the tip should be advanced into the vallecula and then lifted to visualize the glottis. Secretions often obscure visualizations at this step and should be suctioned clear. Once clear visualization of the vocal cords is accomplished, the tube can be placed through the cords. Rapid confirmation of tube placement is essential and should be assessed by as many of the flowing steps as possible: Auscultation of both lung fields as well as the epigastrium for equal breath sounds and good air movement and evaluation of the abdomen for increasing distention should be performed. Adequate bilateral chest expansion and misting inside the tracheal tube with each breath are suggestive of proper tube placement. An increasing heart rate, if heart rate has decreased during the attempt, and a rising or normal pulse oximetry reading are suggestive of successful tube placement. Preoxygenation may significantly delay a drop in SpO_2 with improper tube placement, leading to a significant delay in its recognition. Confirmation of exhaled CO_2 is mandatory. It can be accomplished with use of a disposable colorimetric CO_2 detector or with capnography. In situations of very low pulmonary perfusion, such as cardiac arrest, exhaled CO_2 may not be detected. A chest radiograph should also be obtained to confirm proper placement of the tracheal tube, which should lie roughly halfway between the glottis and the carina (Chapter 62).

Transient Manual Ventilation in the Immediate Preintubation and Postintubation Periods

Establishment of ventilation via bag and mask or bag and tracheal tube is required prior to transport of the patient to a setting

Table 65-7 MEDICATIONS COMMONLY USED FOR INTUBATION

	DRUG	DOSE	ONSET (min)	DURATION (min)	COMMENTS
Sedatives/anesthetics	Midazolam	0.1 mg/kg IV	3-5	60-120	Amnesia Respiratory depression
	Lorazepam	0.1 mg/kg IV	3-5	120-240	Amnesia Respiratory depression
	Ketamine	1-2 mg/kg IV 4-6 mg/kg IM	2-3	10-15	↑ HR, BP, and ICP Bronchodilation
	Propofol	1-3 mg/kg IV	0.5-2	10-15	↓ BP Apnea
	Thiopental	4-7 mg/kg IV	0.5-1	5-10	↓ BP Apnea
Analgesics	Fentanyl	2-5 μg/kg IV	3-5	30-90	Respiratory depression Chest wall rigidity
	Morphine	0.1 mg/kg IV	5-15	120-240	↓ BP Respiratory depression
Neuromuscular blocking agents	Vecuronium	0.1 mg/kg IV	2-3	30-75	↑ HR Renal elimination
	Rocuronium	0.6-1.2 mg/kg IV 1 mg/kg IM	5-15	15-60	↑ HR Renal elimination
	Cisatracurium	0.1 mg/kg IV	2-3	25-30	Histamine release Nonrenal elimination

BP, blood pressure; HR, heart rate; ICP, intracranial pressure; IM, intramuscularly; IV, intravenously.

of continued critical care. The technique of manual ventilation should take into account the underlying pathology. Ventilation of patients with diseases characterized by low FRC (pneumonia, pulmonary edema, ARDS, etc.) should include the application of positive end-expiratory pressure (PEEP) to prevent alveolar derecruitment. This can be accomplished with use of a PEEP valve on a self-inflating ventilation bag or by careful manipulation of exhaust gas using an anesthesia bag. Such diseases are also characterized by a short time constant (Chapter 70) and therefore are best managed with relatively small tidal volumes and high ventilation rates. Diseases characterized by airway obstruction have prolonged time constants and are therefore best managed with relatively slow rates and high tidal volumes.

BIBLIOGRAPHY

Please visit the Nelson Textbook of Pediatrics *website at* *www.expertconsult.com* *for the complete bibliography.*

65.1 Mechanical Ventilation

Ashok P. Sarnaik and Christopher Mastropietro

The decision to institute mechanical ventilation is based mainly on the need to assist lung function; supporting left ventricular performance and treating intracranial hypertension are additional indications. Although there are no absolute criteria for derangement of gas exchange, Pao_2 <60 torr while breathing >60% oxygen, $Paco_2$ >60 torr, and pH <7.25 are often reasons to initiate mechanical ventilation. Clinical impressions of fatigue and impending exhaustion are also indications for ventilatory support even in the presence of adequate gas exchange. Positive pressure ventilation is a powerful means of decreasing left ventricular afterload, and it is used for this purpose in patients with cardiogenic shock resulting from left ventricular dysfunction. Mechanical ventilation is also used in patients whose respirations are unreliable (e.g., unconscious patients, those with neuromuscular dysfunction) and when deliberate hyperventilation is desired, such as in patients with intracranial hypertension.

Mechanical ventilation neither is intended to normalize gas exchange nor is a form of cure. The goals are to maintain sufficient oxygenation and ventilation to ensure tissue viability until the disease process has resolved and to minimize the inevitable complications of the therapeutic intervention itself. Pao_2, $Paco_2$, and pH levels are maintained in ranges that provide a safe environment for the patient while protecting the lungs from damage due to oxygen toxicity, pressure (barotrauma), tidal volume overdistention (volutrauma), atelectotrauma, and cytokine release (biotrauma) (Figs. 65-3 and 65-4).

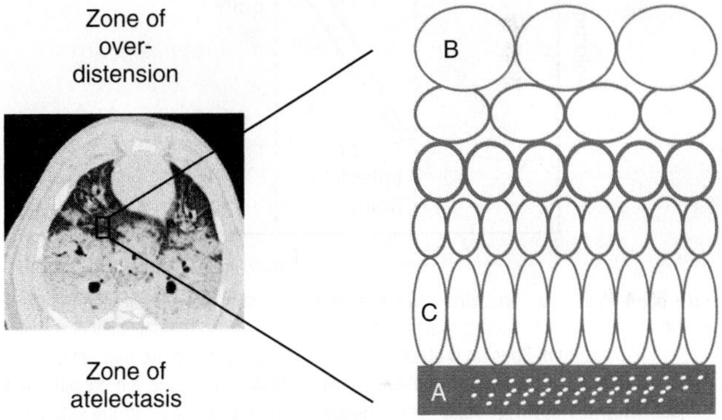

Figure 65-3 Atelectotrauma. The interface between collapsed and consolidated lung (*A*) and overdistended lung units (*B*) is heterogeneous and unstable. Depending on ambient conditions, this region is prone to cyclic recruitment and derecruitment and localized asymmetric stretch of lung units (*C*) immediately apposed to regions of collapsed lung. (From Pinhu L, Whitehead T, Evans T, et al: Ventilator-associated lung injury, *Lancet* 361:332–340, 2003.)

BASIC CONCEPTS OF VENTILATOR MANAGEMENT

Equation of Motion

A pressure gradient is required for air to move from one place to another (Fig. 65-5). During natural spontaneous ventilation, inspiration results from generation of negative intrapleural pressure from contraction of the diaphragm and intercostal muscles, drawing air from the atmosphere across the airways into the alveoli. During mechanical ventilation, inspiration results from positive pressure created by compressed gases through the ventilator, which pushes air across the airways into alveoli. In both spontaneous and mechanical ventilation, exhalation results from alveolar pressure generated by the elastic recoil of the lung and

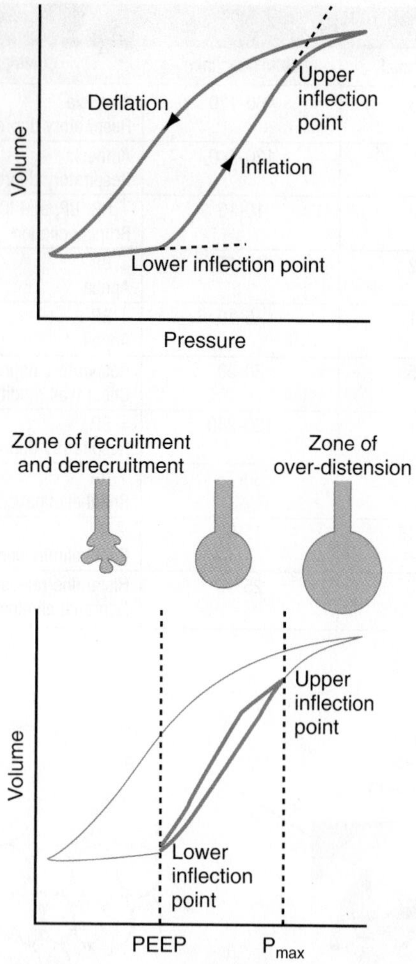

Figure 65-4 Pulmonary pressure-volume relation in a patient with acute lung injury. *Top,* The lower inflection point is typically 12-18 cm H_2O, and the upper inflection point 26-32 cm H_2O. *Bottom,* Specific protective ventilation strategies require that positive end-expiratory pressure is set just above the lower inflection point and the pressure limit (P_{max}) just below the upper inflection point. Hence the lung is ventilated in the safe zone between the zone of recruitment and derecruitment and the zone of overdistention, and both high-volume and low-volume injury are avoided. (From Pinhu L, Whitehead T, Evans T, et al: Ventilator-associated lung injury, *Lancet* 361:332–340, 2003.)

the chest wall. Pressure necessary to move a given amount of air into the lung is determined by two factors: lung and chest wall elastance, and airway resistance. The relationship among pressure gradient, compliance, and resistance is described in Figure 65-5. *Elastance*—defined as the change in pressure (ΔP) divided by the change in volume (ΔV)—refers to the property of a substance to oppose deformation. It is opposite of *compliance* (ΔV ÷ ΔP), the property of a substance to allow distention or lengthening when subjected to pressure. Compliance (C) is therefore expressed as 1/elastance.

The pressure needed to overcome tissue elastance is measured in conditions in which there is no flow (at end-inspiration and end-expiration) and is therefore a reflection of static conditions in the lung. It is influenced by tidal volume and compliance (P = ΔV ÷ C). It is increased with high tidal volume and low compliance. This pressure gradient is used to calculate the static compliance of the respiratory system (C_{STAT}).

Resistance (R) refers to the opposition to generation of flow. It is measured as the amount of pressure needed to generate a unit of flow (Δ P ÷ ΔFlow). Pressure needed to overcome airway resistance is calculated as flow multiplied by resistance. Because this pressure is needed only when the flow is occurring through the airways, it is referred to as the *dynamic component.* Pressure

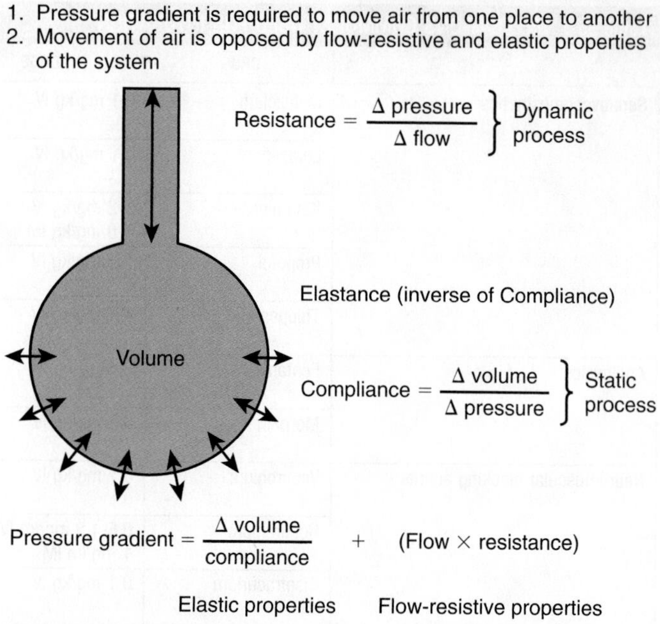

Figure 65-5 Equation of motion. A pressure gradient is required to move air from one place to another. In the lungs, the required pressure gradient must overcome the lung and chest wall elastance (static component) and the flow-resistive properties (dynamic component). The static component is increased in alveolar interstitial diseases and stiff chest wall, whereas the dynamic component is increased with airway obstruction.

to overcome flow-resistive properties is measured when there is maximum flow and is therefore under dynamic conditions. It is increased in conditions with greater airway resistance and flow rate. Flow rate depends on the time allowed for inspiration and expiration. At higher respiratory rates, there is less time available for each inspiration and expiration, necessitating higher flows; therefore higher pressure is required to overcome flow-resistive properties. The pressure gradient necessary to move air from one place to another is the sum of pressure needed to overcome the elastic and flow-resistive properties of the lung. This pressure gradient is taken into account to calculate the dynamic compliance of the respiratory system (C_{DYN}). The difference in change in pressure between static conditions and dynamic conditions is attributable to airway resistance.

Functional Residual Capacity

Also see Chapter 365.

During inspiration, oxygen-enriched gas enters alveoli. During exhalation, oxygen continues to be removed by the pulmonary capillary circulation. *Functional residual capacity* is the volume of gas left in the alveoli at the end of expiration. It is the only source of gas available for gas exchange during exhalation. In diseases with decreased FRC (e.g., ARDS, pulmonary edema), alveolar oxygen concentration declines sharply throughout expiration, resulting in hypoxemia. Two ventilator strategies commonly employed to improve oxygenation in such situations are the application of PEEP and increasing the inspiratory time (TI) (Fig. 65-6). PEEP increases FRC, whereas a longer TI allows longer exposure of pulmonary capillary blood to a higher concentration of O_2 during inspiration.

Time Constant

At the beginning of inspiration, the atmospheric pressure is higher than the pressure in the alveoli, resulting in movement of air into the alveoli. During mechanical ventilation, the ventilator circuit serves as the patient's atmosphere. As alveoli expand with air, the alveolar pressure rises throughout inspiration until it equilibrates with the ventilator pressure, at which time airflow ceases. Expiration starts when the ventilator pressure falls below the alveolar pressure. Alveolar pressure decreases throughout expiration until it reaches the ventilator pressure, at which time no further egress of air from the alveoli occurs. If inspiration or expiration is terminated before pressure equilibration between alveoli and the ventilator is allowed to occur, alveolar expansion during inspiration or alveolar emptying during expiration is incomplete. Incomplete inspiration results in delivery of decreased tidal volume, whereas incomplete expiration is associated with air trapping and the presence of residual PEEP in the alveoli that is greater than the ventilator pressure, referred to as *auto-PEEP*. Some time is required for pressure equilibration to occur between alveoli and the atmosphere, which is reflected in the *time constant* (TC). It takes 3 TCs for 95%, and 5 TCs for 99%, of pressure equilibration to occur. The time constant depends on compliance and resistance, and their relationship is depicted in Figure 65-7. Time constant is calculated as compliance multiplied by resistance ($C \times R$) and is measured in seconds.

Diseases with decreased compliance (increased elastance) are characterized by high elastic recoil pressure, which results in more rapid equilibration of alveolar and ventilator pressures, thereby decreasing TC. Diseases with increased airway resistance are associated with slower flow rates, require longer time for movement of air from one place to another, and therefore have increased TC. Airways expand during inspiration and narrow during expiration (Chapter 365). Therefore, expiratory time constant (TCE) is longer than inspiratory time constant (TCI). In intrathoracic airway obstruction (asthma, bronchiolitis, aspiration syndromes), airway narrowing is much more pronounced during expiration. Therefore, although both TCE and TCI are prolonged in such diseases, TCE is much more prolonged than TCI. Patients with such diseases therefore are best ventilated with slower rates, higher tidal volume, and longer expiratory time than inspiratory time. In diseases characterized by decreased compliance, both TCE and TCI are short; however, the TCE is closer to TCI than in normal lungs because of the stiffer alveoli recoil with greater force. Patients with these diseases are best ventilated with small VT to prevent ventilator-induced lung injury and with a relatively longer inspiratory time in each breath to improve oxygenation.

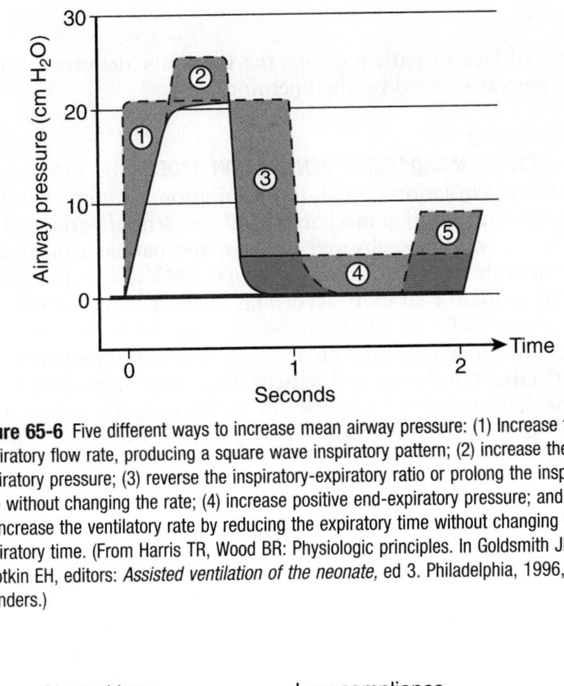

Figure 65-6 Five different ways to increase mean airway pressure: (1) Increase the respiratory flow rate, producing a square wave inspiratory pattern; (2) increase the peak inspiratory pressure; (3) reverse the inspiratory-expiratory ratio or prolong the inspiratory time without changing the rate; (4) increase positive end-expiratory pressure; and (5) increase the ventilatory rate by reducing the expiratory time without changing the inspiratory time. (From Harris TR, Wood BR: Physiologic principles. In Goldsmith JP, Karotkin EH, editors: *Assisted ventilation of the neonate,* ed 3. Philadelphia, 1996, WB Saunders.)

Critical Opening Pressure

Collapsed or atelectatic alveoli require a considerable amount of pressure to open. Once open, the alveoli require relatively less pressure for continued expansion. The process of opening atelectatic alveoli is called *recruitment*. In a normal lung, alveoli remain open at the end of expiration, and therefore the lung requires relatively less pressure to receive its tidal volume. In a disease process in which the alveoli collapse at the end of expiration (e.g., ARDS), a substantial amount of pressure is required to open the alveoli during inspiration. This pressure causes ventilator-induced lung injury via two mechanisms: (1) barotrauma at the terminal airway–alveolar junction and (2) volutrauma due to overdistention of alveoli that are already open (see Figs. 65-3 and 65-4). Although a pulmonary parenchymal disease process is rarely uniform, and each of the millions of alveoli may have its own mechanical characteristics, a composite volume-pressure relationship could be conceptualized for the whole lung (Fig. 65-8).

In these situations, the lower and upper portions of the curve are relatively horizontal, and the middle portion is more vertical. At the beginning of inspiration, atelectatic alveoli are being recruited, requiring high pressure for a relatively small increase in volume. Once they are recruited, further increase in volume requires relatively less pressure. The pressure at which most alveoli are open is called *critical opening pressure;* this point is also referred to as the *lower inflection point* (lower P_{FLEX}). After the lower P_{FLEX}, greater volume can be delivered for relatively less pressure until the upper P_{FLEX} is reached, at which the volume-pressure curve again becomes relatively horizontal. The goal of mechanical ventilation in alveolar interstitial pathology is to deliver a tidal volume between the lower and upper inflection points, the so-called safe zone of ventilation. If tidal volume is delivered with a change in inflation pressure that includes the

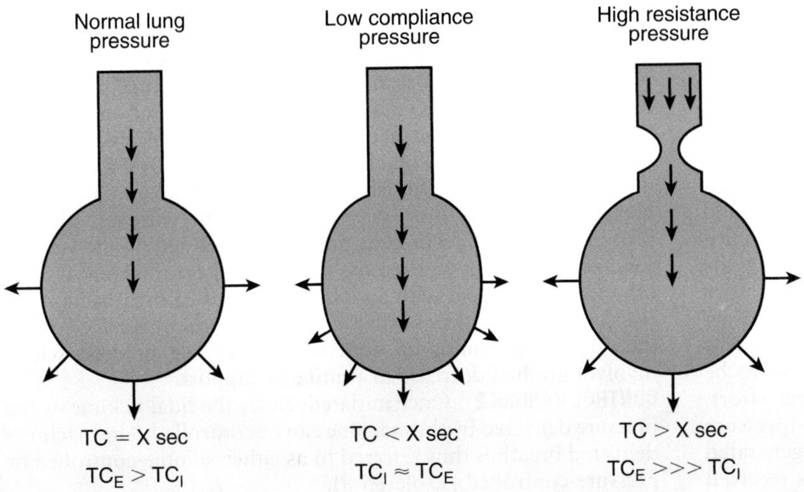

Figure 65-7 Time constant (TC). A certain amount of time is necessary for pressure equilibration (and therefore completion of delivery of gas) to occur between proximal airway and alveoli. TC, a reflection of time required for pressure equilibration, is a product of compliance and resistance. In diseases of decreased lung compliance, less time is needed for pressure equilibration to occur, whereas in diseases of increased airway resistance, more time is required. Expiratory TC is increased much more than inspiratory TC in obstructive airway diseases, because airway narrowing is exaggerated during expiration.

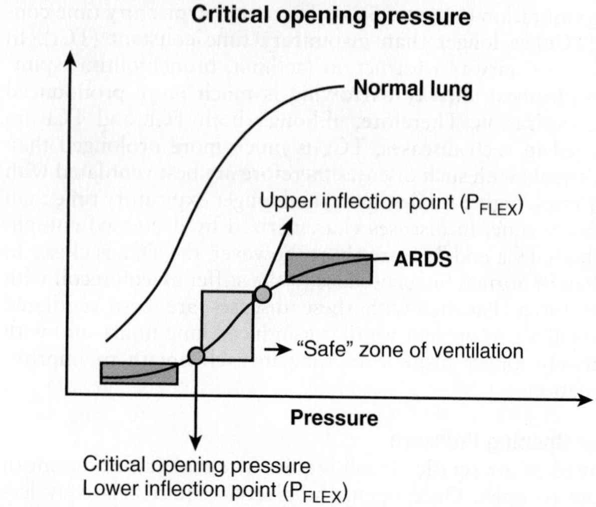

Figure 65-8 Volume-pressure relationship in normal lung and in acute respiratory distress syndrome (ARDS). In ARDS, atelectatic alveoli require a considerable amount of pressure to open. Critical opening pressure, also referred to as lower P_{FLEX}, is the airway pressure above which further alveolar expansion occurs with relatively less pressure. Upper P_{FLEX} is the airway pressure above which further increase in pressure results in less alveolar expansion; this is the area of alveolar overdistention. Keeping tidal volume between upper and lower P_{FLEX} values is considered less injurious to the lung.

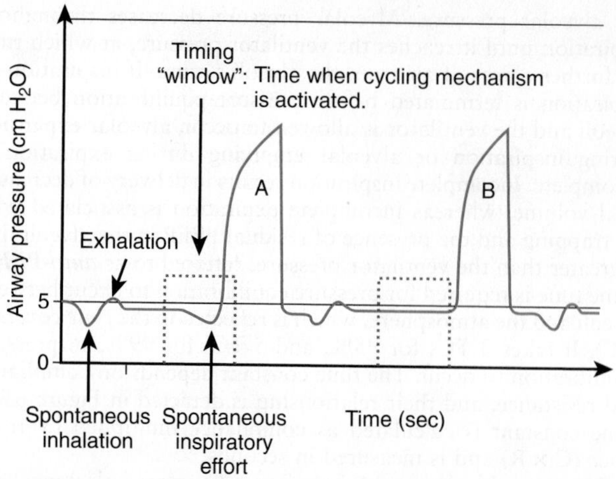

Figure 65-9 Synchronized intermittent mandatory ventilation. At set intervals, the ventilator's timing circuit becomes activated and a timing "window" appears (*shaded area*). If the patient initiates a breath in the timing window, the ventilator delivers a mandatory breath. If no spontaneous effort occurs, the ventilator delivers a mandatory breath at a fixed time after the timing window. (From Banner MJ, Gallagher TJ: Respiratory failure in the adult: ventilatory support. In Kirby RR, Smith RA, Desautels DA, editors: *Mechanical ventilation*, New York, 1985, Churchill Livingstone.)

lower P_{FLEX}, alveoli are likely to open AND close during every breath, a process termed *tidal recruitment* that is injurious to the lung, especially at the terminal airway–alveolar junction. If tidal volume is delivered with a change of pressure that includes the upper P_{FLEX}, overdistention of alveoli is likely to occur, resulting in volutrauma and barotrauma. Keeping tidal ventilation between the upper and lower P_{FLEX} values is accomplished by maintaining a level of PEEP to produce baseline alveolar recruitment and delivering a relatively small (6 mL/kg) tidal volume. Termed "open lung" strategy, this approach has proved to be beneficial in alveolar interstitial diseases such as ARDS.

PHASES OF MECHANICAL VENTILATION

The planning of a ventilatory strategy must consider the four phases of the respiratory cycle separately, taking into account the patient's clinical characteristics. These are: (1) initiation of respiration and a variable that is controlled, often referred to as *mode*; (2) inspiratory phase characteristics, which determine the duration of inspiration and how the pressure or volume is delivered; (3) termination of inspiration, often referred to as *cycle*; and (4) expiratory phase characteristics. Ideally, mechanical ventilation should not completely take over the work of breathing but, rather, should assist the patient's own respiratory effort. In the absence of the patient's effort, respiratory muscle deconditioning may occur, making weaning from mechanical ventilation more difficult.

Initiation of Inspiration and the Control Variable (Mode)

The initiation of inspiration may be set to occur at a predetermined rate and interval regardless of patient effort, or it could be timed in response to patient effort. Once inspiration is initiated, the ventilator breath either is controlled entirely by the ventilator (control mode) or supports the patient's inspiratory effort to a predetermined inspiratory volume or pressure target (support mode). Advances in technology allow for greater patient-ventilator synchrony to occur. The ventilator may be set to be "triggered" by the signal it receives as a result of patient effort. This may be in the form of lowering of either pressure (pressure trigger) or airflow (flow trigger) in the ventilator circuit generated by the patient's inspiratory effort. If no such signal is received because of lack of patient effort, the ventilator delivers a breath at an interval selected by the operator.

Control Modes

INTERMITTENT MANDATORY VENTILATION MODE In intermittent mandatory ventilation (IMV), the inspiration is initiated at a set frequency with a timing mechanism independent of patient effort. In between machine-delivered breaths, the patient can breathe spontaneously from a fresh source of gas. IMV allows for adjustment of ventilator support according to the patient's needs and is therefore useful in the weaning process. Lack of synchrony between machine-delivered breaths and patient efforts may result in ineffective ventilation and patient discomfort, especially when IMV is delivered at a high rate. In such cases, the patient may require sedation and pharmacologic paralysis for efficient delivery of tidal volume. To obviate this problem, *synchronized IMV (SIMV)* is used, whereby the machine-delivered breaths are triggered by the patient's inspiratory efforts (Fig. 65-9). In between the machine-delivered breaths, a fresh source of gas is available for spontaneous patient breaths. In the absence of patient effort, the patient receives a backup rate much like in IMV mode. Even with SIMV, ventilator-patient asynchrony can occur, because tidal volume, inflation pressure, and inspiratory time are determined by the ventilator alone.

ASSIST-CONTROL MODE In assist-control (AC) mode, each and every patient breath is triggered by pressure or flow generated by patient inspiratory effort and "assisted" with either preselected inspiratory pressure or volume. The rate of respirations is therefore determined by the patient's inherent rate. A backup total (patient and ventilator) obligatory rate is set to deliver a minimum number of breaths. On AC mode with a backup rate of 20 breaths/min, all of the breaths of a patient with an inherent respiratory rate of 15 breaths/min will be assisted by the ventilator, and the patient will receive 5 additional breaths/min. On the other hand, a patient with an inherent rate of 25 breaths/min will receive all 25 breaths assisted. Although useful in some patients, the AC mode cannot be used in the weaning process, which involves gradual decrease in ventilator support.

CONTROL VARIABLE Once initiated, either the tidal volume or the pressure delivered by the machine can be controlled. The machine-delivered breath is thus referred to as either volume-controlled or pressure-controlled (Table 65-8).

With *volume-controlled ventilation* (VCV), machine-delivered volume is the primary control, and the inflation pressure generated depends on the respiratory system's compliance and resistance. Changes in respiratory system compliance and resistance are therefore easily detected from changes observed in inflation pressure. In *pressure-controlled ventilation* (PCV), the pressure change above the baseline is the primary control, and the tidal volume delivered to the lungs depends on the respiratory system's compliance and resistance. Changes in respiratory system compliance and resistance do not affect inflation pressure and may therefore go undetected unless the exhaled VT is monitored. VCV and PCV have their own advantages and disadvantages (see Table 65-8). Generally speaking, PCV is more efficient than VCV in terms of amount of tidal volume delivered for a given inflation pressure during ventilation of a lung that has nonuniform time constants, such as asthma. In VCV, relatively less-obstructed airways are likely to receive more of the machine-delivered volume throughout inspiration than relatively more-obstructed airways with longer time constants (Fig. 65-10*A*). This situation would result in uneven ventilation, higher PIP, and a decrease in dynamic compliance. In PCV, because of a constant inflation pressure that is held throughout inspiration, relatively less-obstructed lung units with shorter time constants would achieve pressure equilibration earlier during inspiration than the relatively more-obstructed areas. Thus, units with shorter time constants would attain their final volume earlier in inspiration, and those with longer time constants would continue to receive additional volume later in inspiration (Fig. 65-10*B*). This situation would result in more even distribution of inspired gas, delivery of more tidal volume for the same inflation pressure, and improved dynamic compliance in comparison with VCV.

Table 65-8 CHARACTERISTICS OF PRESSURE-CONTROLLED AND VOLUME-CONTROLLED METHODS OF VENTILATION

	PRESSURE-CONTROLLED VENTILATION	VOLUME-CONTROLLED VENTILATION
Control setting(s)	Inflation pressure Inspiratory time Rise time	VT Flow rate Inspiratory flow pattern (constant vs decelerating)
Machine-delivered volume	Depends on respiratory system compliance and resistance	Constant
Inflation pressure	Constant	Depends on respiratory system compliance and resistance
Endotracheal tube leak	Somewhat compensated	Leaked volume part of VT
Distribution of ventilation	More uniform in lungs with varying time constant units	Less uniform in lungs with varying time constant units
Patient comfort	Possibly compromised	Possibly enhanced
Weaning	Inflation pressure adjustment required to deliver desired VT	VT remains constant, inflation pressure automatically weaned

VT, tidal volume.

Pressure-regulated volume control (PRVC) combines the advantages of VCV and PCV. In this mode, the VT and inspiratory time are controlled as primary variables but the ventilator determines the amount of pressure needed to deliver the desired tidal volume. Inflation pressure is thus adjusted to deliver the prescribed tidal volume over the inspiratory time, depending on the patient's respiratory compliance and resistance.

Support Modes

Pressure support ventilation (PSV) and *volume support ventilation* (VSV) are designed to support the patient's spontaneous respirations. With PSV, initiation of inspiration is triggered by the patient's spontaneous breath, which is then "supported" by a rapid rise in ventilator pressure to a preselected level. The inspiration is continued until the inspiratory flow rate falls to a set level (generally 25% of peak flow rate) as the patient's lungs fill up. Thus, inspiratory time is controlled by the patient's own efforts. PSV can be combined with SIMV so that any breath above the SIMV rate is supported by PSV. Allowing the patient to control as much of the rate, tidal volume, and inspiratory time as possible is considered a gentler form of mechanical ventilation than SIMV, in which the tidal volume (or inflation pressure) and inspiratory time are preset. PSV as the sole source of mechanical ventilator support is often not adequate for patients with severe lung disease; however, it is especially useful in patients in the process of being weaned and in patients who require mechanical ventilation for relatively minor lung disease or for neuromuscular weakness. VSV is similar to PSV, in that all the spontaneous breaths are supported. In VSV, inspiratory pressure to support spontaneous breaths is adjusted to guarantee a preset tidal volume. If there is a change in respiratory mechanics or patient effort, the inspiratory pressure to support the breath initiated by patient effort is automatically adjusted to deliver the set tidal volume.

Inspiratory Phase Characteristics

Inspiratory time, inspiratory flow waveform, and pressure rise time can be adjusted in the inspiratory phase to suit the patient's respiratory mechanics.

In PCV, the duration of *inspiratory time* (TI) is directly set in seconds. In VCV, the inspiratory time can be adjusted by adjusting the inspiratory flow (volume/time). The choice of TI value

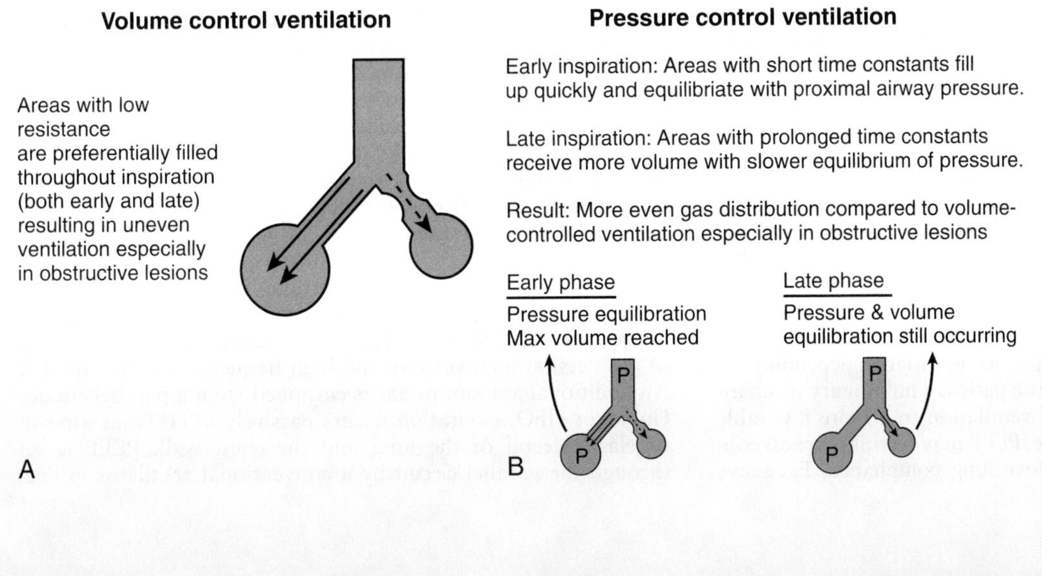

Volume control ventilation
Areas with low resistance are preferentially filled throughout inspiration (both early and late) resulting in uneven ventilation especially in obstructive lesions
A
Pressure control ventilation
Early inspiration: Areas with short time constants fill up quickly and equilibriate with proximal airway pressure.
Late inspiration: Areas with prolonged time constants receive more volume with slower equilibrium of pressure.
Result: More even gas distribution compared to volume-controlled ventilation especially in obstructive lesions
Early phase
Pressure equilibration
Max volume reached
Late phase
Pressure & volume equilibration still occurring
P
B

Figure 65-10 *A,* In volume-controlled ventilation, tidal volume is delivered to the less obstructed areas throughout inspiration. Obstructed areas of the lung therefore receive a lower proportion of tidal volume, resulting in uneven ventilation. *B,* In pressure-controlled ventilation, less obstructed areas equilibrate with inflation pressure and therefore receive most of their tidal volume early during inspiration. More obstructed areas, with prolonged time constants, require longer time for pressure equilibration and therefore continue to receive a portion of their tidal volume later during inspiration. The entire tidal volume is more evenly distributed than with volume-cycled ventilation.

depends on the respiratory rate, which determines the total duration of each breath, and on the estimation of inspiratory and expiratory time constants. Decreasing the flow rate delivery increases T_I, and vice versa. With an increase in T_I, the pulmonary capillary blood is exposed to a higher level of alveolar PO_2 for a longer time. This is beneficial in diseases with decreased FRC, such as ARDS and pulmonary edema. An increase in T_I also increases V_T without increasing inflation pressure in PCV if inspiratory flow is still occurring at the end of expiration. It must be recognized that at a given ventilator rate, an increase in T_I decreases expiratory time (T_E). Therefore, any strategy that employs an increase in the inspiratory component of the respiratory cycle should ensure that the decreased T_E is still sufficient for complete exhalation.

Inspiratory flow waveform can be adjusted in VCV mode as either a constant flow (square waveform) or a decelerating flow (descending ramp waveform). With a square waveform, flow is held constant throughout inspiration. In a descending ramp waveform, the flow is maximum at the start of inspiration and declines throughout its duration. It is debatable which flow pattern is better for a given disease. In PCV and PSV, the prescribed PIP is reached through delivery of airflow. The time required for the ventilator to reach PIP is reflected in the *pressure rise time,* which can be adjusted by control of flow at the beginning of the inspiratory phase. The inspiratory flow rise time is adjusted to provide comfort for a patient who is awake and also to prevent an extremely rapid rise in inspiratory pressure, which might result in barotrauma.

Termination of Inspiration (Cycle)

The two most commonly used inspiratory terminating mechanisms in control modes are time-cycled and volume-cycled. With a time-cycled mechanical breath, inspiration is terminated after a preselected inspiratory time has elapsed, whereas with volume-cycled breath, the inspiration ends after a preselected volume has been delivered by the machine into the ventilator circuit. A time-cycled breath is almost always pressure-limited, with the PIP held constant for the duration of inspiration. A volume-cycled breath can be pressure-limited as a safety mechanism to avoid barotrauma. The inspiration-terminating mechanism is set somewhat differently in support modes. In PSV, the inspiration is set to end after the inspiratory flow decreases below a certain percentage (usually 25%) of peak inspiratory flow. This happens when the patient no longer desires to receive additional tidal volume. Such a breath can be termed *flow-cycled*. In volume support mode, inspiration is terminated when the patient has received the desired tidal volume.

Expiratory Phase Maneuvers

The most useful expiratory phase maneuver is the application of PEEP, which is applied to both the control breath and the assisted breath. The most important clinical benefits of PEEP are to recruit atelectatic alveoli and to increase FRC in patients with alveolar-interstitial diseases and thereby improve oxygenation. There is growing recognition that even a brief disconnection from a ventilator, and therefore having zero end-expiratory pressure, can result in significant alveolar derecruitment and decline in oxygenation. In patients with obstructive lesions in which insufficient exhalation results in air trapping and auto-PEEP, extrinsic PEEP (that applied through a mechanical device) can prevent airway closure during expiration and improve ventilation. Other salutary effects of PEEP include redistribution of extravascular lung water away from gas-exchanging areas, improved ventilation-perfusion relationship, and stabilization of the chest wall. The effect of PEEP on lung compliance is variable, depending on the level of PEEP provided and the patient's pulmonary mechanics. By shifting the tidal volume ventilation to a more favorable part of the pressure-volume curve, PEEP may recruit more alveoli, delay airway closure, and improve lung compliance. Excessive PEEP, on the other hand, may lead to overdistention of alveoli and reduced compliance. The effect of PEEP in individual patients can be ascertained by measuring exhaled tidal volume and calculating dynamic compliance. Other deleterious effects of PEEP include decreased venous return, increased pulmonary vascular resistance, and decreased cardiac output.

ADDITIONAL VENTILATORY MODALITIES

Airway Pressure Release Ventilation

Airway pressure release ventilation (APRV) improves oxygenation in cases of severe hypoxemic respiratory failure resulting from alveolar-interstitial disease. This modality applies a continuous positive airway pressure, designated $CPAP_{HIGH}$, to recruit and maintain FRC with brief intermittent release phases of $CPAP_{LOW}$ to allow alveolar gas to escape. $CPAP_{HIGH}$ is analogous to PIP, and $CPAP_{LOW}$ is similar to setting PEEP. In contrast to the patient receiving conventional mechanical ventilation, a patient receiving APRV spends the majority of time in the $CPAP_{HIGH}$ phase, which may last as long as 3-5 sec with a brief (0.3-0.5 sec) time in the $CPAP_{LOW}$ phase. These atypically long inspiratory times are tolerated because of a floating expiratory valve in the ventilator circuit that permits spontaneous breathing during $CPAP_{HIGH}$ phase. Therefore, even if $CPAP_{HIGH}$ phase can be considered inspiratory and $CPAP_{LOW}$ phase can be considered expiratory as far as the ventilator is concerned, the patient is able to breathe spontaneously during both of these phases. The longer ventilator inspiratory times recruit lung units, and the ability to breathe spontaneously during this phase allows distribution of gas flow to atelectatic lung regions. The outcome benefit of APRV in pediatric hypoxemic respiratory failure has not been proven.

High-Frequency Ventilation

Mechanical ventilation at supraphysiologic rates and low tidal volumes, known as high-frequency ventilation (HFV), improves gas exchange in a selected group of patients who show no response to traditional ventilatory modalities. The mechanism of alveolar ventilation in HFV is very different from that in conventional ventilation, in that HFV is less dependent on tidal volume and more dependent on asymmetric velocities and convective dispersion of inspired gas. Patients with severe persistent hypoxic failure are most likely to benefit from HFV. HFV is also helpful in patients with bronchopleural fistula and persistent air leaks. The main tenet of HFV is to recruit lung volume with a high MAP and produce smaller fluctuations in alveolar pressure during inspiration and expiration, thus maintaining a satisfactory FRC and reducing alveolar stretch. The two most investigated techniques of HFV are high-frequency oscillation (HFO) and high-frequency jet ventilation (HFJV).

The most commonly used HFV modality is HFO, which employs a mechanism to generate to-and-fro air movement. Additional air is dragged in (entrained) through a parallel circuit via a Venturi effect. Air is pushed in during inspiration and actively sucked out during expiration. The main determinants of oxygenation are FIO_2 and MAP, whereas ventilation is determined by changes in pressure (amplitude) from the MAP. Commonly used respiratory frequency varies from 5 Hz (300 breaths/min) in adults and older children, to 6-8 Hz (360-480 breaths/min) in young children, 8-10 Hz (480-600 breaths/min) in infants, and 10-12 Hz (600-720 breaths/min) in newborn and premature babies.

In HFJV, a high-frequency interrupter is interposed between a high-pressure gas source and a small cannula that is incorporated in the endotracheal tube (ET). The cannula propels tiny amounts of gas (jets) at high velocity and high frequency through the ET. An additional amount of gas is entrained from a parallel circuit. Unlike in HFO, expiration occurs passively in HFJV as a result of elastic recoil of the lung and the chest wall. PEEP is set through the parallel circuit by a conventional ventilator in line.

Respiratory rate is generally set at 420 breaths/min. Major determinants of oxygenation are FIO_2 and PEEP, and the major determinant of ventilation is PIP.

CONVENTIONAL VENTILATOR SETTINGS

FIO_2

The shape of the hemoglobin-oxygen dissociation curve dictates that oxygen content in the blood is not linearly related to PaO_2. A PaO_2 value that results in an oxyhemoglobin saturation of 95% is reasonable in most situations, because a higher PaO_2 would cause minimal increase in arterial oxygen content, and a modest (≈10 torr) drop in PaO_2 would result in minimal decrease in oxyhemoglobin saturation. In most cases, a PaO_2 value of 70-75 torr is a reasonable goal. FIO_2 values that are higher than those necessary to attain oxyhemoglobin saturations of 95% expose the patient to unnecessary oxygen toxicity. Whenever possible, FIO_2 values should be decreased to a level ≤0.4 as long as oxyhemoglobin saturation remains 95% or above.

Mode

The choice of mode of ventilation depends on how much ventilator-patient interaction is desired and the disease entity that is being treated. SIMV or AC is chosen as the control mode, PCV, VCV, or PRVC is chosen as the variable that is to be controlled, and PS and VS are the choices for support modes.

Tidal Volume and Rate

As previously discussed, alveolar ventilation, the chief determinant of $PaCO_2$, is calculated using tidal volume, respiratory rate, and dead space volume. A change in V_T results in a corresponding change in V_A without affecting the dead space ventilation. A change in respiratory rate will affect the V_A as well as the dead space ventilation. As mentioned earlier, the choice of V_T and rate depends on the time constant. In a patient with relatively normal lungs, an age-appropriate ventilator rate and a tidal volume of 7-10 mL/kg would be appropriate initial settings. Diseases associated with decreased time constants (decreased static compliance, e.g., ARDS, pneumonia, pulmonary edema) are best treated with small (6 mL/kg) tidal volume and relatively rapid rates (25-40 breaths/min). Diseases associated with prolonged time constants (increased airway resistance, e.g., asthma, bronchiolitis) are best treated with relatively slow rates and higher (10-12 mL/kg) tidal volume. In PCV, the delivered V_T depends on the compliance and resistance of the patient's respiratory system and needs to be monitored to ensure the appropriate amount for a given situation. An inflation pressure of 15 to 25 cm H_2O is sufficient for most patients, but it may need adjustment, depending on the amount of exhaled tidal volume observed. It should be emphasized that achieving a "normal" $PaCO_2$ value is not a requirement for mechanical ventilation. Mild hypercapnia (permissive hypercapnia) should be acceptable, especially when one is attempting to limit injurious inflation pressures or tidal volumes.

Inspiratory Time and Expiratory Time

Inspiratory time and expiratory time are adjusted by setting inspiratory flow rate in VCV and by setting the precise T_I in PCV. Increasing the inspiratory time results in an increase in MAP, improvement in oxygenation in diseases with decreased FRC, and better distribution of tidal volume in obstructive lung disease. Sufficient expiratory time must be provided to ensure adequate emptying of the alveoli.

Positive End-Expiratory Pressure

The best level of PEEP depends on the disease entity that is being treated, and it may change in the same patient from time to time. Decisions are often based on the PaO_2/FIO_2 ratio and the measurement of dynamic compliance.

PATIENT-VENTILATOR ASYNCHRONY

Patient-ventilator asynchrony occurs when the patient's respiratory pattern does not match that of the ventilator. This can occur during all phases of respiration. Adverse effects of patient-ventilator asynchrony include wasted effort, ineffective delivery of desired tidal volume, excessive generation of intrathoracic pressure resulting in barotrauma and adverse effects on cardiac output, increased work of breathing, and patient discomfort. Although several mechanisms exist to facilitate patient-ventilator asynchrony, a certain amount of asynchrony is inevitable unless the patient is pharmacologically sedated and paralyzed.

Triggering the Ventilator

The patient must be able to trigger the ventilator without extraordinary effort. Ventilators can be pressure-triggered or flow-triggered. With pressure triggering, the inspiratory valve opens and flow is delivered when a set negative pressure is generated within the patient-ventilator circuit during both inspiration and expiration. The amount of pressure required to trigger an inspiration depends on the pressure trigger sensitivity. In flow triggering, the ventilator provides a base flow of gas through the ventilator-patient circuit. When a flow sensor on the expiratory limb of the patient-ventilator circuit detects a decrease in flow as a result of the patient's inspiratory effort, the inspiratory valve opens and a ventilator breath is delivered. The degree of change in flow required to trigger an inspiration depends on the flow trigger sensitivity. Flow triggering is considered to be more comfortable, primarily because the patient receives some flow prior to triggering the ventilator, in contrast to pressure triggering, in which no flow is provided until the ventilator breath is triggered. Increasing the trigger sensitivity by decreasing the change in either pressure or flow needed to trigger an inspiration decreases the work of breathing. However, reducing the required pressure or flow excessively could result in accidental triggering and unwanted breaths by turbulence caused by condensation in the ventilator circuit, ET leaks, or cardiac oscillations.

Selection of Appropriate Inspiratory Time

The duration of T_I should match the patient's own inspiratory phase. If T_I is too long, the patient's drive to exhale may begin before the ventilator breath has cycled off. When this occurs, exhalation occurs against inspiratory flow and a closed exhalation valve, resulting in increased work of breathing, excessive rise in intrathoracic pressure, and discomfort. If T_I is too short, the patient may be still inhaling without respirator support. In general terms, T_I is usually initiated at 0.5-0.7 sec for neonates, 0.8-1 sec in older children, and 1-1.2 sec for adolescents and adults. Adjustments need to be made through individual patient observations and according to the type of lung disease present. In patients with severe lung disease (both obstructive and restrictive), unnatural T_I and TE values may have to be selected, as discussed earlier. In such situations, adequate analgesia, sedation, and, in extreme cases, neuromuscular blockade may be needed.

Selection of Inspiratory Flow Pattern

In VCV, inappropriate flow may be another source of patient-ventilator dyssynchrony. After initiation of inspiration, if the set amount of flow is inadequate to meet patient demand, a state of "flow starvation" occurs, resulting in excessive work of breathing and discomfort. Such cases may require a decelerating inspiratory flow pattern, in which a higher flow is provided in the beginning of inspiration and less toward the end as the lungs fill up. On the other hand, such a pattern may be uncomfortable for a patient who desires more gradual alveolar filling. The selection of inspiratory flow pattern should be based on the individual patient's respiratory mechanics. In PCV and PSV, the inspiratory rise time determines the manner in which the airway pressure is raised and tidal volume delivered. Considerations for choosing the appropriate rise time in PCV and PSV are similar to those for choosing the inspiratory flow pattern in VCV.

Use of Support Modes

As much as possible, a conscious patient should be allowed to have spontaneous breaths that are supported by either PSV or VSV. This approach minimizes the mandatory breaths generated by the ventilator that are beyond the patient's control to modulate. Therefore, continued assessments should be made to determine whether the patient is able to maintain ventilatory requirements more in support modes and less in control modes.

Use of Sedation and Pharmacologic Paralysis

Having a conscious but comfortable patient is a desirable goal during mechanical ventilation. Spontaneous breaths with good muscle tone and presence of cough are important for adequate clearance of tracheobronchial secretions. The patient's ability to indicate distress is also important in identifying and preventing potential injurious factors. In certain situations, management of patient-ventilator asynchrony assumes far greater importance when the asynchrony is causing unacceptable derangement of gas exchange and ventilator-induced lung injury. Both alveolar interstitial lung pathology and obstructive airway diseases may necessitate unnatural and uncomfortable settings for respiratory rate, TI, and inflation pressures. In such situations, deep sedation is often necessary. Benzodiazepines and opiates are the agents most commonly used for this purpose. In extreme situations, pharmacologic paralysis with a nondepolarizing agent such as vecuronium is required to abolish any patient effort and respiratory muscle tone. When pharmacologic paralysis is used, deep sedation must be ensured so that the patient does not sense pain and discomfort. Pharmacologic sedation and paralysis can ensure total control of the patient's ventilation by mechanical means and may result in lifesaving improvement in gas exchange with reduction in inflation pressures. However, long-term use of such agents may be associated with undesirable consequences and higher morbidity. The risk of inadequate tracheobronchial secretions and atelectasis is potentially greater. Long-term use of pharmacologic sedation may be associated with chemical dependency and withdrawal manifestations, and prolonged neuromuscular blockade is associated with neuromyopathy in critically ill patients. The benefits of sedation and pharmacologic paralysis therefore should be carefully balanced with the risks, and periodic assessments should be made to determine the need for their continuation.

MONITORING RESPIRATORY MECHANICS

Exhaled Tidal Volume

Exhaled tidal volume (VTE) is measured by a pneumotachometer in the ventilator circuit during exhalation. In VCV, part of the machine-delivered volume may leak out during inspiration and therefore never reach the patient. Measurement of VTE more accurately describes the tidal volume that is contributing to the patient's alveolar ventilation. In PCV, the VTE depends on the patient's respiratory system compliance and resistance, and therefore offers valuable diagnostic clues. A decrease in VTE during PCV is indicative of either decrease in compliance or increase in resistance and is helpful in directing the clinician to appropriate investigation and management. An increase in VTE is indicative of improvement and may require weaning of inflation pressures to adjust the VTE.

Peak Inspiratory Pressure

In VCV and PRVC, the PIP is the secondary variable determined by the patient's respiratory system compliance and resistance. An increase in PIP in these modes is indicative of decreased compliance (e.g., atelectasis, pulmonary edema, pneumothorax) or increased resistance (e.g., bronchospasm, obstructed ET). During VCV and PRVC, decreasing the respiratory rate or prolonging the TI will result in a lower PIP in patients with prolonged time constants because more time will be available for alveoli to fill. In such patients, a decrease in PIP suggests increased compliance or decreased resistance of the respiratory system.

Respiratory System Dynamic Compliance and Static Compliance

The changes in PIP during VCV and PRVC, and in VTE during PCV, are determined by C_{DYN} of the respiratory system (lung and chest wall). Dynamic compliance is calculated as follows:

$$C_{DYN} = V_{TE} \div (PIP - PEEP)$$

It takes into account both the flow-resistive and the elastic properties of the respiratory system. Changes in C_{DYN} can be used to assess effects of different levels of PEEP as tidal ventilation is shifted along the slope of the volume-pressure curve (see Fig. 65-8). After an increase in PEEP in alveolar-interstitial diseases (increased elastance), an increase in C_{DYN} suggests alveolar recruitment, whereas a decrease in C_{DYN} may indicate overdistention. Similarly, in obstructive diseases (increased resistance), adjustment in PEEP levels to ameliorate airway collapse during exhalation can be guided by monitoring C_{DYN}. To assess only the elastic recoil of the lung, measurement of C_{STAT} when there is no airflow is required. This measurement is performed by using an inspiratory hold maneuver with the patient under neuromuscular blockade and observing pressure-time and flow-time waveforms (Fig. 65-11). During this maneuver, inspiratory flow ceases while the expiratory valve continues to remain closed, thus allowing pressure to equilibrate throughout the ventilator circuit and the patient's lungs. This pressure, referred to as the *plateau pressure* (P_{plat}), is reflective of alveolar pressure. C_{STAT} is calculated as follows:

$$C_{STAT} = V_{TE} \div (P_{plat} - PEEP)$$

The difference between C_{DYN} and C_{STAT} is attributable to airway resistance. This difference is minimal in alveolar-interstitial diseases but substantial in airway obstruction.

Assessment of Auto-PEEP

Auto-PEEP is assessed with the use of an expiratory pause maneuver in which inspiration is delayed and alveolar pressure is allowed to equilibrate with the airway. In diseases with airway obstruction, insufficient alveolar emptying may occur if exhalation time is not adequate. The alveolar pressure in excess of the set PEEP at the completion of the expiratory pause is measured as auto-PEEP or intrinsic PEEP. Auto-PEEP can have adverse effects on ventilation and hemodynamic status. It can be managed by decreasing the

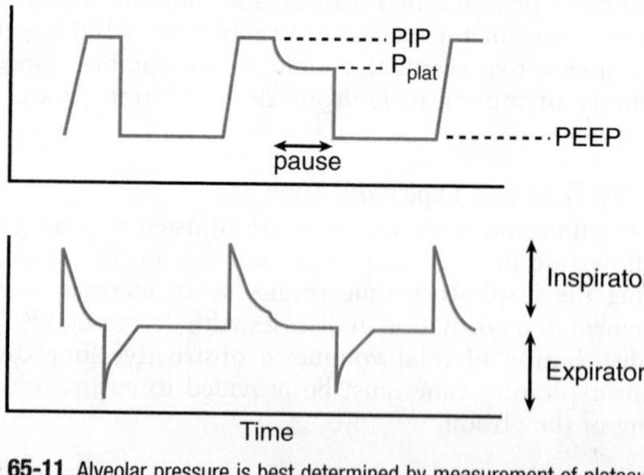

Figure 65-11 Alveolar pressure is best determined by measurement of plateau pressure (P_{plat}). Inspiration is paused for an extended period, and alveolar gas pressure is allowed to equilibrate with the ventilator circuit pressure. Airway pressure at the end of the inspiratory pause is P_{plat}. The difference between peak inspiratory pressure (PIP) and P_{plat} is to overcome flow-resistive properties of the lung, whereas P_{plat} reflects the pressure needed to overcome elastic properties of lung and chest wall.

respiratory rate or inspiratory time and thus allowing greater time for exhalation. Auto-PEEP may also be managed by increasing the set PEEP ("extrinsic" PEEP), thereby delaying airway closure during exhalation and improving alveolar emptying.

Assessment of Dead Space Ventilation

Positive pressure ventilation and application of PEEP may result in a decrease in venous return, cardiac output, and, therefore, also the pulmonary perfusion. Ventilation of poorly perfused alveoli results in dead space ventilation, which does not contribute to gas exchange. The dead space–tidal volume fraction can be calculated with the following equation:

$$V_D/V_T = (Pa_{CO_2} - P_{ECO_2}) \div Pa_{CO_2}$$

Normal V_D/V_T is 0.33. Increased V_D/V_T is indicative of poorly perfused alveoli. Patients with increased V_D/V_T may require intravascular volume infusion or other means of augmenting the cardiac output to improve pulmonary perfusion. The V_D/V_T fraction is calculated and displayed by commercially available capnographs, which measure endotracheal P_{CO_2} continuously.

VENTILATOR-INDUCED LUNG INJURY

Like most medical therapies, mechanical ventilation can be harmful if appropriate principles are not followed. Lung volumes that are too high or too low should be avoided. In attempting to recruit and maintain FRC, the clinician must be careful not to overdistend alveoli. Excessive PIP and V_T can lead to unwelcome stress and strain on alveolar walls. This volutrauma and barotrauma can lead to disruption of tight junctions between alveolar epithelial and capillary endothelial cells, causing fluid and protein transudation in the alveoli. Inflammatory mediators and cytokines are released, exacerbating the injury and promoting exudative fluid formation. Decreased production and inactivation of surfactant result in atelectasis and further impairment of gas exchange. Evidence shows that in patients with severe acute hypoxemic respiratory failure, avoidance of $V_T \geq 10$ mL/kg and $P_{plat} \geq 30$ cm H_2O limits diffuse alveolar damage.

Insufficient PEEP is another important mechanism of ventilator-induced lung injury. Alveoli that are recruited during inspiration must remain open during expiration; if they do not, atelectrauma occurs, which is defined as undesirable shear stress on alveolar walls as they are opened and closed repeatedly. Therefore, the ideal PEEP for a patient should maximize the number of open alveoli and minimize the number of overdistended alveoli. Careful adjustments of PEEP may also permit the clinician to wean a patient from a high inspired oxygen concentration, another potential source of lung injury (oxytrauma). Though most patients receive an inspired oxygen concentration of 100% during endotracheal intubation and at the beginning of mechanical ventilation, increasing PEEP to recruit alveoli without overdistention should be quickly instituted to improve oxygenation and permit weaning of the F_{IO_2}. Although an F_{IO_2} value below which there is no risk of oxygen toxicity is unknown, most clinicians aim for a value <0.6.

Ventilator-Associated Pneumonia

The pathophysiology of ventilator-associated pneumonia (VAP) is multifactorial. Aspiration of oral and/or gastric secretions, colonization of ETs, and suppression of cough reflexes with sedation all play a role. New-onset fever and leukocytosis accompanied by demonstration of an infiltrative process by chest radiographs are consistent with a diagnosis of VAP. This complication can lead to worsened gas exchange, increased duration of ventilation, and even death. Elevation of the head of the bed to 30 degrees after initiation of mechanical ventilation and use of a protocol for oral decontamination during mechanical ventilation are two means of reducing the risk for VAP. The most effective strategy to minimize any of the aforementioned complications is regular assessment of extubation readiness and liberation from mechanical ventilation as soon as clinically possible.

Weaning

Weaning from mechanical ventilation should be considered as a patient's respiratory insufficiency begins to improve. Most pediatricians favor gradual weaning from ventilator support. With SIMV, the ventilator rate is slowly reduced, allowing the patient's spontaneous breaths (typically assisted with pressure or volume support) to assume a larger proportion of the minute ventilation. When the ventilator rate is low (<5 breaths/min) such that its contribution to minute ventilation is minimal, assessment of extubation readiness is performed. An alternative method of gradual weaning is transition to a pressure support mode of ventilation. In this mode, no ventilator rate is set, allowing all triggered breaths to be assisted with pressure support. The clinician reduces the pressure support slowly to a low value (<5-10 cm H_2O), at which point assessment of extubation readiness is performed. During either technique, weaning should be halted if tachypnea, increased work of breathing, hypoxemia, hypercapnia, acidosis, diaphoresis, tachycardia, or hypotension occurs.

The most objective means of assessing extubation readiness is a spontaneous breathing trial (SBT). Prior to performance of an SBT, a patient should be awake with intact airway reflexes, capable of handling oropharyngeal secretions, and with stable hemodynamic status. In addition, gas exchange should be adequate, defined as a Pa_{O_2} >60 mm Hg while receiving an F_{IO_2} <0.4 and PEEP ≤5 cm H_2O. If these criteria are present, a patient should be started on CPAP with minimal or no pressure support (≤5 cm H_2O). If this SBT is tolerated with no episodes of respiratory or cardiovascular decompensation, successful extubation is likely. Some neonates and small children cannot be calmed or consoled long enough to complete the SBT. In this situation, extubation readiness must be assessed on a low level of ventilator support. Data suggest that there is a low risk of extubation failure if the patient is comfortable and has stable hemodynamic status with adequate gas exchange and spontaneous V_T >6.5 mL/kg while receiving <20% of total minute ventilation from the ventilator. Certain patient populations are at increased risk for extubation failure, such as young infants, children mechanically ventilated for >7 days, and patients with chronic respiratory or neurologic conditions. These children often benefit from transition to a noninvasive form of positive pressure ventilation (e.g., high-flow nasal cannula, CPAP, or BiPAP) delivered via nasal prongs or face mask to increase the odds of successful extubation. The likelihood of postextubation upper airway obstruction, the most common cause of extubation failure in children, cannot be predicted on the basis of an SBT result or bedside measurements of physiologic variables. Traumatic endotracheal intubation and subglottic swelling from the ET irritation, especially in patients who exhibit agitation while receiving mechanical ventilation, are common causes of airway narrowing after extubation. Administration of intravenous corticosteroids (dexamethasone 0.5 mg/kg every 6 hours for 4 doses prior to extubation) has been shown to minimize the incidence of postextubation airway obstruction. In patients in whom postextubation airway obstruction develops, the need for re-intubation may be obviated by administration of nebulized racemic epinephrine and helium-oxygen mixture.

BIBLIOGRAPHY

Please visit the Nelson Textbook of Pediatrics *website at* *www.expertconsult.com* *for the complete bibliography.*

65.2 Long-Term Mechanical Ventilation

Ajit Ashok Sarnaik, Matthew J. Gelmini, and Ashok P. Sarnaik

Technology has made mechanical support possible for patients with chronic disorders in various settings outside the intensive care unit (ICU), allowing such patients to live fulfilling lives and even improving their chances of survival. Although short-term mechanical ventilation has allowed many children to survive and to be weaned from life-sustaining therapies, it has also led to an increase in the number of patients who are chronically dependent on technology for survival.

GOALS OF LONG-TERM MECHANICAL VENTILATION

The goals of home mechanical ventilation, based on 2007 American Association of Respiratory Care (AARC) guidelines, are to: sustain and extend life, enhance quality of life, reduce morbidity, enhance growth and development, and provide cost-effective care. Limitations on the use of home mechanical ventilation include FIO_2 requirement of >0.40, positive end-expiratory pressure >10 cm H_2O, inadequate interface (i.e., tracheostomy or noninvasive mask), lack of appropriate discharge plan, and inadequacy of finances, infrastructure, or personnel in the home environment.

The goals should be both optimistic and realistic, and they should be individualized for a given situation. Optimism provides hope and enthusiasm for the care providers, whereas realism avoids unreasonable expectations, unnecessary treatment interventions and pain, as well as disappointment and feelings of anger and hostility. Expected outcomes may range from long-term recovery and liberation from respiratory support to improved patient comfort and a rewarding existence with continued dependence on technology. Patients in whom long-term support of respiration is intended to be a bridge to complete recovery and independence include those with reversible neuropathies, bronchopulmonary dysplasia and pulmonary hypertension, airway abnormalities, and congenital heart disease before or after surgical intervention. Patients for whom the use of long-term respiratory support is intended to prevent morbidity and to allow them to live longer and fulfilling lives include those with congenital myopathies and neuropathies, obstructive sleep apnea, and progressive lung disease.

PATIENT SELECTION AND ETHICAL CONSIDERATIONS

There are several incentives to provide long-term mechanical ventilation to children with chronic respiratory failure at home instead of in the hospital. The cost of home care for these children is significantly less than that of hospital care. The avoidance of hospital-acquired infections and the developmental and psychological benefits of living at home are increasingly recognized. Children who are managed at home become integral parts of their families and may even go to school, participate in social functions, and live near-normal lives. Patients selected for long-term respiratory support either have chronic persistent life-threatening respiratory failure or are at risk for acute deterioration.

Indications

Optimal patient selection for home mechanical ventilation requires identification of the cause of chronic respiratory failure and awareness of the long-term outlook for the patient. Many of the causative conditions have the potential to improve with therapy, time, growth, or age. Some are amenable to surgical correction and have the potential for weaning of the patient from mechanical ventilation after an appropriate intervention is performed. Conditions requiring long-term respiratory support may involve a primary pulmonary parenchymal or airway pathology, neuromuscular or musculoskeletal abnormality, or inadequate CNS control of the respiratory system. In some cases, home mechanical ventilation is indicated to prevent the development of pulmonary hypertension and cor pulmonale from chronic hypoxic pulmonary vasoconstriction (bronchopulmonary dysplasia, obstructive sleep apnea). Other candidates for home ventilation include patients with cardiopulmonary or airway problems who are able to sustain oxygenation and ventilation but are not thriving because of excessive caloric expenditure from increased work of breathing. Tachypnea can also negatively affect oral feeding in infants, further compromising the positive caloric balance needed for growth. This scenario is very common in patients with bronchopulmonary dysplasia and congenital heart disease. Some conditions that cause chronic respiratory failure are slowly progressive and/or irreversible; some patients with these conditions are still excellent candidates for home ventilation. Many children with spinal cord injuries, muscular dystrophy, and type II spinal muscular atrophy enjoy excellent quality of life with long-term ventilation, and some have even graduated from college and become productive members of society. The type of respiratory support needs to be tailored to the individual patient's needs and resources. Availability of resources may depend on local conditions. Also, treatment philosophy and outcome goals vary from patient to patient (Table 65-9).

Conditions for Which Long-Term Ventilation May Be Inappropriate

The decision to employ long-term ventilation must be made judiciously and carefully, weighing the harms against the benefits of the intervention. If the patient has no capacity to participate even minimally in the human experience (e.g., persistent vegetative state, trisomy 18), the harm of continued technologic

Table 65-9 INDICATIONS, PHILOSOPHY OF CARE, OUTCOME GOALS, AND TYPES OF LONG-TERM SUPPORT

INDICATION	TREATMENT PHILOSOPHY	OUTCOME GOALS	INTERVENTION
Central airway obstruction (Pierre-Robin sequence and other causes of midfacial hypoplasia, tracheal stenosis)	Prevention of hypoxic episodes until definitive surgical correction is accomplished	Freedom from extrinsic support after recovery	Tracheostomy, CPAP, mechanical ventilation
Primary pulmonary disease with expectation of recovery (BPD, ARDS)	Enhance growth, prevent pulmonary hypertension, ensure nutrition	Long-term ventilation with weaning as tolerated	Mechanical ventilation
Chest wall deformities, Pickwickian syndrome, obstructive sleep apnea	Prevention of pulmonary hypertension, sleep-related hypoxia, and hypercarbia	Long-term support, possible weaning after treatment	CPAP, mechanical ventilation
Reversible neuropathy (Guillain-Barré syndrome, post–critical care neuropathy)	Support ventilation, prevent atelectasis	Protracted ventilation until recovery	Mechanical ventilation
Slowly progressive neuromyopathy (type II spinal muscular atrophy, muscular dystrophy, mitochondrial myopathy)	Improve quality of life and social experiences, allow developmental and intellectual growth and accomplishments	Long-term ventilation until disease process becomes insufferable	Mechanical ventilation, BiPAP
Static lesion (spinal cord trauma, phrenic palsy, myelomeningocele)	As above	As above	As above
CNS disease: impaired chemoreception (Ondine curse, Arnold-Chiari malformation)	Prevent sleep related hypoventilation	Long-term ventilation	Mechanical ventilation especially during sleep

ARDS, acute respiratory distress syndrome; BiPAP, bilevel positive airway pressure; BPD, bronchopulmonary dysplasia; CNS, central nervous system; CPAP, continuous positive airway pressure.

intervention is unjustified, carrying with it only prolongation of pain and suffering with no net benefit to the patient. Such a patient may have enough rudimentary brain function to sense pain and discomfort. Similarly, patients with rapidly progressive neurodegenerative disease (e.g., Werdnig-Hoffman disease) experience severe weakness and are unable to move, but are able to mentally process every noxious stimulus. Subjecting such patients to long-term ventilation would cause unjustified harm with no long-term benefit; instead, compassionate palliative care should be the goal in such individuals. Although the individual patient's interest is of the utmost importance, adverse effects on family dynamics, allocation of scarce resources, and economic costs to society are also important considerations.

IN-HOSPITAL MANAGEMENT AND DISCHARGE PLANNING

Optimal care of children with chronic respiratory failure begins in the hospital. As soon as the child is identified as one who may need long-term ventilation, there should be open communication between the physician and the family. Many families need time to accept the fact that their children will require therapies at home. Taking the child home for the first time after a prolonged hospital course marks a tremendous life change for the family and often causes emotional and financial strain. The family often needs time to get affairs in order, such as to secure time off from work and to arrange for help in caring for the child and payment for medical care. Because these tasks take time, the planning process must start as early as possible so that the discharge process is organized and expeditious. Ideally, the decision to initiate home mechanical ventilation is made electively. In patients whose neuromuscular weakness is slowly progressive, indicating impending respiratory failure, it would not be beneficial to wait for an episode of acute respiratory failure. This can lead to prolonged hospital and ICU stays and greater morbidity, because these patients are often debilitated from their acute illness. Similarly, physicians should be proactive in initiating mechanical ventilation in a patient who would benefit from its positive effects on caloric balance, instead of waiting until the child fails to thrive. In most children with neuromuscular diseases, home mechanical ventilation is initiated nonelectively, after an acute episode of respiratory failure, and without prior effective discussions of available options. Because these children often have several preceding hospitalizations for episodes of acute respiratory failure, it is evident that health care providers are missing opportunities to adequately prepare their families.

If the best interface for mechanical ventilation is a tracheostomy, a pediatric otolaryngologist must be consulted for the surgical procedure. If the child is not likely to be able to meet caloric demands for growth with oral feeding, a pediatric surgeon is usually consulted for placement of a gastrostomy tube, and the procedure is often performed at the same time as the tracheostomy. Observation in the ICU for approximately 5 days is usually required to allow the tract of the tracheostomy to mature, at which point the tracheostomy tube is replaced.

TEAM STRUCTURE FOR HOME MECHANICAL VENTILATION PROGRAM

For optimal management of the child undergoing home mechanical ventilation, a comprehensive, multidisciplinary approach at a tertiary care center is required (Table 65-10). Indeed, in these cases, life-sustaining therapies are being delivered outside the ICU and often outside the hospital. Several disciplines of health care provision must be involved, and the family must be thoroughly trained to ensure the safety, growth, psychosocial development, and possible clinical improvement of the child.

The team of physicians who will follow a child as an outpatient must become involved while the child is still in the hospital. The primary inpatient physician is usually an intensivist or a neonatologist. A physician leader (usually a pulmonologist) must be identified who is well versed in managing such children and organizing community resources, and who will direct long-term care while remaining in close communication with the family. This arrangement will allow for home ventilator settings to be established and documented before hospital discharge, and long-term reduction of or weaning from mechanical ventilation on an outpatient basis. In many cases, the pulmonologist also serves as the primary care physician, overseeing the child's immunizations, growth, development, and other medical issues. If the family lives far from a tertiary care center, a primary care physician who is willing and qualified to care for the child must be chosen and communicated with prior to the patient's discharge. Even in this situation, a follow-up appointment with a pediatric pulmonologist is required.

Table 65-10 TEAM APPROACH TO INSTITUTIONAL HOME VENTILATION PROGRAM

TASK	PERSON(S) INVOLVED
Decision to institute long-term ventilation	Family, intensivist/neonatologist, pulmonologist
In-hospital management	Intensivist/neonatologist
Assuming overall leadership of long-term care	Pulmonologist or other qualified physician
Medical/surgical issues	Otolaryngologist, general surgeon, neurologist, neurosurgeon, craniofacial surgeon
Training: Suctioning, tracheostomy care, ventilator function and trouble shooting	Respiratory therapist, nurse, medical equipment company, family
Arranging financial and nursing resources	Social worker
Assessment of nutrition, feeding, speech	Dietician, occupational/speech therapist
Primary care: Immunization, growth and development assessment	Primary care physician or pulmonologist
Home medication instructions	Pharmacist, nurse, physician
Follow-up regarding ventilator adjustments	Pulmonologist
Assessment of home suitability	Medical equipment company
Home care	Family, home health nursing company

It cannot be stressed enough how dangerous it would be for a child to receive life-sustaining therapies at home without thorough training of the family, which includes use and troubleshooting of all of the medical equipment, recognition of signs of worsening illness, and cardiopulmonary resuscitation (CPR). Training should begin well in advance of hospital discharge. Generally, a respiratory therapist is responsible for teaching the family how to suction the airway, to change the tracheostomy tube both routinely and emergently, and to connect, use, and troubleshoot the ventilator and oxygen supply. A child who would die without an artificial airway should never be left alone without someone who knows how to change the tube. A dietary plan should be in place prior to hospital discharge, with the child demonstrating tolerance of calories adequate to sustain growth. This may require consultation with occupational or speech therapists to evaluate adequacy of oral feeding skills and with a nutritionist to establish follow-up and adjustment of enteral feeding after discharge.

A social worker should also be involved early in the discharge process to assess the adequacy of the social environment and infrastructure in the home. The family should demonstrate a clear understanding of a daily, weekly, and monthly schedule with respect to home nursing and care of the child. Depending on the complexity of the child's needs, or the work schedules of the family, home nursing may be needed every day. This need requires identification of a home nursing company able to meet these personnel demands, which is difficult in some cases. Arrangements with the health insurance company should also be made, to avoid any delays in hospital discharge. Also, all necessary equipment must be ordered in advance from the medical equipment company.

Follow-up plans with these disciplines and organizations, as well as with services managing the child's other chronic problems, must be made prior to hospital discharge. Ideally, the physician leader would work with the other specialists in a multidisciplinary clinic where other children requiring such care are managed. This arrangement would streamline the care of the child as well as make it more convenient for the family, because transporting such children is very difficult and sometimes even requires an ambulance service. Another approach to address the multidisciplinary needs of a patient, especially one who lives far from the tertiary care center, would be regularly scheduled, short-term hospitalizations every 6-12 months. Such an arrangement would allow for overnight monitoring and adjustment of ventilator settings, if needed, as well as a multidisciplinary assessment, including nutrition, growth, and development.

A well-thought-out plan for emergency care must be established in advance. This process involves interaction with local emergency medical services and emergency departments. Many of the patients requiring long-term ventilation have unique characteristics. A patient with myelomeningocele, for example, may require emergency evaluation of a ventriculoperitoneal shunt, whereas one with a single-ventricle lesion may have special requirements or restrictions for intravascular fluid expansion, oxygen administration, and alveolar inflation pressures. It is useful to have the family always carry a document containing a brief summary of the patient's clinical characteristics and resuscitation requirements along with contact information for subspecialists. Similarly, families of patients who have prepared to forgo resuscitation in their final days of life should have an advanced directive or resuscitation instructions in their possession so that inappropriate and undignified interventions are avoided.

METHODS OF LONG-TERM MECHANICAL VENTILATION

Respiratory Support at Home Through Tracheostomy Interface

Positive pressure ventilation through a tracheostomy is the most commonly employed method of providing home mechanical ventilation. Tracheostomy gives the patient a stable airway for reliable delivery of tidal volume and affords better pulmonary toilet and clearance of secretions. Sudden death can occur from displacement or obstruction of the tracheostomy or from unrecognized disconnection from the ventilator. To ensure patient safety, suctioning equipment and an extra tracheostomy tube should always be immediately available, as well as someone proficient in changing the tube, troubleshooting the equipment, and performing CPR.

The versatility of home ventilators has enabled clinicians to tailor settings to the patient's needs. These features include constant-flow generators, pressure support, flow triggering, and variable rise time adjustment. A leak around the tracheostomy tube is desirable if tolerated by the patient, because it is beneficial for speech development and leads to less irritation of the trachea. Traditional volume-control ventilators cannot provide a consistent minute ventilation with a leak around the tracheostomy, because the degree of leak is often variable and dependent on positioning. Pressure-control ventilators can provide consistent minute ventilation because of leak compensation. The ideal home ventilator is also portable, lightweight, and user-friendly. Alarms for high pressure, low exhaled volume, and patient disconnection should be loud enough to alert the caregiver to an adverse event, with minimal occurrences of false alarms. The primary power source for home ventilators is alternating current (AC). Most models have an internal battery that charges during AC operation and will provide a power source for up to 4 hr when disconnected from the outlet. Oxygen delivery at home is usually in the form of a concentrator, which is limited to a maximum flow rate of 6 L/min.

Noninvasive Home Ventilation

The primary benefit of noninvasive ventilation for respiratory failure in children is avoiding a tracheostomy, which carries risks of tracheal stenosis, tracheitis, and ventilator-associated pneumonia as well as social stigma. Some patients are able to maintain adequate airway patency, oxygenation, and ventilation while awake but need positive pressure ventilation at night because of a decrease in airway tone or respiratory muscle excursion. This subset of patients includes those with obstructive sleep apnea, cystic fibrosis, and neuromuscular disorders.

Appropriate fit of the interface is extremely important, to minimize leaks and discomfort. Interfaces include nasal masks, facial masks covering the nose and mouth, nasal pillows, and mouthpieces. It is important for the child to tolerate and receive time free of mechanical ventilation to avoid facial skin and nasal bridge breakdown, as well as to vent the stomach if necessary. Initiation of the chosen interface method should occur in the inpatient setting, and the patient's tolerance of it must be demonstrated prior to hospital discharge. Ventilators to deliver noninvasive positive pressure ventilation (NIPPV), CPAP or BiPAP machines, are often different from those used in the ICU and invasive home ventilators. CPAP provides airflow at the same level of pressure during inhalation and expiration to keep the airways open throughout the respiratory cycle. Patients eligible for this therapy include those with obstructive sleep apnea, lower airway disease such as tracheomalacia or bronchomalacia, and milder degrees of neuromuscular disease. Patients with more advanced neuromuscular disease may lack the capacity for the respiratory muscle excursion needed for inspiration and would benefit from a higher pressure during inspiration, which can be provided with BiPAP. In the spontaneous BiPAP mode, the difference in pressure between inspiration and expiration is analogous to pressure support in traditional ICU ventilators. Alternatively, BiPAP may be time-cycled to deliver mandatory breaths. One major disadvantage of NIPPV is its impact on airway clearance. It is difficult for patients receiving continuous positive pressure to cough and clear secretions, especially in a weakened state. Secretions may also be forced further down the bronchial tree by the positive pressure. For this reason, patients may benefit from adjunctive airway clearance therapies, such as cough-assistor devices, chest vest vibration, and intermittent positive pressure breathing.

High-flow nasal cannula systems are capable of delivering airflow from 2 to 8 L/min with adequate heat and humidity so as to minimize injury to the respiratory tract. The use of high-flow nasal cannula has increased over the last decade and has been well-studied in the neonatal population. It has been demonstrated in the neonatal population to provide positive distending pressure of 4-5 cm H_2O and respiratory support comparable to that of nasal CPAP. One drawback to this therapy is the variability of the amount of pressure generated, which depends on the fit of the prongs, the flow rate, and the open or closed position of the mouth. In contrast, CPAP devices provide a tight seal and a pressure-release valve to limit the pressure. Therefore, to minimize the risk of excessive pressure, it may be beneficial to choose the smallest high-flow nasal cannula required to provide enough support to the patient.

Diaphragm Pacing

Patients with congenital central hypoventilation syndrome or high cervical spinal cord injury may benefit from electrical stimulation of the phrenic nerves to pace the diaphragm. A surgical procedure is required to implant receivers adjacent to the phrenic nerves, usually bilaterally, and the patient wears a radiofrequency transmitter. The primary benefit of this mode of ventilation is that the transmitter is small and portable enough to give the patient more mobility and freedom from the ventilator for prolonged periods. Risks include diaphragm fatigue, injury to the phrenic nerve from repeated stimulation, and extrathoracic airway obstruction. Because of these concerns, diaphragm pacing is not continuous in most patients, thus requiring CPAP or mechanical ventilation during sleep.

BIBLIOGRAPHY

Please visit the Nelson Textbook of Pediatrics *website at www.expertconsult.com for the complete bibliography.*

Chapter 66
Acute Care of the Victim of Multiple Trauma

Cindy Ganis Roskind, Peter S. Dayan, and Bruce L. Klein

EPIDEMIOLOGY

Injury is a leading cause of death and disability in children throughout the world (Chapter 5.1). According to the World Health Organization report on child injury prevention, unintentional injuries are one of the leading causes of death in children younger than 20 yr and the leading cause of death in children between 10 and 20 yr in the world. Road traffic accidents, drowning, fire-related events, and falls rank among the top causes of death and disability in children. In Asia, injury accounts for more than 50% of deaths in children <18 yr, with drowning accounting for approximately half. In the USA, more than 12,000 children die each year secondary to unintentional injury, with motor vehicle related injuries being the leading cause.

Deaths represent only a small fraction of the total trauma burden. Approximately 9.2 million children are treated in U.S. emergency departments (EDs) each year for injury, most commonly for falls. Many survivors of trauma have permanent or temporary functional limitations. Motor vehicle–related injuries and falls rank among the top 15 causes of disability-adjusted life years in children worldwide.

Trauma is frequently classified according to the number of significantly injured body parts (1 or more), the severity of injury (mild, moderate, or severe), and the mechanism of injury (blunt or penetrating). In childhood, blunt trauma predominates, accounting for the majority of injuries. In adolescence, penetrating trauma increases in frequency, accounting for approximately 15% of injuries, and has a higher case fatality rate.

REGIONALIZATION AND TRAUMA TEAMS

Mortality and morbidity rates have decreased in geographic regions with comprehensive, coordinated trauma systems. Treatment at designated trauma centers is associated with decreased mortality. At the scene of injury, paramedics should administer necessary advanced life support and perform triage (Fig. 66-1; Tables 66-1 and 66-2). It is usually preferable to bypass local hospitals and rapidly transport a seriously injured child directly to a pediatric trauma center (or a trauma center with pediatric commitment). Children have lower mortality rates after severe blunt trauma when they are treated in designated pediatric trauma centers or in hospitals with pediatric intensive care units.

When the receiving ED is notified before the child's arrival, the trauma team should also be mobilized in advance. Each member has defined tasks. A senior surgeon (surgical coordinator) or, sometimes initially, an emergency physician leads the team. Team compositions vary somewhat from hospital to hospital; the model used at Children's National Medical Center (Washington, DC) is shown in Figure 66-2. Consultants,

Table 66-1 CHANGES IN FIELD TRIAGE DECISION SCHEME CRITERIA FROM 1999 TO 2006 VERSION*

STEP ONE: PHYSIOLOGIC CRITERIA
• Add a lower limit threshold for respiratory rate in infants (aged <1 year) of <20 breaths per minute • Remove Revised Trauma Score <11
STEP TWO: ANATOMIC CRITERIA
• Add crushed, degloved, or mangled extremity • Change "open and depressed skull fractures" to "open or depressed skull fractures" • Move combination trauma with burns and major burns to Step Four
STEP THREE: MECHANISM-OF-INJURY CRITERIA
• Add vehicular telemetry data consistent with high risk of injury • Clarify criteria for falls to include: — Adults: fall >20 ft (two stories) — Children aged <15 years: fall >10 ft or two to three times the child's height • Change "high-speed auto crash" to "high-risk auto crash" and modify to include any of the following: — Intrusion >12 inches at occupant site — Intrusion >18 inches at any site — Partial or complete ejection from the vehicle — Death of another passenger in the same passenger compartment — Vehicle telemetry data consistent with high risk for injury • Revise "auto-pedestrian/auto-bicycle injury with significant (>5 mph) impact" and "pedestrian thrown or run over" to "Auto vs. pedestrian/bicyclist thrown, run over, or with significant (>20 mph) impact" • Revise "motorcycle crash >20 mph with separation of rider from bike" to "motorcycle crash >20 mph" • Remove "initial speed >40 mph, major auto deformity >20 inches, extrication time >20 min, and rollover"
STEP FOUR: SPECIAL CONSIDERATIONS
• Add "time-sensitive extremity injury, end-stage renal disease requiring dialysis, and Emergency Medical Service provider judgment" • Add burns from Step Two — Burns without other trauma mechanism: triage to burn facility — Burns with trauma mechanism: triage to trauma center • Clarify aged <5 years or >55 years to read: — Older adults: risk of injury death increases after age 55 years — Children: should be triaged preferentially to pediatric-capable trauma centers • Change "patient with bleeding disorder or patient on anticoagulants" to "anticoagulation and bleeding disorders" • Change "pregnancy" to "pregnancy >20 wks" • Remove "cardiac disease, respiratory disease, insulin-dependent diabetes, cirrhosis, morbid obesity, and immunosuppressed patients"

*Scheme is shown in Fig. 66-1.
Modified from Sasser SM, Hunt RC, Sullivent EE, et al: Guidelines for field triage of injured patients: recommendations of the National Expert Panel on Field Triage, *MMWR Recomm Rep* 58(RR-1):1–35, 2009. http://www.cdc.gov/mmwr/PDF/rr/rr5801.pdf.

especially neurosurgeons and orthopedic surgeons, must be promptly available; the operating room staff should be alerted.

Physiologic status, anatomic locations, and/or mechanism of injury are used for field triage as well as to determine whether to activate the trauma team (see Table 66-2). More importance should be placed on physiologic compromise and less on mechanism of injury. Scoring scales such as the Abbreviated Injury Scale (AIS), Injury Severity Score (ISS), Pediatric Trauma Score, and Revised Trauma Score (Table 66-3) use these parameters to predict patient outcome. The AIS and ISS are used together. First, the AIS is used to numerically score injuries—as 1 minor, 2 moderate, 3 serious, 4 severe, 5 critical, or 6 probably lethal—in each of 6 ISS body regions: head/neck, face, thorax, abdomen, extremity, and external. The ISS is the sum of the squares of the highest 3 AIS region scores.

PRIMARY SURVEY

During the primary survey, the physician quickly assesses and treats any life-threatening injuries. The principal causes of death

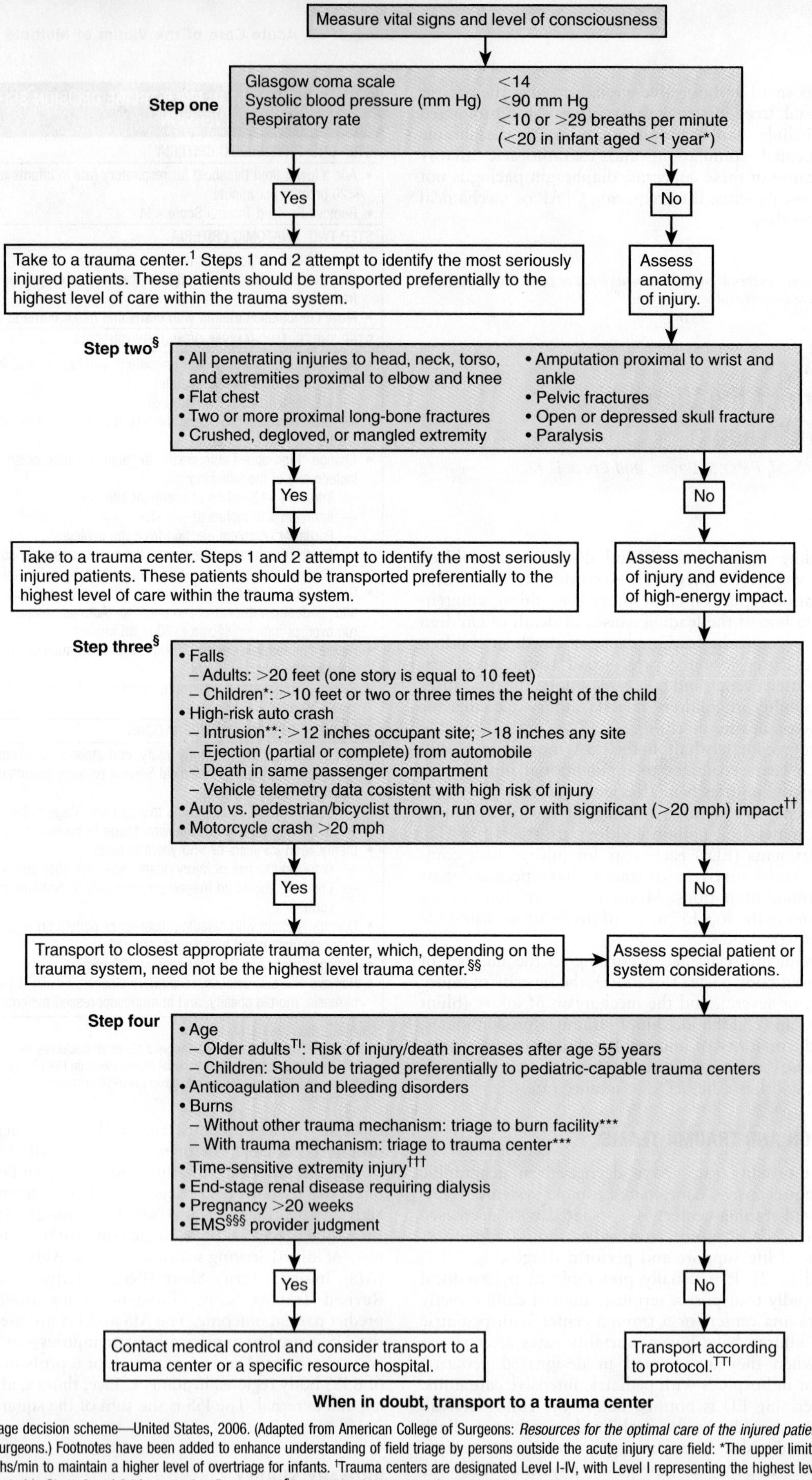

Figure 66-1 Field triage decision scheme—United States, 2006. (Adapted from American College of Surgeons: *Resources for the optimal care of the injured patient,* Chicago, 2006, American College of Surgeons.) Footnotes have been added to enhance understanding of field triage by persons outside the acute injury care field: *The upper limit of respiratory rate in infants is >29 breaths/min to maintain a higher level of overtriage for infants. †Trauma centers are designated Level I-IV, with Level I representing the highest level of trauma care available. §Any injury noted in Steps 2 and 3 triggers a "yes" response. ¶Age <15 yr. ***Intrusion* refers to interior compartment intrusion, as opposed to *deformation,* which refers to exterior damage. ††Includes pedestrians or bicyclists thrown or run over by a motor vehicle or those with estimated impact >20 mph with a motor vehicle. §§Local or regional protocols should be used to determine the most appropriate level of trauma center; appropriate center need not be Level I. ¶¶Age >55 yr. ***Patients with both burns and concomitant trauma for whom the burn injury poses the greatest risk for morbidity and mortality should be transferred to a burn center. If the nonburn trauma presents a greater immediate risk, the patient may be stabilized in a trauma center and then transferred to a burn center. †††Injuries such as an open fracture or fracture with neurovascular compromise. §§§Emergency medical services. ¶¶¶Patients who do not meet any of the triage criteria in Steps 1-4 should be transported to the most appropriate medical facility as outlined in local EMS protocols.

shortly after trauma are airway obstruction, respiratory insufficiency, shock from hemorrhage, and central nervous system injury. The primary survey addresses the ABCDEs: Airway, Breathing, Circulation, neurologic Deficit, and Exposure of the patient and control of the Environment.

Airway/Cervical Spine

Optimizing oxygenation and ventilation while protecting the cervical spine from potential further injury is of paramount importance. Initially, cervical spine injury should be suspected in any child sustaining multiple, blunt trauma. Children are at risk for such injuries because of their relatively large heads, which augment flexion-extension forces, and weak neck muscles, which predispose them to ligament injuries. To prevent additional spinal injury, the current standard is to immobilize the cervical (and thoracic and lumbar) spine in neutral position with a stiff collar, head blocks, tape or cloth placed across the forehead, torso, and thighs to restrain the child, and a rigid backboard.

Table 66-2 CHILDREN REQUIRING PEDIATRIC TRAUMA CENTER CARE

Patients with serious injury to >1 organ or system
Patients with 1-system injury who require critical care or monitoring in an intensive care unit
Patients with signs of shock who require >1 transfusion
Patients with fracture complicated by suspected neurovascular or compartment injury
Patients with fracture of the axial skeleton
Patients with ≥2 long-bone fractures
Patients with potential replantation of an extremity
Patients with suspected or actual spinal cord or column injury
Patients with head injury with any 1 of the following:
Orbital or facial bone fracture
Cerebrospinal fluid leak
Altered state of consciousness
Changing neurologic signs
Open-head injury
Depressed skull fracture
Requiring intracranial pressure monitoring
Patients suspected of requiring ventilator support

Modified from Krug SE: The acutely ill or injured child. In Behrman RE, Kliegman RM, editors: *Nelson essentials of pediatrics*, ed 4, Philadelphia, 2002, WB Saunders, p 96.

Airway obstruction manifests as snoring, gurgling, hoarseness, stridor, and/or diminished breath sounds (even with apparently good respiratory effort). Children are more likely than adults to have airway obstruction because of their smaller oral and nasal cavities, proportionately larger tongues and greater amounts of tonsillar and adenoidal tissue, higher and more anterior glottic openings, and narrower larynxes and tracheas. Obstruction is common in patients with severe head injuries, owing in part to decreased muscle tone, which allows the tongue to fall posteriorly and occlude the airway. With trauma, obstruction can also result from fractures of the mandible or facial bones, secretions such as blood or vomitus, crush injuries of the larynx or trachea, or foreign body aspiration.

If it is necessary to open the airway, a jaw thrust **without head tilt** is recommended. This procedure minimizes cervical spine motion. In an unconscious child, an oropharyngeal airway can be inserted to prevent posterior displacement of the mandibular tissues. A semiconscious child will gag with an oropharyngeal airway but may tolerate a nasopharyngeal airway. *A nasopharyngeal airway is contraindicated when there is a possibility of a cribriform plate fracture.* If these maneuvers plus suctioning do not clear the airway, oral endotracheal intubation is indicated. When endotracheal intubation proves difficult, a laryngeal mask airway can be used as a temporary alternative. A laryngeal mask airway consists of a tube with an inflatable cuff that rests above the larynx and thus does not require placement of the tube into the trachea. Emergency cricothyrotomy is needed in <1% of trauma victims.

Table 66-3 REVISED TRAUMA SCORE*

REVISED TRAUMA SCORE	GLASGOW COMA SCALE SCORE	SYSTOLIC BLOOD PRESSURE (mm Hg)	RESPIRATORY RATE (breaths/min)
4	13-15	>89	10-20
3	9-12	76-89	>29
2	6-8	50-75	6-9
1	4-5	1-49	1-5
0	3	0	0

*A score of 0-4 is given for each variable; then the scores are added (range, 1-12). A total score ≤ 11 indicates potentially important trauma.
From Fitzmaurice LS: Approach to multiple trauma. In Barkin RM, editor: *Pediatric emergency medicine*, ed 2, St Louis, 1997, Mosby, p 224.

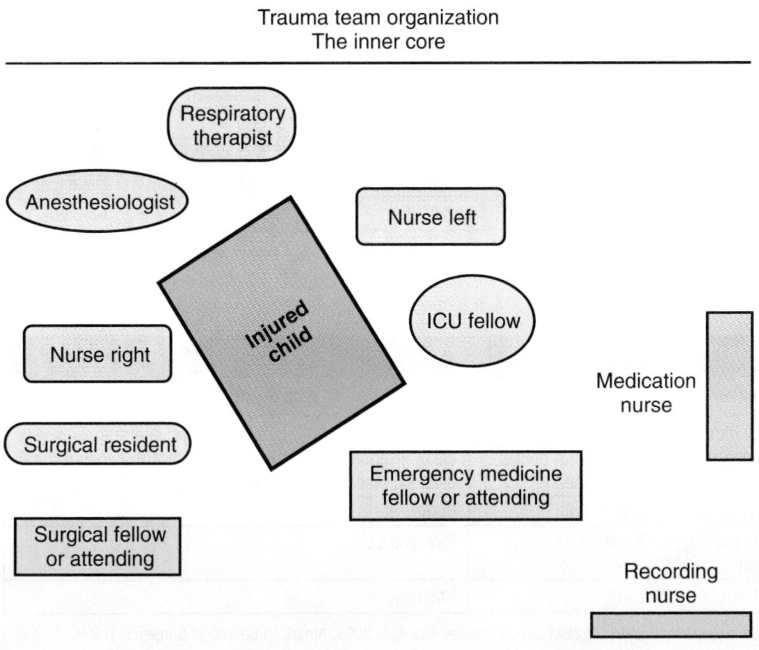

Figure 66-2 Members of the inner core of the trauma team at Children's National Medical Center (Washington, DC). Members of the outer core include a nursing administrator, a social worker, a radiology technician, a transport technician, and a security officer. ICU, intensive care unit.

Breathing

The physician assesses breathing by counting the respiratory rate; visualizing chest wall motion for symmetry, depth, and accessory muscle use; and auscultating breath sounds in both axillae. In addition to looking for cyanosis, pulse oximetry is standard. If ventilation is inadequate, bag-valve-mask ventilation with 100% oxygen must be initiated immediately, followed by endotracheal intubation. End-expiratory carbon dioxide (CO_2) detectors help verify accurate tube placement.

Head trauma is the most common cause of respiratory insufficiency. An unconscious child with a severe head injury may have a variety of breathing abnormalities, including Cheyne-Stokes respirations, slow irregular breaths, and apnea.

Although less common than a pulmonary contusion, tension pneumothorax and massive hemothorax are immediately life-threatening (Tables 66-4 and 66-5). **Tension pneumothorax** occurs when air accumulates under pressure in the pleural space. The adjacent lung is compacted, the mediastinum is pushed toward the opposite hemithorax, and the heart, great vessels, and contralateral lung are compressed or kinked (Chapter 405). Both ventilation and cardiac output are impaired. Characteristic findings include cyanosis, tachypnea, retractions, asymmetric chest rise, contralateral tracheal deviation, diminished breath sounds on the ipsilateral (more than contralateral) side, and signs of shock. Needle thoracentesis, followed by thoracostomy tube insertion, is diagnostic and lifesaving. **Hemothorax** results from injury to the intercostal vessels, lungs, heart, or great vessels. When ventilation is adequate, fluid resuscitation should begin before evacuation, because a large amount of blood may drain through the chest tube, resulting in shock.

Table 66-4 LIFE-THREATENING CHEST INJURIES

TENSION PNEUMOTHORAX
One-way valve leak from the lung parenchyma or tracheobronchial tree Collapse with mediastinal and tracheal shift to the side opposite the leak Compromises venous return and decreases ventilation of the other lung Clinically, manifests as respiratory distress, unilateral absence of breath sounds, tracheal deviation, distended neck veins, tympany to percussion of the involved side, and cyanosis Relieve first with needle aspiration, then with chest tube drainage
OPEN PNEUMOTHORAX (SUCKING CHEST WOUND)
Effect on ventilation depends on size
MAJOR FLAIL CHEST
Usually caused by blunt injury resulting in multiple rib fractures Loss of bone stability of the thoracic cage Major disruption of synchronous chest wall motion Mechanical ventilation and positive end-expiratory pressure required
MASSIVE HEMOTHORAX
Must be drained with a large-bore tube Initiate drainage only with concurrent vascular volume replacement
CARDIAC TAMPONADE **Beck Triad:**
1. Decreased or muffled heart sounds 2. Distended neck veins from increased venous pressure 3. Hypotension with pulsus paradoxus (decreased pulse pressure during inspiration) Must be drained

Modified from Krug SE: The acutely ill or injured child. In Behrman RE, Kliegman RM, editors: *Nelson essentials of pediatrics,* ed 4, Philadelphia, 2002, WB Saunders, p 97.

Circulation

The most common type of shock in trauma is hypovolemic shock due to hemorrhage. Signs of shock include tachycardia; weak pulse; delayed capillary refill; cool, mottled, pale skin; and altered mental status (Chapter 64). Early in shock, blood pressure remains normal because of compensatory increases in heart rate and peripheral vascular resistance (Table 66-6). Some individuals can lose up to 30% of blood volume before blood pressure declines. *It is important to note that 25% of blood volume equals 20 mL/kg, which is only 200 mL in a 10-kg child.* Losses >40% of blood volume cause severe hypotension that, if prolonged, may become irreversible. Direct pressure should be applied to control external hemorrhage. Blind clamping of bleeding vessels, which risks damaging adjacent structures, is not advisable.

Cannulating a larger vein, such as an antecubital vein, is usually the quickest way to achieve intravenous access. A short, large-bore catheter offers less resistance to flow, allowing for more rapid fluid administration. Ideally, a second catheter should be placed within the first few minutes of resuscitation in a severely injured child. If intravenous access is crucial and not rapidly obtainable, an intraosseous catheter should be inserted; all medications and fluids can be administered intraosseously. Other alternatives are central venous access using the Seldinger technique (e.g., in the femoral vein) and, rarely, surgical cutdown (e.g., in the saphenous vein). Ultrasonography can facilitate central venous catheter placement.

Aggressive, intravenous fluid resuscitation is essential early in shock to prevent further deterioration. Isotonic crystalloid solution, such as lactated Ringer's injection or normal saline (20 mL/kg), should be infused rapidly. No consensus exists to support the routine use of colloid or hypertonic (3%) saline solution. When necessary, repeated crystalloid boluses should be given. Most children are stabilized with administration of crystalloid solution alone. However, if the patient remains in shock after

Table 66-5 DIFFERENTIAL DIAGNOSIS OF IMMEDIATELY LIFE-THREATENING CARDIOPULMONARY INJURIES

	TENSION PNEUMOTHORAX	MASSIVE HEMOTHORAX	CARDIAC TAMPONADE
Breath sounds	Ipsilaterally decreased more than contralaterally	Ipsilaterally decreased	Normal
Percussion note	Hyperresonant	Dull	Normal
Tracheal location	Contralaterally shifted	Midline or shifted	Midline
Neck veins	Distended	Flat	Distended
Heart tones	Normal	Normal	Muffled

Modified from Cooper A, Foltin GL: Thoracic trauma. In Barkin RM, editor: *Pediatric emergency medicine,* ed 2, St Louis, 1997, Mosby, p 325.

Table 66-6 SYSTEMIC RESPONSES TO BLOOD LOSS IN PEDIATRIC PATIENTS

SYSTEM	MILD BLOOD LOSS (<30%)	MODERATE BLOOD LOSS (30-45%)	SEVERE BLOOD LOSS (>45%)
Cardiovascular	Increased heart rate; weak, thready peripheral pulses; normal systolic blood pressure; normal pulse pressure	Markedly increased heart rate; weak, thready central pulses; peripheral pulses absent; low normal systolic blood pressure	Tachycardia followed by bradycardia; central pulses very weak or absent; peripheral pulses absent; hypotension; diastolic blood pressure may be undetectable
Central nervous system	Anxiety; irritability; confusion	Lethargy; dulled response to pain	Coma
Skin	Cool, mottled; capillary refill prolonged	Cyanotic; capillary refill markedly prolonged	Pale and cold
Urine output	Low to very low	Minimal	None

Adapted from American College of Surgeons Committee on Trauma: *Advanced trauma life support for doctors: student course manual,* Chicago, 2008, American College of Surgeons, p 234.

boluses totaling 40-60 mL/kg of crystalloid, then 10-15 mL/kg of cross-matched, packed red blood cells should be transfused. Although less desirable, type-specific or O-negative cells can be substituted pending availability of cross-matched blood. When shock persists despite these measures, surgery to stop internal hemorrhage is usually indicated.

Neurologic Deficit

Neurologic status is briefly assessed by determining the level of consciousness and evaluating pupil size and reactivity. The level of consciousness can be classified using the mnemonic AVPU: Alert, responsive to Verbal commands, responsive to Painful stimuli, or Unresponsive.

Head injuries account for approximately 70% of pediatric blunt trauma deaths. Primary direct cerebral injury occurs within seconds of the event and is irreversible. Secondary injury is caused by subsequent anoxia or ischemia. The goal is to minimize secondary injury by ensuring adequate oxygenation, ventilation, and perfusion, and maintaining normal intracranial pressure (ICP). A child with severe neurologic impairment—i.e., with a Glasgow Coma Scale (GCS; see Table 62-3) score of 8 or less—should be intubated.

Signs of increased ICP, including progressive neurologic deterioration and evidence of transtentorial herniation, must be treated immediately. Hyperventilation lowers $PaCO_2$, resulting in cerebral vasoconstriction, reduced cerebral blood flow, and decreased ICP. Brief hyperventilation remains an immediate option for patients with acute increases in ICP. Prophylactic hyperventilation or vigorous or prolonged hyperventilation is not recommended, because the consequent vasoconstriction may excessively decrease cerebral perfusion and oxygenation. Mannitol lowers ICP and may improve survival. Because mannitol acts via osmotic diuresis, it can exacerbate hypovolemia and must be used cautiously. Hypertonic saline may be a useful agent for control of increased ICP in patients with severe head injury and may possibly decrease mortality when compared with mannitol. Neurosurgical consultation is mandatory. If signs of increased ICP persist, the neurosurgeon must decide whether to operate emergently.

Exposure and Environmental Control

All clothing should be cut away to reveal any injuries. Cutting is quickest and minimizes unnecessary patient movement.

Children often arrive mildly hypothermic because of their higher body surface area–mass ratios. They can be warmed with use of radiant heat as well as heated blankets and intravenous fluids.

SECONDARY SURVEY

During the secondary survey, the physician completes a detailed, head-to-toe physical examination.

Head Trauma

A GCS or Pediatric GCS score (see Table 62-3) should be assigned to every child with significant head trauma. This scale assesses eye opening and motor and verbal responses. In the Pediatric GCS, the verbal score is modified for age. The GCS further categorizes neurologic disability, and serial measurements identify improvement or deterioration over time. Patients with low scores 6-24 hr after injuries have poorer prognoses.

In the ED, CT scanning of the head without a contrast agent has become standard to determine the type of injury. Diffuse cerebral injury with edema is a common and serious finding on CT scan in severely brain-injured children. Focal evacuable hemorrhagic lesions (e.g., epidural hematoma) occur less commonly but may require immediate neurosurgical intervention (Fig. 66-3).

Monitoring of ICP should be strongly considered for children with severe brain injury, particularly for those with a GCS score of 8 or less and abnormal head CT findings (Chapter 63). An advantage of an intraventricular catheter over an intraparenchymal device is that cerebrospinal fluid can be drained to treat acute increases in ICP. Hypoxia, hypercarbia, hypotension, and hyperthermia must be aggressively managed to prevent secondary brain injury. Cerebral perfusion pressure should be maintained >40 mm Hg at least (although some experts recommend an even higher minimum).

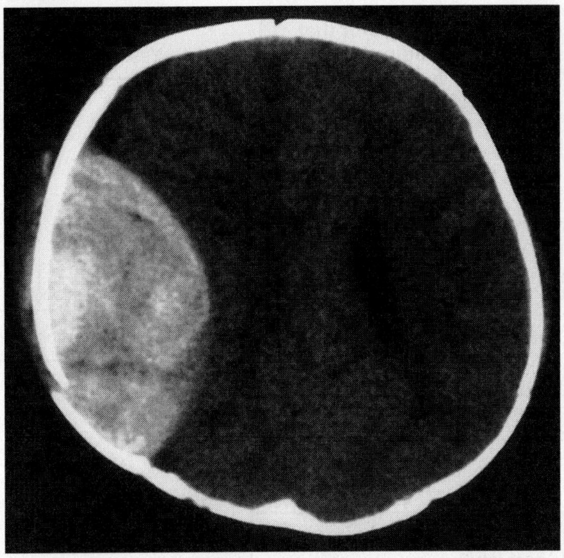

Figure 66-3 According to the history provided, the 7-month-old girl whose head CT scan is shown here did not wake up for her nightly feeding and began vomiting in the morning. The mother's boyfriend reported that the infant had fallen from a chair the previous day. The CT scan shows a large epidural hematoma on the right and marked shift of the midline from right to left. The right lateral ventricle is compressed as a result of the mass effect, and the left lateral ventricle is slightly prominent. The infant underwent emergency surgical evacuation of the epidural hematoma and recovered uneventfully. (From O'Neill JA Jr: *Principles of pediatric surgery,* ed 2, St Louis, 2003, Mosby, p 191.)

A child with a severe brain injury must be treated aggressively in the ED because it is very difficult to accurately predict long-term neurologic outcome. Compared with adults with similar injuries, children are thought to have better functional outcomes.

Cervical Spine Trauma

Cervical spine injuries occur in <3% of children with blunt trauma—with the risk being substantially higher in those with GCS scores ≤8—but they are associated with significant mortality and morbidity. Bony injuries occur mainly from C1 to C4 in children younger than 8 yr. In older children, they occur equally in the upper and lower cervical spine. The mortality rate is significantly higher in patients with upper cervical spine injuries. Spinal cord injury without radiographic (vertebral body) abnormalities (SCIWORA) may be present. Patients with SCIWORA have neurologic symptoms, and spinal cord abnormalities are nearly always noted on MRI. Approximately 30% of all patients with cervical spine injuries have permanent neurologic deficits.

Evaluation begins with a detailed history and neurologic examination. Identifying the mechanism of injury helps in estimating the likelihood of a cervical spine injury. Both the patient and the paramedic should be asked whether any neurologic symptoms or signs, such as weakness or abnormal sensation, were present before arrival in the ED. In a child with neurologic symptoms and normal findings on cervical spine plain radiographs and CT scan, SCIWORA must be considered.

Whenever the history, physical examination, or mechanism of injury suggests a cervical spine injury, radiographs should be obtained after initial resuscitation. In adults, the Canadian

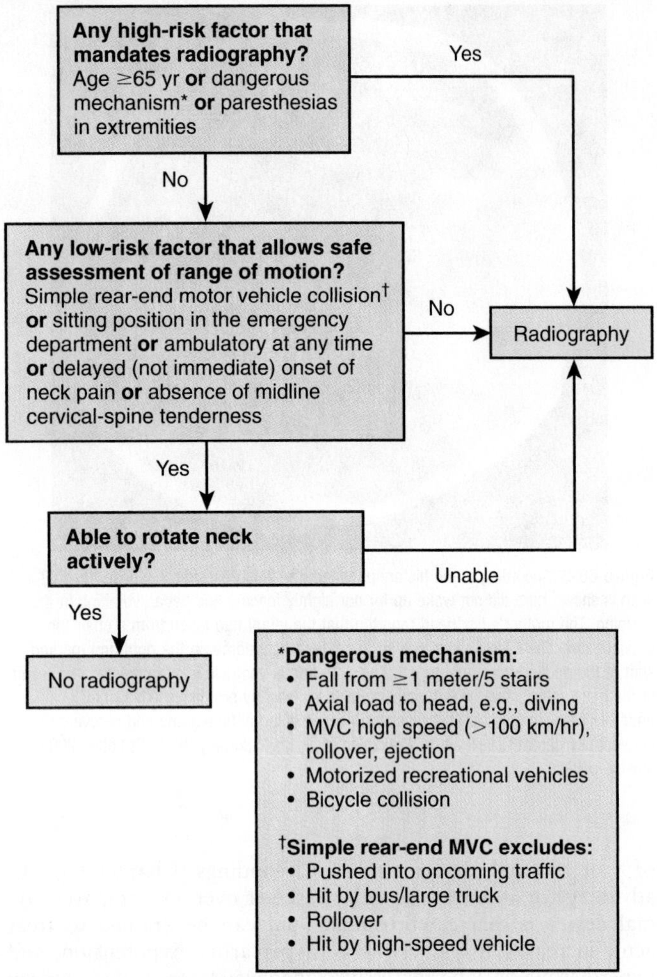

Any high-risk factor that mandates radiography?
Age ≥65 yr or dangerous mechanism* or paresthesias in extremities
Yes
No
Any low-risk factor that allows safe assessment of range of motion?
Simple rear-end motor vehicle collision† or sitting position in the emergency department or ambulatory at any time or delayed (not immediate) onset of neck pain or absence of midline cervical-spine tenderness
No
Radiography
Yes
Able to rotate neck actively?
Unable
Yes
No radiography
*Dangerous mechanism:
• Fall from ≥1 meter/5 stairs
• Axial load to head, e.g., diving
• MVC high speed (>100 km/hr), rollover, ejection
• Motorized recreational vehicles
• Bicycle collision
†Simple rear-end MVC excludes:
• Pushed into oncoming traffic
• Hit by bus/large truck
• Rollover
• Hit by high-speed vehicle

Figure 66-4 The Canadian C-spine rule. For adult patients with trauma who are alert (as indicated by a score of 15 on the Glasgow Coma Scale) and in stable condition and in whom cervical spine injury is a concern, determination of risk factors and physical examination guide the use of cervical spine radiography. MVC, motor vehicle collision. (From Stiell IG, Clement CM, McKnight RD, et al: The Canadian C-spine rule versus the NEXUS low-risk criteria in patients with trauma, *N Engl J Med* 349:2510–2518, 2003.)

C-spine rule helps identify low-risk patients who may not require radiographs (Fig. 66-4). The standard series of plain radiographs includes lateral, anteroposterior, and odontoid views. Some centers use cervical spine CT as the primary diagnostic tool, particularly in patients with abnormal GCS scores and/or significant injury mechanisms, recognizing that CT is more sensitive in detecting bony injury than plain radiographs. CT is also helpful if an odontoid fracture is suspected, because young children typically do not cooperate enough to obtain an "open-mouth" (odontoid) radiographic view. Use of cervical spine CT scan must be balanced with the knowledge that CT exposes thyroid tissue to 90-200 times the amount of radiation from plain films. MRI is indicated in a child with suspected SCIWORA.

Rapid diagnosis of spinal cord injury is essential. Initiating high-dose intravenous methylprednisolone within 8 hr of spinal cord injury has been shown to improve motor outcome and remains standard therapy.

Thoracic Trauma

Pulmonary contusions occur frequently in young children with blunt chest trauma. A child's chest wall is relatively pliable; therefore, less force is absorbed by the rib cage, and more is transmitted to the lungs. Respiratory distress may be noted initially or may develop during the first 24 hr after injury.

Table 66-7 INDICATIONS FOR OPERATION IN THORACIC TRAUMA

THORACOTOMY IMMEDIATELY OR SHORTLY AFTER INJURY
Massive continuing pneumothorax or large air leak from tracheobronchial injury (cannot expand lung and ventilate)
Cardiac tamponade
Open pneumothorax
Esophageal injury
Aortic or other vascular injury
Acute rupture of the diaphragm
DELAYED THORACOTOMY
Chronic rupture of the diaphragm
Clotted hemothorax
Persistent chylothorax
Traumatic intracardiac defects
Evacuation of large foreign bodies
Chronic atelectasis from traumatic bronchial stenosis

Modified from O'Neill JA Jr: *Principles of pediatric surgery,* ed 2, St Louis, 2003, Mosby, p 157.

Table 66-8 FREQUENCY OF ABDOMINAL ORGAN INJURY BY INJURY MECHANISM

BLUNT		PENETRATING	
Organ	%	Organ	%
Spleen	30	Gastrointestinal tract	70
Liver	28	Liver	27
Kidneys	28	Blood vessels	19
Gastrointestinal tract	14	Kidneys	10
Bladder/urethra/ureters	4	Spleen	9
Pancreas	3	Bladder/urethra/ureters	8
Blood vessels	3	Pancreas	6

Modified from O'Neill JA Jr: *Principles of pediatric surgery,* ed 2, St Louis, 2003, Mosby, p 159.

Rib fractures result from significant external force. They are noted in patients with more severe injuries and are associated with a higher mortality rate. Flail chest, which is caused by multiple rib fractures, is rare in children. Indications for operative management in thoracic trauma are listed in Table 66-7. The differential diagnosis of immediately life-threatening cardiopulmonary injuries is shown in Table 66-5.

Abdominal Trauma

Liver and spleen contusions, hematomas, and lacerations account for the majority of intra-abdominal injuries from blunt trauma. The kidneys, pancreas, and duodenum are relatively spared because of their retroperitoneal location. Pancreatic and duodenal injuries are more common after a bicycle handlebar impact or a direct blow to the abdomen (Table 66-8).

Although a thorough examination for intra-abdominal injuries is essential, achieving it often proves difficult. Misleading findings can result from gastric distention after crying or in an uncooperative toddler. Calm reassurance, distraction, and gentle, persistent palpation help with the examination. Important findings include distention, bruises, and tenderness. Specific symptoms and signs give insight into the mechanism of injury and the potential for particular injuries. Pain in the left shoulder may signify splenic trauma. A lap belt mark across the abdomen suggests a bowel or mesentery injury. The presence of certain other injuries, such as lumbar spinal fractures and femur fractures, increases the likelihood of intra-abdominal injury. Other risks are listed in Table 66-9.

An abdominal CT scan with intravenous contrast medium enhancement rapidly identifies structural and functional abnormalities and is the preferred study in a stable child. It has excellent sensitivity and specificity for splenic (Fig. 66-5), hepatic (Fig. 66-6), and renal injuries but is not as sensitive for diaphragmatic,

Table 66-9 PREDICTION RULE FOR IDENTIFICATION OF CHILDREN WITH INTRA-ABDOMINAL INJURIES AFTER BLUNT TORSO TRAUMA

If any one of the following is present, the patient likely has intra-abdominal injury:
Low age-adjusted systolic blood pressure
Abdominal tenderness
Femur fracture
Elevated liver enzymes*
Microscopic hematuria†
Initial hematocrit <30%

*Serum aspartate aminotransferase level >200 U/L or serum alanine aminotransferase level >125 U/L.

†>5 red blood cells/high powered field.

Modified from Holmes JF, Mao A, Awasthi S, et al: Validation of a prediction rule for the identification of children with intra-abdominal injuries after blunt torso trauma, *Ann Emerg Med* 54:528–533, 2009.

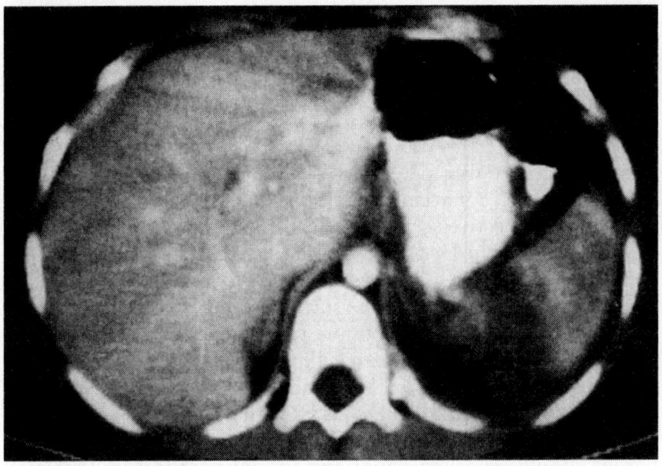

Figure 66-5 CT scan with intravenous and gastrointestinal contrast enhancement shows an isolated splenic rupture that resulted from blunt trauma. This injury responded to nonoperative management, as do most splenic injuries. (From O'Neill JA Jr: *Principles of pediatric surgery,* ed 2, St Louis, 2003, Mosby, p 166.)

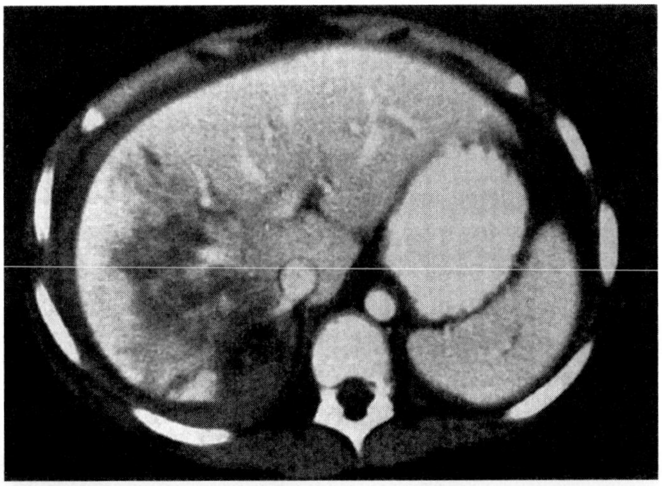

Figure 66-6 CT scan performed after severe blunt injury of the abdomen shows a bursting injury of the liver. The patient was stable, and no operative intervention was required. The decision to perform surgery should be based on the patient's physiologic stability. (From O'Neill JA Jr: *Principles of pediatric surgery,* ed 2, St Louis, 2003, Mosby, p 168.)

pancreatic, or intestinal injuries. Small amounts of free fluid or air or a mesenteric hematoma may be the only sign of an intestinal injury. Administration of an oral contrast agent is not routinely recommended for all abdominal CT scans, but it sometimes aids in identifying an intestinal, especially a duodenal, injury.

Although focused assessment with sonography in trauma (FAST) examination helps detect hemoperitoneum, the variably low sensitivity of this test in children suggests that it should not be used to exclude intra-abdominal injury in patients with a high pretest probability for injury. Serial FAST exams over time may be used by skilled ultrasonographers to rule out injury in need of intervention. FAST is most useful in patients who have blunt trauma and are hemodynamically unstable or patients who require operative intervention for nonabdominal injuries, because in these cases the performance of a CT scan may not be feasible.

Nonoperative treatment has become standard for hemodynamically stable children with splenic, hepatic, and renal injuries from blunt trauma. The majority of such children can be treated nonsurgically. In addition to avoiding perioperative complications, nonoperative treatment decreases the need for blood transfusions and shortens hospital stay. When laparotomy is indicated, splenic repair is preferable to splenectomy.

Pelvic Trauma

Pelvic fractures in children are much less common than in adults, occurring in approximately 5% of children with more severe blunt trauma. Pelvic fractures are typically caused by high forces (e.g., from high-speed motor vehicle crashes or pedestrian impacts) and are often associated with intra-abdominal and/or vascular injuries. The pelvis itself forms a ring, and high-force impacts can lead to disruption of this ring. When the ring is disrupted in more than one location, such as the symphysis pubis and the sacroiliac joint, the ring can become unstable and displaced, potentially injuring large pelvic vessels and leading to massive blood loss. Catheter-directed embolization performed in the radiology department to control bleeding may be required.

The pelvis should be assessed for stability by means of compression-distraction maneuvers. If instability is noted, immediate external fixation with a pelvis-stabilizing device or a sheet should be applied, and orthopedic consultation sought. Most trauma patients should receive an AP pelvic radiograph in the trauma bay. Children without pelvic tenderness, instability, ecchymosis, abrasions, and bleeding, and in whom no is blood coming from the urethra, may be at low risk for significant pelvic fractures.

Lower Genitourinary Trauma

The perineum should be inspected, and the stability of the bones of the pelvis assessed. Urethral injuries are more common in males. Findings suggestive of urethral injury include scrotal or labial ecchymoses, blood at the urethral meatus, gross hematuria, and a superiorly positioned prostate on rectal examination (in an adolescent male). Certain pelvic fractures also increase the risk for potential genitourinary injury. Any of these findings is a contraindication to urethral catheter insertion and warrants consultation with a urologist. Retrograde urethrocystogram and CT scan of the pelvis and abdomen are used to determine the extent of injury.

Extremity Trauma

Extremity fractures may initially be missed as clinicians attend to more life-threatening injuries. Thorough examination of the extremities is essential because extremity fractures are among the most frequently overlooked injuries in children with multiple trauma. All limbs should be inspected for deformity, swelling, and bruises; palpated for tenderness; and assessed for active and passive range of motion, sensory function, and perfusion.

Before radiographs are obtained, suspected fractures and dislocations should be immobilized, and an analgesic administered. Splinting a femur fracture helps alleviate pain and may decrease blood loss. An orthopedic surgeon should be consulted immediately to evaluate children with compartment syndrome, neurovascular compromise, open fracture, and most traumatic amputations.

Radiologic and Laboratory Evaluation

Some authorities recommend ordering multiple studies in the ED that include lateral cervical spine, anteroposterior chest, and anteroposterior pelvis radiographs; arterial blood gas analysis; serum lactate determinations; complete blood cell count; electrolyte measurements; blood glucose and blood urea nitrogen measurements; serum creatinine, amylase, and lipase determinations; liver function tests; prothrombin and partial thromboplastin time determinations; blood typing and cross-matching; and urinalysis. One benefit of standardizing the evaluation of patients with major trauma is that fewer decisions need to be made on an individual basis, possibly expediting ED management.

Some of these studies have prognostic importance. A large base deficit is associated with a higher mortality rate, and elevated lactate values correlate with poor prognosis.

There are limitations of standard tests. The lateral cervical spine radiograph can miss significant injuries. Hemoglobin and hematocrit values provide baseline values in the ED, but they may not have yet equilibrated after a hemorrhage. Abnormal liver function test results or elevated serum amylase and lipase values may be noted in patients with significant abdominal trauma, but most patients with significant trauma to the abdomen already have clinical indications for CT scanning or surgery. The majority of previously healthy children have normal coagulation profiles; these may become abnormal after major head trauma. Although routine urinalysis or dipstick urine testing for blood has been recommended for children, other data suggest that this evaluation may be unnecessary in patients without gross hematuria, hypotension, or other associated abdominal injuries.

Clinical prediction rules that combine patient history with physical exam findings have been developed to identify those at low risk of injury for whom specific radiographic and laboratory studies may not be necessary. The Canadian C-spine rule for adults is one such rule (see Fig. 66-4). In children, a clinical prediction rule for the identification of children with intra-abdominal injuries following blunt trauma has been validated. The presence of any of the risk factors in this prediction rule had a sensitivity of 95% for identifying children with intra-abdominal injury (see Table 66-9). Several clinical prediction rules have also been developed to predict traumatic brain injury following blunt head trauma. These rules, if successfully validated, may allow for more appropriate use of CT in pediatric trauma patients and may potentially reduce unnecessary radiation exposure.

PSYCHOLOGICAL AND SOCIAL SUPPORT

Serious multisystem trauma may result in significant long-term psychologic and social difficulties for the child and family, particularly when there is a major head injury. Like adults, children are at risk for depressive symptoms and post-traumatic stress disorder. Caregivers face persistent stress and have been noted to have more psychologic symptoms. Psychologic and social support, during the resuscitation period and afterwards, is extremely important. Parents often prefer to be offered the choice to be present during resuscitations. A member of the resuscitation team should be made responsible for answering the family's questions and supporting them in the trauma room.

BIBLIOGRAPHY

Please visit the Nelson Textbook of Pediatrics *website at* www.expertconsult.com *for the complete bibliography.*

66.1 Care of Abrasions and Minor Lacerations

Joanna S. Cohen and Bruce L. Klein

LACERATIONS AND CUTS

Lacerations are tears of the skin caused by blunt or shearing forces. A cut (or a stab), in contrast, is an injury inflicted by a sharp object. Although distinguishing between the two can be important for forensic purposes, their evaluation and management are similar. In this chapter, lacerations include cuts and stabs.

Epidemiology

More than half of the 12 million wounds treated annually in U.S. EDs are lacerations. Approximately 30% occur in children younger than 18 yr.

Evaluation

The history should include the mechanism of injury, the amount of force, and the time the injury occurred. The mechanism helps determine whether there may be foreign material in the wound, which would increase the risk for infection. Particularly in children, it is essential to determine whether the injury was inflicted intentionally. If nonaccidental trauma is suspected, the state or local child protective services agency should be notified. The type of force causing the laceration also influences the risk of infection, as a significant crush injury is more likely to become infected than a shearing one. Blunt injury, such as bumping the head, is a common cause of lacerations in children and is less likely to become infected. Theoretically, the amount of bacteria in the wound should increase exponentially with the time from injury to repair; however, the length of time that results in a clinically significant increase in wound infection is unclear. The patient or parent should be asked about any special host factors that may predispose to infection or impede healing, such as diabetes, malnutrition, obesity, and steroid therapy.

The laceration's location also is important with regard to both the risk for infection and the cosmetic outcome. Compared with lacerations in adults, those in children occur more commonly on the face and scalp and less commonly on the upper extremities. Because the face and scalp are more vascular, wounds located there are less likely to become infected. Lacerations overlying joints are more likely to develop wider scars as a result of tension during healing.

Treatment

The goals of treatment are to minimize the risk of infection, to restore skin and underlying tissue integrity, and to produce the most functionally and cosmetically acceptable result possible. In adults, the infection rate for uncomplicated lacerations is approximately 3-7%.

Any significant bleeding must be controlled (with external pressure usually) before a thorough evaluation of the wound can occur. If there is a skin flap, it should be returned to its original position before application of pressure. Clothing over the injury should be removed to minimize wound contamination. Jewelry encircling an injured extremity should be removed to prevent the jewelry from forming a constricting band when the extremity swells.

It is best to administer a local anesthetic early, before exploration and more meticulous cleansing of the wound. This anesthetic can be applied topically (e.g., lidocaine, epinephrine, and tetracaine gel) or infiltrated locally or as a regional nerve block (e.g., lidocaine or bupivacaine), depending on the location of the laceration and the complexity of the repair. Sometimes procedural sedation and analgesia are required for a young uncooperative child. The wound should be examined under proper light to allow identification of foreign bodies or damage to nerves or tendons.

Many lacerations, especially heavily contaminated ones, benefit from irrigation to reduce the risk of infection. It is important to recognize that many traumatic lacerations treated in the ED or office are only minimally contaminated, containing less than 10^2 bacterial colonies. In fact, in one of the few human studies on irrigation, irrigation did not decrease the infection rate of minimally contaminated scalp or facial lacerations in patients who presented to an ED within 6 hours of injury. Another concern is that higher-pressure irrigation may actually increase tissue damage, making the wound and adjacent tissue more susceptible to infection and delaying healing. These caveats notwithstanding, irrigation has benefits, although which technique to use—i.e., which device, what size syringe, what size needle, which solution, how much volume, how much pressure—remains to be determined. These features may vary for different types of lacerations. In heavily contaminated wounds, the benefit of higher-pressure irrigation likely outweighs the harm of tissue damage. For heavily contaminated lacerations, a typical recommendation is to use a 35- to 65-mL syringe attached to a plastic splatter shield, or a 19-gauge needle if a splatter shield is unavailable, and to irrigate with 250-1,000 mL of normal saline. Conversely, for relatively clean wounds, lower-pressure irrigation minimizes tissue damage, which may be more important for outcome than any decrease in bacterial clearance that may ensue. Debridement of devitalized tissue with higher-pressure irrigation, scrubbing, or surgical excision can also be necessary in certain cases, such as crush injuries.

Most lacerations seen in the pediatric ED or office should be closed primarily. Contraindications to primary closure (e.g., certain bite wounds) do exist (Chapter 705). Although it is commonly accepted that the time from injury to repair should be as brief as possible to minimize the risk of infection, there is no universally accepted guideline as to what length of time is too long for primary wound closure. Also, this length of time varies for different types of lacerations. A prudent recommendation is that higher-risk wounds should be closed within 6 hr at most after the injury but that some low-risk wounds (e.g., clean facial lacerations) may be closed as late as 12-24 hr.

Many lacerations can be closed with simple, interrupted, 4-0, 5-0, or 6-0, nonabsorbable sutures. For lacerations under tension, horizontal or vertical mattress sutures—which provide added strength and may evert the wound edges better—can be used instead. For lacerations in cosmetically significant areas, a running intradermal stitch may produce a less conspicuous, more aesthetic scar than simple or mattress skin sutures, which leave unattractive track marks. Deeper lacerations may need repair with an absorbable dermal and/or fascial layer. Other complex lacerations—e.g., those involving the ear, eyelid, nose, lip, tongue, genitalia, or fingertip—sometimes require more advanced techniques as well as subspecialty consultation.

Staples, topical skin adhesives, and surgical tape are acceptable alternatives to sutures, depending on the laceration's location and the health care provider's preference. Staples are particularly useful for lacerations of the scalp, where the appearance of the scar tends to be less important. Topical skin adhesives (e.g., octyl cyanoacrylates or butyl cyanoacrylates) are ideal for linear, relatively superficial lacerations, with easily approximated edges that are not under tension, particularly when these lacerations are located in areas where suture track marks are especially undesirable.

Maintaining a warm, moist, wound environment following repair accelerates wound healing without increasing the risk of infection. A topical antimicrobial ointment (e.g., bacitracin or a bacitracin, neomycin, and polymyxin B combination) and conventional gauze dressing provide such an environment and reduce the infection rate as well. Compared with conventional dressings, occlusive dressings (e.g., hydrocolloids, hydrogels, polyurethane films) may be better at accelerating healing, reducing infection, and decreasing pain but are more expensive; occlusive dressings that adhere (e.g., hydrocolloids or polyurethane films) are impractical for lacerations with protruding sutures. If the laceration overlies or is near a joint, splinting helps limit mobility and can speed healing and minimize dehiscence.

For most routine lacerations evaluated in the ED or office that are repaired early and carefully, prophylactic systemic antibiotics are unnecessary because they do not decrease the rate of infection. Antibiotic prophylaxis is or may be indicated for human and many animal bites, for open fractures and joints, and for grossly contaminated wounds, as well as for wounds in patients who are immunosuppressed or have prosthetic devices. Tetanus prophylaxis should be administered, if indicated, according to Centers for Disease Control and Prevention guidelines (Chapter 203).

ABRASIONS

An *abrasion* is a scrape to the epidermis and sometimes the dermis that is usually caused by friction of the skin against a rough surface. "Road rash" is a colloquial term for abrasions that result from friction of the skin against pavement. Motor vehicle collisions with pedestrians and cycling accidents are common causes of road rash in children. Road rash can be extensive, involving multiple areas on the body. These abrasions also can be deep, and they often contain embedded debris. A "rug burn" is an abrasion sustained by sliding across a carpet. Some abrasions display specific patterns and are called *imprint abrasions*. Ligature marks are a type of imprint abrasion caused by a rope or cord that has been tied around a part of the body and has rubbed against the skin. These injuries should alert the clinician to the likelihood of nonaccidental (including self-inflicted) trauma.

Treatment

All abrasions should be cleansed thoroughly, and any debris or foreign material removed. If debris is not removed, abnormal skin pigmentation, known as post-traumatic tattooing, can occur and can be difficult to treat. A nonadherent occlusive dressing or a topical antibiotic and conventional dressing should be applied. Tetanus prophylaxis should be administered, if indicated (Chapter 203). Large and/or deep abrasions that have not healed in a few weeks require consultation with a plastic surgeon for more advanced care.

BIBLIOGRAPHY

Please visit the Nelson Textbook of Pediatrics *website at* *www.expertconsult.com* *for the complete bibliography.*

Chapter 67
Drowning and Submersion Injury

Elena Shephard and Linda Quan

Drowning is a leading cause of childhood morbidity and mortality in the world. Although the factors that put children at risk of drowning are increasingly well defined, the treatment of drowning has not advanced. Prevention is the most important step to reducing the impact of drowning injury, followed by early initiation of cardiopulmonary resuscitation (CPR) at the scene.

ETIOLOGY

Children are at risk of drowning when they are exposed to a water hazard in their environment. The World Congress of Drowning definition is: "Drowning is the process of experiencing respiratory impairment from submersion/immersion in liquid." The term drowning does not imply the final outcome, death or survival; the outcome should be denoted as fatal or nonfatal drowning. Use of this terminology should improve consistency in reporting and research; the use of confusing descriptive terms such as "near," "wet," "dry," "secondary," "silent," "passive," and "active" should be abandoned.

EPIDEMIOLOGY

In 2006, 4,248 people died from unintentional drowning in the USA. Compared with other types of injuries, drowning has one of the highest case fatality rates. Highest drowning death rates were seen in children aged 1-4 yr and 15-19 yr (2.81 and 1.47/100,000, respectively). In children, drowning is second only to motor vehicle injury as a leading cause of death from unintentional injury. Morbidity in nonfatal cases of drowning is much harder to determine. The ratio of hospitalized survival rate to death rate for drowning varies from 1 : 1 to 1 : 4 by age group and by state. Some estimates indicate that for each child who dies from drowning, 6 more are seen in an emergency department (ED). The Centers for Disease Control and Prevention (CDC) reported that in 2001, 3,372 people suffered fatal drowning and 4,174 were treated in the ED for nonfatal drowning. Estimates of drowning survivors with permanent, severe neurologic damage are not available.

The risk of drowning and the circumstances leading to it vary by age. Drowning risk also relates to male gender, exposure to water, and supervision. These factors are embedded in the context of geography, climate, socioeconomic status, and culture.

Children Younger than 1 Year

Most (71%) drowning deaths in children younger than 1 yr occur in the bathtub, when an infant is left alone or under the "supervision" of an older sibling. Infant tub seats or rings may exacerbate the risk by giving caregivers a false sense of security that the child is safe in the tub. The next major risk to this age group is the large (5-gallon) household bucket, implicated in 16% of infant drowning deaths. These buckets are about 30 cm tall and when half-full can weigh >9 kg. The average 9-mo-old child tends to be top-heavy, so can easily fall head first into a half-full bucket, become stuck, and drown within minutes.

Children 1-4 Years

Drowning rates are consistently highest in 1 to 4 yr old children, likely because of their curious but unaware nature coupled with the rapid progression of their physical capabilities. U.S. rates are highest in the southern regions, in some areas as high as 7.62/100,000, which approaches rates seen in developing countries. A common factor in many of these deaths is a lapse in adult supervision. Most U.S. drownings occur in residential swimming pools. Usually, the child is in his or her own home and the caregiver does not expect the child to be anywhere near the pool. The majority of children who drown are out of their caregivers' sight for <5 min.

In rural areas, children in this age group often drown in irrigation ditches or nearby ponds and rivers. The circumstances are similar to those noted previously, in a body of water that is near the house. Drowning is one of the leading causes of farm injury–related deaths in children.

School-aged Children

School-aged children are at increased risk of drowning in natural bodies of water such as lakes, ponds, rivers, and canals. Although swimming pools account for the majority of nonfatal drownings, open water accounts for a higher death rate from this age group on through adolescence. Unlike for preschool children, swimming or boating activities are important factors in drowning injuries in school-aged children.

Adolescents

The second major peak in drowning death rates occurs in older adolescents, aged 15-19 yr. Almost 70% drown in natural freshwater. In this age group particularly, there are striking disparities in drowning deaths related to gender and race. The drowning rates for adolescent males is nearly 10 times higher than those for adolescent females. The gender gap may likely be related to greater risk-taking behavior and greater alcohol use in males. Males have also reported less perception about risks associated with drowning as well as greater belief in their swimming ability than females. In 2005, as in previous years, drowning rates for black males aged 15-19 yr were nearly double those for white males of the same age. Racial differences are only partially explained by socioeconomic status; other cultural factors contribute. Black children are more likely to drown in unguarded public pools, such as those owned by motels, whereas white children are more likely to drown in residential pools. Hispanic and foreign-born children have significantly higher rates of drowning than their white counterparts. Differences in exposure to swimming lessons and experience around water may contribute to drowning risk.

Underlying Conditions

Several underlying medical conditions are associated with drowning at all ages. A number of studies have found an increased risk, up to 19-fold, in individuals with epilepsy. Drowning risk for children with seizures is greatest in bathtubs and swimming pools. Specific variants of long QT syndrome are associated with drowning; other causes of ventricular arrhythmias, including myocarditis, have been found in some children who die suddenly in the water (Chapters 429 and 430).

Drowning may also be an intentional injury. A history of the event that changes or is inconsistent with the child's developmental stage is the key to recognition of intentional drowning. Physical examination and other physical injuries rarely provide clues. Child abuse is more often recognized in bathtub-related drownings. Suicide usually occurs in lone swimmers in open water.

Alcohol Use

The use of alcohol and drugs greatly increases the risk of drowning. Thirty percent to 40% of teenagers and adults who die have positive blood alcohol levels. Alcohol can impair judgment, leading to riskier behavior, decreased balance and coordination, and blunted response when someone is in trouble. Furthermore, an intoxicated adult may provide less effective supervision of children around water.

Sports and Recreation

The importance of drowning during sports and recreational boating activities is increasingly being recognized. Although the majority of sudden deaths during sports are due to cardiac events, drowning is the leading cause of noncardiac deaths. Surveys confirm that alcohol use is common during water recreation, as is not using a personal flotation device (PFD) during boating activities. Drowning mortalities are significantly increased in people on vacation, probably because of the preceding factors as well as greater participation in risky activities than at home.

Global Impact of Drowning

The World Health Organization (WHO) estimates that 388,000 people died from drowning in 2004. Of these, 175,000 were younger than 20 yr. Deaths in low-income and middle-income countries accounted for the vast majority of these cases (98%). In these countries, drowning surpasses motor vehicle injury as the major cause of injury death. Given the relative size of the pediatric population in many of these countries, drowning is one of the leading causes of death globally. These data exclude any cases of drowning due to intentional harm or assault, accidents of watercraft or water transport, and drowning related to forces of nature/cataclysmic storms, which usually claim large numbers of lives per incident.

Some patterns of pediatric drowning are similar in all countries. By most accounts, the highest rates are seen in males and in children 1-4 yr old.

Whereas bathtubs and places of recreation (i.e., pools, spas) are significant locations for drowning in U.S. children, these are virtually unreported locations for drownings in developing countries. Instead, the predominant locations are near or around the home, involving bodies of water used for activities of daily living. These include water-collecting systems, ponds, ditches, creeks, and watering holes. In tropical areas, death rates increase during monsoon season, when ditches and holes rapidly fill with rain, and are highest during daylight hours, when caregivers are busy with daily chores.

Drowning during natural disasters such as storms and floods is important in all areas of the world. The largest numbers of flood-related deaths occur in developing nations, and most of these are due to drowning during the storm surge. In the USA and much of Europe, advances in weather monitoring and warning systems have reduced such deaths. Analyses of the largest and most recent flooding incidents, including Hurricane Katrina, showed that drowning caused the most deaths, particularly when people became trapped in their vehicles or attempted to rescue others.

PATHOPHYSIOLOGY

Drowning victims drown silently and do not signal distress or call for help. Vocalization is precluded by efforts to achieve maximal lung volume or keep the head above the water, or by aspiration leading to laryngospasm. Young children can struggle for only 10-20 sec before being finally submerged. A swimmer in distress is vertical in the water, pumping the arms up and down. This splashing or efforts to breathe are often misconstrued by nearby persons as merely "playing" in the water until the victim sinks.

Once submersion occurs, all organs and tissues are at risk for hypoxia. In minutes, hypoxia leads to coma and then cardiac arrest, adding ischemia to the succession of events. Global hypoxia is the injury of drowning, with the severity of injury dependent primarily on its duration.

Anoxic-Ischemic Injury

After experimental submersion, a conscious animal initially panics, trying to surface. During this stage, small amounts of water enter the hypopharynx, triggering laryngospasm. There is a progressive decrease in arterial blood oxygen saturation (Sa_{O_2}), and the animal soon loses consciousness from hypoxia. Profound hypoxia and medullary depression lead to terminal apnea. At the same time, the cardiovascular response leads to progressively decreasing cardiac output and oxygen delivery. By 3-4 min, the circulation abruptly fails because of myocardial hypoxia. Ineffective cardiac contractions with electrical activity may occur briefly, but there is no effective perfusion (pulseless electrical activity). Some drowning victims have a primary cardiac arrest secondary to a variant of an inherited prolonged QT syndrome. With early initiation of CPR, spontaneous circulation may initially be successfully restored. The extent of the global hypoxic-ischemic injury becomes more evident over subsequent hours.

With modern intensive care, the cardiorespiratory effects of resuscitated drowning victims are usually manageable and are less often the cause of death than irreversible hypoxic-ischemic central nervous system (CNS) injury (Chapter 63). CNS injury is the most common cause of mortality and long-term morbidity. Although the duration of anoxia before irreversible CNS injury begins is uncertain, it is probably on the order of 3-5 min. Victims with reported submersions of less than 5 min survive and appear normal at hospital discharge.

Several hours after cardiopulmonary arrest, cerebral edema may occur, although the mechanism is not entirely clear. Severe cerebral edema can elevate intracranial pressure (ICP), contributing to further ischemia; intracranial hypertension is an ominous sign of profound CNS damage.

All other organs and tissues may exhibit signs of hypoxic-ischemic injury. In the lung, damage to the pulmonary vascular endothelium can lead to acute respiratory distress syndrome (ARDS; Chapter 65). Aspiration may also compound pulmonary injury. Myocardial dysfunction (so-called stunning), arterial hypotension, decreased cardiac output, arrhythmias, and cardiac infarction may also occur. Acute tubular necrosis, cortical necrosis, and renal failure are common complications of major hypoxic-ischemic events (Chapter 529). Vascular endothelial injury may initiate disseminated intravascular coagulation (DIC), hemolysis, and thrombocytopenia. Many factors contribute to gastrointestinal damage; bloody diarrhea with mucosal sloughing may be seen and often portends a fatal injury. Serum levels of hepatic transaminases and pancreatic enzymes are often acutely increased. Violation of normal mucosal protective barriers predisposes the victim to bacteremia and sepsis.

Pulmonary Injury

Pulmonary aspiration (Chapter 65) occurs in a majority of drowning victims, but the amount aspirated is usually small. Aspirated water does not obstruct airways and is readily moved into the pulmonary circulation with positive pressure ventilation. It can wash out surfactant and cause alveolar instability, ventilation-perfusion mismatch, and intrapulmonary shunting. In humans, aspiration of small amounts (1-3 mL/kg) can lead to marked hypoxemia and a 10-40% reduction in lung compliance. The composition of aspirated material can affect the patient's clinical course: Gastric contents, pathogenic organisms, toxic chemicals, and other foreign matter can injure the lung or cause airway obstruction. Clinical management is not significantly different in saltwater and freshwater aspirations, because most victims do not aspirate enough fluid volume to make a clinical difference. A few children may have massive aspiration, increasing the likelihood of severe pulmonary dysfunction.

Hypothermia

Hypothermia (Chapter 69) is common after submersion. It is often categorized, according to core body temperature measurement, as mild (34-36°C), moderate (30-34°C), or severe (<30°C). Drowning should be differentiated from **cold water immersion** injury, in which the victim remains afloat, keeping the head above water without respiratory impairment. The definition of cold water varies from 60 to 70°F.

Heat loss through conduction and convection is more efficient in water than in air and, if the water is cool, cannot be matched by the body's thermogenic mechanisms (shivering and nonshivering thermogenesis, vasoconstriction, active movements). Children are at increased risk for hypothermia because they have a relatively high ratio of body surface area to mass, decreased subcutaneous fat, and limited thermogenic capacity. Hypothermia can develop as a result of prolonged surface contact with cold water while the head is above water (immersion) or after submersion, which involves the potential additional impact of swallowing or aspirating large quantities of very cold fluid. Hypothermia may develop more quickly with immersion in fast-flowing water as a result of increased convection.

Depending on water and air temperature, insulation, body surface area, thermogenic capacity, and physical condition, heat loss can lead to significant core temperature decreases. As core temperature drops to <35°C, cognition, coordination, and muscle strength become progressively impaired. The likelihood of self-rescue decreases at this point. With progressive hypothermia, there may be loss of consciousness, water aspiration, decreases in heart rate and cardiac output, ineffective breathing, and cardiac arrest.

Immediate effects of cold water immersion are respiratory and cardiovascular. Victims who drown in water <60-70°F also experience **cold water shock**, a dynamic series of cardiorespiratory physiologic responses. In human adults, immersion in icy water results in intense involuntary reflex hyperventilation and to a decrease in breath-holding ability to <10 seconds, which leads to fluid aspiration, contributing to more rapid and deep hypothermia. Severe bradycardia occurs in adults but is transient and rapidly followed by supraventricular and ectopic tachycardias and hypertension. There is no evidence that the diving reflex, or bradycardia that may occur in children after submersion, has any protective effect.

It may theoretically be possible for the brain to rapidly cool to a neuroprotective level, if the water is cold enough, the cooling process is quick, and cardiac output lasts long enough for sufficient heat exchange to occur. Once submersion-associated hypoxia, apnea, and cardiovascular compromise decrease blood circulation, the effect of hypothermia's neuroprotection is mitigated.

After the child is removed from the water, body temperature may continue to fall as a result of cold air, wet clothes, hypoxia, and hospital transport. Hypothermia in pediatric drowning victims is observed even after drowning in relatively warm water and in warm climates. Unrecognized progressive hypothermia can lead to further decompensation. In hypothermic victims, compensatory mechanisms usually attempt to restore normothermia at body temperatures >32°C; at lower temperatures, thermoregulation may fail and spontaneous rewarming will not occur.

With moderate to severe hypothermia, progressive bradycardia, impaired myocardial contractility, and loss of vasomotor tone contribute to inadequate perfusion, hypotension, and possible shock. At body temperature <28°C, extreme bradycardia is usually present, and the propensity for spontaneous ventricular fibrillation (VF) or asystole is high. Central respiratory center depression with moderate to severe hypothermia results in hypoventilation and eventual apnea. A deep coma, with fixed and dilated pupils and absence of reflexes at very low body temperatures (<25-29°C), may give the false appearance of death.

The theoretical benefits, implications, and consequences of hypothermia in drowning victims are areas of controversy. Known adverse effects are associated with hypothermia, and these must be balanced against the potential benefits observed in experimental data. One should clearly differentiate among: (1) controlled hypothermia, such as that used in the operating room before the onset of hypoxia or ischemia, (2) accidental hypothermia, such as occurs in drowning, which is uncontrolled and variable, with onset during or shortly after hypoxia-ischemia, and (3) therapeutic hypothermia, involving the purposeful and controlled lowering and maintenance of body (or brain) temperature at some time after a hypoxic-ischemic event.

In drowning victims with uncontrolled accidental hypothermia associated with icy water submersion, there are a few case reports of good neurologic recovery after prolonged (10-150 min) cardiopulmonary arrest. Almost all of these rare survivors have been in freezing water (<5°C) and had core body temperatures <30°C, often much lower. Presumably, very rapid and sufficiently deep hypothermia developed in these fortunate survivors before irreversible hypoxic-ischemic injury occurred.

Most often hypothermia is a poor prognostic sign, and a neuroprotective effect has not been demonstrated. In King County, Washington, where the water is cold but rarely icy, 92% of drowning survivors with good neurologic outcomes had initial body temperatures ≥34°C, whereas 61% of those who died or had severe neurologic injury had temperatures <34°C. In another study of comatose drowning patients admitted to pediatric intensive care units (PICUs), 65% of hypothermic patients (body temperature <35°C) died, compared with a 27% observed mortality rate in nonhypothermic victims. Similarly, in Finland (where the median water temperature was 16°C), a beneficial effect of hypothermia is not seen in pediatric submersion victims; submersion duration <10 min was most strongly related to good outcome.

MANAGEMENT

The clinical course and outcome for a submersion victim are primarily determined by the circumstances of the incident, the duration of submersion, the speed of the rescue, and the effectiveness of resuscitative efforts. Two groups may be identified on the basis of responsiveness at the scene. The first group consists of children who require minimal resuscitation at the scene and quickly regain spontaneous respiration and consciousness. They have good outcomes and minimal complications. These victims should be transported from the scene to the ED for further evaluation.

The second group comprises children in cardiac arrest who require aggressive or prolonged resuscitation and have a high risk of multiorgan system complications, major neurologic morbidity, or death. Compared with cardiac arrest from other causes, cardiac arrest from drowning has a higher survival rate.

Initial management of drowning victims requires coordinated and experienced prehospital care following the ABCs of emergency resuscitation (Chapter 62). These children often remain comatose and lack brainstem reflexes despite the restoration of oxygenation and circulation. Subsequent ED and PICU care often involve advanced life support strategies and management of multiorgan dysfunction.

Initial Evaluation and Resuscitation

(See Chapter 62.)

Once a submersion has occurred, immediate institution of CPR efforts at the scene is imperative. The goal is to reverse the anoxia from submersion and prevent secondary hypoxic injury after submersion. Every minute that passes without the reestablishment of adequate breathing and circulation dramatically decreases the possibility of a good outcome. When safe for the victim and the rescuer, institution of in-water resuscitation for nonbreathing victims by trained personnel may improve the likelihood of survival. Victims usually need to be extricated from the water as quickly as possible so that effective CPR can be provided. Common themes in children who have good recovery are a short duration of event and initiation of CPR as soon as possible, prior to arrival of emergency medical services (EMS).

Initial resuscitation must focus on rapidly restoring oxygenation, ventilation, and adequate circulation. The airway should be clear of vomitus and foreign material, which may cause obstruction or aspiration. **Abdominal thrusts should not be used** for fluid removal, because many victims have a distended abdomen from swallowed water; abdominal thrusts may increase the risk of regurgitation and aspiration. In cases of suspected airway foreign body, chest compressions or back blows are preferable maneuvers.

The cervical spine should be protected in anyone with potential traumatic neck injury (Chapters 63 and 66). Cervical spine injury is a rare concomitant injury in drowning; only approximately 0.5% of submersion victims have cervical spine injuries. History of the event and victim age guide suspicion of cervical spine injury. Drowning victims with cervical spine injury are usually preteens or teenagers whose drowning event involved diving, a motorized vehicle crash, a fall from a height, a water sport accident, child abuse, or other clinical signs of serious traumatic injury. In such cases, the neck should be maintained in a neutral position and protected with a well-fitting cervical collar. Patients rescued from unknown circumstances may also warrant cervical spine precautions. In low-impact submersions, spinal injuries are exceedingly rare, and routine spinal immobilization is not warranted.

If the victim has ineffective respiration or apnea, ventilatory support must be initiated immediately (Chapter 62). Mouth-to-mouth or mouth-to-nose breathing by trained bystanders often restores spontaneous ventilation. As soon as it is available, supplemental oxygen should be administered to all victims. Positive pressure bag-mask ventilation with 100% inspired oxygen should be instituted in patients with respiratory insufficiency. If apnea, cyanosis, hypoventilation, or labored respiration persists, trained personnel should perform endotracheal tube (ET) intubation as soon as possible. Intubation is also indicated to protect the airway in patients with depressed mental status or hemodynamic instability. Hypoxia must be corrected rapidly to optimize the chance of recovery.

Concurrent with securing of airway control, oxygenation, and ventilation, the child's cardiovascular status must be evaluated and treated according to the usual resuscitation guidelines and protocols. Heart rate and rhythm, blood pressure, temperature, and end-organ perfusion require urgent assessment. CPR should be instituted immediately in pulseless, bradycardic, or severely hypotensive victims. Continuous monitoring of the electrocardiogram (ECG) allows appropriate diagnosis and treatment of arrhythmias. Slow capillary refill, cool extremities, and altered mental status are potential indicators of shock (Chapter 64). Recognition and treatment of hypothermia are the unique aspects of cardiac resuscitation in the drowning victim. Core temperature must be evaluated, especially in children, because moderate to severe hypothermia can depress myocardial function and cause arrhythmias.

Often, IV fluids and cardioactive medications are required to improve circulation and perfusion. Vascular access should be established as quickly as possible for the administration of fluids or pressors. Intraosseous catheter placement is a potentially lifesaving vascular access technique that avoids the delay usually associated with multiple attempts to establish intravenous (IV) access in critically ill children. Epinephrine is usually the initial drug of choice in victims with cardiopulmonary arrest (the IV dose is 0.01 mg/kg of 1:10,000 solution given q3-5min as needed). Epinephrine can be given intratracheally (ET dose is 0.1-0.2 mg/kg of 1:1,000 solution) if no IV access is available. An intravascular bolus of lactated Ringer solution or 0.9% normal saline (10-20 mL/kg) is often used to augment preload; repeated doses may be necessary. Hypotonic or glucose-containing solutions should not be used for intravascular volume administration of drowning victims.

Hospital-Based Evaluation and Treatment

Pediatric drowning victims probably should be observed for at least 6-8 hr, even if they are asymptomatic on presentation to the ED. At a minimum, serial monitoring of vital signs (respiratory rate, heart rate, blood pressure, and temperature) and of oxygenation by pulse oximetry, repeated pulmonary examination, and neurologic assessment should be performed in all drowning victims. Other studies may also be warranted, depending on the specific circumstances (possible abuse or neglect, traumatic injuries, or suspected intoxication). Almost half of asymptomatic or minimally symptomatic alert children (those who do not require advanced life support in the prehospital setting or who have an initial ED Glasgow Coma Scale [GCS] score of ≥13) experience some level of respiratory distress or hypoxemia progressing to pulmonary edema, usually during the 1st 4-8 hr after submersion. Most alert children with early respiratory symptoms respond to oxygen and, despite abnormal initial radiographs, become asymptomatic with a return of normal room air SaO_2 and pulmonary examination by 4-6 hr. Subsequent delayed respiratory deterioration is extremely unlikely in such children. Selected low-risk patients who are alert and asymptomatic with normal physical findings and oxygenation levels may be considered for discharge after 6-8 hr of observation, as long as appropriate follow-up can be ensured.

Cardiorespiratory Management

For children who are not in cardiac arrest, the level of respiratory support should be appropriate to the patient's condition and is a continuation of prehospital management. Frequent assessments are required to ensure that adequate oxygenation, ventilation, and airway control are maintained (Chapter 65). *Hypercapnia should generally be avoided in potentially brain-injured children.* Patients with actual or potential hypoventilation or markedly elevated work of breathing should receive mechanical ventilation to avoid hypercapnia and decrease the energy expenditures of labored respiration.

Measures to stabilize cardiovascular status should also continue. Conditions contributing to myocardial insufficiency include hypoxic-ischemic injury, ongoing hypoxia, hypothermia, acidosis, high airway pressures during mechanical ventilation, alterations of intravascular volume, and electrolyte disorders. Heart failure, shock, arrhythmias, or cardiac arrest may occur. Continuous ECG monitoring is mandatory for recognition and treatment of arrhythmias (Chapter 429).

The provision of adequate oxygenation and ventilation is a prerequisite to improving myocardial function. Fluid resuscitation and inotropic agents are often necessary to improve heart function and restore tissue perfusion (Chapter 62). Increasing preload with IV fluids may be beneficial through improvements in stroke volume and cardiac output. Overzealous fluid administration, especially in the presence of poor myocardial function, can worsen pulmonary edema.

For patients with persistent cardiopulmonary arrest on arrival in the ED after *non–icy water* drowning, the decision to withhold or stop resuscitative efforts can be addressed by review of the history and the response to treatment. Death or severe neurologic sequelae are quite likely in patients with deep coma, apnea, absence of papillary responses, and hyperglycemia in the ED, with submersion durations >10 min, and with failure of response to CPR given for 25 min. In one comprehensive case series, 100% of children with *resuscitation durations* >25 min either died or had severe neurologic morbidity, and all victims with *submersion durations* >25 min died. Because there are reports of good outcome following ongoing CPR in the ED, most drowning victims should be treated aggressively upon presentation. However, for children who do not show ready response to aggressive resuscitative efforts, the need for prolonged ongoing CPR after non–icy water submersion almost invariably predicts death or persistent vegetative state. Consequently, in most cases, discontinuation of CPR in the ED is probably warranted for victims of non–icy water submersion who do not respond to aggressive advanced life support within 25-30 min. Final decisions regarding whether and when to discontinue resuscitative efforts must be individualized, with the understanding that the possibility of good outcome is generally very low with protracted resuscitation efforts.

Neurologic Management

Drowning victims who present to the hospital awake and alert usually have normal neurologic outcomes. In comatose victims, irreversible CNS injury is highly likely. The most critical and effective neurologic intensive care measures after drowning are rapid restoration and maintenance of adequate oxygenation, ventilation, and perfusion. Core body temperature and glucose management may also be important modulators of neurologic injury after hypoxia-ischemia.

Comatose drowning patients are at risk for intracranial hypertension. Although ICP monitoring and therapy to reduce intracranial hypertension would seem likely to preserve cerebral perfusion and prevent herniation, there is little evidence that these measures improve outcomes for drowning victims. Patients with elevated ICP usually have poor outcomes—either death or persistent vegetative state—regardless of ICP management. Children with normal ICP can also have poor outcomes, although less frequently. Conventional neurologic intensive care therapies, such as fluid restriction, hyperventilation, and administration of muscle relaxants, osmotic agents, diuretics, barbiturates, and steroids, have not been shown to benefit the drowning victim, either individually or in combination. Indeed, there is some evidence that these therapies may reduce overall mortality, but only by increasing the number of survivors with severe neurologic morbidity.

Electroencephalographic monitoring has only limited value in the management of drowning victims and is generally not recommended, except to detect seizures or as an adjunct in the clinical evaluation of brain death (Chapter 63). Seizures should be treated if possible, although they tend to be very refractory. There is no evidence that treatment of seizures after drowning improves outcome. Fosphenytoin or phenytoin (loading dose of 10-20 mg of phenytoin equivalents [PE]/kg, followed by maintenance dosing with 5-8 mg of PE/kg/day in 2-3 divided doses; levels should be monitored) may be considered as an anticonvulsant; it may have some neuroprotective effects and may mitigate neurogenic pulmonary edema. Benzodiazepines, barbiturates, and other anticonvulsants may also have some role in seizure therapy.

With optimal management, many initially comatose children can have impressive neurologic improvement, but usually do so within the 1st 24-72 hr. Unfortunately, almost half of deeply comatose drowning victims admitted to the PICU die of their hypoxic brain injury or survive with severe neurologic damage. Many children become brain dead. Deeply comatose drowning victims who do not show substantial improvement on neurologic examination after 24-72 hr and whose coma cannot be otherwise explained should be seriously considered for limitation or withdrawal of support.

Other Management Issues

A few drowning victims may have traumatic injury (Chapter 66), especially if they were participating in water sports involving personal watercraft, boating, diving, or surfing. A high index of suspicion for such injury is required. Spinal precautions should be maintained in victims with altered mental status and suspected traumatic injury. Significant anemia suggests trauma and internal hemorrhage.

Hypoxic-ischemic injury can have multiple systemic effects, although protracted organ dysfunction is uncommon in the absence of severe CNS injury. Hyperglycemia is associated with a poor outcome in pediatric drowning victims. Its etiology is unclear but it is possibly a stress response.

Manifestations of acute renal failure may be seen after hypoxic-ischemic injury (Chapter 529). Diuretics, fluid restriction, and dialysis are occasionally needed to treat fluid overload or electrolyte disturbances; renal function usually normalizes in survivors. Rhabdomyolysis after drowning has been reported.

Profuse bloody diarrhea and mucosal sloughing usually portend a grim prognosis; conservative management includes bowel rest, nasogastric suction, and gastric pH neutralization. Nutritional support for most drowning victims is usually not difficult, because the majority of children either die or recover quickly and resume a normal diet within a few days; enteral tube feeding or parenteral nutrition is occasionally indicated in children who do not recover quickly.

Almost half of drowning victims have a fever during the 1st 48 hr after submersion. Hyperthermia is usually not due to infection and resolves without antibiotics in approximately 80% of patients. Generally, prophylactic antibiotics are not recommended.

Psychiatric and psychosocial sequelae in the family of a pediatric drowning victim are common. Grief, guilt, and anger are common among family members, including siblings. Divorce rates of up to 80% within a few years of the injury have been reported, and parents often report difficulties with employment or substance abuse. Friends and family may blame the parents for the event. Professional counseling, pastoral care, or social work referral should be considered for drowning victims and their families.

Hypothermia Management

Damp clothing should be removed from all drowning victims. Attention to core body temperature starts in the field and continues during transport and in the hospital. The goal is to prevent or treat moderate or severe hypothermia. Rewarming measures are generally categorized as passive, active external, or active internal (Chapter 69). Passive rewarming measures can be applied in the prehospital or hospital setting; they include the provision of dry blankets, a warm environment, and protection from further heat loss. Rewarming measures should be instituted as soon as possible for hypothermic drowning victims who have not had a cardiac arrest.

Full CPR with chest compressions is indicated for hypothermic victims if no pulse can be found or if narrow complex QRS activity is absent on ECG (Chapters 62 and 69). When core body temperature is <30°C, resuscitative efforts should proceed according to the current American Heart Association guidelines for CPR, but IV medications may be given at a lower frequency in moderate hypothermia because of decreased drug clearance. When VF is present in severely hypothermic victims (core temperature <30°C), up to 3 defibrillation attempts should initially be delivered, but further defibrillation attempts should be held until the core temperature is ≥30°C, at which time successful defibrillation may be more likely.

There is significant controversy regarding the discontinuation of prolonged resuscitative efforts in hypothermic drowning victims. Body temperature should be taken into account before resuscitative efforts are terminated. Other considerations include whether the water was icy or the cooling was very rapid with fast-flowing cold water. Victims with profound hypothermia may appear clinically dead, but full neurologic recovery is possible, although rare. Attempts at lifesaving resuscitation should not be withheld on the basis of initial clinical presentation unless the victim is obviously dead (dependent lividity or rigor mortis). Rewarming efforts should usually be continued until the temperature is 32-34°C; if the victim continues to have no effective cardiac rhythm and remains unresponsive to aggressive CPR, then resuscitative efforts may be discontinued.

Complete rewarming is not indicated for all arrest victims before resuscitative efforts are abandoned. Discontinuing resuscitation in victims of non–icy water submersion who remain asystolic despite 30 minutes of CPR is probably warranted. Physicians must use their individual clinical judgment about deciding to stop resuscitative efforts, taking into account the unique circumstances of each incident, including evaluation of the rapidity with which cooling occurred.

Once a drowning victim has undergone successful CPR after a cardiac arrest, temperature management should be carefully considered, and body temperature should be continuously monitored. In victims in whom resuscitation duration was brief and who are awake soon after resuscitation, attempts to restore and maintain normothermia are warranted. Careful monitoring is necessary to prevent unrecognized worsening hypothermia, which can have untoward consequences.

Victims in whom resuscitation duration has been longer are more likely to remain comatose; temperature management in these individuals is an area of controversy. Fever commonly develops within the 1st 24-48 hr of drowning. *There is general consensus that fever or hyperthermia (core body temperature >37.5°C) in comatose drowning victims resuscitated from cardiac arrest should be prevented at all times in the acute recovery period (at least the 1st 24-48 hr).* Hyperthermia after drowning or other types of brain injury may increase the risk of mortality and exacerbate hypoxic-ischemic CNS damage.

For drowning victims who remain comatose after successful CPR, more contentious issues include: (1) rewarming of hypothermic victims and (2) controlled application of therapeutic hypothermia. There are no human trials indicating that hypothermia improves the outcome of drowning patients.

Although there is no consensus of opinion, many investigators now cautiously recommend that hypothermic drowning victims who remain unresponsive because of hypoxic-ischemic encephalopathy after restoration of adequate spontaneous circulation should not be actively rewarmed to normal body temperatures. Active rewarming should be limited to victims with core body temperatures <32°C, but temperatures 32-37.5°C should be allowed without further rewarming efforts.

More controversial is the induction of therapeutic hypothermia in drowning victims who remain comatose because of hypoxic-ischemic encephalopathy after CPR for cardiac arrest. The 2002 World Congress on Drowning recommended that hypothermia (32-34°C) be instituted as soon as possible after resuscitation and sustained for 12-24 hr. These patients should be intubated, mechanically ventilated, and treated with sedatives and/or analgesics (with or without neuromuscular blocking agents) as necessary to prevent shivering and maintain hypothermia. Rewarming after this period should be very gradual.

A specific recommendation for therapeutic hypothermia, especially in children, is not yet generally accepted. The Advanced Life Support Task Force of the International Liaison Committee on Resuscitation (2002) did not recommend therapeutic hypothermia in children resuscitated after cardiopulmonary arrest, citing insufficient evidence and older studies demonstrating a potential deleterious effect in pediatric drowning victims.

PROGNOSIS

The outcomes for drowning victims are remarkably bimodal: The great majority of victims either have a good outcome (intact or mild neurologic injury) or a bad outcome (persistent vegetative state or death), with very few exhibiting intermediate neurologic injury. Of hospitalized pediatric drowning victims, 15% die and as many as 20% survive with severe permanent neurologic damage.

Intact survival or mild neurologic impairment has been seen in 91% of children with submersion duration <5 min and in 87% with resuscitation duration <10 min. Children with normal sinus rhythm, reactive pupils, or neurologic responsiveness at the scene virtually always had good outcomes (99%). For cases requiring advanced CPR, death or severe neurologic morbidity occurred in 93% of patients with submersion duration >10 min and in 100% of victims requiring resuscitation for >25 min. In one study, all victims with submersion duration >25 min died. Similarly, a Finnish study of pediatric drowning showed submersion duration was the best predictor of outcome and water temperature was not. However, there are rare case reports of intact recovery following non–icy water drowning with longer submersion or resuscitation duration. Other studies have looked at factors such as ambulance response time, serum potassium level, gender, rate of rewarming, and initial ECG rhythm. In small numbers of patients, these factors appear to have an association with outcome, but the data are not conclusive, highlighting the difficulty in assigning absolute prognostic classifications the basis of prehospital and ED variables alone.

The GCS score has some limited utility in predicting recovery. Children with a score ≥6 on hospital admission generally have a good outcome, whereas those with a score ≤5 have a much higher probability of poor neurologic outcome. Occasionally, children with a GCS score of 3 or 4 in the ED have complete recovery. Improvement in the GCS score during the first several hours of hospitalization may indicate a better prognosis. Overall, early GCS assessments fail to adequately distinguish children who will survive intact from those with major neurologic injury.

Neurologic examination and progression during the 1st 24-72 hr are currently the best prognosticators of long-term CNS outcome. Children who regain consciousness within 48-72 hr, even after prolonged resuscitation, are unlikely to have serious neurologic sequelae. In a small series of comatose victims of non–icy water submersion, all survivors with a good outcome had spontaneous purposeful movements and normal brainstem function within 24 hr; good recovery did not occur in any child with abnormal brainstem function or absence of purposeful movements at 24 hr. In another small series of drowning victims who remained unconscious >24 hr and survived for at least 1yr, 73% remained in a persistent vegetative state and the rest had severe neurologic impairment. These victims continued to have many complications and a high mortality rate: 45% died during the study's 1-yr follow-up period.

The prognostic value of neurologic responsiveness during the 1st 48-72 hr of hospitalization was also observed in a larger retrospective series of 274 pediatric drowning victims. Of the victims who had an initial GCS score of 3 in the ED, only 14% survived intact. Overall, 67.5% survived intact. Of these, 95% demonstrated purposeful neurologic function within 48 hr. Patients with a documented first purposeful neurologic response within 6 hr all survived intact. Conversely, in only 5.6% of children with poor outcomes (persistent vegetative state or death) was "purposeful" movement documented in the 1st 48 hr. Laboratory and technologic methods to improve prognostication have not yet proved superior to neurologic examination.

Early prognostic certainty in drowning can often be elusive. Serial neurologic evaluations after CPR should be performed over the ensuing 48-72 hr, with consideration given to limitation or withdrawal of support in patients who do not have significant neurologic recovery, even though this may occur before absolute prognostic certainty is achieved.

PREVENTION

The most effective way to decrease the injury burden of drowning is prevention. Drowning is a multifaceted problem, but several preventive strategies are effective. The pediatrician has a prime opportunity to identify and inform families at risk through anticipatory guidance.

A family-centered approach to anticipatory guidance for water safety is to explore and identify the water hazards that each family is exposed to in their environment, with water-related activities, and because of the developmental stage of their child. The practitioner can then discuss the best tools and strategies for prevention that are relevant for the particular family. It is important to identify the risks both in and around the home and in other locations they may frequent, often when vacationing, such as vacation or relatives' homes. For some families the focus may be on bathtubs and bucket safety; for others, home pools or hot tubs may be the major hazards. If the family recreates near or on open water, they also need to learn about safety around boats and open water. In a rural environment, water collection systems and natural bodies of water may pose great risk.

Parents must build layers of water protection around their children. Table 67-1 provides an approach to the hazards and preventive strategies relevant to the most common sources of water involved in childhood drowning. A common preventive strategy for exposure to all water types and all ages is ensuring appropriate supervision. Pediatricians should define for parents what constitutes appropriate supervision at the various developmental levels of childhood. Many parents either underestimate the importance of adequate supervision or are simply unaware of the risks associated with water. Even parents who say that constant supervision is necessary will often admit to brief lapses while their child is alone near water. Parents also overestimate the abilities of older siblings; many bathtub drownings occur when an infant or toddler is left with a child younger than 5 yr.

Supervision of infants and young children means that a responsible adult should be with the child every moment. The caregiver

Table 67-1 APPROACH TO DROWNING-PREVENTION STRATEGIES

	HOME	RECREATION	NEIGHBORHOOD
Water hazards	Swimming pools Ponds Bathtubs Large buckets	Open water swimming or other activities Boating	Irrigation ditches Watering holes Water drainage
Common risks	Lapse in supervision Unexpected toddler exposure Delayed discovery of child Reliance on water wings or pool toys Reliance on sibling or bath seat for bathing supervision	Lapse in supervision Change in weather Unfamiliarity with or change(s) in water conditions: • Steep drop-off • Current/tide • Low temperature Alcohol use Peer pressure	Lapse in supervision, particularly when caregiver is involved with daily chores Risky behavior when with peers
Prevention strategies	Educate families on hazards and risks Provide constant adult supervision of infants and small children Install isolation fencing of pools Install rescue equipment and phone at poolside Learn swimming and water survival skills Individuals with epilepsy should shower and avoid bathtubs Learn first aid and CPR	Provide constant adult supervision Swim in lifeguarded areas Wear U.S. Coast Guard–approved personal flotation devices Avoid alcohol and other drugs Learn swimming and water survival skills Teach children about water safety Recognize limitations of swimming ability Be aware of current weather and water conditions Learn first aid and CPR	Provide constant adult supervision Fence, cover, or fill in ditches to prevent access to water Provide fenced-in "safe area" for children to play

CPR, cardiopulmonary resuscitation.

must be alert, must not be consuming alcohol or other drugs, and must be attentive and focused entirely on watching the child. Even a brief moment of inattention, such as to answer a phone, get a drink, or hold a conversation, can have tragic consequences. If the child does not swim, "touch supervision" is required, meaning that the caregiver should be within arm's reach at all times. Many parents believe that swimming lessons can teach infants and toddlers how to protect themselves in water. However, parents must understand that although such lessons may offer many benefits, they do not result in the need for less supervision of their children near water. Furthermore, a supervising caretaker should be aware of where and how to get help and know how to safely rescue a child in trouble. Because only those trained in water rescue can safely attempt it, families should be encouraged to swim in designated areas only when and where a lifeguard is on duty.

Learning to swim offers another layer of protection. Most children are developmentally ready to learn to swim by age 4 yr. At an earlier age, children may start swim lessons that are developmentally appropriate and aimed at the individual child's readiness and skill level. It is not clear whether lessons provide some level of protection to young children by teaching them swim skills, safer behaviors around water, or simply water awareness. It is also unclear how much risk reduction swim lessons provide. As with any other water safety intervention, parents need to know that swimming lessons and acquisition of swim skills cannot be solely relied on to prevent drowning. No child can be "drown-proof." Children and adolescents should never swim alone regardless of their swimming abilities. Even as they become more independent and participate in recreational activities without their parents, they should be encouraged to seek areas that are watched by lifeguards. It is important to emphasize that even if the child is considered a strong swimmer, the ability to swim in a pool does not translate to being safe in open water, where different water temperature, currents, and underwater obstacles can present additional and unfamiliar challenges. For swimmers, supervision by lifeguards reduces drowning risk, because lifeguards monitor risk behaviors and are trained in the difficult and potentially dangerous task of rescuing drowning victims.

Two of the preventive strategies listed in Table 67-1 deserve special mention. The most vigorously evaluated and effective drowning intervention applies to swimming pools. Isolation fencing that completely surrounds a pool, with a secure, self-locking gate, reduces the risk of drowning. Guidelines for appropriate fencing, provided by the U.S. Consumer Product Safety Commission, are very specific; they were developed through testing of active toddlers in a gymnastics program on their ability to climb barriers of different materials and heights. In families who have a pool on their property, caregivers often erroneously believe that if a child falls into the water there will be a loud noise or splash to alert them. Sadly, these events are usually silent, increasing the time until the child is discovered. This finding highlights the importance of the guideline that the fence actually separate the pool from the house, not just surround the entire property.

The use of U.S. Coast Guard–approved lifejackets or PFDs should be discussed with all families spending time around open water, not just those who consider themselves boaters. This issue is also particularly important for families who will participate in aquatic activities on a vacation. A PFD should be chosen with respect to the weight of the child and the proposed activity. Young children should wear PFDs that will float them head up. Parents should be urged to wear PFDs, too, as their use is associated with greater use by their children. Toys such as water wings and "floaties" should not be relied upon as drowning prevention measures.

Effective preventive efforts must also consider cultural practices. Different ethnic groups may have certain attitudes, beliefs, dress, or other customs that may affect their water safety. The higher drowning risk of minority children needs to be addressed by community-based prevention programs.

In addition to anticipatory guidance, pediatricians can play an active role in drowning prevention by participating in advocacy efforts to improve legislation for pool fencing, PFD use, and alcohol consumption in various water activities. Several counties in the USA, Australia, and New Zealand have laws requiring isolation fencing for pools. Their effectiveness has been limited by a lack of enforcement. Similarly, all states have boating-under-the-influence laws but, similarly, rarely enforce them. Furthermore, efforts at the community level may be needed to ensure the availability of swimming lessons for underserved populations and lifeguarded swim areas.

BIBLIOGRAPHY

Please visit the Nelson Textbook of Pediatrics *website at www.expertconsult.com for the complete bibliography.*

Chapter 68
Burn Injuries

Alia Y. Antoon and Mary K. Donovan

Burns are a leading cause of unintentional death in children, second only to motor vehicle crashes. There has been a decline in the incidence of burn injury requiring medical care over the last decade. This decline has coincided with a stronger focus on burn treatment and prevention, increased fire and burn prevention education, greater availability of regional treatment centers, widespread use of smoke detectors, greater regulation of consumer products and occupational safety, and societal changes such as reductions in smoking and alcohol abuse.

EPIDEMIOLOGY

Approximately 1.2 million people in the USA require medical care for burn injuries each year, with 51,000 requiring hospitalization. Approximately 30-40% of these patients are younger than 15 yr, with an average age of 32 mo. Fires are a major cause of mortality in children, accounting for up to 34% of fatal injuries in those younger than 16 yr. Scald burns account for 85% of total injuries and are most prevalent in children younger than 4 yr. Although the incidence of hot water scalding has been reduced by legislation requiring new water heaters to be preset at 120°F, scald injury remains the leading cause of hospitalization for burns. Steam inhalation used as a home remedy to treat respiratory infections is another potential cause of burns. Flame burns account for 13%; the remaining are electrical and chemical burns. Clothing ignition events have declined since passage of the Federal Flammable Fabric Act requiring sleepwear to be flame-retardant; however, the U.S. Consumer Product Safety Commission has voted to relax the existing children's sleepwear flammability standard. Approximately 18% of burns are the result of child abuse (usually scalds), making it important to assess the pattern and site of injury and their consistency with the patient history (Chapter 37). Friction burns from treadmills are also a problem. Hands are the most commonly injured sites, with deep 2nd-degree friction injury sometimes associated with fractures of the fingers. Anoxia, not the actual burn, is a major cause of morbidity and mortality in house fires.

Review of the history usually shows a common pattern: scald burns to the side of the face, neck, and arm if liquid is pulled from a table or stove; burns in the pant leg area if clothing ignites; burns in a splash pattern from cooking; and burns on the palm of the hand from contact with a hot stove. However, "glove or stocking" burns of the hands and feet, single-area deep burns on the trunk, buttocks, or back, and small, full-thickness burns (cigarette burns) in young children should raise the suspicion of child abuse (Chapter 37).

Burn care involves a range of activities: prevention, acute care and resuscitation, wound management, pain relief, reconstruction, rehabilitation, and psychosocial adjustment. Children with massive burns require early and appropriate psychologic and social support as well as resuscitation. Surgical debridement, wound closure, and rehabilitative efforts should be instituted concurrently to promote optimal rehabilitation. Aggressive surgical removal of devitalized tissue, infection control, and judicious use of antibiotics, as well as early nutrition and cautious use of intubation and mechanical ventilation, are necessary to maximize survival. Children who have sustained burn injuries differ in appearance from their peers, necessitating supportive efforts for reentry to school and social and sporting activities.

PREVENTION

The aim of burn prevention is a continuing reduction in the number of serious burn injuries (Table 68-1). Effective first aid and triage can decrease both the extent (area) and the severity (depth) of injuries. The use of flame-retardant clothing and smoke detectors, control of hot water temperature (thermostat settings) within buildings, and prohibition of cigarette smoking have been partially successful in reducing the incidence of burn injuries. Treatment of children with significant burn injuries in dedicated burn centers facilitates medically effective care, improves survival, and leads to greater cost efficiency. Survival of at least 80% of patients with burns of 90% of the body surface area (BSA) is possible; the overall survival rate of children with burns of all sizes is 99%. Death is more likely in children with irreversible anoxic brain injury sustained at the time of the burn.

Pediatricians can play a major role in preventing the most common burns by educating parents and health care providers. Simple, effective, efficient, and cost-effective preventive measures include the use of appropriate clothing and smoke detectors, and the planning of routes for emergency exit from the home. Child neglect and abuse must be seriously considered when the history of the injury and the distribution of the burn do not match.

ACUTE CARE, RESUSCITATION, AND ASSESSMENT

Indications for Admission

Burns covering >10-15% of total BSA, burns associated with smoke inhalation, burns resulting from high-tension (voltage) electrical injuries, and burns associated with suspected child abuse or neglect should be treated as emergencies, and the child hospitalized (Table 68-2). Small 1st- and 2nd-degree burns of the hands, feet, face, perineum, and joint surfaces also require

Table 68-1 BURN PROPHYLAXIS

PREVENT FIRES
Install and use smoke detectors
Control the hot water thermostat—in public buildings, the maximum water temperature should be 120°F
Keep fire, matches, and lighters out of the reach of children
Avoid cigarette smoking, especially in bed
Do not leave lit candles unattended
Use flame retardant–treated clothing
Use caution when cooking, especially with oil
Keep cloth items off heaters
PREVENT INJURY
Roll, but do not run, if clothing catches fire; wrap in a blanket
Practice escape procedures
Crawl beneath smoke if a fire occurs indoors
Use educational materials*

*National Fire Protection Association pamphlets and videos.

Table 68-2 INDICATIONS FOR HOSPITALIZATION FOR BURNS

Burns affecting >15% of body surface area
3rd-degree burns
Electrical burns caused by high-tension wires or lightening
Chemical burns
Inhalation injury, regardless of the amount of body surface area burned
Inadequate home or social environment
Suspected child abuse or neglect
Burns to the face, hands, feet, perineum, genitals, or major joints
Burns in patients with preexisting medical conditions that may complicate the acute recovery phase
Associated injuries (fractures)
Pregnancy

admission if close follow-up care is difficult to provide. Children who have been in enclosed-space fires and those who have face and neck burns should be hospitalized for at least 24 hr for observation for signs of central nervous system (CNS) effects of anoxia from carbon monoxide poisoning and pulmonary effects from smoke inhalation.

First Aid Measures

Acute care should include the following measures:

1. Extinguish flames by rolling the child on the ground; cover the child with a blanket, coat, or carpet.
2. After determining that the airway is patent, remove smoldering clothing or clothing saturated with hot liquid. Jewelry, particularly rings and bracelets, should be removed or cut away to prevent constriction and vascular compromise during the edema phase in the 1st 24-72 hr after burn injury.
3. In cases of chemical injury, brush off any remaining chemical, if powdered or solid; then use copious irrigation or wash the affected area with water. Call the local poison control center for the neutralizing agent to treat a chemical ingestion.
4. Cover the burned area with clean, dry sheeting and apply cold (not iced) wet compresses to small injuries. Significant large burn injury (>15-20% of BSA) decreases body temperature control and contraindicates the use of cold compresses.
5. If the burn is caused by hot tar, use mineral oil to remove the tar.
6. Administer analgesic medications.

Emergency Care

Life support measures are as follows (Table 68-3):

1. Rapidly review the cardiovascular and pulmonary status and document pre-existing or physiologic lesions (asthma, congenital heart disease, renal or hepatic disease).
2. Ensure and maintain an adequate airway and provide humidified oxygen by mask or endotracheal intubation (Fig. 68-1). The latter may be needed in children who have facial burns

Table 68-3 ACUTE TREATMENT OF BURNS

First aid, including washing of wounds and removal of devitalized tissue
Fluid resuscitation
Provision of energy requirements
Control of pain
Prevention of infection—early excision and grafting
Prevention of excessive metabolic expenditures
Control of bacterial wound flora
Use of biologic and synthetic dressings to close the wound

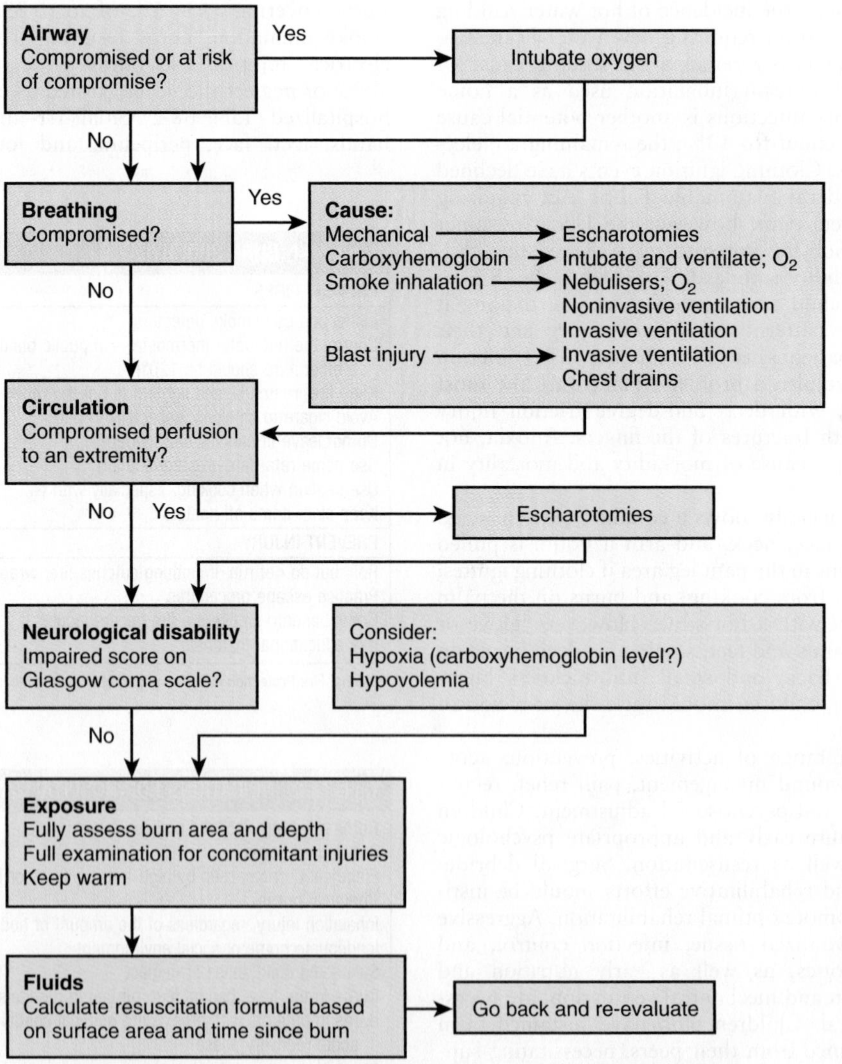

Figure 68-1 Algorithm for the primary survey of a major burn injury. O_2, oxygen. (From Hettiaratchy S, Papini R: Initial management of a major burn I: overview. *BMJ* 328:1555–1557, 2004.)

Table 68-4 CATEGORIES OF BURN DEPTH

	1ST-DEGREE BURN	2ND-DEGREE, OR PARTIAL-THICKNESS, BURN	3RD-DEGREE, OR FULL-THICKNESS, BURN
Surface appearance	Dry, no blisters Minimal or no edema Erythematous Blanches, bleeds	Moist blebs, blisters Underlying tissue is mottled pink and white, with fair capillary refill. Bleeds	Dry, leathery eschar Mixed white, waxy, khaki, mahogany, soot-stained No blanching or bleeding
Pain	Very painful	Very painful	Insensate
Histologic depth	Epidermal layers only	Epidermis, papillary, and reticular layers of dermis May include domes of subcutaneous layers	Down to and may include fat, subcutaneous tissue, fascia, muscle, and bone
Healing time	2-5 days with no scarring	Superficial: 5-21 days with no grafting Deep partial: 21-35 days with no infection; if infected, converts to full-thickness burn	Large areas require grafting, but small areas may heal from the edges after wks

or a burn sustained in an enclosed space, before facial or laryngeal edema becomes evident. If hypoxia or carbon monoxide poisoning is suspected, 100% oxygen should be used (Chapters 62 and 65).

3. Children with burns of >15% of BSA require intravenous (IV) fluid resuscitation to maintain adequate perfusion. All inhalation injuries, regardless of the extent of BSA burn, require venous access to control fluid intake. All high-tension and electrical injuries require venous access to ensure forced alkaline diuresis in case of muscle injury to avoid myoglobinuric renal damage. Lactated Ringer solution, 10-20 mL/kg/hr (normal saline may be used if lactated Ringer solution is not available), is initially infused until proper fluid replacement can be calculated. Consultation with a specialized burn unit should be made to coordinate fluid therapy, the type of fluid, the preferred formula for calculation, and preferences for the use of colloid agents, particularly if transfer to a burn center is anticipated.
4. Evaluate the child for associated injuries, which are common in patients with a history of high-tension electrical burn, especially if there has also been a fall from a height. Injuries to the spine, bones, and thoracic or intra-abdominal organs may occur (Chapter 66). Cervical spine precautions should be observed until this injury is ruled out. There is a very high risk of cardiac abnormalities, including ventricular tachycardia and ventricular fibrillation, resulting from conductivity of the high electric voltage. Cardiopulmonary resuscitation should be instituted promptly at the scene, and cardiac monitoring should be started upon the patient's arrival at the emergency department (ED) (Chapter 62).
5. Children with burns of >15% of BSA should not receive oral fluids (initially), because gastric distention may develop. These children require insertion of a nasogastric tube in the ED to prevent aspiration.
6. A Foley catheter should be inserted to monitor urine output in all children who require IV fluid resuscitation.
7. All wounds should be wrapped with sterile towels until a decision is made about whether to treat the patient on an outpatient basis or refer the patient to an appropriate facility for treatment.
8. A carbon monoxide measurement (carboxyhemoglobin [HbCO]) should be obtained for fire victims, and 100% oxygen administered until the result is known.

Classification of Burns

Proper triage and treatment of burn injury require assessment of the extent and depth of the injury (Table 68-4 and Fig. 68-2). **1st-degree burns** involve only the epidermis and are characterized by swelling, erythema, and pain (similar to mild sunburn). Tissue damage is usually minimal, and there is no blistering. Pain resolves in 48-72 hr; in a small percentage of patients, the damaged epithelium peels off, leaving no residual scars.

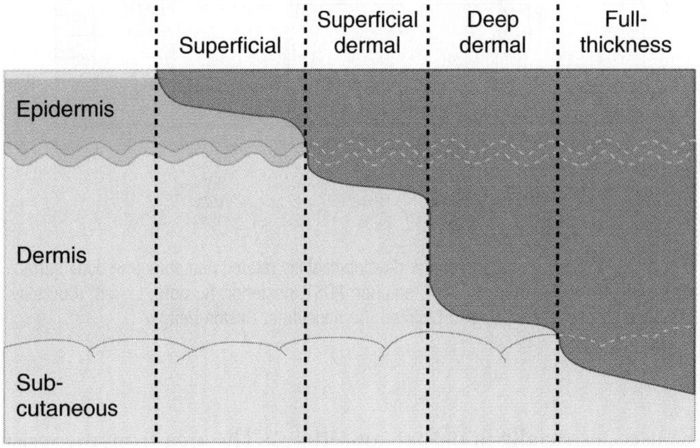

Figure 68-2 Diagram of the different burn depths. (From Hettiaratchy S, Papini R: Initial management of a major burn II: assessment and resuscitation, *BMJ* 329:101–103, 2004.)

A **2nd-degree burn** involves injury to the entire epidermis and a variable portion of the dermal layer (vesicle and blister formation are characteristic). A **superficial** 2nd-degree burn is extremely painful because a large number of remaining viable nerve endings is exposed. Superficial 2nd-degree burns heal in 7-14 days as the epithelium regenerates in the absence of infection. Midlevel to deep 2nd-degree burns also heal spontaneously if wounds are kept clean and infection-free. Pain is less than in more superficial burns because fewer nerve endings remain viable. Fluid losses and metabolic effects of deep dermal (2nd-degree) burns are essentially the same as those of 3rd-degree burns.

Full-thickness, or 3rd-degree, burns involve destruction of the entire epidermis and dermis, leaving no residual epidermal cells to repopulate the damaged area. The wound cannot epithelialize and can heal only by wound contraction or skin grafting. The absence of painful sensation and capillary filling demonstrates the loss of nerve and capillary elements.

Estimation of Body Surface Area for a Burn

Appropriate burn charts for different childhood age groups should be used to accurately estimate the extent of BSA burned. The volume of fluid needed in resuscitation is calculated from the estimation of the extent and depth of burn surface. Mortality and morbidity also depend on the extent and depth of the burn. The variable growth rate of the head and extremities throughout childhood makes it necessary to use BSA charts, such as that modified by Lund and Brower or the chart used at the Shriners Hospital for Children in Boston (Fig. 68-3). The **rule of nines** used in adults may be used only in children older than 14 yr or as a very rough estimate to institute therapy before transfer to a burn center. In small burns, <10% of BSA, the **rule of palm** may

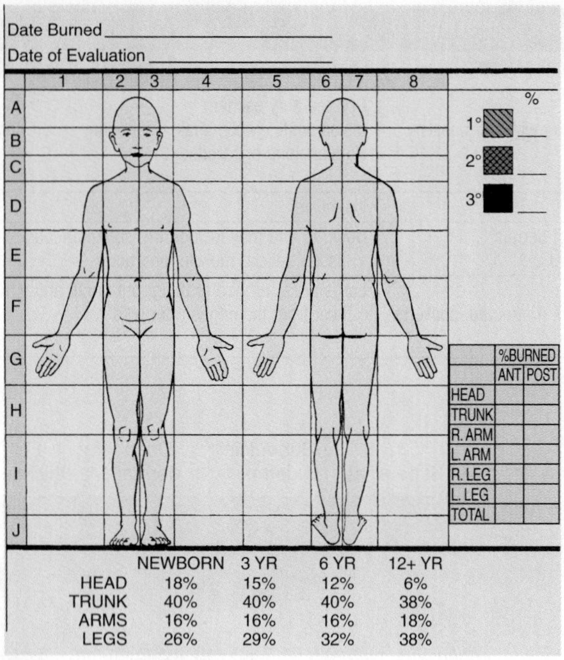

Figure 68-3 Chart to determine the developmentally related percentage of body surface area affected by a burn injury. ANT, anterior; POST, posterior; R., right; L., left. (Courtesy of Shriners Hospital for Crippled Children, Burn Institute, Boston Unit.)

be used, especially in outpatient settings: The area from the wrist crease to the finger crease (the palm) in the child equals 1% of the child's BSA.

TREATMENT

Outpatient Management of Minor Burns

A patient with 1st- and 2nd-degree burns of <10% of BSA may be treated on an outpatient basis unless family support is judged inadequate or there are issues of child neglect or abuse. These outpatients do not require a tetanus booster (unless not truly immunized) or prophylactic penicillin therapy. Blisters should be left intact and dressed with bacitracin or silver sulfadiazine cream (Silvadene). Dressings should be changed once daily, after the wound is washed with lukewarm water to remove any cream left from the previous application. Very small wounds, especially those on the face, may be treated with bacitracin ointment and left open. Debridement of the devitalized skin is indicated when the blisters rupture. A variety of wound dressings/wound membranes are available (e.g., AQUACEL Ag dressing [ConvaTec USA, Skillman, NJ] in a soft feltlike material impregnated with silver ion) may be applied to 2nd-degree burns and wrapped with a dry sterile dressing; similar wound membranes provide pain control, prevention of wound desiccation, and reduction in wound colonization (Table 68-5). These dressings are usually kept on for 7-10 days but are checked twice a week.

Burns to the palm with large blisters usually heal beneath the blisters; they should receive close follow-up on an outpatient basis. The great majority of superficial burns heal in 10-20 days. Deep 2nd-degree burns take longer to heal and may benefit from enzymatic debridement ointment application (collagenase ointment) applied daily on the wound, which aids in the removal of the dead tissue. These ointments should not be applied to the face to avoid the risk of getting them into the eyes.

The depth of scald injuries is difficult to assess early; conservative treatment is appropriate initially, with the depth of the area involved determined before grafting is attempted (Fig. 68-4).

Table 68-5 PARTIAL LISTING OF SOME COMMONLY USED WOUND MEMBRANES—SELECTED CHARACTERISTICS

MEMBRANE	CHARACTERISTIC(S)
Porcine xenograft	Adheres to coagulum Excellent pain control
Biobrane	Bilaminate Fibrovascular in growth into inner layer
Acticoat	Nonadherent dressing that delivers silver
AQUACEL-Ag	Absorptive hydro-fiber that delivers silver
Various semipermeable membranes	Provide vapor and bacterial barrier
Various hydrocolloid dressings	Provide vapor and bacterial barrier Absorb exudates
Various impregnated gauzes	Provide barrier while allowing drainage

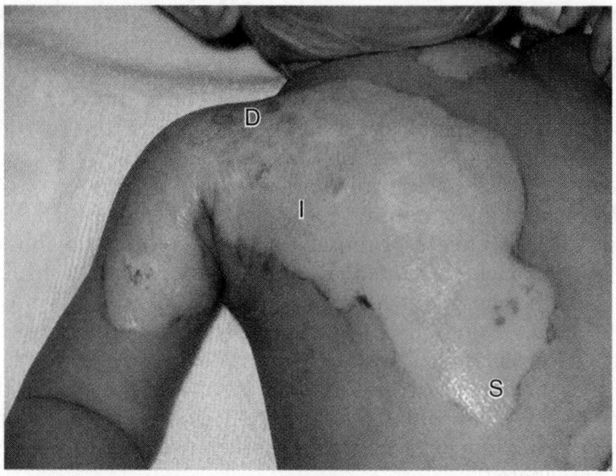

Figure 68-4 Tea scald over the chest and shoulder of a child showing heterogeneity of burn depth. D, deep; I, intermediate; S, superficial. (From Enoch S, Roshan A, Shah M: Emergency and early management of burns and scalds, *BMJ* 338:937–941, 2009.)

This approach obviates the risk of anesthesia and unnecessary grafting.

Fluid Resuscitation

For most children, the Parkland formula is an appropriate starting guideline for fluid resuscitation (4 mL lactated Ringer solution /kg/% BSA burned). Half of the fluid is given over the 1st 8 hr, calculated from the time of onset of injury; the remaining fluid is given at an even rate over the next 16 hr. The rate of infusion is adjusted according to the patient's response to therapy. Pulse and blood pressure should return to normal, and an adequate urine output (>1 mL/kg/hr in children; 0.5-10 mL/kg/hr in adolescents) should be accomplished by varying the IV infusion rate. Vital signs, acid-base balance, and mental status reflect the adequacy of resuscitation. Because of interstitial edema and sequestration of fluid in muscle cells, patients may gain up to 20% over baseline (pre-burn) body weight. Patients with burns of 30% of BSA require a large venous access (central venous line) to deliver the fluid required over the critical 1st 24 hr. Patients with burns of >60% of BSA may require a multilumen central venous catheter; these patients are best cared for in a specialized burn unit. In addition to fluid resuscitation, children should receive standard maintenance fluids (Chapter 53).

During the 2nd 24 hr after the burn, patients begin to reabsorb edema fluid and to experience diuresis. Half of the 1st day's fluid requirement is infused as lactated Ringer solution in 5% dextrose. Children younger than 5 yr may require the addition of 5% dextrose in the 1st 24 hr of resuscitation. Controversy exists as to whether colloid should be provided in the early period of burn resuscitation. One preference is to use colloid replacement concurrently if the burn is >85% of total BSA. Colloid is usually instituted 8-24 hr after the burn injury. In children younger than 12 mo, sodium tolerance is limited; the volume and sodium concentration of the resuscitation solution should be decreased if the urinary sodium level is rising. The adequacy of resuscitation should be constantly assessed by means of vital signs as well as urine output, blood gas, hematocrit, and serum protein measurements. Some patients require arterial and central venous lines, particularly those undergoing multiple excision and grafting procedures, as needed, for monitoring and replacement purposes. Central venous pressure monitoring may be indicated to assess circulation in patients with hemodynamic or cardiopulmonary instability. Femoral vein cannulation is a safe access for fluid resuscitation, especially in infants and children. Burn patients who require frequent blood gas monitoring benefit from radial or femoral arterial catheterization.

Oral supplementation may start as early as 48 hr after burn. Milk formula, artificial feedings, homogenized milk, or soy-based products can be given by bolus or constant infusion through a nasogastric or small bowel feeding tube. As oral fluids are tolerated, IV fluids are decreased proportionately in an effort to keep the total fluid intake constant, particularly if pulmonary dysfunction is present.

A 5% albumin infusion may be used to maintain the serum albumin levels at a desired 2 g/dL. The following rates are effective: For burns of 30-50% of total BSA, 0.3 mL of 5% albumin/kg/% BSA burn is infused over 24 hr; for burns of 50-70% of total BSA, 0.4 mL/kg/% BSA burn is infused over 24 hr; and for burns of 70-100% of total BSA, 0.5 mL/kg/% BSA burn is infused over 24 hr. Infusion of packed red blood cells is recommended if the hematocrit falls to <24% (hemoglobin = 8 g/dL). Some authorities recommend treatment for hematocrit <30% or hemoglobin <10 g/dL in patients with systemic infection, hemoglobinopathy, cardiopulmonary disease, or anticipated (or ongoing) blood loss, if repeated excision and grafting of full-thickness burns is needed. Fresh frozen plasma is indicated if clinical and laboratory assessment shows a deficiency of clotting factors, a prothrombin level >1.5 times control, or a partial thromboplastin time >1.2 times control in children who are bleeding or are scheduled for an invasive procedure or a grafting procedure that could result in an estimated blood loss of more than half of blood volume. Fresh frozen plasma may be used for volume resuscitation within 72 hr of injury in patients younger than 2 yr with burns over 20% of BSA and associated inhalation injury.

Sodium supplementation may be required for children with burns of >20% of BSA if 0.5% silver nitrate solution is used as the topical antibacterial burn dressing. Sodium losses with silver nitrate therapy are regularly as high as 350 mmol/m^2 burn surface area. Oral sodium chloride supplement of 4 g/m^2 burn area/24 hr is usually well tolerated, divided into 4-6 equal doses to avoid osmotic diarrhea. The aim is to maintain serum sodium levels >130 mEq/L and urinary sodium concentration >30 mEq/L. IV potassium supplementation is supplied to maintain a serum potassium level >3 mEq/dL. Potassium losses may be significantly increased when 0.5% silver nitrate solution is used as the topical antibacterial agent or when aminoglycoside, diuretic, or amphotericin therapy is required.

Prevention of Infection and Surgical Management of the Burn Wound

Controversy exists over the prophylactic use of penicillin for all patients hospitalized with acute burn injury and the periodic replacement of central venous catheters to prevent infection. In some units, a 5-day course of penicillin therapy is used for all patients with acute burns; standard-dose crystalline penicillin is given orally or intravenously in 4 divided doses. Erythromycin may be used as an alternative in penicillin-allergic children. Other units have discontinued prophylactic use of penicillin therapy without an increase in the infection rate. Similarly, there is conflicting evidence as to whether relocation of the IV catheter every 48-72 hr decreases or increases the incidence of catheter-related sepsis. Some recommend that the central venous catheter be replaced and relocated every 5-7 days, even if the site is not inflamed and there is no suspicion of catheter-related sepsis.

Mortality related to burn injury is associated not with the toxic effect of thermally injured skin, but with the metabolic and bacterial consequences of a large open wound, reduction of the patient's host resistance, and malnutrition. These abnormalities set the stage for life-threatening bacterial infection originating from the burn wound. Wound treatment and prevention of wound infection also promote early healing and improve aesthetic and functional outcomes. Topical treatment of the burn wound with 0.5% silver nitrate solution, silver sulfadiazine cream, or mafenide acetate (Sulfamylon) cream or topical solution aims at prevention of infection (Table 68-6). These 3 agents have tissue-penetrating capacity. Regardless of the choice of topical antimicrobial agent, it is essential that all 3rd-degree burn tissue be fully excised before bacterial colonization occurs and that the area be grafted as early as possible to prevent deep wound sepsis. Children with a burn of >30% of BSA should be housed in a bacteria-controlled nursing unit to prevent cross-contamination and to provide a temperature- and humidity-controlled environment to minimize hypermetabolism.

Deep 2nd-degree burns of >10% of BSA benefit from early excision and grafting. To improve outcome, sequential excision and grafting of 3rd-degree and deep 2nd-degree burns is required in children with large burns. Prompt excision with immediate wound closure is achieved with autografts, which are often meshed to increase the efficiency of coverings. Alternatives for wound closure, such as allografts, xenografts, and Integra (Integra LifeSciences) and other synthetic skin coverings (bilaminate membrane composed of a porous lattice of cross-linked chondroitin-6-sulfate engineered to induce neovascularization as it is biodegraded), may be important for wound coverage in patients with extensive injury to limit fluid, electrolyte, and protein losses and to reduce pain and minimize temperature loss. Epidermal cultured cells (autologous keratinocytes) are a costly alternative and are not always successful. An experienced burn team can safely carry out early-stage or total excision while burn fluid resuscitation continues. Important keys to success are: (1)

Table 68-6 TOPICAL AGENTS USED FOR BURNS

AGENT	EFFECTIVENESS	EASE OF USE
Silver sulfadiazine	Broad spectrum	Closed dressings
Silvadene cream	Good penetration	Changed twice daily
		Residue *must* be washed off with each dressing change
Mafenide acetate	Broad spectrum, including *Pseudomonas*	Closed dressings Changed twice daily
	Rapid and deep wound penetration	Residue *must* be washed off with each dressing changed
0.5% silver nitrate solution	Bacteriostatic	Closed bulky dressing soaked every 2 hr and changed once daily
	Broad spectrum, including some fungi	
	Superficial penetration	
AQUACEL Ag	Dressing impregnated with silver	Applied directly to 2nd-degree burn; occlusive dressing kept for 10 days
Accuzyme ointment	Topical enzymatic debridement	Applied daily

accurate preoperative and intraoperative determination of burn depth, (2) the choice of excision area and appropriate timing, (3) control of intraoperative blood loss, (4) specific instrumentation, (5) the choice and use of perioperative antibiotics, and (6) the type of wound coverage chosen. This process can accomplish early coverage without the use of recombinant human growth hormone.

Nutritional Support

Supporting the increased energy requirements of a patient with a burn is a high priority. The burn injury produces a hypermetabolic response characterized by both protein and fat catabolism. Depending on the time since the burn, children with a burn of 40% of total BSA require basal energy expenditure (oxygen consumption) approximately 50-100% higher than predicted for their age. Early excision and grafting can decrease the energy requirement. Pain, anxiety, and immobilization increase the physiologic demands. Additional energy expenditure is caused by cold stress if environmental humidity and temperature are not controlled; this is especially true in young infants, in whom the large surface area–mass ratio allows proportionately greater heat loss than in adolescents and adults. Providing environmental temperatures of 28-33°C, adequate covering during transport and liberal use of analgesics and anxiolytics can decrease calorie demands. Special units to control ambient temperature and humidity may be necessary for children with large surface area burns. Appropriate sleep intervals are necessary and should be part of the regimen. Sepsis increases metabolic rates, and early enteral nutrition, initially with high-carbohydrate, high-protein caloric support (1,800 cal/m^2/24 hr maintenance plus 2,200 cal/m^2 of burn/24 hr) reduces metabolic stress.

The objective of caloric supplementation programs is to maintain body weight and minimize weight loss by meeting metabolic demands. This reduces the loss of lean body mass. Calories are provided at approximately 1.5 times the basal metabolic rate, with 3-4 g/kg of protein/day. The focus of nutritional therapy is to support and compensate for the metabolic needs. Multivitamins, particularly the B vitamin group, vitamin C, vitamin A, and zinc, are also necessary.

Alimentation should be started as soon as is practical, both enterally and parenterally, to meet all of the caloric needs and keep the gastrointestinal tract active and intact after the resuscitative phase. Patients with burns of >40% of total BSA need a flexible nasogastric or small bowel feeding tube to facilitate continuous delivery of calories without the risk of aspiration. To decrease the risk of infectious complications, parenteral nutrition is discontinued as soon as is practical, after delivery of sufficient enteral calories is established. Continuous gastrointestinal feeding is essential, even if feeding is interrupted, causing frequent visits to the operating room, until full grafting takes place. The use of anabolic agents (growth hormone, oxandrolone, low-dose insulin) or anticatabolic agents (propranolol) remains controversial, although β-blocking agents may reduce metabolic stress. Burn centers caring for large burns (>50% BSA, 3rd-degree) in patients who might be malnourished have used the anabolic steroid oxandrolone, at a dose of 0.1 to 0.2 mg/kg/day given orally, to promote better protein synthesis while the nutritional support by nasogastric feeding and IV hyperalimentation continues.

Topical Therapy

Topical therapy is widely used and is effective against most burn pathogens (see Table 68-6). A number of topical agents are used: 0.5% silver nitrate solution, sulfacetamide acetate cream or solution, silver sulfadiazine cream, and Accuzyme ointment or AQUACEL Ag$^+$. Accuzyme is an enzymatic debridement agent and may cause a stinging feeling for 15 min after application. Preferences vary among burn units. Each topical agent has advantages and disadvantages in application, comfort, and bacteriostatic spectrum. Sulfacetamide acetate is a very effective broad-spectrum agent with the ability to diffuse through the burn eschar; it is the treatment of choice for injury to cartilaginous surfaces, such as the ears. The carbonic anhydrase inhibition activity of sulfacetamide may cause acid-base imbalance if large surface areas are treated, and adverse reactions to the sulfur-containing agents may produce transient leukopenia. This latter reaction is mostly noted with the use of silver sulfadiazine cream when applied over large surface areas in children younger than 5 yr. This phenomenon is transient, self-limiting, and reversible. No sulfa-containing agent should be used if the child has a history of sulfa allergies.

Inhalational Injury

Inhalational injury is serious in the infant and child, particularly if pre-existing pulmonary conditions are present (Chapter 65). Mortality estimates vary, depending on the criteria for diagnosis, but are 45-60% in adults; exact figures are not available in children. Evaluation aims at early identification of inhalation airway injuries. These may occur from (1) direct heat (greater problems with steam burns), (2) acute asphyxia, (3) carbon monoxide poisoning, and (4) toxic fumes, including cyanides from combustible plastics. Sulfur and nitrogen oxides and alkalis formed during the combustion of synthetic fabrics produce corrosive chemicals that may erode mucosa and cause significant tissue sloughing. Exposure to smoke may cause degradation of surfactant and decrease its production, resulting in atelectasis. Inhalation injury and burn injury are synergistic, and the combined effect can increase morbidity and mortality.

The pulmonary complications of burns and inhalation can be divided into 3 syndromes that have distinct clinical manifestations and temporal patterns:

1. Early carbon monoxide poisoning, airway obstruction, and pulmonary edema are major concerns.
2. The acute respiratory distress syndrome usually becomes clinically evident later, at 24-48 hr, although it can occur even later (Chapter 65).
3. Late complications (days to weeks) include pneumonia and pulmonary emboli.

Inhalation injury should be assessed from the evidence of obvious injury (swelling or carbonaceous material in the nasal passages), wheezing, crackles or poor air entry, and laboratory determinations of (HbCO) and arterial blood gases.

Treatment is initially focused on establishing and maintaining a patent airway through prompt and early nasotracheal or orotracheal intubation and adequate ventilation and oxygenation. Wheezing is common, and β-agonist aerosols or inhaled corticosteroids are useful. Aggressive pulmonary toilet and chest physiotherapy are necessary in patients with prolonged nasotracheal intubation or in the rare patient with a tracheotomy. An endotracheal tube can be maintained for months without the need for tracheostomy. If tracheotomy must be performed, it should be delayed until burns at and near the site have healed, and then it should be performed electively, with the child under anesthesia and the use of optimal tracheal positioning and hemostasis. In children with inhalation injury or burns of the face and neck, upper airway obstruction can develop rapidly; endotracheal intubation becomes a lifesaving intervention. Extubation should be delayed until the patient meets the accepted criteria for maintaining the airway.

Signs of CNS injury from hypoxemia due to asphyxia or carbon monoxide poisoning vary from irritability to depression. Carbon monoxide poisoning may be mild (<20% HbCO), with slight dyspnea, headache, nausea, and decreased visual acuity and higher cerebral functions; moderate (20-40% HbCO), with irritability, agitation, nausea, dimness of vision, impaired judgment, and rapid fatigue; or severe (40-60% HbCO), producing confusion, hallucination, ataxia, collapse, acidosis, and coma. Measurement of HbCO is important for diagnosis and treatment. The PaO_2 value may be normal and the HbCO saturation values misleading because HbCO is not detected by the usual tests of oxygen saturation. Carbon monoxide poisoning is assumed until the tests are performed, and it is treated with 100% oxygen. Significant carbon monoxide poisoning requires hyperbaric oxygen therapy (Chapter 58).

Patients with severe inhalation injury or with other causes of respiratory deterioration that lead to acute respiratory distress syndrome who do not improve with conventional pressure-controlled ventilation (progressive oxygenation failure, as manifested by oxygen saturation <90% while receiving FIO_2 of 0.9-1.0 and positive end-expiratory pressure of at least 12.5 cm H_2O) may benefit from high-frequency ventilation or nitric oxide inhalation treatment. Nitric oxide usually is administered through the ventilator at 5 parts per million (ppm) and increased to 30 ppm. This method of therapy reduces the need for extracorporeal membrane oxygenation.

Pain Relief and Psychologic Adjustment

(See Chapter 71.)

It is important to provide adequate analgesia, anxiolytics, and psychologic support to reduce early metabolic stress, decrease the potential for post-traumatic stress syndrome, and allow future stabilization as well as physical and psychologic rehabilitation. Patients and family members require team support to work through the grieving process and accept long-term changes in appearance.

Children with burn injury show frequent and wide fluctuations in pain intensity. Appreciation of pain depends on the depth of the burn; the stage of healing; the patient's age and stage of emotional development and cognition; the experience and efficiency of the treating team; the use of analgesics and other drugs; the patient's pain threshold; and interpersonal and cultural factors. From the onset of treatment, **preemptive pain control** during dressing changes is of paramount importance. The use of a variety of nonpharmacologic interventions as well as pharmacologic agents must be reviewed throughout the treatment period. Opiate analgesia, prescribed in an adequate dose and timed to cover dressing changes, is essential to comfort management. A supportive person who is consistently present and "knows" the patient profile can integrate and encourage patient participation in burn care. The problem of undermedication is most prevalent in adolescents, in whom fear of drug dependence may inappropriately influence treatment. A related problem is that the child's specific pain experience may be misinterpreted; for anxious patients, those who are confused and alone, or those with preexisting emotional disorders, even small wounds may illicit intense pain. Anxiolytic medication added to the analgesic is usually helpful and has more than a synergistic effect. Equal attention is necessary to decrease stress in the intubated patient. Other modalities of pain and anxiety relief (relaxation techniques) can decrease the physiologic stress response. Oral morphine sulfate (immediate release) is recommended at a consistent schedule at a dose of 0.3-0.6 mg/kg every 4-6 hr initially and until wound cover is accomplished. Morphine sulfate IV bolus at a dose of 0.05-0.1 mg/kg maximum of 2-5 mg every 2 hr is administered. Morphine sulfate rectal suppositories may be useful at a dose of 0.3-0.6 mg/kg every 4 hr when oral administration is not possible. For anxiety, lorazepam is given on a consistent schedule, 0.05-0.1 mg/kg/dose every 6-8 hr. To control pain during a procedure (dressing change or debridement), oral morphine at a dose of 0.3-0.6 mg/kg is given 1-2 hr before the procedure and this is supplemented by a morphine IV bolus at a dose of 0.05-0.1 mg/kg given immediately before the procedure. Lorazepam at a dose of 0.04 mg/kg is given orally or intravenously, if necessary, for anxiety before the procedure. Midazolam (Versed) is also very useful for conscious sedation given at a dose of 0.01-0.02 mg/kg for nonintubated patients and 0.05-0.1 mg/kg for intubated patients, as an intravenous infusion or bolus, and may be repeated in 10 min. During the process of weaning from analgesics, the dose of oral opiates is reduced by 25% over 1-3 days, sometimes with the addition of acetaminophen as opiates are tapered. Antianxiety medications are tapered by reducing the dose of benzodiazepines at 25-50%/dose daily over 1-3 days.

For ventilated patients, pain control is accomplished by using morphine sulfate intermittently as an IV bolus at a dose of 0.05-0.1 mg/kg every 2 hr. Doses may need to be increased gradually, and some children may need continuous infusion; a starting dose of 0.05 mg/kg/hr given as an infusion is increased gradually as the need of the child changes. Naloxone is rarely needed but should be immediately available to reverse the effect of morphine, if necessary; if needed for an airway crisis, it should be given in a dose of 0.1 mg/kg up to a total of 2 mg, either intramuscularly or intravenously. For patients undergoing assisted respiration who require treatment of anxiety, midazolam is used as an intermittent IV bolus (0.04 mg/kg given by slow push every 4-6 hr) or as a continuous infusion. For intubated patients, opiates do not need to be discontinued during the process of weaning from the ventilator. Benzodiazepine should be reduced to approximately half the dose over 24-72 hr before extubation; too-rapid weaning from a benzodiazepine can lead to seizures.

There has been an expansion of the use of psychotropic medication in the care of children with burns, including prescription of selective serotonin reuptake inhibitors (SSRIs) as antidepressants, the use of haloperidol as a neuroleptic in the critical care setting and the treatment of post-traumatic stress disorder (PTSD) with benzodiazepines. Another area of expansion is the use of conscious sedation utilizing ketamine or propofol for major dressing changes.

Reconstruction and Rehabilitation

To ensure maximum cosmetic and functional outcome, occupational and physical therapy must begin on the day of admission, continue throughout hospitalization, and, for some patients, continue after discharge. Physical rehabilitation involves body and limb positioning, splinting, exercises (active and passive movement), assistance with activities of daily living, and gradual ambulation. These measures maintain adequate joint and muscle activity with as normal a range of movement as possible after healing or reconstruction. Pressure therapy is necessary to reduce hypertrophic scar formation; a variety of prefabricated and custom-made garments are available for use in different body areas for prevention of hypertrophic scarring. These custom-made garments deliver consistent pressure on scarred areas; they shorten the time of scar maturation and decrease the thickness of the scar as well as the redness and associated itching. Continued adjustments to scarred areas (scar release, grafting, rearrangement) and multiple minor cosmetic surgical procedures are necessary to optimize long-term function and improve appearance. Replacement of areas of alopecia and scarring has been achieved with the use of tissue expander techniques.

School Reentry and Long-Term Outcome

It is best for the child to return to school immediately after discharge. Occasionally, a child may need to attend a few half-days (because of rehabilitation needs). It is important for the child to return to his or her normal routine of attending school and being with peers. Planning for a return to home and school often requires a *school reentry program* that is individualized to each child's needs. For a school-aged child, planning for the return to school occurs simultaneously with planning for discharge. The

Table 68-7 COMMON LONG-TERM DISABILITIES IN PATIENTS WITH BURN INJURIES

DISABILITIES AFFECTING THE SKIN AND SOFT TISSUE
Hypertrophic scars Susceptibility to minor trauma, chemicals, or cold Dry skin Contractures Itching and neuropathic pain Alopecia Chronic open wounds Skin cancers
ORTHOPEDIC DISABILITIES
Amputations Contractures Heterotopic ossification Osteoporosis
METABOLIC DISABILITIES
Heat exhaustion Obesity
PSYCHIATRIC AND NEUROLOGIC DISABILITIES
Sleep disorders Adjustment disorders Post-traumatic stress syndrome Depression Neuropathy and neuropathic pain Long-term neurologic effects of carbon monoxide poisoning Anoxic brain injury
LONG-TERM COMPLICATIONS OF CRITICAL CARE
Deep-vein thrombosis, venous insufficiency, or varicose veins Tracheal stenosis, vocal cord disorders, or swallowing disorders Renal or adrenal dysfunction Hepatobiliary or pancreatic disease Cardiovascular disease Reactive airway disease or bronchial polyposis
PRE-EXISTING DISABILITIES THAT CONTRIBUTED TO THE INJURIES
Substance abuse Risk-taking behavior Untreated or poorly treated psychiatric disorder

Modified from Sheridan RL, Schultz JT, Ryan CM, et al: Case records of the Massachusetts General Hospital: weekly clinicopathological exercises: case 6-2004: a 35-year-old woman with extensive, deep burns from a nightclub fire, *N Engl J Med* 350:810–821, 2004.

hospital schoolteacher contacts the local school and plans the program with the school faculty, nurses, social workers, recreational/child life therapists, and rehabilitation therapists. This team should work with students and staff to ease anxiety, answer questions, and provide information. Burns and scars evoke fears in those who are not familiar with this type of injury and can result in a tendency to withdraw from or reject the burned child. A school reentry program should be appropriate to a child's development and changing educational needs.

Major advances have made it possible to save the lives of children with massive burns; whereas some children have had lingering physical difficulties, most have a satisfactory quality of life. The comprehensive burn care that includes experienced multidisciplinary aftercare plays an important role in recovery. Long-term complications of burns are listed in Table 68-7.

SPECIAL SITUATIONS

Electrical Burns

There are 3 types of electrical burns. **Minor electrical burns** usually occur as a result of biting on an extension cord. These injuries produce localized burns to the mouth, which usually involve the portions of the upper and lower lips that come in contact with the extension cord. The injury may involve or spare the corners of the mouth. Because these are nonconductive injuries (do not extend beyond the site of injury), hospital admission is not necessary and care is focused on the area of the injury visible in the mouth. Treatment with topical antibiotic creams is sufficient until the patient is seen in a burn unit outpatient department or by a plastic surgeon.

A more serious category of electrical burn is the **high-tension electrical wire burn**, for which children must be admitted for observation, regardless of the extent of the surface area burn. Deep muscle injury is typical and cannot be readily assessed initially. These injuries result from high voltage (>1,000 V) and occur particularly at high-voltage installations, such as electric power stations or railroads; children climb an electric pole and touch an electric box out of curiosity or accidentally touch a high-tension electric wire. Such injuries have a mortality rate of 3-15% for children who arrive at the hospital for treatment. Survivors have a high rate of morbidity, including major limb amputations. Points of entry of current through the skin and the exit site show characteristic features consistent with current density and heat. The majority of entrance wounds involve the upper extremity, with small exit wounds in the lower extremity. The electrical path, from entrance to exit, takes the shortest distance between the 2 points and may produce injury in any organ or tissue in the path of the current. Multiple exit wounds in some patients attest to the possibility of several electrical pathways in the body, placing virtually any structure in the body at risk (Table 68-8). Damage to the abdominal viscera, thoracic structures, and the nervous system in areas remote from obvious extremity injury occurs and must be sought, particularly in injuries with multiple current pathways or those in which the victim falls from a high pole. Sometimes **arcing** occurs and results in concurrent flame burn and clothing fire. Cardiac abnormalities, manifested as ventricular fibrillation or cardiac arrest, are common; patients with high-tension electrical injury need cardiac monitoring until they are stable and have been fully assessed. Higher-risk patients have abnormal electrocardiographic findings and a history of loss of consciousness. Renal damage from deep muscle necrosis and subsequent myoglobinuria is another complication; such patients need forced alkaline diuresis to minimize renal damage. Aggressive removal of all dead and devitalized tissue, even with the risk of functional loss, remains the key to effective management of the electrically damaged extremity. Early debridement facilitates early closure of the wound. Damaged major vessels must be isolated and buried in a viable muscle to prevent exposure. Survival depends on immediate intensive care, whereas a functional result depends on long-term care and delayed reconstructive surgery.

Lightning burns occur when a high-voltage current directly strikes a person (most dangerous) or when the current strikes the ground or an adjacent (in-contact) object. A step voltage burn is observed when lightning strikes the ground and travels up one leg and down the other (the path of least resistance). Lightning burns depend on the current path, the type of clothing worn, the presence of metal, and cutaneous moisture. Entry, exit, and path lesions are possible; the prognosis is poorest for lesions of the head or legs. Internal organ injury along the path is common and does not relate to the severity of the cutaneous burn. Linear burns, usually 1st- or 2nd-degree, are in the locations where sweat is present. Feathering or an arborescent pattern is characteristic of lightning injury. Lightning may ignite clothing or produce serious cutaneous burns from heated metal in the clothing. Internal complications of lightning burns include cardiac arrest caused by asystole, transient hypertension, premature ventricular contractions, ventricular fibrillation, and myocardial ischemia. Most severe cardiac complications resolve if the patient is supported with cardiopulmonary resuscitation (Chapter 62). CNS complications include cerebral edema, hemorrhage, seizures, mood changes, depression, and paralysis of the lower extremities. Rhabdomyolysis and myoglobinuria (with possible renal failure) also occur.

Table 68-8 ELECTRICAL INJURY: CLINICAL CONSIDERATIONS

	CLINICAL MANIFESTATIONS	MANAGEMENT
General	—	Extricate the patient; perform ABCs of resuscitation; immobilize the spine
		History: voltage, type of current
		Complete blood count with platelets, electrolytes, blood urea nitrogen (BUN), creatinine, glucose
Cardiac	Dysrhythmias: asystole, ventricular fibrillation, sinus tachycardia, sinus bradycardia, premature atrial contractions (PACs), premature ventricular contractions (PVCs), conduction defects, atrial fibrillation, ST-T wave changes	Treat dysrhythmias Cardiac monitor, electrocardiogram, and radiographs with suspected thoracic injury
		Creatinine phosphokinase with isoenzyme measurements if indicated
Pulmonary	Respiratory arrest, acute respiratory distress, aspiration syndrome	Protect and maintain the airway
		Mechanical ventilation if indicated, chest radiograph, arterial blood gas levels
Renal	Acute renal failure, myoglobinuria	Provide aggressive fluid management unless a central nervous system injury is present
		Maintain adequate urine output, >1 mL/kg/hr
		Consider central venous or pulmonary artery pressure monitoring
		Measure urine myoglobin; perform urinalysis; measure BUN, creatinine
Neurologic	Immediate: loss of consciousness, motor paralysis, visual disturbances, amnesia, agitation; intracranial hematoma	Treat seizures Provide fluid restriction if indicated
	Secondary: pain, paraplegia, brachial plexus injury, syndrome of inappropriate antidiuretic hormone secretion (SIADH), autonomic disturbances, cerebral edema	Consider spine radiographs, especially cervical
	Delayed: paralysis, seizures, headache, peripheral neuropathy	CT scan of the brain if indicated
Cutaneous/oral	Oral commissure burns, tongue and dental injuries; skin burns resulting from ignition of clothes, entrance and exit burns, and arc burns	Search for the entrance/exit wound Treat cutaneous burns; determine the tetanus status
		Obtain a plastic surgery of ear, nose, and throat consultation if needed
Abdominal	Viscus perforation and solid organ damage; ileus; abdominal injury rare without visible abdominal burns	Place a nasogastric tube if the patient has airway compromise or ileus
		Obtain SGOT (serum glutamate oxaloacetate transaminase or aspartate aminotransferase), SGPT (serum glutamate pyruvate transaminase, alanine aminotransferase), amylase, BUN, and creatinine measurements and, CT scans as indicated
Musculoskeletal	Compartment syndrome from subcutaneous necrosis limb edema and deep burns	Monitor the patient for possible compartment syndrome
	Long bone fractures, spine injuries	Obtain radiographs and orthopedic/general surgery consultations as indicated
Ocular	Visual changes, optic neuritis, cataracts, extraocular muscle paresis	Obtain an ophthalmology consultation as indicated

Modified from Hall ML, Sills RM: Electrical and lightning injuries. In Barkin RM, editor: *Pediatric emergency medicine,* St Louis, 1997, Mosby, p 484.

BIBLIOGRAPHY

Please visit the Nelson Textbook of Pediatrics *website at www.expertconsult.com for the complete bibliography.*

Chapter 69
Cold Injuries

Alia Y. Antoon and Mary K. Donovan

The involvement of children and youth in snowmobiling, mountain climbing, winter hiking, and skiing places them at risk for cold injury. Cold injury may produce either local tissue damage, with the injury pattern depending on exposure to damp cold (frostnip, immersion foot, or trench foot), dry cold (which leads to local frostbite), or generalized systemic effects (hypothermia).

PATHOPHYSIOLOGY

Ice crystals may form between or within cells, interfering with the sodium pump, and may lead to rupture of cell membranes. Further damage may result from clumping of red blood cells or platelets, causing microembolism or thrombosis. Blood may be shunted away from an affected area by secondary neurovascular responses to the cold injury; this shunting often further damages an injured part while improving perfusion of other tissues. The spectrum of injury ranges from mild to severe and reflects the result of structural and functional disturbance in small blood vessels, nerves, and skin.

ETIOLOGY

Body heat may be lost by conduction (wet clothing, contact with metal or other solid conducting objects), convection (wind chill), evaporation, or radiation. Susceptibility to cold injury may be increased by dehydration, alcohol or drug use, substance abuse, impaired consciousness, exhaustion, hunger, anemia, impaired circulation due to cardiovascular disease, and sepsis; it is also greater in very young or aged persons.

Hypothermia occurs when the body can no longer sustain normal core temperature by physiologic mechanisms, such as vasoconstriction, shivering, muscle contraction, and nonshivering thermogenesis. When shivering ceases, the body is unable to maintain its core temperature; when the body core temperature falls to <35°C, the syndrome of hypothermia occurs. Wind chill, wet or inadequate clothing, and other factors increase local injury and may cause dangerous hypothermia, even in the presence of an ambient temperature that is not <17-20°C (50-60°F).

CLINICAL MANIFESTATIONS

Frostnip

Frostnip results in the presence of firm, cold, white areas on the face, ears, or extremities. Blistering and peeling may occur over the next 24-72 hr, occasionally leaving mildly increased hypersensitivity to cold for some days or weeks. Treatment consists of warming the area with an unaffected hand or a warm object before the lesion reaches a stage of stinging or aching and before numbness supervenes.

Immersion Foot (Trench Foot)

Immersion foot occurs in cold weather when the feet remain in damp or wet, poorly ventilated boots. The feet become cold, numb, pale, edematous, and clammy. Tissue maceration and infection are likely, and prolonged autonomic disturbance is common. This autonomic disturbance leads to increased sweating, pain, and hypersensitivity to temperature changes, which may persist for years. The treatment is largely prophylactic and consists of using well-fitting, insulated, waterproof, nonconstricting footwear. Once damage has occurred, patients must choose clothing and footwear that are more appropriate, dry, and well-fitting. The disturbance in skin integrity is managed by keeping the affected area dry and well-ventilated and by preventing or treating infection. Only supportive measures are possible for control of autonomic symptoms.

Frostbite

With frostbite, initial stinging or aching of the skin progresses to cold, hard, white anesthetic and numb areas. On rewarming, the area becomes blotchy, itchy, and often red, swollen, and painful. The injury spectrum ranges from complete normality to extensive tissue damage, even gangrene, if early relief is not obtained.

Treatment consists of warming the damaged area. It is important not to cause further damage by attempting to rub the area with ice or snow; initial warming, as in frostnip, may be tried. The area may be warmed against an unaffected hand, the abdomen, or an axilla during transfer of the patient to a facility where more rapid warming with a water bath is possible. If the skin becomes painful and swelling occurs, anti-inflammatory agents are helpful and an analgesic agent is necessary. Freeze and rethaw cycles are most likely to cause permanent tissue injury, and it may be necessary to delay definitive warming and apply only mild measures if the patient is required to walk on the damaged feet en route to definitive treatment. In the hospital, the affected area should be immersed in warm water (approximately 42°C), with care taken not to burn the anesthetized skin. Vasodilating agents, such as prazosin and phenoxybenzamine, may be helpful. Use of anticoagulants (heparin, dextran) has had equivocal results; results of chemical and surgical sympathectomy have also been equivocal. Oxygen is of help only at high altitudes. Meticulous local care, prevention of infection, and keeping the rewarmed area dry, open, and sterile provide optimal results. Recovery can be complete, and prolonged observation with conservative therapy is justified before any excision or amputation of tissue is considered. Analgesia and maintenance of good nutrition are necessary throughout the prolonged waiting period.

Hypothermia

Hypothermia may occur in winter sports when injury, equipment failure, or exhaustion decreases the level of exertion, particularly if sufficient attention is not paid to wind chill. Immersion in frozen bodies of water and wet wind chill rapidly produce hypothermia. As the core temperature of the body falls, insidious onset of extreme lethargy, fatigue, incoordination, and apathy occurs, followed by mental confusion, clumsiness, irritability, hallucinations, and finally, bradycardia. A number of medical conditions, such as cardiac disease, diabetes mellitus, hypoglycemia, sepsis, β-blocking agent overdose, and substance abuse, may need to be considered in a differential diagnosis. The decrease in rectal temperature to <34°C (93°F) is the most helpful diagnostic feature. Hypothermia associated with drowning is discussed in Chapter 67.

Prevention is a high priority. Of extreme importance for those who participate in winter sports is wearing layers of warm clothing, gloves, socks within insulated boots that do not impede circulation, and a warm head covering, as well as application of adequate waterproofing and protection against the wind. Thirty percent of heat loss for infants occurs from the head. Ample food and fluid must be provided during exercise. Those who participate in sports should be alert to the presence of cold or numbing of body parts, particularly the nose, ears, and extremities, and they should review methods to produce local warming and know to seek shelter if they detect symptoms of local cold injury. Application of petrolatum (Vaseline) to the nose and ears gives certain protection against frostbite.

Treatment at the scene aims at prevention of further heat loss and early transport to adequate shelter. Dry clothing should be provided as soon as practical, and transport should be undertaken if the victim has a pulse. If no pulse is detected at the initial review, cardiopulmonary resuscitation is indicated (Chapter 62; Fig. 69-1). During transfer, jarring and sudden motion should be avoided because these occurrences may cause ventricular arrhythmia. It is often difficult to attain a normal sinus rhythm during hypothermia.

If the patient is conscious, mild muscle activity should be encouraged, and a warm drink offered. If the patient is unconscious, external warming should be undertaken initially with use of blankets and a sleeping bag; wrapping the patient in blankets or sleeping bag with a warm companion may increase the efficiency of warming. On arrival at a treatment center, while a warming bath of 45-48°C (113-118°F) water is prepared, the patient should be warmed through inhalation of warm, moist air or oxygen or with heating pads or thermal blankets. Monitoring of serum chemistry values and an electrocardiogram are necessary until the core temperature rises to >35°C and can be stabilized. Control of fluid balance, pH, blood pressure, and oxygen concentration is necessary in the early phases of the warming period and resuscitation. In severe hypothermia, there may be a combined respiratory and metabolic acidosis. Hypothermia may falsely elevate pH; nonetheless, most authorities recommend warming the arterial blood gas specimen to 37°C before analysis and regarding the result as one from a normothermic patient. In patients with marked abnormalities, warming measures, such as gastric or colonic irrigation with warm saline or peritoneal dialysis, may be considered, but the effectiveness of these measures in treating hypothermia is unknown. In accidental deep hypothermia (core temperature 28°C) with circulatory arrest, rewarming with cardiopulmonary bypass may be lifesaving for previously healthy young individuals.

Chilblain (Pernio)

Chilblain (pernio) is a form of cold injury in which erythematous, vesicular, or ulcerative lesions occur. The lesions are presumed to be of vascular or vasoconstrictive origin. They are often itchy, may be painful, and result in swelling and scabbing. The lesions are most often found on the ears, the tips of the fingers and toes, and exposed areas of the legs. The lesions last for 1-2 wk but may persist for longer. Treatment consists of prophylaxis: avoiding prolonged chilling and protecting potentially susceptible areas with a cap, gloves, and stockings. Prazosin and phenoxybenzamine may be helpful in improving circulation if this is a recurrent problem. For significant itching, local corticosteroid preparations may be helpful.

Cold-Induced Fat Necrosis (Panniculitis)

A common, usually benign injury, cold-induced fat necrosis occurs upon exposure to cold air, snow, or ice and manifests in exposed (or, less often, covered) surfaces as red (or, less often, purple to blue) macular, papular, or nodular lesions. Treatment is with nonsteroidal anti-inflammatory agents. The lesions may last 10 days to 3 wk (Chapter 652) but may persist for longer. There is a possibility of severe coagulopathy associated with poor outcome in some of the severe cold injuries, thus meriting anticoagulation therapy.

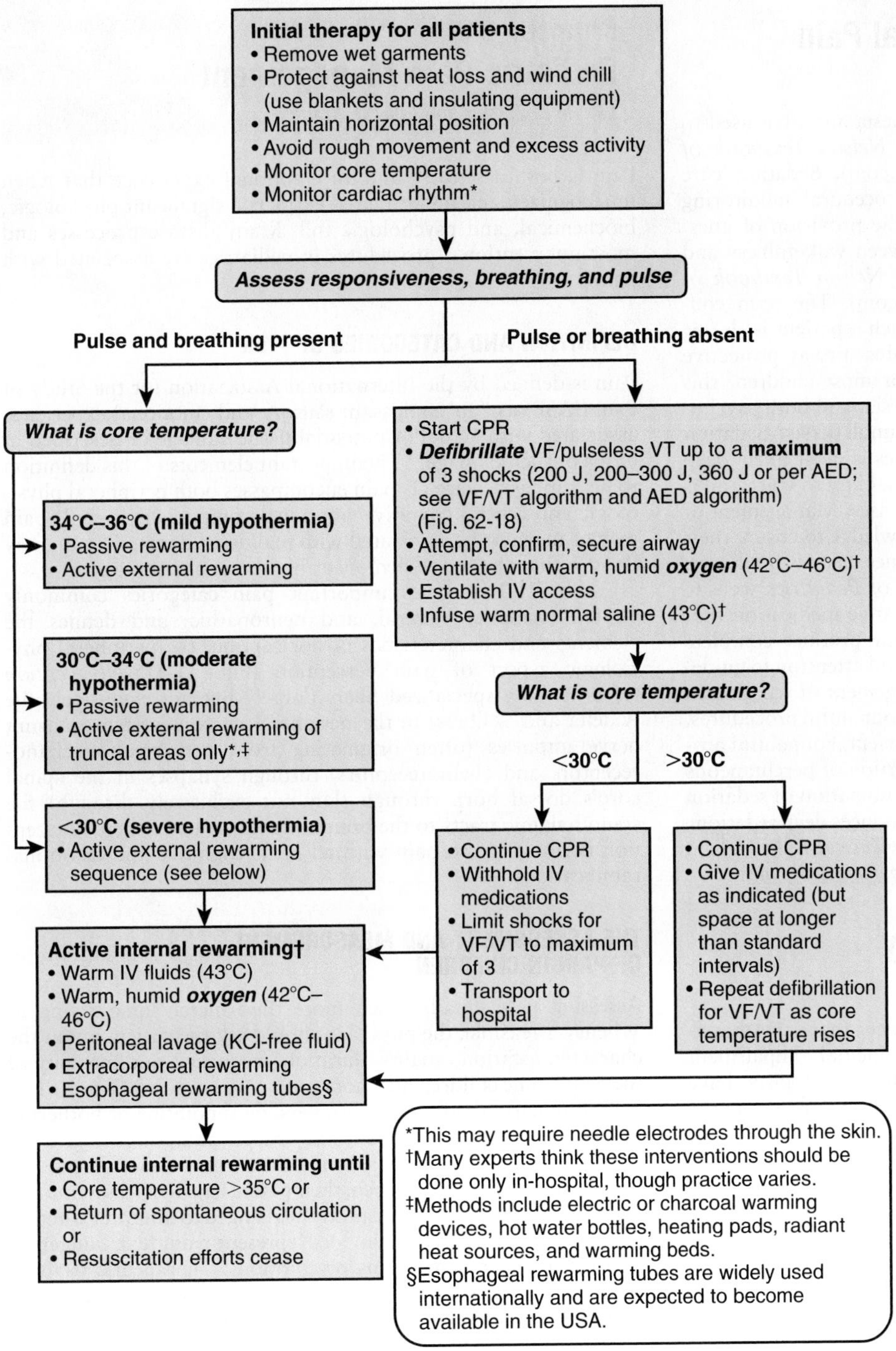
Initial therapy for all patients
• Remove wet garments
• Protect against heat loss and wind chill (use blankets and insulating equipment)
• Maintain horizontal position
• Avoid rough movement and excess activity
• Monitor core temperature
• Monitor cardiac rhythm*
Assess responsiveness, breathing, and pulse
Pulse and breathing present
Pulse or breathing absent
What is core temperature?
34°C–36°C (mild hypothermia)
• Passive rewarming
• Active external rewarming
30°C–34°C (moderate hypothermia)
• Passive rewarming
• Active external rewarming of truncal areas only*,‡
<30°C (severe hypothermia)
• Active external rewarming sequence (see below)
• Start CPR
• Defibrillate VF/pulseless VT up to a maximum of 3 shocks (200 J, 200–300 J, 360 J or per AED; see VF/VT algorithm and AED algorithm) (Fig. 62-18)
• Attempt, confirm, secure airway
• Ventilate with warm, humid oxygen (42°C–46°C)†
• Establish IV access
• Infuse warm normal saline (43°C)†
What is core temperature?
<30°C
>30°C
• Continue CPR
• Withhold IV medications
• Limit shocks for VF/VT to maximum of 3
• Transport to hospital
• Continue CPR
• Give IV medications as indicated (but space at longer than standard intervals)
• Repeat defibrillation for VF/VT as core temperature rises
Active internal rewarming†
• Warm IV fluids (43°C)
• Warm, humid oxygen (42°C–46°C)
• Peritoneal lavage (KCl-free fluid)
• Extracorporeal rewarming
• Esophageal rewarming tubes§
Continue internal rewarming until
• Core temperature >35°C or
• Return of spontaneous circulation or
• Resuscitation efforts cease
*This may require needle electrodes through the skin.
†Many experts think these interventions should be done only in-hospital, though practice varies.
‡Methods include electric or charcoal warming devices, hot water bottles, heating pads, radiant heat sources, and warming beds.
§Esophageal rewarming tubes are widely used internationally and are expected to become available in the USA.

Figure 69-1 Hypothermia treatment algorithm for adult-size children and adolescents. AED, automated external defibrillator; CPR, cardiopulmonary resuscitation; IV, intravenous; VF, ventricular fibrillation; VT, ventricular tachycardia. (From Guidelines 2000 for cardiopulmonary resuscitation and emergency cardiovascular care. Part 8: advanced challenges in resuscitation: section 3: special challenges in ECC. The American Heart Association in collaboration with the International Liaison Committee on Resuscitation, *Circulation* 102:1229–1252, 2000.)

BIBLIOGRAPHY

Please visit the Nelson Textbook of Pediatrics *website at www.expertconsult.com for the complete bibliography.*

Chapter 70
Anesthesia, Perioperative Care, and Sedation

Randall C. Wetzel

The primary purpose of general anesthesia is to suppress the conscious perception of, and physiologic response to, noxious stimuli and to render the patient unconscious. Potent drugs are used to blunt physiologic responses to what would otherwise be life-threatening trauma (surgery). Intraoperatively, the anesthesiologist is responsible for providing analgesia as well as physiologic and metabolic stability (see Table 70-1 on the *Nelson Textbook of Pediatrics* website at www.expertconsult.com). This responsibility is facilitated by obtaining an adequate preanesthesia history (see Table 70-2 on the *Nelson Textbook of Pediatrics* website at www.expertconsult.com). The increased risk of morbidity and mortality in the perioperative period demands the utmost vigilance. The risk is even higher in certain disease states (see Table 70-3 on the *Nelson Textbook of Pediatrics* website at www.expertconsult.com).

For the full continuation of this chapter, please visit the Nelson Textbook of Pediatrics *website at www.expertconsult.com.*

70.1 Sedation and Procedural Pain

Randall C. Wetzel

The same drugs that induce general anesthesia are often used to provide sedation (see Table 70-5 on the *Nelson Textbook of Pediatrics* website at www.expertconsult.com). Sedation care requires a presedation evaluation, intraprocedural monitoring and postsedation recovery, analogous to the provision of anesthesia. Sedation is on the continuum between wakefulness and general anesthesia (see Table 70-4 on the *Nelson Textbook of Pediatrics* website at www.expertconsult.com). The term **conscious sedation** refers to a condition in which a patient is sleepy, comfortable, and cooperative but maintains airway-protective and ventilatory reflexes. Unfortunately, for most children, this level of sedation provides little or no analgesia, and both psychologic and physiologic responses to painful stimuli persist. Sedation that is sufficient to obtund painful responses is most likely deep sedation. **Deep sedation** is a state of unarousability to voice and is accompanied by suppression of reflex responses. Management of sedated children requires vigilance and knowledge to ensure their safety and is governed by the same guidelines as anesthesia care (see Table 70-11 on the *Nelson Textbook of Pediatrics* website at www.expertconsult.com). A dose of sedative medication that causes minimal sedation in one subject may produce complete unconsciousness and apnea in another. Careful attention to guidelines for appropriate monitoring and management of sedation in children is imperative. For threatening and nonpainful procedures, anxiolysis or light sedation is frequently sufficient. For painful procedures (e.g., bone marrow aspiration, insertion of percutaneous IV catheter lines, lumbar punctures), the combination of sedation with analgesia that is required in children produces deep sedation.

For the full continuation of this chapter, please visit the Nelson Textbook of Pediatrics *website at www.expertconsult.com.*

70.2 Anesthetic Neurotoxicity

Randall C. Wetzel

There is compelling experimental evidence that anesthesia-induced neurodegeneration with developmental impairment occurs in neonatal animals. Pediatric anesthesiologists have become deeply concerned by the demonstration of anesthetic-induced apoptotic neuronal cell death, CNS neurodegenerative changes, and their effects on the developing brain. These studies demonstrate both histopathologic changes and developmental defects from both inhalational and IV anesthetics, including isoflurane, ketamine, benzodiazepines, and propofol given to newborn animals. Combinations of drugs may cause more injury. Existing nonclinical data implicate both NMDA and GABA pathways in apoptosis and cell death in neonates.

For the full continuation of this chapter, please visit the Nelson Textbook of Pediatrics *website at www.expertconsult.com.*

Chapter 71
Pediatric Pain Management

Lonnie K. Zeltzer and Elliot J. Krane

Pain is both a sensory and an emotional experience that when unrecognized and undertreated extracts a significant physiologic, biochemical, and psychologic toll. Many disease processes and most interventional procedures in pediatrics are associated with pain.

DEFINITION AND CATEGORIES OF PAIN

Pain is defined by the International Association for the Study of Pain (IASP) as "an unpleasant sensory and emotional experience associated with actual or potential tissue damage or described in terms of such damage." The important elements of this definition to be emphasized are (1) pain encompasses both peripheral physiologic and central cognitive/emotional components and (2) pain may or may not be associated with real tissue damage—pain may exist in the absence of demonstrable somatic pathology.

Table 71-1 specifies important pain categories commonly treated (somatic, visceral, and neuropathic) and defines the elements and characteristics of nociception, the peripheral physiologic aspect of pain perception (Fig. 71-1). *Nociception* refers to how specialized fibers (largely but not exclusively the A delta and C fibers) in the peripheral nervous system transmit nerve impulses (often originating from peripheral mechanoreceptors and chemoreceptors) through synapses in the spinal cord's dorsal horn through (but not exclusively through) the spinothalamic tracts to the brain's higher centers, where nociception is converted to pain with all of its cognitive and emotional ramifications.

THE ASSESSMENT AND MEASUREMENT OF PAIN IN CHILDREN

Assessing pain entails much more than merely quantifying it. Whenever feasible, the physician should ask the patient about the character, location, quality, duration, frequency, and intensity of the pain. Some children may not report pain because of fears (often well-founded), of talking to strangers, disappointing or bothering others, receiving an injection if they report pain, returning to the hospital if they admit to pain, and other negative reinforcers. For infants and nonverbal children, their parents, pediatricians, nurses, and other caregivers are constantly challenged to interpret whether the children's distressed behaviors represent pain, fear, hunger, or a range of other perceptions or emotions. Therapeutic trials of comfort measures (cuddling, feeding) and analgesic medications may be helpful in clarifying such a situation.

Behavior and physiologic signs are useful, but they can be misleading. A toddler may scream and grimace during an ear

Table 71-1 PAIN CATEGORIES AND CHARACTERISTICS

PAIN CATEGORY	DEFINITION AND EXAMPLES	CHARACTERISTICS
Somatic	Pain resulting from injury to or inflammation of tissues (skin, muscle, tendons, bone, joints, fascia, vasculature, etc.) Examples: burns, lacerations, fractures, infections, inflammatory conditions	In skin and superficial structures: sharp; pulsatile; well-localized In deep somatic structures: dull; aching; pulsatile; not well-localized
Visceral	Pain resulting from injury to or inflammation of viscera Examples: angina, hepatic distention, bowel distention or hypermobility, pancreatitis	Aching and cramping; nonpulsatile; poorly localized (e.g., appendiceal pain perceived around umbilicus) or referred to distant locations (e.g., angina perceived in shoulder)
Neuropathic	Pain resulting from injury to, inflammation of, or dysfunction of the peripheral or central nervous systems. Examples: complex regional pain syndrome (CRPS), phantom limb pain, Guillain-Barré syndrome, sciatica	Spontaneous; burning; lancinating or shooting; dysesthesias (pins and needles, electrical sensations); hyperalgesia (amplification of noxious stimuli); hyperpathia (widespread pain in response to a discrete noxious stimulus); allodynia (pain in response to nonpainful stimulation); pain may be perceived distal or proximal to site of injury, usually corresponding to innervation pathways (e.g., sciatica)

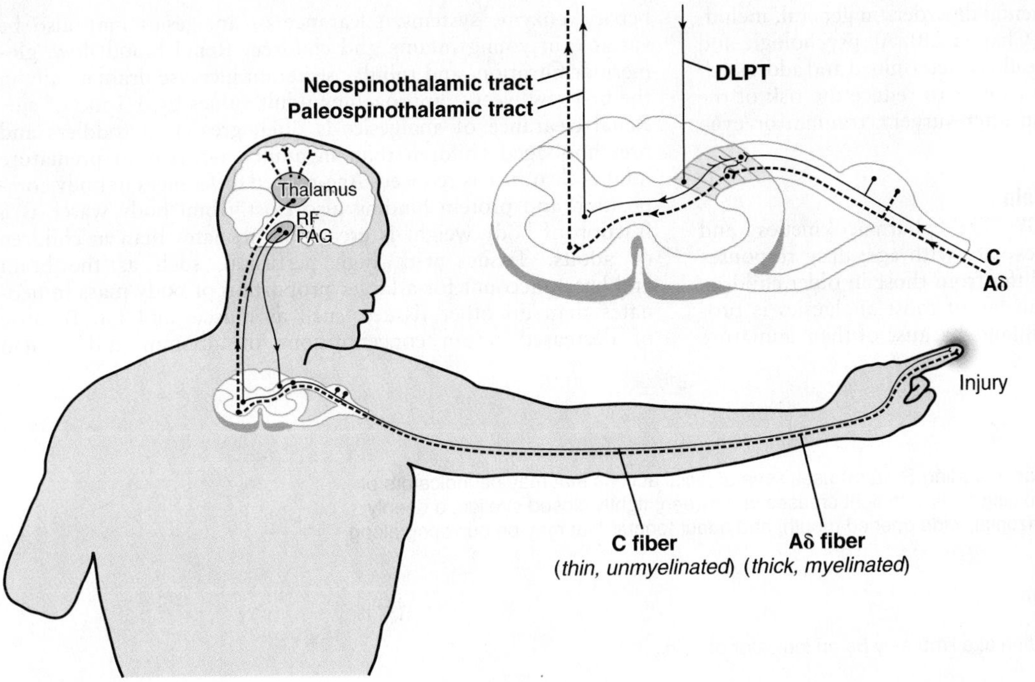

Figure 71-1 The typical neural pathways of nociception, also showing higher projection of nociception to the cortex, where the sensation of nociception is translated to the conscious and emotional phenomenon of pain. DLPT, dorsolateral pontine tegmentum; PAG, periaqueductal gray; RF, reticular formation.

examination because of fear rather than pain. Conversely, children with inadequately relieved persistent pain from cancer, sickle cell disease, trauma, or surgery may withdraw from their surroundings and appear very quiet, leading observers to conclude falsely that they are comfortable or sedated. In these situations, increased dosing of analgesics may make the child become more, not less, interactive and alert. Similarly, neonates and young infants may close their eyes, furrow their brows, and clench their fists in response to pain. Adequate analgesia is often associated with eye opening and increased involvement in the surroundings. A child who is experiencing significant chronic pain may play normally as a way to distract attention from pain. This coping behavior is sometimes misinterpreted as evidence of the child's faking pain at other times.

Age-Specific and Developmentally Specific Measures

Because infants, young children, and nonverbal children cannot express the quantity of pain they experience, several pain scales have been devised in an attempt to quantify pain in these populations (Fig. 71-2; Table 71-2).

THE NEWBORN AND INFANT There are a range of behavioral distress scales for the infant and young child, mostly emphasizing the patient's facial expressions, crying, and body movement. Facial expression measures appear most useful and specific in neonates. Autonomic and vital signs can indicate pain, but because they are nonspecific, they may reflect other processes, including fever, hypoxemia, and cardiac or renal dysfunction.

THE OLDER CHILD Children 3-7 yr old become increasingly articulate in describing the intensity, location, and quality of pain. Pain is occasionally referred to adjacent areas; referral of hip pain to the leg or knee is common in this age range. Self-report measures for children this age include using drawings, pictures of faces, or graded color intensities. Children age 8 yr and older can usually use verbal scales or visual analog pain scales (VASs) accurately (see Fig. 71-2). Verbal numerical ratings are preferred and considered the gold standard; valid and reliable ratings are for children 8 yr and older. The Numerical Rating Scale (NRS) consists of numbers from 0 to 10, in which 0 represents no pain and 10 represents very severe pain. There is debate about the label for the highest pain rating, but the current agreement is NOT to use the worst pain possible, because children can always imagine a greater pain. In the USA, regularly documented pain assessments are required for hospitalized children and children attending outpatient hospital clinics and emergency departments. Pain scores do not always correlate with changes in heart rate or blood pressure.

THE COGNITIVELY IMPAIRED CHILD Measuring pain in cognitively impaired children remains a challenge. Understanding pain expression and experience in this population is important, because behaviors may be misinterpreted as indicating that cognitively impaired children are more insensitive to pain than cognitively competent children. Children with trisomy 21 may express pain less precisely and more slowly than the general population. Pain in children with autism spectrum disorders may be difficult to assess because they may be both *hyposensitive* and *hypersensitive* to many different types of sensory stimuli, and they may have limited communication abilities. Although self-reports of pain can be elicited from some children who are cognitively impaired, observational measures have better validation among these children. The Non-communicating Child's Pain Checklist—Postoperative Version is recommended for children up to 18 yr. Maladaptive behavior and reduction in functions may also indicate pain. Children with severe cognitive impairments experience pain frequently, mostly not because of accidental injury. Children with the fewest abilities experience the most pain.

THE TREATMENT OF PAIN

Both pharmacologic and nonpharmacologic approaches to pain management should be considered for all pain treatment plans. Many simple interventions designed to promote relaxation and patient control can be expected to work synergistically with pain medications for optimal relief of pain and related distress. Psychologic and developmental comorbidities affect the child's experience of pain and ability to tolerate and cope with it. Thus, it is important to assess a child for evidence of situational anxiety and/or anxiety disorders, such as generalized anxiety disorder, post-traumatic stress disorder, social anxiety, separation anxiety, panic disorder, and obsessive-compulsive disorder (Chapter 23). Depression assessment should include current suicidal ideation and intent as well as past history of suicidal gestures or attempts (Chapters 24 and 25). Developmental assessment includes evaluating for specific learning disorders, Asperger disorder, and evidence of pervasive developmental disorders in general, including autism spectrum disorders (Chapter 28). All psychologic and developmental comorbidities should be determined and addressed, to adequately treat the child in pain or to reduce the risk of the child's developing ongoing pain after surgery, trauma, or even invasive medical procedures.

Pharmacologic Treatment of Pain

DEVELOPMENTAL PHARMACOLOGY The pharmacokinetics and pharmacodynamics of analgesics vary with age; drug responses in infants and young children differ from those in older children and adults. The elimination half-life of most analgesics is prolonged in neonates and young infants because of their immature hepatic enzyme systems. Clearance of analgesics may also be variable in young infants and children. Renal blood flow, glomerular filtration, and tubular secretion increase dramatically in the first few weeks, approaching adult values by 3-5 mo of age. Renal clearance of analgesics is often greater in toddlers and preschool-aged children than in adults, whereas in premature infants clearance is reduced. Age-related differences in body composition and protein binding also exist. Total body water as a fraction of body weight is greater in neonates than in children or adults. Tissues with high perfusion, such as the brain and heart, account for a larger proportion of body mass in neonates than do other tissues, such as muscle and fat. Because of decreased serum concentrations of albumin and α_1-acid

Behavioral Indicators

Facial grimacing: The Neonatal Facial Coding System* uses several facial actions that may be indicators of pain. Pain is characterized by a bulging brow with tight creases in between; tightly closed eyelids; a deeply furrowed nasolabial groove; a horizontal, wide opened mouth; and a taut tongue that may be quivering along with the chin.

Crying: May be an indicator of pain.

Activity: Withdrawal or immobilization of a limb may be an indicator of pain.

Response to comfort measures: Feeding, swaddling, holding, and ensuring that the infant is neither wet nor cold may help to discriminate between pain and other conditions.

Physiologic indicators: Alterations in heart rate, blood pressure, SpO_2, respiratory rate, or alterations in pattern of respiration may be nonspecific indicators of pain.

Multidimensional Instrument

FLACC† *Scoring System:* May be used in preverbal, mechanically ventilated, or cognitively impaired patients; it is an acronym that includes five indicators, each scored as a 0, 1, or 2 that forms a ten-point composite scale with a range from "0" (no pain) to "10" (worst pain).

FLACC: Score each category between 0 and 2. The total score may be any number from 0 to 10.

Score:	0	1	2
Face	No expression	Occational action	Frequent action
Legs	Normal	Restless or tense	Kicking, legs withdrawn
Activity	Quiet	Shifting or tense	Rigid, arched, jerking
Cry	None	Moan, whimper	Steady crying, screaming, sobbing, or frequent complaints
Consolability	Content	Consolable	Inconsolable

Self-Report of Pain

Categorical description: Toddlers or young children are asked to say if they are having "a little bit," a "middle amount," or "a lot" of pain.

Faces Scales‡: Children who do not have an appreciation of ordinal numbering are asked to rate their pain based upon cartoons depicting facial indicators of distress.

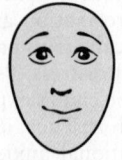

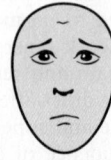

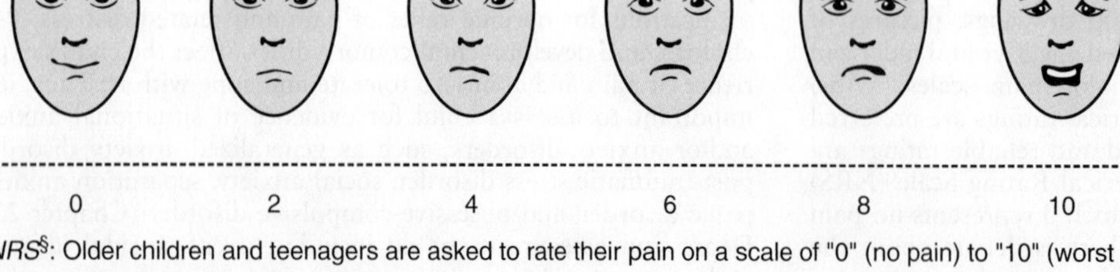

0 2 4 6 8 10

NRS§: Older children and teenagers are asked to rate their pain on a scale of "0" (no pain) to "10" (worst pain).

VAS§: Children or teenagers are asked to move an indicator along a mechanical slide to depict the level of pain; the clinician reads a number along a 10-cm indicator on the back to determine the numeric score.

Figure 71-2 Clinically useful pain assessment tools. (Adapted from Burg FD, Ingelfinger JR, Polin RA, et al, editors: *Current pediatric therapy,* ed 18, Philadelphia, 2006, Saunders/Elsevier, p 16; and Hicks CL, von Baeyer CL, Spafford P, et al: The Faces Pain Scale—revised: toward a common metric in pediatric pain measurement, *Pain* 93:173–183, 2001.)

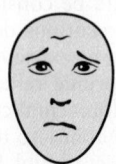

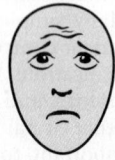

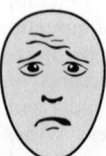

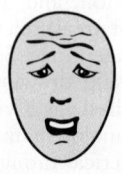

Table 71-2 PAIN MEASUREMENT TOOLS

NAME	FEATURES	AGE RANGE	ADVANTAGES	VALIDATION AND USES	LIMITATIONS
Visual Analog Scale (VAS)	Horizontal 10-cm line; subject marks a spot on the line between anchors of "no pain" (or neutral face) and "most pain imaginable" (or sad face)	6-8 yr and older	Good psychometric properties; validated for research purposes	Acute pain Surgical pain Chronic pain	Cannot be used in younger children or in those with cognitive limitations Requires language skills and numerical processing; upper anchor of "most pain" requires an experiential reference point that is lacking in many children
Likert Scale	Integers from 0 to 10, inclusive, corresponding to a range from no pain to most pain	6-8 yr and older	Good psychometric properties; validated for research purposes	Acute pain Surgical pain Chronic pain	Same as for VAS
Faces Scales (e.g., FACES-R, Wong-Baker, Oucher, Bieri, McGrath scales)	Subjects rate their pain by identifying with line drawings of faces, or photos of children	4 yr and older	Can be used at younger ages than VAS and Likert	Acute pain Surgical pain	Choice of "no pain" face affects responses (neutral vs smiling); not culturally universal
Behavioral or combined behavioral-physiologic scales (e.g., FLACC, N-PASS, CHEOPS, OPS, FACS, NIPS)	Scoring of observed behaviors (e.g., facial expression, limb movement) ± heart rate and blood pressure	Some work for any ages; some work for specific age groups, including preterm infants	May be used in both infants and nonverbal children	FLACC, N-PASS: Acute pain Surgical pain	Nonspecific; over-rates pain in toddlers and preschool children; under-rates persistent pain; some measures are convenient, but others require videotaping and complex processing; vital sign changes unrelated to pain can occur and may affect total score
Autonomic measures (e.g., heart rate, blood pressure, heart rate spectral analyses)	Scores changes in heart rate, blood pressure, or measures of heart rate variability (e.g., "vagal tone")	All ages	Can be used at all ages; useful for patients receiving mechanical ventilation		Nonspecific; vital sign changes unrelated to pain may occur, and may artifactually increase or decrease score
Hormonal-metabolic measures	Plasma or salivary sampling of "stress" hormones (e.g., cortisol, epinephrine)	All ages	Can be used at all ages		Nonspecific; changes unrelated to pain can occur; inconvenient; cannot provide "real-time" information; standard normal values not available for every age bracket

glycoprotein, neonates have reduced protein binding of some drugs, resulting in higher amounts of free, unbound, pharmacologically active drug.

ACETAMINOPHEN, ASPIRIN, AND NONSTEROIDAL ANTI-INFLAMMATORY DRUGS Acetaminophen (APAP) and nonsteroidal anti-inflammatory drugs (NSAIDs) have replaced aspirin as the most commonly used antipyretics and oral, nonopioid analgesics (Table 71-3).

Acetaminophen, a generally safe, nonopioid analgesic and antipyretic, has the advantage of rectal and oral routes of administration, is expected to be available soon also as an intravenous (IV) preparation in the USA, as it is now in Europe. Acetaminophen is not associated with the gastrointestinal or antiplatelet effects of aspirin and NSAIDs, making it a particularly useful drug in patients with cancer. Unlike aspirin and NSAIDs, acetaminophen has only mild anti-inflammatory action. Acetaminophen toxicity can result from either, large single doses or cumulative, excessive dosing over days or weeks (Chapters 58 and 355). A single, massive overdose overwhelms the normal glucuronidation and sulfation metabolic pathways in the liver, whereas long-term overdosing exhausts supplies of the sulfhydryl donor glutathione, leading to alternative cytochrome P-450 catalyzed oxidative metabolism and the production of the hepatotoxic metabolite *N*-acetyl-*p*-benzoquinone imine (NAPQI). Toxicity manifests as fulminant hepatic necrosis and failure in infants, children, and adults. Drug biotransformation processes are immature in neonates, very active in young children, and somewhat less active in adults. Young children are more resistant to acetaminophen-induced hepatotoxicity than adults as a result of metabolism differences: Sulfation predominates over glucuronidation in young children, leading to a reduction in NAPQI production.

Aspirin (ASA) is indicated for certain rheumatologic conditions and for inhibition of platelet adhesiveness, as in the treatment of Kawasaki disease. Concerns about Reye syndrome have resulted in a substantial decline in pediatric aspirin use (Chapter 349).

The **NSAIDs** are used widely to treat pain and fever in children. In children with juvenile rheumatoid arthritis, ibuprofen and aspirin are equally effective, but ibuprofen is associated with fewer side effects and better compliance. NSAIDs used adjunctively in surgical patients reduce opioid requirements (and therefore opioid side effects) by as much as 35-40%. Although NSAIDs can be useful postoperatively, they should be used as an adjunct to, not as a substitute for, opioids in patients with moderate to severe pain.

Ketorolac, an IV NSAID, is useful in treating moderate to severe acute pain in patients who are unable or unwilling to swallow oral NSAIDs. Intravenous ibuprofen is approved in the USA for the management of pain and fever for 5 days or less, although there is no pediatric indication in the package labeling. In Europe, IV ibuprofen is used to treat pediatric pain.

Adverse effects of NSAIDs are uncommon, but they may be serious when they occur. They include gastritis with pain and bleeding; decreased renal blood flow that may reduce glomerular filtration and enhance sodium reabsorption, in some cases leading to tubular necrosis; hepatic dysfunction and liver failure; and inhibition of platelet function. Although the overall incidence of bleeding is very low, NSAIDs should not be used in the child with a bleeding diathesis or at risk for bleeding or when surgical

Table 71-3 COMMONLY USED NONOPIOID MEDICATIONS

MEDICATION	DOSAGE	COMMENT(S)
Acetaminophen	10-15 mg/kg PO q4h 20-30 mg/kg/PR q4h 40 mg/kg/PR q6-8h Maximum daily dosing: 90 mg/kg/24hr (children) 60 mg/kg/24hr (infants) 30-45 mg/kg/24hr (neonates)	Little anti-inflammatory action; no antiplatelet or adverse gastric effects; over-dosing can produce fulminant hepatic failure
Aspirin	10-15 mg/kg PO q4h Maximum daily dosing: 120 mg/kg/24hr (children)	Anti-inflammatory; prolonged antiplatelet effects; may cause gastritis; associated with Reye's syndrome
Ibuprofen	8-10 mg/kg PO q6h	Anti-inflammatory; transient antiplatelet effects; may cause gastritis; extensive pediatric safety experience
Naprosyn	5-7 mg/kg PO q8-12h	Anti-inflammatory; transient antiplatelet effects; may cause gastritis; more prolonged duration than that of ibuprofen
Ketorolac	Loading dose 0.5 mg/kg, then 0.25-0.3 mg/kg IV q6h to a maximum of 5 days; maximum dose 30 mg loading with maximum dosing of 15 mg q6h	Anti-inflammatory; reversible antiplatelet effects; may cause gastritis; useful for short-term situations in which oral dosing is not feasible
Celecoxib	3-6 mg/kg PO q12-24h	Anti-inflammatory; no antiplatelet or gastric effects; cross-reactivity with sulfa allergies
Choline magnesium salicylate	10-20 mg/kg PO q8-12h	Weak anti-inflammatory; lower risk of bleeding and gastritis than with conventional NSAIDs
Nortriptyline, amitriptyline, desipramine	0.1-0.5 mg/kg PO qhs	For neuropathic pain; facilitates sleep; may enhance opioid effect; may be useful in sickle cell pain; risk of dysrhythmia in prolonged QTc syndrome; may cause fatal dysrhythmia in overdose; FDA says agents may enhance suicidal ideation
Gabapentin	100 mg bid or tid titrated to up to 3600 mg/24h	For neuropathic pain; associated with sedation, dizziness, ataxia, headache, and behavioral changes
Quetiapine, risperidone, chlorpromazine, haloperidol	Quetiapine: 6.25 or 12.5 mg PO qd (hs); may use q6hr prn acute agitation with pain. Escalate dose to 25 mg/dose if needed. Risperidone: useful for PDD spectrum or tic disorder and chronic pain; 0.25-1 mg (in 0.25-mg increments) qd or bid; see PDR for other dosing.	Useful when arousal is amplifying pain; often used when patient first starting SSRI and then weaned after at least 2 wk; check for normal QTc before initiating; side effects include extrapyramidal reactions (diphenhydramine may be used to treat) and sedation; in high doses, can lower the seizure threshold
Fluoxetine	10-20 mg PO qd (usually in morning)	SSRI for children with anxiety disorders in which arousal amplifies sensory signaling; useful in PDD spectrum disorders in very low doses; best to use in conjunction with psychiatric evaluation
Sucrose solution via pacifier or gloved finger	*Preterm infants* (gestational age): 28wk: 0.2mL swabbed into mouth 28-32wk: 0.2-2mL, depending on suck/swallow >32wk: 2 mL *Term infants:* 1.5-2 mL PO over 2 min	Allow 2 min before starting procedure; analgesia may last up to 8 min; the dose may be repeated once

FDA, U.S. Food and Drug Administration; IV, intravenous(ly): NSAIDs, nonsteroidal anti-inflammatory drugs; PDD, pervasive developmental disorder; PDR, *Physicians' Desk Reference*; QTc, corrected QT interval on an electrocardiogram; SSRI, selective serotonin reuptake inhibitor.

hemostasis is a prominent concern, such as after tonsillectomy. Renal injury from short-term use of ibuprofen in euvolemic children is quite rare; the risk is increased by hypovolemia or cardiac dysfunction. The safety of both ibuprofen and acetaminophen for short-term use is well established (see Table 71-3).

OPIOIDS Opioids are analgesic substances either derived from the opium poppy (opiates) or synthesized to have a similar chemical structure and mechanism of action (opioids). The older, pejorative term narcotics should not be used for these agents, because it connotes criminality and lacks pharmacologic descriptive specificity. Opioids are administered for moderate and severe pain, such as acute postoperative pain, sickle cell crisis pain, and cancer pain. Opioids can be administered by the oral, rectal, oral transmucosal, transdermal, intranasal, IV, epidural, intrathecal, subcutaneous, or intramuscular route. Historically, infants and young children have been underdosed with opioids for fear of significant respiratory side effects. With proper understanding of the pharmacokinetic and pharmacodynamics of opioids, children can receive effective relief of pain and suffering with a good margin of safety (Tables 71-4 to 71-7).

Opioids act by mimicking the actions of endogenous opioid peptides, binding to receptors in the brain, brainstem, spinal cord, and peripheral nervous system and thus leading to inhibition of nociception. Opioids have dose-dependent respiratory depressant effects, and they blunt ventilatory responses to hypoxia and hypercarbia. These respiratory depressant effects can be increased with co-administration of other sedating drugs, such as benzodiazepines or barbiturates. What was once thought to represent infants' particular sensitivity to the opioids' respiratory depressant effects we now understand to be due to infants' lower metabolic clearance of opioids and higher blood levels with frequent dosing.

Optimal use of opioids requires proactive and anticipatory management of side effects (see Table 71-6). Common side effects include constipation, nausea, vomiting, urinary retention, and pruritus. The most common, troubling but treatable side effect is constipation. Stool softeners and stimulant laxatives should be administered to most patients receiving opioids for more than a few days. Constipation also remains a problem with long-term opioid administration. A peripherally acting opiate μ receptor antagonist, methylnaltrexone, promptly and effectively reverses opioid-induced constipation in patients with chronic pain who are receiving opioids daily. The side effect of nausea typically subsides with long-term dosing, but it may require treatment with antiemetics, such as a phenothiazine, butyrophenones, antihistamines, or a serotonin receptor antagonist such as ondansetron or

Table 71-4 PEDIATRIC DOSAGE GUIDELINES FOR OPIOID ANALGESICS

DRUG	EQUI-ANALGESIC DOSES		PARENTERAL DOSING		IV:PO DOSE RATIO	ORAL DOSING		COMMENTS
	IV	Oral	<50 kg	>50 kg		<50 kg	>50 kg	
Codeine	N/A	20 mg	N/A	N/A	1:2	0.5-1 mg/kg q3-4h	30-60 mg q3-4h	Weak opioid; typically given with acetaminophen; not for severe pain; 33% of patients are not codeine responders
Fentanyl	10 µg	100 µg	0.5-1 µg/kg q1-2h 0.5-1.5 µg/kg/hr	0.5-1 µg/kg q1-2h 0.5-1.5 µg/kg/hr	Oral transmucosal: 1:10 Transdermal: 1:1	Oral transmucosal: 10 µg/kg Transdermal: 12.5-50 µg/hr	Transdermal patches available; patch reaches steady state at 24 hr and should be changed q72h	70-100 times as potent as morphine with rapid onset and shorter duration With high doses and rapid administration, can cause chest-wall rigidity Useful for short procedures; transdermal form should be used only in opioid-tolerant patients with chronic pain
Hydrocodone	N/A	1.5 mg	N/A	N/A	N/A	0.15 mg/kg	10 mg	Weak opioid; preferable to codeine; typically prescribed in form with acetaminophen
Hydromorphone	0.2 mg	0.6 mg	0.01 mg q2-4h 0.002 mg/kg/hr	0.01 mg q2-4h 0.002 mg/kg/hr	1:3	0.04-0.08 mg/kg q3-4h	2-4 mg q3-4h	5× the potency of morphine; no histamine release and fewer adverse events than morphine
Meperidine	10 mg	30 mg	0.5 mg/kg q2-4h	0.5 mg/kg q2-4h	1:4	2-3 mg/kg q3-4h	100-150 mg q3-4h	Primary use in low doses is for treatment of rigors and shivering after anesthesia or with amphotericin or blood products. Not appropriate for repeated dosing.
Methadone	1 mg	2 mg	0.1 mg/kg q8-24h	0.1 mg/kg q8-24h	1:2	0.2 mg/kg q8-12h PO; available as liquid or tablet	5-10 mg q6-8h	Duration 12-24hr; useful in certain types of chronic pain; requires additional vigilance, because it will accumulate over 72 hr and produce delayed sedation When patients who are tolerant to opioids are switched to methadone, they show incomplete cross-tolerance and improved efficacy
Morphine	1 mg	3 mg	0.05 mg/kg q2-4h 0.01-0.03 mg/kg/hr	*Bolus:* 5-8 mg q2-4h	1:3	Immediate release: 0.3 mg/kg q3-4h Sustained release*:* 20-35kg: 10-15 mg q8-12h 35-50kg: 15-30 mg q8-12h	Immediate release: 15-20 mg q3-4h Sustained release: 30-90 mg q8-12h	Potent opioid for moderate/severe pain; may cause histamine release Sustained-release form must be swallowed whole; if crushed, becomes immediate-acting, leading to acute overdose
Oxycodone	N/A	3 mg	N/A	N/A	N/A	0.1-0.2 mg q3-4h; available in liquid (1 mg/mL)	Immediate release: 5-10 mg q4h; Sustained release: 10-120 mg q8-12h	Strong opioid; potent and preferable to hydrocodone. Sustained-release form must be swallowed whole; if crushed, becomes immediate-acting, leading to acute overdose

N/A, not available.

granisetron. Pruritus and other complications during patient-controlled analgesia (PCA) with opioids may be effectively managed by low-dose IV naloxone (see Table 71-6).

One of the potent barriers to effective management of pain with opioids is the unrealistic fear of addiction held by many prescribing pediatricians and parents. Pediatricians should understand the phenomena of tolerance, dependence, withdrawal, and addiction (see Table 71-5) and should know that the rational short- or long-term use of opioids in children does not lead to a predilection or risk of addiction in a child not otherwise at risk by virtue of genetic background and social milieu. It is important for pediatricians to realize that even patients with recognized substance-abuse diagnoses are entitled to effective analgesic management, which often includes the use of opioids. When there are legitimate concerns about addiction in a patient, then safe, effective opioid pain management is often best managed by specialists in pain management and/or addictionology.

There is no longer a reason to administer opioids by intramuscular injection. Continuous IV infusion of opioids is one, effective option that permits more constant plasma concentrations and clinical effects than intermittent IV bolus dosing, without the pain associated with intramuscular injection. The most common approach in pediatric centers is to administer a low-dose basal opioid infusion, while permitting patients to use a PCA device to

Table 71-5 PRACTICAL ASPECTS OF PRESCRIBING OPIOIDS

Morphine, hydromorphone, or fentanyl is regarded as 1st choice for severe pain.
Dosing should be titrated and individualized. There is no "right" dose for everyone.
The right dose is the dose that relieves pain with a good margin of safety.
Dosing should be more cautious in infants, in patients with coexisting diseases that increase risk or impair drug clearance, and with concomitant administration of sedatives.
Anticipate and treat peripheral side effects, including constipation, nausea, and itching.
Give doses at sufficient frequency to prevent the return of severe pain before the next dose.
Use a drug delivery method, such as patient-controlled anesthesia or continuous infusions that avoid the need for "prn" decision-making.
With opioid dosing for more than 1 wk, taper gradually to avoid abstinence syndrome.
When converting between parenteral and oral opioid doses, use appropriate potency ratios (see Table 71-4).
Tolerance refers to decreasing drug effect with continued administration of a drug. Over time a patient will need higher dosing to achieve the same clinical effect; however, tolerance to sedation and respiratory depression develop more rapidly than tolerance to analgesia. Thus, with higher doses, patients do not experience oversedation or respiratory depression.
Dependence refers to the need for continued drug dosing to prevent abstinence syndrome when a drug is abruptly discontinued or its dose reduced. Abstinence syndrome is characterized by irritability, agitation, autonomic arousal, nasal congestion, piloerection, diarrhea and/or jitteriness, and yawning; it is produced by administration of potent opioids for >5-7 days.
Addiction, a psychiatric pathology, refers to psychologic craving, compulsive drug-seeking behavior, and drug use despite medical harm. Addiction has strong genetic determinants. Opioid therapy does not lead to addiction in nonsusceptible individuals, nor does opioid underdosing prevent addiction; it may in fact increase drug-seeking behavior for relief of pain (such as watching the clock), referred to as "pseudo-addiction."

Table 71-6 MANAGEMENT OF OPIOID-INDUCED ADVERSE EFFECTS

Respiratory depression	*Naloxone:* 0.01-0.02 mg/kg up to a full reversal dose of 0.1 mg/kg. May be given IV, IM, SC, or via ET. The full reversal dose should initially be used for apnea in opioid-naive patients. In opioid-tolerant patients, a reduced dose should be given and titrated up slowly to treat symptoms but prevent acute withdrawal. Ventilation may need to be supported during this process. Dose may be repeated every 2 min to a total of 10 mg. Adult maximum dose is 2 mg/dose. Give with caution to patients who are receiving long-term opioid therapy, as it may precipitate acute withdrawal. Duration of effect is 1-4 hr; therefore, close observation for renarcotization is essential.
Excessive sedation without evidence of respiratory depression	*Methylphenidate*:* 0.3 mg/kg per dose PO (typically 10-20 mg/dose to a teenager) before breakfast and lunch. Do not administer to patients receiving clonidine, because dysrhythmias may develop. *Dextroamphetamine:* 2.5-10 mg on awakening and at noon. Not for use in young children or in patients with cardiovascular disease or hypertension. *Modafinil:* Pediatric dose not established. May be useful in selected patients. Typical adult dose: 50-200 mg/day. Change opioid or decrease the dose.
Nausea and vomiting	*Metoclopramide†:* 0.15 mg/kg IV up to 10 mg/dose q6-12h for 24 hr. *Trimethobenzamide:* PO or PR if weight <15 kg, 100 mg q6h; if >15 kg, 200 mg q6h. (N.B.: Suppository contains benzocaine 2%.) Not for use in newborn infants or premature infants. 5-HT_3 blockers: *Ondansetron:* 0.15 mg/kg up to 8 mg IV q6-8h not to exceed 32 mg/day (also available as a sublingual tablet). *Granisetron:* 10 to 20 µg/kg IV q12-24h. *Prochlorperazine** (Compazine): >2 yr or >20 kg, 0.1 mg/kg per dose q8h IM or PO up to 10 mg/dose. Change opioid.
Pruritus	*Diphenhydramine:* 0.5 mg/kg IV or PO q6h. *Hydroxyzine:* 0.5 mg/kg PO q6h. *Nalbuphine:* 0.1 mg/kg IV q6h for pruritus caused by intra-axial opioids, especially fentanyl. Administer slowly over 15-20 min. May cause acute reversal of systemic µ-receptor effects and leave κ-agonism intact. *Naloxone:* 0.003 to 0.1 mg/kg/hr IV infusion (titrate up to decrease pruritus and reduce infusion if pain increases). *Cyproheptadine†:* 0.1-0.2 mg/kg PO q8-12h. Maximum dose 12 mg. Change opioid.

Constipation	Encourage water consumption, high-fiber diet, and vegetable roughage.
	Bulk laxatives: Metamucil, Maltsupex.
	Lubricants: Mineral oil 15-30 mL PO qd as needed (not for use in infants because of aspiration risk).
	Surfactants: Sodium docusate (Colace):
	  <3 yr: 10 mg PO q8h
	  3-6 yr: 15 mg PO q8h
	  6-12 yr: 50 mg PO q8h
	  >12 yr: 100 mg PO q8h
	Stimulants:
	  Bisacodyl suppository (Dulcolax):
	    <2 yr, 5 mg PR qhs
	    >2 yr 10 mg PR qhs
	Senna syrup (218 mg/5mL): >3 yr, 5 mL qhs.
	Enema: Fleet's hypertonic phosphate enema (older children; risk of hyperphosphatemia).
	Electrolytic/osmotic: Milk of magnesia; for severe impaction: polyethylene glycol (GoLYTELY, MiraLax).

Urinary retention	Straight catheterization, indwelling catheter.

*Avoid in patients taking monoamine oxidase inhibitors.
†May be associated with extrapyramidal side effects, which may be more commonly seen in children than in adults.
Modified from Burg FD, Ingelfinger JR, Polin RA, et al, editors: *Current pediatric therapy,* ed 18, Philadelphia, 2006, Saunders/Elsevier, p 16.

Table 71-7 EQUIANALGESIC DOSES AND HALF-LIVES ($T_{1/2\beta}$) OF SOME COMMONLY USED OPIOIDS

OPIOID	IM/IV DOSE (mg)	ORAL DOSE (mg)	$T_{1/2\beta}$ (hr)
Morphine	10	30	2-3
Meperidine (pethidine)	100	400	3-4
Oxycodone	15	20-30	2-3
Codeine	130	200	2-4
Fentanyl	0.15-0.2	—	3-5
Alfentanil	0.75-1.5	—	1-2
Sufentanil	0.02	—	2-3
Diamorphine	5	60	0.5*
Methadone	10	10-15	15-40
Hydromorphone	1.5	7.5	3-4
Tramadol†	100	100	5-7
Buprenorphine	0.4	0.8 (sublingual)	3-5
Pentazocine	60	150	3-5
Nalbuphine	10-20	—	2-4
Butorphanol	2	—	2-3

*Rapidly hydrolyzed to morphine.
†Only part of its analgesic action results from action on μ opioid receptors.
NOTES:
- Published reports vary in the suggested doses considered to be equianalgesic to morphine. Therefore, titration to clinical response in each patient is necessary.
- Suggested doses are the results of single-dose studies only. Therefore, use of the data to calculate total daily dose requirements may not be appropriate.
- There may be incomplete cross-tolerance between these drugs. In patients who have been receiving one opioid for a prolonged period, it is usually necessary to use a dose lower than the expected equianalgesic dose when changing to another opioid, and to titrate to effect.

Modified from Macintyre PE, Ready LB: *Acute pain management: a practical guide,* ed 2, Philadelphia, 2001, WB Saunders, p 19.

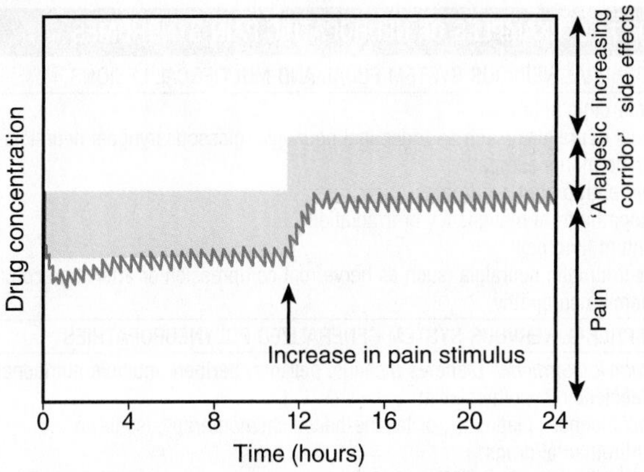

Figure 71-3 Patient-controlled analgesia is more likely to keep blood concentrations of opioid within the "analgesic corridor" and allows rapid titration if there is an increase in pain stimulus requiring higher blood levels of opioid to maintain the analgesia. (From Burg FD, Ingelfinger JR, Polin RA, et al, editors: *Current pediatric therapy,* ed 18. Philadelphia, 2006, Saunders/Elsevier, p 16.)

Table 71-8 CLASSES OF LOCAL ANESTHETIC DRUGS

Amides: Are metabolized in the liver and the elimination half-lives vary from about 1.5 hr to 3.5 hr	Lidocaine (lignocaine) Bupivacaine Prilocaine Dibucaine (cinchocaine) Mepivacaine Etidocaine Ropivacaine
Esters: Are metabolized in plasma (and to a lesser extent the liver) by pseudocholinesterases; thus their half-lives in the circulation are shorter than those of amides	Procaine Chloroprocaine Cocaine Tetracaine (amethocaine) Benzocaine

Modified from Macintyre PE, Ready LB: *Acute pain management: a practical guide,* ed 2, Philadelphia, 2001, WB Saunders, p 19.

titrate the dosage above the infusion (Chapter 70; Fig. 71-3). Compared with children given intermittent intramuscular morphine, children using PCA reported better pain scores. PCA has several other advantages: (1) dosing can be adjusted to account for individual pharmacokinetic and pharmacodynamic variation and for changing pain intensity during the day, (2) psychologically, the patient is more in control, actively coping with the pain, (3) overall opioid consumption is lower, (4) fewer side effects occur, and (5) patient satisfaction is generally much higher. Children as young as 5-6 yr can effectively use PCA. The device can be activated by parents or nurses—the latter practice known as PCA-by-proxy (PCA-P); PCA-P produces analgesia in a safe, effective manner for children who cannot activate the PCA demand button themselves because they are too young or intellectually or physically impaired. PCA overdoses occur when well-meaning, inadequately instructed parents pushed the PCA button in medically complicated situations with or without the use of PCA-P, highlighting the need for patient and family education, the use of protocols, and adequate nursing supervision.

LOCAL ANESTHETICS Local anesthetics are widely used in children for topical application, cutaneous infiltration, peripheral nerve block, epidural neuraxial blocks, intrathecal infusions, and IV infusions (Chapter 70; Table 71-8). Local anesthetics can be used with excellent safety and effectiveness. Excessive systemic concentrations can cause seizures, central nervous system (CNS) depression, arrhythmia, or cardiac depression. Unlike opioids, local anesthetics require a strict maximum dosing schedule. Pediatricians should be aware of the need to calculate these doses and adhere to guidelines. Topical local anesthetic preparations can reduce pain in diverse circumstances: suturing of lacerations, placement of peripheral IV catheters, lumbar punctures, and accessing of indwelling central venous ports. The application of tetracaine, epinephrine, and cocaine (TAC) results in good anesthesia for suturing wounds, but TAC should not be used on mucous membranes. Combinations of tetracaine with phenylephrine and lidocaine-epinephrine-tetracaine are equally as effective as TAC, eliminating the need to use a controlled substance (cocaine). EMLA, a topical eutectic mixture of lidocaine and prilocaine used to anesthetize intact skin, is commonly applied for venipuncture, lumbar puncture, and other needle procedures. EMLA is generally safe for use in neonates, but it has been associated with prilocaine-induced methemoglobinemia. In circumcision, EMLA is more effective than placebo in providing analgesia, but probably less effective than ring block of the penis. EMLA should be used cautiously for circumcision, because its use may cause redness and blistering on the penis. A small area should be tested for hypersensitivity before EMLA is more widely applied. Lidocaine cream, 5%, has replaced EMLA in many pediatric centers. Lidocaine is the most commonly used local anesthetic for cutaneous infiltration. Maximum safe doses of lidocaine are 5 mg/kg without epinephrine and 7 mg/kg with epinephrine. Although concentrated solutions (2%) are commonly available from hospital pharmacies, more dilute solutions such as 0.25% and 0.5% are as equally as effective as 1-2% solutions. The diluted solutions cause less burning discomfort on injection and permit use of larger volumes without achieving toxic doses. In the surgical setting, cutaneous infiltration is more often performed with bupivacaine 0.25% or ropivacaine 0.2% because of the much longer duration of effect. The maximum dose of these long-acting amide anesthetics is 2 to 3 mg/kg.

Neuropathic pain often responds well to the local application of a lidocaine topical patch (Lidoderm) for 12 hr per day (Table 71-9). *Peripheral neuropathic* pain may also respond well to IV lidocaine infusions, which may be used in hospital settings for

Table 71-9 EXAMPLES OF NEUROPATHIC PAIN SYNDROMES

PERIPHERAL NERVOUS SYSTEM FOCAL AND MULTIFOCAL LESIONS
Postherpetic neuralgia Cranial neuralgias (such as trigeminal neuralgia, glossopharyngeal neuralgia) Diabetic mononeuropathy Nerve entrapment syndromes Plexopathy from malignancy or irradiation Phantom limb pain Post-traumatic neuralgia (such as nerve root compression or after thoracotomy) Ischemic neuropathy
PERIPHERAL NERVOUS SYSTEM GENERALIZED POLYNEUROPATHIES
Metabolic/nutritional: Diabetes mellitus, pellagra, beriberi, multiple nutritional deficiency, hypothyroidism *Toxic:* Alcohol-, platinum-, or taxane-based chemotherapy, isoniazid, antiretroviral drugs *Infective/autoimmune:* HIV, acute inflammatory polyneuropathy (Guillain-Barré syndrome), neuroborreliosis (Bannwarth syndrome) *Heriditary:* Fabry disease *Malignancy:* Carcinomatosis *Others:* Idiopathic small fibre neuropathy
CENTRAL NERVOUS SYSTEM LESIONS
Spinal cord injury Prolapsed disc Stroke (brain infarction, spinal infarction) Multiple sclerosis Surgical lesions (such as rhizotomy, cordotomy) Complex neuropathic disorders Complex regional pain syndrome types I and II

Modified from Freynhagen R, Bennett MI: Diagnosis and management of neuropathic pain, *BMJ* 339:b3002, 2009.

Table 71-10 TREATMENT RECOMMENDATIONS FOR CENTRAL NEUROPATHIC PAIN ADAPTED FROM CURRENT EVIDENCE-BASED LITERATURE

MEDICATION CLASS/DRUG	RECOMMENDED STAGE OF TREATMENT
ANTIDEPRESSANTS	
Tricyclics (amitriptyline)	First or second
Serotonin and norepinephrine reuptake inhibitors (duloxetine, venlafaxine)	First or second
ANTICONVULSANTS	
Pregabalin	First or second
Gabapentin	First or second
Lamotrigine	Second or third (in pain after stroke)
Valproate	Third
OPIOIDS*	
Levorphanol	
MISCELLANEOUS	
Cannabinoids	Second (in multiple sclerosis)
Mexiletine	Third

*Second or third (no specification).
From Freynhagen R, Bennett MI: Diagnosis and management of neuropathic pain, *BMJ* 339:b3002, 2009.

refractory pain, complex regional pain syndromes, and pain associated with malignancies or the therapy of malignancies, such as oral mucositis following bone marrow transplantation. In these instances, 1 to 2 mg/kg/hr should be administered, and the infusion titrated to achieve a blood lidocaine level in the 2 to 5 μg/mL range, with use of twice daily therapeutic blood monitoring. Approaches to *central neuropathic pain* are listed in Table 71-10.

UNCONVENTIONAL MEDICATIONS IN PEDIATRIC PAIN *Unconventional analgesic medication* refers to a wide number of drugs that were developed for other indications but that have been found to have analgesic properties. These drugs include some antidepressants, antiepileptic drugs (AEDs), and neurotropic drugs.

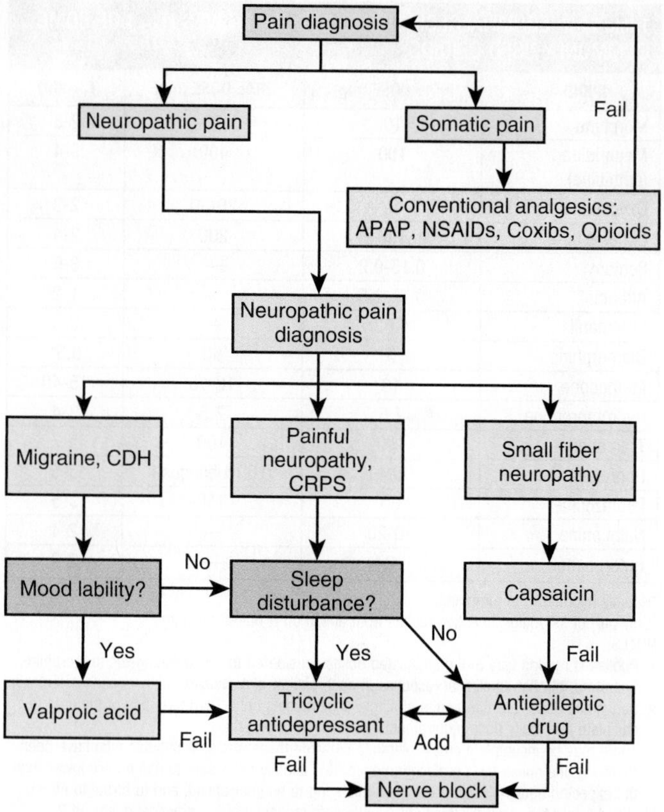

Figure 71-4 A decision tree for the selection of conventional and nonconventional analgesics. APAP, acetaminophen; CDH, chronic daily headaches; CRPS, complex regional pain syndromes; NSAIDs, nonsteroidal anti-inflammatory drugs.

The unconventional analgesics are generally used to manage neuropathic pain conditions, migraine disorders, fibromyalgia syndrome, and some forms of functional chronic abdominal pain syndromes, but they are generally not used to manage surgical, somatic, or musculoskeletal pain. Figure 71-4 presents a decision-making tree that will help the physician select the appropriate analgesic category for various types of pain.

Although several unconventional analgesics have been approved by the U.S. Food and Drug Administration (FDA) for analgesic uses, few have been specifically approved for use in youth with chronic pain. Thus, they should be used with caution, with a focus on mitigating pain to allow a child to participate effectively in therapies and return to normal activity as soon as possible. The use of psychotropic medications should be guided by the principles applied to pharmacologic treatment of any symptom or disease. Target symptoms should be identified, and medication side effects monitored. To determine dosing regimens, the physician should consider the child's weight and the effects that medical condition and other medications, such as psychotropic drugs, may have on the child's metabolism. When available, therapeutic blood level monitoring should be performed. Side effects should be addressed in detail with both parent and child, and specific instructions given for responding to possible adverse events. It may be necessary to directly address concerns about addiction, dependence, and tolerance in order to decrease treatment-related anxiety and improve compliance.

Antidepressant Medications Antidepressant medications are useful in adults with chronic pain, including neuropathic pain, headaches, and rheumatoid arthritis, independent of their effects on depressive disorders. Antidepressants' analgesic properties inhibit norepinephrine reuptake in the CNS. In children, because clinical trials have been limited, the practitioner should use antidepressants cautiously to treat chronic pain or associated depressive or anxiety symptoms. The FDA issued a "black box warning," its strongest warning, to inform the public of a small but significant increase in suicidal thoughts and attempts in children and adolescents receiving antidepressants. A meta-analysis of studies involving children and adolescents receiving antidepressants indicated that no suicides had been completed. The pediatrician should address this issue with parents of patients being treated with antidepressants and should develop monitoring plans consistent with current FDA recommendations.

TRICYCLIC ANTIDEPRESSANTS Tricyclic antidepressants (TCAs), which have been studied most in children with chronic pain, have been found effective in pain relief for symptoms including neuropathic pain, functional abdominal pain, and migraine. TCAs' efficacy may be based on inhibition of the neurochemical pathways involved in norepinephrine and serotonin reuptake and their interference with other neurochemicals involved in the perception or neural conduction of pain. Because sedation is the most common side effect of TCAs, these medications are also effective in treating the sleep disorders that frequently accompany pediatric pain. Biotransformation of TCAs is extensive in healthy children, so the child should be started on a bedtime dose, which should then be titrated to a daily divided dose, with the larger dose given at bedtime. The reader should note that pain symptoms usually remit at lower doses than those recommended or required for the treatment of mood disorders. Most children and adolescents do not require more than 0.25 mg/kg of amitriptyline or nortriptyline once a day at bedtime. Attention should be paid to hepatic microsomal enzyme metabolism, because CYP2D6 inhibitors, such as cimetidine and quinidine, can increase levels of TCAs. Anticholinergic side effects, which are remarkably uncommon in children in comparison with adults, often remit over time. Constipation, orthostatic hypotension, and dental caries due to dry mouth should be addressed by emphasizing the importance of hydration. Other side effects include weight gain, mild bone marrow suppression, and liver dysfunction. Some practitioners recommend monitoring complete blood count (CBC) and liver function values at baseline and periodically during therapy. TCA blood levels can be obtained as well, but therapeutic blood monitoring generally should occur individually, particularly if adherence, overdose, or sudden changes in mental status are an issue. Sudden cardiac death has been reported in children taking TCAs, principally desipramine, leading to concerns about cardiotoxicity. A careful personal and family history focusing on cardiac arrhythmias, heart disease, and syncope should be obtained before the initiation of treatment. If family history is positive for any of these conditions, a baseline electrocardiogram (ECG) should be obtained, with care taken to ensure that the QTc is <445 msec. We recommend that if the dose of amitriptyline or nortriptyline is increased beyond 0.5 mg/kg/day, an ECG should be performed for each dosing increase. With TCAs as with other antidepressants, physical dependence and a known discontinuation syndrome can occur. The discontinuation syndrome includes agitation, sleep disturbances, appetite changes, and gastrointestinal symptoms. These medications should be tapered slowly to assist in distinguishing among symptoms that indicate rebound, withdrawal, or the need for continuing the medication.

SEROTONIN AND SEROTONIN-NOREPINEPHRINE REUPTAKE INHIBITORS Selective serotonin reuptake inhibitors (SSRIs) have minimal efficacy in the treatment of a variety of pain syndromes in adults. SSRIs are very useful when symptoms of depressive or anxiety disorders are present and cannot be addressed adequately by nonpharmacologic means. Although many SSRIs are used in practice with children, only fluoxetine has been approved by the FDA for use in children and adolescents. SSRIs have a significantly milder side effect profile than TCAs (most side effects are transient), and they have no anticholinergic side effects. Chief side effects include gastrointestinal symptoms, headaches, agitation, insomnia, sexual dysfunction, and anxiety. Rarely, hyponatremia, or the syndrome of inappropriate antidiuretic hormone secretion, may occur. Interactions with other medications that have serotonergic effects (tramadol, trazodone, tryptophan, and triptan migraine medication) may also occur. When these medications are used in combination, there is increased likelihood that a life-threatening **serotonergic syndrome** may occur, with associated symptoms of myoclonus, hyperreflexia, autonomic instability, muscle rigidity, and delirium. There is also a **discontinuation syndrome** associated with shorter-acting SSRIs (paroxetine), which includes dizziness, lethargy, paresthesias, irritability, and vivid dreams. Dosages of medications should be tapered slowly over several weeks.

The selective serotonin-norepinephrine reuptake inhibitors (SSNRIs) duloxetine and venlafaxine have demonstrated significant efficacy with chronic neuropathic and other pain syndromes because they inhibit both serotonin and norepinephrine reuptake, and they may directly block associated pain receptors as well. Venlafaxine has no pain indication labeling, but duloxetine is FDA approved for managing neuropathic pain (diabetic neuropathy) and fibromyalgia syndrome.

Because both SSRIs and SSNRIs have fewer anticholinergic side effects than TCAs, adherence to them is better than in psychiatric populations taking TCAs. Side effects of both types of include gastrointestinal symptoms, hyperhidrosis, dizziness, and agitation, but these effects generally wane over time. Hypertension and orthostatic hypotension may occur; in addition, the patient's blood pressure should be closely followed, and appropriate hydration should be stressed. Note that whereas appetite stimulation and weight gain are associated with all TCAs, duloxetine is often associated with weight loss, frequently a desirable side effect, especially in weight-conscious adolescent females.

Antiepileptic Drugs Traditional anticonvulsants, such as carbamazepine and valproic acid, are believed to relieve chronic pain by blocking calcium channels at the cellular neuronal level, thereby suppressing spontaneous electrical activity and restoring the normal threshold to depolarization of hypersensitive nociceptive neurons, without affecting normal nerve conduction. These medications are particularly useful in patients with mood disorders and neuropathic pain. In adults, the FDA has approved carbamazepine for trigeminal neuralgia and valproic acid for migraine prophylaxis. Anticonvulsant medications generally have gastrointestinal side effects in addition to sedation, anemia, ataxia, rash, and hepatotoxicity. Carbamazepine and oxcarbazepine are associated with an increased incidence of Stevens-Johnson syndrome. Liver function values and CBC should be obtained at start of therapy (baseline) and monitored with use of both these agents. These medications have narrow therapeutic windows and may have extreme variability in therapeutic blood medication levels as well as multiple drug-drug interactions; also, they may produce liver disease and renal impairment. Drug levels should be measured with each dose increase and periodically thereafter. Carbamazepine, in particular, causes auto-induction of hepatic microsomal enzymes, which can further complicate obtaining a therapeutic medication level. Frequent pregnancy tests are useful in menstruating female adolescents taking valproic acid, because severe neural tube defects are associated with this medication.

Less toxic AEDs have supplanted the use of valproate and carbamazepine in patients with pain. These newer agents have their own, and sometimes troubling, side effect profiles, but they are far less toxic than their predecessors and they do not require monitoring of liver function, bone marrow function, or therapeutic blood levels. They are also far less lethal in accidental or deliberate overdose.

Gabapentin, the most widely prescribed AED for the management of pain disorders, demonstrates efficacy in treating children with chronic pain, particularly neuropathic pain. Gabapentin has great promise in treating chronic headaches, reflex sympathetic dystrophy, and chronic regional pain syndrome. This agent has a relatively benign side effect profile and few drug interactions. Side effects include somnolence, dizziness, and ataxia. Children occasionally demonstrate side effects not reported in adults—severe impulsive or oppositional behavior, agitation, and, occasionally, depression. These side effects do not seem to be a dose-related.

Another AED, pregabalin, works by mechanisms similar to those of gabapentin but appears to have a better side effect profile. Because it undergoes virtually no hepatic metabolism, pregabalin has no significant drug interactions, a concern in patients with chronic pain, who frequently take multiple medications—for both the pain and the underlying medical condition causing the pain.

Topiramate also demonstrates greater success than traditional anticonvulsants in treating trigeminal neuralgia in adults and in preventing migraines. Its increased efficacy is likely related to its multiple mechanisms of action. Topiramate therapy very frequently results in cognitive dysfunction and short-term memory loss, which are particularly problematic for school-aged children. The pediatrician should also be aware that in female adolescents, topiramate is associated with weight loss, whereas other anticonvulsants are typically associated with significant weight gain.

Benzodiazepines Children and adolescents with chronic pain may have depressive sleep and anxiety disorders, including generalized anxiety disorder, separation anxiety, post-traumatic stress disorder, and panic attacks. Pervasive developmental disorders are also common in this population. Psychologic factors can negatively affect a youth's ability to cope with a pain disorder; a conditioned response to pain may be to feel out of control, leading to increases in anxiety and pain. Conversely, the feeling of helplessness can prime the pain, leading the child to perseverate on the pain, think catastrophically, and feel hopeless, resulting in increased pain experience and development of a depressive disorder.

Benzodiazepines are anxiolytic medications that also have muscle relaxant effects. They are particularly appropriate in acute situations as valuable adjuncts to the management of pain in the hospital setting, because they inhibit painful muscle spasms in surgical patients, but more importantly because they suppress the anxiety that virtually every hospitalized child experiences, anxiety that interferes with restorative sleep and amplifies the child's perception of pain. Benzodiazepines are useful to calm children with anxiety and anticipatory anxiety about planned, painful procedures.

Because dependence, tolerance, and withdrawal may occur with prolonged use, benzodiazepines are generally not recommended for the routine management of *chronic pain*. In concert with psychotherapy, they help control anxiety disorders that amplify the symptoms of the perception of pain. Infrequently, benzodiazepines may cause behavioral disinhibition, psychosis-like behaviors, or, in large doses, respiratory depression. When dosing these medications, the pediatrician should consider that many benzodiazepines are metabolized by the cytochrome P-450 microsomal enzyme system. This issue may be less significant with lorazepam and oxazepam, which undergo first-pass hepatic conjugation. Side effects common to benzodiazepines include sedation, ataxia, anemia, increased bronchial secretions, and depressed mood. If a benzodiazepine is administered for more than several consecutive days, the dosage should be slowly tapered over 2 or more wk; if therapy is abruptly discontinued, autonomic instability, delirium, seizures, and profound insomnia may occur.

Antipsychotics and Major Sedatives Low doses of antipsychotic medications are often used to address more severe anxiety and agitation sometimes associated with chronic pain. The use of these medications is controversial because the associated adverse events may be severe. Typical antipsychotics, including thioridazine (Mellaril), haloperidol, and chlorpromazine, are associated with a decrease in seizure threshold, agranulocytosis, weight gain, cardiac conduction disturbances, tardive dyskinesia, orthostatic hypotension, hepatic dysfunction, and life-threatening laryngeal dystonia. These side effects are generally less severe with atypical antipsychotics. Because they may still occur, the pediatrician should obtain a baseline ECG, liver function values, and CBC. If the pediatrician is using typical antipsychotics, an inventory of movement disturbances, such as the Abnormal Involuntary Movement Scale (AIMS) test, should be performed at baseline and at every follow-up visit, because movement disorders can worsen with abrupt withdrawal of medications or can become irreversible.

Atypical antipsychotics are generally associated with less severe side effect profiles, particularly with regard to side effects such as dyskinesias and dystonias. Use of olanzapine (Zyprexa), which is particularly helpful with insomnia and severe anxiety, requires assessing and monitoring blood levels of glucose, cholesterol, and triglyceride; olanzapine's side effects may include diabetes, hypercholesterolemia, or significant weight gain. The anticholinergic side effects associated with quetiapine (Seroquel) warrant frequent monitoring of blood pressure. Risperidone at doses >6 mg may cause side effects similar to those of typical antipsychotics. Clozapine (Clozaril), which causes increased incidence of life-threatening agranulocytosis, should generally be avoided as a treatment for children and adolescents with chronic pain. Aripiprazole (Abilify) has been used for severe anxiety and/or for treatment-resistant depression. All antipsychotics are associated with the rare, but potentially lethal **neuroleptic malignant syndrome**, which includes severe autonomic instability, muscular rigidity, hyperthermia, catatonia, and altered mental status.

Nonpharmacologic Treatment of Pain

Numerous psychologic and physical treatments for relieving pain, fear, and anxiety as well as enhancing functioning have excellent safety profiles and proven effectiveness. Cognitive-behavioral treatments for childhood chronic headaches are more effective than many pharmacologic treatments, especially because children can apply their learning to new situations, increasing their sense of mastery. In addition, a combination of distraction, cognitive-behavioral interventions, and hypnosis has large effects in children. Psychologic interventions may also be effective for children with musculoskeletal and recurrent abdominal pain.

Nonpharmacologic treatments of pain may be generalized to other treatment needs. A child with cancer who learns self-hypnosis to reduce distress from lumbar punctures may successfully apply this skill to other stressful medical and nonmedical situations. When deciding whether to use nonpharmacologic techniques to treat pain, the practitioner should: (1) pay attention to the patient's environment, optimal positioning, and physical comfort; (2) because nonpharmacologic techniques alone may not work for some children, not withhold appropriate analgesics; (3) give children (and family members) developmentally and situationally appropriate information as to what to expect, given the child's medical condition, procedures, and treatments; (4) include patients and their families in decision-making to ensure an appropriate treatment choice and to optimize adherence to treatment protocols; and (5) above all, develop a **communication plan** among the different therapists, typically with the pediatrician as the case manager, so that the messages to the child and parent are consistent and the modes of therapy are organized into an **integrative team approach.**

Relaxation techniques promote muscle relaxation and reduction of anxiety, which often accompanies and increases pain. Controlled breathing and progressive muscle relaxation are commonly used relaxation techniques for preschool-aged and older children. Asking the child to focus on the breath and pretend to be blowing up a big balloon, while pursing the lips and exhaling slowly, may help induce controlled breathing.

Distraction helps a child of any age shift attention away from pain and onto other activities. Common attention sustainers in the environment include bubbles, music, video games, television, the telephone, conversation, school, and play. Asking children to tell stories, or asking parents to read to the child, and even mutual story-telling can be helpful distracters. Being involved with social, school, physical, or other activities helps the child in chronic pain regain function.

Hypnotherapy helps a child focus on an imaginative experience that is comforting, safe, fun, or intriguing. Hypnotherapy captures the child's attention, alters his sensory experiences, reduces distress, reframes pain experiences, creates time distortions, helps the child dissociate from the pain, and enhances feelings of mastery and self-control. Children with chronic pain can use metaphor, for example, imagining they have overcome something feared because of pain in real life. As the child increases mastery of imagined experiences, the enhanced sense of control can be used during actual pain rehabilitation. Hypnotherapy is best for children of school age or older.

Biofeedback involves controlled breathing, relaxation, or hypnotic techniques with a mechanical device that provides visual or auditory feedback to the child when the desired action is approximated. Common targets of actions include muscle tension, peripheral skin temperature through peripheral vasodilation, and anal control through rectal muscle contraction and relaxation. Biofeedback also enhances the child's sense of mastery and control, especially for the child who needs more "proof" of change than that generated through hypnotherapy alone.

Iyengar yoga was developed to achieve balance in mind, body, and spirit. This form of therapeutic yoga is especially effective for treating chronic pain; improving mood, energy, and sleep; and reducing anxiety. Iyengar yoga involves a series of asanas (body poses) oriented to the specific medical condition or symptoms. It uses props, such as blankets, bolsters, blocks, and belts, to support the body while the patient assumes more healing poses. Yoga promotes a sense of energy, relaxation, strength, balance, and flexibility and, over time, enhances a sense of mastery and control. In more advanced yoga, the child may learn certain types of breathing (pranayama) for added benefit.

Massage therapy involves the therapist's touching and applying varied degrees of pressure on the child's muscles. This massage is very useful for children with chronic pain and especially helpful for those with myofascial pain. There are several types of massage, including craniosacral therapy. For young children, it can be helpful to have parents learn and perform brief massage on their children before bedtime.

Individual psychotherapy can be used to address the cognitive, behavioral, and psychologic contributors to pain and pain behaviors. Assessing and treating such contributors—maladaptive coping, anxiety, depression, learning disorders, social problem-solving deficits, communication problems, relationship issues, unresolved grief or trauma, school avoidance, and other identified problems—can reduce acute distress and chronic stress load on the CNS, thereby reducing excessive arousal and pain.

Family education and/or psychotherapy, particularly cognitive-behavioral family approaches, has been shown to be effective for treating chronic pain. It may help family members to better cope with their child's and their own distress. They can learn the mechanisms and appropriate treatment of pain and alter family patterns that may inadvertently exacerbate pain. A key goal is to develop a plan for the child to manage his/her own symptoms and increase independent functioning. Parents and teachers may need guidance on developing a behavioral incentive plan to help the child return to school, gradually increase attendance, and receive tutoring, after a prolonged, pain-related absence.

Physical therapy can be especially useful for children with chronic, musculoskeletal pain and for those deconditioned from inactivity. Exercise appears to specifically benefit muscle functioning, circulation, and posture, also improving body image, body mechanics, sleep, and mood. The physical therapist and the child can develop a graded exercise plan for enhancing the child's overall function.

Acupuncture involves the placement of needles at specific acupuncture points along a meridian, or energy field, after a diagnosis of excess or deficiency energy in that meridian as the primary cause of the pain is made by the acupuncturist. Acupuncture is a feasible, popular part of a pain management plan for children with chronic pain. Acupuncture alleviates chronic nausea, fatigue, and several chronic pain states, including migraine and chronic daily headaches, abdominal pain, and myofascial pain. Acupuncture also has efficacy in adults with myofascial pain, primary dysmenorrhea, sickle cell crisis pain, and sore throat pain. The acupuncturist must relate well to children so that the experience is not traumatic, because added stress would undo the benefits gained.

Transcutaneous electrical nerve stimulation (TENS) is the use of a battery-operated tool worn on the body to send electrical impulses into the body at certain frequencies set by the machine. TENS is believed to be quite safe and can be tried for many forms of localized pain. Children often find TENS helpful and effective, but there are no randomized clinical trials of TENS for pain in children.

Music and art therapy can be especially helpful for young and nonverbal children who would otherwise have trouble with traditional talk psychotherapies. Also, many creative children can more easily express fears and negative emotions through creative expression and, with the therapist's help, learn about themselves in the process.

Dance, movement, pet therapies, and aromatherapy have also been used and may be very helpful but have not been studied in children for pain control.

Invasive Interventions in Treating Pain

Interventional neuraxial and peripheral nerve blocks provide intraoperative anesthesia, postoperative analgesia (Chapter 70), treatment of acute pain (e.g., long bone fracture and the pain of acute pancreatitis), and contribute to the management of chronic pain (e.g., headaches, abdominal pain, complex regional pain syndromes [CRPS], and cancer pain).

Regional anesthesia provides several benefits: (1) it is an alternative to or augmentation of opioid-based pain control, thereby minimizing the opioid side effects nausea, vomiting, somnolence, respiratory depression, pruritus, and constipation; (2) it generally provides better quality pain relief because it interrupts nociceptive pathways and more profoundly inhibits endocrine stress responses; (3) it results in earlier ambulation in recovering surgical patients; (4) it helps prevent atelectasis in the setting of severe chest pain; and (5) it usually results in earlier discharge from the hospital.

Regional anesthesia is considered safe and effective if performed by trained staff with the proper equipment. Most nerve blocks are performed by an anesthesiologist or pain management physician; a few are easily performed by a non-anesthesiologist with appropriate training.

HEAD AND NECK BLOCKS Primary pain syndromes of the head, such as trigeminal neuralgia, are distinctly unusual in the pediatric population, and few surgical procedures in the head and neck are amenable to regional anesthesia. Pain following tonsillectomies is not amenable to nerve blockade, and neurosurgical incisional pain is usually mitigated by local infiltration of local anesthetic into the wound margins by the surgeon. Headache disorders, very common in the pediatric age group, often respond well to block of the greater and lesser occipital nerves, which provide sensation to most of the scalp, from the anterior hairline to the cervical region. The greater occipital nerve can be blocked adjacent to the occipital artery, which can usually be palpated at the occipital ridge midway between the occipital prominence and the mastoid process. The lesser occipital nerves emerge from deeper layers midway between the greater occipital nerve and the mastoid process, where subcutaneous infiltration is effective.

UPPER EXTREMITY BLOCKS The brachial plexus block controls pain during surgical procedures or other lesions of the upper extremities. This block also protects the extremity from movement, reduces arterial spasm, and blocks sympathetic outflow to the upper extremity. The brachial plexus, responsible for cutaneous and motor innervation of the upper extremity, is an arrangement of nerve fibers originating from spinal nerves C5 through C8 and T1, extending from the neck into the axilla, arm, and hand. The brachial plexus innervates the entire upper limb, except for the trapezius muscle and an area of skin near the axilla. If pain is located proximal to the elbow, the brachial plexus may be blocked above the clavicle (roots and trunks); if the pain is located distal to the elbow, the brachial plexus may be blocked below it (cords). The block may be given as a single injection with a long-acting anesthetic (bupivacaine or ropivacaine) to provide up to 12 hr of analgesia, or given via a catheter (to infuse local anesthetic) attached to a pump that can provide continuous analgesia over days or even weeks.

Anesthesiologists frequently use an IV regional block (IVRA, or Bier block) with a local anesthetic in combination with a vasodilator such as phentolamine and an NSAID (typically ketorolac) to manage the pain of CRPS. The technique requires placement of an IV cannula into the distal part of the affected extremity, exsanguination of the extremity by elevating and wrapping it in an elastic (Esmarch) bandage, and application of a double pneumatic tourniquet, which is then inflated. Local anesthetic with additives as indicated is then injected into the IV cannula, filling the exsanguinated vasculature. The tourniquet must remain inflated for at least 30 minutes to allow fixation of local anesthetic to tissues, which reduces peak blood concentration and toxicity upon tourniquet deflation. Although the anesthetic effect is limited to the time of tourniquet inflation, analgesia for pain disorders usually persists for days, weeks, or months after the block.

TRUNK AND ABDOMINAL VISCERAL BLOCKS Truncal blocks provide somatic and visceral analgesia and anesthesia for pain or surgery of the thorax and abdominal area. Sympathetic, motor, and sensory blockade may be obtained. These blocks are often used in combination to provide optimal relief. Intercostal and paravertebral blocks may be beneficial in those patients for whom an epidural injection or catheter is contraindicated—for example, in the patient with a coagulopathy. Respiratory function is usually well maintained, and the side effects of opioid therapy are eliminated.

The intercostal, paravertebral, rectus sheath, and transverse abdominal plane (TAP) blocks are the most useful ones for pediatric chest and abdominal pain. The celiac plexus block is most useful for visceral pain caused by malignant cancer or pancreatitis. A pediatrician may easily perform an intercostal block, but the other blocks are best performed by an experienced anesthesiologist or pain physician.

The intercostal block is used to block the intercostal nerves, the anterior rami of the thoracic nerves from T1 to T11. These nerves lie inferior and posterior to each rib, with their corresponding vein and artery, where they can be blocked, generally posterior to the posterior axillary line. Ultrasound imaging of the intercostal nerves helps avoid injury to intercostal vessels or insertion of the needle through the pleura, which might result in pneumothorax.

The paravertebral block, an alternative to intercostal nerve block or epidural analgesia, is useful for pain associated with thoracotomy or with unilateral abdominal surgery, such as nephrectomy or splenectomy. Essentially this block causes multiple intercostal blocks with a single injection. The thoracic paravertebral space, lateral to the vertebral column, contains the sympathetic chain, rami communicantes, and dorsal and ventral roots of the spinal nerves. Because it is a continuous space, local anesthetic injection will provide sensory, motor, and sympathetic blockade to several dermatomes. The paravertebral block may be performed as a single injection, or, for a very prolonged effect, as a continuous infusion over several days or weeks via a catheter inserted in the paravertebral space. This block is best performed by an anesthesiologist or interventional pain physician.

Ilioinguinal and iliohypogastric nerve blocks are indicated for surgery for inguinal hernia repair, hydrocele, or orchiopexy repair as well as for chronic pain subsequent to these procedures. The first lumbar nerve divides into the iliohypogastric and ilioinguinal nerves, which emerge from the lateral border of the psoas major muscle. The iliohypogastric nerve supplies the suprapubic area as it pierces the transversus abdominis muscle and runs deep to the internal oblique muscle. The ilioinguinal nerve supplies the upper medial thigh and superior inguinal region as it also pierces the transversus abdominis muscle and runs across the inguinal canal. Ultrasound guidance has made this nerve block nearly always successful.

The **celiac plexus block** is indicated for surgery or pain of the pancreas and upper abdominal viscera. The celiac plexus, located on each side of the L1 vertebral body, contains 1-5 ganglia. The aorta lies posterior, the pancreas anterior, and the inferior vena cava lateral to these nerves. The celiac plexus receives sympathetic fibers from the greater, lesser, and least splanchnic nerves, as well as from parasympathetic fibers from the vagus nerve. Autonomic fibers from the liver, gallbladder, pancreas, stomach, spleen, kidneys, intestines, and adrenal glands originate from the celiac plexus. This block requires CT guidance or fluoroscopy in order to provide direct visualization of the appropriate landmarks and to confirm correct needle placement. The close proximity of structures such as the aorta and vena cava make this a technical procedure best performed by an anesthesiologist, interventional pain physician, or radiologist.

LOWER EXTREMITY BLOCKS Lumbar plexus and sciatic nerve blocks provide pain control for painful conditions or surgical procedures of the lower extremities, with the benefit of providing analgesia to only one extremity while preserving motor and sensory function of the other. Unlike with some caudal or lumbar epidural blocks, the patient may still bear weight bear on the affected leg. The lumbosacral plexus is an arrangement of nerve fibers originating from spinal nerves L2-L4, and S1-S3. The lumbar plexus arises from L2-L4 and divides into the lateral femoral cutaneous, femoral, and obturator nerves. These nerves supply the muscles and sensation of the upper leg, with a sensory branch of the femoral nerve extending below the knee to innervate the medial aspect of the foreleg, ankle, and foot (saphenous nerve). The sacral plexus arises from L4-S3 and divides into the major branches of the sciatic, tibial, and common peroneal nerves. These nerves in turn supply the posterior thigh, lower leg, and foot. Unlike brachial plexus blocks, whose targets are accessible, blockade of the entire lower extremity requires more than one injection because the lumbosacral sheath is not accessible. Separate injections are necessary for the posterior (sciatic) and anterior (lumbar plexus) branches, and the injections can be performed at any of several levels during the course of the nerve, as is clinically expedient. The lumbar plexus can be blocked in the back, resulting in analgesia of the femoral, lateral femoral cutaneous, and obturator nerves. Alternatively, any of these three nerves can be individually anesthetized, depending on the location of the pain. Similarly, the sciatic nerve can be anesthetized proximally as it emerges from the pelvis or more distally in the posterior thigh, or its major branches (the tibial and peroneal nerves) can be individually anesthetized. These nerve blocks are generally best performed by an anesthesiologist, interventional pain physician, or radiologist.

SYMPATHETIC BLOCKS Sympathetic blocks are useful in the diagnosis and treatment of sympathetically mediated pain, CRPS, and other neuropathic pain conditions. The peripheral sympathetic trunk is formed by the branches of the thoracic and lumbar spinal segments, and it extends from the base of the skull to the coccyx. The sympathetic chain, which consists of separate ganglia containing nerves and autonomic fibers with separate plexuses, can be differentially blocked. These separate plexuses include the stellate ganglion in the lower neck and upper thorax, the celiac plexus in the abdomen, the second lumbar plexus for the lower extremities, and the ganglion impar for the pelvis. When blocks of these plexuses are performed, sympathectomy is obtained without attendant motor or sensory anesthesia.

The **stellate ganglion block** is indicated for pain in the face or upper extremity as well as for CRPS, phantom limb pain, amputation stump pain, or circulatory insufficiency of the upper extremities. The stellate ganglion arises from spinal nerves C7-T1 and lies anterior to the first rib. It contains ganglionic fibers to the head and upper extremities. Structures in close proximity include the subclavian and vertebral arteries anteriorly, the recurrent laryngeal nerve, and the phrenic nerve. Chassaignac tubercle, the transverse process of the C6 vertebral body superior to the stellate ganglion, is a useful and easily palpable landmark for the block.

The lumbar sympathetic block addresses pain in the lower extremity, CRPS, phantom limb pain, amputation stump pain, and pain due to circulatory insufficiency. The lumbar sympathetic chain contains ganglionic fibers to the pelvis and lower extremities. It lies along the anterolateral surface of the lumbar vertebral bodies and is most often injected between the L2 and L4 vertebral bodies.

The analgesia produced by peripheral sympathetic blocks usually outlives the duration of the local anesthetic, often persisting for weeks or indefinitely. If analgesia is transient, the blocks may be performed with catheter insertion for continuous local anesthesia of the sympathetic chain over a period of days or weeks. Because precise radiographically guided placement of the needle and/or catheter is required for safety and success, sympathetic blocks are generally best performed by an anesthesiologist, interventional pain physician, or interventional radiologist.

EPIDURAL ANESTHESIA (THORACIC, LUMBAR, AND CAUDAL) Epidural anesthesia and analgesia are indicated for pain below the clavicles, management of CRPS, cancer pain unresponsive to systemic opioids, and pain limited by opioid side effects.

The 3 layers of the spinal meninges—the dura mater (outer), the arachnoid mater (middle), and the pia mater (inner)—envelop the spinal neural tissue. The subarachnoid space contains cerebrospinal fluid between the arachnoid mater and pia mater. The epidural space extends from the foramen magnum to the sacral hiatus. The epidural space, which contains fat, lymphatics, blood vessels, and the spinal nerves as they leave the spinal cord, separates the dura mater from the periosteum of the surrounding vertebral bodies. In children, the fat in the epidural space is not as dense as in adults, predisposing to greater spread of the local anesthetic from the site of injection.

Epidural local anesthetics block both sensory and sympathetic fibers, and if the local anesthetic is of sufficient concentration, they also block motor fibers. Mild hypotension may occur, although it is unusual in children younger than 8 yr. Epidural local anesthetics high in the thoracic spine may also anesthetize the sympathetic nerves to the heart (the cardiac accelerator fibers), producing bradycardia. In addition to using local anesthetics, it is routine to use opioids and α-agonists in the epidural space. These agents have their primary site of action in the spinal cord, to which they diffuse from their epidural depot. Side effects of epidural opioid administration include delayed respiratory depression, particularly when hydrophilic opioids such as morphine are used. The risk of this effect requires that children receiving epidural opioids by intermittent injection or continuous infusion be monitored by continuous pulse oximetry and nursing observation, particularly during the first 24 hr of therapy or after significant dose escalations. Respiratory depression occurring after the first 24 hr of epidural opioid administration is distinctly unusual.

Epidural clonidine, an α_2-agonist with distinct analgesic properties, is associated with minimal risk and side effects. Although product labeling indicates use only in children with severe cancer pain, it is commonly used for routine postoperative pain as well as pain syndromes such as CRPS. Mild sedation is the most common side effect of epidural clonidine, and it is not associated with respiratory depression.

Because performing epidural blockade is technical and may result in spinal cord injury, it is best done by an anesthesiologist or pain physician skilled in the technique.

INTRATHECAL ANALAGESIA Intrathecal catheters infused with opioids, clonidine, ziconotide, and local anesthetics are occasionally applicable in pediatric patients suffering from intractable pain from cancer or other conditions. Typically, intrathecal catheters are attached to an implanted electronic pump containing a drug reservoir sufficient for several months of dosing. The technique is technical and best performed by an experienced pain management physician.

NERVE ABLATION AND DESTRUCTION In infrequent pediatric cases, pain remains refractory in spite of maximal reliance upon oral and IV medications and nerve blockade. In these instances, temporary (ablation) or permanent (lytic) destruction of one or more nerves may be performed. These situations are rather extraordinary in children, and the techniques should be carefully weighed against the consideration of inducing permanent nerve destruction in a growing child with decades of life ahead. On the other hand, when pain is severe in life-limiting disease processes, the long-term considerations are less concerning, and these techniques should be discussed with a pain management specialist skilled in their performance.

CONSIDERATIONS FOR SPECIAL PEDIATRIC POPULATIONS

Pain Perception and Effects of Pain on Newborns and Infants

There are a number of sources of pain in the newborn period. These include acute pain (diagnostic and therapeutic procedures, minor surgery, monitoring), continuous pain (pain from thermal/chemical burns, postsurgical and inflammatory pain), and chronic or disease-related pain (repeated heelsticks, indwelling catheters, necrotizing enterocolitis, nerve injury, chronic conditions, thrombophlebitis). The most common sources of pain in healthy infants are acute procedures, such as heel lances, operations, and, in boys, circumcision.

In premature infants in the neonatal intensive care unit (NICU), there are more procedures. In the 1st first week of life, approximately 94% of preterm infants <28 wk of gestational age are ventilated. Other procedures are heelsticks (the most commonly performed) and airway suctioning. Only a few of these procedures are preceded by any type of analgesia. Repeated handling and acute pain episodes sensitize the neonate to increased reactivity and stress responses to subsequent procedures they undergo as neonates or children. Typical stress responses include increases in heart rate, respiratory rate, blood pressure, and intracranial pressure. Cardiac vagal tone, transcutaneous oxygen saturation, carbon dioxide levels, and peripheral blood flow are decreased. Autonomic signs include changes in skin color, vomiting, gagging, hiccupping, diaphoresis, dilated pupils, and palmar and forehead sweating.

To assess pain in the newborn, it is critical to observe the infant for facial expression, body movements, crying, and any other atypical functional behaviors. The observer must consider the context in which the behavior is experienced. The infant's state (agitated, alert, asleep) and gestational and post-gestational ages also affect behavioral stress responses.

Untreated pain in the newborn has serious short-term and longer-term consequences . There has been a shift in most NICUs to more liberal use of opioids. Nonetheless, morphine, the traditional gold standard of analgesia for acute pain, may not be very effective and may have adverse long-term consequences. No differences have been found in the incidence of severe intraventricular hemorrhage or in the mortality rate when infants receiving morphine are compared with the placebo group, and there are no changes in assessed pain from tracheal suctioning in ventilated infants receiving morphine compared with those receiving a placebo infusion. Morphine may not alleviate acute pain in ventilated preterm neonates, although there are few data on the effects of morphine and fentanyl in nonventilated newborns. The lack of opioid effects for acute pain in neonates may be due to an immaturity of opioid receptors; acute pain may cause the

Table 71-11 WORLD HEALTH ORGANIZATION ANALGESIC LADDER FOR CANCER PAIN
STEP 1
Patients who present with mild to moderate pain should be treated with a nonopioid.
STEP 2
Patients who present with moderate to severe pain or for whom the step 1 regimen fails should be treated with an oral opioid for moderate pain combined with a nonopioid analgesic.
STEP 3
Patients who present with very severe pain or for whom the step 2 regimen fails should be treated with an opioid used for severe pain, with or without a nonopioid analgesic.

uncoupling of μ opioid receptors in the forebrain. Repetitive acute pain may create central neural changes in the newborn that may have long-term consequences for later pain vulnerability, cognitive effects, and opioid tolerance. Most neonatologists use opioids in painful situations. Sucrose and pacifiers are also being used in the NICU. The effects of sucrose (sweet taste) are believed to be opioid-mediated because they are reversed with naloxone; stress and pain relief are integrated through the endogenous opioid system. Sucrose, with or without a pacifier, may be effective for acute pain and stress control. Other nonpharmacologic strategies for stress and pain control include infant care by an individual primary nurse, tactile-kinesthetic stimuli (massage), "kangaroo care," and soothing sensorial saturation.

Children with Cancer Pain

The World Health Organization (WHO) proposed an analgesic therapy model for cancer pain known as the *analgesic ladder* (Table 71-11). Designed to guide therapy in the Third World, this ladder consists of a hierarchy of oral pharmacologic interventions intended to treat pain of increasing magnitude. The hierarchy ignores modalities such as the use of nonconventional analgesics and interventional pain procedures, which are within the capability of physicians to prescribe in developed countries. Nevertheless, because oral medications are simple and efficacious, especially for home use, the ladder presents a framework for rationally using them before applying other drugs and techniques of drug administration.

Oral medications are the first line of analgesic treatment. Because NSAIDs affect platelet adhesiveness, they are typically not used. Opioid therapy is the preferred approach for moderate or severe pain. Nonopioid analgesics are used for mild pain, a weak opioid is added for moderate pain, and strong opioids are administered for more severe pain. Adjuvant analgesics can be added, and side effects and comorbid symptoms are actively managed. Determining the type and sources of the pain will help develop an effective analgesic plan. Certain treatments, such as the chemotherapeutic agent vincristine, are associated with neuropathic pain. Such pain might require anticonvulsants or tricyclic antidepressants. Organ-stretching pain from tumor growth within an organ might require strong opioids and/or radiation therapy if the tumor is radiosensitive. Organ obstruction, such as intestinal obstruction, should be diagnosed to relieve or bypass the obstruction.

It is important to consider both pharmacologic and non-pharmacologic strategies to treat pain in children with cancer.

Children with Pain Associated with Advanced Disease

Patients with advanced diseases, including cancer, AIDS, neurodegenerative disorders, and cystic fibrosis, need palliative care approaches that focus on optimal quality of life. Nonpharmacologic and pharmacologic means of management of pain and other distressing symptoms are palliative care's key components. Differences among these conditions that relate to the progression of underlying illness, associated distressing symptoms, and common emotional responses should shape individual treatment plans (Chapter 40). More than 90% of children and adolescents dying of cancer can be made comfortable by standard escalation of opioids according to the WHO protocol. A small subgroup (5%) has enormous opioid dose escalation to >100 times the standard morphine or other opiate infusion rate. In most of these cases, there is spread of solid tumors to the spinal cord, roots, or plexus, and signs of neuropathic pain are evident. Methadone given orally is often used in palliative care because of its long half-life and its targets at both opioid and *N*-methyl-D-aspartate (NMDA) receptors. The type of pain experienced by the patient (neuropathic, myofascial) should determine the need for adjunctive agents. Complementary measures, such as massage, hypnotherapy, and/or spiritual care, should also be considered in palliative care. Although the oral route of opioid administration should be encouraged, especially to facilitate care at home if possible, some children are unable to take oral opioids. Intravenous infusion with a PCA is the next choice. Small, portable infusion pumps are convenient for home use. If venous access is limited, a useful alternative is to administer opioids (especially morphine or hydromorphone, but not methadone or meperidine) through continuous subcutaneous infusion, with or without a bolus option. A small (e.g., 22-gauge) cannula is placed under the skin and secured on the thorax, abdomen, or thigh. Sites may be changed every 3-7 days, as needed. Alternative routes for opioids include the transdermal and oral transmucosal routes. These latter routes are preferred over IV and subcutaneous drug delivery when the patient is being treated at home.

Examples of Chronic and Recurrent Pain Syndromes

COMPLEX REGIONAL PAIN SYNDROMES Neuropathic pain is caused by abnormal excitability in the peripheral or central nervous system that may persist after an injury heals or inflammation subsides. The pain, which can be acute or chronic, is often described as burning or stabbing and may be associated with cutaneous hypersensitivity (allodynia). Neuropathic pain conditions may be responsible for >35% of referrals to chronic pain clinics, conditions that commonly include post-traumatic and postsurgical peripheral nerve injuries, phantom pain after amputation, pain after spinal cord injury, and pain due to metabolic neuropathies. Neuropathic pain typically responds poorly to opioids. In adults, evidence suggests the efficacy of TCAs (nortriptyline, amitriptyline) and anticonvulsants (gabapentin, pregabalin) for treatment of neuropathic pain (see Tables 71-9 and 71-10).

Complex regional pain syndrome type 1, formerly known as reflex sympathetic dystrophy (RSD), is well-described in the pediatric population. **CRPS type 1** is a syndrome of neuropathic pain that typically follows an antecedent and usually minor injury to an extremity without identifiable nerve injury. The syndrome of CRPS type 1 includes severe spontaneous neuropathic pain, hyperpathia, hyperalgesia, severe cutaneous allodynia to touch and cold, changes in blood flow (typically extremity cyanosis), and sweating. In more advanced cases, symptoms include dystrophic changes of the hair, nails, and skin, immobility of the extremity, and muscle atrophy. In the most advanced cases, symptoms include ankylosis of the joints of the extremity. Specific causal factors in CRPS type 1 in both children and adults remain elusive, although coincidental events may be noted. **CRPS type 2**, formerly referred to as causalgia, is less common.

The syndromes of CRPS type 2 and CRPS type 1 are virtually identical, except that the former is associated with a well-defined peripheral nerve injury. Treatment of CRPS in children has been extrapolated from that in adults, with some low-level evidence for efficacy of physical therapy, cognitive behavioral therapy, nerve blocks, TCAs, gabapentin, and some other related drugs. All experts in pediatric pain management agree on the value of aggressive physical therapy. Some centers provide aggressive therapy without the use of pharmacologic agents or interventional nerve blocks; unfortunately, recurrent episodes may be seen in up to 50% of patients. Physical therapy can be extraordinarily painful for children to endure; it is tolerated only by the most stoic and motivated patients. If children have difficulty enduring the pain, there is a well-established role for using pharmacologic agents with or without peripheral or central neuraxial nerve blocks to render the affected limb sufficiently analgesic so that physical therapy can be tolerated. Pharmacologic interventions include the use of AEDs such as gabapentin and/or TCAs such as amitriptyline (see Fig. 71-4). Although there is clear evidence of a peripheral inflammatory component of CRPS, with release of cytokines and other inflammatory mediators from the peripheral nervous system in the affected limb, the use of anti-inflammatory agents has been disappointing. Commonly used nerve block techniques include sympathetic nerve blocks, IV regional anesthetics, epidural analgesia, and peripheral nerve blocks. In extreme and refractory cases, more invasive strategies have been reported, including surgical sympathectomy and spinal cord stimulation. Although an array of treatments have some benefit, the mainstay of treatment remains physical therapy emphasizing desensitization, strengthening, and functional improvement. Additionally, pharmacologic agents and psychologic and complementary therapies are important components of a treatment plan. Invasive techniques, although not curative, are valuable if they permit the performance of frequent and aggressive physical therapy that cannot be carried out otherwise. Some children with CRPS become so easily sensitized that persistent and bothersome pain may develop at the site of the invasive procedure. A good biopsychosocial evaluation will help determine the orientation of the treatment components.

MYOFASCIAL PAIN DISORDERS AND FIBROMYALGIA Myofascial pain disorders are associated with tender points in the affected muscles as well as with muscle spasms (tight muscles). Treatment is targeted at relaxing the affected muscles through physical therapy, Iyengar yoga, massage, and/or acupuncture. Rarely are pharmacologic muscle relaxants helpful other than for creating tiredness at night for sleep. Dry needling or injections of local anesthetic into the tender points has been advocated, but the data do not support this as a standard treatment. Similarly, although botulinum toxin injections may be used, no data support this practice. Often poor body postures, repetitive use of a part of the body not used to that movement, or carrying heavy backpacks initiates pain. When it becomes widespread with multiples tender points, the diagnosis is juvenile fibromyalgia, which has not been proven through longitudinal studies to subsequently become adult fibromyalgia. Likely there are different subtypes of widespread pain syndromes, and physical therapy is a key component of treatment. Psychologic interventions are important if psychologic comorbidities exist. Any pain rehabilitation plan should enhance return to full function. Because there is a high incidence of chronic pain in parents of children presenting with a chronic pain condition, especially fibromyalgia, family therapy may be needed so that there is no "merging" of the parent and child's pain as a single entity in which the self-fulfilling prophecy of "your pain will become my pain" evolves.

ERYTHROMELALGIA Erythromelalgia in children is generally primary, whereas in adults it may be either primary or secondary to malignancy. Patients with this disorder exhibit red, warm, hyperperfused distal limbs. The disorder is usually bilateral, and it may involve either or both the hands and feet. Patients perceive burning pain and typically seek relief by immersing the affected extremities in ice water, sometimes so often and for so long so that skin pathology results. It is easy to distinguish erythromelalgia (or related syndromes) from CRPS. The limb afflicted with CRPS is typically cold and cyanotic, the disease is typically unilateral, and children with CRPS have cold allodynia, making immersion in cold water exquisitely painful; in erythromelalgia, ice water immersion is analgesic. The evaluation of hyperperfused limbs with burning pain should include genetic testing for Fabry's disease (FD) and screening for hematologic malignancies, with diagnosis of primary erythromelalgia being one of exclusion. The definitive treatment of FD includes enzyme replacement as disease-modifying treatment and administration of neuropathic pain medications, such as gabapentin, although the success of anti–neuropathic pain drugs in small-fiber neuropathies has not been impressive. The treatment of erythromelalgia is far more problematic. Anti–neuropathic pain medications, such as AEDs and TCAs are typically prescribed but rarely helpful (see Fig. 71-4). The pain responds well to regional anesthetic nerve blocks, but it returns immediately when the effects of the nerve block resolve. In contrast, in other neuropathic syndromes, the analgesia usually (and inexplicably) persists well after the resolution of the pharmacologic nerve block. Aspirin and even nitroprusside infusions have been reported to be of benefit with secondary erythromelalgia, but they have not been reported to be helpful in children with primary erythromelalgia. There are case reports in adults and clinical experience in children suggesting that periodic treatment with high-dose capsaicin cream is effective in alleviating the burning pain and disability of erythromelalgia. Capsaicin (essence of chili pepper) cream is a vanilloid receptor (TRPV1) agonist that depletes small-fiber peripheral nerve endings of the neurotransmitter substance P, which are important in the generation and transmission of nociceptive impulses. Once depleted, these nerve endings are no longer capable of generating spontaneous pain until the receptors regenerate, a process that takes many months.

Pain That Is Not the Result of Identifiable or Diagnosable Conditions

When it is concluded that a patient's pain is not specifically disease-related but more likely due to dysregulated neural signaling, perhaps fueled by comorbid anxiety and/or depression, it is very important for the pediatrician to (1) avoid overmedication because this can exacerbate associated disability, (2) maintain an open mind and reassess the diagnosis if the clinical presentation changes, and (3) understand and communicate to the family that pain has a biologic basis (likely related to neural signaling and neurotransmitter dysregulation), and the pain is naturally distressing to the child and family. All patients and families should receive a simple explanation of pain physiology that helps them understand the importance of (1) functional rehabilitation to normalize pain signaling, (2) the low risk of causing further injury with systematic increases in normal functioning, and (3) the risks associated with treating the pain as if it were acute. Because it is counterintuitive for most people to move a part of the body that hurts, many patients with chronic pain have atrophy or contractures of a painful extremity from disuse. Additionally, associated increases in worry and anxiety may exacerbate pain and leave the body even more vulnerable to further illness, injury, and disability. For many children with chronic pain, school absenteeism is a significant problem. A detailed assessment of possible family, cognitive, learning, social, and anxiety, or other emotional problems is indicated to ensure that a successful plan for school reentry can be developed and implemented. Home schooling for these patients has been shown to predict poor outcome and therefore is not recommended as a long-term solution. The physician is often required to intervene with the school system to compel it to develop an Individualized Educational Plan (IEP) to help the child reenter the school system, with appropriate accommodations for the child's pain and resultant disability. Helping the family develop a positive behavioral incentive plan to help their child gradually attend school for increasingly longer periods also facilitates rehabilitation.

BIBLIOGRAPHY

Please visit the Nelson Textbook of Pediatrics *website at* *www.expertconsult.com* *for the complete bibliography.*

PART X Human Genetics

Chapter 72
Integration of Genetics into Pediatric Practice

Brendan Lee

Genetic testing involves analyzing genetic material to obtain information related to a person's health status using chromosomal (cytogenetic) analysis (Chapter 76) or DNA-based testing.

DIAGNOSTIC TESTING

Diagnostic genetic testing helps explain a set of signs and/or symptoms of a disease. The list of disorders for which specific genetic tests is available is extensive. The website *www.genetests.org* provides a database of available tests.

Single-gene disorders can be tested by at least 3 different approaches: linkage analysis, array comparative genomic hybridization (aCGH), and direct mutation (DNA sequence-based) analysis, usually by DNA sequencing (Table 72-1). Linkage analysis is used if the responsible gene is mapped but not yet identified, or if it is impractical to find specific mutations, usually because of the large size and larger number of different mutations in some genes. aCGH can be used to detect large multigene deletions or duplications (copy number variations). However, with increasing resolution, single gene or smaller intragenic deletions or duplications can be detected. Direct DNA mutation analysis is preferred and is possible with the availability of the complete human genome sequence.

Linkage testing involves tracking a genetic trait through a family using closely linked polymorphic markers as a surrogate for the trait (Fig. 72-1). It requires testing an extended family and is vulnerable to several pitfalls, such as genetic recombination, genetic heterogeneity, and incorrect diagnosis in the proband. **Genetic recombination** occurs between any pair of loci, the frequency being proportional to the distance between them. This problem can be ameliorated by using very closely linked markers and, if possible, using markers that flank the specific gene. **Genetic heterogeneity** can be problematic for a linkage-based test if there are multiple distinct genomic loci that can cause the same phenotype, resulting in the risk that the locus tested for is not the one responsible for disease in the family. **Incorrect diagnosis** in the proband also leads to tracking the wrong gene. Linkage testing remains useful for several genetic conditions, though it is increasingly being superseded by the availability of direct DNA sequencing. It is critically important that genetic counseling be provided to the family to explain the complexities of interpretation of test results.

aCGH (Chapter 76) can detect copy number variation in a patient's DNA by comparing it to a standard control DNA. In so doing, it provides a level of genetic resolution between what is available with DNA sequencing and what is available with chromosome analysis. Whereas earlier technologies could only identify large deletions or duplications that might encompass multiple genes, aCGH can resolve deletions or duplications of several kilobases within one gene. In theory, this approach can detect deletion and duplication mutations that would be missed by either chromosome analysis or direct mutation testing by DNA sequencing. However, because the specific resolution and coverage of different aCGH platforms can vary tremendously for different gene regions, the sensitivity for detecting deletions and duplications can vary for different diseases and laboratories.

Direct DNA-based mutation testing avoids the pitfalls of linkage testing by detecting the specific gene mutation (i.e., sequence change). The specific approach used is customized to the biology of the gene being tested. In some disorders, one or a few distinct mutations occur in all affected individuals. This is the case in sickle cell anemia, in which the same single base substitution occurs in everyone with the disorder. In other conditions, there may be many possible mutations that account for the disorder in different individuals. Cystic fibrosis is an example: more than 1,000 distinct mutations have been found in the *CFTR* gene. Mutation analysis is challenging because no single technique can detect all possible mutations. However, with the completion of the human genome sequence and high-throughput DNA sequencing technology, the approach of choice is to directly sequence DNA that is generated by **polymerase chain reaction** (PCR) amplification of DNA isolated from peripheral blood white blood cells. The limitation of this approach is that only DNA that is amplified is sequenced, and usually this is restricted to the coding or *exonic* regions of a gene. Because mutations sometimes occur in the noncoding *intronic* regions, failure to detect a mutation does not exclude the diagnosis. Although DNA sequencing can be highly specific, it is not completely sensitive because of practical limitations of what is commercially available.

Genetic testing is interpreted in light of 3 factors: analytical validity, clinical validity, and clinical utility. **Analytical validity** is test accuracy: Does the test correctly detect the presence or absence of mutation? Most genetic tests have a very high analytical validity, assuming that human error, such as sample mix-up, has not occurred. Such errors are possible, and unlike most medical tests, a genetic test is unlikely to be repeated, because it is assumed that the result will not change over time. Therefore, human errors can go undetected for long periods of time.

Clinical validity is the degree to which the test correctly predicts presence or absence of disease. False-positive and false-negative test results can occur. **False-positive results** are more likely for predictive tests than for diagnostic tests. An important contributing factor is **non-penetrance;** an individual with an at-risk genotype might not clinically express the condition. Another factor is the finding of a genetic variant of unknown significance. Detection of a base sequence variation in an affected patient does not prove that it is the cause of the patient's disorder. Various lines of evidence are used to establish pathogenicity. These include finding the variant only in affected individuals, inferring that the variant alters the function of the gene product, determining whether the amino acid altered by the mutation is conserved in evolution, and determining whether the mutation segregates with disease in the family. In some cases, it is possible to be sure whether the variant is pathogenic or incidental. In spite of all of these approaches, it might still be impossible to definitively assign causality with 100% confidence.

False-negative results reflect an inability to detect a mutation in an affected patient. This occurs principally in disorders where genetic heterogeneity—**allelic** (different mutations occur in one causative gene) heterogeneity or **locus** (more than one gene can cause a disease) heterogeneity—is the rule. It is difficult to detect all possible mutations within a gene, because mutations can be varied in location within the gene and in the type of mutation. Direct sequencing may miss gene deletions or rearrangements, and mutations may be found within noncoding sequences such

Table 72-1 APPROACHES FOR GENETIC TESTING

TYPE OF MUTATION TESTING	RESOLUTION	ADVANTAGES	DISADVANTAGES	SAMPLE REQUIREMENTS
Linkage	Depends on location of polymorphic markers near putative disease gene	Possible when specific disease-causing genetic mutation is not identifiable or found	Can give only diagnostic probability based on likelihood of genetic recombination between presumed DNA mutation and polymorphic markers	Requires multiple family members with documented mendelian pattern of inheritance within family
Array comparative genomic hybridization (aCGH)	Several kilobases to several hundreds of kilobases	Able to detect small deletion or duplications within one or more genes	Can miss small deletions or insertions depending on resolution of the array used	Single patient sample sufficient, though having sample from biological parents can help with interpretation
Direct DNA-based testing (e.g., DNA sequencing)	Single base-pair changes	High specificity if previously described deleterious mutation is found	Can miss deletion or duplication of a segment of gene	Single patient sample sufficient, though having sample from biological parents can help with interpretation

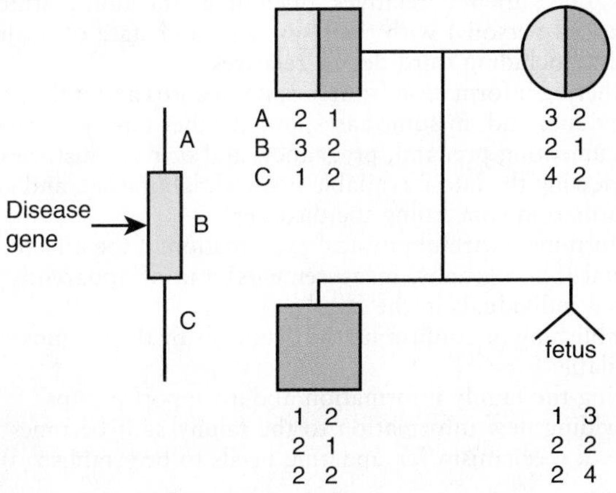

Figure 72-1 Use of linkage analysis in prenatal diagnosis of an autosomal recessive disorder. Both parents are carriers, and they have one affected son. The numbers below the symbols indicate alleles at 3 polymorphic loci: A, B, and C. Locus B resides within the disease gene. The affected son inherited the 1-2-2 chromosome from his father and the 2-1-2 chromosome from his mother. The fetus has inherited the same chromosome from the father, but the 3-2-4 chromosome from the mother and therefore is most likely to be a carrier.

as introns or the promoter; a negative DNA test does not necessarily exclude a diagnosis.

Clinical utility is the degree to which the results of a test guide clinical management. For genetic testing, clinical utility includes establishing a diagnosis that obviates the need for additional workup or guiding surveillance or treatment. Test results may also be used as a basis for genetic counseling. For some disorders, genetic testing is possible but the test results do not add to the clinical assessment. If the diagnosis and genetic implications are already clear, it might not be necessary to pursue genetic testing.

PREDICTIVE TESTING

Predictive genetic testing involves performing a test in a person who is at risk for developing a genetic disorder (**presymptomatic**), usually on the basis of family history, yet who does not manifest signs or symptoms. This is usually done for disorders that display age-dependent penetrance; the likelihood of manifesting signs and symptoms increases with age, as in cancer or Huntington disease.

A major caution with predictive testing is that the presence of a gene mutation does not necessarily mean that the disease will develop. Many of the disorders with age-dependent penetrance display *incomplete penetrance*. A person who inherits a mutation might never develop signs of the disorder. There is concern that a positive DNA test could result in stigmatization of the person and might not provide information that will guide medical management. Stigmatization might include psychological stress, but it could also include discrimination, including denial of health, life, or disability insurance or employment (Chapter 73).

It is generally agreed that predictive genetic tests should be performed for children if the results of the test will benefit the medical management of the child. Otherwise, the test should be deferred until the child has an understanding of the risks and benefits of testing and can provide informed consent. Individual states offer varying degrees of protection from discrimination on the basis of genetic testing. A major milestone in the prevention of genetic discrimination was the passage of the Genetic Information Nondiscrimination Act (GINA) in 2008, which is a federal law that prohibits discrimination in health coverage or employment based on genetic information.

PREDISPOSITIONAL TESTING

It is expected that genetic tests will become available that will predict risk of disease. Common disorders are multifactorial in etiology; there may be many different genes that contribute to risk of any specific condition (Chapter 77). Most of the genetic variants that have been found to correlate with risk of a common disease add small increments of relative risk, probably in most cases too little to guide management. It is possible that further discovery of genes that contribute to common disorders will reveal examples of variants that convey more significant levels of risk. It is also possible that testing several genes together will provide more information about risk than any individual gene variant would confer. The rationale for predispositional testing is that the results would lead to strategies aimed at risk reduction as part of a *personalized approach* to health care maintenance. This might include avoidance of environmental exposures that would increase risk of disease, medical surveillance, or, in some cases, pharmacologic treatment. The value of predispositional testing will need to be critically appraised through outcomes studies as these tests are developed.

PHARMACOGENETIC TESTING

Polymorphisms in drug metabolism genes can result in distinctive patterns of drug absorption, metabolism, excretion, or effectiveness (Chapters 56 and 77). Knowledge of individual genotypes will guide pharmacologic therapy, allowing customization of choice of drug and dosage to avoid toxicity and provide a therapeutic response. An example of this is testing for polymorphisms within the methylenetetrahydrofolate reductase (MTHFR) gene for susceptibility of potentially increased toxicity to methotrexate antimetabolite therapy for treatment of acute lymphoblastic leukemia.

72.1 Genetic Counseling

Brendan Lee

Genetic counseling is a communication process in which the genetic contribution to health is explained, along with specific

Table 72-2 INDICATIONS FOR GENETIC COUNSELING

Advanced parental age
• Maternal age ≥35 yr
• Paternal age ≥50 yr
Previous child with or family history of
• Congenital abnormality
• Dysmorphology
• Mental retardation
• Isolated birth defect
• Metabolic disorder
• Chromosome abnormality
• Single-gene disorder
Adult-onset genetic disease (presymptomatic testing)
• Cancer
• Huntington disease
Consanguinity
Teratogen exposure (occupational, abuse)
Repeated pregnancy loss or infertility
Pregnancy screening abnormality
• Maternal serum α-fetoprotein
• Maternal triple or quad screen or variant of this test
• Fetal ultrasonography
• Fetal karyotype
Heterozygote screening based on ethnic risk
• Sickle cell anemia
• Tay-Sachs, Canavan, Gaucher diseases
• Thalassemias
Follow-up to abnormal neonatal genetic testing

risks of transmission of a trait and options to manage the condition and its inheritance (Table 72-2). The counselor is expected to present information in a neutral, nondirective manner and to provide support to the individual and family to cope with decisions that are made.

Genetic counseling has evolved from a model of care that was developed in the context of prenatal diagnosis and pediatrics (see Table 72-2). For prenatal diagnosis, the task is to assess risk to a couple of having a child with a genetic condition and to advise the couple about options to manage that risk, including reproductive options such as artificial insemination and prenatal or preimplantation genetic diagnosis. In pediatrics, the task is to establish a diagnosis in a child, provide longitudinal care for the child, and advise the parents about risk of recurrence as well as options to deal with that risk.

The genetic counseling role has expanded, particularly with advances in understanding the genetics of adult-onset or common disorders. Genetic counseling has a major role in risk assessment for cancer, especially breast and ovarian cancer or colon cancer, for which well-defined genetic tests are available to assess risk to an individual.

TALKING TO FAMILIES

The type of information provided to a family depends on the urgency of the situation, the need to make decisions, and the need to collect additional information. There are 3 situations in which genetic counseling is particularly important.

The 1st is the **prenatal diagnosis** of a congenital anomaly or genetic disease. The need for information is urgent because a family must often decide whether to continue or to terminate a pregnancy. Risks to the mother must also be considered. The 2nd type of situation occurs when a child is born with a life-threatening congenital anomaly or genetic disease. Decisions must be made immediately with regard to how much support should be provided for the child and whether certain types of therapy should be attempted. The 3rd situation arises later in life when a diagnosis with a genetic implication is made; a couple is planning a family and there is a family history of a genetic problem, including whether one member of a couple carries a translocation or is a carrier of an abnormal gene for an autosomal recessive or X-linked disorder; an adolescent or young adult has a family history of an adult-onset genetic disorder (Huntington disease, breast cancer); unusual features are present and a diagnosis is wanting or not possible; and there is suspected exposure to a toxic substance or teratogen. It is often necessary to have several meetings with a family in this third situation. Urgency is not as much of an issue as being sure that they have as much information and as many options as are available.

GENETIC COUNSELING

Providing accurate information to families requires

- Taking a careful family history and constructing a pedigree that lists the patient's relatives (including abortions, stillbirths, deceased persons) with their sex, age, and state of health, up to and including third-degree relatives
- Gathering information from hospital records about the affected individual and, in some cases, about other family members
- Documenting prenatal, pregnancy, and delivery histories
- Reviewing the latest available medical, laboratory, and genetic information concerning the disorder
- Performing a careful physical examination of the affected individual (photographs, measurements) and of apparently unaffected individuals in the family
- Establishing or confirming the diagnosis by the diagnostic tests available
- Giving the family information about support groups
- Providing new information to the family as it becomes available (a mechanism for updating needs to be established)

Counseling sessions must include the specific condition, knowledge of the diagnosis of the particular condition, the natural history of the condition, the genetic aspects of the condition and the risk of recurrence, prenatal diagnosis and prevention, therapies and referral, support groups, and nondirective counseling.

Specific Condition or Conditions

If a specific diagnosis is made and confirmed, that should be discussed with the family and information should be provided in writing. However, often the disorder fits into a spectrum (e.g., one of many types of arthrogryposis) or the diagnosis is clinical rather than laboratory based. In those situations, the family needs to understand the limits of present knowledge and that additional research will probably lead to better information in the future.

Knowledge of the Diagnosis of the Particular Condition

Although it is not always possible to make an exact diagnosis, having a diagnosis as accurate as possible is important. Estimates of recurrence risk for various family members depend on an accurate diagnosis. When a specific diagnosis cannot be made (as in many cases of multiple congenital anomalies), the various possibilities in the differential diagnosis should be discussed with the family and empirical information should be provided. If specific diagnostic tests are available, they should be discussed. Often, empirical recurrence risks can be given even without a specific laboratory-based diagnosis. At the same time, even negative laboratory testing can further modify this risk.

Natural History of the Condition

It is very important to discuss the natural history of the specific genetic disorder in the family. Affected persons and their families have questions regarding the prognosis and potential therapy that can be answered only with knowledge of the natural history. If there are other possible diagnoses, their natural history may also be discussed. If the disorder is associated with a spectrum of clinical outcomes or complications, the worst and best scenarios, as well as treatment and referral to the appropriate specialist, should be addressed.

Genetic Aspects of the Condition and Recurrence Risk

The genetic aspects and risk of recurrence are important because all family members need to be aware of their reproductive choices. The genetics of the disorder can be explained with visual aids (e.g., diagrams of chromosomes). It is important to provide accurate occurrence and recurrence risks for various members of the family, including unaffected individuals. If a definite diagnosis cannot be made, it is necessary to use empirical recurrence risks. Counseling should give patients the necessary information to understand the various options and let the patients make their own informed decisions regarding pregnancy, adoption, artificial insemination, prenatal diagnosis, screening, carrier detection, and termination of pregnancy. It may be necessary to have more than 1 counseling session.

Prenatal Diagnosis and Prevention

Many different methods of prenatal diagnosis are available, depending on the specific genetic disorder (Chapter 90). The use of ultrasonography allows prenatal diagnosis of anatomic abnormalities such as congenital heart defects. Amniocentesis and chorionic villus sampling are used to obtain fetal tissue for analysis of chromosomal abnormalities, biochemical disorders, and DNA studies. Maternal blood or serum sampling is used for some types of screening. Fetal cells can be retrieved from the umbilical cord or from maternal blood (free fetal DNA) for testing, although mothers might harbor cells from all previous pregnancies.

Therapies and Referral

A number of genetic disorders require the care of a specialist. Girls with Turner syndrome usually need to be evaluated by an endocrinologist. Prevention of known complications is a priority. The psychologic adjustment of the family might require specific intervention. When to discuss the diagnosis of a chronic disease with the patient is always a difficult decision. The decision to do so should always involve the parents and an assessment of the maturity and capacity of the child or adolescent.

Alternative medicines or nontraditional therapies are often brought to attention by parents after exhaustive Internet searches. Such treatments should not necessarily be dismissed out of hand because the physician and counselor should serve as an important resource for helping parents navigate the maze of nonstandard treatments. Instead, the relative merits of treatments should be framed in the context of cost and benefit, scientific rationale, evidence from controlled and/or observational studies, the placebo effect, safety of the treatment, and the gaps on our own scientific knowledge base.

Support Groups

A large number of community lay support groups have been formed to provide information and to fund research on specific genetic and nongenetic conditions. An important part of genetic counseling is to give information about these groups to patients and to suggest a contact person for the families. Many groups have established websites with very helpful information; it is important to stress to families that their individual disease course will be unique.

Follow-up

Families should be encouraged to continue to ask questions and keep up with new information about the specific disorder. New developments often influence the diagnosis and therapy of specific genetic disorders. Lay support groups are a good source of new information.

Nondirective Counseling

Genetic counseling is usually nondirective; choices about reproduction are left to the family to decide what is right for them. The role of the counselor (physician, genetic counselor, nurse, medical geneticist) is to provide information in understandable terms and outline the range of options available.

72.2 Management and Treatment of Genetic Disorders

Brendan Lee

Genetic conditions are often chronic disorders; few are amenable to curative therapies. Nevertheless, many management options are available. All patients and families should be provided information about the disorder, genetic counseling, anticipatory guidance, and appropriate medical surveillance. Surgical management is available for many conditions that are associated with congenital anomalies or predisposition to tumors.

Resources for patients include the National Organization of Rare Disorders (*www.rarediseases.org*), the Genetic Alliance (*www.geneticalliance.org*), the National Library of Medicine (*www.nlm.nih.gov/medlineplus/geneticdisorders.html#specificconditions*), and a large number of disease-specific websites. A curre2nt listing of federally and privately funded clinical trials, including many for genetic diseases, is available at *ClinicalTrials.gov*.

Specific medical therapies for genetic disorders can be classified into physiologic and replacement therapies. Much effort is currently focused in developing gene and cell therapies.

PHYSIOLOGIC THERAPIES

Physiologic therapies attempt to ameliorate the phenotype of a genetic disorder by modifying the physiology of the affected individual. The underlying defect itself is not altered by treatment. Physiologic therapies are used in the treatment of **inborn errors of metabolism** (Chapter 78). These include dietary manipulation, such as avoiding phenylalanine by persons with phenylketonuria; coenzyme supplementation for some patients with methylmalonic acidemia and mitochondrial diseases; stimulation of alternative pathways to excrete ammonia for those with urea cycle disorders; bisphosphonate treatment for those with osteogenesis imperfecta to reduce bone fractures; and avoiding cigarette smoking by persons with α_1-antitrypsin deficiency. Physiologic treatments can be highly effective, but they usually need to be maintained for a lifetime because they do not affect the underlying genetic disorder. Many of these treatments are most effective when begun early in life before irreversible damage has occurred. This is the rationale for comprehensive newborn screening for inborn errors of metabolism.

Many physiologic therapies use small-molecule pharmaceuticals (e.g., to remove ammonia in those with urea cycle disorders). Pharmacologic treatments directly target a defective cellular pathway that is altered by an abnormal or a missing gene product. However, there are relatively few such therapies. One example is the development of imatinib, a small molecule tyrosine kinase inhibitor developed specifically to target the biologic pathway altered in chronic myelogenous leukemia (CML). CML is usually associated with a chromosome 9;22 translocation (the Philadelphia chromosome) that creates a fusion of the BCR protein and the *Abl* oncogene. Imatinib is a small molecule that blocks adenosine triphosphate (ATP) binding in the fusion protein; it is highly effective in treatment of CML and several other malignancies. Other examples include large-molecule biologics such as "humanized" monoclonal antibodies.

REPLACEMENT THERAPIES

Replacement therapies include replacement of a missing metabolite, an enzyme, an organ, or even a specific gene.

Enzyme Replacement

Enzyme replacement therapy (ERT) is a component of the treatment of cystic fibrosis to manage intestinal malabsorption. Pancreatic enzymes are easily administered orally, because they must be delivered to the gastrointestinal tract.

Enzyme replacement strategies are effective for some lysosomal storage disorders. Enzymes are targeted for the lysosome by modification with mannose-6-phosphate, which binds to a specific receptor. This receptor is also present on the cell surface, so lysosomal enzymes with exposed mannose-6-phosphate residues can be infused into the blood and are taken into cells and transported to lysosomes. Enzyme replacement therapies are available for Gaucher disease and Fabry disease, some mucopolysaccharidoses (I, II, VI), Niemann-Pick disease type C, and Pompe disease.

One complication of ERT is antibody response to the enzyme. The magnitude of this response is not always predictable and varies depending on the enzyme preparation and the disease. In most cases, the patient's antibody response does not affect the treatment's efficacy (e.g, in Gaucher disease), but in other situations it may be a significant hurdle (e.g., in Pompe disease).

Transplantation

Cell and organ transplantation are potentially effective approaches to replacement of a defective gene. Aside from transplantation to replace damaged tissues, transplantation of stem cells, liver, or bone marrow is also used for several diseases, mainly inborn errors of metabolism, and hematologic or immunologic disorders. A successful transplant is essentially curative, though there may be significant risks and side effects (Chapters 129-133). Cell and tissue transplantation are effective in many clinical scenarios, but there is always short-term morbidity, often associated with either surgical (liver) or preparative (bone marrow) regimens, and long-term morbidity related to chronic immunosuppression and graft failure. Bone marrow transplantation is the best example of stem cell therapy, but much effort is focused on identifying, characterizing, expanding, and using other tissue stem cells for regenerative therapies.

Alternatively, research since the early 1990s has focused on replacing a defective gene (gene therapy). In theory, if we can target the specific tissue that has a deficiency in the gene or gene product, this can offer a less invasive means of achieving a cure of a genetic disorder. Ultimately, gene therapy depends on the unique interaction of the disease pathophysiology, which is specific to the patient, and the gene delivery vehicle.

Gene-transfer vehicles include viral and nonviral approaches. Most human clinical trials have used viral vectors because of their efficiency of tissue transduction. In some diseases, such as X-linked and adenosine deaminase (ADA)-deficient severe combined immunodeficiency (SCID), clinical gene therapy is a viable and effective option (Chapter 120.1). Preliminary results suggest that gene therapy (intraocular delivery) may be effective for Leber congenital amaurosis.

BIBLIOGRAPHY

Please visit the Nelson Textbook of Pediatrics *website at* *www.expertconsult.com* *for the complete bibliography.*

Chapter 73
The Genetic Approach in Pediatric Medicine

Daryl A. Scott and Brendan Lee

With the completion of the human genome sequence and the haplotype map, investigative and diagnostic tools are available to determine the genetic contributions to uncommon and common disorders. Information about the genetic aspects of all pediatric diseases is readily available on numerous websites and in other locations (Table 73-1).

Table 73-1 USEFUL INTERNET GENETIC REFERENCE SITES

WEB ADDRESS	DATABASE
www.ncbi.nlm.nih.gov	General reference maintained by National Library of Medicine
www.ncbi.nlm.nih.gov/sites/entrez?db=omim	Online Mendelian Inheritance in Man, an extremely useful for clinicians ~20,000 entries of genetic traits indexed by gene name, symptoms, etc
www.ncbi.nlm.nih.gov/genemap	General reference to current efforts to map the human genome
www.ncbi.nlm.nih.gov/Genbank/GenbankOverview.html	Searchable repository of all DNA sequence data
www.ncbi.nlm.nih.gov/ncicgap	Cancer Genome Anatomy Project (National Cancer Institute)
www.genome.gov/	National Human Genome Research Institute; useful information about human genetics and ethics issues
www.hgmd.cf.ac.uk/ac/index.php	Human Gene Mutation Database, a searchable index of all described mutations in human genes with phenotypes and references
www.genetests.org	Directory of clinics and labs for testing genetic disorders GeneReviews contains physician-oriented reviews of common genetic disorders
http://projects.tcag.ca/variation/	A database of chromosomal alterations seen in normal controls
www.geneletter.com	Health, clinical, legal, social, and ethics issues
www.ashg.org	American Society of Human Genetics
www.acmg.net	American College of Medical Genetics
www.aap.org/VISIT/cmte18.htm	Committee on Genetics of the American Academy of Pediatrics: health supervision guidelines for common genetic disorders

THE BURDEN OF GENETIC DISORDERS IN CHILDHOOD

Genetic disorders can appear at any age, but some of the most obvious and severe diseases begin in childhood. It has been estimated that 53/1,000 children and young adults can be expected to have diseases with an important genetic component. If congenital anomalies are included, the rate increases to 79/1,000. In 1978 it was estimated that just over half of admissions to pediatric hospitals were for a genetically determined condition. By 1996, owing to changes in health care delivery and a greater understanding of the genetic basis of many disorders, that percentage rose to 71% in one large pediatric hospital in the USA, and 96% of chronic disorders leading to admission had an obvious genetic component or were influenced by genetic susceptibility. Major categories of genetic disorders include single-gene, genomic, chromosomal, and multifactorial conditions.

Individually, **single-gene disorders** are rare, but collectively they represent an important contribution to childhood disease. The hallmark of a single-gene disorder is that the phenotype is overwhelmingly determined by changes that affect an individual gene. The phenotypes associated with single-gene disorders can vary from one patient to another based on the severity of the change affecting the gene and additional modifications caused by genetic, environmental, and/or stochastic factors. This feature of genetic disease is termed **variable expressivity**. Common single-gene disorders include sickle cell anemia and cystic fibrosis.

Single-gene disorders tend to occur when changes in a gene have a profound effect on the function of the gene product. Such effects can include insufficient product (structural protein, enzyme, metabolites), loss of function, or a harmful gain of function. Testing for single-gene disorders typically involves searching for mutations most often by directly sequencing the gene and, in some cases, looking for small deletions and/or duplications that might affect the causative gene. Single-gene disorders can occur sporadically, owing to occurrence of de novo mutations (mainly true for dominant disorders), but they can also be caused by inherited changes.

The risk of having a child with a single gene disorder can vary from one population to another. In some cases this is due to the **founder effect,** in which a specific change affecting the causative gene achieves relatively high frequency in a population derived from a small number of founders. This frequency is maintained because of restricted interbreeding with persons outside of that population. This is the case for Tay-Sachs disease in Ashkenazi Jews and French Canadians. Other changes may be subject to positive selection when found in the heterozygous carrier state, such as hemoglobin mutations that confer relative resistance to malaria.

Genomic disorders are a group of diseases caused by rearrangements of the genome including deletions (loss of a copy of DNA), duplications (addition of a new copy of DNA), and inversions (altered organization of DNA). When these disorders are caused by rearrangements that affect several adjacent genes that contribute to a specific phenotype they are sometimes referred to as **contiguous gene disorders**. DiGeorge syndrome, which is caused by deletions of genes located on chromosome 22q11, is a common example. Some genomic disorders are associated with distinctive phenotypes that can be recognized clinically, and others produce nondescript phenotypes of developmental impairment with variable effects on intellect as well as growth and physical appearance. Genomic disorders are often identified by fluorescent in situ hybridization (FISH) or by array comparative genome hybridization (aCGH) technologies. Larger changes may be seen on a chromosome (cytogenetic) analysis.

Deletions, duplications, and inversions that affect whole chromosomes, or large portions of a chromosome, are commonly referred to as **chromosomal disorders.** One of the most common chromosomal disorders is Down syndrome, which is most commonly associated with the presence of an extra copy, or **trisomy,** of an entire chromosome 21. When all or a part of a chromosome is missing the disorder is referred to as **monosomy**. In some cases, only a portion of cells that make up a person's body carry the chromosomal defect. This is referred to as **mosaicism**. Translocations are another common type of chromosomal anomaly, in which a piece of one chromosome breaks off and becomes attached to a different, nonhomologous chromosome. Translocations can be balanced, meaning that although there has been a rearrangement, no material has been lost or gained; they can also be unbalanced, when some material (often at the breakpoint connecting DNA from different chromosomes) is deleted or duplicated compared to normal. Chromosomal disorders are typically identified on a chromosome analysis but may also be detected by FISH or aCGH.

Multifactorial disorders are caused by the action of multiple genes and/or gene-environmental effects. Spina bifida and isolated cleft lip or palate are common pediatric disorders that display multifactorial inheritance patterns. These traits can cluster in families but do not have a mendelian pattern of inheritance (Chapter 75). In most cases the causative genes are unknown, and genetic counseling is based on empirical data. The concept of multifactorial inheritance extends to common pediatric disorders, such as asthma and diabetes mellitus.

THE CHANGING PARADIGM OF GENETICS IN MEDICINE

Although specific treatments are not available for most genetic disorders, there are some important exceptions. Inborn errors of metabolism were the first genetic disorders to be recognized, and many are amenable to treatment by dietary manipulation (Chapter 78). These conditions result from genetically determined deficiency of specific enzymes, leading to the buildup of toxic substrates and/or deficiency of critical end products.

Individual metabolic disorders tend to be very rare, but their combined impact on the pediatric population is significant. Tandem mass spectrometry has made it relatively inexpensive to screen for a large number of these disorders in the newborn period. Use of this technology not only dramatically increases the number of metabolic disorders identified within a population but also allows treatment to be initiated at a much earlier stage in development (Chapters 72 and 78).

An area where most progress has been made regarding genetic therapies has been the lysosomal storage disorders. These are a group of metabolic diseases caused by defects in lysosomal function. Lysosomes are cellular organelles that contain specific digestive enzymes. Some of these disorders that were lethal or associated with intractable chronic illness can now be treated using specially modified enzymes that are administered by intravenous infusion. These enzymes are then taken up by cells and incorporated into lysosomes. Conditions such as Gaucher disease and Fabry disease are routinely treated using **enzyme replacement,** and similar therapies are being developed for other lysosomal disorders.

Therapeutic advances are extending to other nonmetabolic genetic disorders as well. Improvements in surgical treatment of congenital anomalies such as heart defects are extending the survival of children with birth defects or conditions such as Down syndrome. The life expectancy of those with cystic fibrosis has steadily increased, largely owing to improvements in antibiotic therapy as well as the management of chronic pulmonary disease and malabsorption. A major consequence of these advances is that an increasing percentage of affected patients are surviving into adulthood, creating a need to transition care from pediatric to adult providers.

Gene-replacement therapies have long been anticipated. However, it has proved difficult to develop safe and effective approaches for inserting genes into diseased tissues in a way that allows physiologically meaningful levels of gene expression to be maintained over long periods. The advent of therapeutics based on stem cells also offers the possibility of treatment for previously intractable disorders.

Long-standing and highly successful carrier screening programs have existed for disorders such as Tay-Sachs disease and many other rare single-gene disorders that are prevalent in specific populations. Couples are commonly offered screening for a variety of conditions, in part based on ancestry (Tay-Sachs disease, hemoglobinopathies, cystic fibrosis). Couples found to be at risk can be offered prepregnancy or prenatal testing, which is based on genetic tests aimed at detecting specific mutations.

Prenatal testing is also offered for chromosomal disorders such as Down syndrome; an increasing number of affected pregnancies are being recognized by noninvasive screening tests of maternal serum in the first and second trimester and by fetal ultrasound. Approaches to noninvasive prenatal diagnosis by sampling of fetal cells or fetal DNA in maternal blood are also being developed. In many cases, prenatal diagnosis can be confirmed by chorionic villus sampling at 10-12 wk or by amniocentesis at 16-18 wk of gestation. When a couple is at risk for a specific genetic defect, **preimplantation genetic diagnosis (PGD)** can sometimes be used to select unaffected early embryos, which are then implanted as part of an in vitro fertilization procedure. It is important that couples understand that although these approaches can be useful in detecting and, in the case of PGD, avoiding affected pregnancies, each has their limitations and none can guarantee the birth of a healthy child.

Genetic testing is increasingly available for a wide variety of both rare and relatively common genetic disorders. Genetic testing is commonly used in pediatric medicine to resolve

Table 73-2 TYPES OF GENETICS PROFESSIONALS

PROFESSIONAL	TRAINING	CERTIFICATION	ROLE
Clinical geneticist	MD or OD and residency in medical genetics	American Board of Medical Genetics	Diagnosis and management of patients with genetic disorders
Medical biochemical geneticist	Clinical geneticist with subspecialty training in biochemical disorders	American Board of Medical Genetics	Care for patients with biochemical (metabolic) disorders
Genetic counselor	MS	American Board of Genetic Counseling	Genetic counseling and coordination of care
Laboratory geneticist	MD, OD, or PhD and 2-yr fellowship	American Board of Medical Genetics	Supervision of laboratory testing in cytogenetics, biochemical genetics, or molecular genetics
Nurse-geneticist	Advanced practice nurse in genetics (master's) or genetics clinical nurse (baccalaureate)	Genetic Nursing Credentialing Commission	Nursing care of patients with genetic disorders

uncertainty regarding diagnosis and provide a basis for genetic counseling; in some instances, it can serve as a prelude for specific treatment. In the future, predictive testing for predisposition to disease could become more common. It is likely that the expansion of such testing will depend, at least in part, on the extent to which such testing can be linked to strategies to prevent disease or improve outcome (Chapter 72).

It is possible that genetic tests will come to underlie a high proportion of all medical decisions and will be seamlessly incorporated into routine medical care. One of the areas in which genetic testing is likely to make a significant impact is on individualized drug treatment. It has long been known that genetic variation in the enzymes involved in drug metabolism underlies differences in the therapeutic effect and toxicity of some drugs. As the genetic changes that underlie these variations are identified, new genetic tests may be developed that will allow physicians to tailor treatments based on individual variations in drug metabolism, responsiveness, and susceptibility to toxicity. Such advances may help to usher in a new era of personalized medical treatment.

GENETICS AND PEDIATRIC PRACTICE

Pediatricians play a critical role in providing and coordinating medical services for families affected by genetic disorders. In this role, pediatricians are likely to come in contact with, or be served by, a variety of genetics professionals. Each of these professionals has undergone a program of training and certification consistent with their clinical role (Table 73-2). In most cases, pediatricians refer children with presumed genetic disorders to a clinical geneticist. Clinical geneticists are physicians who have completed a residency in genetics and are certified by the American Board of Medical Genetics. They can provide expertise in achieving a correct diagnosis, counseling the family regarding natural history and management of the disorder as well as recurrence risk, and implementing a management and treatment plan.

As the number of identifiable genetic disorders and the scope of genetic testing increase, pediatricians and clinical geneticists will be expected to recognize children affected by relatively rare disorders and asymptomatic children who are at risk for genetic disease. Some disorders for which early treatment is critical may be added to newborn or early childhood screening panels; others will be the subject of clinical practice guidelines. It is likely that physicians will come to rely on advances in technology to help them keep pace. Such advances may include the development of computer programs that can aid in the diagnosis of rare disorders and testing panels that can help identify the etiology of genetically heterogeneous disorders—disorders with more than one genetic cause. The usefulness of simple office-based practices such as obtaining an accurate **family history** should not be underestimated.

ETHICS ISSUES

Like all medical care, genetic testing, diagnosis, and treatment should be performed confidentially. Nothing is as personal as one's genetic information, and all efforts should be made to avoid any stigma for the patient. Many people fear that results of genetic testing will put them, or their child, at risk for genetic discrimination. Genetic discrimination occurs when people are treated unfairly because of a difference in their DNA that suggests that they have a genetic disorder or are at an increased risk of developing a certain disease. In the USA, the Genetic Information Nondiscrimination Act of 2008 protects individuals from genetic discrimination at the hands of health insurers and employers but does not extend protection against discrimination from providers of life, disability, or long-term care insurance.

Like all medical decision making, the decisions about genetic testing should be based on a careful evaluation of the potential benefits and risks. In the pediatric setting, these decisions may be more difficult because physicians and parents are often called to make decisions for a child who cannot directly participate in discussions about the testing. Molecular diagnostic tests are often used to diagnose malformation syndromes, mental retardation, or other disabilities wherein there is a clear benefit to the child. In other cases, such as genetic testing for susceptibility to adult-onset diseases, it is appropriate to wait until the child or adolescent is mature enough to weigh the pros and cons and make his or her own decisions about genetic testing.

Policies regarding genetic testing of children have been issued jointly by the American Society of Human Genetics and American College of Medical Genetics (*Am J Hum Genet* 57:1233-1241, 1995) and by the American Academy of Pediatrics (AAP) (*Pediatr* 2001;107:1451-1455, 2001). The AAP recommendations include the following:

- Established newborn screening tests should be reviewed and evaluated periodically to permit modification of the program or elimination of ineffective components. The introduction of new newborn screening tests should be conducted through carefully monitored research protocols.
- Genetic tests, like most diagnostic or therapeutic endeavors for children, require a process of parent's informed consent and the older child's assent. Newborn screening programs are encouraged to evaluate protocols in which informed consent from parents is obtained. The frequency of informed refusals should be monitored. Research to improve the efficiency and effectiveness of informed consent for newborn screening is warranted.
- The AAP does not support the broad use of carrier testing or screening in children or adolescents. Additional research needs to be conducted on carrier screening in children and adolescents. The risks and benefits of carrier screening in the pediatric population should be evaluated in carefully monitored clinical trials before it is offered on a broad scale. Carrier screening for pregnant adolescents or for some adolescents considering pregnancy may be appropriate.
- Genetic testing for adult-onset conditions generally should be deferred until adulthood or until an adolescent interested in testing has developed mature decision-making capacities. The

AAP believes that genetic testing of children and adolescents to predict late-onset disorders is inappropriate when the genetic information has not been shown to reduce morbidity and mortality through interventions initiated in childhood.
- Because genetic screening and testing might not be well understood, pediatricians need to provide parents with the necessary information and counseling about the limits of genetic knowledge and treatment capabilities; the potential harm that may be done by gaining certain genetic information, including the possibilities for psychological harm, stigmatization, and discrimination; and medical conditions and disability and potential treatments and services for children with genetic conditions. Pediatricians can be assisted in managing many of the complex issues involved in genetic testing by collaboration with geneticists, genetics counselors, and prenatal care providers.
- The AAP supports the expansion of educational opportunities in human genetics for medical students, residents, and practicing physicians and the expansion of training programs for genetics professionals.

BIBLIOGRAPHY

Please visit the Nelson Textbook of Pediatrics *website at www.expertconsult.com for the complete bibliography.*

Chapter 74
The Human Genome

Daryl A. Scott and Brendan Lee

The Human Genome Project, culminating in the sequencing of the human genome, made it possible to study virtually any human gene and to explore the roles of genes in both rare and common disorders. It has also become apparent that the genome includes far more than a coded store of information to produce proteins.

For the full continuation of this chapter, please visit the Nelson Textbook of Pediatrics website at www.expertconsult.com.

Chapter 75
Patterns of Genetic Transmission

Daryl A. Scott and Brendan Lee

FAMILY HISTORY AND PEDIGREE NOTATION

The family history remains the most important screening tool for pediatricians in identifying a patient's risk for developing a wide range of diseases, from multifactorial conditions, such as diabetes and attention-deficit disorder, to single-gene disorders such as osteogenesis imperfecta and cystic fibrosis. Through a detailed family history the physician can often ascertain the mode of genetic transmission and the risks to family members. Because not all familial clustering of disease is due to genetic factors, a family history can also identify common environmental and behavioral factors that influence the occurrence of disease. The main goal of the family history is to identify genetic susceptibility, and the cornerstone of the family history is a systematic and standardized pedigree.

A **pedigree** provides a graphic depiction of a family's structure and medical history. It is important when taking a pedigree to be systematic and use standard symbols and configurations (Figs. 75-1, 75-2, 75-3, 75-4) so that anyone can read and understand the information. In the pediatric setting, the **proband** is typically the child or adolescent who is being evaluated. The proband is designated in the pedigree by an arrow.

A 3- to 4-generation pedigree should be obtained for every new patient as an initial screen for genetic disorders segregating within the family. The pedigree can provide clues to the inheritance pattern of these disorders and can aid the clinician in determining the risk to the proband and other family members. The closer the relationship of the proband to the person in the family with the genetic disorder, the greater is the shared genetic complement. **First-degree** relatives, such as a parent, full sibling, or child, share ½ their genetic information on average; 1st cousins share ⅛. Sometimes the person providing the family history may mention a distant relative who is affected with a genetic disorder. In such cases a more extensive pedigree may be needed to identify the risk to other family members. For example, a history of a distant maternally related cousin with mental retardation due to fragile X syndrome can still place a male proband at an elevated risk for this disorder.

MENDELIAN INHERITANCE

There are 3 classic forms of genetic inheritance: **autosomal dominant, autosomal recessive,** and **X-linked.** These are referred to as *mendelian inheritance forms,* after Gregor Mendel, the 19th-century monk whose experiments led to the laws of **segregation of characteristics, dominance,** and **independent assortment.** These remain the foundation of single-gene inheritance.

Autosomal Dominant Inheritance

Autosomal dominant inheritance is determined by the presence of 1 abnormal gene on one of the autosomes (chromosomes 1-22). Autosomal genes exist in pairs, with each parent contributing 1 copy. In an autosomal dominant trait, a change in 1 of the paired genes has an effect on the phenotype; this can refer to physical manifestations, behavioral characteristics, or differences detectable only through laboratory tests, even though the other copy of the gene is functioning correctly.

The pedigree for an autosomal dominant disorder (Fig. 75-5) demonstrates certain characteristics. The disorder is transmitted in a vertical (parent to child) pattern and can appear in multiple generations. This is illustrated by individual I.1 (see Fig 75-5) passing on the changed gene to II.2 and II.5. An affected individual has a 50% (1 in 2) chance of passing on the deleterious gene in *each* pregnancy and, therefore, of having a child affected by the disorder. This is referred to as the **recurrence risk** for the disorder. Unaffected individuals (family members who do not manifest the trait) do not pass the disorder to their children. Males and females are equally affected. Although not a characteristic per se, the finding of male-to-male transmission essentially confirms autosomal dominant inheritance. Vertical transmission can also be seen with X-linked traits. However, because a father passes on his Y chromosome to a son, male-to-male transmission cannot be seen with an X-linked trait. Therefore, male-to-male transmission eliminates X-linked inheritance as a possible explanation. Although male-to-male transmission can occur with Y-linked genes as well, there are very few Y-linked disorders compared with thousands having the autosomal dominant inheritance pattern.

Although parent to child transmission is a characteristic of autosomal dominant inheritance, for many patients with an autosomal dominant disorder there is no history of an affected family member. There are several possible reasons: First, the patient may represent a **new mutation** that occurred in the DNA of the egg or sperm that came together to form that individual. Second, many autosomal dominant conditions demonstrate **incomplete penetrance,** meaning that not all individuals who carry the mutation have phenotypic manifestations. In a pedigree this can appear as a **skipped generation,** in which an unaffected individual links two affected persons (Fig. 75-6). There are many potential

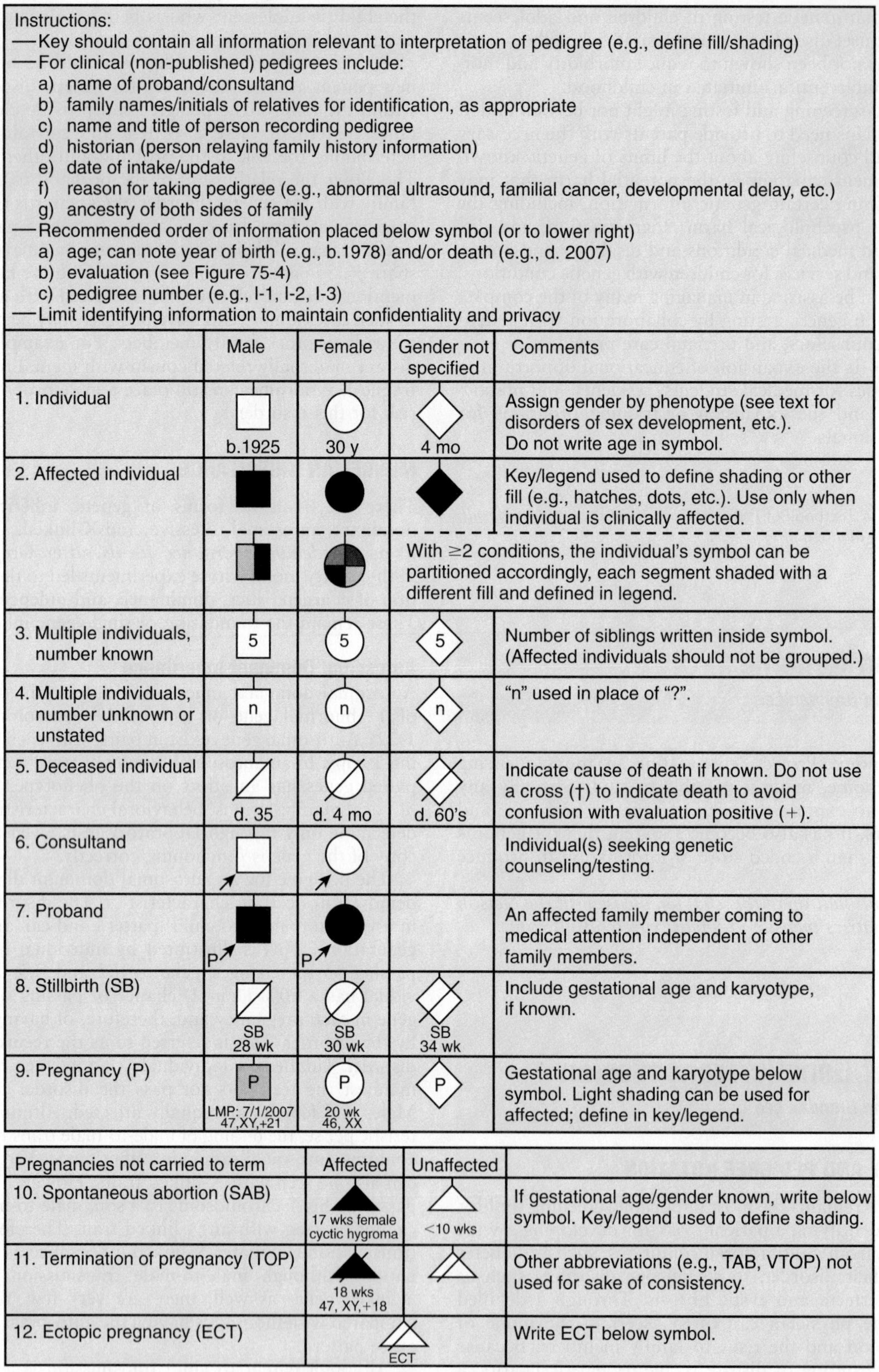
Instructions:
—Key should contain all information relevant to interpretation of pedigree (e.g., define fill/shading)
—For clinical (non-published) pedigrees include:
a) name of proband/consultand
b) family names/initials of relatives for identification, as appropriate
c) name and title of person recording pedigree
d) historian (person relaying family history information)
e) date of intake/update
f) reason for taking pedigree (e.g., abnormal ultrasound, familial cancer, developmental delay, etc.)
g) ancestry of both sides of family
—Recommended order of information placed below symbol (or to lower right)
a) age; can note year of birth (e.g., b.1978) and/or death (e.g., d. 2007)
b) evaluation (see Figure 75-4)
c) pedigree number (e.g., I-1, I-2, I-3)
—Limit identifying information to maintain confidentiality and privacy
Male
Female
Gender not specified
Comments
1. Individual
b.1925
30 y
4 mo
Assign gender by phenotype (see text for disorders of sex development, etc.). Do not write age in symbol.
2. Affected individual
Key/legend used to define shading or other fill (e.g., hatches, dots, etc.). Use only when individual is clinically affected.
With ≥2 conditions, the individual's symbol can be partitioned accordingly, each segment shaded with a different fill and defined in legend.
3. Multiple individuals, number known
5
5
5
Number of siblings written inside symbol. (Affected individuals should not be grouped.)
4. Multiple individuals, number unknown or unstated
n
n
n
"n" used in place of "?".
5. Deceased individual
d. 35
d. 4 mo
d. 60's
Indicate cause of death if known. Do not use a cross (†) to indicate death to avoid confusion with evaluation positive (+).
6. Consultand
Individual(s) seeking genetic counseling/testing.
7. Proband
P
P
An affected family member coming to medical attention independent of other family members.
8. Stillbirth (SB)
SB 28 wk
SB 30 wk
SB 34 wk
Include gestational age and karyotype, if known.
9. Pregnancy (P)
P
LMP: 7/1/2007 47,XY,+21
P
20 wk 46, XX
P
Gestational age and karyotype below symbol. Light shading can be used for affected; define in key/legend.
Pregnancies not carried to term
Affected
Unaffected
10. Spontaneous abortion (SAB)
17 wks female cyctic hygroma
<10 wks
If gestational age/gender known, write below symbol. Key/legend used to define shading.
11. Termination of pregnancy (TOP)
18 wks 47, XY,+18
Other abbreviations (e.g., TAB, VTOP) not used for sake of consistency.
12. Ectopic pregnancy (ECT)
ECT
Write ECT below symbol.

Figure 75-1 Common pedigree symbols, definitions, and abbreviations. (From Bennett RL, French KS, Resta RG, et al: Standardized human pedigree nomenclature: update and assessment of the recommendations of the National Society of Genetic Counselors, *J Genet Counsel* 17:424–433, 2008.)

reasons that a disorder exhibits incomplete penetrance, including the effect of modifier genes, environmental factors, gender, and age. Third, individuals with the same autosomal dominant mutation can manifest the disorder to different degrees. This is termed **variable expression** and is a characteristic of many autosomal dominant disorders. Fourth, some spontaneous genetic mutations occur not in the egg or sperm that forms a child but rather in a cell in the developing embryo. Such events are referred to as **somatic mutations,** and because not all cells are affected, the change is said to be *mosaic.* The resulting phenotype caused by a somatic mutation can be varied, but it is usually milder than if all cells contain the mutation. In **germline mosaicism,** the

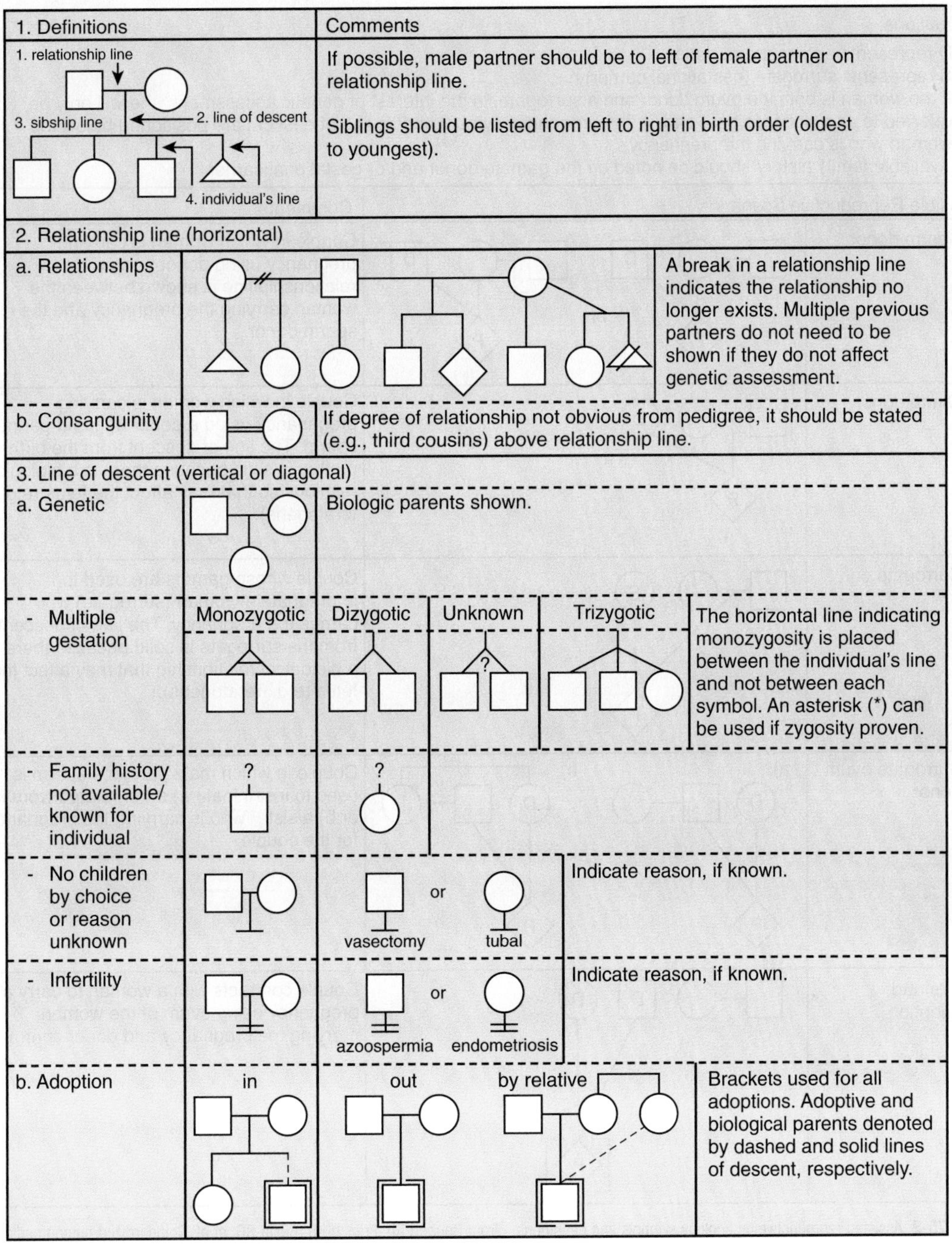

Figure 75-2 Pedigree line definitions. (From Bennett RL, French KS, Resta RG, et al: Standardized human pedigree nomenclature: update and assessment of the recommendations of the National Society of Genetic Counselors, *J Genet Counsel* 17:424–433, 2008.)

mutation occurs in cells that populate the germline that produce eggs or sperm. A germline mosaic might not have any manifestations of the disorder but might produce multiple eggs or sperm that carry the mutation.

Autosomal Recessive Inheritance

Autosomal recessive inheritance involves mutations in both copies of a gene. Examples of autosomal recessive diseases are cystic fibrosis and sickle cell disease. Characteristics of autosomal recessive traits (Fig. 75-7) include **horizontal transmission,** the observation of multiple affected members of a kindred in the same generation, but no affected family members in other generations; recurrence risk of 25% for parents with a previous affected child; males and females being equally affected, although some traits exhibit different expression in males and females and increased incidence, particularly for rare traits, in the offspring of consanguineous parents. **Consanguinity** refers to the existence of a relationship by a common ancestor and increases the chance that both parents carry a gene affected by an identical mutation that they inherited. Consanguinity between parents of a child with a suspected genetic disorder implies (but does not prove) autosomal recessive inheritance. Although consanguineous unions are uncommon in Western society, in other parts of the world (southern India, Japan, and the Middle East) they are common. The risk of a genetic disorder for the offspring of a first-cousin marriage (6-8%) is about double the risk in the general population (3-4%).

Every individual probably has several rare, harmful, recessive mutations. Because most mutations carried in the general population occur at a very low frequency, it does not make economic

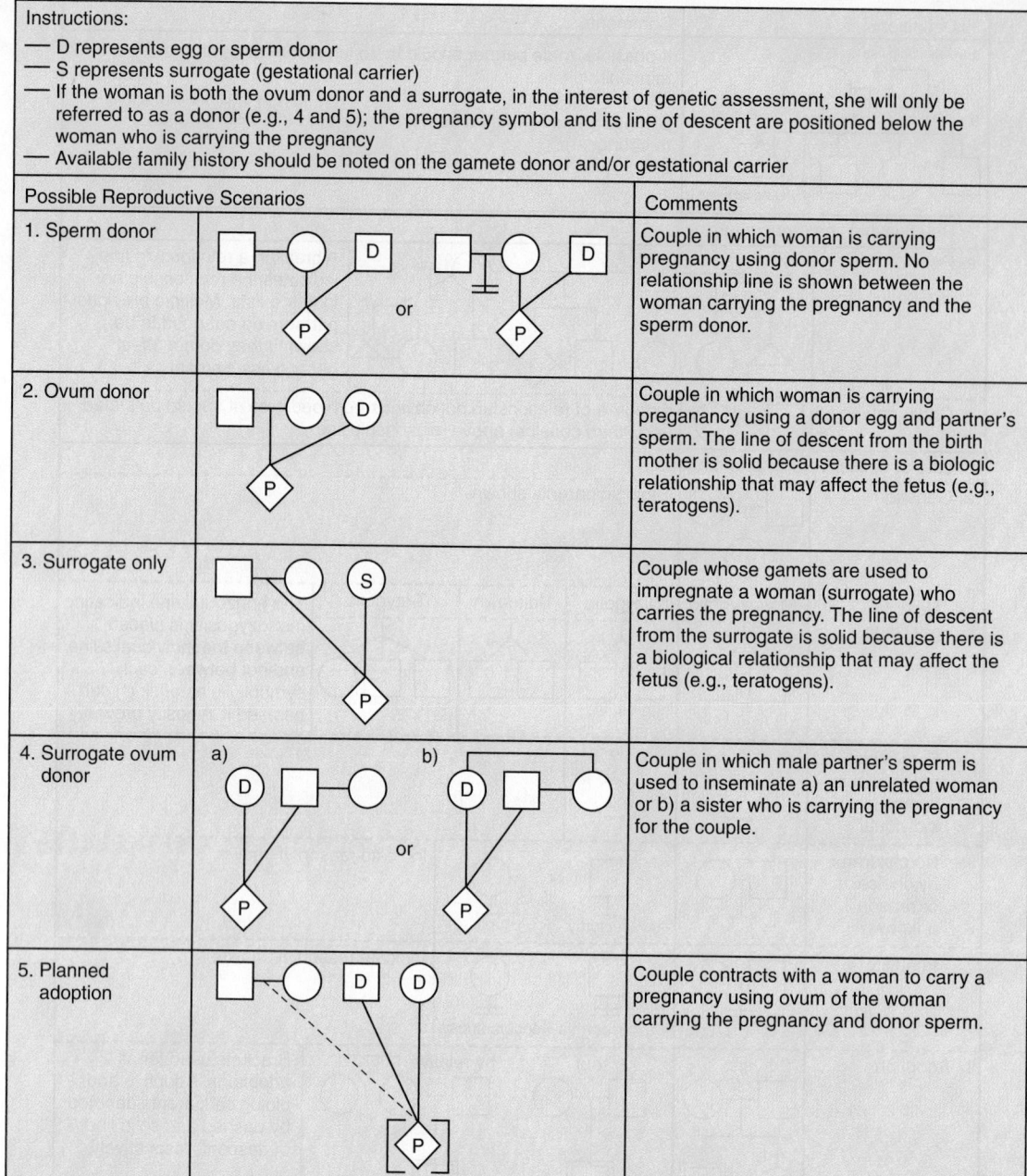

Instructions:
— D represents egg or sperm donor
— S represents surrogate (gestational carrier)
— If the woman is both the ovum donor and a surrogate, in the interest of genetic assessment, she will only be referred to as a donor (e.g., 4 and 5); the pregnancy symbol and its line of descent are positioned below the woman who is carrying the pregnancy
— Available family history should be noted on the gamete donor and/or gestational carrier

Possible Reproductive Scenarios		Comments
1. Sperm donor	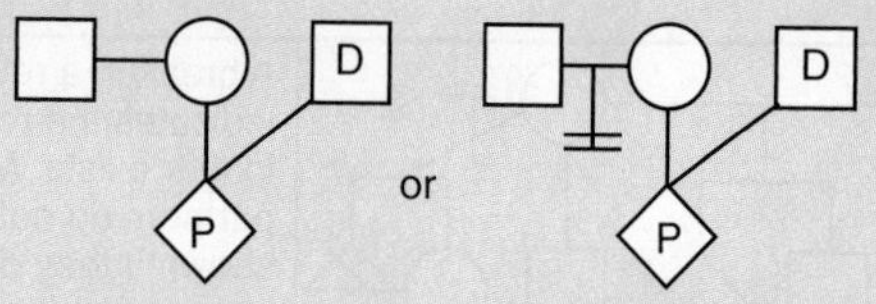	Couple in which woman is carrying pregnancy using donor sperm. No relationship line is shown between the woman carrying the pregnancy and the sperm donor.
2. Ovum donor	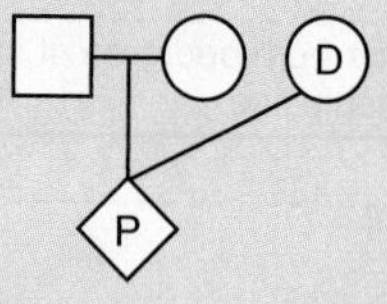	Couple in which woman is carrying preganancy using a donor egg and partner's sperm. The line of descent from the birth mother is solid because there is a biologic relationship that may affect the fetus (e.g., teratogens).
3. Surrogate only	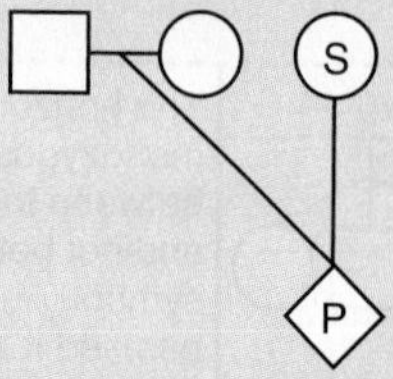	Couple whose gametes are used to impregnate a woman (surrogate) who carries the pregnancy. The line of descent from the surrogate is solid because there is a biological relationship that may affect the fetus (e.g., teratogens).
4. Surrogate ovum donor	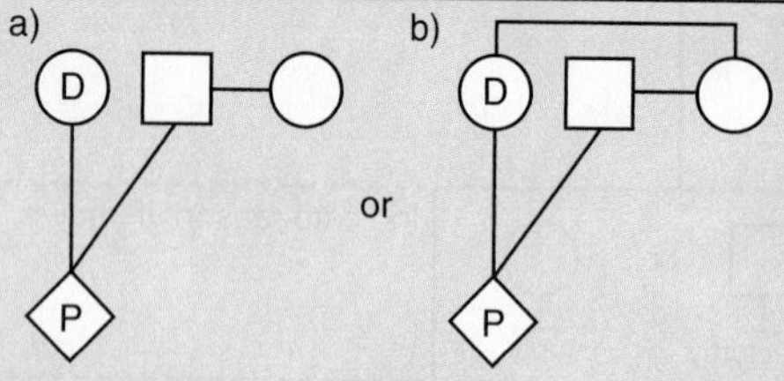	Couple in which male partner's sperm is used to inseminate a) an unrelated woman or b) a sister who is carrying the pregnancy for the couple.
5. Planned adoption	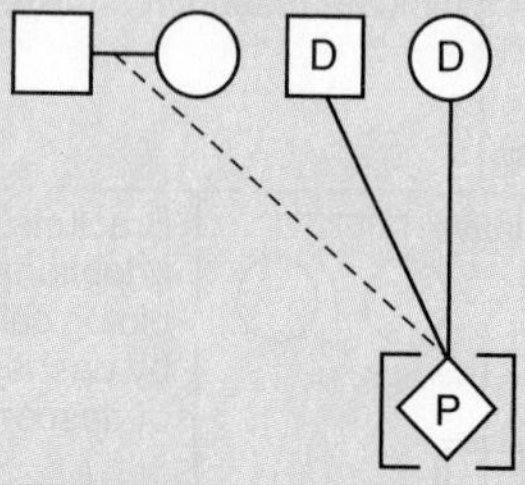	Couple contracts with a woman to carry a pregnancy using ovum of the woman carrying the pregnancy and donor sperm.

Figure 75-3 Assisted reproductive technology symbols and definitions. (From Bennett RL, French KS, Resta RG, et al: Standardized human pedigree nomenclature: update and assessment of the recommendations of the National Society of Genetic Counselors, *J Genet Counsel* 17:424–433, 2008.)

sense to screen the entire population in order to identify the small number of persons who carry these mutations. As a result, these mutations typically remain undetected unless an affected child is born to a couple who both carry mutations affecting the same gene.

However, in some genetic isolates (small populations separated by geography, religion, culture, or language) certain rare recessive mutations are far more common than in the general population. Even though there may be no known consanguinity, couples from these genetic isolates have a greater chance of sharing mutant alleles inherited from a common ancestor. Screening programs have been developed among some such groups to detect persons who carry common disease-causing mutations and therefore are at increased risk for having affected children. For example, a variety of autosomal recessive conditions are more common among Ashkenazi Jews than in the general population. Couples of Ashkenazi Jewish ancestry should be offered prenatal or preconception screening for Gaucher disease type 1 (carrier rate 1:14), cystic fibrosis (1:25), Tay-Sachs disease (1:25), familial dysautonomia (1:30), Canavan disease (1:40), glycogen storage disease type 1A (1:71), maple syrup urine disease (1:81), Fanconi anemia type C (1:89), Niemann-Pick disease type A (1:90), Bloom syndrome (1:100), mucolipidosis IV (1:120), and possibly neonatal familial hyperinsulinemic hypoglycemia.

The prevalence of carriers of certain autosomal recessive genes in some larger populations is unusually high. In such cases, heterozygote advantage is postulated. For example, the carrier frequencies of sickle cell disease in the African population and of cystic fibrosis in the northern European population are much higher than would be expected from new mutations. It is possible that heterozygous carriers have had an advantage in terms of survival and reproduction over noncarriers. In sickle cell disease, the carrier state might confer some resistance to malaria; in cystic fibrosis, the carrier state has been postulated to confer resistance

Instructions:
— E is used for evaluation to represent clinical and/or test information on the pedigree
  a. E is to be defined in key/legend
  b. If more than one evaluation, use subscript (E_1, E_2, E_3) and define in key
  c. Test results should be put in parentheses or defined in key/legend
— A symbol is shaded only when an individual is clinically symptomatic
— For linkage studies, haplotype information is written below the individual. The haplotype of interest should be on left and appropriately highlighted
  Repetitive sequences, trinucleotides, and expansion numbers are written with affected allele first and placed in parentheses
— If mutation known, identify in parentheses

Definition	Symbol	Scenario
1. Documented evaluation (*) Use only if examined/evaluated by you or your research/clinical team or if the outside evaluation has been reviewed and verified.	*	Woman with negative echocardiogram. * E− (echo)
2. Carrier—not likely to manifest disease regardless of inheritance pattern		Male carrier of Tay-Sachs disease by patient report (* not used because results not verified).
3. Asymptomatic/presymptomatic carrier—clinically unaffected at this time but could later exhibit symptoms		Woman age 25 with negative mammogram and positive BRCA1 DNA test. * 25 y E_1− (mammogram) E_2+ (5385insC BRCA1)
4. Uninformative study (u)	Eu	Man age 25 with normal physical exam and uninformative DNA test for Huntington disease (E_2). * 25 y E_1− (physical exam) E_2u (36n/18n)
5. Affected individual with positive evaluation (E+)	E+	Individual with cystic fibrosis and positive mutation study; only one mutation has currently been identified. E+(ΔF508) Eu * E+(ΔF508/u)
		10 week male fetus with a trisomy 18 karyotype. P * 10 wk E+(CVS) 47,XY,+18

Figure 75-4 Pedigree symbols of genetic evaluation and testing information. (From Bennett RL, French KS, Resta RG, et al: Standardized human pedigree nomenclature: update and assessment of the recommendations of the National Society of Genetic Counselors, *J Genet Counsel* 17:424–433, 2008.)

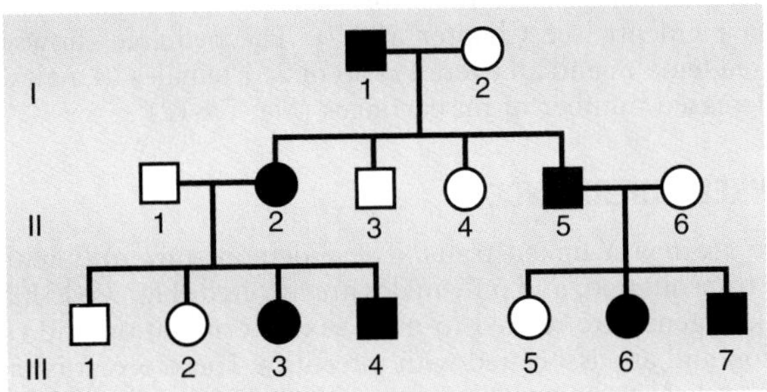

Figure 75-5 Autosomal dominant pedigree. Pedigree showing typical inheritance of a form of achondroplasia *(FGFR3)* inherited as an autosomal dominant trait. *Black,* affected patients.

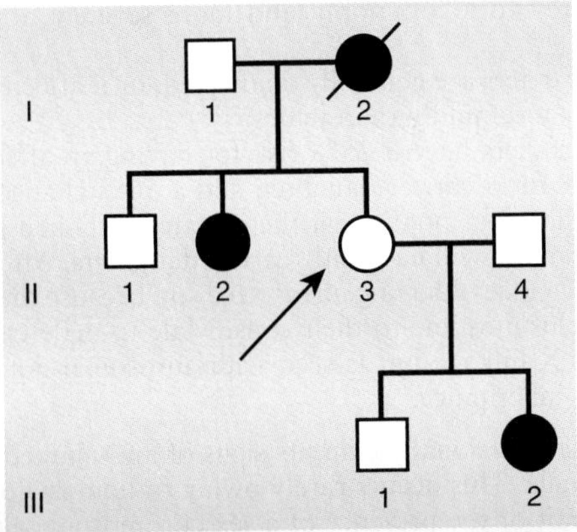

Figure 75-6 Incomplete penetrance. This family segregates a familial cancer syndrome, familial adenomatous polyposis. Individual II.3 is an obligate carrier, but there are no findings to suggest the disorder. This disorder is nonpenetrant in this individual.

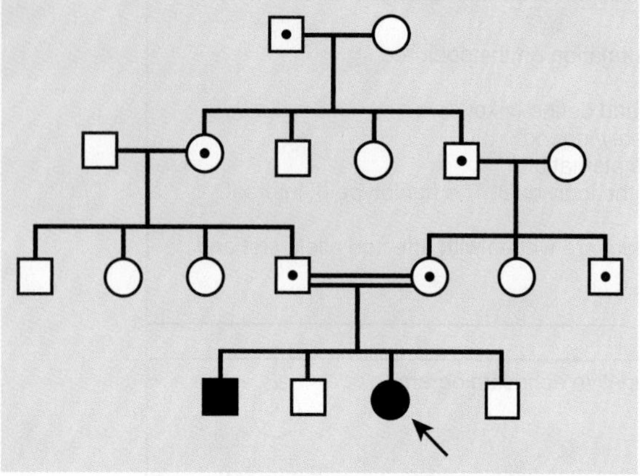

Figure 75-7 Autosomal recessive pedigree with parental consanguinity. *Central dot*, carriers; *black*, affected patients.

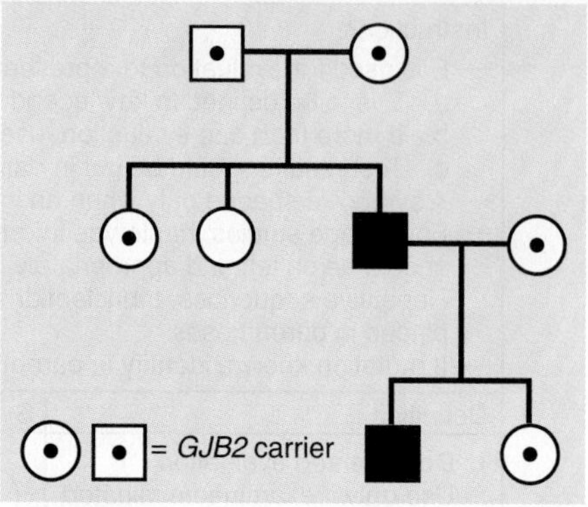

Figure 75-8 Pseudodominant inheritance. *Black*, affected (deaf); *central dot* shows carrier who is asymptomatic (unaffected).

to cholera or enteropathogenic *Escherichia coli* infections. Population-based carrier screening for cystic fibrosis is recommended for persons of northern European and Ashkenazi Jewish ancestry; population-based screening for sickle cell disease is recommended for persons of African ancestry.

If the frequency of an autosomal recessive disease is known, the frequency of the heterozygote or carrier state can be calculated from the **Hardy-Weinberg formula:**

$$p^2 + 2pq + q^2 = 1$$

where p is the frequency of one of a pair of alleles and q is the frequency of the other. For example, if the frequency of cystic fibrosis among white Americans is 1 in 2,500 (p^2), then the frequency of the heterozygote (2pq) can be calculated: If $p^2 = 1/2{,}500$, then $p = 1/50$ and $q = 49/50$; $2pq = 2 \times (1/50) \times (49/50) = 98/2500$ or 3.92%.

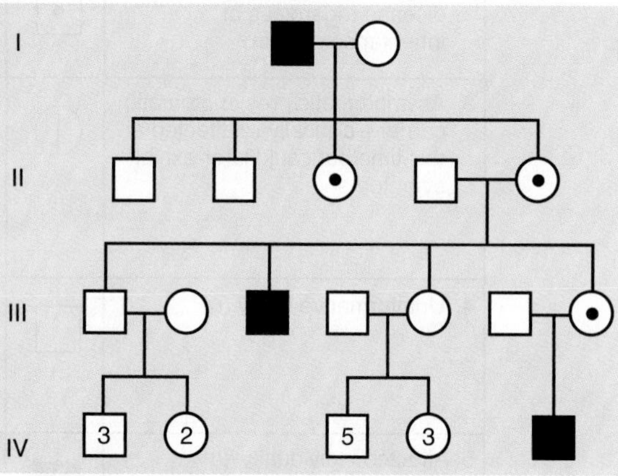

Figure 75-9 Pedigree demonstrating X-linked recessive inheritance.

Pseudodominant Inheritance

Pseudodominant inheritance refers to the observation of apparent dominant (parent to child) transmission of a known autosomal recessive disorder (Fig. 75-8). This occurs when a homozygous affected individual has a partner who is a heterozygous carrier, and it is most likely to occur for relatively common traits, such as sickle cell anemia or nonsyndromic autosomal recessive hearing loss due to mutations in *GJB2*, the gene that encodes Connexin 26.

X-Linked Inheritance

Characteristics of X-linked inheritance (Fig. 75-9) include the following:

- Males are more commonly and more severely affected than females.
- Female carriers are generally unaffected, or if affected, they are affected more mildly than males.
- Female carriers have a 25% risk for having an affected son, a 25% risk for a carrier daughter, and a 50% chance of having a child that does not inherit the mutated X-linked gene.
- Affected males will have only carrier daughters. Affected males have no chance of having an affected son because they will pass their Y chromosome to their sons. Male-to-male transmission excludes X-linkage but is seen with autosomal dominant and Y-linked inheritance.

A female occasionally exhibits signs of an X-linked trait similarly to a male. This occurs rarely owing to homozygosity for an X-linked trait or the presence of a sex chromosome abnormality (45,X or 46,XY female) or skewed or nonrandom X-inactivation. **X chromosome inactivation** occurs early in development and involves random and irreversible inactivation of most genes on one X chromosome in female cells (Fig. 75-10). In some cases, a preponderance of cells inactivates the same X chromosome, resulting in phenotypic expression of an X-linked mutation if it resides on the active chromosome. This can occur owing to chance, selection against cells that have inactivated the X chromosome carrying the normal gene, or X chromosome abnormalities that result in inactivation of the X chromosome carrying the normal gene.

Some X-linked disorders are inherited in an **X-linked dominant** fashion in which female carriers typically manifest abnormal findings. An affected man will have only affected daughters and unaffected sons, and half of the offspring of an affected woman will be affected (Fig. 75-11). Some X-linked dominant conditions are lethal in a high percentage of males. An example is incontinentia pigmenti (see Chapter 589.7). The pedigree shows only affected females and an overall ratio of 2 : 1 females to males with an increased number of miscarriages (Fig. 75-12).

Y-LINKED INHERITANCE

There are few Y-linked traits. These demonstrate *only* male-to-male transmission, and only males are affected (Fig. 75-13). Most Y-linked genes are related to male sex determination and reproduction and are associated with infertility. Therefore, it is rare to see familial transmission of a Y-linked disorder. However, advances in assisted reproductive technologies might make it possible to have familial transmission of male infertility.

Of special note is the pseudoautosomal region on the Y chromosome, the small region of homology that is shared by both Xp and Yp. Very few genes reside in this region. One of the few is *SHOX*. Heterozygous *SHOX* mutations cause **Leri-Weil dyschondrosteosis,** a rare skeletal dysplasia that involves bilateral

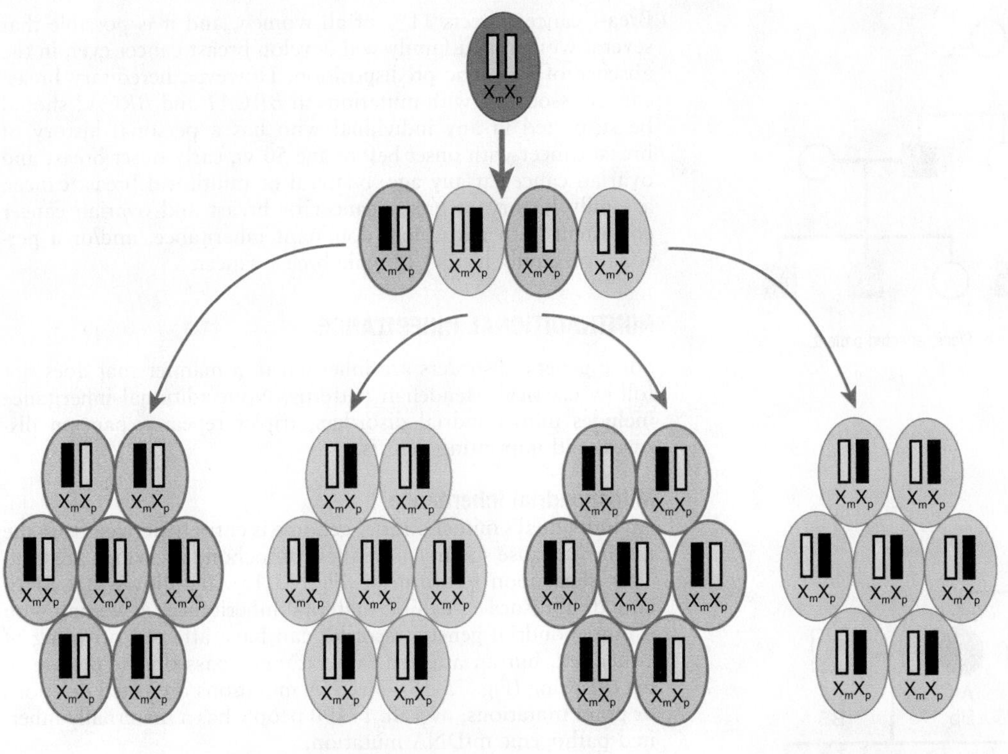

Figure 75-10 X-inactivation. *Black* marks the active X chromosome. Color of the cell represents whether it is the paternal-derived X chromosome (Xp active in *blue cell*) or maternal derived (Xm active in *red cell*).

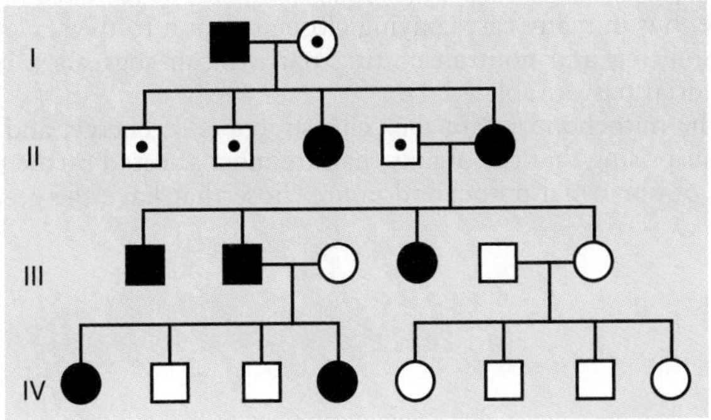

Figure 75-11 Pedigree pattern demonstrating X-linked dominant inheritance. Note there is no father-to-son transmission in this situation, and hemizygosity (i.e., X-linked gene in a male) is not lethal. In some X-linked dominant conditions, X-linked males have a more severe phenotype and might not survive. In that case, only females manifest the disease (see Fig. 75-12).

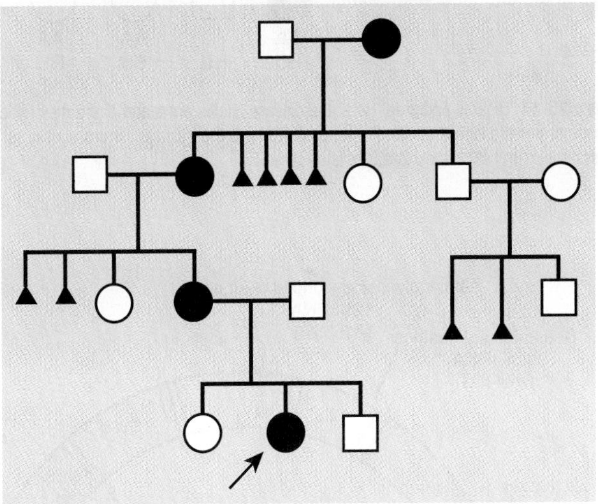

Figure 75-12 Pedigree of an X-linked dominant disorder with male lethality, such as incontinentia pigmenti.

bowing of the forearms with dislocations of the ulna at the wrist and generalized short stature. Homozygous mutations cause the much more severe **Langer mesomelic dwarfism.**

DIGENIC INHERITANCE

Digenic inheritance explains the occurrence of **retinitis pigmentosa** (RP) in children of parents who each carry a mutation in a different RP-associated gene. Both parents have normal vision, as would be expected, but their offspring who are **double heterozygotes**—having inherited both mutations—develop RP. Digenic pedigrees (Fig. 75-14) can exhibit characteristics of both autosomal dominant (vertical transmission) and autosomal recessive inheritance (1 in 4 recurrence risk). For example, a couple in which the two unaffected partners are carriers for mutation in two different RP-associated genes that show digenic inheritance have a 1 in 4 risk of having an affected child similar to what is seen in autosomal recessive inheritance. However, their affected children, and affected children in subsequent generations, have a 1 in 4 risk of transmitting both mutations to their offspring, who would be affected (vertical transmission).

PSEUDOGENETIC INHERITANCE AND FAMILIAL CLUSTERING

Sometimes nongenetic reasons for the occurrence of a particular disease in multiple family members can produce a pattern that mimics genetic transmission. These nongenetic factors can include identifiable environmental factors, teratogenic exposures, or as yet undetermined and/or undefined factors. Examples of identifiable factors might include multiple siblings in a family having asthma due to exposure to cigarette smoke from their parents or having failure to thrive, developmental delay, and unusual facial appearance caused by exposure to alcohol during pregnancy.

In some cases the disease is sufficiently common in the general population that some familial clustering occurs simply by chance.

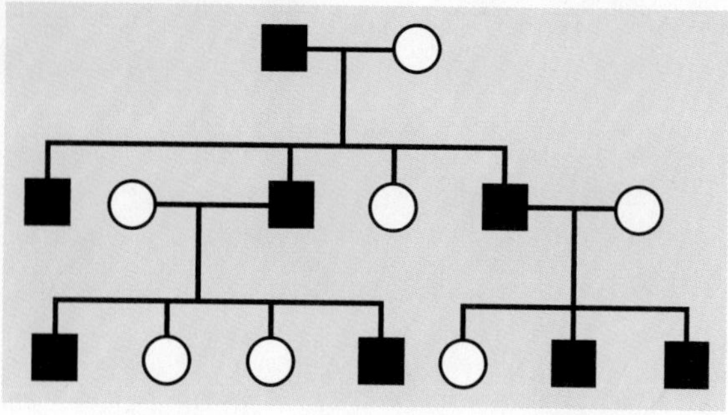

Figure 75-13 Y-linked inheritance. *Black,* affected patient.

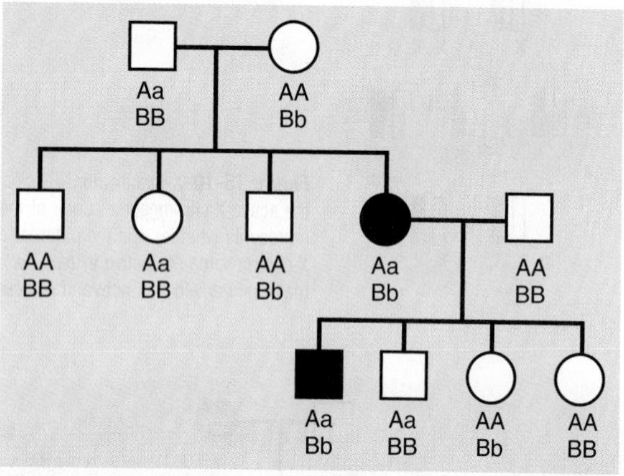

Figure 75-14 Digenic pedigree. Here, the disease alleles are *a* and *b* and they reside on distinct genetic loci or genes. For a person to have the disease, heterozygosity for mutant alleles in both genes (A/a;B/b) is required.

Breast cancer affects 11% of all women, and it is possible that several women in a family will develop breast cancer even in the absence of a genetic predisposition. However, hereditary breast cancer associated with mutations in *BRCA1* and *BRCA2* should be suspected in any individual who has a personal history of breast cancer with onset before age 50 yr, early-onset breast and ovarian cancer at any age, bilateral or multifocal breast cancer, a family history of breast cancer or breast and ovarian cancer consistent with autosomal dominant inheritance, and/or a personal or family history of male breast cancer.

NONTRADITIONAL INHERITANCE

Some genetic disorders are inherited in a manner that does not follow classical Mendelian patterns. Nontraditional inheritance includes mitochondrial disorders, triplet repeat expansion diseases, and imprinting defects.

Mitochondrial Inheritance

An individual's mitochondrial genome is entirely derived from the mother because sperm contain few mitochondria, which are typically shed upon fertilization (Fig. 75-15). It follows that mitochondrial disorders exhibit maternal inheritance. A woman with a mitochondrial genetic disorder can have affected offspring of either sex, but an affected father cannot pass on the disease to his offspring (Fig. 75-16). mtDNA mutations are often deletions or point mutations; overall, 1:400 people has a maternally inherited pathogenic mtDNA mutation.

In individual families, mitochondrial inheritance may be difficult to distinguish from autosomal dominant or X-linked inheritance, but in many cases paying close attention to the sex of the transmitting and nontransmitting parents can suggests a mitochondrial basis (Table 75-1).

The mitochondria are the cell's suppliers of energy, and it is not surprising that the organs that are most affected by the presence of abnormal mitochondria are those that have the greatest

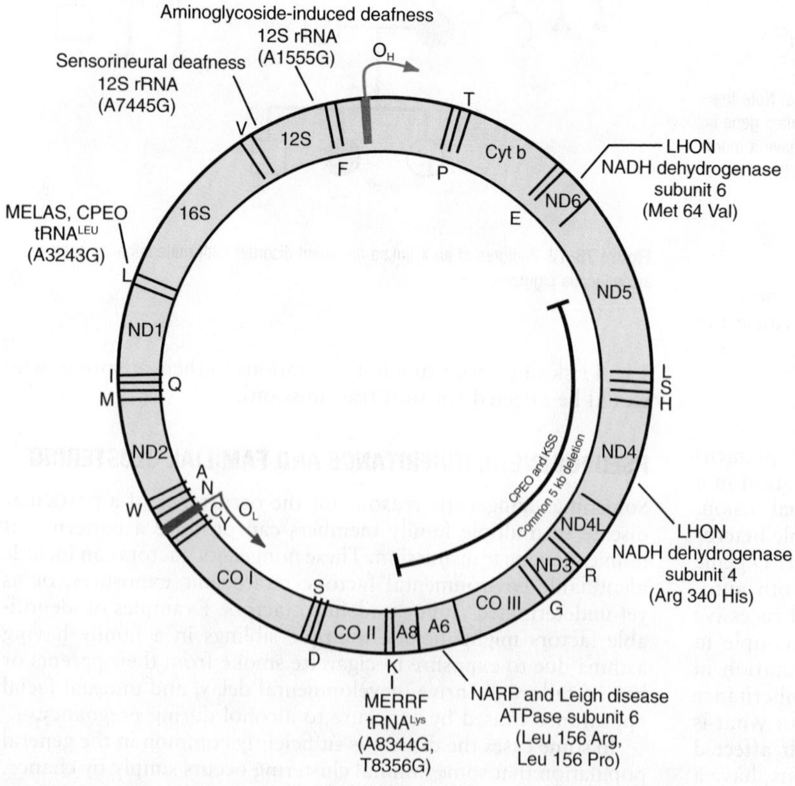

Figure 75-15 The human mitochondrial DNA molecule, showing the location of genes encoding 22 tRNAs, 2 rRNAs, and 13 proteins of the oxidative phosphorylation (OXPHOA) complex. Some of the most common disease-causing substitutions and deletions in the mtDNA genome are also illustrated. OH and OL are the origins of replication of the two DNA strands, respectively; 12S, 12S ribosomal RNA; 16S, 16S ribosomal RNA. The tRNAs are indicated by the single letter code for their corresponding amino acids (e.g., L for leucine, K for lysine). The 13 OXPHOS polypeptides encoded by mtDNA include components of complex I: NADH dehydrogenase (ND1, ND2, ND3, ND4, ND4L, ND5, and ND6); complex III: cytochrome *b* (Cyt *b*); complex IV: cytochrome *c* oxidase I, or Cyt *c* (COI, COII, COIII); and complex V: ATPase 6 (ATP-6, ATP-8). See Table 75-1 for representative diseases. (Adapted from Shoffner JM, Wallace DC: Oxidative phosphorylation disease. In Scriver CR, Beaudet AL, Sly WS, et al, editors: *The metabolic and molecular basis of inherited disease,* ed 7, New York, 1995, McGraw-Hill; and Johns DR: Mitochondrial DNA and disease, *N Engl J Med* 333:638–644, 1995. From Nussbaum RL, McInnes RR, Willard HF: *Thompson & Thompson genetics in medicine,* ed 6, Philadelphia, 2001, WB Saunders.)

energy requirements, such as the brain, muscle, heart, and liver (Chapters 81.4, 353, and 591). Common manifestations include developmental delay, seizures, cardiac dysfunction, decreased muscle strength and tone, and hearing and vision problems. Examples of mitochondrial disorders include **MELAS** (*m*yopathy, *e*ncephalopathy, *l*actic *a*cidosis, and *s*trokelike episodes), **MERRF** (*m*yoclonic *e*pilepsy associated with *r*agged *r*ed *f*ibers), and **Kearns-Sayre syndrome** (ophthalmoplegia, pigmentary retinopathy, and cardiomyopathy) (Chapter 591).

Mitochondrial diseases can be highly variable in clinical manifestation. This is partly because cells can contain multiple mitochondria, each bearing several copies of the mitochondrial genome. Thus, a cell can have a mixture of normal and abnormal mitochondrial genomes, which is referred to as **heteroplasmy.** Unequal segregation of mitochondria carrying normal and abnormal genomes and replicative advantage can result in varying degrees of heteroplasmy in the cells of an affected individual, including the individual ova of an affected female. Because of this, a mother may be asymptomatic and yet have children who are severely affected. The level of heteroplasmy at which disease symptoms typically appear can also vary based on the type of mitochondrial mutation. Detection of mitochondrial genome mutations can require sampling of the affected tissue for DNA analysis; testing for mitochondrial DNA mutations may in some tissues, such as blood, be inadequate because the mutation may be found primarily in affected tissues such as muscle.

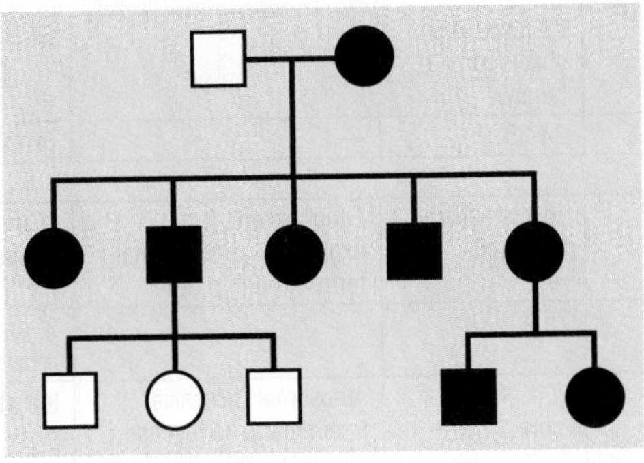

Figure 75-16 Pedigree of a mitochondrial disorder, exhibiting maternal inheritance. *Black,* affected patient.

Triplet Repeat Expansion Disorders

Triplet repeat expansion disorders are distinguished by the special dynamic nature of the disease-causing mutation. Triplet repeat expansion disorders include fragile X syndrome, myotonic dystrophy, Huntington disease, spinocerebellar ataxias, and several others (Table 75-2). These disorders are caused by expansion in the number of 3-bp repeats. The **fragile X gene,** *FMR1,* normally has 5-40 CGG triplets. An error in replication can result in expansion of that number, to a level in the gray zone between 41 and 58 repeats, or to a level referred to as **premutation,** which comprises 59-200 repeats. Some male carriers of the premutation develop fragile X–associated tremor/ataxia syndrome (FXTAS) as adults, and female carriers of the permutation are at risk for *FMR1*-related premature ovarian failure (POF). Persons with a premutation are also at risk for having the gene expand further in subsequent meiosis, hence crossing into the range of full mutation in offspring. In fragile X, the threshold for clinical diagnosis is above 200 repeats. With this number of repeats, the *FMR1* gene becomes hypermethylated, and protein production is lost.

Some triplet expansions associated with other genes can cause disease through a mechanism other than decreased protein production. In **Huntington disease,** the expansion causes the gene product to have a new, toxic effect on the neurons of the basal ganglia. For most triplet-repeat disorders, there is a clinical correlation to the size of the expansion, with a greater expansion causing more severe symptoms and/or earlier age of onset for the disease. The observation of increasing severity of disease and early age of onset in subsequent generations is termed **genetic anticipation** and is a defining characteristic of many triplet-repeat expansion disorders (Fig. 75-17).

Genetic Imprinting

The 2 copies of most autosomal genes are functionally equivalent. However, in some cases only 1 copy of a gene is transcribed and the other copy is silenced. This gene silencing is typically associated with methylation of DNA, which is an **epigenetic modification,** meaning it does not change the nucleotide sequence of the

Table 75-1 REPRESENTATIVE EXAMPLES OF DISORDERS CAUSED BY MUTATIONS IN MITOCHONDRIAL DNA AND THEIR INHERITANCE

DISEASE	PHENOTYPE	MOST FREQUENT MUTATION IN mtDNA MOLECULE	HOMOPLASMY VS HETEROPLASMY	INHERITANCE
Leber hereditary optic neuropathy	Rapid optic nerve death, leading to blindness in young adult life	Substitution Arg340His in *ND1* gene of complex I of electron transport chain; other complex I missense mutations	Homoplasmic (usually)	Maternal
NARP, Leigh disease	*N*europathy, *a*taxia, *r*etinitis *p*igmentosa, developmental delay, mental retardation, lactic acidemia	Point mutations in ATPase subunit 6 gene	Heteroplasmic	Maternal
MELAS	*M*itochondrial *e*ncephalomyopathy, *l*actic *a*cidosis, and *s*trokelike episodes; may manifest only as diabetes mellitus	Point mutation in $tRNA^{Leu}$	Heteroplasmic	Maternal
MERRF	*My*oclonic *e*pilepsy, *r*agged *r*ed *f*ibers in muscle, ataxia, sensorineural deafness	Point mutation in $tRNA^{Lys}$	Heteroplasmic	Maternal
Deafness	Progressive sensorineural deafness, often induced by aminoglycoside antibiotics	A1555G mutation in 12S rRNA	Homoplasmic	Maternal
	Nonsyndromic sensorineural deafness	A7445G mutation in 12S rRNA	Homoplasmic	Maternal
Chronic progressive external ophthalmoplegia (CPEO)	Progressive weakness of extraocular muscles	The common MELAS point mutation in $tRNA^{Lys}$; large deletions similar to KSS	Heteroplasmic	Maternal if point mutations
Pearson syndrome	Pancreatic insufficiency, pancytopenia, lactic acidosis	Large deletions	Heteroplasmic	Sporadic, somatic mutations
Kearns-Sayre syndrome (KSS)	PEO of early onset with heart block, retinal pigmentation	5 kb large deletion	Heteroplasmic	Sporadic, somatic mutations

From Nussbaum RL, McInnes RR, Willard HF, editors: *Thompson and Thompson genetics in medicine,* ed 6, Philadelphia, 2001, WB Saunders, p 246.

Table 75-2 DISEASES ASSOCIATED WITH REPEAT EXPANSIONS

DISEASE	DESCRIPTION	REPEAT SEQUENCE	NORMAL RANGE	ABNORMAL RANGE	PARENT IN WHOM EXPANSION USUALLY OCCURS	LOCATION OF EXPANSION
CATEGORY 1						
Huntington disease	Loss of motor control, dementia, affective disorder	CAG	6-34	36-100 or more	More often through father	Exon
Spinal and bulbar muscular atrophy	Adult-onset motor-neuron disease associated with androgen insensitivity	CAG	11-34	40-62	More often through father	Exon
Spinocerebellar ataxia type 1	Progressive ataxia, dysarthria, dysmetria	CAG	6-39	41-81	More often through father	Exon
Spinocerebellar ataxia type 2	Progressive ataxia, dysarthria	CAG	15-29	35-59	—	Exon
Spinocerebellar ataxia type 3 (Machado-Joseph disease)	Dystonia, distal muscular atrophy, ataxia, external ophthalmoplegia	CAG	13-36	68-79	More often through father	Exon
Spinocerebellar ataxia type 6	Progressive ataxia, dysarthria, nystagmus	CAG	4-16	21-27	—	Exon
Spinocerebellar ataxia type 7	Progressive ataxia, dysarthria, retinal degeneration	CAG	7-35	38-200	More often through father	—
Spinocerebellar ataxia type 17	Progressive ataxia, dementia, bradykinesia, dysmetria	CAG	29-42	47-55	—	Exon
Dentatorubral-pallidoluysian atrophy/Haw River syndrome	Cerebellar atrophy, ataxia, myoclonic epilepsy, choreoathetosis, dementia	CAG	7-25	49-88	More often through father	Exon
CATEGORY 2						
Pseudoachondroplasia, multiple epiphyseal dysplasia	Short stature, joint laxity, degenerative joint disease	GAC	5	6-7	—	Exon
Oculopharyngeal muscular dystrophy	Proximal limb weakness, dysphagia, ptosis	GCG	6	7-13	—	Exon
Cleidocranial dysplasia	Short stature, open skull sutures with bulging calvaria, clavicular hypoplasia, shortened fingers, dental anomalies	GCG, GCT, GCA	17	27 (expansion observed in 1 family)	—	Exon
Synpolydactyly	Polydactyly and syndactyly	GCG, GCT, GCA	15	22-25	—	Exon
CATEGORY 3						
Myotonic dystrophy (DMI; chromosome 19)	Muscle loss, cardiac arrhythmia, cataracts, frontal balding	CTG	5-37	100 to several thousand	Either parent, but expansion to congenital form through mother	3′ untranslated region
Myotonic dystrophy (DM2; chromosome 3)	Muscle loss, cardiac arrhythmia, cataracts, frontal balding	CCTG	<75	75-11,000	—	3′ untranslated region
Friedreich ataxia	Progressive limb ataxia, dysarthria, hypertrophic cardiomyopathy, pyramidal weakness in legs	GAA	7-2	200-900 or more	Autosomal recessive inheritance, so disease alleles are inherited from both parents	Intron
Fragile X syndrome (FRAXA)	Mental retardation, large ears and jaws, macroorchidism in males	CGG	6-52	200-2,000 or more	Exclusively through mother	5′ untranslated region
Fragile site (FRAXE)	Mild mental retardation	GCC	6-35	>200	More often through mother	5′ untranslated region
Spinocerebellar ataxia type 8	Adult-onset ataxia, dysarthria, nystagmus	CTG	16-37	107-127	More often through mother	3′ untranslated region
Spinocerebellar ataxia type 10	Ataxia and seizures	ATTCT	12-16	800-4,500	More often through father	Intron
Spinocerebellar ataxia type 12	Ataxia, eye movement disorders; variable age at onset	CAG	7-28	66-78	—	5′ untranslated region
Progressive myoclonic epilepsy type 1	Juvenile-onset convulsions, myoclonus, dementia	12-bp repeat motif	2-3	30-75	Autosomal recessive inheritance, so transmitted by both parents	5′ untranslated region

From Jorde LB, Carey JC, Bamshad MJ, et al: *Medical genetics*, ed 3, St Louis, 2006, Mosby, p 82.

DNA (Fig. 75-18). In **imprinting,** gene expression depends on the parent of origin of the chromosome (Chapter 76). Imprinting disorders result from an imbalance of active copies of a given gene, which can occur for several reasons. **Prader-Willi** and **Angelman syndromes,** two distinct disorders associated with developmental impairment, are illustrative. Both can be caused by microdeletions of chromosome 15q11-12. The microdeletion in Prader-Willi syndrome is always on the paternally derived chromosome 15, whereas in Angelman syndrome it is on the maternal copy. *UBE3A* is the gene responsible for Angelman syndrome. The paternal copy of *UBE3A* is transcriptionally silenced in the brain and the maternal copy continues to be transcribed. If an individual has a maternal deletion, an insufficient amount of *UBE3A* protein is produced in the brain, resulting in the neurologic deficits seen in Angelman syndrome.

Uniparental disomy (UPD), the rare occurrence of a child inheriting both copies of a chromosome from the same parent, is another genetic mechanism that can cause Prader-Willi and Angelman syndromes. Inheriting both chromosomes 15 from the mother is functionally the same as deletion of the paternal 15q12 and results in Prader-Willi syndrome. About 30% of cases of Prader-Willi syndrome is caused by paternal UPD15, whereas maternal UPD15 accounts for only 3% of Angelman syndrome (Chapter 76).

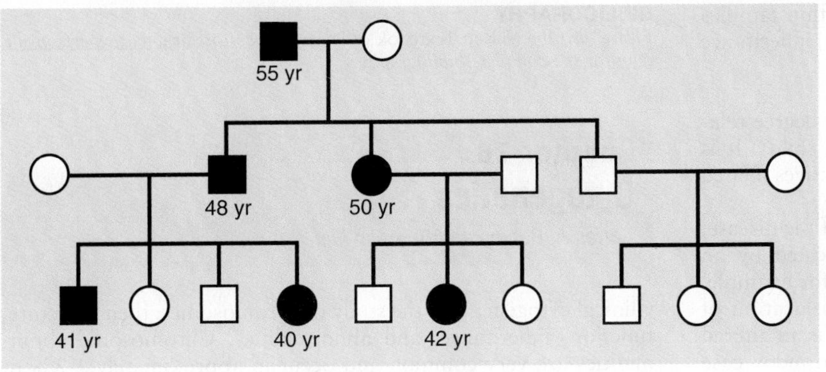

Figure 75-17 Myotonic dystrophy pedigree illustrating anticipation. In this case, the age of onset for family members affected with an autosomal dominant disease is lower in more recent generations. *Black,* affected patients.

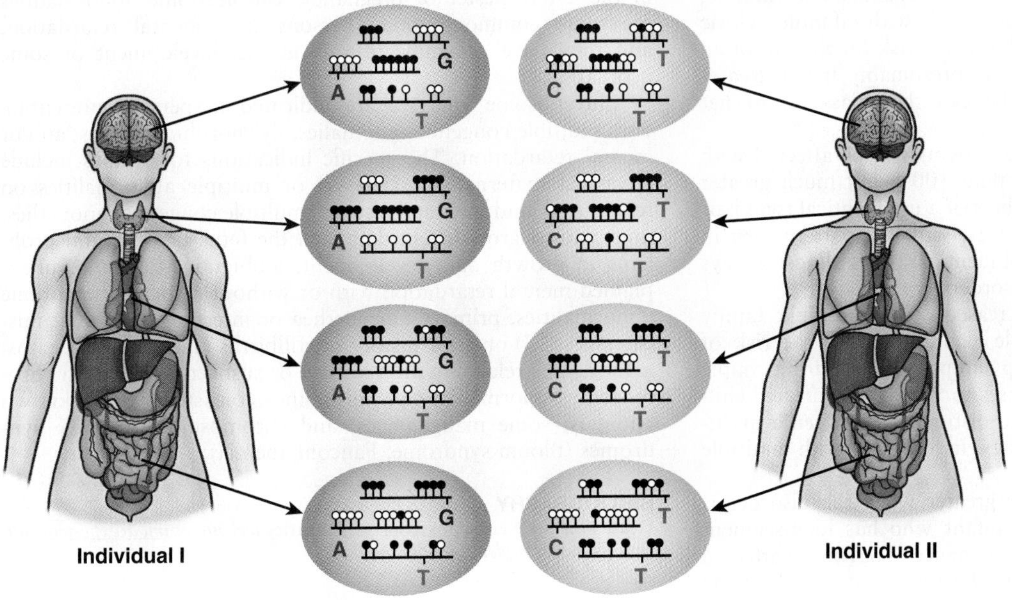

Figure 75-18 Tissue-specific DNA methylation and epigenetic heterogeneity among individuals. A subset of the DNA methylation patterns within a cell is characteristic of that cell type. Cell type–specific and tissue-specific DNA methylation are illustrated by organ-to-organ variations in the clusters of methylated CpGs within the same individual. Despite overall consistency in tissue-specific DNA methylation patterns, variations in these patterns exist among different individuals. Methylated CpGs are indicated by a *filled circle* and unmethylated CpGs by an *open circle.* SNPs are indicated by the corresponding base. (Redrawn from Brena RM, Huang THM, Plass C: Toward a human epigenome, *Nat Genet* 38:1359–1360, 2006.)

A mutation in an imprinted gene is another cause. Mutations in *UBEA3* account for almost 11% of patients with Angelman syndrome and also result in familial transmission. The most uncommon cause is a mutation in the imprinting center, which results in an inability to correctly imprint the *UBE3A*. In a woman, the inability to reset the imprinting on her paternally inherited chromosome 15 imprint results in a 50% risk of passing on an incorrectly methylated copy of *UBE3A* to a child who would then develop Angelman syndrome.

Besides 15q12, other imprinted regions of clinical interest include the short arm of chromosome 11, where the genes for Beckwith-Wiedemann syndrome and nesidioblastosis map, and the long arm of chromosome 7 with maternal uniparental disomy of 7q, which has been associated with some cases of idiopathic short stature and Russell-Silver syndrome.

Imprinting of a gene can occur during gametogenesis or early embryonic development (reprogramming). Genes can become inactive or active by various mechanisms including DNA methylation or demethylation or histone acetylation or deacytylation, with different patterns of (de)methylation noted on paternal or maternal imprintable chromosome regions. Some genes demonstrate tissue-specific imprinting (see Fig. 75-18). Several studies suggest that there may be a small but significantly increased incidence of imprinting disorders, specifically Beckwith-Wiedemann and Angelman syndrome, associated with assisted reproductive technologies such as in vitro fertilization and intracytoplasmic sperm injection. However, the overall incidence of these disorders in children conceived using assisted reproductive technologies is likely to be <1%.

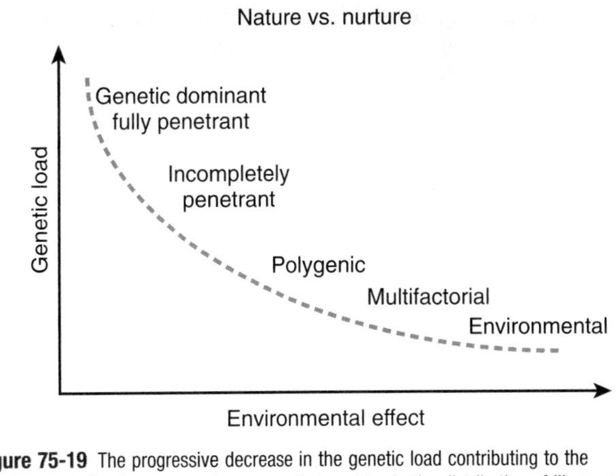

Figure 75-19 The progressive decrease in the genetic load contributing to the development of a disease creates a smooth transition in the distribution of illnesses on an etiologic diagram. In theory, no diseases are completely free from the influence of both genetic and environmental factors. (From Bomprezzi R, Kovanen PE, Martin R: New approaches to investigating heterogeneity in complex traits, *J Med Genet* 40:553–559, 2003. Reproduced with permission from the BMJ Publishing Group.)

MULTIFACTORIAL AND POLYGENIC INHERITANCE

Multifactorial inheritance refers to traits that are caused by a combination of inherited, environmental, and stochastic factors (Fig. 75-19). Multifactorial traits differ from polygenic inheritance, which refers to traits that result from the additive effects of multiple genes. Multifactorial traits segregate within families but do not exhibit a consistent or recognizable inheritance pattern. Characteristics include the following:

- There is a similar rate of recurrence among all 1st-degree relatives (parents, siblings, offspring of the affected child). It is unusual to find a substantial increase in risk for relatives related more distantly than 2nd degree to the index case.
- The risk of recurrence is related to the incidence of the disease.
- Some disorders have a sex predilection, as indicated by an unequal male: female incidence. Pyloric stenosis, for example, is more common in males, whereas congenital dislocation of the hips is more common in females. Where there is an altered sex ratio, the risk is higher for the relatives of an index case whose gender is less commonly affected than relatives of an index case of the more commonly affected gender. For example, the risk to the son of an affected female with infantile pyloric stenosis is 18%, compared with the 5% risk for the son of an affected male. An affected female presumably has a greater genetic susceptibility, which she can then pass on to her offspring.
- The likelihood that both identical twins will be affected with the same malformation is less than 100% but much greater than the chance that both members of a nonidentical twin pair will be affected. This is in contrast with the pattern seen in mendelian inheritance, in which identical twins almost always share fully penetrant genetic disorders.
- The risk of recurrence is increased when multiple family members are affected. A simple example is that the risk of recurrence for unilateral cleft lip and palate is 4% for a couple with 1 affected child and increases to 9% with 2 affected children. It is sometimes difficult to distinguish between a multifactorial and mendelian etiology in families with multiple affected individuals.
- The risk of recurrence may be greater when the disorder is more severe. For example, an infant who has long-segment Hirschsprung disease has a greater chance of having an affected sibling than the infant who has short-segment Hirschsprung disease.

There are 2 types of multifactorial traits. One exhibits continuous variation, with "normal" individuals falling within a statistical range—often defined as having a value 2 standard deviations (SDs) above and/or below the mean—and "abnormals" falling outside that range. Examples include such traits as intelligence, blood pressure, height, and head circumference. For many of these traits, offspring values can be estimated based on a modified average of their parental values, with nutritional and environmental factors playing an important role.

With other multifactorial traits, the distinction between normal and abnormal is based on the presence or absence of a particular trait. Examples include pyloric stenosis, neural tube defects, congenital heart defects, and cleft lip and cleft palate. Such traits follow a threshold model (see Fig. 75-16). A distribution of liability due to genetic and nongenetic factors is postulated in the population. Individuals who exceed a threshold liability develop the trait, and those below the threshold do not.

The balance between genetic and environmental factors is demonstrated by **neural tube defects.** Genetic factors are implicated by the increased recurrence risk for parents of an affected child compared to the general population, yet the recurrence risk is about 3%, less than what would be expected if the trait was caused by a single, fully penetrant mutation. The role of nongenetic environmental factors can be seen in the fact that the recurrence risk can be lowered by up to 87% if the mother-to-be takes 4 mg of folic acid per day starting 3 months before conception.

Many adult-onset diseases behave as if they are caused by multifactorial inheritance. Diabetes, coronary artery disease, and schizophrenia are examples.

BIBLIOGRAPHY

Please visit the Nelson Textbook of Pediatrics *website at* *www.expertconsult.com* *for the complete bibliography.*

Chapter 76
Cytogenetics
Carlos A. Bacino and Brendan Lee

Clinical cytogenetics is the study of chromosomes: their structure, function, inheritance, and abnormalities. Chromosome abnormalities are very common and occur in approximately 1-2% of live births, 5% of stillbirths, and ~50% of early fetal losses in the 1st trimester of pregnancy. Chromosome abnormalities are more common among persons with mental retardation, and they have a significant role in the development of some neoplasias.

Chromosome analyses are indicated in persons presenting with multiple congenital anomalies, dysmorphic features, and/or mental retardation. The specific indications for studies include advanced maternal age (>35 yr) or multiple abnormalities on fetal ultrasound (prenatal testing), multiple congenital anomalies, unexplained growth retardation in the fetus or postnatal problems in growth and development, ambiguous genitalia, unexplained mental retardation with or without associated anatomic abnormalities, primary amenorrhea or infertility, recurrent miscarriages (≥3) or prior history of stillbirths and neonatal deaths, a 1st-degree relative with a known or suspected structural chromosome abnormality, clinical findings consistent with a known anomaly, some malignancies, and chromosome breakage syndromes (Bloom syndrome, Fanconi anemia).

BIBLIOGRAPHY

Please visit the Nelson Textbook of Pediatrics *website at* *www.expertconsult.com* *for the complete bibliography.*

76.1 Methods of Chromosome Analysis
Carlos A. Bacino and Brendan Lee

Cytogenetic studies are usually performed on peripheral blood lymphocytes, although cultured fibroblasts may also be used. Prenatal (fetal) chromosome studies are performed with cells obtained from the amniotic fluid, chorionic villus tissue, and fetal blood or, in the case of preimplantation diagnosis, by analysis of a blastomere. Cytogenetic studies of bone marrow have an important role in tumor surveillance, particularly among patients with leukemia. These are useful to determine induction of remission and success of therapy or, in some cases, the occurrence of relapses.

Chromosome anomalies include abnormalities of number and structure and are the result of errors during cell division. There are 2 types of cell division: mitosis, which occurs in most somatic cells, and meiosis, which is limited to the germ cells. In **mitosis,** 2 genetically identical daughter cells are produced from a single parent cell. DNA duplication has already occurred during **interphase** in the S phase of the cell cycle (DNA synthesis). Therefore, at the beginning of mitosis the chromosomes consist of 2 double DNA strands joined together at the centromere known as *sister chromatids.* Mitosis can be divided into 4 stages: **prophase, metaphase, anaphase,** and **telophase.** Prophase is characterized by condensation of the DNA. Also during prophase, the nuclear membrane and the nucleolus disappear and the mitotic spindle forms. In metaphase, the chromosomes are maximally compacted and are clearly visible as distinct structures. The chromosomes align at the center of the cell and spindle fibers connect to the centromere of each chromosome and extend to centrioles at the

2 poles of the mitotic figure. In anaphase, the chromosomes divide along their longitudinal axes to form 2 daughter chromatids, which then migrate to opposite poles of the cell. Telophase is characterized by formation of 2 new nuclear membranes and nucleoli, duplication of the centrioles, and cytoplasmic cleavage to form the 2 daughter cells.

Meiosis begins in the female oocyte during fetal life and is completed years to decades later. In males, it begins in a particular spermatogonial cell sometime between adolescence and adult life and is completed in a few days. Meiosis is preceded by DNA replication so that at the outset each of the 46 chromosomes consists of 2 chromatids. In meiosis, a **diploid cell** (2n = 46 chromosomes) divides to form **haploid cells** (n = 23 chromosomes). Meiosis consists of 2 major rounds of cell division. In meiosis I, each of the homologous chromosomes pair precisely so that **genetic recombination,** involving exchange between 2 DNA strands (**crossing over**), can occur. This results in a reshuffling of the genetic information on the recombined chromosomes and allows further genetic diversity. Each daughter cell then receives 1 of each of the 23 homologous chromosomes. In oogenesis, 1 of the daughter cells receives most of the cytoplasm and becomes the egg, whereas the other smaller cell becomes the 1st polar body. Meiosis II is similar to a mitotic division but without a preceding round of DNA duplication (replication). Each of the 23 chromosomes divides longitudinally, and the homologous chromatids migrate to opposite poles of the cell. This produces 4 spermatogonia in males, or an egg cell and a 2nd polar body in females, each with a haploid (n = 23) set of chromosomes. Consequently, meiosis fulfills 2 crucial roles: It reduces the chromosome number from diploid (46) to haploid (23) so that upon fertilization a diploid number is restored, and it allows genetic recombination.

Two errors of cell division commonly occur during meiosis or mitosis, and either can result in an abnormal number of chromosomes. The 1st is **nondisjunction,** in which 2 chromosomes fail to separate during meiosis and thus migrate together into 1 of the new cells, producing 1 cell with 2 copies of the chromosome and another with no copy. The 2nd is **anaphase lag,** in which a chromatid or chromosome is lost during mitosis because it fails to move quickly enough during anaphase to become incorporated into 1 of the new daughter cells (Fig. 76-1).

For chromosome analysis, cells are cultured (for varying periods depending on cell type), with or without stimulation, and then artificially arrested in mitosis during metaphase (or prometaphase), later on subjected to a hypotonic solution to allow proper dispersion of the chromosomes for analysis, fixed, banded, and finally stained. The most commonly used banding and staining method is the GTG banding (G-bands trypsin Giemsa) also known as G banding, which produces a unique combination of dark (G-positive) and light (G-negative) bands that permits recognition of all individual 23 chromosome pairs for analysis.

Other banding techniques such as Q-banding using quinacrine, reverse (R-banding) using acridine orange, and C-banding (constitutive heterchromatin) using barium hydroxide are available for use in certain circumstances but are losing ground to molecular technologies. Metaphase chromosome spreads are 1st evaluated microscopically, and then their images are photographed or captured by a video camera and stored on a computer to be later analyzed. Humans have 46 chromosomes or 23 pairs, which are classified as autosomes for chromosomes 1 to 22, and the sex chromosomes, often referred as sex complement: XX for females and XY for males. The homologous chromosomes from a metaphase spread can then be paired and arranged systematically to assemble a karyotype according to well-defined standard conventions like those established by International System for Human Cytogenetic Nomenclature (ISCN), with chromosome 1 being the largest and 22 the smallest. According to nomenclature, the description of the karyotype includes the total number of chromosomes followed by the sex chromosome constitution. A normal karyotype is 46,XX for females and 46,XY for males (Fig. 76-2). Abnormalities are noted after the sex chromosome complement.

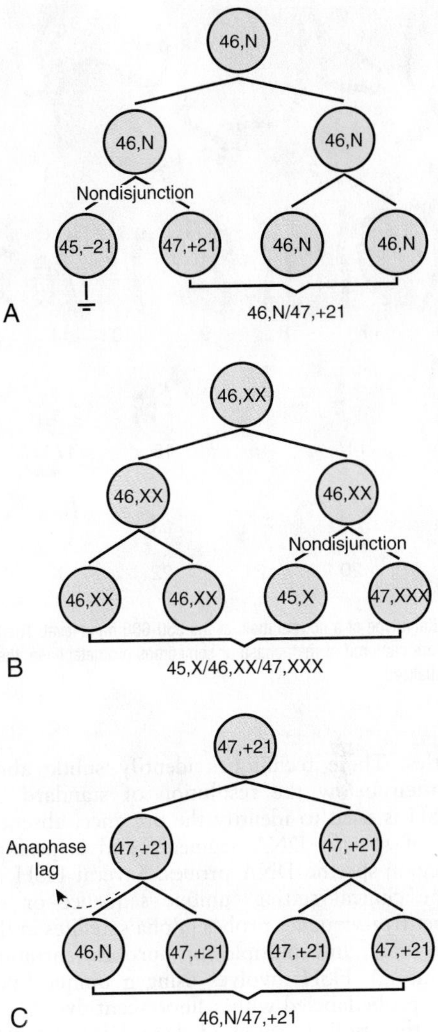

Figure 76-1 Generation of mosaicism. *A,* Postzygotic nondisjunction in an initially normal conceptus. In this example, 1 cell line (monosomic 21) is subsequently lost, with the final karyotype 46,N/47,+21. *B,* Postzygotic nondisjunction in an initially 46,XX conceptus, resulting in 45,X/46,XX/47,XXX mosaicism. *C,* Postzygotic anaphase lag in an initially 47,+21 conceptus. (From Gardner RJM, Sutherland GR: *Chromosome abnormalities and genetic counseling,* ed 3, New York, 2003, Oxford University Press, p 33.)

Although the internationally accepted system for human chromosome classification relies largely on the length and banding pattern of each chromosome, the position of the centromere relative to the ends of the chromosome also is a useful distinguishing feature (Fig. 76-3). The centromere divides the chromosome in 2, with the short arm designated as the **p arm** and the long arm designated as the **q arm.** A plus or minus sign before the number of a chromosome indicate that there is an extra or missing chromosome, respectively. Table 76-1 lists some of the abbreviations used for the descriptions of chromosomes and their abnormalities. A metaphase chromosome spread usually shows 450-550 bands. Prophase and prometaphase chromosomes are longer, are less condensed, and often show 550-850 bands. High-resolution analysis is useful for detecting subtle chromosome abnormalities that might otherwise go unrecognized.

Molecular techniques such as fluorescence in situ hybridization (FISH) and comparative array genomic hybridization studies (conventional CGH and array CGH [aCGH]) have filled a significant void for the diagnosing cryptic chromosomal

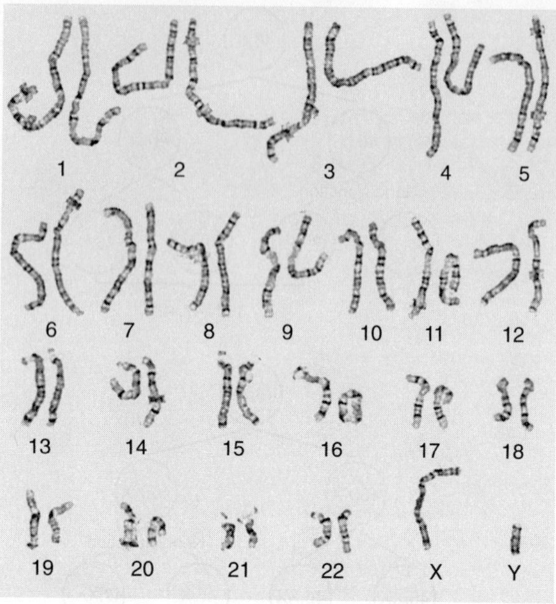

Figure 76-2 Karyotype of a normal male at the 550-600 band level. The longer the chromosomes are captured at metaphase or sometimes prometaphase, the more bands that can be visualized.

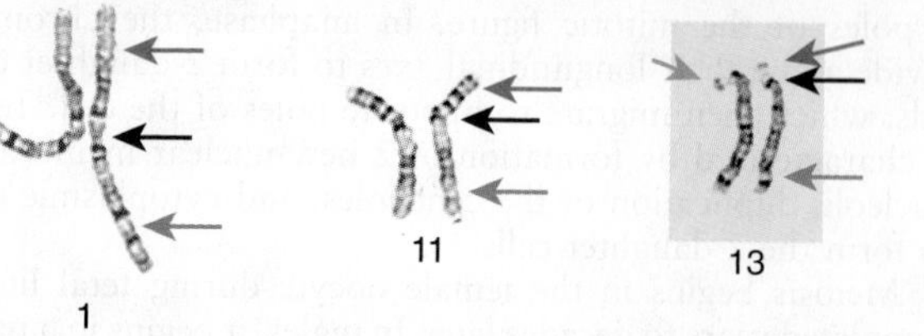

Figure 76-3 Example of different chromosome types according to the position of the centromere. On the *left* is a chromosome 1 pair with the centromere equidistant from the short and long arm (also known as metacentric). In the *center* is a chromosome 11 pair that is submetacentric. On the *right* is a chromosome 13 pair that is an example of an acrocentric chromosome. Acrocentric chromosomes contain a very small short arm, stalks, and satellite DNA. The *black arrow* indicates the position of the centromere. The *blue arrow* shows the long arm of a chromosome. The *red arrow* shows the short arm of a chromosome. The *green arrow* highlights the satellite region, which is made of DNA repeats. The *light area* between the short arm and the satellite is known as the stalk.

abnormalities. These techniques identify subtle abnormalities that are often below the resolution of standard cytogenetic studies. **FISH** is used to identify the presence, absence, or rearrangement of *specific* DNA segments and is performed with gene- or region-specific DNA probes. Several FISH probes are used in the clinical setting: unique sequence or single-copy probes, repetitive-sequence probes (alpha satellites in the pericentromeric regions), and multiple-copy probes (chromosome specific or painting). FISH involves using a unique known DNA sequence or probe labeled with a fluorescent dye that is complementary to the studied region of disease interest. The labeled probe is exposed to the DNA on a microscope slide, typically metaphase or interphase chromosomal DNA, that has been previously treated (denatured) to allow the DNA to become single stranded and to permit hybridization. When the probe pairs with its complementary DNA sequence, it can be then visualized by fluorescence microscopy (Fig. 76-4). In metaphase chromosome spreads, the exact chromosomal location of each probe copy can be documented and often the *number of copies* (deletions, duplications) of the DNA sequence as well, if they are not too close to each other; whereas in interphase cells, only the number of copies of a particular DNA segment can be determined. When the interrogated segments (as in genomic duplications) are close together, only interphase cells can accurately determine the presence of 2 or more copies or signals. In metaphase cells, some duplications might falsely appear as a single signal.

Metaphase and interphase FISH are particularly useful for detecting very small deletions that might escape notice with G-band analysis. In most cases the probe used for identification is used in conjunction with a control probe with a known location nearby the region studied. This allows correct identification of the hybridized signal to the right chromosome, and in some cases identification to the rearranged chromosome. With high-resolution chromosome analysis it is very difficult to recognize deletions of <5 million bp (5 Mb); FISH can reliably detect deletions as small as 50 to 200 kb of DNA. This has allowed the clinical characterization of a number of *microdeletion syndromes*. In addition to gene- or locus-specific probes, complex mixtures of DNA from a chromosome arm or an entire chromosome are available for fluorescence staining of large chromosome sections or entire chromosomes. The probe mixtures are referred to as *chromosome paints* (Fig. 76-5*A* and *B*). Other probes hybridize to repetitive sequences located to the pericentromeric regions. These probes are useful for the rapid identification of certain trisomies in interphase cells of blood smears, or even in the rapid analysis of prenatal samples from cells obtained through amniocentesis. Such probes are available for chromosomes 13, 18, and 21 and for the sex pair X and Y (Fig. 76-5*C* and *D*).

Spectral karyotyping (SKY) and **multicolor FISH** (M-FISH) are similar molecular cytogenetic techniques that use 24 different chromosome painting probes and 5 fluorochromes to simultaneously visualize every chromosome in a metaphase spread. Each of the 24 different chromosome paints is labeled with a different combination of the 5 fluorescent dyes, which emit at different wavelengths. Each of the 22 autosomes and the X and Y chromosomes has its own unique spectrum of wavelengths of fluorescence. Special filters, cameras, and image-processing software are required to identify each chromosome. SKY and M-FISH are especially useful for identifying the complex chromosome rearrangements found in many tumors. This technique requires very special and costly equipment and is being displaced by comparative aCGH.

Comparative genomic hybridization (CGH) is a molecular-based technique that involves differentially labeling the patient's DNA with a fluorescent dye (green) and a normal reference DNA with another fluorescent dye (red) (Fig. 76-6). Equal amounts of the two-label DNA samples are mixed and then used as a painting probe for FISH with normal metaphase chromosomes. The ratio of green:red fluorescence is measured along each chromosome. Regions of amplification of the patient's DNA display an excess of green fluorescence, and regions of loss show excess red fluorescence. If the patient's and the control DNA are equally represented, the green:red ratio is 1:1 and the chromosomes appear yellow.

A modified version of this technology, aCGH, uses DNA spotted onto a slide or microarray grid. In this case, instead of metaphase chromosomes, segments of DNA are represented by BACs (bacterial artificial chromosomes) and PACs (P1 artificial chromosomes) or oligonucleotides (short DNA segments of varied size) distributed in a microarray that resembles the chromosomes in a metaphase. The detection could reach the size of the BACs, PACs, and oligonucleotides and ranges in resolution from approximately 50 to 200 kb (even smaller if using cosmids or shorter polymerase chain reaction (PCR) products used as probes).

There are many advantages of aCGH. They can test all critical disease causing regions in the genome at once; FISH requires the clinical knowledge and tests only 1 area at a time. aCGH can detect duplications and deletions not currently recognized as recurrent disease-causing regions probed by FISH. aCGH can detect single and contiguous gene deletion syndromes. aCGH

Table 76-1 SOME ABBREVIATIONS USED FOR DESCRIPTION OF CHROMOSOMES AND THEIR ABNORMALITIES

ABBREVIATION	MEANING	EXAMPLE	CONDITION
XX	Female	46,XX	Normal female karyotype
XY	Male	46,XY	Normal male karyotype
[##]	Number [#] of cells	46,XY[12]/47,XXY[10]	Number of cells in each clone, typically inside brackets Mosaicism in Klinefelter syndrome with 12 normal cells and 10 cells with an extra X chromosome
cen	Centromere		
del	Deletion	46,XY,del(5p)	Male with deletion of chromosome 5 short arm
der	Derivative	46,XX,der(2),t(2p127q13)	Female with a structurally rearranged chromosome 2 that resulted from a translocation between chromosomes 2 and 7
dup	Duplication	46,XY,dup(15)(q11-13)	Male with interstitial duplication in the long arm of chromosome 15 in the Prader-Willi/Angelman syndrome region
ins	Insertion	46,XY,ins(3)(p13q21q26)	Male with an insertion within chromosome 3 A piece between q21q26 has re-inserted on p13
inv	Inversion	46,XY,inv(2)(p21q31)	Male with pericentric inversion of chromosome 2 with breakpoints at bands p21 and q31
ish	Metaphase FISH	46,XX.ish del(7)(q11.23q11.23)	Female with deletion in the Williams syndrome region detected by in situ hybridization
nuc ish	Interphase FISH	nuc ish(DXZ1 × 3)	Interphase in situ hybridization showing 3 signals for the X chromosome centromeric region
mar	Marker	47,XY,+mar	Male with extra, unidentified chromosome material
mos	Mosaic	mos 45,X[14]/46,XX[16]	Turner syndrome mosaicism (analysis of 30 cells showed that 14 cells were 45,X and16 cells were 46,XX)
p	Short arm	46,XY,del(5)(p12)	Male with a deletion on the short arm of chromosome 5, band p12 (short nomenclature)
q	Long arm	46,XY,del(5)(q14)	Male with a deletion on the long arm of chromosome 5, band 14
r	Ring chromosome	46,X,r(X)(p21q27)	Female with 1 normal X chromosome and a ring X chromosome
t	Translocation	t(2;8)(q33;q24.1)	The interchange of material between chromosomes 2 and 8 with breakpoints at bands 2q33 and 8q24.1
ter	Terminal	46,XY,del(5)(p12-pter)	Male with a deletion of chromosome 5 between p12 and the end of the short arm (long nomenclature)
/	Slash	45,X/46,XY	Separate lines or clones Mosaicism for monosomy X and a male cell line
+	Gain of	47,XX,+21	Female with trisomy 21
–	Loss of	45,XY,–21	Male with monosomy 21

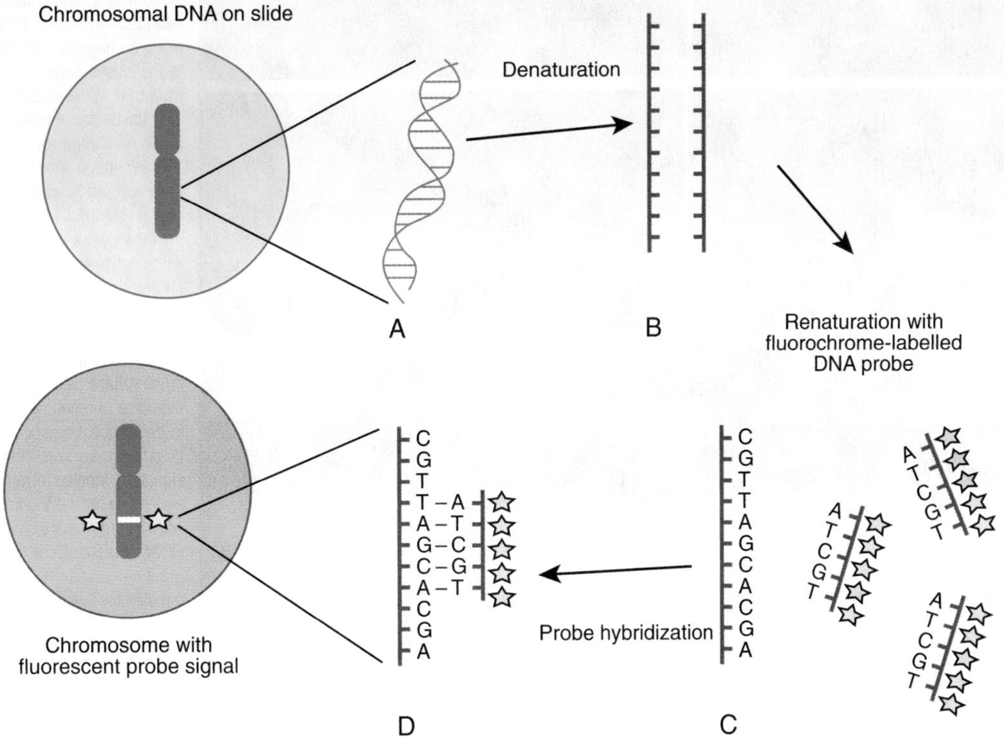

Figure 76-4 Fluorescence in situ hybridization (FISH) involves denaturation of double-stranded DNA as present in metaphase chromosomes or interphase nuclei on cytogenetic slide preparations *(A)* into single-stranded DNA *(B)*. The slide-bound (in situ) DNA is then renatured or reannealed in the presence of excess copies of a single-stranded, fluorochrome-labeled DNA base-pair sequence or probe *(C)*. The probe anneals or "hybridizes" to sites of complementary DNA sequence *(D)* within the chromosomal genome. Probe signal is visualized and imaged on the chromosome by fluorescent microscopy. (From Lin RL, Cherry AM, Bangs CD, et al: FISHing for answers: the use of molecular cytogenetic techniques in adolescent medicine practice. In Hyme HE, Greydanus D, editors: *Genetic disorders in adolescents: state of the art reviews. Adolescent medicine,* Philadelphia, 2002, Hanley and Belfus, pp 305–313.)

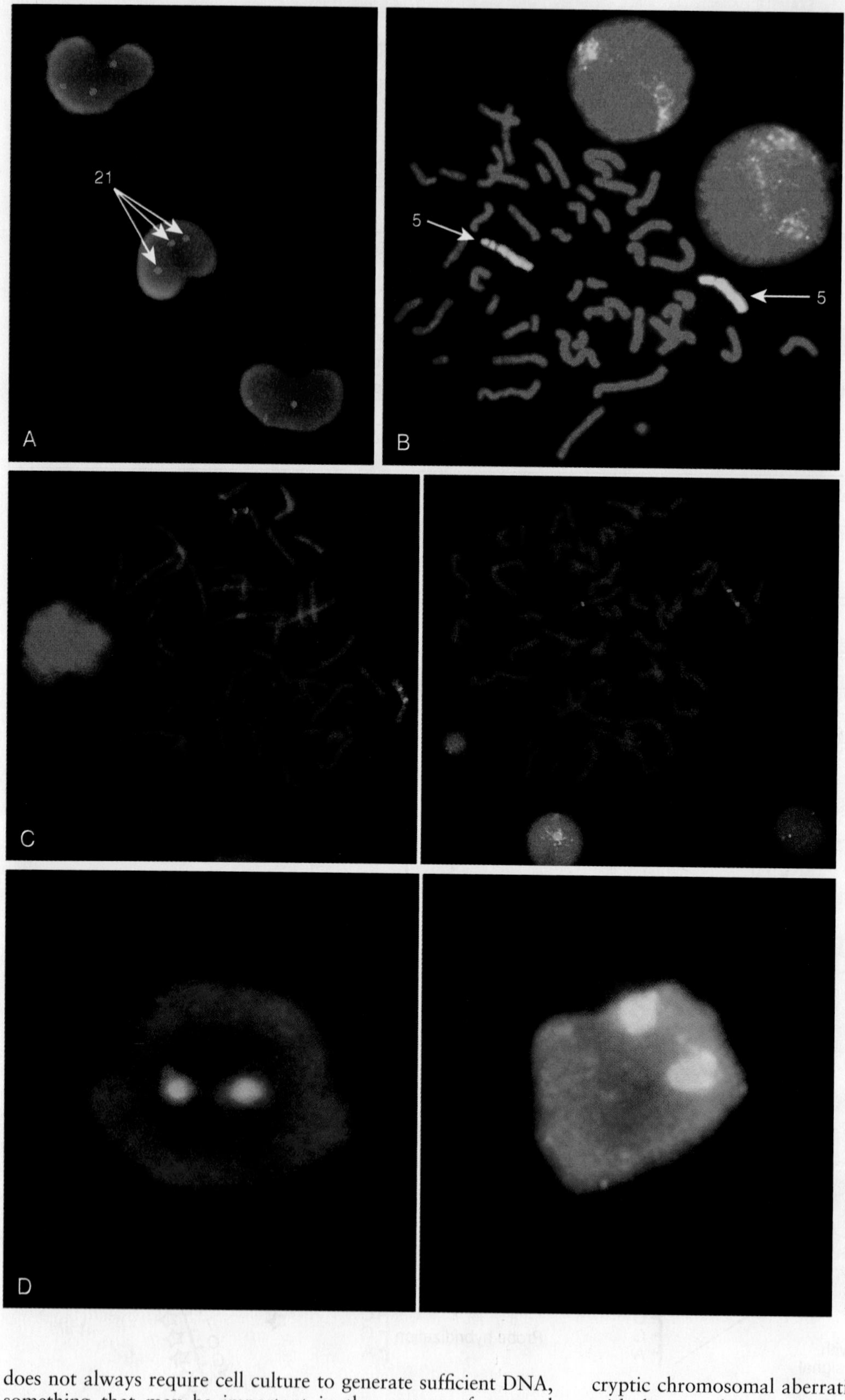

Figure 76-5 *A,* Fluorescence in situ hybridization (FISH) analysis of interphase peripheral blood cells from a patient with Down syndrome using a chromosome 21-specific probe. The 3 red signals mark the presence of 3 chromosomes 21. *B,* FISH analysis of a metaphase chromosome spread from a clinically normal individual using a whole-chromosome paint specific for chromosome 5. Both chromosomes 5 are completely labeled *(yellow)* along their entire length. *C,* Fluorescence in situ hybridization studies (FISH) on metaphase cells using a unique sequence probe that hybridizes to the elastin gene on chromosome 7q11.23, inside the Williams syndrome critical region. The elastin probe is labeled in *red,* and a control probe on chromosome 7 is labeled in *green.* The *left* image shows normal hybridization to chromosome 7, with 2 signals for the elastin region and 2 for the control probe. The *right* image shows a normal chromosome on the *right* with control and elastin signals, and a deleted chromosome 7 on the *left,* evidenced by a single signal for the control probe. This image corresponds to a patient with a Williams syndrome region deletion. *D,* FISH in interphase cells using DNA probes that hybridize to repetitive α-satellite sequences in the pericentromeric region for the sex chromosomes. *Left,* interphase cells with 2 signals, 1 labeled in *red* for the X chromosome and *green* for the Y chromosome, consistent with a normal male chromosome complement. *Right,* interphase cell showing 2 *red* signals for the X chromosome, compatible with a normal female chromosome complement.

does not always require cell culture to generate sufficient DNA, something that may be important in the context of prenatal testing because of timing. There are disadvantages to aCGH: It does not detect balanced translocations, inversions, or very low-levels of mosaicism.

There are 2 different types of aCGH, targeted and whole-genome arrays. aCGH is the equivalent of doing thousands of FISH experiments in a single sample at once. **Targeted aCGH** is an effective and efficient technique for detecting clinically known cryptic chromosomal aberrations, which are typically associated with known disease phenotypes; many of these arrays have expanded detection to areas potentially susceptible to recurring deletion or duplication. **Whole-genome array** targets the entire genome. The advantage of this latter technique is that it allows better and denser coverage of the entire genome in evenly spaced portions; its disadvantage is that interpretation of deletions or duplications may be difficult if it involves areas not previously known to be involved in disease.

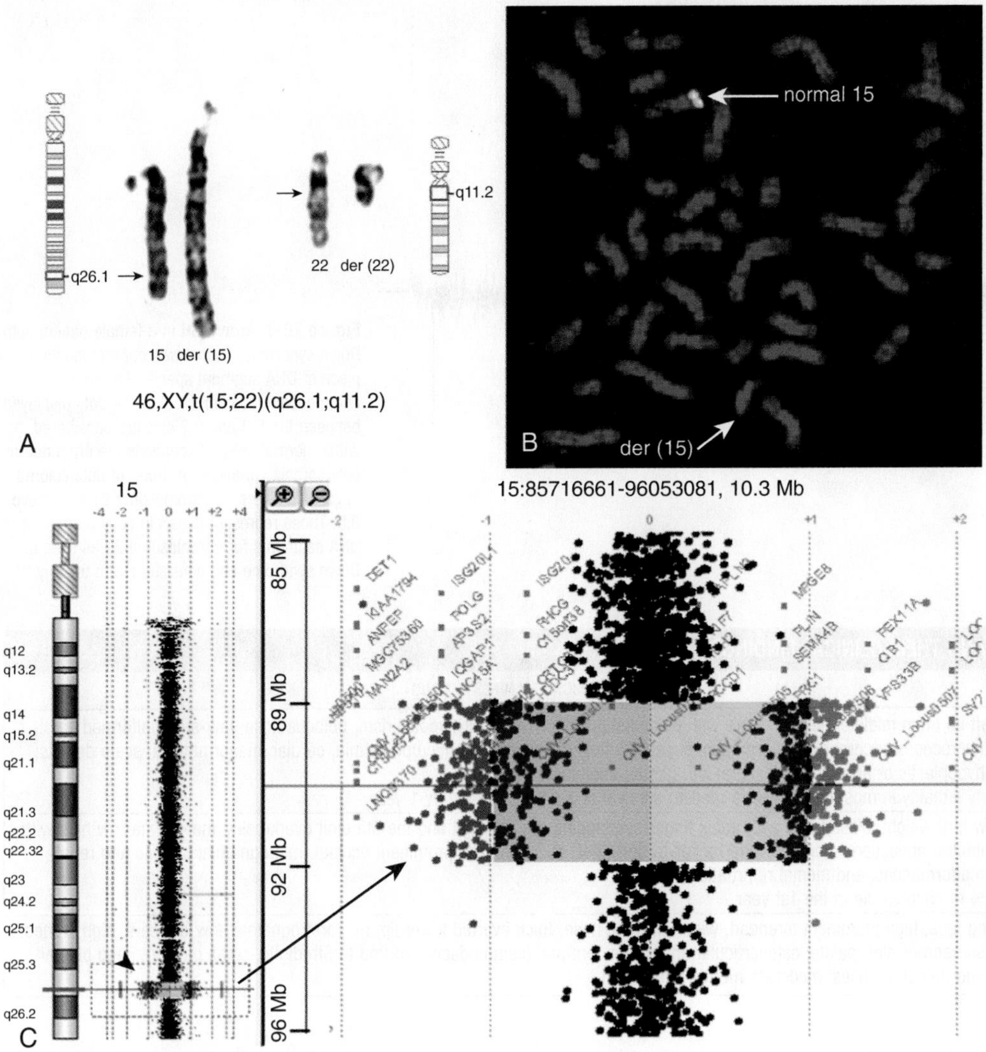

Figure 76-6 An example of a cryptic microdeletion at a translocation breakpoint of an apparently balanced translocation in a patient with DD and growth defect (with permission from the author and the publisher). *A,* Partial karyotype shows t(15;22)(q26.1;q11.2). *B,* FISH with clones 2019 *(green)* and 354M14 *(red)* at 15q26.1; *arrows* indicate signals only present on the normal chromosome 15, suggesting a deletion on the der(15). *C,* Two-color aCGH with dye swap with 244 K oligo probes; *arrowhead* indicates a 3.3-Mb deletion at chromosome 15q26.1-q26.2, *arrow* points to the close-up view of the deletion. (From Li MM, Andersson HC: Clinical application of microarray-based molecular cytogenetics: an emerging new era of genomic medicine, *J Pediatr* 155:311–317, 2009.)

There are many **copy number variations** (**CNVs**) causing deletion or duplication in the human genome. Thus, most detected genetic abnormalities, unless associated with very well known clinical phenotypes, require parental investigations because a detected CNV that is inherited might turn out to be an incidental polymorphic variant. A de novo abnormality (i.e., 1 found only in the child and not the parents) is often more significant if it is associated with an abnormal phenotype and if it involves genes with important functions. aCGH is a very valuable technology alone or when combined with FISH and conventional chromosome studies (Fig. 76-7).

BIBLIOGRAPHY

Please visit the Nelson Textbook of Pediatrics *website at* *www.expertconsult.com* *for the complete bibliography.*

76.2 Down Syndrome and Other Abnormalities of Chromosome Number

Karen Summar and Brendan Lee

ANEUPLOIDY AND POLYPLOIDY

Human cells contain a multiple of 23 chromosomes (n = 23). A haploid cell (n) has 23 chromosomes (typically in the ovum or sperm). If a cell's chromosomes are an exact multiple of 23 (46, 69, 92 in humans), those cells are referred to as euploid. **Polyploid** cells are euploid cells with more than the normal **diploid** number of 46 (2n) chromosomes: 3n, 4n. Polyploid conceptions are usually not viable, but the presence of mosaicism with a karyotypically normal line can allow survival. Mosaicism is an abnormality defined as the presence of 2 or more cell lines in a single individual. Polyploidy is a common abnormality seen in 1st-trimester pregnancy losses. **Triploid cells** are those with 3 haploid sets of chromosomes (3n) and are only viable in a mosaic form. Triploid infants can be liveborn but do not survive long. Triploidy is often the result of fertilization of an egg by 2 sperm (dispermy). Failure of 1 of the meiotic divisions, resulting in a diploid egg or sperm, can also result in triploidy. The phenotype of a triploid conception depends on the origin of the extra chromosome set. If the extra set is of **paternal** origin, it results in a partial hydatidiform mole with poor embryonic development, but triploid conceptions that have an extra set of **maternal** chromosomes results in severe embryonic retardation with a small fibrotic placenta that is typically spontaneously aborted.

Abnormal cells that do not contain a multiple of haploid number of chromosomes are termed **aneuploid** cells. Aneuploidy is the most common and clinically significant type of human chromosome abnormality, occurring in at least 3-4% of all clinically recognized pregnancies. **Monosomies** occur when only 1, instead of the normal 2, of a given chromosome is present in an otherwise diploid cell. In humans, most autosomal monosomies appear to be lethal early in development, and survival is possible in **mosaic forms** or by means of chromosome rescue (restoration

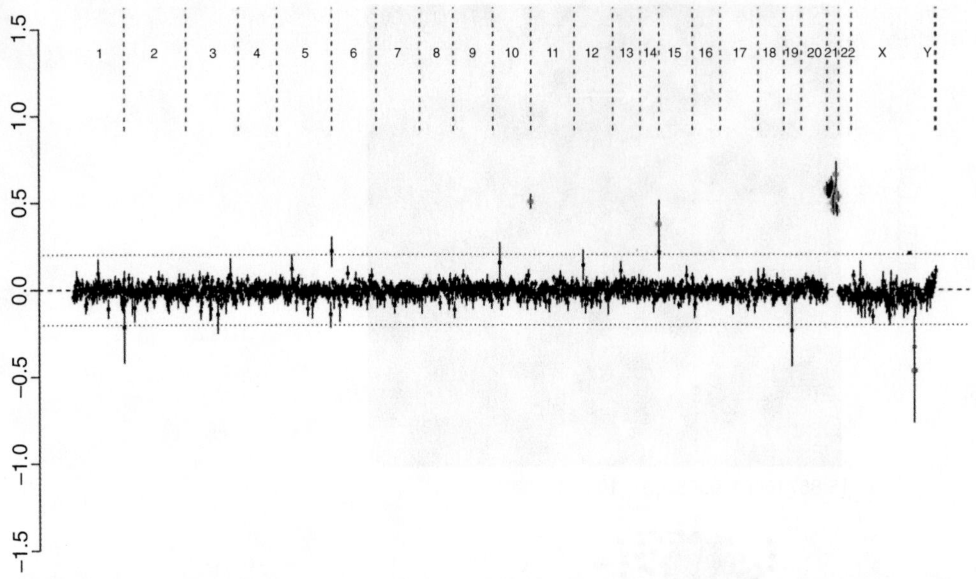

Figure 76-7 Array CGH in a female patient with Down syndrome. Each *black dot* represents a piece of DNA segment specific for different chromosome location. Most of the dots displayed between the 0.0 and 0.2 axis are considered within normal range. Exceptions are often due to polymorphic variations. A group of dots colored in *green* clusters on chromosome 21 and above 0.5. Those represent a *gain* in copy number of DNA segments for chromosome 21 as seen in Down syndrome and consistent with trisomy 21.

Table 76-2 CHROMOSOMAL TRISOMIES AND THEIR CLINICAL FINDINGS

SYNDROME	INCIDENCE	CLINICAL MANIFESTATIONS
Trisomy 13, Patau syndrome	1/10,000 births	Cleft lip often midline; flexed fingers with postaxial polydactyly; ocular hypotelorism, bulbous nose; low-set, malformed ears; microcephaly; cerebral malformation, especially holoprosencephaly; microphthalmia, cardiac malformations; scalp defects; hypoplastic or absent ribs; visceral and genital anomalies Early lethality in most cases, with a median survival of 7 days; 91% die by 1 year
Trisomy 18, Edwards syndrome	1/6,000 births	Low birthweight, closed fists with index finger overlapping the 3rd digit and the 5th digit overlapping the 4th, narrow hips with limited abduction, short sternum, rocker-bottom feet, microcephaly, prominent occiput, micrognathia, cardiac and renal malformations, and mental retardation 95% of children die in the 1st year
Trisomy 8, mosaicism	1/20,000 births	Long face, high prominent forehead, wide upturned nose, thick everted lower lip, microretrognathia, low-set ears, high arched, sometimes cleft palate; osteoarticular anomalies common (camptodactyly of 2nd to 5th digits, small patella); deep plantar and palmar creases; moderate mental retardation

of the normal number by duplication of single monosomic chromosome). An exception to this rule is monosomy for the X chromosome (45,X), seen in Turner syndrome; it has been estimated that the majority of 45,X conceptuses are lost early in pregnancy for as yet unexplained reasons.

The most common cause of aneuploidy is **nondisjunction,** the failure of chromosomes to disjoin normally during meiosis (see Fig. 76-1). Nondisjunction can occur during meiosis I or II or during mitosis. After meiotic nondisjunction, the resulting gamete either lacks a chromosome or has 2 copies instead of 1 normal copy, resulting in a monosomic or trisomic zygote, respectively.

Trisomy is characterized by the presence of 3 chromosomes, instead of the normal 2, of any particular chromosome. Trisomy is the most common form of aneuploidy. Trisomy can occur in all cells or it may be mosaic. Most individuals with trisomy exhibit a consistent and specific phenotype depending on the chromosome involved.

FISH is a technique that can be used for rapid diagnosis in the prenatal detection of common fetal aneuploidies including chromosomes 13, 18, and 21 as well as sex chromosomes (see Fig. 76-5*C* and *D*). The most common numerical abnormalities in liveborn children include trisomy 21 (Down syndrome), trisomy 18 (Edwards syndrome), trisomy 13 (Patau syndrome), and sex chromosomal aneuploidies: Turner syndrome (usually 45,X), Klinefelter syndrome (47,XXY), 47,XXX, and 47,XYY, By far the most common type of trisomy in liveborn infants is trisomy 21 (47,XX,+21 or 47,XY,+21). Trisomy 18 and trisomy 13 are relatively less common and are associated with a characteristic set of congenital anomalies and severe mental retardation (Table 76-2). The occurrence of trisomy 21 and other trisomies increases with advanced maternal age (≥35 yr). Owing to this increased risk, women who are ≥35 yr at the time of delivery should be offered genetic counseling and prenatal diagnosis (including serum screening, ultrasonography, and amniocentesis or chorionic villus sampling; Chapter 90).

DOWN SYNDROME

Trisomy 21 is the most common genetic cause of moderate mental retardation. The incidence of Down syndrome in live births is approximately 1 in 733; the incidence at conception is more than twice that rate; the difference is accounted by early pregnancy losses. In addition to cognitive impairment, Down syndrome is associated with congenital anomalies and characteristic dysmorphic features (Figs. 76-8 and 76-9; Table 76-3). Although there is variability in the clinical features, the constellation of phenotypic features is fairly consistent and permits clinical recognition of trisomy 21. Affected individuals are more prone to congenital heart defects (50%) such as atrioventricular septal defects, ventricular septal defects, isolated secundum atrial septal defects, patent ductus arteriosus, and tetralogy of Fallot. Congenital and acquired gastrointestinal anomalies and hypothyroidism are common (Table 76-4). Other abnormalities include megakaryoblastic leukemia, immune dysfunction, diabetes mellitus, and problems with hearing and vision (see Table 76-4). Alzheimer disease–like dementia is a known complication that occurs as early as the 4th decade and has an incidence 2-3 times higher than sporadic Alzheimer disease. Most males with Down syndrome are sterile, but some females have been able to reproduce, with a 50% chance of having trisomy 21 pregnancies. Two genes

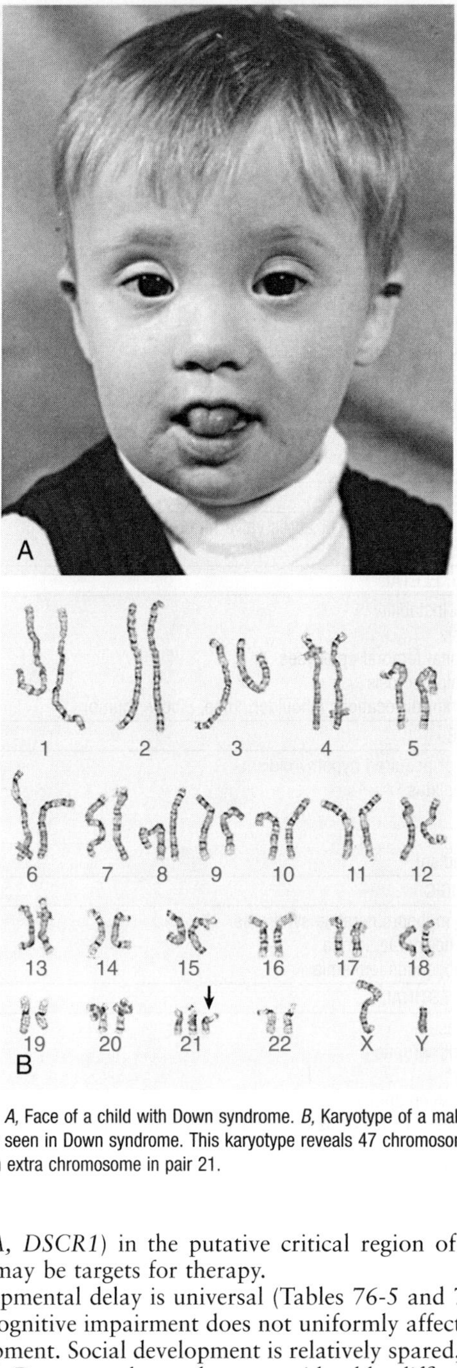

Figure 76-8 *A,* Face of a child with Down syndrome. *B,* Karyotype of a male with trisomy 21 as seen in Down syndrome. This karyotype reveals 47 chromosomes instead of 46, with an extra chromosome in pair 21.

(*DYRK1A, DSCR1*) in the putative critical region of chromosome 21 may be targets for therapy.

Developmental delay is universal (Tables 76-5 and 76-6; Fig. 76-10). Cognitive impairment does not uniformly affect all areas of development. Social development is relatively spared, but children with Down syndrome have considerable difficulty using expressive language. Understanding these individual developmental strengths will maximize the educational process for children with Down syndrome. Persons with Down syndrome often benefit from programs aimed at stimulation, development, and education. These programs are most effective in addressing social skills that often appear advanced for the intellectual delay. Children with Down syndrome also benefit from anticipatory guidance, which establishes the protocol for screening, evaluation, and care for patients with genetic syndromes and chronic disorders (Table 76-7).

The majority of children with Down syndrome do not have behavior problems. It is estimated that psychiatric comorbidity is 18-38% in this population. These estimates are higher than in unaffected children, but they are lower than in children with similar levels of mental retardation from other etiologies. All maladaptive behaviors in persons with Down syndrome are thought to be inherently linked to cognitive impairment.

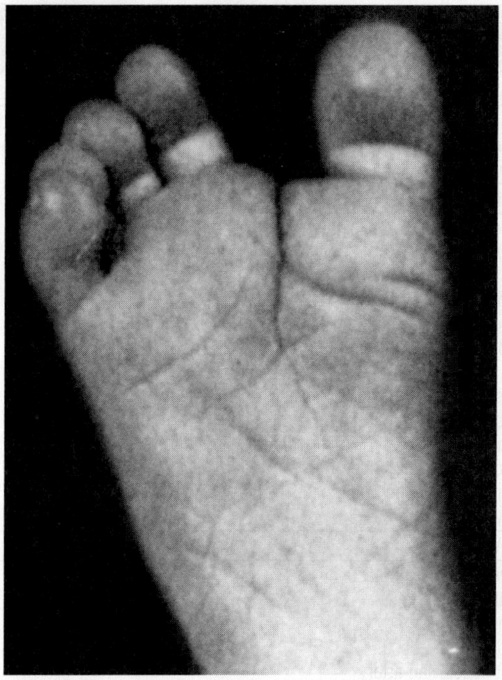

Figure 76-9 Prehensile foot in a 1-mo-old child. (From Wiedemann HR, Kunze J, Dibbern H: *Atlas of clinical syndromes: a visual guide to diagnosis,* ed 3, St Louis, 1989, Mosby.)

Common behavioral difficulties that occur in children with Down syndrome include inattentiveness, stubbornness, and a need for routine and sameness. Aggression and self-injurious behavior are less common in this population. All of these behaviors can respond to educational or pharmacologic interventions.

The life expectancy for children with Down syndrome is reduced and is approximately 50 to 55 yr. Little prospective information about the secondary medical problems of adults with Down syndrome is known. Retrospective studies have shown premature aging and an increased risk of Alzheimer disease in adults with Down syndrome. These studies have also shown unexpected negative associations between Down syndrome and other medical comorbidities. Persons with Down syndrome have fewer than expected deaths caused by solid tumors and ischemic heart disease. This same study reported increased risk of adult deaths due to congenital heart disease, seizures, and leukemia. In 1 large study, leukemias accounted for 60% of all cancers in people with Down syndrome and 97% of all cancers in children with Down syndrome. There was decreased risk of solid tumors in all age groups, including neuroblastomas and nephroblastomas in children with Down syndrome and epithelial tumors in adults with Down syndrome.

Most adults with Down syndrome are able to perform activities of daily living. However, most adults with Down syndrome have difficulty with complex financial, legal, or medical decisions. In most circumstances, a conservator is appointed for the adult with Down syndrome.

This risk of having a child with trisomy 21 is highest in women who conceive at >35 yr of age. Even though younger women have a lower risk, they represent half of all mothers with babies with Down syndrome because of their higher overall birth rate. *All women should be offered screening for Down syndrome* in their 2nd trimester by means of 4 maternal serum tests (free β-human chorionic gonadotropin (β-hCG), unconjugated estriol, inhibin, and α-fetoprotein). This is known as the *quad screen;* it can detect up to 80% of Down syndrome pregnancies compared to 70% in the triple screen. Both tests have a 5% false-positive rate. There is a method of screening during the 1st trimester using fetal nuchal translucency (NT) thickness that can be done alone or

Table 76-3 CLINICAL FEATURES OF DOWN SYNDROME IN THE NEONATAL PERIOD

CENTRAL NERVOUS SYSTEM
Hypotonia* Developmental delay Poor Moro reflex*
CRANIOFACIAL
Brachycephaly with flat occiput Flat face* Upward slanted palpebral fissures* Epicanthal folds Speckled irises (Brushfield spots) Three fontanels Delayed fontanel closure Frontal sinus and midfacial hypoplasia Mild microcephaly Short hard palate Small nose, flat nasal bridge Protruding tongue, open mouth Small dysplastic ears*
CARDIOVASCULAR
Endocardial Cushing defects Ventricular septal defect Atrial septal defect Patent ductus arteriosus Aberrant subclavian artery Pulmonary hypertension
MUSCULOSKELETAL
Joint hyperflexibility* Short neck, redundant skin* Short metacarpals and phalanges Short 5th digit with clinodactyly* Single transverse palmar creases* Wide gap between 1st and 2nd toes Pelvic dysplasia* Short sternum Two sternal manubrium ossification centers
GASTROINTESTINAL
Duodenal atresia Annular pancreas Tracheoesophageal fistula Hirschsprung disease Imperforate anus
CUTANEOUS
Cutis marmorta

*Hall's criteria to aid in diagnosis.

in conjunction with maternal serum β-hCG and pregnancy-associated plasma protein-A (PAPP-A). In the 1st trimester, NT alone can detect ≤70% of Down syndrome pregnancies, but with β-hCG and PAPP-A, the detection goes up to 87%. If both 1st and 2nd trimester screens are combined using NT and biochemical profiles (integrated screen), the detection rate goes up to 95%. If only 1st trimester quad screening is done, α-fetoprotein (MSAFP, which is decreased in affected pregnancies) is recommended as a 2nd trimester follow-up. Detection of fetal DNA in maternal plasma may also be diagnostic. The prenatal screens are also useful for other trisomies, although the detection rates are different from those given for Down syndrome.

In approximately 95% of the cases of Down syndrome there are 3 copies of chromosome 21. The origin of the supernumerary chromosome 21 is maternal in 97% of the cases as a result of errors in meiosis. The majority of these occur in maternal meiosis I (90%). Approximately 1% of persons with trisomy 21 are mosaics, with some cells having 46 chromosomes, and another 4% of have a **translocation** that involves chromosome 21. The majority of translocations in Down syndrome are fusions at the centromere between chromosomes 13, 14, 15, 21, and 22 known as *Robertsonian translocations*. The translocations can be de

Table 76-4 ADDITIONAL FEATURES OF DOWN SYNDROME THAT CAN DEVELOP OR BECOME SYMPTOMATIC WITH TIME

NEUROPSYCHIATRIC
Developmental delay Seizures Autism spectrum disorders Behavioral disorders (disruptive) Depression Alzheimer disease
SENSORY
Congenital or acquired hearing loss Serous otitis media Refractive errors (myopia) Congenital or acquired cataracts Nystagmus Strabismus Glaucoma Blocked tear ducts
CARDIOVASCULAR
Acquired mitral, tricuspid, or aortic valve regurgitation Endocarditis
MUSCULOSKELETAL
Atlantoaxial instability Hip dysplasia Slipped capital femoral epiphyses Avascular hip necrosis Recurrent joint dislocations (shoulder, knee, elbow, thumb)
ENDOCRINE
Congenital or acquired hypothyroidism Diabetes mellitus Infertility Obesity Hyperthyroidism
HEMATOLOGIC
Transient lymphoproliferative syndrome Acute lymphocytic leukemia Acute myelogenous leukemia
GASTROINTESTINAL
Celiac disease Delayed tooth eruption Respiratory Obstructed sleep apnea Frequent infections (sinusitis, nasopharyngitis, pneumonia)
CUTANEOUS
Hyperkeratosis Seborrhea Xerosis Perigenital folliculitis

Table 76-5 DEVELOPMENTAL MILESTONES

MILESTONE	CHILDREN WITH DOWN SYNDROME		UNAFFECTED CHILDREN	
	Average (mo)	Range (mo)	Average (mo)	Range (mo)
Smiling	2	1½-3	1	½-3
Rolling over	6	2-12	5	2-10
Sitting	9	6-18	7	5-9
Crawling	11	7-21	8	6-11
Creeping	13	8-25	10	7-13
Standing	10	10-32	11	8-16
Walking	20	12-45	13	8-18
Talking, words	14	9-30	10	6-14
Talking, sentences	24	18-46	21	14-32

From Levine MD, Carey WB, Crocker AC, editors: *Developmental-behavioral pediatrics*, ed 2, Philadelphia, 1992, Saunders.

novo or inherited. Very rarely is Down syndrome diagnosed in a patient with only a part of the long arm of chromosome 21 in triplicate (**partial trisomy**). Isochromosomes and ring chromosomes are other rarer causes of trisomy 21. Down syndrome patients without a visible chromosome abnormality are the least common. It is not possible to distinguish the phenotypes of persons with full trisomy 21 and those with a translocation. Representative genes on chromosome 21 and their potential effects on development are noted in Table 76-8. Patients who are mosaic tend to have a milder phenotype.

Chromosome analysis is indicated in every person suspected of having Down syndrome. If a translocation is identified, parental chromosome studies must be performed to determine whether 1 of the parents is a translocation carrier, which carries a high recurrence risk for having another affected child. That parent might also have other family members at risk. Translocation (21;21) carriers have a 100% recurrence risk for a chromosomally abnormal child, and other Robertsonian translocations, such as t(14;21), have a 5-7% recurrence risk when transmitted by females. Genomic dosage imbalance contributes through direct and indirect pathways to the Down syndrome phenotype and its phenotypic variation.

Tables 76-9 and 76-10 provide more information on other aneuploidies and partial autosomal aneuploidies (Figs. 76-11 to 76-14).

BIBLIOGRAPHY

Please visit the Nelson Textbook of Pediatrics *website at www.expertconsult.com for the complete bibliography.*

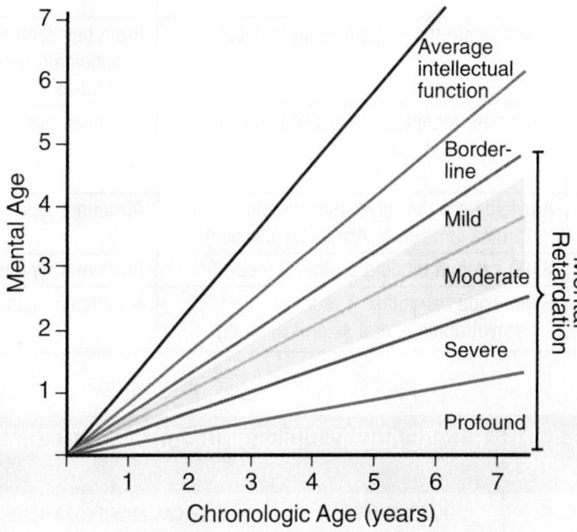

Figure 76-10 The area shaded in yellow denotes the range of intellectual function of the majority of children with Down syndrome. (From Levine MD, Carey WB, Crocker AC, editors: *Developmental-behavioral pediatrics,* ed 2, Philadelphia, 1992, WB Saunders, p 226.)

Table 76-6 SELF-HELP SKILLS

SKILL	DOWN SYNDROME CHILDREN Average (mo)	DOWN SYNDROME CHILDREN Range (mo)	UNAFFECTED CHILDREN Average (mo)	UNAFFECTED CHILDREN Range (mo)
EATING				
Finger feeding	12	8-28	8	6-16
Using spoon/fork	20	12-40	13	8-20
TOILET TRAINING				
Bladder	48	20-95	32	18-60
Bowel	42	28-90	29	16-48
DRESSING				
Undressing	40	29-72	32	22-42
Putting clothes on	58	38-98	47	34-58

From Levine MD, Carey WB, Crocker AC, editors: *Developmental-behavioral pediatrics,* ed 2, Philadelphia, 1992, Saunders.

Table 76-7 HEALTH SUPERVISION FOR CHILDREN WITH DOWN SYNDROME

CONDITION	TIME TO SCREEN	COMMENT
Congenital heart disease	Birth; by pediatric cardiologist Young adult for acquired valve disease	50% risk of congenital heart disease. Increased risk for pulmonary hypertension
Strabismus, cataracts, nystagmus	Birth or by 6 mo; by pediatric ophthalmologist **Check vision annually**	Cataracts occur in 15%, refractive errors in 50%
Hearing impairment or loss	Birth or by 3 mo with auditory brainstem response or otoacoustic emission testing; check hearing q6mo up to 3 yrs if tympanic membrane is not visualized; **annually thereafter**	Risk for congenital hearing loss plus 50-70% risk of serous otitis media.
Constipation	Birth	Increased risk for Hirschsprung disease
Celiac disease	At 2 years or with symptoms	Screen with IgA and tissue transglutaminase antibodies
Hematologic disease	At birth and in adolescence or if symptoms develop	Increased risk for neonatal polycythemia (18%), leukemoid reaction, leukemia (<1%)
Hypothyroidism	Birth; repeat at 6-12 mo and **annually**	Congenital (1%) and acquired (5%)
Growth and development	At each visit Use Down syndrome growth curves	Discuss school placement options Proper diet to avoid obesity
Obstructive sleep apnea	Start at ~1 yr and at each visit	Monitor for snoring, restless sleep
Atlantoaxial subluxation or instability (incidence 10-30%)	At each visit by history and physical exam Radiographs at 3-5 years or when planning to participate in contact sports Radiographs indicated wherever neurologic symptoms are present even if transient (neck pain, torticollis, gait disturbances, weakness) Many are asymptomatic	Special Olympics recommendations are to screen for high risk sports, e.g., diving, swimming, contact sports
Gynecologic care	Adolescent girls	Menstruation and contraception issues
Recurrent infections	When present	Check IgG subclass and IgA levels
Psychiatric, behavioral disorders	At each visit	Depression, anxiety, obsessive compulsive disorder, schizophrenia seem in 10-17% Autism spectrum disorder in 5-10% Early-onset Alzheimer disease

IgA, immunoglobulin A; IgG, immunoglobulin G.
Extracted from Committee on Genetics: Health supervision for children with Down syndrome, *Pediatrics* 107:442–449, 2001; and Baum RA, Spader M, Nash PL, et al: Primary care of children and adolescents with Down syndrome: an update, *Curr Prob Pediatr Adolesc Health Care* 38:235–268, 2008.

Table 76-8 GENES LOCALIZED TO CHROMOSOME 21 THAT POSSIBLY AFFECT BRAIN DEVELOPMENT, NEURONAL LOSS, AND ALZHEIMER TYPE NEUROPATHOLOGY

SYMBOL	NAME	POSSIBLE EFFECT IN DOWN SYNDROME	FUNCTION
SIM2	Single-minded homolog 2	Brain development	Required for synchronized cell division and establishment of proper cell lineage
DYRK1A	Dual-specificity tyrosine-(Y)-phosphorylation regulated kinase 1A	Brain development	Expressed during neuroblast proliferation Believed important homolog in regulating cell-cycle kinetics during cell division
GART	Phosphoribosylglycinamideformyltransferase Phosphoribosylglycinamide synthetase Phosphoribosylaminoimidazole synthetase	Brain development	Expressed during prenatal development of the cerebellum
PCP4	Purkinje cell protein 4	Brain development	Function unknown but found exclusively in the brain and most abundantly in the cerebellum
DSCAM	Down syndrome cell adhesion molecule	Brain development and possible candidate gene for congenital heart disease	Expressed in all molecule regions of the brain and believed to have a role in axonal outgrowth during development of the nervous system
GRIK1	Glutamate receptor, ionotropic kainite1	Neuronal loss	Function unknown, found in the cortex in fetal and early postnatal life and in adult primates, most concentrated in pyramidal cells in the cortex
APP	Amyloid beta (A4) precursor protein (protease nexin-II, Alzheimer disease)	Alzheimer type neuropathy	Seems to be involved in plasticity, neurite outgrowth, and neuroprotection
S100B	S100 calcium binding protein β (neural)	Alzheimer type neuropathy	Stimulates glial formation
SOD1	Superoxide dismutase 1, soluble (amyotrophic lateral sclerosis, adult)	Accelerated aging?	Scavenges free superoxide molecules in the cell and might accelerate aging by producing hydrogen peroxide and oxygen

Table 76-9 OTHER RARE ANEUPLOIDIES AND PARTIAL AUTOSOMAL ANEUPLOIDIES

DISORDER	KARYOTYPE	CLINICAL MANIFESTATIONS
Trisomy 8	47,XX/XY,+8	Growth and mental deficiency are variable The majority of patients are mosaics Deep palmar and plantar furrows are characteristic
Trisomy 9	47,XX/XY,+9	The majority of patients are mosaics Clinical features include craniofacial (high forehead, microphthalmia, low-set malformed ears, bulbous nose) and skeletal (joint contractures) malformations and heart defects (60%)
Trisomy 16	47,XX/XY,+16	The most commonly observed autosomal aneuploidy in spontaneous abortion; the recurrence risk is negligible
Tetrasomy 12p	46,XX[12]/46,XX, +i(12p)[8] (mosaicism for an isochromosome 12p)	Known as Pallister-Killian syndrome. Sparse anterior scalp hair, eyebrows, and eyelashes, prominent forehead, chubby cheeks, long philtrum with thin upper lip and cupid-bow configuration, polydactyly, and streaks of hyper- and hypopigmentation

Table 76-10 FINDINGS THAT MAY BE PRESENT IN TRISOMY 13 AND TRISOMY 18

TRISOMY 13	TRISOMY 18
HEAD AND FACE	
Scalp defects (e.g., cutis aplasia) Microphthalmia, corneal abnormalities Cleft lip and palate in 60%-80% of cases Microcephaly Microphthalmia Sloping forehead Holoprosencephaly (arhinencephaly) Capillary hemangiomas Deafness	Small and premature appearance Tight palpebral fissures Narrow nose and hypoplastic nasal alae Narrow bifrontal diameter Prominent occiput Micrognathia Cleft lip or palate Microcephaly
CHEST	
Congenital heart disease (e.g., VSD, PDA, and ASD) in 80% of cases Thin posterior ribs (missing ribs)	Congenital heart disease (e.g., VSD, PDA, ASD) Short sternum, small nipples
EXTREMITIES	
Overlapping of fingers and toes (clinodactyly) Polydactyly Hypoplastic nails, hyperconvex nails	Limited hip abduction Clinodactyly and overlapping fingers; index over 3rd, 5th over 4th; closed fist Rocker-bottom feet Hypoplastic nails
GENERAL	
Severe developmental delays and prenatal and postnatal growth retardation Renal abnormalities Only 5% live >6 mo	Severe developmental delays and prenatal and postnatal growth retardation Premature birth, polyhydramnios Inguinal or abdominal hernias Only 5% live >1 yr

VSD, ventricular septal defect; PDA, patent ductus arteriosus; ASD, atrial septal defect.
From Behrman RE, Kliegman RM: *Nelson essentials of pediatrics,* ed 4, Philadelphia, 2002, WB Saunders, p 142.

76.3 Abnormalities of Chromosome Structure

Carlos A. Bacino and Brendan Lee

TRANSLOCATIONS

Translocations, which involve the transfer of material from 1 chromosome to another, occur with a frequency of 1/500 liveborn human infants. They may be inherited from a carrier parent or appear de novo, with no other affected family member. Translocations are commonly reciprocal or Robertsonian, involving 2 chromosomes (Fig. 76-15).

Reciprocal translocations are the result of breaks in nonhomologous chromosomes, with reciprocal exchange of the broken segments. Carriers of a reciprocal translocation are

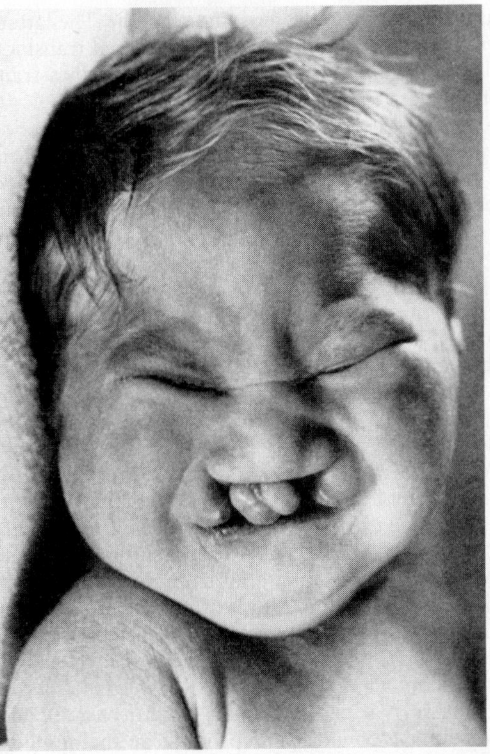

Figure 76-11 Facial appearance of a child with trisomy 13. (From Wiedemann HR, Kunze J, Dibbern H: *Atlas of clinical syndromes: a visual guide to diagnosis,* ed 3, St Louis, 1989, Mosby.)

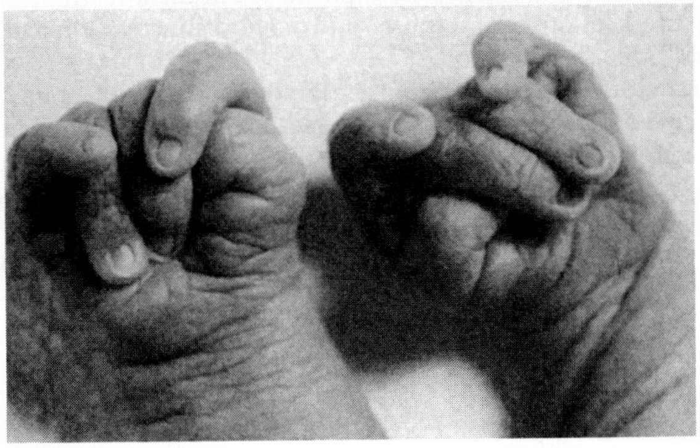

Figure 76-12 Trisomy 18: overlapping fingers and hypoplastic nails. (From Wiedemann HR, Kunze J, Dibbern H: *Atlas of clinical syndromes: a visual guide to diagnosis,* ed 3, St Louis, 1989, Mosby.)

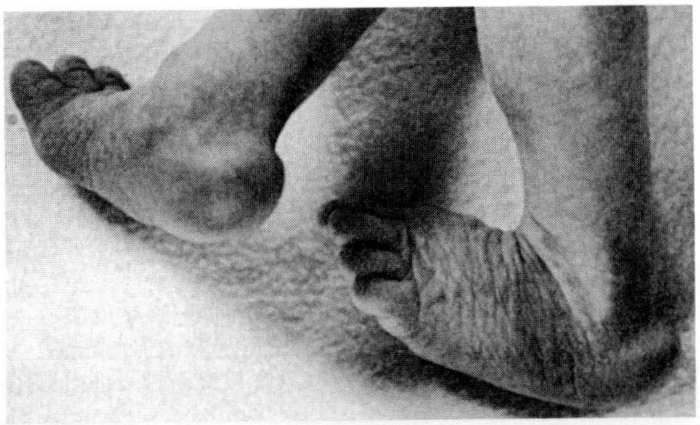

Figure 76-13 Trisomy 18: rocker-bottom feet (protruding calcanei). (From Wiedemann HR, Kunze J, Dibbern H: *Atlas of clinical syndromes: a visual guide to diagnosis,* ed 3, St Louis, 1989, Mosby.)

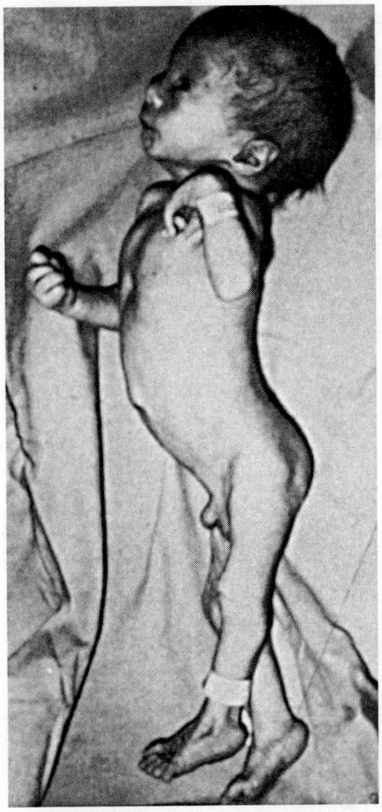

Figure 76-14 Male infant with trisomy 18 at age 4 days. Note prominent occiput, micrognathia, low-set ears, short sternum, narrow pelvis, prominent calcaneus, and flexion abnormalities of the fingers.

usually phenotypically normal but are at an increased risk for miscarriage due to transmission of unbalanced reciprocal translocations and for bearing chromosomally abnormal offspring. Unbalanced translocations are the result of abnormalities in the segregation or crossover of the translocation carrier chromosomes in the germ cells.

Robertsonian translocations involve 2 acrocentric chromosomes (chromosomes 13, 14, 15, 21, and 22) that fuse near the centromeric region with a subsequent loss of the short arms. Because the short arms of all 5 pairs of acrocentric chromosomes have multiple copies of genes for ribosomal RNA, loss of the short arm of 2 acrocentric chromosomes has no deleterious effect. The resulting karyotype has only 45 chromosomes, including the translocated chromosome that is made up of the long arm of the 2 fused chromosomes. Carriers of Robertsonian translocations are usually phenotypically normal. However, they are at increased risk for miscarriage and unbalanced abnormal offspring.

In some rare instances, translocations can involve 3 or more chromosomes, as seen in complex rearrangements. Another, less-common type is the insertional translocation. Insertional translocations result from a piece of chromosome material that breaks away and later is reinserted inside the same chromosome at a different site or inserted in another chromosome.

INVERSIONS

An inversion requires that a single chromosome break at 2 points; the broken piece is then inverted and joined into the same chromosome. Inversions occur in 1/100 live births. There are 2 types of inversions: pericentric and paracentric. In **pericentric inversions,** the breaks are in the 2 opposite arms of the chromosome and include the centromere. They are usually discovered because they change the position of the centromere. The breaks in **paracentric inversions** occur in only 1 arm. Carriers of inversions are usually phenotypically normal, but they are at increased risk for miscarriages, typically in paracentric inversions, and chromosomally abnormal offspring in pericentric inversions.

DELETIONS AND DUPLICATIONS

Deletions involve loss of chromosome material and, depending on their location, they can be classified as **terminal** (at the ends of chromosomes) or **interstitial** (within the arms of a chromosome). They may be isolated or they may occur along with a duplication of another chromosome segment. The latter typically occurs in unbalanced reciprocal chromosomal translocation secondary to abnormal crossover or segregation in a translocation or inversion carrier.

A carrier of a deletion is monosomic for the genetic information of the missing segment. Deletions are usually associated with mental retardation and malformations. The most commonly observed deletions in routine chromosome preparations include 1p-, 4p-, 5p-, 9p-, 11p-, 13q-, 18p-, 18q-, and 21q- (Table 76-11 and Fig. 76-16), all distal or terminal deletions of the short or the long arms of chromosomes. Deletions may be observed in routine chromosome preparations, and deletions and translocations larger than 5-10 Mb are usually visible microscopically.

High-resolution banding techniques, FISH, and molecular studies like aCGH can reveal deletions that are too small to be seen in ordinary or routine chromosome spreads (see Fig. 76-7). **Microdeletions** involve loss of small chromosome regions, the largest of which are detectable only with prophase chromosome studies and/or molecular methods. For submicroscopic deletions, the missing piece can only be detected using molecular methodologies such as FISH or DNA-based studies like aCGH. The presence of extra genetic material from the same chromosome is referred to as **duplication.** Duplications can also be sporadic or result from abnormal segregation in translocation or inversion carriers.

Microdeletions and microduplications usually involve regions that include several genes, so that the affected individuals can have a distinctive phenotype depending on the number of genes involved. When such a deletion involves more than a single gene, the condition is referred to as a **contiguous gene deletion syndrome** (Table 76-12). With the advent of clinically available aCGH, a large number of duplications, most of them microduplications, have been uncovered. Most of those **microduplication syndromes** are the reciprocal duplications of the known deletions or microdeletion counterparts and have distinctive clinical features (Table 76-13).

Subtelomeric regions are often involved in chromosome rearrangements that cannot be visualized using routine cytogenetics. Telomeres, which are the distal ends of the chromosomes, are gene-rich regions. The distal structure of the telomeres is essentially common to all chromosomes, but proximal to those, there are unique regions known as subtelomeres, which typically involved in deletions and most other chromosome rearrangements. Small subtelomeric deletions, duplications, or rearrangements (translocations, inversions) may be relatively common in nonspecific mental retardation with minor anomalies. Subtelomeric rearrangements have been found in 3-7% of children with moderate to mild mental retardation and 0.5% of children with mild mental retardation.

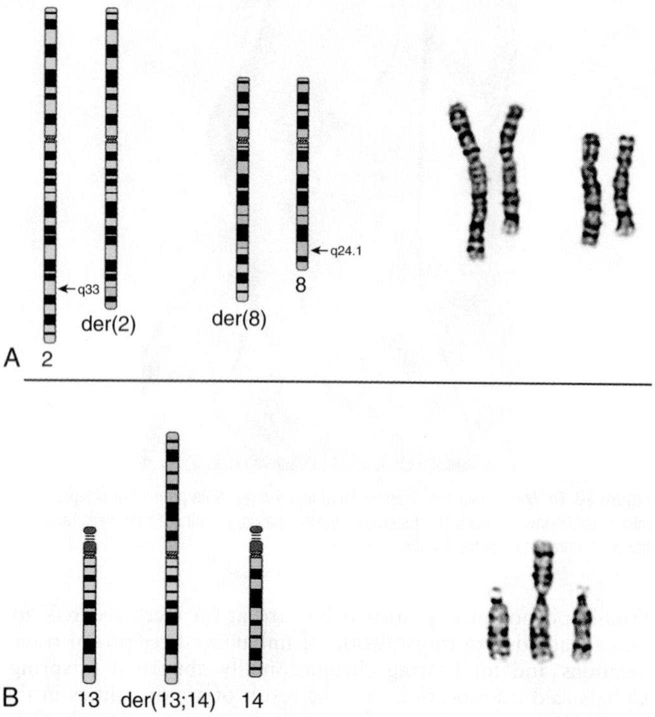

Figure 76-15 *A,* Schematic diagram *(left)* and partial G-banded karyotype *(right)* of a reciprocal translocation between chromosome 2 *(blue)* and chromosome 8 *(pink).* The breakpoints are on the long (q) arm of both chromosomes at bands 2q33 and 8q24.1, with the reciprocal exchange of material between the derivative (der) chromosomes 2 and 8. This translocation is balanced, with no net gain or loss of material. The nomenclature for this exchange is t(2;8)(q33:q24.1). *B,* Schematic diagram *(left)* and partial G-banded karyotype *(right)* of a Robertsonian translocation between chromosomes 13 *(blue)* and 14 *(pink).* The breakpoints are at the centromere (band q10) of both chromosomes, with fusion of the long arms into a single derivative chromosome and loss of the short (p) arm material. The nomenclature for this exchange is der(13;14)(q10;q10).

Table 76-11 COMMON DELETIONS AND THEIR CLINICAL MANIFESTATIONS

DELETION	CLINICAL ABNORMALITIES
4p-	Wolf-Hirschhorn syndrome. The main features are a typical "Greek helmet" facies secondary to ocular hypertelorism, prominent glabella, and frontal bossing; microcephaly, dolichocephaly, hypoplasia of the orbits, ptosis, strabismus, nystagmus, bilateral epicanthic folds, cleft lip and palate, beaked nose with prominent bridge, hypospadias, cardiac malformations, and mental retardation.
5p-	Cri-du-chat syndrome. The main features are hypotonia, short stature, characteristic shrill cry in the first few weeks of life (cat like cry), microcephaly with protruding metopic suture, hypertelorism, bilateral epicanthic folds, high arched palate, wide and flat nasal bridge, and mental retardation.
9p-	The main features are craniofacial dysmorphology with trigonocephaly, slanted palpebral fissures, discrete exophthalmos secondary to supraorbital hypoplasia, arched eyebrows, flat and wide nasal bridge, short neck with low hairline, genital anomalies, long fingers and toes with extra flexion creases, cardiac malformations, and mental retardation.
13q-	The main features are low birthweight, failure to thrive, microcephaly, and severe mental retardation. Facial features include high wide nasal bridge, hypertelorism, ptosis, micrognathia. Ocular malformations are common (retinoblastoma). The hands have hypoplastic or absent thumbs and syndactyly.
18p-	A few patients (15%) are severely affected and have cephalic and ocular malformations: holoprosencephaly, cleft lip and palate, ptosis, epicanthal folds, and varying degrees of mental retardation. Most (80%) have only minor malformations and mild mental retardation.
18q-	Growth deficiency, hypotonia with "froglike" position with the legs flexed, externally rotated, and in hyperabduction. The face is characteristic with depressed midface and apparent protrusion of the mandible, deep-set eyes, short upper lip, everted lower lip ("carplike" mouth); antihelix of the ears is very prominent; varying degrees of mental retardation and belligerent personality. Myelination abnormalities in the CNS.

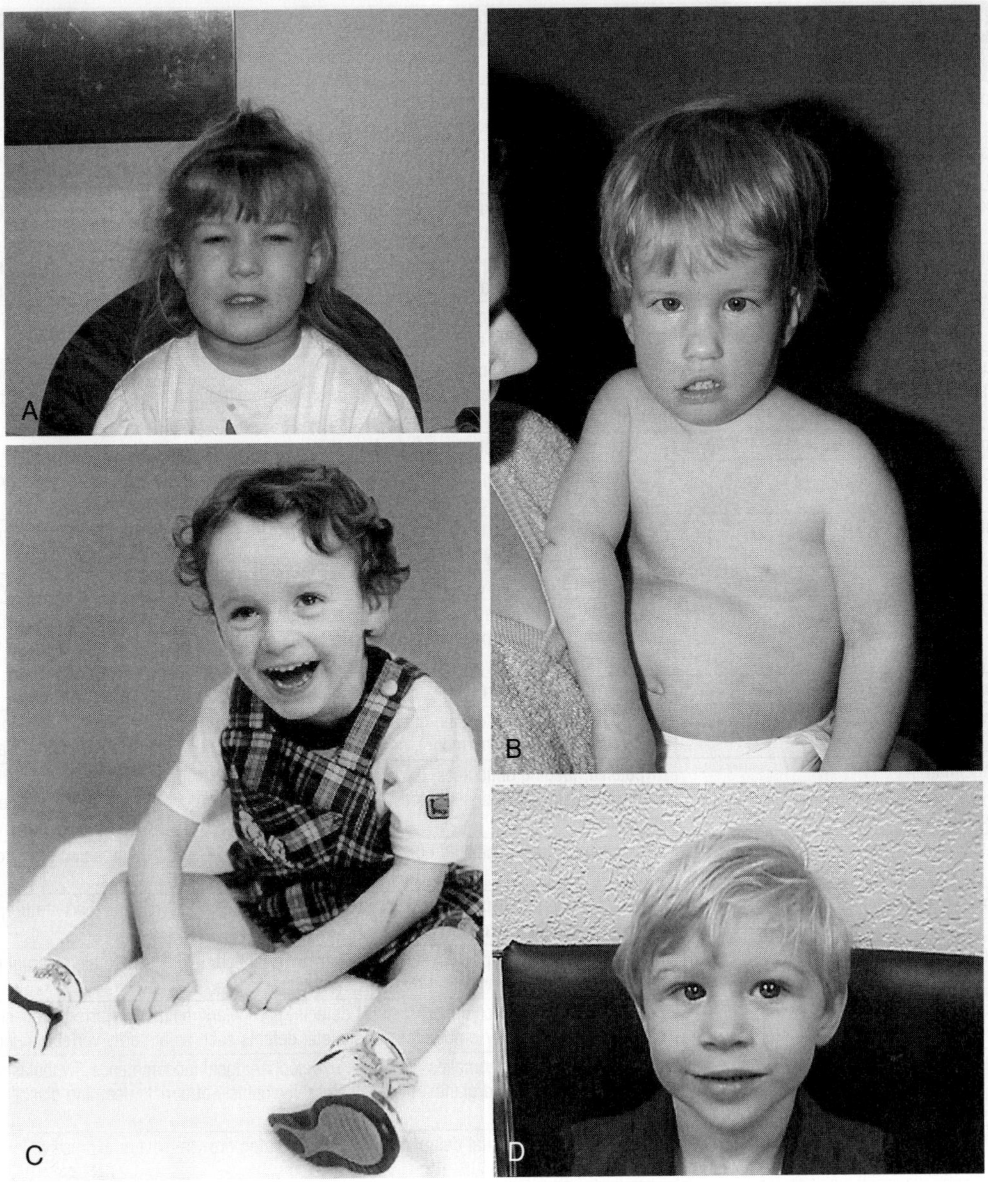

Figure 76-16 *A,* Child with velocardiofacial syndrome (deletion 22q11.2). *B,* Child with Prader-Willi syndrome (deletion 15q11-13). *C,* Child with Angelman syndrome (deletion 15q11-13). *D,* Child with Williams syndrome (deletion 7q11.23). (From Lin RL, Cherry AM, Bangs CD, et al: FISHing for answers: the use of molecular cytogenetic techniques in adolescent medicine practice. In Hyme HE, Greydanus D, editors: *Genetic disorders in adolescents: state of the art reviews. Adolescent medicine,* Philadelphia, 2002, Hanley and Belfus, pp 305–313.)

Clinical features (>30%) include short stature, microcephaly, hypertelorism, nose and ear abnormalities, and cryptorchidism. This group is also characterized by a family history of mental retardation and an increased likelihood of retarded growth beginning in the prenatal period. Telomere mutations have also been associated with dyskeratosis congenita and other aplastic anemia syndromes as well as pulmonary or hepatic fibrosis. Both the subtelomeric rearrangements and the microdeletion and microduplication syndromes are typically diagnosed by molecular techniques like FISH, multiple ligation-dependent primer amplification (MLPA) and/or aCGH. Many studies show that aCGH can detect 14-18% of abnormalities in patients who are previously known to have normal chromosome studies.

INSERTIONS

Insertions occur when a piece of a chromosome broken at 2 points is incorporated into a break in another part of a chromosome. A total of 3 breakpoints are then required, and they can occur between 2 or within 1 chromosome. A form of nonreciprocal translocation, insertions are rare. Insertion carriers are at risk of having offspring with deletions or duplications of the inserted segment.

ISOCHROMOSOMES

Isochromosomes consist of 2 copies of the same chromosome arm joined through a single centromere and forming mirror images of one another. The most commonly reported autosomal isochromosomes tend to involve chromosomes with small arms. Some of the more common chromosome arms involved in this formation include 5p, 8p, 9p, 12p, 18p, and 18q. This is also a common abnormality seen in long arm of the X chromosome and associated with Turner syndrome. Individuals who have 1 isochromosome in 46 chromosomes are monosomic for genes in the lost arm and trisomic for the genes present in the isochromosome.

Table 76-12 MICRODELETION AND CONTIGUOUS GENE SYNDROMES AND THEIR CLINICAL MANIFESTATIONS

DELETION	SYNDROME	CLINICAL MANIFESTATIONS
1p36	1p deletion	Growth retardation, dysmorphic features with midface hypoplasia, straight thin eyebrows, pointy chin, sensorineural hearing loss, progressive cardiomyopathy, hypothyroidism, seizures, mental retardation
5q35	Sotos (50% are deletions of *NSD1* gene in Asians but only 6% in whites)	Overgrowth, macrocephaly, prominent forehead, prominence of extra-axial fluid spaces on brain imaging, large hands and feet, hypotonia, clumsiness, mental disabilities
6p25	Axenfeld-Rieger	Axenfeld-Rieger malformation, hearing loss, congenital heart defects, dental anomalies, developmental delays, facial dysmorphism
7q11.23	Williams	Round face with full cheeks and lips, long philtrum, stellate pattern in iris, strabismus, supravalvular aortic stenosis and other cardiac malformations, varying degrees of mental retardation, friendly personality
8p11	8p11	Kallman syndrome 2 (hypogonadotropic hypogonadism and anosmia), spherocytosis (deletions of ankyrin 1), multiple congenital anomalies, mental retardation
8q24.1-q24.13	Langer-Giedion or trichorhinophalangeal type II	Sparse hair, multiple cone-shaped epiphyses, multiple cartilaginous exostoses, bulbous nasal tip, thickened alar cartilage, upturned nares, prominent philtrum, large protruding ears, mild mental retardation
9q22	Gorlin	Multiple basal cell carcinomas, odontogenic keratocysts, palmoplantar pits, calcification falx cerebri
9q34	9q34 deletion	Distinct face with synophrys, anteverted nares, tented upper lip, protruding tongue, midface hypoplasia, conotruncal heart defects, mental retardation
10p12-p13	DiGeorge 2	Many of the DiGeorge 1 and velocardiofacial 1 features (conotruncal defects, immunodeficiency, hypoparathyroidism, dysmorphic features)
11p11.2	Potocki-Shaffer	Multiple exostoses, parietal foramina, craniosynostosis, facial dysmorphism, syndactyly, mental retardation
11p13	WAGR	Hypernephroma (Wilms tumor), aniridia, male genital hypoplasia of varying degrees, gonadoblastoma, long face, upward slanting palpebral fissures, ptosis, beaked nose, low-set poorly formed auricles, mental retardation
11q24.1-11qter	Jacobsen	Mental and growth retardation, cardiac and digit anomalies, thrombocytopenia
15q11-q13 (pat)	Prader-Willi	Severe hypotonia and feeding difficulties at birth, voracious appetite and obesity in infancy, short stature (responsive to growth hormone), small hands and feet, hypogonadism, mental retardation
15q11-q13 (mat)	Angelman	Hypotonia, feeding difficulties, GE reflux, fair hair and skin, midface hypoplasia, prognathism, seizures, tremors, ataxia, sleep disturbances, inappropriate laughter, poor or absent speech, severe mental retardation
16p13.3	Rubinstein-Taybi	Microcephaly, ptosis, beaked nose with low-lying philtrum, broad thumbs and large toes, mental retardation
17p11.2	Smith-Magenis	Brachycephaly, midfacial hypoplasia, prognathism, myopia, cleft palate, short stature, severe behavioral problems, mental retardation
17p13.3	Miller-Dieker	Microcephaly, lissencephaly, pachygyria, narrow forehead, hypoplastic male external genitals, growth retardation, seizures, profound mental retardation
20p12	Alagille syndrome	Bile duct paucity with cholestasis; heart defects, particularly pulmonary artery stenosis; ocular abnormalities (posterior embryotoxon); skeletal defects such as butterfly vertebrae; long nose
22q11.2	Velocardiofacial-DiGeorge syndrome	Conotruncal cardiac anomalies, cleft palate, velopharyngeal incompetence, hypoplasia or agenesis of the thymus and parathyroid glands, hypocalcemia, hypoplasia of auricle, learning disabilities, psychiatric disorders
22q13.3 deletion		Hypotonia, developmental delay, normal or accelerated growth, severe expressive language deficits, autistic behavior
Xp21.2-p21.3		Duchenne muscular dystrophy, retinitis pigmentosa, adrenal hypoplasia, mental retardation, glycerol kinase deficiency
Xp22.2-p22.3		Ichthyosis, Kallman syndrome, mental retardation, chondrodysplasia punctata
Xp22.3	Microphthalmia with linear defects (MLS)	Microphthalmia, linear skin defects, poikiloderma, congenital heart defects, seizures, mental retardation

pat, paternal; mat, maternal; GE, gastroesophageal.

MARKER AND RING CHROMOSOMES

Marker chromosomes are rare and are usually chromosome fragments that are too small to be identified by conventional cytogenetics; they usually occur in addition to the normal 46 chromosomes. Most are sporadic (70%); mosaicism is often (50%) noted because of the mitotic instability of the marker chromosome. The incidence in newborn infants is 1 in 3,300, and the incidence in persons with mental retardation is 1 in 300. The associated phenotype ranges from normal to severely abnormal depending on the amount of chromosome material and number of genes associated with the fragment.

Ring chromosomes, which are found for all human chromosomes, are rare. A ring chromosome is formed when both ends of a chromosome are deleted and the ends are then joined to form a ring. Depending on the amount of chromosome material that is lacking or in excess (if the ring is in addition to the normal chromosomes), a patient with a ring chromosome can appear normal or nearly normal or can have mental retardation and multiple congenital anomalies.

BIBLIOGRAPHY

Please visit the Nelson Textbook of Pediatrics *website at* *www.expertconsult.com* *for the complete bibliography.*

76.4 Sex Chromosome Aneuploidy

Carlos A. Bacino and Brendan Lee

About 1/400 males and 1/650 females have some form of sex chromosome abnormality. Considered together, sex chromosome abnormalities are the most common chromosome abnormalities

Table 76-13 MICRODUPLICATIONS AND THEIR CLINICAL MANIFESTATIONS

DUPLICATION CHROMOSOME REGION	DISEASE REGION	CLINICAL FEATURES
1q21.1		Macrocephaly, DD, learning disabilities
3q29		Mild to moderate MR, microcephaly
7q11.23	Williams syndrome	DD and severe expressive language disorder, autistic features, subtle dysmorphisms
15q13.3	Prader-Willi/Angelman syndrome region	DD, MR, autistic features in duplications of maternal origin
15q24		Growth retardation, DD, microcephaly, digital anomalies, hypospadias, connective tissue abnormalities
16p11.2		FTT, severe DD, short stature, GH deficiency, dysmorphic features
17p11.2	Potocki-Lupski syndrome	Hypotonia, cardiovascular anomalies, FTT, DD, verbal apraxia, autism, anxiety
17q21.31		Severe DD, microcephaly, short and broad digits, dysmorphic features
22q11.2	Velocardiofacial-DiGeorge syndrome	Cardiovascular defects, velopharyngeal insufficiency
Xq28	*MECP2* gene region (Rett syndrome)	In males: infantile hypotonia, immune deficiency, dysmorphic features, DD, speech delay, autistic behavior, regression in childhood

DD, developmental delay; MR, mental retardation; FTT, failure to thrive; GH, growth hormone.

Table 76-14 SEX CHROMOSOME ABNORMALITIES

DISORDER	KARYOTYPE	APPROXIMATE INCIDENCE
Klinefelter syndrome	47,XXY	1/575-1/1,000 males
	48,XXXY	1/50,000-1/80,000 male births
	Other (48,XXYY; 49,XXXXY; mosaics)	
XYY syndrome	47,XYY	1/800-1,000 males
Other X or Y chromosome abnormalities		1/1,500 males
XX males	46,XX	1/20,000 males
Turner syndrome	45,X	1/2,500-1/5,000 females
	Variants and mosaics	
Trisomy X	47,XXX	1/1,000 females
	48,XXXX and 49,XXXXX	Rare
Other X chromosome abnormalities		1/3,000 females
XY females	46,XY	1/20,000 females

seen in liveborn infants, children, and adults. Sex chromosome abnormalities can be either structural or numerical and can be present in all cells or in a mosaic form. Those affected with these abnormalities might have few or no physical or developmental problems (Table 76-14).

TURNER SYNDROME

Turner syndrome is a condition characterized by complete or partial monosomy of the X chromosome and defined by a combination of phenotypic features (Table 76-15). Half of the patients with Turner syndrome have a 45,X chromosome complement. The other half exhibits mosaicism and varied structural abnormalities of the X or Y chromosome. Maternal age is not a predisposing factor for children with 45,X. Turner syndrome occurs in approximately 1/5,000 female live births. In 75% of patients, the lost sex chromosome is of paternal origin (whether an X or a Y). 45,X is 1 of the chromosome abnormalities most often associated with spontaneous abortion. It has been estimated that 95-99% of 45,X conceptions are miscarried.

Clinical findings in the newborns can include small size for gestational age, webbing of the neck, protruding ears, and lymphedema of the hands and feet, although many newborns are phenotypically normal (Fig. 76-17). Older children and adults have short stature and exhibit variable dysmorphic features. Congenital heart defects (40%) and structural renal anomalies (60%) are common. The most common heart defects are bicuspid aortic valves, coarctation of the aorta, aortic stenosis, and mitral valve prolapse. The gonads are generally streaks of fibrous tissue (**gonadal dysgenesis**). There is primary amenorrhea and lack of secondary sex characters. These children should receive regular endocrinologic testing (Chapter 580). Most patients tend to be of normal intelligence, but mental retardation is seen in 6% of affected children. They are also at increased risk for behavioral problems and deficiencies in spatial and motor perception. Guidelines for health supervision for children with Turner syndrome are published by the American Academy of Pediatrics (AAP).

Patients with **45,X/46,XY mosaicism,** can have Turner syndrome, although this form of mosaicism can also be associated with male pseudohermaphroditism, male or female genitalia in association with mixed gonadal dysgenesis, or a normal male phenotype. This variant is estimated to represent approximately

Table 76-15 SIGNS ASSOCIATED WITH TURNER SYNDROME

Short stature
Congenital lymphedema
Horseshoe kidneys
Patella dislocation
Increased carrying angle of elbow (cubitus valgus)
Madelung deformity (chondrodysplasia of distal radial epiphysis)
Congenital hip dislocation
Scoliosis
Widespread nipples
Shield chest
Redundant nuchal skin (in utero cystic hygroma)
Low posterior hairline
Coarctation of aorta
Bicuspid aortic valve
Cardiac conduction abnormalities
Hypoplastic left heart syndrome and other left heart abnormalities
Gonadal dysgenesis (infertility, primary amenorrhea)
Gonadoblastoma (increased risk if Y chromosome material is present)
Learning disabilities (nonverbal perceptual motor and visuospatial skills) (in 70%)
Developmental delay (in 10%)
Social awkwardness
Hypothyroidism (acquired in 15-30%)
Type 2 diabetes mellitus (insulin resistance)
Strabismus
Cataracts
Red-green colorblindness (as in males)
Recurrent otitis media
Sensorineural hearing loss
Inflammatory bowel disease
Celiac disease (increased incidence)

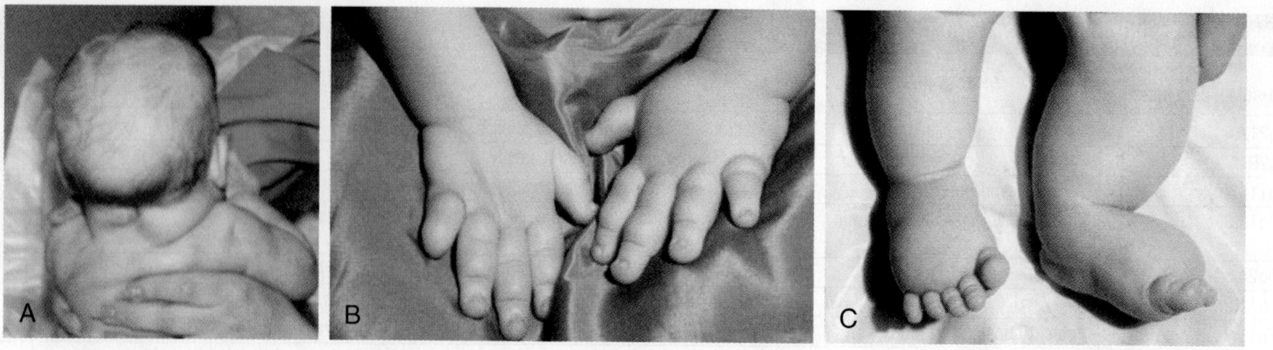

Figure 76-17 Redundant nuchal skin *(A)* and puffiness of the hands *(B)* and feet *(C)* in Turner syndrome. (From Sybert VP, McCauley E: Turner's syndrome, *N Engl J Med* 351:1227–1238, 2004. Copyright © 2004 Massachusetts Medical Society. All rights reserved.)

6% of patients with mosaic Turner syndrome. Some of the patients with Turner syndrome phenotype and a Y cell line exhibit masculinization. Phenotypic females with 45,X/46,XY mosaicism have a 15-30% risk of developing **gonadoblastoma.** The risk for the patients with a male phenotype and external testes is not so high, but tumor surveillance is nevertheless recommended. The AAP has recommended the use of FISH analysis to look for Y-chromosome mosaicism in all 45,X patients. If Y chromosome material is identified, laparoscopic gonadectomy is recommended.

Noonan syndrome shares many clinical features with Turner syndrome, although it is an autosomal dominant disorder resulting from mutations in several genes that are involved in the RAS-MAPK (mitogen activated protein kinase) pathway. The most common of these is *PTPN11* (50%), which encodes a nonreceptor tyrosine kinase (SHP-2) on chromosome 12q24.1. Other genes include *SOS1* in 10-15%, *RAF1* in 3-8%, and *KRAS* in 5%. Features common to Noonan syndrome include short stature, low posterior hairline, shield chest, congenital heart disease, and a short or webbed neck (Table 76-16). In contrast to Turner syndrome, Noonan syndrome affects both sexes and has a different pattern of congenital heart disease typically involving right-sided lesions.

Table 76-16 SIGNS ASSOCIATED WITH NOONAN SYNDROME
Short stature
Failure to thrive
Epicanthal folds
Ptosis
Hypertelorism
Low nasal bridge
Downward-slanting palpebral fissures
Myopia
Nystagmus
Low-set auricles
Dental malocclusion
Low posterior hairline
Short webbed neck, cystic hygroma
Shield chest
Pectus carinatum superiorly
Scoliosis
Cubitus valgus
Pulmonary valve stenosis
Hypertrophic cardiomyopathy
Atrial septal defect, ventricular septal defect
Lymphedema
Cryptorchidism
Small penis
Bleeding disorders, including thrombocytopenia

KLINEFELTER SYNDROME

Persons with Klinefelter syndrome are phenotypically male; this syndrome is the most common cause of hypogonadism and infertility in males and the most common sex chromosome aneuploidy in humans (Chapter 577). Eighty percent of children with Klinefelter syndrome have a male karyotype with an extra chromosome X-47,XXY; the remaining 20% have multiple sex chromosome aneuploidies (48,XXXY; 48,XXYY; 49,XXXXY), mosaicism (46,XY/47,XXY), or structurally abnormal X chromosomes. The greater the aneuploidy, the more severe the mental impairment and dysmorphism. Early studies showed that the birth prevalence is approximately 1/1,000 males. The current prevalence of 47,XXY appears to have increased to approximately 1/580 liveborn boys; the reasons for this are still unknown. Errors in paternal nondisjunction in meiosis I account for half of the cases.

Puberty occurs at the normal age, but the testes remain small. Patients develop secondary sex characters late; 50% develop gynecomastia. They have taller stature. Because many patients with Klinefelter syndrome are phenotypically normal until puberty, the syndrome often goes undiagnosed until they reach adulthood, when their infertility aids in their clinical identification. Patients with 46,XY/47,XXY have a better prognosis for testicular function. Their intelligence shows variability and ranges from above to below average. Persons with Klinefelter syndrome can show behavioral problems, learning disabilities, and deficits in language. Problems with self-esteem are often the case with adolescents and adults. Substance abuse, depression, and anxiety have been reported in adolescents with Klinefelter syndrome. Those who have higher X chromosome counts show impaired cognition. It has been estimated that each additional X chromosome reduces the IQ by 10-15 points, when comparing these persons with their normal siblings. The main effect is seen in language skills and social domains.

47,XYY

The incidence of 47,XYY is approximately 1 in 800-1,000 males, with many cases remaining undiagnosed, because most affected individuals have a normal appearance and normal fertility. The extra Y is the result of nondisjunction at paternal meiosis II (MII). Those with this abnormality have normal intelligence but are at risk for learning disabilities. Behavioral abnormalities including hyperactive behavior, pervasive developmental disorder, and aggressive behavior have been reported. Early reports that assigned stigmata of criminality to this disorder have long been disproved.

BIBLIOGRAPHY

Please visit the Nelson Textbook of Pediatrics *website at* www.expertconsult.com *for the complete bibliography.*

76.5 Fragile Chromosome Sites

Carlos A. Bacino and Brendan Lee

Fragile sites are regions of chromosomes that show a tendency for separation, breakage, or attenuation under particular growth conditions. They appear as a gap in the staining. At least 120 chromosomal loci, many of them heritable, have been identified as fragile sites in the human genome (see Table 75-1).

One fragile site that has clinical significance is the one on the distal long arm of chromosome Xq27.3 associated with the **fragile X syndrome.** Fragile X accounts for 3% of males with mental retardation. There is another fragile site on the X chromosome (FRAXE on Xq28) that has also been implicated in mild mental retardation. The FRA11B (11q23.3) breakpoints are associated with Jacobsen syndrome (condition caused by deletion of the distal long arm of chromosome 11). Fragile sites can also play a role in tumorigenesis.

The main **clinical manifestations** of fragile X syndrome in affected males are mental retardation, autistic behavior, macro-orchidism, and characteristic facial features (Table 76-17). The macro-orchidism may not be evident until puberty. The facial features, which include a long face, large ears, and a prominent square jaw, become more obvious with age. Females affected with fragile X show varying degrees of mental retardation and/or learning disabilities. Diagnosis of fragile X is possible by DNA testing that shows an expansion of a triplet DNA repeat inside the FMR1 gene on the X chromosome. The expansion involves an area of the gene that contains a variable number of trinucleotide (CGG) repeats. The larger the triplet repeat expansion, the more significant the mental retardation. In cases where the expansion is large, females can also manifest different degrees of mental retardation. Therapy of the diverse neuropsychiatric manifestations associated with fragile X syndrome is noted in Table 76-18. Inhibitors of the metabolic glutamate receptor (overexpressed in fragile X) are undergoing clinical trials.

Table 76-17 CLINICAL FEATURES OF FULL AND PREMUTATION *FMR1* ALLELES

DISORDER	PHENOTYPE: Cognitive or Behavioral	PHENOTYPE: Clinical and Imaging Signs	ONSET	PENETRANCE
FULL MUTATION				
FXS	Developmental delay: mean IQ = 42 in M; IQ is higher if significant residual FMRP is produced (e.g., females and mosaic males or unmethylated full mutations) Autism 20-30% ADHD 80% Anxiety 70-100%	Hypothalamic dysfunction: macro-orchidism, 40%* Facial features, 60%,* large cupped ears, elongated face, high arched palate Connective tissue abnormalities: mitral valve prolapse, scoliosis, joint laxity, flat feet Others: seizures (20%), recurrent otitis media (60%), strabismus (8-30%)	Neonate	M 100%
PREMTUTATION				
Female reproductive symptoms		POF (<40 yr)	Adulthood	F 20%†
		Early menopause (<45 yr)		F 30%†
FXTAS	Cognitive decline, dementia, apathy, disinhibition, irritability, depression	Gait ataxia, intention tremor, Parkinsonism, neuropathy, autonomic dysfunction	>50 yr	M 33%‡ F unknown
Neurodevelopmental disorder	ADHD, autism, or developmental delay	Mild features of FXS	Childhood	8% (1/13)*

*Frequency of those signs in prepubertal boys; ⅓ of boys with FXS are without classic facial features. Macro-orchidism is present in 90% of men.
†Maximum penetrance reported for allele size approximately 80-90 CGG repeats.
‡Penetrance is correlated with age and repeat size.
FXS, fragile-X syndrome; M, male; F, female; POF, premature ovarian failure; ADHD, attention-deficit/hyperactivity disorder.
From Jacquemont S, Hagerman RJ, Hagerman PJ, et al: Fragile-X syndrome and fragile X associated tremor/ataxia syndrome: two faces of FMRI, *Lancet Neurol* 6:45–55, 2007 (Table 1).

Table 76-18 THERAPY FOR *FMR1* RELATED DISORDERS

DISORDER	SYMPTOM	THERAPY AND INTERVENTIONS	FUTURE POTENTIAL THERAPY
FULL MUTATION			
FXS*	ADHD	Stimulants	mGluR5 antagonists
	Anxiety, hyperarousal, aggressive outbursts	SSRIs, atypical antipsychotics, occupational therapy, behavioral therapy, counseling	mGluR5 antagonists
	Seizures	Carbamazepine, valproic acid	mGluR5 antagonists
	Cognitive deficit	Occupational therapy, speech therapy, special education support	mGluR5 antagonists
PREMUTATION			
POF	Premature ovarian failure	Reproductive counseling, egg donation	Cryopreservation of ovarian tissue
		Hormone replacement therapy	
FXTAS†	Intention tremor	β-Blockers	
	Parkinsonism	Carbidopa/levodopa	
	Cognitive decline, dementia	Acetylcholinesterase inhibitors	
	Anxiety, apathy, disinhibition, irritability, depression	Venlafaxine, SSRIs	
	Neuropathic pain	Gabapentin	

*These data are based on a survey in 2 large referral centers. Drugs for anxiety were more frequently prescribed than those for neurologic signs.
†There have been no controlled studies to assess drugs for FXTAS. These data were collected through a questionnaire study (n = 56).
ADHD, attention-deficit/hyperactivity disorder; FXS, fragile-X syndrome; FXTAS, fragile X associated tremor/ataxia syndrome; POF, premature ovarian failure; SSRI, selective serotonin reuptake inhibitor.
From Jacquemont S, Hagerman RJ, Hagerman PJ, et al: Fragile-X syndrome and fragile X associated tremor/ataxia syndrome: two faces of FMRI, *Lancet Neurol* 2006:45–55, 2007 (Table 2).

BIBLIOGRAPHY
Please visit the Nelson Textbook of Pediatrics *website at www.expertconsult.com for the complete bibliography.*

76.6 Mosaicism

Carlos A. Bacino and Brendan Lee

Mosaicism describes an individual or tissue that contains ≥2 different cell lines typically derived from a single zygote and the result of mitotic nondisjunction (see Fig. 76-1). Study of placental tissue from chorionic villus samples collected at or before the 10th wk of gestation has shown that 2% or more of all conceptions are mosaic for a chromosome abnormality. With the exception of chromosomes 13, 18, and 21, complete autosomal trisomies are usually nonviable; the presence of a normal cell line might allow these other trisomic conceptions to survive to term. Depending on the point at which the new cell line arises during early embryogenesis, mosaicism may be present in some tissues but not in others. Germline mosaicism, which refers to the presence of mosaicism in the germ cells of the gonad, may be associated with an increased risk for recurrence of an affected child whether the germ cells are affected with a chromosomal abnormality or specific gene mutation.

PALLISTER-KILLIAN SYNDROME

Pallister-Killian syndrome is characterized by coarse facies (prominent full cheeks), abnormal ear lobes, localized alopecia, pigmentary skin anomalies, diaphragmatic hernia, cardiovascular anomalies, supernumerary nipples, seizures, and profound mental retardation. The syndrome is due to mosaicism for an isochromosome 12p. The presence of the isochromosome 12p in cells gives 4 functional copies for the short arm of chromosome 12 in the affected cells. The isochromosome 12p is preferentially cultured from fibroblasts that can be readily obtained from a skin punch biopsy and is seldom present in lymphocytes. The abnormalities seen in affected persons probably reflect the presence of abnormal cells during early embryogenesis.

HYPOMELANOSIS OF ITO

Hypomelanosis of Ito is characterized by unilateral or bilateral macular hypo- or hyperpigmented whorls, streaks, and patches (Chapter 645). Sometimes these pigmentary defects follow the lines of Blaschko. Hair and tooth anomalies are common. Abnormalities of the eyes, musculoskeletal system (growth asymmetry, syndactyly, polydactyly, clinodactyly), and central nervous system (microcephaly, seizures, mental retardation) may also be present. Patients with hypomelanosis of Ito might have 2 genetically distinct cell lines. The mosaic chromosome anomalies that have been observed involve both autosomes and sex chromosomes and have been demonstrated in about 50% of patients. The mosaicism might not be visible in lymphocyte-derived chromosome studies; it is more likely to be found when chromosomes are analyzed from skin fibroblasts. The distinct cell lines might not always be due to observable chromosomal anomalies but might result from single gene mutations or other mechanisms.

76.7 Chromosome Instability Syndromes

Carlos A. Bacino and Brendan Lee

Chromosome instability syndromes, formerly known as chromosome breakage syndromes, are characterized by an increased risk of malignancy and specific phenotypes. They display autosomal recessive inheritance and have an increased frequency of chromosome breakage and/or rearrangement, either spontaneous or induced. They result from specific defects in DNA repair, cell cycle control, and apoptosis. The resulting chromosomal instability leads to the increased risk of developing neoplasms. The classic chromosome instability syndromes are Fanconi anemia, ataxia telangiectasia, Nijmegen syndrome, ICF (immunodeficiency, centromere instability, and facial anomalies) syndrome, Roberts syndrome, Werner syndrome, and Bloom syndrome.

76.8 Uniparental Disomy and Imprinting

Carlos A. Bacino and Brendan Lee

UNIPARENTAL DISOMY

Uniparental disomy (UPD) occurs when both chromosomes of a pair or areas from 1 chromosome in any individual have been inherited from a single parent. UPD can be of 2 types: uniparental isodisomy or uniparental heterodisomy. **Uniparental isodisomy** means that both chromosomes or chromosomal regions are identical (typically the result of monosomy rescue by duplication). **Uniparental heterodisomy** means that the 2 chromosomes are different members of a pair, both of which were still inherited from 1 parent. This results from a trisomy that is later reduced to disomy, leaving 2 copies from 1 parent. The phenotypic result of UPD varies according to the chromosome involved, the parent who contributed the chromosomes, and whether it is isodisomy or heterodisomy. Three types of phenotypic effects are seen in UPD: those related to imprinted genes (i.e., the absence of a gene that is normally expressed only when inherited from a parent of a specific sex), those related to the uncovering of autosomal recessive disorders, and those related to a vestigial aneuploidy producing mosaicism (Chapter 75).

In uniparental isodisomy, both chromosomes or regions (and thus the genes) in the pair are identical. This is particularly important when the parent is a carrier of an autosomal recessive disorder. If the offspring of a carrier parent has UPD with isodisomy for a chromosome that carries an abnormal gene, the abnormal gene will be present in 2 copies and the phenotype will be that of the autosomal recessive disorder; the child has an autosomal recessive disorder even though only 1 parent is a carrier of that recessive disorder. It is estimated that all human beings carry approximately 20 abnormal autosomal recessive genes. Some autosomal recessive disorders like spinal muscular atrophy, cystic fibrosis, cartilage-hair hypoplasia, α- and β-thalassemias, and Bloom syndrome have been reported in cases of UPD. The possibility of uniparental isodisomy should also be considered when a person is affected with >1 recessive disorder because the abnormal genes for both disorders could be carried on the same isodisomic chromosome. Uniparental isodisomy is a *rare* cause of recessively inherited disorders.

Maternal UPD involving chromosomes 2, 7, 14, and 15 and **paternal UPD** involving chromosomes 6, 11, 15, and 20 are associated with phenotypic abnormalities of growth and behavior. UPD maternal 7 is associated with a phenotype similar to Russell-Silver syndrome with intrauterine growth restriction. These phenotypic effects may be related to imprinting (see under Imprinting, next).

UPD for chromosome 15 is seen in some cases of Prader–Willi syndrome and Angelman syndrome. In **Prader-Willi syndrome,** about 25-29% of cases have maternal UPD (missing the paternal chromosome 15). In **Angelman syndrome,** paternal UPD of chromosome 15 is rarer and is observed in approximately 5% of the cases (missing the maternal chromosome 15). The phenotype for Prader-Willi syndrome (Fig. 76-18) and Angelman syndrome in cases of UPD is thought to result from the lack of the functional contribution from a particular parent of chromosome 15. In Prader-Willi syndrome the paternal contribution is missing, and

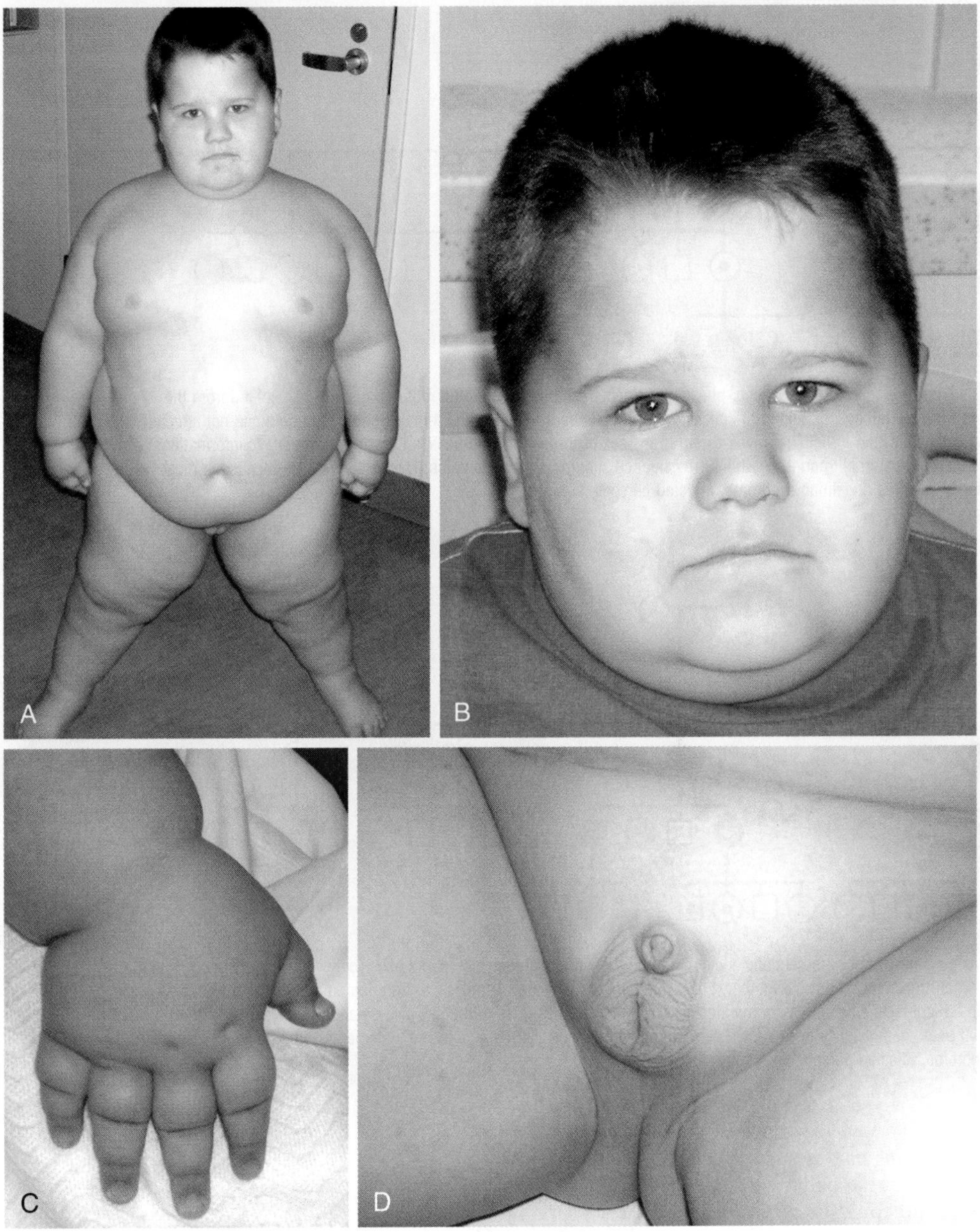

Figure 76-18 *A* and *B*, Individual showing morbid obesity with facial features as shown. *C*, Upper extremities are notable for small hands relative to body size. *D*, External genitalia after laparoscopic orchiopexy at 13 months. Parental informed consent, as approved by the Baylor College of Medicine Institutional Review Board, was obtained to publish the photographs. (From Sahoo T, del Gaudio D, German JR, et al: Prader-Willi phenotype caused by paternal deficiency for the HBII-85 C/D box small nucleolar RNA cluster, *Nat Genet* 40:719–721, 2008.)

the maternal contribution is missing in Angelman syndrome. Prader-Willi may be due to paternal deficiency of HB11-85 snoRNAs (small nucleolar RNAs). These findings suggest that there are differences in function of certain regions of chromosome 15, depending on whether it is inherited from the mother or from the father.

UPD most commonly arises when a pregnancy starts off as a **trisomy by trisomy rescue.** Because most trisomies are lethal, the fetus can only survive if a cell line loses 1 of the extra chromosomes to become disomic. One third of the time, the disomic cell line is uniparental. This is the typical mechanism for Prader-Willi syndrome, and it is often associated with advanced maternal age. The embryo starts off as trisomy 15 secondary to maternal meiosis I nondisjunction, followed by random loss of the paternal chromosome. In this case, the disomic cell line becomes the more viable one and outgrows the trisomic cell line. When mosaic trisomy is found at prenatal diagnosis, care should be taken to determine whether UPD has resulted and whether the chromosome involved is 1 of the disomies known to be associated with phenotypic abnormalities. There must always be concern that some residual cells that are trisomic are present in some tissues, leading to malformations or dysfunction. The presence of aggregates of trisomic cells might account for the spectrum of abnormalities seen in persons with UPD.

IMPRINTING

Traditional genetics has for many years suggested that most genes are equally expressed when inherited from maternal vs. paternal lineages. The only exception to this rule were genes on the X chromosome that are subject to inactivation, and the immunoglobulin genes subject to allelic exclusion, a phenomenon that results in monoallelic expression of a particular immunoglobulin chain by switching on and off expression of parental alleles. Genomic imprinting occurs when the phenotypic expression of a gene depends on the parent of origin for certain genes or in some cases entire chromosome regions. Whether the genetic material is expressed or not depends on the sex of the parent

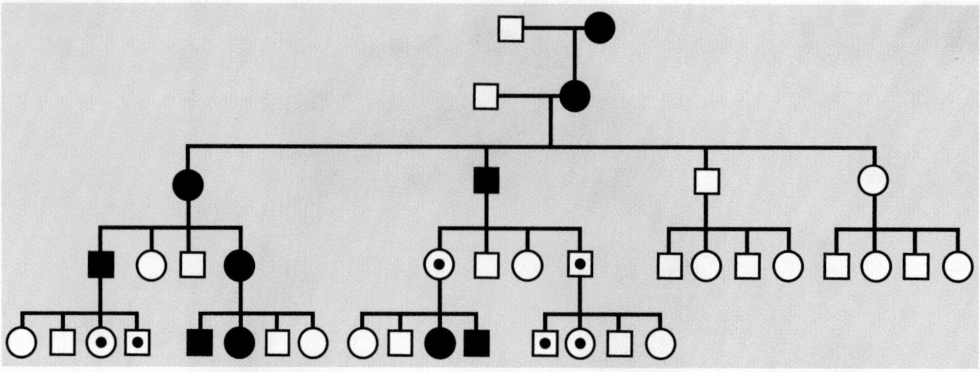

Figure 76-19 In this hypothetical pedigree suggestive of imprinting, phenotypic effects occur only when the mutated gene is transmitted from the mother but not when it is transmitted from the father, i.e., maternal deficiency. Equal numbers of males and females can be affected and not affected phenotypically in each generation. A nonmanifesting transmitter gives a clue to the sex of the parent who passes the expressed genetic information; i.e., in maternal deficiency disorders (also termed paternal imprinting), there are "skipped" nonmanifesting females. This is theoretical, because in most clinical scenarios of maternal deficiency, such as Angelman syndrome, affected persons do not reproduce.

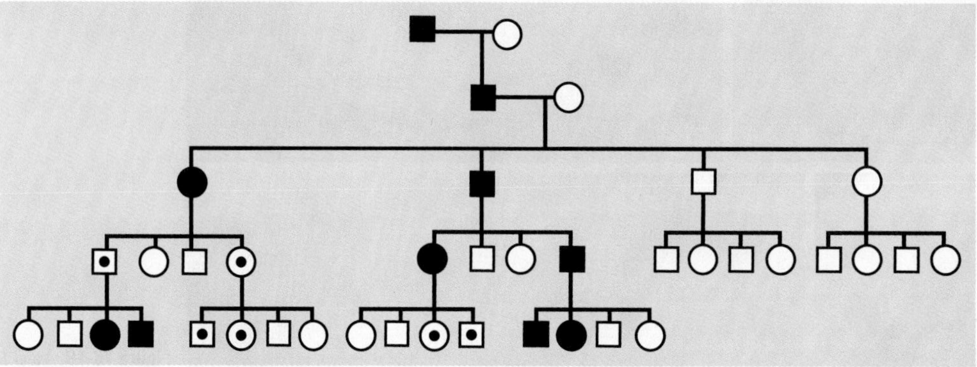

Figure 76-20 In theoretical pedigrees suggestive of paternal deficiency (maternal imprinting), phenotypic effects occur only when the mutated gene is transmitted from the father but not when transmitted from the mother. Equal numbers of males and females can be affected and not affected phenotypically in each generation. In a theoretical situation, a nonmanifesting transmitter gives a clue to the sex of the parent who passes on the expressed genetic information; i.e., in paternal deficiency (also known as maternal imprinting), there are "skipped" nonmanifesting males. In real-life clinical instances of Prader-Willi syndrome, affected persons do not reproduce.

from whom it was derived. Genomic imprinting can be suspected in some cases on the basis of a pedigree. In these pedigrees, the disease is always transmitted from 1 sex and could be passed on silently for several generations by the opposite sex (Figs. 76-19 and 76-20). Imprinting probably occurs in many different parts of the human genome and is thought to be particularly important in gene expression related to development, growth, cancer, and even behavior.

A classic example of imprinting disorder is seen in Prader-Willi syndrome and Angelman syndrome, 2 very different clinical conditions. These syndromes can be associated with deletion of the same region in the proximal long arm of chromosome 15. A deletion on the paternally derived chromosome causes Prader-Willi syndrome, in which the maternally derived copy is still intact but some of the imprinted genes within this region normally remain silent. In contrast, a maternal deletion of the same region causes Angelman syndrome, leaving intact the paternal copy that in this case has genes that are also normally silent. In other situations, UPD can lead to the same diagnosis. Maternal UPD for chromosome 15 results in Prader-Willi syndrome due to lack of the paternal chromosome 15 contribution. In contrast, in Angelman syndrome, the UPD is always paternal, with no maternal contribution. Many other disorders are associated with this type of parent of origin effect, as in some cases of Beckwith-Wiedemann syndrome, Russell-Silver syndrome, and neonatal diabetes.

Chapter 77
Genetics of Common Disorders

John W. Belmont and Brendan Lee

Genetic studies are useful in diagnosing and treating rare pediatric conditions, often alleviating suffering, extending life, and, in the case of neonatal metabolic and presymptomatic screening, preventing injury before symptoms develop. Genetic studies can also contribute to the understanding of more common diseases such as asthma and diabetes. An understanding of the complex and potentially multiple pathways leading to disease is crucial for the development of new therapies and prevention strategies and screening of high-risk children.

For the full continuation of this chapter, please visit the Nelson Textbook of Pediatrics *website at www.expertconsult.com.*

77.1 Major Genetic Approaches to the Study of Common Pediatric Disorders

John W. Belmont and Brendan Lee

A model for the genetic contribution to health is shown in Figure 77-1. Genetic variation that can have an impact on disease

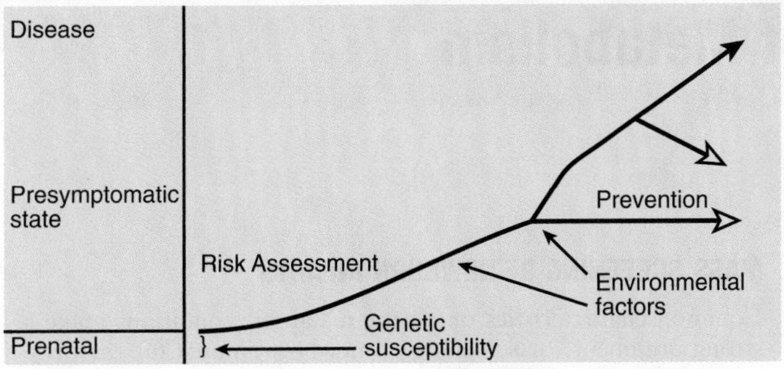

Figure 77-1 Model for the influence of genetics on health. Everyone inherits some genetic liability for disease risk, but for multifactorial disorders this is insufficient to produce disease on its own. Over time, exposure to environmental factors leads from a presymptomatic to a disease state. Identifying the genes responsible for risk can lead to prevention strategies or treatments.

susceptibility is present in every person. Sometimes single gene mutations cause a condition such as cystic fibrosis or sickle cell anemia. But other genetic variations can contribute much less strongly to the emergence of specific medical conditions, and the effect can depend upon exposure to certain environmental factors. One goal in medical genetics is to identify genes that contribute to disease in the hope of preventing the occurrence of disease, either by avoiding inciting environmental factors or by instituting interventions that reduce risk. For persons who cross the threshold of disease, the goal is to better understand the pathogenesis in the hope that this will suggest better approaches to treatment. Common genetic variation can also influence response to medications and the risk of toxicities of various medications and environmental toxins.

For the full continuation of this chapter, please visit the Nelson Textbook of Pediatrics *website at www.expertconsult.com.*

BIBLIOGRAPHY

Please visit the Nelson Textbook of Pediatrics *website at www.expertconsult.com for the complete bibliography.*

77.2 Current Understanding of Genetics of Common Disorders in Children

TYPE 1 DIABETES MELLITUS

See Chapter 583.

OBESITY

See Chapter 44.

ASTHMA

See Chapter 138.

PART XI Genetic Disorders of Metabolism

Chapter 78
An Approach to Inborn Errors of Metabolism

Iraj Rezvani and Geoffrey Rezvani

Many childhood conditions are caused by single gene mutations that encode specific proteins. These mutations can result in the alteration of primary protein structure or the amount of protein synthesized. The function of a protein, whether it is an enzyme, receptor, transport vehicle, membrane, or structural element, may be relatively or seriously compromised. These hereditary biochemical disorders are also termed **inborn errors of metabolism** or **inherited metabolic disorders.**

Most mutations are clinically inconsequential and represent polymorphic differences that set individuals apart *(genetic polymorphism).* Some mutations produce disease states that range from very mild to lethal. Severe forms of these disorders usually become clinically apparent in the newborn period or shortly thereafter.

COMMON CHARACTERISTICS OF GENETIC DISORDERS OF METABOLISM

Although the manifestations of genetic metabolic disorders are quite variable, the following features are shared among most of these conditions:

1. The affected infant is normal at birth and becomes symptomatic later on in life. This differentiates these infants from those who appear sick at birth due to birth trauma, intrauterine insults, chromosomal abnormalities or other genetic diseases.
2. The nature of the mutation that causes the dysfunction of the gene usually varies from family to family. This results in variation in severity of the phenotype in different families. An exception to this is found when a specific mutation has been preserved in an ethnic group primarily due to inbreeding (the founder effect). An example is maple syrup urine disease in Old Order Mennonites in the USA (mainly in Lancaster County, PA), in whom all the affected infants have the same mutation and hence the same phenotype (Chapter 79.6).
3. Mutations causing severe malfunction of the gene or its product result in clinical manifestations shortly after birth. In general, the earlier the appearance of clinical symptoms the more severe is the disease.
4. The majority of conditions are inherited as autosomal recessive traits. Therefore, a history of consanguinity in the parents or of an unexplained death in the neonatal period may raise the question of an inherited metabolic disease in the sick infant.
5. Most of the genetic metabolic conditions can be controlled successfully by some form of therapy, and a few can be potentially cured by the use of bone marrow or liver transplants. These patients can have a normal life if diagnosed and treated early, before irreversible damage to organs, especially to the brain, occurs. This underlines the importance of early diagnosis, which can be achieved through screening of all newborn infants.

MASS SCREENING OF NEWBORN INFANTS

Common characteristics of genetic metabolic conditions make a strong argument for screening all newborn infants for the presence of these conditions. During the past half-century, methods have been developed to screen all infants inexpensively with accurate and fast-yielding results. Tandem mass spectrometry (MS/MS) is the latest technical advance in the field. This method requires a few drops of blood to be placed on a filter paper and mailed to a central laboratory for assay. A large number of genetic conditions can be identified by this method when complemented by a few equally efficient assays for other specific disorders (Tables 78-1 and 78-2). Severe forms of some of these diseases may cause clinical manifestations before the results of the newborn screening become available. It should also be noted that these methods may identify mild forms of inherited metabolic conditions, some of which may never cause clinical disease in the lifetime of the individual. Potential psychosocial implications of such findings can be devastating and deserves serious considerations. An example of this is 3-methylcrotonyl CoA carboxylase deficiency, which has been identified in an unexpectedly high frequency in screening programs using tandem mass spectrometry. The majority of these children have remained asymptomatic (Chapter 79.6).

CLINICAL MANIFESTATIONS OF GENETIC METABOLIC DISEASES

Physicians and other health care providers who care for children should familiarize themselves with early manifestations of genetic metabolic disorders, because (1) severe forms of some of these conditions may cause symptoms before the results of screening studies become available, and (2) the current screening methods, although quite extensive, identify a small number of all inherited metabolic conditions. In the newborn period, the clinical findings are usually nonspecific and similar to those seen in infants with sepsis. A genetic disorder of metabolism should be considered in the differential diagnosis of a severely ill newborn infant, and special studies should be undertaken if the index of suspicion is high (Fig. 78-1).

Signs and symptoms such as lethargy, poor feeding, convulsions, and vomiting may develop as early as a few hours after birth. Occasionally, vomiting may be severe enough to suggest the diagnosis of pyloric stenosis, which is usually not present, although it may occur simultaneously in such infants. Lethargy, poor feeding, convulsions, and coma may also be seen in infants with hypoglycemia (Chapters 86 and 101) or hypocalcemia (Chapters 48 and 565). Measurements of blood concentrations of glucose and calcium and response to intravenous injection of glucose or calcium usually establish these diagnoses. Some of these disorders have a high incidence in specific population groups. Tyrosinemia type 1 is more common among French-Canadians of Quebec than in the general population. Therefore, knowledge of the ethnic background of the patient may be helpful in diagnosis. *Physical examination* usually reveals nonspecific findings; most signs are related to the central nervous system. Hepatomegaly is a common finding in a variety of inborn errors of metabolism. Occasionally, a peculiar odor may offer an invaluable aid to the diagnosis (Table 78-3). A physician caring for a sick infant should smell the patient and his or her excretions; for example, patients with maple syrup urine disease

Table 78-1 DISORDERS RECOMMENDED BY THE AMERICAN COLLEGE OF MEDICAL GENETICS (ACMG) TASK FORCE FOR INCLUSION IN NEWBORN SCREENING ("PRIMARY DISORDERS")*
DISORDERS OF ORGANIC-ACID METABOLISM
Isovaleric acidemia Glutaric aciduria type I 3-Hydroxy-3-methylglutaric aciduria Multiple carboxylase deficiency Methylmalonic acidemia, mutase deficiency form 3-Methylcrotonyl-CoA carboxylase deficiency Methylmalonic acidemia, cblA and cblB forms Propionic acidemia Beta-ketothiolase deficiency
DISORDERS OF FATTY ACID METABOLISM
Medium-chain acyl-CoA dehydrogenase deficiency (MCAD) Very long-chain acyl-CoA dehydrogenase deficiency (VLCAD) Long-chain 3-hydroxy acyl-CoA dehydrogenase deficiency (LCHAD) Trifunctional protein deficiency Carnitine uptake defect
DISORDERS OF AMINO-ACID METABOLISM
Phenylketonuria Maple syrup urine disease Homocystinuria Citrullinemia Argininosuccinic acidemia Tyrosinemia type I
HEMOGLOBINOPATHIES
Sickle cell anemia Hemoglobin S-β-thalassemia Hemoglobin SC disease
OTHER DISORDERS
Congenital hypothyroidism Biotinidase deficiency Congenital adrenal hyperplasia Galactosemia Hearing deficiency Cystic fibrosis

*At this time, there is state-to-state variation in newborn screening; a list of the disorders that are screened for by each state is available at *http://genes-r-us.uthscsa.edu/*.
cblA, cobalamin A defect; cblB, cobalamin B defect; CoA, coenzyme A.

Table 78-2 SECONDARY CONDITIONS RECOMMENDED BY ACMG*
ORGANIC ACID METABOLISM DISORDERS
Methylmalonic acidemia, Cbl C and Cbl D forms 2-Methyl 3-hydroxybutyric aciduria Isobutyryl-CoA dehydrogenase deficiency 2-Methylbutyryl-CoA dehydrogenase deficiency 3-Methylglutaconic aciduria Malonic acidemia
FATTY ACID OXIDATION DISORDERS
Medium-/short-chain 3-OH acyl-CoA dehydrogenase deficiency Short-chain acyl-CoA dehydrogenase deficiency (SCAD) Medium-chain ketoacyl-CoA thiolase deficiency Glutaric acidemia type 2 Carnitine palmitoyltransferase I deficiency Carnitine palmitoyltransferase II deficiency Carnitine acylcarnitine translocase deficiency Dienoyl-CoA reductase deficiency
AMINO ACID METABOLISM DISORDERS
Hyperphenylalaninemia, benign (not PKU) Tyrosinemia type II Tyrosinemia type III Defects of biopterin cofactor biosynthesis Defects of biopterin cofactor regeneration Argininemia Hypermethioninemia Citrullinemia type II
HEMOGLOBINOPATHICS
Hemoglobin variants (including hemoglobin E)
OTHERS
Galactose epimerase deficiency Galactokinase deficiency

*The American College of Medical Genetics task force recommended reporting 25 disorders ("secondary targets") in addition to the primary disorders that can be detected through screening but that do not meet the criteria for primary disorders.

have the unmistakable odor of maple syrup in their urine and on their bodies.

Occasionally, the onset of a genetic metabolic condition may occur months or even years after birth. These children usually have mutations that render the gene partially nonfunctional. *Clinical manifestations* such as mental retardation, motor deficits, developmental regression, convulsions, myopathy, recurrent emesis, and cardiomyopathy in a child beyond the neonatal period should raise the possibility of an inherited metabolic disease. There may be an episodic or intermittent pattern, with episodes of acute clinical manifestations separated by periods of seemingly disease-free states. The episodes are usually triggered by stress or a nonspecific catabolic insult such as an infection. The child may die during one of these acute attacks. A genetic disorder of metabolism should be considered in any child with one or more of the following manifestations: unexplained mental retardation, developmental delay or regression, motor deficit, or convulsions; unusual odor, particularly during an acute illness; intermittent episodes of unexplained vomiting, acidosis, mental deterioration, or coma; hepatomegaly; renal stones; muscle weakness or cardiomyopathy.

Diagnosis usually requires a variety of specific *laboratory studies*. Measurements of serum concentrations of ammonia, bicarbonate, and pH are often very helpful initially in differentiating major causes of genetic metabolic disorders (see Fig. 78-1). Elevation of blood ammonia is usually caused by defects of urea cycle enzymes. Infants with elevated blood ammonia levels from

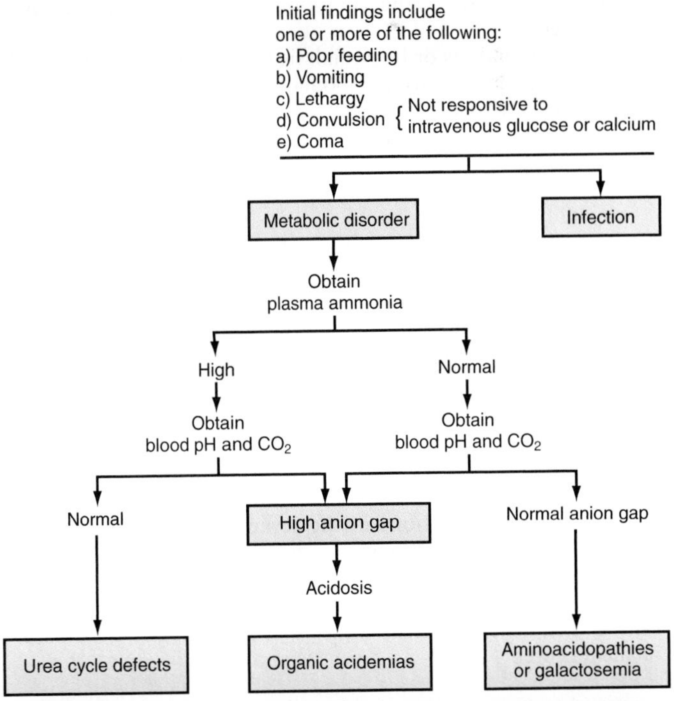

Figure 78-1 Clinical approach to a newborn infant with a suspected genetic metabolic disorder. This schema is a guide to the elucidation of some of the metabolic disorders in newborn infants. Although some exceptions to this schema exist, it is appropriate for most cases.

Table 78-3 INBORN ERRORS OF AMINO ACID METABOLISM ASSOCIATED WITH PECULIAR ODOR

INBORN ERROR OF METABOLISM	URINE ODOR
Glutaric acidemia (type II)	Sweaty feet, acrid
Hawkinsinuria	Swimming pool
3-Hydroxy-3-methylglutaric aciduria	Cat urine
Isovaleric acidemia	Sweaty feet, acrid
Maple syrup urine disease	Maple syrup
Hypermethioninemia	Boiled cabbage
Multiple carboxylase deficiency	Tomcat urine
Oasthouse urine disease	Hops-like
Phenylketonuria	Mousey or musty
Trimethylaminuria	Rotting fish
Tyrosinemia	Boiled cabbage, rancid butter

urea cycle defects commonly have normal serum pH and bicarbonate values; without measurement of blood ammonia, they may remain undiagnosed and succumb to their disease. Elevation of serum ammonia is also observed in some infants with certain organic acidemias. These infants are severely acidotic because of accumulation of organic acids in body fluids.

When blood ammonia, pH, and bicarbonate values are normal, other aminoacidopathies (such as hyperglycinemia) or galactosemia should be considered; galactosemic infants may also manifest cataracts, hepatomegaly, ascites, and jaundice.

TREATMENT

The majority of patients with genetic disorders of metabolism respond to one or all of the following treatments:

1. Special diets play an important role in the treatment of affected children. Dietary changes should be tailored to the pathophysiology of the condition and vary greatly among disorders.
2. Peritoneal dialysis or hemodialysis for expeditious removal of accumulated noxious compounds. This is a very effective modality for treatment of the acute phase of the condition.
3. Administration of the deficient metabolite.
4. Administration of the deficient enzyme.
5. Administration of the cofactor or coenzyme to maximize the residual enzyme activity.
6. Activation of alternate pathways to reduce the noxious compounds accumulated because of the genetic mutation.
7. Bone marrow transplantation.
8. Liver transplantation.

The last two modalities have the potential to cure the metabolic abnormalities. Replacement of the mutant gene with a normal one (gene therapy) is still in the experimental phase.

Treatment of genetic disorders of metabolism is complex and requires medical and technical expertise. The therapeutic regimen often needs to be tailored to the individual patient because of large phenotypic variations in the severity of the disease, even within a single family. Providing education and support for the family is the key to successful long range therapy. Effective treatment is best achieved by a team of specialists (physician specialist, nutritionist, geneticist, neurologist, and psychologist) in a major medical center.

BIBLIOGRAPHY
Please visit the Nelson Textbook of Pediatrics *website at* *www.expertconsult.com* *for the complete bibliography.*

Chapter 79
Defects in Metabolism of Amino Acids

79.1 Phenylalanine

Iraj Rezvani and Joseph John Melvin

Phenylalanine is an essential amino acid. Dietary phenylalanine not utilized for protein synthesis is normally degraded by way of the tyrosine pathway (Fig. 79-1). Deficiency of the enzyme phenylalanine hydroxylase (PAH) or of its cofactor tetrahydrobiopterin (BH_4) causes accumulation of phenylalanine in body fluids and in the brain. The severity of hyperphenylalaninemia depends on the degree of enzyme deficiency and may vary from very high plasma concentrations (>20 mg/dL or >1,200 µmole/L, **classic phenylketonuria [PKU]**) to mildly elevated levels (2-6 mg/dL or 120-360 µmole/L). In affected infants with plasma concentrations >20 mg/dL, excess phenylalanine is metabolized to phenylketones (phenylpyruvate and phenylacetate; see Fig. 79-1) that are excreted in the urine, giving rise to the term *phenylketonuria* (PKU). These metabolites have no role in pathogenesis of central nervous system (CNS) damage in patients with PKU; their presence in the body fluids simply signifies the severity of the condition. The term **hyperphenylalaninemia** implies lower plasma levels (<20 mg/dL) of phenylalanine; these patients may or may not need dietary therapy based on their blood phenylalanine level. The brain is the main organ affected by hyperphenylalaninemia. The CNS damage in affected patients is caused by the elevated concentration of phenylalanine in brain tissue. The high blood levels of phenylalanine in PKU saturate the transport system across the blood-brain barrier causing inhibition of the cerebral uptake of other large neutral amino acids such as tyrosine and tryptophan. The exact mechanism of damage caused by elevated levels of intracerebral phenylalanine remains elusive. There are a few adults with classic PKU and normal intelligence who have never been treated with a phenylalanine-restricted diet. Phenylalanine content of the brain in these individuals was found to be close to that of normal subjects when studied by magnetic resonance spectroscopy (MRS) and imaging (MRI) techniques.

Classic Phenylketonuria

Severe hyperphenylalaninemia (plasma phenylalanine levels >20 mg/dL), if untreated, invariably results in the development of signs and symptoms of classic PKU, except in rare unpredictable cases.

CLINICAL MANIFESTATIONS The affected infant is normal at birth. Profound mental retardation develops gradually if the infant remains untreated. Cognitive delay may not be evident for the 1st few months. In untreated patients, 50-70% will have an IQ below 35, and 88-90% below 65. Only 2-5% of untreated patients will have normal intelligence. Many patients require institutional care if the condition remains untreated. Vomiting, sometimes severe enough to be misdiagnosed as pyloric stenosis, may be an early symptom. Older untreated children become hyperactive with autistic behaviors, including purposeless hand movements, rhythmic rocking, and athetosis.

The infants are lighter in their complexion than unaffected siblings. Some may have a seborrheic or eczematoid rash, which is usually mild and disappears as the child grows older. These children have an unpleasant odor of phenylacetic acid, which has been described as musty or mousey. Neurologic signs include seizures (≈25%), spasticity, hyperreflexia, and tremors; more than 50% have electroencephalographic abnormalities. Microcephaly, prominent maxillae with widely spaced teeth, enamel hypoplasia, and growth retardation are other common findings in untreated children. The clinical manifestations of classic PKU are rarely

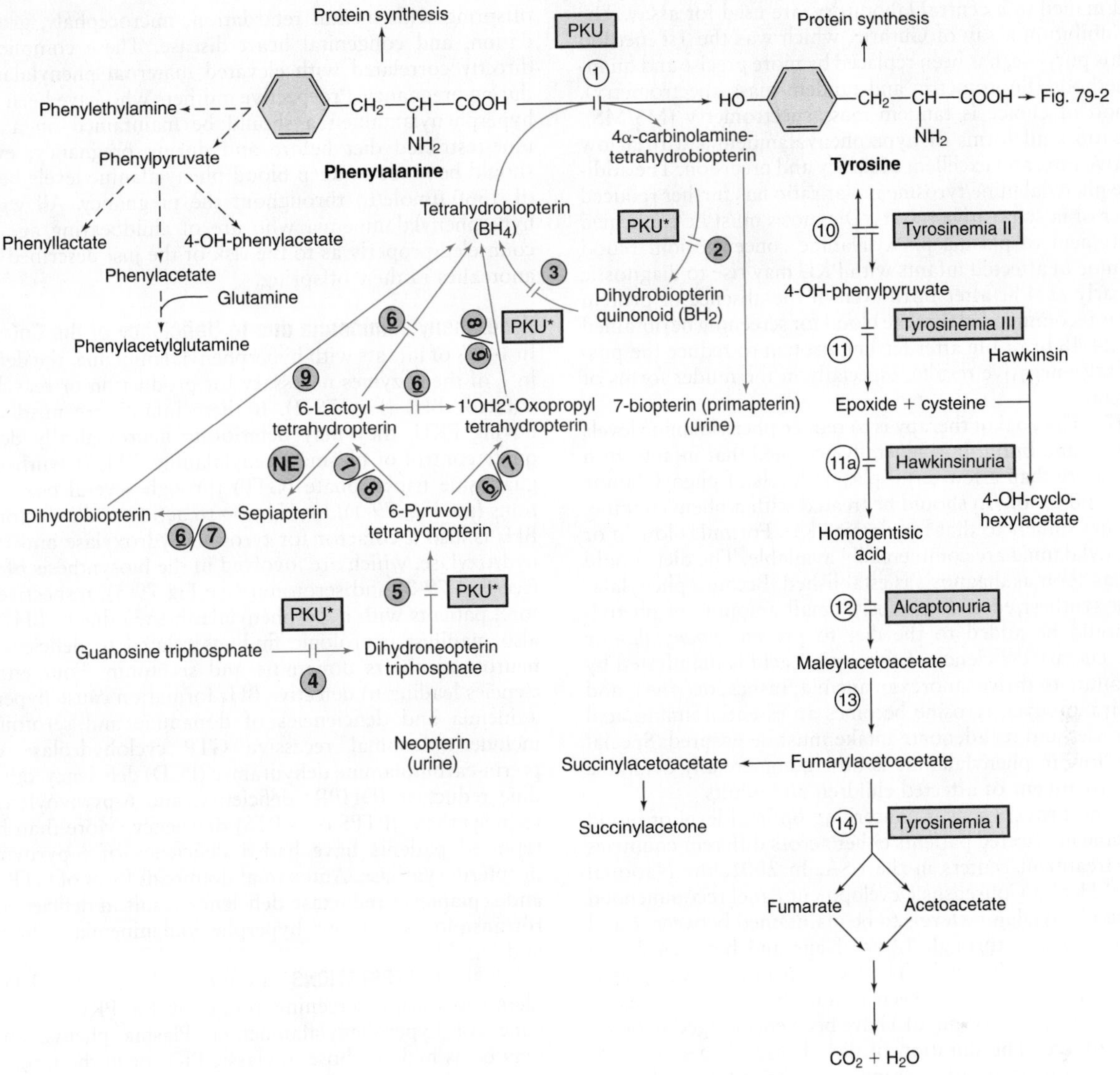

Figure 79-1 Pathways of phenylalanine and tyrosine metabolism. Enzyme defects causing genetic conditions are depicted as horizontal bars crossing the reaction arrow(s). Pathways for synthesis of cofactor BH_4 are shown in purple. PKU* refers to defects of BH_4 metabolism that affect the phenylalanine, tyrosine, and tryptophan hydroxylases (see Figs. 79-2 and 79-5). **Enzymes:** *(1)* phenylalanine hydroxylase (PAH), *(2)* pterin-carbinolamine dehydratase (PCD), *(3)* dihydrobiopterin reductase, *(4)* guanosine triphosphate (GTP) cyclohydrolase, *(5)* 6-pyruvoyltetrahydropterin synthase (6-PTS), *(6)* seriapterin reductase, *(7)* carbonyl reductase, *(8)* aldolase reductase, *(9)* dihydrofolate reductase, *(10)* tyrosine aminotransferase, *(11a)* intramolecular rearrangement, *(11)* 4-hydroxyphenylpyruvate dioxygenase, *(12)* homogentisic acid dioxygenase, *(13)* maleylacetoacetate isomerase, *(14)* fumarylacetoacetate hydroxylase, *(NE)* nonenzymatic.

seen in those countries in which neonatal screening programs for the detection of PKU are in effect.

Milder Forms of Hyperphenylalaninemia, Non-PKU Hyperphenylalaninemias

In any screening program for PKU, a group of infants are identified in whom initial plasma concentrations of phenylalanine are above normal (2 mg/dL, 120 µmole/L) but <20 mg/dL (1,200 µmole/L). These infants do not excrete phenylketones. The term hyperphenylalaninemia implies lower plasma concentration of phenylalanine, but these patients may still require dietary therapy depending on their untreated plasma phenylalanine level. Attempts have been made to classify these patients in different subgroups depending on the degree of hyperphenylalaninemia, but such a practice has little clinical or therapeutic advantage. The possibility of deficiency of BH_4 should be investigated in all infants with the milder forms of hyperphenylalaninemia (see later).

DIAGNOSIS Because of the often gradual development of clinical manifestations, hyperphenylalaninemia is usually diagnosed through mass screening of newborn infants. In infants with positive results from the screen for hyperphenylalaninemia, diagnosis should be confirmed by quantitative measurement of plasma phenylalanine concentration. Identification and measurement of phenylketones in the urine has no place in any screening program. In countries and places where such programs are not in effect, identification of phenylketones in the urine by ferric chloride may offer a simple test for diagnosis of infants with developmental and neurologic abnormalities. Once the diagnosis of hyperphenylalaninemia is established, additional studies for biopterin metabolism should be performed to rule out **biopterin** deficiency as the cause of hyperphenylalaninemia (see later).

NEONATAL SCREENING FOR HYPERPHENYLALANINEMIA Effective and relatively inexpensive methods for mass screening of newborn infants have been developed and are used in the USA and several other countries. A few drops of blood, which are placed on a filter paper and mailed to a central laboratory, are used for assay. The bacterial inhibition assay of Guthrie, which was the 1st method used for this purpose, has been replaced by more precise and quantitative methods (fluorometric and tandem mass spectrometry). The method of choice is tandem mass spectrometry (MS/MS), which identifies all forms of hyperphenyalaninemia with a low false-positive rate, and excellent accuracy and precision. The addition of the phenylalanine/tyrosine molar ratio has further reduced the number of false-positive results. Diagnosis must be confirmed by measurement of plasma phenylalanine concentration. Blood phenylalanine in affected infants with PKU may rise to diagnostic levels as early as 4 hr after birth even in the absence of protein feeding. It is recommended that the blood for screening be obtained in the 1st 24-48 hr of life after feeding protein to reduce the possibility of false-negative results, especially in the milder forms of the condition.

TREATMENT The goal of therapy is to reduce phenylalanine levels in the plasma and brain. It is generally accepted that infants with persistent (more than a few days) plasma levels of phenylalanine >6 mg/dL (360 µmole/L) should be treated with a phenylalanine-restricted diet similar to that for classic PKU. Formulas low in or free of phenylalanine are commercially available. The diet should be started as soon as diagnosis is established. Because phenylalanine is not synthesized endogenously, small amounts of phenylalanine should be added to the diet to prevent *phenylalanine deficiency*. Dietary deficiency of this amino acid is manifested by lethargy, failure to thrive, anorexia, anemia, rashes, diarrhea, and even death; moreover, tyrosine becomes an essential amino acid in this disorder and its adequate intake must be ensured. Special food items low in phenylalanine is now commercially available for dietary treatment of affected children and adults.

There is no firm consensus concerning optimal level of blood phenylalanine in affected patients either across different countries or among treatment centers in the USA. In 2001, the National Institutes of Health Consensus Development Panel recommended that plasma phenylalanine levels to be maintained between 2 and 6 mg/dL in neonates through 12 yr of age and between 2 and 15 mg/dL in older individuals. The fact that brain development continues in adolescence and even in adulthood, lower plasma phenylalanine levels (2-10 mg/dL) have been encouraged strongly after 12 yr of age. The duration of diet therapy is also controversial. Discontinuation of therapy, even in adulthood, may cause deterioration of IQ and cognitive performance. The current recommendation from the 2001 National Institutes of Health Consensus Development Panel is that all patients be kept on a phenylalanine-restricted diet for life.

Given the difficulty of maintaining a strict low-phenylalanine diet, there are continuing attempts to find other modalities for treatment of these patients. Oral administration of tetrahydrobiopterin (BH_4), the cofactor for PAH, may result in reduction of plasma levels of phenylalanine in some patients with PAH deficiency. Plasma levels of phenylalanine in these patients may decrease enough to allow for considerable modification of their dietary restriction. In very rare cases, the diet may be discontinued since the phenylalanine levels remain under 6 mg/dL. The response to BH_4 cannot be predicted consistently on the basis of genotype, especially in compound heterozygous patients. Sapropterin, a synthetic form of BH_4, which acts as a cofactor in patients with residual PAH activity, is approved by the Food and Drug Administration (FDA) to reduce phenylalanine levels in PKU. At a dose of 10 mg/kg/day, it reduces phenylalanine levels in up to 50% of patients.

Long-term care of these patients is best achieved by a team of experienced professionals (physician specialist, nutritionist, neurologist, geneticist, and psychologist) in a regional treatment center.

PREGNANCY IN WOMEN WITH HYPERPHENYLALANINEMIA (MATERNAL PKU) Pregnant women with hyperphenylalaninemia who are not on a phenylalanine-restricted diet have a very high risk of having offspring with mental retardation, microcephaly, growth retardation, and congenital heart disease. These complications are directly correlated with elevated maternal phenylalanine levels during pregnancy. Prospective mothers who have been treated for hyperphenylalaninemia should be maintained on a phenylalanine-restricted diet before and during pregnancy; every effort should be made to keep blood phenylalanine levels below 6 mg/dL (360 µmole/L) throughout the pregnancy. All women with hyperphenylalaninemia who are of childbearing age should be counseled properly as to the risk of the just described congenital anomalies in their offspring.

Hyperphenylalaninemia due to Deficiency of the Cofactor BH_4

In 1-3% of infants with hyperphenylalaninemia, the defect resides in 1 of the enzymes necessary for production or recycling of the cofactor BH_4 (Fig. 79-2). If these infants are misdiagnosed as having PKU, they may deteriorate neurologically despite adequate control of plasma phenylalanine. BH_4 is synthesized from guanosine triphosphate (GTP) through several enzymatic reactions (see Fig. 79-1). In addition to acting as a cofactor for PAH, BH_4 is also a cofactor for tyrosine hydroxylase and tryptophan hydroxylase, which are involved in the biosynthesis of dopamine (see Fig. 79-2) and serotonin (see Fig 79-5), respectively. Therefore, patients with hyperphenylalaninemia due to BH_4 deficiency also manifest neurologic findings related to deficiencies of the neurotransmitters dopamine and serotonin. Four enzyme deficiencies leading to defective BH_4 formation cause hyperphenylalaninemia and deficiencies of dopamine and serotonin. These include autosomal recessive GTP cyclohydrolase deficiency, pterin-carbinolamine dehydratase (PCD) deficiency, dihydropteridine reductase (DHPR) deficiency, and 6-pyruvoyltetrahydropterin synthase (PTPS or 6-PTS) deficiency. More than half of the reported patients have had a deficiency of 6-pyruvoyltetrahydropterin synthase. Autosomal dominant form of GTP deficiency and sepiapterin reductase deficiency result in deficiencies of neurotransmitters without hyperphenylalaninemia (Chapter 79.11 and Fig. 79-1).

CLINICAL MANIFESTATIONS Infants with cofactor deficiency are identified during screening programs for PKU because of evidence of hyperphenylalaninemia. Plasma phenylalanine levels may be as high as those in classic PKU or in the range of milder forms of hyperphenylalaninemia. However, the clinical manifestations of the neurotransmitter disorders differ greatly from those of PKU. Neurologic symptoms of the neurotransmitter disorders often manifest in the 1st few months of life and include extrapyramidal signs with choreoathetotic or dystonic limb movements, axial and truncal hypotonia, hypokinesia, feeding difficulties, and autonomic problems. Mental retardation, seizures, hypersalivation, and swallowing difficulties are also seen. The symptoms are usually progressive and often have a marked diurnal fluctuation.

DIAGNOSIS BH_4 deficiency and the responsible enzyme defect may be diagnosed by the following studies:

1. Measurement of neopterin (oxidative product of dihydroneopterin triphosphate) and biopterin (oxidative product of dihydrobiopterin and tetrahydrobiopterin) in body fluids, especially urine (see Fig. 79-1). In patients with GTP cyclohydrolase deficiency, urinary excretion of both neopterin and biopterin is very low. In patients with 6-pyruvoyltetrahydropterin synthase deficiency, there is a marked elevation of neopterin excretion and a concomitant decrease in biopterin excretion. In patients with dihydropteridine reductase deficiency, neopterin is normal, but biopterin is very high. Excretion of biopterin increases in this enzyme deficiency because the quinonoid dihydrobiopterin cannot be recycled back to BH_4. Patients with pterin-carbinolamine dehydratase deficiency excrete 7-biopterin (an unusual isomer of biopterin) in their urine. In addition, examination of cerebrospinal fluid (CSF) reveals

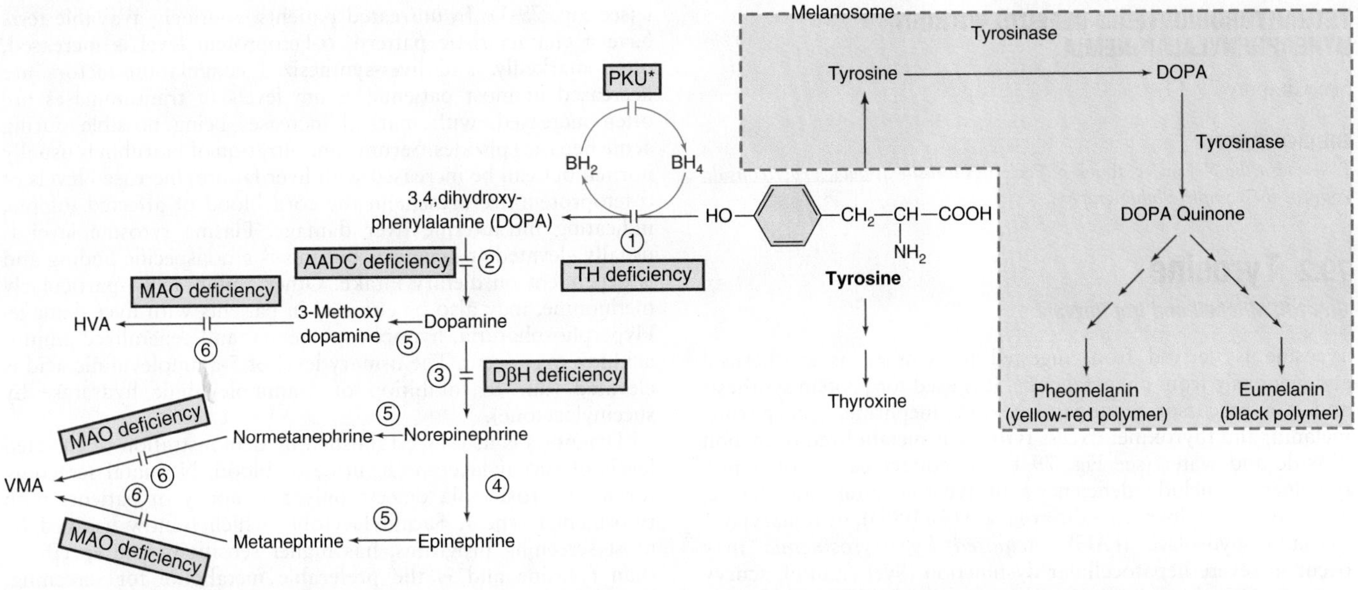

Figure 79-2 Other pathways involving tyrosine metabolism. PKU* indicates hyperphenylalanemia due to tetrahydrobiopterin (BH_4) deficiency (see Fig. 79-1). HVA, homovanillic acid; VMA, vanillylmandelic acid. **Enzymes:** *(1)* tyrosine hydroxylase (TH), *(2)* aromatic L-amino acid decarboxylase (AADC), *(3)* dopamine hydroxylase, *(4)* phenylethanolamine-N-methyltransferase (PNMT), *(5)* catechol *O*-methyltransferase (COMT), *(6)* Monoamine oxidase (MAO).

decreased levels of dopamine, serotonin, and their metabolites in all patients with BH_4 deficiency (Chapter 79.11).

2. BH_4 loading test. An oral dose of BH_4 (20 mg/kg) normalizes plasma phenylalanine in patients with BH_4 deficiency within 4 to 8 hr. The blood phenylalanine should be elevated (>400 µmole/L) to enable interpretation of the results. This may be achieved by discontinuing diet therapy for 2 days before the test or by administering a loading dose of phenylalanine (100 mg/kg) 3 hr before the test. In BH_4-responsive PKU due to PAH deficiency, phenylalanine levels may decrease during the BH_4 loading test but increase later even with BH_4 supplementation. Patients who demonstrate phenylalanine levels within normal range over at least a week without a phenylalanine-restricted diet can be continued on BH_4 supplementation as the sole treatment for the hyperphenylalaninemia. However, it is imperative that plasma phenylalanine levels be monitored prospectively to ensure that phenylalanine levels remain within the normal range.
3. Enzyme assay. The activity of dihydropteridine reductase can be measured in the dry blood spots on the filter paper used for screening purposes. 6-Pyruvoyltetrahydropterin synthase activity can be measured in the liver, kidneys, and erythrocytes. Carbinolamine dehydratase activity can be measured in the liver and kidneys. GTP cyclohydrolase activity can be measured in the liver and in cytokine (interferon-γ) stimulated mononuclear cells or fibroblasts (the enzyme activity is normally very low in unstimulated cells).

TREATMENT The goals of therapy are to correct hyperphenylalaninemia and to restore neurotransmitter deficiencies in the CNS. The control of hyperphenylalaninemia is important in patients with cofactor deficiency, because high levels of phenylalanine interfere with the transport of neurotransmitter precursors (tyrosine, tryptophan) into the brain. Plasma phenylalanine should be maintained as close to normal as possible (<6 mg/dL). This can be achieved by a combination of a low phenylalanine diet and oral supplementation of BH_4. Infants with GTP cyclohydrolase or 6-PTS deficiencies respond more readily to BH_4 therapy (5-10 mg/kg/day) than those with dihydropteridine reductase deficiency. In the latter patients, doses as high as 20 mg/kg/day may be required. BH_4 for replacement therapy is commercially available, although it is expensive.

Lifelong supplementation with **neurotransmitter precursors** such as L-dopa and 5-hydroxytryptophan, along with carbidopa to inhibit degradation of L-dopa before it enters the CNS, is necessary in most of these patients even when treatment with BH_4 normalizes plasma levels of phenylalanine. BH_4 does not readily enter the brain to restore neurotransmitter production. Supplementation with folinic acid is also recommended in patients with dihydropteridine reductase deficiency. Unfortunately, attempting to normalize neurotransmitter levels using neurotransmitter precursors usually does not fully resolve the neurologic symptoms due to the inability to attain normal levels of BH_4 in the brain. Patients often demonstrate mental retardation, fluctuating abnormalities of tone, eye movement abnormalities, poor balance and coordination, decreased ability to ambulate, and seizures in spite of supplementation with neurotransmitter precursors.

Hyperprolactinemia occurs in patients with BH_4 deficiency and may be due to hypothalamic dopamine deficiency. Measurement of serum prolactin levels may be a convenient method for monitoring adequacy of neurotransmitter replacement in affected patients.

Some drugs such as trimethoprim sulfamethoxazole, methotrexate, and other antileukemic agents are known to inhibit dihydropteridine reductase enzyme activity and should be used with great caution in patients with BH_4 deficiency.

GENETICS AND PREVALENCE All defects causing hyperphenylalaninemia are inherited as autosomal recessive traits. The prevalence of PKU in the USA is estimated at 1/14,000 to 1/20,000 live births. The prevalence of non-PKU hyperphenylalaninemia is estimated at 1/50,000. The condition is more common in whites and Native Americans and less prevalent in blacks, Hispanics, and Asians.

The gene for PAH is located on chromosome 12q24.1 and many disease-causing mutations have been identified in different families. The majority of patients are compound heterozygotes for 2 different mutant alleles. The gene for PTP synthase, the most common cause of BH_4 deficiency, resides on chromosome 11q22.3-23.3, the gene for dihydropteridine reductase is located on chromosome 4p15.3, and those of carbinolamine dehydratase and GTP cyclohydrolase are on 10q22 and 14q22.1-22.2, respectively. Many disease-causing mutations of these genes have been identified. Prenatal diagnosis is possible using specific genetic probes in cells obtained from chorionic villi biopsy.

TETRAHYDROBIOPTERIN DEFECTS WITHOUT HYPERPHENYLALANINEMIA

See Chapter 79.11.

BIBLIOGRAPHY

Please visit the Nelson Textbook of Pediatrics *website at www.expertconsult.com for the complete bibliography.*

79.2 Tyrosine

Grant A. Mitchell and Iraj Rezvani

Tyrosine is derived from ingested proteins or is synthesized endogenously from phenylalanine. It is used for protein synthesis and is a precursor of dopamine, norepinephrine, epinephrine, melanin, and thyroxine. Excess tyrosine is metabolized to carbon dioxide and water (see Fig. 79-1). Hereditary causes of hypertyrosinemia include deficiencies of tyrosine aminotransferase, 4-hydroxyphenylpyruvate dioxygenase (4-HPPD), or fumarylacetoacetate hydrolase (FAH). *Acquired hypertyrosinemia* may occur in severe hepatocellular dysfunction (liver failure), scurvy (vitamin C is the cofactor for the enzyme 4-HPPD), and hyperthyroidism. Hypertyrosinemia is common in blood samples obtained soon after eating.

Tyrosinemia Type I (Tyrosinosis, Hereditary Tyrosinemia, Hepatorenal Tyrosinemia)

This severe disease of the liver, kidney, and peripheral nerve, is caused by a deficiency of the enzyme FAH. Organ damage is believed to result from accumulation of metabolites of tyrosine degradation, especially succinylacetone.

CLINICAL MANIFESTATIONS Untreated, the affected infant appears normal at birth and typically presents between 2 and 6 mo of age but rarely may become symptomatic in the 1st mo or appear healthy beyond the 1st yr of life. The earlier the presentation, the poorer is the prognosis. The 1 yr mortality, which is about 60% in infants who develop symptoms before 2 mo of age, decreases to 4% in infants who become symptomatic after 6 mo of age.

An acute **hepatic crisis** commonly heralds the onset of the disease and is usually precipitated by an intercurrent illness that produces a catabolic state. Fever, irritability, vomiting, hemorrhage, hepatomegaly, jaundice, elevated levels of serum transaminases, and hypoglycemia are common. An odor resembling boiled cabbage may be present, due to increased methionine metabolites. Most hepatic crises resolve spontaneously, but may progress to liver failure and death. Between the crises, varying degrees of failure to thrive, hepatomegaly, and coagulation abnormalities often persist. Cirrhosis and eventually hepatocellular carcinoma occur with increasing age. Carcinoma is unusual before 2 yr of age.

Episodes of acute **peripheral neuropathy** resembling acute porphyria occur in ≈40% of affected children. These crises, often triggered by a minor infection, are characterized by severe pain, often in the legs, associated with hypertonic posturing of the head and trunk, vomiting, paralytic ileus, and, occasionally, self-induced injuries of the tongue or buccal mucosa. Marked weakness and paralysis occur in about 30% of episodes, which may lead to respiratory failure requiring mechanical ventilation. Crises typically last 1 to 7 days but recuperation from paralytic crises can be prolonged.

Renal involvement is manifested as a Fanconi-like syndrome with normal anion gap metabolic acidosis, hyperphosphaturia, hypophosphatemia, and vitamin D–resistant rickets. Nephromegaly and nephrocalcinosis may be present on ultrasound examination.

Hypertrophic cardiomyopathy and hyperinsulinism are seen in some infants.

LABORATORY FINDINGS The presence of elevated levels of succinylacetone in serum and urine is diagnostic for tyrosinemia type I (see Fig. 79-1). In untreated patients, routinely available tests have a characteristic pattern. α-Fetoprotein level is increased, often markedly, and liver-synthesized coagulation factors are decreased in most patients; serum levels of transaminases are often increased, with marked increases being possible during acute hepatic episodes. Serum concentration of bilirubin is usually normal but can be increased with liver failure. Increased levels of α-fetoprotein are present in the cord blood of affected infants, indicating intrauterine liver damage. Plasma tyrosine level is usually elevated at diagnosis but this is a nonspecific finding and is dependent on dietary intake. Other amino acids, particularly methionine, may also be elevated in patients with liver damage. Hyperphosphaturia, hypophosphatemia, and generalized aminoaciduria may occur. The urinary level of 5-aminolevulinic acid is elevated (due to inhibition of 5-aminolevulinic hydratase by succinylacetone).

Diagnosis is usually established by demonstration of elevated levels of succinylacetone in urine or blood. Neonatal screening for hypertyrosinemia detects only a minority of patients with tyrosinemia type I. Succinylacetone, which is now assayed by most screening programs, has higher sensitivity and specificity than tyrosine and is the preferable metabolite for screening. Tyrosinemia type I should be differentiated from other causes of hepatitis and hepatic failure in infants, including galactosemia, hereditary fructose intolerance, neonatal iron storage disease, giant cell hepatitis, and citrullinemia type II (Chapter 79.11).

TREATMENT AND OUTCOME A diet low in phenylalanine and tyrosine can slow but does not halt the progression of the condition. The **treatment of choice** is nitisinone (NTBC), which inhibits tyrosine degradation at 4-HPPD (see Fig. 79-1). This treatment prevents acute hepatic and neurologic crises. Although nitisinone stops or greatly slows disease progression, some pretreatment liver damage is not reversible. Therefore, patients must be followed for development of cirrhosis or **hepatocellular carcinoma.** On imaging, the presence of even a single liver nodule usually indicates underlying cirrhosis. Most liver nodules in tyrosinemic patients are benign but current imaging techniques do not accurately distinguish all malignant nodules. Liver transplantation is an effective therapy for tyrosinemia type I and alleviates the risk of hepatocellular carcinoma. The impact of nitisinone treatment on the need for liver transplantation is still under study but the greatest effect is in patients treated early, such as children detected by neonatal screening, prior to the development of clinical symptoms. Rarely, nitisinone-treated patients develop corneal crystals, presumably of tyrosine, which are reversible by strict dietary compliance. This finding, combined with observations of developmental delay in some patients with chronically elevated tyrosine such as tyrosinemia type II, suggests that a diet low in phenylalanine and tyrosine should be continued in patients treated with nitisinone.

GENETICS AND PREVALENCE Tyrosinemia type I is an autosomal recessive trait. The *FAH* gene maps to chromosome 15q; numerous mutations are reported. DNA analysis is useful for molecular prenatal diagnosis and for carrier testing in groups at risk for specific mutations such as French-Canadians from the Saguenay-Lac Saint-Jean region of Quebec. Tyrosinemia type I is panethnic; lack of French-Canadian or Scandinavian ancestry does not exclude the diagnosis. The prevalence of the condition is estimated to be 1/1,846 live births in the Saguenay-Lac Saint-Jean region and ≈1/100,000 worldwide. Prenatal diagnosis is typically performed by measurement of succinylacetone in amniotic fluid, or if the familial mutations are known, by DNA analysis of amniocytes or of chorionic villi.

Tyrosinemia Type II (Richner-Hanhart Syndrome, Oculocutaneous Tyrosinemia)

This rare autosomal recessive disorder is caused by deficiency of tyrosine aminotransferase, resulting in palmar and plantar hyperkeratosis, herpetiform corneal ulcers, and mental retardation (see Fig. 79-1). **Ocular manifestations** include excessive tearing, redness, pain, and photophobia and often occur before skin lesions. Corneal lesions are presumed to be due to tyrosine deposition. In contrast to herpetic ulcers, corneal lesions in tyrosinemia type II stain poorly with fluorescein and often are bilateral. **Skin lesions**, which may develop later in life, include painful, nonpruritic hyperkeratotic plaques on the soles, palms and fingertips. Mental retardation, which occurs in <50% of patients, is usually mild to moderate.

The principal laboratory finding in untreated patients is marked hypertyrosinemia (20-50 mg/dL; 1,100-2,750 µmole/L). Surprisingly, 4-hydroxyphenylpyruvic acid and its metabolites are also elevated in urine despite being downstream from the metabolic block (see Fig. 79-1). This is hypothesized to occur via the action of other transaminases in the presence of high tyrosine concentrations, producing 4HPP in cellular compartments like the mitochondrion in which it is not further degraded. In contrast to tyrosinemia type I, liver and kidney function are normal, as are serum concentrations of other amino acids and succinylacetone. Tyrosinemia type II is due to *TAT* gene mutations, causing deficiency of cytosolic tyrosine aminotransferase activity in liver.

Diagnosis of type II tyrosinemia is established by assay of plasma tyrosine concentration in patients with suggestive findings. Molecular diagnosis is possible. Assay of liver tyrosine aminotransferase activity is rarely indicated.

Treatment with a diet low in tyrosine and phenylalanine improves the biochemical abnormalities and can normalize the skin and eye. The claim that mental retardation may be prevented by early diet therapy is reasonable and is supported by some case reports. The *TAT* gene maps to chromosome 16q and several disease-causing mutations have been identified. About half of reported cases are of Italian descent.

Tyrosinemia Type III (Primary Deficiency of 4-HPPD)

Only a few cases have been reported; most were detected by amino acid chromatography performed for various neurologic findings. Age at presentation has been from 1 to 17 mo. Developmental delay, seizures, intermittent ataxia, and self-destructive behavior are reported. A causal link to 4HPP deficiency is not formally established. Liver or renal abnormalities are absent. Asymptomatic infants with 4-HPPD deficiency have been identified by neonatal screening for hypertyrosinemia.

The diagnosis is suspected in children with sustained moderate increases in plasma levels of tyrosine (typically 350-700 µmole/L on a normal diet) and the presence in urine of 4-hydroxyphenylpyruvic acid and its metabolites 4-hydroxyphenyllactic and 4-hydroxyphenylacetic acids. Diagnosis may be refined by demonstrating the presence of mutations in the gene for 4-HPPD on chromosome 12q, or rarely, by demonstrating a low activity of 4-HPPD enzyme in liver biopsy.

Given the possible association with neurologic abnormalities, dietary reduction of plasma tyrosine levels is prudent. It is also logical to attempt a trial of vitamin C, the cofactor for 4-HPPD. The condition is inherited as an autosomal recessive trait.

Transient Tyrosinemia of the Newborn

In a small number of newborn infants, plasma tyrosine may be as high as 60 mg/dL (3,300 µmole/L) during the 1st 2 weeks of life. Most affected infants are premature and are receiving high-protein diets. Transient tyrosinemia is felt to result from delayed maturation of 4-HPPD (see Fig. 79-1). Lethargy, poor feeding, and decreased motor activity are noted in some patients. Most are asymptomatic and are identified by a high blood phenylalanine or tyrosine level on screening. Laboratory findings include marked elevation of plasma tyrosine with a moderate increase in plasma phenylalanine. The finding of hypertyrosinemia differentiates this condition from PKU. 4-Hydroxyphenylpyruvic acid and its metabolites are present in the urine. Hypertyrosinemia usually resolves spontaneously in the 1st mo of life. It can be corrected promptly by reducing dietary protein to below 2 g/kg/24 hr and by administering vitamin C (200-400 mg/24 hr). Mild intellectual deficits have been reported in some infants that had this condition, but the causal relationship to hypertyrosinemia is not conclusively established.

Hawkinsinuria

This rare autosomal dominant condition is caused by a mutant 4-HPPD enzyme that catalyzes a partial reaction, releasing an intermediate compound used for diagnosis (see Fig. 79-1). This intermediate is either reduced to form 4-hydroxycyclohexylacetic acid (4-HCAA) or reacts with glutathione to form the unusual organic acid hawkinsin (2-L-cysteine-S-yl-1-4-dihydroxycyclohex-5-en-1-yl-acetic acid); secondary glutathione deficiency may occur.

Individuals with this disorder are symptomatic only during infancy. The symptoms usually appear after weaning from breastfeeding with the introduction of a high-protein diet. Severe metabolic acidosis, ketosis, failure to thrive, mild hepatomegaly, and an unusual odor (like that of a swimming pool) are described. Mental development is usually normal.

Affected children and adults excrete the organic acids 4-HCAA, 4-hydroxyphenylpyruvic acid and its metabolites (4-hydroxyphenyllactic and 4-hydroxyphenylacetic acids), 5-oxoproline (owing to secondary glutathione deficiency), and hawkinsin in their urine. Plasma tyrosine level is usually normal.

Treatment consists of a low-protein diet during infancy. Breast feeding is encouraged. A trial with large doses of vitamin C (up to 1,000 mg/24 hr) is also recommended. The same mutation, a substitution of threonine for the normal alanine codon at position 33 of the 4-HPPD gene, has been identified in unrelated patients with hawkinsinuria.

Alcaptonuria

This rare (with an incidence of ≈1/250,000) autosomal recessive disorder is due to a deficiency of homogentisic acid oxidase, which causes large amounts of homogentisic acid to accumulate in the body and then to be excreted in the urine (see Fig. 79-1).

Clinical manifestations of alcaptonuria consist of ochronosis and arthritis in adulthood. The only sign in children is a blackening of the urine on standing, caused by oxidation and polymerization of homogentisic acid. A history of grey- or black-stained diapers should suggest the diagnosis. This sign may never be noted, hence, diagnosis is often delayed until adulthood. *Ochronosis,* which is seen clinically as dark spots on the sclera or ear cartilage, results from the accumulation of the black polymer of homogentisic acid. *Arthritis* can be disabling with advancing age. It involves the large joints (spine, hip, and knee) and is usually more severe in males. Like rheumatoid arthritis, the arthritis has acute exacerbations, but the radiologic findings are typical of osteoarthritis, with characteristic narrowing of the joint spaces and calcification of the intervertebral discs. High incidences of heart disease (mitral and aortic valvulitis, calcification of the heart valves, and myocardial infarction) have been noted.

The diagnosis is confirmed by finding massive excretion of homogentisic acid on urine organic acid testing. Tyrosine levels are normal. The enzyme is expressed only in the liver and kidneys. The gene for alcaptonuria, *HGD*, maps to chromosome 3q. Several disease-causing mutations have been identified. Alcaptonuria is commonest in the Dominican Republic and Slovakia.

Treatment of the arthritis is symptomatic. Nitisinone efficiently reduces homogentisic acid production in alkaptonuria. If presymptomatic individuals are detected, treatment with nitisinone, combined with a phenylalanine- and tyrosine-restricted diet, seems reasonable, although no experience is available regarding long-term efficacy.

Tyrosine Hydroxylase Deficiency

See Chapter 79.11.

Table 79-1 CLASSIFICATION OF ALBINISM

TYPE	GENE	CHROMOSOME
OCULOCUTANEOUS ALBINISM (OCA)		
OCA_1 (tyrosinase deficient)	*TYR*	11q
OCA_1A (severe deficiency)	*TYR*	11q
OCA_1B (mild deficiency)*	*TYR*	11q
OCA_2 (tyrosinase positive)†	*P* (pink-eyed dilution)	15q
OCA_3 (Rufous, red OCA)	*TYRP1*‡	9p
OCA_4	*MATP*	5p13.3
Hermansky-Pudlak syndrome	*HPS1*	10q
Chédiak-Higashi syndrome	*LYST*	1q
OCULAR ALBINISM		
OA_1 (Nettleship-Falls type)	OA	xp
LOCALIZED ALBINISM		
Piebaldism	*KIT*	4q
Waardenburg syndrome I & III	*PAX3*	2q
Waardenburg syndrome II	*MITF*	3p

*This includes Amish, minimal pigment, yellow albinism, and platinum and temperature-sensitive variants.
†Includes brown OCA.
‡Tyrosinase related protein 1.

Albinism

Albinism is due to deficiency of melanin, the main pigment of the skin and eye (Table 79-1). Melanin is synthesized by melanocytes from tyrosine in a membrane-bound intracellular organelle, the melanosome. Melanocytes originate from the embryonic neural crest and migrate to the skin, eyes (choroid and iris), hair follicles, and inner ear. The melanin in the eye is confined to the retinal pigment epithelium, whereas in skin and hair follicles, it is secreted into the epidermis and hair shaft. Albinism can be caused by deficiencies of melanin synthesis, by some hereditary defects of melanosomes, or by disorders of melanocyte migration. Although albinism is a classical example of a biochemical genetic disease, neither the biosynthetic pathway of melanin nor many facets of melanocyte cell biology are completely elucidated (see Fig. 79-2). The end products are 2 pigments: *pheomelanin,* which is a yellow-red pigment; and *eumelanin,* a brown-black pigment.

Clinically, primary albinism can be generalized or localized. Primary generalized albinism can be either ocular or oculocutaneous. Some syndromes feature albinism in association with platelet, immunological, or neurological dysfunction.

In generalized oculocutaneous albinism, hypopigmentation can be either complete or partial. Individuals with complete albinism do not develop detectable skin pigmentation, either generalized (tanning) or localized (pigmented nevi).

The diagnosis of albinism is usually evident, but for some white children whose families are particularly light-skinned, normal variation may be a diagnostic consideration. Such normal fair-skinned children progressively develop pigmentation, the eye manifestations of albinism are absent, and other family members may have had a similar course. The clinical diagnosis of oculocutaneous albinism, as opposed to other types of cutaneous hypopigmentation, requires the presence of characteristic eye findings.

The ocular manifestations of albinism include hypopigmentation, including foveal hypoplasia with reduced visual acuity, refractive errors, nystagmus, alternating strabismus, and a red reflex (diffuse reddish hue of the iris produced during ophthalmoscopic or slit lamp examination of the eye). There is also an abnormality in routing of the optic fibers at the chiasm. Unlike normally pigmented individuals, in patients with albinism the majority of the nerve fibers from the temporal side of the retina cross to the contralateral hemisphere of the brain. This results in lack of biocular (stereoscopic) vision and of depth perception, and in repeated switching of vision from eye to eye, causing alternating strabismus. This abnormality also causes a characteristic pattern of visual evoked potentials. These findings are highly specific for albinism and can be used to formally establish the clinical diagnosis. Regular ophthalmological follow-up is recommended for patients with albinism. For instance, correction of refractive errors can maximize visual function. Normally the alternating strabismus does not result in amblyopia and does not require surgery.

Patients with albinism should be counseled to avoid ultraviolet radiation by wearing protective long-sleeved clothing and by using sunscreens with a sun protection factor (SPF) rating above 30. All forms of oculocutaneous albinism are autosomal recessive traits.

Melanin is also present in the cochlea. Albino individuals may be more susceptible to ototoxic agents such as gentamicin.

Many clinical forms of albinism have been identified. Some of the seemingly distinct clinical forms are caused by different mutations of the same gene. Several genes located on different chromosomes are shown to be involved in melanogenesis (see Table 79-1). Attempts to differentiate types of albinism based on the mode of inheritance, tyrosinase activity, or the extent of hypopigmentation have failed to yield a comprehensive classification. The following classification is based on the distribution of albinism in the body and the type of mutated gene.

Mutation detection is clinically available for most albinism genes (see Table 79-1). Molecular diagnosis is of little use therapeutically in isolated albinism but can be helpful for precise genetic counseling of families.

OCULOCUTANEOUS (GENERALIZED) ALBINISM (OCA) Lack of pigment is generalized, affecting skin, hair, and eyes. Three genetically distinct forms exist: OCA_1, OCA_2 and OCA_3. The lack of pigment is complete in patients with OCA_1 A; the other types may not be clinically distinguishable from one another. All are inherited as autosomal recessive traits.

OCA_1 (Tyrosinase-Deficient Albinism) The defect in these patients resides in the tyrosinase gene, *TYR*, on chromosome 11q. Many mutant alleles have been identified. Most affected individuals are genetic compounds, heterozygous for 2 different mutant alleles. A clinical clue to the diagnosis of OCA_1 is complete lack of pigment at birth. The condition can be subdivided to OCA_1 A and OCA_1 B, based on enzyme activity and later clinical manifestations.

OCA_1 A (Tyrosinase-Negative OCA) In these individuals, both *TYR* alleles have mutations that completely inactivate tyrosinase. Clinically, lack of pigment in the skin (milky white), hair (white hair), and eyes (red gray irides) is evident at birth and remains unchanged throughout life. They do not tan and do not develop pigmented nevi or freckles.

OCA_1 B These patients have *TYR* gene mutations that preserve some residual activity. Clinically they completely lack pigment at birth, but with age become light blond with light blue or hazel eyes. They develop pigmented nevi and freckles and they may tan. OCA_1 B patients, depending on the degree of pigmentation, were once subdivided into different groups and thought to be genetically distinct.

OCA_2 (Tyrosinase-Positive OCA) This is the most common form of generalized OCA, particularly in African blacks. Clinically, patients demonstrate some pigmentation of the skin and eyes at birth and continue to accumulate pigment throughout their lives. The hair is yellow at birth and may darken with age. They have pigmented nevi and freckles but do not tan. They may be clinically indistinguishable from OCA_1 B. These individuals have normal tyrosinase activity in hair bulbs. The defect is in the OCA_2 gene on chromosome 15q, orthologous to the *p* (pink-eyed dilution) gene in the mouse. This gene produces the P protein, a melanosome membrane protein. Patients with Prader-Willi and Angelman syndromes with microdeletion in chromosome 15q12 lack 1 copy of the OCA_2 gene and have mild pigmentary dilution (Chapter 76).

OCA_3 (Rufous Albinism) This form has been identified only in Africans, African-Americans, and natives of New Guinea. Patients have reddish hair and reddish brown skin as adults. The skin color is peculiar to this form. In the young, the coloration may resemble that of OCA_2. Patients with OCA_3 can make pheomelanin but not eumelanin. The mutation is in the tyrosinase related protein 1 (*TYRP1*) gene, the function of which is not understood.

OCA_4 Similar manifestations to OCA_2 have been observed in patients (mostly from Japan) with mutations in *MATP* gene located on chromosome 5p13.3.

OCULAR ALBINISM (OA) Albinism is limited to the eye. All the eye findings of albinism (see earlier) are present. Most cases are X-linked (OA_1). In pedigrees with apparently autosomal recessive OA, OCA_2 with predominant ocular involvement should be considered.

Ocular Albinism 1 (OA_1 Nettleship-Falls Type) Only the hemizygous male has the complete manifestation. Segments of abnormal retinal pigmentation may be present in heterozygous females. An X-linked ocular albinism with late-onset sensorineural deafness has also been reported. The diagnosis of OA_1 is evident in males with the features of albinism in the eye, normal skin pigmentation, and a positive family history suggestive of an X-linked recessive transmission. In patients who are the 1st of their families to be affected, electron microscopic demonstration of characteristic megamelanosomes in skin biopsies or hair root specimens is useful, as is mutation analysis of the *OA_1* gene on chromosome Xp.

SYNDROMIC FORMS OF GENERALIZED ALBINISM

Hermansky-Pudlak Syndrome This group of autosomal recessive disorders is caused by mutations of 1 of 8 genes, *HPS1* to *HPS8*. Hermansky-Pudlak syndrome is suspected in patients with albinism and a bleeding diathesis. Disease subtype can be established with molecular studies.

The HPS genes are necessary for normal structure and function of lysosome-derived organelles, including melanosomes and platelet dense bodies. Patients have a tyrosinase-positive OCA of variable severity associated with platelet dysfunction (owing to the absence of platelet dense bodies). A ceroid-like material accumulates in tissues. Hermansky-Pudlak syndrome is most prevalent in 2 regions of Puerto Rico (types 1 and 3, due to different founder effects). The cutaneous and ocular symptoms of albinism are present. Patients can develop epistaxis, postsurgical bleeding, or abundant menses. Bleeding time is prolonged but platelet count is normal. Major complications are progressive pulmonary fibrosis in young adults and Crohn's-like inflammatory bowel disease in adolescents and young adults. Kidney failure and cardiomyopathy are reported. Neutropenia is described in HPS2. Treatment is symptomatic.

Chédiak-Higashi Syndrome Patients with this rare autosomal recessive condition (Chapter 124) have albinism of variable severity and susceptibility to infection. Bacterial infections of skin and upper respiratory tract are common. Giant peroxidase-positive lysosomal granules can be seen in granulocytes in a blood smear. Patients have a reduced number of melanosomes, which are abnormally large (macromelanosomes). The bleeding tendency is typically mild. The major, life-threatening complication is macrophage activation with hemophagocytic lymphohistiocytosis, manifested by fever, lymphadenopathy, hepatosplenomegaly, cytopenias, and elevated plasma ferritin level. Patients surviving childhood may develop cerebellar atrophy, peripheral neuropathy, and cognitive delay. Mutations in the *LYST* gene on chromosome 1q are the only known cause of this syndrome.

Hypopigmentation is a feature of other syndromes, some with abnormalities of lysosomal biogenesis or melanosome biology, such as Griscelli syndrome (silver-grey hair, pigmentary dilution of skin, and melanosomal clumping in hair shafts and the center of melanocytes, with mental retardation or macrophage activation with hemophagocytosis in different subtypes), Vici syndrome (combined immunodeficiency, mental retardation, agenesis of the corpus callosum, cataracts, and cleft lip and palate), and MAPBPIP protein deficiency (short stature, recurrent infections, neutropenia).

LOCALIZED ALBINISM This term refers to localized patches of hypopigmentation of skin and hair, which may be evident at birth or develop with time. These conditions are caused by abnormal migration of melanocytes during development.

Piebaldism In this autosomal dominant inherited condition, the individual is usually born with a white forelock. The underlying skin is depigmented and devoid of melanocytes. In addition, there are usually white macules on the face, trunk, and extremities. Mutations in the *KIT* gene have been shown in affected patients.

Waardenburg Syndrome In this syndrome, a white forelock is associated with lateral displacement of inner canthi, broad nasal bridge, heterochromia of irides, and sensorineural deafness. This condition is inherited as an autosomal dominant trait. Four major types of this syndrome have been identified. Patients with type I have lateral displacement of inner canthi. The condition is caused by mutations in the *PAX3* gene. Type II patients have normal inner canthal distances, and mutations in the *MITF* gene have been shown in some patients. Patients with type III have all the findings seen in individuals with type I, plus hypoplasia and contractures of the upper limbs. The gene abnormality is in *PAX3*. Type IV, associated with Hirschsprung disease, is heterogeneous. Mutations in different genes (*EDN3, EDNRB*, or *SOX10*) have been identified in different patients.

Other causes of localized hypopigmentation, such as somatic mosaicism for chromosomal abnormalities are dealt with elsewhere (e.g., hypomelanosis of Ito, Chapters 76 and 645; and vitiligo, Chapter 645).

BIBLIOGRAPHY

Please visit the Nelson Textbook of Pediatrics *website at* *www.expertconsult.com* *for the complete bibliography.*

79.3 Methionine

Iraj Rezvani and David S. Rosenblatt

The normal pathway for catabolism of methionine, an essential amino acid, produces S-adenosylmethionine, which serves as a methyl group donor for methylation of a variety of compounds in the body, and cysteine, which is formed through a series of reactions collectively called trans-sulfuration (Fig. 79-3).

Homocystinuria (Homocystinemia)

Normally, most homocysteine, an intermediate compound of methionine degradation, is remethylated to methionine. This methionine-sparing reaction is catalyzed by the enzyme methionine synthase, which requires a metabolite of folic acid (5-methyltetrahydrofolate) as a methyl donor and a metabolite of vitamin B_{12} (methylcobalamin) as a cofactor (see Fig. 79-3). Only 20-30% of total homocysteine (and its dimer homocystine) is in free form in the plasma of normal individuals. The rest is bound to proteins as mixed disulfides. Three major forms of homocystinemia and homocystinuria have been identified.

HOMOCYSTINURIA DUE TO CYSTATHIONINE β-SYNTHASE (CBS) DEFICIENCY (CLASSIC HOMOCYSTINURIA) This is the most common inborn error of methionine metabolism. About 40% of affected patients respond to high doses of vitamin B_6 and usually have milder clinical manifestations than those who are unresponsive to vitamin B_6 therapy. These patients possess some residual enzyme activity.

Infants with this disorder are normal at birth. Clinical manifestations during infancy are nonspecific and may include failure to thrive and developmental delay. The diagnosis is usually made after 3 yr of age, when subluxation of the ocular lens (**ectopia lentis**) occurs. This causes severe myopia and iridodonesis (quivering of the iris). Astigmatism, glaucoma, staphyloma,

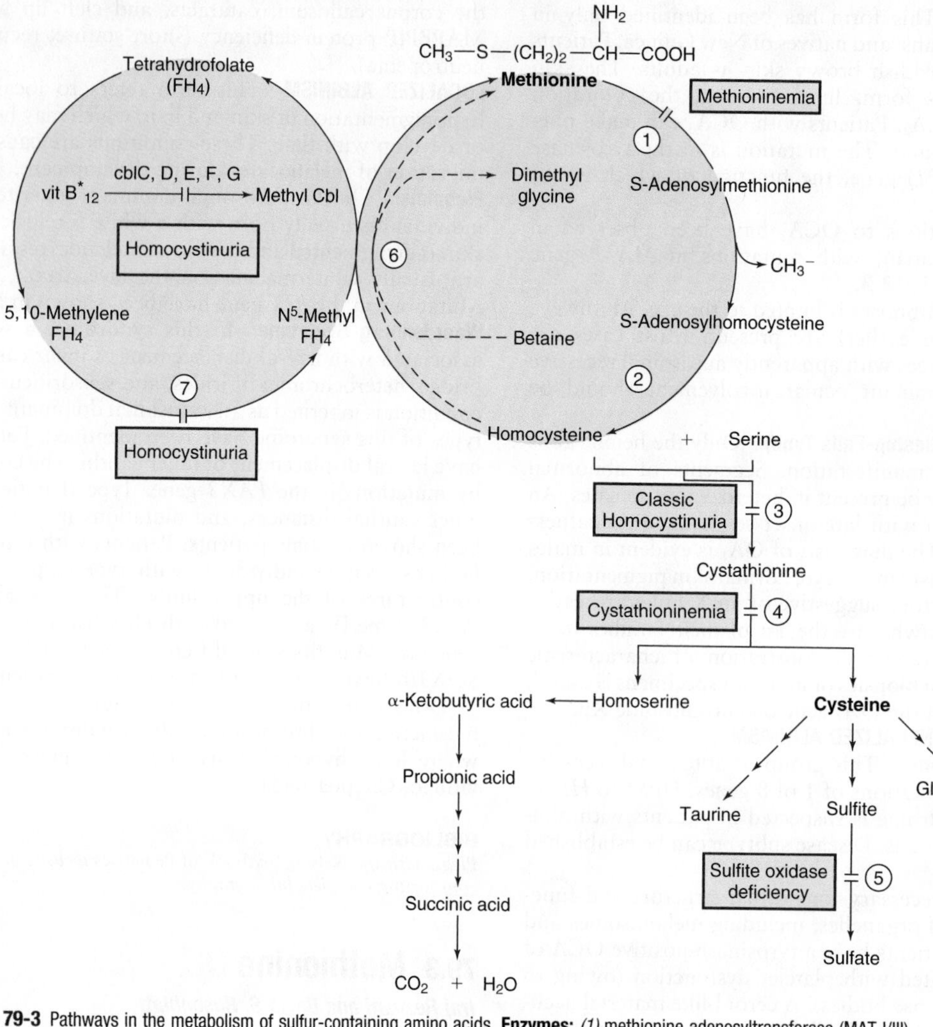

Figure 79-3 Pathways in the metabolism of sulfur-containing amino acids. **Enzymes:** *(1)* methionine adenosyltransferase (MAT I/III), *(2)* adenosylhomocysteine hydrolase, *(3)* cystathionine synthase, *(4)* cystathionase, *(5)* sulfite oxidase, *(6)* betaine homocysteine methyltransferase, *(7)* methylene tetrahydrofolate reductase.

cataracts, retinal detachment, and optic atrophy may develop later in life. Progressive **mental retardation** is common. Normal intelligence has been reported. In an international survey of >600 patients, IQ scores ranged from 10 to 135. Higher IQ scores are seen in vitamin B_6 responsive patients. **Psychiatric and behavioral disorders** have been observed in >50% of affected patients. Convulsions occur in about 20% of patients. Affected individuals with homocystinuria manifest **skeletal abnormalities** resembling those of Marfan syndrome (Chapter 693); they are usually tall and thin, with elongated limbs and arachnodactyly. Scoliosis, pectus excavatum or carinatum, genu valgum, pes cavus, high arched palate, and crowding of the teeth are commonly seen. These children usually have fair complexions, blue eyes, and a peculiar malar flush. Generalized osteoporosis, especially of the spine, is the main roentgenographic finding. **Thromboembolic episodes** involving both large and small vessels, especially those of the brain, are common and may occur at any age. Optic atrophy, paralysis, cor pulmonale, and severe hypertension (due to renal infarcts) are among the serious consequences of thromboembolism, which is caused by changes in the vascular walls and increased platelet adhesiveness secondary to elevated homocystine levels. The risk of thromboembolism increases after surgical procedures. Spontaneous pneumothorax and acute pancreatitis are rare complications.

Elevations of both methionine and homocystine (or homocysteine) in body fluids are the diagnostic laboratory findings. Freshly voided urine should be tested for homocystine because this compound is unstable and may disappear as the urine is stored. Cystine is low or absent in plasma. The diagnosis may be established by assay of the enzyme in liver biopsy specimens, cultured fibroblasts, or phytohemagglutinin-stimulated lymphocytes or by DNA analysis.

Treatment with high doses of vitamin B_6 (200-1,000 mg/24 hr) causes dramatic improvement in most patients who are responsive to this therapy. The degree of response to vitamin B_6 treatment may be different in different families. Some patients may not respond because of folate depletion; a patient should not be considered unresponsive to vitamin B_6 until folic acid (1-5 mg/24 hr) has been added to the treatment regimen. Restriction of methionine intake in conjunction with cysteine supplementation is recommended for patients who are unresponsive to vitamin B_6. The need for dietary restriction and its extent remains controversial in patients with vitamin B_6 responsive form. In some patients with this form, addition of betaine may obviate the need for any dietary restriction. Betaine (trimethylglycine, 6-9 g/24 hr for adults or 200-250 mg/kg/day for children) lowers homocysteine levels in body fluids by remethylating homocysteine to methionine (see Fig. 79-3); this may result in further elevation of plasma methionine levels. This treatment has produced clinical improvement (preventing vascular events) in patients who are unresponsive to vitamin B_6 therapy. Cerebral edema has occurred in a patient with vitamin B_6 nonresponsive homocystinuria and dietary noncompliance during betaine therapy. Administration of large doses of vitamin C (1 g/day) has improved the endothelial function; long-term clinical efficacy is not known.

More than 100 pregnancies in women with the classic form of homocystinuria have been reported with favorable outcomes for both mothers and infants. The majority of infants were full term and normal. Postpartum thromboembolic events occurred in a few mothers. All but 1 of the 38 affected male patients has had normal offspring.

The screening of newborn infants for classic homocystinuria has been performed worldwide and a prevalence of 1/200,000 to 1/350,000 has been estimated. The condition seems more common in New South Wales, Australia (1/60,000), and Ireland. Early treatment of patients identified by the screening process has produced favorable results. The mean IQ of 16 patients with vitamin B_6 unresponsive form treated in early infancy was 94 ± 4. Dislocation of the lens seemed to be prevented in some patients.

Homocystinuria is inherited as an autosomal recessive trait. The gene for cystathionine β-synthase is located on chromosome 21q22.3. Prenatal diagnosis is feasible by performing an enzyme assay of cultured amniotic cells or chorionic villi or by DNA analysis. Many disease-causing mutations have been identified in different families. The majority of affected patients are compound heterozygotes for 2 different alleles. Heterozygous carriers are usually asymptomatic; thromboembolic events and coronary heart disease are more common in these individuals than in the normal population.

HOMOCYSTINURIA DUE TO DEFECTS IN METHYLCOBALAMIN FORMATION Methylcobalamin is the cofactor for the enzyme methionine synthase, which catalyzes remethylation of homocysteine to methionine. There are at least 5 distinct defects in the intracellular metabolism of cobalamin that may interfere with the formation of methylcobalamin. To better understand the metabolism of cobalamin, see methylmalonic acidemia (Fig. 79-4; Chapter 79.6 and Fig. 79-3). The 5 defects are designated as *cbl*C, *cbl*D (including *cbl*D variant 1), *cbl*E *(methionine synthase reductase)*, *cbl*G *(methionine synthase)*, and *cbl*F. Patients with *cbl*C, *cbl*D (not those with *cbl*D variant 2), and *cbl*F defects have methylmalonic acidemia in addition to homocystinuria because formation of both adenosylcobalamin and methylcobalamin is impaired (Chapter 79.6).

Patients with *cbl*E and *cbl*G defects are unable to form methylcobalamin and develop homocystinuria without methylmalonic acidemia (see Fig. 79-4); fewer than 40 patients are known with each of these diseases.

The clinical manifestations are similar in patients with all of these defects. Vomiting, poor feeding, lethargy, hypotonia, and developmental delay may occur in the 1st few months of life. One patient with the *cbl*G defect was not symptomatic (except for mild developmental delay) until she was 21 yr old, however, when she developed difficulty in walking and numbness of the hands. Laboratory findings include megaloblastic anemia, homocystinuria, and hypomethioninemia. The presence of megaloblastic anemia differentiates these defects from homocystinuria due to methylenetetrahydrofolate reductase deficiency (see later). The presence of hypomethioninemia differentiates both of these conditions from cystathionine β-synthase deficiency (see earlier).

Diagnosis is established by complementation studies performed in cultured fibroblasts. Prenatal diagnosis has been accomplished by studies in amniotic cell cultures. All of these conditions are inherited as autosomal recessive traits. The gene for *cbl*E (*MTRR*) is on chromosome 5p15.3-p15.2 and that for *cbl*G (*MTR*) is on chromosome 1q43; several disease-causing mutations, including a common missense mutation (P1173L) in the *MTR* gene, have been described.

Treatment with vitamin B_{12} in the form of hydroxycobalamin (1-2 mg/24 hr) is used to correct the clinical and biochemical findings. Results vary among both diseases and sibships.

HOMOCYSTINURIA DUE TO DEFICIENCY OF METHYLENETETRAHYDROFOLATE REDUCTASE (MTHFR) This enzyme reduces 5,10-methylenetetrahydrofolate to form 5-methyltetrahydrofolate, which provides the methyl group needed for remethylation of homocysteine to methionine (see Fig. 79-3).

The severity of the enzyme defect and of the clinical manifestations varies considerably in different families. Clinical findings vary from apnea, seizure, microcephaly, coma, and death to developmental delay, ataxia, and motor abnormalities or even psychiatric manifestations. Premature vascular disease or peripheral neuropathy has been reported as the only manifestation of this enzyme deficiency in some patients. Adults with severe enzyme deficiency may even be completely asymptomatic. Exposure to the anesthetic nitrous oxide (which inhibits methionine synthase) in patients with MTHFR deficiency may result in neurologic deterioration and death.

Laboratory findings include moderate homocystinemia and homocystinuria. The methionine concentration is low or low normal. This finding differentiates this condition from classic homocystinuria caused by cystathionine synthase deficiency. Absence of megaloblastic anemia distinguishes this condition from homocystinuria caused by methylcobalamin formation (see earlier). Thromboembolism of vessels has also been observed in these patients. Diagnosis may be confirmed by the enzyme assay in cultured fibroblasts or leukocytes or by finding causal mutation in the *MTHR* gene.

A number of polymorphisms have been described in the *MTHR* gene. Two of these (677C → T and 1298A → C) may affect levels of plasma total homocysteine and have been studied as possible risk factors for a wide variety of medical conditions, ranging from birth defects to vascular disease and even cancer, Alzheimer disease, and death from leukemia. To date, the best data support a role for 677C → T polymorphism as a risk factor for neural tube defects. Although a clinical test for this polymorphism is widely available, its predictive value in any given individual has yet to be determined.

Treatment of severe MTHFR deficiency with a combination of folic acid, vitamin B_6, vitamin B_{12}, methionine supplementation, and betaine has been tried. Of these, early treatment with betaine seems to have the most beneficial effect.

The condition is inherited as an autosomal recessive trait; the gene for the enzyme has been located on chromosome 1p36.3 and many disease-causing mutations have been reported. Prenatal diagnosis can be offered by measuring MTHFR enzyme activity in cultured chorionic villi cells or amniocytes, by linkage analysis in informative families, or by DNA analysis of the mutation.

Hypermethioninemia

Secondary hypermethioninemia occurs in liver disease, tyrosinemia type I, and classic homocystinuria. Hypermethioninemia has also been found in premature and some full-term infants receiving high-protein diets, in whom it may represent delayed maturation of the enzyme methionine adenosyltransferase. Lowering the protein intake usually resolves the abnormality. **Primary hypermethioninemia** caused by the deficiency of hepatic methionine adenosyltransferase (MAT I/III; MAT II, which is present in other tissues, is not affected; see Fig. 79-3) has been reported in approximately 60 patients. The majority of these patients have been diagnosed in the neonatal period through screening for homocystinuria. Affected individuals with residual enzyme activity remain asymptomatic throughout life despite persistent hypermethioninemia. Some complain of unusual odor to their breath (boiled cabbage). A few patients with complete enzyme deficiency have had neurologic abnormalities related to demyelination (mental retardation, dystonia, dyspraxia). Normal pregnancies producing normal offspring have been reported in mothers with methionine adenoslytransferase deficiency. The condition is inherited as an autosomal recessive trait. The gene

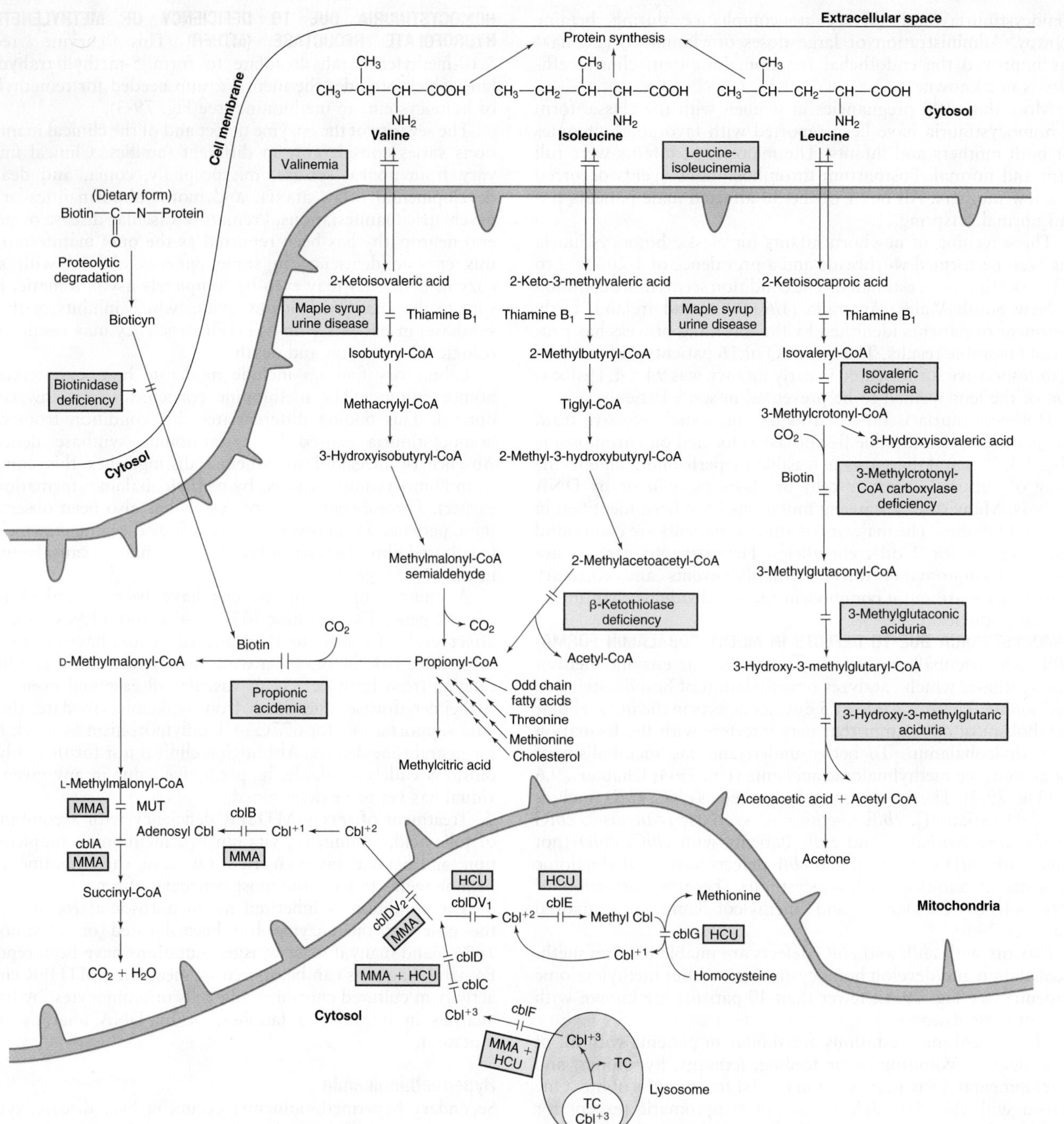

Figure 79-4 Pathways in the metabolism of the branched-chain amino acids, biotin, and vitamin B_{12} (cobalamin). MMA, methylmalonic acidemia; HCU, homocystinuria; Cbl, cobalamin; OHCbl, hydroxycobalamin; cbl, defect in metabolism of cobalamin; cblDV$_1$, cblD variant 1; cblDV$_2$, cblD variant 2; TC, transcobalamin.

for hepatic methionine adenosyltransferase is on chromosome 10q22 and several disease-causing mutations have been identified. A novel defect, glycine N-methyltransferase deficiency, also causes isolated hypermethioninemia.

Cystathioninemia (Cystathioninuria)

Secondary cystathioninuria occurs in patients with vitamin B_6 or B_{12} deficiency, liver disease (particularly damage caused by galactosemia), thyrotoxicosis, hepatoblastoma, neuroblastoma, ganglioblastoma, or defects in remethylation of homocysteine.

Cystathionase deficiency results in massive cystathioninuria and mild to moderate cystathioninemia; cystathionine is not normally detectable in blood. Deficiency of this enzyme is inherited as an autosomal recessive trait and its prevalence is estimated to be about 1/14,000 live births. Affected subjects with a wide variety of clinical manifestations have been reported. Lack of a consistent clinical picture and the presence of cystathioninuria in a number of normal persons suggest that cystathionase deficiency may be of no clinical significance. A majority of reported cases are responsive to oral administration of large doses of vitamin B_6

(≥100 mg/24 hr). When cystathioninuria is discovered in a patient, vitamin B_6 treatment seems indicated, but its beneficial effect has not been established. The gene encoding for cystathionase is located on chromosome 16.

BIBLIOGRAPHY
Please visit the Nelson Textbook of Pediatrics *website at www.expertconsult.com for the complete bibliography.*

79.4 Cysteine/Cystine

Iraj Rezvani

Cysteine is a sulfur-containing nonessential amino acid that is synthesized from methionine (see Fig. 79-3). In the presence of oxygen, 2 molecules of cysteine are oxidized to form cystine. The most common disorders of cysteine/cystine metabolism, cystinuria (Chapter 541) and cystinosis (Chapter 523.3).

SULFITE OXIDASE DEFICIENCY (MOLYBDENUM COFACTOR DEFICIENCY)

At the last step in cysteine metabolism, sulfite is oxidized to sulfate by sulfite oxidase, and the sulfate is excreted in the urine (see Fig. 79-3). This enzyme requires a molybdenum-pterin complex named molybdenum cofactor. This cofactor is also necessary for the function of 2 other enzymes in humans: xanthine dehydrogenase (which oxidizes xanthine and hypoxanthine to uric acid) and aldehyde oxidase. Three enzymes, encoded by 3 different genes, are involved in the synthesis of the cofactor. The genes are mapped to chromosomes 14q24, 6p21.3, and 5q11. Deficiency of any of the 3 enzymes causes cofactor deficiency with identical phenotype. Most patients who were originally diagnosed as having sulfite oxidase deficiency have been proven to have molybdenum cofactor deficiency. Both conditions are inherited as autosomal recessive traits. The gene for sulfite oxidase is on chromosome 12.

The enzyme and the cofactor deficiencies produce identical clinical manifestations. Refusal to feed, vomiting, severe intractable seizures (tonic, clonic, myoclonic), and severe developmental delay may develop within a few weeks after birth. Bilateral dislocation of ocular lenses is a common finding in patients who survive the neonatal period.

These children excrete large amounts of sulfite, thiosulfate, S-sulfocysteine, xanthine, and hypoxanthine in their urine. Urinary and serum levels of uric acid and urinary concentration of sulfate are diminished. Fresh urine should be used for screening purposes and for quantitative measurements of sulfite, because oxidation at room temperature may produce false-negative results.

Diagnosis is confirmed by measurement of sulfite oxidase and molybdenum cofactor in fibroblasts and liver biopsies, respectively. Prenatal diagnosis is possible by performing an assay of sulfite oxidase activity in cultured amniotic cells or in samples of chorionic villi.

No effective treatment is available, and most children die in the 1st 2 yr of life. The prevalence of these deficiencies in the general population is not known.

BIBLIOGRAPHY
Please visit the Nelson Textbook of Pediatrics *website at www.expertconsult.com for the complete bibliography.*

79.5 Tryptophan

Iraj Rezvani

Tryptophan is an essential amino acid and a precursor for nicotinic acid (niacin) and serotonin (Fig. 79-5). The genetic disorders of metabolism of serotonin, 1 of the major neurotransmitters, are discussed in Chapter 79.11.

Hartnup Disorder

In this autosomal recessive disorder, named after the 1st affected family to be reported, there is a defect in the transport of monoamino-monocarboxylic amino acids (neutral amino acids), including tryptophan, by the intestinal mucosa and renal tubules. Decreased intestinal absorption of tryptophan in conjunction with its increased renal loss is believed to cause reduced availability of tryptophan for niacin synthesis. Most children with Hartnup defect remain asymptomatic. The major clinical manifestation in the rare symptomatic patient is cutaneous photosensitivity. The skin becomes rough and red after moderate exposure to the sun, and with greater exposure, a pellagra-like rash may develop. The rash may be pruritic, and a chronic eczema may appear. The skin changes have been reported in affected infants as young as 10 days of age. Some patients may have intermittent ataxia manifested as an unsteady, wide-based gait. The ataxia may last a few days and usually recovers spontaneously. Mental development is usually normal. Two individuals in the original kindred were mentally retarded. Episodic psychologic changes, such as irritability, emotional instability, depression, and suicidal tendencies, have been observed; these changes are usually associated with bouts of ataxia. Short stature and atrophic glossitis are seen in some patients.

Most children diagnosed with Hartnup disorder by neonatal screening have remained asymptomatic. This indicates that other factors are also involved in pathogenesis of the clinical condition.

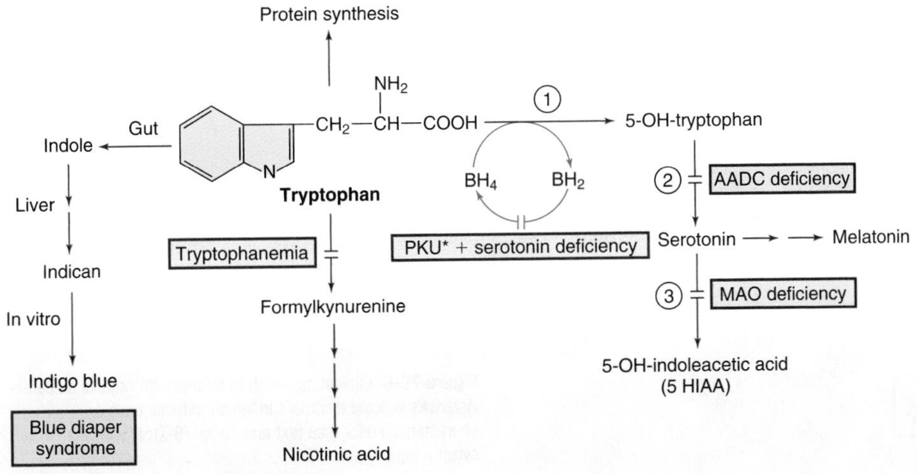

Figure 79-5 Pathways in the metabolism of tryptophan. PKU* indicates hyperphenylalanemia due to tetrahydrobiopterin deficiency (see Fig. 79-1). **Enzymes:** *(1)* tryptophan hydroxylase, *(2)* aromatic L-amino acid decarboxylase (AADC), *(3)* monoamine oxidase (MAO).

The main laboratory finding is aminoaciduria, which is restricted to neutral amino acids (alanine, serine, threonine, valine, leucine, isoleucine, phenylalanine, tyrosine, tryptophan, histidine). Urinary excretion of proline, hydroxyproline, and arginine remains normal. This finding differentiates Hartnup disorder from other causes of generalized aminoaciduria, such as Fanconi syndrome. Plasma concentrations of neutral amino acids are usually normal. This seemingly unexpected finding is because these amino acids are absorbed as dipeptides and the transport system for small peptides is intact in Hartnup disorder. The indole derivatives (especially indican) may be found in large amounts in some patients, owing to bacterial breakdown of unabsorbed tryptophan in the intestines.

Diagnosis is established by the striking intermittent nature of symptoms and the just described urinary findings.

Treatment with nicotinic acid or nicotinamide (50-300 mg/24 hr) and a high-protein diet results in a favorable response in symptomatic patients. Because of the intermittent nature of the clinical manifestations, the efficacy of these treatments is difficult to evaluate. The prevalence of the disorder is estimated to be 1/20,000 to 1/30,000. Normal outcome both for mother and fetus is reported in affected pregnant women. The gene (*SLC6A19*) for this condition is on chromosome 5p15.33.

BIBLIOGRAPHY

Please visit the Nelson Textbook of Pediatrics *website at* *www.expertconsult.com* *for the complete bibliography.*

79.6 Valine, Leucine, Isoleucine, and Related Organic Acidemias

Iraj Rezvani and David S. Rosenblatt*

The early steps in the degradation of these 3 essential amino acids, the **branched-chain amino acids**, are similar (see Fig. 79-4). The intermediate metabolites are all organic acids, and deficiency of any of the degradative enzymes, except for the transaminases, causes acidosis; in such instances, the organic acids before the enzymatic block accumulate in body fluids and are excreted in the urine. These disorders commonly cause metabolic acidosis, which usually occurs in the 1st few days of life. Although most of the clinical findings are nonspecific, some manifestations may provide important clues to the nature of the enzyme deficiency. An approach to infants suspected of having an organic acidemia is presented in Figure 79-6. Definitive diagnosis is usually established by identifying and measuring specific organic acids in body fluids (blood, urine), by the enzyme assay, and by identification of the mutant gene.

Organic acidemias are not limited to defects in the catabolic pathways of branched-chain amino acids. Disorders causing accumulation of other organic acids include those derived from lysine (Chapter 79.14), those associated with lactic acid (Chapter 81), and dicarboxylic acidemias associated with defective fatty acid degradation (Chapter 80.1).

Maple Syrup Urine Disease (MSUD)

Decarboxylation of leucine, isoleucine, and valine is accomplished by a complex enzyme system (branched-chain α-ketoacid dehydrogenase) using thiamine pyrophosphate (vitamin B_1) as a coenzyme. This mitochondrial enzyme consists of 4 subunits: $E_{1\alpha}$, $E_{1\beta}$, E_2, and E_3. The E_3 subunit is shared with 2 other dehydrogenases in the body, namely pyruvate dehydrogenase and α-ketoglutarate dehydrogenase. Deficiency of this enzyme system causes MSUD (see Fig. 79-4), named after the sweet odor of maple syrup found in body fluids, especially urine. Based on clinical findings and response to thiamine administration, 5 phenotypes of MSUD have been identified.

CLASSIC MSUD This form has the most severe clinical manifestations. Affected infants who are normal at birth develop poor feeding and vomiting in the 1st wk of life; lethargy and coma may ensue within a few days. Physical examination reveals hypertonicity and muscular rigidity with severe opisthotonos. Periods of hypertonicity may alternate with bouts of flaccidity. Neurologic findings are often mistaken for generalized sepsis and meningitis. Cerebral edema may be present; convulsions occur in most infants, and hypoglycemia is common. In contrast to most hypoglycemic states, correction of the blood glucose concentration does not improve the clinical condition. Routine laboratory findings are usually unremarkable, except for metabolic acidosis. Death usually occurs in untreated patients in the 1st few weeks or months of life.

Diagnosis is often suspected because of the peculiar odor of maple syrup found in urine, sweat, and cerumen (see Fig. 79-6). It is usually confirmed by amino acid analysis showing marked elevations in plasma levels of leucine, isoleucine, valine, and alloisoleucine (a stereoisomer of isoleucine not normally found in blood) and depression of alanine. Leucine levels are usually

*David S. Rosenblatt contributed to the section on methylmalonic acidemia.

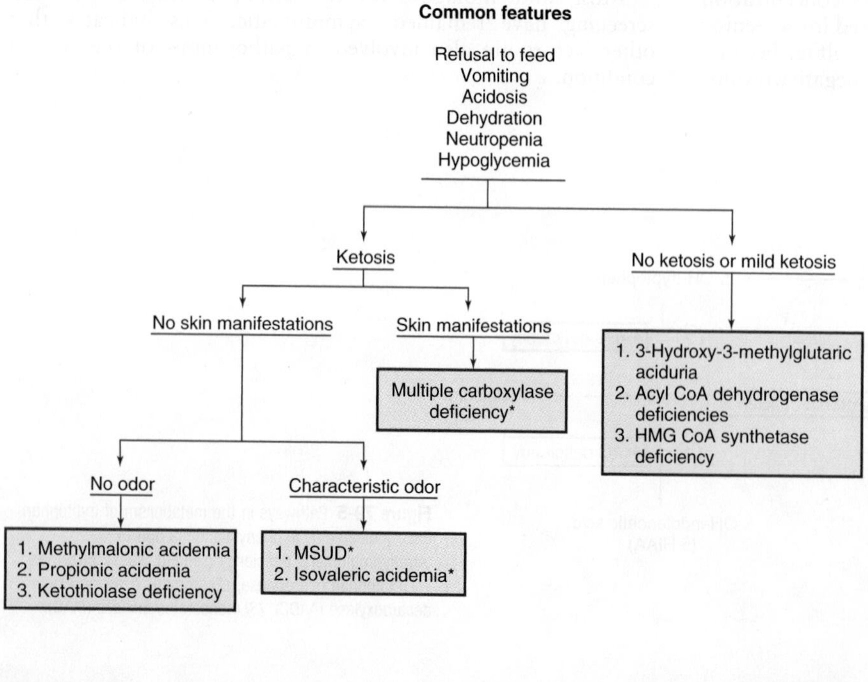

Figure 79-6 Clinical approach to infants with organic acidemia. *Asterisks* indicate disorders in which patients have a characteristic odor (see text and Table 79-2). MSUD, maple syrup urine disease.

higher than those of the other 3 amino acids. Urine contains high levels of leucine, isoleucine, and valine and their respective ketoacids. These ketoacids may be detected qualitatively by adding a few drops of 2,4-dinitrophenylhydrazine reagent (0.1% in 0.1 N HCl) to the urine; a yellow precipitate of 2,4-dinitrophenylhydrazone is formed in a positive test. Neuroimaging during the acute state may show cerebral edema, which is most prominent in the cerebellum, dorsal brainstem, cerebral peduncle, and internal capsule. After recovery from the acute state and with advancing age, hypomyelination and cerebral atrophy may be seen in neuroimaging of the brain. The enzyme activity can be measured in leukocytes and cultured fibroblasts.

Treatment of the acute state is aimed at hydration and rapid removal of the branched-chain amino acids and their metabolites from the tissues and body fluids. Because renal clearance of these compounds is poor, hydration alone may not produce a rapid improvement. Peritoneal dialysis or hemodialysis is the most effective mode of therapy in critically ill infants and should be instituted promptly; significant decreases in plasma levels of leucine, isoleucine, and valine are usually seen within 24 hr of institution of treatment. Providing sufficient calories and nutrients intravenously or orally should reverse the patient's catabolic state. Cerebral edema may need to be treated with mannitol, diuretics (e.g., furosemide), or hypertonic saline.

Treatment after recovery from the acute state requires a diet low in branched-chain amino acids. Synthetic formulas devoid of leucine, isoleucine, and valine are available commercially. Because these amino acids cannot be synthesized endogenously, small amounts of them should be added to the diet; the amount should be titrated carefully by performing frequent analyses of the plasma amino acids. A clinical condition resembling **acrodermatitis enteropathica** occurs in affected infants whose plasma isoleucine concentration becomes very low; addition of isoleucine to the diet causes a rapid and complete recovery. Patients with MSUD should remain on the diet for the rest of their lives. Liver transplantation has been performed in a number of patients with classic MSUD with promising results. These children have been able to tolerate a normal diet.

The long-term prognosis of affected children remains guarded. Severe ketoacidosis, cerebral edema, and death may occur during any stressful situation such as infection or surgery, especially in mid-childhood. Mental and neurologic deficits are common sequelae.

INTERMITTENT MSUD In this form of MSUD, seemingly normal children develop vomiting, odor of maple syrup, ataxia, lethargy, and coma during any stress or catabolic state such as infection or surgery. During these attacks, laboratory findings are indistinguishable from those of the classic form, and death may occur. **Treatment** of the acute attack of intermittent MSUD is similar to that of the classic form. After recovery, although a normal diet is tolerated, a diet low in branched-chain amino acids is recommended. Activity of dehydrogenase in patients with the intermittent form is higher than in the classic form and may reach 5-20% of the normal activity.

MILD (INTERMEDIATE) MSUD In this form, affected children develop milder disease after the neonatal period. Clinical manifestations are insidious and limited to the CNS. Patients have mild to moderate mental retardation (usually after 5 mo of age) with or without seizures. They have the odor of maple syrup and excrete moderate amounts of the branched-chain amino acids and their ketoacid derivatives in the urine. Plasma concentrations of leucine, isoleucine, and valine are moderately increased whereas those of lactate and pyruvate are normal. These children are commonly diagnosed during an intercurrent illness when signs and symptoms of classic MSUD may occur. The dehydrogenase activity is 3-30% of normal. Because patients with thiamine-responsive MSUD usually have manifestations similar to those seen in the mild form, a trial of thiamine therapy is recommended. Diet therapy, similar to that of classic MSUD, is needed.

THIAMINE-RESPONSIVE MSUD Some children with mild or intermediate forms of MSUD who are treated with high doses of thiamine have dramatic clinical and biochemical improvement. Although some respond to treatment with thiamine at 10 mg/24 hr, others may require as much as 200 mg/24 hr for at least 3 wk before a favorable response is observed. These patients also require diets deficient in branched-chain amino acids. The enzymatic activity in these patients is 2-40% of normal.

MSUD DUE TO A DEFICIENCY OF E_3 SUBUNIT (DIHYDROLIPOYL DEHYDROGENASE) This is a very rare disorder. Patients develop lactic acidosis in addition to signs and symptoms similar to those of intermediate MSUD because the E_3 subunit is also a component of pyruvate dehydrogenase and α-ketoglutarate dehydrogenase. Progressive neurologic impairment manifested by hypotonia and developmental delay occurs after 2 mo of age. Abnormal movements progress to ataxia. Death may occur in early childhood.

Laboratory findings include persistent lactic acidosis with high levels of plasma lactate, pyruvate, and alanine. Plasma concentrations of branched-chain amino acids are moderately increased. Patients excrete large amounts of lactate, pyruvate, α-glutarate, and the 3 branched-chain ketoacids in their urine.

No effective treatment is available. Dietary restriction of branched-chain amino acids and treatment with high doses of thiamine, biotin, and lipoic acid have been ineffective.

GENETICS AND PREVALENCE OF MSUD All forms of MSUD are inherited as an autosomal recessive trait. The gene for each subunit resides on different chromosomes. The gene for $E_{1\alpha}$ is on chromosome 19q13.1-q13.2; that for $E_{1\beta}$ is on chromosome q14; the gene for E_2 is on chromosome 1p31; and that for E_3 is on chromosome 7q31-q32. Many different disease-causing mutations have been identified in patients with different forms of MSUD. A given phenotype is caused by a variety of genotypes; patients from different pedigrees with the classic form of MSUD have been shown to have mutations in genes for $E_{1\alpha}$, $E_{1\beta}$, or E_2. Most patients are compound heterozygotes inheriting 2 different mutant alleles. Mutations in genes for $E_{1\beta}$ (38%) and $E_{1\alpha}$ (33%) account for about 70% of cases.

The prevalence is estimated at 1/185,000. The classic form of MSUD is more prevalent in the Old Order Mennonites in the USA, with estimated prevalence of 1/358. Affected patients in this population are homozygous for a specific mutation (Y393N) in the $E_{1\alpha}$ subunit gene.

Early detection of MSUD is feasible by mass screening of newborn infants. Prenatal diagnosis has been accomplished by enzyme assay of the cultured amniocytes, cultured chorionic villi tissue, or direct assay of the chorionic villi samples and by identification of the mutant gene.

Several successful pregnancies have occurred in women with different forms of MSUD. No ill effects have been observed in the offspring of these patients. Episodes of metabolic decompensations have occurred in the mothers during pregnancy and the postpartum period.

Isovaleric Acidemia

This rare condition is due to the deficiency of isovaleryl coenzyme A (CoA) dehydrogenase (see Fig. 79-5).

Clinical manifestations in the *acute form* include vomiting and severe acidosis in the 1st few days of life. Lethargy, convulsions, and coma may ensue, and death may occur if proper therapy is not initiated. The vomiting may be severe enough to suggest pyloric stenosis. The characteristic odor of "sweaty feet" may be present (see Fig. 79-6). Infants who survive this acute episode will go on to have the chronic intermittent form later on in life. A milder form of the disease *(chronic intermittent form)* also exists; in this, the 1st clinical manifestation (vomiting, lethargy, acidosis or coma) may not appear until the child is a few months or a few years old. In both forms, acute episodes of metabolic decompensations may occur during a catabolic state such as an infection. Sensitive methods for newborn screening have identified yet a milder and potentially asymptomatic phenotype of the condition; a few older siblings of these affected newborns were found to have identical genotype and biochemical abnormalities without any clinical manifestations.

Laboratory findings during the acute attacks include ketoacidosis, neutropenia, thrombocytopenia, and occasionally pancytopenia. Hypocalcemia, hyperglycemia, and moderate to severe hyperammonemia may be present in some patients. Increases in plasma ammonia may suggest a defect in the urea cycle. In urea cycle defects the infant is not acidotic (see Fig. 79-6).

Diagnosis is established by demonstrating marked elevations of isovaleric acid and its metabolites (isovalerylglycine, 3-hydroxyisovaleric acid) in body fluids, especially urine. The main compound in plasma is isovalerylcarnitine, which can be measured even in a few drops of dried blood on a filter paper. Measuring the enzyme in cultured skin fibroblasts confirms the diagnosis.

Treatment of the acute attack is aimed at hydration, reversal of the catabolic state (by providing adequate calories orally or intravenously), correction of metabolic acidosis (by infusing sodium bicarbonate), and removal of the excess isovaleric acid. Because isovalerylglycine has a high urinary clearance, administration of glycine (250 mg/kg/24 hr) is recommended to enhance formation of isovalerylglycine. L-carnitine (100 mg/kg/24 hr orally) also increases removal of isovaleric acid by forming isovalerylcarnitine, which is excreted in the urine. In patients with significant hyperammonemia (blood ammonia >200 µM), measures that reduce blood ammonia should be employed (Chapter 79.12). Exchange transfusion and peritoneal dialysis may be needed if the just described measures fail to induce significant clinical and biochemical improvement. After recovery from the acute attack, the patient should receive a low-protein diet (1.0-1.5 g/kg/24 hr) and should be given glycine and carnitine supplements. Pancreatitis (acute or recurrent forms) has been reported in survivors. Normal development can be achieved with early and proper treatment.

Prenatal diagnosis may be accomplished by measuring isovalerylglycine in amniotic fluid, by enzyme assay in cultured amniocytes, or by identification of the mutant gene. Successful pregnancy with favorable outcomes both for the mother and the infant has been reported. Mass screening of newborn infants is in use in the USA and other countries. Isovaleric acidemia is inherited as an autosomal recessive trait. The gene has been mapped to chromosome 15q14q15 and many disease-causing mutations have been identified. The prevalence of the condition is estimated from 1/62,500 (in parts of Germany) to 1/250,000 (in the USA).

Multiple Carboxylase Deficiencies (Defects in Utilization of Biotin)

Biotin is a water-soluble vitamin that is a cofactor for all 4 carboxylase enzymes in humans: pyruvate carboxylase, acetyl CoA carboxylase, propionyl CoA carboxylase, and 3-methylcrotonyl CoA carboxylase. The latter 2 are involved in the metabolic pathways of leucine, isoleucine, and valine (see Fig. 79-4).

Dietary biotin is bound to proteins; free biotin is generated in the intestine by the action of digestive enzymes, by intestinal bacteria, and perhaps by biotinidase. The latter enzyme, which is found in serum and most tissues in the body, is also essential for the recycling of biotin in the body by releasing it from the apoenzymes (carboxylases, see Fig. 79-4). Free biotin must form a covalent peptide bond with the apoprotein of the 4 carboxylases to activate them (holocarboxylase). This binding is catalyzed by holocarboxylase synthetase. Deficiencies in this enzyme or in biotinidase result in malfunction of all the carboxylases and in organic acidemia.

HOLOCARBOXYLASE SYNTHETASE DEFICIENCY (MULTIPLE CARBOXYLASE DEFICIENCY—INFANTILE OR EARLY FORM) Infants with this rare autosomal recessive disorder become symptomatic in the 1st few weeks of life. Symptoms may appear as early as a few hours after birth to 21 mo of age. Clinically, the affected infants who seem normal at birth develop breathing difficulties (tachypnea and apnea) shortly after birth. Feeding problems, vomiting, and hypotonia are also commonly present. If the condition remains untreated, generalized erythematous rash with exfoliation and alopecia (partial or total), failure to thrive, irritability, seizures, lethargy, and even coma may occur. Developmental delay is common. Immune deficiency manifests with susceptibility to infection. The urine may have a peculiar odor, which has been described as similar to tomcat urine. The rash, when present, differentiates this condition from other organic acidemias (see Fig. 79-6).

Laboratory findings include metabolic acidosis, ketosis, hyperammonemia, and the presence of a variety of organic acids, which include lactic acid, propionic acid, 3-methylcrotonic acid, 3-methylcrotonylglycine, tiglylglycine, methylcitrate, and 3-hydroxyisovaleric acid in body fluids. Diagnosis is confirmed by the enzyme assay in lymphocytes or cultured fibroblasts. The mutant enzyme usually has an increased K_m value for biotin; the enzyme activity may be restored by the administration of large doses of biotin.

Treatment with biotin (10 mg/day orally) usually results in an improvement in clinical manifestations and may normalize the biochemical abnormalities. Early diagnosis and treatment are critical to prevent irreversible neurologic damage. In some patients, however, complete resolution may not be achieved even with large doses (up to 80 mg/day) of biotin.

The gene for holocarboxylase synthetase is located on chromosome 21q22.1 and many disease-causing mutations have been identified in different families. Prenatal diagnosis has been accomplished by assaying enzyme activity in cultured amniotic cells and by measurement of intermediate metabolites (3-hydroxyisovalerate and methylcitrate) in amniotic fluid. Pregnant mothers who had previous offspring with holocarboxylase synthetase deficiency have been treated with biotin late in pregnancy. Affected infants were normal at birth, but the efficacy of the treatment as related to the outcome remains unclear.

BIOTINIDASE DEFICIENCY (MULTIPLE CARBOXYLASE DEFICIENCY—JUVENILE OR LATE FORM) The absence of biotinidase results in biotin deficiency. Infants with this deficiency may develop clinical manifestations similar to those seen in infants with holocarboxylase synthetase deficiency, but, unlike the latter, symptoms may appear later, when the child is several months or several years old; symptoms may develop as early as 1 wk of age. Therefore, the term "late form" does not apply to all cases and can be misleading. The delay is presumably because of the presence of sufficient free biotin derived from the mother or the diet. Atopic or seborrheic dermatitis, alopecia, ataxia, myoclonic seizures, hypotonia, developmental delay, sensorineural hearing loss, and immunodeficiency (from T-cell abnormalities) may occur. A small number of children with intractable seborrheic dermatitis and partial (15-30% activity) deficiency of the enzyme, in whom the dermatitis resolved with biotin therapy, has been reported; these children were otherwise asymptomatic. Asymptomatic children and adults with this enzyme deficiency have been identified in screening programs. Most of these individuals have shown to have partial deficiency of the enzyme activity.

Laboratory findings and the pattern of organic acids in body fluids resemble those associated with holocarboxylase synthetase deficiency (see earlier). Diagnosis can be established by measurement of the enzyme activity in the serum. A simplified method for mass screening of newborn infants is now available and is in use in the USA and around the world.

Treatment with free biotin (5-20 mg/24 hr) results in a dramatic clinical and biochemical response. Treatment with biotin is also suggested for individuals with partial biotinidase deficiency.

The prevalence of this autosomal recessive trait is estimated at 1/60,000. The gene for biotinidase is located on chromosome 3p25 and many disease-causing mutations have been identified in different families. Prenatal diagnosis is possible by the measurement of the enzyme activity in the amniotic cells or by identification of the mutant gene.

MULTIPLE CARBOXYLASE DEFICIENCY DUE TO DIETARY BIOTIN DEFICIENCY Acquired deficiency of biotin may occur in infants receiving total parenteral nutrition without added biotin, in patients receiving prolonged anticonvulsant drugs (phenytoin, primidone, carbamazepine) or in children with short bowel syndrome or chronic diarrhea who are receiving formulas low in biotin. Excessive ingestion of raw eggs may also cause biotin deficiency because the protein avidin in egg white binds biotin and makes it unavailable for absorption. Infants with biotin deficiency develop dermatitis, alopecia, and candidal skin infections.

Isolated 3-Methylcrotonyl CoA Carboxylase Deficiency

This enzyme is 1 of 4 carboxylase enzymes in the body that require biotin as a cofactor (see Fig. 79-4). An isolated deficiency of this enzyme must be differentiated from disorders of biotin metabolism (multiple carboxylase deficiency), which cause diminished activity of all 4 carboxylases. 3-Methylcrotonyl CoA carboxylase is a heteromeric enzyme consisting of α (biotin containing) and β subunits.

Clinical manifestations are highly variable, ranging from fatal neonatal onset with acidosis, severe hypotonia, and seizures to completely asymptomatic individuals. In the severe form of the condition, the affected infant who has been seemingly normal develops an acute episode of vomiting, hypotonia, lethargy, and convulsions after a minor infection. Death may occur during the acute episode.

Laboratory findings during acute episodes include mild to moderate acidosis, ketosis, severe hypoglycemia, hyperammonemia, and elevated serum levels of liver transaminases. Large amounts of 3-hydroxyisovaleric acid and 3-methylcrotonylglycine are found in the urine. Urinary excretion of 3-methylcrotonic acid is not usually increased in this condition because the accumulated 3-methylcrotonyl CoA is converted to 3-hydroxyisovaleric acid. Severe secondary carnitine deficiency is common. The condition should be differentiated biochemically from multiple carboxylase deficiency (see above) in which lactic acid and metabolites of propionic acid are present in body fluids in addition to 3-hydroxyisovaleric acid. Diagnosis may be confirmed by measurement of the enzyme activity in cultured fibroblasts. Documentation of normal activities of other carboxylases is necessary for definitive diagnosis.

Aggressive **treatment** of acute episodes with hydration, intravenous infusion of glucose, and alkali is recommended. These patients are unresponsive to biotin therapy. Patients who in earlier reports were found to be biotin responsive were most probably suffering from multiple carboxylase deficiency due to biotinidase deficiency (see above). Long-term treatment includes a diet restricted in leucine in conjunction with the oral administration of L-carnitine (75-100 mg/kg/24 hr) and the prevention of catabolic states. Normal growth and development are expected in these patients.

The condition is inherited as an autosomal recessive trait. The gene for α subunit (*MCC1*) is located on chromosome 3q25-27 and that for the β subunit (*MCC2*) is mapped to chromosome 5q12-13. Mutation in either of these genes may result in the deficiency of the enzyme activity. Similar phenotype may be caused by different genotype. Several disease-causing mutations in either gene have been identified in different families. Newborn screening programs using tandem mass spectrometry have identified an unexpectedly high number of infants with 3-methylcrotonyl CoA carboxylase deficiency (1 : 50,000). Only a small number (<10%) of the affected infants become symptomatic; none of the symptoms reported so far could be clearly attributed to the enzyme deficiency. These findings have questioned the advisability of including this condition in the routine newborn screening programs because the psychological and financial burdens may outweigh the potential benefits.

3-Methylglutaconic Aciduria

At least 3 inherited conditions are known to be associated with excessive excretion of 3-methylglutaconic acid in the urine. Deficiency of the enzyme 3-methylglutaconyl CoA hydratase (see Fig. 79-4) has been documented in only 1 condition (type I). In the other 2 conditions, the enzyme activity is normal despite a modest 3-methylglutaconic aciduria.

3-METHYLGLUTACONIC ACIDURIA TYPE I (3-METHYLGLUTACONYL COA HYDRATASE DEFICIENCY) (SEE FIG. 79-4) This very rare autosomal recessive condition may manifest by speech retardation, choreoathetoid movements, optic atrophy, mild psychomotor delay, and the development of metabolic acidosis during a catabolic state. Asymptomatic affected children and adults have also been reported. Patients excrete large amounts of 3-methylglutaconic acid and moderate amounts of 3-hydroxyisovaleric and 3-methylglutaric acids. Deficiency of 3-methylglutaconyl CoA hydratase has been shown in cultured fibroblasts and lymphoblasts. **Treatment** with a low-protein diet has been suggested. Beneficial effects of this therapy on the clinical course of the disease remain doubtful. Administration of L-carnitine has resulted in clinical improvement in 1 patient. The gene for the enzyme (*AUH*) is mapped to chromosome 9.

3-METHYLGLUTACONIC ACIDURIA TYPE II (X-LINKED CARDIOMYOPATHY, NEUTROPENIA, GROWTH RETARDATION, AND 3-METHYLGLUTACONIC ACIDURIA WITH NORMAL 3-METHYLGLUTACONYL COA HYDRATASE, BARTH SYNDROME) Clinical manifestations of this condition, which usually occur shortly after birth in a male infant, include dilated cardiomyopathy (manifested as respiratory distress and heart failure), hypotonia, growth retardation, and moderate to severe neutropenia. Mild lactic aciduria and/or hypoglycemia have been reported in some patients. If patients survive infancy, relative improvement may occur with advancing age. Cognitive development is usually normal despite delayed motor function.

Laboratory findings include mild to moderate increases in urinary excretion of 3-methylglutaconic, 3-methylglutaric, and 2-ethylhydracrylic acids. Neutropenia is a common finding. Lactic acidosis, hypoglycemia, and abnormal mitochondrial ultrastructure have been shown in some patients. Unlike 3-methylglutaconic aciduria type I, urinary excretion of 3- hydroxyisovaleric acid is not elevated. Total cardiolipin and subclasses of cardiolipin are very low in skin fibroblast cultures from these patients. This finding may be useful for establishing the diagnosis.

The condition is inherited as an X-linked recessive trait. The gene has been mapped to chromosome Xq28 and several disease-causing mutations have been identified. The activity of the enzyme 3-methylglutaconyl CoA hydratase is normal. The reason for the increased excretion of the herein described organic acids is not yet understood. No effective treatment is available.

3-METHYLGLUTACONIC ACIDURIA TYPE III (COSTEFF OPTIC ATROPHY SYNDROME) Clinical manifestations in these patients include early onset optic atrophy and later development of choreoathetoid movements, spasticity, ataxia, dysarthria, and mild developmental delay. All reported patients except 1 were Iraqi Jews living in Israel. These patients excrete moderate amounts of 3-methylglutaconic and 3-methylglutaric acids. As in 3-methylglutaconic aciduria type II, the reason for the increased excretion of these organic acids has not been elucidated. Activity of the enzyme 3-methylglutaconyl CoA hydratase has been normal. The condition is inherited as an autosomal recessive trait. The gene for this condition (*OPA3*) is mapped to chromosome 19q13.2-q13.3. No effective treatment is available.

β-Ketothiolase (3-Oxothiolase) Deficiency (Mitochondrial Acetoacetyl CoA Thiolase [T_2] Deficiency)

This reversible mitochondrial enzyme cleaves 2-methylacetoacetyl CoA (see Fig. 79-4) or acetoacetyl CoA in 1 direction and synthesizes these compounds in a reverse action (Fig. 79-7).

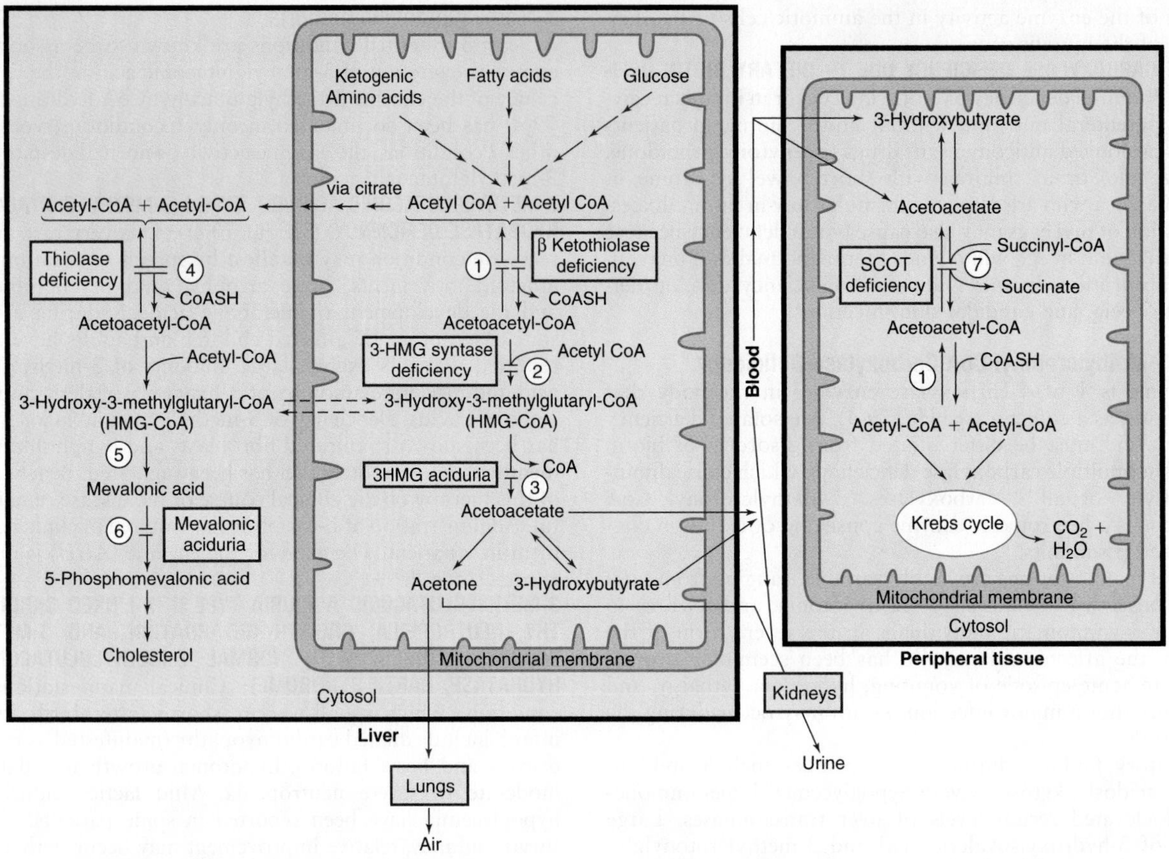

Figure 79-7 Formation (liver) and metabolism (peripheral tissues) of ketone bodies and cholesterol synthesis. **Enzymes:** *(1)* mitochondrial acetoacetyl CoA thiolase, *(2)* HMG-CoA synthase, *(3)* HMG-CoA lyase, *(4)* cytosolic acetoacetyl CoA thiolase, *(5)* HMG-CoA reductase, *(6)* mevalonic kinase, *(7)* succinyl CoA:3-ketoacid CoA transferase (SCOT).

Clinical manifestations are quite variable, ranging from an asymptomatic course in an adult to severe episodes of acidosis starting in the 1st yr of life. These children have intermittent episodes of unexplained ketosis and acidosis. These episodes usually occur after an intercurrent infection and respond quickly to intravenous fluids and bicarbonate therapy. Mild to moderate hyperammonemia may also be present during attacks. Both hypoglycemia and hyperglycemia have been reported in isolated cases. The child may be completely asymptomatic between episodes and may tolerate a normal protein diet well. Mental development is normal in most children. The episodes may be misdiagnosed as salicylate poisoning because of the similarity of clinical findings and the interference of elevated blood levels of acetoacetate with the colorimetric assay for salicylate.

Laboratory findings during the acute attack include acidosis, ketosis, and hyperammonemia. The urine contains large amounts of 2-methylacetoacetate and its decarboxylation product butanone, 2-methyl-3-hydroxybutyrate, and tiglylglycine. Lower concentrations of these urinary metabolites persist during the seemingly well periods. Mild hyperglycinemia may also be present. The clinical and biochemical findings should be differentiated from those seen with propionic and methylmalonic acidemias (see later). Diagnosis may be established by assay of the enzyme in leukocytes, cultured fibroblasts, or identification of the mutant gene.

Treatment of acute episodes includes hydration and infusion of bicarbonate to correct the acidosis; a 10% glucose solution with the appropriate electrolytes and intravenous lipids may be used to minimize the catabolic state. Restriction of protein intake (1-2 g/kg/24 hr) is recommended for long-term therapy. Oral L-carnitine (50-100 mg/kg/24 hr) is also recommended to prevent possible secondary carnitine deficiency. Long-term prognosis for achieving normal life seems very favorable. Three patients graduated from high school and 1 has attended college. All patients continued to have abnormal metabolites in body fluids. Successful pregnancy with normal outcomes for both mother and infant has been reported.

The pathogenesis of ketosis in this condition is not adequately explained because, in this enzyme deficiency, one expects impaired ketone formation (see Fig. 79-7). It is postulated that excess acetoacetyl CoA produced from other sources is used as a substrate for 3-hydroxy-3-methylglutaryl (HMG) CoA synthesis in the liver.

This condition is inherited as an autosomal recessive trait and may be more prevalent than has been appreciated. It is most prevalent in Tunisia. The gene (*ACAT1*) for this enzyme (T_2) is located on chromosome 11q22.3-q23.1.

Cytosolic Acetoacetyl CoA Thiolase ($ACAT_2$) Deficiency

This enzyme catalyzes the cytosolic production of acetoacetyl CoA from 2 moles of acetyl CoA (see Fig. 79-7). Cytosolic acetoacetyl CoA is the precursor of hepatic cholesterol synthesis. Cytosolic acetoacetyl CoA thiolase is a completely different enzyme from that of mitochondrial thiolase (see earlier and Fig. 79-4). Clinical manifestations in patients with this rare enzyme deficiency are similar to those in patients with mevalonic acidemia (see later). Severe progressive developmental delay, hypotonia, and choreoathetoid movements develop in the 1st few months of life. Laboratory findings are nonspecific; elevated levels of lactate, pyruvate, acetoacetate, and 3-hydroxybutyrate may be found in blood and urine. One patient had normal levels of acetoacetate and 3-hydroxybutyrate. Diagnosis can be established by demonstrating a deficiency in cytosolic thiolase activity in liver biopsy or in cultured fibroblasts or by DNA analysis. No effective treatment is available. The gene for this condition is mapped to chromosome 6q25.3-q26.

Mitochondrial 3-Hydroxy-3-Methylglutaryl (HMG) CoA Synthase Deficiency

This enzyme catalyzes synthesis of HMG-CoA from acetoacetyl CoA in the mitochondria. This is a critical step in ketone body synthesis in the liver (see Fig. 79-7). A few patients with deficiency of this enzyme have been reported. All patients have had similar presentations and outcomes. Signs and symptoms of acute hypoglycemia have occurred after an acute illness (gastroenteritis). Age at presentation has ranged from 18 mo to 6 yr. All children were asymptomatic before the episodes and remained normal after the recovery (except for mild hepatomegaly with fatty infiltration). None of the patients has had a 2nd episode, perhaps as a result of preventive measures to avoid prolonged fasting during ensuing intercurrent illnesses. Hepatomegaly was a consistent physical finding in all patients. Laboratory findings included hypoglycemia, acidosis with mild or no ketosis, elevation of liver function tests, and massive dicarboxylic aciduria. The clinical and laboratory findings may be confused with those of patients with defects in fatty acid metabolism (see Chapter 80.1). In contrast to the latter, blood concentrations of acylcarnitine conjugates are normal in patients with HMG-CoA synthase deficiency. Fasting of these patients has produced the abovementioned clinical and biochemical abnormalities.

Treatment consisted of provision of adequate calories and avoidance of prolonged periods of fasting. No dietary protein restriction was needed.

The condition is inherited as an autosomal recessive trait. The gene for this condition is located on chromosome 1p13-p12 and several disease-causing mutations have been identified. The condition should be considered in any child with fasting hypoglycemia and is perhaps more common than appreciated.

3-Hydroxy-3-Methylglutaric Aciduria

This condition is due to a deficiency of HMG-CoA lyase (see Fig. 79-4). This enzyme catalyzes the conversion of HMG-CoA to acetoacetate and is a rate-limiting enzyme for ketogenesis (see Fig. 79-7). Clinically, >60% of patients become symptomatic between 3 and 11 mo of age, whereas about 30% develop symptoms in the 1st few days of life. One child remained asymptomatic until 15 yr of age. Episodes of vomiting, severe hypoglycemia, hypotonia, acidosis with mild or no ketosis, and dehydration may rapidly lead to lethargy, ataxia, and coma. These episodes often occur during a catabolic state such as fasting or an intercurrent infection. Hepatomegaly is common. These manifestations may be mistaken for Reye syndrome or medium-chain acyl CoA dehydrogenase (MCAD) deficiency. Patients are usually clinically asymptomatic between the attacks; 1 patient died of acute cardiomyopathy at age 7 mo during a febrile illness. Development is usually normal, but mental retardation and seizure with abnormalities of white matter (shown by MRI) have been observed in patients with prolonged episodes of hypoglycemia.

Laboratory findings include hypoglycemia, moderate to severe hyperammonemia, and acidosis. There is mild or no ketosis (see Fig. 79-7). Urinary excretion of 3-hydroxy-3-methylglutaric acid and other proximal intermediate metabolites of leucine catabolism (3-methylglutaconic acid and 3-hydroxyisovaleric acid) is markedly increased causing the urine to smell like cat urine. These organic acids are excreted in the urine as carnitine conjugates, resulting in secondary carnitine deficiency. Glutaric and adipic acids may also be increased in urine during acute attacks. Diagnosis may be confirmed by enzyme assay in cultured fibroblasts, leukocytes, or liver specimens or by identification of the mutant gene. Prenatal diagnosis is possible by the assay of the enzyme in cultured amniocytes or a chorionic villi biopsy or by DNA analysis.

Treatment of acute episodes includes hydration, infusion of glucose to control hypoglycemia, provision of adequate calories, and administration of bicarbonate to correct acidosis. Hyperammonemia should be treated promptly (Chapter 79.12). Exchange transfusion and peritoneal dialysis may be required in patients with severe hyperammonemia. Restriction of protein and fat intake is recommended for long-term management. Oral administration of L-carnitine (50-100 mg/kg/24 hr) prevents secondary carnitine deficiency. Prolonged fasting should be avoided. One child died after routine immunization. The condition is inherited as an autosomal recessive trait. The gene for HMG-CoA lyase resides on chromosome 1pter-p33 and several disease-causing mutations have been identified in different families. The gene defect appears to be more common in the Arabic population, especially in Saudi Arabia.

Succinyl CoA:3-Ketoacid CoA Transferase (SCOT) Deficiency

This enzyme is necessary for the metabolism of ketone bodies (acetoacetate and 3-hydroxybutyrate) in peripheral tissue (see Fig. 79-7). A deficiency of this enzyme results in the underutilization and accumulation of ketone bodies and ketoacidosis. Only a few patients with SCOT deficiency have been reported to date; the condition may not be rare because many cases are undiagnosed.

The presentation is an acute episode of unexplained severe ketoacidosis in an infant who had been growing and developing normally. About half of the patients present in the 1st wk of life and all before 2 yr. The acute episode is often precipitated by an intercurrent infection or a catabolic state. Death may occur during these episodes. A chronic subclinical ketosis usually persists between the attacks. Development is usually normal.

Laboratory findings during the acute episode are nonspecific and include metabolic acidosis and ketonuria with high levels of acetoacetate and 3-hydroxybutyrate in blood and urine. No other organic acids are found in the blood or in the urine. Blood glucose levels are usually normal, but hypoglycemia has been reported in 2 newborn infants with severe ketoacidosis. Plasma amino acids are usually normal. Diagnosis can be established by demonstrating a deficiency of enzyme activity in cultured fibroblasts or by DNA analysis.

Treatment of acute episodes consists of hydration, correction of acidosis, and the provision of a diet adequate in calories. Long-term treatment with a high-carbohydrate diet and avoidance of catabolic states is recommended. *This condition should be considered in any infant with unexplained bouts of ketoacidosis.* The condition is inherited as an autosomal recessive trait. The gene for this enzyme is located on chromosome 5p13, and several disease-causing mutations have been found in different families.

Mevalonic Aciduria

Mevalonic acid, an intermediate metabolite of cholesterol synthesis, is converted to 5-phosphomevalonic acid by the action of the enzyme mevalonate kinase (MVK) (see Fig. 79-7). Based on clinical manifestations, 2 forms of this condition have been recognized.

MEVALONIC ACIDURIA, SEVERE FORM Clinical manifestations include mental retardation, failure to thrive, growth retardation, hypotonia, ataxia, hepatosplenomegaly, cataracts, and facial dysmorphism (dolichocephaly, frontal bossing, low-set ears, downward slanting of the eyes, and long eyelashes). Recurrent crises, characterized by fever, vomiting, diarrhea, arthralgia, edema, lymphadenopathy, further enlargement of liver and spleen, and morbilliform rash have been observed in all patients. These episodes last 4-5 days and recur up to 25 times/yr. Death may occur during these crises.

Laboratory findings include marked elevation of mevalonic acid in urine; the concentration may be as high as 56,000 µmole/mole of creatinine (normal <0.3). Plasma levels of mevalonic acid are also greatly increased (as high as 54 µmole/dL; normal <0.004). This is the only abnormal organic acid found in these patients. The level of mevalonic acid tends to correlate with the severity of the condition and increases during crises. Serum cholesterol concentration is normal or mildly decreased. Serum concentration of creatine kinase (CK) is markedly increased. Sedimentation rate and serum leukotriene-4 are increased during the crises. Serial examination of the brain by MRI reveals progressive atrophy of the cerebellum.

Diagnosis may be confirmed by assay of MVK activity in lymphocytes or in cultured fibroblasts. No effective therapy is available. **Treatment** with high doses of prednisone (2 mg/kg/24 hr) causes improvement of the acute crises. The condition is inherited as an autosomal recessive trait. Prenatal diagnosis is possible by measurement of mevalonic acid in the amniotic fluid, by assay of the enzyme activity in cultured amniocytes or chorionic villi samples or by demonstration of the mutant gene. The gene for MVK is on chromosome 12q24.

PERIODIC FEVER WITH HYPERIMMUNOGLOBULINEMIA D (MEVALONIC ACIDURIA, MILD FORM) Some mutations of mevalonic kinase gene (MVK) cause mild deficiencies of the enzyme and produce the clinical picture of periodic fever with hyperimmunogobulinemia D (Chapter 157). These patients have periodic bouts of fever associated with abdominal pain, vomiting, diarrhea, arthralgia, arthritis, hepatosplenomegaly, lymphadenopathy, and morbilliform rash (even petechia and purpura), which usually start before 1 yr of age. The attacks can be produced by vaccination, minor trauma, or stress; usually occur every 1-2 mo and last 2-7 days. Patients are free of symptoms between acute attacks. The diagnostic laboratory finding is elevation of serum immunoglobulin gamma D (IgD); IgA is also elevated in 80% of patients. During acute attacks, leukocytosis, increased C-reactive protein, and mild mevalonic aciduria may be present. High concentration of serum IgD differentiates this condition from familial Mediterranean fever.

Treatment of acute attacks remains symptomatic and includes corticosteroids. Anakinra or etanercept and eventually bone marrow transplantation may be needed in more severely affected children. The condition is inherited as an autosomal recessive trait; most patients are white and are from western European countries (60% are either Dutch or French). The enzyme activity is usually about 5-15% of normal. The pathogenesis of the condition remains unclear. Several disease-causing mutations of the gene (located on chromosome 12q24) have been identified, but 1 mutation (V377I) is present in 50-80% of patients. Long-term prognosis is usually good, but amyloidosis has occurred in a few patients.

Propionic Acidemia (Propionyl CoA Carboxylase Deficiency)

Propionic acid is an intermediate metabolite of isoleucine, valine, threonine, methionine, odd-chain fatty acids, and cholesterol catabolism. It is normally carboxylated to methylmalonic acid by the mitochondrial enzyme propionyl CoA carboxylase, which requires biotin as a cofactor (see Fig. 79-4). The enzyme is composed of 2 nonidentical subunits, α and β. Biotin is bound to the α subunit.

Clinical findings are nonspecific. In the severe form of the condition, patients develop symptoms in the 1st few days or weeks of life. Poor feeding, vomiting, hypotonia, lethargy, dehydration, and clinical signs of severe ketoacidosis progress rapidly to coma and death. Seizures occur in approximately 30% of affected infants. If an infant survives the 1st attack, similar episodes may occur during an intercurrent infection or constipation or after ingestion of a high-protein diet. Moderate to severe mental retardation and neurologic manifestations indicating extrapyramidal (dystonia, choreoathetosis, tremor), and pyramidal (paraplegia) dysfunction are common sequelae in the older survivors. These abnormalities, which usually occur after an episode of metabolic decompensation, have been shown by neuroimaging to be due to the destruction of basal ganglia, especially that of the globus pallidus. This phenomenon has been referred to in the literature as **metabolic stroke**. In the milder forms, the older infant may have mental retardation without acute attacks of ketosis. Some affected children may have episodes of unexplained severe ketoacidosis separated by periods of seemingly normal health. Mass screening of newborn infants has identified milder forms of the condition; a few of theses infants were completely asymptomatic at diagnosis. The severity of clinical manifestations may also be variable within a family; in 1 kindred, a brother was diagnosed at 5 yr of age whereas his 13 yr old sister, with the same level of enzyme deficiency, was asymptomatic.

Laboratory findings during the acute attack include severe metabolic acidosis with a large anion gap, ketosis, neutropenia, thrombocytopenia, and hypoglycemia. Moderate to severe hyperammonemia is common; plasma ammonia concentrations usually correlate with the severity of the disease. Measurement of plasma ammonia is especially helpful in planning therapeutic strategy during episodes of exacerbation in a patient whose diagnosis has been established. Pathogenesis of hyperammonemia is not well understood. Hyperglycinemia is a common finding. Elevations in plasma and urinary levels of glycine have also been observed in patients with methylmalonic acidemia. These disorders were collectively referred to as *ketotic hyperglycinemia* before the specific enzyme deficiencies were elucidated. Concentrations of propionic acid and methylcitric acid (presumably made by the condensation of propionyl CoA with oxaloacetic acid) are markedly elevated in the plasma and urine of infants with propionic acidemia. 3-Hydroxypropionic acid, propionylglycine, and other intermediate metabolites of isoleucine catabolism, such as tiglic acid, tiglylglycine, and 2-methyloacetoacetic acid, are also found in urine. Moderate elevations in blood levels of ammonia, glycine, and previously mentioned organic acids usually persist between the acute attacks. CT scan and MRI of the brain may reveal cerebral atrophy, demyelination, and abnormalities in the globus pallidus and basal ganglia as the evidence of a metabolic stroke in this condition (see earlier).

The diagnosis of propionic acidemia should be differentiated from multiple carboxylase deficiencies (see earlier and Fig. 79-6). Infants with the latter condition may have skin manifestations and excrete large amounts of lactic acid, 3-methylcrotonic acid, and 3-hydroxyisovaleric acid in addition to propionic acid. The presence of hyperammonemia may suggest a genetic defect in the urea cycle enzymes. Infants with defects in the urea cycle are usually not acidotic (see Fig. 79-1). Definitive diagnosis of propionic acidemia can be established by measuring the enzyme activity in leukocytes or cultured fibroblasts.

Treatment of acute attacks includes hydration, correction of acidosis, and amelioration of the catabolic state by provision of adequate calories through parenteral hyperalimentation. Minimal amounts of protein (0.25 g/kg/24 hr), preferably a protein deficient in propionate precursors, should be provided in the hyperalimentation fluid very early in the course of treatment. To curtail the possible production of propionic acid by intestinal bacteria, sterilization of the intestinal tract flora by antibiotics (oral neomycin, or metronidazole) should be promptly initiated. Constipation should also be treated. Patients with propionic acidemia may develop carnitine deficiency, presumably as a result of urinary loss of propionylcarnitine formed from the accumulated organic acid. Administration of L-carnitine (50-100 mg/kg/24 hr orally or 10 mg/kg/24 hr intravenously) normalizes fatty acid oxidation and improves acidosis. In patients with concomitant hyperammonemia, measures to reduce blood ammonia should be employed (Chapter 79.12). Very ill patients with severe acidosis and hyperammonemia require peritoneal dialysis or hemodialysis to remove ammonia and other toxic compounds efficiently. Although infants with true propionic acidemia are rarely responsive to biotin, this compound should be administered (10 mg/24 hr orally) to all infants during the 1st attack and until the diagnosis is established.

Long-term treatment consists of a low-protein diet (1.0-1.5 g/kg/24 hr) and administration of L-carnitine (50-100 mg/kg/24 hr orally). Synthetic proteins deficient in propionate precursors (isoleucine, valine, methionine, and threonine) may be used to increase the amount of dietary protein (to 1.5-2.0 g/kg/24 hr) while causing minimal change in propionate production. Excessive supplementation with these proteins may cause a deficiency of the essential amino acids. To avoid this problem, natural proteins should comprise most of the dietary protein (50-75%). Some patients may require chronic alkaline therapy to correct chronic acidosis. The concentration of ammonia in the blood usually normalizes between attacks, and chronic treatment of hyperammonemia is not usually needed. Catabolic states that may trigger acute attacks (infections, constipation) should be treated promptly and aggressively. Close monitoring of blood pH, amino acids, urinary content of propionate and its metabolites, and growth parameters is necessary to ensure the proper balance of the diet and the success of therapy.

Long-term prognosis is guarded. Death may occur during an acute attack. Normal psychomotor development is possible, especially in the mild forms identified through screening programs; most children identified clinically manifest some degree of permanent neurodevelopmental deficit such as tremor, dystonia, chorea, and pyramidal signs despite adequate therapy. These neurologic findings may be sequelae of a metabolic stroke occurring during an acute decompensation (see earlier).

Prenatal diagnosis is achieved by measuring the enzyme activity in cultured amniotic cells or in samples of uncultured chorionic villi, by measurement of methylcitrate in amniotic fluid, or by identification of the mutant gene.

The condition is inherited as an autosomal recessive trait and can be identified by mass screening of newborns. It is more prevalent in Saudi Arabia (1:2,000 to 1:5,000). The gene for the α subunit (*PCCA* gene) is located on chromosome 13q32 and that of the β subunit (*PCCB* gene) is mapped to the chromosome 3q21-q22. Many mutations in either gene have been identified in different patients. Pregnancy with normal outcome has been reported in affected females.

Methylmalonic Acidemia

Methylmalonic acid, a structural isomer of succinic acid, is normally derived from propionic acid as part of the catabolic pathways of isoleucine, valine, threonine, methionine, cholesterol, and odd-chain fatty acids. Two enzymes are involved in the conversion of D-methylmalonic acid to succinic acid: methylmalonyl CoA racemase, which forms the L-isomer; and methylmalonyl CoA mutase, which converts the L-methylmalonic acid to succinic acid (see Fig. 79-4). The latter enzyme requires adenosylcobalamin, a metabolite of vitamin B_{12}, as a coenzyme. Deficiency of either the mutase or its coenzyme causes the accumulation of methylmalonic acid and its precursors in body fluids. A deficiency of the racemase can be associated with mild elevations of methylmalonic acid, but the clinical consequence of racemase deficiency is not known.

At least 2 forms of mutase apoenzyme deficiencies have been identified. These are designated *mut*^{0}, meaning no detectable enzyme activity, and *mut*$^-$, indicating residual, although abnormal, mutase activity. The majority of reported patients with methylmalonic acidemia have a deficiency of the mutase apoenzyme (*mut*^{0} or *mut*$^-$). These patients are not responsive to vitamin B_{12} therapy. In the remaining patients with methylmalonic acidemia, the defect resides in the formation of adenosylcobalamin.

DEFECTS IN METABOLISM OF VITAMIN B_{12} (COBALAMIN, CBL) Dietary vitamin B_{12} requires intrinsic factor (IF), a glycoprotein secreted by the gastric parietal cells, for absorption in the terminal ileum. It is transported in the blood by haptocorrin (TCI) and transcobalamin II (TC). The complex of transcobalamin II-cobalamin (TC-Cbl) is recognized by a specific receptor on the cell membrane and enters the cell by endocytosis. The TC-Cbl complex is hydrolyzed in the lysosome, and free cobalamin is released into the cytosol (see Fig. 79-4). The cobalt of the molecule is reduced in the cytosol from 3 valences (cob[III]alamin) to 2 (cob[II]alamin) before it enters the mitochondria, where further reduction to cob(I)alamin occurs. The latter compound reacts with adenosine to form adenosylcobalamin (coenzyme for methylmalonyl CoA mutase). The free cobalamin in the cytosol may also undergo a series of poorly understood enzymatic steps to form methylcobalamin (coenzyme for methionine synthase, see Fig. 79-3).

Seven different defects in the intracellular metabolism of cobalamin have been identified. These are designated *cbl*A through *cbl*G (*cbl* stands for a defect in any step of cobalamin metabolism). *cbl*A, *cbl*B, and *cbl*D variant 2 cause methylmalonic acidemia only; *cbl*B is caused by a deficiency of adenosylcobalamin transferase. In patients with *cbl*C, classic *cbl*D, and *cbl*F defects, synthesis of both adenosylcobalamin and methylcobalamin is impaired, causing homocystinuria in addition to methylmalonic acidemia. The *cbl*D variant 1, *cbl*E, and the *cbl*G defects involve only the synthesis of methylcobalamin, resulting in homocystinuria without methylmalonic aciduria but usually with megaloblastic anemia.

Clinical manifestations of patients with methylmalonic acidemia due to *mut*^{0}, *mut*$^-$, *cbl*A, *cbl*B, and *cblD* variant 2 are similar. There are wide variations in clinical presentation, ranging from very sick newborn infants to asymptomatic adults, regardless of the nature of the enzymatic defect or the biochemical abnormalities. In severe forms, lethargy, feeding problems, vomiting, tachypnea (due to acidosis), and hypotonia may develop in the 1st few days of life and may progress to coma and death if untreated. Infants who survive the 1st attack may go on to develop similar acute metabolic episodes during a catabolic state (such as infection) or after ingestion of a high-protein diet. Between the acute attacks, the patient commonly continues to exhibit hypotonia and feeding problems with failure to thrive. In milder forms, patients may present later in life with hypotonia, failure to thrive, and developmental delay. Asymptomatic patients with typical biochemical abnormalities of methylmalonic acidemia are also reported. It is important to note that mental development and IQ of patients with methylmalonic acidemia may remain within the normal range despite repeated acute attacks and regardless of the nature of the enzyme deficiency. In 1 study of patients with different forms of the condition, developmental retardation was noted in only 47%. One adolescent girl with a *mut*$^-$ deficiency had an IQ of 129.

The episodic nature of the condition and its biochemical abnormalities may be confused with those of ethylene glycol (antifreeze) ingestion. The peak of propionate in a blood sample from an infant with methylmalonic acidemia has been mistaken for ethylene glycol when the sample was assayed by gas chromatography without mass spectrometry.

Laboratory findings include ketosis, acidosis, anemia, neutropenia, thrombocytopenia, hyperglycinemia, hyperammonemia, hypoglycemia, and the presence of large quantities of methylmalonic acid in body fluids (see Fig. 79-6). Propionic acid and its metabolites 3-hydroxypropionate and methylcitrate are also found in the urine. Hyperammonemia may suggest the presence of genetic defects in the urea cycle enzymes; patients with defects in urea cycle enzymes are not acidotic (see Fig. 79-12). The reason for hyperammonemia is not well understood.

Diagnosis can be confirmed by measuring propionate incorporation and performing complementation analysis in cultured fibroblasts, by measuring the specific activity of the mutase enzyme in biopsies or cell extracts or by identifying the mutations in the causal gene.

Treatment of acute attacks is similar to that of attacks in patients with propionic acidemia (see earlier), except that large doses (1 mg/24 hr) of vitamin B_{12} are used instead of biotin. Long-term treatment consists of administration of a low-protein diet (1.0-1.5 g/kg/24 hr), L-carnitine (50-100 mg/kg/24 hr orally), and vitamin B_{12} (1 mg/24 hr for patients with defects in vitamin B_{12} metabolism; the dose can be decreased depending on the clinical response). The protein composition of the diet is similar to that prescribed for patients with propionic acidemia. Chronic alkaline therapy is usually required to correct chronic acidosis, especially during infancy and early childhood. Blood levels of ammonia usually normalize between the attacks, and chronic treatment of hyperammonemia is rarely needed. Stressful situations that may trigger acute attacks (such as infection) should be treated promptly.

Inadequate oral intake secondary to poor appetite is a common and bothersome complication in long-term management of these patients. Consequently, enteral feeding (through a nasogastric tube or gastrostomy) should be considered early in the course of the treatment. Close monitoring of blood pH, amino acid levels, blood and urinary concentrations of methylmalonate, and growth parameters is necessary to ensure proper balance in the diet and the success of therapy. Glutathione deficiency, responsive to high doses of ascorbate, has been described. Liver, kidney, and combined liver and kidney transplantations have been attempted in a small number of affected patients. Liver transplantation reduced but did not eliminate the metabolic abnormalities and did not prevent the occurrence of metabolic stroke. Kidney transplantation alone restored the renal function but caused only minor improvement in the methylmalonic acidemia.

Prognosis depends on the severity of symptoms and the occurrence of complications (see later). In general, patients with complete deficiency of mutase apoenzyme (*mut*^{0}) have the least favorable prognosis and those with *mut*$^-$ and *cbl*A defects have a better outcome than those with *cbl*B.

Complications have been noted in survivors. Metabolic strokes (see earlier) have been reported in a few patients during an acute episode of metabolic decompensation. These patients have survived with major extrapyramidal (tremor, dystonia) and pyramidal (paraplegia) sequelae. The pathogenesis of this complication also remains unclear.

Chronic renal failure necessitating renal transplant has been reported in a number of older patients with the condition. This complication has been observed in all genetic forms of the condition. **Tubulointerstitial nephritis** has been documented in some of these patients and is thought to be the major cause of renal failure. The pathogenesis remains unclear.

Acute and recurrent pancreatitis has been reported in the affected patients as young as 13 mo of age. This complication may account for a fair number of hospitalizations of these children.

The prevalence of all forms of methylmalonic aciduria is estimated to be in the range of 1/48,000. All defects causing methylmalonic acidemia are inherited as autosomal recessive traits. Successful mass screening of newborns has been achieved by the tandem mass spectrometry method. The gene for the mutase (*MUT*) is on the short arm of chromosome 6, and over 150 different mutations have been identified including a number of ethnic-specific mutations. Neonates with methylmalonic acidemia and severe diabetes due to the absence of β cells who have paternal uniparental isodisomy of chromosome 6 have been reported. Mutations in the gene for *cbl*A (*MMAA*, on chromosome 4q31-q31.2), *cbl*B (*MMAB*, on chromosome 12q24), and all forms of *cbl*D (*MMADHC*, on chromosome 2q23.2) have been identified in affected patients. The previously described *cbl*H group has been shown to be identical to *cbl*D variant 2.

Successful pregnancy with normal outcomes for both the mother and the baby has been reported.

Combined Methylmalonic Aciduria and Homocystinuria (*cbl*C, *cbl*D, and *cbl*F Defects)

Over 300 patients with methylmalonic acidemia and homocystinuria due to *cbl*C have been reported. Indeed with the advent of expanded newborn screening, *cbl*C may be as common as mutase deficiency. The *cbl*D, and *cbl*F defects are much rarer with less than a dozen patients known with each (see Figs. 79-3 and 79-4). Neurologic findings are prominent in patients with *cbl*C and *cbl*D defects. Most patients with the *cbl*C defect present in the 1st yr of life because of failure to thrive, lethargy, poor feeding, mental retardation, and seizures. However, late-onset defects with sudden development of dementia and myelopathy have been reported, even with presentation is adulthood. Megaloblastic anemia was a common finding in patients with *cbl*C defect. Mild to moderate increases in concentrations of methylmalonic acid and homocysteine were found in body fluids. Unlike patients with classic homocystinuria, plasma levels of methionine are low to normal in these defects. Neither hyperammonemia nor hyperglycinemia is present in these patients. The clinical findings in the *cbl*F defect are quite variable; the 1st 2 patients had poor feeding, growth and developmental delay, and persistent stomatitis manifesting in the 1st 3 wk of life. One patient was not diagnosed until age 10 yr and had findings suggestive of rheumatoid arthritis, a pigmented skin abnormality, and encephalopathy. Vitamin B_{12} malabsorption has been noted in patients with *cbl*F defect.

Experience with **treatment** of patients with *cbl*C, *cbl*D, and *cbl*F defects is limited. Large doses of hydroxycobalamin (OHCbl; 1-2 mg/24 hr) in conjunction with betaine (6-9 g/24 hr) seem to produce biochemical improvement with little clinical effect. Unexplained severe hemolytic anemia, hydrocephalus, and congestive heart failure have been major complications in patients with *cbl*C defect. The *cbl*C disorder is caused by mutations in the *MMACHC* gene on chromosome 1p34.1 and there are a number of common mutations and ones that are more common in specific ethnic groups. The *cbl*D disorder is caused by mutations in the *MMADHC* gene on chromosome 2q23.2. Mutations resulting in the variant 1 (homocystinuria) affect the C-terminal domain of the gene product; those resulting in the variant 2 (methylmalonic aciduria) affect the N terminal. The classical form of *cbl*D with both homocystinuria and methylmalonic aciduria had mutations resulting in decreased protein expression. The *cbl*F disorder has been found to be due to mutations in the *LMBRD1* gene on chromosome 6p13 coding for the lysosomal cobalamin transporter.

Patients with *cbl*D variant 1, *cbl*E and *cbl*G defects do not have methylmalonic acidemia (Chapter 79.3).

BIBLIOGRAPHY

Please visit the Nelson Textbook of Pediatrics *website at* *www.expertconsult.com* *for the complete bibliography.*

79.7 Glycine

Iraj Rezvani

Glycine is a nonessential amino acid synthesized mainly from serine and threonine. Structurally, it is the simplest amino acid. It is involved in many reactions in the body, especially in the nervous system where it functions as a neurotransmitter (excitatory in the cortex, inhibitory in the brainstem and the spinal cord; Chapter 79.11). Its main catabolic pathway requires the complex glycine cleavage enzyme to cleave the first carbon of glycine and convert it to carbon dioxide (Fig. 79-8). The glycine cleavage protein, a mitochondrial multienzyme, is composed of 4 proteins: P protein (glycine decarboxylase), H protein, T protein, and L protein, which are encoded by 4 different genes.

Hypoglycinemia

Defects in the biosynthetic pathway of serine (Chapter 79.8) cause deficiency of glycine in addition to that of serine in body fluids, especially in the CSF. Isolated primary deficiency of glycine has not been reported.

Hyperglycinemia

Elevated levels of glycine in body fluids occur in propionic acidemia and methylmalonic acidemia that are collectively referred

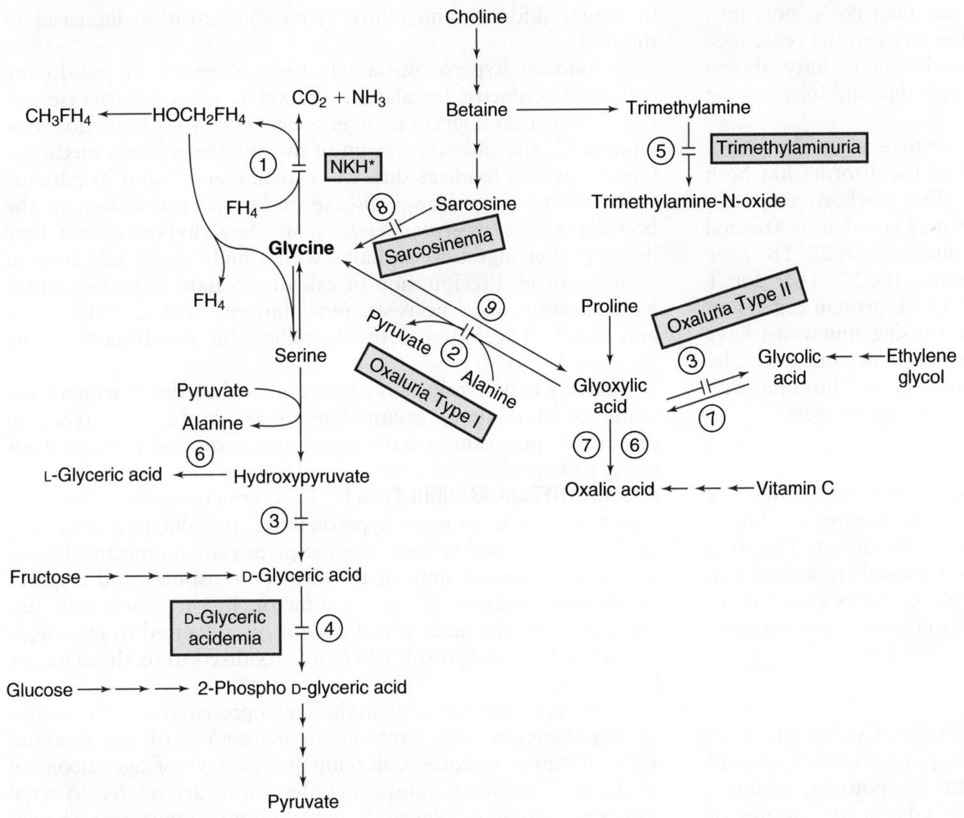

Figure 79-8 Pathways in the metabolism of glycine and glyoxylic acid. **Enzymes:** *(1)* glycine cleavage enzyme, *(2)* alanine: glyoxylate aminotransferase, *(3)* D-glyceric acid dehydrogenase, *(4)* glycerate kinase, *(5)* trimethylamine oxidase, *(6)* lactate dehydrogenase, *(7)* glycolate oxidase, *(8)* sarcosine Dehydrogenase, *(9)* glycine oxidase. FH_4, tetrahydrofolate; NkH*, nonketotic hyperglycinemia.

to as ketotic hyperglycinemia because episodes of severe acidosis and ketosis occur. The pathogenesis of hyperglycinemia in these disorders is not fully understood, but inhibition of the glycine cleavage enzyme system by the various organic acids has been shown to occur in some of the patients. The term **nonketotic hyperglycinemia** (NKH) is reserved for the clinical condition caused by the genetic deficiency of the glycine cleavage enzyme system (see Fig. 79-8). In this condition, hyperglycinemia is present without ketosis.

Nonketotic Hyperglycinemia, Glycine Encephalopathy

Four forms of this condition have been identified: neonatal, infantile, late onset, and transient.

NEONATAL HYPERGLYCEMIA This is the most common form of NKH. Clinical manifestations develop in the 1st few days of life (between 6 hr and 8 days after birth). Poor feeding, failure to suck, lethargy, and profound hypotonia may progress rapidly to a deep coma, apnea, and death. Convulsions, especially myoclonic seizures and hiccups, are common.

Laboratory findings reveal moderate to severe hyperglycinemia (as high as 8 times normal) and hyperglycinuria. The unequivocal elevation of glycine concentration in the spinal fluid (15 to 30 times normal) and the high ratio of glycine concentration in spinal fluid to that in plasma (a value >0.08) are diagnostic of NKH. Serum pH is normal; plasma serine levels are usually low.

About 30% of affected infants die despite supportive therapy. Those who survive develop profound psychomotor retardation and intractable seizure disorders (myoclonic and/or grand mal seizures). Hydrocephalus, requiring shunting, and pulmonary hypertension have been noted in some survivors.

INFANTILE NKH These previously normal infants develop signs and symptoms of neonatal NKH (see earlier) after 6 mo of age. Seizures are the common presenting signs. This condition appears to be a milder form of neonatal hyperglycinemia; infants usually survive and mental retardation is not as profound as in the neonatal form.

Laboratory findings in these patients are identical to those seen in the neonatal form.

LATE-ONSET NKH, MILD EPISODIC FORM Progressive spastic diplegia, optic atrophy, and choreoathetotic movements are the main clinical manifestations. Age of onset has been between 2 and 33 yr. Symptoms of delirium, chorea, and vertical gaze palsy may occur episodically in some patients during an intercurrent infection. Mental development is usually normal, but mild retardation has been reported in some patients. Seizures have occurred in only 1 patient.

Laboratory findings are similar to but not as pronounced as in the neonatal form.

TRANSIENT NKH Most clinical and laboratory manifestations of this form are indistinguishable from those of the neonatal form. By 2 to 8 wk of age, however, the elevated glycine levels in plasma and CSF normalize and a complete clinical recovery may occur. Most of these patients develop normally with no neurologic sequelae, but mental retardation has been noted in some. The etiology of this condition is not known, but it is believed to be due to immaturity of the enzyme system.

All forms of NKH should be differentiated from ketotic hyperglycinemia, D-glyceric aciduria (see later), and ingestion of valproic acid. The latter compound causes a moderate increase in blood and urinary concentrations of glycine. Repeat assays after discontinuation of the drug should establish the diagnosis.

Diagnosis can be established by assay of the enzyme in liver or brain specimens or by identification of the mutation. Enzyme activity in the neonatal form is close to zero, whereas in the other forms, some residual activity is present. In most patients with the neonatal form, the enzyme defect resides in the P protein; defects in the T protein account for the rest. The enzyme assay in 3 patients with the infantile and late-onset forms has revealed 2 patients with a defect in the T protein and 1 with a defect in the H protein.

No effective **treatment** is known. Exchange transfusion, dietary restriction of glycine, and administration of sodium benzoate or folate have not altered the neurologic outcome. Drugs that counteract the effect of glycine on neuronal cells, such as strychnine, diazepam, and dextromethorphan, have shown some beneficial effects only in patients with the mild forms of the condition.

NKH is inherited as an autosomal recessive trait. The prevalence is not known, but high frequency of the disorder has been noted in northern Finland (1/12,000). The newborn screening method using tandem mass spectrometry may not identify affected infants. The gene for P protein is on chromosome 9p22. The gene for H protein is mapped to chromosome 16q24. That for T protein is on chromosome 3p21-p21.1. The L protein gene is on chromosome 7q31-q32. Several disease-causing mutations have been identified. Prenatal diagnosis has been accomplished by performing an assay of the enzyme activity in chorionic villi biopsy specimens or by identification of the mutant gene.

Sarcosinemia

Increased concentrations of sarcosine (N-methylglycine) are observed in both blood and urine, but no consistent clinical picture has been attributed to this metabolic defect. This is a recessively inherited metabolic condition caused by a defect in sarcosine dehydrogenase, the enzyme that converts sarcosine to glycine (see Fig. 79-8). The gene for this enzyme is on chromosome 9q33-q34.

D-Glyceric Aciduria

D-Glyceric acid is an intermediate metabolite of serine and fructose metabolism (see Fig. 79-8). In this rare condition, clinical manifestations of severe encephalopathy (hypotonia, seizures, and mental and motor deficits) and the laboratory findings of hyperglycinemia and hyperglycinuria were suggestive of NKH. These patients excreted large quantities of D-glyceric acid. This compound is not normally detectable in urine. Enzyme studies indicated a deficiency of glycerate kinase in 1 patient and decreased activity of D-glyceric dehydrogenase in another.

No effective therapy is available. Restriction of fructose reduced the incidence of seizures in 1 patient. The gene for glycerate kinase is on chromosome 3p21.

Trimethylaminuria

Trimethylamine is normally produced in the intestine from the breakdown of dietary choline and trimethylamine oxide by bacteria. Egg yolk and liver are the main sources of choline, and fish is the major source of trimethylamine oxide. Trimethylamine is absorbed and oxidized in the liver by trimethylamine oxidase (flavin-containing monooxygenases) to trimethylamine oxide, which is odorless and excreted in the urine (see Fig. 79-8). Deficiency of this enzyme results in massive excretion of trimethylamine in urine. Several asymptomatic patients with trimethylaminuria have been reported; there is a foul body odor that resembles that of a rotten fish, which may have significant social and psychosocial ramifications. Restriction of fish, eggs, liver, and other sources of choline (such as nuts and grains) in the diet significantly reduce the odor. Treatment with short courses of oral metronidazole, neomycin or lactulose cause temporary reduction in the body odor. The gene for trimethylamine oxidase has been mapped to chromosome 1q23-q25.

Hyperoxaluria and Oxalosis

Normally, oxalic acid is derived mostly from oxidation of glyoxylic acid, and to a lesser degree, from oxidation of ascorbic acid (see Fig. 79-8). Glyoxylic acid is formed from the oxidation of glycolic acid and the deamination of glycine in the peroxisomes. The source of glycolic acid is poorly understood. Foods containing oxalic acid, such as spinach and rhubarb, are the main exogenous sources of this compound. Oxalic acid cannot be further metabolized in humans and is excreted in the urine as oxalates. Calcium oxalate is relatively insoluble in water and precipitates in tissues (kidneys and joints) if its concentration increases in the body.

Secondary hyperoxaluria has been observed in pyridoxine deficiency (cofactor for alanine-glyoxylate aminotransferase; see Fig. 79-8) after ingestion of ethylene glycol or high doses of vitamin C, after administration of the anesthetic agent methoxyflurane (which oxidizes directly to oxalic acid), and in patients with inflammatory bowel disease or extensive resection of the bowel *(enteric hyperoxaluria)*. Acute, fatal hyperoxaluria may develop after ingestion of plants with a high oxalic acid content such as sorrel. Precipitation of calcium oxalate in tissues causes hypocalcemia, liver necrosis, renal failure, cardiac arrhythmia, and death. The lethal dose of oxalic acid is estimated to be between 5 and 30 g.

Primary hyperoxaluria is a rare genetic disorder in which large amounts of oxalates accumulate in the body. Two types of primary hyperoxaluria have been identified. The term **oxalosis** refers to deposition of calcium oxalate in parenchymal tissue.

PRIMARY HYPEROXALURIA TYPE I This rare condition is the most common form of primary hyperoxaluria. It is due to a deficiency of the peroxisomal enzyme alanine-glyoxylate aminotransferase, which is expressed only in the liver peroxisomes and requires pyridoxine (vitamin B_6) as its cofactor. In the absence of this enzyme, glyoxylic acid, which cannot be converted to glycine, is transferred to the cytosol, where it is oxidized to oxalic acid (see Fig. 79-8).

There is a wide variation in the age of presentation. The majority of patients become symptomatic before 5 yr of age. In about 10% of cases, symptoms develop before 1 yr of age (neonatal oxaluria). The initial clinical manifestations are related to renal stones and nephrocalcinosis. Renal colic and asymptomatic hematuria lead to a gradual deterioration of renal function, manifested by growth retardation and uremia. Most patients die before 20 yr of age from renal failure if the disorder is untreated. Acute arthritis is a rare manifestation and may be misdiagnosed as gout because uric acid is usually elevated in patients with type I hyperoxaluria. Late forms of the disease presenting during adulthood have also been reported. Crystalline retinopathy and optic neuropathy causing visual loss have occurred in a few patients.

A marked increase in urinary excretion of oxalate (normal excretion 10-50 mg/24 hr) is the most important laboratory finding. The presence of oxalate crystals in urinary sediment is rarely helpful for diagnosis because such crystals are often seen in normal individuals. Urinary excretion of glycolic acid and glyoxylic acid is increased. Diagnosis can be confirmed by performing an assay of the enzyme in liver specimens or by identification of the mutant gene.

Treatment has been largely unsuccessful. In some patients (especially those whose condition is due to mistargeting of the enzyme to the mitochondria; see later) administration of large doses of pyridoxine reduces urinary excretion of oxalate. Renal transplantation in patients with renal failure has not improved the outcome in most cases, because oxalosis has recurred in the transplanted kidney. Combined liver and kidney transplants have resulted in a significant decrease in plasma and urinary oxalate in a few patients, and this may be the most effective treatment of this disorder.

The condition is inherited as an autosomal recessive trait. The gene for this enzyme is mapped to chromosome 2q36-q37. Several mutations of the gene have been described in patients with this condition. The most common mutation results in the mistargeting of the enzyme to the mitochondria instead of the peroxisomes. The in vitro enzyme activity in these patients may reach the level found in obligate heterozygotes. In vivo function remains defective, however. About 30% of patients with hyperoxaluria type 1 are estimated to have this defect.

Prenatal diagnosis has been achieved by the measurement of fetal hepatic enzyme activity obtained by needle biopsy or by DNA analysis of chorionic villi samples.

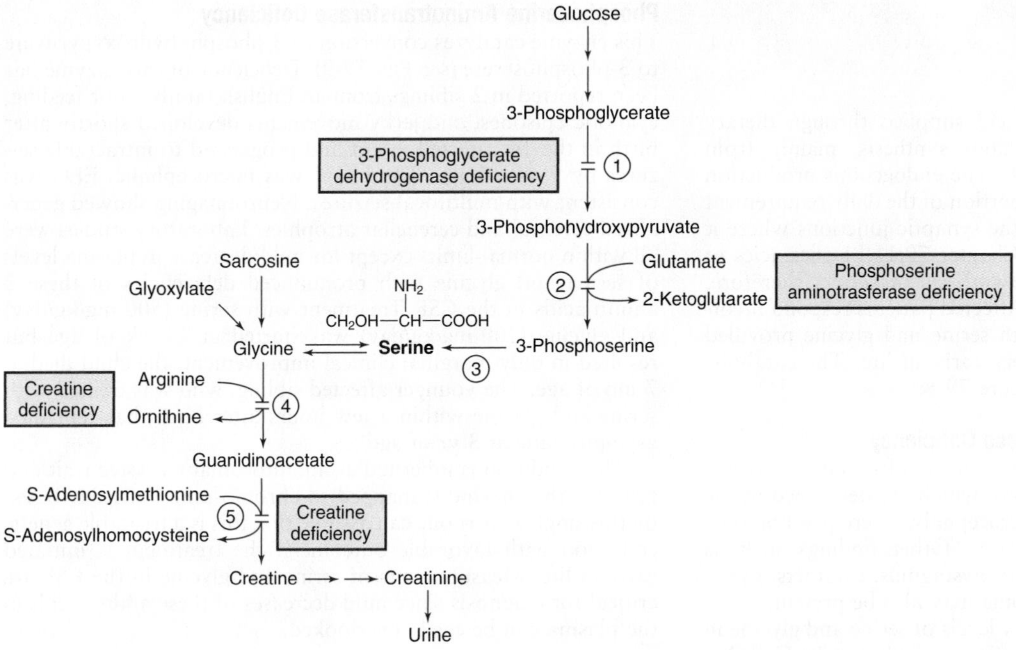

Figure 79-9 Pathways for the synthesis of serine and creatine. **Enzymes:** *(1)* 3-phosphoglycerate dehydrogenase, *(2)* phosphoserine amidinotransferase, *(3)* phosphoserine phosphatase, *(4)* arginine:glycine amidinotransferase (AGAT). *(5)* guanidinoacetate methyltransferase (GAMT).

PRIMARY HYPEROXALURIA TYPE II (L-GLYCERIC ACIDURIA) This rare condition is due to a deficiency of D-glycerate dehydrogenase (hydroxypyruvate reductase)/glyoxylate reductase enzyme complex (see Fig. 79-8). A deficiency in the activity of this enzyme results in an accumulation of 2 intermediate metabolites, hydroxypyruvate (the ketoacid of serine) and glyoxylic acid. Both these compounds are further metabolized by lactate dehydrogenase (LDH) to L-glyceric acid and oxalic acid, respectively. About 30% of reported patients are from the Saulteaux-Ojibway Indians of Manitoba.

These patients are indistinguishable from those with hyperoxaluria type I. Renal stones presenting with renal colic and hematuria may develop before age 2 yr. Renal failure is less common in this condition than in hyperoxaluria type I; the urine contains large amounts of L-glyceric acid in addition to high levels of oxalate. L-glyceric acid is not normally present in urine. Urinary excretion of glycolic acid and glyoxylic acid is not increased. The presence of L-glyceric acid without increased levels of glycolic and glyoxylic acids in urine differentiates this type from type I hyperoxaluria. The gene is mapped to chromosome 9cen.

No effective therapy is available. Experience with liver transplantation is very limited at this time.

CREATINE DEFICIENCY

Creatine is synthesized in the liver, pancreas, and kidneys from arginine and glycine (Fig. 79-9) and is transported to muscles and the brain, in which there is high activity of the enzyme creatine kinase. Phosphorylation and dephosphorylation of creatine in conjunction with adenosine triphosphate and diphosphate (ATP and ADP), respectively, provide high-energy phosphate transfer reactions in these organs. Creatine is nonenzymatically metabolized to creatinine at a constant daily rate and is excreted in the urine. Three genetic conditions are known to cause creatine deficiency in tissues. Two are due to deficiency of the enzymes involved in the biosynthesis of creatine. The enzymes are arginine:glycine amidinotransferase (AGAT) and guanidinoacetate methyltransferase (GAMT) (see Fig. 79-9). Both conditions respond well to creatine supplementation. The third condition is caused by the defect in the creatinine transporter (CRTR) and is not responsive to creatine administration.

Clinical manifestations of the 3 defects are similar, relate to the brain and muscles, and may appear in the 1st few weeks or months of life. Developmental delay, mental retardation, speech delay, hypotonia, ataxia, and seizures are common. Dystonic hyperkinetic movements are seen in severe GAMT deficiency.

Laboratory findings include decreased creatine and creatinine in blood and urine in patients with AGAT and GAMT defects. Urinary ratio of creatine to creatinine is increased in patients with CRTR defect. Marked elevations of guanidinoacetate in blood, urine, and especially in CSF are diagnostic of GAMT defects. Low levels of guanidinoacetate are found with the AGAT defect. Absence of creatine and creatine phosphate (in all 3 defects) and high levels of guanidinoacetate (with GAMT defects) can be demonstrated in the brain by magnetic resonance spectroscopy (MRS). MRI of the brain shows signal hyperintensity of the globus pallidus. Diagnosis of AGAT or GAMT defects may be confirmed by measurement of the enzyme in the liver, cultured fibroblasts, or stimulated lymphoblasts or by DNA analysis of the gene. Diagnosis of CRTR is confirmed by genetic analysis or creatine uptake by fibroblasts.

Treatment with creatine monohydrate (350 mg-2 g/kg/day) orally has resulted in a dramatic improvement in muscle tone and overall mental development and has normalized MRI and electroencephalographic findings in patients with AGAT and GAMT defects. It is believed that early treatment may assure normal development. No therapy is available for the CRTR defect.

AGAT and GAMT defects are inherited as autosomal recessive traits. The gene for AGAT is on chromosome 15q15.3 and that for GAMT is on chromosome 19q13.3. CRTR is an X-linked trait (Xq28). The respective prevalences of these enzyme deficiencies are not known; 4 patients with GAMT defects (3 from 1 family) were identified among 180 institutionalized patients with severe mental handicap. In another study, of 188 children with mental retardation, 4 patients (all males) had a CRTR defect and 1 patient had GAMT deficiency. Creatine deficiency must be considered in any patient with concomitant brain and muscle dysfunction, as treatment can produce a dramatic response.

BIBLIOGRAPHY

Please visit the Nelson Textbook of Pediatrics *website at* *www.expertconsult.com* *for the complete bibliography.*

79.8 Serine

Iraj Rezvani

Serine is a nonessential amino acid supplied through dietary sources and through its endogenous synthesis, mainly from glucose and glycine (see Fig. 79-9). The endogenous production of serine comprises an important portion of the daily requirement of this amino acid, especially in the synaptic junctions where it functions as a neurotransmitter (Chapter 79.11). Deficiencies of the enzymes involved in the biosynthesis of serine, therefore, cause neurologic manifestations. Affected patients respond favorably to oral supplementation with serine and glycine provided that the treatment is initiated very early in life. The catabolic pathway of serine is shown in Figure 79-8.

3-Phosphoglycerate Dehydrogenase Deficiency

Deficiency of this enzyme causes deficiencies of serine and glycine in the body. Clinical manifestations, which are developed in the 1st few months of life, include microcephaly, severe psychomotor retardation, and intractable seizures. Other findings such as failure to thrive, spastic tetraplegia, nystagmus, cataracts, hypogonadism, and megaloblastic anemia may also be present.

Laboratory findings include low levels of serine and glycine in plasma and very low levels of serine and glycine in CSF. No abnormal organic acid is found in the urine. MRI of the brain shows significant attenuation of white matter and incomplete myelination.

Diagnosis can be confirmed by measurement of the enzyme activity in cultured fibroblasts and by DNA analysis.

Treatment with serine (200-600 mg/kg/24 hr, orally) alone or in conjunction with glycine (200-300 mg/kg/24 hr) normalizes the serine levels in the blood and CSF. This treatment produces significant improvement in all clinical findings except for the psychomotor retardation; seizure activity subsides within a few days of therapy and may be halted completely. Microcephaly improves in young affected infants. There is evidence to indicate that psychomotor retardation may be prevented if the treatment starts in the 1st few days of life.

The condition is inherited as an autosomal recessive trait. The gene for 3-phosphoglycerate dehydrogenase enzyme has been mapped to chromosome 1q12 and a few disease-producing mutations have been identified in different families. Prenatal diagnosis has been achieved by DNA analysis in a family with previously affected offspring; administration of serine to the mother corrected the microcephaly in the affected fetus as evidenced by ultrasound imaging. The favorable response of this condition to a simple treatment makes this diagnosis an important consideration in any child with microcephaly and neurologic defects such as psychomotor delay or a seizure disorder.

Phosphoserine Aminotransferase Deficiency

This enzyme catalyzes conversion of 3-phosphohydroxypyruvate to 3-phosphoserine (see Fig. 79-9). Deficiency of this enzyme has been reported in 2 siblings from an English family. Poor feeding, cyanotic episodes, and jerky movements developed shortly after birth in the 1st affected infant and progressed to intractable seizures by 9 wk of age. The infant was microcephalic. EEG was consistent with multifocal seizures. Neuroimaging showed generalized cerebral and cerebellar atrophies. Laboratory studies were all within normal limits except for mild decrease in plasma levels of serine and glycine with pronounced deficiencies of these 2 amino acids in the CSF. Treatment with serine (500 mg/kg/day) and glycine (200 mg/kg/day) was started at 11 wk of age but resulted in only marginal clinical improvement; the child died at 7 mo of age. The younger affected sibling, who was treated with serine and glycine within a few hours after birth, has remained asymptomatic at 3 yr of age.

The condition is inherited as an autosomal recessive trait and gene for the enzyme is mapped to chromosome 9q21.31. Based on this single report one can assume that this is a treatable genetic condition with favorable outcome if the treatment is initiated early in life. Measurements of serine and glycine in the CSF are critical for diagnosis since mild decreases of these amino acids in the plasma can be easily overlooked.

BIBLIOGRAPHY

Please visit the Nelson Textbook of Pediatrics *website at* *www.expertconsult.com* *for the complete bibliography.*

79.9 Proline

Iraj Rezvani

Proline is a nonessential amino acid synthesized endogenously from glutamic acid, ornithine, and arginine (Fig. 79-10). Proline and hydroxyproline are found in high concentrations in collagen. Neither of these amino acids is normally found in urine in the free form except in early infancy. Excretion of proline and hydroxyproline as iminopeptides (dipeptides and tripeptides containing proline or hydroxyproline) reflects collagen turnover and is increased in disorders of accelerated collagen turnover, such as rickets or hyperparathyroidism. Proline is also found at synaptic junctions and functions as a neurotransmitter (Chapter 79.11).

Hyperprolinemia

Two types of primary hyperprolinemia have been described.

HYPERPROLINEMIA TYPE I This rare autosomal recessive condition is due to deficiency of proline oxidase (proline dehydrogenase, see Fig. 79-10). Clinical manifestations are variable; some affected

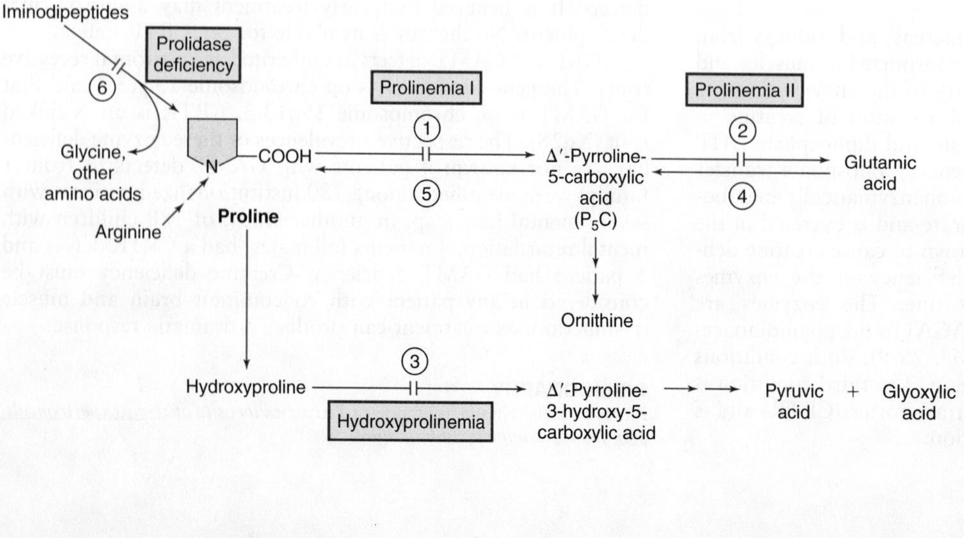

Figure 79-10 Pathways in the metabolism of proline. **Enzymes:** *(1)* proline oxidase (dehydrogenase), *(2)* Δ^1-pyrroline-5-carboxylic acid (P5C) dehydrogenase, *(3)* hydroxyproline oxidase, *(4)* Δ^1-pyrroline-5-carboxylic acid synthase, *(5)* Δ^1-pyrroline-5-carboxylic acid reductase, *(6)* prolidase.

individuals are asymptomatic but patients with severe psychomotor retardation and seizures have been reported. Schizophrenia is a common finding in these patients. The gene for proline oxidase is located on chromosome 22q11.2 and several disease-causing mutations have been identified. Microdeletions involving this region of chromosome 22 cause velocardiofacial (DiGeorge, Shprintzen) syndrome; approximately 50% of patients with this syndrome have been reported to have hyperprolinemia type I. Therefore, all patients with hyperprolinemia type I should be screened (by FISH analysis) for presence of DiGeorge syndrome.

Laboratory studies reveal high concentrations of proline in plasma, urine, and in the CSF. About 30% of obligate heterozygous individuals (parents, siblings) also have hyperprolinemia. Increased urinary excretion of hydroxyproline and glycine is also present; this is due to saturation of the shared tubular reabsorption mechanism by massive prolinuria.

No effective treatment has yet emerged. Restriction of dietary proline causes modest improvement in plasma proline with no proven clinical benefit.

HYPERPROLINEMIA TYPE II This is a rare autosomal recessive condition caused by the deficiency of pyrroline-carboxylic acid dehydrogenase (aldehyde dehydrogenase 4, ALDH4; see Fig. 79-10). Psychomotor retardation (modest to severe) and seizures (usually precipitated by an intercurrent infection) have been reported in most affected children, but asymptomatic patients have also been reported.

Laboratory studies reveal increased concentrations of proline and Δ^1-pyrroline-5-carboxylic acid (P5C) in blood, urine, and the CSF. Increased excretion of xanthurenic acid has also been reported in this condition. The presence of P5C differentiates this condition from hyperprolinemia type I (see earlier). Increased levels of P5C in body fluids, especially in the CNS, cause inactivation of vitamin B_6 and generate a state of vitamin B_6 dependency (Chapter 79.14). Deficiency of vitamin B_6 is perhaps the main cause of neurologic findings in this condition and may explain the variability in clinical manifestations in different patients. **Treatment** with high doses of vitamin B_6 in conjunction with a diet low in proline is recommended but the experience remains very limited because of paucity of patients. The gene for P5C dehydrogenase (ALDH4) is on chromosome 1p36.

Prolidase Deficiency

During collagen degradation, imidodipeptides (dipeptides containing proline such as glycylproline) are released and are normally cleaved by tissue prolidase. This enzyme requires manganese for its proper activity. Deficiency of prolidase, which is inherited as an autosomal recessive trait, results in the accumulation of imidodipeptides in body fluids.

The clinical manifestations of this rare condition and the age at onset are quite variable (19 mo to 19 yr) and include recurrent, painful skin ulcers, which are typically on hands and legs. Other skin lesions that may precede ulcers by several years may include scaly erythematous maculopapular rash, purpura, and telangiectasia. Most ulcers become infected. Healing of the ulcers may take 4 to 7 mo. Mild to severe mental and motor deficits and susceptibility to infections are also present in most patients (recurrent otitis media, sinusitis, respiratory infection, splenomegaly). Infection is the cause of death. Some patients may have some craniofacial abnormalities such as ptosis, ocular proptosis, and prominent cranial sutures. Asymptomatic cases have also been reported. Development of systemic lupus erythematosus (SLE) has been noted in affected children of 1 family; young patients with SLE should be screened for prolidase deficiency. High levels of urinary excretion of imidodipeptides are diagnostic. Enzyme assay may be performed in erythrocytes or cultured skin fibroblasts.

Oral supplementation with proline, ascorbic acid, and manganese and the topical use of proline and glycine result in an improvement in leg ulcers. These treatments have not been found to be consistently effective in all patients.

The gene for prolidase enzyme has been mapped to chromosome 19cen-q13.11 and several disease-causing mutations have been identified in different families.

BIBLIOGRAPHY

Please visit the Nelson Textbook of Pediatrics *website at www.expertconsult.com for the complete bibliography.*

79.10 Glutamic Acid

Iraj Rezvani

Glutamic acid and its aminated derivative glutamine have a wide range of functions in the body. One of the major products of glutamic acid is glutathione (γ-glutamylcysteinylglycine). This ubiquitous tripeptide, with its function as the major antioxidant in the body, is synthesized and degraded through a complex cycle called the γ-glutamyl cycle (Fig. 79-11). Because of its free sulfhydryl (-SH) group and its abundance in the cell, glutathione protects other sulfhydryl-containing compounds (such as enzymes and CoA) from oxidation. It is also involved in the detoxification of peroxides, including hydrogen peroxide, and in keeping the intracellular milieu in a reduced state. The common consequence of glutathione deficiency is hemolytic anemia. Glutathione also participates in amino acid transport across the cell membrane through the γ-glutamyl cycle. Glutamic acid is also the precursor of γ-aminobutyric acid (GABA), a major neurotransmitter in the nervous system (Chapter 79.11).

Glutathione Synthetase Deficiency (See Fig. 79-11)

Three forms of this condition have been reported. In the **severe form**, which is due to generalized deficiency of the enzyme, severe acidosis and massive 5-oxoprolinuria are the rule. In the **mild form**, in which the enzyme deficiency causes glutathione deficiency only in erythrocytes, neither 5-oxoprolinuria nor acidosis has been observed. A **moderate form** has also been observed in which the hemolytic anemia is associated with variable degrees of acidosis and 5-oxoprolinuria. In all forms, patients have hemolytic anemia secondary to glutathione deficiency. All forms are rare; a total of 65 patients have been reported.

GLUTATHIONE SYNTHETASE DEFICIENCY, SEVERE FORM (PYROGLUTAMIC ACIDEMIA, SEVERE 5-OXOPROLINURIA) AND MODERATE FORM Clinical manifestations of this rare condition occur in the 1st few days of life and include metabolic acidosis, jaundice, and mild to moderate hemolytic anemia. Chronic acidosis continues after recovery. Similar episodes of life-threatening acidosis may occur during gastroenteritis or an infection or after a surgical procedure. Progressive neurologic damage, manifested by mental retardation, spastic tetraparesis, ataxia, tremor, dysarthria, and seizures, develops with age. Susceptibility to infection, presumably due to granulocyte dysfunction, is observed in some patients. Patients with the moderate form have milder acidosis and less 5-oxoprolinuria than is seen in the severe form; neurologic manifestations are also absent.

Laboratory findings include metabolic acidosis, mild to moderate degrees of hemolytic anemia, and 5-oxoprolinuria. High concentrations of 5-oxoproline are also found in blood. The glutathione content of erythrocytes is markedly decreased. Increased synthesis of 5-oxoproline in this disorder is believed to be due to the conversion of γ-glutamylcysteine to 5-oxoproline by the enzyme γ-glutamyl cyclotransferase (see Fig. 79-11). γ-Glutamylcysteine production increases greatly because the normal inhibitory effect of glutathione on the γ-glutamylcysteine synthetase enzyme is removed. A deficiency of glutathione synthetase has been demonstrated in a variety of cells including erythrocytes.

Treatment of acute attack includes hydration, correction of acidosis (by infusion of sodium bicarbonate), and measures to correct anemia and hyperbilirubinemia. Chronic administration

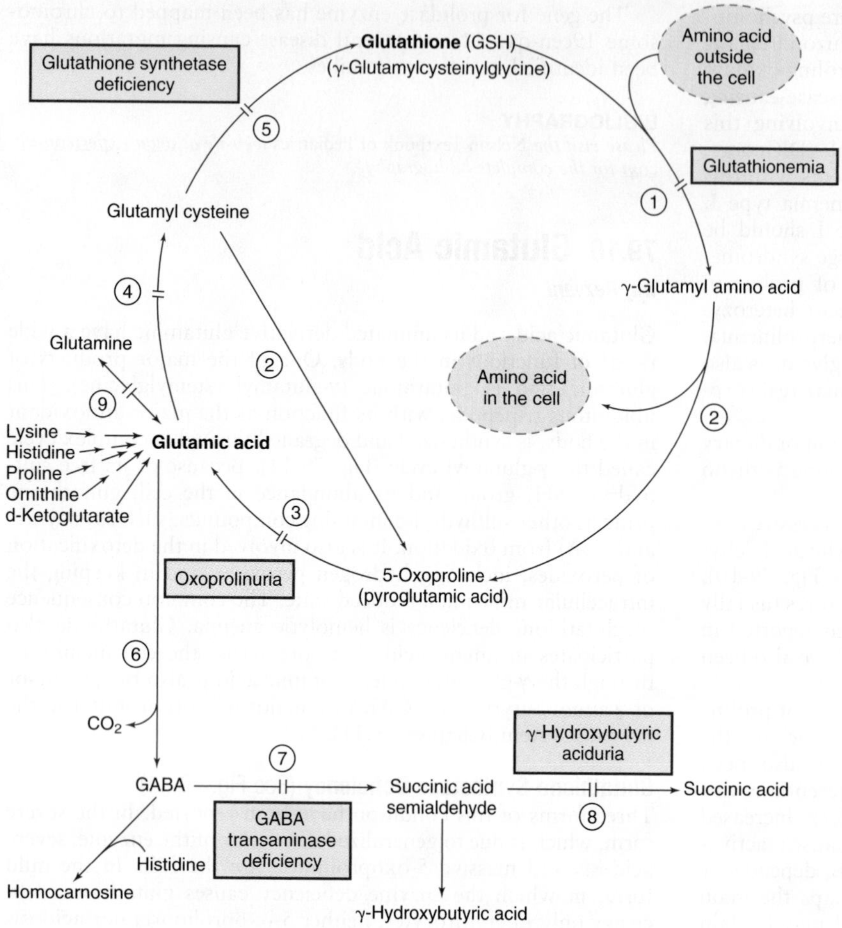

Figure 79-11 The γ-glutamyl cycle. Defects of the glutathione synthesis and degradation are noted. **Enzymes:** *(1)* γ-glutamyl transpeptidase, *(2)* γ-glutamyl cyclotransferase, *(3)* 5-oxoprolinase, *(4)* γ-glutamyl-cysteine synthetase, *(5)* glutathione synthetase, *(6)* glutamic acid decarboxylase, *(7)* GABA transaminase, *(8)* succinic semialdehyde dehydrogenase, *(9)* glutamine synthase.

of alkali is usually needed indefinitely. Administration of large doses of vitamins C and E has been recommended. Drugs and oxidants that are known to cause hemolysis and stressful catabolic states should be avoided. Oral administration of glutathione analogs has been tried with variable success.

Prenatal diagnosis can be achieved by the measurement of 5-oxoproline in amniotic fluid, by enzyme analysis in cultured amniocytes or chronic villi samples, or by DNA analysis of the gene. Successful pregnancy in an affected female (moderate form) with favorable outcomes for both mother and infant has been reported.

GLUTATHIONE SYNTHETASE DEFICIENCY, MILD FORM This form has been reported in only a few patients. Mild to moderate hemolytic anemia has been the only clinical finding in these patients. Splenomegaly has been reported in some patients. Mental development is normal; metabolic acidosis and increased concentrations of 5-oxoproline do not occur. Similar to other types of glutathione synthase deficiency, this form is due to mutations in the gene that encodes the enzyme. These mutations, however, decrease the half-life and increase the rate of turnover of the protein, but do not affect its catalytic function. The expedited rate of enzyme turnover caused by these mutations is of no consequence for tissues with protein synthetic capability. However, mature erythrocytes do not synthesize protein, and this results over time in a deficiency of the more rapidly degraded enzyme and a consequent deficiency of glutathione. **Treatment** is that of hemolytic anemia and avoidance of drugs and oxidants that can trigger the hemolytic process.

All forms of the condition are inherited as an autosomal recessive trait. The gene for this enzyme is located on chromosome 20q11.2. Several disease-causing mutations have been identified in different families.

5-OXOPROLINASE DEFICIENCY (5-OXOPROLINURIA) The main cause of massive 5-oxoprolinuria is glutathione synthetase deficiency (see above). Moderate 5-oxoprolinuria has been found in a variety of metabolic and acquired conditions, such as in patients with severe burns, Stevens-Johnson syndrome, homocystinuria, urea cycle defects, and tyrosinemia type I.

A few individuals with moderate 5-oxoprolinuria (4-10 g/day) due to 5-oxoprolinase deficiency have been identified. No specific clinical picture has yet emerged. Moderate to severe mental retardation has been reported in 2 patients. Asymptomatic individuals with the enzyme deficiency have also been identified, however. It is, therefore, not clear whether 5-oxoprolinase deficiency is of any clinical consequence. No treatment has been recommended.

γ-GLUTAMYLCYSTEINE SYNTHETASE DEFICIENCY Only a few patients with this enzyme deficiency have been reported. The most consistent clinical manifestation has been mild chronic hemolytic anemia. Acute attacks of hemolysis have occurred after exposure to sulfonamides. Peripheral neuropathy and progressive spinocerebellar degeneration have been noted in 2 siblings in adulthood. Laboratory findings of chronic hemolytic anemia were present in all patients. Generalized aminoaciduria is also present because the γ-glutamyl cycle is involved in amino acid transport in cells (see Fig. 79-11). **Treatment** is that of hemolytic anemia and avoidance of drugs and oxidants that may trigger the hemolytic process. The condition is inherited as an autosomal recessive trait.

Glutathionemia (γ-Glutamyl Transpeptidase [GGT] Deficiency)

This enzyme is present in any cell that has secretory or absorptive functions. It is especially abundant in the kidneys, pancreas, intestines, and liver. The enzyme is also present in the bile.

Measurement of this enzyme in the blood is commonly performed to evaluate liver and bile duct diseases.

Deficiency of this enzyme causes elevation in glutathione concentrations in body fluids, but the cellular levels remain normal. Only a few patients with enzyme deficiency have been reported; therefore, the scope of clinical manifestations has not yet been defined. Mild to moderate mental retardation and severe behavioral problems were observed in 3 patients. One of the 2 sisters with this condition had normal intelligence as an adult, however, and the other had Prader-Willi syndrome.

Laboratory findings include marked elevations in urinary concentrations of glutathione (up to 1 g/day), γ-glutamylcysteine, and cysteine. None of the reported patients has had generalized aminoaciduria, a finding that would have been expected to occur in this enzyme deficiency (see Fig. 79-11).

Diagnosis can be confirmed by measurement of the enzyme activity in leukocytes or cultured skin fibroblasts. No effective treatment is available.

The condition is inherited as an autosomal recessive trait. The enzyme GGT is a complex protein and is encoded by at least seven genes.

Genetic Disorders of Metabolism of γ-Aminobutyric Acid (Chapter 79.11)

CONGENITAL GLUTAMINE DEFICIENCY This rare disorder is due to a deficiency of glutamine synthase. Glutamine is absent in plasma, urine, and CSF, but plasma levels of glutamic acid remain normal. Manifestations include cerebral malformations (abnormal gyration, white matter lesions), multiorgan failure including respiratory failure, and neonatal death. It may be inherited as an autosomal trait; the gene is mapped to chromosome 1q31.

BIBLIOGRAPHY

Please visit the Nelson Textbook of Pediatrics *website at* *www.expertconsult.com* *for the complete bibliography.*

79.11 Genetic Disorders of Neurotransmitters

Iraj Rezvani and K. Michael Gibson

Neurotransmitters are released from the axonal end of excited neurons at the synaptic junctions and cause propagation and amplification or inhibition of neural impulses. A number of amino acids and their metabolites comprise the bulk of neurotransmitters. Mutations in genes responsible for the synthesis or degradation of these substances may cause conditions that are usually manifested by neurologic and/or psychiatric abnormalities (Table 79-2). Previously, affected children have been diagnosed with cerebral palsy, seizure disorder, parkinsonism, or dystonia. Correct diagnosis is important because most of these conditions respond favorably to therapy. Diagnosis requires specialized laboratory studies of the CSF in most cases because some of the neurotransmitters generated in the CNS (dopamine and serotonin) do not cross the blood-brain barrier and are therefore not detected in the serum or urine. An ever-growing number of these conditions are being identified; diseases that were once thought to be very rare are now diagnosed with increasing frequency.

Table 79-2 GENETIC DISORDERS OF NEUROTRANSMITTERS IN CHILDREN

TRANSMITTER	SYNTHESIS DEFECTS	DEGRADATION DEFECTS
MONOAMINES		
Dopamine	TH deficiency	MAO deficiency
Serotonin and dopamine	AADC deficiency	MAO deficiency
	BH_4 deficiency With hyperphe Without hyperphe	
Norepinephrine	DβH deficiency	MAO deficiency
GABA	GAD deficiency?	GABA transaminase deficiency GHB aciduria
Histamine	HDC deficiency	?
AMINO ACIDS		
Proline	?	Hyperprolinemia
Serine	3-PGD, PSAT deficiencies	?
Glycine	3-PDG, PSAT deficiencies	NKH

TH, tyrosine hydroxylase; MAO, monoamine oxidase; AADC, aromatic L-amino acid decarboxylase; BH_4, tetrahydrobiopterin; Hyperphe, hyperphenylalaninemia; DβH, dopamine β-hydroxylase; GABA, γ-aminobutyric acid; GAD, glutamic acid decarboxylase; GHB, γ-hydroxybutyric; HDC, histidine decarboxylase; 3-PGD, 3-phosphoglycerate dehydrogenase; PSAT, phosphoserine aminotransferase; NKH, nonketotic hyperglycinemia.

TYROSINE HYDROXYLASE DEFICIENCY (INFANTILE PARKINSONISM, AUTOSOMAL RECESSIVE DOPA-RESPONSIVE DYSTONIA)

Tyrosine hydroxylase catalyzes the formation of L-dopa from tyrosine (see Fig. 79-2). Deficiency of this enzyme has been reported in a few children with dystonia and parkinsonism. The clinical picture resembles that of autosomal dominant dystonia due to GTP cyclohydrolase deficiency (see later). The spectrum of the condition is not fully appreciated.

Clinical manifestations such as involuntary movements of the limbs associated with spasticity and muscle rigidity, dystonia, expressionless face, ptosis, drooling, oculogyric crises, and parkinsonism may start in early infancy. Psychomotor retardation has been seen in some patients. No diurnal variation of the symptoms has been noted.

Laboratory findings include reduced levels of dopamine and its metabolite homovanillic acid (HVA), and normal concentrations of tetrahydrobiopterin and neopterin in the CSF. Serum prolactin levels are usually elevated.

Diagnosis may be established by gene study.

Treatment with L-dopa/carbidopa results in significant clinical improvement in most patients. The condition, however, is progressive and usually lethal if it remains untreated. It is inherited as an autosomal recessive trait. The gene for tyrosine hydroxylase is mapped to chromosome 11p.

AROMATIC L-AMINO ACID DECARBOXYLASE DEFICIENCY

Aromatic L-amino acid decarboxylase (AADC) enzyme catalyzes decarboxylation of both 5-hydroxytryptophan (to form serotonin, see Fig. 79-5) and L-dopa (to generate dopamine, see Fig. 79-2). Clinical manifestations of this relatively rare enzyme deficiency are related to underproduction of both dopamine and serotonin. Poor feeding, lethargy, hypotension, hypothermia, eye rolling (oculogyric crises), and ptosis have been observed in affected neonates. Clinical findings in infants and older children include developmental delay, truncal hypotonia with hypertonia of limbs, oculogyric crises, extrapyramidal movements (choreoathetosis, dystonia, myoclonus), and autonomic abnormalities (sweating, salivation, irritability, temperature instability, hypotension). Laboratory findings include decreased concentrations of dopamine and serotonin and their metabolites (homovanillic acid, 5-hydroxyindoleacetic acid, vanillylmandelic acid and norepinephrine), and increased levels of 5-hydroxytryptophan, L-dopa and its metabolite (3-O-methyldopa) in body fluids, especially in CSF. Elevated serum concentrations of prolactin (due to dopamine deficiency) have also been observed. The electroencephalogram and imaging of the brain are usually normal but progressive cerebral atrophy may be present in older patients. Patients with

AADC enzyme deficiency may be misdiagnosed as having cerebral palsy, epilepsy, mitochondrial cytopathy, myasthenia gravis or dystonia. The condition should also be differentiated from other neurotransmitter disorders such as tyrosine hydroxylase deficiency and Segawa disease. **Treatment** with neurotransmitter precursors has produced limited clinical improvement. Dopamine and serotonin have no therapeutic value because of their inability to cross the blood-brain barrier. Dopamine agonists (L-dopa/carbidopa, bromocriptine), monoamine oxidase (MAO) inhibitors (tranylcypromine), serotonergic agents and high doses of pyridoxine (cofactor for AADC enzyme) have been tried. No treatment of choice has yet emerged because of the paucity of patients. The condition is inherited as an autosomal recessive trait and several disease-producing mutations have been identified in different families. The condition seems to be more severe in females. The gene for the enzyme is mapped to chromosome 7p11.

TETRAHYDROBIOPTERIN (BH_4) DEFICIENCY (CHAPTER 79.1)

Tetrahydrobiopterin is the cofactor for PAH (see Fig. 79-1), tyrosine hydroxylase (see Fig. 79-2), tryptophan hydroxylase (see Fig. 79-5), and nitric oxide synthase. It is synthesized from GTP in many tissues of the body (see Fig. 79-1). Deficiencies of enzymes involved in the biosynthesis of BH_4 result in inadequate production of this cofactor which in turn causes deficiencies of the neurotransmitters serotonin and dopamine with or without concomitant hyperphenylalaninemia.

BH_4 Deficiency with Hyperphenylalalinemia

See Chapter 79.1.

BH_4 Deficiency Without Hyperphenylalaninemia

Hereditary progressive dystonia, autosomal dominant dopa-responsive dystonia, Segawa disease (Chapter 590.3).

This form of dystonia, first described in Japan, is caused by GTP cyclohydrolase I deficiency. It is inherited as an autosomal dominant trait and is more common in females than males (4:1).

Clinical manifestations usually start in early childhood and are heralded by tremors and dystonia of the lower limbs (toe gait), which may spread to all extremities within a few years. Torticollis, dystonia of the arms, and poor coordination may precede dystonia of the lower limbs in some patients. Early development is generally normal. The symptoms usually have an impressive diurnal variation, becoming worse by the end of the day and improving with sleep. Autonomic instability is not uncommon. Parkinsonian signs may also be present or develop subsequently with advancing age. Late presentation in adult life has also been reported.

Laboratory findings show no hyperphenylalaninemia, but reduced levels of BH_4 and neopterin are found in the CSF. Dopamine and its metabolite (homovanillic acid) may also be reduced in the spinal fluid. The serotonergic pathway is less affected by this enzyme deficiency; thus, concentrations of serotonin and its metabolites are usually normal. Plasma phenylalanine is normal but an oral phenylalanine loading test (100 mg/kg) produces an abnormally high plasma phenylalanine level with a high ratio of phenylalanine to tyrosine. It is believed that the enzyme deficiency in this condition is less severe than that of the autosomal recessive form of GTP cyclohydrolase I deficiency, which is associated with hyperphenylalaninemia (Chapter 79.1). The existence of asymptomatic carriers indicates that other factors or genes may play a role in the pathogenesis of the phenotype. The asymptomatic carrier may be identified by the phenylalanine loading test (see earlier).

Diagnosis may be confirmed by reduced levels of BH_4 and neopterin in the spinal fluid, by measurement of the enzyme activity, and by identification of the gene defect (Chapter 79.1). Clinically, the condition should be differentiated from other causes of dystonias and childhood parkinsonism, especially tyrosine hydroxylase, sepiapterin reductase, and aromatic amino acid decarboxylase deficiencies.

Treatment with L-dopa/carbidopa usually produces dramatic clinical improvement. Oral administration of BH_4 is also effective but is rarely used. The gene for the GTP cyclohydrolase I enzyme is located on chromosome 14q22.1-22.2.

Sepiapterin Reductase Deficiency

Sepiapterin reductase is 1 of the enzymes that is involved in conversion of 6-pyruvoyl-tetrahydropterin to tetrahydrobiopterin (BH_4). It also participates in the salvage pathway of tetrahydrobiopterin synthesis (see Fig. 79-1). Deficiency of this enzyme results in accumulation of 6-lactoyl-tetrahydropterin, which is converted to sepiapterin nonenzymatically. Most of the sepiapterin is metabolized to tetrahydrobiopterin through the salvage pathway in peripheral tissues (see Fig. 79-1), but because of the low enzyme activity of dihydrofolate reductase (DHFR) in the human brain, the amount of BH_4 remains inadequate for proper synthesis of dopamine and serotonin in the CNS. This explains the lack of hyperphenylalaninemia in this condition. Fewer than 40 patients with this disorder have been identified but the condition may be underdiagnosed since the diagnosis requires highly specialized assays of the CSF.

Clinical manifestations appear within a few months of life and are similar to those of Segawa disease and tyrosine hydroxylase deficiency. Progressive psychomotor retardation, truncal hypotonia with limb hypertonia, dystonia, abnormal eye movements (that can be mistaken for seizures), and hyperreflexia are common findings. The symptoms usually have a diurnal variation, becoming worse by the end of the day and improving with sleep. Growth is normal.

Diagnosis is established by measurement of neurotransmitters and pterin metabolites in the CSF which reveals decreased concentrations of homovanillic acid, 5-hydroxyindoleacetic acid and markedly elevated levels of sepiapterin and dihydrobiopterin (BH_2). The serum concentration of serotonin is low and that of prolactin is elevated. The plasma concentration of phenylalanine and the ratio of phenylalanine to tyrosine are normal but rise abnormally after the phenylalanine loading test (see earlier). The EEG and imaging of the brain are usually normal. Diagnosis may be confirmed by assay of the enzyme activity in fibroblast culture or by DNA analysis.

Treatment with slowly increasing doses of L-dopa/carbidopa and 5-hydroxytryptophan usually produces dramatic clinical improvement.

The condition is inherited as an autosomal recessive trait; heterozygous carriers are normal. The gene for the enzyme is on chromosome 2p12-14 and several disease-causing mutations have been reported in different families.

DOPAMINE β-HYDROXYLASE DEFICIENCY (SEE FIG. 79-2)

The condition has been reported in only a few adult subjects with clinical manifestations of orthostatic hypotension. Past histories of these subjects have revealed ptosis, hypotension, hypothermia, and hypoglycemia in the neonatal period. Spontaneous abortion and stillbirth have been also documented in the mothers of affected patients. It is thought that most mutations for this enzyme are lethal and surviving affected adults have a mild form of the condition. Laboratory findings include absence of norepinephrine and epinephrine and their metabolites with elevated levels of dopamine and its metabolite in plasma, CSF, and urine. **Treatment** with dihydroxyphenylserine that is converted to norepinephrine directly in vivo by the action of aromatic L-amino acid decarboxylase (AADC) leads to significant improvement in orthostatic hypotension and normalizes noradrenaline and its metabolites in the body. The condition is inherited as an autosomal recessive trait and the gene for the enzyme resides on chromosome 9q34.

MONOAMINE OXIDASE (MAO) DEFICIENCY

There are 2 monoamine oxidase isoenzymes, MAO A and MAO B. Both enzymes catalyze oxidative deamination of most biogenic amines in the body including serotonin (see Fig 79-5), norepinephrine, epinephrine, and dopamine (see Fig. 79-2). The genes for both isoenzymes are on chromosome X (Xp11.23). The deficiencies of these enzymes, therefore, are expected to be of clinical significance mainly in hemizygous males. Deficiency of MAO A has been reported in a large Dutch kindred. All affected males showed mild mental retardation with aggressive, violent behavior. MAO B deficiency has been found in patients with Norrie disease (Chapter 614); the importance of the enzyme deficiency in the pathogenesis of this condition is not known. Isolated MAO B deficiency has not been reported. Etiologic contribution of the deficiency of these enzymes to psychiatric diseases has been postulated but has not been supported by clinical studies. Diagnosis is established by elevated levels of norepinephrine, dopamine, serotonin, in conjunction with low levels of their metabolites in body fluids. No effective therapy has yet emerged.

γ-AMINOBUTYRIC ACID (GABA)

γ-Aminobutyric acid (GABA) is the main inhibitory neurotransmitter, which is synthesized in the synapses through decarboxylation of glutamic acid by glutamic acid decarboxylase (GAD). The same pathway is responsible for production of GABA in other organs, especially the kidneys and the β cells of the pancreas. GABA is metabolized to succinic acid by 2 enzymes, GABA transaminase and succinic semialdehyde dehydrogenase (SSADH) (see Fig. 79-11).

Glutamic Acid Decarboxylase (GAD) Deficiency (See Fig. 79-11)

GAD enzyme requires pyridoxine (vitamin B_6) as a cofactor. Two GAD enzymes (GAD_{65} and GAD_{67}) have been identified. GAD_{67} is the main enzyme in the brain and GAD_{65} is the major enzyme in the β cells. Antibodies against GAD_{65} and GAD_{67} are the major markers for type 1 diabetes and **stiff-man syndrome**, respectively. Deficiency of this enzyme has not been reported in humans. An association of mutations in GAD_{67} gene with cleft lip with and without cleft palate in human has been shown in 1 study. The gene for GAD_{65} is on chromosome 10p11.23 and that for GAD_{67} is on chromosome 2q31.

GABA Transaminase Deficiency (See Fig. 79-11)

This is a very rare autosomal recessive condition that has been reported in 2 infants from a single family. Clinical manifestations included severe psychomotor retardation, hypotonia, hyperreflexia, lethargy, refractory seizures, and increased linear growth. Increased concentrations of GABA and β-alanine were found in the spinal fluid. Evidence of leukodystrophy was noted in the postmortem examination of the brain. GABA transaminase deficiency is demonstrated in the brain and lymphocytes. No effective treatment is available. Treatment with vitamin B_6 has been ineffective. The gene for this enzyme is located on chromosome 16p13.3.

γ-Hydroxybutyric Aciduria (Succinic Semialdehyde Dehydrogenase Deficiency)

This is the most common genetic disorder of neurotransmitters. More than 350 patients with this enzyme deficiency (see Fig. 79-11) have been identified. Clinical manifestations, which usually begin in early infancy, include mild to moderate mental retardation, delayed speech, marked hypotonia, neuropsychiatric symptoms (sleep disturbances, anxiety, inattention, hyperactivity), nonprogressive ataxia, and seizures. Other associated findings are autistic features, hallucinations, and aggressive behavior.

Laboratory studies reveal marked elevations in γ-hydroxybutyric acid concentrations in the blood (up to 200-fold), spinal fluid (up to 1,200-fold), and urine (up to 800-fold). There is no acidosis. Urinary excretion of γ-hydroxybutyric acid decreases with age. About half of the affected subjects show EEG abnormalities. MRI of the brain may show increased T2 signal in the globus pallidus with cerebral and cerebellar atrophy.

Diagnosis can be confirmed by measurement of the enzyme activity in lymphocytes. Prenatal diagnosis has been achieved by measurement of γ-hydroxybutyric acid in the amniotic fluid and assay of the enzyme activity in the amniocytes or in biopsy specimens of chorionic villi.

Treatment has been largely ineffective; vigabatrin has produced some improvement in ataxia and mental status in some patients.

The condition is inherited as an autosomal recessive trait. The gene for succinic semialdehyde dehydrogenase is on chromosome 6p22; several disease-causing mutations have been identified in different families.

The role of γ-hydroxybutyric acid in the pathogenesis of this condition remains unclear, since administration of this compound to humans and animals has produced variably conflicting effects. γ-Hydroxybutyrate (GHB) has been used illicitly as a recreational drug with anesthetic effect and is 1 of the date-rape drugs (Chapter 108).

Histidine Decarboxylase Deficiency

Decarboxylation of histidine by histidine decarboxylase produces histamine, which functions as a neurotransmitter in the brain. Deficiency of this enzyme (expressed mainly in the posterior hypothalamus) results in deficiency of histamine in the central nervous system and has been shown to cause autosomal dominant form of Tourette syndrome in one family.

HYPERPROLINEMIA

Psychomotor retardation and seizures are common findings in most patients with hyperprolinemia type I and type II. Patients with type I hyperprolinemia also have an increased risk of developing schizophrenia. The contribution of increased concentration of proline to the pathogenesis of these conditions, however, remains unclear. The neurologic abnormalities observed in hyperprolinemia type II is now believed to be mainly due to development of vitamin B_6 dependency in this condition (Chapter 79.9).

3-PHOSPHOGLYCERATE DEHYDROGENASE DEFICIENCY

See Chapter 79.8.

PHOSPHOSERINE AMINOTRANSFERASE DEFICIENCY

See Chapter 79.8.

NONKETOTIC HYPERGLYCINEMIA

See Chapter 79.7.

BIBLIOGRAPHY

Please visit the Nelson Textbook of Pediatrics *website at www.expertconsult.com for the complete bibliography.*

79.12 Urea Cycle and Hyperammonemia (Arginine, Citrulline, Ornithine)

Iraj Rezvani and Marc Yudkoff

Catabolism of amino acids results in the production of free ammonia, which, in high concentration, is extremely toxic to

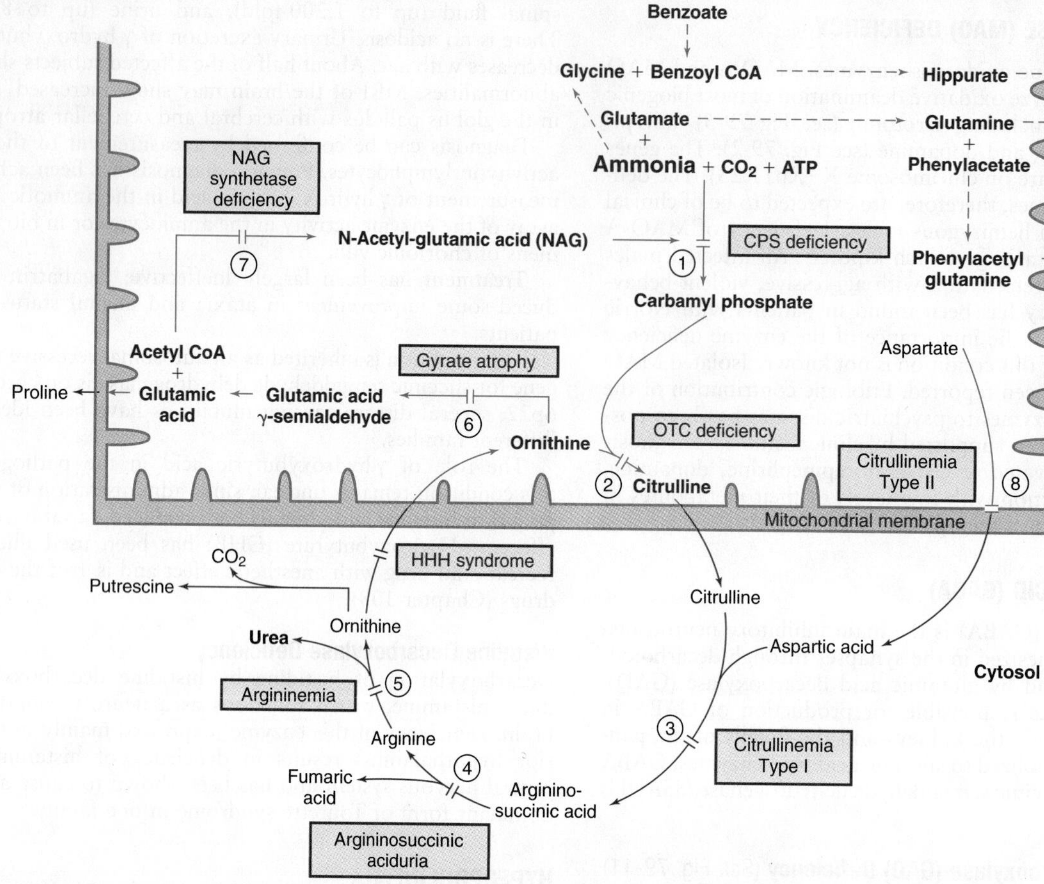

Figure 79-12 Urea cycle: pathways for ammonia disposal and ornithine metabolism. Reactions occurring in the mitochondria are depicted in *purple*. Reactions shown with *interrupted arrows* are the alternate pathways for the disposal of ammonia. **Enzymes:** *(1)* carbamyl phosphate synthetase (CPS), *(2)* ornithine transcarbamylase (OTC), *(3)* argininosuccinic acid synthetase (AS), *(4)* argininosuccinic acid lyase (AL), *(5)* arginase, *(6)* ornithine 5-aminotransferase, *(7)* *N*-acetylglutamate (NAG) synthetase, *(8)* citrin. HHH syndrome, hyperammonemia-hyperornithinemia-homocitrullinemia.

the CNS. In mammals ammonia is detoxified to urea via the urea cycle (Fig. 79-12). Five enzymes are involved in the synthesis of urea: carbamyl phosphate synthetase (CPS), ornithine transcarbamylase (OTC), argininosuccinate synthetase (AS), argininosuccinate lyase (AL), and arginase. A 6th enzyme, *N*-acetylglutamate synthetase, is also required for synthesis of *N*-acetylglutamate, which is an activator (effector) of the CPS enzyme. Individual deficiencies of these enzymes have been observed and, with an overall estimated prevalence of 1/30,000 live births, they are the most common genetic causes of hyperammonemia in infants.

Genetic Causes of Hyperammonemia

In addition to genetic defects of the urea cycle enzymes, a marked increase in plasma level of ammonia is observed in other genetic disorders of metabolism (Table 79-3); the pathogenesis for hyperammonemia in some of these conditions is not fully understood.

Clinical Manifestations of Hyperammonemia

In the **neonatal period**, symptoms and signs are mostly related to brain dysfunction and are similar regardless of the cause of the hyperammonemia. The affected infant is normal at birth but becomes symptomatic within a few days of protein feeding. Refusal to eat, vomiting, tachypnea, and lethargy can quickly progress to a deep coma. Convulsions are common. Physical examination may reveal hepatomegaly in addition to the neurologic signs of deep coma. Hyperammonemia can trigger increased intracranial pressure that may be manifested with bulging fontanel and dilated pupils.

Table 79-3 INBORN ERRORS OF METABOLISM CAUSING HYPERAMMONEMIA

Deficiencies of the urea cycle enzymes
Carbamyl phosphate synthetase (CPS)
Ornithine transcarbamylase (OTC)
Argininosuccinate synthetase (AS)
Argininosuccinate lyase (AL)
Arginase
N-Acetylglutamate synthetase
Organic acidemias
Propionic acidemia
Methylmalonic acidemia
Isovaleric acidemia
β-Ketothiolase deficiency
Multiple carboxylase deficiencies
Medium-chain fatty acid acyl CoA dehydrogenase deficiency
Glutaric acidemia type II
3-Hydroxy-3-methylglutaric aciduria
Lysinuric protein intolerance
Hyperammonemia-hyperornithinemia-homocitrullinemia syndrome
Transient hyperammonemia of the newborn
Congenital hyperinsulinism with hyperammonemia

In **infants and older children** acute hyperammonemia is manifested by vomiting and neurologic abnormalities such as ataxia, mental confusion, agitation, irritability, and combativeness. These manifestations may alternate with periods of lethargy and somnolence that may progress to coma.

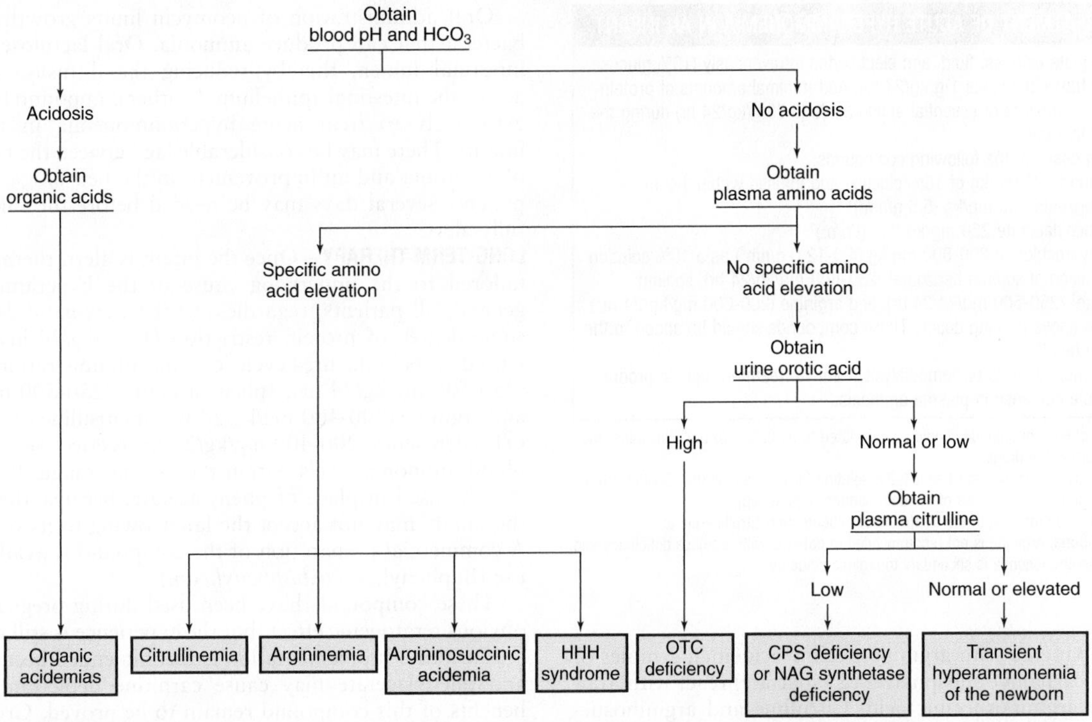

Figure 79-13 Clinical approach to a newborn infant with symptomatic hyperammonemia. CPS, carbamyl phosphate synthetase; HHH syndrome, hyperammonemia-hyperornithinemia-homocitrullinemia; NAG, *N*-acetylglutamate; OTC, ornithine transcarbamylase.

Routine laboratory studies show no specific findings when hyperammonemia is due to defects of the urea cycle enzymes. Blood urea nitrogen is usually low in these patients; serum pH is usually normal or mildly elevated. There may be mild increases in serum transaminases (ALT, AST) since ammonia can cause swelling of hepatic mitochondria. In infants with organic acidemias, hyperammonemia is commonly associated with severe acidosis as well as ketonuria. Newborn infants with hyperammonemia are often misdiagnosed as having sepsis; they may succumb without a correct diagnosis. Neuroimaging may reveal cerebral edema. Autopsy is usually unremarkable. It is imperative to measure plasma ammonia levels in any ill infant whose clinical manifestations cannot be explained by an obvious infection.

Diagnosis

The main criterion for diagnosis is hyperammonemia. Each clinical laboratory should establish its own normal values for blood ammonia; some variation is common. In the older child and adult, the normal limit is typically <35 µmole/L. Blood concentrations in healthy newborn infants often are higher (as high as 100 µmole/L in a full-term baby and 150 µmole/L in a premature infant). An approach to the differential diagnosis of hyperammonemia in the newborn infant is illustrated in Figure 79-13. Plasma amino acids reveal abnormalities that may help the diagnosis. In patients with deficiencies of either CPS, OTC, or *N*-acetylglutamate (NAG) synthetase frequent findings are elevations in plasma glutamine and alanine with concurrent decrements in citrulline and arginine. These disorders cannot be differentiated from one another by the plasma amino acid levels alone. A marked increase in urinary orotic acid in patients with OTC deficiency differentiates this defect from CPS deficiency. Differentiation between the CPS deficiency and the NAG synthetase deficiency may require an assay of the respective enzymes. Clinical improvement occurring after oral administration of carbamylglutamate, however, may suggest NAG synthetase deficiency. Patients with deficiencies of AS, AL, or arginase have marked increases in the plasma levels of citrulline, argininosuccinic acid, or arginine, respectively. Indeed, the combination of hyperammonemia and marked hypercitrullinemia or argininosuccinic acidemia is virtually pathognomonic for these disorders.

Treatment of Acute Hyperammonemia

The outcome for patients with hyperammonemic episodes depends mainly on the severity and duration of the hyperammonemia. Serious neurologic sequelae are highly likely in newborn infants with severe elevations in blood ammonia (>300 µmole/L) for more than 12 hr. Thus, hyperammonemia should be treated promptly and vigorously. The goal of therapy is to lower the concentration of ammonia in the body. This is accomplished in two ways: (1) by removal of ammonia from the body in a form other than urea, and (2) by provision of adequate calories and essential amino acids to minimize the endogenous protein degradation and favor protein synthesis (Table 79-4). Fluid, electrolytes, glucose (5-15%), and lipids (1-2 g/kg/24 hr) should be infused intravenously together with a minimal amount of protein (0.25 g/kg/24 hr), preferably in the form of essential amino acids. As soon as the clinical condition of the patient allows, oral feeding with a low-protein formula (0.5-1.0 g/kg/24 hr) through a nasogastric tube should be started.

An important advance in treatment of hyperammonemia has been the advent of acylation therapy in which exogenously administered organic acids form acyl adducts with endogenous nonessential amino acids. These adducts are nontoxic compounds with high renal clearances. The main organic acids used for this purpose are sodium salts of benzoic acid and phenylacetic acid. Benzoate forms hippuric acid with endogenous glycine in the liver (see Fig. 79-12). Each mole of benzoate removes 1 mole of ammonia as glycine. Phenylacetate conjugates with glutamine to form phenylacetylglutamine, which is readily excreted in the urine. One mole of phenylacetate removes 2 moles of ammonia as glutamine from the body (see Fig. 79-12).

Arginine administration is effective in the treatment of hyperammonemia that is due to most defects of the urea cycle because it supplies the urea cycle with ornithine and NAG (see Fig. 79-12). In patients with citrullinemia, 1 mole of arginine reacts with 1 mole of ammonia (as carbamyl phosphate) to form

Table 79-4 TREATMENT OF ACUTE HYPERAMMONEMIA IN AN INFANT

1. Provide adequate calories, fluid, and electrolytes intravenously (10% glucose, NaCl* and intravenous lipids 1 g/kg/24 hr). Add minimal amounts of protein preferably as a mixture of essential amino acids (0.25 g/kg/24 hr) during the 1st 24 hr of therapy.
2. Give priming doses of the following compounds:
   - To be added to 20 mL/kg of 10% glucose and infused within 1-2 hr
   - Sodium benzoate 250 mg/kg (5.5 g/nm^2)†
   - Sodium phenylacetate 250 mg/kg (5.5 g/nm^2)†
   - Arginine hydrochloride 200-600 mg/kg (4.0-12.0 g/nm^2) as a 10% solution
3. Continue infusion of sodium benzoate† (250-500 mg/kg/24 hr), sodium phenylacetate† (250-500 mg/kg/24 hr), and arginine (200-600 mg/kg/24 hr‡) following the above priming doses. These compounds should be added to the daily intravenous fluid.
4. Initiate peritoneal dialysis or hemodialysis if above treatment fails to produce an appreciable decrease in plasma ammonia.

*The concentration of sodium chloride should be calculated to be 0.45% to 0.9% including the amount of the sodium in the drugs.
†These compounds are usually prepared as a 1-2% solution for intravenous use. Sodium from these drugs should be included as part of the daily sodium requirement.
‡The higher dose is recommended in the treatment of patients with citrullinemia and argininosuccinic aciduria. Arginine is not recommended in patients with arginase deficiency and in those whose hyperammonemia is secondary to organic acidemia.

citrulline. In patients with argininosuccinic acidemia, 2 moles of ammonia (as carbamyl phosphate and aspartate) react with arginine to form argininosuccinic acid. Citrulline and argininosuccinic acid are far less toxic and more readily excreted by the kidneys than ammonia. In patients with CPS or OTC deficiency, arginine administration is indicated because arginine becomes an essential amino acid in these disorders. Patients with OTC deficiency benefit from supplementation with citrulline (200 mg/kg/24 hr), which reacts with 1 mole of ammonia (as aspartic acid) to form arginine. **Administration of arginine or citrulline is contraindicated in patients with arginase deficiency**, a rare condition in which the presenting clinical picture is one of spastic diplegia rather than hyperammonemia (see later). Furthermore, arginine therapy is of no benefit if hyperammonemia is secondary to an organic acidemia. However, in a newborn infant with a 1st attack of hyperammonemia, arginine should be used until the diagnosis is established.

Benzoate, phenylacetate, and arginine may be administered together for maximal therapeutic effect. A priming dose of these compounds is followed by continuous infusion until recovery from the acute state occurs (see Table 79-4). Both benzoate and phenylacetate are usually supplied as concentrated solutions and should be properly diluted (1-2% solution) for intravenous use. The recommended therapeutic doses of both compounds deliver a substantial amount of sodium to the patient that should be calculated as part of the daily sodium requirement. A commercial preparation of sodium benzoate plus sodium phenylacetate is available for intravenous use (Ammonul; *www.ammonul.com*). Benzoate and phenylacetate should be used with caution in newborn infants with hyperbilirubinemia because they may displace bilirubin from albumin. However, despite this theoretical risk, no documented case of kernicterus (Chapter 96.4) has yet been reported in neonates with hyperammonemia who have received such therapies.

If the foregoing therapies fail to produce any appreciable change in the blood ammonia level within a few hours, peritoneal dialysis, or preferably, hemodialysis should be used. Exchange transfusion has little effect on reducing total body ammonia. It should be used only if dialysis cannot be employed promptly or when the patient is a newborn infant with hyperbilirubinemia. Hemodialysis is the most effective measure, but if it is unavailable or technically unfeasible, peritoneal dialysis can decrease the plasma ammonia level within hours. When hyperammonemia is due to an organic acidemia, dialysis effectively removes both the offending organic acid and ammonia from the body.

Oral administration of neomycin limits growth of intestinal bacteria that can produce ammonia. Oral lactulose acidifies the intestinal lumen, thereby reducing the diffusion of ammonia across the intestinal epithelium. Neither compound has been used extensively to treat acute hyperammonemia in the newborn infants. There may be considerable lag between the normalization of ammonia and an improvement in the neurologic status of the patient. Several days may be needed before the infant becomes fully alert.

LONG-TERM THERAPY Once the infant is alert, therapy should be tailored to the underlying cause of the hyperammonemia. In general, all patients, regardless of the enzymatic defect, require some degree of protein restriction (1-2 g/kg/24 hr). In patients with defects in the urea cycle, chronic administration of benzoate (250-500 mg/kg/24 hr), phenylacetate (250-500 mg/kg/24 hr), and arginine (200-400 mg/kg/24 hr) or citrulline (in patients with OTC deficiency, 200-400 mg/kg/24 hr) is effective in maintaining blood ammonia levels within the normal range. Phenylbutyrate may be used in place of phenylacetate, because the patient and the family may not accept the latter owing to its offensive odor. A commercial preparation of the compound is available for oral use (Buphenyl; *www.buphenyl.com*).

These compounds have been used during pregnancy without obvious teratogenic effect, but the experience is still quite limited.

Carnitine supplementation is recommended because benzoate and phenylacetate may cause carnitine depletion; the clinical benefits of this compound remain to be proved. Growth parameters, especially head circumference and nutritional indices (blood albumin, prealbumin, pH, electrolytes, amino acids, zinc, selenium), should be followed closely. Long-term care of these patients is best achieved by a team of experienced professionals (physician specialist, nutritionist, neurologist, geneticist). Skin lesions resembling **acrodermatitis enteropathica** have been noted in a few patients with different types of urea cycle defects, presumably due to deficiency of essential amino acids, especially arginine, caused by overzealous dietary protein restriction. Catabolic states (infections, fasting) triggering hyperammonemia should be avoided or treated vigorously. It is important that all children with hyperammonemia syndromes avoid valproic acid (Depakote) as an anticonvulsant or mood stabilizer because this drug tends to cause elevation of blood ammonia even in healthy subjects. Liver transplant has been beneficial in some patients if no prior severe hyperammonemic crisis occurred.

Carbamyl Phosphate Synthetase (CPS) and N-Acetylglutamate (NAG) Synthetase Deficiencies (See Fig. 79-12)

Deficiencies of these 2 enzymes produce similar clinical and biochemical manifestations. There is a wide variation in severity of symptoms and in the age of presentation. In near complete enzymatic deficiency, symptoms appear during the 1st few days or even hours of life with signs and symptoms of hyperammonemia (refusal to eat, vomiting, lethargy, convulsion, and coma). Increased intracranial pressure is a frequent finding. Late forms (as late as 32 yr of age) may present as an acute bout of hyperammonemia (lethargy, headache, seizures, psychosis) in a seemingly normal individual. Coma and death may occur during these episodes (a previously asymptomatic 26 yr old female died from hyperammonemia during childbirth). Diagnostic confusion with migraine is frequent. Intermediate forms with mental retardation and chronic subclinical hyperammonemia interspersed with bouts of acute hyperammonemia have also been observed.

Laboratory findings include hyperammonemia. The plasma aminogram commonly shows a marked increase of glutamine and alanine with a relatively low levels of citrulline and arginine. Urinary orotic acid is usually low or may be absent (see Fig. 79-13).

Treatment of acute hyperammonemic attacks and the long-term therapy of the condition is outlined earlier (see Table 79-4). Patients with NAG synthetase deficiency benefit from oral administration of carbamylglutamate. It is therefore important to differentiate between CPS and NAG synthetase deficiencies by assay of the enzyme activities in liver biopsy specimens. Deficiency of NAG synthetase is rare in North America.

CPS deficiency is inherited as an autosomal recessive trait; the enzyme is normally present in the liver and intestine. The gene is on chromosome 2q35. Several disease-causing mutations have been found in different families. The prevalence of the condition is not known.

Ornithine Transcarbamylase (OTC) Deficiency (See Fig. 79-12)

In this X-linked partially dominant disorder, the hemizygote males are more severely affected than heterozygote females. The heterozygous females may have a mild form of the disease, but the majority (75%) is asymptomatic, although subtle neurologic defects may be present in women without a frank history of hyperammonemia. This is the most common form of all the urea cycle disorders, comprising about 40% of all cases.

Clinical manifestations in male newborn infants are usually those of severe hyperammonemia (see earlier) occurring in the 1st few days of life. Milder forms of the condition are commonly seen in heterozygous females and in some affected males. **Mild** forms characteristically have episodic manifestations, which may occur at any age (usually after infancy). Episodes of hyperammonemia (manifested by vomiting and neurologic abnormalities such as ataxia, mental confusion, agitation, and combativeness) are separated by periods of wellness. These episodes usually occur after ingestion of a high-protein diet or as a result of a catabolic state such as infection. Hyperammonemic coma, cerebral edema, and death may occur during 1 of these attacks. Mental development may proceed normally. Mild to moderate mental retardation, however, is common. Gallstones have been seen in the survivors; the mechanism remains unclear.

The major laboratory finding during the acute attack is hyperammonemia accompanied by marked elevations of plasma concentrations of glutamine and alanine with low levels of citrulline and arginine. Blood level of urea (BUN) is usually low. A marked increase in the urinary excretion of orotic acid differentiates this condition from CPS deficiency (see Fig. 79-13). Orotates may precipitate in urine as pink gravel. In the mild form, these laboratory abnormalities may revert to normal between attacks. This form should be differentiated from all the episodic conditions of childhood. In particular, patients with lysinuric protein intolerance (Chapter 79.13) may demonstrate some features of OTC deficiency, but the former can be differentiated by increased urinary excretion of lysine, ornithine, and arginine and elevated blood concentrations of citrulline.

The diagnosis may be confirmed by performing an assay of enzyme activity that is normally present only in the liver or by mutational analysis of the gene. Several commercial laboratories now offer sequencing of the OTC gene, although as many as 20% of affected patients demonstrate a normal sequence, perhaps because the mutation involves an intron or a leader sequence. Prenatal diagnosis has been achieved by means of fetal liver biopsy or by analysis of DNA in amniocytes or in chorionic villi samples. An oral protein load, which increases plasma ammonia and urinary orotic acid levels, may identify asymptomatic heterozygous female carriers. A marked increase in urinary excretion of orotidine after an allopurinol loading test also detects obligate female carriers. The importance of a detailed family history should be emphasized. A history of migraine or protein aversion is common in maternal female relatives of the proband. Indeed, careful scrutiny of the family history may reveal a pattern of unexplained deaths in male newborns in the maternal lineage.

Treatment of acute hyperammonemic attacks and the long-term therapy of the condition were outlined earlier. Citrulline is used in place of arginine in patients with OTC deficiency. Liver transplantation is a successful and definite treatment that has been utilized even in infants.

The gene for OTC is on Xp21.1. Many disease-causing mutations (>300) have been identified in different patients. The degree of enzyme deficiency determines severity of the phenotype in most cases. Mothers of affected infants are expected to be carriers of the mutant gene unless a de novo mutation has occurred. A mother who gave birth to 2 affected male offspring was found to have normal genotype, suggesting gonadal mosaicism in the mother.

Argininosuccinate Synthetase (AS) Deficiency (Citrullinemia) (See Fig. 79-12)

Two clinically and genetically distinct forms of citrullinemia have been identified. The classic form (type I) is due to the deficiency of the AS enzyme. The adult form (type II) is due to deficiency of a mitochondrial transport protein named citrin.

CITRULLINEMIA TYPE I (CLASSIC CITRULLINEMIA, CTLN 1) This condition is caused by the deficiency of AS (see Fig. 79-12) and has variable clinical manifestation depending on the degree of the enzyme deficiency. Two major forms of the condition have been identified. The **severe** or **neonatal form**, which is most common, appears in the 1st few days of life with signs and symptoms of hyperammonemia (see earlier). In the **subacute** or **mild form**, clinical findings such as failure to thrive, frequent vomiting, developmental delay, and dry, brittle hair appear gradually after 1 yr of age. Acute hyperammonemia, triggered by an intercurrent catabolic state, may bring the diagnosis to light.

Laboratory findings are similar to those found in patients with OTC deficiency except that the plasma citrulline concentration is markedly elevated (50-100 times normal) in citrullinemia type I (see Fig. 79-13). Urinary excretion of orotic acid is moderately increased; crystalluria due to precipitation of orotates may also occur. The diagnosis is confirmed by enzyme assay in cultured fibroblasts or by DNA analysis. Prenatal diagnosis is feasible with the assay of the enzyme activity in cultured amniotic cells or by DNA analysis of chorionic villi biopsy.

Treatment of acute hyperammonemic attacks and the long-term therapy of the condition are outlined above. Plasma concentration of citrulline remains elevated at all times and may increase further after administration of arginine. Although prognosis is poor for symptomatic neonates, patients with the mild disease usually do well on a protein-restricted diet in conjunction with sodium benzoate, phenylbutyrate and arginine therapy. Mild to moderate mental deficiency is common, even in a well-treated patient.

Citrullinemia is inherited as an autosomal recessive trait. The gene is located on chromosome 9q34.1. Several disease-causing mutations have been identified in different families. The majority of patients are compound heterozygotes for 2 different alleles. The prevalence of the condition is not known. The recent introduction of neonatal screening for urea cycle defects has disclosed affected patients who are ostensibly asymptomatic, even with ingestion of a regular diet. Long-term follow-up is needed to be certain that these individuals do not sustain neurologic sequelae.

CITRULLINEMIA DUE TO CITRIN DEFICIENCY (CITRULLINEMIA TYPE II, CLTN 2) Citrin (aspartate-glutamate carrier, AGC2) is a mitochondrial transport protein encoded by a gene (*SLC25A13*) on chromosome 7q21.3. The major function of this protein is to transport aspartate from mitochondria to cytoplasm; aspartate is required for converting citrulline to argininosuccinic acid (see Fig. 79-12). If aspartate is unavailable to the cytoplasmic component of the urea cycle, urea will not be formed at a normal rate and citrulline will accumulate in the body. AS activity is deficient in the liver of these patients, but no mutation in the gene for AS has been found. It is postulated that citrin deficiency or its mutated gene interferes with translation of mRNA for AS enzyme in the liver. The condition initially was reported among Japanese individuals but a few non-Japanese patients have also been identified. Two forms of citrin deficiency have been described.

NEONATAL INTRAHEPATIC CHOLESTASIS (CITRULLINEMIA TYPE II-NEONATAL FORM) Clinical and laboratory manifestations, which usually start before 1 yr of age, include cholestatic jaundice with mild to moderate direct (conjugated) hyperbilirubinemia, marked hypoproteinemia, clotting dysfunction (increased prothrombin time and partial thromboplastin times), and increased serum γ-glutamyltranspeptidase (GGTP) and alkaline phosphatase activities; liver transaminases are usually normal. Plasma concentrations of ammonia and citrulline are usually normal, but moderate elevations are reported. There may be increases in plasma concentrations of methionine, tyrosine, alanine, and threonine. Elevated levels of serum galactose may occur, but all enzymes involved in galactose metabolism are normal. The reason for hypergalactosemia is not known. Marked elevation in serum level of α-fetoprotein is also present. These findings resemble those of tyrosinemia type I, but unlike the latter condition, urinary excretion of succinylacetone is not elevated (Chapter 79.2). Liver biopsy shows fatty infiltration, cholestasis with dilated canaliculi, and a moderate degree of fibrosis. The condition is usually self-limiting and the majority of infants recover spontaneously by 1 yr of age with only supportive and symptomatic treatment. Hyperammonemia and hypercitrullinemia, if present, should be treated with low-protein diet and other appropriate measures (see earlier). Hepatic failure requiring liver transplantation has occurred in a few cases. The diagnosis should be considered in cases of unexplained neonatal hepatitis with cholestasis. Data on the long-term prognosis and the natural history of the condition are limited; development into the adult form of the condition after several years of seemingly asymptomatic hiatus has been observed.

Citrullinemia Type II, Adult Form (Adult-Onset Citrullinemia, Citrullinemia Type II-Mild Form) This form starts suddenly in a previously normal individual and manifests with neuropsychiatric symptoms such as disorientation, delirium, delusion, aberrant behavior, tremors, and frank psychosis. Moderate degrees of hyperammonemia and hypercitrullinemia are present. The age of onset is usually between 20 and 40 yr (range 11 to 79 yr). Patients who recover from the 1st episode may have recurrent attacks and most will die within a few years of diagnosis mainly from cerebral edema. Pancreatitis, hyperlipidemia, and hepatoma are major complications among the survivors. **Treatment** of an acute attack is mainly supportive and symptomatic. Administration of large amounts of glucose and restriction of dietary protein, both of which seem intuitively beneficial, may have deleterious effects by aggravating cytosolic aspartate deficiency. Liver transplantation is the most effective therapy and should be considered soon after recovery from the first attack.

Several disease-causing mutations of the gene have been identified. The pathogenesis of citrullinemia type II (neonatal and adult forms) remains enigmatic. Although the frequency of the disease-causing gene is quite high in Japan (1:20,000 homozygosity), the clinical condition has a frequency of only 1:100,000. This indicates that a substantial number of homozygous individuals remain asymptomatic.

Argininosuccinate Lyase (AL) Deficiency (Argininosuccinic Aciduria) (See Fig. 79-12)

The severity of the clinical and biochemical manifestations varies considerably. In the **neonatal form**, signs and symptoms of severe hyperammonemia (see earlier) develop in the 1st few days of life and mortality is usually high. Survivors manifest a **subacute or late form** that is characterized by mental retardation, failure to thrive and hepatomegaly. Abnormalities of the hair characterized by dryness and brittleness are of special diagnostic value (trichorrhexis nodosa). Gallstones have been seen in some of the survivors. Acute attacks of severe hyperammonemia commonly occur during a catabolic state.

Laboratory findings include hyperammonemia, moderate elevations in liver enzymes, nonspecific increases in plasma levels of glutamine and alanine, moderate increase in plasma levels of citrulline (less than that seen in citrullinemia), and marked increase in plasma levels of argininosuccinic acid (see Fig. 79-13). In most amino acid analyzers, argininosuccinic acid appears as series of anhydrides within the isoleucine or methionine region, which may cause confusion in the diagnosis. Argininosuccinic acid can also be found in large amounts in urine and spinal fluid. The levels in the spinal fluid are usually higher than those in plasma. The enzyme is normally present in erythrocytes, the liver, and cultured fibroblasts. Prenatal diagnosis is possible by measurement of the enzyme activity in cultured amniotic cells or by identification of the mutant gene. Argininosuccinic acid is also elevated in the amniotic fluid of affected fetuses.

Treatment of acute hyperammonemic attacks and the long-term therapy of the condition were outlined earlier. Mental retardation, persistent hepatomegaly with mild increases in liver enzymes, and bleeding tendencies due to abnormal clotting factors are common sequelae. This deficiency is inherited as an autosomal recessive trait with a prevalence of ≈1/70,000 live births. The gene is located on chromosome 7cen-q11.2

Arginase Deficiency (Hyperargininemia) (See Fig. 79-12)

This defect is inherited as an autosomal recessive trait. There are 2 genetically distinct arginases in humans. One is cytosolic (A1) and is expressed in the liver and erythrocytes, and the other (A2) is found in the renal and brain mitochondria. The gene for cytosolic enzyme, which is the 1 deficient in patients with arginase deficiency, is mapped to chromosome 6q23. The role of the mitochondrial enzyme is not well understood; its activity increases in patients with argininemia but has no protective effect. Several disease-causing mutations have been identified in different families.

The clinical manifestations of this rare condition are quite different from those of other urea cycle enzyme defects. The onset is insidious; the infant usually remains asymptomatic in the 1st few months or, sometimes, years of life. A **progressive spastic diplegia** with scissoring of the lower extremities, choreoathetotic movements, and loss of developmental milestones in a previously normal infant may suggest a degenerative disease of the CNS. Two children were treated for several years as cerebral palsy before the diagnosis of arginase deficiency was confirmed. Mental retardation is progressive; seizures are common, but episodes of severe hyperammonemia are not usually seen in this disorder. Hepatomegaly may be present. The acute neonatal form with intractable seizures, cerebral edema, and death has also been reported.

Laboratory findings include marked elevations of arginine in plasma and CSF (see Fig. 79-13). Urinary orotic acid is moderately increased. Plasma ammonia levels may be normal or mildly elevated. Urinary excretions of arginine, lysine, cystine, and ornithine are usually increased, but normal levels have also been noted. Therefore, determination of amino acids in plasma is a critical step in the diagnosis of argininemia. The guanidino compounds (α-keto-guanidinovaleric acid, argininic acid) are markedly increased in urine. The diagnosis is confirmed by assaying arginase activity in erythrocytes.

Treatment consists of a low-protein diet devoid of arginine. Administration of a synthetic protein made of essential amino acids usually results in a dramatic decrease in plasma arginine concentration and an improvement in neurologic abnormalities. The composition of the diet and the daily intake of protein should be monitored by frequent plasma amino acid determinations. Sodium benzoate (250-375 mg/kg/24 hr) is also effective in controlling hyperammonemia, when present; lowering of plasma arginine levels has been noted with this treatment. Mental retardation is a common sequela of the condition. One patient developed type 1 diabetes at age 9 yr while his argininemia was under good control.

Transient Hyperammonemia of the Newborn

Blood concentration of ammonia in some healthy full-term infants may be as high as 100 μmole/L, or 2 to 3 times higher than that of the older child or adult. In premature infants the upper limit of normal for blood ammonia may be as high as 150 µmole/L. Blood levels approximate the adult normal values after a few weeks of life. These infants are asymptomatic, and follow-up studies up to 18 mo of age have not revealed any significant neurologic deficits.

Severe transient hyperammonemia has been observed in newborn infants. The majority of affected infants is premature and has mild respiratory distress syndrome. Hyperammonemic coma may develop within 2-3 days of life, and the infant may succumb to the disease if treatment is not started immediately. Laboratory studies reveal marked hyperammonemia (plasma ammonia as high as 4,000 µmole/L) with moderate increases in plasma levels of glutamine and alanine. Plasma concentrations of urea cycle intermediate amino acids are usually normal. The cause of the disorder is unknown. Urea cycle enzyme activities are normal. **Treatment** of hyperammonemia should be initiated promptly and continued vigorously (see above). Recovery without sequelae is common, and hyperammonemia does not recur even with a normal protein diet.

Ornithine

Ornithine is 1 of the intermediate metabolites of the urea cycle that is not incorporated into natural proteins. Rather, it is generated in the cytosol from arginine and must be transported into the mitochondria where it is used as a substrate for the enzyme OTC to form citrulline. Excess ornithine is catabolized by 2 enzymes, ornithine 5-aminotransferase, which is a mitochondrial enzyme and converts ornithine to a proline precursor, and ornithine decarboxylase, which resides in the cytosol and converts ornithine to putrescine (see Fig. 79-12). Two genetic disorders result in hyperornithinemia: gyrate atrophy of the retina and hyperammonemia-hyperornithinemia-homocitrullinemia syndrome.

GYRATE ATROPHY OF THE RETINA AND CHOROID This is a rare autosomal recessively inherited disorder caused by the deficiency of the enzyme ornithine 5-aminotransferase (see Fig. 79-12). About 30% of the reported cases are from Finland. Clinical manifestations are limited to the eyes and include night blindness, myopia, loss of peripheral vision, and posterior subcapsular cataracts. These eye changes start between 5 and 10 yr of age and progress to complete blindness by the 4th decade of life. Atrophic lesions in the retina resemble cerebral gyri. These patients usually have normal intelligence. There is a 10- to 20-fold increase in plasma levels of ornithine (400-1,400 µmole/L). There are no hyperammonemia and no increases in any other amino acids; plasma levels of glutamate, glutamine, lysine, creatine, and creatinine are moderately decreased. Some patients respond partially to high doses of pyridoxine (500-1,000 mg/24 hr). Arginine-restricted diet in conjunction with supplemental lysine, proline, and creatine has been successful in reducing plasma ornithine concentration and has produced some clinical improvements. The gene for ornithine 5-aminotransferase is on chromosome 10q26. Many (at least 60) disease-causing mutations have been identified in different families.

Hyperammonemia-Hyperornithinemia-Homocitrullinemia (HHH) Syndrome

In this rare autosomal recessively inherited disorder, the defect is in the transport system of ornithine from the cytosol into the mitochondria, resulting in accumulation of ornithine in the cytosol and its deficiency in the mitochondria. The former causes hyperornithinemia and the latter results in disruption of the urea cycle and hyperammonemia (see Fig. 79-12). Homocitrulline is presumably formed from the reaction of mitochondrial carbamyl phosphate with lysine, which occurs because of the intramitochondrial deficiency of ornithine. Clinical manifestations of hyperammonemia may develop shortly after birth or may be delayed until adulthood. Acute episodes of hyperammonemia manifest as refusal to feed, vomiting, and lethargy; coma may occur during infancy. Progressive neurologic signs, such as lower limb weakness, increased deep tendon reflexes, spasticity, clonus, seizures, and varying degrees of psychomotor retardation may develop if the condition remains undiagnosed. No clinical ocular findings have been observed in these patients.

Laboratory findings reveal marked increases in plasma levels of ornithine and homocitrulline in addition to hyperammonemia. Restriction of protein intake improves hyperammonemia. Ornithine supplementation may produce clinical improvement in some patients. The gene for this disorder (*SLC25A15*) is on chromosome 13q14.

BIBLIOGRAPHY

Please visit the Nelson Textbook of Pediatrics *website at www.expertconsult.com for the complete bibliography.*

79.13 Histidine

Iraj Rezvani

Histidine is an essential amino acid only during infancy. Its biosynthetic pathway in older children and adults is poorly understood. Histidine is degraded through the urocanic acid pathway to glutamic acid. Several genetic biochemical aberrations involving the degradative pathway of histidine have been reported, but none has any clinical consequence.

Decarboxylation of histidine by histidine decarboxylase produces histamine. Deficiency of this enzyme has been shown to be the cause of familial form of Tourette's syndrome (Chapter 79.11).

BIBLIOGRAPHY

Please visit the Nelson Textbook of Pediatrics *website at www.expertconsult.com for the complete bibliography.*

79.14 Lysine

Iraj Rezvani

Lysine is catabolized through 2 pathways. In the first pathway, lysine is condensed with α-ketoglutaric acid to form saccharopine. Saccharopine is then metabolized to α-aminoadipic acid semialdehyde and glutamic acid. These 1st 2 steps are catalyzed by α-aminoadipic semialdehyde synthase, which has 2 activities: lysine-ketoglutarate reductase, and saccharopine dehydrogenase (Fig. 79-14). In the second pathway, lysine is first transaminated and then condensed to its cyclic forms, pipecolic acid and piperidine-6-carboxylic acid. The latter compound and its linear form, α-aminoadipic acid semialdehyde, are oxidized to α-aminoadipic acid by the enzyme antiquitin. This is the major pathway for D-lysine in the body and for the L-lysine in the brain (see Fig. 79-14).

Hyperlysinemia, *α-aminoadipic acidemia*, and *α-ketoadipic acidemia* are 3 biochemical conditions that are due to inborn errors of metabolism of lysine. Individuals with these conditions are usually asymptomatic.

Pyridoxine (Vitamin B_6)-Dependent Epilepsy

Pyridoxal 5′-phosphate, the active form of pyridoxine, is the cofactor for many enzymes including those involved in the metabolism of neurotransmitters. Intracellular deficiency of pyridoxal 5′-phosphate in the brain may result in a seizure disorder that is responsive to high doses of pyridoxine. This pyridoxine-dependent epilepsy is seen in the following genetic metabolic conditions:

ANTIQUITIN (α-AMINOADIPIC SEMIALDEHYDE DEHYDROGENASE) DEFICIENCY This is the most common cause of pyridoxine-dependent epilepsy. Deficiency of antiquitin (named because of preservation of its structure from garden pea to human) results in

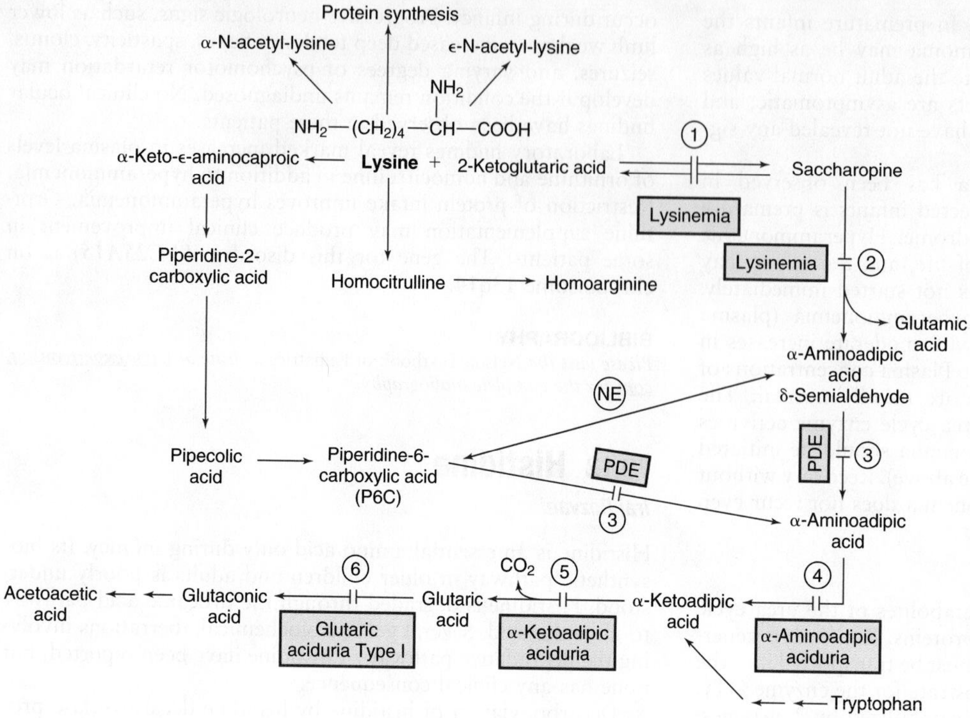

Figure 79-14 Pathways in the metabolism of lysine. **Enzymes:** *(1)* lysine ketoglutarate reductase, *(2)* saccharopine dehydrogenase, *(3)* α-aminoadipic semialdehyde/piperidine-6-carboxylic acid (P6C) dehydrogenase (antiquitin) *(4)* α-aminoadipic acid transferase, *(5)* α-ketoadipic acid dehydrogenase, *(6)* glutaryl CoA dehydrogenase. NE, nonenzymatic; PDE, pyridoxine dependent epilepsy.

accumulation of Δ^1-piperidine-6-carboxylic acid (P6C) in brain tissue (see Fig. 79-14); P6C reacts with pyridoxal 5′-phosphate and renders it inactive. Large doses of pyridoxine are, therefore, needed to overcome this inactivation.

HYPERPROLINEMIA TYPE II In this condition, accumulation of Δ^1-pyrroline-5-carboxylic acid (P5C) in brain tissue causes inactivation of pyridoxal 5′-phosphate and hence pyridoxine dependency (Chapter 79.9 and Fig. 79-10).

HYPOPHOSPHATASIA Pyridoxal 5′-phosphate is the main circulating form of pyridoxine. Alkaline phosphatase is required for dephosphorylation of pyridoxal 5′-phosphate to generate free pyridoxine which is the only form of vitamin B_6 that can cross the blood-brain barrier and enter the brain cells. Pyridoxine is rephosphorylated intracellularly to form pyridoxal 5′-phosphate. In the infantile form of hypophosphatasia, marked deficiency of tissue nonspecific alkaline phosphatase causes intracellular deficiency of pyridoxine and, therefore, pyridoxine-dependent epilepsy (Chapter 696).

The main clinical manifestation of **pyridoxine-dependent epilepsy** due to antiquitin deficiency is generalized seizures, which usually occur in the 1st few hours of life and are unresponsive to anticonvulsant therapy. Some mothers of affected fetuses report abnormal intrauterine fluttering movements. The seizures are usually tonic-clonic in nature but can be almost any type. Other manifestations such as dystonia, respiratory distress, and abdominal distension with vomiting, hepatomegaly, and hypothermia may be present. Late onset forms of the condition (as late as 5 yr of age) have been reported. A trial with vitamin B_6, therefore, is recommended in any infant with intractable convulsions.

Laboratory studies reveal increased concentrations of α-aminoadipic semialdehyde and pipecolic acid in the CSF, plasma, and urine. EEG shows abnormalities corresponding to the seizures; these changes usually normalize after treatment. Neuroimaging may be normal but cerebellar and cerebral atrophy, periventricular hyperintensity, intracerebral hemorrhage, and hydrocephalus may be present.

Treatment with large doses of vitamin B_6 (5 to 100 mg/kg) usually results in a dramatic improvement of both seizures and the EEG abnormalities. The dependency and hence the therapy are lifelong. Learning problems and speech delay are common sequelae. The condition is inherited as an autosomal recessive trait; the gene for antiquitin (*ALDH7A1*) is on chromosome 5q31.

Glutaric Aciduria Type I

Glutaric acid is an intermediate in the degradation of lysine (see Fig. 79-14), hydroxylysine, and tryptophan. Glutaric aciduria type I, a disorder caused by a deficiency of glutaryl CoA dehydrogenase, should be differentiated from glutaric aciduria type II, a distinct clinical and biochemical disorder caused by defects in the electron transport system (Chapter 80.1).

CLINICAL MANIFESTATIONS Affected infants with glutaric aciduria type I may develop normally up to 2 yr of life; macrocephaly is a common finding in these infants. Symptoms of hypotonia, loss of head control, choreoathetosis, seizures, generalized rigidity, opisthotonos, and dystonia may occur suddenly in a seemingly normal infant after a minor infection. Recovery from the 1st attack usually occurs slowly, but some residual neurologic abnormalities, especially dystonia and extrapyramidal movements, may persist. Additional acute episodes resembling the 1st one usually occur during an intercurrent infection. In other patients, these signs and symptoms may develop gradually in the 1st few years of life and hypotonia and choreoathetosis may gradually progress into rigidity and dystonia. Acute episodes of metabolic decompensation with vomiting, ketosis, seizures, and coma also commonly occur in these patients after infection or other catabolic states. Death usually occurs in the 1st decade of life during one of these episodes. The intellectual abilities usually remain relatively normal in most patients.

LABORATORY FINDINGS During acute episodes, mild to moderate metabolic acidosis and ketosis may occur. Hypoglycemia, hyperammonemia, and elevations of serum transaminases are seen in some patients. High concentrations of glutaric acid are usually found in urine, blood, and CSF. 3-Hydroxyglutaric acid may also be present in the urine. Plasma amino acid concentrations are usually within normal limits. Laboratory findings may be unremarkable between attacks. Severely affected children without glutaric aciduria have also been reported. In some of these patients, the glutaric acid is elevated only in the spinal fluid. In any child with progressive dystonia and dyskinesia, activity of the enzyme glutaryl CoA dehydrogenase should be measured in leukocytes or cultured fibroblasts. Neuroimaging of the brain may reveal macrocephaly, increased extra-axial (particularly frontal) fluid, striatal lesions, dilated lateral ventricles, cortical atrophy and fibrosis.

TREATMENT A low-protein diet (especially a diet restricted in lysine and tryptophan) and high doses (200-300 mg/24 hr) of riboflavin (the coenzyme for glutaryl CoA dehydrogenase) and L-carnitine (50-100 mg/kg/24 hr orally) produce a dramatic decrease in the levels of glutaric acid in body fluids, but their effects on the clinical outcome have been variable. Early diagnosis (through newborn screening) with prevention and aggressive treatment of intercurrent catabolic states (infections) are shown to minimize striatal insults and assure a more favorable prognosis. The addition of a GABA analog (baclofen) and valproic acid to the therapeutic regimen produces improvement in some affected children.

The condition is inherited as an autosomal recessive trait. The prevalence is not known. The condition is more prevalent in Sweden and among the Old Order Amish population in the USA. The gene is located on chromosome 19p13.2 and many disease-causing mutations have been reported in different families. A single mutation (*A421V*) accounts for all the patients from Lancaster County Old Order Amish.

Prenatal diagnosis may be accomplished by demonstrating increased concentrations of glutaric acid in amniotic fluid, by the assay of the enzyme activity in amniocytes or chorionic villi samples, or by identification of the mutant gene.

Lysinuric Protein Intolerance (Familial Protein Intolerance)

This rare autosomal recessive disorder is due to a defect in the transport of the cationic amino acids lysine, ornithine, and arginine in both kidneys and intestine. Unlike patients with cystinuria, urinary excretion of cystine is not increased in these patients. About half of the reported cases have been from Finland, where the prevalence has been estimated to be 1/60,000.

Clinical manifestations consist of refusal to feed, nausea, aversion to protein, vomiting, and mild diarrhea, which may result in failure to thrive, wasting, and hypotonia. Breast-fed infants usually remain asymptomatic until shortly after weaning. This may be due to the low protein content of breast milk. Episodes of hyperammonemia may occur after ingestion of a high-protein diet. Mild to moderate hepatosplenomegaly, osteoporosis, sparse brittle hair, thin extremities with moderate centripetal adiposity, and growth retardation are common physical findings in patients whose condition has remained undiagnosed. Mental development is usually normal, but moderate mental retardation has been observed in 20% of patients. **Interstitial pneumonitis** manifesting with fever, fatigue, cough, and dyspnea occur as an acute episode or as a chronic progressive process. Some patients have remained undiagnosed until the appearance of pulmonary manifestations. Radiographic evidence of pulmonary fibrosis has been observed in up to 65% of patients without clinical manifestations of pulmonary involvement. Acute pulmonary proteinosis with renal involvement resembling glomerulonephritis has occurred in older patients and may cause death.

Laboratory findings may reveal hyperammonemia and an elevated concentration of urinary orotic acid, which develop only after protein feeding. Fasting blood ammonia and urinary orotic acid excretion are usually normal. Plasma concentrations of lysine, arginine, and ornithine are usually mildly decreased, but urinary levels of these amino acids, especially lysine, are greatly increased. The mechanism producing hyperammonemia is not clear. All enzymes of the urea cycle are normal. Hyperammonemia may be related to a disturbance of the urea cycle secondary to a deficiency of arginine and ornithine. However, in patients with cystinuria who also have defects in the transport of lysine, arginine, and ornithine in both intestine and kidneys, hyperammonemia is not observed. Plasma concentrations of alanine, glutamine, serine, glycine, proline, and citrulline are usually increased. These abnormalities may be secondary to hyperammonemia and are not specific to this disorder.

Mild anemia and increased serum levels of ferritin, lactic dehydrogenase (LDH), and thyroxine-binding globulin have also been observed in these patients. This condition should be differentiated from hyperammonemia due to urea cycle defects (Chapter 79.11), especially in heterozygous females with OTC deficiency. Increased urinary excretion of lysine, ornithine, and arginine and elevated blood levels of citrulline are not seen in patients with OTC deficiency.

The transport defect in this condition resides in the basolateral (antiluminal) membrane of enterocytes and renal tubular epithelia. This explains the observation that cationic amino acids are unable to cross these cells even when administered as dipeptides. Lysine in the form of dipeptide crosses the luminal membrane of the enterocytes but hydrolyzes to free lysine molecules in the cytoplasm. Free lysine, unable to cross the basolateral membrane of the cells, diffuses back into the lumen.

Treatment with a low-protein diet (1.0-1.5 g/kg/24 hr) supplemented with citrulline (3-8 g/day) has produced biochemical and clinical improvements. Episodes of hyperammonemia should be treated promptly (Chapter 79.12). Supplementation with lysine is not useful because it is poorly absorbed and tends to produce diarrhea and abdominal pain. Treatment with high doses of prednisone and bronchoalveolar lavage has been effective in the management of acute pulmonary complications.

The gene for lysinuric protein intolerance (*SLC7A7*) is mapped to chromosome 14q11.2 and several disease-causing mutations have been identified in different families. Pregnancies in affected mothers have been complicated by anemia, thrombocytopenia, toxemia, and bleeding, but offspring have been normal.

BIBLIOGRAPHY

Please visit the Nelson Textbook of Pediatrics *website at* *www.expertconsult.com* *for the complete bibliography.*

79.15 Aspartic Acid (Canavan Disease)

Amanda A. Trott, Kimberlee M. Matalon, Marie Michelle Grino, and Reuben K. Matalon

N-Acetylaspartic acid, a derivative of aspartic acid, is synthesized in the brain and is found in a high concentration, similar to that of glutamic acid. Its function is unknown, but it serves as reservoir for acetate, which is needed for myelin synthesis. Excessive amounts of *N*-acetylaspartic acid in urine and deficiency of the enzyme aspartoacylase that cleaves the *N*-acetyl group from *N*-acetylaspartic acid are associated with Canavan disease.

Canavan Disease

Canavan disease, an autosomal recessive disorder characterized by spongy degeneration of the white matter of the brain, leads to a severe form of leukodystrophy. It is more prevalent in individuals of Ashkenazi Jewish descent than in other ethnic groups.

ETIOLOGY AND PATHOLOGY The deficiency of the enzyme aspartoacylase leads to the accumulation of *N*-acetylaspartic acid in the brain, especially in white matter, and massive urinary excretion of this compound. Excessive amounts of *N*-acetylaspartic acid are also present in the blood and CSF. There is striking vacuolization and astrocytic swelling in white matter. Electron microscopy reveals distorted mitochondria. As the disease progresses, the ventricles enlarge, owing to cerebral atrophy.

CLINICAL MANIFESTATIONS The severity of Canavan disease covers a wide spectrum. Infants usually appear normal at birth and may not manifest symptoms of the disease until 3-6 mo of age, when they develop progressive macrocephaly, severe hypotonia, and persistent head lag. As the infant grows older, delayed milestones become evident. These children become hyperreflexic and hypertonic; joint "stiffness" and contractures may be encountered, as is commonly seen in cerebral palsy. As these patients grow older, seizures and optic atrophy develop. Feeding difficulties, poor weight gain, and gastroesophageal reflux may occur in the 1st yr of life; swallowing deteriorates in the 2nd and 3rd yr of life, and nasogastric feeding or permanent gastrostomy may be required. Most patients die in the 1st decade of life; with improved nursing care, they may survive through the 2nd decade.

ATYPICAL CANAVAN DISEASE Mildly affected patients with Canavan disease have mutations that are less severe in their biochemical effects. These include (Y288C), a substitution of tyrosine with cysteine, or (R71H), a substitution of arginine with histidine, and others. Such patients have very mild delays and are often not suspected of having Canavan disease. However, the urinary excretion of *N*-acetylaspartic acid is moderately increased, which raises the question of Canavan disease. Brain MRI demonstrates increased signal intensity in the basal ganglia rather than global white matter disease, sometimes leading to confusion with mitochondrial disease. In the very young patient with typical Canavan disease, as well, severe white matter disease may not be seen in the white matter of the brain, and mitochondrial disease may be suspected. However, the diagnosis will be reached by determining the level of *N*-acetylaspartic acid in urine or after magnetic resonance spectroscopy (MRS) of the brain.

DIAGNOSIS In a typical patient with Canavan disease, CT scan and MRI reveal diffuse white matter degeneration, primarily in the cerebral hemispheres, with less involvement of the cerebellum and brainstem (Fig. 79-15). Repeated evaluations may be required. MRS performed at the time MRI is done can show the high peak of *N*-acetylaspartic acid, suggesting Canavan disease. The differential diagnosis of Canavan disease should include Alexander disease, which is another leukodystrophy associated with macrocephaly. Progression is usually slower in Alexander disease; hypotonia is not as pronounced as it is in Canavan disease. Brain biopsies of patients with Canavan disease show spongy degeneration of the myelin fibers, astrocytic swelling, and elongated mitochondria. Definitive diagnosis can be established by finding elevated amounts of *N*-acetylaspartic acid in the urine or blood. A deficiency of aspartoacylase can be found in cultured skin fibroblasts. The biochemical method is the preferred choice for diagnosis. *N*-acetylaspartic acid is found only in trace amounts (24 ± 16 μmol/mmol creatinine) in the urine of unaffected individuals, whereas in patients with Canavan disease its concentration is in the range of 1,440 ± 873 μmol/mmol creatinine. High levels of *N*-acetylaspartic acid can also be detected in plasma, CSF, and brain tissue. The activity of aspartoacylase in the fibroblasts of obligate carriers is less than or equal to half of the activity found in normal individuals.

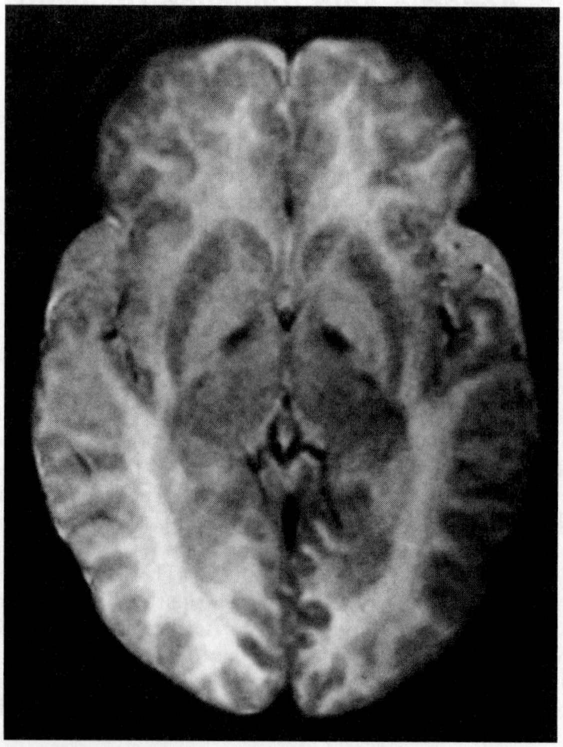

Figure 79-15 Axial T weighted MRI of a 2 yr old patient with Canavan disease. Extensive thickening of the white matter is seen.

The gene for aspartoacylase has been cloned, and mutations leading to Canavan disease have been identified. There are 2 mutations predominant in the Ashkenazi Jewish population. The 1st is an amino acid substitution (E285A) in which glutamic acid is substituted for alanine. This mutation is the most frequent and encompasses 83% of 100 mutant alleles examined in Ashkenazi Jewish patients. The second common mutation is a change from tyrosine to a nonsense mutation, leading to a stop in the coding sequence (Y231X). This mutation accounts for 13% of the 100 mutant alleles. In the non-Jewish population, more diverse mutations have been observed, and the 2 mutations common in Jewish people are rare. A different mutation (A305E), substitution of alanine for glutamic acid, accounts for 40% of 62 mutant alleles in non-Jewish patients. There have been more than 50 mutations described in the non-Jewish population. With Canavan disease, it is important to obtain a molecular diagnosis because this will lead to accurate counseling and prenatal guidance for the family. If the mutations are not known, prenatal diagnosis relies on the level of *N*-acetylaspartic acid in the amniotic fluid. In Ashkenazi Jewish patients, the carrier frequency can be as high as 1:36, which is close to that of Tay-Sachs disease. Carrier screening for Canavan disease is now in practice for Jewish individuals.

TREATMENT AND PREVENTION No specific treatment is available. Feeding problems and seizures should be treated on an individual basis. Genetic counseling, carrier testing, and prenatal diagnosis are the only methods of prevention. Gene therapy for Canavan disease has been attempted but not yet successful. There are currently ongoing trials of glycerol-triacetate as a supplement for acetate deficiency; the results of these trials are not yet available. There are also ongoing attempts to deliver aspartoacylase across the blood-brain barrier. These experiments have shown promise in the Canavan mouse and need to be confirmed in humans with Canavan disease.

BIBLIOGRAPHY

Please visit the Nelson Textbook of Pediatrics *website at* *www.expertconsult.com* *for the complete bibliography.*

Chapter 80
Defects in Metabolism of Lipids

80.1 Disorders of Mitochondrial Fatty Acid β-Oxidation

Charles A. Stanley and Michael J. Bennett

Mitochondrial β-oxidation of fatty acids is an essential energy-producing pathway. It is a particularly important pathway during prolonged periods of starvation, and during periods of reduced caloric intake due to gastrointestinal illness or increased energy expenditure during febrile illness. Under these conditions, the body switches from using predominantly carbohydrate to predominantly fat as its major fuel. Fatty acids are also important fuels for exercising skeletal muscle and are the preferred substrate for the heart. In these tissues, fatty acids are completely oxidized to carbon dioxide and water. The end products of hepatic fatty acid oxidation are the ketone bodies β-hydroxybutyrate and acetoacetate. These cannot be oxidized by the liver but serve as important fuels in peripheral tissues, particularly the brain.

Genetic defects have been identified in nearly all of the known steps in the fatty acid oxidation pathway; all are recessively inherited (Table 80-1).

Clinical manifestations characteristically involve the tissues with a high β-oxidation flux including liver, skeletal, and cardiac muscle. The most common presentation is an acute episode of life-threatening coma and hypoglycemia induced by a period of fasting due to defective hepatic ketogenesis. Other manifestations include chronic cardiomyopathy and muscle weakness or exercise-induced acute rhabdomyolysis. The fatty acid oxidation defects can be asymptomatic during periods when there is no fasting stress. Acutely presenting disease may be misdiagnosed as Reye

Table 80-1 MITOCHONDRIAL FATTY ACID OXIDATION DISORDERS—CLINICAL AND BIOCHEMICAL FEATURES

ENZYME DEFICIENCY	GENE	CLINICAL PHENOTYPE	LABORATORY FINDINGS
Carnitine transporter	*OCTN2*	Cardiomyopathy, skeletal myopathy, liver disease, sudden death, endocardial fibroelastosis, prenatal and NB screening diagnosis reported	↓ Total and free carnitine, normal acylcarnitines, acylglycine, and organic acids
Long-chain fatty acid transporter	*FATP1-6*	Rare, acute liver failure in childhood requiring liver transplantation	Reduced intracellular C_{14}-C_{18} fatty acids, reduced fatty acid oxidation
Carnitine palmitoyl transferase-I	*CPT-IA*	Liver failure, renal tubulopathy, and sudden death. Prenatal and NB screening diagnosis reported, maternal preeclampsia, HELLP syndrome association described in a few patients.	Normal or ↑ free carnitine, normal acylcarnitines, acylglycine, and organic acids
Carnitine acylcarnitine translocase	*CACT*	Chronic progressive liver failure, persistent ↑ NH_3, hypertrophic cardiomyopathy. NB screening diagnosis reported	Normal or ↓ free carnitine, abnormal acylcarnitine profile
Carnitine palmitoyl transferase-II	*CPT-II*	Early and late onset types. Liver failure, encephalopathy, skeletal myopathy, cardiomyopathy, renal cystic changes, NB screening diagnosis reported.	Normal or ↓ free carnitine, abnormal acylcarnitine profile
Short-chain acyl CoA dehydrogenase	*SCAD*	Clinical phenotype is unclear. Many individuals appear to be normal. Others have a variety of inconsistent signs and symptoms.	Normal or ↓ free carnitine, elevated urine ethylmalonic acid, inconsistently abnormal acylcarnitine profile
Medium-chain acyl CoA dehydrogenase	*MCAD*	Hypoglycemia, hepatic encephalopathy, sudden death. NB screening diagnosis possible, maternal preeclampsia, HELLP syndrome association described rarely.	Normal or ↓ free carnitine, ↑ plasma acylglycine, plasma C_6-C_{10} free fatty acids, ↑ C_8-C_{10} acyl-carnitine
Very long chain acyl CoA dehydrogenase	*VLCAD*	Dilated cardiomyopathy, arrhythmias, hypoglycemia, and hepatic steatosis. Late-onset, stress-induced rhabdomyolysis, episodic myopathy. Prenatal and NB screening diagnosis possible.	Normal or ↓ free carnitine, ↑ plasma $C_{14:1}$, C_{14} acylcarnitine, ↑ plasma C_{10}-C_{16} free fatty acids
ETF dehydrogenase*	*ETF-DH*	Nonketotic fasting hypoglycemia, congenital anomalies, milder forms of liver disease, cardiomyopathy, and skeletal myopathy.	Normal or ↓ free carnitine, increased ratio of acyl to free carnitine, ↑ acyl-carnitine, urine organic acid and acylglycines
Electron transport flavoprotein-α*	*α-ETF*	Nonketotic fasting hypoglycemia, congenital anomalies, liver disease, cardiomyopathy, and skeletal myopathy also described	Normal or ↓ free carnitine, increased ratio of acyl to free carnitine, ↑ acyl-carnitine, urine organic acid and acylglycines
Electron transport flavoprotein-β*	*β-ETF*	Fasting hypoglycemia, congenital anomalies, liver disease, cardiomyopathy, and skeletal myopathy also described	Normal or ↓ free carnitine, increased ratio of acyl to free carnitine, ↑ acyl-carnitine, urine organic acid and acylglycines
Short-chain L-3-hydroxyacyl CoA dehydrogenase	*SCHAD*	Hypoglycemia, hyperinsulinemia, cardiomyopathy, myopathy. NB screening diagnosis possible.	Normal or ↓ free carnitine, elevated free fatty acids, inconsistently abnormal urine organic acid and plasma acylcarnitines
Long-chain L-3-hydroxyacyl CoA dehydrogenase	*LCHAD*	NB screening diagnosis possible, maternal preeclampsia, HELLP syndrome, and AFLP association described frequently. See also *MTP* below for clinical manifestations.	Normal or ↓ free carnitine, increased ratio of acyl to free carnitine, ↑ free fatty acids, ↑ C_{16}-OH and C_{18}-OH carnitines
Mitochondrial trifunctional protein	*MTP*	Severe cardiac and skeletal myopathy, hypoglycemia, acidosis, hyper NH_3, sudden death, elevated liver enzymes, retinopathy. Maternal preeclampsia, HELLP syndrome, and AFLP association described frequently.	Normal or ↓ free carnitine, increased ratio of acyl to free carnitine, ↑ free fatty acids, ↑ C_{16}-OH and C_{18}-OH carnitines
Long-chain 3-ketoacyl-CoA thiolase	*LKAT*	Severe neonatal presentation, hypoglycemia, acidosis, ↑ creatine kinase, cardiomyopathy, neuropathy, and early death.	Normal or ↓ free carnitine, increased ratio of acyl to free carnitine, ↑ free fatty acids, ↑ 2-trans, 4-cis-decadienoylcarnitine
2,4-Dienoyl-CoA reductase	*DECR1*	Only one patient described, hypotonia in the newborn, mainly severe skeletal myopathy and respiratory failure. Hypoglycemia rare.	Normal or ↓ free carnitine, ↑ acyl to free carnitine ratio, normal urine organic acids and acylglycines
HMG CoA synthetase	*HMGCS2*	Hypoketosis and hypoglycemia, rarely myopathy	Elevated total plasma fatty acids, enzyme studies in biopsied liver may be diagnostic, genetic testing is preferred
HMG CoA lyase	*HMGCL*	Hypoketosis and hypoglycemia, rarely myopathy	Normal free carnitine, ↑ C_5-OH, and methylglutaryl-carnitine, enzymes studies in fibroblasts may be diagnostic

*Also known as glutaric acidemia type II or multiple acyl-CoA dehydrogenase deficiency (MADD).
HELLP, hemolysis, elevated liver enzymes, low platelets; NB, newborn.
From Shekhawat PS, Matern D, Strauss AW: Fetal fatty oxidation disorders, their effect on maternal health and neonatal outcome: impact of expanded newborn screening on their diagnosis and management, *Pediatr Res* 57:78R–84R, 2005.

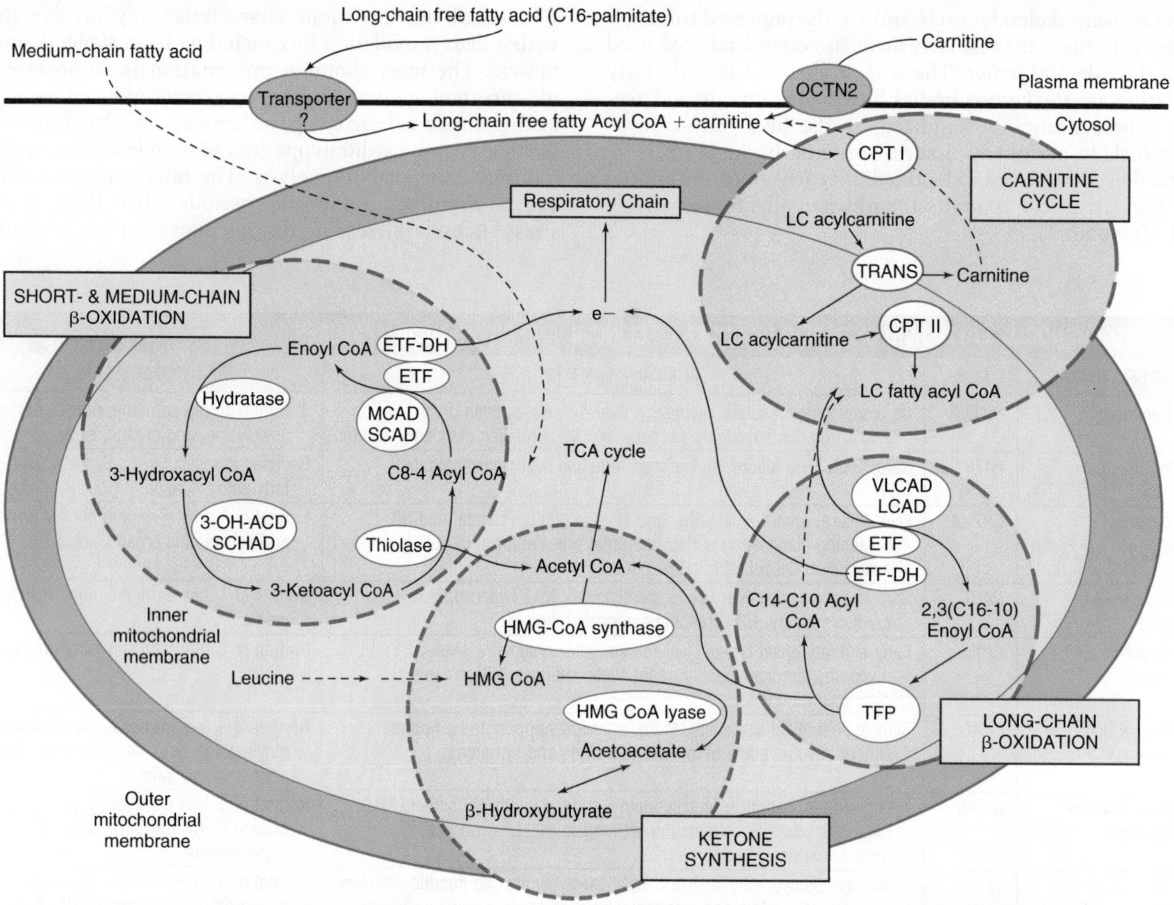

Figure 80-1 Mitochondrial fatty acid oxidation. Carnitine enters the cell through the action of the organic cation/carnitine transporter (OCTN2). Palmitate, a typical 16-carbon long-chain fatty acid, is transported across the plasma membrane and can be activated to form a long-chain (LC) fatty acyl coenzyme A (CoA). It then enters into the carnitine cycle, where it is transesterified by carnitine palmitoyltransferase-I (CPT-I), translocated across the inner mitochondrial membrane by carnitine/acylcarnitine translocase (TRANS), and then reconverted into a long-chain fatty acyl CoA by carnitine palmitoyltransferase-II (CPT-II) to undergo β-oxidation. Very long chain acyl CoA dehydrogenase (VLCAD/LCAD) leads to the production of (C16-10) 2,3 enoyl CoA. Trifunctional protein (TFP) contains the activities of enoyl CoA hydratase (hydratase), 3-OH-hydroxyacyl CoA dehydrogenase (3-OH-ACD), and β-ketothiolase (thiolase). Acetyl CoA, FADH, and NADH are produced. Medium- and short-chain fatty acids (C8-4) can enter the mitochondrial matrix independent of the carnitine cycle. Medium-chain acyl CoA dehydrogenase (MCAD), short-chain acyl CoA dehydrogenase (SCAD), and short-chain hydroxy acyl CoA dehydrogenase (SCHAD) are required. Acetyl CoA can then enter the Krebs (TCA) cycle. Electrons are transported from FADH to the respiratory chain via the electron transfer flavoprotein (ETF) and the electron transfer flavoprotein dehydrogenase (ETF-DH). NADH enters the electron transport chain through complex I. Acetyl CoA can be converted into hydroxymethylglutaryl (HMG) CoA by β-hydroxy-β-methylglutaryl CoA synthase (HMG CoA synthase) and then the ketone body acetoacetate by the action of β-hydroxy-β-methylglutaryl CoA lyase (HMG CoA lyase).

syndrome or, if fatal, as sudden unexpected infant death. Fatty acid oxidation disorders are easily overlooked because the only specific clue to the diagnosis may be the finding of inappropriately low concentrations of urinary ketones in an infant who has hypoglycemia. Genetic defects in ketone body utilization may be overlooked because ketosis is an expected finding with fasting hypoglycemia. In some circumstances, clinical manifestations appear to arise from toxic effects of fatty acid metabolites rather than inadequate energy production. These include disorders (LCHAD, CPT-IA, TFP) in which the presence of a homozygous affected fetus increases the risk of a life-threatening illness in the heterozygote mother, resulting in acute fatty liver of pregnancy or preeclampsia with HELLP (hemolysis, elevated liver enzymes, low platelets) syndrome. Malformations of the brain and kidneys have been described in severe electron transfer flavoprotein (ETF), ETF dehydrogenase (ETF-DH), and carnitine palmitoyltransferase-2 (CPT-II) deficiencies that might reflect in utero toxicity of fatty acid metabolites. Progressive retinal degeneration, peripheral neuropathy and chronic progressive liver disease have been identified in LCHAD and TFP deficiency. Newborn screening programs using tandem mass spectrometry (MS/MS) detect characteristic acylcarnitines seen in many of these disorders and permit presymptomatic diagnosis. Screening programs have provided evidence that all the fatty acid oxidation disorders combined are among the most common inborn errors of metabolism.

Figures 80-1 and 80-2 outline the steps involved in the oxidation of a typical long-chain fatty acid. In the *carnitine cycle*, fatty acids are transported across the barrier of the inner mitochondrial membrane as acylcarnitine esters. Within the mitochondria, successive turns of the 4-step β-oxidation cycle convert the coenzyme A (CoA)-activated fatty acid to acetyl CoA units. Two to three different chain-length specific isoenzymes are needed for each of these β-oxidation steps to accommodate the different-sized fatty acyl CoA species. The electron transfer pathway carries electrons generated in the 1st β-oxidation step (acyl CoA dehydrogenase) to the *electron transport chain* for adenosine triphosphate (ATP) production, while electrons generated from the third step (3-hydroxyacyl CoA dehydrogenase) enter the *respiratory chain* at the level of complex 1. Most of the acetyl CoA generated from hepatic β-oxidation flows through the *pathway of ketogenesis* to form β-hydroxybutyrate and acetoacetate.

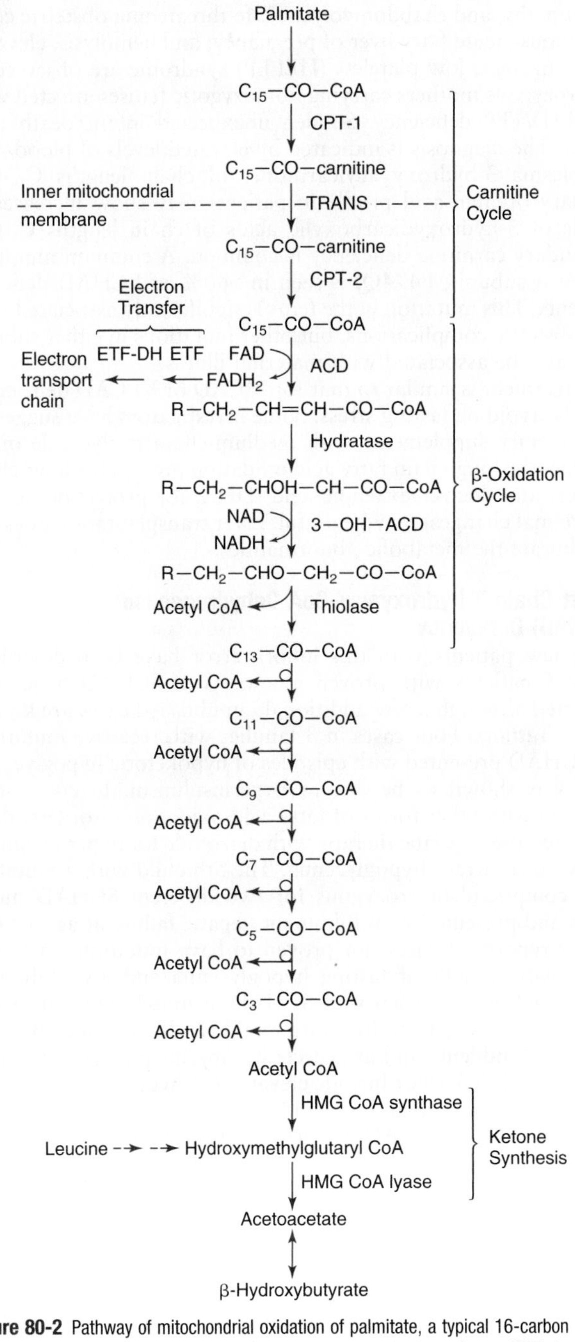

Figure 80-2 Pathway of mitochondrial oxidation of palmitate, a typical 16-carbon long-chain fatty acid. Enzyme steps include carnitine palmitoyltransferase (CPT) 1 and 2, carnitine/acylcarnitine translocase (TRANS), electron transfer flavoprotein (ETF), ETF dehydrogenase (ETF-DH), acyl CoA dehydrogenase (ACD), enoyl CoA hydratase (hydratase), 3-hydroxy-acyl CoA dehydrogenase (3-OH-ACD), β-ketothiolase (thiolase), β-hydroxy-β-methylglutaryl CoA (HMG CoA) synthase, and lyase.

DEFECTS IN THE β-OXIDATION CYCLE

Medium-Chain Acyl CoA Dehydrogenase (MCAD) Deficiency

MCAD deficiency is the most common fatty acid oxidation disorder. The disorder shows a strong founder effect; most patients have a northwestern European ancestry, and the majority of patients are homozygous for a single common missense mutation, an A-G transition at cDNA position 985 that changes a lysine to glutamic acid at residue 329 (K329E).

CLINICAL MANIFESTATIONS Affected patients usually present in the 1st 3 mo-5 yr of life with episodes of acute illness triggered by prolonged fasting (longer than 12-16 hr). Signs and symptoms include vomiting and lethargy, which rapidly progress to coma or seizures and cardiorespiratory collapse. Sudden unexpected infant death may occur. The liver may be slightly enlarged with fat deposition. Attacks are rare until the infant is beyond the 1st few months of life, presumably due to more frequent feedings at a younger age. Affected older infants are at higher risk of illness as they begin to fast through the night or are exposed to fasting stress during an intercurrent childhood illness. Presentation in the 1st days of life with neonatal hypoglycemia, has been reported in newborns that were fasted inadvertently. Diagnosis of MCAD has occasionally been documented in previously healthy teenage and adult individuals, indicating that even patients who have been asymptomatic in infancy are still at risk for metabolic decompensation if exposed to sufficient periods of fasting. An unknown number may remain asymptomatic.

LABORATORY FINDINGS During acute episodes, hypoglycemia is usually present. Plasma and urinary ketone concentrations are inappropriately low (**hypoketotic hypoglycemia**). Because of the relative hypoketonemia, there is little or no metabolic acidemia. Tests of liver function are abnormal, with elevations of liver enzymes (ALT, AST), elevated blood ammonia, and prolonged prothrombin (PT) and partial thromboplastin times (PTT). Liver biopsy at times of acute illness shows microvesicular or macrovesicular steatosis due to triglyceride accumulation. During fasting stress or at times of acute illness, urinary organic acid profiles by gas chromatography/mass spectrometry show inappropriately low concentrations of ketones and elevated levels of medium-chain dicarboxylic acids (adipic, suberic, and sebacic acids) that derive from microsomal and peroxisomal omega oxidation of fatty acids. Plasma and tissue concentrations of total carnitine are reduced to 25-50% of normal, and the fraction of total esterified carnitine is increased. This pattern of **secondary carnitine deficiency** is seen in most fatty acid oxidation defects and reflects competition between increased acylcarnitine levels and free carnitine transport at the plasma membrane. Significant exceptions to this rule are the plasma membrane carnitine transporter, CPT-IA and β-hydroxy-β-methylglutaryl CoA (HMG CoA) synthase deficiencies.

Diagnostic patterns include increased plasma $C_{8:0}$, $C_{10:0}$, and $C_{10:1}$ acylcarnitine species and increased urinary acylglycines including hexanoyl-, suberyl- and 3-phenylpropionyl glycines. Newborn screening programs using tandem mass spectrometry which almost all babies born in the USA receive can diagnose presymptomatic MCAD deficiency based on the detection of the abnormal acylcarnitines in filter paper blood spots. In many cases, the diagnosis can be confirmed by finding the common A985G mutation. A second common variant, T199C, has been detected in infants with characteristic acylcarnitines in newborn screening tests. Interestingly, this allele has not been seen to date in symptomatic MCAD patients; it may represent a mild mutation.

TREATMENT Acute illnesses should be promptly treated with intravenous fluids containing 10% dextrose to treat or prevent hypoglycemia and to suppress lipolysis as rapidly as possible (Chapter 86). Chronic therapy consists of avoiding fasting. This usually requires simply adjusting the diet to ensure that overnight fasting periods are limited to <10-12 hr. Restricting dietary fat or treatment with carnitine is controversial. The necessity for active therapeutic intervention for individuals with the T199C variant has not yet been established.

PROGNOSIS Up to 25% of unrecognized patients may die during their 1st attack of illness. There is frequently a history of a previous sibling death due to unrecognized MCAD deficiency. Some patients may develop permanent brain injury during an attack of profound hypoglycemia. The prognosis for survivors without brain damage is excellent because cognitive impairment or cardiomyopathy does not occur in MCAD deficiency. Muscle pain and reduced exercise tolerance may become evident with increasing age. Fasting tolerance improves with age and the risk of illness decreases. As many as 35% of affected patients have never had an episode; therefore, testing of siblings of affected patients is important to detect asymptomatic family members.

Very Long Chain Acyl CoA Dehydrogenase (VLCAD) Deficiency

VLCAD deficiency is the second most commonly diagnosed disorder of fatty acid oxidation. It was originally termed LCAD deficiency before the existence of the inner mitochondrial membrane-bound VLCAD was known. *All patients previously diagnosed as having LCAD deficiency have VLCAD enzyme deficiency.* Patients with VLCAD deficiency are usually more severely affected than those with MCAD deficiency, presenting earlier in infancy and having more chronic problems with muscle weakness or episodes of muscle pain and rhabdomyolysis. Cardiomyopathy may be present during acute attacks associated with fasting. The left ventricle may be hypertrophic or dilated and show poor contractility on echocardiography. Sudden unexpected death has occurred in several patients, but most who survived the initial episode showed improvement, including normalization of cardiac function. Other physical and routine laboratory features are similar to those of MCAD deficiency, including secondary carnitine deficiency. The urinary organic acid profile shows a nonketotic dicarboxylic aciduria. Increased levels of $C_{6\text{-}12}$ dicarboxylic acids may be noted in the urine. Diagnosis may be suggested by an abnormal acylcarnitine profile with plasma or blood spot $C_{14:1,14:0}$ acylcarnitine species, but the specific diagnosis requires assay of enzyme activities of VLCAD in cultured fibroblasts or direct mutational analysis of the VLCAD gene. Treatment is based primarily on avoidance of fasts for >10-12 hr. Continuous intragastric feeding is useful in some patients.

Short-Chain Acyl CoA Dehydrogenase (SCAD) Deficiency

A small number of patients with two clear null mutations in the SCAD gene have been described with variable phenotype. Most individuals classified as being SCAD deficient have been shown to have polymorphic DNA changes in the SCAD gene. The two common polymorphisms are G185S and R147W, which are present in 7% of the population. Some investigators argue that these may be susceptibility changes, which require a second, as yet unknown, genetic mutation to express a clinical phenotype; while others believe that SCAD deficiency is a harmless biochemical condition. This autosomal recessive disorder presents with neonatal hypoglycemia and may have normal levels of ketone bodies. The diagnosis is indicated by elevated levels of butyrylcarnitine on blood spots or plasma and increased excretion of urinary ethylmalonic acid and butyrylglycine. These metabolic abnormalities are most pronounced in patients with null mutations and variably present in patients who are homozygous for the polymorphisms.

The necessity for treatment in SCAD deficiency has not yet been established. It has been proposed that long-term evaluation of symptomless individuals is necessary to determine whether this is or is not a real disease.

Long-Chain 3-Hydroxyacyl CoA Dehydrogenase (LCHAD)/Mitochondrial Trifunctional Protein (TFP) Deficiency

The LCHAD enzyme is part of a mitochondrial trifunctional protein (TFP), which also contains two other steps in β-oxidation, long-chain enoyl CoA hydratase and long-chain β-ketothiolase. It is a hetero-octameric protein composed of 4 α and 4 β chains that derive from distinct contiguous genes with a common promoter region. In some patients, only the LCHAD activity of the TFP is affected (LCHAD deficiency), whereas others have deficiencies of all 3 activities (TFP deficiency).

Clinical manifestations include attacks of acute hypoketotic hypoglycemia similar to MCAD deficiency; patients often show evidence of more severe disease, including cardiomyopathy, muscle cramps and weakness, and abnormal liver function (cholestasis). Toxic effects of fatty acid metabolites may produce pigmented retinopathy, progressive liver failure, peripheral neuropathy, and rhabdomyolysis. Life-threatening obstetric complications; acute fatty liver of pregnancy; and hemolysis, elevated liver enzymes, low platelets (HELLP) syndrome are observed in heterozygous mothers carrying homozygotic fetuses affected with LCHAD/TFP deficiency. Sudden unexpected infant death may occur. The diagnosis is indicated by elevated levels of blood spot or plasma 3-hydroxy acylcarnitines of chain lengths C_{16}-C_{18}. Urinary organic acid profile in patients may show increases in levels of 3-hydroxydicarboxylic acids of chain lengths C_6-C_{14}. Secondary carnitine deficiency is common. A common mutation in the α subunit, E474Q, is seen in >60% of LCHAD deficient patients. This mutation in the fetus is significantly associated with the obstetric complications, but other mutations in either subunit may also be associated with maternal illness.

Treatment is similar to that for MCAD or VLCAD deficiency; that is, avoiding fasting stress. Some investigators have suggested that dietary supplements with medium-chain triglyceride oil to by-pass the long-chain fatty acid oxidation process for long-chain defects and docosahexaenoic acid (DHA, for protection against the retinal changes) may be useful. Liver transplantation does not ameliorate the metabolic abnormalities.

Short-Chain 3-Hydroxyacyl-CoA Dehydrogenase (SCHAD) Deficiency

Very few patients with this inborn error have been described. Only 5 patients with proven mutations of SCHAD have been reported although a few additional unpublished cases are known to the authors. Four cases in 3 families with recessive mutations of SCHAD presented with episodes of hypoketotic hypoglycemia that was shown to be due to hyperinsulinism. In contrast to patients with other forms of fatty acid oxidation disorders, these cases required specific therapy with diazoxide for hyperinsulinism to avoid recurrent hypoglycemia. The 5th child with a mutation was compound heterozygous for two different SCHAD mutations and presented with fulminant hepatic failure at age 10 mo. Other reports of cases not proven to have mutations include a child with attacks of fasting hypoglycemia and myoglobinuria associated with deficiency of SCHAD in muscle but not in cultured fibroblasts, 3 children with fatal liver disease, and an infant who died suddenly and unexpectedly. Specific metabolic markers for SCHAD deficiency include elevated C4-hydroxy acylcarnitine and urine 3-hydroxyglutaric acid.

Treatment of SCHAD deficient patients with hyperinsulinism is with diazoxide.

DEFECTS IN THE CARNITINE CYCLE

Plasma Membrane Carnitine Transport Defect (Primary Carnitine Deficiency)

Primary carnitine deficiency is the only genetic defect in which carnitine deficiency is the cause, rather than the consequence, of impaired fatty acid oxidation. The most common presentation is progressive **cardiomyopathy** with or without skeletal muscle weakness beginning at 1-4 yr of age. A smaller number of patients may present with fasting hypoketotic hypoglycemia in the 1st yr of life before the cardiomyopathy becomes symptomatic. The underlying defect involves the plasma membrane sodium gradient-dependent carnitine transporter that is present in heart, muscle, and kidney. This transporter is responsible both for maintaining intracellular carnitine concentrations 20- to 50-fold higher than plasma concentrations and for renal conservation of carnitine.

Diagnosis of the carnitine transporter defect is aided by the fact that patients have extremely reduced carnitine levels in plasma and muscle (1-2% of normal). Heterozygote parents have plasma carnitine levels approximately 50% of normal. Fasting ketogenesis may be normal because liver carnitine transport is normal, but it may be impaired if dietary carnitine intake is interrupted. The fasting urinary organic acid profile may show a hypoketotic dicarboxylic aciduria pattern if hepatic fatty acid oxidation is impaired, but it is otherwise unremarkable. The defect in carnitine transport can be demonstrated clinically by severe reduction in renal carnitine threshold or in vitro by assay of carnitine uptake using cultured fibroblasts or lymphoblasts. Mutations in the organic cation/carnitine transporter (*OCTN2*) underlie this disorder. Treatment of this disorder with pharmacologic doses of oral carnitine (100-200 mg/kg/day) is highly effective in correcting the cardiomyopathy and muscle weakness as well as any impairment in fasting ketogenesis. Muscle total carnitine concentrations remain <5% of normal on treatment.

Carnitine Palmitoyltransferase-IA (CPT-IA) Deficiency

Several dozen infants and children have been described with a deficiency of the liver and kidney isozyme of CPT-IA. Clinical manifestations include fasting hypoketotic hypoglycemia, occasionally with markedly abnormal liver function tests and, rarely, with renal tubular acidosis. The heart and skeletal muscle are not involved because the muscle isozyme is unaffected. Fasting urinary organic acid profile shows a hypoketotic C_6-C_{12} dicarboxylic aciduria but may be normal. Plasma acylcarnitine analysis demonstrates mostly free carnitine with very little acylated carnitine. This observation has been used to establish CPT-IA diagnosis on newborn screening by tandem mass spectrometry. CPT-IA deficiency is the only fatty acid oxidation disorder in which plasma total carnitine levels are elevated to 150-200% of normal. This may be explained by the fact that the inhibitory effects of long-chain acylcarnitines on the renal tubular carnitine transporter are absent in CPT-IA deficiency. The enzyme defect can be demonstrated in cultured fibroblasts or lymphoblasts. CPT-IA deficiency in the fetus has been associated with acute fatty liver of pregnancy in the mother in a single case report. A common variant in the CPT1A gene has been identified in individuals of Inuit background in the USA and First Nations tribes in Canada. The variant results in a positive newborn screen and 20% residual enzyme activity which is unregulated. It has not been established if this is a pathological DNA variant or an adaptive process to ancient Inuit and First Nations lifestyles. Treatment for the severe CPT1A deficiency is similar to that for MCAD deficiency with avoidance of situations where fasting ketogenesis is necessary.

Carnitine-Acylcarnitine Translocase (CACT) Deficiency

This defect of the inner mitochondrial membrane carrier protein for fatty acylcarnitines blocks the entry of long-chain fatty acids into the mitochondria for oxidation. The clinical phenotype of this disorder is characterized by a severe and generalized impairment of fatty acid oxidation. Most newborn patients present with attacks of fasting-induced hypoglycemia, hyperammonemia, and cardiorespiratory collapse. All symptomatic newborns have had evidence of cardiomyopathy and muscle weakness. Several patients with a partial translocase deficiency and milder disease without cardiac involvement have also been identified. No distinctive urinary or plasma organic acids are noted, although increased levels of plasma long-chain acylcarnitines are reported. Diagnosis can be made using cultured fibroblasts or lymphoblasts. The human gene has been cloned, and mutations have been identified in affected patients. Treatment is similar to that of other long-chain fatty acid oxidation disorders.

Carnitine Palmitoyltransferase-II (CPT-II) Deficiency

Three forms of CPT-II deficiency have been described. The antenatal presentation of this disorder is associated with a profound enzyme deficiency, and neonatal death has been reported in several newborns with dysplastic kidneys, cerebral malformations, and mild facial anomalies. A severe deficiency of enzyme activity is associated with an infantile-onset form. This form shares all the clinical and laboratory features of CACT deficiency. A milder defect is associated with an adult presentation of episodic rhabdomyolysis. The 1st episode usually does not occur until late childhood or early adulthood. Attacks may be precipitated by prolonged exercise. There is aching muscle pain and myoglobinuria that may be severe enough to cause renal failure. Serum levels of creatine kinase are elevated to 5,000-100,000 U/L. Fasting hypoglycemia has not been described, but fasting may contribute to attacks of myoglobinuria. Muscle biopsy shows increased deposition of neutral fat. The myopathic presentation of CPT-II deficiency is associated with a common mutation S113L. This mutation produces a heat-labile protein that is unstable to increased muscle temperature due to exercise resulting in the myopathic presentation. An intermediate form of CPT-II deficiency presents in infancy/early childhood with fasting-induced hepatic failure, cardiomyopathy, and skeletal myopathy with hypoketotic hypoglycemia but does not have the severe developmental changes seen in the neonatal presentation. This pattern is more like that seen in VLCAD deficiency and management is identical. Patients are generally heterozygous for one of the severe mutations and one of the milder mutations.

Diagnosis of all forms of CPT-II deficiency can be made by demonstrating deficient enzyme activity in muscle or other tissues and in cultured fibroblasts. Mutation analysis is available.

DEFECTS IN ELECTRON TRANSFER PATHWAY

Electron Transfer Flavoprotein (ETF) and Electron Transfer Flavoprotein Dehydrogenase (ETF-DH) Deficiencies (GLUTARIC Aciduria Type 2, Multiple Acyl CoA Dehydrogenation Deficiencies)

ETF and ETF-DH function to transfer electrons into the mitochondrial electron transport chain from dehydrogenation reactions catalyzed by VLCAD, MCAD, and SCAD, as well as glutaryl CoA dehydrogenase and at least four enzymes involved in branch-chain amino acid oxidation. Deficiencies of ETF or ETF-DH produce illness that combines the features of impaired fatty acid oxidation and impaired oxidation of several amino acids. Complete deficiencies of either protein are associated with severe illness in the newborn period, characterized by acidosis, hypoglycemia, coma, hypotonia, cardiomyopathy, and an unusual odor of sweaty feet due to isovaleryl CoA dehydrogenase inhibition. Some affected neonates have had facial dysmorphism and polycystic kidneys similar to that seen in severe CPT-II deficiency, which suggests that toxic effects of accumulated metabolites may occur in utero.

Diagnosis can be made from the urinary organic acid profile, which shows abnormalities corresponding to blocks in oxidation of fatty acids (ethylmalonate and C_6-C_{10} dicarboxylic acids), lysine (glutarate), and branched-chain amino acids (isovaleryl-, isobutyryl-, and α-methylbutyryl-glycine). Most severely affected infants do not survive the neonatal period.

Partial deficiencies of ETF and ETF-DH produce a disorder that may mimic MCAD deficiency or other milder fatty acid oxidation defects. These patients have attacks of fasting hypoketotic coma. The urinary organic acid profile reveals primarily elevations of dicarboxylic acids and ethylmalonate, derived from short-chain fatty acid intermediates. Secondary carnitine deficiency is present. Some patients with mild forms of ETF/ETF-DH deficiency benefit from treatment with high doses of riboflavin, which is a cofactor for the pathway of electron transfer.

DEFECTS IN KETONE SYNTHESIS PATHWAY

β-Hydroxy-β-Methylglutaryl CoA (HMG CoA) Synthase Deficiency (Chapter 79.6)

HMG CoA synthase is the rate-limiting step in the conversion of acetyl CoA derived from fatty acid β-oxidation in the liver to ketones. Several patients with this defect have recently been identified. The presentation is one of fasting hypoketotic hypoglycemia without evidence of impaired cardiac or skeletal muscle function. Urinary organic acid profile showed only a hypoketotic dicarboxylic aciduria. Plasma and tissue carnitine levels are normal, in contrast to all the other disorders of fatty acid oxidation. A separate synthase enzyme, present in cytosol for cholesterol biosynthesis, is not affected. The HMG CoA synthase defect is expressed only in the liver and cannot be demonstrated in cultured fibroblasts. The gene has been cloned, and mutations in the affected patients have been characterized. Avoiding fasting is usually a successful treatment.

β-Hydroxy-β-Methylglutaryl CoA Lyase Deficiency

See Chapter 79.6.

DEFECTS IN KETONE UTILIZATION

The ketones β-hydroxybutyrate and acetoacetate are the end products of hepatic fatty acid oxidation and are important as metabolic fuels for the brain during fasting. Two defects in utilization of ketones in brain and other peripheral tissues present as episodes of "hyperketotic" coma, with or without hypoglycemia.

Succinyl-CoA: 3-Ketoacid CoA Transferase (SCOT) Deficiency (Chapter 79.6)

Several patients with SCOT deficiency have been reported. Characteristic presentation is an infant with recurrent episodes of severe ketoacidosis induced by fasting. Plasma acylcarnitine and urine organic acid abnormalities do not distinguish from other causes of ketoacidosis. Treatment of episodes requires infusion of glucose and large amounts of bicarbonate until metabolically stable. All patients exhibit inappropriate hyperketonemia even between catabolic episodes. SCOT is responsible for activating acetoacetate in peripheral tissues using succinyl CoA as a donor to form acetoacetyl CoA. Deficient activity can be demonstrated in brain, muscle, and fibroblasts from affected patients. The gene has been cloned, and numerous mutations have been characterized.

β-Ketothiolase Deficiency

See Chapter 79.6.

BIBLIOGRAPHY

Please visit the Nelson Textbook of Pediatrics *website at www.expertconsult.com for the complete bibliography.*

80.2 Disorders of Very Long Chain Fatty Acids

*Hugo W. Moser**

PEROXISOMAL DISORDERS

The peroxisomal diseases are genetically determined disorders caused either by the failure to form or maintain the peroxisome or by a defect in the function of a single enzyme that is normally located in this organelle. These disorders cause serious disability in childhood and occur more frequently and present a wider range of phenotype than has been recognized in the past.

Etiology

Peroxisomal disorders are subdivided into 2 major categories (Table 80-2).

Table 80-2 CLASSIFICATION OF PEROXISOMAL DISORDERS

A: DISORDERS OF PEROXISOME IMPORT
A1: Zellweger syndrome
A2: Neonatal adrenoleukodystrophy
A3: Infantile Refsum disease
A4: Rhizomelic chondrodysplasia punctata
B: DEFECTS OF SINGLE PEROXISOMAL ENZYME
B1: X-linked adrenoleukodystrophy
B2: Acyl CoA oxidase deficiency
B3: Bifunctional enzyme deficiency
B4: Peroxisomal thiolase deficiency
B5: Classic Refsum disease
B6: 2-Methylacyl CoA racemase deficiency
B7: DHAP acyltransferase deficiency
B8: Alkyl-DHAP synthase deficiency
B9: Mevalonic aciduria
B10: Glutaric aciduria type III
B11: Hyperoxaluria type I
B12: Acatalasemia

In category A, the **peroxisomal biogenesis disorders** (PBD), the basic defect is the failure to import one or more proteins into the organelle. In category B, **defects affect a single peroxisomal protein.** The peroxisome is present in all cells except mature erythrocytes and is a subcellular organelle surrounded by a single membrane; >50 peroxisomal enzymes are identified. Some enzymes are involved in the production and decomposition of hydrogen peroxide; others are concerned with lipid and amino acid metabolism. Most peroxisomal enzymes are first synthesized in their mature form on free polyribosomes and enter the cytoplasm. Proteins that are destined for the peroxisome contain specific peroxisome targeting sequences (PTS). Most peroxisomal matrix proteins contain PTS1, a 3-amino acid sequence at the carboxyl terminus. PTS2 is an amino-terminal sequence that is critical for the import of enzymes involved in plasmalogen and branched-chain fatty acid metabolism. Import of proteins involves a complex series of reactions that involves at least 23 distinct proteins. These proteins are referred to as peroxins encoded by *PEX* genes. Table 80-3 summarizes the *PEX* genes that are defective in human disease states.

Epidemiology

Except for X-linked adrenoleukodystrophy (X-ALD), all the peroxisomal disorders in Table 80-2 are autosomal recessive traits. X-ALD is the most common peroxisomal disorder, with an estimated incidence of 1/17,000. The combined incidence of the other peroxisomal disorders is estimated to be 1/50,000.

Pathology

Absence or reduction in the number of peroxisomes is pathognomonic for disorders of peroxisome biogenesis. In most disorders, there are membranous sacs that contain peroxisomal integral membrane proteins, which lack the normal complement of matrix proteins; these are peroxisome "ghosts." Pathologic changes are observed in many organs and include profound and characteristic defects in neuronal migration; micronodular cirrhosis of the liver; renal cysts; chondrodysplasia punctata; corneal clouding, congenital cataracts, glaucoma, and retinopathy; congenital heart disease; and dysmorphic features.

Pathogenesis

It is likely that all pathologic changes are secondary to the peroxisome defect. Multiple peroxisomal enzymes fail to function in the PBD (Table 80-4). The enzymes that are diminished or absent are synthesized but are degraded abnormally fast because they may

*This chapter has been extensively evaluated by Drs. Charles Stanley and Michael Bennett and the reference list has been updated to reflect more recent articles. However, Drs. Stanley and Bennett find that there have been no substantive diagnostic pathophysiological or therapeutic advances in this field since the previous version was written and, with deep respect to the late Dr. Moser, consider that no textual modifications are required for this present edition of the text book.

Table 80-3 PEROXISOME BIOGENESIS FACTORS (PEX) AND THEIR ALTERATIONS IN HUMAN PEROXISOMAL BIOGENESIS DISORDERS (PBD)

PEROXIN #	CHARACTERISTIC	COMPLEMENTATION GROUP			NO. OF PATIENTS STUDIED AT KKI	PHENOTYPE	CHROMOSOME
		KKI	Japan	Ams	KKI		
1	143-kd AAA ATPase	1	E	2	99	ZS, NALD, IRD	7q21-22
2	C_3HC_4 zinc binding integral peroxisomal membrane protein 35-52 kd	10	F	5	2	ZS	
3	51-52 kd Integral peroxisomal membrane protein						
4	21-24 kd Peroxisomal associated ubiquitin-conjugating enzyme						
5	PTS 1 receptor	2		4	2	ZS, NALD	12p13.3
6	12-127 kd AAA ATPase	4	C	3	16	ZS, NALD	6p21.1
7	PTS 2 receptor	11		1	43	RCDP	6q22-24
8	71-81 kd Peroxisomal associated protein						
9	42-kd Integral peroxisomal membrane protein						
10	C_3HC_4 zinc-binding integral peroxisomal membrane protein	7	B		5	ZS, NALSD	8q21.1
11	27-32 kd Peroxisomal membrane protein involved in peroxisomal proliferation						
12	48-kd C_3HC_4 zinc binding integral peroxisomal membrane protein	3			6	ZS, NALSD, IRD	
13	SH-3 containing 40-43-kd peroxisomal integral peroxisomal membrane protein		H		2	ZS, NALSD	
14	41-kd Integral membrane protein						
15	48-kd Cytosolic protein						
16	39-kd Peripheral peroxisomal membrane protein	9	D		1	ZS	
17	27-30 kd Peroxisomal? intrinsic membrane protein						
18	35-39 kd Peroxisomal membrane protein zinc finger motif						
19	Peroxisomal membrane protein, prenylated		J			ZS	
		8	A		7	ZS, NALSD, IRD	
			G			ZS	
26	? Docking factor for Pex1p and Pex6p						

Ams, Amsterdam; KKI, Kennedy Krieger Institute.
From Moser HW: Genotype-phenotype correlations in disorders of peroxisome biogenesis, *Mol Genet Metab* 68:316, 1999.

Table 80-4 ABNORMAL LABORATORY FINDINGS COMMON TO DISORDERS OF PEROXISOME BIOGENESIS

Peroxisomes absent to reduced in number
Catalase in cytosol
Deficient synthesis and reduced tissue levels of plasmalogens
Defective oxidation and abnormal accumulation of very long chain fatty acids
Deficient oxidation and age-dependent accumulation of phytanic acid
Defects in certain steps of bile acid formation and accumulation of bile acid intermediates
Defects in oxidation and accumulation of L-pipecolic acid
Increased urinary excretion of dicarboxylic acids

be unprotected outside of the peroxisome. It is not clear how defective peroxisome functions lead to the widespread pathologic manifestations.

The PBD are associated with genetically determined import defects. The PBD have been subdivided into 12 complementation groups. The molecular defects have been defined in 10 of these groups (see Table 80-3). The pattern and severity of pathologic features vary with the nature of the import defects and the degree to which import is impaired. These gene defects lead to disorders that were named before their relationship to the peroxisome was recognized, namely, Zellweger syndrome (ZS), neonatal adrenoleukodystrophy (NALD), infantile Refsum disease (IRD), and rhizomelic chondrodysplasia punctata (RCDP). The first 3 disorders are considered to form a clinical continuum, with ZS the most severe, IRD the least severe, and NALD intermediate. They can be caused by 11 different gene defects, which involve mainly the import of proteins that contain the PTS1 targeting signal; the gene defects cannot be distinguished on the basis of clinical features. The clinical severity varies with the degree to which protein import is impaired. Mutations that abolish import completely are often associated with the ZS phenotype, whereas a missense mutation, in which some degree of import function is retained, leads to the somewhat milder phenotypes. A defect in *PEX7*, which involves the import of proteins that utilize PTS2, is associated with RCDP. *PEX7* defects that leave import partially intact are associated with milder phenotypes, some of which resemble classic Refsum disease.

The genetic disorders that involve single peroxisomal enzymes usually have clinical manifestations that are more restricted and present subsequent to the neonatal period and not infrequently in adolescents or adults. The clinical manifestations may be related to the biochemical defect. The primary adrenal insufficiency of X-ALD is caused by accumulation of very long chain fatty acids (VLCFA) in the adrenal cortex, and the peripheral neuropathy in Refsum disease is caused by the accumulation of phytanic acid in Schwann cells and myelin.

PBD WITH MILDER OR ATYPICAL PHENOTYPES Newborn infants with **Zellweger syndrome** show striking and consistent, recognizable abnormalities. Of central diagnostic importance are the typical facial appearance (high forehead, unslanting palpebral fissures, hypoplastic supraorbital ridges, and epicanthal folds; Fig. 80-3), severe weakness and hypotonia, neonatal seizures, and eye abnormalities (cataracts, glaucoma, corneal clouding, Brushfield spots, pigmentary retinopathy, and nerve dysplasia). Because of the hypotonia and "mongoloid" appearance, Down syndrome may be suspected. Infants with Zellweger syndrome rarely live more than a few months. More than 90% show postnatal growth failure. Table 80-5 lists the main clinical abnormalities.

Patients with **neonatal ALD** show fewer and, occasionally, no dysmorphic features. Neonatal seizures occur frequently. Some degree of psychomotor development is present; function remains in the severely or profoundly retarded range, and development may regress after 3-5 yr of age, probably from a progressive leukodystrophy. Several patients are now in a stable, albeit disabled, state in their 3rd or 4th decade. Hepatomegaly, impaired liver function, pigmentary degeneration of the retina, and severely impaired hearing are invariably present. Adrenocortical function

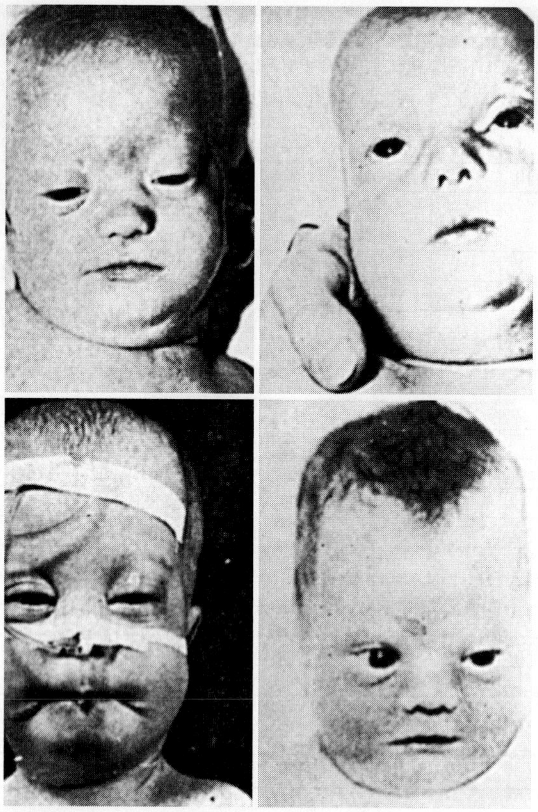

Figure 80-3 Four patients with Zellweger cerebrohepatorenal syndrome. Note the high forehead, epicanthal folds, and hypoplasia of supraorbital ridges and midface. (Courtesy of Hans Zellweger, MD.)

is usually impaired, but overt Addison disease is rare. Chondrodysplasia punctata and renal cysts are absent.

Patients with **infantile Refsum disease** have survived to the 2nd decade or longer. They are able to walk, although gait may be ataxic and broad based. Cognitive function is in the severely retarded range. All have sensorineural hearing loss and pigmentary degeneration of the retina. They have moderately dysmorphic features that may include epicanthal folds, a flat bridge of the nose, and low-set ears. Early hypotonia and hepatomegaly with impaired function are common. Levels of plasma cholesterol and high- and low-density lipoprotein are often moderately reduced. Chondrodysplasia punctata and renal cortical cysts are absent. Postmortem study in infantile Refsum disease reveals micronodular liver cirrhosis and small hypoplastic adrenals. The brain shows no malformations, except for severe hypoplasia of the cerebellar granule layer and ectopic locations of the Purkinje cells in the molecular layer. The mode of inheritance is autosomal recessive.

Some patients with PBD disorders have milder and atypical phenotypes. They may present with peripheral neuropathy or with retinopathy, impaired vision, or cataracts in childhood, adolescence, or adulthood and have been diagnosed to have Charcot-Marie-Tooth disease or Usher syndrome. Some patients have survived to the 5th decade. Defects in *PEX7*, which most commonly lead to the RCDP phenotype, may also lead to a milder phenotype with clinical manifestations similar to those of classical Refsum disease (phytanoyl CoA hydroxylase deficiency).

RHIZOMELIC CHONDRODYSPLASIA PUNCTATA (RCDP) This disorder is characterized by the presence of stippled foci of calcification within the hyaline cartilage and is associated with dwarfing, cataracts (72%), and multiple malformations due to contractures. Vertebral bodies have a coronal cleft filled by cartilage that is a result of an embryonic arrest. Disproportionate short stature affects the proximal parts of the extremities (Fig. 80-4*A*). Radiologic abnormalities consist of shortening of the proximal limb bones, metaphyseal cupping, and disturbed ossification (Fig. 80-4*B*). Height, weight, and head circumference are less than the 3rd percentile, and these children are severely retarded mentally. Skin changes such as those observed in ichthyosiform erythroderma are present in about 25% of patients.

Table 80-5 MAIN CLINICAL ABNORMALITIES IN ZELLWEGER SYNDROME

ABNORMAL FEATURE	CASES IN WHICH INFORMATION ABOUT THE FEATURE WAS AVAILABLE No.	%	CASES IN WHICH THE FEATURE WAS PRESENT No.	%
High forehead	60	53	58	97
Flat occiput	16	14	13	81
Large fontanelle(s), wide sutures	57	50	55	96
Shallow orbital ridges	33	29	33	100
Low/broad nasal bridge	23	20	23	100
Epicanthus	36	32	33	92
High arched palate	37	32	35	95
External ear deformity	40	35	39	97
Micrognathia	18	16	18	100
Redundant skin fold of neck	13	11	13	100
Brushfield spots	6	5	5	83
Cataract/cloudy cornea	35	31	30	86
Glaucoma	12	11	7	58
Abnormal retinal pigmentation	15	13	6	40
Optic disc pallor	23	20	17	74
Severe hypotonia	95	83	94	99
Abnormal Moro response	26	23	26	100
Hyporeflexia or areflexia	57	50	56	98
Poor sucking	77	68	74	96
Gavage feeding	26	23	26	100
Epileptic seizures	61	54	56	92
Psychomotor retardation	45	39	45	100
Impaired hearing	21	18	9	40
Nystagmus	37	32	30	81

From Heymans HAS: *Cerebro-hepato-renal (Zellweger) syndrome: clinical and biochemical consequences of peroxisomal dysfunctions.* Thesis, University of Amsterdam, 1984.

ISOLATED DEFECTS OF PEROXISOMAL FATTY ACID OXIDATION The disorders labeled B1 through B3 (see Table 80-2) each involve 1 of 3 enzymes involved in peroxisomal fatty acid oxidation. Their clinical manifestations resemble those of the Zellweger syndrome/neonatal ALD/infantile Refsum disease continuum; they can be distinguished from disorders of peroxisome biogenesis by laboratory tests. Defects of bifunctional enzyme are common and are found in about 15% of patients with the Zellweger syndrome/neonatal ALD/infantile Refsum disease phenotype. Patients with isolated acyl CoA oxidase deficiency have a somewhat milder phenotype that resembles that of neonatal ALD.

ISOLATED DEFECTS OF PLASMALOGEN SYNTHESIS Plasmalogens are lipids in which the 1st carbon of glycerol is linked to an alcohol rather than a fatty acid. They are synthesized through a complex series of reactions, the 1st two steps of which are catalyzed by the peroxisomal enzymes dihydroxyacetone phosphate alkyl transferase and synthase. Deficiency of either of these enzymes (B4 and B5 in Table 80-2) leads to a phenotype that is clinically indistinguishable from the peroxisomal import disorder RCDP. This latter disorder is caused by a defect in *PEX7*, the receptor for peroxisome targeting sequence 2. It shares the severe deficiency of plasmalogens with disorders B4 and B5 but, in addition, has defects of phytanic oxidation. The fact that disorders B4 and

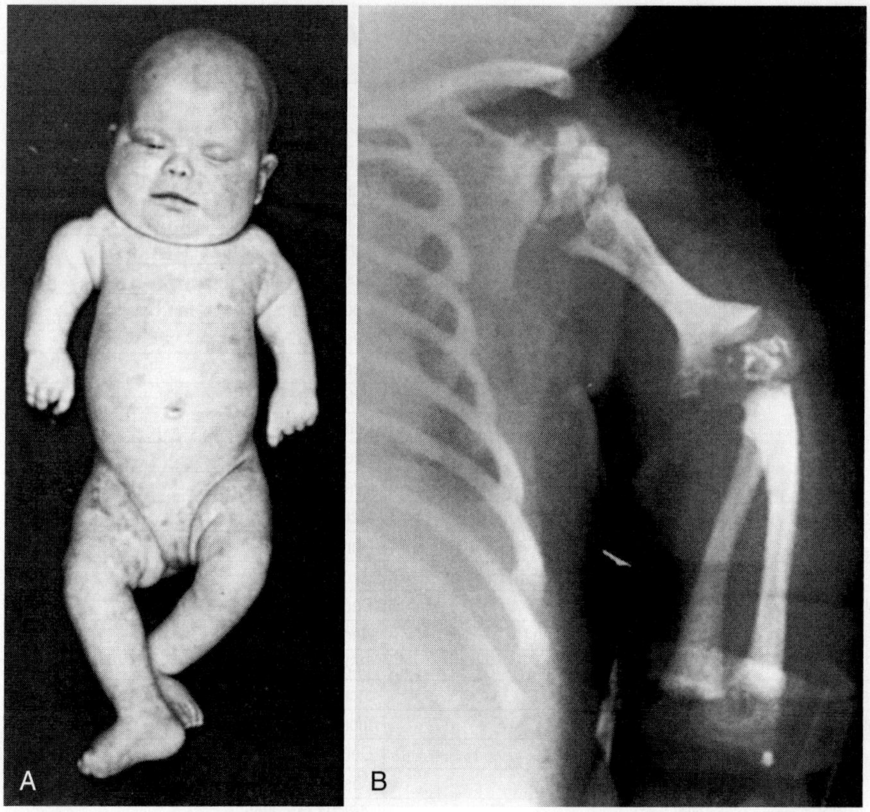

Figure 80-4 *A,* Newborn infant with rhizomelic chondrodysplasia punctata (RCDP). Note the severe shortening of the proximal limbs, the depressed bridge of the nose, hypertelorism, and widespread scaling skin lesions. *B,* Note the marked shortening of the humerus and epiphyseal stippling at the shoulder and elbow joints. (Courtesy of John P. Dorst, MD.)

B5 are associated with the full phenotype of RCDP suggests that a deficiency of plasmalogens is sufficient to produce it.

CLASSIC REFSUM DISEASE The defective enzyme (phytanoyl CoA oxidase) is localized to the peroxisome. The manifestation of classic Refsum disease includes impaired vision from retinitis pigmentosa, ichthyosis, peripheral neuropathy, ataxia, and, occasionally, cardiac arrhythmias. In contrast to infantile Refsum disease, cognitive function is normal and there are no congenital malformations. Classic Refsum disease often does not manifest until young adulthood, but visual disturbances such as night blindness, ichthyosis, and peripheral neuropathy may already be present in childhood and adolescence. Early diagnosis is important because institution of a phytanic acid-restricted diet can reverse the peripheral neuropathy and prevent the progression of the visual and central nervous system manifestations. The classical Refsum disease phenotype may also be caused by defects in *PEX7*.

2-METHYLACYL COA RACEMASE DEFICIENCY This disorder is caused by an enzyme defect that leads to the accumulation of the branched-chain fatty acids (phytanic and pristanic acid) and bile acids. Patients present with adult-type peripheral neuropathy and may also have pigmentary degeneration of the retina.

Laboratory Findings

Laboratory tests for peroxisomal disorders can be viewed at three levels of complexity.

LEVEL 1: DOES THE PATIENT HAVE A PEROXISOMAL DISORDER? This can be resolved by noninvasive tests that are generally available (Table 80-6). Measurement of plasma VLCFA is the most commonly used assay. Whereas plasma VLCFA levels are elevated in many patients with peroxisomal disorders, this is not always the case. The most important exceptions are RCDP, in which VLCFA levels are normal, but plasma phytanic acid levels are increased and red blood cell plasmalogen levels are reduced. In some other peroxisomal disorders, the biochemical abnormalities are still more restricted. Therefore, a panel of tests is recommended and includes plasma levels of VLCFA and phytanic, pristanic, and pipecolic acids and red blood cell levels of plasmalogens. Tandem mass spectrometry techniques also permit convenient quantitation of bile acids in plasma and urine. This panel of tests can be performed on 2 mL samples of venous blood and permits detection of most peroxisomal disorders. Furthermore, normal results make the presence of a peroxisomal disorder unlikely.

LEVEL 2: WHAT IS THE PRECISE NATURE OF THE PEROXISOMAL DISORDER? Table 80-6 lists the main biochemical abnormalities in the various peroxisomal disorders. When combined with the clinical presentation, the panel of level 1 tests (see earlier) is often sufficient to identify the precise nature of the defect. Elevated plasma VLCFA levels permit the precise diagnosis of X-ALD in male patients. Marked reduction of erythrocyte plasmalogen levels combined with elevated plasma phytanic acid permits precise diagnosis in a patient with the clinical features of RCDP. Classic Refsum disease can be diagnosed by demonstration of increased plasma phytanic acid combined with normal or reduced levels of pristanic acid levels, while in D-bifunctional enzyme deficiency and 2-methylacyl CoA racemase deficiency, the levels of pristanic and phytanic acid are both increased. Precise identification of some peroxisomal disorders may require more extensive studies in cultured skin fibroblasts. This may be required for the differentiation of PBD from defects in bifunctional enzyme. In PBD, the patient's peroxisomes are absent and catalase is in the soluble fraction, whereas in bifunctional enzyme defect, peroxisomes are present and catalase is in the particulate fraction. Fibroblast studies are required to identify the nature of the molecular defect in PBD. Whether such specialized studies are clinically warranted depends on individual circumstances. Precise definition of the defect in a proband may improve the precision of prenatal diagnosis in at-risk pregnancies, and it is required for carrier detection. It is also of value in setting prognosis. Precise characterization is of prognostic value in patients with *PEX1*

Table 80-6 PEROXISOMAL DISORDERS THAT INVOLVE FATTY ACID OXIDATION: DIAGNOSTIC ASSAYS

DISEASE	ASSAY		FINDING
Zellweger syndrome	Plasma	VLCFA	Increased
Neonatal adrenoleukodystrophy		Phytanic acid	Age-dependent increase
Infantile Refsum disease		Pristanic acid	Age-dependent increase
		Pipecolic acid	Increased
		Bile acid	Increased, abnormal pattern
	RBCs	Plasmalogen levels	Variably decreased
	Fibroblasts	VLCFA levels	Increased
		VLCFA oxidation	Decreased
		Plasmalogen synthesis	Decreased
		Phytanic, pristanic oxidation	Decreased
		Catalase localization	Cytosolic
		Immunocytochemistry	Peroxisomes absent
		Complementation	See Table 80-1
		DNA	See Table 80-1
Rhizomelic chondrodysplasia punctata	Plasma	Phytanic acid	Increased
		VLCFA	Normal
	RBCs	Plasmalogen levels	Decreased
	Fibroblasts	Plasmalogen synthesis	Decreased
		Phytanic acid oxidation	Decreased
		DNA	*PEX7* defect
X-linked ALD hemizygote	Plasma	VLCFA	Increased
	Fibroblasts	VLCFA levels	Increased
		VLCFA oxidation	Decreased
		ALDP immunoreactivity	Absent 70%
		DNA	*ABCD1* mutation
X-linked ALD heterozygote	Plasma	VLCFA	Variable increase in 85%
	Fibroblasts	VLCFA levels	Variable increase in 90%
		ALDP immunoreactivity	Variable decrease
		DNA	*ABCD1* mutation
Bifunctional enzyme defect	Plasma	VLCFA	Increased
		Phytanic acid	Increased
		Pristanic acid	Increased
		Bile acids	Increased, abnormal pattern
	Fibroblasts	VLCFA levels	Increased
		Pristanic acid oxidation	Decreased
		Catalase localization	Peroxisomal
		Enzyme	D-bifunctional protein deficiency
Acyl CoA oxidase deficiency	Plasma Fibroblasts	VLCFA	Increased
		VLCFA levels	Increased
		VLCFA oxidation	Decreased
		Enzyme	Acyl CoA oxidase defect
2-Methyl acyl CoA racemase deficiency	Plasma	Pristanic acid	Increased
		Bile acids	Increased, abnormal pattern
	Fibroblasts	Pristanic acid oxidation	Decreased
		Enzyme	2-Methyl acyl CoA oxidase defect
Classic Refsum disease	Plasma	Phytanic acid	Increased
		Pristanic acid	Decreased
	Fibroblasts	Enzyme	Phytanoyl CoA deficiency

ALD, adrenoleukodystrophy; VLCFA, very long chain fatty acids.

defects. This defect is present in approximately 60% of PBD patients, and about half of the *PEX1* defects have the G843D allele, which is associated with a significantly milder phenotype than is found in other mutations.

LEVEL 3: WHAT IS THE MOLECULAR DEFECT? Table 80-3 shows that the molecular defects in most of the PBD have been defined. Definition of the molecular defect in the proband, which is now offered in several laboratories, is essential for carrier detection and speeds prenatal diagnosis.

Diagnosis

There are several noninvasive laboratory tests that permit precise and early diagnosis of peroxisomal disorders (see Table 80-6). The challenge in PBD is to differentiate them from the large variety of other conditions that can cause hypotonia, seizures, failure to thrive, or dysmorphic features. Experienced clinicians can readily recognize classic Zellweger syndrome by its clinical manifestations. PBD patients often do not show the full clinical spectrum of disease and may be identifiable only by laboratory assays. Clinical features that may serve as indications for these diagnostic assays include severe psychomotor retardation; weakness and hypotonia; dysmorphic features; neonatal seizures; retinopathy, glaucoma, or cataracts; hearing deficits; enlarged liver and impaired liver function; and chondrodysplasia punctata. The presence of one or more of these abnormalities increases the likelihood of this diagnosis. Atypical milder forms presenting as peripheral neuropathy have also been described.

Some patients with the isolated defects of peroxisomal fatty acid oxidation (group B) resemble those with group A disorders and can be detected by the demonstration of abnormally high levels of VLCFA.

Patients with RCDP must be distinguished from patients with other causes of chondrodysplasia punctata. In addition to warfarin embryopathy and Zellweger syndrome, these disorders include the milder autosomal dominant form of chondrodysplasia punctata (Conradi-Hünermann syndrome), which is characterized by longer survival, absence of severe limb shortening, and usually intact intellect; an X-linked dominant form; and an X-linked recessive form associated with a deletion of the terminal portion of the short arm of the X chromosome. RCDP is suspected clinically because of the shortness of limbs, psychomotor retardation, and ichthyosis. The most decisive laboratory test is the demonstration of abnormally low plasmalogen levels in red blood cells and an impaired capacity to synthesize plasmalogens in cultured skin fibroblasts. These biochemical defects are not present in other types of chondrodysplasia punctata. Chondrodysplasia punctata may also be associated with a defect of 3β-hydroxysteroid-Δ^8,Δ^7-isomerase, an enzyme involved in biosynthesis of cholesterol.

Complications
Patients with Zellweger cerebrohepatorenal syndrome have multiple disabilities involving muscle tone, swallowing, cardiac abnormalities, liver disease, and seizures. These conditions are treated symptomatically, but the prognosis is poor, and most patients succumb in the 1st few months of life. Patients with RCDP may develop quadriparesis owing to compression at the base of the brain.

Treatment
The most effective therapy is the dietary treatment of classic Refsum disease with a phytanic acid-restricted diet.

For patients with the somewhat milder variants of the peroxisome import disorders, success has been achieved with multidisciplinary early intervention, including physical and occupational therapy, hearing aids, alternative communication, nutrition, and support for the parents. Although most patients continue to function in the profoundly or severely retarded range, some make significant gains in self-help skills, and several are in stable condition in their teens or even early 20s.

Studies to mitigate some of the secondary biochemical abnormalities include the oral administration of docosahexaenoic acid in a dosage of 50-100 mg/24 hr either as the ethyl ester or in the form of a triglyceride in which one of the fatty acids has been replaced by docosahexaenoic acid. The levels of this substance are greatly reduced in patients with disorders of peroxisome biogenesis because the last step of its synthesis takes place in the peroxisome. This therapy normalizes the plasma and erythrocyte levels of this substance, which has important physiologic functions in retina and brain. There are anecdotal reports of clinical improvement. The oral administration of cholic acid and chenodeoxycholic acid in a dosage of 100-250 mg/24 hr, with the aim of reducing the levels of presumably toxic bile acid intermediates, may be effective as well.

Genetic Counseling
All the peroxisomal disorders, except hyperoxaluria type 1, can be diagnosed prenatally in the 1st or 2nd trimester. The tests are similar to those described for postnatal diagnosis (see Table 80-6) and use chorionic villus sampling or amniocytes. More than 300 pregnancies have been monitored, and more than 60 affected fetuses have been identified without diagnostic error. Because of the 25% recurrence risk, couples with an affected child must be advised about the availability of prenatal diagnosis. Heterozygotes can be identified in X-ALD and in those disorders in which the molecular defect has been identified (see Table 80-3).

ADRENOLEUKODYSTROPHY (X-LINKED)

X-ALD is a genetically determined disorder associated with the accumulation of saturated VLCFA and a progressive dysfunction of the adrenal cortex and central and peripheral nervous system white matter.

Etiology
The key biochemical abnormality is the tissue accumulation of unbranched saturated VLCFA, with a carbon chain length of 24 or more. Excess hexacosanoic acid (C26:0) is the most striking and characteristic feature. This accumulation of fatty acids is caused by genetically deficient peroxisomal degradation of fatty acid. The key biochemical defect involves the impaired function of peroxisomal lignoceroyl CoA ligase, the enzyme that catalyzes the formation of the CoA derivative of VLCFA. The gene that is defective (*ABCD1*) codes for a peroxisomal membrane (ALDP). More than 400 distinct mutations have been identified, and most families have a mutation that is "private" (unique to that kindred) and are updated on the website, *www.x-ald.nl*. The gene has been mapped to chromosome Xq28. The mechanism by which the ALDP defect leads to VLCFA accumulation and the pathology of X-ALD is unknown.

Epidemiology
The minimum incidence of X-ALD in males is 1/21,000, and the combined incidence of X-ALD males and heterozygous females in the general population is estimated to be 1/17,000. All races are affected. The various phenotypes often occur in members of the same kindred.

Pathology
Characteristic lamellar cytoplasmic inclusions can be demonstrated with the electron microscope in adrenocortical cells, testicular Leydig cells, and nervous system macrophages. These inclusions probably consist of cholesterol esterified with VLCFA. They are most prominent in cells of the zona fasciculata of the adrenal cortex, which at first are distended with lipid and later atrophy.

The nervous system can display 2 types of lesions. In the severe childhood cerebral form and in the rapidly progressive adult forms, demyelination is associated with an inflammatory response manifested by the accumulation of perivascular lymphocytes that is most intense in the parieto-occipital region. In the slowly progressive adult form, **adrenomyeloneuropathy** (**AMN**), the main finding is a distal axonopathy that affects the long tracts in the spinal cord. The inflammatory response is mild or absent.

Pathogenesis
The adrenal dysfunction is probably a direct consequence of the accumulation of VLCFA. The cells in the zona fasciculata are distended with abnormal lipids. Cholesterol esterified with VLCFA is relatively resistant to adrenocorticotropic hormone (ACTH)-stimulated cholesterol ester hydrolases, and this limits the capacity to convert cholesterol to active steroids. In addition, C26:0 excess increases the viscosity of the plasma membrane and this may interfere with receptor and other cellular functions.

There is no correlation between the neurologic phenotype and the nature of the mutation or the severity of the biochemical defect as assessed by plasma levels of VLCFA or between the degree of adrenal involvement and nervous system involvement. The severity of the illness and rate of progression correlate with the intensity of the inflammatory response. The inflammatory response may be cytokine mediated and may involve an autoimmune response triggered in an unknown way by the excess of VLCFA. A CD1 lipid antigen has been implicated. Mitochondrial damage and oxidative stress also contribute. Approximately half of the patients do not experience the inflammatory response. A modifier gene that sets the "thermostat" for the inflammatory response is postulated.

Clinical Manifestations

There are 5 relatively distinct phenotypes, 3 of which are present in childhood with symptoms and signs. In all the phenotypes, development is usually normal in the 1st 3-4 yr of life.

In the **childhood cerebral form** of ALD, symptoms are first noted most commonly between the ages of 4 and 8 yr (21 mo is the earliest onset reported). The most common initial manifestations are hyperactivity, which is often mistaken for an attention deficit disorder, and worsening school performance in a child who had previously been a good student. **Auditory discrimination** is often impaired, although tone perception is preserved. This may be evidenced by difficulty in using the telephone and greatly impaired performance on intelligence tests in items that are presented verbally. Spatial orientation is often impaired. Other initial symptoms are disturbances of vision, ataxia, poor handwriting, seizures, and strabismus. Visual disturbances are often due to involvement of the cerebral cortex, which leads to variable and seemingly inconsistent visual capacity. **Seizures** occur in nearly all patients and may represent the 1st manifestation of the disease. Some patients present with increased intracranial pressure or with unilateral mass lesions. Impaired cortisol response to ACTH stimulation is present in 85% of patients, and mild hyperpigmentation is noted. In most patients with this phenotype, adrenal dysfunction is recognized only after the condition is diagnosed because of the cerebral symptoms. Cerebral childhood ALD tends to progress rapidly with increasing spasticity and paralysis, visual and hearing loss, and loss of ability to speak or swallow. The mean interval between the 1st neurologic symptom and an apparently vegetative state is 1.9 yr. Patients may continue in this apparently vegetative state for 10 yr or more.

Adolescent ALD designates patients who experience neurologic symptoms between the ages of 10 and 21 yr. The manifestations resemble those of childhood cerebral ALD except that progression is slower. About 10% of patients present acutely with status epilepticus, adrenal crisis, acute encephalopathy, or coma.

Adrenomyeloneuropathy first manifests in late adolescence or adulthood as a progressive paraparesis caused by long tract degeneration in the spinal cord. Approximately half of the patients also have involvement of the cerebral white matter.

The **"Addison only"** phenotype is an important and underdiagnosed condition. Of male patients with Addison disease, 25% may have the biochemical defect of ALD. Many of these patients have intact neurologic systems, whereas others have subtle neurologic signs. Many acquire adrenomyeloneuropathy in adulthood.

The term "asymptomatic ALD" is applied to persons who have the biochemical defect of ALD but are free of neurologic or endocrine disturbances. Nearly all persons with the gene defect eventually become neurologically symptomatic. A few have remained asymptomatic even in the 6th or 7th decade.

Approximately 50% of female heterozygotes acquire a syndrome that resembles adrenomyeloneuropathy but is milder and of later onset. Adrenal insufficiency is rare.

Laboratory and Radiographic Findings

The most specific and important laboratory finding is the demonstration of abnormally high levels of VLCFA in plasma, red blood cells, or cultured skin fibroblasts. The test should be performed in a laboratory that has experience with this specialized procedure. Positive results are obtained in all male patients with X-ALD and in about 85% of female carriers of X-ALD. Mutation analysis is the most reliable method for the identification of carriers.

CT AND MRI Patients with childhood cerebral or adolescent ALD show cerebral white matter lesions that are characteristic with respect to location and attenuation patterns on MRI. In 80% of patients, the lesions are symmetric and involve the periventricular white matter in the posterior parietal and occipital lobes. About 50% show location of a garland of accumulated contrast material adjacent and anterior to the posterior hypodense lesions (Fig. 80-5*A*). This zone corresponds to the zones of intense perivascular lymphocytic infiltration where the blood-brain barrier breaks down. In 12% of patients, the initial lesions are frontal. Unilateral lesions that produce a mass effect suggestive of a brain tumor may occur. MRI provides a clearer delineation of normal and abnormal white matter than does CT and may demonstrate abnormalities missed by CT (Fig. 80-5*B*).

IMPAIRED ADRENAL FUNCTION More than 85% of patients with the childhood form of ALD have elevated levels of ACTH in plasma and a subnormal rise of cortisol levels in plasma following intravenous injection of 250 μg of ACTH (Cortrosyn).

Diagnosis and Differential Diagnosis

The earliest manifestations of childhood cerebral ALD are difficult to distinguish from the more common attention-deficit disorders or learning disabilities. Rapid progression, signs of dementia, or difficulty in auditory discrimination suggest ALD. Even in early stages, CT or MRI may show strikingly abnormal changes. Other leukodystrophies (Chapters 592 and 605.10) or multiple sclerosis (Chapter 593.1) may mimic these radiographic findings. Definitive diagnosis depends on demonstration of VLCFA excess, which occurs only in X-ALD and the other peroxisomal disorders. The latter may be distinguished from X-ALD by their clinical presentation during the neonatal period.

Cerebral forms of ALD may present as increased intracranial pressure and unilateral mass lesions. These have been misdiagnosed as gliomas, even after brain biopsy, and several patients have received radiotherapy before the correct diagnosis was made. Measurement of VLCFA in plasma or brain biopsy specimens is the most reliable differentiating test.

Adolescent or adult cerebral ALD can be confused with psychiatric disorders, dementing disorders, or epilepsy. The 1st clue to the diagnosis of ALD may be the demonstration of white matter lesions by CT or MRI; assays of VLCFA are confirmatory.

ALD cannot be distinguished clinically from other forms of Addison disease; it is recommended that assays of VLCFA levels be performed in all male patients with Addison disease. ALD patients do not usually have antibodies to adrenal tissue in their plasma.

Complications

An avoidable complication is the occurrence of adrenal insufficiency. The most difficult neurologic problems are those related to bed rest, contracture, coma, and swallowing disturbances. Other complications involve behavioral disturbances and injuries associated with defects of spatial orientation, impaired vision and hearing, and seizures.

Treatment

Corticosteroid replacement for adrenal insufficiency or adrenocortical hypofunction is effective (Chapter 569). It may be lifesaving and increase general strength and well-being, but it does not alter the course of the neurologic disability.

BONE MARROW TRANSPLANTATION Bone marrow transplantation (BMT) benefits patients who show early evidence of the inflammatory demyelination that is characteristic of the rapidly

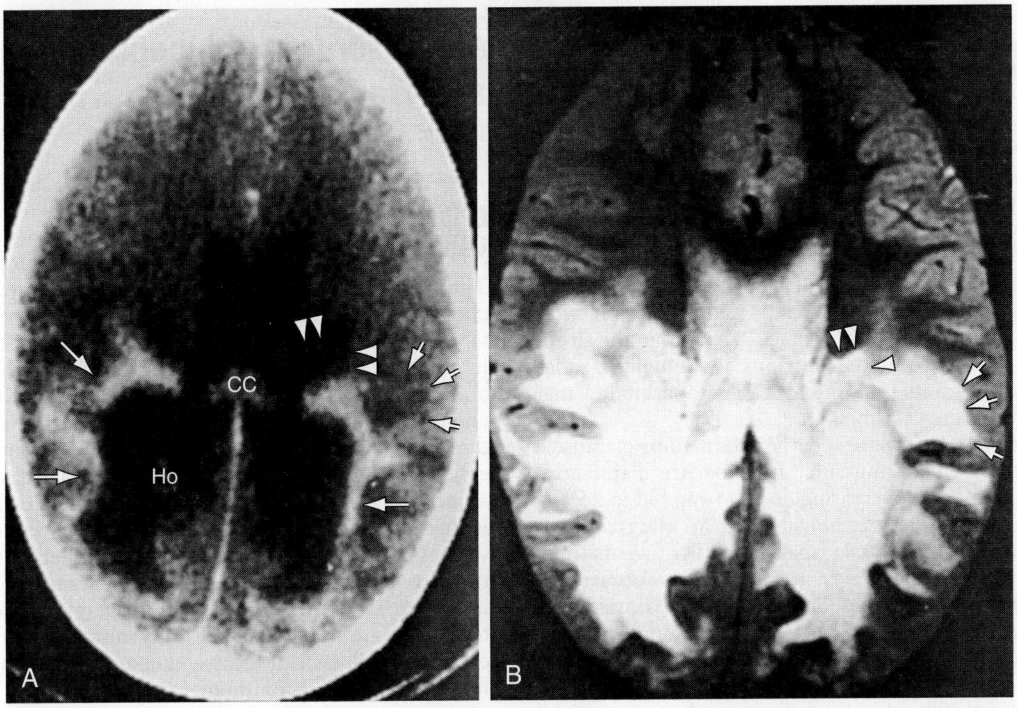

Figure 80-5 *A,* Contrast enhanced CT abnormalities in adrenoleukodystrophy (ALD) with typical parieto-occipital location, showing symmetric bilateral hypodense inactive zones (Ho). The enhancing active periphery zone of hypodensity is demarcated by *arrows.* Compare the anterior zone of hypodensity *(arrowheads)* with that on the MRI in *B.* CC, corpus callosum. *B,* MRI of the same pattern and area shown by CT. MRI T2 weighted image shows a high-intensity signal of the abnormally bright parieto-occipital white matter. Subcortical involvement is better identified on MRI. Separation of active zones may be better appreciated by CT, because both inactive and active zones are seen at high-signal areas on MRI. It is assumed, however, that such major distinctions afforded by CT will also be demonstrable when IV enhancement (paramagnetic enhancement) becomes readily available. Note the hypodense involvement of CT (*arrowheads* and *arrows* in *A*) compared with the well-resolved lesions on MRI in *B.* (From Kumar AJ, Rosenbaum WE, Naidu S, et al: Adrenoleukodystrophy: corresponding MR imaging with CT, *Radiology* 165:497–504, 1987.)

progressive neurologic disability in boys and adolescents with the cerebral X-ALD phenotype. BMT is a high-risk procedure, and patients must be selected with great care. The mechanism of the beneficial effect is incompletely understood. Bone marrow-derived cells do express ALDP, the protein that is deficient in X-ALD; approximately 50% of brain microglial cells are bone marrow derived. It is possible that replacement of affected cells by cells that contain the normal gene changes the brain milieu sufficiently to correct the brain metabolic disturbance. The favorable effect may also be caused by modification of the brain inflammatory response. Five to 10 yr follow-up of boys and adolescents who had early cerebral involvement has shown stabilization and, in some instances, improvement. On the other hand, BMT has not shown favorable effects in patients who had already severe brain involvement and may accelerate disease progression under these circumstances. The nonverbal IQ has been found to be of predictive value, and transplant is not recommended in patients with nonverbal IQ significantly below 80. Unfortunately, in more than half the patients who are diagnosed because of neurologic symptoms, the illness is so advanced that they are not candidates for transplant.

Consideration of BMT is most relevant in neurologically asymptomatic or mildly involved patients. Screening at-risk relatives of symptomatic patients identifies these patients most frequently. Screening by measurement of plasma VLCFA levels in patients with Addison disease may also identify candidates for BMT. Because of its risk (10-20% mortality) and the fact that up to 50% of untreated patients with X-ALD do not develop inflammatory brain demyelination, transplant is not recommended in patients who are free of demonstrable brain involvement. The MRI is also of key importance for the crucial decision of whether transplant should be performed. MRI abnormalities precede clinically evident neurologic or neuropsychologic abnormalities. The brain MRI should be monitored at 6 mo to 1 yr intervals in neurologically asymptomatic boys and adolescents between the ages of 3 and 15 yr. If the MRI is normal, BMT is not indicated. If brain MRI abnormalities develop, the patient should be evaluated at 3 mo intervals to determine if the abnormality is progressive, in combination with careful neurologic and neuropsychologic evaluation; and if early progressive involvement is confirmed, transplant should be considered. Magnetic resonance spectroscopy improves the capacity to determine whether the brain involvement is progressive. It is not known whether BMT has a favorable effect on the noninflammatory spinal cord involvement in adults with the adrenomyeloneuropathy phenotype.

LORENZO'S OIL THERAPY The administration of Lorenzo's oil to asymptomatic boys reduces the risk of developing the childhood cerebral phenotype by a factor of 2 or more. Lorenzo's oil (4:1 mixture of glyceryl trioleate and glyceryl trierucate) combined with a dietary regimen is recommended for neurologically asymptomatic boys who have a normal brain MRI and are younger than 8 yr old, but must be supervised carefully. Adrenal function and brain MRI must be monitored. Patients who develop progressive MRI abnormalities are evaluated for hematopoietic stem cell transplant when changes are still in an early phase. Lorenzo's oil has not been shown to alter disease progression in patients who already have cerebral involvement.

SUPPORTIVE THERAPY The progressive behavioral and neurologic disturbances associated with the childhood form of ALD are extremely difficult for the family. ALD patients require the establishment of a comprehensive management program and partnership among the family, physician, visiting nursing staff, school authorities, and counselors. In addition, parent support groups are often helpful (United Leukodystrophy Foundation, 2304 Highland Drive, Sycamore, IL 60178). Communication with school authorities is important because under the provisions of Public Law 94-142, children with ALD qualify for special services as "other health impaired" or "multihandicapped." Depending on the rate of progression of the disease, special needs might range from relatively low-level resource services within a regular school program to home- and hospital-based teaching programs for children who are not mobile.

Management challenges vary with the stage of the illness. The early stages are characterized by subtle changes in affect, behavior, and attention span. Counseling and communication with school authorities are of prime importance. Changes in the sleep-wake cycle can be benefited by the judicious use at night of sedatives such as chloral hydrate (10-50 mg/kg), pentobarbital (5 mg/kg), or diphenhydramine (2-3 mg/kg).

As the leukodystrophy progresses, the modulation of muscle tone and support of bulbar muscular function are major concerns. Baclofen in gradually increasing doses (5 mg bid to 25 mg qd) is the most effective pharmacologic agent for the treatment of acute episodic painful muscle spasms. Other agents may also be used, with care being taken to monitor the occurrence of side effects and drug interactions. As the leukodystrophy progresses, bulbar muscular control is lost. Although initially this can be managed by changing the diet to soft and pureed foods, most patients eventually require a nasogastric tube or a gastrostomy. At least 30% of patients have focal or generalized seizures that usually readily respond to standard anticonvulsant medications.

Genetic Counseling and Prevention

Genetic counseling and primary and secondary prevention of X-ALD are of crucial importance. Extended family screening should be offered to all at-risk relatives of symptomatic patients; one program led to the identification of more than 250 asymptomatic affected males and 1,200 women heterozygous for X-ALD. The plasma assay permits reliable identification of affected males in whom plasma VLCFA levels are increased already on the day of birth. Identification of asymptomatic males permits institution of steroid replacement therapy when appropriate and prevents the occurrence of adrenal crisis, which may be fatal. Monitoring of brain MRI also permits identification of patients who are candidates for BMT at a stage when this procedure has the greatest chance of success. Plasma VLCFA assay is recommended in all male patients with Addison disease. X-ALD has been shown to be the cause of adrenal insufficiency in >25% of boys with Addison disease of unknown cause. Identification of women heterozygous for X-ALD is more difficult than that of affected males. Plasma VLCFA levels are normal in 15-20% of heterozygous women, and failure to note this has led to serious errors in genetic counseling. If VLCFA levels are normal both in plasma and cultured skin fibroblasts, the risk of false-negative results is reduced but not eliminated. DNA analysis permits accurate identification of carriers, provided that the mutation has been defined in a family member, and is the procedure recommended for the identification of heterozygous women. Mutation analysis is available on a service basis.

Prenatal diagnosis of affected male fetuses can be achieved by measurement of VLCFA levels in cultured amniocytes or chorionic villus cells and by mutation analysis. Whenever a new patient with X-ALD is identified, a detailed pedigree should be constructed and efforts should be made to identify all at-risk female carriers and affected males. These investigations should be accompanied by careful and sympathetic attention to social, emotional, and ethical issues during counseling.

BIBLIOGRAPHY

Please visit the Nelson Textbook of Pediatrics *website at www.expertconsult.com for the complete bibliography.*

80.3 Disorders of Lipoprotein Metabolism and Transport

William A. Neal

EPIDEMIOLOGY OF BLOOD LIPIDS AND CARDIOVASCULAR DISEASE

The relationship between dietary fat consumption and plasma cholesterol was demonstrated nearly a century ago. The Seven Countries Study of geographic, social class, and ethnic differences in coronary heart disease (CHD) around the world found strong associations between average intake of saturated fats, plasma cholesterol, and mortality from CHD. Of all common chronic diseases, none is so clearly influenced by both environmental and genetic factors as CHD. This multifactorial disorder is strongly associated with increasing age and male gender, though it is increasingly apparent that heart disease is under recognized in women. Tobacco use confers a 2-fold higher lifetime risk. Sedentary activity and high intake of saturated fats leading to adiposity increase risk through differences in the plasma levels of lipoproteins that are atherogenic. Family history is a reflection of the combined influence of lifestyle and genetic predisposition to early heart disease. Risk of premature heart disease associated with positive family history is 1.7 times higher than in families with no such history.

The pathogenesis of atherosclerosis begins during childhood. The Johns Hopkins Precursors Study demonstrated that white male medical students with blood cholesterol levels in the lowest quartile showed only a 10% incidence of CHD 3 decades later, whereas those in the highest quartile had a 40% incidence. The Pathobiological Determinants of Atherosclerosis in Youth (PDAY) Study demonstrated a significant relationship between the weight of the abdominal fat pad and the extent of atherosclerosis found at autopsy on subjects 15-34 yr of age. The Bogalusa Heart Study of >3,000 black and white children and adolescents has provided the most comprehensive longitudinal data relating the presence and severity of CHD risk factors with semiquantifiable severity of atherosclerosis.

The "fetal origins hypothesis" is based on the observation that infants born with low birthweight have a higher incidence of heart disease as adults. Epidemiologic studies support the idea that prenatal and early postnatal conditions may affect adult health status. Children who are large for gestational age at birth and exposed to an intrauterine environment of either diabetes or maternal obesity are at increased risk of eventually developing the "metabolic syndrome" (insulin resistance, type II diabetes, obesity, CHD). Breast-feeding preterm infants confers a long-term cardioprotective benefit 13-16 yr later. Those adolescents who were breast-fed as infants had lower C-reactive protein concentrations and a 14% lower LDL to HDL ratio compared to those fed infant formulas.

In addition, secondary causes of hyperlipidemia may be the result of drugs (cyclosporine, steroids, isotretinoin, protease inhibitors, alcohol, thiazide diuretics, beta blocking agents, valproate), or various diseases (nephrotic syndrome, hypothyroidism, Cushing syndrome, anorexia nervosa, obstructive jaundice).

BLOOD LIPIDS AND ATHEROGENESIS

Numerous epidemiologic studies have demonstrated the association of hypercholesterolemia, referring to elevated total blood cholesterol, with atherosclerotic disease. The ability to measure subcomponents within classes of lipid particles, as well as markers of inflammation, have further elucidated the process of atherogenesis and plaque rupture leading to acute coronary syndromes.

Atherosclerosis affects primarily the coronary arteries but also often involves the aorta, arteries of the lower extremities, and carotid arteries.

The early stage of development of atherosclerosis is thought to begin with vascular endothelial dysfunction and intima media thickness, which has been shown to occur in preadolescent children with risk factors such as obesity or familial hypercholesterolemia. The complex process of penetration of the intimal lining of the vessel may be due to a variety of insults, including the presence of highly toxic oxidized LDL particles. Lymphocytes and monocytes penetrate the damaged endothelial lining, where they become macrophages laden with LDL lipids and then become foam cells. Such accumulation is counterbalanced by HDL particles capable of removing lipid deposits from the vessel wall. Fundamental to plaque formation is an inflammatory process (elevated C-reactive protein) involving macrophages and the arterial wall. The deposition of lipid within the subendothelial lining of the arterial wall appears macroscopically as fatty streaks, which may to some degree be reversible. A later stage of plaque development involves disruption of arterial smooth muscle cells stimulated by the release of tissue cytokines and growth factors. The atheroma is composed of a core of fatty substance separated from the lumen by collagen and smooth muscle (Fig. 80-6). Growth of the atherosclerotic plaque may result in ischemia of the tissue supplied by the artery. Chronic inflammation within the atheroma, perhaps caused by infectious agents such as *Chlamydia pneumoniae,* results in plaque instability and subsequent rupture. Platelet adherence leads to clot formation at the site of rupture, resulting in myocardial infarction or a cerebrovascular event.

PLASMA LIPOPROTEIN METABOLISM AND TRANSPORT

Abnormalities of lipoprotein metabolism are associated with diabetes mellitus and premature atherosclerosis. Lipoproteins are soluble complexes of lipids and proteins that effect transport of fat absorbed from the diet, or synthesis by the liver and adipose tissues, for utilization and storage. Dietary fat is transported from the small intestine as chylomicrons. Lipids synthesized by the liver as very low density lipoproteins (VLDL) are catabolized to intermediate density lipoproteins (IDL) and low-density lipoproteins (LDL). High-density lipoproteins (HDL) are fundamentally involved in VLDL and chylomicron metabolism and cholesterol transport. Nonesterified free fatty acids (FFAs) are metabolically active lipids derived from lipolysis of triglycerides stored in adipose tissue bound to albumin for circulation in the plasma (Fig. 80-7).

Lipoproteins consist of a central core of triglycerides and cholesteryl esters (CE) surrounded by phospholipids, cholesterol, and proteins (Fig. 80-8). The density of the several classes of lipoproteins is inversely proportional to the ratio of lipid to protein (Fig. 80-9).

Constituent proteins are known as apolipoproteins (Table 80-7). They are responsible for a variety of metabolic functions in addition to their structural role, including cofactors or inhibitors of enzymatic pathways, and mediators of lipoprotein binding to cell surface receptors. ApoA is the major apoliprotein of HDL. ApoB is present in LDL, VLDL, IDL, and chylomicrons. ApoB-100 is derived from the liver, whereas apoB-48 comes from the small intestine. ApoC-I, C-II, and C-III are small peptides important in triglyceride metabolism. Likewise, apoE, which is present in VLDL, HDL, chylomicrons, and chylomicron remnants, plays an important role in the clearance of triglycerides.

Transport of Exogenous (Dietary) Lipids

All dietary fat with the exception of medium-chain triglycerides is efficiently carried into the circulation by way of lymphatic drainage from the intestinal mucosa. Triglyceride (TG) and CE combine with apoA and apoB-48 in the intestinal mucosa to form chylomicrons, which are carried into the peripheral circulation via the lymphatic system. HDL particles contribute apoC-II to the chylomicrons, required for the activation of lipoprotein lipase (LPL) within the capillary endothelium of adipose, heart, and skeletal muscle tissue. Free fatty acids are oxidized, resterified for storage as triglycerides, or released into the circulation bound to albumin for transport to the liver. After hydrolysis of the TG core from the chylomicron, apoC particles are recirculated back to HDL. The subsequent contribution of apoE from HDL to the remnant chylomicron facilitates binding of the particle to hepatic LDL receptors (LDL-R). Within the hepatocyte, the chylomicron remnant may be incorporated into membranes, re-secreted as lipoprotein back into the circulation, or secreted as bile acids. Normally, all dietary fat is disposed of within 8 hr after the last meal, an exception being individuals with a disorder of chylomicron metabolism. Postprandial hyperlipidemia is a risk factor for atherosclerosis. Abnormal transport of chylomicrons and their remnants may result in their absorption into the blood vessel wall as foam cells, caused by the ingestion of CE by macrophages, the earliest stage in the development of fatty streaks.

Transport of Endogenous Lipids from the Liver

The formation and secretion of VLDL from the liver and its catabolism to IDL and LDL particles describe the endogenous lipoprotein pathway. Fatty acids used in the hepatic formation of VLDL are derived primarily by uptake from the circulation. VLDL appears to be transported from the liver as rapidly as it is synthesized, and it consists of triglycerides, cholesteryl esters, phospholipids, and apoB-100. Nascent particles of VLDL secreted

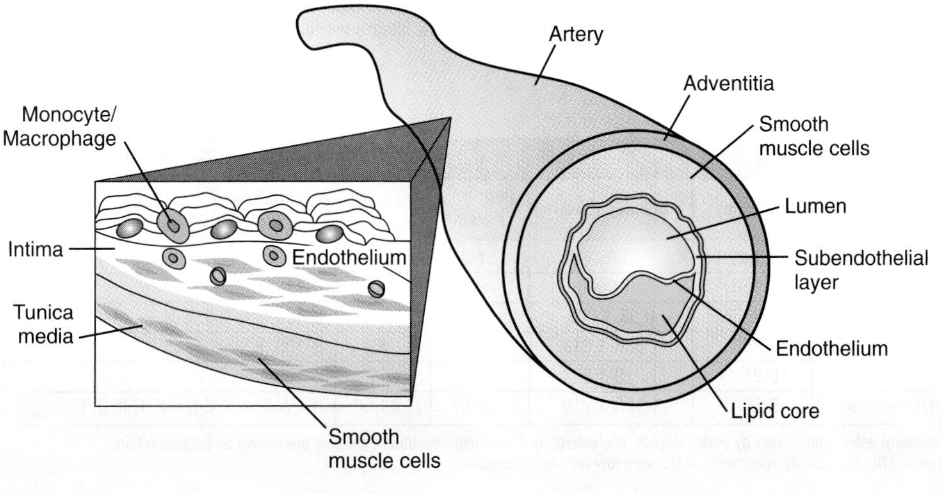

Figure 80-6 The early stage of development of atherosclerosis begins with penetration of the intimal lining of the vessel by inflammatory cells. Deposition of lipid within the subendothelial lining of the arterial wall eventually leads to disruption of smooth muscle cells to form an atheromatous lipid core that impinges on the lumen. Chronic inflammation leads to plaque instability, setting the stage for plaque rupture and complete occlusion of the vessel lumen by clot formation.

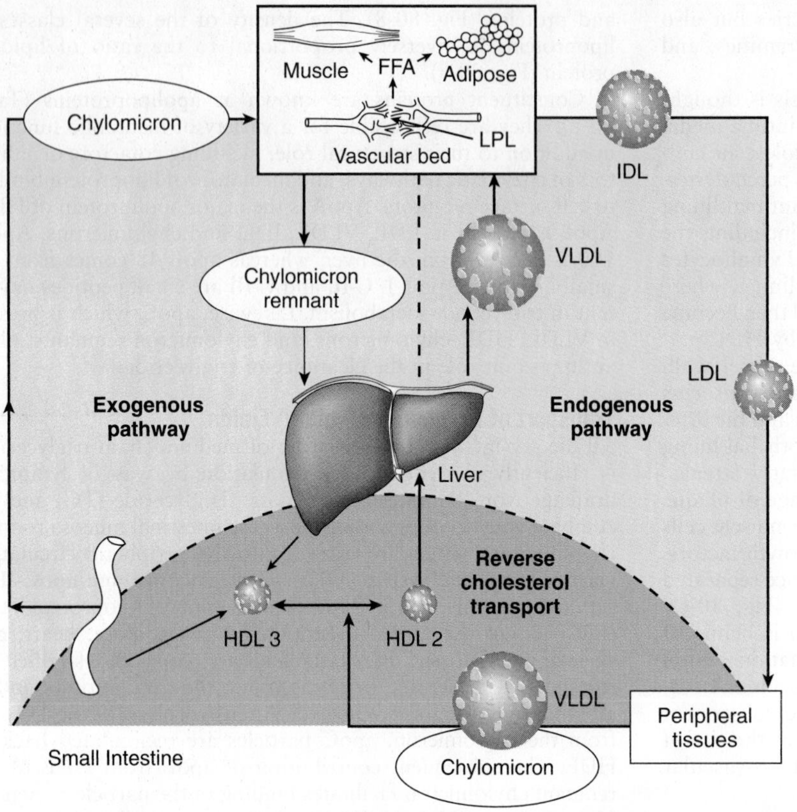

Figure 80-7 The exogenous, endogenous, and reverse cholesterol pathways. The exogenous pathway transports dietary fat from the small intestine as chylomicrons to the periphery and the liver. The endogenous pathway denotes the secretion of very low density lipoprotein (VLDL) from the liver and its catabolism to intermediate density lipoprotein (IDL) and low-density lipoprotein (LDL). Triglycerides are hydrolyzed from the VLDL particle by the action of lipoprotein lipase (LPL) in the vascular bed, yielding free fatty acids (FFAs) for utilization and storage in muscle and adipose tissue. High-density lipoprotein (HDL) metabolism is responsible for the transport of excess cholesterol from the peripheral tissues back to the liver for excretion in the bile. Nascent HDL-3 particles derived from the liver and small intestine are esterified to more mature HDL-2 particles by enzyme-mediated movement of chylomicron and VLDL into the HDL core, which is removed from the circulation by endocytosis.

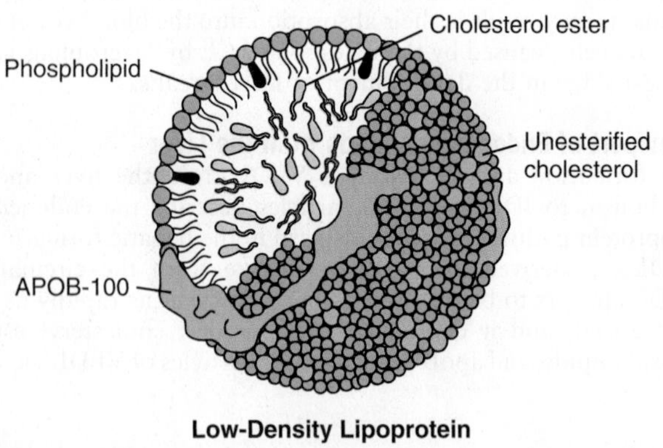

Figure 80-8 Schematic model of low-density lipoprotein (LDL). Lipoprotein consists of a central core of cholesteryl esters, surrounded by phospholipids, cholesterol, and protein.

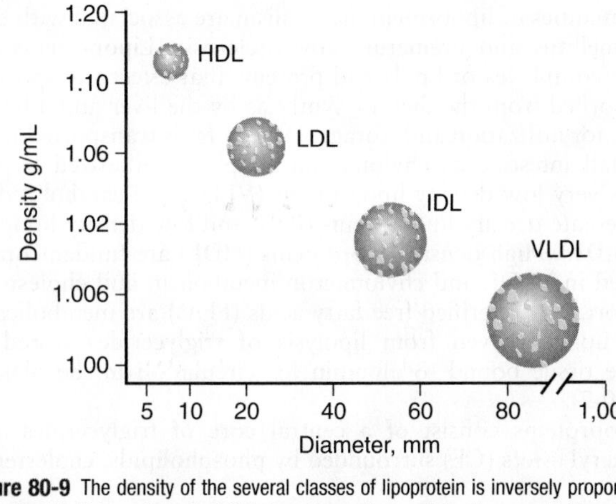

Figure 80-9 The density of the several classes of lipoprotein is inversely proportional to the ratio of lipid to protein. As lipid is less dense than protein, the more lipid contained in the particle increases its size and decreases its density. HDL, high-density lipoprotein; LDL, low-density lipoprotein; IDL, intermediate density lipoprotein; VLDL, very low density lipoprotein.

Table 80-7 CHARACTERISTICS OF THE MAJOR LIPOPROTEINS

LIPOPROTEIN*	SOURCE	SIZE (nm)	DENSITY (g/mL)	COMPOSITION %		
				Protein	Lipid	APOLIPOPROTEINS*
Chylomicrons	Intestine	80-1,200	<0.95	1-2	98-99	C-I, C-II, C-III, E, A-I, A-II, A-IV, B-48
Chylomicron remnants	Chylomicrons	40-150	<1.0006	6-8	92-94	B-48, E
VLDL	Liver, intestine	30-80	0.95-1.006	7-10	90-93	B-100, C-I, C-II, C-III
IDL	VLDL	25-35	1.006-1.019	11	89	B-100, E
LDL	VLDL	18-25	1.019-1.063	21	79	B-100
HDL	Liver, intestine VLDL, Chylomicrons	5-20	1.125-1.210	32-57	43-68	A-I, A-II, A-IV C-I, C-II, C-III D, E

*Lipoproteins consist of a central core of triglycerides and cholestenyl esters surrounded by phospholipids, cholesterol, and proteins. Constituent proteins are known as apolipoproteins.
HDL, high-density lipoprotein; IDL, intermediate density lipoprotein; LDL, low-density lipoprotein; VLDL, very low density lipoprotein.

into the circulation combine with apoliproteins Cs and E. The size of the VLDL particle is determined by the amount of triglyceride present, progressively shrinking in size as TG is hydrolyzed by the action of LPL, yielding free fatty acids for utilization or storage in muscle and adipose tissue. Hydrolysis of about 80% of the TG present in VLDL particles produces IDL particles containing an equal amount of cholesterol and TG. The remaining remnant IDL is converted to LDL for delivery to peripheral tissues or to the liver. ApoE is attached to the remnant IDL particle to allow binding to the cell and subsequent incorporation into the lysosome. Individuals with deficiency of either apoE2 or hepatic triglyceride lipase (HTGL) accumulate IDL in the plasma.

LDL particles account for approximately 70% of the plasma cholesterol in normal individuals. LDL receptors are present on the surfaces of nearly all cells. Most LDL is taken up by the liver, and the rest is transported to peripheral tissues such as the adrenal glands and gonads for steroid synthesis. Dyslipidemia is greatly influenced by LDL-R activity. The efficiency with which VLDL is converted into LDL is also important in lipid homeostasis.

HDL and Reverse Cholesterol Transport

As hepatic secretion of lipid particles into the bile is the only mechanism by which cholesterol can be removed from the body, transport of excess cholesterol from the peripheral cells is a vitally important function of HDL. HDL is heavily laden with apoA-I containing lipoproteins, which is nonatherogenic in contrast to B lipoproteins. Cholesterol-poor nascent HDL particles secreted by the liver and small intestine are esterified to more mature HDL-2 particles by the action of the enzyme lecithin-cholesterol acyltransferase (LCAT), which facilitates movement of chylomicrons and VLDL into the HDL core. HDL-2 may transfer cholesteryl esters back to apoB lipoproteins mediated by cholesteryl ester transfer protein (CETP), or the cholesterol-rich particle may be removed from the plasma by endocytosis, completing reverse cholesterol transport. Low HDL may be genetic (deficiency of apoA-I) or secondary to increased plasma TG.

HYPERLIPOPROTEINEMIAS

Hypercholesterolemia (Table 80-8)

FAMILIAL HYPERCHOLESTEROLEMIA (FH) FH is a monogenic autosomal co-dominant disorder caused by mutations affecting the LDL receptor. It is characterized by strikingly elevated LDL cholesterol, premature cardiovascular disease (CVD), and tendon xanthomas. There are five classes of mutations affecting the ability of LDL cholesterol to bind with the LDL receptor. Of the nearly 800 mutations described, some result in failure of synthesis of the LDL receptor (receptor negative) and others cause defective binding or release at the lipoprotein-receptor interface. Receptor negative mutations result in more severe phenotypes than receptor defective mutations.

HOMOZYGOUS FH FH homozygotes inherit 2 abnormal LDL receptor genes, resulting in markedly elevated plasma cholesterol levels ranging between 500 and 1,200 mg/dL. Triglyceride levels are normal to mildly elevated, and HDL levels may be slightly decreased. The condition occurs in 1/1,000,000 persons. Receptor negative patients have <2% normal LDL receptor activity, whereas those who are receptor defective may have as much 25% normal activity and a better prognosis.

The prognosis is poor regardless of the specific LDL receptor aberration. Severe atherosclerosis involving the aortic root and coronary arteries is present by early- to mid-childhood. These children usually present with xanthomas, which may cause thickening of the Achilles tendon or extensor tendons of the hands, or cutaneous lesions on the hands, elbows, knees, or buttocks (Figs. 80-10, 80-11, and 80-12). Corneal arcus may be present. Family history is informative because premature heart disease is strongly prevalent among relatives of both parents. The diagnosis may be confirmed by measuring LDL receptor activity in cultured skin fibroblasts. Phenotypic expression of the disease may also be assessed by measuring receptor activity on the surface of lymphocytes by using cell sorting techniques.

Untreated homozygous patients rarely survive to adulthood. Symptoms of coronary insufficiency may occur; sudden death is common. LDL apheresis to selectively remove LDL particles from the circulation is recommended for many children and has been shown to slow the progression of atherosclerosis. Liver transplantation has also been successful in decreasing LDL cholesterol levels, but complications related to immunosuppression are common. HMG CoA reductase inhibitors are often effective

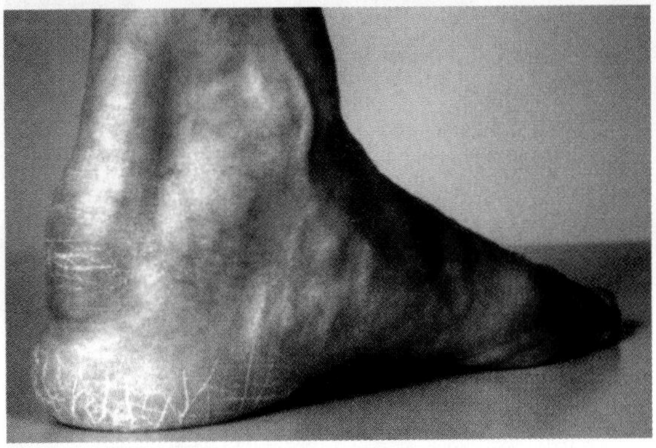

Figure 80-10 Achilles tendon xanthoma (heterozygous familial hypercholesterolemia). (From Durrington P: Dyslipidaemia, *Lancet* 362:717–731, 2003.)

Table 80-8 HYPERLIPOPROTEINEMIAS

DISORDER	LIPOPROTEINS ELEVATED	CLINICAL FINDINGS	GENETICS	ESTIMATED INCIDENCE
Familial hypercholesterolemia	LDL	Tendon xanthomas, CHD	AD	1/500
Familial defective ApoB-100	LDL	Tendon xanthomas, CHD	AD	1/1,000
Autosomal recessive hypercholesterolemia	LDL	Tendon xanthomas, CHD	AR	<1/1,000,000
Sitosterolemia	LDL	Tendon xanthomas, CHD	AR	<1/1,000,000
Polygenic hypercholesterolemia	LDL	CHD		1/30?
Familial combined hyperlipidemia (FCHL)	LDL, TG	CHD	AD	1/200
Familial dysbetalipoproteinemia	LDL, TG	Tubereruptive xanthomas, peripheral vascular disease	AD	1/10,000
Familial chylomicronemia (Frederickson type I)	TG↑↑	Eruptive xanthomas, hepatosplenomegaly, pancreatitis	AR	1/1,000,000
Familial hypertriglyceridemia (Frederickson type IV)	TG↑	±CHD	AD	1/500
Familial hypertriglyceridemia (Frederickson type V)	TG↑↑	Xanthomas ± CHD	AD	
Familial hepatic lipase deficiency	VLDL	CHD	AR	<1/1,000,000

AD, autosomal dominant; AR, autosomal recessive; CHD, coronary heart disease; LDL, low-density lipoproteins, TG, triglycerides; VLDL, very low density lipoproteins.

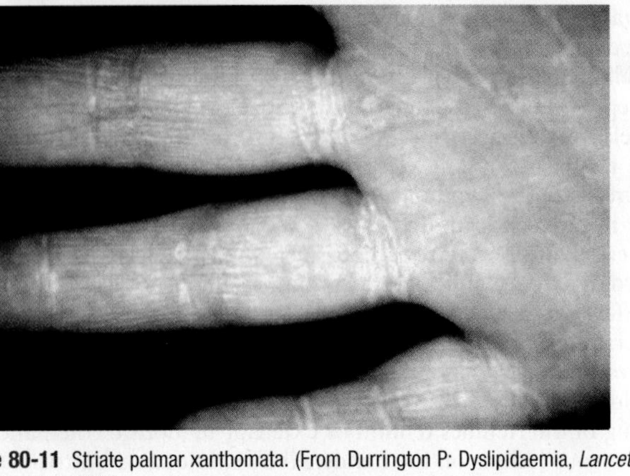

Figure 80-11 Striate palmar xanthomata. (From Durrington P: Dyslipidaemia, *Lancet* 362:717–731, 2003.)

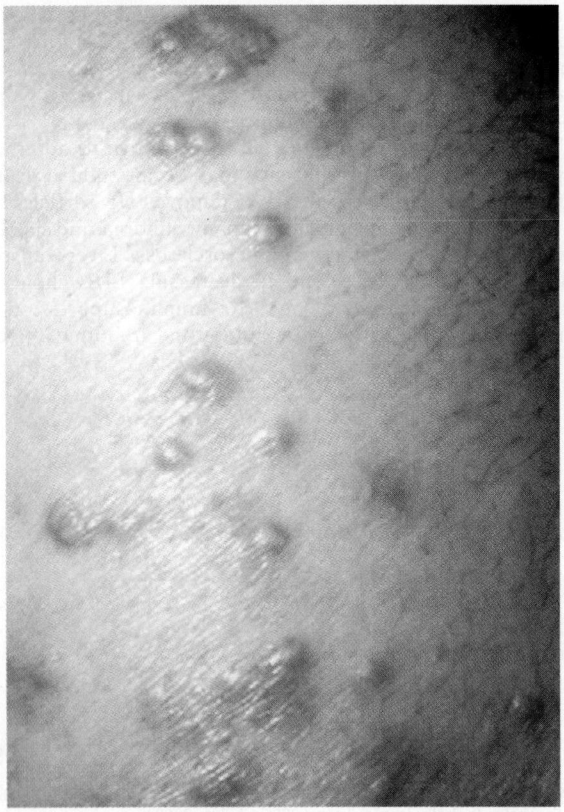

Figure 80-12 Eruptive xanthomata on extensor surface of forearm. (From Durrington P: Dyslipidaemia, *Lancet* 362:717–731, 2003.)

depending on the specific class of LDL receptor defect present. Combination therapy with ezetimibe, selectively blocking cholesterol adsorption in the gut, usually results in further modest decline in LDL levels; it has largely replaced the use of bile acid sequestrants.

HETEROZYGOUS FH Heterozygous FH is one of the most common single gene mutations associated with acute coronary syndromes and atherosclerotic CHD in adults. Its prevalence is approximately 1/500 individuals worldwide, but the frequency may be as high as 1/250 in selected populations such as French-Canadians, Afrikaners, and Christian Lebanese due to the founder effect of unique new mutations.

Heart disease accounts for more than half of all deaths in Western society. The pathogenesis of CHD is both environmental and genetic, and the complex interrelationship between the two determines the phenotypic expression of disease. Chinese people with heterozygous FH living in China have a mean LDL cholesterol of 168 mg/dL, whereas immigrant Chinese with the disease living in Canada average 288 mg/dL. This dramatic disparity in lipoprotein levels between geographic locations is expected to narrow as dietary and physical activity practices in China approximate those of the industrialized West.

Because heterozygous FH is a co-dominant condition with nearly full penetrance 50% of first-degree relatives of affected individuals will have the disease, as will 25% of second-degree relatives. An estimated 10 million people have FH worldwide. Symptoms of CHD usually occur at the mean age of 45-48 yr in males, and a decade later in females.

The World Health Organization (WHO) has targeted FH for individualized intervention strategies because of its large effect on morbidity and mortality. A relatively small percentage of the population accounts for a disproportionately high share of the burden of CVD. The clinical expression of the disease is straightforward and treatment is effective.

One cannot overemphasize the importance of family history for suspecting the possibility of FH. Indeed, the whole basis for deciding which children should have blood cholesterol testing is determined by a family history of premature CHD and/or parental hypercholesterolemia.

Plasma levels of LDL cholesterol do not allow unequivocal diagnosis of FH heterozygotes, but values are generally twice normal for age because of one absent or dysfunctional allele. The U.S. MED-PED ("make early diagnosis-prevent early death") Program based in Utah has formulated diagnostic criteria. Similar criteria with minor variation exist in the United Kingdom and Holland. The diagnosis within well-defined FH families is predictable according to LDL cut points. More stringent criteria are required to establish the diagnosis in previously undiagnosed families, requiring strong evidence of an autosomal inheritance pattern and higher LDL cut points. At a total cholesterol level of 310 mg/dL, only 4% of persons in the general population would have FH, whereas 95% of persons who were first-degree relatives of known cases would have the disease. The mathematical probability of FH, verified by molecular genetics, is derived from a U.S. population cohort and may not be applicable to other countries.

Very high cholesterol levels in children should prompt extensive screening of adult first- and second-degree relatives ("reverse" cholesterol screening). A child younger than 18 yr with total plasma cholesterol of 270 mg/dL and/or LDL-C of 200 mg/dL has an 88% chance of having FH. If there is a first-degree relative with proven FH, the diagnosis in the child is virtually certain (Table 80-9). Conversely, criteria for diagnosing probable FH in a child whose first-degree relative has known FH require only modest elevation of total cholesterol to 220 mg/dL (LDL-C 155 mg/dL).

Treatment of children with FH should begin with a rather rigorous low-fat diet (see later). Diet alone is rarely sufficient for decreasing blood cholesterol levels to acceptable levels (LDL-C <130 mg/dL). The Expert Panel on Blood Cholesterol Levels in Children and Adolescents (National Cholesterol Education Program) has promulgated guidelines for the consideration of cholesterol lowering medication in children at least 10 yr of age. Such consideration should be given if the LDL-C is >160 mg/dL in the presence of a strong history of premature heart disease in the family; or >190 mg/dL even in the absence of a positive family history, for example, if the child is adopted and family history is not available.

Ezetimibe blocks cholesterol adsorption in the gastrointestinal tract and has a low risk of side effects. Preliminary data suggest that ezetimibe will lower total cholesterol by 20-30 mg/dL. This medication has not been evaluated by controlled clinical trials in children. HMG CoA reductase inhibitors have become the drug of choice for treatment of FH because of their remarkable effectiveness and acceptable risk profile. There is sufficient clinical experience with this class of drugs in children to document that they are as effective in children as adults, and the risks of elevated hepatic enzymes and myositis are no greater than in adults.

Table 80-9 PERCENTAGE OF YOUTHS UNDER AGE 18 YR EXPECTED TO HAVE FH ACCORDING TO CHOLESTEROL LEVELS AND CLOSEST RELATIVE WITH FH

TOTAL CHOL (mg/dL)	LDL CHOL (mg/dL)	PERCENTAGE WITH FH AT THAT LEVEL — DEGREE OF RELATIVE			
		First	Second	Third	General Population
180	122	7.2	2.4	0.9	0.01
190	130	13.5	5.0	2.2	0.03
200	138	26.4	10.7	4.9	0.07
210	147	48.1	23.6	11.7	0.19
220	155	73.1	47.5	27.9	0.54
230	164	90.0	75.0	56.2	1.8
240	172	97.1	93.7	82.8	6.3
250	181	99.3	97.6	95.3	22.2
260	190	99.9	99.5	99.0	57.6
270	200	100.0	99.9	99.8	88.0
280	210	100.0	100.0	100.0	97.8
290	220	100.0	100.0	100.0	99.6
300	230	100.0	100.0	100.0	99.9
310	210	100.0	100.0	100.0	100.0

Chol, cholesterol; FH, familial hypercholesterolemia; LDL, low-density lipoprotein.
From Williams RR, Hunt SC, Schumacher MC, et al: Diagnosing heterozygous familial hypercholesterolemia using new practical criteria validated by molecular genetics, *Am J Cardiol* 72:171–176, 1993.

FAMILIAL DEFECTIVE APOB-100 (FDB) FDB is an autosomal dominant condition that is indistinguishable from heterozygous FH. LDL cholesterol levels are increased, triglycerides are normal, adults often develop tendon xanthomas, and premature CHD occurs. FDB is caused by mutation in the receptor binding region of apoB-100, the ligand of the LDL receptor, with an estimated frequency of 1/700 people in Western cultures. It is usually caused by substitution of glutamine for arginine in position 3500 in apoB-100, which results in reduced ability of the LDL receptor to bind LDL cholesterol, thus impairing its removal from the circulation. Specialized laboratory testing can distinguish FDB from FH, but this is not necessary, except in research settings, because treatment is the same.

AUTOSOMAL RECESSIVE HYPERCHOLESTEROLEMIA (ARH) This rare condition, caused by a defect in LDL receptor mediated endocytosis in the liver, clinically presents with severe hypercholesterolemia at levels intermediate between those found in homozygous and heterozygous FH. It is disproportionately present among Sardinians, and is modestly responsive to treatment with HMG CoA reductase inhibitors.

SITOSTEROLEMIA A rare autosomal recessive condition characterized by excessive intestinal adsorption of plant sterols, sitosterolemia is caused by mutations in the ATP-binding cassette transporter system, which is responsible for limiting adsorption of plant sterols in the small intestine and promotes biliary excretion of the small amounts adsorbed. Plasma cholesterol levels may be severely elevated, resulting in tendon xanthomas and premature atherosclerosis. Diagnosis can be confirmed by measuring elevated plasma sitosterol levels. Treatment with HMG CoA reductase inhibitors is not effective, but cholesterol adsorption inhibitors such as ezetimibe and bile acid sequestrants are effective.

POLYGENIC HYPERCHOLESTEROLEMIA Primary elevation in LDL cholesterol among children and adults is most often polygenic; the small effects of many genes are impacted by environmental influences (diet). Plasma cholesterol levels are modestly elevated; triglyceride levels are normal. Polygenic hypercholesterolemia aggregates in families sharing a common lifestyle but does not follow predictable hereditary patterns found in single gene lipoprotein defects. Treatment of children with polygenic hypercholesterolemia is directed toward adoption of a healthy lifestyle: reduced total and saturated fat consumption and at least 1 hr of physical activity daily. Cholesterol lowering medication is rarely necessary.

Hypercholesterolemia with Hypertriglyceridemia

FAMILIAL COMBINED HYPERLIPIDEMIA (FCHL) This is an autosomal dominant condition characterized by moderate elevation in plasma LDL cholesterol and triglycerides, and reduced plasma HDL cholesterol. It is the most common primary lipid disorder, occurring in approximately 1/200 people. No single metabolic aberration has been identified linking FCHL with atherogenesis, but it is well documented that about 20% of individuals who develop CHD by 60 yr of age have FCHL. Family history of premature heart disease is typically positive; the formal diagnosis requires that at least two first-degree relatives have evidence of one of three variants of dyslipidemia: (1) >90th percentile plasma LDL cholesterol; (2) >90th percentile LDL cholesterol and triglycerides; and (3) >90th percentile triglycerides. Individuals switch from one phenotype to another. Xanthomas are not a feature of FCHL. Elevated plasma apoB levels with increased small dense LDL particles support the diagnosis.

Children and adults with FCHL have co-existing adiposity, hypertension, and hyperinsulinemia, suggesting the presence of the *metabolic syndrome.* Formal diagnosis of this multiplex syndrome as defined by the NCEP's Adult Treatment Panel III (ATP III) identifies 6 major components: abdominal obesity, atherogenic dyslipidemia, hypertension, insulin resistance with or without impaired glucose tolerance, evidence of vascular inflammation, and prothrombotic state. It is estimated that 30% of overweight adults fulfill criteria for the diagnosis of metabolic syndrome, including 65% of those with FCHL. Hispanics and South Asians from the Indian subcontinent are especially susceptible.

The mechanisms associating visceral adiposity with the metabolic syndrome and type II diabetes are not fully understood. A plausible unifying principal is that obesity causes endoplasmic reticulum stress, leading to suppression of insulin receptor signaling and thus insulin resistance and heightened inflammatory response. How this relates to atherogenesis is unclear. It is assumed that hypercholesterolemia and, with less certainty, hypertriglyceridemia confer risk for CVD in patients with FCHL. When features of the metabolic syndrome are included in logistic models shared etiologic features such as increased visceral adiposity become apparent. Visceral adiposity increases with age and its importance in children as a risk factor for heart disease and diabetes is limited by the relative paucity of data. Though longitudinal measurement of waist circumference and the presence of intra-abdominal fat as determined by MRI is being conducted in the research setting, body mass index (BMI) remains the surrogate for adiposity in the pediatric clinical setting.

The metabolic syndrome is a dramatic illustration of the interaction of genetics and the environment. Genetic susceptibility is essential as an explanation for premature heart disease in individuals with FCHL. Unhealthy lifestyle, poor diet, and physical inactivity contribute to obesity and attendant features of the metabolic syndrome.

The cornerstone of management is lifestyle modification. This includes a diet low in saturated fats, trans fats, and cholesterol, as well as reduced consumption of simple sugars. Increased dietary intake of fruits and vegetables is important, as is 1 hr of moderate physical activity daily. Compliance among children and their parents is often a problem, but small incremental steps are more likely to succeed than aggressive weight-loss strategies. It is very important that the child's caregivers participate in the process. Plasma triglyceride levels are usually quite responsive to dietary restriction, especially reduction in the amount of sweetened drinks consumed. Blood cholesterol levels may decrease by 10-15%, but if LDL cholesterol remains >160 mg/dL, drug therapy should be considered.

FAMILIAL DYSBETALIPOPROTEINEMIA (FDBL, TYPE III HYPERLIPOPROTEINEMIA) FDBL is caused by mutations in the gene for apolipoprotein E (apoE), which when exposed to environmental influences such as high fat, high caloric diet, or excessive alcohol intake, results in a mixed type of hyperlipidemia. Patients tend to have elevated plasma cholesterol and triglycerides to a relatively similar degree. HDL cholesterol is typically normal in contrast to other causes of hypertriglyceridemia associated with low HDL. This rare disorder affects about 1/10,000 persons. ApoE mediates removal of chylomicron and VLDL remnants from the circulation by binding to hepatic surface receptors. The polymorphic *apoE* gene expresses in three isoforms: *apoE3, apoE2*, and *apoE4. E4* is the "normal" allele present in the majority of the population. The *apoE2* isoform has lower affinity for the LDL receptor and its frequency is about 7%. About 1% of the population is homozygous for *apoE2/E2*, the most common mutation associated with FDBL, but only a minority express the disease. Expression requires precipitating illnesses such as diabetes, obesity, renal disease, or hypothyroidism. Individuals homozygous for *apoE4/E4* are at risk for late-onset Alzheimer disease.

Most patients with FDBL present in adulthood with distinctive xanthomas. Tuberoeruptive xanthomas resemble small grapelike clusters on the knees, buttocks, and elbows. Prominent orange-yellow discoloration of the creases of the hands (palmar xanthomas) is also typically present. Atherosclerosis, often presenting with peripheral vascular disease, usually occurs in the 4th or 5th decade. Children may present with a less distinctive rash and generally have precipitating illnesses.

The diagnosis of FDBL is established by lipoprotein electrophoresis, which demonstrates a broad beta band containing remnant lipoproteins. Direct measurement of VLDL by ultracentrifugation can be performed in specialized lipid laboratories. A VLDL/total triglyceride ratio >0.30 supports the diagnosis. *ApoE* genotyping for *apoE2* homozygosity can be performed, confirming the diagnosis in the presence of the distinctive physical findings. A negative result does not necessarily rule out the disease as other mutations in *apoE* may cause even more serious manifestations.

Pharmacologic treatment of FDBL is necessary to decrease the likelihood of symptomatic atherosclerosis in adults. HMG CoA reductase inhibitors, nicotinic acid, and fibrates are all effective. FDBL is quite responsive to recommended dietary restriction.

Hypertriglyceridemias

The familial disorders of triglyceride-rich lipoproteins include both common and rare variants of the Frederickson classification system. These include chylomicronemia (type I), familial hypertriglyceridemia (type IV), and the more severe combined hypertriglyceridemia and chylomicronemia (type V). Hepatic lipase (HL) deficiency also results in a similar combined hyperlipidemia.

FAMILIAL CHYLOMICRONEMIA (TYPE I HYPERLIPIDEMIA) This rare single gene defect, like familial hypercholesterolemia, is due to mutations affecting clearance of apoB-containing lipoproteins. Deficiency or absence of lipoprotein lipase (LPL) or its cofactor apoC-II, which facilitates lipolysis by LPL, causes severe elevation of triglyceride rich plasma chylomicrons. HDL cholesterol levels are decreased. As clearance of these particles is markedly delayed, the plasma is noted to have a turbid appearance even after prolonged fasting (Fig. 80-13). Chylomicronemia caused by LPL deficiency is associated with modest elevation in triglycerides, whereas this is not the case when the cause is deficient or absent apoC-II. Both are autosomal recessive conditions with a frequency of approximately 1/1,000,000. The disease usually presents during childhood with acute pancreatitis. Eruptive xanthomas on the arms, knees, and buttocks may be present, and there may be hepatosplenomegaly. The diagnosis is established by assaying triglyceride lipolytic activity. Treatment of chylomicronemia is by vigorous dietary fat restriction supplemented by fat-soluble vitamins. Medium-chain triglycerides that are adsorbed into the portal venous system may augment total fat intake, and administration of fish oils may also be beneficial.

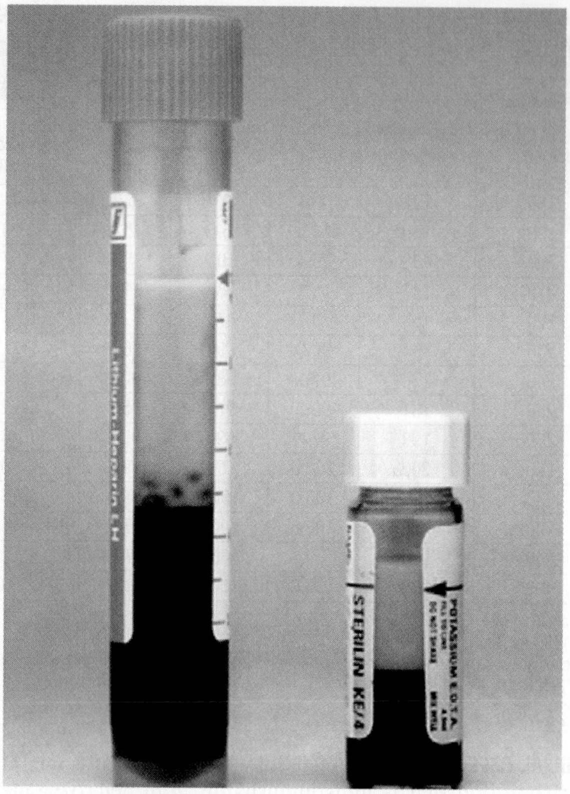

Figure 80-13 Milky plasma from patient with acute abdominal pain. (From Durrington P: Dyslipidaemia, *Lancet* 362:717–731, 2003.)

Familial Hypertriglyceridemia (FHTG, Type IV Hyperlipidemia)

FHTG is an autosomal dominant disorder of unknown etiology, which occurs in about 1/500 individuals. It is characterized by elevation of plasma triglycerides >90th percentile (250-1,000 mg/dL range), often accompanied by slight elevation in plasma cholesterol and low HDL. FHTG does not usually manifest until adulthood, though it is expressed in about 20% of affected children. In contrast to FCHL, FHTG is not thought to be highly atherogenic. It is most likely caused by defective breakdown of VLDL, or less often by overproduction of this class of lipoproteins.

The diagnosis should include the presence of at least one first-degree relative with hypertriglyceridemia. FHTG should be distinguished from FCHL and FDBL, as the latter require more vigorous treatment to prevent coronary or peripheral vascular disease. The differentiation is usually possible on clinical grounds, in that lower LDL cholesterol levels accompany FHTG, but measurement of normal apoB levels in FHTG may be helpful in ambiguous situations.

A more severe hypertriglyceridemia characterized by increased levels of chylomicrons as well as VLDL particles (Frederickson type V) may occasionally be encountered. Triglyceride levels are often >1,000 mg/dL. The disease is rarely seen in children. In contrast to chylomicronemia (Frederickson type I), LPL or apoC-II deficiency is not present. These patients often develop eruptive xanthomas in adulthood, whereas type IV hypertriglyceridemia individuals do not. Acute pancreatitis may be the presenting illness. As with other hypertriglyceridemias, excessive alcohol consumption and estrogen therapy can exacerbate the disease.

Secondary causes of transient hypertriglyceridemia should be ruled out before making a diagnosis of FHTG. A diet high in simple sugars and carbohydrates, or excessive alcohol consumption as well as estrogen therapy may exacerbate hypertriglyceridemia. Adolescents and adults should be questioned about excessive consumption of soda and other sweetened drinks, as it is common to encounter people who drink supersized drinks or multiple 12 oz cans of sweetened drinks daily. Cessation of this practice often results in dramatic fall in triglyceride levels as well as weight among those who are obese. HDL cholesterol levels will tend to rise as BMI stabilizes.

Pediatric diseases associated with hyperlipidemia include hypothyroidism, nephrotic syndrome, biliary atresia, glycogen storage disease, Niemann-Pick disease, Tay-Sachs disease, systemic lupus erythematosus, hepatitis, and anorexia nervosa (Table 80-10). Certain medications exacerbate hyperlipidemia, including isotretinoin (Accutane), thiazide diuretics, oral contraceptives, steroids, β-blockers, immunosuppressants, and protease inhibitors used in the treatment of HIV.

Treatment of hypertriglyceridemia in children rarely requires medication unless levels >1,000 mg/dL persist after dietary restriction of fats, sugars, and carbohydrates, accompanied by increased physical activity. In such cases, the aim is to prevent episodes of pancreatitis. The common use of fibrates (fenofibric acid) and niacin in adults with hypertriglyceridemia is not recommended in children. HMG CoA reductase inhibitors are reasonably effective in lowering triglyceride levels, and there is considerably more experience documenting the safety and efficacy of this class of lipid lowering medications in children.

HEPATIC LIPASE DEFICIENCY Hepatic lipase deficiency is a very rare autosomal recessive condition causing elevation in both plasma cholesterol and triglycerides. Hepatic lipase (HL) hydrolyzes triglycerides and phospholipids in VLDL remnants and IDL, preventing their conversion to LDL. HDL cholesterol levels tend to be increased rather than decreased, suggesting the diagnosis. Laboratory confirmation is established by measuring HL activity in heparinized plasma.

Table 80-10 SECONDARY CAUSES OF HYPERLIPIDEMIA

HYPERCHOLESTEROLEMIA
Hypothyrodism
Nephrotic syndrome
Cholestasis
Anorexia nervosa
Drugs: progesterone, thiazides, tegretol, cyclosporine
HYPERTRIGLYCERIDEMIA
Obesity
Type II diabetes
Alcohol
Renal failure
Sepsis
Stress
Cushing syndrome
Pregnancy
Hepatitis
AIDS, protease inhibitions
Drugs: anabolic steroids, β blockers, estrogen, thiazides
REDUCED HIGH-DENSITY LIPOPROTEIN
Smoking
Obesity
Type II diabetes
Malnutrition
Drugs: β Blockers, anabolic steroids

Disorders of HDL Metabolism

PRIMARY HYPOALPHALIPOPROTEINEMIA Isolated low HDL cholesterol is a familial condition that often follows a pattern suggestive of autosomal dominant inheritance but may occur independent of family history. It is the most common disorder of HDL metabolism. It is defined as HDL cholesterol <10th percentile for gender and age with normal plasma triglycerides and LDL cholesterol. Whether it is associated with more rapid atherosclerosis is uncertain. It appears to be related to a reduction in apoA-I synthesis and increased catabolism of HDL. Secondary causes of low HDL cholesterol, such as the metabolic syndrome, and rare diseases such as LCAT deficiency and Tangier disease must be ruled out.

FAMILIAL HYPERALPHALIPOPROTEINEMIA This is an unusual condition conferring deceased risk for CHD among family members. Plasma levels of HDL cholesterol exceed 80 mg/dL.

FAMILIAL APOA-I DEFICIENCY Mutations in the *apoA-I* gene may result in complete absence of plasma HDL. Nascent HDL is produced in the liver and small intestine. Free cholesterol from peripheral cells is esterified by LCAT, enabling formation of mature HDL particles. ApoA-I is required for normal enzymatic functioning of LCAT. The resultant accumulation of free cholesterol in the circulation eventually leads to corneal opacities, planar xanthomas, and premature atherosclerosis. Some patients, however, may have mutations of *apoA-I* that result in very rapid catabolism of the protein not associated with atherogenesis, despite HDL cholesterol levels in the 15-30 mg/dL range.

TANGIER DISEASE This is an autosomal co-dominant disease associated with levels of HDL cholesterol <5 mg/dL. It is caused by mutations in ABCA1, a protein that facilitates the binding of cellular cholesterol to apoA-I. This results in free cholesterol accumulation in the reticuloendothelial system manifested by tonsillar hypertrophy of a distinctive orange color and hepatosplenomegaly. Intermittent peripheral neuropathy may occur from cholesterol accumulation in Schwann cells. Diagnosis should be suspected in children with enlarged orange tonsils and extremely low HDL cholesterol levels.

FAMILIAL LECITHIN–CHOLESTEROL ACYLTRANSFERASE (LCAT) DEFICIENCY Mutations affecting LCAT interfere with the esterification of cholesterol, thereby preventing formation of mature HDL particles. This is associated with rapid catabolism of apoA-I. Free circulating cholesterol in the plasma is greatly increased, which leads to corneal opacities and HDL cholesterol levels <10 mg/dL. Partial LCAT deficiency is known as "fish-eye" disease. Complete deficiency causes hemolytic anemia and progressive renal insufficiency early in adulthood. This rare disease is not thought to cause premature atherosclerosis. Laboratory confirmation is based on demonstration of decreased cholesterol esterification in the plasma.

CHOLESTERYL ESTER TRANSFER PROTEIN (CETP) DEFICIENCY Mutations involving the CETP gene are localized to chromosome 16y21. CETP facilitates the transfer of lipoproteins from mature HDL to and from VLDL and chylomicron particles, thus ultimately regulating the rate of cholesterol transport to the liver for excretion in the bile. About half of mature HDL2 particles are directly removed from the circulation by HDL receptors on the surface of the liver. The other half of cholesteryl esters in the core of HDL exchange with triglycerides in the core of apoB lipoproteins (VLDL, IDL, LDL) for transport to the liver. Homozygous deficiency of CETP has been observed in subsets of the Japanese population with extremely high HDL cholesterol levels (>150 mg/dL).

Conditions Associated with Low Cholesterol

Disorders of apoB-containing lipoproteins and intracellular cholesterol metabolism are associated with low plasma cholesterol.

ABETALIPOPROTEINEMIA This rare autosomal recessive disease is caused by mutations in the gene encoding microsomal triglyceride transfer protein necessary for the transfer of lipids to nascent chylomicrons in the small intestine and VLDL in the liver. This results in absence of chylomicrons, VLDL, LDL, and apoB, and very low levels of plasma cholesterol and triglycerides. Fat malabsorption, diarrhea, and failure to thrive present in early childhood. Spinocerebellar degeneration, secondary to vitamin E deficiency, manifests in loss of deep tendon reflexes progressing to ataxia and lower extremity spasticity by adulthood. Patients with abetalipoproteinemia also acquire a progressive pigmented retinopathy associated with decreased night and color vision and eventual blindness. The neurologic symptoms and retinopathy may be mistaken for Friedreich ataxia. Differentiation from Friedreich ataxia is suggested by the presence of malabsorption and acanthocytosis on peripheral blood smear in abetalipoproteinemia. Many of the clinical manifestations of the disease are a result of malabsorption of fat-soluble vitamins, such as vitamins E, A, and K. Early treatment with supplemental vitamins, especially E, may significantly slow the development of neurologic sequelae. Vitamin E is normally transported from the small intestine to the liver by chylomicrons, where it is dependent on the endogenous VLDL pathway for delivery into the circulation and peripheral tissues. Parents of children with abetalipoproteinemia have normal blood lipid and apoB levels.

FAMILIAL HYPOBETALIPOPROTEINEMIA Familial homozygous hypobetalipoproteinemia is associated with symptoms very similar to those of abetalipoproteinemia, but the inheritance pattern is autosomal co-dominant. The disease is caused by mutations in the gene encoding apoB-100 synthesis. It is distinguishable from abetalipoproteinemia in that heterozygous parents of probands have plasma LDL cholesterol and apoB levels less than half normal. There are no symptoms or sequelae associated with the heterozygous condition.

The selective inability to secrete apoB-48 from the small intestine results in a condition resembling abetalipoproteinemia or homozygous hypobetalipoproteinemia. Sometimes referred to as Anderson disease, the failure of chylomicron absorption causes steatorrhea and fat-soluble vitamin deficiency. The blood level of apoB-100, derived from normal hepatocyte secretion, is normal in this condition.

SMITH-LEMLI-OPITZ SYNDROME (SLOS) Patients with SLOS often have multiple congenital anomalies and developmental delay caused by low plasma cholesterol and accumulated precursors (Tables 80-11 and 80-12). Family pedigree analysis has revealed its autosomal recessive inheritance pattern. Mutations in the *DHCR7* (7-dehydrocholesterol-Δ^7 reductase) gene result in deficiency of the microsomal enzyme DHCR7, which is necessary to complete the final step in cholesterol synthesis. It is not known why defects in cholesterol synthesis result in congenital malformations, but as cholesterol is a major component of myelin and a contributor to signal transduction in the developing nervous system, neurodevelopment is severely impaired. The incidence of SLOS is estimated to be 1/20,000-60,000 births among whites, with a somewhat higher frequency in Hispanics and lower incidence in individuals of African descent.

Spontaneous abortion of SLOS fetuses may occur. Type II SLOS often leads to death by the end of the neonatal period. Survival is unlikely when the plasma cholesterol level is <20 mg/dL. Laboratory measurement should be performed by gas chromatography, as standard techniques for lipoprotein assay include measurement of cholesterol precursors, which may yield a false positive result. Milder cases may not present until late childhood. Phenotypic variance ranges from microcephaly, cardiac and brain malformation, and multiple organ-system failure to only subtle dysmorphic features and mild developmental delay. Treatment includes supplemental dietary cholesterol (egg yolk) and HMG CoA reductase inhibition to prevent the synthesis of toxic precursors proximal to the enzymatic block.

Disorders of Intracellular Cholesterol Metabolism

CEREBROTENDINOUS XANTHOMATOSIS This autosomal recessive disorder presents clinically in late adolescence with tendon xanthomas, cataracts, and progressive neurodegeneration. It is caused

Table 80-11 MAJOR CLINICAL CHARACTERISTICS OF SMITH-LEMLI-OPITZ SYNDROME: FREQUENT ANOMALIES (>50% OF PATIENTS)

CRANIOFACIAL
Microcephaly
Blepharoptosis
Anteverted nares
Retromicrognathia
Low-set, posteriorly rotated ears
Midline cleft palate
Broad maxillary alveolar ridges
Cataracts (<50%)
SKELETAL ANOMALIES
Syndactyly of toes II/III
Postaxial polydactyly (<50%)
Equinovarus deformity (<50%)
GENITAL ANOMALIES
Hypospadias
Cryptorchidism
Sexual ambiguity (<50%)
DEVELOPMENT
Pre- and postnatal growth retardation
Feeding problems
Mental retardation
Behavioral abnormalities

From Haas D, Kelley RI, Hoffmann GF: Inherited disorders of cholesterol biosynthesis, *Neuropediatrics* 32:113–122, 2001.

Table 80-12 CHARACTERISTIC MALFORMATIONS OF INTERNAL ORGANS IN SEVERELY AFFECTED SMITH-LEMLI-OPITZ PATIENTS

CENTRAL NERVOUS SYSTEM
Frontal lobe hypoplasia
Enlarged ventricles
Agenesis of corpus callosum
Cerebellar hypoplasia
Holoprosencephaly
CARDIOVASCULAR
Atrioventricular canal
Secundum atrial septal defect
Patent ductus arteriosus
Membranous ventricular septal defect
URINARY TRACT
Renal hypoplasia or aplasia
Renal cortical cysts
Hydronephrosis
Ureteral duplication
GASTROINTESTINAL
Hirschsprung disease
Pyloric stenosis
Refractory dysmotility
Cholestatic and noncholestatic progressive liver disease
PULMONARY
Pulmonary hypoplasia
Abnormal lobation
ENDOCRINE
Adrenal insufficiency

From Haas D, Kelley RI, Hoffmann GF: Inherited disorders of cholesterol biosynthesis, *Neuropediatrics* 32:113–122, 2001.

by tissue accumulation of bile acid intermediates shunted into cholestanol resulting from mutations in the gene for sterol 27-hydroxylase. This enzyme is necessary for normal mitochondrial synthesis of bile acids in the liver. Early treatment with chenodeoxycholic acid reduces cholesterol levels and prevents the development of symptoms.

WOLMAN DISEASE AND CHOLESTEROL ESTER STORAGE DISEASE (CESD) These autosomal recessive disorders are caused by lack of lysosomal acid lipase. After LDL cholesterol is incorporated into the cell by endocytosis, it is delivered to lysosomes where it is hydrolyzed by lysosomal lipase. Failure of hydrolysis because of complete absence of the enzyme causes accumulation of cholesteryl esters within the cells. Hepatosplenomegaly, steatorrhea, and failure to thrive occur during early infancy, leading to death by the age of 1 yr. In CESD, a less severe form than Wolman disease, there is low but detectable acid lipase activity.

NIEMANN-PICK DISEASE TYPE C This is a disorder of intracellular cholesterol transport characterized by accumulation of cholesterol and sphingomyelin in the central nervous and reticuloendothelial systems. Death from this autosomal recessive neurologic disease usually occurs by adolescence.

Lipoprotein Patterns in Children and Adolescents

Table 80-13, derived primarily from the Lipid Research Clinics Population Studies, shows the distribution of lipoprotein levels in American youth at various ages. Total plasma cholesterol rises rapidly from a mean of 68 mg/dL at birth to a level approximately twice that by the end of the neonatal period. A very gradual rise in total cholesterol level occurs until puberty, at which time the mean level reaches 160 mg/dL. Total cholesterol falls transiently during puberty, in males due to a small decrease in HDL cholesterol, and in females secondary to a slight fall in LDL cholesterol. Blood cholesterol levels track reasonably well as individuals age. High blood cholesterol tends to aggregate in families, a reflection of genetic and environmental influences.

Acceptable total cholesterol among children and adolescents is <170 mg/dL; borderline is 170-199 mg/dL; and high >200 mg/dL. Acceptable LDL cholesterol is <110 mg/dL; borderline 110-129 mg/dL; and high >130 mg/dL. HDL cholesterol should be >40 mg/dL.

Blood Cholesterol Screening

Guidelines for cholesterol measurement in children were updated by the American Academy of Pediatricians in 2008. A *targeted* approach to cholesterol screening for children remains in effect:

- Screen children and adolescents whose parents or grandparents have documented coronary artery disease before the age of 55 yr.
- Screen the offspring of a parent who has been found to have high blood concentrations of cholesterol (>240 mg/dL).
- Screen children and adolescents for whom family history is unobtainable, particularly those with other risk factors such as obesity, hypertension, or diabetes mellitus.

Whereas Lipid Research Clinics data referenced in the original NCEP guidelines predicted that selective blood cholesterol screening of children would apply to a quarter of American youth, more recent population-based studies such as the National Health and Nutrition Examination Surveys (NHANES), predict that nearly half of children fulfill criteria for screening. The increase is likely due to the worrisome rise in youth obesity.

Being overweight confers special risk of CVD because of the strong association with the insulin resistance syndrome (metabolic syndrome). Though there is no single definition of metabolic syndrome defined for youth, it is likely that half of all severely obese children are insulin resistant. Among a large cohort of 5th grade school children who had comprehensive screening of CVD risk factors conducted by the Coronary Artery Risk Detection in Appalachian Communities (CARDIAC) Project, 49% of those with the hyperpigmented rash, acanthosis nigricans, had 3 or more risk factors for the metabolic syndrome, including insulin resistance, hypertension, and abnormal lipid levels (triglycerides >150 mg/dL; HDL-C <40 mg/dL) (Chapter 44).

Reliance on family history of premature heart disease, or known parental hypercholesterolemia greater than 240 mg/dL, is considered by some to be too insensitive and difficult to apply. Indeed, over half of children with hypercholesterolemia will be missed by the targeted approach to screening. It was predicted that those with severe genetic predisposition to premature heart disease, such as familial hypercholesterolemia (FH), would be identified by application of selective criteria for screening. However, data from the CARDIAC Project found that universal screening of youth identified just as many children with severe dyslipidemia who did not fulfill criteria as those who did.

It is possible that, in the future, guidelines regarding blood cholesterol screening in childhood may be liberalized further to include all children because of newer information and changing

Table 80-13 PLASMA CHOLESTEROL AND TRIGLYCERIDE LEVELS IN CHILDHOOD AND ADOLESCENCE: MEANS AND PERCENTILES

	TOTAL TRIGLYCERIDE (mg/dL)					TOTAL CHOLESTEROL (mg/dL)					LOW-DENSITY LIPOPROTEIN CHOLESTEROL (mg/dL)					HIGH-DENSITY LIPOPROTEIN CHOLESTEROL (mg/dL)*				
	5th	Mean	75th	90th	95th	5th	Mean	75th	90th	95th	5th	Mean	75th	90th	95th	5th	10th	25th	Mean	95th
Cord	14	34	—	—	84	42	68	—	—	103	17	29	—	—	50	13	—	—	35	60
1-4 yr																				
Male	29	56	68	85	99	114	155	170	190	203	—	—	—	—	—	—	—	—	—	—
Female	34	64	74	95	112	112	156	173	188	200	—	—	—	—	—	—	—	—	—	—
5-9 yr																				
Male	28	52	58	70	85	125	155	168	183	189	63	93	103	117	129	38	42	49	56	74
Female	32	64	74	103	126	131	164	176	190	197	68	100	115	125	140	36	38	47	53	73
10-14 yr																				
Male	33	63	74	94	111	124	160	173	188	202	64	97	109	122	132	37	40	46	55	74
Female	39	72	85	104	120	125	160	171	191	205	68	97	110	126	136	37	40	45	52	70
15-19 yr																				
Male	38	78	88	125	143	118	153	168	183	191	62	94	109	123	130	30	34	39	46	63
Female	36	73	85	112	126	118	159	176	198	207	59	96	111	29	137	35	38	43	52	74

*Note that different percentiles are listed for HDL cholesterol.

Data for cord blood from Strong W: Atherosclerosis: its pediatric roots. In Kaplan N, Stamler J, editors: *Prevention of coronary heart disease,* Philadelphia, 1983, WB Saunders. Data for children 1-4 yr from Tables 6, 7, 20 and 21, and all other data from Tables 24, 25, 32, 33, 36, and 37 in *Lipid research clinics population studies data book, Vol. 1, The prevalence study,* NIH publication No. 80-1527. Washington, DC, 1980, National Institutes of Health.

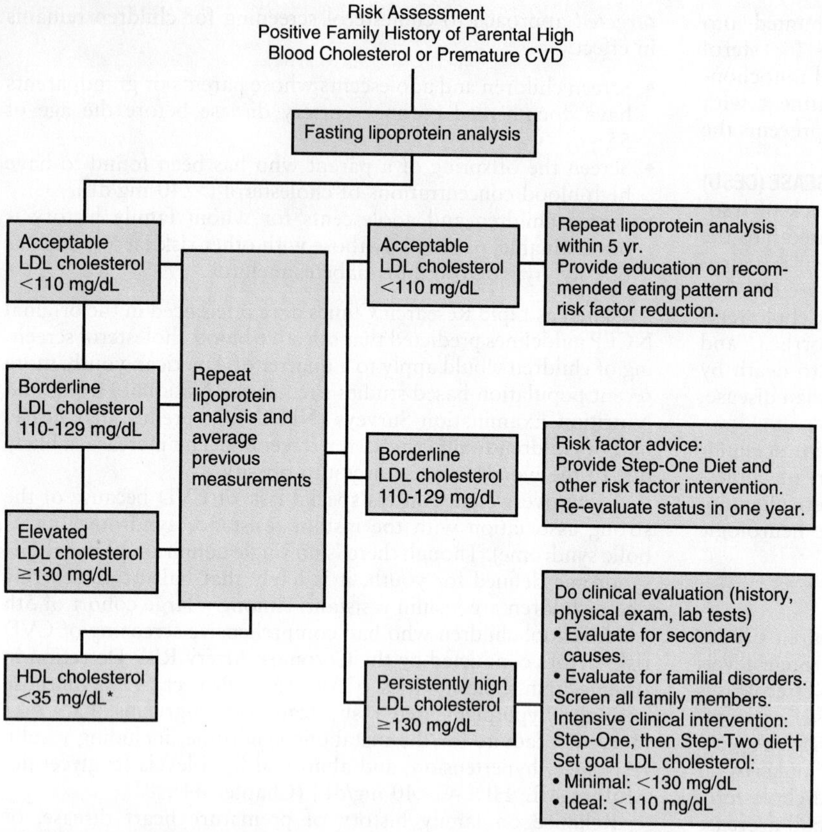
Risk Assessment
Positive Family History of Parental High Blood Cholesterol or Premature CVD
Fasting lipoprotein analysis
Acceptable LDL cholesterol <110 mg/dL
Borderline LDL cholesterol 110-129 mg/dL
Elevated LDL cholesterol ≥130 mg/dL
HDL cholesterol <35 mg/dL*
Repeat lipoprotein analysis and average previous measurements
Acceptable LDL cholesterol <110 mg/dL
Repeat lipoprotein analysis within 5 yr. Provide education on recommended eating pattern and risk factor reduction.
Borderline LDL cholesterol 110-129 mg/dL
Risk factor advice: Provide Step-One Diet and other risk factor intervention. Re-evaluate status in one year.
Persistently high LDL cholesterol ≥130 mg/dL
Do clinical evaluation (history, physical exam, lab tests)
• Evaluate for secondary causes.
• Evaluate for familial disorders. Screen all family members.
Intensive clinical intervention: Step-One, then Step-Two diet†
Set goal LDL cholesterol:
• Minimal: <130 mg/dL
• Ideal: <110 mg/dL

*If low HDL cholesterol is detected, then patients should be counseled regarding cigarette smoking, low saturated fat diet, physical activity, and weight management (if overweight).
†For patients ≥10 yr old and with LDL-C >190 mg/dL (or >160 mg/dL with additional risk factors), if diet does not achieve the goal, then pharmacologic intervention should be considered.

Figure 80-14 Flow chart of classification, education, and follow-up of children based on low-density lipoprotein (LDL) cholesterol levels. CVD, cardiovascular disease; HDL, high-density lipoprotein. (From Williams CL, Hagman LL, Daniels SR, et al: Cardiovascular health in childhood, *Circulation* 106:143–160, 2002.)

circumstances. It is well documented that many parents are unaware of their own cholesterol levels, making the criteria problematic. The evidence that cholesterol screening of children may cause psychological harm to the child is less than compelling, as is the concern that universal screening might lead to overuse of cholesterol lowering medication by practitioners. Finally, the epidemic of childhood obesity, approaching 50% in some disadvantaged high-risk populations, supports broader screening to identify those with the metabolic syndrome. A fasting lipid profile is recommended in order to detect hypertriglyceridemia and/or low HDL cholesterol often found in this pre-diabetic condition. The AAP guidelines recommend that blood cholesterol testing occur sometime after age 2 yr but no later than age 10 yr.

Risk Assessment and Treatment of Hyperlipidemia

The National Cholesterol Education Program (NCEP) recommends a population-based approach toward healthy lifestyle applicable to all children, and an individualized approach directed at those children at high risk (Fig. 80-14). The important focus on maintenance of a healthy lifestyle rather than aggressive weight reduction is recommended by the AAP.

The AHA Step I diet, with updated dietary recommendations based on new U.S. Department of Agriculture guidelines, is still applicable to most children older than 2 yr:

- Calories consumed as fat should not exceed 30% of total calories consumed per day.
- Calories consumed as saturated fat should equal no more than 10% of total calories per day.
- Total cholesterol intake should be limited to less than 300 mg/dL per day.
- Intake of trans fatty acids should be limited to <1% of total calories.

Persistence of an elevated LDL cholesterol >130 mg/dL indicates the need for more comprehensive evaluation and lifestyle modification. History and physical examination and additional laboratory tests aimed at ruling out secondary causes of hyperlipidemia (see Table 80-10) should be performed. Other family members should have blood cholesterol screening. If the LDL cholesterol level does not achieve the minimal goal of <130 mg/dl the AHA Step II diet should be recommended. This diet allows the same average fat consumption of no more than 30% of total calories, but restricts saturated fats to <7-8% of total calories and cholesterol intake to <200 mg per day. Follow-up lab tests, measurement of height and weight for the calculation of body mass index (BMI), and dietary history should be scheduled at 3-6 mo intervals.

The 2004 revision of the NCEP Adult Treatment Panel III raised the minimal acceptable level of HDL cholesterol from 35 mg/dL to 40 mg/dL. If low HDL cholesterol is present, counseling directed toward weight management, tobacco avoidance, and daily physical activity should be provided.

No restriction of fat or cholesterol is recommended for infants less than 2 yr of age because of rapid growth and development, especially involving the central nervous system. Overfeeding should be discouraged as increasingly infants and toddlers are exceeding weight for height standards published by the U.S. Centers for Disease Control and Prevention. The myth that "a bigger baby is a healthier baby" persists.

The safety of a heart healthy diet among children 3-19 yr has been established by the National Health and Nutrition

Examination Survey (NHANES III). Despite a decrease in the average level of fat intake from the second survey there was no evidence of poor growth or compromised nutritional status. The prospective, well-controlled Dietary Intervention Study in Children (DISC) compared children consuming a low-fat Step I diet with subjects consuming the "usual" diet containing 33-34% of calories as fat, and 13% as saturated fat. No differences between groups with regard to height, weight, micronutrients, or psychological well-being were observed. Children on the low-fat diet had lower LDL cholesterol levels.

The Committee on Nutrition of the American Academy of Pediatrics suggests that as children older than 2 yr consume fewer calories from fat, they should eat more grain product, fruits, vegetables, low-fat milk products, beans, lean meats, poultry, fish, and other protein-rich foods. Low-carbohydrate, high-fat diets have become popular over the last decade as a means to achieve weight reduction. Unlimited fat intake is strongly discouraged, as is unrestricted sugar and carbohydrate consumption. Carbohydrates should comprise about 55% of calories, achieved by consuming complex carbohydrates such as pasta, some vegetables, potatoes, legumes, and whole grain cereals and bread.

Protein should provide about 15-20% of calories, and should contain all of the essential fatty acids. The exclusion of meat or fish from the diet necessitates a healthy mixture of plant proteins in order to achieve appropriate nutrient balance. Thus foods high in fiber, such as fruits, vegetables, and whole grains are recommended because of their excellent nutrient content as components of a low saturated fat eating pattern. Children should eat 5 or more fruits and vegetables daily. Canned and frozen vegetables and soups should be selected for low sodium content.

If followed, these dietary recommendations provide adequate calories for optimal growth and development without promoting obesity. Compliance on the part of children and their caregivers is challenging in today's society. Children learn eating habits from their parents. Successful adoption of a healthier diet is far more likely to occur if meals and snacks in the home are applicable to the entire family rather than an individual child. A regular time for meals together as a family is desirable. Grandparents and other nonparental caregivers sometimes need to be reminded not to indulge the child who is on a restricted diet. The rise in obesity is prompting some school districts to restrict sweetened drink availability, and offer more nutritious cafeteria selections.

The rise in sedentary activity among our youth is contributing to the increase in obesity nationwide, in turn increasing the prevalence of other risk factors such as dyslipidemia and hypertension. The National Association for Sport and Physical Education (NASPE) recommends that children should accumulate at least 60 min of age-appropriate physical activity on most days of the week. Extended periods (2 hr or more) of daytime inactivity are discouraged, as is more than 2 hr of television and other forms of screen time.

DRUG THERAPY (TABLES 80-14 AND 80-15) The AAP has slightly modified the original 1992 NCEP guidelines in that consideration be given to pharmacologic treatment of hyperlipidemia if the child is at least 8 yr of age and an adequate period of dietary restriction has not achieved therapeutic goals. Drug therapy should be considered when:

- LDL cholesterol remains >190 mg/dL;
- LDL cholesterol remains >160 mg/dL, and other risk factors are present, including obesity, hypertension, or cigarette smoking or positive family history of premature CVD; and
- LDL cholesterol is >130 mg/dL in children with diabetes mellitus.

These arbitrary but sensible guidelines are based on the statistical probability of the child having an inherited form of dyslipidemia such as heterozygous familial hypercholesterolemia (FH). Pharmacologic treatment of children less than 8 yr of age should be reserved for the rare child with homozygous FH and LDL cholesterol levels exceeding 500 mg/dL.

Table 80-14 DRUGS USED FOR THE TREATMENT OF HYPERLIPIDEMIA

DRUG	MECHANISM OF ACTION	INDICATION	STARTING DOSE
HMG CoA reductase inhibitors (statins)	↓ Cholesterol and VLDL synthesis	Elevated LDL	5-80 mg qhs
	↑ Hepatic LDL receptors		
Bile acid sequestrants:	↑ Bile and excretion	Elevated LDL	
Cholestyramine			4-32 g daily
Colestipol			5-40 g daily
Nicotinic acid	↓ Hepatic VLDL synthesis	Elevated LDL	100-2,000 mg tid
		Elevated TG	
Fibric acid derivatives:	↑ LPL	Elevated TG	600 mg bid
Gemfibrozil	↓ VLDL		
Fish oils	↓ VLDL production	Elevated TG	3-10 g daily
Cholesterol absorption inhibitors:			
Ezetimibe	↓ Intestinal absorption cholesterol	Elevated LDL	10 mg daily

LDL, low-density lipoprotein; LPL, lipoprotein lipase; TG, triglyceride; VLDL, very low density lipoprotein.

Considerable experience with drug therapy in children and adolescents with hyperlipidemia over the past 15 yr has expanded therapeutic options, improved compliance, and enhanced efficacy. In the past, the mainstay of drug therapy was bile acid sequestrants such as cholestyramine and colestipol because they were not systemically absorbed. Interruption of the enterohepatic circulation of bile acids promotes synthesis in the liver of new bile acids from cholesterol. Gastrointestinal side effects and taste resulted in less than desirable compliance, even when there were few viable options.

HMG-CoA reductase inhibitors, known also as "statins" are remarkably effective in lowering LDL cholesterol levels and reducing plaque inflammation, thereby reducing the likelihood of a sudden coronary event in an at-risk adult within weeks of starting the medication. As a class they work by blocking the intrahepatic biosynthesis of cholesterol, thereby stimulating the production of more LDL receptors on the cell surface. The NCEP Adult Treatment Panel now advocates aggressive lowering of LDL to below 70 mg/dL in individuals with known coronary heart disease. This information is relevant because children who fulfill criteria for consideration of cholesterol lowering medication will almost always have inherited the condition from one of his or her parents. Not infrequently when providing care for the child questions come up about screening and treatment of parents or grandparents. Statins are equally effective in children, capable of lowering LDL cholesterol levels by half when necessary. They also will effect modest reduction in triglycerides and inconsistent increase in HDL cholesterol. Their side-effect profile, mainly liver dysfunction and rarely rhabdomyolysis with secondary renal failure, should be taken into consideration before prescribing the drug. However, there has been no evidence to date that complications are any more frequent in children than adults, and skeletal muscle discomfort seems to be somewhat less of a problem. Statins are contraindicated in patients with active liver disease and during pregnancy and lactation. Children should have liver enzymes monitored regularly, and creatine phosphokinase (CPK) measured if muscle aches or weakness occurs. Liver enzymes may be allowed to rise threefold before discontinuing the drug. It should be reemphasized that children with modest elevations in cholesterol, such as that seen in polygenic hypercholesterolemia,

Table 80-15 SIDE EFFECTS OF LIPID-LOWERING DRUGS

DRUG AND SITE OR TYPE OF EFFECT	EFFECT
STATINS	
Skin	Rash
Nervous system	Loss of concentration, sleep disturbance, headache, peripheral neuropathy
Liver	Hepatitis, loss of appetite, weight loss, and increases in serum aminotransferases to two to three times the upper limit of the normal range
Gastrointestinal tract	Abdominal pain, nausea, diarrhea
Muscles	Muscle pain or weakness, myositis (usually with serum creatine kinase >1,000U/L), rhabdomyolysis with renal failure
Immune system	Lupus-like syndrome (lovastatin, simvastatin, or fluvastatin)
Protein binding	Diminished binding of warfarin (lovastatin, simvastatin, fluvastatin)
BILE ACID-BINDING RESINS	
Gastrointestinal tract	Abdominal fullness, nausea, gas, constipation, hemorrhoids, anal fissure, activation of diverticulitis, diminished absorption of vitamin D in children
Liver	Mild serum aminotransferase elevations, which can be exacerbated by concomitant treatment with a statin
Metabolic system	Increases in serum triglycerides of ≈10% (greater increases in patients with hypertriglyceridemia)
Electrolytes	Hyperchloremic acidosis in children and patients with renal failure (cholestyramine)
Drug interactions	Binding of warfarin, digoxin, thiazide diuretics, thyroxine, statins
NICOTINIC ACID	
Skin	Flushing, dry skin, pruritus, ichthyosis, acanthosis nigricans
Eyes	Conjunctivitis, cystoid macular edema, retinal detachment
Respiratory tract	Nasal stuffiness
Heart	Supraventricular arrhythmias
Gastrointestinal tract	Heartburn, loose bowel movements or diarrhea
Liver	Mild increase in serum aminotransferases, hepatitis with nausea and fatigue
Muscles	Myositis
Metabolic system	Hyperglycemia (incidence, ≈5% higher in patients with diabetes), increase of 10% in serum uric acid
FIBRATES	
Skin	Rash
Gastrointestinal tract	Stomach upset, abdominal pain (mainly gemfibrozil), cholesterol-saturated bile, increase of 1-2% in gallstone incidence
Genitourinary tract	Erectile dysfunction (mainly clofibrate)
Muscles	Myositis with impaired renal function
Plasma proteins	Interference with binding of warfarin, requiring reduction in the dose of warfarin by ≈30%
Liver	Increased serum aminotransferases

From Knopp RH: Drug treatment of lipid disorders, *N Engl J Med* 341:498–512, 1999.

are not candidates for statins as a rule because of their side-effect profile.

Other cholesterol lowering medications such as nicotinic acid and fibrates have been used far less often in children than bile acid sequestrants and statins. Nicotinic acid has been used selectively in children with marked hypertriglyceridemia at risk for acute pancreatitis, though dietary restriction of complex sugars and carbohydrates will usually result in significant lowering of triglyceride levels.

Ezetimibe has proven to be especially useful in the pediatric population because of its efficacy and low side-effect profile. Ezetimibe reduces plasma LDL cholesterol by blocking sterol absorption in enterocytes. The drug is marketed as an adjunct to statins when adult subjects are not achieving sufficient blood lipid lowering with statins alone. Not surprisingly, large clinical trials of ezetimibe used as monotherapy in children have not been conducted because the potential market in the pediatric age group is small. Nevertheless there are sufficient reports in the literature documenting the impressive effectiveness of this medication without worrisome side-effects that one can feel on relatively safe grounds recommending it instead of a statin when moderate hypercholesterolemia is encountered. The dose is 10 mg taken once daily. Parents concerned about the possibility of lifelong use of statins as a treatment are generally much more receptive to the use of ezetimibe. Regardless of which drug is selected for a given child or adolescent in need of pharmacologic treatment, the goal is to decrease the LDL cholesterol to <130 mg/dL, or more ideally <110 mg/dL. There is no reason to push LDL levels lower as is recommended in high-risk adults.

BIBLIOGRAPHY

Please visit the Nelson Textbook of Pediatrics *website at www.expertconsult.com for the complete bibliography.*

80.4 Lipidoses (Lysosomal Storage Disorders)

Margaret M. McGovern and Robert J. Desnick

The lysosomal lipid storage diseases are diverse disorders each due to an inherited deficiency of a lysosomal hydrolase leading to the intralysosomal accumulation of the enzyme's particular substrate (Tables 80-16 and 80-17). With the exception of Wolman disease and cholesterol ester storage disease, the lipid substrates share a common structure that includes a ceramide backbone (2-N-acylsphingosine) from which the various sphingolipids are derived by substitution of hexoses, phosphorylcholine, or one or more sialic acid residues on the terminal hydroxyl group of the ceramide molecule. The pathway of sphingolipid metabolism in nervous tissue (Fig. 80-15) and in visceral organs (Fig. 80-16) is known; each catabolic step, with the exception of the catabolism of lactosylceramide, has a genetically determined metabolic defect and a resultant disease. Because sphingolipids

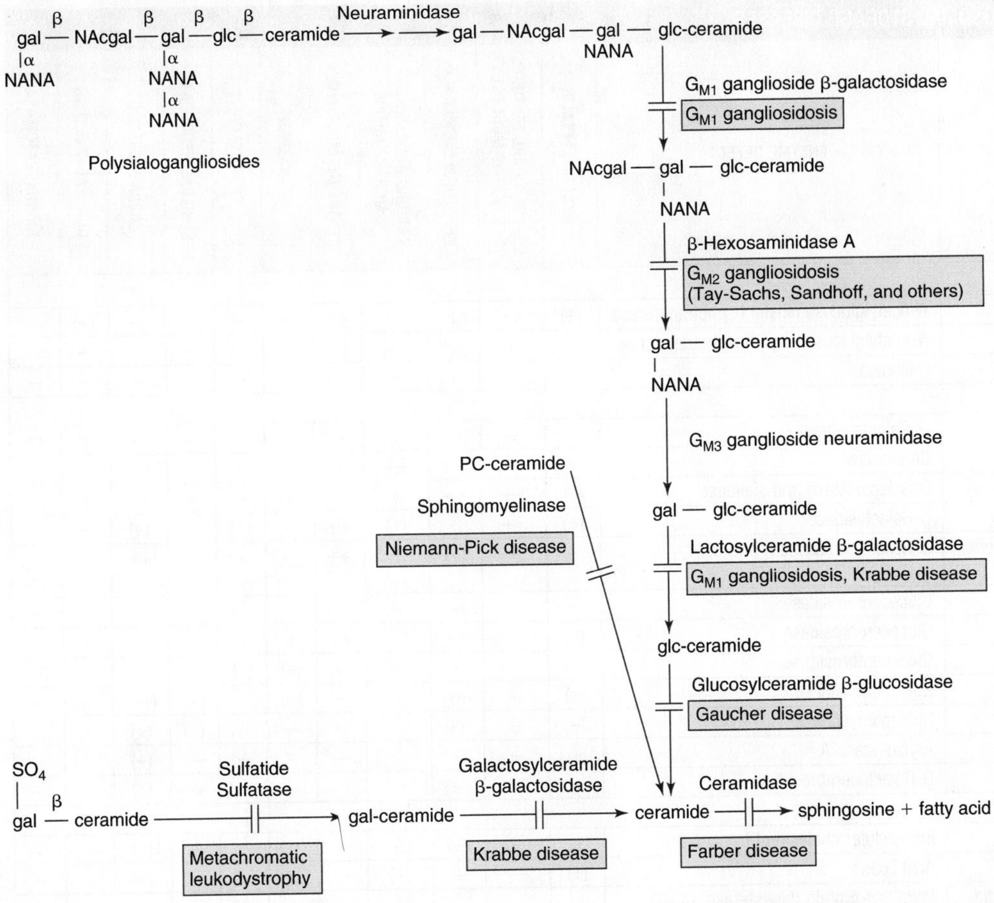

Figure 80-15 Pathways in the metabolism of sphingolipids found in nervous tissues. The name of the enzyme catalyzing each reaction is given with the name of the substrate acted on. Inborn errors are depicted as *bars* crossing the reactions *arrows,* and the name of the associated defect or defects is given in the nearest *box.* The gangliosides are named according to the nomenclature of Svennerholm. Anomeric configurations are given only at the largest starting a compound. Gal, galactose; glc, glucose; NAcgal, N-acetylgalactosamine; NANA, N-acetylneuraminic acid; PC, phosphorylcholine.

are essential components of all cell membranes, the inability to degrade these substances and their subsequent accumulation results in the physiologic and morphologic alterations and characteristic clinical manifestations of the lipid storage disorders (see Table 80-16). Progressive lysosomal accumulation of glycosphingolipids in the central nervous system leads to neurodegeneration, whereas storage in visceral cells can lead to organomegaly, skeletal abnormalities, pulmonary infiltration, and other manifestations. The storage of a substrate in a specific tissue is dependent on its normal distribution in the body.

Diagnostic assays for the identification of affected individuals rely on the measurement of the specific enzymatic activity in isolated leukocytes or cultured fibroblasts or lymphoblasts. An approach to differentiating these disorders is noted in Figure 80-17. For most disorders, carrier identification and prenatal diagnosis are available; a specific diagnosis is essential to permit genetic counseling. The characterization of the genes that encode the specific enzymes required for sphingolipid metabolism permit the development of therapeutic options, such as recombinant enzyme replacement therapy, as well as the potential of cell or gene therapy. Identification of specific disease-causing mutations improves diagnosis, prenatal detection, and carrier identification. For several disorders (Gaucher, Fabry, and Niemann-Pick disease), it has been possible to make genotype-phenotype correlations that predict disease severity and allow more precise genetic counseling. Inheritance is autosomal recessive except for X-linked Fabry disease.

GM_1 Gangliosidosis

GM_1 gangliosidosis most frequently presents in early infancy, but has been described in patients with a juvenile and onset subtypes. Inherited as an autosomal recessive trait, each subtype results from a different gene mutation that leads to the deficient activity of β-galactosidase, a lysosomal enzyme encoded by a gene on chromosome 3 (3p21.33). Although the disorder is characterized by the pathologic accumulation of GM_1 gangliosides in the lysosomes of both neural and visceral cells, GM_1 ganglioside accumulation is most marked in the brain. In addition, keratan sulfate, a mucopolysaccharide, accumulates in liver and is excreted in the urine of patients with GM_1 gangliosidosis. The β-galactosidase gene has been isolated and sequenced; mutations causing the disease subtypes have been identified.

The clinical manifestations of the infantile form of GM_1 gangliosidosis may be evident in the newborn as hepatosplenomegaly, edema, and skin eruptions (**angiokeratoma**). It most frequently presents in the first 6 mo of life with developmental delay followed by progressive psychomotor retardation and the onset of tonic-clonic seizures. A typical facies is characterized by low-set ears, frontal bossing, a depressed nasal bridge, and an abnormally long philtrum. Up to 50% of patients have a **macular cherry red spot.** Hepatosplenomegaly and skeletal abnormalities similar to those of the mucopolysaccharidoses, including anterior beaking of the vertebrae, enlargement of the sella turcica, and thickening of the calvarium, are present. By the end of the first year of life, most patients are blind and deaf, with severe neurologic impairment characterized by decerebrate rigidity. Death usually occurs by 3-4 yr of age. The juvenile-onset form of GM_1 gangliosidosis is clinically distinct, with a variable age at onset. Affected patients present primarily with neurologic symptoms including ataxia, dysarthria, mental retardation, and spasticity. Deterioration is slow; patients may survive through the 4th decade of life. These patients lack the visceral involvement, facial abnormalities, and skeletal features seen in type 1 disease. Adult-onset patients have been described who present with gait and speech abnormalities, dystonia and mild skeletal abnormalities. There is no specific treatment for either form of GM_1 gangliosidosis.

Table 80-16 CLINICAL FINDINGS IN LYSOSOMAL STORAGE DISEASES

NOMENCLATURE	ENZYME DEFECT	HYDROPS FETALIS	COARSE FACIAL FEATURES DYSOSTOSIS MULTIPLEX	HEPATOSPLENOMEGALY	CARDIAC INVOLVEMENT CARDIAC FAILURE	MENTAL DETERIORATION	MYOCLONUS	SPASTICITY	PERIPHERAL NEUROPATHY	CHERRY-RED SPOT	CORNEAL CLOUDING	ANGIOKERATOMATA
MUCOLIPIDOSES												
Mucolipidoses II, I-cell disease	*N*-Acetylglucosaminylphosphotransferase	(+)	++	+	++	++	–	–	–	–	(+)	–
Mucolipidosis III, Pseudo-Hurler	*N*-Acetylglucosaminylphosphotransferase	–	+	(+)	–	(+)	–	–	–	–	+	–
Mucolipidosis IV	Unknown	–	–	+	–	(+)	–	–	–	–	–	–
SPHINGOLIPIDOSES												
Fabry disease	α-Galactosidase	–	–	–	+	–	–	–	–	–	+	++
Farber disease	Ceramidase	–	–	(+)	++	+	–	–	+	(+)	–	–
Galactosialidosis	β-Galactosidase and sialidase	(+)	++	++	+	++	(+)	+	–	+	+	+
G_{M1} gangliosidosis	β-Galactosidase	(+)	++	+	(+)	++	–	(+)	–	(+)	+	+
G_{M2} gangliosidosis (Tay-Sachs disease, Sandhoffc disease)	β-Hexosaminidases A and B	–	–	(+)	–	++	+	+	–	++	–	–
Gaucher type I	Glucocerebrosidase	–	–	++	–	–	–	–	–	–	–	–
Gaucher type II	Glucocerebrosidase	(+)	–	++	–	++	+	+	–	–	–	–
Gaucher type III	Glucocerebrosidase	(+)	–	+	–	+	(+)	(+)	–	–	–	–
Niemann-Pick type A	Sphingomyelinase	(+)	–	++	–	+	(+)	–	(+)	(++)	–	–
Niemann-Pick type B	Sphingomyelinase	–	–	++	–	–	–	–	(+)	(+)	–	–
Metachromatic leukodystrophy	Arylsulfatase A	–	–	–	–	++	–	+	++	(+)	–	–
Krabbe disease	β-Galactocerebrosidase	–	–	–	–	++	–	+	++	(+)	–	–
LIPID STORAGE DISORDERS												
Niemann-Pick type C	Intracellular cholesterol transport	–	–	(+)	–	+	–	–	–	(+)	–	–
Wolman disease	Acid lipase	(+)	–	+	(+)	–	–	–	–	(+)	–	–
Ceroid lipofuscinosis, infantile (Santavuori-Hantia)	Palmitoyl-protein thioesterase (CLN1)	–	–	–	–	+	+	+	–	–	–	–
Ceroid lipofuscinosis, late infantile (Jansky-Bielschowsky)	Pepstatin-insensitive peptidase (CLN2). Variants in Finland (CLN5), Turkey (CLN7), and Italy (CLN6)	–	–	–	–	+	+	+	–	–	–	–
Ceroid lipofuscinosis, juvenile (Spielmeyer-Vogt)	CLN3, membrane protein	–	–	–	–	+	–	(+)	–	–	–	–
Ceroid lipofuscinosis, adult (Kufs, Parry)	CLN4, probably heterogeneous	(+)	–	–	–	+	–	–	–	–	–	–
OLIGOSACCHARIDOSES												
Aspartylglucosaminuria	Aspartylglucosaminase	–	+	(+)	(+)	+	–	–	–	–	(+)	(+)
Fucosidosis	α-Fucosidase	–	++	(+)	+	++	+	+	–	–	–	(+)
α-Mannosidosis	α-Mannosidase	–	++	+	–	++	–	(+)	–	–	++	(+)
β-Mannosidosis	β-Mannosidase	–	+	(+)	–	+	–	+	+	–	–	(+)
Schindler disease	α-*N*-Acetylgalactosaminidase	–	–	–	–	+	+	+	–	–	–	–
Sialidosis I	Sialidase	(+)	–	–	–	–	++	+	+	++	(+)	–
Sialidosis II	Sialidase	(+)	++	+	+	++	(+)	–	–	++	–	+

++, prominent; +, often present, (+), inconstant or occurring later in the disease course; –, not present.
GAG, glycosaminoglycans.
Modified from Hoffmann GF, Nyhan WL, Zschoke J, et al: *Storage disorders in inherited metabolic diseases*, Philadelphia, 2002, Lippincott Williams & Wilkins, pp 346–351.

The diagnosis of GM_1 gangliosidosis should be suspected in infants with typical clinical features and is confirmed by the demonstration of the deficiency of β-galactosidase activity in peripheral leukocytes. Other disorders that share some of the features of the GM_1 gangliosidoses include Hurler disease (mucopolysaccharidosis type I), I-cell disease, and Niemann-Pick disease (NPD) type A, which can each be distinguished by the demonstration of their specific enzymatic deficiencies. Carriers of the disorder are detected by the measurement of the enzymatic activity in peripheral leukocytes or by identifying the specific gene mutations; prenatal diagnosis is accomplished by determination of the enzymatic activity in cultured amniocytes or chorionic villi. Currently only supportive therapy is available for patients with GM_1 gangliosidosis.

The GM_2 Gangliosidoses

The GM_2 gangliosidoses include **Tay-Sachs disease** and **Sandhoff disease**; each results from the deficiency of β-hexosaminidase activity and the lysosomal accumulation of GM_2 gangliosides, particularly in the central nervous system. Both disorders have been classified into infantile-, juvenile-, and adult-onset forms based on the age at onset and clinical features. β-Hexosaminidase occurs as 2 isozymes: β-hexosaminidase A, which is composed of 1 α and 1 β subunit, and β-hexosaminidase B, which has 2 β subunits. β-Hexosaminidase A deficiency results from mutations in the α subunit and causes Tay-Sachs disease, whereas mutations in the β-subunit gene result in the deficiency of both β-hexosaminidases A and B and cause Sandhoff disease. Both are autosomal recessive traits, with Tay-Sachs disease having a

Table 80-17 SYMPTOMS ENCOUNTERED IN PATIENTS WITH LYSOSOMAL STORAGE DISORDERS

System	Manifestations
Neurologic	Hypotonia
	Floppy-infant syndrome
	Trismus
	Strabismus
	Opisthotonus
	Spasticity
	Seizures
	Peripheral neuropathy
	Developmental delay
	Irritability
	Extrapyramidal movement disorder
	Hydrocephalus
Respiratory	Congenital lobar emphysema
	Impaired cough
	Recurrent respiratory infections
	Hoarseness
Endocrine	Osteopenia
	Metabolic bone disease
	Secondary hyperparathyroidism
	Congenital adrenal hyperplasia
Cardiovascular	Cardiomegaly
	Congenital heart failure
	Arrhythmias
	Wolff-Parkinson-White syndrome
	Cardiomyopathy
Dysmorphology	
Head and neck	Microcephaly
	Enlarged nuchal translucency
	Microstomia
	Micrognathia/microretrognathia
	Long philtrums
Limbs	Bilateral broad thumbs and toes
	Bilateral club feet
	Eversed lips
	Flattened nasal bridge
	Short nasal columella
Oral	Macroglossia
	Molar hypoplasia
	Hypertrophic gums
	Absent nasal septum
	Bilateral epicanthal inferior orbital creases
	Palpebral edema
	Hypertelorism
Facial	Coarse facies
	Low-set ears
Gastrointestinal	Hepatosplenomegaly
	Neonatal cholestasis
Bones and joints	Lytic bone lesions
	Joint contractures
	Dysostosis multiplex
	Hyperphosphatasemia
	Vertebral breaking
	Broadening of tubular bones
	Punctuate epiphysis
	Craniosynostosis
	Painful joint swelling
Skin	Congenital ichthyosis
	Collodion infant
	Hypopigmentation
	Telangiectasias
	Extended Mongolian spots
Ocular	Corneal clouding
	Megalocornea
	Glaucoma
	Cherry-red spots
	Fundi hypopigmentation
	Bilateral cataracts
Hematologic	Anemia
	Thrombocytopenia
Hydrops fetalis	NIHF
	Congenital ascites
Recurrent fetal losses	

From Staretz-Chacham O, Lang TC, LaMarca ME, et al: Lysosomal storage disorders in the newborn, *Pediatrics* 123:1191–1207, 2009.

predilection for the Ashkenazi Jewish population, where the carrier frequency is about 1/25.

More than 50 mutations have been identified; most are associated with the infantile forms of disease. Three mutations account for >98% of mutant alleles among Ashkenazi Jewish carriers of Tay-Sachs disease, including one allele associated with the adult-onset form. Mutations that cause the subacute or chronic forms result in enzyme proteins with residual enzymatic activities, the levels of which correlate with the severity of the disease.

Patients with the infantile form of Tay-Sachs disease have clinical manifestations in infancy including loss of motor skills, increased startle reaction, and macular pallor and **retinal cherry red spots** (see Table 80-16). Affected infants usually develop normally until 4-5 mo of age when decreased eye contact and an exaggerated startle response to noise (**hyperacusis**) are noted. **Macrocephaly**, not associated with hydrocephalus, may develop. In the 2nd yr of life, seizures develop which may be refractory to anticonvulsant therapy. Neurodegeneration is relentless, with death occurring by the age of 4 or 5 yr. The juvenile and later-onset forms initially present with ataxia and dysarthria and may not be associated with a macular cherry red spot.

The clinical manifestations of **Sandhoff** disease are similar to those for Tay-Sachs disease. Infants with Sandhoff disease have hepatosplenomegaly, cardiac involvement, and mild bony abnormalities. The juvenile form of this disorder presents as ataxia, dysarthria, and mental deterioration, but without visceral enlargement or a macular cherry red spot. There is no treatment available for Tay-Sachs disease or Sandhoff disease, although experimental approaches are being evaluated.

The diagnosis of infantile Tay-Sachs disease and Sandhoff disease is usually suspected in an infant with neurologic features and a cherry red spot. Definitive diagnosis is made by determination of β-hexosaminidase A and B activities in peripheral leukocytes. The two disorders are distinguished by the enzymatic assay, because in Tay-Sachs disease only the β-hexosaminidase A isozyme is deficient, whereas in Sandhoff disease both the β-hexosaminidase A and B isozymes are deficient. Future at-risk pregnancies for both disorders can be prenatally diagnosed by determining the enzyme levels in fetal cells obtained by amniocentesis or chorionic villus sampling. Identification of carriers in families is also possible by β-hexosaminidases A and B determination. Indeed, for Tay-Sachs disease, carrier screening of all couples in which at least one member is of Ashkenazi Jewish descent is recommended before the initiation of pregnancy to identify couples at risk. These studies can be conducted by the determination of the level of β-hexosaminidase A activity in peripheral

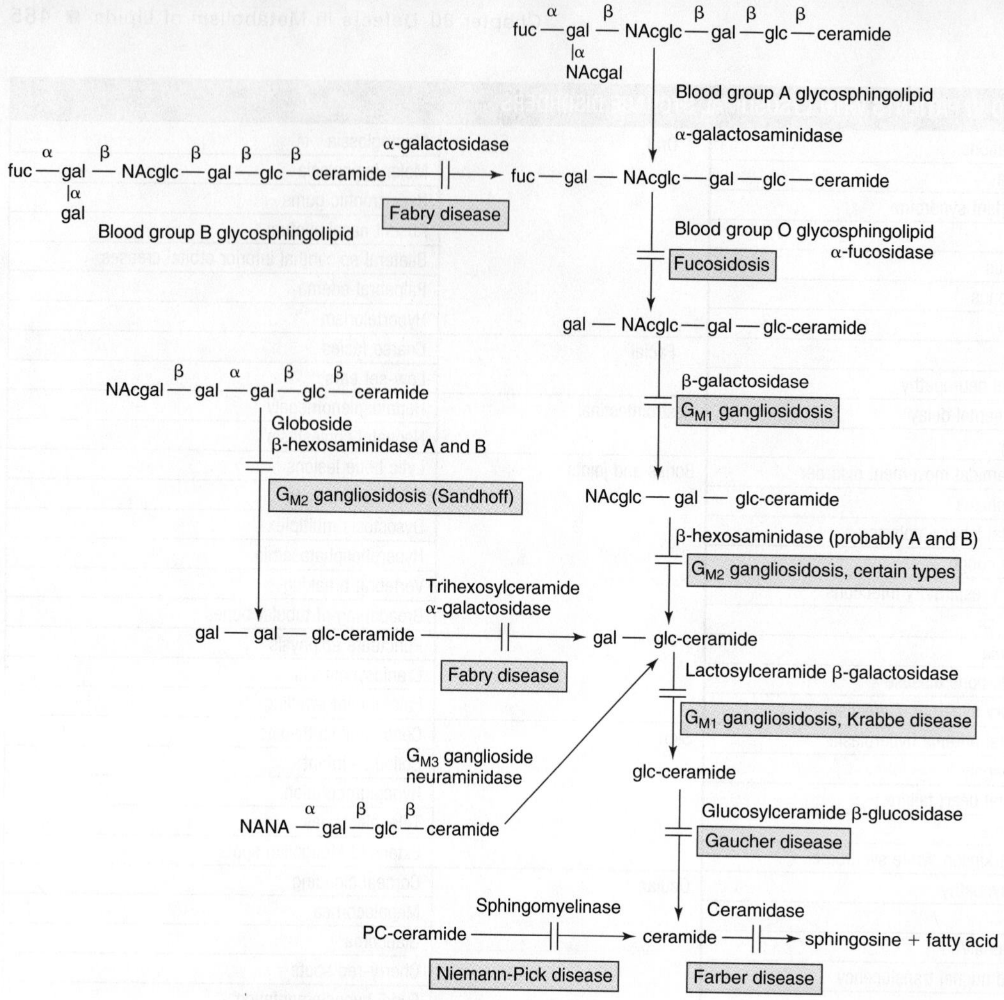

Figure 80-16 Pathways in the degradation of sphingolipids found in visceral organs and red or white blood cells. See also the legend for Figure 80-15. Fuc, fucose; NAcglc, N-acetylglucosamine.

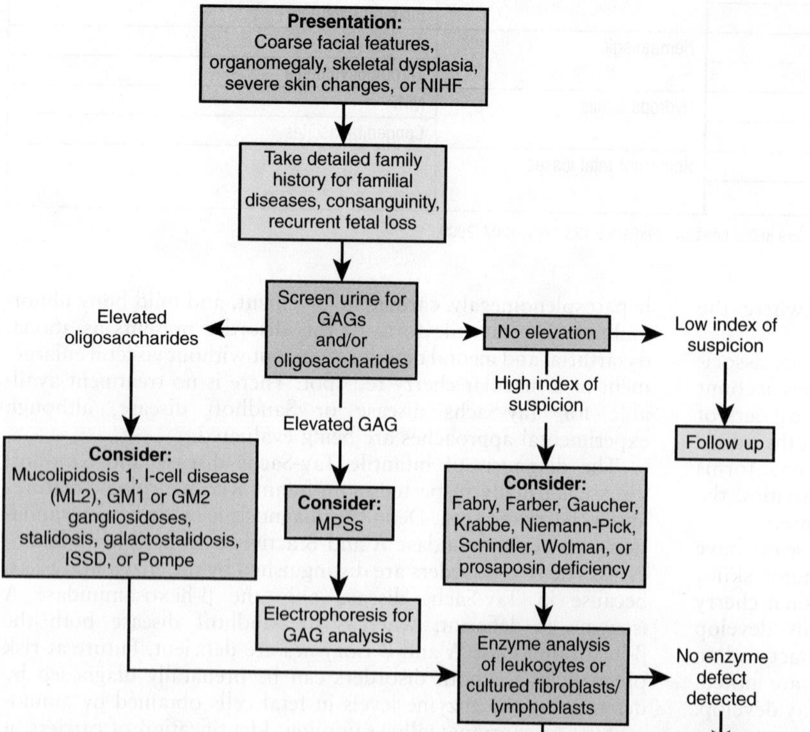

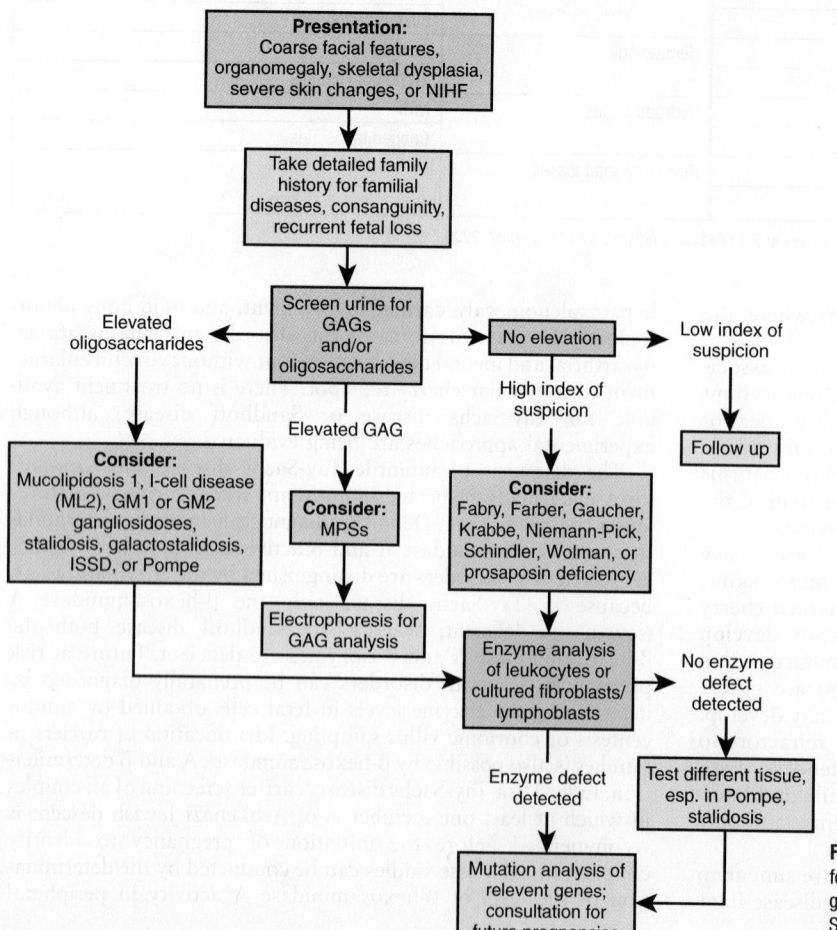

Figure 80-17 Algorithm of the clinical evaluation recommended for an infant with a suspected lysosomal storage disease. GAGs, glycosaminoglycans; NIHF, nonimmune hydrops fetalis. (From Staretz-Chacham O, Lang TC, LaMarca ME, et al: Lysosomal storage disorders in the newborn, *Pediatrics* 123:1191–1207, 2009.)

leukocytes or plasma. Molecular studies to identify the exact molecular defect in enzymatically identified carriers should also be performed to permit more specific identification of carriers in the family and to allow prenatal diagnosis in at-risk couples by both enzymatic and genotype determinations. The incidence of Tay-Sachs disease has been markedly reduced since the introduction of carrier screening programs in the Ashkenazi Jewish population. Newborn screening may be possible by measuring specific glycosphingolipid markers, or the relevant enzymatic activities in dried blood spots.

Gaucher Disease

This disease is a multisystemic lipidosis characterized by hematologic abnormalities, organomegaly, and skeletal involvement, the latter usually manifesting as bone pain and pathologic fractures (see Table 80-16). It is the most common lysosomal storage disease and the most prevalent genetic defect among Ashkenazi Jews. There are 3 clinical subtypes delineated by the absence or presence and progression of neurologic manifestations: type 1 or the adult, non-neuronopathic form; type 2, the infantile or acute neuronopathic form; and type 3, the juvenile or subacute neuronopathic form. All are autosomal recessive traits. Type 1, which accounts for 99% of cases, has a striking predilection for Ashkenazi Jews, with an incidence of about 1/1,000 and a carrier frequency of about 1/18.

Gaucher disease results from the deficient activity of the lysosomal hydrolase, acid β-glucosidase, which is encoded by a gene located on chromosome 1q21-q31. The enzymatic defect results in the accumulation of undegraded glycolipid substrates, particularly glucosylceramide, in cells of the reticuloendothelial system. This progressive deposition results in infiltration of the bone marrow, progressive hepatosplenomegaly, and skeletal complications. Four mutations—N370S, L444P, 84insG, and IVS2—account for about 95% of mutant alleles among Ashkenazi Jewish patients, permitting screening for this disorder in this population. Genotype-phenotype correlations have been noted, providing the molecular basis for the clinical heterogeneity seen in Gaucher disease type 1. Patients who are homozygous for the N370S mutation tend to have later onset, with a more indolent course than patients with one copy of N370S and another common allele.

Clinical manifestations of type 1 Gaucher disease have a variable age at onset, from early childhood to late adulthood, with most symptomatic patients presenting by adolescence. At presentation, patients may have bruising from thrombocytopenia, chronic fatigue secondary to anemia, hepatomegaly with or without elevated liver function test results, splenomegaly, and bone pain. Occasional patients have pulmonary involvement at the time of presentation. Patients presenting in the first decade frequently are not Jewish and have growth retardation and a more malignant course. Other patients may be discovered fortuitously during evaluation for other conditions or as part of routine examinations; these patients may have a milder or even a benign course. In symptomatic patients, splenomegaly is progressive and can become massive. Most patients develop radiologic evidence of skeletal involvement, including an Erlenmeyer flask deformity of the distal femur. Clinically apparent bony involvement, which occurs in most patients, can present as bone pain, a pseudo-osteomyelitis pattern or pathologic fractures. Lytic lesions can develop in the long bones, including the femur, ribs, and pelvis; osteosclerosis may be evident at an early age. Bone crises with severe pain and swelling can occur. Bleeding secondary to thrombocytopenia may manifest as epistaxis or bruising and is frequently overlooked until other symptoms become apparent. With the exception of the severely growth-retarded child, who may experience developmental delay secondary to the effects of chronic disease, development and intelligence are normal.

The pathologic hallmark of Gaucher disease is the Gaucher cell in the reticuloendothelial system, particularly in the bone

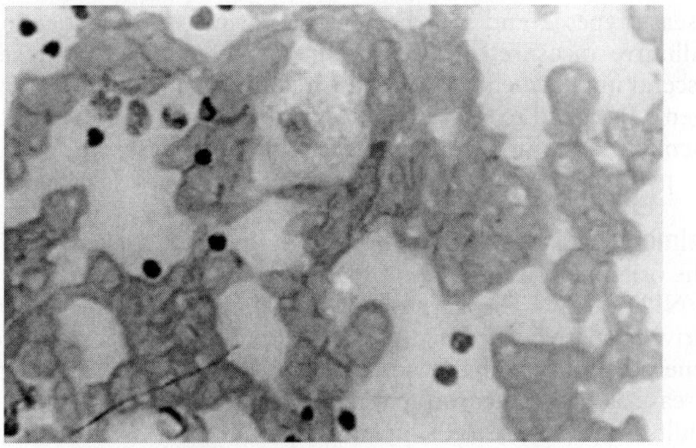

Figure 80-18 Cells from the spleen of a patient with Gaucher disease. A characteristic spleen cell is shown engorged with glucocerebroside.

marrow (Fig. 80-18). These cells, which are 20-100 μm in diameter, have a characteristic wrinkled paper appearance resulting from the presence of intracytoplasmic substrate inclusions. The cytoplasm of the Gaucher cell reacts strongly positive with the periodic acid–Schiff stain. The presence of this cell in bone marrow and tissue specimens is highly suggestive of Gaucher disease, although it also may be found in patients with granulocytic leukemia and myeloma.

Gaucher disease type 2 is much less common and does not have an ethnic predilection. It is characterized by a rapid neurodegenerative course with extensive visceral involvement and death within the first years of life. It presents in infancy with increased tone, strabismus, and organomegaly. Failure to thrive and stridor caused by laryngospasm are typical. After a several-year period of psychomotor regression, death occurs secondary to respiratory compromise. **Gaucher disease type 3** presents as clinical manifestations that are intermediate to those seen in types 1 and 2, with presentation in childhood and death by age 10-15 yr. It has a predilection for the Swedish Norrbottnian population, among which the incidence is about 1/50,000. Neurologic involvement is present. Type 3 disease is further classified as types 3a and 3b based on the extent of neurologic involvement and whether there is progressive myotonia and dementia (type 3a) or isolated supranuclear gaze palsy (type 3b).

Gaucher disease should be considered in the differential diagnosis of patients with unexplained organomegaly, who bruise easily, have bone pain, or have a combination of these conditions. Bone marrow examination usually reveals the presence of Gaucher cells. All suspected diagnoses should be confirmed by determination of the acid β-glucosidase activity in isolated leukocytes or cultured fibroblasts. In Ashkenazi Jewish individuals the identification of carriers can be achieved best by molecular testing for the common mutations. Testing should be offered to all family members, keeping in mind that heterogeneity, even among members of the same kindred, can be so great that nonsymptomatic affected individuals may be diagnosed. Prenatal diagnosis is available by determination of enzyme activity and/or the specific family mutations in chorionic villi or cultured amniotic fluid cells.

Treatment of patients with Gaucher disease type 1 includes enzyme replacement therapy, with recombinant acid β-glucosidase (imiglucerase). Most extraskeletal symptoms (organomegaly, hematologic indices) are reversed by enzyme (60 IU/kg) administered by intravenous infusion every other week. Monthly maintenance enzyme replacement improves bone structure, decreases bone pain, and induces compensatory growth in affected children. A small number of patients have undergone bone marrow transplantation, which is curative but results in significant morbidity and mortality from the procedure, making the selection of appropriate candidates limited. Although enzyme replacement does not alter the neurologic progression of patients with Gaucher disease types 2 and 3, it has been used in selected patients as a palliative measure, particularly in type 3 patients with severe visceral involvement. Alternative treatments, including the use of agents designed to decrease the synthesis of glucosylceramide by chemical inhibition of glucosylceramide synthase, are available for patients who cannot be treated by enzyme replacement.

Neimann-Pick Disease (NPD)

The original description of NPD was what is now known as **type A NPD**, a fatal disorder of infancy characterized by failure to thrive, hepatosplenomegaly, and a rapidly progressive neurodegenerative course that leads to death by 2-3 yr of age. **Type B** disease is a non-neuronopathic form observed in children and adults. **Type C** disease is a neuronopathic form that results from defective cholesterol transport. All subtypes are inherited as autosomal recessive traits and display variable clinical features (see Table 80-16).

NPD types A and B result from the deficient activity of acid sphingomyelinase, a lysosomal enzyme encoded by a gene on chromosome 11 (11p15.1-p15.4). The enzymatic defect results in the pathologic accumulation of sphingomyelin, a ceramide phospholipid, and other lipids in the monocyte-macrophage system the primary pathologic site. The progressive deposition of sphingomyelin in the central nervous system results in the neurodegenerative course seen in type A, and in non-neural tissue in the systemic disease manifestations of type B, including progressive lung disease in some patients. A variety of mutations in the acid sphingomyelinase gene that cause types A and B NPD have been identified.

The clinical manifestations and course of type A NPD is uniform and is characterized by a normal appearance at birth. Hepatosplenomegaly, moderate lymphadenopathy, and psychomotor retardation are evident by 6 mo of age, followed by neurodevelopmental regression and death by 3 yr. With advancing age, the loss of motor function and the deterioration of intellectual capabilities are progressively debilitating; and in later stages, spasticity and rigidity are evident. Affected infants lose contact with their environment. In contrast to the stereotyped type A phenotype, the clinical presentation and course of patients with type B disease are more variable. Most are diagnosed in infancy or childhood when enlargement of the liver or spleen, or both, is detected during a routine physical examination. At diagnosis, type B NPD patients usually have evidence of mild pulmonary involvement, usually detected as a diffuse reticular or finely nodular infiltration on the chest radiograph. **Pulmonary symptoms** usually present in adults. In most patients, hepatosplenomegaly is particularly prominent in childhood, but with increasing linear growth, the abdominal protuberance decreases and becomes less conspicuous. In mildly affected patients, the splenomegaly may not be noted until adulthood, and there may be minimal disease manifestations.

In some type B patients, decreased pulmonary diffusion caused by alveolar infiltration becomes evident in late childhood or early adulthood and progresses with age. Severely affected individuals may experience significant pulmonary compromise by 15-20 yr of age. Such patients have low Po_2 values and dyspnea on exertion. Life-threatening bronchopneumonias may occur, and cor pulmonale has been described. Severely affected patients may have liver involvement leading to life-threatening cirrhosis, portal hypertension, and ascites. Clinically significant pancytopenia due to secondary **hypersplenism** may require partial or complete splenectomy; this should be avoided if possible because splenectomy frequently causes progression of pulmonary disease, which can be life-threatening. In general, type B patients do not have neurologic involvement and have a normal IQ. Some patients with type B disease have cherry red maculae or haloes and subtle neurologic symptoms (peripheral neuropathy).

Type C NPD patients often present with prolonged neonatal jaundice, appear normal for 1-2 yr, and then experience a slowly progressive and variable neurodegenerative course. Their hepatosplenomegaly is less severe than that of patients with types A or B NPD, and they may survive into adulthood. The underlying biochemical defect in type C patients is an abnormality in cholesterol transport, leading to the accumulation of sphingomyelin and cholesterol in their lysosomes and a secondary partial reduction in acid sphingomyelinase activity (Chapter 80.3).

In type B NPD patients, splenomegaly is usually the first manifestation detected. The splenic enlargement is noted in early childhood; in very mild disease, the enlargement may be subtle and detection may be delayed until adolescence or adulthood. The presence of the characteristic NPD cells in bone marrow aspirates supports the diagnosis of type B NPD. Patients with type C NPD, however, also have extensive infiltration of NPD cells in the bone marrow and, thus, all suspected cases should be evaluated enzymatically to confirm the clinical diagnosis by measuring the acid sphingomyelinase activity level in peripheral leukocytes, cultured fibroblasts, or lymphoblasts, or a combination of these cells. Patients with types A and B NPD have markedly decreased levels (1-10%), whereas patients with type C NPD have normal or somewhat decreased acid sphingomyelinase activities. The enzymatic identification of NPD carriers is problematic. In families in which the specific molecular lesion has been identified, however, family members can be accurately tested for heterozygote status by DNA analysis. Prenatal diagnosis of types A and B NPD can be made reliably by the measurement of acid sphingomyelinase activity in cultured amniocytes or chorionic villi; molecular analysis of fetal cells can provide the specific diagnosis or serve as a confirmatory test. The clinical diagnosis of type C NPD can be supported by the demonstration of filipin stain positivity in cultured fibroblasts and/or by identifying a specific mutation in the *NPC* gene.

Currently there is no specific treatment for NPD. Orthotopic liver transplantation in an infant with type A disease and amniotic cell transplantation in several type B NPD patients have been attempted with little or no success. Bone marrow transplantation in a small number of type B NPD patients has been shown to be successful in reducing the spleen and liver volumes, the sphingomyelin content of the liver, the number of Niemann-Pick cells in the marrow, and radiologically detected infiltration of the lungs. In one patient, liver biopsies taken up to 33 mo post transplantation showed only a moderate reduction in stored sphingomyelin. To date, lung transplantation has not been performed in any severely compromised patient with type B disease, although two patients who underwent whole lung lavages with variable results have been reported. A phase I trial of enzyme replacement therapy for type B NPD has been completed and further clinical studies to evaluate effectiveness of this approach are planned. Clinical trials of miglustat (Acetelion, Basel, Switzerland) have been performed and the drug has been approved in Europe for the treatment of type C disease. Treatment of type A disease by bone marrow transplantation has not been successful presumably due to the severe neurologic involvement.

Fabry Disease

This condition is an X-linked inborn error of glycosphingolipid metabolism characterized by angiokeratomas (telangiectatic skin lesions), hypohidrosis, corneal and lenticular opacities, acroparesthesias, and vascular disease of the kidney, heart, and/or brain (see Table 80-16). The classic phenotype is due to the deficient activity of the enzyme α-galactosidase A and has an estimated prevalence of approximately 1/50,000 males. Later-onset affected males with residual α-galactosidase A activity may present with cardiac and/or renal disease including hypertrophic cardiomyopathy and renal failure and is more prevalent than the classic phenotype. Heterozygous females for the classic phenotype can be asymptomatic or as severely affected as the males, the variability due to random X-inactivation. The disease results from mutations in the α-galactosidase A gene located on the long arm

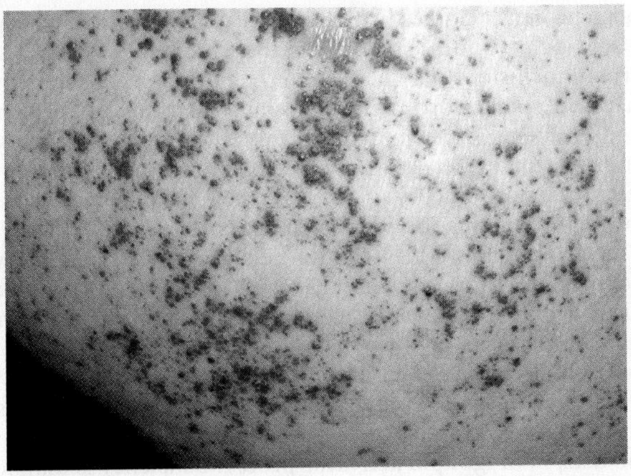

Figure 80-19 Typical angiokeratomas. Angiokeratomas are quite large and easily recognizable, but if only a few lesions exist or they are restricted only to the genitalia or umbilical regions, they can be easily missed. (From Zarate VA, Hopkin RJ: Fabray's disease, *Lancet* 372:1427, 2008.)

of the X chromosome (Xq22). The enzymatic defect leads to the systemic accumulation of neutral glycosphingolipids, primarily globotriaosylceramide, particularly in the plasma and lysosomes of vascular endothelial and smooth muscle cells. The progressive vascular glycosphingolipid deposition in classically affected males results in ischemia and infarction, leading to the major disease manifestations. The cDNA and genomic sequences encoding α-galactosidase A have identified more than 500 different mutations in the α-galactosidase A gene that are responsible for this lysosomal storage disease, including amino acid substitutions, gene rearrangements, and mRNA splicing defects.

Affected males with the classic phenotype have the skin lesions, acroparesthesias, hypohidrosis, and ocular changes, whereas males with the later onset phenotypes lack these findings and present with cardiac and/or renal disease in adulthood. The classic **angiokeratomas** usually occur in childhood and may lead to early diagnosis (Fig. 80-19). They increase in size and number with age and range from barely visible to several mm in diameter. The lesions are punctate, dark red to blue-black, and flat or slightly raised. They do not blanch with pressure, and the larger ones may show slight hyperkeratosis. Characteristically, the lesions are most dense between the umbilicus and knees, in the "bathing trunk area," but may occur anywhere, including the oral mucosa. The hips, thighs, buttocks, umbilicus, lower abdomen, scrotum, and glans penis are common sites, and there is a tendency toward symmetry. Variants without skin lesions have been described. Sweating is usually decreased or absent. Corneal opacities and characteristic lenticular lesions, observed under slit-lamp examination, are present in affected males as well as in about 90% of heterozygotes. Conjunctival and retinal vascular tortuosity is common and results from the systemic vascular involvement.

Pain is the most debilitating symptom in childhood and adolescence. **Fabry crises**, lasting from minutes to several days, consist of agonizing, burning pain in the hands, feet, and proximal extremities and are usually associated with exercise, fatigue, fever, or a combination of these factors. These painful acroparesthesias usually become less frequent in the 3rd and 4th decades of life, although in some men, they may become more frequent and severe. Attacks of abdominal or flank pain may simulate appendicitis or renal colic.

The major morbid symptoms result from the progressive involvement of the vascular system. Early in the course of the disease, casts, red cells, and lipid inclusions with characteristic birefringent "Maltese crosses" appear in the urinary sediment. Proteinuria, isosthenuria, and gradual deterioration of renal function and development of azotemia occur in the 2nd through 4th decades. Cardiovascular findings may include hypertension, left ventricular hypertrophy, anginal chest pain, myocardial ischemia or infarction, and heart failure. Mitral insufficiency is the most common valvular lesion. Abnormal electrocardiographic and echocardiographic findings are common. Cerebrovascular manifestations result from multifocal small vessel involvement. Other features may include chronic bronchitis and dyspnea, lymphedema of the legs without hypoproteinemia, episodic diarrhea, osteoporosis, retarded growth, and delayed puberty. Death most often results from uremia or vascular disease of the heart or brain. Before hemodialysis or renal transplantation, the mean age at death for affected men was 40 yr. Patients with the later onset phenotype with residual α-galactosidase A activity have cardiac and/or renal disease. The cardiac manifestations include hypertrophy of the left ventricular wall and interventricular septum, and electrocardiographic abnormalities consistent with cardiomyopathy. Others have had hypertrophic cardiomyopathy or myocardial infarction, or both.

The diagnosis in classically affected males is most readily made from the history of painful acroparesthesias, hypohidrosis, the presence of characteristic skin lesions, and the observation of the characteristic corneal opacities and lenticular lesions. The disorder is often misdiagnosed as rheumatic fever, erythromelalgia, or neurosis. The skin lesions must be differentiated from the benign angiokeratomas of the scrotum (Fordyce disease) or from angiokeratoma circumscriptum. **Angiokeratomas** identical to those of Fabry disease have been reported in fucosidosis, aspartylglycosaminuria, late-onset GM_1 gangliosidosis, galactosialidosis, α-N-acetylgalactosaminidase deficiency, and sialidosis. Later onset patients have been identified among patients on hemodialysis and among patients with hypertrophic cardiomyopathy or who have suffered cryptogenic strokes. Later-onset patients lack the early classic manifestations such as the angiokeratomas, acroparesthesias, hypohidrosis, and corneal opacities. The diagnosis of classic and later-onset patients is confirmed biochemically by the demonstration of markedly decreased α-galactosidase A activity in plasma, isolated leukocytes, or cultured fibroblasts or lymphoblasts.

Heterozygous females may have corneal opacities, isolated skin lesions, and intermediate activities of α-galactosidase A in plasma or cells. Rare female heterozygotes may have manifestations as severe as those in affected males. Asymptomatic at-risk females in families affected by Fabry disease, however, should be optimally diagnosed by the direct analysis of their family's specific mutation. Prenatal detection of affected males can be accomplished by the demonstration of deficient α-galactosidase A activity or the family's specific gene mutation in chorionic villi obtained in the 1st trimester or in cultured amniocytes obtained by amniocentesis in the 2nd trimester of pregnancy. Fabry disease can be detected by newborn screening and pilot studies have been conducted in Italy and Taiwan.

Treatment for Fabry disease may include the use of phenytoin and/or carbamazepine to decrease the frequency and severity of the chronic acroparesthesias and the periodic crises of excruciating pain. Renal transplantation and long-term hemodialysis are lifesaving procedures for patients with renal failure.

Recombinant α-galactosidase (Fabrazyme, Genzyme Corporation, Cambridge, Mass; Replagal, Shire, UK) is a safe and effective enzyme replacement therapy of choice for Fabry disease at a dose of 1 mg/kg every other week. It has been shown to clear microvascular endothelial deposits of globotriaosylceramide from the kidneys, heart, and skin in patients with Fabry disease with stabilization of renal disease, regression of hypertrophic cardiomyopathy, reduction of pain, and improvement in quality of life.

Fucosidosis

This is a rare autosomal recessive disorder caused by the deficient activity of α-fucosidase and the accumulation of fucose-containing glycosphingolipids, glycoproteins, and oligosaccharides in the lysosomes of the liver, brain, and other organs (see Table 80-16). The α-fucosidase gene is on chromosome 1 (1p24), and specific mutations are known. Although the disorder is panethnic, most affected patients are from Italy and the USA. There is wide variability in the clinical phenotype, with the most severely affected patients presenting in the first year of life with developmental delay and somatic features similar to those of the mucopolysaccharidoses. These features include frontal bossing, hepatosplenomegaly, coarse facial features, and macroglossia. The central nervous system storage results in a relentless neurodegenerative course, with death in childhood. Patients with milder disease have angiokeratomas and longer survival. No specific therapy exists for the disorder, which can be diagnosed by the demonstration of deficient α-fucosidase activity in peripheral leukocytes or cultured fibroblasts. Carrier identification studies and prenatal diagnosis are possible by determination of the enzymatic activity or the specific family mutations.

Schindler Disease

This is an autosomal recessive neurodegenerative disorder that results from the deficient activity of α-N-acetylgalactosaminidase and the accumulation of sialylated and asialoglycopeptides and oligosaccharides (see Table 80-16). The gene for the enzyme is located on chromosome 22 (22q11). The disease is clinically heterogeneous, and two major phenotypes have been identified. Type I disease is an infantile-onset neuroaxonal dystrophy. Affected infants have normal development for the 1st 9-15 mo of life followed by a rapid neurodegenerative course that results in severe psychomotor retardation, cortical blindness, and frequent myoclonic seizures. Type II disease is characterized by a variable age at onset, mild retardation, and angiokeratomas. There is no specific therapy for either form of the disorder. The diagnosis is by demonstration of the enzymatic deficiency in leukocytes or cultured skin fibroblasts or specific gene mutations.

Metachromatic Leukodystrophy (MLD)

This is an autosomal recessive white matter disease caused by a deficiency of arylsulfatase A (ASA), which is required for the hydrolysis of sulfated glycosphingolipids. Another form of MLD is caused by a deficiency of a sphingolipid activator protein (SAP1), which is required for the formation of the substrate-enzyme complex. The deficiency of this enzymatic activity results in the white matter storage of sulfated glycosphingolipids, which leads to demyelination and a neurodegenerative course. The ASA gene is on chromosome 22 (22q13.31qter); specific mutations are known to fall into two groups that correlate with disease severity.

The clinical manifestations of the late **infantile** form of MLD, which is most common, usually presents between 12 and 18 mo of age as irritability, inability to walk, and hyperextension of the knee, causing genu recurvatum. The clinical progression of the disease relates to the pathological involvement of both central and peripheral nervous system, giving a mixture of upper and lower motor neuron and cognitive and psychiatric signs. Deep tendon reflexes are diminished or absent. Gradual muscle wasting, weakness, and hypotonia become evident and lead to a debilitated state. As the disease progresses, nystagmus, myoclonic seizures, optic atrophy, and quadriparesis appear, with death in the 1st decade of life (see Table 80-16). The **juvenile** form of the disorder has a more indolent course with onset that may occur as late as 20 yr of age. This form of the disease presents with gait disturbances, mental deterioration, urinary incontinence, and emotional difficulties. The **adult** form, which presents after the 2nd decade, is similar to the juvenile form in its clinical manifestations, although emotional difficulties and psychosis are more prominent features. Dementia, seizures, diminished reflexes, and optic atrophy also occur in both the juvenile and adult forms. The pathologic hallmark of MLD is the deposition of metachromatic bodies, which stain strongly positive with periodic acid–Schiff and Alcian blue, in the white matter of the brain. Neuronal inclusions may be seen in the midbrain, pons, medulla, retina, and spinal cord; demyelination occurs in the peripheral nervous system. Bone marrow transplantation has resulted in normal enzymatic levels in peripheral blood, but no clear evidence for clinical efficacy in terms of the neurologic course; supportive care remains the primary intervention.

The diagnosis of MLD should be suspected in patients with the clinical features of leukodystrophy. Decreased nerve conduction velocities, increased cerebrospinal fluid protein, metachromatic deposits in sampled segments of sural nerve, and metachromatic granules in urinary sediment are all suggestive of MLD. Confirmation of the diagnosis is based on the demonstration of the reduced activity of ASA in leukocytes or cultured skin fibroblasts. Sphingolipid activator protein deficiency is diagnosed by measuring the concentration of SAP1 in cultured fibroblasts using a specific antibody to the protein. Carrier detection and prenatal diagnosis is available for all forms of the disorder.

Multiple Sulfatase Deficiency

This is an autosomal recessive disorder that results from the enzymatic deficiency of at least 9 sulfatases including arylsulfatases A, B, and C, and iduronate-2-sulfatase. The specific defect has been shown to be an enzyme in the C-α-formylglycine generating system (whose gene is located at 3p26), which introduces a common post-translational modification in all of the affected sulfatases and explains the occurrence of these multiple enzyme defects. Due to the deficiency of these enzymes, sulfatides, mucopolysaccharides, steroid sulfates, and gangliosides accumulate in the cerebral cortex and visceral tissues, resulting in a clinical phenotype with features of **leukodystrophy** as well as those of the **mucopolysaccharidoses**. Severe ichthyosis may also occur. Carrier testing and prenatal diagnosis by measurement of the enzymatic activities can be performed. There is no specific treatment for multiple sulfatase deficiency other than supportive care.

Krabbe Disease

This condition, also called globoid cell leukodystrophy, is an autosomal recessive fatal disorder of infancy. It results from the deficiency of the enzymatic activity of galactocerebrosidase (GALC) and the white matter accumulation of galactosylceramide, which is normally found almost exclusively in the myelin sheath. Both peripheral and central myelin are affected, resulting in spasticity and cognitive impairment coupled with deceptively normal or even absent deep tendon reflexes. The galactocerebrosidase gene is on chromosome 14 (14q31), and specific disease-causing mutations are known. The **infantile** form of Krabbe disease is rapidly progressive and patients present in early infancy with irritability, seizures, and hypertonia (see Table 80-16). Optic atrophy is evident in the 1st yr of life, and mental development is severely impaired. As the disease progresses, optic atrophy and severe developmental delay become apparent; affected children exhibit opisthotonos and die before 3 yr of age. A 2nd, **late infantile** form of Krabbe disease also exists and patients present after the age of 2 yr. Affected individuals have a disease course similar to that of the early infantile form.

The diagnosis of Krabbe disease relies on the demonstration of the specific enzymatic deficiency in white blood cells or cultured skin fibroblasts. Causative gene mutations have been identified. Carrier identification and prenatal diagnosis are available. The development of methods to measure GALC activity on dried blood spots has led to the inclusion of Krabbe disease in the newborn screening programs of some states. Treatment of infants with Krabbe disease with umbilical cord blood cell transplantation has been reported in prenatally identified asymptomatic newborns and symptomatic infants. The long term outcome of umbilical cord blood cell transplantation is being evaluated;

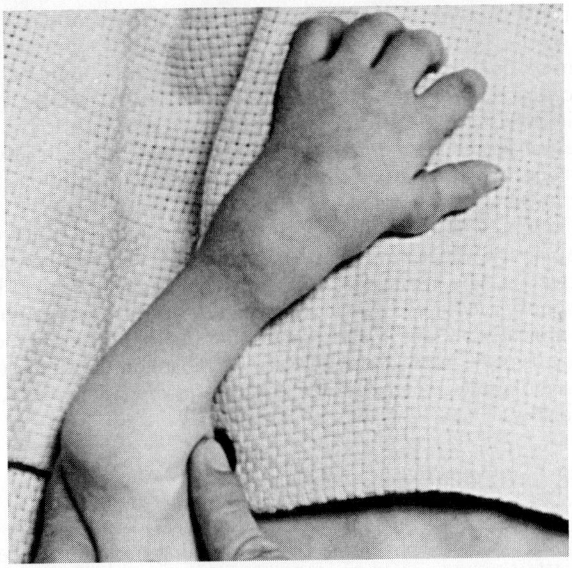

Figure 80-20 Forearm of an 18 mo old girl with Farber disease. Note the painful joint swelling and the nodule formation. The infant was suspected of having rheumatoid arthritis.

transplanted infants develop neurologic manifestations at a slower rate but succumb to a neurologic demise.

Farber Disease

This is a rare autosomal recessive disorder that results from the deficiency of the lysosomal enzyme acid ceramidase and the accumulation of ceramide in various tissues, especially the joints. Symptoms can begin as early as the 1st year of life with painful joint swelling and nodule formation (Fig. 80-20), which is sometimes diagnosed as rheumatoid arthritis. As the disease progresses, nodule or granulomatous formation on the vocal cords can lead to hoarseness and breathing difficulties; failure to thrive is common. In some patients, moderate central nervous system dysfunction is present (see Table 80-16). Patients may die of recurrent pneumonias in their teens; there is currently no specific therapy. The diagnosis of this disorder should be suspected in patients who have nodule formation over the joints but no other findings of rheumatoid arthritis. In such patients, ceramidase activity should be determined in cultured skin fibroblasts or peripheral leukocytes. Various disease causing mutations have been identified in the acid ceramidase gene. Carrier detection and prenatal diagnosis are available.

Wolman Disease and Cholesterol Ester Storage Disease (CESD)

These are autosomal recessive lysosomal storage diseases that result from the deficiency of acid lipase and the accumulation of cholesterol esters and triglycerides in histiocytic foam cells of most visceral organs. The gene for lysosomal acid lipase is on chromosome 10 (10q24-q25). Wolman disease is the more severe clinical phenotype and is a fatal disorder of infancy. Clinical features become apparent in the 1st wk of life and include failure to thrive, relentless vomiting, abdominal distention, steatorrhea, and hepatosplenomegaly (see Table 80-16). There usually is hyperlipidemia. Hepatic dysfunction and fibrosis may occur. **Calcification of the adrenal glands** is pathognomonic for the disorder. Death usually occurs within 6 mo.

Cholesterol ester storage disease is a less severe disorder that may not be diagnosed until adulthood. Hepatomegaly can be the only detectable abnormality, but affected individuals are at significant risk for premature atherosclerosis. Adrenal calcification is not a feature.

Diagnosis and carrier identification are based on measuring acid lipase activity in peripheral leukocytes or cultured skin fibroblasts. Disease causing mutations have been identified in the acid ceramide gene. Prenatal diagnosis depends on measuring decreased enzyme levels or identifying specific mutations in cultured chorionic villi or amniocytes. There is no specific therapy available for either disorder, although pharmacologic agents to suppress cholesterol synthesis, in combination with cholestyramine and diet modification, have been used in patients with cholesterol ester storage disease (see Chapter 80.3).

BIBLIOGRAPHY

Please visit the Nelson Textbook of Pediatrics *website at www.expertconsult.com for the complete bibliography.*

80.5 Mucolipidoses

Margaret M. McGovern and Robert J. Desnick

I-cell disease (mucolipidosis II [ML-II]) and **pseudo-Hurler polydystrophy (mucolipidosis III [ML-III])** are rare autosomal recessive disorders that share some clinical features with Hurler syndrome (Chapter 82). These diseases result from the abnormal transport of newly synthesized lysosomal enzymes that are normally targeted to the lysosome by the presence of mannose-6-phosphate residues and recognized by specific lysosomal membrane receptors. These mannose-6-phosphate recognition markers are synthesized in a 2-step reaction that occurs in the Golgi apparatus and is mediated by 2 enzymatic activities. The enzyme that catalyzes the 1st step, the UDP-N-acetylglucosamine:lysosomal enzyme *N*-acetylglucosamine-1-phosphotransferase, is defective in both ML-II and ML-III, which are allelic disorders resulting from mutations in the GlcNAc-phosphotransferase alpha/beta-subunits precursor gene (GNPTAB). This enzyme deficiency results in abnormal targeting of the lysosomal enzymes that are consequently secreted into the extracellular matrix. Because the lysosomal enzymes require the acidic medium of the lysosome to function, patients with this defect accumulate a variety of different substrates due to the intracellular deficiency of all lysosomal enzymes. The diagnosis of ML-II and ML-III can be made by the determination of the serum lysosomal enzymatic activities, which are elevated, or by the demonstration of reduced enzymatic activity levels in cultured skin fibroblasts. Direct measurement of the phosphotransferase activity is possible as well. Prenatal diagnosis is available for both disorders by measurement of lysosomal enzymatic activities in amniocytes or chorionic villus cells; carrier identification studies are available for both disorders using cultured skin fibroblasts. Neonatal screening by tandem mass spectroscopy may detect I-cell disease.

I-Cell Disease

This disorder shares many of the clinical manifestations of Hurler syndrome (Chapter 82), although there is no mucopolysacchariduria and the presentation is earlier (see Table 80-16). Some patients have clinical features evident at birth, including coarse facial features, craniofacial abnormalities, restricted joint movement, and hypotonia. Nonimmune hydrops may be present in the fetus. The remainder of patients present in the first year with severe psychomotor retardation, coarse facial features, and skeletal manifestations that include kyphoscoliosis and a lumbar gibbus. Patients may also have congenital dislocation of the hips, inguinal hernias, and gingival hypertrophy. Progressive, severe psychomotor retardation leads to death in early childhood. No treatment is available.

Pseudo-Hurler Polydystrophy

Pseudo-Hurler polydystrophy is a less severe disorder than I-cell disease, with later onset and survival to adulthood reported. Affected children may present around the age of 4 or 5 yr with joint stiffness and short stature. Progressive destruction of the hip joints and moderate dysostosis multiplex are evident.

Radiographic evidence of low iliac wings, flattening of the proximal femoral epiphyses with valgus deformity of the femoral head, and hypoplasia of the anterior third of the lumbar vertebrae are characteristic findings. Ophthalmic findings include corneal clouding, retinopathy, and astigmatism; visual complaints are uncommon (see Table 80-16). Some patients have learning disabilities or mental retardation. Treatment, which should include orthopedic care, is symptomatic.

BIBLIOGRAPHY

Please visit the Nelson Textbook of Pediatrics *website at www.expertconsult.com for the complete bibliography.*

Chapter 81

Defects in Metabolism of Carbohydrates

Priya S. Kishnani and Yuan-Tsong Chen

Carbohydrate synthesis and degradation provide the energy required for most metabolic processes. The important carbohydrates include 3 monosaccharides—glucose, galactose, and fructose—and a polysaccharide, glycogen. The relevant biochemical pathways of these carbohydrates are shown in Figure 81-1. Glucose is the principal substrate of energy metabolism. A continuous source of glucose from dietary intake, gluconeogenesis, and glycogenolysis of glycogen maintains normal blood glucose levels. Metabolism of glucose generates adenosine triphosphate (ATP) via glycolysis (conversion of glucose or glycogen to pyruvate), mitochondrial oxidative phosphorylation (conversion of pyruvate to carbon dioxide and water), or both. Dietary sources of glucose come from ingesting polysaccharides, primarily starch and disaccharides, including lactose, maltose, and sucrose. Oral intake of glucose is intermittent and unreliable. Glucose made de novo from amino acids, primarily alanine (gluconeogenesis), contributes to maintaining the euglycemic state, but this process requires time. The breakdown of hepatic glycogen provides the rapid release of glucose, which maintains a constant blood glucose concentration. Glycogen is also the primary stored energy source in muscle, providing glucose for muscle activity during exercise. Galactose and fructose are monosaccharides that provide fuel for cellular metabolism; their role is less significant than that of glucose. Galactose is derived from lactose (galactose + glucose), which is found in milk and milk products. Galactose is an important energy source in infants, but it is 1st metabolized to glucose. Galactose (exogenous or endogenously synthesized from glucose) is also an important component of certain glycolipids, glycoproteins, and glycosaminoglycans. The dietary sources of fructose are sucrose (fructose + glucose, sorbitol) and fructose itself, which is found in fruits, vegetables, and honey.

Defects in glycogen metabolism typically cause an accumulation of glycogen in the tissues, hence the name **glycogen storage disease** (Table 81-1). Defects in gluconeogenesis or the glycolytic pathway, including galactose and fructose metabolism, do not result in an accumulation of glycogen (see Table 81-1). The defects in pyruvate metabolism in the pathway of the conversion of pyruvate to carbon dioxide and water via mitochondrial oxidative phosphorylation are more often associated with **lactic acidosis** and some tissue glycogen accumulation.

81.1 Glycogen Storage Diseases

Priya S. Kishnani and Yuan-Tsong Chen

The disorders of glycogen metabolism, the glycogen storage diseases (GSDs), result from deficiencies of various enzymes or transport proteins in the pathways of glycogen metabolism (see Fig. 81-1). The glycogen found in these disorders is abnormal in quantity, quality, or both. GSDs are categorized by numeric type in accordance with the chronological order in which these enzymatic defects were identified. This numeric classification is still widely used, at least up to number VII. The GSDs can also be classified by organ involvement and clinical manifestations into liver and muscle glycogenoses (see Table 81-1).

There are more than 12 forms of glycogenoses. Glucose-6-phosphatase deficiency (type I), lysosomal acid α-glucosidase deficiency (type II), debrancher deficiency (type III), and liver phosphorylase kinase deficiency (type IX) are the most common that typically present in early childhood; myophosphorylase deficiency (type V, McArdle disease) is the most common in adolescents and adults. The frequency of all forms of GSD is ≈1/20,000 live births.

LIVER GLYCOGENOSES

The GSDs that principally affect the liver include glucose-6-phosphatase deficiency (type I), debranching enzyme deficiency (type III), branching enzyme deficiency (type IV), liver phosphorylase deficiency (type VI), phosphorylase kinase deficiency (type IX, formerly termed GSD VIa), glycogen synthetase deficiency (type 0), and glucose transporter-2 defect. Because hepatic carbohydrate metabolism is responsible for plasma glucose homeostasis, this group of disorders typically causes fasting hypoglycemia and hepatomegaly. Some (type III, type IV, type IX) can be associated with liver cirrhosis. Other organs can also be involved and may manifest as renal dysfunction in type I, myopathy (skeletal and/or cardiomyopathy) in types III and IV, as well as in some rare forms of phosphorylase kinase deficiency, and neurological involvement in types II (the brain, anterior horns cells), III (peripheral nerves), and IV (some patients can present with diffuse central and peripheral nervous system dysfunction).

Type I Glycogen Storage Disease (Glucose-6-Phosphatase or Translocase Deficiency, Von Gierke Disease)

Type I GSD is caused by the absence or deficiency of glucose-6-phosphatase activity in the liver, kidney, and intestinal mucosa. It can be divided into two subtypes: type Ia, in which the glucose-6-phosphatase enzyme is defective; and type Ib, in which a translocase that transports glucose-6-phosphate across the microsomal membrane is defective. The defects in both type Ia and type Ib lead to inadequate hepatic conversion of glucose-6-phosphate to glucose through normal glycogenolysis and gluconeogenesis and make affected individuals susceptible to fasting hypoglycemia.

Type I GSD is an autosomal recessive disorder. The structural gene for glucose-6-phosphatase is located on chromosome 17q21; the gene for translocase is on chromosome 11q23. Common mutations responsible for the disease are known. Carrier detection and prenatal diagnosis are possible with the DNA-based diagnosis.

CLINICAL MANIFESTATIONS Patients with type I GSD may present in the neonatal period with hypoglycemia and lactic acidosis; they more commonly present at 3-4 mo of age with hepatomegaly, hypoglycemic seizures, or both. These children often have **doll-like faces** with fat cheeks, relatively thin extremities, short stature, and a protuberant abdomen that is due to massive hepatomegaly; the kidneys are also enlarged, whereas the spleen and heart are normal.

The biochemical hallmarks of the disease are hypoglycemia, lactic acidosis, hyperuricemia, and hyperlipidemia. Hypoglycemia and lactic acidosis can develop after a short fast. Hyperuricemia is present in young children; gout rarely develops before puberty. Despite marked hepatomegaly, the liver transaminase levels are usually normal or only slightly elevated. Intermittent diarrhea may occur in GSD I. In patients with GSD Ib, the loss of mucosal barrier function due to inflammation, which is likely

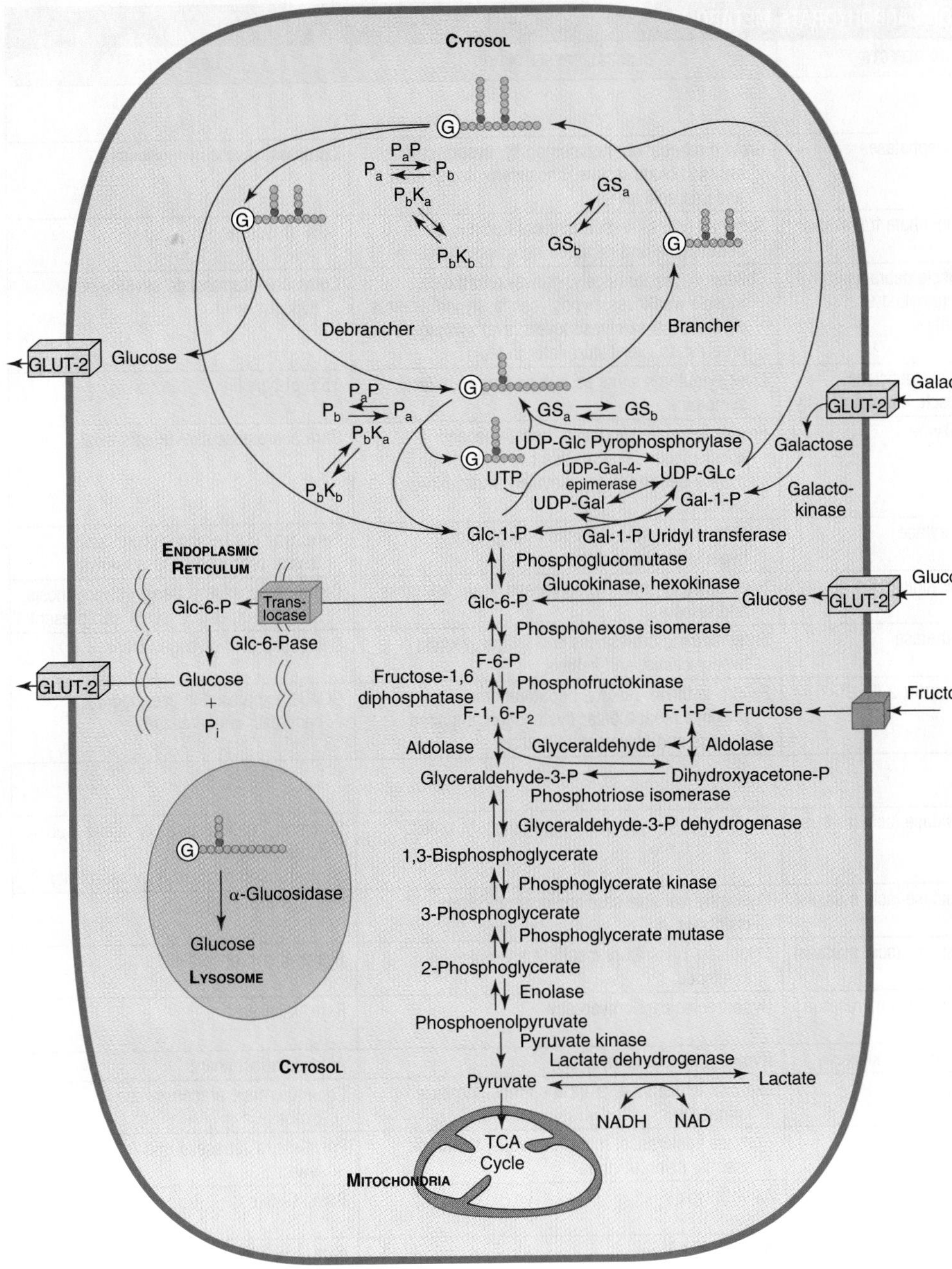

Figure 81-1 Pathway related to glycogen storage diseases and galactose and fructose disorders. GSa, active glycogen synthetase; GSb, inactive glycogen synthetase; Pa, active phosphorylase; Pb, inactive phosphorylase; PaP, phosphorylase a phosphatase; PbKa, active phosphorylase b kinase; PbKb, inactive phosphorylase b kinase; G, glycogen, the primer for glycogen synthesis; UDP, uridine diphosphate; GLUT-2, glucose transporter 2; NAD/NADH, nicotinamide-adenine dinucleotide. (Modified from Beaudet AR: Glycogen storage disease. In Harrison TR, Isselbacher KJ, editors: *Harrison's principles of internal medicine,* ed 13, New York, 1994, McGraw-Hill. Reproduced with permission of The McGraw-Hill Companies.)

related to the disturbed neutrophil function, seems to be the main cause of diarrhea. Easy bruising and epistaxis are common and are associated with a prolonged bleeding time as a result of impaired platelet aggregation and adhesion.

The plasma may be "milky" in appearance as a result of a striking elevation of triglyceride levels. Cholesterol and phospholipids are also elevated, but less prominently. The lipid abnormality resembles type IV hyperlipidemia and is characterized by increased levels of very low density lipoprotein, low-density lipoprotein, and a unique apolipoprotein profile consisting of increased levels of apo B, C, and E, with relatively normal or reduced levels of apo A and D. The histologic appearance of the liver is characterized by a universal distention of hepatocytes by glycogen and fat. The lipid vacuoles are particularly large and prominent. There is little associated fibrosis.

All these findings apply to both type Ia and type Ib GSD, but **type Ib** has additional features of recurrent bacterial infections from **neutropenia** and impaired neutrophil function. Gut mucosa ulceration culminating in GSD enterocolitis is also common. Exceptional cases of type Ib without neutropenia and type Ia with neutropenia have been reported.

Although type I GSD affects mainly the liver, multiple organ systems are involved. Puberty is often delayed. Virtually all females have ultrasound findings consistent with **polycystic ovaries;** other features of polycystic ovary syndrome (acne, hirsuitism) are not seen. Nonetheless, fertility appears to be normal, as evidenced in several reports of successful pregnancy in women with GSD I. Increased bleeding during menstrual cycles, including life-threatening menorrhagia, has been noted and could be related to the impaired platelet aggregation. Symptoms of gout usually start around puberty from long-term hyperuricemia. Secondary to the lipid abnormalities, there is an increased risk of **pancreatitis.** The dyslipidemia, together with elevated erythrocyte aggregation, predisposes these patients to atherosclerosis. Premature atherosclerosis has not yet been clearly documented except for rare cases. Impaired platelet aggregation and increased antioxidative defense to prevent lipid peroxidation may function as a protective mechanism to help reduce the risk of atherosclerosis.

Table 81-1 FEATURES OF THE DISORDERS OF CARBOHYDRATE METABOLISM

DISORDERS	BASIC DEFECTS	CLINICAL PRESENTATION	COMMENTS
LIVER GLYCOGENOSES **Type/Common Name**			
Ia/Von Gierke	Glucose-6-phosphatase	Growth retardation, hepatomegaly, hypoglycemia; elevated blood lactate, cholesterol, triglyceride, and uric acid levels	Common, severe hypoglycemia
Ib	Glucose-6-phosphate translocase	Same as type Ia, with additional findings of neutropenia and impaired neutrophil function	10% of type Ia
IIIa/Cori or Forbes	Liver and muscle debrancher deficiency (amylo-1,6 glucosidase)	Childhood: hepatomegaly, growth retardation, muscle weakness, hypoglycemia, hyperlipidemia, elevated transaminase levels; liver symptoms can progress to liver failure later in life	Common, intermediate severity of hypoglycemia
IIIb	Liver debrancher deficiency; normal muscle enzyme activity	Liver symptoms same as in type IIIa; no muscle symptoms	15% of type III
IV/Andersen	Branching enzyme	Failure to thrive, hypotonia, hepatomegaly, splenomegaly, progressive cirrhosis (death usually before 5th yr), elevated transaminase levels	Rare neuromuscular variants exist
VI/Hers	Liver phosphorylase	Hepatomegaly, typically mild hypoglycemia, hyperlipidemia, and ketosis	Rare, typically benign glycogenosis; severe presentation also known
Phosphorylase kinase deficiency	Phosphorylase kinase	Hepatomegaly, mild hypoglycemia, hyperlipidemia, and ketosis	Common, typically a benign glycogenosis, severe progressive forms also present
Glycogen synthetase deficiency	Glycogen synthetase	Early morning drowsiness and fatigue, fasting hypoglycemia, and ketosis	Decreased liver glycogen store
Fanconi-Bickel syndrome	Glucose transporter 2 (GLUT-2)	Failure to thrive, rickets, hepatorenomegaly, proximal renal tubular dysfunction, impaired glucose and galactose utilization	GLUT-2 expressed in liver, kidney, pancreas, and intestine
MUSCLE GLYCOGENOSES **Type/Common Name**			
II/Pompe Infantile	Acid α-glucosidase (acid maltase)	Cardiomegaly, hypotonia, hepatomegaly; onset: birth to 6 mo	Common, cardiorespiratory failure leading to death by age 2 yr; Minimal to no residual enzyme activity
Juvenile	Acid α-glucosidase (acid maltase)	Myopathy, variable cardiomyopathy; onset: childhood	Residual enzyme activity
Adult	Acid α-glucosidase (acid maltase)	Myopathy, respiratory insufficiency; onset: adulthood	Residual enzyme activity
Danon disease	Lysosome-associated membrane protein 2 (LAMP2)	Hypertrophic cardiomyopathy	Rare, X-linked
PRKAG2 deficiency	AMP-activated protein kinase γ	Hypertrophic cardiomyopathy	Autosomal dominant
V/McArdle	Myophosphorylase	Exercise intolerance, muscle cramps, increased fatigability	Common, male predominance
VII/Tarui	Phosphofructokinase	Exercise intolerance, muscle cramps, hemolytic anemia, myoglobinuria	Prevalent in Japanese and Ashkenazi Jews
Phosphoglycerate kinase deficiency	Phosphoglycerate kinase	As with type V	Rare, X-linked
Phosphoglycerate mutase deficiency	M subunit of phosphoglycerate mutase	As with type V	Rare, majority of patients are African-American
Lactate dehydrogenase deficiency	M subunit of lactate dehydrogenase	As with type V	Rare
GALACTOSE DISORDERS			
Galactosemia with transferase deficiency	Galactose-1-phosphate uridyltransferase	Vomiting, hepatomegaly, cataracts, aminoaciduria, failure to thrive	African-American patients tend to have milder symptoms
Galactokinase deficiency	Galactokinase	Cataracts	Benign
Generalized uridine diphosphate galactose-4-epimerase deficiency	Uridine diphosphate galactose-4-epimerase	Similar to transferase deficiency with additional findings of hypotonia and nerve deafness	A benign variant also exists
FRUCTOSE DISORDERS			
Essential fructosuria	Fructokinase	Urine reducing substance	Benign
Hereditary fructose intolerance	Fructose-1-phosphate aldolase	Acute: vomiting, sweating, lethargy Chronic: failure to thrive, hepatic failure	Prognosis good with fructose restriction
DISORDERS OF GLUCONEOGENESIS			
Fructose-1,6-diphosphatase deficiency	Fructose-1,6-diphosphatase	Episodic hypoglycemia, apnea, acidosis	Good prognosis, avoid fasting
Phosphoenolpyruvate carboxykinase deficiency	Phosphoenolpyruvate carboxykinase	Hypoglycemia, hepatomegaly, hypotonia, failure to thrive	Rare

Table 81-1 FEATURES OF THE DISORDERS OF CARBOHYDRATE METABOLISM—cont'd

DISORDERS	BASIC DEFECTS	CLINICAL PRESENTATION	COMMENTS
DISORDERS OF PYRUVATE METABOLISM			
Pyruvate dehydrogenase complex defect	Pyruvate dehydrogenase	Severe fatal neonatal to mild late onset, lactic acidosis, psychomotor retardation, and failure to thrive	Most commonly due to E1 α subunit, defect X-linked
Pyruvate carboxylase deficiency	Pyruvate carboxylase	Same as above	Rare, autosomal recessive
Respiratory chain defects (oxidative phosphorylation disease)	Complex I to V, many mitochondrial DNA mutations	Heterogeneous with multisystem involvement	Mitochondrial inheritance
DISORDERS IN PENTOSE METABOLISM			
Pentosuria	L-Xylulose reductase	Urine reducing substance	Benign
Transaldolase deficiency	Transaldolase	Liver cirrhosis and failure, cardiomyopathy	Autosomal recessive
Ribose-5-phosphate isomerase deficiency	Ribose-5-phosphate isomerase	Progressive leukoencephalopathy and peripheral neuropathy	

Frequent fractures and radiographic evidence of **osteopenia** are common; bone mineral content is reduced even in prepubertal patients.

By the 2nd or 3rd decade of life, most patients with type I GSD exhibit **hepatic adenomas** that can hemorrhage and, in some cases, become malignant. **Pulmonary hypertension** has been seen in some long-term survivors of the disease.

Renal disease is another complication, and most patients with type I GSD who are >20 yr of age have proteinuria. Many also have hypertension, renal stones, nephrocalcinosis, and altered creatinine clearance. Glomerular hyperfiltration, increased renal plasma flow, and microalbuminuria are often found in the early stages of renal dysfunction and can occur before the onset of proteinuria. In younger patients, hyperfiltration and hyperperfusion may be the only signs of renal abnormalities. With the advancement of renal disease, focal segmental glomerulosclerosis and interstitial fibrosis become evident. In some patients, renal function has deteriorated and progressed to failure, requiring dialysis and transplantation. Other renal abnormalities include amyloidosis, a Fanconi-like syndrome, hypocitraturia, hypercalciuria, and a distal renal tubular acidification defect.

DIAGNOSIS The diagnosis of type I GSD is suspected on the basis of clinical presentation and the laboratory findings of hypoglycemia, lactic acidosis, hyperuricemia, and hyperlipidemia. Neutropenia is noted in GSD Ib patients, typically after the 1st 2-3 yr of life. Administration of glucagon or epinephrine results in little or no rise in blood glucose level, but the lactate level rises significantly. Before the glucose-6-phosphatase and glucose-6-phosphate translocase genes were cloned, a definitive diagnosis required a liver biopsy. Gene-based mutation analysis provides a noninvasive way of diagnosis for most patients with types Ia and Ib disease.

TREATMENT Treatment is designed to maintain normal blood glucose levels and is achieved by continuous nasogastric infusion of glucose or oral administration of uncooked cornstarch. Nasogastric drip feeding can be introduced in early infancy from the time of diagnosis. It can consist of an elemental enteral formula or contain only glucose or a glucose polymer to provide sufficient glucose to maintain normoglycemia during the night. Frequent feedings with high-carbohydrate content are given during the day.

Uncooked cornstarch acts as a slow-release form of glucose and can be introduced at a dose of 1.6 g/kg every 4 hr for infants <2 yr of age. The response of young infants is variable. As the child grows older, the cornstarch regimen can be changed to every 6 hr at a dose of 1.75-2.5 g/kg of body weight. New starch products, which are currently being developed, are thought to be longer acting, better tolerated, and more palatable. A short-term double-blind crossover pilot study comparing uncooked, physically modified cornstarch to traditional cornstarch showed that the majority of GSD patients treated with the new starch had better short-term metabolic control and longer duration of euglycemia; however, more extensive studies replicating these results are necessary at this time. Because fructose and galactose cannot be converted directly to glucose in GSD type I, these sugars are restricted in the diet. Sucrose (table sugar, cane sugar, other ingredients), fructose (fruit, juice, high fructose corn syrup), lactose (dairy foods), and sorbitol should be avoided or limited. Due to these dietary restrictions, vitamins and minerals such as calcium and vitamin D may be deficient and supplementation is required to prevent nutritional deficiencies. Dietary therapy improves hyperuricemia, hyperlipidemia, and renal function, slowing the development of renal failure. This therapy fails, however, to normalize blood uric acid and lipid levels completely in some individuals, despite good metabolic control, especially after puberty. The control of hyperuricemia can be further augmented by the use of allopurinol, a xanthine oxidase inhibitor. The hyperlipidemia can be reduced with lipid-lowering drugs such as HMG-CoA reductase inhibitors and fibrate (Chapter 80). Microalbuminuria, an early indicator of renal dysfunction in type I disease, is treated with angiotensin-converting enzyme (ACE) inhibitors. Citrate supplements can be beneficial for patients with hypocitraturia by preventing or ameliorating nephrocalcinosis and development of urinary calculi. Growth hormone should be used with extreme caution and limited to only those with a documented growth hormone deficiency. Even in those cases, there should be close monitoring of metabolic parameters and presence of adenomas.

In patients with type Ib GSD, granulocyte and granulocyte-macrophage colony–stimulating factors are successful in correcting the neutropenia, decreasing the number and severity of bacterial infections, and improving the chronic inflammatory bowel disease.

Orthotopic liver transplantation is a potential cure of type I GSD, but the inherent short- and long-term complications leave this as a treatment of last resort, usually for patients with liver malignancy, multiple liver adenomas, metabolic derangements refractory to medical management, and/or liver failure. Large adenomas (>2 cm) that are rapidly increasing in size and/or number may require partial hepatic resection. Smaller adenomas (<2 cm) can be treated with percutaneous ethanol injection or transcatheter arterial embolization. A challenge is the recurrence of liver adenomas with potential for malignant transformation in these patients, ultimately requiring a liver transplant. Bone marrow transplantation has been reported to correct the neutropenia of type Ib.

Before any surgical procedure, the bleeding status must be evaluated and good metabolic control established. Prolonged bleeding times can be normalized by the use of intensive intravenous glucose infusion for 24-48 hr before surgery. Use of 1-deamino-8-D-arginine vasopressin (DDAVP) can reduce

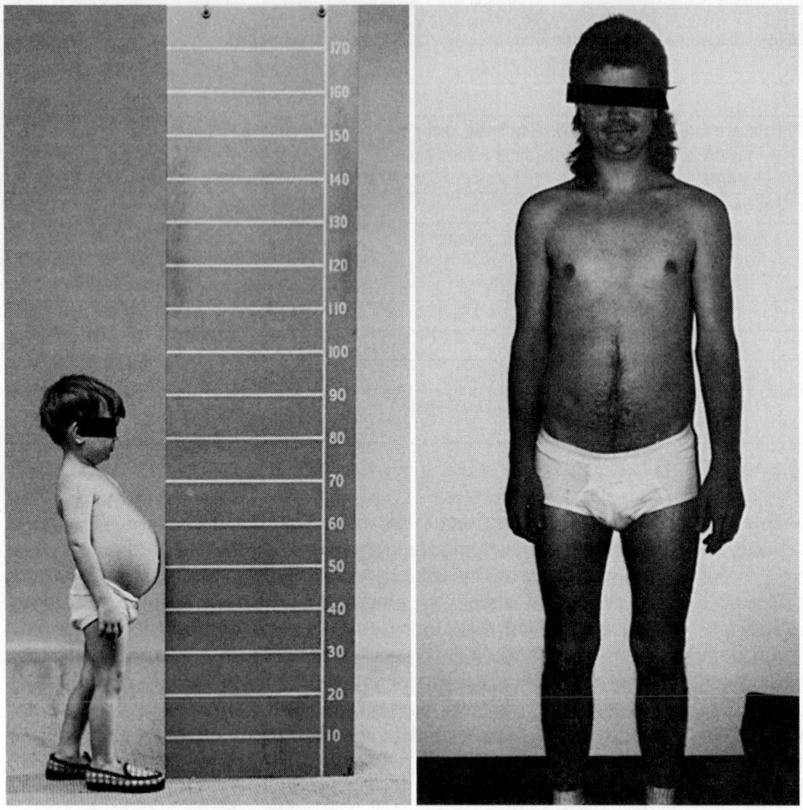

Figure 81-2 Growth and development in a patient with type IIIb glycogen storage disease. The patient has debrancher deficiency in liver but normal activity in muscle. As a child, he had hepatomegaly, hypoglycemia, and growth retardation. After puberty, he no longer had hepatomegaly or hypoglycemia, and his final adult height is normal. He had no muscle weakness or atrophy; this is in contrast to type IIIa patients, in whom a progressive myopathy is seen in adulthood.

bleeding complications. Lactated ringer solution should be avoided because it contains lactate and no glucose. Glucose levels should be maintained in the normal range throughout surgery with the use of 10% dextrose.

PROGNOSIS Previously, many patients with type I GSD died at a young age, and the prognosis was guarded for those who survived. The long-term complications occur mostly in adults whose disease was not adequately treated during childhood. Early diagnosis and effective treatment have improved the outcome; renal disease and formation of hepatic adenomas with potential risk for malignant transformation remain serious complications.

Type III Glycogen Storage Disease (Debrancher Deficiency, Limit Dextrinosis)

Type III GSD is caused by a deficiency of glycogen debranching enzyme activity. Debranching enzyme, together with phosphorylase, is responsible for complete degradation of glycogen. When debranching enzyme is defective, glycogen breakdown is incomplete and an abnormal glycogen with short outer branch chains and resembling limit dextrin accumulates. Deficiency of glycogen debranching enzyme causes hepatomegaly, hypoglycemia, short stature, variable skeletal myopathy, and variable cardiomyopathy. The disorder usually involves both liver and muscle and is termed type IIIa GSD. In approximately 15% of patients, the disease appears to involve only liver and is classified as type IIIb.

Type III glycogenosis is an autosomal recessive disease that has been reported in many different ethnic groups; the frequency is relatively high in Sephardic Jews from North Africa. The gene for debranching enzyme is located on chromosome 1p21. More than 30 different mutations are identified; 2 exon 3 mutations (17delAG and Q6X) are specifically associated with glycogenosis IIIb. Carrier detection and prenatal diagnosis are possible using DNA-based linkage or mutation analysis.

CLINICAL MANIFESTATIONS During infancy and childhood, the disease may be indistinguishable from type I GSD, because hepatomegaly, hypoglycemia, hyperlipidemia, and growth retardation are common (Fig. 81-2). Splenomegaly may be present, but the kidneys are not enlarged. Remarkably, hepatomegaly and hepatic symptoms in most patients with type III GSD improve with age and usually resolve after puberty. Progressive liver cirrhosis and failure can occur. **Hepatocellular carcinoma** has also been reported, more typically in patients with progressive liver cirrhosis. The frequency of adenomas in individuals with GSD III is far less, compared to GSD I. Furthermore, the relationship of hepatic adenomas and malignancy in GSD III is unclear. A single case of malignant transformation at the site of adenomas has been noted. In patients with muscular involvement (type IIIa), muscle weakness can present in childhood but can become severe after the 3rd or 4th decade of life, as evidenced by slowly progressive weakness and wasting. Because patients with GSD III can have decreased bone density, they are at an increased risk of potential fracture. Myopathy does not follow any particular pattern of involvement; both proximal and distal muscles are involved. Electromyography reveals a widespread myopathy; nerve conduction studies are often abnormal. Ventricular hypertrophy is a frequent finding, but overt cardiac dysfunction is rare. There have been some reports of life-threatening arrhythmia and need for heart transplant in some GSD III patients. Hepatic symptoms in some patients may be so mild that the diagnosis is not made until adulthood, when the patients show symptoms and signs of neuromuscular disease. The initial diagnosis has been confused with Charcot-Marie-Tooth disease. Polycystic ovaries are common; some patients can develop hirsutism, irregular menstrual cycles, and other features of polycystic ovarian syndrome. Fertility does not appear to be reduced; successful pregnancies in patients with GSD III have been reported.

Hypoglycemia and hyperlipidemia are common. In contrast to type I GSD, elevation of liver transaminase levels and fasting ketosis are prominent, but blood lactate and uric acid concentrations are usually normal. Serum creatine kinase levels can be useful to identify patients with muscle involvement; normal levels do not rule out muscle enzyme deficiency. The administration of glucagon 2 hr after a carbohydrate meal provokes a normal increase in blood glucose; after an overnight fast, glucagon may provoke no change in blood glucose level.

DIAGNOSIS The histologic appearance of the liver is characterized by a universal distention of hepatocytes by glycogen and the presence of fibrous septa. The fibrosis and the paucity of fat distinguish type III glycogenosis from type I. The fibrosis, which ranges from minimal periportal fibrosis to micronodular cirrhosis, appears in most cases to be nonprogressive. Overt cirrhosis has been seen in some patients with GSD III.

Patients with myopathy and liver symptoms have a generalized enzyme defect (type IIIa). The deficient enzyme activity can be demonstrated not only in liver and muscle, but also in other tissues such as heart, erythrocytes, and cultured fibroblasts. Patients with hepatic symptoms without clinical or laboratory evidence of myopathy have debranching enzyme deficiency only in the liver, with enzyme activity retained in the muscle (type IIIb). Definite diagnosis requires enzyme assay in liver, muscle, or both. Mutation analysis can provide a noninvasive method for diagnosis and subtype assignment in the majority of patients; however, the large size of the gene and the distribution of mutations across the entire gene present a challenge.

TREATMENT Dietary management is less demanding than in type I GSD. Patients do not need to restrict dietary intake of fructose and galactose. If hypoglycemia is present, frequent meals high in carbohydrates with cornstarch supplements or nocturnal gastric drip feedings are usually effective. A high-protein diet during the daytime plus overnight protein enteral infusion can also be effective in preventing hypoglycemia and preventing endogenous protein breakdown because protein can be used as a substrate for gluconeogenesis, a pathway that is intact in type III GSD. There is no satisfactory treatment for the progressive myopathy other than recommending a high-protein diet and an exercise program. Liver transplantation has been performed in patients with end-stage cirrhosis and/or hepatic carcinoma.

Type IV Glycogen Storage Disease (Branching Enzyme Deficiency, Amylopectinosis, or Andersen Disease)

Deficiency of branching enzyme activity results in accumulation of an abnormal glycogen with poor solubility. The disease is referred to as type IV GSD or amylopectinosis because the abnormal glycogen has fewer branch points, more α 1-4 linked glucose units, and longer outer chains, resulting in a structure resembling amylopectin.

Type IV GSD is an autosomal recessive disorder. The glycogen branching enzyme gene is located on chromosome 3p21. Mutations responsible for type IV GSD have been identified, and their characterization in individual patients can be useful in predicting the clinical outcome. Some mutations are associated with a good prognosis and lack of progression of liver disease.

CLINICAL MANIFESTATIONS This disorder is clinically variable. The most common and classic form is characterized by progressive cirrhosis of the liver and is manifested in the 1st 18 mo of life as hepatosplenomegaly and failure to thrive. The cirrhosis progresses to portal hypertension, ascites, esophageal varices, and liver failure that usually leads to death by 5 yr of age. Rare patients survive without progression of liver disease; these patients have a milder hepatic form and do not require a liver transplant.

A **neuromuscular** form of the disease has been reported; there are 4 main variants recognized based on age of presentation. The perinatal form presents as a fetal akinesia deformation sequence and death in the perinatal period. The congenital form presents at birth with severe hypotonia, muscle atrophy, and neuronal involvement with death in the neonatal period; some patients have cardiomyopathy. The childhood form presents primarily with myopathy or cardiomyopathy. The adult form presents with diffuse central and peripheral nervous system dysfunction accompanied by accumulation of polyglucosan material in the nervous system (**adult polyglucosan body disease**). For adult polyglucosan disease, a leukocyte or nerve biopsy is needed to establish the diagnosis because the branching enzyme deficiency is limited to those tissues.

DIAGNOSIS Tissue deposition of amylopectin-like materials can be demonstrated in liver, heart, muscle, skin, intestine, brain, spinal cord, and peripheral nerve. The hepatic histologic findings are characterized by micronodular cirrhosis and faintly stained basophilic inclusions in the hepatocytes. The inclusions consist of coarsely clumped, stored material that is periodic acid–Schiff positive and partially resistant to diastase digestion. Electron microscopy shows, in addition to the conventional α and β glycogen particles, accumulation of the fibrillar aggregations that are typical of amylopectin. The distinct staining properties of the cytoplasmic inclusions, as well as electron microscopic findings, could be diagnostic. However, polysaccharidoses with histologic features reminiscent of type IV disease, but without enzymatic correlation, have been observed. The definitive diagnosis rests on the demonstration of the deficient branching enzyme activity in liver, muscle, cultured skin fibroblasts, or leukocytes, or on the identification of disease-causing mutations in the glycogen branching enzyme (*GBE*) gene. Prenatal diagnosis is possible by measuring the enzyme activity in cultured amniocytes, chorionic villi, or mutation analysis.

TREATMENT There is no specific treatment for type IV GSD. Unlike patients with the other liver GSDs (I, III, VI, IX), those with GSD IV do not have hypoglycemia, which is only seen when there is overt liver cirrhosis. Liver transplantation has been performed for patients with progressive hepatic failure, but because it is a multisystem disorder involving many organ systems, the long-term success of liver transplantation is unknown. Caution should be taken in selecting type IV patients for liver transplantation because these patients have variable phenotypes, which include a nonprogressive form of the liver disease and in some cases, extrahepatic manifestations of the disease.

Type VI Glycogen Storage Disease (Liver Phosphorylase Deficiency, Hers Disease)

There are few patients with documented liver phosphorylase deficiency. Such patients usually have a benign course and present with hepatomegaly and growth retardation in early childhood; however, some cases are more severe. Hypoglycemia, hyperlipidemia, and hyperketosis are of variable severity. Lactic acid and uric acid levels are normal. The heart and skeletal muscles are not involved. The hepatomegaly and growth retardation improve with age and usually disappear around puberty; however, patients with severe hepatomegaly, recurrent severe hypoglycemia, hyperketosis, and postprandial lactic acidosis have recently been reported. Treatment is symptomatic. A high-carbohydrate diet and frequent feeding are effective in preventing hypoglycemia; most patients require no specific treatment. GSD VI is an autosomal recessive disease. Diagnosis rests on enzyme analysis of the liver biopsy. The liver phosphorylase gene (*PYGL*) is on chromosome 14q21-22 and has 20 exons. Many mutations are known in this gene; a splice site mutation in intron 13 has been identified in the Mennonite population.

Type IX Glycogen Storage Disease (Phosphorylase Kinase Deficiency)

This disorder represents a heterogeneous group of glycogenoses. Phosphorylase, the rate-limiting enzyme of glycogenolysis, is activated by a cascade of enzymatic reactions involving adenylate cyclase, cyclic adenosine monophosphate–dependent protein kinase (protein kinase A), and phosphorylase kinase. The latter enzyme has 4 subunits (α, β, γ, δ), each encoded by different genes on different chromosomes and differentially expressed in various tissues. This cascade of reactions is stimulated primarily by glucagon. This glycogenosis could be the result of any enzyme deficiency along this pathway; the most common is the deficiency of phosphorylase kinase. The phenotypic variability within each subtype is being uncovered with the availability of molecular testing.

The numeric classification of phosphorylase kinase deficiency is confusing, ranging from type VIa to VIII to IX. It is advisable to refrain from such a designation and to classify the various disorders according to organ involvement and mode of inheritance.

X-Linked Liver Phosphorylase Kinase Deficiency

X-linked liver phosphorylase kinase deficiency is the most common form of liver glycogenoses. In addition to liver, enzyme activity can also be deficient in erythrocytes, leukocytes, and fibroblasts; it is normal in muscle. Typically, a 1-5 yr old male presents with growth retardation, an incidental finding of hepatomegaly, and a slight delay in motor development. Cholesterol, triglycerides, and liver enzymes are mildly elevated. Ketosis may occur after fasting. Lactate and uric acid levels are normal. Hypoglycemia is typically mild, if present. The response in blood glucose to glucagon is normal. Hepatomegaly and abnormal blood chemistries gradually improve and can normalize with age. Most adults achieve a normal final height and are usually asymptomatic despite a persistent phosphorylase kinase deficiency. Liver histologic appearance shows glycogen-distended hepatocytes. The accumulated glycogen (β particles, rosette form) has a frayed or burst appearance and is less compact than the glycogen seen in type I or type III GSD. Fibrous septal formation and low-grade inflammatory changes may be present.

The structural gene for the common liver isoform of the phosphorylase kinase subunit, liver α subunit, is on the X chromosome (αL at Xp22.2). Several missense, nonsense, and splice-site mutations of this gene are known.

Autosomal Liver and Muscle Phosphorylase Kinase Deficiency

Several patients have been reported with phosphorylase kinase deficiency in liver and blood cells and an autosomal mode of inheritance. As with the X-linked form, hepatomegaly and growth retardation apparent in early childhood are the predominant symptoms. Some patients also exhibit muscle hypotonia. When measured in a few cases, reduced activity of the enzyme has been demonstrated in muscle. Mutations causing autosomally transmitted liver and muscle phosphorylase kinase deficiency are found in the autosomal β subunit gene of the PK gene (chromosome 16q12-q13). Several nonsense mutations, a single-base insertion, a splice-site mutation, and a large intragenic mutation have been identified. In addition, a missense mutation was discovered in an atypical patient with normal blood cell phosphorylase kinase activity.

Autosomal Liver Phosphorylase Kinase Deficiency

This form of phosphorylase kinase deficiency is due to mutations in the testis/liver isoform of the γ subunit of the gene (TL, PHKG2). In contrast to X-linked phosphorylase kinase deficiency, patients with mutations in the *PHKG2* gene typically have more severe phenotypes with recurrent hypoglycemia and often develop progressive liver cirrhosis. *PHKG2* maps to chromosome 16p12.1 and many disease-causing mutations are known for this gene.

Muscle-Specific Phosphorylase Kinase Deficiency

A few cases of phosphorylase kinase deficiency restricted to muscle are known. Patients, both male and female, present either with muscle cramps and myoglobinuria with exercise or with progressive muscle weakness and atrophy. Phosphorylase kinase activity is decreased in muscle but normal in liver and blood cells. There is no hepatomegaly or cardiomegaly. The structural gene for the muscle specific form α subunit (αM) is located at Xq12. Mutations of this gene have been found in male patients with this disorder. The gene for muscle γ subunit (γM, PHKG1) is on chromosome 7p12.[29] No mutations in this gene have been reported so far.

Phosphorylase Kinase Deficiency Limited to Heart

These patients present with **cardiomyopathy** in infancy and rapidly progress to heart failure and death. Phosphorylase kinase deficiency is demonstrated in the heart with normal enzyme activity in skeletal muscle and liver. Studies have questioned the existence of cardiac-specific primary phosphorylase kinase deficiency because they did not find any mutations in the 8 genes encoding the phosphorylase kinase subunits.

DIAGNOSIS Definitive diagnosis of phosphorylase kinase deficiency requires demonstration of the enzymatic defect in affected tissues. Phosphorylase kinase can be measured in leukocytes and erythrocytes, but because the enzyme has many isozymes, the diagnosis can be missed without studies of liver, muscle, or heart in certain instances. Mutation analysis is necessary in many cases to determine the disease's subtype.

The *PHKA2* gene encoding the α subunit is most commonly involved, followed by the *PHKB* gene encoding the β subunit, regardless of the presence of deficiency in erythrocytes. Mutations in the *PHKG2* gene underlying γ-subunit deficiency are typically associated with severe liver involvement with recurrent hypoglycemia and liver fibrosis.

TREATMENT The treatment for liver phosphorylase kinase deficiency includes a high-carbohydrate diet and frequent feedings to prevent hypoglycemia; most patients require no specific treatment. Prognosis for the X-linked and certain autosomal forms is good. Patients with mutations in the γ subunit typically have a more severe clinical course with progressive liver disease. There is no treatment for the fatal form of isolated cardiac phosphorylase kinase deficiency other than heart transplantation.

Glycogen Synthetase Deficiency (GSD 0)

Deficiency of hepatic glycogen synthetase (*GYS2*) activity leads to a marked decrease of glycogen stored in the liver. The disease appears to be very rare in humans, and in the true sense, this is not a type of GSD because the deficiency of the enzyme leads to decreased glycogen stores.

The patients present in infancy with early-morning (before eating breakfast) drowsiness, pallor, emesis, and fatigue and sometimes convulsions associated with hypoglycemia and hyperketonemia. Blood lactate and alanine levels are low, and there is no hyperlipidemia or hepatomegaly. Prolonged hyperglycemia, glycosuria, and elevation of lactate with normal insulin levels after administration of glucose or a meal suggest a possible diagnosis of deficiency of glycogen synthetase. Definitive diagnosis requires a liver biopsy to measure the enzyme activity or identification of mutations in the liver glycogen synthetase gene, located on chromosome 12p12.2. Treatment consists of frequent meals, rich in protein, and nighttime supplementation with uncooked cornstarch. Most children with GSD 0 are cognitively and developmentally normal. Short stature and osteopenia are common features. The prognosis seems good for patients who survive to adulthood, including resolution of hypoglycemia, except during pregnancy.

MUSCLE GLYCOGEN SYNTHASE DEFICIENCY This GSD results from muscle glycogen synthase (glycogen synthase I, *GYS1*) deficiency.

It is extremely rare and was reported in 3 children of consanguineous parents of Syrian origin. Muscle biopsies showed lack of glycogen, predominantly oxidative fibers, and mitochondrial proliferation. Glucose tolerance was normal. Molecular study revealed a homozygous stop mutation (R462→ter) in the muscle glycogen synthase gene. The phenotype was variable in the 3 siblings and ranged from sudden cardiac arrest, muscle fatigability, hypertrophic cardiomyopathy, an abnormal heart rate, and hypotension while exercising, to mildly impaired cardiac function at rest.

Hepatic Glycogenosis with Renal Fanconi Syndrome (Fanconi-Bickel Syndrome)

This rare autosomal recessive disorder is caused by defects in the facilitative glucose transporter 2 (GLUT-2), which transports glucose in and out of hepatocytes, pancreatic β cells, and the basolateral membranes of intestinal and renal epithelial cells. The disease is characterized by proximal renal tubular dysfunction, impaired glucose and galactose utilization, and accumulation of glycogen in liver and kidney.

The affected child typically presents in the 1st yr of life with failure to thrive, rickets, and a protuberant abdomen from hepatomegaly and nephromegaly. The disease may be confused with type I GSD because a Fanconi-like syndrome can develop in type I disease patients.

Laboratory findings include glucosuria, phosphaturia, generalized aminoaciduria, bicarbonate wasting, hypophosphatemia, increased serum alkaline phosphatase levels, and radiologic findings of rickets. Mild fasting hypoglycemia and hyperlipidemia may be present. Liver transaminase, plasma lactate, and uric acid levels are usually normal. Oral galactose or glucose tolerance tests show intolerance, which could be explained by the functional loss of GLUT-2 preventing liver uptake of these sugars.

Tissue biopsy results show marked accumulation of glycogen in hepatocytes and proximal renal tubular cells, presumably owing to the altered glucose transport out of these organs. Diffuse glomerular mesangial expansion along with glomerular hyperfiltration and microalbuminuria similar to nephropathy in GSD Ia and diabetes have been reported.

Fanconi-Bickel syndrome is rare. Seventy percent of patients with a detectable GLUT-2 mutation have consanguineous parents. Most patients are homozygous for the disease-related mutations; some patients are compound heterozygotes. The majority of mutations detected thus far predict a premature termination of translation. The resulting loss of the C-terminal end of the GLUT-2 protein predicts a nonfunctioning glucose transporter with an inward-facing substrate-binding site.

There is no specific treatment. Growth retardation persists through adulthood. Symptomatic replacement of water, electrolytes, and vitamin D; restriction of galactose intake; and a diet similar to that used for diabetes mellitus presented in frequent and small meals with an adequate caloric intake may improve growth.

MUSCLE GLYCOGENOSES

The role of glycogen in muscle is to provide substrates for the generation of ATP for muscle contraction. The muscle GSDs are broadly divided into 2 groups. The 1st group is characterized by hypertrophic cardiomyopathy, progressive skeletal muscle weakness and atrophy, or both, and includes deficiencies of acid α-glucosidase, a lysosomal glycogen degrading enzyme (type II GSD), and deficiencies of lysosomal-associated membrane protein 2 (LAMP2) and AMP-activated protein kinase γ2 (PRKAG2). The 2nd group comprises muscle energy disorders characterized by muscle pain, exercise intolerance, myoglobinuria, and susceptibility to fatigue. This group includes myophosphorylase deficiency (McArdle disease, type V) and deficiencies of phosphofructokinase (type VII), phosphoglycerate kinase, phosphoglycerate mutase, and lactate dehydrogenase. Some of these latter enzyme deficiencies can also be associated with compensated hemolysis, suggesting a more generalized defect in glucose metabolism.

Type II Glycogen Storage Disease (Lysosomal Acid α-1,4-Glucosidase Deficiency, Pompe Disease)

Pompe disease, also referred to as GSD type II or acid maltase deficiency, is caused by a deficiency of acid α-1,4-glucosidase (acid maltase), an enzyme responsible for the degradation of glycogen in lysosomes. This enzyme defect results in lysosomal glycogen accumulation in multiple tissues and cell types, with cardiac, skeletal, and smooth muscle cells being the most seriously affected. The disease is characterized by accumulation of glycogen in lysosomes, as opposed to its accumulation in cytoplasm in the other glycogenoses.

Pompe disease is an autosomal recessive disorder with an incidence of approximately 1/40,000 live births. The gene for acid α-glucosidase is on chromosome 17q25.2. Multiple pathogenic mutations have been identified that could be helpful in delineating the phenotypes. An example is a splice site mutation (IVS1-13T → G), commonly seen in late-onset patients of white racial groups.

CLINICAL MANIFESTATIONS The disorder encompasses a range of phenotypes, each including myopathy but differing in age at onset, organ involvement, and clinical severity. **Infantile Pompe disease** was uniformly lethal without enzyme replacement therapy. Affected infants present in the 1st few months of life with hypotonia, a generalized muscle weakness with a "floppy infant" appearance, neuropathic bulbar weakness, feeding difficulties, macroglossia, hepatomegaly, and a hypertrophic cardiomyopathy followed by death from cardiorespiratory failure or respiratory infection usually by 1 yr of age. **Juvenile and adult-onset disease** (late-onset Pompe disease) is characterized by a lack or absence of severe cardiac involvement and a less severe short-term prognosis. Symptoms can start at any age and are related to progressive dysfunction of skeletal muscles. The clinical picture is dominated by slowly progressive proximal muscle weakness with truncal involvement and greater involvement of the lower limbs than the upper limbs. The pelvic girdle, paraspinal muscles, and diaphragm are the muscle groups most seriously affected. These patients often present with proximal or limb girdle muscle weakness. With disease progression, patients become confined to wheelchairs and require artificial ventilation. The initial symptoms in some patients may be respiratory insufficiency manifested by somnolence, morning headache, orthopnea, and exertional dyspnea, which eventually lead to sleep-disordered breathing and respiratory failure. Respiratory failure is the cause of significant morbidity and mortality in this form of the disease. The age of death varies from early childhood to late adulthood, depending on the rate of disease progression and the extent of respiratory muscle involvement.

LABORATORY FINDINGS These include elevated levels of serum creatine kinase, aspartate aminotransferase, and lactate dehydrogenase. In the infantile form a chest x-ray showing massive cardiomegaly is frequently the 1st symptom detected. Electrocardiographic findings include a high-voltage QRS complex and a shortened PR interval. Echocardiography reveals thickening of both ventricles and/or the intraventricular septum and/or left ventricular outflow tract obstruction. Muscle biopsy shows the presence of vacuoles that stain positively for glycogen; acid phosphatase is increased, presumably from a compensatory increase of lysosomal enzymes. Electron microscopy reveals glycogen accumulation within the membranous sac and in the cytoplasm. Electromyography reveals myopathic features with excessive electrical irritability of muscle fibers and pseudomyotonic discharges. Serum creatine kinase is not always elevated in adult patients. Depending on the muscle sampled or tested, the muscle histologic appearance and electromyography may not be abnormal. It is prudent to examine the affected muscle.

Some patients with infantile Pompe disease who had peripheral nerve biopsies demonstrated glycogen accumulation in the neurons and Schwann cells, too. Infantile Pompe disease may manifest both myopathic and neuropathic clinical signs. Generally, the former predominate.

DIAGNOSIS The confirmatory step for a diagnosis of Pompe disease is enzyme assay demonstrating deficient acid α-glucosidase or gene sequencing showing 2 pathogenic mutations in the GAA gene. The enzyme assay is usually done in muscle, cultured skin fibroblasts, dried blood spots, leukocytes, or blood mononuclear cells using maltose, glycogen, or 4-methylumbelliferyl-α-D-glucopyranoside (4MUG) as a substrate. Deficiency is usually more severe in the infantile form than in the late onset forms. The skin fibroblast assay is usually preferred to muscle biopsy because it is a less invasive procedure with the advantage of maintaining a cell line for future use and providing information on residual enzyme activity. Blood-based assays, especially dried blood spots have the advantage of a rapid turn-around time. A muscle biopsy can yield faster results and provide additional information about glycogen content and site of glycogen storage within and outside the lysosomes of muscle cells. A major limitation of a muscle biopsy in late-onset patients is the variable pathology and glycogen accumulation in different muscles and within muscle fibers; muscle histology and glycogen content can vary depending on the site of muscle biopsy. There is also a risk from anesthesia; EKG can be helpful in making the diagnosis in suspected cases of the infantile form and should be done in patients suspected of having Pompe disease before any procedure requiring anesthesia, including muscle biopsy, is performed. Prenatal diagnosis using amniocytes or chorionic villi is available in the infantile form.

TREATMENT Treatment options were once limited to supportive or palliative care. Specific enzyme replacement therapy (ERT) with recombinant human acid α-glucosidase (alglucosidase alfa, [Myozyme]) is available for treatment of Pompe disease. Recombinant acid α-glucosidase is capable of preventing deterioration or reversing abnormal cardiac and skeletal muscle functions (Fig. 81-3). ERT should be initiated as soon as possible and preferably <6 mo of age; the dose is 20 mg/kg given every 2 wk. A high-protein diet and exercise therapy may also be beneficial. Nocturnal ventilatory support, when indicated, should be used. It has been shown to improve the quality of life and is particularly beneficial during a period of respiratory decompensation.

Glycogen Storage Diseases Mimicking Hypertrophic Cardiomyopathy

Deficiencies of lysosomal-associated membrane protein 2 (LAMP2, also called Danon disease) and AMP-activated protein kinase γ2 (PRKAG2) result in accumulation of glycogen in the heart and skeletal muscle. These patients present primarily as a hypertrophic cardiomyopathy, but can be distinguished from the usual causes of hypertrophic cardiomyopathy due to defects in sarcomere protein genes by their electrophysiologic abnormalities, particularly ventricular pre-excitation and conduction defects. The onset of cardiac symptoms, including chest pain, palpitation, syncope, and cardiac arrest, can occur between the ages of 8 and 15 yr for LAMP2 deficiency, younger than the average age for patients with PRKAG2 deficiency, which is 33 yr. Danon disease is transmitted as a X-linked trait and *PRKAG2* mutations as a dominant trait.

The prognosis for LAMP2 deficiency is poor with progressive end-stage heart failure early in adulthood. Cardiomyopathy due to PRKAG2 mutations is compatible with long-term survival, although some patients may necessitate the implantation of a pacemaker and aggressive control of arrhythmias. A congenital form presents in early infancy with severe hypertrophic cardiomyopathy and a rapidly fatal course.

Type V Glycogen Storage Disease (Muscle Phosphorylase Deficiency, Mcardle Disease)

This is caused by the deficiency of muscle phosphorylase activity. Lack of this enzyme limits muscle ATP generation by glycogenolysis, resulting in muscle glycogen accumulation, and is the prototype of muscle energy disorders. A deficiency of myophosphorylase impairs the cleavage of glucosyl molecules from the straight chain of glycogen.

CLINICAL MANIFESTATIONS Symptoms usually 1st develop in late childhood or as an adult and are characterized by exercise intolerance with muscle cramps and pain. Two types of activity tend to cause symptoms: brief exercise of great intensity, such as sprinting or carrying heavy loads; and less intense but sustained activity, such as climbing stairs or walking uphill. Moderate exercise, such as walking on level ground, can be performed by most patients for long periods. Many patients experience a characteristic "second wind" phenomenon. If they slow down or pause briefly at the 1st appearance of muscle pain, they can resume exercise

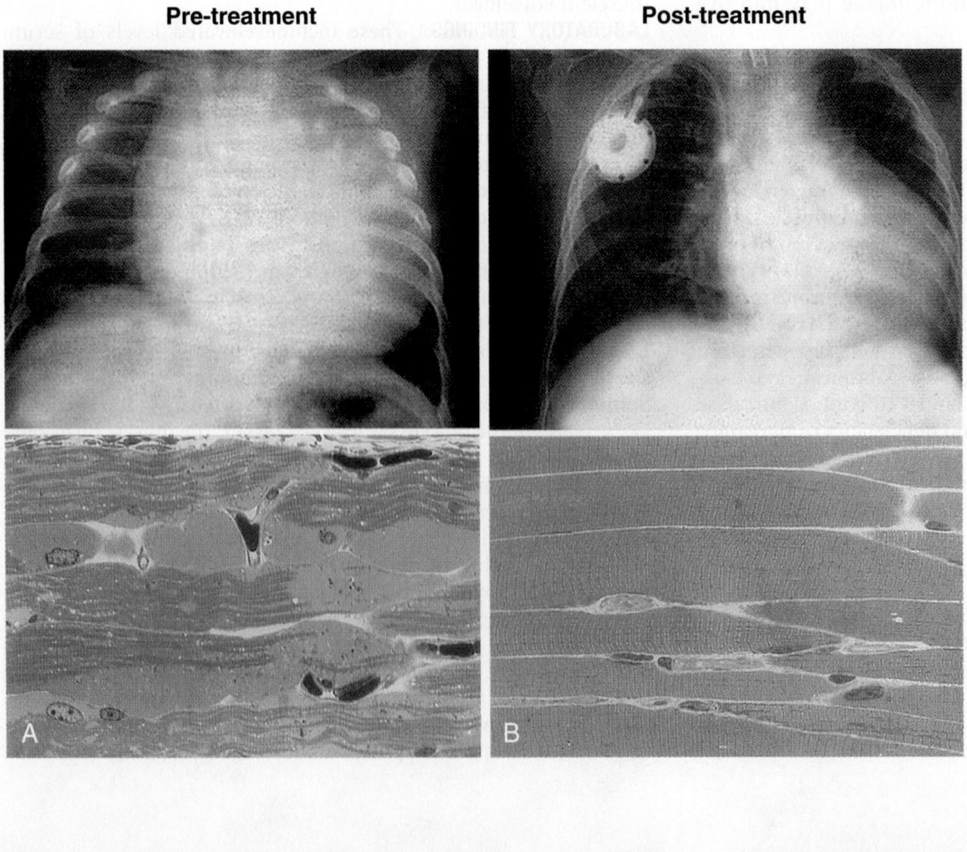

Figure 81-3 Chest x-ray and muscle histology findings of an infantile-onset Pompe disease patient before *(A)* and after *(B)* enzyme replacement therapy. Note the decrease in heart size and muscle glycogen with the therapy. (Modified from Amalfitano A, Bengur AR, Morse RP, et al: Recombinant human acid alpha-glucosidase enzyme therapy for infantile glycogen storage disease type II: results of a phase I/II clinical trial, *Genet Med* 3:132–138, 2001.)

with more ease. Due to the underlying myopathy, these patients may be at risk for statin-induced myopathy and rhabdomyolysis. While patients typically experience episodic muscle pain and cramping due to exercise, 35% of patients with McArdle disease report permanent pain that has a serious impact on sleep and other activities.

About 50% of patients report burgundy-colored urine after exercise, which is the consequence of exercise-induced **myoglobinuria** secondary to **rhabdomyolysis.** Intense myoglobinuria after vigorous exercise may cause acute renal failure. In rare cases, electromyographic findings may suggest an inflammatory myopathy and the diagnosis can be confused with polymyositis.

The level of serum creatine kinase is usually elevated at rest and increases more after exercise. Exercise also increases the levels of blood ammonia, inosine, hypoxanthine, and uric acid. The latter abnormalities are attributed to accelerated recycling of muscle purine nucleotides owing to insufficient ATP production. Type V GSD is an autosomal recessive disorder. The gene for muscle phosphorylase (*PYGM*) has been mapped to chromosome 11q13.

Clinical heterogeneity is uncommon in type V GSD, but late-onset disease with no symptoms as late as the 8th decade and an early-onset, fatal form with hypotonia, generalized muscle weakness, and progressive respiratory insufficiency have been described.

DIAGNOSIS An ischemic exercise test offers a rapid diagnostic screening for patients with a metabolic myopathy. Lack of an increase in blood lactate levels and exaggerated blood ammonia elevations indicate muscle glycogenosis and suggest a defect in the conversion of muscle glycogen or glucose to lactate. The abnormal ischemic exercise response is not limited to type V GSD. Other muscle defects in glycogenolysis or glycolysis produce similar results (deficiencies of muscle phosphofructokinase, phosphoglycerate kinase, phosphoglycerate mutase, or lactate dehydrogenase).

Phosphorus magnetic resonance imaging (^{31}P MRI) allows for the noninvasive evaluation of muscle metabolism. Patients with type V GSD have no decrease in intracellular pH and have excessive reduction in phosphocreatine in response to exercise. The diagnosis should be confirmed by enzymatic evaluation of muscle. A common nonsense mutation R49X in exon 1 is found in 90% of white patients, and a deletion of a single codon in exon 17 is found in 61% of Japanese patients. The R49X mutation represents 55% of alleles in Spanish patients, whereas the W797R mutation represents 14% and the G204S represents 9% of mutant alleles in the Spanish population.

TREATMENT Avoidance of strenuous exercise prevents the symptoms; however, regular and moderate exercise is recommended to improve exercise capacity. Glucose or sucrose given before exercise or injection of glucagon can markedly improve tolerance in these patients. A high-protein diet may increase muscle endurance and creatine supplement has been shown to improve muscle function in some patients. Vitamin B_6 supplementation reduces exercise intolerance and muscle cramps. Longevity is not generally affected.

Type VII Glycogen Storage Disease (Muscle Phosphofructokinase Deficiency, Tarui Disease)

Type VII GSD is caused by a deficiency of muscle phosphofructokinase, which catalyzes the ATP-dependent conversion of fructose-6-phosphate to fructose-1,6-diphosphate and is a key regulatory enzyme of glycolysis. Phosphofructokinase is composed of 3 isoenzyme subunits (M [muscle], L [liver], and P [platelet]) that are encoded by different genes and differentially expressed in tissues. Skeletal muscle contains only the M subunit, and red blood cells contain a hybrid of L and M forms. Type VII disease is due to a defective M isoenzyme, which causes a complete enzyme defect in muscle and a partial defect in red blood cells.

Type VII GSD is an autosomal recessive disorder and is prevalent among Japanese people and Ashkenazi Jews. The gene for muscle phosphofructokinase is located on chromosome 12q13.3. A splicing defect and a nucleotide deletion in the muscle phosphofructokinase gene account for 95% of mutant alleles in Ashkenazi Jews. Diagnosis based on molecular testing is thus possible in this population.

CLINICAL MANIFESTATIONS Six features of type VII are distinctive: (1) Exercise intolerance, usually evident in childhood, is more severe than in type V disease and may be associated with nausea, vomiting, and severe muscle pain; vigorous exercise causes severe muscle cramps and myoglobinuria. (2) Compensated hemolysis occurs as evidenced by an increased level of serum bilirubin and an elevated reticulocyte count. (3) Hyperuricemia is common and exaggerated by muscle exercise to a more severe degree than that observed in type V or III GSD. (4) An abnormal polysaccharide is present in muscle fibers; it is periodic acid–Schiff positive but resistant to diastase digestion. (5) Exercise intolerance is particularly acute after meals that are rich in carbohydrates because glucose cannot be utilized in muscle and because glucose inhibits lipolysis and thus deprives muscle of fatty acid and ketone substrates. In contrast, patients with type V disease can metabolize blood-borne glucose derived from either liver glycogenolysis or exogenous glucose; indeed, glucose infusion improves exercise tolerance in type V patients. (6) There is no spontaneous second-wind phenomenon because of the inability to metabolize blood glucose.

Other rare type VII variants occur. One variant presents in infancy with hypotonia and limb weakness and proceeds to a rapidly progressive myopathy that leads to death by 4 yr of age. There is a 2nd variant that occurs in infancy and results in congenital myopathy and arthrogryposis with a fatal outcome. A 3rd variant presents in infancy with hypotonia, mild developmental delay and seizures. An additional presentation is hereditary nonspherocytic hemolytic anemia. While these patients do not experience muscle symptoms, it remains unclear whether these symptoms will develop later in life. One variant presents in adults and is characterized by a slowly progressive, fixed muscle weakness rather than cramps and myoglobinuria.

DIAGNOSIS To establish a diagnosis, a biochemical or histochemical demonstration of the enzymatic defect in the muscle is required. The absence of the M isoenzyme of phosphofructokinase can also be demonstrated in blood cells and fibroblasts.

TREATMENT There is no specific treatment. Avoidance of strenuous exercise is advisable to prevent acute attacks of muscle cramps and myoglobinuria.

Other Muscle Glycogenoses with Muscle Energy Impairment

Six additional defects in enzymes—phosphoglycerate kinase, phosphoglycerate mutase, lactate dehydrogenase, fructose-1,6- bisphosphate aldolase A, muscle pyruvate kinase, and β-enolase in the pathway of the terminal glycolysis—cause symptoms and signs of muscle energy impairment similar to those of types V and VII GSD. The failure of blood lactate to increase in response to exercise is a useful diagnostic test and can be used to differentiate muscle glycogenoses from disorders of lipid metabolism, such as carnitine palmitoyl transferase II deficiency and very long chain acyl-CoA dehydrogenase deficiency, which also cause muscle cramps and myoglobinuria. Muscle glycogen levels can be normal in the disorders affecting terminal glycolysis and assaying the muscle enzyme activity is needed to make a definite diagnosis. There is no specific treatment. Avoidance of strenuous exercise prevents acute attacks of muscle cramps and myoglobinuria. Avoidance of drugs such as statins, and malignant hyperthermia precautions for patients undergoing anesthesia should be followed.

BIBLIOGRAPHY

Please visit the Nelson Textbook of Pediatrics *website at www.expertconsult.com for the complete bibliography.*

81.2 Defects in Galactose Metabolism

Priya S. Kishnani and Yuan-Tsong Chen

Milk and dairy products contain lactose, the major dietary source of galactose. The metabolism of galactose produces fuel for cellular metabolism through its conversion to glucose-1-phosphate (see Table 81-1). Galactose also plays an important role in the formation of galactosides, which include glycoproteins, glycolipids, and glycosaminoglycans. Galactosemia denotes the elevated level of galactose in the blood and is found in 3 distinct inborn errors of galactose metabolism defective in 1 of the following enzymes: galactose-1-phosphate uridyl transferase, galactokinase, and uridine diphosphate galactose-4-epimerase. The term *galactosemia,* although adequate for the deficiencies in any of these disorders, generally designates the transferase deficiency.

Galactose-1-Phosphate Uridyl Transferase Deficiency Galactosemia

Two forms of the deficiency exist: Infants with complete or near complete deficiency of the enzyme (classic galactosemia) and those with partial transferase deficiency. **Classic galactosemia** is a serious disease with onset of symptoms typically by the 2nd half of the 1st wk of life. The incidence is 1/60,000. The newborn infant receives high amounts of lactose (up to 40% in breast milk and certain formulas), which consists of equal parts of glucose and galactose. Without the transferase enzyme, the infant is unable to metabolize galactose-1-phosphate, the accumulation of which results in injury to kidney, liver, and brain. This injury may begin prenatally in the affected fetus by transplacental galactose derived from the diet of the heterozygous mother or by endogenous production of galactose in the fetus.

CLINICAL MANIFESTATIONS The diagnosis of uridyl transferase deficiency should be considered in newborn or young infants with any of the following features: jaundice, hepatomegaly, vomiting, hypoglycemia, seizures, lethargy, irritability, feeding difficulties, poor weight gain or failure to regain birth weight, aminoaciduria, nuclear cataracts, vitreous hemorrhage, hepatic failure, liver cirrhosis, ascites, splenomegaly, or mental retardation. Symptoms are milder and improve when milk is temporarily withdrawn and replaced by intravenous or lactose-free nutrition. Patients with galactosemia are at increased risk for *Escherichia coli* neonatal sepsis; the onset of sepsis often precedes the diagnosis of galactosemia. Pseudotumor cerebri can occur and cause a bulging fontanel. Death from liver and kidney failure and sepsis may follow within days. When the diagnosis is not made at birth, damage to the liver (cirrhosis) and brain (mental retardation) becomes increasingly severe and irreversible.

Partial transferase deficiency is generally asymptomatic. It is more frequent than classic galactosemia and is diagnosed in newborn screening because of moderately elevated blood galactose and/or low transferase activity. Galactosemia should be considered for the newborn or young infant who is not thriving or who has any of the preceding findings. Light and electron microscopy of hepatic tissue reveals fatty infiltration, the formation of pseudoacini, and eventual macronodular cirrhosis. These changes are consistent with a metabolic disease but do not indicate the precise enzymatic defect.

DIAGNOSIS The preliminary diagnosis of galactosemia is made by demonstrating a reducing substance in several urine specimens collected while the patient is receiving human milk, cow's milk, or any other formula containing lactose. The reducing substance found in urine by Clinitest (glucose, galactose, others) can be identified by chromatography or by an enzymatic test specific for galactose. Galactosuria is present, provided the last milk feed does not date back more than a few hours and the child is not vomiting excessively. Clinistix urine test results are usually negative because the test materials rely on the action of glucose oxidase, which is specific for glucose and is nonreactive with galactose. Owing to a proximal renal tubular syndrome, the acutely ill baby may also excrete glucose together with amino acids. Because galactose is injurious to persons with galactosemia, diagnostic challenge tests dependent on administering galactose orally or intravenously should not be used. Direct enzyme assay using erythrocytes establishes the diagnosis. One needs to confirm that the patient did not receive a blood transfusion before the collection of the blood sample, as a diagnosis could be missed. Deficient activity of galactose-1-phosphate uridyl transferase is demonstrable in hemolysates of erythrocytes, which also exhibit increased concentrations of galactose-1-phosphate.

GENETICS Transferase deficiency galactosemia is an autosomal recessive disorder. There are several enzymatic variants of galactosemia. The *Duarte variant*, a single amino acid substitution (N314D), has diminished red cell enzyme activity (50% of normal), but usually no clinical significance. This variant is the most common, with a carrier frequency of 12% in the general population. Some African-American patients have milder symptoms despite the absence of measurable transferase activity in erythrocytes; these patients retain 10% enzyme activity in liver and intestinal mucosa, whereas most white patients have no detectable activity in any of these tissues. In African-Americans, 62% of alleles are represented by the S135L mutation, a mutation that is responsible for a milder disease course. In the white population, 70% of alleles are represented by the Q188R and K285N missense mutations and are associated with severe disease. Carrier testing and prenatal diagnosis can be performed by direct enzyme analysis of amniocytes or chorionic villi; testing can also be DNA based.

TREATMENT AND PROGNOSIS Because of newborn screening for galactosemia, patients are being identified and treated early. Various non–lactose containing milk substitutes are available (casein hydrolysates, soybean-based formula). Elimination of galactose from the diet reverses growth failure and renal and hepatic dysfunction. Cataracts regress, and most patients have no impairment of vision. Early diagnosis and treatment have improved the prognosis of galactosemia; however, on long-term follow-up, patients still manifest ovarian failure with primary or secondary amenorrhea, decreased bone mineral density, developmental delay, and learning disabilities that increase in severity with age. Hypergonadotrophic hypogonadism is reported in 80% to over 90% of female patients with classic galactosemia. Although most women with classic galactosemia are infertile when they reach childbearing age, a small number have given birth. Most patients manifest speech disorders, whereas a smaller number demonstrate poor growth and impaired motor function and balance (with or without overt ataxia). The relative control of galactose-1-phosphate levels does not always correlate with long-term outcome, leading to the belief that other factors, such as elevated galactitol, decreased uridine diphosphate galactose (UDP-galactose, a donor for galactolipids and proteins), and endogenous galactose production may be responsible.

Galactokinase Deficiency

The deficient enzyme is galactokinase, which normally catalyzes the phosphorylation of galactose. The principal metabolites accumulated are galactose and galactitol. Two genes have been reported to encode galactokinase: GK1 on chromosome 17q24 and GK2 on chromosome 15. Cataracts are usually the sole manifestation of galactokinase deficiency; pseudotumor cerebri is a rare complication. The affected infant is otherwise asymptomatic. Heterozygote carriers may be at risk for presenile cataracts. Affected patients have an increased concentration of blood galactose levels, provided they have been fed a lactose-containing formula. The diagnosis is made by demonstrating an absence of galactokinase activity in erythrocytes or fibroblasts. Transferase activity is normal. Treatment is dietary restriction of galactose.

Uridine Diphosphate Galactose-4-Epimerase Deficiency

The abnormally accumulated metabolites are similar to those in transferase deficiency; however, there is also an increase in cellular UDP-galactose. There are 2 distinct forms of epimerase deficiency. The 1st is a benign form discovered incidentally through neonatal screening programs. Affected persons are healthy and without problems; the enzyme deficiency is limited to leukocytes and erythrocytes. No treatment is required. The 2nd form of epimerase deficiency is severe, and clinical manifestations resemble transferase deficiency, with the additional symptoms of hypotonia and nerve deafness. The enzyme deficiency is generalized, and clinical symptoms respond to restriction of dietary galactose. Although this form of galactosemia is rare, it must be considered in a symptomatic patient with measurable galactose-1-phosphate who has normal transferase activity. Diagnosis is confirmed by the assay of epimerase in erythrocytes.

Patients with the severe form of epimerase deficiency cannot synthesize galactose from glucose and are galactose dependent. Because galactose is an essential component of many nervous system structural proteins, patients are placed on a galactose-restricted diet rather than a galactose-free diet.

Infants with the mild form of epimerase deficiency have not required treatment. It is advisable to follow urine specimens for reducing substances and exclude aminoaciduria within a few weeks of diagnosis while the infant is still on lactose-containing formula.

The gene for UDP-galactose-4-epimerase is located on chromosome 1 at 1p36. Carrier detection is possible by measurement of epimerase activity in the erythrocytes. Prenatal diagnosis for the severe form of epimerase deficiency, using an enzyme assay of cultured amniotic fluid cells, is possible.

BIBLIOGRAPHY

Please visit the Nelson Textbook of Pediatrics *website at* *www.expertconsult.com* *for the complete bibliography.*

81.3 Defects in Fructose Metabolism

Priya S. Kishnani and Yuan-Tsong Chen

Two inborn errors are known in the specialized pathway of fructose metabolism: benign or essential fructosuria and hereditary fructose intolerance (HFI). Fructose-1,6-bisphosphatase deficiency, although strictly speaking not a defect of the specialized fructose pathway, is discussed in Chapter 81.4.

Deficiency of Fructokinase (Essential or Benign Fructosuria)

Deficiency of fructokinase is not associated with any clinical manifestations. It is an accidental finding usually made because the asymptomatic patient's urine contains a reducing substance. No treatment is necessary and the prognosis is excellent. Inheritance is autosomal recessive with an incidence of 1/120,000. The gene encoding fructokinase is located on chromosome 2p23.3.

Fructokinase catalyzes the 1st step of metabolism of dietary fructose: conversion of fructose to fructose-1-phosphate (see Fig. 81-1). Without this enzyme, ingested fructose is not metabolized. Its level is increased in the blood, and it is excreted in urine because there is practically no renal threshold for fructose. Clinitest results reveal the urinary-reducing substance, which can be identified as fructose by chromatography.

Deficiency of Fructose-1,6-Bisphosphate Aldolase (Aldolase B, Hereditary Fructose Intolerance)

Deficiency of fructose-1,6-bisphosphate aldolase is a severe condition of infants that appears with the ingestion of fructose-containing food and is caused by a deficiency of fructose aldolase B activity in the liver, kidney, and intestine. The enzyme catalyzes the hydrolysis of fructose-1,6-bisphosphate into triose phosphate and glyceraldehyde phosphate. The same enzyme also hydrolyzes fructose-1-phosphate. Deficiency of this enzyme activity causes a rapid accumulation of fructose-1-phosphate and initiates severe toxic symptoms when exposed to fructose.

EPIDEMIOLOGY AND GENETICS The true incidence of HFI is unknown but may be as high as 1/26,000. The gene for aldolase B is on chromosome 9q22.3. Several mutations causing HFI are known. A single missense mutation, a G→C transversion in exon 5 resulting in the normal alanine at position 149 being replaced by a proline, is the most common mutation identified in northern Europeans. This mutation, plus 2 other point mutations (A174D and N334K), account for 80-85% of HFI in Europe and the USA. Diagnosis of HFI can be made by direct DNA analysis.

CLINICAL MANIFESTATIONS Patients with HFI are asymptomatic until fructose or sucrose (table sugar) is ingested (usually from fruit, fruit juice, or sweetened cereal). Symptoms may occur early in life, soon after birth if foods or formulas containing these sugars are introduced into the diet. Certain patients are very sensitive to fructose, whereas others can tolerate moderate intakes (up to 250 mg/kg/day). The average intake of fructose in Western societies is 1-2 g/kg/day. Early clinical manifestations resemble galactosemia and include jaundice, hepatomegaly, vomiting, lethargy, irritability, and convulsions. There may also be a higher incidence of celiac disease in HFI patients (>10%) than in the general population (1-3%). Laboratory findings include a prolonged clotting time, hypoalbuminemia, elevation of bilirubin and transaminase levels, and proximal tubular dysfunction. Acute fructose ingestion produces symptomatic hypoglycemia; the higher the intake, the more severe is the clinical picture. Chronic ingestion results in failure to thrive and hepatic disease. If the intake of the fructose persists, hypoglycemic episodes recur, and liver and kidney failure progress, eventually leading to death.

DIAGNOSIS Suspicion of the enzyme deficiency is fostered by the presence of a reducing substance in the urine during an episode.

The fructose challenge although an effective method of diagnosis, causes a rapid fall, first of serum phosphate and then of blood glucose, and a subsequent increase in uric acid and magnesium. Due to high risks to the patient who can become acutely ill after the oral tolerance test, it should not be performed. Definitive diagnosis is made by assay of fructaldolase B activity in the liver. Gene-based diagnosis is available for most patients with this disease; a common mutation (substitution of *Pro* for *Ala* at position 149) accounts for 53% of HFI alleles worldwide.

TREATMENT Treatment consists of the complete elimination of all sources of sucrose, fructose, and sorbitol from the diet. It may be difficult because these sugars are widely used additives, found even in most medicinal preparations. With treatment, liver and kidney dysfunction improves, and catch-up in growth is common. Intellectual development is usually unimpaired. As the patient matures, symptoms become milder even after fructose ingestion; the long-term prognosis is good. Because of voluntary dietary avoidance of sucrose, affected patients have few dental caries.

BIBLIOGRAPHY

Please visit the Nelson Textbook of Pediatrics *website at* *www.expertconsult.com* *for the complete bibliography.*

81.4 Defects in Intermediary Carbohydrate Metabolism Associated with Lactic Acidosis

Priya S. Kishnani and Yuan-Tsong Chen

Lactic acidosis occurs with defects of carbohydrate metabolism that interfere with the conversion of pyruvate to glucose via the pathway of gluconeogenesis or to carbon dioxide and water via the mitochondrial enzymes of the Krebs cycle. Figure 81-4 depicts

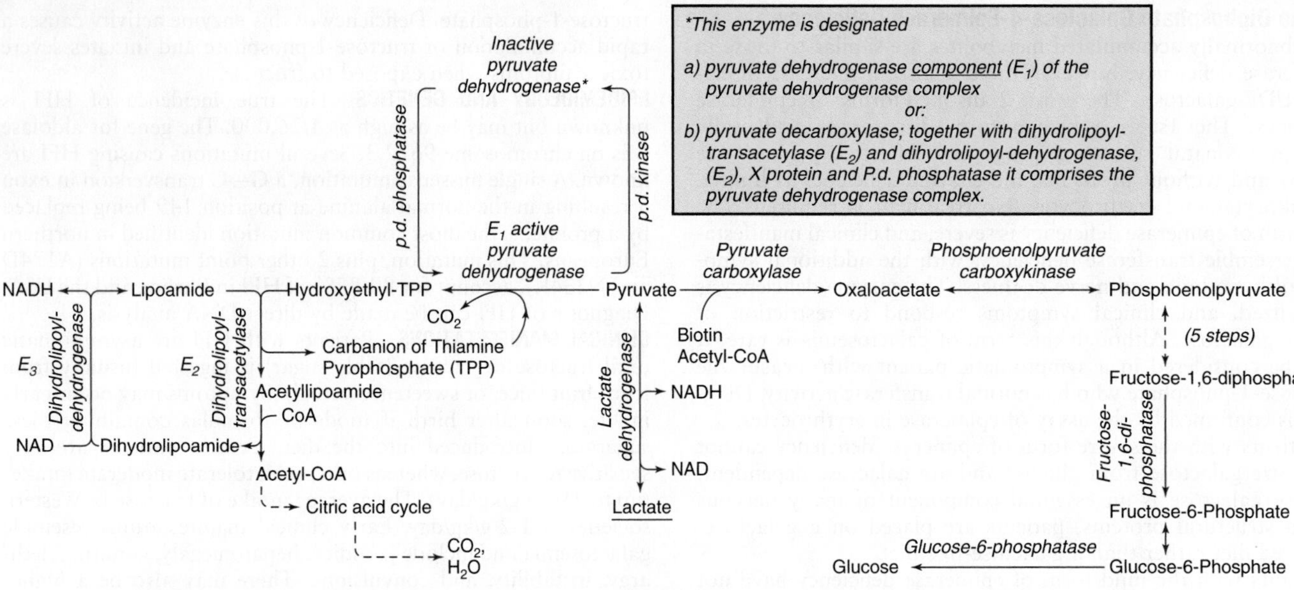

Figure 81-4 Enzymatic reactions of carbohydrate metabolism, deficiencies of which can give rise to lactic acidosis, pyruvate elevations, or hypoglycemia. The pyruvate dehydrogenase complex comprises, in addition to E_1, E_2, and E_3, an extra lipoate-containing protein (not shown), called protein X, and pyruvate dehydrogenase phosphatase.

the relevant metabolic pathways. Type I GSD, fructose-1,6-diphosphatase deficiency, and phosphoenolpyruvate carboxylase deficiency are disorders of gluconeogenesis associated with lactic acidosis. Pyruvate dehydrogenase complex deficiency, respiratory chain defects, and pyruvate carboxylase deficiency are disorders in the pathway of pyruvate metabolism causing lactic acidosis. Lactic acidosis can also occur in defects of fatty acid oxidation, organic acidurias (Chapters 79.6, 79.10, and 80.1), or biotin utilization diseases. These disorders are easily distinguishable by the presence of abnormal acylcarnitine profiles, amino acids in the blood, and unusual organic acids in the urine. Blood lactate, pyruvate, and acylcarnitine profiles and the presence of these unusual urine organic acids should be determined in infants and children with unexplained acidosis, especially if there is an increase of anion gap.

Lactic acidosis unrelated to an enzymatic defect occurs in hypoxemia. In this case, as well as in defects in the respiratory chain, the serum pyruvate concentration may remain normal (<1.0 mg/dL with an increased lactate : pyruvate ratio), whereas pyruvate is usually increased when lactic acidosis results from an enzymatic defect in gluconeogenesis or pyruvate dehydrogenase complex (both lactate and pyruvate are increased and the ratio is normal). Lactate and pyruvate should be measured in the same blood specimen and on multiple blood specimens obtained when the patient is symptomatic because lactic acidosis can be intermittent. An algorithm for the differential diagnosis of lactic acidosis is shown in Figure 81-5.

DISORDERS OF GLUCONEOGENESIS

Deficiency of Glucose-6-Phosphatase (Type I Glycogen Storage Disease)

Type I GSD is the only glycogenosis associated with significant lactic acidosis. The chronic metabolic acidosis predisposes these patients to osteopenia; after prolonged fasting, the acidosis associated with hypoglycemia is a life-threatening condition (Chapter 81.1).

Fructose-1,6-Diphosphatase Deficiency

Fructose-1,6-diphosphatase deficiency impairs the formation of glucose from all gluconeogenic precursors, including dietary fructose. Hypoglycemia occurs when glycogen reserves are limited or exhausted. The clinical manifestations are characterized by life-threatening episodes of acidosis, hypoglycemia, hyperventilation, convulsions, and coma. In about half of the cases, the deficiency presents in the 1st wk of life. In infants and small children, episodes are triggered by febrile infections and gastroenteritis if oral food intake decreases. The frequency of the attacks decreases with age. Laboratory findings include low blood glucose, high lactate and uric acid levels, and metabolic acidosis. In contrast to HFI, there is usually no aversion to sweets; renal tubular and liver functions are normal.

The diagnosis is established by demonstrating an enzyme deficiency in either liver or intestinal biopsy. The enzyme defect can also be demonstrated in leukocytes in some cases. The gene coding for fructose-1,6-diphosphatase is located on chromosome 9q22; mutations are characterized, making carrier detection and prenatal diagnosis possible. Treatment of acute attacks consists of correction of hypoglycemia and acidosis by intravenous glucose infusion; the response is usually rapid. Avoidance of fasting, aggressive management of infections and restriction of fructose and sucrose from the diet can prevent further episodes. For long-term prevention of hypoglycemia, a slowly released carbohydrate such as cornstarch is useful. Patients who survive childhood develop normally.

Phosphoenolpyruvate Carboxykinase (PEPCK) Deficiency

PEPCK is a key enzyme in gluconeogenesis. It catalyzes the conversion of oxaloacetate to phosphoenolpyruvate (see Fig. 81-4). PEPCK deficiency is both a mitochondrial enzyme deficiency and a cytosolic enzyme deficiency, encoded by 2 distinct genes.

The disease has been reported in only a few cases. The clinical features are heterogeneous, with hypoglycemia, lactic acidemia, hepatomegaly, hypotonia, developmental delay, and failure to thrive as the major manifestations. There may be multisystem involvement, with neuromuscular deficits, hepatocellular damage, renal dysfunction, and cardiomyopathy. The diagnosis is based on the reduced activity of PEPCK in liver, fibroblasts, or lymphocytes. Fibroblasts and lymphocytes are not suitable for diagnosing the cytosolic form of PEPCK deficiency because these tissues possess only mitochondrial PEPCK. To avoid hypoglycemia, patients should be treated with slow-release carbohydrates such as cornstarch, and fasting should be avoided.

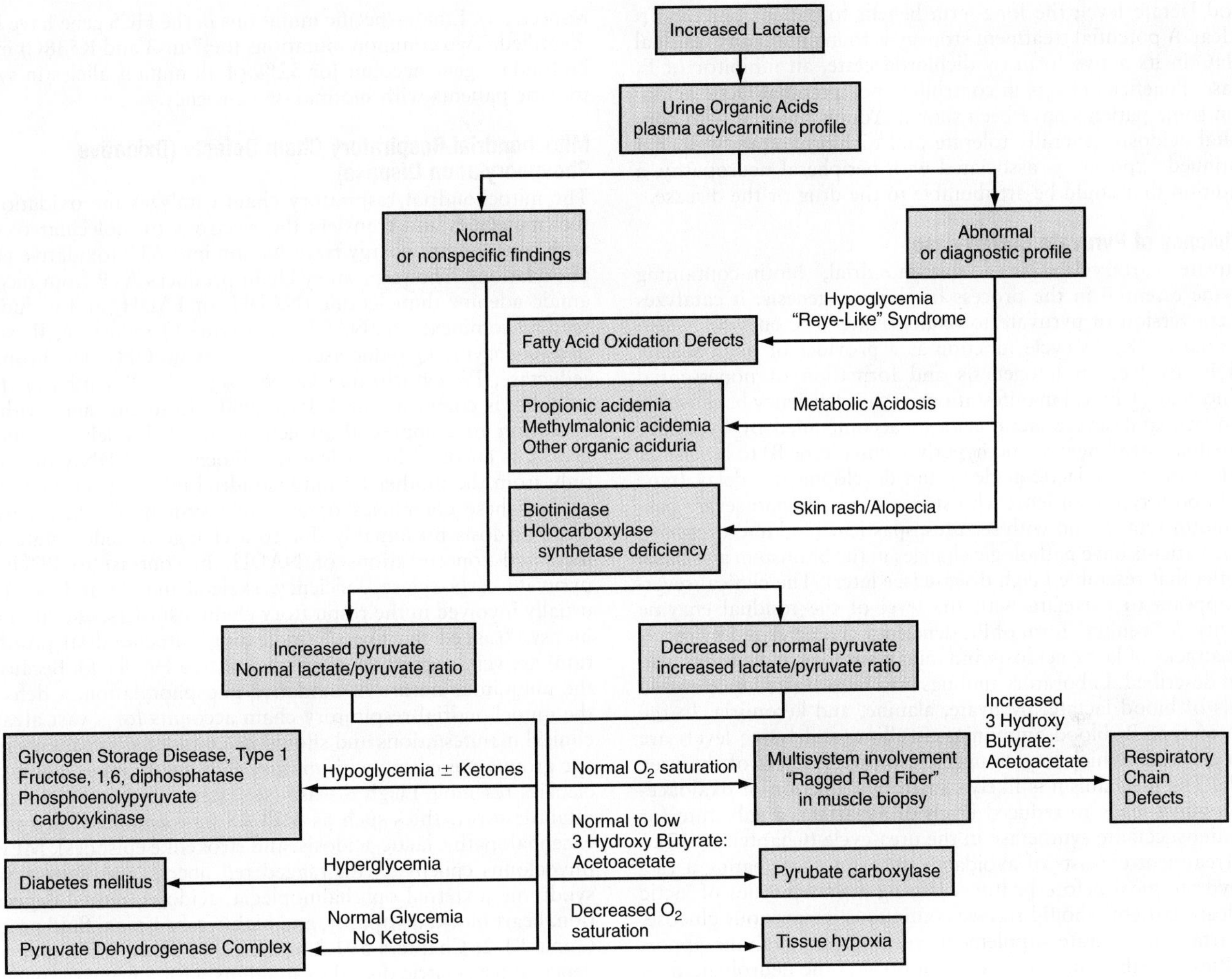

Figure 81-5 Algorithm of the differential diagnosis of lactic acidosis.

DISORDERS OF PYRUVATE METABOLISM

Pyruvate is formed from glucose and other monosaccharides, from lactate, and from alanine. It is metabolized through 4 main enzyme systems: lactate dehydrogenase, alanine aminotransferase, pyruvate carboxylase, and pyruvate dehydrogenase complex. Deficiency of the M subunit of lactate dehydrogenase causes exercise intolerance and myoglobinuria (Chapter 81.1). Genetic deficiency of alanine aminotransferase has not been reported in humans.

Pyruvate Dehydrogenase Complex Deficiency

After entering the mitochondria, pyruvate is converted into acetyl coenzyme A (acetyl CoA) by the pyruvate dehydrogenase complex (PDHC), which catalyzes the oxidation of pyruvate to acetyl CoA, which then enters the tricarboxylic acid cycle for ATP production. The complex comprises 5 components: E_1, an α-keto acid decarboxylase; E_2, a dihydrolipoyl transacylase; E_3, a dihydrolipoyl dehydrogenase; protein X, an extra lipoate-containing protein; and pyruvate dehydrogenase phosphatase. The most common is a defect in the E_1 (see Fig. 81-4).

Deficiency of the PDHC is the most common of the disorders leading to lactic acidemia and central nervous system dysfunction. The central nervous system dysfunction is because the brain obtains its energy primarily from oxidation of glucose. Brain acetyl CoA is synthesized nearly exclusively from pyruvate.

The E_1 defects are caused by mutations in the gene coding for E_1 α subunit, which is X-linked. Although X-linked, its deficiency is a problem in both males and females even though only 1 E_1 α allele in females carries a mutation.

CLINICAL MANIFESTATIONS The disease has a wide spectrum of presentations from the most severe neonatal presentation to a mild late-onset form. The **neonatal onset** is associated with lethal lactic acidosis, white matter cystic lesions, agenesis of the corpus callosum, and the most severe enzyme deficiency. **Infantile onset** can be lethal or associated with psychomotor retardation and chronic lactic acidosis, cystic lesions in the brainstem and basal ganglia, and pathologic features resembling **Leigh disease** (see later). Older children, usually boys, may have less acidosis, have greater enzyme activity, and manifest ataxia with high-carbohydrate diets. Intelligence may be normal. Patients of all ages may have facial dysmorphology, features similar to those of fetal alcohol syndrome.

The E_2 and protein X-lipoate defects are rare and result in severe psychomotor retardation. The E_3 lipoamide dehydrogenase defect leads to deficient activity not only in the PDHC, but also in the α-ketoglutarate and branched-chain keto acid dehydrogenase complexes. Pyruvate dehydrogenase phosphatase deficiency has also been reported. These other PDHC defects have clinical manifestations within the variable spectrum associated with PDHC deficiency due to E_1 deficiency.

TREATMENT The general prognosis is poor except in rare cases in which mutation is associated with altered affinity for thiamine pyrophosphate, which may respond to thiamine supplementation. Because carbohydrates can aggravate lactic acidosis, a ketogenic diet is recommended. The diet has been found to lower the blood lactate level; the long-term benefit to patient outcome is unclear. A potential treatment strategy is to maintain any residual PDHC in its active form by **dichloroacetate,** an inhibitor of E_1 kinase. Beneficial effects in controlling postprandial lactic acidosis in some patients have been shown. Young children with congenital acidosis generally tolerate oral dichloroacetate well, but continued exposure is associated with peripheral neuropathy, a condition that could be attributable to the drug or the disease.

Deficiency of Pyruvate Carboxylase

Pyruvate carboxylase is a mitochondrial, biotin-containing enzyme essential in the process of gluconeogenesis; it catalyzes the conversion of pyruvate to oxaloacetate. The enzyme is also essential for Krebs cycle function as a provider of oxaloacetate and is involved in lipogenesis and formation of nonessential amino acids. Clinical manifestations of this deficiency have varied from neonatal severe lactic acidosis accompanied by hyperammonemia, citrullinemia, and hyperlysinemia (**type B**) to late-onset mild to moderate lactic acidosis and developmental delay (**type A**). In both types, patients who survived usually had severe psychomotor retardation with seizures, spasticity, and microcephaly. Some patients have pathologic changes in the brainstem and basal ganglia that resemble **Leigh disease** (see later). The clinical severity appears to correlate with the level of the residual enzyme activity. A "benign" form of PC deficiency characterized by recurrent attacks of lactic acidosis and mild neurologic deficits has also been described. Laboratory findings are characterized by elevated levels of blood lactate, pyruvate, alanine, and ketonuria. In the case of type B, blood ammonia, citrulline, and lysine levels are also elevated, which might suggest a primary defect of the urea cycle. The mechanism is likely caused by depletion of oxaloacetate, which leads to reduced levels of aspartate, a substrate for argininosuccinate synthetase in the urea cycle (Chapter 79.12).

Treatment consists of avoidance of fasting, and eating a carbohydrate meal before bedtime. During acute episodes of lactic acidosis, patients should receive continuous intravenous glucose. Aspartate and citrate supplements restore the metabolic abnormalities; whether this treatment can prevent the neurologic deficits is not known. Liver transplantation has been attempted; its benefit remains unknown. Diagnosis of pyruvate carboxylase deficiency is made by the measurement of enzyme activity in liver or cultured skin fibroblasts and must be differentiated from holocarboxylase synthetase or biotinidase deficiency.

Deficiency of Pyruvate Carboxylase Secondary to Deficiency of Holocarboxylase Synthetase or Biotinidase

Deficiency of either holocarboxylase synthetase (HCS) or biotinidase, which are enzymes of biotin metabolism, result in multiple carboxylase deficiency (pyruvate carboxylase and other biotin-requiring carboxylases and metabolic reactions) and in clinical manifestations associated with the respective deficiencies, as well as rash, lactic acidosis, and alopecia (Chapter 79.6). The course of HCS or biotinidase deficiency can be protracted, with intermittent exacerbation of chronic lactic acidosis, failure to thrive, seizures, and hypotonia leading to spasticity, lethargy, coma, and death. Auditory and optic nerve dysfunction can lead to deafness and blindness, respectively. Late-onset milder forms have also been reported. Laboratory findings include metabolic acidosis and abnormal organic acids in the urine. In HCS deficiency, biotin concentrations in plasma and urine are normal. Diagnosis can be made in skin fibroblasts or lymphocytes by assay for HCS activity, and in the case of biotinidase, in the serum by a screening blood spot.

Treatment consists of biotin supplementation, 5-20 mg/day, and is generally effective if treatment is started before the development of brain damage. Patients identified through newborn screening and treated with biotin have remained asymptomatic.

Both enzyme deficiencies are autosomal recessive traits. HCS and biotinidase are located on chromosome 21q22 and 3p25, respectively. Ethnic-specific mutations in the HCS gene have been identified. Two common mutations (del7/ins3 and R538C) in the biotinidase gene account for 52% of all mutant alleles in symptomatic patients with biotinidase deficiency.

Mitochondrial Respiratory Chain Defects (Oxidative Phosphorylation Disease)

The mitochondrial respiratory chain catalyzes the oxidation of fuel molecules and transfers the electrons to molecular oxygen with concomitant energy transduction into ATP (oxidative phosphorylation). The respiratory chain produces ATP from nicotinamide adenine dinucleotide (NADH) or $FADH_2$ and includes 5 specific complexes (I: NADH–coenzyme Q reductase; II: succinate–coenzyme Q reductase; III: coenzyme QH_2 cytochrome C reductase; IV: cytochrome C oxidase; V: ATP synthase). Each complex is composed of 4-35 individual proteins and, with the exception of complex II (which is encoded solely by nuclear genes), is encoded by nuclear or mitochondrial DNA (inherited only from the mother by mitochondrial inheritance). Defects in any of these complexes or assembly systems produce chronic lactic acidosis presumably due to a change of redox state with increased concentrations of NADH. In contrast to PDHC or pyruvate carboxylase deficiency, skeletal muscle and heart are usually involved in the respiratory chain disorders, and in muscle biopsy, "ragged red fibers" (indicating mitochondrial proliferation) are very suggestive when present (see Fig. 81-5). Because of the ubiquitous nature of oxidative phosphorylation, a defect of the mitochondrial respiratory chain accounts for a vast array of clinical manifestations and should be considered in patients in all age groups presenting with multisystem involvement. Some deficiencies resemble **Leigh disease** (see later), whereas others cause infantile myopathies such as **MELAS** (mitochondrial myopathy, encephalopathy, lactic acidosis, and strokelike episodes), **MERRF** (myoclonus epilepsy, with ragged red fibers), and **Kearns-Sayre syndrome** (external ophthalmoplegia, acidosis, retinal degeneration, heart block, myopathy, and high cerebrospinal fluid protein) (Table 81-2; Chapters 591.2 and 603.4). There is a higher incidence of psychiatric disorders in adults with a primary oxidative phosphorylation disease than in the general population. Diagnosis requires demonstration of abnormalities of oxidative phosphorylation enzyme complex activities in tissues or of mitochondrial DNA (mtDNA) or a nuclear gene coding form mitochondrial functions, or both (Fig. 81-6). Analysis of oxidative phosphorylation complexes I-IV from intact mitochondria isolated from fresh skeletal muscle is the most sensitive assay for mitochondrial disorders. Specific criteria may assist in making a diagnosis (Table 81-3). Clues to the diagnosis of mitochondrial diseases are noted in Table 81-4.

Treatment remains largely symptomatic and does not significantly alter the outcome of disease. Some patients appear to respond to cofactor supplements, typically coenzyme Q_{10} plus L-carnitine at pharmacologic doses. The addition of creatine monohydrate and alpha-lipoic acid supplementation may add a significant benefit.

Leigh Disease (Subacute Necrotizing Encephalomyelopathy)

Leigh disease is a heterogenous neurologic disease that remains a neuropathologic description characterized by demyelination, gliosis, necrosis, relative neuronal sparing, and capillary proliferation in specific brain regions. In decreasing order of severity, the affected areas are the basal ganglia, brainstem cerebellum, and cerebral cortex (Chapter 591). The classic presentation is of an infant who presents with central hypotonia, developmental regression or arrest, and signs of brainstem or basal ganglia involvement. The clinical presentation is highly variable. Diagnosis is usually confirmed by radiologic or pathologic evidence of symmetric lesions affecting the basal ganglia, brainstem, and subthalamic nuclei. Patients with Leigh disease have defects in several enzyme complexes. Dysfunction in cytochrome C oxidase

Table 81-2 CLINICAL AND GENETIC HETEROGENEITY OF DISORDERS RELATED TO MUTATIONS IN MITOCHONDRIAL DNA (mtDNA)*

SYMPTOMS, SIGNS, AND FINDINGS	GIANT DELETIONS IN mtDNA			MUTATION IN TRANSFER RNA		MUTATION IN RIBOSOMAL RNA	MUTATION IN MESSENGER RNA		
	KSS	PEO	PS	MERRF	MELAS	AID	NARP	MILS	LHON
CENTRAL NERVOUS SYSTEM									
Seizures	–	–	–	⊞	+	–	–	+	–
Ataxia	+	–	–	+	+	⊞	+	±	–
Myoclonus	–	–	–	+	±	–	–	–	–
Psychomotor retardation	–	–	–	–	–	–	–	+	–
Psychomotor regression	+	–	–	±	+	–	–	–	–
Hemiparesis and hemianopia	–	–	–	–	⊞	–	–	–	–
Cortical blindness	–	–	–	–	+	–	–	–	–
Migraine-like headaches	–	–	–	–	+	–	–	–	–
Dystonia	–	–	–	–	+	–	–	+	±
PERIPHERAL NERVOUS SYSTEM									
Peripheral neuropathy	±	–	–	±	±	–	⊞	–	–
MUSCLE									
Weakness and exercise intolerance	+	⊞	–	+	+	–	+	+	–
Ophthalmoplegia	+	+	±	–	–	–	–	–	–
Ptosis	⊞	+	–	–	–	–	–	–	–
EYE									
Pigmentary retinopathy	⊞	–	–	–	–	–	⊞	±	–
Optic atrophy	–	–	–	–	–	–	±	±	⊞
BLOOD									
Sideroblastic anemia	±	–	⊞	–	–	–	–	–	–
ENDOCRINE SYSTEM									
Diabetes mellitus	±	–	–	–	±	–	–	–	–
Short stature	+	–	–	+	+	–	–	–	–
Hypoparathyroidism	±	–	–	–	–	–	–	–	–
HEART									
Conduction disorder	⊞	⊟	–	–	±	–	–	–	±
Cardiomyopathy	±	–	–	–	±	⊞	–	±	–
GASTROINTESTINAL SYSTEM									
Exocrine pancreatic dysfunction	±	–	⊞	–	–	–	–	–	–
Intestinal pseudo-obstruction	–	–	–	–	+	–	–	–	–
EAR, NOSE, AND THROAT									
Sensorineural hearing loss	±	–	–	+	+	⊞	±	–	–
KIDNEY									
Fanconi syndrome	⊞	–	⊞	–	⊞	–	–	–	–
LABORATORY FINDINGS									
Lactic acidosis	+	±	+	+	+	–	–	±	–
Ragged-red fibers on muscle biopsy	+	+	±	+	+	–	–	–	–
MODE OF INHERITANCE									
Maternal	–	–	–	+	+	–	+	+	+
Sporadic	+	+	+	–	–	–	–	–	–

*Characteristic constellations of symptoms and signs are boxed.

+, Presence of a symptom, sign, or finding; –, absence of a symptom, sign, or finding; ±, possible presence of a symptom, sign, or finding; AID, aminoglycoside-induced deafness; KSS, Kearns-Sayre syndrome; LHON, Leber's hereditary optic neuropathy; MELAS, mitochondrial encephalomyopathy, lactic acidosis, and strokelike episodes; MERRE, myoclonic epilepsy with ragged-red fibers; MILS, maternally inherited Leigh syndrome; NARP, neuropathy, ataxia, and retinitis pigmentosa; PEO, progressive external ophthalmoplegia; PS, Pearson syndrome.

From DiMauro S, Schon EA: Mitochondrial respiratory-chain diseases, *N Engl J Med* 348:2656–2668, 2003.

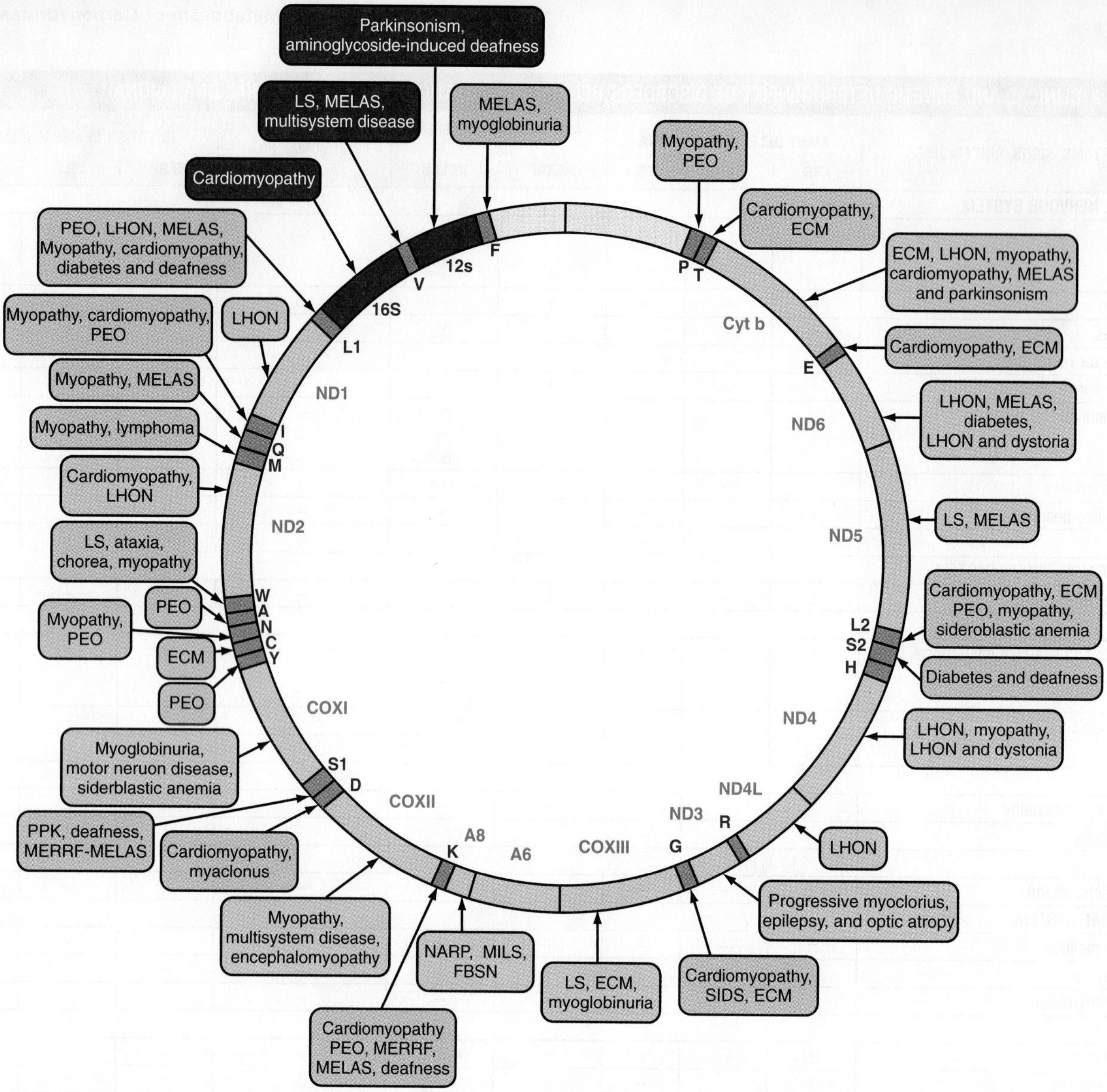

Figure 81-6 Mutations in the human mitochondrial genome that are known to cause disease. Disorders that are frequently or prominently associated with mutations in a particular gene are shown in *bold.* Diseases due to mutations that impair mitochondrial protein synthesis are shown in *blue.* Diseases due to mutations in protein-coding genes are shown in *red.* ECM, encephalomyopathy; FBSN, familial bilateral striatal necrosis; LHON, Leber hereditary optic neuropathy; LS, Leigh syndrome; MELAS, mitochondrial encephalomyopathy, lactic acidosis, and strokelike episodes; MERRF, myoclonic epilepsy with ragged-red fibers; MILS, maternally inherited Leigh syndrome; NARP, neuropathy, ataxia, and retinitis pigmentosa; PEO, progressive external ophthalmoplegia; PPK, palmoplantar keratoderma; and SIDS, sudden infant death syndrome. (From DiMauro S, Schon EA: Mitochondrial respiratory-chain diseases, *N Engl J Med* 348:2656–2668, 2003.Copyright © 2003 Massachusetts Medical Society. All rights reserved.)

Table 81-3 MODIFIED WALKER CRITERIA APPLIED TO CHILDREN REFERRED FOR EVALUATION OF MITOCHONDRIAL DISEASE

	MAJOR CRITERIA	MINOR CRITERIA
Clinical	Clinically complete RC encephalomyopathy* or a mitochondrial cytopathy defined as fulfilling 3 criteria†	Symptoms compatible with an RC defect‡
Histology	>2% ragged red fibers (RRF) in skeletal muscle	Smaller numbers of RRF, SSAM, or widespread electron microscopy abnormalities of mitochondria
Enzymology	Cytochrome c oxidase–negative fibers or residual activity of an RC complex <20% in a tissue; <30% in a cell line, or <30% in 2 or more tissues	Antibody-based demonstration of an RC defect or residual activity of an RC complex 20-30% in a tissue, 30-40% in a cell line, or 30-40% in 2 or more tissues
Functional	Fibroblast ATP synthesis rates >3 SD below mean	Fibroblast ATP synthesis rates 2-3 SD below mean, or fibroblasts unable to grow in galactose media
Molecular	Nuclear or mtDNA mutation of undisputed pathogenicity	Nuclear or mtDNA mutation of probable pathogenicity
Metabolic		One or more metabolic indicators of impaired metabolic function

*Leigh disease, Alpers disease, LIMD, Pearson syndrome, Kearns-Sayre syndrome, MELAS, MERRF, NARP, MNGIE, and LHON.

†(1) Unexplained combination of multisystemic symptoms that is essentially pathognomonic for an RC disorder, (2) a progressive clinical course with episodes of exacerbation or a family history strongly indicative of an mtDNA mutation, and (3) other possible metabolic or nonmetabolic disorders have been excluded by appropriate testing.

‡Added pediatric features: stillbirth associated with a paucity of intrauterine movement, neonatal death or collapse, movement disorder, severe failure to thrive, neonatal hypotonia, and neonatal hypertonia as minor clinical criteria.

ATP, adenosine triphosphate; RC, respiratory chain; SSAM, subsarcolemmal accumulation of mitochondria.

From Scaglia F, Towbin JA, Craigen WJ, et al: Clinical spectrum, morbidity and mortality in 113 pediatric patients with mitochondrial disease, *Pediatrics* 114:925–931, 2004.

Table 81-4 CLUES TO THE DIAGNOSIS OF MITOCHONDRIAL DISEASE

NEUROLOGIC
Cerebral strokelike lesions in a nonvascular pattern
Basal ganglia disease
Encephalopathy: recurrent or with low/moderate dosing of valproate
Neurodegeneration
Epilepsia partialis continua
Myoclonus
Ataxia
MRI findings consistent with Leigh disease
Characteristic MRS peaks
Lactate peak at 1.3 ppm TE (time to echo) at 35 and 135
Succinate peak at 2.4 ppm
CARDIOVASCULAR
Hypertrophic cardiomyopathy with rhythm disturbance
Unexplained heart block in a child
Cardiomyopathy with lactic acidosis (>5 mM)
Dilated cardiomyopathy with muscle weakness
Wolff-Parkinson-White arrhythmia
OPHTHALMOLOGIC
Retinal degeneration with signs of night blindness, color vision deficits, decreased visual acuity, or pigmentary retinopathy
Ophthalmoplegia/paresis
Fluctuating, dysconjugate eye movements
Ptosis
Sudden- or insidious-onset optic neuropathy/atrophy
GASTROENTEROLOGIC
Unexplained or valproate-induced liver failure
Severe dysmotility
Pseudo-obstructive episodes
OTHER
A newborn, infant, or young child with unexplained hypotonia, weakness, failure to thrive, and a metabolic acidosis (particularly lactic acidosis)
Exercise intolerance that is not in proportion to weakness
Hypersensitivity to general anesthesia
Episodes of acute rhabdomyolysis

From Haas RH, Parikh S, Falk MJ, et al: Mitochondrial disease: a practical approach for primary care physicians, *Pediatrics* 120:1326–1333, 2007, Table 1, p 1327.

(complex IV) is the most commonly reported defect, followed by NADH-coenzyme Q reductase (complex I), PDHC, and pyruvate carboxylase. Mutations in the nuclear SURF1 gene, which encodes a factor involved in the biogenesis of cytochrome C oxidase and mitochondrial DNA mutations in the ATPase 6 coding region, are common molecular findings in patients with Leigh disease. Patients with Leigh disease frequently present with developmental delay, seizures, altered consciousness, failure to thrive, pericardial effusion, and dilated cardiomyopathy. The prognosis for Leigh syndrome is poor. In a study of 14 cases, there were 7 fatalities before the age of 1.5 yr.

BIBLIOGRAPHY

Please visit the Nelson Textbook of Pediatrics *website at www.expertconsult.com for the complete bibliography.*

81.5 Defects in Pentose Metabolism

Priya S. Kishnani and Yuan-Tsong Chen

About 90% of glucose metabolism in the body is via the glycolytic pathway, with the remaining 10% via the hexose monophosphate pathway. The hexose monophosphate shunt leads to formation of pentoses, as well as providing NADH. One of the metabolites is ribose-5-phosphate, which is used in the biosynthesis of ribonucleotides and deoxyribonucleotides. Through the transketolase and transaldolase reactions, the pentose phosphates can be converted back to fructose-6-phosphate and glucose-6-phosphate.

For the full continuation of this chapter, please visit the Nelson Textbook of Pediatrics *website at www.expertconsult.com.*

81.6 Disorders of Glycoprotein Degradation and Structure

Margaret M. Mcgovern and Robert J. Desnick

The disorders of glycoprotein degradation and structure include several lysosomal storage diseases that result from defects in glycoprotein degradation, and the congenital disorders of glycosylation (CDGs), which are pathophysiologically unrelated. Glycoproteins are macromolecules that are composed of oligosaccharide chains linked to a peptide backbone. They are synthesized by 2 pathways: the glycosyltransferase pathway, which synthesizes oligosaccharides linked O-glycosidically to serine or threonine residues; and the dolichol, lipid-linked pathway, which synthesizes oligosaccharides linked N-glycosidically to asparagine.

For the full continuation of this chapter, please visit the Nelson Textbook of Pediatrics *website at www.expertconsult.com.*

Chapter 82
Mucopolysaccharidoses

Jürgen Spranger

Mucopolysaccharidoses are hereditary, progressive diseases caused by mutations of genes coding for lysosomal enzymes needed to degrade glycosaminoglycans (acid mucopolysaccharides). Glycosaminoglycan (GAG) is a long-chain complex carbohydrate composed of uronic acids, amino sugars, and neutral sugars. The major GAGs are chondroitin-4-sulfate, chondroitin-6-sulfate, heparan sulfate, dermatan sulfate, keratan sulfate, and hyaluronan. These substances are synthesized and, with the exception of hyaluronan, linked to proteins to form proteoglycans, major constituents of the ground substance of connective tissue, as well as nuclear and cell membranes. Degradation of proteoglycans starts with the proteolytic removal of the protein core followed by the stepwise degradation of the GAG moiety. Failure of this degradation due to absent or grossly reduced activity of mutated lysosomal enzymes results in the intralysosomal accumulation of GAG fragments (Fig. 82-1). Distended lysosomes accumulate in the cell, interfere with cell function, and lead to a characteristic pattern of clinical, radiologic, and biochemical abnormalities (Table 82-1, Fig. 82-2). Within this pattern, specific diseases can be recognized that evolve from the intracellular accumulation of different degradation products (Table 82-2). As a general rule, the impaired degradation of heparan sulfate is more closely associated with mental deficiency and the impaired degradation of dermatan sulfate, chondroitin sulfates, and keratan sulfate with mesenchymal abnormalities. Variable expression within a given entity results from allelic mutations and varying residual activity of mutated enzymes. Allelic mutations of the gene encoding L-iduronidase may result in severe Hurler disease with early death or in mild Scheie disease manifesting only with limited joint mobility, mild skeletal abnormalities, and corneal opacities. Mucopolysaccharidoses are autosomal recessive disorders, with the exception of Hunter disease, which is X-linked recessive. Their overall frequency is between 3.5/100,000 and 4.5/100,000. The most common subtype is MPS-III, followed by MPS-I and MPS-II.

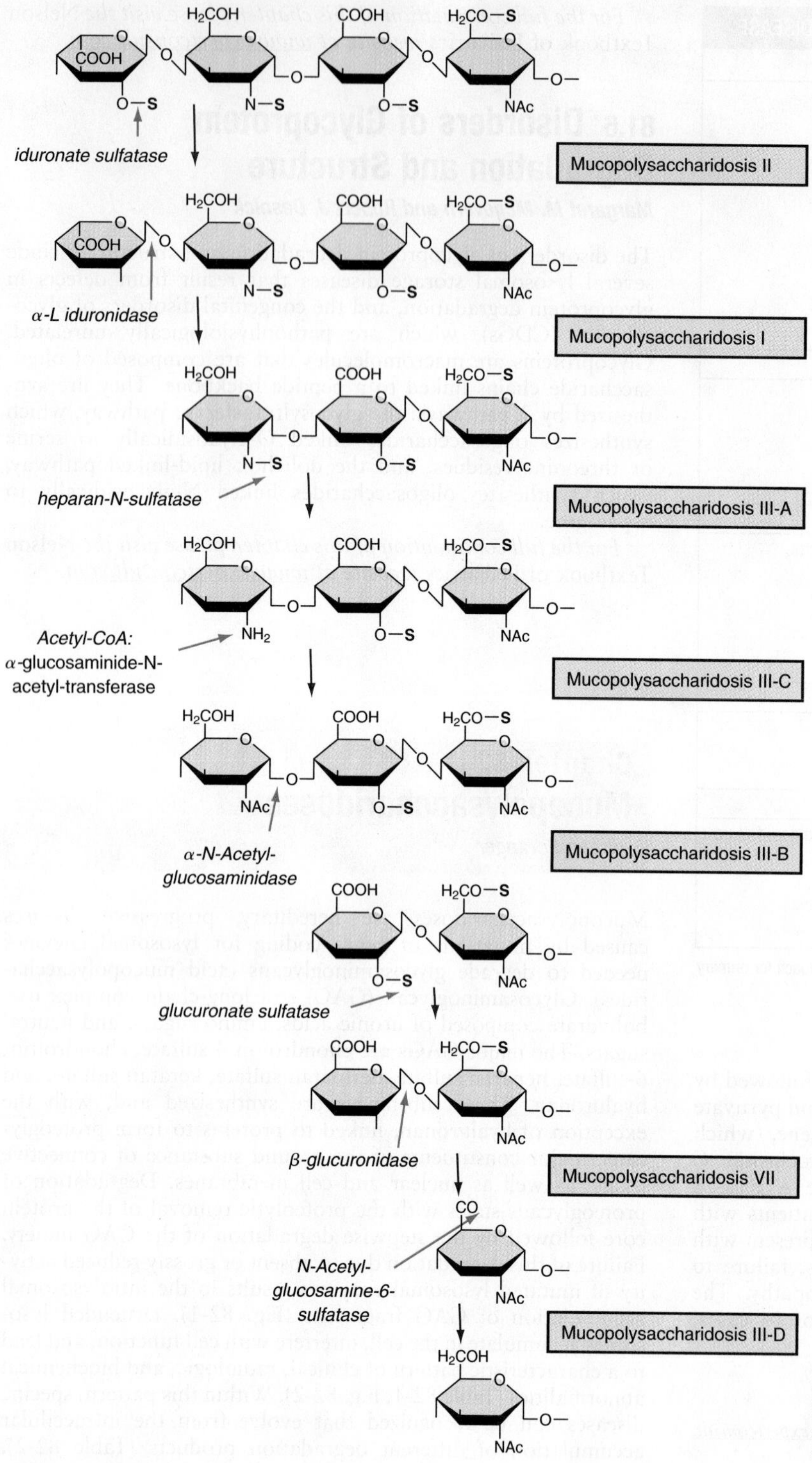

Figure 82-1 Degradation of heparan sulfate and mucopolysaccharidoses resulting from the deficiency of individual enzymes. Some of the enzymes are also involved in the degradation of other glycosaminoglycans (not shown).

CLINICAL ENTITIES

Mucopolysaccharidosis I

MPS I is caused by mutations of the *IUA* gene on chromosome 4p16.3 encoding α-L-iduronidase. Mutation analysis reveals 2 major alleles, W402X and Q70X, that account for more than ½ the MPS-I alleles in the white population. The mutations introduce stop codons with ensuing absence of functional enzyme (null alleles); homozygosity or compound heterozygosity gives rise to Hurler disease. Other mutations occur in only one or a few individuals.

Deficiency of α-L-iduronidase results in a broad clinical spectrum, from severe **Hurler** disease to mild **Scheie** diseases. Homozygous or double heterozygous nonsense mutations result in severe forms of MPS I, whereas missense mutations are more likely to preserve some residual enzyme activity associated with a milder form of the disease. Varying efficacy of GAG synthesis may also influence the prognosis.

HURLER DISEASE This form of MPS I (MPS I-H) is a severe, progressive disorder with multiple organ and tissue involvement that results in premature death, usually by 10 yr of age. An infant with Hurler syndrome appears normal at birth, but inguinal

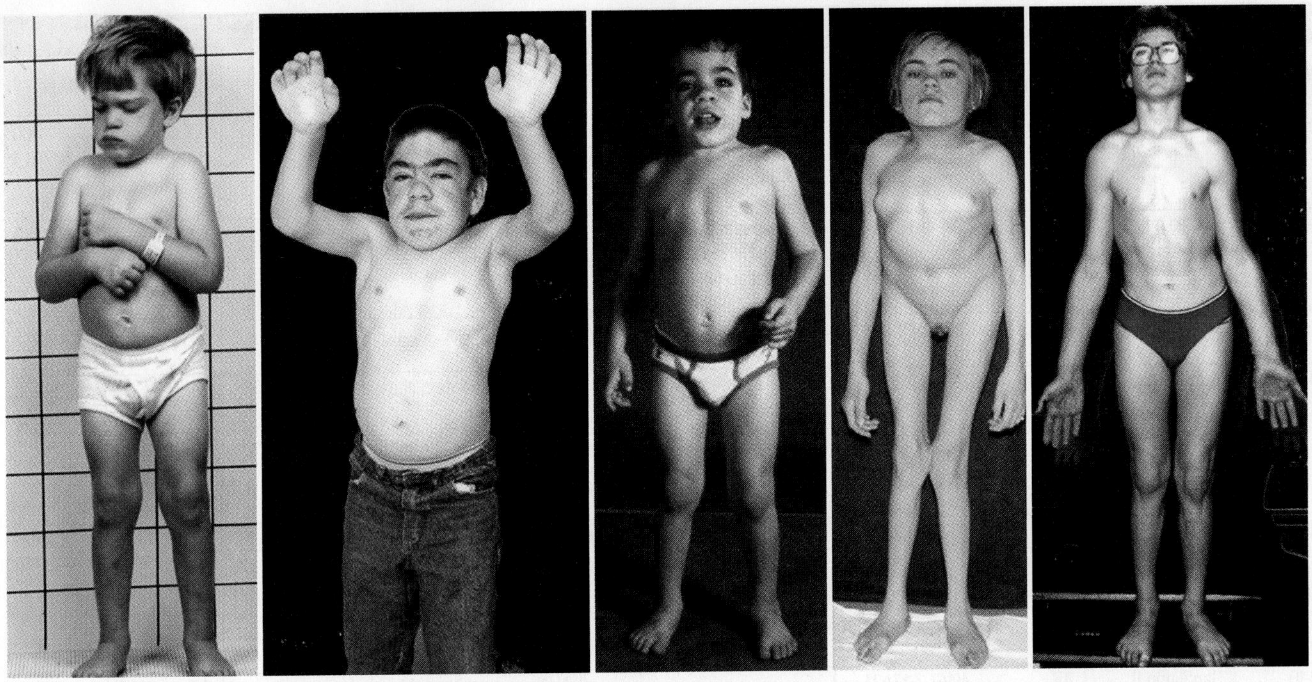

MPS-I MPS-II MPS-III MPS-IV MPS-VI

Figure 82-2 Patients with various types of mucopolysaccharidoses. I: Hurler disease, 3 yr; II: Hunter disease, 12 yr; III: Sanfilippo disease, 4 yr; IV: Morquio disease, 10 yr; VI: Maroteaux-Lamy disease, 15 yr.

Table 82-1 RECOGNITION PATTERN OF MUCOPOLYSACCHARIDOSES

MANIFESTATIONS	MUCOPOLYSACCHARIDOSIS TYPE						
	I-H	I-S	II	III	IV	VI	VII
Mental deficiency	+	−	±	+	−	−	±
Coarse facial features	+	(+)	+	+	−	+	±
Corneal clouding	+	+	−	−	(+)	+	±
Visceromegaly	+	(+)	+	(+)	−	+	+
Short stature	+	(+)	+	−	+	+	+
Joint contractures	+	+	+	−	−	+	+
Dysostosis multiplex	+	(+)	+	(+)	+	+	+
Leucocyte inclusions	+	(+)	+	+	−	+	+
Mucopolysacchariduria	+	+	+	+	+	+	+

I-H, Hurler disease; I-S, Scheie disease; II, Hunter disease; III, Sanfilippo disease; IV, Morquio disease; VI, Maroteaux-Lamy disease; VII, Sly disease.

hernias are often present. Diagnosis is usually made between 6 and 24 mo of age with evidence of hepatosplenomegaly, coarse facial features, corneal clouding, large tongue, prominent forehead, joint stiffness, short stature, and skeletal dysplasia (see Fig. 82-2). Acute cardiomyopathy has been found in some infants <1 yr of age. Most patients have recurrent upper respiratory tract and ear infections, noisy breathing, and persistent copious nasal discharge. Valvular heart disease with incompetence, notably of the mitral and aortic valves, regularly develops, as does coronary artery narrowing. Obstructive airway disease, notably during sleep, may necessitate tracheotomy. Obstructive airway disease, respiratory infection, and cardiac complications are the common causes of death.

Most children with Hurler syndrome acquire social but only limited language skills because of developmental delay, combined conductive and neurosensory hearing loss, and an enlarged tongue. Progressive ventricular enlargement with increased intracranial pressure caused by communicating hydrocephalus may be responsible for headache and sleep disturbance. Corneal clouding, glaucoma, and retinal degeneration are common. Radiographs show a characteristic skeletal dysplasia known as **dysostosis multiplex** (Figs. 82-3 and 82-4). The earliest radiographic signs are thick ribs and ovoid vertebral bodies. Skeletal abnormalities in addition to those shown in the figures include enlarged, coarsely trabeculated diaphyses of the long bones with irregular metaphyses and epiphyses. With progression of the disease, macrocephaly develops, with thickened calvarium, premature closure of lambdoid and sagittal sutures, shallow orbits, enlarged J-shaped sella, and abnormal spacing of teeth with dentigenous cysts.

HURLER-SCHEIE DISEASE The clinical phenotype of MPS I-H/S is intermediate between Hurler and Scheie diseases and is characterized by progressive somatic involvement, including dysostosis multiplex with little or no intellectual dysfunction. The onset of symptoms is usually observed between 3 and 8 yr of age; survival to adulthood is common. Cardiac involvement and upper airway obstruction contribute to clinical morbidity. Some patients have spondylolisthesis, which may cause cord compression.

SCHEIE DISEASE MPS I-S is a comparatively mild disorder characterized by joint stiffness, aortic valve disease, corneal clouding, and mild dysostosis multiplex. Onset of significant symptoms is usually after the age of 5 yr, with diagnosis made between 10 and 20 yr of age. Patients with Scheie disease have normal intelligence and stature but have significant joint and ocular involvement. A carpal tunnel syndrome often develops. Ophthalmic features include corneal clouding, glaucoma, and retinal degeneration. Obstructive airway disease, causing sleep apnea, develops in some patients, necessitating tracheotomy. Aortic valve disease is common and has required valve replacement in some patients.

Mucopolysaccharidosis II

Hunter disease (MPS II) is an X-linked disorder caused by the deficiency of iduronate-2-sulfatase (IDS). The gene encoding IDS is mapped to Xq28. Point mutations of the *IDS* gene have been detected in about 80% of patients with MPS II. Major deletions or rearrangements of the *IDS* gene have been found in the rest; these are usually associated with a more severe clinical phenotype

Table 82-2 MUCOPOLYSACCHARIDOSES: CLINICAL, MOLECULAR, AND BIOCHEMICAL ASPECTS

MPS TYPE	EPONYM	GENE Inheritance	Chromosome	MAIN CLINICAL FEATURES	DEFECTIVE ENZYME	ASSAY	MIM NUMBER
I-H	Pfaundler-Hurler	AR	*IDA* 4p16.3	Severe Hurler phenotype, mental deficiency, corneal clouding, death usually before age 14 yr	α-L-Iduronidase	L,F,Ac,Cv	252800 607014
I-S	Scheie	AR	*IDA* 4p16.4	Stiff joints, corneal clouding, aortic valve disease, normal intelligence, survive to adulthood	α-L-Iduronidase	L,F,Ac,Cv	607016
I-HS	Hurler-Scheie	AR	*IDA* 4p16.4	Phenotype intermediate between I-H and I-S	α-L-Iduronidase	L,F,Ac,Cv	607015
II	Hunter	XLR	*IDS* Xq27.3-28	Severe course similar to I-H but clear corneas. Mild course: less pronounced features, later manifestation, survival to adulthood with mild or no mental deficiency	Iduronate sulfate sulfatase	S,F,Af,Ac,Cv	309900
III-A	Sanfilippo A	AR	*HSS* 17q25.3	Behavioral problems, sleeping disorder, aggression, progressive dementia, mild dysmorphism, coarse hair, clear corneas, survival to adulthood possible	Heparan-S-sulfamidase	L,F,Ac,Cv	252900 605270
II-IB	Sanfilippo B	AR	*NAGLU* 17q21		N-Ac-α-glucosaminidase	S,F,Ac,Cv	252920
III-C	Sanfilippo C	AR	*HGSNAT 8p11-q13*		Ac-CoA-glucosaminide-N-acetyltransferase	F,Ac	252930
III-D	Sanfilippo D	AR	*GNS* 12q14		N-Ac-glucosaminine-6-sulfate sulfatase	F,Ac	252940 607664
IV-A	Morquio A	AR	*GALNS* 16q24.3	Short-trunk dwarfism, fine corneal opacities, characteristic bone dysplasia; final height <125 cm	N-Ac-galactosamine-6-sulfate sulfatase	L,F,Ac	253000
IV-B	Morquio B	AR	*GLB1* 3p21.33	Same as IV-A, but milder; adult height >120 cm	β-Galactosidase	L,F,Ac,Cv	253010 230500
VI	Maroteaux-Lamy	AR	*ARSB* 5q11-q13	Hurler phenotype with marked corneal clouding but normal intelligence; mild, moderate, and severe expression in different families	N-Ac-galactos-amine-α-4-sulfate sulfatase (arylsulfatase B)	L,F,Ac	253200
VII	Sly	AR	*GUSB* 7q21.11	Varying from fetal hydrops to mild dysmorphism; dense inclusions in granulocytes	β-Glucuronidase	S,F,Ac,Cv	253220
IX	Hyaluronidase deficiency	AR	*HYAL1* 3p21.3	Periarticular masses, no Hurler phenotype	Hyaluronidase 1	S	601492

Ac, cultured amniotic cells; Af, amniotic fluid; Cv, chorionic villi; F, cultured fibroblasts; L, leukocytes; MIM, Mendelian Inheritance in Man Catalog; S, serum.

(see Fig. 82-2). Hunter disease manifests almost exclusively in males; it has been observed in a few females and this is explained by skewed inactivation of the X chromosome carrying the normal gene.

Marked molecular heterogeneity explains the wide clinical spectrum of Hunter disease. Patients with severe MPS II have features similar to those of Hurler disease except for the lack of corneal clouding and the somewhat slower progression of somatic and central nervous system (CNS) deterioration. Coarse facial features, short stature, dysostosis multiplex, joint stiffness, and mental retardation manifest between 2 and 4 yr of age. Grouped skin papules are present in some patients. Extensive Mongolian spots have been observed in African and Asian patients since birth and may be an early marker of the disease. Storage in gastrointestinal cells may produce chronic diarrhea. Communicating hydrocephalus and spastic paraplegia may develop due to thickened meninges. In severely affected patients, extensive, slowly progressive neurologic involvement precedes death, which usually occurs between 10 and 15 yr of age.

Patients with the mild form have a prolonged life span, minimal CNS involvement, and slow progression of somatic deterioration with preservation of intelligence in adult life. Survival to ages 65 and 87 yr has been reported; some patients had children. Somatic features are Hurler-like but milder with a greatly reduced rate of progression. Adult height may exceed 150 cm. Airway involvement, valvular cardiac disease, hearing impairment, carpal tunnel syndrome, and joint stiffness are common and can result in significant loss of function in both the mild and severe forms.

Mucopolysaccharidosis III

Sanfilippo disease (MPS III) makes up a genetically heterogeneous but clinically similar group of 4 recognized types. Each type is caused by a different enzyme deficiency involved in the degradation of heparan sulfate (see Fig. 82-1). Mutations have been found in all the MPS III disorders for which the genes have been isolated.

Phenotypic variation exists in MPS III patients but to a lesser degree than in other MPS disorders. Patients with Sanfilippo

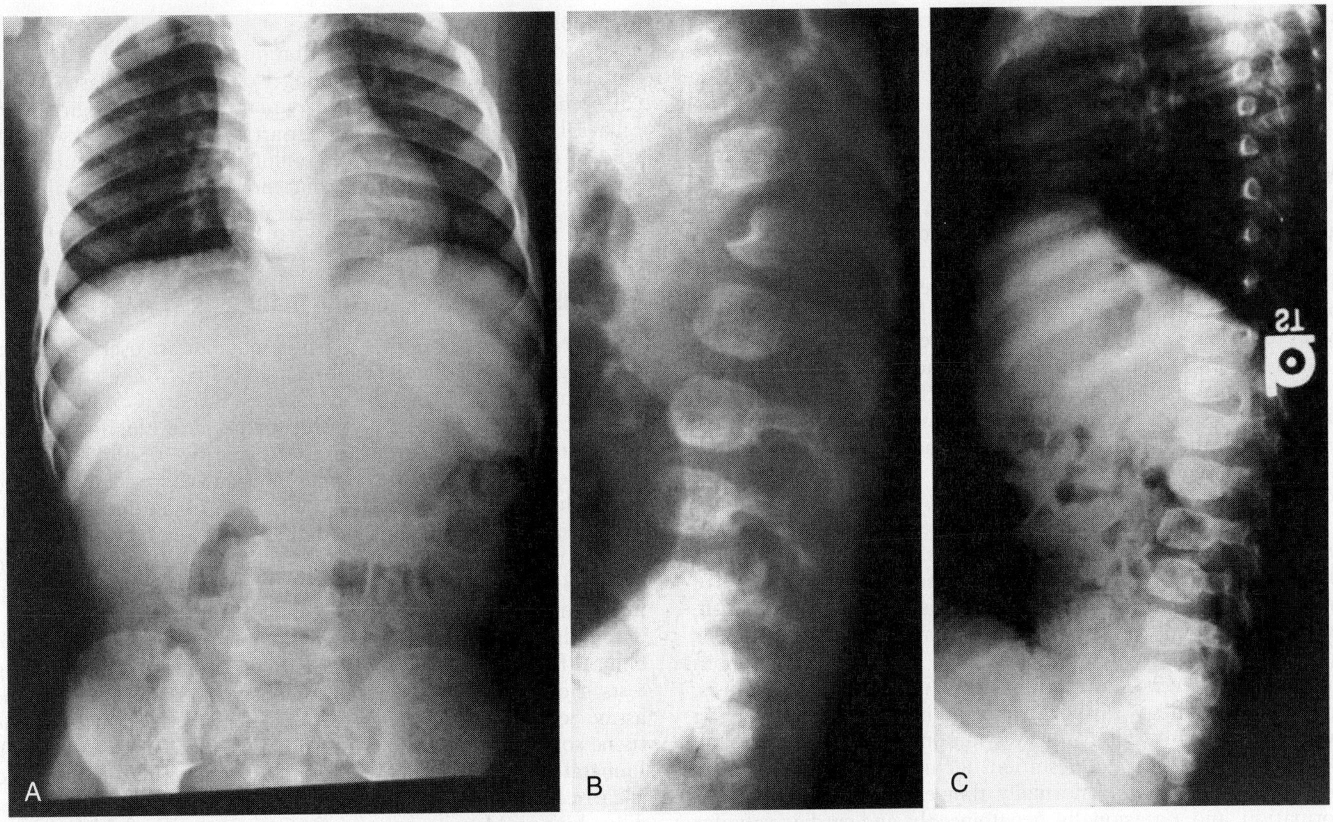

Figure 82-3 Dysostosis multiplex. *A,* Sanfilippo disease, 4 yr: The ribs are wide. *B,* Sanfilippo disease, 4 yr: immature, ovoid configuration of the vertebral bodies. *C,* Hurler disease, 18 mo: anterior-superior hypoplasia of L-1 resulting in hook-shaped appearance.

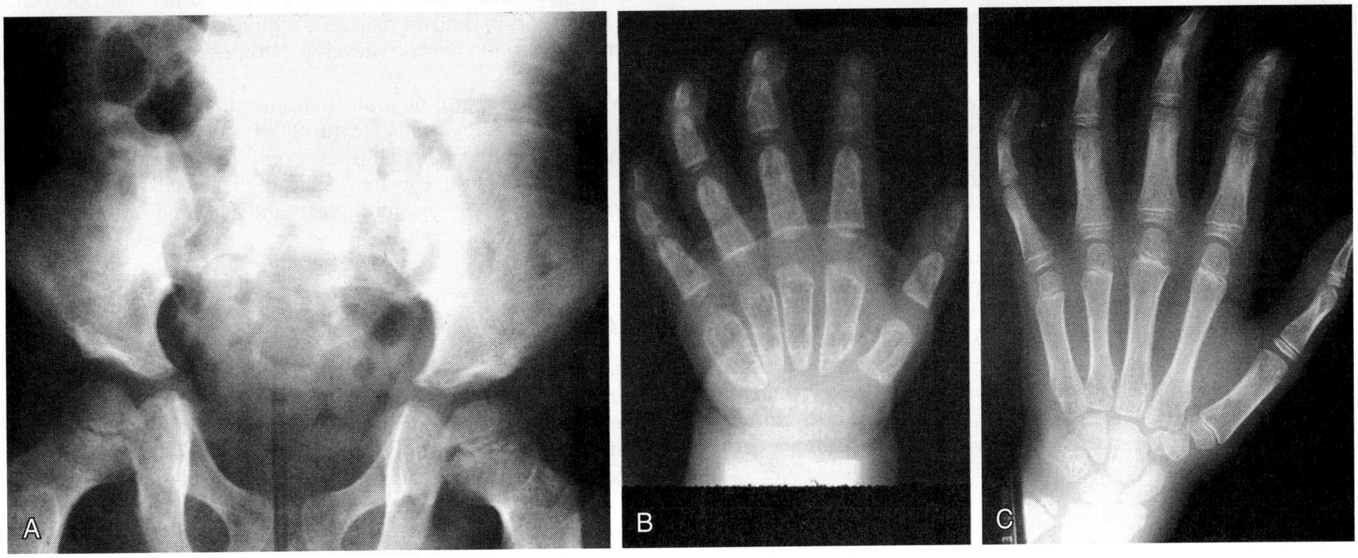

Figure 82-4 Dysostosis multiplex. *A,* Mucopolysaccharidosis (MPS) I-H, 10 yr. The inferior portions of the ilia are hypoplastic with resulting iliac flare and shallow acetabular fossae. The femoral necks are in valgus position. *B,* MPS I-H, 4 yr. Metacarpals and phalanges are abnormally short, wide, and deformed with proximal pointing of the metacarpals and bullet-shaped phalanges. Bone trabeculation is coarse and the cortices are thin. *C,* MPS I-S, 13 yr. The carpal bones are small leading to a V-shaped configuration of the digits. The short tubular bones are well modeled. Flexion of the middle and distal phalanges II-V is caused by joint contractures.

disease are characterized by slowly progressive, severe CNS involvement with mild somatic disease. Such disproportionate involvement of the CNS is unique to MPS III. Onset of clinical features usually occurs between 2 and 6 yr in a child who previously appeared normal. Presenting features include delayed development, hyperactivity with aggressive behavior, coarse hair, hirsutism, sleep disorders, and mild hepatosplenomegaly (see Fig. 82-2). Delays in diagnosis of MPS III are common due to the mild physical features, hyperactivity, and slowly progressive neurologic disease. Severe neurologic deterioration occurs in most patients by 6-10 yr of age, accompanied by rapid deterioration of social and adaptive skills. Severe behavior problems such as sleep disturbance, uncontrolled hyperactivity, temper tantrums, destructive behavior, and physical aggression are common. Profound mental retardation and behavior problems often occur in patients with normal physical strength, making management particularly difficult.

Mucopolysaccharidosis IV

Morquio disease (MPS IV) is caused by a deficiency of N-acetylgalactosamine-6-sulfatase (MPS IV-A) or of β-galactosidase (MPS IV-B). Both result in the defective degradation of keratan sulfate. The gene encoding N-acetylgalactosamine-6-sulfatase is on chromosome 16q24.3 and the gene encoding β-galactosidase, *GLB1,* on chromosome 3p21.33. β-Galactosidase catalyzes G_{M1} ganglioside in addition to keratan sulfate, and most mutations of *GLB1* result in generalized gangliosidosis, a spectrum of neurodegenerative disorders associated with dysostosis multiplex. A W273L mutation of the *GLB1* gene, either in the homozygous state or as part of compound heterozygosity, commonly results in Morquio B disease.

Both types of Morquio disease are characterized by short-trunk dwarfism, fine corneal deposits, a skeletal dysplasia that is distinct from other mucopolysaccharidoses, and preservation of intelligence. MPS IV-A is usually more severe than MPS IV-B, with adult heights of <125 cm in the former and >150 cm in the latter. There is considerable variability of expression in both subtypes, however. The appearance of genua valga, kyphosis, growth retardation with short trunk and neck, and waddling gait with a tendency to fall are early symptoms of MPS IV (see Fig. 82-2). Extra skeletal manifestations include mild corneal clouding, small teeth with abnormally thin enamel, frequent caries formation, and, occasionally, hepatomegaly, and cardiac valvular lesions. Instability of the odontoid process and ligamentous laxity are regularly present and can result in life-threatening atlanto-axial instability and dislocation. Surgery to stabilize the upper cervical spine, usually by posterior spinal fusion before the development of cervical myelopathy, can be lifesaving.

Mucopolysaccharidosis VI

Maroteaux-Lamy disease (MPS VI) is caused by mutations of the *ARSB* gene on chromosome 5q11-13 encoding N-acetylgalactosamine-4-sulfatase (arylsulfatase B). It is characterized by severe to mild somatic involvement, as seen in MPS I, but with preservation of intelligence. The somatic involvement of the severe form of MPS VI is characterized by corneal clouding, coarse facial features, joint stiffness, valvular heart disease, communicating hydrocephalus, and dysostosis multiplex (see Fig. 82-2). In the severe form, growth can be normal for the 1st few years of life but seems virtually to stop after age 6-8 yr. The mild to intermediate forms of Maroteaux-Lamy disease can be easily confused with Scheie syndrome. Spinal cord compression from thickening of the dura in the upper cervical canal with resultant myelopathy is a frequent occurrence in patients with MPS VI.

Mucopolysaccharidosis VII

Sly syndrome (MPS VII) is caused by mutations of the *GUSB* gene located on chromosome 7q21.11. Mutations result in a deficiency of β-glucuronidase, intracellular storage of GAG fragments and a very wide range of clinical involvement. The most severe form presents as lethal nonimmune fetal hydrops and may be detected in utero by ultrasound. Some severely affected newborns survive for some months and have, or develop, signs of lysosomal storage including thick skin, visceromegaly, and dysostosis multiplex. Less severe forms of MPS VII present in the 1st years of life with features of MPS-I but slower progression. Corneal clouding varies. Patients with manifestation after 4 yr of life have skeletal abnormalities of dysostosis multiplex but normal intelligence and usually clear corneae. They may be found incidentally on the basis of a blood smear that shows coarse granulocytic inclusions.

Mucopolysaccharidosis IX

The disorder is caused by a mutation in the *HYAL1* gene on chromosome 3p21.2-21.2 encoding 1 of 3 hyaluronidases. Clinical findings in the only known patient, a 14 yr old girl, were bilateral nodular soft tissue periarticular masses, lysosomal storage of GAGs in histiocytes, mildly dysmorphic craniofacial features, short stature, normal joint movement, and normal intelligence. Small erosions in both acetabulae were the only radiographic findings.

DIAGNOSIS AND DIFFERENTIAL DIAGNOSIS

Radiographs of chest, spine, pelvis, and hands are useful to detect early signs of dysostosis multiplex (see Figs. 82-3 and 82-4). Semiquantitative spot tests for increased urinary GAG excretion are quick, inexpensive, and useful for initial evaluation but are subject to both false-positive and false-negative results. Chemical quantification of uronic acid–containing substances is required to assess the total urinary excretion of GAG. Quantitative analysis of single GAG by various methods, or of oligosaccharides by tandem mass spectrometry, reveals type-specific profiles. Morquio disease is often missed in urinary assays but can reliably be diagnosed in serum using monoclonal antibodies to keratan sulfate. Any individual who is suspected of an MPS disorder based on clinical features, radiographic results, or urinary GAG screening tests should have a definitive diagnosis established by enzyme assay. Serum, leukocytes, or cultured fibroblasts are used as the tissue source for measuring lysosomal enzymes (see Table 82-2). Prenatal diagnosis is available for all mucopolysaccharidoses and is carried out on cultured cells from amniotic fluid or chorionic villus biopsy. Measurement of GAGs in amniotic fluid is unreliable. Carrier testing in Hunter syndrome, an X-linked disorder, requires analysis of the *IDS* gene once the specific mutation or chromosome arrangement in the family under consideration is known. Molecular analysis in patients with other mucopolysaccharidoses or in known carriers requires a specific rationale. Attempts are being made to develop methods for routine newborn screening.

Mucolipidoses and oligosaccharidoses manifest with the same clinical and radiographic features as mucopolysaccharidoses (Chapters 80.4 and 80.5). In these conditions, the urinary excretion of GAGs is not elevated. Hurler-like facial features, joint contractures, dysostosis multiplex, and elevated urinary GAG excretion differentiate the mucopolysaccharidoses from other neurodegenerative and dwarfing conditions.

TREATMENT

Hematopoietic stem cell transplantation results in significant clinical improvement of somatic disease in MPS I, II, and VI. Clinical effects include increased life expectancy, resolution or improvement of growth failure, upper airway obstruction, hepatosplenomegaly, joint stiffness, facial appearance, pebbly skin changes in MPS II, obstructive sleep apnea, heart disease, communicating hydrocephalus, and hearing loss. Enzyme activity in serum and urinary GAG excretion normalize. Transplantation prevents neurocognitive degeneration but does not correct existent cerebral damage. Hence, the main target group are young children with severe MPS I, anticipated neurodegeneration, who undergo transplantation before 24 mo of age and have a baseline mental development index >70. In children with anticipated normal neurodevelopment the benefits of transplantation must be weighed against its complications, including transplantation-related death or primary graft failure, which occurs in ≈30% of the patients.

Stem cell transplantation does not correct skeletal and ocular anomalies; they have to be treated with appropriate orthopedic and ophthalmologic procedures.

Enzyme replacement using recombinant enzymes is approved for patients with MPS I, MPS II, and MPS VI. It reduces organo-

Table 82-3 MANAGEMENT OF MUCOPOLYSACCHARIDOSES

PROBLEM	PREDOMINANTLY IN	MANAGEMENT
NEUROLOGIC		
Hydrocephalus	MPS I, II, VI, VII	Fundoscopy, CT scan, ventriculoperitoneal shunting
Chronic headaches	All	See behavioral disturbances
Behavioral disturbance	MPS III	Behavioral or medication therapy, sometimes CT scan, ventriculoperitoneal shunting
Disturbed sleep/wake circle	MPS III	Melatonin
Seizures	MPS I, II, III	EEG, anticonvulsants
Odontoid hypoplasia	MPS IV	Cervical MRI, upper cervical fusion
Spinal cord compression	All	Laminectomy, dural excision
OPHTHALMOLOGIC		
Corneal opacity	MPS I, VI, VII	Corneal transplant
Glaucoma	MPS I, VI, VII	Medication, surgery
Retinal degeneration	MPS I, II	Night light
EARS, AIRWAYS		
Recurrent otitis media	MPS I, II, VI, VII	Ventilating tubes
Impaired hearing	All except MPS IV	Audiometry, hearing aids
Obstruction	All except MPS III	Adenotomy, tonsillectomy, bronchodilator therapy, CPAP at night, laser excision of tracheal lesions, tracheotomy
CARDIAC		
Cardiac valve disease	MPS I, II, VI, VII	Endocarditis prevention, valve replacement
Coronary insufficiency	MPS I, II, VI, VII	Medical therapy
Arrhythmias	MPS I, II, VI, VII	Antiarrhythmic medication, pacemaker
ORAL, GASTROINTESTINAL		
Hypertrophic gums, poor teeth	MPS I, II, VI, VII	Dental care
Chronic diarrhea	MPS II	Diet modification, loperamide
MUSCULOSKELETAL		
Joint stiffness	All except MPS IV	Physical therapy
Weakness	All	Physical therapy, wheelchair
Gross long bone malalignment	All	Corrective osteotomies
Carpal tunnel syndrome	MPS I, II, VI, VII	Electromyography, surgical decompression
ANESTHESIA	All except III	Avoid atlantoaxial dislocation, use angulated videointubation laryngoscope and small endotracheal tubes

CPAP, continuous positive air pressure.

Table 82-4 RECOMMENDED MINIMAL SCHEDULE OF ASSESSMENTS FOR ALL PATIENTS WITH MPS I

	INITIAL ASSESSMENTS	EVERY 6 MO	EVERY 12 MO	EVERY OTHER YEAR
GENERAL				
Demographic characteristics	X			
Patient diagnosis	X			
Medical history	X	X		
Physical examination	X	X		
General appearance	X	X		
CLINICAL ASSESSMENTS				
Neurologic/central nervous system				
Computed tomographic or MRI scans of brain	X			X
MRI scans of spine	X			X
Median nerve conduction velocity	X			X
Cognitive testing (DQ/IQ)	X		X	
Auditory				
Audiometry	X		X	
Ophthalmologic				
Visual acuity	X		X	
Retinal examination	X		X	
Corneal examination	X		X	
Respiratory				
Forced vital capacity/forced expiratory volume	X	X		
Sleep study	X		X	
Cardiac				
Echocardiography	X			X
Electrocardiography	X			X

Continued

Table 82-4 RECOMMENDED MINIMAL SCHEDULE OF ASSESSMENTS FOR ALL PATIENTS WITH MPS I—cont'd

	INITIAL ASSESSMENTS	EVERY 6 MO	EVERY 12 MO	EVERY OTHER YEAR
Musculoskeletal				
Skeletal survey with radiographs*	X			X
Gastrointestinal				
Spleen volume†	X			X‡
Liver volume†	X			X‡
VITAL SIGNS AND LABORATORY TESTS				
Height and weight	X	X		
Head circumference*	X	X		
Blood pressure	X	X		
Enzyme activity level	X			
Urinary glycosaminoglycan level	X	X‡		
Urinalysis	X	X‡		
FUNCTIONAL OUTCOME MEASUREMENTS				
Mucopolysaccharidosis Health Assessment Questionnaire or other tools exploring functional ability and quality of life§	X		X	

This schedule of assessments addresses the core MPS I–related disease manifestations that are assessed to stage disease progression over the lifelong course of the disease. The schedule was adapted from the report by Pastores et al,[13] with permission. Physicians should determine the actual frequency of necessary assessments according to each patient's need for medical care and routine follow-up monitoring. See text for additional guidance on individualization of routine follow-up assessments. All tests requiring sedation are recommended only if sedation is considered to be safe for the patient.

*Studies are only for pediatric patients, unless determined otherwise by the treating physician.

†The recommended method for determining organ volumes is MRI or CT, to enable quantitative analysis. If it is unsafe to sedate the patient, in the opinion of the clinician, then ultrasonography may be substituted.

‡Studies are only for patients treated with ERT, unless determined otherwise by the treating physician.

§Assessment may not be possible for uncooperative patients or patients younger than 5 to 6 yr.

From Muenzer J, Wraith JE, Clare LA, et al: Mucopolysaccharidosis I: management and treatment guidelines, *Pediatrics* 123:19–29, 2009.

megaly and ameliorates rate of growth, joint mobility, and physical endurance. It also reduces the number of episodes of sleep apnea and urinary GAG excretion. The enzymes do not cross the blood-brain barrier and do not prevent deterioration of neurocognitive involvement. Consequently, this therapy is the domain for patients with mild central nervous involvement. To stabilize extraneural manifestations, it is also recommended in young patients before stem cell transplantation. The combination of enzyme replacement therapy and early stem cell transplantation may offer the best treatment. Recombinant iduronate-2-sulfatase ameliorates the non-neurologic manifestations of Hunter disease, and recombinant N-Ac-gal4-sulfatase has been successfully tested in patients with MPS VI.

Primary prevention through genetic counseling and tertiary prevention to avoid or treat complications remains the mainstay of supportive pediatric care. Multidisciplinary attention to respiratory and cardiovascular complications, hearing loss, carpal tunnel syndrome, spinal cord compression, hydrocephalus, and other problems can greatly improve the quality of life for patients and their families (Table 82-3). The progressive nature of clinical involvement in MPS patients dictates the need for specialized and coordinated evaluation (Table 82-4).

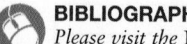

BIBLIOGRAPHY

Please visit the Nelson Textbook of Pediatrics *website at www.expertconsult.com for the complete bibliography.*

Chapter 83
Disorders of Purine and Pyrimidine Metabolism
James C. Harris

The inherited disorders of purine and pyrimidine metabolism cover a broad spectrum of illnesses with various presentations. These include hyperuricemia, acute renal failure, renal stones, gout, unexplained neurologic deficits (seizures, muscle weakness, choreoathetoid and dystonic movements), developmental disability, intellectual disability, compulsive self-injury and aggression, autistic-like behavior, unexplained anemia, failure to thrive, susceptibility to recurrent infection (immune deficiency), and deafness. When such disorders are identified, all family members should be screened.

For the full continuation of this chapter, please visit the Nelson Textbook of Pediatrics *website at www.expertconsult.com.*

Chapter 84
Progeria
Michael J. Painter

The Hutchinson-Gilford progeria syndrome (HGPS) is a rare, fatal, sporadic, autosomal dominant disorder with an incidence of ≈1/4,000,000 live births. HGPS is regarded as the most prominent of the senile-like appearance syndromes. Sexual maturation is incomplete and these patients do not reproduce. Parent to child transmission has not occurred. The most prominent features of HGPS are changes that simulate accelerated aging, the recognition of which establishes the diagnosis. Genetic diagnosis is available; HGPS is caused by a single base mutation in *LMNA*, which results in the production of a mutant lamin A, progerin. Progerin is found in increased concentration in fibroblasts of normal older compared to younger individuals, suggesting a role in normal aging. The mean age of survival of children with HGPS is 13 yr, with a range of 5 to 20 yr, such that there are approximately 40 patients world wide at any point in time. A study of 15 patients, about 40% of the world's population, revealed that all were heterozygous for the G608G mutation.

For the full continuation of this chapter, please visit the Nelson Textbook of Pediatrics *website at www.expertconsult.com.*

Chapter 85
The Porphyrias

Karl E. Anderson, Chul Lee, Manisha Balwani, and Robert J. Desnick

Porphyrias are metabolic diseases resulting from altered activities of specific enzymes of the heme biosynthetic pathway. These enzymes are most active in bone marrow and liver. Erythropoietic porphyrias, in which overproduction of heme pathway intermediates occurs primarily in bone marrow erythroid cells, usually present at birth or in early childhood with cutaneous photosensitivity, or in the case of congenital erythropoietic porphyria, even in utero as nonimmune hydrops. Most porphyrias are hepatic, with overproduction and initial accumulation of porphyrin precursors or porphyrins occurring 1st in the liver. Regulatory mechanisms for heme biosynthesis in liver are distinct from those in the bone marrow and appear to account for activation of hepatic porphyrias during adult life rather than childhood. Homozygous forms of the hepatic porphyrias may manifest clinically prior to puberty, and asymptomatic heterozygous children may present with nonspecific and unrelated symptoms. Parents often request advice about long-term prognosis and information about management of these disorders and drugs that can be taken safely to treat other common conditions.

For the full continuation of this chapter, please visit the Nelson Textbook of Pediatrics *website at www.expertconsult.com.*

Chapter 86
Hypoglycemia

Mark A. Sperling

Glucose has a central role in fuel economy and is a source of energy storage in the form of glycogen, fat, and protein (Chapter 81). Glucose, an immediate source of energy, provides 38 mol of adenosine triphosphate (ATP) per mol of glucose oxidized. It is essential for cerebral energy metabolism because it is usually the preferred substrate and its utilization accounts for nearly all the oxygen consumption in the brain. Cerebral glucose uptake occurs through a glucose transporter molecule or molecules that are not regulated by insulin. Cerebral transport of glucose is a carrier-mediated, facilitated diffusion process that is dependent on blood glucose concentration. Deficiency of brain glucose transporters can result in seizures because of low cerebral and cerebrospinal fluid (CSF) glucose concentrations (hypoglycorrhachia) despite normal blood glucose levels. To maintain the blood glucose concentration and prevent it from falling precipitously to levels that impair brain function, an elaborate regulatory system has evolved.

The defense against hypoglycemia is integrated by the autonomic nervous system and by hormones that act in concert to enhance glucose production through enzymatic modulation of glycogenolysis and gluconeogenesis while simultaneously limiting peripheral glucose utilization. Hypoglycemia represents a defect in one or several of the complex interactions that normally integrate glucose homeostasis during feeding and fasting. This process is particularly important for neonates, in whom there is an abrupt transition from intrauterine life, characterized by dependence on transplacental glucose supply, to extrauterine life, characterized ultimately by the autonomous ability to maintain euglycemia. Because prematurity or placental insufficiency may limit tissue nutrient deposits, and genetic abnormalities in enzymes or hormones may become evident in the neonate, hypoglycemia is common in the neonatal period.

DEFINITION

In neonates, there is not always an obvious correlation between blood glucose concentration and the classic clinical manifestations of hypoglycemia. The absence of symptoms does not indicate that glucose concentration is normal and has not fallen to less than some optimal level for maintaining brain metabolism. There is evidence that hypoxemia and ischemia may potentiate the role of hypoglycemia in causing permanent brain damage. Consequently, the lower limit of accepted normality of the blood glucose level in newborn infants with associated illness that already impairs cerebral metabolism has not been determined (Chapter 101). Out of concern for possible neurologic, intellectual, or psychologic sequelae in later life, most authorities recommend that any value of blood glucose <50 mg/dL in neonates be viewed with suspicion and vigorously treated. This is particularly applicable after the initial 2-3 hr of life, when glucose normally has reached its nadir; subsequently, blood glucose levels begin to rise and achieve values of 50 mg/dL or higher after 12-24 hr. In older infants and children, a whole blood glucose concentration of <50 mg/dL (10-15% higher for serum or plasma) represents hypoglycemia.

SIGNIFICANCE AND SEQUELAE

Metabolism by the adult brain accounts for the majority of total basal glucose turnover. Most of the endogenous hepatic glucose production in infants and young children can be accounted for by brain metabolism.

Because the brain grows most rapidly in the 1st yr of life and because the larger proportion of glucose turnover is used for brain metabolism, sustained or repetitive hypoglycemia in infants and children can retard brain development and function. Transient isolated and asymptomatic hypoglycemia of short duration does not appear to be associated with these severe sequelae. In the rapidly growing brain, glucose may also be a source of membrane lipids and, together with protein synthesis it can provide structural proteins and myelination that are important for normal brain maturation. Under conditions of severe and sustained hypoglycemia, these cerebral structural substrates may become degraded to energy-usable intermediates such as lactate, pyruvate, amino acids, and ketoacids, which can support brain metabolism at the expense of brain growth. The capacity of the newborn brain to take up and oxidize ketone bodies is about 5-fold greater than that of the adult brain. The capacity of the liver to produce ketone bodies may be limited in the newborn period, especially in the presence of hyperinsulinemia, which acutely inhibits hepatic glucose output, lipolysis, and ketogenesis, thereby depriving the brain of any alternate fuel sources. Although the brain may metabolize ketones, these alternate fuels cannot completely replace glucose as an essential central nervous system (CNS) fuel. The deprivation of the brain's major energy source during hypoglycemia and the limited availability of alternate fuel sources during hyperinsulinemia have predictable adverse consequences on brain metabolism and growth: decreased brain oxygen consumption and increased breakdown of endogenous structural components with destruction of functional membrane integrity.

The major long-term sequelae of severe, prolonged hypoglycemia are mental retardation, recurrent seizure activity, or both. Subtle effects on personality are also possible but have not been clearly defined. Permanent neurologic sequelae are present in 25-50% of patients with severe recurrent symptomatic hypoglycemia who are younger than 6 mo of age. These sequelae may be reflected in pathologic changes characterized by atrophic gyri, reduced myelination in cerebral white matter, and atrophy in the cerebral cortex. These sequelae are more likely when alternative fuel sources are limited, as occurs with hyperinsulinemia, when the episodes of hypoglycemia are repetitive or prolonged, or when they are compounded by hypoxia. There is no precise knowledge relating the duration or severity of hypoglycemia to subsequent neurologic development of children in a predictable manner. Although less common, hypoglycemia in older children may also produce long-term neurologic defects through neuronal death mediated, in part, by cerebral excitotoxins released during hypoglycemia.

SUBSTRATE, ENZYME, AND HORMONAL INTEGRATION OF GLUCOSE HOMEOSTASIS

In the Newborn (Chapter 101)

Under nonstressed conditions, fetal glucose is derived entirely from the mother through placental transfer. Therefore, fetal glucose concentration usually reflects but is slightly lower than maternal glucose levels. Catecholamine release, which occurs with fetal stress such as hypoxia, mobilizes fetal glucose and free fatty acids (FFAs) through β-adrenergic mechanisms, reflecting β-adrenergic activity in fetal liver and adipose tissue. Catecholamines may also inhibit fetal insulin and stimulate glucagon release.

The acute interruption of maternal glucose transfer to the fetus at delivery imposes an immediate need to mobilize endogenous glucose. Three related events facilitate this transition: changes in hormones, changes in their receptors, and changes in key enzyme activity. There is a 3- to 5-fold abrupt increase in glucagon concentration within minutes to hours of birth. The level of insulin usually falls initially and remains in the basal range for several days without demonstrating the usual brisk response to physiologic stimuli such as glucose. A dramatic surge in spontaneous catecholamine secretion is also characteristic. Epinephrine can also augment growth hormone secretion by α-adrenergic mechanisms; growth hormone levels are elevated at birth. Acting in concert, these hormonal changes at birth mobilize glucose via glycogenolysis and gluconeogenesis, activate lipolysis, and promote ketogenesis. As a result of these processes, plasma glucose concentration stabilizes after a transient decrease immediately after birth, liver glycogen stores become rapidly depleted within hours of birth, and gluconeogenesis from alanine, a major gluconeogenic amino acid, can account for about 10% of glucose turnover in the human newborn infant by several hours of age. FFA concentrations also increase sharply in concert with the surges in glucagon and epinephrine and are followed by rises in ketone bodies. Glucose is thus partially spared for brain utilization while FFAs and ketones provide alternative fuel sources for muscle as well as essential gluconeogenic factors such as acetyl coenzyme A (CoA) and the reduced form of nicotinamide-adenine dinucleotide (NADH) from hepatic fatty acid oxidation, which is required to drive gluconeogenesis.

In the early postnatal period, responses of the endocrine pancreas favor glucagon secretion so that blood glucose concentration can be maintained. These adaptive changes in hormone secretion are paralleled by similarly striking adaptive changes in hormone receptors. Key enzymes involved in glucose production also change dramatically in the perinatal period. Thus, there is a rapid fall in glycogen synthase activity and a sharp rise in phosphorylase after delivery. Similarly, the amount of rate-limiting enzyme for gluconeogenesis, phosphoenolpyruvate carboxykinase, rises dramatically after birth, activated in part by the surge in glucagon and the fall in insulin. This framework can explain several causes of neonatal hypoglycemia based on inappropriate changes in hormone secretion and unavailability of adequate reserves of substrates in the form of hepatic glycogen, muscle as a source of amino acids for gluconeogenesis, and lipid stores for the release of fatty acids. In addition, appropriate activities of key enzymes governing glucose homeostasis are required (see Fig. 81-1).

In Older Infants and Children

Hypoglycemia in older infants and children is analogous to that of adults, in whom glucose homeostasis is maintained by glycogenolysis in the immediate postfeeding period and by gluconeogenesis several hours after meals. The liver of a 10 kg child contains 20-25 g of glycogen, which is sufficient to meet normal glucose requirements of 4-6 mg/kg/min for only 6-12 hr. Beyond this period, hepatic gluconeogenesis must be activated. Both glycogenolysis and gluconeogenesis depend on the metabolic pathway summarized in Figure 81-1. Defects in glycogenolysis or gluconeogenesis may not be manifested in infants until the frequent feeding at 3-4 hr intervals ceases and infants sleep through the night, a situation usually present by 3-6 mo of age. The source of gluconeogenic precursors is derived primarily from muscle protein. The muscle bulk of infants and small children is substantially smaller relative to body mass than that of adults, whereas glucose requirements/unit of body mass are greater in children, so the ability to compensate for glucose deprivation by gluconeogenesis is more limited in infants and young children, as is the ability to withstand fasting for prolonged periods. The ability of muscle to generate alanine, the principal gluconeogenic amino acid, may also be limited. Thus, in normal young children, the blood glucose level falls after 24 hr of fasting, insulin concentrations fall appropriately to levels of <5-10 μU/mL, lipolysis and ketogenesis are activated, and ketones may appear in the urine.

The switch from glycogen synthesis during and immediately after meals to glycogen breakdown and later gluconeogenesis is governed by hormones, of which insulin is of central importance. Plasma insulin concentrations increase to peak levels of 50-100 μU/mL after meals, which serve to lower the blood glucose concentration through the activation of glycogen synthesis, enhancement of peripheral glucose uptake, and inhibition of glucose production. In addition, lipogenesis is stimulated, whereas lipolysis and ketogenesis are curtailed. During fasting, plasma insulin concentrations fall to ≤5-10 μU/mL, and together with other hormonal changes, this fall results in activation of gluconeogenic pathways (see Fig. 81-1). Fasting glucose concentrations are maintained through the activation of glycogenolysis and gluconeogenesis, inhibition of glycogen synthesis, and activation of lipolysis and ketogenesis. It should be emphasized that a plasma insulin concentration of >5 μU/mL, in association with a blood glucose concentration of ≤40 mg/dL (2.2 mM), is abnormal, indicating a **hyperinsulinemic state** and failure of the mechanisms that normally result in suppression of insulin secretion during fasting or hypoglycemia.

The hypoglycemic effects of insulin are opposed by the actions of several hormones whose concentration in plasma increases as blood glucose falls. These **counter-regulatory hormones**, glucagon, growth hormone, cortisol, and epinephrine, act in concert by increasing blood glucose concentrations via activating glycogenolytic enzymes (glucagon, epinephrine); inducing gluconeogenic enzymes (glucagon, cortisol); inhibiting glucose uptake by muscle (epinephrine, growth hormone, cortisol); mobilizing amino acids from muscle for gluconeogenesis (cortisol); activating lipolysis and thereby providing glycerol for gluconeogenesis and fatty acids for ketogenesis (epinephrine, cortisol, growth hormone, glucagon); and inhibiting insulin release and promoting growth hormone and glucagon secretion (epinephrine).

Congenital or acquired deficiency of any one of these hormones is uncommon but will result in hypoglycemia, which occurs when endogenous glucose production cannot be mobilized to meet energy needs in the postabsorptive state, that is, 8-12 hr after meals or during fasting. Concurrent deficiency of several hormones (**hypopituitarism**) may result in hypoglycemia that is more severe or appears earlier during fasting than that seen with isolated hormone deficiencies. Most of the causes of hypoglycemia in infancy and childhood reflect inappropriate adaptation to fasting.

CLINICAL MANIFESTATIONS (CHAPTER 101)

Clinical features generally fall into 2 categories. The 1st includes symptoms associated with the activation of the autonomic

Table 86-1 MANIFESTATIONS OF HYPOGLYCEMIA IN CHILDHOOD

FEATURES ASSOCIATED WITH ACTIVATION OF AUTONOMIC NERVOUS SYSTEM AND EPINEPHRINE RELEASE*
Anxiety†
Perspiration†
Palpitation (tachycardia)†
Pallor
Tremulousness
Weakness
Hunger
Nausea
Emesis
Angina (with normal coronary arteries)
FEATURES ASSOCIATED WITH CEREBRAL GLUCOPENIA
Headache†
Mental confusion†
Visual disturbances (↓ acuity, diplopia)†
Organic personality changes†
Inability to concentrate†
Dysarthria
Staring
Paresthesias
Dizziness
Amnesia
Ataxia, incoordination
Somnolence, lethargy
Seizures
Coma
Stroke, hemiplegia, aphasia
Decerebrate or decorticate posture

*Some of these features will be attenuated if the patient is receiving β-adrenergic blocking agents.
†Common.

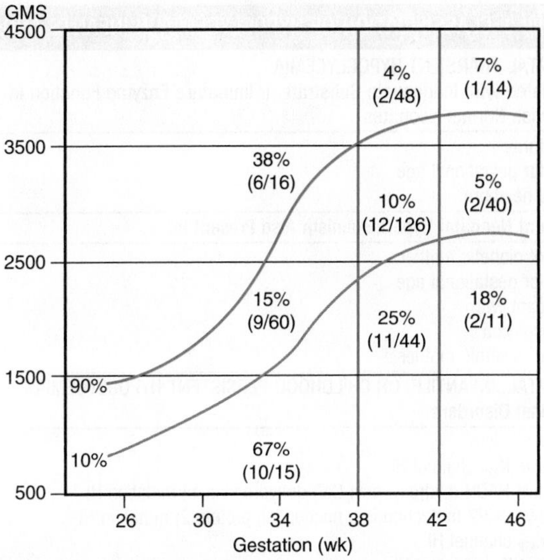

Figure 86-1 Incidence of hypoglycemia by birthweight, gestational age, and intrauterine growth. (From Lubchenco LO, Bard H: Incidence of hypoglycemia in newborn infants classified by birthweight and gestational age, *Pediatrics* 47:831–838, 1971.)

nervous system and epinephrine release, usually seen with a rapid decline in blood glucose concentration (Table 86-1). The 2nd category includes symptoms due to decreased cerebral glucose utilization, usually associated with a slow decline in blood glucose level or prolonged hypoglycemia (see Table 86-1). Although these classic symptoms occur in older children, the symptoms of hypoglycemia in infants may be subtler and include cyanosis, apnea, hypothermia, hypotonia, poor feeding, lethargy, and seizures. Some of these symptoms may be so mild that they are missed. Occasionally, hypoglycemia may be asymptomatic in the immediate newborn period. Newborns with hyperinsulinemia are often large for gestational age; older infants with hyperinsulinemia may eat excessively because of chronic hypoglycemia and become obese. In childhood, hypoglycemia may present as behavior problems, inattention, ravenous appetite, or seizures. It may be misdiagnosed as epilepsy, inebriation, personality disorders, hysteria, and retardation. A blood glucose determination should always be performed in sick neonates, who should be vigorously treated if concentrations are <50 mg/dL. At any age level, hypoglycemia should be considered a cause of an initial episode of convulsions or a sudden deterioration in psychobehavioral functioning.

Many neonates have asymptomatic (chemical) hypoglycemia. The incidence of symptomatic hypoglycemia is highest in small for gestational age infants (Fig. 86-1). The exact incidence of symptomatic hypoglycemia has been difficult to establish because many of the symptoms in neonates occur **together** with other conditions such as infections, especially sepsis and meningitis; central nervous system anomalies, hemorrhage, or edema; hypocalcemia and hypomagnesemia; asphyxia; drug withdrawal; apnea of prematurity; congenital heart disease; or polycythemia.

The onset of symptoms in neonates varies from a few hr to a wk after birth. In approximate order of frequency, symptoms include jitteriness or tremors, apathy, episodes of cyanosis, convulsions, intermittent apneic spells or tachypnea, weak or high-pitched cry, limpness or lethargy, difficulty feeding, and eye rolling. Episodes of sweating, sudden pallor, hypothermia, and cardiac arrest and failure also occur. Frequently, a clustering of episodic symptoms may be noted. Because these clinical manifestations may result from various causes, it is critical to measure serum glucose levels and determine whether they disappear with the administration of sufficient glucose to raise the blood sugar to normal levels; if they do not, other diagnoses must be considered.

CLASSIFICATION OF HYPOGLYCEMIA IN INFANTS AND CHILDREN

Classification is based on knowledge of the control of glucose homeostasis in infants and children (Table 86-2).

Neonatal, Transient, Small for Gestational Age, and Premature Infants (Chapter 101)

The estimated incidence of symptomatic hypoglycemia in newborns is 1-3/1,000 live births. This incidence is increased severalfold in certain high-risk neonatal groups (see Table 86-2 and Fig. 86-1). The premature and small for gestational age (SGA) infants are vulnerable to the development of hypoglycemia. The factors responsible for the high frequency of hypoglycemia in this group, as well as in other groups outlined in Table 86-2, are related to the inadequate stores of liver glycogen, muscle protein, and body fat needed to sustain the substrates required to meet energy needs. These infants are small by virtue of prematurity or impaired placental transfer of nutrients. Their enzyme systems for gluconeogenesis may not be fully developed. Transient hyperinsulinism responsive to diazoxide has also been reported as contributing to hypoglycemia in asphyxiated, SGA, and premature newborn infants. This form of hyperinsulinism associated with perinatal asphyxia, intrauterine growth restriction (IUGR), maternal toxemia and other perinatal stressors, is probably the most common cause of hyperinsulinemic hypoglycemia in neonates and may be quite severe. In most cases, the condition resolves quickly, but it may persist to 7 mo of life or more. A genetic cause of this form of dysregulated insulin secretion has not been established.

In contrast to deficiency of substrates or enzymes, the hormonal system appears to be functioning normally at birth in most low-risk neonates. Despite hypoglycemia, plasma concentrations of alanine, lactate, and pyruvate are higher, implying their

Table 86-2 CLASSIFICATION OF HYPOGLYCEMIA IN INFANTS AND CHILDREN

NEONATAL TRANSIENT HYPOGLYCEMIA
Associated with Inadequate Substrate or Immature Enzyme Function in Otherwise Normal Neonates
Prematurity
Small for gestational age
Normal newborn
Transient Neonatal Hyperinsulinism Also Present in:
Infant of diabetic mother
Small for gestational age
Discordant twin
Birth asphyxia
Infant of toxemic mother
NEONATAL, INFANTILE, OR CHILDHOOD PERSISTENT HYPOGLYCEMIAS
Hormonal Disorders
Hyperinsulinism
Recessive K_{ATP} channel HI
Recessive HADH (hydroxyl acyl CoA dehydrogenase) mutation HI
Recessive UCP2 (mitochondrial uncoupling protein 2) mutation HI
Focal K_{ATP} channel HI
Dominant K_{ATP} channel HI
Dominant glucokinase HI
Dominant glutamate dehydrogenase HI (hyperinsulinism/hyperammonemia syndrome)
Dominant mutation in HNF4A (hepatic nuclear factor 4 alpha) HI with MODY later in life
Dominant mutation in SLC16A1(the pyruvate transporter)-exercise-induced hypoglycemia
Acquired islet adenoma
Beckwith-Wiedemann syndrome
Insulin administration (Munchausen syndrome by proxy)
Oral sulfonylurea drugs
Congenital disorders of glycosylation
Counter-Regulatory Hormone Deficiency
Panhypopituitarism
Isolated growth hormone deficiency
Adrenocorticotropic hormone deficiency
Addison disease
Epinephrine deficiency
Glycogenolysis and Gluconeogenesis Disorders
Glucose-6-phosphatase deficiency (GSD 1a)
Glucose-6-phosphate translocase deficiency (GSD 1b)
Amylo-1,6-glucosidase (debranching enzyme) deficiency (GSD 3)
Liver phosphorylase deficiency (GSD 6)
Phosphorylase kinase deficiency (GSD 9)
Glycogen synthetase deficiency (GSD 0)
Fructose-1,6-diphosphatase deficiency
Pyruvate carboxylase deficiency
Galactosemia
Hereditary fructose intolerance
Lipolysis Disorders
Fatty Acid Oxidation Disorders
Carnitine transporter deficiency (primary carnitine deficiency)
Carnitine palmitoyltransferase-1 deficiency
Carnitine translocase deficiency
Carnitine palmitoyltransferase-2 deficiency
Secondary carnitine deficiencies
Very long, long-, medium-, short-chain acyl CoA dehydrogenase deficiency
OTHER ETIOLOGIES
Substrate-Limited
Ketotic hypoglycemia
Poisoning—drugs
Salicylates
Alcohol
Oral hypoglycemic agents
Insulin
Propranolol
Pentamidine
Quinine
Disopyramide
Ackee fruit (unripe)—hypoglycin
Vacor (rate poison)
Trimethoprim-sulfamethoxazole (with renal failure)
Liver Disease
Reye syndrome
Hepatitis
Cirrhosis
Hepatoma
Amino Acid and Organic Acid Disorders
Maple syrup urine disease
Propionic acidemia
Methylmalonic acidemia
Tyrosinosis
Glutaric aciduria
3-Hydroxy-3-methylglutaric aciduria
Systemic Disorders
Sepsis
Carcinoma/sarcoma (secreting—insulin-like growth factor II)
Heart failure
Malnutrition
Malabsorption
Anti-insulin receptor antibodies
Anti-insulin antibodies
Neonatal hyperviscosity
Renal failure
Diarrhea
Burns
Shock
Postsurgical
Pseudohypoglycemia (leukocytosis, polycythemia)
Excessive insulin therapy of insulin-dependent diabetes mellitus
Factitious
Nissen fundoplication (dumping syndrome)
Falciparum malaria

GSD, glycogen storage disease; HI, hyperinsulinemia; K_{ATP}, regulated potassium channel.

diminished rate of utilization as substrates for gluconeogenesis. Infusion of alanine elicits further glucagon secretion but causes no significant rise in glucose. During the initial 24 hr of life, plasma concentrations of acetoacetate and β-hydroxybutyrate are lower in SGA infants than in full-term infants, implying diminished lipid stores, diminished fatty acid mobilization, impaired ketogenesis, or a combination of these conditions. Diminished lipid stores are most likely because fat (triglyceride) feeding of newborns results in a rise in the plasma levels of glucose, FFAs, and ketones. For infants with perinatal asphyxia and some SGA newborns who have transient hyperinsulinemia, hypoglycemia and diminished concentrations of FFAs are the hallmark of hyperinsulinemia.

The role of FFAs and their oxidation in stimulating neonatal gluconeogenesis is essential. The provision of FFAs as triglyceride feedings from formula or human milk together with gluconeogenic precursors may prevent the hypoglycemia that usually ensues after neonatal fasting. For these and other reasons, milk feedings are introduced early (at birth or within 2-4 hr) after delivery. In the hospital setting, when feeding is precluded by virtue of respiratory distress or when feedings alone cannot maintain blood glucose concentrations at levels >50 mg/dL, intravenous glucose at a rate that supplies 4-8 mg/kg/min should be started. Infants with transient neonatal hypoglycemia can usually maintain the blood glucose level spontaneously after 2-3 days of life, but some require longer periods of support. In these latter infants, insulin values >5 μU/ml at the time of hypoglycemia should be treated with diazoxide.

Infants Born to Diabetic Mothers (Chapter 101)

Of the transient hyperinsulinemic states, infants born to diabetic mothers are the most common. Gestational diabetes affects some 2% of pregnant women, and ≈1/1,000 pregnant women have insulin-dependent diabetes. At birth, infants born to these mothers may be large and plethoric, and their body stores of glycogen, protein, and fat are replete.

Hypoglycemia in infants of diabetic mothers is mostly related to hyperinsulinemia and partly related to diminished glucagon secretion. Hypertrophy and hyperplasia of the islets is present, as is a brisk, biphasic, and typically mature insulin response to glucose; this insulin response is absent in normal infants. Infants born to diabetic mothers also have a subnormal surge in plasma glucagon immediately after birth, subnormal glucagon secretion in response to stimuli, and, initially, excessive sympathetic activity that may lead to adrenomedullary exhaustion as reflected by decreased urinary excretion of epinephrine. The normal plasma hormonal pattern of low insulin, high glucagon, and high catecholamines is reversed to a pattern of high insulin, low glucagon, and low epinephrine. As a consequence of this abnormal hormonal profile, the endogenous glucose production is significantly inhibited compared with that in normal infants, thus predisposing them to hypoglycemia.

Mothers whose diabetes has been well controlled during pregnancy, labor, and delivery generally have infants near normal size who are less likely to develop neonatal hypoglycemia and other complications formerly considered typical of such infants (Chapter 101). In supplying exogenous glucose to these hypoglycemic infants, it is important to avoid hyperglycemia that evokes a prompt exuberant insulin release, which may result in rebound hypoglycemia. When needed, glucose should be provided at continuous infusion rates of 4-8 mg/kg/min, but the appropriate dose for each patient should be individually adjusted. During labor and delivery, maternal hyperglycemia should be avoided because it results in fetal hyperglycemia, which predisposes to hypoglycemia when the glucose supply is interrupted at birth. Hypoglycemia persisting or occurring after 1 wk of life requires an evaluation for the causes listed in Table 86-2.

Infants born with **erythroblastosis fetalis** may also have hyperinsulinemia and share many physical features, such as large body size, with infants born to diabetic mothers. The cause of the hyperinsulinemia in infants with erythroblastosis is not clear.

PERSISTENT OR RECURRENT HYPOGLYCEMIA IN INFANTS AND CHILDREN

Hyperinsulinism

Most children with hyperinsulinism that causes hypoglycemia present in the neonatal period or later in infancy; hyperinsulinism is the most common cause of persistent hypoglycemia in early infancy. Hyperinsulinemic infants may be macrosomic at birth, reflecting the anabolic effects of insulin in utero. There is no history or biochemical evidence of maternal diabetes. The onset is from birth to 18 mo of age, but occasionally it is 1st evident in older children. Insulin concentrations are inappropriately elevated at the time of documented hypoglycemia; with non-hyperinsulinemic hypoglycemia, plasma insulin concentrations should be <5 μU/mL and no higher than 10 μU/mL. In affected infants, plasma insulin concentrations at the time of hypoglycemia are commonly >5-10 μU/mL. Some authorities set more stringent criteria, arguing that any value of insulin >2 μU/mL with hypoglycemia is abnormal. The insulin (μU/mL):glucose (mg/dL) ratio is commonly >0.4; plasma insulin-like growth factor binding protein-1 (IGFBP-1), ketones, and FFA levels are low with hyperinsulinemia. Macrosomic infants may present with hypoglycemia from the 1st days of life. Infants with lesser degrees of hyperinsulinemia may manifest hypoglycemia after the 1st few weeks to months, when the frequency of feedings has been decreased to permit the infant to sleep through the night and hyperinsulinism prevents the mobilization of endogenous glucose. Increasing appetite and demands for feeding, wilting spells, jitteriness, and frank seizures are the most common presenting features. Additional clues include the rapid development of fasting hypoglycemia within 4-8 hr of food deprivation compared with other causes of hypoglycemia (Tables 86-3 and 86-4); the need for high rates of exogenous glucose infusion to prevent hypoglycemia, often at rates >10-15 mg/kg/min; the absence of ketonemia or acidosis; and elevated C-peptide or proinsulin levels at the time of hypoglycemia. The latter insulin-related products are absent in **factitious hypoglycemia** from exogenous administration of insulin as a form of child abuse (Munchausen by proxy syndrome) (Chapter 37.2). Hypoglycemia is invariably provoked by withholding feedings for several hours, permitting simultaneous measurement of glucose, insulin, ketones, and FFAs in the same sample at the time of clinically manifested hypoglycemia. This is termed the "**critical sample.**" The glycemic response to glucagon at the time of hypoglycemia reveals a brisk increment in glucose concentration of at least 40 mg/dL, which implies that glucose mobilization has been restrained by insulin but that glycogenolytic mechanisms are intact (Tables 86-5, 86-6, and 86-7).

Table 86-3 HYPOGLYCEMIA IN INFANTS AND CHILDREN: CLINICAL AND LABORATORY FEATURES

GROUP	AGE AT DIAGNOSIS (mo)	GLUCOSE (mg/dL)	INSULIN (μU/mL)	FASTING TIME TO HYPOGLYCEMIA (hr)
HYPERINSULINEMIA (*N* = 12)				
Mean	7.4	23.1	22.4	2.1
SEM	2.0	2.7	3.2	0.6
NONHYPERINSULINEMIA (*N* = 16)				
Mean	41.8	36.1	5.8	18.2
SEM	7.3	2.4	0.9	2.9

Adapted from Antunes JD, Geffner ME, Lippe BM, et al: Childhood hypoglycemia: differentiating hyperinsulinemic from nonhyperinsulinemic causes, *J Pediatr* 116:105–108, 1990.

The measurement of serum IGFBP-1 concentration may help diagnose hyperinsulinemia. The secretion of IGFBP-1 is acutely inhibited by insulin; IGFBP-1 concentrations are low during hyperinsulinism-induced hypoglycemia. In patients with spontaneous or fasting-induced hypoglycemia with a low insulin level (ketotic hypoglycemia, normal fasting), IGFBP-1 concentrations are significantly higher.

The differential diagnosis of endogenous hyperinsulinism includes **diffuse β-cell hyperplasia or focal β-cell microadenoma.** The distinction between these 2 major entities is important because the former, if unresponsive to medical therapy requires near total pancreatectomy, despite which hypoglycemia may persist or diabetes mellitus may ensue at some later time. By contrast, focal adenomas diagnosed preoperatively or intraoperatively permit localized curative resection with subsequent normal glucose metabolism. About 50% of the autosomal recessive or sporadic forms of neonatal/infantile hyperinsulinism are due to focal microadenomas, which may be distinguished from the diffuse form by the pattern of insulin response to selective insulin secretagogues infused into an artery supplying the pancreas with sampling via the hepatic vein. However, these invasive and difficult procedures have been largely abandoned in favor of positron emission tomography (PET scanning) using 18-fluoro-L-dopa.

Table 86-4 CORRELATION OF CLINICAL FEATURES WITH MOLECULAR DEFECTS IN PERSISTENT HYPERINSULINEMIC HYPOGLYCEMIA IN INFANCY

TYPE	MACROSOMIA	HYPOGLYCEMIA/ HYPERINSULINEMIA	FAMILY HISTORY	MOLECULAR DEFECTS	ASSOCIATED CLINICAL, BIOCHEMICAL, OR MOLECULAR FEATURES	RESPONSE TO MEDICAL MANAGEMENT	RECOMMENDED SURGICAL APPROACH	PROGNOSIS
Sporadic	Present at birth	Moderate/severe in 1st days to weeks of life	Negative	? *SUR1*/K_{IR}6.2 Mutations not always identified in diffuse hyperplasia	Loss of heterozygosity in microadenomatous tissue	Generally poor; may respond better to somatostatin than to diazoxide	Partial pancreatectomy if frozen section shows β-cell crowding with small nuclei—suggests microadenoma Subtotal >95% pancreatectomy if frozen section shows giant nuclei in β-cells—suggests diffuse hyperplasia	Excellent if focal adenoma is removed, thereby curing hypoglycemia and retaining sufficient pancreas to avoid diabetes Guarded if subtotal (>95%) pancreatectomy is performed because diabetes develops in ½, and hypoglycemia persists in ⅓
Autosomal recessive	Present at birth	Severe in 1st days to weeks of life	Positive	*SUR*/K_{IR}6.2	Consanguinity a feature in some populations	Poor	Subtotal pancreatectomy	Guarded
Autosomal dominant	Unusual	Moderate onset usually post 6 mo of age	Positive	Glucokinase (activating) Some cases gene unknown	None	Very good to excellent	Surgery usually not required Partial pancreatectomy only if medical management fails	Excellent
Autosomal dominant	Unusual	Moderate onset usually post 6 mo of age	Positive	Glutamate dehydrogenase (activating)	Modest hyperammonemia	Very good to excellent	Surgery usually not required	Excellent
Beckwith-Wiedemann syndrome	Present at birth	Moderate, spontaneously resolves post 6 mo of age	Negative	Duplicating/ imprinting in chromosome 11p15.1	Macroglossia, omphalocele, hemihypertrophy	Good	Not recommended	Excellent for hypoglycemia; embryonal tumors (Wilms hepatoblastoma)
Congenital disorders of glycosylation	Not usual	Moderate/onset post 3 mo of age	Negative	Phosphomannose isomerase deficiency	Hepatomegaly, vomiting, intractable diarrhea	Good with mannose supplement	Not recommended	Fair

Table 86-5 ANALYSIS OF CRITICAL BLOOD SAMPLE DURING HYPOGLYCEMIA AND 30 MINUTES AFTER GLUCAGON*

SUBSTRATES	HORMONES
Glucose	Insulin
Free fatty acids	Cortisol
Ketones	Growth hormone
Lactate	Thyroxine, thyroid-stimulating hormone
Uric acid	IGFBP-1†
Ammonia	

IGFBP-1, insulin-like growth factor binding protein-1.
*Glucagon 50 μg/kg with maximum of 1 mg IV or IM.
†Measure once only before or after glucagon administration. Rise in glucose of ≥40 mg/dL after glucagon given at the time of hypoglycemia strongly suggests a hyperinsulinemic state with adequate hepatic glycogen stores and intact glycogenolytic enzymes. If ammonia is elevated to 100-200 μM, consider activating mutation of glutamate dehydrogenase.

Table 86-6 CRITERIA FOR DIAGNOSING HYPERINSULINISM BASED ON "CRITICAL" SAMPLES (DRAWN AT A TIME OF FASTING HYPOGLYCEMIA: PLASMA GLUCOSE <50 MG/DL)

1. Hyperinsulinemia (plasma insulin >2 μU/mL)*
2. Hypofattyacidemia (plasma free fatty acids <1.5 mmol/L)
3. Hypoketonemia (plasma β-hydroxybutyrate: <2.0 mmol/L)
4. Inappropriate glycemic response to glucagon, 1 mg IV (delta glucose >40 mg/dL)

*Depends on sensitivity of insulin assay.
From Stanley CA, Thomson PS, Finegold DN, et al: Hypoglycemia in infants and neonates. In Sperling MA, editor: *Pediatric endocrinology*, ed 2, Philadelphia, 2002, WB Saunders, pp 135–159.

This technique can distinguish the diffuse form (uniform fluorescence throughout the pancreas) from the focal form (focal uptake of 18-fluoro-L-dopa and localized fluorescence) with an extremely high degree of reliability, success, specificity, and sensitivity (see below).

Insulin-secreting macroadenomas are rare in childhood and may be diagnosed preoperatively via CT or MRI. The plasma levels of insulin alone, however, cannot distinguish the aforementioned entities. The diffuse or microadenomatous forms of islet cell hyperplasia represent a variety of genetic defects responsible for abnormalities in the endocrine pancreas characterized by autonomous insulin secretion that is not appropriately reduced when blood glucose declines spontaneously or in response to provocative maneuvers such as fasting (see Tables 86-4, 86-7, and 86-8 and Fig. 86-2). Clinical, biochemical, and molecular genetic approaches now permit classification of congenital hyperinsulinism, formerly termed **nesidioblastosis,** into distinct entities. **Persistent hyperinsulinemic hypoglycemia of infancy (PHHI)** may be inherited or sporadic, is severe, and is caused by mutations in the regulation of the potassium channel intimately involved in insulin secretion by the pancreatic β cell (Fig. 86-2). Normally, glucose entry into the β cell is enabled by the non–insulin-responsive glucose transporter GLUT-2. On entry, glucose

Table 86-7 DIAGNOSIS OF ACUTE HYPOGLYCEMIA IN INFANTS AND CHILDREN

ACUTE SYMPTOMS PRESENT
1. Obtain blood sample before and 30 min after glucagon administration. 2. Obtain urine as soon as possible. Examine for ketones; if not present and hypoglycemia confirmed, suspect hyperinsulinemia or fatty acid oxidation defect; if present, suspect ketotic, hormone deficiency, inborn error of glycogen metabolism, or defective gluconeogenesis. 3. Measure glucose in the original blood sample. If hypoglycemia is confirmed, proceed with substrate-hormone measurement as in Table 86-5. 4. If glycemic increment after glucagon exceeds 40 mg/dL above basal, suspect hyperinsulinemia. 5. If insulin level at time of confirmed hypoglycemia is >5 μU/mL, suspect endogenous hyperinsulinemia; if >100 μU/mL, suspect factitious hyperinsulinemia (exogenous insulin injection). Admit to hospital for supervised fast. 6. If cortisol is <10 μg/dL or growth hormone is <5 ng/mL, or both, suspect adrenal insufficiency or pituitary disease, or both. Admit to hospital for hormonal testing and neuroimaging.
HISTORY SUGGESTIVE: ACUTE SYMPTOMS NOT PRESENT
1. Careful history for relation of symptoms to time and type of food intake, bearing in mind age of patient. Exclude possibility of alcohol or drug ingestion. Assess possibility of insulin injection, salt craving, growth velocity, intracranial pathology. 2. Careful examination for hepatomegaly (glycogen storage disease; defect in gluconeogenesis); pigmentation (adrenal failure); stature and neurologic status (pituitary disease) 3. Admit to hospital for provocative testing: a. 24 hr fast under careful observation; when symptoms provoked, proceed with steps 1-4 as when acute symptoms present b. Pituitary-adrenal function using arginine-insulin stimulation test if indicated 4. Liver biopsy for histologic and enzyme determinations if indicated 5. Oral glucose tolerance test (1.75 g/kg; max 75 g) if reactive hypoglycemia suspected (dumping syndrome, etc.).

is phosphorylated to glucose-6-phosphate by the enzyme glucokinase, enabling glucose metabolism to generate ATP. The rise in the molar ratio of ATP relative to adenosine diphosphate (ADP) closes the ATP-sensitive potassium channel in the cell membrane (K_{ATP} channel). This channel is composed of two subunits, the K_{IR} 6.2 channel, part of the family of inward-rectifier potassium channels, and a regulatory component in intimate association with K_{IR} 6.2 known as the sulfonylurea receptor (SUR). Together, K_{IR} 6.2 and SUR constitute the potassium-sensitive ATP channel K_{ATP}. Normally, the K_{ATP} is open, but with the rise in ATP and closure of the channel, potassium accumulates intracellularly, causing depolarization of the membrane, opening of voltage-gated calcium channels, influx of calcium into the cytoplasm, and secretion of insulin via exocytosis. The genes for both SUR and K_{IR} 6.2 are located close together on the short arm of chromosome 11, the site of the insulin gene. **Inactivating** mutations in the gene for SUR or, less often, K_{IR} 6.2 prevent the potassium channel from opening. It remains essentially variably closed with constant depolarization and, therefore, constant inward flux of calcium; hence, insulin secretion is continuous. A milder autosomal dominant form of these defects is also reported. Likewise, an **activating** mutation in glucokinase or glutamate dehydrogenase results in closure of the potassium channel through overproduction of ATP and hyperinsulinism. Recently, genetic defects in fatty acid metabolism, in the insulin transcription factor HNF4alpha, and in the uncoupling protein UCP-2 of the mitochondrial gene complex also have been involved in hyperinsulinemic hypoglycemia. **Inactivating** mutations of the glucokinase gene or **activating** mutations of the ATP regulated potassium channel which prevent or limit closure of the channel, are responsible for inadequate insulin secretion and form the basis of some forms of maturity-onset diabetes of youth or of neonatal diabetes mellitus (Chapter 583).

The familial forms of PHHI are more common in certain populations, notably Arabic and Ashkenazi Jewish communities, where it may reach an incidence of about 1/2,500, compared with the sporadic rates in the general population of ≈1/50,000. These **autosomal recessive forms** of PHHI typically present in the immediate newborn period as macrosomic newborns with a weight >4.0 kg and severe recurrent or persistent hypoglycemia manifesting in the initial hours or days of life. Glucose infusions as high as 15-20 mg/kg/min and frequent feedings fail to maintain euglycemia. Diazoxide, which acts by opening K_{ATP} channels (see Fig. 86-2), fails to control hypoglycemia adequately. Somatostatin, which also opens K_{ATP} and inhibits calcium flux, may be partially effective in about 50% of patients (see Fig. 86-2). Calcium channel blocking agents have had inconsistent effects. When affected patients are unresponsive to these measures, pancreatectomy is strongly recommended to avoid the long-term neurologic sequelae of hypoglycemia. If surgery is undertaken, preoperative CT or MRI rarely reveals an isolated adenoma, which would then permit local resection. Intraoperative ultrasonography may identify a small impalpable adenoma, permitting local resection. Adenomas often present in late infancy or early childhood.

Distinguishing between **focal** and **diffuse** cases of **persistent hyperinsulinism** has been attempted in several ways. Preoperatively, transhepatic portal vein catheterization and selective pancreatic venous sampling to measure insulin may localize a focal lesion from the step-up in insulin concentration at a specific site. Selective catheterization of arterial branches supplying the pancreas, followed by infusion of a secretagogue such as calcium and portal vein sampling for insulin concentration (arterial stimulation-venous sampling) may localize a lesion. Both approaches are highly invasive, restricted to specialized centers, and not uniformly successful in distinguishing the focal from the diffuse forms, hence, these techniques are not recommended. 18F-labeled L-dopa combined with PET scanning is a highly promising means to distinguish the focal from the diffuse lesions of hyperinsulinism unresponsive to medical management (Fig. 86-3). The "gold standard" remains intraoperative histologic characterization. Diffuse hyperinsulinism is characterized by large β cells with abnormally large nuclei, whereas focal adenomatous lesions display small and normal β cell nuclei. Although *SUR1* mutations are present in both types, the focal lesions arise by a random loss of a maternally imprinted growth-inhibitory gene on maternal chromosome 11p in association with paternal transmission of a mutated *SUR1* or K_{IR} 6.2 paternal chromosome 11p. Thus the focal form represents a double hit-loss of maternal repressor and transmission of a paternal mutation. Local excision of focal adenomatous islet cell hyperplasia results in a cure with little or no recurrence. For the diffuse form, near-total resection of 85-90% of the pancreas is recommended. The near-total pancreatectomy required for the diffuse hyperplastic lesions is, however, often associated with persistent hypoglycemia with the later development of hyperglycemia or frank, insulin-requiring diabetes mellitus.

Further resection of the remaining pancreas may occasionally be necessary if hypoglycemia recurs and cannot be controlled by medical measures, such as the use of somatostatin or diazoxide.

Experienced pediatric surgeons in medical centers equipped to provide the necessary preoperative and postoperative care, diagnostic evaluation, and management should perform surgery. In some patients who have been managed medically, hyperinsulinemia and hypoglycemia regress over months. This is similar to what occurs in children with the hyperinsulinemic hypoglycemia seen in **Beckwith-Wiedemann syndrome.**

If hypoglycemia 1st manifests between 3 and 6 mo of age or later, a therapeutic trial using medical approaches with diazoxide, somatostatin, and frequent feedings can be attempted for up to 2-4 wk. Failure to maintain euglycemia without undesirable side effects from the drugs may prompt the need for surgery. Some success in suppressing insulin release and correcting hypoglyce-

Table 86-8 CLINICAL MANIFESTATIONS AND DIFFERENTIAL DIAGNOSIS IN CHILDHOOD HYPOGLYCEMIA

CONDITION	HYPOGLYCEMIA	URINARY KETONES OR REDUCING SUGARS	HEPATOMEGALY	SERUM		EFFECT OF 24-36 HR FAST ON PLASMA					GLYCEMIC RESPONSE TO GLUCAGON		GLYCEMIC RESPONSE TO INFUSION OF	
				Lipids	Uric Acid	Glucose	Insulin	Ketones	Alanine	Lactate	Fed	Fasted	Alanine	Glycerol
Normal	0	0	0	Normal	Normal	↓	↓	↑	↓	Normal	↑	↓		Not indicated
Hyperinsulinemia	Recurrent severe	0	0	Normal or ↑	Normal	↓↓	↑↑	↓↓	Normal	Normal	↑	↑		Not indicated
Ketotic hypoglycemia	Severe with missed meals	Ketonuria +++	0	Normal	Normal	↓↓	↓	↑↑	↓↓	Normal	↑	↓↓		Not indicated
Fatty acid oxidation disorder	Severe with missed meals	Absent	0 to + Abnormal liver function test results	Abnormal	↑		Contraindicated				↑	↓		Not indicated
Hypopituitarism	Moderate with missed meals	Ketonuria ++		Normal	Normal	↓↓	↓	↑↑	↓↓	Normal	↑	↓↓	↑	↑
Adrenal insufficiency	Severe with missed meals	Ketonuria ++	0	Normal	Normal	↓↓	↓	↑↑	↓↓	Normal	↑	↓↓	↑	↑
Enzyme deficiencies	Severe-constant	Ketonuria +++	+++	↑↑	↑↑	↓↓	↓	↑↑	↑↑	↑↑	0	0-↓↓	0	0
Glucose-6-phosphatase debrancher	Moderate with fasting	++	++	Normal	Normal	↓↓	↓	↑↑	↓↓	Normal	↑	0-↓↓	↑	↑
Phosphorylase	Mild-moderate	Ketonuria ++	+	Normal	Normal	↓	↓	↑↑	↓↓	Normal	0-↑	0-↓↓	↑	↑
Fructose-1, 6-diphosphatase	Severe with fasting	Ketonuria +++	+++	↑↑	↑↑	↓↓	↓	↑↑	↑↑	↑↑	↑	0-↓↓	↓	↓
Galactosemia	After milk or milk products	0 Ketones;(s) +	+++	Normal	Normal	↓	↓	↑	↓	Normal	↑	0-↓↓	↑	↑
Fructose intolerance	After fructose	0 Ketones;(s) +	+++	Normal	Normal	↓	↓	↑	↓	Normal	↑	0-↓↓	↑	↑

Details of each condition are discussed in the text. 0, absence; ↑ or ↓ indicates respectively small increase or decrease; ↑↑ or ↓↓ indicates respectively large increase or decrease.

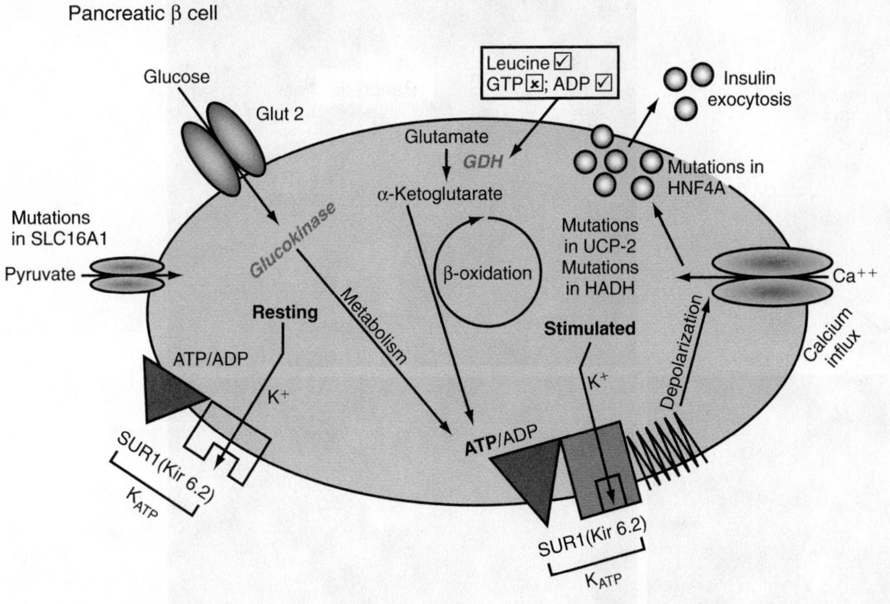

Figure 86-2 Schematic representation of the pancreatic cell with some important steps in insulin secretion. The membrane-spanning, adenosine triphosphate (ATP)-sensitive potassium (K^+) channel (K_{ATP}) consists of 2 subunits: the sulfonylurea receptor (SUR) and the inward rectifying K channel (K_{IR} 6.2). In the resting state, the ratio of ATP to adenosine diphosphate (ADP) maintains K_{ATP} in an open state, permitting efflux of intracellular K^+. When blood glucose concentration rises, its entry into the β cell is facilitated by the GLUT-2 glucose transporter, a process not regulated by insulin. Within the β cell, glucose is converted to glucose-6-phosphate by the enzyme glucokinase and then undergoes metabolism to generate energy. The resultant increase in ATP relative to ADP closes K_{ATP}, preventing efflux of K^+, and the rise of intracellular K^+ depolarizes the cell membrane and opens a calcium (Ca^{2+}) channel. The intracellular rise in Ca^{2+} triggers insulin secretion via exocytosis. Sulfonylureas trigger insulin secretion by reacting with their receptor (SUR) to close K_{ATP}; diazoxide inhibits this process, whereas somatostatin, or its analog octreotide, inhibits insulin secretion by interfering with calcium influx. Genetic mutations in *SUR* or K_{IR} 6.2 that prevent K_{ATP} from being open, tonically maintain inappropriate insulin secretion and are responsible for autosomal recessive forms of persistent hyperinsulinemic hypoglycemia of infancy (PHHI). One form of autosomal dominant PHHI is due to an activating mutation in glucokinase. The amino acid leucine also triggers insulin secretion by closure of K_{ATP}. Metabolism of leucine is facilitated by the enzyme glutamate dehydrogenase (GDH), and overactivity of this enzyme in the pancreas leads to hyperinsulinemia with hypoglycemia, associated with hyperammonemia from overactivity of GDH in the liver. Mutations in the pyruvate channel SLC16A1 can cause ectopic expression in the beta cell and permit pyruvate, accumulated during exercise, to induce insulin secretion and hence exercise-induced hypoglycemia. Mutations in the mitochondrial uncoupling protein 2 (UCP2) and hydroxyl acyl CoA dehydrogenase (HADH) are associated with hyperinsulinism (HI) by mechanisms yet to be defined. Mutations in the transcription factor hepatic nuclear factor (HNF) 4 alpha can be associated with neonatal macrosomia and HI, but progress to monogenic diabetes of youth (MODY) later in life. √, stimulation; GTP, guanosine triphosphate; X, inhibition.

mia in patients with PHHI has been reported with the use of the long-acting somatostatin analog octreotide. Most cases of neonatal PHHI are sporadic; familial forms permit genetic counseling on the basis of anticipated autosomal recessive inheritance.

A 2nd form of familial PHHI suggests **autosomal dominant inheritance.** The clinical features tend to be less severe, and onset of hypoglycemia is most likely, but not exclusively, to occur beyond the immediate newborn period and usually beyond the period of weaning at an average age at onset of about 1 yr. At birth, macrosomia is rarely observed, and response to diazoxide is almost uniform. The initial presentation may be delayed and rarely occur as late as 30 yr, unless provoked by fasting. The genetic basis for this autosomal dominant form has not been delineated; it is not always linked to K_{IR} 6.2/*SUR1*. The activating mutation in glucokinase is transmitted in an autosomal dominant manner. If a family history is present, genetic counseling for a 50% recurrence rate can be given for future offspring.

A 3rd form of persistent PHHI is associated with **mild and asymptomatic hyperammonemia,** usually as a sporadic occurrence, although dominant inheritance occurs. Presentation is more like the autosomal dominant form than the autosomal recessive form. Diet and diazoxide control symptoms, but pancreatectomy may be necessary in some cases. The association of hyperinsulinism and hyperammonemia is caused by an inherited or de novo gain-of-function mutation in the enzyme glutamate dehydrogenase. The resulting increase in glutamate oxidation in the pancreatic β cell raises the ATP concentration and, hence, the ratio of ATP:ADP, which closes K_{ATP}, leading to membrane depolarization, calcium influx, and insulin secretion (see Fig. 86-2). In the liver, the excessive oxidation of glutamate to β-ketoglutarate may generate ammonia and divert glutamate from being processed to *N*-acetylglutamate, an essential cofactor for removal of ammonia through the urea cycle via activation of the enzyme carbamoyl phosphate synthetase. The hyperammonemia is mild, with concentrations of 100-200 μM/L, and produces no CNS symptoms or consequences, as seen in other hyperammonemic states. Leucine, a potent amino acid for stimulating insulin secretion and implicated in leucine-sensitive hypoglycemia, acts by allosterically stimulating glutamate dehydrogenase. Thus, **leucine-sensitive hypoglycemia** may be a form of the hyperinsulinemia-hyperammonemia syndrome or a potentiation of mild disorders of the K_{ATP} channel; it need not always be associated with a modest increase in serum ammonia.

Hypoglycemia associated with hyperinsulinemia is also seen in about 50% of patients with the **Beckwith-Wiedemann syndrome.** This syndrome is characterized by omphalocele, gigantism, macroglossia, microcephaly, and visceromegaly (Fig. 86-4). Distinctive lateral earlobe fissures and facial nevus flammeus are present; hemihypertrophy occurs in many of these infants. Diffuse islet cell hyperplasia occurs in infants with hypoglycemia. The diagnostic and therapeutic approaches are the same as those discussed previously, although microcephaly and retarded brain development may occur independently of hypoglycemia. Patients with the Beckwith-Wiedemann syndrome may acquire tumors, including Wilms tumor, hepatoblastoma, adrenal carcinoma,

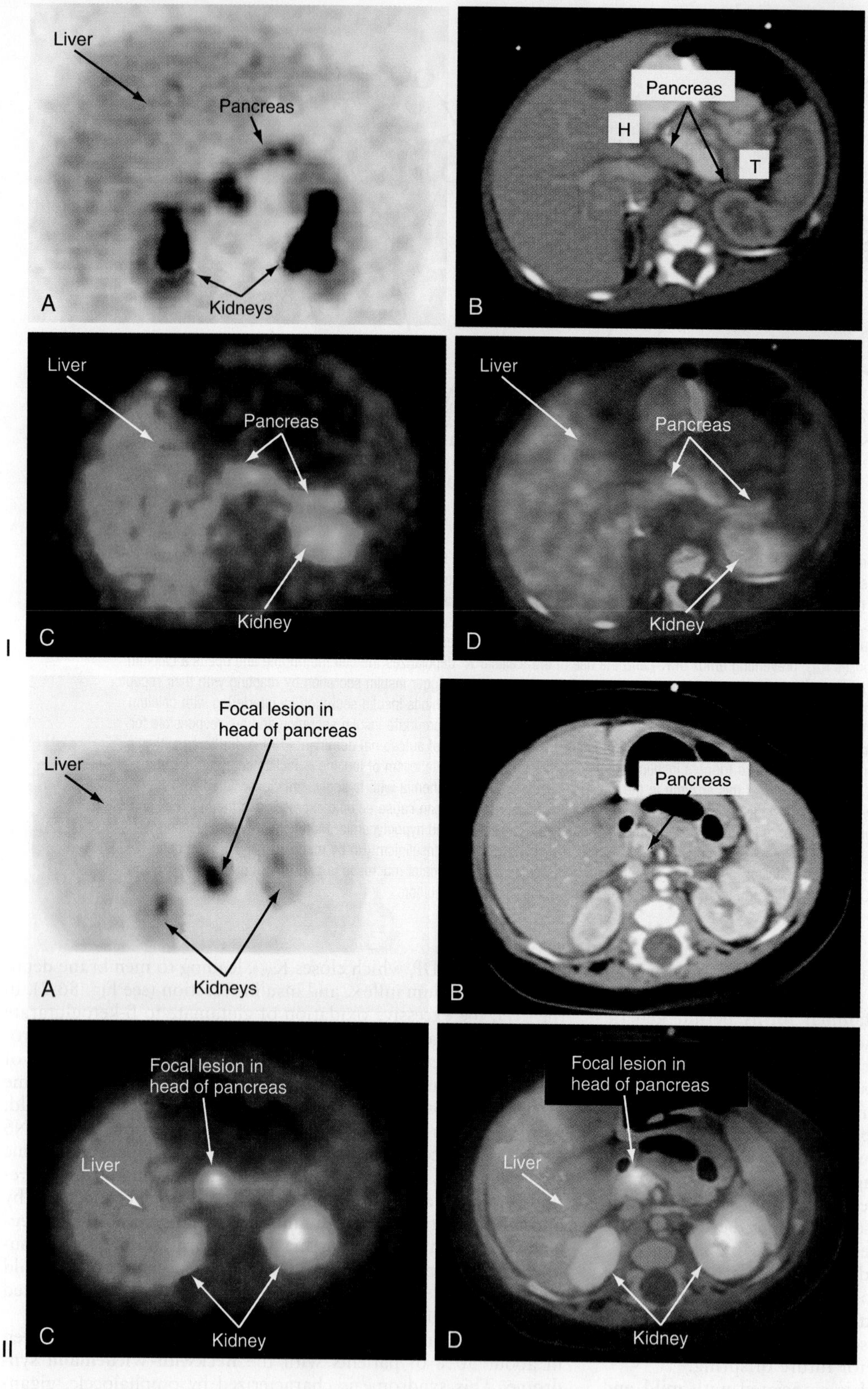

Figure 86-3 Congenital hyperinsulinism. **I** panels (Diffuse): [18F]-DOPA PET of patient with diffuse form of congenital hyperinsulinism. *A,* Diffuse uptake of [18F]-DOPA is visualized throughout the pancreas. Transverse views show *B,* normal pancreatic tissue on abdominal CT; *C,* diffuse uptake of [18F]-DOPA in pancreas; and *D,* confirmation of pancreatic uptake of [18F]-DOPA with coregistration. H, head of pancreas; T, tail of pancreas. **II** panels (Focal): [18F]-DOPA PET of patient with focal form of congenital hyperinsulinism. *A,* Discrete area of increased [18F]-DOPA uptake is visualized in the head of the pancreas. The intensity of this area is greater than that observed in the liver and neighboring normal pancreatic tissue. Transverse views show *B,* normal pancreatic tissue on abdominal CT; *C,* focal uptake of [18F]-DOPA in pancreatic head; and *D,* confirmation of [18F]-DOPA uptake in the pancreatic head with coregistration. (Courtesy of Dr Olga Hardy, Children's Hospital of Philadelphia.)

gonadoblastoma, and rhabdomyosarcoma. This overgrowth syndrome is caused by mutations in the chromosome 11p15.5 region close to the genes for insulin, SUR, K_{IR} 6.2, and IGF-2. Duplications in this region and genetic imprinting from a defective or absent copy of the maternally derived gene are involved in the variable features and patterns of transmission. Hypoglycemia may resolve in weeks to months of medical therapy. Pancreatic resection may also be needed.

Hyperinsulinemic hypoglycemia in infancy is reported as a manifestation of one form of congenital disorder of glycosylation. Disorders of protein glycosylation usually present with neurologic symptoms but may also include liver dysfunction with hepatomegaly, intractable diarrhea, protein-losing enteropathy, and hypoglycemia (Chapter 81.6). These disorders are often underdiagnosed. One entity associated with hyperinsulinemic hypoglycemia is caused by phosphomannose isomerase deficiency, and

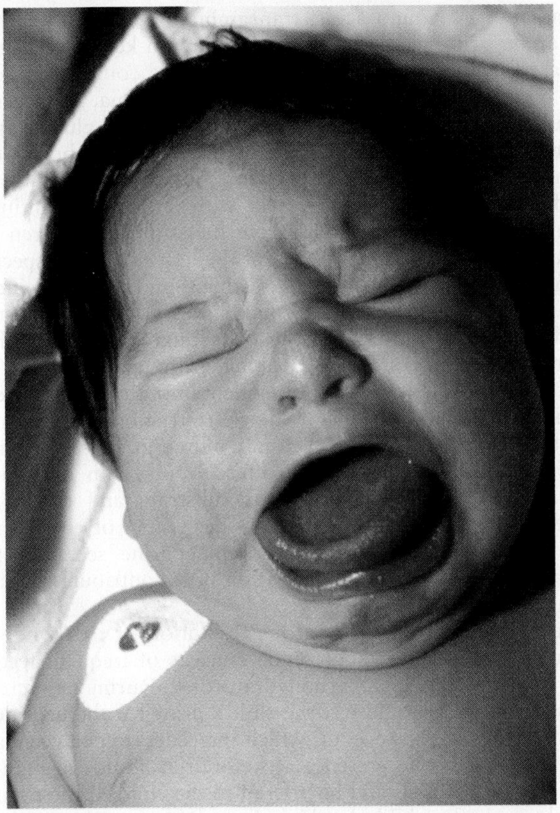

Figure 86-4 Beckwith-Wiedemann syndrome. (Courtesy of Dr. Michael Cohen, Dalhousie University, Halifax, Nova Scotia. From Jones KL: *Smith's recognizable patterns of human malformation*, ed 6, Philadelphia, 2006, Saunders.)

clinical improvement followed supplemental treatment with oral mannose at a dose of 0.17 g/kg 6 times per day.

After the 1st 12 mo of life, hyperinsulinemic states are uncommon until islet cell adenomas reappear as a cause after the patient is several years of age. Hyperinsulinemia due to **islet cell adenoma** should be considered in any child 5 yr or older presenting with hypoglycemia. Islet cell adenomas do not "light up" during scanning with L-dopa labeled with fluorine-18. An islet cell adenoma in a child should arouse suspicion of the possibility of **multiple endocrine neoplasia** type 1 (Wermer syndrome), which involves mutations in the menin gene and may be associated with hyperparathyroidism and with pituitary tumors. The diagnostic approach is outlined in Tables 86-7 and 86-8. Fasting for up to 24-36 hr usually provokes hypoglycemia; coexisting hyperinsulinemia confirms the diagnosis, provided that factitious administration of insulin by the parents, a form of **Munchausen syndrome by proxy,** is excluded. Occasionally, provocative tests may be required. Exogenously administered insulin can be distinguished from endogenous insulin by simultaneous measurement of C-peptide concentration. If C-peptide levels are elevated, endogenous insulin secretion is responsible for the hypoglycemia; if C-peptide levels are low but insulin values are high, exogenous insulin has been administered, perhaps as a form of child abuse. Islet cell adenomas at this age are treated by surgical excision. Antibodies to insulin or the insulin receptor (insulin mimetic action) are also rarely associated with hypoglycemia. Some tumors produce insulin-like growth factors, thereby provoking hypoglycemia by interacting with the insulin receptor. The astute clinician must also consider the possibility of deliberate or accidental ingestion of drugs such as a sulfonylurea or related compound that stimulates insulin secretion. In such cases, insulin and C-peptide concentrations in blood will be elevated. Inadvertent substitution of an insulin secretagogue by a dispensing error should be considered in those taking medications who suddenly develop documented hypoglycemia.

A rare form of hyperinsulinemic hypoglycemia has been reported after exercise. Whereas glucose and insulin remain unchanged in most people after moderate, short-term exercise, rare patients manifest severe hypoglycemia with hyperinsulinemia 15-50 min after the same standardized exercise. This form of exercise-induced hyperinsulinism is caused by an abnormal responsiveness of β-cell insulin release in response to pyruvate generated during exercise. The gene responsible for this syndrome, SLC16A1, regulates a transporter, MCT1R, that controls the entry of pyruvate into cells. Dominant mutations in SLC16A1 that increase the ectopic expression of MCTR1 transporter in pancreatic beta cells permit excessive entry of pyruvate into beta cells and act to increase insulin secretion with resultant hypoglycemia during exercise.

Hypoglycemia with so-called nesidioblastosis has also rarely been reported after bariatric surgery for obesity. The mechanism for this form of hyperinsulinemic hypoglycemia remains to be defined.

Infants and children with **Nissen fundoplication,** a relatively common procedure used to ameliorate gastroesophageal reflux, frequently have an associated "dumping" syndrome with hypoglycemia. Characteristic features include significant hyperglycemia of up to 500 mg/dL 30 min postprandially and severe hypoglycemia (average 32 mg/dL in 1 series) 1.5-3.0 hr later. The early hyperglycemia phase is associated with brisk and excessive insulin release that causes the rebound hypoglycemia. Glucagon responses have been inappropriately low in some. Although the physiologic mechanisms are not always clearly apparent, and attempted treatments not always effective, **acarbose,** an inhibitor of glucose absorption, has been reported to be successful in one small series.

Endocrine Deficiency

Hypoglycemia associated with endocrine deficiency is usually caused by adrenal insufficiency with or without associated growth hormone deficiency (Chapters 551 and 569). In panhypopituitarism, isolated adrenocorticotropic hormone (ACTH) or growth hormone deficiency, or combined ACTH deficiency plus growth hormone deficiency, the incidence of hypoglycemia is as high as 20%. In the newborn period, hypoglycemia may be the presenting feature of hypopituitarism; in males, a microphallus may provide a clue to a coexistent deficiency of gonadotropin. Newborns with hypopituitarism often have a form of "hepatitis" associated with cholestatic jaundice and hypoglycemia. The combination of hypoglycemia and cholestatic jaundice requires exclusion of hypopituitarism as a cause, since the jaundice resolves with replacement treatment of growth hormone, cortisol, and thyroid as required. This constellation is often associated with the syndrome of **septo-optic dysplasia.** When adrenal disease is severe, as in congenital adrenal hyperplasia caused by cortisol synthetic enzyme defects, adrenal hemorrhage, or congenital absence of the adrenal glands, disturbances in serum electrolytes with hyponatremia and hyperkalemia or ambiguous genitals may provide diagnostic clues (Chapter 570). In older children, failure of growth should suggest growth hormone deficiency. Hyperpigmentation may provide the clue to Addison disease with increased ACTH levels or adrenal unresponsiveness to ACTH owing to a defect in the adrenal receptor for ACTH. The frequent association of Addison disease in childhood with hypoparathyroidism (hypocalcemia), chronic mucocutaneous candidiasis, and other endocrinopathies should be considered. Adrenoleukodystrophy should also be considered in the differential diagnosis of primary Addison disease in older male children (Chapter 80.2).

Hypoglycemia in cortisol–growth hormone deficiency may be caused by decreased gluconeogenic enzymes with cortisol deficiency, increased glucose utilization due to a lack of the antagonistic effects of growth hormone on insulin action, or failure to supply endogenous gluconeogenic substrate in the form of alanine and lactate with compensatory breakdown of fat and generation of ketones. Deficiency of these hormones results in reduced gluconeogenic substrate, which resembles the syndrome of ketotic hypoglycemia. Investigation of a child with hypoglycemia, therefore, requires exclusion of ACTH-cortisol or growth hormone deficiency and, if diagnosed, its appropriate replacement with cortisol or growth hormone.

Epinephrine deficiency could theoretically be responsible for hypoglycemia. Urinary excretion of epinephrine has been diminished in some patients with spontaneous or insulin-induced hypoglycemia in whom absence of pallor and tachycardia was also noted, suggesting that failure of catecholamine release, due to a defect anywhere along the hypothalamic-autonomic-adrenomedullary axis, might be responsible for the hypoglycemia. This possibility has been challenged, owing to the rarity of hypoglycemia in patients with bilateral adrenalectomy, provided that they receive adequate glucocorticoid replacement, and because diminished epinephrine excretion is found in normal patients with repeated insulin-induced hypoglycemia. Many of the patients described as having hypoglycemia with failure of epinephrine excretion fit the criteria for ketotic hypoglycemia. Also, repetitive hypoglycemia leads to diminished cortisol plus epinephrine responses, as seen most commonly in insulin-treated diabetes mellitus and the syndrome of hypoglycemia unawareness.

Glucagon deficiency in infants or children may theoretically be associated with hypoglycemia but has never been fully documented.

Substrate Limited

KETOTIC HYPOGLYCEMIA Ketotic hypoglycemia is the **most common** form of *childhood* hypoglycemia. This condition usually presents between the ages of 18 mo and 5 yr and commonly remits spontaneously by the age of 8-9 yr. Hypoglycemic episodes typically occur during periods of intercurrent illness when food intake is limited. The classic history is of a child who eats poorly or completely avoids the evening meal, is difficult to arouse from sleep the following morning and hence eats poorly again, and may have a seizure or be comatose by mid-morning. Another common presentation occurs when parents sleep late and the affected child is unable to eat breakfast, thus prolonging the overnight fast.

At the time of documented hypoglycemia, there is associated ketonuria and ketonemia; plasma insulin concentrations are appropriately low, ≤5-10 µU/mL, thus excluding hyperinsulinemia. A ketogenic provocative diet, formerly used as a diagnostic test, is no longer used to establish the diagnosis because fasting alone provokes a hypoglycemic episode with ketonemia and ketonuria within 12-18 hr in susceptible individuals. Normal children of similar age can withstand fasting without hypoglycemia developing during the same period, although even normal children may acquire these features by 36 hr of fasting.

Children with ketotic hypoglycemia have plasma alanine concentrations that are markedly reduced in the basal state after an overnight fast and decline even further with prolonged fasting. Alanine, produced in muscle, is a major gluconeogenic precursor. Alanine is the only amino acid that is significantly lower in these children, and infusions of alanine (250 mg/kg) produce a rapid rise in plasma glucose without causing significant changes in blood lactate or pyruvate levels, indicating that the entire gluconeogenic pathway from the level of pyruvate is intact, but that there is a deficiency of substrate. Glycogenolytic pathways are also intact because glucagon induces a normal glycemic response in affected children in the fed state. The levels of hormones that counter hypoglycemia are appropriately elevated, and insulin is appropriately low.

The etiology of ketotic hypoglycemia may be a defect in any of the complex steps involved in protein catabolism, oxidative deamination of amino acids, transamination, alanine synthesis, or alanine efflux from muscle. Children with ketotic hypoglycemia are frequently smaller than age-matched controls and often have a history of transient neonatal hypoglycemia. Any decrease in muscle mass may compromise the supply of gluconeogenic substrate at a time when glucose demands per unit of body weight are already relatively high, thus predisposing the patient to the rapid development of hypoglycemia, with ketosis representing the attempt to switch to an alternative fuel supply. Children with ketotic hypoglycemia may represent the low end of the spectrum of children's capacity to tolerate fasting. Similar relative intolerance to fasting is present in normal children, who cannot maintain blood glucose after 30-36 hr of fasting, compared with the adult's capacity for prolonged fasting. Although the defect may be present at birth, it may not be evident until the child is stressed by more prolonged periods of calorie restriction. Moreover, the spontaneous remission observed in children at age 8-9 yr might be explained by the increase in muscle bulk with its resultant increase in supply of endogenous substrate and the relative decrease in glucose requirement per unit of body mass with increasing age. Impaired norepinephrine secretion from immaturity of autonomic innervation may contribute to ketotic hypoglycemia.

In anticipation of spontaneous resolution of this syndrome, treatment of ketotic hypoglycemia consists of frequent feedings of a high-protein, high-carbohydrate diet. During intercurrent illnesses, parents should test the child's urine for the presence of ketones, the appearance of which precedes hypoglycemia by several hours. In the presence of ketonuria, liquids of high carbohydrate content should be offered to the child. If these cannot be tolerated, the child should be cared for in a hospital with intravenous glucose administration.

BRANCHED-CHAIN KETONURIA (MAPLE SYRUP URINE DISEASE) (CHAPTER 79.6) The hypoglycemic episodes were once attributed to high levels of leucine, but evidence indicates that interference with the production of alanine and its availability as a gluconeogenic substrate during calorie deprivation is responsible for hypoglycemia.

Glycogen Storage Disease

See Chapter 81.1.

GLUCOSE-6-PHOSPHATASE DEFICIENCY (TYPE I GLYCOGEN STORAGE DISEASE) Affected children usually display a remarkable tolerance to their chronic hypoglycemia; blood glucose values in the range of 20-50 mg/dL are not associated with the classic symptoms of hypoglycemia, possibly reflecting the adaptation of the CNS to ketone bodies as an alternative fuel.

AMYLO-1,6-GLUCOSIDASE DEFICIENCY (DEBRANCHER ENZYME DEFICIENCY; TYPE III GLYCOGEN STORAGE DISEASE) See Chapter 81.

LIVER PHOSPHORYLASE DEFICIENCY (TYPE VI GLYCOGEN STORAGE DISEASE) (CHAPTER 81) Low hepatic phosphorylase activity may result from a defect in any of the steps of activation; a variety of defects have been described. Hepatomegaly, excessive deposition of glycogen in liver, growth retardation, and occasional symptomatic hypoglycemia occur. A diet high in protein and reduced in carbohydrate usually prevents hypoglycemia.

GLYCOGEN SYNTHETASE DEFICIENCY (CHAPTER 81) The inability to synthesize glycogen is rare. There is hypoglycemia and hyperketonemia after fasting because glycogen reserves are markedly diminished or absent. After feeding, however, hyperglycemia with glucosuria may occur because of the inability to assimilate some of the glucose load into glycogen. During fasting hypoglycemia, levels of the counter-regulatory hormones, including catecholamines, are appropriately elevated or normal, and insulin levels are appropriately low. The liver is not enlarged. Protein-rich feedings at frequent intervals result in dramatic clinical improvement, including growth velocity. This condition mimics the syndrome of ketotic hypoglycemia and should be considered in the differential diagnosis of that syndrome.

Disorders of Gluconeogenesis

FRUCTOSE-1,6-DIPHOSPHATASE DEFICIENCY (CHAPTER 81.3) A deficiency of this enzyme results in a block of gluconeogenesis from all possible precursors below the level of fructose-1,6-diphosphate. Infusion of these gluconeogenic precursors results in lactic acidosis without a rise in glucose; acute hypoglycemia may be provoked by inhibition of glycogenolysis. Glycogenolysis remains intact, and glucagon elicits a normal glycemic response in the fed, but not in the fasted, state. Accordingly, affected individuals have hypoglycemia only during caloric deprivation, as in fasting, or during intercurrent illness. As long as glycogen stores remain normal, hypoglycemia does not develop. In affected families, there may be a history of siblings with known hepatomegaly who died in infancy with unexplained metabolic acidosis.

DEFECTS IN FATTY ACID OXIDATION (CHAPTER 80) The important role of fatty acid oxidation in maintaining gluconeogenesis is underscored by examples of congenital or drug-induced defects in fatty acid metabolism that may be associated with fasting hypoglycemia.

Various congenital enzymatic deficiencies causing defective carnitine or fatty acid metabolism occur. A severe and relatively common form of fasting hypoglycemia with hepatomegaly, cardiomyopathy, and hypotonia occurs with long- and medium-chain fatty acid coenzyme-A dehydrogenase deficiency (LCAD and MCAD). Plasma carnitine levels are low, ketones are not present in urine, but dicarboxylic aciduria is present. Clinically, patients with **acyl CoA dehydrogenase deficiency** present with a Reye-like syndrome (Chapter 353), recurrent episodes of severe fasting hypoglycemic coma, and cardiorespiratory arrest (sudden infant death syndrome-like events). Severe hypoglycemia and metabolic acidosis without ketosis also occur in patients with multiple acyl CoA dehydrogenase disorders. Hypotonia, seizures, and acrid odor are other clinical clues. Survival depends on whether the defects are severe or mild; diagnosis is established from studies of enzyme activity in liver biopsy tissue or in cultured fibroblasts from affected patients. Tandem mass spectrometry can be employed for blood samples, even those on filter paper, for screening of congenital inborn errors. The frequency of this disorder is at least 1/10,000-15,000 births. Avoidance of fasting and supplementation with carnitine may be lifesaving in these patients who generally present in infancy.

Interference with fatty acid metabolism also underlies the fasting hypoglycemia associated with Jamaican vomiting sickness, with atractyloside, and with the drug valproate. In **Jamaican vomiting sickness,** the unripe ackee fruit contains a water-soluble toxin, hypoglycin, which produces vomiting, CNS depression, and severe hypoglycemia. The hypoglycemic activity of hypoglycin derives from its inhibition of gluconeogenesis secondary to its interference with the acyl CoA and carnitine metabolism essential for the oxidation of long-chain fatty acids. The disease is almost totally confined to Jamaica, where ackee forms a staple of the diet for the poor. The ripe ackee fruit no longer contains this toxin. *Atractyloside* is a reagent that inhibits oxidative phosphorylation in mitochondria by preventing the translocation of adenine nucleotides, such as ATP, across the mitochondrial membrane. Atractyloside is a perhydrophenanthrenic glycoside derived from *Atractylis gummifera.* This plant is found in the Mediterranean basin; ingestion of this "thistle" is associated with hypoglycemia and a syndrome similar to Jamaican vomiting sickness. The anticonvulsant drug **valproate** is associated with side effects, predominantly in young infants, which include a Reye-like syndrome, low serum carnitine levels, and the potential for fasting hypoglycemia. In all these conditions, hypoglycemia *is not associated with ketonuria.*

ACUTE ALCOHOL INTOXICATION The liver metabolizes alcohol as a preferred fuel, and generation of reducing equivalents during the oxidation of ethanol alters the NADH:NAD ratio, which is essential for certain gluconeogenic steps. As a result, gluconeogenesis is impaired and hypoglycemia may ensue if glycogen stores are depleted by starvation or by pre-existing abnormalities in glycogen metabolism. In toddlers who have been unfed for some time, even the consumption of small quantities of alcohol can precipitate these events. The hypoglycemia promptly responds to intravenous glucose, which should always be considered in a child who presents initially with coma or seizure, after taking a blood sample to determine glucose concentration. The possibility of the child's ingesting alcoholic drinks must also be considered if there was a preceding adult evening party. A careful history allows the diagnosis to be made and may avoid needless and expensive hospitalization and investigation.

SALICYLATE INTOXICATION (CHAPTER 58) Both hyperglycemia and hypoglycemia occur in children with salicylate intoxication. Accelerated utilization of glucose, resulting from augmentation of insulin secretion by salicylates, and possible interference with gluconeogenesis may contribute to hypoglycemia. Infants are more susceptible than are older children. Monitoring of blood glucose levels with appropriate glucose infusion in the event of hypoglycemia should form part of the therapeutic approach to salicylate intoxication in childhood. Ketosis may occur.

PHOSPHOENOL PYRUVATE CARBOXYKINASE DEFICIENCY Deficiency of this rate-limiting gluconeogenic enzyme is associated with severe fasting hypoglycemia and variable onset after birth. Hypoglycemia may occur within 24 hr after birth, and defective gluconeogenesis from alanine can be documented in vivo. Liver, kidney, and myocardium demonstrate fatty infiltration, and atrophy of the optic nerve and visual cortex may occur. Hypoglycemia may be profound. Lactate and pyruvate levels in plasma have been normal, but a mild metabolic acidosis may be present. The fatty infiltration of various organs is caused by increased formation of acetyl CoA, which becomes available for fatty acid synthesis. Diagnosis of this rare entity can be made with certainty only through appropriate enzymatic determinations in liver biopsy material. Avoidance of periods of fasting through frequent feedings rich in carbohydrate should be helpful because glycogen synthesis and breakdown are intact.

PYRUVATE CARBOXYLASE DEFICIENCY (CHAPTER 81)

Other Enzyme Defects

GALACTOSEMIA (GALACTOSE-1-PHOSPHATE URIDYL TRANSFERASE DEFICIENCY) See Chapter 81.

FRUCTOSE INTOLERANCE (FRUCTOSE-1-PHOSPHATE ALDOLASE DEFICIENCY) (CHAPTER 81) Acute hypoglycemia is due to the inhibition by fructose-1-phosphate of glycogenolysis via the phosphorylase system and of gluconeogenesis at the level of fructose-1,6-diphosphate aldolase. Affected individuals usually learn spontaneously to eliminate fructose from their diet.

Defects in Glucose Transporters

GLUT-1 DEFICIENCY Two infants with a seizure disorder were found to have low cerebrospinal fluid (CSF) glucose concentrations despite normal plasma glucose. Lactate concentrations in CSF were also low, suggesting decreased glycolysis rather than bacterial infection, which causes low CSF glucose with high lactate. The erythrocyte glucose transporter was defective, suggesting a similar defect in the brain glucose transporter responsible for the clinical features. A ketogenic diet reduced the severity of seizures by supplying an alternate source of brain fuel that bypassed the defect in glucose transport.

GLUT-2 DEFICIENCY Children with hepatomegaly, galactose intolerance, and renal tubular dysfunction (**Fanconi-Bickel syndrome**) have been shown to have a deficiency of the GLUT-2 glucose transporter of plasma membranes. In addition to liver and kidney tubules, GLUT-2 is also expressed in pancreatic β cells. Hence, the clinical manifestations reflect impaired glucose release from liver and defective tubular reabsorption of glucose plus phosphaturia and aminoaciduria.

Systemic Disorders

Several systemic disorders are associated with hypoglycemia in infants and children. Neonatal sepsis is often associated with

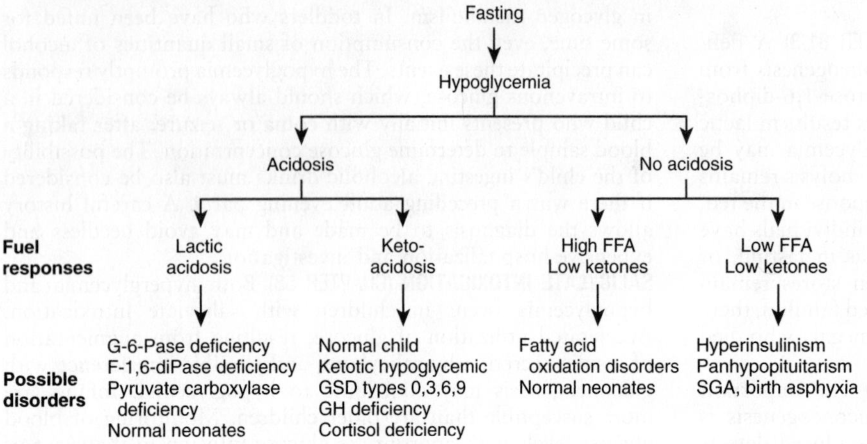

Figure 86-5 Algorithm for diagnosis of hypoglycemia based on fasting fuel responses. F1,6-diPase, fructose-1,6-diphosphatase; FFA, free fatty acid; G-6Pase, glucose-6-phosphatase; GH, growth hormone; GSD, glycogen storage disease; SGA, small for gestational age. (From Kliegman RM, Greenbaum LA, Lye PS, editors: *Practical strategies in pediatric diagnosis and therapy*, ed 2, Philadelphia, 2004, Elsevier Saunders.)

hypoglycemia, possibly as a result of diminished caloric intake with impaired gluconeogenesis. Similar mechanisms may apply to the hypoglycemia found in severely malnourished infants or those with severe malabsorption. Hyperviscosity with a central hematocrit of >65% is associated with hypoglycemia in at least 10-15% of affected infants. **Falciparum malaria** has been associated with hyperinsulinemia and hypoglycemia. Heart and renal failure have also been associated with hypoglycemia, but the mechanism is obscure.

DIAGNOSIS AND DIFFERENTIAL DIAGNOSIS

Table 86-8 and Figure 86-5 list the pertinent clinical and biochemical findings in the common childhood disorders associated with hypoglycemia. A careful and detailed history is essential in every suspected or documented case of hypoglycemia (see Table 86-7). Specific points to be noted include age at onset, temporal relation to meals or caloric deprivation, and a family history of prior infants known to have had hypoglycemia or of unexplained infant deaths. In the 1st wk of life, the majority of infants have the transient form of neonatal hypoglycemia either as a result of prematurity/intrauterine growth restriction or by virtue of being born to diabetic mothers. The absence of a history of maternal diabetes, but the presence of macrosomia and the characteristic large plethoric appearance of an "infant of a diabetic mother" should arouse suspicion of hyperinsulinemic hypoglycemia of infancy probably due to a K_{ATP} channel defect that is familial (autosomal recessive) or sporadic; plasma insulin concentrations >5-10 μU/mL in the presence of documented hypoglycemia confirm this diagnosis. The presence of hepatomegaly should arouse suspicion of an enzyme deficiency; if non–glucose-reducing sugar is present in the urine, galactosemia is most likely. In males, the presence of a microphallus suggests the possibility of hypopituitarism, which also may be associated with jaundice in both sexes.

Past the newborn period, clues to the cause of persistent or recurrent hypoglycemia can be obtained through a careful history, physical examination, and initial laboratory findings. The temporal relation of the hypoglycemia to food intake may suggest that the defect is one of gluconeogenesis, if symptoms occur 6 hr or more after meals. If hypoglycemia occurs shortly after meals, galactosemia or fructose intolerance is most likely, and the presence of reducing substances in the urine rapidly distinguishes these possibilities. The autosomal dominant forms of hyperinsulinemic hypoglycemia need to be considered, with measurement of glucose, insulin, and ammonia, and careful history for other affected family members of any age. Measurement of IGFBP-1 may be useful; it is low in hyperinsulinemia states and high in other forms of hypoglycemia. The presence of hepatomegaly suggests one of the enzyme deficiencies in glycogen breakdown or in gluconeogenesis, as outlined in Table 86-8. The absence of ketonemia or ketonuria at the time of initial presentation strongly suggests hyperinsulinemia or a defect in fatty acid oxidation. In most other causes of hypoglycemia, with the exception of galactosemia and fructose intolerance, ketonemia and ketonuria are present at the time of fasting hypoglycemia. At the time of the hypoglycemia, serum should be obtained for determination of hormones and substrates, followed by repeated measurement after an intramuscular or intravenous injection of glucagon, as outlined in Table 86-7. Interpretation of the findings is summarized in Table 86-8. Hypoglycemia with ketonuria in children between ages 18 mo and 5 yr is most likely to be ketotic hypoglycemia, especially if hepatomegaly is absent. The ingestion of a toxin, including alcohol or salicylate, can usually be excluded rapidly by the history. Inadvertent or deliberate drug ingestion and errors in dispensing medicines should also be considered.

When the history is suggestive, but acute symptoms are not present, a 24-36 hr supervised fast can usually provoke hypoglycemia and resolve the question of hyperinsulinemia or other conditions (see Table 86-8). Such a fast is contraindicated if a fatty acid oxidation defect is suspected; other approaches such as mass tandem spectrometry or molecular diagnosis, or both, should be considered. Because adrenal insufficiency may mimic ketotic hypoglycemia, plasma cortisol levels should be determined at the time of documented hypoglycemia; increased buccal or skin pigmentation may provide the clue to primary adrenal insufficiency with elevated ACTH (melanocyte-stimulating hormone) activity. Short stature or a decrease in the growth rate may provide the clue to pituitary insufficiency involving growth hormone as well as ACTH. Definitive tests of pituitary-adrenal function such as the arginine-insulin stimulation test for growth hormone IGF-1, IGFBP-1, and cortisol release may be necessary.

In the presence of hepatomegaly and hypoglycemia, a presumptive diagnosis of the enzyme defect can often be made through the clinical manifestations, presence of hyperlipidemia, acidosis, hyperuricemia, response to glucagon in the fed and fasted states, and response to infusion of various appropriate precursors (see Tables 86-7 and 86-8). These clinical findings and investigative approaches are summarized in Table 86-8. Definitive diagnosis of the glycogen storage disease may require an open liver biopsy (Chapter 81). Occasional patients with all the manifestations of glycogen storage disease are found to have normal enzyme activity. These definitive studies require special expertise available only in certain institutions.

TREATMENT

The prevention of hypoglycemia and its resultant effects on CNS development are important in the newborn period. For neonates with hyperinsulinemia not associated with maternal diabetes, subtotal or focal pancreatectomy may be needed, unless hypoglycemia can be readily controlled with long-term diazoxide or somatostatin analogs.

Treatment of **acute symptomatic** neonatal or infant hypoglycemia includes intravenous administration of 2 mL/kg of D_{10} W, followed by a continuous infusion of glucose at 6-8 mg/kg/min, adjusting the rate to maintain blood glucose levels in the normal range. If hypoglycemic seizures are present, some recommend a 4 mL/kg bolus of D_{10} W.

The management of **persistent** neonatal or infantile hypoglycemia includes increasing the rate of intravenous glucose infusion to 10-15 mg/kg/min or more, if needed. This may require a central venous or umbilical venous catheter to administer a hypertonic 15-25% glucose solution. If hyperinsulinemia is present, it should be medically managed initially with diazoxide and then somatostatin analogs. If hypoglycemia is unresponsive to intravenous glucose plus diazoxide (maximal doses up to 20 mg/kg/day) and somastostatin analogs, surgery via partial or near-total pancreatectomy should be considered.

Oral diazoxide, 5-15 mg/kg/24 hr given in divided doses twice daily, may reverse hyperinsulinemic hypoglycemia but may also produce hirsutism, edema, nausea, hyperuricemia, electrolyte disturbances, advanced bone age, IgG deficiency, and, rarely, hypotension with prolonged use. A long-acting somatostatin analog (octreotide, formerly SMS 201-995) is sometimes effective in controlling hyperinsulinemic hypoglycemia in patients with islet cell disorders not caused by genetic mutations in K_{ATP} channel and islet cell adenoma. Octreotide is administered subcutaneously every 6-12 hr in doses of 20-50 µg in neonates and young infants. Potential but unusual complications include poor growth due to inhibition of growth hormone release, pain at the injection site, vomiting, diarrhea, and hepatic dysfunction (hepatitis, cholelithiasis). Octreotide is usually employed as a temporizing agent for various periods before subtotal pancreatectomy for K_{ATP} channel disorders. It may be particularly useful for the treatment of refractory hypoglycemia despite subtotal pancreatectomy. Total pancreatectomy is not optimal therapy, owing to the risks of surgery, permanent diabetes mellitus, and exocrine pancreatic insufficiency. Continued prolonged medical therapy without pancreatic resection if hypoglycemia is controllable is worthwhile because some children have a spontaneous resolution of the hyperinsulinemic hypoglycemia. This should be balanced against the risk of hypoglycemia-induced CNS injury and the toxicity of drugs.

PROGNOSIS

The prognosis is good in asymptomatic neonates with hypoglycemia of short duration. Hypoglycemia recurs in 10-15% of infants after adequate treatment. Recurrence is more common if intravenous fluids are extravasated or discontinued too rapidly before oral feedings are well tolerated. Children in whom ketotic hypoglycemia later develops have an increased incidence of neonatal hypoglycemia.

The prognosis for normal intellectual function must be guarded because prolonged, recurrent, and severe symptomatic hypoglycemia is associated with neurologic sequelae. Symptomatic infants with hypoglycemia, particularly low-birthweight infants, those with persistent hyperinsulinemic hypoglycemia, and severely hypoglycemic infants born to poorly controlled diabetic mothers, have a poorer prognosis for subsequent normal intellectual development than asymptomatic infants do.

BIBLIOGRAPHY

Please visit the Nelson Textbook of Pediatrics *website at www.expertconsult.com for the complete bibliography.*

PART XII The Fetus and the Neonatal Infant

Chapter 87
Overview of Mortality and Morbidity

Waldemar A. Carlo

The risk for mortality in fetuses and neonates is very high around the time of birth. The perinatal period is most often defined as the period from the 28th wk of gestation through the 7th day after birth. The neonatal period is defined as the 1st 28 days after birth and may be further subdivided into the very early (birth to less than 24 hr), early (birth to <7 days), and late neonatal periods (7 days to <28 days). Infancy is defined as the 1st year after birth.

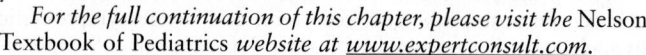

For the full continuation of this chapter, please visit the Nelson Textbook of Pediatrics *website at* www.expertconsult.com.

Chapter 88
The Newborn Infant (See Also Chapter 7)

Waldemar A. Carlo

The neonatal period is a highly vulnerable time for an infant, who is completing many of the physiologic adjustments required for extrauterine existence. The high neonatal morbidity and mortality rates attest to the fragility of life during this period; of all deaths occurring in the 1st yr of life in the USA, two thirds are in the neonatal period. The annual rate of deaths during the 1st yr is unequaled by the rate in any other period of life until the 7th decade.

An infant's transition from intrauterine to extrauterine life requires many biochemical and physiologic changes. Many of a newborn infant's special problems are related to poor adaptation because of asphyxia, premature birth, life-threatening congenital anomalies, or the adverse effects of delivery.

88.1 History in Neonatal Pediatrics

Waldemar A. Carlo

The perinatal history should include the following information:

- Demographic and social data: socioeconomic status, age, race
- Past medical illnesses in the mother and family, including previous siblings: cardiopulmonary disorders, infectious diseases, genetic disorders, anemia, jaundice, diabetes mellitus
- Previous maternal reproductive problems: stillbirth, prematurity, blood group sensitization
- Events occurring in the present pregnancy: preterm labor, fetal assessments, vaginal bleeding, medications, acute illness, duration of rupture of membranes
- Description of the labor (duration, fetal presentation, fetal distress, fever) and delivery (cesarean section, anesthesia or sedation, use of forceps, Apgar scores, need for resuscitation)

88.2 Physical Examination of the Newborn Infant

Waldemar A. Carlo

Many physical and behavioral characteristics of a normal newborn infant are described in Chapters 7 and 584.

The **initial examination** of a newborn infant should be performed as soon as possible after delivery. Temperature, pulse, respiratory rate, color, type of respiration, tone, activity, and level of consciousness of infants should be monitored frequently until stabilization. For high-risk deliveries, this examination should take place in the delivery room and should focus on congenital anomalies, maturation and growth, and pathophysiologic problems that may interfere with normal cardiopulmonary and metabolic adaptation to extrauterine life. Congenital anomalies of varying degrees of severity may be present in 3-5% of infants. After a stable delivery room course, a 2nd and more detailed examination should be performed within 24 hr of birth. If an infant remains in the hospital longer than 48 hr, a **discharge examination** should be performed within 24 hr of discharge. For a healthy infant, the mother should be present during this examination; even minor, seemingly insignificant anatomic variations may worry a family and should be explained. The explanation must be careful and skillful so that otherwise unworried families are not unduly alarmed. Infants should not be discharged from the hospital without a final examination because certain abnormalities, particularly heart murmurs, often appear or disappear in the immediate neonatal period; in addition, evidence of disease that has just been acquired may be noted. The pulse (normal, 120-160 beats/min), respiratory rate (normal, 30-60 breaths/min), temperature, weight, length, head circumference, and dimensions of any visible or palpable structural abnormality should be assessed. Blood pressure is determined if a neonate appears ill or has a heart murmur. Pulse oximetry is performed by some clinicians to screen for serious ductus arteriosus–dependent congenital heart disease.

Examining a newborn requires patience, gentleness, and procedural flexibility. Thus, if the infant is quiet and relaxed at the beginning of the examination, palpation of the abdomen or auscultation of the heart should be performed 1st, before other, more disturbing manipulations are attempted.

GENERAL APPEARANCE

Physical activity may be absent during normal sleep, or it may be decreased by the effects of illness or drugs; an infant may be either lying with the extremities motionless, to conserve energy for the effort of difficult breathing, or vigorously crying, with accompanying activity of the arms and legs. Both active and passive muscle tone and any unusual posture should be noted. Coarse, tremulous movements with ankle or jaw **myoclonus** are more common and less significant in newborn infants than at any other age. Such movements tend to occur when an infant is active, whereas convulsive twitching usually occurs in a quiet state. **Edema** may produce a superficial appearance of good nutrition. Pitting after applied pressure may or may not be noted, but the skin of the fingers and toes lacks the normal fine wrinkles when filled with fluid. Edema of the eyelids commonly results from irritation caused by the administration of silver nitrate. Generalized edema may occur with prematurity, hypoproteinemia secondary to severe erythroblastosis fetalis, nonimmune hydrops, congenital nephrosis, Hurler syndrome, and from unknown causes. Localized edema suggests a congenital malformation of the lymphatic system; when confined to one or more extremities of a female infant, it may be the initial sign of Turner syndrome (Chapters 76 and 580).

SKIN

Vasomotor instability and peripheral circulatory sluggishness are revealed by deep redness or purple lividity in a crying infant, whose color may darken profoundly with closure of the glottis preceding a vigorous cry, and by harmless cyanosis (**acrocyanosis**) of the hands and feet, especially when they are cool. Mottling, another example of general circulatory instability, may be associated with serious illness or related to a transient fluctuation in skin temperature. An extraordinary division of the body from the forehead to the pubis into red and pale halves is known as **harlequin color change**, a transient and harmless condition. Significant **cyanosis** may be masked by the pallor of circulatory failure or anemia; alternatively, the relatively high hemoglobin content of the 1st few days and the thin skin may combine to produce an appearance of cyanosis at a higher PaO_2 than in older children. Localized cyanosis is differentiated from ecchymosis by the momentary blanching pallor (with cyanosis) that occurs after pressure. The same maneuver also helps in demonstrating icterus. **Pallor** may be due to anemia, asphyxia, shock, or edema. Early recognition of anemia may lead to a diagnosis of erythroblastosis fetalis, subcapsular hematoma of the liver or spleen, subdural hemorrhage, or fetal-maternal or twin-twin transfusion. Without being anemic, postmature infants tend to have paler and thicker skin than term or premature infants. The ruddy appearance of plethora is seen with polycythemia.

The vernix and common transitory macular capillary hemangiomas of the eyelids and neck are described in Chapter 639. Cavernous hemangiomas are deeper, blue masses that, if large, may trap platelets and produce disseminated intravascular coagulation or interfere with local organ function. Scattered petechiae may be seen on the presenting part (usually the scalp or face) after a difficult delivery. Slate-blue, well-demarcated areas of pigmentation are seen over the buttocks, back, and sometimes other parts of the body in more than 50% of black, Native American, and Asian infants and occasionally in white ones. These benign patches have no known anthropologic significance despite their name, **Mongolian spots**; they tend to disappear within the 1st year. The vernix, skin, and especially the cord may be stained brownish yellow if the amniotic fluid has been colored by the passage of meconium during or before birth.

The skin of premature infants is thin and delicate and tends to be deep red; in extremely premature infants, the skin appears almost gelatinous and translucent. Fine, soft, immature hair, **lanugo**, frequently covers the scalp and brow and may also cover the face of premature infants. Lanugo has usually been lost or replaced by vellus hair in term infants. **Tufts of hair** over the lumbosacral spine suggest an underlying abnormality such as occult spina bifida, a sinus tract, or a tumor. The nails are rudimentary in very premature infants, but they may protrude beyond the fingertips in infants born past term. Post-term infants may have a peeling, parchment-like skin (Fig. 88-1), a severe degree of which suggests ichthyosis congenita (Chapter 650).

In many neonates, small, white papules on an erythematous base develop 1-3 days after birth. This benign rash, **erythema toxicum**, persists for as long as 1 wk, contains eosinophils, and is usually distributed on the face, trunk, and extremities (Chapter 639). **Pustular melanosis**, a benign lesion seen predominantly in black neonates, contains neutrophils and is present at birth as a vesiculopustular eruption around the chin, neck, back, extremities, and palms or soles; it lasts 2-3 days. Both lesions need to be distinguished from more dangerous vesicular eruptions such as herpes simplex (Chapter 244) and staphylococcal disease of the skin (Chapter 174.1).

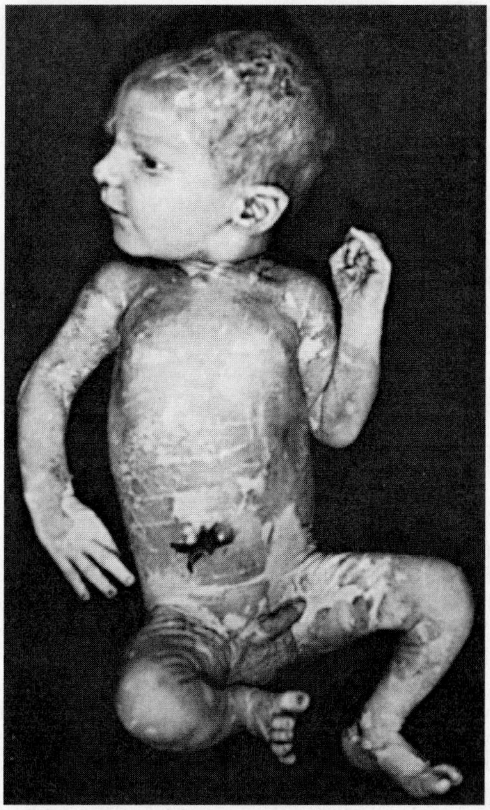

Figure 88-1 Infant with intrauterine growth retardation as a result of placental insufficiency. Note the long, thin appearance with peeling, parchment-like dry skin, alert expression, meconium staining of the skin, and long nails. (From Clifford S: *Advances in pediatrics*, vol 9, Chicago, 1962, Year Book.)

Amniotic bands may disrupt the skin, extremities (amputation, ring constriction, syndactyly), face (clefts), or trunk (abdominal or thoracic wall defects). Their cause is uncertain but may be related to amniotic membrane rupture or vascular compromise with fibrous band formation. Excessive skin fragility and extensibility with joint hypermobility suggest Ehlers-Danlos syndrome, Marfan syndrome, congenital contractural arachnodactyly, and other disorders of collagen synthesis.

SKULL

The head circumference of all infants should be charted. The skull may be molded, particularly if the infant is the first-born and if the head has been engaged in the pelvic canal for a considerable time. The parietal bones tend to override the occipital and frontal bones. The head of an infant born by cesarean section or from a breech presentation is characterized by its roundness. The suture lines and the size and fullness of the anterior and posterior fontanels should be determined digitally by palpation. Premature fusion of sutures (**cranial synostosis**) is identified as a hard nonmovable ridge over the suture and an abnormally shaped skull. Great variation in the size of the **fontanels** exists at birth; if small, the anterior fontanel usually tends to enlarge during the 1st few months of life. The persistence of excessively large anterior (normal, 20 ± 10 mm) and posterior fontanels has been associated with several disorders (Table 88-1). Persistently small fontanels suggest microcephaly, craniosynostosis, congenital hyperthyroidism, or wormian bones; presence of a 3rd fontanel suggests trisomy 21 but is seen in preterm infants. Soft areas (**craniotabes**) are occasionally found in the parietal bones at the vertex near the sagittal suture; they are more common in premature infants and

Table 88-1 DISORDERS ASSOCIATED WITH A LARGE ANTERIOR FONTANEL
Achondroplasia
Apert syndrome
Athyrotic hypothyroidism
Cleidocranial dysostosis
Congenital rubella syndrome
Hallermann-Streiff syndrome
Hydrocephaly
Hypophosphatasia
Intrauterine growth retardation
Kenny syndrome
Osteogenesis imperfecta
Prematurity
Pyknodysostosis
Russell-Silver syndrome
Trisomies 13-, 18-, and 21
Vitamin D deficiency rickets

in infants who have been exposed to uterine compression. Though such soft areas are usually insignificant, their possible pathologic cause should be investigated if they persist. Soft areas in the occipital region suggest the irregular calcification and wormian bone formation associated with osteogenesis imperfecta, cleidocranial dysostosis, lacunar skull, cretinism, and, occasionally, Down syndrome. Transillumination of an abnormal skull in a dark room followed by ultrasound or computed tomography will rule out hydranencephaly and hydrocephaly (Chapter 585). An excessively large head (megalencephaly) suggests hydrocephaly, storage disease, achondroplasia, cerebral gigantism, neurocutaneous syndromes, or inborn errors of metabolism, or may be familial. The skull of a premature infant may suggest hydrocephaly because of the relatively larger brain growth in comparison with growth of other organs. Depression of the skull (indentation, fracture, ping-pong ball deformity) is usually of prenatal onset and due to prolonged focal pressure by the bony pelvis. Atrophic or alopecic scalp areas may represent aplasia cutis congenita, which may be sporadic or autosomal dominant or associated with trisomy 13, chromosome 4 deletion, or Johanson-Blizzard syndrome. Deformational plagiocephaly may be due to in utero positioning forces on the skull and manifests as an asymmetric skull and face with ear malalignment. It is associated with torticollis and vertex positioning. Any significant and persistent abnormality in shape or size of the skull should be evaluated by cranial CT.

FACE

The general appearance of the face should be noted with regard to dysmorphic features, such as epicanthal folds, widely or narrowly spaced eyes, microphthalmos, asymmetry, long philtrum, and low-set ears, which are often associated with congenital syndromes. The face may be asymmetric as a result of a 7th nerve palsy, hypoplasia of the depressor muscle at the angle of the mouth, or an abnormal fetal posture (Chapter 102); when the jaw has been held against a shoulder or an extremity during the intrauterine period, the mandible may deviate strikingly from the midline. Symmetric facial palsy suggests absence or hypoplasia of the 7th nerve nucleus (**Möbius syndrome**).

Eyes

The eyes often open spontaneously if the infant is held up and tipped gently forward and backward. This maneuver, a result of labyrinthine and neck reflexes, is more successful for inspecting the eyes than is forcing the lids apart. Conjunctival and retinal hemorrhages are usually benign. Retinal hemorrhages are more common with vacuum-assisted deliveries (75%) than after cesarean section (7%). They resolve in most infants by 2 wk of age (85%) and in all infants by 4 wk. **Pupillary reflexes** are present after 28-30 wk of gestation. The iris should be inspected for colobomas and heterochromia. A cornea >1cm in diameter in a term infant (with photophobia and tearing) suggests congenital glaucoma and requires prompt ophthalmologic consultation. The presence of bilateral red reflexes suggests the absence of cataracts and intraocular pathology (Chapters 611, 619-625). **Leukokoria** (white pupillary reflex) suggests cataracts, tumor, chorioretinitis, retinopathy of prematurity, or a persistent hyperplastic primary vitreous and warrants an immediate ophthalmologic consultation.

Ears

Deformities of the pinnae are occasionally seen. Unilateral or bilateral preauricular skin tags occur frequently; if pedunculated, they can be tightly ligated at the base, resulting in dry gangrene and sloughing. The tympanic membrane, easily seen otoscopically through the short, straight external auditory canal, normally appears dull gray.

Nose

The nose may be slightly obstructed by mucus accumulated in the narrow nostrils. The nares should be symmetric and patent. Dislocation of the nasal cartilage from the vomerian groove results in asymmetric nares. Anatomic obstruction of the nasal passages secondary to unilateral or bilateral choanal atresia results in respiratory distress.

Mouth

A normal mouth may rarely have precocious dentition, with natal (present at birth) or neonatal (eruption after birth) teeth in the lower incisor position or aberrantly placed; these teeth are shed before the deciduous ones erupt (Chapter 299). Alternatively, such teeth occur in Ellis-van Creveld, Hallermann-Streiff, and other syndromes. Extraction is not usually indicated. Premature eruption of deciduous teeth is even more unusual. The soft and hard palate should be inspected and palpated for a complete or submucosal cleft, and the contour noted if the arch is excessively high or the uvula is bifid. On the hard palate on either side of the raphe, there may be temporary accumulations of epithelial cells called **Epstein pearls**. Retention cysts of similar appearance may also be seen on the gums. Both disappear spontaneously, usually within a few weeks of birth. Clusters of small white or yellow follicles or ulcers on erythematous bases may be found on the anterior tonsillar pillars, most frequently on the 2nd or 3rd day of life. Of unknown cause, they clear without treatment in 2-4 days.

Neonates do not have active salivation. The tongue appears relatively large; the frenulum may be short, but its shortness (**tongue-tied** or **ankyloglossia**) is rarely a reason for cutting it. If there are problems with feedings (breast or bottle) and the frenulum is short, frenulotomy may be indicated. The sublingual mucous membrane occasionally forms a prominent fold. The cheeks have fullness on both the buccal and the external aspects as a result of the accumulation of fat making up the sucking pads. These pads, as well as the labial tubercle on the upper lip (**sucking callus**), disappear when suckling ceases. A marble-sized buccal mass is usually due to benign idiopathic fat necrosis.

The throat of a newborn infant is hard to see because of the low arch of the palate; it should be clearly viewed because posterior palatal or uvular clefts are easy to miss. The tonsils are small.

NECK

The neck appears relatively short. Abnormalities are not common but include goiter, cystic hygroma, branchial cleft rests, teratoma, hemangioma, and lesions of the sternocleidomastoid muscle that are presumably traumatic or due to a fixed positioning in utero that produces either a hematoma or fibrosis, respectively. Congenital **torticollis** causes the head to turn toward and the face to turn away from the affected side. Plagiocephaly, facial asymmetry, and hemihypoplasia may develop if it is untreated (Chapter 672.1). Redundant skin or webbing in a female infant suggests intrauterine lymphedema and Turner syndrome (Chapters 76 and 580). Both clavicles should be palpated for fractures.

CHEST

Breast hypertrophy is common, and milk may be present (but should not be expressed). Asymmetry, erythema, induration, and tenderness suggest mastitis or a breast abscess. Supernumerary nipples, inverted nipples, or widely spaced nipples with a shield-shaped chest may be seen; the last finding suggests Turner syndrome.

LUNGS

Much can be learned by observing breathing. Variations in rate and rhythm are characteristic and fluctuate according to the infant's physical activity, the state of wakefulness, or the presence of crying. Because fluctuations are rapid, the respiratory rate should be counted for a full minute with the infant in the resting state, preferably asleep. Under these circumstances, the usual rate for normal term infants is 30-60 breaths/min; in premature infants the rate is higher and fluctuates more widely. A rate consistently over 60 breaths/min during periods of regular breathing usually indicates pulmonary, cardiac, or metabolic disease (acidosis). Premature infants may breathe with a Cheyne-Stokes rhythm, known as periodic respiration, or with complete irregularity. Irregular gasping, sometimes accompanied by spasmodic movements of the mouth and chin, strongly indicates serious impairment of the respiratory centers.

The breathing of newborn infants at rest is almost entirely diaphragmatic, so during inspiration, the soft front of the thorax is usually drawn inward while the abdomen protrudes. If the baby is quiet, relaxed, and of good color, this "paradoxic movement" does not necessarily signify insufficient ventilation. On the other hand, labored respiration with retractions is important evidence of respiratory distress syndrome, pneumonia, anomalies, or mechanical disturbance of the lungs. A weak persistent or intermittent groaning, whining cry, or **grunting** during expiration signifies potentially serious cardiopulmonary disease or sepsis and warrants immediate attention. When benign, the grunting resolves between 30 and 60 min after birth. Flaring of the alae nasi and retraction of the intercostal muscles and sternum are common signs of pulmonary pathology.

Normally, the breath sounds are bronchovesicular. Suspicion of pulmonary pathology because of diminished breath sounds, rales, retractions, or cyanosis should always be verified with a chest radiograph.

HEART

Normal variation in the size and shape of the chest makes it difficult to estimate the size of the heart. The location of the heart should be determined to detect dextrocardia. Transitory murmurs usually represent a closing ductus arteriosus. Although congenital heart disease may not initially produce a murmur, a substantial portion of infants in whom persistent murmurs are detected during routine neonatal examination have underlying malformation. Evaluation of the heart by echocardiography is essential when the possibility of a significant lesion exists. Oxygen saturation measurements can be used to screen for serious congenital heart disease. Oxygen saturation value < 96% 24 hours after birth has been used as a cutoff for suspicion of serious congenital heart disease.

The pulse may vary normally from 90 beats/min in relaxed sleep to 174 beats/min during activity. The still higher rate of supraventricular tachycardia (>220 beats/min) may be determined better with a cardiac monitor or electrocardiogram than by ear. Premature infants, whose resting heart rate is usually 140-150 beats/min, may have a sudden onset of sinus bradycardia. On both admission to and discharge from the nursery, the infant's pulses should be palpated in the upper and lower extremities to detect coarctation of the aorta.

Blood pressure measurements may be a valuable diagnostic aid in ill infants (Chapter 419). The oscillometric method is the easiest and most accurate noninvasive method available. Continuous or intermittent direct measurement of blood pressure with an umbilical artery catheter may be indicated in special circumstances for infants who are under close observation in an intensive care unit (Fig. 88-2).

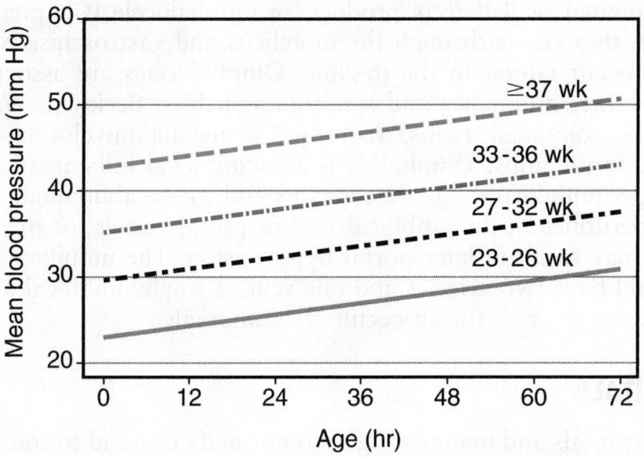

Figure 88-2 Nomogram for mean blood pressure (BP) in neonates with gestational ages of 23-43 wk derived from continuous arterial BP measurements obtained from 103 infants admitted to the neonatal intensive care unit. The graph shows the predicted mean BP of neonates of different gestational ages during the 1st 72 hours of life. Each *line* represents the lower limit of the 80% confidence interval (two-tail) of the mean BP for each gestational age group; 90% of infants for each gestational age group will be expected to have a mean BP value equal to or above the value indicated by the corresponding line, the lower limit of the confidence interval. (From Nuntnarumit P, Yang W, Bada-Ellzey SB: Blood pressure measurements in the newborn, *Clin Perinatol* 26:976–996, 1999.)

ABDOMEN

The liver is usually palpable, sometimes as much as 2 cm below the rib margin. Less commonly, the tip of the spleen may be felt. The approximate size and location of each kidney can usually be determined on deep palpation. At no other period of life does the amount of air in the gastrointestinal tract vary so much, nor is it usually so great under normal circumstances. Gas should normally be present in the rectum on roentgenogram by 24 hr of age. The abdominal wall is normally weak (especially in premature infants), and diastasis recti and umbilical hernias are common, particularly among black infants.

Unusual masses should be investigated immediately with ultrasonography. Renal pathology is the cause of most neonatal abdominal masses. **Cystic abdominal masses** include hydronephrosis, multicystic-dysplastic kidneys, adrenal hemorrhage, hydrometrocolpos, intestinal duplication, and choledochal, ovarian, omental, or pancreatic cysts. **Solid masses** include neuroblastoma, congenital mesoblastic nephroma, hepatoblastoma, and teratoma. A solid flank mass may be caused by **renal vein thrombosis**, which becomes clinically apparent with hematuria, hypertension, and thrombocytopenia. Renal vein thrombosis in infants is associated with polycythemia, dehydration, maternal diabetes, asphyxia, sepsis, nephrosis, and hypercoagulable states such as antithrombin III and protein C deficiency.

Abdominal distention at birth or shortly afterward suggests either obstruction or perforation of the gastrointestinal tract, often as a result of meconium ileus; later distention suggests lower bowel obstruction, sepsis, or peritonitis. A scaphoid abdomen in a newborn suggests diaphragmatic hernia.

Abdominal wall defects produce an omphalocele (Chapter 99) when they occur through the umbilicus and gastroschisis when they occur lateral to the midline. Omphaloceles are associated with other anomalies and syndromes such as Beckwith-Wiedemann, conjoined twins, trisomy 18, meningomyelocele, and imperforate anus. **Omphalitis** is an acute local inflammation of the periumbilical tissue that may extend to the abdominal wall, the peritoneum, the umbilical vein or portal vessels, or the liver and may result in later portal hypertension. The umbilical cord should have two arteries and one vein. A single umbilical artery increases the risk for an occult renal anomaly.

GENITALS

The genitals and mammary glands normally respond to transplacentally acquired maternal hormones to produce enlargement and secretion of the breasts in both sexes and prominence of the genitals in females, often with considerable nonpurulent discharge. These transitory manifestations require no intervention.

An imperforate hymen may result in **hydrometrocolpos** and a lower abdominal mass. A normal scrotum at term is relatively large; its size may be increased by the trauma of breech delivery or by a transitory hydrocele, which is distinguished from a hernia by palpation and transillumination. The testes should be in the scrotum or should be palpable in the canals in term infants. Black male infants usually have dark pigmentation of the scrotum before the rest of the skin assumes its permanent color.

The prepuce of a newborn infant is normally tight and adherent. Severe hypospadias or epispadias should always lead one to suspect either that abnormal sex chromosomes are present (Chapter 76) or that the infant is actually a masculinized female with an enlarged clitoris, because this finding may be the 1st evidence of adrenogenital syndrome (Chapter 570). Erection of the penis is common and has no significance. Urine is usually passed during or immediately after birth; a period without voiding may normally follow. Most neonates void by 12 hr, and about 95% of preterm and term infants void within 24 hr.

ANUS

Some passage of meconium usually occurs within the 1st 12 hr after birth; 99% of term infants and 95% of premature infants pass meconium within 48 hr of birth. Imperforate anus is not always visible and may require evidence obtained by gentle insertion of the examiner's little finger or a rectal tube. Radiographic study is required. Passage of meconium does not rule out an imperforate anus if a rectal-vaginal fistula is present. The dimple or irregularity in skinfold often normally present in the sacrococcygeal midline may be mistaken for an actual or potential neurocutaneous sinus.

EXTREMITIES

During examination of the extremities, the effects of fetal posture (Chapter 664) should be noted so that their cause and usual transitory nature can be explained to the mother. Such explanations are particularly important after breech presentations. A fracture or nerve injury associated with delivery can be detected more commonly by observation of the extremities in spontaneous or stimulated activity than by any other means. The hands and feet should be examined for polydactyly, syndactyly, and abnormal dermatoglyphic patterns such as a simian crease.

The hips of all infants should be examined with specific maneuvers to rule out congenital dislocation (Chapter 670.1).

NEUROLOGIC EXAMINATION (CHAPTERS 7 AND 584)

In utero neuromuscular diseases associated with limited fetal motion produce a constellation of signs and symptoms that are independent of the specific disease. Severe positional deformation and contractures produce arthrogryposis. Other manifestations of fetal neuromuscular disease include breech presentation, polyhydramnios, failure to breathe at birth, pulmonary hypoplasia, dislocated hips, undescended testes, thin ribs, and clubfoot. Many congenital disorders manifest as hypotonia, hypertonia, or seizures.

BIBLIOGRAPHY

Please visit the Nelson Textbook of Pediatrics *website at www.expertconsult.com for the complete bibliography.*

88.3 Routine Delivery Room and Initial Care

Waldemar A. Carlo

Low-risk infants may initially be placed head downward after delivery to allow gravity to clear the mouth, pharynx, and nose of fluid, mucus, blood, and amniotic debris; wiping of the mouth with a cloth or gentle suction with a bulb syringe or soft catheter may also be helpful if there is an excessive amount of fluid in the mouth or nares. Most healthy infants who appear to be in satisfactory condition should be given directly to their mothers for immediate bonding and nursing. If respiratory distress is a concern, infants should be placed under warmers for observation.

The **Apgar score** is a practical method of systematically assessing newborn infants immediately after birth (Table 88-2). A low score may be due to fetal distress but may also be due to a number of factors, including prematurity and drugs given to the mother during labor (Table 88-3). The Apgar score was not designed to predict neurologic outcome. Indeed, the score is normal in most patients in whom cerebral palsy subsequently develops, and the incidence of cerebral palsy is low in infants with Apgar scores of 0-3 at 5 min (but higher than in infants with Apgar scores of 7-10). Low Apgar scores and umbilical artery blood pH predict neonatal death. An Apgar score of 0-3 at 5 min is uncommon but is a better predictor of neonatal death (in both term and preterm infants) than an umbilical artery pH ≤ 7.0; the presence of both variables increases the relative risk of neonatal mortality in term and preterm infants (Table 88-4). Infants who fail to initiate respiration should receive prompt resuscitation and close observation (Chapter 94).

MAINTENANCE OF BODY HEAT

Newborn infants are at risk for heat loss and hypothermia for several reasons. Relative to body weight, the body surface area

Table 88-2 APGAR EVALUATION OF NEWBORN INFANTS*

SIGN	0	1	2
Heart rate	Absent	Below 100	Over 100
Respiratory effort	Absent	Slow, irregular	Good, crying
Muscle tone	Limp	Some flexion of extremities	Active motion
Response to catheter in nostril (tested after oropharynx is clear)	No response	Grimace	Cough or sneeze
Color	Blue, pale	Body pink, extremities blue	Completely pink

*Sixty sec after complete birth of the infant (disregarding the cord and placenta), the five objective signs listed here are evaluated, and each is given a score of 0, 1, or 2. A total score of 10 indicates an infant in the best possible condition. An infant with a score of 0-3 requires immediate resuscitation.

Modified from Apgar V: A proposal for a new method of evaluation of the newborn infant, *Res Anesth Analg* 32:260–267, 1953.

Table 88-3 FACTORS AFFECTING THE APGAR SCORE*

FALSE-POSITIVE (NO FETAL ACIDOSIS OR HYPOXIA; LOW APGAR SCORE)
Prematurity
Analgesics, narcotics, sedatives
Magnesium sulfate
Acute cerebral trauma
Precipitous delivery
Congenital myopathy
Congenital neuropathy
Spinal cord trauma
Central nervous system anomaly
Lung anomaly (diaphragmatic hernia)
Airway obstruction (choanal atresia)
Congenital pneumonia and sepsis
Previous episodes of fetal asphyxia (recovered)
Hemorrhage-hypovolemia
FALSE-NEGATIVE (ACIDOSIS; NORMAL APGAR SCORE)
Maternal acidosis
High fetal catecholamine levels
Some full-term infants

*Regardless of the etiology, a low Apgar score because of fetal asphyxia, immaturity, central nervous system depression, or airway obstruction identifies an infant needing immediate resuscitation.

Table 88-4 INCIDENCE OF NEONATAL DEATH IN 132,228 SINGLETON INFANTS BORN AT TERM (37TH WEEK OF GESTATION OR LATER) IN RELATION TO APGAR SCORES AT 5 MINUTES OF AGE*

5-MIN APGAR SCORE	NO. OF LIVE BIRTHS	NO. NEONATAL DEATHS (PER 1,000 BIRTHS)	RELATIVE RISK (95% CI)
0-3	86	21 (244)	1,460 (835-2,555)
4-6	561	5 (9)	53 (20-140)
7-10	131,581	22 (0.2)	1

*Infants with 5-min Apgar scores of 7-10 served as the reference group.
CI, confidence interval.
From Casey BM, McIntire DD, Leveno KJ: The continuing value of the Apgar score for the assessment of newborn infants, *N Engl J Med* 344:467–471, 2001.

of a newborn infant is approximately three times that of an adult. Generation of body heat depends in large part on body weight, but heat loss depends on surface area. In low birthweight and preterm infants, the insulating layer of subcutaneous fat is thin. The estimated rate of heat loss in a newborn is approximately four times that of an adult. Under the usual delivery room conditions (20-25°C), an infant's skin temperature falls approximately 0.3°C/min and deep body temperature decreases approximately 0.1°C/min during the period immediately after delivery; these rates generally result in a cumulative loss of 2-3°C in deep body temperature (corresponding to a heat loss of approximately 200 kcal/kg). The heat loss occurs by four mechanisms: (1) **convection** of heat energy to the cooler surrounding air, (2) **conduction** of heat to the colder materials touching the infant, (3) **heat radiation** from the infant to other nearby cooler objects, and (4) **evaporation** from skin and lungs.

Metabolic acidosis, hypoxemia, hypoglycemia, and increased renal excretion of water and solutes may develop in term infants exposed to cold after birth because of their effort to compensate for heat loss. Heat production is augmented by increasing the metabolic rate and oxygen consumption in part by releasing norepinephrine, which results in nonshivering thermo-genesis through oxidation of fat, particularly brown fat. In addition, muscular activity may increase. Hypoglycemic or hypoxic infants cannot increase their oxygen consumption when exposed to a cold environment, and their central temperature decreases. After labor and vaginal delivery, many newborn infants have mild to moderate metabolic acidosis, for which they may compensate by hyperventilating, a response that is more difficult for infants with central nervous system depression (asphyxia, drugs) and infants exposed to cold stress in the delivery room. Therefore, to reduce heat loss, it is desirable to ensure that infants are dried and either wrapped in blankets or placed under radiant warmers. **Skin-to-skin contact** with the mother is the optimal method of maintaining temperature in the stable newborn. Because carrying out resuscitative measures on a covered infant or one enclosed in an incubator is difficult, a radiant heat source should be used to warm the baby during resuscitation.

ANTISEPTIC SKIN AND CORD CARE

Careful removal of blood from the skin shortly after birth may reduce the risk of infection with blood-borne agents. Once a healthy infant's temperature has stabilized, the entire skin and cord should be cleansed with warm water or a mild nonmedicated soap solution and rinsed with water to reduce the incidence of skin and periumbilical colonization with pathogenic bacteria and subsequent infectious complications. To avoid heat loss, the infant is then dried and wrapped in clean blankets. To reduce colonization with *Staphylococcus aureus* and other pathogenic bacteria, the umbilical cord may be treated daily with a bactericidal or antimicrobial agents such as triple dye or bacitracin. One application of triple dye followed by twice-daily alcohol swabbing (until the cord falls off) reduces colonization, exudates, and foul odor of the umbilicus in comparison with dry care (soap and water when soiled). Alternatively, chlorhexidine washing or, on rare occasion during *S. aureus* epidemics, a single hexachlorophene bath may be used. Topical ointments should not be applied to preterm infants in neonatal intensive care units because this treatment increases the risk of bacterial sepsis. Routine or repeated total body exposure to hexachlorophene may be neurotoxic, particularly in low-birthweight infants, and is thus contraindicated. Nursery personnel should use chlorhexidine or iodophor-containing antiseptic soaps for routine handwashing before caring for each infant. Rigid enforcement of hand-to-elbow washing for 2 min in the initial wash and 15-30 sec in the 2nd wash is essential for staff and visitors entering the nursery. Equally thorough washes between handling infants are also required.

OTHER MEASURES

The eyes of all infants, including those born by cesarean section, must be protected against gonococcal ophthalmia neonatorum by instillation of 1% silver nitrate drops or erythromycin (0.5%) or tetracycline (1.0%) sterile ophthalmic ointments. This procedure may be delayed during the initial short-alert period after birth to promote bonding, but once applied, drops should not be rinsed out (Chapters 185 and 218.3).

Although hemorrhage in newborn infants can be due to factors other than vitamin K deficiency, an intramuscular injection of 1 mg of water-soluble vitamin K_1 (phytonadione) is recommended for all infants immediately after birth to prevent hemorrhagic disease of the newborn (Chapter 97.4). Oral vitamin K may also be useful but is not as effective as the parenteral dosage. Administration of vitamin K to the mother during labor is not recommended because of unpredictable placental transfer.

Hepatitis B immunization before discharge from the nursery is recommended for newborns with weight >2 kg irrespective of maternal hepatitis status.

Neonatal screening is available for various genetic, metabolic, hematologic, and endocrine disorders. All states in the USA have neonatal screening programs, although the specific tests required vary (Chapter 78). The expanded newborn screening, which consists of a panel of approximately 29 disorders, is estimated to increase by 32% the number of affected children identified. The most commonly identified disorders (and their rates) include hypothyroidism (52/100,000 births), cystic fibrosis

(30/100,000), hemoglobinopathies (26/100,000), medium-chain acyl–coenzyme A dehydrogenase deficiency (6/100,000), galactosemia (5/100,000), and phenylketonuria (5/100,000), and adrenal hyperplasia (5/100,000). To be effective in the timely identification and prompt management of treatable diseases, screening programs must include not only high-quality laboratory tests but also follow-up of infants with abnormal test results; education, counseling, and psychologic support for families; and prompt referral of the identified neonate for accurate diagnosis and therapy.

Hearing impairment, a serious morbidity that affects speech and language development, may be severe in 2/1,000 births and overall affects 5/1,000 births. Universal screening of infants is recommended to ensure early detection of hearing loss and appropriate, timely intervention.

Routine measurement of the hematocrit or blood glucose value is not necessary in the absence of risk factors. Screening for hyperbilirubinemia should include risk assessment in all infants with measurement of serum or transcutaneous bilirubin levels as indicated.

BIBLIOGRAPHY

Please visit the Nelson Textbook of Pediatrics *website at www.expertconsult.com for the complete bibliography.*

88.4 Nursery Care

Waldemar A. Carlo

Non–high-risk, healthy infants may be taken to the "regular" (normal) newborn nursery or may be placed in the mother's room if the hospital has rooming-in facilities.

The bassinet, preferably of clear plastic to allow for easy visibility and care, should be cleaned frequently. All professional care should be given to the infant in the bassinet, including the physical examination, clothing changes, temperature taking, skin cleansing, and other procedures that, if performed elsewhere, would establish a common contact point and possibly provide a channel for cross infection. The clothing and bedding should be minimal, only enough needed for an infant's comfort; the nursery temperature should be kept at approximately 22-26°C (72-78°F). The infant's temperature should be taken by axillary measurement. Although the interval between temperature measurements depends on many circumstances, it need not be shorter than 4 hr during the 1st 2-3 days and 8 hr thereafter. Axillary temperatures of 36.4-37.0°C (97.0-98.5°F) are within normal limits. Weighing at birth and daily thereafter is sufficient. Healthy infants should be placed supine to reduce the risk of sudden infant death syndrome.

Vernix is spontaneously shed within 2-3 days, much of it adhering to the clothing, which should be completely changed daily. The diaper should be checked before and after feeding and when the baby cries; it should be changed when wet or soiled. The perineal area can be cleaned with baby wipes or with mild soap and warm water. Meconium or feces should be cleansed from the buttocks with sterile cotton moistened with sterile water. The foreskin of a male infant should not be retracted. Circumcision is an elective procedure. Circumcision may decrease phimosis, urinary tract infections in infancy, penile cancer, and acquisition of some sexually transmitted infections, including HIV. Parents should make a determination in the interest of the baby until firm recommendations are provided.

Early discharge (<48 hr) or very early discharge (<24 hr) of a neonate may increase the risk of rehospitalization for hyperbilirubinemia, sepsis, failure to thrive, dehydration, and missed congenital anomalies. Early discharge requires careful ambulatory follow-up at home (by a visiting nurse) or in the office within 48 hr. Additional criteria for the early discharge of term neonates have been developed by the American Academy of Pediatrics and American College of Obstetrics and Gynecology (Table 88-5).

Table 88-5 RECOMMENDATIONS FOR EARLY DISCHARGE FROM THE NORMAL NEWBORN NURSERY*

Uncomplicated antepartum, intrapartum, postpartum courses
Vaginal delivery
Singleton at 38-42 wk: appropriate for gestational age
Normal vital signs including respiratory rate <60 breaths/min; axillary temperature 36.1-37°C (97.0-98.6°F) in open crib
Physical examination reveals no abnormalities requiring continued hospitalization
Urination; stool × 1
At least two uneventful, successful feedings
No excessive bleeding after (2 hr) circumcision
No jaundice within 24 hr of birth; if jaundice, appropriate management and follow-up are in place
Evidence of parental knowledge, ability, and confidence to care for the baby at home:
Feeding
Cord, skin, genital care
Recognition of illness (jaundice, poor feeding, lethargy, fever, etc.)
Infant safety (car seat, supine sleep position, etc.)
Availability of family and physician support (physician follow-up)
Laboratory evaluation:
Syphilis
Hepatitis B surface antigen and vaccination or appointment for vaccination
Coombs' test and blood type if clinically indicated
Expanded metabolic screening: phenylketonuria, thyroid, galactosemia, sickle cell
Hearing screening
No social risks:
Substance abuse
History of child abuse
Domestic violence
Mental illness
Teen mother
Homelessness
Barriers to follow-up
Source of continuing medal care is identified

*It is not likely that all these criteria will be met before 48 hr of age.

Adapted from American Academy of Pediatrics, American College of Obstetricians and Gynecologists: *Guidelines for perinatal care*, ed 5, Elk Grove Village, IL, 2002, American Academy of Pediatrics.

BIBLIOGRAPHY

Please visit the Nelson Textbook of Pediatrics *website at www.expertconsult.com for the complete bibliography.*

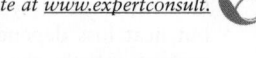

88.5 Parent-Infant Bonding (See Also Chapter 7)

Waldemar A. Carlo

Normal infant development depends partly on a series of affectionate responses exchanged between a mother and her newborn infant that binds them psychologically and physiologically. This bonding is facilitated and reinforced by the emotional support of a loving family. The attachment process may be important in enabling some mothers to provide loving care during the neonatal period and subsequently during childhood. The power of this attachment is so great that it enables the mother and the father to make unusual sacrifices necessary for the day-to-day care of the infant, care night after night, giving feedings 24 hours a day, attending to crying, and so on. The sacrifices continue for many years as parents dedicate much of their lives to their children.

Parent-infant bonding is initiated before birth with the planning and confirmation of the pregnancy. Subsequently, there is a growing awareness of the baby as an individual, starting usually with the remarkably powerful event of "quickening" or sensation of fetal movements. After delivery and during the ensuing weeks, sensory (visual, auditory, olfactory) and physical contact between the mother and baby triggers various mutually rewarding and pleasurable interactions, such as the mother touching the infant's extremities and face with her fingertips and encompassing and gently massaging the infant's trunk with her hands. Touching an infant's cheek elicits responsive turning toward the mother's face or toward the breast with nuzzling and licking of the nipple, a powerful stimulus for prolactin secretion. An infant's initial quiet alert state provides the opportunity for eye-to-eye contact, which is particularly important in stimulating the loving and possessive feelings of many parents for their babies. An infant's crying elicits the maternal response of touching the infant and speaking in a soft, soothing, higher-toned voice. Initial contact between the mother and infant should take place in the delivery room, and opportunities for extended intimate contact and breast-feeding should be provided within the 1st hours after birth. Delayed or abnormal maternal-infant bonding, as occurs because of prematurity, infant or maternal illness, birth defects, or family stress, may harm infant development and maternal caretaking ability. Hospital routines should be designed to encourage parent-infant contact. Open nurseries, rooming-in arrangements, care by parents, and family-centered care increase the opportunities for better parent-infant interaction.

NURSERIES AND BREAST-FEEDING

See Chapter 42 for full discussions of breast-feeding and formula feeding. Hospital practices that encourage successful breast-feeding include antepartum education and encouragement, immediate postpartum mother-infant contact with suckling, rooming-in arrangements, demand feeding, inclusion of fathers in prenatal breast-feeding education, and support from experienced women. Nursing at first for least 5 min at each breast is reasonable, allows a baby to obtain most of the available breast contents, and provides effective stimulation for increasing the milk supply. Nursing episodes should then be extended according to the comfort and desire of the mother and infant. A confident and relaxed mother, supported by an encouraging home and hospital environment, is likely to nurse well. The Baby-Friendly Hospital Initiative, a

Table 88-6 TEN STEPS TO SUCCESSFUL BREAST-FEEDING

Every facility providing maternity services and care for newborn infants should accomplish the following:

1. Have a written breast-feeding policy that is routinely communicated to all health care staff.
2. Train all health care staff in the skills necessary to implement this policy.
3. Inform all pregnant women about the benefits and management of breast-feeding.
4. Help mothers initiate breast-feeding within a half hour of birth.
5. Show mothers how to breast-feed and how to maintain lactation even if they should be separated from their infants.
6. Give newborn infants no food or drink other than breast milk unless *medically* indicated.
7. Practice rooming-in (allow mothers and infants to remain together) 24 hr a day.
8. Encourage breast-feeding on demand.
9. Give no artificial teats or pacifiers (also called *dummies* or *soothers*) to breast-feeding infants.
10. Foster the establishment of breast-feeding support groups and refer mothers to them on discharge from the hospital or clinic.

From *Protecting, promoting and supporting breastfeeding: the special role of maternity services. A joint WHO/UNICEF statement.* Geneva, 1989, World Health Organization.

Table 88-7 DRUGS AND BREAST-FEEDING

CONTRAINDICATED	AVOID OR GIVE WITH CAUTION	PROBABLY SAFE
Amphetamines	Alcohol	Acetaminophen
Antineoplastic agents	Amiodarone	Acyclovir
Bromocriptine	Anthroquinones (laxatives)	Aldomet
Chloramphenicol	Aspirin (salicylates)	Anesthetics
Clozapine	Atropine	Antibiotics (not chloramphenicol)
Cocaine	β-adrenergic blocking agents	Antiepileptics
Cyclophosphamide	Birth control pills	Antihistamines*
Diethylstilbestrol	Bromides	Antithyroid (not methimazole)
Doxorubicin	Calciferol	Bishydroxycoumarin
Ergots	Cascara	Chlorpromazine*
Gold salts	Ciprofloxacin	Codeine*
Heroin	Danthron	Cyclosporine
Immunosuppressants	Dihydrotachysterol	Depo-Provera
Iodides	Domperidone	Digoxin
Lithium	Estrogens	Dilantin (phenytoin)
Methimazole	Metoclopramide	Diuretics
Methylamphetamine	Metronidazole	Fluoxetine
Phencyclidine (PCP)	Meperidine	Furosemide
Radiopharmaceuticals	Phenobarbital*	Haloperidol*
Thiouracil	Primidone	Hydralazine
	Psychotropic drugs	Indomethacin, other nonsteroidal anti-inflammatory drugs
	Reserpine	Low molecular weight heparins
	Salicylazosulfapyridine (sulfasalazine)	Metformin
		Methadone*
		Morphine
		Muscle relaxants
		Paroxetine
		Prednisone
		Propranolol
		Propylthiouracil
		Sedatives*
		Sertraline
		Theophylline
		Vitamins
		Warfarin

*Watch for sedation.

Table 88-8 SUMMARY OF INFECTIOUS AGENTS DETECTED IN MILK AND NEWBORN DISEASE

INFECTIOUS AGENT	DETECTED IN BREAST MILK?	BREAST MILK REPORTED AS CAUSE OF NEWBORN DISEASE?	MATERNAL INFECTION CONTRAINDICATION TO BREAST-FEEDING?
BACTERIA			
Mastitis/*Staphylococcus aureus*	Yes	No	No, unless breast abscess present
Mycobacterium tuberculosis:			
Active disease	Yes	No	Yes, because of aerosol spread, or TB mastitis
Purified protein derivative skin test result positive, chest radiograph findings negative	No	No	No
Escherichia coli, other gram-negative rods	Yes, stored	Yes, stored	—
Group B streptococci	Yes	Yes	No*
Listeria monocytogenes	Yes	Yes	No*
Coxiella burnetii	Yes	Yes	No*
Syphilis	No	No	No[†]
VIRUSES			
HIV	Yes	Yes	Yes, developed countries
Cytomegalovirus:			
Term infant	Yes	Yes	No
Preterm infant	Yes	Yes	Evaluate on an individual basis
Hepatitis B virus	Yes, surface antigen	No	No, developed countries[‡]
Hepatitis C virus	Yes	No	No[§]
Hepatitis E virus	Yes	No	No
Human T-cell leukemia virus (HTLV)-1	Yes	Yes	Yes, developed countries
HTLV-2	Yes	?	Yes, developed countries
Herpes simplex virus	Yes	No/?yes	No, unless breast vesicles present
Rubella			
Wild type	Yes	Yes, rare	No
Vaccine	Yes	No	No
Varicella-zoster virus	Yes	No	No, cover active lesions[¶]
Epstein-Barr virus	Yes	No	No
Human herpesvirus (HHV)-6	No	No	No
HHV-7	Yes	No	No
West Nile virus	Possible	Possible	Unknown
PARASITES			
Toxoplasma gondii	Yes	Yes, one case	No

*Provided that the mother and child are taking appropriate antibiotics.
[†]Treat mother and child if active disease.
[‡]Immunize and immune globulin at birth.
[§]Provided that the mother is HIV-seronegative. Mothers should be counseled that breast milk transmission of hepatitis C virus has not been documented, but is theoretically possible.
[¶]Provide appropriate antivaricella therapy or prophylaxis to newborn.
Modified from Jones CA: Maternal transmission of infectious pathogens in breast milk, *J Paediatr Child Health* 37:576–582, 2001.

global effort (sponsored by the World Health Organization and the United Nations Children's Fund) to promote breast-feeding, recommends 10 steps to successful breast-feeding (Table 88-6). Some hospital practices contribute to difficulties in breast-feeding by enforcing 4-hr feeding schedules, limiting nursing time, using only one breast at a feeding, washing nipples with substances other than water, delaying the 1st feeding, providing formula supplements, and using heavy intrapartum sedation.

DRUGS AND BREAST-FEEDING

Maternal medications may affect the production and safety of breast milk (Table 88-7). Although most commonly used medications are safe, the safety of any new drug to be used while a woman is breast-feeding must be confirmed before the drug is initiated and/or breast-feeding is continued. Maternal sedatives may result in sedation of the infant. Maternal drugs that are weak acids, composed of large molecules, plasma bound, or poorly absorbed from the maternal or neonatal intestine are less likely to affect a neonate.

Medical contraindications to breast-feeding in the USA include infection with HIV, human T-cell leukemia virus types 1 and 2, cytomegalovirus (preterm infants), active tuberculosis (until appropriately treated ≥2wk and not considered contagious), and hepatitis B virus (until an infant receives hepatitis B immune globulin and vaccine) (Table 88-8).

BIBLIOGRAPHY

Please visit the Nelson Textbook of Pediatrics *website at www.expertconsult.com for the complete bibliography.*

Chapter 89
High-Risk Pregnancies

Waldemar A. Carlo

High-risk pregnancies are those that increase the likelihood of abortion, fetal death, premature delivery, intrauterine growth restriction, poor cardiopulmonary or metabolic transitioning at birth, fetal or neonatal disease, congenital malformations, mental retardation, or other handicaps (see Table 89-1 on the *Nelson Textbook of Pediatrics* website at www.expertconsult.com;

Chapter 90). Some factors, such as ingestion of a teratogenic drug in the 1st trimester, are causally related to the risk; others, such as hydramnios, are associations that alert a physician to determine the etiology and avoid the inherent risks associated with excessive amniotic fluid. On the basis of their history, 10-20% of pregnant women can be identified as being at high risk; nearly half of all perinatal mortality and morbidity is associated with these high-risk pregnancies. Although assessing antepartum risk is important in reducing perinatal mortality and morbidity, some pregnancies become high risk only during labor and delivery; therefore, careful monitoring is critical throughout the intrapartum course.

For the full continuation of this chapter, please visit the Nelson Textbook of Pediatrics *website at www.expertconsult.com.*

Chapter 90
The Fetus
Waldemar A. Carlo

The major emphasis in fetal medicine involves (1) assessment of fetal growth and maturity, (2) evaluation of fetal well-being or distress, (3) assessment of the effects of maternal disease on the fetus, (4) evaluation of the effects of drugs administered to the mother on the fetus, and (5) identification and treatment of fetal disease or anomalies. Increasing knowledge of fetal physiology has paved the way for effective fetal therapy, intervention during fetal distress, and improved adaptation of a newborn infant to extrauterine life, particularly a premature infant. Some aspects of human fetal growth and development are summarized in Chapter 6.

90.1 Fetal Growth and Maturity
Waldemar A. Carlo

Ultrasonography of the fetus, a common obstetric procedure, is both safe and accurate. Indications for antenatal ultrasonography include estimation of gestational age (unknown dates, discrepancy between uterine size and dates or suspected growth restriction), assessment of amniotic fluid volume, estimation of fetal weight, determination of the location of the placenta and the number and position of fetuses, and identification of congenital anomalies.

Fetal growth can be assessed by ultrasonography as early as 6-8 wk. The most accurate assessment of gestational age is by 1st-trimester ultrasound measurement of crown-rump length. The biparietal diameter is used to assess gestational age beginning in the 2nd trimester. Through 30 weeks the biparietal diameter accurately estimates gestation to within ± 10 days. Later in gestation, accuracy falls to ± 3 wk. Methods used to assess gestational age at term include measurement of abdominal circumference and femoral length. If a single ultrasound examination is performed, the most information can be obtained with a scan at 18-20 wk, when both gestational age and fetal anatomy can be evaluated. Serial scans may be useful in assessing fetal growth. Two patterns of fetal growth restriction have been identified: continuous fetal growth 2 standard deviations (SD) below the mean for gestational age or a normal fetal growth curve that abruptly slows or flattens later in gestation (Fig. 90-1).

Fetal maturity and dating are usually assessed by history (last menstrual period), physical examination, auscultation of fetal heart sounds at 16-18 wk, maternal perception of fetal movements at 18-20 wk, fundal height, and ultrasound (growth). Lung maturation may be estimated by determining the surfactant content of amniotic fluid (Chapter 95.3).

BIBLIOGRAPHY
Please visit the Nelson Textbook of Pediatrics *website at www.expertconsult.com for the complete bibliography.*

90.2 Fetal Distress
Waldemar A. Carlo

Fetal compromise may occur during the antepartum or intrapartum period; it may be asymptomatic in the antenatal period. Antepartum fetal surveillance is warranted for women at increased risk for fetal death, including those with a history of stillbirth, intrauterine growth restriction (IUGR), oligohydramnios or

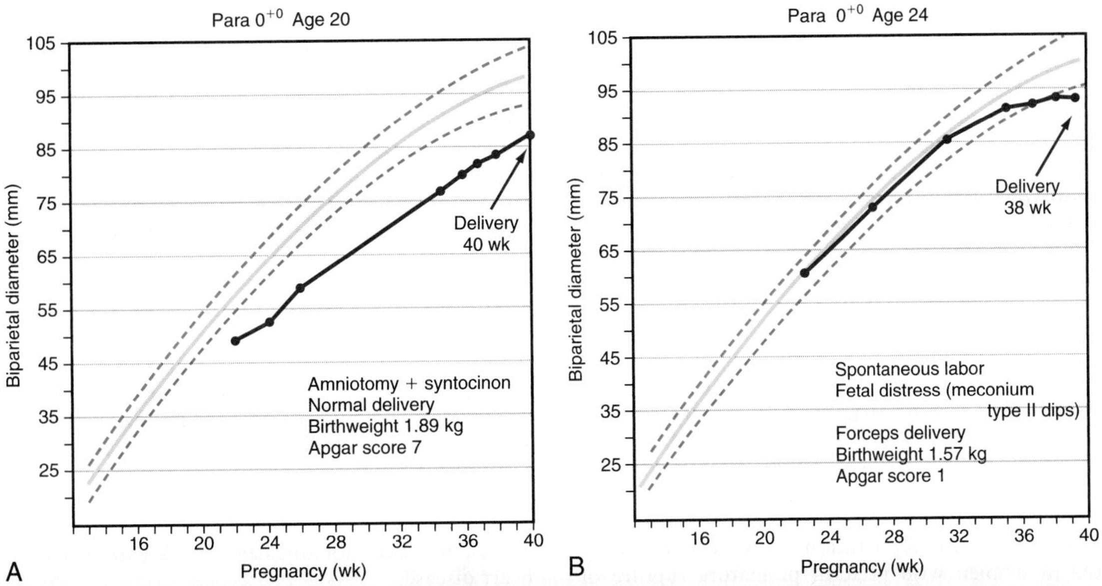

Figure 90-1 *A,* Example of a "low-profile" growth retardation pattern in an uneventful pregnancy and labor. The baby cried at 1 min and hypoglycemia did not develop. Birthweight was below the 5th percentile for gestational age. *B,* Example of a "late-flattening" growth retardation pattern. The mother had a typical history of preeclampsia, and the infant had intrapartum fetal distress, a low Apgar score, and postnatal hypoglycemia. Birthweight was below the 5th percentile for gestational age. (From Campbell S: Fetal growth, *Clin Obstet Gynecol* 1:41–65, 1974.)

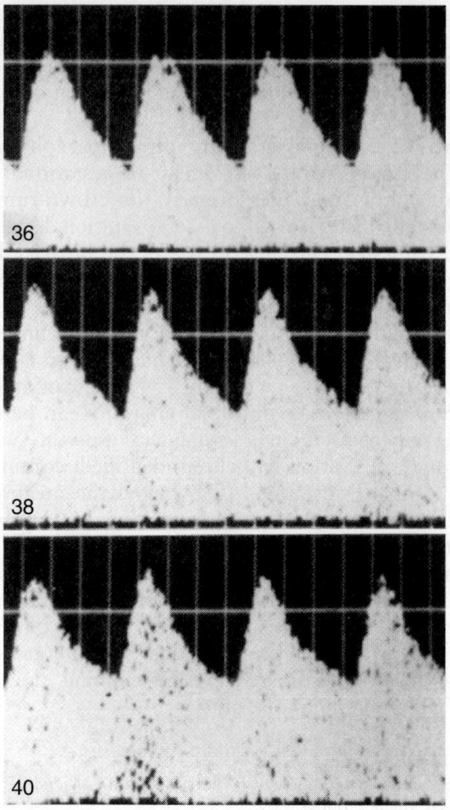

Figure 90-2 Normal Doppler velocity in sequential studies of fetal umbilical artery flow velocity waveforms from one normal pregnancy. Note the systolic peak flow with lower but constant heart flow during diastole. The systolic : diastolic ratio can be determined and, in normal pregnancies, is less than 3 after the 30th wk of gestation. The *numbers* indicate the weeks of gestation. (From Trudinger B: Doppler ultrasound assessment of blood flow. In Creasy RK, Resnik R, editors: *Maternal-fetal medicine: principles and practice,* ed 5, Philadelphia, 2004, WB Saunders.)

polyhydramnios, multiple gestation, rhesus sensitization, hypertensive disorders, diabetes mellitus or other chronic maternal disease, decreased fetal movement, and post-term pregnancy. The predominant cause of antepartum fetal distress is uteroplacental insufficiency, which may manifest clinically as IUGR, fetal hypoxia, increased vascular resistance in fetal blood vessels (Figs. 90-2 and 90-3), and, when severe, mixed respiratory and metabolic (lactic) acidosis. The goals of antepartum fetal surveillance are to prevent intrauterine fetal demise, to prevent hypoxic brain injury, and to either prolong gestation in women at risk for preterm delivery when such prolongation is safe or deliver a fetus when it is in jeopardy. Methods for assessing fetal well-being are listed in Table 90-1.

The most commonly used noninvasive tests are the nonstress test (NST), the full and modified biophysical profile (BPP), and less commonly, the contraction stress test (CST). The **NST** monitors the presence of fetal heart rate accelerations that follow fetal movement. A reactive (normal) NST result demonstrates two fetal heart rate accelerations of at least 15 beats/min lasting 15 sec. A nonreactive NST result suggests fetal compromise and requires further assessment with a CST or the BPP. A **CST** observes the fetal heart rate response to spontaneous, nipple-stimulated, or oxytocin-stimulated uterine contractions. Fetal compromise is suggested when the majority of contractions in 10 min are followed by late decelerations. A CST is relatively contraindicated in women with preterm premature rupture of membranes, a previous uterine scar from a classic cesarean section, multiple gestations, incompetent cervix, and placenta previa. The goals of fetal monitoring are to prevent intrauterine fetal demise and hypoxic brain injury. Although the CST and

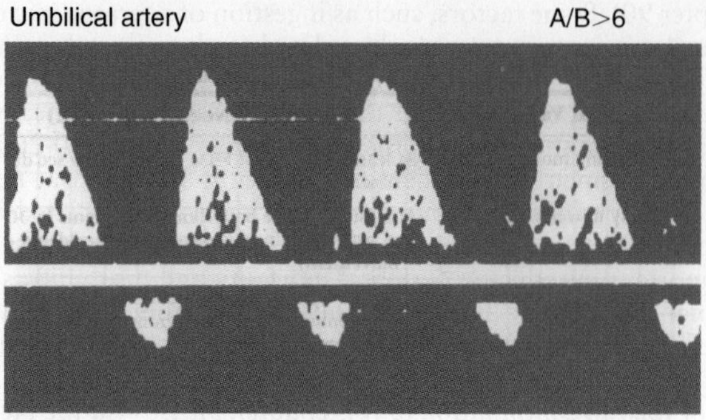

Figure 90-3 Abnormal umbilical artery Doppler in which the diastolic component shows flow in a reverse direction. This finding occurs in severe intrauterine hypoxia and intrauterine growth restriction. (From Trudinger C: Doppler ultrasound assessment of blood flow. In Creasy RK, Resnik R, editors: *Maternal-fetal medicine: principles and practice,* ed 5, Philadelphia, 2004, WB Saunders.)

NST have low false-negative rates, both have high false-positive rates. The full **BPP** assesses fetal breathing, body movement, tone, heart rate, and amniotic fluid volume, and it is used to improve the accurate and safe identification of fetal compromise (Table 90-2). A score of 2 is given for each observation present. A total score of 8-10 is reassuring; a score of 6 is equivocal, and retesting should be done in 12-24 hr; and a score of 4 or less warrants immediate evaluation and possible delivery. The BPP has good negative predictive value. The modified BPP consists of the combination of an ultrasound estimate of amniotic fluid volume (the amniotic fluid index) and the NST. When results of both are normal, fetal compromise is very unlikely. Signs of progressive compromise seen on Doppler ultrasonography include reduced, absent, or reversed diastolic waveform velocity in the fetal aorta or umbilical artery (see Fig. 90-3 and Table 90-1). High-risk fetuses often have combinations of abnormalities, such as oligohydramnios, reversed diastolic Doppler umbilical artery blood flow velocity, and a low BPP.

Fetal compromise *during labor* may be detected by monitoring the fetal heart rate, uterine pressure, and fetal scalp blood pH (Fig. 90-4). **Continuous fetal heart rate monitoring** detects abnormal cardiac patterns by instruments that compute the beat-to-beat fetal heart rate from a fetal electrocardiographic signal. Signals are derived from an electrode attached to the fetal presenting part, from an ultrasonic transducer placed on the maternal abdominal wall to detect continuous ultrasonic waves reflected from the contractions of the fetal heart, or from a phonotransducer placed on the mother's abdomen. Uterine contractions are simultaneously recorded from an amniotic fluid catheter and pressure transducer or from a tocotransducer applied to the maternal abdominal wall overlying the uterus. Fetal heart rate patterns show various characteristics, some of which suggest fetal compromise. The baseline fetal heart rate is the average rate between uterine contractions, which gradually decreases from about 155 beats/min in early pregnancy to about 135 beats/min at term; the normal range at term is 110-160 beats/min. **Tachycardia** (>160 beats/min) is associated with early fetal hypoxia, maternal fever, maternal hyperthyroidism, maternal β-sympathomimetic drug or atropine therapy, fetal anemia, infection, and some fetal arrhythmias. The last do not generally occur with congenital heart disease and may resolve spontaneously at birth. **Fetal bradycardia** (<110 beats/min) may be normal (e.g., 105-110 beats/min) but may occur with fetal hypoxia, placental transfer of local anesthetic agents and β-adrenergic blocking agents, and, occasionally, heart block with or without congenital heart disease.

Normally, the baseline fetal heart rate is variable. **Variability** is classified as follows: **absence of variability**, if an amplitude change is undetectable; **minimal variability** if amplitude range is ≤ 5 beats/min (beats/min); **moderate variability** if amplitude range

Table 90-1 FETAL DIAGNOSIS AND ASSESSMENT

METHOD	COMMENT(S) AND INDICATION(S)
Imaging:	
Ultrasound (real-time)	Biometry (growth), anomaly (morphology) detection Biophysical profile Amniotic fluid volume, hydrops
Ultrasound (Doppler)	Velocimetry (blood flow velocity) Detection of increased vascular resistance secondary to fetal hypoxia
Embryoscopy	Early diagnosis of limb anomaly
Fetoscopy	Detection of facial, limb, cutaneous anomalies
MRI	Defining of lesions before fetal surgery
Fluid analysis:	
Amniocentesis	Fetal maturity (L:S ratio), karyotype (cytogenetics), biochemical enzyme analysis, molecular genetic DNA diagnosis, bilirubin, or α-fetoprotein determination Bacterial culture, pathogen antigen, or genome detection
Fetal urine	Prognosis of obstructive uropathy
Cordocentesis (percutaneous umbilical blood sampling)	Detection of blood type, anemia, hemoglobinopathies, thrombocytopenia, acidosis, hypoxia, polycythemia, immunoglobulin M antibody response to infection Rapid karyotyping and molecular DNA genetic diagnosis Fetal therapy (see Table 90-5)
Fetal tissue analysis:	
Chorionic villus biopsy	Karyotype, molecular DNA genetic analysis, enzyme assays
Skin biopsy	Hereditary skin disease*
Liver biopsy	Enzyme assay*
Circulating fetal cells or DNA in maternal blood or plasma	Molecular DNA genetic analysis
Maternal serum α-fetoprotein concentration:	
Elevated	Twins, neural tube defects (anencephaly, spina bifida), intestinal atresia, hepatitis, nephrosis, fetal demise, incorrect gestational age
Reduced	Trisomies, aneuploidy
Maternal cervix:	
Fetal fibronectin	Indicates risk of preterm birth
Bacterial culture	Identifies risk of fetal infection (group B streptococcus, *Neisseria gonorrhoeae*)
Fluid	Determination of premature rupture of membranes
Antepartum biophysical monitoring:	
Nonstress test	Fetal distress; hypoxia
Contraction stress test	Fetal distress; hypoxia
Biophysical profile and modified biophysical profile	Fetal distress; hypoxia
Intrapartum fetal heart rate monitoring	See Fig. 90-4

*DNA genetic analysis on chorionic villus samples, amniocytes from amniocentesis, or fetal cells recovered from the maternal circulation may obviate the need for direct fetal tissue biopsy if the gene or genetic marker is available (e.g., the gene for Duchenne muscular dystrophy).

Table 90-2 BIOPHYSICAL PROFILE SCORING: TECHNIQUE AND INTERPRETATION

BIOPHYSICAL VARIABLE	NORMAL SCORE (2)	ABNORMAL SCORE (0)
Fetal breathing movements (FBMs)	At least 1 episode of FBM of at least 30 sec duration in 30 min observation	Absence of FBM or no episode ≥30 sec in 30 min
Gross body movement	At least 3 discrete body/limb movements in 30 min (episodes of active continuous movement considered a single movement)	2 or fewer episodes of body/limb movements in 30 min
Fetal tone	At least 1 episode of active extension with return to flexion of fetal limb(s) or trunk Opening and closing of hand considered evidence of normal tone	Either slow extension with return to partial flexion or movement of limb in full extension or absence of fetal movement with the hand held in complete or partial deflection
Reactive fetal heart rate (FHR)	At least 2 episodes of FHR acceleration of ≥15 beats/min and at least 15 sec in duration associated with fetal movement in 30 min	Less than 2 episodes of acceleration of FHR or acceleration of <15 beats/min in 30 min
Qualitative amniotic fluid (AF) volume *	At least 1 pocket of AF that measures at least 2 cm in 2 perpendicular planes	Either no AF pockets or a pocket <2 cm in 2 perpendicular planes

*Modification of the criteria for reduced amniotic fluid from less than 1 cm to less than 2 cm would seem reasonable. Ultrasound is used for biophysical assessment of the fetus.
From Creasy RK, Resnik R, Iams JD, editors: *Maternal-fetal medicine: principles and practice*, ed 5, Philadelphia, 2004, Saunders.

is 6-25 beats/min; **marked variability** if amplitude range is > 25 beats/min. Variability may be decreased or lost with fetal hypoxemia or the placental transfer of drugs such as atropine, diazepam, promethazine, magnesium sulfate, and most sedative and narcotic agents. Prematurity, the sleep state, and fetal tachycardia may also diminish beat-to-beat variability.

Periodic accelerations or decelerations of the fetal heart rate in response to uterine contractions may also be monitored (see Fig. 90-4). An **acceleration** is an abrupt increase in fetal heart rate of ≥15 beats/min in ≥15 sec. The presence of accelerations or moderate variability reliably predicts the absence of fetal metabolic acidemia. However, their absence does not reliably predict

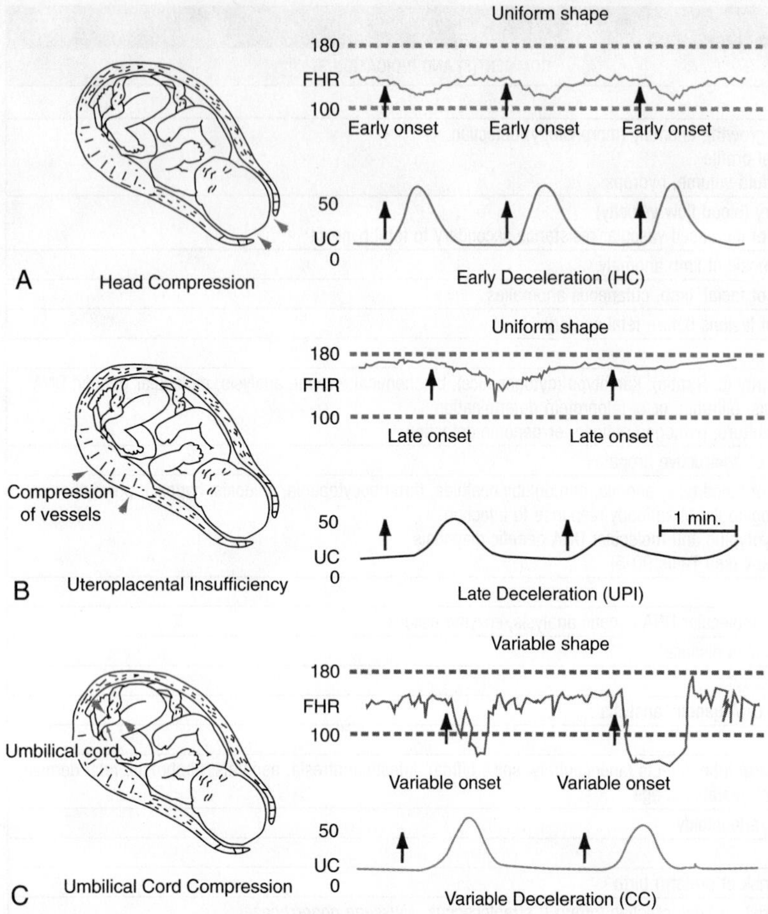

Figure 90-4 Patterns of periodic fetal heart rate (FHR) deceleration. The tracing in *A* shows early deceleration occurring during the peak of uterine contractions as a result of pressure on the fetal head. *B,* Late deceleration caused by uteroplacental insufficiency. *C,* Variable deceleration as a result of umbilical cold compression. *Arrows* denote the time relationship between the onset of FHR changes and uterine contractions. (From Hon EH: *An atlas of fetal heart rate patterns,* New Haven, CT, 1968, Harty Press.)

fetal acidemia or hypoxemia. **Early deceleration** associated with head compression is a repetitive pattern of gradual decrease and return of the fetal heart rate that is coincidental with the uterine contraction (Table 90-3). **Variable deceleration** (associated with cord compression) is characterized by variable shape, abrupt onset and occurrence with consecutive contractions, and return to baseline at or after the conclusion of the contraction. **Late deceleration,** associated with fetal hypoxemia, occurs repetitively after a uterine contraction is well established and persists into the interval following contractions. The late deceleration pattern is usually associated with maternal hypotension or excessive uterine activity, but it may be a response to any maternal, placental, umbilical cord, or fetal factor that limits effective oxygenation of the fetus. Reflex late decelerations with normal beat-to-beat variability are associated with chronic compensated fetal hypoxia, and they occur during uterine contractions that temporarily impede oxygen transport to the heart. Nonreflex late decelerations are more ominous and indicate severe hypoxic depression of myocardial function.

If late decelerations are unresponsive to oxygen supplementation, hydration, discontinuation of labor stimulation, and position changes, prompt delivery is indicated. A three-tier system has been developed by a panel of experts for interpretation of fetal heart rate tracings (Table 90-4). **Category I tracings** are normal and are strongly predictive of normal fetal acid-base status at the time of the observation. **Category II tracings** are not predictive of abnormal fetal status, but there is insufficient evidence to categorize them as category I or III; further evaluation, surveillance, and reevaluation are indicated. **Category III tracings** are abnormal and predictive of abnormal fetal acid-base status at the time of observation. Category III tracings require prompt evaluation and efforts to expeditiously resolve the abnormal fetal heart rate as previously discussed for late decelerations.

Fetal scalp blood sampling during labor through a slightly dilated cervix may aid in confirming fetal distress suspected on the basis of variations in fetal heart rate or the presence of meconium in amniotic fluid. The proper use of this technique may result in earlier delivery of depressed infants, who thus have a better chance of successful resuscitation, increased survival, and less morbidity. Alternatively, when continuous fetal heart rate monitoring or general clinical evaluation suggests that a fetus is at risk, a normal fetal scalp blood sample may help avert obstetric intervention.

Fetal scalp blood pH in normal labor decreases from about 7.33 early in labor to approximately 7.25 at the time of vaginal delivery; the base deficit is about 4-6 mEq/L. Changes in the buffer base may be particularly helpful in assessing fetal status, because they correspond to the accumulation of fetal lactic acid. A pH <7.25 suggests fetal distress, and a pH <7.20 is an indication for further assessment and intervention. Determination of the lactate concentration in fetal scalp blood is another tool for monitoring the condition of the fetus.

Umbilical cord blood samples obtained at the time of delivery are useful to document fetal acid-base status. Although the exact cord blood pH value that defines significant fetal acidemia is unknown, an umbilical artery pH <7.0 has been associated with greater need for resuscitation and a higher incidence of respiratory, gastrointestinal, cardiovascular, and neurologic complications. Nonetheless, in many cases, even when a low pH is detected, newborn infants are neurologically normal.

Intrapartum fetal pulse oximetry is another measure of fetal status. Even though initial data suggested that intrapartum fetal pulse oximetry could help identify fetuses with a nonreassuring status, a large randomized controlled trial showed that intrapartum fetal pulse oximetry does not lead to a reduction in cesarean section rates or improvement in the condition of newborns at birth.

Table 90-3 CHARACTERISTICS OF DECELERATIONS OF THE FETAL HEART RATE

LATE DECELERATION
• Visually apparent, usually symmetric *gradual* decrease and return of the fetal heart rate (FHR) associated with a uterine contraction. • A *gradual* FHR decrease is defined as duration of ≥ 30 sec from the onset to the nadir of the FHR. • The decrease in FHR is calculated from the onset to the nadir of the deceleration. • The deceleration is delayed in timing, with the nadir of the deceleration occurring after the peak of the contraction. • In most cases, the onset, nadir, and recovery of the deceleration occur after the beginning, peak, and ending of the contraction, respectively.
EARLY DECELERATION
• Visually apparent, usually symmetric *gradual* decrease and return of the FHR associated with a uterine contraction. • A *gradual* FHR decrease is defined as duration of ≥ 30 sec from the onset to the FHR nadir. • The decrease in FHR is calculated from the onset to the nadir of the deceleration. • The nadir of the deceleration occurs at the same time as the peak of the contraction. • In most cases, the onset, nadir, and recovery of the deceleration are coincident with the beginning, peak, and ending of the contraction, respectively.
VARIABLE DECELERATION
• Visually apparent, *abrupt* decrease in FHR. • An *abrupt* FHR decrease is defined as duration < 30 sec from the onset of the deceleration to the beginning of the FHR nadir of. • The decrease in FHR is calculated from the onset to the nadir of the deceleration. • The decrease in FHR is ≥ 15 beats/ min, lasting ≥ 15 sec, and < 2 min in duration. • When variable decelerations are associated with uterine contractions, their onset, depth, and duration commonly vary with successive uterine contractions.

From Macones GA, Hankins GDV, Spong CY, et al: The 2008 National Institute of Child Health and Human Development workshop report on electronic fetal monitoring: update on definitions, interpretation, and research guidelines, *Obstet Gynecol* 112:661–666, 2008.

Table 90-4 THREE-TIER FETAL HEART RATE INTERPRETATION SYSTEM

CATEGORY I
Category I fetal heart rate (FHR) tracings include all of the following: • Baseline rate: 110-160 beats per minute (beats/min) • Baseline FHR variability: moderate • Late or variable decelerations: absent • Early decelerations: present or absent • Accelerations: present or absent
CATEGORY II
Category II FHR tracings include all FHR tracings not categorized as category I or category III. Category II tracings may represent an appreciable fraction of those encountered in clinical care. Examples of category II FHR tracings include any of the following:
Baseline Rate
• Bradycardia not accompanied by absence of baseline variability • Tachycardia
Baseline FHR Variability
• Minimal baseline variability • Absence of baseline variability not accompanied by recurrent decelerations • Marked baseline variability
Accelerations
• Absence of induced accelerations after fetal stimulation
Periodic or Episodic Decelerations
• Recurrent variable decelerations accompanied by minimal or moderate baseline variability • Prolonged deceleration, ≥ 2 minutes but < 10 minutes • Recurrent late decelerations with moderate baseline variability • Variable decelerations with other characteristics, such as slow return to baseline, "overshoots," and "shoulders"
CATEGORY III

Category III FHR tracings include either:
• Absence of baseline FHR variability and any of the following:
  • Recurrent late decelerations
  • Recurrent variable decelerations
  • Bradycardia
• Sinusoidal pattern

From Macones GA, Hankins GDV, Spong CY, et al: The 2008 National Institute of Child Health and Human Development workshop report on electronic fetal monitoring: update on definitions, interpretation, and research guidelines, *Obstet Gynecol* 112:661–666, 2008.

BIBLIOGRAPHY

Please visit the Nelson Textbook of Pediatrics *website at* *www.expertconsult.com* *for the complete bibliography.*

90.3 Maternal Disease and the Fetus

Waldemar A. Carlo

INFECTIOUS DISEASES (SEE TABLE 89-3)

Almost any maternal infection with severe systemic manifestations may result in miscarriage, stillbirth, or premature labor. Whether these results are due to infection of the fetus or are secondary to maternal illness is not always clear. Maternal hyperthermia may be associated with an increased incidence of congenital anomalies, including neural tube defects (NTDs). Regardless of the severity of the maternal infection, certain agents frequently infect the fetus and have serious sequelae. Fetuses of mothers infected with these agents are often small for gestational age but also microcephalic. Some infections, such as rubella, may also produce congenital malformations if they occur during the period of organogenesis. Intrauterine infection/chorioamnionitis may be an important risk factor for cerebral white matter injury and subsequent cerebral palsy. Infections that affect maternal nutrition (e.g., hookworm) may also result in IUGR.

NONINFECTIOUS DISEASES (SEE TABLE 89-2)

Maternal diabetes increases the risk for neonatal hypoglycemia, hypocalcemia, respiratory distress syndrome and other respiratory problems, polycythemia, macrosomia, myocardial dysfunction, jaundice, and congenital malformations (Chapter 101.1). There is increased risk for incidence of uteroplacental insufficiency, polyhydramnios, and intrauterine death in poorly controlled diabetic mothers. **Eclampsia-preeclampsia** of pregnancy, **chronic hypertension,** and **chronic renal disease** can result in IUGR, prematurity, and intrauterine death, all probably caused by diminished uteroplacental perfusion. Uncontrolled maternal **hypothyroidism** or **hyperthyroidism** is responsible for relative infertility, spontaneous abortion, premature labor, and fetal death. Hypothyroidism in pregnant women (even if mild or asymptomatic) can adversely affect neurodevelopment of the child. Maternal **immunologic diseases** such as idiopathic thrombocytopenic purpura, systemic lupus erythematosus, myasthenia gravis, and Graves disease, all of which are mediated by immunoglobulin (Ig) G autoantibodies that can cross the placenta, frequently cause transient illness in the newborn. Maternal autoantibodies to the folate receptor are associated with NTDs, whereas maternal immunologic sensitization to paternal antigens may be associated with neonatal hemochromatosis. Untreated maternal **phenylketonuria** results in miscarriage, congenital cardiac malformations, and injury to the brain of a non-phenylketonuric heterozygotic fetus.

BIBLIOGRAPHY

Please visit the Nelson Textbook of Pediatrics *website at* *www.expertconsult.com* *for the complete bibliography.*

90.4 Maternal Medication and Toxin Exposure and the Fetus

Waldemar A. Carlo

The use of medications or herbal remedies during pregnancy is potentially harmful to the fetus. Consumption of medications occurs during the majority of pregnancies. The average mother has taken 4 drugs other than vitamins or iron during pregnancy. Almost 40% of pregnant women receive a drug for which human safety during pregnancy has not been established (category C pregnancy risk; see later). Moreover, many women are exposed to potential reproductive toxins, such as occupational, environmental, or household chemicals, including solvents, pesticides, and hair products. The effects of drugs taken by the mother vary considerably, especially in relation to the time in pregnancy when they are taken and the fetal genotype for drug-metabolizing enzymes. Miscarriage or congenital malformations result from the maternal ingestion of teratogenic drugs during the period of organogenesis. Maternal medications taken later, particularly during the last few weeks of gestation or during labor, tend to affect the function of specific organs or enzyme systems, and they adversely affect the neonate rather than the fetus (Tables 90-5 and 90-6).

The effects of drugs may be evident immediately in the delivery room or later in the neonatal period, or they may be delayed even longer. The administration of diethylstilbestrol during pregnancy, for instance, resulted in vaginal adenocarcinoma in the female offspring in the 2nd or 3rd decade of life.

Evidence has confirmed an interaction between genetic factors and susceptibility to certain drugs or environmental toxins. Phenytoin teratogenesis may be mediated by genetic differences in the enzymatic production of epoxide metabolites; specific genes may

Table 90-5 AGENTS ACTING ON PREGNANT WOMEN THAT MAY ADVERSELY AFFECT THE STRUCTURE OR FUNCTION OF THE FETUS AND NEWBORN

DRUG	EFFECT ON FETUS
Accutane (isotretinoin)	Facial-ear anomalies, heart disease, CNS anomalies
Alcohol	Congenital cardiac, CNS, limb anomalies; IUGR; developmental delay; attention deficits; autism
Aminopterin	Abortion, malformations
Amphetamines	Congenital heart disease, IUGR, withdrawal
Azathioprine	Abortion
Busulfan (Myleran)	Stunted growth; corneal opacities; cleft palate; hypoplasia of ovaries, thyroid, and parathyroids
Carbamazepine	Spina bifida, possible neurodevelopmental delay
Carbimazole	Scalp defects, choanal atresia, esophageal atresia, developmental delay
Carbon monoxide	Cerebral atrophy, microcephaly, seizures
Chloroquine	Deafness
Chorionic villus sampling	Probably no effect, possibly limb reduction
Cigarette smoking	Low birthweight for gestational age
Cocaine/crack	Microcephaly, LBW, IUGR, behavioral disturbances
Cyclophosphamide	Multiple malformations
Danazol	Virilization
17α-Ethinyl testosterone (Progestoral)	Masculinization of female fetus
Hyperthermia	Spina bifida
Lithium	Ebstein anomaly, macrosomia
6-Mercaptopurine	Abortion
Methyl mercury	Minamata disease, microcephaly, deafness, blindness, mental retardation
Methyltestosterone	Masculinization of female fetus
Misoprostol	Arthrogryposis, cranial neuropathies (Möbius syndrome), equinovarus
Mycophenolate mofetil	Craniofacial, limb, cardiovascular, CNS anomalies
Norethindrone	Masculinization of female fetus
Penicillamine	Cutis laxa syndrome
Phenytoin	Congenital anomalies, IUGR, neuroblastoma, bleeding (vitamin K deficiency)
Polychlorinated biphenyls	Skin discoloration—thickening, desquamation, LBW, acne, developmental delay
Prednisone	Oral clefts
Progesterone	Masculinization of female fetus
Quinine	Abortion, thrombocytopenia, deafness
Selective serotonin reuptake inhibitors	Small increased risk of congenital anomalies
Statins	IUGR, limb deficiencies, VACTERAL
Stilbestrol (diethylstilbestrol [DES])	Vaginal adenocarcinoma in adolescence
Streptomycin	Deafness
Tetracycline	Retarded skeletal growth, pigmentation of teeth, hypoplasia of enamel, cataract, limb malformations
Thalidomide	Phocomelia, deafness, other malformations
Toluene (solvent abuse)	Craniofacial abnormalities, prematurity, withdrawal symptoms, hypertonia
Trimethadione and paramethadione	Abortion, multiple malformations, mental retardation
Valproate	CNS (spina bifida), facial and cardiac anomalies, limb defects, impaired neurologic function
Vitamin D	Supravalvular aortic stenosis, hypercalcemia
Warfarin (Coumadin)	Fetal bleeding and death, hypoplastic nasal structures

CNS, central nervous system; IUGR, intrauterine growth restriction; LBW, low birthweight. VACTERAL, vertebral, anal, cardiac, tracheoesophagcal fistula, renal, arterial, limb.

Table 90-6 AGENTS ACTING ON PREGNANT WOMEN THAT MAY ADVERSELY AFFECT THE NEWBORN INFANT

Acebutolol—IUGR, hypotension, bradycardia
Acetazolamide—metabolic acidosis
Amiodarone—bradycardia, hypothyroidism
Anesthetic agents (volatile)—CNS depression
Adrenal corticosteroids—adrenocortical failure (rare)
Ammonium chloride—acidosis (clinically inapparent)
Aspirin—neonatal bleeding, prolonged gestation
Atenolol—IUGR, hypoglycemia
Baclofen—withdrawal
Blue cohosh herbal tea—neonatal heart failure
Bromides—rash, CNS depression, IUGR
Captopril, enalapril—transient anuric renal failure, oligohydramnios
Caudal-paracervical anesthesia with mepivacaine (accidental introduction of anesthetic into scalp of baby)—bradypnea, apnea, bradycardia, convulsions
Cholinergic agents (edrophonium, pyridostigmine)—transient muscle weakness
CNS depressants (narcotics, barbiturates, benzodiazepines) during labor—CNS depression, hypotonia
Cephalothin—positive direct Coombs test reaction
Dexamethasone—periventricular leukomalacia
Fluoxetine and other SSRIs—transient neonatal withdrawal, hypertonicity, minor anomalies, preterm birth, prolonged QT interval
Haloperidol—withdrawal
Hexamethonium bromide—paralytic ileus
Ibuprofen—oligohydramnios, pulmonary hypertension
Imipramine—withdrawal
Indomethacin—oliguria, oligohydramnios, intestinal perforation, pulmonary hypertension
Intravenous fluids during labor (e.g., salt-free solutions)—electrolyte disturbances, hyponatremia, hypoglycemia
Iodide (radioactive)—goiter
Iodides—goiter
Lead—reduced intellectual function
Magnesium sulfate—respiratory depression, meconium plug, hypotonia
Methimazole—goiter, hypothyroidism
Morphine and its derivatives (addiction)—withdrawal symptoms (poor feeding, vomiting, diarrhea, restlessness, yawning and stretching, dyspnea and cyanosis, fever and sweating, pallor, tremors, convulsions)
Naphthalene—hemolytic anemia (in G6PD-deficient infants)
Nitrofurantoin—hemolytic anemia (in G6PD-deficient infants)
Oxytocin—hyperbilirubinemia, hyponatremia
Phenobarbital—bleeding diathesis (vitamin K deficiency), possible long-term reduction in IQ, sedation
Primaquine—hemolytic anemia (in G6PD-deficient infants)
Propranolol—hypoglycemia, bradycardia, apnea
Propylthiouracil—goiter, hypothyroidism
Pyridoxine—seizures
Reserpine—drowsiness, nasal congestion, poor temperature stability
Sulfonamides—interfere with protein binding of bilirubin; kernicterus at low levels of serum bilirubin, hemolysis with G6PD deficiency
Sulfonylurea agents—refractory hypoglycemia
Sympathomimetic (tocolytic β-agonist) agents—tachycardia
Thiazides—neonatal thrombocytopenia (rare)
Valproate—developmental delay
Zolpidem (Ambien)—low birth weight

CNS, central nervous system; G6PD, glucose-6-phosphate dehydrogenase; IUGR, intrauterine growth restriction; SSRI, selective serotonin reuptake inhibitor.

influence the adverse effects of benzene exposure during pregnancy. Polymorphisms of genes encoding enzymes that metabolize the polycyclic aromatic hydrocarbons in cigarette smoke influence the growth-restricting effects of smoking on the fetus.

Often the risk of controlling maternal disease must be balanced with the risk of possible complications in the fetus. The majority of women with epilepsy have normal fetuses. Nonetheless, several commonly used antiepileptic drugs are associated with congenital malformations. Infants exposed to valproic acid may have multiple anomalies, including NTDs, hypospadias, facial anomalies, cardiac anomalies, and limb defects. In addition, they have lower developmental index scores than unexposed infants and infants exposed to other commonly used antiepileptic drugs.

Methotrexate is used for medical termination of pregnancy; surviving exposed infants may be at higher risk for congenital anomalies, IUGR, hypotonia, and developmental delay.

Moderate or high alcohol intake (≥7 drinks per week or ≥3 drinks on multiple occasions) is a risk for fetal alcohol syndrome. The exposed fetuses are at risk for growth failure, central nervous system abnormalities, cognitive defects, and behavioral problems. Smoking during pregnancy is associated with IUGR and facial clefts.

In view of the limits of current knowledge about the fetal effects of maternal medication, drugs and herbal agents should not be prescribed during pregnancy without weighing of maternal need against the risk of fetal damage. All women should be specifically counseled to abstain from the use of alcohol, tobacco, and illicit drugs during pregnancy.

BIBLIOGRAPHY

Please visit the Nelson Textbook of Pediatrics *website at www.expertconsult.com for the complete bibliography.*

90.5 Teratogens

Waldemar A. Carlo

When an infant or child has a congenital malformation or is developmentally delayed, the parents often wrongly blame themselves and attribute the child's problems to events that occurred during pregnancy. Because benign infections occur and several nonteratogenic drugs are often taken during many pregnancies, the pediatrician must evaluate the presumed viral infections and the drugs ingested to help parents understand their child's birth defect. The causes of approximately 40% of congenital malformations are unknown. Although only a relatively few agents are recognized to be teratogenic in humans (see Tables 90-5 and 90-6), new agents continue to be identified. Overall, only 10% of anomalies are due to recognizable teratogens (Chapter 102). The time of exposure is usually at less than 60 days of gestation during organogenesis. Specific agents produce predictable lesions. Some agents have a dose or threshold effect; below the threshold, no alterations in growth, function, or structure occur. Genetic variables such as the presence of specific enzymes may metabolize a benign agent into a more toxic-teratogenic form (e.g., phenytoin conversion to its epoxide). In many circumstances, the same agent and dose may not consistently produce the lesion.

Reduced enzyme activity of the folate methylation pathway, particularly the formation of 5-methyltetrahydrofolate, may be responsible for neural tube or other birth defects. The common thermolabile mutation of 5,10-methylene tetrahydrofolate reductase may be one of the enzymes responsible. Folate supplementation for all pregnant women (by direct fortification of cereal grains, mandatory in the USA), and oral folic acid tablets taken during organogenesis may overcome this genetic enzyme defect, thus reducing the incidence of neural tube and perhaps other birth defects.

The U.S. Food and Drug Administration (FDA) classifies drugs into five pregnancy risk categories. **Category A** drugs pose no risk on the basis of evidence from controlled human studies. For **category B** drugs, either no risk has been shown in animal studies but no adequate studies in humans *or* some risk has been shown in animal studies but these results are not confirmed by human studies. For **category C** drugs, either definite risk has been shown in animal studies but no adequate human studies have been performed *or* no data is available from either animal or human studies. **Category D** includes drugs with some risk but with a benefit that may exceed that risk for the treated life-threatening condition, such as streptomycin for tuberculosis. **Category X** is for drugs that are contraindicated in pregnancy on the basis of animal and human evidence and for which the risk exceeds the benefits.

The specific mechanism of action is known or postulated for very few teratogens. Warfarin, an anticoagulant because it is a vitamin K antagonist, prevents the carboxylation of γ-carboxyglutamic acid, which is a component of osteocalcin and other vitamin K–dependent bone proteins. The teratogenic effect of warfarin on developing cartilage, especially nasal cartilage, appears to be avoided if the pregnant woman's anticoagulation treatment is switched from warfarin to heparin for the period between weeks 6 and 12 of gestation. Hypothyroidism in the fetus may be caused by the maternal ingestion of an excessive amount of iodides or propylthiouracil; each interferes with the conversion of inorganic to organic iodides. Phenytoin may be teratogenic because of the accumulation of a metabolite as a result of deficiency of epoxide hydrolase.

Recognition of teratogens offers the opportunity to prevent related birth defects. If a pregnant woman is informed of the potentially harmful effects of alcohol on her unborn infant, she may be motivated to avoid alcohol consumption during pregnancy. A woman with insulin-dependent diabetes mellitus may significantly decrease her risk for having a child with birth defects by achieving good control of her disease before conception.

BIBLIOGRAPHY

Please visit the Nelson Textbook of Pediatrics *website at* *www.expertconsult.com* *for the complete bibliography.*

90.6 Radiation (See Also Chapter 699)

Waldemar A. Carlo

Accidental exposure of a pregnant woman to radiation is a common cause for anxiety about whether her fetus will have genetic abnormalities or birth defects. It is unlikely that exposure to diagnostic radiation will cause gene mutations; no increase in genetic abnormalities has been identified in the offspring exposed as unborn fetuses to the atomic bomb explosions in Japan in 1945.

A more realistic concern is whether the exposed human fetus will show birth defects or a higher incidence of malignancy. The estimated radiation dose for most radiographs is less than 0.1 rad, and for most CT scans it is less than 5 rad. Imaging studies with high radiation exposure (such as CT scans) can be modified to ensure that radiation doses are kept as low as possible. Thus, single diagnostic studies do not result in radiation doses high enough to affect the embryo or fetus. Therapeutic abortion should not be recommended, given the low likelihood for high radiation exposure. Most of the evidence suggests that usual fetal radiation exposure does not increase the risk of childhood leukemia and other cancers. The limited data on human fetuses show that large doses of radiation (20-50 rad) may cause fetal death (the most sensitive period is the 3rd and 4th post-conception wk) as well as microcephaly, severe mental retardation, and growth retardation (the most sensitive period is 4th to 15th wk). The available data suggest no harmful fetal effect of diagnostic MRI or ultrasonography.

BIBLIOGRAPHY

Please visit the Nelson Textbook of Pediatrics *website at* *www.expertconsult.com* *for the complete bibliography.*

90.7 Intrauterine Diagnosis of Fetal Disease (See Table 90-1 and Chapter 90.2)

Waldemar A. Carlo

Diagnostic procedures are used to identify fetal diseases when abortion is being considered, when direct fetal treatment is possible, or when a decision is made to deliver a viable but premature infant to avoid intrauterine fetal demise. Fetal assessment is also indicated in a broader context when the family, medical, or reproductive history of the mother suggests the presence of a high-risk pregnancy or a high-risk fetus (Chapters 89 and 90.3).

Various methods are used for identifying fetal disease (see Table 90-1). Fetal ultrasonographic imaging may detect fetal growth abnormalities (by biometric measurements of biparietal diameter, femoral length, or head or abdominal circumference) or fetal malformations (Fig. 90-5). Although 89% of fetuses whose biparietal diameter is 9.5 cm or more are at least in the 37th wk of gestation, the lungs of these fetuses may not be mature. Serial determinations of growth velocity and the head-to-abdomen circumference ratio enhance the ability to detect IUGR. Real-time ultrasonography may identify placental abnormalities (abruptio placentae, placenta previa) and fetal anomalies such as hydrocephalus, NTDs, duodenal atresia, diaphragmatic hernia, renal agenesis, bladder outlet obstruction, congenital heart disease, limb abnormalities, sacrococcygeal teratoma, cystic hygroma, omphalocele, gastroschisis, and hydrops (Table 90-7).

Real-time ultrasonography also facilitates performance of cordocentesis and the BPP by imaging fetal breathing, body movements, tone, and amniotic fluid volume (see Table 90-2). Doppler velocimetry assesses fetal arterial blood flow (vascular resistance) (see Figs. 90-2 and 90-3). Roentgenographic examination of the fetus has been replaced by real-time ultrasonography, MRI, and fetoscopy.

Amniocentesis, the transabdominal withdrawal of amniotic fluid during pregnancy for diagnostic purposes (see Table 90-1), is frequently performed to determine the timing of delivery of fetuses with erythroblastosis fetalis or the need for fetal transfusion. It is also done for genetic indications, usually between the 15th and 16th wk of gestation, with results available within 1-2 wk. The most common indication for genetic amniocentesis is advanced maternal age (the risk for chromosome abnormality at age 21 years is 1:526, vs 1:8 at age 49). The amniotic fluid may be directly analyzed for amino acids, enzymes, hormones, and abnormal metabolic products, and amniotic fluid cells may be cultivated to permit detailed cytologic analysis for prenatal detection of chromosomal abnormalities and DNA-gene or enzymatic analysis for the detection of inborn metabolic errors. Analysis of amniotic fluid may also help in identifying NTDs (elevation of α-fetoprotein), adrenogenital syndrome (elevation of 17-ketosteroids and pregnanetriol), and thyroid dysfunction. Chorionic villus biopsy (transvaginal or transabdominal) performed in the 1st trimester also provides fetal cells but may pose a slightly increased risk for fetal loss and limb reduction defects. Fetal cells circulating in maternal blood and fetal DNA in maternal plasma are potential noninvasive sources of material for prenatal diagnosis. This technology may eliminate the need for amniocentesis or chorionic villus sampling.

The best available chemical indices of fetal maturity are provided by determination of amniotic fluid creatinine and lecithin levels, which reflect the maturity of the fetal kidneys and lungs, respectively. Lecithin is produced in the lungs by type II alveolar cells and eventually reaches the amniotic fluid via the effluent from the trachea. Until the middle of the 3rd trimester, its concentration nearly equals that of sphingomyelin; thereafter, the sphingomyelin concentration remains constant in amniotic fluid while the lecithin concentration increases. By 35 wk, the lecithin : sphingomyelin (L:S) ratio averages about 2:1, indicative of lung maturity.

Earlier lung maturation may occur in the presence of severe premature separation of the placenta, premature rupture of the fetal membranes, narcotic addiction, or maternal hypertensive and renal vascular disease. A delay in pulmonary maturation may be associated with hydrops fetalis or maternal diabetes without vascular disease. The likelihood of hyaline membrane disease is greatly reduced with L:S ratios of 2:1 or more, although hypoxia, acidosis, and hypothermia may increase the risk despite this

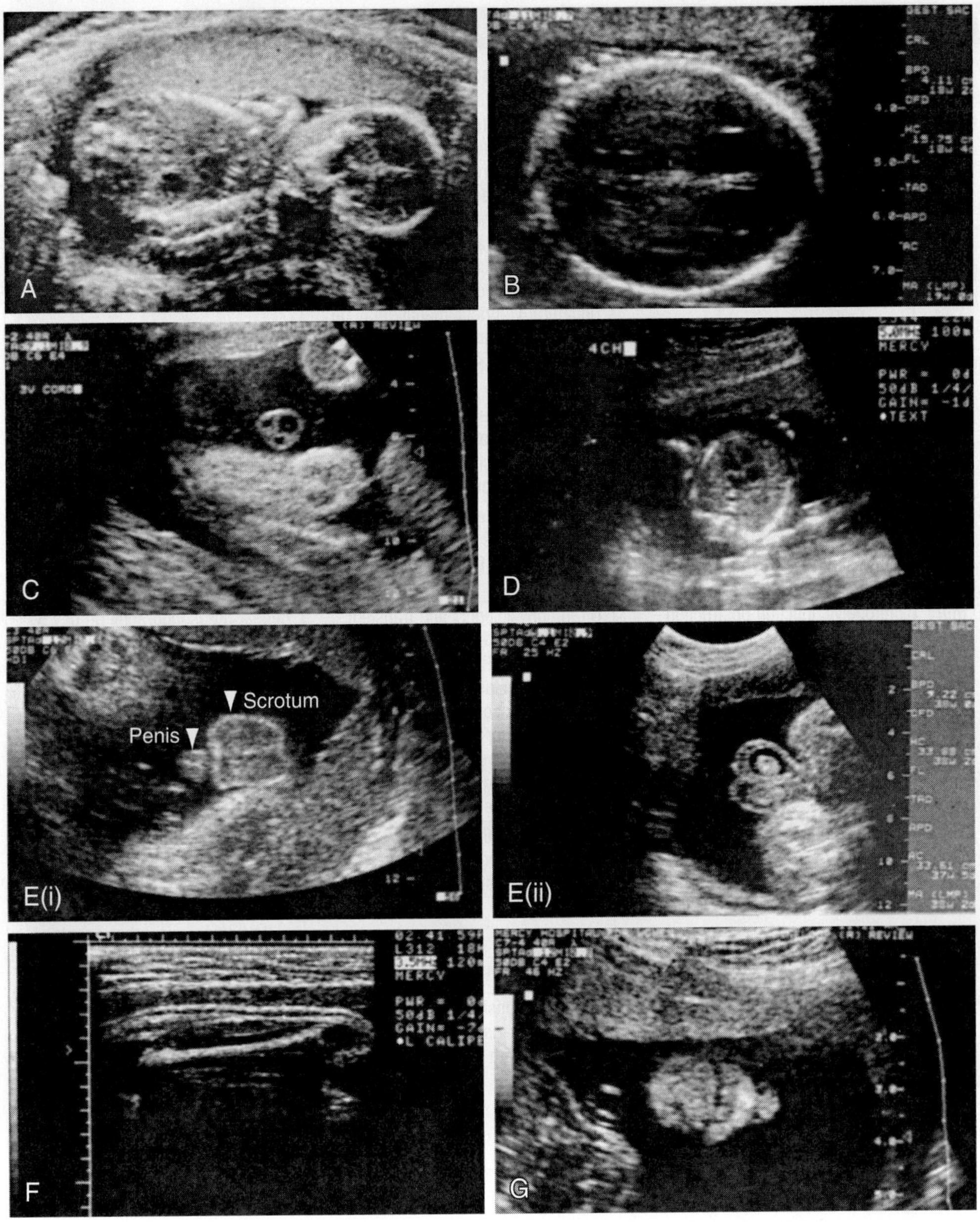

Figure 90-5 Assessment of fetal anatomy. *A,* Overall view of the uterus at 24 wk showing a longitudinal section of the fetus and an anterior placenta. *B,* Transverse section at the level of the lateral ventricle at 18 wk showing (*on the right*) prominent anterior horns of the lateral ventricles on either side of the midline echo of the falx. *C,* Cross section of the umbilical cord showing that the lumen of the umbilical vein is much wider than that of the two umbilical arteries. *D,* Four-chambered view of the heart at 18 wk with equal-sized atria. *E(i),* normal male genitals near term. *E(ii),* Hydrocele outlining a testicle within the scrotum projecting into a normal-sized pocket of amniotic fluid at 38 wk. Approximately 2% of male infants after birth have clinical evidence of a hydrocele that is often bilateral, not to be confused with subcutaneous edema occurring during vaginal breech birth. *F,* Section of a thigh near term showing thick subcutaneous tissue (4.6 mm between markers) above the femur of a fetus with macrosomia. *G,* Fetal face viewed from below, showing (*from right to left*) the nose, alveolar margin, and chin at 20 wk. (From Special investigative procedures. In Beischer NA, Mackay EV, Colditz PB, editors: *Obstetrics and the newborn,* ed 3, Philadelphia, 1997, WB Saunders.)

"mature" L:S ratio. Maternal and fetal blood have an L:S ratio of about 1:4; thus, contamination will not alter the significance of a ratio of 2:1 or more. Meconium contamination, sample storage, and sample centrifugation may reduce the reliability of the L:S ratio.

Saturated phosphatidylcholine or phosphatidylglycerol concentrations in amniotic fluid may be more specific and sensitive predictors of pulmonary maturity, especially in high-risk pregnancies such as those occurring in women with diabetes (Chapters 89 and 101.1).

Amniocentesis can be carried out with little discomfort to the mother, but even in experienced hands, the procedure entails some small risk, such as direct damage to the fetus, placental puncture and bleeding with secondary damage to the fetus, stimulation of uterine contraction and premature labor, amnionitis, and maternal sensitization to fetal blood. The earlier in gestation that amniotic puncture is done, the greater the risk to the fetus. Using ultrasound for placental and fetal localization can reduce the risk of complications. The procedure should be limited to cases in which the potential benefits of the findings will outweigh the risk.

Cordocentesis, or percutaneous umbilical blood sampling, is used to diagnose fetal hematologic abnormalities, genetic disorders, infections, and fetal acidosis (see Table 90-1). Under direct ultrasonographic visualization, a long needle is passed into the umbilical vein at its entrance to the placenta or fetal abdominal wall. Umbilical blood may be withdrawn to determine fetal hemoglobin, platelet concentration, lymphocyte DNA, the presence of infection, or Pa_{O_2}, pH, P_{CO_2}, and lactate levels.

Transfusion or administration of drugs can be performed through the umbilical vein (Table 90-8). Serum screening is offered to pregnant women at midgestation to evaluate the risk for Down syndrome (trisomy 21) and congenital malformations known to cause elevations of various markers, including abdominal wall and NTDs. A combination of these biochemical markers (including α-fetoprotein, inhibin A, estriol, pregnancy-associated plasma protein A, and β-HCG [human chorionic gonadotropin]) and ultrasound increases the positive predictive value of these screening tests. Additionally, families with a known genetic syndrome may be offered prenatal genetic testing from amniotic fluid or amniocytes obtained via amniocentesis or chorionic villus sampling.

Table 90-7 SIGNIFICANCE OF FETAL ULTRASONOGRAPHIC ANATOMIC FINDINGS

PRENATAL OBSERVATION	DEFINITION	DIFFERENTIAL DIAGNOSIS	SIGNIFICANCE	POSTNATAL EVALUATION
Dilated cerebral ventricles	Ventriculomegaly ≥10 mm	Hydrocephalus Hydranencephalus Dandy-Walker cyst Agenesis of corpus callosum	Transient isolated ventriculomegaly is common and usually benign Persistent or progressive ventriculomegaly more worrisome Identify associated cranial and extracranial anomalies Bilateral ventriculomegaly increases risk of developmental delay Unilateral ventriculomegaly may be normal variant	Serial head US or CT Evaluate for extracranial anomalies
Choroid plexus cysts	Size ~10 mm: unilateral or bilateral 1-3% incidence	Abnormal karyotype (trisomy 18, 21) Aneuploidy risk 1:100 if isolated. ↑ Risk (1:3) with other anomalies. Risk ↑ if large, complex, or bilateral cysts or advanced maternal age	Often isolated, benign; resolves by 24-28 wk Fetus should be examined for other organ anomalies; then amniocentesis should be performed for karyotype	Head US or CT Examine for extracranial anomalies; karyotype if indicated
Nuchal pad thickening	≥6 mm at 15-20 wk	Cystic hygroma Trisomy 21, 18 Turner syndrome (XO) Nonchromosomal syndromes Normal (~25%)	≈50% of affected fetuses have chromosome abnormalities Amniocentesis for karyotype needed	Evaluate for multiple organ malformations; karyotype if indicated
Dilated renal pelvis	Pyelectasis ≥ 5 to 10 mm 0.6-1% incidence	Uteropelvic junction obstruction Vesicoureteral reflux Posterior ureteral valves Entopic ureterocele Large-volume nonobstruction	Often "physiologic" and transient Reflux is common If dilation is >10 mm or associated with caliectasis, pathologic cause should be considered If large bladder present, posterior urethral valves and megacystics-megaduodenum syndrome should be considered	Repeat ultrasonography on day 5 and at 1 mo; voiding cystourethrogram, prophylactic antibiotics
Echogenic bowel	0.6% incidence	CF, meconium peritonitis, trisomy 21 or 18, other chromosomal abnormalities cytomegalovirus, toxoplasmosis, GI obstruction	Often normal (65%) 10% of affected fetuses have CF; 1.5% have aneuploidy	Sweat chloride and DNA testing Karyotype Surgery for obstruction Evaluation for TORCH (toxoplasmosis, other agents, rubella, CMV, herpes simplex) syndrome
Stomach appearance	Small or absent or with double bubble	Upper GI obstruction (esophageal atresia) Double bubble signifies duodenal atresia Abnormal karyotype Polyhydramnios Stomach in chest signifies diaphragmatic hernia	Must also consider neurologic disorders that reduce swallowing Over 30% with double bubble have trisomy 21	Chromosomes, kidney, ureter, and bladder radiograph if indicated, upper GI series, neurologic evaluation

CF, cystic fibrosis; GI, gastrointestinal.

BIBLIOGRAPHY

Please visit the Nelson Textbook of Pediatrics *website at* *www.expertconsult.com* *for the complete bibliography.*

90.8 Treatment and Prevention of Fetal Disease

Waldemar A. Carlo

Management of a fetal disease depends on coordinated advances in diagnostic accuracy and knowledge of the disease's natural history; an understanding of fetal nutrition, pharmacology, immunology, and pathophysiology; the availability of specific active drugs that cross the placenta; and therapeutic procedures. Progress in providing specific treatments for accurately diagnosed diseases has improved with the advent of real-time ultrasonography and cordocentesis (see Tables 90-1 and 90-8).

The incidence of sensitization of Rh-negative women by Rh-positive fetuses has been reduced by prophylactic administration of Rh(D) immunoglobulin to mothers early in pregnancy and after each delivery or abortion, thus reducing the frequency of hemolytic disease in their subsequent offspring. Fetal erythroblastosis (Chapter 97.2) may be accurately diagnosed by amniotic fluid analysis and treated with intrauterine intraperitoneal or, more often, intraumbilical vein transfusions of packed Rh-negative blood cells to maintain the fetus until it is mature enough to have a reasonable chance of survival.

Fetal hypoxia or distress may be diagnosed with moderate success. Treatment, however, remains limited to supplying the mother with high concentrations of oxygen, positioning the uterus to avoid vascular compression, and initiating operative delivery before severe fetal injury occurs.

Pharmacologic approaches to fetal immaturity (e.g., administration of steroids to the mother to accelerate fetal lung maturation and decrease the incidence of respiratory distress syndrome [Chapter 95.3] in prematurely delivered infants) are successful. Inhibiting labor with tocolytic agents is unfortunately not successful in most patients with premature labor. Management of definitively diagnosed fetal genetic disease or congenital anomalies consists of parental counseling or abortion; rarely, high-dose vitamin therapy for a responsive inborn error of metabolism (biotin-dependent disorders) or fetal transfusion (with red blood cells or platelets) may be indicated. Fetal surgery (see Table 90-8) remains an experimental approach to therapy and is available

Table 90-8 FETAL THERAPY

DISORDER	POSSIBLE TREATMENT
HEMATOLOGIC	
Anemia with hydrops (erythroblastosis fetalis)	Umbilical vein packed red blood cell transfusion
Thalassemia	Fetal stem cell transplantation
Isoimmune thrombocytopenia	Umbilical vein platelet transfusion, maternal IVIG
Autoimmune thrombocytopenia (ITP)	Maternal steroids and IVIG
Chronic granulomatous disease	Fetal stem cell transplantation
METABOLIC-ENDOCRINE	
Maternal phenylketonuria (PKU)	Phenylalanine restriction
Fetal galactosemia	Galactose-free diet (?)
Multiple carboxylase deficiency	Biotin if responsive
Methylmalonic acidemia	Vitamin B_{12} if responsive
21-Hydroxylase deficiency	Dexamethasone
Maternal diabetes mellitus	Tight insulin control during pregnancy, labor, and delivery
Fetal goiter	Maternal hyperthyroidism—maternal propylthiouracil
	Fetal hypothyroidism—intra-amniotic thyroxine
Bartter syndrome	Maternal indomethacin may prevent nephrocalcinosis and postnatal sodium losses
FETAL DISTRESS	
Hypoxia	Maternal oxygen, position
Intrauterine growth restriction	Maternal oxygen, position, improve macronutrients and micronutrients if deficient
Oligohydramnios, premature rupture of membranes with variable deceleration	Amnioinfusion (antepartum and intrapartum)
Polyhydramnios	Amnioreduction (serial), indomethacin (if due to increased urine output) if indicated
Supraventricular tachycardia	Maternal digoxin,* flecainide, procainamide, amiodarone, quinidine
Lupus anticoagulant	Maternal aspirin, prednisone
Meconium-stained fluid	Amnioinfusion
Congenital heart block	Dexamethasone, pacemaker (with hydrops)
Premature labor	Magnesium sulfate, antibiotics sympathomimetics, indomethacin
RESPIRATORY	
Pulmonary immaturity	Betamethasone
Bilateral chylothorax—pleural effusions	Thoracentesis, pleuroamniotic shunt
CONGENITAL ABNORMALITIES†	
Neural tube defects	Folate, vitamins (prevention); fetal surgery‡
Obstructive uropathy (with oligohydramnios but without renal dysplasia)	>24 wk <32 wk of gestation, vesicoamniotic shunt plus amnioinfusion
Cystic adenomatoid malformation (with hydrops)	Pleuroamniotic shunt or resection‡
Fetal neck masses	Secure an airway with EXIT procedure‡
INFECTIOUS DISEASE	
Group B streptococcus colonization	Ampicillin, penicillin
Chorioamnionitis	Antibiotics
Toxoplasmosis	Spiramycin, pyrimethamine, sulfadiazine, and folic acid
Syphilis	Penicillin
Tuberculosis	Antituberculosis drugs
Lyme disease	Penicillin, ceftriaxone
Parvovirus	Intrauterine red blood cell transfusion for hydrops, severe anemia
Chlamydia trachomatis	Erythromycin
HIV-AIDS	Zidovudine (AZT) plus protease inhibitors
Cytomegalovirus	Ganciclovir by umbilical vein
OTHER	
Nonimmune hydrops (anemia)	Umbilical vein packed red blood cell transfusion
Narcotic abstinence (withdrawal)	Maternal low-dose methadone
Severe combined immunodeficiency disease	Fetal stem cell transplantation
Sacrococcygeal teratoma (with hydrops)	In utero resection or catheter directed vessel obliteration
Twin-twin transfusion syndrome	Repeated amniocentesis, yttrium-aluminum-garnet (YAG) laser photocoagulation of shared vessels
Twin reversed arterial perfusion (TRAP) syndrome	Digoxin, indomethacin, cord occlusion
Multifetal gestation	Selective reduction
Neonatal hemochromatosis	Maternal IVIG

*Drug of choice (may require percutaneous umbilical cord sampling and umbilical vein administration if hydrops is present). Most drug therapy is given to the mother, with subsequent placental passage to the fetus.

†Detailed fetal ultrasonography is needed to detect other anomalies; karyotype is also indicated.

‡EXIT permits surgery and other procedures.

EXIT, Ex utero intrapartum treatment; IVIG, intravenous immunoglobulin; (?), possible but not proved efficacy.

only in a few highly specialized perinatal centers. The nature of the defect and its consequences, as well as ethical implications for the fetus and the parents, must be considered.

Folic acid supplementation decreases the incidence and recurrence of (NTDs). Because the neural tube closes within the 1st 28 days of conception, periconceptional supplementation is needed for prevention. It is recommended that women without a prior history of a NTD ingest 400 µg/day of folic acid throughout their reproductive years. Women with a history of a prior pregnancy complicated by an NTD or a 1st-degree relative with an NTD should have preconceptional counseling and should ingest 4 mg/day of supplemental folic acid beginning at least 1 mo before conception. Fortification of cereal grain flour with folic acid is established policy in the USA and some other countries. The optimal concentration of folic acid in enriched grains is somewhat controversial. The incidence of NTD in the USA and other countries has decreased significantly since these public health initiatives were implemented. Use of some antiepileptic drugs (valproate, carbamazepine) during pregnancy is associated with an increased risk of NTD. Women taking these medications should ingest 1-5 mg of folic acid/day in the preconception period.

BIBLIOGRAPHY

Please visit the Nelson Textbook of Pediatrics *website at www.expertconsult.com for the complete bibliography.*

Chapter 91
The High-Risk Infant

Waldemar A. Carlo

Neonates at risk should be identified as early as possible to decrease neonatal morbidity and mortality (Chapter 87). The term high-risk infant designates an infant who should be under close observation by experienced physicians and nurses. Factors that define infants as being high-risk are listed in Table 91-1. Approximately 9% of all births require special or neonatal intensive care. Usually needed for only a few days, such observation may last from a few hours to several months. Some institutions find it advantageous to provide a special or transitional care nursery for high-risk infants, often within the labor and delivery suite. This facility should be equipped and staffed like a neonatal intensive care area.

Examination of the fresh **placenta, cord,** and **membranes** may alert the physician to a newborn infant at high risk and may help confirm a diagnosis in a sick infant. **Fetal blood loss** may be indicated by placental pallor, retroplacental hematoma, and tears in the velamentous cords or chorionic blood vessels supplying the succenturiate lobes. Placental edema and secondary possible immunoglobulin G deficiency in a newborn may be associated with fetofetal transfusion syndrome, hydrops fetalis, congenital nephrosis, or hepatic disease. **Amnion nodosum** (granules on the amnion) and **oligohydramnios** are associated with pulmonary hypoplasia and renal agenesis, whereas small whitish nodules on the cord suggest a candidal infection. Short cords and noncoiled cords occur with chromosome abnormalities and omphalocele. True umbilical cord knots are seen in approximately 1% of births and are associated with a long cord, small fetal size, polyhydramnios, monoamniotic twinning, fetal demise, and low Apgar scores.

Chorioangiomas are associated with prematurity, abruptio placentae, polyhydramnios, and intrauterine growth restriction (IUGR). **Meconium staining** suggests in utero stress, and opacity of the fetal surface of the placenta suggests infection. Single umbilical arteries are associated with an increased incidence of congenital renal abnormalities and syndromes.

Table 91-1 HIGH-RISK INFANTS

DEMOGRAPHIC SOCIAL FACTORS
Maternal age <16 or >40 yr
Illicit drug, alcohol, cigarette use
Poverty
Unmarried
Emotional or physical stress
PAST MEDICAL HISTORY
Genetic disorders
Diabetes mellitus
Hypertension
Asymptomatic bacteriuria
Rheumatologic illness (systemic lupus erythematosus)
Long-term medication (see Tables 90-5 and 90-6)
PREVIOUS PREGNANCY
Intrauterine fetal demise
Neonatal death
Prematurity
Intrauterine growth restriction
Congenital malformation
Incompetent cervix
Blood group sensitization, neonatal jaundice
Neonatal thrombocytopenia
Hydrops
Inborn errors of metabolism
PRESENT PREGNANCY
Vaginal bleeding (abruptio placentae, placenta previa)
Sexually transmitted infections (colonization: herpes simplex, group B streptococcus, chlamydia, syphilis, hepatitis B, HIV)
Multiple gestation
Preeclampsia
Premature rupture of membranes
Short interpregnancy time
Poly/oligohydramnios
Acute medical or surgical illness
Inadequate prenatal care
Familial or acquired hypercoagulable states
Abnormal fetal ultrasonographic findings
Treatment of infertility
LABOR AND DELIVERY
Premature labor (<37 wk)
Postdates pregnancy (≥42 wk)
Fetal distress
Immature lethicin:sphingomyelin ratio; absence of phosphatidylglycerol
Breech presentation
Meconium-stained fluid
Nuchal cord
Cesarean section
Forceps delivery
Apgar score <4 at 1 min
NEONATE
Birthweight <2,500 or >4,000 g
Birth <37 or ≥42 wk of gestation
Small or large for gestational age
Respiratory distress, cyanosis
Congenital malformation
Pallor, plethora, petechiae

For many infants who are born prematurely, are small for gestational age (SGA), have significant perinatal asphyxia, are breech, or are born with life-threatening congenital anomalies, there are no previously identified risk factors. For any given duration of gestation, the lower the birthweight, the higher the neonatal mortality; for any given birthweight, the shorter the gestational duration, the higher the neonatal mortality (Fig. 91-1). The highest risk of neonatal mortality occurs in infants who weigh <1,000 g at birth and whose gestation was <28 wk. The lowest risk of neonatal mortality occurs in infants with a birthweight of 3,000-4,000 g and a gestational age of 38-42 wk. As birthweight increases from 500 to 3,000 g, a logarithmic

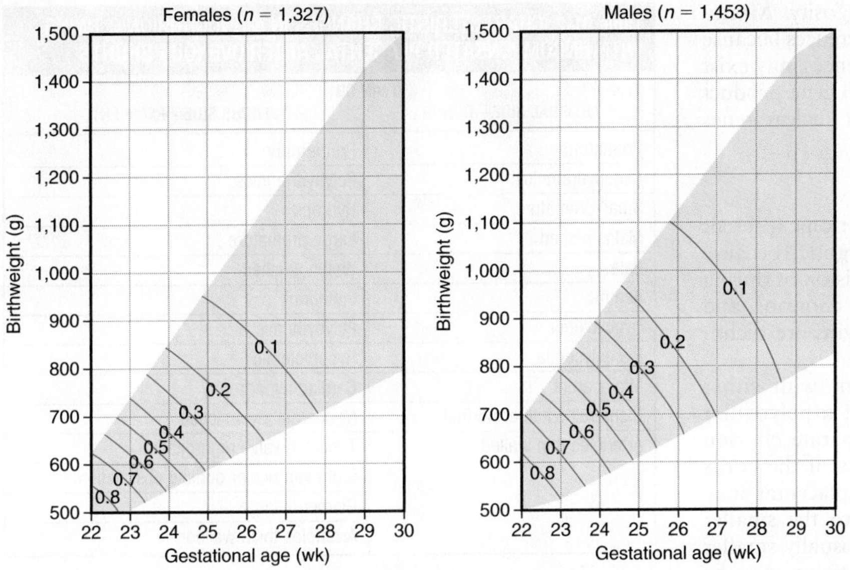

Figure 91-1 Estimated mortality risk by birthweight and gestational age based on singleton infants in National Institute of Child Health and Human Development (NICHD) Neonatal Research Network centers between January 1, 1995, and December 31, 1996. (From Lemons JA, Bauers CR, Oh W, et al: Very low birthweight outcomes of the National Institute of Child Health and Human Development Neonatal Research Network, January 1995 through December 1996, *Pediatrics* 107:2001; available at www.pediatrics.org.cgi/content/full/107/1/el.)

decrease in neonatal mortality occurs; for every week of increase in gestational age from the 25th to the 37th wk, the neonatal mortality rate decreases by approximately half. Nevertheless, approximately 40% of all perinatal deaths occur after 37 wk of gestation in infants weighing 2,500 g or more; many of these deaths take place in the period immediately before birth and are more readily preventable than those of smaller and more immature infants. Neonatal mortality rates rise sharply for infants weighing over 4,000 g at birth and for those whose gestational period is 42 wk or longer. Because neonatal mortality largely depends on birthweight and gestational age, Figure 91-1 can be used to help identify high-risk infants quickly. This analysis is based on total live births and therefore describes the mortality risk only at birth. Because most neonatal mortality occurs within the 1st hours and days after birth, the outlook improves dramatically with increasing postnatal survival.

BIBLIOGRAPHY

Please visit the Nelson Textbook of Pediatrics *website at www.expertconsult.com for the complete bibliography.*

91.1 Multiple Gestation Pregnancies

Waldemar A. Carlo

INCIDENCE

The reported incidence of spontaneous twinning is highest among blacks and East Indians, followed by northern European whites, and is lowest in the Asian races. Specific rates are 1/56 in Belgium, 1/70 among American blacks, 1/86 in Italy, 1/88 among American whites, 1/130 in Greece, 1/150 in Japan, and 1/300 in China. Differences in the incidence of twins mainly involve fraternal (polyovular) dizygotic twins. Triplets are estimated to occur in 1 in 86^2 pregnancies and quadruplets in 1 in 86^3 pregnancies in the USA. The incidence of monozygotic twins (3-5/1,000) is unaffected by racial or familial factors. The incidence of twins detected by ultrasonography at 12 wk of gestation (3-5%) is much higher than that occurring later in pregnancy; the **vanishing twin syndrome** results in a singleton fetus. Although the incidence of spontaneous multifetal gestation has been stable over the years, the overall incidence of multifetal gestation is increasing as a result of treatment of infertility with ovarian stimulants (clomiphene, gonadotropins) and in vitro fertilization. Twins account for about 2.5% of births but about 20% of very low birthweight (VLBW) infants.

ETIOLOGY

The occurrence of monovular twins appears to be independent of genetic influence. Polyovular pregnancies are more frequent beyond the 2nd pregnancy, in older women, and in families with a history of polyovular twins. They may result from simultaneous maturation of multiple ovarian follicles, but follicles containing two ova have been described as a genetic trait leading to twin pregnancies. Twin-prone women have higher levels of gonadotropin. Polyovular pregnancies occur in many women treated for infertility.

Conjoined twins (Siamese twins—incidence 1/50,000) probably result from relatively late monovular separation, as does the presence of two separate embryos in one amniotic sac. The latter condition has a high fatality rate owing to obstruction of the circulation secondary to intertwining of the umbilical cords. The prognosis for conjoined twins depends on the possibility of surgical separation, which in turn depends on the extent to which vital organs are shared. The site of connections varies: thoraco-omphalopagus (28% of conjoined twins), thoracopagus (18%), omphalopagus (10%), craniopagus (6%), and incomplete duplication (10%). Difficult-to-separate conjoined twins have occasionally survived to adulthood. Most conjoined twins are female.

Superfecundation, or fertilization of an ovum by an insemination that takes place after one ovum has already been fertilized, and **superfetation**, or fertilization and subsequent development of an embryo when a fetus is already present in the uterus, have been proposed as uncommon explanations for differences in size and appearance of certain twins at birth.

A prenatal diagnosis of pregnancy with twins is suggested by a uterine size that is greater than that expected for gestational age, auscultation of two fetal hearts, and elevated maternal serum α-fetoprotein or human chorionic gonadotropin levels, and it is confirmed by ultrasonography. Ninety percent of twins are detected before delivery.

MONOZYGOTIC VERSUS DIZYGOTIC TWINS

Identifying twins as monozygotic or dizygotic (monovular or polyovular) is important because studying monozygotic twins is useful in determining the relative influence of heredity and environment on human development and disease. Twins of widely discrepant size are usually monochorionic. Twins not of the same sex are dizygotic. In twins of the same sex, zygosity should be determined and recorded at birth through careful examination of the placenta. Detailed blood typing, gene analysis, or tissue

(HLA) typing can also be used to determine zygosity. Monozygotic twins may have physical and cognitive differences because their in utero environment may be different; differences may exist in the mitochondrial genome, in post-translational gene product modification, and in the epigenetic modification of nuclear genes in response to environmental factors.

Examination of the Placenta

If the placentas are separate, they are always dichorionic (present in 75%), but the twins are not necessarily dizygotic, because initiation of monovular twinning at the 1st cell division or during the morula stage may result in two amnions, two chorions, and even two placentas. One third of monozygotic twins are dichorionic and diamnionic.

An apparently single placenta may be present with either monovular or polyovular twins; yet inspection of a polyovular placenta usually reveals that each twin has a separate chorion that crosses the placenta between the attachments of the cords and two amnions. Separate or fused dichorionic placentas may be disproportionate in size. The fetus attached to the smaller placenta or the smaller portion of the placenta is usually smaller than its twin or is malformed. **Monochorionic twins** may be presumed to be monovular. They are usually diamnionic, and almost invariably, the placenta is a single mass.

Problems of twin gestation include polyhydramnios, hyperemesis gravidarum, preeclampsia, premature rupture of membranes, vasa previa, velamentous insertion of the umbilical cord, abnormal presentations (breech), and premature labor. When compared with the first-born twin, the 2nd twin is at increased risk for respiratory distress syndrome and asphyxia. Twins are at risk for IUGR, twin-twin transfusion, and congenital anomalies, which occur predominantly in monozygotic twins. Anomalies are due to compression deformation of the uterus from crowding (hip dislocation), vascular communication with embolization (ileal atresia, porencephaly, cutis aplasia) or without embolization (acardiac twin), and unknown factors that cause twinning (conjoined twins, anencephaly, meningomyelocele).

Placental vascular anastomoses occur with high frequency only in monochorionic twins. In monochorionic placentas, the fetal vasculature is usually joined, sometimes in a very complex manner. The vascular anastomoses in monochorionic placentas may be artery to artery, vein to vein, or artery to vein. They are usually balanced so that neither twin suffers. Artery-to-artery communications cross over placental veins, and when anastomoses are present, blood can readily be stroked from one fetal vascular bed to the other. Vein-to-vein communications are similarly recognized but are less common. A combination of artery-to-artery and vein-to-vein anastomoses is associated with the condition of **acardiac fetus.** This rare lethal anomaly (1/35,000) is secondary to the **TRAP** (twin reversed arterial perfusion) **syndrome**—In utero neodynium:yttrium-aluminum-garnet (Nd:YAG) laser ablation of the anastomosis or cord occlusion can be used to treat heart failure in the surviving twin. In rare cases, one umbilical cord may arise from the other after leaving the placenta. In such cases, the twin attached to the secondary cord usually is malformed or dies in utero.

In the **fetal transfusion syndrome,** an artery from one twin acutely or chronically delivers blood that is drained into the vein of the other. The latter becomes plethoric and large, and the former is anemic and small. Generally, with chronicity, 5 g/dL hemoglobin and 20% body weight differences can be noted in this syndrome. Maternal hydramnios in a twin pregnancy suggests fetal transfusion syndrome. Anticipating this possibility by preparing to transfuse the donor twin or bleed the recipient twin may be lifesaving. Death of the donor twin in utero may result in generalized fibrin thrombi in the smaller arterioles of the recipient twin, possibly as the result of transfusion of thromboplastin-rich blood from the macerating donor fetus. Disseminated intravascular coagulation may develop in the surviving twin.

Table 91-2 CHARACTERISTIC CHANGES IN MONOCHORIONIC TWINS WITH UNCOMPENSATED PLACENTAL ARTERIOVENOUS SHUNTS

TWIN ON: ARTERIAL SIDE—DONOR	VENOUS SIDE—RECIPIENT
Prematurity	Prematurity
Oligohydramnios	Polyhydramnios
Small premature	Hydrops
Malnourished	Large premature
Pale	Well nourished
Anemic	Plethoric
Hypovolemia	Polycythemic
Hypoglycemia	Hypervolemic
Microcardia	Cardiac hypertrophy
Glomeruli small or normal	Myocardial dysfunction
Arterioles thin walled	Tricuspid valve regurgitation
	Right ventricular outflow obstruction
	Glomeruli large
	Arterioles thick walled

Table 91-2 lists the more frequent changes associated with a large uncompensated arteriovenous shunt from the placenta of one twin to that of the other. Treatment of this highly lethal problem includes maternal digoxin, aggressive amnioreduction for polyhydramnios, selective twin termination, and Nd:YAG laser or fetoscopic ablation of the anastomosis.

Postnatal Identification

The following physical criteria can be used to determine whether twins are monovular: (1) both must be of the same sex; (2) their features, including ears and teeth, must be obviously alike (but they need not resemble each other more than the lateral halves of one individual); (3) their hair must be identical in color, texture, natural curl, and distribution; (4) their eyes must be of the same color and shade; (5) their skin must be of the same texture and color (nevi may be differently apportioned and distributed); (6) their hands and feet must be of the same conformation and of similar size; and (7) their anthropometric values must show close agreement.

PROGNOSIS

Most twins are born prematurely, and maternal complications of pregnancy are more common than with single pregnancies. The risk for twins is most often associated with twin-twin transfusion, assisted reproductive technology, and early-onset discordant growth. Although monochorionic twins have a significantly higher perinatal mortality, there is no significant difference between the neonatal mortality rates of twin births and single births in comparable weight and gestational age groups (Fig. 91-2). Because most twins are premature, their overall mortality is higher than that of single-birth infants. The perinatal mortality of twins is about four times that of singletons. Monoamnionic twins have an increased likelihood of entangling the cords, which may lead to asphyxia. Theoretically, the 2nd twin is more subject to anoxia than the 1st because the placenta may separate after birth of the 1st twin and before birth of the 2nd. In addition, delivery of the 2nd twin may be difficult because it may be in an abnormal presentation (breech, entangled), uterine tone may be decreased, or the cervix may begin to close after the 1st twin's birth. The mortality for multiple gestations with four or more fetuses is excessively high for each fetus. Because of this poor prognosis, selective fetal reduction (with transabdominal intrathoracic fetal injection of KCl) to two to three fetuses has been offered as a treatment option. Monozygotic twins have an increased risk of one twin dying in utero. The surviving twin has a greater risk for cerebral palsy and other neurodevelopmental sequelae.

TREATMENT

Prenatal diagnosis enables the obstetrician and pediatrician to anticipate the birth of infants who are at high risk because of twinning. Close observation is indicated during labor and in the immediate neonatal period so that prompt treatment of asphyxia or fetal transfusion syndrome can be initiated. The decision to perform an immediate blood transfusion in a severely anemic "donor twin" or to perform a partial exchange transfusion of a "recipient twin" must be based on clinical judgment.

BIBLIOGRAPHY

Please visit the Nelson Textbook of Pediatrics *website at www.expertconsult.com for the complete bibliography.*

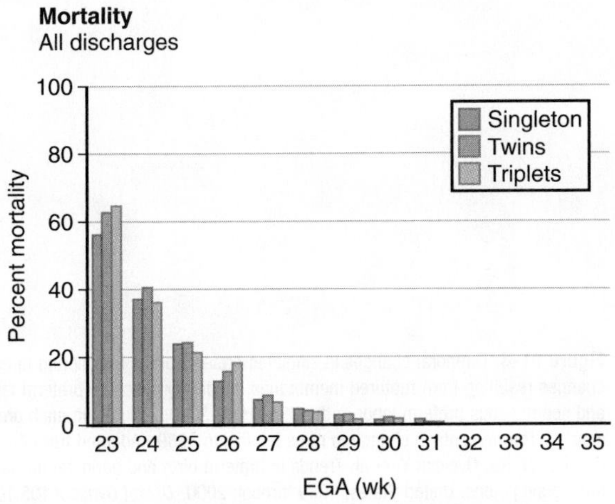

Figure 91-2 Mortality, all discharges, The neonatal mortality rate for all babies who died during the original hospitalization at each week of gestational age is given. The *bars on the left* represent singletons; the *middle bars* represent twins, and the *bars on the right* represent triplets. There are no differences among singleton births, twin births, and triplet births. EGA, estimated gestational age. (From Garite TJ, Clark RH, Elliott JP, et al: Twins and triplets: the effect of plurality and growth on neonatal outcome compared with singleton infants, *Am J Obstet Gynecol* 191:700–707, 2004.)

91.2 Prematurity and Intrauterine Growth Restriction

Waldemar A. Carlo

DEFINITIONS

Liveborn infants delivered before 37 wk from the 1st day of the last menstrual period are termed premature by the World Health Organization. LBW (birthweight of 2,500 g or less) is due to prematurity, poor intrauterine growth (IUGR, also referred to as SGA), or both. Prematurity and IUGR are associated with increased neonatal morbidity and mortality. Ideally, definitions of LBW for individual populations should be based on data that are as genetically and environmentally homogeneous as possible. As previously mentioned, Figure 91-1 presents variations in mortality based on birthweight, gestational age, and gender.

INCIDENCE

There is an increasing percentage of deaths in children <5 yr of age that occur in the neonatal period. Approximately 57% of deaths in this age group occur within the 1st mo of life, of which approximately 36% are attributable to premature birth. In 2008, 8.2% of liveborn neonates in the USA weighed <2,500 g; the rate for blacks was almost twice that for whites. Over the past 2 decades, the LBW rate has increased primarily because of an increased number of preterm births. Women whose 1st births are delivered before term are at increased risk for recurrent preterm delivery. Approximately 30% of LBW infants in the USA have IUGR and are born after 37 wk. At LBW rates >10%, the contribution of IUGR increases and that of prematurity decreases. In developing countries, approximately 70% of LBW infants have IUGR. Infants with IUGR have greater morbidity and mortality than do appropriately grown, gestational age–matched infants (see Fig. 91-1). Although U.S. infant mortality rates have fallen since 1971, the ethnic disparity between black infants and white or Hispanic infants remains unchanged. Black infants have higher neonatal mortality rates and comprise a larger percentage of low birthweight births in the USA.

The incidence of preterm births in the USA continues to rise (Fig. 91-3) and is due in part to multiple gestation pregnancies. In single births, the overall incidence has been stable, but premature births due to medically indicated deliveries have increased,

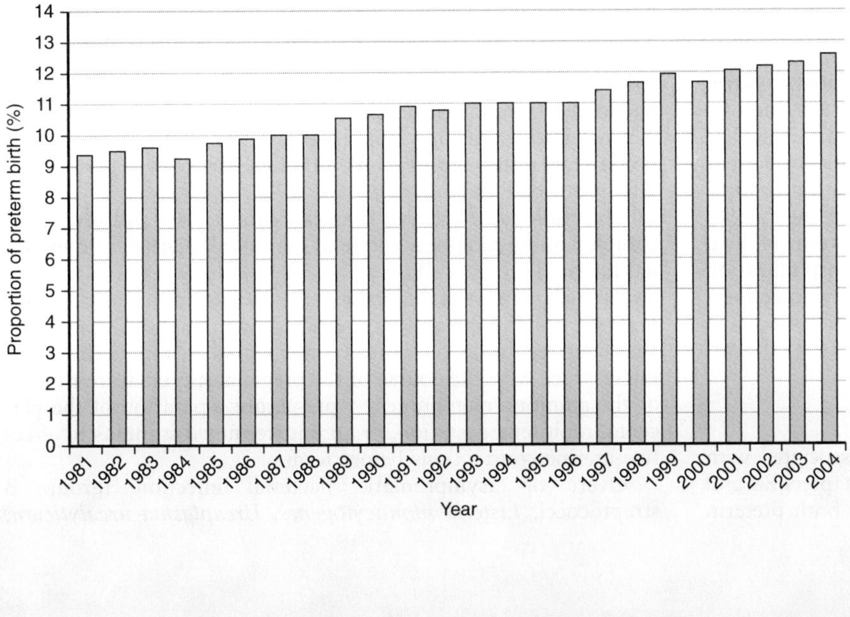

Figure 91-3 Percentage of all births classified as preterm in the USA, 1981-2004. (From Martin JA, Kochanek KD, Strobino DM, et al: Annual summary of vital statistics—2003, *Pediatrics* 115:619–634, 2005.)

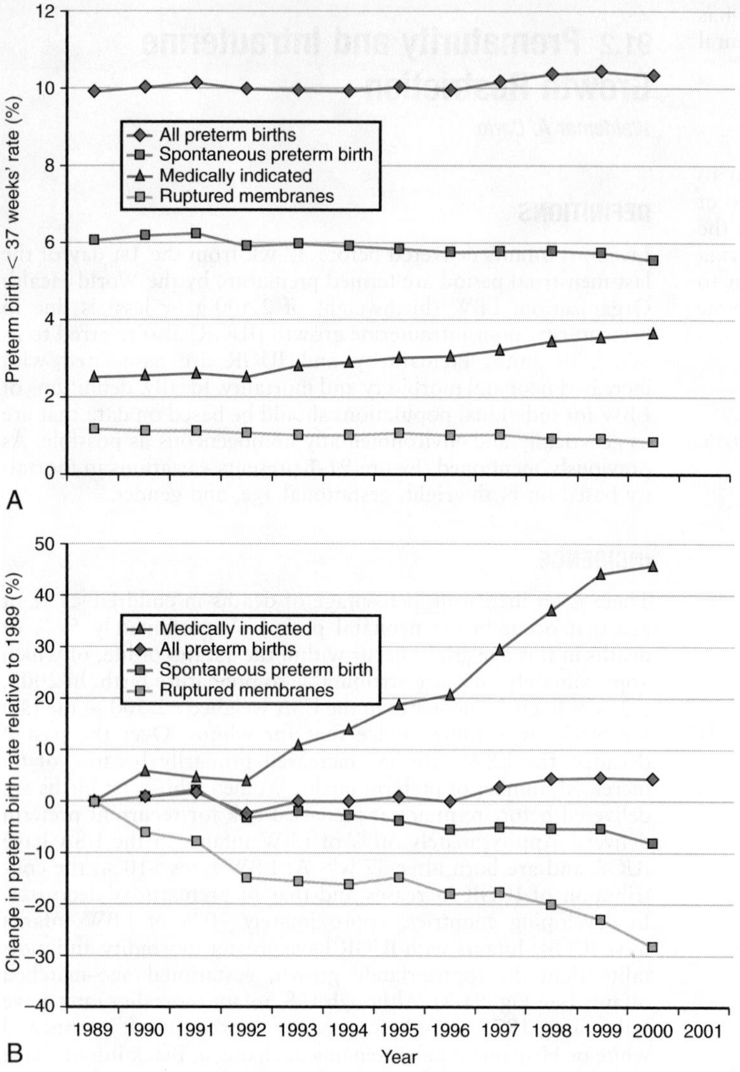

Figure 91-4 Temporal changes in singleton preterm births overall and temporal changes resulting from ruptured membranes, medically indicated preterm labor, and spontaneous preterm labor in the USA, 1989-2000. *A,* Rates in each group by year. *B,* The percentage change in rates relative to 1989. (Adapted from Ananth CV, Joseph KS, Oyelese Y, et al: Trends in preterm birth and perinatal mortality among singletons: United States, 1989 through 2000, *Obstet Gynecol* 105:1084–1091, 2005.)

whereas premature births due to spontaneous preterm birth or ruptured membranes have declined (Fig. 91-4).

VERY LOW BIRTHWEIGHT INFANTS

VLBW infants weigh <1,500 g and are predominantly premature. In the USA in 2008, the VLBW rates were approximately 1.46% overall, 3.01% among blacks, and 1.18% among whites. The VLBW rate is an accurate predictor of the infant mortality rate. VLBW infants account for over 50% of neonatal deaths and 50% of handicapped infants; their survival is directly related to birthweight, with approximately 20% of those between 500 and 600 g and >90% of those between 1,250 and 1,500 g surviving. The VLBW rate has remained unchanged for black Americans but has increased among whites, perhaps because of a rise in multiple births among whites. Perinatal care has improved the rate of survival of VLBW infants. When compared with term infants, VLBW neonates have a higher incidence of rehospitalization during the 1st yr of life for sequelae of prematurity, infections, neurologic complications, and psychosocial disorders.

FACTORS RELATED TO PREMATURE BIRTH AND LOW BIRTHWEIGHT

It is difficult to separate completely the factors associated with prematurity from those associated with IUGR (Chapters 88 and 89). A strong positive correlation exists between both preterm birth and IUGR and low socioeconomic status. Families of low socioeconomic status have higher rates of maternal undernutrition, anemia, and illness; inadequate prenatal care; drug misuse; obstetric complications; and maternal history of reproductive inefficiency (abortions, stillbirths, premature or LBW infants). Other associated factors, such as single-parent families, teenage pregnancies, short interpregnancy interval, and mothers who have borne more than four previous children, are also encountered more frequently in such families. Systematic differences in fetal growth have also been described in association with maternal size, birth order, sibling weight, social class, maternal smoking, and other factors. The degree to which the variance in birthweight among various populations is due to environmental (extrafetal) rather than genetic differences in growth potential is difficult to determine.

The etiology of preterm birth is multifactorial and involves a complex interaction between fetal, placental, uterine, and maternal factors (Table 91-3).

Premature birth of infants whose LBW is appropriate for their preterm gestational age is associated with medical conditions characterized by an inability of the uterus to retain the fetus, interference with the course of the pregnancy, premature rupture of the amniotic membranes or premature separation of the placenta, multifetal gestation, or an undetermined stimulus to effective uterine contractions before term.

Overt or asymptomatic bacterial infection (group B streptococci, *Listeria monocytogenes*, *Ureaplasma urealyticum*,

Table 91-3 IDENTIFIABLE CAUSES OF PRETERM BIRTH

FETAL
Fetal distress Multiple gestation Erythroblastosis Nonimmune hydrops
PLACENTAL
Placental dysfunction Placenta previa Abruptio placentae
UTERINE
Bicornuate uterus Incompetent cervix (premature dilatation)
MATERNAL
Preeclampsia Chronic medical illness (cyanotic heart disease, renal disease) Infection (*Listeria monocytogenes*, group B streptococcus, urinary tract infection, bacterial vaginosis, chorioamnionitis) Drug abuse (cocaine)
OTHER
Premature rupture of membranes Polyhydramnios Iatrogenic Trauma

Table 91-4 FACTORS OFTEN ASSOCIATED WITH INTRAUTERINE GROWTH RESTRICTION

FETAL
Chromosomal disorders (autosomal trisomies) Chronic fetal infections (cytomegalic inclusion disease, congenital rubella, syphilis) Congenital anomalies—syndrome complexes Irradiation Multiple gestation Pancreatic hypoplasia Insulin deficiency (production or action of insulin) Insulin-like growth factor type I deficiency
PLACENTAL
Decreased placental weight, cellularity, or both Decrease in surface area Villous placentitis (bacterial, viral, parasitic) Infarction Tumor (chorioangioma, hydatidiform mole) Placental separation Twin transfusion syndrome
MATERNAL
Toxemia Hypertension or renal disease, or both Hypoxemia (high altitude, cyanotic cardiac or pulmonary disease) Malnutrition (micronutrient or macronutrient deficiencies) Chronic illness Sickle cell anemia Drugs (narcotics, alcohol, cigarettes, cocaine, antimetabolites)

Mycoplasma hominis, Chlamydia, Trichomonas vaginalis, Gardnerella vaginalis, Bacteroides spp.) of the amniotic fluid and membranes (chorioamnionitis) may initiate preterm labor. Bacterial products may stimulate the production of local inflammatory mediators (interleukin-6, prostaglandins), which may induce premature uterine contractions or a local inflammatory response with focal amniotic membrane rupture. Appropriate antibiotic therapy reduces the risk of fetal infection and may prolong gestation.

IUGR is associated with medical conditions that interfere with the circulation and efficiency of the placenta, with the development or growth of the fetus, or with the general health and nutrition of the mother (Table 91-4). Many factors are common to both prematurely born and LBW infants with IUGR. IUGR is associated with decreased insulin production or insulin (or insulin-like growth factor [IGF]) action at the receptor level. Infants with IGF-I receptor defects, pancreatic hypoplasia, or transient neonatal diabetes have IUGR. Genetic mutations affecting the glucose-sensing mechanisms of the pancreatic islet cells that result in decreased insulin release (loss of function of the glucose-sensing glucokinase gene) give rise to IUGR.

IUGR may be a normal fetal response to nutritional or oxygen deprivation. Therefore, the issue is not the IUGR but rather the ongoing risk of fetal malnutrition or hypoxia. Similarly, some preterm births signify a need for early delivery from a potentially disadvantageous intrauterine environment. IUGR is often classified as reduced growth that is symmetric (head circumference, length, and weight equally affected) or asymmetric (with relative sparing of head growth) (see Fig. 90-1). **Symmetric IUGR** often has an earlier onset and is associated with diseases that seriously affect fetal cell number, such as conditions with chromosomal, genetic, malformation, teratogenic, infectious, or severe maternal hypertensive etiologies. It is important to assess gestational age carefully in infants suspected to have symmetric IUGR because incorrect overestimation of gestational age may lead to the diagnosis of symmetric IUGR. **Asymmetric IUGR** is often of late onset, demonstrates preservation of Doppler waveform velocity to the carotid vessels, and is associated with poor maternal nutrition or with late onset or exacerbation of maternal vascular disease (preeclampsia, chronic hypertension). Problems of infants with IUGR are noted in Table 91-5.

Table 91-5 PROBLEMS OF INFANTS SMALL FOR GESTATIONAL AGE OR WITH INTRAUTERINE GROWTH RETARDATION*

PROBLEM	PATHOGENESIS
Intrauterine fetal demise	Hypoxia, acidosis, infection, lethal anomaly
Perinatal asphyxia	↓ Uteroplacental perfusion during labor ± chronic fetal hypoxia-acidosis; meconium aspiration syndrome
Hypoglycemia	↓ Tissue glycogen stores, ↓ gluconeogenesis, hyperinsulinism, ↑ glucose needs of hypoxia, hypothermia, large brain
Polycythemia-hyperviscosity	Fetal hypoxia with ↑ erythropoietin production
Reduced oxygen consumption/hypothermia	Hypoxia, hypoglycemia, starvation effect, poor subcutaneous fat stores
Dysmorphology	Syndrome anomalads, chromosomal-genetic disorders, oligohydramnios-induced deformation, TORCH (*t*oxoplasmosis, *o*ther agents, *r*ubella, *c*ytomegalovirus, *h*erpes simplex) infection

*Other problems include pulmonary hemorrhage and those common to the gestational age-related risks of prematurity if born at less than 37 wk.
↓, Decreased; ↑, increased.

ASSESSMENT OF GESTATIONAL AGE AT BIRTH

When compared with a premature infant of appropriate weight, an infant with IUGR has a reduced birthweight and may appear to have a disproportionately larger head relative to body size; infants in both groups lack subcutaneous fat. Neurologic maturity (nerve conduction velocity), in the absence of asphyxia, correlates with gestational age despite reduced fetal weight. Physical signs may be useful in estimating gestational age at birth. Commonly used, the Ballard scoring system is accurate to ±2 wk (Figs. 91-5 to 91-7). An infant should be presumed to be at high risk for mortality or morbidity if a discrepancy exists between the estimation of gestational age by physical examination, the mother's estimated date of her last menstrual period, and fetal ultrasonographic evaluation.

Physical maturity

	−1	0	1	2	3	4	5
Skin	Sticky, friable, transparent	Gelatinous, red, translucent	Smooth, pink, visible veins	Superficial peeling and/or rash, few veins	Cracking, pale areas, rare veins	Parchment, deep cracking, no vessels	Leathery, cracked, wrinkled
Lanugo	None	Sparse	Abundant	Thinning	Bald areas	Mostly bald	
Plantar surface	Heel-toe 40-50 mm:–1 <40 mm: –2	<50 mm, no crease	Faint red marks	Anterior transverse crease only	Creases on ant. 2/3	Creases over entire sole	
Breast	Imperceptible	Barely perceptible	Flat areola–no bud	Stippled areola, 1-2 mm bud	Raised areola, 3-4 mm bud	Full areola, 5-10 mm bud	
Eye/ear	Lids fused loosely (–1), tightly (–2)	Lids open, pinna flat, stays folded	Slightly curved pinna; soft; slow recoil	Well-curved pinna, soft but ready recoil	Formed and firm, instant recoil	Thick cartilage, ear stiff	
Genitals, male	Scrotum flat, smooth	Scrotum empty, faint rugae	Testes in upper canal, rare rugae	Testes descending, few rugae	Testes down, good rugae	Testes pendulous, deep rugae	
Genitals, female	Clitoris prominent, labia flat	Prominent clitoris, small labia minora	Prominent clitoris, enlarging minora	Majora and minora equally prominent	Majora large, minora small	Majora cover clitoris and minora	

Figure 91-5 Physical criteria for maturity. The expanded New Ballard score includes extremely premature infants and has been refined to improve accuracy in more mature infants. (From Ballard JL, Khoury JC, Wedig K, et al: New Ballard score, expanded to include extremely premature infants, *J Pediatr* 119:417–423, 1991.)

Neuromuscular maturity

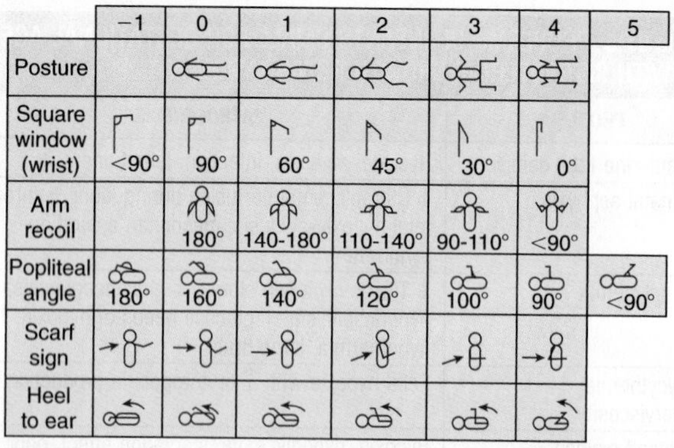
−1
0
1
2
3
4
5
Posture
Square window (wrist)
<90°
90°
60°
45°
30°
0°
Arm recoil
180°
140-180°
110-140°
90-110°
<90°
Popliteal angle
180°
160°
140°
120°
100°
90°
<90°
Scarf sign
Heel to ear

Figure 91-6 Neuromuscular criteria for maturity. The expanded New Ballard score includes extremely premature infants and has been refined to improve accuracy in more mature infants. (From Ballard JL, Khoury JC, Wedig K, et al: New Ballard score, expanded to include extremely premature infants, *J Pediatr* 119:417–423, 1991.)

Maturity Rating

Score	Weeks
− 10	20
− 5	22
0	24
5	26
10	28
15	30
20	32
25	34
30	36
35	38
40	40
45	42
50	44

Figure 91-7 Maturity rating. The physical and neurologic scores are added to calculate gestational age. (From Ballard JL, Khoury JC, Wedig K, et al: New Ballard score, expanded to include extremely premature infants, *J Pediatr* 119:417–423, 1991.)

SPECTRUM OF DISEASE IN LOW-BIRTHWEIGHT INFANTS

Immaturity increases the severity but reduces the distinctiveness of the clinical manifestations of most neonatal diseases. Immature organ function, complications of therapy, and the specific disorders that caused the premature onset of labor contribute to the neonatal morbidity and mortality associated with premature, LBW infants (Table 91-6). Among VLBW infants, morbidity is inversely related to birthweight. Respiratory distress syndrome is noted in approximately 80% of infants weighing 501-750 g; in 65% of those 751-1,000 g; in 45% of those 1,001-1,250 g; and in 25% of those 1,251-1,500 g. Severe intraventricular hemorrhage (IVH) is noted in approximately 25% of infants weighing 501-750 g; in 12% of those 751-1,000 g; in 8% of those 1,001-1,250 g; and in 3% of those 1,251-1,500 g. Overall, the risk of late sepsis (24%), bronchopulmonary dysplasia (23%), severe IVH (11%), necrotizing enterocolitis (7%), and prolonged hospitalization (45-125 days) is high in VLBW infants. Problems associated with IUGR LBW infants are noted in Table 91-5; these added problems are often superimposed on those noted in Table 91-6 if an infant with IUGR is also premature. Poor postnatal growth is an important problem for both preterm and IUGR infants.

NURSERY CARE

At birth, the measures needed to clear the airway, initiate breathing, care for the umbilical cord and eyes, and administer vitamin K are the same for immature infants as for those of normal weight and maturity (Chapter 88). Special care is required to maintain a patent airway. Additional considerations are the need for (1)

Table 91-6 NEONATAL PROBLEMS ASSOCIATED WITH PREMATURE INFANTS

RESPIRATORY
Respiratory distress syndrome (hyaline membrane disease)* Bronchopulmonary dysplasia Pneumothorax, pneumomediastinum; interstitial emphysema Congenital pneumonia Apnea*
CARDIOVASCULAR
Patent ductus arteriosus* Hypotension Bradycardia (with apnea)*
HEMATOLOGIC
Anemia (early or late onset)
GASTROINTESTINAL
Poor gastrointestinal function—poor motility* Necrotizing enterocolitis Hyperbilirubinemia—direct and indirect* Spontaneous gastrointestinal isolated perforation
METABOLIC-ENDOCRINE
Hypocalcemia* Hypoglycemia* Hyperglycemia* Late metabolic acidosis Hypothermia* Euthyroid but low thyroxine status
CENTRAL NERVOUS SYSTEM
Intraventricular hemorrhage* Periventricular leukomalacia Seizures Retinopathy of prematurity Deafness Hypotonia*
RENAL
Hyponatremia* Hypernatremia* Hyperkalemia* Renal tubular acidosis Renal glycosuria Edema
OTHER
Infections* (congenital, perinatal, nosocomial: bacterial, viral, fungal, protozoal)

*Common.

thermal control and monitoring of the heart rate and respiration, (2) oxygen therapy, and (3) special attention to the details of fluid requirements and nutrition. Safeguards against infection can never be relaxed. Routine procedures that disturb these infants may result in hypoxia. The need for regular and active participation by the parents in the infant's care in the nursery, the need to instruct the mother in at-home care of her infant, and the question of prognosis for later growth and development require special consideration.

Thermal Control

The survival rate of LBW and sick infants is higher when they are cared for at or near their **neutral thermal environment.** This environment is a set of thermal conditions, including air and radiating surface temperatures, relative humidity, and airflow, at which heat production (measured experimentally as oxygen consumption) is minimal and the infant's core temperature is within the normal range. The neutral thermal environment is a function of the size and postnatal age of an infant; larger, older infants require lower environmental temperatures than smaller, younger infants do. Incubators or radiant warmers can be used to maintain body temperature. Body heat is conserved through provision of a warm environment and humidity. The optimal environmental temperature for minimal heat loss and oxygen consumption for an unclothed infant is one that maintains the infant's core temperature at 36.5-37.0°C. It depends on an infant's size and maturity; the smaller and more immature the infant, the higher the environmental temperature required. An additional acrylic resin (Plexiglas) heat shield or head cap and body clothing may be required to keep an extremely LBW (ELBW) preterm infant warm. Infant warmth can be maintained by heating the air to a desired temperature or by servo-controlling the infant's body temperature at a desired set point. Continuous monitoring of the infant's temperature is required so that the environmental temperature can be adjusted to maintain optimal body temperature. **Kangaroo mother care** with direct skin-to-skin contact and a hat and blanket covering the infant is a safe alternative, with careful monitoring to avoid the risk of serious hypothermia when incubators are unavailable or when the infant is stable and the parents desire close contact with their infant.

Maintaining a relative humidity of 40-60% aids in stabilizing body temperature by reducing heat loss at lower environmental temperatures; by preventing drying and irritation of the lining of respiratory passages, especially during the administration of oxygen and after or during endotracheal intubation (usually 100% humidity); and by thinning viscid secretions and reducing insensible water loss from the lungs. An infant should be weaned and then removed from the incubator or radiant warmer only when the gradual change to the atmosphere of the nursery does not result in a significant change in the infant's temperature, color, activity, or vital signs.

Administering oxygen to reduce the risk of injury from hypoxia and circulatory insufficiency must be balanced against the risk of hyperoxia to the eyes (retinopathy of prematurity) and oxygen injury to the lungs. Oxygen should be administered via a head hood, nasal cannula, continuous positive airway pressure apparatus, or endotracheal tube to maintain stable and safe inspired oxygen concentrations. Although cyanosis must be treated immediately, oxygen is a drug, and its use must be carefully regulated to maximize benefit and minimize potential harm. The concentration of inspired oxygen must be adjusted in accordance with the oxygen tension of arterial blood (PaO_2) or a noninvasive method such as continuous pulse oximetry or transcutaneous oxygen measurements. Capillary blood gas determinations are inadequate for estimating arterial oxygen levels.

Fluid Requirements

Fluid needs vary according to gestational age, environmental conditions, and disease states. Assuming minimal water loss in the stool of infants not receiving oral fluids, their water needs are equal to their insensible water loss, excretion of renal solutes, growth, and any unusual ongoing losses. Insensible water loss is indirectly related to gestational age; very immature preterm infants (<1,000 g) may lose as much as 2-3 mL/kg/hr, partly because of immature skin, lack of subcutaneous tissue, and a large exposed surface area. Insensible water loss is increased under radiant warmers, during phototherapy, and in febrile infants. High humidity can be used to reduce insensible water losses. The loss is diminished when an infant is clothed, is covered by an acrylic resin inner heat shield, breathes humidified air, or is of advanced postnatal age. A larger premature infant (2,000-2,500 g) nursed in an incubator may have an insensible water loss of approximately 0.6-0.7 mL/kg/hr.

Adequate fluid intake is essential for excretion of the urinary solute load (urea, electrolytes, phosphate). The amount varies with dietary intake and the anabolic or catabolic state of nutrition. Formulas with a high solute load, high protein intake, and catabolism increase the end products that require urinary excretion and thus increase the requirement for water. **Renal solute loads** may vary between 7.5 and 30 mOsm/kg. Newborn infants, especially VLBW ones, are also less able to concentrate urine, so they need higher fluid intake to excrete solutes.

Fluid intake in term infants is usually begun at 60-70 mL/kg on day 1 and increased to 100-120 mL/kg by days 2-3. Smaller, more premature infants may need to start with 70-80 mL/kg on day 1 and advance gradually to 150 mL/kg/day. Fluid volumes should be titrated individually, although it is unusual to exceed 150 mL/kg/24 hr. Infants weighing <750 g in the 1st wk of life have immature skin and a large surface area, characteristics that lead to a high rate of transepidermal fluid loss, at times requiring higher rates of intravenous fluids. Daily weights, urine output, and serum urea nitrogen and sodium levels should be monitored carefully to determine water balance and fluid needs. Clinical observation and physical examination are poor indicators of the state of hydration of premature infants. Conditions that increase fluid loss, such as glycosuria, the polyuric phase of acute tubular necrosis, and diarrhea, may place additional strain on kidneys that have not yet acquired their maximal capacity to conserve water and electrolytes, the result of which may be severe dehydration. Alternatively, fluid overload may lead to edema, heart failure, patent ductus arteriosus, and bronchopulmonary dysplasia.

Total Parenteral Nutrition

Before complete enteral feeding has been established or when enteral feeding is impossible for prolonged periods, total intravenous alimentation may provide sufficient fluid, calories, amino acids, electrolytes, and vitamins to sustain the growth of ill infants. This technique has been lifesaving for VLBW and preterm infants and infants who have had intractable diarrheal syndromes or extensive bowel resection. Infusions may be administered through a percutaneously or, less often, surgically placed indwelling central venous catheter or through a peripheral vein. The umbilical vein may also be used for up to 2 wk.

The goal of parenteral alimentation is to deliver sufficient calories from glucose, protein, and lipids to promote optimal growth. The infusate should contain 2.5-3.5 g/dL of synthetic amino acids and usually 10-15 g/dL of glucose, in addition to appropriate quantities of electrolytes, trace minerals, and vitamins. If a peripheral vein is used, it is advisable to keep the glucose concentration below 12.5 g/dL. If a central vein is used, glucose concentrations as high as 25 g/dL may be used (rarely). Intravenous fat emulsions such as Intralipid 20% (2.2 kcal/mL) may be administered to provide calories without an appreciable osmotic load, thereby decreasing the need for infusion of the higher concentrations of glucose by central or peripheral vein while preventing the development of essential fatty acid deficiency. A 20% fat emulsion may be initiated at 0.5 g/kg/24 hr and advanced to 3 g/kg/24 hr, if triglyceride levels remain normal; 0.5 g/kg/24 hr is sufficient to prevent essential fatty acid deficiency. Electrolytes, trace minerals, and vitamin additives are included in amounts approximating established intravenous maintenance requirements. The content of each day's infusate should be determined after careful assessment of the infant's clinical and biochemical status. Slow and continuous infusion is advisable. A well-trained pharmacist should mix all solutions under a laminar flow hood.

After a caloric intake of >100 kcal/kg/24 hr is established by total parenteral intravenous nutrition, the infants can be expected to gain about 15 g/kg/24 hr, with a positive nitrogen balance of 150-200 mg/kg/24 hr, in the absence of episodes of sepsis, surgical procedures, and other severe stress. This goal can usually be achieved (and the catabolic tendency during the 1st wk of life reversed, with subsequent weight gain) by peripheral vein infusion of 2.5-3.5 g/kg/24 hr of an amino acid mixture, 10 g/dL of glucose, and 2-3 g/kg/24 hr of a 20% fat emulsion.

Complications of intravenous alimentation are related to both the catheter and the metabolism of the infusate. Sepsis, the most important problem of central vein infusions, can be minimized only by meticulous catheter care and aseptic preparation of the infusate; a vancomycin-heparin solution also reduces the risk of line sepsis. Coagulase-negative staphylococcus is the most common infecting organism. Treatment includes appropriate antibiotics. If an infection persists (repeatedly positive blood culture results while the infant is receiving appropriate antibiotics), the line must be removed. Thrombosis, extravasation of fluid, and accidental dislodgment of catheters have also occurred. Although sepsis is less often attributable to peripheral vein infusion, phlebitis, cutaneous sloughing, and superficial infection may occur. Metabolic complications of parenteral nutrition include hyperglycemia from the high glucose concentration of the infusate, which may lead to osmotic diuresis and dehydration; azotemia; a possible increased risk of nephrocalcinosis; hypoglycemia from sudden accidental cessation of the infusate; hyperlipidemia and possibly hypoxemia from intravenous lipid infusions; and hyperammonemia, which may be due to high levels of certain amino acids. Metabolic bone disease and/or cholestatic jaundice and liver disease may develop in infants who require long-term parenteral nutrition and receive no enteral nutrition. Biochemical and physiologic monitoring of infants receiving intravenous alimentation is indicated because of the frequency and seriousness of complications.

Feeding

The method of feeding each LBW or preterm infant should be individualized. It is important to avoid fatigue and aspiration of food through regurgitation or the feeding process. No feeding method averts these problems unless the person feeding the infant has been well trained in the method. Oral feeding (nipple) should not be initiated or should be discontinued in infants with respiratory distress, hypoxia, circulatory insufficiency, excessive secretions, gagging, sepsis, central nervous system depression, severe immaturity, or signs of serious illness. These high-risk infants require parenteral nutrition or gavage feeding to supply calories, fluid, and electrolytes. The process of oral alimentation requires, in addition to a strong sucking effort, coordination of swallowing, epiglottal and uvular closure of the larynx and nasal passages, and normal esophageal motility, a synchronized process that is usually absent before 34 wk of gestation.

Preterm infants at 34 wk of gestation or more can often be fed by bottle or at the breast. Because the effort of sucking is usually the limiting factor, direct breast-feeding is less likely to succeed in very preterm infants until they mature. Bottle-feeding of expressed breast milk may be a temporary alternative. In bottle-feeding, the infant's effort may be reduced by use of special small, soft nipples with large holes. Smaller or less vigorous infants should be fed by gavage: A soft plastic tube with No. 5 French external and approximately 0.05 cm internal diameters and with a rounded atraumatic tip and two holes on alternate sides is preferable. The tube is passed through the nose until approximately 2.5 cm (1 inch) of the lower end is in the stomach. The free end of the tube has an adapter into which the tip of a syringe is fitted, and a measured amount of fluid is given by pump or by gravity. Such a tube may be left in place for 3-7 days before being replaced by a similar tube through the other nostril. Infants occasionally have enough local irritation from an indwelling tube that they may gag or troublesome secretions may gather around it in the nasopharynx. In such cases, a catheter may be passed through the mouth by a skilled person and removed at the end of each feeding.

The infant may be fed with intermittent bolus feedings or continuous feeding. In the occasional infant with feeding intolerance, nasojejunal feeding may be successful. Intestinal perforation is a risk with nasojejunal feeding. A change to breast- or bottle-feeding may be instituted gradually as soon as an infant displays general vigor adequate for oral feeding without fatigue.

Gastrostomy feeding is not usually indicated in premature or LBW infants except as an adjunct to surgical management of specific gastrointestinal conditions or in patients with permanent neurologic injuries who are unable to suck and swallow normally.

Initiation of Feeding

The optimal time to introduce enteral feeding to a sick premature or LBW infant is controversial. **Trophic feeding** is the practice of feeding very small amounts of enteral nourishment to VLBW preterm infants to stimulate development of the immature gastrointestinal tract. The benefits of trophic feeding include enhanced gut motility, improved growth, decreased need for parenteral nutrition, fewer episodes of sepsis, and shortened hospital stay. Once the infant is stable, small-volume feedings are given in addition to intravenous fluids/nutrition. Feeding is gradually advanced, and parenteral nutrition decreased. This approach may reduce the incidence of necrotizing enterocolitis. The main principle in feeding premature infants is to proceed cautiously and gradually. Careful early feeding of breast milk or formula tends to reduce the risk of hypoglycemia, dehydration, and hyperbilirubinemia without the additional risk of aspiration, provided that there is no indication for withholding oral feedings, such as the presence of respiratory distress or other disorders.

If an infant is well, is making sucking movements, and is in no distress, oral feeding may be attempted, although most infants weighing <1,500 g require tube feeding because they are unable to coordinate breathing, sucking, and swallowing. Intestinal tract readiness for feeding may be determined by active bowel sounds, passage of meconium, and the absence of abdominal distention, bilious gastric aspirates, and emesis. For infants <1,000 g, the initial trophic feedings can be given at 10-20 mL/kg/24 hr as a continuous nasogastric tube drip (or given by intermittent gavage every 2-3 hr) for 5-10 days. If the initial feedings are tolerated, the volume is increased by 20-30 mL/kg/24 hr. Once a volume of 150 mL/kg/24 hr has been achieved, the caloric content may be increased to 24 or 27 kcal/oz. With high caloric density, infants are at risk for dehydration, edema, lactose intolerance, diarrhea, flatus, and delayed gastric emptying with emesis. Intravenous fluids are needed until feedings provide approximately 120 mL/kg/24 hr. The feeding protocol for premature infants weighing >1,500 g is initiated at a volume of 20-30 mL/kg/24 hr with increments in total daily formula volume of 20-30 mL/kg/24 hr. The expected weight increments for premature infants of various birthweights are projected from Figure 91-8. Infants with IUGR may not demonstrate the marked initial weight loss noted in premature infants.

Regurgitation, vomiting, abdominal distention, or gastric residuals from previous feedings should arouse suspicion of sepsis, necrotizing enterocolitis, or intestinal obstruction; these conditions are indications to stop feedings, at least temporarily, and to increase subsequent feedings slowly only as tolerated or to change to intravenous alimentation and evaluate the infant for more serious problems (Chapter 96.2). Weight gain may not be achieved for 10-12 days. Alternatively, in infants whose feeding schedule is advanced successfully in calories or volume, weight gain may appear within a few days.

When tube feeding is used, the contents of the stomach should be aspirated before each feeding. If only air or small amounts of mucus are obtained, the feeding is given as planned. If all or a substantial part of the previous feeding is aspirated, it is advisable to withhold feedings or to reduce the amount of the feeding and proceed more gradually with subsequent increases, depending on the physical findings and other evidence of feeding intolerance.

The digestive enzyme systems of infants older than 28 wk of gestation are mature enough to permit adequate digestion and absorption of protein and carbohydrate. Fat is less well absorbed, primarily because of inadequate amounts of bile salt; unsaturated fats and the fat of human milk are absorbed better than the fat of cow's milk. The weight gain of infants weighing <2,000 g at birth should be adequate when either human milk or "humanized" milk premature formula (40% casein and 60% whey) with a protein intake of 2.25-2.75 g/kg/24 hr is fed. These two alternatives should provide all amino acids essential for premature infants, including tyrosine, cystine, and histidine. Higher protein intake may be well tolerated and is generally safe, especially in older, rapidly growing infants. Protein intake >4-5 g/kg/24 hr may be hazardous. Although they may promote linear growth, high-protein formulas may cause abnormal plasma aminogram results; elevations in blood urea nitrogen, ammonia, and sodium concentrations; metabolic acidosis (cow's milk formulas); and untoward effects on neurologic development. Furthermore, the high protein and mineral contents of balanced cow's milk formulas with a high caloric content constitute a large solute load for the kidneys, a fact important in maintaining water balance, especially in infants with diarrhea or fever.

Breast milk from their mothers is the preferred milk for all infants, including VLBW infants. In addition to nutritional advantages, the benefits of breast milk include protection against a wide range of infections (through both specific and nonspecific anti-infective factors in breast milk and beneficial effects on intestinal flora), a decreased risk of necrotizing enterocolitis in preterm infants, a lower risk of sudden infant death syndrome, and possible long-term effects, including a lower risk of childhood/

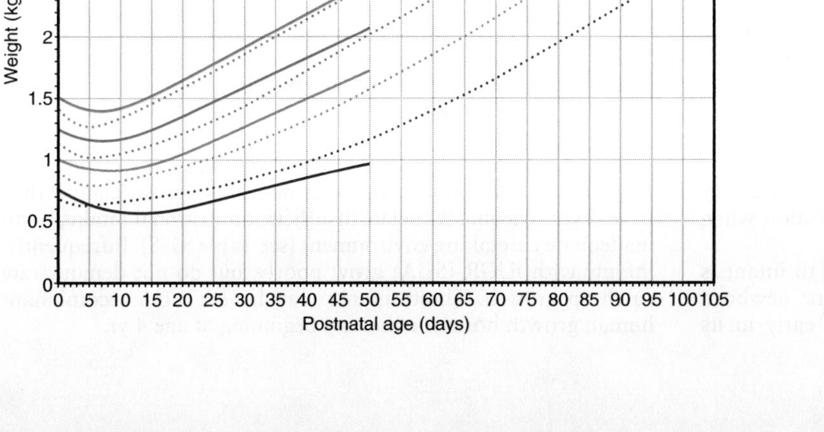

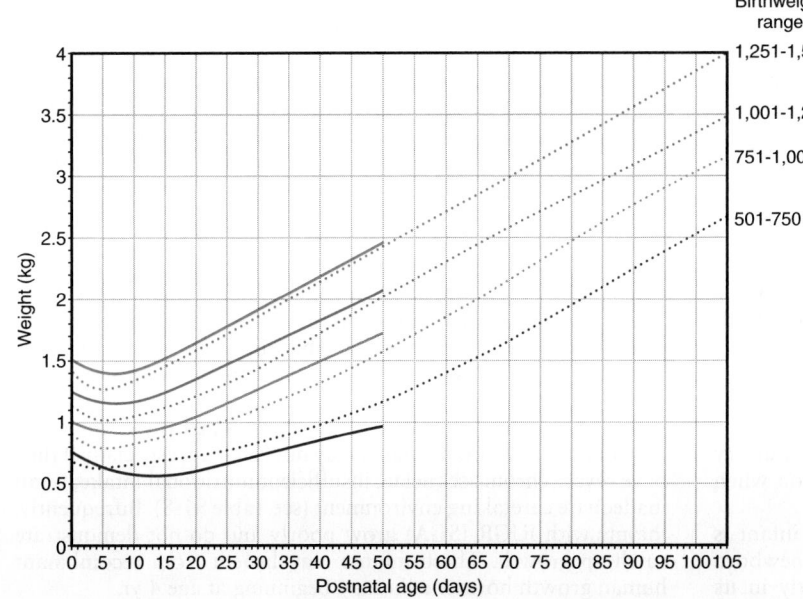

Figure 91-8 Average daily weight vs postnatal age for infants with birthweight ranges of 501-750 g, 751-1,000 g, 1,001-1,250 g, and 1,251-1,500 g (*dotted lines*), plotted with the curves from Dancis and colleagues for infants with birthweights of 750 g, 1,000 g, 1,250 g, and 1,500 g (*solid lines*). (From Wright K, Dawson JP, Fallis D, et al: New postnatal growth grids for very low birth weight infants, *Pediatrics* 91:922–926, 1993.)

adolescent obesity and improved neurodevelopmental outcome. Once a premature infant takes 120 mL/kg/24 hr, **breast milk fortifiers** are added to supplement breast milk with protein, calcium, and phosphorus. If breast milk is unavailable, special preterm formulas should be used.

Properly fed premature infants may have from 1 to 8 daily stools of semisolid consistency; a sudden increase in their number, the appearance of occult or gross blood, or change to a watery consistency is more reason for concern than any arbitrarily stated stooling frequency.

Vitamins

Although formula in amounts necessary for adequate growth probably contains adequate quantities of all vitamins, the volume of milk sufficient to satisfy these requirements may not be ingested for several weeks. Therefore, LBW and preterm infants should be given supplemental vitamins. Because requirements for these infants have not been precisely established, the recommended daily allowances for term infants should be given (Chapter 41). Furthermore, infants may have a special need for certain vitamins. Intermediary metabolism of phenylalanine and tyrosine depends, in part, on vitamin C. Decreased fat absorption with increased fecal fat loss may be associated with decreased absorption of vitamin D, other fat-soluble vitamins, and calcium in premature infants. VLBW infants are particularly prone to the development of osteopenia, but their total intake of vitamin D should not exceed 1,500 IU/24 hr. Folic acid is essential for the formation of DNA and production of new cells; serum and erythrocyte levels decrease in preterm infants during the 1st few wk of life and remain low for 2-3 mo. Therefore, folic acid supplementation is recommended, although it does not result in improved growth or an increased hemoglobin concentration. Deficiency of vitamin E is uncommon but is associated with increased hemolysis and, if severe, with anemia and edema in premature infants. Vitamin E functions as an antioxidant to prevent the peroxidation of excessive polyunsaturated fatty acids in red blood cell membranes; its need may increase because of the higher membrane content of these fatty acids when formulas with high polyunsaturated fatty acids are used. Vitamin A supplementation reduces bronchopulmonary dysplasia in ELBW infants. Vitamin K deficiency is discussed in Chapter 97.4.

In LBW and premature infants, **physiologic anemia** due to postnatal suppression of erythropoiesis is exacerbated by smaller fetal iron stores and greater expansion of blood volume from the more rapid growth than that of term infants; therefore, the anemia develops earlier and reaches a lower ultimate level. Fetal or neonatal blood loss accentuates this problem. Iron stores, even in a VLBW neonate, are usually adequate until an infant's birthweight has doubled; iron supplementation (2 mg/kg/24 hr) should then be started. If erythropoietin is used, iron supplementation is also required.

Prevention of Infection

Premature infants have an increased susceptibility to infection, and thus meticulous attention to infection control is required. Prevention strategies include strict compliance with handwashing and universal precautions, minimizing the risk of catheter contamination and duration, meticulous skin care, encouraging early appropriate advancement of enteral feeding, education and feedback to staff, and surveillance of nosocomial infection rates in the nursery. Although no one with an active infection should be permitted in the nursery, the risks of infection must be balanced against the disadvantages of limiting the infant's contact with the family. Early and frequent participation by parents in the nursery care of their infant does not increase the risk of infection when preventive precautions are maintained.

Preventing transmission of infection from infant to infant is difficult because often neither term nor premature newborn infants have clear clinical evidence of an infection early in its course. When epidemics occur within a nursery, cohort nursing and isolation rooms should be used. Universal precautions require gloves to be worn with all patient contact. Because premature infants have immature immune function, some will develop nosocomial infection even when all precautions are followed.

Routine immunizations should be given on the regular schedule at standard doses (Chapter 165).

IMMATURITY OF DRUG METABOLISM

Renal clearance of almost all substances excreted in the urine is diminished in newborn infants, but more so in premature ones. The glomerular filtration rate rises with increasing gestational age; therefore drug dosing recommendations vary with age. Intervals between doses may therefore need to be extended with administration of drugs excreted chiefly by the kidneys. Longer intervals are required for many drugs administered to preterm infants. Drugs that are detoxified in the liver or require chemical conjugation before renal excretion should also be given with caution and in doses smaller than usual.

When possible, blood levels should be determined for potentially toxic drugs, especially if renal or hepatic dysfunction is present. Decisions about the choice and dose of antibacterial agents and the route of administration should be made on an individual basis rather than routinely because of the dangers of (1) development of infections with organisms resistant to antibacterial agents, (2) inhibition of intestinal bacteria that manufacture significant amounts of essential vitamins (vitamin K and thiamine), and (3) harmful interference in important metabolic processes.

Many drugs apparently safe for adults on the basis of toxicity studies may be harmful to newborn infants, especially premature ones. Oxygen and a number of drugs have proved toxic to premature infants in amounts not harmful to term infants (Table 91-7). Thus, administering any drug, particularly in high doses, that has not undergone pharmacologic testing in premature infants should be undertaken carefully after risks have been weighed against benefits.

PROGNOSIS

Infants born weighing 1,501-2,500 g have a 95% or greater chance of survival, but those weighing still less have significantly higher mortality (see Fig. 91-1). Intensive care has extended the period during which a VLBW infant is at increased risk of dying of complications of prematurity, such as bronchopulmonary dysplasia, necrotizing enterocolitis, and nosocomial infection (Table 91-8). The postdischarge mortality rate of LBW infants is higher than that of term infants during the 1st 2 yr of life. Because many of the deaths are attributable to infection (e.g., respiratory syncytial virus [RSV]), they are at least theoretically preventable. In addition, premature infants have an increased incidence of failure to thrive, sudden infant death syndrome, child abuse, and inadequate maternal-infant bonding. The biologic risk associated with poor cardiorespiratory regulation due to immaturity or complications of underlying perinatal disease and the social risk associated with poverty also contribute to the high mortality and morbidity of these infants. Congenital anomalies are present in approximately 3-7% of LBW infants.

In the absence of congenital abnormalities, central nervous system injury, VLBW, or marked IUGR, the **physical growth** of LBW infants tends to approximate that of term infants by the 2nd yr; the approximation occurs earlier in premature infants with larger birth size. VLBW infants may not catch up, especially if they have severe chronic sequelae, insufficient nutritional intake, or an inadequate caretaking environment (see Table 91-8). Infrequently, infants with IUGR (SGA) grow poorly and do not demonstrate catch-up growth. These infants may benefit from recombinant human growth hormone therapy beginning at age 4 yr.

Table 91-7 POTENTIAL ADVERSE REACTIONS TO DRUGS ADMINISTERED TO PREMATURE INFANTS

DRUG	REACTION(S)
Oxygen	Retinopathy of prematurity, bronchopulmonary dysplasia
Sulfisoxazole	Kernicterus
Chloramphenicol	Gray baby syndrome—shock, bone marrow suppression
Vitamin K analogs	Jaundice
Novobiocin	Jaundice
Hexachlorophene	Encephalopathy
Benzyl alcohol	Acidosis, collapse, intraventricular bleeding
Intravenous vitamin E	Ascites, shock
Phenolic detergents	Jaundice
$NaHCO_3$	Intraventricular hemorrhage
Amphotericin	Anuric renal failure, hypokalemia, hypomagnesemia
Reserpine	Nasal stuffiness
Indomethacin	Oliguria, hyponatremia, intestinal perforation
Cisapride	Prolonged QTc interval
Tetracycline	Enamel hypoplasia
Tolazoline	Hypotension, gastrointestinal bleeding
Calcium salts	Subcutaneous necrosis
Aminoglycosides	Deafness, renal toxicity
Enteric gentamicin	Resistant bacteria
Prostaglandins	Seizures, diarrhea, apnea, hyperostosis, pyloric stenosis
Phenobarbital	Altered state, drowsiness
Morphine	Hypotension, urine retention, withdrawal
Pancuronium	Edema, hypovolemia, hypotension, tachycardia, vecuronium contractions, prolonged hypotonia
Iodine antiseptics	Hypothyroidism, goiter
Fentanyl	Seizures, chest wall rigidity, withdrawal
Dexamethasone	Gastrointestinal bleeding, hypertension, infection, hyperglycemia, cardiomyopathy, reduced growth
Furosemide	Deafness, hyponatremia, hypokalemia, hypochloremia, nephrocalcinosis, biliary stones
Heparin (not low-dose prophylactic use)	Bleeding, intraventricular hemorrhage, thrombocytopenia
Erythromycin	Pyloric stenosis

Table 91-8 SEQUELAE OF LOW BIRTHWEIGHT

IMMEDIATE	LATE
Hypoxia, ischemia	Mental retardation, spastic diplegia, microcephaly, seizures, poor school performance
Intraventricular hemorrhage	Mental retardation, spasticity, seizures, hydrocephalus
Sensorineural injury	Hearing, visual impairment, retinopathy of prematurity, strabismus, myopia
Respiratory failure	Bronchopulmonary dysplasia, cor pulmonale, bronchospasm, malnutrition, subglottic stenosis
Necrotizing enterocolitis	Short-bowel syndrome, malabsorption, malnutrition, infectious diarrhea
Cholestatic liver disease	Cirrhosis, hepatic failure, malnutrition
Nutrient deficiency	Osteopenia, fractures, anemia, growth failure
Social stress	Child abuse or neglect, failure to thrive, divorce
Other	Sudden infant death syndrome, infections, inguinal hernia, cutaneous scars (chest tube, patent ductus arteriosus ligation, intravenous infiltration), gastroesophageal reflux, hypertension, craniosynostosis, cholelithiasis, nephrocalcinosis, cutaneous hemangiomas

Premature birth in itself may adversely affect later development. The greater the immaturity and the lower the birthweight, the greater the likelihood of intellectual and neurologic deficit; as many as 50% of 500-750 g infants have significant neurodevelopmental impairment (mental retardation, cerebral palsy, blindness, deafness). Small head circumference at birth may be related to a poor neurobehavioral prognosis. Many surviving LBW infants have hypotonia before 8 mo corrected age, which improves by the time they are 8 mo to 1 yr old. This transient hypotonia is not a poor prognostic sign. Thirty percent to 50% of VLBW children have poor school performance at 7 yr of age (repeating of grades, special classes, learning disorders, poor speech and language), despite a normal IQ. Factors posing a risk for poor academic performance include birthweight below 750 g, severe IVH, periventricular leukomalacia, bronchopulmonary dysplasia, cerebral atrophy, posthemorrhagic hydrocephalus, IUGR, low socioeconomic status, and, possibly, low thyroxine levels. Antenatal exposure to magnesium sulfate may have neuroprotective effects and may reduce the incidence of cerebral palsy in high-risk neonates. Adolescents who were VLBW report satisfactory health; 94% are integrated in regular classes despite neurosensory disabilities (hearing, vision, cerebral palsy, cognition) in 24%.

Both premature and IUGR infants are at risk for significant metabolic conditions (obesity, type II diabetes) and cardiovascular disorders (ischemic heart disease, hypertension) as adults. This **fetal origins** hypothesis of adult morbidities may involve insulin resistance, which may be evident in early childhood.

PREDICTING NEONATAL MORTALITY

Birthweight and gestational age have traditionally been used as strong indicators for the risk of neonatal death. Indeed, survival at 22 wk of gestation is poor, particularly in those infants requiring aggressive resuscitation in the delivery room. With increasing gestational age, survival rates rise to approximately 15% at 23 wk, 56% at 24 wk, and 79% at 25 wk. The survival of infants of <24 wk gestation, weighing <750 g, and with a 1-min Apgar score <3 is 30%. Antenatal steroids to increase lung maturation, female sex, and singleton pregnancy increase the chance for survival. However, extremely premature infants are also at risk for poor neurodevelopmental outcome.

Birthweight-specific neonatal diseases such as intraventricular hemorrhage, group B streptococcal sepsis/pneumonia, and pulmonary hypoplasia also contribute to a poor outcome. **Scoring systems** that have been developed take into consideration physiologic abnormalities (hypotension-hypertension, acidosis, hypoxia, hypercapnia, anemia, neutropenia), as in the **Score for Neonatal Acute Physiology (SNAP)**, or clinical parameters (gestational age, birthweight, anomalies, acidosis, Fio_2), as in the **Clinical Risk Index for Babies (CRIB)**. CRIB includes six parameters collected in the 1st 12 hr after birth, and SNAP has 26 variables collected in the 1st 24 hr. Prediction models can be used before birth, but additional data from throughout the hospitalization improve the identification of infants at high risk for death or neurodevelopmental impairment. Combining a physician's judgment and an objective score may produce a more accurate assessment of the risk of death.

DISCHARGE FROM THE HOSPITAL

Before discharge, a premature infant should be taking all nutrition by nipple, either bottle or breast (Table 91-9). Some medically fragile infants may be discharged home while receiving gavage feedings after the parents have received appropriate training and education. Growth should be occurring at steady increments of approximately 30 g/day. Temperature should be stabile in an open crib. Infants should have had no recent episodes of apnea or bradycardia, and parenteral drug administration should have been discontinued or converted to oral dosing. Stable infants

Table 91-9 RECOMMENDATIONS FOR THE DISCHARGE OF HIGH-RISK LOW-BIRTHWEIGHT INFANTS

Resolution of acute life-threatening illnesses
Ongoing follow-up for chronic but stable problems:
Bronchopulmonary dysplasia
Intraventricular hemorrhage
Necrotizing enterocolitis after surgery or recovery
Ventricular septal defect, other cardiac lesions
Anemia
Retinopathy of prematurity
Hearing problems
Apnea
Cholestasis
Stable temperature regulation
Gain of weight with oral feedings:
Breast-feeding
Bottle-feeding
Gastric tube
Free of significant apnea; home monitoring for apnea if needed
Appropriate immunizations and planning for respiratory syncytial virus prophylaxis if indicated
Hearing screenings
Ophthalmologic examination if <27 wk of gestation or <1,250 g at birth
Mother's knowledge, skill, confidence documented in:
Administration of medications (diuretics, methylxanthines, aerosols, etc.)
Use of oxygen, apnea monitors, oximeters
Nutritional support:
Timing
Volume
Mixing concentrated formulas
Recognition of illness and deterioration
Basic cardiopulmonary resuscitation
Infant safety (see Table 91-1)
Scheduling of referrals:
Primary care provider
Neonatal follow-up clinic
Occupational therapy/physical therapy
Imaging (head ultrasound)
Assessment of and solution to social risks (see Table 91-1)

Adapted from American Academy of Pediatrics, American College of Obstetricians: *Guidelines for perinatal care,* ed 5, Elk Grove Village, IL, 2002, American Academy of Pediatrics.

recovering from bronchopulmonary dysplasia may be discharged on a regimen of oxygen given by nasal cannula as long as careful follow-up is arranged with frequent pulse oximetry monitoring and outpatient visits. All infants with birthweight <1,500 g and those with birthweights between 1,500 and 2,000 g with an unstable clinical course requiring oxygen should undergo an eye examination to screen for retinopathy of prematurity. All infants should have a hearing test prior to discharge. In those who had indwelling umbilical arterial catheters, blood pressure should be measured to check for renal vascular hypertension. The hemoglobin level or hematocrit should be determined to evaluate for possible anemia. If all major medical problems have resolved and the home setting is adequate, premature infants may then be discharged when their weight approaches 1,800-2,100 g; close follow-up plus easy access to health care providers is essential for early discharge protocols. Alternatively, if the medical or social environment is not ideal, high-risk neonates who have been transported to neonatal intensive care units and whose major illnesses have resolved may be returned to their hospital of birth for an additional period of hospitalization. Standard vaccinations with full doses should commence after discharge or, if infants are still in the hospital, with vaccines that do not contain live viruses. For RSV prophylaxis, see Chapter 252.

HOME CARE

While the infant is in the hospital, the mother should receive instruction on how to care for the baby after discharge and should be allowed to provide infant care in the hospital. Ideally, a home care program should include at least one home visit by someone capable of evaluating domestic arrangements and advising about any needed improvements. Early developmental intervention programs focused on parent-infant relationship and/or infant development after discharge improve cognitive development in the short to medium term (up to preschool) but do not improve motor outcomes. However these benefits are not sustained at school age.

BIBLIOGRAPHY

Please visit the Nelson Textbook of Pediatrics *website at www.expertconsult.com for the complete bibliography.*

91.3 Post-Term Infants

Waldemar A. Carlo

Post-term infants are those born after 42 completed weeks of gestation, as calculated from the mother's last menstrual period, regardless of weight at birth. Historically, about 12% of pregnancies ended after the 294th day. Obstetric interventions often occur earlier, and the rate of post-term births is decreasing. The cause of post-term birth or postmaturity is unknown.

For the full continuation of this chapter, please visit the Nelson Textbook of Pediatrics *website at www.expertconsult.com.*

91.4 Large-for-Gestational-Age Infants

Waldemar A. Carlo

See also Chapter 101.1.

For the full continuation of this chapter, please visit the Nelson Textbook of Pediatrics *website at www.expertconsult.com.*

91.5 Infant Transport

Waldemar A. Carlo

With the advent of regionalized care of high-risk neonates, increasing numbers of high-risk mothers and sick infants are transported to hospitals with neonatal intensive care units. Neonatal transport should include consultation about the infant's problem and care before transport, ease of access to the transport team, and transport and stabilization by the team before moving the infant. Securing an airway, providing oxygen, assisting with infant ventilation, providing antimicrobial therapy, maintaining the circulation, providing a warmed environment, and placing intravenous or arterial lines or chest tubes should be initiated, if indicated, before transport. Infant and maternal records and laboratory reports should also be provided. Before departure of an infant, the mother should be briefly reassured and allowed to see her stabilized infant; the father should enter his car and follow the transport vehicle to the unit. The transport officer or nurse should also call ahead to inform the receiving unit about the nature of the patient's illness.

For the full continuation of this chapter, please visit the Nelson Textbook of Pediatrics *website at www.expertconsult.com.*

Chapter 92
Clinical Manifestations of Diseases in the Newborn Period

Waldemar A. Carlo

The wide varieties of disorders that affect the newborn originate in utero, during birth, or in the immediate postnatal period. These disorders may be due to prematurity, genetic mutations, chromosomal aberrations, or acquired diseases and injuries. Recognizing disease in newborn infants depends on knowledge of the disorder and evaluation of a limited number of relatively nonspecific clinical signs and symptoms.

For the full continuation of this chapter, please visit the Nelson Textbook of Pediatrics *website at www.expertconsult.com.*

Chapter 93
Nervous System Disorders
Waldemar A. Carlo

Central nervous system (CNS) disorders are important causes of neonatal mortality and both short- and long-term morbidity. The CNS can be damaged as a result of hypoxia, asphyxia, hemorrhage, trauma, hypoglycemia, or direct cytotoxicity. The etiology of CNS damage is often multifactorial and includes acute perinatal complications, postnatal hemodynamic instability, and developmental abnormalities that may be genetic and/or environmental. Predisposing factors for brain injury include chronic and acute maternal illness resulting in uteroplacental dysfunction, intrauterine infection, macrosomia/dystocia, malpresentation, prematurity, and intrauterine growth restriction. Acute and often unavoidable emergencies during the delivery process frequently result in mechanical and/or hypoxic-ischemic brain injury.

93.1 The Cranium
Waldemar A. Carlo

Erythema, abrasions, ecchymoses, and subcutaneous fat necrosis of facial or scalp soft tissues may be noted after a normal delivery or after forceps or vacuum-assisted deliveries. Their location depends on the area of contact with the pelvic bones or of application of the forceps. Traumatic hemorrhage may involve any layer of the scalp as well as intracranial contents (Fig. 93-1).

Caput succedaneum is a diffuse, sometimes ecchymotic, edematous swelling of the soft tissues of the scalp involving the area presenting during vertex delivery (see Fig. 93-1). It may extend across the midline and across suture lines. The edema disappears within the 1st few days of life. Molding of the head and overriding of the parietal bones are frequently associated with caput succedaneum and become more evident after the caput has receded; they disappear during the 1st weeks of life. Rarely, a hemorrhagic caput may result in shock and require blood transfusion. Analogous swelling, discoloration, and distortion of the face are seen in face presentations. No specific treatment is needed, but if extensive ecchymoses are present, hyperbilirubinemia may develop.

Cephalohematoma (Fig. 93-2) is a subperiosteal hemorrhage, hence always limited to the surface of one cranial bone. Cephalohematomas occur in 1-2% of live births. No discoloration of the overlying scalp occurs, and swelling is not usually visible for several hours after birth because subperiosteal bleeding is a slow process. The lesion becomes a firm tense mass with a palpable rim localized over one area of the skull. Most cephalohematomas are resorbed within 2 wk-3 mo, depending on their size. They may begin to calcify by the end of the 2nd week. A few remain for years as bony protuberances and are detectable on radiographs as widening of the diploic space; cystlike defects may persist for months or years. An underlying skull fracture, usually linear and not depressed, may be associated with 10-25% of cases. A sensation of central depression suggesting but not indicative of an underlying fracture or bony defect is usually encountered on palpation of the organized rim of a cephalohematoma. Cephalohematomas require no treatment, although phototherapy may be necessary to treat hyperbilirubinemia. Infection of the hematoma is a very rare complication.

A **subgaleal hemorrhage** is a collection of blood beneath the aponeurosis that covers the scalp the entire length of the occipitofrontalis muscle. Bleeding can be very extensive into this large potential space and may even dissect into the subcutaneous tissues of the neck. There is often an association with vacuum-assisted delivery. The mechanism of injury is most likely secondary to a linear skull fracture, suture diastasis or fragmentation of the superior margin of the parietal bone, and/or rupture of the emissary vein. Extensive subgaleal bleeding is occasionally secondary to a hereditary coagulopathy (hemophilia). A subgaleal hemorrhage manifests as a firm fluctuant mass that increases in size after birth. Many patients have a consumptive coagulopathy owing to massive blood loss. Patients should be monitored for hypotension and the development of hyperbilirubinemia. These lesions typically resolve over 2-3 weeks.

Fractures of the skull may occur as a result of pressure from forceps or from the maternal symphysis pubis, sacral promontory, or ischial spines. Linear fractures, the most common, cause no symptoms and require no treatment. Depressed fractures are usually indentations of the calvaria similar to the dents in a ping-pong ball; they are generally a complication of forceps delivery or fetal compression. Affected infants may be asymptomatic unless they have associated intracranial injury; it is advisable to elevate severe depressions to prevent cortical injury from sustained pressure. Fracture of the occipital bone with separation of the basal and squamous portions almost invariably causes fatal

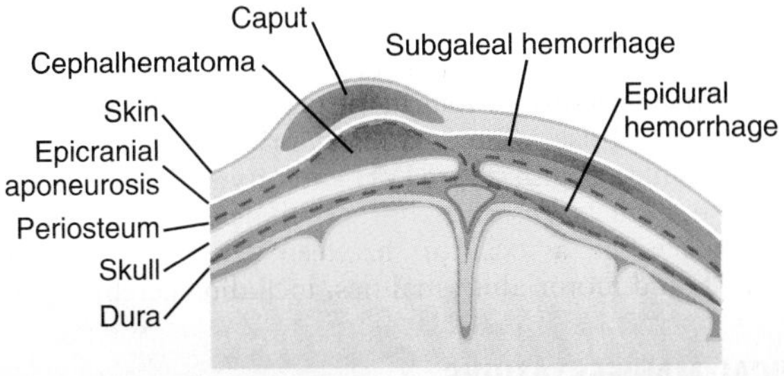

Figure 93-1 Sites of extracranial (and extradural) hemorrhages in the newborn. Schematic diagram of important tissue planes from skin to dura. (From Volpe JJ: *Neurology of the newborn*, ed 4, Philadelphia, 2001, WB Saunders.)

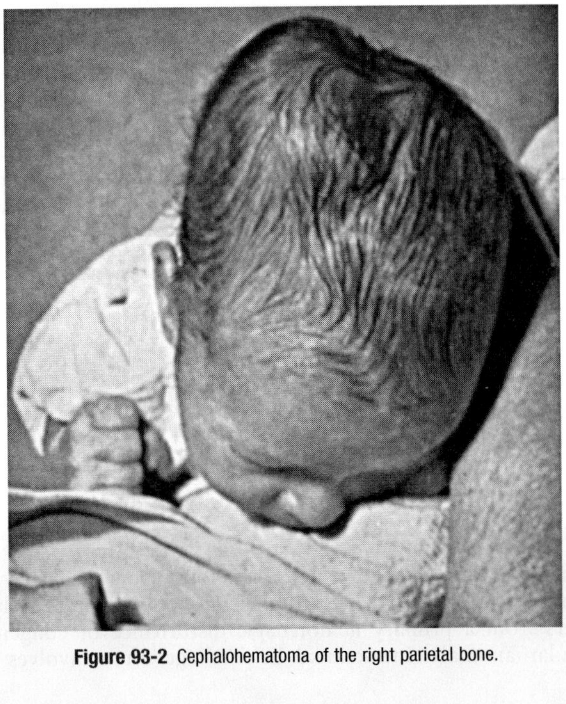

Figure 93-2 Cephalohematoma of the right parietal bone.

hemorrhage because of disruption of the underlying vascular sinuses. Such fractures may result during breech deliveries from traction on the hyperextended spine of the infant while the head is fixed in the maternal pelvis.

Subconjunctival and **retinal hemorrhages** are frequent; petechiae of the skin of the head and neck are also common. All are probably secondary to a sudden increase in intrathoracic pressure during passage of the chest through the birth canal. Parents should be assured that these hemorrhages are temporary and the result of normal events of delivery. The lesions resolve rapidly within the 1st 2 wk of life.

93.2 Traumatic, Epidural, Subdural, and Subarachnoid Hemorrhage

Waldemar A. Carlo

Traumatic **epidural, subdural, or subarachnoid hemorrhage** is especially likely when the fetal head is large in proportion to the size of the mother's pelvic outlet, with prolonged labor, in breech or precipitous deliveries, or as a result of mechanical assistance with delivery. Massive **subdural hemorrhage,** often associated with tears in the tentorium cerebelli or, less frequently, in the falx cerebri, is rare but is encountered more often in full-term than in premature infants. Patients with massive hemorrhage caused by tears of the tentorium or falx cerebri rapidly deteriorate and may die soon after birth. The majority of **subdural and epidural hemorrhages** resolve without intervention; consultation with a neurosurgeon is recommended. The diagnosis of subdural hemorrhage may be delayed until the chronic subdural fluid volume expands and produces megalocephaly, frontal bossing, a bulging fontanel, anemia, and, sometimes, seizures. CT scan and MRI are useful imaging techniques to confirm these diagnoses. Symptomatic subdural hemorrhage in large term infants should be treated by removal of the subdural fluid collection with a needle placed through the lateral margin of the anterior fontanelle. In addition to birth trauma, child **abuse** must be suspected in all infants with subdural effusion after the immediate neonatal period.

Subarachnoid hemorrhage (SAH) is rare and typically is clinically silent. The anastomoses between the penetrating leptomeningeal arteries or the bridging veins are the most likely source of the bleeding. The majority of affected infants have no clinical symptoms, but the SAH may be detected because of an elevated number of red blood cells in a lumbar puncture sample. Some infants experience benign seizures, which tend to occur on the 2nd day of life. Rarely, an infant has a life-threatening catastrophic hemorrhage and dies. There are usually no neurologic abnormalities during the acute episode or on follow-up. Significant neurologic findings should suggest an arteriovenous malformation; this lesion can easily be detected on CT or MRI; ultrasonography is a less sensitive tool.

93.3 Intracranial-Intraventricular Hemorrhage and Periventricular Leukomalacia

Waldemar A. Carlo

ETIOLOGY

Intracranial hemorrhage usually develops spontaneously; less commonly, it may be due to trauma or asphyxia, and rarely, it occurs from a primary hemorrhagic disturbance or congenital vascular anomaly. Intracranial hemorrhage often involves the ventricles (**intraventricular hemorrhage** [IVH]) of premature infants delivered spontaneously without apparent trauma. Primary hemorrhagic disturbances and vascular malformations are rare and usually give rise to subarachnoid or intracerebral hemorrhage. In utero hemorrhage associated with maternal idiopathic or, more often, fetal alloimmune thrombocytopenia may occur as severe cerebral hemorrhage or a porencephalic cyst after resolution of a fetal cortical hemorrhage. Intracranial bleeding may be associated with disseminated intravascular coagulopathy, isoimmune thrombocytopenia, and neonatal vitamin K deficiency, especially in infants born to mothers receiving phenobarbital or phenytoin.

EPIDEMIOLOGY

The overall incidence of IVH has decreased over the past decades as a result of improved perinatal care and increased use of antenatal corticosteroids, surfactant to treat respiratory distress syndrome (RDS), and, possibly, prophylactic indomethacin; however, it continues to be an important cause of morbidity in preterm infants. Approximately 30% of premature infants <1,500 g have IVH. The risk is inversely related to gestational age and birthweight, with the smallest and most immature infants being at the highest risk; 7% of infants 1,001-1,500 g have a severe IVH (grade III or IV), compared with 14% of infants 751-1,000 g and 24% of infants ≤750 g. In 3% of infants <1,000 g, **periventricular leukomalacia (PVL)** develops.

PATHOGENESIS

The major neuropathologic lesions associated with VLBW infants are IVH and PVL. IVH in premature infants occurs in the gelatinous subependymal germinal matrix. This periventricular area is the site of origin for embryonal neurons and fetal glial cells, which migrate outwardly to the cortex. Immature blood vessels in this highly vascular region of the developing brain combined with poor tissue vascular support predispose premature infants to hemorrhage. The germinal matrix involutes as the infant approaches full-term gestation and the tissue's vascular integrity improves; therefore IVH is much less common in the term infant. **Periventricular hemorrhagic infarction** often develops after a grade IV IVH owing to venous congestion. Predisposing factors for IVH include prematurity, respiratory distress syndrome, hypoxic-ischemic or hypotensive injury, reperfusion injury of damaged vessels, increased or decreased cerebral blood flow, reduced vascular integrity, increased venous pressure, pneumothorax, thrombocytopenia, hypervolemia, and hypertension.

Understanding of the pathogenesis of PVL is evolving, and it appears to involve both intrauterine and postnatal events. A complex interaction exists between the development of the cerebral vasculature and the regulation of cerebral blood flow (both of which are gestational age dependent), disturbances in the oligodendrocyte precursors required for myelination, and maternal/fetal infection and/or inflammation. Similar factors (hypoxia-ischemia), venous obstruction from an IVH, or undetected fetal stress may result in decreased perfusion to the brain, leading in turn to periventricular hemorrhage and necrosis. PVL is characterized by focal necrotic lesions in the periventricular white matter and/or more diffuse white matter damage. The risk for PVL increases in infants with severe IVH and/or ventriculomegaly. The corticospinal tracts descend through the periventricular white matter, hence the association between cerebral white matter injury/PVL and motor abnormalities, including cerebral palsy.

CLINICAL MANIFESTATIONS

The majority of patients with IVH, including some with moderate to severe hemorrhages, have no clinical symptoms. Some premature infants in whom severe IVH develops may have acute deterioration on the 2nd or 3rd day of life. Hypotension, apnea, pallor, or cyanosis; poor suck; abnormal eye signs; a high-pitched, shrill cry; convulsions, or decreased muscle tone; metabolic acidosis; shock; and a decreased hematocrit or failure of the hematocrit to increase after transfusion may be the 1st clinical indications. IVH may rarely manifest at birth; 50% of cases are diagnosed within the 1st day of life, and up to 75% within the 1st 3 days. A small percentage of infants have late hemorrhage, between days 14 and 30. IVH as a primary event is rare after the 1st month of life.

PVL is usually clinically asymptomatic until the neurologic sequelae of white matter damage become apparent in later infancy as spastic motor deficits. PVL may be present at birth but usually occurs later as an early echodense phase (3-10 days of life), followed by the typical echolucent (cystic) phase (14-20 days of life).

The severity of hemorrhage may be defined on CT scans by the location and degree of ventricular dilatation. In a **grade I** hemorrhage, bleeding is isolated to the subependymal area. In **Grade II** hemorrhage, there is bleeding within the ventricle but without evidence of ventricular dilatation. **Grade III** hemorrhage consists of IVH with ventricular dilatation. In **Grade IV** hemorrhage, there is intraventricular and parenchymal hemorrhage. Another grading system describes 3 levels of increasing severity of IVH detected on ultrasound: In **grade I,** bleeding is confined to the germinal matrix–subependymal region or to <10% of the ventricle (≈35% of IVH cases); **grade II** is defined as intraventricular bleeding with 10-50% filling of the ventricle (≈40% of IVH cases) and in **grade III,** more than 50% of the ventricle is involved, with dilated ventricles (Fig. 93-3). **Ventriculomegaly** is defined as mild (0.5-1 cm), moderate (1.0-1.5 cm), or severe (>1.5 cm).

DIAGNOSIS

Intracranial hemorrhage is suspected on the basis of the history, clinical manifestations, and knowledge of the birthweight-specific risks for IVH. The associated clinical signs of IVH are typically nonspecific or absent; therefore, it is recommended that premature infants <32 wk of gestation be evaluated with routine real-time cranial ultrasonography through the anterior fontanel to screen for IVH. Infants <1,000 g are at highest risk and should undergo cranial ultrasonography within the 1st 3-7 days of age, when approximately 75% of lesions will be detectable. Ultrasonography is the preferred imaging technique for screening because it is noninvasive, portable, reproducible, and sensitive and specific for detection of IVH. All at-risk infants should undergo follow-up ultrasonography at 36-40 wk of postmenstrual age to evaluate adequately for PVL, because cystic changes related to perinatal injury may not be visible for at least 2-4 wk. In one study, 29% of LBW infants who later experienced cerebral palsy did not have radiographic evidence of PVL until after 28 days of age. Ultrasonography also detects the precystic and cystic symmetric lesions of PVL and the asymmetric intraparenchymal echogenic lesions of cortical hemorrhagic infarction. Furthermore, the delayed development of cortical atrophy, porencephaly, and the severity, progression, or regression of posthemorrhagic hydrocephalus can be determined by serial ultrasonographic examinations.

Approximately 3-5% of VLBW infants have **posthemorrhagic hydrocephalus** and require ventriculoperitoneal shunt insertion; if the initial ultrasonography findings are abnormal, additional interval ultrasonographic studies are indicated to monitor for the development of hydrocephalus.

IVH represents only one facet of brain injury in the term or preterm infant. MRI is a more sensitive tool for evaluation of extensive periventricular injury and may be more predictive of adverse long-term outcome. CT or, more reliably, diffusion-weighted MRI is indicated for term infants in whom brain injury or stroke is suspected, because ultrasonography may not reveal edema or intraparenchymal hemorrhage and infarction.

PROGNOSIS

The degree of IVH and the presence of PVL are strongly linked to neurodevelopmental impairment. For infants with birthweight <1,000 g, the incidences of severe neurologic impairment (defined as mental developmental index <70, psychomotor development index <70, cerebral palsy, blindness, or deafness) are about 50%, 55%, and 70% for infants with grade II, grade III, and grade IV IVH, respectively (Table 93-1). In contrast, the rate of neurodevelopmental impairment is approximately 40% in infants without IVH and those with grade I IVH. PVL, cystic PVL, and progressive hydrocephalus requiring shunt insertion are each independently associated with a poorer prognosis.

Most infants with IVH and acute ventricular distention do not have **posthemorrhagic hydrocephalus (PHH).** Ten percent to 15% of LBW neonates with IVH demonstrate hydrocephalus, which may initially be present without clinical signs, such as an enlarging head circumference, lethargy, a bulging fontanel or widely split sutures, apnea, and bradycardia. In infants in whom symptomatic hydrocephalus develops, clinical signs may be delayed 2-4 wk despite progressive ventricular distention with compression and thinning of the cerebral cortex. Many infants

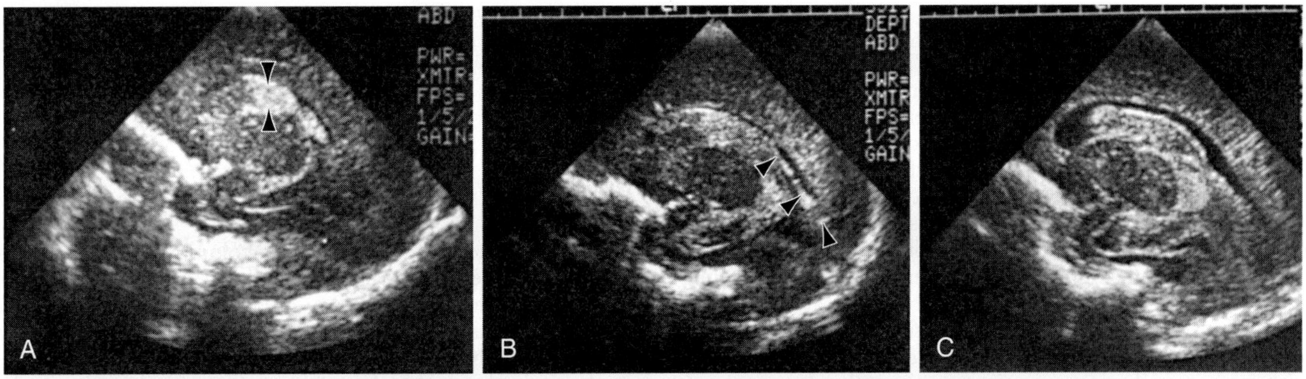

Figure 93-3 Grading the severity of germinal matrix intraventricular hemorrhage with parasagittal ultrasound scans. *A,* Grade I: Note the echogenic blood in the germinal matrix *(arrowheads)* just anterior to the anterior tip of the choroid plexus, which (normally) is also echogenic. *B,* Grade II: Note the echogenic blood *(arrowheads)* filling <50% of the ventricular area. *C,* Grade III: Note the large blood clot nearly completely filling and distending the entire lateral ventricle. (From Intracranial hemorrhage: germinal matrix-intraventricular hemorrhage of the premature infant. In Volpe JJ: *Neurology of the newborn,* ed 4, Philadelphia, 2001, WB Saunders.)

Table 93-1 PERCENTAGE OF INFANTS WITH EACH NEUROLOGIC OUTCOME AT 18 TO 22 MONTHS CORRECTED AGE BY HEAD ULTRASOUND FINDINGS*

HEAD ULTRASOUND VARIABLE	NDI (N = 929)	MDI >70 (N = 174)	PDI <70 (N = 478	CEREBRAL PALSY (N = 478)	BLINDNESS (N = 66)	DEAFNESS (N = 42)	NON-INDEPENDENT WALKING (N = 260)	NON-INDEPENDENT FEEDING (N = 318)
Normal (n=1308)	39.4	31.9	18.8	10.1	1.6	1.5	7.7	12.8
Intracranial hemorrhage:								
Grade 1 (n = 244)	40.6	31.5	18.0	17.2	2.9	1.2	10.7	13.9
Grade 2 (n = 151)	51.0	36.9	22.3	17.2	4.0	3.3	9.3	13.9
Grade 3 (n = 215)	55.4	43.3	36.7	31.3	7.0	2.8	25.1	23.4
Grade 4 (n = 145)	69.7	52.6	55.5	51.4	11.2	4.9	42.4	28.5
Periventricular leukomalacia (n = 134)	72.4	60.3	52.8	50.0	10.5	3.7	44.0	29.1
Cystic periventricular leukomalacia (n = 50)	76.0	60.4	64.6	64.0	18.0	6.3	50.0	32.0

*All infants were counted only once and were assigned the highest grade of intracranial hemorrhage/leukomalacia from either head ultrasound scan. Missing values in either the row or column variable were excluded from the analysis.

MDI, Mental Developmental Index; NDI, neurodevelopment impairment; PDI, Psychomotor Developmental Index.

Data from Broitman E, Ambalavanan N, Higgins RD, et al: Clinical data predict neurodevelopmental outcome better than head ultrasound in extremely low birth weight infants, *J Pediatr* 151:500–505, 2007.

with PHH have spontaneous regression; 3-5% of VLBW infants with PHH require shunt insertion. Infants with PHH requiring shunt insertion have lower cognitive and psychomotor performance at 18-22 mo.

PREVENTION

Improved perinatal care is imperative to minimize traumatic brain injury and decrease the risk of preterm delivery. The incidence of traumatic intracranial hemorrhage may be reduced by judicious management of cephalopelvic disproportion and operative (forceps, vacuum) delivery. Fetal or neonatal hemorrhage caused by maternal idiopathic thrombocytopenic purpura or alloimmune thrombocytopenia may be reduced by maternal treatment with steroids, intravenous immunoglobulin, fetal platelet transfusion, or cesarean section. Tenacious care of the LBW infant's respiratory status and fluid and electrolyte management—including avoidance of acidosis, hypocarbia, hypoxia, hypotension, wide fluctuations in neonatal blood pressure or P_{CO_2}, and pneumothorax—are important factors that may affect the risk for development of IVH and PVL.

A single course of antenatal corticosteroids is recommended in pregnancies 24-34 wk of gestation that are at risk for preterm delivery. Antenatal steroids decrease the risk of death, grade III and IV IVH, and PVL in the neonate. The prophylactic administration of low-dose indomethacin (0.1 mg/kg/day for 3 days) to VLBW preterm infants reduces the incidence of severe IVH.

TREATMENT

Although no treatment is available for IVH, it may be associated with other complications that require therapy. Seizures should be treated with anticonvulsant drugs. Anemia and coagulopathy require transfusion with packed red blood cells or fresh frozen plasma. Shock and acidosis are treated with the judicious and slow administration of sodium bicarbonate and fluid resuscitation.

Insertion of a ventriculoperitoneal shunt is the preferred method to treat progressive and symptomatic posthemorrhagic hydrocephalus; some infants require temporary cerebrospinal fluid diversion before a permanent shunt can be safety inserted. Diuretics and acetazolamide are not effective. Serial lumbar punctures, ventricular taps or reservoirs, and externalized ventricular drains are potential temporizing interventions; they have an associated risk of infection and of "puncture porencephaly" owing to injury to the surrounding parenchyma. A ventriculosubgaleal shunt inserted from the ventricle into a surgically created subgaleal pocket provides a closed system for constant ventricular

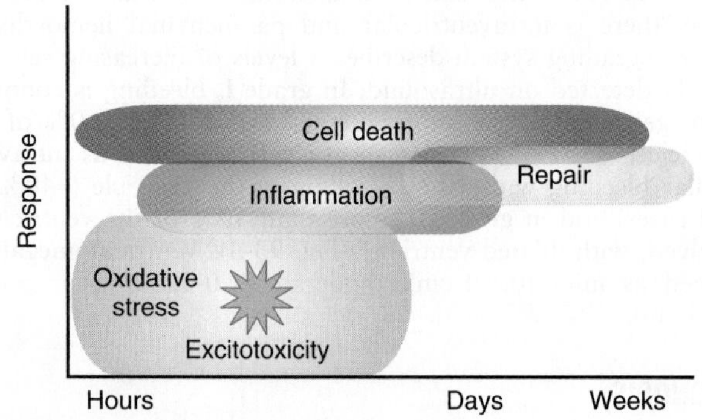

Figure 93-4 Mechanisms of brain injury in the term neonate. Oxidative stress and excitotoxicity, through downstream intracellular signaling, produce both inflammation and repair. Cell death begins immediately and continues during a period of days to weeks. The cell-death phenotype changes from an early necrotic morphology to a pathology resembling apoptosis. This evolution is called the necrosis-apoptosis continuum. (From Ferriero DM: Neonatal brain injury, *N Engl J Med* 351:1985–1995, 2004.Copyright © 2004 Massachusetts Medical Society. All rights reserved.)

decompression without these additional risk factors. Decompression is regulated by the pressure gradient between the ventricle and the subgaleal pocket.

BIBLIOGRAPHY

Please visit the Nelson Textbook of Pediatrics *website at* *www.expertconsult.com* *for the complete bibliography.*

93.4 Brain Injury from Inflammation, Infection, and Medications

Waldemar A. Carlo

Severe IVH and PVL are the most commonly associated risk factors for adverse outcome in the VLBW infant. Other factors are also involved in the etiology of perinatal brain injury. Cytokines and prenatal or postnatal infection or inflammation may contribute to brain injury. A systemic inflammatory response syndrome in the mother, fetus, or infant may induce the production of various inflammatory mediators that are directly cytotoxic or cause decreased CNS perfusion (Fig. 93-4). Preterm infants with evidence (often subclinical) of intrauterine or postnatal infection or maternal chorioamnionitis are more likely than uninfected infants to have adverse neurodevelopmental outcome including cerebral palsy.

In utero infections may involve the developing CNS and directly impair cell growth or produce cell neurosis, resulting in microcephaly, developmental delay, mental retardation, or cerebral palsy. These specific congenital or perinatal acquired infections include those due to cytomegalovirus (Chapter 247), toxoplasmosis (Chapter 282), herpes simplex (Chapter 244), syphilis (Chapter 210), rubella (Chapter 239), and human immunodeficiency virus (Chapter 268). Postnatal acquired bacterial meningitis in the 1st year, but even more so in the 1st month of life, is another major risk factor for CNS injury and associated adverse neurodevelopmental outcome (Chapter 595).

Long-term adverse neurodevelopmental outcomes are also associated with high-dose postnatal corticosteroid use in VLBW infants. Early postnatal exposure to dexamethasone, within the 1st wk of life, is associated with metabolic derangements, poor growth, increased risk for sepsis, and an increased risk of spontaneous bowel perforation. Infants exposed to postnatal steroids after the 1st wk of life have an increased risk of cerebral palsy and developmental delay. The risk may be increased with prolonged steroid use (>6 wk). At 8 yr of age, dexamethasone-treated children are smaller, have smaller head circumferences, poorer motor skills and coordination, more difficulty with visual motor integration, and lower full-scale verbal IQ and performance IQ scores. The American Academy of Pediatrics (AAP) recommends that postnatal corticosteroid use in VLBW infants be limited to exceptional clinical circumstances and that parents of infants in whom corticosteroids are used be informed of the potential adverse side effects, including increased risk for developmental delay, cerebral palsy, and impaired growth.

Necrotizing enterocolitis (NEC) affects approximately 9-14% of LBW infants and is associated with significant morbidity and mortality (Chapter 96.2). Patients with NEC requiring surgery are more likely to have Mental Developmental Index (MDI) scores <70, Psychomotor Developmental Index (PDI) scores <70, and evidence of overall neurodevelopmental impairment. Infants with severe NEC are reported to have a higher incidence of PVL, postnatal infections, and poor growth.

BIBLIOGRAPHY

Please visit the Nelson Textbook of Pediatrics *website at www.expertconsult.com for the complete bibliography.*

93.5 Hypoxic-Ischemic Encephalopathy

Namasivayam Ambalavanan and Waldemar A. Carlo

Anoxia is a term used to indicate the consequences of complete lack of oxygen as a result of a number of primary causes. **Hypoxemia** refers to decreased arterial concentration of oxygen. **Hypoxia** refers to a decreased oxygenation to cells or organs. **Ischemia** refers to blood flow to cells or organs that is insufficient to maintain their normal function. **Hypoxic-ischemic encephalopathy** (HIE) is an important cause of permanent damage to CNS tissues that may result in neonatal death or manifest later as cerebral palsy or developmental delay. About 20-30% of infants with HIE die in the neonatal period, and ≈ 33-50% of survivors are left with permanent neurodevelopmental abnormalities (cerebral palsy, mental retardation). The greatest risk of adverse outcome is seen in infants with severe fetal acidosis (pH <6.7) (90% death/impairment) and a base deficit >25 mmol/L (72% mortality). Multiorgan failure and insult can occur (Table 93-2).

ETIOLOGY

Most neonatal encephalopathic or seizure disorders, in the absence of major congenital malformations or syndromes, appear to be due to perinatal events. Brain MRI or autopsy findings in full-term neonates with encephalopathy demonstrate that 80% have acute injuries, <1% have prenatal injuries, and 3% have non–hypoxic-ischemic diagnoses. Fetal hypoxia may be caused by various disorders in the mother, including (1) inadequate oxygenation of maternal blood from hypoventilation during anesthesia, cyanotic heart disease, respiratory failure, or carbon monoxide poisoning; (2) low maternal blood pressure from acute blood loss, spinal anesthesia, or compression of the vena cava and aorta by the gravid uterus; (3) inadequate relaxation of the uterus to permit placental filling as a result of uterine tetany caused by the administration of excessive oxytocin; (4) premature separation of the placenta; (5) impedance to the circulation of blood through the umbilical cord as a result of compression or knotting of the cord; and (6) placental insufficiency from toxemia or postmaturity.

Table 93-2 MULTIORGAN SYSTEMIC EFFECTS OF ASPHYXIA

SYSTEM	EFFECT(S)
Central nervous system	Hypoxic-ischemic encephalopathy, infarction, intracranial hemorrhage, seizures, cerebral edema, hypotonia, hypertonia
Cardiovascular	Myocardial ischemia, poor contractility, cardiac stunning, tricuspid insufficiency, hypotension
Pulmonary	Pulmonary hypertension, pulmonary hemorrhage, respiratory distress syndrome
Renal	Acute tubular or cortical necrosis
Adrenal	Adrenal hemorrhage
Gastrointestinal	Perforation, ulceration with hemorrhage, necrosis
Metabolic	Inappropriate secretion of antidiuretic hormone, hyponatremia, hypoglycemia, hypocalcemia, myoglobinuria
Integument	Subcutaneous fat necrosis
Hematology	Disseminated intravascular coagulation

Placental insufficiency often remains undetected on clinical assessment. Intrauterine growth restriction may develop in chronically hypoxic fetuses without the traditional signs of fetal distress. Doppler umbilical waveform velocimetry (demonstrating increased fetal vascular resistance) and cordocentesis (demonstrating fetal hypoxia and lactic acidosis) identify a chronically hypoxic infant (Chapter 90). Uterine contractions may further reduce umbilical oxygenation, depressing the fetal cardiovascular system and CNS and resulting in low Apgar scores and respiratory depression at birth.

After birth, hypoxia may be caused by (1) failure of oxygenation as a result of severe forms of cyanotic congenital heart disease or severe pulmonary disease; (2) severe anemia (severe hemorrhage, hemolytic disease); (3) or shock severe enough to interfere with the transport of oxygen to vital organs from overwhelming sepsis, massive blood loss, and intracranial or adrenal hemorrhage.

PATHOPHYSIOLOGY AND PATHOLOGY

The topography of injury typically correlates with areas of decreased cerebral blood flow. After an episode of hypoxia and ischemia, anaerobic metabolism occurs and generates increased amounts of lactate and inorganic phosphates. Excitatory and toxic amino acids, particularly glutamate, accumulate in the damaged tissue. Increased amounts of intracellular sodium and calcium may result in tissue swelling and cerebral edema. There is also increased production of free radicals and nitric oxide in these tissues. The initial circulatory response of the fetus is increased shunting through the ductus venosus, ductus arteriosus, and foramen ovale, with transient maintenance of perfusion of the brain, heart, and adrenals in preference to the lungs, liver, kidneys, and intestine.

The pathology of hypoxia-ischemia depends on the affected organ and the severity of the injury. Early congestion, fluid leak

Table 93-3 TOPOGRAPHY OF BRAIN INJURY IN TERM INFANTS WITH HYPOXIC-ISCHEMIC ENCEPHALOPATHY AND CLINICAL CORRELATES

AREA OF INJURY	LOCATION OF INJURY	CLINICAL CORRELATE(S)	LONG-TERM SEQUELA(E)
Selective neuronal necrosis	Entire neuroaxis, deep cortical area, brainstem and pentocubicular	Stupor or coma Seizures Hypotonia Oculomotor abnormalities Suck/swallow abnormalities	Cognitive delay Cerebral palsy Dystonia Seizure disorder Ataxia Bulbar and pseudobulbar palsy
Parasagittal injury	Cortex and subcortical white matter Parasagittal regions, especially posterior	Proximal limb weakness Upper extremities affected more than lower extremities	Spastic quadriparesis Cognitive delay Visual and auditory processing difficulty
Focal ischemic necrosis	Cortex and subcortical white matter Vascular injury (usually middle cerebral artery distribution)	Unilateral findings Seizures common and typically focal	Hemiparesis Seizures Cognitive delays
Periventricular injury	Injury to motor tracts, especially lower extremity	Bilateral and symmetric weakness in lower extremities More common in preterm infants	Spastic diplegia

Modified from Volpe JJ: *Neurology of the newborn*, ed 4, Philadelphia, 2001, WB Saunders.

from increased capillary permeability, and endothelial cell swelling may then lead to signs of coagulation necrosis and cell death. Congestion and petechiae are seen in the pericardium, pleura, thymus, heart, adrenals, and meninges. Prolonged intrauterine hypoxia may result in inadequate perfusion of the periventricular white matter, resulting, in turn, in PVL. Pulmonary arteriole smooth muscle hyperplasia may develop, which predisposes the infant to pulmonary hypertension (Chapter 95.7). If fetal distress produces gasping, the amniotic fluid contents (meconium, squames, lanugo) are aspirated into the trachea or lungs.

The combination of chronic fetal hypoxia and acute hypoxic-ischemic injury around the time of birth results in gestational age–specific neuropathology (Table 93-3). Term infants demonstrate neuronal necrosis of the cortex (later, cortical atrophy) and parasagittal ischemic injury. Preterm infants demonstrate PVL (later, spastic diplegia), status marmoratus of the basal ganglia, and IVH. Term more often than preterm infants have focal or multifocal cortical infarcts that manifest clinically as focal seizures and hemiplegia.

CLINICAL MANIFESTATIONS

Intrauterine growth restriction with increased vascular resistance may be the 1st indication of fetal hypoxia. During labor, the fetal heart rate slows and beat-to-beat variability declines. Continuous heart rate recording may reveal a variable or late deceleration pattern (see Fig. 90-4). Particularly in infants near term, these signs should lead to the administration of high concentrations of oxygen to the mother and consideration of immediate delivery to avoid fetal death and CNS damage.

At delivery, the presence of meconium-stained amniotic fluid is evidence that fetal distress has occurred. At birth, affected infants may be depressed and may fail to breathe spontaneously. During the ensuing hours, they may remain hypotonic or change from a hypotonic to a hypertonic state, or their tone may appear normal (Tables 93-4 and 93-5). Pallor, cyanosis, apnea, a slow heart rate, and unresponsiveness to stimulation are also signs of HIE. Cerebral edema may develop during the next 24 hr and result in profound brainstem depression. During this time, seizure activity may occur; it may be severe and refractory to the usual doses of anticonvulsants. Though most often a result of the HIE, seizures in asphyxiated newborns may also be due to hypocalcemia, hypoglycemia, or infection.

In addition to CNS dysfunction, heart failure and cardiogenic shock, persistent pulmonary hypertension, respiratory distress syndrome, gastrointestinal perforation, hematuria, and acute tubular necrosis are associated with perinatal asphyxia secondary to inadequate perfusion (see Table 93-2).

Table 93-4 PREDICTOR VARIABLES, ODDS RATIOS, AND SCORES ASSIGNED TO EACH VARIABLE FOR DEATH/DISABILITY SCORING IN INFANTS WITH HYPOXIC-ISCHEMIC ENCEPHALOPATHY

VARIABLE	LEVEL OF VARIABLE	ODDS RATIO	SCORE*
Posture	Normal	0.037	1
	Distal flexion	0.401	11
	Decerebrate	1	27
Spontaneous activity	Normal/decreased	0.147	1
	None	1	7
Base deficit of 1st postnatal blood gas analysis	<15 mmol/L	0.073	1
	15-22 mmol/L	0.304	4
	>22 mmol/L	1	14
Apgar score at 5 min	7-10	0.082	14
	4-6	0.676	8
	0-3	1	12
Chronic hypertension/ preeclampsia/eclampsia	Yes	0.2	1
	No	1	5

*The total score is obtained by adding the scores for each of the variables. Interpretation of the total score is as follows: <23: no death or moderate/severe disability even without hypothermia; 23-28: probable benefit from hypothermia; 29-52: possible benefit; >52: death/disability likely despite hypothermia. =172.

From Ambalavanan, N, Carlo WA, Shankaran S, et al; National Institute of Child Health and Human Development Neonatal Research Network: Predicting outcomes of neonates diagnosed with hypoxemic-ischemic encephalopathy, *Pediatrics* 118:2084–2093, 2006.

The severity of neonatal encephalopathy depends on the duration and timing of injury. Symptoms develop over a series of days, making it important to perform serial neurologic examinations (see Tables 93-4 and 93-5). During the initial hours after an insult, infants have a depressed level of consciousness. Periodic breathing with apnea or bradycardia is present, but cranial nerve functions are often spared with intact pupillary responses and spontaneous eye movement. Seizures are common with extensive injury. Hypotonia is also common as an early manifestation.

DIAGNOSIS

Diffusion-weighted MRI is the preferred imaging modality in neonates with HIE because of its increased sensitivity and specificity early in the process and its ability to outline the topography of the lesion (Figs. 93-5 to 93-8). CT scans are helpful in identifying focal hemorrhagic lesions, diffuse cortical injury, and damage to the basal ganglia; CT has limited ability to identify cortical injury during the 1st few days of life. Ultrasonography has limited utility in evaluation of hypoxic injury in the term infant; it is the preferred modality in evaluation of the preterm infant.

Table 93-5 HYPOXIC-ISCHEMIC ENCEPHALOPATHY IN TERM INFANTS

SIGNS	STAGE 1	STAGE 2	STAGE 3
Level of consciousness	Hyperalert	Lethargic	Stuporous, coma
Muscle tone	Normal	Hypotonic	Flaccid
Posture	Normal	Flexion	Decerebrate
Tendon reflexes/clonus	Hyperactive	Hyperactive	Absent
Myoclonus	Present	Present	Absent
Moro reflex	Strong	Weak	Absent
Pupils	Mydriasis	Miosis	Unequal, poor light reflex
Seizures	None	Common	Decerebration
Electroencephalographic findings	Normal	Low voltage changing to seizure activity	Burst suppression to isoelectric
Duration	<24 hr if progresses; otherwise, may remain normal	24 hr-14 days	Days to weeks
Outcome	Good	Variable	Death, severe deficits

Modified from Sarnat HB, Sarnat MS: Neonatal encephalopathy following fetal distress: a clinical and electroencephalographic study, *Arch Neurol* 33:696–705, 1976. Copyright 1976, American Medical Association.

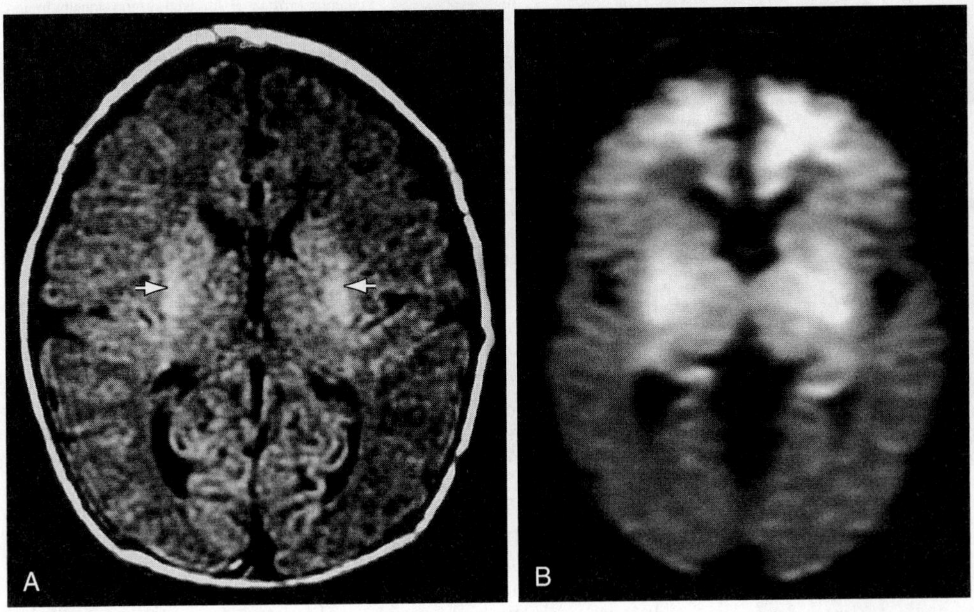

Figure 93-5 MR images of selective neuronal injury. The infant experienced intrapartum asphyxia and had seizures on the 1st postnatal day. MRI was performed on the 5th postnatal day. *A,* An axial, fluid-attenuated inversion recovery image shows increased signal in the putamen bilaterally (*arrows*) but no definite abnormality in the cerebral cortex. *B,* By contrast, a diffusion-weighted image shows striking increased signal intensity (i.e., decreased diffusion) in the frontal cortex (in addition to a more pronounced basal ganglia abnormality). (From Volpe JJ, editor: *Neurology of the newborn*, ed 5, Philadelphia, 2008, Saunders/Elsevier, p 420.)

Amplitude-integrated electroencephalography (aEEG) may help to determine which infants are at highest risk for long-term brain injury. A single-channel tracing is generated from 2 electrodes placed in the biparietal area. A filter is used to filter and attenuate the signal between 2 Hz and 15 Hz. This technique is simple to perform and correlates with standard EEG. It has good reliability, a positive predictive value of 85%, and a negative predictive value of 91-96% for infants who will have adverse neurodevelopmental outcome. The technique provides information quickly within the window during which intervention is most likely to be useful. Also, aEEG is able to detect seizure activity, which is common in patients with HIE. Continuous aEEG monitoring detects subclinical seizure activity during the subacute phase.

TREATMENT

Selective cerebral or whole body (systemic) therapeutic hypothermia reduces mortality or major neurodevelopmental impairment in term and near-term infants with HIE. Hypothermia decreases the rate of apoptosis and suppresses production of mediators known to be neurotoxic, including extracellular glutamate, free radicals, nitric oxide, and lactate. The neuroprotective effects are thought to be secondary to downregulation of the secondary mediators of injury resulting from cerebral edema, accumulation of cytokines, and seizures. Animal data suggest that the intervention is most effective when implemented within 6 hr of the event.

Several clinical trials and a meta-analysis demonstrate that either isolated cerebral cooling or systemic hypothermia to a core temperature of 33.5°C within the 1st 6 hr after birth reduces mortality and major neurodevelopmental impairment at 18 mo of age. Systemic hypothermia may result in more uniform cooling of the brain and deeper CNS structures. Infants treated with systemic hypothermia have a lower incidence of cortical neuronal injury on MRI.

Phenobarbital, the drug of choice for seizures, is given with an intravenous loading dose (20 mg/kg); additional doses of 5-10 mg/kg (up to 40-50 mg/kg total) may be needed. Phenytoin (20 mg/kg loading dose) or lorazepam (0.1 mg/kg) may be needed for refractory seizures. Phenobarbital levels should be monitored 24 hr after the loading dose has been given and maintenance therapy (5 mg/kg/24hr) is begun. Therapeutic phenobarbital levels are 20-40 µg/mL. There is some clinical evidence that high-dose prophylactic phenobarbital may decrease neurodevelopmental impairment in infants with HIE.

Additional therapy for infants with HIE includes supportive care directed at management of organ system dysfunction. Hyperthermia has been found to be associated with impaired

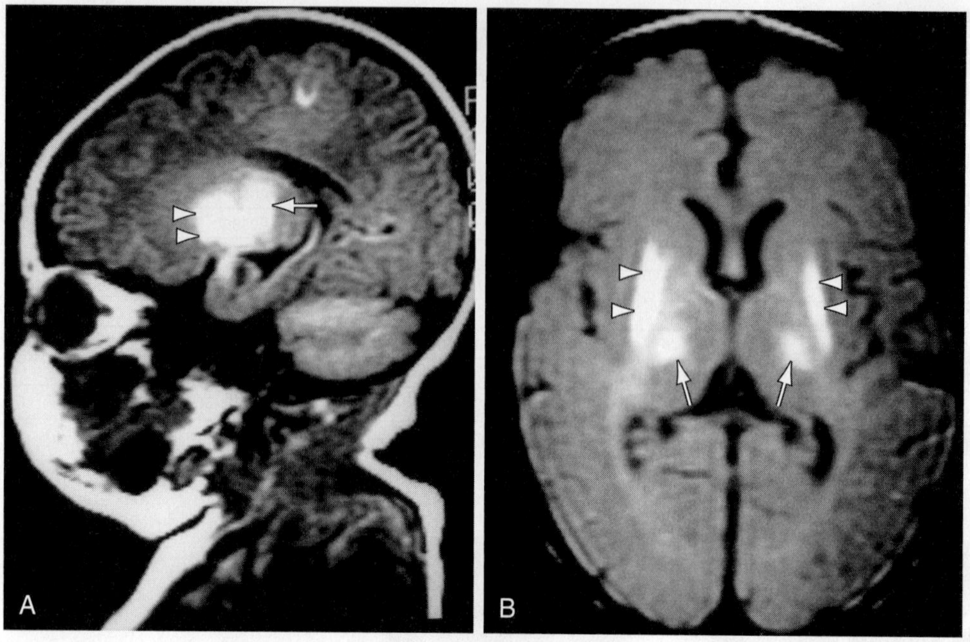

Figure 93-6 MR images of hypoxic-ischemic injury to basal ganglia and thalamus. MRI was performed in a 5-day-old infant who experienced severe perinatal asphyxia. *A,* Note, in this parasagittal T1-weighted image, the markedly increased signal intensity in the basal ganglia, especially the putamen (*arrowheads*) and the thalamus (*arrow*). *B,* An axial proton density image also demonstrates the injury well in the same distribution. (From Volpe JJ, editor: *Neurology of the newborn,* ed 5, Philadelphia, 2008, Saunders/Elsevier, p 420.)

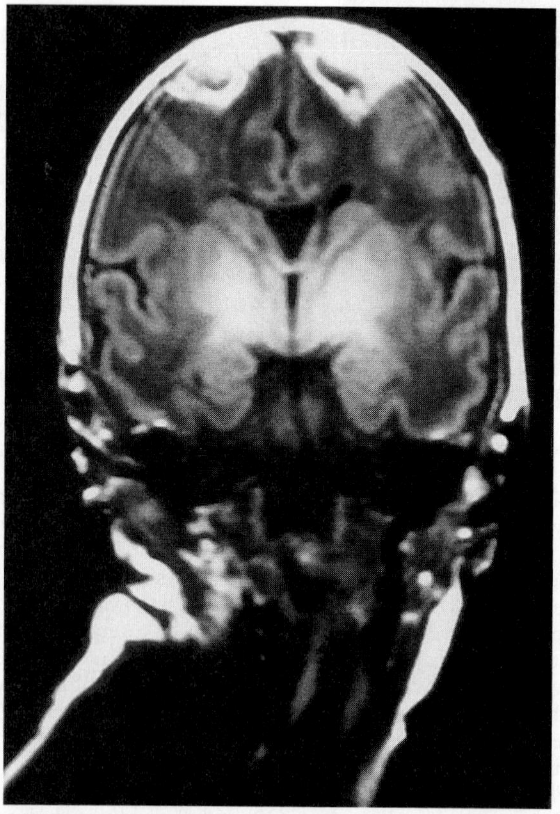

Figure 93-7 MR image of a parasagittal cerebral injury. A coronal T1-weighted image, obtained on the 5th postnatal day in an asphyxiated term infant, shows striking triangular lesions in the parasagittal areas bilaterally; increased signal intensity is also apparent in the basal ganglia and thalamus bilaterally. (From Volpe JJ, editor: *Neurology of the newborn,* ed 5, Philadelphia, 2008, Saunders/Elsevier, p 421.)

neurodevelopment, so it is important to prevent hyperthermia before initiation of hypothermia. Careful attention to ventilatory status and adequate oxygenation, blood pressure, hemodynamic status, acid-base balance, and possible infection is important. Secondary hypoxia or hypotension due to complications of HIE must be prevented. Aggressive treatment of seizures is critical and may necessitate continuous EEG monitoring.

PROGNOSIS

The outcome of HIE, which correlates with the timing and severity of the insult, ranges from complete recovery to death. The prognosis varies depending on the severity of the insult and the treatment. Infants with initial cord or initial blood pH <6.7 have a 90% risk for death or severe neurodevelopmental impairment at 18 mo of age. In addition, infants with Apgar scores of 0-3 at 5 min, high base deficit (>20-25 mmol/L), decerebrate posture, and lack of spontaneous activity are also at increased risk for death or impairment. These predictor variables can be combined to determine a score that helps with prognosis (see Table 93-4). Infants with the highest risk are likely to die or have severe disability despite aggressive treatment including hypothermia. Those with intermediate scores are likely to benefit from treatment. In general, severe encephalopathy, characterized by flaccid coma, apnea, absence of oculocephalic reflexes, and refractory seizures, is associated with a poor prognosis (see Table 93-5). A low Apgar score at 20 min, absence of spontaneous respirations at 20 min of age, and persistence of abnormal neurologic signs at 2 wk of age also predict death or severe cognitive and motor deficits. The combined use of early EEG and MRI is useful in predicting outcome in term infants with HIE. Normal MRI and EEG findings are associated with a good recovery, whereas severe MRI and EEG abnormalities predict a poor outcome. Microcephaly and poor head growth during the 1st year of life also correlate with injury to the basal ganglia and white matter and adverse developmental outcome at 12 mo. All survivors of moderate to severe encephalopathy require comprehensive high-risk medical and developmental follow-up. Early identification of neurodevelopmental problems allows prompt referral for developmental, rehabilitative, neurologic care, and early intervention services so that the best possible outcome can be achieved.

Brain death after neonatal HIE is diagnosed from the clinical findings of coma unresponsive to pain, auditory, or visual stimulation; apnea with P_{CO_2} rising from 40 to >60 mm Hg without ventilatory support; and absence of brainstem reflexes (pupillary, oculocephalic, oculovestibular, corneal, gag, sucking) (Chapter 63.1). These findings must occur in the absence of hypothermia,

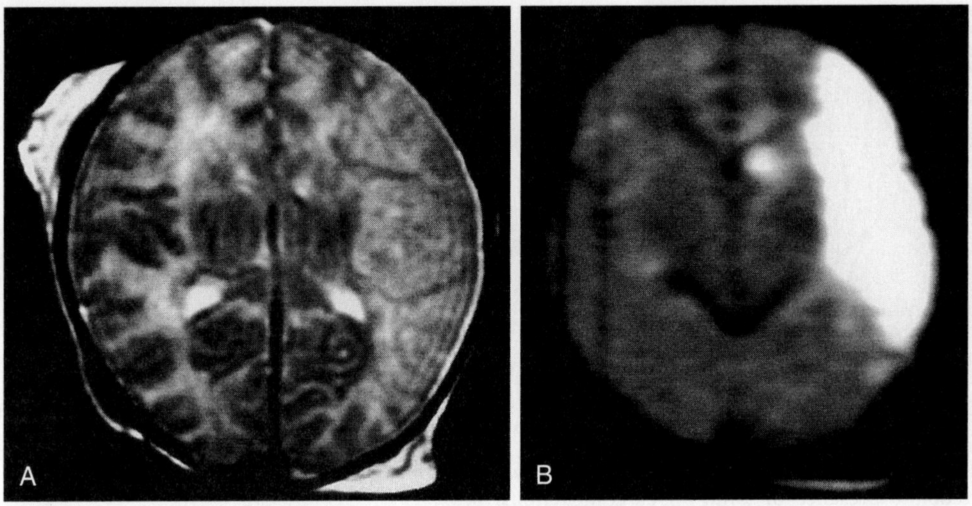

Figure 93-8 MR images of focal ischemic cerebral injury. MRI was performed on the 3rd postnatal day. *A,* An axial T2-weighted image shows a lesion in the distribution of the main branch of the left middle cerebral artery. *B,* A diffusion-weighted image demonstrates the lesion more strikingly. (From Volpe JJ, editor: *Neurology of the newborn*, ed 5, Philadelphia, 2008, Saunders/Elsevier, p 422.)

hypotension, and elevations of depressant drugs (phenobarbital). An absence of cerebral blood flow on radionuclide scans and of electrical activity on EEG (electrocerebral silence) is inconsistently observed in clinically brain-dead neonatal infants. Persistence of the clinical criteria for 2 days in term infants and 3 days in preterm infants predicts brain death in most asphyxiated newborns. Nonetheless, no universal agreement has been reached regarding the definition of neonatal brain death. Consideration of withdrawal of life support should include discussions with the family, the health care team, and, if there is disagreement, an ethics committee. The best interest of the infant involves judgments about the benefits and harm of continuing therapy or avoiding ongoing futile therapy.

BIBLIOGRAPHY
Please visit the Nelson Textbook of Pediatrics *website at www.expertconsult.com for the complete bibliography.*

93.6 Spine and Spinal Cord

Waldemar A. Carlo

Injury to the spine/spinal cord during birth is rare but can be devastating. Strong traction exerted when the spine is hyperextended or when the direction of pull is lateral, or forceful longitudinal traction on the trunk while the head is still firmly engaged in the pelvis, especially when combined with flexion and torsion of the vertical axis, may produce fracture and separation of the vertebrae. Such injuries are most likely to occur when difficulty is encountered in delivering the shoulders in cephalic presentations and the head in breech presentations. The injury occurs most commonly at the level of the 4th cervical vertebra with cephalic presentations and the lower cervical–upper thoracic vertebrae with breech presentations. Transection of the cord may occur with or without vertebral fractures; hemorrhage and edema may produce neurologic signs that are indistinguishable from those of transection except that they may not be permanent. Areflexia, loss of sensation, and complete paralysis of voluntary motion occur below the level of injury, although the persistence of a withdrawal reflex mediated through spinal centers distal to the area of injury is frequently misinterpreted as representing voluntary motion. If the injury is severe, the infant, who from birth may be in poor condition because of respiratory depression, shock, or hypothermia, may deteriorate rapidly to death within several hours before any neurologic signs are obvious. Alternatively, the course may be protracted, with symptoms and signs appearing at birth or later in the 1st wk; immobility, flaccidity, and associated brachial plexus injuries may not be recognized for several days. Constipation may also be present. Some infants survive for prolonged periods, their initial flaccidity, immobility, and areflexia being replaced after several weeks or months by rigid flexion of the extremities, increased muscle tone, and spasms. Apnea on day 1 and poor motor recovery by 3 mo are poor prognostic signs.

The **differential diagnosis** of spine/spinal cord injury includes amyotonia congenita and myelodysplasia associated with spina bifida occulta. Ultrasonography or, more often, MRI confirms the diagnosis. Treatment of the survivors is supportive, including home ventilation; patients often remain permanently disabled. When a fracture or dislocation is causing spinal compression, the prognosis is related to the time elapsed before the compression is relieved.

BIBLIOGRAPHY
Please visit the Nelson Textbook of Pediatrics *website at www.expertconsult.com for the complete bibliography.*

93.7 Peripheral Nerve Injuries

Waldemar A. Carlo

BRACHIAL PALSY

Brachial plexus injury is a common problem, with an incidence of 0.6-4.6/1,000 live births. Injury to the brachial plexus may cause paralysis of the upper part of the arm with or without paralysis of the forearm or hand or, more commonly, paralysis of the entire arm. These injuries occur in macrosomic infants and when lateral traction is exerted on the head and neck during delivery of the shoulder in a vertex presentation, when the arms are extended over the head in a breech presentation, or when excessive traction is placed on the shoulders. Approximately 45% of brachial plexus injuries are associated with shoulder dystocia. In **Erb-Duchenne paralysis**, the injury is limited to the 5th and 6th cervical nerves. The infant loses the power to abduct the arm from the shoulder, rotate the arm externally, and supinate the forearm. The characteristic position consists of adduction and internal rotation of the arm with pronation of the forearm. Power to extend the forearm is retained, but the biceps reflex is absent; the Moro reflex is absent on the affected side (Fig. 93-9). The outer aspect of the arm may have some sensory impairment.

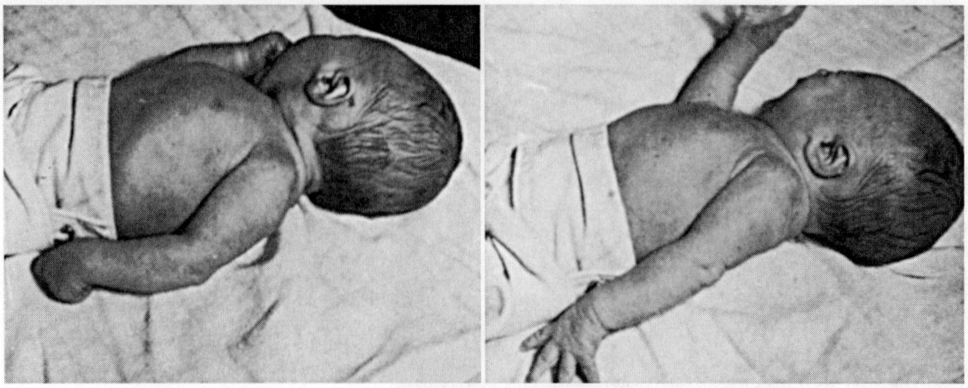

Figure 93-9 Brachial palsy of the left arm (asymmetric Moro reflex).

Power in the forearm and hand grasps is preserved unless the lower part of the plexus is also injured; the presence of hand grasp is a favorable prognostic sign. When the injury includes the phrenic nerve, alteration in diaphragmatic excursion may be observed with ultrasonography or fluoroscopy. **Klumpke paralysis** is a rare form of brachial palsy, in which injury to the 7th and 8th cervical nerves and the 1st thoracic nerve produces a paralyzed hand and ipsilateral ptosis and miosis (**Horner syndrome**) if the sympathetic fibers of the 1st thoracic root are also injured. Mild cases may not be detected immediately after birth. Differentiation must be made from cerebral injury; from fracture, dislocation, or epiphyseal separation of the humerus; and from fracture of the clavicle. MRI demonstrates nerve root rupture or avulsion.

Full recovery occurs in most patients; prognosis depends on whether the nerve was merely injured or was lacerated. If the paralysis was due to edema and hemorrhage about the nerve fibers, function should return within a few months; if it was due to laceration, permanent damage may result. Involvement of the deltoid is usually the most serious problem and may result in shoulder drop secondary to muscle atrophy. In general, paralysis of the upper part of the arm has a better prognosis than paralysis of the lower part.

Treatment consists of initial conservative management with monthly follow-up and a decision for surgical intervention by three months if function has not improved. Partial immobilization and appropriate positioning are used to prevent the development of contractures. In upper arm paralysis, the arm should be abducted 90 degrees with external rotation at the shoulder, full supination of the forearm, and slight extension at the wrist with the palm turned toward the face. This position may be achieved with a brace or splint during the 1st 1-2 wk. Immobilization should be intermittent throughout the day while the infant is asleep and between feedings. In lower arm or hand paralysis, the wrist should be splinted in a neutral position, and padding placed in the fist. When the entire arm is paralyzed, the same treatment principles should be followed. Gentle massage and range-of-motion exercises may be started by 7-10 days of age. Infants should be closely monitored with active and passive corrective exercises. If the paralysis persists without improvement for 3 months, neuroplasty, neurolysis, end-to-end anastomosis, and nerve grafting offer hope for partial recovery.

The type of treatment and the prognosis depend on the mechanism of injury and the number of nerve roots involved. The mildest injury to a peripheral nerve (neurapraxia) is due to edema and heals spontaneously within a few weeks. Axonotmesis is more severe and is due to nerve fiber disruption with an intact myelin sheath; function usually returns in a few months. Total disruption of nerves (neurotmesis) or root avulsion is the most severe, especially if it involves C5-T1; microsurgical repair may be indicated. Fortunately, most (75%) injuries are at the root level C5-C6, involve neurapraxia and axonotmesis, and should heal spontaneously. Botulism toxin may be used to treat biceps-triceps co-contractions.

PHRENIC NERVE PARALYSIS

Phrenic nerve injury (3rd, 4th, 5th cervical nerves) with diaphragmatic paralysis must be considered when cyanosis and irregular and labored respirations develop. Such injuries, usually unilateral, are associated with ipsilateral upper brachial palsy. Because breathing is thoracic in type, the abdomen does not bulge with inspiration. Breath sounds are diminished on the affected side. The thrust of the diaphragm, which may often be felt just under the costal margin on the normal side, is absent on the affected side. The diagnosis is established by ultrasonographic or fluoroscopic examination, which reveals elevation of the diaphragm on the paralyzed side and seesaw movements of the 2 sides of the diaphragm during respiration.

No specific treatment is available; infants should be placed on the involved side and given oxygen if necessary. Initially, intravenous feedings may be needed; later, progressive gavage or oral feeding may be started, depending on the infant's condition. Pulmonary infections are a serious complication. Recovery usually occurs spontaneously by 1-3 mo; rarely, surgical plication of the diaphragm may be indicated.

FACIAL NERVE PALSY

Facial palsy is usually a peripheral paralysis that results from pressure over the facial nerve in utero, from efforts during labor, or from forceps use during delivery. Rarely, it may result from nuclear agenesis of the facial nerve. Peripheral paralysis is flaccid and, when complete, involves the entire side of the face, including the forehead. When the infant cries, movement occurs only on the nonparalyzed side of the face, and the mouth is drawn to that side. On the affected side the forehead is smooth, the eye cannot be closed, the nasolabial fold is absent, and the corner of the mouth droops. The forehead wrinkles on the affected side with central paralysis because only the lower ⅔ of the face is involved. The infant also usually has other manifestations of intracranial injury, most commonly 6th nerve palsy. The prognosis depends on whether the nerve was injured by pressure or the nerve fibers were torn. Improvement occurs within a few weeks in the former instance. Care of the exposed eye is essential. Neuroplasty may be indicated when the paralysis is persistent. Facial palsy may be confused with absence of the depressor muscles of the mouth, which is a benign problem.

Other peripheral nerves are seldom injured in utero or at birth except when they are involved in fractures or hemorrhage.

BIBLIOGRAPHY

Please visit the Nelson Textbook of Pediatrics *website at* www.expertconsult.com *for the complete bibliography.*

Chapter 94
Delivery Room Emergencies
Waldemar A. Carlo

Most infants complete the transition to extrauterine life without difficulty; however, a small percentage requires resuscitation after birth. The most common delivery room emergency for neonates is secondary to failure to initiate and maintain effective respirations. Less frequent, but of major importance, are shock (Chapter 92), severe anemia (Chapter 97.1), plethora (Chapter 97.3), convulsions (Chapter 586.7), and management of life-threatening congenital malformations (Chapter 92). Improved perinatal care and prenatal diagnosis of fetal anomalies allow for appropriate maternal transports for high-risk deliveries.

RESPIRATORY DISTRESS AND FAILURE

Disorders of respiration in newborn infants can be categorized as either central nervous system (CNS) failure, representing depression or failure of the respiratory center, or peripheral respiratory difficulty, indicating interference with the alveolar exchange of oxygen and carbon dioxide. Cyanosis occurs in both groups (see Table 92-1). Respiratory problems encountered in the delivery room are most frequently those of airway obstruction and depression of the CNS (maternal medications, asphyxia) with an absence of adequate respiratory effort. Respiratory distress in the presence of good respiratory effort should lead to an immediate consideration of the underlying cause and is an indication for radiographic examination of the chest.

If respiratory movements are made with the mouth closed but the infant fails to move air in and out of the lungs, bilateral **choanal atresia** (Chapter 368) or other obstruction of the upper respiratory tract should be suspected. The mouth should be opened, and the mouth and posterior of the pharynx cleared of secretions with gentle suction. An oropharyngeal airway should be inserted, and the source of the obstruction sought immediately. If effective respiratory flow is not produced by opening the infant's mouth and clearing the airway, laryngoscopy is indicated. With obstructive malformations of the mandible, epiglottis, larynx, or trachea, an endotracheal tube should be inserted; prolonged endotracheal intubation or tracheostomy may be required. Respiratory failure caused by CNS depression or injury may require continuous mechanical ventilation.

Hypoplasia of the mandible (Pierre Robin, DiGeorge, and other syndromes; Chapters 300 and 303) with posterior displacement of the tongue may result in symptoms similar to those of choanal atresia and may be temporarily relieved by pulling the tongue or mandible forward or placing the infant in the prone position. A scaphoid abdomen suggests a **diaphragmatic hernia** or **eventration,** as does asymmetry in contour or movement of the chest or a shift of the apical impulse of the heart; these latter manifestations are also compatible with **tension pneumothorax.** A pneumothorax can be the presenting symptom in infants with pulmonary hypoplasia, renal malformations, or both.

Pulmonary causes of respiratory difficulty are discussed in Chapter 95.

FAILURE TO INITIATE OR SUSTAIN RESPIRATION

Failure to initiate or sustain respiratory effort is common at birth. Infants with **primary apnea** respond to stimulation by establishing normal breathing. Infants with secondary apnea need ventilatory assistance. **Secondary apnea** usually originates in the CNS as a result of asphyxia or peripherally because of neuromuscular disorders. Prematurity alone is seldom a causative factor, except in infants weighing <1,500 g. Intrapulmonary problems, such as respiratory distress syndrome, pulmonary hypoplasia associated with oligohydramnios as in Potter syndrome or neuromuscular diseases, bilateral pleural effusions (hydrops fetalis), pneumothorax, and severe intrauterine pneumonia, may at times result in poor ventilation despite strong respiratory efforts. The lungs in affected infants may be noncompliant, and efforts to begin respirations may be inadequate to initiate sufficient ventilation.

Narcosis results from administration of morphine, meperidine, fentanyl, barbiturates, or tranquilizers to the mother shortly before delivery or from maternal anesthesia given during the 2nd stage of labor. This sequela should be avoided by the use of appropriate analgesic and anesthetic practices. Treatment includes initial physical stimulation and securing of a patent airway. If effective ventilation is not initiated, artificial breathing with a bag and mask must be instituted. At the same time, if the respiratory depression is due to an opiate, naloxone hydrochloride (Narcan), 0.1mg/kg, should be given intravenously or intramuscularly. Naloxone is contraindicated in infants born to mothers with opiate addiction because it precipitates acute neonatal withdrawal with severe seizures. If depression is due to other anesthetics or analgesics, artificial respiration should be continued until the infant is able to sustain ventilation. CNS-stimulant drugs should not be used because they are ineffective and may be harmful. External cardiac massage, correction of acidosis, and circulatory support with drugs may be important adjuncts to ventilation in the severely asphyxiated infant.

NEONATAL RESUSCITATION

Although the majority of babies undergo a smooth physiologic transition and breathe effectively after delivery, 5-10% require active intervention to establish normal cardiorespiratory function. The goals of neonatal resuscitation are to prevent the morbidity and mortality associated with hypoxic-ischemic tissue (brain, heart, kidney) injury and to reestablish adequate spontaneous respiration and cardiac output. High-risk situations should be anticipated from the history of the pregnancy, labor, and delivery and identification of signs of fetal distress. Infants who are born limp, cyanotic, apneic, or pulseless require immediate resuscitation before assignment of the 1-min Apgar score. Rapid and appropriate resuscitative efforts improve the likelihood of preventing brain damage and achieving a successful outcome.

Guidelines for neonatal resuscitation propose an "integrated" assessment/response approach for the initial evaluation of an infant, consisting of simultaneous assessment of infant color, general appearance, and risk factors. The fundamental principles include evaluation of the airway, establishing effective respiration and adequate circulation; the guidelines also highlight the assessment and response to the neonatal heart rate and the management of infants with meconium-stained amniotic fluid.

Immediately after birth, an infant in need of resuscitation should be placed under a radiant heater and dried (to avoid hypothermia), positioned with the head down and slightly extended; the airway should be cleared by suctioning, and gentle tactile stimulation provided (slapping the foot, rubbing the back). Simultaneously, the infant's color, heart rate, and respiratory effort should be assessed (Fig. 94-1).

The steps in neonatal resuscitation follow the ABCs: **A,** anticipate and establish a patent airway by suctioning and, if necessary, performing endotracheal intubation; **B,** initiate breathing by using tactile stimulation or positive-pressure ventilation with a bag and mask or through an endotracheal tube; **C,** maintain the circulation with chest compression and medications, if needed. Steps to follow for immediate neonatal evaluation and resuscitation are outlined in Figure 94-1 (Chapter 62).

If no respirations are noted or if the heart rate is <100 beats/min, positive pressure ventilation is given through a tightly fitted face bag and mask for 15-30 sec. In infants with severe

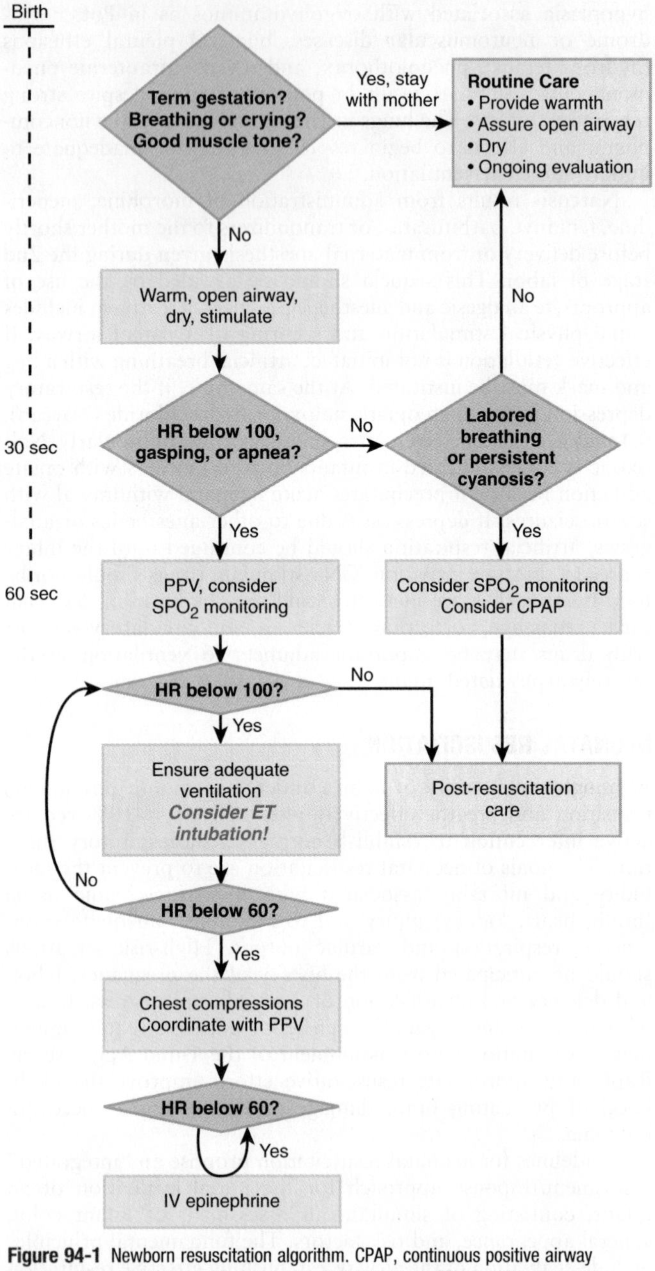

Figure 94-1 Newborn resuscitation algorithm. CPAP, continuous positive airway pressure; ET, endotracheal; HR, heart rate; IV, intravenous; PPV, positive pressure ventilation. (From Perlman JM, Wyllie J, Kattwinkel J, et al: Part 11: Neonatal resuscitation: 2010 International Consensus on Cardiopulmonary Resuscitation and Emergency Cardiovascular Care Science with Treatment Recommendations, *Circulation* 122:S517, 2010.)

respiratory depression that does not respond to positive-pressure ventilation via bag and mask, endotracheal intubation should be performed. Many authorities recommend early intubation for extremely low birthweight (ELBW) preterm infants. Guidelines for endotracheal tube size and depth of insertion in infants with different birthweights are shown in Table 94-1. If the heart rate does not improve after 30 sec with bag and mask (or endotracheal) ventilation and remains below 100 beats/min, ventilation is continued and chest compression should be initiated over the lower third of the sternum at a rate of 120 beats/min. The ratio of compressions to ventilation is 3:1. If the heart rate remains <60 beats/min despite effective compressions and ventilation, administration of epinephrine should be considered. Persistent bradycardia in neonates is usually due to hypoxia resulting from respiratory arrest and often responds rapidly to effective ventilation alone. Persistent bradycardia despite what appears to be adequate resuscitation suggests more severe cardiac compromise or inadequate ventilation technique. Poor response to ventilation may be due to a loosely fitted mask, poor positioning of the endotracheal tube, intraesophageal intubation, airway obstruction, insufficient pressure, pleural effusions, pneumothorax, excessive air in the stomach, asystole, hypovolemia, diaphragmatic hernia, or prolonged intrauterine asphyxia.

Table 94-1 GUIDELINES FOR TRACHEAL TUBE SIZE AND DEPTH OF INSERTION

TUBE SIZE (mm internal diameter)	DEPTH OF INSERTION FROM UPPER LIP (cm)	WEIGHT (g)	GESTATION (wk)
2.5	6.5-7	<1,000	<28
3	7-8	1,000-2,000	28-34
3/3.5	8-9	2,000-3,000	34-38
3.5/4.0	≥9	>3,000	>38

From Kattwinkel J, Niermeyer S, Nadkarni V, et al: ILCOR advisory statement: resuscitation of the newly born infant: an advisory statement from the Pediatric Working Group of the International Liaison Committee on Resuscitation, *Circulation* 99:1927–1938, 1999. By permission of the American Heart Association, Inc.

Traditionally, the inspired gas for neonatal resuscitation has been 100% oxygen. Resuscitation with room air (or 30%) is equally effective and may reduce the risk of hyperoxia, which is associated with decreased cerebral blood flow and generation of oxygen free radicals. Currently, 100% O_2 is recommended. Room air (or 30%) may become the preferred initial gas for neonatal resuscitation in the future; if the neonate does not achieve normal oxygen saturation levels within 90 sec, increasing concentrations of oxygen should be blended in (up to 100% oxygen) until normal oxygen saturation levels are achieved. If pulmonary hypertension is suspected (meconium aspiration, diaphragmatic hernia) one may consider 100% oxygen as the initial gas for resuscitation. Particular attention is required during the resuscitation of very LBW (VLBW) neonates, to monitor oxygen saturation so as to minimize the risk of hyperoxia.

Although the 1st breath normally requires pressures as low as 15-20 cm H_2O, pressures as high as 30-40 cm H_2O may be needed. Subsequent breaths are given at a rate of 40-60/min with a pressure of 15-20 cm H_2O. Noncompliant stiff lungs secondary to respiratory distress syndrome, congenital pneumonia, pulmonary hypoplasia, or meconium aspiration may require higher pressures. Successful ventilation is signified by adequate chest rise, symmetric breath sounds, improved pink color, heart rate >100 beats/min, spontaneous respirations, presence of end-tidal CO_2, and improved tone. Various devices to detect exhaled CO_2 and to confirm accurate placement of an endotracheal tube are available commercially. A laryngeal mask airway may be an effective tool to establish an airway, especially if bag and mask ventilation is ineffective or intubation is unsuccessful.

If the infant has respiratory depression and the mother has received an analgesic narcotic drug within 4 hr prior to delivery, naloxone hydrochloride (0.1 mg/kg) is given while adequate ventilation is maintained. Breathing in the depressed infant should be maintained until a response to naloxone is noted. Continuous observation of the infant is important because repeated doses of naloxone may be needed even after the infant has been transferred to the nursery owing to the short half-life of naloxone.

Medications are rarely required but should be administered when the heart rate is <60 beats/min after 30 sec of combined ventilation and chest compressions or during asystole. The umbilical vein can generally be readily cannulated and used for immediate administration of medications during neonatal resuscitation (Fig. 94-2). The endotracheal tube may be used for the administration of epinephrine if intravenous access is not

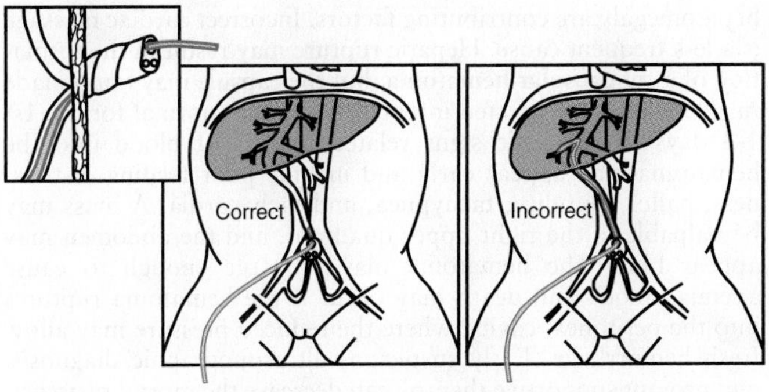

Figure 94-2 Use of the umbilical vein for administration of medications during neonatal resuscitation. (From Kattwinkel J, Bloom RS, editors: *Neonatal resuscitation textbook,* ed 5, Elk Grove, IL, 2006, American Academy of Pediatrics, American Heart Association.)

available and/or for naloxone. Epinephrine (0.1-0.3 mL/kg of a 1:10,000 solution, given intravenously or intratracheally) is given for asystole or for failure to respond to 30 sec of combined resuscitation. The dose may be repeated every 3-5 min. Data in neonates are insufficient to recommend higher doses in infants who are unresponsive to the standard dose. Emergency volume expansion is accomplished with 10-20 mL/kg of an isotonic crystalloid solution or type O Rh-negative red blood cells (in acute hemorrhage). Volume infusions should be used cautiously during the resuscitation of a VLBW infant. Sodium bicarbonate (2 mEq/kg, 0.5 mEq/mL of a 4.2% solution) is often given and should be administered slowly (1 mEq/kg/min) if metabolic acidosis has been documented and the resuscitation is prolonged. Sodium bicarbonate should be given only after effective ventilation has been established, because such therapy may increase the blood CO_2 concentration and produce respiratory acidosis, complicating an existing metabolic acidosis. Restoration of oxygenation and tissue perfusion is the main treatment of metabolic acidosis associated with asphyxia.

Severe asphyxia may also depress myocardial function and cause cardiogenic shock despite the recovery of heart and respiratory rates. Dopamine or dobutamine administered as a continuous infusion (5-20 μg/kg/min) and fluids should be started after the initial resuscitation effort, to improve cardiac output in an infant with poor peripheral perfusion, weak pulses, hypotension, tachycardia, and poor urine output. Epinephrine (0.1-1.0 μg/kg/min) may be indicated for infants in severe shock that does not respond to dopamine or dobutamine (Chapter 62).

Less severe degrees of poor cardiopulmonary transition in the delivery room can usually be managed by brief periods of bag and mask ventilation. Chest compression and medications are not needed for most neonates who have mild to moderate birth depression. Regardless of the severity of asphyxia or the response to resuscitation, asphyxiated infants should be monitored closely for signs of multiorgan hypoxic-ischemic tissue injury (see Table 93-1).

MECONIUM

Meconium staining of the amniotic fluid may be an indication of fetal stress; therefore, personnel skilled at endotracheal intubation and resuscitation should be present at the delivery. Previously the decision to intubate a neonate was based on the presence and thickness/consistency of the meconium-stained fluid; current evidence no longer supports this practice. If any meconium staining is present in the amniotic fluid, the obstetrician should suction the mouth, nose, and hypopharynx immediately after delivery of the head but before delivery of the shoulders. If the infant is vigorous with good respiratory effort and a heart rate >100 beats/min, tracheal intubation to aspirate meconium should not be attempted, and the mouth and nose should be suctioned with a bulb or suction catheter. If the infant is depressed with poor muscle tone and/or a heart rate <100 beats/min, tracheal intubation and suctioning should be performed. The endotracheal tube should be attached to a suction device, and free-flow oxygen should be provided throughout the procedure.

SHOCK

Circulatory insufficiency may be present at birth as a result of severe asphyxia or hemorrhage during gestation, labor, or delivery. Causes of blood loss include hemolysis; placental abruption or tear, placenta previa; traumatic injury to the umbilical cord or internal organs; and intracranial bleeding. Clinical manifestations include signs of respiratory distress, cyanosis, pallor, flaccidity, cold mottled skin, tachycardia or bradycardia, hepatosplenomegaly, and, rarely, convulsions. Edema and hepatosplenomegaly suggest hydrops fetalis or heart failure without shock. Shock from overwhelming infection may be present immediately after birth.

Supportive treatment with type O Rh-negative blood or normal saline is indicated for hemorrhage or hypovolemia, respectively. Oxygen should be administered and the metabolic acidosis corrected with sodium bicarbonate. A sympathomimetic agent such as dopamine or dobutamine may be needed to support cardiac output and blood pressure. The diagnosis and treatment of erythroblastosis fetalis are discussed in Chapter 97.2. If infection is present, appropriate antibiotics must be started as soon as possible.

After supportive measures have stabilized the infant's condition, a specific diagnosis should be established, and appropriate continuing treatment instituted.

PNEUMOTHORAX

Infants may experience pneumothorax in the delivery room, resulting in respiratory distress and hypoxia. Approximately 1-2% of infants have pneumothorax after birth; only 0.05-0.07% have symptoms (Chapter 95.12). The risk is higher in infants requiring positive pressure ventilation or those with meconium-stained amniotic fluid. Rarely, an infant has a congenital malformation that results in lung hypoplasia, such as congenital diaphragmatic hernia or renal agenesis. Clinically, the infant demonstrates respiratory distress and has diminished breath sounds on the affected side. Transillumination may be helpful to confirm the diagnosis, particularly in the LBW infant. Emergency evacuation of a pneumothorax without radiographic confirmation is indicated in an infant who is unresponsive to resuscitation efforts, and has asymmetric breath sounds, bradycardia, and cyanosis. A 23-gauge butterfly needle or angiocatheter attached to a stopcock and syringe should be inserted perpendicular to the chest wall above the rib in the 4th intercostal space at the level of the nipple (Fig. 94-3). The air is evacuated. The catheter is then inserted with constant negative pressure, and the air evacuated.

AIRWAY OBSTRUCTION

Critical fetal and then neonatal airway obstruction represents an emergency in the delivery room. The ex utero intrapartum treatment procedure (**EXIT procedure**) allows time to secure the airway in an infant known to have airway obstruction for a variety of causes, including laryngeal atresia or stenosis, teratomas, hydromas, and oral tumors, before the infant is separated from the placenta. Uteroplacental gas exchange is maintained throughout the procedure. High-risk perinatal care has led to more frequent prenatal diagnosis of many disorders known to cause the critical high airway obstruction syndrome (CHAOS) (Fig. 94-4).

ABDOMINAL WALL DEFECTS

Appropriate management of patients with abdominal wall defects (omphalocele, gastroschisis) in the delivery room prevents excessive fluid loss and minimizes the risk for injury to the exposed viscera. Gastroschisis is the more common defect and typically the intestines are not covered by a membrane. The exposed intestines should be gently placed in a sterile clear plastic bag after delivery. A membrane often covers an omphalocele, and care should be taken to prevent its rupture. The infant should be transferred to a tertiary referral center for surgical consultation and evaluation for other associated anomalies (Chapter 99).

INJURY DURING DELIVERY

Central Nervous System

See Chapter 93.

Viscera

The **liver** is the only internal organ other than the brain that is injured with any frequency during the delivery process. Damage usually results from pressure on the liver during delivery of the head in breech presentations. Large infant size, intrauterine asphyxia, coagulation disorders, extreme prematurity, and hepatomegaly are contributing factors. Incorrect cardiac massage is a less frequent cause. Hepatic rupture may result in the formation of a **subcapsular hematoma,** but the capsule may tamponade further bleeding. Affected infants may appear normal for the 1st 1-3 days. Nonspecific signs related to loss of blood into the hematoma may appear early and include poor feeding, listlessness, pallor, jaundice, tachypnea, and tachycardia. A mass may be palpable in the right upper quadrant, and the abdomen may appear blue. The hematoma may be large enough to cause anemia. Shock and death may occur if the hematoma ruptures into the peritoneal cavity, where the reduced pressure may allow fresh hemorrhage. Early suspicion, ultrasonographic diagnosis, and prompt supportive therapy can decrease the mortality associated with this disorder. Surgical repair of a laceration may be required. Rupture of the spleen may occur alone or in connection with rupture of the liver. The causes, complications, treatment, and prevention are similar.

Although **adrenal hemorrhage** occurs with some frequency, especially after breech delivery, in infants who are large for gestational age or have diabetic mothers, its cause is often undetermined; it may be due to trauma, anoxia, or severe stress, as in overwhelming infection. Ninety percent of adrenal hemorrhages are unilateral; 75% are right-sided. Calcified central hematomas of the adrenal, identified on radiographs or at autopsy in older infants and children, suggest that not all adrenal hemorrhages are immediately fatal. In severe cases, the diagnosis is usually made at postmortem examination. The symptoms are profound shock and cyanosis. A mass may be present in the flank along with overlying skin discoloration; jaundice may also develop. If adrenal hemorrhage is suspected, abdominal ultrasonography may be helpful, and treatment of acute adrenal failure may be indicated (Chapter 569).

Fractures

CLAVICLE The clavicle is fractured during labor and delivery more frequently than any other bone; it is particularly vulnerable with difficult delivery of the shoulder in vertex presentations and the extended arms in breech deliveries. The infant characteristically does not move the arm freely on the affected side; crepitus and bony irregularity may be palpated, and discoloration is occasionally visible over the fracture site. The Moro reflex is absent on the affected side, and spasm of the sternocleidomastoid muscle with obliteration of the supraclavicular depression at the site of the fracture can be noted. Infants with greenstick clavicle fractures may not have any limitation of movement, and the Moro reflex may be present. The prognosis for this fracture is excellent. **Treatment,** if any, consists of immobilization of the arm and shoulder on the affected side. A remarkable degree of

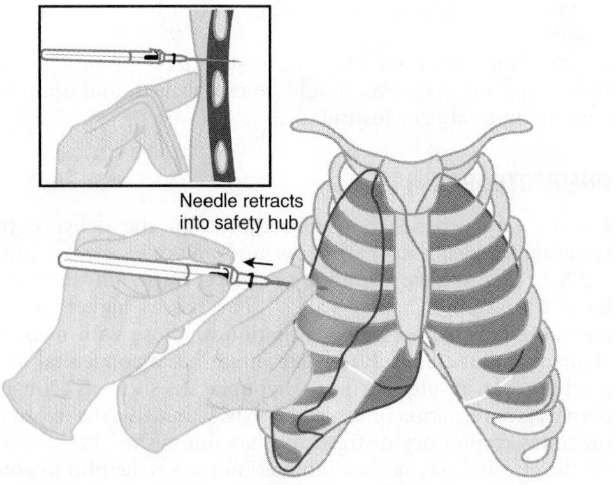

Figure 94-3 Decompression of a pneumothorax. (From Kattwinkel J, Bloom RS, editors: *Neonatal resuscitation textbook,* ed 5, Elk Grove, IL, 2006, American Academy of Pediatrics, American Heart Association.)

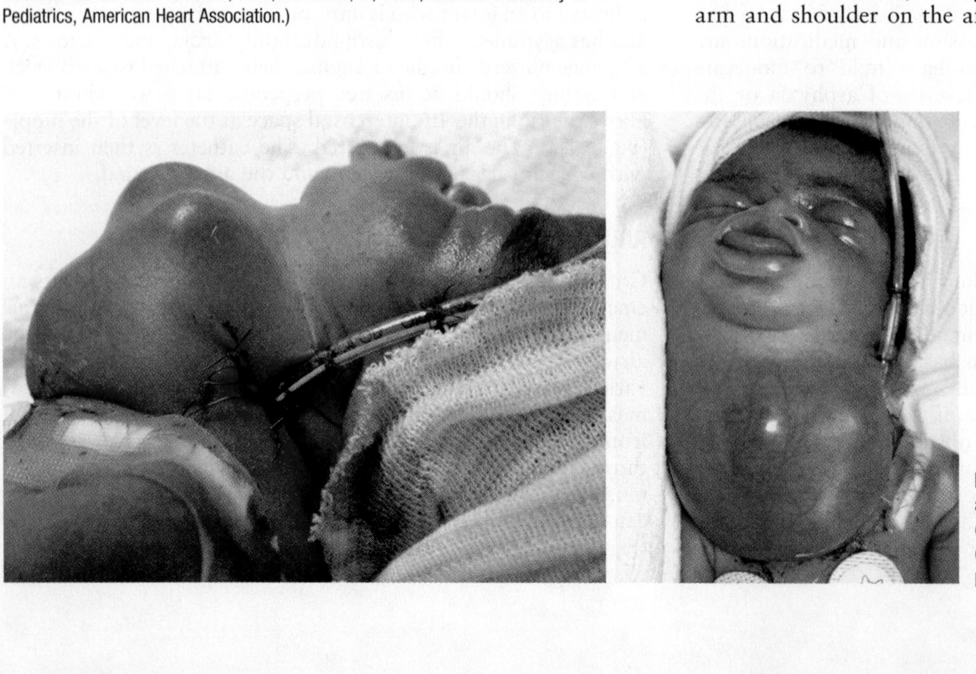

Figure 94-4 EXIT procedure. Baby with teratoma and critical high airway obstruction syndrome (CHAOS). Trachea is displaced to the lateral neck. (Photograph compliments of Dr. Mark Wulkan, pediatric surgeon at Emory University.)

palpable callus develops at the site within a week and may be the initial evidence of the fracture. Fracture of the humerus or brachial palsy may also be responsible for limitation of movement of an arm and absence of a Moro reflex on the affected side.

EXTREMITIES In fractures of the long bones, spontaneous movement of the extremity is usually absent (**pseudoparalysis**). The Moro reflex is often absent from the involved extremity. Associated nerve involvement may occur. Satisfactory results of treatment of a fractured humerus are obtained with 2-4 wk of immobilization, during which the arm is strapped to the chest, a triangular splint and a Velpeau bandage are applied, or a cast is applied. For fracture of the femur, good results are achieved with traction-suspension of both lower extremities, even if the fracture is unilateral; the legs are immobilized in a spica cast. Splints are effective for treatment of fractures of the forearm or leg. Healing is usually accompanied by excess callus formation. The prognosis is excellent for fractures of the extremities. Fractures in VLBW infants may be related to osteopenia (Chapter 100).

Dislocations and epiphyseal separations rarely result from birth trauma. The upper femoral epiphysis may be separated by forcible manipulation of the infant's leg as, for example, in breech extraction or after version. The affected leg shows swelling, slight shortening, limitation of active motion, painful passive motion, and external rotation. The diagnosis is established roentgenographically. The prognosis is good for milder injuries, but coxa vara frequently results from extensive displacement.

NOSE The most prevalent injury to the nose is dislocation of the cartilaginous portion of the septum from the vomerine groove and the columella. The affected infant may have difficulty nursing and some impairment of nasal respiration. On physical examination, the nares appear asymmetric and the nose is flattened. An oral airway is rarely needed, and surgical consultation should be obtained for definitive treatment.

BIBLIOGRAPHY

Please visit the Nelson Textbook of Pediatrics *website at www.expertconsult.com for the complete bibliography.*

Chapter 95
Respiratory Tract Disorders

Waldemar A. Carlo

Respiratory disorders are the most frequent cause of admission for neonatal intensive care in both term and preterm infants. Signs and symptoms of respiratory distress include cyanosis, grunting, nasal flaring, retractions, tachypnea, decreased breath sounds with or without rales and/or rhonchi, and pallor. A wide variety of pathologic lesions may be responsible for respiratory disturbances, including pulmonary, airway, cardiovascular, central nervous, and other disorders (Fig. 95-1).

It is occasionally difficult to distinguish respiratory from nonrespiratory etiologies on the basis of clinical signs alone. Any sign of respiratory distress is an indication for a physical examination and diagnostic evaluation, including a blood gas or pulse oximetry determination and radiograph of the chest. Timely and appropriate therapy is essential to prevent ongoing injury and improve outcome. As a result of important advances in treatment respiratory disease as well as in understanding of its pathophysiology, neonatal and infant deaths from early respiratory disease have declined markedly. The challenge is not only to continue to improve survival but also to reduce short- and long-term complications related to early lung disease.

95.1 Transition to Pulmonary Respiration

Waldemar A. Carlo

Successful establishment of adequate lung function at birth depends on airway patency, functional lung development, and maturity of respiratory control. Fetal lung fluid must be removed and replaced with gas. This process begins before birth as active sodium transport across the pulmonary epithelium drives liquid from the lung lumen into the interstitium with subsequent absorption into the vasculature. Increased levels of circulating catecholamines, vasopressin, prolactin, and glucocorticoids enhance lung fluid adsorption and trigger the change in lung epithelia from a

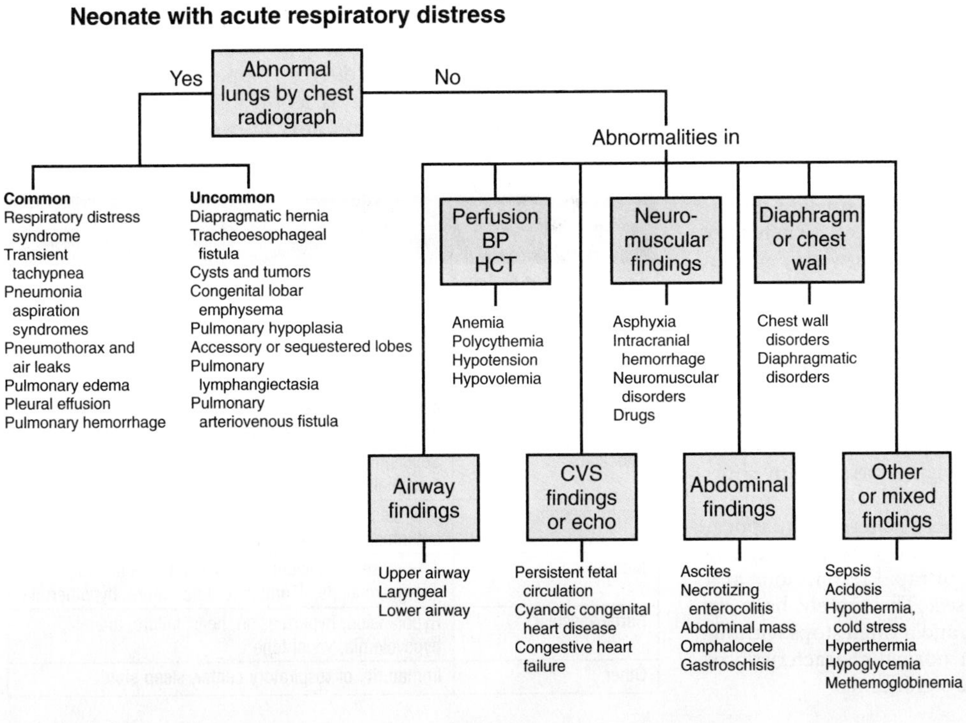

Figure 95-1 Neonate with acute respiratory distress. BP, blood pressure; CVS, cardiovascular system; HCT, hematocrit. (From Battista MA, Carlo WA: Differential diagnosis of acute respiratory distress in the neonate. In Frantz ID, editor: *Tufts University of School of Medicine and Floating Hospital for Children reports on neonatal respiratory diseases,* vol 2, issue 3, Newtown, PA, 1992, Associates in Medical Marketing Co.)

chloride-secretory to a sodium-reabsorptive mode. Functional residual capacity (FRC) must be established and maintained in order to develop a ventilation-perfusion relationship that will provide optimal exchange of oxygen and carbon dioxide between alveoli and blood (Chapter 415).

THE FIRST BREATH

During vaginal delivery, intermittent compression of the thorax facilitates removal of lung fluid. Surfactant lining the alveoli enhances the aeration of gas-free lungs by reducing surface tension, thereby lowering the pressure required to open alveoli. Although spontaneously breathing infants do not need to generate an opening pressure to create airflow, infants requiring positive pressure ventilation at birth need an opening pressure of 13-32 cm H_2O and are more likely to establish FRC if they generate a spontaneous, negative pressure breath. Expiratory esophageal pressures associated with the 1st few spontaneous breaths in term newborns range from 45 to 90 cm H_2O. This high pressure, due to expiration against a partially closed glottis, may aid in the establishment of FRC but would be difficult to mimic safely with use of artificial ventilation. The higher pressures needed to initiate respiration are required to overcome the opposing forces of surface tension (particularly in small airways) and the viscosity of liquid remaining in the airways, as well as to introduce about 50 mL/kg of air into the lungs, 20-30 mL/kg of which remains after the 1st breath to establish FRC. Air entry into the lungs displaces fluid, decreases hydrostatic pressure in the pulmonary vasculature, and increases pulmonary blood flow. The greater blood flow, in turn, increases the blood volume of the lung and the effective vascular surface area available for fluid uptake. The remaining fluid is removed via the pulmonary lymphatics, upper airway, mediastinum, and pleural space. Fluid removal may be impaired after cesarean section or as a result of surfactant deficiency, endothelial cell damage, hypoalbuminemia, high pulmonary venous pressure, or neonatal sedation.

Initiation of the 1st breath is due to a decline in $Pa{O_2}$ and pH and a rise in $Pa{CO_2}$ as a result of interruption of the placental circulation, a redistribution of cardiac output, a decrease in body temperature, and various tactile and sensory inputs. The relative contributions of these stimuli to the onset of respiration are uncertain.

When compared with term infants, the low birthweight (LBW) infant who has a very compliant chest wall may be at a disadvantage in establishing FRC. The FRC is lowest in the most immature infants because of the decrease in alveolar number. Abnormalities in ventilation-perfusion ratio are greater and persist for longer periods in LBW infants and may lead to hypoxemia and hypercarbia as a result of atelectasis, intrapulmonary shunting, hypoventilation, and gas trapping. The smallest immature infants have the most profound disturbances, which may resemble respiratory distress syndrome (RDS). However, even in healthy term infants, oxygenation is impaired soon after birth, and oxygen saturation improves to exceed 90% at around 5 minutes.

BREATHING PATTERNS IN NEWBORNS

During sleep in the 1st months of life, normal full-term infants may have episodes when regular breathing is interrupted by short pauses. This **periodic breathing** pattern, which shifts from a regular rhythmicity to cyclic brief episodes of intermittent apnea, is more common in premature infants, who may have apneic pauses of 5-10 sec followed by a burst of rapid respirations at a rate of 50-60 breaths/min for 10-15 sec. They rarely have an associated change in color or heart rate, and it often stops without apparent reason. Periodic breathing, a normal characteristic of neonatal respiration, has no prognostic significance.

95.2 Apnea

Waldemar A. Carlo

Apnea is a common problem in preterm infants that may be due to prematurity or an associated illness. In term infants, apnea is always worrisome and demands immediate diagnostic evaluation. Periodic breathing must be distinguished from prolonged apneic pauses, because the latter may be associated with serious illnesses. Apnea is a feature of many primary diseases that affect neonates (Table 95-1). These disorders produce apnea by direct depression of the central nervous system's control of respiration (hypoglycemia, meningitis, drugs, hemorrhage, seizures), disturbances in oxygen delivery (shock, sepsis, anemia), or ventilation defects (obstruction of the airway, pneumonia, muscle weakness).

Idiopathic apnea of prematurity occurs in the absence of identifiable predisposing diseases. Apnea is a disorder of respiratory control and may be obstructive, central, or mixed. **Obstructive apnea** (pharyngeal instability, neck flexion) is characterized by absence of airflow but persistent chest wall motion. Pharyngeal collapse may follow the negative airway pressures generated during inspiration, or it may result from incoordination of the tongue and other upper airway muscles involved in maintaining airway patency. In **central apnea,** which is caused by decreased central nervous system (CNS) stimuli to respiratory muscles, airflow and chest wall motion are absent. Gestational age is the most important determinant of respiratory control, with the frequency of apnea being inversely related to gestational age. The immaturity of the brainstem respiratory centers is manifested by an attenuated response to carbon dioxide and a paradoxical response to hypoxia that results in apnea rather than the hyperventilation observed after the 1st months of life. The most common pattern of idiopathic apnea in preterm neonates is **mixed apnea** (50-75% of cases), with obstructive apnea preceding (usually) or following central apnea. Short episodes of apnea are usually central, whereas prolonged ones are often mixed. Apnea depends on the sleep state; its frequency increases during active (rapid eye movement) sleep.

CLINICAL MANIFESTATIONS

The incidence of idiopathic apnea of prematurity varies inversely with gestational age. The onset of idiopathic apnea can be during the 1st 1-2 weeks after birth but is often delayed if there is RDS or other causes of respiratory distress. Apneic episodes have been noted to be as frequent on day 1 as throughout the 1st week in premature infants without respiratory disease. In preterm infants,

Table 95-1 POTENTIAL CAUSES OF NEONATAL APNEA AND BRADYCARDIA

Central nervous system	Intraventricular hemorrhage, drugs, seizures, hypoxic injury, herniation, neuromuscular disorders, Leigh syndrome, brainstem infarction or anomalies (e.g., olivopontocerebellar atrophy), after general anesthesia
Respiratory	Pneumonia, obstructive airway lesions, upper airway collapse, atelectasis, extreme prematurity, laryngeal reflex, phrenic nerve paralysis, pneumothorax, hypoxia
Infectious	Sepsis, meningitis (bacterial, fungal, viral), respiratory syncytial virus, pertussis
Gastrointestinal	Oral feeding, bowel movement, necrotizing enterocolitis, intestinal perforation
Metabolic	↓ Glucose, ↓ calcium, ↓/↑ sodium, ↑ ammonia, ↑ organic acids, ↑ ambient temperature, hypothermia
Cardiovascular	Hypotension, hypertension, heart failure, anemia, hypovolemia, vagal tone
Other	Immaturity of respiratory center, sleep state

serious **apnea** is defined as cessation of breathing for longer than 20 sec or for any duration if accompanied by cyanosis and bradycardia. The incidence of associated bradycardia increases with the length of the preceding apnea and correlates with the severity of hypoxia. Short apnea episodes (10 sec) are rarely associated with bradycardia, whereas longer episodes (>20 sec) have a higher incidence of bradycardia. Bradycardia follows the apnea by 1-2 sec in more than 95% of cases and is most often sinus, but on occasion it can be nodal. Vagal responses and, rarely, heart block are causes of bradycardia without apnea. Short oxygen desaturation episodes noted with oxygen saturation monitoring are normal in neonates, and treatment is not necessary.

TREATMENT

Infants at risk for apnea should be started on cardiorespiratory monitoring. Gentle tactile stimulation is often adequate therapy for mild and intermittent episodes. The onset of apnea in a previously well premature neonate after the 2nd wk of life or in a term infant at any time is a critical event that warrants immediate investigation. Recurrent apnea of prematurity may be treated with theophylline or caffeine. Methylxanthines increase central respiratory drive by lowering the threshold of response to hypercapnia as well as enhancing contractility of the diaphragm and preventing diaphragmatic fatigue. Theophylline and caffeine are as effective, but caffeine has fewer side effects (tachycardia, feeding intolerance). Loading doses of 5-7 mg/kg of theophylline (orally) or aminophylline (intravenously) should be followed by doses of 1-2 mg/kg given every 6-12 hr by the oral or intravenous route. Loading doses of 20 mg/kg of **caffeine citrate** are followed 24 hr later by maintenance doses of 5 mg/kg/24 hr qd, either orally or intravenously. These doses should be monitored through observation of vital signs and clinical response. Serum drug determinations (therapeutic levels: theophylline, 6-10 µg/mL; caffeine, 8-20 µg/mL) are optional because important side effects of these agents are rare. Higher doses of methylxanthines are more effective, do not result in frequent side effects, and tend to reduce major neurodevelopmental disabilities. Withholding respiratory stimulants in infants with RDS may result in ventilator dependency, increased bronchopulmonary dysplasia (BPD), and death. Doxapram, known to be a potent respiratory stimulant, acts predominantly on peripheral chemoreceptors and is effective in neonates with apnea of prematurity that is unresponsive to methylxanthines. Transfusion of packed red blood cells to reduce the incidence of idiopathic apnea is reserved for severely anemic infants. Gastroesophageal reflux is common in neonates, but data do not support a causal relationship between gastroesophageal reflux and apneic events or the use of antireflux medications to reduce the frequency of apnea in preterm infants.

Nasal continuous positive airway pressure (continuous positive airway pressure [CPAP], 2-5 cm H_2O) and high-flow humidification using nasal cannula (1-2.5 L/min) are therapies for mixed or obstructive apnea, but CPAP is preferred because of its proven efficacy and safety. The efficacy of CPAP is related to its ability to splint the upper airway and prevent airway obstruction.

PROGNOSIS

Apnea of prematurity does not alter an infant's prognosis unless it is severe, recurrent, and refractory to therapy. The associated problems of intraventricular hemorrhage (IVH), BPD, and retinopathy of prematurity are critical in determining the prognosis for apneic infants. Apnea of prematurity usually resolves by 36 wk of postconceptional age (PCA) and does not predict future episodes of sudden infant death syndrome (SIDS). Some infants with persistent apnea are discharged as long as cardiorespiratory monitoring can be performed at home. In the absence of significant events, home monitoring can be safely discontinued after 44 wk PCA.

APNEA AND SUDDEN INFANT DEATH SYNDROME

Although preterm infants are at higher risk for SIDS, apnea of prematurity is not a risk factor for SIDS. The epidemiologic evidence that positioning the babies to sleep on their backs reduces the rate of SIDS deaths by more than 50% suggests that position, and not prematurity, has been the primary cause of SIDS. Avoidance of cigarette smoking exposure and of overheating the infant are also important in the prevention of SIDS.

BIBLIOGRAPHY

Please visit the Nelson Textbook of Pediatrics *website at* *www.expertconsult.com* *for the complete bibliography.*

95.3 Respiratory Distress Syndrome (Hyaline Membrane Disease)

Waldemar A. Carlo and Namasivayam Ambalavanan

INCIDENCE

Respiratory distress syndrome occurs primarily in premature infants; its incidence is inversely related to gestational age and birthweight. It occurs in 60-80% of infants <28 wk of gestational age, in 15-30% of those between 32 and 36 wk, and rarely in those >37 wk. The risk for development of RDS increases with maternal diabetes, multiple births, cesarean delivery, precipitous delivery, asphyxia, cold stress, and a maternal history of previously affected infants. The incidence is highest in preterm male or white infants. The risk of RDS is reduced in pregnancies with chronic or pregnancy-associated hypertension, maternal heroin use, prolonged rupture of membranes, and antenatal corticosteroid prophylaxis.

ETIOLOGY AND PATHOPHYSIOLOGY

Surfactant deficiency (decreased production and secretion) is the primary cause of RDS. The failure to attain an adequate FRC and the tendency of affected lungs to become atelectatic correlate with high surface tension and the absence of pulmonary surfactant. The major constituents of surfactant are dipalmitoyl phosphatidylcholine (lecithin), phosphatidylglycerol, apoproteins (surfactant proteins SP-A, SP-B, SP-C, and SP-D), and cholesterol (Fig. 95-2). With advancing gestational age, increasing amounts of phospholipids are synthesized and stored in type II alveolar cells (Fig. 95-3). These surface-active agents are released into the alveoli, where they reduce surface tension and help maintain alveolar stability by preventing the collapse of small air spaces at end-expiration. Because of immaturity, the amounts produced or released may be insufficient to meet postnatal demands. Surfactant is present in high concentrations in fetal lung homogenates by 20 wk of gestation, but it does not reach the surface of the lungs until later. It appears in amniotic fluid between 28 and 32 wk. Mature levels of pulmonary surfactant are present usually after 35 wk. Though rare, genetic disorders may contribute to respiratory distress. Abnormalities in surfactant protein B and C genes as well as a gene responsible for transporting surfactant across membranes (ABC transporter 3 *[ABCA3]*) are associated with severe and often lethal familial respiratory disease. Other familial causes of neonatal respiratory distress (not RDS) include alveolar capillary dysplasia, acinar dysplasia, pulmonary lymphangiectasia, and mucopolysaccharidosis.

Synthesis of surfactant depends in part on normal pH, temperature, and perfusion. Asphyxia, hypoxemia, and pulmonary ischemia, particularly in association with hypovolemia, hypotension, and cold stress, may suppress surfactant synthesis. The epithelial lining of the lungs may also be injured by high oxygen concentrations and the effects of respirator management, thereby resulting in a further reduction in surfactant.

Alveolar atelectasis, hyaline membrane formation, and interstitial edema make the lungs less compliant in RDS, so greater pressure is required to expand the alveoli and small airways. In affected infants, the lower part of the chest wall is pulled in as the diaphragm descends, and intrathoracic pressure becomes negative, thus limiting the amount of intrathoracic pressure that can be produced; the result is the development of atelectasis. The chest wall of the preterm infant, which is highly compliant, offers less resistance than that of the mature infant to the natural tendency of the lungs to collapse. Thus, at end-expiration, the volume of the thorax and lungs tends to approach residual volume, and atelectasis may develop.

Deficient synthesis or release of surfactant, together with small respiratory units and a compliant chest wall, produces atelectasis and results in perfused but not ventilated alveoli, causing **hypoxia.** Decreased lung compliance, small tidal volumes, increased physiologic dead space, and insufficient alveolar ventilation eventually result in **hypercapnia.** The combination of hypercapnia, hypoxia, and acidosis produces pulmonary arterial vasoconstriction with increased right-to-left shunting through the foramen ovale and ductus arteriosus and within the lung itself. Pulmonary blood flow is reduced and ischemic injury both to the cells producing surfactant and to the vascular bed results in an effusion of proteinaceous material into the alveolar spaces (Fig. 95-4).

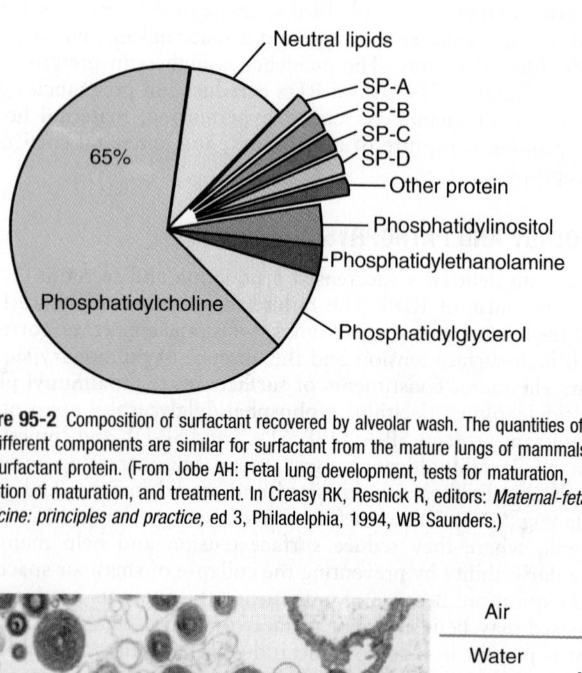

Figure 95-2 Composition of surfactant recovered by alveolar wash. The quantities of the different components are similar for surfactant from the mature lungs of mammals. SP, surfactant protein. (From Jobe AH: Fetal lung development, tests for maturation, induction of maturation, and treatment. In Creasy RK, Resnick R, editors: *Maternal-fetal medicine: principles and practice,* ed 3, Philadelphia, 1994, WB Saunders.)

CLINICAL MANIFESTATIONS

Signs of RDS usually appear within minutes of birth, although they may not be recognized for several hours in larger premature infants until rapid, shallow respirations have increased to 60 breaths/min or greater. A late onset of tachypnea should suggest other conditions. Some patients require resuscitation at birth because of intrapartum asphyxia or initial severe respiratory distress (especially with a birthweight < 1,000 g). Characteristically, tachypnea, prominent (often audible) grunting, intercostal and subcostal retractions, nasal flaring, and cyanosis are noted. Breath sounds may be normal or diminished with a harsh tubular quality, and on deep inspiration, fine rales may be heard. The natural course of untreated RDS is characterized by progressive worsening of cyanosis and dyspnea. If the condition is inadequately treated, blood pressure may fall; cyanosis and pallor increase, and grunting decreases or disappears, as the condition worsens. Apnea and irregular respirations are ominous signs requiring immediate intervention. Patients may also have a mixed respiratory-metabolic acidosis, edema, ileus, and oliguria. Respiratory failure may occur in infants with rapid progression of the disease. In most cases, the symptoms and signs reach a peak within 3 days, after which improvement is gradual. Improvement is often heralded by spontaneous diuresis and improved blood gas values at lower inspired oxygen levels and/or lower ventilator support. Death can be due to severe impairment of gas exchange, alveolar air leaks (interstitial emphysema, pneumothorax), pulmonary hemorrhage, or IVH. Death may be delayed by weeks or months if BPD develops in infants with severe RDS.

DIAGNOSIS

The clinical course, chest radiographic findings, and blood gas and acid-base values help establish the clinical diagnosis. On radiographs, the lungs may have a characteristic but not pathognomonic appearance that includes a fine reticular granularity of the parenchyma and air bronchograms, which are often more prominent early in the left lower lobe because of superimposition of the cardiac shadow (Fig. 95-5). The initial radiographic appearance is occasionally normal, with the typical pattern developing at 6-12 hr. Considerable variation in film findings may be seen, depending on the phase of respiration (inspiratory vs expiratory radiograph) and the use of CPAP or positive end-expiratory pressure (PEEP); this variation often results in poor correlation between radiographic findings and the clinical course. Laboratory findings are characterized initially by hypoxemia and later by progressive hypoxemia, hypercapnia, and variable metabolic acidosis.

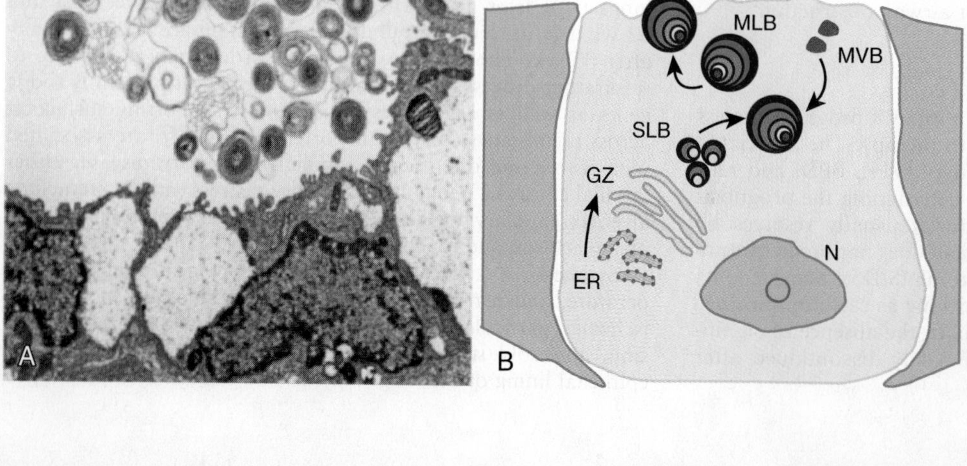

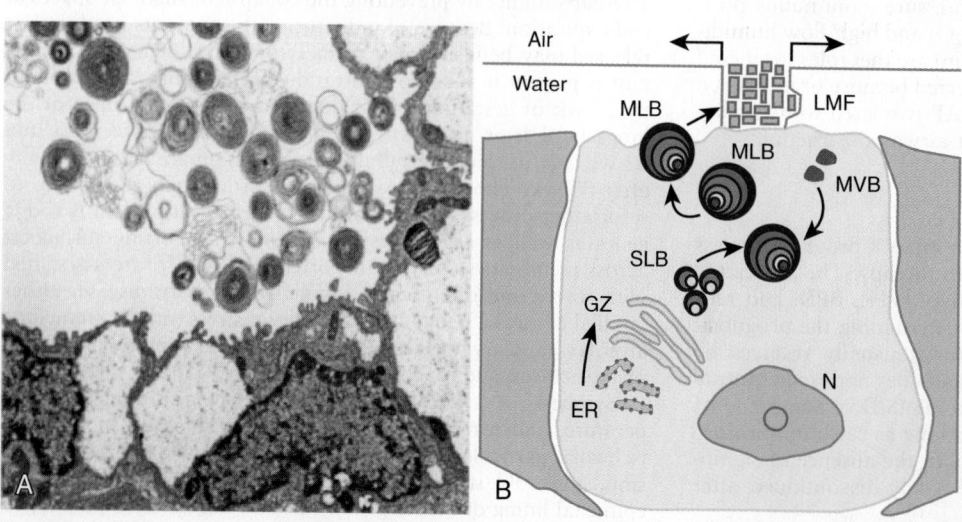

Figure 95-3 *A,* Fetal rat lung (low magnification), day 20 (term, day 22) showing developing type II cells, stored glycogen *(pale areas),* secreted lamellar bodies, and tubular myelin. (Courtesy of Mary Williams, MD, University of California, San Francisco.) *B,* Possible pathway for transport, secretion, and reuptake of surfactant. ER, endoplasmic reticulum; GZ, Golgi zone; LMF, lattice (tubular) myelin figure; MLB, mature lamellar body; MVB, multivesicular body; N, nucleus; SLB, small lamellar body. (From Hansen T, Corbet A: Lung development and function. In Taeusch HW, Ballard RA, Avery MA, editors: *Schaffer and Avery's diseases of the newborn,* ed 6, Philadelphia, 1991, WB Saunders.)

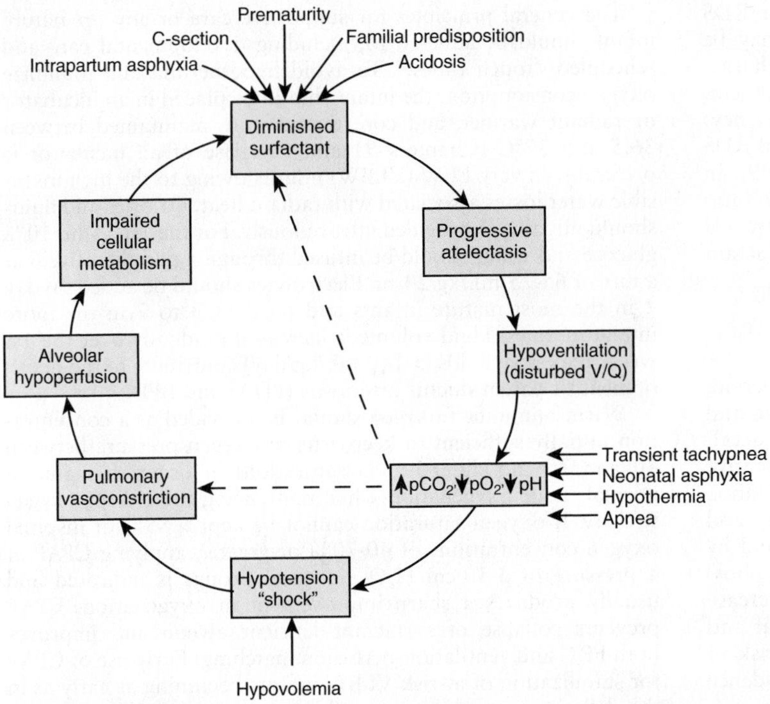

Figure 95-4 Contributing factors in the pathogenesis of hyaline membrane disease. The potential "vicious circle" perpetuates hypoxia and pulmonary insufficiency. (From Farrell P, Zachman R: Pulmonary surfactant and the respiratory distress syndrome. In Quilligan EJ, Kretchmer N, editors: *Fetal and maternal medicine,* New York, 1980, Wiley. Reprinted by permission of John Wiley and Sons, Inc.)

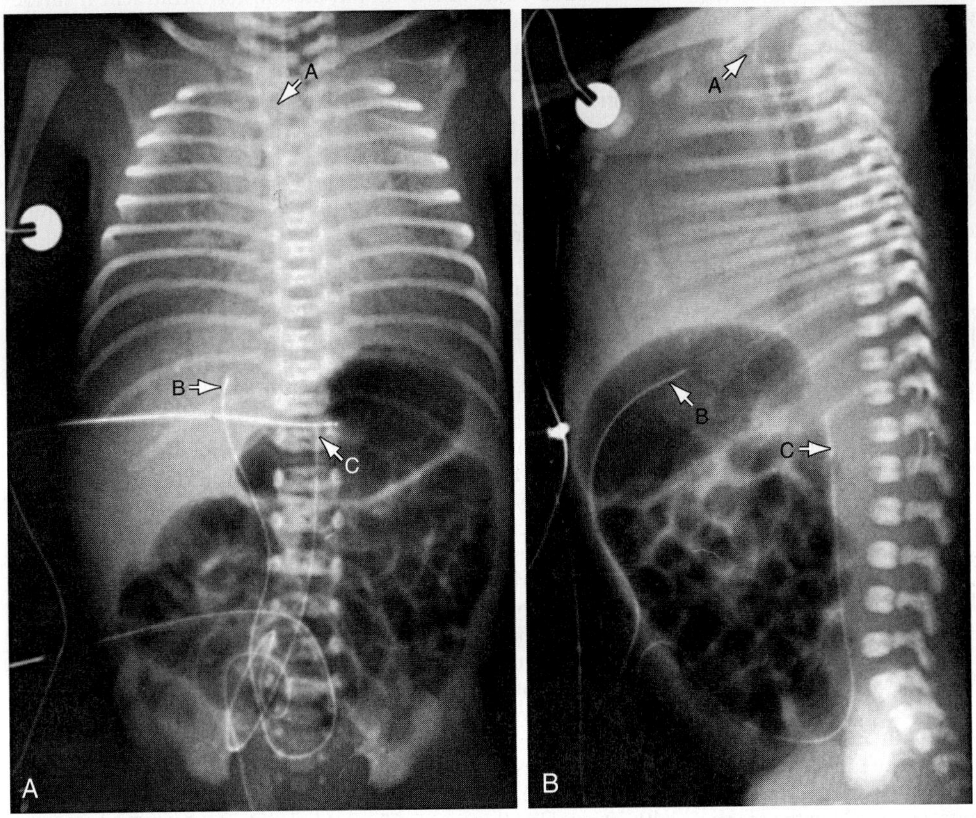

Figure 95-5 Infant with respiratory distress syndrome. Note the granular lungs, air bronchogram, and air-filled esophagus. Anteroposterior *(A)* and lateral *(B)* roentgenograms are needed to distinguish the umbilical artery from the vein catheter and to determine the appropriate level of insertion. The lateral view clearly shows that the catheter has been inserted into an umbilical vein and is lying in the portal system of the liver. A indicates endotracheal tube; B indicates the umbilical venous catheter at the junction of the umbilical vein, ductus venosus, and portal vein; C indicates the umbilical artery catheter passed up the aorta to T12. (Courtesy of Walter E. Berdon, Babies Hospital, New York City.)

In the differential diagnosis, **early-onset sepsis** may be indistinguishable from RDS. In **pneumonia** manifested at birth, the chest roentgenogram may be identical to that for RDS. Maternal group B streptococcal colonization, identification of organisms on gram staining of gastric or tracheal aspirates or a buffy coat smear, and/or the presence of marked neutropenia may suggest the diagnosis of early-onset sepsis. **Cyanotic heart disease** (total anomalous pulmonary venous return) can also mimic RDS both clinically and radiographically. Echocardiography with color-flow imaging should be performed in infants who show no response to surfactant replacement, to rule out cyanotic congenital heart disease as well as ascertain patency of the ductus arteriosus and assess pulmonary vascular resistance (PVR). **Persistent pulmonary hypertension, aspiration (meconium, amniotic fluid) syndromes, spontaneous pneumothorax, pleural effusions,** and **congenital anomalies** such as cystic adenomatoid malformation, pulmonary lymphangiectasia, diaphragmatic hernia, and lobar emphysema must be considered in patients with an atypical clinical course but can generally be differentiated from RDS through radiographic evaluation. **Transient tachypnea** may be distinguished by its short and mild clinical course and is characterized by low or no need for oxygen supplementation. Congenital alveolar proteinosis (congenital surfactant protein B deficiency) is a rare familial disease that manifests as severe and lethal RDS in predominantly term and near-term infants (Chapter 399). In atypical cases of RDS, a lung profile (lecithin:sphingomyelin ratio and phosphatidylglycerol determination) performed on a tracheal aspirate can be helpful in establishing a diagnosis of surfactant deficiency.

PREVENTION

Avoidance of unnecessary or poorly timed cesarean section, appropriate management of high-risk pregnancy and labor, and prediction of pulmonary immaturity with possible in utero acceleration of maturation (Chapter 90) are important preventive strategies. In timing of cesarean section or induction of labor, estimation of fetal head circumference by ultrasonography and determination of the lecithin concentration in amniotic fluid by the lecithin:sphingomyelin ratio (particularly useful with phosphatidylglycerol measurement in diabetic pregnancies) decrease the likelihood of delivering a premature infant. Antenatal and intrapartum fetal monitoring may similarly decrease the risk of fetal asphyxia; asphyxia is associated with an increased incidence and severity of RDS.

Administration of antenatal corticosteroids to women between 24 and 34 wk of gestation significantly reduces the incidence and mortality of RDS as well as overall neonatal mortality. Antenatal steroids also reduce (1) the need for and duration of ventilatory support and admission to a neonatal intensive care unit (NICU) and (2) the incidence of severe IVH, necrotizing enterocolitis, early-onset sepsis, and developmental delay. Postnatal growth is not adversely affected. Antenatal steroids do not increase the risk of maternal death, chorioamnionitis, or puerperal sepsis. Corticosteroid administration is recommended for all women in preterm labor (24-34 wk of gestation) who are likely to deliver a fetus within 1 wk. Repeated weekly doses of betamethasone until 32 wk may reduce neonatal morbidities and the duration of mechanical ventilation. Antenatal glucocorticoids act synergistically with postnatal exogenous surfactant therapy so they should be given even though surfactant therapy is so effective. Betamethasone and dexamethasone have been used antenatally. Dexamethasone may result in a lower incidence of IVH than betamethasone, but further research is needed to determine whether one of these steroids is superior for antenatal treatment.

Administration of a 1st dose of surfactant into the trachea of symptomatic premature infants immediately after birth (prophylactic) or during the 1st few hours of life (early rescue) reduces air leak and mortality from RDS but does not alter the incidence of BPD.

TREATMENT

The basic defect requiring treatment in RDS is inadequate pulmonary exchange of oxygen and carbon dioxide; metabolic acidosis and circulatory insufficiency are secondary manifestations. Early supportive care of premature infants, especially in the treatment of acidosis, hypoxia, hypotension (Chapter 92), and hypothermia, may lessen the severity of RDS. Therapy requires careful and frequent monitoring of heart and respiratory rates, oxygen saturation, Pa_{O_2}, Pa_{CO_2}, pH, serum bicarbonate, electrolytes, glucose, and hematocrit, blood pressure, and temperature. Arterial catheterization is frequently necessary. Because most cases of RDS are self-limited, the goal of treatment is to minimize abnormal physiologic variations and superimposed iatrogenic problems. Treatment of infants with RDS is best carried out in the NICU.

The general principles for supportive care of any premature infant should be adhered to, including developmental care and scheduled "touch times." To avoid hypothermia and minimize oxygen consumption, the infant should be placed in an incubator or radiant warmer, and core temperature maintained between 36.5 and 37°C (Chapters 91 and 92). Use of an incubator is preferable in very LBW (VLBW) infants owing to the high insensible water losses associated with radiant heat. Calories and fluids should initially be provided intravenously. For the 1st 24 hr, 10% glucose and water should be infused through a peripheral vein at a rate of 65-75 mL/kg/24 hr. Electrolytes should be added on day 2 in the most mature infants and on days 3 to 7 in the more immature ones. Fluid volume is increased gradually over the 1st week. Excessive fluids (> 140 mL/kg/day) contribute to the development of patent ductus arteriosus (PDA) and BPD.

Warm humidified oxygen should be provided at a concentration initially sufficient to keep arterial oxygen pressure between 40 and 70 mm Hg (85-95% saturation) in order to maintain normal tissue oxygenation while minimizing the risk of oxygen toxicity. If oxygen saturation cannot be kept > 85% at inspired oxygen concentrations of 40-70% or greater, applying CPAP at a pressure of 5-10 cm H_2O via nasal prongs is indicated and usually produces a sharp improvement in oxygenation. CPAP prevents collapse of surfactant-deficient alveoli and improves both FRC and ventilation-perfusion matching. Early use of CPAP for stabilization of at-risk VLBW infants beginning as early as in the delivery room reduces ventilatory needs. Another approach is to intubate the VLBW infant, administer intratracheal surfactant, and then extubate the infant and begin CPAP. The amount of CPAP required usually decreases after about 72 hr of age, and most infants can be weaned from CPAP shortly thereafter. If an infant with RDS undergoing CPAP cannot keep oxygen saturation > 85% while breathing 40-70% oxygen, assisted ventilation and surfactant are indicated.

Infants with respiratory failure or persistent apnea require assisted mechanical ventilation. Reasonable measures of respiratory failure are: (1) arterial blood pH <7.20, (2) arterial blood P_{CO_2} of 60 mmHg or higher, and (3) oxygen saturation <85% at oxygen concentrations of 40-70% and CPAP of 5-10 cm H_2O. Infants with persistent apnea also need mechanical ventilation. Intermittent positive pressure ventilation delivered by time-cycled, pressure-limited, continuous flow ventilators is a common method of conventional ventilation for newborns. Other methods of conventional ventilation are synchronized intermittent mandatory ventilation (the set rate and pressure synchronized with the patient's own breaths), pressure support (the patient triggers each breath and a set pressure is delivered), and volume ventilation (a mode in which a specific tidal volume is set and the delivered pressure varies), and combinations thereof. Assisted ventilation for infants with RDS should always include PEEP (Chapter 65.1). High ventilatory rates (60/min) result in fewer air leaks. With use of high ventilatory rates, sufficient expiratory time should be allowed to avoid the administration of inadvertent PEEP.

The **goal of mechanical ventilation** is to improve oxygenation and elimination of carbon dioxide without causing pulmonary injury or oxygen toxicity. Acceptable ranges of blood gas values, after the risks of hypoxia and acidosis are balanced against those of mechanical ventilation, vary among institutions: Pa_{O_2} 40-70 mmHg, Pa_{CO_2} 45-65 mmHg, and pH 7.20-7.35. During mechanical ventilation, **oxygenation** is improved by increasing either the fraction of inspired oxygen (F_{IO_2}) or the mean airway pressure. The latter can be increased by raising the peak inspiratory pressure, PEEP gas flow, or inspiratory-expiratory ratio. Pressure changes are usually most effective. However, excessive PEEP may impede venous return, thereby reducing cardiac output and decreasing oxygen delivery despite improvement in Pa_{O_2}. PEEP levels of 4-6 cm H_2O are usually safe and effective. **Carbon dioxide elimination** is achieved by increasing the peak inspiratory pressure (tidal volume) or the rate of the ventilator.

A strategy to minimize ventilator-associated lung injury is the use of CPAP instead of endotracheal intubation. The decreased need for ventilator support with the use of CPAP may allow lung inflation to be maintained but may prevent volutrauma due to overdistention and/or atelectasis. However, controlled trials do not report benefits of early CPAP. Interestingly, nasal intermittent mandatory ventilation (vs nasal CPAP) reduces extubation failure in small trials; this method could be an alternative by which to avoid intubation.

The strategy most evaluated with conventional mechanical ventilation is the use of high rates and presumably small tidal volumes as $Paco_2$ levels were kept in comparable ranges. Meta-analyses of the randomized controlled trials comparing high (>60 per min) and low (usually 30-40 per min) rates (and presumed low vs. high tidal volumes, respectively) revealed that the high ventilatory rate strategy led to fewer air leaks and a trend for increased survival.

If mechanical ventilation is needed, a ventilatory approach using small tidal volumes and permissive hypercapnia can be employed. **Permissive hypercapnia** is a strategy for the management of patients receiving ventilatory support in which priority is given to the prevention or limitation of lung injury from the ventilator by tolerating relatively high levels of $Paco_2$ rather than maintenance of normal blood gas values. A multicenter trial of infants ≤1,000 g reported that permissive hypercapnia (target $Paco_2$ >50 mm Hg) during the 1st 10 days led to a trend for lower rates of BPD or death at 36 wk. Furthermore, the strategy of permissive hypercapnia reduced severity of BPD, as evidenced by a decreased need for ventilator support at 36 wk, from 16% to 1%. A large multi-center randomized controlled trial of permissive hypercapnia with emphasis on the use of CPAP revealed that this is an effective and maybe preferred approach to the standard strategy of intubation and surfactant administration to preterm infants with RDS. Volume-targeted ventilation allows the clinician to set a tidal volume that may prevent volutrama. There are limited data on volume-targeted ventilation, but this mode of ventilation may decrease the rates of pneumothorax and BPD.

Hyperoxia may also contribute to lung injury in preterm infants. Thus, permissive hypoxemia is another strategy that may reduce BPD. Trials to target different levels of oxygen saturation performed for treatment of retinopathy of prematurity or BPD revealed that the groups with lower saturation targets (89-94% or 91-94%, respectively) had less need for oxygen supplementation and lower rates of BPD or BPD exacerbation. Even lower oxygen saturation targets (85-89%) reduced retinopathy of prematurity significantly and tended to reduce BPD but increased mortality rates in a large multi-center randomized controlled trial. Thus, optimal target saturations are still not determined but some restriction of oxygen appears beneficial.

Many ventilated neonates receive sedation or pain relief with benzodiazepines or opiates (morphine, fentanyl), respectively. Midazolam is approved for use in neonates and has demonstrated sedative effects. Adverse hemodynamic effects and myoclonus have been associated with its use in neonates. If it is used, a continuous infusion or administration of individual doses over at least 10 min is recommended to reduce these risks. Data are insufficient to assess the efficacy and safety of lorazepam. Diazepam is not recommended owing to its long half-life, its long-acting metabolites, and concern about the benzyl alcohol content of diazepam injection. Continuous infusion of morphine in VLBW neonates requiring mechanical ventilation does not reduce mortality rates, severe IVH, or periventricular leukomalacia (PVL). The need for additional doses of morphine is associated with poor outcome.

High-frequency ventilation (**HFV**) achieves desired alveolar ventilation by using smaller tidal volumes and higher rates (300-1,200 breaths/min or 5-20 Hz). HFV may improve the elimination of carbon dioxide and improve oxygenation in patients who show no response to conventional ventilators and who have severe RDS, interstitial emphysema, recurrent pneumothoraces, or meconium aspiration pneumonia. High-frequency oscillatory ventilation (HFOV) and high-frequency jet ventilation (HFJV) are the most frequently used methods of HFV. HFOV reduces BPD but increases air leaks and may raise the risk for IVH and PVL. HFOV strategies that promote lung recruitment, combined with surfactant therapy, may improve gas exchange. HFJV facilitates resolution of air leaks. Elective use of either method, in comparison with conventional ventilation, generally does not offer advantages if used as the initial ventilation strategy to treat infants with RDS.

Surfactant deficiency is the primary pathophysiology of RDS. Immediate effects of surfactant replacement therapy include improved alveolar-arterial oxygen gradients, reduced ventilatory support, increased pulmonary compliance, and improved chest radiograph appearance . **Treatment** is initiated as soon as possible in the hours after birth. Repeated dosing is given via the endotracheal tube every 6-12 hr for a total of 2 to 4 doses, depending on the preparation. Exogenous surfactant should be given by a physician who is qualified in neonatal resuscitation and respiratory management and who is able to care for the infant beyond the 1st hr of stabilization. Additional on-site staff support required includes nurses and respiratory therapists experienced in the ventilatory management of premature infants. Appropriate monitoring equipment (radiology, blood gas laboratory, pulse oximetry) must also be available. Complications of surfactant therapy include transient hypoxia, hypercapnia, bradycardia and hypotension, blockage of the endotracheal tube, and pulmonary hemorrhage (Chapter 95.13).

A number of surfactant preparations are available, including synthetic surfactants and natural surfactants derived from animal sources. Exosurf is a synthetic surfactant. Natural surfactants include Survanta (bovine), Infasurf (calf), and Curosurf (porcine). Surfactant replacement therapy is one of the major advances in the care of preterm infants. Prophylactic and rescue administrations of synthetic and natural surfactants have reduced adverse outcomes, including mortality. Specifically, neonatal mortality is lower with prophylactic (vs rescue) administration of both synthetic and natural surfactants. Prophylactic administration of both types of surfactants decreases the risk for pneumothorax and pulmonary interstitial emphysema. The lack of reduction in BPD rates following surfactant replacement is probably, in part, due to the survival of infants with severe RDS who would have died without surfactant administration.

In more mature preterm infants, a policy of prophylactic administration of surfactant may result in many infants' receiving surfactant unnecessarily, and it is possible that early rather than prophylactic surfactant administration may be sufficiently effective. However, the time of rescue surfactant administration in the prophylactic trials varied widely. Early (< 2 hr) rather than delayed rescue surfactant administration resulted in decreased risk for neonatal mortality. Early rescue administration of surfactant reduced rates of both pneumothorax (from 14% to 12%) and pulmonary interstitial emphysema (from 15% to 10%). An alternative to early surfactant administration in many infants is to treat infants with surfactant before ventilation is needed. Temporary endotracheal intubation for surfactant administration in infants requiring only CPAP reduces the subsequent need for mechanical ventilation and may reduce mortality and/or BPD.

Head-to-head trials of natural and synthetic surfactants report superiority of the natural surfactants. Use of natural (vs synthetic) surfactants resulted in lower rates of pneumothorax (12% vs 7%) and mortality (18% vs. 16%) than use of synthetic surfactants. Natural surfactants are superior because of their surfactant-associated protein content, their more rapid onset, and their lower risk of pneumothorax and improved survival. Surfaxin, formerly known as KL4 surfactant, is a novel synthetic lung surfactant containing phospholipids and an engineered peptide, sinapultide, designed to mimic the actions of human SP-B. Use of Surfaxin for the prevention and treatment of RDS demonstrates equivalency to use of the natural surfactants Survanta and Curosurf. Initial protocols for surfactant administration used single-dose therapies. However, compared with a strategy of a single dose of surfactant, administration of multiple doses of surfactant when indicated according to the protocol resulted in lower pneumothorax risk (18% vs 9%) and a trend for lower mortality. A review of all the current evidence supports the use of prophylactic or early use of natural surfactants as early as when infants require CPAP. More than one dose of surfactant should be administered if indicated to optimize the benefits of this therapy.

Premature infants requiring ventilator support after 1 wk of age experience transient episodes of surfactant dysfunction associated with deficiencies of SP-B and SP-C, which are temporally associated with episodes of infection and respiratory deterioration.

Inhaled nitric oxide (iNO) decreases the need for extracorporeal membrane oxygenation (ECMO) in term and near-term infants with hypoxic respiratory failure or persistent pulmonary hypertension of the neonate. The response to iNO is equivalent to that to HFOV in term or near-term infants with hypoxic respiratory failure. A positive response to combined therapy suggests that alveolar recruitment by HFOV may allow iNO gas to reach the pulmonary resistance vessels. A reduction in the rate of death or BPD in infants <1,000 g treated with iNO was observed in one study but not in others.

Strategies for weaning infants from ventilators vary widely and are influenced by lung mechanics as well as the availability of ventilatory modes (pressure support). Once extubated, many infants are transitioned to nasal CPAP to avoid postextubation atelectasis and reduce re-intubation. Synchronized nasal intermittent ventilation decreases the need for re-intubation in premature infants. High flow (1-2 L/min) or warmed, humidified high-flow (2-8 L/min) nasal cannula oxygen is commonly used to support term and near-term infants following extubation and to wean premature infants from nasal CPAP. Preloading with methylxanthines may enhance the success of extubation.

Pharmacologic Therapies

Several pharmacologic options are available to the clinician for the treatment of RDS and prevention of its complications. Selected treatments are reviewed here.

Vitamin A supplementation given largely to infants < 1,000 g resulted in a decrease in death and/or BPD at 36 wk (from 66% to 60%) and trends for less nosocomial sepsis and retinopathy of prematurity.

Systemic corticosteroids have been used to treat infants with RDS, to selectively treat infants who continue to require respiratory support, and to treat those in whom BPD develops. Mortality and/or BPD at 36 wk decrease (from 72% to 45%) with moderately early (7-14 days) administration of corticosteroids. Early (<96 hr) and delayed (> 2-3 wk) administration of systemic steroids has also been assessed with meta-analyses, and the results are qualitatively similar. However, there are **short-term adverse** effects, including hyperglycemia, hypertension, gastrointestinal bleeding, gastrointestinal perforation, hypertrophic obstructive cardiomyopathy, poor weight gain, poor growth of the head, and a trend toward a higher incidence of PVL. Furthermore, data showing an increased incidence of neurodevelopmental delay and cerebral palsy in infants randomly assigned to receive systemic corticosteroids raise serious concerns about adverse long-term outcomes of this therapy. Thus, routine use of systemic corticosteroids for the prevention or treatment of BPD is not recommended by the Consensus Group of the American Academy of Pediatrics and the Canadian Pediatric Society. Administration of inhaled steroids to ventilated preterm infants during the 1st 2 wk after birth reduced the need for systemic steroids (from 45% to 35%) and tended to decrease rates of death and/or BPD at 36 wk without an increase in adverse effects.

Inhaled NO has been evaluated in preterm infants following the observation of its effectiveness in term and near-term infants with hypoxemic respiratory failure. Despite optimistic results from a large randomized controlled trial, trials in preterm infants report heterogeneous effects on BPD, mortality, and other important outcomes. The most current data do not support the routine administration of iNO in preterm infants with hypoxemic respiratory failure.

Prevention of extubation failure has been attempted with use of various pharmacologic approaches. Methylaxanthines appear to have a large effect on reducing extubation (from 51% to 25%). Similarly, use of systemic steroids before extubation reduces the need for re-intubation (from 10% to 1%). In contrast, administration of racemic epinephrine after extubation does not improve pulmonary function or the rate of extubation failure.

Metabolic acidosis in RDS may be a result of perinatal asphyxia and hypotension and is often encountered when an infant has required resuscitation (Chapter 94). Sodium bicarbonate, 1-2 mEq/kg, may be administered over 15-20 min through a peripheral or umbilical vein, followed by an acid-base determination within 30 min, or it may be administered over several hours. Often, sodium bicarbonate is administered on an emergency basis through an umbilical venous catheter. Alkali therapy may result in skin slough from infiltration, increased serum osmolarity, hypernatremia, hypocalcemia, hypokalemia, and liver injury when concentrated solutions are administered rapidly through an umbilical vein catheter wedged in the liver.

Monitoring of aortic blood pressure through an umbilical or peripheral arterial catheter or by oscillometric technique is useful in managing the shock-like state that may occur during the 1st hr or so in premature infants who have been asphyxiated or have severe RDS (see Fig. 94-2). The position of a radiopaque umbilical catheter should be checked roentgenographically after insertion (see Fig. 95-5). The tip of an umbilical artery catheter should lie just above the bifurcation of the aorta (L3-L5) or above the celiac axis (T6-T10). Preferred sites for peripheral catheters are the radial or posterior tibial arteries. The placement and supervision should be carried out by skilled and experienced personnel. Catheters should be removed as soon as patients no longer have any indication for their continued use—usually when an infant is stable and the FIO_2 is < 40%. Hypotension and low flow in the superior vena cava (SVC) have been associated with higher rates of CNS morbidity and mortality and should be treated with cautious administration of volume (crystalloid) and early use of vasopressors. Dopamine is more effective in raising blood pressure than dobutamine. Hypotension may be refractory to pressors, but responsive to glucocorticoids, especially in neonates < 1,000 g. This hypotension may be due to transient adrenal insufficiency in the ill premature infant. It should be treated with intravenous hydrocortisone (Solu-Cortef) at 1-2 mg/kg/dose q6-12 hr (Chapter 92).

Periodic **monitoring of Pao_2, $Paco_2$, and pH** is an important part of the management; if assisted ventilation is being used, such monitoring is essential. Oxygenation may be assessed continuously from transcutaneous electrodes or pulse oximetry (oxygen saturation). Capillary blood samples are of limited value for determining Po_2 but may be useful for evaluating Pco_2 and pH.

Because of the difficulty of distinguishing **group B streptococcal** or other bacterial infections from RDS, empirical antibiotic therapy is indicated until the results of blood cultures are available. Penicillin or ampicillin with an aminoglycoside is suggested, although the choice of antibiotics should be based on the recent pattern of bacterial sensitivity in the hospital where the infant is being treated (Chapter 103).

COMPLICATIONS OF RESPIRATORY DISTRESS SYNDROME AND INTENSIVE CARE

The most serious complications of **tracheal intubation** are pneumothorax and other air leaks, asphyxia from obstruction or dislodgment of the tube, bradycardia during intubation or suctioning, and the subsequent development of subglottic stenosis. Other complications include bleeding from trauma during intubation, posterior pharyngeal pseudodiverticula, need for tracheostomy, ulceration of the nares due to pressure from the tube, permanent narrowing of the nostril as a result of tissue damage and scarring from irritation or infection around the tube, erosion of the palate, avulsion of a vocal cord, laryngeal ulcer, papilloma of a vocal cord, and persistent hoarseness, stridor, or edema of the larynx.

Measures to reduce the incidence of these complications include skillful intubation, adequate securing of the tube, use of polyvinyl endotracheal tubes, use of the smallest tube that will provide effective ventilation in order to reduce local pressure necrosis and ischemia, avoidance of frequent changes and motion of the tube in situ, avoidance of too frequent or too vigorous suctioning, and prevention of infection through meticulous cleanliness and frequent sterilization of all apparatus attached to or passed through the tube. The personnel inserting and caring for the endotracheal tube should be experienced and skilled in such care.

Risks associated with **umbilical arterial catheterization** include vascular embolization, thrombosis, spasm, and vascular perforation; ischemic or chemical necrosis of abdominal viscera; infection; accidental hemorrhage; hypertension; and impairment of circulation to a leg with subsequent gangrene. Aortography has demonstrated that clots form in or about the tips of 95% of catheters placed in an umbilical artery. Aortic ultrasonography can also be used to investigate for the presence of thrombosis. The risk of a serious clinical complication resulting from umbilical catheterization is probably between 2% and 5%.

Transient blanching of the leg may occur during catheterization of the umbilical artery. It is usually due to reflex arterial spasm, the incidence of which is lessened by using the smallest available catheter, particularly in very small infants. The catheter should be removed immediately; catheterization of the other artery may then be attempted. Persistent spasm after removal of the catheter may be relieved by topical nitroglycerin paste applied to the affected area or, rarely, by warming the other leg. Blood sampling from a radial artery may similarly result in spasm or thrombosis, and the same treatment is indicated. Intermittent severe spasm or unrelieved spasm may respond to the cautious use of topical nitroglycerin. Spasm or thrombosis unresponsive to treatment may result in gangrene of the organ or area supplied by the vessel.

Serious hemorrhage upon removal of the catheter is rare. Thrombi may form in the artery or in the catheter, the incidence of which can be lowered by using a smooth-tipped catheter with a hole only at its end, by rinsing the catheter with a small amount of saline solution containing heparin, or by continuously infusing a solution containing 1-2 units/mL of heparin. The risk of thrombus formation with potential vascular occlusion can also be reduced by removing the catheter when early signs of thrombosis, such as narrowing of pulse pressure and disappearance of the dicrotic notch, are noted. Some authorities prefer to use the umbilical artery for blood sampling only and to leave the catheter filled with heparinized saline between samplings. **Renovascular hypertension** may occur days to weeks after umbilical arterial catheterization in a small proportion of neonates.

Umbilical vein catheterization is associated with many of the same risks as umbilical artery catheterization. Additional risks are cardiac perforation and pericardial tamponade, which can occur if the catheter is incorrectly placed in the right atrium; portal hypertension can develop from portal vein thrombosis, especially in the presence of omphalitis.

Air leaks are a common complication of the management of infants with RDS (Chapter 95.12).

Some neonates with RDS may have clinically significant shunting through a **patent ductus arteriosus.** Delayed closure of the PDA is associated with hypoxia, acidosis, increased pulmonary pressure secondary to vasoconstriction, systemic hypotension, immaturity, and local release of prostaglandins, which dilate the ductus. Shunting through the PDA may initially be bidirectional or right-to-left. As RDS resolves, PVR decreases, and left-to-right shunting may occur, leading to left ventricular volume overload and pulmonary edema. Manifestations of PDA may include (1) a hyperdynamic precordium, bounding peripheral pulses, wide pulse pressure, and a continuous or systolic murmur with or without extension into diastole or an apical diastolic murmur, or multiple clicks resembling the shaking of dice; (2) radiographic evidence of cardiomegaly and increased pulmonary vascular markings; (3) hepatomegaly; (4) increasing oxygen dependence; and (5) carbon dioxide retention. The **diagnosis** is confirmed by echocardiographic visualization of a PDA with Doppler flow imaging that demonstrates left-to-right or bidirectional shunting. Prophylactic "closure" before symptoms or signs of a PDA, closure of the asymptomatic but clinically detected PDA, and closure of the symptomatic PDA are three strategies to manage a PDA. Interventions include fluid restriction, the use of cyclooxygenase inhibitors (indomethacin or ibuprofen) to close the ductus, and surgical closure. Short-term benefits have to be balanced against adverse effects such as transient renal dysfunction and a possible increase in the risk of intestinal perforation with indomethacin. Much uncertainty about "best practice" in the management of a PDA remains. Many cases respond to general supportive measures, including fluid restriction. Medical and/or surgical ductal closure is indicated in the premature infant with a large PDA when there is a delay in clinical improvement or deterioration after initial clinical improvement of RDS. Intravenous indomethacin (0.1-0.2 mg/kg/dose) is given in three doses every 12-24 hr; treatment may be repeated once. A second course may be needed in a few symptomatic patients. If closure does not occur in a symptomatic patient, surgical ligation is usually the next step. Prophylactic low-dose indomethacin given soon after birth reduces the incidence of both IVH and PDA and improves the rate of permanent ductus closure even in the most immature infants. **Contraindications** to indomethacin include thrombocytopenia (<50,000 platelets/mm^3), bleeding disorders, oliguria (urine output <1 mL/kg/hr), necrotizing enterocolitis, isolated intestinal perforation, and an elevated plasma creatinine value (>1.8 mg/dL). The infant whose symptomatic PDA fails to close with indomethacin or who has contraindications to indomethacin is a candidate for surgical closure. Surgical mortality is very low even in the extremely LBW infants. Complications of surgery include Horner syndrome, injury to the recurrent laryngeal nerve, chylothorax, transient hypertension, pneumothorax, and bleeding from the surgical site. Inadvertent ligation of the left pulmonary artery or the transverse aortic arch has been reported.

Intravenous ibuprofen may be an alternative to indomethacin; it can be as effective in closing a PDA without reducing cerebral, mesenteric, or renal blood flow velocity. Compared with indomethacin, therapeutic ibuprofen has a lower risk of oliguria.

Bronchopulmonary dysplasia is a result of lung injury in infants requiring mechanical ventilation and supplemental oxygen. The clinical, radiographic, and lung histology of **classic BPD** described in 1967, in an era before the widespread use of antenatal steroids and postnatal surfactant, was a disease of more mature preterm infants with RDS who were treated with positive pressure ventilation and oxygen. The **new BPD** is a disease primarily of infants with birthweight <1,000 g born at less than 28 wk gestation, some of whom have little or no lung disease at birth but experience progressive respiratory failure over the 1st few weeks of life.

The morphometric features currently found in infants with the new BPD include alveolar hypoplasia, variable saccular wall fibrosis, and minimal airway disease. Some specimens also have decreased pulmonary microvasculature development. The histopathology of BPD indicates interference with normal lung

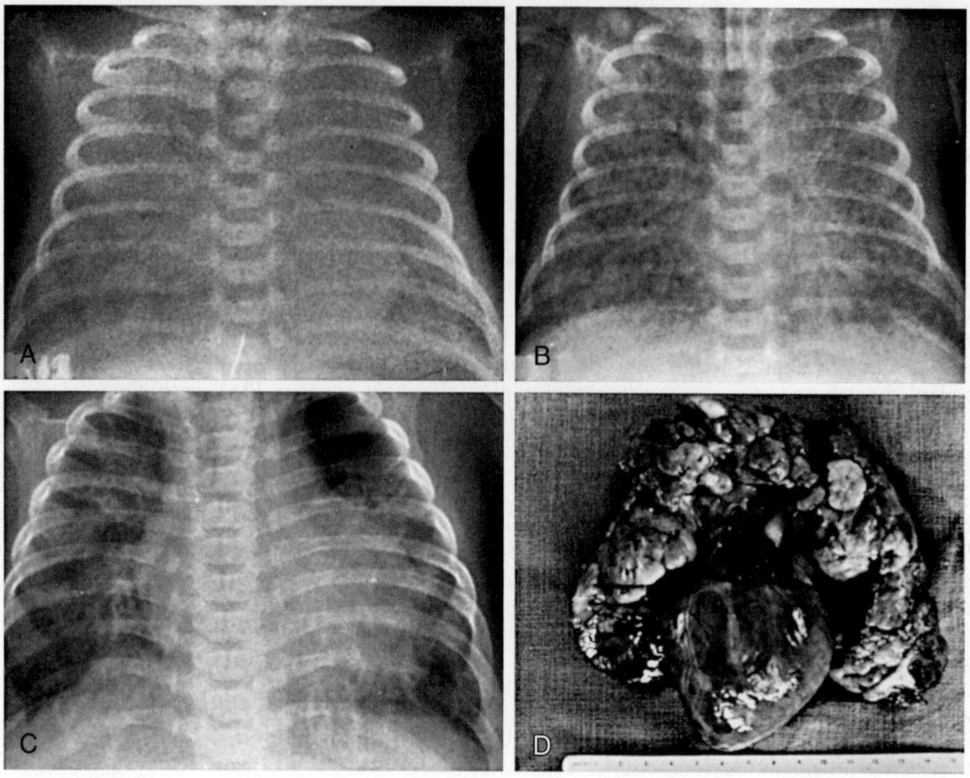

Figure 95-6 Pulmonary changes in infants treated with prolonged, intermittent positive pressure breathing with air containing 80-100% oxygen in the immediate postnatal period for the clinical syndrome of hyaline membrane disease. *A,* A 5-day-old infant with nearly complete opacification of the lungs. *B,* A 13-day-old infant with "bubbly lungs" simulating the roentgenographic appearance of the Wilson-Mikity syndrome. *C,* A 7-mo-old infant with irregular, dense strands in both lungs, hyperinflation, and cardiomegaly suggestive of chronic lung disease. *D,* Large right ventricle and a cobbly, irregular aerated lung of an infant who died at 11 mo of age. This infant also had a patent ductus arteriosus. (From Northway WH Jr, Rosan RC, Porter DY: Pulmonary disease following respirator therapy of hyaline-membrane disease, *N Engl J Med* 276:357–368, 1967.)

anatomic maturation, which may prevent subsequent lung growth and development. The pathogenesis of BPD is multifactorial and affects both the lungs and the heart. RDS is a disease of progressive alveolar collapse. Alveolar collapse (**atelectotrauma**) due to surfactant deficiency, together with ventilator-induced phasic overdistention of the lung (**volutrauma**), promotes injury. Oxygen induces injury by producing free radicals that cannot be metabolized by the immature antioxidant systems of VLBW neonates. Mechanical ventilation and oxygen injure the lung through their effect on alveolar and vascular development. Inflammation (detected with measurement of circulating neutrophils, neutrophils and macrophages in alveolar fluid, and pro-inflammatory cytokines) contributes to the progression of lung injury. Several clinical factors, including immaturity, chorioamnionitis, infection, symptomatic PDA, and malnutrition, contribute to the development of BPD.

The occurrence of BPD is inversely related to gestational age. Additional associations include the presence of interstitial emphysema, male sex, low $Paco_2$ during the treatment of RDS, PDA, high peak inspiratory pressure, increased airway resistance in the 1st wk of life, increased pulmonary artery pressure, and, possibly, a family history of atopy or asthma. Genetic polymorphisms may increase the risk for development of BPD. In some VLBW infants without RDS who require mechanical ventilation for apnea or respiratory insufficiency, BPD that does not follow the classic pattern may develop. Overhydration during the 1st days of life may also contribute to the development of BPD. Vitamin A supplementation (5,000 IU intramuscularly 3 times/wk for 4 wk) in VLBW infants reduces the risk of BPD (1 case prevented for every 14-15 infants treated). Early use of nasal CPAP and rapid extubation with transition to nasal CPAP are associated with a decreased risk of BPD.

Instead of showing improvement on the 3rd or 4th day, which would be consistent with the natural course of RDS, some infants demonstrate an increased need for oxygen and ventilatory support. Respiratory distress persists or worsens and is characterized by hypoxia, hypercapnia, oxygen dependence, and, in severe cases, the development of right-sided heart failure. The chest roentgenogram may reveal pulmonary interstitial emphysema, wandering atelectasis with concomitant hyperinflation, and cyst formation (Fig. 95-6). Four distinct pathologic stages of classic BPD have been identified: acute lung injury, exudative bronchiolitis, proliferative bronchiolitis, and obliterative fibroproliferative bronchiolitis. Histologic study at this stage (10-20 days) shows residual hyaline membrane formation, progressive alveolar coalescence with atelectasis of the surrounding alveoli, interstitial edema, coarse focal thickening of the basement membrane, and widespread bronchial and bronchiolar mucosal metaplasia and hyperplasia. These findings correspond to a severe maldistribution of ventilation. Pathologic examination of infants who die later in the course of BPD reveals cardiac enlargement and pulmonary changes consisting of focal areas of emphysema with hypertrophy of the peribronchial smooth muscle of the tributary bronchioles, perimucosal fibrosis, widespread metaplasia of the bronchiolar mucosa, thickening of basement membranes, and separation of the capillaries from the alveolar epithelial cells.

BPD can be classified according to the need for oxygen supplementation (Table 95-2). Neonates receiving positive pressure support or ≥30% supplemental oxygen at 36 wk or at discharge (whichever occurs 1st) are diagnosed as having severe BPD. Those needing supplementation with 22-29% oxygen at this age are diagnosed as having moderate BPD. Those who need oxygen supplementation for >28 days but are breathing room air at 36 wk or at discharge are diagnosed as having mild BPD. Those receiving <30% oxygen should undergo a stepwise 2% reduction in supplemental oxygen to room air while under continuous observation and with oxygen saturation monitoring to determine whether they can be weaned off oxygen. This test is highly reliable and correlated with discharge home on oxygen, length of hospital stay, and hospital readmissions in the 1st yr of life.

Severe BPD requires prolonged mechanical ventilation. Gradual weaning should be attempted despite elevations in $Paco_2$, because hypercapnia may be the result of gas trapping rather than inadequate minute ventilation. Acceptable blood gas concentrations include hypercapnia with pH >7.20 and a Pao_2 of 50-70 mm Hg with an oxygen saturation of 88-95%. Lower

Table 95-2 DEFINITION OF BRONCHOPULMONARY DYSPLASIA: DIAGNOSTIC CRITERIA*

	GESTATIONAL AGE	
	<32 Wk	≥32 Wk
Time point of assessment	36 wk postmenstrual age or discharge home, whichever comes 1st Treatment with >21% oxygen for at least 28 days **plus**	>28 days but <56 days postnatal age or discharge home, whichever comes 1st Treatment with >21% oxygen for at least 28 days **plus**
Mild BPD	Breathing room air at 36 wk postmenstrual age or discharge home, whichever comes 1st	Breathing room air by 56 days postnatal age or discharge home, whichever comes 1st
Moderate BPD	Need† for <30% oxygen at 36 wk postmenstrual age or discharge home, whichever comes 1st	Need† for <30% oxygen at 56 days postnatal age or discharge home, whichever comes 1st
Severe BPD	Need† for ≥30% oxygen and/or positive pressure (PPV or NCPAP) at 36 wk postmenstrual age or discharge home, whichever comes 1st	Need† for ≥30% oxygen and/or positive pressure (PPV or NCPAP) at 56 days postnatal age or discharge home, whichever comes 1st

*BPD usually develops in neonates being treated with oxygen and PPV for respiratory failure, most commonly respiratory distress syndrome. Persistence of the clinical features of respiratory disease (tachypnea, retractions, crackles) is considered common to the broad description of BPD and has not been included in the diagnostic criteria describing the severity of BPD. Infants treated with > 21% oxygen and/or PPV for nonrespiratory disease (e.g., central apnea or diaphragmatic paralysis) do not have BPD unless parenchymal lung disease also develops and they have clinical features of respiratory distress. A day of treatment with > 21% oxygen means that the infant received > 21% oxygen for more than 12 hr on that day. Treatment with > 21% oxygen and/or PPV at 36 wk postmenstrual age or at 56 days postnatal age or discharge should not reflect an "acute" event, but should rather reflect the infant's usual daily therapy for several days preceding and after 36 wk postmenstrual age, 56 days postnatal age, or discharge.

†A physiologic test confirming that the oxygen requirement at the assessment time point remains to be defined. This assessment may include a pulse oximetry saturation range.

BPD, bronchopulmonary dysplasia; NCPAP, nasal continuous positive airway pressure; PPV, positive pressure ventilation.

From Jobe AH, Bancalari E: Bronchopulmonary dysplasia, *Am J Respir Crit Care Med* 163:1723–1729, 2001.

levels of Pao_2 may exacerbate pulmonary hypertension with resultant cor pulmonale, so the lower limit of oxygenation targets in neonates with BPD are higher than those in neonates with RDS. Airway obstruction in BPD may be due to mucus and edema production, bronchospasm, and airway collapse from acquired tracheobronchomalacia. These events may contribute to "blue spells." Alternatively, blue spells may be due to acute pulmonary vasospasm or right ventricular dysfunction.

Treatment of BPD includes nutritional support, fluid restriction, drug therapy, maintenance of adequate oxygenation, and prompt treatment of infection. Growth must be monitored because recovery depends on the growth of lung tissue and remodeling of the pulmonary vascular bed. Nutritional supplementation to provide added calories (24-30 calories/30 mL formula), protein (3-3.5 g/kg/24 hr), and fat (3 g/kg/24 hr) is needed for growth. Diuretic therapy results in a short-term improvement in lung mechanics and may lead to decreased oxygen and ventilatory requirements. Furosemide (1 mg/kg/dose intravenously twice daily [bid] or 2 mg/kg/dose orally bid) is the treatment of choice for acute fluid overload in infants with BPD. This loop diuretic has been demonstrated to decrease pulmonary interstitial emphysema (PIE) and PVR, improve pulmonary function, and facilitate weaning from mechanical ventilation and oxygen. Adverse effects of long-term diuretic therapy are common and include hyponatremia, hypokalemia, alkalosis, azotemia, hypocalcemia, hypercalciuria, cholelithiasis, renal stones, nephrocalcinosis, and ototoxicity. Potassium chloride supplementation is often necessary. Hyponatremia should be treated with fluid restriction and a decrease in the dose or frequency of furosemide. Sodium chloride supplementation should be avoided. Thiazide diuretics with inhibitors of aldosterone have been used in infants with BPD. Several trials of thiazide diuretics combined with spironolactone have shown increased urine output with or without improvement in pulmonary mechanics in infants with BPD. Adverse effects include electrolyte imbalance.

Inhaled bronchodilators improve lung mechanics by decreasing airway resistance. Albuterol is a specific β2-agonist used to treat bronchospasm in infants with BPD. Albuterol may improve lung compliance by decreasing airway resistance secondary to smooth muscle cell relaxation. Changes in pulmonary mechanics may last as long as 4-6 hr. Adverse effects include hypertension and tachycardia. Ipratropium bromide is a muscarinic antagonist related to atropine, but with more potent bronchodilator effects. Improvements in pulmonary mechanics have been demonstrated in BPD after ipratropium bromide inhalation. Combination therapy using albuterol and ipratropium bromide may be more effective than either agent alone. Few adverse effects have been noted. With current aerosol administration strategies, exactly how much medication is delivered to the airways and lungs of infants with BPD, especially if they are ventilator dependent, is unclear. Because significant smooth muscle relaxation does not appear to occur within the 1st few weeks of life, aerosol therapy in the early stages of BPD is not indicated. Methylxanthines are used to increase respiratory drive, decrease apnea, and improve diaphragmatic contractility. Methylxanthines may also decrease PVR and increase lung compliance in infants with BPD, probably through direct smooth muscle relaxation. They also exhibit diuretic effects. These effects may accelerate weaning from mechanical ventilation. Synergy between theophylline and diuretics has been demonstrated. Theophylline has a half-life of 30-40 hr, is metabolized primarily to caffeine in the liver and may have adverse effects, such as tachycardia, gastroesophageal reflux, agitation, and seizures. Caffeine has a longer half-life than theophylline. Both are available in intravenous and enteral formulations.

Preventive therapy of BPD with postnatal dexamethasone may reduce the time to extubation and may decrease the risk of BPD but is associated with substantial short- and long-term risks, including hypertension, hyperglycemia, gastrointestinal bleeding and perforation, hypertrophic cardiomyopathy, sepsis, and poor weight gain and head growth. Survival is not improved, and infants who have been treated with dexamethasone have an increased risk of neurodevelopmental delay and cerebral palsy. The use of dexamethasone for the prevention of BPD is not recommended unless an infant has severe pulmonary disease, for example is ventilator dependent for at least 1 to 2 wk after birth. A rapid tapering course of therapy, starting at 0.25 mg/kg/day and lasting for 5-7 days, may be adequate. Inhaled beclomethasone does not prevent BPD but does decrease the need for systemic steroids. Inhaled corticosteroids facilitate earlier extubation of ventilated infants with BPD.

Physiologic abnormalities of the pulmonary circulation in BPD include elevated PVR and abnormal vasoreactivity. Acute exposure to even modest levels of hypoxemia causes large elevations in pulmonary artery pressure in infants with BPD with pulmonary hypertension. Higher oxygen saturations are effective in lowering pulmonary artery pressure. The current recommendation for treatment of patients with BPD and pulmonary hypertension is to avoid oxygen saturation values <88% and, in those with established pulmonary hypertension, to maintain oxygen saturation values in the 90-95% range.

Low-dose iNO has no acute effects on lung function, cardiac function, or oxygenation in evolving BPD. The use of low-dose iNO may improve oxygenation in some infants with severe BPD, allowing decreased FIO_2 and ventilator support.

PROGNOSIS

Early provision of intensive observation and care of high-risk newborn infants can significantly reduce the morbidity and mortality associated with RDS and other acute neonatal illnesses. Antenatal steroids, postnatal surfactant use, and improved modes of ventilation have resulted in low mortality from RDS (≈10%). Mortality increases with decreasing gestational age. Optimal results depend on the availability of experienced and skilled personnel, care in specially designed and organized regional hospital units, proper equipment, and lack of complications such as severe asphyxia, intracranial hemorrhage, or irremediable congenital malformation. Surfactant therapy has reduced mortality from RDS approximately 40%, but the incidence of BPD has not been measurably affected.

Although 85-90% of all infants surviving RDS after requiring ventilatory support with respirators are normal, the outlook is much better for those weighing > 1,500 g. The long-term prognosis for normal pulmonary function in most infants surviving RDS is excellent. Survivors of severe neonatal respiratory failure may have significant pulmonary and neurodevelopmental impairment.

Prolonged ventilation, IVH, pulmonary hypertension, cor pulmonale, and oxygen dependence beyond 1 yr of life are poor prognostic signs. Mortality in infants with BPD ranges from 10% to 25% and is highest in infants who remain ventilator dependent for longer than 6 mo. Cardiorespiratory failure associated with cor pulmonale and acquired infection (respiratory syncytial virus) are common causes of death. Survivors with BPD often go home on a regimen of oxygen, diuretics, and bronchodilator therapy.

Noncardiorespiratory complications of BPD include growth failure, psychomotor retardation, and parental stress as well as sequelae of therapy such as nephrolithiasis, osteopenia, and electrolyte imbalance. Airway problems, such as tonsillar and adenoidal hypertrophy, vocal cord paralysis, subglottic stenosis, and tracheomalacia, are common and may aggravate or cause pulmonary hypertension. Subglottic stenosis may require tracheotomy or an anterior cricoid split procedure to relieve upper airway obstruction. Cardiac complications of BPD include pulmonary hypertension, cor pulmonale, systemic hypertension, left ventricular hypertrophy, and the development of aortopulmonary collateral vessels, which, if large, may cause heart failure. Pulmonary function slowly improves in most survivors owing to continued lung and airway growth and healing. Rehospitalization for impaired pulmonary function is most common during the 1st 2 yr of life. There is a gradual decrease in symptom frequency in children aged 6-9 yr from the frequency during the 1st 2 yr of life. Persistence of respiratory symptoms and abnormal pulmonary function test results are present in children aged 7-10 yr. Airway obstruction and hyperactivity and hyperinflation are noted in some adolescent and adult survivors of BPD. High-resolution chest CT scanning or MRI studies in children and adults with a history of BPD reveal lung abnormalities that correlate directly with the degree of pulmonary function abnormality.

BIBLIOGRAPHY

Please visit the Nelson Textbook of Pediatrics *website at* *www.expertconsult.com* *for the complete bibliography.*

95.4 Transient Tachypnea of the Newborn

Namasivayam Ambalavanan and Waldemar A. Carlo

Transient tachypnea usually follows uneventful preterm or term vaginal delivery or cesarean delivery. It is characterized by the early onset of tachypnea, sometimes with retractions, or expiratory grunting and, occasionally, cyanosis that is relieved by minimal oxygen supplementation (<40%). Most infants recover rapidly, within 3 days. The chest generally sounds clear without rales or rhonchi, and the chest radiograph shows prominent pulmonary vascular markings, fluid in the intralobar fissures, overaeration, flat diaphragms, and, rarely, small pleural effusions. Hypercapnia and acidosis are uncommon. Distinguishing the disease from RDS and other respiratory disorders (e.g., pneumonia) may be difficult, and transient tachypnea is frequently a diagnosis of exclusion; the distinctive features of transient tachypnea are rapid recovery of the infant and the absence of radiographic findings for RDS (hypoaeration, diffuse reticulogranular pattern, air bronchograms) and other lung disorders. The syndrome is believed to be secondary to slow absorption of fetal lung fluid, resulting in decreased pulmonary compliance and tidal volume and increased dead space. In severe cases, retained fetal lung fluid may interfere with the normal postnatal fall in PVR, resulting in persistent pulmonary hypertension. Treatment is supportive. There is no evidence supporting the use of oral furosemide in this disorder.

Severe respiratory morbidity and mortality have been reported in infants born by elective cesarean section who initially present with signs and symptoms of transient tachypnea. These infants demonstrate refractory hypoxemia due to pulmonary hypertension and require ECMO support. The term "malignant TTN" has been used to describe this condition.

BIBLIOGRAPHY

Please visit the Nelson Textbook of Pediatrics *website at* *www.expertconsult.com* *for the complete bibliography.*

95.5 Aspiration of Foreign Material (Fetal Aspiration Syndrome, Aspiration Pneumonia)

Waldemar A. Carlo

During prolonged labor and difficult deliveries, infants often initiate vigorous respiratory movements in utero because of interference with the supply of oxygen through the placenta. Under such circumstances, the infant may aspirate amniotic fluid containing vernix caseosa, epithelial cells, meconium, blood, or material from the birth canal, which may block the smallest airways and interfere with alveolar exchange of oxygen and carbon dioxide. Pathogenic bacteria may accompany the aspirated material, and pneumonia may ensue, but even in noninfected cases, respiratory distress accompanied by roentgenographic evidence of aspiration is seen (Fig. 95-7).

Postnatal pulmonary aspiration may also occur in newborn infants as a result of prematurity, tracheoesophageal fistula, esophageal and duodenal obstruction, gastroesophageal reflux, improper feeding practices, and administration of depressant medicines. To avoid aspiration of gastric contents, the stomach should be aspirated using a soft catheter just before surgery or other major procedures that require anesthesia or conscious sedation. The treatment of aspiration pneumonia is symptomatic and may include respiratory support and systemic antibiotics (Chapters 103.8 and 389). Gradual improvement generally occurs over 3-4 days.

95.6 Meconium Aspiration

Namasivayam Ambalavanan and Waldemar A. Carlo

Meconium-stained amniotic fluid is found in 10-15% of births and usually occurs in term or post-term infants. Meconium aspiration syndrome (MAS) develops in 5% of such infants; 30% require

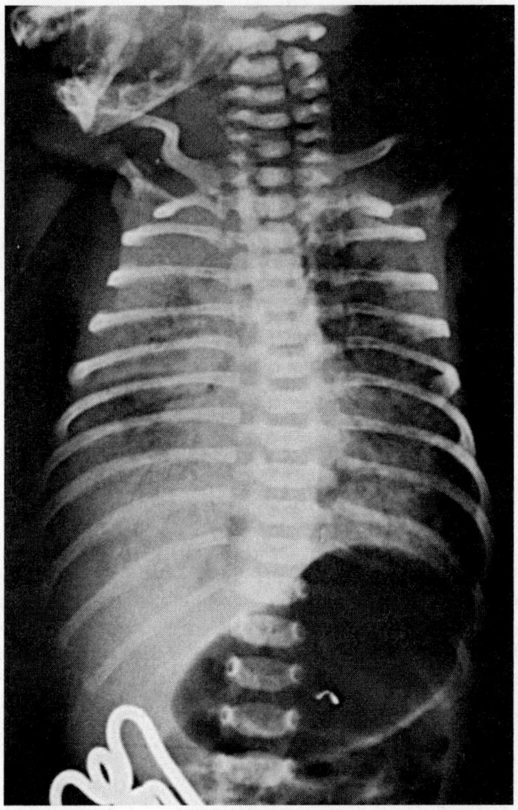

Figure 95-7 Fetal aspiration syndrome (aspiration pneumonia). Note the coarse granular pattern with irregular aeration typical of fetal distress from the aspiration of material contained in amniotic fluid, such as vernix caseosa, epithelial cells, and meconium. (From Goodwin SR, Grave SA, Haberkern CM: Aspiration in intubated premature infants, *Pediatrics* 75:85–88, 1985.)

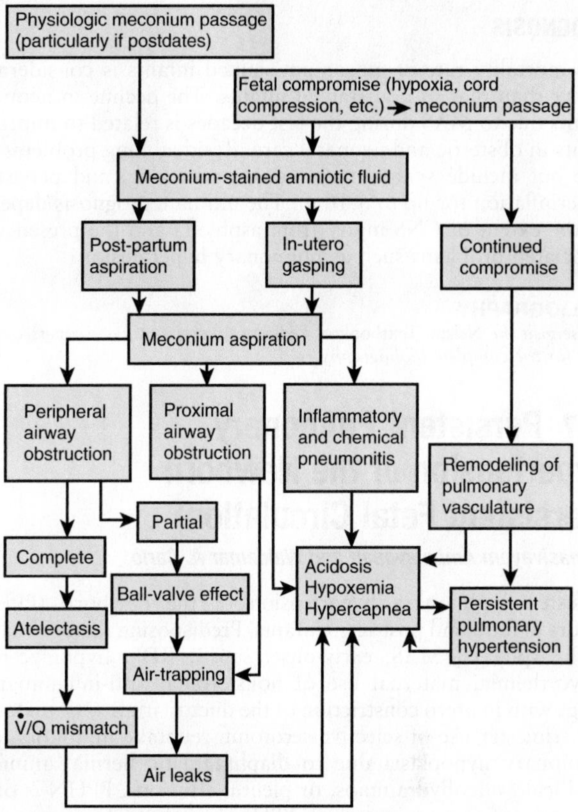

Figure 95-8 Pathophysiology of meconium passage and the meconium aspiration syndrome. $\dot{V}/\dot{Q}$, ventilation-perfusion ratio. (From Wiswell TE, Bent RC: Meconium staining and the meconium aspiration syndrome: unresolved issues, *Pediatr Clin North Am* 40:955–981, 1993.)

mechanical ventilation, and 3-5% die. Usually, but not invariably, fetal distress and hypoxia occur before the passage of meconium into amniotic fluid. The infants are meconium stained and may be depressed and require resuscitation at birth. The pathophysiology is shown in Figure 95-8. Infants with MAS are at increased risk of persistent pulmonary hypertension (Chapter 95.7).

CLINICAL MANIFESTATIONS

Either in utero or with the 1st breath, thick, particulate meconium is aspirated into the lungs. The resulting small airway obstruction may produce respiratory distress within the 1st hours, with tachypnea, retractions, grunting, and cyanosis observed in severely affected infants. Partial obstruction of some airways may lead to pneumomediastinum, pneumothorax, or both. Overdistention of the chest may be prominent. The condition usually improves within 72 hr, but when its course requires assisted ventilation, it may be severe with a high risk for mortality. Tachypnea may persist for many days or even several weeks. The typical chest roentgenogram is characterized by patchy infiltrates, coarse streaking of both lung fields, increased anteroposterior diameter, and flattening of the diaphragm. A normal chest roentgenogram in an infant with severe hypoxemia and no cardiac malformation suggests the diagnosis of pulmonary hypertension (Chapter 95.7).

PREVENTION

The risk of meconium aspiration may be decreased by rapid identification of fetal distress and initiation of prompt delivery in the presence of late fetal heart rate (FHR) deceleration or poor beat-to-beat FHR variability. Despite initial enthusiasm for amnioinfusion, it does not reduce the risk of MAS, cesarean delivery, or other major indicators of maternal or neonatal morbidity. Nasopharyngeal suctioning of a meconium-stained infant after delivery of the head was once considered a low-risk method of reducing the incidence of MAS. However, routine intrapartum nasopharyngeal suctioning in infants with meconium-stained amniotic fluid does not reduce the risk for MAS.

TREATMENT

Routine intubation to aspirate the lungs of vigorous infants born through meconium-stained fluid is not effective in reducing MAS or other major adverse outcomes. Depressed infants (those with hypotonia, bradycardia, or decreased respiratory effort) are at higher risk of MAS and may benefit from endotracheal intubation and suction to remove meconium from the airway before the 1st breath in the delivery room. The risk associated with laryngoscopy and endotracheal intubation (bradycardia, laryngospasm, hypoxia) is less than the risk of MAS in meconium-stained infants who are depressed at birth.

Treatment of MAS includes supportive care and standard management for respiratory distress. The beneficial effect of mean airway pressure on oxygenation must be weighed against the risk of pneumothorax. Administration of exogenous surfactant and/or iNO to infants with MAS and hypoxemic respiratory failure or pulmonary hypertension requiring mechanical ventilation decreases the need for ECMO support, which is needed by the most severely affected infants who show no response to therapy. Severe meconium aspiration may be complicated by persistent pulmonary hypertension. Patients with MAS that is refractory to conventional mechanical ventilation may benefit from HFV or ECMO (Chapter 95.7).

PROGNOSIS

The mortality rate of meconium-stained infants is considerably higher than that of non-stained infants. The decline in neonatal deaths due to MAS during the last decades is related to improvements in obstetric and neonatal care. Residual lung problems are rare but include symptomatic cough, wheezing, and persistent hyperinflation for up to 5-10 yr. The ultimate prognosis depends on the extent of CNS injury from asphyxia and the presence of associated problems such as pulmonary hypertension.

BIBLIOGRAPHY

Please visit the Nelson Textbook of Pediatrics *website at www.expertconsult.com for the complete bibliography.*

95.7 Persistent Pulmonary Hypertension of the Newborn (Persistent Fetal Circulation)

Namasivayam Ambalavanan and Waldemar A. Carlo

Persistent pulmonary hypertension of the newborn (PPHN) occurs in term and post-term infants. Predisposing factors include birth asphyxia, MAS, early-onset sepsis, RDS, hypoglycemia, polycythemia, maternal use of nonsteroidal anti-inflammatory drugs with in utero constriction of the ductus arteriosus, maternal late trimester use of selective serotonin reuptake inhibitors, and pulmonary hypoplasia due to diaphragmatic hernia, amniotic fluid leak, oligohydramnios, or pleural effusions. PPHN is often idiopathic. Some patients with PPHN have low plasma arginine and NO metabolite concentrations and polymorphisms of the carbamoyl phosphate synthase gene, findings suggestive of a possible subtle defect in NO production. The incidence is 1/500-1,500 live births with a wide variation among clinical centers.

PATHOPHYSIOLOGY

Persistence of the fetal circulatory pattern of right-to-left shunting through the PDA and foramen ovale after birth is due to excessively high PVR. Fetal PVR is usually elevated relative to fetal systemic or postnatal pulmonary pressure. This fetal state normally permits shunting of oxygenated umbilical venous blood to the left atrium (and brain) through the foramen ovale, from which it bypasses the lungs through the ductus arteriosus and passes to the descending aorta. After birth, PVR normally declines rapidly as a consequence of vasodilation secondary to filling of the lungs with gas, a rise in postnatal Pao_2, a reduction in $Paco_2$, increased pH, and release of vasoactive substances. Increased neonatal PVR may be (1) maladaptive from an acute injury (not demonstrating normal vasodilation in response to increased oxygen and other changes after birth); (2) the result of increased pulmonary artery medial muscle thickness and extension of smooth muscle layers into the usually nonmuscular, more peripheral pulmonary arterioles in response to chronic fetal hypoxia; (3) due to pulmonary hypoplasia (diaphragmatic hernia, Potter syndrome); or (4) obstructive as a result of polycythemia or total anomalous pulmonary venous return, or of alveolar capillary dysplasia, which is a lethal autosomal recessive disorder characterized by thickened alveolar septa, increased muscularization of the pulmonary arterioles, a reduced number of capillaries, and misalignment of the intrapulmonary veins. Regardless of etiology, profound hypoxemia from right-to-left shunting and normal or elevated $Paco_2$ are present (Fig. 95-9).

CLINICAL MANIFESTATIONS

Infants with PPHN become ill in the delivery room or within the 1st 12 hr of life. PPHN related to polycythemia, idiopathic causes, hypoglycemia, or asphyxia may result in severe cyanosis with tachypnea, although initial signs of respiratory distress may be minimal. Infants who have PPHN associated with meconium aspiration, group B streptococcal pneumonia, diaphragmatic hernia, or pulmonary hypoplasia usually exhibit cyanosis, grunting, flaring, retractions, tachycardia, and shock. Multiorgan involvement may be present (see Table 92-1). Myocardial ischemia, papillary muscle dysfunction with mitral and tricuspid regurgitation, and biventricular dysfunction produce cardiogenic shock with decreases in pulmonary blood flow, tissue perfusion, and oxygen delivery. The hypoxemia is often labile and out of proportion to the findings on chest roentgenograms.

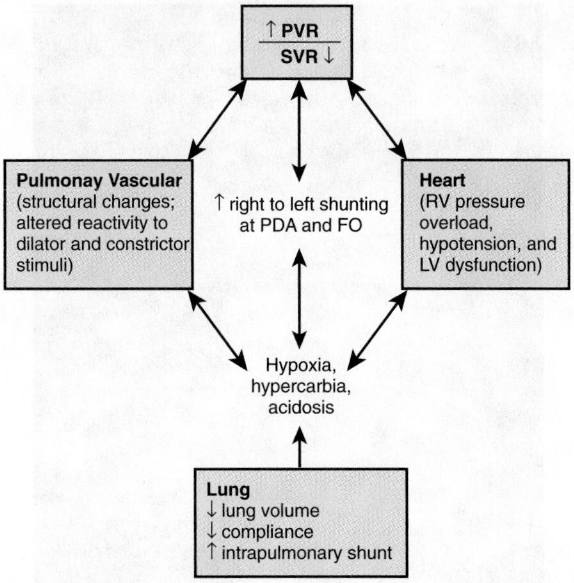

Figure 95-9 Cardiopulmonary interactions in persistent pulmonary hypertension of the newborn (PPHN). FO, foramen ovale; LV, left ventricular; PDA, patent ductus arteriosus; PVR, pulmonary vascular resistance; RV, right ventricular; SVR, systemic vascular resistance. (From Kinsella JP, Abman SH: Recent developments in the pathophysiology and treatment of persistent pulmonary hypertension of the newborn, *J Pediatr* 126:853–864, 1995.)

DIAGNOSIS

PPHN should be suspected in all term infants who have cyanosis with or without a history of fetal distress, intrauterine growth restriction, meconium-stained amniotic fluid, hypoglycemia, polycythemia, diaphragmatic hernia, pleural effusions, and birth asphyxia. Hypoxemia is universal and is unresponsive to 100% oxygen given by oxygen hood, but it may respond transiently to hyperoxic hyperventilation administered after endotracheal intubation or to the application of a bag and mask. A Pao_2 gradient between a preductal (right radial artery) and a postductal (umbilical artery) site of blood sampling >20 mm Hg suggests right-to-left shunting through the ductus arteriosus, as does an oxygenation saturation gradient >5% between preductal and postductal sites on pulse oximetry. Real-time echocardiography combined with Doppler flow imaging studies demonstrates right-to-left or bidirectional shunting across a patent foramen ovale and a ductus arteriosus. Deviation of the intra-atrial septum into the left atrium is seen in severe PPHN. Tricuspid or mitral insufficiency may be noted on auscultation as a holosystolic murmur and can be visualized echocardiographically together with poor contractility when PPHN is associated with myocardial ischemia. The degree of tricuspid regurgitation can be used to estimate pulmonary artery pressure. The 2nd heart sound is accentuated and not split. In asphyxia-associated and idiopathic PPHN, chest roentgenogram findings are normal, whereas in PPHN associated with pneumonia and diaphragmatic hernia, parenchymal opacification and bowel and/or liver in the chest, respectively, are seen. The **differential diagnosis** of PPHN includes cyanotic heart disease (especially obstructed total anomalous pulmonary venous return) and the associated etiologic entities that predispose to PPHN (hypoglycemia, polycythemia, sepsis).

TREATMENT

Therapy is directed toward correcting any predisposing condition (hypoglycemia, polycythemia) and improving poor tissue oxygenation. The response to therapy is often unpredictable, transient, and complicated by the adverse effects of drugs or mechanical ventilation. Initial management includes oxygen administration and correction of acidosis, hypotension, and hypercapnia. Persistent hypoxemia should be managed with intubation and mechanical ventilation.

The optimal approach to mechanical ventilation is controversial. In the pre-NO era, one approach to the treatment of severe PPHN consisted of instituting mechanical ventilation with or without the use of muscle relaxants; ventilator settings were adjusted to achieve a $Pa{O_2}$ of 50-70 mm Hg and a $Pa{CO_2}$ of 50-60 mm Hg. Tolazoline (1 mg/kg), a nonselective α-adrenergic antagonist, was sometimes used as an adjunct to nonselectively vasodilate the pulmonary arterial system, but its use also usually resulted in systemic hypotension, which was treated with volume expansion and dopamine. Another approach incorporated hyperventilation to reduce pulmonary vasoconstriction by lowering the $Pa{CO_2}$ (≈25 mm Hg) and increasing the pH (7.50-7.55). This strategy required high peak inspiratory pressures and rapid respiratory rates, often necessitating the use of muscle relaxants for control of ventilation. Ventilator settings were adjusted to achieve a $Pa{O_2}$ between 90 and 100 mm Hg. Alkalinization with sodium bicarbonate was also used to elevate serum pH.

Forced alkalosis using sodium bicarbonate and hyperventilation were popular therapies because of their ability to produce acute pulmonary vasodilation and rapid increases in $Pa{O_2}$. Hypocarbia constricts the cerebral vasculature and reduces cerebral blood flow. Extreme alkalosis and hypocarbia are associated with later neurodevelopmental deficits, including cerebral palsy and neurosensory hearing loss. Other complications of hyperventilation included air trapping, reduced cardiac output due to decreased venous return, barotrauma, pneumothorax, increased fluid requirements, and edema. Sodium bicarbonate and tromethamine (Tham) infusions, on the other hand, require careful monitoring of serum electrolytes and blood gases to ensure that ventilation is adequate to allow carbon dioxide clearance. The use of alkali infusions is associated with an increased need for ECMO and an increased rate of chronic lung disease. Currently, infants with PPHN are often managed without hyperventilation and/or alkalinization. In skilled hands, "gentle ventilation" with normocarbia or permissive hypercarbia results in excellent outcomes and a low incidence of chronic lung disease.

Because of their lability and ability to fight the ventilator, newborns with PPHN usually require sedation. Fentanyl may decrease sympathetic tone during stressful interventions and maintain a more relaxed pulmonary vascular bed. The use of paralytic agents is controversial and reserved for the newborn who cannot be treated with sedatives alone. Muscle relaxants may promote atelectasis of dependent lung regions and ventilation-perfusion mismatch. Paralysis may be associated with an increased risk of death. In survivors of congenital diaphragmatic hernia (CDH), prolonged administration of pancuronium during the neonatal period is associated with sensorineural hearing loss as well as an acute myopathy.

Inotropic therapy is frequently needed to support blood pressure and perfusion. Whereas dopamine is frequently used as a 1st-line agent, other agents, such as dobutamine, epinephrine, and milrinone, may be helpful when myocardial contractility is poor. Some of the sickest newborns with PPHN demonstrate hypotension refractory to vasopressor administration. This results from desensitization of the cardiovascular system to catecholamines by overwhelming illness and relative adrenal insufficiency. Hydrocortisone rapidly upregulates cardiovascular adrenergic receptor expression and serves as a hormone substitute in cases of adrenal insufficiency.

NO gas is an endothelium-derived signaling molecule that relaxes vascular smooth muscle and can be delivered to the lung by inhalation. Use of iNO reduces the need for ECMO support by approximately 40%. The optimal starting dose is 20 ppm. Higher doses have not been shown to be more effective and are associated with side effects including methemoglobinemia and increased levels of nitrogen dioxide, a pulmonary irritant. Most newborns require iNO for < 5 days. Although NO has been used as long-term therapy in children and adults with primary pulmonary hypertension, prolonged dependency is rare in neonates and suggests the presence of lung hypoplasia, congenital heart disease, or alveolar capillary dysplasia. The maximal safe duration of iNO therapy is unknown. The dose can be weaned to 5 ppm after 6-24 hr of therapy. The dose can then be weaned slowly and discontinued when the $Fi{O_2}$ is < 0.6 and the iNO dose is 1 ppm. Abrupt discontinuation should be avoided as it may cause rebound pulmonary hypertension. Inhaled NO should be used only at institutions that offer ECMO support or have the capability of transporting an infant on iNO therapy if a referral for ECMO is necessary. Some cases of PPHN do not respond adequately to iNO. Therapy with continuous inhaled or intravenous prostacyclin (prostaglandin I_2) has improved oxygenation and outcome in infants with PPHN. Intravenous continuous prostacyclin is also effective in treating older children with primary pulmonary hypertension. Oral sildenafil (a type 5 phosphodiesterase inhibitor) improves exercise tolerance in adults with moderately severe pulmonary artery hypertension. The safety and efficacy of intravenous sildenafil in newborns with PPHN is under investigation; initial results are promising.

Extracorporeal Membrane Oxygenation

In 5-10% of patients with PPHN (approximately 1/4,000 births), the response to 100% oxygen, mechanical ventilation, and drugs is poor. In such patients, two parameters have been used to predict mortality, the alveolar-arterial oxygen gradient ($PA{O_2} - Pa{O_2}$), which is roughly, at sea level, 760 − 47, and the oxygenation index (OI), which is calculated as follows:

$$OI = (\text{Mean airway pressure} \times Fi{O_2} \times 100)/\text{Postductal } Pa{O_2}$$

An alveolar-arterial gradient >620 for 8-12 hr and an OI >40 that is unresponsive to iNO predict a high mortality rate (>80%) and are indications for ECMO. ECMO is used to treat carefully selected, severely ill infants with hypoxemic respiratory failure caused by RDS, meconium aspiration pneumonia, congenital diaphragmatic hernia, PPHN, or sepsis.

ECMO is a form of cardiopulmonary bypass that augments systemic perfusion and provides gas exchange. Most experience has been with venoarterial bypass, which requires carotid artery ligation and the placement of large catheters in the right internal jugular vein and carotid artery. Venovenous bypass avoids carotid artery ligation and provides gas exchange, but it does not support cardiac output. Blood is initially pumped through the ECMO circuit at a rate that approximates 80% of the estimated cardiac output, 150-200 mL/kg/min. Venous return passes through a membrane oxygenator, is rewarmed, and returns to the aortic arch in venoarterial ECMO and to the right atrium in venovenous ECMO. Venous oxygen saturation values are used to monitor tissue oxygen delivery and subsequent extraction for infants undergoing venoarterial ECMO, whereas arterial oxygen saturation values are used to monitor oxygenation for infants receiving venovenous ECMO. The rate of ECMO flow is adjusted to achieve satisfactory venous oxygen saturation (>65%) and cardiovascular stability with venoarterial ECMO and an arterial saturation of 85-95% with venovenous ECMO. When ECMO is started in an infant, the FiO_2 is gradually changed over to room air and ventilatory settings are minimized to reduce the risk of oxygen toxicity and barotrauma, thus permitting time for the lungs to rest and heal.

Because ECMO requires complete heparinization to prevent clotting in the circuit, it cannot be used in patients with or at high risk for IVH (weight <2 kg, gestational age <34 wk). In addition, infants for whom ECMO is being considered should have reversible lung disease, no signs of systemic bleeding, an absence of severe asphyxia or lethal malformations, and they should have been ventilated for less than 10 days. Complications of ECMO include thromboembolism, air embolization, bleeding, stroke, seizures, atelectasis, cholestatic jaundice, thrombocytopenia, neutropenia, hemolysis, infectious complications of blood transfusions, edema formation, and systemic hypertension.

The number of neonatal respiratory ECMO cases has shown a progressive decline from a high of 1,500/year in 1992 to 750/year in 2004. The probable reasons for this decline are improved perinatal management and neonatal care, including the use of lung-protective ventilation and iNO.

PROGNOSIS

Survival in patients with PPHN varies with the underlying diagnosis. The long-term outcome for infants with PPHN is related to the associated hypoxic-ischemic encephalopathy and the ability to reduce PVR. The long-term prognosis for infants who have PPHN and who survive after treatment with hyperventilation is comparable to that for infants who have underlying illnesses of equivalent severity (birth asphyxia, hypoglycemia, polycythemia). The outcome for infants with PPHN who are treated with ECMO is also favorable; 70-80% survive, and 60-75% of survivors appear normal at 1-3.5 yr of age. Survival of infants born with CDH has increased over the past 10 yr to 67%; benchmark institutions are reporting survival rates > 80%. Those infants with CDH who require ECMO continue to have a lower survival than the general neonatal population undergoing ECMO (52%).

BIBLIOGRAPHY

Please visit the Nelson Textbook of Pediatrics *website at www.expertconsult.com for the complete bibliography.*

95.8 Diaphragmatic Hernia

Akhil Maheshwari and Waldemar A. Carlo

A diaphragmatic hernia is defined as a communication between the abdominal and thoracic cavities with or without abdominal contents in the thorax (Fig. 95-10). The etiology may be congenital or traumatic. The symptoms and prognosis depend on the location of the defect and associated anomalies. The defect may be at the esophageal hiatus (hiatal), paraesophageal (adjacent to the hiatus), retrosternal (Morgagni), or at the posterolateral (Bochdalek) portion of the diaphragm. The term *congenital diaphragmatic hernia* typically refers to the Bochdalek form. These lesions may cause significant respiratory distress at birth, can be associated with other congenital anomalies, and have significant mortality and long-term morbidity. The overall survival from the CDH Study Group is 67%. The Bochdalek hernia accounts for up to 90% of the hernias seen in the newborn period, with 80-90% occurring on the left side. The Morgagni hernia accounts for 2-6% of congenital diaphragmatic defects. The size of the defect is highly variable, ranging from a small hole to complete agenesis of this area of the diaphragm.

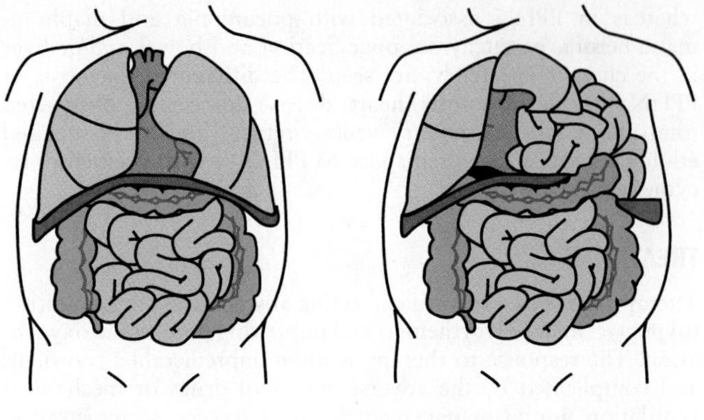

Figure 95-10 *A,* A normal diaphragm separating the abdominal and thoracic cavity. *B,* Diaphragmatic hernia with a small lung and abdominal contents in the thoracic cavity.

CONGENITAL DIAPHRAGMATIC HERNIA (BOCHDALEK)

Pathology and Etiology

Although CDH is characterized by a structural diaphragmatic defect, a major limiting factor for survival is the associated **pulmonary hypoplasia.** Lung hypoplasia was initially thought to be due solely to the compression of the lung from the herniated abdominal contents, which impaired lung growth. However, emerging evidence indicates that pulmonary hypoplasia, at least in some cases, may precede the development of the diaphragmatic defect.

Pulmonary hypoplasia is characterized by a reduction in pulmonary mass and the number of bronchial divisions, respiratory bronchioles, and alveoli. The pathology of pulmonary hypoplasia and CDH includes abnormal septa in the terminal saccules, thickened alveoli, and thickened pulmonary arterioles. Biochemical abnormalities include relative surfactant deficiencies, increased glycogen in the alveoli, and decreased levels of phosphatidylcholine, total DNA, and total lung protein, all of which contribute to limited gas exchange.

Epidemiology

The incidence of CDH is between 1/2,000 and 1/5,000 live births, with females affected twice as often as males. Defects are more common on the left (85%) and are occasionally (<5%) bilateral. Pulmonary hypoplasia and malrotation of the intestine are part of the lesion, not associated anomalies. Most cases of CDH are sporadic, but familial cases have been reported. In one study, complete agenesis of the diaphragm had an autosomal recessive pattern of inheritance; in the majority of cases, genetic factors are multifactorial. Associated anomalies have been reported in up to 30% of cases; these include CNS lesions, esophageal atresia, omphalocele, and cardiovascular lesions. CDH is recognized as part of several chromosomal syndromes: trisomy 21, trisomy 13, trisomy 18, Fryns, Brachmann-de Lange, Pallister-Killian, and Turner.

Diagnosis and Clinical Presentation

CDH can be diagnosed on prenatal ultrasonography (between 16 and 24 wk of gestation) in > 50% of cases. High-speed fetal MRI can further define the lesion. Findings on ultrasonography may include polyhydramnios, chest mass, mediastinal shift, gastric bubble or a liver in the thoracic cavity, and fetal hydrops. Certain imaging features may predict outcome; these include lung to head size ratio (LHR). Nonetheless, no definitive characteristic reliably

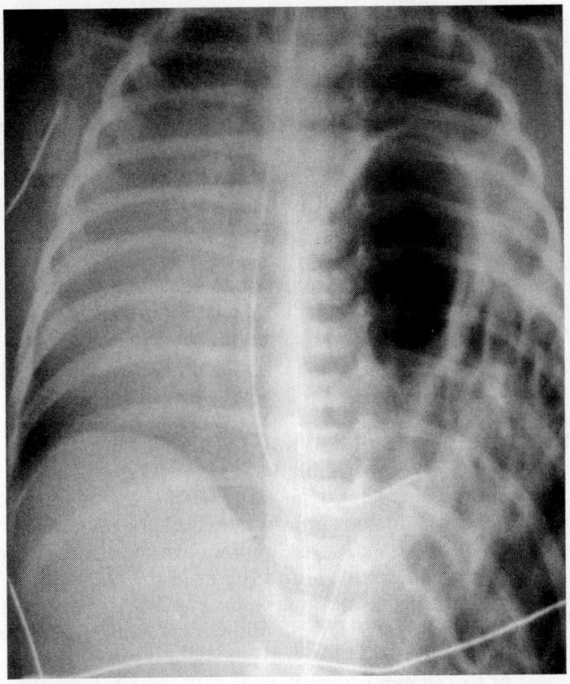

Figure 95-11 This chest radiograph shows a stomach, nasogastric tube, and small bowel contents in the thoracic cavity, consistent with a congenital diaphragmatic hernia (CDH).

predicts outcome. After delivery, a chest radiograph is needed to confirm the diagnosis (Fig. 95-11). In some infants with an echogenic chest mass, further imaging is required. The **differential diagnosis** may include a cystic lung lesion (pulmonary sequestration, cystic adenomatoid malformation) requiring a CT scan or an upper gastrointestinal radiographic series to confirm the diagnosis.

Arriving at the diagnosis early in pregnancy allows for prenatal counseling, possible fetal interventions, and planning for postnatal care. A referral to a center providing high-risk obstetrics, pediatric surgery, and tertiary care neonatology is advised. Careful evaluation for other anomalies should include echocardiography and amniocentesis. To avoid unnecessary pregnancy termination and unrealistic expectations, an experienced multidisciplinary group must carefully counsel the parents of a child diagnosed with a diaphragmatic hernia.

Respiratory distress is a cardinal sign in babies with CDH. It may occur immediately after birth, or there may be a "honeymoon" period of up to 48 hr during which the baby is relatively stable. Early respiratory distress, within 6 hr of life, is thought to be a poor prognostic sign. Respiratory distress is characterized clinically by tachypnea, grunting, use of accessory muscles, and cyanosis. *Children with CDH also have a scaphoid abdomen and increased chest wall diameter.* Bowel sounds may also be heard in the chest with decreased breath sounds bilaterally. The point of maximal cardiac impulse may be displaced away from the side of the hernia if mediastinal shift has occurred. A chest radiograph and passage of a nasal gastric tube are all that is usually required to confirm the diagnosis.

A small group of infants with CDH present beyond the neonatal period. Patients with a delayed presentation may experience vomiting as a result of intestinal obstruction or mild respiratory symptoms. Delayed presentation of a diaphragmatic hernia (often right-sided) after a documented episode of group B streptococcal sepsis is well described. Occasionally, incarceration of the intestine proceeds to ischemia with sepsis and shock. Unrecognized diaphragmatic hernia is a rare cause of sudden death in infants and toddlers.

Treatment

INITIAL MANAGEMENT Aggressive respiratory support is often needed in children with CDH. This includes rapid endotracheal intubation, sedation, and possibly paralysis. Arterial (preductal and postductal) and central venous (umbilical) lines are mandated, as are a urinary catheter and nasogastric tube. A preductal arterial oxygen saturation (Sao_2) value ≥85% should be the minimum goal. *Prolonged mask ventilation in the delivery room, which enlarges the stomach and small bowel and thus makes oxygenation more difficult, must be avoided.* Barotrauma is a significant problem; therefore, peak inspiratory pressure (PIP) must be carefully monitored and kept below 25 cm H_2O. Permissive hypercapnia with a $Paco_2$ of 45-60 mm Hg is helpful as long the pH is > 7.3. Gentle ventilation with **permissive hypercapnia** reduces lung injury and mortality. Factors that contribute to pulmonary hypertension (hypoxia, acidosis, hypothermia) should be avoided. Echocardiography is a critically important imaging study that guides therapeutic decisions by measuring pulmonary and system vascular pressures and defining the presence of cardiac dysfunction. Routine use of inotropes is indicated in the presence of left ventricular dysfunction. Babies with CDH may be surfactant deficient. Although surfactant is commonly used, no study has proven that it is beneficial in treatment of CDH.

VENTILATION STRATEGIES Conventional mechanical ventilation, HFOV, and ECMO are the 3 main strategies to support respiratory failure in the newborn with CDH. The goal is to maintain oxygenation without inducing barotrauma. The 1st modality to be used is conventional ventilation. Pressure-limited ventilation with the rate set between 30 and 60 breaths/min and a PIP ≤25 cm H_2O reduces the risk of lung injury. Hyperventilation to induce alkalosis and decrease ductal shunting has not proved effective and should be avoided. Permissive hypercapnia has reduced lung injury and mortality rates in several studies. HFOV was initially used as a high-pressure strategy to recruit alveolar units. It was unsuccessful because it resulted in increased barotrauma because the newborn with CDH has a nonrecruitable lung. The most logical approach to HFOV is to use it early, thus allowing ventilation at lower mean airway pressures.

NO is a selective pulmonary vasodilator. Its use reduces ductal shunting and pulmonary pressures and results in improved oxygenation. Although it has been helpful in PPHN, randomized trials have not demonstrated improved survival or reduced need for ECMO when NO is used in newborns with CDH. Nonetheless, it is used in patients with CDH before ECMO is started (Chapter 95.7).

EXTRACORPOREAL MEMBRANE OXYGENATION The availability of ECMO and the utility of preoperative stabilization have improved survival of babies with CDH. ECMO combined with paralysis and nasogastric suction may produce a dramatic reduction of the volume of herniated viscera. ECMO is the therapeutic option in children in whom conventional ventilation or conventional ventilation and HFOV fail. ECMO is most commonly used before repair of the defect. Several objective criteria for ECMO have been developed (Chapter 95.7).

Birthweight and the 5-min Apgar score may be the best predictors of outcome in patients treated with ECMO. The lower limit of weight for ECMO is 2,000 g. ECMO modes may be venoarterial (VA) or venovenous (VV), although VA is used most commonly (85%).

The duration of ECMO for neonates with diaphragmatic hernia is significantly longer (7-14 days) than for those with persistent fetal circulation or meconium aspiration, and may last up to 2-4 wk. Timing of repair of the diaphragm while the infant receives ECMO is controversial; some centers prefer early repair to allow a greater duration of ECMO after the repair, whereas many centers defer repair until the infant has demonstrated the ability to tolerate weaning from ECMO. The recurrence of pulmonary hypertension is associated with a high mortality, and weaning from ECMO support should be cautious. If the patient cannot be weaned from ECMO after repair of CDH, options include discontinuing support and, in rare cases, lung transplantation.

NOVEL STRATEGIES FOR INFANTS WITH CONGENTIAL DIAPHRAGMATIC HERNIA There are no reliable prenatal prognosticators of outcomes in children with CDH. The most widely studied is fetal ultrasonography. A prospective study using this modality at 24-26 wk compared fetal LHR values. There were no survivors when the LHR was <1, and all babies with LHR >1.4 survived. A second important consideration was the presence of liver in the thoracic cavity, which is a poor prognostic feature. Human studies have shown no benefit for in utero repair of CDH.

Tracheal occlusion in utero is based on the observation that in utero fetal lung fluid plays a critical role in lung growth and maturity. A deficiency of lung fluid results in pulmonary hypoplasia. Initial studies in affected fetuses have not demonstrated success, but preliminary reports from an ongoing European study are showing some efficacy. Partial liquid ventilation (PLV) after birth is an experimental therapy under investigation in adults and children with severe respiratory failure. PLV increases FRC by recruiting collapsed alveoli, thereby improving ventilation-perfusion mismatches and compliance. It also may reduce lung injury and increase surfactant production. A study is under way to evaluate the role of PLV in neonates with CDH.

SURGICAL REPAIR The ideal time to repair the diaphragmatic defect is under debate. Most centers wait at least 48 hr after stabilization and resolution of the pulmonary hypertension. Good relative indicators of stability are the requirement for conventional ventilation only, a low PIP, and a FIO_2 <50. If the newborn was on HFOV, repair is delayed until the child can return to conventional ventilation. If the newborn was on ECMO, an ability to be weaned from this support should be a consideration before surgical repair. In some centers, the repair is done with the cannulas in place; in other centers, the cannulas are removed. A subcostal approach is the most frequently used (Fig. 95-12). This allows for good visualization of the defect and, if the abdominal cavity cannot accommodate the herniated contents, a polymeric silicone (Silastic) patch can be placed. Both laparoscopic and thoracoscopic repairs have been reported, but these should be reserved for only the most stable infants.

The defect size and amount of native diaphragm present are variable. Whenever possible, a primary repair using native tissue is performed. If the defect is too large, a porous polytetrafluoroethylene (GORE-TEX) patch is used.

There is a higher recurrence rate of CDH among children with patches (the patch does not grow as the child grows) than among those with repairs with native tissue. A loosely fitted patch may reduce the recurrence rates. Pulmonary hypertension must be monitored carefully, and in some instances, a postoperative course of ECMO is needed. Other recognized complications include bleeding, chylothorax, and bowel obstruction.

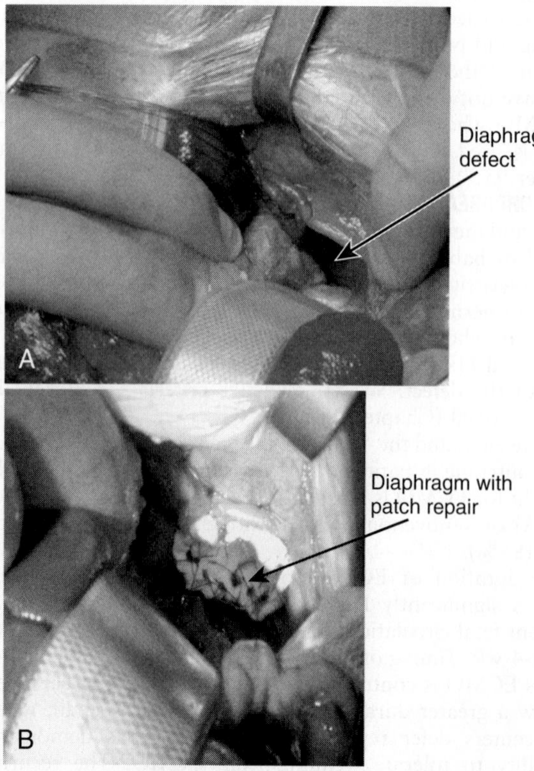

Figure 95-12 *A,* An intraoperative picture of a congenital diaphragmatic hernia (CDH) before repair. *B,* An intraoperative picture of a patch repair of a CDH.

Outcome and Long-Term Survival

Overall survival of liveborn infants with CDH is 67%. The incidence of spontaneous fetal demise is 7-10%. Relative predictors of a poor prognosis include an associated major anomaly, symptoms before 24 hr of age, severe pulmonary hypoplasia, herniation to the contralateral lung, and the need for ECMO.

Pulmonary problems continue to be a source of morbidity for long-term survivors of CDH. Children receiving CDH repair who were studied at 6-11 yr of age demonstrated significant decreases in forced expiratory flow at 50% of vital capacity and decreased peak expiratory flow. Both obstructive and restrictive patterns can occur. Those without severe pulmonary hypertension and barotrauma do the best. Those at highest risk include children who required ECMO and patch repair, but the data clearly show that CDH survivors who did not require ECMO also need frequent attention to pulmonary issues. At discharge, up to 20% of infants require oxygen, but only 1-2% require oxygen past 1 yr of age. **BPD** is frequently documented radiographically but will improve as more alveoli develop and the child ages.

Gastroesophageal reflux disease (GERD) is reported in more than 50% of children with CDH. It is more common in those children whose diaphragmatic defect involves the esophageal hiatus. Approximately 25% of cases of GERD in children with CDH are refractory to medical management and require an antireflux procedure. Intestinal obstruction is reported in up to 20% of children. This condition could be due to a midgut volvulus, adhesions, or a recurrent hernia that became incarcerated. Recurrent diaphragmatic hernia is reported in 5-20% in most series. Children with patch repairs are at highest risk.

Children with CDH typically have **delayed growth** in the 1st 2 yr of life. Contributing factors include poor intake, GERD, and a caloric requirement that may be higher because of the energy required to breathe. Many children normalize and "catch up" in growth by the time they are 2 yr old.

Neurocognitive defects are common and may be due to the disease or the interventions. The incidence of neurologic abnormalities is higher in infants who require ECMO (67% vs 24% of those who do not). The abnormalities are similar to those seen in neonates treated with ECMO for other diagnoses and include transient and permanent developmental delay, abnormal hearing or vision, and seizures. Serious hearing loss may occur in up to 28% of children who underwent ECMO. The majority of neurologic abnormalities are classified as mild to moderate.

Other long-term problems occurring in this population include pectus excavatum and scoliosis. Survivors of CDH repair, particularly those requiring ECMO support, have a variety of long-term abnormalities that appear to improve with time but require close monitoring and multidisciplinary support.

BIBLIOGRAPHY

Please visit the Nelson Textbook of Pediatrics *website at* *www.expertconsult.com* *for the complete bibliography.*

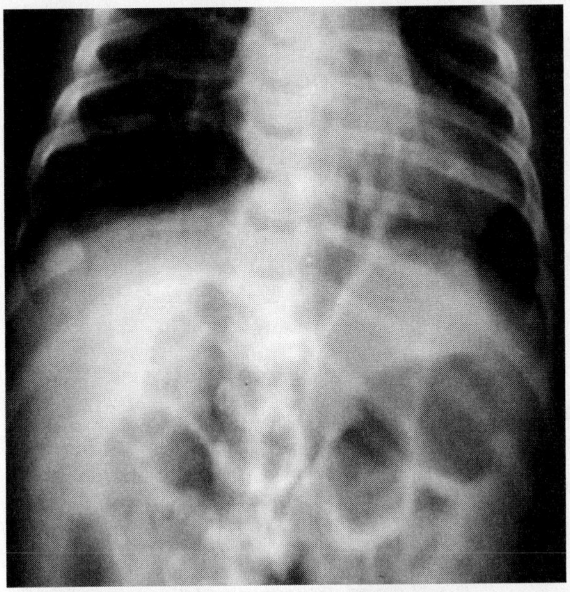

Figure 95-13 A chest radiograph demonstrating a Morgagni hernia.

95.9 Foramen of Morgagni Hernia

Akhil Maheshwari and Waldemar A. Carlo

The anteromedial diaphragmatic defect through the foramen of Morgagni accounts for 2-6% of diaphragmatic hernias. Failure of the sternal and crural portions of the diaphragm to meet and fuse produces this defect. These defects are usually small, with a greater transverse than anteroposterior diameter, and are more commonly right-sided (90%) but may be bilateral (Fig. 95-13). The transverse colon or small intestine or liver is usually contained in the hernial sac. The majorities of children with these defects are asymptomatic and are diagnosed beyond the neonatal period. The diagnosis is usually made on chest radiograph when a child is evaluated for another reason. Theanteroposterior radiograph shows a structure behind the heart, and a lateral film localizes the mass to the retrosternal area. Chest CT will confirm the diagnosis. When symptoms occur, they can be recurrent respiratory infections, cough, vomiting, or reflux; in rare instances, incarceration may occur. Repair is recommended for all patients, in view of the risk of bowel strangulation, and can be accomplished laparoscopically or by an open approach. Prosthetic material is rarely required.

95.10 Paraesophageal Hernia

Akhil Maheshwari and Waldemar A. Carlo

Paraesophageal hernia is differentiated from hiatal hernia in that the gastroesophageal junction is in the normal location. The herniation of the stomach alongside or adjacent to the gastroesophageal junction is prone to incarceration with strangulation and perforation. A previous Nissen fundoplication and other diaphragmatic procedures are risk factors. This unusual diaphragmatic hernia should be repaired promptly after identification.

95.11 Eventration

Akhil Maheshwari and Waldemar A. Carlo

Eventration of the diaphragm is an abnormal elevation, consisting of a thinned diaphragmatic muscle that causes elevation of the entire hemidiaphragm or, more commonly, the anterior aspect of the hemidiaphragm. This elevation produces a paradoxical motion of the affected hemidiaphragm. Most eventrations are asymptomatic and do not require repair. A congenital form is the result of either incomplete development of the muscular portion or central tendon or abnormal development of the phrenic nerves. Congenital eventration may affect lung development, but it has not been associated with pulmonary hypoplasia. The **differential diagnosis** includes diaphragmatic paralysis, diaphragmatic hernia, traction injury, and iatrogenic injury after heart surgery. Eventration is also associated with pulmonary sequestration, congenital heart disease, and chromosomal trisomies. Most eventrations are asymptomatic and do not require repair. The indications for surgery include continued need for mechanical ventilation, recurrent infections, and failure to thrive. Large or symptomatic eventrations can be repaired by plication through an abdominal or thoracic approach that is minimally invasive.

BIBLIOGRAPHY

Please visit the Nelson Textbook of Pediatrics *website at www.expertconsult.com for the complete bibliography.*

95.12 Extrapulmonary Air Leaks (Pneumothorax, Pneumomediastinum, Pulmonary Interstitial Emphysema, Pneumopericardium)

Waldemar A. Carlo

Asymptomatic pneumothorax, usually unilateral, is estimated to occur in 1-2% of all newborn infants; symptomatic pneumothorax and pneumomediastinum are less common (Chapter 94). The incidence of pneumothorax is increased in infants with lung diseases such as meconium aspiration and RDS; in those who have undergone vigorous resuscitation or are receiving assisted ventilation, especially if high ventilator support is necessary; and in infants with urinary tract anomalies or oligohydramnios.

ETIOLOGY AND PATHOPHYSIOLOGY

The most common cause of pneumothorax is overinflation resulting in alveolar rupture. It may be "spontaneous" or may be due to underlying pulmonary disease, such as lobar emphysema or rupture of a congenital lung cyst or pneumatocele, to trauma, or to a "ball-valve" type of bronchial or bronchiolar obstruction resulting from aspiration.

Pneumothorax associated with **pulmonary hypoplasia** is common, tends to occur during the 1st hours after birth, and is due to reduced alveolar surface area and poorly compliant lungs. It is associated with disorders of decreased amniotic fluid volume (Potter syndrome, renal agenesis, renal dysplasia, chronic amniotic fluid leak), decreased fetal breathing movement (oligohydramnios, neuromuscular disease), pulmonary space-occupying lesions (diaphragmatic hernia, pleural effusion, chylothorax), and thoracic abnormalities (asphyxiating thoracic dystrophies).

Gas from a ruptured alveolus escapes into the interstitial spaces of the lung, where it may cause interstitial emphysema or dissect along the peribronchial and perivascular connective tissue sheaths to the hilum of the lung. If the volume of escaped air is great enough, it may collect in the mediastinal space (**pneumomediastinum**) or rupture into the pleural space (**pneumothorax**), subcutaneous tissue (**subcutaneous emphysema**), peritoneal cavity (**pneumoperitoneum**), and/or pericardial sac (**pneumopericardium**). Rarely, increased mediastinal pressure may compress the pulmonary veins at the hilum and thereby interfere with pulmonary venous return to the heart and cardiac output. On occasion, air may embolize into the circulation (**pulmonary air embolism**) and produce cutaneous blanching, air in intravascular catheters, an air-filled heart and vessels on chest roentgenograms, and death.

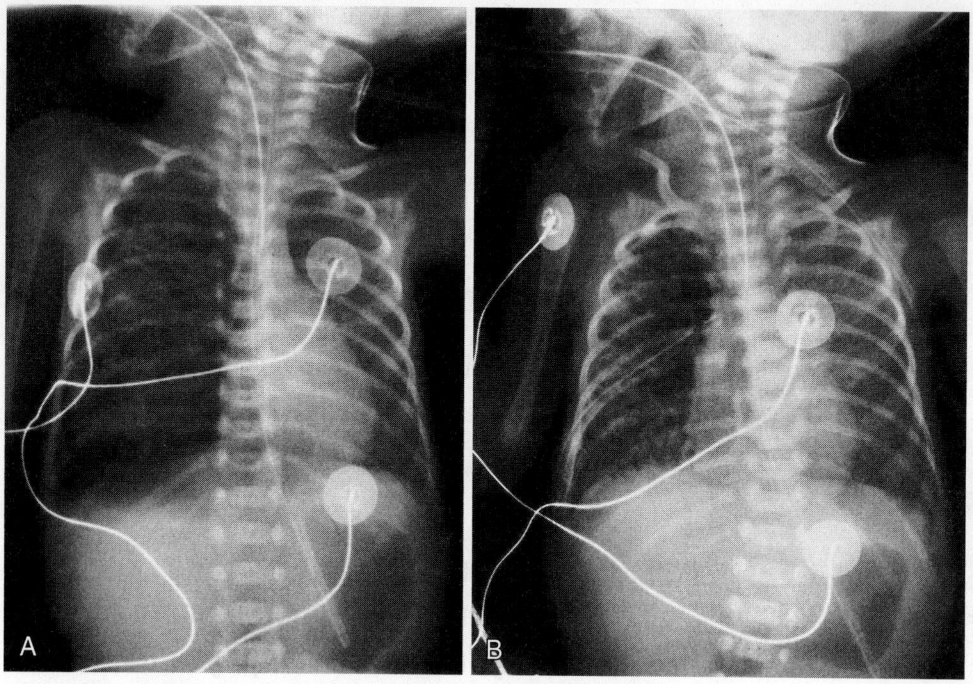

Figure 95-14 *A,* Right-sided tension pneumothorax and widespread right lung pulmonary interstitial emphysema in a preterm infant receiving intensive care. *B,* Resolution of pneumothorax with a chest tube in place. Pulmonary interstitial emphysema (PIE) persists. (From Meerstadt PWD, Gyll C: *Manual of neonatal emergency x-ray interpretation,* Philadelphia, 1994, WB Saunders, p 73.)

Tension pneumothorax occurs if an accumulation of air within the pleural space is sufficient to elevate intrapleural pressure above atmospheric pressure. Unilateral tension pneumothorax results in impaired ventilation not only in the ipsilateral lung but also in the contralateral lung owing to a shift in the mediastinum toward the contralateral side. Compression of the vena cava and torsion of the great vessels may interfere with venous return.

CLINICAL MANIFESTATIONS

The physical findings of a clinically asymptomatic **pneumothorax** are hyperresonance and diminished breath sounds over the involved side of the chest with or without tachypnea.

Symptomatic pneumothorax is characterized by respiratory distress, which varies from merely high respiratory rate to severe dyspnea, tachypnea, and cyanosis. Irritability and restlessness or apnea may be the earliest signs. The onset is usually sudden but may be gradual; an infant may rapidly become critically ill. The chest may appear asymmetric with an increased anteroposterior diameter and bulging of the intercostal spaces on the affected side; other signs may be hyperresonance and diminished or absence of breath sounds. The heart is displaced toward the unaffected side, resulting in displacement of the cardiac apex and point of maximal impulse (PMI) of the heart. The diaphragm is displaced downward, as is the liver with right-sided pneumothorax, and may result in abdominal distention. Because pneumothorax may be bilateral in approximately 10% of patients, symmetry of findings does not rule it out. In tension pneumothorax, signs of shock may be noted.

Pneumomediastinum occurs in at least 25% of patients with pneumothorax and is usually asymptomatic. The degree of respiratory distress depends on the amount of trapped gas. If it is great, bulging of the midthoracic area is observed, the neck veins are distended, and blood pressure is low. The last two findings are a result of tamponade of the systemic and pulmonary veins. Although often asymptomatic, subcutaneous emphysema in newborn infants is almost pathognomonic of pneumomediastinum.

Pulmonary interstitial emphysema may precede the development of a pneumothorax or may occur independently and lead to increasing respiratory distress as a result of decreased compliance, hypercapnia, and hypoxia. The last is due to an increased alveolar-arterial oxygen gradient and intrapulmonary shunting. Progressive enlargement of blebs of gas may result in cystic dilatation and respiratory deterioration resembling pneumothorax. In severe cases, PIE precedes the development of BPD. Avoidance of high inspiratory or mean airway pressures may prevent the development of PIE. Treatment may include bronchoscopy in patients with evidence of mucous plugging, selective intubation and ventilation of the uninvolved bronchus, oxygen, general respiratory care, and HFV.

DIAGNOSIS

Pneumothorax and other air leaks should be suspected in newborn infants who show signs of respiratory distress, are restless or irritable, or have a sudden change in condition. The diagnosis of pneumothorax is established by radiography, with the edge of the collapsed lung standing out in relief against the pneumothorax (Fig. 95-14); pneumomediastinum is signified by hyperlucency around the heart border and between the sternum and the heart border (Fig. 95-15). Transillumination of the thorax is often helpful in the emergency diagnosis of pneumothorax; the affected side transmits excessive light. Associated renal anomalies are identified by ultrasonography. Pulmonary hypoplasia is suggested by signs of uterine compression (extremity contractures), a small thorax on chest roentgenograms, severe hypoxia with hypercapnia, and signs of the primary disease (hypotonia, diaphragmatic hernia, Potter syndrome).

Pneumopericardium may be asymptomatic, requiring only general supportive treatment, but it usually manifests as sudden shock with tachycardia, muffled heart sounds, and poor pulses suggesting tamponade. **Pneumoperitoneum** from air dissecting through the diaphragmatic apertures during mechanical ventilation may be confused with intestinal perforation. Paracentesis can be helpful in differentiating the two conditions. The presence of organisms on Gram stain of intestinal contents suggests the latter. Occasionally, pneumoperitoneum can result in an abdominal compartment syndrome requiring decompression.

TREATMENT

Without a continued air leak, asymptomatic and mildly symptomatic small pneumothoraces require only close observation. Conservative management of a pneumothorax is effective even in

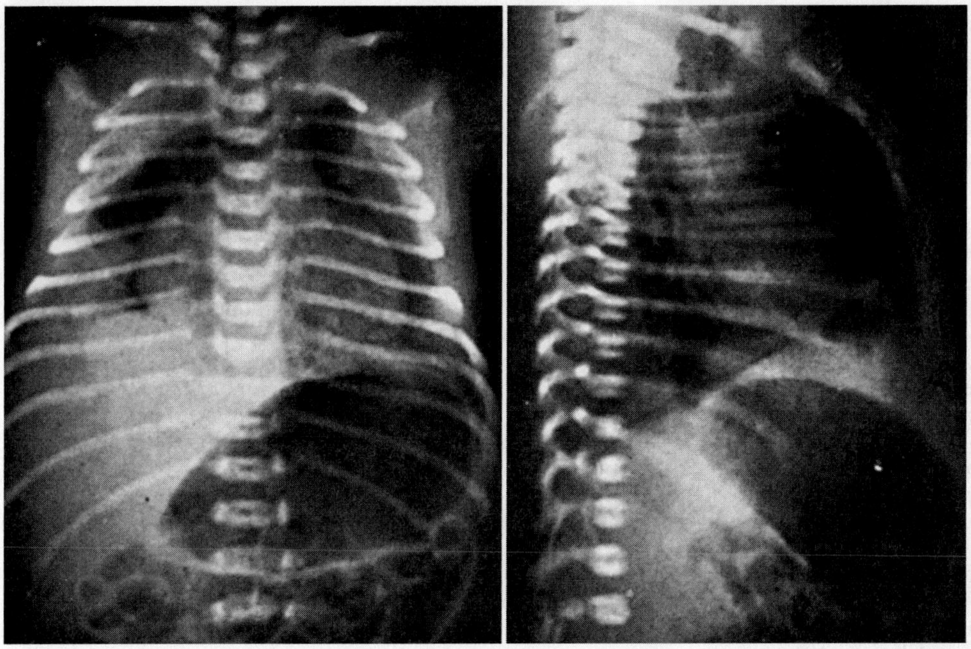

Figure 95-15 Pneumomediastinum in a newborn infant. The anteroposterior view (*left*) demonstrates compression of the lungs, and the lateral view (*right*) shows bulging of the sternum, each resulting from distention of the mediastinum by trapped air.

selected infants requiring ventilatory support. Frequent small feedings may prevent gastric dilatation and minimize crying, which can further compromise ventilation and worsen the pneumothorax. Breathing 100% oxygen in term infants accelerates the resorption of free pleural air into blood by reducing the nitrogen tension in blood and producing a resultant nitrogen pressure gradient from the trapped gas in the blood, but the clinical effectiveness is not proven and the benefit must be weighed against the risks of oxygen toxicity. With severe respiratory or circulatory embarrassment, emergency aspiration using a soft small catheter introduced with a needle is indicated. Either immediately or after catheter aspiration, a chest tube should be inserted and attached to underwater seal drainage (see Fig. 95-14). If the air leak is ongoing, continuous suction (–5 to –20 cm H_2O) may be needed to evacuate the pneumothorax completely. A pneumopericardium requires prompt evacuation of entrapped air. Severe localized interstitial emphysema may respond to selective bronchial intubation. Judicious use of sedation in an infant fighting a ventilator may reduce the risk of pneumothorax. Surfactant therapy for RDS reduces the incidence of pneumothorax.

BIBLIOGRAPHY

Please visit the Nelson Textbook of Pediatrics *website at www.expertconsult.com for the complete bibliography.*

95.13 Pulmonary Hemorrhage

Namasivayam Ambalavanan and Waldemar A. Carlo

Massive pulmonary hemorrhage is a relatively uncommon, but catastrophic complication with a high risk of morbidity and mortality. Some degree of pulmonary hemorrhage occurs in about 10% of extremely preterm infants. However, massive pulmonary hemorrhage is less common and can be fatal. Autopsy demonstrates massive pulmonary hemorrhage in 15% of neonates who die in the 1st 2 wk of life. The reported incidence at autopsy varies from 1 to 4/ 1,000 live births. About 75% of affected patients weigh <2,500 g at birth. Prophylactic indomethacin in ELBW infants reduces the incidence of pulmonary hemorrhage.

Most infants with pulmonary hemorrhage have had symptoms of respiratory distress that are indistinguishable from those of RDS. The onset may occur at birth or may be delayed several days. Hemorrhagic pulmonary edema is the source of blood in many cases and is associated with significant ductal shunting and high pulmonary blood flow or severe left-sided heart failure resulting from hypoxia. In severe cases, cardiovascular collapse, poor lung compliance, profound cyanosis, and hypercapnia may be present. Radiographic findings are varied and nonspecific, ranging from minor streaking or patchy infiltrates to massive consolidation.

The incidence of pulmonary hemorrhage is increased in association with acute pulmonary infection, severe asphyxia, RDS, assisted ventilation, PDA, congenital heart disease, erythroblastosis fetalis, hemorrhagic disease of the newborn, thrombocytopenia, inborn errors of ammonia metabolism, and cold injury. Pulmonary hemorrhage is the only severe complication whose rate is *increased* with surfactant treatment. Pulmonary hemorrhage is seen with all surfactants; the incidence ranges from 1-5% of treated infants and is higher with natural surfactant. Bleeding is predominantly alveolar in about 65% of cases and interstitial in the rest. Bleeding into other organs is observed at autopsy of severely ill neonates, suggesting the possibility of an additional bleeding diathesis such as disseminated intravascular coagulation.

Treatment of pulmonary hemorrhage includes blood replacement, suctioning to clear the airway, intratracheal administration of epinephrine, and, in some cases, HFV. Although surfactant treatment has been associated with the development of pulmonary hemorrhage, administration of exogenous surfactant after the bleeding has occurred can improve lung compliance, because the presence of intra-alveolar blood and protein can inactivate surfactant.

Acute pulmonary hemorrhage may rarely occur in previously healthy full-term infants. The cause is unknown. Pulmonary hemorrhage may manifest as hemoptysis or blood in the nasopharynx or airway with no evidence of upper respiratory or gastrointestinal bleeding. Patients present with acute, severe respiratory failure requiring mechanical ventilation. Chest radiographs usually demonstrate bilateral alveolar infiltrates. The condition usually responds to intensive supportive treatment (Chapter 401).

BIBLIOGRAPHY

Please visit the Nelson Textbook of Pediatrics *website at www.expertconsult.com for the complete bibliography.*

Chapter 96
Digestive System Disorders

Akhil Maheshwari and Waldemar A. Carlo

VOMITING

Vomiting or, more often, regurgitation is a relatively frequent symptom during the neonatal period. In the 1st few hours after birth, infants may vomit mucus, occasionally blood streaked. This vomiting rarely persists after the 1st few feedings; it may be due to irritation of the gastric mucosa by material swallowed during delivery. If vomiting is protracted, gastric lavage with physiologic saline solution may relieve it.

When vomiting occurs shortly after birth and is persistent, the possibilities of intestinal obstruction, metabolic disorders, and increased intracranial pressure must be considered. A history of maternal polyhydramnios suggests upper gastrointestinal (esophageal, duodenal, ileal) atresia. Bile-stained emesis suggests intestinal obstruction beyond the duodenum but may also be idiopathic. Abdominal radiographs (kidney-ureter-bladder [KUB] and cross-table lateral views) should be performed in neonates with persistent emesis and in all infants with bile-stained emesis to detect air-fluid levels, distended bowel loops, characteristic patterns of obstruction (double bubble: duodenal atresia), and pneumoperitoneum (intestinal perforation). A contrast swallow roentgenogram with small bowel follow-through is indicated in the presence of bilious emesis.

Obstructive lesions of the digestive tract are the most frequent gastrointestinal anomalies (Chapters 311, 321, 322, and 324). Vomiting (and drooling) from esophageal obstruction occurs with the 1st feeding. The diagnosis of esophageal atresia can be suspected if unusual drooling from the mouth is observed and if resistance is encountered during an attempt to pass a catheter into the stomach. The diagnosis should be made before the infant has trouble with oral feedings and aspiration pneumonia develops. Infantile achalasia (cardiospasm), a rare cause of vomiting in newborn infants, is demonstrable radiographically as obstruction at the cardiac end of the esophagus without organic stenosis. Regurgitation of feedings because of continuous relaxation of the esophageal-gastric sphincter, or chalasia, is a cause of vomiting. Keeping the infant in a semi-upright position, thickening the feeding, or administering prokinetic drugs can control it.

Vomiting due to obstruction of the small intestine usually begins on the 1st day of life and is frequent, persistent, usually nonprojectile, copious, and, unless the obstruction is above the ampulla of Vater, bile-stained; it is associated with abdominal distention, visible deep peristaltic waves, and reduction or absence of bowel movements. Malrotation with obstruction from **midgut volvulus** is an acute emergency that must be not only considered but also urgently evaluated by an upper gastrointestinal contrast radiographic series. Radiographs of the abdomen show the distribution of air in the intestine, which may point to the anatomic location of an obstruction; malrotation can be identified only by contrast studies. Normally, air can be demonstrated by radiographs in the jejunum by 15-60 min, in the ileum by 2-3 hr, and in the colon by 3 hr after birth. Absence of rectal gas at 24 hr is abnormal. Persistent vomiting may occur with congenital diaphragmatic hernia. The vomiting associated with pyloric stenosis may begin any time after birth but does not assume its characteristic pattern before the 2nd-3rd wk. Vomiting with obstipation is a common early sign of **Hirschsprung disease.** Vomiting may occur with many other disturbances that do not obstruct the digestive tract, such as milk allergy, adrenal hyperplasia of the salt-losing variety, galactosemia, hyperammonemias, organic acidemias, increased intracranial pressure, septicemia, meningitis, and urinary tract infection. In many infants, it is simply regurgitation from overfeeding or from failure to permit the infant to eructate swallowed air. (See Chapter 315 for a discussion of gastric emptying and gastroesophageal reflux.)

DIARRHEA

See Chapters 332 and 333.

CONSTIPATION

More than 90% of full-term newborn infants pass meconium within the 1st 24 hr. The possibility of intestinal obstruction should be considered in any infant who does not pass meconium by 24-36 hr. Intestinal atresia, stricture, or stenosis; Hirschsprung disease; milk bolus obstruction; meconium ileus; or meconium plugs may manifest as constipation or, more often, obstipation. About 20% of very low birthweight (VLBW) infants do not pass meconium within the 1st 24 hr. Constipation not present from birth but appearing during the 1st mo of life may be a sign of short-segment congenital aganglionic megacolon, hypothyroidism, strictures after necrotizing enterocolitis (NEC), or anal stenosis. It must be kept in mind that infrequent bowel movements do not necessarily mean constipation. A breast-fed infant usually has frequent bowel movements, whereas a formula-fed infant may have 1-2 movements a day or every other day.

MECONIUM PLUGS

Lower colonic or anorectal plugs (Fig. 96-1) with a lower than normal water content may cause intestinal obstruction. Rarely, a firm mass of meconium may form elsewhere in the intestine and cause intrauterine intestinal obstruction and meconium peritonitis unrelated to cystic fibrosis (CF). Anorectal plugs may also cause mucosal ulceration and intestinal perforation. **Meconium plugs** are associated with small left colon syndrome in infants of diabetic mothers and with CF, rectal aganglionosis, maternal opiate use, and magnesium sulfate therapy for preeclampsia. The plug may be evacuated by glycerin suppository or rectal irrigation with isotonic saline. Enemas with the iodinated contrast medium Gastrografin usually induce passage of the plug, presumably because the high osmolarity (1,900 mOsm/L) of the solution draws fluid rapidly into the intestinal lumen and loosens inspissated material. Such rapid loss of fluid into the bowel may result in acute dehydration and shock, so it is advisable to dilute the contrast material with an equal amount of water, correct any existing dehydration, and provide intravenous fluids during and for several hours after the procedure. After removal of a

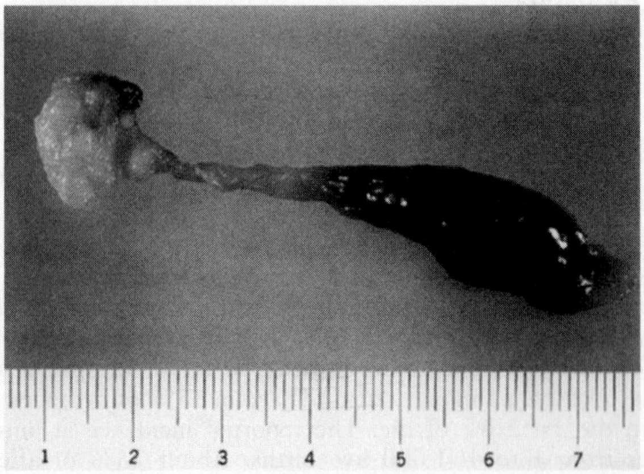

Figure 96-1 This plug of meconium and mucus (scale in cm) caused bowel obstruction in a premature infant. A radiograph showed marked gaseous distention and multiple fluid levels at 30 hr of age. Dramatic improvement occurred when the plug was passed after an enema. (From: The abnormal fetus. In Beischer NA, Mackay EV, Colditz PB, editors: *Obstetrics and the newborn*, ed 3, Philadelphia, 1997, WB Saunders.)

meconium plug, the infant should be observed closely for the possible presence of congenital aganglionic megacolon.

96.1 Meconium Ileus in Cystic Fibrosis

Akhil Maheshwari and Waldemar A. Carlo

Impaction of meconium causes intestinal obstructions and may be associated with CF. The absence of fetal pancreatic enzymes in CF limits normal digestive activities in the intestine, and meconium becomes viscid and mucilaginous. It clings to the intestinal wall and moves with difficulty. The inspissated and impacted meconium fills the intestinal canal but is most concentrated in the lower part of the ileum. Clinically, the pattern is that of congenital intestinal obstruction with or without intestinal perforation. Abdominal distention is prominent, and vomiting becomes persistent. Infrequently, one or more inspissated meconium stools may be passed shortly after birth.

The **differential diagnosis** involves other causes of intestinal obstruction, including intestinal pseudo-obstruction and other causes of pancreatic insufficiency (Chapter 341). A presumptive diagnosis can be made on the basis of a history of CF in a sibling, via palpation of doughy or cordlike masses of intestines through the abdominal wall, and from the radiographic appearance. In contrast to the generally evenly distended intestinal loops above an atresia, the loops may vary in width and are not as evenly filled with gas. At points of heaviest meconium concentration, the infiltrated gas may create a bubbly granular appearance (Figs. 96-2 and 96-3). It is technically difficult to perform a sweat test in a neonate. Genetic testing confirms the diagnosis of CF.

Treatment for meconium ileus is high Gastrografin enema as described previously for meconium plugs. If the procedure unsuccessful or perforation of the bowel wall is suspected, laparotomy is performed, and the ileum opened at the point of greatest diameter of the impaction. Approximately 50% of these infants have associated intestinal atresia, stenosis, or volvulus that requires surgery. The inspissated meconium is removed by gentle and patient irrigation with warm isotonic sodium chloride or acetylcysteine (Mucomyst) solution through a catheter passed between the impaction and the bowel wall. Most infants with meconium ileus survive the neonatal period. If meconium ileus is associated with CF, the long-term prognosis depends on the severity of the underlying disease (Chapter 395).

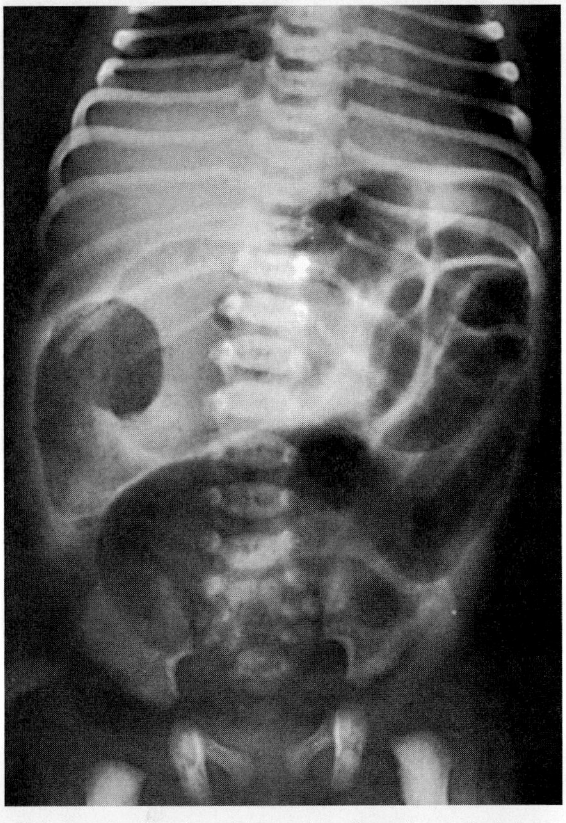

Figure 96-2 Meconium ileus. Impacted meconium with small amounts of air interspersed can be seen in loops of intestine on the right side of the abdomen. The intestinal loops above this impaction are greatly distended.

MECONIUM PERITONITIS

Perforation of the intestine may occur in utero or shortly after birth. Frequently, the intestinal perforation seals naturally with relatively little meconium leakage into the peritoneal cavity. In some cases, with long-standing perforation, meconium peritonitis is more pronounced. Perforations occur most often as a complication of meconium ileus in infants with CF but are occasionally due to a meconium plug or in utero intestinal obstruction of another cause. Cases at the most severe end of the spectrum may be diagnosed on prenatal ultrasonography with fetal ascites, polyhydramnios, bowel dilatation, intra-abdominal calcifications, and hydrops fetalis. At the other end are cases in which an intestinal perforation may seal spontaneously with only a minor meconium leak, so the event may never be detected except when meconium becomes calcified and is later discovered on radiographs of the abdomen. Alternatively, the clinical picture may be dominated by the signs of intestinal obstruction (as in meconium ileus) or chemical peritonitis. Characteristic clinical findings include abdominal distention, vomiting, and absence of stools. Treatment consists primarily of elimination of the intestinal obstruction and drainage of the peritoneal cavity.

96.2 Neonatal Necrotizing Enterocolitis

Akhil Maheshwari and Waldemar A. Carlo

NEC is the most common life-threatening emergency of the gastrointestinal tract in the newborn period. The disease is characterized by various degrees of mucosal or transmural necrosis of the intestine. The cause of NEC remains unclear but is most likely multifactorial. The incidence of NEC is 1-5% of infants in neonatal intensive care units (NICUs). Both incidence and case

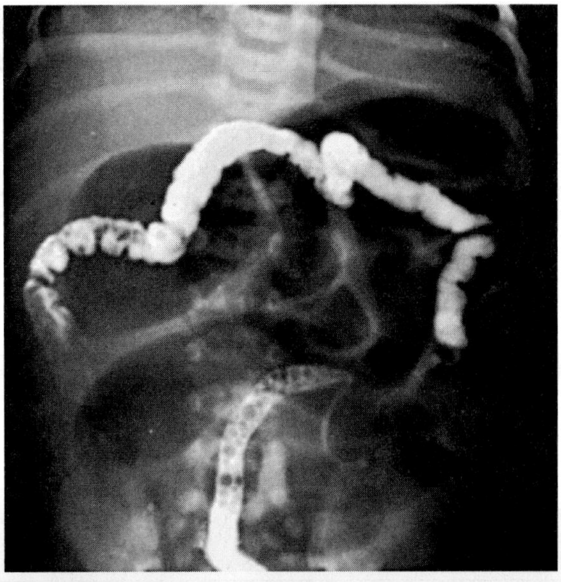

Figure 96-3 Meconium ileus. The colon, outlined by contrast material, is small because meconium has not reached it.

fatality rates increase with decreasing birthweight and gestational age. Because very small, ill preterm infants are particularly susceptible to NEC, a rising incidence may reflect improved survival of this high-risk group of patients.

PATHOLOGY AND PATHOGENESIS

Many factors may contribute to the development of a necrotic segment of intestine, gas accumulation in the submucosa of the bowel wall (**pneumatosis intestinalis**), and progression of the necrosis to perforation, peritonitis, sepsis, and death. The distal part of the ileum and the proximal segment of colon are involved most frequently; in fatal cases, gangrene may extend from the stomach to the rectum. Although NEC is a multifactorial disease primarily associated with intestinal immaturity, the concept of "risk factors" for NEC is controversial. The triad of intestinal ischemia (injury), enteral nutrition (metabolic substrate), and bacterial translocation has classically been linked to NEC. The greatest risk factor for NEC is prematurity. The disorder probably results from an interaction between loss of mucosal integrity due to a variety of factors (ischemia, infection, inflammation) and the host's response to that injury (circulatory, immunologic, inflammatory), leading to necrosis of the affected area. Coagulation necrosis is the characteristic histologic finding in intestinal specimens. Clustering of cases suggests a primary role for an infectious agent. Various bacterial and viral agents, including *Escherichia coli, Klebsiella, Clostridium perfringens, Staphylococcus epidermidis,* astrovirus, norovirus, and rotavirus, have been recovered from cultures. Nonetheless, in most situations, no pathogen is identified. NEC rarely occurs before the initiation of enteral feeding and is much less common in infants fed human milk. Aggressive enteral feeding may predispose to the development of NEC.

Although nearly 90% of all cases of NEC occur in premature infants, the disease can occur in full-term neonates. NEC in term infants is often a "secondary" disease, seen more frequently in infants with history of birth asphyxia, Down syndrome, congenital heart disease, rotavirus infections, and Hirschsprung disease.

CLINICAL MANIFESTATIONS

Infants with NEC have a variety of signs and symptoms and may have an insidious or sudden catastrophic onset (Table 96-1). The onset of NEC is usually in the 2nd or 3rd week of life but can be as late as 3 mo in VLBW infants. Age of onset is inversely related to gestational age. The 1st signs of impending disease may be nonspecific, including lethargy and temperature instability, or related to gastrointestinal pathology, such as abdominal distention and gastric retention. Obvious bloody stools are seen in 25% of patients. Because of nonspecific signs, sepsis may be suspected before NEC. The spectrum of illness is broad, ranging from mild disease with only guaiac-positive stools to severe illness with bowel perforation, peritonitis, systemic inflammatory response syndrome, shock, and death. Progression may be rapid, but it is unusual for the disease to progress from mild to severe after 72 hr.

Table 96-1 SIGNS AND SYMPTOMS ASSOCIATED WITH NECROTIZING ENTEROCOLITIS

GASTROINTESTINAL
Abdominal distention
Abdominal tenderness
Feeding intolerance
Delayed gastric emptying
Vomiting
Occult/gross blood in stool
Change in stool pattern/diarrhea
Abdominal mass
Erythema of abdominal wall
SYSTEMIC
Lethargy
Apnea/respiratory distress
Temperature instability
"Not right"
Acidosis (metabolic and/or respiratory)
Glucose instability
Poor perfusion/shock
Disseminated intravascular coagulopathy
Positive results of blood cultures

From Kanto WP Jr, Hunter JE, Stoll BJ: Recognition and medical management of necrotizing enterocolitis, *Clin Perinatol* 21:335–346, 1994.

DIAGNOSIS

A very high index of suspicion in treating preterm at-risk infants is crucial. Plain abdominal radiographs are essential to make a diagnosis of NEC. The finding of pneumatosis intestinalis (air in the bowel wall) confirms the clinical suspicion of NEC and is diagnostic; 50-75% of patients have pneumatosis when treatment is started (Fig. 96-4). Portal venous gas is a sign of severe disease, and pneumoperitoneum indicates a perforation (Figs. 96-4 and 96-5). Hepatic ultrasonography may detect portal venous gas despite normal abdominal roentgenograms.

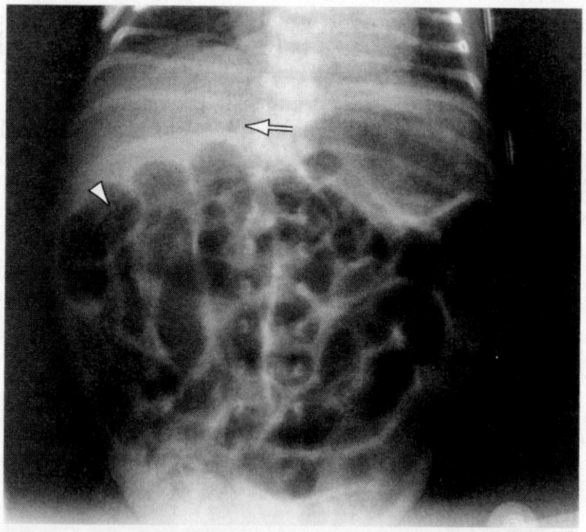

Figure 96-4 Necrotizing enterocolitis. A kidney-ureter-bladder film demonstrates abdominal distention, hepatic portal venous gas *(arrow)*, and a bubbly appearance of pneumatosis intestinalis (*arrowhead;* right lower quadrant). The latter two signs are thought to be pathognomonic for neonatal necrotizing enterocolitis.

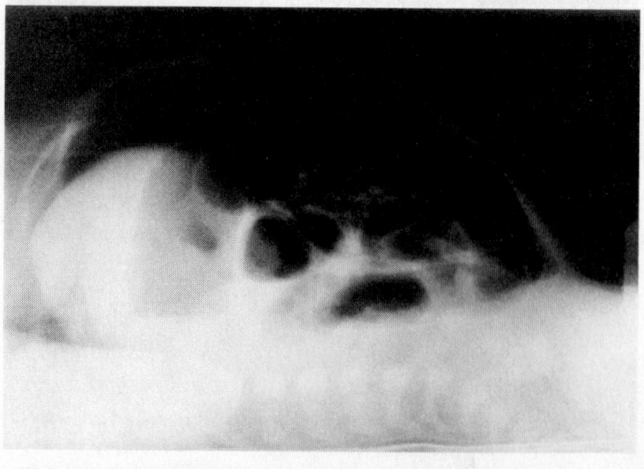

Figure 96-5 Intestinal perforation. A cross-table abdominal roentgenogram in a patient with a neonatal necrotizing enterocolitis demonstrates marked distention and massive pneumoperitoneum as evidenced by the free air below the anterior abdominal wall.

The **differential diagnosis** of NEC includes specific infections (systemic or intestinal), gastrointestinal obstruction, volvulus, and isolated intestinal perforation. Idiopathic focal intestinal perforation can occur spontaneously or after the early use of postnatal steroids and indomethacin. Pneumoperitoneum develops in such patients, but they are usually less ill than those with NEC.

TREATMENT

Rapid initiation of therapy is required for suspected as well as proven cases of NEC. There is no definitive treatment for established NEC, so, therapy is directed at giving supportive care and preventing further injury with cessation of feeding, nasogastric decompression, and administration of intravenous fluids. Careful attention to respiratory status, coagulation profile, and acid-base and electrolyte balances are important. Once blood has been drawn for culture, systemic antibiotics (with broad coverage based on the antibiotic sensitivity patterns of the gram-positive, gram-negative, and anaerobic organisms in the particular NICU) should be started immediately. If present, umbilical catheters should be removed, but good intravenous access is maintained. Ventilation should be assisted in the presence of apnea or if abdominal distention is contributing to hypoxia and hypercapnia. Intravascular volume replacement with crystalloid or blood products, cardiovascular support with fluid boluses and/or inotropes, and correction of hematologic, metabolic, and electrolyte abnormalities are essential to stabilize the infant with NEC.

The patient's course should be monitored closely by means of frequent physical assessments; sequential anteroposterior and cross-table lateral or lateral decubitus abdominal radiographs to detect intestinal perforation; and serial determinations of hematologic, electrolyte, and acid-base status. Gown and glove isolation and grouping of infants at similar increased risks into cohorts separate from other infants should be instituted to contain an epidemic.

A surgeon should be consulted early in the course of treatment. **Indications for surgery** include evidence of perforation on abdominal roentgenograms (pneumoperitoneum) or positive result of abdominal paracentesis (stool or organism on Gram stain preparation from peritoneal fluid). Failure of medical management, a single fixed bowel loop on radiographs, abdominal wall erythema, and a palpable mass are relative indications for exploratory laparotomy. Ideally, surgery should be performed after intestinal necrosis develops but before perforation and peritonitis occur. In unstable premature infants with perforated NEC, **peritoneal drainage** can be cautiously considered as an alternative to **exploratory laparotomy**, although the best surgical approach in these infants remains unresolved. The type of surgical operation did not influence survival or other clinically important early outcomes in one multicenter study, but another large randomized trial showed that a majority of infants who were initially treated with peritoneal drains required a delayed secondary laparotomy. There are also some concerns about the long-term outcome (death or neurodevelopmental outcome) for infants treated with peritoneal drainage.

Patients with isolated intestinal perforation tend to have a lower birthweight, are less likely to be receiving oral feeding, and are prone to perforation at an earlier postnatal age than are patients with perforation related to NEC. In many patients with isolated intestinal perforation treated by drainage, no further surgical procedure is needed; a small subgroup may require later surgery to repair an intestinal stricture or fistula.

PROGNOSIS

Medical management fails in about 20-40% of patients with pneumatosis intestinalis at diagnosis; of these, 10-30% die. Early postoperative complications include wound infection, dehiscence, and stomal problems (prolapse, necrosis). Later complications include **intestinal strictures**, which develop at the site of the necrotizing lesion in about 10% of surgically or medically managed patients. Resection of the obstructing stricture is curative. After massive intestinal resection, complications from postoperative NEC include **short-bowel syndrome** (malabsorption, growth failure, malnutrition), complications related to central venous catheters (sepsis, thrombosis), and cholestatic jaundice. Premature infants with NEC who require surgical intervention or who have concomitant bacteremia are at increased risk for adverse growth and neurodevelopmental outcome.

PREVENTION

Newborns exclusively breast-fed have a reduced risk of NEC. There have been concerns about early and aggressive increase in feeding volumes in raising the risk of NEC in VLBW infants, although a safe feeding regimen remains unknown. Gut stimulation protocols consisting of minimal enteral feeds followed by judicious volume advancement decreased the incidence of NEC in smaller study cohorts, but significant benefits were not detected in a meta-analysis of all randomized studies. Prophylactic enteral antibiotics can reduce the risk of NEC, although concerns about adverse outcomes persist, particularly related to the development of resistant bacteria. Probiotic preparations may also decrease the incidence of NEC; enteral supplementation of probiotics reduces the risk of severe NEC (stage II or higher) and mortality in preterm infants. The safety and efficacy of these supplements needs further evaluation in infants <1,000 g birthweight.

BIBLIOGRAPHY

Please visit the Nelson Textbook of Pediatrics *website at www.expertconsult.com for the complete bibliography.*

96.3 Jaundice and Hyperbilirubinemia in the Newborn

Namasivayam Ambalavanan and Waldemar A. Carlo

Hyperbilirubinemia is a common and, in most cases, benign problem in neonates. Jaundice is observed during the 1st wk of life in approximately 60% of term infants and 80% of preterm infants. The yellow color usually results from the accumulation of unconjugated, nonpolar, lipid-soluble bilirubin pigment in the skin. This unconjugated bilirubin (designated **indirect-acting** by nature of the Van den Bergh reaction) is an end product of hemeprotein catabolism from a series of enzymatic reactions by hemeoxygenase and biliverdin reductase and nonenzymatic reducing agents in the reticuloendothelial cells. It may also be due in part to deposition of pigment from conjugated bilirubin, the end product from indirect, unconjugated bilirubin that has undergone conjugation in the liver cell microsome by the enzyme uridine diphosphoglucuronic acid (UDP)–glucuronyl transferase to form the polar, water-soluble glucuronide of bilirubin (**direct-reacting**). Although bilirubin may have a physiologic role as an antioxidant, elevations of indirect, unconjugated bilirubin are potentially neurotoxic. Even though the conjugated form is not neurotoxic, direct hyperbilirubinemia indicates a potentially serious hepatic disorders or a systemic illness.

ETIOLOGY

During the neonatal period, metabolism of bilirubin is in transition from the fetal stage, during which the placenta is the principal route of elimination of the lipid-soluble, unconjugated bilirubin, to the adult stage, during which the water-soluble conjugated form is excreted from hepatic cells into the biliary system and gastrointestinal tract. Unconjugated hyperbilirubinemia may be caused or increased by any factor that (1) increases the load of bilirubin to be metabolized by the liver (hemolytic anemias, polycythemia, bruising or internal hemorrhage, shortened red blood cell life as a result of immaturity or transfusion of cells, increased enterohepatic circulation, infection); (2) damages or reduces the activity of the transferase enzyme or other related enzymes (genetic deficiency, hypoxia, infection, thyroid deficiency); (3) competes for or blocks the transferase enzyme (drugs and other substances requiring glucuronic acid conjugation); or (4) leads to an absence or decreased amounts of the enzyme or to reduction of bilirubin uptake by liver cells (genetic defect, and prematurity). The toxic effects of elevated serum concentrations of unconjugated bilirubin are increased by factors that reduce the retention of bilirubin in the circulation (hypoproteinemia, displacement of bilirubin from its binding sites on albumin by competitive binding of drugs such as sulfisoxazole and moxalactam, acidosis, and increased free fatty acid concentration secondary to hypoglycemia, starvation, or hypothermia). Neurotoxic effects are directly related not only to the permeability of the blood-brain barrier and nerve cell membranes but also to neuronal susceptibility to injury, all of which are adversely influenced by asphyxia, prematurity, hyperosmolality, and infection. Early and frequent feeding decreases, whereas breast-feeding and dehydration increase, serum levels of bilirubin. Delay in passage of meconium, which contains 1 mg bilirubin/dL, may contribute to jaundice by enterohepatic recirculation after deconjugation by intestinal glucuronidase (Fig. 96-6). Drugs such as oxytocin (in the mother) and chemicals used in the nursery such as phenolic detergents may also produce unconjugated hyperbilirubinemia. Risk factors for unconjugated hyperbilirubinemia are listed in Table 96-2. Additional risk factors include polycythemia, infection, prematurity, and having a diabetic mother.

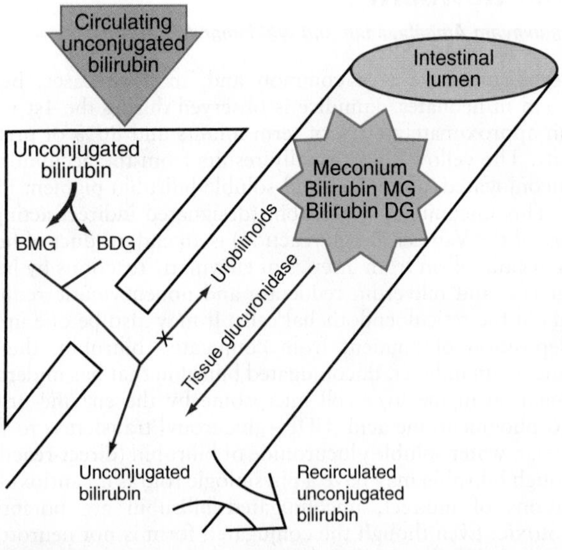

Figure 96-6 The neonatal production rate of bilirubin is 6-8 mg/kg/24 hr (in contrast to 3-4 mg/kg/24 hr in adults). Water-insoluble bilirubin is bound to albumin. At the plasma-hepatocyte interface, a liver membrane carrier (bilitranslocase) transports bilirubin to a cytosolic binding protein (ligandin or Y protein, now known to be glutathione S-transferase), which prevents back-absorption to plasma. Bilirubin is converted to bilirubin monoglucuronide (BMG). Neonates excrete more BMG than adults do. In the fetus, conjugated lipid-insoluble BMG and bilirubin diglucoronide (BDG) must be deconjugated by tissue β-glucuronidases to facilitate placental transfer of lipid-soluble unconjugated bilirubin across the placental lipid membranes. After birth, intestinal or milk-containing glucuronidases contribute to the enterohepatic recirculation of bilirubin and possibly to the development of hyperbilirubinemia.

CLINICAL MANIFESTATIONS

Jaundice may be present at birth or may appear at any time during the neonatal period, depending on etiology. Jaundice usually becomes apparent in a cephalocaudal progression, starting on the face and progressing to the abdomen and then the feet, as serum levels increase. Dermal pressure may reveal the anatomic progression of jaundice (face, ≈5 mg/dL; mid-abdomen, ≈15 mg/dL; soles, ≈20 mg/dL), but clinical examination cannot be depended on to estimate serum levels. Jaundice to the mid-abdomen, signs or symptoms, high-risk factors that suggest nonphysiologic jaundice, or hemolysis must be evaluated further (Tables 96-2 and 96-3). Noninvasive techniques for transcutaneous measurement of bilirubin (TcB) that correlate with serum levels may be used to screen infants, but determination of serum bilirubin level is indicated in patients with elevated age-specific transcutaneous bilirubin measurement, progressing jaundice, or risk for either hemolysis or sepsis. Whereas jaundice from deposition of indirect bilirubin in the skin tends to appear bright yellow or orange, jaundice of the obstructive type (direct bilirubin) has a greenish or muddy yellow cast. Infants with severe hyperbilirubinemia may present with lethargy and poor feeding and, without treatment, can progress to acute bilirubin encephalopathy (kernicterus) (Chapter 96.4).

DIFFERENTIAL DIAGNOSIS

Jaundice, consisting of either indirect or direct bilirubin, that is present at birth or appears within the 1st 24 hr of life requires immediate attention and may be due to erythroblastosis fetalis, concealed hemorrhage, sepsis, or congenital infections, including syphilis, cytomegalovirus, rubella, and toxoplasmosis. Hemolysis is suggested by a rapid rise in serum bilirubin concentration (>0.5 mg/dL/hr), anemia, pallor, reticulocytosis,

Table 96-2 RISK FACTORS FOR DEVELOPMENT OF SEVERE HYPERBILIRUBINEMIA IN INFANTS ≥35 WEEKS OF GESTATION (IN APPROXIMATE ORDER OF IMPORTANCE)

MAJOR RISK FACTORS
Predischarge TSB or TcB level in the high-risk zone (see Fig. 96-8)
Jaundice observed in the first 24 hr
Blood group incompatibility with positive direct antiglobulin test, other known hemolytic disease (glucose-6-phosphate dehydrogenase deficiency), elevated end-title CO concentration
Gestational age 35-36 wk
Previous sibling received phototherapy
Cephalohematoma or significant bruising
Exclusive breast-feeding, particularly if nursing is not going well and weight loss is excessive
East Asian race*
MINOR RISK FACTORS
Predischarge TSB or TcB level in the high intermediate-risk zone
Gestational age 37-38 wk
Jaundice observed before discharge
Previous sibling with jaundice
Macrosomic infant of a diabetic mother
Maternal age ≥25 yr
Male gender
DECREASED RISK (these factors are associated with decreased risk of significant jaundice, listed in order of decreasing importance)
TSB or TcB level in the low-risk zone (see Fig. 96-8)
Gestational age ≥41 wk
Exclusive bottle-feeding
Black race
Discharge from hospital after 72 hr

*Race as defined by mother's description.
TcB, transcutaneous bilirubin; TSB, total serum bilirubin.
From AAP Subcommittee on Hyperbilirubinemia: Management of hyperbilirubinemia in the newborn infant 35 or more weeks of gestation, *Pediatrics* 114:297–316, 2004.

hepatosplenomegaly, and a positive family history. An unusually high proportion of direct-reacting bilirubin may characterize jaundice in infants who have received intrauterine transfusions for erythroblastosis fetalis. Jaundice that first appears on the 2nd or 3rd day is usually **physiologic** but may represent a more severe form. Familial nonhemolytic icterus (**Crigler-Najjar syndrome**) and early-onset breast-feeding jaundice are seen initially on the 2nd or 3rd day. Jaundice appearing after the 3rd day and within the first week suggests bacterial sepsis or urinary tract infection; it may also be due to other infections, notably syphilis, toxoplasmosis, cytomegalovirus, and enterovirus. Jaundice secondary to extensive ecchymosis or blood extravasation may occur during the 1st day or later, especially in premature infants. Polycythemia may also lead to early jaundice.

There is a long differential diagnosis for jaundice first recognized *after* the 1st wk of life, including breast milk jaundice, septicemia, congenital atresia or paucity of the bile ducts, hepatitis, galactosemia, hypothyroidism, cystic fibrosis, and congenital hemolytic anemia crises related to red blood cell morphology and enzyme deficiencies (Fig. 96-7). The differential diagnosis for persistent jaundice during the first month of life includes hyperalimentation-associated cholestasis, hepatitis, cytomegalic inclusion disease, syphilis, toxoplasmosis, familial nonhemolytic icterus, congenital atresia of the bile ducts, galactosemia, and inspissated bile syndrome following hemolytic disease of the newborn. Rarely, physiologic jaundice may be prolonged for several weeks, as in infants with hypothyroidism or pyloric stenosis.

Full-term, low-risk, asymptomatic infants with jaundice may be evaluated by monitoring of total serum bilirubin (TSB) levels. Regardless of gestation or time of appearance of jaundice, patients with significant hyperbilirubinemia and those with symptoms or signs require a complete diagnostic evaluation, which includes determination of direct and indirect bilirubin fractions, hemoglobin, reticulocyte count, blood type, Coombs test, and examination of a peripheral blood smear. Indirect hyperbilirubinemia, reticulocytosis, and a smear with evidence of red blood cell destruction suggest hemolysis (see Table 96-3). In the absence of blood group incompatibility, nonimmunologically induced hemolysis should be considered. If the reticulocyte count, Coombs test result, and direct bilirubin value are normal, physiologic or pathologic indirect hyperbilirubinemia may be present (see Fig. 96-7). If direct hyperbilirubinemia is present, hepatitis, congenital bile duct disorders (atresia, paucity, Byler disease), cholestasis, inborn errors of metabolism, cystic fibrosis, and sepsis are diagnostic possibilities.

PHYSIOLOGIC JAUNDICE (ICTERUS NEONATORUM)

Under normal circumstances, the level of indirect bilirubin in umbilical cord serum is 1-3 mg/dL and rises at a rate of <5 mg/dL/24 hr; thus, jaundice becomes visible on the 2nd or 3rd day, usually peaking between the 2nd and 4th days at 5-6 mg/dL and decreasing to <2 mg/dL between the 5th and 7th days of life. Jaundice associated with these changes is designated *physiologic* and is believed to be the result of increased bilirubin production from the breakdown of fetal red blood cells combined with transient limitation in the conjugation of bilirubin by the immature neonatal liver.

Overall, 6-7% of full-term infants have indirect bilirubin levels >13 mg/dL and less than 3% have levels >15 mg/dL. Risk

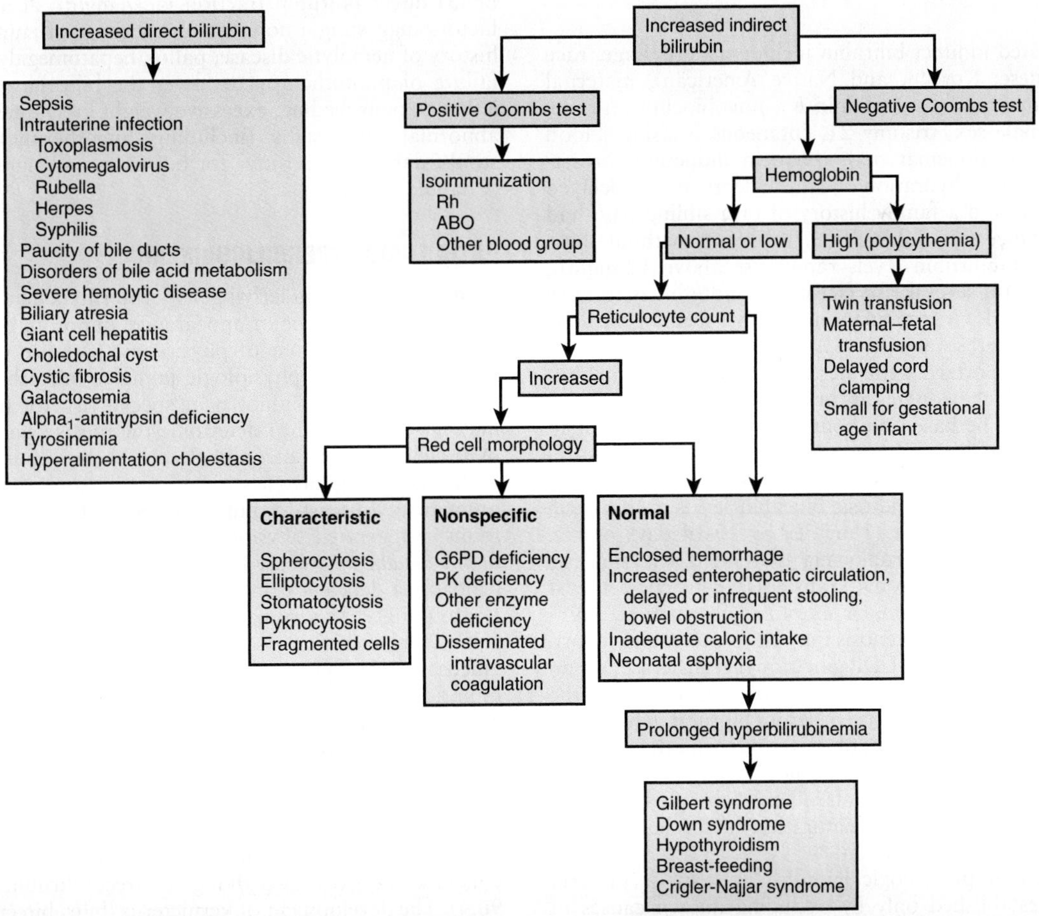

Figure 96-7 Schematic approach to the diagnosis of neonatal jaundice. G6PD, glucose-6-phosphate dehydrogenase; PK, pyruvate kinase. (From Oski FA: Differential diagnosis of jaundice. In Taeusch HW, Ballard RA, Avery MA, editors: *Schaffer and Avery's diseases of the newborn,* ed 6, Philadelphia, 1991, WB Saunders.)

Table 96-3 LABORATORY EVALUATION OF THE JAUNDICED INFANT ≥35 WEEKS OF GESTATION

INDICATIONS	ASSESSMENTS
Jaundice in first 24 hr	Measure TcB and/or TSB
Jaundice appears excessive for infant's age	Measure TcB and/or TSB
Infant receiving phototherapy or TSB rising rapidly (i.e., crossing percentiles [see Fig. 96-8]) and unexplained by history and physical examination	Blood type and Coombs test, if not obtained with cord blood Complete blood count and smear Measure direct or conjugated bilirubin It is an option to perform reticulocyte count, G6PD, and $ETCO_C$, if available Repeat TSB in 4-24 hr depending on infant's age and TSB level
TSB concentration approaching exchange levels or not responding to phototherapy	Perform reticulocyte count, G6PD, albumin, $ETCO_C$, if available
Elevated direct (or conjugated) bilirubin level	Do urinalysis and urine culture Evaluate for sepsis if indicated by history and physical examination
Jaundice present at or beyond age 3 wk, or sick infant	Total and direct (or conjugated) bilirubin level If direct bilirubin elevated, evaluate for causes of cholestasis Check results of newborn thyroid and galactosemia screen, and evaluate infant for signs or symptoms of hypothyroidism

$ETCO_C$, end tidal carbon monoxide concentration; G6PD, glucose-6-phosphate dehydrogenase; TcB, transcutaneous bilirubin; TSB, total serum bilirubin.
From AAP Subcommittee on Hyperbilirubinemia: Management of hyperbilirubinemia in the newborn infant 35 or more weeks of gestation, *Pediatrics* 114:297–316, 2004.

factors for elevated indirect bilirubin include maternal age, race (Chinese, Japanese, Korean, and Native American), maternal diabetes, prematurity, drugs (vitamin K_3, novobiocin), altitude, polycythemia, male sex, trisomy 21, cutaneous bruising, blood extravasation (cephalohematoma), oxytocin induction, breast-feeding, weight loss (dehydration or caloric deprivation), delayed bowel movement, and a family history of or a sibling who had physiologic jaundice (see Table 96-2). In infants without these variables, indirect bilirubin levels rarely rise above 12 mg/dL, whereas infants with several risk factors are more likely to have higher bilirubin levels. A combination of breast-feeding, variant-glucuronosyl transferase activity (1A1), and alterations of the organic anion transporter 2 gene increases the risk in Asian children. Predicting which neonates are at risk for exaggerated physiologic jaundice can be based on hour-specific bilirubin levels in the first 24-72 hr of life (Fig. 96-8). Transcutaneous measurements of bilirubin are linearly correlated with serum levels and can be used for screening. Indirect bilirubin levels in full-term infants decline to adult levels (1 mg/dL) by 10-14 days of life. Persistent indirect hyperbilirubinemia beyond 2 wk suggests hemolysis, hereditary glucuronyl transferase deficiency, breast milk jaundice, hypothyroidism, or intestinal obstruction. Jaundice associated with pyloric stenosis may be due to caloric deprivation, deficiency of hepatic UDP-glucuronyl transferase, or an increase in the enterohepatic circulation of bilirubin from the ileus. In premature infants, the rise in serum bilirubin tends to be the same or somewhat slower but of longer duration than in term infants. Peak levels of 8-12 mg/dL are not usually reached until the 4th-7th day, and jaundice is infrequently observed after the 10th day, corresponding to the maturation of mechanisms for bilirubin metabolism and excretion.

The diagnosis of physiologic jaundice in term or preterm infants can be established only by excluding known causes of jaundice on the basis of the history, clinical findings, and laboratory data (Table 96-4). In general, a search to determine the cause of jaundice should be made if (1) it appears in the first

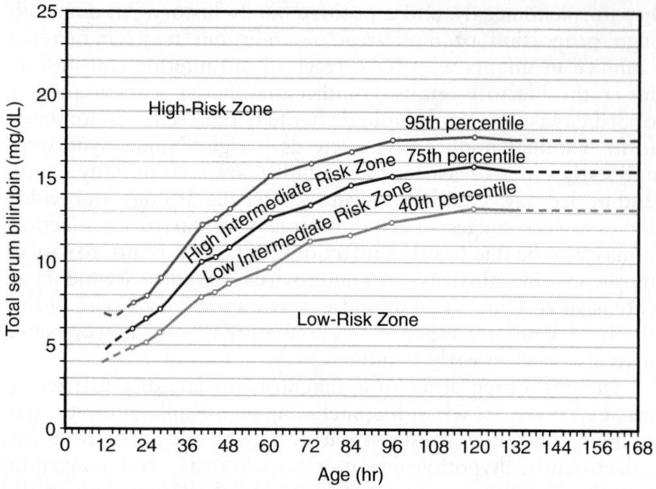

Figure 96-8 Risk designation of term and near-term well newborns based on their hour-specific serum bilirubin values. The high-risk zone is subdivided by the 95th percentile track. The intermediate -risk zone is subdivided into upper and lower risk zones by the 75th percentile track. The low-risk zone has been electively and statistically defined by the 40th percentile track. (From Bhutani VK, Johnson L, Sivieri EM: Predictive ability of a predischarge hour-specific serum bilirubin for subsequent significant hyperbilirubinemia in healthy term and near-term newborns, *Pediatrics* 103:6–14, 1999.)

24-36 hr of life, (2) serum bilirubin is rising at a rate faster than 5 mg/dL/24 hr, (3) serum bilirubin is >12 mg/dL in a full-term infant (especially in the absence of risk factors) or 10-14 mg/dL in a preterm infant, (4) jaundice persists after 10-14 days of life, or (5) direct bilirubin fraction is >2 mg/dL at any time. Other factors suggesting a nonphysiologic cause of jaundice are family history of hemolytic disease, pallor, hepatomegaly, splenomegaly, failure of phototherapy to lower the bilirubin level, vomiting, lethargy, poor feeding, excessive weight loss, apnea, bradycardia, abnormal vital signs (including hypothermia), light-colored stools, dark urine positive for bilirubin, and signs of kernicterus (Chapter 96.4).

PATHOLOGIC HYPERBILIRUBINEMIA

Jaundice and its underlying hyperbilirubinemia are considered pathologic if the time of appearance, duration, or pattern varies significantly from that of physiologic jaundice or if the course is compatible with physiologic jaundice but other reasons exist to suspect that the infant is at special risk for neurotoxicity. It may not be possible to determine the precise cause of an abnormal elevation of unconjugated bilirubin, but many infants with this finding have associated risk factors such as Asian race, prematurity, breast-feeding, and weight loss. Frequently, the terms *exaggerated physiologic jaundice* and *hyperbilirubinemia of the newborn* are used in infants whose primary problem is probably a deficiency or inactivity of bilirubin glucuronyl transferase (Gilbert syndrome) rather than an excessive load of bilirubin for excretion (see Table 96-2). The combination of glucose-6-phosphate dehydrogenase (G6PD) deficiency and a mutation of the promoter region of UDP-glucuronyl transferase-1 produces indirect hyperbilirubinemia in the absence of signs of hemolysis. Nonphysiologic hyperbilirubinemia may also be caused by mutations in the gene for bilirubin UDP-glucuronyl transferase.

The greatest risk associated with indirect hyperbilirubinemia is the development of bilirubin-induced neurologic dysfunction, which typically occurs with high indirect bilirubin levels (Chapter 96.4). The development of kernicterus (bilirubin encephalopathy) depends on the level of indirect bilirubin, duration of exposure to bilirubin elevation, the cause of jaundice, and the infant's well-being. Neurologic injury including kernicterus may occur at

Table 96-4 DIAGNOSTIC FEATURES OF THE VARIOUS TYPES OF NEONATAL JAUNDICE

DIAGNOSIS	NATURE OF VAN DEN BERGH REACTION	JAUNDICE Appears	JAUNDICE Disappears	PEAK BILIRUBIN CONCENTRATION mg/dL	PEAK BILIRUBIN CONCENTRATION Age in Days	BILIRUBIN RATE OF ACCUMULATION (mg/dL/day)	REMARKS
"Physiologic jaundice":							Usually relates to degree of maturity
Full-term	Indirect	2-3 days	4-5 days	10-12	2-3	<5	
Premature	Indirect	3-4 days	7-9 days	15	6-8	<5	
Hyperbilirubinemia due to metabolic factors:							Metabolic factors: hypoxia, respiratory distress, lack of carbohydrate
Full-term	Indirect	2-3 days	Variable	>12	1st wk	<5	Hormonal influences: cretinism, hormones, Gilbert syndrome
Premature	Indirect	3-4 days	Variable	>15	1st wk	<5	Genetic factors: Crigler-Najjar syndrome, Gilbert syndrome Drugs: vitamin K, novobiocin
Hemolytic states and hematoma	Indirect	May appear in 1st 24 hr	Variable	Unlimited	Variable	Usually >5	Erythroblastosis: Rh, ABO, Kell Congenital hemolytic states: spherocytic, nonspherocytic Infantile pyknocytosis Drugs: vitamin K Enclosed hemorrhage—hematoma
Mixed hemolytic and hepatotoxic factors	Indirect and direct	May appear in 1st 24 hr	Variable	Unlimited	Variable	Usually >5	Infection: bacterial sepsis, pyelonephritis, hepatitis, toxoplasmosis, cytomegalic inclusion disease, rubella, syphilis Drugs: vitamin K
Hepatocellular damage	Indirect and direct	Usually 2-3 days; may appear by 2nd wk	Variable	Unlimited	Variable	Variable, can be >5	Biliary atresia; paucity of bile ducts, familial cholestasis, galactosemia; hepatitis and infection

From Brown AK: Neonatal jaundice, *Pediatr Clin North Am* 9:575–603, 1962.

lower bilirubin levels in preterm infants and in the presence of asphyxia, intraventricular hemorrhage, hemolysis, or drugs that displace bilirubin from albumin. The exact serum indirect bilirubin level that is harmful for VLBW infants is unclear.

JAUNDICE ASSOCIATED WITH BREAST-FEEDING

Significant elevation in unconjugated bilirubin (breast milk jaundice) develops in an estimated 2% of breast-fed term infants after the 7th day of life, with maximal concentrations as high as 10-30 mg/dL reached during the 2nd-3rd week. If breast-feeding is continued, the bilirubin gradually decreases but may persist for 3-10 wk at lower levels. If nursing is discontinued, the serum bilirubin level falls rapidly, reaching normal range within a few days. With resumption of breast-feeding, bilirubin seldom returns to previously high levels. Phototherapy may be of benefit (Chapter 96.4). Although uncommon, kernicterus can occur in patients with breast milk jaundice. The etiology of breast milk jaundice is not entirely clear but may be attributed to the presence of glucuronidase in some breast milk.

This syndrome should be distinguished from an early-onset, accentuated unconjugated hyperbilirubinemia known as breast-feeding jaundice, which occurs in the 1st week of life in breast-fed infants, who normally have higher bilirubin levels than formula-fed infants (Fig. 96-9). Hyperbilirubinemia (>12 mg/dL) develops in 13% of breast-fed infants in the 1st wk of life and may be due to decreased milk intake with dehydration and/or reduced caloric intake. Prophylactic supplements of glucose water to breast-fed infants are associated with higher bilirubin levels, in part because of reduced intake of the higher–caloric density breast milk. Frequent breast-feeding (>10/24 hr), rooming-in with night feeding, and ongoing lactation support may reduce the incidence of early breast-feeding jaundice. Even when breast-feeding jaundice develops, breast-feeding should be continued if possible. It is an option to temporarily interrupt breast-feedings and substitute formula for a day or two. In addition, frequent feeding and supplementation with formula or expressed breast milk is

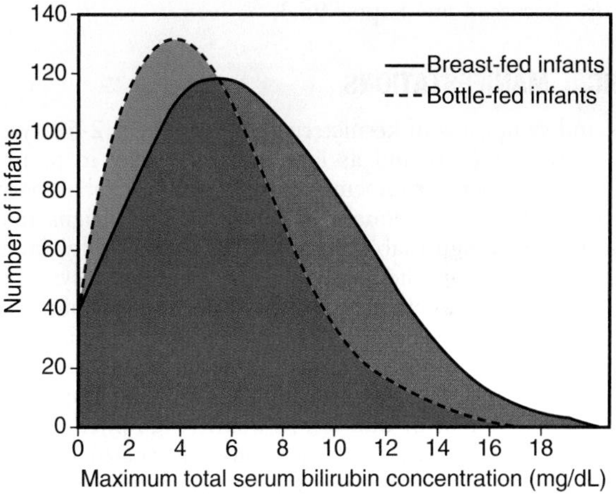

Figure 96-9 Distribution of maximal bilirubin levels during the first wk of life in breast-fed and formula-fed white infants weighing more than 2,500 g. (From Maisels MJ, Gifford K: Normal serum bilirubin levels in the newborn and the effect of breast-feeding, *Pediatrics* 78:837–843, 1986.)

appropriate if the intake seems inadequate, weight loss is excessive, or the infant appears dehydrated.

NEONATAL HEPATITIS

See Chapter 348.1.

CONGENITAL ATRESIA OF THE BILE DUCTS

See Chapter 348.1. Jaundice persisting for more than 2 wk or associated with acholic stools and dark urine suggests biliary atresia. All infants with such findings must undergo an immediate diagnostic evaluation, including determination of direct bilirubin.

INSPISSATED BILE SYNDROME

See Late Complications in Chapter 97.3.

BIBLIOGRAPHY

Please visit the Nelson Textbook of Pediatrics *website at www.expertconsult.com for the complete bibliography.*

96.4 Kernicterus

Namasivayam Ambalavanan and Waldemar A. Carlo

Kernicterus, or bilirubin encephalopathy, is a neurologic syndrome resulting from the deposition of unconjugated (indirect) bilirubin in the basal ganglia and brainstem nuclei. The pathogenesis of kernicterus is multifactorial and involves an interaction between unconjugated bilirubin levels, albumin binding and unbound bilirubin levels, passage across the blood-brain barrier, and neuronal susceptibility to injury. Disruption of the blood-brain barrier by disease, asphyxia, and other factors and maturational changes in blood-brain barrier permeability affect risk.

The precise blood level above which indirect-reacting bilirubin or free bilirubin will be toxic for an individual infant is unpredictable, but in a large series, kernicterus occurred only in infants with a bilirubin >20 mg/dL. Ninety percent of the infants in whom kernicterus developed were in previously healthy, predominantly breast-fed term and near-term infants. The duration of exposure to high bilirubin levels needed to produce toxic effects are unknown. The more immature the infant is, the greater the susceptibility to kernicterus. Factors that potentiate the movement of bilirubin across the blood-brain barrier and into brain cells are discussed in Chapter 96.3.

CLINICAL MANIFESTATIONS

Signs and symptoms of kernicterus usually appear 2-5 days after birth in term infants and as late as the 7th day in premature infants, but hyperbilirubinemia may lead to encephalopathy at any time during the neonatal period. The early signs may be subtle and indistinguishable from those of sepsis, asphyxia, hypoglycemia, intracranial hemorrhage, and other acute systemic illnesses in a neonate. Lethargy, poor feeding, and loss of the Moro reflex are common initial signs. Subsequently, the infant may appear gravely ill and prostrate, with diminished tendon reflexes and respiratory distress. Opisthotonos with a bulging fontanel, twitching of the face or limbs, and a shrill high-pitched cry may follow. In advanced cases, convulsions and spasm occur, with affected infants stiffly extending their arms in an inward rotation with the fists clenched (Table 96-5). Rigidity is rare at this late stage.

Many infants who progress to these severe neurologic signs die; the survivors are usually seriously damaged but may appear to recover and for 2-3 mo show few abnormalities. Later in the 1st yr of life, opisthotonos, muscle rigidity, irregular movements, and convulsions tend to recur. In the 2nd yr, the opisthotonos and seizures abate, but irregular, involuntary movements, muscle rigidity, or, in some infants, hypotonia increase steadily. By 3 yr of age, the complete neurologic syndrome is often apparent; it consists of bilateral choreoathetosis with involuntary muscle spasms, extrapyramidal signs, seizures, mental deficiency, dysarthric speech, high-frequency hearing loss, squinting, and defective upward eye movements. Pyramidal signs, hypotonia, and ataxia occur in a few infants. In mildly affected infants, the syndrome may be characterized only by mild to moderate neuromuscular incoordination, partial deafness, or "minimal brain dysfunction," occurring singly or in combination; these problems may be inapparent until the child enters school (see Table 96-5).

Table 96-5 CLINICAL FEATURES OF KERNICTERUS

ACUTE FORM
Phase 1 (1st 1-2 days): poor suck, stupor, hypotonia, seizures Phase 2 (middle of 1st wk): hypertonia of extensor muscles, opisthotonos, retrocollis, fever Phase 3 (after the 1st wk): hypertonia
CHRONIC FORM
1st year: hypotonia, active deep tendon reflexes, obligatory tonic neck reflexes, delayed motor skills After 1st yr: movement disorders (choreoathetosis, ballismus, tremor), upward gaze, sensorineural hearing loss

From Dennery PA, Seidman DS, Stevenson DK: Neonatal hyperbilirubinemia, *N Engl J Med* 344:581–590, 2001.

INCIDENCE AND PROGNOSIS

By pathologic criteria, kernicterus develops in 30% of infants (all gestational ages) with untreated hemolytic disease and bilirubin levels >25-30 mg/dL. The incidence at autopsy in hyperbilirubinemic premature infants is 2-16% and is related to the risk factors discussed in Chapter 96.3. Reliable estimates of the frequency of the clinical syndrome are not available because of the wide spectrum of manifestations. Overt neurologic signs have a grave prognosis; more than 75% of infants die, and 80% of affected survivors have bilateral choreoathetosis with involuntary muscle spasms. Mental retardation, deafness, and spastic quadriplegia are common.

PREVENTION

Although kernicterus has been thought to be a disease of the past, there are reports of neurotoxic effects of bilirubin in term and near-term infants who were discharged as healthy newborns. Some but not all experts recommend universal screening for hyperbilirubinemia in the 1st 24-48 hr of life to detect infants at high risk for severe jaundice and bilirubin-induced neurologic dysfunction.

Effective prevention requires ongoing vigilance and a practical, system-based approach in order to distinguish infants with benign newborn jaundice from those whose course may be less predictable and potentially harmful. Protocols using the hour-specific bilirubin nomogram (see Fig. 96-8), physical examination, and clinical risk factors have been successful in identifying patients at risk for hyperbilirubinemia and candidates for targeted management. The American Academy of Pediatrics (AAP) has identified potentially preventable causes of kernicterus, as follows: (1) early discharge (<48 hr) with no early follow-up (within 48 hr of discharge); this problem is particularly important in near-term infants (35-37 wk of gestation); (2) failure to check the bilirubin level in an infant noted to be jaundiced in the first 24 hr; (3) failure to recognize the presence of risk factors for hyperbilirubinemia; (4) underestimation of the severity of jaundice by clinical (visual) assessment; (5) lack of concern regarding the presence of jaundice; (6) delay in measuring the serum bilirubin level despite marked jaundice or delay in initiating phototherapy in the presence of elevated bilirubin levels; and (7) failure to respond to parental concern regarding jaundice, poor feeding, or lethargy. An evidence-based management algorithm for infants is shown in Figure 96-10. In addition, it is recommended to determine before discharge each infant's risk factors from established protocols (see Table 96-2).

The following approach is further recommended: (1) any infant who is jaundiced before 24 hr requires measurement of serum bilirubin level and, if it is elevated, evaluation for possible hemolytic disease and (2) follow-up should be provided within 2-3 days of discharge to all neonates discharged earlier than 48 hr after birth. Early follow-up is particularly important for

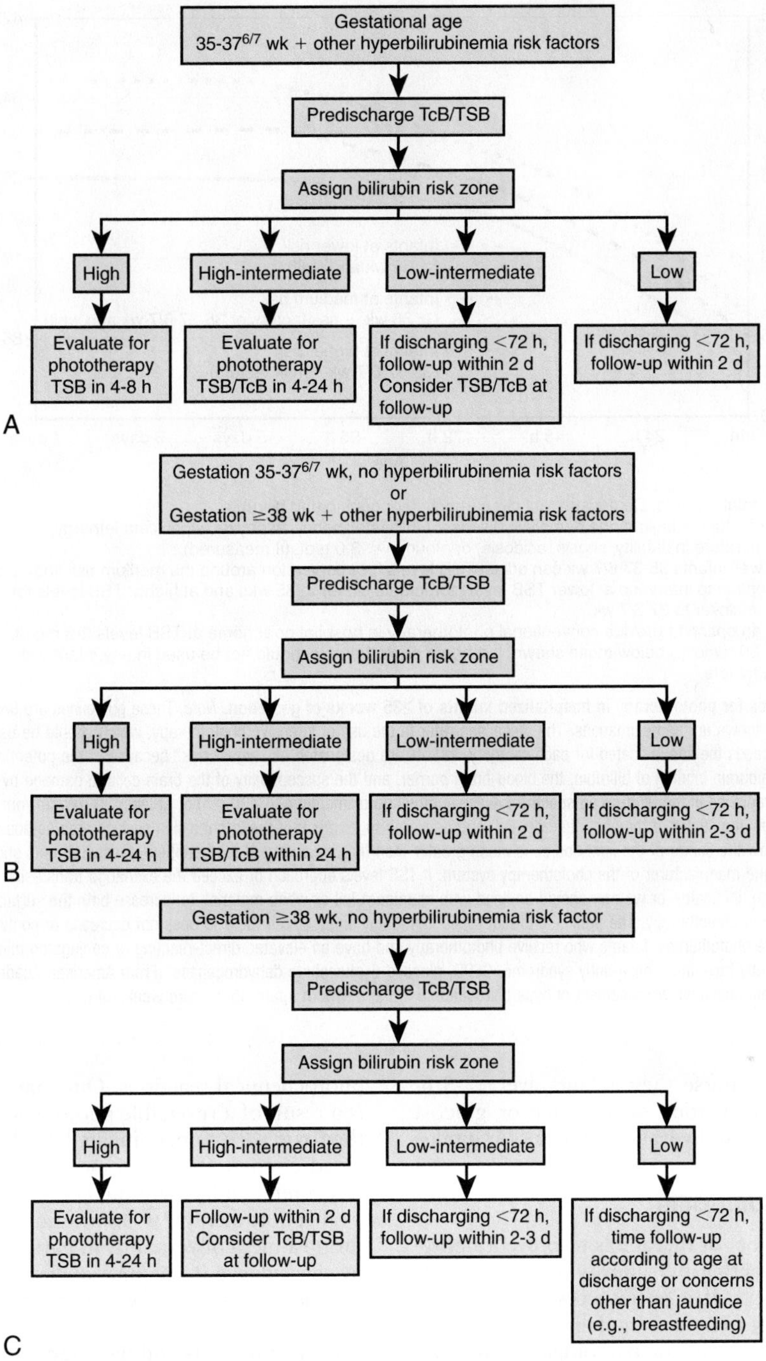

- Provide lactation evaluation and support for all breastfeeding mothers.
- Recommendation for timing of repeat TSB measurement depends on age at measurement and how far the TSB level is above the 95th percentile. Higher and earlier initial TSB levels require an earlier repeat TSB measurment.
- Perform standard clinical evaluation at all follow-up visits.
- For evaluation of jaundice see 2004 AAP guideline.
- In hospital or as outpatient. Follow-up recommendations can be modified according to level of risk for hyperbilirubinemia; depending on the circumstances in infants at low risk, later follow-up can be considered.

Figure 96-10 Algorithm providing recommendations for management and follow-up according to predischarge bilirubin measurements, gestation, and risk factors for subsequent hyperbilirubinemia. TcB, transcutaneous bilirubin; TSB, total serum bilirubin. (From Maisels MJ, Bhutani VK, Bogen D, et al: Hyperbilirubinemia in the newborn infant ≥ 35 weeks' gestation: an update with clarifications, *Pediatrics* 124:1193–1198, 2009.)

infants younger than 38 wk of gestation. The timing of follow-up depends on the age at discharge and the presence of risk factors. In some cases, follow-up within 24 hr is necessary. Post-discharge follow-up is essential for early recognition of problems related to hyperbilirubinemia and disease progression. Parental communication with regard to concerns about infant's skin color and behavioral activities should be addressed early and frequently, including education about potential risks and neurotoxicity. Ongoing lactation promotion, education, support, and follow-up services are essential throughout the neonatal period.

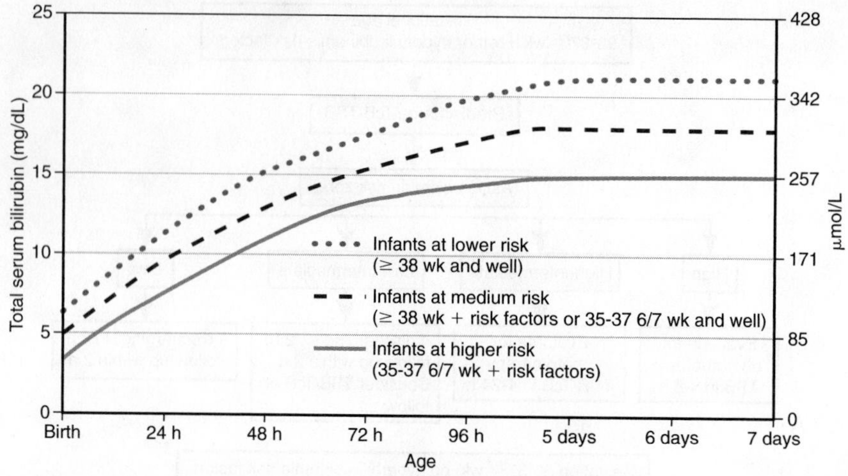

- Use total bilirubin. Do not subtract direct reacting or conjugated bilirubin.
- Risk factors = isoimmune hemolytic disease, G6PD deficiency, asphyxia, significant lethargy, temperature instability, sepsis, acidosis, or albumin < 3.0 g/dL (if measured).
- For well infants 35-37 6/7 wk can adjust TSB levels for intervention around the medium risk line. It is an option to intervene at lower TSB levels for infants closer to 35 wks and at higher TSB levels for those closer to 37 6/7 wk.
- It is an option to provide conventional phototherapy in hospital or at home at TSB levels 2-3 mg/dL (35-50 mmol/L) below those shown, but home phototherapy should not be used in any infant with risk factors.

Figure 96-11 Guidelines for phototherapy in hospitalized infants of ≥35 weeks of gestation. *Note:* These guidelines are based on limited evidence, and the levels shown are approximations. The guidelines refer to the use of intensive phototherapy, which should be used when the total serum bilirubin (TSB) exceeds the line indicated for each category. Infants are designated as "higher risk" because of the potential negative effects of the conditions listed on albumin binding of bilirubin, the blood-brain barrier, and the susceptibility of the brain cells to damage by bilirubin. "Intensive phototherapy" implies irradiance in the blue-green spectrum (wavelengths approximately 430-490 nm) of at least 30 $\mu W/cm^2/nm$ (measured at the infant's skin directly below the center of the phototherapy unit) and delivered to as much of the infant's skin surface area as possible. Note that irradiance measured below the center of the light source is much greater than that measured at the periphery. Measurements should be made with a radiometer specified by the manufacturer of the phototherapy system. If TSB levels approach or exceed the exchange transfusion line (see Fig. 96-12), the sides of the bassinette, incubator, or warmer should be lined with aluminum foil or white material, to increase both the surface area of the infant exposed and the efficacy of phototherapy. The presence of hemolysis is strongly suggested if the TSB does not decrease or continues to rise in an infant who is receiving intensive phototherapy. Infants who receive phototherapy and have an elevated direct-reacting or conjugated bilirubin value (cholestatic jaundice) may inconsistently have the bronze-baby syndrome. G6PD, glucose-6-phosphate dehydrogenase. (From American Academy of Pediatrics Subcommittee on Hyperbilirubinemia: Management of hyperbilirubinemia in the newborn infant 35 or more weeks of gestation, *Pediatrics* 114:297–316, 2004.)

Mothers should be advised to nurse their infants every 2-3 hr and to avoid routine supplementation with water or glucose water in order to ensure adequate hydration and caloric intake.

TREATMENT OF HYPERBILIRUBINEMIA

Regardless of the cause, the goal of therapy is to prevent neurotoxicity related to indirect-reacting bilirubin while not causing undue harm. Phototherapy and, if it is unsuccessful, exchange transfusion remain the primary treatment modalities used to keep the maximal total serum bilirubin below pathologic levels (Figs. 96-11 and 96-12; Table 96-6). The risk of injury to the central nervous system from bilirubin must be balanced against the potential risk of treatment. There is lack of consensus regarding the exact bilirubin level at which to initiate phototherapy. Because phototherapy may require 6-12 hr to have a measurable effect, it must be started at bilirubin levels below those indicated for exchange transfusion. When identified, underlying medical causes of elevated bilirubin and physiologic factors that contribute to neuronal susceptibility should be treated, with antibiotics for septicemia and correction of acidosis (Table 96-7).

Phototherapy

Clinical jaundice and indirect hyperbilirubinemia are reduced by exposure to a high intensity of light in the visible spectrum. Bilirubin absorbs light maximally in the blue range (420-470 nm). Broad-spectrum white, blue, and special narrow-spectrum (super) blue lights have been effective in reducing bilirubin levels. Bilirubin in the skin absorbs light energy, causing several photochemical reactions. One major product from phototherapy is a result of a reversible photo-isomerization reaction converting the toxic native unconjugated 4Z,15Z-bilirubin into an unconjugated configurational isomer, 4Z,15E-bilirubin, which can then be excreted in bile without conjugation. The other major product from phototherapy is lumirubin, which is an irreversible structural isomer converted from native bilirubin that can be excreted by the kidneys in the unconjugated state.

The therapeutic effect of phototherapy depends on the light energy emitted in the effective range of wavelengths, the distance between the lights and the infant, and the surface area of exposed skin, as well as the rate of hemolysis and in vivo metabolism and excretion of bilirubin. Available commercial phototherapy units vary considerably in spectral output and the intensity of radiance emitted; therefore, the wattage can be accurately measured only at the patient's skin surface. Dark skin does not reduce the efficacy of phototherapy. Maximal intensive phototherapy should be used when indirect bilirubin levels approach those noted in Figure 96-11 and Table 96-7. Such therapy includes using "special blue" fluorescent tubes, placing the lamps within 15-20 cm of the infant, and putting a fiberoptic phototherapy blanket under the infant's back to increase the exposed surface area. Aggressive phototherapy may improve neurodevelopmental outcome in infants <1,000 g.

The use of phototherapy has decreased the need for exchange transfusion in term and preterm infants with hemolytic and nonhemolytic jaundice. When indications for exchange transfusion are present, phototherapy should not be used as a substitute; however, phototherapy may reduce the need for repeated exchange

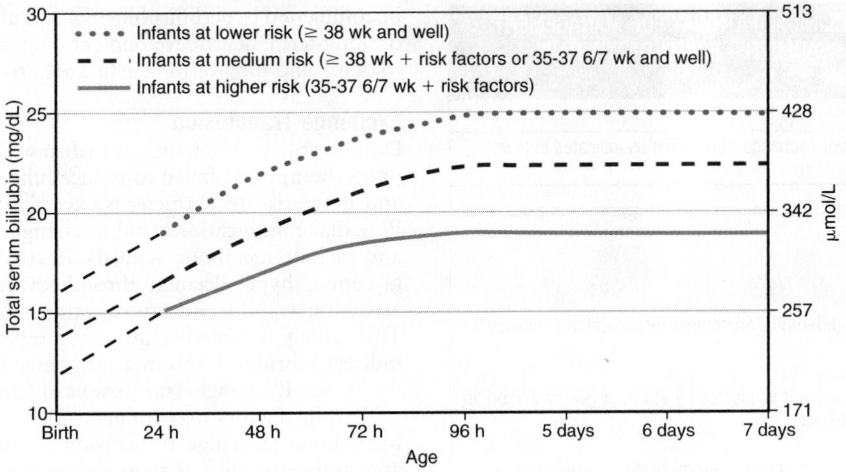

- The dashed lines for the first 24 hours indicate uncertainty due to a wide range of clinical circumstances and a range of responses to phototherapy.
- Immediate exchange transfusion is recommended if infant shows signs of acute bilirubin encephalopathy (hypertonia, arching, retrocollis, opisthotonos, fever, high pitched cry) or if TSB is ≥ 5 mg/dL (85 μmol/L) above these lines.
- Risk factors = isoimmune hemolytic disease, G6PD deficiency, asphyxia, significant lethargy, temperature instability, sepsis, acidosis.
- Measure serum albumin and calculate B/A ratio (see legend).
- Use total bilirubin. Do not subtract direct reacting or conjugated bilirubin.
- If infant is well and 35-37 6/7 wk (median risk), can individualize TSB levels for exchange based on actual gestational age.

Figure 96-12 Guidelines for exchange transfusion in hospitalized infants of ≥35 weeks of gestation. *Note:* These suggested levels represent a consensus of most of the committee but are based on limited evidence, and the levels shown are approximations. During birth hospitalization, exchange transfusion is recommended if the total serum bilirubin (TSB) rises to these levels despite intensive phototherapy. In a readmitted infant, if the TSB level is above the exchange level, TSB measurement should be repeated every 2-3 hr; exchange transfusion should be considered if the TSB remains above the levels indicated after intensive phototherapy for 6 hr. The following B/A ratios can be used together with, but not in lieu of, the TSB level as an additional factor in determining the need for exchange transfusion. G6PD, glucose-6-phosphate dehydrogenase. (From American Academy of Pediatrics Subcommittee on Hyperbilirubinemia: Management of hyperbilirubinemia in the newborn infant 35 or more weeks of gestation, *Pediatrics* 114:297–316, 2004.)

Table 96-6 SUGGESTED MAXIMAL INDIRECT SERUM BILIRUBIN CONCENTRATIONS (mg/dL) IN PRETERM INFANTS

BIRTHWEIGHT (g)	UNCOMPLICATED*	COMPLICATED*
<1,000	12-13	10-12
1,000-1,250	12-14	10-12
1,251-1,499	14-16	12-14
1,500-1,999	16-20	15-17
2,000-2,500	20-22	18-20

*Complications include perinatal asphyxia, acidosis, hypoxia, hypothermia, hypoalbuminemia, meningitis, intraventricular hemorrhage, hemolysis, hypoglycemia, or signs of kernicterus. Phototherapy is usually started at 50-70% of the maximal indirect level. If values greatly exceed this level, if phototherapy is unsuccessful in reducing the maximal bilirubin level, or if signs of kernicterus are evident, exchange transfusion is indicated.

transfusions in infants with hemolysis. Conventional phototherapy is applied continuously, and the infant is turned frequently for maximal skin surface area exposure. It should be discontinued as soon as the indirect bilirubin concentration has reduced to levels considered safe with respect to the infant's age and condition. Serum bilirubin levels and hematocrit should be monitored every 4-8 hr in infants with hemolytic disease and those with bilirubin levels near toxic range for the individual infant. Others, particularly older infants, may be monitored less frequently. Serum bilirubin monitoring should continue for at least 24 hr after cessation of phototherapy in patients with hemolytic disease, because unexpected rises in bilirubin may occur, requiring further treatment. Skin color cannot be relied on for evaluating the effectiveness of phototherapy; the skin of babies exposed to light may appear to be almost without jaundice in the presence of marked hyperbilirubinemia. Although not necessary for all affected infants, intravenous fluid supplementation added to oral feedings may be beneficial in dehydrated patients or infants with bilirubin levels nearing those requiring exchange transfusion.

Complications associated with phototherapy include loose stools, erythematous macular rash, purpuric rash associated with transient porphyrinemia, overheating, dehydration (increased insensible water loss, diarrhea), hypothermia from exposure, and a benign condition called bronze baby syndrome (which occurs in the presence of direct hyperbilirubinemia; see later). Phototherapy is contraindicated in the presence of porphyria. Before phototherapy is initiated, the infant's eyes should be closed and adequately covered to prevent light exposure and corneal damage. Body temperature should be monitored, and the infant should be shielded from bulb breakage. Irradiance should be measured directly. In infants with hemolytic disease, care must be taken to monitor for the development of anemia, which may require transfusion. Anemia may develop despite lowering of bilirubin levels. Clinical experience suggests that long-term adverse biologic effects of phototherapy are absent, minimal, or unrecognized.

The term **bronze baby syndrome** refers to a sometimes-noted dark, grayish brown skin discoloration in infants undergoing phototherapy. Almost all infants observed with this syndrome have had significant elevation of direct-reacting bilirubin and other evidence of obstructive liver disease. The discoloration may be due to photo-induced modification of porphyrins, which are often present during cholestatic jaundice and may last for many months. Despite the bronze baby syndrome, phototherapy can continue if needed.

Intravenous Immunoglobulin

The administration of intravenous immunoglobulin is an adjunctive treatment for hyperbilirubinemia due to isoimmune

Table 96-7 EXAMPLE OF A CLINICAL PATHWAY FOR MANAGEMENT OF THE NEWBORN INFANT READMITTED FOR PHOTOTHERAPY OR EXCHANGE TRANSFUSION

TREATMENT
Use intensive phototherapy and/or exchange transfusion as indicated in Figs. 96-11 and 96-12
LABORATORY TESTS
TSB and direct bilirubin levels Blood type (ABO, Rh) Direct antibody test (Coombs) Serum albumin Complete blood cell count with differential and smear for red cell morphology Reticulocyte count End-tidal CO concentration (if available) Glucose-6-phosphate dehydrogenase if suggested by ethnic or geographic origin or if poor response to phototherapy Urine for reducing substances If history and/or presentation suggest sepsis, perform blood culture, urine culture, and cerebrospinal fluid for protein, glucose, cell count, and culture
INTERVENTIONS
If TSB ≥25 mg/dL (428 µmol/L) or ≥20 mg/dL (342 µmol/L) in a sick infant or infant <38 wk gestation, obtain a type and crossmatch, and request blood in case an exchange transfusion is necessary. In infants with isoimmune hemolytic disease and TSB level rising in spite of intensive phototherapy or within 2-3 mg/dL (34-51 µmol/L) of exchange level (Fig. 96-12), administer intravenous immunoglobulin 0.5-1 g/kg over 2 hr and repeat in 12 hr if necessary. If infant's weight loss from birth is >12% or there is clinical or biochemical evidence of dehydration, recommend formula or expressed breast milk. If oral intake is in question, give intravenous fluids.
FOR INFANTS RECEIVING INTENSIVE PHOTOTHERAPY:
Breast-feed or bottle-feed (formula or expressed breast milk) every 2-3 hr If TSB ≥25 mg/dL (428 µmol/L), repeat TSB within 2-3 hr If TSB 20-25 mg/dL (342-428 µmol/L), repeat within 3-4 hr. If TSB <20 mg/dL (342 µmol/L), repeat in 4-6 hr. If TSB continues to fall, repeat in 8-12 hr. If TSB is not decreasing or is moving closer to level for exchange transfusion or the TSB/albumin ratio exceeds levels shown in Fig. 96-12, consider exchange transfusion (see Fig. 96-12 for exchange transfusion recommendations). When TSB is <13-14 mg/dL (239 µmol/L), discontinue phototherapy. Depending on the cause of the hyperbilirubinemia, it is an option to measure TSB 24 hr after discharge to check for rebound.

TSB, total serum bilirubin.
From AAP Subcommittee on Hyperbilirubinemia: Management of hyperbilirubinemia in the newborn infant 35 or more weeks of gestation, *Pediatrics* 114:297–316, 2004.

hemolytic disease. Its use is recommended when serum bilirubin is approaching exchange levels despite maximal interventions including phototherapy. Intravenous immunoglobulin (0.5-1.0 g/kg/dose; repeat in 12 hr) has been shown to reduce the need for exchange transfusion in both ABO and Rh hemolytic disease, presumably by reducing hemolysis.

Metalloporphyrins

A potentially important alternative therapy is the use of metalloporphyrins for hyperbilirubinemia. The metalloporphyrin Sn-mesoporphyrin (SnMP) offers promise as a drug candidate. The proposed mechanism of action is competitive enzymatic inhibition of the rate-limiting conversion of heme-protein to biliverdin (an intermediate metabolite in the production of unconjugated bilirubin) by heme-oxygenase. A single intramuscular dose on the 1st day of life may reduce the need for subsequent phototherapy. Such therapy may be beneficial when jaundice is anticipated, particularly in patients with ABO incompatibility or G6PD deficiency or when blood products are objected to, as with Jehovah's Witness patients. Complications from metalloporphyrins include transient erythema if the infant is receiving phototherapy. Administration of SnMP may reduce bilirubin levels and decrease both the need for phototherapy and the duration of hospital stay; however, it remains unclear whether treatment with metalloporphyrins for unconjugated hyperbilirubinemia will alter the risk of kernicterus or long-term neurodevelopment impairment. Data on efficacy, toxicity, and long-term benefit are currently being evaluated.

Exchange Transfusion

Double-volume exchange transfusion is performed if intensive phototherapy has failed to reduce bilirubin levels to a safe range and if the risk of kernicterus exceeds the risk of the procedure. Potential complications from exchange transfusion are not trivial and include metabolic acidosis, electrolyte abnormalities, hypoglycemia, hypocalcemia, thrombocytopenia, volume overload, arrhythmias, NEC, infection, graft versus host disease, and death. This widely accepted treatment is repeated if necessary to keep indirect bilirubin levels in a safe range (see Fig. 96-12 and Table 96-7). See Exchange Transfusion in Chapter 97.

Various factors may influence the decision to perform a double-volume exchange transfusion in an individual patient. The appearance of clinical signs suggesting kernicterus is an indication for exchange transfusion at any level of serum bilirubin. A healthy full-term infant with physiologic or breast milk jaundice may tolerate a concentration slightly higher than 25 mg/dL with no apparent ill effect, whereas kernicterus may develop in a sick premature infant at a significantly lower level. A level approaching that considered critical for the individual infant may be an indication for exchange transfusion during the 1st or 2nd day of life when a further rise is anticipated, but not typically on the 4th day in a term infant or on the 7th day in a premature infant because an imminent fall may be anticipated as the hepatic conjugating mechanism becomes more effective.

BIBLIOGRAPHY

Please visit the Nelson Textbook of Pediatrics *website at www.expertconsult.com for the complete bibliography.*

Chapter 97
Blood Disorders

97.1 Anemia in the Newborn Infant

Akhil Maheshwari and Waldemar A. Carlo

Hemoglobin increases with advancing gestational age: at term, cord blood hemoglobin is 16.8 g/dL (14-20 g/dL); hemoglobin levels in very low birthweight (VLBW) infants are 1-2 g/dL below those in term infants (Fig. 97-1). A hemoglobin value less than the normal range of hemoglobin for birthweight and postnatal age is defined as anemia (Table 97-1). A "physiologic" decrease in hemoglobin content is noticed at 8-12 wk in term infants (hemoglobin, 11 g/dL) and at about 6 wk in premature infants (7-10 g/dL).

Infants born by cesarean section may have a lower hematocrit (Hct) than those born vaginally. **Anemia at birth** is manifested as pallor, heart failure, or shock (Fig. 97-2). It may be due to acute or chronic fetal blood loss, hemolysis, or underproduction of erythrocytes. Specific causes include hemolytic disease of the newborn, tearing or cutting of the umbilical cord during delivery, abnormal cord insertion, communicating placental vessels, placenta previa or abruptio, nuchal cord, incision into the placenta, internal hemorrhage (liver, spleen, intracranial), α-thalassemia, congenital parvovirus infection or other hypoplastic anemias, and twin-twin transfusion in monozygotic twins with arteriovenous placental connections (Chapter 92).

Transplacental hemorrhage with bleeding from the fetal into the maternal circulation has been reported in 5-15% of pregnancies, but, unless severe, it is not usually sufficient to cause clinically apparent anemia at birth. The cause of transplacental hemorrhage is not clear, but its occurrence has been proven by

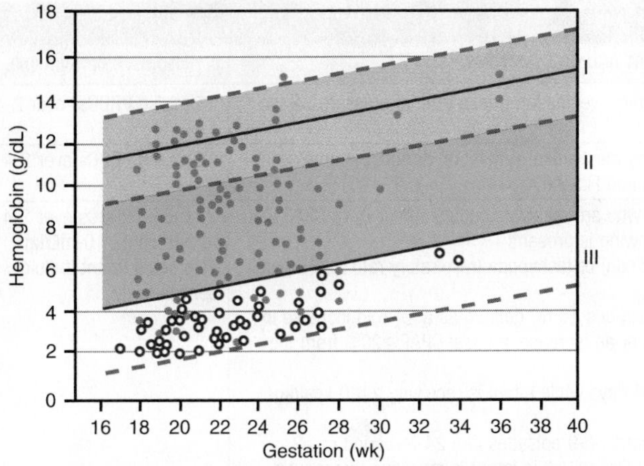

Figure 97-1 Range (mean and 95% confidence limits) of hemoglobin concentration from 10 to 40 wk of gestational age in normal (zone I) fetuses obtained by cordocentesis (percutaneous umbilical blood sample). *Solid circles* depict maternal red blood cell isoimmunization; *open circles* indicate hemoglobin levels in fetuses with ultrasonographic evidence of hydrops (zone III). (From Soothill PW: Cordocentesis: role in assessment of fetal condition, *Clin Perinatol* 16:755–770, 1989.)

Table 97-1 NORMAL RED BLOOD CELL VALUES FROM 18 WEEKS OF GESTATION TO 14 WEEKS OF LIFE

AGE	HEMOGLOBIN (g/dL)	HEMATOCRIT (%)	MCV (μ³)	RETICULOCYTES (%)
GESTATIONAL (wk)				
18-20*	11.5 ± 0.8	36 ± 3	134 ± 8.8	N/A
21-22*	12.3 ± 0.9	39 ± 3	130 ± 6.2	N/A
23-25*	12.4 ± 0.8	39 ± 2	126 ± 6.2	N/A
26-27	19.0 ± 2.5	62 ± 8	132 ± 14.4	9.6 ± 3.2
28-29	19.3 ± 1.8	60 ± 7	131 ± 13.5	7.5 ± 2.5
30-31	19.1 ± 2.2	60 ± 8	127 ± 12.7	5.8 ± 2.0
32-33	18.5 ± 2.0	60 ± 8	123 ± 15.7	5.0 ± 1.9
34-35	19.6 ± 2.1	61 ± 7	122 ± 10.0	3.9 ± 1.6
36-37	19.2 ± 1.7	64 ± 7	121 ± 12.5	4.2 ± 1.8
38-40	19.3 ± 2.2	61 ± 7	119 ± 9.4	3.2 ± 1.4
POSTNATAL (DAYS)				
1	19.0 ± 2.2	61 ± 7	119 ± 9.4	3.2 ± 1.4
2	19.0 ± 1.9	60 ± 6	115 ± 7.0	3.2 ± 1.3
3	18.7 ± 3.4	62 ± 9	116 ± 5.3	2.8 ± 1.7
4	18.6 ± 2.1	57 ± 8	114 ± 7.5	1.8 ± 1.1
5	17.6 ± 1.1	57 ± 7	114 ± 8.9	1.2 ± 0.2
6	17.4 ± 2.2	54 ± 7	113 ± 10.0	0.6 ± 0.2
7	17.9 ± 2.5	56 ± 9	118 ± 11.2	0.5 ± 0.4
POSTNATAL (wk)				
1-2	17.3 ± 2.3	54 ± 8	112 ± 19.0	0.5 ± 0.3
2-3	15.6 ± 2.6	46 ± 7	111 ± 8.2	0.8 ± 0.6
3-4	14.2 ± 2.1	43 ± 6	105 ± 7.5	0.6 ± 0.3
4-5	12.7 ± 1.6	36 ± 5	101 ± 8.1	0.9 ± 0.8
5-6	11.9 ± 1.5	36 ± 6	102 ± 10.2	1.0 ± 0.7
6-7	12.0 ± 1.5	36 ± 5	105 ± 12.0	1.2 ± 0.7
7-8	11.1 ± 1.1	33 ± 4	100 ± 13.0	1.5 ± 0.7
8-9	10.7 ± 0.9	31 ± 3	93 ± 12.0	1.8 ± 1.0
9-10	11.2 ± 0.9	32 ± 3	91 ± 9.3	1.2 ± 0.6
10-11	11.4 ± 0.9	34 ± 2	91 ± 7.7	1.2 ± 0.7
11-12	11.3 ± 0.9	33 ± 3	88 ± 7.9	0.7 ± 0.3
12-14	11.9	37	86.8	0.9

*Based on samples collected in utero. Results expressed as mean value ± 1 standard deviation from the mean except for postnatal weeks 12-14 in which only the mean value is given.
From Bizzarro MJ, Colson E, Ehrenkranz RA: Differential diagnosis and management of anemia in the newborn, *Pediatr Clin North Am* 51:1087–1107, 2004.

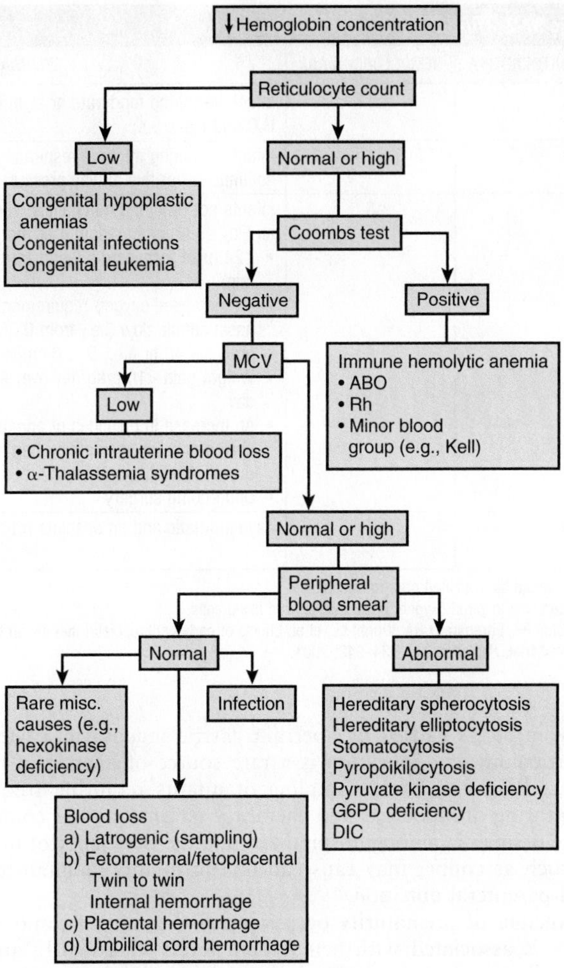

Figure 97-2 Diagnostic approach to anemia in newborn infants. DIC, disseminated intravascular coagulation; G6PD, glucose-6-phosphate dehydrogenase; MCV, mean corpuscular volume. (Modified from Blanchette VS, Zipursky A: Assessment of anemia in newborn infants, *Clin Perinatol* 11:489–510, 1984.)

demonstration of significant amounts of fetal hemoglobin and red blood cells (RBCs) in maternal blood on the day of delivery by the **Kleihauer-Betke** test or by flow cytometry methods to detect fetal cells in maternal blood. If the infant has severe anemia with heart failure, emergency exchange transfusion to restore Hct and oxygen-carrying capacity may be needed.

Acute blood loss usually results in severe distress at birth, initially with a normal hemoglobin level, no hepatosplenomegaly, and early onset of shock. In contrast, chronic blood loss in utero produces marked pallor, less distress, a low hemoglobin level with microcytic indices, and, if severe, heart failure.

Anemia appearing in the first few days after birth is also most frequently a result of hemolytic disease of the newborn. Other causes are hemorrhagic disease of the newborn, bleeding from an improperly tied or clamped umbilical cord, large cephalohematoma, intracranial hemorrhage, and subcapsular bleeding from rupture of the liver, spleen, adrenals, or kidneys. Rapid decreases in hemoglobin or Hct values during the first few days of life may be the initial clue to these conditions.

Later in the neonatal period, delayed anemia may develop as a result of hemolytic disease of the newborn, with or without exchange transfusion or phototherapy. Congenital hemolytic anemia (spherocytosis) occasionally appears during the 1st mo of life, and hereditary nonspherocytic hemolytic anemia has been described during the neonatal period secondary to deficiency of glucose-6-phosphate dehydrogenase (G6PD) and pyruvate kinase. Bleeding from hemangiomas of the upper gastrointestinal tract

Table 97-2 TRANSFUSION PROTOCOL

HEMATOCRIT (%)	HEMOGLOBIN (g/dL)	RESPIRATORY SUPPORT AND/OR SYMPTOMS	TRANSFUSION VOLUME
≤35	≤11	Infants requiring moderate or significant mechanical ventilation (mean arterial pressure >8 cm H_2O and FIO_2 >0.4)	15 mL/kg PRBCs* over 2-4 hr
≤30	≤10	Infants requiring minimal respiratory support (any mechanical ventilation or endotracheal/nasal continuous positive airway pressure >6 cm H_2O and FIO_2 ≤0.4)	15 mL/kg PRBCs over 2-4 hr
≤25	≤8	Infants not requiring mechanical ventilation but who are receiving supplemental O_2 or CPAP with an FIO_2 ≤0.4 and in whom 1 or more of the following is present: • ≤24 hr of tachycardia (heart rate >180 beats/min) or tachypnea (respiratory rate >80 breaths/min) • An increased oxygen requirement from the previous 48 hr, defined as a ≥4-fold increase in nasal canula flow (i.e., from 0.25 to 1 L/min) or an increase in nasal CPAP ≥20% from the previous 48 hr (i.e., 5 to 6 cm H_2O) • Weight gain <10 g/kg/day over the previous 4 days while infant is receiving ≥100 kcal/kg/day • An increase in episodes of apnea and bradycardia (>9 episodes in a 24-hr period or ≥2 episodes in 24 hr requiring bag and mask ventilation) while infant is receiving therapeutic doses of methylxanthines • Undergoing surgery	20 mL/kg PRBCs over 2-4 hr (divide into 2 10-mL/kg volumes if infant is fluid sensitive)
≤20	≤7	Asymptomatic and an absolute reticulocyte count <100,000 cells/µL	20 mL/kg PRBCs over 2-4 hr (2 10-mL/kg volumes)

*RBCs should be irradiated prior to transfusion.
FIO_2, fractional inspired oxygen; PRBC, packed red blood cells.
From Ohls RK, Ehrenkranz RA, Wright LL, et al: Effects of early erythropoietin therapy on the transfusion requirements of preterm infants below 1250 grams birth weight: a multicenter, randomized, controlled trial, *Pediatrics* 108:934–942, 2001.

or from ulcers caused by aberrant gastric mucosa in a Meckel diverticulum or duplication is a rare source of anemia in newborns. Repeated blood sampling of infants requiring frequent monitoring of blood gas and chemistry parameters is a common cause of anemia among hospitalized infants. Deficiency of minerals such as copper may cause anemia in infants maintained on total parenteral nutrition.

Anemia of prematurity occurs in LBW infants 1-3 mo after birth, is associated with hemoglobin levels <7-10 g/dL, and is clinically manifested as pallor, poor weight gain, decreased activity, tachypnea, tachycardia, and feeding problems. Repeated phlebotomy for blood tests, shortened RBC survival, rapid growth, and the physiologic effects of the transition from fetal (low PaO_2 and hemoglobin saturation) to neonatal life (high PaO_2 and hemoglobin saturation) contribute to anemia of prematurity. The oxygen available to neonatal tissue is lower than that in adults, but a neonate's erythropoietin response is attenuated for the degree of anemia, and as a result, hemoglobin and reticulocyte levels are low. In VLBW infants, delayed clamping of the umbilical cord with the infant held below the level of the placenta may enhance placental-infant transfusion and reduce postnatal transfusion needs. This maneuver should not delay any needed resuscitation and may lead to hyperviscosity.

Delayed cord clamping (≈1-2 min or after cessation of cord pulsation) may be beneficial in otherwise well newborns in preventing anemia in full-term infants, with effects extending beyond the neonatal period. The benefits of delayed cord clamping persist for 2-6 mo as improved hematocrit, iron status as measured by ferritin concentration and stored iron, and a clinically important reduction in the risk of anemia in infancy. Late clamping may result in delivery of an extra 20-40 mL of blood and 30-35 mg of iron to the newborn. Polycythemia is a risk with delayed clamping but is often asymptomatic.

Treatment of neonatal anemia by blood transfusion depends on the severity of symptoms, the hemoglobin level, and the presence of co-morbid diseases (bronchopulmonary dysplasia, cyanotic congenital heart disease, respiratory distress syndrome) that interfere with oxygen delivery. The need for treatment with blood should be balanced against the risks of transfusion, including hemolytic transfusion reactions, exposure to blood product preservatives and other potential toxins, volume overload, possible increased risk of retinopathy of prematurity and necrotizing enterocolitis, graft-versus-host (GVH) reaction, and transfusion-acquired infection (cytomegalovirus [CMV], HIV, parvovirus, hepatitis B and C) (Chapter 468). The risk of CMV infection can be almost eliminated by the use of leukoreduced blood. In the infant <1,500 g, CMV antibody-negative leukoreduced blood should be used. The risk of acquiring HIV and hepatitis B and C viruses is reduced but not eliminated by antibody screening of donated blood. Blood banking techniques that limit multiple donor exposure should be encouraged.

Although transfusion guidelines for preterm infants have been proposed (Table 97-2), they have not been subjected to rigorous clinical study. Nonetheless, these guidelines have led to a decline in the number of unnecessary transfusions. The use of restrictive vs more liberal transfusion guidelines has been examined in two randomized trials, one conducted at University of Iowa and a second multicentric trial known as the PINT (Premature Infants in Need of Transfusion) study. The restrictive guidelines in the two groups were generally similar. In the Iowa trial, the transfusion thresholds in the liberal- and restrictive-transfusion groups were <46% and <34%, respectively, in tracheally intubated infants receiving assisted ventilation; <38% and <28%, respectively, in infants receiving nasal continuous positive airway pressure or supplemental oxygen; and <30% and <22%, respectively, in infants breathing room air. The transfusion thresholds for the liberal groups were higher in the Iowa trial than in the PINT study. In both trials, the use of restrictive thresholds resulted in fewer transfusions and also increased the number of infants who received no transfusions at all. However, in the Iowa trial (but not in the PINT study), restrictive transfusion thresholds were associated with increases in major cranial ultrasonographic abnormalities and in the frequency of apneic spells. Although these findings need further evaluation in clinical studies, the issue of finding an appropriate transfusion threshold in premature infants remains unresolved.

Asymptomatic full-term infants with a hemoglobin level of 10 g/dL may be monitored, whereas symptomatic neonates born after abruptio placentae or with severe hemolytic disease of the newborn need immediate transfusion. Preterm infants who have repeated episodes of apnea and bradycardia despite theophylline therapy and a hemoglobin level ≤8 g/dL may benefit from RBC transfusion. In addition, infants with respiratory distress syndrome or severe bronchopulmonary dysplasia may need hemoglobin levels of 12-14 g/dL to improve oxygen delivery. No transfusion is needed to replace blood removed for testing or for mild asymptomatic anemia. Asymptomatic neonates with reticulocytopenia and hemoglobin levels ≤7 g/dL may require transfusion; if a transfusion is not provided, close observation is essential. Packed RBC transfusion (10-20 mL/kg) is given at a rate of 2-3 mL/kg/hr to raise the hemoglobin concentration; 2 mL/kg raises the hemoglobin level 0.5-1 g/dL. Hemorrhage should be treated with whole blood if available; alternatively, fluid resuscitation is initiated, followed by packed RBC transfusion.

Recombinant human erythropoietin (r-HuEPO) may be considered in the treatment of chronic or anticipated anemia in an attempt to decrease or eliminate transfusions when families, for religious reasons, request all possible measures to avoid transfusions. Therapy with r-HuEPO must be supplemented with oral iron. Doses and regimens vary. In anemia of prematurity, r-HuEPO does not provide a major reduction in transfusion requirements or the number of donors; therefore, *routine* use of erythropoietin in VLBW infants is not recommended. Early initiation of r-HuEPO therapy may produce a small reduction in the total transfusion volume per infant. There were concerns about an increased risk of severe retinopathy of prematurity in the r-HuEPO group. The effects of *late* initiation of r-HuEPO (≥8 days) have also been associated with small reductions in the total blood volume transfused per infant and the number of transfusions per infant.

BIBLIOGRAPHY

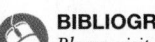

Please visit the Nelson Textbook of Pediatrics *website at* *www.expertconsult.com* *for the complete bibliography.*

97.2 Hemolytic Disease of the Newborn (Erythroblastosis Fetalis)

Akhil Maheshwari and Waldemar A. Carlo

Erythroblastosis fetalis is caused by the transplacental passage of maternal antibody active against paternal RBC antigens of the infant and is characterized by an increased rate of RBC destruction. It is an important cause of anemia and jaundice in newborn infants despite the development of a method of preventing maternal isoimmunization by Rh antigens. Although more than 60 different RBC antigens are capable of eliciting an antibody response, significant disease is associated primarily with the D antigen of the Rh group and with incompatibility of ABO factors. Rarely, hemolytic disease may be caused by C or E antigens or by other RBC antigens, such as C^W, C^X, D^U, K (Kell), M, Duffy, S, P, MNS, Xg, Lutheran, Diego, and Kidd. Anti-Lewis antibodies do not cause disease.

HEMOLYTIC DISEASE OF THE NEWBORN CAUSED BY RH INCOMPATIBILITY

The Rh antigenic determinants are genetically transmitted from each parent, determine the Rh type, and direct the production of a number of blood group factors (C, c, D, d, E, and e). Each factor can elicit a specific antibody response under suitable conditions; 90% are due to D antigen and the remainder to C or E antigens.

Pathogenesis

Isoimmune hemolytic disease from D antigen is approximately three times more frequent among white persons than among black persons. When Rh-positive blood is infused into an Rh-negative woman through error or when small quantities (usually > 1 mL) of Rh-positive fetal blood containing D antigen inherited from an Rh-positive father enter the maternal circulation during pregnancy, with spontaneous or induced abortion, or at delivery, antibody formation against D antigen may be induced in the unsensitized Rh-negative recipient mother. Once sensitization has taken place, considerably smaller doses of antigen can stimulate an increase in antibody titer. Initially, a rise in immunoglobulin (Ig) M antibody occurs, which is later replaced by IgG antibody; the latter readily crosses the placenta to cause hemolytic manifestations.

Hemolytic disease rarely occurs during a first pregnancy because transfusion of Rh-positive fetal blood into an Rh-negative mother occurs near the time of delivery, too late for the mother to become sensitized and transmit antibody to her infant before delivery. The facts that 55% of Rh-positive fathers are heterozygous (D/d) and may have Rh-negative offspring and that fetal-to-maternal transfusion occurs in only 50% of pregnancies reduce the chance of sensitization, as does small family size, in which the opportunities for its reoccurrence are reduced. The disparity between the numbers of incompatible vs alloimmunized maternal-fetal pairs can also be due to a threshold effect of fetomaternal transfusions (a certain amount of the immunizing blood cell antigen is required to activate the maternal immune system), the type of antibody response (IgG antibodies are more efficiently transferred across the placenta to the fetus), differential immunogenicity of blood group antigens, and differences in maternal immune response, presumably related to differences in the efficiency of antigen presentation by various major histocompatibility loci. Thus, the overall incidence of isoimmunization of Rh-negative mothers at risk is low, with antibody to antigen D detected in >10% of those studied, even after five or more pregnancies; only about 5% ever have babies with hemolytic disease.

When the mother and fetus are also incompatible with respect to group A or B, the mother is partially protected against sensitization by the rapid removal of Rh-positive cells from her circulation by her preexisting anti-A or anti-B antibodies, which are IgM antibodies and do not cross the placenta. Once a mother has been sensitized, her infant is likely to have hemolytic disease. The severity of Rh illness worsens with successive pregnancies. The possibility that the first affected infant after sensitization may represent the end of the mother's childbearing potential for Rh-positive infants argues urgently for the prevention of sensitization. *The injection of anti-D gamma globulin (RhoGAM) into the mother immediately after the delivery of each Rh-positive infant has been a successful strategy to reduce Rh hemolytic disease (see later).*

Clinical Manifestations

A wide spectrum of hemolytic disease occurs in affected infants born to sensitized mothers, depending on the nature of the individual immune response. The severity of the disease may range from only laboratory evidence of mild hemolysis (15% of cases) to severe anemia with compensatory hyperplasia of erythropoietic tissue leading to massive enlargement of the liver and spleen. When the compensatory capacity of the hematopoietic system is exceeded, profound anemia occurs and results in pallor, signs of cardiac decompensation (cardiomegaly, respiratory distress), massive anasarca, and circulatory collapse. This clinical picture of excessive abnormal fluid in two or more fetal compartments (skin, pleura, pericardium, placenta, peritoneum, amniotic fluid), termed **hydrops fetalis,** frequently results in death in utero or shortly after birth. With the use of anti-D gamma globulin to prevent Rh sensitization, nonimmune (nonhemolytic) conditions have become frequent causes of hydrops (Table 97-3). The severity of hydrops is related to the level of anemia and the degree of reduction in serum albumin (oncotic pressure), which is due in part to hepatic dysfunction. Alternatively, heart failure may increase right heart pressure, with the subsequent development of edema and ascites. Failure to initiate spontaneous effective ventilation because of pulmonary edema or bilateral pleural effusions results in birth asphyxia; after successful resuscitation, severe respiratory distress may develop. Petechiae, purpura, and

Table 97-3 ETIOLOGY OF HYDROPS FETALIS*

CATEGORY	DISORDER(S)
Anemia	Immune (Rh, Kell) hemolysis
	α-Thalassemia
	Red blood cell enzyme deficiencies (glucose-6-phosphate dehydrogenase)
	Fetomaternal hemorrhage
	Donor in twin-to-twin transfusion
	Diamond-Blackfan syndrome
Cardiac dysrhythmias	Supraventricular tachycardia
	Atrial flutter
	Congenital heart block
Structural heart lesions	Premature closure of foramen ovale
	Tricuspid insufficiency
	Hypoplastic left heart
	Endocardial cushion defect
	Cardiomyopathy
	Endocardial fibroelastosis
	Tuberous sclerosis with cardiac rhabdomyoma
	Pericardial teratoma
Vascular	Chorioangioma of placenta, chorionic vessels, or umbilical vessels
	Umbilical artery aneurysm
	Angiomyxoma of umbilical cord
	True knot of umbilical cord
	Hepatic hemangioma
	Cerebral arteriovenous malformation (aneurysm of vein of Galen)
	Angiosteohypertrophy (Klippel-Trénaunay syndrome)
	Thrombosis of renal or umbilical vein or inferior vena cava
	Recipient in twin-to-twin transfusion
Lymphatic	Lymphangiectasia
	Cystic hygroma
	Chylothorax, chylous ascites
	Noonan syndrome
	Multiple pterygium syndrome
Central nervous system	Absent corpus callosum
	Encephalocele
	Intracranial hemorrhage
	Holoprosencephaly
Thoracic lesions	Cystic adenomatoid malformation of lung
	Mediastinal teratoma
	Diaphragmatic hernia
	Sequestered lung
Teratomas	Choriocarcinoma
	Sacrococcygeal teratoma
Tumors and storage diseases	Neuroblastoma
	Hepatoblastoma
	Gaucher disease
	Niemann-Pick disease
	Mucolipidosis
	GM_1 gangliosidosis
	Mucopolysaccharidosis
Chromosome abnormalities	Trisomy 13, 15, 16, 18, 21
	XX/XY, 45XO
	Partial duplication of chromosome 11, 15, 17, 18
	Partial deletion of chromosome 13, 18
	Triploidy
	Tetraploidy
Bone diseases	Osteogenesis imperfecta
	Asphyxiating thoracic dystrophy
	Skeletal dysplasias
Congenital infections	Cytomegalovirus
	Parvovirus
	Rubella
	Toxoplasmosis
	Syphilis
	Leptospirosis
	Chagas disease
Others	Bowel obstruction with perforation and meconium peritonitis, volvulus
	Hepatic fibrosis
	Beckwith-Wiedemann syndrome
	Prune-belly syndrome
	Congenital nephrosis
	Infant of a diabetic mother
	Myotonic dystrophy
	Neu-Laxova syndrome
	Maternal therapy with indomethacin
	Fetal akinesia
Idiopathic	Multiple congenital anomaly syndromes

*The incidence of nonimmune (nonhemolytic) hydrops fetalis is 1/2,000-1/3,500 births.
Modified from Phibbs R. In Polin N, Fox W, editors: *Fetal and neonatal physiology,* ed 2, Philadelphia, 1998, WB Saunders.

thrombocytopenia may also be present in severe cases as a result of decreased platelet production or the presence of concurrent disseminated intravascular coagulation.

Jaundice may be absent at birth because of placental clearance of lipid-soluble unconjugated bilirubin, but in severe cases, bilirubin pigments stain the amniotic fluid, cord, and vernix caseosa yellow. Jaundice is generally evident on the 1st day of life because the infant's bilirubin-conjugating and excretory systems are unable to cope with the load resulting from massive hemolysis. Indirect-reacting bilirubin therefore accumulates postnatally and may rapidly reach extremely high levels and present a significant risk of bilirubin encephalopathy. The risk of development of kernicterus from hemolytic disease is greater than from comparable nonhemolytic hyperbilirubinemia, although the risk in an individual patient may be affected by other complications (hypoxia, acidosis). Hypoglycemia occurs frequently in infants with severe isoimmune hemolytic disease and may be related to hyperinsulinism and hypertrophy of the pancreatic islet cells in these infants.

Infants born after intrauterine transfusion for prenatally diagnosed erythroblastosis may be severely affected because the indications for transfusion are evidence of already severe disease in utero (hydrops, fetal anemia). Such infants usually have very high (but extremely variable) cord levels of bilirubin, reflecting the severity of the hemolysis and its effects on hepatic function. Infants treated with intraumbilical vein transfusions in utero may also have a benign postnatal course if the anemia and hydrops resolve before birth. Anemia from continuing hemolysis may be masked by the previous intrauterine transfusion, and the clinical manifestations of erythroblastosis may be superimposed on various degrees of immaturity resulting from spontaneous or induced premature delivery.

Laboratory Data

Before treatment, the direct Coombs test result is usually positive and anemia is generally present. The cord blood hemoglobin content varies and is usually proportional to the severity of the disease; with hydrops fetalis it may be as low as 3-4 g/dL. Alternatively, despite hemolysis, it may be within the normal range because of compensatory bone marrow and extramedullary hematopoiesis. The blood smear typically shows polychromasia and a marked increase in nucleated RBCs. The reticulocyte count is increased. The white blood cell count is usually normal but may be elevated; thrombocytopenia may develop in severe cases. Cord bilirubin is generally between 3 and 5 mg/dL; the direct-reacting (conjugated) bilirubin content may also be elevated, especially if there was an intrauterine transfusion. Indirect-reacting bilirubin content rises rapidly to high levels in the 1st 6 hr of life.

After intrauterine transfusions, cord blood may show a normal hemoglobin concentration, negative direct Coombs test result, predominantly type O Rh-negative adult RBCs, and relatively normal smear findings.

Diagnosis

Definitive diagnosis of erythroblastosis fetalis requires demonstration of blood group incompatibility and corresponding antibody bound to the infant's RBCs.

ANTENATAL DIAGNOSIS In Rh-negative women, a history of previous transfusions, abortion, or pregnancy should suggest the possibility of sensitization. Expectant parents' blood types should be tested for potential incompatibility, and the maternal titer of IgG antibodies to D antigen should be assayed at 12-16, 28-32, and 36 wk of gestation. Fetal Rh status may be determined by isolating fetal cells or fetal DNA (plasma) from the maternal circulation. The presence of elevated antibody titers at the beginning of pregnancy, a rapid rise in titer, or a titer of 1:64 or greater suggests significant hemolytic disease, although the exact titer correlates poorly with the severity of disease. If a mother is found to have antibody against D antigen at a titer of 1:16 (15 IU/mL in Europe) or greater at any time during a subsequent pregnancy, the severity of fetal disease should be monitored by Doppler ultrasonography of the middle cerebral artery and then percutaneous umbilical blood sampling (PUBS) if indicated (Chapter 90). If the mother has a history of a previously affected infant or a stillbirth, an Rh-positive infant is usually equally or more severely affected than the previous infant, and the severity of disease in the fetus should be monitored.

Assessment of the fetus may require information obtained from ultrasonography and PUBS. Real-time ultrasonography is used to detect the progression of disease, with hydrops defined as skin or scalp edema, pleural or pericardial effusions, and ascites. Early ultrasonographic signs of hydrops include organomegaly (liver, spleen, heart), the double–bowel wall sign (bowel edema), and placental thickening. Progression to polyhydramnios, ascites, pleural or pericardial effusions, and skin or scalp edema may then follow. If pleural effusions precede ascites and hydrops by a significant time, causes other than fetal anemia should be suspected (see Table 97-4). Extramedullary hematopoiesis and, less so, hepatic congestion compress the intrahepatic vessels and produce venous stasis with portal hypertension, hepatocellular dysfunction, and decreased albumin synthesis.

Hydrops is present with a fetal hemoglobin level <5 g/dL, frequent with a level <7 g/dL, and variable with levels between 7 and 9 g/dL. Real-time ultrasonography predicts fetal well-being by means of the biophysical profile (see Table 90-2), whereas Doppler ultrasonography assesses fetal distress by demonstrating increased vascular resistance in fetal arteries (middle cerebral). In pregnancies with ultrasonographic evidence of hemolysis (hepatosplenomegaly), early or late hydrops, or fetal distress, further and more direct assessment of fetal hemolysis should be performed.

Amniocentesis was classically used to assess fetal hemolysis. Hemolysis of fetal RBCs produces hyperbilirubinemia before the onset of severe anemia. Bilirubin is cleared by the placenta, but a significant proportion enters the amniotic fluid and can be measured by spectrophotometry. Ultrasonographically guided transabdominal aspiration of amniotic fluid may be performed as early as 18-20 wk of gestation. Spectrophotometric scanning of amniotic fluid wavelengths demonstrates a positive optical density (OD) deviation of absorption for bilirubin from normal at 450 nm. Amniocentesis and cordocentesis are invasive procedures with risks to both the fetus and mother, including fetal death, bleeding, or bradycardia, worsening of alloimmunization, premature rupture of membranes, preterm labor, and chorioamnionitis. Noninvasive measurements to detect fetal anemia are desirable. In fetuses without hydrops, moderate to severe anemia can be detected noninvasively by demonstration of an increase in the peak velocity of systolic blood flow in the middle cerebral artery by Doppler ultrasonography.

PUBS is the standard approach to assessment of the fetus if Doppler and real-time ultrasonography findings suggest that the fetus has erythroblastosis fetalis. PUBS is performed to determine fetal hemoglobin levels and to transfuse packed RBCs in those with serious fetal anemia (Hct 25-30%).

POSTNATAL DIAGNOSIS Immediately after the birth of any infant to an Rh-negative woman, blood from the umbilical cord or from the infant should be examined for ABO blood group, Rh type, Hct and hemoglobin, and reaction to the direct Coombs test. If the Coombs test result is positive, a baseline serum bilirubin level should be measured, and a commercially available RBC panel should be used to identify RBC antibodies present in the mother's serum, both tests being performed not only to establish the diagnosis but also to ensure selection of the most compatible blood for exchange transfusion should it be necessary. The direct Coombs test result is usually strongly positive in clinically affected infants and may remain so for a few days up to several months.

Treatment

The main goals of therapy are to (1) prevent intrauterine or extrauterine death from severe anemia and hypoxia, and (2) avoid neurotoxicity from hyperbilirubinemia.

TREATMENT OF AN UNBORN INFANT Survival of severely affected fetuses has been improved by the use of fetal ultrasonography to identify the need for in utero transfusion. Intravascular (umbilical vein) transfusion of packed RBCs is the treatment of choice for fetal anemia, replacing intrauterine transfusion into the fetal peritoneal cavity. Hydrops or fetal anemia (Hct < 30%) is an indication for umbilical vein transfusion in infants with pulmonary immaturity (see Fig. 97-1). **Intravascular fetal transfusion** is facilitated by maternal and hence fetal sedation with diazepam and by fetal paralysis with pancuronium. Packed RBCs are given by slow-push infusion after being cross-matched against the mother's serum. The cells should be obtained from a CMV-negative donor and irradiated to kill lymphocytes to avoid GVH disease. Of note, leukoreduction alone (without irradiation) does not prevent GVH disease. Transfusions should achieve a post-transfusion Hct of 45-55% and can be repeated every 3-5 wk. Indications for delivery include pulmonary maturity, fetal distress, complications of PUBS, and 35-37 wk of gestation. The survival rate for intrauterine transfusions is 89%; the complication rate is 3%. Complications include rupture of the membranes and preterm delivery, infection, fetal distress requiring emergency cesarean section, and perinatal death.

TREATMENT OF A LIVEBORN INFANT The birth should be attended by a physician skilled in neonatal resuscitation. Fresh, low-titer, group O, leukoreduced, and irradiated Rh-negative blood cross-matched against maternal serum should be immediately available.

If clinical signs of severe hemolytic anemia (pallor, hepatosplenomegaly, edema, petechiae, ascites) are evident at birth, immediate resuscitation and supportive therapy, temperature stabilization, and monitoring before proceeding with exchange transfusion may save some severely affected infants. Such therapy should include correction of acidosis with 1-2 mEq/kg of sodium bicarbonate; a small transfusion of compatible packed RBCs to correct anemia; volume expansion for hypotension, especially in those with hydrops; and provision of assisted ventilation for respiratory failure.

EXCHANGE TRANSFUSION When an infant's clinical condition at birth does not require an immediate full or partial exchange transfusion, the decision to perform one should be based on a judgment that the infant has a high risk of rapid development of a dangerous degree of anemia or hyperbilirubinemia. Cord hemoglobin value of 10 g/dL or less and bilirubin concentration of 5 mg/dL or more suggest severe hemolysis but inconsistently predict the need for exchange transfusion. Some physicians consider previous kernicterus or severe erythroblastosis in a sibling, reticulocyte counts >15%, and prematurity to be additional factors supporting a decision for early exchange transfusion (Chapters 96.3 and 96.4). Intrauterine, intravascular transfusions have decreased the need for exchange transfusion.

The hemoglobin concentration, Hct, and serum bilirubin level should be measured at 4-6 hr intervals initially, with extension to longer intervals if and as the rate of change diminishes. The decision to perform an exchange transfusion is based on the likelihood that the trend of bilirubin levels plotted against hours of age indicates that serum bilirubin will reach the levels indicated in Figure 96-12 and Table 96-7. Term infants with bilirubin levels ≥20 mg/dL have an increased risk of kernicterus. Ordinary transfusions of compatible Rh-negative, leukoreduced, and irradiated RBCs may be necessary to correct anemia at any stage of the disease up to 6-8 wk of age, when the infant's own blood-forming mechanism may be expected to take over. Weekly determinations of hemoglobin or Hct values should be performed until a spontaneous rise has been demonstrated.

Careful monitoring of the serum bilirubin level is essential until a falling trend has been demonstrated in the absence of phototherapy (Chapter 96.3). Even then, an occasional infant, particularly if premature, may experience an unpredicted significant rise in serum bilirubin as late as the 7th day of life. Attempts to predict the attainment of dangerously high levels of serum bilirubin on the basis of observed levels exceeding 6 mg/dL in the 1st 6 hr or 10 mg/dL in the 2nd 6 hr of life or on rates of rise exceeding 0.5-1.0 mg/dL/hr can be unreliable. Measurement of unbound bilirubin may be a more sensitive predictor of the risk associated with hyperbilirubinemia.

Blood for exchange transfusion should be as fresh as possible. Heparin or citrate-phosphate-dextrose-adenine solution may be used as an anticoagulant. If the blood is obtained before delivery, it should be taken from a type O, Rh-negative donor with a low titer of anti-A and anti-B antibodies and should be determined compatible with the mother's serum by the indirect Coombs test. After delivery, blood should be obtained from an Rh-negative donor whose cells are compatible with both the infant's and the mother's sera; when possible, type O donor cells are generally used, but cells of the infant's ABO blood type may be used when the mother has the same type. A complete cross match, including an indirect Coombs test, should be performed before the 2nd and subsequent transfusions. Blood should be gradually warmed and maintained at a temperature between 35 and 37°C throughout the exchange transfusion. It should be kept well mixed by gentle squeezing or agitation of the bag to avoid sedimentation; otherwise, the use of supernatant serum with a low RBC count at the end of the exchange will leave the infant anemic. Whole blood or packed leukoreduced and irradiated RBCs reconstituted with fresh frozen plasma to an Hct of 40% should be used. The infant's stomach should be emptied before transfusion to prevent aspiration, and body temperature should be maintained and vital signs monitored. A competent assistant should be present to help monitor, tally the volume of blood exchanged, and perform emergency procedures.

With strict aseptic technique, the umbilical vein is cannulated with a polyvinyl catheter to a distance no greater than 7 cm in a full-term infant. When free flow of blood is obtained, the catheter is usually in a large hepatic vein or the inferior vena cava. Alternatively, the exchange may be performed through peripheral arterial (drawn out) and venous (infused in) lines. The exchange should be carried out over 45-60 min, with aspiration of 20 mL of infant blood alternating with infusion of 20 mL of donor blood. Smaller aliquots (5-10 mL) may be indicated for sick and premature infants. The goal should be an isovolumetric exchange of approximately two blood volumes of the infant (2 × 85 mL/kg).

Infants with acidosis and hypoxia from respiratory distress, sepsis, or shock may be further compromised by the significant acute acid load contained in citrated blood, which usually has a pH between 7 and 7.2. The subsequent metabolism of citrate may result in metabolic alkalosis later if citrated blood is used. Fresh heparinized blood avoids this problem. During the exchange, blood pH and Pa_{O_2} should be serially monitored because infants often become acidotic and hypoxic during exchange transfusions. Symptomatic hypoglycemia may occur before or during an exchange transfusion in moderately to severely affected infants; it may also occur 1-3 hr after exchange. Acute complications, noted in 5-10% of infants, include transient bradycardia with or without calcium infusion, cyanosis, transient vasospasm, thrombosis, apnea with bradycardia requiring resuscitation, and death. Infectious risks include CMV, HIV, and hepatitis. Necrotizing enterocolitis is a rare complication of exchange transfusion.

The risk of death from an exchange transfusion performed by an experienced physician is 0.3/100 procedures. With the decreasing use of this procedure because of the use of phototherapy and prevention of sensitization, the general level of physician competence is diminishing. Thus, it is best if this procedure is performed in experienced neonatal referral centers.

After exchange transfusion, the bilirubin level must be determined at frequent intervals (every 4-8 hr) because bilirubin may rebound 40-50% within hours. Repeated exchange transfusions should be carried out to keep the indirect fraction from exceeding the levels indicated in Table 96-7 for preterm infants and 20 mg/dL for term infants. Symptoms suggestive of kernicterus are mandatory indications for exchange transfusion at any time.

INTRAVENOUS IMMUNOGLOBULIN Early administration of intravenous immunoglobulin (IVIG) may reduce hemolysis, peak serum bilirubin levels, and the need for exchange transfusions. IVIG administration reduces the need for exchange transfusion, the duration of phototherapy, and the length of hospitalization. A dose of 0.5-1 gm/kg may be used.

Late Complications

Infants who have hemolytic disease or who have had an exchange or an intrauterine transfusion must be observed carefully for the development of anemia and cholestasis. **Late anemia** may be hemolytic or hyporegenerative. Treatment with supplemental iron, blood transfusion, or erythropoietin may be indicated. A mild GVH reaction may manifest as diarrhea, rash, hepatitis, or eosinophilia.

Inspissated bile syndrome refers to the rare occurrence of persistent icterus in association with significant elevations in direct and indirect bilirubin levels in infants with hemolytic disease. The cause is unclear, but the jaundice clears spontaneously within a few weeks or months.

Portal vein thrombosis and portal hypertension may occur in children who have been subjected to exchange transfusion as newborn infants. It is probably associated with prolonged, traumatic, or septic umbilical vein catheterization.

Prevention of Rh Sensitization

The risk of initial sensitization of Rh-negative mothers has been reduced to less than 1% by the intramuscular injection of 300 µg of human anti-D globulin (1 mL of RhoGAM) within 72 hr of delivery of an Rh-positive infant, ectopic pregnancy, abdominal trauma in pregnancy, amniocentesis, chorionic villus biopsy, or abortion. This quantity is sufficient to eliminate ≈ 10 mL of potentially antigenic fetal cells from the maternal circulation. Large fetal-to-maternal transfers of blood may require proportionately more human anti-D globulin. RhoGAM Administration of human anti-D globulin at 28-32 wk and again at birth (40 wk) is more effective than a single dose. The use of this technique, combined with improved methods of detecting maternal sensitization and measuring the extent of fetal-to-maternal transfusion, plus the use of fewer obstetric procedures that increase the risk of such fetal-to-maternal bleeding (version, manual separation of the placenta), should further reduce the incidence of erythroblastosis fetalis.

HEMOLYTIC DISEASE OF THE NEWBORN CAUSED BY BLOOD GROUP A AND B INCOMPATIBILITY

ABO incompatibility is the most common cause of hemolytic disease of the newborn. Approximately 15% of live births are at risk, but manifestations of disease develop in only 0.3-2.2%. Major blood group incompatibility between the mother and fetus generally results in milder disease than Rh incompatibility does. Maternal antibody may be formed against B cells if the mother is type A or against A cells if the mother is type B. Usually, the mother is type O and the infant is type A or B. Although ABO incompatibility occurs in 20-25% of pregnancies, hemolytic disease develops in only 10% of the offspring in such pregnancies, and the infants are generally type A_1, which is more antigenic than A_2. Low antigenicity of the ABO factors in the fetus and newborn infant may account for the low incidence of severe ABO hemolytic disease relative to the incidence of incompatibility between the blood groups of the mother and child. Although antibodies against A and B factors occur without previous immunization ("natural" antibodies), they are usually IgM antibodies that do not cross the placenta. However, IgG antibodies to A antigen may be present and these do cross the placenta, so A-O isoimmune hemolytic disease may be found in first-born infants. Mothers who have become immunized against A or B factors from a previous incompatible pregnancy also exhibit IgG antibody. These "immune" antibodies are the primary mediators in ABO isoimmune disease.

Clinical Manifestations

Most cases are mild, with jaundice being the only clinical manifestation. The infant is not generally affected at birth; pallor is not present, and hydrops fetalis is extremely rare. The liver and spleen are not greatly enlarged, if at all. Jaundice usually appears during the 1st 24 hr. Rarely, it may become severe, and symptoms and signs of kernicterus develop rapidly.

Diagnosis

A presumptive diagnosis is based on the presence of ABO incompatibility, a weakly to moderately positive direct Coombs test result, and spherocytes in the blood smear, which may at times suggest the presence of hereditary spherocytosis. Hyperbilirubinemia is often the only other laboratory abnormality. The hemoglobin level is usually normal but may be as low as 10-12 g/dL. Reticulocytes may be increased to 10-15%, with extensive polychromasia and increased numbers of nucleated RBCs. In 10-20% of affected infants, the unconjugated serum bilirubin level may reach 20 mg/dL or more unless phototherapy is administered.

Treatment

Phototherapy may be effective in lowering serum bilirubin levels (Chapter 96.4). In severe cases, IVIG administration can reduce the rate of hemolysis and the need for exchange transfusion. Exchange transfusions with type O blood of the same Rh type as the infant may be needed in some cases to correct dangerous degrees of anemia or hyperbilirubinemia. Indications for this procedure are similar to those previously described for hemolytic disease due to Rh incompatibility. Some infants with ABO hemolytic disease may require transfusion of packed RBCs at several weeks of age because of slowly progressive anemia. Post-discharge monitoring of hemoglobin or Hct is essential in newborns with ABO hemolytic disease.

OTHER FORMS OF HEMOLYTIC DISEASE

Blood group incompatibilities other than Rh or ABO account for < 5% of hemolytic disease of the newborn. The direct Coombs test result is invariably positive, and exchange transfusion may be indicated for hyperbilirubinemia and anemia. Hemolytic disease, anemia, and hydrops fetalis as a result of anti-Kell antibodies are not predictable from the previous obstetric history, amniotic fluid bilirubin determinants, or the maternal antibody titer. Erythroid suppression may contribute to the anemia; PUBS is beneficial in actually measuring the fetal Hct. Kell-alloimmunized infants often have inappropriately low numbers of circulating reticulocytes in comparison with other forms of hemolytic disease, which can cause difficulties in the laboratory confirmation of the hemolytic etiology of hyperbilirubinemia. The clinical characteristics of hemolytic disease due to Rh, ABO, and Kell antigen systems are summarized in Table 97-4.

BIBLIOGRAPHY

Please visit the Nelson Textbook of Pediatrics *website at www.expertconsult.com for the complete bibliography.*

97.3 Plethora in the Newborn Infant (Polycythemia) (See Also Chapter 461)

Akhil Maheshwari and Waldemar A. Carlo

Plethora, a ruddy, deep red-purple appearance associated with a high Hct, is often due to polycythemia, defined as a central Hct of 65% or higher. Peripheral (heelstick) Hct values are higher than central values, whereas Coulter counter results are lower than Hct values determined by microcentrifugation. The incidence of neonatal polycythemia is increased at high altitudes (5% in Denver vs 1.6% in Texas); in postmature (3%) vs term (1-2%) infants; in small for gestational age (SGA; 8%) vs large for gestational age (LGA; 3%) vs average for gestational age (1-2%) infants; during the 1st day of life (peak, 2-3 hr); in the recipient infant of a twin-twin transfusion; after delayed clamping of the umbilical cord; in infants of diabetic mothers; in trisomy 13, 18, or 21; in adrenogenital syndrome; in neonatal Graves disease; in hypothyroidism; in infants of hypertensive mothers or those on propranolol; and in Beckwith-Wiedemann syndrome. Infants of diabetic or hypertensive mothers and those with growth restriction may have been exposed to chronic fetal hypoxia, which stimulates erythropoietin production and increases RBC production.

Clinical manifestations include irritability, lethargy, tachypnea, respiratory distress, cyanosis, feeding disturbances, hyperbilirubinemia, hypoglycemia, and thrombocytopenia. Severe complications include seizures, stroke, pulmonary hypertension, necrotizing enterocolitis, renal vein thrombosis, and renal failure. *Many affected infants are asymptomatic.* Hyperviscosity is present in many infants with central Hct values of 65% or higher and accounts for the symptoms of polycythemia. Hyperviscosity determined at constant shear rates (11.5 sec^{-1}) is present when whole blood viscosity is >18 cycles/sec. Hyperviscosity is accentuated because neonatal RBCs have decreased deformability and filterability, which predispose to stasis in the microcirculation.

Table 97-4 HEMOLYTIC DISEASE OF THE NEWBORN

	Rh	ABO	KELL
BLOOD GROUPS			
Mother	Rh-negative	O (occasionally B)	K1-negative
Infant	Positive (D, sometimes C)	A (sometimes B)	K1-positive
CLINICAL FEATURES OF HEMOLYTIC DISEASE IN THE NEWBORN			
Occurrence in first-born	5%	40-50%	Rare
Severity in subsequent pregnancies:	Predictable	Difficult to predict	Somewhat predictable
Stillbirth/hydrops	Frequent	Rare	10%
Severe anemia	Frequent	Rare	Frequent
Jaundice	Prominent, severe	Mild-moderate	Mild
LABORATORY TESTS:			
Direct Coombs' test result (infant)	Positive	Positive or negative	Positive or negative
Reticulocyte count	High	High	May not be high
Maternal antibodies	Usually detectable Maternal antibody titers can help predict the severity of fetal disease	May not be detectable Titers may not correlate with fetal disease	Usually detectable Titers may not correlate with fetal disease; fetus affected at titers lower than for Rh-mediated hemolysis

Treatment of symptomatic polycythemic newborns is partial exchange transfusion (with normal saline). A partial exchange transfusion should be considered if the Hct is ≥70-75% or even lower if signs of hyperviscosity are present. Partial exchange transfusion lowers the Hct and viscosity and improves acute symptoms. The volume to be exchanged is calculated from the following formula:

$$\text{Volume of exchange (mL)} = \text{Blood volume} \times (\text{Observed} - \text{Desired hematocrit})/\text{Observed hematocrit}$$

The long-term prognosis of polycythemic infants is unclear. Reported adverse outcomes include speech deficits, abnormal fine motor control, reduced IQ, school problems, and other neurologic abnormalities. The underlying etiology (chronic intrauterine hypoxia) and hyperviscosity is thought to contribute to adverse outcomes. It is unclear whether partial exchange transfusion improves the long-term outcome. Most asymptomatic infants develop normally.

BIBLIOGRAPHY

Please visit the Nelson Textbook of Pediatrics *website at* *www.expertconsult.com* *for the complete bibliography.*

97.4 Hemorrhage in the Newborn Infant

Akhil Maheshwari and Waldemar A. Carlo

HEMORRHAGIC DISEASE OF THE NEWBORN

A moderate decrease in factors II, VII, IX, and X normally occurs in all newborn infants by 48-72 hr after birth, with a gradual return to birth levels by 7-10 days of age. This transient deficiency of vitamin K–dependent factors is probably due to lack of free vitamin K from the mother and absence of the bacterial intestinal flora normally responsible for the synthesis of vitamin K. Rarely in term infants and more frequently in premature infants, accentuation and prolongation of this deficiency between the 2nd and 7th days of life result in spontaneous and prolonged bleeding. Breast milk is a poor source of vitamin K, but hemorrhagic complications are more frequent in breast-fed than in formula-fed infants. This classic form of hemorrhagic disease of the newborn, which is responsive to and prevented by vitamin K therapy, must be distinguished from disseminated intravascular coagulopathy and from the more infrequent congenital deficiencies of one or more of the other factors that are unresponsive to vitamin K (Chapter 470). Early-onset life-threatening vitamin K deficiency–induced bleeding (onset from birth to 24 hr) also occurs if the mother has been treated with drugs (phenobarbital, phenytoin) that interfere with vitamin K function. Late onset (>2 wk) is often associated with vitamin K malabsorption, as noted in neonatal hepatitis or biliary atresia (Table 97-5).

Hemorrhagic disease of the newborn resulting from severe transient deficiencies in vitamin K–dependent factors is characterized by bleeding that tends to be gastrointestinal, nasal, subgaleal, intracranial, or post-circumcision. Prodromal or warning signs (mild bleeding) may occur before serious intracranial hemorrhage. The prothrombin time (PT), blood coagulation time, and partial thromboplastin time (PTT) are prolonged, and levels of prothrombin (II) and factors VII, IX, and X are decreased. Vitamin K facilitates post-transcriptional carboxylation of factors II, VII, IX, and X. In the absence of carboxylation, such factors form PIVKA (protein induced in vitamin K absence), which is a sensitive marker for vitamin K status. Bleeding time, fibrinogen, factors V and VIII, platelets, capillary fragility, and clot retraction are normal for maturity.

Intramuscular administration of 1 mg of vitamin K at the time of birth **prevents** the decrease in vitamin K–dependent factors in full-term infants, but it is not uniformly effective in the prophylaxis of hemorrhagic disease of the newborn, particularly in breast-fed and in premature infants. The disease may be effectively **treated** with a slow intravenous infusion of 1-5 mg of vitamin K_1, with improvement in coagulation defects and cessation of bleeding noted within a few hours. Serious bleeding, particularly in premature infants or those with liver disease, may require a transfusion of **fresh frozen plasma** or whole blood. The mortality rate is low in treated patients.

A particularly severe form of deficiency of vitamin K–dependent coagulation factors has been reported in infants born to mothers receiving anticonvulsive medications (phenobarbital and phenytoin) during pregnancy. The infants may have severe bleeding, with onset within the 1st 24 hr of life; the bleeding is usually corrected by vitamin K_1, although in some the response is poor or delayed. A PT should be measured in cord blood, and the infant given 1-2 mg of vitamin K intravenously. If the PT is greatly prolonged and fails to improve, 10 mL/kg of fresh frozen plasma should be administered.

The routine use of intramuscular vitamin K for prophylaxis in the United States is safe and is not associated with an increased risk of childhood cancer or leukemia. Although oral vitamin K (birth, discharge, 3-4 wk: 1-2 mg) has been suggested as an

Table 97-5 HEMORRHAGIC DISEASE OF THE NEWBORN

	EARLY-ONSET DISEASE	CLASSIC DISEASE	LATE-ONSET DISEASE
Age	0-24 hr	2-7 days	1-6 mo
Site of hemorrhage	Cephalohematoma	Gastrointestinal	Intracranial
	Subgaleal	Ear-nose-throat-mucosal	Gastrointestinal
	Intracranial	Intracranial	Cutaneous
	Gastrointestinal	Circumcision	Ear-nose-throat-mucosal
	Umbilicus	Cutaneous	Injection sites
	Intra-abdominal	Gastrointestinal	Thoracic
		Injection sites	
Etiology/risks	Maternal drugs (phenobarbital, phenytoin, warfarin, rifampin, isoniazid) that interfere with vitamin K	Vitamin K deficiency Breast-feeding	Cholestasis—malabsorption of vitamin K (biliary atresia, cystic fibrosis, hepatitis)
	Inherited coagulopathy		Abetalipoprotein deficiency Idiopathic in Asian breast-fed infants Warfarin ingestion
Prevention	Possibly, administrations of vitamin K to infant at birth or to mother (20 mg) before birth Avoid high-risk medications	Prevented by parenteral vitamin K at birth Oral vitamin K regimens require repeated dosing over time	Prevented by parenteral and high-dose oral vitamin K during periods of malabsorption or cholestasis
Incidence	Very rare	≈2% if infant not given vitamin K	Dependent on primary disease

alternative, oral vitamin K is less effective in preventing the late onset of bleeding due to vitamin K deficiency and thus cannot be recommended for routine therapy. The intramuscular route remains the method of choice.

Other forms of bleeding may be clinically indistinguishable from hemorrhagic disease of the newborn responsive to vitamin K, but they are neither prevented nor successfully treated with vitamin K. A clinical pattern identical to that of hemorrhagic disease of the newborn may also result from any of the congenital defects in blood coagulation (Chapters 470 and 471). Hematomas, melena, and post-circumcision and umbilical cord bleeding may be present; only 5-35% of cases of factor VIII and IX deficiency become clinically apparent in the newborn period. Treatment of the rare congenital deficiencies of coagulation factors requires fresh frozen plasma or specific factor replacement.

Disseminated intravascular coagulopathy in newborn infants results in consumption of coagulation factors and bleeding. Affected infants are often premature; the clinical course is frequently characterized by asphyxia, hypoxia, acidosis, shock, hemangiomas, or infection. Treatment is directed at correcting the primary clinical problem, such as infection, interrupting consumption of clotting factors, and replacing them (Chapter 477).

Infants with central nervous system or other bleeding posing an immediate threat to life should receive fresh frozen plasma, vitamin K, and blood if needed as soon as possible after a blood specimen has been obtained for coagulation studies, which should include a determination of the number of platelets.

The **swallowed blood syndrome,** in which blood or bloody stools are passed, usually on the 2nd or 3rd day of life, may be confused with hemorrhage from the gastrointestinal tract. The blood may be swallowed during delivery or from a fissure in the mother's nipple. Differentiation from gastrointestinal hemorrhage is based on the fact that the infant's blood contains mostly fetal hemoglobin, which is alkali-resistant, whereas swallowed blood from a maternal source contains adult hemoglobin, which is promptly changed to alkaline hematin after the addition of alkali. Apt devised the following test for this differentiation: (1) Rinse a blood-stained diaper or some grossly bloody (red) stool with a suitable amount of water to obtain a distinctly pink supernatant hemoglobin solution; (2) centrifuge the mixture and decant the supernatant solution; (3) add 1 part of 0.25 N (1%) sodium hydroxide to 5 parts of the supernatant fluid. Within 1-2 min, a color reaction takes place: A yellow-brown color indicates that the blood is maternal in origin; a persistent pink indicates that it is from the infant. A control test with known adult or infant blood, or both, is advisable.

Widespread subcutaneous ecchymoses in premature infants at or immediately after birth are apparently a result of fragile superficial blood vessels rather than a coagulation defect. Administering vitamin K_1 to the mother during labor has no effect on the incidence of ecchymoses. Occasionally, an infant is born with petechiae or a generalized bluish suffusion limited to the face, head, and neck, probably as a result of venous obstruction by a nuchal cord or sudden increases in intrathoracic pressure during delivery. It may take 2-3 wk for such suffusions to disappear.

NEONATAL THROMBOCYTOPENIC PURPURA

See Chapter 478.

BIBLIOGRAPHY

Please visit the Nelson Textbook of Pediatrics *website at www.expertconsult.com for the complete bibliography.*

Chapter 98
Genitourinary System (See Also Part XXIV)

Waldemar A. Carlo

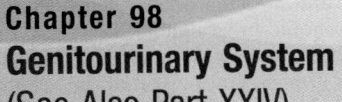

Urinary tract anomalies (hydronephrosis, dysplasia, agenesis, cystic or solitary kidney) can be identified by prenatal ultrasonography (see Table 90-1). After birth, the presence/extent of anomalies needs to be confirmed and followed by detailed evaluation and appropriate management. Multicystic and polycystic forms of kidney disease have high risk for mortality and renal morbidity. In contrast, the majority of mild dilatations have no clinical consequences but cause unnecessary anxiety in many cases.

For the full continuation of this chapter, please visit the Nelson Textbook of Pediatrics *website at www.expertconsult.com.*

Chapter 99
The Umbilicus
Waldemar A. Carlo

UMBILICAL CORD

The umbilical cord contains the two umbilical arteries, the umbilical vein, the rudimentary allantois, the remnant of the omphalomesenteric duct, and a gelatinous substance called Wharton jelly. The sheath of the umbilical cord is derived from the amnion. The muscular umbilical arteries contract readily, but the vein does not. The vein retains a fairly large lumen after birth. The normal cord at term is 55 cm long. Abnormally short cords are associated with antepartum abnormalities, including fetal hypotonia, oligohydramnios, and uterine constraint, and with increased risk for complications of labor and delivery for both mother and infant. Long cords (>70 cm) increase risk for true knots, wrapping around fetal parts (neck, arm), and/or prolapse. Straight untwisted cords are associated with fetal distress, anomalies, and intrauterine fetal demise.

For the full continuation of this chapter, please visit the Nelson Textbook of Pediatrics *website at www.expertconsult.com.*

Chapter 100
Metabolic Disturbances
Waldemar A. Carlo

HYPERTHERMIA IN THE NEWBORN

Elevations in temperature (38-39°C [100-103°F]) are occasionally noted on the 2nd or 3rd day of life in infants whose clinical course has been otherwise satisfactory. This disturbance is especially likely to occur in breast-fed infants whose intake of fluid has been particularly low or in infants who are overdressed or are exposed to high environmental temperatures, either in an incubator, in a bassinette near a radiator, or in the sun.

The infant may lose weight. A consistent relationship may not be seen between the fever and the extent of weight loss or inadequacy of fluid intake. Urinary output and the frequency of voiding diminish. The fontanel may be depressed. The infant takes fluids avidly, but the apparent vigor of the infant contrasts with the usual appearance of "being sick" from an infection. The rise in temperature may be associated with increases in serum levels of protein and sodium and in hematocrit. The possibility of local or systemic infection should be evaluated. Lowering the environmental temperature leads to prompt reduction of the fever and alleviation of symptoms. Oral hydration should be accomplished with additional nursing or formula and not with pure water, because of the risk of hyponatremia.

A more severe form of neonatal hyperthermia occurs in both newborn and older infants when they are warmly dressed. The diminished sweating capacity of newborn infants is a contributing factor. Warmly dressed infants left near stoves or radiators, traveling in well-heated automobiles, or left with bright sunlight shining directly on them through the windows of a closed room or automobile are likely to be victims. Body temperature may become as high as 41-44°C (106-111°F). The skin is hot and dry, and initially the infant usually appears flushed and apathetic. The extremities are warm. Tachypnea and irritability may be noted. This stage may be followed by stupor, grayish pallor, coma, and convulsions. Hypernatremia may contribute to the convulsions. Mortality and morbidity (brain damage) rates are high. Hyperthermia has been associated with sudden infant death, **hemorrhagic shock, and encephalopathy syndrome** (Chapter 64). The condition is prevented by dressing infants in clothing suitable for the temperature of the immediate environment. In newborn infants, exposure of the body to usual room temperature or immersion in tepid water usually suffices to bring the temperature back to normal levels. Older infants may require cooling for a longer time by repeated immersion. Attention to possible fluid and electrolyte disturbance is essential.

Hyperthermia a few days after birth can be due to infection, particularly herpes sepsis. Infants with infection appear ill with cold extremities, in contrast to those in whom hyperthermia is due to environmental causes.

NEONATAL COLD INJURY

Neonatal cold injury usually occurs in abandoned infants, infants in inadequately heated homes during cold spells when the outside temperature is in the freezing range, and in preterm infants (Chapter 69). The initial features are apathy, refusal of food, oliguria, and coldness to touch. The body temperature is usually between 29.5 and 35°C (85-95°F), and immobility, edema, and redness of the extremities, especially the hands and feet, and of the face are observed. Bradycardia and apnea may also occur. The facial erythema frequently gives a false impression of health and delays recognition that the infant is ill. Local hardening over areas of edema may lead to confusion with scleredema. Hypoglycemia and acidosis are common. Hemorrhagic manifestations are frequent; massive pulmonary hemorrhage is a common finding at autopsy. Hypothermia in preterm infants can be prevented with special plastic wraps that reduce evaporation and heat loss. Because of their high ratio of surface area to body mass, preterm infants are very vulnerable to evaporation heat loss. Infants at <28-30 wk should be placed inside a clear polyethylene bag without prior drying. Neonatal cold injury in preterm infants occurs in the developing world and can be prevented with skin-to-skin (kangaroo mother) care. **Treatment** consists of warming and paying scrupulous attention to recognition and correction of hypotension and metabolic imbalances, particularly hypoglycemia. Prevention consists of providing adequate environmental heat. The mortality rate is about 10%; about 10% of survivors have evidence of brain damage.

EDEMA

Generalized edema occurs in association with **hydrops fetalis** (Chapter 97.2) and in the offspring of diabetic mothers. In premature infants, edema is often a consequence of a decreased ability to excrete water or sodium, although some have considerable edema without identifiable cause. Infants with respiratory distress syndrome may become edematous without heart failure. Edema of the face and scalp may be caused by pressure from the umbilical cord around the neck, and transient localized swelling of the hands or feet may similarly be due to intrauterine pressure. Edema may be associated with heart failure. A lag in renal excretion of electrolytes and water may result in edema after a sudden large increase in intake of electrolytes, particularly with feeding of concentrated cow's milk formulas. High-protein formulas may also cause edema as a result of the excessive renal solute load, particularly in premature infants. Rarely, idiopathic hypoproteinemia with edema lasting weeks or months is observed in term infants. The cause is unclear, and the disturbance is benign. Persistent edema of 1 or more extremities may represent congenital lymphedema (Milroy disease) or, in females, Turner syndrome. Generalized edema with hypoproteinemia may be seen in the neonatal period with congenital nephrosis and rarely with Hurler syndrome or after feeding hypoallergenic formulas to infants with cystic fibrosis of the pancreas. Sclerema is described in Chapter 639.

HYPOCALCEMIA (TETANY) (CHAPTER 48)

Metabolic Bone Disease

Metabolic bone disease is a common complication in very low birthweight (VLBW) preterm infants. The smallest, sickest infants are at greatest risk. Progressive osteopenia with demineralized bones and, occasionally, pathologic fractures may develop. The major cause is inadequate intake of calcium and phosphorus to meet the requirements for growth. Poor intake of vitamin D is an additional risk factor. Contributing factors include prolonged parenteral nutrition, vitamin D and calcium malabsorption, intake of unsupplemented human milk, immobilization, and urinary calcium losses from long-term diuretic use. The serum alkaline phosphatase level is used to monitor metabolic bone disease and can be > 1,000 U/L in severe cases. Fortified human milk and formulas designed for preterm infants provide higher amounts of calcium, phosphorus, and vitamin D; promote bone mineralization; and may prevent metabolic bone disease. Many extremely LBW infants will require additional oral supplements of calcium and phosphorus. Treatment of fractures requires immobilization and administration of calcium, phosphorus, and, if needed, vitamin D (not more than 1,000 IU/day unless severe cholestasis or vitamin D resistance is present). See also Chapters 48 and 564.

HYPOMAGNESEMIA

Rarely, hypomagnesemia of unknown cause may occur in newborn infants, usually in association with hypocalcemia. It may also be associated with insufficient stores of skeletal magnesium secondary to deficient placental transfer, decreased intestinal absorption, neonatal hypoparathyroidism, hyperphosphatemia, renal loss (primary or secondary to drugs, e.g., amphotericin B), a defect in magnesium and calcium homeostasis, or iatrogenic deficiency caused by loss incurred during exchange transfusion or insufficient replacement during total intravenous alimentation. Infants of diabetic mothers may have lower than normal serum magnesium levels. The clinical manifestations of hypomagnesemia are indistinguishable from those of hypocalcemia and tetany and may, in fact, contribute to the accompanying hypocalcemia.

Hypomagnesemia occurs when serum magnesium levels fall below 1.5 mg/dL (0.62 mmol/L), although clinical signs do not usually develop until serum magnesium levels fall below 1.2 mg/dL. During exchange transfusion with citrated blood, which is low in magnesium because of binding by citrate, serum magnesium decreases about 0.5 mg/dL (0.2 mmol/L); approximately 10 days are required for return to normal. In non-iatrogenic hypomagnesemia, the serum magnesium level may be <0.5 mg/dL. Serum calcium in either instance is usually at levels noted in hypocalcemic tetany, but the serum phosphorus value is normal or high. Because the hypocalcemia accompanying hypomagnesemia is inadequately corrected by administration of calcium alone, hypomagnesemia should also be suspected in any patient with tetany not responding to calcium therapy.

Immediate **treatment** consists of intramuscular injection of magnesium sulfate. For newborn infants, 25-50 mg/kg/dose every 8 hr for 3-4 doses usually suffices. The accompanying hypocalcemia usually corrects itself as the hypomagnesemia resolves. The same daily dose can be given for oral maintenance therapy. Four to 5 times higher doses may be required in malabsorptive states. In most cases, the metabolic defect is transient, and treatment can be discontinued after 1-2 wk. A few patients appear to have a permanent form of the disease that requires continuous oral supplementation with magnesium to prevent recurrence of hypomagnesemia. No residual damage to the central nervous system is evident after prompt treatment.

HYPERMAGNESEMIA

Hypermagnesemia may occur in newborn infants of mothers treated with magnesium sulfate during labor. At high serum levels, the central nervous system is depressed and infants have respiratory depression that may require mechanical ventilation. Lower levels may result in hypoventilation, lethargy, flaccidity, hyporeflexia, and poor sucking. Hypermagnesemia may be associated with failure to pass meconium. The upper limit of normal magnesium is 2.8 mg/dL (1.15 mmol/L), but serious symptoms rarely occur at levels < 5 mg/dL (2.1 mmol/L). In most cases, no specific therapy (beyond supportive care and maintenance of respiratory support) is required. Intravenous calcium and diuresis will reduce the magnesium levels. In rare cases, exchange transfusion has been used for rapid removal of magnesium ion from the blood.

SUBSTANCE ABUSE AND NEONATAL ABSTINENCE (WITHDRAWAL)

Substance abuse during pregnancy is a serious problem for both the mother and her newborn. The mother may suffer adverse consequences of her addiction, including episodes of drug withdrawal during pregnancy and illnesses related to high-risk behavior. Effects on the fetus and newborn include chronic or intermittent drug exposure, poor maternal nutrition, acute withdrawal shortly after birth, and long-term effects on physical growth and neurodevelopment. Because infants with in utero drug exposure often have social and environmental risk factors and may have been exposed to multiple substances, it may be difficult to evaluate the effects of specific in utero drug exposure on long-term neurodevelopmental outcome.

Pregnancies in women who use illegal drugs or alcohol are high risk. Prenatal care is usually inadequate, and these women have a higher incidence of sexually transmitted infections, including syphilis, HIV, and hepatitis. In addition, the risk of preterm labor, intrauterine growth restriction, premature rupture of membranes, and perinatal morbidity and mortality is higher. Physiologic addiction to narcotics occurs in most infants born to actively addicted mothers because opiates cross the placenta. Withdrawal may manifest even before birth as increased activity of the fetus when the mother feels a need for the drug or withdrawal symptoms develop. Heroin and methadone are the drugs most frequently associated with withdrawal syndromes, but such syndromes may also occur with alcohol, nicotine, phenobarbital, pentazocine, codeine, propoxyphene, hydroxyzine, amphetamines, neuroleptics, antidepressants, and benzodiazepines.

Heroin addiction results in a 50% incidence of LBW infants, half of whom are small for gestational age. Chronic infections, maternal undernutrition, and a direct fetal growth–inhibiting effect are possible causes. The rate of stillbirths is increased, but not the incidence of congenital anomalies. Clinical manifestations of withdrawal occur in 50-75% of infants, usually beginning within the 1st 48 hr, depending on the daily maternal dose (<6 mg/24 hr is associated with no or mild symptoms), the duration of addiction (duration > 1 yr has a > 70% incidence of withdrawal), and the time of the last maternal dose (the incidence is higher if the last dose was taken within 24 hr of birth). Rarely, symptoms may appear as late as 4-6 wk of age. The incidence of respiratory distress syndrome and hyperbilirubinemia may be decreased in preterm infants of heroin users; accelerated production of pulmonary surfactant may explain the former, and enzyme induction of hepatic glucuronyl transferase the latter.

Tremors and hyperirritability are the most prominent symptoms. The tremors may be fine or jittery and indistinguishable from those of hypoglycemia, but they are more often coarse, “flapping,” and bilateral; the limbs are frequently rigid, hyperreflexic, and resistant to flexion and extension. Irritability and hyperactivity are generally marked and may lead to skin abrasions. Other signs include wakefulness, hyperacusis, hypertonicity, tachypnea, diarrhea, vomiting, high-pitched cry, fist sucking, poor feeding with weight loss (disorganized sucking), and fever. Sneezing, yawning, hiccups, myoclonic jerks, convulsions, abnormal sleep cycles, nasal stuffiness, apnea, flushing alternating rapidly with pallor, and lacrimation are less common. The Neonatal Intensive Care Unit Network Neurobehavioral Scale (NNNS) is a useful way to evaluate neonates exposed to opiates or other drugs (Table 100-1). The risk of sudden infant death syndrome is higher in such neonates. The diagnosis is generally established from the history and clinical findings. Examining the urine for opiates may reveal only low levels during withdrawal, but quinine, which is often mixed with heroin, may be present in higher concentrations. Meconium testing is more accurate than neonatal urine drug testing. Hypoglycemia and hypocalcemia should be excluded.

Methadone addiction is associated with severe withdrawal symptoms, the incidence varying from 20 to 90%. Mothers taking methadone usually have better prenatal care than those taking heroin; these mothers have a high incidence of polysubstance abuse, including alcohol, barbiturates, and tranquilizers, and they are often heavy smokers. The incidence of congenital anomalies is not increased. The average birthweight of infants of mothers taking methadone is higher than that of infants of heroin-addicted mothers; the clinical manifestations are similar, except that the former group has a higher incidence of seizures (10-20%) and later onset (2-6 wk of age) of withdrawal. Women who continue to abuse heroin, even if they enter a methadone program, are more likely to have preterm and/or low birthweight infants than those born to women who stop using heroin. They are also more likely to suffer withdrawal and have a higher risk of neonatal mortality

Alcohol withdrawal is uncommon. Infants of women who have been drinking immediately before delivery may have alcohol on their breath for several hours because it rapidly crosses the placenta. Blood levels in the infant are similar to those in the mother. Hypoglycemia and metabolic acidosis may be present. Infants in whom withdrawal symptoms develop often become agitated and hyperactive, with marked tremors lasting 72 hr, followed by about 48 hr of lethargy before return to normal activity. Seizures may develop.

Phenobarbital withdrawal usually occurs in infants of mothers addicted to the drug. Symptoms begin at a median age of 7 days (range, 2-14 days). Infants may have a brief acute stage consisting of irritability, constant crying, sleeplessness, hiccups, and mouthing movements, followed by a subacute stage consisting of voracious appetite, frequent regurgitation and gagging, episodic irritability, hyperacusis, sweating, and a disturbed sleep pattern, all of which may last 2-4 mo.

Cocaine abuse in pregnant women is common, but withdrawal in their infants is unusual; the pregnancy may be complicated by premature labor, abruptio placentae, and fetal asphyxia. Infants may have intrauterine growth restriction and neurobehavioral deficits characterized by impaired state regulation, impaired auditory information processing, developmental delay, and learning disabilities. At 24 mo of age, they score lower on the mental portion of the Bayley Scales of Infant Development and are twice as likely to have developmental delay. Family disorganization, polysubstance abuse, sexually transmitted infections, and child abuse and neglect may also be present. At 4 yr of age, children exposed prenatally to cocaine demonstrate specific cognitive impairments (visual-spatial and math skills; general knowledge) and are less likely to have an IQ above the normative mean. With a more enriching home environment, IQ scores of cocaine-exposed children are similar to those of nonexposed children.

Table 100-1 NEUROBEHAVIORAL SCALE

DOMAIN	ITEMS
Physiological	Labored breathing
	Nasal flaring
Autonomic	Sweating
	Spit-up
	Hiccoughing
	Sneezing
	Nasal stuffiness
	Yawning
CNS	Abnormal sucking
	Choreiform movements
	Athetoid postures and movements
	Tremors
	Cogwheel movements
	Startles
	Hypertonia
	Back arching
	Fisting
	Cortical thumb
	Myoclonic jerks
	Generalized seizures
	Abnormal posture
Skin	Pallor
	Mottling
	Lividity
	Overall cyanosis
	Circumoral cyanosis
	Periocular cyanosis
Visual	Gaze aversion during orientation
	Pull-down during orientation
	Fuss/cry during orientation
	Obligatory following during orientation
	End point nystagmus during orientation
	Sustained spontaneous nystagmus
	Visual locking
	Hyperalertness
	Setting sun sign
	Roving eye movements
	Strabismus
	Tight blinking
	Other abnormal eye signs
Gastrointestinal	Gagging/choking
	Loose stools, watery stools
	Excessive gas, bowel sounds
State	High-pitched cry
	Monotone-pitch cry
	Weak cry
	No cry
	Extreme irritability
	Abrupt state changes
	Inability to achieve quiet awake state (state 4)

CNS, central nervous system.
From Lester BM, Tronick EZ, Brazelton TB: The Neonatal Intensive Care Unit Network Neurobehavioral Scales procedures, *Pediatrics* 113:641–667, 2004.

Treatment

The decision to use drug therapy for neonatal drug withdrawal should be based on the presence of signs of withdrawal. Infants with confirmed drug exposure who do not have signs of withdrawal do not require pharmacologic treatment. Drug withdrawal is a self-limiting process. However, withdrawal from sedative-hypnotic drugs or narcotics can be life-threatening. Indications for drug treatment include seizures, poor feeding, diarrhea, excessive vomiting, inability to sleep, and fever. Several methods to assess severity of the withdrawal are available.

Infants who are undergoing opiate withdrawal require care in a quiet environment with reduction of external stimuli and swaddling. Treatment of heroin and methadone withdrawal using methadone has been successful. Methadone withdrawal may require larger amounts of medication for longer periods to control clinical manifestations than are needed for heroin withdrawal. Paregoric at a beginning dose of 0.05-0.1 mL/kg is given every 3-4 hr and increased by 0.05 mL every 4 hr if necessary, depending on the size and response of the infant. Paregoric abolishes most withdrawal symptoms, especially diarrhea. Tincture of opium (10 mg/mL) diluted 25-fold results in the same morphine equivalency as paregoric. The recommended dose of diluted tincture of opium is 0.1 mL/kg (≈2 drops/kg) with feedings every 4 hr. The dose may be increased by 2 drops every 4 hr if needed. The dose and duration of therapy may be adjusted according to the clinical response. A combination of an opiate plus phenobarbital may be the most effective approach to an opiate withdrawal. Parenteral administration of fluids may be necessary to prevent aspiration or dehydration until the symptoms are brought under control. Buprenorphine, rather than methadone, treatment during pregnancy reduces the severity and duration of withdrawal.

Mortality from withdrawal is <5% and may be negligible with early recognition and treatment. The prognosis for normal development is affected by the adverse circumstances of high-risk pregnancy and delivery and by the environment to which the infant is returned after recovery, as well as by the effects of the particular drug on fetal and subsequent neonatal development.

BIBLIOGRAPHY

Please visit the Nelson Textbook of Pediatrics *website at www.expertconsult.com for the complete bibliography.*

100.1 Maternal Selective Serotonin Reuptake Inhibitors and Neonatal Behavioral Syndromes

Waldemar A. Carlo

Women of childbearing age have a combined incidence of depression and anxiety of approximately 19%. Selective serotonin reuptake inhibitors (SSRIs; fluoxetine, paroxetine, sertraline, citalopram, fluvoxamine) and, less often, serotonin norepinephrine reuptake inhibitors (SNRIs; venlafaxine, duloxetine) have been used to treat pregnant women with depression or anxiety disorders. Exposure to these agents during pregnancy may inconsistently produce congenital malformations (Chapter 90). In addition, poor neonatal adaptation has been noted with the use of many of these agents but most often with paroxetine and fluoxetine.

It is unclear whether poor neonatal adaptation is due to serotonin overstimulation (**serotonin syndrome**) or to withdrawal (**serotonin discontinuation syndrome**). Indeed, both conditions may occur with different agents. Paroxetine has a short half-life and few if any active metabolites and is also a potent muscarinic blocking agent. Serum paroxetine levels after birth decline rapidly. Neonatal adaptive symptoms after late pregnancy exposure to paroxetine may be withdrawal with cholinergic overdrive. Symptoms may also be delayed. In contrast, fluoxetine and its active metabolite (nor-fluoxetine) have long half-lives and may produce a serotonin syndrome of acute toxicity. Onset may be at birth or in the 1st 24 hr of life. The cord blood level of fluoxetine is equal to blood level in the mother. All agents cross the placental and blood-brain barriers.

A neonatal behavioral syndrome that has features of both direct serotonin toxicity and withdrawal (cholinergic overdrive) is noted in Figure 100-1 and is characterized by central nervous system (irritability, excess or restless sleep), motor (agitation, tremor, hyperreflexia, rigidity, hypotonia or hypertonia), respiratory (nasal congestion, respiratory distress, tachypnea), gastrointestinal (diarrhea, emesis, poor feeding) and systemic (hypothermia or hyperthermia, hypoglycemia) manifestations. Most infants have only mild symptoms that resolve within 2 wk; a severe syndrome characterized by seizures, dehydration, weight loss, hyperpyrexia, and respiratory failure is present in 1%. No deaths have been reported.

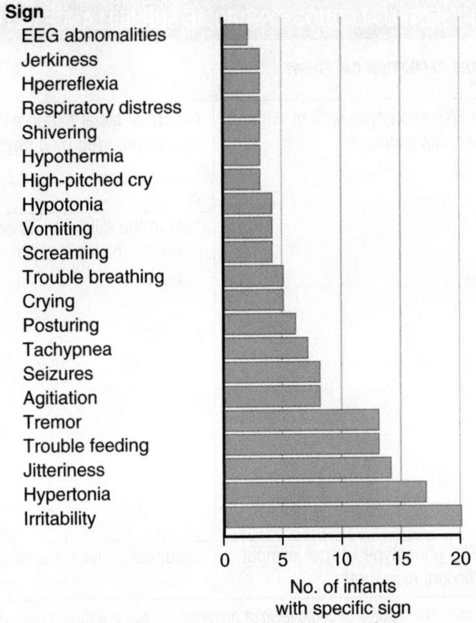

Figure 100-1 Neonatal signs after late in utero exposure to serotonin reuptake inhibitors. Frequencies of specific signs reported to the U.S. Food and Drug Administration (FDA) Adverse Events Reporting System. Ordered by frequency of occurrence ($n = 57$ infants). EEG, electroencephalographic. (From Moses-Kolko EL, Bogen D, Perel J, et al: Neonatal signs after late in utero exposure to serotonin reuptake inhibitors, *JAMA* 293:2372–2383, 2005.)

Treatment is directed at the individual manifestations and accompanied by supportive therapies. A method of prevention of neonatal SSRI withdrawal has been proposed that consists of weaning the mother from the SSRI in the 3rd trimester of pregnancy. The advantages of this approach for the fetus must be weighed against the risk for the mother of recurrence of psychiatric symptoms during the last trimester and postpartum period.

BIBLIOGRAPHY

Please visit the Nelson Textbook of Pediatrics *website at www.expertconsult.com for the complete bibliography.*

100.2 Fetal Alcohol Syndrome

Waldemar A. Carlo

High levels of alcohol ingestion during pregnancy can be damaging to embryonic and fetal development. A specific pattern of malformation identified as *fetal alcohol syndrome* has been documented, and major and minor components of the syndrome are expressed in 1-2 infants/1,000 live births (see Table 100-2). Both moderate and high levels of alcohol intake during early pregnancy may result in alterations in growth and morphogenesis of the fetus; the greater the intake, the more severe the signs. The risk of abnormality for infants born to heavy drinkers is twice that for infants born to moderate drinkers; in one study, 32% of infants born to heavy drinkers had congenital anomalies, compared with 9% of those born to abstinent mothers and 14% of those born to moderate drinkers. Additional maternal risk factors associated with fetal alcohol syndrome are advanced maternal

Table 100-2 FETAL ALCOHOL SYNDROME SURVEILLANCE NETWORK CASE DEFINITION CATEGORIES

CASE DEFINITION CATEGORY	PHENOTYPE POSITIVE Face	Central Nervous System	Growth
Confirmed FAS phenotype with or without maternal alcohol exposure*	Abnormal facial features consistent with FAS as reported by a physician	Frontal-occipital circumference ≤10th percentile at birth or any age	Intrauterine weight or height corrected for gestational age ≤10th percentile
	or	*or*	*or*
	Two of the following: Short palpebral fissures, abnormal philtrum, thin upper lip	Standardized measure of intellectual function ≤1 SD below the mean	Postnatal weight or height ≤10th percentile for age
		or	*or*
		Standardized measure of developmental delay ≤1 SD below the mean	Postnatal weight for height ≤10th percentile
		or	
		Developmental delay or mental retardation diagnosed by a qualified examiner (e.g., psychologist or physician)	
		or	
		Attention deficit disorder diagnosed by a qualified evaluator	
Probable FAS phenotype with or without maternal alcohol exposure*	Required; facial features same as above	Must meet either central nervous system or growth criteria as outlined above	

*Documentation in the records of some level of maternal alcohol use during the index pregnancy.
FAS, fetal alcohol syndrome; SD, standard deviation.
From Fetal alcohol syndrome—Alaska, Arizona, Colorado and New York, 1995-1997, *MMWR Morb Mortal Wkly Rep* 51:433–435, 2002.

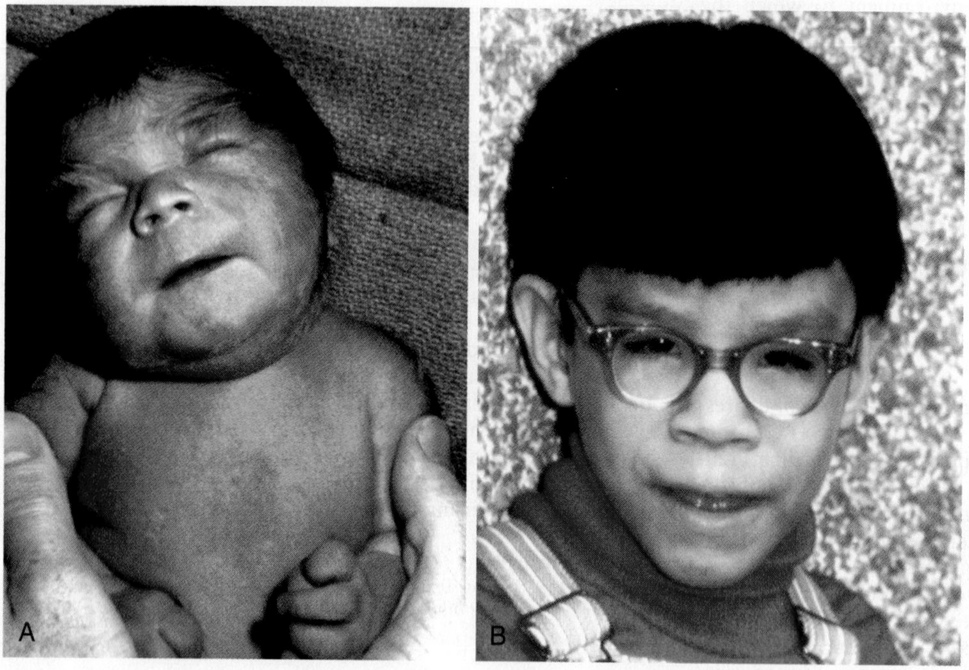

Figure 100-2 At birth *(A)* and at 4 yr of age *(B)*. Note the short palpebral fissures; long, smooth philtrum with vermillion border; and hirsutism in the newborn. (From Jones KL, Smith DW: Recognition of the fetal alcohol syndrome in early infancy, *Lancet* 2:999–1001, 1973.)

age, low socioeconomic status, poor psychologic indicators, and binge drinking.

Characteristics of fetal alcohol syndrome include (1) prenatal onset and persistence of growth deficiency for length, weight, and head circumference; (2) facial abnormalities, including short palpebral fissures, epicanthal folds, maxillary hypoplasia, micrognathia, smooth philtrum, and a thin, smooth upper lip (Fig. 100-2); (3) cardiac defects, primarily septal defects; (4) minor joint and limb abnormalities, including some restriction of movement and altered palmar crease patterns; and (5) delay of development and mental deficiency varying from borderline to severe (Table 100-2). Fetal alcohol syndrome is a common identifiable cause of mental retardation. The severity of dysmorphogenesis may range from severely affected infants with full manifestations of fetal alcohol syndrome to those mildly affected with only a few manifestations.

The detrimental effects may be due to the alcohol itself or to one of its breakdown products. Some evidence suggests that alcohol may impair placental transfer of essential amino acids and zinc, both of which are necessary for protein synthesis, an effect that may account for the intrauterine growth restriction.

Treatment of infants with fetal alcohol syndrome is difficult because no specific therapy exists. These infants may remain hypotonic and tremulous despite sedation, and the prognosis is poor. Counseling with regard to recurrence is important. Prevention is achieved by eliminating alcohol intake after conception.

BIBLIOGRAPHY

Please visit the Nelson Textbook of Pediatrics *website at www.expertconsult.com for the complete bibliography.*

Chapter 101 The Endocrine System

Waldemar A. Carlo

The endocrinopathies are discussed in detail in Part XXVI.

Pituitary dwarfism is not usually apparent at birth, although male infants with panhypopituitarism may have neonatal hypoglycemia, hyperbilirubinemia, and micropenis. Conversely, constitutional dwarfs usually have length and weight suggestive of prematurity when born after a normal gestational period; otherwise, their physical appearance is normal.

Primary hypothyroidism occurs in approximately 1/4,000 births (Chapter 559). Because most infants with serious and treatable disease are asymptomatic at birth, all states screen for it. Thyroid deficiency may also be apparent at birth in genetically determined cretinism or in infants of mothers treated with antithyroid medications or during a pregnancy complicated by maternal hyperthyroidism. Constipation, prolonged jaundice, goiter, lethargy, or poor peripheral circulation as shown by persistently mottled skin or cold extremities should suggest cretinism. Early diagnosis and treatment of congenital thyroid hormone deficiency improve intellectual outcome and are facilitated by screening of all newborn infants for this deficiency.

Transient hypothyroxinemia of prematurity is most common in ill and very premature infants. These infants are probably chemically euthyroid, as suggested by normal levels of serum thyrotropin and other tests of the pituitary-hypothalamic axis. Because the relationship between low thyroid levels and neurodevelopmental outcome is unclear, it remains uncertain whether premature infants with this transient problem should be treated with thyroid hormone.

Transient hyperthyroidism may occur at birth in infants of mothers with hyperthyroidism or in infants whose mothers have been receiving thyroid medication.

Transient hypoparathyroidism may manifest as tetany of the newborn (Chapter 565).

The adrenal glands are subject to numerous disturbances, which may become apparent and require lifesaving treatment during the neonatal period. Acute **adrenal hemorrhage** and failure may occur after breech or other traumatic deliveries or in association with overwhelming infection. Signs of adrenal insufficiency and shock can occur. **Congenital adrenal hyperplasia** is suggested by vomiting, diarrhea, dehydration, hyperkalemia, hyponatremia, shock, ambiguous genitals, or clitoral enlargement. Some infants have ambiguous genitals and hypertension. Because the condition is genetically determined, newborn siblings of patients with the salt-losing variety of adrenocortical hyperplasia should be closely observed for manifestations of adrenal insufficiency. Newborn screening and early diagnosis and therapy for this disorder may prevent severe salt wasting and adverse outcomes. Congenitally hypoplastic adrenal glands may also give rise to adrenal insufficiency during the 1st few weeks of life.

Female infants with webbing of the neck, lymphangiectatic edema, hypoplasia of the nipples, cutis laxa, low hairline at the nape of the neck, low-set ears, high-arched palate, deformities of the nails, cubitus valgus, and other anomalies should be suspected of having gonadal dysgenesis.

Transient diabetes mellitus (Chapter 583) is rare and is encountered only in newborns. It usually manifests as dehydration, loss of weight, or acidosis in infants who are small for gestational age.

BIBLIOGRAPHY

Please visit the Nelson Textbook of Pediatrics *website at* *www.expertconsult.com for the complete bibliography.*

101.1 Infants of Diabetic Mothers

Waldemar A. Carlo

Women with diabetes in pregnancy (type 1, type 2, and gestational) are at increased risk for adverse pregnancy outcomes. Adequate glycemic control before and during pregnancy is crucial to improving outcome.

Diabetic mothers have a high incidence of polyhydramnios, preeclampsia, pyelonephritis, preterm labor, and chronic hypertension; their fetal mortality rate is greater than that of nondiabetic mothers, especially after 32 wk of gestation. Fetal loss throughout pregnancy is associated with poorly controlled maternal diabetes (especially ketoacidosis) and congenital anomalies. Most infants born to diabetic mothers are large for gestational age. If the diabetes is complicated by vascular disease, infants may be growth restricted, especially those born after 37 wk of gestation. The neonatal mortality rate is >5 times that of infants of nondiabetic mothers and is higher at all gestational ages and in every birthweight for gestational age category.

PATHOPHYSIOLOGY

The probable pathogenic sequence is that maternal hyperglycemia causes fetal hyperglycemia, and the fetal pancreatic response leads to fetal hyperinsulinemia; fetal hyperinsulinemia and hyperglycemia then cause increased hepatic glucose uptake and glycogen synthesis, accelerated lipogenesis, and augmented protein synthesis (Fig. 101-1). Related pathologic findings are hypertrophy and hyperplasia of the pancreatic islet β cells, increased weight of the placenta and infant organs except for the brain, myocardial hypertrophy, increased amount of cytoplasm in liver cells, and extramedullary hematopoiesis. Hyperinsulinism and

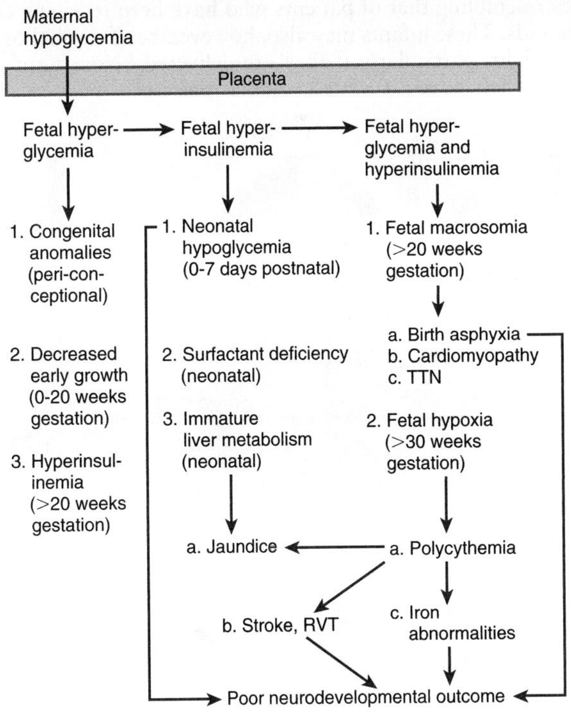

Figure 101-1 The fetal and neonatal events attributable to fetal hyperglycemia (column 1), fetal hyperinsulinemia (column 2), or both in synergy (column 3). Time of risk is denoted in *parentheses.* RVT, renal vein thrombosis; TTN, transient tachypnea of the newborn. (From Nold JL, Georgieff MK: Infants of diabetic mothers, *Pediatr Clin North Am* 51:619–637, 2004.)

hyperglycemia produce fetal acidosis, which may result in an increased rate of stillbirth. Separation of the placenta at birth suddenly interrupts glucose infusion into the neonate without a proportional effect on the hyperinsulinism, and hypoglycemia and attenuated lipolysis develop during the first hours after birth.

Hyperinsulinemia has been documented in infants of mothers with gestational diabetes and in those of mothers with insulin-dependent diabetes (diabetic mothers) without insulin antibodies. The former group also has significantly higher fasting plasma insulin levels than normal newborns do despite similar glucose levels; they also respond to glucose with an abnormally prompt elevation in plasma insulin and assimilate a glucose load more rapidly. After arginine administration, they also have an enhanced insulin response and increased disappearance rates of glucose in comparison with normal infants. In contrast, fasting glucose production and utilization rates are diminished in infants of mothers with gestational diabetes. The lower free fatty acid levels in infants of mothers with insulin-dependent diabetes reflect their hyperinsulinemia. With good prenatal diabetic control, the incidence of macrosomia and hypoglycemia has decreased.

Although hyperinsulinism is probably the main cause of hypoglycemia, the diminished epinephrine and glucagon responses that occur may be contributing factors. Congenital anomalies correlate with poor metabolic control during the periconception and organogenesis periods and may be due to hyperglycemia-induced teratogenesis. Chronic fetal hypoxia, indicated by elevated amniotic fluid erythropoietin values, is associated with increased fetal and neonatal morbidity.

CLINICAL MANIFESTATIONS

Infants of mothers with diabetic and those of mothers with gestational diabetes often bear a surprising resemblance to each other (Fig. 101-2). They tend to be large and plump as a result of increased body fat and enlarged viscera, with puffy, plethoric facies resembling that of patients who have been receiving corticosteroids. These infants may also, however, be of normal or low birthweight, particularly if they are delivered before term or if their mothers have associated vascular disease.

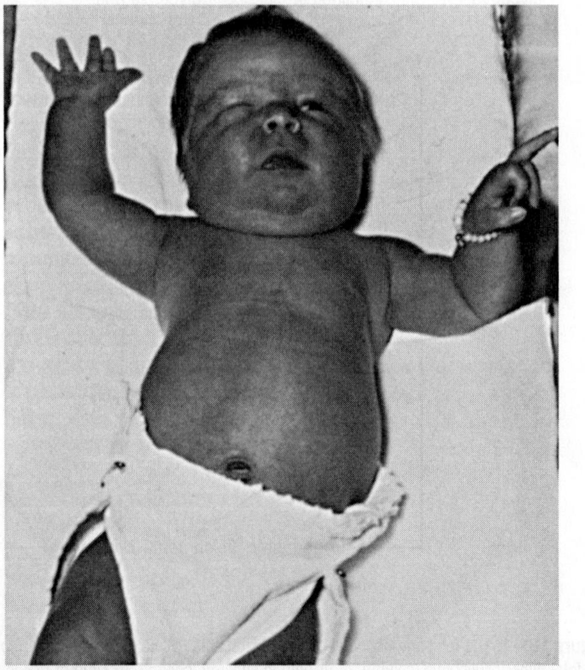

Figure 101-2 Large, plump, plethoric infant of a mother with gestational diabetes. The baby was born at 38 wk of gestation but weighed 9 lb, 11 oz (4,408 g). Mild respiratory distress was the only symptom other than appearance.

Hypoglycemia develops in about 25-50% of infants of diabetic mothers and 15-25% of infants of mothers with gestational diabetes, but only a small percentage of these infants become symptomatic. The probability that hypoglycemia will develop in such an infant increases, and glucose levels are likely to be lower with higher cord or maternal fasting blood glucose levels. The nadir in an infant's blood glucose concentration is usually reached between 1 and 3 hr; spontaneous recovery may begin by 4-6 hr.

The infants tend to be jittery, tremulous, and hyperexcitable during the 1st 3 days of life, although hypotonia, lethargy, and poor sucking may also occur. They may have any of the diverse manifestations of hypoglycemia. Early appearance of these signs is more likely to be related to hypoglycemia, and their later appearance to hypocalcemia; these abnormalities may also occur together. Perinatal asphyxia may produce similar signs. Hypomagnesemia may be associated with the hypocalcemia. These manifestations may also occur in the absence of hypoglycemia, hypocalcemia, and asphyxia.

Tachypnea develops in many infants of diabetic mothers during the 1st 2 days of life and may be a manifestation of hypoglycemia, hypothermia, polycythemia, cardiac failure, transient tachypnea, or cerebral edema from birth trauma or asphyxia. Infants of diabetic mothers have a higher incidence of **respiratory distress syndrome** than do infants of nondiabetic mothers born at comparable gestational age; the greater incidence is possibly related to an antagonistic effect of insulin on stimulation of surfactant synthesis by cortisol.

Cardiomegaly is common (30%), and heart failure occurs in 5-10% of infants of diabetic mothers. Asymmetric septal hypertrophy may occur and may manifest like transient idiopathic hypertrophic subaortic stenosis. Inotropic agents worsen the obstruction and are contraindicated. Congenital heart disease is more common in infants of diabetic mothers. Birth trauma is also a common sequela of fetal macrosomia.

Neurologic development and ossification centers tend to be immature and to correlate with brain size (which is not increased) and gestational age rather than total body weight. In addition, these infants have an increased incidence of hyperbilirubinemia, polycythemia, and renal vein thrombosis; the last should be suspected in the infant with a flank mass, hematuria, and thrombocytopenia.

The incidence of **congenital anomalies** is increased threefold in infants of diabetic mothers; cardiac malformations (ventricular or atrial septal defect, transposition of the great vessels, truncus arteriosus, double-outlet right ventricle, tricuspid atresia, coarctation of the aorta) and lumbosacral agenesis are most common. Additional anomalies include neural tube defects, hydronephrosis, renal agenesis and dysplasia, duodenal or anorectal atresia, situs inversus, double ureter, and holoprosencephaly. These infants may also demonstrate abdominal distention caused by a transient delay in development of the left side of the colon, the small left colon syndrome.

PROGNOSIS

The subsequent incidence of diabetes mellitus in infants of diabetic mothers is higher than that in the general population. Physical development is normal, but oversized infants may be predisposed to childhood obesity that may extend into adult life. Disagreement persists about whether these infants have a slightly increased risk of impaired intellectual development unrelated to hypoglycemia; symptomatic hypoglycemia increases the risk, as does maternal ketonuria.

TREATMENT

Treatment of infants of diabetic mothers should be initiated before birth by means of frequent prenatal evaluation of all pregnant women with overt or gestational diabetes, evaluation of fetal maturity, biophysical profile, Doppler velocimetry, and planning of the delivery of these infants in hospitals where expert obstetric and pediatric care is continuously available. Periconception glucose control reduces the risk of anomalies and other adverse outcomes, and glucose control during labor reduces the incidence of neonatal hypoglycemia. Women with type 1 diabetes who have tight glucose control during pregnancy (average daily glucose levels < 95 mg/dL) deliver infants with birthweights and anthropomorphic features similar to those of infants of nondiabetic mothers. Treatment of gestational diabetes also reduces complications; dietary advice, glucose monitoring, metformin, and insulin therapy as needed decrease the rate of serious perinatal outcomes (death, shoulder dystocia, bone fracture, or nerve palsy). Women with gestational diabetes may also be treated successfully with glyburide, which may not cross the placenta. In these mothers, the incidence of macrosomia and neonatal hypoglycemia is similar to that in mothers with insulin-treated gestational diabetes.

Regardless of size, all infants of diabetic mothers should initially receive intensive observation and care. Asymptomatic infants should undergo blood glucose determination within 1 hr of birth and then every hour for the next 6-8 hr; for an infant found to be clinically well and normoglycemic, oral or gavage feeding with breast milk or formula should be started as soon as possible and continued at 3-hr intervals. If any question arises about an infant's ability to tolerate oral feeding, peripheral intravenous infusion at a rate of 4-8 mg/kg/min should be given. Hypoglycemia should be treated, even in asymptomatic infants, by frequent feeding and/or intravenous infusion of glucose. Bolus injections of hypertonic glucose should be avoided because they may cause further hyperinsulinemia and potentially produce rebound hypoglycemia.

Managing hypoglycemia in sick or symptomatic infants is discussed in the following section. For treatment of hypocalcemia and hypomagnesemia, see Chapter 100; for respiratory distress syndrome treatment, see Chapter 95.3; for treatment of polycythemia, see Chapter 97.3.

BIBLIOGRAPHY

Please visit the Nelson Textbook of Pediatrics *website at www.expertconsult.com for the complete bibliography.*

Chapter 102
Dysmorphology

Anthony Wynshaw-Boris and Leslie G. Biesecker

Dysmorphology is the study of abnormalities of human form and the mechanisms that cause them. It is estimated that 1 in 40, or 2.5% of newborns, have a recognizable malformation or malformations at birth. In about half of these newborns, a single isolated malformation is found, whereas in the other half there are multiple malformations. It is estimated that 10% of pediatric hospital admissions involve known genetic conditions, 18% involve congenital defects of unknown etiology, and 40% of surgical admissions are of patients with congenital malformations. Twenty percent to 30% of infant deaths and 30-50% of deaths after the neonatal period are due to congenital abnormalities (*http://www.marchofdimes.com/peristats/*). In 2001, birth defects accounted for 1 in 5 infant deaths in the United States, with a rate of 137.6 deaths per 100,000 live births, which is higher than other causes such as preterm/low birthweight (109.5/100,000), sudden infant death syndrome (55.5/100,000), maternal complications of pregnancy (37.3/100,000), and respiratory distress syndrome (25.3/100,000).

For the full continuation of this chapter, please visit the Nelson Textbook of Pediatrics *website at www.expertconsult.com.*

Chapter 103
Infections of the Neonatal Infant

103.1 Pathogenesis and Epidemiology

Barbara J. Stoll

Infections are a frequent and important cause of neonatal and infant morbidity and mortality. As many as 2% of fetuses are infected in utero, and up to 10% of infants have infections in the 1st mo of life. Neonatal infections are unique in several ways:

1. Infectious agents can be transmitted from the mother to the fetus or newborn infant by diverse modes.
2. Newborn infants are less capable of responding to infection because of 1 or more immunologic deficiencies.
3. Coexisting conditions often complicate the diagnosis and management of neonatal infections.
4. The clinical manifestations of newborn infections vary and include subclinical infection, mild to severe manifestations of focal or systemic infection, and, rarely, congenital syndromes resulting from in utero infection. The timing of exposure, inoculum size, immune status, and virulence of the etiologic agent influence the expression of disease.
5. Maternal infection that is the source of transplacental fetal infection is often undiagnosed during pregnancy because the mother was either asymptomatic or had nonspecific signs and symptoms at the time of acute infection.
6. A wide variety of etiologic agents infect the newborn, including bacteria, viruses, fungi, protozoa, and mycoplasmas.
7. Immature, very low birthweight (VLBW) newborns have improved survival but remain in the hospital for a long time in an environment that puts them at continuous risk for acquired infections.

BIBLIOGRAPHY

Please visit the Nelson Textbook of Pediatrics *website at www.expertconsult.com for the complete bibliography.*

103.2 Modes of Transmission and Pathogenesis

Barbara J. Stoll

PATHOGENESIS OF INTRAUTERINE INFECTION

Intrauterine infection is a result of clinical or subclinical maternal infection with a variety of agents (cytomegalovirus [CMV], *Treponema pallidum, Toxoplasma gondii,* rubella virus, varicella virus, parvovirus B19) and hematogenous transplacental transmission to the fetus. Transplacental infection may occur at any time during gestation, and signs and symptoms may be present at birth or may be delayed for months or years (Fig. 103-1). Infection may result in early spontaneous abortion, congenital malformation, intrauterine growth restriction, premature birth, stillbirth, acute or delayed disease in the neonatal period, or asymptomatic persistent infection with sequelae later in life. In some cases, no apparent effects are seen in the newborn infant.

The timing of infection during gestation affects the outcome. First-trimester infection may alter embryogenesis, with resulting congenital malformations (congenital rubella) (Chapter 239). Third-trimester infection often results in active infection at the time of delivery (toxoplasmosis, syphilis) (Chapters 282 and

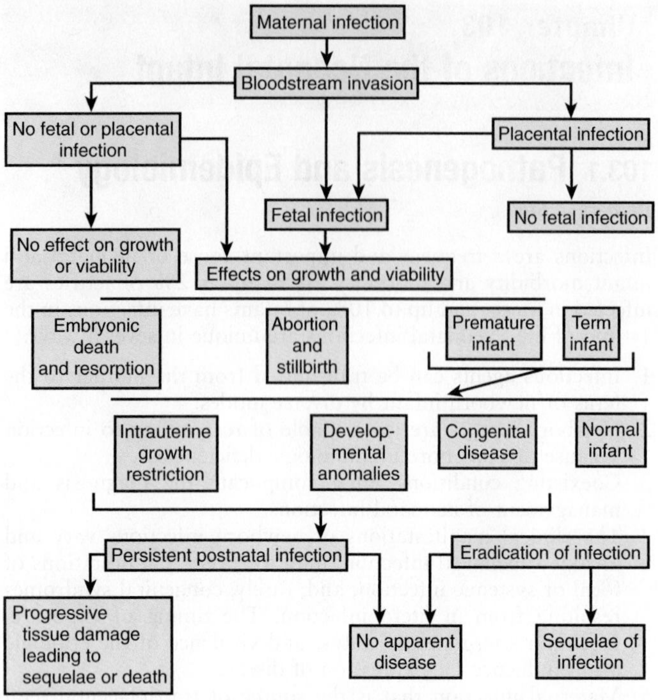

Figure 103-1 Pathogenesis of hematogenous transplacental infections. (From Klein JO, Remington JS: Current concepts of infections of the fetus and newborn infant. In Remington JS, Klein JO, editors: *Infectious diseases of the fetus and newborn infant*, ed 5, Philadelphia, 2002, WB Saunders.)

210). Infections that occur late in gestation may lead to a delay in clinical manifestations until some time after birth (syphilis).

Maternal infection is a necessary prerequisite for transplacental infection. For some etiologic agents (rubella), maternal immunity is effective and antibody is protective for the fetus. For other agents (CMV), maternal antibody may ameliorate the outcome of infection or may have no effect (Chapter 247). Even without maternal antibody, transplacental transmission of infection to a fetus is variable because the placenta may function as an effective barrier.

PATHOGENESIS OF ASCENDING BACTERIAL INFECTION

In most cases, the fetus or neonate is not exposed to potentially pathogenic bacteria until the membranes rupture and the infant passes through the birth canal and/or enters the extrauterine environment. The human birth canal is colonized with aerobic and anaerobic organisms that may result in ascending amniotic infection and/or colonization of the neonate at birth. Vertical transmission of bacterial agents that infect the amniotic fluid and/or vaginal canal may occur in utero or, more commonly, during labor and/or delivery (Fig. 103-2). **Chorioamnionitis** results from microbial invasion of amniotic fluid, often as a result of prolonged rupture of the chorioamniotic membrane. Amniotic infection may also occur with apparently intact membranes or with a relatively brief duration of membrane rupture. The term *chorioamnionitis* refers to the clinical syndrome of intrauterine infection, which includes maternal fever, with or without local or systemic signs of chorioamnionitis (uterine tenderness, foul-smelling vaginal discharge/amniotic fluid, maternal leukocytosis, maternal and/or fetal tachycardia). Chorioamnionitis may also be asymptomatic, diagnosed only by amniotic fluid analysis or pathologic examination of the placenta. The rate of histologic chorioamnionitis is inversely related to gestational age at birth (Fig. 103-3) and directly related to duration of membrane rupture. Rupture of membranes for longer than 24 hr was once

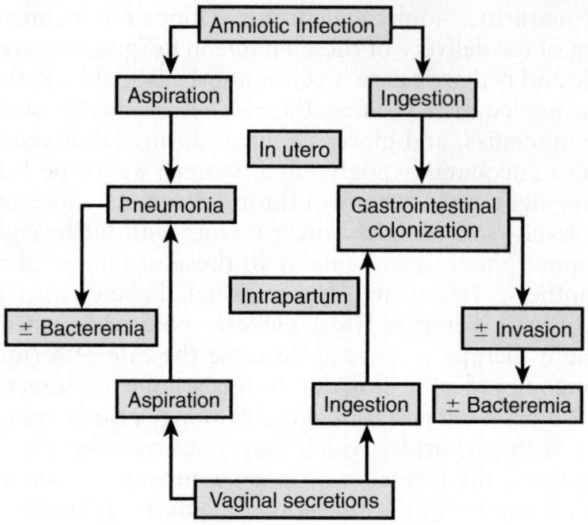

Figure 103-2 Pathways of ascending or intrapartum infection.

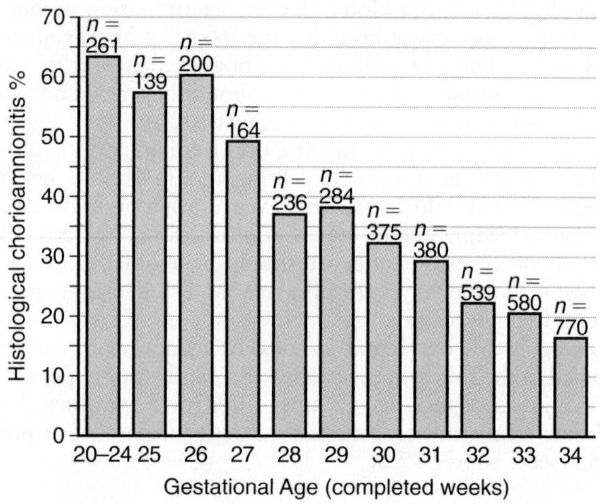

Figure 103-3 Histologic chorioamnionitis in liveborn preterm babies by gestational age (n = 3,928 babies). (From Lahra MM, Jeffery HE: A fetal response to chorioamnionitis is associated with early survival after preterm birth, *Am J Obstet Gynecol* 190:147–151, 2004.)

considered prolonged because microscopic evidence of inflammation of the membranes is uniformly present when the duration of rupture exceeds 24 hr. At 18 hr of membrane rupture, however, the incidence of early-onset disease with group B streptococcus (GBS) increases significantly; 18 hr is the appropriate cutoff for increased risk of neonatal infection.

Bacterial colonization does not always result in disease. Factors influencing which colonized infant will experience disease are not well understood but include prematurity, underlying illness, invasive procedures, inoculum size, virulence of the infecting organism, genetic predisposition, the innate immune system, host response, and transplacental maternal antibodies (Fig. 103-4). Aspiration or ingestion of bacteria in amniotic fluid may lead to congenital pneumonia or systemic infection, with manifestations becoming apparent before delivery (fetal distress, tachycardia), at delivery (failure to breathe, respiratory distress, shock), or after a latent period of a few hours (respiratory distress, shock). Aspiration or ingestion of bacteria during the birth process may lead to infection after an interval of 1-2 days.

Resuscitation at birth, particularly if it involves endotracheal intubation, insertion of an umbilical vessel catheter, or both, is associated with an increased risk of bacterial infection. Explanations include the presence of infection at the time of birth or acquisition of infection during the invasive procedures associated with resuscitation.

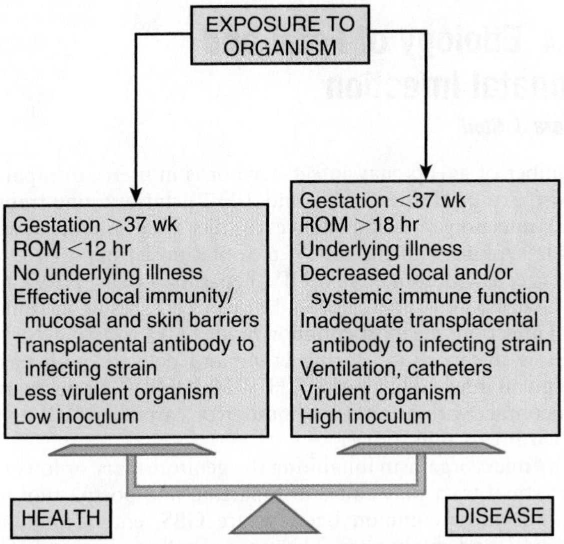

Figure 103-4 Factors influencing the balance between health and disease in neonates exposed to a potential pathogen. ROM, rupture of membranes. (Adapted from Baker CJ: Group B streptococcal infections, *Clin Perinatol* 24:59–70, 1997.)

PATHOGENESIS OF LATE-ONSET POSTNATAL INFECTIONS

After birth, neonates are exposed to infectious agents in the nursery or in the community. Postnatal infections may be transmitted by direct contact with hospital personnel, the mother, or other family members; from breast milk (HIV, CMV); or from inanimate sources such as contaminated equipment. The most common source of postnatal infections in hospitalized newborns is hand contamination of health care personnel.

Most cases of meningitis result from hematogenous dissemination. Less often, meningitis results from contiguous spread as a result of contamination of open neural tube defects, congenital sinus tracts, or penetrating wounds from fetal scalp sampling or internal fetal electrocardiographic monitors. Abscess formation, ventriculitis, septic infarcts, hydrocephalus, and subdural effusions are complications of meningitis that occur more often in newborn infants than in older children.

BIBLIOGRAPHY

Please visit the Nelson Textbook of Pediatrics *website at* *www.expertconsult.com* *for the complete bibliography.*

103.3 Immunity

Barbara J. Stoll

Decreased function of neutrophils and other cells involved in the response to infection has been demonstrated in both term and preterm infants. Preterm infants may also have low concentrations of immunoglobulins. Both preterm and term infants have quantitative and qualitative defects of the complement system. Despite these alterations in immune function, the rate of systemic infection in newborns is low. All newborns enter an unsterile environment, but infection develops in only a few.

IMMUNOGLOBULINS

Immunoglobulin (Ig) G is actively transported across the placenta, with concentrations in a full-term infant comparable to or higher than those in the mother. The specificity of IgG antibody in cord blood depends on the mother's previous antigenic exposure and immunologic response. In premature infants, cord IgG levels are directly proportional to gestational age. Studies of type-specific IgG antibodies to GBS have shown that the ratio of cord to maternal serum concentrations is 1.0 at term, 0.5 at 32 wk of gestation, and 0.3 at 28 wk. Levels of maternally derived IgG fall rapidly after birth. Infants with birthweights <1,500 g become significantly hypogammaglobulinemic, with mean plasma IgG concentrations in the range of 200-300 mg/dL in the 1st wk of life. Other classes of immunoglobulins are not transferred across the placenta, although a fetus can synthesize IgA and IgM in response to intrauterine infection.

The presence of passively transferred specific IgG antibody in adequate concentration provides neonates protection against infections to which protection is mediated by that antibody (tetanus, encapsulated bacteria such as GBS). Specific bactericidal and opsonic antibodies against enteric gram-negative bacteria are predominantly in the IgM class. Newborn infants usually lack antibody-mediated protection against *Escherichia coli* and other *Enterobacteriaceae.*

COMPLEMENT

The complement system mediates bactericidal activity against certain organisms such as *E. coli* and functions as an opsonin with antibody in the phagocytosis of bacteria such as GBS. No transplacental passage of complement from the maternal circulation takes place. A fetus begins to synthesize complement components as early as the 1st trimester. Full-term newborn infants have slightly diminished classical pathway complement activity and moderately diminished alternative pathway activity. Considerable variability, however, is seen in both the concentration and activity of complement components. Premature infants have lower levels of complement components and less complement activity than full-term newborns do. These deficiencies contribute to diminished complement-derived chemotactic activity and to a lesser ability to opsonize certain organisms in the absence of antibody. Opsonization of *Staphylococcus aureus* is normal in neonatal sera, but various degrees of impairment have been noted with GBS and *E. coli.*

NEUTROPHILS

Quantitative and qualitative deficiencies of the phagocyte system contribute to the newborn's susceptibility to infection. Neutrophil migration (chemotaxis) is abnormal at birth in both term and preterm infants. Neonatal neutrophils have decreases in adhesion, aggregation, and deformability, all of which may delay the response to infection. Abnormal expression of cell membrane adhesion molecules (the β_2 integrins and selectins) and abnormalities in the neonatal neutrophil cytoskeleton contribute to abnormal chemotaxis. With adequate opsonization, phagocytosis and killing by neutrophils are comparable in newborn infants and adults. In the presence of infectious or noninfectious stress (respiratory distress syndrome), however, the ability of neonatal neutrophils to phagocytose gram-negative (but not gram-positive) bacteria is decreased. Impairment of the oxidative respiratory burst of neonatal neutrophils is a factor in the increased risk of sepsis, especially in preterm infants.

The number of circulating neutrophils is elevated after birth in both term and preterm infants, with a peak at 12 hr that returns to normal by 22 hr. Band neutrophils constitute less than 15% in normal newborns and may increase in newborns with infection and other stress responses, such as asphyxia.

Neutropenia, which is frequently observed in preterm infants and infants with intrauterine growth restriction, increases the risk for sepsis. The neutrophil storage pool in newborn infants is 20-30% of that in adults and is more likely to be depleted in the face of infection. Mortality is increased when sepsis is associated with severe sepsis-induced neutropenia and bone marrow depletion. Granulocyte colony–stimulating factor (G-CSF) and granulocyte-macrophage CSF (GM-CSF) are cytokines that play important roles in the proliferation, differentiation, functional activation, and survival of phagocytes. These cytokines stimulate myeloid progenitor cells, increase the bone marrow neutrophil storage pool, induce peripheral blood neutrophilia, and influence neutrophil function, including enhancement of bactericidal activity. Although these myeloid colony-stimulating factors influence neutrophil number and function, their clinical utility in the treatment and/or prevention of neonatal sepsis remains undetermined.

MONOCYTE-MACROPHAGE SYSTEM

The monocyte-macrophage system consists of circulating monocytes and tissue macrophages, particularly in the liver, spleen, and lung. Activated macrophages are involved in antigen presentation, phagocytosis, and immune modulation. The number of circulating monocytes in neonatal blood is normal, but the mass or function of macrophages in the reticuloendothelial system is diminished, particularly in preterm infants. In both term and preterm infants, chemotaxis of monocytes is impaired; this impairment affects the inflammatory response in tissues and the results of delayed hypersensitivity skin tests. Monocytes from neonates ingest and kill microorganisms as well as monocytes from adults.

NATURAL KILLER CELLS

Natural killer (NK) cells are a subgroup of lymphocytes that are cytolytic against cells infected with viruses. NK cells also lyse cells coated with antibody in a process called antibody-dependent cell-mediated cytotoxicity (ADCC). NK cells appear early in gestation and are present in cord blood in numbers equivalent to those in adults; neonatal NK cells have decreased cytotoxic activity and ADCC in comparison with adult cells. The diminished cytotoxicity against herpes simplex virus (HSV)–infected cells may predispose to disseminated HSV infection in newborns (Chapter 249).

CYTOKINES/INFLAMMATORY MEDIATORS

The patient's response to infection and clinical outcome involves a balance between pro-inflammatory and anti-inflammatory cytokines. Several adverse neonatal outcomes, including brain injury, necrotizing enterocolitis (NEC), and bronchopulmonary dysplasia, may be mediated by the cytokine response to infection in the mother, fetus, or newborn. The mediators that have been studied in newborns include tumor necrosis factor-α (TNFα), interleukin 1 (IL-1), IL-4, IL-6, IL-8, IL-10, IL-12, platelet-activating factor, and the leukotrienes. The release of various inflammatory mediators in response to infection offers the potential opportunity to facilitate an early laboratory diagnosis of infection. Potential surrogate markers for bacterial sepsis, pneumonia, and NEC include TNFα, IL-6, and IL-8.

Innate immunity involves nonspecific cellular and humoral responses to an infectious agent without previous exposure. Recognition of pathogens is initiated by soluble components in plasma (including mannose-binding lectin) and by recognition of receptors on monocytes and other cells. Toll-like receptors play an important role in pathogen recognition. Genetic polymorphisms (mutations) of various proteins involved in the immune response may increase the risk and severity of neonatal infections. The neutrophil is another important cellular component of innate immunity. Neutrophil granules contain many enzymes; one protein, bactericidal/permeability-increasing protein (BPI), binds to the endotoxin in the cell wall of gram-negative bacteria. This protein facilitates opsonization and prevents the inflammatory response to endotoxin. BPI activity may be decreased in neonates.

BIBLIOGRAPHY

Please visit the Nelson Textbook of Pediatrics *website at www.expertconsult.com for the complete bibliography.*

103.4 Etiology of Fetal and Neonatal Infection

Barbara J. Stoll

A number of agents may infect newborns in utero, intrapartum, or postpartum (Tables 103-1 and 103-2). Intrauterine transplacental infections of significance to the fetus and/or newborn include syphilis, rubella, CMV, toxoplasmosis, parvovirus B19, and varicella. Although HSV, HIV, hepatitis B virus (HBV), hepatitis C virus, and tuberculosis (TB) can each result in transplacental infection, the most common mode of transmission for these agents is intrapartum, during labor and delivery with passage through an infected birth canal (HIV, HSV, HBV), or postpartum, from contact with an infected mother or caretaker (TB) or with infected breast milk (HIV).

Any microorganism inhabiting the genitourinary or lower gastrointestinal tract may cause intrapartum and postpartum infection. The most common bacteria are GBS, enteric organisms, gonococci, and chlamydiae. The more common viruses are CMV, HSV, enteroviruses, and HIV.

Agents that commonly cause **nosocomial** infection are coagulase-negative staphylococci, gram-negative bacilli *(E. coli, Klebsiella pneumoniae, Salmonella, Enterobacter, Citrobacter, Pseudomonas aeruginosa, Serratia)*, enterococci, *S. aureus*, and *Candida*. Viruses contributing to nosocomial neonatal infection include enteroviruses, CMV, hepatitis A, adenoviruses, influenza,

Table 103-1 BACTERIAL CAUSES OF SYSTEMIC NEONATAL INFECTIONS

BACTERIA	EARLY ONSET	LATE ONSET		
		Maternal Origin	Nosocomial	Community-Acquired
GRAM POSITIVE				
Clostridia	+		+	*
Enterococci	+		++	
Group B streptococcus	+++	+	+	+
Listeria monocytogenes	+	+		
Other streptococci	++			+
Staphylococcus aureus	+		++	+
Staphylococcus, coagulase-negative	+		+++	
Streptococcus pneumoniae	+			++
Viridans streptococcus	+		++	
GRAM NEGATIVE				
Bacteroides	+		+	
Campylobacter	+			
Citrobacter			+	+
Enterobacter			+	
Escherichia coli	+++		+	++
Haemophilus influenzae	+			+
Klebsiella			+	
Neisseria gonorrhoeae	+			
Neisseria meningitidis	+		+	
Proteus			+	
Pseudomonas			+	
Salmonella		+		+
Serratia			+	
OTHERS				
Treponema pallidum	+	+		
Mycobacterium tuberculosis		+		

**Clostridium tetani* in some developing countries.
+, relative frequency.

respiratory syncytial virus (RSV), rhinovirus, parainfluenza, HSV, and rotavirus. Community-acquired pathogens such as *Streptococcus pneumoniae* may also cause infection in newborn infants after discharge from the hospital.

Congenital pneumonia may be caused by CMV, rubella virus, and *T. pallidum* and, less commonly, by the other agents producing transplacental infection (Table 103-3). Microorganisms causing pneumonia acquired during labor and delivery include GBS, gram-negative enteric aerobes, *Listeria monocytogenes*, genital *Mycoplasma, Chlamydia trachomatis,* CMV, HSV, and *Candida* species.

Bacteria responsible for most cases of nosocomial pneumonia typically include staphylococcal species, gram-negative enteric aerobes, and occasionally, *Pseudomonas.* Fungi are responsible for an increasing number of systemic infections acquired during prolonged hospitalization of preterm neonates. Respiratory viruses cause isolated cases and outbreaks of nosocomial pneumonia. These viruses, usually endemic during the winter months and acquired from infected hospital staff or visitors to the nursery, include RSV, parainfluenza virus, influenza viruses, and adenovirus. Respiratory viruses are the single most important cause of community-acquired pneumonia and are usually contracted from infected household contacts.

The most common bacterial causes of **neonatal meningitis** are GBS, *E. coli*, and *L. monocytogenes. S. pneumoniae,* other streptococci, non-typable *Haemophilus influenzae,* both coagulase-positive and coagulase-negative staphylococci, *Klebsiella, Enterobacter, Pseudomonas, T. pallidum,* and *Mycobacterium tuberculosis* may also produce meningitis.

Table 103-2 NONBACTERIAL CAUSES OF SYSTEMIC NEONATAL INFECTIONS

VIRUSES
Adenovirus
Cytomegalovirus
Enteroviruses
Parechoviruses
Hepatitis B virus
Herpes simplex virus
Human immunodeficiency virus
Parvovirus
Rubella virus
Varicella-zoster virus
MYCOPLASMA
M. *hominis*
Ureaplasma urealyticum
FUNGI
Candida species
Malassezia species
PROTOZA
Plasmodia
Toxoplasma gondii
Trypanosoma cruzi

Table 103-3 ETIOLOGIC AGENTS OF NEONATAL PNEUMONIA ACCORDING TO TIMING OF ACQUISITION

TRANSPLACENTAL
Cytomegalovirus
Herpes simplex virus
Mycobacterium
Tuberculosis
Rubella virus
Treponema pallidum
Varicella-zoster virus
PERINATAL
Anaerobic bacteria
Chlamydia
Cytomegalovirus
Enteric bacteria
Group B streptococci
Haemophilus influenzae
Herpes simplex virus
Listeria monocytogenes
Mycoplasma
POSTNATAL
Adenovirus
Candida species*
Coagulase-negative staphylococci
Cytomegalovirus
Enteric bacteria*
Enteroviruses
Influenza viruses A, B
Parainfluenza
*Pseudomonas**
Respiratory syncytial virus
Staphylococcus aureus
Mycobacterium tuberculosis

*More likely with mechanical ventilation or indwelling catheters, or after abdominal surgery.

BIBLIOGRAPHY

Please visit the Nelson Textbook of Pediatrics *website at* www.expertconsult.com *for the complete bibliography.*

103.5 Epidemiology of Early- and Late-Onset Neonatal Infections

Barbara J. Stoll

The terms *early-onset infection* and *late-onset infection* refer to the different ages at onset of infection in the neonatal period (Table 103-4). Although these disorders were originally divided arbitrarily into infections occurring before and after 1 wk of life, it is more useful to separate early- and late-onset infections according to peripartum pathogenesis. Early-onset infections are acquired before or during delivery (vertical mother-to-child transmission). Late-onset infections develop after delivery from organisms acquired in the hospital or the community. The age at onset depends on the timing of exposure and virulence of the infecting organism. Very-late-onset infections (onset after 1 mo of life) may also occur, particularly in VLBW preterm infants or term infants requiring prolonged neonatal intensive care.

The incidence of neonatal bacterial sepsis varies from 1 to 4/1,000 live births in developed countries, with considerable fluctuation over time and with geographic variation. Studies suggest that term male infants have a higher incidence of sepsis than term females. This sex difference is less clear in preterm LBW infants. Attack rates of neonatal sepsis increase significantly in LBW infants in the presence of maternal chorioamnionitis, congenital immune defects, mutations of genes involved in the innate immune system, asplenia, galactosemia *(E. coli),* and malformations leading to high inocula of bacteria (obstructive uropathy).

A study from the National Institute of Child Health and Human Development (NICHD) Neonatal Research Network documented rates of early-onset sepsis among approximately 200,000 live births at Network centers. The overall rate of early-onset sepsis was 1.2 cases per 1000 live births with rates inversely related to birthweight (401-1500 g BW, 12.33/1000; 1501-2500 g BW, 1.96/1000; >2500 g BW, 0.71/1000) (Table 103-5).

Intrapartum antibiotics are used to reduce vertical transmission of GBS as well as to lessen neonatal morbidity after preterm rupture of membranes. With introduction of selective intrapartum antibiotic prophylaxis to prevent perinatal transmission of GBS, rates of early-onset neonatal GBS infection in the USA declined from 1.7/1,000 live births to 0.32/ 1,000, according to

Table 103-4 NEONATAL INFECTION ACCORDING TO AGE AT ONSET

CHARACTERISTICS	EARLY ONSET	LATE ONSET	VERY LATE (NOSOCOMIAL) ONSET
Age at onset	Birth to 7 days usually <72 hr	7-30 days	>30 days
Maternal obstetric complications	Common	Uncommon	Varies
Prematurity	Frequent	Varies	Usual
Organism source	Maternal genital tract	Maternal genital tract/environment	Environment/community
Manifestation	Multisystem	Multisystem or focal	Multisystem or focal
Site	Normal nursery, NICU, community	NICU, community	NICU, community

NICU, neonatal intensive care unit.

Table 103-5 RATES OF EARLY-ONSET SEPSIS PER 1,000 LIVE BIRTHS: NICHD NEONATAL RESEARCH NETWORK/CDC SURVEILLANCE STUDY OF EARLY-ONSET SEPSIS

	BIRTHWEIGHT (g)			
	401-1,500	1,501-2,500	>2,500	All
All	10.96	1.38	0.57	0.98
Group B streptococcus	2.08	0.38	0.35	0.41
Escherichia coli	5.09	0.54	0.07	0.28

Modified from Stoll BJ, Hansen NI, Sanchez PJ, et al: Early onset neonatal sepsis: the burden of group B streptococcal and *E. coli* disease continues, *Pediatrics* 127(5):817–826, 2011.

U.S. Centers for Disease Control and Prevention (CDC) surveillance data. Intrapartum chemoprophylaxis does not reduce the rates of late-onset GBS disease and has no effect on the rates of infection with non-GBS pathogens. Of concern is a possible increase in gram-negative infections (especially *E. coli*) in VLBW and possibly term infants in spite of a reduction in early GBS sepsis by intrapartum antibiotics.

The incidence of meningitis is 0.2-0.4/1,000 live births in newborn infants and is higher in preterm infants. Bacterial meningitis may be associated with sepsis or may occur as a local meningeal infection. One third of VLBW infants with late-onset meningitis have negative blood culture results. The discordance between results of blood and cerebrospinal fluid (CSF) cultures suggests that meningitis may be underdiagnosed among VLBW infants and emphasizes the need for culture of CSF in VLBW infants when late-onset sepsis is suspected and in all infants who have positive blood culture results.

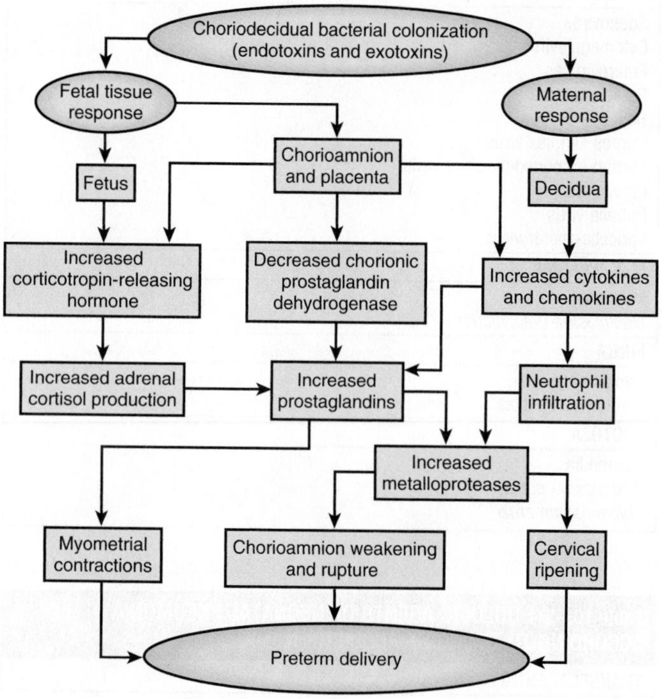

Figure 103-5 Potential pathways from choriodecidual bacterial colonization to preterm delivery. (From Goldenberg RL, Hauth JA, Andrews WW: Intrauterine infection and preterm delivery, *N Engl J Med* 342:1500–1507, 2000. Copyright 2000, Massachusetts Medical Society.)

PREMATURITY

The most important neonatal factor predisposing to infection is prematurity or LBW. Preterm LBW infants have a 3- to 10-fold higher incidence of infection than full-term normal birthweight infants. Possible explanations are as follows: (1) maternal genital tract infection is considered to be an important cause of preterm labor, with an increased risk of vertical transmission to the newborn (Figs. 103-5 and 103-6); (2) the frequency of intra-amniotic infection is inversely related to gestational age (see Fig. 103-3); (3) premature infants have documented immune dysfunction; and (4) premature infants often require prolonged intravenous access, endotracheal intubation, or other invasive procedures that provide a portal of entry or impair barrier and clearance mechanisms.

NOSOCOMIAL INFECTIONS

Nosocomial (hospital-acquired) infections are responsible for significant morbidity and late mortality in hospitalized newborns. Many experts define nosocomial infections in newborns as infections occurring after 3 days of life that are not directly acquired from the mother's genital tract. For the purposes of surveillance in the acute care setting, the CDC National Healthcare Safety Network (NHSN) defines health care–associated infections in newborns as those that result from passage through the birth canal as well as infections that occur from exogenous sources such as health care personnel, visitors, and equipment/devices in the health care environment. This surveillance definition includes any infection occurring after admission to the neonatal intensive care unit (NICU) that was not transplacentally acquired. Rates of nosocomial infection in healthy term infants who are either rooming-in with their mothers or staying in the well baby nursery are low (<1%). The majority of nosocomial infections occur in preterm or term infants who require intensive care. Risk factors for nosocomial infection in these infants include prematurity, LBW, invasive procedures, indwelling vascular catheters, parenteral nutrition with lipid emulsions, endotracheal tubes, ventricular shunts, alterations in the skin and/or mucous membrane barriers, frequent use of broad-spectrum antibiotics, and prolonged hospital stay. The most frequent nosocomial infections are bloodstream infections associated with an intravascular catheter and pneumonia, especially ventilator-associated pneumonia. Nonetheless, nosocomial sepsis may occur in the absence of a catheter or ventilator. In addition, infants receiving intensive care in the NICU are at risk to acquire community or hospital associated infections during seasonal epidemics (rotavirus, RSV, influenza).

Almost one quarter of VLBW infants (<1,500 g BW) experience nosocomial infections. Rates of infections increase with

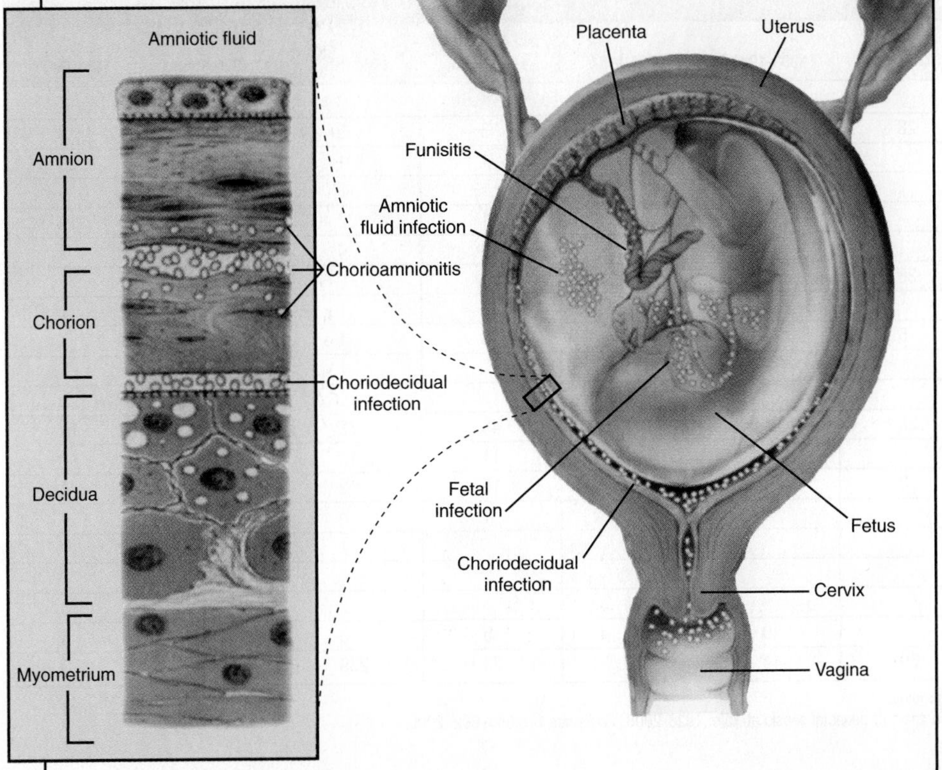

Figure 103-6 Potential sites of bacterial infection within the uterus. (From Goldenberg RL, Hauth JA, Andrews WW: Intrauterine infection and preterm delivery, *N Engl J Med* 342:1500–1507, 2000. Copyright 2000, Massachusetts Medical Society.)

decreasing gestational age and birthweight. The NICHD Neonatal Research Network has reported rates of 43% for infants 401-750 g; 28% for those 751-1,000 g; 15% for those 1,001-1,250 g; and 7% for those 1,251-1,500 g. The CDC NHSN monitors device-associated nosocomial infection rates. Rates are inversely related to birthweight, and in level III NICUs, they range from 3.7 infections per 1,000 central line days for infants < 750 g to 2.0 infections per 1,000 central line days for those weighing > 2,500 g. The widespread differences in practice regarding the inclusion of lumbar puncture (LP) in the diagnostic evaluation of an infant with suspected sepsis make it more difficult to determine rates of late-onset meningitis.

Various bacterial and fungal agents colonize hospitalized infants, health care workers, and visitors. Pathogenic agents can be transmitted by direct contact or indirectly via contaminated equipment, intravenous fluids, medications, blood products, or enteral feedings. Colonization of the infant's skin, umbilicus, and respiratory or gastrointestinal tract with pathogenic agents often precedes the development of infection. Antibiotic use interferes with colonization by normal flora, thereby facilitating colonization with more virulent pathogens.

Coagulase-negative staphylococci are the most frequent neonatal nosocomial pathogens. In a cohort of 6,215 VLBW infants in the NICHD Neonatal Research Network, gram-positive agents were associated with 70%, gram-negative with 18%, and fungi with 12% of cases of late-onset sepsis (Table 103-6). Coagulase-negative staphylococcus, the single most common organism, was isolated in 48% of these infections. The emergence of nosocomial bacterial pathogens resistant to multiple antibiotics is a growing concern. Among NICU patients, methicillin-resistant *S. aureus*, vancomycin-resistant enterococci, and multidrug-resistant gram-negative pathogens are particularly alarming. Organisms responsible for all categories of neonatal sepsis and meningitis may change with time (Table 103-7).

Viral organisms may also cause nosocomial infection in the NICU; they include RSV, varicella, influenza, rotavirus, and

Table 103-6 DISTRIBUTION OF PATHOGENS ASSOCIATED WITH THE 1ST EPISODE OF LATE-ONSET SEPSIS IN VERY LOW BIRTHWEIGHT INFANTS*

ORGANISM†	N	%
Gram-positive organisms:	**922**	**70.2**
Staphylococcus—coagulase negative	629	47.9
Staphylococcus aureus	103	7.8
Enterococcus spp.	43	3.3
Group B streptococci	30	2.3
Other	117	8.9
Gram-negative organisms:	**231**	**17.6**
Escherichia coli	64	4.9
Klebsiella	52	4.0
Pseudomonas	35	2.7
Enterobacter	33	2.5
Serratia	29	2.2
Other	18	1.4
Fungi:	**160**	**12.2**
Candida albicans	76	5.8
Candida parapsilosis	54	4.1
Other	30	2.3
TOTAL	**1,313**	**100**

*National Institute of Child Health and Human Development Neonatal Research Network, September 1, 1998, through August 31, 2000.

†Patients with dual infections and patients with presumed coagulase-negative staphylococci (CONS) contaminants excluded. According to the definitions in text, 276 (44%) CONS were definite infections and 353 (56%) were possible infections.

From Stoll BJ, Hansen N, Fanaroff AA, et al: Late-onset sepsis in very low birthweight neonates: the experience of the NICHD Neonatal Research Network, *Pediatrics* 110:285–291, 2002.

Table 103-7 NEONATAL INBORN SEPSIS, 1928-2003

	% IN EACH STUDY*						
	1928-1932	1933-1943	1944-1957	1958-1965	1966-1978	1979-1988	1989-2003
GRAM-POSITIVE AEROBIC BACTERIA							
Staphylococcus aureus	28	9	13	3	5	3	8
Coagulase-negative staphylococcus				1	1	8	29
β-hemolytic streptococci							
Group B		5	6	1	32	37	12
Group D			2	10	4	8	9
Nongrouped and other	38	36	10				
Viridans streptococci		2		3	1	3	1
Streptococcus pneumoniae	5	11	5	3	1	1	
Listeria monocytogenes		2	2		1	1	<1
GRAM-NEGATIVE AEROBIC BACTERIA							
Escherichia coli	26	25	37	45	32	20	11
Klebsiella-Enterobacter				11	12	3	11
Pseudomonas	3		21	15	2	3	3
Haemophilus				1	4	5	1
Salmonella			2		1	1	
GRAM-NEGATIVE ANAEROBIC BACTERIA					1	3	
Fungi					2	1	8
Other		9	3	5	5	1	6
n	39	44	62	73	239	147	520

*Percentages do not always sum up to 100% as a result of rounding.
From Bizzarro MJ, Raskind C, Baltimore RS, et al: Seventy-five years of neonatal sepsis at Yale: 1928-2003, *Pediatrics* 116:595–602, 2005.

enteroviruses. For viral as well as bacterial infections, nursery outbreaks may occur in addition to individual cases. Hospital infection control policies are essential to prevent and/or contain nursery infection outbreaks.

The mean age at onset of the 1st episode of late-onset nosocomial sepsis is 2-3 wk, independent of the infecting pathogen. Nosocomial infections increase the risk of adverse outcomes, including prolonged hospitalization and mortality.

Active surveillance for nosocomial infection is essential in monitoring overall rates of infection, rates of infection with specific pathogens, and antibiotic susceptibility patterns and in identifying clusters of cases or true infectious outbreaks. Surveillance is based on the ongoing review of nursery infections and data from the microbiology laboratory; routine surveillance to detect colonization is not indicated. Culture results should indicate the bacterial isolate and the antimicrobial sensitivity pattern. Assessment of other microbial markers (biotype, serotype, DNA fingerprint) is helpful in epidemics. During epidemics, investigation of possible reservoirs of infection, modes of transmission, and risk factors is necessary. Identification of colonized infants and nursery personnel is also helpful.

Infections acquired by newborns after discharge from the nursery are usually community acquired. They have the same epidemiologic considerations as other community-acquired infections in infants and children, except for protection provided by maternal antibody.

BIBLIOGRAPHY

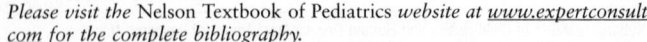

Please visit the Nelson Textbook of Pediatrics *website at www.expertconsult.com for the complete bibliography.*

103.6 Clinical Manifestations of Transplacental Intrauterine Infections

Barbara J. Stoll

Infection with agents that cross the placenta (CMV, *T. pallidum, T. gondii,* rubella, parvovirus B19) may be asymptomatic at birth or may cause a spectrum of disease ranging from relatively mild symptoms to multisystem involvement with severe and life-threatening complications. For some agents, disease is characterized by chronicity, recurrence, or both, and the agent may cause ongoing injury. Clinical signs and symptoms do not help make a specific etiologic diagnosis but, rather, raise suspicion of an intrauterine infection and help distinguish these infections from acute bacterial infections that occur during labor and delivery. The following signs and symptoms are common to many of these agents (Table 103-8): intrauterine growth restriction, microcephaly or hydrocephalus, intracranial calcifications, chorioretinitis, cataracts, myocarditis, pneumonia, hepatosplenomegaly, direct hyperbilirubinemia, anemia, thrombocytopenia, hydrops fetalis, and skin manifestations. Many of these agents cause late sequelae, even if the infant is asymptomatic at birth. These adverse outcomes include sensorineural hearing loss, visual disturbances (including blindness), seizures, and neurodevelopmental abnormalities.

BACTERIAL SEPSIS

Neonates with bacterial sepsis may have either nonspecific signs and symptoms or focal signs of infection (Tables 103-9 and 103-10), including temperature instability, hypotension, poor perfusion with pallor and mottled skin, metabolic acidosis, tachycardia or bradycardia, apnea, respiratory distress, grunting, cyanosis, irritability, lethargy, seizures, feeding intolerance, abdominal distention, jaundice, petechiae, purpura, and bleeding. International criteria for bacterial sepsis are listed in Table 103-11. The initial manifestation may involve only limited symptomatology and only 1 system, such as apnea alone or tachypnea with retractions or tachycardia, or it may be an acute catastrophic manifestation with multiorgan dysfunction. Infants should be reevaluated over time to determine whether the symptoms have progressed from mild to severe. Later complications of sepsis include respiratory failure, pulmonary hypertension, cardiac failure, shock, renal failure, liver dysfunction, cerebral edema or thrombosis, adrenal hemorrhage and/or insufficiency, bone marrow dysfunction (neutropenia,

Table 103-8 CLINICAL MANIFESTATIONS OF TRANSPLACENTAL INFECTIONS

MANIFESTATION	PATHOGEN
Intrauterine growth restriction	CMV, *Plasmodium,* rubella, toxoplasmosis, *Treponema pallidum, Trypanosoma cruzi,* VZV
Congenital anatomic defects:	
Cataracts	Rubella
Heart defects	Rubella
Hydrocephalus	HSV, lymphocytic choriomeningitis virus, rubella, toxoplasmosis
Intracranial calcification	CMV, HIV, toxoplasmosis, *T. cruzi*
Limb hypoplasia	VZV
Microcephaly	CMV, HSV, rubella, toxoplasmosis
Microphthalmos	CMV, rubella, toxoplasmosis
Neonatal organ involvement:	
Anemia	CMV, parvovirus, *Plasmodium,* rubella, toxoplasmosis, *T. cruzi, T. pallidum*
Carditis	Coxsackieviruses, rubella, *T. cruzi*
Encephalitis	CMV, enteroviruses, HSV, rubella, toxoplasmosis, *T. cruzi, T. pallidum*
Hepatitis	CMV, enteroviruses, HSV
Hepatosplenomegaly	CMV, enteroviruses, HIV, HSV, *Plasmodium,* rubella, *T. cruzi, T. pallidum*
Hydrops	Parvovirus, *T. pallidum,* toxoplasmosis
Lymphadenopathy	CMV, HIV, rubella, toxoplasmosis, *T. pallidum*
Osteitis	Rubella, *T. pallidum*
Petechiae, purpura	CMV, enteroviruses, rubella, *T. cruzi*
Pneumonitis	CMV, enteroviruses, HSV, measles, rubella, toxoplasmosis, *T. pallidum,* VZV
Retinitis	CMV, HSV, lymphocytic choriomeningitis virus, rubella, toxoplasmosis, *T. pallidum,* West Nile virus
Rhinitis	Enteroviruses, *T. pallidum*
Skin lesions	Entroviruses, HSV, measles, rubella, *T. pallidum,* VZV
Thrombocytopenia	CMV, enteroviruses, HIV, HSV, rubella, toxoplasmosis, *T. pallidum*
Late sequelae:	
Convulsions	CMV, enteroviruses, rubella, toxoplasmosis
Deafness	CMV, rubella, toxoplasmosis
Dental/skeletal problems	Rubella, *T. pallidum*
Endocrinopathies	Rubella, toxoplasmosis
Eye pathology	HSV, rubella, toxoplasmosis, *T. cruzi, T. pallidum.* VZV
Hepatitis	Hepatitis B
Mental retardation	CMV, HIV, HSV, rubella, toxoplasmosis, *T. cruzi,* VZV
Nephrotic syndrome	*Plasmodium, T. pallidum*

CMV, cytomegalovirus; HSV, herpes simplex virus; VZV, varicella-zoster virus.

thrombocytopenia, anemia), and disseminated intravascular coagulopathy (DIC).

A variety of noninfectious conditions can occur together with neonatal infection or can make the diagnosis of infection more difficult. Respiratory distress syndrome (RDS) secondary to surfactant deficiency can coexist with bacterial pneumonia. Because bacterial sepsis can be rapidly progressive, the physician must be alert to the signs and symptoms of possible infection and must initiate diagnostic evaluation and empirical therapy in a timely manner. The **differential diagnosis** of many of the signs and symptoms that suggest infection is extensive; these noninfectious disorders must also be considered (Table 103-12).

Table 103-9 INITIAL SIGNS AND SYMPTOMS OF INFECTION IN NEWBORN INFANTS

GENERAL
Fever, temperature instability "Not doing well" Poor feeding Edema
GASTROINTESTINAL SYSTEM
Abdominal distention Vomiting Diarrhea Hepatomegaly
RESPIRATORY SYTEM
Apnea, dyspnea Tachypnea, retractions Flaring, grunting Cyanosis
RENAL SYSTEM
Oliguria
CARDIOVASCULAR SYSTEM
Pallor; mottling; cold, clammy skin Tachycardia Hypotension Bradycardia
CENTRAL NERVOUS SYSTEM
Irritability, lethargy Tremors, seizures Hyporeflexia, hypotonia Abnormal Moro reflex Irregular respirations Full fontanel High-pitched cry
HEMATOLOGIC SYSTEM
Jaundice Splenomegaly Pallor Petechiae, purpura Bleeding

SYSTEMIC INFLAMMATORY RESPONSE SYNDROME

The clinical manifestations of infection depend on the virulence of the infecting organism and the body's inflammatory response. The term *systemic inflammatory response syndrome (SIRS)* is most frequently used to describe this unique process of infection and the subsequent systemic response (Chapter 64). In addition to infection, SIRS may result from trauma, hemorrhagic shock, other causes of ischemia, NEC, and pancreatitis.

Patients with SIRS have a spectrum of clinical symptoms that represent progressive stages of the pathologic process. In adults, SIRS is defined by the presence of 2 or more of the following: (1) fever or hypothermia, (2) tachycardia, (3) tachypnea, and (4) abnormal white blood cell (WBC) count or an increase in immature forms. In neonates and pediatric patients, SIRS manifests as temperature instability, respiratory dysfunction (altered gas exchange, hypoxemia, acute respiratory distress syndrome [ARDS]), cardiac dysfunction (tachycardia, delayed capillary refill, hypotension), and perfusion abnormalities (oliguria, metabolic acidosis) (Table 103-13). Increased vascular permeability results in capillary leak into peripheral tissues and the lungs, with resultant pulmonary and peripheral edema. DIC results in the more severely affected cases. The cascade of escalating tissue injury may lead to multisystem organ failure and death.

Fever

Only about 50% of infected newborn infants have a temperature higher than 37.8°C (axillary) (Chapter 100). Fever in newborn

Table 103-10 MANIFESTATIONS OF NEONATAL BACTERIAL INFECTIONS

	TIME		OCCURRENCE	
	Early Onset	Late Onset	Common	Uncommon
ABDOMEN				
Peritonitis	+	+	+	
Hepatitis	+	+		+
Adrenal abscess	+	+		+
Gallbladder hydrops	+	+		+
BRAIN				
Meningitis	+	+	+	
Abscess		+	+	
Subdural empyema		+	+	
Cerebritis	+	+	+	
Ventriculitis		+	+	
CARDIOVASCULAR				
Endovascular infection		+	+	
Endocarditis	+	+		+
Pericarditis	+	+		+
Myocarditis	+	+		+
OCULAR				
Conjunctivitis	+	+	+	
Endophthalmitis	+	+		+
Chorioretinitis		+		+
OSTEOARTICULAR				
Arthritis	+	+		+
Osteomyelitis		+		+
Dactylitis		+		+
RESPIRATORY TRACT				
Pneumonia	+	+	+	
Ethmoiditis	+	+		+
Otitis media		+		+
Mastoiditis		+		+
Salivary glands		+		+
Retropharyngeal cellulitis		+		+
Empyema	+	+	+	
SKIN, SOFT TISSUE				
Breast abscess	+	+	+	
Facial cellulitis	+	+		+
Adenitis		+		+
Fasciitis	+	+		+
Impetigo		+	+	
Purpura fulminans	+	+		+
Omphalitis		+		+
Scalp abscess	+	+		+
Abscess of cystic hygroma		+		+
Urinary tract infection	+	+	+	
NO FOCUS				
Bacteremia	+	+	+	
Sepsis	+	+	+	

infants does not always signify infection; it may be caused by increased ambient temperature, isolette or radiant warmer malfunction, dehydration, central nervous system (CNS) disorders, hyperthyroidism, familial dysautonomia, or ectodermal dysplasia. A single temperature elevation is infrequently associated with infection; fever sustained over 1 hr is more likely to be due to infection. Most febrile infected infants have additional signs compatible with infection, although a focus of infection is not always apparent. Acute febrile illnesses occurring later in the neonatal period may be caused by urinary tract infection, meningitis, pneumonia, osteomyelitis, or gastroenteritis, in addition to sepsis, thus

Table 103-11 CLINICAL CRITERIA FOR THE DIAGNOSIS OF SEPSIS

	IMCI CRITERIA FOR SEVERE BACTERIAL INFECTION*	WHO YOUNG INFANT STUDY GROUP†
Convulsions	X	X
Respiratory rate >60 breaths/min	X	X (divided by age group)
Severe chest indrawing	X	X
Nasal flaring	X	
Grunting	X	
Bulging fontanel	X	
Pus draining from the ear	X	
Redness around umbilicus extending to the skin	X	
Temperature >37.7°C (or feels hot) or <35.5°C (or feels cold)	X	X
Lethargic or unconscious	X	X (not aroused by minimal stimulus)
Reduced movements	X	X (change in activity)
Not able to feed	X	X (not able to sustain such)
Not attaching to the breast	X	
No suckling at all	X	
Crepitations		X
Cyanosis		X
Reduced digital capillary refill time		X

*Any of the signs listed implies high suspicion for serious bacterial infection.
†Each symptom or sign is associated with a score. The score indicates the probability of disease.
IMCI, Integrated Management of Childhood Illness; WHO, World Health Organization.
From Vergnano S, Sharland M, Kazembe P, et al: Neonatal sepsis: an international perspective, *Arch Dis Child Fetal Neonatal Ed* 90:F220–F224, 2005.

Table 103-12 SERIOUS SYSTEMIC ILLNESS IN NEWBORNS: DIFFERENTIAL DIAGNOSIS OF NEONATAL SEPSIS

CARDIAC
Congenital: hypoplastic left heart syndrome, other structural disease, persistent pulmonary hypertension of the newborn (PPHN) Acquired: myocarditis, hypovolemic or cardiogenic shock, PPHN
GASTROINTESTINAL
Necrotizing enterocolitis Spontaneous gastrointestinal perforation Structural abnormalities
HEMATOLOGIC
Neonatal purpura fulminans Immune-mediated thrombocytopenia Immune-mediated neutropenia Severe anemia Malignancies (congenital leukemia) Hereditary clotting disorders
METABOLIC
Hypoglycemia Adrenal disorders: Adrenal hemorrhage, adrenal insufficiency, congenital adrenal hyperplasia Inborn errors of metabolism: Organic acidurias, lactic acidoses, urea cycle disorders, galactosemia
NEUROLOGIC
Intracranial hemorrhage: spontaneous, due to child abuse Hypoxic-ischemic encephalopathy Neonatal seizures Infant botulism
RESPIRATORY
Respiratory distress syndrome Aspiration pneumonia: amniotic fluid, meconium, or gastric contents Lung hypoplasia Tracheoesophageal fistula Transient tachypnea of the newborn

Table 103-13 DEFINITIONS OF SYSTEMIC INFLAMMATORY RESPIRATORY RESPONSE SYNDROME AND SEPSIS IN PEDIATRIC PATIENTS

SIRS: The systemic inflammatory response to a variety of clinical insults, manifested by 2 or more of the following conditions:
Temperature instability <35°C or >38.5°C
Respiratory dysfunction:
Tachypnea >2 SD above the mean for age
Hypoxemia (PaO_2 <70 mm Hg on room air)
Cardiac dysfunction:
Tachycardia >2 SD above the mean for age
Delayed capillary refill >3 sec
Hypotension >2 SD below the mean for age
Perfusion abnormalities:
Oliguria (urine output <0.5 mL/kg/hr)
Lactic acidosis (elevated plasma lactate and/or arterial pH <7.25)
Altered mental status
Sepsis: The systemic inflammatory response to an infectious process

From Adams-Chapman I, Stoll BJ: Systemic inflammatory response syndrome, *Semin Pediatr Infect Dis* 12:5–16, 2001.

underscoring the importance of a diagnostic evaluation that includes blood culture, urine culture, LP, and other studies as indicated (see later). Many agents may cause these late infections, including HSV, enteroviruses, RSV, and bacterial pathogens. In premature infants, hypothermia or temperature instability requiring increasing ambient (isolette, warmer) temperatures is more likely to accompany infection.

Rash

Cutaneous manifestations of infection include impetigo, cellulitis, mastitis, omphalitis, and subcutaneous abscesses. **Ecthyma gangrenosum** is indicative of infection with *Pseudomonas* species. The presence of small salmon-pink papules suggests *L. monocytogenes* infection. A vesicular rash is consistent with herpesvirus infection. The mucocutaneous lesions of *Candida albicans* are discussed elsewhere (Chapter 226.1). Petechiae and purpura may have an infectious cause. Purple papulonodular lesions are referred to as "blueberry muffin" rash and represent dermal erythropoiesis. Causes include congenital viral infections (CMV, rubella, and parvovirus), congenital neoplastic disease, and Rh hemolytic disease.

Omphalitis

Omphalitis is a neonatal infection resulting from inadequate care of the umbilical cord, which continues to be a problem, particularly in developing countries. The umbilical stump is colonized by bacteria from the maternal genital tract and the environment (Chapter 99). The necrotic tissue of the umbilical cord is an excellent medium for bacterial growth. Omphalitis may remain a localized infection or may spread to the abdominal wall, the peritoneum, the umbilical or portal vessels, or the liver. Abdominal wall cellulitis or necrotizing fasciitis with associated sepsis and a high mortality rate may develop in infants with omphalitis. Prompt diagnosis and treatment are necessary to avoid serious complications.

Tetanus (Chapter 203)

Neonatal tetanus is a serious neonatal infection in developing countries. It results from unclean delivery and unhygienic management of the umbilical cord in an infant born to a mother who has not been immunized against tetanus. The surveillance **case definition** of neonatal tetanus requires the ability of a newborn to suck at birth and for the 1st few days of life, followed by an inability to suck starting between 3 and 10 days of age, difficulty swallowing, spasms, stiffness, seizures, and death. Bronchopneumonia, presumably resulting from aspiration, is a common complication and cause of death. Neonatal tetanus is a preventable disease. It can be prevented by immunizing mothers before or during pregnancy and by ensuring a clean delivery, sterile cutting of the umbilical cord, and proper cord care after birth.

Pneumonia

Early signs and symptoms of pneumonia may be nonspecific; they include poor feeding, lethargy, irritability, cyanosis, temperature instability, and the overall impression that the infant is not well. Respiratory symptoms include grunting, tachypnea, retractions, flaring of the alae nasi, cyanosis, apnea, and progressive respiratory failure. If the infant is premature, signs of progressive respiratory distress may be superimposed upon RDS or bronchopulmonary dysplasia (BPD). For infants on mechanical ventilation, need for increased ventilating support may indicate infection.

Signs of pneumonia on physical examination, such as dullness to percussion, change in breath sounds, and the presence of rales or rhonchi, are very difficult to appreciate in a neonate. Radiographs of the chest may reveal new infiltrates or an effusion, but if the neonate has underlying RDS or BPD, it is very difficult to determine whether the radiographic changes represent a new process or worsening of the underlying disease.

The progression of neonatal pneumonia can be variable. Fulminant infection is most commonly associated with pyogenic organisms such as GBS (Chapter 177). Onset may occur during the 1st hours or days of life, with the infant often manifesting rapidly progressive circulatory collapse and respiratory failure. With early-onset pneumonia, the clinical course and radiographs of the chest may be indistinguishable from those with severe RDS.

In contrast to the rapid progression of pneumonia due to pyogenic organisms, an indolent course may be seen in nonbacterial infection. The onset can be preceded by upper respiratory tract symptoms or conjunctivitis. The infant may demonstrate a nonproductive cough, and the degree of respiratory compromise is variable. Fever is usually absent, and radiographic examination of the chest shows focal or diffuse interstitial pneumonitis. Infection is generally caused by *C. trachomatis*, CMV, *Ureaplasma urealyticum*, or one of the respiratory viruses. Although *Pneumocystis carinii* was implicated in the original description of this syndrome, its etiologic role is now in doubt, except in newborns infected with HIV.

BIBLIOGRAPHY

Please visit the Nelson Textbook of Pediatrics *website at* *www.expertconsult.com* *for the complete bibliography.*

103.7 Diagnosis

Barbara J. Stoll

The maternal history may provide important information about the mother's exposure to infection, immunity (natural or acquired), and colonization as well as about obstetric risk factors (prematurity, prolonged ruptured membranes, maternal chorioamnionitis) (see Tables 89-2 and 89-3).

Sexually transmitted infections (STIs) that infect a pregnant woman are of particular concern to the fetus and newborn because of the possibility for intrauterine or perinatal transmission. All pregnant women and their partners should be queried about a history of STIs. Women should also be counseled about the need for timely diagnosis and therapy for infections during pregnancy. The CDC recommends the following screening tests and appropriate treatment of infected mothers:

1. All pregnant women should be offered voluntary and confidential HIV testing at the 1st prenatal visit. For women at high risk of infection during pregnancy (multiple sexual partners or STIs during pregnancy, intravenous drug use), repeat testing in the 3rd trimester is recommended.
2. A serologic test for syphilis should be performed on all pregnant women at the 1st prenatal visit. Repeat screenings early

in the 3rd trimester and again at delivery are recommended for women in whom syphilis test results in the 1st trimester were positive and for those at high risk for infection during pregnancy.

3. Serologic testing for hepatitis B surface antigen (HBsAg) should be performed at the 1st prenatal visit and repeated late in pregnancy in women in whom the first test results were negative but who are at high risk for infection.
4. A maternal genital culture for *C. trachomatis* should be performed at the 1st prenatal visit. Young women (< 25 yr) and those at increased risk for infection (new or multiple partners during pregnancy) should be retested during the 3rd trimester.
5. A maternal genital culture for *Neisseria gonorrhoeae* should be performed at the 1st prenatal visit for women at risk and for those who live in areas with a high prevalence of gonorrhea. Repeat testing in the 3rd trimester is recommended for those at continued risk.
6. Evaluation for bacterial vaginosis should be considered at the 1st prenatal visit for asymptomatic women at high risk for preterm labor.
7. The CDC has recommended universal screening for rectovaginal GBS colonization of all pregnant women at 35-37 wk of gestation and a screening-based approach to selective intrapartum antibiotic prophylaxis against GBS (Table 103-14 and Figs. 103-7 and 103-8; Chapter 177). The approach to the infant born after intrapartum antibiotic prophylaxis is shown in Figure 103-9.

SUSPECTED INTRAUTERINE INFECTION

The acronym *TORCH* refers to toxoplasmosis, other agents (syphilis, varicella, parvovirus B19, many more), rubella, CMV, and HSV. Although the term may be helpful in remembering some of the etiologic agents of intrauterine infection, the TORCH battery of serologic tests has a poor diagnostic yield, and specific diagnostic studies should be selected for each etiologic agent

Table 103-14 INDICATIONS FOR INTRAPARTUM ANTIBIOTIC PROPHYLAXIS TO PREVENT EARLY-ONSET GBS DISEASE

INTRAPARTUM GBS PROPHYLAXIS INDICATED	INTRAPARTUM GBS PROPHYLAXIS NOT INDICATED
Previous infant with invasive GBS disease	Colonization with GBS during a previous pregnancy (unless an indication for GBS prophylaxis is present for current pregnancy)
GBS bacteriuria during any trimester of the current pregnancy	GBS bacteriuria during previous pregnancy (unless another indication for GBS prophylaxis is present for current pregnancy)
Positive GBS screening culture during current pregnancy (unless a cesarean delivery is performed before onset of labor or amniotic membrane rupture)	Cesarean delivery before onset of labor or amniotic membrane rupture, regardless of GBS colonization status or gestational age
Unknown GBS status at the onset of labor (culture not done, incomplete, or results unknown) and any of the following: Delivery at <37 weeks' gestation* Amniotic membrane rupture ≥18 hr Intrapartum temperature ≥100.4°F (≥38.0°C)† Intrapartum NAAT‡ positive for GBS	Negative vaginal and rectal GBS screening culture in late gestation during the current pregnancy, regardless of intrapartum risk factors

*Recommendations for the use of intrapartum antibiotics for prevention of early-onset GBS disease in the setting of threatened preterm delivery are presented in Figures 103-7 and 103-8.

†If amnionitis is suspected, broad-spectrum antibiotic therapy that includes an agent known to be active against GBS should replace GBS prophylaxis.

‡If intrapartum NAAT is negative for GBS but any other intrapartum risk factor (delivery at <37 weeks' gestation, amniotic membrane rupture ≥18 hr, or temperature ≥100.4°F [≥38.0°C]) is present, then intrapartum antibiotic prophylaxis is indicated.

GBS, group B streptococcus; NAAT, nucleic acid amplification test.

From Verani J, McGee L, Schrag S: Prevention of perinatal group B streptococcal disease—revised guidelines from CDC, 2010, *MMWR Recomm Rep* 59(RR-10):1–36, 2010.

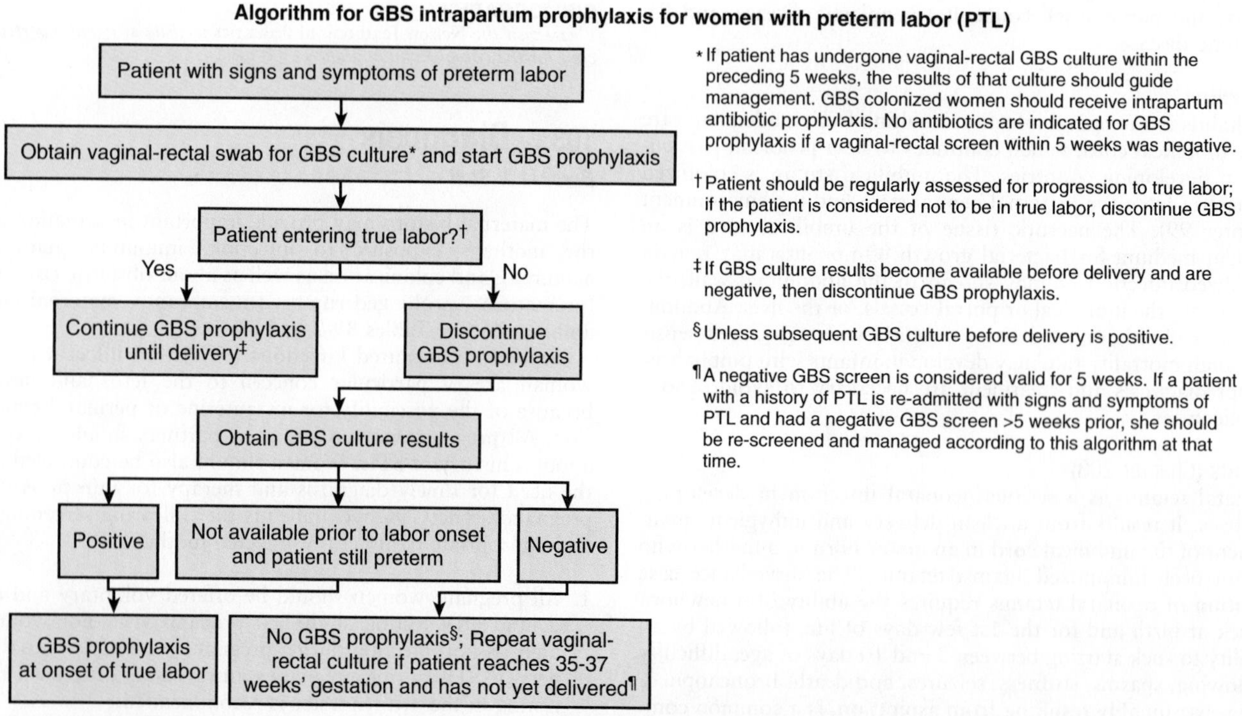
Algorithm for GBS intrapartum prophylaxis for women with preterm labor (PTL)
Patient with signs and symptoms of preterm labor
Obtain vaginal-rectal swab for GBS culture* and start GBS prophylaxis
Patient entering true labor?†
Yes
No
Continue GBS prophylaxis until delivery‡
Discontinue GBS prophylaxis
Obtain GBS culture results
Positive
Not available prior to labor onset and patient still preterm
Negative
GBS prophylaxis at onset of true labor
No GBS prophylaxis§; Repeat vaginal-rectal culture if patient reaches 35-37 weeks' gestation and has not yet delivered¶
* If patient has undergone vaginal-rectal GBS culture within the preceding 5 weeks, the results of that culture should guide management. GBS colonized women should receive intrapartum antibiotic prophylaxis. No antibiotics are indicated for GBS prophylaxis if a vaginal-rectal screen within 5 weeks was negative.
† Patient should be regularly assessed for progression to true labor; if the patient is considered not to be in true labor, discontinue GBS prophylaxis.
‡ If GBS culture results become available before delivery and are negative, then discontinue GBS prophylaxis.
§ Unless subsequent GBS culture before delivery is positive.
¶ A negative GBS screen is considered valid for 5 weeks. If a patient with a history of PTL is re-admitted with signs and symptoms of PTL and had a negative GBS screen >5 weeks prior, she should be re-screened and managed according to this algorithm at that time.

Figure 103-7 Algorithm for group B streptococcus (GBS) intrapartum prophylaxis for women with preterm labor. (From Verani J, McGee L, Schrag S: Prevention of perinatal group B streptococcal disease—revised guidelines from CDC, 2010, *MMWR Recomm Rep* 59[RR-10]:1–36, 2010.)

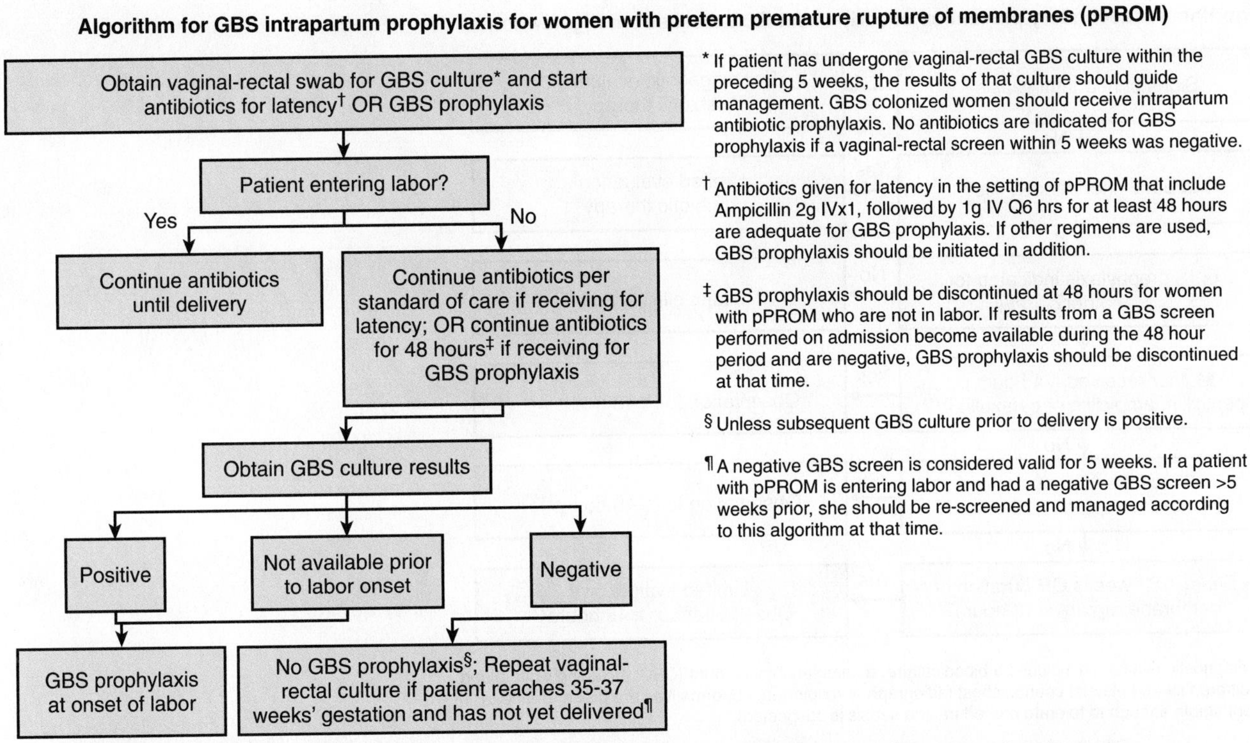

Figure 103-8 Algorithm for group B streptococcus (GBS) intrapartum prophylaxis for women with preterm premature rupture of membranes. (From Verani J, McGee L, Schrag S: Prevention of perinatal group B streptococcal disease—revised guidelines from CDC, 2010, *MMWR Recomm Rep* 59[RR-10]:1–36, 2010.)

under consideration. CMV and HSV require culture or polymerase chain reaction (PCR) methods; toxoplasmosis is diagnosed by serologic tests and PCR, whereas syphilis and rubella are diagnosed by serologic methods (Table 103-15).

In most cases of suspected fetal infection, concern is not raised until the pregnant woman has been ill for several weeks or, in retrospect, after delivery. At this time, the maternal immune response to the suspected pathogen may no longer reflect an acute infection; that is, the specific IgM response is no longer detectable and the IgG response has already reached a plateau. Many of the pathogen-specific IgM serologic assays require considerable skill to perform and tend to be less reliable than the more common IgG assays. As a result, IgM assay results can be either falsely negative or falsely positive.

Neonatal antibody titers are often difficult to interpret because (1) IgG is acquired from the mother by transplacental passage and (2) determination of neonatal IgM titers to specific pathogens is technically difficult to perform and is not universally available. IgM titers to specific pathogens have high specificity but only moderate sensitivity; they should not be used to preclude infection. Paired maternal and fetal-neonatal IgG titers showing higher newborn IgG levels or rising IgG titers during infancy may be used to diagnose some congenital infections (syphilis). Total cord blood IgM or IgA (neither is actively transported across the placenta to the fetus) and the presence of IgM–rheumatoid factor in neonatal serum are nonspecific tests for intrauterine infection.

If the likelihood of maternal infection with a known teratogenic agent is high, fetal ultrasound examination is recommended. If the examination demonstrates either a physical abnormality or delayed growth for gestational age, examination of a fetal blood sample may be warranted. **Cordocentesis** can provide a sufficient sample for both total and pathogen-specific IgM assays, for PCR, or for culture. The total IgM value is important because the normal fetal IgM level is <5 mg/dL. Any elevation in total IgM may indicate an underlying fetal infection. Specific IgM antibody tests are available for CMV, *T. pallidum*, parvovirus B19, and toxoplasmosis. IgM tests are useful only when the results are strongly positive. A negative pathogen-specific IgM finding does not rule out that pathogen as a cause of fetopathy.

If maternal serologic studies point to a specific pathogen, it is sometimes possible to detect the organism in amniotic fluid or fetal blood (culture, PCR). Amniocentesis can be performed and the fluid sent for analysis. The presence of CMV, *Toxoplasma*, or parvovirus in amniotic fluid indicates that the fetus is infected and at high risk, but it does not always mean that the fetus will have severe sequelae. In contrast, HSV and varicella-zoster virus (VZV) are rarely isolated from amniotic fluid samples. CMV, *Toxoplasma*, and parvovirus can also be identified from cordocentesis sampling.

Parvovirus does not grow in the cell cultures commonly available in the virology laboratory. An IgM response is not always detectable in women with primary infection. When fetal parvovirus infection is suspected, testing of fetal blood or amniotic fluid by PCR is recommended in addition to testing for a specific IgM response in the fetus. PCR may also be used for the diagnosis of toxoplasmosis, CMV, HSV, rubella, and syphilis.

Neonatal infections with CMV, *Toxoplasma*, rubella, HSV, and syphilis present a diagnostic dilemma because (1) their clinical features overlap and may initially be indistinguishable; (2) disease may be inapparent; (3) maternal infection is often asymptomatic; (4) special laboratory studies may be needed; and (5) appropriate treatment of toxoplasmosis, syphilis, cytomegalovirus, and HSV, which may reduce significant long-term morbidity, is predicated on an accurate diagnosis. Common shared features that should suggest the diagnosis of an intrauterine infection include intrauterine growth restriction, hematologic involvement (anemia, neutropenia, thrombocytopenia, petechiae, purpura), ocular signs (chorioretinitis, cataracts, keratoconjunctivitis, glaucoma, microphthalmos), CNS signs (microcephaly, aseptic meningitis, hydrocephaly, intracranial calcifications), other organ system involvement (pneumonia, myocarditis, nephritis, hepatitis with hepatosplenomegaly, jaundice), and nonimmune hydrops.

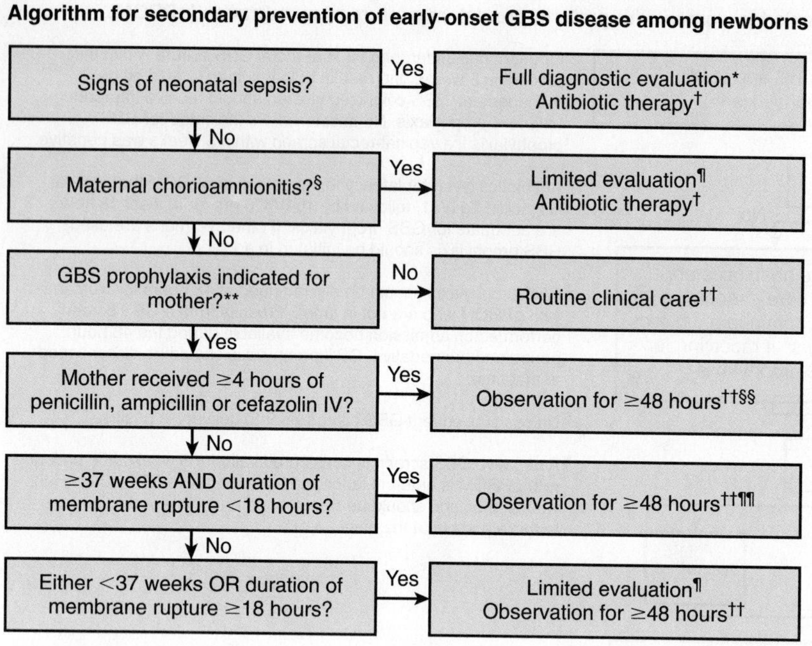

* Full diagnostic evaluation includes a blood culture, a complete blood count (CBC) including white blood cell differential and platelet counts, chest radiograph (if respiratory abnormalities are present), and LP (if patient stable anough to tolerate procedure and sepsis is suspected).

† Antibiotic therapy should be directed toward the most common causes of neonatal sepsis including intravenous ampicillin for GBS and coverage for other organisms (including *Escherichia coli* and other gram-negative pathogens), and should take into account local antibiotic resistance patterns.

§ Consultation with obstetric providers is important to determine the level of clinical suspicion for chorioamnionitis. Chorioamnionitis is diagnosed clinically and some of the signs are nonspecific.

¶ Limited evaluation includes blood culture (at birth), and CBC with differential and platelets (at birth and/or at 6-12 hours of life).

** GBS prophylaxis indicated in one or more of the following: (1) mother GBS positive within preceding 5 weeks, (2) GBS status unknown with one or more intrapartum risk factors including <37 weeks' gestation, ROM ≥18 hours or T ≥100.4°F (38.0°C), (3) GBS bacteriuria during current pregnancy, (4) history of a previous infant with GBS disease.

†† If signs of sepsis develop, a full diagnostic evaluation should be done and antibiotic therapy initiated.

§§ If ≥37 weeks' gestation, observation may occur at home after 24 hours if other discharge criteria have been met, there is ready access to medical care, and a person who is able to comply fully with instructions for home observation will be present. If any of these conditions is not met, the infant should be observed in the hospital for at least 48 hours and until discharge criteria are achieved.

¶¶ Some experts recommend a CBC with differential and platelets at 6-12 hours of age.

Figure 103-9 Algorithm for secondary prevention of early-onset group B streptococcus (GBS) disease among newborns. (From Verani J, McGee L, Schrag S: Prevention of perinatal group B streptococcal disease—revised guidelines from CDC, 2010, *MMWR Recomm Rep* 59[RR-10]:1–36, 2010.)

Diagnostic studies in newborns with suspected chronic intrauterine infection should specifically test for each diagnostic consideration. Systemic infections with CMV, HSV, and enteroviruses frequently involve the liver; if these infections are suspected, liver function tests should be performed. Neonatal HSV CNS disease may be confirmed by viral culture or by PCR identification from CSF. Given that approximately 50% of infants infected with HSV do not have CNS disease, cultures of skin, eyes, and mouth should also be performed in all infants with suspected HSV disease.

SUSPECTED BACTERIAL OR FUNGAL INFECTIONS

Bacterial or fungal infection is diagnosed by isolating the etiologic agent from a normally sterile body site (blood, CSF, urine, joint fluid). Obtaining 2 blood culture specimens by venipuncture from different sites avoids confusion caused by skin contamination and increases the likelihood of bacterial detection. Samples should be obtained from an umbilical catheter only at the time of initial insertion. A peripheral venous sample should also be obtained when blood is drawn for culture from central venous catheters. Although blood cultures are usually the basis for a diagnosis of bacterial infection, the bacteremic phase of the illness may be missed by poor timing or inadequate blood sample size. Low-level bacteremia (<10 colony-forming units/mL) has been observed in some infants from birth to 2 mo of age with positive culture results. Automated blood culture systems (BACTEC, Becton Dickinson; BacT/Alert, Organon Teknika), which continuously monitor blood cultures by checking each bottle every few minutes, have led to earlier detection of bacterial growth. After positive signaling in the automated system, the specific pathogen is identified by biochemical tests. PCR technology is emerging for more rapid accurate identification of a number of viral and bacterial agents.

Documentation of a positive blood culture result is the first diagnostic criterion that must be met for sepsis (see Table 103-15). It is important to note, however, that some patients with bacterial infection may have negative blood culture results ("clinical infection"), and other approaches to identification of infection are needed. A variety of diagnostic markers of infection are

Table 103-15 EVALUATION OF A NEWBORN FOR INFECTION OR SEPSIS

HISTORY (SPECIFIC RISK FACTORS)
Maternal infection during gestation or at parturition (type and duration of antimicrobial therapy):
Urinary tract infection
Chorioamnionitis
Maternal colonization with group B streptococci, *Neisseria gonorrhoeae*, herpes simplex
Gestational age/birthweight
Multiple birth
Duration of membrane rupture
Complicated delivery
Fetal tachycardia (distress)
Age at onset (in utero, birth, early postnatal, late)
Location at onset (hospital, community)
Medical intervention:
Vascular access
Endotracheal intubation
Parenteral nutrition
Surgery
EVIDENCE OF OTHER DISEASES*
Congenital malformations (heart disease, neural tube defect)
Respiratory tract disease (respiratory distress syndrome, aspiration)
Necrotizing enterocolitis
Metabolic disease, e.g., galactosemia
EVIDENCE OF FOCAL OR SYSTEMIC DISEASE
General appearance, neurologic status
Abnormal vital signs
Organ system disease
Feeding, stools, urine output, extremity movement
LABORATORY STUDIES
Evidence of Infection
Culture from a normally sterile site (blood, CSF, other)
Demonstration of a microorganism in tissue or fluid
Molecular detection (blood, urine, CSF)
Maternal or neonatal serology (syphilis, toxoplasmosis)
Autopsy
Evidence of Inflammation
Leukocytosis, increased immature/total neutrophil count ratio
Acute-phase reactants: C-reactive protein, erythrocyte sedimentation rate
Cytokines: interleukin-6, interleukin-B, tumor necrosis factor
Pleocytosis in CSF or synovial or pleural fluid
Disseminated intravascular coagulation: fibrin degradation products, D dimer
Evidence of Multiorgan System Disease
Metabolic acidosis: pH, P_{CO_2}
Pulmonary function: P_{O_2}, P_{CO_2}
Renal function: blood urea nitrogen, creatinine
Hepatic injury/function: bilirubin, alanine aminotransferase, aspartate aminotransferase , ammonia, prothrombin time, partial thromboplastin time
Bone marrow function: neutropenia, anemia, thrombocytopenia

*Diseases that increase the risk of infection or may overlap with signs of sepsis.
CSF, cerebrospinal fluid.

being evaluated. Although the total WBC count and differential counts and the ratio of immature to total neutrophils have limitations in sensitivity and specificity, an immature-to-total neutrophil ratio of ≥0.2 suggests bacterial infection. Neutropenia is more common than neutrophilia in severe neonatal sepsis, but neutropenia also occurs in association with maternal hypertension, preeclampsia, and intrauterine growth restriction. Thrombocytopenia is a nonspecific indicator of infection. Tests to demonstrate an inflammatory response include determinations of C-reactive protein, procalcitonin, haptoglobin, fibrinogen, proteomic markers in amniotic fluid, inflammatory cytokines (including IL-6, IL-8, and TNFα), and cell surface markers. It is unclear which surrogate markers for infection are most helpful.

When the clinical findings suggest an acute infection and the site of infection is unclear, laboratory studies should be performed, including blood cultures, LP, urine examination, and a chest radiograph. Urine should be collected by catheterization or suprapubic aspiration; urine culture for bacteria can be omitted in suspected early-onset infections because hematogenous spread to the urinary tract is rare at this point. Examination of the buffy coat with Gram or methylene blue stain may demonstrate intracellular pathogens. Demonstration of bacteria and inflammatory cells in gram-stained gastric aspirates on the 1st day of life may reflect maternal amnionitis, which is a risk factor for early-onset infection. Stains of endotracheal secretions in infants with early-onset pneumonia may demonstrate intracellular bacteria, and cultures may reveal either pathogens or upper respiratory tract flora. Careful examination of the placenta can be helpful in the diagnosis of both chronic and acute intrauterine infections.

Diagnostic evaluation (including blood culture) is indicated for asymptomatic infants born to mothers with chorioamnionitis. The probability of neonatal infection correlates with the degree of prematurity and bacterial contamination of the amniotic fluid. Some experts recommend presumptive treatment with antibiotics. By contrast, all symptomatic infants should be treated with antibiotics after blood cultures are obtained. There is controversy over whether an LP is necessary for all term infants with suspected early-onset sepsis. If the blood culture result is positive or if the infant becomes symptomatic, LP should definitely be performed. If the mother has been treated with antibiotics for chorioamnionitis, the newborn's blood culture result may be negative, and the clinician must rely on clinical observation and other laboratory tests (see Fig. 103-9).

The diagnosis of pneumonia in a neonate is usually presumptive; microbiologic proof of infection is generally lacking because lung tissue is not easily cultured. CDC definitions of pneumonia do not target newborns, particularly the high-risk group of VLBW infants on mechanical ventilation. Although some clinicians rely on the results of bacteriologic culture of material obtained from the trachea as "proof" of cause, interpretation of such cultures has many pitfalls. These cultures often reflect upper respiratory tract commensal organisms and may have no etiologic significance. Even cultures performed on material obtained by bronchoalveolar lavage in a neonate are unreliable because the small bronchoscopes used in neonates cannot be protected from contamination as they are introduced into the distal airways. Short of tissue obtained by lung biopsy, the only reliable bacteriologic cultures are those performed on specimens obtained from blood or pleural fluid. Unfortunately, blood culture results are usually negative, and sufficient pleural fluid for culture is rarely present.

Interpretation of fungal cultures is associated with the same problems as that of bacterial cultures. Cultures of respiratory secretions for *U. urealyticum* and other genital *Mycoplasma* species are of little value because normal neonates are often colonized with these agents as a result of contamination with secretions from the maternal genital tract. Cultures for respiratory viruses and *C. trachomatis* may be valuable; these organisms are never indigenous flora, and isolation of them therefore suggests an etiologic role.

Other tests of potential value in evaluating neonates with possible infectious pneumonitis are discussed under diagnosis of infections (Chapter 164). The **differential diagnosis** of pneumonitis in neonates is broad and includes RDS, meconium aspiration syndrome, persistent pulmonary hypertension, diaphragmatic hernia, transient tachypnea of the newborn, congenital heart disease, and BPD.

The diagnosis of meningitis is confirmed by examination of CSF and identification of a bacterium, virus, or fungus by culture, antigen, or the use of PCR. The importance of the LP as part of the diagnostic evaluation of the neonate with suspected sepsis has been the subject of debate; clinical practice varies. For term infants with suspected early-onset sepsis, many clinicians start with a blood culture and a complete blood count, because 70-85% of term neonates with bacterial meningitis have positive blood culture results. Examination and culture of CSF are undertaken in term infants with symptoms and/or bacteremia. Many clinicians defer the LP in severely ill infants with suspected early-onset infection because of the fear of respiratory and/or cardiovascular compromise. In these situations, blood culture should be performed and treatment initiated for presumed meningitis until LP can be safely performed.

Normal, uninfected infants from 0-4 wk of age may have the following elevated CSF findings: protein 84 ± 45 mg/dL, glucose 46 ± 10 mg/dL, and leukocyte count 11 ± 10 mm^3 with the 90th percentile being 22. The proportion of polymorphonuclear leukocytes is 2.2 ± 3.8% with the 90th percentile being 6. Elevated CSF protein values and leukocyte counts and hypoglycorrhachia may develop in preterm infants after intraventricular hemorrhage. Many nonpyogenic congenital infections (toxoplasmosis, CMV, HSV, syphilis producing an aseptic meningitis) can also produce alterations in CSF protein value and leukocyte count.

Gram staining of CSF yields a positive result in most patients with bacterial meningitis. The leukocyte count is usually elevated, with a predominance of neutrophils (>70-90%); the number is often >1,000 but may be <100 in infants with neutropenia or early in the disease. Microorganisms are recovered from most patients who have not been pretreated with antibiotics. Bacteria have also been isolated from CSF that did not have an abnormal number of cells (<25) or an abnormal protein level (<200 mg/dL), thus underscoring the importance of performing a culture and Gram stain on all CSF specimens. Contamination of CSF by bacteremia after traumatic LP may occur rarely. Culture-negative meningitis may be seen with antibiotic pretreatment, a brain abscess, or infection with *Mycobacterium hominis, U. urealyticum, Bacteroides fragilis,* enterovirus, or HSV. Use of PCR has improved the ability to detect viruses in CSF. Head ultrasonography or, more often, CT with contrast enhancement may be helpful in diagnosing ventriculitis and brain abscess.

BIBLIOGRAPHY

Please visit the Nelson Textbook of Pediatrics *website at* www.expertconsult.com *for the complete bibliography.*

103.8 Treatment

Barbara J. Stoll

Treatment of suspected bacterial infection is determined by the pattern of disease and the organisms that are common for the age of the infant and the flora of the nursery. Once appropriate culture specimens have been obtained, intravenous or, less often, intramuscular antibiotic therapy should be instituted immediately. Initial empirical treatment of early-onset bacterial infections should consist of ampicillin and an aminoglycoside (usually gentamicin). Nosocomial infections acquired in a NICU are more likely to be caused by staphylococci, various Enterobacteriaceae, *Pseudomonas* species, or *Candida* species. Thus, an antistaphylococcal drug (oxacillin or nafcillin for *S. aureus* or, more often, vancomycin for coagulase-negative staphylococci or methicillin-resistant *S. aureus*) should be substituted for ampicillin. A history of recent antimicrobial therapy or the presence of antibiotic-resistant infections in the NICU suggests the need for a different agent. When the history or the presence of necrotic skin lesions suggests *Pseudomonas* infection, initial therapy should consist of piperacillin, ticarcillin, or ceftazidime and an aminoglycoside. Some experts recommend antifungal prophylaxis with fluconazole for particularly high-risk newborns—that is, those of extremely LBW (<1000 g) and low gestational age (<27 wk). Doses of commonly used antibiotics are provided in Table 103-16. Peak and trough levels of gentamicin (peak, 5-10 µg/mL; trough, <2 µg/mL) and vancomycin (peak, 25-40 µg/mL; trough, <10 µg/mL) are useful to ensure therapeutic levels and minimize toxicity if the agent is administered for more than 2-3 days. The use of antifungal therapy should be considered in VLBW infants who have had previous antibiotic therapy, may have mucosal colonization with *C. albicans,* and are at high risk for invasive disease (Chapter 226.1).

Once the pathogen has been identified and its antibiotic sensitivities determined, the most appropriate drug or drugs should be selected. For most gram-negative enteric bacteria, ampicillin and an aminoglycoside or a 3rd-generation cephalosporin (cefotaxime or ceftazidime) should be used. Enterococci should be treated with both a penicillin (ampicillin or piperacillin) and an aminoglycoside because the synergy of both drugs is needed. Ampicillin alone is adequate for *L. monocytogenes,* and penicillin suffices for GBS. Clindamycin or metronidazole is appropriate for anaerobic infections.

Third-generation cephalosporins such as cefotaxime are valuable additions for treating documented neonatal sepsis and meningitis because (1) the minimal inhibitory concentrations of these agents needed for treatment of gram-negative enteric bacilli are much lower than those of the aminoglycosides, (2) excellent penetration into CSF occurs, and (3) much higher doses can be given. The end result is much higher bactericidal titers in serum and CSF than achievable with ampicillin-aminoglycoside combinations. However, the *routine* use of 3rd-generation cephalosporins for suspected sepsis in NICU patients is inappropriate because of the potential for rapid emergence of resistant organisms and a possible link with *Candida* sepsis.

The emergence of antibiotic resistance among pathogens that infect newborns is of great concern. Vancomycin-resistant enterococci and vancomycin-insensitive *S. aureus* are worrisome. Guidelines to limit the use of vancomycin must be followed. Although the use of vancomycin use cannot be avoided in neonatal units where methicillin-resistant *S. aureus* is endemic, its use can be reduced by limiting empirical therapy to patients with a high suspicion of severe infection with coagulase-negative staphylococci (severely ill neonate with an indwelling intravascular catheter) and by discontinuing therapy after 2-3 days when blood culture results are negative. The rational use of antibiotics in neonates involves using narrow-spectrum drugs when possible, treating infection and not colonization, and limiting the duration of therapy. Antibiotic stewardship programs promote the appropriate use of antibiotics (choice of drug, dose, duration, route) with the aim to improve clinical outcome and reduce emergence of antimicrobial resistance.

Therapy for most bloodstream infections should be continued for a total of 7-10 days, or for at least 5-7 days after a clinical response has occurred. Blood culture of a specimen taken 24-48 hr after initiation of therapy should yield negative results. If the blood culture result remains positive, the possibility of an infected indwelling catheter, endocarditis, an infected thrombus, an occult abscess, subtherapeutic antibiotic levels, or resistant organisms should be considered. A change in antibiotics, longer duration of therapy, or removal of the catheter may be indicated.

Treatment of newborn infants whose mothers received antibiotics during labor should be individualized. If early-onset sepsis is thought to be likely, treatment of the infant should be continued until it is shown that no infection has occurred (the infant remains asymptomatic for 24-72 hr) or clinical and laboratory evidence of recovery is apparent. Furthermore, in the context of intrapartum antibiotic use, it is important to consider that the organism causing infection may be resistant to the antibiotic given to the mother, a possibility that may influence choice of antibiotic use in the infant.

For pneumonia developing in the 1st 7-10 days of life, a combination of ampicillin and an aminoglycoside or cefotaxime is appropriate. Nosocomial pneumonia, which generally manifests after this time, can be treated empirically with methicillin or vancomycin and an aminoglycoside or a 3rd-generation cephalosporin. *Pseudomonas* pneumonia should be treated with an aminoglycoside combined with ticarcillin or ceftazidime. Pneumonia caused by *C. trachomatis* is treated with either erythromycin or

Table 103-16 SUGGESTED DOSAGE SCHEDULES FOR ANTIBIOTICS USED IN NEWBORNS

ANTIBIOTIC	ROUTE	DOSAGE (mg/kg) AND INTERVAL OF ADMINISTRATION				
		Weight < 1,200 g*	Weight 1,200-2,000 g		Weight > 2,000 g	
		Age 0-4 wk	*Age 0-7 Days*	*Age > 7 Days*	*Age 0-7 Days*	*Age > 7 Days*
Amikacin†:						
SDD	IV, IM	7.5 q12h	7.5 q12h	7.5 q8h	10 q12h	10 q8h
ODD	IV, IM	18 q48h	16 q36h	15 q24h	15 q24h	15 q24h
Ampicillin:	IV, IM					
Meningitis		50 q12h	50 q12h	50 q8h	50 q8h	50 q6h
Other infections		25 q12h	25 q12h	25 q8h	25 q8h	25 q6h
Aztreonam	IV, IM	30 q12h	30 q12h	30 q8h	30 q8h	30 q6h
Cefazolin	IV, IM	20 q12h	20 q12h	20 q12h	20 q12h	20 q8h
Cefepime	IV, IM	50 q12h	50 q12h	50 q8h	50 q12h	50 q8h
Cefotaxime	IV, IM	50 q12h	50 q12h	50 q8h	50 q12h	50 q8h
Ceftazidime	IV, IM	50 q12h	50 q12h	50 q8h	50 q8h	50 q8h
Ceftriaxone	IV, IM	50 q24h	50 q24h	50 q24h	50 q24h	75 q24h
Cephalothin	IV	20 q12h	20 q12h	20 q8h	20 q8h	20 q6h
Chloramphenicol†	IV, PO	25 q24h	25 q24h	25 q24h	25 q24h	25 q12h
Ciprofloxacin‡	IV	—	—	10-20 q24h	—	20-30 q12h
Clindamycin	IV, IM, PO	5 q12h	5 q12h	5 q8h	5 q8h	5 q6h
Erythromycin	PO	10 q12h	10 q12h	10 q8h	10 q12h	10 q8h
Gentamicin†:						
SDD	IV, IM	2.5 q18h	2.5 q12h	2.5 q8h	2.5 q12h	2.5 q8h
ODD	IV, IM	5 q48h	4 q36h	4 q24h	4 q24h	4 q24h
Imipenem	IV, IM	—	20 q12h	20 q12h	20 q12h	20 q8h
Linezolid	IV	—	10 q12h	10 q8h	10 q12h	10 q8h
Methicillin:						
Meningitis	IV, IM	50 q12h	50 q12h	50 q8h	50 q8h	50 q6h
Other infections	IV, IM	25 q12h	25 q12h	25 q8h	25 q8h	25 q6h
Metronidazole§	IV, PO	7.5 q48h	7.5 q24h	7.5 q12h	7.5 q12h	15 q12h
Mezlocillin	IV, IM	75 q12h	75 q12h	75 q8h	75 q12h	75 q8h
Meropenem¶	IV, IM	—	20 q12h	20 q12h	20 q12h	20 q8h
Nafcillin	IV	25 q12h	25 q12h	25 q8h	25 q8h	37.5 q6h
Netilmicin:						
SDD†	IV, IM	2.5 q18h	2.5 q12h	2.5 q8h	2.5 q12h	2.5 q8h
ODD	IV, IM	Same as for gentamicin				
Oxacillin	IV, IM	25 q12h	25 q12h	25 q8h	25 q8h	37.5 q6h
Penicillin G (units):						
Meningitis	IV	50,000 q12h	50,000 q12h	50,000 q8h	50,000 q8h	50,000 q6h
Other infections	IV	25,000 q12h	25,000 q12h	25,000 q8h	25,000 q8h	25,000 q6h
Penicillin benzathine (units)	IM	—	50,000 (one dose)	50,000 (one dose)	50,000 (one dose)	50,000 (one dose)
Penicillin procaine (units)	IM		50,000 q24h	50,000 q24h	50,000 q24h	50,000 q24h
Piperacillin	IV, IM	—	50-75 q12h	50-75 q8h	50-75 q8h	50-75 q6h
Piperacillin/tazobactam	Same as for piperacillin					
Rifampin	PO, IV	—	10 q24h	10 q24h	10 q24h	10 q24h
Ticarcillin	IV, IM	75 q12h	75 q12h	75 q8h	75 q8h	75 q6h
Ticarcillin-clavulanate	Same as for ticarcillin					
Tobramycin:						
SDD†	IV, IM	2.5 q18h	2 q12h	2 q8h	2 q12h	2 q8h
ODD	IV, IM	Same as for gentamicin				
Vancomycin†	IV	15 q24h	10 q12h	10 q12h	10 q8h	10 q8h

*Data from Prober CG, Stevenson DK, Benitz WE: The use of antibiotics in neonates weighing less than 1200 grams, *Pediatr Infect Dis J* 9:111, 1990.
†Adjustments of further dosing intervals should be based on aminoglycoside half-lives calculated after serum peak and trough concentration measurements.
‡Doses suggested are based on anecdotal clinical experience.
§A loading intravenous dose of 15 mg/kg followed 24 hr later (term infants) or 48 hr later (preterm infants) by 7.5 mg/kg q12h has been suggested by other investigators.
¶Dosages of meropenem suggested are the same as those of imipenem.
IM, intramuscular; IV, intravenous; ODD, once-daily dosing; PO, oral; SDD, standard daily dosing.
Adapted from Sáez-Llorens X, McCraken GH Jr: Clinical pharmacology of antibacterial agents. In Remington JS, Klein JO, Wilson CB, et al, editors: *Infectious diseases of the fetus and newborn infant,* ed 6, Philadelphia, 2005, Elsevier.

trimethoprim-sulfamethoxazole; *U. urealyticum* infection is treated with erythromycin.

Presumptive antimicrobial therapy for bacterial meningitis should include ampicillin in doses used for meningitis and cefotaxime or gentamicin unless staphylococci are likely, which is an indication for vancomycin. Susceptibility testing of gram-negative enteric organisms is important because their resistance to cephalosporins and aminoglycosides is common. Most aminoglycosides administered by parenteral routes do not achieve sufficiently high antibiotic levels in the lumbar CSF or ventricles to inhibit the growth of gram-negative bacilli. Therefore, some experts recommend a combination of intravenous ampicillin and a 3rd-generation cephalosporin for the treatment of neonatal gram-negative meningitis. Cephalosporins should not be used as empirical monotherapy because *L. monocytogenes* and enterococcus are resistant to cephalosporins.

Meningitis caused by GBS usually responds within 24-48 hr and should be treated for 14-21 days. Gram-negative bacilli may continue to grow from repeated CSF samples for 72-96 hr after therapy despite the use of appropriate antibiotics. Treatment of gram-negative meningitis should be continued for 21 days or for at least 14 days after sterilization of the CSF, whichever is longer. *P. aeruginosa* meningitis should be treated with ceftazidime. Metronidazole is the treatment of choice for infection caused by *B. fragilis*. Prolonged antibiotic administration, with or without drainage for treatment and diagnosis, is indicated for neonatal cerebral abscesses. CT scans are recommended for patients with suspected ventriculitis, hydrocephalus, or cerebral abscess (initial and follow-up assessments) and for those with an unexpectedly complicated course (prolonged coma, focal neurologic deficits, persistent or recurrent fever). Neonatal herpes meningoencephalitis should be treated with acyclovir, and empirical therapy should be considered in symptomatic infants with a CSF mononuclear pleocytosis. Pleconaril is the treatment of choice for severe enteroviral infections such as meningoencephalitis, carditis, and hepatitis. Treatment of candidal meningitis is discussed in Chapter 226.

Treatment of sepsis and meningitis may be divided into antimicrobial therapy for the suspected or known pathogen and supportive care. Careful attention to respiratory and cardiovascular status is mandatory. Adequate oxygenation of tissues should be maintained; ventilatory support is frequently necessary for respiratory failure caused by sepsis, pneumonia, pulmonary hypertension, or ARDS. Refractory hypoxia and shock may require extracorporeal membrane oxygenation, which has reduced mortality rates in full-term infants with respiratory failure. Shock and metabolic acidosis should be identified and managed with fluid resuscitation and inotropic agents as needed. Corticosteroids should be administered only for adrenal insufficiency. Fluids, electrolytes, and glucose levels should be monitored carefully with correction of hypovolemia, hyponatremia, hypocalcemia, and hypoglycemia/hyperglycemia. Hyperbilirubinemia should be monitored and treated aggressively with phototherapy and/or exchange transfusion, because the risk of kernicterus increases in the presence of sepsis and meningitis. Seizures should be treated with anticonvulsants. Parenteral nutrition is needed for any infant who cannot sustain enteral feeding.

DIC may complicate neonatal septicemia. Platelet counts, hemoglobin levels, and clotting times should be monitored. DIC is treated by management of the underlying infection, but if bleeding occurs, DIC may require fresh frozen plasma, platelet transfusions, or whole blood.

Because neutrophil storage pool depletion has been associated with a poor prognosis, therapies that increase the number or improve the quality of neutrophils have been studied, including granulocyte transfusions, GM-CSF, and G-CSF. The use of G-CSF or GM-CSF abolishes sepsis-induced neutropenia, but the effect of these cytokines on sepsis-related mortality is unproven. Modern leukapheresis techniques and the use of G-CSF to mobilize polymorphonuclear cells in healthy donors for use in granulocyte transfusion is a promising approach that needs further study. The use of intravenous immunoglobulin (IVIG) has been shown to decrease mortality in patients with sepsis; a meta-analysis of several trials recommended administration of a single dose of 500-750 mg/kg as adjunctive therapy. Selected IVIG preparations containing specific monoclonal antibodies are being studied. Other potential immunomodulatory agents are pentoxifylline, probiotics, and human breast milk.

It is important to remember that nonbacterial infectious agents can produce the syndrome of neonatal sepsis. HSV infection requires immediate specific treatment, as does systemic *Candida* infection. Treatment and other aspects of various nonbacterial infections are discussed in detail in other sections: TB (Chapter 207), syphilis (Chapter 210), genital mycoplasmas (Chapter 216), *C. trachomatis* (Chapter 218), *Candida* (Chapter 221), rubella (Chapter 239), enteroviruses (Chapter 242), parvovirus B19 (Chapter 243), HSV (Chapter 244), VZV (Chapter 245), and CMV (Chapter 247).

BIBLIOGRAPHY

Please visit the Nelson Textbook of Pediatrics *website at* *www.expertconsult.com* *for the complete bibliography.*

103.9 Complications and Prognosis

Barbara J. Stoll

Complications of bacterial or fungal infections may be divided into those related to the acute inflammatory process and those that underlie neonatal problems such as respiratory distress and fluid and electrolyte abnormalities.

Complications of bacteremic infections include endocarditis, septic emboli, abscess formation, septic joints with residual disability, and osteomyelitis and bone destruction. Recurrent bacteremia is rare (<5% of patients). Candidemia may lead to vasculitis, endocarditis, and endophthalmitis as well as abscesses in the kidneys, liver, lungs, and brain. Sequelae of sepsis may result from septic shock, DIC, or organ failure.

Mortality rates from the sepsis syndrome depend on the definition of sepsis. In adults, the mortality rate approaches 50%, and the rate in newborn infants is probably at least that high. Reported mortality rates in neonatal sepsis are as low as 10% because all bacteremic infections are included in the definition. Several studies have documented that the sepsis case fatality rate is highest for gram-negative and fungal infections (Table 103-17).

The case fatality rate for neonatal bacterial meningitis is between 20% and 25%. Many of these patients have associated sepsis. Risk factors for death or for moderate or severe disability include seizure duration >72 hr, coma, need for inotropic agents, and leukopenia. Immediate complications of meningitis include ventriculitis, cerebritis, and brain abscess. Late complications of meningitis occur in 40-50% of survivors and include hearing loss, abnormal behavior, developmental delay, cerebral palsy, focal motor disability, seizure disorders, and hydrocephalus. Advanced imaging (CT, MRI) has demonstrated cerebritis, brain abscess, infarct, subdural effusions, cortical atrophy, and diffuse encephalomalacia in newborns surviving meningitis. A number of these sequelae may be encountered in infants with sepsis but without meningitis, as a result of cerebritis or septic shock. Extremely LBW infants (<1,000 g) with sepsis are at increased risk for poor neurodevelopmental and growth outcomes in early childhood.

BIBLIOGRAPHY

Please visit the Nelson Textbook of Pediatrics *website at* *www.expertconsult.com* *for the complete bibliography.*

Table 103-17 INFECTING PATHOGEN VERSUS DEATH RATE IN LATE-ONSET SEPSIS IN VERY LOW BIRTHWEIGHT INFANTS*

ORGANISM†	N	DEATH N‡
All gram-positive organisms	**905**	**101 (11.2%)**
Staphylococcus—coagulase negative	606	55 (9.1%)
Staphylococcus aureus	99	17 (17.2%)
Group B streptococcus	32	7 (21.9%)
All other streptococci	65	7 (10.8%)
All gram-negative organisms	**257**	**93 (36.2%)**
Escherichia coli	53	18 (34.0%)
Klebsiella	62	14 (22.6%)
Pseudomonas	43	32 (74.4%)
Enterobacter	41	11 (26.8%)
Serratia	39	14 (35.9%)
All fungal organisms	**151**	**48 (31.8%)**
Candida albicans	82	36 (43.9%)
Candida parapsilosis	44	7 (15.9%)

*From late-onset sepsis review in VLBW infants, National Institute of Child Health and Human Development Neonatal Research Network, September 1, 1998, through August 31, 2000.
†Organisms found on the last positive blood culture before death or discharge.
‡The odds ratios for death, with control for gestational age, study center, race, and sex, were as follows: gram-positive vs other infections, 0.26 (0.19-0.35), $P<.001$; gram-negative vs other infections, 3.5 (2.5-4.9), $P<.001$; and fungi vs other infections, 2.0 (1.3-3.0), $P<.01$.
From Stoll BJ, Hansen N, Fanaroff AA, et al: Late-onset sepsis in very low birthweight neonates: the experience of the NICHD Neonatal Research Network, *Pediatrics* 110:285–291, 2002.

Table 103-18 PRINCIPLES FOR THE PREVENTION OF NOSOCOMIAL INFECTION IN THE NEONATAL INTENSIVE CARE UNIT

Observe recommendations for universal precautions with all patient contact:
- Gloves
- Gowns, mask, and isolation as indicated

Nursery design engineering:
- Appropriate nursing: patient ratio
- Avoid overcrowding and excessive workload
- Readily accessible sinks, antiseptic solutions, soap, and paper towels

Handwashing:
- Improve handwashing compliance
- Wash hands before and after each patient encounter
- Appropriate use of soap, alcohol-based preparations, or antiseptic solutions
- Alcohol-based antiseptic solution at each patient bedside
- Provide emollients for nursery staff
- Education and feedback for nursery staff

Minimizing risk of CVC contamination:
- Maximal sterile barrier precautions during CVC insertion
- Local antisepsis with chlorhexidine gluconate
- Minimize repeated entry into the line for laboratory tests
- Aseptic technique when entering the line
- Minimize CVC days
- Sterile preparation of all fluids to be administered via a CVC

Meticulous skin care

Encourage early and appropriate advancement of enteral feeding

Education and feedback for nursery personnel

Continuous monitoring and surveillance of nosocomial infection rates in the neonatal intensive care unit

CVC, central venous catheter.
From Adams-Chapman I, Stoll BJ: Prevention of nosocomial infections in the neonatal intensive care unit, *Curr Opin Pediatr* 14:157–164, 2002.

103.10 Prevention

Barbara J. Stoll

Maternal immunization protects the mother against vaccine-preventable diseases that can cause intrauterine infections (rubella, hepatitis B, VZV) and may also protect the infant via passive transfer of protective maternal antibodies (tetanus). CMV vaccines are under study. Toxoplasmosis is preventable with appropriate diet and avoidance of exposure to cat feces. Malaria during pregnancy can be minimized with chemoprophylaxis and use of insecticide-treated bed nets. Congenital syphilis is preventable by timely diagnosis and appropriate early treatment of infected pregnant women.

Aggressive management of suspected maternal chorioamnionitis with antibiotic therapy during labor, along with rapid delivery of the infant, reduces the risk of early-onset neonatal sepsis. Vertical transmission of GBS (Chapter 177) is significantly reduced by selective intrapartum chemoprophylaxis. Neonatal infection with *Chlamydia* can be prevented by identification and treatment of infected pregnant women (Chapter 218). Mother-to-child transmission of HIV is significantly reduced by maternal antiretroviral therapy during pregnancy, labor, and delivery, cesarean section delivery prior to rupture of membranes, and antiretroviral treatment of the infant after birth (Chapter 268).

PREVENTION OF NOSOCOMIAL INFECTION

Principles for the prevention of nosocomial infection include adherence to universal precautions with all patient contact, avoiding nursery crowding and limiting nurse-to-patient ratios, strict compliance with handwashing, meticulous neonatal skin care, minimizing the risk of catheter contamination, decreasing the number of venipunctures and heelsticks, reducing the duration of catheter and mechanical ventilation days, encouraging appropriate advancement of enteral feedings, providing education and feedback to nursery personnel, and ongoing monitoring and surveillance of nosocomial infection rates in the NICU (Table 103-18).

Most nosocomial infections in the NICU are bloodstream infections associated with intravascular catheters. Catheters used in neonates include peripheral intravenous catheters, umbilical catheters, peripherally inserted central catheters, and surgically placed central venous catheters (CVCs). Efforts to reduce catheter-related infections include proper antisepsis of the skin before insertion of the catheter, sterile precautions during catheter insertion, aseptic technique when entering the line, minimizing repeated entry into the line for blood sampling, sterile preparation of fluids to be used with a CVC, and, finally, minimizing the number of catheter days.

The skin is an important mechanical barrier to infection. VLBW infants are born with an ineffective epidermal barrier that results in increases in transepidermal water loss and risk for infection. Efforts to reduce traumatic injury to this immature skin are important, including a reduction in the number of heelsticks.

Handwashing remains the most important and effective means of reducing nosocomial infections. Several expert groups have established guidelines for effective handwashing. Antimicrobial soaps or alcohol-based preparations are recommended. Proper handwashing is essential before entry into the NICU and before each patient contact. Barriers to compliance with handwashing include overcrowding, excessive patient-to-nurse ratios, poorly located sinks and inadequate supplies, lack of easy-to-use alcohol-based products at the bedside, concern about skin irritation, and inadequate knowledge, including the mistaken belief that the use of gloves obviates the need for handwashing. Ongoing education of staff regarding practices that are likely to reduce nosocomial infections and active surveillance of infection rates are important components of nosocomial infection control.

Neonatal immunization, commonly used in the USA to protect the newborn against hepatitis B infection and in other countries to protect against TB, is a promising strategy for a number of postnatal infections and deserves further study. Neonatal immunization is particularly attractive because the infant's birth hospitalization is the most reliable point of health care contact.

Oral administration of bovine lactoferrin either alone or with a probiotic *(Lactobacillus rhamnosus GG)* for 30 days in LBW infants has been demonstrated to reduce the incidence of late-onset bacterial and fungal sepsis; probiotics have also reduced the incidence of NEC (Chapter 96.2).

BIBLIOGRAPHY

Please visit the Nelson Textbook of Pediatrics *website at* *www.expertconsult.com* *for the complete bibliography.*

PART XIII Adolescent Medicine

Chapter 104 Adolescent Development

See also Part XII and Chapters 555 and 556.

104.1 Adolescent Physical and Social Development

Barbara Cromer

Young people undergo rapid changes in body structure and physiologic, psychological, and social functioning between the ages of approximately 9 to 10 and 20 yr. Adolescence consists of 3 distinct periods—early, middle, and late—each marked by a characteristic set of biologic, psychological, and social issues (Table 104-1). Hormones set this developmental agenda together with social structures designed to foster the transition from childhood to adulthood. Although individual variation is substantial, in both the timing of somatic changes and the quality of the experience, pubertal changes follow a predictable sequence. Gender and subculture profoundly affect the developmental course, as do physical and social stressors.

EARLY ADOLESCENCE

Biologic Development

Adolescence is defined as a period of development; *puberty* is the biologic process in which a child becomes an adult. These changes include appearance of the secondary sexual characteristics, increase to adult size, and development of reproductive capacity. Adrenal production of androgen (chiefly dehydroepiandrosterone sulfate [DHEAS]) may occur as early as 6 yr of age, with development of underarm odor and faint genital hair (adrenarche). Levels of luteinizing hormone (LH) and follicle-stimulating hormone (FSH) rise progressively throughout middle childhood without dramatic effect. Rapid pubertal changes begin with increased sensitivity of the pituitary to gonadotropin-releasing hormone (GnRH); pulsatile release of GnRH, LH, and FSH during sleep; and corresponding increases in gonadal androgens and estrogens. The triggers for these changes are incompletely understood, but may involve ongoing neuronal development throughout middle childhood and adolescence.

Data regarding the timing for the onset of puberty in girls are controversial (Table 104-2). Several studies from 1948 to 1981 identified the average age for the onset of breast development to range from 10.6-11.2 yr of age. Multiple reports since 1997 suggest a significantly earlier onset of breast development, ranging from 8.9-9.5 yr in African-American girls and 10.0-10.4 yr in white girls. There also appears to be a small secular trend toward decreasing ages for the onset of pubic hair development and menarche. The reasons for the larger decrease in age for breast development may include the epidemic of childhood obesity as well as exposure to estrogen-like toxins in the environment that include certain pesticides, plastics, phytoestrogens, and industrial compounds along with beef fattened with subcutaneous estrogen pellets.

It is less clear whether there is also a secular trend for decreasing age for onset of puberty in boys (Table 104-3). It appears that, over the past 40 yr, the average age for the onset of genital and pubic hair development may have decreased by about a year. The onset of puberty in African-American boys precedes that in white boys by at least 6 mo.

Once the onset of puberty has begun, the resulting sequence of somatic and physiologic changes gives rise to the **sexual maturity rating (SMR)**, or **Tanner stages**. Figures 104-1 and 104-2 depict the somatic changes used in the SMR scale; Tables 104-4 and 104-5 also describe these changes. Figures 104-3 and 104-4 depict the typical sequence of pubertal changes in boys and girls, respectively. The range of normal progress through sexual maturation is wide.

In girls, the 1st visible sign of puberty and the hallmark of SMR2 is the appearance of breast buds, between 8 and 12 yr of age. Menses typically begins 2-2½ yr later, during SMR3-4 (median age, 12 yr; normal range, 9-16 yr) (see Fig. 104-4). Less obvious changes include enlargement of the ovaries, uterus, labia, and clitoris, and thickening of the endometrium and vaginal mucosa.

In boys, the 1st visible sign of puberty and the hallmark of SMR2 is testicular enlargement, beginning as early as 9½ yr. This is followed by penile growth during SMR3. Peak growth occurs when testis volumes reach approximately 9-10 cm^3 during SMR4. Under the influence of LH and testosterone, the seminiferous tubules, epididymis, seminal vesicles, and prostate enlarge. The left testis normally is lower than the right. Some degree of breast hypertrophy, typically bilateral, occurs in 40-65% of boys during SMR2-3 due to a relative excess of estrogenic stimulation.

Growth acceleration begins in early adolescence for both sexes, but peak growth velocities are not reached until SMR3-4. Boys typically peak 2-3 yr later than girls, begin this growth at a later SMR stage (Fig. 104-5), and continue their linear growth for approximately 2-3 yr after girls have stopped. The asymmetric growth spurt begins distally, with enlargement of the hands and feet, followed by the arms and legs, and finally, the trunk and chest, giving young adolescents a gawky appearance. Rapid enlargement of the larynx, pharynx, and lungs leads to changes in vocal quality, typically preceded by vocal instability (voice cracking). Elongation of the optic globe often results in nearsightedness. Dental changes include jaw growth, loss of the final deciduous teeth, and eruption of the permanent cuspids, premolars, and finally, molars (Chapter 299). Orthodontic appliances may be needed, secondary to growth exacerbations of bite disturbances.

Cognitive and Moral Development (See Also Chapter 6)

While adolescence has traditionally been described as the time of transition from concrete operational thinking to formal **logical thinking** (abstract thought), other processes include the important but distinct contributions of **reasoning** (cognitive abilities) and **judgment** (the process of thinking through the consequences of alternative decisions or actions). Because these processes may develop at very different rates, young adolescents may be able to apply formal logical thinking to schoolwork, but not to personal dilemmas. When emotional stakes are high, adolescents may regress to more concrete operational and/or magical thinking. This can interfere with higher-order cognition and ultimately affect the ability to perceive long-term outcomes of current decision-making. The development of **moral thinking** roughly but imperfectly parallels cognitive development. Whereas younger children view relationships with adults in terms of power and fear of punishment, preadolescents begin to perceive right and wrong as absolute and unquestionable. During mid-adolescence most adolescents become more multidimensional in their thinking

Table 104-1 CENTRAL ISSUES IN EARLY, MIDDLE, AND LATE ADOLESCENCE

VARIABLE	EARLY ADOLESCENCE	MIDDLE ADOLESCENCE	LATE ADOLESCENCE
Sexual maturity rating*	1-2	3-5	5
Somatic	Secondary sex characteristics Beginning of rapid growth Awkward appearance	Height growth peaks Body shape and composition change Acne and odor Menarche/spermarche	Physically mature Slower growth
Cognitive and moral	Concrete operations Unable to perceive long-term outcome of current decision-making Conventional morality	Emergence of abstract thought (formal operations) May perceive future implications, but may not apply in decision-making Questioning mores	Future-oriented with sense of perspective Idealism; absolutism Able to think things through independently
Self-concept/identity formation	Preoccupied with changing body Self-consciousness about appearance and attractiveness Fantasy and present-oriented	Concern with attractiveness Increasing introspection "Stereotypical adolescent"	More stable body image Attractiveness may still be of concern Emancipation complete Firmer identity
Family	Increased need for privacy Increased bid for independence	Conflicts over control and independence Struggle for acceptance of greater autonomy	Emotional and physical separation from family Increased autonomy
Peers	Seeks same-sex peer affiliation to counter instability	Intense peer group involvement Preoccupation with peer culture Peers provide behavioral example	Peer group and values recede in importance Intimacy/possible commitment takes precedence
Sexual	Increased interest in sexual anatomy Anxieties and questions about genital changes, size Limited dating and intimacy	Testing ability to attract partner Initiation of relationships and sexual activity Questions of sexual orientation	Consolidation of sexual identity Focus on intimacy and formation of stable relationships Planning for future and commitment
Relationship to society	Middle school adjustment	Gauging skills and opportunities	Career decisions (e.g., college, work)

*See text and Figures 104-1 and 104-2.

Table 104-2 REPORTED MEAN AGES ± SD (YEARS) FOR FEMALE SEXUAL MATURATION IN THE UK AND THE USA

	NUMBER OF SUBJECTS (AGE RANGE IN YR)	BREASTS AT TANNER STAGE 2	MENARCHE	PUBIC HAIR AT TANNER STAGE 2
Marshall and Tanner (UK) (1969)	192 (8 up)	11.15 ± 1.10	13.47 ± 1.02	–
Reynolds and Wines (USA) (1948)	49 (8-18)	10.8 ± 1.1	12.9 ± 1.4	11.0 ± 1.1
Nicolson and Hanley (USA) (1953)	252	10.6	12.8	11.6
Lee (USA) (1980)	18 (8.6-17.8)	11.2 ± 1.6	13.3 ± 1.3	11.9 ± 1.5
Billewicz et al (UK) (1981)	788 (9-17)	10.8 ± 1.6	13.4 ± 1.1	
Roche et al (USA) (1995)	67 (9.5-17)	11.2 ± 0.7 8.87 ± 1.93 Whites 9.96 ± 1.82	African-Americans 12.16 ± 1.21 Whites 12.88 ± 1.20	African-Americans 8.78 ± 2.0 Whites 10.51 ± 1.67
Sun et al (USA) (2002)	1215 (8-19)	African-Americans 9.48 Whites 10.38	–	African-Americans 9.43 Whites 10.57
Wu et al (USA) (2002)	1623-1168 (8-16)	African-Americans 9.5 Whites 10.3	African-Americans 12.2 Whites 12.6	African-Americans 9.5 Whites 10.6
Freedman et al (USA) (2002)				
Data collected 1973-1974	1398 (7-16)	–	African-Americans 12.9 Whites 12.7	–
Data collected 1992-1994	1230 (7-16)	–	African-Americans 12.1 Whites 12.5	–
Chumlea et al (USA) (2003)	2510 (8-20)	–	African-Americans 12.06 Whites 12.55	–
Anderson et al (USA) (2003)				
Data collected 1963-1970	3272 (10-15)	–	African-Americans 12.48 Whites 12.8	–
Data collected 1988-1994	1326 (10-15)	–	African-Americans 12.14 Whites 12.60	–

Table 104-3 REPORTED MEAN AGES ± SD (YEARS) FOR MALE SEXUAL MATURATION IN THE UK AND THE USA

	NUMBER OF SUBJECTS (AGE RANGE IN YEARS)	GENITALIA TANNER STAGE 2	PUBIC HAIR TANNER STAGE 2
Marshall and Tanner (UK) (1970)	228	11.64 ± 1.07	(13.44 ± 1.09)
Lee (USA) (1980)	36 (9-17.5)	11.9 ± 1.1	12.3 ± 0.8
Roche et al (USA) (1995)	78 (9.5-17)	11.2 ± 0.7	11.2 ± 0.8
Biro et al. (USA) (1995)	515 (10-15)	12.2	–
Herman-Giddens et al (USA) (2001)	2114 (8-19)	African-Americans 9.5 Whites 10.1	African-Americans 11.2 Whites 12.0
Sun et al (USA) (2002)	500 (8-19)	African-Americans 9.20 Whites 10.03	African-Americans 11.16 Whites 11.98

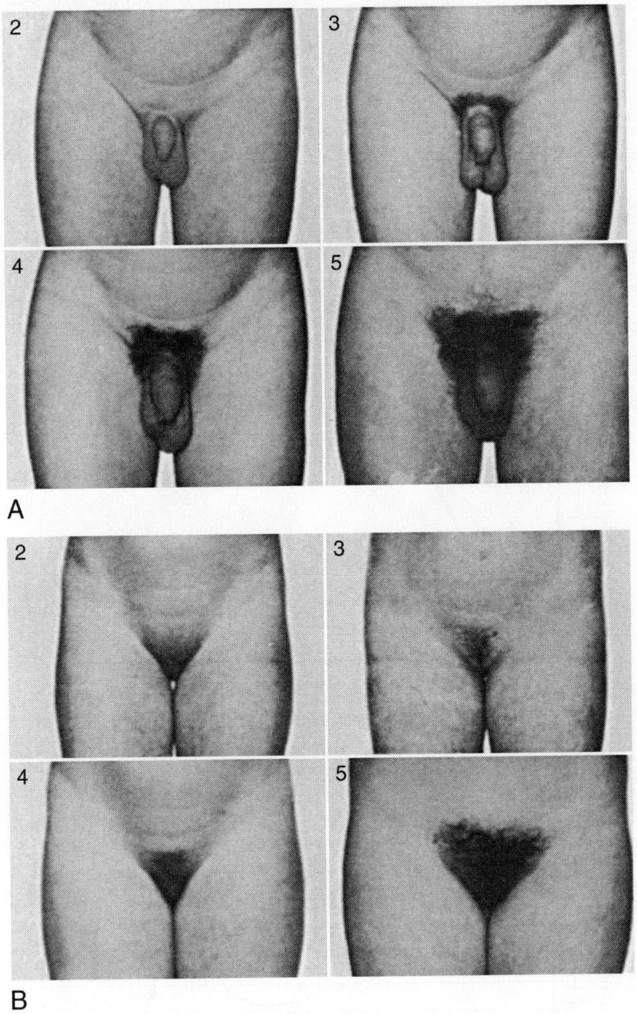

Figure 104-1 Sexual maturity ratings (2 to 5) of pubic hair changes in adolescent boys *(A)* and girls *(B)* (see Tables 104-4 and 104-5). (Courtesy of J.M. Tanner, MD, Institute of Child Health, Department for Growth and Development, University of London, London, England.)

and are better able to contemplate hypothetical situations and the relationship between varied actions or decisions and differing outcomes. Despite their increasing abilities for complex decision-making, adolescent decision-making remains particularly susceptible to emotions.

Neuroimaging has enabled greater insight into changes in developing brains that help explain variations in decision-making capacities. Some theorists argue that the transition from concrete to formal operations follows from quantitative increases in knowledge, experience, and cognitive efficiency rather than from a qualitative reorganization of thinking. Consistent with this view is a steady rise in cognitive processing speed from late childhood through early adulthood, associated with a reduction in synaptic number (pruning of less-used pathways) and continued myelination of neurons. Adolescents also experience the development of the dorsolateral prefrontal cortex and the superior temporal gyrus, areas responsible for higher-order associations, including the ability to inhibit impulses, weigh the consequences of decisions, prioritize, and strategize. It is unclear whether the hormonal changes of puberty directly affect cognitive development. Related to neurobehavioral maturation, adolescents may experience an increased intensity of emotion and/or greater inclination to seek experiences that create such high-intensity emotions. Cognitive development also differs by gender, with girls developing at earlier ages than boys.

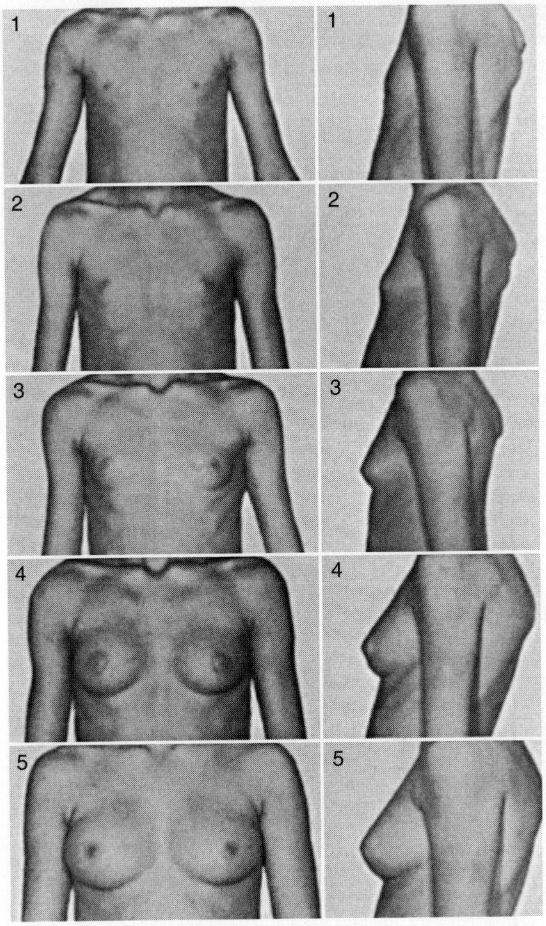

Figure 104-2 Sexual maturity ratings (1 to 5) of breast changes in adolescent girls. (Courtesy of J.M. Tanner, MD, Institute of Child Health, Department for Growth and Development, University of London, London, England.)

Table 104-4 CLASSIFICATION OF SEXUAL MATURITY STATES IN GIRLS

SMR STAGE	PUBIC HAIR	BREASTS
1	Preadolescent	Preadolescent
2	Sparse, lightly pigmented, straight, medial border of labia	Breast and papilla elevated as small mound; diameter of areola increased
3	Darker, beginning to curl, increased amount	Breast and areola enlarged, no contour separation
4	Coarse, curly, abundant, but less than in adult	Areola and papilla form secondary mound
5	Adult feminine triangle, spread to medial surface of thighs	Mature, nipple projects, areola part of general breast contour

SMR, sexual maturity rating.
From Tanner JM: *Growth at adolescence*, ed 2, Oxford, England, 1962, Blackwell Scientific.

Self-Concept

Self-consciousness increases exponentially in response to the somatic transformations of puberty. Self-awareness at this age centers on external characteristics, in contrast to the introspection of later adolescence. It is normal for early adolescents to be preoccupied with their body changes, scrutinize their appearance, and feel that everyone else is staring at them (Elkind's imaginary audience).

The media, with its overrepresentation of sex, violence, and substance use, has a profound influence on cultural norms and an adolescents' sense of identity. Adolescents use, on average, 7 hr

Table 104-5 CLASSIFICATION OF SEX MATURITY STATES IN BOYS

SMR STAGE	PUBIC HAIR	PENIS	TESTES
1	None	Preadolescent	Preadolescent
2	Scanty, long, slightly pigmented	Minimal change/ enlargement	Enlarged scrotum, pink, texture altered
3	Darker, starting to curl, small amount	Lengthens	Larger
4	Resembles adult type, but less quantity; coarse, curly	Larger; glans and breadth increase in size	Larger, scrotum dark
5	Adult distribution, spread to medial surface of thighs	Adult size	Adult size

SMR, sexual maturity rating.
From Tanner JM: *Growth at adolescence*, ed 2, Oxford, England, 1962, Blackwell Scientific.

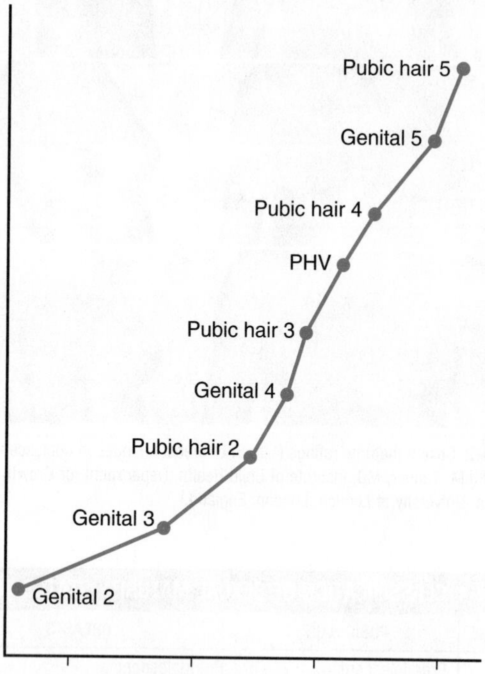

Figure 104-3 Sequence of pubertal events in males. PHV, peak height velocity. (From Root AW: Endocrinology of puberty, *J Pediatr* 83:1, 1973.)

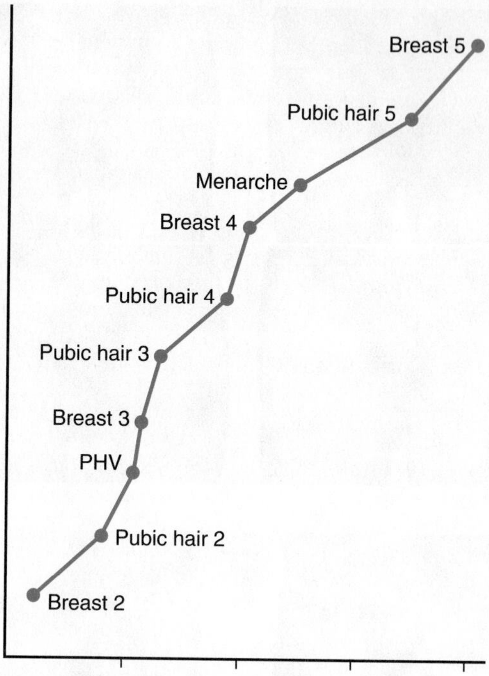

Figure 104-4 Sequence of pubertal events in females. PHV, peak height velocity. (From Root AW: Endocrinology of puberty, *J Pediatr* 83:1, 1973.)

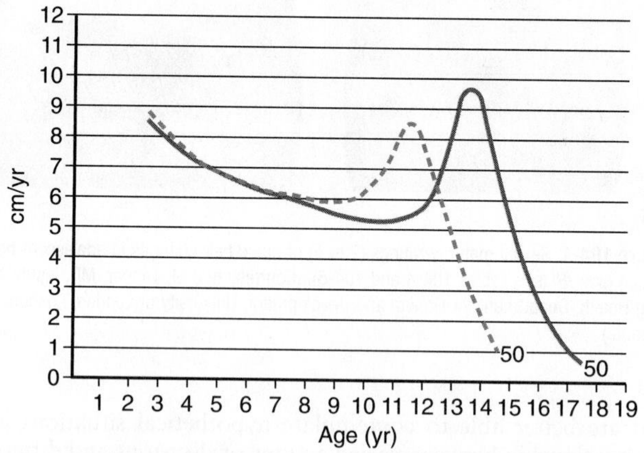

Figure 104-5 Height velocity curves for American boys *(solid line)* and girls *(dashed line)* who have their peak height velocity at the average age (i.e., average growth tempo). (From Tanner JM, Davies PSW: Clinical longitudinal standards for height and height velocity for North American children, *J Pediatr* 107:317, 1985.)

of media per day (e.g., television, Internet). Over half of all high school students have a television in their bedrooms, 70% live in homes with a personal computer, and the proportion with Internet access is approximately 75%. The advent (and ubiquity) of cell phones with texting capability and social networking sites have greatly enhanced communication among adolescents of all ages.

This exposure may cause girls to develop a distorted sense of femininity, and they may be at risk for viewing themselves as overweight, leading to eating disorders and depression (Chapter 26). Similarly, boys may have difficulties with self-image. Images of masculinity may be confusing, leading to self-doubt, insecurity, and misleading conceptions about male behavior. Adolescents who develop earlier than their peers, especially girls, may have higher rates of school difficulty, body dissatisfaction, and depression. These adolescents look like adults and may have adult expectations placed on them, but are not cognitively or psychologically mature.

Relationships with Family, Peers, and Society

In early adolescence, young teens become less interested in parental activities and more interested in the peer group, typically with peers of the same sex. Early adolescents often disregard parents' advice about safety, appearance, etiquette, and overall comportment and display markedly different values, tastes, and interests. Superficial differences may spark conflicts that are truly about power or difficulty accepting separation. Other core individual characteristics, like sexual identity, might become a source of conflict with potentially damaging and long-lasting consequences for the entire family. Adolescents also seek more privacy, which may contribute to family discord.

The trend toward separation from family often involves selecting adults outside of the family as role models and developing close relationships with particular teachers or the parents of other children. Organizations such as scouting or sports teams can also provide an important sense of extrafamilial belonging.

Early adolescents often socialize in same-sex peer groups. Deepening relationships with peers contributes importantly to their gradual individuation and independence from families of origin. Indicative of increasing sexual awareness, teasing directed against the other gender, homophobic comments and acts, and sexually-related gossip are common, albeit inappropriate, means to cope with personal insecurities and seek social approval. Belonging is all important. In one-to-one friendships, boys and girls differ in important ways. Female friendships may center on emotional intimacy, whereas male relationships may focus more on activities.

An early adolescent's relationship to society centers on school. The shift from elementary school to middle school or junior high school entails giving up the protection of a single classroom in exchange for the additional stimulation and responsibility involved in moving from class to class. This change in school structure mirrors and reinforces the changes involved in separating from the family.

Sexuality

Anxiety and interest in sex and sexual anatomy increase during early puberty. It is normal for young adolescents to compare themselves with others. In boys, ejaculation occurs for the 1st time, usually during masturbation and later as nocturnal emissions, and may be a cause of anxiety. Early adolescents sometimes masturbate together; isolated incidents of mutual sexual exploration are not necessarily a sign of homosexuality. The prevalence of other forms of sexual behavior, other than masturbation, varies by culture but generally are less common in early adolescents.

Implications for Pediatricians and Parents

Parents may have concerns that they are hesitant to discuss. Parents can be interviewed separately from the adolescent to avoid undermining the adolescent's trust. When interviewing and examining an adolescent, health care providers should keep in mind that physical maturation correlates with sexual maturity, whereas psychosocial development correlates more closely with chronological age. Early adolescents typically need reassurance that the somatic changes they are experiencing are common and normal.

The pediatrician needs to help parents differentiate between the normal discomforts of the age and truly concerning behaviors. Bids for autonomy, such as avoiding family activities, demanding privacy, and increasing argumentativeness, are normal; extreme withdrawal or antagonism may be dysfunctional. Bewilderment and dysphoria at the start of junior high school are normal; continued failure to adapt several weeks to months later suggests a more serious problem. Risk-taking is limited in early adolescence; escalation of risk-taking behaviors is problematic. Parents must adapt discipline measures to the changing abilities of the adolescent, who can think through problems, assess consequences, and problem solve. Thus, the development of negotiation strategies is critical. Children and adolescents raised by parents who use negotiating as part of child rearing have more positive outcomes than those raised by parents who use more authoritarian or permissive styles.

MIDDLE ADOLESCENCE

Biologic Development

Growth accelerates above the prepubertal rate of 6-7 cm (3 in) per year during middle adolescence. In the average girl, the growth spurt peaks at 11.5 yr at a top velocity of 8.3 cm (3.8 in) per year and then slows to a stop at 16 yr (see Fig. 104-5). In the average boy, the growth spurt starts later, peaks at 13.5 yr at 9.5 cm (4.3 in) per year, and then slows to a stop at 18 yr. Weight gain parallels linear growth, with a delay of several months, so that adolescents seem first to stretch and then to fill out. Muscle mass also increases, followed approximately 6 mo later by an increase in strength; boys show greater gains in both. Lean body mass, approximately 80% in the average prepubertal child, increases to 90% in boys and decreases to 75% in girls as subcutaneous fat accumulates.

Boys with SMR3 pubic hair and SMR4 genitals normally have their peak growth spurts ahead of them; girls at the same SMR are usually past their peaks (see Figs. 104-3 and 104-4). Widening of the shoulders in boys and the hips in girls is also hormonally determined. Other changes include a doubling in heart size and lung vital capacity. Blood pressure, blood volume, and hematocrit rise, particularly in boys. Androgenic stimulation of sebaceous and apocrine glands results in acne and body odor. Physiologic changes in sleep patterns and requirements may be mistaken for laziness; adolescents have difficulty falling asleep and waking up, especially for early school start times as opposed to typical self-regulated or preferred sleep schedules.

Menarche is achieved by 30% of girls by SMR3 and by 90% by SMR4 (95% of girls reach menarche at 10.5-14.5 yr of age). Menarche usually follows approximately 1 yr after the growth spurt begins. It is very common for cycles to be **anovulatory** during the 1st 2 yr after menarche (approximately 50%). The timing of menarche, which is not completely understood, appears to be determined by genetics as well as by factors such as adiposity, chronic illness, nutritional status, type and amount of exercise, and emotional well-being. Before menarche, the uterus achieves a mature configuration, vaginal lubrication increases, and a clear vaginal discharge appears (physiologic leukorrhea). In boys, the phallus lengthens and widens during SMR3, and sperm are usually apparent in semen.

Cognitive and Moral Development

With the transition to formal logical thinking, middle adolescents start to question and analyze extensively. Young people now have the cognitive ability to understand the intricacy of the world they live in, self-reflect, see beyond themselves, and to begin to understand their own actions in a moral and legal context. Questioning of moral conventions fosters the development of personal codes of ethics, which may be similar to or different from those of their parents. An adolescent's new flexibility of thought can have pervasive effects on relationships with the self and others.

Self-Concept

Middle adolescents are more accepting of their own body changes and become preoccupied with idealism in exploring future options. Affiliation with a peer group is an important step in confirming one's identity and self-image. It is normal for middle adolescents to experiment with different personas, changing styles of dress, groups of friends, and interests from month to month. Many philosophize about the meaning of life and wonder, "Who am I?" and "Why am I here?" Intense feelings of inner turmoil and misery are common. Girls may tend to characterize themselves and their peers according to interpersonal relationships ("I am a girl with close friends"), whereas boys may focus on abilities ("I am good at sports"). Adolescents of both genders, but especially boys, who develop later than their peers may experience poorer self-image and have higher rates of difficulty in school.

Relationships with Family, Peers, and Society

Middle adolescence refers to "stereotypical adolescence." Relationships with parents become more strained and distant due to redirected energies toward peer relationships and separation from the family. Dating can become a lightning rod for parent-child battles, in which the real issue may be the separation from parents rather than the particulars of "with whom" or "how late." The majority of teenagers progress through adolescence with minimal difficulties rather than experiencing the stereotypical "storm and stress." It is the minority of adolescents (approximately 20-30%) who *do* experience stress and struggle through this period who require support. Adolescents with visible differences are also at risk for problems, such as not developing adequate social skills and confidence and having more difficulty establishing satisfying relationships.

As part of middle adolescents' exploration of future options, they begin to think seriously about what they want to do as adults, a question that formerly had been comfortably hypothetical. The process involves self-assessment and exploration of available opportunities. The presence or absence of realistic role models, as opposed to the idealized ones of earlier periods, can be crucial.

Sexuality

Dating becomes a normative activity as middle adolescents assess their ability to attract others. The degree of sexual activity and its onset vary widely by race, ethnicity, and nation. In the USA, by age 17 yr about 30% of Asians (females 28%, males 33%), about 50% of whites (58% females, 53% males) and Hispanic females (59%), and about 75% of African-Americans (74% females, 82% males) and Hispanic males (69%) have initiated sex. Among youth in rural Africa the median age of sexual debut was 18.5 yr for women and 19.2 yr for men; age at 1st sexual intercourse among Rwandan youth is 20 yr for both males and females. Gay, lesbian, bisexual, and transgender youth often acknowledge their attractions and sexual identity during this period.

In addition to sexual orientation, middle adolescents begin to sort out other important aspects of sexual identity, including beliefs about love, honesty, and propriety. Relationships at this age are often superficial and emphasize attractiveness and sexual experimentation rather than intimacy. Adolescents tend to follow several characteristic patterns of sexual behavior: abstinence, serial monogamy, or polyamory. Most have some knowledge of the risks of pregnancy, HIV, and other sexually transmitted infections, but knowledge does not consistently control behavior. Many sexually active adolescents use condoms consistently with or without other contraceptives; up to 70% of adolescents used some form of contraception or prophylaxis for sexually transmitted infections (STIs) at their 1st intercourse.

Implications for Pediatricians and Parents

Middle adolescence is a time when the opportunity to talk confidentially with a nonjudgmental, informed adult can be particularly appreciated and helpful in the midst of significant psychologic and biologic change.

Adolescents vary greatly in their rate of physical and social progress and in the resolution of central conflicts about autonomy and self-esteem. Questions about family and peer relationships can help locate a child along the developmental continuum and facilitate individualized counseling. Early- and late-maturing adolescents are at risk for psychologic problems. Anticipatory guidance with parents or guardians and appropriate referral to mental health professionals of these adolescents may be warranted.

In asking about dating and sex, *do not assume heterosexuality*; this approach is sure to preempt further discussion of sexual identity and any associated questions or concerns. Intention to have sex and whether close friends are sexually active are good indications that a youth may be initiating sexual activity shortly. Parental connectedness and close supervision or monitoring of the youth's activities and peer group can be protective against early onset of sexual activity and involvement in other risk-taking behaviors, and can foster positive youth development. Parents should also assume an active role in their adolescent's transition to adulthood to ensure that their child receives appropriate preventive health services.

LATE ADOLESCENCE

Biologic Development

The somatic changes in this period are modest by comparison to earlier periods. The final stages of breast, penile, and pubic hair development occur by 17-18 yr of age in 95% of males and females. Minor changes in hair distribution often continue for several years in males, including the growth of facial and chest hair and the onset of male pattern baldness in a few. Acne occurs in the majority of adolescents, particularly males.

Psychosocial Development

Slowing physical changes permit the emergence of a more stable body image. Cognition tends to be less self-centered, with increasing thoughts about concepts such as justice, patriotism, and history. Older adolescents are more future-oriented and able to act on long-term plans, delay gratification, compromise, set limits, and think independently. Older adolescents are often idealistic but may also be absolutist and intolerant of opposing views. Religious or political groups that promise answers to complex questions may hold great appeal. With impending emancipation, older adolescents begin the transition to adult roles in work and their relationships.

They also have more constancy in their emotions. The peer group and peer values recede in importance. Individual, particularly intimate relationships take precedence, providing an important component of identity for many older adolescents. In contrast to the often superficial dating relationships of middle adolescence, these relationships increasingly involve love and commitment. Career decisions become pressing because an adolescent's self-concept is increasingly bound up in his or her emerging role in society.

Implications for Pediatricians and Parents

Erikson identified the crucial task of adolescence as the establishment of a stable sense of identity, including emotional and physical separation from the family of origin, initiation of intimacy, and realistic planning for economic independence. The relationship changes from one of parent-child to an adult-adult model. In lieu of equal treatment under the law, adolescents who do not identify as heterosexual face structural barriers in transition to adulthood, such as formal exclusion or discrimination in the military service and in many workplaces and faith-based organizations, legislation prohibiting marriage of same-sex partners, and ineligibility for associated legal and financial benefits in health care and insurance, workers' compensation, family medical leave, foster- and adoptive-parenting, and consumer benefits for heterosexual families. When no such barriers exist, lack of progress toward adult autonomy may indicate a need for professional counseling. Adolescents who become parents may have the added difficulty of achieving appropriate developmental milestones prior to assuming adult responsibilities.

BIBLIOGRAPHY

Please visit the Nelson Textbook of Pediatrics *website at www.expertconsult.com for the complete bibliography.*

104.2 Sexual Identity Development

Walter Bockting

TERMS AND DEFINITIONS

Sex and Sexual Identity

Sex is multifaceted and has at least 9 components: chromosomal sex, gonadal sex, fetal hormonal sex (prenatal hormones produced by the gonads), internal morphologic sex (internal genitalia), external morphologic sex (external genitalia), hypothalamic sex (sex of the brain), sex of assignment and rearing, pubertal hormonal sex, and gender identity and role. *Sexual identity* is a self-perceived identification distilled from any or all aspects of sexuality, and has at least 4 components: sex assigned at birth, gender identity, social sex role, and sexual orientation.

Sex Assigned at Birth

A newborn is assigned a sex before (ultrasound) or at the time of birth based on the external genitalia. In case of a *disorder of sex development*, these genitalia may appear ambiguous, and additional components of sex (e.g., chromosomal, gonadal, hormonal sex) are assessed. In consultation with specialists, parents assign the child a sex that they believe is most likely to be consistent with gender identity, which cannot be assessed until later in life (Chapter 582).

Gender Identity, Gender Role, and Social Sex Role

Gender identity refers to a person's basic sense of being a boy/man, girl/woman, or other gender (e.g., transgender). *Gender role* refers to one's role in society, typically either the male or female role. Gender identity needs to be distinguished from *social sex role* (also referred to as gender role behavior), which refers to characteristics in personality, appearance, and behavior that are, in a given culture and time, considered masculine or feminine. Gender role is about one's presentation as a boy/man or girl/woman, whereas social sex role is about the masculine and/or feminine characteristics one exhibits in a given gender role. Both boys/men, girls/women, and transgender persons can be masculine and/or feminine to varying degrees; gender identity and social sex role are not necessarily congruent. A child or adolescent might be *gender role nonconforming*, that is, a predominantly feminine boy or a predominantly masculine girl.

Sexual Orientation and Behavior

Sexual orientation refers to attractions, behaviors, fantasies, and emotional attachments toward men, women, or both. *Sexual behavior* refers to any sensual activity to pleasure oneself or another person sexually.

Gender Variant and Transgender

Gender variant refers to any gender identity or role that varies from what is typically associated with one's sex assigned at birth. Sometimes the term *gender variant identity* is used to refer to variation in gender identity and in that case is synonymous with transgender. *Transgender* people are a diverse group of individuals who cross or transcend culturally defined categories of gender. They include *transsexuals* (who typically live in the cross-gender role and seek hormonal and/or surgical interventions to modify primary or secondary sex characteristics); *cross-dressers* or *transvestites* (who wear clothing and adopt behaviors associated with the other sex for emotional or sexual gratification and may spend part of the time in the cross-gender role); *drag queens* and *kings* (female and male impersonators); and individuals identifying as *bigender* (both man and woman) or *gender queer* (gender variant). Transgender individuals may be attracted to men, women, or other transgender persons.

FACTORS THAT INFLUENCE SEXUAL IDENTITY DEVELOPMENT

During prenatal sexual development, a gene located on the Y chromosome (*XRY*) induces the development of testes. The hormones produced by the testes direct sexual differentiation in the male direction resulting in the development of male internal and external genitalia. In the absence of this gene in XX chromosomal females, ovaries develop and sexual differentiation proceeds in the female direction resulting in female internal and external genitalia. These hormones may also play a role in sexual differentiation of the brain. In disorders of sex development, chromosomal and prenatal hormonal sex varies from this typical developmental pattern and may result in ambiguous genitalia at birth (Chapter 582).

Gender identity develops early in life and is typically fixed by 2-3 yr of age. Children first learn to identify their own and others' sex (*gender labeling*), then learn that gender is stable over time (*gender constancy*), and finally learn that gender is permanent (*gender consistency*). What determines gender identity remains largely unknown, but it is thought to be an interaction of biologic, environmental, and sociocultural factors.

Some evidence has been found for the impact of biologic and environmental factors on social sex role and gender role behavior, while their impact on gender identity remains less clear. Animal research has shown the influence of prenatal hormones on sexual differentiation of the brain. In humans, prenatal exposure to unusually high levels of androgens in girls with congenital adrenal hyperplasia (CAH) has been associated with more masculine gender role behavior, gender variant identity, and same-sex sexual orientation, but cannot account for all of the variance found (Chapter 570). Research on environmental factors has focused on the influence of sex-typed socialization. Social sex role stereotypes develop early in life. Until later in adolescence, boys and girls are typically socially segregated by gender, reinforcing sex-typed characteristics such as boys' focus on rough-and-tumble play and asserting dominance, and girls focus on verbal communication and creating relationships. Parents, other adults, teachers, peers, and the media serve as gender socializing role models and agents by treating boys and girls differently.

For information on the development of sexual orientation, see Chapter 104.3.

GENDER VARIANCE/GENDER ROLE NONCONFORMITY AMONG CHILDREN AND ADOLESCENTS

Prevalence

Gender variance and gender role nonconformity need to be distinguished from a gender variant or transgender identity. The former operate on the level of social sex role, whereas the latter is about variation in core gender identity. Gender role nonconformity is more common among girls (7%) than boys (5%), but boys are referred more often than girls for concerns regarding gender identity and role. This is likely due to parents, teachers, and peers being less tolerant of gender variant behaviors in boys than in girls.

Gender variance as part of exploring one's gender identity and role is part of normal sexual development. Gender variance in childhood may or may not persist into adolescence. Marked gender variance in adolescence often persists into adulthood. Only a minority of gender variant children develop an adult transgender identity; most develop a gay or lesbian identity and some, a heterosexual identity.

Etiology of Gender Variant Behavior

Prenatal hormones play a role in the development of gender role nonconformity, but cannot completely account for all of the variance. In addition, a heritable component of gender variant behavior exists, but twin studies indicate that genetic factors do not account for all of the variance. Family of origin factors hypothesized to play a role in the development of gender variance lack empirical support. Maternal psychopathology and emotional absence of the father are the only factors shown to be associated with gender variance, yet it is unclear whether these factors are cause or effect.

Stigma, Stigma Management, and Advocacy

Children with gender variance are subject to ostracism from peers, which may negatively impact their psychosocial adjustment and lead to social isolation, loneliness, low self esteem, and behavioral problems. To assist children and families, individual stigma management strategies as well as interventions to change the environment can be offered. Stigma management might involve consultation with a health professional to provide support and education, normalizing the gender variant behavior and encouraging the child and family to build on the child's strengths and interests to foster self esteem. It might also involve making choices about certain preferences (e.g., a boy who likes to wear head bands) to limit these to times and environments that are more accepting. Most health professionals agree that too much focus on curtailing gender variant behavior leads to increased shame and undermines the child's self esteem.

The health professional and family can also assist the child or adolescent to find others with similar interests (within and beyond the gender related interests) to strengthen positive peer support. Equally important are interventions in school and society to raise awareness and promote accepting and positive attitudes, take a stand against bullying and abuse, and implement anti-bullying policies and initiatives. Gay, lesbian, bisexual, transgender, and straight alliance groups are helpful in providing a haven for gender variant youth as well as recognizing them as part of diversity to be respected and embraced within the school system.

GENDER VARIANT IDENTITY/TRANSGENDER CHILDREN AND ADOLESCENTS

Prevalence

About 1.3% of parents of 4-5 yr old boys report that their son wished to be of the opposite sex, and 0% for 12-13 yr olds; for girls these percentages are 5% for 4-5 yr olds and 2.7% for 12-13 yr olds.

Boys are referred by caregivers more often than girls for concerns regarding gender identity. Only a minority of children's gender identity concerns persist into adolescence (20% in 1 study of boys). Persistence of gender identity concerns from adolescence into adulthood is higher; the majority identify as transgender in adulthood and may pursue sex reassignment. On the basis of adults enrolled in a national sex reassignment program in the Netherlands, the prevalence of adult transsexualism is estimated at 1:11,900 for male-to-females and 1:30,400 for female-to-males.

Etiology of a Gender Variant Identity

The etiology of a gender variant or transgender identity remains unknown. Factors hypothesized to play a role in the development of a gender variant identity include environmental and biologic factors. Gender variant children seem to have more trouble than other children with basic cognitive concepts concerning their gender. They may experience emotional distance from their father. Whether these factors are cause or effect remains unclear. Another hypothesis that has been examined is that boys with a gender variant identity are more physically attractive and hence solicit a different response from parental identification figures.

There may be an influence of prenatal and perinatal hormones on sexual differentiation of the brain. Some girls with CAH develop a male gender identity, yet most do not. The size of the sex-dimorphic central part of the red nucleus of the stria terminalis (BSTc) in the hypothalamus of male-to-female transsexuals is smaller than in males and within the range of nontranssexual women; the opposite is true for a female-to-male transsexuals. This structure is regulated by hormones in animals, but in humans no evidence yet exists of a direct relationship between prenatal and perinatal hormones and the sexually dimorphic nature of this nucleus.

Clinical Presentation

Children with a gender variant identity may experience 2 sources of stress: distress inherent to the incongruence between sex assigned at birth and gender identity (gender dysphoria) or distress associated with social stigma. The 1st source of distress is reflected in discomfort with the developing primary and secondary sex characteristics and the gender role assigned at birth. The 2nd source of distress relates to feeling different, not fitting in, peer ostracism, and social isolation, and may result in shame, low self-esteem, anxiety, or depression.

Boys with a gender variant identity may at an early age identify as a girl, expect to grow up female, or express the wish to do so. They may experience distress about being a boy and/or having a male body, prefer to urinate in a sitting position, and express a specific dislike of their male genitals and even want to cut off their genitals. They may dress up in girls' clothes as part of playing dress up or in private. Girls may identify as a boy, expect or wish to grow up male. They may experience distress about being a girl and/or having a female body, pretend to have a penis, or expect to grow one. Girls may express a dislike of feminine clothing and hairstyles. In early childhood, children may spontaneously express these concerns, yet depending on the response of the environment, these feelings may go "underground" and be kept more private. The distress may intensify by the onset of puberty; the physical changes of puberty are described by many transsexual adolescents and adults as traumatic.

Children and adolescents with a gender variant identity may struggle with a number of general behavior problems. Both boys and girls have a predominance of internalizing (anxious and depressed) as opposed to externalizing behavioral difficulties. Compared to controls, gender variant boys are more prone to anxiety, have more negative emotions and a higher stress response, and are rated lower in self-worth, social competence, and psychologic well-being. Gender variant children have more peer relationship difficulties than controls. Both femininity in boys and masculinity in girls are socially stigmatized, although the former seems to carry a higher level of stigma. Boys have been shown to be teased more than girls; teasing for boys increases with age. Poor peer relations is the strongest predictor of behavior problems in both boys and girls who are gender variant.

Gender variant adolescents may struggle with a number of adjustment problems as a result of social stigma and lack of access to transgender-specific health care. Gender variant youth, especially those of color, are vulnerable to verbal and physical abuse, academic difficulties, school dropout, illicit hormone and silicone use, substance use, difficulty finding employment, homelessness, sex work, forced sex, incarceration, HIV/STIs, and suicide. Parental support can buffer against psychologic distress, yet many parents still react negatively to their child's gender variance, although mothers tend to be more supportive than fathers.

The Diagnosis of Gender Identity Disorder: Criteria and Critique

Gender identity disorder is classified as a mental disorder in the *Diagnostic and Statistical Manual of Mental Disorders* (DSM) and *International Classification of Diseases,* which, particularly for children, is controversial. Diagnostic criteria conflate gender variant identity with gender variant behavior. A child could receive the DSM diagnosis without having indicated "a repeated stated desire to be or insistence that he or she is, the other sex," because only 4 of the 5 A category criteria need to be met (Table 104-6). Critics have argued that the distress children experience is mainly the result of social stigma rather than "a manifestation of a behavioral, psychological, or biological dysfunction in the individual" and hence would not meet the definition of a mental disorder. Critics have also expressed concern about children with normal variation in gender role being labeled with a mental disorder perpetuating social stigma, yet there is a tendency of clinicians to underdiagnose rather than overdiagnose children whose gender variance goes beyond behavior and who report gender dysphoria. These children could potentially benefit from the diagnosis to receive early treatment in the form of support, education, advocacy, and, in case of persistent and severe gender dysphoria, puberty-delaying hormone therapy as a reversible precursor to feminizing or masculinizing hormone therapy.

Transgender Identity Development

A stage model of "coming out" might be helpful to understand the experience and potential challenges transgender youth might face. In the *pre–coming out* stage, the individual is aware that their gender identity is different from that of most boys and girls.

Table 104-6 SUMMARY OF DSM IV DIAGNOSTIC CRITERIA FOR GENDER IDENTITY DISORDER (AMERICAN PSYCHIATRIC ASSOCIATION, 2000)

A. STRONG AND PERSISTENT CROSS-GENDER IDENTIFICATION				
In children (302.6), manifested by four (or more) of the following:				
1. Repeatedly stated desire to be, or insistence that he or she is, the other sex	2. In boys, preference for cross-dressing or simulating female attire; in girls, insistence on wearing only stereotypical masculine clothing	3. Strong and persistent preferences for cross-sex roles in make-believe play or persistent fantasies of being the other sex	4. Intense desire to participate in the stereotypical games and pastimes of the other sex	5. Strong preference for playmates of the other sex
In adolescents and adults (302.85), manifested by symptoms such as:				
A stated desire to be the other sex	Frequent passing as the other sex	Desire to live or be treated as the other sex	The conviction that he or she has the typical feelings and reactions of the other sex	
B. PERSISTENT DISCOMFORT WITH HIS OR HER SEX OR SENSE OF INAPPROPRIATENESS IN THE GENDER ROLE OF THAT SEX				
In children (302.6), manifested by any of the following:				
In boys, assertion that his penis or testes are disgusting or will disappear, or assertion that it would be better not to have a penis	In boys, aversion toward rough-and-tumble play and rejection of male stereotypical toys, games, and activities	In girls, rejection of urinating in a sitting position	In girls, assertion that she has or will grow a penis, or assertion that she does not want to grow breasts or menstruate	In girls, marked aversion toward normative feminine clothing
In adolescents and adults (302.85), manifested by symptoms such as:				
Preoccupation with getting rid of primary and secondary sex characteristics	Belief that he or she was born the wrong sex			
C. THE DISTURBANCE IS NOT CONCURRENT WITH A PHYSICAL INTERSEX CONDITION (IN THAT CASE, USE 302.6, GENDER IDENTITY NOT OTHERWISE SPECIFIED)				
D. THE DISTURBANCE CAUSES CLINICALLY SIGNIFICANT DISTRESS OR IMPAIRMENT IN SOCIAL, OCCUPATIONAL, OR OTHER IMPORTANT AREAS OF FUNCTIONING				

In addition to a gender identity that varies from sex assigned at birth, some of these children are also gender role nonconforming while others are not. Those who are also gender role nonconforming cannot hide their transgender identity, are noticed for who they are, and may face teasing, ridicule, abuse, and rejection. They must learn to cope with these challenges at an early age and usually proceed quickly to the next stage of *coming out*. Children who are not visibly gender role nonconforming are able to avoid stigma and rejection by hiding their transgender feelings. They often experience a split between their gender identity cherished in private and expressed in a fantasy world, and a "false self" presented outwardly to fit in and meet gendered expectations. These individuals often times proceed to coming out later in life.

Coming out involves acknowledging one's transgender identity to self and others (parents, other caregivers, trusted health providers, peers). An open and accepting attitude is essential; rejection can perpetuate stigma and its negative emotional consequences. By accessing transgender community resources, including peer support (either online or offline), the transgender youth can then proceed to the *exploration* stage. This is a time of learning as much as possible about being transgender, getting to know similar others, and experimenting with various options for gender expression. Changes in gender role are carefully considered, as are medical interventions to masculinize or feminize the body to alleviate dysphoria. Successful resolution of this stage is a sense of pride in being transgender and comfort with gender role.

Once gender dysphoria has been alleviated, the individual can proceed with other human development tasks, including dating and relationships in the *intimacy* stage. As a result of social stigma and rejection, transgender individuals may struggle with feeling unlovable. Sexual development has often been compromised by gender and genital dysphoria. Now that greater comfort has been achieved with gender identity and role, dating and sexual intimacy have a greater chance of succeeding. Finally, in the *integration* stage, transgender is no longer the most important signifier of identity but one of several important parts of overall identity.

Interventions and Treatment

Health providers can assist gender variant children, adolescents, and their families by directing them to resources and by helping them to make informed decisions about changes in gender role and the available medical interventions to reduce intense and persistent gender dysphoria. To alleviate socially induced distress, interventions focus on stigma management and stigma reduction. It might be in the child's best interest to set reasonable limits on gender variant expression contributing to teasing and ridicule. The main goal of these interventions is not to change the child's gender variant behavior but to assist families, schools, and the wider community to create a supportive environment in which the child can thrive and safely explore his or her gender identity and expression. Decisions to change gender roles, particularly in school, are not to be taken lightly and are best carefully anticipated and planned in consultation with parents, child, teachers, school counselor, and other providers involved in the adolescent's care. Medical interventions are available as early as Tanner Stage 2. Such treatment is guided by the Standards of Care set forth by the World Professional Association for Transgender Health. Although some controversy still exists about the appropriateness of early medical intervention, follow up studies of adolescents treated in accordance with these guidelines show it to be effective in alleviating intense and persistent gender dysphoria. Care needs to be taken not to foreclose the child's exploration of identity.

Pediatricians who encounter transgender youth in their practice should be careful not to make assumptions about gender and sexual identity, but rather ask youth how they would describe themselves. This includes asking if they like being a boy or girl, have ever questioned this, or wished they were born the other sex; have a preferred nickname or pronoun (he or she; if not sure, avoid pronouns); and how they feel about their maturing body and sex characteristics, and what they would change about that if they could. Extra caution should be exercised during physical and genital exams because transgender youth may be particularly uncomfortable with their anatomy. When considering contraceptive options for female-to-males, alternatives to feminizing agents should be explored. For transgender-specific medical interventions, transgender youth should be referred to specialists in the treatment of gender dysphoria (see World Professional Association for Transgender Health, *www.wpath.org*). For other health concerns, ensure referral to transgender or gay, lesbian, bisexual, transgendered (GLBT) friendly providers, especially in the case of gender segregated treatment facilities. Advocates for Youth (*www.advocatesforyouth.org*) and Parents, Families and Friends of Lesbians and Gays (*www.pflag.org*) offer excellent support resources for transgender youth and their families.

BIBLIOGRAPHY

Please visit the Nelson Textbook of Pediatrics *website at* *www.expertconsult.com* *for the complete bibliography.*

104.3 Adolescent Homosexuality

Gary Remafedi

Sexual orientation is a persistent pattern of physical and/or emotional attraction to members of the same or the opposite sex. It encompasses different aspects of sexuality, including sexual fantasy, emotional attraction, sexual behavior, self-identification, and cultural affiliation. The heterosexual or homosexual direction of these different dimensions may be inconsistent, defying the simple categorization of individuals as heterosexual, homosexual, or bisexual. Sexual orientation can be viewed as a continuum between absolute heterosexuality and homosexuality. *Homosexuality* refers to a persistent pattern of same-sex arousal, accompanied by weak or absent heterosexual arousal; and *bisexuality* refers to attractions for both genders. Most homosexual people refer to themselves as *gay* men and *lesbian* women; and many young people refer to themselves as "queer," "curious," and "questioning." *Homosexual* refers to both males and females, whereas the term *gay* applies specifically to men and *lesbian* to women.

Epidemiology

Homosexuality has existed in all societies and cultures and in all times. Prevalence estimates vary according to the time, place, and definitions. Many youths begin adolescence unsure of their sexual orientation, but uncertainty generally resolves with advancing age and sexual experience. In a large state-wide sample of public high school students in the USA, reported homosexual attractions (4.5%) exceeded fantasies, the latter being more common in girls (3.1%) than in boys (2.2%). Overall, 1.1% of students described themselves as predominantly homosexual or bisexual. The prevalence of reported homosexual experiences remained constant (0.9%) among girls, but increased from 0.4-2.8% in boys between the ages of 12 and 18 yr. Only about 30% of the teens reporting homosexual experiences or fantasies identified themselves as homosexual or bisexual.

Etiology

Males and females develop and experience sexual orientation in very different ways. Biology influences sexual orientation development to some degree and possibly affects males and females differently. Factors yet to be identified might organize and activate key areas of the brain early in life to shape sexual response. Neuroanatomic, neurophysiologic, and functional differences (e.g., left-handedness) related to sexual orientation in men and in women point to centrally mediated biologic effects.

Yet, the underlying activating mechanism puzzles scientists. Having a greater number of older brothers, the "fraternal birth order effect," is a robust correlate of homosexuality in males (but not females). In females, the apparent association between homosexuality and in utero exposure to androgens implicates hormones. The relative concordance of homosexuality in monozygotic twins, as compared to dizygotic and non-twin sibships, highlights the role of genetic make-up, especially in males. A candidate gene for an X-linked type of male homosexuality is under investigation.

Also uncertain are the ways biology might interact with environment and experience in shaping sexual identity. Hypothetically, environment modulates the expression of one's fundamental biologic predisposition by influencing social norms and the visibility of homosexual people. There are no differences in the familial and social backgrounds of homosexual and heterosexual men and women, nor is there evidence that homosexuality is related to abnormal parenting, sexual abuse, or other traumatic events.

Development of a Homosexual Identity

The timing and tempo of sexual orientation development varies among individuals based on demographic, cultural, social, historical, and maturational factors. The process typically unfolds with an initial awareness of same-sex attractions as early as the 1st decade in life, followed by sexual orientation identification, sexual debut, and possibly disclosure to others during adolescence and young adulthood. Sexual attractions might be the earliest and best indicator of ultimate sexual identity.

Awareness of attractions is a well-recognized and necessary precursor of disclosure; but self-identification can precede sexual behavior, and vice versa. The developmental process seldom is direct and easy. Misinformation and stigma can lead to significant inner turmoil and anxiety. Volitional disclosure usually starts with telling close friends before parents, and with mothers before fathers; but disclosure can happen unwittingly or prematurely, creating considerable distress. Successful resolution of the developmental process, characterized by personal acceptance and healthy intimate relationships, depends on many factors, such as maturity, access to accurate information, positive role models, and social support. Many adolescents reach adulthood without event, whereas others have a much more challenging transition.

IMPLICATIONS FOR HEALTH

Homophobia

The psychosocial problems among gay and lesbian youths are best understood in the context of homophobia. *Homophobia* is an irrational fear, hatred, or otherwise distorted perception of homosexuality that can manifest in personal discomfort, stereotypes, prejudice, and violence. At a time in life when peers play a critical role in healthy personal and social development, isolation and stigma can be highly traumatic. Compared with classmates, homosexual students are more likely to fear for their safety and to be attacked and injured. With repeated exposure, homosexual youths might internalize negative stereotypes and engage in self-defeating behaviors.

Social Issues

Academic underachievement, truancy, and dropping out are common consequences of abuse and violence at school. Some parents are unable to adopt a supportive attitude, and a substantial number of homosexual children run away or are evicted. Homosexual young people are overrepresented in homeless and runaway populations across the USA. Life on the streets exposes them to drugs and sexual abuse and promotes illegal conduct for survival.

Mental Health Issues

Substance abuse, anxiety, depression, suicide attempts, and disordered eating behaviors are prevalent. Compared with heterosexual peers, homosexual youths initiate tobacco use at younger ages and are more likely to smoke regularly. A study of 13-21 yr old gay and bisexual male adolescents found that 24.5% of participants reported frequent (>40 times/yr) use of alcohol; 8.4%, cannabis; and 2.4%, cocaine or crack. More than 4% had used intravenous drugs in the last year alone. Methamphetamine and other "club" drug use may be fueling the spread of HIV infection.

Rates of attempted suicide among homosexual youths, especially males, are consistently higher than expected in the general population of adolescents, ranging from 20-42%. Identified risk factors include gender nonconformity, early awareness of homosexuality, gay-related stress, victimization by violence, lack of social support, school drop-out, family problems, suicide attempts by friends or relatives, and homelessness.

Data on disordered eating behavior are sparse and conflicting. As compared to young heterosexuals of the same sex, lesbians generally have better body image and are more likely to be overweight, while young gay men have worse body image and are more likely to restrict eating and/or engage in compensatory weight loss strategies.

Medical Threats to Health

Homosexual adolescents generally have the same medical concerns as heterosexual youths. Risky sexual behaviors, not sexual orientation, endanger health. The most common and serious sexually-related conditions arise from unprotected anal intercourse. The epithelial surfaces of the fragile rectal mucosa can be easily damaged during sex, facilitating the transmission of pathogens. Rectal intercourse has been shown to be the most efficient route of infection by hepatitis B (Chapter 350), cytomegalovirus (Chapter 247), and HIV (Chapter 268). Oral-anal or digital-anal contact can transmit enteric pathogens, such as the hepatitis A virus. Unprotected oral sex also can lead to oropharyngeal disease in the receptive partner and gonococcal and non-gonococcal urethritis for the insertive partner. Certain STIs, particularly ulcerative diseases, such as syphilis and herpes simplex virus infection, facilitate the spread of HIV.

Among U.S. adolescents and young adults, young men who have sex with men (YMSM) continue to have the greatest toll of HIV/AIDS for various reasons, including misinformation, noncommunication with partners about risk reduction, potentially false assumptions about partners' serostatus, substance use, and impaired reasoning and judgment. Although possible, female-to-female sexual transmission of HIV is inefficient, and women who only engage in same-sex behavior are less likely than other youths to acquire a STI.

RECOMMENDATIONS FOR CARE

The American Academy of Pediatrics recognizes physicians' responsibility to provide comprehensive, nonjudgmental health care and guidance to gay and lesbian adolescents and to others who are struggling with sexual orientation issues. The goal of care for homosexual adolescents is promoting normal adolescent development, social and emotional well-being, and physical health.

Clinicians who are unable to offer nonjudgmental care and information should refer patients to better resources. Placed in a waiting area, written material about sexual orientation, support groups, and community resources signal that the staff is open to discussing sexuality. Use of well-designed comprehensive health history forms, like the American Medical Association's Guidelines for Adolescent Prevention Services Questionnaire, can trigger conversation about sexual identity and related issues. Privacy, confidentiality, sensitivity, and patience are the cornerstones of effective communication.

Evaluation

Providers should be aware of potential threats to the medical and psychosocial health of homosexual teenagers and screen for them appropriately. Classifying an adolescent's sexual orientation seldom is necessary, but a thoughtful assessment of emotional, social, and physical health can uncover risks and direct further evaluation and treatment. Questions in the sexual history should avoid heterosexual assumptions, asking instead about the direction of romantic interests and partners. With some exceptions noted below, the physical examination and laboratory evaluation of homosexual adolescents are the same as for any teenagers.

Prevention, Treatment, and Referrals

Special emphasis should be placed on education and counseling to prevent the spread of HIV and STIs through safer sexual behavior, including limiting the numbers of sexual partners, avoiding anal intercourse, staying sober in sexual situations, and consistently using condoms. Young men who meet sexual partners online, as opposed to face-to-face, may have more partners; but they do not necessarily have riskier sex. The use of dental dams, cut open latex condoms, or plastic wrap during oral sex, and the use of latex condoms for sexual appliances are recommended for lesbians. Given the fact that some homosexual adolescents engage in sex with the opposite sex, pregnancy prevention should be addressed.

According to the Centers for Disease Control and Prevention (CDC), vaccination against hepatitis A and B is recommended for all men who have sex with men (MSM) in whom previous infection or immunization cannot be documented. Preimmunization serologic testing can reduce the cost of vaccinating MSM who are already immune to these infections but should not delay vaccination. The CDC recommends that sexually active MSM, regardless of condom use history, obtain the following tests at least annually:

- HIV serology, if prior status is negative or unknown
- Syphilis serology
- A test for urethral infection with *Neisseria gonorrhoeae* and *Chlamydia trachomatis* for men who have had insertive intercourse
- A culture or another approved test for rectal infection with *N. gonorrhoeae* and *C. trachomatis* for men who have had receptive anal intercourse
- A culture or another approved test for pharyngeal infection with *N. gonorrhoeae* in men who have had receptive oral sex; testing for *C. trachomatis* pharyngeal infection is not recommended.

In addition, though firm recommendations are pending, some specialists routinely obtain type-specific serologic tests for herpes simplex virus-2 and vaccinate gay adolescents and other young MSM with Gardasil preventatively. For treatment of STIs, see Chapter 114. Complicated STIs and HIV infection warrant referral to medical subspecialists.

Many minor psychosocial problems can be handled by referral to social support groups, sometimes known as gay–straight alliances. In some localities, specialized social service agencies can help with social, educational, vocational, housing, and other unmet needs. Adolescents with serious psychiatric symptoms, such as suicidal ideation, depression, and chemical dependency, should be referred to mental health specialists with experience treating homosexual adolescents. Individual or family therapy might be indicated for personal, family, or environmental adjustment difficulties. Not only is it ineffective, so-called reparative therapy aiming to change sexual orientation is contraindicated because of its potential to heighten guilt and anxiety.

Well-informed professionals can help adolescents and their parents to explore their feelings and learn about topics related to homosexuality and its etiology, psychologic normalcy, spiritual and cultural implications, disclosure to a significant other, preventive care, and community resources. With appropriate support from families, school, and communities, homosexual youths have the same potential as others to lead happy, healthy, and productive lives.

BIBLIOGRAPHY

Please visit the Nelson Textbook of Pediatrics *website at www.expertconsult.com for the complete bibliography.*

Chapter 105
The Epidemiology of Adolescent Health Problems

Gale R. Burstein

Circumstances impacting adolescent lives vary across the globe. In countries at war, adolescents may be serving as soldiers. In countries deeply affected by AIDS, youth may be at the demographic epicenter of the epidemic and/or assuming the role as primary provider for younger siblings in the aftermath of parent death. In low income nations, youth may be laboring long hours in rural fields near their homes or in distant cities as urban migrants, while in middle and high income nations, they are more likely to be in school. Health promoting behaviors also vary; among youth ages 11, 13, and 15 yr from 29 countries, 54% of U.S. females and 74% of U.S. males exercise on 2 or more occasions per week. Among the remaining 28 countries, rates of exercise twice a week for males range from 90% in Northern Ireland to 60% in Greenland, and for females, rates range from 66% in Germany and the Czech Republic to a low of 37% in Greenland. Among females in all 29 countries, there is a decline in this proportion with age; this trend is not seen among males.

Health outcomes also vary. About 16 million women aged 15-19 yr old give birth annually, accounting for 10% of births worldwide. The average adolescent birthrate in low-income countries is 5-fold that of high-income countries. Complications from pregnancy and childbirth are the leading cause of death among adolescents in developing countries; death as an outcome of pregnancy is rare in developed countries. Perceptions of feeling healthy also vary greatly by country as shown in Figure 105-1; those who do not feel healthy increases proportionately with age.

Despite these variations by geographic region and level of economic development, there are many similarities in adolescent health issues. In all nations, adolescence is a time of immense biologic, psychologic, and social change (Chapter 104). Many of the psychologic changes have a biologic substrate in the development and eventual maturation of the central nervous system, particularly the frontal lobe areas responsible for executive functioning (Fig. 105-2). In addition to cognitive development, there are both risk and protective factors for adverse adolescent health behaviors that are dependent on the social environment as well as the mental health of an adolescent (Table 105-1).

Geographic similarities are reflected in many adolescent health outcomes. Suicide is the 3rd leading cause of death among adolescents worldwide. In the USA, an estimated 13.8% of high school students seriously considered attempting suicide, and 6.3% had actually attempted suicide in the previous 12 mo. Experimentation with new behaviors leads to an increase in risky behaviors among adolescents in the USA (Fig. 105-3) and globally. The Global Youth Tobacco Survey, initiated by the World Health Organization (WHO) in 1999, reveals that tobacco use is a major problem among adolescents ages 13-15 yr in all 6 regions of the globe (Africa, Americas, Eastern Mediterranean, Europe, Southeast Asia, and Western Pacific), averaging 17% globally, with a low of 11% in the Western Pacific region and a high of 22% in the Americas. Alcohol and illicit drugs are a major cause of concern in high-income countries and have also been estimated by the WHO to contribute 4% of the disease burden in adolescents and young adults in low- and middle-income countries. Adolescents and young adults worldwide have high rates of most common sexually transmitted infections in their countries. Persons in this age group in the USA have been estimated to account for nearly half of all incidents of sexually transmitted infections, although they represent only 25% of the sexually active population. A study of 9 developed countries revealed a similar pattern in many of the nations: >50% of cases of syphilis

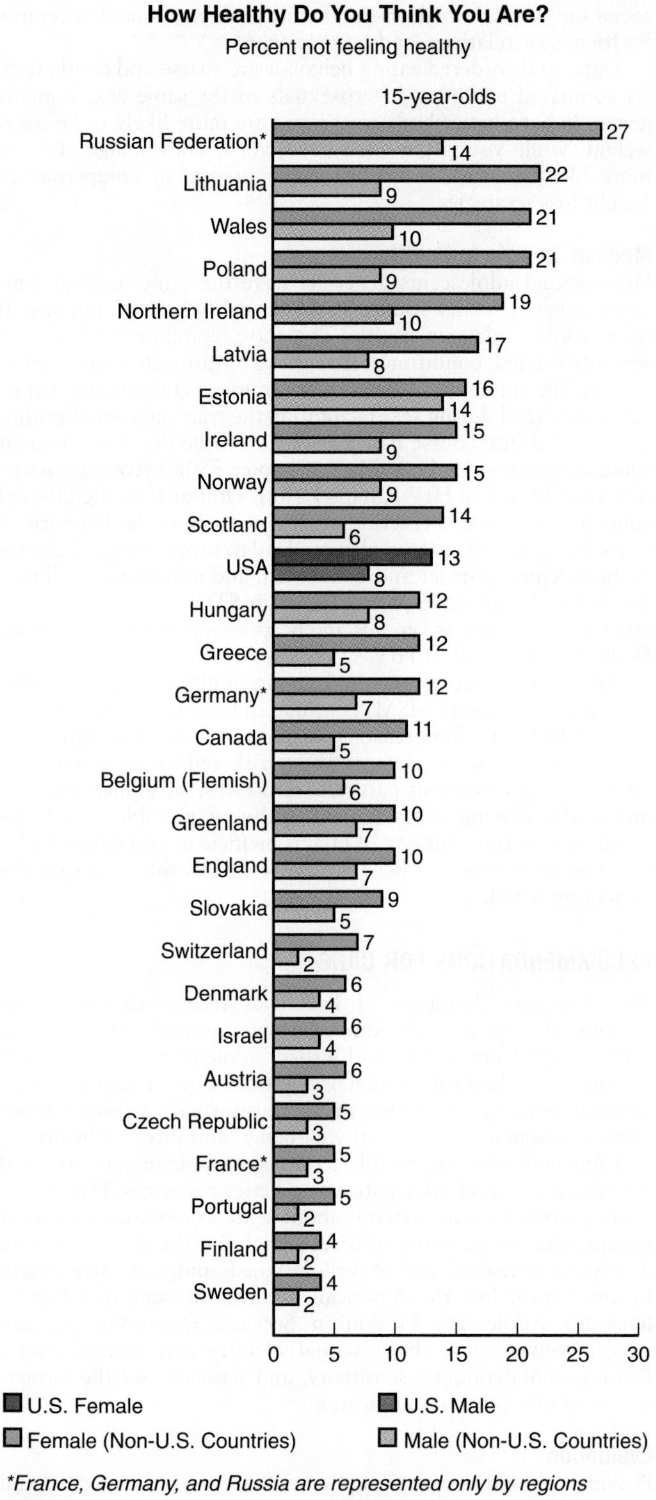

Figure 105-1 Proportion of 15 yr old youth from 28 nations who report not feeling healthy. (From Health Resources and Services Administration, Maternal and Child Health Bureau: *U.S. teens in our world. Understanding the health of U.S. youth in comparison to youth in other countries* (website). www.mchb.hrsa.gov/mchirc/_pubs/us_teens/main_pages/ch_1.htm. Accessed April 16, 2010.)

occurred among youth 15-24 yr in Romania and the Russian Federation; >50% of cases of gonorrhea occurred in this age group in Romania, the Russian Federation, the Slovak Republic, Canada, England and Wales, and the USA; and in 6 countries, youth this age were responsible for >50% of annually reported chlamydia cases.

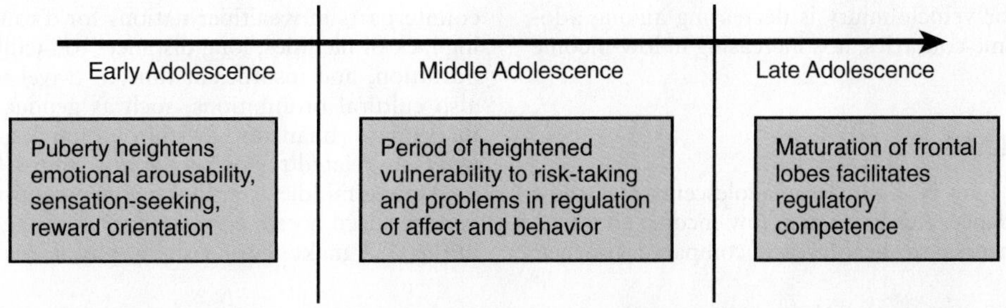

Figure 105-2 It has been speculated that the impact of puberty on arousal and motivation occurs before the maturation of the frontal lobes is complete. This gap may create a period of heightened vulnerability to problems in the regulation of affect and behavior, which might help to explain the increased potential in adolescence for risk taking, recklessness, and the onset of emotional and behavioral problems. (From Steinberg L: Cognitive and affective development in adolescence, *Trends Cogn Sci* 9:69–74, 2005.)

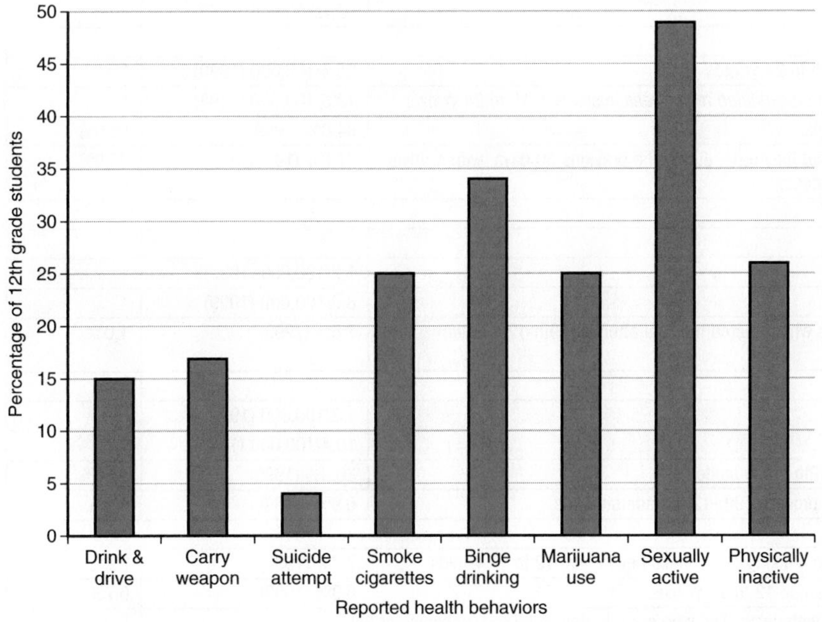

Figure 105-3 Selected health risk behaviors among 12th grade high school students. (Data from Centers for Disease Control and Prevention: *2009 youth risk surveillance system* (website). www.cdc.gov/HealthyYouth/yrbs/index.htm. Accessed February 20, 2011.)

Table 105-1 IDENTIFIED RISK AND PROTECTIVE FACTORS FOR ADOLESCENT HEALTH BEHAVIORS

BEHAVIOR	RISK FACTORS	PROTECTIVE FACTORS
Smoking	Depression and other mental health problems, alcohol use, disconnectedness from school or family, difficulty talking with parents, minority ethnicity, low school achievement, peer smoking	Family connectedness, perceived healthiness, higher parental expectations, low prevalence of smoking in school
Alcohol and drug misuse	Depression and other mental health problems, low self-esteem, easy family access to alcohol, working outside school, difficulty talking with parents, risk factors for transition from occasional to regular substance misuse (smoking, availability of substances, peer use, other risk behaviors)	Connectedness with school and family, religious affiliation
Teenage pregnancy	Deprivation, city residence, low educational expectations, lack of access to sexual health services, drug and alcohol use	Connectedness with school and family, religious affiliation
Sexually transmitted infections	Mental health problems, substance misuse	Connectedness with school and family, religious affiliation

Adapted from McIntosh N, Helms P, Smyth R, editors: *Forfar and Arneils textbook of paediatrics,* ed 6, Edinburgh, 2003, Churchill Livingstone, pp 1757–1768; and Viner R, Macfarlane A: Health promotion, *Br Med J* 330:527–529, 2005.

In the USA, injuries cause more than twice as many deaths among adolescents as do natural causes; motor vehicle traffic–related injuries and firearm-related injuries are the 2 leading causes of injury death among adolescents 10-19 yr of age (Chapter 5). Although infectious diseases remain important causes of death for adolescents in some low-income countries, adolescents worldwide are increasingly exposed to risk-taking behavior including violence. Worldwide, motor vehicle accidents are the greatest cause of death and disability among men ages 15-19 yr. For all causes of mortality resulting from unintentional injury there is an inverse relationship between mortality rates and per capita income except for motor vehicle traffic among adolescents and young adults; for this category, mortality is higher in high-income countries compared to low-income countries. Though mortality due to motor vehicle injury is decreasing among adolescents in higher income countries, it is increasing in low-income countries.

ACCESS TO HEALTH CARE

Access to health care may be limited for adolescents regardless of the country of residence. Adolescents in low-income countries experience reduced access to health care compared to their counterparts in wealthier nations for a range of reasons, including lack of facilities, long distances to facilities, inadequate transportation, and insufficient time to travel to facilities. There are also cultural prohibitions, such as gender, poor education, and inadequate financing. Within countries, access is generally inversely related to socioeconomic status (Chapter 1).

Among middle- and high-income countries, adolescents often have reduced access compared to other age groups. Adolescents in the USA make fewer visits to physicians for ambulatory office

Table 105-2 TWENTY-ONE CRITICAL HEALTH OBJECTIVES FOR ADOLESCENTS AND YOUNG ADULTS

OBJ. #	OBJECTIVE	BASELINE (YEAR)	2010 TARGET
16-03. (a,b,c)	*Reduce deaths of adolescents and young adults.*		(per 100,000)
	10 to 14 yr olds	21.5/100,000 (1998)	16.8
	15 to 19 yr olds	69.5/100,000 (1998)	39.8
	20 to 24 yr olds	92.7/100,000 (1998)	49.0
UNINTENTIONAL INJURY			
15-15. (a)	*Reduce deaths caused by motor vehicle crashes;* 15 to 24 yr olds	25.6/100,000 (1999)	*
26-01. (a)	*Reduce deaths and injuries caused by alcohol- and drug-related motor vehicle crashes;* 15 to 24 yr olds	13.5/100,000 (1998)	*
15-19.	Increase use of safety belts. 9th-12th grade students	84.0% (1999)	92.0%
26-06.	Reduce the proportion of adolescents who report that they rode, during the previous 30 days, with a driver who had been drinking alcohol; 9th-12th grade students	33.0% (1999)	30.0%
VIOLENCE			
18-01.	*Reduce the suicide rate.*		
	10 to 14 yr olds	1.2/100,000 (1999)	*
	15 to 19 yr olds	8.0/100,000 (1999)	*
18-02.	Reduce the rate of suicide attempts by adolescents who required medical attention; 9th-12th grade students	2.6% (1999)	1.0%
15-32.	*Reduce homicides.*		
	10 to 14 yr olds	1.2/100,000 (1999)	*
	15 to 19 yr olds	10.4/100,000 (1999)	*
15-38.	Reduce physical fighting among adolescents; 9th-12th grade students	36.0% (1999)	32.0%
15-39.	Reduce weapon carrying by adolescents on school property; 9th-12th grade students	6.9% (1999)	4.9%
SUBSTANCE ABUSE AND MENTAL HEALTH			
26-11. (d)	Reduce the proportion of persons engaging in binge drinking of alcoholic beverages; 12 to 17 yr olds	7.7% (1998)	2.0%
26-10. (b)	Reduce past-month use of illicit substances (marijuana); 12 to 17 yr olds	8.3% (1998)	0.7%
06-02.	Reduce the proportion of children and adolescents with disabilities who are reported to be sad, unhappy, or depressed; 4 to 17 yr olds	†	†
18-07.	Increase the proportion of children with mental health problems who receive treatment	59.0% (2001)	66.0%
REPRODUCTIVE HEALTH			
09-07.	*Reduce pregnancies among adolescent females;* 15 to 17 yr olds	68.0/1000 females (1996)	43.0/1000
13-05.	*Reduce the number of new cases of HIV/AIDS diagnosed among adolescents and adults;* 13 to 24 yr olds	16,479 (1998)‡	§
25-01. (a,b,c)	*Reduce the proportion of adolescents and young adults with Chlamydia trachomatis infections;* 15 to 24 yr olds		
	Females attending family-planning clinics	5.0% (1997)	3.0%
	Females attending sexually transmitted disease clinics	12.2% (1997)	3.0%
	Males attending sexually transmitted disease clinics	15.7% (1997)	3.0%
25-11. (a,b,c)	Increase the proportion of adolescents (9th-12th grade students) who:		
	Have never had sexual intercourse	50.0% (1999)	56.0%
	If sexually experienced, are not currently sexually active	27.0% (1999)	30.0%
	If currently sexually active, used a condom the last time they had sexual intercourse	58.0% (1999)	65.0%
CHRONIC DISEASES			
27-02. (a)	Reduce tobacco use by adolescents; 9th-12th grade students	40.0% (1999)	21.0%
19-03. (b)	*Reduce the proportion of children and adolescents who are overweight or obese,* 12 to 19 yr olds	11.0% (1988-1994)	5.0%
22-07.	Increase the proportion of adolescents who engage in vigorous physical activity that promotes cardiorespiratory fitness ≥3 days per week for ≥20 min per occasion; 9th-12th grade students	65.0% (1999)	85.0%

The 21 Critical Health Objectives represent the most serious health and safety issues facing adolescents and young adults (aged 10-24 yr): mortality, unintentional injury, violence, substance abuse and mental health, reproductive health, and the prevention of chronic diseases during adulthood.
Note: Critical health outcomes are italicized, and behaviors that substantially contribute to important health outcomes are in normal type.
*2010 target not provided for adolescent/young adult age group.
†Baseline and target inclusive of age groups outside of adolescent/young adult age parameters.
‡Proposed baseline is shown but has not yet been approved by the *Healthy People 2010* Steering Committee.
§Development objective: baseline and 2010 target to be provided by 2005.
From U.S. Department of Health and Human Services: *Healthy People 2010,* 1 and 2. Washington, DC, U.S. Government Printing Office, November 2000. This information can also be accessed at *http://wonder.cdc.gov/data2010/.*

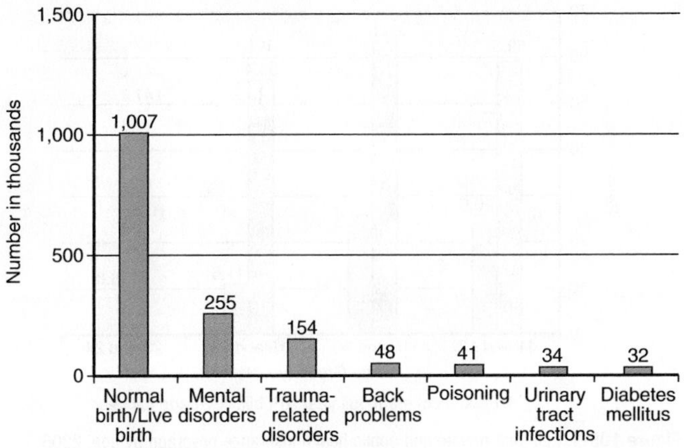

Figure 105-4 Number of hospital inpatient stays by condition, ages 12-24 yr, 2004. (Adapted from National Adolescent Health Information Center: *2008 fact sheet on health care access & utilization: adolescents & young adults*, San Francisco, 2008, University of California, San Francisco. Source: Medical Expenditure Panel Survey, Household Component Summary Tables, 2007.)

visits than does any other age group; school-aged children and adolescents are more likely than younger children to have unmet health needs and delayed medical care. Adolescents and young adults are less likely to be insured than all other age groups. Young adults 18-24 yr are more likely to be uninsured because until the passage in 2010 of America's Affordable Health Choices Act, many were no longer eligible to receive benefits from their parents' health plans or public insurance programs. In addition, health insurance status differs based on income and race/ethnicity. Adolescents and young adults who are near poor (100-199% federal poverty level [FPL]) and poor (below 100% FPL) are less likely to have health insurance coverage than those with higher family incomes; and Hispanic and black adolescents and young adults are less likely to have health insurance coverage than their non-Hispanic white and Asian peers. Uninsured children and adolescents are less likely to receive preventive visits and have a regular source of care than the insured, and are more likely to go without treatment of symptoms.

Adolescents who actually receive preventive care may still not have access to time alone with their provider or discuss important confidential health issues, such as sexually transmitted infections, HIV, or pregnancy prevention. Less than half (40%) of adolescents have time alone with their health care provider during a preventive health care visit; sexually experienced teens report sexual health discussions more often than nonsexually experienced teens, but the frequency is still low at 64% and 33.5% for sexually experienced females and males, respectively.

In 2002-2004, adolescents 10-19 yr of age in the USA had about 13 million emergency department (ED) visits annually. ED visit rates increase with age for both male and female adolescents. Female ED visit rates more than double between ages 10-13 yr and 18-19 yr, in part because of pregnancy and sexual activity–related conditions. Among adolescents and young adults ages 15-24 yr in 2005, females and blacks had higher ED visit rates than their peers. Injuries are a major cause of ED visits. In 2002-2004, initial injury-related ED visits comprised 42% of all ED visits for 10-19 yr olds and were higher among male than female adolescents. Other principal ED diagnoses among adolescents 10-19 yr of age include asthma, upper respiratory conditions, and abdominal or gastrointestinal conditions. Among female adolescents, ED visits for symptomatic sexually transmitted infections, urinary tract infections, and pregnancy-related conditions are also high and increase substantially with age.

Adolescents are among the least likely of all age groups to be hospitalized. In 2004, childbirth was the leading cause of inpatient hospitalizations for adolescents and young adults ages 12-24 yr, followed by mental health disorders and trauma-related disorders, such as open wounds and fractures (Fig. 105-4).

The National Initiative to Improve Adolescent Health by the Year 2010 has identified 21 critical health objectives for adolescents and young adults as a strategy to focus state and community resources and health professionals on improving the health status of U.S. youths (Table 105-2). Progress to date includes significant improvement in incidence of teen pregnancy and tobacco use, small increments of improvement in some areas (i.e., physical fighting, weapon carrying, safety belt use), and worsening trends for others such as motor vehicle crashes, chlamydial infections, and obesity. These health objectives are applicable to adolescents throughout the world.

BIBLIOGRAPHY

Please visit the Nelson Textbook of Pediatrics *website at www.expertconsult.com for the complete bibliography.*

Chapter 106
Delivery of Health Care to Adolescents

Gale R. Burstein and Barbara Cromer

Adolescence provides a unique opportunity to prevent health conditions and behaviors that develop in the second decade of life and that can lead to substantial morbidity and mortality, such as trauma, cardiovascular and pulmonary disease, type 2 diabetes, reproductive health disease, and cancer. Health care providers play an important role in nurturing healthy behaviors among adolescents because the leading causes of death and disability among adolescents are preventable. Access to developmentally appropriate, affordable, high-quality health care during the adolescent years sets the stage for a lifetime of good health.

The Society for Adolescent Medicine identified 10 program and policy characteristics to ensure comprehensive and high-quality care to adolescents. **Health insurance coverage** that is affordable, continuous, and not subject to exclusion for preexisting conditions should be available for all adolescents and young adults who have no access to private insurance. **Comprehensive, coordinated benefits** should meet the developmental needs of adolescents, particularly for reproductive, mental health, dental, and substance abuse services. **Safety net providers and programs,** such as school-based health centers, community health centers, family planning services, and clinics that treat sexually transmitted infections (STIs) in adolescents and young adults, need to have assured funding for viability and sustainability. **Quality of care** data should be collected and analyzed by age so that the performance measures for age-appropriate health care needs of adolescents are monitored. **Affordability** is important for access to preventive services. Family involvement should be encouraged, but **confidentiality** and adolescent consent are critically important. Health plans and providers should be adequately **compensated** to support the range and intensity of services required to address the developmental and health service needs of adolescents. **Health care providers, trained and experienced,** to care for adolescents should be available in all communities. The creation and dissemination of provider education about adolescent preventive health guidelines have been demonstrated to improve the content of recommended care (Table 106-1). The ease of recognition or expectation that an adolescent's needs can be addressed in a setting relates to the **visibility and flexibility** of sites and services. Staff at sites should be approachable, linguistically capable, and culturally competent. Health services should be **coordinated** to respond to goals for adolescent health at the local, state, and national levels. The coordination should address service financing and delivery in a manner that reduces disparities in care.

Table 106-1 BRIGHT FUTURES/AMERICAN ACADEMY OF PEDIATRICS RECOMMENDATIONS FOR PREVENTIVE HEALTH CARE FOR 11-21 YEAR OLDS

	PERIODICITY AND INDICATIONS
HISTORY	Annual
MEASUREMENTS	
Body mass index	Annual
Blood pressure	Annual
SENSORY SCREENING	
Vision	At 11, 15, and 18 year visits or if risk assessment positive
Hearing	If risk assessment positive
DEVELOPMENTAL/BEHAVIORAL ASSESSMENT	
Developmental surveillance	Annual
Psychosocial/behavioral assessment	Annual
Alcohol and drug use assessment	If risk assessment positive
PHYSICAL EXAMINATION	Annual
PROCEDURES	
Immunization*	Annual
Hematocrit or hemoglobin	If risk assessment positive
Tuberculin test	If risk assessment positive
Dyslipidemia screening	If risk assessment positive
STI screening	If sexually active
Cervical dysplasia screening†	Annual beginning at age 21 yr
ORAL HEALTH	Annual refer to dental home or administer oral health risk assessment
ANTICIPATORY GUIDANCE	Annual‡

*Schedules as per the AAP Committee on Infectious Diseases, published annually in the January issue of *Pediatrics*.
†American College of Obstetrics and Gynecology: Cervical cytology screening. ACOG Practice Bulletin No. 109, *Obstet Gynecol* 114:1409–1420, 2009.
‡Refer to specific guidance by age as listed in *Bright Futures* Guidelines.
Adapted from American Academy of Pediatrics and Bright Futures Periodicity Schedule. In Hagan JF, Shaw JS, Duncan PM, editors: *Bright futures: guidelines for health supervision of infants, children, and adolescents*, ed 3, Elk Grove Village, IL, 2008, American Academy of Pediatrics. *brightfutures.aap.org/pdfs/Guidelines_PDF/20-Appendices_PeriodicitySchedule.pdf.* Accessed April 16, 2010.

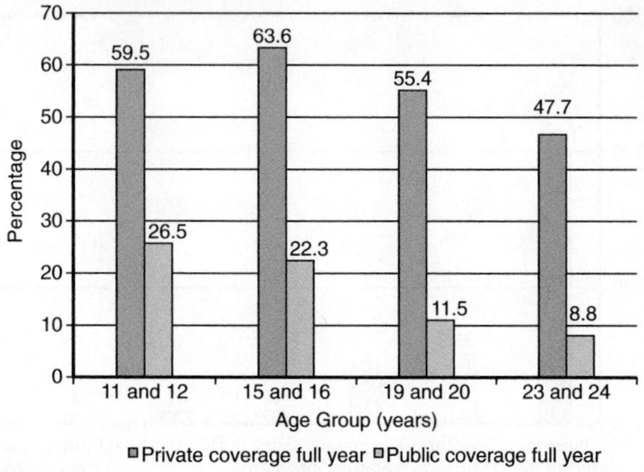

Figure 106-1 Full-year private and public health insurance coverage by age, 2006. (Data from Public Policy Analysis and Education Center for Middle Childhood, Adolescent and Young Adults Health. National Health Interview Survey, 2006. Adapted from Mulye TP, Park MJ, Nelson CD, et al: Trends in adolescent and young adult health in the United States, *J Adolesc Health* 45:8-24, 2009.)

Adolescents have the lowest annual rate of visits to office-based physicians compared with all other age groups. Adolescents 10-19 yr of age are less likely to have had a recent health care visit than children <10 yr of age. In 2005, 83% of adolescents had one or more contacts with a health care professional compared with 91% of children <10 yr of age. Uninsured adolescents are the least likely to receive care. In 2005, the proportion of adolescents without health insurance who had not visited a health care provider in the past year was more than 3 times as high as insured adolescents. Older teens and young adults are more likely to be uninsured (Fig. 106-1). In 2006, while 86% of 11-12 yr olds were covered by either public or private health insurance, only 67% of 19-20 yr olds and 56.5% of 23-24 yrs olds had were covered by health care insurance. Even for insured adolescents and young adults, health care expenses present a barrier to care. In 2004, 80% of adolescents 10-21 yr of age incurred out-of-pocket expenses for health care; on average, this was $1,514 annually. Adolescents with health insurance were considerably more likely to have incurred out-of-pocket expenses and the average annual out-of-pocket amount spent was higher for insured compared to uninsured adolescents.

The complexity and interaction of physical, cognitive, and psychosocial developmental processes during adolescence require sensitivity and skill on the part of the health professional (Chapter 104). Health education and promotion as well as disease prevention should be the focus of every visit. In 2008, the American Academy of Pediatrics in collaboration with the U.S. Department of Health and Human Services, Health Resources and Services Administration, Maternal and Child Health Bureau, published the 3rd edition of *Bright Futures: Guidelines for Health Supervision of Infants, Children, and Adolescents*, that offers providers a strategy for delivery of adolescent preventive health services with screening and counseling recommendations for early, middle, and late adolescence (Table 106-2). Bright Futures is rooted in the philosophy of preventive care and reflects the concept of caring for children in a "medical home." These guidelines emphasize effective partnerships with parents and the community to support the adolescent's health and development.

The Centers for Disease Control and Prevention's Advisory Committee on Immunization Practices (ACIP) currently recommends 3 routine adolescent vaccines, tetanus–diphtheria–acellular pertussis vaccine (Tdap), the meningococcal conjugate vaccine (MCV4) and the human papillomavirus (HPV) vaccine, for universal administration beginning at the 11-12 yr old visit or as soon as possible (Chapter 165). ACIP recommends a second varicella vaccine, annual influenza vaccination, and hepatitis A vaccination in states or communities where routine hepatitis A vaccination has been implemented and for travelers, men who have sex with men, injection drug users, and those with chronic liver disease or clotting factor disorders.

The time spent on various elements of the screening will vary with the issues that surface during the assessment. For gay and lesbian youth (Chapter 104.3), emotional and psychologic issues related to their experiences, from fear of disclosure to the trauma of homophobia, may direct the clinician to spend more time assessing emotional and psychologic supports in the young person's environment. For youths with chronic illnesses or special needs, the assessment of at-risk behaviors should not be omitted or de-emphasized by assuming they do not experience the "normal" adolescent vulnerabilities.

BIBLIOGRAPHY

Please visit the Nelson Textbook of Pediatrics *website at www.expertconsult.com for the complete bibliography.*

106.1 Legal Issues

Gale R. Burstein

The rights of an individual including those of adolescents vary widely between nations. In the USA, the right of a minor to consent to treatment without parental knowledge differs between states and is governed by state-specific minor consent laws. Some

Table 106-2 BRIGHT FUTURES ADOLESCENT SCREENING RECOMMENDATIONS

		11-14 YEAR OLD VISIT	15-17 YEAR OLD VISIT	19-21 YEAR OLD VISIT
UNIVERSAL SCREENING		**ACTION**	**ACTION**	**ACTION**
Vision (once during each of 3 adolescent age groups)		Snellen test	Snellen test	Snellen test
Dyslipidemia (once in late adolescence)		NA	NA	Fasting lipid profile
SELECTIVE SCREENING	**RISK ASSESSMENT**	**ACTION IF RA+**	**ACTION IF RA+**	**ACTION IF RA+**
Vision at other ages	+ on risk screening questions	Snellen test	Snellen test	Snellen test
Hearing	+ on risk screening questions	Audiometry	Audiometry	Audiometry
Anemia	+ on risk screening questions	Hemoglobin or hematocrit	Hemoglobin or hematocrit	Hemoglobin or hematocrit
Tuberculosis	+ on risk screening questions	Tuberculin skin test	Tuberculin skin test	Tuberculin skin test
Dyslipidemia	+ on risk screening questions and not previously screened with normal results	Lipid screen	Lipid screen	Lipid screen if not age 20, + on risk screening questions and not previously screened with normal results
STIs	Sexually active	Chlamydia and gonorrhea screen (use tests appropriate for population and clinical setting)	Chlamydia and gonorrhea screen (use tests appropriate for population and clinical setting)	Chlamydia and gonorrhea screen (use tests appropriate for population and clinical setting)
	Sexually active and + on risk screening questions	Syphilis test HIV test*	Syphilis test HIV test*	Syphilis test HIV test*
Pregnancy	Sexually active, without contraception, late menses or amenorrhea	Urine hCG	Urine hCG	Urine hCG
Cervical dysplasia†	NA	NA	NA	Pap smear, conventional slide or liquid-based at age 21 yr
Alcohol or drug use	+ on risk screening questions	Administer alcohol and drug screening tool	Administer alcohol and drug screening tool	Administer alcohol and drug screening tool

*CDC has recently recommended universal, voluntary HIV screening of all sexually active people, beginning at age 13 years. At the time of publication, the AAP and other groups had not yet commented on the CDC recommendation, nor recommended screening criteria or techniques. The health care professional's attention is drawn to the voluntary nature of screening and that the CDC offers an opt-out in communities where the HIV rate is <0.1%. The management of positives and false positives must be considered before testing.

†American College of Obstetrics and Gynecology: Cervical cytology screening. ACOG Practice Bulletin No. 109, *Obstet Gynecol* 114:1409–1420, 2009.

RA, risk assessment; NA, not applicable; hCG, human chorionic gonadotropin.

Adapted from American Academy of Pediatrics: *Bright futures guidelines priorities and screening tables* (PowerPoint presentation). brightfutures.aap.org/Presentations/Bright%20Futures%20Priority%20and%20Screening%20Tables%200308.ppt. Accessed April 16, 2010.

minor consent laws are based on a minor's status, such as minors who are emancipated, parents, married, pregnant, in the armed services, or mature. Minors can be considered *emancipated* if they are or have served in the armed services or are living apart from parents and are economically independent through gainful employment. A *mature minor* is a minor who is emotionally and intellectually mature enough to give informed consent and who lives under the supervision of a parent or guardian. Courts have held that if a minor is mature, a physician is not liable for providing beneficial treatment. There is no formal process for recognition of a mature minor. The determination is made by the health care provider.

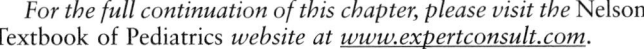

For the full continuation of this chapter, please visit the Nelson Textbook of Pediatrics *website at* *www.expertconsult.com*.

106.2 Screening Procedures

Gale R. Burstein

Interviewing the Adolescent

The preparation for a successful interview with an adolescent patient varies based on the history of the relationship with the patient. Patients (and their parents) who are going from preadolescence to adolescence while seeing the same provider, should be guided through the transition. Although the rules for confidentiality are the same for new and continuing patients, the change in the physician-patient relationship, allowing more privacy during the visit and more autonomy in the health process, may be threatening for the parent as well as the adolescent. For new patients, the initial phases of the interview are more challenging given the need to establish rapport rapidly with the patient in order to meet the goals of the encounter. Issues of confidentiality and privacy should be explicitly stated along with the conditions under which that confidentiality may need to be altered, that is, in life- or safety-threatening situations. For new patients, the parents should be interviewed with the adolescent or before the adolescent to ensure that the adolescent does not perceive a breach of confidentiality. The clinician who takes time to listen avoids judgmental statements and the use of street jargon and shows respect for the adolescent's emerging maturity will have an easier time communicating with him or her. The use of open-ended questions, rather than closed-ended questions, will further facilitate history taking. (The closed-ended question "Do you get along with your father?" leads to the answer "yes" or "no," in contrast to the question, "What would you like to change in your relationship with your mother?" which may lead to an answer such as "I would like her to stop always worrying about me.")

The goals of the interview or clinical encounter are to establish an information base, identify problems and issues from the patient's perspective, and identify problems and issues from the perspective of the clinician based on knowledge of the health and other issues relevant to the adolescent age group. The adolescent should be given an opportunity to express concerns and the reasons for seeking medical attention. The adolescent as well as the parent should be given an opportunity to express the strengths and successes of the adolescent, in addition to communicating problems.

Barriers to an effective interview occur when the interviewer is distracted by other events or individuals in the office, when there are extreme time limitations obvious to either party, or when there is expressible discomfort with either the patient or the interviewer. The need for an interpreter when a patient is hearing impaired or if the patient and interviewer are not language compatible provides a challenge but not necessarily a barrier under most circumstances (Chapter 4). Observations during the interview can be useful to the overall assessment of the patient's maturity, presence or absence of depression, and the parent-adolescent relationship. Given the key role of a successful interview in the screening process, adequate training and experience should be sought by clinicians wishing to give comprehensive care to adolescent patients.

Psychosocial Assessment

A few questions should be asked to detect the adolescent who is having difficulty with peer relationships ("Do you have a best friend with whom you can share even the most personal secret?"), self-image ("Is there anything you would like to change about yourself?"), depression ("What do you see yourself doing 5 yr from now?"), school ("How are your grades this year compared with last year?"), personal decisions ("Are you feeling pressured to engage in any behavior for which you do not feel you are ready?"), and an eating disorder ("Do you ever feel that food controls you rather than vice versa?"). Bright Futures materials provide questions and patient encounter forms to structure the assessments that are available at their website *(brightfutures.aap.org/index.html)*. The **HEADS/SF/FIRST** mnemonic, basic or expanded, can be useful in guiding the interview if encounter forms are not available (Table 106-4). Based on the assessments, appropriate counseling or referrals are recommended for more thorough probing or for in-depth interviewing.

PHYSICAL EXAMINATION

Audiometry

Highly amplified music of the kind enjoyed by many adolescents may result in hearing loss (Chapter 629). A hearing screening is recommended by the Bright Futures guidelines for adolescents who are exposed to loud noises regularly, have had recurring ear infections, or report problems.

Table 106-4 HEADS/SF/FIRST
Home. Space, privacy, frequent geographic moves, neighborhood.
Education/School. Frequent school changes, repetition of a grade/in each subject, teachers' reports, vocational goals, after-school educational clubs (language, speech, math, etc.), learning disabilities.
Abuse. Physical, sexual, emotional, verbal abuse; parental discipline.
Drugs. Tobacco, alcohol, marijuana, inhalants, "club drugs," "rave" parties, others. Drug of choice, age at initiation, frequency, mode of intake, rituals, alone or with peers, quit methods, and number of attempts.
Safety. Seat belts, helmets, sports safety measures, hazardous activities, driving while intoxicated.
Sexuality/Sexual Identity. Reproductive health (use of contraceptives, presence of sexually transmitted infections, feelings, pregnancy)
Family and Friends. Family: Family constellation, genogram, single/married/separated/divorced/blended family, family occupations and shifts; history of addiction in 1st- and 2nd-degree relatives, parental attitude toward alcohol and drugs, parental rules; chronically ill physically or mentally challenged parent. **Friends:** peer cliques and configuration ("preppies," "jocks," "nerds," "computer geeks," cheerleaders), gang or cult affiliation.
Image. Height and weight perceptions, body musculature and physique, appearance (including dress, jewelry, tattoos, body piercing as fashion trends or other statement).
Recreation. Sleep, exercise, organized or unstructured sports, recreational activities (television, video games, computer games, Internet and chat rooms, church or community youth group activities [e.g., Boy/Girl Scouts; Big Brother/Sister groups, campus groups]). How many hours per day, days per week involved?
Spirituality and Connectedness. Use HOPE* or FICA† acronym; adherence, rituals, occult practices, community service or involvement.
Threats and Violence. Self-harm or harm to others, running away, cruelty to animals, guns, fights, arrests, stealing, fire setting, fights in school.

*HOPE: **h**ope or security for the future; **o**rganized religion; **p**ersonal spirituality and practices; **e**ffects on medical care and end of life issues.
†FICA: **f**aith beliefs; **i**mportance and influence of faith; **c**ommunity support.
From Dias PJ: Adolescent substance abuse. Assessment in the office, *Pediatr Clin North Am* 49:269–300, 2002.

Vision Testing

The pubertal growth spurt may involve the optic globe, resulting in its elongation and myopia in genetically predisposed individuals. Vision testing should, therefore, be performed in order to detect this problem before it affects school performance.

Blood Pressure Determination

Criteria for a diagnosis of hypertension are based on age-specific norms that increase with pubertal maturation (Chapter 439). An individual whose blood pressure exceeds the 95th percentile for his or her age is suspect for having hypertension, regardless of the absolute reading. Those adolescents with blood pressure between the 90th and 95th percentiles should receive appropriate counseling relative to weight and have a follow-up examination in 6 mo. Those with blood pressure above the 90th percentile should have their blood pressure measured on three separate occasions to determine the stability of the elevation before moving forward with an intervention strategy. The technique is important; false-positive results may be obtained if the cuff covers less than two thirds of the upper arm. The patient should be seated, and an average should be taken of the 2nd and 3rd consecutive readings, using the change rather than the disappearance as the diastolic pressure. Most adolescents with elevations of blood pressure have labile hypertension. If the blood pressure is below 2 standard deviations for age, anorexia nervosa and Addison disease should be considered.

Scoliosis (Chapter 671)

Approximately 5% of male and 10-14% of female adolescents have a mild curvature of the spine. This is 2 to 4 times the rate in younger children. Scoliosis is typically manifested during the peak of the height velocity curve, at approximately 12 yr in females and 14 yr in males. Curves measuring greater than 10 degrees should be monitored by an orthopedist until growth is complete.

Breast Examination (Chapters 109 and 545)

Examination of the female adolescent's breasts is performed to detect masses, evaluate progression of sexual maturation, provide reassurance about development, and teach the technique of self-examination with the hope that this practice will continue into the higher risk later years. However, there is disagreement on the justification for promoting this routinely, given the rare instances of malignant breast masses in this age group.

Scrotum Examination

The peak incidence of germ cell tumors of the testes is in late adolescence and early adulthood. Palpation of the testes may have an immediate yield and should serve as a model for instruction of self-examination. Because varicoceles often appear during puberty, the examination also provides an opportunity to explain and reassure the patient about this entity (Chapter 539).

Pelvic Examination

See Chapter 542.

Laboratory Testing

The increased incidence of iron-deficiency anemia after menarche mandates the performance of a hematocrit annually in young women with moderate to heavy menses. The reference standard for this test changes with progression of puberty, as estrogen suppresses erythropoietin (Chapter 440). Populations with nutritional risk should also have the hematocrit monitored. Androgens have the opposite effect, causing the hematocrit to rise during male puberty; Sexual Maturity Rating 1 males (Chapter 104) have an average hematocrit of 39%, whereas those who have completed puberty (Sexual Maturity Rating 5; Chapter 104) have an average value of 43%. Tuberculosis testing on an annual basis is important in adolescents with risk factors, such as an adolescent with HIV, living in the household with someone with HIV, the incarcerated adolescent, or those with other risk factors, because puberty has been shown to activate this disease in those not previously treated. Hepatitis C virus screening should be offered to adolescents who report risk factors, such as injection drug use, received blood products or organ donation before 1992, long-term hemodialysis, or high prevalence setting (i.e., correctional facilities or STI clinics).

Sexually active adolescents should undergo screening for STIs regardless of symptoms (Chapter 114). There are clear indications for chlamydia and gonorrhea screening of females 25 yr old and younger, but less sufficient evidence to support routine screening in young men. Screening young men is a clinical option and with newer noninvasive testing. HIV screening should be discussed with those who are sexually active, especially men who have sex with men, and injection drug users. Syphilis screening is recommended for pregnant adolescents and those at increased risk of infection. For sexually active females, the guidelines for Pap smears for cervical cancer screening suggest that annual screening can be delayed safely up to 3 yr after the onset of sexual activity or age 21 yr, whichever is earlier; HPV DNA testing should not be used routinely for females 29 yr and younger since the results would not influence management.

BIBLIOGRAPHY

Please visit the Nelson Textbook of Pediatrics *website at www.expertconsult.com for the complete bibliography.*

106.3 Health Enhancement

Gale R. Burstein

Adolescence is a critical period for developing behaviors that create a strong foundation for healthy living over the full life span. Health care providers play an important role in fostering healthy behaviors among adolescents by applying principles of prevention and anticipatory guidance. Since adolescents may not utilize routine preventive health care, incorporating these services into the episodic "sick visit" optimizes comprehensive adolescent health care delivery. Offering needed immunizations at any adolescent visit will maximize protection against vaccine-preventable diseases. STI and pregnancy prevention are important issues to address with both male and female adolescents and a discussion should be integrated into all visits with sexually active adolescents. Prevention of illicit drug and alcohol use and the potential for related consequences should be reviewed. Prevention of behaviors that can lead to substantial morbidity and mortality, such as motor vehicle accidents, violence, and tobacco use, should also be discussed. All adolescents should be screened for mental health care needs and provided with appropriate care either in the primary care site or through specialty referral. Facilitating an optimal health outcome for the adolescent patient also includes supporting him or her in successfully negotiating adolescence through school, job, and personal and family relations.

BIBLIOGRAPHY

Please visit the Nelson Textbook of Pediatrics *website at www.expertconsult.com for the complete bibliography.*

106.4 Transitioning to Adult Care

Barbara Cromer

Transition to adult care is a crucial aspect of the health of all adolescents. The transition is especially important for those young people with chronic medical conditions. Delayed transition or transfer to an inappropriate adult health service may result in disrupted care, nonadherence to treatment, and adverse health outcomes. With improved survival into adulthood among children with complex medical conditions resulting from improved technology and medical therapy, there has been increasing focus on designing effective programs for optimizing the transition process to adult care.

For the full continuation of this chapter, please visit the Nelson Textbook of Pediatrics *website at www.expertconsult.com.*

Chapter 107
Violent Behavior

Margaret M. Stager

The World Health Organization (WHO) recognizes violence as a leading worldwide public health problem and defines violence as "The intentional use of physical force or power, threatened or actual, against oneself, another person, or against a group or community that either results in or has a high likelihood of resulting in injury, death, psychologic harm, maldevelopment or deprivation" (Chapter 36). Youths may be perpetrators of violence, victims of violence, or observers of violence with varying severity of impact on the individual, family, or larger community. A number of risk factors have been identified that may increase the risk of a youth to engage in violence such as poverty, substance abuse, mental health disorders, and poor family functioning.

EPIDEMIOLOGY

In 2006, homicide in the USA was the second leading cause of death for 10-24 yr olds totaling 5,958 deaths, which were largely males (87%) killed by a handgun (84%) in a gang-related incident (Table 107-1). The WHO reports that other than the USA, where the youth and young adult homicide rate was 11 per 100,000, most countries with homicide rates above 10 per 100,000 are developing nations or countries with rapid socioeconomic changes. However, while rates of violent deaths among adolescents are higher in the USA compared to other developed countries, rates are increasing; in Israel, France, and Norway, firearms are the second leading mechanism of death in 15-24 yr olds. Although the prevalence of behaviors that contribute to violence has decreased from 1991 to 2007, fighting and weapon carrying remain prevalent among U.S. youth (Table 107-2). In 2007, 668,000 youths were treated in U.S. emergency departments for violence-related injuries such as stab wounds, gunshot wounds, broken bones, and lacerations. The rate of homicide by

Table 107-1 HOMICIDE TYPE BY AGE, 1976-2005

	VICTIM'S AGE (YR) Under 18	18-34	OFFENDER'S AGE (YR) Under 18	18-34
All homicides	9.8%	52.7%	10.9%	65.0%
VICTIM/OFFENDER RELATIONSHIP				
Intimate	1.5%	46.7%	1.0%	46.2%
Family	19.6%	31.9%	6.0%	49.1%
CIRCUMSTANCES				
Felony murder	7.6%	46.9%	14.8%	72.9%
Sex related	19.6%	45.1%	10.7%	73.6%
Drug related	5.4%	71.4%	10.6%	76.9%
Gang related	24.2%	68.4%	28.9%	69.2%
Argument	5.5%	56.1%	6.9%	60.2%

From Federal Bureau of Investigation: *Supplementary homicide reports, 1976-2005.* www.ojp.usdoj.gov/homicide.

Table 107-2 TRENDS (% OF YOUTH) IN THE PREVALENCE OF BEHAVIORS THAT CONTRIBUTE TO VIOLENCE (1991-2007)

1991	1993	1995	1997	1999	2001	2003	2005	2007	CHANGES FROM 1991 TO 2007*
CARRIED A WEAPON (FOR EXAMPLE, A GUN, KNIFE, OR CLUB ON AT LEAST 1 DAY DURING THE 30 DAYS BEFORE THE SURVEY)									
26.1 (23.7-28.5)†	22.1 (19.8-24.6)	20.0 (18.8-21.4)	18.3 (16.5-20.2)	17.3 (15.4-19.3)	17.4 (15.5-19.5)	17.1 (15.4-19.0)	18.5 (16.9-20.2)	18.0 (16.3-19.8)	Decreased, 1991-1999 No change, 1999-2007
CARRIED A GUN (ON AT LEAST 1 DAY DURING THE 30 DAYS BEFORE THE SURVEY)									
NA‡	7.9 (6.9-9.3)	7.6 (6.5-8.7)	5.9 (5.1-6.8)	4.9 (3.8-6.3)	5.7 (4.8-6.8)	6.1 (5.1-7.2)	5.4 (4.6-6.3)	5.2 (4.4-6.0)	Decreased, 1993-1999 No change, 1999-2007
IN A PHYSICAL FIGHT (ONE OR MORE TIMES DURING THE 12 MONTHS BEFORE THE SURVEY)									
42.5 (40.0-45.0)	41.8 (39.8-43.8)	38.7 (36.5-40.9)	36.6 (34.7-38.7)	35.7 (33.4-38.1)	33.2 (31.8-34.7)	33.0 (31.1-35.1)	35.9 (34.3-37.4)	35.5 (34.0-37.1)	Decreased, 1991-2003 Increased, 2003-2007
INJURED IN A PHYSICAL FIGHT WITH INJURIES THAT HAD TO BE TREATED BY A DOCTOR OR NURSE (ONE OR MORE TIMES DURING THE 12 MONTHS BEFORE THE SURVEY)									
4.4 (3.6-5.3)	4.0 (3.2-5.0)	4.2 (3.6-4.8)	3.5 (3.0-4.1)	4.0 (3.3-4.8)	4.0 (3.6-4.5)	4.2 (3.4-5.3)	3.6 (3.2-4.0)	4.2 (3.7-4.7)	No change, 1991-2007

*Based on trend analyses using a logistic regression model controlling for sex, race/ethnicity, and grade.
†95% confidence interval.
‡Not available.
From Eaton DK, Kann L, Kinchen S, et al: Youth risk behavior surveillance—United States, 2007, *MMWR Surveill Summ* 57(SS-4):1–131, 2008.

handgun is considerably higher than homicide by other weapon type, suggesting that access to firearms may play a major role in youth injuries and deaths (Fig. 107-1). A cross-sectional, nationally representative survey of ~21,000 youth at ages 11.5, 13.5, and 15.5 yr in 5 countries (Ireland, Israel, Portugal, Sweden, and the USA) revealed that the rates of fighting, weapon carrying, and fighting injury were similar among the countries while bullying frequency varied widely, from 15% in Sweden to 43% in Israel (Table 107-3).

Violence at schools in the USA and elsewhere remains a significant problem with 12.4% of students reported being in a fight on school property in the preceding 30 days. The 2007 Youth Risk Behavior Surveillance System reported 18% youths overall carried a weapon such as a gun, knife, or club in the last 30 days; 6% carried the weapon to school; and 8% reported being threatened or injured with a type of weapon on school property. Males are more likely than females to carry a gun or weapon and therefore may need increased monitoring at home and at school. Physical fighting remains prevalent at schools; 12.4% of students report having been in a physical fight on school property in the preceding 12 mo. These violence-related behaviors at school affect the students' perception of safety. Five percent of students did not go to school on 1 or more days in the preceding 30 days because they felt it unsafe at school. Dating violence (having been hit, slapped, or physically hurt intentionally by a boyfriend or girlfriend) is reported by 9.9% of students, with highest prevalence rates seen in African-American students (14.2%) and older students (10.6%, 11th graders; 12.1%, 12th graders). School-based prevention programs initiated at the elementary school level have been found to decrease violent behaviors in students. Increased surveillance of students is warranted both on and around school property to improve student safety.

Advancements of technology are being used by youths as a vehicle to inflict aggression of a different nature. The Centers for Disease Control and Prevention (CDC) defines electronic aggression as *any type of harassment or bullying (teasing, telling lies, making fun of someone, making rude or mean comments, spreading rumors, or making threatening or aggressive comments) that occurs through e-mail, chat rooms, instant messaging, blogs, test messaging or videos or photos posted on a website or sent via cell phone* (Chapter 36.1). In 2005, 9% of youth surveyed reported being a victim of online harassment via instant messaging (67%), e-mail (24%), and text messages (15%). Of the youth surveyed, 7-14% reported being both a victim and a perpetrator, suggesting that there is a related behavioral link between the 2 roles.

Parents can provide the primary prevention with filters on the home computer, increased monitoring of their teen's use of electronic interactions, and setting limits on texting and instant messaging. Many schools have established cyber-bullying policies and are increasingly involved with teaching youth about guidelines for appropriate online interactions, and monitoring for cyber-bullying problems. About 12 states have enacted legislation that allows schools to take action in response to electronic aggression or cyber-bullying against a student, whether it takes place on or off school grounds.

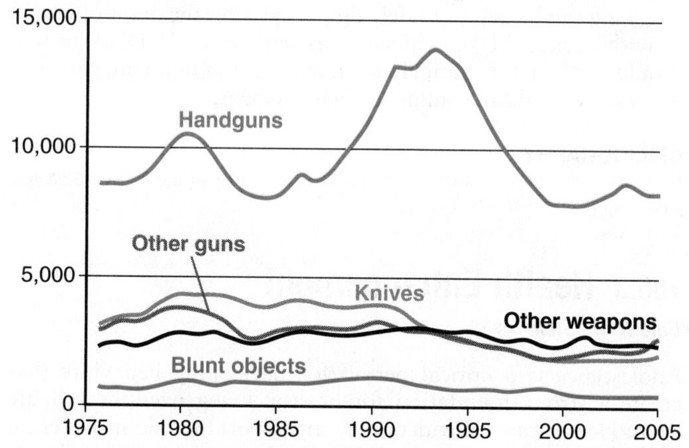

Figure 107-1 Number of victims of homicides by weapon type, 1976-2005. (From U.S. Department of Justice, Office of Justice Programs, Bureau of Justice Statistics: *Homicide trends in the U.S.* www.ojp.usdoj.gov/bjs/homicide/teens.htm. Accessed June 2009.)

ETIOLOGY

The WHO places youth violence in a model within the context of 3 larger types of violence: self-inflicted, interpersonal, and collective. **Interpersonal violence** is subdivided into violence largely between family members or partners and includes child abuse. **Community violence** occurs between individuals who are unrelated. **Collective violence** incorporates violence by people who are members of an identified group against another group of individuals with social, political, or economic motivation. The types of violence in this model have behavioral links, in that child abuse victims are more likely to experience violent and aggressive interpersonal behavior as adolescents and adults. Overlapping risk factors exist for the types of violence, such as firearm availability, alcohol use, and socioeconomic inequalities. The benefit

Table 107-3 DISTRIBUTION OF VIOLENCE INDICATORS FOR ALL COUNTRIES (%)

VIOLENCE INDICATOR	ISRAEL	IRELAND	UNITED STATES	SWEDEN	PORTUGAL	TOTAL
PHYSICAL FIGHTING, TIMES PER YEAR						
0	54.6	55.5	60.2	61.2	68.8	59.7
1	1.5	19.9	17.1	14.2	15.8	13.6
2	26.9	9.9	9.4	9.3	7.4	12.8
3	6.4	4.8	4.8	5.6	3.2	5.0
≥4	10.7	9.8	8.5	9.7	4.8	8.9
WEAPON CARRYING, DAYS PER MONTH						
0	84.0	89.6	89.6	NA	94.4	89.2
1	1.0	3.7	3.3		2.0	2.6
2-3	8.7	2.3	2.4		1.1	3.6
4-5	2.0	0.8	0.9		0.5	1.0
≥6	4.3	3.3	3.8		1.9	3.5
INJURIES FROM FIGHTING, TIMES PER YEAR						
0	82.1	82.4	84.5	NA	87.8	84.2
1	10.6	14.2	12.5		10.6	11.9
2	3.5	1.4	1.4		0.8	1.8
3	1.6	0.6	0.5		0.2	0.8
≥4	2.2	1.3	1.1		0.5	1.3
HAVE BULLIED, TIMES PER SCHOOL TERM						
None	57.0	75.5	60.8	85.2	63.8	66.2
Once or twice	24.1	18.7	24.3	10.9	24.5	21.6
Sometimes	12.3	3.8	8.8	2.4	9.2	8.0
Once a week	3.0	0.8	2.5	0.6	1.0	1.8
Several times a week	3.5	1.2	3.6	0.9	1.5	2.3

NA, not applicable.
Adapted from Table 2 in Smith-Khuri E, Iachan R , Scheidt PC, et al: A cross-national study of violence-related behaviors in adolescents, *Arch Pediatr Adolesc Med* 158(6):539–544, 2004.

to identifying common risk factors for the types of violence lies in the potential for intervening with prevention efforts and gaining positive outcomes for more than one type of violent behavior. The model further acknowledges 4 categories that explore the potential nature of violence as involving physical, sexual, or psychologic force, or deprivation.

There may be 2 types of antisocial youths: one that is life course persistent and one that is life course limited. **Adolescent-limited offenders** have no childhood aberrant behaviors and are more likely to commit status offenses such as vandalism, running away, and other behaviors symbolic of their struggle for autonomy from parents. **Life course–persistent offenders** exhibit aberrant behavior in childhood, such as problems with temperament, behavioral development, and cognition; as adolescents they participate in more victim-oriented crimes. The public health model emphasizes the environment and other external influences. A 3rd theoretical model examines violent behaviors across the spectrum occurring within and outside the family and is referred to as the **cycle of violence.** This hypothesis proposes that precursors such as child abuse and neglect, a child witnessing violence, adolescent sexual and physical abuse, and adolescent exposure to violence and violent assaults predispose youths to outcomes of violent behavior, violent crime, delinquency, violent assaults, suicide, or premature death. An additional common paradigm for high-risk violence behavior poses a balance of risk and protective factors at the individual, family, and community levels. None of these theories successfully explains interpersonal or self-inflicted violent behavior. Although the media influence violence through a modeling effect on aggressive behavior, many questions still remain about the causes of violent behavior.

CLINICAL MANIFESTATIONS

There are several identified risk factors for youth violence, including poverty, association with delinquent peers, poor school performance/low education status, disconnection from adult role models or mentors, prior history of violence or victimization, poor family functioning, childhood abuse, substance abuse, and certain mental health disorders. The most common disorders associated with aggressive behavior in adolescents are mental retardation, learning disabilities, moderately severe language disorders, and mental disorders such as attention-deficit/hyperactivity and mood disturbances. Of note, the link between severe mental illness and violent behaviors is most strongly linked for those with co-occurring alcohol or substance abuse or dependence.

Inability to master prosocial skills such as the establishment and maintenance of positive family and peer relations and poor resolution of conflict may put adolescents with these disorders at higher risk of physical violence and other risky behaviors. **Conduct disorder** and **oppositional defiant disorder** are specific psychiatric diagnoses whose definitions are associated with violent behavior (Table 107-4). They occur co-morbidly with other disorders such as attention-deficit/hyperactivity disorder and increase an adolescent's vulnerability for juvenile delinquency, substance use or abuse, sexual promiscuity, adult criminal behavior, incarceration, and antisocial personality disorder. Other co-occurring risk factors for youth violence include use of anabolic steroids, gang tattoos, belief in one's premature death, preteen alcohol use, and placement in a juvenile detention center.

DIAGNOSIS

The assessment of an adolescent at risk, or with a history of violent behavior or victimization should be a part of the health maintenance visit of all adolescents. The answers to questions about recent history of involvement in a physical fight, carrying a weapon, or firearms in the household, as well as concerns that the adolescent may have about his or her personal safety may suggest a problem requiring a more in-depth evaluation. The **FISTS** mnemonic provides guidance for structuring the

Table 107-4 OPPOSITIONAL DEFIANT DISORDER, CONDUCT DISORDER, AND JUVENILE DELINQUENCY

PSYCHIATRIC DISORDER LABELS		
Oppositional Defiant Disorder	**Conduct Disorder**	**LEGAL LABEL JUVENILE DELINQUENCY**
Recurrent pattern of negativistic, defiant, disobedient, and hostile behavior toward authority figures that has a significant adverse effect on functioning (e.g., social, academic, occupational)	Repetitive and persistent pattern of behavior that violates the basic rights of others or major age-appropriate societal norms or rules	Offenses that are illegal because of age; illegal acts
Examples: losing temper; arguing with adults; defying or refusing to comply with request or rules of adults; annoying behavior; blaming others; and being irritable, spiteful, resentful	Examples: physical fighting, deceitfulness, stealing, destruction of property, threatening or causing physical harm to people or animals, driving without a license, prostitution, rape (even if not adjudicated in the legal system)	Examples: single or multiple instances of being arrested or adjudicated for any of the following: stealing, destruction of property, threatening or causing physical harm to people or animals, driving without a license, prostitution, rape
Diagnosed by a mental health clinician	Diagnosed by a mental health practitioner	Adjudicated in the legal system

From Greydanus DE, Pratt HD, Patel DR, et al: The rebellious adolescent, *Pediatr Clin North Am* 44:1460, 1997.

Table 107-5 FISTS MNEMONIC TO ASSESS AN ADOLESCENT'S RISK OF VIOLENCE

F: Fighting (How many fights were you in last year? What was the last?)
I: Injuries (Have you ever been injured? Have you ever injured someone else?)
S: Sex (Has your partner hit you? Have you hit your partner? Have you ever been forced to have sex?)
T: Threats (Has someone with a weapon threatened you? What happened? Has anything changed to make you feel safer?)
S: Self-defense (What do you do if someone tries to pick a fight? Have you carried a weapon in self-defense?)

From Knox L: *Connecting the dots to prevent youth violence: a training and outreach guide for physicians and other health professionals,* Chicago, 2002, American Medical Association, p 24.

Table 107-6 PUBLIC HEALTH APPROACH TO YOUTH VIOLENCE PREVENTION MODEL WITH EXAMPLES

	VICTIM (HOST)	PERPETRATOR (VECTOR)	FIREARM (AGENT)	SOCIAL ENVIRONMENT	PHYSICAL ENVIRONMENT
Primary prevention	Conflict resolution Violence anticipatory guidance	Substance abuse treatment Home visiting programs for new and single parents	Handgun and assault weapons ban Firearm registration	Job opportunities Adult-supervised activities	Better lighting Zoning-enforced limits in liquor licenses
Secondary prevention	Medical services Psychologic services	Job training Psychosocial rehabilitation	Handgun locks Public education on risks of ownership	School incident debriefing Safe havens	Increased police presence Graffiti removal
Tertiary prevention	Physical rehabilitation Psychosocial services	Incarceration Educational-psychosocial rehabilitation	Firearm surveillance	Foster care Alternative schools	Urban planning, e.g., decrease population density in public housing and mixture of income levels

From Calhoun AD, Clark-Jones F: Theoretical frameworks: developmental psychopathology, the public health approach to violence, and the cycle of violence, *Pediatr Clin North Am* 45:287, 1998.

assessment (Table 107-5). The additional factors of physical or sexual abuse, serious problems at school, poor school performance and attendance, multiple incidents of trauma, substance use, and symptoms associated with mental disorders are indications for evaluation by a mental health professional. In a situation of acute trauma, assault victims are not always forthcoming about the circumstances of their injuries for fear of retaliation or police involvement. Stabilization of the injury or the gathering of forensic evidence in sexual assault is the treatment priority; however, once this is achieved, addressing a more comprehensive set of issues surrounding the assault is appropriate.

TREATMENT

In the instance of acute injury secondary to violent assault, the treatment plan should follow standards established by the American Academy of Pediatrics model protocol, which includes, but is not limited to, the stabilization of the injury, evaluation and treatment of the injury, evaluation of the assault circumstance, psychologic evaluation and support, social service evaluation of the circumstance surrounding the assault, and a treatment plan on discharge that is designed to protect the adolescent from subsequent injury episodes and minimize the development of psychologic disability. Victims as well as witnesses of violence are at risk for post-traumatic stress disorder, and future aggressive and/or violent behavior.

Multiple treatment modalities are used simultaneously in managing adolescents with persistent violent and aggressive behavior and range from cognitive-behavioral therapy involving the individual and family to specific family interventions (parent management training, multisystemic treatment) and pharmacotherapy. Treatment of existing co-morbid conditions such as attention-deficit/hyperactivity disorder, depression, and substance abuse appears to reduce aggressive behavior.

PREVENTION

The WHO report recognizes a multifactorial approach to prevention: individual approaches, relationship approaches, community approaches, and societal approaches (Table 107-6). **Individual approaches** concentrate on changing attitudes and behaviors to avoid aggressive and violent behavior as well as teaching coping strategies and nonviolent conflict resolution for all children as well as youths who have already displayed some violent tendencies. **Relationship approaches** focus more on victims, families, and peer relationships, especially those with the potential to trigger aggressive or violent responses. Solutions include improving skills in coping or problem solving in recent perceived crises, interpersonal conflicts, and close relationships. Family-based programs provide training for parents in areas of effective communication, child development, and solving problems in nonviolent methods. **Community-based approaches** raise public awareness in an effort to stimulate action by community members to reduce violence and protect vulnerable community members. Universal school-based violence prevention programs have been found to be effective in reducing violent and aggressive behaviors. Interventions beginning as early as preschool have been found to have positive outcomes years later. **Societal approaches** include broader advocacy and legislative actions, as well as changing the cultural norm toward violent behaviors. A specific prevention strategy can incorporate several approaches, such as the handgun/firearm prevention recommendations that include gun-lock safety, public education, and legislative advocacy. Other efforts are directed toward establishing a national database to track and define the problem of youth violence. The National Violent Death Reporting System (NVDRS) collects and analyzes violent death data from 17 states and aims to improve surveillance of current trends, to share information state to state, to build partnerships among state and community organizations, and to develop and implement prevention and intervention programs. Ultimately the NVDRS will be expanded to include all 50 states. The CDC characterizes specific successful programs and summarizes program content on its website *(www.cdc.gov)*.

BIBLIOGRAPHY

Please visit the Nelson Textbook of Pediatrics *website at www.expertconsult.com for the complete bibliography.*

Chapter 108
Substance Abuse

Margaret M. Stager

Adolescents are influenced by a complex interaction between biologic and psychosocial development, environmental messages, and societal attitudes about the use of substances such as alcohol, tobacco, or marijuana. Occasional or situational use of certain substances such as alcohol may be viewed as "normative" given the proportion of youths who report some experience with these substances. Others view the potential for adverse outcomes even with occasional use in immature adolescents, such as motor vehicle crashes and other injuries, sufficient justification to consider any drug use in younger adolescents a considerable risk.

Individuals who initiate drug use at an early age are at a greater risk for becoming addicted than those who try drugs in early adulthood. Drug use in younger, less experienced adolescents can act as a substitute for developing age-appropriate coping strategies and enhance vulnerability to poor decision-making. The first use of the most commonly used drugs occurs before age 18 yr, with 88% of people reporting first alcohol use <21 yr old, the legal drinking age in the USA. Inhalants have been identified as a popular first drug for youth in grade 8. When drug use begins to negatively alter functioning in adolescents at school and at home, and risk-taking behavior is seen, intervention is warranted. Serious drug use is not an isolated phenomenon. It occurs across every segment of the population and is one of the most challenging public health problems facing society. The challenge to the clinician is to identify youths at risk for substance abuse and offer early intervention. The challenge to the community and society is to create norms that decrease the likelihood of adverse health outcomes for adolescents and promote and facilitate opportunities for adolescents to choose healthier and safer options. Recognizing those drugs with the greatest *harm*, and at times focusing on *harm reduction* with or without abstinence, is an important modern approach to adolescent substance abuse (Figs. 108-1, 108-2).

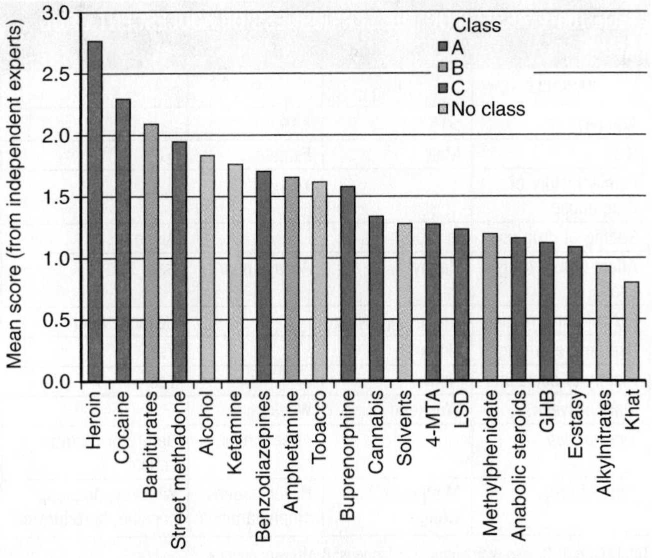

Figure 108-1 Mean harm scores for 20 substances as determined by an expert panel based on 3 criteria: physical harm to user; potential for dependence; and effect on family, community, and society. Classification under the Misuse of Drugs Act, when appropriate, is shown by the color of each bar. Class A drugs are deemed potentially most dangerous; class C least dangerous. (From Nutt D, King LA, Saulsbury W, et al: Development of a rational scale to access the harm of drugs of potential misuse, *Lancet* 369:1047–1053, 2007.)

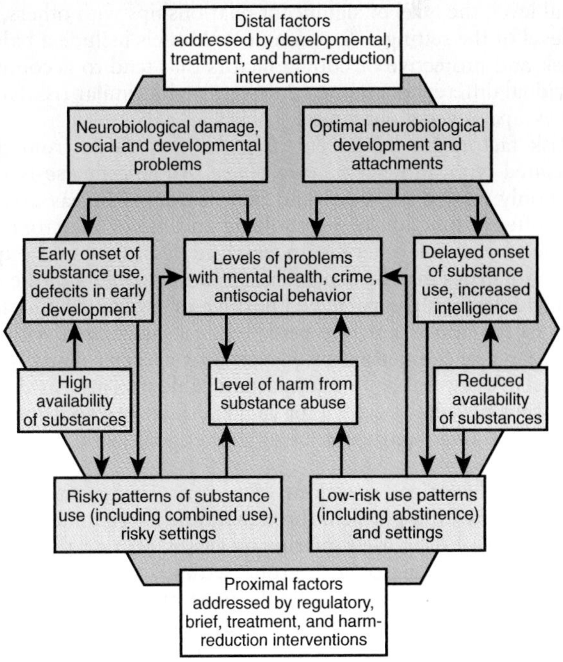

Figure 108-2 Protection and risk model for distal and proximal determinants of risky substance use and related harms. (From Toumbourou JW, Stockwell T, Neighbors C, et al: Interventions to reduce harm associated with adolescent substance use, *Lancet* 369:1391–1401, 2007.)

ETIOLOGY

Substance abuse is biopsychosocially determined (see Fig. 108-2). Biologic factors, including genetic predisposition, are established contributors. Behaviors such as rebelliousness, poor school performance, delinquency, and criminal activity and personality traits such as low self-esteem, anxiety, and lack of self-control are frequently associated with or predate the onset of drug use. Psychiatric disorders are often co-morbidly associated with adolescent substance use. Conduct disorders and antisocial personality

Table 108-1 ASSESSING THE SERIOUSNESS OF ADOLESCENT DRUG ABUSE

VARIABLE	0	+1	+2
Age (yr)	>15	<15	
Sex	Male	Female	
Family history of drug abuse		Yes	
Setting of drug use	In group		Alone
Affect before drug use	Happy	Always poor	Sad
School performance	Good, improving		Recently poor
Use before driving	None		Yes
History of accidents	None		Yes
Time of week	Weekend	Weekdays	
Time of day		After school	Before or during school
Type of drug	Marijuana, beer, wine	Hallucinogens, amphetamines	Whiskey, opiates, cocaine, barbiturates

Total score: 0-3, less worrisome; 3-8, serious; 8-18, very serious.

Table 108-2 STAGES OF ADOLESCENT SUBSTANCE ABUSE

STAGE	DESCRIPTION
1	Potential for abuse • Decreased impulse control • Need for immediate gratification • Available drugs, alcohol, inhalants • Need for peer acceptance
2	Experimentation: learning the euphoria • Use of inhalants, tobacco, marijuana, and alcohol with friends • Few, if any, consequences • Use may increase to weekends regularly • Little change in behavior
3	Regular use: seeking the euphoria • Use of other drugs, e.g., stimulants, LSD, sedatives • Behavioral changes and some consequences • Increased frequency of use; use alone • Buying or stealing drugs
4	Regular use: preoccupation with the "high" • Daily use of drugs • Loss of control • Multiple consequences and risk-taking • Estrangement from family and "straight" friends
5	Burnout: use of drugs to feel normal • Polysubstance use/cross-addiction • Guilt, withdrawal, shame, remorse, depression • Physical and mental deterioration • Increased risk-taking, self-destructive, suicidal

disorders are the most common diagnoses coexisting with substance abuse, particularly in males. Teens with depression (Chapter 24), attention deficit disorder (Chapter 30), and eating disorders (Chapter 26) have high rates of substance use. The determinants of adolescent substance use and abuse are explained using a number of theoretical models, with factors at the individual level, the level of significant relationships with others, and the level of the setting or environment. Models include a balance of risk and protective or coping factors that tend to account for individual differences among adolescents with similar risk factors who escape adverse outcomes.

Risk factors for adolescent *drug use* may differ from those associated with adolescent *drug abuse*. Adolescent *use* is more commonly related to social and peer factors, whereas *abuse* is more often a function of psychologic and biologic factors. The likelihood that an otherwise normal adolescent would experiment with drugs may be dependent on the availability of the drug to the adolescent, the perceived positive or otherwise functional value to the adolescent, the perceived risk associated with use, and the presence or absence of restraints as determined by the adolescent's cultural or other important value systems. An abusing adolescent may have genetic or biologic factors coexisting with dependence on a particular drug for coping with day-to-day activities.

Specific historical questions can assist in determining the severity of the drug problem through a rating system (Table 108-1). The type of drug used (marijuana versus heroin), the circumstances of use (alone or in a group setting), the frequency and timing of use (daily before school versus rarely on a weekend), the premorbid mental health status (depressed versus happy), as well as the teenager's general functional status should all be considered in evaluating any youngster found to be abusing a drug. The stage of drug use/abuse should also be considered (Table 108-2). A teen may spend months or years in the experimentation phase trying a variety of illicit substances including the most common drugs, cigarettes, alcohol, and marijuana. It is not until regular use of drugs resulting in negative consequences (problem use) that the teen typically become identified as having a problem, either by parents, teachers, or a physician. Certain protective factors play a part in buffering the risk factors as well as assisting in anticipating the long-term outcome of experimentation. Having emotionally supportive parents with open communication styles, involvement in organized school activities, having mentors or role models outside of the home, and recognition of the importance of academic achievement are examples of the important protective factors.

EPIDEMIOLOGY

The National Survey on Drug Use and Health is an annual survey of persons(s) from a randomly selected set of households in the USA but does not capture those who refuse to participate in the survey. School-based surveys (Monitoring the Future study and Youth Risk Behavior Surveillance) are limited to those youth enrolled and attending school and do not capture school dropouts or those youth in the juvenile detention system. The rates of drug use across surveys are not dramatically different and certain observations are consistent across surveys.

In the USA, alcohol and cigarettes and marijuana are the most commonly reported substances used among teens (Table 108-3). The prevalence of substance use and associated risky behaviors vary by age, gender, race/ethnicity, and other sociodemographic factors. Younger teenagers tend to report less use of drugs than do older teenagers, with the exception of inhalants (in 2008, 15.7% in 8th grade, 12.8% in 10th grade, 9.9% in 12th grade). Males have higher rates of both licit and illicit drug use than females, with greatest differences seen in their higher rates of frequent use of smokeless tobacco, cigars, and anabolic steroids. In school surveys, drug use patterns of Hispanics tend to fall in between whites and African-Americans, with the exception of 12th grade Hispanics reporting highest rates of crack cocaine, heroin (injected), and crystal methamphetamine use. African-Americans report less use of drugs across all drug categories with dramatically lower levels of cigarette use in comparison to whites.

In examining trends in drug use, positive findings are that fewer students reported cigarette, alcohol, or stimulant use than in the previous 5 yr. Marijuana use has leveled off after a general decline. (Past year use of marijuana in 2008: 10.9% in 8th graders, 23.9% in 10th graders, 32.4% in 12th graders.) Prescription drug abuse is increasing in prevalence with 15.4% of high school seniors reported taking a prescription drug nonmedically in the last yr (Table 108-4). For many adolescents and young adults, **prescription drug use** is the most common abused category of drugs and includes opioids, drugs that treat ADHD, antianxiety agents, dextromethorphan, antihistamines, sedatives, and tranquilizers. Many of these agents can be found in the parents' home, some are over-the-counter, while others are

Table 108-3 THIRTY DAY PREVALENCE USE OF ALCOHOL, CIGARETTES, MARIJUANA, AND INHALANTS IN 8TH GRADERS, 10TH GRADERS, AND 12TH GRADERS, 2005 AND 2008

	8TH GRADERS (%)	10TH GRADERS (%)	12TH GRADERS (%)
ALCOHOL			
2005	17.1	33.2	47.0
2008	15.9	{28.8}*	43.1
CIGARETTES (ANY USE)			
2005	9.3	14.9	23.2
2008	6.8	12.3	20.4
SMOKELESS TOBACCO			
2005	3.3	5.6	7.6
2008	3.5	5.0	6.5
MARIJUANA/HASHISH			
2005	6.6	15.2	19.8
2008	5.8	13.8	19.4
INHALANTS			
2005	4.2	2.2	2.0
2008	4.1	2.1	1.4
STEROIDS			
2005	0.5	0.6	0.9
2008	0.5	0.5	1.0

*Data in brackets indicate statistically significant change from the previous year.
National Institute of Drug Abuse: *2008 Monitoring the Future Study, NIDA InfoFacts.* www.drugabuse.gov.

purchased from drug dealers at schools and colleges. Many users believe that these drugs are benign because they are obtained by prescription or purchased at a pharmacy. Club drugs, commonly used at all-night dance parties, are increasingly popular among older adolescents and young adults (Table 108-5). These drugs have significant side effects especially if taken in combination with alcohol or other drugs. Anterograde amnesia, impaired learning ability, disassociation, and breathing difficulties may occur. Repeated use may lead to tolerance, cravings for the drug, and withdrawal effects including anxiety, tremors, and sweating.

The European School Survey Project on Alcohol and other Drugs results (4 surveys over 12 yr among European students) demonstrate declines in smoking in most of the surveyed nations; since 1995 the overall average of "smoked in the last 30 days" declined 4% to the current level of 29%. Average alcohol use in the past 12 mo (82%) remains essentially stable but heavy episodic drinking appears to have increased somewhat. There is substantial between-country variation in alcohol use. Marijuana remains the primary illicit drug used; overall in 2007 19% of youth reported ever having used marijuana, compared to only 7% reporting use of other illicit drugs.

CLINICAL MANIFESTATIONS

Although manifestations vary by the specific substance of use, adolescents who use drugs often present in an office setting with

Table 108-4 SELECTED PRESCRIPTION DRUGS WITH POTENTIAL FOR ABUSE

Selected Prescription Drugs With Potential for Abuse
Visit NIDA at www.drugabuse.gov

NIDA NATIONAL INSTITUTE ON DRUG ABUSE
U.S. Department of Health and Human Services
National Institutes of Health

Substances: Category and Name	Examples of *Commercial* and Street Names	DEA Schedule*/ How Administered**	*Intoxication Effects*/Potential Health Consequences
Depressants			*reduced pain and anxiety; feeling of well-being; lowered inhibitions; slowed pulse and breathing; lowered blood pressure; poor concentration*/confusion, fatigue; impaired coordination, memory, judgment; respiratory depression and arrest, addiction *Also, for barbiturates—sedation, drowsiness*/depression, unusual excitement, fever, irritability, poor judgment, slurred speech, dizziness *for benzodiazepines—sedation, drowsiness*/dizziness *for flunitrazepam*—visual and gastrointestinal disturbances, urinary retention, memory loss for the time under the drug's effects
barbiturates	*Amytal, Nembutal, Seconal, Phenobarbital;* barbs, reds, red birds, phennies, tooies, yellows, yellow jackets	II, III, V/injected, swallowed	
benzodiazepines (other than flunitrazepam)	*Ativan, Halcion, Librium, Valium, Xanax;* candy, downers, sleeping pills, tranks	IV/swallowed	
flunitrazepam****	*Rohypnol;* forget-me pill, Mexican Valium, R2, Roche, roofies, roofinol, rope, rophies	IV/swallowed, snorted	
Dissociative Anesthetics			*increased heart rate and blood pressure, impaired motor function*/memory loss; numbness; nausea/vomiting *Also, for ketamine—at high doses, delirium, depression, respiratory depression and arrest*
ketamine	*Ketalar SV;* cat Valium, K, Special K, vitamin K	III/injected, snorted, smoked	
Opioids and Morphine Derivatives			*pain relief, euphoria, drowsiness*/respiratory depression and arrest, nausea, confusion, constipation, sedation, unconsciousness, coma, tolerance, addiction *Also, for codeine—less analgesia, sedation, and respiratory depression than morphine*
codeine	*Empirin with Codeine, Fiorinal with Codeine, Robitussin A-C, Tylenol with Codeine;* Captain Cody, Cody, schoolboy; (with glutethimide) doors & fours, loads, pancakes and syrup	II, III, IV/injected, swallowed	
fentanyl	*Actiq, Duragesic, Sublimaze;* Apache, China girl, China white, dance fever, friend, goodfella, jackpot, murder 8, TNT, Tango and Cash	II/injected, smoked, snorted	
morphine	*Roxanol, Duramorph;* M, Miss Emma, monkey, white stuff	II, III/injected, swallowed, smoked	
opium	laudanum, paregoric; big O, black stuff, block, gum, hop	II, III, V/swallowed, smoked	
other opioid pain relievers (oxycodone, meperidine, hydromorphone, hydrocodone, propoxyphene)	*Tylox, OxyContin, Percodan, Percocet;* oxy 80s, oxycotton, oxycet, hillbilly heroin, percs *Demerol, meperidine hydrochloride;* demmies, pain killer *Dilaudid;* juice, dillies *Vicodin, Lortab, Lorcet; Darvon, Darvocet*	II, III, IV/swallowed, injected, suppositories, chewed, crushed, snorted	
Stimulants			*increased heart rate, blood pressure, metabolism; feelings of exhilaration, energy, increased mental alertness*/rapid or irregular heart beat; reduced appetite, weight loss, heart failure *Also, for amphetamines—rapid breathing; hallucinations*/tremor, loss of coordination; irritability, anxiousness, restlessness, delirium, panic, paranoia, impulsive behavior, aggressiveness, tolerance, addiction *for cocaine—increased temperature*/chest pain, respiratory failure, nausea, abdominal pain, strokes, seizures, headaches, malnutrition *for methamphetamine—aggression, violence, psychotic behavior*/memory loss, cardiac and neurological damage; impaired memory and learning, tolerance, addiction *for methylphenidate—increase or decrease in blood pressure, psychotic episodes*/digestive problems, loss of appetite, weight loss
amphetamines	*Biphetamine, Dexedrine;* bennies, black beauties, crosses, hearts, LA turnaround, speed, truck drivers, uppers	II/injected, swallowed, smoked, snorted	
cocaine	*Cocaine hydrochloride;* blow, bump, C, candy, Charlie, coke, crack, flake, rock, snow, toot	II/injected, smoked, snorted	
methamphetamine	*Desoxyn;* chalk, crank, crystal, fire, glass, go fast, ice, meth, speed	II/injected, swallowed, smoked, snorted	
methylphenidate	*Ritalin;* JIF, MPH, R-ball, Skippy, the smart drug, vitamin R	II/injected, swallowed, snorted	
Other Compounds			*no intoxication effects*/hypertension, blood clotting and cholesterol changes, liver cysts and cancer, kidney cancer, hostility and aggression, acne; adolescents, premature stoppage of growth; in males, prostate cancer, reduced sperm production, shrunken testicles, breast enlargement; in females, menstrual irregularities, development of beard and other masculine characteristics
anabolic steroids	*Anadrol, Oxandrin, Durabolin, Depo-Testosterone, Equipoise;* roids, juice	III/injected, swallowed, applied to skin	

**Schedule I and II drugs have a high potential for abuse. They require greater storage security and have a quota on manufacturing, among other restrictions. Schedule I drugs are available for research only and have no approved medical use; Schedule II drugs are available only by prescription (unrefillable) and require a form for ordering. Schedule III and IV drugs are available by prescription, may have five refills in 6 months, and may be ordered orally. Most Schedule V drugs are available over the counter.*

***Taking drugs by injection can increase the risk of infection through needle contamination with staphylococci, HIV, hepatitis, and other organisms.*

****Associated with sexual assaults.*

†Not available by prescription in U.S.

Printed September 2002, Revised April 2005

Continued

Table 108-4 SELECTED PRESCRIPTION DRUGS WITH POTENTIAL FOR ABUSE—cont'd

Facts About Prescription Drug Abuse

Medications can be effective when they are used properly, but some can be addictive and dangerous when misused. This chart provides a brief look at some prescribed medications that—when used in ways other than they are prescribed—have the potential for abuse and even addiction.

Fortunately, most Americans take their medications responsibly. Addiction to prescription drugs is rare. However, in 2003, approximately 15 million Americans reported using a prescription drug for nonmedical reasons at least once during the year.

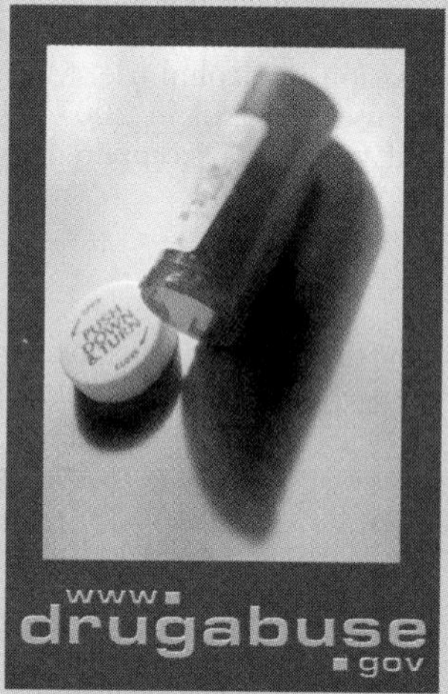

Order NIDA publications from NCADI: 1-800-729-6686 or TDD, 1-800-487-4889

What types of prescription drugs are misused or abused?

Three types of drugs are misused or abused most often:

- Opioids—prescribed for pain relief
- CNS depressants—barbiturates and benzodiazepines prescribed for anxiety or sleep problems (often referred to as sedatives or tranquilizers)
- Stimulants—prescribed for attention-deficit hyperactivity disorder (ADHD), the sleep disorder narcolepsy, or obesity.

How can you help prevent prescription drug misuse or abuse?

- Keep your doctor informed about all medications you are taking, including over-the-counter medications.
- Take your medication(s) as prescribed.
- Read the information your pharmacist provides before starting to take medications.
- Ask your doctor or pharmacist about your medication, especially if you are unsure about its effects.

More than 6.3 Million Americans Reported Current Use of Prescription Drugs for Nonmedical Purposes in 2003

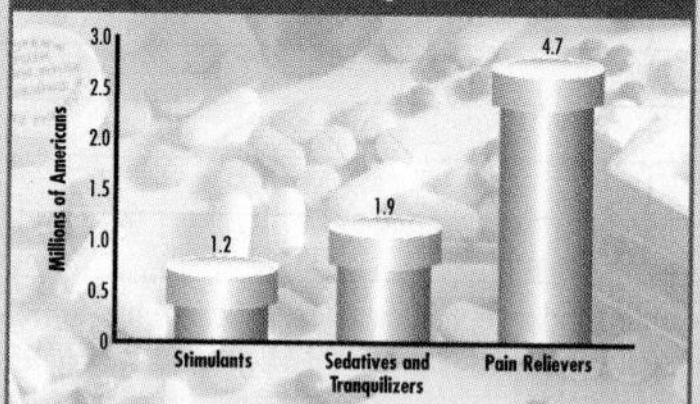

Source: Office of Applied Studies, Substance Abuse and Mental Health Services Administration. National Survey on Drug Use and Health, 2004.

Past Month Use of Selected Illicit Drugs Among Youths, by Age: 2003

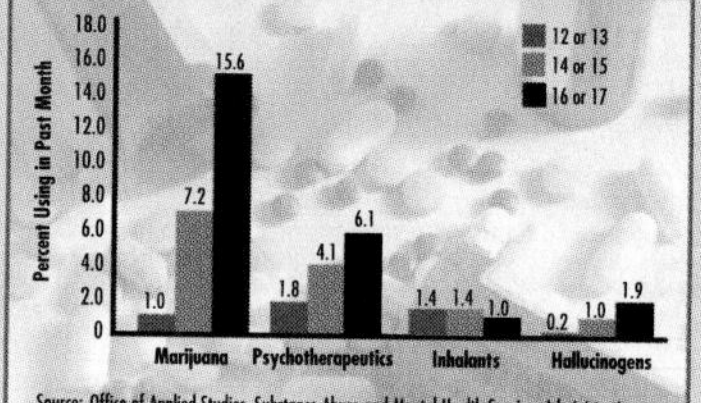

Source: Office of Applied Studies, Substance Abuse and Mental Health Services Administration. National Survey on Drug Use and Health, 2004.

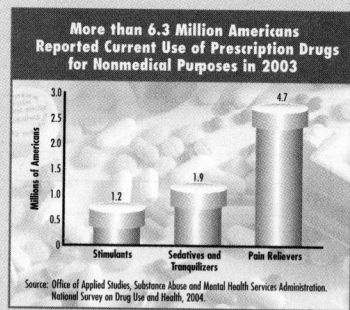

Courtesy of the National Institute on Drug Abuse, U.S. Department of Health and Human Services, National Institutes of Health, *www.drugabuse.gov*, 2005.

no obvious physical findings. Drug use is more frequently detected in adolescents who experience trauma such as motor vehicle crashes, bicycle injuries, or violence. Eliciting appropriate historical information regarding substance use, followed by blood alcohol and urine drug screens is recommended in emergency settings. An adolescent presenting to an emergency setting with an impaired sensorium should be evaluated for substance use as a part of the differential diagnosis (Table 108-6). Screening for substance use is recommended for patients with psychiatric and behavioral diagnoses. Other clinical manifestations of substance use are associated with the route of use; intravenous drug use is associated with venous "tracks" and needle marks, while nasal mucosal injuries are associated with nasal insufflation of drugs. Seizures can be a direct effect of drugs such as cocaine and amphetamines or an effect of drug withdrawal in the case of barbiturates or tranquilizers.

SCREENING FOR SUBSTANCE ABUSE DISORDERS

In a primary care setting the annual health maintenance examination provides an opportunity for identifying adolescents with substance use or abuse issues. The direct questions as well as the assessment of school performance, family relationships, and peer activities may necessitate a more in-depth interview if there are suggestions of difficulties in those areas. Additionally there are several self-report screening questionnaires available with varying degrees of standardization, length, and reliability. The **CRAFFT mnemonic** is specifically designed to screen for adolescents' substance use in the primary setting (Table 108-7). Privacy and confidentiality need to be considered when asking the teen about specifics of their substance experimentation or use. Interviewing the parents can provide additional perspective on early warning signs that go unnoticed or disregarded by the teen. Examples of early warning signs of teen substance use are change in mood, appetite, or sleep pattern; decreased interest in school or school performance; loss of weight; secretive behavior about social plans; or valuables such as money or jewelry missing from the home. The use of urine drug screening is recommended when select circumstances are present: (1) psychiatric symptoms to rule out co-morbidity or dual diagnoses, (2) significant changes in school performance or other daily behaviors, (3) frequently occurring accidents, (4) frequently occurring episodes of respiratory problems, (5) evaluation of serious motor vehicular or other injuries, and (6) as a monitoring procedure for a recovery program. Table 108-8 demonstrates the types of tests commonly used for detection by substance, along with the approximate

Table 108-5 COMMON NAMES AND SALIENT FEATURES OF CLUB DRUGS USED RECREATIONALLY

	MDMA	EPHEDRINE	γ-HYDROXYBUTYRATE	γ-BUTYROLACTONE	1,4-BUTANEDIOL	KETAMINE	FLUNITRAZEPAM	NITRITES
Common name	Ecstasy, XTC, E, X, adam, hug drug	Herbal Ecstasy, herbal fuel, zest	Liquid Ecstasy, goop soap, Georgia homeboy, grievous bodily harm	Blue nitro, longevity, revivarant, GH revitalizer, gamma G, nitro, insom-X, remforce, firewater, invigorate	Thunder nectar, serenity, pine needle extract, zen, enliven, revitalise plus, lemon drops	K, special K, vitamin K, ket, kat	Roofies, circles, rophies, rib, roche, roaches, forget pill, R2, Mexican valium, roopies ruffies	Poppers, ram, rock hard, thrust, TNT
Duration of action	4-6 hr	4-6 hr	1.5-3.5 hr	1.5-3.5 hr	1.5-3.5 hr	1-3 hr	6-12 hr	Minutes
Elimination half-life	8-9 hr	5-7 hr	27 min	ND	ND	2 hr	9-25 hr	ND
Peak plasma concentration	1-3 hr	2-3 hr	20-60 min*	15-45 min	15-45 min	20 min	1 hr	Seconds
Physical dependence	No	No	Yes	Yes	Yes	No	Yes	No
Antidote	No	No	No	No	No	No	Yes	No
DEA schedule	I	None	III	None	None	III	IV	None
Detection with routine drug screen	Yes†	Yes†	No	No	No	No‡	No‡	No
Best detection method (time frame)	GC/MS (4 hr-2 days)	GC/MS (4 hr-2 days)	GC/MS (1-12 hr)	GC/MS (1-12 hr)	GC/MS (1-12 hr)	GC/MS (1 day)	GC/MS (1-12 hr)	GC/MS (1-12 hr)

*Depends on dose.
†Concentrations that are sufficiently high can give positive results for amphetamine because of cross reactions.
‡Flunitrazepam can give positive results for benzodiazepines; ketamine can give positive results for phencyclidine.
DEA, U.S. Drug Enforcement Agency, currently reviewing possibility of flunitrazepam being placed into schedule of the U.S. Controlled Substance Act; GC/MS, gas chromatography–mass spectroscopy. Duration, half-life, and peak plasma are probably different after high or sequential doses because of nonlinear kinetics; ND, not determined in human beings.
From Ricaurte GA, McCann UD: Recognition and management of complications of new recreational drug use, *Lancet* 365:2137–2145, 2005.

Table 108-6 THE MOST COMMON TOXIC SYNDROMES

ANTICHOLINERGIC SYNDROMES	
Common signs	Delirium with mumbling speech, tachycardia, dry, flushed skin, dilated pupils, myoclonus, slightly elevated temperature, urinary retention, and decreased bowel sounds. Seizures and dysrhythmias may occur in severe cases.
Common causes	Antihistamines, antiparkinsonian medication, atropine, scopolamine, amantadine, antipsychotic agents, antidepressant agents, antispasmodic agents, mydriatic agents, skeletal muscle relaxants, and many plants (notably jimson weed and *Amanita muscaria*).
SYMPATHOMIMETIC SYNDROMES	
Common signs	Delusions, paranoia, tachycardia (or bradycardia if the drug is a pure α-adrenergic agonist), hypertension, hyperpyrexia, diaphoresis, piloerection, mydriasis, and hyperreflexia. Seizures, hypotension, and dysrhythmias may occur in severe cases.
Common causes	Cocaine, amphetamine, methamphetamine (and its derivatives 3,4-methylenedioxyamphetamine, 3,4-methylenedioxymethamphetamine, 3,4-methylenedioxyethamphetamine, and 2,5-dimethoxy-4-bromoamphetamine), and over-the-counter decongestants (phenylpropanolamine, ephedrine, and pseudoephedrine). In caffeine and theophylline overdoses, similar findings, except for the organic psychiatric signs, result from catecholamine release.
OPIATE, SEDATIVE, OR ETHANOL INTOXICATION	
Common signs	Coma, respiratory depression, miosis, hypotension, bradycardia, hypothermia, pulmonary edema, decreased bowel sounds, hyporeflexia, and needle marks. Seizures may occur after overdoses of some narcotics, notably propoxyphene.
Common causes	Narcotics, barbiturates, benzodiazepines, ethchlorvynol, glutethimide, methyprylon, methaqualone, meprobamate, ethanol, clonidine, and guanabenz.
CHOLINERGIC SYNDROMES	
Common signs	Confusion, central nervous system depression, weakness, salivation, lacrimation, urinary and fecal incontinence, gastrointestinal cramping, emesis, diaphoresis, muscle fasciculations, pulmonary edema, miosis, bradycardia or tachycardia, and seizures.
Common causes	Organophosphate and carbamate insecticides, physostigmine, edrophonium, and some mushrooms.

From Kulig K: Initial management of ingestions of toxic substances, *N Engl J Med* 326:1678, 1992.

Table 108-7 CRAFFT MNEMONIC TOOL

- Have you ever ridden in a **C**ar driven by someone (including yourself) who was high or had been using alcohol or drugs?
- Do you ever use alcohol or drugs to **R**elax, feel better about yourself or fit in?
- Do you ever use alcohol or drugs while you are by yourself (**A**lone)?
- Do you ever **F**orget things you did while using alcohol or drugs?
- Do your **F**amily or **F**riends ever tell you that you should cut down on your drinking or drug use?
- Have you ever gotten into **T**rouble while you were using alcohol or drugs?

Adapted from Anglin TM: Evaluation by interview and questionnaire. In Schydlower M, editor: *Substance abuse: a guide for health professionals*, ed 2, Elk Grove Village, IL, 2002, American Academy of Pediatrics, p 69.

Table 108-8 URINE SCREENING FOR DRUGS COMMONLY ABUSED BY ADOLESCENTS

DRUG	MAJOR METABOLITE	INITIAL	FIRST CONFIRMATION	SECOND CONFIRMATION	APPROXIMATE RETENTION TIME
Alcohol (blood)	Acetaldehyde	GC	IA		7-10 hr
Alcohol (urine)	Acetaldehyde	GC	IA		10-13 hr
Amphetamines		TLC	IA	GC, GC/MS	48 hr
Barbiturates		IA	TLC	GC, GC/MS	Short-acting (24 hr); long-acting (2-3 wk)
Benzodiazepines		IA	TLC	GC, GC/MS	3 days
Cannabinoids	Carboxy- and hydroxymetabolites	IA	TLC	GC/MS	3-10 days (occasional user); 1-2 mo (chronic user)
Cocaine	Benzoylecgonine	IA	TLC	GC/MS	2-4 days
Methaqualone	Hydroxylated metabolites	TLC	IA	GC/MS	2 wk
Opiates					
Heroin	Morphine	IA	TLC	GC, GC/MS	2 days
	Glucuronide				
Morphine	Morphine	IA	TLC	GC, GC/MS	2 days
	Glucuronide				
Codeine	Morphine	IA	TLC	GC, GC/MS	2 days
	Glucuronide				
Phencyclidine		TLC	IA	GC, GC/MS	8 days

GC, gas chromatography; IA, immunoassay; MS, mass spectrometry; TLC, thin-layer chromatography.
Modified from Drugs of abuse—urine screening [physician information sheet]. Los Angeles, Pacific Toxicology. From MacKenzie RG, Kipke MD: Substance use and abuse. In Friedman SB, Fisher M, Schonberg SK, editors: *Comprehensive adolescent health care*, St Louis, 1998, Mosby.

retention time between the use and the identification of the substance in the urine. Most initial screening uses an immunoassay method such as the enzyme-multiplied immunoassay technique followed by a confirmatory test using highly sensitive, highly specific gas chromatography–mass spectrometry. The substances that can cause false-positive results should be considered, especially when there is a discrepancy between the physical findings and the urine drug screen result. In 2007 the American of Academy of Pediatrics released guidelines that strongly discourage home-based or school-based testing.

DIAGNOSIS

Substance abuse is characterized by a maladaptive pattern of use indicated by continued use despite serious consequences or physical harm. *Chemical dependence* can be defined as a chronic and progressive disease process characterized by loss of control over use, compulsion, and the establishment of an altered state where one requires continued administration of a psychoactive substance in order to feel good or to avoid feeling bad. Diagnosing substance abuse rests on the realization that all children and adolescents are at risk but that some are at substantially more risk than others. Specific diagnostic codes are assigned to substance abuse and substance dependence (Table 108-9). These criteria are used in adults and have limitations in use with adolescents due to differing patterns of use, developmental implications, and other age-related consequences; an additional adolescent-sensitive set of criteria specifically for diagnostic use has not been developed. Adolescents who meet diagnostic criteria should be referred to a program for substance abuse treatment unless the primary care physician has additional training in addiction medicine.

COMPLICATIONS

Substance use in adolescence is associated with co-morbidities and acts of juvenile delinquency. Youth may engage in other high risk behaviors such as robbery, burglary, drug dealing, or prostitution for the purpose of acquiring the money necessary to buy drugs or alcohol. Regular use of any drug eventually diminishes judgment and is associated with unprotected sexual activity with its consequences of pregnancy and sexually transmitted infections, including HIV, as well as physical violence and trauma. Drug and alcohol use is closely associated with trauma in the adolescent population. Several studies of adolescent trauma victims have identified cannabinoids and cocaine in blood and urine samples in significant proportions (40%), in addition to the more common identification of alcohol. Any use of injected substances involves the risk of hepatitis B and C viruses as well as HIV.

Table 108-9 DSM-IV-TR DIAGNOSTIC CRITERIA FOR SUBSTANCE ABUSE AND SUBSTANCE DEPENDENCE

SUBSTANCE ABUSE: A maladaptive pattern of substance use leading to clinical significant impairment of distress as manifested by one or more of the following criteria:

- Recurrent substance use resulting in a failure to fulfill major role obligations at work, school, or home (e.g., substance-related absences or suspensions from school, being fired from a job)
- Recurrent substance use in circumstances that are physically hazardous (e.g., driving an automobile, skiing, swimming, rock climbing, riding a bicycle, scooter or skateboard, or operating machinery while impaired by a substance's effects)
- Recurrent substance-related legal problems (e.g., arrest for driving under the influence, disorderly conduct, or vandalism, while impaired by a substance's effects)
- Continued substance use despite persistent or recurrent social or interpersonal problems caused or exacerbated by the effects of the substance (e.g., physical fights or unpleasant argument, damaging furniture or punching holes in the wall, sexual behavior that is later regretted)

From American Psychiatric Association: *Diagnostic and statistical manual of mental disorders, fourth edition, text revision,* Washington, DC, 2000, American Psychiatric Association.

TREATMENT

Adolescent drug abuse is a complex condition requiring a multidisciplinary approach that attends to the needs of the individual, not just drug use. Three decades of research analyzing effective drug abuse treatment have yielded 13 fundamental principles for treatment. In brief these include accessibility to treatment; utilizing a multidisciplinary approach; employing individual or group counseling; offering mental health services; monitoring of drug use while in treatment; and understanding that recovery from drug abuse/addiction may involve multiple relapses. For most patients, remaining in treatment for a minimum period of 3 mo will result in a significant improvement.

PROGNOSIS

For adolescent substance abusers who have been referred to a drug treatment program, positive outcomes are directly related to regular attendance in post-treatment groups. For males with learning problems or conduct disorder, their outcomes are poorer than those without such disorders. Peer use patterns and parental use have a major influence on outcome for males. For females, factors such as self-esteem and anxiety are more important influences on outcomes. The chronicity of a substance use disorder makes relapse an issue that must always be kept in mind when managing patients after treatment, and appropriate assistance from a health professional qualified in substance abuse management should be obtained.

PREVENTION

Preventing drug use among children and teens requires prevention efforts aimed at the individual, family, school, and community levels. The National Institute on Drug Abuse (NIDA) has identified essential principles of successful prevention programs. Programs should enhance protective factors (parent support) and reduce risk factors (poor self-control); should address all forms of drug abuse (legal and illegal); should address the specific type(s) of drug abuse within an identified community; and should be culturally competent to improve effectiveness. See Table 108-10 for examples of risk factors and protective factors within those domains. The highest risk periods for substance use in children and adolescents are during life transitions such as the move from elementary school to middle school, or from middle school to high school. Prevention programs need to target these emotionally and socially intense times for teens in order to adequately anticipate potential substance use or abuse. Examples of effective research-based drug abuse prevention programs featuring a variety of strategies are listed on the NIDA website (*www.drugabuse.gov*), and on the Center for Substance Abuse Prevention website (*www.prevention.samhsa.gov*).

Table 108-10 DOMAINS OF RISK AND PROTECTIVE FACTORS FOR SUBSTANCE ABUSE PREVENTION

RISK FACTORS	DOMAIN	PROTECTIVE FACTORS
Early aggressive behavior	Individual	Self-control
Lack of parental supervision	Family	Parental monitoring
Substance abuse	Peer	Academic competence
Drug availability	School	Anti–drug use policies
Poverty	Community	Strong neighborhood attachment

From National Institute on Drug Abuse: *Preventing drug use among children and adolescents. A research based guide for parents, educators, and community leaders.* NIH publication No. 04-4212(B), ed 2, Bethesda, MD, 2003, National Institute on Drug Abuse.

BIBLIOGRAPHY
Please visit the Nelson Textbook of Pediatrics *website at* *www.expertconsult.com* *for the complete bibliography.*

108.1 Alcohol

Margaret M. Stager

Alcohol is the most popular drug among teens. By 12th grade, close to 75% of adolescents in U.S. high schools report ever having an alcoholic drink, with 24% having their first drink before age 13 yr; rates are even higher among European youth. Multiple factors can affect a young teen's risk of developing a drinking problem at an early age (Table 108-11). Moreover, 30% of high school seniors admit to combining drinking behaviors with other risky behaviors such as driving or taking additional substances. Binge drinking remains especially problematic among the older teens and young adults. Thirty-six percent of high school seniors report having 5 or more drinks in a row in the last 30 days. Teens with binge drinking patterns are more likely to be assaulted, engage in high risk sexual behaviors, have academic problems, and acquire injuries than those teens without binge drinking patterns.

Alcohol contributes to more deaths in young individuals than all the illicit drugs combined. Among studies of adolescent trauma victims, alcohol is reported to be present in 32-45% of hospital admissions. Motor vehicle crashes are the most frequent type of event associated with alcohol use, but the injuries spanned several types including self-inflicted wounds.

Table 108-11 RISK FACTORS FOR A TEEN DEVELOPING A DRINKING PROBLEM

FAMILY RISK FACTORS
• Low parental supervision • Poor parent to teen communication • Family conflicts • Severe or inconsistent family discipline • Having a parent with an alcohol or drug problem
INDIVIDUAL RISK FACTORS
• Poor impulse control • Emotional instability • Thrill seeking behaviors • Behavioral problems • Perceived risk of drinking is low • Begins drinking before age 14 years

PHARMACOLOGY AND PATHOPHYSIOLOGY

Alcohol (ethyl alcohol or ethanol) is rapidly absorbed in the stomach and is transported to the liver and metabolized by 2 pathways. The primary metabolic pathway contributes to the excess synthesis of triglycerides, a phenomenon that is responsible for producing a **fatty liver,** even in those who are well nourished. Engorgement of hepatocytes with fat causes necrosis, triggering an inflammatory process (**alcoholic hepatitis**), which is later followed by fibrosis, the hallmark of **cirrhosis.** Early hepatic involvement may result in elevation in γ-glutamyl transpeptidase and serum glutamic-pyruvic transaminase. The second metabolic pathway, which is utilized at high serum alcohol levels, involves the microsomal enzyme system of the liver, in which the cofactor is reduced nicotinamide-adenine dinucleotide phosphate. The net effect of activation of this pathway is to decrease metabolism of drugs that share this system and to allow for their accumulation, enhanced effect, and possible toxicity.

CLINICAL MANIFESTATIONS

Alcohol acts primarily as a central nervous system depressant. It produces euphoria, grogginess, talkativeness, impaired short-term memory, and an increased pain threshold. Alcohol's ability to produce vasodilation and hypothermia is also centrally mediated. At very high serum levels, respiratory depression occurs. Its inhibitory effect on pituitary antidiuretic hormone release is responsible for its diuretic effect. The gastrointestinal complications of alcohol use can occur from a single large ingestion. The most common is acute erosive **gastritis,** which is manifested by epigastric pain, anorexia, vomiting, and heme-positive stools. Less commonly, vomiting and midabdominal pain may be caused by acute alcoholic **pancreatitis;** diagnosis is confirmed by the finding of elevated serum amylase and lipase levels.

DIAGNOSIS

Primary care settings provide opportunity to screen teens for alcohol use or problem behaviors. Brief alcohol screening instruments (CRAFFT [see Table 108-7] or AUDIT [Alcohol Use Disorders Identification Test, Table 108-12]) perform well in a clinical setting as techniques to identify *Diagnostic and Statistical Manual of Mental Disorders,* 4th edition (DSM-IV)–defined adolescents with alcohol use disorders (Table 108-13). A score of ≥8 on the AUDIT questionnaire identifies people who drink excessively and who would benefit from reducing or ceasing drinking (see Table 108-12). Teenagers in the early phases of alcohol use exhibit few physical findings. Recent use of alcohol may be

Table 108-12 ALCOHOL USE DISORDERS IDENTIFICATION TEST (AUDIT)

	SCORE (0-4)*
1. How often do you have a drink containing alcohol?	Never (0) to more than four per week (4)
2. How many drinks containing alcohol do you have on a typical day?	One or two (0) to more than ten (4)
3. How often do you have six or more drinks on one occasion?	Never (0) to daily or almost daily (4)
4. How often during the last year have you found that you were not able to stop drinking once you had started?	Never (0) to daily or almost daily (4)
5. How often during the last year have you failed to do what was normally expected from you because of drinking?	Never (0) to daily or almost daily (4)
6. How often during the last year have you needed a first drink in the morning to get yourself going after a heavy drinking session?	Never (0) to daily or almost daily (4)
7. How often during the last year have you had a feeling of guilt or remorse after drinking?	Never (0) to daily or almost daily (4)
8. How often during the last year have you been unable to remember what happened the night before because you had been drinking?	Never (0) to daily or almost daily (4)
9. Have you or someone else been injured as a result of your drinking?	No (0) to yes, during the last year (4)
10. Has a relative, friend, doctor or other health worker been concerned about your drinking or suggested that you should cut down?	No (0) to yes, during the last year (4)

*Score ≥8 = problem drinking.
From Schuckit MA: Alcohol-use disorders, *Lancet* 373:492–500, 2009, Table 1.

Table 108-13 CRITERIA FOR DIAGNOSIS OF ALCOHOL DEPENDENCE, ACCORDING TO DIAGNOSTIC AND STATISTICAL MANUAL (DSM-IV) AND INTERNATIONAL CLASSIFICATION OF DISEASES (ICD-10)

DIAGNOSTIC AND STATISTICAL MANUAL (DSM-IV)
• Tolerance to alcohol • Withdrawal syndrome • Greater alcohol use than intended* • Desire to use alcohol and inability to control use • Devotion of large proportion of time to getting and using alcohol, and recovering from alcohol use • Neglect of social, work, or recreational activities • Continued alcohol use despite physical or psychological problems
INTERNATIONAL CLASSIFICATION OF DISEASES (ICD-10)
• Strong desire or compulsion to use alcohol • Inability to control use • Withdrawal syndrome • Tolerance to alcohol • Neglect of pleasures or interests • Continued alcohol use despite physical or psychological problems Alcohol dependence is defined as three or more of these criteria in a 12-month period.

reflected in elevated gamma-glutamyl transferase (GGT) and amino transferase (AST).

In acute care settings, the **alcohol overdose syndrome** should be suspected in any teenager who appears disoriented, lethargic, or comatose. Although the distinctive aroma of alcohol may assist in diagnosis, confirmation by analysis of blood is recommended. At levels >200 mg/dL, the adolescent is at risk of death, and levels >500 mg/dL (median lethal dose) are usually associated with a fatal outcome. When the level of obtundation appears excessive for the reported blood alcohol level, head trauma, hypoglycemia, or ingestion of other drugs should be considered as possible confounding factors.

TREATMENT

The usual mechanism of death from the alcohol overdose syndrome is respiratory depression, and artificial ventilatory support must be provided until the liver can eliminate sufficient amounts of alcohol from the body. In a patient without alcoholism, it generally takes 20 hr to reduce the blood level of alcohol from 400 mg/dL to zero. Dialysis should be considered when the blood level is >400 mg/dL. As a follow-up to acute treatment, referral for treatment of the alcohol use disorder is indicated. Group counseling, individualized counseling, and multifamily educational intervention have been found to be quite effective interventions for teens.

BIBLIOGRAPHY

Please visit the Nelson Textbook of Pediatrics *website at* www.expertconsult.com *for the complete bibliography.*

108.2 Tobacco

Margaret M. Stager

CIGARETTES

Nearly 5 million persons die annually from smoking across the globe; the number of deaths is roughly equal between developing nations and industrialized nations. Compared to all other substances and firearms, tobacco kills more individuals in the USA each yr than all these other causes combined. The average smoker in the USA starts at age 12 yr, and most are regular smokers by age 14 yr. More than 90% of adolescent smokers become adult smokers. Factors associated with youth tobacco use include exposure to smokers (friends, parents), availability of tobacco, low socioeconomic status, poor school performance, low self-esteem, lack of perceived risk of use, and lack of skills to resist influences to tobacco use.

Current smoking rates among high school students have trended downward over the last decade for lifetime cigarette use (from 20.0% to 12.4%) and current frequent cigarette use (from 16.8% to 8.1%). Overall, more whites report current tobacco use (29.9%) than Hispanics (20.1%) or blacks (16.0%). Clove cigarettes (kreteks) and flavored cigarettes (bidis) are popular with younger students. Both types of flavored cigarettes contain tobacco with other additives and deliver more nicotine and other harmful substances because they are unfiltered. Cigar or mini-cigar (cigarillo) use is reported most frequently by older male students (26.2%). Tobacco use is linked to other high risk behaviors. Teens who smoke are more likely than nonsmokers to use alcohol and engage in unprotected sex, are 8 times more likely to use marijuana, and are 22 times more likely to use cocaine.

Tobacco is used by teens in all regions of the world, although the form of tobacco used differs. In the Americas and Europe, cigarette smoking prevalence is higher than other tobacco use, although cigars and smokeless tobacco are also used; in the Eastern Mediterranean, shisha (flavored tobacco smoked in hookah pipes) is prevalent; in Southeast Asia, smokeless tobacco products are used; in the Western Pacific, betel nut is chewed with tobacco; and pipe, snuff, and rolled tobacco leaves are used in Africa.

PHARMACOLOGY

Nicotine, the primary active ingredient in cigarettes, is addictive. Nicotine is absorbed by multiple sites in the body, including the lungs, skin, gastrointestinal tract, and buccal and nasal mucosa. The action of nicotine is mediated through nicotinic acetylcholine receptors located on noncholinergic presynaptic and postsynaptic sites in the brain and causes increased levels of dopamine. Nicotine also stimulates the adrenal glands to release epinephrine, causing an immediate elevation in blood pressure, respiration and heart rate. The average nicotine content of 1 cigarette is 10 mg and the average nicotine intake per cigarette ranges from 1.0 to 3 mg. Nicotine, as delivered in cigarette smoke, has a half-life of about 2 hr. **Cotinine** is the major metabolite of nicotine via C-oxidation. It has a biologic half-life of 19-24 hr and can be detected in urine, serum, and saliva.

CLINICAL MANIFESTATIONS

Adverse health effects from regular smoking include an increased prevalence of chronic cough, sputum production, and wheezing. Smoking during pregnancy is associated with an average decrease in fetal weight of 200 g; this decrease, added to the already smaller size of infants born to teenagers, increases perinatal morbidity and mortality. Tobacco smoke induces hepatic smooth endoplasmic reticulum enzymes and, as a result, may also influence metabolism of drugs such as phenacetin, theophylline, and imipramine. Withdrawal symptoms can occur when adolescents try to quit. Irritability, decreased concentration, increased appetite, and strong cravings for tobacco are common withdrawal symptoms. Nicotine dependence is defined in Table 108-14.

TREATMENT

The approach to smoking cessation in adolescents includes the 5 A's (**Ask, Advise, Assess, Assist, and Arrange**) and use of nicotine replacement therapy in addicted teens who are motivated to quit and are not using smokeless tobacco (SLT). Consensus panels recommend the 5 A's although evidence of efficacy in adolescents

Table 108-14 CHARACTERISTICS OF NICOTINE DEPENDENCE BASED ON THE DIAGNOSTIC AND STATISTICAL MANUAL VERSION IV (DSM-IV) AND THE INTERNATIONAL CLASSIFICATION OF DISEASES REVISION 10 (ICD-10)

DSM-IV CRITERIA
Three or more of the following at any time in the same 12-month period: • Tolerance—smoker needs increased amounts of nicotine to achieve desired effect, or diminished effect with continued use of same amount • Withdrawal symptoms • Nicotine often taken in larger amounts or over a longer period than intended • Persistent or unsuccessful efforts to cut down or control use • Great deal of time spent in activities necessary to obtain nicotine or recover from its effects • Important social, occupational, or recreational activities given up or reduced because of nicotine use • Nicotine use continued despite knowledge of having a persistent or recurrent physical or psychological problem that is likely to have been caused or exacerbated by it
ICD-10 CRITERIA
A cluster of behavioral, cognitive, and psychologic occurrences that develop after repeated use: • Increased tolerance • Sometimes physical withdrawal symptoms • A strong desire to take nicotine • Difficulty controlling use • Higher priority given to nicotine use than to other activities and obligations • Persisting use despite harmful effects

From American Psychiatric Association: *Diagnostic and statistical manual of mental disorders, fourth edition, text revision,* Washington, DC, 2000, American Psychiatric Association.

is limited. Nicotine patch studies to date in adolescents suggest a positive effect on reducing withdrawal symptoms and that pharmacotherapy should be combined with behavioral therapy to reach higher cessation and lower relapse rates. Nicotine is also available as a gum, inhaler, nasal spray, lozenge, or microtab. Medications such as bupropion are not approved for use under 18 yr old; some pilot studies in adolescents report cessation efficacy with 150 mg or 300 mg of bupropion daily. Varenicline has successfully been used in adults but may be associated with a risk of suicide. Additional options may be available through formal smoking cessation programs offered by community agencies.

SMOKELESS TOBACCO

Surveys in the late 1980s and 1990s indicating the increased use of SLT prompted the National Cancer Institute to lead the U.S. federal government's effort to prevent SLT use, especially in adolescents. Surveys indicate that from the early to mid 1990s to 2008, lifetime prevalence of SLT use continues to decline in 8th, 10th, and 12th graders. It remains more popular with boys than girls (13.4% versus 2.3%). While it is less lethal, SLT carries risks of addiction and oral problems such as receding gums/gingivitis and precancerous leukoplakia.

BIBLIOGRAPHY

Please visit the Nelson Textbook of Pediatrics *website at www.expertconsult.com for the complete bibliography.*

108.3 Marijuana

Margaret M. Stager

Marijuana (THC, "pot," "weed," "hash," "grass"), derived from the *Cannabis sativa* hemp plant, is the most commonly abused illicit drug. The main active chemical, tetrahydrocannabinol (THC), is responsible for its hallucinogenic properties. THC is absorbed rapidly by the nasal or oral routes, producing a peak of subjective effect at 10 min and 1 hr, respectively. Marijuana is generally smoked as a cigarette ("reefer" or "joint") or in a pipe.

Table 108-15 ACUTE AND CHRONIC ADVERSE EFFECTS OF CANNABIS USE

ACUTE ADVERSE EFFECTS
• Anxiety and panic, especially in naive users • Psychotic symptoms (at high doses) • Road crashes if a person drives while intoxicated
CHRONIC ADVERSE EFFECTS
• Cannabis dependence syndrome (in around one in ten users) • Chronic bronchitis and impaired respiratory function in regular smokers • Psychotic symptoms and disorders in heavy users, especially those with a history of psychotic symptoms or a family history of these disorders • Impaired educational attainment in adolescents who are regular users • Subtle cognitive impairment in those who are daily users for 10 years or more

From Hall W, Degenhardt L: Adverse health effects of non-medical cannabis use, *Lancet* 374:1383–1390, 2009.

Although there is much variation in content, each cigarette contains 8-10% THC. Another popular form that is smoked, a "blunt," is a hollowed-out small cigar refilled with marijuana. Hashish is the concentrated THC resin in a sticky black liquid or oil. While marijuana use by teens has declined in the last decade, 32.4% of U.S. high school seniors report past-year use; 19% of European students reported use of marijuana at least once during their lifetime. Worldwide, including sub-Saharan Africa and Asia, it represents the majority of illicit drug use by youth.

CLINICAL MANIFESTATIONS

In addition to the "desired" effects of elation and euphoria, marijuana may cause impairment of short-term memory, poor performance of tasks requiring divided attention (e.g., those involved in driving), loss of critical judgment, decreased coordination, and distortion of time perception (Table 108-15). Visual hallucinations and perceived body distortions occur rarely, but there may be "flashbacks" or recall of frightening hallucinations experienced under marijuana's influence that usually occur during stress or with fever.

Smoking marijuana for a minimum of 4 days/wk for 6 mo appears to result in dose-related suppression of plasma testosterone levels and spermatogenesis, prompting concern about the potential deleterious effect of smoking marijuana before completion of pubertal growth and development. There is an antiemetic effect of oral THC or smoked marijuana, often followed by appetite stimulation, which is the basis of the drug's use in patients receiving cancer chemotherapy. Although the possibility of teratogenicity has been raised because of findings in animals, there is no evidence of such effects in humans. An **amotivational syndrome** has been described in long-term marijuana users who lose interest in age-appropriate behavior, yet proof of the causative relationship remains equivocal. Chronic use is associated with increased anxiety and depression, learning problems, poor job performance, and respiratory problems such as pharyngitis, sinusitis, bronchitis, and asthma (see Table 108-15).

The increased THC content of marijuana of 5- to 15-fold in the 1990s, as compared to the 1970s, is related to the observation of a **withdrawal syndrome,** occurring 24 to 48 hr after discontinuing the drug. Heavy users experience malaise, irritability, agitation, insomnia, drug craving, shakiness, diaphoresis, night sweats, and gastrointestinal disturbance. The symptoms peak by the 4th day, and they resolve in 10-14 days. Certain drugs may interact with marijuana to potentiate sedation (alcohol, diazepam), potentiate stimulation (cocaine, amphetamines), or be antagonistic (propranolol, phenytoin).

Behavioral interventions, including cognitive-behavioral therapy and motivational incentives, have shown to be effective in treating marijuana dependency.

BIBLIOGRAPHY
Please visit the Nelson Textbook of Pediatrics *website at* *www.expertconsult.com* *for the complete bibliography.*

108.4 Inhalants

Margaret M. Stager

Inhalants, found in many common household products, comprise a diverse group of volatile substances whose vapors can be inhaled to produce psychoactive effects. The practice of inhalation is popular among younger adolescents and decreases with age. Young adolescents are attracted to these substances because of their rapid action, easy availability, and low cost. Products that are abused as inhalants include volatile solvents (paint thinners, glue), aerosols (spray paint, hair spray), gases (propane tanks, lighter fluid), and nitrites ("poppers" or "video head cleaner"). The most popular inhalants among young adolescents are glue, shoe polish, and spray paint. The various products contain a wide range of chemicals with serious adverse health effects (Table 108-16). **Huffing,** the practice of inhaling fumes can be accomplished using a paper bag containing a chemical-soaked cloth, spraying aerosols directly into the nose/mouth, or using a balloon, plastic bag, or soda can filled with fumes. The percentage of adolescents using inhalants continues to decline, with 3.9% of high school students reported having used inhalants in the preceding 30-day period (2008); 9% of European youth reported ever using inhalants. Inhalant use has been high among Native American youth perhaps resulting from isolation and lower educational levels; Eskimo youth living in 14 isolated villages in the Bering Strait reported a lifetime of inhalant use of 48%.

CLINICAL MANIFESTATIONS

The major effects of inhalants are psychoactive (Table 108-17). The intoxication lasts only a few minutes, so a typical user will huff repeatedly over an extended period of time (hours) in order to maintain the high. The immediate effects of inhalants are similar to alcohol: euphoria, slurred speech, decreased coordination, and dizziness. Toluene, the main ingredient in model airplane glue and some rubber cements, causes relaxation and pleasant hallucinations for up to 2 hr. Euphoria is followed by violent excitement or coma may result from prolonged or rapid inhalation. Volatile nitrites, such as amyl nitrite, butyl nitrite, and related compounds marketed as room deodorizers, are used as euphoriants, enhancers of musical appreciation, and sexual enhancements among older adolescents and young adults. They may result in headaches, syncope, and lightheadedness; profound hypotension and cutaneous flushing followed by vasoconstriction and tachycardia; transiently inverted T waves and depressed ST segments on electrocardiography; methemoglobinemia; increased bronchial irritation; and increased intraocular pressure.

COMPLICATIONS

Model airplane glue is responsible for a wide range of complications, related to chemical toxicity, to the method of administration (in plastic bags, with resultant suffocation), and to the often dangerous setting in which the inhalation occurs (inner-city roof tops). Common neuromuscular changes reported in chronic inhalant abusers include difficulty coordinating movement, gait disorders, muscle tremors, and spasticity, particularly in the legs (Table 108-18). Moreover, chronic use may cause pulmonary hypertension, restrictive lung defects or reduced diffusion capacity, peripheral neuropathy, hematuria, tubular acidosis, and possibly cerebral and cerebellar atrophy. Chronic inhalant abuse has long been linked to widespread brain damage and cognitive abnormalities that can range from mild impairment (poor memory, decreased learning ability) to severe dementia. Death in the acute phase may result from cerebral or pulmonary edema or myocardial involvement (see Table 108-18).

DIAGNOSIS

Diagnosis of inhalants is difficult because of the ubiquitous nature of the products and decreased parental awareness of their dangers. In the primary care setting, providers need to enquire of parents if they have witnessed any unusual behaviors in their teen; noticed high-risk products in their bedrooms; seen paint on the teen's hands, nose, or mouth; or found paint coated or chemical coated rags. Complete blood counts, coagulation studies, and hepatic and renal function studies may identify the complications. In extreme intoxication, a user may manifest symptoms of restlessness, general muscle weakness, dysarthria, nystagmus, disruptive behavior, and occasionally hallucinations. Toluene is excreted

Table 108-16 HAZARDS OF CHEMICALS FOUND IN COMMONLY ABUSED INHALANTS

Amyl nitrite, butyl nitrite *("poppers," "video head cleaner")*: sudden sniffing death syndrome, suppressed immunologic function, injury to red blood cells (interfering with oxygen supply to vital tissues)
Benzene *(found in gasoline)*: bone marrow injury, impaired immunologic function, increased risk of leukemia, reproductive system toxicity
Butane, propane *(found in lighter fluid, hair and paint sprays)*: sudden sniffing death syndrome via cardiac effects, serious burn injuries (because of flammability)
Freon *(used as a refrigerant and aerosol propellant)*: sudden sniffing death syndrome, respiratory obstruction and death (from sudden cooling/cold injury to airways), liver damage
Methylene chloride *(found in paint thinners and removers, degreasers)*: reduction of oxygen-carrying of blood, changes to the heart muscle and heartbeat
Nitrous oxide *("laughing gas")*, **hexane**: death from lack of oxygen to the brain, altered perception and motor coordination, loss of sensation, limb spasms, blackouts caused by blood pressure changes, depression of heart muscle functioning
Toluene *(found in gasoline, paint thinners and removers, correction fluid)*: brain damage (loss of brain tissue mass, impaired cognition, gait disturbance, loss of coordination, loss of equilibrium, limb spasms, hearing and vision loss), liver and kidney damage
Trichlorethylene *(found in spot removers, degreasers)*: sudden sniffing death syndrome, cirrhosis of the liver, reproductive complications, hearing and vision damage

Table 108-17 STAGES IN SYMPTOM DEVELOPMENT

STAGE	SYMPTOMS
1: Excitatory	Euphoria, excitation, exhilaration, dizziness, hallucinations, sneezing, coughing, excess salivation, intolerance to light, nausea and vomiting, flushed skin and bizarre behavior
2: Early CNS depression	Confusion, disorientation, dullness, loss of self-control, ringing or buzzing in the head, blurred or double vision, cramps, headache, insensitivity to pain, and pallor or paleness
3: Medium CNS depression	Drowsiness, muscular uncoordination, slurred speech, depressed reflexes, and nystagmus or rapid involuntary oscillation of the eyeballs
4: Late CNS depression	Unconsciousness that may be accompanied by bizarre dreams, epileptiform seizures, and EEG changes

CNS, central nervous system; EEG, electroencephalogram.
From Harris D: Volatile substance abuse, *Arch Dis Child Educ Pract Ed* 91:ep93-ep100, 2006, Table 1.

Table 108-18 DOCUMENTED CLINICAL PRESENTATIONS OF VOLATILE SUBSTANCE ABUSE (VSA)

CLINICAL PRESENTATIONS OF ACUTE AND CHRONIC VSA	
Ventricular fibrillation	Muscle weakness
Asystolic cardiac arrest	Abdominal pain
Myocardial infarction	Cough
Ataxia	Aspiration pneumonia
Agitation	Chemical pneumonitis
Limb and trunk uncoordination	Coma
Tremor	Visual and auditory hallucinations
Visual loss	Acute delusions
Tinnitus	Nausea and vomiting
Dysarthria	Pulmonary edema
Vertigo	Photophobia
Hyperreflexia	Rash
Acute confusional state	Jaundice
Conjunctivitis	Anorexia
Acute paranoia	Slurred speech
Depression	Diarrhea
Oral and nasal mucosal ulceration	Weight loss
Halitosis	Epistaxis
Convulsions/fits	Rhinitis
Headache	Cerebral edema
Peripheral neuropathy	Visual loss
Methemoglobinemia	Burns
Acute trauma	Renal tubular acidosis

From Harris D: Volatile substance abuse, *Arch Dis Child Edu Pract Ed* 91:ep93-ep100, 2006, Table 2.

rapidly in the urine as hippuric acid, with the residual detectable in the serum by gas chromatography.

TREATMENT

Treatment is generally supportive and directed toward control of arrhythmia and stabilization of respirations and circulation. Withdrawal symptoms do not usually occur.

BIBLIOGRAPHY

Please visit the Nelson Textbook of Pediatrics *website at* *www.expertconsult.com* *for the complete bibliography.*

108.5 Hallucinogens

Margaret M. Stager

Several naturally occurring and synthetic substances are used by adolescents for their hallucinogenic properties. They have chemical structures similar to neurotransmitters such as serotonin, yet their exact mechanism of action remains unclear. Lysergic acid diethylamide (LSD) and methylenedioxymethamphetamine (MDMA) or Ecstasy are the most commonly reported hallucinogens used.

LYSERGIC ACID DIETHYLAMIDE

LSD (acid, big "d," blotters) is a very potent hallucinogen that is made from lysergic acid found in ergot, a fungus that grows on rye and other grains. Its high potency allows effective doses to be applied to absorbent paper, or it can be taken as a liquid or a tablet. The onset of action can be between 30 and 60 min, and it peaks between 2 and 4 hr. By 10-12 hr, an individual returns to the predrug state. Four percent of U.S. 12th graders report trying LSD at least once.

CLINICAL MANIFESTATIONS

The effects of LSD can be divided into 3 categories: somatic (physical effects), perceptual (altered changes in vision and hearing), and psychic effects (changes in sensorium). The common somatic symptoms are dizziness, dilated pupils, nausea, flushing, elevated temperature, and tachycardia. The sensation of synesthesia, or "seeing" smells and "hearing" colors, as well as major distortions of time and self have been reported with high doses of LSD. Delusional ideation, body distortion, and suspiciousness to the point of toxic psychosis are the more serious of the psychic symptoms. LSD is not considered to be an addictive drug since it does not typically produce drug-seeking behavior.

TREATMENT

An individual is considered to have a "bad trip" when the sensory experiences causes the user to become terrified or panicked. These episodes should be treated by removing the individual from the aggravating situation and placing him in a quiet room with a calming friend. In situations of extreme agitation or seizures, use of benzodiazepines may be warranted. "Flashbacks" or LSD-induced states after the drug has worn off and tolerance to the effects of the drug are additional complications of its use.

METHYLENEDIOXYMETHAMPHETAMINE

MDMA ("X," Ecstasy), a phenylisopropylamine hallucinogen, is a synthetic compound similar to hallucinogenic mescaline and the stimulant methamphetamine. Like other hallucinogens, this drug is proposed to interact with serotoninergic neurons in the central nervous system (CNS). It is the preferred drug at "raves," all-night dance parties, and is also known as one of the "club drugs" along with γ-hydroxybutyrate (GHB) and ketamine (see Table 108-5). Between 2005 and 2008, past-year use of MDMA increased among both 10th and 12th graders. Six percent of 12th graders report having tried MDMA at least once. Similar increases were seen among European youth; the European School Survey Project on Alcohol and Other Drugs reported that in 2007, 3% of European students report having tried ecstasy during their lifetime, with 5 countries reporting ever-use rates of 6-7%.

CLINICAL MANIFESTATIONS

Euphoria, a heightened sensual awareness, and increased psychic and emotional energy are acute effects. Compared to other hallucinogens, MDMA is less likely to produce emotional lability, depersonalization, and disturbances of thought. Nausea, jaw clenching, teeth grinding, and blurred vision are somatic symptoms, whereas anxiety, panic attacks, and psychosis are the adverse psychiatric outcomes. A few deaths have been reported after ingestion of the drug. In high doses, MDMA can interfere with the body's ability to regulate temperature. The resultant hyperthermia in association with vigorous dancing at a "rave" has resulted in severe liver, kidney, and cardiovascular system failure and death. There are no specific treatment regimens recommended for acute toxicity. Chronic MDMA use can lead to changes in brain function, affecting cognitive tasks and memory. These symptoms may occur because of MDMA's effects on neurons that use serotonin as a neurotransmitter. The serotonin system plays an important role in regulating mood, aggression, sexual activity, sleep, and sensitivity to pain. A high rate of dependence has been found among MDMA users. MDMA exposure may be associated with long-term neurotoxicity and damage to serotonin-containing neurons. In nonhuman primates, exposure to MDMA for only 4 days caused damage to serotonin nerve terminals that was evident 6-7 yr later. There are no specific pharmacologic treatments for MDMA addiction. Drug abuse recovery groups are recommended.

PHENCYCLIDINE

Phencyclidine (PCP) (sternyl, angel dust, "hog," "peace pill," "sheets") is an arylcyclohexalamine whose popularity is related, in part, to its ease of synthesis in home laboratories. One of the by-products of home synthesis causes cramps, diarrhea, and hematemesis. It is a "dissociative drug" that produces feelings of detachment from the surrounding environment and self. The drug is thought to potentiate adrenergic effects by inhibiting neuronal reuptake of catecholamines. PCP is available as a tablet, liquid, or powder, which may be used alone or sprinkled on cigarettes ("joints"). The powders and tablets generally contain 2-6 mg of PCP, whereas joints average 1 mg for every 150 mg of tobacco leaves, or approximately 30-50 mg per joint.

CLINICAL MANIFESTATIONS

The clinical manifestations are dose related and produce alterations of perception, behavior, and autonomic functions. Euphoria, nystagmus, ataxia, and emotional lability occur within 2-3 min after smoking 1-5 mg and last for 4-6 hr. At these low doses the user is likely to experience shallow breathing, flushing, generalized numbness of extremities, and loss of motor coordination. Hallucinations may involve bizarre distortions of body image that often precipitate panic reactions. With doses of 5-15 mg, a toxic psychosis may occur, with disorientation, hypersalivation, and abusive language lasting for >1 hr. Hypotension, generalized seizures, and cardiac arrhythmias commonly occur with plasma concentrations from 40-200 mg/dL. Death has been reported during psychotic delirium, from hypertension, hypotension, hypothermia, seizures, and trauma. The coma of PCP may be distinguished from that of the opiates by the absence of respiratory depression; the presence of muscle rigidity, hyperreflexia, and nystagmus; and lack of response to naloxone. PCP psychosis may be difficult to distinguish from schizophrenia. In the absence of a history of use, analysis of urine must be depended on for diagnosis.

TREATMENT

Management of the PCP-intoxicated patient includes placement in a darkened, quiet room on a floor pad, safe from injury. Acute alcohol intoxication may be present also. For recent oral ingestion, gastric absorption is poor and induction of emesis or gastric lavage is useful. Diazepam, in a dose of 5-10 mg orally or 2-5 mg intravenously, may be helpful if the patient is agitated and not comatose. Rapid excretion of the drug is promoted by acidification of the urine. Supportive therapy of the comatose patient is indicated with particular attention to hydration, which may be compromised by PCP-induced diuresis. Inpatient and/or behavioral treatments can be helpful for chronic PCP users.

BIBLIOGRAPHY

Please visit the Nelson Textbook of Pediatrics *website at www.expertconsult.com for the complete bibliography.*

108.6 Cocaine

Margaret M. Stager

Cocaine, an alkaloid extracted from the leaves of the South American *Erythroxylon coca,* is supplied as the hydrochloride salt in crystalline form. With "snorting" it is rapidly absorbed into the bloodstream from the nasal mucosa, detoxified by the liver, and excreted in the urine as benzoylecgonine. Smoking the cocaine alkaloid ("freebasing") involves inhaling the cocaine vapors in pipes, or cigarettes mixed with tobacco or marijuana. Accidental burns are potential complications of this practice. With crack cocaine, the crystallized rock form, the smoker feels "high" in <10 sec. The risk of addiction with this method is higher and more rapidly progressive than from snorting cocaine. Tolerance develops and the user must increase the dose or change the route of administration, or both, to achieve the same effect. In order to sustain the high, cocaine users repeatedly use cocaine in short periods of time known as "binges." Drug dealers often place cocaine in plastic bags or condoms and swallow these containers during transport. Rupture of a container produces a sympathomimetic crisis (see Table 108-6). Cocaine use among high school students has remained unchanged in the last decade, with 7.2% of 12th graders having tried the drug (any route) at least once. Average use rates are somewhat lower among European students.

CLINICAL MANIFESTATIONS

Cocaine is a strong central nervous system stimulant that increases dopamine levels by preventing reuptake. Cocaine produces euphoria, increased motor activity, decreased fatigability, and mental alertness. Its sympathomimetic properties are responsible for pupillary dilatation, tachycardia, hypertension, and hyperthermia. Snorting cocaine chronically results in loss of sense of smell, nosebleeds, and chronic rhinorrhea. Injecting cocaine increases risk for HIV infection. Chronic abusers experience anxiety, irritability, and sometimes paranoid psychosis. Lethal effects are possible, especially when cocaine is used in combination with other drugs, such as heroin, in an injectable form known as a "speedball." Cocaine, when taken with alcohol, is metabolized by the liver to produce cocaethylene, a substance that enhances the euphoria and is associated with a greater risk of sudden death than cocaine alone. Pregnant adolescents who use cocaine place their fetus at risk of premature delivery, complications of low birthweight, and possibly developmental disorders.

TREATMENT

There are no FDA-approved medications for treatment of cocaine addiction. Cognitive-behavioral therapy has been shown to be effective when provided in combination with additional services and social support.

BIBLIOGRAPHY

Please visit the Nelson Textbook of Pediatrics *website at www.expertconsult.com for the complete bibliography.*

108.7 Amphetamines

Margaret M. Stager

Stimulants, particularly amphetamines, are among the most frequently reported illicit drugs, other than marijuana used by high school seniors. Methamphetamine, commonly known as "ice," accounted for >25% of stimulant use. Methamphetamine, a nervous system stimulant and schedule II drug, has a high potential for abuse. Most of the methamphetamine currently abused is produced in illegal laboratories. It is a white, odorless, bitter tasting powder that is particularly popular among adolescents and young adults because of its potency and ease of absorption. It can be ingested orally, by smoking, needle injection, or absorption across mucous membranes. Amphetamines have multiple CNS effects, among them the release of neurotransmitters and an indirect catecholamine agonist effect. In recent years there has been a general decline of methamphetamine use among high school students. In the 2008 Monitoring the Future Study, 2.8% of 12th graders report using methamphetamine at least once. In the 2007 European School Survey Project on Alcohol and Other Drugs, 3% of European students reported lifetime use of amphetamines.

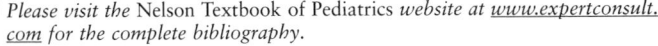

Table 108-19 SIGNS AND SYMPTOMS OF INTOXICATION AND WITHDRAWAL

	OPIATES	AMPHETAMINES/COCAINE	BENZODIAZEPINES
INTOXICATION			
Behavior	Apathy and sedation; disinhibition; psychomotor retardation; impaired attention and judgment	Euphoria and sensation of increased energy; hypervigilance; grandiosity, aggression, argumentative; labile mood; repetitive stereotyped behaviors; hallucinations, usually with intact orientation; paranoid ideation; interference with personal functioning	Euphoria; apathy and sedation; abusiveness or aggression; labile mood; impaired attention; anterograde amnesia; impaired psychomotor performance; interference with personal functioning
Signs	Drowsiness; slurred speech; pupillary constriction (except anoxia due to severe overdose—dilatation); decreased level of consciousness	Dilated pupils; tachycardia (occasionally bradycardia, cardiac arrhythmias); hypertension; nausea/vomiting; sweating and chills; evidence of weight loss; dilated pupils; chest pain; convulsions	Unsteady gait; difficulty in standing; slurred speech; nystagmus; decreased level consciousness; erythematous skin lesions or blisters
Overdose	Respiratory depression; hypothermia		Hypotension; hyperthermia; depression of gag reflex; coma
Withdrawal	Craving to use; lacrimation; yawning; rhinorrhea/sneezing; muscle aches or cramps; abdominal cramps; nausea/vomiting/diarrhoea; sweating; dilated pupils; anorexia; irritability; tremor; piloerection/chills; restlessness; disturbed sleep	Dysphoric mood (sadness/anhedonia); lethargy and fatigue; psychomotor retardation or agitation; craving; increased appetite; insomnia or hypersomnia; bizarre or unpleasant dreams	Tremor of tongue, eyelids, or outstretched hands; nausea or vomiting; tachycardia; postural hypotension; psychomotor agitation; headache; insomnia; malaise or weakness; transient visual, tactile, or auditory hallucinations or illusions; paranoid ideation; grand mal convulsions

From Haber PS, Demirkol A, Lange K, et al: Management of injecting drug users admitted to hospital, *Lancet* 374:1284–1292, 2009, Table 2.

CLINICAL MANIFESTATIONS

Methamphetamine rapidly increases the release and blocks the reuptake of dopamine, a powerful "feel good" neurotransmitter (Table 108-19). The effects of amphetamines can be dose related. In small amounts amphetamine effects resemble other stimulants: increased physical activity, rapid and/or irregular heart rate, increased blood pressure and decreased appetite. High doses produce slowing of cardiac conduction in the face of ventricular irritability. Hypertensive and hyperpyrexic episodes can occur as seizures (see Table 108-6). Binge effects result in the development of psychotic ideation with the potential for sudden violence. Cerebrovascular damage, psychosis, severe receding of the gums with tooth decay, and infection with HIV and hepatitis B and C can result from long-term use. There is a withdrawal syndrome associated with amphetamine use, with early, intermediate, and late phases. The early phase is characterized as a "crash" phase with depression, agitation, fatigue, and desire for more of the drug. Loss of physical and mental energy, limited interest in the environment, and anhedonia mark the intermediate phase. In the final phase, drug craving returns, often triggered by particular situations or objects.

TREATMENT

Acute agitation and delusional behaviors can be treated with haloperidol or droperidol. Phenothiazines are contraindicated and may cause a rapid drop in blood pressure or seizure activity. Other supportive treatment consists of a cooling blanket for hyperthermia and treatment of the hypertension and arrhythmias, which may respond to sedation with lorazepam or diazepam. For the chronic user, comprehensive cognitive-behavioral interventions have been shown to effective treatment options.

BIBLIOGRAPHY
Please visit the Nelson Textbook of Pediatrics *website at* *www.expertconsult.com* *for the complete bibliography.*

108.8 Opiates

Margaret M. Stager

Heroin is a highly addictive synthetic opiate drug made from a naturally occurring substance (morphine) in the opium poppy plant. It is a white or brown powder that can be injected (intravenously or subcutaneously), snorted/sniffed, or smoked. Intravenous injection produces an immediate effect, whereas effects from the subcutaneous route occur in minutes, and from snorting, 30 minutes. After injection, heroin crosses the blood-brain barrier, is converted to morphine, and binds to opiate receptors. Tolerance develops to the euphoric effect, and the chronic user must use more heroin to achieve the same intense effect. Heroin use among teens peaked in the mid-1990s but is resurgent in some suburban communities, as is the use of prescription opioids found in the home. Approximately 1.5% of high school seniors report having tried heroin at least once; similar rates are reported among European students.

CLINICAL MANIFESTATIONS

The clinical manifestations are determined by the purity of the heroin or its adulterants, combined with the route of administration. The immediate effects include euphoria, diminution in pain, flushing of the skin, and pinpoint pupils (Table 108-19). An effect on the hypothalamus is suggested by the lowering of body temperature. The most common dermatologic lesions are the "tracks," the hypertrophic linear scars that follow the course of large veins. Smaller, discrete peripheral scars, resembling healed insect bites, may be easily overlooked. The adolescent who injects heroin subcutaneously may have fat necrosis, lipodystrophy, and atrophy over portions of the extremities. Attempts to conceal these stigmata may include amateur tattoos in unusual sites. Skin abscesses secondary to unsterile techniques of drug administration are commonly found. There is a loss of libido; the mechanism is unknown. The chronic heroin user may resort to prostitution to support the habit, thus increasing the risk of sexually transmitted diseases (including HIV), pregnancy, and other infectious diseases. Constipation results from decreased smooth muscle propulsive contractions and increased anal sphincter tone. The absence of sterile technique in injection may lead to cerebral microabscesses or endocarditis, usually caused by *Staphylococcus aureus*. Abnormal serologic reactions are also common, including false-positive Venereal Disease Research Laboratory and latex fixation tests.

WITHDRAWAL

After a period of ≥8 hr without heroin, the addicted individual undergoes, during a 24-36 hr period, a series of physiologic disturbances referred to collectively as "withdrawal" or the **abstinence syndrome** (see Table 108-19). The earliest sign is yawning, followed by lacrimation, mydriasis, restlessness, insomnia, "goose flesh," cramping of the voluntary musculature, bone pain, hyperactive bowel sounds and diarrhea, tachycardia, and systolic hypertension. While the administration of methadone has been the most common method of detoxification, the addition of buprenorphine, an opiate agonist-antagonist, is available for detoxification and maintenance treatment of heroin and other opiates. This medication has the advantage in that it offers less risk of addiction and overdose, and withdrawal effects and can be dispensed in the privacy of a physician's office. Combined with behavioral interventions, it has a greater success rate of detoxification. A combination drug, buprenorphine/naloxone has been formulated to minimize abuse during detoxification.

OVERDOSE SYNDROME

The overdose syndrome is an acute reaction after the administration of an opiate. It is the leading cause of death among drug users. The clinical signs include stupor or coma, seizures, miotic pupils (unless severe anoxia has occurred), respiratory depression, cyanosis, and pulmonary edema. The differential diagnosis includes CNS trauma, diabetic coma, hepatic (and other) encephalopathy, Reye syndrome, as well as overdose of alcohol, barbiturates, PCP, or methadone. Diagnosis of opiate toxicity is facilitated by intravenous administration of the opiate antagonist naloxone, 0.01 mg/kg (2 mg is a common initial dose for an adolescent), which causes dilation of pupils constricted by the opiate. Diagnosis is confirmed by the finding of morphine in the serum.

TREATMENT

Treatment of acute heroin overdose consists of maintaining adequate oxygenation and continued administration of naloxone, a pure opioid antagonist. It may be given intravenously, intramuscularly, subcutaneously, or through the endotracheal tube. Naloxone has an ultrarapid onset of action (1 min) and a duration of action of 20-60 min. If there is no response then other etiologies for the respiratory depression must be explored. Naloxone may have to be continued for 24 hr if methadone, rather than shorter acting heroin, has been taken. Admission to the intensive care unit is indicated for patients who require continuous naloxone infusions (rebound coma, respiratory depression), and for those with life-threatening arrhythmias, shock, and seizures.

BIBLIOGRAPHY

Please visit the Nelson Textbook of Pediatrics *website at www.expertconsult.com for the complete bibliography.*

108.9 Anabolic Steroids

See Chapter 683.

Chapter 109
The Breast

Barbara Cromer

Breast development is one of the first obvious signs of puberty in the adolescent female. It is clinically important to distinguish normal progression of breast development, some variation in that progression, or a definable disorder. Normal breast development during puberty is described using a Sex Maturity Rating scale of 1-5, as the breast becomes more mature (Chapter 104).

For the full continuation of this chapter, please visit the Nelson Textbook of Pediatrics *website at www.expertconsult.com.*

Chapter 110
Menstrual Problems

Barbara Cromer

See also Chapter 544.

Menstrual dysfunction occurs at some time in about 50% of adolescent females. Although most of the problems are minor, severe dysmenorrhea or prolonged menstrual bleeding can be both frightening and debilitating. Adolescents with mild dysfunction that does not require medical intervention should have their condition explained to them and should be reassured regarding their reproductive health.

NORMAL MENSTRUATION

In 2008, the majority of an expert panel convened by the U.S. Environmental Protection Agency confirmed a secular trend toward an earlier age of menarche among U.S. girls, concluding that age at menarche has decreased by 2.5 to 4 mo in the past quarter century. The age of normal menarche, or first menses, varies according to the racial/ethnic background of the population and possibly socioeconomic status. In surveys conducted since 2000, in the USA, the age at menarche was 12.52 yr for non-Hispanic whites, 12.06 yr for non-Hispanic blacks, and 12.09 yr for Mexican Americans. In China, the median age of menarche was 12.8 yr in the urban area and 13.2 yr in the rural area. A study in Mozambique found that girls living in more affluent areas recalled a median age of 13.35 yr while those in a slum area reported 14.51 yr. There is a close concordance of the age at menarche between mother and daughter, suggesting that genetic factors are also determinants of menarche along with individual factors, such as diet, percent of body fat, and environmental factors, such as stress.

Menarche usually occurs about 2.3 yr after the initiation of puberty, with a range of 1-3 yr; periods become regular 2-2.5 yr after menarche. The length of the menstrual cycle from the 1st day of menses of 1 cycle to the 1st day of the next cycle can range from 21 to 45 days, although the average is about 28 days. Anovulatory cycles are generally longer. The average blood flow usually results in about 40 mL of blood loss, with a range of 25-70 mL. The later the age at which menarche occurs, the longer it is until the ovulatory cycles are established.

The onset and continuation of normal menstrual cycling depend on the functional and anatomic integrity of (1) the hypothalamus together with higher centers, including possibly the pineal gland; (2) the anterior pituitary; (3) the ovary; and (4) the uterus. It is a relatively fragile axis that is easily interrupted by a variety of individual and external factors.

MENSTRUAL IRREGULARITIES

Menstrual cycle irregularities are described according to variation in frequency of menses, amount, and both frequency and amount (Table 110-1). Most menstrual cycle abnormalities are explained by maturation of the hypothalamic-pituitary-ovarian axis, although organic pathology should be considered and excluded in a logical and cost-effective manner. A complete history for evaluating a patient with menstrual dysfunction should include questions specifically related to puberty and menstrual patterns, a family history of gynecologic problems and maternal onset of menarche, and a medical history noting hospitalizations, chronic illness, medication or substance use, and infections. The related associations of weight change, nutrition, exercise, and sports participation can be critically important in considering a differential diagnosis. Regardless of the age of the adolescent, an appropriate history of any type of sexual activity should be elicited, and the pediatrician should be cognizant of the need to rule

Table 110-1 TERMS FOR MENSTRUAL CYCLE IRREGULARITIES
VARIATIONS IN FREQUENCY
Polymenorrhea: frequent regular or irregular bleeding at <21-day intervals **Oligomenorrhea:** infrequent irregular bleeding at >45-day intervals **Primary amenorrhea:** no menstrual flow by age 16 yr **Secondary amenorrhea:** absence of vaginal bleeding for >3 mo **Irregular menses:** bleeding at varying intervals, ≥21-day intervals but <45-day intervals
VARIATIONS IN AMOUNT
Hypomenorrhea: decreased menstrual flow at regular intervals **Hypermenorrhea:** profuse menstrual flow of normal duration at regular intervals
VARIATIONS IN AMOUNT AND DURATION
Metrorrhagia: intermenstrual irregular bleeding between regular periods **Menorrhagia:** excessive amount and increased duration of uterine bleeding occurring regularly **Menometrorrhagia:** frequent irregular, excessive, and prolonged episodes of uterine bleeding **Dysfunctional uterine bleeding:** prolonged excessive menstrual bleeding associated with irregular periods; usually due to immaturity of reproductive axis in adolescence if within first 2 yr of menarche

From Blythe MI: Common menstrual problems of adolescence, *Adolesc Med* 8:87–109, 1997.

out sexual abuse as an issue in very young adolescents when other findings suggest sexual activity.

In addition to the basic growth parameters of weight, height, blood pressure, heart rate, and body mass index, signs of excess androgen should be assessed, such as hirsutism and acne. A careful external and internal pelvic examination is sometimes necessary to eliminate anatomic defects and to obtain additional specimens for the evaluation. In the young adolescent, someone with expertise in this age group should perform the examination with the proper size equipment.

Psychogenic factors have been implicated in amenorrhea. It is often difficult to separate psychologic from nutritional factors because weight loss is a common confounding variable in many of these situations, such as depression (Chapter 24), anorexia nervosa (Chapter 26), or stress.

BIBLIOGRAPHY

Please visit the Nelson Textbook of Pediatrics *website at www.expertconsult.com for the complete bibliography.*

110.1 Amenorrhea

Barbara Cromer

Differential Diagnosis

In *primary amenorrhea*, defined as failure for menstruation to begin, chromosomal or congenital abnormalities, such as gonadal dysgenesis, triple X syndrome, isochromosomal abnormalities, testicular feminization syndrome, and, rarely, true hermaphroditism, should be considered in addition to the conditions that cause secondary amenorrhea (Table 110-2). Elevated levels of follicle-stimulating hormone (FSH) and luteinizing hormone (LH) suggest primary gonadal failure, and chromosome analysis often elucidates its cause. When primary amenorrhea occurs with otherwise normal progression of pubertal development, a structural anomaly of the *müllerian duct system* (Chapter 548) should be suspected. Imperforate hymen is most the common disorder of müllerian duct descent and is associated with recurrent (monthly) abdominal pain and, after some time has passed, a midline, lower abdominal mass, which is the blood-filled vagina, and is called hematocolpos. Diagnosis is made by inspection of the introitus, revealing a bulging hymen with bluish discoloration. If the obstruction is at the level of the cervix, the blood-filled uterus (hematometrium) is apparent on bimanual examination or ultrasonography. Agenesis of the cervix or uterus is rare but occurs in association with sacral agenesis.

Primary or secondary amenorrhea may also be caused by chronic illness, particularly that associated with malnutrition or tissue hypoxia, such as diabetes mellitus, inflammatory bowel disease, cystic fibrosis, or cyanotic congenital heart disease. In most cases, the illness has been diagnosed previously, but, occasionally, the amenorrhea is its first manifestation. *Pregnancy is a common cause of secondary and occasionally primary amenorrhea.* **Polycystic ovarian syndrome** (PCOS) (Chapter 580.2) is one of the most common endocrine disorders affecting 4-6% of premenopausal women and presents with menstrual abnormalities that range from amenorrhea to dysfunctional uterine bleeding. The criterion for the diagnosis of PCOS is menstrual irregularity in the face of androgen excess with either hirsutism, acne, or increased serum androgens. When the androgen excess is coupled with insulin resistance and acanthosis nigricans, the term **HAIR-AN syndrome** is used. A central nervous system (CNS) tumor, most commonly a craniopharyngioma, may present with amenorrhea. **Prolactinomas,** although rare, are the most common pituitary tumor in adolescence. Abnormalities of the thyroid gland, typically hyperthyroidism, may first be suspected by delayed sexual maturation or amenorrhea, even in the absence of other signs and symptoms. Hypothyroidism may cause precocious puberty but may also be associated with delayed puberty or abnormal uterine bleeding. Anorexia nervosa, which may present with either primary or secondary amenorrhea, is occasionally confused with hyperthyroidism because of weight loss, hyperactivity, and personality changes seen in both entities. Amenorrhea is one of the components of the **female athlete triad** in association with disordered eating and low bone mass (Chapter 682). Ballerinas, gymnasts, and runners may be at disproportionate risk of this triad. Ingestion of drugs, both legal and illegal, may cause amenorrhea and, in the case of phenothiazines, even a false-positive urine pregnancy test. Some drugs, including phenothiazines and certain antihypertensive agents, may cause galactorrhea, further mimicking pregnancy. Pertinent findings on physical exam include signs of androgen excess, such as obesity, acne, hirsutism, and clitoromegaly, along with excessive thinness, galactorrhea, and thyromegaly. Adolescents with amenorrhea who diet, whether or not they meet diagnostic criteria for anorexia nervosa, are at risk for low bone density.

Laboratory Findings

The approach to the clinical evaluation of amenorrhea follows a stepwise progression initiated by the history and physical examination. The pregnancy test, usually a qualitative measure of urinary chorionic gonadotropin, is the key laboratory test to perform in the evaluation of amenorrhea regardless of the history or sexual activity given by the patient (Fig. 110-1). The next step for laboratory determinations follows the scheme in which gonadotropin levels. The measurement of FSH is critical in determining whether chromosomal abnormalities (with FSH elevation >25 mIU/mL) or other endocrinopathies or CNS tumors (with normal or low FSH <5 mIU/mL) are present. Prolonged amenorrhea (>6 mo) or persistent oligomenorrhea (<6 menses in past year) without an explanation should prompt the measurement of thyroid-stimulating hormone, FSH, LH, and prolactin levels, even in the face of a normal progesterone challenge. Elevated LH and normal FSH levels require the measurement of androgen excess even in the absence of virilization. An LH:FSH ratio >3 and elevated free testosterone and DHEAS (dihydroepiandrosterone sulfate) levels are common in adolescents with PCOS. Hyperinsulinemia is a characteristic feature of PCOS, and there is an increased risk of type 2 diabetes mellitus. Elevated DHEAS may indicate the source of excess androgen to disorders in the adrenal gland. An elevated prolactin level or other clinical features suggesting a CNS tumor should be followed up with cranial CT scan or, preferably, MRI.

Table 110-2 CONGENITAL ANATOMIC CAUSES OF PRIMARY AMENORRHEA WITH NORMAL BREAST DEVELOPMENT*

DIAGNOSIS	MÜLLERIAN AGENESIS	ANDROGEN INSENSITIVITY (AI)	TRANSVERSE VAGINAL SEPTUM	IMPERFORATE HYMEN
Patients with primary amenorrhea†	15%	1%	3%	1%
Patients with primary amenorrhea and apparent obstruction or absence of vagina†	75%	5%	15%	5%
Chromosomes‡	46,XX	46,XY	46,XX	46,XX
Gonads	Ovaries	Testes	Ovaries	Ovaries
Serum testosterone‡	Normal female level	Normal male level (high)	Normal female level	Normal female level
Vagina	Absent or shallow	Absent or shallow	Obstructed by septum which may be thick or thin, high or low	Obstructed by thin membrane, which may look blue from hematocolpos
Axillary/pubic hair	+	Absent unless AI is incomplete	+	+
Cyclic pain	±	–	+	+
Uterus	Absent or rudimentary	–	+	+
Mass	–	–	+ Can present with acute urinary retention as hematocolpos mass obstructs urethra	+ Can present with acute urinary retention
Introitus bulges with Valsalva maneuver	–	–	–	+
Associated anomalies	Urinary tract and skeletal	Inguinal hernias; gonadal malignancy in adulthood	Major urinary tract abnormalities in 15%	Possibly some increase in urinary tract abnormalities
Treatment	Vaginal dilation or surgical neovagina	Gonadectomy after age 16-18 yr Vaginal dilation or surgical neovagina	Surgical approach depends on extent and location of septum; may be extensive; should be done as soon as possible	Excision of hymen as soon as possible; diagnostic needle aspiration contraindicated because of risk of infection
Fertility	Advanced reproductive technology required; in vitro fertilization surrogate with uterus to gestate pregnancy	Not fertile	Variable, low septa have a better prognosis than do high septa	Usually fertile

*Cervix not visible on pelvic examination. Short vagina; may be absent or obstructed.
†Data from Reindollar RH, Byrd JR, McDonough PG: Delayed sexual development: a study of 252 patients, *Am J Obstet Gynecol* 140:371, 1981.
‡Sometimes useful in differentiating müllerian agenesis from androgen insensitivity.
+, present; –, absent; ±, may be present or absent.
From Kliegman RM, Greenbaum LA, Lye PS: *Practical strategies in pediatric diagnosis and therapy*, ed 2, Philadelphia, 2004, Elsevier, p 505.

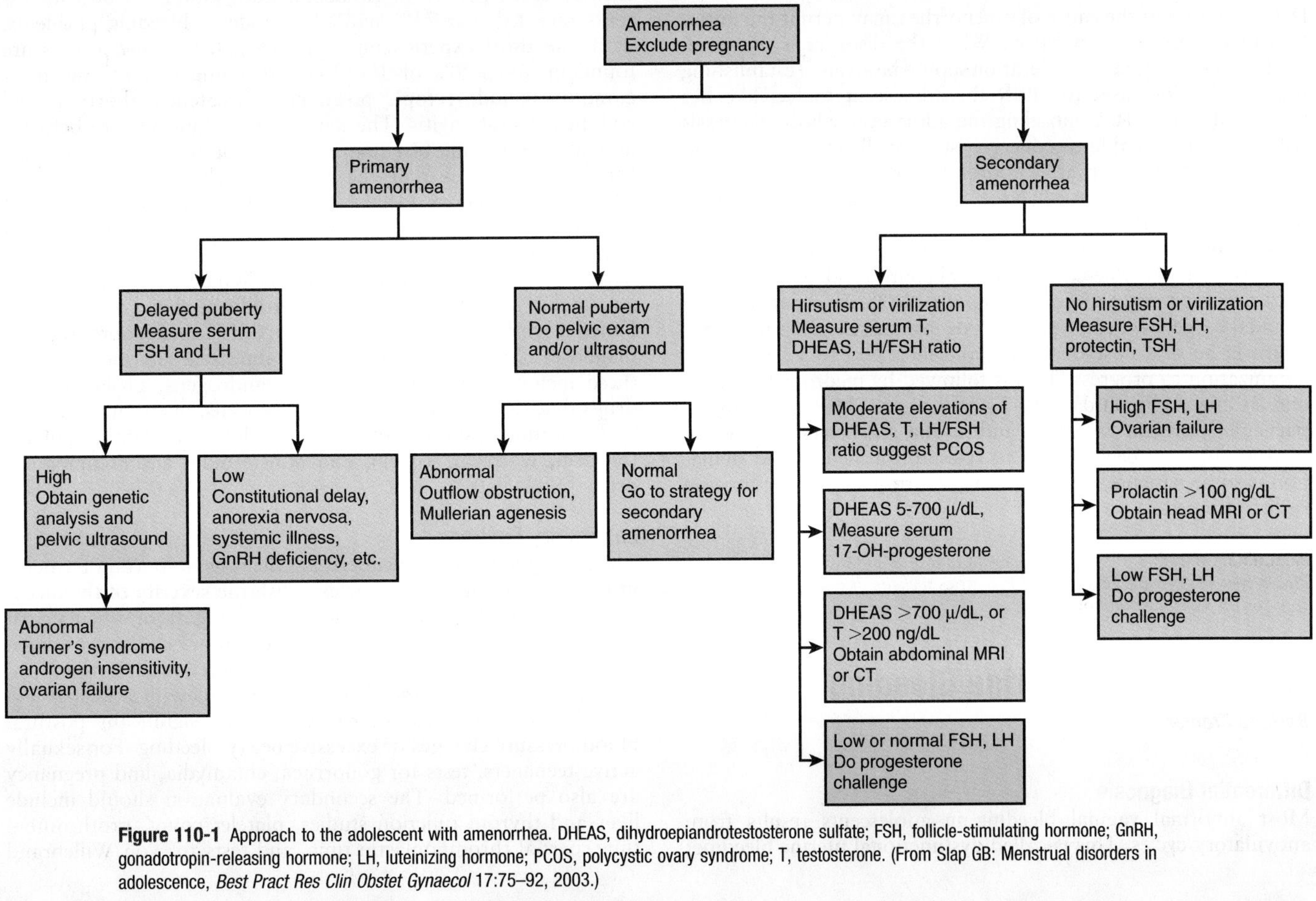

Figure 110-1 Approach to the adolescent with amenorrhea. DHEAS, dihydroepiandrotestosterone sulfate; FSH, follicle-stimulating hormone; GnRH, gonadotropin-releasing hormone; LH, luteinizing hormone; PCOS, polycystic ovary syndrome; T, testosterone. (From Slap GB: Menstrual disorders in adolescence, *Best Pract Res Clin Obstet Gynaecol* 17:75–92, 2003.)

Table 110-3 HORMONE REPLACEMENT OPTIONS FOR AMENORRHEIC CONDITIONS*

	HORMONE REPLACEMENT	BENEFITS OF THERAPY	RISKS OF THERAPY
Chronic anovulation (estrogen present)	Progestin therapy with medroxyprogesterone acetate, 5-10 mg/day PO or 5 mg norethindrone acetate 12 days/mo every 1-3 mo	Diminishes risk of sudden menorrhagia and of endometrial hyperplasia/cancer later in life; creates predictable normal menses	Some premenstrual symptoms may occur while the patient is taking progestin; does not provide contraception or address cause of amenorrhea; does not suppress androgens to treat hirsutism
	Low-dose oral contraceptive pills (20-35 μg estrogen) or contraceptive patch	Same as for progestin therapy; provides contraception; improves hirsutism by suppressing ovarian androgens	Does not address cause of amenorrhea; some parents object to their daughters taking oral contraceptives; side effects can include nausea, headache, and breakthrough bleeding
Hypogonadism (low-estrogen state)†	Oral medroxyprogesterone acetate 5-10 mg/day or 2.5-5 mg norethindrone acetate on days 1-12 of the month (by calendar) plus oral conjugated estrogens, 0.625 mg/day	Prevents low bone mass,‡ heart disease, and atrophic vaginal changes; eliminates hot flashes if present	Does not address cause of amenorrhea; does not provide contraception (if ovulation is possible, given the diagnosis); premenstrual symptoms may occur while the patient is taking progestins; some adolescents prefer oral contraceptives to "medications"
	Low-dose oral contraceptive pills (20-35 μg estrogen)	Same as HRT; provides contraception in case of spontaneous ovulation (if that is a possibility); many adolescents prefer taking oral contraceptives to taking "medications"	Same as risks of oral contraceptives for chronic anovulation

*These options may need modification according to the individual's response.
†See Chapter 580 for treatment of pubertal delay.
‡Estrogen therapy may not prevent bone loss in girls with amenorrhea and low body weight.
HRT, hormone replacement therapy.
From Kliegman RM, Greenbaum LA, Lye PS: *Practical strategies in pediatric diagnosis and therapy*, ed 2, Philadelphia, 2004, Elsevier, p 508.

Endometrial status can be assessed as part of the evaluation when other endocrinologic parameters are normal by a progesterone challenge in which 5 or 10 mg oral medroxyprogesterone acetate is given for 5-10 days. Withdrawal bleeding should occur 2-7 days thereafter when normal endometrium is present. If bleeding does not occur, one must consider insufficient estrogenic priming of the endometrium, an abnormal uterus, or an outflow tract obstruction.

Treatment

Determination of the cause of amenorrhea may permit the initiation of corrective intervention. When the disorder is not amenable to remediation, consideration should be given to establishing regular pseudomenses to allow the adolescent to feel like her peers (Table 110-3). Counseling the adolescent whose diagnosis will render her unable to conceive is especially challenging, and support and follow-up are important. If the result of a vaginal smear is positive for estrogen effect, regular cycling can be accomplished using medroxyprogesterone in a dose of 10 mg orally for 10-12 days at least every other month. Combination norgestimate- or drospirenone-containing oral contraceptives can also be used for this purpose in patients with PCOS. In a patient with gonadal dysgenesis, conjugated estrogens must be given first (Premarin in an oral dose of 0.3 mg and increased to 1.25 mg) for feminization to progress. This is followed by medroxyprogesterone, 10 mg orally on days 10-21 of the cycle. Lifestyle changes, particularly weight reduction and insulin sensitizers, specifically metformin, have been shown to re-establish menses and ovulation is some patients, but symptoms return when the medication is discontinued.

BIBLIOGRAPHY
Please visit the Nelson Textbook of Pediatrics *website at www.expertconsult.com for the complete bibliography.*

110.2 Abnormal Uterine Bleeding

Barbara Cromer

Differential Diagnosis

Most abnormal vaginal bleeding in adolescents results from anovulatory cycles. This is called **dysfunctional uterine bleeding;** this term is used when no demonstrable organic lesion is identified to account for the abnormal bleeding. When it occurs during the 1st 2 yr after menarche, dysfunctional uterine bleeding usually reflects an immaturity of the hypothalamic-pituitary-ovarian axis; specifically, the mid-cycle LH surge is not in place, leading to anovulation and, hence, potential for irregular bleeding.

Among U.S. adolescents admitted to the hospital for menorrhagia, anovulation was the most common cause (46%), followed by hematologic causes (33%), infection (11%), and chemotherapy (11%). In Sweden, a study among ~1,000 adolescents revealed that 73% had ≥1 episode of bleeding problems, with one third experiencing menorrhagia. Organic lesions are found in about 9% of 10-20 yr old young women; the most common include ectopic pregnancy, threatened abortion, and endometritis/salpingitis. The key distinguishing feature between anovulatory uterine bleeding and that due to organic disorders listed previously is that the latter are characterized by pain whereas anovulatory bleeding is usually painless. Table 110-4 lists the extensive differential diagnosis; studies of severe cases that require hospitalization report coagulation disorders (idiopathic thrombocytopenic purpura, von Willebrand disease, Glanzmann disease, leukemia), hypothyroidism, thalassemia major, Fanconi syndrome, and rheumatoid arthritis as the more frequent diagnoses. Medications may cause abnormal uterine bleeding; these include estrogens, progestins, androgens, prolactin, and drugs that cause prolactin release (estrogens, phenothiazines, tricyclic antidepressants, metoclopramide), and anticoagulants (heparin, warfarin, aspirin, and nonsteroidal antiinflammatory drugs [NSAIDs]).

Laboratory Findings

The hemoglobin and hematocrit are the most important elements in the initial evaluation. They establish the **severity of the bleeding,** with levels less than a hemoglobin of 9 g/dL or a hematocrit of 27% considered severe, 9-11 g/dL and 27-33% considered moderate, and >11 g/dL and >33% considered mild. Hospitalization is generally recommended for adolescents with a hemoglobin <7 g/dL or a hemoglobin <10 g/dL with significant postural blood pressure changes or excessive heavy bleeding. For sexually active teenagers, tests for gonorrhea, chlamydia, and pregnancy are also performed. The secondary evaluation should include liver and thyroid function studies, platelet count, prothrombin time, partial thromboplastin time, and tests for von Willebrand

Table 110-4 DIFFERENTIAL DIAGNOSIS OF ABNORMAL VAGINAL BLEEDING IN ADOLESCENTS

	BLEEDING PATTERN MR	MMR	IB	EVALUATION Suggestive Finding; *Diagnostic Finding*	TREATMENT
SOURCE: UTERUS				**COMMON CAUSES**	
Anovulation	+	+		No extrauterine source of bleeding seen on examination	See text
				Responds appropriately to treatment	
Coagulopathy	+			More commonly found in cases of severe bleeding especially if onset at menarche; family history, ROS suggestive of clotting disorder; ecchymoses, petechiae may be seen on examination	Treat coagulopathy; oral contraceptives may help with menorrhagia; complete menstrual suppression sometimes required
				Abnormal PT, PTT, platelet count, bleeding time, or test for von Willebrand disease	See Chapters 470-478
Complication of pregnancy		+		History of late period; pregnancy symptoms (nausea, breast tenderness)	See Chapter 112
				Positive urine or blood pregnancy test	
SOURCE: VAGINA				**UNCOMMON CAUSES**	
Injury			+	History *Visible laceration*	Surgical or topical hemostasis; suture or allow to heal by secondary intention
Foreign body (e.g., retained tampon or contraceptive sponge)			+	History, foul discharge *Visible foreign body*	Removal
Cancer			+	Lesion seen, ±abnormal cytologic findings	Referral to specialist; therapy chosen per type and stage of tumor
			+	*Biopsy*	
SOURCE: CERVIX				**LESS COMMON CAUSES**	
Neoplasia					
Dysplasia/carcinoma			+	Bleeding point on cervix; abnormal cytology	LEEP, laser, cryotherapy, or cone biopsy
				Colposcopy with directed biopsies	
Cervical polyp			+	Polyp seen	Grasp with clamp or ring forceps and twirl off polyp in office; send specimen to pathologist
Hemangioma			+	Lesion seen	Conservative versus excision or ablation
Infection (cervicitis) (Chapter 114)					
Herpes simplex (Chapter 244)			+	Cervical vesicles ± ulceration, ± pelvic pain, tenderness; Pap smear sometimes shows multinucleated giant cells	If primary infection, consider oral famcyclovir, 250 mg b.i.d. × 7-10 days
				Culture positive for herpes	
Human papillomavirus (HPV) (Chapter 258)			+	Flat or raised warts seen on cervix	Laser, LEEP, cryotherapy, trichloroacetic acid or 5-fluorouracil cream after Pap smear and colposcopy; treat for dysplasia or symptoms
				Pap smear + colposcopy necessary to differentiate from dysplasia; HPV typing may determine risk of cancer	
Trichomonas (Chapter 276)			+	Friable inflamed cervix; yellow-green vaginal discharge, pH 7-8	Metronidazole, 2 g orally once each for patient and sexual partners
				Saline preparation: motile flagellates	
SOURCE: UTERUS				**LESS COMMON CAUSES**	
Neoplasia					
Fibroid	±		±	± Enlarged uterus on examination; palpable fibroids *Abnormal findings on ultrasound and/or hysteroscopy*	NSAID sometimes helpful for menorrhagia; myomectomy via hysteroscope or laparoscope or laparotomy may be needed
Endometrial polyps			+	History of spotting superimposed on normal menstrual cycle	D&C or hysteroscopic excision
				Hysteroscopy, saline sonogram, and/or D&C	
Malignant uterine tumor		±	±	Abnormal Pap smear, enlarged uterus, tissue at cervical os	Surgery determined by type of tumor and stage
				Biopsy	
Ovarian tumor producing estrogen (bleeding is uterine)		+		Adnexal mass on examination or ultrasonography *Surgical diagnosis and staging*	Surgery
Foreign body					
IUD	+		+	No other cause of bleeding (patient ovulatory, not pregnant, no PID) *IUD in uterus; responds to therapy*	NSAID sometimes useful for menorrhagia; removal if PID coexists or if necessary to control bleeding

Continued

Table 110-4 DIFFERENTIAL DIAGNOSIS OF ABNORMAL VAGINAL BLEEDING IN ADOLESCENTS—cont'd

	BLEEDING PATTERN MR	MMR	IB	EVALUATION Suggestive Finding; *Diagnostic Finding*	TREATMENT
Infection					
PID	+		+	Tender uterus and adnexae; purulent cervical discharge ± ↑ WBC count, ESR, or fever *Clinical diagnosis, tests often positive for gonorrhea, chlamydia*	CDC guidelines (Chapter 114)
Postpartum or postabortal endometritis ± retained products of conception			+	± ↑ WBC count, ESR, fever *Recent pregnancy; tender uterus*	D&C if retained tissue seen on sonogram; broad-spectrum antibiotics, methergine
Congenital partially obstructed hemivagina or uterine horn			+	Foul, dark blood after menses *Abnormal pelvic examination and/or pelvic ultrasonography*	Refer for surgical treatment

CDC, Centers for Disease Control and Prevention; D&C, dilation and curettage; ESR, erythrocyte sedimentation rate; IB, intermenstrual bleeding; IUD, intrauterine device; LEEP, loop electroexcisional procedure; MMR, menometrorrhagia; MR, menorrhagia; NSAID, nonsteroidal antiinflammatory drug; Pap, Papanicolaou; PID, pelvic inflammatory disease; PT, prothrombin time; PTT, partial thromboplastin time; ROS, review of systems; WBC, white blood cell.

From Kliegman RM, Greenbaum LA, Lye PS: *Practical strategies in pediatric diagnosis and therapy*, ed 2, Philadelphia, 2004, Elsevier, pp 497–498.

disease. If these studies are not performed at the first visit, they must be performed before any estrogen therapy is initiated that might interfere with interpreting the results.

Treatment

In **mild** cases, iron supplementation is recommended, and the patient should keep a menstrual calendar to follow the subsequent flow patterns. With **moderate** disturbances, cycling with oral contraceptives, barring any contraindications, should be considered along with monitoring the iron status and oral iron therapy. **Severe** bleeding, not requiring hospitalization, can usually be stopped with hormonal therapy, either medroxyprogesterone acetate (Provera) 10 mg/24 hr for 10-14 days or a combination oral contraceptive using 2-4 pills per day until the bleeding stops, and then 1 pill per day for the remainder of the cycle. Once a patient is hospitalized, Premarin 25 mg every 4 hr up to 2 to 3 doses given intravenously is required. At the same time, the combination oral contraceptive regimen or Depo-Provera (medroxyprogesterone acetate [DMPA]), 150 mg IM every 12 wk, required for maintenance, can be initiated. These estrogen doses are high, prompting some concern about the risk of thromboembolism, but no complications have been reported from short-term use. For severe cases, transfusion of packed red blood cells may be needed.

In the rare case of a patient whose bleeding cannot be controlled by one of these methods, an endometrial curettage may be indicated. Although this procedure is frequently undertaken in adult women with menometrorrhagia, the rarity of endometrial carcinoma and the usual efficacy of hormonal therapy in adolescence make this procedure unnecessarily invasive in this age group.

BIBLIOGRAPHY

Please visit the Nelson Textbook of Pediatrics *website at* *www.expertconsult.com* *for the complete bibliography.*

110.3 Dysmenorrhea

Barbara Cromer

Painful menstrual cramps are experienced by nearly 65% of postmenarchal teenagers in the USA. More than 10% of this group suffers sufficiently to miss school, making dysmenorrhea the leading cause of short-term school absenteeism in female adolescents. Dysmenorrhea may be primary or secondary. **Primary dysmenorrhea** is characterized by the absence of any specific pelvic pathologic condition and is the more commonly occurring form (Table 110-5). Prostaglandins F_2 and E_2, produced by the endometrium, stimulate local vasoconstriction and myometrial contractions, thereby producing pain. **Secondary dysmenorrhea** results from an underlying **structural abnormality** of the cervix or uterus, a **foreign body** such as an intrauterine device, **endometriosis,** or **endometritis.** Endometriosis is a condition in which implants of endometrial tissue are found at ectopic locations within the peritoneal cavity. Characteristically, there is severe pain at the time of menses; its specific location depends on the site of the implants.

With its very high prevalence, primary dysmenorrhea should be presumed on initial presentation. Because adolescents suffering from dysmenorrhea have high levels of prostaglandins, they experience symptomatic relief when prostaglandin synthetase inhibitors are administered (Table 110-6). If given before a menstrual period (or shortly after it begins), administration of a rapidly absorbed prostaglandin synthetase inhibitor, such as naproxen sodium, is effective in reducing prostaglandin production before they cause pain (2 tablets of 275 mg each taken with the onset of menses and 1 tablet taken every 6-8 hr after that for the 1st 24 hr). Medication is rarely needed beyond the 1st day. For the teenager with dysmenorrhea who requires contraception, combined hormonal therapy in the form of oral contraceptives, the contraceptive patch, or vaginal ring may be indicated. It is not certain whether the beneficial effect of such use derives from the ability of oral contraceptives to inhibit ovulation and thus eliminate progesterone production from the corpus luteum or from their ability to limit endometrial proliferation and therefore the production of prostaglandins.

In adolescent patients with **endometriosis,** danazol, an antigonadotropin, is rarely prescribed because of the unacceptable side effects of weight gain, irregular menses, edema, acne, oily skin, hirsutism, and a deep voice change. The use of gonadotropin-releasing hormone (GnRH) agonists such as nafarelin and leuprolide are often used with the goal of the creation of an acyclic, low-estrogen environment. This prevents bleeding at the site of the implants and further seeding of the pelvis during retrograde menstruation. GnRH agonist can be given as a nasal spray or IM injection every 3 mo. Depot-leuprolide can be given at a dose of 11.25 mg every 3 mo. To reduce the risk of decreased bone density, a long-term side effect of GnRH analog therapy, prescriptions for courses of therapy lasting longer than 6 consecutive mo are not recommended. "Add back" hormonal therapy with norethindrone or conjugated estrogen has been shown to reduce bone and lipid metabolism side effects. Although there is insufficient

Table 110-5 DIFFERENTIAL DIAGNOSIS OF DYSMENORRHEA

	DESCRIPTION OF PAIN	OCCURRENCE OF DYSMENORRHEA IN ANOVULATORY CYCLES	DIAGNOSIS	TREATMENT
Primary	Crampy lower abdominal/low back pain ± radiation to upper thighs ± nausea, vomiting, diarrhea, headache; begins at time of menstrual flow; lasts 1-3 days	No	Normal abdominal and pelvic examination; internal pelvic examination can be reserved for sexually active girls and older teenagers; rectoabdominal examination assesses pelvic pathology	NSAIDs and/or oral contraceptives; see Table 110-6
Secondary				
Congenital partial outflow obstruction (e.g., rudimentary uterine horn, obstructed hemivagina)	Pain begins at or shortly after menarche and occurs with bleeding	Yes	Pelvic examination ± ultrasonography ± laparoscopy; found in 8% of adolescents who underwent laparoscopy for pain	Surgical relief of obstruction
Endometriosis	Increasingly severe dysmenorrhea ± chronic pelvic pain exacerbated during menses	No	Found in 16-70% of adolescents who underwent laparoscopy for pelvic pain; pelvic examination finding may be normal or there may be tenderness of the uterosacral ligaments/cul-de-sac and/or ovarian masses; although congenital obstruction of menstrual outflow increases chance of endometriosis, most teenagers with endometriosis have normal anatomy; diagnosis is by laparoscopy	Surgical and/or hormonal therapy; post-treatment prophylaxis with oral contraceptives
Atypical secondary dysmenorrhea				
Pelvic inflammatory disease	Pain during or immediately after menses	Yes	Pelvic examination: tender uterus and adnexa, ± cervicitis, ± ↑ WBC count, ± ↑ ESR, ± fever	Follow CDC recommendations (Chapter 114)
Pregnancy complication	Pain and bleeding may coincide and may be interpreted by the patient as a painful menstrual period	N/A	UCG, or serum hCG	See Table 112-2

CDC, Centers for Disease Control and Prevention; ESR, erythrocyte sedimentation rate; hCG, human chorionic gonadotropin, N/A, not applicable; NSAIDs, nonsteroidal antiinflammatory drugs; UCG, urinary chorionic gonadotropin; WBC, white blood cell.
From Kliegman RM, Greenbaum LA, Lye PS: *Practical strategies in pediatric diagnosis and therapy*, ed 2, Philadelphia, 2004, Elsevier, p 509.

Table 110-6 TREATMENT OF PRIMARY DYSMENORRHEA

	MEDICATION	REGIMEN	COMMENTS
NSAID	Ibuprofen, 200 mg	2 tablets PO q4-6h	Over-the-counter
	Naproxen sodium, 275 mg	2 tablets to start, then 1 PO q6h	Over-the-counter
	Naproxen sodium, 550 mg	1 tablet PO q12h	12-hr regimen is appealing to patients
	Mefenamic acid, 250 mg	2 tablets to start, then 1 PO q6h	Suggested in some studies as most effective drug
Oral contraceptives or contraceptive patch	Any low-dose pill (≤35 µg of estrogen) or ortho Evra	Cyclic	Particularly useful if birth control method is needed; a few cycles may be needed to reach maximum effectiveness

Aspirin has not been shown to be better than placebo in the treatment of primary dysmenorrhea. NSAID treatment is effective if started at the onset of cramping and bleeding.
NSAID, nonsteroidal antiinflammatory drug; PO, per os (orally).
From Kliegman RM, Greenbaum LA, Lye PS: *Practical strategies in pediatric diagnosis and therapy*, ed 2, Philadelphia, 2004, Elsevier, p 510.

evidence to support a role for acupuncture in management of this condition, there is evidence supporting the use of some Chinese herbal medicines for primary dysmenorrhoea.

BIBLIOGRAPHY

Please visit the Nelson Textbook of Pediatrics *website at* *www.expertconsult.com* *for the complete bibliography.*

110.4 Premenstrual Syndrome

Barbara Cromer

Premenstrual syndrome (PMS), or the late luteal phase syndrome, is a complex of physical signs and behavioral symptoms occurring during the 2nd half of the menstrual cycle, which may resolve with the onset of menses. **Clinical manifestations** may include breast fullness and tenderness; bloating; fatigue; headache; increased appetite, especially for sweets and salty foods; irritability and mood swings; depression; inability to concentrate; tearfulness; and violent tendencies. About 30% of women in the reproductive age group and ≥20% adolescents experience PMS; the absence of objective findings makes this difficult to corroborate. It does not relate to the presence of dysmenorrhea, which is much more common in this age group. For the diagnosis of PMS, documentation of symptoms using a special calendar for 2-3 mo should demonstrate the pattern of association with menses. Nonsteroidal antiinflammatory drugs (NSAIDs), particularly mefenamic acid, diuretics, and agnus castus fruit extract have demonstrated some therapeutic efficacy in small trials. **Premenstrual dysphoric disorder** occurs less commonly, in 3-8% of women of reproductive age and is a more severe form of premenstrual syndrome (Table 110-7), requiring more intensive therapy (Table 110-8).

Table 110-7 CRITERIA FOR PREMENSTRUAL DYSPHORIC DISORDER*

In most menstrual cycles during the past year, presence of ≥5 of the following symptoms for most of the last week of the luteal phase, with remission beginning within a few days after the onset of the follicular phase and absence of symptoms during the week after menses; inclusion of ≥1 of the first 4 symptoms: Markedly depressed mood, feelings of hopelessness, or self-deprecating thoughts Marked anxiety, tension, feelings of being "keyed up" or "on edge" Marked affective lability (e.g., feeling suddenly sad or tearful or having increased sensitivity to rejection) Persistent and marked anger or irritability or increased interpersonal conflicts Decreased interest in usual activities (e.g., work, school, friends, and hobbies) Subjective sense of difficulty in concentrating Lethargy, easy fatigability, or marked lack of energy Marked change in appetite, overeating, or specific food cravings Hypersomnia or insomnia Subjective sense of being overwhelmed or out of control Other physical symptoms, such as breast tenderness or swelling, headache, joint or muscle pain, a sensation of "bloating," weight gain
Marked interference with work or school or with usual social activities and relationships with others (e.g., avoidance of social activities or decreased productivity and efficiency at work or school)
Disturbance not a mere exacerbation of the symptoms of another disorder, such as major depressive disorder, panic disorder, dysthymic disorder, or a personality disorder (although possibly superimposed on any of these disorders)
Confirmation of 3 criteria above by prospective daily ratings during at least 2 consecutive symptomatic menstrual cycles (diagnosis may be made provisionally before such confirmation)

*The criteria are from the *Diagnostic and Statistical Manual of Mental Disorders, Fourth Edition, Text Revision.* In menstruating women, the luteal phase corresponds to the period between ovulation and the onset of menses, and the follicular phase begins with menses. In nonmenstruating women (e.g., women who have had a hysterectomy), determination of the timing of the luteal and follicular phases are variable.

From Grady-Weliky TA: Premenstrual dysphoric disorder, *N Engl J Med* 348:433–438, 2003.

Table 110-8 RECOMMENDED TREATMENT STRATEGIES FOR PREMENSTRUAL DYSPHORIC DISORDER*

MEDICATION	STARTING DOSE (MG)	THERAPEUTIC DOSE (MG)	COMMON SIDE EFFECTS
FIRST-LINE: SELECTIVE SEROTONIN REUPTAKE INHIBITORS			
Fluoxetine	10-20	20	Sexual dysfunction (anorgasmia and decreased libido), sleep alterations (insomnia, sedation, or hypersomnia), and gastrointestinal distress (nausea and diarrhea)
Sertraline	25-50	50-150	Same as fluoxetine
Paroxetine	10-20	20-30	Same as fluoxetine
Citalopram	10-20	20-30	Same as fluoxetine
SECOND-LINE			
Clomipramine	25	50-75	Dry mouth, fatigue, vertigo, sweating, headache, nausea
Alprazolam	0.50-0.75	1.25-2.25	Drowsiness, sedation
THIRD-LINE			
Leuprolide	3.75	3.75	Hot flashes, night sweats, headache, nausea

*For selective serotonin reuptake inhibitors and clomipramine, the starting and therapeutic doses are administered once daily and are the same with luteal-phase and continuous administration. For luteal-phase administration, the medication should be intiated at time of ovulation (usually approximately 2 wk before the expected onset of menses) and discontinued on the 1st day of menses. The therapeutic doses given for selective serotonin reuptake inhibitors are those that were reported in the randomized clinical trials. However, clinical experience has shown that a subgroup of patients with premenstrual dysphoric disorder may require slightly higher doses (up to 60 mg fluoxetine; up to 150 mg sertraline; up to 40 mg paroxetine; and up to 40 mg citalopram). If a patient is taking another selective serotonin reuptake inhibitor and tolerating it well but has a partial response at the doses listed, it would be appropriate to increase the dose of the specific selective serotonin reuptake inhibitor before switching to another agent. Alprazolam is administered 3 times a day; treatment should begin at 0.25 mg 3 times a day. Clinical trials of leuprolide used the depot form: leuprolide should be administered intramuscularly each month.

From Grady-Weliky TA: Premenstrual dysphoric disorder, *N Engl J Med* 384:433–438, 2003.

BIBLIOGRAPHY

Please visit the Nelson Textbook of Pediatrics *website at* *www.expertconsult.com* *for the complete bibliography.*

Chapter 111 Contraception

Barbara Cromer

Adolescents bear a disproportionate risk of the adverse consequences of sexual activity, sexually transmitted infections (STIs) (Chapter 114), and early, unintended pregnancy (Chapter 112). Adolescents often do not seek reproductive health care for 6 to 12 mo after initiating sex; many will become pregnant and/or acquire an STI during this interval. Youth who plan sexual initiation are 75% more likely to use contraception at sexual debut. Early adolescents are concrete thinkers, which may limit their ability to plan; most contraception requires some planning. Appropriate educational interventions with adolescents including the health care provider bringing up the topic of prevention can decrease sexual risk behavior.

EPIDEMIOLOGY

Sexual Activity

The median age at 1st intercourse varies greatly across the globe. Among participants ranging in age from 16 to above 65 yr representing all educational levels from 26 middle- and high-income nations, age of sexual debut was 18.9 yr for women and 19.5 yr for men, with an overall range of 23.0 yr in Malaysia to 17.3 yr in Austria (18.0 yr in the USA) (Fig. 111-1). Among developing nations, there is greater diversity; 73% of Liberian women ages

15-19 yr have had intercourse, compared to 53% of Nigerian, 49% of Ugandan, and 32% of Botswanan women. Only 7% of Chinese university students report being sexually experienced. Among U.S. high schools students in 2007, 7% report having initiated sex before age 13 yr, including 16% of African-American, 8% of Hispanic, and 4% of white youth; 48% of high school students are sexually experienced, including 67% African-American, 52% Hispanic, and 44% white.

Factors associated with early sexual activity in nations worldwide include lower expectations for education, poor perception of life options, low school grades, and involvement in other high-risk behaviors. For those who have never had intercourse, being against their religion and morals, avoiding pregnancy or a sexually transmitted infection, and waiting for the right person were the most frequent reasons adolescents report for abstaining.

Despite decreases in adverse outcomes of adolescent sexual activity in the USA for the decade at the end of the 20th and beginning of the 21st century, this trend may be reversing. The annual rate of AIDS diagnoses reported among males aged 15-19 yr doubled in the past from 1.3 cases per 100,000 population in 1997 to 2.5 cases in 2006; and rates of gonorrhea and syphilis also increased. Birthrates among adolescents aged 15-19 yr decreased each year from 1991-2005 but increased from 40.5 live births per 1,000 females in 2005 to 42.5 in 2007. The USA has the highest rate of teen pregnancy in the western industrialized world. Of the >750,000 pregnancies among women aged 15-19 yr annually, ~ 80% are unintended (of which 30% are aborted). Consistent with these decreases and subsequent increases in adverse outcomes, the Centers for Disease Control and Prevention "Youth Risk Behavior Survey" reported that among high school students the rate of "ever had intercourse" declined from 54.1% in 1991 to 46.7% in 2005. From 2005 to 2007 there was no further decline; rather, albeit insignificant statistically, all 3 categories of sexual activity (ever had sex, number of partners, currently sexually active) showed increasing trends and both contraception reports (use a condom, use birth control) showed decreasing trends (Table 111-1).

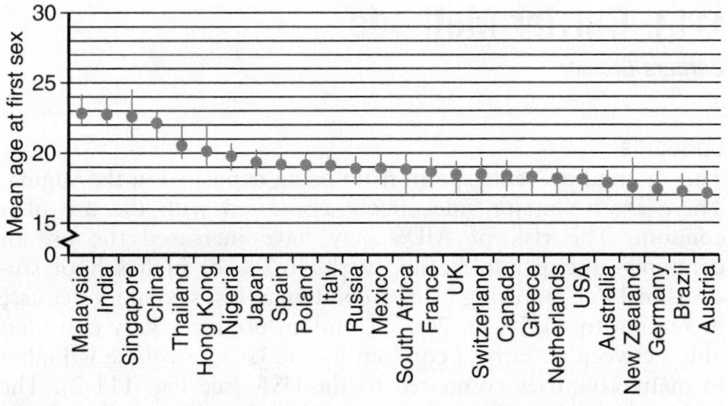

Figure 111-1 Mean age at first sex by country. (From Durex Network: *The face of global sex 2007. First sex: opportunity of a lifetime,* Cambridge, UK, 2007, SSL International, p 13. www.durexnetwork.org/en-GB/research/faceofglobalsex/Pages/Home.aspx. Accessed April 22, 2010.)

Contraceptive Use

Use of contraception at first sex has increased over the past half-century. Among the residents of 26 middle- and high-income countries listed in Figure 111-2, individuals >65 yr were 8-fold more likely to have used no contraception for their sexual debut, compared to youth currently 16-19 yr of age (among whom 75% used contraception). Females compared to males were 25% more likely to use some form of contraception when they made their sexual debut. Factors increasing the use of contraception at sexual debut include: increasing age among teens up to age 17 yr; spending some time at college; and planning their sexual debut (75% more likely to have used contraception than those who did not plan it). Among U.S. men, data from the National Center for Health Statistics reveals that 48% of those 15-44 yr report using a condom the 1st time they had sex, while 71% of sexually experienced men age 15-19 yr report using a condom the 1st time they have sex. Use of a condom at last episode of intercourse

Table 111-1 TRENDS IN THE PREVALENCE OF SEXUAL BEHAVIORS: NATIONAL YRBS: 1991-2007

1991	1993	1995	1997	1999	2001	2003	2005	2007	CHANGES FROM 1991-2007*	CHANGES FROM 2005-2007†
EVER HAD SEXUAL INTERCOURSE										
54.1 (50.5-57.8)‡	53.0 (50.2-55.8)	53.1 (48.4-57.7)	48.4 (45.2-51.6)	49.9 (46.1-53.7)	45.6 (43.2-48.1)	46.7 (44.0-49.4)	46.8 (43.4-50.2)	47.8 (45.1-50.6)	Decreased, 1991-2007	No change
HAD SEXUAL INTERCOURSE WITH FOUR OR MORE PERSONS DURING THEIR LIFE										
18.7 (16.6-21.0)	18.7 (16.8-20.9)	17.8 (15.2-20.7)	16.0 (14.6-17.5)	16.2 (13.7-19.0)	14.2 (13.0-15.6)	14.4 (12.9-16.1)	14.3 (12.8-15.8)	14.9 (13.4-16.5)	Decreased, 1991-2007	No change
CURRENTLY SEXUALLY ACTIVE (HAD SEXUAL INTERCOURSE WITH AT LEAST ONE PERSON DURING THE 3 MONTHS BEFORE THE SURVEY)										
37.5 (34.3-40.7)	37.5 (35.4-39.7)	37.9 (34.4-41.5)	34.8 (32.6-37.2)	36.3 (32.7-40.0)	33.4 (31.3-35.5)	34.3 (32.1-36.5)	33.9 (31.4-36.6)	35.0 (32.8-37.2)	Decreased, 1991-2007	No change
USED A CONDOM DURING LAST SEXUAL INTERCOURSE (AMONG STUDENTS WHO WERE CURRENTLY SEXUALLY ACTIVE)										
46.2 (42.8-49.6)	52.8 (50.0-55.6)	54.4 (50.7-58.0)	56.8 (55.2-58.4)	58.0 (53.6-62.3)	57.9 (55.6-60.1)	63.0 (60.5-65.5)	62.8 (60.6-64.9)	61.5 (59.4-63.6)	Increased, 1991-2003 No change, 2003-2007	No change
USED BIRTH CONTROL PILLS BEFORE LAST SEXUAL INTERCOURSE (TO PREVENT PREGNANCY, AMONG STUDENTS WHO WERE CURRENTLY SEXUALLY ACTIVE)										
20.8 (18.5-23.2)	18.4 (16.3-20.7)	17.4 (15.2-19.8)	16.6 (14.7-18.8)	16.2 (13.6-19.0)	18.2 (16.5-20.0)	17.0 (14.7-19.4)	17.6 (15.1-20.5)	16.0 (14.2-17.9)	No change, 1991-2007	No change
DRANK ALCOHOL OR USED DRUGS BEFORE LAST SEXUAL INTERCOURSE (AMONG STUDENTS WHO WERE CURRENTLY SEXUALLY ACTIVE)										
21.6 (18.7-24.8)	21.3 (19.3-23.5)	24.8 (22.1-27.8)	24.7 (22.9-26.7)	24.8 (21.8-28.0)	25.6 (23.8-27.4)	25.4 (23.2-27.8)	23.3 (21.1-25.6)	22.5 (20.7-24.5)	Increased, 1991-2001 Decreased, 2001-2007	No change
EVER TAUGHT IN SCHOOL ABOUT AIDS OR HIV INFECTION										
83.3 (80.1-86.0)	86.1 (83.4-88.4)	86.3 (79.0-91.3)	91.5 (90.3-92.5)	90.6 (89.1-91.9)	89.0 (87.6-90.3)	87.9 (85.8-89.7)	87.9 (85.8-89.7)	89.5 (88.1-90.7)	Increased, 1991-1997 Decreased, 1997-2007	No change

*Based on trend analyses using a logistic regression model controlling for sex, race/ethnicity, and grade.
†Based on t-test analyses, $p > .05$.
‡95% confidence interval.
From http://www.cdc.gov/HealthyYouth/yrbs/pdf/yrbs07_us_sexual_Behaviors_trend.pdf.

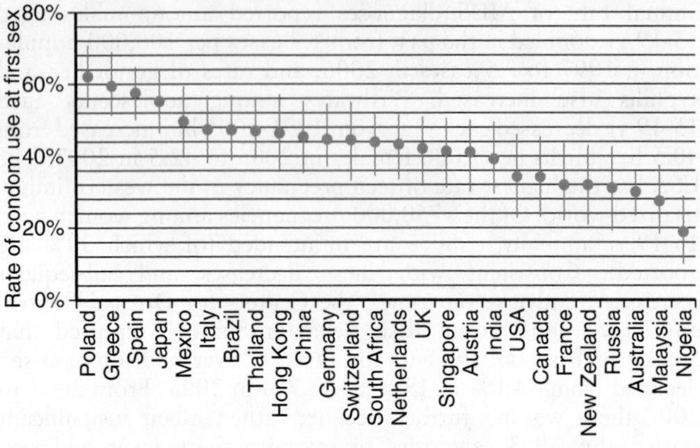

Figure 111-2 Rate of condom use at first sex by country. (From Durex Network: *The face of global sex 2007. First sex: opportunity of a lifetime*, Cambridge, UK, 2007, SSL International. www.durexnetwork.org/en-GB/research/faceofglobalsex/Pages/Home.aspx. Accessed April 22, 2010.)

increased from 46% in 1991 to 63% in 2003; in 2007 61.5% reported using a condom; use of birth control pills was 20.8% in 1991 and 16% in 2007 (see Table 111-1). Condoms were the most frequently used method, with dramatic increases from 1995-2002 in non-Hispanic white females (40.8% to 60.8%) and non-Hispanic black males (71% to 86.1%). The type of hormonal method selected also varies by ethnicity, with non-Hispanic white women more likely to select pills (40.7%); black women use pills as the first choice, and use the injectable method twice as much as white women.

Teens in the USA used medical methods at last intercourse less frequently compared to other teens; 52% in U.S. teens, 56% in Swedish 18-19 yr olds, 67% of French 15-19 yr olds, 72% of British 16-19 yr olds, and 73% of Canadian 15-19 yr olds. A higher likelihood of contraceptive use in women is associated with older age at sexual initiation, aspirations for higher academic achievement, acceptance of one's own sexuality, and a positive attitude toward contraception.

Contraceptive Counseling

The health screening interview during the adolescent preventive visit offers the opportunity both to support the adolescent who is abstinent to continue to be so and to identify the sexually active adolescent who has unsafe sexual practices (Chapter 106). Adolescents with chronic diseases are particularly vulnerable to having these issues omitted from the health maintenance visit (Chapter 39). There may be particular cautions related to concurrent medication to be noted for these chronically ill teenagers; sexuality and contraceptive issues do need to be addressed. The goals of a counseling intervention with the adolescent are to understand the adolescent's perceptions and misperceptions about contraceptives, help him or her put the risk of unprotected intercourse in a personal perspective, and educate the adolescent regarding the real risk and contraindications for the various methods available.

The likelihood that an adolescent will use a contraceptive method depends on such factors as the developmental level of the adolescent, the reproductive history, the involvement in other high-risk behaviors, and the degree of readiness for using contraception. **Readiness to use contraception** progresses in stages, from (1) precontemplative, not thinking about using contraception; (2) contemplative, giving it some thought, but having no immediate plans; (3) preparative, wanting to try a method in the near future; to (4) active, using contraception. The adolescent should also be made aware of the "perfect" use failure rates versus the "typical" failure rates based on the correct and consistent use of the method (Table 111-2). The pregnancy risk for use of withdrawal as a contraceptive method is probably underestimated in adolescents, and its low efficacy rate should be specifically addressed with young adolescents. Once an adolescent chooses a method, the provider and youth must discuss recognition of the common side effects, with clear plans on management; communication with the provider about the realistic expectation for failure; a contingency plan for that possibility; and strategies for close follow-up (see Table 111-2). A pelvic examination is not required for provision of a contraceptive method. Guidelines from the American College of Obstetrics and Gynecology stipulate that a routine pelvic exam with Pap smear be initiated 3 yr after onset of sexual activity. After this event, annual urine screening for STIs is advised. Confidentiality and consent issues related to contraceptive management are discussed in Chapter 106.

BIBLIOGRAPHY

Please visit the Nelson Textbook of Pediatrics *website at www.expertconsult.com for the complete bibliography.*

111.1 Barrier Methods

Barbara Cromer

Condoms

This method prevents sperm from being deposited in the vagina. There are no major side effects associated with the use of a condom. The risk of AIDS may have increased the use of condoms among adolescents, with 46.2% of high school students in 1991 reporting using a condom at last sexual intercourse increasing to 61.5% in 2007. Condom use rates vary considerably between countries; condom use at 1st intercourse is higher in many countries compared to the USA (see Fig. 111-2). The main advantages of condoms are their low price, availability without prescription, little need for advance planning, and, most important for this age group, their effectiveness in preventing transmission of STIs, including HIV and human papillomavirus (HPV). Latex condoms are recommended as protection against STIs, to be used along with all nonbarrier medical methods for adolescents. A female condom is available over the counter in single size disposable units. It is a 2nd choice over the male latex condom because of the complexity of properly using the device, its low typical efficacy rate, and the lack of studies in humans demonstrating its effectiveness against STIs. Most adolescents would require intensive education and hands-on practice to use it effectively.

Diaphragm and Cervical Cap

These methods have few side effects but are much less likely to be used by teenagers. Adolescents tend to object to the messiness of the jelly or to the fact that the insertion of a diaphragm may interrupt the spontaneity of sex, or they may express discomfort about touching their genitals.

111.2 Spermicides

Barbara Cromer

A variety of agents containing the spermicide nonoxynol-9 are available as foams, jellies, creams, films, or effervescent vaginal suppositories. They must be placed in the vaginal cavity shortly before intercourse and reinserted before each subsequent ejaculation in order to be effective. Rare side effects consist of contact vaginitis. There has been some concern regarding the vaginal and cervical mucosal damage observed with nonoxynol-9, and the overall impact on HIV transmission is unknown. The finding that nonoxynol-9 is gonococcicidal and spirocheticidal has not been substantiated in randomized clinical trials. Spermicides should be used in combination with condoms.

Table 111-2 CONTRACEPTIVE METHODS

METHOD	FAILURE RATE (%) Perfect Use	FAILURE RATE (%) Typical Use	DOSING	MECHANISM OF ACTION	POTENTIAL SIDE EFFECTS	ADVANTAGES
HORMONAL CONTRACEPTIVES						
The patch	0.7	0.9	Weekly for 3 wk (off on 4th wk) 20 μg ethinyl estradiol 150 μg norelgestromin released daily	Combined hormonal method: thickens cervical mucus, inhibits ovulation, inhibits sperm's ability to fertilize egg, slows tubal mobility, disrupts ovum transport, induces endometrial atrophy	Breakthrough bleeding, nausea, headaches, breast tenderness, skin site reaction, less effective if patient >90 kg (198 lb)	Similar to OCPs but less frequent dosing
Oral contraceptive (the pill) combination	0.1	5	Daily Varies 20-50 μg estrogen Varies 0.15-1 μg progestogen	Combined hormonal method: (see above)	Breakthrough bleeding, nausea, headaches, breast tenderness	Decrease in: PID risk, ectopic pregnancy risk, menstrual blood loss, dysmenorrheal, acne
Progestin only	0.5	5	Daily (within 3-hr period) 0.35 mg norethindrone or 0.075 mg norgestrel	Progestin-only hormonal method: inhibits ovulation, thickens and decreases cervical mucus, atrophies endometrium	Irregular bleeding, breast tenderness, depression	No estrogen
Contraceptive injections progestin-only injection (Depo-Provera)	0.3	0.3	3 mo 150 mg depot medroxyprogesterone per injection	Progestin-only hormonal method: (see above)	Irregular bleeding or amenorrhea, weight gain, breast tenderness, acne, depression, possible decrease in bone density	No estrogen, decrease in: menstrual blood loss, dysmenorrhea, PID risk
Progestin-releasing IUD (Mirena)	0.1	0.1	5 yr Releases 20 μg/day levonorgestrel	Progestin-only hormonal effect and IUD effect of preventing sperm from fertilizing ovum	Breakthrough bleeding in first 3-6 mo, then hypo-, or amenorrhea	No estrogen, easy to use, long-acting Decrease in: menstrual blood loss, dysmenorrheal, (possible) PID risk
Vaginal ring (NuvaRing)	0.65	N/A	Monthly (insert for 3 wk of each month) Serum levels of 15 μg ethinyl estradiol Releases 150 μg norelgestromin daily	Combined hormonal method: (see above)	Vaginal irritation, vaginal discharge, headache	Similar to OCs but less frequent dosing
Implant (Implanon)	0%	N/A	Insertion of implant once every 3 yr	Suppression of ovulation; thickening of cervical mucous	Rare insertion complications, possible weight gain, uterine bleeding changes	High efficacy, discreetness, relief of dysmenorrheal, reduced risk of ectopic pregnancy, reversibility, high acceptability and continuation rates
NONHORMONAL CONTRACEPTIVES						
Male condom	3	14	Every act of intercourse	Barrier method: blocks passage of semen	Latex allergy	Recommended to be used in addition to another contraceptive; only method that decreased STD, HIV risk
Female condom	5	21	Every act of intercourse	Barrier method: lines the vagina fully and perineum partially	Vaginal discomfort, partner penile irritation	Provides some protection against STD, HIV
IUD copper-containing (ParaGard)	0.6	0.8	10 yr 36 × 22 mm, copper wire wound around vertical stem of T	IUD: prevents sperm from fertilizing ova	Heavier menses	Easy to use, long-acting nonhormonal
Spermicides	18	29	Every act of intercourse nonoxynol-9 (in USA). Dose varies by formulation, e.g., gel, suppository, from 52.5 to 150 mg	Kills sperm by destroying sperm cell membrane	Allergy or sensitivity to ingredients, recurrent urinary tract infections	Recommended to be used in addition to another barrier contraceptive

IUD, intrauterine device; OCs, oral contraceptives; PID, pelvic inflammatory disease; STD, sexually transmitted disease.
From As-Sanie S, Gantt A, Rosenthal MS: Pregnancy prevention in adolescents, *Am Fam Physician* 70:1517–1524, 2004; and Hatcher RA, Trussell J, et al, editors: *Contraceptive technology,* New York, 2007, Ardent Media.

111.3 Combination Methods

Barbara Cromer

The conjoint use of the condom by the male and spermicidal foam by the female adolescent is extremely effective; the failure rate is 2% (perfect use), without any of the potential side effects and complications associated with the use of other forms of contraception having comparable efficacy. This combination also prevents STIs, including HIV and HPV.

BIBLIOGRAPHY

Please visit the Nelson Textbook of Pediatrics *website at www.expertconsult.com for the complete bibliography.*

111.4 Hormonal Methods

Barbara Cromer

Hormonal methods employ either an estrogenic substance in combination with a progestin or a progestin alone. The major mechanism of action of both the estrogen-progestin combination and the progestin-only methods, is to prevent the surge of luteinizing hormone and, as a result, to inhibit ovulation. Additional effects to the reproductive tract, which may add to contraceptive efficacy, include thickening of the cervical mucus in such a way that prevents sperm penetration.

Combination Oral Contraceptives

Oral contraceptives (OCs) are commonly referred to as "the pill" and contain 35, 30, or 20 µg of estrogenic substance, typically ethinyl estradiol, and a progestin. The pill is one of the most reliable contraceptive methods available; typical-use failure rates in 15-19 yr old women have ranged up to 18.1%. Thrombophlebitis, hepatic adenomas, myocardial infarction, and carbohydrate intolerance are some of the more serious potential complications of exogenous estrogen use. These disorders are exceedingly rare in adolescents. Even though teenage smokers who use OCs have a relative risk of more than 2.0 for myocardial infarction, the likelihood of its occurrence is very small, and thus clinically insignificant, compared to the risk of dying from pregnancy-related complications. Some long-range beneficial effects of estrogen use include decreased risks of benign breast disease, ovarian disease, and anemia.

The short-term adverse effects of OCs, such as nausea and weight gain, often interfere with compliance in adolescent patients. These effects are usually transient and may be overshadowed by the beneficial effects of a shortened menses and the relief of dysmenorrhea. The inhibition of ovulation or the suppressant effect of estrogens on prostaglandin production by the endometrium makes OCs effective in preventing dysmenorrhea (Chapter 110). An initial thought for younger adolescents regarding the potentially unknown effect of estrogens on epiphyseal growth is no longer a concern. Acne may be worsened by some and improved by other OC preparations. The pills with nonandrogenic progestins are particularly effective in reducing acne and hirsutism. Drospirenone, a progestin with antimineralocorticoid activity, has been shown to reduce premenstrual symptomatology, but the potential for hyperkalemia as a side effect eliminates patients with renal, liver, or adrenal diseases and patients on certain medications. A beneficial cardiovascular effect occurs for adolescents taking estrogen-containing OCs; these young women have higher levels of cardioprotective high-density lipoproteins than controls. Although women <35 yr old who smoke are at less risk of cardiovascular complications, adolescents on OCs should be encouraged to stop smoking.

Extended cycling of OCs for adolescents has some anticipated benefits with increased ovarian activity suppression and improved contraceptive efficacy during treatment with drugs that reduce OC efficacy. Seasonale (0.15 mg levonorgestrel/30 µg ethinyl estradiol) was approved by the U.S. Food and Drug Administration (FDA) in September 2003 for extended cycling with 84 active pills and 7 placebo pills, resulting in a cycle of 91 days. The most common side effect is intermenstrual bleeding and/or spotting with the total days of bleeding over the 1st year of treatment being similar for Seasonale subjects and subjects on a 28-day cycle. The unscheduled bleeding pattern diminishes over time. Other advantages include diminished frequency of hormonal withdrawal (premenstrual) effects including headaches and migraines, mood changes, and heavy monthly bleeding.

The first extended-cycle oral contraceptive that supplies continuously throughout the year, Lybrel (90 µg of levonorgestrel and 20 µg of ethinyl estradiol) causes cessation of menstruation for an entire year.

Contraindications to the use of estrogen-containing OCs include hepatocellular disease, migraine headaches, breast disease, any condition in which hypercoagulability may be a problem (replaced cardiac valve, thrombophlebitis, sickle cell anemia) because of the increased levels of factor VIII and decreased production of antithrombin III, and known or suspected pregnancy (Table 111-3). The risks of pregnancy must be balanced against the benefits of reliable contraception in patients with chronic diseases such as diabetes, epilepsy, and sickle cell disease. The initial history taken before prescribing OCs should specifically address these risks. The World Health Organization ranks multiple medical eligibility criteria for safety with the use of hormonal contraception from 4, precluding use, to 1, conditions raising no concerns, and provides a thorough listing for reference purposes.

Missed Contraceptive Pills

The effectiveness of OC is dependent on compliance, and unfortunately adolescent women may forget to take a pill each day. A pill is considered missed if it is 12 hr late from the designated daily time. If 3 pills are missed, back up contraception is required and if intercourse has occurred, emergency contraception (EC) is indicated (Fig. 111-3). Rules for missed pills are noted in Table 111-4.

Other Combination Methods

The *transdermal patch* (Ortho Evra) releases 20 µg ethinyl estradiol and 150 µg norelgestromin daily and is applied to the lower

Table 111-3 CONTRAINDICATIONS TO COMBINED HORMONAL CONTRACEPTIVES

ABSOLUTE CONTRAINDICATIONS (CLASS 4 IN THE WHO CLASSIFICATION)
Pregnancy
Undiagnosed genital bleeding
Breast cancer
Past or present circulatory disease (for example, arterial or venous thrombosis, ischemic heart disease, and cerebral hemorrhage)
Thrombophilia
Pill induced hypertension
Migraine with aura
Active liver disease, cholestatic jaundice, Dubin-Johnson syndrome, acute porphyria
Systemic lupus erythematosus
Hemolytic-uremic syndrome
Thrombotic thrombocytopenic purpura
RELATIVE CONTRAINDICATIONS (CLASS 2 OR 3 IN THE WHO CLASSIFICATION)
Smoker aged over 35 years
Hypertension (blood pressure above 140/90 mm Hg)
Diabetes
Hyperprolactinemia
Gall bladder disease
Migraine without aura
Otosclerosis
Sickle cell disease

From Amy JJ, Tripathi V: Contraception for women: an evidence based overview, *BMJ* 339:563–568, 2009.

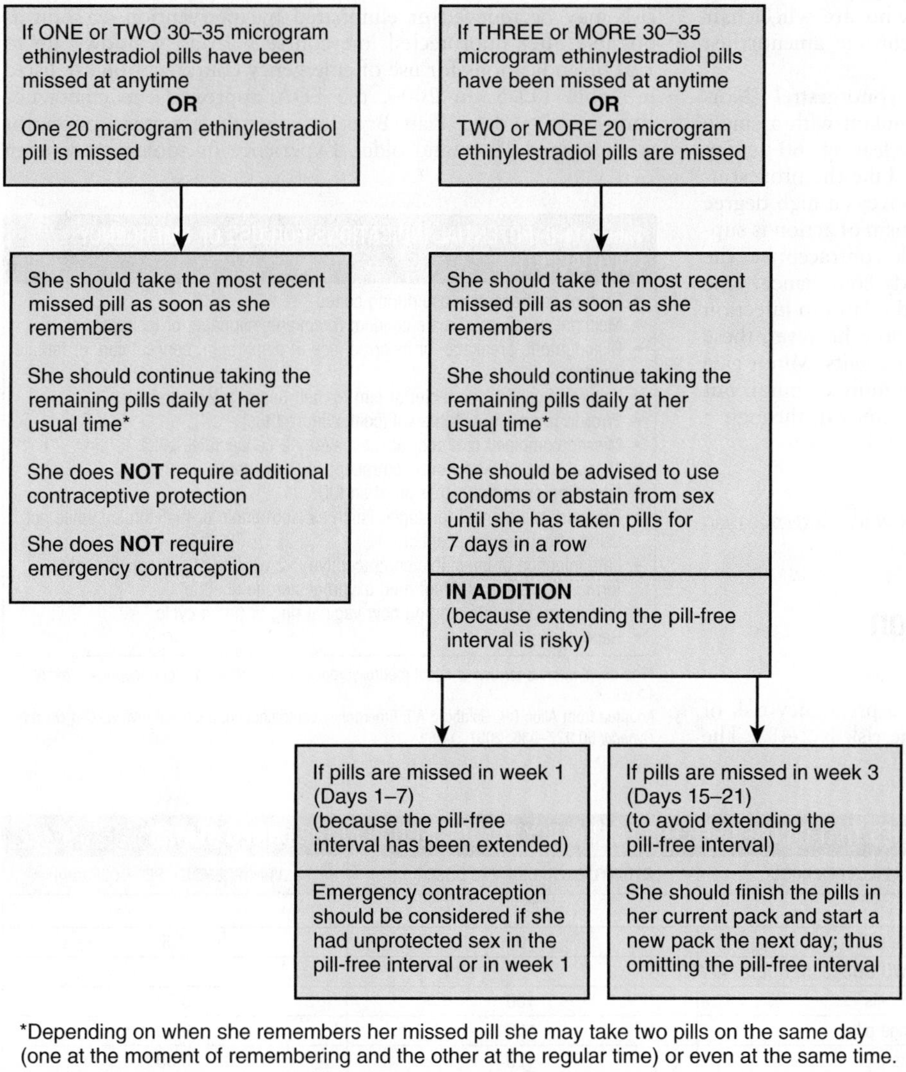
If ONE or TWO 30–35 microgram ethinylestradiol pills have been missed at anytime
OR
One 20 microgram ethinylestradiol pill is missed
If THREE or MORE 30–35 microgram ethinylestradiol pills have been missed at anytime
OR
TWO or MORE 20 microgram ethinylestradiol pills are missed
She should take the most recent missed pill as soon as she remembers
She should continue taking the remaining pills daily at her usual time*
She does NOT require additional contraceptive protection
She does NOT require emergency contraception
She should take the most recent missed pill as soon as she remembers
She should continue taking the remaining pills daily at her usual time*
She should be advised to use condoms or abstain from sex until she has taken pills for 7 days in a row
IN ADDITION
(because extending the pill-free interval is risky)
If pills are missed in week 1 (Days 1–7) (because the pill-free interval has been extended)
Emergency contraception should be considered if she had unprotected sex in the pill-free interval or in week 1
If pills are missed in week 3 (Days 15–21) (to avoid extending the pill-free interval)
She should finish the pills in her current pack and start a new pack the next day; thus omitting the pill-free interval
*Depending on when she remembers her missed pill she may take two pills on the same day (one at the moment of remembering and the other at the regular time) or even at the same time.

Figure 111-3 Advice for women missing combined oral contraceptives (30-35 µg and 20 µg ethinyl estradiol formulations). (From Faculty of Family Planning and Reproductive Health Care Effectiveness Unit: *FFPRHC Guidance [July 2006]. First prescription of combined oral contraception.* The full statement is available at www.ffprhc.org.uk.)

Table 111-4 MISSED PILL RULES

- Whenever a woman realizes that she missed pills, the essential advice is "**just keep going.**" She should take a pill as soon as possible and then resume her usual pill-taking schedule.
- **Also**, if the missed pills are in **wk 3**, she should **omit the pill-free interval**.
- **Also**, a back-up method (usually condoms) or abstinence should be used for 7 days if the following numbers of pills are missed:
- **Two for 20** (if two or more 20 µg ethinylestradiol pills are missed)
- **Three for 30** (if three or more 30-35 µg ethinylestradiol pills are missed)

From Faculty of Family Planning and Reproductive Health Care Clinical Effectiveness Unit: *Missed pills: new recommendations*, April 2005. www.ffprhc.org.uk/admin/uploads/MissedPillRules%20.pdf. Accessed April 23, 2010.

abdomen, buttocks, or upper body. It is worn continuously for 1 wk and changed weekly for a total of 3 wk, then removed to allow menstrual bleeding (see Table 111-2). It should not be applied to the breast. Limited studies in adolescents suggest higher rates of partial or full detachment compared to adults, with high patient satisfaction and 50-83% continuation rates from 3-18 mo of use.

The *vaginal contraceptive ring* (NuvaRing) is a flexible, transparent, colorless vaginal ring that measures about 2.1 inches in diameter and is inserted into the vagina by the patient. It releases 15 µg ethinyl estradiol and 120 µg etonogestrel per day and remains in place for 3 wk, during which time these hormones are absorbed. If the ring is accidentally expelled, it should be reinserted; however, if it is out of place for more than 3 hr, a back-up method of contraception should be used.

All these methods have contraindications similar to those to oral contraceptives (see Table 111-3).

All-Progestin Contraceptives

Progestin-only oral contraceptives are available for the adolescent in whom the use of estrogen is potentially deleterious: those with liver disease, replaced cardiac valves, or hypercoagulable states. These agents ("mini-pills") are less reliable in inhibiting ovulation and are associated with a 0.5%/yr pregnancy rate (perfect use). Acceptance by adolescents is limited by the necessity of taking the pill daily, the higher incidence of amenorrhea, and increased breakthrough bleeding.

An *injectable progestin,* medroxyprogesterone acetate (Depo-Provera, DMPA), is highly effective as birth control in a dose of 150 mg as a deep intramuscular injection, with failure rates typically at 0.3-0.4% (see Table 111-2). DMPA is particularly attractive for adolescents who have difficulty with compliance, are intellectually impaired, and are chronically ill or have a relative contraindication to estrogen use. Although concern has been directed toward the potential for loss in bone mineral density in adolescents, thereby potentially increasing their risk for osteoporosis later in life, recent studies have found that bone density is recovered after discontinuation of the method. Health care providers may want to consider a contraceptive containing estrogen in teens who are already at high risk for low bone density, such as those who have chronic renal disease, who are wheelchair bound, or who have eating disorders or chronic amenorrhea (Chapter 698).

The *long-acting progestational agent* levonorgestrel (Norplant) is not available in the USA. A 3-yr implant with a single rod containing etonogestrel (Implanon) releasing 60 µg/day received FDA approval in the USA in 2006. Like the progestin-only injectable contraceptive, the implant conveys a high degree of contraceptive efficacy and its main mechanism of action is suppression of ovulation. Also like the injectable contraceptive, the implant does not require daily or even weekly compliance. One potential unique complication of this method relates to infection and other serious side effects after implantation; however, these events are rare, occurring in less than 1% of patients. Minor side effects, such as bruising or skin irritation are more common but tend to resolve without treatment. Implant removal, through a minor surgical procedure, occurs at the end of 3 years.

BIBLIOGRAPHY

Please visit the Nelson Textbook of Pediatrics *website at* *www.expertconsult.com* *for the complete bibliography.*

111.5 Emergency Contraception

Barbara Cromer

Unprotected intercourse at mid-cycle carries a pregnancy risk of 20-30%. At other times during the cycle, the risk is 2-4%. The risk may be reduced or eliminated by intervention as soon as possible after unprotected intercourse with a "window" up to 120 hr. Indications for use of emergency contraception are listed in Table 111-5. In 2006, the FDA approved the emergency contraceptive drug Plan B as an over-the-counter option for women aged 18 yr and older. Experience in adolescent women

Table 111-5 POTENTIAL INDICATIONS FOR USE OF EMERGENCY CONTRACEPTION

- Lack of contraceptive use during coitus
- Mechanical failure of male condom (breakage, slippage, or leakage)
- Dislodgment, breakage, or incorrect use of diaphragm, cervical cap, or female condom
- Failure of spermicide tablet or film to melt before intercourse
- Error in practicing withdrawal (coitus interruptus)
- Missed combined oral contraceptives (any 2 consecutive pills)
- Missed progestin-only oral contraceptive (1 or more)
- Expulsion or partial expulsion of an IUD
- Exposure to potential teratogen (such as isotretinoin or thalidomide while not using effective contraception)
- Late injection of injectable contraceptive (>2 wk late of a progestin-only formulation such as depot medroxyprogesterone acetate)*
- 2 or more days late starting new vaginal ring or patch cycle
- Rape

*The usual interval for use of depot medroxyprogesterone acetate as contraception is every 12 wk.

Adapted from Allen RH, Goldberg AB: Emergency contraception: a clinical review, *Clin Obstet Gynecol* 50:927–936, 2007.

Table 111-6 TWENTY-THREE ORAL CONTRACEPTIVES THAT CAN BE USED FOR EMERGENCY CONTRACEPTION IN THE UNITED STATES*

BRAND	COMPANY	PILLS PER DOSE†	ETHINYL ESTRADIOL PER DOSE (µg)	LEVONORGESTREL PER DOSE (mg)‡
PROGESTIN-ONLY PILLS: TAKE ONE DOSE†				
Plan B	Barr/Duramed	2 white pills	0	1.5
COMBINED PROGESTIN AND ESTROGEN PILLS: TAKE TWO DOSES 12 HOURS APART				
Alesse	Wyeth-Ayerst	5 pink pills	100	0.50
Aviane	Barr/Duramed	5 orange pills	100	0.50
Cryselle	Barr/Duramed	4 white pills	120	0.60
Enpresse	Barr/Duramed	4 orange pills	120	0.50
Jolessa	Barr/Duramed	4 pink pills	120	0.60
Lessina	Barr/Duramed	5 pink pills	100	0.50
Levlen	Berlex	4 light-orange pills	120	0.60
Levlite	Berlex	5 pink pills	100	0.50
Levora	Watson	4 white pills	120	0.60
Lo/Ovral	Wyeth-Ayerst	4 white pills	120	0.60
Low-Ogestrel	Watson	4 white pills	120	0.60
Lutera	Watson	5 white pills	100	0.50
Nordette	Wyeth-Ayerst	4 light-orange pills	120	0.60
Ogestrel	Watson	2 white pills	100	0.50
Ovral	Wyeth-Ayerst	2 white pills	100	0.50
Portia	Barr/Duramed	4 pink pills	120	0.60
Quasense	Watson	4 white pills	120	0.60
Seasonale	Barr/Duramed	4 pink pills	120	0.60
Seasonique	Barr/Duramed	4 light blue-green pills	120	0.60
Tri-Levlen	Berlex	4 yellow pills	120	0.50
Triphasil	Wyeth-Ayerst	4 yellow pills	120	0.50
Trivora	Watson	4 pink pills	120	0.50

*Plan B is the only dedicated product specifically marketed for emergency contraception. Alesse, Aviane, Cryselle, Enpresse, Jolessa, Lessina, Levlen, Levora, Lo/Ovral, Low-Ogestrel, Lutera, Nordette, Ogestrel, Ovral, Portia, Quasense, Seasonale, Seasonique, Tri-Levlen, Triphasil and Trivora have been declared safe and effective for use as emergency contraceptive pills (ECPs) by the U.S. FDA. Worldwide, about 50 ECPs are specifically packaged, labeled, and marketed. For example, Gedeon Richter and HRA Pharma are marketing in many countries the levonorgestrel-only products Postinor-2 and Norlevo, respectively, each consisting of a 2-pill strip with each pill containing 0.75 mg levonorgestrel. Levonorgestrel-only ECPs are available either over-the-counter or from a pharmacist without having to see a clinician in 43 countries.

†The label for Plan B says to take 1 pill within 72 hours after unprotected intercourse, and another pill 12 hours later. However, recent research has found that both Plan B pills can be taken at the same time. Research has also shown that all of the brands listed here are effective when used within 120 hr after unprotected sex.

‡The progestin in Crysell, Lo/Ovral, Low-Ogestrel, Ogestrel, and Ovral is norgestrel, which contains two isomers, only one of which (levonorgestrel) is bioactive; the amount of norgestrel in each tablet is twice the amount of levonorgestrel.

demonstrates more effective use of EC with advance provision and is not associated with more frequent unprotected intercourse or less condom or pill use.

The **Yuzpe method** is commonly used in the USA, consisting of combination pills totaling 200 µg ethinyl estradiol and 2.0 mg norgestrel or 1.0 mg levonorgestrel. Pills that can be utilized for this method are shown in Table 111-6. The high-dose combination OCs disrupt the luteal phase hormone pattern, creating an unstable and unsuitable uterine lining for implantation. If used mid-cycle, when ovulation is about to occur, the high-dose estrogen and progestin blunt the luteinizing hormone surge and impair ovulation. This method is effective in reducing the risk of pregnancy by 75%. The most common side effects are nausea (50%) and vomiting (20%), prompting some clinicians to prescribe or recommend antiemetics along with the OCs. A urine pregnancy test is usually required prior to dispensing the pills to rule out an existing pregnancy. There is some controversy about the need to do this, since there is no evidence to suggest that OCs used in this manner affect early fetal development and the dose as prescribed would not disrupt a previously undetected pregnancy. The EC kit prepackaged for this method (Preven) was withdrawn from the market in 2004. A progestin-only EC kit was FDA approved in 1999 and contains 2 tablets, each with 0.75 mg levonorgestrel. Nausea and vomiting are uncommon side effects, and in a recent comparison, levonorgestrel proved more effective at preventing pregnancy than the Yuzpe method.

Mifepristone (RU-486) is an antiprogestin agent that blocks the binding of progestin to its receptor. It prevents ovulation or interferes with the luteal phase of the menstrual cycle and is as effective as Plan B for emergency contraception.

Teens can access EC information through a hotline at 1-888-NOT-2-LATE. A 2-wk follow-up appointment is recommended following any of the methods to determine the effectiveness of treatment and to diagnose a possible early pregnancy. The visit also provides an opportunity to counsel the adolescent, explore the situation leading up to the unprotected intercourse, test for STDs, and initiate continuing contraception when appropriate. Pap smear screening is not initiated until 21 yr of age.

BIBLIOGRAPHY

Please visit the Nelson Textbook of Pediatrics *website at www.expertconsult.com for the complete bibliography.*

111.6 Intrauterine Devices

Barbara Cromer

Intrauterine devices (IUDs) are small, flexible, plastic objects introduced into the uterine cavity through the cervix. They differ in size, shape, and the presence or absence of pharmacologically active substances (copper or progesterone). The mechanism of action of the TCu380A IUD is uncertain, although they render the endometrium unsuitable for implantation by inducing a local polymorphonuclear leukocyte response and production of prostaglandin. The levonorgestrel IUD may also have various contraceptive actions, from thickening of cervical mucus and inhibiting sperm survival to suppressing the endometrium. Both types of IUDs are effective in preventing pregnancy in 97-99% of women. Although early studies suggested an increased risk for upper genital tract infection due theoretically to the presence of a foreign body in the cervix, more recent work has refuted these earlier concerns. Because of this clinicians have been encouraged to reconsider use of IUDs in adolescents despite relatively high prevalence rates of STIs.

BIBLIOGRAPHY

Please visit the Nelson Textbook of Pediatrics *website at www.expertconsult.com for the complete bibliography.*

Chapter 112
Adolescent Pregnancy

Dianne S. Elfenbein and Marianne E. Felice

EPIDEMIOLOGY

In 2006, there were approximately 442,000 births in the USA to young women under the age of 20 yr. This figure represents a birthrate of 41.9 births per 1,000 young women ages 15-19 yr and is a 3% increase over the birthrate in 2005 (40.5). This is the 1st time in the last 15 yr that teen birthrates have increased in the USA.

Before 2006, adolescent birthrates in the USA had steadily decreased since the early 1990s for all ages, races, and ethnic groups (Table 112-1), with the most dramatic decreases noted in African-American teens. In spite of the 3% increase from 2005 to 2006, the 2006 birthrate for teens ages 15-19 yr is considerably lower than the 1991 rate of 61.8. Pregnancy rates, which include births, miscarriages, stillbirths, and induced abortions, also decreased during this time frame, indicating that the decline in birthrates was not due to an increase in pregnancy terminations. The improvement in U.S. teen birthrates is attributed to 3 factors: more teens are delaying the onset of sexual intercourse, more teens are using some form of contraception when they begin to have sexual intercourse, and there is increased use of the new, long-lasting hormonal contraceptives.

In spite of the decrease in teen births in the last decade, the USA has the highest teen birthrate among all industrialized countries. U.S. teen birthrates are twice the rates in Great Britain and Canada and nearly 4 times the rates in France and Sweden. Two thirds of teen births are to 18-19 yr old women who technically have reached the age of majority.

ETIOLOGY

In industrialized countries with policies supporting access to protection against pregnancy and sexually transmitted infections (STIs), older adolescents are more likely to use hormonal contraceptives and condoms, resulting in lowered risk of unplanned pregnancy. Younger teenagers are likely to be less deliberate and logical about their sexual decisions and their sexual activity is likely to be sporadic or even coercive, contributing to inconsistent contraceptive use and a greater risk of unplanned pregnancy. Better hopes for employment and higher educational goals are associated with lowered probability of childbearing. In

Table 112-1 TEEN BIRTH RATES (BIRTHS PER 1,000 FEMALES) IN THE USA

AGE (YR)	1940	1950	1960	1970	1980	1990	2000	2001	2002	2003	2004	2005	2006
15-19	54.1	81.6	89.1	68.3	53.0	59.9	47.7	45.9	43.0	41.7	41.2	40.5	41.9
15-17	–	–	43.9	38.8	32.5	37.5	26.9	25.3	23.2	22.4	22.1	21.4	22.0
18-19	–	–	166.7	114.7	82.1	88.6	78.1	75.8	72.8	70.8	70.8	70.8	73.0

Adapted from *Facts at a glance*, Washington, DC, 2008, Child Trends.

nonindustrialized countries, laws permitting marriage of young and mid-adolescents, poverty, and limited female education are associated with increased adolescent pregnancy rates.

CLINICAL MANIFESTATIONS

Adolescents may experience the traditional symptoms of pregnancy: morning sickness (vomiting, nausea that may also occur any time of the day), swollen tender breasts, weight gain, and amenorrhea. Often the presentation is less classic. Headache, fatigue, abdominal pain, dizziness, and scanty or irregular menses are common presenting complaints.

In the pediatric office, some teens are reluctant to divulge concerns of pregnancy. Denial of sexual activity and menstrual irregularity should not preclude the diagnosis in face of other clinical or historical information. An unanticipated request for a complete checkup or a visit for contraception may uncover a suspected pregnancy. Pregnancy is still the most common diagnosis when an adolescent presents with **secondary amenorrhea.**

DIAGNOSIS (TABLE 112-2)

On physical examination, the findings of an enlarged uterus, cervical cyanosis (**Chadwick sign**), a soft uterus (**Hegar sign**), or a soft cervix (**Goodell sign**) are highly suggestive of an intrauterine pregnancy. A confirmatory pregnancy test is always recommended, either *qualitative* or *quantitative*. Modern **qualitative** urinary detection methods are efficient at detecting pregnancy, whether performed at home or in the office. These tests are based on detection of the beta subunit of human chorionic gonadotropin (HCG). While claims for over-the-counter home pregnancy tests may indicate 98% detection on the day of the 1st missed menstrual period, sensitivity and accuracy vary considerably. Office or point of care tests have increased standardization and generally have increased sensitivity, with the possibility of detecting a pregnancy within 3-4 days after implantation. However, in any menstrual cycle, ovulation may be delayed and in any pregnancy, the day of implantation may vary considerably as may rate of production of HCG. This variability, along with variation of urinary concentration, may affect test sensitivity. **Therefore, each negative test should be repeated in 1-4 wk if there is a heightened suspicion of pregnancy.** The most sensitive pregnancy detection test is a serum **quantitative** beta HCG radioimmunoassay in which results are reliable within 7 days after fertilization. This more expensive test is used primarily during evaluations for ectopic pregnancy, to detect retained placenta after pregnancy termination, or in the management of a molar pregnancy. It is generally used when serial measurements are necessary in clinical management.

Though not generally used for primary diagnosis of pregnancy, pelvic or vaginal ultrasound can be used to detect and date a pregnancy. Pelvic ultrasound will detect a gestational sac at about 5-6 wk (dated from last menstrual period) and vaginal ultrasound at 4.5-5 wk. This tool may also be used to distinguish diagnostically between intrauterine and ectopic pregnancies.

Table 112-2 DIAGNOSIS OF PREGNANCY DATED FROM FIRST DAY OF LAST MENSTRUAL CYCLE

CLASSIC SYMPTOMS
Missed menses, breast tenderness, nipple sensitivity, nausea, vomiting, fatigue, abdominal and back pain, weight gain, urinary frequency
Teens may present with unrelated symptoms that enable them to visit the doctor and maintain confidentiality
LABORATORY DIAGNOSIS
Tests for human chorionic gonadotropin in urine or blood may be positive 7-10 days after fertilization, depending on sensitivity
Irregular menses make ovulation/fertilization difficult to predict. Home pregnancy tests have a high error rate.
PHYSICAL CHANGES
2-3 wk after implantation: cervical softening and cyanosis
8 wk: uterus size of orange
12 wk: uterus size of grapefruit and palpable suprapubically
20 wk: uterus at umbilicus
If physical findings are not consistent with dates, ultrasound will confirm

PREGNANCY COUNSELING AND INITIAL MANAGEMENT

After the diagnosis of pregnancy is made, it is important to begin addressing the psychosocial, as well as the medical, aspects of the pregnancy. The patient's response to the pregnancy should be assessed and her emotional issues addressed. It should not be assumed that the pregnancy was unintended. Discussion of the patient's options should be initiated. These options include (1) releasing the child to an adoptive family, (2) electively terminating the pregnancy, or (3) raising the child herself with the help of family, father, friends, and/or other social resources. Options should be presented in a supportive, informative, nonjudgmental fashion; they may need to be discussed over several visits for some young women. Physicians who are uncomfortable in presenting options to their young patients should refer their patients to a provider who can provide this service expeditiously. Pregnancy terminations implemented early in the pregnancy are generally less risky and less expensive than those initiated later. Other issues that may need discussion are how to inform and involve the patient's parents and the father of the infant; implementing strategies for insuring continuation of the young mother's education; discontinuation of tobacco, alcohol, and illicit drug use; discontinuance and avoidance of any medications that may be considered teratogenic; starting folic acid, calcium, and iron supplements; proper nutrition, and testing for STIs. Especially in younger adolescents, the possibility of **coercive sex** (Chapter 113) should be considered and appropriate social work/legal referrals made if abuse has occurred, though most pregnancies are not a result of coercive sex. Patients who elect to continue their pregnancies should be referred as soon as possible to an adolescent-friendly obstetric provider.

CHARACTERISTICS OF TEEN PARENTS

Young women who become parents as teenagers often come from economically disadvantaged families. Although birthrates among black and Hispanic teens have decreased in the past decade, their rates are more than double those for non-Hispanic whites. Parenting teens frequently have poor school performance prior to becoming pregnant, and they often have a family history of low educational attainment. Learning disabilities are not uncommon. Teen mothers frequently come from single-parent families where their own mother gave birth during adolescence. A large majority (84%) of teen mothers have a baby outside of marriage. They may view pregnancy as having a positive social value and as not interfering with their long-term goals.

Teenage men who become fathers as adolescents also have poorer educational achievement than their age-matched peers. They are more likely than peers to have been involved with illegal activities and with the use of illegal substances. Adult men who father the children of teen mothers are poorer and educationally less advanced than their age-matched peers and tend to be 2-3 yr older than the mother; any combination of age differences may exist. Younger teen mothers are more likely to have a greater age difference between themselves and the father of their child, raising the issue of coercive sex or statutory rape (Chapter 113).

Male partners have a significant influence on the young woman's decision/desire to become pregnant and to parent her child. Sensitively and appropriately including the male partner in discussions of fertility planning, contraception, and pregnancy options may be a useful strategy in improving outcomes for all.

MEDICAL COMPLICATIONS OF MOTHERS AND BABIES

Although pregnant teens are at higher than average risk of some complications of pregnancy, most teenagers have pregnancies that are without major medical complications, delivering healthy infants. The miscarriage/stillbirth risk for adolescents is estimated at 15% and the pregnancy termination rate has been fairly stable at approximately 33% since 1995. As expected, teen mothers have low rates of age-related chronic disease (diabetes or hypertension) that might affect the outcomes of a pregnancy. They also have lower rates of twin pregnancies than older women. They tolerate childbirth well with few operative interventions. However, as compared with 20-39 yr old mothers, teens have higher incidences of low birthweight infants, preterm infants, neonatal deaths, passage of moderate to heavy fetal meconium during parturition, and infant deaths within 1 yr after birth. The highest rates of these poor outcomes occur in the youngest and most economically deprived mothers. Gastroschisis, though very rare, has a markedly higher incidence in infants of teen mothers for reasons that are not yet clear. Teen mothers also have higher rates of anemia, pregnancy-associated hypertension, and eclampsia, with the youngest teens having rates of pregnancy-associated hypertension 40% higher than the rates of women in their 20s and 30s. The youngest teens also have a higher incidence of poor weight gain (<16 lb) during their pregnancy. This correlates with a decrease in the birthweights of their infants. Poor maternal weight gain also correlates strongly with teens' late entrance into prenatal care and with inadequate utilization of prenatal care. Sexually active teens have higher rates of STIs than older sexually active women.

Many young women who become pregnant have been exposed to violence or abuse in some form during their lives. There is some evidence that teenage women have the highest rates of **violence** during pregnancy of any group. Violence has been associated with injuries and death as well as preterm births, low birthweight, bleeding, substance abuse, and late entrance into prenatal care. An analysis of the Pregnancy Mortality Surveillance System indicates that from 1991 to 1999, homicide was the 2nd leading cause of injury-related deaths in pregnant and postpartum women. Women ages 19 yr and younger had the highest pregnancy-related homicide rate (Chapter 107).

Prematurity and low birthweight increase the perinatal morbidity and mortality for infants of teen mothers. These infants also have higher than average rates of sudden infant death syndrome (Chapter 367), possibly because of less use of the supine sleep position, and are at higher risk of both intentional and unintentional injury (Chapter 37). One study shows the risk of homicide to be 9 to 10 times higher if a child born to a teen mother is not the mother's firstborn as compared with the risk to a firstborn of a woman age 25 yr or older. The perpetrator is often the father, stepfather, or boyfriend of the mother.

After childbirth, **depressive symptoms** may occur in as many as 40-50% of teenaged mothers. Depression seems to be greater with additional social stressors and with decreased social supports. Support from the infant's father and the teen's mother seems to be especially important in preventing depression. Pediatricians who care for parenting teens should be sensitive to the possibility of depression as well as to inflicted injury to mother or child; appropriate diagnosis, treatment, and referral to mental health or social agencies should be offered and facilitated.

PSYCHOSOCIAL OUTCOMES/RISKS FOR MOTHER AND CHILD

Educational

Teenage mothers often do poorly in school and drop out prior to becoming pregnant. After childbirth many choose to defer completion of their education for some time. High school graduation or an equivalency degree is generally achieved eventually. Mothers who have given birth as teens generally remain 2 yr behind their age-matched peers in formal educational attainment at least through their 3rd decade. Maternal lack of education limits the income of many of these young families (Chapter 1).

Substance Use

Teenagers who abuse drugs, alcohol, and tobacco have higher pregnancy rates than their peers. Most substance-abusing mothers appear to decrease or stop their substance use while pregnant. Use begins to increase again about 6 mo postpartum, complicating the parenting process and the mother's return to school.

Repeat Pregnancy

Approximately 20% of all births to adolescent mothers (15-19 yr) are second order or higher. Prenatal care is begun even later with a 2nd pregnancy, and the 2nd infant is at higher risk of poor outcome than the 1st birth. Mothers at risk of early repeat pregnancy include those who do not initiate long-acting contraceptives after the index birth, those who do not return to school within 6 mo of the index birth, those who are married or living with the infant's father, or those who are no longer involved with the baby's father and who meet a new boyfriend who wants to have a child. To reduce repeat pregnancy rates in these teens, programs must be tailored for this population, preferably offering comprehensive health care for both the young mother and her child (Table 112-3).

Behavioral, Educational, and Social Outcomes of Infants

Many infants born to teen mothers have behavioral problems seen as early as the preschool period. Many drop out of school early (33%), become adolescent parents (25%), or, if male, are incarcerated (16%). Explanations for these poor outcomes include poverty, parental learning difficulties, negative parenting styles of teen parents, maternal depression, parental immaturity, poor parental modeling, social stress, exposure to surrounding violence, and conflicts with grandparents, especially grandmothers. Continued positive paternal involvement throughout the child's life may be somewhat protective against negative outcomes. Many of these poor outcomes appear to be due to the socioeconomic/demographic situation in which the teen pregnancy has occurred, not solely to maternal age. Even when socioeconomic status and demographics are controlled, infants of teen mothers have lower achievement scores, lower high school graduation rates, increased risk of teen births themselves, and, at least in Illinois (where records include age of birth mother), a higher probability of abuse and neglect.

Comprehensive programs focused on supporting adolescent mothers and infants utilizing life skills training, medical care, and psychosocial support demonstrate, at least in the short term, higher employment rates, higher income, and less welfare dependency in adolescents exposed to the programs. These may be helpful in improving the infants' outcomes.

Prevention of Teen Pregnancies

Adolescent pregnancy is a multifaceted problem that requires multifactorial solutions. The provision of contraception and education about fertility risk from the primary care physician is important, but insufficient to address the problem fully. Family and community involvement are also needed. Strategies for primary prevention (preventing 1st births) are different from the strategies needed for secondary prevention (preventing 2nd or more births).

Abstinence-only sexual education aims to teach adolescents to wait until marriage to initiate sexual activity but unfortunately does not mention contraception. Abstinence education is

Table 112-3 2001 AMERICAN ACADEMY OF PEDIATRICS POLICY STATEMENT RECOMMENDATIONS FOR CARE OF ADOLESCENT PARENTS AND THEIR CHILDREN

Create a medical home for adolescent parents and their children	Involve both adolescent mothers and co-parenting father Emphasize anticipatory guidance, parenting, and basic child care–giving skills
Provide comprehensive, multidisciplinary care	Access community resources such as special Supplemental Nutrition Program for Women, Infants, and Children Provide medical and developmental services to low-income parents and children Facilitate coordination of services
Contraceptive counseling	Emphasize condom use Encourage long-acting contraceptive methods
Encourage breast-feeding	Support breast-feeding in home, work, and school settings
Encourage high school completion	
Assess risk of domestic violence	
Encourage adolescent parenting	Work with other involved adults such as grandparents to encourage developmental growth of adolescent as parent as well as optimize infant developmental outcomes
Adapt counseling to developmental level of adolescent	Utilize school-, home-, and office-based interventions Consider use of support groups
Awareness and monitoring of developmental progression of infant and adolescent parent	Advocate for high-quality community resources for adolescents, including developmental resources, child care, and parenting classes Facilitate access to Head Start and education resources for individuals with disability
Provide positive reinforcement for success	Educational achievements Parenting achievements, such as compliance with well child care and immunizations Avoidance of drugs, alcohol, or nicotine Maintenance of breast-feeding and other healthy behaviors

From Beers LAS, Hollo RE: Approaching the adolescent-headed family: a review of teen parenting, *Curr Probl Pediatr Adolesc Health Care* 39:215–234, 2009.

sometimes coupled with "virginity pledges" in which teenagers pledge to remain abstinent until they marry. Other educational programs emphasize HIV and STI prevention and in the process prevent pregnancy, while others include both abstinence and contraception in their curricula. Sex education and teaching about contraception do not lead to an increase in sexual activity. Teenagers who participate in programs that have comprehensive sex education components generally have lower rates of pregnancy than those teenagers who have exposure to abstinence-only programs or no sex education at all.

In many communities, programs that engage youth in community service and/or combine sex education and youth development are also successful in deterring pregnancy. Programs vary in their sites of service from schools, to social agencies, to health clinics, to youth organizations, to churches. Other countries have taken different approaches. In Sweden, family life and sex education have been taught in schools since the 1950s, and since 1975, abortion has been free on demand. Contraceptive counseling is free and readily available at family planning and youth health clinics along with STI screening.

Secondary prevention programs are fewer in number. In the USA, some communities have tried to "pay" young mothers to not become pregnant again, but these efforts have not always been fruitful. Home visiting by nurses has been successful in some areas, and many communities have developed "Teen Tot" Clinics that provide a "one-stop shopping model" for health care for both the teen mother and the baby in the same site at the same time. Both of these latter types of programs have reported some successes.

In the practice setting, the identification of the sexually active adolescent through a confidential clinical interview is a 1st step in pregnancy prevention. The primary care physician should provide the teenager with factual information in a nonjudgmental manner and then guide him or her in the decision-making process of choosing a contraceptive. In addition, the practice setting is an ideal setting to support the teenager who chooses to remain abstinent.

BIBLIOGRAPHY

Please visit the Nelson Textbook of Pediatrics *website at* *www.expertconsult.com* *for the complete bibliography.*

Chapter 113
Adolescent Rape

Christine E. Barron and Marianne E. Felice

Rape is coercive sexual intercourse involving physical force or psychologic manipulation of a female or a male. Rape is defined as penetration of any genital, oral, or anal orifice by a part of the assailant's body or any object. *Rape is an act of violence, not an act of sex.*

EPIDEMIOLOGY

Exact figures on the incidence of rape are unavailable because many rapes are not reported. Females exceed males as reported rape victims by nearly 10:1, but male rape may be more underreported than female rape. In the USA, the annual rates of sexual victimization per 1,000 persons were reported in 2008 by the U.S. Department of Justice, National Crime Victimization Survey to be 1.6 for ages 12-15 yr, 2.2 for ages 16-19 yr, and 2.1 for ages 20-24 yr. The highest annual rate of sexual victimization has continued to be among 16-19 yr old adolescents. Rape occurs worldwide and is especially prevalent in war. An estimated one fourth to one half million adolescent and older women were raped during the 1994 conflict in Rwanda. During the Balkan conflict, with teenage girls particularly targeted, at least 20,000 girls and women were raped. In East Timor, 23% of adolescent and adult women reported being sexually assaulted during the 1999 armed conflict, declining to 10% during the post crisis period. In the context of the war in the Democratic Republic of the Congo, there were 20,517 female rape survivors in the 3 yr period 2005-2007.

Female adolescents and young adults account for the highest rates of rape compared to any other age group. The normal developmental growth tasks of adolescence may contribute to this vulnerability in the following ways: (1) the emergence of independence from parents and the establishment of relationships outside the family may expose adolescents to environments with which they are unfamiliar and situations that they are unprepared to handle; (2) dating and becoming comfortable with one's

Table 113-1 ADOLESCENTS AT HIGH RISK OF RAPE VICTIMIZATION
MALE AND FEMALE ADOLESCENTS
Drug and alcohol use
Runaways
Intellectual disability or developmental delay
Street youths
Youths with a parental history of sexual abuse
PRIMARILY FEMALES
Survivors of prior sexual assault
Newcomers to a town or college
PRIMARILY MALES
Institutionalized settings (detention centers, prison)
Young male homosexuals

sexuality may result in activities that are unwanted, but the adolescent is too inexperienced to stop the unwanted actions; and (3) young adolescents may be naïve and more trusting than they should be. Many teens are computer competent, which gives sexual perpetrators access to unsuspecting vulnerable populations who were previously beyond their reach. Chat rooms represent a major risk for adolescents, resulting in correspondence with individuals unknown to them or protective family members, while simultaneously providing a false sense of security due to remote electronic communications. A determined perpetrator can obtain specific information to identify the adolescent and arrange for a meeting that is primed for sexual victimization.

Some adolescents are at higher risk of being victims of rape than others (Table 113-1).

TYPES OF RAPE

Acquaintance rape (by a person known to the victim) is the most common form of rape for victims between 16 and 24 yr of age. The acquaintance may be a neighbor, classmate, or friend of the family. The victim-assailant relationship may cause conflicting loyalties in families, and the teen's report may be received with disbelief and/or skepticism by her or his family. Adolescent acquaintance rape differs from adult acquaintance rape because weapons are less often used, and victims are less likely to sustain physical injuries. Victims of acquaintance rape are also more likely to delay seeking medical care, may never report the crime (males greater than females), and are less likely to proceed with criminal prosecution even after reporting the incident(s).

Date rape (by a person dating the victim) is often drug facilitated and is prevalent in adolescent populations. Date rape drugs are pharmaceuticals administered in a clandestine manner to potential victims. γ-Hydroxybutyric acid (GHB), flunitrazepam (Rohypnol), and ketamine hydrochloride are the leading agents used for these illegal purposes (Chapter 108). The pharmacologic properties of these drugs make them suitable for this use as they have simple modes of administration, are easily concealed (colorless, odorless, tasteless), have rapid onsets of action with resulting induction of anterograde amnesia, and have rapid eliminations due to short half-lives. Detection of these drugs requires a high index of suspicion and medical evaluation within 8-12 hr, prompting specific testing because routine toxicology screening is insufficient.

Date rape victims are often new to a specific environment (college freshman, newcomer to a town) and lack strong social support. Victims may not be assertive in establishing boundaries or limits with their dates and may be intoxicated when the incident takes place. The date rape assailant may engage in more sexual activities than other men his age and often has a history of aggressive behavior toward women. He may interpret passivity as assent and deny the charge of coercion or force; he may also be intoxicated at the time of the assault.

A date rape victim often experiences long-term issues of trust, self-blame, and guilt. She may lose confidence in her judgment concerning men in the future. She is nearly always ashamed of the incident and is less likely to report the rape. She is reluctant to talk about the rape to family, friends, or a counselor and may never heal from the psychologic scars that ensue.

Male rape generally refers to same-sex rape of male teens by other males. Specific subgroups of young men are at high risk of being victims of rape (see Table 113-1). Male rape is most prevalent within institutional settings. Male rape that occurs outside of institutional settings typically involves coercion of the male teen by someone considered an authority figure, either male or female. Male rape victims often experience conflicted sexual identity whether or not they are homosexual. Issues of loss of control and powerlessness are particularly bothersome for male rape victims, and these young men commonly have symptoms of anxiety, depression, sleep disturbance, and suicidal ideation. Males are less likely than females to report rape and less likely to seek professional help.

Gang rape usually occurs when a group of young men rape a solitary female victim. This type of rape may be part of a ritualistic activity or rite of passage for some male group (gangs, college fraternity) or be displaced rage on the part of the assailants.

Female victims of gang rape may find it difficult to return to the environment in which the rape occurred for fear of confrontation with the assailants (college setting or place of employment) and may insist on moving away from the locale entirely.

Statutory rape refers to sexual activity between an adult and an adolescent under the age of legal consent, as defined by individual state law. Statutory rape laws are based on the premise that below a certain age, an individual is not legally capable of giving consent to engage in sexual intercourse. In some states in the USA, statutory rape laws apply to sexual contact or intercourse occurring between a minor and another individual with a specific age difference even when both are minors and both assert that the sexual act was voluntary (an 18 yr old male who has sexual intercourse with a 14 yr old female). The intent of such laws is to protect youths from being victimized, but they may inadvertently lead a teenager to withhold pertinent sexual information from a clinician for fear that their sexual partner will be reported to the law. A clinician must be familiar with the laws of the state or province in which they are practicing medicine.

Stranger rape occurs less frequently within the adolescent population and is most similar to adult rape. Such rapes frequently occur with an abduction, use of weapons, and increased risk of physical injuries. These rapes are more likely to be reported and prosecuted.

Clinical Manifestations

The adolescent's acute presentation following a rape may vary considerably, from histrionics to near-mute withdrawal. Even if they do not seem to be afraid, most victims are extremely fearful and very anxious about the incident, the rape report, examination, and the entire process including potential repercussions. Since adolescents are between the developmental lines of childhood and adulthood their responses to rape may have elements of both child and adult behaviors. Many teens, particularly young adolescents, may experience some level of cognitive disorganization.

Adolescents may be reluctant to report rape for a variety of reasons, including self-blame, fear, embarrassment, or in the circumstances of drug-facilitated rape, uncertainty of event details. Adolescent victims, unlike child victims who elicit sympathy and support, are often faced with intense scrutiny regarding their credibility and inappropriately misplaced societal blame for the assault. This view is baseless and should not be used during an evaluation of any teenage victim, including acquaintance rape.

When adolescents do not report a rape, they may present at a future date with symptoms of post-traumatic stress disorder, such as sleep disturbances, nightmares, mood swings, and flashbacks. Other teens may present with psychosomatic complaints or difficulties with schoolwork; all adolescents should be screened for the possibility of sexual abuse at nearly all health examination visits.

Interview and Physical Examination

Although many teens delay seeking medical care, others present to a medical facility within 72 hr of the rape, at which time forensic evidence collection should be completed. Experienced clinicians with training and knowledge of forensic evidence collection and medical-legal procedures should complete the rape evaluation or supervise the evaluation when possible.

The clinician's responsibilities are to provide support, to obtain the history in a nonjudgmental manner, to conduct a complete examination without re-traumatizing the victim, and to collect forensic evidence. The clinician must complete laboratory testing, administer prophylaxis treatment for STIs and emergency contraception, arrange for counseling services, and file a report to appropriate authorities. It is not the clinician's responsibility to decide whether a rape has occurred; the legal system will do so.

Ideally a clinician trained in forensic interviewing should obtain the history. If that is not possible the history should be obtained asking only open-ended questions to obtain information about (1) what happened? (2) where did it happen? (3) when did it happen? and (4) who did it? After obtaining a concise history including details of the physical contact that occurred between the victim and the assailant, the clinician should conduct a thorough and complete physical examination and document all injuries. Clinicians should provide sensitive, nonjudgmental support during the entire evaluation, as the adolescent victim has experienced a major trauma and is susceptible to re-traumatization during this process. Each component of the evaluation should be explained in detail to the victim, allowing the adolescent as much control as possible, including refusal to complete any part or all of the forensic evidence collection process. It is often useful to permit a trusted supportive person, such as a family member, friend or rape crisis advocate, to be present during the evaluation if that is the adolescent's wish.

The examining clinician should be familiar with the **forensic evidence collection** kit prior to initiating the examination. In the USA, each state's forensic evidence kit is different, but most include some or all of the following components: forensic evidence of semen deposits detected by a fluorescent lamp with a wavelength near 490 nm (many Woods lamps are inadequate), swabs of bite mark impressions to collect genetic markers (DNA, ABO group), swabs of any penetrated orifice, and documentation of acute cutaneous injuries utilizing body diagram charts and/or photographs with visible standard measurements. Areas of restraint should be carefully inspected for injuries; these areas include extremities, neck, and the inner aspect of the oral mucosa where a dentition impression may be seen.

The genital examination of a female rape victim should be undertaken with the patient in the lithotomy position. The genital examination of a male rape victim should be undertaken with the patient in supine position. The clinician's examination should include careful inspection of the entire pelvic, genital, and perianal areas. The clinician should document any acute injuries such as edema, erythema, petechiae, hemorrhage, or tearing. Aqueous solution of toluidine blue (1%), which adheres to nucleated cells, may be used during the acute examination to improve visualization of microtrauma in the perianal area. Additionally, a colposcope may be used to provide magnification and photodocumentation of injuries.

Laboratory Data

The forensic evidence kit should be completed when clinically indicated and if the patient is evaluated within 72 hr of sexual assault. Additional laboratory studies required during initial evaluation are noted in Table 113-2. Follow-up evaluations should be scheduled to repeat these laboratory studies.

Treatment

Medical treatment includes prophylaxis treatment for STIs (Chapter 114) and emergency contraception (Chapter 111.5). The Centers for Disease Control and Prevention estimates that the risk for acquiring STIs following a sexual assault in adults is 6-12% for *Neisseria gonorrhoeae,* 4-17% for *Chlamydia trachomatis,* and 0.5-3.0% for syphilis. Antimicrobial prophylaxis is recommended for adolescent rape victims due to the risk of acquiring an STI and the risk of pelvic inflammatory disease (Table 113-3). HIV postexposure prophylaxis should be considered and consultation with an infectious disease specialist sought if higher transmission risk factors are identified (e.g., knowing that the perpetrator is HIV-positive, significant mucosal injury of the victim) to prescribe a triple antiretroviral regimen. Clinicians should review the importance for patient's compliance with medical and psychological treatment and follow-up.

Table 113-2 LABORATORY DATA FOR EVALUATION OF RAPE VICTIMS

WITHIN 8-12 HR (IF INDICATED BY HISTORY)
Urine and blood for date rape drugs (GHB, Rohypnol, and ketamine)
WITHIN 72 HR
Forensic evidence kit
Urinalysis
Pregnancy test
Hepatitis B screen
Syphilis (RPR, VDRL)
Herpes simplex virus titers (I & II)
HIV
Wet mount for the detection of spermatozoa, *Trichomonas vaginalis,* and bacterial vaginosis
Cultures obtained based on history of physical contact for: Oropharynx: *Neisseria gonorrhoeae* Rectal: *N. gonorrhoeae* and *Chlamydia* Urethral (male): *N. gonorrhoeae* and *Chlamydia* Endocervical (female): *N. gonorrhoeae* and *Chlamydia*

GHB, γ-hydroxybutyric acid; RPR, rapid plasma reagin; VDRL, Venereal Disease Research Laboratory.

Table 113-3 PROPHYLAXIS TREATMENT FOR RAPE VICTIMS

*Neisseria gonorrhoeae**	Ceftriaxone 250 mg IM × 1 dose or Cefixime 400 mg PO × 1 dose for anogenital but not oral exposure
*Chlamydia trachomatis**	Azithromycin 1 g PO × 1 dose or Doxycycline 100 mg PO BID × 7 days
*Trichomonas vaginalis and bacterial vaginosis**	Metronidazole 2 g PO × 1 dose
HIV†	Combivir 1 tab PO bid × 28 days
Hepatitis B	Complete immunizations
Human papillomavirus	Complete immunizations
Emergency contraception‡	Ovral 2 tabs (0.05 mg ethinyl estradiol, 0.50 mg norgestrel) and 2nd dose in 12 hr Plan B 1 tab (0.75 mg levonorgestrel) and 2nd dose in 12 hr, or both pills together as one dose

*Prophylaxis is recommended for all three STIs.
†HIV postexposure prophylaxis is provided for patients with penetration and when the assailant is known to be HIV positive or at high risk due to a history of incarceration, intravenous drug use, or multiple sexual partners. If provided, follow-up must be arranged.
‡Provided for patients with negative urine pregnancy screen. In addition, provide antiemetic (Compazine, Zofran) for patients receiving emergency contraception medication other than Plan B.

At the time of presentation, the clinician should address the need for follow-up care including psychologic counseling. Adolescent victims are at increased risk of post-traumatic stress disorder, depression, self-abusive behaviors, suicidal ideation, delinquency, substance abuse, eating disorders, and sexual revictimization. It is important for the adolescent victim and parents to understand the value of timely counseling services to decrease these potential long-term sequelae. Counseling services should be arranged during the initial evaluation, with follow-up arranged with the primary care physician to improve compliance. Counseling services for family members of the victim may improve their ability to provide appropriate support to the adolescent victim. Caution parents not to use the assault as a validation of their parental guidance, as it will only serve to place blame inappropriately on the adolescent victim.

Prevention

Primary prevention may be accomplished through education of preadolescents and adolescents on the issues of rape, healthy relationships, Internet dangers, and drug-facilitated rape. Prevention messages should be targeted to both males and females at high schools and colleges. Particular emphasis on prevention efforts during college orientation is highly recommended. High-risk situations that may increase the likelihood of a sexual assault (use of drugs or alcohol) should be discouraged. **Secondary prevention** includes informing adolescents of the benefits of timely medical evaluations when rape has occurred. Individual clinicians should ask adolescents about past experiences of forced and unwanted sexual behaviors and offer help in dealing with those experiences. The importance of prevention cannot be overstated since adolescents are disproportionately affected by rape and they are particularly vulnerable to long-term consequences.

BIBLIOGRAPHY

Please visit the Nelson Textbook of Pediatrics *website at www.expertconsult.com for the complete bibliography.*

Chapter 114
Sexually Transmitted Infections
Gale R. Burstein

When controlled for sexual activity, age-specific rates of many sexually transmitted infections (STIs) are highest among sexually experienced adolescents. Some STI pathogens present as STI syndromes with a specific constellation of symptoms, but most are asymptomatic and only detected by a laboratory test. The approach to prevention and control of these infections lies in education, screening, and early diagnosis and treatment.

ETIOLOGY

The risk of contracting an STI exists in any adolescent who has had oral, vaginal, or anal sexual intercourse. Physical, behavioral, and social factors contribute to the adolescent's higher risk (Table 114-1). Adolescents who initiate sex at a younger age are at higher risk for STIs, along with youth residing in detention facilities, youth attending sexually transmitted diseases (STD) clinics, young men having sex with men (YMSM), and youth who are injecting-drug users (IDUs). Adolescence-increased STI risk may in part be attributed to risky behaviors, such as sex with multiple concurrent partners or multiple sequential partners of limited duration, failure to use barrier protection consistently and correctly, and increased biological susceptibility to infection. Although all 50 states and the District of Columbia explicitly allow minors to consent for their own sexual health services, many adolescents encounter multiple obstacles to accessing this care. Adolescents who are victims of sexual assault may not consider themselves "sexually active," given the context of the encounter, and need reassurance, protection, and appropriate intervention when these circumstances are uncovered.

Table 114-1 CIRCUMSTANCES CONTRIBUTING TO ADOLESCENTS' SUSCEPTIBILITY TO SEXUALLY TRANSMITTED INFECTIONS

PHYSICAL
Younger age at puberty
Cervical ectopy
Smaller introitus leading to traumatic sex
Asymptomatic nature of sexually transmitted infection
Uncircumcised penis
BEHAVIOR LIMITED BY COGNITIVE STAGE OF DEVELOPMENT
Early adolescence: have not developed ability to think abstractly
Middle adolescence: develop belief of uniqueness and invulnerability
SOCIAL FACTORS
Poverty
Limited access to "adolescent friendly" health care services
Adolescent health-seeking behaviors (forgoing care because of confidentiality concerns or denial of health problem)
Sexual abuse and violence
Homelessness
Young adolescent females with older male partners

From Shafii T, Burstein G: An overview of sexually transmitted infections among adolescents, *Adolesc Med Clin* 15:207, 2004.

EPIDEMIOLOGY

In the USA, STI prevalence varies by age, gender, and race/ethnicity. Adolescents and young adults less than 25 yr of age have the highest reported prevalence of gonorrheal (Chapter 185) and chlamydial (Chapter 218) infection; among females, rates are highest in the 15-19 yr old age group, and among males, rates are highest for 20-24 yr olds. In 2008, females 15-19 yr of age had the highest reported chlamydia rate (3,275.8 per 100,000 population), followed by females 20 to 24 years of age (3,179.9 per 100,000 population) (Fig. 114-1). The reported 2008 chlamydia rate for 15-19 yr old females was almost 5 times higher than for 15-19 yr old males. Chlamydia is common among all races and ethnic groups; however, African-American, Native American/Alaska Native, and Hispanic women are disproportionately affected. In 2008, black females 15-19 yr of age had the highest chlamydia rate of any group (10,513.4), followed by black females 20-24 yr of age (9,373.9). Data from the 1999-2002 National Health and Nutrition Examination Survey estimate the prevalence of chlamydia among the U.S. population was highest among African-Americans across all ages, including adolescents (Fig. 114-2).

Reported rates of other bacterial STIs are also high among adolescents. In 2008, 15-19 yr old females had the highest (636.8 per 100,000 population) and 20-24 yr old females had the second highest gonorrhea rates (608.6 per 100,000 population) compared to any other age/sex group (Chapter 185). Gonorrhea rates among 15-24 yr old females have increased for the past 5 years. Primary and secondary (P&S) syphilis rates among 15-19 yr old females have increased annually since 2004 from 1.5 cases per 100,000 population to 3.0 per 100,000 population in 2008 (Chapter 210). Rates in women have been the highest each year in the 20-24 yr age group (5.1 cases per 100,000 population in 2008). P&S syphilis rates among 15-19 yr old males are much lower than those in older males. However, these rates have increased since 2002 from 1.3 cases per 100,000 population to 5.3 in 2008. Pelvic inflammatory disease (PID) rates are highest in females aged 15-24 yr when compared to older women.

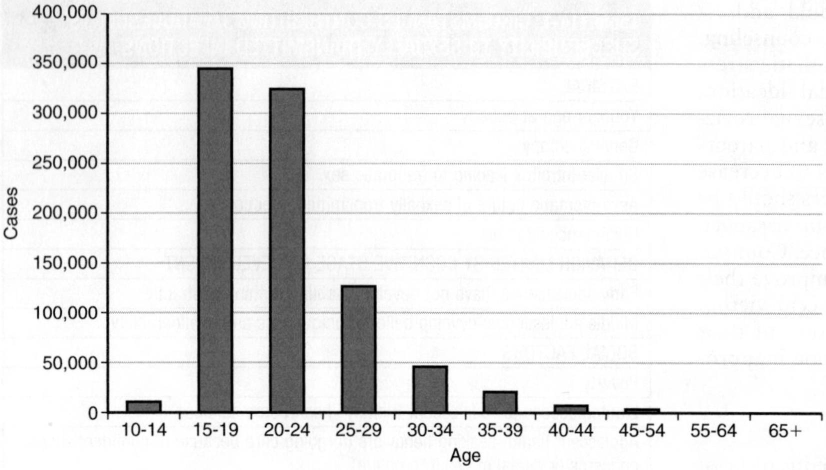

Figure 114-1 Reported *Chlamydia trachomatis* cases among females by age, USA, 2008. (Adapted from the Centers for Disease Control and Prevention: *Sexually transmitted diseases in the United States, 2008* [website]. www.cdc.gov/std/stats08/trends.htm. Accessed June 22, 2010.)

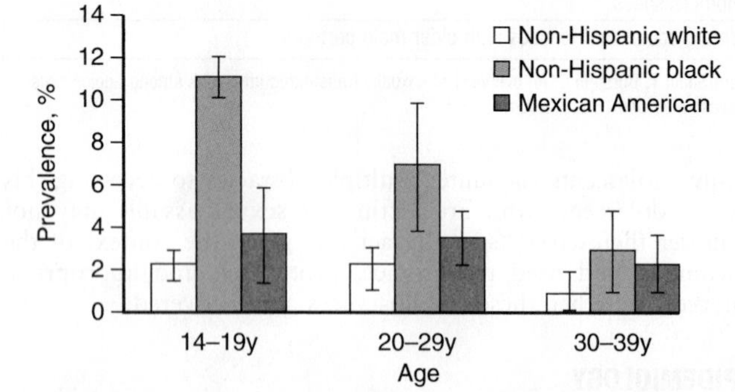

Figure 114-2 *Chlamydia trachomatis* prevalence by age group and race/ethnicity from a national survey, 1999-2002. Error bars indicate 95% confidence intervals. (Adapted from Centers for Disease Control and Prevention: *Chlamydia. Sexually transmitted disease surveillance 2008* (slide presentation). www.cdc.gov/std/stats08/slides/chlamydia.ppt. Accessed June 22, 2010.)

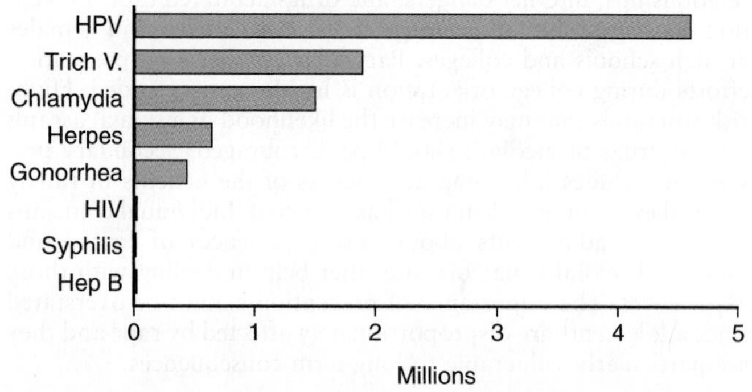

Figure 114-3 Estimated incidence of sexually transmitted infections among American youth ages 15 to 24 years, 2000. (Adapted from Weinstock H, Berman S, Cates W: Sexually transmitted diseases among American youth: incidence and prevalence estimates, 2000, *Perspect Sex Reprod Health* 36:6–10, 2004.)

Adolescents also suffer from a large burden of viral STIs. Young people in the USA are at persistent risk for HIV infection (Chapter 268). This risk is especially notable for youth of minority races and ethnicities. In 2004 in the 35 areas with long-term, confidential name-based HIV reporting, an estimated 4,883 young people aged 13-24 yr received a diagnosis of HIV infection or AIDS, representing about 13% of the persons given a diagnosis during that year. As of April 2008, all 50 states, the District of Columbia, and 5 dependent areas use the same confidential name-based reporting system to collect HIV and AIDS data. Surveillance data on HIV infections provide a more complete picture of the HIV/AIDS epidemic and the need for prevention and care services than does the picture provided by AIDS data alone.

The STI with the highest estimated incidence in the USA is HPV. The 2003-2004 National Health and Nutrition Examination Survey (NHANES) found a third of females aged 14-24 yr were actively infected with HPV. The highest HPV infection prevalence was among females aged 20-24 yr (44.8%; 95% CI, 36.3-55.3%) (Chapter 258). Among sexually active females, half of 20-24 yr olds were HPV-infected. Although HPV infection is common, studies suggest approximately 90% of infections clear within 2 years.

Herpes simplex virus-2 (HSV-2) is the most prevalent viral STI (Chapter 244). HSV-2 prevalence rates among adolescents in the USA and young adults appear to be decreasing. The 2005-2008 NHANES estimates that 1.4% (95% CI, 1.0-2.0) of adolescents age 14-19 yr are infected with HSV-2, which is about a 76% decrease observed from the 1988-1994 NHANES and 10.5% (95% CI, 9.0-12.3) of 20-29 yr olds are HSV-2 seropositive, which is about a 39% decrease compared to the 1988-1994 NHANES (Fig. 114-3).

Pathogenesis

During puberty, increasing levels of estrogen cause the vaginal epithelium to thicken and cornify and the cellular glycogen content to rise, the latter causing the vaginal pH to fall. These changes increase the resistance of the vaginal epithelium to penetration by certain organisms (including *Neisseria gonorrhoeae*) and increase the susceptibility to others (*Candida albicans* and *Trichomonas*, Chapter 276). The transformation of the vaginal cells leaves columnar cells on the ectocervix, forming a border of the 2 cell types on the ectocervix, known as the squamocolumnar junction. The appearance is referred to as **ectopy** (Fig. 114-4). With maturation, this tissue involutes. Prior to involution, it represents a unique vulnerability to infection for adolescent females. A 15 yr old sexually active girl with endocervical colonization has a 1:8 chance of developing PID compared to the 1:80 chance for a 24 yr old. As a result of these physiologic changes, gonococcal infection becomes primarily cervical and susceptibility to ascending infection is greatest during menses, when the pH is 6.8-7.0. The association of early sexual debut and younger gynecologic age with increased risk of sexually transmitted infections supports this explanation of the pathogenesis of infection in young adolescents.

STI Screening

Early detection and treatment are the primary STI control strategies. Some of the most common STIs in adolescents, including HPV, HSV, chlamydia, and gonorrhea, are usually asymptomatic

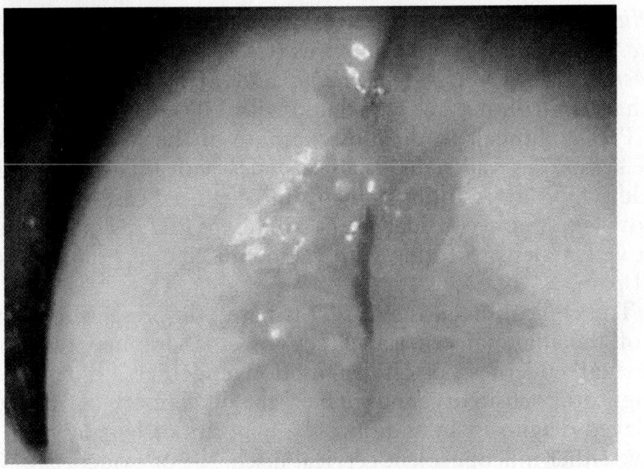

Figure 114-4 Cervical ectopy. (From the Seattle STD/HIV Prevention Training Center at the University of Washington: Claire E. Stevens.)

and if undetected can be spread inadvertently by the infected host. Screening initiatives for chlamydial infections have demonstrated reductions in PID cases by up to 40%. Although federal and professional medical organizations recommend annual chlamydia screening for sexually active females 24 yr and younger, in 2007, less than half (42%) of the sexually active females enrolled in commercial and Medicaid health plans were screened. The lack of a dialogue about STIs or the provision of STI services at annual preventive service visits to adolescents who are sexually experienced are missed opportunities for screening and education. Comprehensive, confidential, reproductive health services including STI screening should be offered to all sexually experienced adolescents (Table 114-2).

Table 114-2 ROUTINE LABORATORY SCREENING RECOMMENDATIONS FOR SEXUALLY TRANSMITTED INFECTIONS IN SEXUALLY ACTIVE ADOLESCENTS AND YOUNG ADULTS

Chlamydia trachomatis* AND *Neisseria gonorrhoeae
• Routinely screening for *C. trachomatis* and *N. gonorrhoeae* of all sexually active females aged ≤25 yr is recommended annually • Routinely screening for asymptomatic *C. trachomatis* infection in young men has not been recommended because studies have not yet demonstrated efficacy in decreasing prevalence or preventing disease outcomes in women by screening for chlamydial infection in men. Screening of sexually active young men *should be considered* in clinical settings with a high chlamydia prevalence rates (e.g., adolescent or school-based clinics, correctional facilities, Job Corps, and STD clinics).
HIV
• HIV screening should be discussed with all adolescents and encouraged for those who are sexually active and injection drug using
SYPHILIS
• Syphilis screening should be offered to sexually active adolescents reporting risk factors • The majority of U.S. syphilis cases occurring among YMSM and many early syphilis cases are identified from correctional facilities • Providers should consult with their local health department regarding local syphilis prevalence and associated risk factors that are associated with syphilis acquisition
HEPATITIS C VIRUS
• Screening adolescents for hepatitis C virus who report risk factors, i.e., injection drug use, MSM, received blood products or organ donation before 1992, received clotting factor concentrates before 1987, long term hemodialysis, or high prevalence setting, i.e., correctional facilities or STD clinics
NO RECOMMENDATIONS
• Although prevalent among adolescent populations, currently there are no recommendations to routinely screen adolescents who are asymptomatic for infections, such as trichomoniasis, bacterial vaginosis, genital herpes infection, HPV, HAV, or HBV • Young MSM and pregnant adolescent females may require more thorough evaluations and assessments

STD, sexually transmitted diseases; HIV, human immunodeficiency virus; YMSM, young men who have sex with men; HPV, human papillomavirus; HAV, hepatitis A virus; HBV, hepatitis B virus.
From Centers for Disease Control and Prevention: Sexually transmitted diseases treatment guidelines, 2010, *MMWR* 59(No. RR-12):1-110, 2010.

Definitions, Etiology, and Clinical Manifestations

STI syndromes are generally characterized by the location of the manifestation (vaginitis) or the type of lesion (genital ulcer). Certain constellations of presenting symptoms suggest the inclusion of a possible STI in the differential diagnosis.

URETHRITIS Urethritis is an STI syndrome characterized by inflammation of the urethra, usually due to an infectious etiology. Urethritis may present with urethral discharge, urethral itching, dysuria, or urinary frequency. Urgency, frequency of urination, erythema of the urethral meatus, and scrotal pain are less common clinical presentations. Many patients are completely asymptomatic at the time of diagnosis. On examination, the classic finding is mucoid or purulent discharge from the urethral meatus (Fig. 114-5). If no discharge is evident on exam, providers may attempt to express discharge by applying gentle pressure to the urethra from the base distally to the meatus 3-4 times. *Chlamydia trachomatis* and *N. gonorrhoeae* are the most commonly identified pathogens. *Mycoplasma genitalium* and *Ureaplasma urealyticum* are considered potential pathogens in nongonococcal urethritis (NGU) when chlamydia is not confirmed. NGU caused by these pathogens may be less responsive to usual NGU therapy. *Trichomonas vaginalis* and HSV should also be considered in the NGU differential diagnosis. Sensitive diagnostic tests for these NGU pathogens are not available but should be considered when NGU is not responsive to treatment. Noninfectious causes of urethritis include urethral trauma or foreign body. Unlike in females, urinary tract infections are fairly rare in males who have no past genitourinary medical history. In the typical sexually active adolescent male, dysuria and urethral discharge suggest the presence of an STI unless proven otherwise. Laboratory evaluation is essential to identify the involved pathogens to determine treatment, partner notification, and disease control.

EPIDIDYMITIS The inflammation of the epididymis in adolescent males is most often associated with an STI, most frequently *C. trachomatis* or *N. gonorrhoeae*. The presentation of unilateral

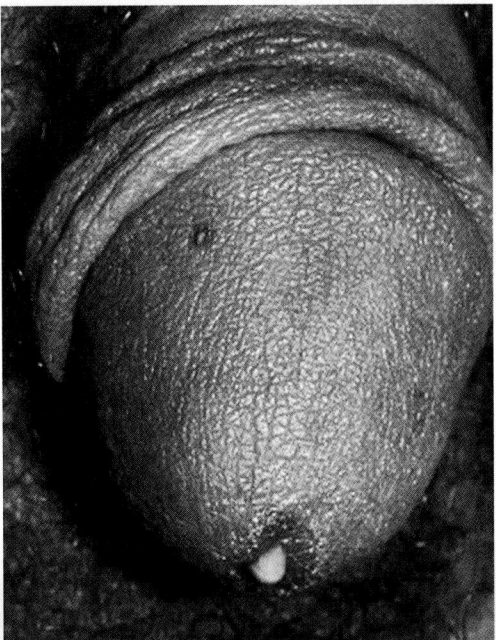

Figure 114-5 Gonococcal urethral discharge. (From the Seattle STD/HIV Prevention Training Center at the University of Washington: Connie Celum and Walter Stamm.)

scrotal swelling and tenderness, often accompanied by a hydrocele and palpable swelling of the epididymis, associated with the history of urethral discharge, constitute the presumptive diagnosis of epididymitis. Testicular torsion, a surgical emergency usually presenting with sudden onset of severe testicular pain, should be considered in the differential diagnosis (Chapter 539). Males who practice insertive anal intercourse are also vulnerable to *Escherichia coli* infection.

VAGINITIS Vaginitis is a superficial infection of the vaginal mucosa frequently presenting as a vaginal discharge, with or without vulvar involvement (Chapter 543). Bacterial vaginosis, vulvovaginal candidiasis (VVC), and trichomoniasis are the predominant infections associated with vaginal discharge. Bacterial vaginosis is replacement of the normal H_2O_2–producing *Lactobacillus* sp. vaginal flora by an overgrowth of anaerobic microorganisms as well as *Gardnerella vaginalis, Ureaplasma*, and *Mycoplasma*. Although bacterial vaginosis is not categorized as a STI, sexual activity is associated with increased frequency of vaginosis. VVC, usually caused by *C. albicans*, can trigger vulvar pruritus, pain, swelling, and redness and dysuria. Findings on vaginal exam include vulvar edema, fissures, excoriations, or thick curdy vaginal discharge. Trichomoniasis is caused by the protozoan *T. vaginalis*. Infected females may present with symptoms characterized by a diffuse, malodorous, yellow-green vaginal discharge with vulvar irritation or may be diagnosed by screening an asymptomatic patient. Cervicitis can sometimes cause a vaginal discharge. Laboratory confirmation is recommended because clinical presentations may vary and patients may be infected with more than 1 pathogen.

CERVICITIS The inflammatory process in cervicitis involves the deeper structures in the mucous membrane of the cervix uteri. Vaginal discharge can be a manifestation of cervicitis, if the cervical discharge is profuse. Less subtle clinical manifestations of cervicitis are irregular or postcoital bleeding, mucopurulent discharge from the os, and a friable cervix. The cervical changes associated with cervicitis must be distinguished from cervical ectopy in the younger adolescent to avoid the over diagnosis of inflammation (Fig. 114-6; see Fig. 114-4). The pathogens identified most commonly with cervicitis are *C. trachomatis* and *N. gonorrhoeae*, although no pathogen is identified in the majority of cases. HSV is a less common pathogen associated with ulcerative and necrotic lesions on the cervix.

PELVIC INFLAMMATORY DISEASE PID encompasses a spectrum of inflammatory disorders of the female upper genital tract, including endometritis, salpingitis, tubo-ovarian abscess, and pelvic peritonitis, usually in combination rather than as separate entities. *N. gonorrhoeae* and *C. trachomatis* predominate as the involved pathogenic organisms in younger adolescents, although PID should be approached as multiorganism etiology, including pathogens such as anaerobes, *G. vaginalis, Haemophilus influenzae*, enteric gram-negative rods, and *Streptococcus agalactiae*. In addition, cytomegalovirus (CMV) (Chapter 247), *Mycoplasma hominis, U. urealyticum*, and *Mycoplasma genitalium* (Chapter 216), may be associated with PID.

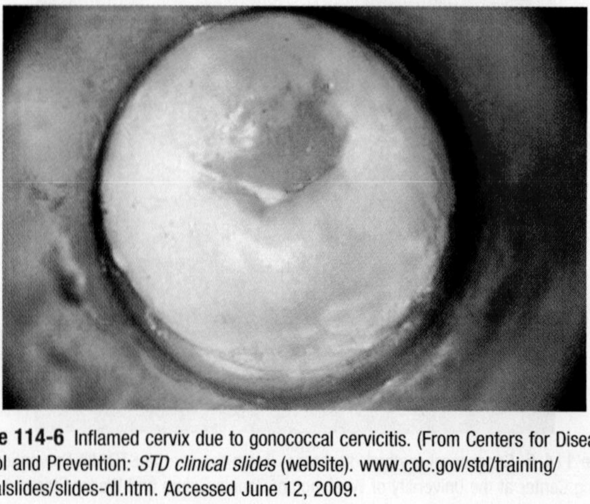

Figure 114-6 Inflamed cervix due to gonococcal cervicitis. (From Centers for Disease Control and Prevention: *STD clinical slides* (website). www.cdc.gov/std/training/clinicalslides/slides-dl.htm. Accessed June 12, 2009.

PID is difficult to diagnose because of the wide variation in the symptoms and signs. Many females with PID have subtle or mild symptoms resulting in many unrecognized cases. Health care providers should consider the possibility of PID in young sexually active females presenting with vaginal discharge and/or abdominal pain.

The clinical diagnosis of PID is based on presence of at least 1 of the minimal criteria, either lower abdominal tenderness, adnexal tenderness, or cervical motion tenderness, to increase the diagnostic sensitivity and reduce the likelihood of missed or delayed diagnosis. In addition, the majority of females with PID have either mucopurulent cervical discharge or evidence of WBC on a microscopic evaluation of a vaginal fluid saline preparation. If the cervical discharge appears normal and no WBCs are observed on the wet prep of vaginal fluid, the diagnosis of PID is unlikely, and alternative causes of pain should be investigated. Specific, but not always practical, criteria for PID include evidence of endometritis on biopsy, transvaginal sonography or MRI evidence of thickened, fluid-filled tubes, or Doppler evidence of tubal hyperemia or laparoscopic evidence of PID.

GENITAL ULCER SYNDROMES An ulcerative lesion in a mucosal area exposed to sexual contact is the unifying characteristic of infections associated with these syndromes. These lesions are most frequently seen on the penis and vulva, but also occur on oral and rectal mucosa depending on the adolescent's sexual practices. HSV, *Treponema pallidum* (syphilis), and *Haemophilus ducreyi* (chancroid) are the most common organisms associated with genital ulcer syndromes.

Genital herpes, the most common ulcerative STI among adolescents, is a chronic, life-long viral infection. Two sexually transmitted HSV types have been identified, HSV-1 and HSV-2. The majority of cases of recurrent genital herpes are caused by HSV-2. Most HSV-2–infected persons are unaware of their diagnosis because they experience mild or unrecognized infections but continue to shed virus intermittently in the genital tract. Therefore, the majority of genital herpes infections are transmitted by asymptomatic persons who are unaware of their infection.

Although the initial herpetic lesion is a vesicle, by the time the patient presents clinically, the vesicle most often has ruptured spontaneously, leaving a shallow, painful ulcer. Up to 50% of first genital herpes episodes are caused by HSV-1, but recurrences and subclinical shedding are much more frequent for genital HSV-2 infection.

Syphilis and chancroid are less common causes of genital ulcers in adolescents than in adults. Lymphogranuloma venereum due to *C. trachomatis* serovars L1-L3, and donovanosis are rare infections in the USA and other industrialized countries, although outbreaks of lymphogranuloma venereum do occur in MSM. In these circumstances, genital ulcerations with inflamed inguinal lymph nodes (buboes) are unusual; proctitis or proctocolitis is the usual manifestation. HIV is present in affected men.

Clinical characteristics differentiating the lesions of the most common infections associated with genital ulcers are presented in Table 114-3, along with the required laboratory diagnosis to identify the causative agent accurately. The differential diagnosis includes Behçet disease (Chapter 155), Crohn disease (Chapter 328), and **acute genital ulcers (AGU)** due to Epstein-Barr virus (Chapter 246). AGU often follows a flu or mononucleosis-like illness in an immunocompetent female and is unrelated to sexual activity. The lesions are 0.5-2.5 cm in size, bilateral, symmetric, multiple, painful and necrotic, and are associated with inguinal lymphadenopathy. This primary infection is also associated with fever and malaise. The diagnosis may require EBV titers, or PCR testing. Treatment is supportive care including pain management.

Table 114-3 SIGNS, SYMPTOMS, AND PRESUMPTIVE AND DEFINITIVE DIAGNOSES OF GENITAL ULCERS

SIGNS/SYMPTOMS	HERPES SIMPLEX VIRUS	SYPHILIS (PRIMARY)	CHANCROID
Ulcers	Vesicles rupture to form shallow ulcers	Ulcer with well-demarcated indurated borders and a clean base (chancre)	Unindurated and undermined borders and a purulent base
Painful	Painful	Painless*	Painful
Number of lesions	Usually multiple	Usually single	Multiple
Inguinal lymphadenopathy	First-time infections may cause constitutional symptoms and lymphadenopathy	Usually mild and minimally tender	Unilateral or bilateral painful adenopathy in >50% Inguinal bubo formation and rupture may occur
Presumptive diagnosis	Typical lesions; positive HSV-2 type-specific antibody test	Early syphilis: a typical chancre plus a reactive nontreponemal test (RPR, VDRL) and no history of syphilis or a 4-fold increase in a quantitative nontreponemal test in a person with a history of syphilis; positive treponemal EIA with reactive nontreponemal test (RPR, VDRL) and no prior history of syphilis treatment	Exclusion of other causes of ulcers in the presence of (1) typical ulcers and lymphadenopathy, (2) a typical Gram stain and a history of contact with a high-risk individual (prostitute) or living in an endemic area
Definitive diagnosis	Detection of HSV by culture or polymerase chain reaction from ulcer scraping or aspiration of vesicle fluid	Identification *T. pallidum,* from a chancre or lymph node aspirate, on dark-field microscopy or by DFA	Detection of *H. ducreyi* by culture

*Primary syphilitic ulcers may be painful if they become co-infected with bacteria or 1 of the other organisms responsible for genital ulcers.
DFA, direct fluorescent antibody; HSV, herpes simplex virus; EIA, enzyme immunoassay; RPR, rapid plasma reagin; VDRL, Venereal Disease Research Laboratory.
Data from Centers for Disease Control and Prevention: Sexually transmitted diseases treatment guidelines, 2010, *MMWR* 59(No. RR-12):1-110, 2010.

GENITAL LESIONS AND ECTOPARASITES Lesions that present as outgrowths on the surface of the epithelium and other limited epidermal lesions are included under this categorization of syndromes. HPV can cause genital warts and genital cervical abnormalities that can lead to cancer. Genital HPV types are classified according to their association with cervical cancer. Infections with low-risk types, such as HPV types 6 and 11, can cause benign or low-grade changes in cells of the cervix, genital warts, and recurrent respiratory papillomatosis. High-risk HPV types can cause cervical, anal, vulvar, vaginal, and head and neck cancers. High-risk HPV types 16 and 18 are detected in approximately 70% of cervical cancers. Persistent infection increases the risk of cervical cancer. Molluscum contagiosum and condyloma lata associated with secondary syphilis complete the classification of genital lesion syndromes. As a result of the close physical contact during sexual contact, common ectoparasitic infestations of the pubic area occur as pediculosis pubis or the papular lesions of scabies (Chapter 660).

HIV DISEASE AND HEPATITIS B HIV and hepatitis B present as an asymptomatic, unexpected occurrences in most infected adolescents. Risk factors identified in the history or routine screening during prenatal care are much more likely to result in suspicion of infection, leading to the appropriate laboratory screening, than are clinical manifestations in this age group (Chapters 268 and 350).

Diagnosis

Most adolescents infected with viral and bacterial STI pathogens usually do not report symptoms suggestive of infection. With the increased use of very sensitive, noninvasive, **nucleic acid amplification tests** (**NAAT**), providers are finding that most genital infections in females as well as many males are asymptomatic. Therefore, a good sexual history is key to identifying adolescents who should be screened for STIs and for identifying those who require a laboratory diagnostic evaluation for an STD syndrome.

When eliciting a sexual health history, discussions should be appropriate for the patient's developmental level. In addition to questions regarding vaginal or urethral discharge, genital lesions, and lower abdominal pain among females, one should ask about prior treatment of any STI symptoms, including self-treatment using over-the-counter medications. **Dyspareunia** is a consistent symptom in adolescents with PID. Providers must ask about oral or anal sexual activity to determine sites for specimen collection.

Urethritis should be objectively documented by either (1) mucoid or purulent urethral discharge, (2) ≥5 WBC per high-power field on microscopic examination of a urethral secretions Gram stain, (3) ≥10 WBC per high-power field on microscopic examination of first-void urine (FVU) specimen, or (4) positive FVU leukocyte esterase test. The presence of gram-negative intracellular diplococci on microscopy confirms the diagnosis of gonococcal urethritis. Patient complaint without objective clinical or laboratory evidence does not fulfill diagnostic criteria. All patients with complaints, whether or not diagnostic criteria are fulfilled, should be tested for gonorrhea and chlamydia.

An essential component of the diagnostic evaluation of vaginal, cervical or urethral discharge is a chlamydia and gonorrhea NAAT. NAATs are the most sensitive chlamydia tests available and allow for noninvasive STI testing via urine and self-collected vaginal swabs in addition to testing endocervical and urethral specimens (Table 114-4). Gonorrhea and chlamydia NAATs perform well on rectal and oropharyngeal specimens and can be performed by most commercial laboratories.

Evaluation of adolescent females with vaginitis includes laboratory data. The cause of vaginal symptoms usually can be determined by pH and microscopic examination of the discharge. Using pH paper, an elevated pH (i.e., >4.5) is common with BV or trichomoniasis. For microscopic exam, a slide can be made with the discharge diluted in 1-2 drops of 0.9% normal saline solution and another slide with discharge diluted in 10% potassium hydroxide (KOH) solution. Examining the saline specimen slide under a microscope may reveal motile or dead *T. vaginalis* or *clue cells* (epithelial cells with borders obscured by small bacteria), which are characteristic of bacterial vaginosis. WBCs without evidence of trichomonads or yeast are usually suggestive of cervicitis. The yeast or pseudohyphae of *Candida* species are more easily identified in the KOH specimen (Fig. 114-7). The sensitivity of microscopy is approximately 60-70% and requires immediate evaluation of the slide for optimal results. Therefore, lack of findings does not eliminate the possibility of infection. *T. vaginalis* culture is more sensitive than microscopy. Objective signs of vulvar inflammation in the absence of vaginal pathogens, along with a minimal amount of discharge, suggest the possibility of mechanical, chemical, allergic, or other noninfectious irritation of the vulva (Table 114-5).

Table 114-4 AMPLIFIED GONORRHEA AND CHLAMYDIA TESTS AND APPROVED SPECIMENS FOR TESTING*

TEST TECHNOLOGY AND NAME (MANUFACTURER)	SPECIMENS APPROVED FOR TESTING
POLYMERASE CHAIN REACTION	
COBAS AMPLICOR (CT/NG) Test (Roche Diagnostics, Indianapolis, IN)	**Female**: cervical, urine (NOT approved for *Neisseria gonorrhoeae* female urine testing) **Male**: urethral (NOT approved for asymptomatic *N. gonorrhoeae* male urethral swab testing), urine
Abbott RealTime CT/NG Assay (Abbott Laboratories, Abbott Park, IL)	**Female:** cervical, urine, vaginal (including self-collected in health-care setting) **Male:** urethral, urine
TRANSCRIPTION MEDIATED AMPLIFICATION	
APTIMA COMBO 2 Assay (GenProbe, San Diego, CA)	**Female**: cervical, urine, vaginal (including self-collected in health-care setting), liquid pap specimen **Male**: urethral, urine
STRAND DISPLACEMENT AMPLIFICATION	
BDProbeTec ET *Chlamydia trachomatis* and *N. gonorrhoeae* Amplified DNA Assays	**Female:** cervical, urine **Male:** urethral, urine
BDProbeTec CT/GC Q^x Amplified DNA Assays (Becton Dickinson, Sparks, MD)	**Female:** cervical, urine, vaginal (including self-collected in health care setting) **Male:** urethral, urine
NUCLEIC ACID HYBRIDIZATION WITH SIGNAL AMPLIFICATION	
digene HC2 CT/GC DNA Test (QIAGEN, Gaithersburg, MD)	**Female:** swab, cytobrush

*Specimens approved for testing as of June 22, 2010.

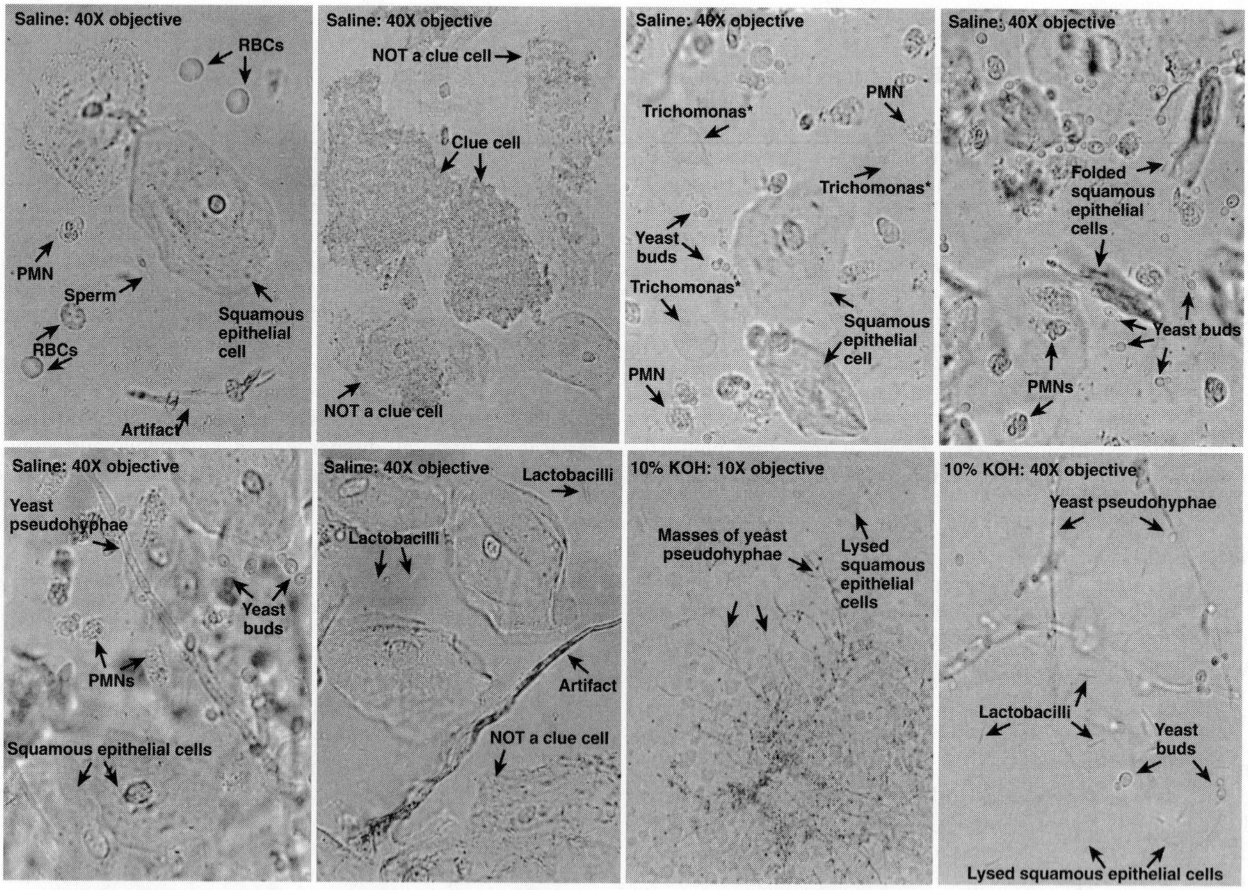

Figure 114-7 Common normal and abnormal microscopic findings during examination of vaginal fluid. KOH, potassium hydroxide solution; PMN, polymorphonuclear leukocyte; RBC, red blood cell. (From *Adolescent medicine: state of the art reviews*, vol 14, no 2, Philadelphia, 2003, Hanley & Belfus, pp 350–351.)

In settings where microscopy is not available, alternative tests may be used to diagnose vaginitis. The OSOM Trichomonas Rapid Test (Genzyme Diagnostics, Cambridge, MA), an immunochromatographic capillary flow dipstick technology, is Clinical Laboratory Improvement Amendments (CLIA)-waived and results are available in 10 min. The Affirm VPIII (Becton Dickenson, San Jose, CA), a nucleic acid probe test that evaluates for *T. vaginalis*, *G. vaginalis*, and *C. albicans*, is a moderate complexity laboratory test and results are available within 45 min. Both tests have a sensitivity >83% and a specificity >97% and are point-of-care diagnostics.

The **definitive diagnosis of PID** is difficult based on clinical findings alone. Clinical diagnosis is imprecise and no single historical, physical, or laboratory finding is both sensitive and specific for the diagnosis of acute PID. Clinical criteria have a positive predictive value of only 65-90% compared with laparoscopy. Although health care providers should maintain a low threshold for the diagnosis of PID, additional criteria to enhance specificity of diagnosis, such as transvaginal ultrasonography, can be considered (Table 114-6).

Isolation of HSV in cell culture is the preferred virologic test for genital ulcers, but culture sensitivity is low and false negatives do occur due to intermittent viral shedding. HSV PCR assays are more sensitive and can be used instead of viral culture. The Tzanck test is insensitive and nonspecific and should not be relied on.

Accurate type-specific HSV serologic assays are based on the HSV-specific glycoprotein G2 (HSV-2) and glycoprotein G1 (HSV-1). Both laboratory-based and point-of-care tests are available. Because nearly all HSV-2 infections are sexually acquired, the presence of type-specific HSV-2 antibody implies anogenital infection. The presence of HSV-1 antibody alone is more difficult to interpret because of the frequency of oral HSV infection acquired during childhood. Type-specific HSV serologic assays might be useful in the following scenarios: (1) recurrent genital symptoms or atypical symptoms with negative HSV cultures; (2) a clinical diagnosis of genital herpes without laboratory confirmation; and (3) a partner with genital herpes, especially if considering suppressive antiviral therapy to prevent transmission.

For syphilis screening more laboratories are now using treponemal enzyme immunoassay (EIA) tests. A positive treponemal EIA test identifies both previously treated and untreated or incompletely treated syphilis. False-positive results can occur, particularly among populations with low syphilis prevalence. Persons with a positive treponemal screening test should have a standard nontreponemal test with titer, such as an RPR or VDRL to guide patient management decisions.

Adolescents with STIs should be offered HIV testing. Rapid HIV testing with the availability of results in 10-20 min can be useful in settings in which the likelihood of adolescents returning for their results is low. Point-of-care, CLIA-waived tests for whole blood finger-stick and oral fluid specimen testing are available. Clinical studies have demonstrated that the rapid HIV test performance is comparable to those of EIAs. Because some reactive test results may be false-positive, every reactive rapid test must be confirmed by a more specific test, such as a Western blot.

Table 114-5 PATHOLOGIC VAGINAL DISCHARGE

INFECTIVE DISCHARGE	OTHER REASONS FOR DISCHARGE
COMMON CAUSES	**COMMON CAUSES**
Organisms	Retained tampon or condom
Candida albicans	Chemical irritation
Trichomonas vaginalis	Allergic responses
Chlamydia trachomatis	Ectropion
Neisseria gonorrhoeae	Endocervical polyp
Conditions	Intrauterine device
Bacterial vaginosis	Atrophic changes
Acute pelvic inflammatory disease	**LESS COMMON CAUSES**
Postoperative pelvic infection	Physical trauma
Postabortal sepsis	Vault granulation tissue
Puerperal sepsis	Vesicovaginal fistula
LESS COMMON CAUSES	Rectovaginal fistula
Mycoplasma genitalium	Neoplasia
Ureaplasma urealyticum	Cervicitis
Syphilis	
Escherichia coli	

From Mitchell H: Vaginal discharge—causes, diagnosis, and treatment, *Br Med J* 328:1306–1308, 2004.

Treatment

See Part XVI for chapters on the treatment of specific microorganisms and Tables 114-7 to 114-9. Treatment regimens using over-the-counter products for candida vaginitis and pediculosis reduce financial and access barriers to rapid treatment for adolescents, but there are potential risks for inappropriate self-treatment and complications from untreated more serious infections that must be considered before using this approach. Minimizing noncompliance with treatment, finding and treating the sexual partners, addressing prevention and contraceptive issues, offering available vaccines to prevent STIs and making every effort to preserve fertility are additional physician responsibilities. Repeat testing in 3-4 mo is recommended for patients with chlamydial and gonorrheal infections. Some experts also recommend repeat testing for trichomonas infection. Once an infection is diagnosed, partner evaluation, testing, and treatment are recommended for sexual contacts within 60 days of symptoms or diagnosis or the most recent partner if sexual contact was >60 days, even if the partner is asymptomatic. Abstinence is recommended for at least 7 days after both patient and partner are treated. A test for pregnancy should be performed for all females with suspected PID, since the test outcome will affect management.

Table 114-6 EVALUATION FOR PELVIC INFLAMMATORY DISEASE (PID)

2010 CENTERS FOR DISEASE CONTROL AND PREVENTION DIAGNOSTIC CRITERIA
Minimal Criteria
Additional Criteria to Enhance Specificity of the Minimal Criteria
• Oral temperature >101°F (>38.3°C) • Abnormal cervical or vaginal mucopurulent discharge* • Presence of abundant numbers of white blood cells on saline microscopy of vaginal secretions* • Elevated ESR or C-reactive protein • Laboratory documentation of cervical *Neisseria gonorrhoeae* or *Chlamydia trachomatis* infection
Most Specific Criteria to Enhance the Specificity of the Minimal Criteria
• Transvaginal sonography or MRI techniques showing thickened, fluid-filled tubes, with or without free pelvic fluid or tubo-ovarian complex, or Doppler studies suggesting pelvic infection (e.g., tubal hyperemia) • Endometrial biopsy with histopathologic evidence of endometritis • Laparoscopic abnormalities consistent with PID
DIFFERENTIAL DIAGNOSIS (PARTIAL LIST)
GI: appendicitis, constipation, diverticulitis, gastroenteritis, inflammatory bowel disease, irritable bowel syndrome GYN: ovarian cyst (intact, ruptured, or torsed), endometriosis, dysmenorrhea, ectopic pregnancy, mittelschmerz, ruptured follicle, septic or threatened abortion, tubo-ovarian abscess Urinary tract: cystitis, pyelonephritis, urethritis, nephrolithiasis

*If the cervical discharge appears normal and no WBCs are observed on the wet prep of vaginal fluid, the diagnosis of PID is unlikely and alternative causes of pain should be investigated.
SR, erythrocyte sedimentation rate; GI, gastrointestinal; GYN, gynecologic; WBC, white blood cell.
Adapted from Centers for Disease Control and Prevention: Sexually transmitted diseases treatment guidelines, 2010, *MMWR* 59(No. RR-12):1-110, 2010.

Table 114-7 MANAGEMENT GUIDELINES FOR UNCOMPLICATED BACTERIAL STIS IN ADOLESCENTS AND ADULTS

PATHOGEN	RECOMMENDED REGIMENS	ALTERNATIVE REGIMENS AND SPECIAL CONSIDERATIONS
Chlamydia trachomatis	Azithromycin 1 g orally once OR Doxycycline 100 mg orally twice daily for 7 days	For pregnancy: Azithromycin 1 g orally once OR Amoxicillin 500 mg orally 3 times a day for 7 days
Neisseria gonorrhoeae (cervix, urethra, and rectum)	Ceftriaxone 250 mg IM in a single dose OR, IF NOT AN OPTION Cefixime 400 mg orally in a single dose OR Single-dose injectable cephalosporin (e.g., ceftizoxime 500 mg IM, cefoxitin 2 g IM with probenecid 1 g orally, and cefotaxime 500 mg IM) PLUS Treatment for Chlamydia infection if not ruled out with NAAT	Alternative: Cefpodoxime 400 mg orally in a single dose Cephalosporin allergy: Azithromycin 2 g orally in a single dose
Neisseria gonorrhoeae (pharynx)	Ceftriaxone 250 mg IM in a single dose PLUS Treatment for *Chlamydia* infection if not ruled out with NAAT	
Gonococcal conjunctivitis	Ceftriaxone 1 g IM in a single dose	
Treponema pallidum (primary and secondary syphilis or early latent syphilis, i.e., infection <12 mo)	Benzathine penicillin G 2.4 million units IM in 1 dose	Penicillin allergy: Doxycycline 100 mg orally twice daily for 14 days OR Tetracycline 500 mg 4 times daily for 14 days. Some experts recommend ceftriaxone 1 g daily either IM or IV for 8-10 days or azithromycin 2 g orally in a single dose
Treponema pallidum (late latent syphilis or syphilis of unknown duration)	Benzathine penicillin G 7.2 million units total, administered as 3 doses of 2.4 million units IM each at 1 wk intervals	Penicillin allergy: Doxycycline 100 mg orally twice daily or Tetracycline 500 mg orally 4 times daily, both for 28 days in conjunction with close serologic and clinical follow-up
Haemophilus ducreyi (chancroid: genital ulcers, lymphadenopathy)	Azithromycin 1 g orally in a single dose OR Ceftriaxone 250 mg IM in a single dose OR Ciprofloxacin 500 mg orally twice a day for 3 days OR Erythromycin base 500 mg orally 3 times a day for 7 days	
Chlamydia trachomatis serovars L1, L2, or L3 (lymphogranuloma venereum)	Doxycycline 100 mg orally twice daily for 21 days	Alternative: Erythromycin base 500 mg orally 4 times a day for 21 days OR Azithromycin 1.0 g orally once weekly for 3 wk
Calymmatobacterium granulomatis (donovanosis or granuloma inguinale)	Doxycycline 100 mg orally twice daily for at least 3 weeks and until all lesions have healed	Alternative regimens should be taken at least until all lesions have completely healed: Azithromycin 1 g orally once per week for at least 3 weeks OR Ciprofloxacin 750 mg orally twice a day for at least 3 wk OR Erythromycin base 500 mg orally 4 times a day for at least 3 wk OR Trimethoprim-sulfamethoxazole 1 double-strength (160 mg/800 mg) tablet orally twice a day for at least 3 wk

IM, intramuscular; IV, intravenous; NAAT, nucleic acid amplification test.
Adapted for Centers for Disease Control and Prevention: *2010 Sexually transmitted diseases treatment guidelines*, 2010 *MMWR* 59(No. RR-12):1-110, 2010.

Table 114-8 MANAGEMENT GUIDELINES FOR UNCOMPLICATED MISCELLANEOUS SEXUALLY TRANSMITTED INFECTIONS IN ADOLESCENTS AND ADULTS

PATHOGEN	RECOMMENDED REGIMENS	ALTERNATIVE REGIMENS
Trichomonas vaginalis	Metronidazole 2 g orally in a single dose OR Tinidazole 2 g orally in a single dose	Metronidazole 500 mg orally twice daily for 7 days
Phthirus pubis (pubic lice)	Permethrin 1% cream rinse applied to affected areas and washed off after 10 min OR Pyrethrins with piperonyl butoxide applied to affected areas and washed off after 10 min Launder clothing and bedding	Malathion 0.5% lotion applied for 8-12 hr and washed off OR Ivermectin 250 μg/kg PO, repeat in 2 wk
Sarcoptes scabiei (scabies)	Permethrin 5% cream applied to all areas from the neck down, washed off after 8-14 hr OR Ivermectin 200 μg/kg orally, repeated in 2 wk Launder clothing and bedding	Lindane (1%) 1 oz of lotion or 30 g of cream in thin layer to all areas of body from neck down; wash off in 8 hr

Adapted for Centers for Disease Control and Prevention: *2010 Sexually transmitted diseases treatment guidelines*, 2010 *MMWR* 59(No. RR-12):1-110, 2010.

Table 114-9 MANAGEMENT GUIDELINES FOR UNCOMPLICATED GENITAL WARTS AND GENITAL HERPES IN ADOLESCENTS AND ADULTS

PATHOGEN	RECOMMENDED REGIMENS	ALTERNATIVE REGIMENS
Human papillomaviruses external genital warts	Patient-applied: Podofilox 0.5% solution or gel self-applied to warts twice daily for 3 consecutive days each wk followed by 4 days of no therapy. May be repeated for up to 4 cycles. OR Imiquimod 5% cream self-applied to warts once daily at bedtime 3 times wkly for up to 16 wk; washed off after 6-10 hr OR Sinecatechins 15% ointment self-applied 3 times daily for up to 16 wk. Does not need to be washed off. Provider-administered: Cryotherapy with liquid nitrogen or cryoprobe. Repeat applications every 1-2 weeks. OR Podophyllin resin 10-25% in a compound tincture of benzoin. A small amount should be applied to each wart and allowed to air dry. Can be repeated weekly, if necessary. May wash off 1-4 hr after application to reduce irritation. OR Trichloroacetic acid (TCA) or bichloroacetic acid (BCA) 80-90%. A small amount should be applied only to the warts and allowed to dry, at which time a white "frosting" develops. Can be repeated weekly, if necessary. OR Surgical removal either by tangential scissor excision, tangential shave excision, curettage, or electrosurgery	Intralesional interferon OR Photodynamic therapy and topical ciclovir Safety of podofilox, imiquimod, sinecatechins or podophyllin resin during pregnancy has not been established.
Human papillomaviruses Cervical warts	Refer to specialist for oncologic evaluation	
Human papillomaviruses Vaginal warts	**Cryotherapy** with liquid nitrogen. Avoid use of a cryoprobe. OR TCA or BCA 80-90% applied to warts. A small amount should be applied only to warts and allowed to dry, at which time a white "frosting" develops. Can be repeated weekly, if necessary.	
Human papillomaviruses Urethral meatal warts	Cryotherapy with liquid nitrogen OR Podophyllin 10-25% in compound tincture of benzoin. Treatment area must be dry before contact with normal mucosa. Can be repeated weekly, if necessary.	
Human papillomaviruses Anal warts	Cryotherapy with liquid nitrogen OR TCA or BCA 80-90% applied to warts. A small amount should be applied only to warts and allowed to dry, at which time a white "frosting" develops. Can be repeated weekly, if necessary. OR Surgical removal	Warts on the rectal mucosa should be managed in consultation with a specialist. Persons with anal warts should have rectal mucosa inspected by digital examination or anoscopy.
Herpes simplex virus (genital herpes): First clinical episode	Treat for 7-10 days with 1 of the following: Acyclovir 400 mg orally 3 times daily OR Acyclovir 200 mg orally 5 times daily OR Famciclovir 250 mg orally 3 times daily OR Valacyclovir 1 g orally twice daily	Consider extending treatment if healing is incomplete after 10 days of therapy.
Herpes simplex virus (genital herpes): Episodic therapy for recurrences	Acyclovir 400 mg orally 3 times daily for 5 days OR Acyclovir 800 mg orally twice daily for 5 days OR Acyclovir 800 mg orally 3 times daily for 2 days OR Famciclovir 125 mg orally twice daily for 5 days OR Famciclovir 1000 mg orally twice daily for 1 day OR Famciclovir 500 mg orally once then 250 mg twice daily for 2 days OR Valacyclovir 500 mg orally twice daily for 3 days OR Valacyclovir 1000 mg orally once daily for 5 days	Effective episodic treatment of recurrences requires initiation of therapy within 1 day of lesion onset or during the prodrome that precedes some outbreaks. The patient should be provided with a supply or a prescription for the medication with instructions to initiate treatment immediately when symptoms begin.
Herpes simplex virus (genital herpes): Suppressive therapy for recurrences	Acyclovir 400 mg orally twice daily OR Famciclovir 250 mg orally twice daily OR Valacyclovir 500 mg orally once daily or 1 g orally once daily	All patients should be counseled regarding suppressive therapy availability, regardless of number of outbreaks per year. Since the frequency of recurrent outbreaks diminishes over time in many patients, periodically, providers should discuss the need to continue therapy.

Adapted from Centers for Disease Control and Prevention: STD Treatment Guidelines 2010, *MMWR* 59(No. RR-12):1-110, 2010.

Diagnosis and therapy are often necessarily carried out within the context of a confidential relationship between the physician and the patient. Therefore, the need to report certain STIs to health department authorities should be clarified at the outset. Health departments are HIPAA-exempt and will not violate confidentiality. Health department role is to assure that treatment and case finding have been accomplished and that sexual partners have been notified of their STI exposure. **Expedited partner therapy (EPT)**, where the patient delivers the medication or a prescription for the medication to the partner for treatment without a clinical assessment, is a strategy to reduce further transmission of infection, particularly for male partners of women with gonorrhea and/or chlamydia who are otherwise unlikely to seek care for STI exposure. In randomized trials, EPT has reduced the rates of persistent or recurrent gonorrhea and chlamydia infection. Serious adverse reactions are rare with recommended chlamydia and gonorrhea treatment regimens, such as doxycycline, azithromycin, and cefixime. Transient gastrointestinal side effects are more common but rarely result in severe morbidity. Many states expressly permit EPT or may potentially allow its practice. Resources for information regarding EPT and state laws are available at the Centers for Disease Control and Prevention website *(www.cdc.gov/std/ept/)*.

Prevention

Health care providers should integrate sexuality education into clinical practice with children from early childhood through adolescence. Providers should counsel adolescents regarding sexual behaviors associated with risk of STI acquisition and should educate using evidence-based prevention strategies, which include a discussion of abstinence and other risk reduction strategies, such as consistent and correct condom use. The U.S. Preventative Task Force recommends high-intensity behavioral counseling to prevent STIs for all sexually active adolescents. The HPV vaccine series with either the bivalent (HPV types 16 and 18) or quadrivalent (HPV types 16, 18, 11, and 6) vaccine is routinely recommended for 11 and 12 yr old females, although it can be given at 9 yr of age. Catch-up vaccination is recommended for 13 through 26 yr old females who have not yet received or completed the vaccine series. The quadrivalent HPV may also be given to males aged 9 through 26 to reduce their likelihood of acquiring genital warts.

BIBLIOGRAPHY

Please visit the Nelson Textbook of Pediatrics *website at www.expertconsult.com for the complete bibliography.*

Chapter 115
Chronic Fatigue Syndrome

James F. Jones and Hal B. Jenson

GENERAL

Chronic fatigue syndrome (chronic mononucleosis, chronic Epstein-Barr virus infection, myalgic encephalomyelitis, immune dysfunction syndrome) describes the syndrome of unusual fatigability associated with mild to debilitating somatic symptoms. This syndrome was formally defined by the Centers for Disease Control and Prevention (CDC) in 1988 as *chronic fatigue syndrome* (CFS) because persistent and unexplained fatigue was considered the principal and invariable physical symptom. It results in severe impairment of daily functioning and is associated with a variety of physical symptoms. The fatigue does not require exertion by the patient, nor does rest relieve it. The current definition was created in 2003 to exclude psychiatric cases. CFS is a complex, diverse illness requiring fatigue, impairment in function, and selected symptoms for diagnosis. A definitive identifiable infectious agent does not cause it, although the differential diagnosis includes many infectious and inflammatory diseases. It is not a single disease with consistent physiologic or pathologic abnormalities but rather the measurable experience of symptoms that occur with various clinical conditions of somatic, psychologic, and mixed causes. The understanding of this condition is largely from studies among adults and adolescents, with limited descriptions of chronic fatiguing illness among young children.

For the full continuation of this chapter, please visit the Nelson Textbook of Pediatrics *website at www.expertconsult.com.*

PART XIV Immunology

Section 1 EVALUATION OF THE IMMUNE SYSTEM

Chapter 116 Evaluation of Suspected Immunodeficiency

Rebecca H. Buckley

Recurrent infections or fevers in children are among the most frequent clinical dilemmas for primary care physicians. The number of children suspected of having primary or secondary immunodeficiency far exceeds the number of actual cases, as most patients with recurrent infections do not have an identifiable immunodeficiency disorder. A major reason for the apparent high rate of recurrent infections among children is repeated exposure to common and usually benign infectious agents in child care and other group settings.

Primary care physicians must have a high index of suspicion if defects of the immune system are to be diagnosed early enough that appropriate treatment can be instituted before irreversible damage develops. Diagnosis is difficult because primary immunodeficiency diseases are not screened for at any time during life and most affected do not have abnormal physical features. Screening for SCID (T-cell lymphopenia) has become incorporated as part of the newborn screening programs in a few states. Extensive use of antibiotics may mask the classic presentation of many primary immunodeficiency diseases. Evaluation of immune function should be initiated in those rare infants or children who do have clinical manifestations of a specific immune disorder and in all who have unusual, chronic, or recurrent infections such as (1) 1 or more systemic bacterial infections (sepsis, meningitis); (2) 2 or more serious respiratory or documented bacterial infections (cellulitis, abscesses, draining otitis media, pneumonia, lymphadenitis) within 1 yr; (3) serious infections occurring at unusual sites (liver, brain abscess); (4) infections with unusual pathogens *(Pneumocystis jiroveci, Aspergillus, Serratia marcescens, Nocardia, Burkholderia cepacia);* and (5) infections with common childhood pathogens but of unusual severity (Table 116-1). Additional clues to immunodeficiency include: failure to thrive with or without chronic diarrhea, persistent infections after receiving live vaccines, and chronic oral or cutaneous moniliasis. Certain clinical features suggestive of immunodeficiency syndromes are noted in Tables 116-2 and 116-3.

Children with defects in antibody production, phagocytic cells, or complement proteins have recurrent infections with encapsulated bacteria and may grow and develop normally despite their recurring infections, unless they develop bronchiectasis from repeated lower respiratory tract bacterial infections or persistent enteroviral infections of the central nervous system. Patients with only repeated benign viral infections (with the exception of persistent enterovirus infections) are not as likely to have an immunodeficiency. By contrast, patients with deficiencies in T-cell function usually develop opportunistic infections or serious illnesses from common viral agents early in life, and they fail to thrive (Table 116-4).

The initial evaluation of immunocompetence includes a thorough history, physical examination, and family history (Table 116-5). Most immunologic defects can be excluded at minimal cost with the proper choice of screening tests, which should be broadly informative, reliable, and cost-effective (Table 116-6 and Fig. 116-1). A complete blood count (CBC), manual differential count, and erythrocyte sedimentation rate (ESR) are among the most cost-effective screening tests. If the ESR is normal, chronic bacterial or fungal infection is unlikely. If an infant's neutrophil count is persistently elevated in the absence of any signs of infection, a leukocyte adhesion deficiency should be suspected. If the absolute neutrophil count is normal, congenital and acquired neutropenias and leukocyte adhesion defects are excluded. If the absolute lymphocyte count is normal, the patient is not likely to have a severe T-cell defect, because T cells normally constitute 70% of circulating lymphocytes and their absence results in striking lymphopenia. Normal lymphocyte counts are higher in infancy and early childhood than later in life (Fig. 116-2). Knowledge of normal values for absolute lymphocyte counts at various ages in infancy and childhood (Chapter 708) is crucial in the detection of T-cell defects. At 9 mo of age, an age when infants affected with severe T-cell immunodeficiency are likely to present, the lower limit of normal is 4,500 lymphocytes/mm^3. Absence of Howell-Jolly bodies or pitted erythrocytes by microscopic examination of erythrocytes rules against congenital asplenia. Normal platelet size or count excludes Wiskott-Aldrich syndrome. If a CBC and a manual differential were performed on the cord blood of all infants, severe combined immunodeficiency (SCID) could be detected at birth by the identification of **lymphopenia**, and lifesaving immunologic reconstitution could then be provided to all affected infants shortly after birth and before they become infected.

Patients found to have abnormalities on any screening tests should be characterized as fully as possible before any type of immunologic treatment is begun, unless there is a life-threatening illness (Table 116-7). Some "abnormalities" may prove to be laboratory artifacts and, conversely, an apparently straightforward diagnosis may prove to be a much more complex disorder. For patients with recurrent or unusual bacterial infections, evaluation of T-cell and phagocytic cell functions is indicated even if results of initial screening tests including the CBC and manual differential, immunoglobulin levels, and CH_{50} are normal.

Because of the lack of screening, the true incidence and prevalence of primary immunodeficiency diseases are unknown, although the incidence has been estimated to be 1:10,000 births (Table 116-8). If true, this is higher than some disorders that are part of the newborn metabolic screening program (phenylketonuria [PKU] is 1:16,000) (Chapter 79.1). Approximately 80% of the mutated genes causing the more than 150 known primary immunodeficiency diseases are known, information that is crucial for genetic counseling and that could eventually be used in neonatal screening. Newborn or early childhood screening would be extremely valuable so that timely initiation of appropriate therapy can be initiated before infections develop. Currently it is likely that many affected patients die before a diagnosis is determined.

B CELLS

Antibody production by B cells is easily evaluated by measuring serum immunoglobulin levels and determining antibody titers to protein and polysaccharide antigens.

Table 116-1 PREDISPOSITION TO SPECIFIC INFECTIONS IN HUMANS

PATHOGEN	PRESENTATION	AFFECTED GENE/ CHROMOSOMAL REGION	FUNCTIONAL DEFECT	NOTES
BACTERIA				
Streptococcus pneumoniae	Invasive disease	*IRAK-4, MyD88*	Impaired production of inflammatory cytokines following TLR stimulation	Also susceptible to other pyogenic bacteria such as *Staphylococcus aureus*
Neisseria	Invasive disease	MAC components (C5, C6, C7, C8A, C8B, C8G, C9)	MAC deficiency	
	Invasive disease, poor prognosis	*PFC*	Properdin deficiency	
Mycobacteria	MSMD	*IL12B, IL12RB1, IKBKG*	Impaired IFN-γ response to IL-12/23	Also susceptible to *Salmonella typhi* infections
		IFNGR1, IFNGR2, STAT1	Impaired cellular response to IFN-γ	
Mycobacterium leprae	Leprosy	*PARK2*	Unknown	Possible E3-ubiquitin ligase dysfunction
		LTA	Unknown	
VIRUSES				
Herpes simplex (type 1)	Herpes simplex encephalitis	*UNC93B1, TLR3*	Impaired production of type 1 IFNs	STAT1 and NEMO deficiency also predispose to HSV infections, amongst other infections
Epstein-Barr virus	XLP	*SH2DIA*	SAP deficiency	Fulminant infectious mononucleosis, malignant and nonmalignant lymphoproliferative disorders, dysgammaglobulinemia, autoimmunity
		XIAP/BIRC4	XIAP deficiency	
Human papillomaviruses	Epidermodysplasia verruciformis WHIM	*EVER1/TMC6* *EVER2/TMC8* *CXCR4*	EVER1 deficiency EVER2 deficiency Truncated CXCR4	Altered neutrophil mobilization, T-cell lymphopenia, recurrent bacterial respiratory infections chronic cutaneous/genital papillomavirus disease
PARASITES				
Plasmodium falciparum	Malaria fever episodes Severe malaria Severe malaria	10p15 *GNAS* *IFNR1*	Unknown Unknown Unknown	Linkage studies SNP association studies SNP association studies
Schistosoma mansoni	Intensity of infection Hepatic fibrosis	5q311-q33 6q22-q23, *IFNR1*	Unknown Unknown	
Leishmania donovani	Visceral leishmaniasis (kala-azar)	22q12, 2q35 (*NRAMP1*)	Unknown	
YEAST				
Candida	APECED, Chronic candidiasis	Aire	Unknown	APS-1 chronic candidiasis, chronic hyperthyroidism, Addison's disease

APECED, autoimmune, polyendocrinopathy, candidiasis, ectodermal dystrophy; IFN, interferon; MAC, membrane attack complex; MSMD, mendelian susceptibility to mycobacterial disease; NEMO, nuclear factor kappa B essential modulator; SAP, SLAM-associated protein; SNP, single nucleotide polymorphism; TLR, Toll-like receptor; WHIM, warts, hypogammaglobulinemia, infections, and myelokathexis syndrome; XIAP, X-linked inhibitor of apoptosis; XLP, X-linked lymphoproliferative disease.

Modified from Pessach I, Walter J, Notarangelo LD: Recent advances in primary immunodeficiencies: identification of novel genetic defects and unanticipated phenotypes, *Pediatr Res* 65:3R–12R, 2009.

Table 116-2 CHARACTERISTIC CLINICAL PATTERNS IN SOME PRIMARY IMMUNODEFICIENCIES

FEATURES	DIAGNOSIS
IN NEWBORNS AND YOUNG INFANTS (0 TO 6 MONTHS)	
Hypocalcemia, unusual facies and ears, heart disease	DiGeorge anomaly
Delayed umbilical cord detachment, leukocytosis, recurrent infections	Leukocyte adhesion defect
Persistent thrush, failure to thrive, pneumonia, diarrhea	Severe combined immunodeficiency
Bloody stools, draining ears, atopic eczema	Wiskott-Aldrich syndrome
Pneumocystis jiroveci pneumonia, neutropenia, recurrent infections	X-linked hyper-IgM syndrome
IN INFANCY AND YOUNG CHILDREN (6 MONTHS TO 5 YEARS)	
Severe progressive infectious mononucleosis	X-linked lymphoproliferative syndrome
Recurrent staphylococcal abscesses, staphylococcal pneumonia with pneumatocele formation, coarse facial features, pruritic dermatitis	Hyper-IgE syndrome
Persistent thrush, nail dystrophy, endocrinopathies	Chronic mucocutaneous candidiasis
Short stature, fine hair, severe varicella	Cartilage hair hypoplasia with short-limbed dwarfism
Oculocutaneous albinism, recurrent infection	Chédiak-Higashi syndrome
Abscesses, suppurative lymphadenopathy, antral outlet obstruction, pneumonia, osteomyelitis	Chronic granulomatous disease
IN OLDER CHILDREN (OLDER THAN 5 YEARS) AND ADULTS	
Progressive dermatomyositis with chronic enterovirus encephalitis	X-linked agammaglobulinemia
Sinopulmonary infections, neurologic deterioration, telangiectasia	Ataxia-telangiectasia
Recurrent neisserial meningitis	C6, C7, or C8 deficiency
Sinopulmonary infections, splenomegaly, autoimmunity, malabsorption	Common variable immunodeficiency

Modified from Stiehm ER, Ochs HD, Winkelstein JA: *Immunologic disorders in infants and children,* ed 5, Philadelphia, 2004, Elsevier/Saunders.

Table 116-3 COMMON CLINICAL FEATURES OF IMMUNODEFICIENCY

Usually present	Recurrent upper respiratory infections
	Severe bacterial infections
	Persistent infections with incomplete or no response to therapy
	Paucity of lymph nodes and tonsils
Often present	Persistent sinusitis or mastoiditis (*Streptococcus pneumoniae, Haemophilus, Pneumocystis jiroveci, Staphylococcus aureus, Pseudomonas* spp.)
	Recurrent bronchitis or pneumonia
	Failure to thrive or growth retardation for infants or children; weight loss for adults
	Intermittent fever
	Infection with unusual organisms
	Skin lesions: rash, seborrhea, pyoderma, necrotic abscesses, alopecia, eczema, telangiectasia
	Recalcitrant thrush
	Diarrhea and malabsorption
	Hearing loss due to chronic otitis
	Chronic conjunctivitis
	Arthralgia or arthritis
	Bronchiectasis
	Evidence of autoimmunity, especially autoimmune thrombocytopenia or hemolytic anemia
	Hematologic abnormalities: aplastic anemia, hemolytic anemia, neutropenia, thrombocytopenia
	History of prior surgery, biopsy
Occasionally present	Lymphadenopathy
	Hepatosplenomegaly
	Severe viral disease (e.g., EBV, CMV, adenovirus, varicella, herpes simplex)
	Chronic encephalitis
	Recurrent meningitis
	Deep infections: cellulitis, osteomyelitis, organ abscesses
	Chronic gastrointestinal disease, infections, lymphoid hyperplasia, sprue-like syndrome, atypical inflammatory bowel disease
	Autoimmune disease such as autoimmune thrombocytopenia, hemolytic anemia, rheumatologic disease, alopecia, thyroiditis, pernicious anemia
	Pyoderma gangrenosum
	Adverse reaction to vaccines
	Delayed umbilical cord detachment
	Chronic stomatitis or peritonitis

EBV, Epstein-Barr virus; CMV, cytomegalovirus.
Modified from Goldman L, Ausiello D: *Cecil textbook of medicine,* ed 22, Philadelphia, 2004, Saunders, p 1598.

Table 116-4 CHARACTERISTIC FEATURES OF PRIMARY IMMUNODEFICIENCY

CHARACTERISTIC	PREDOMINANT T-CELL DEFECT	PREDOMINANT B-CELL DEFECT	GRANULOCYTE DEFECT	COMPLEMENT DEFECT
Age at the onset of infection	Early onset, usually 2-6 mo of age	Onset after maternal antibodies diminish, usually after 5-7 mo of age, later childhood to adulthood	Early onset	Onset at any age
Specific pathogens involved	Bacteria: common gram-positive and gram-negative bacteria and mycobacteria	Bacteria: pneumococci, streptococci, staphylococci, *Haemophilus, Campylobacter, Mycoplasma*	Bacteria: staphylococci, *Pseudomonas, Serratia, Klebsiella, Salmonella*	Bacteria: pneumococci, *Neisseria*
	Viruses: CMV, EBV, adenovirus, parainfluenza 3, varicella, enterovirus	Viruses: enterovirus*		
	Fungi: *Candida* and *Pneumocystis jiroveci*	Fungi and parasites: giardia, cryptosporidia	Fungi and parasites: *Candida, Nocardia, Aspergillus*	
Affected organs	Extensive mucocutaneous candidiasis, lungs, failure to thrive, protracted diarrhea	Recurrent sinopulmonary infections, chronic gastrointestinal symptoms, malabsorption, arthritis, enteroviral meningoencephalitis*	Skin: abscesses, impetigo, cellulitis Lymph nodes: suppurative adenitis Oral cavity: gingivitis, mouth ulcers Internal organs: abscesses, osteomyelitis	Infections: meningitis, arthritis, septicemia, recurrent sinopulmonary infections
Special features	Graft-versus-host disease caused by maternal engraftment or nonirradiated blood transfusion Postvaccination disseminated BCG or varicella Hypocalcemic tetany in infancy†	Autoimmunity Lymphoreticular malignancy: lymphoma, thymoma Postvaccination paralytic polio	Prolonged attachment of umbilical cord, poor wound healing	Autoimmune disorders: SLE, vasculitis, dermatomyositis, scleroderma, glomerulonephritis, angioedema

*X-linked (Bruton) agammaglobulinemia.
†DiGeorge anomaly.
BCG, bacille Calmette-Guérin; CMV, cytomegalovirus; EBV, Epstein-Barr virus; PCP, *Pneumocystis carinii*; SLE, systemic lupus erythematosus.
Modified from Woroniecka M, Ballow M: Office evaluation of children with recurrent infection, *Pediatr Clin North Am* 47:1211–1224, 2000.

Table 116-5 SPECIAL PHYSICAL FEATURES ASSOCIATED WITH IMMUNODEFICIENCY DISORDERS

CLINICAL FEATURES	DISORDERS
DERMATOLOGIC	
Eczema	Wiskott-Aldrich syndrome, IPEX
Sparse and/or hypopigmented hair	Cartilage hair hypoplasia, Chédiak-Higashi syndrome, Griscelli syndrome
Ocular telangiectasia	Ataxia-telangiectasia
Oculocutaneous albinism	Chédiak-Higashi syndrome
Severe dermatitis	Omenn syndrome
Recurrent abscesses with pulmonary pneumatoceles	Hyper-IgE syndrome
Recurrent organ abscesses, liver and rectum especially	Chronic granulomatous disease
Recurrent abscesses or cellulitis	Chronic granulomatous disease, hyper-IgE syndrome, leukocyte adhesion defect
Oral ulcers	Chronic granulomatous disease, severe combined immunodeficiency, congenital neutropenia
Periodontitis, gingivitis, stomatitis	Neutrophil defects
Oral or nail candidiasis	T-cell immune defects, combined defects, mucocutaneous candidiasis, hyper-IgE syndrome
Vitiligo	B-cell defects, mucocutaneous candidiasis
Alopecia	B-cell defects, mucocutaneous candidiasis
Chronic conjunctivitis	B-cell defects
EXTREMITIES	
Clubbing of the nails	Chronic lung disease due to antibody defects
Arthritis	Antibody defects, Wiskott-Aldrich syndrome, hyper-IgM syndrome
ENDOCRINOLOGIC	
Hypoparathyroidism	DiGeorge syndrome, mucocutaneous candidiasis
Endocrinopathies (autoimmune)	Mucocutaneous candidiasis
Growth hormone deficiency	X-linked agammaglobulinemia
Gonadal dysgenesis	Mucocutaneous candidiasis
HEMATOLOGIC	
Hemolytic anemia	B- and T-cell immune defects, ALPS
Thrombocytopenia, small platelets	Wiskott-Aldrich syndrome
Neutropenia	Hyper-IgM syndrome, Wiskott-Aldrich variant
Immune thrombocytopenia	B-cell immune defects, ALPS
SKELETAL	
Short-limb dwarfism	Short-limb dwarfism with T- and/or B-cell immune defects
Bony dysplasia	ADA deficiency, cartilage hair hypoplasia

ADA, adenosine deaminase deficiency; AID, activation-induced cytidine deaminase; ALPS, autoimmune lymphoproliferative syndrome; GVHD, graft-versus-host disease; Ig, immunoglobulin; IPEX, X-linked immune dysfunction enteropathy polyendocrinopathy; SCID, severe combined immunodeficiency.
From Goldman L, Ausiello D: *Cecil textbook of medicine,* ed 22, Philadelphia, 2004, Saunders, p 1599.

Table 116-6 INITIAL IMMUNOLOGIC TESTING OF THE CHILD WITH RECURRENT INFECTIONS

COMPLETE BLOOD COUNT, MANUAL DIFFERENTIAL, AND ERYTHROCYTE SEDIMENTATION RATE
Absolute lymphocyte count (normal result [Chapter 709] rules against T-cell defect) Absolute neutrophil count (normal result [Chapter 709] rules against congenital or acquired neutropenia and [usually] both forms of leukocyte adhesion deficiency, in which elevated counts are present even between infections) Platelet count (normal result excludes Wiskott-Aldrich syndrome) Howell-Jolly bodies (absence rules against asplenia) Erythrocyte sedimentation rate (normal result indicates chronic bacterial or fungal infection unlikely)
SCREENING TESTS FOR B-CELL DEFECTS
IgA measurement; if abnormal, IgG and IgM measurement Isohemagglutinins Antibody titers to blood group substances, tetanus, diphtheria, *Haemophilus influenzae,* and pneumococcus
SCREENING TESTS FOR T-CELL DEFECTS
Absolute lymphocyte count (normal result indicates T-cell defect unlikely) *Candida albicans* intradermal skin test: 0.1 mL of a 1 : 1,000 dilution for patients ≥6 yr, 0.1 mL of a 1 : 100 dilution for patients <6 yr
SCREENING TESTS FOR PHAGOCYTIC CELL DEFECTS
Absolute neutrophil count Respiratory burst assay
SCREENING TEST FOR COMPLEMENT DEFICIENCY
CH_{50}

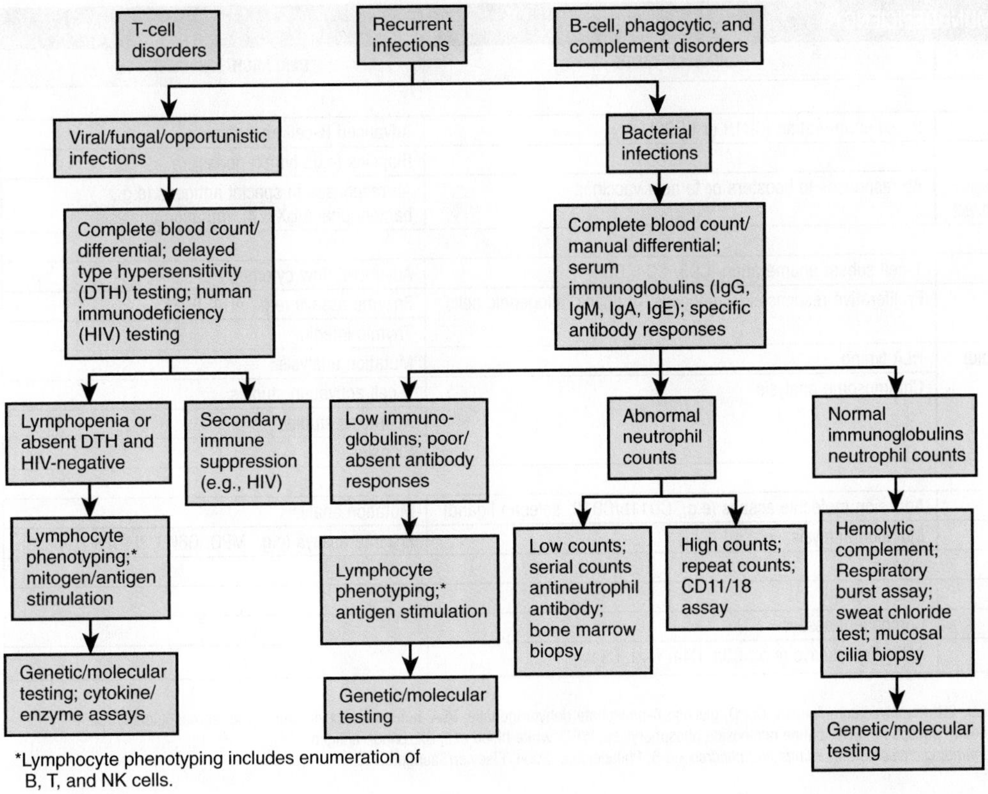

Figure 116-1 A diagnostic testing algorithm for primary immunodeficiency diseases. DTH, delayed type hypersensitivity. (From Lindegren ML, Kobrynski L, Rasmussen SA: Applying public health strategies to primary immunodeficiency diseases: a potential approach to genetic disorders, *MMWR Recomm Rep* 53[RR-1]:1–29, 2004.)

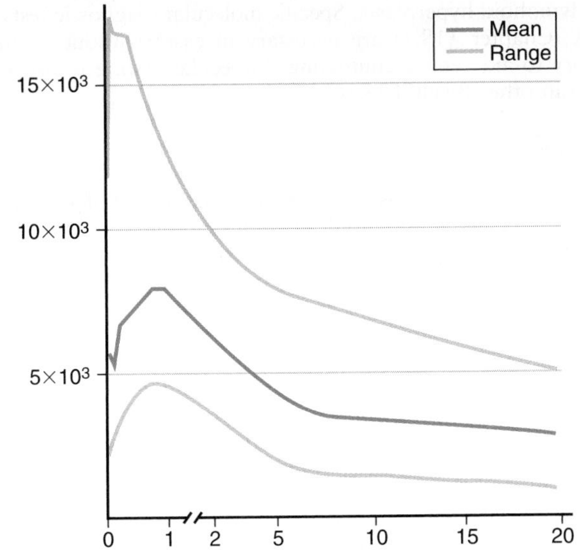

Figure 116-2 Absolute lymphocyte counts in normal individual during maturation. (Data graphed from Altman PL: *Blood and other body fluids.* Prepared under the auspices of the Committee on Biological Handbooks. Washington, DC, Federation of American Societies for Experimental Biology, 1961.)

A simple screening test for B-cell defects is the measurement of serum IgA. If the IgA level is normal, selective IgA deficiency, which is the most common B-cell defect, is excluded, as are most of the permanent types of hypogammaglobulinemia, since IgA is usually very low or absent in those conditions. If IgA is low, IgG and IgM should also be measured. Patients who are receiving corticosteroids or who have protein-losing states (nephrosis, protein-losing enteropathy) often have low serum IgG concentrations but produce antibodies normally. Thus, if immunoglobulins are low, it is crucial before starting intravenous immunoglobulin (IVIG) therapy that antibody titers to specific antigens are obtained to determine whether the levels are low because of inadequate antibody synthesis or due to protein loss. Antibody titers are not interpretable after the patient has received a blood transfusion or IVIG, which contains antibodies from a minimum of 60,000 normal donors.

One of the most useful tests for B-cell function is to determine the presence and titer of **isohemagglutinins,** or antibodies to type A and B red blood cell polysaccharide antigens. This test measures predominantly IgM antibodies. Isohemagglutinins may be absent normally in the 1st 2 yr of life and are always absent if the patient is blood type AB.

Because most infants and children are immunized with diphtheria-tetanus-pertussis (DTaP), conjugated *Haemophilus influenzae* type b (Hib), and pneumococcal conjugate vaccine (PCV7), it is often informative to test for specific antibodies to diphtheria, tetanus, *H. influenzae* polyribose phosphate, and pneumococcal antigens. If the titers are low, measurement of antibodies to diphtheria or tetanus toxoids before and 2 wk after a pediatric DTaP or DT booster is helpful in assessing the capacity to form IgG antibodies to protein antigens. To evaluate a patient's ability to respond to polysaccharide antigens, anti-pneumococcal antibodies can be measured before and 3 wk after immunization with pneumococcal polysaccharide vaccine (PPV23) in patients >2-3 yr old. Antibodies detected in these tests are of the IgG isotype. These antibody studies can be performed in several different laboratories, but it is important to choose a reliable laboratory and to use the same laboratory for preimmunization and post-immunization samples. In children <2 yr of age with low anti-pneumococcal antibody titers, it is useful to boost with conjugate pneumococcal vaccine twice, 1 mo apart, before giving a polysaccharide pneumococcal vaccine 1 mo later and then measuring antibody titers 3 wk later. Patients with significant or permanent B-cell defects do not produce either IgM or IgG antibodies normally. If results of these tests prove to be normal and the immunoglobulins remain low, studies should be performed to evaluate

Table 116-7 LABORATORY TESTS IN IMMUNODEFICIENCY

SCREENING TESTS	ADVANCED TESTS	RESEARCH/SPECIAL TESTS
B-CELL DEFICIENCY		
IgG, IgM, IgA, and IgE levels	B-cell enumeration (CD19 or CD20)	Advanced B-cell phenotyping
Isohemagglutinin titers		Biopsies (e.g., lymph nodes)
Ab response to vaccine antigens (e.g., tetanus, diphtheria, pneumococci, *Haemophilus influenzae*)	Ab responses to boosters or to new vaccines	Ab responses to special antigens (e.g., bacteriophage ϕX174), mutation analysis
T-CELL DEFICIENCY		
Lymphocyte count	T-cell subset enumeration (CD3, CD4, CD8)	Advanced flow cytometry
Chest x-ray examination for thymic size*	Proliferative responses to mitogens, antigens, allogeneic cells	Enzyme assays (e.g., ADA, PNP)
		Thymic imaging
Delayed skin tests (e.g., *Candida,* tetanus toxoid)	HLA typing	Mutation analysis
	Chromosome analysis	T-cell activation studies
		Apoptosis studies
		Biopsies
PHAGOCYTIC DEFICIENCY		
WBC count, morphology	Adhesion molecule assays (e.g., CD11b/CD18, selectin ligand)	Mutation analysis
Respiratory burst assay	Mutation analysis	Enzyme assays (e.g., MPO, G6PD, NADPH oxidase)
COMPLEMENT DEFICIENCY		
CH_{50} activity	AH50, activity	
C3 level	Component assays	
C4 level	Activation assays (e.g., C3a, C4a, C4d, C5a)	

*In infants only.

Ab, antibody; ADA, adenosine deaminase; C, complement; CH, hemolytic complement; G6PD, glucose-6-phosphate dehydrogenase; HLA, human leukocyte antigen; Ig, immunoglobulin; MPO, myeloperoxidase; NADPH, nicotinamide adenine dinucleotide phosphate; PNP, purine nucleoside phosphorylase; WBC, white blood cell; ϕX, phage antigen.

Modified from Stiehm ER, Ochs HD, Winkelstein JA: *Immunologic disorders in infants and children,* ed 5, Philadelphia, 2004, Elsevier/Saunders.

the possible loss of immunoglobulins through the urinary or gastrointestinal tracts (nephrotic syndrome, protein-losing enteropathies, intestinal lymphangiectasia). Very high serum concentrations of 1 or more immunoglobulin classes suggest HIV infection, chronic granulomatous disease, chronic inflammation, or autoimmune lymphoproliferative syndrome (ALPS).

IgG subclass measurements are seldom helpful in assessing immune function in children with recurrent infections. It is difficult to know the biologic significance of the various mild to moderate deficiencies of IgG subclasses, particularly when completely asymptomatic individuals have been described as totally lacking IgG1, IgG2, IgG4, and/or IgA1 owing to immunoglobulin heavy chain gene deletions. Many healthy children have been described as having low levels of IgG2 but normal responses to polysaccharide antigens when immunized. When children with low IgG2 subclass levels and histories of frequent infections were studied in depth, they were found to have broader immunologic dysfunction, including poor responses to protein antigens, suggesting that they may have been in the process of developing into **common variable immunodeficiency (CVID).** Only when profound antibody deficiencies are detected despite normal levels of immunoglobulins are IgG subclass measurements occasionally helpful. Children who completely lack IgG2 are usually unable to make antibodies to polysaccharide antigens, although this may occur among individuals with normal IgG2. Thus, specific antibody measurements are far more cost-effective than IgG subclass determinations.

Patients found to be **agammaglobulinemic** should have their blood B cells enumerated by **flow cytometry** using dye-conjugated monoclonal antibodies to B-cell–specific CD antigens (usually CD19 or CD20). Normally, approximately 8-10% of circulating lymphocytes are B cells. B cells are absent in X-linked agammaglobulinemia (XLA), and present in CVID, IgA deficiency, and hyper-IgM syndromes. This distinction is important, because children with hypogammaglobulinemia from XLA and CVID can have different clinical problems, and the 2 conditions clearly have different inheritance patterns. Patients with XLA have a heightened susceptibility to persistent enteroviral infections, whereas those with CVID have more problems with autoimmune diseases and lymphoid hyperplasia. Specific molecular diagnostic tests for XLA (Chapter 118.1) are necessary in cases without a family history to aid genetic counseling. Molecular testing is also indicated in other B-cell defects.

T CELLS

The ***Candida* skin test** is the most cost-effective test of T-cell function. Adults and children older than 6 yr of age should be tested by intradermal injection with 0.1 mL of a 1:1,000 dilution of a known potent *Candida albicans* extract. If the test result is negative at 24 hr, 48 hr, and 72 hr, a 1:100 dilution should be used, which can also be used for the initial testing of children <6 yr of age. If the *Candida* skin test result is positive, as defined by erythema and induration of ≥10 mm at 48 hr and that is greater than at 24 hr, all primary T-cell defects are precluded, which obviates the need for more expensive in vitro tests such as lymphocyte phenotyping or assessments of responses to mitogens.

T cells and T-cell subpopulations can be enumerated by **flow cytometry** using dye-conjugated monoclonal antibodies recognizing CD antigens present on T cells (i.e., CD2, CD3, CD4, and CD8). This is a particularly important test to perform on any infant who is lymphopenic, because $CD3^+$ T cells usually constitute 70% of peripheral lymphocytes. Infants with SCID are unable to produce T cells so are lymphopenic at birth. SCID is a pediatric emergency that can be successfully treated by stem cell marrow transplantation in >94% of cases if diagnosed before serious, untreatable infections develop. Normally, there are roughly twice as many $CD4^+$ (helper) T cells as there are $CD8^+$ (cytotoxic) T cells. Because there are examples of severe immunodeficiency in which phenotypically normal T cells are present, tests of T-cell function are far more informative and cost-effective than enumeration of T-cell subpopulations by flow cytometry. T cells are normally stimulated through their T-cell receptors (TCRs) by antigen present in the groove of major histocompatibility complex (MHC) molecules. The TCR can also be stimulated directly with **mitogens** such as phytohemagglutinin (PHA), concanavalin A

Table 116-8 2003 MODIFIED IUIS CLASSIFICATION OF PRIMARY AND SECONDARY IMMUNODEFICIENCIES

GROUPS AND DISEASES	INHERITANCE
A. PREDOMINANTLY ANTIBODY DEFICIENCIES	
XL agammaglobulinemia	XL
AR agammaglobulinemia	AR
Hyper-IgM syndromes	XL
a. XL	XL
b. AID defect	AR
c. CD40 defect	AR
d. UNG defect	AR
e. Other AR defects	AR
Ig heavy-chain gene deletions	AR
κ chain deficiency mutations	AR
Selective IgA deficiency	AD
Common variable immunodeficiency	AD
B. SEVERE COMBINED IMMUNODEFICIENCIES	
$T^-B^+NK^-$ SCID	
a. X-linked (γc deficiency)	XL
b. Autosomal recessive (Jak3 deficiency)	AR
$T^-B^+NK^+$ SCID	
a. IL-7 Rα deficiency	AR
b. CD3δ, CD3ε, or CD3ζ deficiencies	AR
c. CD45 deficiency	AR
$T^-B^-NK^+$ SCID	
a. RAG-1/2 deficiency	AR
b. Artemis defect	AR
Omenn syndrome	
a. RAG-1/2 deficiency	AR
b. IL-2Rα deficiency	AR
c. γc deficiency	XL
Combined Immunodeficiencies	
a. Purine nucleoside phosphorylase deficiency	AR
b CD8 deficiency (ZAP-70 defect)	AR
c. MHC class II deficiency	AR
d. MHC class I deficiency caused by TAP-1/2 mutations	AR
Reticular dysgenesis	AR
C. OTHER CELLULAR IMMUNODEFICIENCIES	
Wiskott-Aldrich syndrome	XL
Ataxia-telangiectasia	AR
DiGeorge anomaly	?
D. DEFECTS OF PHAGOCYTIC FUNCTION	
Chronic granulomatous disease	
a. XL	XL
b. AR	AR
1. p22 phox deficiency	
2. p47 phox deficiency	
3. p67 phox deficiency	
Leukocyte adhesion defect 1	AR
Leukocyte adhesion defect 2	AR
Neutrophil G6PD deficiency	XL
Myeloperoxidase deficiency	AR
Secondary granule deficiency	AR
Shwachman syndrome	AR
Severe congenital neutropenia (Kostmann)	AR
Cyclic neutropenia (elastase defect)	AR
Leukocyte mycobacterial defects	AR
IFN-γR1 or R2 deficiency	AR
IFN-γR1 deficiency	AD
IL-12Rβ1 deficiency	AR
IL-12p40 deficiency	AR
STAT1 deficiency	AD
E. IMMUNODEFICIENCIES ASSOCIATED WITH LYMPHOPROLIFERATIVE DISORDERS	
Fas deficiency	AD
Fas ligand deficiency	
FLICE or caspase 8 deficiency	
Unknown (caspase 3 deficiency)	
F. COMPLEMENT DEFICIENCIES	
C1q deficiency	AR
C1r deficiency	AR
C4 deficiency	AR
C2 deficiency	AR
C3 deficiency	AR
C5 deficiency	AR
C6 deficiency	AR
C7 deficiency	AR
C8α deficiency	AR
C8β deficiency	AR
C9 deficiency	AR
C1 inhibitor	AD
Factor I deficiency	AR
Factor H deficiency	AR
Factor D deficiency	AR
Properdin deficiency	XL
G. IMMUNODEFICIENCY ASSOCIATED WITH OR SECONDARY TO OTHER DISEASES	
Chromosomal Instability or Defective Repair	
Bloom syndrome	
Fanconi anemia	
ICF syndrome	
Nijmegen breakage syndrome	
Seckel syndrome	
Xeroderma pigmentosum	
Chromosomal Defects	
Down syndrome	
Turner syndrome	
Chromosome 18 rings and deletions	
Skeletal Abnormalities	
Short-limbed skeletal dysplasia	
Cartilage-hair hypoplasia	
Immunodeficiency with Generalized Growth Retardation	
Schimke immuno-osseous dysplasia	
Immunodeficiency with absent thumbs	
Dubowitz syndrome	
Growth retardation, facial anomalies, and immunodeficiency	
Progeria (Hutchinson-Gilford syndrome)	
Immunodeficiency with Dermatologic Defects	
Partial albinism	
Dyskeratosis congenita	
Netherton syndrome	
Acrodermatitis enteropathica	
Anhidrotic ectodermal dysplasia	
Papillon-Lefèvre syndrome	
Hereditary Metabolic Defects	
Transcobalamin 2 deficiency	
Methylmalonic acidemia	
Type 1 hereditary orotic aciduria	
Biotin-dependent carboxylase deficiency	
Mannosidosis	
Glycogen storage disease, type 1b	
Chédiak-Higashi syndrome	
Hypercatabolism of Immunoglobulin	
Familial hypercatabolism	
Intestinal lymphangiectasia	
H. OTHER IMMUNODEFICIENCIES	
Hyper-IgE syndrome	AD and AR
Chronic mucocutaneous candidiasis	
Chronic mucocutaneous candidiasis with polyendocrinopathy (APECED)	AR
Hereditary or congenital hyposplenia or asplenia	
Ivemark syndrome	
IPEX syndrome	XL
Ectodermal dysplasia (NEMO defect)	XL

AD, autosomal dominant; ADA, adenosine deaminase; AID, activation-induced cytidine deaminase; APECED, autoimmune, polyendocrinopathy, candidiasis, ectodermal dystrophy; AR, autosomal recessive; caspase, cysteinyl aspartate specific proteinase; FLICE, Fas-associating protein with death domain–like IL-1–converting enzyme; G6PD, glucose 6-phosphate dehydrogenase; ICF, immunodeficiency, centromeric instability, facial anomalies; IFN, interferon; Ig, immunoglobulin; IL, interleukin; IPEX, immune dysregulation, polyendocrinopathy, enteropathy; MHC, major histocompatibility complex; NEMO, nuclear factor B essential modulator; SCID, severe combined immunodeficiency; TAP-2, transporter associated with antigen presentation; XL, X-linked.

Modified from (no authors listed) Primary immunodeficiency diseases. Report of an International Union of Immunological Studies Scientific Committee, *Clin Exp Immunol* 118:1–28, 1999; Chapel H, Geha R, Rosen F: IUIS PID (Primary Immunodeficiencies) Classification committee: Primary immunodeficiency diseases: an update, *Clin Exp Immunol* 132:9–15, 2003; Stiehm ER, Ochs HD, Winkelstein JA: *Immunologic disorders in infants and children,* ed 5, Philadelphia, 2004, Elsevier/Saunders.

(Con A), or pokeweed mitogen (PWM). After 3-5 days of incubation with the mitogen, the proliferation of T cells is measured by the incorporation of radiolabeled thymidine into DNA. Other stimulants that can be used to assess T-cell function in the same type of assay include antigens (*Candida*, tetanus toxoid) and allogeneic cells (see Table 116-6).

NK CELLS

Natural killer (NK) cells can be enumerated by flow cytometry using monoclonal antibodies to NK-specific CD antigens, CD16 and CD56. NK function is assessed by a radiolabeled chromium-release assay, using the cell line K562, which is readily killed by NK cells.

PHAGOCYTIC CELLS

Killing defects of phagocytic cells, which should be suspected if a patient has recurrent staphylococcal abscesses or gram-negative infections, can be evaluated by screening tests measuring the neutrophil respiratory burst after phorbol ester stimulation. The most reliable and useful test of this type is a flow cytometric assessment of the respiratory burst using rhodamine dye, which has replaced the nitroblue tetrazolium (NBT) dye test, which was plagued by technical problems with reproducibility. Leukocyte adhesion deficiencies can be easily diagnosed by flow cytometric assays of blood lymphocytes or neutrophils, using monoclonal antibodies to CD18 or CD11 (LAD1) or to CD15 (LAD2).

Phagocytic cell defects can be further defined according to their molecular cause. Mutations in the genes encoding 4 different components of the electron transport chain have been discovered in various patients with chronic granulomatous disease (CGD). It is important to identify the specific molecular type of CGD to provide appropriate genetic counseling, as 1 type is X linked and the other 3 types are autosomal recessive. Early diagnosis of leukocyte adhesion deficiency (LAD) is of crucial importance because stem cell transplantation can be lifesaving.

COMPLEMENT

The most effective screening test for complement defects is a CH_{50} assay, a bioassay that measures the intactness of the entire complement pathway and yields abnormal results if complement has been consumed from the specimen for any reason. Genetic deficiencies in the complement system are usually characterized by extremely low CH_{50} values. The most common cause of an abnormal CH_{50} result, however, is a delay in or improper transport of the specimen to the laboratory. Specific immunoassays for C3 and C4 are commercially available, but further identification of other complement component deficiencies is usually possible only in research laboratories. Nevertheless, it is extremely important to identify which component is missing, because there are different disease susceptibilities depending on whether there are deficiencies of early or late components (Chapter 128). Identifying the mode of inheritance is also important for genetic counseling. Properdin deficiency is X linked, but all of the other complement deficiencies are autosomal. Measurement of C4 can be helpful in assessing suspected hereditary angioedema.

BIBLIOGRAPHY

Please visit the Nelson Textbook of Pediatrics *website at www.expertconsult.com for the complete bibliography.*

Section 2 THE T-, B-, AND NK-CELL SYSTEMS

Chapter 117
T Lymphocytes, B Lymphocytes, and Natural Killer Cells

Rebecca H. Buckley

Defense against infectious agents is secured through a combination of anatomic physical barriers including the skin, mucous membranes, mucous blanket, and ciliated epithelial cells, as well as the various components of the immune system. The **immune system** of vertebrates integrates 2 fundamental response mechanisms. **Innate (natural) immunity** responds to infection regardless of previous exposure to the agent and includes polymorphonuclear leukocytes, dendritic and mononuclear phagocytic cells, various receptors that recognize common pathogen antigens (Toll-like receptors) and the complement system. **Acquired (adaptive) immunity** is a highly specific response that includes T lymphocytes, B lymphocytes, and natural killer (NK) cells. The immune system also helps protect against malignancy and autoimmunity.

For the full continuation of this chapter, please visit the Nelson Textbook of Pediatrics *website at www.expertconsult.com.*

Chapter 118
Primary Defects of Antibody Production

Rebecca H. Buckley

Of all of the primary immunodeficiency diseases, those affecting antibody production are most frequent. Selective absence of serum and secretory IgA is the most common defect, with rates ranging from 1/333 to 1/18,000 persons among different races. By contrast, agammaglobulinemia is estimated to occur with a frequency of only 1/10,000 to 1/50,000 persons. Patients with antibody deficiency are usually recognized because they have recurrent infections with encapsulated bacteria predominantly in the upper and lower respiratory tracts; some individuals with selective IgA deficiency or infants with transient hypogammaglobulinemia may have few or no infections (see Table 116-4). The defective gene products for many primary antibody deficiency disorders have been identified (Table 118-1) and localized (Fig. 118-1). Sometimes the defect is not in the B cell itself but in T cells, which are required for complete B-cell function.

Table 118-1 GENETIC BASIS OF PRIMARY ANTIBODY DEFICIENCY DISORDERS

CHROMOSOME AND REGION	GENE PRODUCT	DISORDER	FUNCTIONAL DEFICIENCIES
2p11	κ chain	κ chain deficiency	Absence of immunoglobulins bearing κ chains
2q33	Inducible co-stimulator (ICOS)	ICOS-deficient CVID (common variable immunodeficiency)	Low or absent concentrations of all immunoglobulins
6p21.3	Unknown	Selective IgA deficiency; CVID	Low or absent IgA; low concentrations of all immunoglobulins in CVID
12p13	Activation-induced cytidine deaminase (AICDA)*	Autosomal recessive hyper-IgM syndrome (HIGM2)	Failure to produce IgG, IgA, and IgE antibodies
12q23-q24.1	Uracil DNA glycosylase (UNG)	Autosomal recessive hyper-IgM syndrome (HIGM5)	Failure to produce IgG, IgA, and IgE antibodies
14q32.3	Immunoglobulin heavy chains*	B-cell–negative agammaglobulinemia; in others, selective isotype deficiencies	Absence of antibody production, lack of B cells, in μ heavy chain mutations; in others, subclasses missing but B cells present
16p11.2	CD19	CD19 deficient CVID	Low or absent concentrations of all immunoglobulins
17p11.2	TACI* (transmembrane activator calcium-modulator, and cyclophilin ligand interactor)	TACI–deficient CVID	Low or absent concentrations of all immunoglobulins
20	CD40*	Autosomal recessive hyper IgM syndrome type 3 (HIGM3)	Failure to produce IgG, IgA, and IgE antibodies
22q13.1-q13.31	BAFF-R (B-cell–activating factor of the TNF family receptor)	BAFF-R–deficient CVID	Low or absent concentrations of all immunoglobulins
Xq22	Bruton tyrosine kinase (Btk)*	X-linked agammaglobulinemia (XLA, or Bruton agammaglobulinemia)	Absence of antibody production, lack of B cells
Xq25	SLAM-associated protein (SH2D1A)*	X-linked lymphoproliferative disease (XLP)	Lack of anti-EBNA (Epstein-Barr virus nuclear antigen) and long-lived T-cell immunity; low immunoglobulins
Xq26	CD154 (CD40 ligand)*	X-linked hyper-IgM syndrome type 1 (HIGM1)	Failure to produce IgG, IgA, and IgE antibodies
Xq28	Nuclear factor κB essential modulator (NEMO)*	Anhidrotic ectodermal dysplasia with immunodeficiency	Hyper IgM or IgG subclass and anti-polysaccharide antibody deficiencies

*The gene has been cloned and sequenced.

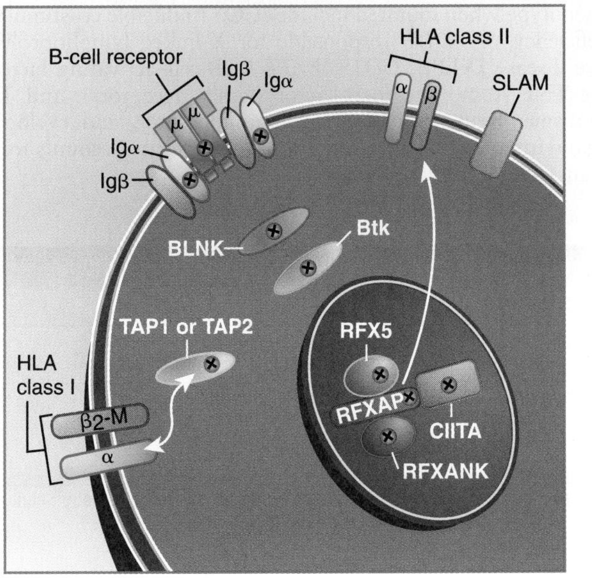

Figure 118-1 Locations of mutant proteins *(X)* in B cells identified in primary immunodeficiency diseases. β_2m, β_2 microglobulin; BLNK, B-cell linker adaptor protein; Btk, Bruton tyrosine kinase; HLA, human leukocyte antigen; Ig, immunoglobulin; RFX, RFXAP and CIITA transcription factors; SLAM, signaling lymphocyte activation molecule; TAP1 and TAP2, transporters of processed antigen. (From Buckley RH: Primary immunodeficiency diseases due to defects in lymphocytes, *N Engl J Med* 343:1313–1324, 2000.)

X-LINKED AGAMMAGLOBULINEMIA (XLA)

Patients with X-linked agammaglobulinemia (XLA), or **Bruton agammaglobulinemia,** have a profound defect in B-lymphocyte development resulting in severe hypogammaglobulinemia, an absence of circulating B cells, small to absent tonsils, and no palpable lymph nodes.

Genetics and Pathogenesis

The abnormal gene in XLA maps to q22 on the long arm of the X chromosome and encodes the B-cell protein tyrosine kinase **Btk (Bruton tyrosine kinase).** Btk is a member of the Tec family of cytoplasmic protein tyrosine kinases and is expressed at high levels in all B-lineage cells, including pre–B cells. It appears to be necessary for pre–B-cell expansion and maturation into surface Ig-expressing B cells, but probably has a role at all stages of B-cell development; it has also been found in cells of the myeloid series. More than 500 different mutations in the human *Btk* gene are recognized; they encompass most parts of the coding portions of the gene. There is not a clear correlation between the location of the mutation and the clinical phenotype (Fig. 118-2). Carriers are detected by mutation analysis, and prenatal diagnosis of affected male fetuses is possible if the mutation is known in the family.

The expression of Btk in cells of myeloid lineage is of interest because boys with XLA often have neutropenia at the height of an acute infection. It is conceivable that Btk is only one of the signaling molecules participating in myeloid maturation and that neutropenia is observed in XLA only when rapid production of such cells is needed. Some pre–B cells are found in the bone marrow; the percentage of peripheral blood B lymphocytes is <1%. The percentage of T cells is increased, ratios of T-cell subsets are normal, and T-cell function is intact. The thymus is normal.

Six autosomal recessive defects have also been shown to result in agammaglobulinemia with an absence of circulating B cells (see Fig. 118-2), including mutations in the genes encoding: (1) the μ heavy chain gene; (2) the Igα and Igβ signaling molecules; (3) B-cell linker adaptor protein (BLNK); (4) the surrogate light chain, λ5/14.1; and (5) leucine-rich repeat-containing 8 (LRRC8).

Clinical Manifestations

Most boys afflicted with XLA remain well during the 1st 6-9 mo of life by virtue of maternally transmitted IgG antibodies. Thereafter, they acquire infections with extracellular pyogenic organisms, such as *Streptococcus pneumoniae* and *Haemophilus influenzae,* unless they are given prophylactic antibiotics or immunoglobulin therapy. Infections include sinusitis, otitis media, pneumonia, or, less often, sepsis or meningitis. Infections with *Mycoplasma* are also particularly problematic. Chronic fungal infections are seen; *Pneumocystis jiroveci* pneumonia rarely occurs. Viral infections are usually handled normally with the exceptions of hepatitis viruses and enteroviruses. There were several examples of **paralysis** when live polio vaccine was administered to these patients and chronic, eventually fatal, central nervous system infections with various echoviruses and coxsackieviruses have occurred in a significant number of them. Echovirus-associated **myositis** resembling dermatomyositis has also been observed. These observations suggest a primary role for antibody, particularly secretory IgA, in host defense against enteroviruses. Growth hormone deficiency has also been reported in association with XLA.

Diagnosis

The diagnosis of XLA should be suspected if **lymphoid hypoplasia** is found on physical examination (minimal or no tonsillar tissue and no palpable lymph nodes), and serum concentrations of IgG, IgA, IgM, and IgE are far below the 95% confidence limits for appropriate age- and race-matched controls (Chapter 708), usually with total immunoglobulins <100 mg/dL. Levels of natural antibodies to type A and B red blood cell polysaccharide antigens (isohemagglutinins) and antibodies to antigens given during routine immunizations are abnormally low in this disorder, whereas they are normal in transient hypogammaglobulinemia of infancy. **Flow cytometry** is an important test to demonstrate the absence of circulating B cells, which will distinguish this disorder from common variable immunodeficiency, the hyper-IgM syndrome and transient hypogammaglobulinemia of infancy.

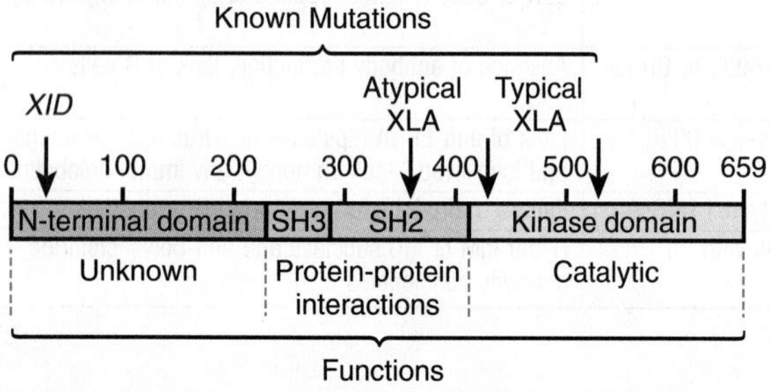

Figure 118-2 Location of mutations in the functional domains of the Bruton tyrosine kinase (Btk) protein. Deletion and point mutations in Btk identified to date in many boys with classic X-linked agammaglobulinemia (XLA) are in the kinase domain, whereas CBA/N XID mice with a less severe B-cell defect have a point mutation at position 28 in the N-terminal domain. More recently, however, boys with classic XLA are also reported to have mutations at the XID mutation site and in the SH2 domain. (From Buckley RH: Breakthroughs in the understanding and therapy of primary immunodeficiency, *Pediatr Clin North Am* 41:665–690, 1994.)

COMMON VARIABLE IMMUNODEFICIENCY

Common variable immunodeficiency (CVID) is a syndrome characterized by hypogammaglobulinemia with phenotypically normal B cells. It has also been called **"acquired hypogammaglobulinemia"** because of a generally later age of onset of infections. CVID patients may appear similar clinically to those with XLA in the types of infections experienced and bacterial etiologic agents involved, except that echovirus meningoencephalitis is rare in patients with CVID (Table 118-2). In contrast to XLA, the sex distribution in CVID is almost equal, the age of onset is later (although it may be present in infancy), and infections may be less severe.

Genetics and Pathogenesis

Most patients have no identified molecular diagnosis. CVID is a category of primary immunodeficiency disorders that likely consists of several different genetic defects with autosomal recessive or dominant inheritance. Genes known to produce the CVID phenotype when mutated include *ICOS* (inducible co-stimulator) deficiency, *SH2DIA* (responsible for X-linked lymphoproliferative disease [XLP]), *CD19, BAFF-R* (B-cell–activating factor of the TNF [tumor necrosis factor] family receptors), and *TACI* (transmembrane activator, calcium-modulator, and cyclophilin ligand interactor). These mutations in aggregate accounts for less than 10% of all cases of CVID.

Table 118-2 DIFFERENTIAL DIAGNOSIS FOR PATIENTS WITH SUSPECTED CVID (HYPOGAMMAGLOBULINEMIA WITH RECURRENT INFECTIONS)*

	LABORATORY FEATURES	CLINICAL FEATURES	FURTHER TESTING
Selective IgA deficiency	Low titers of or absent IgA with normal IgG and IgM concentrations	Usually asymptomatic	Needed if symptomatic
Selective IgG subclass deficiency	Low titers of one or more of the IgG subclasses (G1, G2, G3, and G4); normal total IgG concentrations unless IgG1 is affected	Usually asymptomatic	Needed if symptomatic
X-linked agammaglobulinemia	Modest to profound hypogammaglobulinemia with low numbers or absence of peripheral-blood B cells	Recurrent infections	Btk protein expression by flow cytometry†; gene sequencing† if protein absent
X-linked lymphoproliferative syndrome	Hypogammaglobulinemia, EBV infection is usually the trigger	Aberrant response to EBV, lymphoproliferative disease	SH2D1A protein expression by flow cytometry,† confirmation by SH2D1A gene sequencing†
Autosomal recessive agammaglobulinemia	Profound hypogammaglobulinemia with absent or very low numbers of peripheral B cells	Tends to manifest early in infancy or childhood, recurrent and severe infections	Gene sequencing of six genes identified (Igμ heavy chain, *IgVκA2, CD79A, CD79B,* λ5 surrogate light chain, *BLNK*)‡
Hyper-IgM syndromes	Normal to high titers of IgM with low titers of IgG and IgA, very low numbers or absent class-switched memory B cells	Recurrent opportunistic sinopulmonary infections, patients with NEMO defects have hypohidrotic ectodermal dysplasia and susceptibility to recurrent mycobacterial infections	Protein expression by flow cytometry for CD40L on activated T cells and CD40 on B cells, receptor-binding function for CD40L, confirmation by gene sequencing is available for the five genes implicated *(CD40L, NEMO, CD40, AID, and UNG)*†

*Drugs, hematological malignancies, and other clinical phenotypes that can cause secondary hypogammaglobulinemia are described in the text.
†Tests available clinically in specialized reference laboratories.
‡Tests available only in the research setting.
Btk, Bruton tyrosine kinase; EBV, Epstein-Barr virus; CD40L, CD40 ligand; NEMO, NF-κB essential modulator; AID, activation-induced cytidine deaminase; UNG, uracil DNA glycosylase.
From Park MA, Li JT, Hagan JB, et al: Common variable immunodeficiency: a new look at an old disease, *Lancet* 372:489–502, 2008, p 491, Table 1.

Because CVID occurs in 1st-degree relatives of patients with selective IgA deficiency, and some patients with IgA deficiency later become panhypogammaglobulinemic, a large subtype of CVID may have a common genetic basis with IgA deficiency. The high incidence of abnormal immunoglobulin concentrations, autoantibodies, autoimmune disease, and malignancy in both CVID and IgA deficiency and in other members of their families also suggests a shared hereditary influence. This concept is supported by the discovery of a high incidence of C4-A gene deletions and C2 rare gene alleles in the class III major histocompatibility complex (MHC) region in individuals with either IgA deficiency or CVID, suggesting that a common susceptibility gene is on chromosome 6. Only a few human leukocyte antigen (HLA) haplotypes are shared by individuals affected with IgA deficiency and CVID, with at least 1 of 2 particular haplotypes being present in 77% of those affected. In 1 large family with 13 members, 2 had IgA deficiency and 3 had CVID. All of the immunodeficient patients in the family had at least 1 copy of an MHC haplotype that is abnormally frequent in IgA deficiency and CVID: HLA-DQB1 *0201, HLA-DR3, C4B-Sf, C4A-deleted, G11-15, Bf-0.4, C2a, HSP70-7.5, TNFa-5, HLA-B8, and HLA-A1. In a study of 83 multiply affected families with IgA deficiency and CVID, increased allele sharing at chromosome 6p21 in the proximal part of the MHC was observed in a susceptibility locus now designated as *IGAD1*. More sensitive genetic analysis in 101 multiple-case and 110 single-case families further localized the defect to the *HLADQ/DR* locus. Environmental factors, particularly drugs such as phenytoin, D-penicillamine, gold, and sulfasalazine are suspected to be triggers for disease expression in individuals with the permissive genetic background.

Most cases of CVID are sporadic or follow an autosomal dominant pattern of inheritance. Patients who lack inducible costimulator (ICOS), a surface protein on activated T cells, have an autosomal recessive pattern of inheritance. Nine such patients from 6 families in the Black Forest of Germany have been found to have identical homozygous large genomic deletions of the *ICOS* gene, suggesting a founder effect. Those who have XLP have an X-linked pattern of inheritance and those with autosomally inherited *TACI* defects may have heterozygous or homozygous mutations.

Despite normal numbers of circulating immunoglobulin-bearing B lymphocytes and the presence of lymphoid cortical follicles, blood B lymphocytes from CVID patients do not differentiate normally into immunoglobulin-producing cells when stimulated with pokeweed mitogen (PWM) in vitro, even when co-cultured with normal T cells. CVID B cells from some patients can be stimulated both to switch isotype and to synthesize and secrete some immunoglobulin when stimulated with anti-CD40 and IL-4 or IL-10. T cells and T-cell subsets are usually present in normal percentages, although T-cell function is depressed in some patients.

Clinical Manifestations

The serum immunoglobulin and antibody deficiencies in CVID may be as profound as in XLA. Patients with CVID often have autoantibody formation and normal-sized or enlarged tonsils and lymph nodes, and ≈25% of patients have splenomegaly. CVID has also been associated with a sprue-like syndrome with or without nodular follicular lymphoid hyperplasia of the intestine, thymoma, alopecia areata, hemolytic anemia, gastric atrophy, achlorhydria, thrombocytopenia, and pernicious anemia. Lymphoid interstitial pneumonia, pseudolymphoma, B-cell lymphomas, amyloidosis, and noncaseating sarcoid-like granulomas of the lungs, spleen, skin, and liver also occur. There is a 438-fold increase in lymphomas among affected women in the 5th and 6th decades of life. CVID has been reported to resolve transiently or permanently in patients who acquire human immunodeficiency virus (HIV) infection.

Recurrent or chronic infections include pneumonia, sinusitis, otitis media, and diarrhea (bacterial, giardiasis). Repeated pulmonary infections may produce bronchiectasis, while live polio virus vaccines may produce paralysis. Sepsis and meningitis with encapsulated bacteria occur more frequently than the general population. There is often a delay in the diagnosis of 5-10 yr between the 1st infections and a definitive diagnosis.

SELECTIVE IgA DEFICIENCY

An isolated absence or near absence (<10 mg/dL) of serum and secretory IgA is the most common well-defined immunodeficiency disorder, with a disease frequency as high as 0.33% in some populations. This condition is also occasionally associated with ill health.

The basic defect resulting in IgA deficiency is unknown. Phenotypically normal blood B cells are present. IgA deficiency occasionally remits spontaneously or after discontinuation of phenytoin (Dilantin) therapy. The occurrence of IgA deficiency in both males and females and in members of successive generations within families suggests autosomal dominant inheritance with variable expressivity. This defect also occurs commonly in pedigrees containing individuals with CVID. Indeed, IgA deficiency may evolve into CVID, and the finding of rare alleles and deletions of MHC class III genes in both conditions suggests that the susceptibility gene common to these 2 conditions may reside in the MHC class III region on chromosome 6. IgA deficiency is noted in patients treated with the same drugs associated with producing CVID (phenytoin, D-penicillamine, gold, and sulfasalazine), suggesting that environmental factors may trigger this disease in a genetically susceptible person.

Clinical Manifestations

Infections occur predominantly in the respiratory, gastrointestinal, and urogenital tracts. Bacterial agents responsible are the same as in other antibody deficiency syndromes. Intestinal giardiasis is common. Children with IgA deficiency vaccinated intranasally with killed poliovirus produce local IgM and IgG antibodies. Serum concentrations of other immunoglobulins are usually normal in patients with selective IgA deficiency, although IgG2 (and other) subclass deficiency has been reported, and IgM (usually elevated) may be monomeric.

Patients with IgA deficiency often have IgG antibodies against cow's milk and ruminant serum proteins. These antiruminant antibodies may cause false-positive results in immunoassays for IgA that use goat (but not rabbit) antisera. IgA deficiency is associated with a sprue-like syndrome, which may or may not respond to a gluten-free diet. The incidence of autoantibodies, autoimmune diseases, and malignancy is increased. Serum antibodies to IgA are reported in as many as 44% of patients with selective IgA deficiency. If these antibodies are of the IgE isotype, they can cause severe or fatal anaphylactic reactions after intravenous administration of blood products containing IgA. Only 5-times washed (in 200-mL volumes) normal donor erythrocytes (frozen blood would have this done routinely), or blood products from other IgA-deficient individuals, should be administered to patients with IgA deficiency. Administration of intravenous immunoglobulin (IVIG), which is >99% IgG, is not indicated because most IgA-deficient patients make IgG antibodies normally. Many IVIG preparations contain sufficient IgA to cause anaphylactic reactions.

IgG SUBCLASS DEFICIENCIES

Some patients have deficiencies of 1 or more of the 4 subclasses of IgG despite normal or elevated total IgG serum concentration. Some patients with absent or very low concentrations of IgG2 also have IgA deficiency. Other patients with IgG2 deficiency have gone on to develop CVID, suggesting that the presence of IgG subclass deficiency may be a marker for more generalized immune dysfunction. The biologic significance of the numerous moderate deficiencies of IgG subclasses that have been reported is difficult to assess, particularly because commercial laboratory measurement of IgG subclasses is problematic. IgG subclass measurement is not cost-effective in evaluating immune function in the child with recurrent infection. The more relevant issue is a patient's capacity to make specific antibodies to protein and polysaccharide antigens, because profound deficiencies of antipolysaccharide antibodies have been noted even in the presence of normal concentrations of IgG2. IVIG should not be administered to patients with IgG subclass deficiency unless they are shown to have a deficiency of antibodies to a broad array of antigens.

IMMUNOGLOBULIN HEAVY- AND LIGHT-CHAIN DELETIONS

Some completely asymptomatic individuals have been documented to have a total absence of IgG1, IgG2, IgG4, and/or IgA1 due to gene deletions. These abnormalities were discovered fortuitously in 16 individuals, 15 of whom had no history of undue susceptibility to infection, and all of whom produced antibodies of all other isotypes in normal quantities. These patients illustrate the importance of assessing specific antibody formation before deciding to initiate IVIG therapy in IgG subclass-deficient patients.

HYPER-IgM SYNDROME

The hyper-IgM syndrome is genetically heterogeneous and characterized by normal or elevated serum IgM levels associated with low or absent IgG, IgA, and IgE serum levels, indicating a defect in the class-switch recombination (CSR) process. Causative mutations have been identified in 2 genes on the X chromosome, the CD40 ligand (hyper-IgM syndrome type 1, HIGM1) and NEMO (nuclear factor κB [NF-κB] essential modulator, XHM-ED) genes; and 3 genes on autosomal chromosomes, the AICDA gene (hyper-IgM type 2, HIGM2) on chromosome 12, the uracil DNA glycosylase gene (UNG, hyper-IgM type 5, HIGM5) , on chromosome 12, and the CD40 gene (hyper-IgM type 3, HIGM3) on chromosome 20. Distinctive clinical features permit presumptive recognition of the type of mutation in these patients, thereby aiding proper choice of therapy. All such patients should undergo molecular analysis to ascertain the affected gene for purposes of genetic counseling, carrier detection, and decisions regarding definitive therapy.

X-Linked Hyper-IgM Caused by Mutations in the CD40 Ligand: Hyper-IgM Type 1 (HIGM1)

HIGM1 is caused by mutations in the gene that encodes the CD40 ligand (CD154, CD40L), which is expressed on activated T helper cells. Boys with this syndrome have very low serum concentrations of IgG and IgA, with a usually normal or sometimes elevated concentration of polyclonal IgM, may or may not have small tonsils, usually have no palpable lymph nodes, and often profound **neutropenia**.

GENETICS AND PATHOGENESIS B cells from boys with the CD40 ligand defect are capable of synthesizing not only IgM but also IgA and IgG when co-cultured with normal activated T helper cells, indicating that the B cells are actually normal in this condition and that the defect is in the T cells. The abnormal gene is localized to Xq26, and the gene product, CD154 (CD40L), is the ligand for CD40, which is present on B cells and monocytes. CD154 is upregulated on activated T cells. Mutations in CD154 result in an inability to signal B cells to undergo isotype switching, and thus the B cells produce only IgM. The failure of T cells to interact with B cells through this receptor-ligand pair also causes a failure of upregulation of the B cell and monocyte surface molecules CD80 and CD86 that interact with CD28/CTLA4 on T cells, resulting in failure of "cross talk" between immune system cells. The failure of interaction of the molecules of those pathways results in a propensity for tolerogenic T-cell signaling and defective recognition of tumor cells. More than 73 distinct point mutations or deletions in the gene encoding CD154 have been identified in 87 unrelated families, giving rise to frame shifts, premature stop codons, and single amino acid substitutions, most of which are clustered in the domain with homology to TNF, located in the carboxy-terminal region.

CLINICAL MANIFESTATIONS Similar to patients with XLA, boys with the CD40 ligand defect become symptomatic during the 1st or 2nd yr of life with recurrent pyogenic infections, including otitis media, sinusitis, pneumonia, and tonsillitis. Lymph node histology shows only abortive germinal center formation with severe depletion and phenotypic abnormalities of follicular dendritic cells. These patients have normal numbers of circulating B lymphocytes, marked susceptibility to *P. jiroveci* pneumonia, and are frequently profoundly neutropenic. Circulating T cells are also present in normal number and in vitro responses to mitogens are normal, but there is decreased antigen-specific T-cell function. In a study of patients with the CD40 ligand defect, 23.3% had died at a mean age at death of 11.7 yr. In addition to opportunistic infections such as *P. jiroveci* pneumonia, there is an increased incidence of extensive verruca vulgaris lesions, *Cryptosporidium* enteritis, subsequent liver disease, and increased risk of malignancy. Because of the poor prognosis, the treatment of choice is an HLA-identical stem cell transplant at an early age. Alternative treatment for this condition is monthly infusion of IVIG. In patients with severe neutropenia, the use of G-CSF (granulocyte colony stimulating factor) has been beneficial.

X-Linked Hyper-IgM Caused by Mutations in the Gene Encoding Nuclear Factor κB (NF-κB) Essential Modulator (NEMO, OR IKKγ); XHM-ED

This syndrome in males is characterized most often clinically as **anhydrotic ectodermal dysplasia with associated immunodeficiency (EDA-ID)**. The condition results from missense mutations in the IKBKG gene at position 28q on the X chromosome that encodes **nuclear factor κB (NF-κB) essential modulator (NEMO)**, a regulatory protein required for the activation of the transcription factor NF-κB. Germ line loss-of-function mutations cause the X-linked dominant condition incontinentia pigmenti in females and are lethal in male fetuses. Mutations in the coding region of IKBKG are associated with EDA-ID. The immunodeficiency is variable, with most patients showing impaired antibody responses to polysaccharide antigens. Some patients with EDA-ID have hyper-IgM. Pharmacologic inhibitors of NF-κB activation have been shown to downregulate CD154 mRNA and protein levels, suggesting the mechanism of hyper-IgM in this condition. The hyper-IgM patients with this defect should be easily recognizable because of the presence of ectodermal dysplasia, although there is a report of this condition without ectodermal dysplasia.

Autosomal Recessive Hyper-IgM Caused by Mutations in the Gene for Activation-Induced Cytidine Deaminase (AICDA): Hyper-IgM Type 2 (HIGM2)

An autosomal recessive form of hyper-IgM syndrome is caused by mutations in the gene for activation-induced cytidine deaminase (AICDA).

GENETICS AND PATHOGENESIS Patients with autosomal hyper-IgM usually have normal numbers of circulating B lymphocytes, but, in contrast to patients with the CD40 ligand defect, B cells from these patients are not able to switch from IgM-secreting to IgG-, IgA-, or IgE-secreting cells, even when co-cultured with monoclonal antibodies to CD40 and a variety of cytokines. When their B cells are cultured in vitro, they spontaneously secrete large amounts of IgM, but this is not further augmented by the addition of IL-4 or anti-CD40 with IL-4 or other cytokines. Thus, in these patients, there is truly an intrinsic B-cell abnormality. The defect in many such patients has been identified as due to mutations in a gene on chromosome 12p13 that encodes AICDA. AICDA is a single-stranded (SS) DNA deaminase required for somatic hypermutation (SHM) and CSR of immunoglobulin genes. Histologic examination of the enlarged lymph nodes reveals the presence of giant germinal centers (5-10 times larger than normal) filled with highly proliferating B cells. Proliferating B cells co-express IgM, IgD, and CD38, a phenotype previously described for a small B-cell subset corresponding to germinal center (GC) founder cells. These cells are thought to correspond to a transitional stage between follicular mantle and GC B cells, at the onset of somatic mutation of the Ig variable region gene and antigen-driven selection. Deficiency of AICDA results in impaired terminal differentiation of B cells, a failure of CSR, and lack of immunoglobulin gene SHM.

CLINICAL MANIFESTATIONS Concentrations of serum IgG, IgA, and IgE are very low in AICDA deficiency. In contrast to the CD40 ligand defect, however, the serum IgM concentration in patients with AICDA deficiency is usually markedly elevated and polyclonal. Patients with this form of hyper-IgM have lymphoid hyperplasia, are generally older at age of onset, do not have susceptibility to *P. jiroveci* pneumonia, often do have isohemagglutinins, and are much less likely to have neutropenia unless it occurs on an autoimmune basis. They have a tendency, however, to develop autoimmune and inflammatory disorders including diabetes mellitus, polyarthritis, autoimmune hepatitis, hemolytic anemia, immune thrombocytopenia, Crohn disease, and chronic uveitis. With early diagnosis and monthly infusions of IVIG, as well as good management of infections with antibiotics, patients with AICDA mutations generally have a more benign course than do boys with the CD40 ligand defect.

Autosomal Recessive Hyper-IgM Caused by Mutations in the Gene for Uracil DNA Glycosylase (UNG); Hyper-IgM Type 5 (HIGM5)

Another cause of the hyper-IgM syndrome is a deficiency of uracil DNA glycosylase.

GENETICS AND PATHOGENESIS AICDA deaminates cytosine into uracil in targeted DNA, which is followed by uracil removal by UNG. Profoundly impaired class-switch recombination was found in 3 hyper-IgM patients reported to have UNG deficiency. Their clinical characteristics were similar to those with AICDA deficiency, with increased susceptibility to bacterial infections and lymphoid hyperplasia. The patients had a markedly elevated serum IgM and profoundly decreased serum IgG and IgA concentrations. Their B cells had an intrinsic defect in CSR when stimulated with anti-CD40 and IL-4 and constitutively produced high quantities of IgM. They had only a partial defect in SHM, however.

Autosomal Recessive Hyper-IgM Caused by Mutations in CD40: Hyper-IgM Type 3 (HIGM3)

Patients with autosomal recessive hyper-IgM who failed to express CD40 on their B-cell surfaces, resulting from mutations in the CD40 gene, were identified.

GENETICS AND PATHOGENESIS CD40 is a type I integral membrane glycoprotein encoded by a gene on chromosome 20 and belonging to the TNF and nerve growth factor receptor superfamily. It is expressed on B cells, macrophages, dendritic cells, and a few other types of cells. Mutations in the CD40 gene cause an autosomal recessive form of hyper-IgM syndrome that is clinically indistinguishable from HIGM1, resulting from the X-linked CD40 ligand (CD154) defect. In contrast to the CD40 ligand defect, however, the B cells in the autosomal recessive condition are intrinsically abnormal and cannot isotype switch. The T cells are normal except to the extent that they cannot cause upregulation of CD80 and CD86 on B cells and macrophages to interact with CD28/CTLA4 on T cells.

Hyper-IgM Type 4 (HIGM4)

The defective gene in a 4th autosomal recessive form of hyper-IgM syndrome has not yet been identified, but appears to be in a gene downstream of AICDA. These patients all have defective class-switch recombination with preserved SHM.

X-LINKED LYMPHOPROLIFERATIVE DISEASE

X-linked lymphoproliferative (XLP) disease, also referred to as **Duncan disease** after the original kindred in which it was described, is an X-linked recessive trait characterized by an inadequate immune response to infection with Epstein-Barr virus (EBV).

GENETICS AND PATHOGENESIS The defective gene in XLP was localized to Xq25, cloned, and the gene product was initially named SAP (for SLAM-associated protein), but is now known officially as SH2D1A. SLAM (signaling lymphocyte activation molecule) is an adhesion molecule that is upregulated on both T and B cells with infection and other stimulation. SH2D1A is highly expressed in thymocytes and peripheral blood T and NK cells, with a prevalent expression on Th1 cells. Its presence on B lymphocytes is unclear. Thus, although antibody deficiency is frequently present, this is really a T- and NK-cell defect. SH2D1A competes with SHP-2 for binding to SLAM and, as such, is a regulatory molecule (see Fig. 119-1). In XLP patients, the absence of SH2D1A can lead to an uncontrolled cytotoxic T-cell immune response to EBV. The SH2D1A protein associates permissively with 2B4 on NK cells; thus, selective impairment of 2B4-mediated NK-cell activation also contributes to the immunopathology of XLP.

XLP type 2 is less common and is due to a mutation in *XIAP* (X-linked inhibitor of apoptosis protein); disease manifestations are similar to XLP.

CLINICAL MANIFESTATIONS Affected males are usually healthy until they acquire EBV infection. The mean age of presentation is <5 yr. There are 3 major clinical phenotypes: (1) fulminant, often fatal, infectious mononucleosis (50% of cases); (2) lymphomas, predominantly involving B-lineage cells (25%); or (3) acquired hypogammaglobulinemia (25%). There is a marked impairment in production of antibodies to the EBV nuclear antigen (EBNA), whereas titers of antibodies to the viral capsid antigen (VCA) have ranged from absent to markedly elevated. XLP has an unfavorable prognosis; 70% of affected boys die by age 10 yr. Only 2 XLP patients are known to have survived beyond 40 yr of age. Unless there is a family history of XLP, diagnosis prior to the onset of complications is difficult because affected individuals are asymptomatic initially. Using mutation analysis, it is possible to identify affected males within identified kindreds before they develop primary EBV infection. Approximately half of the few patients with XLP given HLA-identical related or unrelated stem cell transplants are currently surviving without signs of the disease.

Two pedigrees have been reported in which boys in one arm of each pedigree were diagnosed with CVID, whereas those in the other arms had fulminant infectious mononucleosis. The family members with CVID never gave a history of infectious mononucleosis. All affected members of each pedigree had the same distinct SH2D1A mutation, however, despite the different clinical phenotypes. Because the SH2D1A mutation was the same but the phenotype varied in these families, XLP should be considered in all males with a diagnosis of CVID, particularly if there is more than one male family member with this phenotype.

BIBLIOGRAPHY

Please visit the Nelson Textbook of Pediatrics *website at www.expertconsult.com for the complete bibliography.*

118.1 Treatment of B-Cell Defects

Rebecca H. Buckley

Except for the CD40 ligand defect and XLP, for which stem cell transplantation is recommended, judicious use of antibiotics to treat documented infections and regular administration of intravenous immunoglobulins are the only effective treatments for primary B-cell disorders. The most common forms of replacement therapy are either intravenous or subcutaneous immunoglobulin (IVIG or SCIG). Broad antibody deficiency should be carefully documented before such therapy is initiated. The rationale for the use of IVIG or SCIG is to provide missing antibodies, not to raise the serum IgG or IgG subclass level. The development of safe and effective immunoglobulin preparations is a major advance in the treatment of patients with severe antibody deficiencies, although it is expensive and there have been national shortages. Almost all commercial preparations are isolated from normal plasma by the Cohn alcohol fractionation method or a modification of this method. Cohn fraction II is then further treated to remove aggregated IgG. Additional stabilizing agents such as sugars, glycine, and albumin are added to prevent reaggregation and protect the IgG molecule during lyophilization. The ethanol used in preparation of immunoglobulin inactivates HIV; and an organic solvent/detergent step inactivates hepatitis B and C viruses. Some preparations are also nanofiltered to remove infectious agents. Most commercial lots are produced from plasma pooled from more than 60,000 donors and therefore contain a broad spectrum of antibodies. Each pool must contain adequate levels of antibody to antigens in various vaccines, such as tetanus and measles. However, there is no standardization based on titers of antibodies to more clinically relevant organisms, such as *Streptococcus pneumoniae* and *Haemophilus influenzae* type b.

The IVIG and SCIG preparations available in the USA have similar efficacy and safety. Rare transmission of hepatitis C virus has occurred in the past, but the potential transmission of hepatitis C virus has been resolved by additional treatment with an organic solvent/detergent mixture. There has been no documented transmission of HIV by any of these preparations. **IVIG or SCIG at a dose of 400 mg/kg/mo** achieves trough IgG levels close to the normal range. Systemic reactions may occur, but rarely are these true anaphylactic reactions. Anaphylactic reactions caused by a patient's IgE antibodies to IgA in the IVIG or SCIG preparation may occur in patients with CVID or IgA deficiency. Newly diagnosed patients with CVID should be screened through the American Red Cross for anti-IgA antibodies. If anti-IgA antibodies are detected, IVIG therapy should consist of the one available immunoglobulin preparations containing almost no IgA (Gammagard S/D, Baxter).

BIBLIOGRAPHY

Please visit the Nelson Textbook of Pediatrics *website at www.expertconsult.com for the complete bibliography.*

Chapter 119
Primary Defects of Cellular Immunity

Rebecca H. Buckley

In general, patients with defects in T-cell function have infections or other clinical problems that are more severe than in patients with antibody deficiency disorders (see Table 116-4). The defective gene products for some primary T-cell diseases are identified (Table 119-1). These individuals rarely survive beyond infancy or childhood. Transplantation of thymic tissue, or of major histocompatibility complex (MHC)-compatible sibling or haploidentical (half-matched) parental hematopoietic stem cell, is the treatment of choice for patients with primary T-cell defects (Chapter 129).

THYMIC HYPOPLASIA (DIGEORGE SYNDROME)

Thymic hypoplasia results from dysmorphogenesis of the 3rd and 4th pharyngeal pouches during early embryogenesis, leading to hypoplasia or aplasia of the thymus and parathyroid glands. Other structures forming at the same age are also frequently affected, resulting in anomalies of the great vessels (right-sided aortic arch), esophageal atresia, bifid uvula, congenital heart disease (conotruncal, atrial, and ventricular septal defects), a short philtrum of the upper lip, hypertelorism, an antimongoloid slant to the eyes, mandibular hypoplasia, and low-set, often notched ears (Chapters 76 and 102). The diagnosis is often first suggested by hypocalcemic seizures during the neonatal period.

Genetics and Pathogenesis

DiGeorge syndrome occurs in both males and females. Microdeletions of specific DNA sequences from chromosome 22q11.2, the **DiGeorge chromosomal region (DGCR)**, are found in a majority of cases. Several candidate genes have been identified in this region. A T-box transcription family member, TBX1, has been implicated as an etiology for most of the major signs of DGS. There appears to be an excess of 22q11.2 deletions of maternal origin. Polymerase chain reaction (PCR)-based genotyping using microsatellite DNA markers located within the commonly deleted region permits rapid detection of such microdeletions. Conotruncal heart defects and 22q deletions are observed in DiGeorge syndrome, velocardiofacial syndrome (VCFS), and conotruncal anomaly face syndrome (CTAFS). The **CATCH 22 syndrome** (*c*ardiac, *a*bnormal facies, *t*hymic hypoplasia, *c*left palate, *h*ypocalcemia) includes the broad clinical spectrum of conditions with 22q11.2 deletions. Other deletions

Table 119-1 GENETIC BASIS OF PRIMARY CELLULAR IMMUNODEFICIENCY DISEASES

CHROMOSOME AND REGION	GENE PRODUCT	DISORDER	FUNCTIONAL DEFICIENCIES
1p35-p34.3	Lck*	T-cell-activation defect	Impaired T-cell function
2p12	CD8α*	CD8 deficiency	Lack of cytotoxic T cells
2q12	ZAP-70*	CD8 deficiency	Failure of CD4 T cells to respond to usual signals
10p13	Unknown	Thymic hypoplasia (DiGeorge syndrome, velocardiofacial syndrome)	Low number of T cells and impaired T-cell function
11q23	CD3*	CD3 deficiency	Poor T-cell responses to mitogens; lack of cytotoxic T cells; IgG subclass deficiency
21q22.3	Autoimmune regulator (AIRE)	APECED, chronic mucocutaneous candidiasis, parathyroid and adrenal antoimmunity	Poor response to candida antigen; autoimmune responses
22q11.22	?TBX1	Thymic hypoplasia (DiGeorge syndrome, velocardiofacial syndrome)	Low number of T cells and impaired T-cell function

*The gene has been cloned and sequenced.
APECED, autoimmune polyendocrinopathy-candidiasis ectodermal dysplasia; ZAP-70, zeta-associated protein 70.

associated with DiGeorge and velocardiofacial syndromes have been identified on chromosome 10p13 (Chapter 76).

Variable hypoplasia of the thymus and parathyroid glands defines **partial DiGeorge syndrome,** which is more frequent than total aplasia; aplasia is present in <1% of patients with DiGeorge syndrome and defines **complete DiGeorge syndrome.** Slightly less than half of patients with complete DiGeorge syndrome are hemizygous at chromosome 22q11. Approximately 15% are born to diabetic mothers. Another 15% of infants have no identified risk factors. Approximately one third of infants with complete DiGeorge syndrome have **CHARGE association** (*c*oloboma, *h*eart defect, choanal *a*tresia, growth or developmental *r*etardation, genital hypoplasia, and *e*ar anomalies including deafness). Mutations in the chromodomain helicase DNA binding protein 7 (CHD7) gene on chromosome 8q12.2 are found in approximately 60-65% of individuals with CHARGE syndrome. Concentrations of serum immunoglobulins in DiGeorge syndrome are usually normal, but IgA may be diminished and IgE elevated. Other laboratory findings vary depending on the degree of thymic dysfunction.

Absolute lymphocyte counts are usually only moderately low for age. The CD3 T-cell counts are variably decreased in number, corresponding to the degree of thymic hypoplasia, resulting in an increased percentage of B cells. Lymphocyte responses to mitogen stimulation are absent, reduced, or normal, depending on the degree of thymic deficiency. Thymic tissue, when found, contains Hassall corpuscles, normal density of thymocytes, and corticomedullary distinction. Lymphoid follicles are usually present, but lymph node paracortical areas and thymus-dependent regions of the spleen show variable degrees of depletion.

Clinical Manifestations

Children with partial thymic hypoplasia may have little trouble with infections and grow normally. Patients with complete DiGeorge syndrome resemble patients with severe combined immunodeficiency (SCID) in their susceptibility to infections with low-grade or opportunistic pathogens, including fungi, viruses, and *Pneumocystis jiroveci*, and to graft versus host disease (GVHD) from nonirradiated blood transfusions. Patients with complete DiGeorge syndrome can develop an atypical phenotype in which oligoclonal T-cell populations appear in the blood associated with rash and lymphadenopathy. These atypical patients appear phenotypically to be similar to patients with Omenn syndrome or maternal lymphocyte engraftment.

It is critical to confirm the diagnosis of complete DiGeorge syndrome in a timely manner because this disease is fatal without treatment. A T-cell count should be obtained on all infants born with primary hypoparathyroidism, CHARGE syndrome, truncus arteriosus, and interrupted aortic arch type B. If a patient has findings consistent with DiGeorge syndrome and also has rash and lymphadenopathy, the patient should be referred to an immunologist for evaluation.

Treatment

The immune deficiency in the complete DiGeorge syndrome is correctable primarily by cultured unrelated thymic tissue transplants or non-irradiated unfractionated bone marrow or peripheral blood transplantation from an HLA-identical sibling (Chapter 129).

DEFECTIVE EXPRESSION OF THE T-CELL RECEPTOR–CD3 COMPLEX (Ti-CD3)

The first type of this disorder was found in two brothers in a Spanish family. The proband presented with severe infections and died at 31 mo of age with autoimmune hemolytic anemia and viral pneumonia. His lymphocytes had responded poorly to mitogens and to anti-CD3 in vitro and could not be stimulated to develop cytotoxic T cells. His antibody responses to protein antigens had been normal, indicating normal T-helper-cell function. His 12 yr old brother was healthy but had almost no CD3-bearing T cells and had IgG2 deficiency similar to his sibling. The defect in this family was due to mutations in the gene encoding the CD3γ chain (Fig. 119-1).

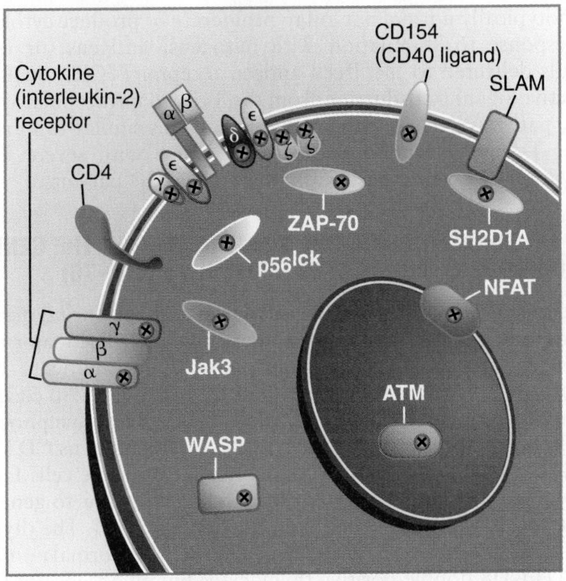

Figure 119-1 Locations of mutant proteins *(X)* in activated CD4 T cells identified in primary immunodeficiency diseases. ZAP-70, zeta-associated protein 70; SLAM, signaling lymphocyte activation molecule; SH2D1A, SLAM-associated protein; ATM, ataxia telangiectasia mutation; NFAT, nuclear factor of activated T cells; Jak3, Janus kinase 3; WASP, Wiskott-Aldrich syndrome protein. (From Buckley RH: Primary immunodeficiency diseases due to defects in lymphocytes, *N Engl J Med* 343:1313–1324, 2000.)

The second type of this disorder was diagnosed in a 4 yr old French boy who had recurrent *Haemophilus influenzae* pneumonia and otitis media in early life but is now healthy. He had a partial defect in expression of Ti-CD3, and thus the percentage of CD3 cells was about half-normal, but the level of expression is markedly decreased. The defect was shown to be due to two independent CD3ε gene mutations, leading to defective CD3ε chain synthesis. There was a splice site mutation on one allele that did not totally abrogate the normal intron 7 splicing, thus there was partial expression of CD3 on the T cells. His T cells did not proliferate normally in response to anti-CD3 or anti-CD2, but did respond normally to stimulation with anti-CD28 or antigens, such as tetanus toxoid. Thus, this mutation did not result in failure of T-cell development, whereas mutations in the portions of the gene that encode the extracellular component of CD3ε result in a profound deficiency of circulating mature CD3 T cells (Chapter 120).

DEFECTIVE CYTOKINE PRODUCTION

IL-12, which is produced by activated antigen-presenting cells, promotes the development of Th1 responses and is a powerful inducer of IFN-γ production by T and natural killer (NK) cells. A child with bacille Calmette-Guérin (BCG) and *Salmonella enteritidis* infections had a large homozygous deletion within the IL-12 p40 subunit gene precluding expression of functional IL-12 p70 cytokine by activated dendritic cells and phagocytes. IFN-γ production by the child's lymphocytes was therefore markedly impaired. IL-12 may be essential for protective immunity to intracellular bacteria such as *Mycobacterium* and *Salmonella.*

T-CELL ACTIVATION DEFECTS

T-cell activation defects are characterized by the presence of normal or elevated numbers of blood T cells that appear phenotypically normal but fail to proliferate or produce cytokines in response to stimulation with mitogens, antigens, or other signals delivered to the T-cell antigen receptor (TCR), owing to defective signal transduction from the TCR to intracellular metabolic pathways. These patients have problems similar to those of other T-cell–deficient individuals, and some with severe T-cell activation defects may clinically resemble SCID patients.

CD8 LYMPHOCYTOPENIA DUE TO MUTATIONS IN THE GENE ENCODING ZETA-ASSOCIATED PROTEIN 70 (ZAP-70)

Patients with this T-cell activation defect present during infancy with severe, recurrent, and often fatal infections. The majority of cases are reported among Mennonites. These patients have normal or elevated numbers of blood B cells and low to elevated serum immunoglobulin concentrations. Their blood lymphocytes exhibit normal expression of the T-cell surface antigens CD3 and CD4, but CD8 cells are almost totally absent. These cells fail to respond to mitogens or to allogeneic cells in vitro or to generate cytotoxic T lymphocytes. NK cell activity is normal. The thymus of one patient exhibited normal architecture with normal numbers of CD4:CD8 double-positive thymocytes but an absence of CD8 single-positive thymocytes. This condition is due to mutations in the gene encoding **zeta-associated protein** 70 (ZAP-70), a non-src family protein tyrosine kinase important in T-cell signaling that is localized to chromosome 2q12 (see Fig. 119-1). The normal number of CD4:CD8 double-positive T cells results because the thymocytes can use the other member of the same tyrosine kinase family, Syk, to facilitate positive selection. Syk is present at fourfold higher levels in thymocytes than in peripheral T cells, possibly accounting for the lack of normal responses by the CD4 blood T cells.

Another condition that can result in CD8 deficiency is a mutation in the gene that encodes CD8α. There is a deficiency of cytotoxic T cells in that condition, but the functional immune defect is mild compared to that of ZAP-70 deficiency.

P56 LCK DEFICIENCY

A 2 mo old male infant who presented with bacterial, viral, and fungal infections was found to be lymphopenic and hypogammaglobulinemic. B and NK cells were present, but there was a low number of CD4 T cells. Mitogen responses were variable. The T cells failed to express the activation marker CD69 when stimulated through the T-cell receptor but did when stimulated with phorbol myristate acetate and a calcium ionophore, suggesting a proximal signaling defect. Molecular studies revealed an alternatively spliced transcript for p56 lck that lacked the kinase domain.

AUTOIMMUNE POLYENDOCRINOPATHY-CANDIDIASIS ECTODERMAL DYSPLASIA (APECED)

Patients with this syndrome present with chronic mucocutaneous candidiasis and autoimmune polyendocrinopathy, usually producing hypoparathyroidism and Addison disease. Additional features include hypogonadism, chronic active hepatitis, alopecia, vitiligo, pernicious anemia, and Sjögren syndrome. APECED, or autoimmune polyendocrinopathy syndrome type I (APS1), is due to a mutation in the autoimmune regulator *(AIRE)* gene. The gene product, AIRE, is expressed at high levels in purified human thymic medullary stromal cells and is thought to regulate the cell surface expression of tissue-specific proteins such as insulin and thyroglobulin. Expression of these self-proteins allows for the negative selection of autoreactive T cells during their development. Failure of negative selection results in organ-specific autoimmune destruction. The overall significance of AIRE in the establishment and maintenance of T-cell self-tolerance is not well understood.

Most pediatric patients are identified by the presence of mucocutaneous candidiasis and hypoparathyroidsim and later develop insidious signs of Addison disease (Chapter 565).

BIBLIOGRAPHY

Please visit the Nelson Textbook of Pediatrics *website at* *www.expertconsult.com* *for the complete bibliography.*

Chapter 120
Primary Combined Antibody and Cellular Immunodeficiencies

Rebecca H. Buckley

Patients with combined antibody and cellular defects have severe, frequently opportunistic infections that lead to death in infancy or childhood unless they are provided hematopoietic stem cell transplantation early in life. These are thought to be rare defects, although the true incidences are unknown because there has been no newborn screening for any of these defects. It is possible that many affected children die of infection during infancy without being diagnosed. The defective gene products for many combined immunodeficiencies are identified (Table 120-1). Because life threatening infection may occur in infancy, screening for SCID has been recommended by the U.S. Secretary of Health and Human Services to be included in the state newborn screening programs. Live, vaccine-derived infections have occurred during this time of life and knowledge of SCID status could prevent these infections. In addition, early identification and subsequent bone marrow transplantation before life-threatening infections and end organ injury is the best approach to therapy.

120.1 Severe Combined Immunodeficiency (SCID)

Rebecca H. Buckley

The syndromes of SCID are caused by diverse genetic mutations that lead to absence of all adaptive immune function and, in some, a lack of natural killer (NK) cells. Patients with this group of disorders have the most severe immunodeficiency.

Pathogenesis

SCID results from mutations in any 1 of 13 known genes that encode components of the immune system crucial for lymphoid cell development (Table 120-2). All patients with SCID have very small thymuses (<1 g) that usually fail to descend from the neck, contain no thymocytes, and lack corticomedullary distinction or Hassall corpuscles. The thymic epithelium appears histologically normal. Both the follicular and paracortical areas of the spleen are depleted of lymphocytes. Lymph nodes, tonsils, adenoids, and Peyer patches are absent or extremely underdeveloped.

Clinical Manifestations

Affected infants present within the 1st few months of life with recurrent or persistent diarrhea, pneumonia, otitis media, sepsis, and cutaneous infections. Growth may appear normal initially, but extreme wasting usually ensues after diarrhea and infections begin. Persistent infections with opportunistic organisms including *Candida albicans, Pneumocystis jiroveci,* parainfluenza 3 virus, adenovirus, respiratory syncytial virus, rotavirus vaccine virus, cytomegalovirus (CMV), Epstein-Barr virus (EBV), varicella-zoster virus, measles virus, MMR-V vaccine virus, or bacillus Calmette-Guérin (BCG) lead to death. Affected infants also lack the ability to reject foreign tissue and are therefore at risk for severe or fatal graft versus host disease (GVHD) from T lymphocytes in

Table 120-1 GENETIC BASIS OF COMBINED IMMUNODEFICIENCY DISORDERS

CHROMOSOME AND REGION	GENE PRODUCT	DISORDER	FUNCTIONAL DEFICIENCIES
1q	RFX5*	MHC class II antigen deficiency	Low immunoglobulins, lack of T-cell responses to antigens, CD4 deficiency
1q31-q32	CD45*	T–B+NK+ SCID	Absence of T- and B-cell functions
5p13	IL-7Rα*	T–B+NK+ SCID	Absence of T- and B-cell functions
6p21.3	TAP1,* TAP2*	MHC class I antigen deficiency	Marked deficiency of CD8 T cells; combined B- and T-cell defects
6q22-q23	IFN-γR1* IFN-γR2* IL-12Rβ1*	Disseminated mycobacterial infections	Failure of macrophages and other cells to produce TNF-α in response to IFN–
9p21-p13	Endoribonuclease RNase MRP*	Cartilage-hair hypoplasia	Combined B- and T-cell defects of varying severity
10p13	Artemis*	T–B–NK+ SCID	Absence of T- and B-cell functions
10p14-p15	IL-2Rα*	Lymphoproliferative syndrome	Poor T-cell responses; impaired apoptosis; increased bcl-2; autoimmunity
11p13	RAG1* or RAG2*	T–B–NK+ SCID	Absence of T- and B-cell functions
11q22.3	DNA-dependent kinase*	Ataxia-telangiectasia	Selective IgA deficiency; T-cell deficiency
11q23	CD3δ or CD3ζ*	T–B+NK+ SCID	Absence of T- and B-cell functions
13q	RFXAP*	MHC class II antigen deficiency	Low immunoglobulins, lack of T-cell responses to antigens, CD4 deficiency
14q13.1	Purine nucleosidase*	PNP deficiency	Severe T-cell deficiency; may have immunoglobulins
16p13	CIITA*	MHC class II antigen deficiency	Low immunoglobulins, lack of T-cell responses to antigens, CD4 deficiency
19p13.1	Jak3*	T–B+NK– SCID	Absence of T-, B-, and NK-cell functions
20q13.11	ADA*	T–B–NK– SCID	Absence of T- and B-cell functions
Xp11.23	WASP*	Wiskott-Aldrich syndrome	Thrombocytopenia; poor antibody production to polysaccharides; T-cell deficiency
Xq13.1	Common γ chain (γ_c) for several cytokine receptors (including IL-2, IL-4, IL-7, IL-9, IL-15, and IL-21)*	T–B+NK– SCID	Absence of T-, B-, and NK-cell functions

*The gene has been cloned and sequenced.
ADA, adenosine deaminase; CIITA, class II transactivator; IFN-γR1, interferon receptor chain 1; IL-2Rα, interleukin 2 receptor α chain; IL-7Rα, interleukin 7 receptor α chain; IL-12Rβ1, interleukin 12 receptor β1 chain; Jak3, Janus kinase 3; MHC, major histocompatibility complex; PNP, purine nucleoside phosphorylase; RAG1 and RAG2, recombinase activating genes 1 and 2; SCID, severe combined immunodeficiency; TAP, transporter of antigenic peptide; TH1, T-helper cell type 1; TH2, T-helper cell type 2; WASP, Wiskott-Aldrich syndrome protein.

Table 120-2 PATHOPHYSIOLOGY MECHANISMS THAT ACCOUNT FOR SEVERE COMBINED IMMUNE DEFICIENCY (SCID)

DISEASE MECHANISM	GENE DEFECTS
Increased apoptosis	
• Due to mitochondrial energy failure	*AK2*
• Due to accumulation of toxic metabolites	*ADA*
• Due to abnormal actin polymerization	*CORO1A*
Impaired cytokine-mediated signaling	
• Due to defects of the common γ chain	*IG2RG* (X-linked SCID)
• Due to defects of the IL-7R α chain	*IL7R*
• Due to defects of Jak3	*JAK3*
Impaired signaling through the pre–T cell receptor	
• Due to defective V(D)J recombination	*RAG1, RAG2, DCLRE1C, LIG4,* PRKDC*
• Due to impaired expression of CD3 subunits	*CD3D, CD3E, CD3Z*
Impaired signaling in the periphery	ORA1
Unknown mechanism	RMRP*

*These gene defects are most often associated with a milder clinical phenotype than SCID.
From Pessach I, Walter J, Notarangelo LD: Recent advances in primary immunodeficiencies: identification of novel genetic defects and unanticipated phenotypes, *Pediatr Res* 65:3R–12R, 2009.

nonirradiated blood products or in allogeneic stem cell transplants or less severe GVHD from maternal immunocompetent T cells that crossed the placenta while the infant was in utero.

Because all molecular types of SCID lack T cells, infants with SCID have **lymphopenia** (<2,500/mm^3) that is present at birth, indicating that the condition could be diagnosed in all affected infants if white blood cell counts with manual differential counts were routinely performed on all cord bloods and the absolute lymphocyte count calculated. These infants also have an absence of lymphocyte proliferative responses to mitogens, antigens, and allogeneic cells in vitro. Patients with adenosine deaminase (ADA) deficiency have the lowest absolute lymphocyte counts, usually <500/mm^3. Serum immunoglobulin concentrations are low or absent, and no antibodies are formed after immunizations. Analyses of lymphocyte populations and subpopulations demonstrate distinctive phenotypes for the various genetic forms of SCID (see Table 120-2). T cells are extremely low or absent in all types; when detected, in most cases they are transplacentally derived maternal T cells.

Treatment

SCID is a true pediatric emergency. Unless immunologic reconstitution is achieved through stem cell transplantation, death usually occurs during the 1st yr of life and almost invariably before 2 yr of age. If diagnosed at birth or within the 1st 3.5 mo of life, >94% of cases can be treated successfully with HLA-identical or T-cell–depleted haploidentical (half-matched) parental hematopoietic stem cell transplantation without the need for pretransplant chemoablation or post-transplant GVHD prophylaxis. ADA-deficient SCID and X-linked SCID have been treated with somatic gene therapy; although serious adverse events occurred in the case of X-SCID. These successes offer hope for gene therapy eventually becoming the treatment of choice for all forms of SCID for which the gene has been identified. ADA-deficient SCID is also managed with repeated injections of polyethylene glycol modified bovine adenosine deaminase (PEG-ADA).

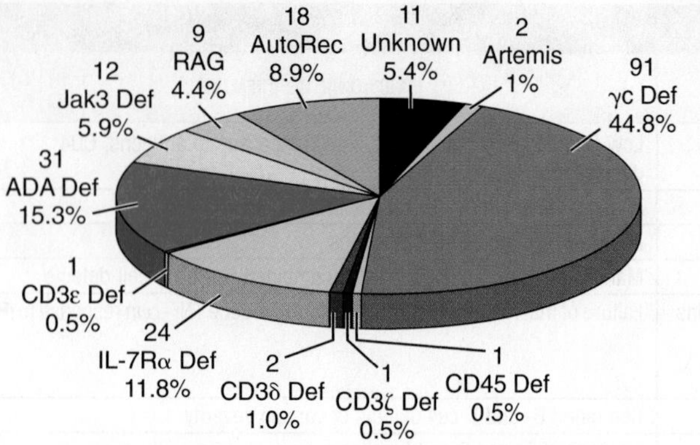

Figure 120-1 Relative frequencies of the different genetic types among 203 patients with severe combined immunodeficiency seen consecutively over 4 decades. RAG, recombinase activating gene; Jak3, Janus kinase 3; ADA, adenosine deaminase; IL-7Rα, interleukin 7 receptor α chain.

X-LINKED SEVERE COMBINED IMMUNODEFICIENCY (SCIDX1) DUE TO MUTATIONS IN THE GENE ENCODING THE COMMON CYTOKINE RECEPTOR γ CHAIN (γ_c)

X-linked SCID (X-SCD) is the most common form of SCID in the USA, accounting for 47% of cases (Fig. 120-1). Clinically, immunologically, and histopathologically, affected individuals appear similar to those with other forms of SCID except for having uniformly **low percentages of T and NK cells** and an **elevated percentage of B cells** (T–, B+, NK–), a characteristic feature shared only with Janus kinase 3 (Jak3)–deficient SCID. The abnormal gene in X-SCD was mapped to Xq13, cloned, and found to encode the common γ chain (γ_c) for several cytokine receptors, including IL-2, IL-4, IL-7, IL-9, IL-15, and IL-21. The shared γ_c functions both to increase the affinity of the receptor for the respective cytokine and to enable the receptors to mediate intracellular signaling. Incapacitation of the receptors for all of these developmentally crucial cytokines by genetic mutations in γ_c provides an explanation for the severity of the immunodeficiency in SCIDX1. In the 1st 136 patients studied, 95 distinct mutations spanning all 8 IL2RG exons were identified, most of them consisting of small changes at the level of 1 to a few nucleotides. These mutations resulted in abnormal γ_c chains in two thirds of the cases and absent γ_c protein in the remainder. Carriers can be detected by demonstrating nonrandom X-chromosome inactivation or the deleterious mutation in their T, B, or NK lymphocytes. Unless donor B or NK cells develop, patients with X-SCID lack B- and NK-cell function after bone marrow transplantation because the abnormal γ_c persists in those host cells, despite excellent reconstitution of T-cell function by donor-derived T cells.

AUTOSOMAL RECESSIVE SEVERE COMBINED IMMUNODEFICIENCY

This pattern of inheritance of SCID is less common in the USA than in Europe. Mutated genes on autosomal chromosomes have been identified in 12 forms of SCID: ADA deficiency; Jak3 deficiency; IL-7 receptor α chain (IL-7Rα) deficiency; RAG1 or RAG2 deficiency; Artemis deficiency; ligase 4 deficiency; DNA–protein kinase catalytic subunit (DNA-PKcs) deficiency; CD3δ, CD3ε, CD3ζ deficiency; and CD45 deficiency (see Fig. 120-1).

ADA Deficiency

An absence of the enzyme adenosine deaminase (ADA) is observed in approximately 15% of patients, the second most common form of SCID, resulting from various point and deletional mutations in the ADA gene on chromosome 20q13-ter. Marked accumulations of adenosine, 2′-deoxyadenosine, and 2′-O-methyladenosine lead directly or indirectly to T-cell apoptosis, which causes the immunodeficiency. ADA-deficient patients usually have a much more profound **lymphopenia** than do infants with other types of SCID, with mean absolute lymphocyte counts of <500/mm³; the absolute numbers of T, B, and NK cells are very low. NK function is normal. After T-cell function is conferred by hematopoietic stem cell transplantation without pretransplant chemotherapy, there is generally excellent B-cell function despite the fact that the B cells are of host origin. This is because ADA deficiency affects primarily T-cell function. Milder forms of ADA deficiency have led to delayed diagnosis of immunodeficiency, even to adulthood. Other **distinguishing features** of ADA-deficient SCID include the presence of rib cage abnormalities similar to a rachitic rosary and numerous skeletal abnormalities of chondro-osseous dysplasia, which occur predominantly at the costochondral junctions, at the apophyses of the iliac bones, and in the vertebral bodies where a "bone-in-bone" effect is observed.

As with other types of SCID, ADA deficiency can be cured by HLA-identical or haploidentical T-cell–depleted stem cell transplantation without the need for pre- or post-transplant chemotherapy; this remains the treatment of choice. Enzyme replacement therapy should not be initiated if stem cell transplantation is possible because it confers graft-rejection capability. Enzyme replacement provides protective immunity but over time there is a decline of lymphocyte counts and mitogenic proliferative responses. Fifteen infants with ADA deficiency have become immune reconstituted by gene therapy; in all cases, PEG-ADA was withheld. Spontaneous reversion to normal of a mutation in the ADA gene has also been reported.

Jak3 Deficiency

Patients with this autosomal recessive defect resemble all other types of SCID patients clinically. They have a lymphocyte phenotype similar only to that of patients with X-SCID, with an elevated percentage of B cells and very low or no T and NK cells. Because Jak3 is the only signaling molecule known to be associated with γ_c, it was a candidate gene for mutations leading to autosomal recessive SCID. Jak3 deficiency accounts for 6% of SCID cases. Even after successful T-cell reconstitution by transplantation of haploidentical stem cells, patients with Jak3-deficient SCID fail to develop NK cells or normal B-cell function owing to the defective function of those host cells that bear abnormal cytokine receptors that share γ_c.

IL-7Rα Deficiency

Patients with IL-7Rα-deficient SCID have a distinctive lymphocyte phenotype in that, though lacking T cells, they have normal or elevated numbers of both B and NK cells (T–, B+, NK+). This is the **third most common** form of SCID, accounting for 12% of cases in the USA (see Fig. 120-1). In contrast to patients with γ_c- and Jak3-deficient SCID, the immunologic defect in these patients is completely correctable by bone marrow stem cell transplantation, as the host B and NK cells appear to be normal.

RAG1 or RAG2 Deficiencies

Infants with these causes of SCID have a different lymphocyte phenotype from those of patients with SCID due to γ_c, Jak3, IL-7Rα, or ADA deficiencies in that they lack both B and T lymphocytes and have primarily NK cells in their circulation (T–, B–, NK+). This suggested a problem with their antigen receptor genes, which led to the discovery of mutations in recombinase-activating genes, *RAG1* or *RAG2*. Such mutations result in a functional inability to form antigen receptors through genetic recombination. **Omenn syndrome** is an autosomal recessive, fatal condition characterized by profound susceptibility to infection with clonal T-cell infiltration of skin, intestines, liver, and spleen leading to an exfoliative erythroderma, lymphadenopathy, hepatosplenomegaly, and intractable diarrhea. Mutations in the recombinase activating genes, *RAG1* and *RAG2*, have also been found in patients with this condition. These infants have persistent leukocytosis with marked eosinophilia and lymphocytosis; elevated serum IgE; low IgG, IgA, and IgM; and low or absent B cells. There is dominance of clonal TH2-like cells with severely impaired T-cell function due to the restricted heterogeneity of the host T-cell repertoire.

Artemis Deficiency

Another cause of SCID is a deficiency of a novel V(D)J recombination/DNA repair factor that belongs to the metallo-β-lactamase superfamily, which is encoded on chromosome 10p by a gene called *Artemis*. Deficiency of this factor results in an inability to repair DNA after double-stranded cuts by the *RAG1* or *RAG2* gene products in rearranging antigen receptor genes from their germ line configuration. Similar to RAG1- and RAG2-deficient SCID, this defect results in failure to develop T and B cells and is, therefore, another form of T–, B–, NK+ SCID, also called **Athabascan SCID.** There is increased radiation sensitivity of both skin fibroblasts and bone marrow cells of those affected with this type of SCID as well as with DNA-PKcs deficiency.

CD45 Deficiency

Other molecular defects causing SCID are mutations in the gene encoding the common leukocyte surface protein CD45. This hematopoietic cell–specific transmembrane protein tyrosine phosphatase functions to regulate src kinases required for T- and B-cell antigen receptor signal transduction. A 2 mo old male infant presented with a clinical picture of SCID and was found to have a very low number of T cells but a normal number of B cells. The T cells failed to respond to mitogens, and serum immunoglobulins diminished with time. He was found to have a large deletion on 1 CD45 allele and a point mutation causing an alteration of the intervening sequence 13 donor splice site on the other allele. A 2nd case of SCID due to CD45 deficiency has been reported, and the author has evaluated and treated a 3rd case.

CD3δ, CD3ε, and CD3ζ Deficiencies

Other causes of autosomal recessive SCID are deficiencies of components of the T-cell receptor (CD3δ, CD3ε, and CD3ζ chains). Mutations in the portions of these genes that encode the extracellular components of the proteins result in a profound deficiency of circulating mature CD3 T cells. Thus, CD3δ, CD3ε, and CD3ζ appear to be essential for intrathymic development of T cells. Since only T-cell development is affected in these defects, both B and NK cells are normal. Thus, the lymphocyte phenotype resembles that of SCID infants with IL-7Rα chain deficiency (T–B+NK+).

RETICULAR DYSGENESIS

Reticular dysgenesis was 1st described in identical twin boys who exhibited a total lack of both lymphocytes and granulocytes in their peripheral blood and bone marrow. Of 8 infants with this defect, 7 died between 3 and 119 days of age as a result of overwhelming infections; 7 infants have been cured by bone marrow transplantation. The thymus glands have all weighed <1 g, have no Hassall corpuscles, and have few or no thymocytes. Reticular dysgenesis is considered a variant of SCID. The molecular basis of this autosomal recessive disorder has recently been found to be due to mutations in the gene encoding adenylate kinase 2.

120.2 Combined Immunodeficiency (CID)

Rebecca H. Buckley

CID is distinguished from SCID by the presence of low but not absent T-cell function. Similar to SCID, CID is a syndrome of diverse genetic causes. Patients with CID have recurrent or chronic pulmonary infections, failure to thrive, oral or cutaneous candidiasis, chronic diarrhea, recurrent skin infections, gram-negative bacterial sepsis, urinary tract infections, and severe varicella in infancy. Although they usually survive longer than infants with SCID, they fail to thrive and die early in life. Neutropenia and eosinophilia are common. Serum immunoglobulins may be normal or elevated for all classes, but selective IgA deficiency, marked elevation of IgE, and elevated IgD levels occur in some cases. Although antibody-forming capacity is impaired in most patients, it is not absent.

Studies of cellular immune function show lymphopenia, profound deficiencies of T cells, and extremely low but not absent lymphocyte proliferative responses to mitogens, antigens, and allogeneic cells in vitro. Peripheral lymphoid tissues demonstrate paracortical lymphocyte depletion. The thymus is very small with a paucity of thymocytes and usually no Hassall corpuscles. An autosomal recessive pattern of inheritance is common.

PURINE NUCLEOSIDE PHOSPHORYLASE DEFICIENCY

More than 40 patients with CID have been found to have purine nucleoside phosphorylase (PNP) deficiency. Point mutations identified in the PNP gene on chromosome 14q13.1 account for these deficiencies. In contrast to ADA deficiency, no characteristic physical or skeletal abnormalities have been noted, but serum and urinary uric acid are usually markedly deficient. Deaths result from generalized vaccinia, varicella, lymphosarcoma, or GVHD mediated by allogeneic T cells in nonirradiated blood or bone marrow. Two thirds of patients have neurologic abnormalities, and one third of patients have autoimmune diseases. Lymphopenia is striking, primarily because of a marked deficiency of T cells; T-cell function is decreased to various degrees. The proportion of circulating NK cells is increased. Prenatal diagnosis is possible. Bone marrow transplantation is the only successful form of therapy.

INTERLEUKIN 2 RECEPTOR α CHAIN (IL-2Rα [CD25]) MUTATION

An infant boy born of a consanguineous union developed CMV pneumonia, persistent candidiasis, adenoviral gastroenteritis, failure to thrive, lymphadenopathy, hepatosplenomegaly, and chronic inflammation of his lungs and mandible. Biopsy specimens revealed extensive lymphocytic infiltration of his lung, liver, intestines, and bone. Serum IgA level was low. He had T-cell lymphopenia, and the T cells responded poorly to anti-CD3, phytohemagglutinin (PHA) and other mitogens, and IL-2. He was found to have a mutation in the gene encoding the IL-2 receptor α chain (IL-2Rα [CD25]), leading to truncation of the protein. He had no CD1 in his thymus, and an elevation of the anti-apoptotic protein bcl-2. This defect reveals that some components of cytokine receptors normally serve a negative regulatory role. Mutations in those components can result in unchecked lymphoproliferation and autoimmunity in addition to immunodeficiency.

CARTILAGE HAIR HYPOPLASIA

Cartilage hair hypoplasia (CHH) is an unusual form of **short-limbed dwarfism** with frequent and severe infections. It occurs predominantly among the Pennsylvania Amish, but non-Amish patients have been described.

Genetics and Pathogenesis

CHH is an autosomal recessive condition. Numerous mutations that co-segregate with the CHH phenotype have been identified in the untranslated RNase MRP gene, which has been mapped to chromosome 9p21-p13 in Amish and Finnish families (see Table 120-1). The RNase MRP endoribonuclease consists of an RNA molecule bound to several proteins and has at least two functions: cleavage of RNA in mitochondrial DNA synthesis and nucleolar cleaving of pre-RNA. Mutations in RMRP cause CHH by disrupting a function of RNase MRP RNA that affects multiple organ systems. In vitro studies show decreased numbers of T cells and defective T-cell proliferation due to an intrinsic defect related to the G1 phase, resulting in a longer cell cycle for individual cells. NK cells are increased in number and function.

Clinical Manifestations

Clinical features include short, pudgy hands; redundant skin; hyperextensible joints of hands and feet but an inability to extend the elbows completely; and fine, sparse, light hair and eyebrows. Severe and often fatal varicella infections, progressive vaccinia, and vaccine-associated poliomyelitis have been observed. Associated conditions include deficient erythrogenesis, Hirschsprung disease, and an increased risk of malignancies. The bones radiographically show scalloping and sclerotic or cystic changes in the metaphyses and flaring of the costochondral junctions of the ribs. Three patterns of immune dysfunction have emerged: defective antibody-mediated immunity, CID (most common), and SCID. The severity of the immunodeficiency varies; in 1 series, 11 of 77 patients died before age 20 yr, but 2 were still alive at age 76 yr. Stem cell transplantation has resulted in immunologic reconstitution in some CHH patients with the SCID phenotype.

DEFECTIVE EXPRESSION OF MAJOR HISTOCOMPATIBILITY COMPLEX ANTIGENS

The 2 main forms of immunodeficiency and abnormalities of expression of the major histocompatibility complex (MHC) are MHC class I (HLA-A, -B, and -C) antigen deficiency and MHC class II (HLA-DR, -DQ, and -DP) antigen deficiency. The associated defects of both B- and T-cell immunity and of HLA expression emphasize the important biologic role for HLA determinants in effective immune cell cooperation.

MHC Class I Antigen Deficiency

Isolated deficiency of MHC class I (HLA-A, -B, and -C) antigens, the **bare lymphocyte syndrome,** is rare. The resulting immunodeficiency is much milder than in SCID, contributing to a later age of presentation. Sera from affected children contain normal quantities of MHC class I antigens and β_2-microglobulin, but MHC class I antigens are not detected on any cells in the body. There is a deficiency of CD8 but not CD4 T cells. Mutations have been found in 2 genes within the MHC locus on chromosome 6 that encode the peptide transporter proteins TAP1 and TAP2 (see Fig. 118-1). TAP functions to transport antigenic peptides from the cytoplasm across the Golgi apparatus membrane to join the α chain of MHC class I antigens and β_2-microglobulin. All these are then assembled into a MHC class I complex that can then move to the cell surface. If the assembly of the complex cannot be completed because there is no antigenic peptide, the MHC class I complex is destroyed in the cytoplasm.

MHC Class II Antigen Deficiency

Many affected with MHC class II (HLA-DR, -DQ, and -DP) deficiency are of North African descent. Patients present in early infancy with persistent diarrhea that is often associated with cryptosporidiosis and enteroviral infections (e.g., poliovirus, coxsackievirus). They also have an increased frequency of infections with herpesviruses and other viruses, oral candidiasis, bacterial pneumonia, *P. jiroveci* pneumonia, and septicemia. The immunodeficiency is not as severe as in SCID, as evidenced by their failure to develop disseminated infection after BCG vaccination or GVHD from nonirradiated blood transfusions.

Four different molecular defects resulting in impaired expression of MHC class II antigens have been identified (see Table 120-1 and Fig. 118-1). One form is a mutation in the gene on chromosome 1q that encodes a protein called RFX5, a subunit of RFX, which is a multiprotein complex that binds the X box motif of MHC-II promoters. A second form is caused by mutations in a gene on chromosome 13q that encodes a second 36-kD subunit of the RFX complex, called RFX-associated protein (RFXAP). The most common cause of MHC class II defects is mutation in RFXANK, the gene encoding a 3rd subunit of RFX. In a 4th type, there is a mutation in the gene on chromosome 16p13 that encodes a novel MHC class II transactivator (CIITA), a non–DNA-binding co-activator that controls the cell-type specificity and inducibility of MHC-II expression. All 4 of these defects cause impairment in the coordinate expression of MHC class II molecules on the surface of B cells and macrophages.

MHC class II–deficient patients have a very low number of CD4 T cells but normal or elevated numbers of CD8 T cells. Lymphopenia is only moderate. The MHC class II antigens HLA-DP, DQ, and DR are undetectable on blood B cells and monocytes, even though B cells are present in normal number. Patients are hypogammaglobulinemic owing to impaired antigen-specific responses caused by the absence of these antigen-presenting molecules. In addition, MHC antigen-deficient B cells fail to stimulate allogeneic cells in mixed leukocyte culture. Lymphocyte proliferation studies show normal responses to mitogens but no response to antigens. The thymus and other lymphoid organs are severely hypoplastic, and the lack of class II molecules results in abnormal thymic selection with circulating CD4 T cells that have altered CDR3 profiles.

IMMUNODEFICIENCY WITH THROMBOCYTOPENIA AND ECZEMA (WISKOTT-ALDRICH SYNDROME)

Wiskott-Aldrich syndrome, an X-linked recessive syndrome, is characterized by atopic dermatitis, thrombocytopenic purpura with normal-appearing megakaryocytes but small defective platelets, and undue susceptibility to infection.

Genetics and Pathogenesis

The abnormal gene, on the proximal arm of the X chromosome at Xp11.22-11.23 near the centromere, encodes a 501–amino acid proline-rich cytoplasmic protein restricted in its expression to hematopoietic cell lineages. The Wiskott-Aldrich syndrome protein (WASP) (see Fig. 119-1) binds CDC42H2 and rac, members of the Rho family of guanosine triphosphatases. WASP appears to control the assembly of actin filaments required for microvesicle formation downstream of protein kinase C and tyrosine kinase signaling. Carriers can be detected by nonrandom X-chromosome inactivation in several hematopoietic cell lineages or by demonstration of the deleterious mutation.

Clinical Manifestations

Patients often have prolonged bleeding from the circumcision site or bloody diarrhea during infancy. The thrombocytopenia is not initially due to antiplatelet antibodies. Atopic dermatitis and recurrent infections usually develop during the 1st yr of life. *Streptococcus pneumoniae* and other bacteria having polysaccharide capsules cause otitis media, pneumonia, meningitis, and sepsis. Later, infections with agents such as *P. jiroveci* and the herpesviruses become more frequent. Survival beyond the teens is rare; infections, bleeding, and EBV-associated malignancies are major causes of death.

Patients with this defect uniformly have an impaired humoral immune response to polysaccharide antigens, as evidenced by absent or markedly diminished isohemagglutinins, and poor or absent antibody responses after immunization with polysaccharide vaccines. IgG2 subclass concentrations, surprisingly, are normal. Anamnestic responses to protein antigens are poor or absent. There is an accelerated rate of synthesis as well as hypercatabolism of albumin, IgG, IgA, and IgM, resulting in highly variable concentrations of different immunoglobulins, even within the same patient. The predominant immunoglobulin pattern is a low serum level of IgM, elevated IgA and IgE, and a normal or slightly low IgG concentration. Because of their profound antibody deficiencies, these patients should be given monthly infusions of intravenous immunoglobulin (IVIG) regardless of their serum levels of the different immunoglobulin isotypes. Percentages of T cells are moderately reduced, and lymphocyte responses to mitogens are variably depressed.

Treatment

Good supportive care includes appropriate nutrition, routine IVIG, use of killed vaccines, aggressive management of eczema and associated cutaneous infections, platelet transfusion for serious bleeding episodes, splenectomy, and high-dose IVIG with systemic steroids for autoimmune complications. Bone marrow or cord blood transplantation is the treatment of choice and is usually curative.

ATAXIA-TELANGIECTASIA

Ataxia-telangiectasia is a complex syndrome with immunologic, neurologic, endocrinologic, hepatic, and cutaneous abnormalities.

Genetics and Pathogenesis

The mutated gene responsible for this defect, ataxia telangiectasia mutation (*ATM*), was mapped to the long arm of chromosome 11 (11q22-23) and has been cloned (see Fig. 119-1). The gene product is a DNA-dependent protein kinase localized predominantly to the nucleus and involved in mitogenic signal transduction, meiotic recombination, and cell cycle control. Cells from patients as well as those of heterozygous carriers have increased sensitivity to ionizing radiation, defective DNA repair, and frequent chromosomal abnormalities.

In vitro tests of lymphocyte function have generally shown moderately depressed proliferative responses to T- and B-cell mitogens. Percentages of CD3 and CD4 T cells are moderately reduced, with normal or increased percentages of CD8 and elevated numbers of Tiγ/δ T cells. Studies of immunoglobulin synthesis have shown both T-helper-cell and intrinsic B-cell defects. The thymus is very hypoplastic, exhibits poor organization, and lacks Hassall corpuscles.

Clinical Manifestations

The most prominent clinical features are progressive cerebellar ataxia, oculocutaneous telangiectasias, chronic sinopulmonary disease, a high incidence of malignancy, and variable humoral and cellular immunodeficiency. Ataxia typically becomes evident soon after these children begin to walk and progresses until they are confined to a wheelchair, usually by the age of 10-12 yr. The telangiectasias begin to develop at 3-6 yr of age. The most frequent humoral immunologic abnormality is the selective absence of IgA, which occurs in 50-80% of these patients. Hypercatabolism of IgA also occurs. IgE concentrations are usually low, and the IgM may be of the low molecular weight variety. IgG2 or total IgG levels may be decreased, and specific antibody titers may be decreased or normal. Recurrent sinopulmonary infections occur in approximately 80% of these patients. Although common viral infections have not usually resulted in untoward sequelae, fatal varicella has occurred. The malignancies associated with ataxia-telangiectasia are usually of the lymphoreticular type, but adenocarcinomas also occur. Unaffected relatives have an increased incidence of malignancy.

120.3 Defects of Innate Immunity

Rebecca H. Buckley

A number of defects in non–antigen-specific immunity (innate immunity) affect antigen-specific immune responses, as there is interaction between the adaptive and innate immune systems.

INTERFERON-γ RECEPTOR 1 AND 2 AND IL-12 RECEPTOR β1 MUTATIONS

Disseminated BCG and other severe nontuberculosis mycobacterial infections (sepsis, osteomyelitis) occur in patients with severe T-cell defects; however, no specific host defect is identified in approximately half of such cases. The 1st report was a 2.5 mo old Tunisian girl with fatal idiopathic disseminated BCG infection; 4 children from Malta had disseminated atypical mycobacterial infections in the absence of a recognized immunodeficiency. There was consanguinity in all, and all had a functional defect in the upregulation of tumor necrosis factor α (TNF-α) production by their blood macrophages in response to stimulation with interferon-γ (IFN-γ). All also had a mutation in the gene on chromosome 6q22-q23 that encodes the IFN-γ receptor 1 (IFN-γR1). IFN-γR1 deficiency may be inherited as a complete autosomal recessive (early onset ≈3 yr of age, more episodes, more severe disease, and higher mortality) or partial dominant (onset ≈10 yr of age) disease. Patients with mutations in the IFN-γR2 have also been identified. A 3rd type of defect was found in other patients who had disseminated mycobacterial infections, who have mutations in the β1 chain of the IL-12 receptor (IL-12Rβ1). IL-12 is a powerful inducer of IFN-γ production by T and NK cells, and the mutated receptor chain gene resulted in unresponsiveness of the cells of these patients to IL-12 and inadequate IFN-γ production. The children deficient in IFN-γR1, IFN-γR2, or IL-12Rβ1 appeared not to be susceptible to infection with many agents other than mycobacteria (occasionally *Salmonella, Listeria, Histoplasma*). TH1 responses appeared to be normal in these patients, and the susceptibility to mycobacterial infections thus apparently results from an intrinsic impairment of the IFN-γ pathway response to these particular intracellular pathogens, showing that IFN-γ is obligatory for efficient macrophage antimycobacterial activity.

GERM LINE STAT 1 MUTATION

Interferons induce the formation of 2 transcriptional activators: gamma-activating factor (GAF) and interferon-stimulated gamma factor 3 (ISGF3). A natural heterozygous dominant germ line *STAT-1* mutation associated with susceptibility to mycobacterial but not viral disease was found in 2 unrelated patients with unexplained mycobacterial disease. This mutation caused a loss of GAF and ISGF3 activation but was dominant for 1 cellular phenotype and recessive for the other. The mutation impaired the nuclear accumulation of GAF but not of ISGF3 in cells stimulated by interferons, implying that the antimycobacterial but not the antiviral effects of human interferons are mediated by GAF. More recently, 2 patients have been identified with homozygous *STAT-1* mutations who developed both post–BCG vaccination disseminated disease and lethal viral infections. The mutations in these patients caused a complete lack of STAT-1 and resulted in a lack of formation of both GAF and ISGF3.

IL-1R–ASSOCIATED KINASE 4 (IRAK4) DEFICIENCY

Members of interleukin-1 receptor (IL-1R) and the Toll-like receptor (TLR) superfamily share an intracytoplasmic Toll-IL-1 receptor (TIR) domain, which mediates recruitment of the interleukin-1 receptor-associated kinase (IRAK) complex via TIR-containing adapter molecules. Three unrelated otherwise healthy children with recurrent pyogenic infections due to pneumococci and staphylococci had normal immunocompetence by standard immune studies. They had normal titers of anti-pneumococcal antibodies. Their blood and fibroblast cells did not activate nuclear factor κB (NF-κB), and mitogen-activated protein kinase (MAPK) and failed to induce downstream cytokines in response to any of the known ligands of TIR-bearing receptors. All were found to have an inherited deficiency of IRAK-4. The TIR-IRAK signaling pathway appears to be crucial for protective immunity

Table 120-3 CLINICAL FEATURES OF AUTOSOMAL DOMINANT HYPER IgE SYNDROME (AD-HIES)

IMMUNOLOGIC (APPROXIMATE % FREQUENCY)
Peak serum IgE >2000 IU/mL (97)
Recurrent pneumonias (87)
Parenchymal lung abnormalities (bronchiectasis/pneumatocele) (70)
Boils (87)
Moderate-severe eczema (95)
Newborn rash (80)
Mucocutaneous candidiasis (83)
Recurrent sinusitis or otitis (80)
Eosinophilia (90)
Lymphoma (5)
SOMATIC (APPROXIMATE % FREQUENCY)
Characteristic face (85)
Hyperextensibility (70)
Retained primary teeth (70)
Minimal trauma fractures (65)
Scoliosis >10 degrees (60)
Coronary vasculature anomalies (60)
Arnold-Chiari I malformations (40)
Focal hyperintensities on brain MRI (75)

From Freeman AF, Holland SM: Clinical manifestations, etiology, and pathogenesis of the hyper-IgE syndromes, *Pediatr Res* 65:32R–37R, 2009.

against specific bacteria but is redundant against most other microorganisms.

HYPER-IgE SYNDROME

The hyper-IgE syndrome is a relatively rare primary immunodeficiency syndrome characterized by recurrent severe staphylococcal abscesses of the skin, lungs, and other viscera as well as sinusitis, mastoiditis, and markedly elevated levels of serum IgE (Table 120-3). *C. albicans* is the second most common pathogen. More than 200 patients with hyper-IgE syndrome have been reported. The most common form of this condition (autosomal dominant) is now known to be caused by mutations in the gene encoding STAT-3. These mutations result in a dominant negative effect on the expression of STAT-3 by the other nonmutated gene. Rarely, autosomal recessive forms of the hyper-IgE syndrome have been reported, mainly in Turkey, and a mutation in the gene encoding Tyk2 was found in one such patient but not in the others.

Clinical Manifestations

The characteristic clinical features of the autosomal dominant form of the hyper-IgE syndrome are staphylococcal abscesses, pneumatoceles, osteopenia, and unusual facial features. There is often history from infancy of recurrent staphylococcal abscesses involving the skin, lungs, joints, and other sites. Persistent pneumatoceles develop as a result of recurrent pneumonia. The pruritic dermatitis that occurs is not typical atopic eczema and does not always persist. Allergic respiratory symptoms are usually absent. The 1st 2 reported patients were described as having **coarse facial features,** including a prominent forehead, deep-set wide-spaced eyes, a broad nasal bridge, a wide fleshy nasal tip, mild prognathism, facial asymmetry, and hemihypertrophy. In older children, delay in shedding primary teeth, recurrent fractures, and scoliosis occur.

These patients demonstrate an exceptionally high serum IgE concentration; an elevated serum IgD concentration; usually normal concentrations of IgG, IgA, and IgM; pronounced blood and sputum eosinophilia; abnormally low anamnestic antibody responses; and poor antibody and cell-mediated responses to neoantigens. In vitro studies show normal percentages of blood T, B, and NK lymphocytes, with the exception of a decreased percentage of T cells with the memory (CD45RO) phenotype. Recently, several laboratories have reported that there is an absence or deficiency of TH17 T cells. The latter cells produce IL-17, a cytokine that acts on monocytes to induce secretion of proinflammatory mediators such as IL-8, TNF, and GM-CSF. It is not clear exactly how the STAT3 mutation causes all parts of the syndrome, but it is thought that the IL-17 deficiency may account in part for the susceptibility to infection. Most patients have normal T-lymphocyte proliferative responses to mitogens but very low or absent responses to antigens or allogeneic cells from family members. Blood, sputum, and histologic sections of lymph nodes, spleen, and lung cysts show striking eosinophilia. Hassall corpuscles and thymic architecture are normal. Phagocytic cell ingestion, metabolism, killing, and total hemolytic complement activity are normal in all patients, and results of chemotaxis studies have been mostly normal.

Autosomal recessive hyper-IgE syndrome presents with recurrent viral infections such as molluscum contagiosum, herpes zoster, and herpes simplex infections, in addition to staphylococcal skin infections. Other features that distinguish this form from the autosomal dominant form include frequent central nervous system abnormalities and vasculitis, a higher mortality, a lack of tendency to pneumatocele formation, delayed shedding of the primary teeth, or osteopenia. Distinctive laboratory findings in the autosomal recessive form include poor T-cell responses to mitogens and absent responses to antigens.

The most effective **therapy** for the hyper-IgE syndrome is long-term administration of therapeutic doses of a penicillinase-resistant antistaphylococcal antibiotic, adding other agents as required for specific infections. IVIG should be administered to antibody-deficient patients, and appropriate thoracic surgery should be provided for superinfected pneumatoceles or those persisting beyond 6 mo. Bone marrow transplantation has been unsuccessful in this condition.

120.4 Treatment of Cellular or Combined Immunodeficiency

Rebecca H. Buckley

Good supportive care including prevention and treatment of infections is critical while patients await more definitive therapy (Table 120-4). Having knowledge of the pathogens causing disease with specific immune defects is also useful (see Table 120-4).

Transplantation of MHC-compatible sibling or haploidentical (half-matched) parental hematopoietic stem cells is the treatment of choice for patients with fatal T-cell or combined T- and B-cell defects. The major risk to the recipient from transplants of bone marrow or peripheral blood stem cells is GVHD. The development of techniques to deplete all post-thymic T cells from donor marrow permits safe and successful use of haploidentical related donor stem cells for the correction of SCID and other fatal immunodeficiency syndromes. Patients with less severe forms of cellular immunodeficiency, including some forms of CID, Wiskott-Aldrich syndrome, cytokine deficiency, and MHC antigen deficiency, reject even HLA-identical marrow grafts unless chemoablative treatment is given before transplantation. Several patients with these conditions have been treated successfully with HLA-identical stem cell transplantation after conditioning.

More than 90% of patients with primary immunodeficiency transplanted with HLA-identical related marrow will survive with immune reconstitution. T-cell–depleted haploidentical related marrow transplants in patients with primary immunodeficiency have a 55% survival rate worldwide. The greatest success has been in patients with SCID, who do not require pre-transplant conditioning or GVHD prophylaxis; 80-95% of patients with SCID will survive after T-cell–depleted parental marrow is given without pre-transplant chemotherapy or post-transplant GVHD prophylaxis, depending on whether the

Table 120-4 INFECTION IN THE HOST COMPROMISED BY B- AND T-CELL IMMUNODEFICIENCY SYNDROMES

IMMUNODEFICIENCY SYNDROME	OPPORTUNISTIC ORGANISMS ISOLATED MOST FREQUENTLY	APPROACH TO TREATMENT OF INFECTIONS	PREVENTION OF INFECTIONS
B-cell immunodeficiencies	Encapsulated bacteria (*Streptococcus pneumoniae, Staphylococcus aureus, Haemophilus influenzae,* and *Neisseria meningitidis*), *Pseudomonas aeruginosa, Campylobacter* sp., enteroviruses, rotaviruses, *Giardia lamblia, Crytosporidium* sp., *Pneumocystis jiroveci, Ureaplasma urealyticum,* and *Mycoplasma pneumoniae*	1. IVIG 200-800 mg/kg 2. Vigorous attempt to obtain specimens for culture before antimicrobial therapy 3. Incision and drainage if abscess present 4. Antibiotic selection on the basis of sensitivity data	1. Maintenance IVIG for patients with quantitative and qualitative defects in IgG metabolism (400-800 mg/kg q3-5 wk) 2. In chronic recurrent respiratory disease, vigorous attention to postural drainage 3. In selected cases (recurrent or chronic pulmonary or middle ear), prophylactic administration of ampicillin, penicillin, or trimethoprim-sulfamethoxazole
T-cell immunodeficiencies	Encapsulated bacteria (*S. pneumoniae, H. influenzae, S. aureus*), facultative intracellular bacteria (*Mycobacterium tuberculosis,* other *Mycobacterium* sp., and *Listeria monocytogenes*); *Escherichia coli; Pseudomonas aeruginosa; Enterobacter* sp.; *Klebsiella* sp.; *Serratia marcescens; Salmonella* sp.; *Nocardia* sp.; viruses (cytomegalovirus, herpes simplex virus, varicella-zoster virus, Epstein-Barr virus, rotaviruses, adenoviruses, enteroviruses, respiratory syncytial virus, measles virus, vaccinia virus, and parainfluenza viruses); protozoa (*Toxoplasma gondii* and *Cryptosporidium* sp.); and fungi (*Candida* sp., *Cryptococcus neoformans, Histoplasma capsulatum,* and *Pneumocystis jiroveci*)	1. Vigorous attempt to obtain specimens for culture before antimicrobial therapy 2. Incision and drainage if abscess present 3. Antibiotic selection on the basis of sensitivity data 4. Early antiviral treatment for herpes simplex, cytomegalovirus, and varicella-zoster viral infections 5. Topical and nonadsorbable antimicrobial agents frequently are useful	1. Prophylactic administration of trimethoprim-sulfamethoxazole for prevention of *P. jiroveci* pneumonia 2. Oral nonadsorbable antimicrobial agents to lower concentration of gut flora 3. No live virus vaccines or bacillus Calmette-Guérin vaccine 4. Careful tuberculosis screening

IVIG, intravenous immunoglobulin.
From Stiehm ER, Ochs HD, Winkelstein JA: *Immunologic disorders in infants and children,* ed 5, Philadelphia, 2004, Elsevier/Saunders.

transplant can be performed soon after birth when the infant is healthy or after several months when the infant presents with serious infections. Until somatic cell gene therapy is more fully developed, bone marrow transplantation remains the most important and effective therapy for these inborn errors of the immune system. There was remarkable success with gene therapy in immunologically reconstituting 9 infants with X-linked SCID. Unfortunately, leukemic-like clonal T cells or lymphomas developed in 4 of the children. Insertional mutagenesis caused by retroviral insertion of the IL2RG cDNA near the LMO-2 gene produced these serious complications of gene therapy. Efforts are being focused on ways to prevent this problem, but for now gene therapy is on hold except in ADA-deficient SCID, where there has been outstanding success without insertional oncogenesis.

Table 120-5 ALPS CASE CRITERIA AND ALPS CLASSIFICATION

REQUIRED
1. Chronic nonmalignant lymphoproliferation 2. Defective lymphocyte apoptosis in vitro 3. ≥1% TCR α/β^+ $CD4^-$ $CD8^-$ T cells (α/β^+-DNT cells) in peripheral blood and/or presence of DNT cells in lymphoid tissue
SUPPORTING
4. Autoimmunity/autoantibodies 5. Mutations in *TNFRSF6,* FasL, or caspase 10 genes
ALPS Ia = due to mutation in *TNFRSF6*
ALPS Ib = due to mutation in the gene for Fas ligand
ALPS II = due to mutation in the gene for caspase 10
ALPS III = ALPS without defined genetic cause

From Straus SE, Sneller M, Lenardo MJ, et al: An inherited disorder of lymphocyte apoptosis: the autoimmune lymphoproliferative syndrome, *Ann Intern Med* 130:591–601, 1999; Bleesing JJH, Straus SE, Fleisher TA: Autoimmune lymphoproliferative syndrome: a human disorder of abnormal lymphocyte survival, *Pediatr Clin North Am* 47:1291–1310, 2000.

120.5 Immune Dysregulation with Autoimmunity or Lymphoproliferation

Rebecca H. Buckley

AUTOIMMUNE LYMPHOPROLIFERATIVE SYNDROME (ALPS)

ALPS, also known as Canale-Smith syndrome, is a disorder of abnormal lymphocyte apoptosis leading to polyclonal populations of T cells (double-negative T cells), which express CD3 and α/β antigen receptors but do not have CD4 or CD8 co-receptors (CD3 + T cell receptor α/β^+ $CD4^-$ $CD8^-$). These T cells respond poorly to antigens or mitogens and do not produce growth or survival factors (interleukin 2). The genetic deficit in most patients is a germ line or somatic mutation in the Fas gene, which produces a cell surface receptor of the tumor necrosis factor receptor superfamily (TNFRSF6), which, when stimulated by its ligand, will produce programmed cell death (Table 120-5). Persistent survival of these lymphocytes leads to immune dysregulation and autoimmunity.

Clinical Manifestations

ALPS is characterized by autoimmunity, chronic persistent or recurrent lymphadenopathy, splenomegaly, hepatomegaly (in 50%), and hypergammaglobulinemia (IgG, IgA). Many patients present in the 1st yr of life, and most are symptomatic by yr 5. Lymphadenopathy can be striking (Fig. 120-2). Splenomegaly may produce hypersplenism with cytopenias. Autoimmunity also produces anemia (Coombs positive hemolytic anemia) or thrombocytopenia or a mild neutropenia. Lymphoproliferative process (lymphadenopathy, splenomegaly) may regress over time, but autoimmunity does not and is characterized by frequent exacerbations and recurrences. Other autoimmune features include urticaria, uveitis, glomerulonephritis, hepatitis, vasculitis, glomulonephritis, vasculitis, panniculitis, arthritis, and central nervous system involvement (seizures, headaches, encephalopathy).

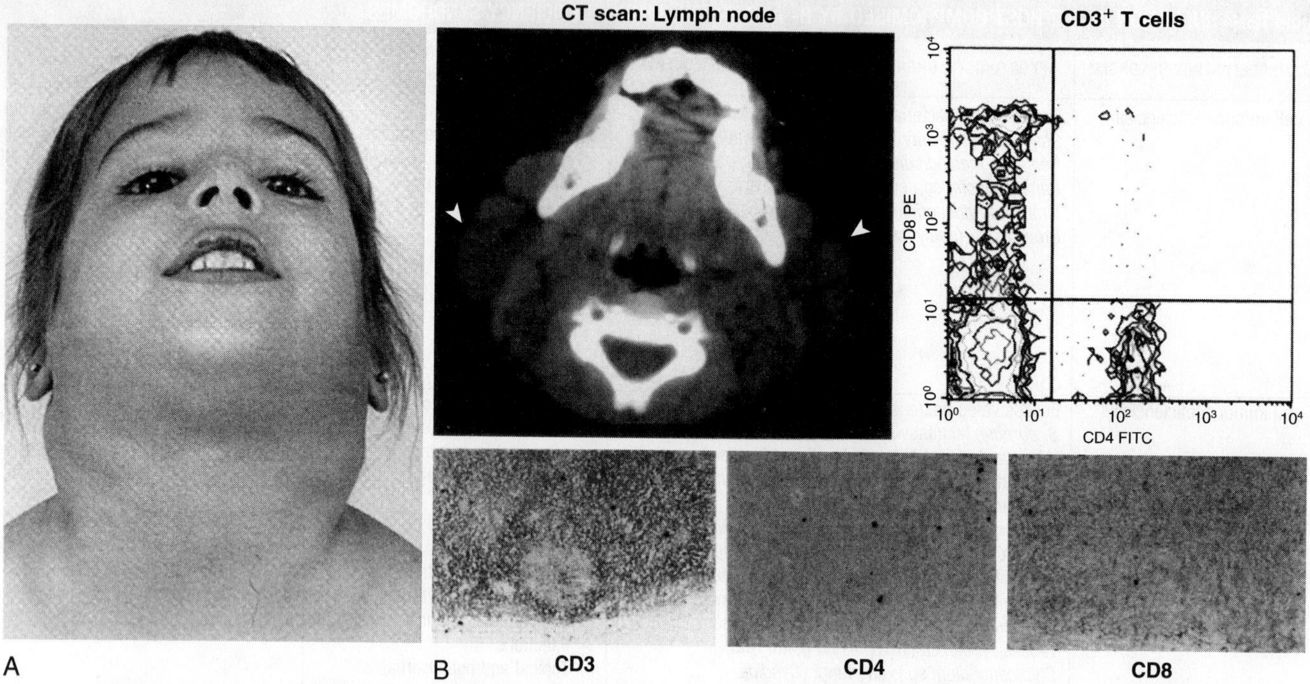

Figure 120-2 Clinical, radiographic, immunologic, and histologic characteristics of the autoimmune lymphoproliferative syndrome. *A,* Front view of the National Institutes of Health patient. *B, Top middle,* a CT scan of the neck is shown demonstrating enlarged preauricular, cervical, and occipital lymph nodes. *Arrowheads* denote the most prominent lymph nodes. The *top right* panels show the flow-cytometric analysis of peripheral blood T cells from a patient with autoimmune lymphoproliferative syndrome (ALPS), with CD8 expression on the vertical axis and CD4 on the horizontal axis. The *lower left quadrant* contains CD4-CD8 (double-negative) T cells, which are usually present at <1% of T cells expressing the αβ TCR. The *bottom panels* show CD3, CD4, and CD8 staining on serial sections of a lymph node biopsy specimen from a patient with ALPS and also shows that large numbers of DNCD3+ CD4-CD8 (double-negative) T cells are present in the interfollicular areas of the lymph node. (Adapted from Siegel RM, Fleisher TA: The role of Fas and related death receptors in autoimmune and other disease states, *J Allergy Clin Immunol* 103:729–738, 1999; with permission.)

Malignancies are also more common in patients with ALPS and include Hodgkin and non-Hodgkin lymphomas and solid tissue tumors of thyroid, skin, heart, or lung.

Diagnosis
Laboratory abnormalities depend on the lymphoproliferative organ response (hypersplenism) or the degree of autoimmunity (anemia, thrombocytopenia). There may be lymphocytosis or lymphopenia. Criteria for the diagnosis are noted in Table 120-5. Flow cytometry helps identify the lymphocyte type (see Fig. 120-2). Functional genetic analysis for the *TNFRSF6* gene often reveals a heterozygous mutation.

Treatment
Lymphoproliferative manifestations have been managed with corticosteroids and immunosuppressive agents (Cytoxan [cyclophosphamide], methotrexate, azathioprine); once weaned, the manifestation recurs. Hypersplenism may require splenectomy. Malignancies can be treated with the usual protocols used in patients unaffected by ALPS. Stem cell transplantation is another possible option in treating the autoimmune manifestations of ALPS.

IMMUNE-DYSREGULATION, POLYENDOCRINOPATHY, ENTEROPATHY, X-LINKED (IPEX) SYNDROME

This immune dysregulation syndrome is characterized by onset within the 1st weeks or months of life with watery diarrhea, an eczematous rash, insulin-dependent diabetes mellitus, hyperthyroidism or hypothyroidism, and other autoimmune disorders (Coombs positive hemolytic anemia, thrombocytopenia, neutropenia, alopecia).

IPEX is due to a mutation in the *FOXP3* gene, which encodes a forkhead-winged helix transcription factor (scurfin) involved in the function and development of CD4+CD25+ regulatory T cells. The absence of regulatory cells may predispose to abnormal activation of effector T cells.

Clinical Manifestations
Watery diarrhea with intestinal villous atrophy leads to failure to thrive in most patients. Cutaneous lesions (usually eczema) and insulin-dependent diabetes begin in infancy. Lymphadenopathy and splenomegaly are also present. Serious bacterial infections (meningitis, sepsis, pneumonia, osteomyelitis) may be related to neutropenia, malnutrition, or immune dysregulation. Laboratory features reflect the associated autoimmune diseases, dehydration, and malnutrition. In addition, serum IgE levels are elevated with normal levels of IgM, IgG, and IgA. The diagnosis is made clinically and by mutational analysis of the *FOXP3* gene.

Treatment
Inhibition of T-cell activation by cyclosporine, tacrolimus, or sirolimus with steroids is the treatment of choice, along with the specific care of the endocrinopathy and other manifestations of autoimmunity. Stem cell transplantation is the only possibility for curing IPEX. Overall, the combination of the risks for serious bacterial infection in the untreated condition and the risks of immunosuppression and bone marrow transplantation gives IPEX a poor prognosis. Untreated, most die by 2 yr of age.

BIBLIOGRAPHY
Please visit the Nelson Textbook of Pediatrics *website at www.expertconsult.com for the complete bibliography.*

Section 3 THE PHAGOCYTIC SYSTEM

Chapter 121
Neutrophils

Peter E. Newburger and Laurence A. Boxer

THE PHAGOCYTIC INFLAMMATORY RESPONSE

The phagocyte system includes both granulocytes (neutrophils, eosinophils, and basophils) and mononuclear phagocytes (monocytes and tissue macrophages). Neutrophils and mononuclear phagocytes share primary functions, including the defining properties of large particle ingestion and microbial killing. Phagocytes participate primarily in the innate immune response but also help initiate acquired immunity. Mononuclear phagocytes, including tissue macrophages and circulating monocytes, are discussed in Chapter 122.

For the full continuation of this chapter, please visit the Nelson Textbook of Pediatrics *website at www.expertconsult.com.*

Chapter 122
Monocytes, Macrophages, and Dendritic Cells

Richard B. Johnston, Jr.

Mononuclear phagocytes (monocytes, macrophages) are distributed across all body tissues and play a central role in maintaining homeostasis. They are essential for innate host defense against infection, tissue repair and remodeling, and the antigen-specific adaptive immune response. No human has been identified as having congenital absence of this cell line, probably because macrophages are required to remove primitive tissues during fetal development as new tissues develop to replace them. Monocytes and tissue macrophages in their various forms (see Table 122-1 on the *Nelson Textbook of Pediatrics* website at www.expertconsult.com) constitute the **mononuclear phagocyte system.** These cells are a system because of their location, common origin, similar morphology, shared surface markers, and common functions, particularly phagocytosis. Conventional **dendritic cells** are specialized derivatives of this system that develop from a common monocyte-dendritic cell precursor.

For the full continuation of this chapter, please visit the Nelson Textbook of Pediatrics *website at www.expertconsult.com.*

Chapter 123
Eosinophils

Laurence A. Boxer and Peter E. Newburger

Eosinophils are distinguished from other leukocytes by their morphology, constituent products, and association with specific diseases. Eosinophils are nondividing fully-differentiated cells with a diameter of ≈8 µm and a bilobed nucleus. They differentiate from stem cell precursors in the bone marrow under the control of T cell–derived interleukin (IL)-3, granulocyte-macrophage colony-stimulating factor (GM-CSF), and, especially, IL-5. Their characteristic membrane-bound specific granules stain reddish brown with eosin and consist of a crystalline core made up of major basic protein (MBP) surrounded by a matrix containing the eosinophil cationic protein (ECP), eosinophil peroxidase (EPO), and eosinophil-derived neurotoxin (EDN). These basic proteins are cytotoxic for the larval stages of helminthic parasites such as *Schistosoma mansoni* and are also thought to contribute to much of the inflammation associated with asthma, causing sloughing of epithelial cells and contributing to clinical dysfunction (Chapter 138).

Both eosinophil MBP and ECP are also present in large quantities in the airways of patients who have died of asthma and are thought to inflict epithelial cell damage leading to airway hyperresponsiveness. Eosinophil granule contents also contribute to Loeffler endocarditis associated with hypereosinophilic syndrome. MBP has the potential to activate other proinflammatory cells, including mast cells, basophils, neutrophils, and platelets. Eosinophils have the capacity to generate large amounts of the lipid mediators platelet-activating factor and leukotriene-C4, both of which can cause vasoconstriction, smooth muscle contraction, and mucus hypersecretion. Eosinophils are a source of a number of proinflammatory cytokines, including IL-1, IL-3, IL-4, IL-5, IL-9, IL-13, and GM-CSF; they can also function as antigen-presenting cells. Thus, eosinophils have considerable potential to initiate and sustain inflammatory response of the innate and acquired immune systems.

Eosinophil migration from the vasculature into the extracellular tissue is mediated by the binding of leukocyte adhesion receptors to their ligands or counterstructures on the postcapillary endothelium. Similar to neutrophils (see Fig. 121-2), transmigration begins as the eosinophil selectin receptor binds to the endothelial carbohydrate ligand in loose association, which promotes eosinophils rolling along the endothelial surface until they encounter a priming stimulus such as a chemotactic mediator. Eosinophils then establish a high-affinity bond between integrin receptors and their corresponding immunoglobulin-like ligand. Unlike neutrophils, which become flattened before transmigrating between the tight junctions of the endothelial cells, eosinophils can use unique integrins, known as VLA-4, to bind to vascular cell adhesion molecule (VCAM)-1, which enhances eosinophil adhesion and transmigration through endothelium. Eosinophils are recruited to tissues in inflammatory states by the chemokine **eotaxin.** These unique pathways account for selective accumulation of eosinophils in allergic and inflammatory disorders. Eosinophils normally dwell primarily in tissues, especially tissues with an epithelial interface with the environment, including the respiratory, gastrointestinal, and lower genitourinary tracts. The life span of eosinophils may extend for weeks within tissues.

IL-5 selectively enhances eosinophil production, adhesion to endothelial cells, and function. Considerable evidence shows that IL-5 has a pivotal role in promoting eosinophil accumulation. It is the predominant cytokine in allergen-induced pulmonary late-phase reaction, and antibodies against IL-5 block eosinophil infiltration into the lungs in animal models associated with airway hyperresponsiveness following allergen challenge. Eosinophils also bear unique receptors for several chemokines, including RANTES, eotaxin, monocyte chemotactic protein (MCP)–3, and MCP-4. These chemokines appear to be key mediators in the induction of tissue eosinophilia.

Blood eosinophil numbers do not always reflect the extent of eosinophil involvement in disease-affected tissues. Eosinopenia occurs after corticosteroid administration and with some bacterial and viral infections.

DISEASES ASSOCIATED WITH EOSINOPHILIA

The **absolute eosinophilia count** is used to quantitate eosinophilia. Calculated as the white blood cell (WBC) count/µL ×

Table 123-1 CAUSES OF EOSINOPHILIA
ALLERGIC DISORDERS
Allergic rhinitis
Asthma
Acute and chronic urticaria
Pemphigoid
Hypersensitivity drug reactions
INFECTIOUS DISEASES
Tissue-Invasive Helminth Infections
Trichinosis
Toxocariasis
Strongyloidosis
Ascariasis
Filariasis
Schistosomiasis
Echinococcosis
Pneumocystis carinii
Toxoplasmosis
Scarlet fever
Amebiasis
Malaria
Bronchopulmonary aspergillosis
Coccidioidomycosis
Scabies
MALIGNANT DISORDERS
Brain tumors
Hodgkin disease and T-cell lymphoma
Acute myelogenous leukemia
Myeloproliferative disorders
Eosinophilic leukemia
GASTROINTESTINAL DISORDERS
Inflammatory bowel disease
Peritoneal dialysis
Eosinophilic gastroenteritis
Milk precipitin disease
Chronic active hepatitis
RHEUMATOLOGIC DISEASE
Rheumatoid arthritis
Eosinophilic fasciitis
Scleroderma
IMMUNODEFICIENCY DISEASE
Hyper-IgE syndrome
Wiskott-Aldrich syndrome
Graft-versus-host disease
Omenn syndrome
Severe congenital neutropenia
Hypersensitivity pneumonia
MISCELLANEOUS
Thrombocytopenia with absent radii
Vasculitis
Postirradiation of abdomen
Histiocytosis with cutaneous involvement

percent of eosinophils, it is usually <450 cells/µL and varies diurnally, with eosinophil numbers higher in the early morning and diminishing as endogenous glucocorticoid levels rise.

Many diseases are associated with moderate (1,500-5,000 cells/µL) or severe (>5,000 cells/µL) eosinophilia (Table 123-1). Patients with sustained blood eosinophilia may develop organ damage, especially cardiac damage as found in the idiopathic hypereosinophilic syndrome, and should be monitored for evidence of cardiac disease. Many cases of moderately severe eosinophilia often have no clear etiology.

Allergic Diseases

Allergy is the most common cause of eosinophilia in children in the USA. Acute allergic reactions may cause eosinophilic leukemoid responses with absolute eosinophil counts >20,000 cells/µL; chronic allergy is rarely associated with absolute eosinophil counts of >2,000 cells/µL. Hypersensitivity drug reactions can elicit eosinophilia with or without drug fever or organ dysfunction. Various skin diseases have also been associated with eosinophilia, including atopic dermatitis, eczema, pemphigus, urticaria, and toxic epidermal necrolysis.

Infectious Diseases

Eosinophilia is often associated with infection with multicellular helminthic parasites, which are the most common cause in developing countries. Severe eosinophilia in children is most commonly due to **visceral larva migrans.** The level of eosinophilia tends to parallel the magnitude and extent of tissue invasion, especially by larvae. Eosinophilia often *does not* occur in established parasitic infections that are well contained within tissues or are solely intraluminal in the gastrointestinal tract, such as *Giardia lamblia* and *Enterobius vermicularis* infection.

In evaluating patients with unexplained eosinophilia, the dietary history and geographic or travel history may indicate potential exposures to helminthic parasites. It is frequently necessary to examine the stool for ova and larvae at least 3 times. Additionally, the diagnostic parasite stages of many of the helminthic parasites that cause eosinophilia never appear in feces. Thus, normal results of stool examinations do not absolutely preclude a helminthic cause of eosinophilia; diagnostic blood tests or tissue biopsy may be needed. *Toxocara* causes visceral larva migrans usually in toddlers with pica (Chapter 290). Most young children are asymptomatic, but some develop fever, pneumonitis, hepatomegaly, and hypergammaglobulinemia accompanied by severe eosinophilia. Isohemagglutinins are frequently elevated. Serology can establish the diagnosis.

Two fungal diseases may be associated with eosinophilia: aspergillosis in the form of allergic bronchopulmonary aspergillosis (Chapter 229.1) and coccidioidomycosis (Chapter 232) following primary infection, especially in conjunction with erythema nodosum.

Hypereosinophilic Syndrome

The idiopathic hypereosinophilic syndrome is a heterogeneous group of disorders characterized by sustained overproduction of eosinophils. The 3 diagnostic criteria for this disorder are (1) eosinophilia >1,500 cells/µL persisting for ≥6 mo, (2) absence of another diagnosis to explain the eosinophilia, and (3) signs and symptoms of organ involvement. The clinical signs and symptoms of hypereosinophilic syndrome can be heterogeneous because of the diversity of potential organ (pulmonary, cutaneous, neurologic, serosal, gastrointestinal) involvement. Loeffler endocarditis, one of the most serious and life-threatening complications, can cause heart failure due to endomyocardial thrombosis and fibrosis. Eosinophilic leukemia, a clonal myeloproliferative variant, may be distinguished from idiopathic hypereosinophilic syndrome by demonstrating a clonal interstitial deletion on chromosome 4q12 that fuses the platelet-derived growth factor receptor-alpha (PDGFRA) and FIP1-like-1 (FIP1L1) genes; this disorder is treated with imatinib mesylate, which helps target the fusion oncoprotein.

Therapy is aimed at suppressing eosinophilia and is initiated with corticosteroids. Imatinib mesylate, a tyrosine kinase inhibitor, may be effective in F1P1L1-PDGFRA negative patients. Hydroxyurea may be beneficial in patients unresponsive to corticosteroids. Specific anti IL-5 monoclonal antibodies (mepolizumab) targets this cytokine, which has a central role in eosinophil differentiation, mobilization and activity. With therapy, the eosinophil count declines and corticosteroid doses may be reduced. For patients with prominent organ involvement who fail to respond to therapy, the mortality is ≈75% after 3 yr.

Miscellaneous Diseases

Eosinophilia is observed in many patients with primary immunodeficiency syndromes, especially hyper-IgE syndrome (Chapter

116), Wiskott-Aldrich syndrome, and Omenn syndrome. Eosinophilia is also frequently present in the syndrome of thrombocytopenia with absent radii and in familial reticuloendotheliosis with eosinophilia. Mild eosinophilia is found in 20% of patients with Hodgkin disease and in gastrointestinal disorders including ulcerative colitis, Crohn disease during symptomatic phases, gastroenteritis that is associated with milk precipitins, and chronic hepatitis. Primary eosinophilic gastroenteritis usually involves the esophagus and stomach.

BIBLIOGRAPHY

Please visit the Nelson Textbook of Pediatrics *website at* *www.expertconsult.com* *for the complete bibliography.*

Chapter 124
Disorders of Phagocyte Function

Laurence A. Boxer and Peter E. Newburger

Neutrophils are particularly important in protecting the skin, the lining of the respiratory and gastrointestinal tracts, and other mucous membranes as part of the 1st line of defense against microbial invasion. During the critical 2-4 hr after microbial invasion, these phagocytes arrive at the site of inflammation to contain the infection and prevent hematogenous dissemination.

Immunologic evaluation of patients with suspected immunodeficiency (Chapter 116) should focus on disorders of phagocyte function (Table 124-1) in patients with recurrent or unusual bacterial infections (Fig. 124-1).

Chemotaxis, the direct migration of cells into sites of infection, involves a complex series of events (Chapter 121). Studies of defective in vitro chemotaxis of neutrophils obtained from children having various clinical conditions have not established whether frequent infections arise from a primary chemotactic abnormality or occur as secondary medical complications of the underlying disorder. For example, variable but at times severe abnormalities in neutrophil motility accompany the hyper-IgE syndrome, which is characterized by markedly elevated levels of IgE, chronic dermatitis, and recurrent sinopulmonary infections, as well as coarse facial features, retention of primary teeth, and a propensity for recurrent bone fractures (Chapter 123).

LEUKOCYTE ADHESION DEFICIENCY

Leukocyte adhesion deficiency 1 (LAD-1), 2 (LAD-2), and 3 (LAD-3) are rare autosomal recessive disorders of leukocyte function. LAD-1 affects about 1 per 10 million individuals and is characterized by recurrent bacterial and fungal infections and depressed inflammatory responses despite striking blood neutrophilia.

Genetics and Pathogenesis

LAD-1 results from mutations of the gene on chromosome 21q22.3 encoding CD18, the 95-kD β_2 leukocyte integrin subunit. Normal neutrophils express 4 heterodimeric adhesion molecules: LFA-1 (CD11a/CD18), Mac-1 (CD11b/CD18, also known as CR3 or iC3b receptor), p150,95 (CD11c/CD18), and αd β_2 (CD11d/CD18). These 4 transmembrane adhesion molecules are composed of unique α_1 subunits of 185 kD, 190 kD, 150 kD, and 160 kD, respectively, encoded on chromosome 16, and share a common β_2 subunit. This group of leukocyte integrins is responsible for the tight adhesion of neutrophils to the endothelial cell surface, egress from the circulation, and adhesion to iC3b-coated microorganisms, which promotes phagocytosis and particulate activation of the phagocyte NADPH oxidase.

Mutations in the CD18 gene either impair gene expression or affect the structure of the synthesized CD18 peptide, leading to functionally abnormal CD11/CD18. Some mutations of CD11/CD18 allow a low level of assembly and activity of integrin molecules. These children retain some neutrophil integrin adhesion function and have a moderate phenotype. Failure of neutrophils to bear the β_2-integrins leads to inability to migrate to sites of inflammation outside the blood vessel lumen because of their inability to adhere firmly to surfaces and undergo transendothelial migration. Failure of the CD11/CD18–deficient neutrophils to undergo transendothelial migration occurs because the β_2-integrins bind to intercellular adhesion molecules 1 (ICAM-1) and 2 (ICAM-2) expressed on inflamed endothelial cells (Chapter 121). Neutrophils that do arrive at inflammatory sites by CD11/CD18–independent processes fail to recognize microorganisms opsonized with complement fragment iC3b, an important stable opsonin formed by the cleavage of C3b. Hence, other neutrophil functions such as degranulation and oxidative metabolism normally triggered by iC3b binding are also markedly compromised in LAD-1 neutrophils, resulting in impaired phagocytic function and high risk for serious and recurrent bacterial infections.

Monocyte function is also impaired, with poor fibrinogen-binding function, an activity that is promoted by the CD11/CD18 complex. Consequently, such cells are unable to participate effectively in wound healing.

Children with **LAD-2** share the clinical features of LAD-1 but have normal CD11/CD18 integrins. Features unique to LAD-2 include neurologic defects, cranial facial dysmorphism, and absence of the erythrocyte ABO blood group antigen (Bombay phenotype). LAD-2 (also known as congenital disorder of glycosylation IIc) derives from mutations in the gene encoding a specific GDP-L-fucose transporter of the Golgi apparatus. This abnormality prevents the incorporation of fucose into various cell surface glycoproteins, which are expressed on cell surface membranes. These include the erythrocyte carbohydrate blood group markers and neutrophil the carbohydrate structure sialyl Lewis X. Absence of this selectin ligand renders the cells incapable of rolling adhesion to activated endothelial cells, an initial step necessary for subsequent integrin-mediated activation, spreading, and transendothelial migration. Infections in LAD-2 are milder than that in LAD-1.

LAD-3 is characterized by a Glanzmann thrombasthenia-like bleeding disorder, delayed separation of the umbilical cord as well as serious skin and soft tissue infections similar to that seen in LAD-1, and failure of leukocytes to undergo β_2 and β_1 integrin mediated adhesion and migration. Mutations in *KINDLIN3* affect integrin activation.

Clinical Manifestations

Patients with the severe clinical form of LAD-1 express <0.3% of the normal amount of the β_2-integrin molecules, whereas patients with the moderate phenotype may express 2-7% of the normal amount. Children with severe disease present in infancy with recurrent, indolent bacterial infections of the skin, mouth, respiratory tract, lower intestinal tract, and genital mucosa. They may have a history of delayed separation of the umbilical cord, usually with associated infection (omphalitis) of the cord stump. However, 10% of healthy infants can have cord separation at age 3 wk or later, so this sign alone should not be sufficient to raise suspicion of LAD-1. Skin infection may progress to large chronic ulcers with polymicrobial infection, including anaerobic organisms. The ulcers heal slowly, need months of antibiotic treatment, and often require plastic surgical grafting. Severe gingivitis can lead to early loss of primary and secondary teeth.

The pathogens infecting patients with LAD-1 are similar to those affecting patients with severe neutropenia (Chapter 125) and include *Staphylococcus aureus* and enteric gram-negative organisms such as *Escherichia coli.* These patients are also susceptible to opportunistic infection by fungi such as *Candida* and *Aspergillus.* Typical signs of inflammation such as swelling, erythema, and warmth may be absent. Pus does not form, and few

Table 124-1 CLINICAL DISORDERS OF NEUTROPHIL FUNCTION

DISORDER	ETIOLOGY	IMPAIRED FUNCTION	CLINICAL CONSEQUENCE
DEGRANULATION ABNORMALITIES			
Chédiak-Higashi syndrome	Autosomal recessive; disordered coalescence of lysosomal granules; responsible gene is *CHSI/LYST*, which encodes a protein hypothesized to regulate granule fusion.	Decreased neutrophil chemotaxis, degranulation, and bactericidal activity; platelet storage pool defect; impaired NK function, failure to disperse melanosomes	Neutropenia; recurrent pyogenic infections, propensity to develop marked hepatosplenomegaly as a manifestation of the hemophagocytic syndrome
Specific granule deficiency	Autosomal recessive; functional loss of myeloid transcription factor arising from a mutation or arising from reduced expression of *Gfi-1* or *C/EBP*, which regulates specific granule formation	Impaired chemotaxis and bactericidal activity; bilobed nuclei in neutrophils; defensins, gelatinase, collagenase, vitamin B_{12}–binding protein, and lactoferrin	Recurrent deep-seated abscesses
ADHESION ABNORMALITIES			
Leukocyte adhesion deficiency I	Autosomal recessive; absence of CD11/CD18 surface adhesive glycoproteins (β_2 integrins) on leukocyte membranes most commonly arising from failure to express CD18 mRNA	Decreased binding of C3bi to neutrophils and impaired adhesion to ICAM1 and ICAM2	Neutrophilia; recurrent bacterial infection associated with a lack of pus formation
Leukocyte adhesion deficiency II	Autosomal recessive; loss of fucosylation of ligands for selectins and other glycol-conjugates arising from mutations of the GDP-fucose transporter	Decreased adhesion to activated endothelium expressing ELAM	Neutrophilia; recurrent bacterial infection without pus
Leukocyte adhesion deficiency III (LAD-1 variant syndrome)	Autosomal recessive; impaired integrin function arising from mutations of *FERMT3* which encodes kindlin-3 in hematopoietic cells; kindlin-3 binds to β-integrin and thereby transmits integrin activation.	Impaired neutrophil adhesion and platelet activation	Recurrent infections, neutropenia, bleeding tendency
DISORDERS OF CELL MOTILITY			
Enhanced motile responses; FMF	Autosomal recessive gene responsible for FMF on chromosome 16 which encodes for a protein called pyrin; pyrin regulates caspase-1 and thereby IL-1β secretion; mutated pyrin may lead to heightened sensitivity to endotoxin, excessive IL-1β production, and impaired monocyte apoptosis.	Excessive accumulation of neutrophils at inflamed sites, which may be the result of excessive IL-1β production	Recurrent fever, peritonitis, pleuritis, arthritis, and amyloidosis
DEPRESSED MOTILE RESPONSES			
Defects in the generation of chemotactic signals	IgG deficiencies; C3 and properdin deficiency can arise from genetic or acquired abnormalities; mannose-binding protein deficiency predominantly in neonates	Deficiency of serum chemotaxis and opsonic activities	Recurrent pyogenic infections
Intrinsic defects of the neutrophil, e.g., leukocyte adhesion deficiency, Chédiak-Higashi syndrome, specific granule deficiency, neutrophil actin dysfunction, neonatal neutrophils	In the neonatal neutrophil there is diminished ability to express β_2- integrins, and there is a qualitative impairment in β_2-integrin function.	Diminished chemotaxis	Propensity to develop pyogenic infections.
Direct inhibition of neutrophil mobility, e.g., drugs	Ethanol, glucocorticoids, cyclic AMP	Impaired locomotion and ingestion; impaired adherence	Possible cause for frequent infections; neutrophilia seen with epinephrine arises from cyclic AMP release from endothelium
Immune complexes	Bind to Fc receptors on neutrophils in patients with rheumatoid arthritis, systemic lupus erythematosus, and other inflammatory states	Impaired chemotaxis	Recurrent pyogenic infections
Hyper-IgE syndrome	Autosomal dominant; responsible gene is *Stat3*	Impaired chemotaxis at times; impaired regulation of cytokine production	Recurrent skin and sinopulmonary infections, eczema, mucocutaneous candidiasis, eosinophilia, retained primary teeth, minimal trauma fractures, scoliosis, and characteristic facies
Hyper-IgE syndrome–AR	Autosomal recessive; more then one gene likely contributes to its etiology.	High IgE levels, impaired lymphocyte activation to staphylococcal antigens	Recurrent pneumonia without pneumatoceles sepsis, enzyme, boils, mucocutaneous candidiasis, neurologic symptoms, eosinophilia
MICROBICIDAL ACTIVITY			
Chronic granulomatous disease	X-linked and autosomal recessive; failure to express functional gp91^{phox} in the phagocyte membrane in p22^{phox} (autosomal recessive). Other autosomal recessive forms of CGD arise from failure to express protein p47^{phox} or p67^{phox}.	Failure to activate neutrophil respiratory burst leading to failure to kill catalase-positive microbes	Recurrent pyogenic infections with catalase-positive microorganisms
G6PD deficiency	Less than 5% of normal activity of G6PD	Failure to activate NADPH-dependent oxidase, and hemolytic anemia	Infections with catalase-positive microorganisms
Myeloperoxidase deficiency	Autosomal recessive; failure to process modified precursor protein arising from missense mutation	H_2O_2-dependent antimicrobial activity not potentiated by myeloperoxidase	None
Rac-2 deficiency	Autosomal dominant; dominant negative inhibition by mutant protein of Rac-2 mediated functions	Failure of membrane receptor mediated O_2^- generation and chemotaxis	Neutrophilia, recurrent bacterial infections
Deficiencies of glutathione reductase and glutathione synthetase	Autosomal recessive; failure to detoxify H_2O_2	Excessive formation of H_2O_2	Minimal problems with recurrent pyogenic infections

AMP, adenosine monophosphate; AR, autosomal recessive; C, complement; CD, cluster of differentiation; CGD, chronic granulomatous disease; FMF, familial Mediterranean fever; G6PD, glucose-6-phosphate dehydrogenase; ICAM, intracellular adhesion molecule; IL-1, interleukin-1; LAD, leukocyte adhesion deficiency; NADPH, nicotinamide adenine dinucleotide phosphate; NK, natural killer.
Modified from Curnutte JT, Boxer LA: Clinically significant phagocytic cell defects. In Remington JS, Swartz MN, editors: *Current clinical topics in infectious disease*, ed 6, New York, 1985, McGraw-Hill, p 144.

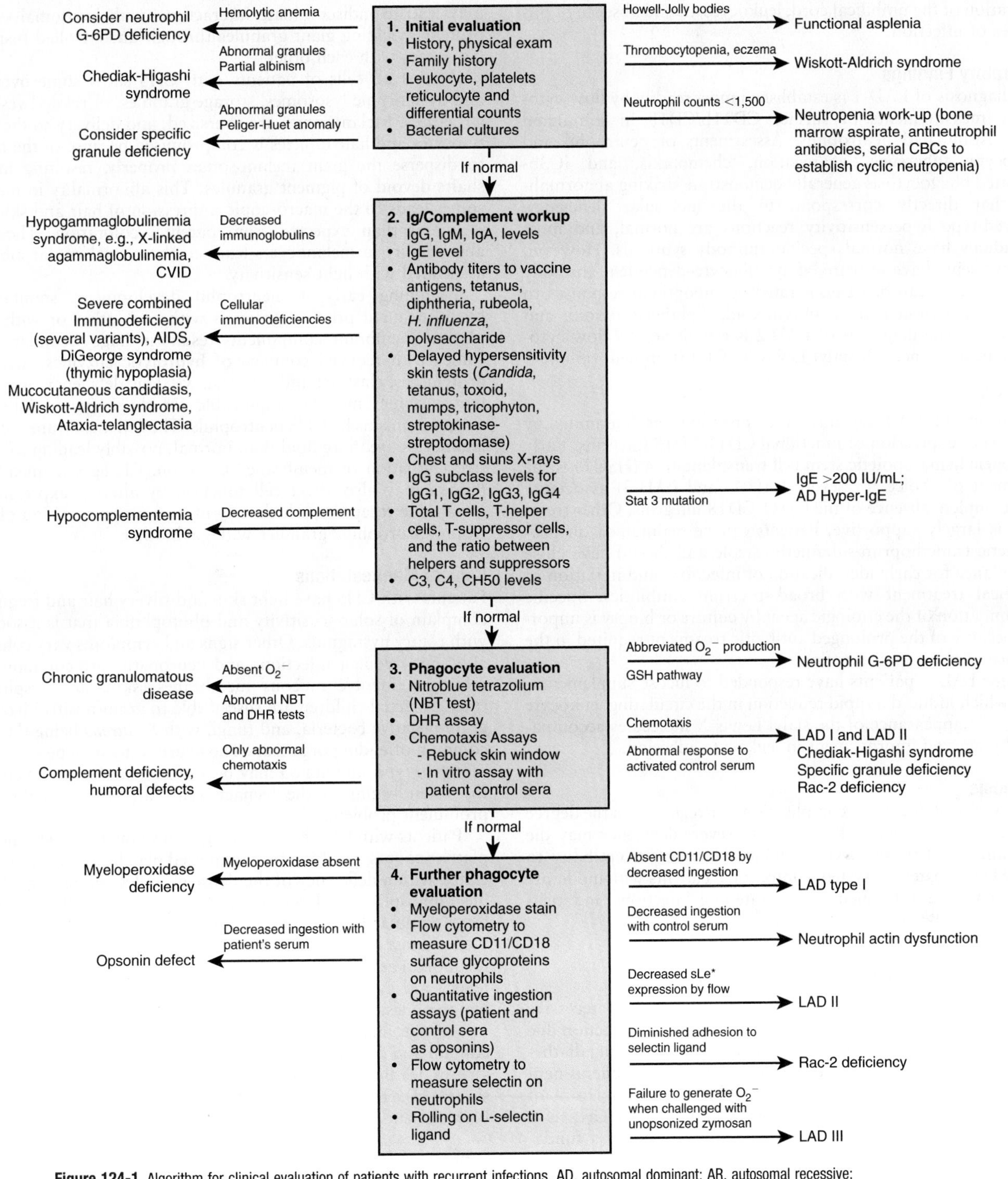

Figure 124-1 Algorithm for clinical evaluation of patients with recurrent infections. AD, autosomal dominant; AR, autosomal recessive; C, complement; CBC, complete blood count; CD, cluster of differentiation; CVID, common variable immunodeficiency; DHR, dihydrorhodamine; G-6PD, glucose-6-phosphate dehydrogenase; Ig, immunoglobulin; LAD, leukocyte adhesion deficiency; NK, natural killer; X, X-linked. (Modified from Curnutte JT, Boxer LA: Clinically significant phagocyte cell defects. In Remington JS, Swartz MN, editors: *Current clinical topics in infectious diseases,* ed 6, New York, 1985, McGraw-Hill, p 144.)

neutrophils are identified microscopically in biopsy specimens of infected tissues. Despite the paucity of neutrophils within the affected tissue, the circulating neutrophil count during infection typically exceeds 30,000/μL and can surpass 100,000/μL. During intervals between infections, the peripheral blood neutrophil count may chronically exceed 12,000/μL. LAD-1 genotypes producing moderate amounts of functional integrins at the surface of the neutrophil significantly reduce the severity and frequency of infections compared to children with the severe form.

Similar clinical syndromes have been reported in patients with endothelial cell E-selectin deficiency, which manifests with delayed separation of the umbilical cord and omphalitis, and in a child with an autosomal dominant mutation of Rac2 (a Rho GTPase needed to regulate actin organization and superoxide production). **Rac2 deficiency** is characterized by delayed separation of the umbilical cord, leukocytosis, and absence of pus at sites of infection.

Laboratory Findings
The diagnosis of LAD-1 is established most readily by **flow cytometric** measurements of surface CD11b/CD18 in stimulated and unstimulated neutrophils. Assessments of neutrophil and monocyte adherence, aggregation, chemotaxis, and iC3b-mediated phagocytosis generally demonstrate striking abnormalities that directly correspond to the molecular deficiency. Delayed-type hypersensitivity reactions are normal, and most individuals have normal specific antibody synthesis. However, some patients have impaired T lymphocyte–dependent antibody responses that can be demonstrated by suboptimal responses to repeat vaccination with tetanus toxoid, diphtheria toxoid, and poliovirus. The diagnosis of LAD-2 is established by flow cytometric measurement of sialyl Lewis X (CD15) on neutrophils.

Treatment
Treatment of LAD-1 depends on the phenotype as determined by the level of expression of functional CD11/CD18 integrins. Early **allogeneic hematopoietic stem cell transplantation (HSCT)** is the treatment of choice for severe LAD-1 (and LAD-3) associated with complete absence of the CD11/CD18 integrins. Other treatment is largely supportive. Patients can be maintained on prophylactic trimethoprim-sulfamethoxazole and should have close surveillance for early identification of infections and initiation of empirical treatment with broad-spectrum antibiotics. Specific determination of the etiologic agent by culture or biopsy is important because of the prolonged antibiotic treatment required in the absence of neutrophil function.

Some LAD-2 patients have responded to fucose supplementation, which induced a rapid reduction in the circulating leukocyte count and appearance of the sialyl Lewis X molecules accompanied by marked improvement in leukocyte adhesion.

Prognosis
The severity of infectious complications correlates with the degree of β_2-integrin deficiency. Patients with severe deficiency may die in infancy, and those surviving infancy have a susceptibility to severe life-threatening systemic infections. Patients with moderate deficiency have infrequent life-threatening infections and relatively long survival.

CHÉDIAK-HIGASHI SYNDROME

Chédiak-Higashi syndrome (CHS) is a rare autosomal recessive disorder characterized by increased susceptibility to infection due to defective degranulation of neutrophils, a mild bleeding diathesis, partial oculocutaneous albinism, progressive peripheral neuropathy, and a tendency to develop a life-threatening form of hemophagocytic lymphohistiocytosis (Chapter 501). CHS is a disorder of generalized cellular dysfunction caused by a fundamental defect in granule morphogenesis that results in abnormally large granules in multiple tissues. Pigmentary dilution involving the hair, skin, and ocular fundi results from pathologic aggregation of melanosomes. Neurologic deficits are associated with a failure of decussation of the optic and auditory nerves. Patients exhibit an increased susceptibility to infection that can be explained in part by defects in neutrophil chemotaxis, degranulation, and bactericidal activity. Giant granules in the neutrophils probably interfere with the cells' ability to traverse the narrow passages between endothelial cells into tissue.

Genetics and Pathogenesis
LYST (for lysosomal traffic regulator), the gene mutated in CHS, is located at chromosome 1q2-q44. The LYST/CHS protein is thought to regulate vesicle transport by mediating protein-protein interaction and protein-membrane associations. Loss of function may lead to indiscriminate interactions with lysosomal surface proteins, yielding giant granules through uncontrolled fusion of lysosomes with each other.

Almost all cells of patients with CHS show some oversized and dysmorphic lysosomes, storage granules, or related vesicular structures. Melanosomes are oversized, and delivery to the keratinocytes and hair follicles is compromised because of the failure to disperse the giant melanosomes properly, resulting in hair shafts devoid of pigment granules. This abnormality in melanosomes leads to the macroscopic impression of hair and skin that is lighter than expected from parental coloration. The same abnormality in melanocytes leads to the partial ocular albinism associated with light sensitivity.

Beginning early in neutrophil development, spontaneous fusion of giant primary granules with each other or with cytoplasmic membrane components results in huge secondary lysosomes with reduced contents of hydrolytic enzymes, including proteinases, elastase, and cathepsin G. This deficiency of proteolytic enzymes may be responsible for the impaired killing of microorganisms by CHS neutrophils. The cell membranes of CHS leukocytes are more fluid than normal, possibly leading to defective regulation of membrane activation. Changes in membrane fluidity may also affect cell function by altering expression of membrane receptors, which may in turn promote fusion of neutrophil azurophilic granules with each other.

Clinical Manifestations
Patients with CHS have light skin and silvery hair and frequently complain of solar sensitivity and photophobia that is associated with rotary nystagmus. Other signs and symptoms vary considerably, but frequent infections and neuropathy are common. The infections involve mucous membranes, skin, and respiratory tract. Affected children are susceptible to gram-positive bacteria, gram-negative bacteria, and fungi, with *S. aureus* being the most common offending organism. The **neuropathy** may be sensory or motor in type, and ataxia may be a prominent feature. Neuropathy often begins in the teenage years and becomes the most prominent problem.

Patients with CHS have prolonged bleeding times with normal platelet counts, resulting from impaired platelet aggregation associated with a deficiency of the dense granules containing adenosine diphosphate and serotonin. Natural killer cell function of large granular lymphocytes is also impaired.

The most life-threatening complication of CHS is the development of an accelerated phase characterized by pancytopenia, high fever, and lymphohistiocytic infiltration of liver, spleen, and lymph nodes. The onset of the accelerated phase, which can occur at any age, may be related to the inability of these patients to contain and control Epstein-Barr virus infection, as well as other viruses, leading to features of **hemophagocytic lymphohistiocytosis (HLH)**. The accelerated phase is associated with secondary bacterial and viral infections and usually results in death.

Laboratory Findings
The diagnosis of CHS is established by finding large inclusions in all nucleated blood cells. These can be seen on Wright-stained blood films and are accentuated by a peroxidase stain. Because of impaired egress from the bone marrow, cells containing the large inclusions may be missed on peripheral blood smear but readily identified on bone marrow examination.

Treatment
High-dose ascorbic acid (200 mg/day for infants, 2,000 mg/day for adults) improves the clinical status of some children in the stable phase. Although controversy surrounds the efficacy of ascorbic acid, given the safety of the vitamin, it is reasonable to administer ascorbic acid to all patients.

The only curative therapy to prevent the accelerated phase is **HSCT**. Normal stem cells reconstitute hematopoietic and immunologic function, correct the natural killer cell deficiency, and prevent conversion to the accelerated phase, but can not correct or prevent the peripheral neuropathy. If the patient is in the accelerated phase with active HLH, HSCT often fails to prevent death.

MYELOPEROXIDASE DEFICIENCY

Myeloperoxidase (MPO) deficiency is an autosomal recessive disorder of oxidative metabolism and is one of the most common inherited disorders of phagocytes, occurring at a frequency approaching 1 per 2,000 individuals. MPO is a green heme protein located in the azurophilic lysosomes of neutrophils and monocytes and is the basis for the greenish tinge to pus accumulated at a site of infection. Most individuals with the trait do not have an increased rate of infection or other clinical manifestations of disease.

Genetics and Pathogenesis

Mutations in the MPO gene causing this defect provide insight into the post-translational processing of this granule protein. MPO mRNA is transcribed exclusively during the promyelocytic stage of granulopoiesis. MPO deficiency is caused by a missense mutation in the MPO gene that results in an MPO precursor that does not incorporate heme. Although this mutation is the most common cause of MPO deficiency, many patients are compound heterozygotes with 1 allele bearing the common mutation and the other possessing a mutation not yet identified. A partial deficiency results if only 1 allele is normal.

Partial or complete MPO deficiency leads to diminished production of hypochlorous acid (HOCl) and HOCl-derived chloramines. The deficiency in HOCl leads to early depression of gram-positive and gram-negative bacterial rates of killing in vitro that normalizes after 1 hr incubation. These data indicate that deficient cells use an MPO-independent microbicidal system that is slower to kill pathogens than the MPO-H_2O_2-halide system used by normal neutrophils.

Clinical Manifestations

MPO deficiency is usually clinically silent. Rarely, patients may have disseminated candidiasis, usually in conjunction with diabetes mellitus. Acquired partial MPO deficiency can develop in acute myelogenous leukemia and in myelodysplastic syndromes.

Laboratory Findings

Deficiency of neutrophil and monocyte MPO can be identified by histochemical analysis.

Treatment

There is no specific therapy. Aggressive treatment with antifungal agents should be provided for candidal infections. The prognosis is usually excellent.

CHRONIC GRANULOMATOUS DISEASE

Chronic granulomatous disease (CGD) is characterized by neutrophils and monocytes capable of normal chemotaxis, ingestion, and degranulation, but unable to kill **catalase-positive microorganisms** because of a defect in the generation of microbicidal oxygen metabolites. CGD is a rare disease with an incidence of 4 to 5 per million individuals, caused by 4 genes, 1 X-linked and 3 autosomal recessive in inheritance.

Genetics and Pathogenesis

Activation of the phagocyte NADPH oxidase requires stimulation of the neutrophils and involves assembly from cytoplasmic and integral membrane subunits (see Fig. 121-3). Oxidase activation initiates with phosphorylation of a cationic cytoplasmic protein, $p47^{phox}$ (47-kd phagocyte oxidase protein). Phosphorylated $p47^{phox}$, together with 2 other cytoplasmic components of the oxidase, $p67^{phox}$ and the low molecular weight GTPase Rac-2, translocates to the membrane where they combine with the cytoplasmic domains of the transmembrane flavocytochrome b_{558} to form the active oxidase complex (see Fig. 121-3). The flavocytochrome is a heterodimer composed of $p22^{phox}$ and highly glycosylated $gp91^{phox}$. Current models predict that 3 transmembrane domains within the N-terminus of the flavocytochrome contain the histidines that coordinate heme binding. The $p22^{phox}$ component is required for stability of $gp91^{phox}$ and provides a docking site for the cytoplasmic subunits. The $gp91^{phox}$ glycoprotein catalyzes electron transport through its NADPH-binding, flavin-binding, and heme-binding domains. The cytoplasmic $p47^{phox}$, $p67^{phox}$, and Rac-2 components appear to serve as regulatory elements for activation of cytochrome b_{558}. An addition protein, $p40^{phox}$, stabilizes the preactivation cytoplasmic complex of $p67^{phox}$ and $p47^{phox}$ and protects $p67^{phox}$ from degradation. Defects in any of these NADPH oxidase components can lead to CGD.

Approximately 65% of patients with CGD are males who inherit their disorder as a result of mutations in *CYBB*, an X-chromosome gene encoding $gp91^{phox}$. About 35% of patients inherit CGD in an autosomal recessive fashion resulting from mutations in the *NCF1* gene on chromosome 7, encoding $p47^{phox}$. Defects in the genes encoding $p67^{phox}$ (*NCF2* on chromosome 1) and $p22^{phox}$ (*CYBA* on chromosome 16) are inherited in an autosomal recessive manner and account for about 5% of cases of CGD.

The metabolic deficiency of the CGD neutrophil predisposes the host to infection. The CGD phagocytic vacuoles lack microbicidal reactive oxygen species and remain acidic, so bacteria are not killed or digested properly (Fig. 124-2). Hematoxylin-eosin–stained sections from patients' tissues show multiple granulomas that give CGD its descriptive name; the macrophages may contain a golden pigment that reflects an abnormal accumulation of ingested material and contributes to granuloma formation. The metabolic impairment in the CGD neutrophil leads to delayed

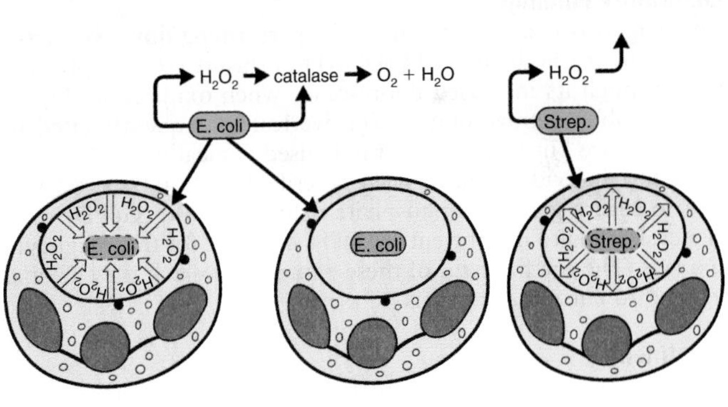

Figure 124-2 The pathogenesis of chronic granulomatous disease (CGD). The manner in which the metabolic deficiency of the CGD neutrophil predisposes the host to infection is shown schematically. Normal neutrophils stimulate hydrogen peroxide in the phagosome containing ingested *Escherichia coli.* Myeloperoxidase is delivered to the phagosome by degranulation, as indicated by the *closed circles.* In this setting, hydrogen peroxide acts as a substrate for myeloperoxidase to oxidize halide to hypochlorous acid and chloramines that kill the microbes. The quantity of hydrogen peroxide produced by the normal neutrophil is sufficient to exceed the capacity of catalase, a hydrogen peroxide-catabolizing enzyme of many aerobic microorganisms, including *Staphylococcus aureus,* most gram-negative enteric bacteria, *Candida albicans,* and *Aspergillus.* When organisms such as *E. coli* gain entry into CGD neutrophils, they are not exposed to hydrogen peroxide because the neutrophils do not produce it, and the hydrogen peroxide generated by microorganisms themselves is destroyed by their own catalase. When CGD neutrophils ingest streptococci, which lack catalase, the organisms generate enough hydrogen peroxide to result in a microbicidal effect. As indicated *(middle),* catalase-positive microbes such as *E. coli* can survive within the phagosome of the CGD neutrophil. (Modified from Boxer LA: Quantitative abnormalities of granulocytes. In Beutler E, Lichtman MA, Coller BS, et al, editors: *Williams hematology,* ed 6, New York, 2001, McGraw-Hill, p 845.)

neutrophil apoptosis and subsequent clearance of degenerating neutrophils by macrophages, which in turn leads to ongoing local tissue damage from release of proteases and other granule proteins.

Clinical Manifestations

Although the clinical presentation is variable, several features suggest the diagnosis of CGD. Any patient with recurrent pneumonia, lymphadenitis, hepatic or other abscesses, osteomyelitis at multiple sites, a family history of recurrent infections, or any infection with an unusual catalase-positive organism requires evaluation. Residual NADPH oxidase may attenuate CGD.

The onset of clinical signs and symptoms may occur from early infancy to young adulthood. The attack rate and severity of infections are exceedingly variable. The most common pathogen is *S. aureus,* although any catalase-positive microorganism may be involved. Other organisms frequently causing infections include *Serratia marcescens, Burkholderia cepacia, Aspergillus, Candida albicans, Nocardia,* and *Salmonella.* There may also be increased susceptibility to mycobacterium including the BCG vaccine. Pneumonia, lymphadenitis, osteomyelitis, and skin infections are the most common illnesses encountered. Bacteremia or fungemia occur but are much less common than focal infections. Patients may suffer from the sequelae of chronic infection, including anemia of chronic disease, poor growth, lymphadenopathy, hepatosplenomegaly, chronic purulent dermatitis, restrictive lung disease, gingivitis, hydronephrosis, and pyloric outlet narrowing. Perirectal abscesses and recurrent skin infections, including folliculitis, cutaneous granulomas, and discoid lupus erythematosus also suggest the possibility of CGD. **Granuloma formation** and inflammatory processes are a hallmark of CGD and may be the presenting symptoms that prompt testing for CGD if they cause pyloric outlet obstruction, bladder outlet or ureter obstruction, or rectal fistulae and granulomatous colitis simulating Crohn disease.

Laboratory Findings

The diagnosis is most often made by performing **flow cytometry** using dihydrorhodamine 123 (DHR) to measure oxidant production through its increased fluorescence when oxidized by H_2O_2. The nitroblue tetrazolium (NBT) dye test is frequently cited in the literature but is now only rarely used clinically.

A few individuals have been described with apparent CGD due to severe glucose-6-phosphate dehydrogenase (G6PD) deficiency, leading to insufficient NADPH substrate for the phagocyte oxidase. The erythrocytes of these patients also lack the enzyme, leading to chronic hemolysis.

Treatment

HSCT is the only known **cure** for CGD. For supportive care, patients with CGD should be given daily oral trimethoprim-sulfamethoxazole and an antifungal drug, such as itraconazole (see later), for prophylaxis of infections. Cultures must be obtained as soon as infection is suspected. Most abscesses require surgical drainage for therapeutic and diagnostic purposes. Prolonged use of antibiotics is often required. *Aspergillus* or *Candida* infection requires treatment with intravenous antifungal drugs. Granulocyte transfusions may be necessary if antibiotics are ineffective. If fever occurs without an obvious focus, it is advisable to consider the use of radiographs of the chest and skeleton as well as CT scans of the liver to determine if pneumonia, osteomyelitis, or liver abscesses are present. The cause of fever cannot always be established, and empirical treatment with broad-spectrum parenteral antibiotics is often required. The erythrocyte sedimentation rate (ESR) may be used to help determine the duration of antibiotic treatment.

Corticosteroids may also be useful for the treatment of children with antral and urethral obstruction or severe granulomatous colitis. Granulomas may be sensitive to low doses of prednisone (0.5 mg/kg/day); treatment should be tapered over several weeks. Inhibitors of tumor necrosis factor alpha pathways, such as infliximab, should be avoided if possible due to the very high risk of invasive fungal infection.

Interferon-γ (IFN-γ) 50 μg/m² 3 times/wk reduces the number of hospitalizations and serious infections. The mechanism of action of IFN-γ therapy in CGD is unknown. **Itraconazole** (200 mg/day for patients >50 kg and 100 mg/day for patients <50 kg and ≤5 yr of age) administered prophylactically reduces the frequency of fungal infections.

Genetic Counseling

Identifying a patient's specific genetic subgroup is useful primarily for genetic counseling and prenatal diagnosis. In cases of suspected X-linked CGD, further analysis is not necessary if the fetus is initially demonstrated to be a 46,XX female. Fetal blood sampling and oxidase function analysis of fetal neutrophils can be used for prenatal diagnosis of CGD. DNA analysis of amniotic fluid cells or chorionic villus biopsy is an option for early prenatal diagnosis in families in which the specific mutation is known.

Prognosis

The overall mortality rate for CGD is about 2 patient deaths/yr/100 cases, with the highest mortality among young children. The development of effective infection prophylactic regimens, close surveillance for signs of infections, and aggressive surgical and medical interventions has improved the prognosis.

BIBLIOGRAPHY

Please visit the Nelson Textbook of Pediatrics *website at www.expertconsult.com for the complete bibliography.*

Chapter 125
Leukopenia

Peter E. Newburger and Laurence A. Boxer

Marked developmental changes in normal values for the total white blood cell (WBC) count occur during childhood (Chapter 708). The mean WBC count at birth is high, followed by a rapid fall beginning at 12 hr until the end of the 1st wk. Thereafter, values are stable until 1 yr of age. A slow, steady decline in the WBC count continues throughout childhood until reaching the adult value during adolescence. **Leukopenia** in adolescents and adults is defined as a total WBC count <4,000/μL. Evaluation of patients with leukopenia, neutropenia, or lymphopenia begins with a thorough history, physical examination, family history, and screening laboratory tests (Table 125-1).

NEUTROPENIA

Neutropenia is an **absolute neutrophil count** (ANC), calculated as the WBC count × % of neutrophils and bands, more than 2 standard deviations below the normal mean. Normal neutrophil counts must be stratified for age and race. For whites over the age of 12 mo, the lower limit of normal for the neutrophil count is 1,500/μL, and for blacks over 12 mo old, the lower limit of normal is 1,200/μL. The relatively lower limit in blacks probably reflects a relative decrease in neutrophils in the storage compartment of the bone marrow. Neutropenia may be characterized as **mild neutropenia,** with an ANC of 1,000-1,500/μL; **moderate neutropenia,** with an ANC of 500-1,000/μL; or **severe neutropenia,** with an ANC <500/μL. This stratification aids in predicting the risk of pyogenic infection; only patients with severe neutropenia have significantly increased susceptibility to life-threatening infections.

Table 125-1 DIAGNOSTIC APPROACH FOR PATIENTS WITH LEUKOPENIA

EVALUATION	ASSOCIATED CLINICAL DIAGNOSES
INITIAL EVALUATION	
• History of acute or chronic leukopenia	
• General medical history	Congenital syndromes (Shwachman-Diamond, Wiskott-Aldrich, Fanconi anemia, dyskeratosis congenita, glycogen storage disease type Ib, disorders of vesicular transport)
• Physical examination: stomatitis, gingivitis, dental defects, congenital anomalies	
• Spleen size	Hypersplenism
• History of drug exposure	Drug-associated neutropenia
• Complete blood count with differential and reticulocyte counts	Neutropenia, aplastic anemia, autoimmune cytopenias
IF ANC <1,000/µL	
EVALUATION OF ACUTE ONSET NEUTROPENIA	
• Repeat blood counts in 3-4 weeks	Transient myelosuppression (e.g., viral)
• Serology and cultures for infectious agents	Active or chronic infection with viruses (e.g., EBV, CMV), bacteria, mycobacteria, rickettsia
• Discontinue drug(s) associated with neutropenia	Drug-associated neutropenia
• Test for antineutrophil antibodies	Autoimmune neutropenia
• Measure quantitative immunoglobulins (G, A, and M), lymphocyte subsets	Neutropenia associated with disorders of immune function
IF ANC <500/µL ON 3 SEPARATE TESTS	
• Bone marrow aspiration and biopsy, with cytogenetics	Severe congenital neutropenia, Shwachman-Diamond syndrome, myelokathexis; chronic benign or idiopathic neutropenia
• Serial CBCs (3/week for 6 weeks)	Cyclic neutropenia
• Exocrine pancreatic function	Shwachman-Diamond syndrome
• Skeletal radiographs	Shwachman-Diamond syndrome, cartilage-hair hypoplasia, Fanconi anemia
IF ABSOLUTE LYMPHOCYTE COUNT <1000/µL	
• Repeat blood counts in 3-4 weeks	Transient leukopenia (e.g., viral)
IF ALC <1000/µL ON 3 SEPARATE TESTS	
• HIV-1 antibody test	HIV-1 infection, AIDS
• Quantitative immunoglobulins (G, A, and M), lymphocyte subsets	Congenital or acquired disorders of immune function
IF THERE IS PANCYTOPENIA	
• Bone marrow aspiration and biopsy	Bone marrow replacement by malignancy, fibrosis, granulomata, storage cells
• Bone marrow cytogenetics	Myelodysplasia, leukemia
• Vitamin B_{12} and folate levels	Vitamin deficiencies

ANC, absolute neutrophil count; CBC, complete blood count; CMV, cytomegalovirus; EBV, Epstein-Barr virus.

Table 125-2 CAUSES OF NEUTROPENIA EXTRINSIC TO MARROW MYELOID CELLS

CAUSE	ETIOLOGIC FACTORS/AGENTS	ASSOCIATED FINDINGS
Infection	Viruses, bacteria, protozoa, rickettsia, fungi	Redistribution from circulating to marginating pools, impaired production, accelerated destruction
Drug-induced	Phenothiazines, sulfonamides, anticonvulsants, penicillins, aminopyrine	Hypersensitivity reaction (fever, lymphadenopathy, rash, hepatitis, nephritis, pneumonitis, aplastic anemia), antineutrophil antibodies
Immune neutropenia	Alloimmune, autoimmune	Variable arrest from metamyelocyte to segmented neutrophils in bone marrow
Reticuloendothelial sequestration	Hypersplenism	Anemia, thrombocytopenia, neutropenia
Bone marrow replacement	Malignancy (lymphoma, metastatic solid tumor, etc.)	Presence of immature myeloid and erythroid precursors in peripheral blood
Cancer chemotherapy or radiation therapy to bone marrow	Suppression of myeloid cell production	Bone marrow hypoplasia, anemia, thrombocytosis

Etiology

Acute neutropenia evolving over a few days often occurs when neutrophil use is rapid and production is compromised. **Chronic neutropenia** lasting months or years can arise from reduced production, increased destruction, or excessive splenic sequestration of neutrophils. Neutropenia may be classified by whether it arises secondary to factors extrinsic to marrow myeloid cells (Table 125-2), which is common; as an acquired disorder of myeloid progenitor cells (Table 125-3), which is less common; or, more rarely, as an intrinsic defect affecting proliferation and maturation of myeloid progenitor cells (Table 125-4).

INFECTIOUS CAUSES Transient neutropenia often accompanies or follows viral infections (Table 125-5). Neutropenia associated with common childhood viral disease occurs during the 1st 1-2 days of illness and may persist for 3-8 days. It usually corresponds to a period of acute viremia and is related to virus-induced redistribution of neutrophils from the circulating to the marginating pool. Neutrophil sequestration possibly occurs after virus-induced tissue damage. Moderate to severe neutropenia may also be associated with a wide variety of other infectious causes. Bacterial sepsis is a particularly serious cause of neutropenia and neonates are particularly vulnerable to developing neutropenia

Table 125-3 ACQUIRED DISORDERS OF MYELOID CELLS

CAUSE	ETIOLOGIC FACTORS/AGENTS	ASSOCIATED FINDINGS
Aplastic anemia	Stem cell destruction and depletion	Pancytopenia
Vitamin B_{12} or folate deficiency	Malnutrition; congenital deficiency of B_{12} absorption, transport, and storage; vitamin avoidance	Megaloblastic anemia, hypersegmented neutrophils
Acute leukemia, chronic myelogenous leukemia	Bone marrow replacement with malignant cells	Pancytopenia, leukocytosis
Myelodysplasia	Dysplastic maturation of stem cells	Bone marrow hypoplasia with megaloblastoid red cell precursors, thrombocytopenia
Prematurity with birthweight <2 kg	Impaired regulation of myeloid proliferation and reduced size of postmitotic pool	Maternal preeclampsia
Chronic idiopathic neutropenia	Impaired myeloid proliferation and/or maturation	None
Paroxysmal nocturnal hemoglobinuria	Acquired stem cell defect secondary to mutation of *PIG-A* gene	Pancytopenia, thrombosis

Table 125-4 INTRINSIC DISORDERS OF MYELOID PRECURSOR CELLS

SYNDROME	INHERITANCE *(GENE)*	CLINICAL FEATURES (INCLUDING STATIC NEUTROPENIA UNLESS OTHERWISE NOTED)
PRIMARY DISORDERS OF MYELOPOIESIS		
Cyclic neutropenia	AD (*ELA2*)	Periodic oscillation (21-day cycles) in ANC
Severe congenital neutropenia	AD (*ELA2, GFI1, others*)	Risk of MDS and AML
	X-linked (*WAS*)	Neutropenic variant of Wiskott-Aldrich syndrome
Kostmann syndrome	AR (*HAX1*)	Neurological abnormalities, risk of MDS and AML
DISORDERS OF RIBOSOMAL FUNCTION		
Shwachman-Diamond syndrome	AR (*SBDS*)	Pancreatic insufficiency, variable neutropenia, other cytopenias, metaphysical dysostosis
Dyskeratosis congenita	Telomerase defects: XL (*DKC1*), AD (*TERC*), AR (*TERT*)	Nail dystrophy, leukoplakia, reticulated hyperpigmentation of the skin; 30-60% develop bone marrow failure
DISORDERS OF GRANULE SORTING		
Chédiak-Higashi syndrome	AR (*LYST*)	Partial albinism, giant granules in myeloid cells, platelet storage pool defect, impaired natural killer cell function, hemophagocytic lymphohistiocytosis
Griscelli syndrome, type II	AR (*RAB27a*)	Partial albinism, impaired natural killer cell function, hemophagocytic lymphohistiocytosis
Cohen syndrome	AR (*COH1*)	Partial albinism
Hermansky-Pudlak syndrome, type II	AR (*AP3P1*)	Cyclic neutropenia, partial albinism
p14 deficiency	probable AR (*MAPBPIP*)	Partial albinism, decreased B and T cells
DISORDERS OF METABOLISM		
Glycogen storage disease, type 1b	AR (*G6PT1*)	Hepatic enlargement, growth retardation, impaired neutrophil motility
G6Pase, catalytic subunit 3, deficiency	AR (*G6PC3*)	Structural heart defects, urogenital abnormalities, venous angiectasia
Barth syndrome	XL (*TAZ1*)	Episodic neutropenia, dilated cardiomyopathy, methylglutaconic aciduria
Pearson's syndrome	Mitochondrial (DNA deletions)	Episodic neutropenia, pancytopenia; defects in exocrine pancreas, liver, and kidneys
NEUTROPENIA IN DISORDERS OF IMMUNE FUNCTION		
Common variable immunodeficiency	Familial, sporadic (*TNFRSF13B*)	Hypogammaglobulinemia, other immune system defects
IgA deficiency	Unknown (Unknown or TNFRSF13B)	Decreased IgA
Severe combined immunodeficiency	AR, XL (multiple loci)	Absent humoral and cellular immune function
Hyper-IgM syndrome	XL (*HIGM1*)	Absent IgG, elevated IgM, autoimmune cytopenia
WHIM syndrome	AD (*CXCR4*)	Warts, hypogammaglobulinemia, infections, myelokathexis
Cartilage-hair hyperplasia	AR (*RMKP*)	Lymphopenia, short-limbed dwarfism, metaphysical chondrodysplasia, fine sparse hair
Schimke immuno-osseous dysplasia	probable AR (*SMARCAL1*)	Lymphopenia, pancytopenia, spondyloepiphyseal dysplasia, growth retardation, renal failure

AD, autosomal dominant; AML, acute myelogenous leukemia; ANC, absolute neutrophil count; AR, autosomal recessive; MDS, myelodysplasia; XL, X-linked.

because of a deficient pool of reserve neutrophils in the bone marrow.

Chronic neutropenia often accompanies infection with Epstein-Barr virus, cytomegalovirus, or HIV. The neutropenia associated with AIDS probably arises from a combination of impaired neutrophil production, the accelerated destruction of neutrophils mediated by antineutrophil antibodies, and sometimes effects of antiretroviral or other drugs.

DRUG-INDUCED NEUTROPENIA Drugs constitute one of the most common causes of neutropenia (Table 125-6). The incidence of drug-induced neutropenia increases dramatically with age; only 10% of cases occur among children and young adults, and the majority of cases among adults over age 65 yr. Drug-induced neutropenia has several underlying mechanisms (immune-mediated, toxic, idiosyncratic, hypersensitivity reactions) that are distinct from the severe neutropenia that predictably occurs after administration of cytoreductive cancer drugs or radiotherapy.

Drug-induced neutropenia due to immune mechanisms usually develops abruptly, is accompanied by fever, and lasts for about 1 wk after discontinuation of the drug. The process likely arises from effects of drugs such as propylthiouracil or penicillin that act as haptens to stimulate antibody formation, or drugs such as quinine that induce immune complex formation. Other drugs, including the antipsychotic drugs such as the phenothiazines, can cause neutropenia when given in toxic amounts, but some individuals, such as those with pre-existing neutropenia, may be susceptible to levels at the high end of the usual therapeutic range. Late-onset neutropenia can occur after rituximab therapy. Idiosyncratic reactions, for example to chloramphenicol, are unpredictable with regard to dose or duration of use. Hypersensitivity reactions are rare and may involve arene oxide metabolites of aromatic anticonvulsants. Fever, rash, lymphadenopathy, hepatitis, nephritis, pneumonitis, and aplastic anemia are often associated with hypersensitivity-induced neutropenia. Acute hypersensitivity reactions such as those caused by phenytoin or phenobarbital may last for only a few days if the offending drug is discontinued. Chronic hypersensitivity may last for months to years. Drug-induced neutropenia may occasionally be asymptomatic despite severely reduced numbers of neutrophils and is noted only because of regular monitoring of WBC counts during drug therapy.

Neutropenia commonly and predictably follows the use of anticancer drugs or radiation therapy, especially radiation therapy directed at the pelvis or vertebrae, secondary to cytotoxic effects on rapidly replicating myeloid precursors. A decline in the WBC count typically occurs 7-10 days after administration of the anticancer drug and may persist for 1-2 wk. The neutropenia accompanying malignancy or following cancer chemotherapy is frequently associated with compromised cellular immunity, thereby predisposing patients to a much greater risk of infection (Chapter 171) than found in disorders associated with isolated neutropenia.

Table 125-5 INFECTIONS THAT ARE ASSOCIATED WITH NEUTROPENIA

VIRAL
Respiratory syncytial virus
Dengue fever
Colorado tick fever
Mumps
Viral hepatitis
Infectious mononucleosis (Epstein-Barr virus)
Influenza
Measles
Rubella
Varicella
Cytomegalovirus
Human immunodeficiency virus
Sandfly fever
BACTERIAL
Pertussis
Typhoid fever
Paratyphoid fever
Tuberculosis (disseminated)
Brucellosis
Tularemia
Gram-negative sepsis
Psittacosis
FUNGAL
Histoplasmosis (disseminated)
PROTOZOA
Malaria
Leishmaniasis (kala-azar)
RICKETTSIAL
Rocky Mountain spotted fever
Typhus fever
Rickettsialpox

From Boxer LA, Blackwood RA: Leukocyte disorders: quantitative and qualitative disorders of the neutrophil, part 1, *Pediatr Rev* 17:19–28, 1996.

BONE MARROW REPLACEMENT Various acquired bone marrow disorders lead to neutropenia, usually accompanied by anemia and thrombocytopenia. Hematologic malignancies, including leukemia and lymphoma, and metastatic solid tumors (e.g., neuroblastoma, rhabdomyosarcoma, and Ewing sarcoma) suppress myelopoiesis by infiltrating the bone marrow. Neutropenia may also accompany myelodysplastic disorders or preleukemic syndromes, which are characterized by peripheral cytopenias and macrocytic blood cells associated with impaired survival of myeloid precursors. Aplastic anemia arising from damage (generally immune-mediated) and depletion of stem cells also causes neutropenia in the setting of pancytopenia.

RETICULOENDOTHELIAL SEQUESTRATION Splenic enlargement resulting from intrinsic splenic disease (e.g., storage disease), portal hypertension, or systemic causes of splenic hyperplasia (e.g., inflammation, neoplasia) can lead to neutropenia. The neutropenia is usually mild to moderate and accompanied by corresponding degrees of thrombocytopenia and anemia, and may be corrected by successfully treating the underlying disease. The reduced neutrophil survival corresponds to the size of the spleen, and the extent of the neutropenia is inversely proportional to bone marrow compensatory mechanisms. In selected cases, splenectomy may be necessary to restore the neutrophil count to normal but results in increased risk of infections by encapsulated bacterial organisms.

IMMUNE NEUTROPENIA Immune neutropenias are usually associated with the presence of circulating antineutrophil antibodies, which may mediate neutrophil destruction by complement-mediated lysis or splenic phagocytosis of opsonized neutrophils, or by accelerated apoptosis of mature neutrophils or myeloid precursors.

Alloimmune Neonatal Neutropenia

This form of neonatal neutropenia occurs after transplacental transfer of maternal alloantibodies directed against antigens on the infant's neutrophils, analogous to Rh hemolytic disease. Prenatal sensitization induces maternal IgG antibodies to neutrophil antigens on fetal cells. The antibodies are usually complement

Table 125-6 CHARACTERISTICS OF DRUG-INDUCED NEUTROPENIA

CHARACTERISTIC	IMMUNOLOGIC FORM	TOXIC FORM	HYPERSENSITIVITY FORM
Paradigm drugs	Aminopyrine, propylthiouracil, penicillin	Phenothiazine	Phenytoin, phenobarbital
Time to onset	Days to weeks	Weeks to months	Weeks to months
Clinical appearance	Acute, often explosive symptoms	Often asymptomatic or insidious onset	May be associated with fever, rash, nephritis, pneumonitis, or aplastic anemia
Rechallenge	Prompt recurrence with small test dose	Latent period; high doses required	Latent period; high doses required
Laboratory findings	Antibody test results positive	Evidence of direct toxicity to cells	Evidence of metabolite-mediated damage to cells

From Boxer LA: Approach to the patient with leukopenia. In Humes H, editor: *Kelley's textbook of internal medicine*, ed 4, Philadelphia, 2000, Lippincott Williams & Wilkins, p 1579.

activating and are frequently directed to neutrophil-specific antigens. Symptomatic infants may present with delayed separation of the umbilical cord, mild skin infections, fever, and pneumonia within the 1st 2 wk of life. The neutropenia is often severe and associated with fever and infections due to the usual microbes that cause neonatal disease. By 7 wk of age, the neutrophil count usually returns to normal, reflecting the decay of maternal antibodies in the infant's circulation. **Treatment** consists of supportive care and appropriate antibiotics for clinical infections.

Neonatal Passive Autoimmune Neutropenia

Mothers with autoimmune disease may give birth to infants who develop transient neutropenia. The duration of the neutropenia depends on the time required for the infant to clear the maternally transferred circulating IgG antibody. It persists in most cases for a few weeks to a few months. Neonates almost always remain asymptomatic.

Autoimmune Neutropenia

Autoimmune neutropenia is analogous to autoimmune hemolytic anemia and thrombocytopenia. Antibodies causing neutropenia have been detected in patients who have no other signs of autoimmune disease, in patients who have additional antibodies against red blood cells and/or platelets, and in patients who have a connective tissue disorder. Autoimmune neutropenia is distinguished from other forms of neutropenia only by the demonstration of antineutrophil antibodies and the appearance of myeloid hyperplasia on bone marrow examination. Antineutrophil antibody assays are quite prone to false-negative and false-positive results. Autoimmune neutropenia may occur in children with congenital or acquired immune deficiencies, including common variable immunodeficiency, dysgammaglobulinemias, or in the settings of systemic lupus erythematosus or autoimmune lymphoproliferative syndrome.

Treatment with recombinant human granulocyte colony–stimulating factor (rhG-CSF; filgrastim [Neupogen]) is generally effective at raising the ANC and preventing infection. Often, very low doses (<1-2 μg/kg/day) are effective, and administration of "standard" doses can lead to severe bone pain due to marrow expansion.

Autoimmune Neutropenia of Infancy (ANI)

This benign condition is diagnosed more frequently as techniques for detection of antineutrophil antibodies have become more available. The exact incidence of ANI remains unknown, but because of its benign nature, the disorder may be more common than currently appreciated. In 1 study, ANI occurred with an annual incidence of approximately 1/100,000 among children between infancy and 10 yr. All patients recognized as having ANI have severe neutropenia on presentation, with an ANC usually <500/μL, but the total WBC count is generally within normal limits. Monocytosis or eosinophilia may occur but does not affect the low rate of infection. The age at diagnosis is usually between 5 and 15 mo, with a female to male ratio of 6:4. None of the affected children has evidence of other autoimmune diseases. Children with ANI present with minor infections such as otitis media, gingivitis, respiratory tract infections, gastroenteritis, and cellulitis. The diagnosis often is considered only after the blood count reveals neutropenia. Occasionally, children may present with more severe infections, including pneumonia, sepsis, or abscesses. Longitudinal studies of infants with ANI demonstrate a median duration of disease of ≈7-24 mo. The diagnosis is established by the presence of antineutrophil antibodies in serum.

Treatment is not generally necessary, but rhG-CSF may be useful in providing temporary remission in infants with severe infections or requiring surgical intervention.

INEFFECTIVE MYELOPOIESIS

Extrinsic Disorders

Ineffective myelopoiesis may result from congenital or acquired vitamin B_{12} or folic acid deficiency. Megaloblastic pancytopenia also can result from extended use of antibiotics such as trimethoprim-sulfamethoxazole, which inhibit folic acid metabolism, and from the use of phenytoin, which may impair folate absorption in the small intestine. Neutropenia also occurs with starvation and marasmus in infants, with anorexia nervosa, and occasionally among patients receiving prolonged parenteral feedings without vitamin supplementation.

Intrinsic Disorders of Myeloid Precursors

The isolated disorders of proliferation and maturation of myeloid precursor cells are rare. Table 125-4 presents a classification based on genetics and molecular mechanisms; selected disorders are discussed in the next sections.

Primary Disorders of Granulocytopoiesis

Cyclic neutropenia, an autosomal dominant disorder, is characterized by regular, periodic oscillation in the number of peripheral neutrophils from normal to neutropenic values with a mean oscillatory period of 21 ± 3 days. During the neutropenic phase, most patients suffer from fever, stomatitis or pharyngitis, and occasionally lymph node enlargement. Serious infections may occur at the ANC nadirs, including pneumonia, periodontitis, and recurrent ulcerations of the oral, vaginal, and rectal mucosa, leading to life-threatening clostridial sepsis. Cyclic neutropenia arises from a regulatory abnormality involving early hematopoietic precursor cells and is associated with mutations in the neutrophil elastase gene, *ELA2*, that lead to accelerated apoptosis due to abnormal protein folding. Many patients experience abatement of symptoms with age. The cycles tend to become less noticeable in older patients, and the hematologic picture often begins to resemble that of chronic neutropenia. **Treatment** with rhG-CSF elevates the neutrophil counts and improves outcome.

Severe congenital neutropenia is characterized by an arrest in myeloid maturation at the promyelocyte stage in the bone marrow, resulting in consistent ANCs <200/μL. This disorder occurs sporadically or with autosomal dominant or recessive inheritance. The dominant form is caused most often by mutations in *ELA2*, while the recessive form (**Kostmann disease**) arises from mutations in *HAX1*, which protects cells against apoptosis. Patients typically show monocytosis and eosinophilia and suffer from recurrent, severe pyogenic infections, especially of the skin, mouth, and rectum. Anemia of chronic inflammation is often present. Approximately 20% of patients develop acute myelogenous leukemia or myelodysplasia associated with monosomy 7 and sometimes preceded by acquisition of mutations in the gene encoding the G-CSF receptor. Before the advent of **treatment** with rhG-CSF, most of these patients died of fatal infections before reaching adolescence.

Disorders of Ribosomal Function

Shwachman-Diamond syndrome is an autosomal recessive disorder characterized by pancreatic insufficiency and neutropenia. Shwachman-Diamond syndrome is caused by pro-apoptotic mutations of the *SBDS* gene, which encodes a protein that may play a role in ribosome biogenesis or RNA processing. The initial symptoms are usually diarrhea and failure to thrive because of malabsorption, which develops in almost all infants by 4 mo of age. Some patients have respiratory problems with pneumonia and frequent otitis media, as well as eczema. Virtually all patients with Shwachman-Diamond syndrome have neutropenia, with the ANC periodically <1,000/μL associated with hypoplastic myelopoiesis. Some children have been reported to have a chemotactic defect that may contribute to the increased susceptibility to pyogenic infection. The illness may progress to bone marrow hypoplasia with moderate thrombocytopenia and anemia. Myelodysplasia and acute myelogenous leukemia associated with monosomy 7 have also been reported in this syndrome. The neutropenia responds to treatment with rhG-CSF.

Granule Sorting Disorders

This constellation of very rare autosomal recessive disorders combine neutropenia with partial oculocutaneous albinism, immunodeficiencies, and other features, all derived from defects in formation or trafficking of lysosome-related organelles (see Table 125-4). **Treatment** usually includes hematopoietic stem cell transplantation.

Chédiak-Higashi syndrome, best known for the characteristic giant cytoplasmic granules in neutrophils, monocytes, and lymphocytes, is a disorder of subcellular vesicular dysfunction due to mutations in the *LYST* gene, with resultant fusion of cytoplasmic granules in all granule-bearing cells. Patients have increased susceptibility to infections, mild bleeding diathesis, progressive peripheral neuropathy, and predisposition to life-threatening hemophagocytic syndrome. The only curative treatment remains allogeneic stem cell transplantation.

Griscelli syndrome type II also features neutropenia, albinism, and a high risk of hemophagocytic syndrome, but peripheral blood granulocytes do not show giant granules. The autosomal recessive disorder is caused by mutations in *RAB27a*, which encodes a small GTPase that regulates granule secretory pathways.

Disorders of Metabolism

Recurrent infections with neutropenia are a distinctive feature of **glycogen storage disease (GSD) type Ib**. Both classic von Gierke glycogen storage disease (GSDIa) and GSDIb cause massive enlargement of liver and severe growth retardation (Chapter 81.1). In contrast to GSDIa, glucose-6-phosphatase (G6Pase) enzyme activity is normal, but mutations in the G6P transporter 1, *G6PT1*, inhibit glucose transport in GSDIb, resulting in both defective neutrophil motility and increased apoptosis associated with neutropenia and recurrent bacterial infections. **Treatment** with rhG-CSF can correct the neutropenia.

Metabolically related but phenotypically distinct mutations in *G6PC3*, encoding glucose-6-phosphatase, catalytic subunit 3, result in neutropenia with heart defects, urogenital abnormalities, and venous angiectasia but not symptomatic disruption of glucose transport.

NEUTROPENIA IN DISORDERS OF IMMUNE FUNCTION

Congenital immunologic disorders that have severe neutropenia as a clinical feature include common variable immunodeficiency, the severe combined immunodeficiencies, hyper-IgM syndrome, WHIM syndrome, and a number of even rarer immunodeficiency syndromes (see Table 125-4).

Unclassified Disorders

Acquired **idiopathic chronic neutropenia** is characterized by onset of neutropenia after 2 yr of age. Patients with an ANC persistently <500/µL are afflicted with recurrent pyogenic infections involving the skin, mucous membranes, lungs, and lymph nodes. Bone marrow examination reveals variable patterns of myeloid formation with arrest generally occurring between the myelocyte and band forms (see Table 125-3). Often there is overlap with the diagnoses of chronic benign or autoimmune neutropenias.

Chronic benign neutropenia of childhood represents a common group of disorders characterized by mild to moderate neutropenia that does not lead to an increased risk of pyogenic infections. Spontaneous remissions are often reported, although these may represent misdiagnosis of autoimmune neutropenia of infancy, in which remissions occur commonly during childhood. Chronic benign neutropenia may be inherited in either a dominant or recessive form. An autosomal recessive form of benign neutropenia is encountered in Yemenite Jews. Because of the relatively low risk of serious infection, patients should be not subjected to the potentially toxic therapy.

Clinical Manifestations of Neutropenia

Individuals with neutrophil counts <500/µL are at substantial risk for developing infections, primarily from their endogenous flora as well as from nosocomial organisms. Some patients with isolated chronic neutropenia with an ANC <200/µL may not experience many serious infections, probably because the remainder of the immune system remains intact. In contrast, children whose neutropenia is secondary to acquired disorders of production such as with cytotoxic therapy, immunosuppressive drugs, or radiation therapy are likely to develop serious bacterial infections because many arms of the immune system are markedly compromised.

Neutropenia associated with leukopenia, that is, additional monocytopenia or lymphocytopenia, is more highly associated with serious infection than neutropenia alone. The integrity of skin and mucous membranes, the vascular supply to tissues, and nutritional status also influence the risk of infection.

The most common **clinical presentation of profound neutropenia** includes fever >38°C, aphthous stomatitis and gingivitis, cellulitis, furunculosis, perirectal inflammation, colitis, sinusitis, and otitis media are also frequent accompaniments of profound neutropenia in children. Other clinical manifestations of profound neutropenia include hepatic abscesses, recurrent pneumonias, and septicemia. Isolated neutropenia does not heighten a patient's susceptibility to parasitic or viral infections or to bacterial meningitis.

The most common pathogens causing infections in neutropenic patients are *Staphylococcus aureus* and gram-negative bacteria. The usual signs and symptoms of local infection and inflammation such as exudate, fluctuance, and regional lymphadenopathy are generally diminished in the absence of neutrophils because of the inability to form pus. Patients with complete agranulocytosis still experience fever and feel pain at sites of inflammation.

Laboratory Findings

Isolated absolute neutropenia has a limited number of causes (see Tables 125-1 through 125-4). The duration and severity of the neutropenia greatly influence the extent of laboratory evaluation. Patients with chronic neutropenia since infancy and a history of recurrent fevers and chronic gingivitis should have WBC counts and differential counts determined 3 times weekly for 6 wk to evaluate the periodicity suggestive of cyclic neutropenia. Bone marrow aspiration and biopsy should be performed on selected patients to assess cellularity. Additional marrow studies such as cytogenetic analysis and special stains for detecting leukemia and other malignant disorders should be obtained for patients with suspected intrinsic defects in the myeloid progenitors and for patients with suspected malignancy. Selection of further laboratory tests is determined by the duration and severity of the neutropenia and the associated findings on physical examination (see Table 125-1).

Treatment

The management of acquired transient neutropenia associated with malignancies, myelosuppressive chemotherapy, or immunosuppressive chemotherapy differs from that of congenital or chronic forms of neutropenia. In the former situation, infections sometimes are heralded only by fever, and sepsis is a major cause of death. Early recognition and treatment of infections may be lifesaving (Chapter 171).

Therapy of severe chronic neutropenia is dictated by the clinical manifestations. Patients with benign neutropenia and no evidence of repeated bacterial infections or chronic gingivitis require no specific therapy. Superficial infections in children with mild to moderate neutropenia may be treated with appropriate oral antibiotics. In patients who have invasive or life-threatening infections, broad-spectrum intravenous antibiotics should be started promptly.

Subcutaneously administered rhG-CSF can provide effective treatment of severe chronic neutropenia including severe congenital neutropenia, chronic symptomatic idiopathic neutropenia, and cyclic neutropenia. Doses ranging from 2 to over 100 µg/kg/day lead to dramatic increases in neutrophil counts, resulting in marked attenuation of infection and inflammation. rhG-CSF, often at very low doses, may also benefit patients who have immune or drug-induced neutropenias. The long-term effects of rhG-CSF therapy are unknown but include a propensity for the development of moderate splenomegaly, thrombocytopenia, and, occasionally, vasculitis. Autoimmune neutropenia may be responsive to intermittent corticosteroids, especially if it is part of an underlying disease process such as systemic lupus erythematosus.

Patients with severe congenital neutropenia or Shwachman-Diamond syndrome who develop myelodysplasia or acute myelogenous leukemia respond only to allogeneic stem cell transplantation. Chemotherapy is ineffective. Hematopoietic stem cell transplantation is also the treatment of choice for aplastic anemia or hemophagocytic lymphohistiocytosis complicating syndromes discussed earlier.

Table 125-7 CAUSES OF LYMPHOCYTOPENIA

ACQUIRED CAUSES
Infectious Diseases
AIDS
Viral hepatitis
Influenza
Tuberculosis
Typhoid fever
Sepsis
Iatrogenic
Immunosuppressive therapy
Corticosteroids
High-dose PUVA therapy
Cytotoxic chemotherapy
Radiation
Thoracic duct drainage
Systemic and Other Diseases
Systemic lupus erythematosus
Myasthenia gravis
Hodgkin disease
Protein-losing enteropathy
Renal failure
Sarcoidosis
Thermal injury
Aplastic anemia
Dietary Deficiency
Dietary deficiency associated with ethanol abuse
INHERITED CAUSES
Aplasia of lymphopoietic stem cells
Severe combined immunodeficiency
Ataxia-telangiectasia
Wiskott-Aldrich syndrome
Immunodeficiency with thymoma
Cartilage-hair hypoplasia
Idiopathic CD4 T lymphocytopenia

ADA, adenosine deaminase; IL-2, interleukin 2; PNP, purine nucleoside phosphorylase; PUVA, psoralen and ultraviolet A irradiation.
From Boxer LA: Approach to the patient with leukopenia. In Humes HD, editor: *Kelley's textbook of internal medicine*, ed 4, Philadelphia, 2000, Lippincott Williams & Wilkins, p 1580.

LYMPHOPENIA

Lymphopenia by itself usually causes no symptoms and is often detected in the evaluation of other illnesses, particularly recurrent viral, fungal, and parasitic infections. Lymphocyte subpopulations can be measured by multiparameter flow cytometry, which uses the pattern of antigen expression to classify and characterize these cells.

Inherited Causes of Lymphocytopenia

Inherited immunodeficiency disorders may have a quantitative or qualitative stem cell abnormality resulting in ineffective lymphocytopoiesis (Table 125-7). Other disorders such as Wiskott-Aldrich syndrome may have associated lymphocytopenia arising from accelerated destruction of T cells. A similar mechanism is present in patients with adenosine deaminase deficiency and purine nucleoside phosphorylase deficiency. Lymphocyte counts may also be decreased in some forms of inherited bone marrow failure, such as reticular dysgenesis, severe congenital neutropenia secondary to *GFI1* mutation, or dyskeratosis congenita.

Acquired Lymphocytopenia

AIDS is the most common infectious disease associated with lymphocytopenia, which results from destruction of CD4 T cells infected with HIV-1 or HIV-2. Other viral and bacterial diseases may be associated with lymphocytopenia. In some instances of acute viremia with other viral infections, lymphocytes may undergo accelerated destruction from intracellular viral replication, become trapped in the spleen or nodes, or migrate to the respiratory tract.

Systemic autoimmune diseases such as systemic lupus erythematosus are associated with lymphocytopenia. Other conditions such as protein-losing enteropathy and aberrant or surgical drainage of the thoracic duct are associated with lymphocyte depletion. Iatrogenic lymphocytopenia may be caused by cytotoxic chemotherapy, radiation therapy, and administration of antilymphocyte globulin. Long-term treatment of psoriasis with psoralen and ultraviolet irradiation may also destroy T lymphocytes. Corticosteroids can cause lymphopenia through increased cell destruction.

BIBLIOGRAPHY

Please visit the Nelson Textbook of Pediatrics *website at www.expertconsult.com for the complete bibliography.*

Chapter 126 Leukocytosis

Laurence A. Boxer and Peter E. Newburger

Leukocytosis is an elevation in the total leukocyte, or white blood cell (WBC), count that is 2 standard deviations above the mean count for a particular age (Chapter 708). The various causes of leukocytosis are categorized by the class of leukocyte that is elevated and whether the process is acute, chronic, or lifelong. To evaluate the patient with leukocytosis, it is critical to determine which class of WBCs is elevated, and also the duration and extent of the leukocytosis. Each blood count should be evaluated with regard to the absolute number of cells/µL and the normal range for the patient's age.

For the full continuation of this chapter, please visit the Nelson Textbook of Pediatrics *website at www.expertconsult.com.*

Section 4 THE COMPLEMENT SYSTEM

Chapter 127
The Complement System
Richard B. Johnston, Jr.

Complement was originally defined as the nonspecific, heat-labile complementary principle required with specific antibody to lyse bacteria. The 1st 4 components were numbered in the order of their discovery and are termed the classical pathway. Unfortunately, the components fix to the immune complex in a different order, C1423. Beyond this confusing start, complement is a logical, exquisitely balanced, and highly influential system that is fundamental to the clinical expression of host defense and inflammation.

For the full continuation of this chapter, please visit the Nelson Textbook of Pediatrics *website at www.expertconsult.com.*

Chapter 128
Disorders of the Complement System

128.1 Evaluation of the Complement System
Richard B. Johnston, Jr.

Testing for **total hemolytic complement activity** (CH_{50}) effectively screens for most of the diseases of the complement system. A normal result in this assay depends on the ability of all 11 components of the classical pathway and membrane attack complex to interact and lyse antibody-coated sheep erythrocytes. The dilution of serum that lyses 50% of the cells determines the endpoint. In **congenital deficiencies** of C1 through C8, the CH_{50} value is 0 or close to 0; in C9 deficiency, the value is approximately half-normal. Values in the acquired deficiencies vary with the type and severity of the underlying disorder. This assay does not detect deficiency of mannose-binding lectin (MBL), factors D or B of the alternative pathway, or properdin. Deficiency of factors I or H permits consumption of C3, with partial reduction in the CH_{50} value. When clotted blood or serum sits at room temperature or warms, CH_{50} activity begins to decline, which leads to values that are falsely low but not zero. It is important to separate the serum and freeze it at −70°C by no more than an hour after blood draw.

In **hereditary angioedema,** depression of C4 and C2 during an attack significantly reduces the CH_{50}. Typically, C4 is low and C3 normal or slightly decreased. Concentrations of C1 inhibitor protein will be normal in 15% of cases; but C1 acts as an esterase, and the diagnosis can be established by showing increased capacity of patients' sera to hydrolyze synthetic esters.

A decrease in serum concentration of both C4 and C3 suggests activation of the **classical pathway** by immune complexes. Decreased C3 and normal C4 levels suggest activation of the **alternative pathway.** This difference is particularly useful in distinguishing nephritis secondary to immune complex deposition from that due to NeF (nephritic factor). In the latter condition and in deficiency of factor I or H, factor B is consumed and C3 serum concentration is low. Alternative pathway activity can be measured with a relatively simple and reproducible hemolytic assay that depends on the capacity of rabbit erythrocytes to serve as both an activating (permissive) surface and a target of alternative pathway activity. This assay (AP_{50}) detects deficiency of properdin, factor D, and factor B. Immunochemical methods can be used to quantify individual components of all 3 pathways, guided by results of the screening hemolytic assays. It is possible to analyze the genes encoding many of the components.

A defect of complement function should be considered in any patient with recurrent angioedema, autoimmune disease, chronic nephritis, hemolytic-uremic syndrome (HUS), or partial lipodystrophy, or with recurrent pyogenic infections, disseminated meningococcal or gonococcal infection, or a second episode of bacteremia at any age. A previously well adolescent or young adult with meningococcal meningitis due to an uncommon serotype (not A, B, or C) should undergo screening for a late-component or alternative pathway deficiency with CH_{50} and AP_{50} assays.

BIBLIOGRAPHY

Please visit the Nelson Textbook of Pediatrics *website at www.expertconsult.com for the complete bibliography.*

128.2 Genetic Deficiencies of Complement Components
Richard B. Johnston, Jr.

Congenital deficiencies of all 11 components of the classical-membrane attack pathway and of factor D and properdin of the alternative pathway are described (Table 128-1). All of the components of the classical and alternative pathways except properdin are inherited as autosomal recessive co-dominant traits. Each parent transmits a gene that codes for synthesis of half the serum level of the component. Deficiency results from inheritance of 1 null gene from each parent; the hemizygous parents typically have CH_{50} levels that are low normal. Properdin deficiency is transmitted as an X-linked trait.

Most patients with primary **C1q deficiency** have systemic lupus erythematosus (SLE), an SLE-like syndrome without typical SLE serology, a chronic rash that has shown an underlying vasculitis on biopsy, or membranoproliferative glomerulonephritis (MPGN). Some C1q-deficient children have serious infections, including septicemia and meningitis. Individuals with **C1r, C1s, combined C1r/C1s, C4, C2,** or **C3 deficiency** also have a high incidence of autoimmune syndromes (see Table 128-1), especially SLE or an SLE-like syndrome in which antinuclear antibody level is not elevated.

C4 is encoded by 2 genes, termed C4A and C4B. **C4 deficiency** represents absence of both gene products. Complete deficiency of only C4A, present in about 1% of the population, also predisposes to SLE, though C4 levels are only partially reduced. Patients with only C4B deficiency may be predisposed to infection. A few patients with **C5, C6, C7,** or **C8 deficiency** have SLE, but recurrent meningococcal infections are much more likely to be the major problem.

The reason for the concurrence of deficiencies of complement components, especially C1, C4, C2, or C3 deficiency, and autoimmune-immune complex diseases is not entirely clear, but deposition of C3 on autoimmune complexes facilitates their removal from the circulation through binding to complement receptor 1

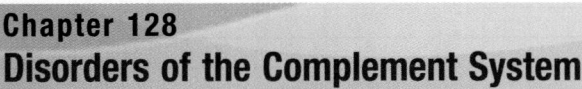

Table 128-1 GENETIC DEFICIENCIES OF PLASMA COMPLEMENT COMPONENTS AND ASSOCIATED CLINICAL FINDINGS

DEFICIENT COMPONENT	INFECTION* Very Common	Common	Occasional	AUTOIMMUNE/IMMUNE COMPLEX DISEASE* Very Common	Common	Occasional
CLASSICAL PATHWAY						
C1q			Pneumococcal B/M, other pyogenic	SLE	GN	DV/DLE
C1r, C1s, C1rs		Other pyogenic	Pneumococcal B/M, DGI	SLE	Other AD	GN
C4		Other pyogenic		SLE	GN, other AD	
C2		Other pyogenic, pneumococcal B/M, meningococcal M			SLE, GN, DV/DLE, other AD	
C3	Other pyogenic	Pneumococcal B/M, meningococcal M			GN, DV/DLE	SLE, other AD
C5	Meningococcal M	DGI	Other pyogenic			SLE, GN
C6	Meningococcal M	DGI	Other pyogenic			SLE, GN, other AD
C7	Meningococcal M		DGI, other pyogenic		SLE, other AD	
C8	Meningococcal M	DGI	Other pyogenic			SLE, GN
C9		Meningococcal M				
LECTIN PATHWAY						
MBL			Other pyogenic, fungal, HIV			SLE
MASP-2			Pneumococcal pneumonia			SLE
Ficolin-3			Other pyogenic			
ALTERNATIVE PATHWAY						
Factor D	DGI, meningococcal M, other pyogenic					
CONTROL PROTEINS						
C1 INH	Hereditary angioedema†					SLE
Factor I	Other pyogenic, meningococcal M	Pneumococcal B/M				
Factor H		Meningococcal B/M	Other pyogenic		GN, aHUS	SLE
Properdin		Meningococcal M	Pneumococcal B/M, other pyogenic		DV/DLE	
C4-binding protein						Other AD

*A finding was reported as "very common" if it occurred in 50% or more of reported cases, "common" if reported in about 5-50% of cases, and "occasional" if present in one or two cases or <5% of the more frequent deficiencies.

†Hereditary angioedema is not typically associated with infection or autoimmunity.

aHUS, atypical hemolytic-uremic syndrome; B/M, bacteremia and/or meningitis; DGI, disseminated gonococcal infection; DV/DLE, dermal vasculitis or typical discoid lupus erythematosus; GN, glomerulonephritis in various forms, often membranoproliferative; HIV, human immunodeficiency virus; M, meningitis; MASP, MBL-associated serine protease; MBL, mannose-binding lectin; other AD, autoimmune disease (almost all possible diagnoses have been reported); other pyogenic, serious deep or systemic infection due to, or typically caused by, a pyogenic bacterium (abscess, osteomyelitis, pneumonia, bacteremia other than pneumococcal, meningitis other than meningococcal or pneumococcal, cellulitis, myopericarditis, and peritonitis); SLE, typical systemic lupus erythematosus or an SLE-like syndrome without characteristic serologic findings.

Data from Figueroa JE, Densen P: Infectious diseases associated with complement deficiencies, *Clin Microbiol Rev* 4:359–395, 1991; Ross SC, Densen P: Complement deficiency states and infection: epidemiology, pathogenesis and consequences of neisserial and other infections in an immune deficiency, *Medicine* 63:243–273, 1984; and other cases and series reported to date.

(CR1) on erythrocytes and transport to the spleen and liver. The early components, particularly C1q and C3, expedite the clearance of necrotic and apoptotic cells, which are sources of autoantigens. Inefficiency of either or both of these processes might explain the concurrence of autoimmune disease and complement deficiency.

Individuals with **C2 deficiency** are predisposed to life-threatening septicemic illnesses, most commonly due to pneumococci. Most have not had problems with increased susceptibility to infection, presumably because of the protective function of the alternative pathway. The genes for C2, factor B, and C4 are situated close to each other on chromosome 6, and a partial depression of factor B levels can occur in conjunction with C2 deficiency. Persons with a deficiency of both proteins may be at particular risk.

Because C3 can be activated by C142 or by the alternative pathway, a defect in the function of either pathway can be compensated for, at least to some extent. Without C3, however, opsonization of bacteria is inefficient, and the chemotactic fragment from C5 (C5a) is not generated. Some organisms must be well opsonized in order to be cleared, and genetic **C3 deficiency** has been associated with recurrent, severe pyogenic infections due to pneumococci and meningococci.

More than half of the individuals reported to have congenital **C5, C6, C7,** or **C8 deficiency** have had meningococcal meningitis or extragenital gonococcal infection. Patients with **C9 deficiency** retain about one-third normal CH_{50} titers; some of these patients have also had *Neisseria* disease. In studies of patients ≥10 yr of age with systemic meningococcal disease, 3-15% have had a genetic deficiency of C5, C6, C7, C8, C9, or properdin. Among patients with infections caused by the uncommon *Neisseria meningitidis* serogroups (X, Y, Z, W135, 29E, or nongroupable; not A, B, or C), 33-45% have an underlying complement deficiency. It is not clear why patients with a deficiency of 1 of the late-acting components suffer a particular predisposition to *Neisseria* infections. It may be that serum bacteriolysis is uniquely important in defense against this organism. Many persons with such a deficiency have no significant illness.

A few individuals have been identified with **deficiency of factor D** of the alternative pathway, all with recurrent infections, most often neisserial. Hemolytic complement activity and C3 levels in their serum were normal, but alternative pathway activity was markedly deficient or absent. Complete factor B deficiency has not been described.

Mutations in the structural gene encoding MBL or polymorphisms in the promoter region of the gene result in pronounced interindividual variation in the level of circulating MBL. More than 90% of individuals with **MBL deficiency** do not express a predisposition to infection. Those with a very low level of MBL have a predisposition to recurrent respiratory infections in infancy and to serious pyogenic and fungal infections if there is another underlying defect of host defense. **MASP-2 deficiency** has been reported with SLE-like symptoms and recurrent pneumococcal pneumonia. Homozygous **ficolin-3 deficiency** has been associated with repeated pneumonia since early childhood, cerebral abscesses, and bronchiectasis.

BIBLIOGRAPHY

Please visit the Nelson Textbook of Pediatrics *website at* *www.expertconsult.com* *for the complete bibliography.*

128.3 Deficiencies of Plasma, Membrane, or Serosal Complement Control Proteins

Richard B. Johnston, Jr.

Congenital deficiencies of 5 plasma complement control proteins have been described (see Table 128-1). **Factor I deficiency** was reported originally as a deficiency of C3 resulting from hypercatabolism. The 1st patient described had suffered a series of severe pyogenic infections similar to those associated with agammaglobulinemia or congenital deficiency of C3. Factor I is an essential regulator of both pathways. Its deficiency permits prolonged existence of C3b in the C3 convertase of the alternative pathway, C3bBb, resulting in constant activation of the alternative pathway and cleavage of more C3 to C3b, in circular fashion. Intravenous infusion of plasma or purified factor I induced a prompt rise in serum C3 concentration in the patient and a return to normal of in vitro C3-dependent functions such as opsonization.

The effects of **factor H deficiency** are like those of factor I deficiency because factor H assists in dismantling the alternative pathway C3 convertase. Levels of C3, factor B, total hemolytic activity, and alternative pathway activity have been low or undetectable in these patients. Patients have sustained systemic infections due to pyogenic bacteria, particularly *N. meningitidis.* Many have had glomerulonephritis or atypical HUS (aHUS) (Chapter 512). Mutations in genes encoding membrane cofactor protein (MCP), factors I or B, C3, or the endothelial anti-inflammatory protein thrombomodulin, or autoantibodies to factor H, have also been associated with aHUS. The few patients thus far reported as having **C4-binding protein deficiency** have about 25% of the normal levels of the protein and no typical disease presentation, although one had angioedema and Behçet disease.

Persons with **properdin deficiency** have a striking predisposition to *N. meningitidis* meningitis. All reported patients have had been male. The predisposition to infection in these patients demonstrates clearly the need for the alternative pathway in defense against bacterial infection. Serum hemolytic complement activity is normal in these patients, and if the patient has specific antibacterial antibody, the need for the alternative pathway and properdin is greatly reduced. Several patients have had dermal vasculitis or discoid lupus.

Hereditary angioedema occurs in persons unable to synthesize normal levels of active C1 inhibitor (C1 INH). In 85% of affected families, the patient has markedly reduced concentrations of inhibitor, averaging 30% of normal; the other 15% have normal or elevated concentrations of an immunologically cross-reacting but nonfunctional protein. Both forms of the disease are transmitted as autosomal dominant traits. C1 INH suppresses the complement proteases C1rs and MASP-2 and the activated proteases of the contact and fibrinolysis systems. In doing so, C1 INH, is consumed as a "suicide inhibitor." Thus, in the absence of full C1 INH function, activation of any of these proteases tips the balance toward the protease. This activation leads to uncontrolled C1 and kallikrein activity with breakdown of C4 and C2 and release of bradykinin, which interacts with vascular endothelial cells to cause vasodilation and localized, nonpitting edema. The biochemical triggers that induce attacks of angioedema in these patients are not clearly defined.

Swelling of the affected part progresses rapidly, without urticaria, itching, discoloration, or redness and often without severe pain. Swelling of the intestinal wall, however, can lead to intense abdominal cramping, sometimes with vomiting or diarrhea. Concomitant subcutaneous edema is often absent, and patients have undergone abdominal surgery or psychiatric examination before the true diagnosis was established. Laryngeal edema can be fatal. Attacks last 2-3 days and then gradually abate. They may occur at sites of trauma, especially dental, after vigorous exercise, or with menses, fever, or emotional stress. Attacks can begin in the 1st two years of life but are usually not severe until late childhood or adolescence. **Acquired C1 INH deficiency** can occur in association with B-cell cancer or autoantibody to C1 INH. SLE and glomerulonephritis have been reported in patients with the congenital disease.

Three of the membrane complement control proteins—CR1, membrane cofactor protein (CD46), and decay-accelerating factor (DAF)—prevent the formation of the full C3-cleaving enzyme, C3bBb, which is triggered by C3b deposition. CD59 (membrane inhibitor of reactive lysis) prevents the full development of the membrane attack complex that creates the "hole." **Paroxysmal nocturnal hemoglobinuria** (PNH) is a hemolytic anemia that occurs when DAF and CD59 are not expressed on the erythrocyte surface. The condition is acquired as a somatic mutation in a hematopoietic stem cell of the *PIG-A* gene on the X chromosome. The product of this gene is required for normal synthesis of a glycosyl-phosphatidylinositol molecule that anchors about 20 proteins to cell membranes, including DAF and CD59. One patient with **genetic isolated CD59 deficiency** had a mild PNH-like disease in spite of normal expression of membrane DAF. In contrast, **genetic isolated DAF deficiency** has not resulted in hemolytic anemia.

BIBLIOGRAPHY

Please visit the Nelson Textbook of Pediatrics *website at* *www.expertconsult.com* *for the complete bibliography.*

128.4 Secondary Disorders of Complement

Richard B. Johnston, Jr.

Partial deficiency of C1q has occurred in patients with severe combined immunodeficiency disease or hypogammaglobulinemia, apparently secondary to the deficiency of IgG, which normally binds reversibly to C1q and prevents its rapid catabolism.

Chronic membranoproliferative glomerulonephritis (MPGN) can be due to **nephritic factor** (NeF), an IgG autoantibody to the C3-cleaving enzyme of the alternative pathway, C3bBb, which protects the enzyme from inactivation and promotes overactivation of the alternative pathway. The result is increased consumption of C3 and decreased concentration of serum C3. Pyogenic infections, including meningitis, may occur if the serum C3 level drops to <10% of normal. This disorder has been found in children and adults with **partial lipodystrophy**. Adipocytes are the main source of factor D and synthesize C3 and factor B; exposure to NeF induces their lysis. An IgG nephritic factor that binds to and protects C42, the classical pathway C3 convertase, has been described in acute postinfectious nephritis and in SLE. The consumption of C3 that characterizes poststreptococcal nephritis and SLE could be due to this factor, to complement activation by immune complexes, or to both.

Newborn infants have mild to moderate reductions in all plasma components of the complement system. Opsonization and generation of chemotactic activity in serum from full-term newborns can be markedly deficient through either the classical or alternative pathway. Complement activity is even lower in preterm infants. Patients with severe chronic cirrhosis of the liver, hepatic failure, malnutrition, or anorexia nervosa can have significant deficiency of complement components and functional activity. Synthesis of components is depressed in these conditions, and serum from some patients with malnutrition also contains immune complexes that could accelerate depletion.

Patients with **sickle cell disease** have normal activity of the classical pathway, but some have defective function of the alternative pathway in opsonization of pneumococci, in bacteriolysis and opsonization of *Salmonella,* and in lysis of rabbit erythrocytes. Deoxygenation of erythrocytes from patients with sickle cell disease alters their membranes to increase exposure of phospholipids that can activate the alternative pathway and consume its components. This activation is accentuated during painful crisis. An alternative pathway defect has been described in about 10% of individuals who have undergone splenectomy, and in some patients with β-thalassemia major. The underlying mechanism for this defect in these last 2 conditions is not known. Children with nephrotic syndrome may have decreased serum levels of factors B and D and subnormal serum opsonizing activity.

Immune complexes initiated by microorganisms or their byproducts can induce complement consumption. Activation occurs primarily through fixation of C1 and initiation of the classical pathway. Formation of immune complexes and consumption of complement have been demonstrated in lepromatous leprosy, bacterial endocarditis, infected ventriculojugular shunts, malaria, infectious mononucleosis, dengue hemorrhagic fever, and acute hepatitis B. Nephritis or arthritis can develop as a result of deposition of immune complexes and activation of complement in these infections. In SLE, immune complexes activate C142, and C3 is deposited at sites of tissue damage, including kidneys and skin; depressed synthesis of C3 is also noted. The syndrome of recurrent urticaria, angioedema, eosinophilia, and hypocomplementemia secondary to activation of the classical pathway may be due to autoantibody to C1q and circulating immune complexes. Circulating immune complexes and decreased C3 have been reported in some patients with dermatitis herpetiformis, celiac disease, primary biliary cirrhosis, and Reye syndrome.

Circulating bacterial products in sepsis or tissue factors released after severe trauma can initiate activation of the classical and alternative pathways, leading to respiratory distress syndrome and multiple organ failure. Intravenous injection of iodinated roentgenographic contrast medium can trigger a rapid and significant activation of the alternative pathway, which may explain the occasional reactions that occur in patients undergoing this procedure.

Burns can induce massive activation of the complement system, especially the alternative pathway, within a few hours after injury. Resulting generation of C3a and C5a stimulates neutrophils and induces their sequestration in the lungs, leading to shock lung. Cardiopulmonary bypass, ECMO, plasma exchange, or hemodialysis using cellophane membranes may be associated with a similar syndrome due to activation of plasma complement, with release of C3a and C5a. In patients with erythropoietic protoporphyria or porphyria cutanea tarda, exposure of the skin to light of certain wavelengths activates complement, generating chemotactic activity. This chemotactic activity results in lysis of capillary endothelial cells, mast cell degranulation, and the appearance of neutrophils in the dermis.

Some tumor cells can avoid complement-mediated lysis by overexpressing DAF, MCP, CD59, CR1, or factor H or by secreting proteases that cleave tumor-bound C3b. Microorganisms have evolved similar evasive mechanisms; for example, HIV-1 particles budding from infected cells acquire the membrane proteins DAF and CD59.

BIBLIOGRAPHY

Please visit the Nelson Textbook of Pediatrics *website at* www.expertconsult.com *for the complete bibliography.*

128.5 Treatment of Complement Disorders

Richard B. Johnston, Jr.

No specific therapy is available at present for genetic deficiencies of the complement system except hereditary angioedema, but much can be done to protect patients with any of these disorders from serious complications. Management of hereditary angioedema starts with avoidance of precipitating factors, usually trauma. Infusion of C1 INH concentrate or a kallikrein inhibitor are approved in the USA for use in adolescents and adults for long-term prophylaxis, preparation of surgery or dental procedures, or treatment of acute attacks. The synthetic androgen oxandrolone increases the level of functional C1 INH severalfold and is approved for cautious use in children. Antihistamines, adrenalin, and corticosteroids have no effect. Agents that block the bradykinin receptor or inhibit kallikrein are under development.

Effective supportive management is available for other primary diseases of the complement system, and identification of a specific defect in the complement system can have an important impact on management. Concern for the associated complications such as autoimmune disease and infection should encourage vigorous diagnostic efforts and earlier institution of therapy. Individuals with SLE and a complement defect generally respond as well to therapy as those without complement deficiency. With the onset of unexplained fever, cultures should be obtained and antibiotic therapy instituted more quickly and with less stringent indications than in a normal child. The parent or patient should be given letters describing any predisposition to systemic bacterial infection or autoimmune disease associated with the patient's deficiency, along with the recommended approach to management, for possible use by school, camp, or emergency room physicians. The patient and close household contacts should be immunized against *Haemophilus influenzae, Streptococcus pneumoniae,* and *N. meningitidis.* High titers of specific antibody might opsonize effectively without the full complement system, and immunization of household members could reduce the risk of exposing patients to these particularly threatening pathogens. Repeat immunization of patients is advisable since complement deficiency can be associated with a blunted or shorter-lived antibody response than normal.

Considering the many conditions in which complement is a central mediator of disease, there is an intensive effort to develop therapeutic complement inhibitors. These include soluble CR1 and inhibitors of C5 convertase and C3a and C5a binding. Heparin, which inhibits both classical and alternative pathways, has been used to prevent "post-pump syndrome."

Section 5 HEMATOPOIETIC STEM CELL TRANSPLANTATION

Chapter 129
Principles and Clinical Indications

Andrea Velardi and Franco Locatelli

Thousands of children have received an infusion of either **allogeneic** or **autologous** (from the same individual) hematopoietic stem cells to cure both malignant and nonmalignant disorders. **Autologous** transplantation is employed as a rescue strategy after delivering otherwise lethal doses of radiotherapy and chemotherapy in children with hematological malignancies or solid tumors. **Allogeneic** transplantation is used to treat children with genetic diseases of blood cells, such as thalassemia and primary immunodeficiency diseases, as well as hematologic malignancies, such as leukemia and lymphoma. Bone marrow has traditionally represented the source of hematopoietic progenitors employed. Growth factor (G-CSF)-mobilized peripheral blood hematopoietic stem cells and umbilical cord blood hematopoietic progenitors have been introduced in the clinical practice to perform hematopoietic stem cell transplantation (HSCT).

In addition, a human leukocyte antigen (HLA)-matched sibling had been the only type of donor employed. Currently, matched unrelated volunteers, full-haplotype mismatched family members, and unrelated cord blood donors have also been employed to transplant patients lacking an HLA-identical relative.

Protocols for allogeneic HSCT consist of 2 parts: the preparative regimen and transplantation itself. During the **preparative conditioning regimen,** chemotherapy, often associated with irradiation, is administered to destroy the patient's hematopoietic system and to suppress the immune system, especially T cells, so that graft rejection is prevented. In patients with malignancies, the preparative regimen also serves to significantly reduce the tumor burden. The patient then receives an intravenous infusion of hematopoietic cells from the donor. The intrabone injection of cord blood cells has been pioneered to optimize stem cells homing in the marrow niches.

The immunology of HSCT is distinct from that of other types of transplant because, in addition to stem cells, the graft contains mature blood cells of donor origin, including T cells, natural killer (NK) cells, and dendritic cells. These cells repopulate the recipient's lympho-hematopoietic system and give rise to a new immune system, which helps eliminate residual leukemia cells that survive the conditioning regimen. This effect is known as the **graft versus leukemia (GVL) effect.**

The donor immune system exerts its T cell–mediated GVL effect through alloreactions directed against not shared recipient histocompatibility antigens displayed on recipient leukemia cells. Because some of these histocompatibility antigens are also displayed on tissues, however, T cell–mediated alloreactions may ensue. Specifically, donor alloreactive cytotoxic CD8+ effector T cells may attack recipient tissues—in particular, the skin, gastrointestinal tract, and liver—causing acute graft versus host disease (GVHD), a condition of varying severity, that, in some cases, can be life-threatening (Chapter 131).

The success of allogeneic HSCT is undermined by diversity between donors and recipients in major and minor histocompatibility antigens. Major histocompatibility complex (MHC) molecules, the HLA-A, HLA-B, and HLA-C MHC class I molecules, present peptides to CD8+ T cells, while the HLA-DR, HLA-DQ, and HLA-DP MHC class II molecules present peptides to CD4+ T cells. There are hundreds of variant forms of each class I and class II molecule, and even small differences can provoke alloreactive T-cell responses that mediate graft rejection and/or GVHD. Disparities for HLA-A, -B, -C, or -DRB1 alleles in the donor-recipient pair are independent risk factors for both acute and chronic GVHD.

Minor histocompatibility antigens derive from differences between the HLA-matched recipient and donor in peptides that are presented by the same HLA allotype. They are due to polymorphisms of non-HLA proteins, to differences in the level of expression of proteins, or to genome differences between males and females. An example of the latter is represented by the H-Y antigens encoded by the Y chromosome, which can stimulate GVHD when a female donor is employed to transplant to an HLA-identical recipient. Thus, GVHD may occur even when the donor and recipient are HLA identical.

The optimal donor for any patient undergoing HSCT is an HLA-identical sibling. Because polymorphic HLA genes are closely linked and usually constitute a single genetic locus, any pair of siblings has a 25% chance of being HLA identical. Thus, also in view of the limited family size in the developed countries, approximately only 25-30% of patients in need of an allograft can receive their transplant from an HLA-identical sibling.

HSCT FROM AN HLA-IDENTICAL SIBLING DONOR

Allogeneic HSCT from an HLA-compatible sibling is the treatment of choice for children with hematological malignancies and congenital diseases (Table 129-1). Best results are achieved in patients with congenital or acquired nonmalignant disorders because the risk of disease recurrence is low and the cumulative transplant-related mortality is lower than in children transplanted for hematological malignancies.

Acute Lymphoblastic Leukemia (ALL)

Allogeneic HSCT is used for pediatric patients with acute lymphoblastic leukemia (ALL), either in the 1st complete remission when a child is considered to be at high risk of leukemia recurrence (such as, for example, those with Ph+ ALL or with high levels of minimal residual disease), or in 2nd or further complete remission after previous marrow relapse. ALL is the most common indication for HSCT in childhood (Chapter 489). Several patient-, donor-, disease-, and transplant-related variables may influence the outcome of patients with ALL given an allogeneic HSCT. The long-term probabilities of event-free survival for patients with ALL transplanted in the 1st or 2nd complete remission is 60-70% and 50%, respectively. Inferior results are obtained in patients transplanted in more advanced disease phases. The use of radiotherapy, total body irradiation (TBI), during the preparative regimen offers an advantage in terms of better event-free survival compared to a regimen consisting of cytotoxic drugs alone (Fig. 129-1). Less intensive GVHD prophylaxis is also associated with a better outcome. Bone marrow is still the preferred source of stem cells to be employed for transplantation.

Acute Myeloid Leukemia (AML)

Allogeneic HSCT from an HLA-identical sibling is largely employed as postremissional treatment of pediatric patients with acute myeloid leukemia (AML) (Chapter 489). Many studies have shown that children with AML in 1st complete remission given allogeneic HSCT as consolidation therapy have a better probability of event-free survival as compared to those treated with either chemotherapy alone or with autologous transplantation. Results obtained in patients given HSCT from an HLA-identical sibling

Table 129-1 INDICATIONS FOR ALLOGENEIC HEMATOPOIETIC STEM CELL TRANSPLANTATION FOR PEDIATRIC DISEASES

- Acute lymphoblastic leukemia
  - First complete remission for patients at very high risk of relapse
    - Translocation t(9;22) or t(4;11)
    - Nonresponder after 1 wk of corticosteroid therapy *and*
      - T-immunophenotype *or*
      - >100,000 cells/μL at diagnosis
    - Not in remission at the end of the induction phase
    - High levels of minimal residual disease at the end of induction therapy
  - Second complete remission
  - Third or later complete remission
- Acute myeloid leukemia in first complete remission *or* in advanced disease phase
- Philadelphia chromosome-positive chronic myeloid leukemia
- Myelodysplastic syndromes
- Hodgkin and non-Hodgkin lymphomas
- Selected solid tumours
  - Metastatic neuroblastoma
  - Rhabdomyosarcoma refractory to conventional treatment
  - Very high risk Ewing sarcoma
- Severe acquired aplastic anemia
- Fanconi anemia
- Congenital dyskeratosis
- Diamond-Blackfan anemia
- Thalassemia major
- Sickle cell disease
- Variants of severe combined immunodeficiency (SCID)
- Hyper-IgM syndrome
- Leukocyte adhesion deficiency
- Omenn syndrome
- Wiskott-Aldrich syndrome
- Chédiak-Higashi syndrome
- Kostmann syndrome (infantile malignant agranulocytosis), chronic granulomatous disease, and other severe neutrophil defects
- X-linked lymphoproliferative disease (Duncan syndrome)
- Hemophagocytic lymphohistiocytosis
- Selected severe variants of platelet function disorders (e.g., Glanzmann thromboasthenia, congenital amegakaryocytic thrombocytopenia, or Bernard-Soulier syndrome)
- Selected types of mucopolysaccharidosis (Hurler disease) or other liposomal/peroxisomal disorders (Krabbe disease, adrenoleukodystrophy)
- Infantile malignant osteopetrosis
- Life-threatening cytopenia unresponsive to conventional treatments

after either a TBI-containing or a chemotherapy-based preparative regimen are similar, the probability of event-free survival being on the order of 60-70%. Children with acute promyelocytic leukemia in molecular remission at the end of treatment with chemotherapy and all-trans retinoic acid or with AML and either translocation t(8;21) or inversion of chromosome 16 (inv.16) are no longer considered eligible for allogeneic HSCT in 1st complete remission in view of their excellent prognosis with alternative treatments. Around 40% of pediatric patients with AML in the 2nd complete remission can be rescued by an allograft from an HLA-identical sibling.

Chronic Myelogenous Leukemia (CML)

Allogeneic HSCT is considered to be the only proven curative treatment for children with Philadelphia positive (Ph+) CML. Leukemia-free survival of CML patients after an allograft is 45-80%, the phase of disease (chronic phase, accelerated phase, blast crisis), recipient age, type of donor employed (either related or unrelated), and time interval between diagnosis and HSCT being the main factors influencing the outcome. The best results are obtained in children transplanted during the chronic phase from an HLA-identical sibling within 1 yr from diagnosis. Treatment with the specific Bcr-Abl tyrosine protein kinase inhibitors (imatinib mesylate, dasatinib, nilotinib), which target the enzymatic activity of the Bcr-Abl fusion protein, could modify the natural history of the disease and, thus, the indications for

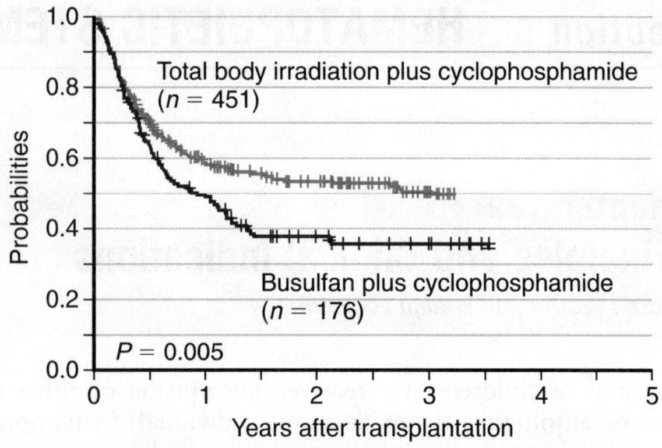

Figure 129-1 Cumulative probability of leukemia-free survival after human leukocyte antigen–identical sibling bone marrow transplantation for childhood acute lymphoblastic leukemia, by pretransplant conditioning regimen of total body irradiation (TBI) plus cyclophosphamide (CY) *(upper line)* or busulfan (Bu) plus cyclophosphamide *(lower line)*. There was superior survival with the total body irradiation plus cyclophosphamide regimen. (Data from Davies S, Ramsay NK, Klein JP, et al: Comparison of preparative regimens in transplants for children with acute lymphoblastic leukemia, *J Clin Oncol* 18:340–347, 2000.)

transplantation. Infusion of **donor leukocytes** can re-induce a state of complete remission in a large proportion of patients experiencing leukemia relapse.

Juvenile Myelomonocytic Leukemia (JMML)

This is a rare hematopoietic malignancy of early childhood, representing 2-3% of all pediatric leukemias. JMML is characterized by hepatosplenomegaly and organ infiltration, with excessive proliferation of cells of monocytic and granulocytic lineages. Hypersensitivity to granulocyte-macrophage colony-stimulating factor (GM-CSF) and pathologic activation of the RAS-RAF-MAP (mitogen-activated protein) kinase signaling pathway play an important role in the pathophysiology. JMML usually runs an aggressive clinical course, with a median duration of survival for untreated children <12 mo from diagnosis. HSCT is able to cure approximately 50% of patients with JMML. Patients transplanted from an unrelated donor have comparable outcome to those given HSC from an HLA-compatible related donor. Leukemia recurrence represents the main cause of treatment failure in children with JMML after HSCT, the relapse rate being as high as 40-50%. Because children with JMML frequently have massive spleen enlargement, splenectomy has been performed before transplantation. Spleen size at the time of HSCT and splenectomy before HSCT do not appear to affect the posttransplant outcome. While donor leukocyte infusion is not useful for rescuing patients experiencing disease recurrence, a 2nd allograft can induce sustained remission in around one third of children with JMML relapsing after a 1st HSCT.

Myelodysplastic Syndromes Other Than JMML

Myelodysplastic syndromes are a heterogeneous group of clonal disorders characterized by ineffective hematopoiesis leading to peripheral blood cytopenia and a propensity to evolve toward AML. HSCT is the treatment of choice for children with refractory anemia with excess of blasts (RAEB) and for those with RAEB in transformation (RAEB-t). The probability of survival without evidence of disease for these children is 50-60% if the donor is an HLA-identical sibling, whereas that of patients transplanted from an alternative donor is slightly lower. It is still unclear whether patients with myelodysplastic syndromes and a blast percentage >20% benefit from pretransplant chemotherapy. HSCT from an HLA-identical sibling is also the preferred treatment for all children with refractory cytopenia. Transplantation from an alternative donor is also employed in children with refractory cytopenia associated to either monosomy 7, complex karyotype, life-threatening infections, or transfusion dependency. For children with refractory cytopenia, the probability of event-free survival after HSCT may be as high as 80%, disease recurrence being rarely observed. This observation has provided the rationale for testing reduced-intensity regimens in these patients.

Non-Hodgkin Lymphoma and Hodgkin Disease

Childhood non-Hodgkin lymphoma (NHL) and Hodgkin disease (HD) are quite responsive to conventional chemoradiotherapy, but some of these patients are at high risk for relapse. HSCT can cure a proportion of patients with relapsed NHL and HD and should be offered early after relapse, while the disease is still sensitive to therapy. If an HLA-identical sibling is available, allogeneic transplant should be offered to take advantage from the GVL effect. Patients with sensitive disease and limited tumor burden have favorable outcomes, with event-free survival rates of 50-60%.

Acquired Aplastic Anemia

HSCT from an HLA-identical sibling is the treatment of choice for children with the severe form of acquired aplastic anemia, defined as two of the following: platelet count <20,000/mm^3, absolute neutrophil count <500/mm^3, or reticulocyte count <1% when anemia is present, together with hypoplastic bone marrow (<20% total cellularity) (Chapter 463). The probability of survival with sustained donor engraftment for these patients is >80%, with younger patients having even better outcomes. Every child diagnosed with severe acquired aplastic anemia should undergo HLA-typing as early as possible in order to identify a suitable HLA-compatible family donor. Graft rejection represents the most important cause of treatment failure. Blood transfusion should be avoided whenever possible because sensitization to blood products increases the likelihood of graft rejection. GVHD prophylaxis combining cyclosporine and short-term methotrexate is associated with a better outcome as compared to cyclosporine alone (Fig. 129-2). Some studies have suggested that the addition of antithymocyte globulin to the classical conditioning regimen consisting of cyclophosphamide (200 mg/kg) can reduce the risk of graft rejection, particularly in patients with previous heavy sensitization to blood products. The use of G-CSF mobilized peripheral blood progenitors has provided inferior results with respect to the infusion of bone marrow cells.

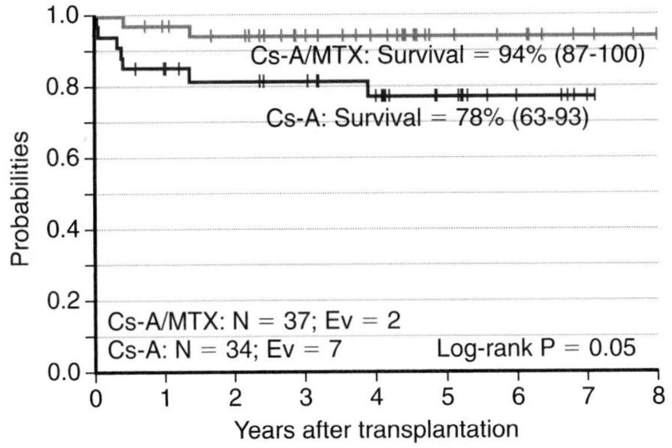

Figure 129-2 Cumulative probability of survival after human leukocyte antigen–identical sibling bone marrow transplantation (BMT) for aplastic anemia, by graft versus host disease (GVHD) prophylaxis with cyclosporin alone *(dotted line)* or cyclosporine plus methotrexate *(continuous line)*. GVHD prophylaxis combining cyclosporin and short-term methotrexate was associated with superior outcome compared to cyclosporin alone. EV, number of events occurring in each arm of randomization; N, number of patients in each arm of randomization. (From Locatelli F, Bruno B, Zecca M, et al: Cyclosporin A and short-term methotrexate versus cyclosporin A as graft versus host disease prophylaxis I patients with severe aplastic anemia given allogeneic bone marrow transplantation from an HLA-identical sibling: results of a GITMO/EMBT randomized trial, *Blood* 96:1690–1697, 2000.)

Constitutional Aplastic Anemia

Fanconi anemia and **dyskeratosis congenita** are genetic disorders associated with a high risk of developing pancytopenia (Chapter 462). Fanconi anemia is an autosomal recessive disease characterized by spontaneous chromosomal fragility, which is increased after exposure of peripheral blood lymphocytes to DNA cross-linking agents, including clastogenic compounds, such as diepoxybutane, mitomycin C, and melphalan. Besides being at risk of pancytopenia, patients with Fanconi anemia show a high propensity to develop clonal disorders of hematopoiesis, such as myelodysplastic syndromes and acute myeloid leukemia. HSCT can rescue aplastic anemia and prevent the occurrence of clonal hematopoietic disorders. In view of their defects in DNA repair mechanisms, which are responsible for the chromosomal fragility, Fanconi anemia patients have an exquisite sensitivity to alkylating agents. Thus, they must be prepared for the allograft with reduced doses of cyclophosphamide. Many patients were once successfully transplanted after receiving low-dose cyclophosphamide and thoraco-abdominal irradiation. However, the use of this regimen is associated with an increased incidence of post-transplant head and neck cancers. Either reduced doses of cyclophosphamide alone or low-dose cyclophosphamide with fludarabine are currently employed for preparing Fanconi anemia patients to the allograft. Using these regimens, the success rate of HSCT from an HLA-identical sibling is on the order of 70-80%.

Allogeneic HSCT remains the only potentially curative approach for severe bone marrow failure associated with dyskeratosis congenita, a rare congenital syndrome characterized also by atrophy and reticular pigmentation of the skin, nail dystrophy, and leukoplakia of mucosa membrane. Results of allograft in these patients have been relatively poor, due to occurrence of both early and late complications, reflecting increased sensitivity of endothelial cells to radiotherapy and alkylating agents.

Thalassemia

Conventional treatment (blood transfusion and iron chelation therapy) has dramatically improved both the survival and quality of life of patients with thalassemia, changing a previously fatal disease with early death to a chronic, slowly progressive disease compatible with prolonged survival (Chapter 456.9). HSCT remains the only curative treatment for patients with thalassemia. In these patients the risk of dying from transplant-related complications is primarily dependent on patient age, iron overload, and concomitant hepatic viral infections. Adults, especially when affected by chronic active hepatitis, have a poorer outcome than children. Among children, 3 classes of risk have been identified on the basis of 3 parameters, namely regularity of previous iron chelation, liver enlargement, and presence of portal fibrosis. In pediatric patients without liver disease who have received regular iron chelation (class 1 patients), the probability of survival with transfusion independence is >90%, whereas for patients with low compliance with iron chelation and signs of severe liver damage (class 3 patients), the probability of survival is 60% (Fig. 129-3). As in other nonmalignant disorders the best pharmacologic combinations (such as that including cyclosporine A and methotrexate) should be employed to prevent GVHD.

Sickle Cell Disease

Disease severity varies greatly among patients with sickle cell disease (SCD), with 5-20% of the overall population suffering significant morbidity from vaso-occlusive crises and pulmonary, renal, or neurologic damage (Chapter 456.1). Despite the fact that hydroxyurea, an agent favoring the synthesis of HbF, has been demonstrated to reduce the frequency and severity of vaso-occlusive crises and to improve the quality of life for patients with sickle cell disease, allogeneic HSCT is the only curative treatment for this disease. Although HSCT can cure homozygous HbS disease, selecting appropriate candidates for transplantation is difficult. Patients with SCD may survive for decades, but some

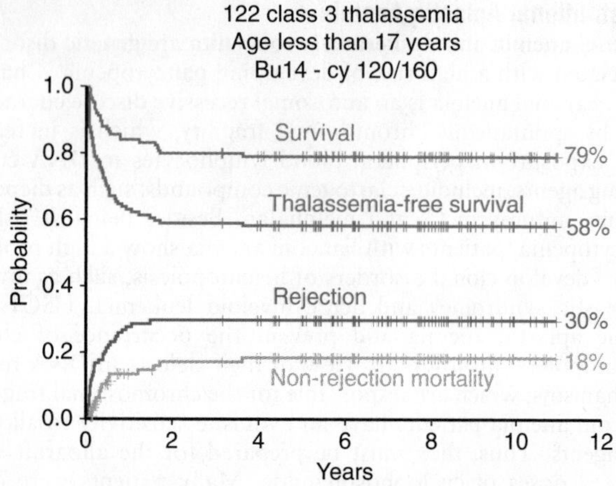

Figure 129-3 Kaplan-Meier estimates of survival and thalassemia-free survival, and cumulative incidences of rejection and nonrejection mortality for 122 thalassemic patients <17 yr of age given a myeloablative preparative regimen including busulfan and cyclophosphamide. (Courtesy of Dr. Emanuele Angelucci.)

patients have a poor quality of life, with repeated hospitalizations for painful vaso-occlusive crises and central nervous system infarcts. The main **indications for** performing HSCT in patients with sickle cell disease are history of strokes, magnetic resonance imaging of central nervous system lesions associated with impaired neuropsychologic function, failure to respond to hydroxyurea as shown by recurrent acute chest syndrome, and/or recurrent vaso-occlusive crises and/or severe anemia and/or osteonecrosis. The results of HSCT are best, with a probability of cure of 80-90%, when performed in children with an HLA-identical sibling. The use of antithymocyte globulin during the preparative regimen has been shown to improve patient outcomes, preventing graft failure.

Immunodeficiency Disorders

HSCT is the **treatment of choice** for children affected by severe combined immunodeficiency (SCID) and other inherited immunodeficiencies (see Table 129-1). With an HLA-identical sibling, the probability of survival approaches 100%, with less favorable results for patients transplanted from an unrelated volunteer or an HLA-partially matched relative. Some children with SCID may be transplanted without receiving any preparative regimen, in particular those without residual NK activity or maternal T-cell engraftment. Sustained donor engraftment is more difficult to achieve in children with Omenn syndrome, hemophagocytic lymphohistiocytosis, or leukocyte adhesion deficiency. Life-threatening opportunistic fungal and viral infections occurring before the allograft adversely affect the patient's outcome after HSCT. Patients with the most severe immunodeficiencies must be transplanted as early as possible.

BIBLIOGRAPHY

Please visit the Nelson Textbook of Pediatrics *website at www.expertconsult.com for the complete bibliography.*

Chapter 130

HSCT from Alternative Sources and Donors

Andrea Velardi and Franco Locatelli

Two thirds of patients who need allogeneic hematopoietic stem cell transplantation (HSCT) do not have an available human leukocyte antigen (HLA)-identical sibling. Alternative donor sources of hematopoietic stem cells are being increasingly used and include matched unrelated donors (MUDs), unrelated umbilical cord blood (UCB), and HLA-haploidentical relatives. Each of these options has advantages and limitations, but rather than being considered competing alternatives, they should be regarded as complementary alternatives to be chosen after a careful evaluation of the relative risks and benefits in the individual patient. The choice of the donor will depend on various factors related to urgency of transplantation, center experience, and patient-, disease-, and transplant-related factors.

For the full continuation of this chapter, please visit the Nelson Textbook of Pediatrics *website at www.expertconsult.com.*

Chapter 131

Graft Versus Host Disease (GVHD) and Rejection

Andrea Velardi and Franco Locatelli

The major cause of mortality and morbidity after allogeneic hematopoietic stem cell transplantation (HSCT) is graft versus host disease (GVHD), which is caused by engraftment of immunocompetent donor lymphocytes in an immunologically compromised host that shows histocompatibility differences with the donor. These differences between the donor and the host may result in donor T-cell activation against recipient major histocompatibility complex (MHC) antigens or minor histocompatibility antigens. GVHD is usually subdivided in 2 forms: acute GVHD, which occurs within 3 mo after transplantation, and chronic GVHD, which, though related, is a different disease occurring later and displaying some clinical and pathological features that resemble those observed in selected autoimmune disorders (systemic sclerosis, Sjögren syndrome, etc.).

ACUTE GVHD

Acute GVHD is caused by the alloreactive, donor-derived T cells contained in the graft, which attack nonshared recipient's antigens on target tissues. A 3-step process generates the clinical syndrome. First, conditioning-induced tissue damage activates recipient antigen-presenting cells (APC), which present recipient alloantigens to the donor T cells transferred with the graft and secrete cytokines, such as interleukin 12, favoring the polarization of T-cell response in the type 1 direction. Second, in response to recipient antigens, donor T cells become activated, proliferate, expand, and generate cytokines such as tumor necrosis factor-α (TNF-α), interleukin 2 (IL-2), and interferon-γ (IFN-γ). In the 3rd step of the process, these cytokines cause tissue damage and promote differentiation of cytotoxic CD8+ T cells, which together with macrophages kill recipient cells and further disrupt tissues.

Acute GVHD usually develops from 2-5 wk post-transplantation. The primary **manifestations** are an erythematous maculopapular rash, persistent anorexia, vomiting and/or diarrhea, and liver disease with increased serum levels of bilirubin, alanine aminotransferase, aspartate aminotransferase, and alkaline phosphatase (Table 131-1). Diagnosis may benefit from skin, liver, or endoscopic biopsy for confirmation. Endothelial damage and lymphocytic infiltrates are seen in all affected organs. The epidermis and hair follicles of the skin are damaged, the hepatic small bile ducts show segmental disruption, and there is destruction of the crypts and mucosal ulceration of the gastrointestinal tract. Grade I acute GVHD (skin rash alone) has a favorable prognosis and often does not require treatment (Fig. 131-1). Grade II GVHD is a moderately severe multiorgan disease requiring therapy. Grade III GVHD is a severe multiorgan disease, and grade IV GVHD is a life-threatening, often fatal condition. The standard **prophylaxis** of GVHD relies mainly on post-transplant administration of immunosuppressive drugs such as cyclosporine or tacrolimus, often in combination with methotrexate or prednisone, anti–T-cell antibodies, mycophenolate mofetil, or other immunosuppressive agents. An alternative approach that has been widely used in clinical practice is the removal of T lymphocytes from the graft (T-cell depletion). Any form of GVHD prophylaxis in itself may impair post-transplant immunologic reconstitution, increasing the risk of infection-related deaths. T-cell depletion of the graft has also been associated with an increased risk of leukemia recurrence in patients transplanted from an HLA-identical sibling or an unrelated volunteer.

Despite prophylaxis, significant acute GVHD develops in ≈30% of recipients of HSCT from matched siblings and in as many as 60% of HSCT recipients from unrelated donors. The risk of acute GVHD is increased by factors such as diagnosis of malignant disease, older donor and recipient ages, and, in patients given an unmanipulated allograft, GVHD prophylaxis with only 1 drug. However, the most important risk factor for acute GVHD is the present of disparities for HLA-molecules in the donor/recipient pair. Acute GVHD is usually treated with glucocorticoids; about 40-50% of patients show a complete response to steroids. The risk of transplantation-related mortality is much higher in patients who did not respond to steroids than in those showing a complete response. Antithymocyte globulin, mycophenolate mofetil, pentostatin, extracorporeal photopheresis, or monoclonal antibodies targeting molecules expressed on T cells or cytokines during the inflammatory cascade, which underlies the physiopathology of GVHD, have been used in patients with steroid-resistant acute GVHD. There are no clear data showing the superiority of 1 of these approaches over the others. Promising results in children with steroid-resistant acute GVHD have been recently obtained using mesenchymal stromal cells (MSCs).

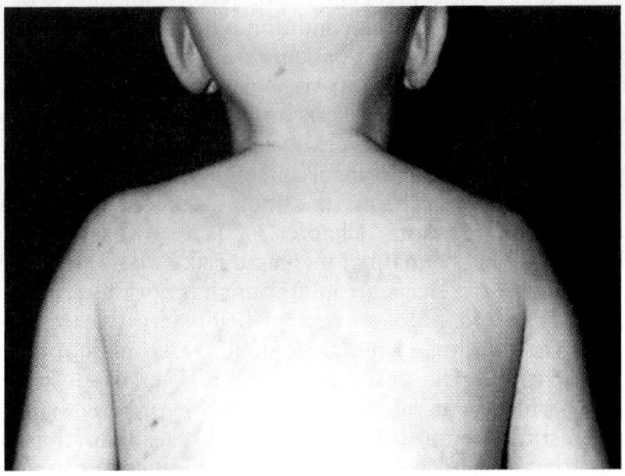

Figure 131-1 Acute graft versus host disease of the skin with ear, arm, shoulder, and trunk involvement. (Courtesy of Evan Farmer, MD.)

CHRONIC GVHD

Chronic GVHD develops or persists >3 mo post-transplant and is the most frequent late complication of allogeneic HSCT, with an incidence of ≈25% in pediatric patients. Chronic GVHD is the major cause of nonrelapse mortality and morbidity in long-term HSCT survivors. Acute GVHD has been recognized as the most important factor predicting the development of the chronic form of the disease. The use of matched unrelated volunteers as donors, and of peripheral blood as the stem cell source, has increased the incidence and severity of chronic GVHD. Other factors that predict occurrence of chronic GVHD include older donor and recipient ages, female donor for male recipient, diagnosis of malignancy, and use of total body irradiation (TBI) as part of the preparative regimen.

Chronic GVHD is a disorder of immune regulation characterized by autoantibody production, increased collagen deposition and fibrosis, and clinical symptoms similar to those seen in patients with autoimmune diseases. The predominant cytokines involved in the pathophysiology of chronic GVHD are usually type II cytokines such as IL-4, IL-5, and IL-13. IL-4 and IL-5 contribute to eosinophilia and B-cell hyperactivity with elevated IgM, IgG, and IgE titers. Associated monoclonal gammopathies indicate clonal dysregulation. Chronic GVHD is dependent on the development and persistence of donor T cells that are not tolerant to the recipient. They could well derive from the original donor inoculum and/or the recipient thymus that has been damaged by acute GVHD. Maturation of transplanted stem cells within a damaged thymus could lead to errors in negative selection and production of cells that have not been tolerized to recipient antigens and are therefore autoreactive or, more accurately, **recipient reactive.** This ongoing immune reactivity results in clinical features resembling a systemic autoimmune disease with lichenoid and sclerodermatous skin lesions, malar rash, sicca syndrome, arthritis, joint contractures, obliterative bronchiolitis, and bile duct degeneration with cholestasis.

Patients with chronic GVHD involving only the skin and liver have a favorable course (Fig. 131-2). Extensive multiorgan disease may be associated with a very poor quality of life, recurrent infections associated with prolonged immunosuppressive regimens to control GVHD, and a high mortality rate. Morbidity and mortality are highest in patients with a **progressive onset** of chronic GVHD that directly follows acute GVHD, intermediate in those with a **quiescent onset** after resolution of acute GVHD, and lowest in patients with **de novo onset** in the absence of acute GVHD. Single-agent prednisone is standard treatment at present, although other agents, including extracorporeal photopheresis, mycophenolate mofetil, anti-CD20 monoclonal antibody, and pentostatin, have been employed with variable success. Treatment

Table 131-1 CLINICAL STAGING AND GRADING OF GRAFT VERSUS HOST DISEASE (GVHD)

STAGE	SKIN	LIVER	INTESTINAL TRACT
+	Maculopapular rash <25% of body surface	Bilirubin 2-3 mg/dL	>500 mL diarrhea/day
++	Maculopapular rash 25-50% of body surface	Bilirubin 3-6 mg/dL	>1,000 mL diarrhea/day
+++	Generalized erythroderma	Bilirubin 6-15 mg/dL	>1,500 mL diarrhea/day
++++	Generalized erythroderma with bullous formation and desquamation	Bilirubin >15 mg/dL	Severe abdominal pain with or without ileus

GVHD GRADE	SKIN STAGE	LIVER STAGE	INTESTINAL TRACT STAGE	DECREASE IN CLINICAL PERFORMANCE
I	+ to ++	0	0	None
II	+ to +++	+	+	Mild
III	++ to +++	++ to ++++	++ to +++	Marked
IV	++ to ++++	++ to ++++	++ to ++++	Extreme

Adapted from Thomas ED, Storb R, Clift RA, et al: Bone marrow transplantation, *N Engl J Med* 292:832–843, 895–902, 1975.

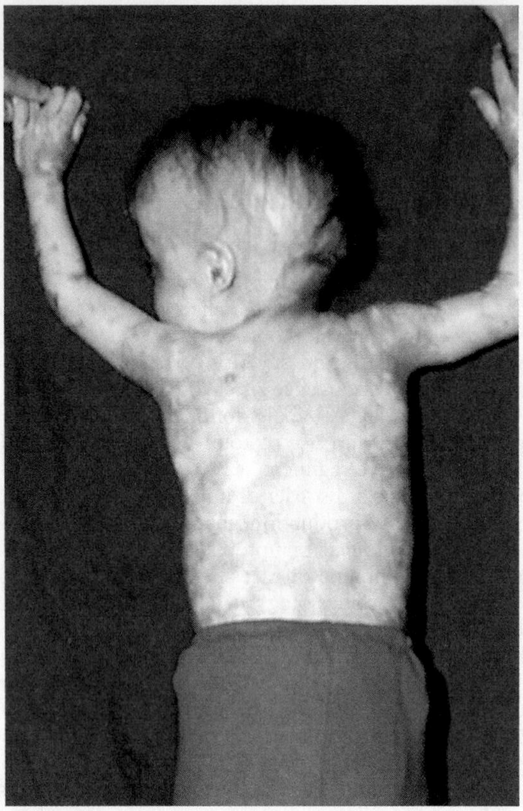

Figure 131-2 Chronic graft versus host disease of the skin with sclerodermoid changes. See also color plates. (Courtesy of Evan Farmer, MD.)

with imatinib mesylate, which inhibits the synthesis of collagen, has been effective in patients with chronic GVHD and sclerotic features. As a consequence of prolonged immunosuppression, patients with chronic GVHD are particularly susceptible to infections and should receive appropriate antibiotic prophylaxis, including trimethoprim-sulfamethoxazole. Chronic GVHD resolves in most patients but may require 1-3 yr of immunosuppressive therapy before the drugs can be withdrawn without the disease recurring. Chronic GVHD also promotes the development of secondary neoplasms.

Graft failure is a serious complication exposing patients to a high risk of fatal infection. **Primary graft failure** is defined as failure to achieve a neutrophil count of $0.2 \times 10^9/L$ by 21 days post-transplant. **Secondary graft failure** is loss of peripheral blood counts following initial transient engraftment of donor cells. Causes of graft failure after autologous and allogeneic transplantation include transplant of an inadequate stem cell dose (more frequently observed in children given cord blood transplantation), and viral infections such as with cytomegalovirus (CMV) or human herpesvirus type 6 (HHV6), which are often associated with activation of recipient macrophages. However, graft failure after allogeneic transplantation is mainly caused by immunologically mediated rejection of the graft by residual recipient-type T cells that survive the conditioning regimen. **Diagnosis** of graft failure resulting from immunologic mechanisms is based on examination of peripheral blood and marrow aspirate and biopsy, along with molecular analysis of chimerism status. Persistence of lymphocytes of host origin in allogeneic transplant recipients with graft failure indicates immunologic rejection. The risk of immune-mediated graft rejection is higher in patients given HLA-disparate, T-cell–depleted grafts, reduced-intensity conditioning regimens, and transplantation of low numbers of stem cells, and in recipients who are sensitized toward HLA antigens or, less frequently, minor histocompatibility antigens. Allosensitization develops as a consequence of preceding blood product transfusions and is observed particularly in recipients with aplastic anemia, sickle cell disease, and thalassemia. In HSCT for nonmalignant diseases, such as mucopolysaccharidoses, graft failure is also facilitated by the absence of previous treatment with cytotoxic and immunosuppressive drugs. In thalassemia, graft failure is promoted by expansion of hematopoietic cells. GVHD prophylaxis with methotrexate, an antimetabolite, and anti-infective prophylaxis with trimethoprim-sulfamethoxazole or ganciclovir may also delay engraftment.

Treatment of graft failure usually requires removing all potentially myelotoxic agents from the treatment regimen and attempting a short trial of hematopoietic growth factors, such as G-CSF. A second transplant, usually preceded by a highly immune-suppressive regimen, has to be frequently employed to rescue patients experiencing graft failure. High-intensity regimens are generally tolerated poorly if administered within 100 days of a 1st transplant because of cumulative toxicities.

BIBLIOGRAPHY

Please visit the Nelson Textbook of Pediatrics *website at www.expertconsult.com for the complete bibliography.*

Chapter 132
Infectious Complications of HSCT

Andrea Velardi and Franco Locatelli

Hematopoietic stem cell transplantation (HSCT) recipients experience a transient but profound state of immune deficiency. Immediately after transplantation, patients are particularly susceptible to bacterial and fungal infections, because neutrophils are absent. Consequently, most centers start prophylactic antibiotic or antifungal treatment during the conditioning regimen. Despite these prophylactic measures, most patients will develop fever and signs of infection in the early post-transplant period. The common pathogens include enteric bacteria and fungi such as *Candida* and *Aspergillus*. An indwelling central venous line is a significant risk factor for bacterial and fungal infections with staphylococcal species and *Candida* being the most frequent pathogens in catheter-related infections (Chapter 172).

HSCT recipients remain at increased risk of developing severe infections even after the neutrophil count has normalized, because T-cell number and function remain below normal for months after transplantation. Unrelated donor transplant recipients are at increased risk of developing graft versus host disease (GVHD), which is an additional risk factor for fungal and viral opportunistic infections. After cord blood transplantation, infections are the consequence of the slow neutrophil engraftment and donor T-cell naïveté. In haploidentical transplantation, the increased risk of infection observed in the 1st 4-6 mo after the allograft is the consequence of T-cell depletion of the graft.

Among HSCT recipients, invasive aspergillosis, cytomegalovirus (CMV) infection and Epstein-Barr virus (EBV)–related lymphoproliferative disorders represent life-threatening complications that significantly affect patient's outcome.

Invasive **aspergillosis** remains a significant cause of infectious morbidity and mortality in HSCT recipients. Despite prompt and aggressive administration of potent antifungal agents, proven cases of aspergillosis remain difficult to treat, with case fatality rates of 80-90%. The annual incidence of invasive aspergillosis has risen with use of stem cells from alternative sources. The incidence has been reported to be 7.3% in recipients of a human leukocyte antigen (HLA)-matched related donor transplant and 10.5% in patients given the allograft from either an HLA-mismatched family donor or an unrelated donor volunteer. Most cases of aspergillosis are diagnosed from 40 to 180 days after HSCT, with 30% diagnosed <40 days and 17% >6 mo after transplantation. The risk of developing aspergillosis is mainly influenced by the duration of neutropenia, GVHD occurrence, use of corticosteroid therapy, post-transplant CMV infection, viral respiratory tract infections, older age, and T-cell depletion of the graft. Patients with a previous history of invasive aspergillosis are at particular risk.

Aspergillus infection often originates from the upper airway mucosa. Early lesions in the nose should be sought in patients with neutropenia who have fever and minimal epistaxis. Rapid extension into the adjacent paranasal sinuses, orbit, or face is usual, with or without the appearance of lung lesions. In the lung, invasive aspergillosis generally presents as an acute, rapidly progressive, densely consolidated pulmonary infiltrate. Infection progresses by direct extension across tissue and by hematogenous dissemination to brain and other organs. One or more small pulmonary nodules are the earliest finding on CT scan. As a nodule enlarges, the dense central core of infarcted tissue becomes surrounded by edema or hemorrhage, forming a hazy rim, the **halo sign.** This rim disappears in a few days as the dense core enlarges. In neutropenic patients, when bone marrow function recovers, the infarcted central core cavitates, creating the **crescent sign.** Antifungal prophylaxis includes isolation of the patient in a laminar air flow or positive pressure room. Liposomal amphotericin B, azole compounds (itraconazole, voriconazole), and echinocandins (caspofungin, micafungin, anidulafungin) are useful for both preventing and treating the fungal infection. Voriconazole represents the treatment of choice for patients with invasive apsergillosis. However, often aspergillosis does not respond satisfactorily to antifungal agents alone, and patients remain at risk until T-cell counts and function recover. This observation provides the rationale for developing strategies to accelerate the recovery of pathogen-specific immune responses.

Cytomegalovirus (CMV) infection remains the most common and potentially severe viral complication in patients given allogeneic HSCT. Seropositivity for CMV is an independent risk factor for mortality, even in recipients of matched sibling or unrelated donor transplants. CMV is itself immunosuppressive, as it impairs dendritic cell and T-lymphocyte function. Moreover, ganciclovir, the most frequently used anti-CMV agent, may cause leukopenia and T-cell immune suppression.

The period of maximal risk for CMV infection is 1-4 mo after transplantation. Until CMV-specific T-cell responses develop several months after transplant, CMV infection may result in a variety of syndromes, including fever, leukopenia, thrombocytopenia, hepatitis, pneumonitis, esophagitis, gastritis, and colitis. CMV pneumonia is the most life-threatening complication related to viral infection and has been reported to occur in up to 15-20% of bone marrow transplant recipients, with a case fatality rate of 85%. The risk is greatest between 5 and 13 wk after transplantation. Risk factors include T-cell depletion of the graft, donor seronegative status, recipient seropositive status, acute GVHD, and patient older age.

Tachypnea, hypoxia, and unproductive cough signals respiratory involvement. Chest x-ray often reveals bilateral interstitial or reticulonodular infiltrates, which begin in the periphery of the lower lobes and spread centrally and superiorly. The differential diagnosis includes infection with *Pneumocystis jiroveci* or other fungal, viral, or bacterial pathogens; pulmonary hemorrhage; and injury secondary to irradiation or to treatment with cytotoxic drugs. Gastrointestinal CMV involvement may lead to ulcers of the esophagus, stomach, small intestine, and colon that may result in bleeding or perforation.

Fatal CMV infections are often associated with persistent viremia and multiorgan involvement. CMV disease has largely been **prevented** through prophylaxis and a preemptive approach. Prophylaxis is based on administration of antiviral drugs to all transplanted patients for a median duration of 3 mo after transplantation. Preemptive (presymptomatic) therapy aims at treating only patients who experience CMV reactivation and, thus, are at risk of developing overt disease; it starts only upon detection of CMV in blood by any assay. The most widely used assays detect CMV antigenemia (pp65) or CMV DNA in blood and have been used to decide inception of treatment when they either become positive or reach a predetermined threshold. While in the past treatment usually started after one of these assays became positive, nowadays therapy is usually initiated when a certain viral load is reached. Moreover, quantification of CMV DNA in blood provides a more reliable approach for deciding interruption of treatment. The major drawback of this strategy is the need for serial monitoring that is required for the period in which patients are at risk of developing CMV disease. In this regard, approaches able to reliably prove the restoration of virus-specific immunity have been developed recently. Ganciclovir or sometimes foscarnet is usually used for prophylaxis and preemptive treatment of CMV infection.

Epstein-Barr virus (EBV)–related **lymphoproliferative** disease (EBV-LPD) is a major complication in HSCT and solid organ transplantation. In patients receiving HSCT, selective procedures of T-cell depletion sparing B lymphocytes and use of HLA partially matched family and unrelated donors are risk factors for the development of EBV-LPD. These disorders usually present in the 1st 4-6 mo after transplantation as high-grade diffuse large cell B-cell lymphomas, which are oligoclonal or monoclonal, express the full array of EBV antigens, and are of donor origin. High levels of EBV-DNA in blood and in vitro spontaneous growth of EBV-lymphoblastoid cell lines predict development of EBV-LPD.

In immunocompromised hosts, EBV-LPD originates from a deficiency of virus-specific cytotoxic T lymphocytes (CTL), which control outgrowth of EBV-infected B cells. This finding provided the original rationale for developing strategies of adoptive cell therapy to restore EBV-specific immune competence. Unselected donor leukocyte infusion (DLI), the first attempt at EBV-directed adoptive immunotherapy in humans, can induce EBV-LPD remission but exposes patients to a high risk of developing clinically relevant GVHD and is not suitable for patients transplanted from an HLA-mismatched donor. A safer approach is infusion of in vitro generated EBV-specific CTL lines of donor origin containing both CD8+ and CD4+ T lymphocytes. These CTL lines prevent lymphoproliferative disorders in patients considered at high risk, such as patients given T-cell depleted HSCT from HLA-disparate donors, and cure clinically overt LPD. In recent years, use of monoclonal antibodies directed against CD20, a molecule expressed on B cells, has significantly contributed to reduce the incidence and severity of EBV-related LPD, although it can be associated with the emergence of neoplasms in which cells are CD19+ but CD20 negative, thus rendering patients no longer susceptible to the treatment with the monoclonal antibody.

BIBLIOGRAPHY

Please visit the Nelson Textbook of Pediatrics *website at* *www.expertconsult.com* *for the complete bibliography.*

Chapter 133
Late Effects of HSCT

Andrea Velardi and Franco Locatelli

Many children who receive hematopoietic stem cell transplantation (HSCT) become long-term survivors. Besides chronic graft versus host disease (GVHD), long-term complications include impaired growth, neuroendocrine dysfunction, delayed puberty, infertility, second malignancies, cataracts and other ocular complications, leukoencephalopathy, and cardiac and pulmonary dysfunction (see Table 133-1 on the *Nelson Textbook of Pediatrics* website at www.expertconsult.com).

For the full continuation of this chapter, please visit the Nelson Textbook of Pediatrics *website at* *www.expertconsult.com*.

PART XV Allergic Disorders

Chapter 134
Allergy and the Immunologic Basis of Atopic Disease

Donald Y.M. Leung and Cezmi A. Akdis

Allergic or atopic patients have an altered state of reactivity to common environmental and food antigens that do not cause clinical reactions in most people. Patients with clinical allergy usually produce immunoglobulin (Ig) E antibodies to the antigens that trigger their illness. The term allergy represents the clinical expression of IgE-mediated allergic diseases that have a familial predisposition and that manifest as hyperresponsiveness in target organs such as the lung, skin, gastrointestinal tract, and nose. There has been a significant increase in the prevalence of allergic diseases during the last few decades. This increase is attributed to changes in environmental factors (exposure to tobacco smoke, air pollution, indoor and outdoor allergens, respiratory viruses, obesity).

For the full continuation of this chapter, please visit the Nelson Textbook of Pediatrics *website at www.expertconsult.com.*

Chapter 135
Diagnosis of Allergic Disease

Dan Atkins and Donald Y.M. Leung

Allergic diseases arise from the acute or chronic exposure of a sensitized individual to a specific allergen by inhalation, ingestion, contact, or injection. Symptoms most often involve the nose, eyes, lungs, skin, or gastrointestinal tract either individually or in combination. A carefully obtained history, including environmental exposures, and the appropriate laboratory tests or allergen challenges, is critical for an accurate diagnosis.

ALLERGY HISTORY

Obtaining a complete history from the allergic patient involves eliciting a description of all symptoms along with their timing and duration, exposure to common allergens, and responses to previous therapies. Because patients often suffer from more than one allergic disease, the presence or absence of other allergic diseases, including allergic rhinitis, allergic conjunctivitis, asthma, food allergy, and atopic dermatitis, should be determined. A family history of allergic disease is common and is one of the most important factors predisposing a child to the development of allergies. The risk of allergic disease in a child approaches 50% when one parent is allergic and 66% when both parents are allergic.

Several characteristic behaviors are often seen in allergic children. Because of nasal pruritus and rhinorrhea, children with allergic rhinitis often perform the **allergic salute** by rubbing their nose upward with the palm of their hand. This maneuver gives rise to the **nasal crease**, a horizontal wrinkle over the bridge of the nose. Characteristic vigorous **grinding** of the eyes with the thumb and side of the fist is frequently observed in children with allergic conjunctivitis. The **allergic cluck** is produced when the tongue is placed against the roof of the mouth to form a seal and withdrawn rapidly in an effort to scratch the palate. The presence of other symptoms, such as fever, unilateral nasal obstruction, and purulent nasal discharge, suggests other diagnoses.

The timing of onset and the progression of symptoms are relevant. The onset of recurrent or persistent nasal symptoms coinciding with placement in a daycare center might suggest recurrent infection rather than allergy. When patients present with a history of episodic acute symptoms, it is important to review the setting in which symptoms occur as well as the activities and exposures that immediately precede their onset. Symptoms associated with lawn mowing suggest allergy to grass pollen or fungi, whereas if the symptoms always occur in homes with pets, then animal dander sensitivity is an obvious consideration. Reproducible reactions after the ingestion of a specific food raise the possibility of food allergy. When symptoms wax and wane but evolve gradually and are more chronic in duration, a closer look at whether the timing and progression of symptoms correlate with exposure to a seasonal aeroallergen is warranted.

Aeroallergens such as pollens and fungal spores, the concentrations of which in outdoor air fluctuate seasonally, are prominent causes of allergic disease. Correlating symptoms with the seasonal pollination patterns of indigenous plants along with information provided by local pollen counts can aid in identifying the allergen to which the patient is sensitized. Throughout most of the USA, trees pollinate in the early spring. Grasses pollinate in the late spring and early summer, whereas weeds pollinate in late summer through the fall. The presence of fungal spores in the atmosphere follows a seasonal pattern in the northern USA, with spore counts rising with the onset of warmer weather and peaking in the late summer months, only to recede again with the onset of colder weather in the late fall through the winter. In warmer regions of the southern USA, fungal spores and grass pollens may cause symptoms on a perennial basis.

Rather than experiencing seasonal symptoms, some patients suffer allergic symptoms year-round. In these patients, sensitization to sources of perennial allergens usually found indoors, such as dust mites, animal dander, cockroaches, and fungi, warrants consideration. Species of certain fungi, such as *Aspergillus* and *Penicillium,* are found indoors, whereas *Alternaria* is found in both indoor and outdoor environments. Cockroach allergens are often problematic in inner city environments. Patients sensitive to perennial allergens often also become sensitized to seasonal allergens and experience baseline symptoms year-round with worsening during the spring and fall pollen seasons.

The age of the patient is an important consideration in identifying potential allergens. Infants and young children are first sensitized to allergens that are in their environment on a continuous basis, such as dust mites, animal dander, and fungi. Clinically relevant sensitization to seasonal allergens usually takes several seasons of exposure to develop. Food allergies are more common in infants and young children, resulting primarily in cutaneous, gastrointestinal, and, less frequently, respiratory symptoms.

Complete information from all previous evaluations and prior treatments for allergic disease should be reviewed, including the response to all medications that have been used and the duration and impact of allergen immunotherapy. Improvement in symptoms during treatment with medications or therapies used to treat allergic disease provides additional evidence that the symptoms are the result of an allergic process.

A thorough environmental survey should be performed, with attention to potential sources of allergen and/or irritant exposure. The age and type of the dwelling, how it is heated and cooled, the use of humidifiers or air filtration units (either central or portable), and any history of flooding or water damage should be noted. Forced hot air heating may repeatedly stir up dust mite, fungi, and animal allergens. The irritant effects of wood-burning stoves, fireplaces, and kerosene heaters may provoke respiratory symptoms in allergic patients. Increased humidity or water damage in the home is often associated with greater exposure to dust mites and fungi. Carpeting serves as a reservoir for dust mites, fungi, and animal dander. The number of domestic pets and their movements about the house, including where they sleep, should be ascertained. Special attention should be focused on the bedroom, where a child spends a significant portion of time. The age and type of bedding, the number of stuffed animals, window treatments, and accessibility of the room to pets should be reviewed. The number of smokers in the home and where they smoke is useful information. Hobbies that might result in exposure to allergens or respiratory irritants such as paint fumes, cleansers, sawdust, latex, or glues should be identified. Similar information should be obtained in regard to other environments where the child spends large portions of time, such as a relative's home, the classroom, or a daycare center.

PHYSICAL EXAMINATION

In patients with **asthma,** a peak flow analysis or spirometry should be performed for evidence of airway obstruction. If respiratory distress is observed, pulse oximetry should be performed. The child presenting with a chief complaint of rhinitis or rhinoconjunctivitis should be observed for mouth breathing, paroxysms of sneezing, sniffing, and rubbing of the nose and eyes. Infants should be observed during feeding for nasal obstruction severe enough to interfere with feeding as well as for evidence of aspiration or gastroesophageal reflux. The frequency and nature of coughing that occurs during the interview and any positional increase in coughing or wheezing should be noted. Children with asthma should be observed for congested cough, tachypnea at rest, retractions, and audible wheezes. Patients with atopic dermatitis should be monitored for repetitive scratching and the extent of skin involvement.

Because children with severe asthma as well as those receiving oral corticosteroids may suffer growth suppression, an accurate height should be plotted at regular intervals. Poor weight gain in a child with chronic chest symptoms should prompt consideration of cystic fibrosis. The blood pressure should be measured to evaluate for steroid-induced hypertension. The patient with acute asthma may present with **pulsus paradoxus,** defined as a drop in systolic blood pressure during inspiration >10 mm Hg. Moderate to severe airways obstruction is indicated by a decrease of >20 mm Hg. An increased heart rate may be the result of an asthma flare or the use of a β-agonist or decongestant. Fever is not caused by allergy alone and should prompt consideration of an infectious process, which may exacerbate asthma.

Parents of allergic children are often concerned about blue-gray to purple discolorations beneath the lower eyelids, attributed to venous stasis and referred to as **allergic shiners.** They are found in up to 60% of allergic patients and almost 40% of patients without allergic disease. They are often accompanied by **Dennie lines (Dennie-Morgan folds),** which are prominent symmetric skin folds that extend in an arc from the inner canthus beneath and parallel to the lower lid margin.

In most patients with **allergic conjunctivitis,** involvement of the eyes is bilateral. Examination of the conjunctiva reveals varying degrees of conjunctival injection and edema. In severe cases, periorbital edema may involve primarily the lower eyelids be observed. The classic discharge associated with allergic conjunctivitis is usually described as "stringy" or "ropy." In children with vernal conjunctivitis, examination of the tarsal conjunctiva may reveal cobblestoning. Children repeatedly receiving large doses of oral corticosteroids for management of severe asthma are at risk for development of posterior subcapsular cataracts. **Keratoconus,** or protrusion of the cornea, may occur in patients with atopic dermatitis as a result of repeated trauma produced by persistent rubbing of the eyes.

The external ear should be examined for eczematous changes in patients with atopic dermatitis. Because otitis media with effusion is common in children with allergic rhinitis, pneumatic otoscopy should be performed to evaluate for the presence of fluid in the middle ear and to exclude infection.

Examination of the nose in allergic patients often reveals the presence of a transverse nasal crease on top of the nose at the junction of the cartilaginous and bony portions of the nasal bridge, which is caused by frequent rubbing of the nose. Nasal patency should be assessed, and the nose examined for structural abnormalities affecting nasal airflow, such as a septal deviation, turbinate hypertrophy, septal spurs, and nasal polyps. Decrease or absence of the sense of smell should raise concern about the presence of nasal polyps, a feature of cystic fibrosis. The nasal mucosa in allergic rhinitis is classically described as pale to purple in comparison with the beefy red mucosa of patients with nonallergic rhinitis. Allergic nasal secretions are typically thin and clear. Purulent secretions suggest another cause of rhinitis. The frontal and maxillary sinuses should be palpated to identify tenderness to pressure that might be associated with sinusitis.

Examination of the lips may reveal cheilitis caused by drying of the lips from continuous mouth breathing and repeated licking of the lips in an attempt to replenish moisture and relieve discomfort. Tonsillar and adenoidal hypertrophy along with a history of impressive snoring raises the possibility of obstructive sleep apnea. The posterior pharynx should be examined for the presence of postnasal drip and posterior pharyngeal lymphoid hyperplasia.

Chest findings in asthmatic children vary significantly, depending on disease duration, severity, and activity. In a child with mild or well-controlled asthma, the chest may appear entirely normal on examination between asthma exacerbations. Examination of the same child during an acute episode of asthma may reveal hyperinflation, tachypnea, cyanosis, use of accessory muscles, wheezing, and decreased air exchange with a prolonged expiratory time. Tachycardia may be caused by the asthma exacerbation or accompanied by jitteriness and caused by treatment with β-agonists. Decreased airflow or rhonchi and wheezes over the right chest may be noted in children with mucus plugging and right middle lobe atelectasis. Unilateral wheezing after an episode of coughing and choking in a small child without a history of previous respiratory illness suggests **aspiration of a foreign body.** Wheezing limited to the larynx in association with inspiratory stridor is seen in older children and adolescents with **vocal cord dysfunction.** In children with chronic asthma, an increased anteroposterior diameter of the chest suggests significant air trapping. In infants and younger children with significant asthma, a groove along the lower ribs at the site of attachment of the diaphragm may be present. Digital clubbing is rarely seen in patients with uncomplicated asthma and should prompt further evaluation to rule out other potential chronic diagnoses.

The skin of the allergic patient should be examined for evidence of urticaria/angioedema or atopic dermatitis. **Xerosis,** or dry skin, is the most common skin abnormality of allergic children. Keratosis pilaris, often found on the extensor surfaces of the upper arms and thighs, is characterized by roughness of the skin caused by keratin plugs lodged in the openings of hair follicles. Examination of the skin of the palms and feet reveals exaggerated palmar and plantar creases in some allergic children.

DIAGNOSTIC TESTING

The laboratory evaluation of the child in whom allergic disease is suspected should focus on obtaining objective evidence to support the diagnosis, documenting sensitivity to allergens implicated by the history, and ruling out other potential diagnoses.

In Vitro Tests

Allergic diseases are often associated with increased numbers of eosinophils circulating in the peripheral blood and invading the tissues and secretions of target organs. Eosinophilia, defined as the presence of >450 eosinophils/µL in peripheral blood, is the most common hematologic abnormality of allergic patients. Seasonal increases in the number of circulating eosinophils may be observed in sensitized patients after exposure to allergens such as tree, grass, and weed pollens. The number of circulating eosinophils can be suppressed by certain infections and systemic corticosteroids. In certain pathologic conditions, such as drug reactions and eosinophilic pneumonias, significantly increased numbers of eosinophils may be present in the target organ in the absence of peripheral blood eosinophilia. Increased numbers of eosinophils are observed in a wide variety of disorders in addition to allergy (Table 135-1) (Chapter 123).

Nasal and bronchial secretions are often examined for the presence of eosinophils. The presence of eosinophils in the sputum of asthmatic patients is classic. An increased number of eosinophils in a smear of nasal mucus stained with Hansel stain is a more sensitive indicator of nasal allergies than peripheral blood eosinophilia and aids in distinguishing allergic rhinitis from other causes of rhinitis. In young children, nasal eosinophilia is defined as the presence of >4% eosinophils in nasal mucus smears, whereas a finding of >10% eosinophils is required in adolescents and adults. Nasal mucus eosinophilia also has therapeutic implications, predicting a higher probability of responsiveness to topical nasal corticosteroid sprays.

An elevated immunoglobulin (Ig) E value is often found in the serum of allergic patients, because IgE is the primary antibody associated with allergic reactions. IgE values are measured in international units (IU), with 1 IU equal to 2.4 ng of IgE. Maternal IgE does not cross the placenta. Although the fetus is capable of producing IgE as early as the 11th wk of gestation, infants in developed countries produce little IgE in utero, owing to the lack of stimulation by allergens. Serum IgE levels gradually rise over the first years of life to peak in the teen years and decrease steadily thereafter. A variety of factors in addition to age, such as genetic influences, race, gender, certain diseases, and exposure to cigarette smoke and allergens, affects serum IgE levels. Serum IgE levels may increase twofold to fourfold in allergic patients during and immediately after the pollen season, and then gradually decline until the next pollen season. Comparison of total serum IgE levels among patients with allergic disease reveals that those with atopic dermatitis tend to have the highest levels, whereas patients with allergic asthma generally have higher levels than those with allergic rhinitis. Although average total serum IgE levels are higher in populations of allergic patients than in comparable populations without allergic disease, the overlap in levels is such that the diagnostic value of a total serum IgE level is poor. Approximately one half of patients with allergic disease have total serum IgE levels in the normal range. Total serum IgE measurement is indicated when the diagnosis of **allergic bronchopulmonary aspergillosis** is suspected; total serum IgE concentration >1,000 ng/mL is a criterion for diagnosis of this disorder (Chapter 229.1). Continued monitoring of the total serum IgE in patients with allergic bronchopulmonary aspergillosis is encouraged because serum IgE levels decrease with appropriate therapy and rise again during exacerbations of the disease. The total serum IgE value is also elevated in several nonallergic diseases (Table 135-2).

The presence of IgE specific for a particular allergen can be documented in vivo by skin testing or in vitro by the measurement of allergen-specific IgE (as-IgE) levels in the serum (Table 135-3). The first test for documenting the presence of as-IgE was called the **radioallergosorbent test (RAST)** because it used a radiolabeled anti-IgE antibody. The RAST has been replaced by an improved generation of as-IgE assays that use enzyme-conjugated rather than radiolabeled anti-IgE. These assays use solid-phase supports to which allergens of an individual allergen extract are bound. A small amount of the patient's serum is incubated with the allergen-coated support, resulting in binding of the patient's as-IgE to the allergens on the support. Next, the allergen-coated support to which the patient's as-IgE is bound is incubated with enzyme conjugated antihuman-IgE that then binds to the patient's as-IgE. Incubation of this complex with a fluorescent substrate of the conjugated enzyme results in the generation of fluorescence that is proportional to the amount of as-IgE in the serum sample. The amount of as-IgE in the serum sample is calculated by interpolation from a standard calibration

Table 135-1 DIFFERENTIAL DIAGNOSIS OF CHILDHOOD EOSINOPHILIA

PHYSIOLOGIC
Prematurity
Infants receiving hyperalimentation
Familial
INFECTIOUS
Parasitic (with tissue-invasive helminths, e.g., trichinosis, strongyloidiasis, pneumocystosis, filariasis, cysticercosis, cutaneous and visceral larva migrans, echinococcosis)
Bacterial (brucellosis, tularemia, cat-scratch disease, *Chlamydia*)
Fungal (histoplasmosis, blastomycosis, coccidioidomycosis, allergic bronchopulmonary aspergillosis)
Mycobacterial (tuberculosis, leprosy)
Viral (hepatitis A, hepatitis B, hepatitis C, Epstein-Barr virus)
PULMONARY
Allergic (rhinitis, asthma)
Loeffler syndrome
Hypersensitivity pneumonitis
Eosinophilic pneumonia
Pulmonary interstitial eosinophilia
DERMATOLOGIC
Atopic dermatitis
Pemphigus
Dermatitis herpetiformis
Infantile eosinophilic pustular folliculitis
Episodic angioedema and urticaria
Eosinophilic fasciitis (Schulman syndrome)
Eosinophilic cellulitis (Well syndrome)
Kimura disease
ONCOLOGIC
Neoplasm (lung, gastrointestinal, uterine)
Hodgkin disease
Leukemia
Myelofibrosis
IMMUNOLOGIC
T-cell immunodeficiencies
Hyperimmunoglobulin E (Job) syndrome
Wiskott-Aldrich syndrome
Graft versus host disease
Drug hypersensitivity
Post-irradiation
Post-splenectomy
ENDOCRINE
Post-adrenalectomy
Addison disease
Panhypopituitarism
CARDIOVASCULAR
Loeffler disease (fibroplastic endocarditis)
Congenital heart disease
Hypersensitivity vasculitis
GASTROINTESTINAL
Milk protein allergy
Inflammatory bowel disease
Eosinophilic esophagitis
Eosinophilic gastroenteritis

Table 135-2 NONALLERGIC DISEASES ASSOCIATED WITH INCREASED SERUM IMMUNOGLOBULIN E (IgE) CONCENTRATIONS

PARASITIC INFESTATIONS
Ascariasis
Capillariasis
Echinococcosis
Fascioliasis
Filariasis
Hookworm
Onchocerciasis
Paragonimiasis
Schistosomiasis
Strongyloidiasis
Trichinosis
Visceral larva migrans
INFECTIONS
Allergic bronchopulmonary aspergillosis
Candidiasis, systemic
Coccidioidomycosis
Cytomegalovirus mononucleosis
Infectious mononucleosis (Epstein-Barr virus)
Leprosy
IMMUNODEFICIENCY
Hyper-IgE (Job) syndrome
IgA deficiency, selective
Nezelof syndrome
Thymic hypoplasia (DiGeorge anomaly)
Wiskott-Aldrich syndrome
NEOPLASTIC DISEASES
Hodgkin disease
IgE myeloma
OTHER DISEASES AND DISORDERS
Burns
Cystic fibrosis
Dermatitis, chronic acral
Erythema nodosum, streptococcal infection
Guillain-Barré syndrome
Hemosiderosis, primary pulmonary
Intestinal nephritis, drug-induced
Kawasaki disease
Liver disease
Pemphigus, bullous
Polyarteritis nodosa, infantile
Rheumatoid arthritis

Table 135-3 DETERMINATION OF SPECIFIC IMMUNOGLOBULIN E (IgE) BY SKIN TESTING VERSUS IN VITRO TESTING

VARIABLE	SKIN TEST*	ALLERGEN-SPECIFIC IgE ASSAY
Risk of allergic reaction	Yes	No
Relative sensitivity†	High	Less
Affected by antihistamines	Yes	No
Affected by corticosteroids	Usually not	No
Affected by extensive dermatitis or dermographism	Yes	No
Convenience, less patient anxiety	No	Yes
Broad selection of antigens	Yes	No
Immediate results	Yes	No
Expensive	No	Yes
Semiquantitative	No	Yes
Lability of allergens	Yes	No
Results evident to patient	Yes	No

*Skin testing may be the prick test or intradermal injection. Prick testing tends to be quicker, easier to perform and interpret, and more amenable to testing of infants.
†Because skin tests are more sensitive, they are more reliable than allergen-specific IgE assays in confirming life-threatening anaphylactic conditions if maximal sensitivity is required, such as for penicillin or Hymenoptera hypersensitivity.

curve and reported in arbitrary mass units (kilo-IU of allergen-specific antibody per unit volume of sample [kUa/L]).

The primary advantages of these assays in comparison with allergen skin testing are their safety and that the results are not influenced by skin disease or medications. Overall, the results of these tests correlate well with those obtained by skin testing and provocation challenges. The as-IgE assays are not as sensitive as the skin test. In patients with histories of life-threatening reactions to foods, insect stings, drugs, or latex, skin testing is still required because of its higher sensitivity even if the as-IgE assay result is negative.

In Vivo Tests

Allergen skin testing is the primary in vivo procedure for the diagnosis of allergic disease. Mast cells with allergen-specific IgE antibodies attached to high-affinity receptors on their surfaces reside in the skin of allergic patients. The introduction of minute amounts of an allergen to which the patient is allergic into the skin results in cross linking by the allergen of allergen-specific IgE antibodies on the mast cell surface, thereby triggering mast cell activation. Once activated, these mast cells release a variety of preformed and newly generated mediators that act on surrounding tissues. Histamine is the mediator most responsible for the immediate wheal and flare reactions observed in skin testing. Examination of the site of a positive skin test result reveals a pruritic wheal surrounded by an area of erythema. The time course of these reactions is rapid in onset, reaching a peak within ≈20 min and usually resolving over the next 20-30 min. In some patients, however, a larger area of less distinctly demarcated edema on an erythematous base develops at the skin test site over the next 6-12 hr. This reaction, the **late-phase response,** usually resolves by 24 hr. Biopsy of the site of a late-phase response reveals the presence of an inflammatory infiltrate consisting of T cells, neutrophils, and eosinophils. These reactions are thought to be similar to the late-phase responses observed in other organs, such as the nose and lungs, after provocation challenges.

Skin testing in children is usually first performed using the **prick/puncture technique.** With this technique, a small drop of allergen is applied to the skin surface, and a tiny amount is introduced into the epidermis by lightly pricking or puncturing the skin through the drop of extract with a small needle. When the prick/puncture skin test result is negative and the history is suggestive, selective skin testing using the **intradermal technique** may be performed. This technique involves using a 26-gauge needle to inject 0.01-0.02 mL of a dilute allergen extract into the dermis of the arm. This technique is more sensitive than the prick/puncture technique, and the allergen extracts used are 1,000- to 100-fold less concentrated than extracts used for prick/puncture testing. Intradermal skin tests are not recommended for use with food allergens because of the risk of triggering anaphylaxis. Irritant rather than allergic reactions can occur with intradermal skin testing if higher concentrations of extracts, such as 1:100 weight:volume, are used. Although prick/puncture testing is less sensitive than intradermal skin testing, positive prick/puncture skin test results tend to correlate better with symptoms on natural exposure to the allergen.

Panels of skin tests that include the appropriate allergens for a given geographic area in addition to common indoor allergens are often applied; the number of skin tests performed should be individualized, with the allergens suggested by the history taken into account. A positive and negative control skin test, using histamine and saline, respectively, is performed with each set of skin tests. A negative control is necessary to ensure that the patient is not dermatographic and that reactions caused merely by applying pressure to overly sensitive skin are not interpreted as due to allergen sensitivity. A positive control is necessary to establish the presence of a cutaneous response to histamine. Medications with antihistaminic properties in addition to adrenergic agents such as ephedrine and epinephrine suppress skin test responses and should be avoided for appropriate intervals (≈3-10 days) before the performance of skin tests. Prolonged courses of systemic corticosteroids may suppress cutaneous reactivity by decreasing the number of tissue mast cells as well as their ability to release mediators.

Under certain circumstances, **provocation testing** is performed to examine the association between allergen exposure and the development of symptoms. Provocation challenges involving exposure of the skin, conjunctiva, nasal mucosa, oral mucosa, gastrointestinal tract, or lungs to allergens are performed in a variety of clinical and research settings. Bronchial provocation challenges are performed by having patients inhale increasingly concentrated solutions of nebulized allergen extracts and monitoring for airways obstruction by clinical observation and the performance of pulmonary function testing. Results of bronchial provocation challenges correlate well with other clinical data obtained by skin testing or in vitro testing. Although a large number of bronchial provocation challenges to allergens have been performed safely, the possibility of a severe reaction and the time, expense, and expertise required for the performance of these tests limit their performance to a research setting.

The bronchial provocation test most frequently performed is to methacholine, which causes potent bronchoconstriction of asthmatic but not of normal airways. **Methacholine challenge testing** is performed to document the presence and degree of bronchial hyperreactivity in a patient in whom asthma is suspected. After baseline spirometry values are obtained, increasing concentrations of nebulized methacholine are inhaled until a specified drop in lung function, such as a 20% decrease in FEV_1 (forced expiratory volume in the first second of expiration), occurs or the patient is able to tolerate the inhalation of a set concentration of methacholine, such as 25 mg/mL, without a significant decrease in lung function.

Oral **food challenges** are performed to determine whether a specific food causes symptoms or whether a suspected food can be added to the diet. Food challenges are performed for those foods incriminated by the history and results of skin tests and/or in vitro testing. These challenges may be performed in an open, single-blind, double-blind, or double-blind placebo-controlled fashion and involve the ingestion of gradually increasing amounts of the suspected food at set time intervals until the patient either experiences a reaction or tolerates a normal portion of the food openly. Because of the potential for significant allergic reactions, these challenges should be performed only in an appropriately equipped facility with personnel experienced in the performance of food challenges and the treatment of anaphylaxis, including cardiopulmonary resuscitation.

BIBLIOGRAPHY

Please visit the Nelson Textbook of Pediatrics *website at www.expertconsult.com for the complete bibliography.*

Chapter 136
Principles of Treatment of Allergic Disease

Dan Atkins and Donald Y.M. Leung

The basic principles of the treatment of allergic disease include the avoidance of exposure to allergens and irritants that trigger symptoms and the pharmacologic management of symptoms caused by unavoidable acute and chronic allergen exposures. In selected patients with allergic disease refractory to avoidance measures and optimal pharmacologic management, allergen immunotherapy may be considered.

ENVIRONMENTAL CONTROL MEASURES

Children spend the majority of their time in indoor environments, including the home. In an effort to save energy, houses and buildings have been built more tightly and with more insulation with fewer air exchanges. These factors have led to an increase in indoor humidity and higher concentrations of allergens and irritants in indoor air. Examination of indoor environments suggests that house dust mite, cat, and cockroach allergens are the most common significant triggers of allergic disease in these settings; exposures to allergens from other pets, pests, fungi, and respiratory irritants such as cigarette smoke are also a problem.

More than 30,000 species of mites have been identified, but the term *dust mites* usually refers to the pyroglyphid mites *Dermatophagoides pteronyssinus, Dermatophagoides farinae,* and *Euroglyphus maynei,* which are the major sources of allergen in house dust. Respiration and water vapor exchange occur through the skin of dust mites, rendering them sensitive to decreases in humidity and temperature extremes. The regular use of humidifiers and swamp coolers promotes dust mite survival. Mites do not survive with relative humidity <50%. They feed on animal and human skin scales and other debris, which is why they exist in large numbers in mattresses and bedding, carpet, and upholstered furniture. They are also found in flour and mixes for baked goods. Anaphylaxis has been reported following the ingestion of baked goods such as waffles and pancakes prepared with flour infested with dust mites. Dust mite fecal pellets are a major source of allergens. They consist of partially digested food combined with digestive enzymes encased in a permeable membrane, which keeps the fecal pellets intact. These fecal pellets have been likened to pollen grains, given their similarities in size (10-40 µm), the amount of allergen they contain, and their ability to release allergens rapidly on contact with moist mucous membranes. Mites can persist in imported furnishings for at least 2 yr; mite allergens have been shown to remain stable under domestic conditions for periods of at least 4 yr. Dust mite allergens become airborne during normal household activities; a vigorous disturbance such as vacuuming without a vacuum bag or shaking a bed sheet can launch significant amounts of dust mite allergens into the air. Once airborne, dust mite allergen particles settle out of the air relatively rapidly because of their size and weight. Nonetheless, dust mite allergen exposure likely occurs during sleep on mite-infested pillows and mattresses and during normal household activities when dust mite concentrations in the home are high enough. Levels of dust mite allergens as low as 2 µg/g of house dust can lead to sensitization, whereas levels of 10 µg/g of house dust are associated with symptoms.

Appropriate environmental control measures can significantly reduce exposure to dust mite allergens (Table 136-1). Major emphasis should be placed on reducing exposure to dust mite allergens in the bedroom and the bed because of the large amount of time the child spends there. Encasements impermeable to dust mite allergens should be placed on all pillows, the mattress, and the box spring. Dust should be removed from the surfaces of these covers and the bed frame by vacuuming weekly. The sheets and mattress pad should be washed weekly in hot water at a temperature of >130°F. Minimizing the number of items in the room that collect dust, such as books, drapes, toys, stuffed animals, and any clutter, is recommended. Major reservoirs of dust mite allergen that are often more difficult to deal with include the carpet and upholstered furniture, which should be vacuumed weekly with an efficient double-thickness-bagged vacuum cleaner. Although the application of acaricides or denaturing agents to carpets and upholstered furniture has been advised, the actual benefit remains unclear, and the amount of effort required may be more than most families are willing to invest. If possible, carpet removal, at least in the bedroom, may prove a better choice for eliminating a large reservoir of dust mite allergen. Other measures for dust mite allergen control include

Table 136-1 ENVIRONMENTAL CONTROL OF ALLERGEN EXPOSURE

ALLERGEN	CONTROL MEASURES
Dust mites	Encase bedding in airtight, allergen-impermeable covers Wash bedding weekly in water at temperatures >130°F Remove wall-to-wall carpeting Replace curtains with blinds Remove upholstered furniture Reduce indoor humidity
Animal dander	Avoid furred pets Keep animals out of patient's bedroom
Cockroaches	Control available food and water sources Keep kitchen/bathroom surfaces dry and free of standing water Seal cracks in walls Use professionally extermination services; safe pesticide should be used in baits
Mold	Repair moisture-prone areas Avoid high humidity in patient's bedroom Use high-efficiency particulate air (HEPA) filters in living areas Repair water leaks Replace carpets with hardwood floors Regularly check basements, attics, and crawl spaces for standing water and mold
Pollen	Keep automobile and house windows closed Control timing of outdoor exposure Restrict camping, hiking, and leaf raking Drive in an air-conditioned automobile Air-condition the home Install portable HEPA filters

Modified from Leung DYM, Sampson HA, Geha RS, et al: *Pediatric allergy principles and practice*, St Louis, 2003, Mosby, p 294.

maintaining the indoor relative humidity at <50% and keeping the air conditioning set at the lowest level during the warmer months.

In many countries, more than half of the households have pets, the most common of which are cats and dogs. The major sources of allergens from cats, dogs, horses, and cattle are hair, dander, and saliva, whereas the major source of allergens from rodents is urine. Studies of airborne cat allergen have shown that a significant portion is found on small particles that behave aerodynamically like spheres <7 μm in diameter. As much as 30% of airborne cat allergen may reside on particles <5 μm. Particles this small may not be adequately filtered by the nose and could potentially be deposited in the airways. Their small size enables these particles to remain airborne for longer periods and to be suspended repeatedly by air currents from heating and ventilation systems or just by walking across the carpet or sitting in an upholstered chair. **Fel d 1,** the major cat allergen, is a highly charged protein that readily sticks to a variety of surfaces, including walls, carpeting, and upholstered furniture. Owing to this adhesiveness, cat allergens bind to the cat owner's clothing and are routinely transported to public buildings, including schools, where they have been measured in moderately high amounts. From these sites, significant amounts of cat allergen can subsequently be carried into homes without cats. Analysis of house dust from homes with cats reveals levels of Fel d 1 ranging from 8 μg to 1.5 mg/g of house dust. Levels of Fel d 1 in homes without cats vary from 0.2 to 80 μg/g of house dust. Sensitization to cat allergen has been associated with levels ranging from 1 to 8 μg/g of house dust. Carpets, upholstered furniture, and bedding serve as reservoirs of cat allergens, resulting in the persistence of significant amounts in the home for months after a cat has been removed. Complete avoidance of cat allergen is virtually impossible, although significant reduction in exposure to cat allergens is achievable.

Removing the pet from the home is obviously the most effective means of reducing exposure to animal allergens, although it has been demonstrated that without other interventions, such as removing carpeting and upholstered furniture and wiping down walls, it takes 6 months or more for the levels of cat allergen to drop to a level found in houses without a cat. As a result, cat owners who remove their pets from their homes should be informed not to expect immediate results. Unfortunately, advice to remove a pet from the home or keep it outdoors is often ignored. In contrast to dust mite allergens, cat allergen is light and remains suspended in the air for long periods. As a result, **air cleaners with high-efficiency particulate air (HEPA) filters** are helpful in reducing the amount of airborne cat allergen. Other suggested methods include washing the cat regularly and maintaining a cat allergen–free bedroom from which the cat is excluded and where mattress covers and air-filtering devices are used. The cat should also be restricted from other living areas where the sensitized child spends large amounts of time, such as the family room and other play areas (see Table 136-1). Regular vacuuming with a HEPA-filtered and double–thickness bag vacuum cleaner is also encouraged. Similar measures are suggested for the control of exposure to other animal allergens, although whether these measures reduce exposure to levels resulting in clinical improvement as demonstrated by decreased symptoms, improved peak flows, or decreases in bronchial hyperreactivity remains to be documented by appropriately controlled studies.

Infestation of the home by insects and other pests such as mice and rats is another potential source of significant allergen exposure in the indoor environment. Studies have identified the importance of exposure to cockroach allergens as a major risk factor for the development of asthma in inner-city children. Once sensitized, inner-city cockroach-sensitive asthmatic children with continued exposure to high levels of cockroach allergens in their bedrooms are at higher risk for urgent care visits and hospitalization than inner-city asthmatic children who are not allergic to cockroaches. Recommended methods to decrease cockroach allergen exposure include reducing cockroaches' access to the home by sealing cracks in the flooring and walls and removing sources of food and water by repairing leaky pipes, putting away food, and frequent cleaning (see Table 136-1). Regular extermination using baits or chemical treatment of infested areas is also advised.

Efforts to improve indoor air quality should also encompass reducing exposure to respiratory irritants. Passive exposure to environmental tobacco smoke worsens asthma and increases nasal symptoms in patients with allergic nasal disease. Smoking cessation should be repeatedly encouraged, and smoking indoors should never be permitted. The use of wood-burning stoves and fireplaces and of kerosene heaters should be discouraged.

Although exposure to pollens and fungi occurs primarily outdoors, these allergens are detectable indoors during the warmer months, when their indoor levels often reflect their prevalence in the outdoor environment. During the winter, when the outdoor levels of other fungi are lowest, the indoor fungi *Aspergillus* and *Penicillium* are the most prevalent. Fungi are often found in damp basements and thrive in conditions associated with increased moisture in the home, such as water leaks, flooding, and increased humidity promoted by the excessive use of humidifiers or swamp coolers. Exposure to indoor fungal allergens can be reduced by maintaining the indoor relative humidity at < 50%, removing contaminated carpets, and wiping down washable surfaces prone to fungal growth, such as shower stalls, shower curtains, sinks, drip trays, and garbage pails, with the use of solutions of detergent and 5% bleach (see Table 136-1). Dehumidifiers should be placed in damp basements. Standing water at any site in the home should be eliminated, and the cause addressed. Removing all items from the home that are prone to fungal contamination and growth is also encouraged. Keeping the windows and doors closed and using air conditioning to filter outdoor air can keep both indoor pollen and fungi levels to a minimum during the warmer months, when outdoor levels of these allergens are at their peak. The use of window or attic fans is to be avoided.

Laundry should be dried in a dryer rather than on a clothesline. Measures to avoid pollens and fungal spores when out of the house include closing the windows and using the air conditioner when traveling in the car, avoiding moldy vegetation, and wearing a mask when these materials cannot be avoided. Outdoor activities during periods of high pollen counts should be kept to a minimum. Someone other than the sensitized patient should mow the lawn and rake leaves. Frequent handwashing after outdoor play is suggested to avoid transferring pollens from the hands to the eyes and nose. At the end of the day, showering and shampooing are suggested to avoid contamination of the bed with allergens. During the day, the bed should remain covered with a bedspread.

PHARMACOLOGIC THERAPY

Adrenergic Agents

Adrenergic agents exert their effects through the stimulation of cell surface α- and β-adrenergic receptors in a variety of target tissues. These receptors belong to the G protein–coupled superfamily of receptors. In general, α-adrenergic receptor stimulation results in excitatory responses such as vasoconstriction, whereas β-adrenergic stimulation leads to inhibitory responses such as bronchodilation. The α-adrenergic receptors have been classified into α_1- and α_2-adrenergic receptors. Further studies of these receptors in humans have identified 3 subtypes of α_1-adrenergic receptors and 3 subtypes of α_2-adrenergic receptors. The β-adrenergic receptors are further divided into 3 subtypes: β_1, β_2, and β_3. Each of these adrenergic receptors exhibits a distinctive tissue distribution. The physiologic response in a given tissue to the administration of an adrenergic agent depends on the specific receptor-binding characteristics of the drug as well as the numbers and distribution of the various types of adrenergic receptors in the tissue. Epinephrine remains the drug of choice for the treatment of anaphylaxis because of its combined α- and β-adrenergic effects.

The α-adrenergic agents are effective in the treatment of allergic nasal disease because of their decongestant effects (see Tables 137-2 and 137-4). In the nose, stimulation of α_1-adrenergic receptors on postcapillary venules and of α_2-adrenergic receptors on precapillary arterioles leads to vasoconstriction, resulting in a reduction in nasal congestion. The oral decongestants currently in clinical use include pseudoephedrine and phenylephrine. These medications are available individually or in combination with antihistamines in liquid and tablet forms, including sustained-release preparations. Phenylpropanolamine and all combination products containing this sympathomimetic amine similar in structure to pseudoephedrine have been taken off the market in the USA by the U.S. Food and Drug Administration (FDA) because of concerns about the risk of hemorrhagic stroke and the inability to predict who is at risk. Pseudoephedrine is rapidly and thoroughly absorbed, whereas phenylephrine, the less effective of the two drugs, is incompletely absorbed, resulting in a significantly lower bioavailability of ≈ 38%. Peak plasma concentrations of these drugs are reached between 30 min and 2 hr of administration, but the decongestant effect has not been directly correlated to the plasma concentration. Pseudoephedrine is excreted essentially unchanged by the kidney. The use of oral decongestants should be avoided in patients with hypertension, coronary artery disease, glaucoma, or metabolic disorders such as diabetes and hyperthyroidism. Reported **adverse effects** of oral decongestants include excitability, headache, nervousness, palpitations, tachycardia, arrhythmias, hypertension, nausea, vomiting, and urinary retention. Decongestants available as topical nasal sprays include phenylephrine, oxymetazoline, naphthazoline, tetrahydrozoline, and xylometazoline. Given their efficacy and rapid onset of action, the potential for excessive use of topical nasal decongestants resulting in rebound nasal congestion is high. When this occurs, refraining from the use of these sprays for 2-3 days is necessary for recovery.

Drugs that stimulate β-adrenergic receptors have been used for years in the treatment of asthma because of their potent bronchodilator effects (see Table 138-11). The subclassification of β-adrenergic receptors into β_1 and β_2 subtypes led to the development of drugs selective for the β_2-adrenergic receptor, such as albuterol, that have the advantage of producing significant bronchodilation with less cardiac stimulation. The long-acting inhaled β_2-adrenergic agonists (LABAs) salmeterol and formoterol, with a 12-hr duration of action, are approved for use in children ≥ 4 yr of age. LABAs are not recommended for the treatment of acute asthma exacerbations because of their relatively slow onset of action. Concern about an apparent increased risk of asthma-related adverse events is why LABAs are not recommended as monotherapy for the long-term control of persistent asthma but are promoted as best used in conjunction with an inhaled steroid. Dry powder inhaled and metered-dose inhaler preparations combining a LABA with an inhaled corticosteroid have had significant impact on the treatment of children with moderate persistent asthma. In addition to their bronchodilating effects, β_2-adrenergic agonists have been reported to improve mucociliary clearance, decrease microvascular permeability, inhibit cholinergic nerve transmission, and reduce mediator release in mast cells, basophils, and eosinophils. The β-adrenergic agonists can be delivered orally, by inhalation, or by injection. The inhaled route is preferred because of the rapid onset of action and fewer adverse effects. Reported **adverse effects** of β-adrenergic agents include tremor, palpitations, tachycardia, arrhythmias, central nervous system stimulation, hyperglycemia, hypokalemia, hypomagnesemia, and a transient increase in hypoxia, which is attributed to an increase in perfusion to inadequately ventilated areas of the asthmatic lung. In some studies, levalbuterol, a single isomer of albuterol developed to reduce the adverse effects of short-acting β-agonists, has been reported to exhibit a bronchodilatory effect clinically comparable to that of racemic albuterol at a lower dose and with a preferable safety profile. Levalbuterol is available as a nebulized preparation and a metered-dose inhaler preparation.

Anticholinergic Agents

Anticholinergic drugs inhibit vagally mediated reflexes by antagonizing the action of acetylcholine at muscarinic receptors. Of the available anticholinergic agents, **ipratropium bromide** is the most commonly used. It is a quaternary amine that is poorly absorbed across mucosal surfaces and does not readily cross the blood-brain barrier. As a bronchodilator, it has a slower onset of action than short-acting inhaled β_2-agonists and takes longer to reach maximal effect, making it less effective as a rescue medication. Ipratropium is available by prescription as a metered-dose inhaler delivering 17 µg/spray and as a 0.02% nebulized solution (500 µg/2.5 mL). Inhaled anticholinergics have very few adverse effects, although they occasionally trigger coughing.

Ipratropium given as a nasal spray (0.03-0.06%) has been shown to be effective in the reduction of rhinorrhea resulting from perennial nonallergic rhinitis, the common cold, and other triggers such as exposure to irritants or cold air. The use of ipratropium is limited in the treatment of moderate to severe allergic rhinitis because it does not alter other common allergic nasal symptoms, such as sneezing, nasal congestion, and pruritus. Nasal dryness and epistaxis are occasionally encountered with use of the nasal spray.

Antihistamines

The release of histamine and its effects on surrounding tissues is central to the development of symptoms classically associated with the allergic response. As a result, antihistamines are frequently used for the treatment of allergic disease. Histamine exerts its effects through binding with one of its four receptors, as H_1-, H_2-, H_3-, or H_4-receptor. Histamine effects triggered through H_1-receptor binding are those most relevant to allergic

Table 136-2 CLASSIFICATION OF ANTIHISTAMINES (H_1-ANTAGONISTS)

CLASS	EXAMPLES
ETHYLENEDIAMINES	
First-generation	Antazoline, pyrilamine, tripelennamine
TYPE II ETHANOLAMINES	
First-generation	Carbinoxamine, clemastine, diphenhydramine
TYPE III ALKYLAMINES	
First-generation	Brompheniramine, chlorpheniramine, triprolidine
Second-generation	Acrivastine
TYPE IV PIPERAZINES	
First-generation	Cyclizine, hydroxyzine, meclizine
Second-generation	Cetirizine
TYPE V PIPERIDINES	
First-generation	Azatadine, cyproheptadine
Second-generation	Fexofenadine, loratadine
TYPE VI PHENOTHIAZINES	
First-generation	Methdilazine, promethazine

inflammation, and include pain, pruritus, vasodilation, increased vascular permeability, smooth muscle contraction, mucus production, and the stimulation of parasympathetic nerve endings and reflexes. The human H_1-receptor gene has been mapped to the distal short arm of chromosome 3. The antimuscarinic effect of some of the early H_1-type antihistamines may be explained by the reported 45% homology of the H_1-receptor with the human muscarinic receptor. The H_1-type antihistamines prevent the effects of H_1-receptor activation through reversible, competitive inhibition of histamine by binding to the H_1-receptor. As a result, antihistamines work best in preventing rather than reversing the actions of histamine and are most effective when given at doses and dosing intervals resulting in the persistent saturation of target organ tissue histamine receptors.

The H_1-type antihistamines are traditionally divided into six classes on the basis of differences in their chemical structures (Tables 136-2 and 137-2). These antihistamines are further divided into first-generation antihistamines, which, because of their lipophilicity, cross the blood-brain barrier to exert effects on the central nervous system, and second-generation antihistamines, which exert minimal, if any, central nervous system effects because of their inability to cross the blood-brain barrier owing to their size, charge, and lipophilicity. The sedative effects and cognitive impairment associated with the use of first-generation antihistamines are well documented. Thus, one of the primary advantages of second-generation antihistamines is that they are nonsedating or much less sedating than first-generation antihistamines. Both first- and second-generation antihistamines are available in oral preparations. A number of first-generation antihistamines are available over the counter, whereas loratadine and cetirizine are currently the second-generation antihistamines available without a prescription. Other first-generation and second-generation antihistamines require a prescription. The only antihistamines available as an intranasal spray are azelastine and olopatadine, which is also a mast cell stabilizer. The benefit of this form of administration is the potential for a rapid onset of action, within 15-30 min. Azelastine, which is systemically absorbed and can cross the blood-brain barrier, has central nervous system effects in some patients and is not currently approved for use in children <12 yr of age.

Orally administered antihistamines are well absorbed and reach peak serum concentrations within ~2 hr. High tissue concentrations of antihistamines are usually achieved, likely accounting for the sustained suppression of wheal and flare reactions even after serum levels have significantly declined. Most antihistamines are metabolized by the hepatic cytochrome P450 enzyme system. Elimination of antihistamines may be reduced in patients with hepatic impairment or by the simultaneous ingestion of inhibitors of this pathway, such as erythromycin and other macrolide antibiotics, ciprofloxacin, ketoconazole, itraconazole, and certain antidepressants, such as nefazodone and fluvoxamine. Some antihistamines, such as hydroxyzine and loratadine, are converted to clinically active metabolites. Clearance of fexofenadine and cetirizine is reduced in patients with impaired renal function. Cetirizine clearance is also reduced in patients with hepatic dysfunction.

The efficacy of antihistamines in the treatment of seasonal and perennial allergic rhinoconjunctivitis is well documented (Chapter 137). Compared with other medications in regard to the relief of allergic nasal symptoms, antihistamines are more effective than cromolyn sodium but significantly less effective than intranasal corticosteroids. Improvement in symptom relief in patients with allergic rhinitis has been reported when an antihistamine is given in combination with a decongestant or with an intranasal steroid. Numerous formulations combining antihistamines and decongestants are available. Antihistamines have also been shown to be beneficial in the treatment of acute and chronic urticaria/angioedema. With regard to asthma, a significant clinical effect of antihistamines at conventional doses is difficult to document, other than the possible improvement offered by better control of allergic nasal symptoms.

The second-generation antihistamines are preferable for the treatment of allergic disease in children because of negligible sedative and anticholinergic effects in comparison with first-generation antihistamines without a sacrifice in efficacy. Most second-generation antihistamines are effective with once-daily dosing, which, because of the convenience, may improve therapy adherence. The widespread availability of first-generation antihistamines and their lower cost account for their continued use. The **adverse effects** most often encountered with second-generation agents include the performance impairment and anticholinergic effects noted with first-generation antihistamines. The anticholinergic adverse effects encountered may include drying of the mouth and eyes, urinary retention, constipation, excitation, nervousness, palpitations, and tachycardia. Prolongation of the QT interval and ventricular tachycardia (Torsades de pointes) were reported in association with the use of two second-generation antihistamines that have since been removed from the market; those currently in use have not been associated with concerning cardiac effects.

Chromones

Cromolyn sodium, the disodium salt of 1,3-bis (2-carboxychromon-5-yloxy)-2-hydroxypropane, and nedocromil sodium, a pyranoquinoline dicarboxylic acid, are the two chromones used to treat allergic disorders. Neither cromolyn nor nedocromil is absorbed well orally, with only 1% of the swallowed dose absorbed. Absorbed drug is not metabolized but is rapidly eliminated in approximately equal amounts by the kidneys and liver. These drugs must be applied topically to the mucosal surface of the target organ to be effective. Both drugs inhibit mast cell degranulation and mediator release. They suppress the activation of a variety of cells, such as eosinophils, neutrophils, macrophages, and epithelial cells. They also suppress the activity of afferent C-type sensory nerve fibers of the nonadrenergic, noncholinergic nervous system. Both drugs inhibit the intracellular increase in free calcium after mast cell activation and phosphorylate a mast cell protein resembling moesin, which is thought to be involved in terminating mediator release. Despite these findings, the molecular mechanism of action of these drugs remains to be completely defined.

Cromolyn and nedocromil prevent early- and late-phase allergic responses when administered before allergen exposure. They block allergen-induced increases in bronchial hyperresponsiveness as well as seasonal increases in nonspecific bronchial hyperresponsiveness. With prolonged use, both drugs are capable of reducing bronchial hyperresponsiveness. These drugs have no bronchodilator properties but can inhibit the bronchoconstrictive effects of a variety of stimuli, such as allergen challenge, exercise, hyperventilation with cold air, ultrasonically nebulized distilled water, and exposure to atmospheric and industrial pollutants.

Cromolyn and nedocromil are used as alternative, but not preferred, therapy for the treatment of mild persistent asthma. Because of their lack of bronchodilator properties, neither drug is useful for the treatment of acute asthma, although both may be used as preventive treatment before vigorous exercise or unavoidable known allergen exposure. Nedocromil is the more potent of the two. Cromolyn is available for the treatment of asthma by prescription as a 1% solution (20 mg/2 mL) for nebulization and in a metered-dose inhaler (800 µg/actuation). The suggested dose for the treatment of asthma is 20 mg of cromolyn 2 to 4 times/24 hr by nebulization or 1.6 mg 2 to 4 times/24 hr by metered-dose inhaler. In numerous studies, cromolyn has been found useful in the treatment of allergic rhinitis and allergic conjunctivitis. Preparations for the nasal and ocular administration of cromolyn are available without a prescription. The suggested dose for the treatment of allergic rhinitis is one spray in each nostril 3 to 4 times daily of a nasal spray containing 5.2 mg of cromolyn per spray (see Table 137-4). For the treatment of allergic conjunctivitis, the suggested dose is 1 drop in each eye 4 to 6 times a day of a 4% ophthalmic solution. Nedocromil is not available in a nebulized form but is available in a metered-dose inhaler. The recommended dose for the treatment of asthma is 3.5 mg (1.75 mg/puff) 2 to 4 times/24 hr. A 2% solution of nedocromil is available by prescription for the treatment of allergic conjunctivitis at a suggested dose of 1-2 drops in each eye twice daily.

The safety of these drugs, even with prolonged administration, is well documented. Dry throat and transient bronchoconstriction have been the most frequently reported adverse effects of cromolyn use for the treatment of asthma, with only rare reports of patients becoming sensitized to the drug. Some patients using nedocromil complain about its taste. Infrequently reported adverse effects of nedocromil include coughing, sore throat, rhinitis, headache, and nausea.

Glucocorticoids

Glucocorticoids are widely used in the treatment of allergic disorders because of their potent anti-inflammatory properties. The diverse anti-inflammatory actions of glucocorticoids are mediated via the glucocorticoid receptor, which is present in all inflammatory effector cells, as well as by direct inhibition of cytokines and mediators. Glucocorticoids are administered topically in ophthalmic preparations, nasal sprays, creams and ointments, metered-dose inhalers, and as a solution for nebulization. Systemic administration is accomplished orally or parenterally. The proper use and efficacy of glucocorticoids in the treatment of allergic disease along with the adverse effects associated with their use are presented in discussions of individual allergic diseases (Chapters 137-146).

Leukotriene-Modifying Agents

Drugs that alter the leukotriene pathway exert their clinical effects either by inhibiting leukotriene production or by blocking receptor binding. These agents possess mild anti-inflammatory properties and exhibit bronchodilator effects. In addition to inhibiting the early- and late-phase allergic responses to inhaled allergen, they diminish bronchoconstriction induced by exercise and exposure to allergen, aspirin, and cold air. These agents have some use in the treatment of asthma (Chapter 138) and are modestly effective in the treatment of allergic rhinitis (Chapter 137).

Theophylline

Because of its bronchodilating effects, theophylline (1,3-dimethyxanthine) has been used for years for the treatment of acute and chronic asthma. Nonspecific inhibition of phosphodiesterase isozymes and antagonism of adenosine receptors occur at achievable serum concentrations of the drug. The bronchodilator effect of theophylline is likely caused by its action as a phosphodiesterase inhibitor, whereas its ability to antagonize adenosine receptors may play a role in other effects, such as the attenuation of diaphragmatic muscle fatigue and diminishing adenosine-enhanced mast cell mediator release. Theophylline inhibits the immediate- and late-phase pulmonary responses to allergen challenge and exhibits modest protective effects. Selected anti-inflammatory and immunomodulatory effects of this drug are also documented. Theophylline is available by prescription as both rapidly absorbed and slow-release formulations. It is often administered intravenously when used for the treatment of severe acute asthma. The therapeutic and toxic effects of theophylline are related to the serum concentration, with the incidence of toxic effects significantly increasing as the serum levels approach and exceed 20 µg/mL. A variety of conditions and medications are capable of increasing or decreasing theophylline metabolism. The **toxic effects** of theophylline, ranging from mild nausea, insomnia, irritability, tremors, and headache to cardiac arrhythmias, seizures, and death, necessitate the routine monitoring of theophylline serum levels. Because of the introduction of other effective therapies for the treatment of acute and chronic asthma, the need to monitor drug serum levels routinely, and the potential for significant toxicity, the role of theophylline in the treatment of asthma has contracted significantly (Chapter 138).

Lodoxamide Tromethamine

A mast cell stabilizer, lodoxamide tromethamine is more effective than topical cromolyn sodium in alleviating signs and symptoms of allergic ocular disease (Chapter 141). It is used in children >2 yr of age for vernal keratoconjunctivitis, vernal conjunctivitis, and vernal keratitis. Occasional adverse effects have included transient burning or stinging after instillation.

Olopatadine Hydrochloride

Olopatadine hydrochloride is both a mast cell stabilizer and an H_1-receptor antagonist effective in relieving signs and symptoms of allergic conjunctivitis after topical instillation. It is labeled for use in children at least 3 yr of age. Headaches have occurred in 7% of patients treated; burning and stinging have occurred in <5%.

Anti–Immunoglobulin E

Monoclonal anti–immunoglobulin E antibodies (anti-IgE) bind to circulating IgE at a site that prevents its subsequent attachment to the high-affinity receptors for IgE on the mast cell surface. The parenteral administration of anti-IgE reduces free serum IgE concentrations, inhibits skin test responses in allergic patients, suppresses early- and late-phase responses to allergens, and decreases sputum eosinophilia in asthmatic persons. Anti-IgE has a beneficial effect in the treatment of patients with allergic rhinitis and asthma. An anti-IgE preparation (**omalizumab**) is available for the treatment of children ≥12 yr of age with documented allergen-induced asthma that is inadequately controlled by inhaled corticosteroids. Although this agent is usually well tolerated, local reactions at the injection site and rare episodes of anaphylaxis have been reported. Anti-IgE may also be beneficial in the treatment of other allergic disorders, such as anaphylaxis and food allergy. One monoclonal antibody preparation of anti-IgE used in the treatment of adults with peanut allergy resulted in a significant increase in the symptom threshold dose of peanuts. The cost of anti-IgE therapy requires careful patient selection, special consideration being given to those patients with persistent symptoms despite aggressive pharmacotherapy, significant adverse effects of current therapy, and more than one allergic disorder.

New Therapies

Several strategies for inhibiting the actions of proinflammatory cytokines are under investigation. Approaches include the use of recombinant soluble receptors that attach to a specific cytokine and inhibit subsequent binding to cell surface receptors, the development of specific cytokine receptor antagonists, and the administration of humanized monoclonal anti-cytokine antibodies. Recombinant soluble interleukin-4 (IL-4) receptor antagonists exert their effects by binding to and inactivating IL-4 before it can attach to its cell surface receptor. Although initial studies of an inhaled soluble IL-4 receptor in patients with moderate asthma requiring inhaled corticosteroids suggested a beneficial clinical effect, subsequent clinical studies of the effects of anti–IL-4 drugs in the treatment of asthma revealed these therapies to be safe, but clinical efficacy was lacking. Clinical trials of humanized monoclonal anti–IL-5 antibodies administered by injection to asthmatic patients revealed a decrease in circulating eosinophils and sputum eosinophilia, but a lesser reduction of eosinophils from the bronchial submucosa, and this effect was unaccompanied by a reduction in methacholine reactivity or a suppression of the early- or late-phase response to allergen.

The use of cytokines with anti-inflammatory effects in the treatment of allergic disorders is under investigation. Unfortunately, initial studies have not demonstrated a beneficial effect of IL-10 or interferons in the treatment of asthma. Although studies have documented that IL-12 administration is associated with a decrease in eosinophil accumulation in response to allergen challenge, inhibition of early- and late-phase responses to allergen and decreases in bronchial hyperreactivity have not been observed. In addition, the high incidence of significant adverse effects encountered with IL-12 administration limits its potential as a viable therapeutic option.

ALLERGEN IMMUNOTHERAPY

Allergen immunotherapy involves administering gradually increasing doses of allergens to a person with allergic disease for the purpose of reducing or eliminating the patient's adverse clinical response to subsequent natural exposure to those allergens. When properly administered to an appropriate candidate, allergen immunotherapy is a safe, effective form of therapy capable not only of reducing or preventing symptoms but also of potentially altering the natural history of the disease by minimizing disease duration and preventing disease progression. Conventional allergen immunotherapy is given subcutaneously under the direction of an experienced allergist.

Indications and Contraindications

Allergen immunotherapy is reserved for patients with an allergic disease demonstrated to respond to this form of therapy, such as seasonal or perennial allergic rhinoconjunctivitis, asthma triggered by allergen exposures, and insect venom sensitivity. Proof of the efficacy of conventional allergen immunotherapy for the treatment of food allergy, atopic dermatitis, latex allergy, and acute or chronic urticaria is lacking and, therefore, allergen immunotherapy is not recommended for the treatment of these disorders. Before allergen immunotherapy is considered, sensitivity of the patient to the allergens to be administered should be documented by a positive skin test result or an in vitro test revealing an increased serum level of allergen-specific IgE. The clinical relevance of these allergens should be supported by a history of symptoms upon known exposure or a timing of symptoms that correlates well with suspected allergen exposure, such as the presence of allergic nasal and ocular symptoms throughout the late summer and fall in a child with a large positive ragweed skin test response. The duration and severity of the patient's symptoms should warrant the expense, effort, and risk associated with the administration of allergen immunotherapy. The presence of disabling symptoms in spite of a trial of allergen avoidance and appropriate medications at a suitable dose should be documented. For patients sensitized to seasonal allergens, more than two consecutive seasons of symptoms are usually required before allergen immunotherapy is recommended, unless the symptoms are unusually severe or the adverse effects of medication are unacceptable. The obvious exception to this rule is the child with insect sting anaphylaxis, who should be started on venom immunotherapy once the sensitivity is correctly diagnosed (Chapter 140).

Other factors that may affect the decision to institute allergen immunotherapy include quality of life issues, such as the amount of school missed or medical resource utilization, the age of the patient, and other logistical factors. With the exception of venom immunotherapy, few data for the efficacy of allergen immunotherapy in children <5 yr of age are available. Allergen immunotherapy is not recommended for children <5 yr of age because of their increased risk of systemic reactions, the special expertise required to treat anaphylaxis in this age group, their potential inability to communicate clearly with the physician in the event of an allergic reaction, and their age-related potential for emotional distress with frequent injections. Other important logistic factors include the willingness of the patient to comply with a schedule of frequent injections over the course of several years, cost considerations, and the availability of an appropriate setting for administering allergen immunotherapy.

Allergen immunotherapy is **contraindicated** in children undergoing β-blocker therapy as well as those with certain immunologic or autoimmune disorders, allergic bronchopulmonary aspergillosis, hypersensitivity pneumonitis, severe psychiatric disturbance, or a medical condition that would impair the ability to survive an allergic reaction. Pregnancy is a contraindication to the initiation of allergen immunotherapy or dosing increases, although a pregnant adolescent can continue to receive her usual maintenance dose. Patients with unstable asthma should not be started on allergen immunotherapy because of their increased risk for fatal anaphylaxis. Allergen immunotherapy is not used for the treatment of allergic bronchopulmonary aspergillosis or hypersensitivity pneumonitis because it has no benefit. Children receiving β-blockers should be switched to another form of therapy before allergen immunotherapy is considered, because of an increased intensity of allergic reactions and a poor response of conventional therapy to these reactions with β-blocker therapy. Allergen immunotherapy is usually avoided in patients with autoimmune disorders because of the potential for unanticipated stimulation of the immune system, which might result in disease activation.

Allergen Extracts

The potency of the aqueous extracts used in allergen immunotherapy is affected by numerous factors. Allergens from weed and grass pollens are more easily extracted in aqueous solutions and, as a result, are more potent than extracts obtained from other sources, such as molds, tree pollens, and dust mites. Owing to their complexity, allergen extracts from fungal allergens are more variable than extracts from pollen allergens. Refrigeration and appropriate handling of allergen extracts used in allergen immunotherapy are important, because degradation of many allergen extracts, such as those from tree, grass, and weed pollens and dust mites, may occur at higher temperatures. Dilute extracts are more susceptible to loss of potency resulting from adherence of allergen to the glass vial than are more concentrated extracts. To combat this effect, human serum albumin is sometimes added to dilute allergen extracts. Some allergen extracts, such as those from cockroaches, dust mites, and fungi, contain proteases capable of degrading other allergens in the extract. As a result, it is often recommended that these allergens not be mixed with those from tree, grass, and weed pollens. Insect venoms are never mixed with other allergens. When available, the use of standardized allergen extracts is preferred to ensure consistency in dosing and to avoid the variability in allergen content encountered with nonstandardized allergen extracts.

Allergen Extract Administration

The goal of allergen immunotherapy is to increase gradually the dose of allergen extract administered until the injection of an "optimal" maintenance dose containing 4-12 μg of each major allergen in the extract is reached. The mixture of allergen extracts administered during the course of allergen immunotherapy is individually formulated for each patient on the basis of his or her documented sensitivities. Although various dosing schedules are used, initial injections are most often given at 5- to 10-day intervals year-round. Schedules of allergen administration are selected according to the sensitivity of the patient to the allergens in the extract. The most sensitive patients are advanced to a maintenance dose more gradually. Doses of allergen immunotherapy are increased according to a set schedule, although the reaction to the previous injection is also taken into account. A systemic reaction to the previous dose would result in a significant reduction in the next dose, whereas reducing the dose solely on the basis of a local reaction does not reduce the rate of systemic reactions. Usually 5-6 mo of weekly injections is required to reach the maintenance dose, although it may take longer in patients with marked sensitivity. Unique schedules for the administration of insect venoms, which differ from those for the administration of other allergens (Chapter 140), are used. Once the maintenance dose is reached and well tolerated, the interval between injections is increased to a few weeks or a month. Because allergen extracts gradually lose potency, the first dose from a fresh replacement vial of maintenance allergen extract is reduced by 25-75% and is then increased in increments weekly until the usual maintenance dose is reached. The recommended length for a course of allergen immunotherapy is 3-5 yr. Insect venom immunotherapy may be continued longer in patients with a history of life-threatening anaphylaxis. Patients who have not shown improvement after 1 yr of receiving maintenance doses of an appropriate allergen extract are unlikely to benefit, and their allergen immunotherapy should be discontinued. Most patients enjoy a sustained improvement after allergen immunotherapy, whereas others experience a gradual return of symptoms. Those who experience a relapse may have response to another course of treatment.

Rush immunotherapy is the administration of multiple injections either in a single day or over several days in an attempt to reach maintenance dose more rapidly. The risk of adverse reactions, including systemic reactions, is higher than with traditional allergen immunotherapy schedules. Patients to undergo rush immunotherapy are often pretreated with antihistamines and corticosteroids. Children are at even greater risk for adverse reactions with rush immunotherapy, so the benefits and risks should be fully considered. Pre-administration of omalizumab has been shown to reduce the incidence of systemic reactions associated with the use of this form of immunotherapy.

Although allergen immunotherapy is regarded as safe, the potential for anaphylaxis always exists when patients are injected with extracts containing allergens to which they are sensitized. Allergen immunotherapy should be offered in only medical settings where a physician with access to emergency equipment and medications required for the treatment of anaphylaxis is available (Chapter 143). Allergy shots should never be given at home or by untrained personnel. The patient should remain in the office for 30 min after the injection because most reactions to allergen immunotherapy begin within this time frame. Fatal anaphylaxis triggered by allergen immunotherapy, although rare, is estimated to occur at an incidence of 1 per 2 million injections. The risk of an adverse reaction is increased by dosage errors and the use of rush immunotherapy schedules. Particular caution is warranted when injections from a new vial are given. Patients with exquisite sensitivity or unstable asthma and those experiencing exacerbations of allergic rhinitis or asthma are also at increased risk for adverse reactions to allergen immunotherapy. Precautions to reduce significant adverse reactions include using standardized extracts, allowing only trained personnel to administer injections, paying careful attention to detail when giving injections, ensuring beforehand that the patient is medically stable, having appropriate medications and equipment available, and requiring the patient to remain in the office for 30 min after each injection. Checking peak flow or spirometry values before an injection is advisable for some asthmatic patients.

A desire to decrease the likelihood of allergic reactions induced by the administration of aqueous allergens led to the development of alum-precipitated extracts, in which the proteins are precipitated with aluminum hydroxide and alum-precipitated, pyridine-extracted extracts. Because of the smaller number of available extracts, the use of this type of extract remains limited. Another method developed to reduce allergenicity while maintaining immunogenicity is the polymerization of allergen extracts with glutaraldehyde. When polymerized extracts are used, the maintenance dose can be reached within 2 mo with a markedly reduced incidence of systemic reactions. Polymerized allergen extracts have not yet been approved for use in the USA. Other approaches to immunotherapy are under investigation; they include chemical or genetic manipulation of the allergen and linking of the principle allergenic moiety of a relevant allergen to a highly active adjuvant, such as an immunostimulatory sequence mimicking patterns of bacterial DNA.

Local nasal immunotherapy is administered by having the patient spray allergen solutions into the nose at scheduled intervals. Although symptom amelioration has been noted, a lack of a significant systemic immunologic response has decreased interest in pursuing this form of therapy. Sublingual immunotherapy (SLIT) involves the sublingual administration of high-dose allergen, which is then swallowed. The use of SLIT is expected to increase significantly because of its favorable safety profile and convenience of administration.

Efficacy

The positive impact of allergen immunotherapy on seasonal or perennial allergic rhinitis or rhinoconjunctivitis is well documented. In regard to the treatment of allergic rhinitis, birch, mountain cedar, grass, ragweed, and *Cladosporium* are allergens for which the efficacy of allergen immunotherapy has been effective. Effectiveness of allergen immunotherapy with other allergens commonly used for the treatment of allergic rhinitis is inconclusive. As with allergic rhinitis, most of the controlled trials examining the effects of allergen immunotherapy on seasonal or perennial allergic asthma also report favorable results. A meta-analysis of 20 trials examining the effects of allergen immunotherapy on allergic asthma revealed a significant increase in the odds for improvement after treatment along with fewer symptoms, improved pulmonary functions, less need for medication, and a reduction in bronchial hyperreactivity. The most convincing data for the benefit of allergen immunotherapy in the treatment of allergic asthma are available for birch, mountain cedar, grass, ragweed, and dust mite, with less conclusive, but suggestive data available for *Cladosporium, Alternaria,* and cat allergens. Studies examining the effects of allergen immunotherapy in the treatment of patients with allergic rhinitis and allergic asthma have usually documented increases in circulating allergen-specific IgG and decreases in allergen-specific IgE after treatment. Reductions in sensitivity to administered allergens have been demonstrated in nasal and bronchial challenges. These studies have often shown that the late-phase response after allergen challenge is ablated or significantly reduced. The protective benefit as well as the safety of venom immunotherapy in patients with sensitivity to *Hymenoptera* venoms has also been well documented in several large studies. The efficacy of allergen immunotherapy for the treatment of atopic dermatitis, urticaria, and latex allergy has not been documented. Studies using oral immunotherapy (OIT), involving the oral administration of gradually increasing doses of a food allergen under close medical observation followed by a prolonged maintenance phase of daily fixed-dose food allergen administration at home, have documented the safety of this approach and suggested promise as a viable form of treatment. Although still under investigation, OIT and perhaps SLIT may provide a much awaited therapeutic approach to the treatment of food allergy in the future.

BIBLIOGRAPHY

Please visit the Nelson Textbook of Pediatrics *website at www.expertconsult.com for the complete bibliography.*

Chapter 137
Allergic Rhinitis

Henry Milgrom and Donald Y.M. Leung

Allergic rhinitis (AR) is an inflammatory disorder of the nasal mucosa characterized by nasal congestion, rhinorrhea, and itching, often accompanied by sneezing and conjunctival irritation. Its categorization as a major chronic respiratory disease of children is predicated on its high prevalence, detrimental effects on quality of life and school performance, and co-morbidities. Children with AR often have related sinusitis, conjunctivitis, otitis media, serous otitis, hypertrophic tonsils and adenoids, and eczema. Childhood allergic rhinitis is associated with at least twofold increase in risk for asthma at an older age. Over the past 40 yr an upsurge in AR has taken place throughout the world, sparing rural and underdeveloped regions. In prosperous societies, 20-40% of children suffer from AR. Its symptoms may appear in infancy, with the diagnosis generally established by the time the child reaches age 6 yr. The prevalence peaks late in childhood. Risk factors include family history of atopy and serum immunoglobulin (Ig) E higher than 100 IU/mL before age 6 yr. The risk increases in children introduced to foods or formula early in infancy, those whose mothers smoke heavily, especially before the children are 1 yr old, and those with heavy exposure to indoor allergens. A critical period appears to exist early in infancy when the genetically susceptible individual is at greatest risk of sensitization. Breast-feeding of high-risk infants and exposure to dogs, cats, and endotoxin early in childhood protect against atopy and early wheezing. Delivery by cesarean section is associated with allergic rhinitis and atopy among children with a parental history of asthma or allergies. This association may be explained by the lack of exposure to maternal vaginal/fecal flora during delivery. Children between 2 and 3 yr old who have elevated anti-cockroach and anti-mouse IgE are at increased risk of wheezing, rhinitis, and atopic dermatitis. The occurrence of 3 or more episodes of rhinorrhea in the first year of life is associated with allergic rhinitis at age 7 yr. Early life exposures or their absence have a profound influence on the development of the allergic phenotype.

ETIOLOGY

Two factors necessary for expression of AR are sensitivity to an allergen and the presence of an allergen in the environment. AR is currently classified as **seasonal (SAR)** or **perennial (PAR)**, although these terms may soon be replaced by **intermittent allergic rhinitis (IAR)** and **persistent rhinitis (PER)**. The 2 sets of terms are based on different premises, but inhalant allergens are the main cause of all forms of rhinitis irrespective of the terminology. SAR follows a well-defined course of cyclical exacerbation, whereas PAR causes year-round symptoms. Approximately 20% of cases are strictly seasonal, 40% perennial, and 40% mixed (perennial with seasonal exacerbations). In temperate climates, airborne pollens responsible for SAR appear in distinct phases: trees pollinate in the spring, grasses in the early summer, and weeds in the late summer. In temperate climates, mold spores persist outdoors only in the summer, and in warm climates, mold spores persist throughout the year. Symptoms of seasonal allergies cease with the appearance of frost. Knowledge of the occurrence of seasonal symptoms, of the regional patterns of pollination and mold sporulation, and of the patient's specific IgE is necessary to recognition of the cause of SAR. PAR is most often associated with the indoor allergens: house dust mites, animal danders, mice, and cockroaches. Cat and dog allergies are of major importance in the United States. The allergens from the saliva and sebaceous secretions may remain airborne for a prolonged time. The ubiquitous major cat allergen, Fel d 1, may be carried on cat owners' clothing into such "cat-free" settings as schools and hospitals.

PATHOGENESIS

The exposure of an atopic host to an allergen leads to specific IgE production. The clinical reactions on re-exposure to the allergen have been designated as early-phase and late-phase allergic responses (EPRs and LPRs). Bridging of the IgE molecules on the surface of mast cells by allergen initiates EPR, characterized by degranulation of mast cells and release of preformed and newly generated inflammatory mediators including histamine, prostaglandin 2, and the cysteinyl leukotrienes. LPR arises 4 to 8 hr following allergen exposure. Inflammatory cells, including basophils, eosinophils, neutrophils, mast cells, and mononuclear cells, infiltrate the nasal mucosa. Eosinophils release proinflammatory mediators, including cysteinyl leukotrienes, cationic proteins, eosinophil peroxidase, and major basic protein, and serve as a source of interleukin-3 (IL-3), IL-5, granulocyte-macrophage colony-stimulating factor (GM-CSF), and IL-13. Repeated intranasal introduction of allergens causes "priming"—a brisk response to reduced provocation. Over the course of an allergy season a multifold increase in epithelial and submucosal mast cells takes place. These cells were once thought to have a role exclusively in the EPR but now appear to have an important function in sustaining chronic allergic disease. Allergens, autoantigens, and components of superimposed infectious agents activate the immune system. Immune regulation in the lymphatic organs and in the tissue has an important role in the control and suppression of allergic disease in all stages of the inflammatory process, such as inflammatory cell migration to tissues, inflammatory cell–mediated destruction in tissues, and inflammatory cell interaction with resident tissue cells to enhance inflammation.

CLINICAL MANIFESTATIONS

Symptoms of AR are often ignored or are mistakenly attributed to a respiratory infection. Older children blow their noses, but younger children tend to sniff and snort. Nasal itching brings on grimacing, twitching, and picking of the nose that may result in epistaxis. Children with AR often perform the allergic salute, an upward rubbing of the nose with an open palm or extended index finger. This maneuver relieves itching and briefly unblocks the airway. It also gives rise to the nasal crease, a horizontal skin fold over the bridge of the nose. The diagnosis of AR is based on symptoms in the absence of an upper respiratory tract infection and structural abnormalities. Typical complaints include intermittent nasal congestion, itching, sneezing, clear rhinorrhea, and conjunctival irritation. Symptoms increase with greater exposure to the responsible allergen. The patients may lose their senses of smell and taste. Some experience headaches, wheezing, and coughing. Nasal congestion is often more severe at night, causing mouth-breathing and snoring, interfering with sleep, and inciting irritability.

Signs on physical exam include abnormalities of facial development, dental malocclusion, and the "allergic gape" or continuous open-mouth breathing, chapped lips, "allergic shiners" (dark circles under the eyes), and the transverse nasal crease. Conjunctival edema, itching, tearing, and hyperemia are frequent findings. A nasal exam performed with a source of light and a speculum may reveal clear nasal secretions; edematous, boggy, and bluish mucus membranes with little or no erythema; and swollen turbinates that may block the nasal airway. It may be necessary to use a topical decongestant to perform an adequate examination. Thick, purulent nasal secretions indicate the presence of infection.

DIFFERENTIAL DIAGNOSIS

Evaluation of AR calls for a thorough history, including details of the patient's environment and diet and family history of allergic conditions such as eczema, asthma, and AR, physical examination, and laboratory evaluation. The history and laboratory findings provide clues to the provoking factors. Symptoms that include sneezing, rhinorrhea, nasal itching, and congestion and the laboratory findings of elevated IgE, specific IgE antibodies, and positive allergy skin test results typify AR. SAR differs from PAR by history and skin test results. Nonallergic rhinitides cause sporadic symptoms and may resemble PAR. Their causes are often unknown. Nonallergic inflammatory rhinitis with eosinophils (NARES) imitates AR in presentation and response to treatment, but without elevated IgE antibodies. Vasomotor rhinitis is characterized by excessive responsiveness of the nasal mucosa to physical stimuli. Other nonallergic conditions, such as infectious rhinitis, structural problems including nasal polyps and septal deviation, rhinitis medicamentosa (due to the overuse of topical vasoconstrictors), hormonal rhinitis associated with pregnancy or hypothyroidism, neoplasms, vasculitides, and granulomatous disorders may mimic AR (Table 137-1).

COMPLICATIONS

AR is frequently associated with complications and co-morbid conditions. Children with AR experience frustration over their appearance. Chronic sinusitis is a common complication of AR, sometimes associated with purulent infection, but in the majority of patients, marked mucosal thickening, sinus opacification, and nasal polyposis with inflammation but negative culture results develop. The inflammatory process is characterized by marked eosinophilia. Allergens, possibly fungal, may be the inciting agents. The sinusitis of triad asthma (asthma, sinusitis with nasal polyposis, and aspirin sensitivity) often responds poorly to therapy. Patients who undergo repeated endoscopic surgery derive diminishing benefit with each successive procedure.

Rhinitis that coexists with asthma may be taken too lightly or completely overlooked. Up to 78% of patients with asthma have AR, and 38% of patients with AR have asthma. Aggravation of AR coincides with exacerbation of asthma, and treatment of nasal inflammation reduces bronchospasm, asthma-related emergency department visits, and hospitalizations. Postnasal drip associated with AR commonly causes persistent or recurrent cough. Eustachian tube obstruction and middle ear effusion are frequent complications. Chronic allergic inflammation causes hypertrophy of adenoids and tonsils that may be associated with eustachian tube obstruction, serous effusion, otitis media, and obstructive sleep apnea. AR is strongly associated with snoring in children. The association between rhinitis and sleep abnormalities and subsequent daytime fatigue is well documented, but the mechanisms remain poorly understood.

Quality of life indices have been developed to explore the effects of the disease and of therapeutic interventions. The Pediatric Rhinoconjunctivitis Quality of Life Questionnaire (PRQLQ) is suitable for children from 6 to 12 yr old, and the Adolescent RQLQ is appropriate for patients between 12 and 17. Studies using the PRQLQ in children with rhinitis have documented anxiety and physical, social, and emotional issues that affect learning and the ability to integrate with peers. The disorder contributes to headaches and fatigue, limits daily activities, and interferes with sleep. There is evidence of impaired cognitive functioning and learning that may be further threatened by the adverse effects of sedating medications. Rhinitis is an important cause of lost school attendance, resulting in more than 2 million absent days in the United States annually. A classification based on severity is shown in Figure 137-1.

Table 137-1 CAUSES OF RHINITIS

Allergic rhinitis
Seasonal
Perennial
Perennial with seasonal exacerbation
Nonallergic rhinitis
Structural/mechanical factors:
Deviated septum/septal wall anomalies
Hypertrophic turbinates
Adenoidal hypertrophy
Foreign bodies
Nasal tumors:
Benign
Malignant
Choanal atresia
Infectious:
Acute
Chronic
Inflammatory/immunologic:
Wegener granulomatosis
Sarcoidosis
Midline granuloma
Systemic lupus erythematosus
Sjögren syndrome
Nasal polyposis
Physiologic:
Ciliary dyskinesia syndrome
Atrophic rhinitis
Hormonally induced:
Hypothyroidism
Pregnancy
Oral contraceptives
Menstrual cycle
Exercise
Atrophic
Drug induced:
Rhinitis medicamentosa
Oral contraceptives
Antihypertensive therapy
Aspirin
Nonsteroidal anti-inflammatory drugs
Reflex induced:
Gustatory rhinitis
Chemical or irritant induced
Posture reflexes
Nasal cycle
Environmental factors:
Odors
Temperature
Weather/barometric pressure
Occupational
Nonallergic rhinitis with eosinophilia syndrome
Perennial nonallergic rhinitis (vasomotor rhinitis)
Emotional factors

From Leung DYM, Sampson HA, Geha RS, et al: *Pediatric allergy principles and practice*, St Louis, 2003, Mosby, p 290.

LABORATORY FINDINGS

Epicutaneous skin tests provide the best method for detection of allergen-specific IgE (positive predictive value of 48.7% for the epidemiologic diagnosis of allergic rhinitis). They are inexpensive and sensitive, and the risks and discomfort are minimal. Responses to seasonal respiratory allergens are rare before two seasons of exposure, and children younger than 1 yr rarely display positive skin test responses to these allergens. To avoid false-negative results, montelukast should be withheld for 1 day, most sedating antihistamine preparations for 3-4 days, and nonsedating antihistamines for 5-7 days. Serum immunoassays for IgE to allergens provide a suitable alternative (positive predictive value 43.5%) for patients with dermatographism or extensive dermatitis, patients taking medications that interfere with mast cell degranulation, others at high risk for anaphylaxis, and some who cannot cooperate with the procedure. Presence of eosinophils in nasal smear supports the diagnosis of AR, and that of neutrophils, of infectious rhinitis. Eosinophilia and measurements of total serum IgE concentrations have relatively low sensitivity. Improved methods for objective evaluation are still needed to assess the effects of treatment and to guide future developments.

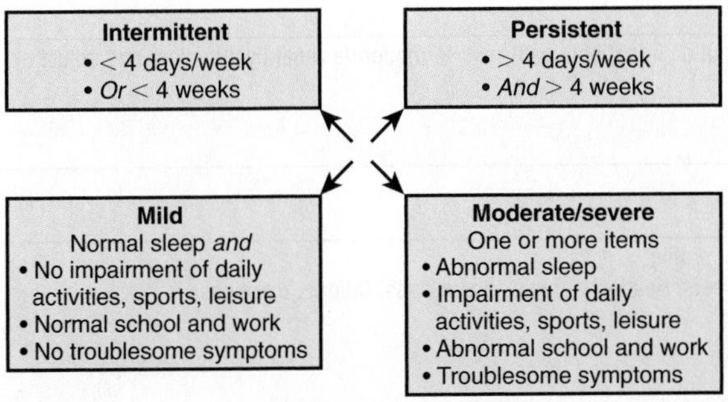

Figure 137-1 Allergic Rhinitis and Its Impact on Asthma (ARIA) classification of allergic rhinitis. (From Adkinson NF Jr, Bochner BS, Busse WW, et al, editors: *Middleton's allergy principles and practice,* ed 7, Philadelphia, 2009, Mosby/Saunders, p 977.)

TREATMENT

Safe and effective prevention or relief of symptoms is the goal of treatment. Specific measures to reduce indoor allergen exposure may reduce the risk of sensitization and symptoms of allergic respiratory disease, although existing studies report contradictory results. Sealing the patient's mattress, pillow, and covers in allergen-proof encasings reduces the exposure to mite allergen. Bed linen and blankets should be washed every week in hot water (>130°F). The only effective measure for avoiding animal allergens in the home is the removal of the pet. Avoidance of pollen and outdoor molds can be accomplished by staying in a controlled environment. Air conditioning allows for keeping windows and doors closed, reducing the pollen exposure. HEPA filters lower the counts of airborne mold spores.

The direct costs of allergic rhinitis have increased substantially since the introduction of second-generation antihistamines and intranasal corticosteroids (Tables 137-2 through 137-4). Oral antihistamines administered as needed constitute acceptable pharmacotherapy of mild, intermittent symptoms; however, first- and second-generation antihistamines available over the counter (OTC) may be associated with adverse effects on cognitive function and learning as a result of their sedative properties. Antihistamines relieve sneezing and rhinorrhea. Second-generation antihistamines are preferred because they cause less sedation. Five second-generation oral preparations are currently available:

Cetirizine: 6-12 mo: 2.5 mg qd; 1-2 yr: 2.5 mg qd, dosage may be increased to 2.5 mg bid; 2-5 yr: 2.5 mg/day, dosage may be increased to a maximum of 5 mg/day given either as a

Table 137-2 ANTIHISTAMINES AND PSEUDOEPHEDRINE

DRUG AND TRADE NAME(S)	INDICATIONS (I), MECHANISM OF ACTION (M), AND DOSING*	COMMENTS, CAUTIONS, AND ADVERSE EVENTS
Diphenhydramine (OTC):	*I:* Allergic rhinitis, atopic dermatitis, urticaria, night-time sedation. *M:* Histamine H_1-receptor antagonist.	Diphenhydramine has marked anticholinergic and sedating properties. Chewable tablets contain phenylalanine. New product labeling for OTC antihistamines will state, "Do not use in children under four years of age." *Adverse effects:* Hypotension, tachycardia, drowsiness, paradoxical excitement, dry mouth.
Benadryl	2-6 yr: 6.25 mg q4-6h; max 37.5 mg/24 hr 6-12 yr: 12.5-25 mg q4-6h; max 150 mg/24 hr >12 yr: 25-50 mg q4-6h; max 300 mg/24 hr	
Chlorpheniramine (OTC):	*I:* Allergic rhinitis, atopic dermatitis, urticaria, night-time sedation. *M:* Histamine H_1 receptor antagonist.	Chlorpheniramine is available in many preparations recommended for cough and cold. Its use for treatment of upper respiratory infections is unfounded. Chlorpheniramine has anticholinergic and sedating properties. New product labeling for OTC antihistamines will state, "Do not use in children under four years of age." *Adverse effects:* Slight to moderate drowsiness, headache, excitability, fatigue, nervousness, dizziness.
Chlor-Trimeton	2-6 yr: 1 mg q4-6h; max 6 mg/24 hr 6-12 yr: 2 mg q4-6h; max 12 mg/24 hr >12 yr: 4 mg q4-6h; max 24 mg/ 24 hr Sustained-release preparation: 6-12 yr: 8 mg hs >12 yr: 8-12 mg q8-12h	
Brompheniramine (OTC):	*I:* Allergic rhinitis. *M:* Histamine H_1 receptor antagonist.	Brompheniramine is used primarily in combination preparations, most commonly with pseudoephedrine, recommended for cough and cold. Base the dose of combined preparations containing pseudoephedrine on pseudoephedrine. The use of brompheniramine for treatment of upper respiratory infections is unfounded. Brompheniramine has anticholinergic and sedating properties. New product labeling for OTC antihistamines will state, "Do not use in children under four years of age." *Adverse events attributable to the brompheniramine component:* Slight to moderate drowsiness, headache, excitability, fatigue, nervousness, dizziness.
Dimetapp	<6 yr: 0.125 mg/kg/dose q6h; max 1 mg/24 hr 6-12 yr: 2-4 mg/dose q6-8h; max 12 mg/24 hr >12 yr: 4-8 mg/dose q4-6h; max 24 mg/24 hr	
Loratadine (OTC):	*I:* Allergic rhinitis, urticaria. *M:* Long-acting tricyclic antihistamine with selective peripheral histamine H_1-receptor antagonistic properties.	Do not exceed recommended dose. *Note:* Dimetapp Children's ND contains loratadine. New product labeling for OTC antihistamines will state, "Do not use in children under four years of age." *Adverse effects:* Nervousness, fatigue, malaise, hyperkinesia, rash, abdominal pain.
Claritin, Alavert, Dimetapp Children's ND	2-5 yr: 5 mg qd >6 yr: 10 mg qd	

Continued

Table 137-2 ANTIHISTAMINES AND PSEUDOEPHEDRINE—cont'd

DRUG AND TRADE NAME(S)	INDICATIONS (I), MECHANISM OF ACTION (M), AND DOSING*	COMMENTS, CAUTIONS, AND ADVERSE EVENTS
Desloratadine (Rx):	*I:* Allergic rhinitis, urticaria. *M:* Desloratadine, a major metabolite of loratadine, is a long-acting tricyclic antihistamine with selective peripheral histamine H_1-receptor antagonistic properties.	Orally disintegrating tablets contain phenylalanine. *Adverse effects:* Headache, fatigue, somnolence, dizziness.
Clarinex	6-12 mo: 1 mg qd 1-5 yr: 1.25 mg qd 6-12 yr: 2.5 mg qd >12 yr: 5 mg qd	
Cetirizine (Rx and OTC):	*I:* Allergic rhinitis, urticaria. *M:* Histamine H_1-receptor antagonist.	Doses > 10 mg/day may cause significant drowsiness. *Adverse effects:* Headache, somnolence, insomnia, abdominal pain.
Zyrtec	6-24 mo: 2.5 mg qd (in children 12-24 mo, dose may be increased to 2.5 mg bid) 2-6 yr: 2.5-5 mg qd >6 yr: 5-10 mg qd	
Levocetirizine (Rx):	*I:* Allergic rhinitis, urticaria. *M:* Levocetirizine is the R-enantiomer of cetirizine; it is a histamine H_1-receptor antagonist.	Use with caution in patients with mild to moderate renal dysfunction, and adjust dosage.
Xyzal	6-12 yr; 2.5 mg qd in the evening >12 yr: 5 mg qd in the evening	
Fexofenadine (Rx):	*I:* Allergic rhinitis, urticaria. *M:* Fexofenadine is an active metabolite of terfenadine; it is a histamine H_1-receptor antagonist.	Good safety profile. *Adverse effects:* Headache, fever, drowsiness, fatigue, dizziness.
Allegra	For chronic idiopathic urticaria: 6 mo–<2 yr: 15 mg bid 2-11 yr: 30 mg bid ≥12 yr: Refer to adult dosing. For allergic rhinitis: 2-11 yr: 30 mg bid ≥12 yr: Refer to adult dosing.	
Pseudoephedrine (OTC):	*I:* Temporary symptomatic relief of nasal congestion due to common cold, allergic rhinitis, and sinusitis. *M:* α-Agonist, decongestant.	Dosing errors and accidental ingestions are an important cause of rare adverse events in children. Use with caution in patients with hyperthyroidism, hypertension, diabetes, arrhythmias, or heart disease. Chewable tablets contain phenylalanine. OTC and prescribed antihistamines may be formulated in combination with pseudoephedrine. For combination preparations containing pseudoephedrine and an antihistamine, base the dose on pseudoephedrine. Pseudoephedrine serves as the raw ingredient in the illicit production of methamphetamine. *Adverse effects:* Tachycardia, palpitations, arrhythmias, nervousness, excitability, dizziness, insomnia, drowsiness, headache, seizures, hallucinations, nausea, vomiting, tremor, weakness, diaphoresis.
Sudafed	<2 yr: 4 mg/kg/dose q6h 2-5 yr: 15 mg q6h; max 60 mg/24 hr 6-12 yr: 30 mg q6h; max 120 mg/24 hr <12 yr: 60 mg q6h ≥12 yr: 120 mg q12h *or* 240 mg qd; max 240 mg/24 hr	

*All of these agents are administered orally.
OTC, available over the counter (nonprescription); Rx, prescription required.

Table 137-3 INTRANASAL INHALED CORTICOSTEROIDS

DRUG, TRADE NAME(S), AND FORMULATIONS	INDICATIONS (I), MECHANISM(S) OF ACTION (M), AND DOSING	COMMENTS, CAUTIONS, ADVERSE EVENTS, AND MONITORING
Beclomethasone:	*I:* Allergic rhinitis. *M:* Anti-inflammatory, immune modulator.	Shake container before use; blow nose; occlude one nostril, administer dose to the other nostril. *Adverse effects:* Burning and irritation of nasal mucosa, epistaxis. Monitor growth.
Beconase AQ (42 μg/spray)	6-12 yr: 1 spray in each nostril bid >12 yr: 1 or 2 spray in each nostril bid	
Flunisolide	6-14 yr: 1 spray each nostril 3 times daily *or* 2 sprays in each nostril twice daily; not to exceed 4 sprays/day in each nostril ≥15 yr: 2 sprays each nostril twice daily (morning and evening); may increase to 2 sprays 3 times daily; maximum dose: 8 sprays/day in each nostril (400 μg/day)	Shake container before use; blow nose; occlude one nostril, administer dose to the other nostril. *Adverse effects:* Burning and irritation of nasal mucosa, epistaxis. Monitor growth.
Nasarel (25 μg/spray)	≥6 yr: initial dose 1 spray tid or 2 sprays in each nostril bid; reduce to lowest effective dose	
Triamcinolone:	*I:* Allergic rhinitis. *M:* Anti-inflammatory, immune modulator.	Shake container before use; blow nose; occlude one nostril, administer dose to the other nostril. *Adverse effects:* Burning and irritation of nasal mucosa, epistaxis. Monitor growth.
Nasacort HFA (55 μg/spray), Nasacort AQ (55 μg/spray)	2-6 yr; 1 spray in each nostril qd 6-12 yr: 1-2 sprays in each nostril qd ≥12 yr: 2 sprays in each nostril qd	

Table 137-3 INTRANASAL INHALED CORTICOSTEROIDS—cont'd

DRUG, TRADE NAME(S), AND FORMULATIONS	INDICATIONS (I), MECHANISM(S) OF ACTION (M), AND DOSING	COMMENTS, CAUTIONS, ADVERSE EVENTS, AND MONITORING
Fluticasone:	*I:* Allergic rhinitis. *M:* Anti-inflammatory, immune modulator.	Shake container before use; blow nose; occlude one nostril, administer dose to the other nostril. Ritonavir significantly increases fluticasone serum concentrations and may result in systemic corticosteroid effects. Use fluticasone with caution in patients receiving ketoconazole or other potent cytochrome P450 3A4 isoenzyme inhibitors. *Adverse effects:* Burning and irritation of nasal mucosa, epistaxis. Monitor growth.
Fluticasone propionate (available as a generic preparation):		
Flonase (50 μg/spray)	≥4 yr: 1-2 sprays in each nostril qd	
Fluticasone furoate:		
Veramyst (27.5 μg/spray)	2-12 yr: Initial dose: 1 spray (27.5 μg/spray) per nostril once daily (55 μg/day). Patients who do not show adequate response may use 2 sprays per nostril once daily (110 μg/day). Once symptoms are controlled, dosage may be reduced to 55 μg once daily. Total daily dosage should not exceed 2 sprays in each nostril (110 μg)/day. ≥12 yr and adolescents: Initial dose: 2 sprays (27.5 μg/spray) per nostril once daily (110 μg/day). Once symptoms are controlled, dosage may be reduced to 1 spray per nostril once daily (55 μg/day). Total daily dosage should not exceed 2 sprays in each nostril (110 μg)/day.	
Mometasone:	*I:* Allergic rhinitis. *M:* Anti-inflammatory, immune modulator.	Mometasone and its major metabolites are undetectable in plasma after nasal administration of recommended doses. Preventive treatment of seasonal allergic rhinitis should begin 2-4 wk prior to pollen season. Shake container before use; blow nose; occlude one nostril, administer dose to the other nostril. *Adverse effects:* Burning and irritation of nasal mucosa, epistaxis. Monitor growth.
Nasonex (50 μg/spray)	2-12 yr: 1 spray in each nostril qd >12 yr: 2 sprays in each nostril qd	
Budesonide:	*I:* Allergic rhinitis. *M:* Anti-inflammatory, immune modulator.	Shake container before use; blow nose; occlude one nostril, administer dose to the other nostril. *Adverse effects:* Burning and irritation of nasal mucosa, epistaxis. Monitor growth.
Rhinocort AQ (32 μg/spray)	>6 yr: 1 spray in each nostril qd 6-12 yr: 2 sprays in each nostril qd >12 yr: up to 4 sprays in each nostril qd (maximum dose)	
Ciclesonide:	*I:* Allergic rhinitis. *M:* Anti-inflammatory, immune modulator.	Prior to initial use, gently shake, then prime the pump by actuating eight times. If the product is not used for 4 consecutive days, gently shake and reprime with one spray or until a fine mist appears.
Omnaris (50 μg/spray)	>6 yr: 2 sprays in each nostril qd	

single dose or divided into 2 doses; >6 yr: 5-10 mg/day as a single dose or divided into 2 doses.

Levocetirizine: 6-11 yr: 2.5 mg PO once daily; >12 yr: 5 mg PO once daily.

Loratadine (available OTC): 2-5 yr: 5 mg qd; >6 yr: 10 mg qd.

Fexofenadine: 6-11 yr: 30 mg PO bid; >12 yr: 60 mg bid or 180 mg PO qd.

Desloratadine: 6-11 mo: 1 mg qd; 1-5 yr: 1.25 mg qd; 6-11 yr: 2.5 mg qd; >12 yr: 5 mg qd.

Azelastine is a topically active antihistamine available as a nasal spray (5-12 yr: 1 spray per nostril bid; >12 yr :2 sprays/nostril bid) and as eye drops (>3 yr: 1 drop in each affected eye bid). Pseudoephedrine (available OTC, generally in combination with OTC antihistamines) is an oral vasoconstrictor known to cause irritability and insomnia and to be associated with infant mortality. The anticholinergic nasal spray ipratropium bromide (2 sprays/nostril bid or tid; use 0.03% preparation) is effective for the treatment of serous rhinorrhea. Intranasal decongestants should be used for less than 5 days, not to be repeated more than once a month. Sodium cromoglycate (available OTC) is effective but requires frequent administration, q4h. Leukotriene-modifying agents have a modest effect on rhinorrhea and nasal blockage. Nasal saline irrigation is a good adjunctive option with all other treatment of allergic rhinitis.

Patients with more persistent, severe symptoms require treatment with intranasal corticosteroids, the most effective therapy for AR. These agents reduce all symptoms of AR with eosinophilic inflammation but not those of rhinitis associated with neutrophils or free of inflammation. The older drugs beclomethasone, triamcinolone, and flunisolide are absorbed from the gastrointestinal (GI) tract as well as from the respiratory tract. New corticosteroid preparations—budesonide, fluticasone propionate, mometasone furoate, and ciclesonide—have been developed that offer greater topical activity with lower systemic exposure. Fluticasone (>4 yr: 1-2 sprays/nostril qd), mometasone (2-11 yr: 1 spray/nostril qd; >12 yr: 2 sprays/nostril qd), budesonide (>6 yr: 1 spray/nostril qd, dose may be increased if needed; maximum

Table 137-4 MISCELLANEOUS INTRANASAL SPRAYS

DRUG, TRADE NAME(S), AND FORMULATIONS	INDICATIONS (I), MECHANISM(S) OF ACTION (M), AND DOSING	COMMENTS, CAUTIONS, ADVERSE EVENTS, AND MONITORING
Ipratropium bromide:	*I:* Symptomatic relief of rhinorrhea. *M:* Anticholinergic.	Atrovent inhalation aerosol is contraindicated in patients with hypersensitivity to soy lecithin. Safety and efficacy of use beyond 4 days in patients with the common cold have not been established. *Adverse effects:* Epistaxis, nasal dryness, nausea.
Atrovent nasal spray (0.06%)	Colds (symptomatic relief of rhinorrhea): 5-12 yr: 2 sprays in each nostril 3 times/day ≥12 yr and adults: 2 sprays in each nostril 3-4 times/day	
Azelastine:	*I:* Treatment of rhinorrhea, sneezing, and nasal pruritus. *M:* Antagonism of histamine H_1-receptor.	May cause drowsiness. *Adverse effects:* Headache, somnolence, bitter taste.
Astelin	6-12 yr: 1 spray bid >12 yr: 1-2 sprays bid	
Cromolyn sodium:	*I:* Allergic rhinitis. *M:* Inhibition of mast cell degranulation.	Not effective immediately; requires frequent administration.
Nasalcrom	>2 yr: 1 spray tid-qid; max 6 ×/day	
Oxymetazoline:	*I:* Symptomatic relief of nasal mucosal congestion. *M:* Adrenergic agonist, vasoconstricting agent.	Excessive dosage may cause profound CNS depression. Use in excess of 3 days may result in severe rebound nasal congestion. Do not repeat more than once a month. Use with caution in patients with hyperthyroidism, heart disease, hypertension, and diabetes. *Adverse effects:* Hypertension, palpitations, reflex bradycardia, nervousness, dizziness, insomnia, headache, CNS depression, convulsions, hallucinations, nausea, vomiting, mydriasis, elevated intraocular pressure, blurred vision.
Afrin, Nōstrilla	0.05% solution: Instill 2-3 sprays into each nostril twice daily; therapy should not exceed 3 days	
Phenylephrine:	*I:* Symptomatic relief of nasal mucosal congestion. *M:* Adrenergic, vasoconstricting agent.	Use in excess of 3 days may result in severe rebound nasal congestion. Do not repeat more than once a month. 0.16% and 0.125% solutions are not commercially available. *Adverse effects:* Reflex bradycardia, excitability, headache, anxiety, and dizziness.
Neo-Synephrine	2-6 yr: 1 drop every 2-4 hr of 0.125% solution as needed. *Note:* Therapy should not exceed 3 continuous days. 6-12 yr: 1-2 sprays or 1-2 drops every 4 hr of 0.25% solution as needed. *Note:* Therapy should not exceed 3 continuous days. >12 yr: 1-2 sprays or 1-2 drops every 4 hr of 0.25% to 0.5% solution as needed; 1% solution may be used in adults with extreme nasal congestion. *Note:* Therapy should not exceed 3 continuous days.	

dose for children <12 yr: 2 sprays/nostril qd, and for children >12 yr: 4 sprays/nostril qd), and ciclesonide (>6 yr with SAR and >12 yr with PAR: 2 sprays/nostril qd) have lower systemic bioavailability and better safety profiles. More severely affected patients may benefit from simultaneous treatment with antihistamines and intranasal corticosteroids.

Specific allergen immunotherapy administered by subcutaneous injection should be considered for children in whom IgE-mediated allergic symptoms cannot be adequately controlled by avoidance and medication, especially in the presence of co-morbid conditions. Allergen immunotherapy interferes with IgE production and allergic symptoms. It has been found to be effective in the treatment of allergic rhinitis. Locally applied immunotherapy, which may be oral, sublingual, or nasal, has been used successfully in Europe and South America. Sublingual immunotherapy holds promise for the treatment for allergic rhinitis, but it is currently considered investigational in the USA until formulations approved by the U.S. Food and Drug Administration are available. Studies have now shown that anti-IgE reduces allergic responses in the nose. Treatment strategies that incorporate both anti-IgE and immunotherapy hold promise for the future.

PROGNOSIS

Therapy with nonsedating antihistamines and intranasal corticosteroids significantly improves health-related quality of life measures in patients of all ages with AR, provided that they continue to take their medications. The reported rates of remission among children are between 10% and 23%. However, prognosis for the future is much brighter. It includes exciting measures to prevent atopy, induce immune tolerance, and hold back the expression of the allergic phenotype. Pharmacotherapy will target cells and cytokines involved in inflammation and treat allergy as a systemic process.

BIBLIOGRAPHY

Please visit the Nelson Textbook of Pediatrics *website at www.expertconsult.com for the complete bibliography.*

Chapter 138
Childhood Asthma

Andrew H. Liu, Ronina A. Covar, Joseph D. Spahn, and Donald Y.M. Leung

Asthma is a chronic inflammatory condition of the lung airways resulting in episodic airflow obstruction. This chronic inflammation heightens the twitchiness of the airways—**airways hyperresponsiveness** (AHR)—to provocative exposures. Asthma management is aimed at reducing airways inflammation by minimizing proinflammatory environmental exposures, using daily controller anti-inflammatory medications, and controlling co-morbid conditions that can worsen asthma. Less inflammation typically leads to better asthma control, with fewer exacerbations and decreased need for quick-reliever asthma medications. Nevertheless, exacerbations can still occur. Early intervention with systemic corticosteroids greatly reduces the severity of such episodes. Advances in asthma management and, especially, pharmacotherapy enable all but the uncommon child with severe asthma to live normally.

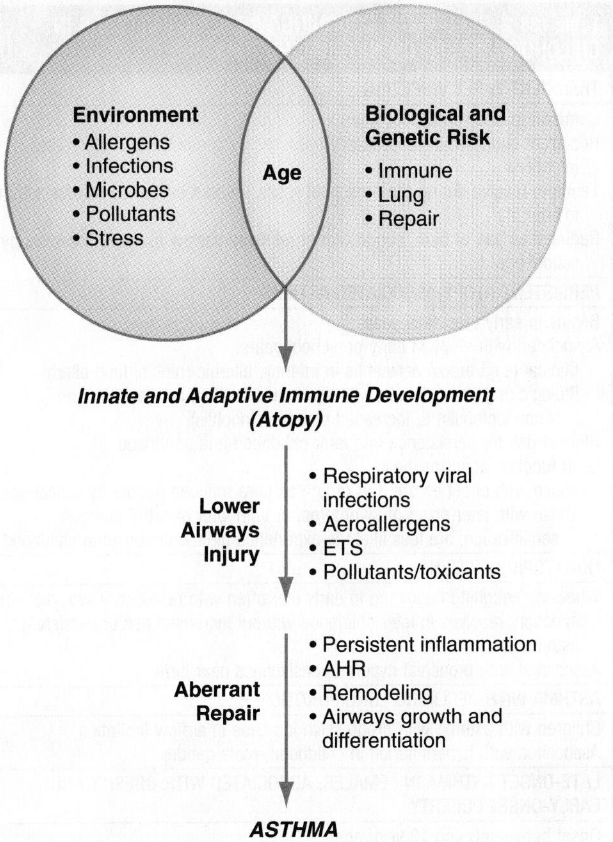

Figure 138-1 Etiology and pathogenesis of asthma. A combination of environmental and genetic factors in early life shape how the immune system develops and responds to ubiquitous environmental exposures. Respiratory microbes, inhaled allergens, and toxins that can injure the lower airways target the disease process to the lungs. Aberrant immune and repair responses to airways injury underlie persistent disease. AHR, airways hyperresponsiveness; ETS, environmental tobacco smoke.

ETIOLOGY

Although the cause of childhood asthma has not been determined, contemporary research implicates a combination of environmental exposures and inherent biologic and genetic vulnerabilities (Fig. 138-1). Respiratory exposures in this causal environment include inhaled allergens, respiratory viral infections, and chemical and biologic air pollutants such as environmental tobacco smoke. In the predisposed host, immune responses to these common exposures can be a stimulus for prolonged, pathogenic inflammation and aberrant repair of injured airways tissues. Lung dysfunction (i.e., AHR and reduced airflow) develops. These pathogenic processes in the growing lung during early life adversely affect airways growth and differentiation, leading to altered airways at mature ages. Once asthma has developed, ongoing exposures appear to worsen it, driving disease persistence and increasing the risk of severe exacerbations.

Genetics

More than 100 genetic loci have been linked to asthma. Although the genetic linkages to asthma have sometimes differed between cohorts, asthma has been consistently linked with loci containing proallergic, proinflammatory genes (the interleukin [IL]-4 gene cluster on chromosome 5). Genetic variation in receptors for different asthma medications is associated with variation in biologic response to these medications (polymorphisms in the β_2-adrenergic receptor). Other candidate genes include *ADAM-33* (member of the metalloproteinase family), the gene for the prostanoid DP receptor, and genes located on chromosome 5q31 (possibly IL-12).

Environment

Recurrent wheezing episodes in early childhood are associated with common respiratory viruses, including respiratory syncytial virus, rhinovirus, influenza virus, adenovirus, parainfluenza virus, and human metapneumovirus. This association implies that host features affecting immunologic host defense, inflammation, and the extent of airways injury from ubiquitous viral pathogens underlie susceptibility to recurrent wheezing in early childhood. Furthermore, injurious viral infections of the airways that manifest as pneumonia or bronchiolitis requiring hospitalization are risk factors for persistent asthma in childhood. Other airways exposures can also exacerbate ongoing airways inflammation, increase disease severity, and drive asthma persistence. Indoor and home allergen exposures in sensitized individuals can initiate airways inflammation and hypersensitivity to other irritant exposures, and are strongly linked to disease severity and persistence. Consequently, eliminating the offending allergen(s) can lead to resolution of asthma symptoms and can sometimes "cure" asthma. Environmental tobacco smoke and air pollutants (ozone, sulfur dioxide) aggravate airways inflammation and increase asthma severity. Cold dry air and strong odors can trigger bronchoconstriction when airways are irritated but do not worsen airways inflammation or hyperresponsiveness.

EPIDEMIOLOGY

Asthma is a common chronic disease, causing considerable morbidity. In 2007, 9.6 million children (13.1%) had been diagnosed with asthma in their lifetimes. Of this group, 70% had asthma currently, and 3.8 million children (5.2%), nearly 60% of those with current asthma, had experienced at least one asthma attack in the prior year. Boys (14% vs 10% girls) and children in poor families (16% vs 10% not poor) are more likely to have asthma.

In the USA, childhood asthma is among the most common causes of childhood emergency department visits, hospitalizations, and missed school days, accounting in 2004 for 12.8 million missed school days, 750,000 emergency department visits, 198,000 hospitalizations, and 186 childhood deaths. A disparity in asthma outcomes links high rates of asthma hospitalization and death with poverty, ethnic minorities, and urban living. In the past 2 decades, African-American children had 2 to 4 times more emergency department visits, hospitalizations, and deaths due to asthma than white children. For ethnic minority asthmatic patients living in U.S. inner-city low-income communities, a combination of biologic, environmental, economic, and psychosocial risk factors is believed to increase the likelihood of severe asthma exacerbations. Although current asthma prevalence is higher in black than in non-black U.S. children (12.8%, in 2003-2005, vs 7.9% for white and 7.8% for Latino children), prevalence differences cannot fully account for this disparity in asthma outcomes.

Worldwide, childhood asthma appears to be increasing in prevalence, despite considerable improvements in our management and pharmacopeia to treat asthma. Numerous studies conducted in different countries have reported an increase in asthma prevalence of about 50% per decade. Globally, childhood asthma prevalence varies widely in different locales. A large international survey study of childhood asthma prevalence in 97 countries (International Study of Asthma and Allergies in Childhood) found a wide range in the prevalence of current wheeze, 0.8-37.6%. Asthma prevalence correlated well with reported allergic rhinoconjunctivitis and atopic eczema prevalence. Childhood asthma seems more prevalent in modern metropolitan locales and more affluent nations, and it is strongly linked with other allergic conditions. In contrast, children living in rural areas of developing countries and farming communities are less likely to experience asthma and allergy, although childhood asthma in less affluent nations seems more severe.

Table 138-1 EARLY CHILDHOOD RISK FACTORS FOR PERSISTENT ASTHMA
Parental asthma
Allergy:
Atopic dermatitis (eczema)
Allergic rhinitis
Food allergy
Inhalant allergen sensitization
Food allergen sensitization
Severe lower respiratory tract infection:
Pneumonia
Bronchiolitis requiring hospitalization
Wheezing apart from colds
Male gender
Low birthweight
Environmental tobacco smoke exposure
Possible use of acetaminophen (paracetamol)
Exposure to chlorinated swimming pools:
Reduced lung function at birth

Approximately 80% of all asthmatic patients report disease onset prior to 6 yr of age. However, of all young children who experience recurrent wheezing, only a minority go on to have persistent asthma in later childhood. Early childhood risk factors for persistent asthma have been identified (Table 138-1). Prediction of asthma includes major (parent asthma, eczema, inhalant allergen sensitization) and minor (allergic rhinitis, wheezing apart from colds, ≥4% eosinophils, food allergen sensitization) risk factors. Allergy in young children has emerged as a major risk factor for the persistence of childhood asthma.

Types of Childhood Asthma

Asthma is considered to be a common clinical presentation of intermittent, recurrent wheezing and/or coughing, resulting from different airways pathologic processes underlying different types of asthma. There are 2 main types of childhood asthma: (1) **recurrent wheezing** in early childhood, primarily triggered by common viral infections of the respiratory tract, and (2) **chronic asthma** associated with allergy that persists into later childhood and often adulthood. A 3rd type of childhood asthma typically emerges in females who experience obesity and early-onset puberty (by 11 yr of age). Some children may be hypersensitive to common air pollutants (environmental tobacco smoke, ozone, endotoxin) such that exposures to these pollutants might not only make existing asthma worse but may also have a causal role in the susceptible. The most common persistent form of childhood asthma is associated with allergy and susceptibility to common respiratory virus–induced exacerbations (Table 138-2).

PATHOGENESIS

Airflow obstruction in asthma is the result of numerous pathologic processes. In the small airways, airflow is regulated by smooth muscle encircling the airways lumens; bronchoconstriction of these bronchiolar muscular bands restricts or blocks airflow. A cellular inflammatory infiltrate and exudates distinguished by eosinophils, but also including other inflammatory cell types (neutrophils, monocytes, lymphocytes, mast cells, basophils), can fill and obstruct the airways and induce epithelial damage and desquamation into the airways lumen. Helper T lymphocytes and other immune cells that produce proallergic, proinflammatory cytokines (IL-4, IL-5, IL-13), and chemokines (eotaxin) mediate this inflammatory process. Pathogenic immune responses and inflammation may also result from a breach in normal immune regulatory processes (such as regulatory T lymphocytes that produce IL-10 and transforming growth factor [TGF]-β) that dampen effector immunity and inflammation when they are no longer needed. Hypersensitivity or susceptibility to a

Table 138-2 RECURRENT COUGHING/WHEEZING PATTERNS IN CHILDHOOD, BASED ON NATURAL HISTORY
TRANSIENT EARLY WHEEZING
Common in early preschool years Recurrent cough/wheeze, primarily triggered by common respiratory viral infections Tends to resolve during the preschool years, without increased risk for asthma in later life Reduced airflow at birth, suggestive of relativity narrow airways, improves by school age
PERSISTENT ATOPY-ASSOCIATED ASTHMA
Begins in early preschool years Associated with atopy in early preschool years: Clinical (e.g., atopic dermatitis in infancy, allergic rhinitis, food allergy) Biologic (e.g., early inhalant allergen sensitization, increased serum immunoglobulin E, increased blood eosinophils) Highest risk for persistence into later childhood and adulthood Lung function abnormalities: Those with onset before 3 yr of age acquire reduced airflow by school age Those with later onset of symptoms, or with later onset of allergen sensitization, are less likely to experience airflow limitation in childhood
NONATOPIC WHEEZING
Wheezing/coughing beginning in early life, often with respiratory syncytial virus infection; resolves in later childhood without increased risk of persistent asthma Associated with bronchial hyperresponsiveness near birth
ASTHMA WITH DECLINING LUNG FUNCTION
Children with asthma with progressive increase in airflow limitation Associated with hyperinflation in childhood, male gender
LATE-ONSET ASTHMA IN FEMALES, ASSOCIATED WITH OBESITY AND EARLY-ONSET PUBERTY
Onset between 8 and 13 yr of age Associated with obesity and early-onset puberty; specific for females
OCCUPATIONAL-TYPE ASTHMA IN CHILDREN
Children with asthma associated with occupational-type exposures known to trigger asthma in adults in occupational settings (e.g., endotoxin exposure in children raised on farms)

From Taussig LM, Landau LI, et al, editors: *Pediatric respiratory medicine,* ed 2, Philadelphia, 2008, Mosby/Elsevier, p 822.

variety of provocative exposures or triggers (Table 138-3) can lead to airways inflammation, AHR, edema, basement membrane thickening, subepithelial collagen deposition, smooth muscle and mucous gland hypertrophy, and mucus hypersecretion—all processes that contribute to airflow obstruction (Chapter 134).

CLINICAL MANIFESTATIONS AND DIAGNOSIS

Intermittent dry coughing and expiratory wheezing are the most common chronic symptoms of asthma. Older children and adults report associated shortness of breath and chest tightness; younger children are more likely to report intermittent, nonfocal chest pain. Respiratory symptoms can be worse at night, especially during prolonged exacerbations triggered by respiratory infections or inhalant allergens. Daytime symptoms, often linked with physical activities or play, are reported with greatest frequency in children. Other asthma symptoms in children can be subtle and nonspecific, including self-imposed limitation of physical activities, general fatigue (possibly due to sleep disturbance), and difficulty keeping up with peers in physical activities. Asking about previous experience with asthma medications (bronchodilators) may provide a history of symptomatic improvement with treatment that supports the diagnosis of asthma. Lack of improvement with bronchodilator and corticosteroid therapy is inconsistent with underlying asthma and should prompt more vigorous consideration of asthma-masquerading conditions.

Asthma symptoms can be triggered by numerous common events or exposures: physical exertion and hyperventilation

Table 138-3 ASTHMA TRIGGERS

Common viral infections of the respiratory tract
Aeroallergens in sensitized asthmatic patients:
Animal dander
Indoor allergens
Dust mites
Cockroaches
Molds
Seasonal aeroallergens:
Pollens (trees, grasses, weeds)
Seasonal molds
Environmental tobacco smoke
Air pollutants:
Ozone
Sulfur dioxide
Particulate matter
Wood- or coal-burning smoke
Endotoxin, mycotoxins
Dust
Strong or noxious odors or fumes:
Perfumes, hairsprays
Cleaning agents
Occupational exposures:
Farm and barn exposures
Formaldehydes, cedar, paint fumes
Cold air, dry air
Exercise
Crying, laughter, hyperventilation
Co-morbid conditions:
Rhinitis
Sinusitis
Gastroesophageal reflux

(laughing), cold or dry air, and airways irritants (see Table 138-3). Exposures that induce airways inflammation, such as infections (rhinovirus, respiratory syncytial virus, metapneumovirus, torque teno virus, parainfluenza virus, influenza virus, adenovirus, *Mycoplasma pneumonia, Chlamydia pneumoniae*), and inhaled allergens, also increase AHR to irritant exposures. An environmental history is essential for optimal asthma management (Chapter 135).

The presence of risk factors, such as a history of other allergic conditions (allergic rhinitis, allergic conjunctivitis, atopic dermatitis, food allergies), parental asthma, and/or symptoms apart from colds, supports the diagnosis of asthma. During routine clinic visits, children with asthma commonly present without abnormal signs, emphasizing the importance of the medical history in diagnosing asthma. Some may exhibit a dry, persistent cough. The chest findings are often normal. Deeper breaths can sometimes elicit otherwise undetectable wheezing. In clinic, quick resolution (within 10 min) or convincing improvement in symptoms and signs of asthma with administration of a short-acting inhaled β-agonist (SABA; e.g., albuterol) is supportive of the diagnosis of asthma.

During asthma exacerbations, expiratory wheezing and a prolonged expiratory phase can usually be appreciated by auscultation. Decreased breath sounds in some of the lung fields, commonly the right lower posterior lobe, are consistent with regional hypoventilation owing to airways obstruction. Crackles (or rales) and rhonchi can sometimes be heard, resulting from excess mucus production and inflammatory exudate in the airways. The combination of segmental crackles and poor breath sounds can indicate lung segmental atelectasis that is difficult to distinguish from bronchial pneumonia and can complicate acute asthma management. In severe exacerbations, the greater extent of airways obstruction causes labored breathing and respiratory distress, which manifests as inspiratory and expiratory wheezing, increased prolongation of exhalation, poor air entry, suprasternal and intercostal retractions, nasal flaring, and accessory respiratory muscle use. In extremis, airflow may be so limited that wheezing cannot be heard (Table 138-4).

DIFFERENTIAL DIAGNOSIS

Many childhood respiratory conditions can present with symptoms and signs similar to those of asthma (Table 138-5). Besides asthma, other common causes of chronic, intermittent coughing include gastroesophageal reflux (GER) and rhinosinusitis. Both GER and chronic sinusitis can be challenging to diagnose in children. Often, GER is clinically silent in children, and children with chronic sinusitis do not report sinusitis-specific symptoms, such as localized sinus pressure and tenderness. In addition, both GER and rhinosinusitis are often co-morbid with childhood asthma and, if not specifically treated, may make asthma difficult to manage.

In early life, chronic coughing and wheezing can indicate recurrent aspiration, tracheobronchomalacia, a congenital anatomic abnormality of the airways, foreign body aspiration, cystic fibrosis, or bronchopulmonary dysplasia.

In older children and adolescents, **vocal cord dysfunction (VCD)** can manifest as intermittent daytime wheezing. In this condition, the vocal cords involuntarily close inappropriately during inspiration and sometimes exhalation, producing shortness of breath, coughing, throat tightness, and often audible laryngeal wheezing and/or stridor. In most cases of VCD, spirometric lung function testing reveals "truncated" and inconsistent inspiratory and expiratory flow-volume loops, a pattern that differs from the reproducible pattern of airflow limitation in asthma that improves with bronchodilators. VCD can coexist with asthma. Flexible rhinolaryngoscopy in the patient with symptomatic VCD can reveal paradoxical vocal cord movements with anatomically normal vocal cords. This condition can be well managed with specialized speech therapy training in the relaxation and control of vocal cord movement. Furthermore, treatment of underlying causes of vocal cord irritability (e.g., high gastroesophageal reflux/aspiration, allergic rhinitis, rhinosinusitis, asthma) can improve VCD. During acute VCD exacerbations, in addition to relaxation breathing techniques in conjunction with inhalation of heliox (a mixture of 70% helium and 30% oxygen) can relieve vocal cord spasm and VCD symptoms.

In some locales, hypersensitivity pneumonitis (farming communities, homes of bird owners), pulmonary parasitic infestations (rural areas of developing countries), or tuberculosis may be common causes of chronic coughing and/or wheezing. Rare asthma-masquerading conditions in childhood include bronchiolitis obliterans, interstitial lung diseases, primary ciliary dyskinesias, humoral immune deficiencies, allergic bronchopulmonary mycoses, congestive heart failure, mass lesions in or compressing the larynx, trachea, or bronchi, and coughing and/or wheezing that is an adverse effect of medication. Chronic pulmonary diseases often produce clubbing, but clubbing is a very unusual finding in childhood asthma.

LABORATORY FINDINGS

Lung function tests can help to confirm the diagnosis of asthma and to determine disease severity.

Pulmonary Function Testing

Forced expiratory airflow measures are helpful in diagnosing and monitoring asthma and in assessing efficacy of therapy. Lung function testing is particularly helpful in children with asthma who are poor perceivers of airflow obstruction or when physical signs of asthma do not occur until airflow obstruction is severe.

Many asthma guidelines promote spirometric measures of airflow and lung volumes during forced expiratory maneuvers as standard for asthma assessment. **Spirometry** is helpful as an

Table 138-4 FORMAL EVALUATION OF ASTHMA EXACERBATION SEVERITY IN THE URGENT OR EMERGENCY CARE SETTING*

	MILD	MODERATE	SEVERE	SUBSET: RESPIRATORY ARREST IMMINENT
SYMPTOMS				
Breathlessness	While walking	While at rest (infant—softer, shorter cry, difficulty feeding)	While at rest (infant—stops feeding)	
	Can lie down	Prefers sitting	Sits upright	
Talks in	Sentences	Phrases	Words	
Alertness	May be agitated	Usually agitated	Usually agitated	Drowsy or confused
SIGNS				
Respiratory rate†	Increased	Increased	Often >30 breaths/min	
Use of accessory muscles; suprasternal retractions	Usually not	Commonly	Usually	Paradoxical thoracoabdominal movement
Wheeze	Moderate; often only end-expiratory	Loud; throughout exhalation	Usually loud; throughout inhalation and exhalation	Absence of wheeze
Pulse rate (beats/min)‡	<100	100-120	>120	Bradycardia
Pulsus paradoxus	Absent <10 mm Hg	May be present 10-25 mm Hg	Often present >25 mm Hg (adult) 20-40 mm Hg (child)	Absence suggests respiratory muscle fatigue
FUNCTIONAL ASSESSMENT				
Peak expiratory flow (value predicted or personal best)	≥70%	Approx. 40-69% or response lasts <2 hr	<40%	<25%§
Pao_2 (breathing air) *and/or*	Normal (test not usually necessary)	≥60 mm Hg (test not usually necessary)	<60 mm Hg; possible cyanosis	
Pco_2	<42 mm Hg (test not usually necessary)	<42 mm Hg (test not usually necessary)	≥42 mm Hg; possible respiratory failure	
Sao_2 (breathing air) at sea level	>95% (test not usually necessary)	90-95% (test not usually necessary)	<90%	
	Hypercapnia (hypoventilation) develops more readily in young children than in adults and adolescents			

*Notes:
- The presence of several parameters, but not necessarily all, indicates the general classification of the exacerbation.
- Many of these parameters have not been systematically studied, especially as they correlate with each other. Thus, they serve only as general guides.
- The emotional impact of asthma symptoms on the patient and family is variable but must be recognized and addressed and can affect approaches to treatment and follow-up.

†Normal breathing rates in awake children by age: <2 mo, <60 breaths/min; 2-12 mo, <50 breaths/min; 1-5 yr, <40 breaths/min; 6-8 yr, <30 breaths/min.
‡Normal pulse rates in children by age: 2-12 mo, <160 beats/min; 1-2 yr, <120 beats/min; 2-8 yr, <110 beats/min.
§Peak expiratory flow testing may not be needed in very severe attacks.
Modified from EPR—3. Expert panel report 3: guidelines for the diagnosis and management of asthma, NIH Publication No. 07-4051, Bethesda, MA, 2007, U.S. Department of Health and Human Services; National Institutes of Health, National Heart, Lung, and Blood Institute; National Asthma Education and Prevention Program. www.nhlbi.nih.gov/guidelines/asthma/asthgdln.htm.

objective measure of airflow limitation (Fig. 138-2). Knowledgeable personnel are needed to perform and interpret findings of spirometry tests. Valid spirometric measures depend on a patient's ability to properly perform a full, forceful, and prolonged expiratory maneuver, usually feasible in children > 6 yr of age (with some younger exceptions). Reproducible spirometric efforts are an indicator of test validity; if the **FEV_1** (forced expiratory volume in 1 sec) is within 5% on 3 attempts, then the *highest* FEV_1 effort of the 3 is used. This standard utilization of the highest of 3 reproducible efforts is indicative of the effort dependence of reliable spirometric testing.

In asthma, airways blockage results in reduced airflow with forced exhalation and smaller partial-expiratory lung volumes (see Fig. 138-2). Because asthmatic patients typically have hyperinflated lungs, FEV_1 can be simply adjusted for full expiratory lung volume—the forced vital capacity (FVC)—with an FEV_1/FVC ratio. Generally, an FEV_1/FVC ratio <0.80 indicates significant airflow obstruction (Table 138-6). Normative values for FEV_1 have been determined for children on the basis of height, gender, and ethnicity. Abnormally low FEV_1 as a percentage of predicted norms is 1 of 6 criteria used to determine asthma severity in the National Institutes of Health (NIH)–sponsored asthma guidelines.

Such measures of airflow alone are not diagnostic of asthma, because numerous other conditions can cause airflow reduction. Bronchodilator response to an inhaled β-agonist (e.g., albuterol) is greater in asthmatic patients than nonasthmatic persons; an improvement in FEV_1 ≥12% or >200 mL is consistent with asthma. **Bronchoprovocation challenges** can be helpful in diagnosing asthma and optimizing asthma management. Asthmatic airways are hyperresponsive and therefore more sensitive to inhaled methacholine, histamine, and cold or dry air. The degree of AHR to these exposures correlates to some extent with asthma severity and airways inflammation. Although bronchoprovocation challenges are carefully dosed and monitored in an investigational setting, their use is rarely practical in a general practice setting. **Exercise challenges** (aerobic exertion or "running" for 6-8 min) can help to identify children with **exercise-induced bronchospasm.** Although the airflow response of non-asthmatic persons to exercise is to increase functional lung volumes and improve FEV_1 slightly (5-10%), exercise often provokes airflow obstruction in persons with inadequately treated asthma. Accordingly, in asthmatic patients, FEV_1 typically decreases during or after exercise by >15% (see Table 138-6). The onset of exercise-induced bronchospasm is usually within 15 min after a vigorous exercise challenge and can spontaneously resolve within 30-60 min. Studies of exercise challenges in school-aged children typically identify an additional 5-10% with exercise-induced bronchospasm and previously unrecognized asthma. There are two caveats regarding exercise challenges: first, treadmill challenges in the clinic are not completely reliable and can miss exertional asthma that can be demonstrated on the playing field; and second, treadmill challenges can induce severe exacerbations in at-risk patients. Careful patient selection for exercise challenges and preparedness for severe asthma exacerbations are required.

Measuring **exhaled nitric oxide** (FE_{NO}), a marker of airway inflammation in allergy-associated asthma, has been thought to

Table 138-5 DIFFERENTIAL DIAGNOSIS OF CHILDHOOD ASTHMA

UPPER RESPIRATORY TRACT CONDITIONS
Allergic rhinitis*
Chronic rhinitis*
Sinusitis*
Adenoidal or tonsillar hypertrophy
Nasal foreign body
MIDDLE RESPIRATORY TRACT CONDITIONS
Laryngotracheobronchomalacia*
Laryngotracheobronchitis (e.g., pertussis)*
Laryngeal web, cyst, or stenosis
Vocal cord dysfunction*
Vocal cord paralysis
Tracheoesophageal fistula
Vascular ring, sling, or external mass compressing on the airway (e.g., tumor)
Foreign body aspiration*
Chronic bronchitis from environmental tobacco smoke exposure*
Toxic inhalations
LOWER RESPIRATORY TRACT CONDITIONS
Bronchopulmonary dysplasia (chronic lung disease of preterm infants)
Viral bronchiolitis*
Gastroesophageal reflux*
Causes of bronchiectasis:
Cystic fibrosis
Immune deficiency
Allergic bronchopulmonary mycoses (e.g., aspergillosis)
Chronic aspiration
Immotile cilia syndrome, primary ciliary dyskinesia
Bronchiolitis obliterans
Interstitial lung diseases
Hypersensitivity pneumonitis
Pulmonary eosinophilia, Churg-Strauss vasculitis
Pulmonary hemosiderosis
Tuberculosis
Pneumonia
Pulmonary edema (e.g., congestive heart failure)
Medications associated with chronic cough:
Acetylcholinesterase inhibitors
β-Adrenergic antagonists
Angiotensin-converting enzyme inhibitors

*More common asthma masqueraders.

Table 138-6 LUNG FUNCTION ABNORMALITIES IN ASTHMA

Spirometry (in clinic):
Airflow limitation:
Low FEV_1 (relative to percentage of predicted norms)
FEV_1/FVC ratio <0.80
Bronchodilator response (to inhaled β-agonist):
Improvement in FEV_1 ≥12% and ≥200 mL*
Exercise challenge:
Worsening in FEV_1 ≥15%*
Daily peak flow or FEV_1 monitoring: day to day and/or AM-to-PM variation ≥20%*

*Main criteria consistent with asthma.
FEV_1, forced expiratory volume in 1 sec; FVC, forced vital capacity.

help with anti-inflammatory management and in confirming the diagnosis of asthma.

Peak expiratory flow (PEF) monitoring devices provide simple and inexpensive home-use tools to measure airflow and can be helpful in a number of circumstances (Fig. 138-3). "Poor perceivers" of airflow obstruction due to asthma can benefit by monitoring PEFs daily to assess objectively airflow as an indicator of asthma control or problems that would be more sensitive than their symptom perception. PEF devices vary in the ability to detect airflow obstruction: they are generally less sensitive than spirometry to airflow obstruction such that, in some patients, PEF values decline only when airflow obstruction is severe. Therefore, PEF monitoring should be started by measuring morning and evening PEFs (best of 3 attempts) for several weeks for patients to practice the technique, to determine a "personal best," and to correlate PEF values with symptoms (and ideally spirometry). PEF variation >20% is consistent with asthma (see Fig. 138-3 and Table 138-6).

Radiology

The findings of chest radiographs (posteroanterior and lateral views) in children with asthma often appear to be normal, aside from subtle and nonspecific findings of hyperinflation (flattening of the diaphragms) and peribronchial thickening (Fig. 138-4). Chest radiographs can be helpful in identifying abnormalities that are hallmarks of **asthma masqueraders** (aspiration pneumonitis, hyperlucent lung fields in bronchiolitis obliterans), and complications during asthma exacerbations (atelectasis, pneumomediastinum, pneumothorax). Some lung abnormalities can be better appreciated with high-resolution, thin-section chest CT scans. **Bronchiectasis,** which is sometimes difficult to appreciate on chest radiograph but is clearly seen on CT scan, implicates an asthma masquerader, such as cystic fibrosis, allergic bronchopulmonary mycoses (aspergillosis), ciliary dyskinesias, or immune deficiencies.

Other tests, such as allergy testing to assess sensitization to inhalant allergens, help with the management and prognosis of asthma. In a comprehensive U.S. study of 5-12 yr old asthmatic children (Childhood Asthma Management Program [CAMP]), 88% of the subjects had inhalant allergen sensitization according to results of allergy prick skin testing.

TREATMENT

The *National Asthma Education and Prevention Program's Expert Panel Report 3 (EPR3): Guidelines for the Diagnosis and Management of Asthma 2007* is available online (www.nhlbi.nih.gov/guidelines/asthma/asthgdln.htm), and the highlights of significant changes from the previous version of the guidelines have been published. The key components to optimal asthma management are specified (Fig. 138-5). **Management** of asthma should have the following components: (1) assessment and monitoring of disease activity; (2) provision of education to enhance the patient's and family's knowledge and skills for self-management; (3) identification and management of precipitating factors and co-morbid conditions that may worsen asthma; and (4) appropriate selection of medications to address the patient's needs. The long-term goal of asthma management is attainment of optimal asthma control.

Component 1: Regular Assessment and Monitoring

Regular assessment and monitoring are based on the concepts of asthma severity, asthma control, and responsiveness to therapy. **Asthma severity** is the intrinsic intensity of disease, and assessment is generally most accurate in patients not receiving controller therapy. Hence, assessing asthma severity directs the initial level of therapy. The 2 general categories are **intermittent** asthma and **persistent** asthma, the latter further subdivided into **mild, moderate**, and **severe**. Asthma severity is to be assessed only once, during a patient's initial evaluation, and only in patients who are not yet using a daily controller agent. In contrast, **asthma control** refers to the degree to which symptoms, ongoing functional impairments, and risk of adverse events are minimized and goals of therapy are met. In children receiving controller therapy, asthma control is to be assessed. Assessment of asthma control is important in adjusting therapy and is categorized in 3 levels: well-controlled, not well-controlled, and very poorly controlled. **Responsiveness to therapy** is the ease with which asthma control is attained by treatment. It can also encompass monitoring for adverse effects related to medication use.

Classification of asthma severity and control is based on the domains of **Impairment** and **Risk.** These domains may not correlate with each other and may respond differently to treatment.

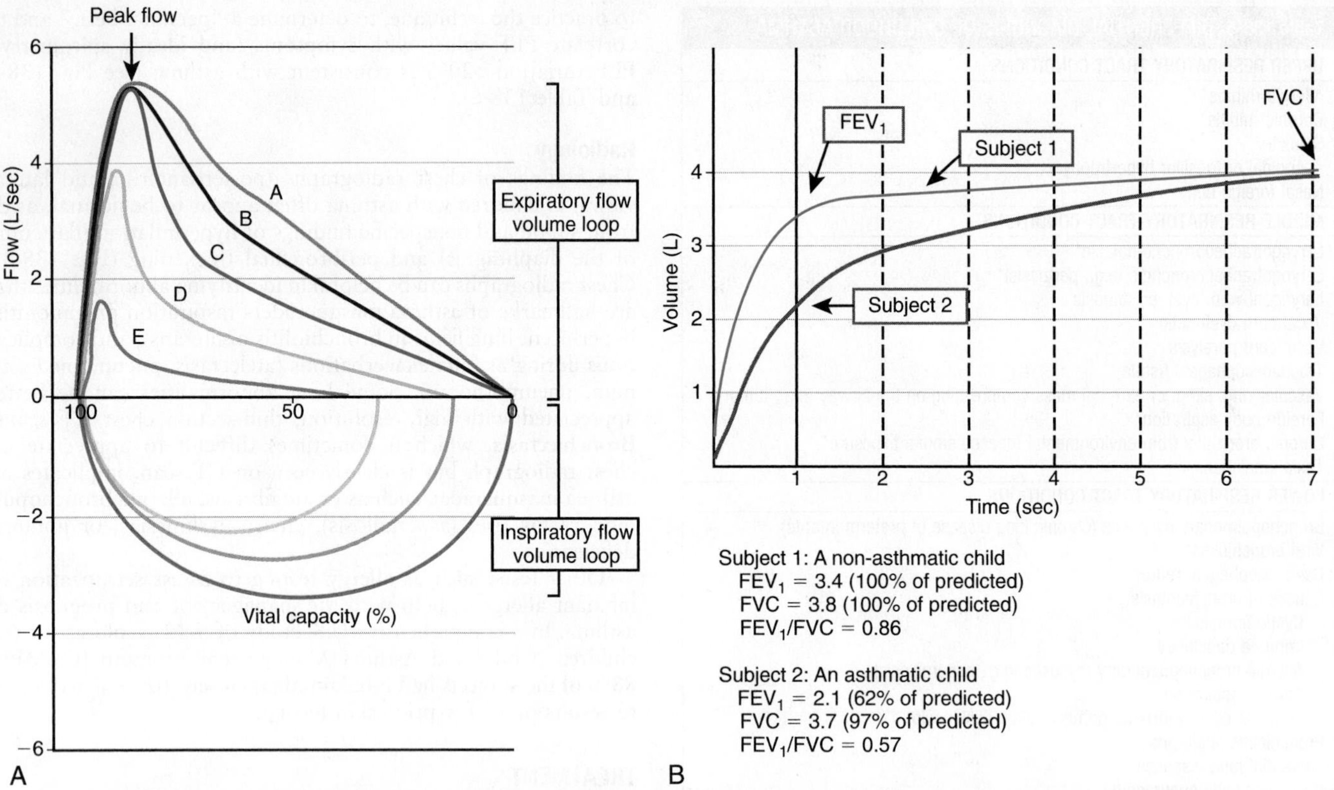

Figure 138-2 Spirometry. *A,* Spirometric flow-volume loops. A is an expiratory flow-volume loop of a nonasthmatic person without airflow limitation. B through E are expiratory flow-volume loops in asthmatic patients with increasing degrees of airflow limitation (B is mild; E is severe). Note the "scooped" or concave appearance of the asthmatic expiratory flow-volume loops; with increasing obstruction, there is greater "scooping." *B,* Spirometric volume-time curves. Subject 1 is a nonasthmatic person; subject 2 is an asthmatic patient. Note how the FEV_1 and FVC lung volumes are obtained. The FEV_1 is the volume of air exhaled in the 1st sec of a forced expiratory effort. The FVC is the total volume of air exhaled during a forced expiratory effort. Note that subject 2's FEV_1 and FEV_1/FVC ratio are smaller than subject 1's, demonstrating airflow limitation. Also, subject 2's FVC is very close to what is expected. FEV_1, forced expiratory volume in 1 sec; FVC, forced vital capacity.

The NIH guidelines have criteria for 3 age groups—0-4 yr, 5-11 yr, and ≥12 yr—for the evaluation of both severity (Table 138-7) and control (Table 138-8). The level of asthma severity or control is based on the most severe impairment or risk category. In assessing asthma severity, **impairment** consists of an assessment of the patient's recent symptom frequency (daytime and nighttime with subtle differences in numeric cutoffs between the 3 age groups), need for short-acting β_2-agonists for quick relief, ability to engage in normal or desired activities, and airflow compromise, which is evaluated with spirometry in children 5 yr and older. **Risk** refers to an evaluation of the likelihood of developing asthma exacerbations for the individual patient. Of note, in the absence of frequent symptoms, persistent asthma should be considered, and therefore long-term controller therapy should be initiated for infants or children who have risk factors for asthma (see earlier) and 4 or more episodes of wheezing over the past year that lasted longer than 1 day and affected sleep, or 2 or more exacerbations in 6 months requiring systemic corticosteroids.

Asthma management can be optimized through regular clinic visits every 2-6 wk until good asthma control is achieved. For children already on controller medication therapy, management is tailored to the child's level of control. The NIH guidelines provide tables for evaluating asthma control for the 3 age groups (see Table 138-8). In evaluation of asthma control, as in severity assessment, impairment includes an assessment of the patient's symptom frequency (daytime and nighttime), need for short-acting β_2-agonists for quick relief, ability to engage in normal or desired activities, and, for older children, airflow measurements. In addition, determination of quality of life measures for older children is included. Furthermore, with respect to risk assessment, besides considering severity and frequency of exacerbations requiring systemic corticosteroids, tracking of lung growth in older children and monitoring of untoward effects of medications are also warranted. As already mentioned, the degree of impairment and risk are used to determine the patient's level of asthma control as well-controlled, not well-controlled, or very poorly controlled. Children with *well-controlled asthma* have: daytime symptoms ≤2 days/week and need a rescue bronchodilator ≤2 days/week; an FEV_1 of >80% of predicted (and FEV_1/FVC ratio >80% for children 5-11 yr of age); no interference with normal activity; and <2 exacerbations in the past year. The impairment criteria vary slightly depending on age group: there are different thresholds in the frequency of nighttime awakenings; addition of FEV_1/FVC ratio criteria for children 5-11 yr old, and addition of validated questionnaires in evaluating quality of life for older children. Children whose status does not meet all of the criteria defining well-controlled asthma are determined to have either not well-controlled or very poorly controlled asthma, which is determined by the single criterion with the lowest rating.

Two to four asthma checkups per year are recommended for reassessing and maintaining good asthma control. During these visits, asthma control can be assessed by determining the: (1) frequency of asthma symptoms during the day, at night, and with physical exercise; (2) frequency of "rescue" SABA medication use and refills; (3) quality of life for youths with an assessment tool; (4) lung function measurements for older children and youths; (5) number and severity of asthma exacerbations; and (6) presence of medication adverse effects since the last visit (see Fig. 138-5). Lung function testing (spirometry) is recommended at least annually and more often if asthma is inadequately

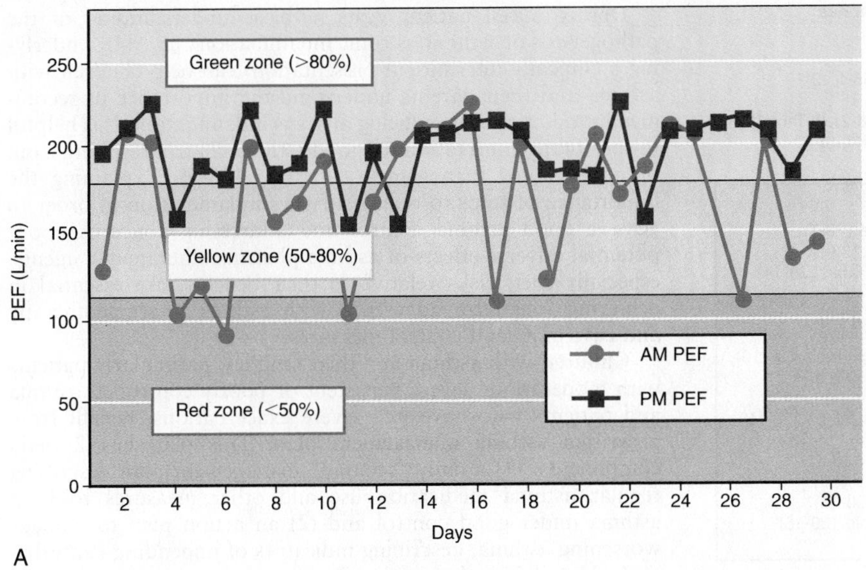

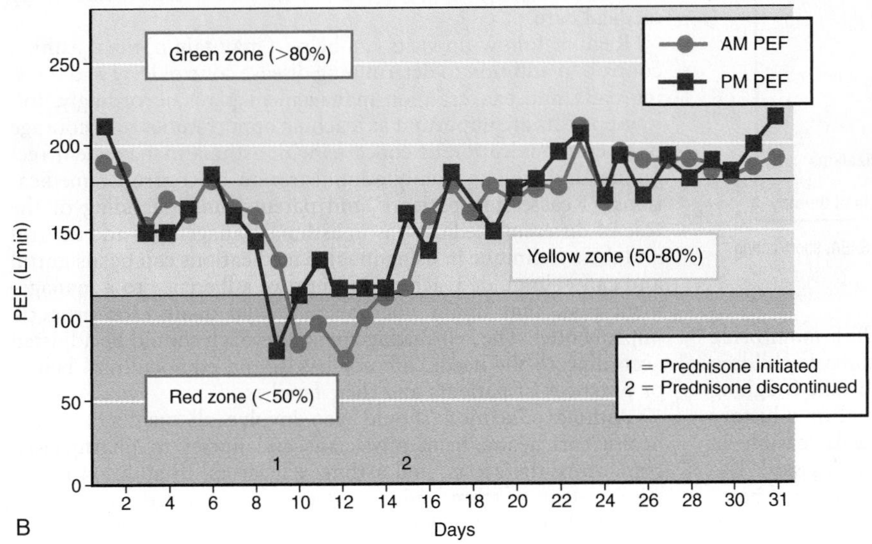

Figure 138-3 An example of the role of peak flow monitoring in childhood asthma. *A,* Peak expiratory flows (PEFs) performed and recorded twice daily, in the morning (AM) and evening (PM), over 1 mo in an asthmatic child. This child's "personal best" PEF value is 220 L/min; therefore, the green zone (>80-100% of best) is 175-220 L/min; the yellow zone (50-80%) is 110-175 L/min; and the red zone (<50%) is <110 L/min. Note that this child's PM PEF values are almost always in the green zone, whereas his AM PEFs are often in the yellow or red zone. This pattern illustrates the typical diurnal AM-to-PM variation of inadequately controlled asthma. *B,* PEFs performed twice daily, in the morning (AM) and evening (PM), over 1 mo in an asthmatic child in whom an asthma exacerbation developed from a viral respiratory tract infection. Note that the child's PEF values were initially in the green zone. A viral respiratory tract infection led to asthma worsening, with a decline in PEF to the yellow zone that continued to worsen until PEF values were in the red zone. At that point, a 4-day prednisone course was administered, followed by improvement in PEF back to the green zone.

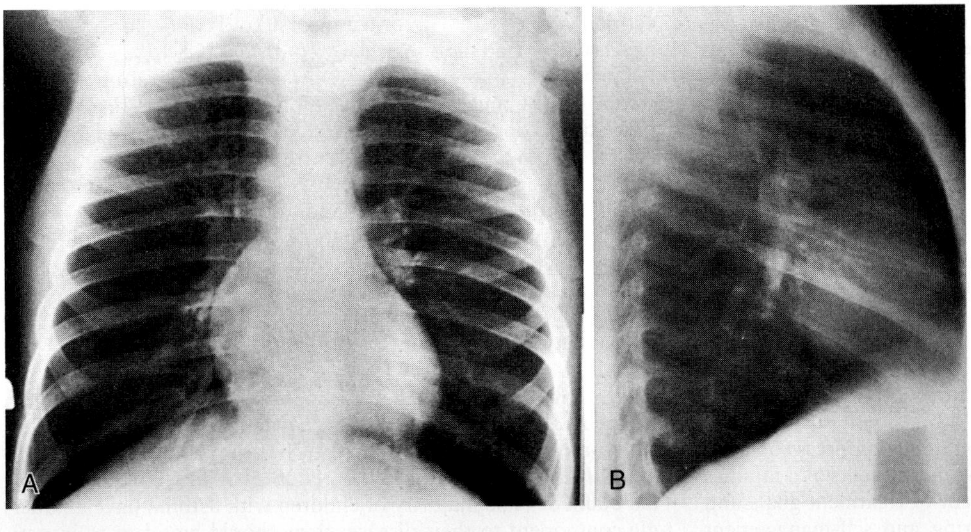

Figure 138-4 A 4-year-old boy with asthma. Frontal *(A)* and lateral *(B)* radiographs show pulmonary hyperinflation and minimal peribronchial thickening. No asthmatic complication is apparent.

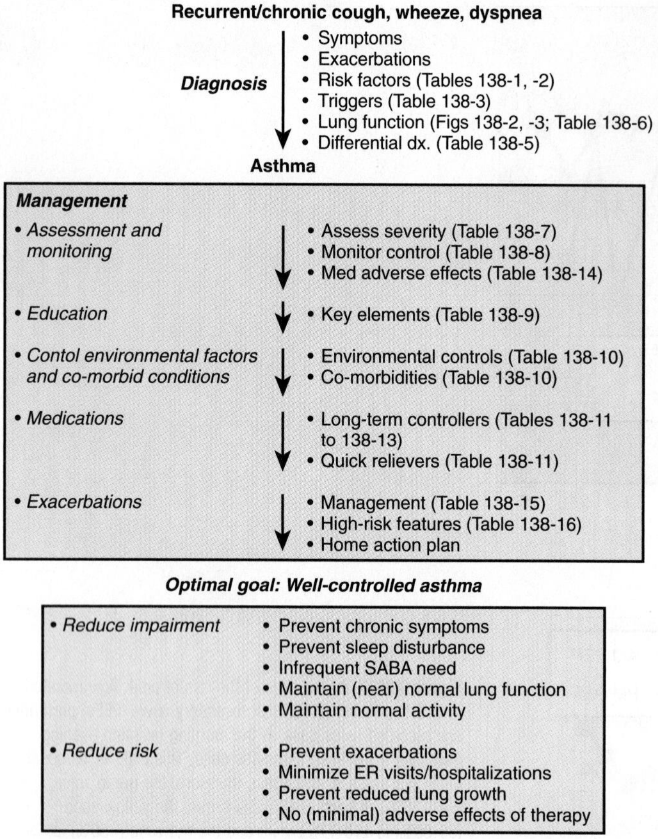

Recurrent/chronic cough, wheeze, dyspnea
Diagnosis
• Symptoms
• Exacerbations
• Risk factors (Tables 138-1, -2)
• Triggers (Table 138-3)
• Lung function (Figs 138-2, -3; Table 138-6)
• Differential dx. (Table 138-5)
Asthma
Management
• Assessment and monitoring
• Assess severity (Table 138-7)
• Monitor control (Table 138-8)
• Med adverse effects (Table 138-14)
• Education
• Key elements (Table 138-9)
• Contol environmental factors and co-morbid conditions
• Environmental controls (Table 138-10)
• Co-morbidities (Table 138-10)
• Medications
• Long-term controllers (Tables 138-11 to 138-13)
• Quick relievers (Table 138-11)
• Exacerbations
• Management (Table 138-15)
• High-risk features (Table 138-16)
• Home action plan
Optimal goal: Well-controlled asthma
• Reduce impairment
• Prevent chronic symptoms
• Prevent sleep disturbance
• Infrequent SABA need
• Maintain (near) normal lung function
• Maintain normal activity
• Reduce risk
• Prevent exacerbations
• Minimize ER visits/hospitalizations
• Prevent reduced lung growth
• No (minimal) adverse effects of therapy

Figure 138-5 The key elements to optimal asthma management. SABA, short-acting β-agonist.

controlled or lung function is abnormally low. PEF monitoring at home can be helpful in the assessment of asthmatic children with poor symptom perception, other causes of chronic coughing in addition to asthma, moderate to severe asthma, or a history of severe asthma exacerbations. PEF monitoring is feasible in children as young as 4 yr who are able to master this skill. Use of a **stoplight zone system** tailored to each child's "personal best" PEF values can optimize effectiveness and interest (see Fig 138-3): The green zone (80-100% of personal best) indicates good control; the yellow zone (50-80%) indicates less than optimal control and necessitates increased awareness and treatment; the red zone (<50%) indicates poor control and greater likelihood of an exacerbation, requiring immediate intervention. In actuality, these ranges are approximate and may need to be adjusted for many asthmatic children by raising the ranges that indicate inadequate control (in the yellow zone, 70-90%). The NIH guidelines recommend at least once-daily PEF monitoring, preferably in the morning when peak flows are typically lower.

Component 2: Patient Education

Specific educational elements in the clinical care of children with asthma are believed to make an important difference in home management and in adherence of families to an optimal plan of care and eventually impacting patient outcomes (Table 138-9). Every visit presents an important opportunity to educate the child and family, allowing them to become knowledgeable partners in asthma management, because optimal management depends on their daily assessments and implementation of any management plan. Effective communications take into account sociocultural and ethnic factors of children and their families, address concerns about asthma and its treatment, and include patients and families as active participants in the development of treatment goals and selection of medications. Self-monitoring and self-management skills should be reinforced regularly.

During initial patient visits, a basic understanding of the pathogenesis of asthma (chronic inflammation and AHR underlying a clinically intermittent presentation) can help children with asthma and their parents understand the importance of recommendations aimed at reducing airways inflammation. It is helpful to specify the expectations of good asthma control resulting from optimal asthma management (see Fig. 138-5). Explaining the importance of steps to reduce airways inflammation in order to achieve good asthma control and addressing concerns about potential adverse effects of asthma pharmacotherapeutic agents, especially their risks relative to their benefits, are essential in achieving long-term adherence with asthma pharmacotherapy and environmental control measures.

Children with asthma and their families, particularly patients with moderate or severe persistent or poorly controlled asthma and patients who have had severe exacerbations, benefit from a **written asthma management plan.** This plan has 2 main components: (1) a daily "routine" management plan describing regular asthma medication use and other measures to keep asthma under good control and (2) an action plan to manage worsening asthma, describing indicators of impending exacerbations, identifying what medications to take, and specifying when to contact the regular physician and/or obtain urgent/emergency medical care.

Regular follow-up visits can help to maintain optimal asthma control. In addition to determining disease control level and revising daily and exacerbation management plans accordingly, follow-up visits are important as teaching opportunities to encourage open communication of concerns with asthma management recommendations (e.g., daily administration of controller medications). Reassessing patients' and parents' understanding of the role of different medications in asthma management and control and their technique in using inhaled medications can be insightful and can help guide teaching to improve adherence to a management plan that might not have been adequately or properly implemented. The self-management approach should be adjusted according to the needs, literacy levels, and ethnocultural beliefs or practices of patients and their families.

Asthma education should also involve all members of the health care team, from physicians and nurses to pharmacists, respiratory therapists, and asthma educators. In addition to the clinic setting, asthma education can be provided in patients' homes, pharmacies, emergency rooms and hospitals, schools, and communities.

ADHERENCE Asthma is a chronic condition that is often best managed with daily controller medication. Adherence to a daily regimen is commonly suboptimal; inhaled corticosteroids (ICSs) are underused 60% of the time. In one study, children with asthma who required an oral corticosteroid course for an asthma exacerbation had used their daily controller ICS 15% of the time. Adherence is poorer when prescribed administration is more frequent (3-4 times/day). Medication formulations for once- or twice-daily dosing can improve patient adherence. Misconceptions about controller medication efficacy and safety often underlie poor adherence and can be addressed by asking about such concerns at each visit. In addition, choosing treatment that is tailored to the patient or family's expected outcomes and preferences will provide an incentive to improve adherence to the action plan.

Component 3: Control of Factors Contributing to Asthma Severity

Controllable factors that can significantly worsen asthma can be generally grouped as (1) environmental exposures and (2) co-morbid conditions (Table 138-10).

ELIMINATING AND REDUCING PROBLEMATIC ENVIRONMENTAL EXPOSURES The majority of children with asthma have an allergic component to their disease; steps should be taken to investigate and minimize allergen exposures in sensitized asthmatic

Table 138-7 ASSESSING ASTHMA SEVERITY AND INITIATING TREATMENT FOR PATIENTS WHO ARE NOT CURRENTLY TAKING LONG-TERM CONTROL MEDICATIONS*

	CLASSIFICATION OF ASTHMA SEVERITY			
	Intermittent	Persistent: Mild	Persistent: Moderate	Persistent: Severe
COMPONENTS OF SEVERITY				
Impairment				
Daytime symptoms	≤2 days/wk	>2 days/wk but not daily	Daily	Throughout the day
Nighttime awakenings:				
Age 0-4 yr	0	1-2×/mo	3-4×/mo	>1×/wk
Age ≥5 yr	≤2×/mo	3-4×/mo	>1×/wk but not nightly	Often 7×/wk
Short-acting β_2-agonist use for symptoms (not for prevention of exercise-induced bronchospasm)	≤2 days/wk	>2 days/wk but not daily, and not more than 1× on any day	Daily	Several times per day
Interference with normal activity	None	Minor limitation	Some limitation	Extreme limitation
Lung function:				
FEV_1 % predicted, age ≥5 yr	Normal FEV_1 between exacerbations >80% predicted	≥80% predicted	60-80% predicted	<60% predicted
FEV_1/FVC ratio[†]:				
Age 5- 11 yr	>85%	>80%	75-80%	<75%
Age ≥12 yr	Normal	Normal	Reduced 5%	Reduced >5%
Risk				
Exacerbations requiring systemic corticosteroids: Age 0-4 yr	0-1/yr (see notes)	≥ 2 exacerbations in 6 mo requiring systemic corticosteroids *or* ≥ 4 wheezing episodes/yr lasting >1 day *and* risk factors for persistent asthma		
Age ≥ 5 yr	0-1/yr (see notes)	≥2/yr (see notes)	≥2/yr (see notes)	≥2/yr (see notes)
Consider severity and interval since last exacerbation. Frequency and severity may fluctuate over time for patients in any severity category. Relative annual risk of exacerbations may be related to FEV_1.				
RECOMMENDED STEP FOR INITIATING THERAPY				
All ages	Step 1	Step 2		
Age 0-4 yr			Step 3	Step 3
Age 5-11 yr			Step 3, medium-dose ICS option	Step 3, medium-dose ICS option *or* Step 4
Age ≥12 yr			Consider a short course of systemic corticosteroids	Consider a short course of systemic corticosteroids
	In 2-6 wk, evaluate level of asthma control that is achieved and adjust therapy accordingly. If no clear benefit is observed within 4-6 wk, consider adjusting therapy or alternative diagnoses.			

*Notes:

- The stepwise approach is meant to assist, not replace, the clinical decision-making required to meet individual patient needs.
- Level of severity is determined by both impairment and risk. Assess impairment domain by patient's/caregiver's recall of previous 2-4 wk. Symptom assessment for longer periods should reflect a global assessment, such as inquiring whether a patient's asthma is better or worse since the last visit. Assign severity to the most severe category in which any feature occurs.
- At present, there are inadequate data to correspond frequencies of exacerbations with different levels of asthma severity. For treatment purposes, patients who had ≥ 2 exacerbations requiring oral systemic corticosteroids in the past 6 mo, or ≥ 4 wheezing episodes in the past year, and who have risk factors for persistent asthma may be considered the same as patients who have persistent asthma, even in the absence of impairment levels consistent with persistent asthma.

[†]Normal FEV_1/FVC: 8-19 yr, 85%; 20-39 yr, 80%.

FEV_1, forced expiratory volume in 1 sec; FVC, forced vital capacity; ICS, inhaled corticosteroids.

Adapted from the National Asthma Education and Prevention Program: Expert Panel Report 3 (EPR 3): Guidelines for the diagnosis and management of asthma—summary report 2007, *J Allergy Clin Immunol* 120(Suppl):S94–S138, 2007.

patients. For sensitized asthmatic patients, reduced exposure to perennial allergens in the home decreases asthma symptoms, medication requirements, AHR, and asthma exacerbations. The important home allergens that are linked to asthma worsening differ between locales and even between homes. Common perennial allergen exposures include furred or feathered animals as pets (cats, dogs, ferrets, birds) or as pests (mice, rats) and occult indoor allergens such as dust mites, cockroaches, and molds. Although some sensitized children may report an increase in asthma symptoms on exposure to the allergen source, improvement from allergen avoidance may not become apparent without a sustained period of days to weeks away from the offending exposure. Tobacco, wood and coal smoke, dusts, strong odors, and noxious fumes can all aggravate asthma. These airways irritants should be eliminated from or reduced in the homes and automobiles used by children with asthma. School classrooms and daycare settings can also be sites of asthma-worsening environmental exposures. Eliminating or minimizing these exposures (e.g., furred or feathered pets in classrooms of sensitized children with asthma) can reduce asthma symptoms, disease severity, and the amount of medication needed to achieve good asthma control. Annual influenza vaccination continues to be recommended for all children with asthma (except for those with egg allergy), although influenza is not responsible for the large majority of virus-induced asthma exacerbations experienced by children.

TREAT CO-MORBID CONDITIONS Rhinitis, sinusitis, and gastroesophageal reflux often accompany asthma and can mimic asthma symptoms and worsen disease severity. Indeed, these conditions with asthma are the most common causes of chronic coughing. Effective management of these co-morbid conditions may improve asthma symptoms and disease severity, such that less asthma medication is needed to achieve good asthma control.

Table 138-8 ASSESSING ASTHMA CONTROL AND ADJUSTING THERAPY IN CHILDREN*

	CLASSIFICATION OF ASTHMA CONTROL		
	Well-Controlled	**Not Well-Controlled**	**Very Poorly Controlled**
COMPONENTS OF CONTROL **Impairment**			
Symptoms	≤2 days/wk but not more than once on each day	>2 days/wk or multiple times on ≤2 days/wk	Throughout the day
Nighttime awakenings:			
Age 0-4 yr	≤1×/mo	>1×/mo	>1×/wk
Age 5-11 yr	≤1×/mo	≥2×/mo	≥2×/wk
Age ≥12 yr	≤2×/mo	1-3×/wk	≥4×/wk
Short-acting β_2-agonist use for symptoms (not for exercise-induced bronchos8pasm pretreatment)	≤2 days/wk	>2 days/wk	Several times per day
Interference with normal activity	None	Some limitation	Extremely limited
Lung function:			
Age 5-11 yr:			
FEV_1 (% predicted or peak flow)	>80% predicted or personal best	60-80% predicted or personal best	<60% predicted or personal best
FEV_1/FVC:	>80%	75-80%	<75%
Age ≥ 12 yr:			
FEV_1 (% predicted or peak flow)	>80% predicted or personal best	60-80% predicted or personal best	<60% predicted or personal best
Validated questionnaires†:			
Age ≥ 12 yr:			
ATAQ	0	1-2	3-4
ACQ	≤0.75	≤1.5	N/A
ACT	≥220	16-19	≤15
Risk			
Exacerbations requiring systemic corticosteroids:			
Age 0-4 yr	0-1/yr	2-3/yr	>3/yr
Age ≥5 yr	0-1/yr	≥2/yr (see notes)	
	Consider severity and interval since last exacerbation.		
Treatment-related adverse effects	Medication side effects can vary in intensity from none to very troublesome and worrisome. The level of intensity does not correlate to specific levels of control but should be considered in the overall assessment of risk.		
Reduction in lung growth *or* progressive loss of lung function	Evaluation requires long-term follow-up care.		
RECOMMENDED ACTION FOR TREATMENT			
	Maintain current step. Regular follow-up every 1-6 mo to maintain control. Consider step down if well-controlled for at least 3 mo.	Step up‡ (1 step) and reevaluate in 2-6 wk. If no clear benefit in 4-6 wk, consider alternative diagnoses or adjusting therapy. For side effects, consider alternative options.	Consider short course of oral corticosteroids. Step up§ (1-2 steps) and reevaluate in 2 weeks. If no clear benefit in 4-6 wk, consider alternative diagnoses or adjusting therapy. For side effects, consider alternative options.

*Notes:
- The stepwise approach is meant to assist, not replace, the clinical decision-making required to meet individual patient needs.
- The level of control is based on the most severe impairment or risk category. Assess impairment domain by caregiver's recall of previous 2-4 wk. Symptom assessment for longer periods should reflect a global assessment such as inquiring whether the patient's asthma is better or worse since the last visit.
- At present, there are inadequate data to correspond frequencies of exacerbations with different levels of asthma control. In general, more frequent and intense exacerbations (e.g., requiring urgent, unscheduled care, hospitalization, or intensive care unit admission) indicate poorer disease control. For treatment purposes, patients who had ≥2 exacerbations requiring oral systemic corticosteroids in the past year may be considered the same as patients who have not-well-controlled asthma, even in the absence of impairment levels consistent with not-well-controlled asthma.

†Validated questionnaires for the impairment domain (the questionnaires do not assess lung function or the risk domain) and definition of minimal important difference (MID) for each:
- ATAQ, Asthma Therapy Assessment Questionnaire; MID = 1.0
- ACQ, Asthma Control Questionnaire; MID = 0.5
- ACT, Asthma Control Test; MID not determined

‡ACQ values of 0.76-1.40 are indeterminate regarding well-controlled asthma.

§Before step- up therapy: (1) review adherence to medications, inhaler technique, and environmental control; (2) if alternative treatment option was used in a step, discontinue it and use preferred treatment for that step.

FEV_1, forced expiratory volume in 1 sec; FVC, forced vital capacity.

Adapted from the National Asthma Education and Prevention Program: Expert Panel Report 3 (EPR 3): Guidelines for the diagnosis and management of asthma—summary report 2007, *J Allergy Clin Immunol* 120(Suppl):S94–S138, 2007.

Table 138-9 KEY ELEMENTS OF PRODUCTIVE CLINIC VISITS FOR ASTHMA

Specify goals of asthma management
Explain basic facts about asthma:
Contrast normal vs asthmatic airways
Link airways inflammation, "twitchiness," and bronchoconstriction
Long-term-control and quick-relief medications
Address concerns about potential adverse effects of asthma pharmacotherapy
Teach, demonstrate, and have patient show proper technique for:
Inhaled medication use (spacer use with metered-dose inhaler)
Peak flow measures
Investigate and manage factors that contribute to asthma severity:
Environmental exposures
Co-morbid conditions
Written two-part asthma management plan:
Daily management
Action plan for asthma exacerbations
Regular follow-up visits:
Twice yearly (more often if asthma not well-controlled)
Monitor lung function annually

Table 138-10 CONTROL OF FACTORS CONTRIBUTING TO ASTHMA SEVERITY

Eliminate or reduce problematic environmental exposures:
Environmental tobacco smoke elimination or reduction:
In home and automobiles
Allergen exposure elimination or reduction in sensitized asthmatic patients:
Animal danders:
Pets (cats, dogs, rodents, birds)
Pests (mice, rats)
Dust mites
Cockroaches
Molds
Other airway irritants:
Wood- or coal-burning smoke
Strong chemical odors and perfumes (e.g., household cleaners)
Dusts
Treat co-morbid conditions:
Rhinitis
Sinusitis
Gastroesophageal reflux
Annual influenza vaccination (unless patient is egg-allergic)

Gastroesophageal reflux is more common, with a reported incidence of GER-related asthma symptoms in up to 64% of asthmatic patients. GER may worsen asthma through 2 postulated mechanisms: (1) aspiration of refluxed gastric contents (micro- or macro-aspiration); and (2) vagally-mediated reflex bronchospasm. Occult GER should be suspected in individuals with difficult-to-control asthma, especially patients who have prominent asthma symptoms while eating or sleeping (in a horizontal position) or who prop themselves up in bed to reduce nocturnal symptoms. GER can be demonstrated by reflux of barium into the esophagus during a barium swallow procedure or by esophageal pH monitoring. Because radiographic studies lack sufficient sensitivity and specificity, extended esophageal pH monitoring is the method of choice for diagnosing GER. If significant GER is noted, reflux precautions should be instituted (no food 2 hr before bedtime, head of the bed elevated 6 in., avoidance of caffeinated foods and beverages) and medications such as proton pump inhibitors (omeprazole, lansoprazole) or H_2-receptor antagonists (cimetidine, ranitidine) administered for 8 to 12 wk. Proton pump inhibition did not improve asthma control in one study of adults with asthma and GER.

Rhinitis is usually co-morbid with asthma, detected in ≈90% of children with asthma. Rhinitis can be seasonal and/or perennial, with allergic and nonallergic components. Rhinitis complicates and worsens asthma via numerous direct and indirect mechanisms. Nasal breathing may improve asthma and reduce exercise-induced bronchospasm by humidifying and warming inspired air and filtering out allergens and irritants that can trigger asthma and increase AHR. Reduction of nasal congestion and obstruction can help the nose to perform these humidifying, warming, and filtering functions. In asthmatic patients, improvement in rhinitis is also associated with improvement in AHR, lower airways inflammation, asthma symptoms, and asthma medication use. Optimal rhinitis management in children is similar to asthma management in regard to the importance of interventions to reduce nasal inflammation (Chapter 137).

Radiographic evidence for sinus disease is common in patients with asthma. There is usually significant improvement in asthma control in patients diagnosed and treated for sinus disease. A coronal, "screening" or "limited" CT scan of the sinuses is the gold standard test for sinus disease and is often helpful if recurrent sinusitis has been suspected and treated without such evidence. If the patient with asthma has clinical and radiographic evidence for sinusitis, topical therapy to include nasal saline irrigations and possibly intranasal corticosteroids should be instituted, and a 2- to 3-wk course of antibiotics administered.

Component 4: Principles of Asthma Pharmacotherapy

The current version of NIH asthma guidelines (2007) proposes an expanded stepwise treatment approach to assist, not replace, the clinical decision-making required to meet individual patient needs. The recommendations vary by age groups and are based on current evidence (Table 138-11). The goals of therapy are to reduce the components of both impairment (e.g., preventing chronic and troublesome symptoms, allowing infrequent need of quick-reliever medications, maintaining "normal" lung function, maintaining normal activity levels including physical activity and school attendance, meeting families' expectations and satisfaction with asthma care) and risk (e.g., preventing recurrent exacerbations, reduced lung growth, and medications' adverse effects). The choice of initial therapy is based on assessment of asthma severity, and for patients who are already using controller therapy, modification of treatment is based on assessment of asthma control and responsiveness to therapy. A major objective of this approach is to identify and treat all "persistent" and uncontrolled asthma with anti-inflammatory controller medication. Daily controller therapy is not recommended for children with "intermittent asthma." Management of intermittent asthma is simply the use of a short-acting inhaled β-agonist as needed for symptoms and for pre-treatment in those with exercise-induced bronchospasm (Step 1 therapy; see Table 138-11).

The preferred treatment for all patients with persistent asthma is daily ICS therapy, as monotherapy or in combination with adjunctive therapy. The type(s) and amount(s) of daily controller medications to be used are determined by the asthma severity and control rating. Alternative medications for Step 2 therapy include a leukotriene receptor antagonist (montelukast), nonsteroidal anti-inflammatory agents (cromolyn and nedocromil), and theophylline (for youths). For young children (≤4 r of age) with moderate or severe persistent asthma, medium-dose ICS monotherapy is recommended (Step 3); combination therapy is recommended only as a Step 4 treatment for uncontrolled asthma.

Along with medium-dose ICSs, combination therapy with an ICS plus any of the following adjunctive therapies (depending on age group) is recommended as Step 4 treatment for moderate persistent asthma, or as step-up therapy for uncontrolled persistent asthma: long-acting inhaled β_2-agonists (LABAs), leukotriene-modifying agents, cromones, and theophylline. Children with severe persistent asthma (Treatment Steps 5 and 6) should receive high-dose ICS, an LABA, and long-term administration of oral corticosteroids if required. In addition, omalizumab can be used in older children (≥12 yr old) with severe allergic asthma. A rescue course of systemic corticosteroids may be necessary at any step.

Table 138-11 STEPWISE APPROACH FOR MANAGING ASTHMA IN CHILDREN*

AGE	THERAPY†	INTERMITTENT ASTHMA	PERSISTENT ASTHMA: DAILY MEDICATION				
			STEP DOWN if possible (and asthma is well controlled at least 3 months)		ASSESS CONTROL	STEP UP if needed (first check inhaler technique, adherence, environmental control, and comorbid condition)	
		Step 1	Step 2	Step 3	Step 4	Step 5	Step 6
0-4 yr	Preferred	SABA prn	Low-dose ICS	Medium-dose ICS	Medium dose ICS + *either* LABA *or* LTRA	High-dose ICS + *either* LABA *or* LTRA	High-dose ICS + *either* LABA *or* LTRA *and* Oral corticosteroid
	Alternative		Cromolyn or montelukast				
5-11 yr	Preferred	SABA prn	Low dose ICS	*Either* low-dose ICS ± LABA, LTRA, or theophylline *or* Medium-dose ICS	Medium-dose ICS + LABA	High-dose ICS + LABA	High dose ICS + LABA *and* Oral corticosteroid
	Alternative		Cromolyn, LTRA, nedocromil, or theophylline		Medium-dose ICS + *either* LTRA *or* Theophylline	High-dose ICS + *either* LTRA *or* Theophylline	High-dose ICS + *either* LTRA *or* Theophylline *and* Oral corticosteroid
≥12 yr	Preferred	SABA prn	Low-dose ICS	Low-dose ICS + LABA *or* Medium-dose ICS	Medium-dose ICS + LABA	High-dose ICS + LABA *and* Consider omalizumab for patients with allergies	High-dose ICS + LABA + oral corticosteroid *and* Consider omalizumab for patients with allergies
	Alternative		Cromolyn, LTRA, nedocromil, or theophylline	Low-dose ICS + LTRA, theophylline, or zileuton	Medium-dose ICS + LTRA, theophylline, or zileuton		
	Each step: Patient education, environmental control, and management of comorbidities. Age ≥5 yr: Steps 2-4: Consider subcutaneous allergen immunotherapy for patients who have allergic asthma.						
	QUICK-RELIEF MEDICATION FOR ALL PATIENTS						
	SABA as needed for symptoms. Intensity of treatment depends on severity of symptoms: up to 3 treatments at 20-min intervals as needed. Short course of oral systemic corticosteroids may be needed. *Caution:* Use of SABA >2 days/wk for symptom relief (not prevention of exercise-induced bronchospasm) generally indicates inadequate control and the need to step up treatment. For ages 0-4 yr: With viral respiratory infection: SABA q4-6h up to 24 hr (longer with physician consult). Consider short course of systemic corticosteroids if exacerbation is severe or patient has history of previous severe exacerbations.						

*Notes:

- The stepwise approach is meant to assist, not replace, the clinical decision-making required to meet individual patient needs.
- If alternative treatment is used and response is inadequate, discontinue it and use the preferred treatment before stepping up.
- If clear benefit is not observed within 4-6 wk and patient/family medication technique and adherence are satisfactory, consider adjusting therapy or alternative diagnosis.
- Studies on children aged 0-4 yr are limited. The stepwise approach is meant to assist, not replace, the clinical decision-making required to meet individual patient needs.
- Clinicians who administer immunotherapy or omalizumab should be prepared and equipped to identify and treat anaphylaxis that may occur.
- Theophylline is a less desirable alternative due to the need to monitor serum concentration levels.
- Zileuton is less desirable alternative due to limited studies as adjunctive therapy and the need to monitor liver function.

†Alphabetical order is used when more than one treatment option is listed within either preferred or alternative therapy.

ICS, inhaled corticosteroid; LABA, inhaled long-acting β_2-agonist; LTRA, leukotriene receptor antagonist; prn, as needed; SABA, inhaled short-acting β_2-agonist.

Adapted from the National Asthma Education and Prevention Program: Expert Panel Report 3 (EPR 3): Guidelines for the diagnosis and management of asthma—summary report 2007, *J Allergy Clin Immunol* 120(Suppl):S94–S138, 2007.

For children 5 yr and older with allergic asthma requiring Steps 2-4 care, allergen immunotherapy can be considered.

"STEP-UP, STEP-DOWN" APPROACH The NIH guidelines emphasize initiating higher-level controller therapy at the outset to establish prompt control, with measures to "step down" therapy once good asthma control is achieved. Initially, airflow limitation and the pathology of asthma may limit the delivery and efficacy of ICS such that stepping up to higher doses and/or combination therapy may be needed to gain asthma control. Furthermore, ICS requires weeks to months of daily administration for optimal efficacy to occur. Combination pharmacotherapy can achieve relatively immediate improvement while also providing daily ICS to improve long-term control.

Asthma therapy can be stepped down after good asthma control has been achieved and ICS has had time to achieve optimal efficacy, by determining the lowest number or dose of daily controller medications that can maintain good control, thereby reducing the potential for medication adverse effects. If a child has had well-controlled asthma for at least 3 months, the guidelines suggest decreasing the dose or number of the child's controller medication(s) to establish the minimum required medications to maintain well-controlled asthma. Regular follow-up is still emphasized because the variability of asthma's course is well recognized. In contrast, if a child has not well-controlled asthma, the therapy level should be increased by 1 step and close monitoring is recommended. For a child with very poorly controlled asthma, the recommendations are that treatment go up 2 steps and/or a short course of oral corticosteroid therapy be given, with evaluation within 2 wk. As step-up therapy is being considered at any point, it is important to check inhaler technique and adherence, implement environmental control measures, and identify and treat comorbid conditions.

REFERRAL TO ASTHMA SPECIALIST Referral to an asthma specialist for consultation or co-management is recommended if there are difficulties in achieving or maintaining control. For children younger than 4 yr, referral is recommended for moderate persistent asthma or if the patient requires at least Step 3 care, and should be considered if the patient requires Step 2 care. For children 5 yr of age and older, consultation with a specialist is recommended if the patient requires step 4 care or higher, and should be considered if Step 3 is required. Referral is also recommended if allergen immunotherapy or anti-IgE therapy is being considered.

Long-Term Controller Medications

All levels of persistent asthma should be treated with daily medications to improve long-term control (see Table 138-11). Such medications include ICSs, LABAs, leukotriene modifiers, nonsteroidal anti-inflammatory agents, and sustained-release theophylline. An anti-IgE preparation, omalizumab (Xolair), has been approved by the U.S. Food and Drug Administration (FDA) for use as an add-on therapy in children ≥12 yr who have moderate to severe allergic asthma that is difficult to control. Corticosteroids are the most potent and most effective medications used to treat both the acute (administered systemically) and chronic (administered by inhalation) manifestations of asthma. They are available in inhaled, oral, and parenteral forms (Tables 138-12 and 138-13).

INHALED CORTICOSTEROIDS The NIH guidelines recommend daily ICS therapy as the treatment of choice for all patients with persistent asthma (see Table 138-11). ICS therapy has been shown to improve lung function as well as to reduce asthma symptoms, AHR, and use of "rescue" medications; most important, it has been found to reduce urgent care visits, hospitalizations, and prednisone use for asthma exacerbations by about 50%. ICS therapy may lower the risk of death due to asthma. It can achieve all of the goals of asthma management and, as a result, is viewed as first-line treatment for persistent asthma.

Currently, 6 ICSs are approved for use in children by the FDA, and the NIH guidelines provide an equivalence classification (see Table 138-13), although direct comparisons of efficacy and safety outcomes in children are lacking. ICSs are available in metered-dose inhalers (MDIs), in dry powder inhalers (DPIs), or in suspension for nebulization. Fluticasone propionate, mometasone furoate, ciclesonide, and, to a lesser extent, budesonide are considered "2nd-generation" ICSs, in that they have greater anti-inflammatory potency and diminished systemic bioavailability for potential adverse effects, owing to extensive first-pass hepatic metabolism. The selection of the initial ICS dose is based on the determination of disease severity. A fraction of the initial ICS dose is often sufficient to maintain good control after this goal has been achieved.

Although ICS therapy has been widely used in adults with persistent asthma, its application in children has lagged because of concerns about the potential for adverse effects with long-term use. Generally, clinically significant adverse effects that occur with long-term systemic corticosteroid therapy have not been seen or have only very rarely been reported in children receiving ICSs in recommended doses. The risk of adverse effects from ICS therapy is related to the dose and frequency with which ICSs are given (Table 138-14). High doses (≥1,000 µg/day in children) and frequent administration (4 times/day) are more likely to have local and systemic adverse effects. Children who receive maintenance therapy with higher ICS doses are also likely to require systemic corticosteroid courses for asthma exacerbations, further increasing the risk of corticosteroid adverse effects.

The most commonly encountered **adverse effects** of ICSs are local: oral candidiasis (thrush) and dysphonia (hoarse voice). Thrush results from propellant-induced mucosal irritation and local immunosuppression. Dysphonia occurs from vocal cord myopathy. These effects are dose-dependent and are most common in individuals receiving high-dose ICS and/or oral corticosteroid therapy. The incidence of these local effects can be greatly minimized by using a spacer with an MDI ICS, because spacers reduce oropharyngeal deposition of the drug and propellant. Mouth rinsing using a "swish and spit" technique after ICS use is also recommended.

The potential for growth suppression and osteoporosis with long-term ICS use has been a concern. In the long term, prospective NIH-sponsored CAMP study of children with mild to moderate asthma, after ≈4.3 yr of ICS therapy and 5 yr after the trial, there was a significant 1.7-cm decrease in height in girls, but not in boys. There was also a slight dose-dependent effect of ICS therapy on bone mineral accretion in boys, but not girls. A greater effect on bone mineral accretion was observed with increasing numbers of courses of oral corticosteroid burst therapy for asthma, as well as an increase in risk for osteopenia, again limited to boys. Although this study cannot predict a significant effect of ICS therapy in childhood on osteoporosis in later adulthood, improved asthma control with ICS therapy may result in a need for fewer courses of oral corticosteroid burst therapy over time. These findings were with use of budesonide at doses of about 400 µg/day; higher ICS doses, especially of agents with increased potency, have a greater potential for adverse effects. Hence, corticosteroid adverse effects screening and osteoporosis prevention measures are recommended for patients receiving higher ICS doses, as these patients are also likely to require systemic courses for exacerbations (see Table 138-14).

SYSTEMIC CORTICOSTEROIDS ICS therapy has allowed the large majority of children with asthma to maintain good disease control without maintenance oral corticosteroid therapy. Oral corticosteroids are used primarily to treat asthma exacerbations and, rarely, in patients with severe disease who remain symptomatic despite optimal use of other asthma medications. In these severely asthmatic patients, every attempt should be made to exclude any co-morbid conditions and to keep the oral corticosteroid dose at ≤20 mg qod. Doses exceeding this amount are associated with numerous adverse effects (Chapter 571). To determine the need for continued oral corticosteroid therapy, tapering of the oral corticosteroid dose (over several weeks to months) should be considered, with close monitoring of the patient's symptoms and lung function.

When administered orally, prednisone, prednisolone, and methylprednisolone are rapidly and completely absorbed, with peak plasma concentrations occurring within 1-2 hr. Prednisone is an inactive prodrug that requires biotransformation via first-pass hepatic metabolism to prednisolone, its active form. Corticosteroids are metabolized in the liver into inactive compounds, with the rate of metabolism influenced by drug interactions and disease states. Anticonvulsants (phenytoin, phenobarbital, carbamazepine) increase the metabolism of prednisolone, methylprednisolone, and dexamethasone, with methylprednisolone most significantly affected. Rifampin also enhances the clearance of corticosteroids and can result in diminished therapeutic effect. Other medications (ketoconazole, oral contraceptives) can significantly delay corticosteroid metabolism. Macrolide antibiotics (erythromycin, clarithromycin, troleandomycin) delay the clearance of only methylprednisolone.

Children who require long-term oral corticosteroid therapy are at risk for development of associated adverse effects over

Table 138-12 USUAL DOSAGES FOR LONG-TERM CONTROL MEDICATIONS

MEDICATION	AGE		
	0-4 yr	5-11 yr	≥12 yr
INHALED CORTICOSTEROIDS (also see Table 138-13)			
Methylprednisolone: 2-, 4-, 8-, 16-, 32-mg tablets Prednisolone: 5-mg tablets; 5 mg/5 mL, 15 mg/5 mL Prednisone: 1-, 2.5-, 5-, 10-, 20-, 50-mg tablets; 5 mg/mL, 5 mg/5 mL	• 0.25-2 mg/kg daily in single dose in AM or qod as needed for control • Short-course "burst": 1-2 mg/kg/day; maximum 30 mg/day for 3-10 days	• 0.25-2 mg/kg daily in single dose in AM or qod as needed for control • Short-course "burst": 1-2 mg/kg/day; maximum 60 mg/day for 3-10 days	• 7.5-60 mg daily in a single dose in AM or qod as needed for control • Short-course "burst" to achieve control: 40-60 mg/day as single or 2 divided doses for 3-10 days
Salmeterol: DPI 50 mg/blister	NA	1 blister q 12 hr	1 blister q 12 hr
Formoterol: DPI 12 mg/single-use capsule	NA	1 capsule q 12 hr	1 capsule q 12 hr
Fluticasone/salmeterol:	NA		
DPI: 100, 250 , or 500 mg/50 mg		1 inhalation bid; dose depends on level of severity or control	1 inhalation bid; dose depends on level of severity or control
HFA: 45 μg/21 μg, 115 μg/21 μg, 230 μg/21 μg		2 inhalations bid; dose depends on level of severity or control	2 inhalations bid; dose depends on level of severity or control
Budesonide/formoterol: HFA: 80 μg/4.5 μg, 160 μg/4.5 μg	NA	2 inhalations bid; dose depends on level of severity or control	2 inhalations bid; dose depends on level of severity or control
Cromolyn: MDI 0.8 mg/puff	NA	2 puffs qid	2 puffs qid
Nebulizer 20 mg/ampule	1 ampule qid; NA < 2 yr of age	1 ampule qid	1 ampule qid
Nedocromil: MDI 1.75 mg/puff	NA < 6 yr of age	2 puffs qid	2 puffs qid
Leukotriene receptor antagonists: Montelukast: 4- or 5-mg chewable tablet 4-mg granule packets 10-mg tablet	4 mg qhs (1-5 yr of age)	5 mg qhs (6-14 yr)	10mg qhs
Zafirlukast: 10- or 20-mg tablet	NA	10 mg bid (7-11 yr)	40 mg daily (20-mg tablet bid)
5-lipoxygenase inhibitor: Zileuton: 600-mg tablet	NA	NA	2,400 mg daily (give tablets qid)
Theophylline: Liquids, sustained-release tablets, and capsules	Starting dose 10 mg/kg/day; usual max: • < 1 yr of age: 0.2 (age in wk) + 5 = mg/kg/day • >1 yr of age: 16 mg/kg/day	Starting dose 10 mg/kg/day; usual maximun: 16 mg/kg/day	Starting dose 10 mg/kg/day up to 300 mg maximum; usual maximum 800 mg/day
Immunomodulators: Omalizumab (anti-IgE): Subcutaneous injection, 150 mg/1.2 mL after reconstitution with 1.4 mL sterile water for injection	NA	NA	150-375 mg SC q 2-4 wk, depending on body weight and pretreatment serum IgE level

bid, twice a day; DPI, dry powder inhaler; HFA, hydrofluoroalkane Ig, immunoglobulin; MDI, metered-dose inhaler; q, every; qhs, every night; qid, 4 times a day; qod, every other day; SC, subcutaneous.

time. Essentially all major organ systems can be adversely affected by long-term oral corticosteroid therapy (Chapter 571). Some of these effects occur immediately (metabolic effects). Others can develop insidiously over several months to years (growth suppression, osteoporosis, cataracts). Most adverse effects occur in a cumulative dose- and duration-dependent manner. Children who require routine or frequent short courses of oral corticosteroids, especially with concurrent high-dose ICSs, should receive corticosteroid adverse effects screening (see Table 138-14) and osteoporosis preventive measures (Chapter 698).

LONG-ACTING INHALED β-AGONISTS LABAs (salmeterol, formoterol) are considered to be daily controller medications, *not intended* for use as "rescue" medication for acute asthma symptoms or exacerbations, nor as monotherapy for persistent asthma. Controller formulations that combine an ICS with an LABA (fluticasone/salmeterol, budesonide/formoterol) are available and recommended, in lieu of separate inhaler delivery devices. Salmeterol has a prolonged onset of action, with maximal bronchodilation about 1 hr after administration, whereas formoterol has an onset of action within 5-10 min. Both medications have a prolonged duration of effect, at least 12 hr. Given their long duration of action, they are well suited for patients with nocturnal asthma and for individuals who require frequent SABA use during the day to prevent exercise-induced bronchospasm. Their major role is as an add-on agent in patients whose asthma is suboptimally controlled with ICS therapy alone. For those patients, several studies have found the addition of an LABA to ICS therapy to be superior to doubling the dose of ICS, especially on day and nocturnal symptoms. Of note, the FDA requires all LABA-containing medications to be labeled with a warning of an increase in severe asthma episodes associated with these agents. Some studies have reported a higher number of asthma-related deaths among patients receiving LABA therapy in addition to their usual asthma care than in patients not receiving LABAs. This notice

Table 138-13 ESTIMATED COMPARATIVE INHALED CORTICOSTEROID DOSES

DRUG	LOW DAILY DOSE PER AGE			MEDIUM DAILY DOSE PER AGE			HIGH DAILY DOSE PER AGE		
	0-4 yr	5-11 yr	≥12 yr	0-4 yr	5-11 yr	≥ 12 yr	0-4 yr	5-11 yr	≥ 12 yr
Beclomethasone HFA, 40 or 80 µg/puff	NA	80-160 µg	80-240 µg	NA	>160-320 µg	>240-480 µg	NA	>320 µg	>480 µg
Budesonide DPI 90, 180, or 200 mcg/inhalation	NA	180-400 µg	180-600 µg	NA	>400-800 µg	>600-1200 µg	NA	>800 µg	>1200 µg
Budesonide inhaled suspension for nebulization, 0.25-, 0.5-, and 1.0-mg dose	0.25-0.5 mg	0.5 mg	NA	>0.5-1.0 mg	1.0 mg	NA	>1.0 mg	2.0 mg	NA
Flunisolide, 250 mcg/puff	NA	500-750 µg	500-1000 µg	NA	1000-1250 µg	>1000-2000 µg	NA	>1250 µg	>2000 µg
Flunisolide HFA, 80 µg/puff	NA	160 µg	320 µg	NA	320 µg	>320-640 µg	NA	≥640 µg	>640 µg
Fluticasone HFA/MDI: 44, 110, or 220 µg/puff	176 µg	88-176 µg	88-264 µg	>176-352 µg	>176-352 µg	>264-440 µg	>352 µg	>352 µg	>440 µg
Fluticasone DPI, 50, 100, or 250 µg /inhalation	NA	100-200 µg	100-300 µg	NA	>200-400 µg	>300-500 µg	NA	>400 µg	>500 µg
Mometasone DPI, 220 µg/ inhalation	NA	NA	220 µg	NA	NA	440 µg	NA	NA	>440 µg
Triamcinolone acetonide, 75 µg/puff	NA	300-600 µg	300-750 µg	NA	>600-900 µg	>750-1500 µg	NA	>900 µg	>1500 µg

DPI, dry powder inhaler; HFA, hydrofluoroalkane; MDI, metered-dose inhaler; NA, not approved and no data available for this age group.
Adapted, from the National Asthma Education and Prevention Program: Expert Panel Report 3 (EPR 3): Guidelines for the diagnosis and management of asthma—summary report 2007, *J Allergy Clin Immunol* 120(Suppl):S94–S138, 2007.

Table 138-14 RISK ASSESSMENT FOR CORTICOSTEROID ADVERSE EFFECTS

	CONDITIONS	RECOMMENDATIONS
Low risk	(≤ 1 risk factor*) Low- to medium-dose ICS (see Table 138-11)	• Monitor blood pressure and weight with each physician visit • Measure height annually (stadiometry); monitor periodically for declining growth rate and pubertal developmental delay • Encourage regular physical exercise • Ensure adequate dietary calcium and vitamin D with additional supplements for daily calcium if needed • Avoid smoking and alcohol • Ensure TSH status if patient has history of thyroid abnormality
Medium risk	(if > 1 risk factor,* consider evaluating as high risk) High-dose ICS (see Table 138-11) At least 4 courses oral corticosteroid/yr	As above, plus: • Yearly ophthalmologic evaluations to monitor for cataracts or glaucoma • Baseline bone densitometry (DEXA scan) • Consider patient at increased risk for adrenal insufficiency, especially with physiologic stressors (e.g., surgery, accident, significant illness)
High risk	Chronic systemic corticosteroids (>7.5 mg daily or equivalent for >1 mo) ≥ 7 oral corticosteroid burst treatments/year Very-high-dose ICS (e.g., fluticasone propionate ≥800 µg/day)	As above, plus: • DEXA scan: if DEXA Z score ≤1.0, recommend close monitoring (every 12 mo) • Consider referral to a bone or endocrine specialist • Bone age assessment • Complete blood count • Serum calcium, phosphorus, alkaline phosphatase determinations • Urine calcium and creatinine measurements • Measurements of testosterone in males, estradiol in amenorrheic premenopausal women, vitamin D (25-OH and 1,25-OH vitamin D), parathyroid hormone, and osteocalcin • Urine telopeptides for those receiving long-term systemic or frequent oral corticosteroid treatment • Assume adrenal insufficiency for physiologic stressors (e.g., surgery, accident, significant illness)

***Risk factors for osteoporosis:** Presence of other chronic illness(es), medications (corticosteroids, anticonvulsants, heparin, diuretics), low body weight, family history of osteoporosis, significant fracture history disproportionate to trauma, recurrent falls, impaired vision, low dietary calcium and vitamin D intake, and lifestyle factors (decreased physical activity, smoking, and alcohol intake).
DEXA, dual-energy x-ray absorptiometry; ICS, inhaled corticosteroid; TSH, thyroid-stimulating hormone.

reinforces the appropriate use of LABAs in the management of asthma. Specifically, LABA products should not be initiated as first-line or sole asthma therapy without the concomitant use of an ICS, used with worsening wheezing, or used for acute control of bronchospasm. LABAs should be stopped once asthma control is achieved, and the asthma should be maintained with the use of an asthma controller agent (ICS). Fixed-dose preparations (with an ICS) are recommended to ensure compliance with these guidelines.

LEUKOTRIENE-MODIFYING AGENTS Leukotrienes are potent proinflammatory mediators that can induce bronchospasm, mucus secretion, and airways edema. Two classes of leukotriene modifiers have been developed: inhibitors of leukotriene synthesis and leukotriene receptor antagonists (LTRAs). Zileuton, the only leukotriene synthesis inhibitor, is not approved for use in children <12 yr of age. Because zileuton requires administration 4 times daily, can result in elevated liver function enzyme values in 2-4% of patients, and interacts with medications metabolized via the cytochrome P450 system, it is rarely prescribed for children with asthma.

LTRAs have bronchodilator and targeted anti-inflammatory properties and reduce exercise-, aspirin-, and allergen-induced bronchoconstriction. They are recommended as alternative treatment for mild persistent asthma and as add-on medication with ICS for moderate persistent asthma. Two LTRAs are FDA-approved for use in children: montelukast and zafirlukast. Both medications improve asthma symptoms, decrease the need for rescue β-agonist use, and improve lung function. Montelukast is FDA-approved for use in children ≥1 yr of age and is administered once daily. Zafirlukast is FDA-approved for use in children ≥5 yr of age and is administered twice daily. Although incompletely studied in children with asthma, LTRAs appear to be less effective than ICSs in patients with moderate persistent asthma. In general, ICSs improve lung function by 5-15%, whereas LTRAs improve lung function by 2-7.5%. LTRAs are not thought to have significant adverse effects, although case reports described a Churg-Strauss–like vasculitis (pulmonary infiltrates, eosinophilia, cardiomyopathy) in adults with corticosteroid-dependent asthma treated with LTRAs. It remains to be determined whether these patients have a primary eosinophilic vasculitis masquerading as asthma, which was "unmasked" as the oral corticosteroid dose was tapered, or whether the disease is a very rare adverse effect of LTRA.

NONSTEROIDAL ANTI-INFLAMMATORY AGENTS Cromolyn and nedocromil are nonsteroidal anti-inflammatory agents that can inhibit allergen-induced asthmatic responses and reduce exercise-induced bronchospasm. According to the NIH guidelines, both drugs are considered alternative anti-inflammatory drugs for children with mild persistent asthma. Although largely devoid of adverse effects, these medications must be administered frequently (2-4 times/day) and are not nearly as effective daily controller medications as ICSs and leukotriene-modifying agents. Because they inhibit exercise-induced bronchospasm, they can be used in place of SABAs, especially in children who develop unwanted adverse effects with β-agonist therapy (tremor and elevated heart rate). Cromolyn and nedocromil can also be used in addition to a SABA in a combination pretreatment for exercise-induced bronchospasm in patients who continue to experience symptoms with use of SABA pretreatment alone.

THEOPHYLLINE In addition to its bronchodilator effects, theophylline has anti-inflammatory properties as a phosphodiesterase inhibitor, although the extent of its clinical relevance has not been clearly established. When used long term, theophylline can reduce asthma symptoms and the need for rescue SABA use. Although it is considered an alternative monotherapy controller agent for older children and adults with mild persistent asthma, it is no longer considered a first-line agent for young children, in whom there is significant variability in the absorption and metabolism of different theophylline preparations, necessitating frequent dose monitoring (drug blood levels) and adjustments. Because theophylline may have some corticosteroid-sparing effects in individuals with oral corticosteroid–dependent asthma, it is still sometimes used in this group of asthmatic children. Theophylline has a narrow therapeutic window; therefore, when it is used, serum theophylline levels need to be routinely monitored, especially if the patient has a viral illness associated with a fever or is started on a medication known to delay theophylline clearance, such as a macrolide antibiotic, cimetidine, an oral antifungal agent, an oral contraceptive, a leukotriene synthesis inhibitor, or ciprofloxacin. Theophylline overdosage and elevated theophylline levels have been associated with headaches, vomiting, cardiac arrhythmias, seizures, and death.

ANTI–IMMUNOGLOBULIN E (OMALIZUMAB) Omalizumab is a humanized monoclonal antibody that binds IgE, thereby preventing its binding to the high-affinity IgE receptor and blocking IgE-mediated allergic responses and inflammation. Because it is unable to bind IgE that is already bound to high-affinity IgE receptors, the risk of anaphylaxis via direct IgE cross linking by the drug is circumvented. It is FDA-approved for patients >12 yr old with moderate to severe asthma, documented hypersensitivity to a perennial aeroallergen, and inadequate disease control with inhaled and/or oral corticosteroids. Omalizumab is given every 2-4 wk subcutaneously, the dosage based on body weight and serum IgE levels. Its clinical efficacy as an add-on therapy for patients with moderate to severe allergic asthma has been demonstrated in large clinical trials, with asthmatic patients receiving omalizumab having fewer asthma exacerbations and symptoms while able to reduce their ICS and/or oral corticosteroid doses. This agent is generally well tolerated, although local injection site reactions can occur. Hypersensitivity reactions (including anaphylaxis) and malignancies have been very rarely associated with omalizumab use. The FDA requires packaging of omalizumab to contain a black box warning of potentially serious and life-threatening anaphylactic reactions with omalizumab treatment. On the basis of reports from approximately 39,500 patients, anaphylaxis following omalizumab treatment occurred in at least 0.1% of treated people. Although most of these reactions occurred within 2 hr of omalizumab injection, there were also reports of serious delayed reactions 2-24 hr or even longer after injections. Anaphylaxis occurred after any omalizumab dose (including the first dose). Omalizumab-treated patients should be observed in the facility for an extended period after the drug is given, and medical providers who administer the injection should be prepared to manage life-threatening anaphylactic reactions. Patients who receive omalizumab should be fully informed about the signs and symptoms of anaphylaxis, their chance of development of delayed anaphylaxis following each injection and how to treat it, including the use of autoinjectable epinephrine.

Mepolizumab, an anti–interleukin-5 antibody, has been shown to improve asthma control, reduce prednisone dose and lower sputum and blood eosinophil events in adults with prednisone-dependent asthma who also had sputum eosinophils.

Quick-Reliever Medications

Quick-reliever or "rescue" medications (SABAs, inhaled anticholinergics, and short-course systemic corticosteroids) are used in the management of acute asthma symptoms (Table 138-15).

SHORT-ACTING INHALED β-AGONISTS Given their rapid onset of action, effectiveness, and 4- to 6-hr duration of action, SABAs (albuterol, levalbuterol, terbutaline, pirbuterol) are the drugs of choice for acute asthma symptoms ("rescue" medication) and for preventing exercise-induced bronchospasm. β-Agonists cause bronchodilation by inducing airway smooth muscle relaxation, reducing vascular permeability and airways edema, and improving mucociliary clearance. Levalbuterol, or the R-isomer of albuterol, is associated with less tachycardia and tremor, which can be bothersome to some asthmatic patients. Overuse of β-agonists is associated with an increased risk of death or near-death episodes from asthma. This is a major concern for some patients with asthma who rely on the frequent use of SABAs as a "quick fix" for their asthma, rather than using controller medications in a preventive manner. It is helpful to monitor the frequency of SABA use, in that use of at least 1 MDI/mo or at least 3 MDIs/year (200 inhalations/MDI) indicates inadequate asthma control and necessitates improving other aspects of asthma therapy and management.

ANTICHOLINERGIC AGENTS As bronchodilators, the anticholinergic agents (ipratropium bromide) are much less potent than the β-agonists. Inhaled ipratropium is used primarily in the treatment of acute severe asthma. When used in combination with albuterol, ipratropium can improve lung function and reduce the rate of hospitalization in children who present to the emergency department with acute asthma. Ipratropium is the anticholinergic formulation of choice for children because it has few central nervous system adverse effects and it is available in both MDI and nebulizer formulations. Although widely used in children with asthma exacerbations of all ages, it is approved by the FDA for use in children >12 yr of age.

Delivery Devices and Inhalation Technique

Inhaled medications are delivered in aerosolized form in a metered-dose inhaler, as a dry powder inhaler formulation, or in a suspension or solution form delivered via a nebulizer. In the past, MDIs, which require coordination and use of a spacer

TABLE 138-15 MANAGEMENT OF ASTHMA EXACERBATION (STATUS ASTHMATICUS)

RISK ASSESSMENT ON ADMISSION		
Focused history	• Onset of current exacerbation • Frequency and severity of daytime and nighttime symptoms and activity limitation • Frequency of rescue bronchodilator use • Current medications and allergies • Potential triggers • History of systemic steroid courses, emergency department visits, hospitalization, intubation, or life-threatening episodes	
Clinical assessment	• Physical examination findings: vital signs, breathlessness, air movement, use of accessory muscles, retractions, anxiety level, alteration in mental status • Pulse oximetry • Lung function (defer in patients with moderate to severe distress or history of labile disease)	
Risk factors for asthma morbidity and death	See Table 138-16	
TREATMENT		
DRUG AND TRADE NAME	**MECHANISMS OF ACTION AND DOSING**	**CAUTIONS AND ADVERSE EFFECTS**
Oxygen (mask or nasal cannula)	Treats hypoxia	• Monitor pulse oximetry to maintain O_2 saturation >92% • Cardiorespiratory monitoring
Inhaled short-acting β-agonists:	Bronchodilator	• During exacerbations, frequent or continuous doses can cause pulmonary vasodilation, $\dot{V}/\dot{Q}$ mismatch, and hypoxemia • Adverse effects: palpitations, tachycardia, arrhythmias, tremor, hypoxemia
Albuterol nebulizer solution (5 mg/mL concentrate; 2.5 mg/3 mL, 1.25 mg/3 mL, 0.63 mg/3 mL)	Nebulizer: 0.15 mg/kg (minimum: 2.5 mg) as often as every 20 min for 3 doses as needed, then 0.15-0.3 mg/kg up to 10 mg every 1-4 hr as needed, or up to 0.5 mg/kg/hr by continuous nebulization	• Nebulizer: when giving concentrated forms, dilute with saline to 3 mL total nebulized volume
Albuterol MDI (90 μg/puff)	2-8 puffs up to every 20 min for 3 doses as needed, then every 1-4 hr as needed	• For MDI: use spacer/holding chamber
Levalbuterol (Xopenex) nebulizer solution (1.25 mg/0.5 mL concentrate; 0.31 mg/3 mL, 0.63 mg/3mL, 1.25 mg/3 mL)	0.075 mg/kg (minimum: 1.25 mg) every 20 min for 3 doses, then 0.075-0.15 mg/kg up to 5 mg every 1-4 hr as needed, or 0.25 mg/kg/hr by continuous nebulization	• Levalbuterol 0.63 mg is equivalent to 1.25 mg of standard albuterol for both efficacy and side effects
Systemic corticosteroids:	Anti-inflammatory	• If patient has been exposed to chickenpox or measles, consider passive immunoglobulin prophylaxis; also, risk of complications with herpes simplex and tuberculosis • For daily dosing, 8 AM administration minimizes adrenal suppression • Children may benefit from dosage tapering if course exceeds 7 days • Adverse effects monitoring: Frequent therapy bursts risk numerous corticosteroid adverse effects (Chapter 571); see Table 138-14 for adverse effects screening recommendations
Prednisone: 1-, 2.5-, 5-, 10-, 20-, 50-mg tablets Methylprednisolone (Medrol): 2-, 4-, 8-, 16-, 24-, 32-mg tablets Prednisolone: 5-mg tablets; 5 mg/5 mL and 15 mg/5 mL solution	0.5-1 mg/kg every 6-12 hr for 48 hr, then 1-2 mg/kg/day bid (maximum: 60 mg/day)	
Depo-Medrol (IM); Solu-Medrol (IV)	Short-course "burst" for exacerbation: 1-2 mg/kg/day qd or bid for 3-7 days	
Anticholinergics:	Mucolytic/bronchodilator	• Should not be used as first-line therapy; added to β_2-agonist therapy
Ipratropium: Atrovent (nebulizer solution 0.5 mg/2.5 mL; MDI 18 μg/inhalation)	Nebulizer: 0.5 mg q6-8h (tid-qid) as needed MDI: 2 puffs qid	
Ipratropium with albuterol: DuoNeb nebulizer solution (0.5 mg ipratropium + 2.5 mg albuterol/3-mL vial)	1 vial by nebulizer qid	• Nebulizer: may mix ipratropium with albuterol

Continued

TABLE 138-15 MANAGEMENT OF ASTHMA EXACERBATION (STATUS ASTHMATICUS)—cont'd

DRUG AND TRADE NAME	MECHANISMS OF ACTION AND DOSING	CAUTIONS AND ADVERSE EFFECTS
Injectable sympathomimetic epinephrine:	Bronchodilator	• For extreme circumstances (e.g., impending respiratory failure despite high-dose inhaled SABA, respiratory failure)
Adrenalin 1 mg/mL (1 : 1000) EpiPen autoinjection device (0.3 mg; EpiPen Jr 0.15 mg)	SC or IM: 0.01 mg/kg (max dose 0.5 mg); may repeat after 15-30 min	
Terbutaline:		• Terbutaline is β-agonist–selective relative to epinephrine • Monitoring with continuous infusion: cardiorespiratory monitor, pulse oximetry, blood pressure, serum potassium • Adverse effects: tremor, tachycardia, palpitations, arrhythmia, hypertension, headaches, nervousness, nausea, vomiting, hypoxemia
Brethine 1 mg/mL	Continuous IV infusion (terbutaline only): 2-10 μg/kg loading dose, followed by 0.1-0.4 μg/kg/min Titrate in 0.1-0.2 μg/kg/min increments every 30 min, depending on clinical response	
RISK ASSESSMENT FOR DISCHARGE		
Medical stability	Discharge to home if there has been sustained improvement in symptoms and bronchodilator treatments are at least 3 hr apart, physical findings are normal, PEF >70% of predicted or personal best, and oxygen saturation >92% when breathing room air	
Home supervision	Capability to administer intervention and to observe and respond appropriately to clinical deterioration	
Asthma education	See Table 138-9	

IM, intramuscular; MDI, metered-dose inhaler; PEF, peak expiratory flow; SABA, short-acting β-agonist; SC, subcutaneous; $\dot{V}/\dot{Q}$, ventilation-perfusion.

device, have dominated the market. MDIs are now using hydrofluoroalkane propellant for its ozone-friendly properties, rather than chlorofluorocarbon. Spacer devices, recommended for the administration of all MDI medications, are simple and inexpensive tools that: (1) decrease the coordination required to use MDIs, especially in young children; (2) improve the delivery of inhaled drug to the lower airways; and (3) minimize the risk of propellant-mediated adverse effects (thrush). Optimal inhalation technique for each puff of MDI-delivered medication is a slow (5-sec) inhalation, then a 5- to 10-sec breath-hold. No waiting time between puffs of medication is needed. Young, preschool-aged children cannot perform this inhalation technique. MDI medications can also be delivered with a spacer and mask, using a different technique: Each puff is administered with regular breathing for about 30 sec or 5-10 breaths, a tight seal must be maintained, and talking, coughing, or crying will blow the medication out of the spacer. This technique will not deliver as much medication per puff as the optimal MDI technique used by older children and adults.

DPI devices (e.g. Diskus, Flexhaler Autohaler, Twisthaler, Aerolizer) are popular because of their simplicity of use, albeit adequate inspiratory flow is needed. They are breath-actuated (the drug comes out only as it is breathed in) and spacers are not needed. Mouth rinsing is recommended after ICS use to rinse out ICS deposited on the oral mucosa and reduce the swallowed ICS and the risk of thrush.

Nebulizers have been the mainstay of aerosol treatment for infants and young children. An advantage of using nebulizers is the simple technique required of relaxed breathing. The preferential nasal breathing, small airways, low tidal volume, and high respiratory rate of infants markedly increase the difficulty of inhaled drug therapy targeting the lung airways. Disadvantages of nebulizers include need for a power source, inconvenience in that treatments take about 5 min, expense, and potential for bacterial contamination.

Asthma Exacerbations and Their Management

Asthma exacerbations are acute or subacute episodes of progressively worsening symptoms and airflow obstruction. Airflow obstruction during exacerbations can become extensive, resulting in life-threatening respiratory insufficiency. Often, asthma exacerbations worsen during sleep (between midnight and 8 AM), when airways inflammation and hyperresponsiveness are at their peak. Importantly, SABAs, which are first-line therapy for asthma symptoms and exacerbations, increase pulmonary blood flow through obstructed, unoxygenated areas of the lungs with increasing dosage and frequency. When airways obstruction is not resolved with SABA use, ventilation-perfusion mismatching can cause significant hypoxemia, which can perpetuate bronchoconstriction and further worsen the condition. Severe, progressive asthma exacerbations need to be managed in a medical setting, with administration of supplemental oxygen as first-line therapy and close monitoring for potential worsening. Complications that can occur during severe exacerbations include atelectasis and air leaks in the chest (pneumomediastinum, pneumothorax).

A severe exacerbation of asthma that does not improve with standard therapy is termed **status asthmaticus.** Immediate management of an asthma exacerbation involves a rapid evaluation of the severity of obstruction and assessment of risk for further clinical deterioration (see Tables 138-14 and 138-15). For most patients, exacerbations improve with frequent bronchodilator treatments and a course of systemic (oral or intravenous) corticosteroid. However, the optimal management of a child with an asthma exacerbation should include a more comprehensive assessment of the events leading up to the exacerbation and the underlying disease severity. Indeed, the frequency and severity of asthma exacerbations help define the severity of a patient's asthma. Whereas most children who experience life-threatening asthma episodes have moderate to severe asthma by other criteria, some children with asthma appear to have mild disease

Table 138-16 RISK FACTORS FOR ASTHMA MORBIDITY AND MORTALITY

BIOLOGIC
Previous severe asthma exacerbation (intensive care unit admission, intubation for asthma)
Sudden asphyxic episodes (respiratory failure, arrest)
Two or more hospitalizations for asthma in past year
Three or more emergency department visits for asthma in past year
Increasing and large diurnal variation in peak flows
Use of >2 canisters of short-acting β-agonists per month
Poor response to systemic corticosteroid therapy
Male gender
Low birthweight
Nonwhite (especially black) ethnicity
Sensitivity to *Alternaria*
ENVIRONMENTAL
Allergen exposure
Environmental tobacco smoke exposure
Air pollution exposure
Urban environment
ECONOMIC AND PSYCHOSOCIAL
Poverty
Crowding
Mother <20 yr old
Mother with less than high school education
Inadequate medical care:
Inaccessible
Unaffordable
No regular medical care (only emergency)
Lack of written asthma action plan
No care sought for chronic asthma symptoms
Delay in care of asthma exacerbations
Inadequate hospital care for asthma exacerbation
Psychopathology in the parent or child
Poor perception of asthma symptoms or severity
Alcohol or substance abuse

except when they suffer severe, even near-fatal exacerbations. The biologic, environmental, economic, and psychosocial risk factors associated with asthma morbidity and death can further guide this assessment (Table 138-16).

Asthma exacerbations characteristically vary among individuals but tend to be similar in the same patient. Severe asthma exacerbations, resulting in respiratory distress, hypoxia, hospitalization, and/or respiratory failure, are the best predictors of future life-threatening exacerbations or a fatal asthma episode. In addition to distinguishing such high-risk children, some experience exacerbations that come on over days, with airflow obstruction resulting from progressive inflammation, epithelial sloughing, and cast impaction of small airways. When such a process is extreme, respiratory failure due to fatigue can ensue, necessitating mechanical ventilation for numerous days. In contrast, some children experience abrupt-onset exacerbations that may result from extreme AHR and physiologic susceptibility to airways closure. Such exacerbations, when extreme, are asphyxial in nature, often occur outside medical settings, are initially associated with very high arterial P_{CO_2} levels, and tend to require only brief periods of supportive ventilation. Recognizing the characteristic differences in asthma exacerbations is important for optimizing their early management.

Home Management of Asthma Exacerbations

Families of all children with asthma should have a **written action plan** to guide their recognition and management of exacerbations, along with the necessary medications and tools to manage them. Early recognition of asthma exacerbations in order to intensify treatment early can often prevent further worsening and keep exacerbations from becoming severe. A written home action plan can reduce the risk of asthma death by 70%. The NIH guidelines recommend immediate treatment with "rescue" medication (inhaled SABA, up to 3 treatments in 1 hr). A good response is characterized by resolution of symptoms within 1hr, no further symptoms over the next 4 hr, and improvement in PEF value to at least 80% of personal best. The child's physician should be contacted for follow-up, especially if bronchodilators are required repeatedly over the next 24-48 hr. If the child has an incomplete response to initial treatment with rescue medication (persistent symptoms and/or a PEF value < 80% of personal best), a short course of oral corticosteroid therapy (prednisone 1-2 mg/kg/day [not to exceed 60 mg/day] for 4 days) in addition to inhaled β-agonist therapy should be instituted. The physician should also be contacted for further instructions. Immediate medical attention should be sought for severe exacerbations, persistent signs of respiratory distress, lack of expected response or sustained improvement after initial treatment, further deterioration, or high-risk factors for asthma morbidity or mortality (previous history of severe exacerbations). For patients with severe asthma and/or a history of life-threatening episodes, especially if abrupt-onset in nature, providing an injectable form of epinephrine (EpiPen) and, possibly, portable oxygen at home should be considered. Use of either of these extreme measures for home management of asthma exacerbations would be an indication to call 911 for emergency support services.

Emergency Department Management of Asthma Exacerbations

In the emergency department, the primary goals of asthma management include correction of hypoxemia, rapid improvement of airflow obstruction, and prevention of progression or recurrence of symptoms. Interventions are based on clinical severity on arrival, response to initial therapy, and presence of risk factors that are associated with asthma morbidity and mortality (see Table 138-16). Indications of a severe exacerbation include breathlessness, dyspnea, retractions, accessory muscle use, tachypnea or labored breathing, cyanosis, mental status changes, a silent chest with poor air exchange, and severe airflow limitation (PEF or FEV_1 value <50% of personal best or predicted values). Initial treatment includes supplemental oxygen, inhaled β-agonist therapy every 20 min for 1 hr, and, if necessary, systemic corticosteroids given either orally or intravenously (see Table 138-15). Inhaled ipratropium may be added to the β-agonist treatment if no significant response is seen with the 1st inhaled β-agonist treatment. An intramuscular injection of epinephrine or other β-agonist may be administered in severe cases. Oxygen should be administered and continued for at least 20 min after SABA administration to compensate for possible ventilation-perfusion abnormalities caused by SABAs.

Close monitoring of clinical status, hydration, and oxygenation are essential elements of immediate management. A poor response to intensified treatment in the 1st hour suggests that the exacerbation will not remit quickly. The patient may be discharged to home if there is sustained improvement in symptoms, normal physical findings, PEF >70% of predicted or personal best, an oxygen saturation >92% while the patient is breathing room air for 4 hr. Discharge medications include administration of an inhaled β-agonist up to every 3-4 hr plus a 3-to 7-day course of an oral corticosteroid. Optimizing controller therapy before discharge is also recommended. The addition of ICS to a course of oral corticosteroid in the emergency department setting reduces the risk of exacerbation recurrence over the subsequent month.

Hospital Management of Asthma Exacerbations

For patients with moderate to severe exacerbations that do not adequately improve within 1-2 hr of intensive treatment, observation and/or admission to the hospital, at least overnight, is likely to be needed. Other indications for hospital admission include high-risk features for asthma morbidity or death (see Table 138-16). Admission to an intensive care unit is indicated for patients with severe respiratory distress, poor response to therapy, and concern for potential respiratory failure and arrest.

Supplemental oxygen, frequent or continuous administration of an inhaled bronchodilator, and systemic corticosteroid therapy are the conventional interventions for children admitted to the hospital for status asthmaticus (see Table 138-15). Supplemental oxygen is administered because many children hospitalized with acute asthma have or eventually have hypoxemia, especially at night and with increasing SABA administration. SABAs can be delivered frequently (every 20 min to 1 hr) or continuously (at 5-15 mg/hr). When administered continuously, significant systemic absorption of β-agonist occurs and, as a result, continuous nebulization can obviate the need for intravenous β-agonist therapy. Adverse effects of frequently administered β-agonist therapy include tremor, irritability, tachycardia, and hypokalemia. Patients requiring frequent or continuous nebulized β-agonist therapy should have ongoing cardiac monitoring. Because frequent β-agonist therapy can cause ventilation-perfusion mismatch and hypoxemia, oximetry is also indicated. Inhaled ipratropium bromide is often added to albuterol every 6 hr if patients do not show a remarkable improvement, although there is little evidence to support its use in hospitalized children receiving aggressive inhaled β-agonist therapy and systemic corticosteroids. In addition to its potential to provide a synergistic effect with a β-agonist agent in relieving severe bronchospasm, ipratropium bromide may be beneficial in patients who have mucous hypersecretion or are receiving β-blockers.

Short-course systemic corticosteroid therapy is recommended for use in moderate to severe asthma exacerbations to hasten recovery and prevent recurrence of symptoms. Corticosteroids are effective as single doses administered in the emergency department, short courses in the clinic setting, and both oral and intravenous formulations in hospitalized children. Studies in children hospitalized with acute asthma have found corticosteroids administered orally to be as effective as intravenous corticosteroids. Accordingly, oral corticosteroid therapy can often be used, although children with sustained respiratory distress who are unable to tolerate oral preparations or liquids are obvious candidates for intravenous corticosteroid therapy.

Patients with persistent severe dyspnea and high-flow oxygen requirements require additional evaluations, such as complete blood cell counts, measurements of arterial blood gases and serum electrolytes, and chest radiograph, to monitor for respiratory insufficiency, co-morbidities, infection, and/or dehydration. Hydration status monitoring is especially important in infants and young children, whose increased respiratory rate (insensible losses) and decreased oral intake put them at higher risk for dehydration. Further complicating this situation is the association of increased antidiuretic hormone (ADH) secretion with status asthmaticus. Administration of fluids at or slightly below maintenance fluid requirements is recommended. Chest physical therapy, incentive spirometry, and mucolytics are **not** recommended during the early acute period of asthma exacerbations as they can trigger severe bronchoconstriction.

Despite intensive therapy, some asthmatic children remain critically ill and at risk for respiratory failure, intubation, and mechanical ventilation. Complications (air leaks) related to asthma exacerbations increase with intubation and assisted ventilation; every effort should be made to relieve bronchospasm and prevent respiratory failure. Several therapies, including parenterally administered epinephrine, β-agonists, methylxanthines, magnesium sulfate (25-75 mg/kg, maximum dose 2.5 g, given intravenously over 20 min), and inhaled heliox have demonstrated some benefit as adjunctive therapies in patients with severe status asthmaticus. Administration of either methylxanthine or magnesium sulfate requires monitoring of serum levels and cardiovascular status. Parenteral (subcutaneous, intramuscular, or intravenous) epinephrine or terbutaline sulfate may be effective in patients with life-threatening obstruction that is not responding to high doses of inhaled β-agonists, because in such patients, inhaled medication may not reach the lower airway.

Rarely, a severe asthma exacerbation in a child results in respiratory failure, and intubation and mechanical ventilation become necessary. Mechanical ventilation in severe asthma exacerbations requires the careful balance of enough pressure to overcome airways obstruction while reducing hyperinflation, air trapping, and the likelihood of barotrauma (pneumothorax, pneumomediastinum) (Chapter 65.1). To minimize the likelihood of such complications, mechanical ventilation should be anticipated, and asthmatic children at risk for the development of respiratory failure should be managed in a pediatric intensive care unit (ICU). Elective tracheal intubation with rapid-induction sedatives and paralytic agents is safer than emergency intubation. Mechanical ventilation aims to achieve adequate oxygenation while tolerating mild to moderate hypercapnia (P_{CO_2} 50-70 mm Hg) to minimize barotrauma. Volume-cycled ventilators, using short inspiratory and long expiratory times, 10-15 mL/kg tidal volume, 8-15 breaths/min, peak pressures < 60 cm H_2O, and without positive end-expiratory pressure are starting mechanical ventilation parameters that can achieve these goals. As measures to relieve mucous plugs, chest percussion and airways lavage are not recommended because they can induce further bronchospasm. One must consider the nature of asthma exacerbations leading to respiratory failure; those of rapid or abrupt onset tend to resolve quickly (hours to 2 days), whereas those that progress gradually to respiratory failure can require days to weeks of mechanical ventilation. Such prolonged cases are further complicated by muscle atrophy and, when combined with corticosteroid-induced myopathy, can lead to severe muscle weakness requiring prolonged rehabilitation. This myopathy should not be confused with the rare occurrence of an asthma-associated flaccid paralysis (Hopkins syndrome), which is of unknown etiology but prolongs the intensive care stay.

In children, management of severe exacerbations in medical centers is usually successful, even when extreme measures are required. Consequently, asthma deaths in children rarely occur in medical centers; most occur at home or in community settings before lifesaving medical care can be administered. This point highlights the importance of home and community management of asthma exacerbations, early intervention measures to keep exacerbations from becoming severe, and steps to reduce asthma severity. A follow-up appointment within 1 to 2 wk of a child's discharge from the hospital after resolution of an asthma exacerbation should be used to monitor clinical improvement and to reinforce key educational elements, including action plans and controller medications.

SPECIAL MANAGEMENT CIRCUMSTANCES

Management of Infants and Young Children Recurrent wheezing episodes in preschool-aged children are very common, occurring in as much as one third of this population. Of them, most improve and even become asymptomatic during the prepubescent school-age years, whereas others have lifelong persistent asthma. All require management of their recurrent wheezing problems (see Tables 138-5, 138-6, and 138-11). The updated NIH guidelines recommend risk assessment to identify preschool-aged children who are likely to have persistent asthma. One implication of this recommendation is that these at-risk children may be candidates for conventional asthma management, including daily controller therapy and early intervention with exacerbations (see Tables 138-7, 138-8, and 138-11). Nebulized budesonide and montelukast appear to be more effective than cromolyn. For young children with a history of moderate to severe exacerbations, nebulized budesonide is FDA-approved, and its use as a controller medication could prevent subsequent exacerbations.

Using aerosol therapy in infants and young children with asthma presents unique challenges. There are 2 delivery systems for inhaled medications for this age group, the nebulizer and the MDI with spacer/holding chamber and face mask. Multiple studies have demonstrated the effectiveness of both nebulized albuterol in acute episodes and nebulized budesonide in the treatment of recurrent wheezing in infants and young children. In such young children, inhaled medications administered via MDI with spacer and face mask may be acceptable, although perhaps not preferred owing to limited published information and lack of FDA approval for children <4yr of age.

Asthma Management in Pregnancy Asthma management in pregnancy essentially follows the NIH clinical practice guidelines. The goals of asthma management during pregnancy should include prevention of exacerbations and control of chronic symptoms through the use of medications that pose minimal risk to the mother and fetus because most drugs cross the placenta. It is considered safer for pregnant asthmatic women to be treated with controller medications than it is to have uncontrolled symptoms and severe exacerbations. Albuterol is the preferred SABA for use during pregnancy. There is reassuring efficacy and safety data from prospective cohort studies supporting ICS use in pregnant women with asthma. Budesonide is currently the preferred ICS for pregnant women, attaining an FDA Pregnancy Category B rating because of substantial reassuring safety data. Nonmedication approaches to improve asthma control are encouraged. A multidisciplinary approach with monthly evaluations (including pulmonary function tests when not contraindicated) and ongoing consultation with the obstetrician and asthma specialist is recommended. Frequent fetal and maternal surveillance is especially important for adolescents with suboptimal asthma control, those with moderate to severe asthma, and those with a recent exacerbation.

Asthma Management During Surgery Patients with asthma are at risk from disease-related complications from surgery, such as bronchoconstriction and asthma exacerbation, atelectasis, impaired coughing, respiratory infection, and latex exposure, that may induce asthma complications in patients with latex allergy. All patients with asthma should be evaluated before surgery, and those who are inadequately controlled should allow time for intensified treatment in order to improve asthma stability before surgery if possible. A systemic corticosteroid course may be indicated for the patient who is having symptoms and/or FEV_1 or PEF values <80% of the patient's personal best. In addition, patients who have received >2 wk of systemic corticosteroid and/or moderate- to high-dose ICS therapy may be at risk for intraoperative adrenal insufficiency. For these patients, anesthesia services should be alerted to provide "stress" replacement doses of systemic corticosteroid for the surgical procedure and possibly the postoperative period if needed.

PROGNOSIS

Recurrent coughing and wheezing occurs in 35% of preschool-aged children. Of these, approximately one third continue to have persistent asthma into later childhood, and approximately two thirds improve on their own through their teen years. Asthma severity by the ages of 7-10 yr of age is predictive of asthma persistence in adulthood. Children with moderate to severe asthma and with lower lung function measures are likely to have persistent asthma as adults. Children with milder asthma and normal lung function are likely to improve over time, with some becoming periodically asthmatic (disease-free for months to years); however, complete remission for 5 yr in childhood is uncommon.

PREVENTION

Although chronic airways inflammation may result in pathologic remodeling of lung airways, conventional anti-inflammatory interventions—the cornerstone of asthma control—do not help children "outgrow" their asthma. Although controller medications reduce asthma morbidities, most children with moderate to severe asthma continue to have symptoms into young adulthood. Investigations into the environmental and lifestyle factors responsible for the lower prevalence of childhood asthma in rural areas and farming communities suggest that early immunomodulatory intervention might prevent asthma development. A "hygiene hypothesis" purports that naturally occurring microbial exposures in early life might drive early immune development away from allergic sensitization, persistent airways inflammation, and remodeling. If these natural microbial exposures truly have an asthma-protective effect, without significant adverse health consequences, then these findings may foster new strategies for asthma prevention.

Several nonpharmacotherapeutic measures with numerous positive health attributes—avoidance of environmental tobacco smoke (beginning prenatally), prolonged breastfeeding (>4 mo), an active lifestyle, and a healthy diet—might reduce the likelihood of asthma development. Immunizations are currently not considered to increase the likelihood of development of asthma; therefore, all standard childhood immunizations are recommended for children with asthma, including varicella and annual influenza vaccines.

BIBLIOGRAPHY

Please visit the Nelson Textbook of Pediatrics *website at* *www.expertconsult.com* *for the complete bibliography.*

Chapter 139
Atopic Dermatitis (Atopic Eczema)

Donald Y.M. Leung

Atopic dermatitis (AD), or eczema, is the most common chronic relapsing skin disease seen in infancy and childhood. It affects 10-30% of children worldwide and frequently occurs in families with other atopic diseases, such as asthma, allergic rhinitis, and food allergy. Infants with AD are predisposed to development of allergic rhinitis and/or asthma later in childhood, a process called "the atopic march."

ETIOLOGY

AD is a complex genetic disorder that results in a defective skin barrier, reduced skin innate immune responses, and exaggerated T-cell responses to environmental allergens and microbes that lead to chronic skin inflammation.

PATHOLOGY

Acute AD skin lesions are characterized by **spongiosis,** or marked intercellular edema, of the epidermis. In AD, dendritic antigen-presenting cells (APCs) in the epidermis, such as Langerhans cells (LCs), exhibit surface-bound immunoglobulin (Ig) E molecules. These APCs play an important role in cutaneous allergen presentation to T helper type 2 (Th2) cells (Chapter 134). There is a marked perivenular T-cell infiltrate with occasional monocyte-macrophages in acute AD lesions. Mast cells are found in normal numbers but in different stages of degranulation. Chronic, lichenified AD is characterized by a hyperplastic epidermis with hyperkeratosis, and minimal spongiosis. There are predominantly IgE-bearing LCs in the epidermis, and macrophages in the dermal mononuclear cell infiltrate. Mast cell and eosinophil numbers are increased. Eosinophils contribute to allergic inflammation by secreting cytokines and mediators that augment inflammatory responses and induce tissue injury in AD through the production of reactive oxygen intermediates and release of toxic granule proteins.

PATHOGENESIS

Two forms of AD have been identified. **Atopic eczema** is associated with IgE-mediated sensitization (at onset or during the course of eczema) and occurs in 70-80% of patients with AD. **Nonatopic eczema** is not associated with IgE-mediated sensitization and is seen in 20-30% of patients with AD. Both forms of AD are associated with eosinophilia. In atopic eczema, circulating T cells expressing the skin homing receptor **cutaneous lymphocyte-associated antigen** (CLA) produce increased levels of Th2 cytokines, including interleukin-4 (IL-4) and IL-13, which induce isotype switching to IgE synthesis. Another cytokine, IL-5, plays an important role in eosinophil development and survival. These CLA+ T cells also produce abnormally low levels of interferon-γ (IFN-γ), a Th1 cytokine known to inhibit Th2 cell function. Nonatopic eczema is associated with lower IL-4 and IL-13 production than is atopic eczema. Another Th2 cytokine, IL-31, induces marked pruritus in experimental animals.

Compared with the skin of healthy subjects, both unaffected skin and acute skin lesions of patients with AD have an increased number of cells expressing IL-4 and IL-13; however, acute AD does not involve significant numbers of cells that express IFN-γ or IL-12. Chronic AD skin lesions, by contrast, have significantly fewer cells that express IL-4 and IL-13 but increased numbers of cells that express IL-5, granulocyte-macrophage colony-stimulating factor (GM-CSF), IL-12, and IFN-γ than acute AD lesions. Thus, chronic AD, unlike acute AD, is characterized by a shift from a Th2-dominant to a Th1-dominant profile. The increased expression of IL-12 in eosinophils, inflammatory dendritic epidermal cells, and macrophages in chronic AD skin lesions may play a role in initiating this switch to Th1 cell development. Persistent skin inflammation may be associated with a relative lack of T-regulatory cells in the skin of AD subjects and increased expression of IL-17.

The development of AD skin lesions is orchestrated by local tissue expression of proinflammatory cytokines and chemokines. Cytokines, such as tumor necrosis factor-α (TNF-α) and IL-1 from keratinocytes, mast cells, and dendritic cells, bind to receptors on vascular endothelium. The ligand-receptor pair activates cellular signaling, including the NF-κB pathway, and induces expression of vascular endothelial cell adhesion molecules (VCAM). These events proceed from tethering, activation, and adhesion to the endothelium, followed by extravasation of inflammatory cells. Once the inflammatory cells infiltrate the tissue, they respond to chemotactic gradients established by chemokines, which are released at sites of injury or infection. Chemokines play a central role in defining the nature of the inflammatory infiltrate in AD. The chemotactic protein, CCL27, is highly upregulated in AD and preferentially attracts CLA+ T cells to the skin. Other C-C chemokines, RANTES ("regulated on activation, normal T expressed and secreted"), monocyte chemotactic protein-4 (MCP-4), and eotaxin are increased in AD skin lesions, resulting in chemotaxis of eosinophils, macrophages, and Th2 lymphocytes expressing their receptor (CCR3). Selective recruitment of CCR4-expressing Th2 cells into skin affected by AD may also be mediated by macrophage-derived chemokine (MDC) and TARC (expand), which are increased in AD. Elevated IL-5 and GM-CSF in chronic AD may lead to enhanced survival of eosinophils and monocyte-macrophages as well as LCs.

Research has identified the mechanisms leading to barrier dysfunction in AD. In healthy people, the skin acts as a protective barrier against external irritants, moisture loss, and infection. Proper function of the skin depends on adequate moisture and lipid content, functional immune responses, and structural integrity. Severely dry skin is a hallmark of AD. This is a result of compromise of the physical and chemical structures of the epidermal barrier, which leads to excess transepidermal water loss. Filaggrin, a component of the cytoskeleton, and its breakdown products are critical to skin barrier function. Genetic mutations in the filaggrin gene family have been identified in up to 50% of severe patients with AD. Such patients have increased risk of bacterial, viral, and fungal infection related to impairment of innate immunity, including a loss of barrier function and impaired generation of antimicrobial peptides.

CLINICAL MANIFESTATIONS

AD typically begins in infancy. Approximately 50% of patients experience symptoms in the 1st year of life, and an additional 30% are diagnosed between 1 and 5 yr of age. Intense **pruritus**, especially at night, and **cutaneous reactivity** are the cardinal features of AD. Scratching and excoriation cause increased skin inflammation that contributes to the development of more pronounced eczematous skin lesions. Foods (cow milk, egg, peanut, tree nuts, soy, wheat, fish, shellfish), inhalant allergens, bacterial infection, reduced humidity, excessive sweating, and irritants (wool, acrylic, soaps, toiletries, fragrances, detergents) can exacerbate (trigger) pruritus and scratching.

Acute AD skin lesions are intensely pruritic with erythematous papules (Figs. 139-1 and 139-2). Subacute dermatitis manifests as erythematous, excoriated, scaling papules. In contrast, chronic AD is characterized by **lichenification** (Fig. 139-3), or thickening of the skin with accentuated surface markings, and **fibrotic papules (prurigo nodularis)**. In chronic AD, all three types of skin reactions may coexist in the same individual. Most patients with AD have dry, lackluster skin irrespective of their stage of illness. Skin reaction pattern and distribution vary with the patient's age and disease activity. AD is generally more acute in infancy and involves the face, scalp, and extensor surfaces of the extremities. The diaper area is usually spared. Older children and children with chronic AD have lichenification and localization of the rash to the flexural folds of the extremities. AD often goes into remission as the patient grows older, leaving an adolescent or adult with skin prone to itching and inflammation when exposed to exogenous irritants.

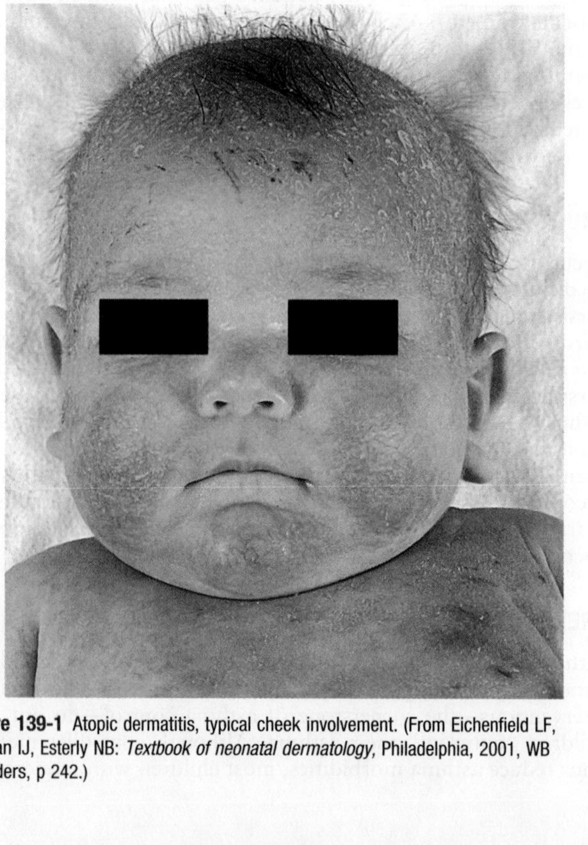

Figure 139-1 Atopic dermatitis, typical cheek involvement. (From Eichenfield LF, Friedan IJ, Esterly NB: *Textbook of neonatal dermatology*, Philadelphia, 2001, WB Saunders, p 242.)

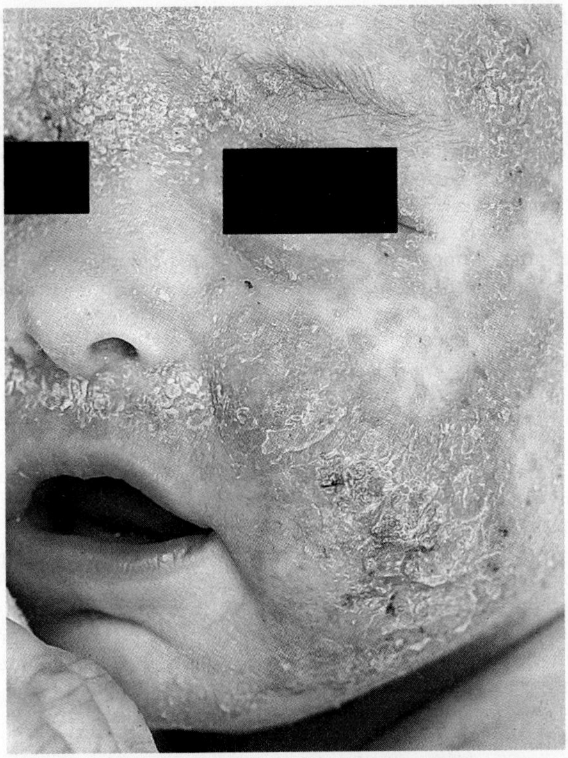

Figure 139-2 Crusted lesions of atopic dermatitis on the face. (From Eichenfield LF, Friedan IJ, Esterly NB: *Textbook of neonatal dermatology,* Philadelphia, 2001, WB Saunders, p 242.)

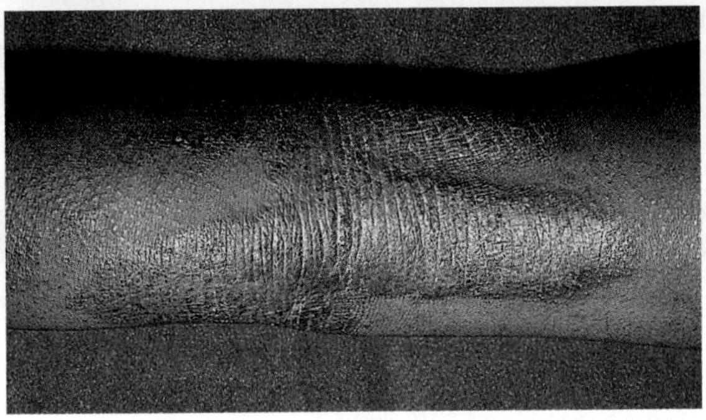

Figure 139-3 Lichenification of the popliteal fossa from chronic rubbing of the skin in atopic dermatitis. (From Weston WL, Lane AT, Morelli JG: *Color textbook of pediatric dermatology,* ed 2, St Louis, 1996, Mosby, p 33.)

LABORATORY FINDINGS

There are no specific laboratory tests to diagnose AD. Many patients have peripheral blood eosinophilia and increased serum IgE levels. Serum IgE measurement or prick skin testing can identify the allergens to which patients are sensitized. The diagnosis of clinical allergy to these allergens requires confirmation by history and environmental challenges.

DIAGNOSIS AND DIFFERENTIAL DIAGNOSIS

AD is diagnosed on the basis of 3 major features: pruritus, an eczematous dermatitis that fits into a typical presentation, and a chronic or chronically relapsing course (Table 139-1). Associated features, such as a family history of asthma, hay fever, elevated IgE, and immediate skin test reactivity, are variably present.

Many inflammatory skin diseases, immunodeficiencies, skin malignancies, genetic disorders, infectious diseases, and infestations share symptoms with AD and should be considered and excluded before a diagnosis of AD is established (Table 139-2). Severe combined immunodeficiency syndrome (Chapter 120.1) should be considered for infants presenting in the 1st year of life with diarrhea, failure to thrive, generalized scaling rash, and recurrent cutaneous and/or systemic infection. Histiocytosis (Chapter 501) should be excluded in any infant with AD and

Table 139-1 CLINICAL FEATURES OF ATOPIC DERMATITIS

MAJOR FEATURES
Pruritus
Facial and extensor eczema in infants and children
Flexural eczema in adolescents
Chronic or relapsing dermatitis
Personal or family history of atopic disease
ASSOCIATED FEATURES
Xerosis
Cutaneous infections (*Staphylococcus aureus,* group A streptococcus, herpes simplex, vaccinia, molluscum, warts)
Nonspecific dermatitis of the hands or feet
Ichthyosis, palmar hyperlinearity, keratosis pilaris
Nipple eczema
White dermatographism and delayed blanch response
Anterior subcapsular cataracts, keratoconus
Elevated serum immunoglobulin E levels
Positive results of immediate-type allergy skin tests
Early age at onset
Dennie lines (Dennie-Morgan infraorbital folds)
Facial erythema or pallor
Course influenced by environmental and/or emotional factors

Table 139-2 DIFFERENTIAL DIAGNOSIS OF ATOPIC DERMATITIS

CONGENITAL DISORDERS
• Netherton syndrome • Familial keratosis pilaris
CHRONIC DERMATOSES
• Seborrheic dermatitis • Contact dermatitis (allergic or irritant) • Nummular eczema • Psoriasis • Ichthyoses
INFECTIONS AND INFESTATIONS
• Scabies • HIV-associated dermatitis • Dermatophytosis • Insect bites • Onchocerciasis
MALIGNANCIES
• Cutaneous T-cell lymphoma (mycosis fungoides/Sézary syndrome) • Letterer-Siwe disease
AUTOIMMUNE DISORDERS
• Dermatitis herpetiformis • Pemphigus foliaceus • Graft vs host disease • Dermatomyositis
IMMUNODEFICIENCIES
• Wiskott-Aldrich syndrome • Severe combined immunodeficiency syndrome • Hyper–immunoglobulin E syndrome • Immunodysregulation polyendocrinopathy enteropathy X-linked (IPEX) syndrome
METABOLIC DISORDERS
• Zinc deficiency • Pyridoxine (vitamin B_6) and niacin • Multiple carboxylase deficiency • Phenylketonuria

From Leung DYM, Sampson HA, Geha RS, et al: *Pediatric allergy principles and practice,* St Louis, 2003, Mosby, p 562.

failure to thrive. Wiskott-Aldrich syndrome (Chapter 120.2), an X-linked recessive disorder associated with thrombocytopenia, immune defects, and recurrent severe bacterial infections, is characterized by a rash almost indistinguishable from that in AD. Hyper-IgE syndrome (Chapter 120.2) is characterized by markedly elevated serum IgE values, recurrent deep-seated bacterial infections, chronic dermatitis, and refractory dermatophytosis.

Adolescents who present with an eczematous dermatitis but no history of childhood eczema, respiratory allergy, or atopic family history may have allergic **contact dermatitis** (Chapter 647). A contact allergen may be the problem in any patient whose AD does not respond to appropriate therapy. Sensitizing chemicals, such as parabens and lanolin, can be irritants for patients with AD and are commonly found as vehicles in therapeutic topical agents. Topical glucocorticoid contact allergy has been reported in patients with chronic dermatitis who are undergoing topical corticosteroid therapy. Eczematous dermatitis has also been reported with HIV infection as well as with a variety of infestations such as scabies. Other conditions that can be confused with AD include psoriasis, ichthyoses, and seborrheic dermatitis.

TREATMENT

The treatment of AD requires a systematic, multifaceted approach that incorporates skin hydration, topical anti-inflammatory therapy, identification and elimination of flare factors, and, if necessary, systemic therapy. Assessment of the severity also helps direct therapy (Table 139-3).

Cutaneous Hydration

Because patients with AD have impaired skin barrier function from reduced lipid levels, they present with diffuse, abnormally dry skin, or **xerosis.** Lukewarm soaking baths for 15-20 min followed by the application of an occlusive emollient to retain moisture provide symptomatic relief. Hydrophilic ointments of varying degrees of viscosity can be used according to the patient's preference. Occlusive ointments are sometimes not well tolerated because of interference with the function of the eccrine sweat ducts and may induce the development of folliculitis. In these cases, less occlusive agents should be used.

Hydration by baths or wet dressings promotes transepidermal penetration of topical glucocorticoids. Dressings may also serve as effective barriers against persistent scratching, in turn promoting healing of excoriated lesions. Wet dressings are recommended for use on severely affected or chronically involved areas of dermatitis refractory to skin care. It is critical that wet dressing therapy be followed by topical emollient application to avoid potential drying and fissuring from the therapy. Wet dressing therapy can be complicated by maceration and secondary infection and should be closely monitored by a physician.

Topical Corticosteroids

Topical corticosteroids are the cornerstone of anti-inflammatory treatment for acute exacerbations of AD. Patients should be carefully instructed on their use of topical glucocorticoids in order to avoid potential adverse effects. There are 7 classes of topical glucocorticoids, ranked according to their potency as determined by vasoconstrictor assays (Table 139-4). Because of their potential adverse effects, the ultra-high-potency glucocorticoids should not be used on the face or intertriginous areas and should be used only for very short periods on the trunk and extremities. Mid-potency glucocorticoids can be used for longer periods to treat chronic AD involving the trunk and extremities. Long-term control can be maintained with twice-weekly applications of topical fluticasone or mometasone to areas that have healed but are prone to relapse, once control of AD is achieved after a daily regimen of topical corticosteroids. Compared with creams, ointments have a greater potential to occlude the epidermis, resulting in enhanced systemic absorption. Adverse effects of topical glucocorticoids can be divided into local adverse effects and systemic adverse effects, the latter of which result from suppression of the hypothalamic-pituitary-adrenal axis. Local adverse effects include the development of striae and skin atrophy. Systemic adverse effects are related to the potency of the topical corticosteroid, site of application, occlusiveness of the preparation, percentage of the body surface area covered, and length of use. The potential for adrenal suppression from potent topical corticosteroids is greatest in infants and young children with severe AD requiring intensive therapy.

Topical Calcineurin Inhibitors

The nonsteroidal topical calcineurin inhibitors are effective in reducing AD skin inflammation. Pimecrolimus cream 1% (Elidel) is indicated for mild to moderate AD. Tacrolimus ointment 0.1% and 0.03% (Protopic) is indicated for moderate to severe AD. Both are approved for short-term or intermittent long-term treatment of AD in patients ≥2 yr whose disease is unresponsive to or who are intolerant of other conventional therapies or for whom these therapies are inadvisable owing to potential risks. Topical calcineurin inhibitors may be better than topical corticosteroids

Table 139-3 CATEGORIZATION OF PHYSICAL SEVERITY OF ATOPIC ECZEMA

Clear—Normal skin, with no evidence of atopic eczema
Mild—Areas of dry skin, infrequent itching (with or without small areas of redness)
Moderate—Areas of dry skin, frequent itching, redness (with or without excoriation and localized skin thickening)
Severe—Widespread areas of dry skin, incessant itching, redness (with or without excoriation, extensive skin thickening, bleeding, oozing, cracking, and alteration of pigmentation)

From Lewis-Jones S, Mugglestone MA; Guideline Development Group: Management of atopic eczema in children aged up to 12 years: summary of NICE guidance, *BMJ* 335:1263–1264, 2007.

Table 139-4 SELECTED TOPICAL CORTICOSTEROID PREPARATIONS*

GROUP 1
Clobetasol propionate (Temovate) 0.05% ointment/cream Betamethasone dipropionate (Diprolene) 0.05% ointment/cream
GROUP 2
Mometasone furoate (Elocon) 0.1% ointment Halcinonide (Halog) 0.1% cream Fluocinonide (Lidex) 0.05% ointment/cream Desoximetasone (Topicort) 0.25% ointment/cream
GROUP 3
Fluticasone propionate (Cutivate) 0.005% ointment Halcinonide (Halog) 0.1% ointment Betamethasone valerate (Valisone) 0.1% ointment
GROUP 4
Mometasone furoate (Elocon) 0.1% cream Triamcinolone acetonide (Kenalog) 0.1% ointment/cream Fluocinolone acetonide (Synalar) 0.025% ointment
GROUP 5
Fluocinolone acetonide (Synalar) 0.025% cream Hydrocortisone valerate (Westcort) 0.2% ointment
GROUP 6
Desonide (DesOwen) 05% ointment/cream/lotion Alclometasone dipropionate (Aclovate) 0.05% ointment/cream
GROUP 7
Hydrocortisone (Hytone) 2.5% & 1% ointment/cream

*Representative corticosteroids are listed by group from 1 (superpotent) through 7 (least potent).

Adapted from Stoughton RB: Vasoconstrictor assay-specific applications. In Malbach HI, Surber C, editors: *Topical corticosteroids,* Basel, Switzerland, 1992, Karger, pp 42–53.

in the treatment of patients whose AD is poorly responsive to topical steroids, of patients with steroid phobia, and of patients with face and neck dermatitis, in which ineffective, low-potency topical corticosteroids are usually used because of fears of steroid-induced skin atrophy.

Tar Preparations

Coal tar preparations have antipruritic and anti-inflammatory effects on the skin; however, the anti-inflammatory effects are usually not as pronounced as those of topical glucocorticoids or calcineurin inhibitors. Tar preparations are useful in reducing the potency of topical glucocorticoids required in long-term maintenance therapy of AD. Tar shampoos can be particularly beneficial for scalp dermatitis. Adverse effects associated with tar preparations include skin irritation, folliculitis, and photosensitivity.

Antihistamines

Systemic antihistamines act primarily by blocking the histamine H_1 receptors in the dermis, thereby reducing histamine-induced pruritus. Histamine is only one of many mediators that induce pruritus of the skin, so patients may derive minimal benefit from antihistaminic therapy. Because pruritus is usually worse at night, sedating antihistamines (hydroxyzine, diphenhydramine) may offer an advantage with their soporific side effects when used at bedtime. Doxepin hydrochloride has both tricyclic antidepressant and H_1- and H_2-receptor blocking effects. Short-term use of a sedative to allow adequate rest may be appropriate in cases of severe nocturnal pruritus. Studies of newer nonsedating antihistamines have shown variable effectiveness in controlling pruritus in AD, although they may be useful in the small subset of patients with AD and concomitant urticaria.

Systemic Corticosteroids

Systemic corticosteroids are rarely indicated in the treatment of chronic AD. The dramatic clinical improvement that may occur with systemic corticosteroids is frequently associated with a severe rebound flare of AD after therapy discontinuation. Short courses of oral corticosteroids may be appropriate for an acute exacerbation of AD while other treatment measures are being instituted in parallel. If a short course of oral corticosteroids is given, it is important to taper the dosage and begin intensified skin care, particularly with topical corticosteroids and frequent bathing followed by application of emollients, to prevent rebound flaring of AD.

Cyclosporine

Cyclosporine is a potent immunosuppressive drug that acts primarily on T cells by suppressing cytokine gene transcription. Cyclosporine forms a complex with an intracellular protein, cyclophilin, and this complex in turn inhibits calcineurin, a phosphatase required for activation of NFAT (nuclear factor of activated T cells), a transcription factor necessary for cytokine gene transcription. Cyclosporine (5 mg/kg/day) for short-term and long-term (1 yr) use has been beneficial for children with severe, refractory AD. Possible adverse effects include renal impairment and hypertension.

Phototherapy

Natural sunlight is often beneficial to patients with AD as long as sunburn and excessive sweating are avoided. Many phototherapy modalities are effective for AD, including ultraviolet A-1, ultraviolet B (UVB), narrow-band UVB, and psoralen plus ultraviolet A (PUVA). Phototherapy is generally reserved for patients in whom standard treatments fail. Maintenance treatments are usually required for phototherapy to be effective. Short-term adverse effects with phototherapy include erythema, skin pain, pruritus, and pigmentation. Long-term adverse effects include predisposition to cutaneous malignancies.

Unproven Therapies

Other therapies that may be considered in patients with refractory AD are as follows.

INTERFERON-γ IFN-γ is known to suppress Th2-cell function. Several studies, including a multicenter, double-blind, placebo-controlled trial and several open trials, have demonstrated that treatment with recombinant human IFN-γ results in clinical improvement of AD. Reduction in clinical severity of AD correlated with the ability of IFN-γ to decrease total circulating eosinophil counts. Influenza-like symptoms are commonly observed side effects during the treatment course.

OMALIZUMAB Treatment of patients who have severe AD and elevated serum IgE values with monoclonal anti-IgE may be considered in those with allergen-induced flares of AD. However, there have been no published double-blind, placebo-controlled trials of its use. Most reports have been case studies and show inconsistent responses to anti-IgE.

ALLERGEN IMMUNOTHERAPY In contrast to its acceptance for treatment of allergic rhinitis and extrinsic asthma, immunotherapy with aeroallergens in the treatment of AD is controversial. There are reports of both disease exacerbation and improvement. Studies suggest specific immunotherapy in patients with AD sensitized to dust mite allergen showed improvement in severity of skin disease as well as reduction in topical steroid use. However, well-controlled studies are still required to determine the role for immunotherapy with this disease, particularly in children.

PROBIOTICS Perinatal administration of the probiotic *Lactobacillus rhamnosus* strain GG has been shown to reduce the incidence of AD in at-risk children during the first 2 yr of life. The treatment response has been found to be more pronounced in patients with positive skin prick test results and elevated IgE values. Other studies have not demonstrated a benefit.

CHINESE HERBAL MEDICATIONS Several placebo-controlled clinical trials have suggested that patients with severe AD may benefit from treatment with traditional Chinese herbal therapy. The subjects had significantly reduced skin disease and decreased pruritus. The beneficial response of Chinese herbal therapy is often temporary, and effectiveness may wear off despite continued treatment. The possibility of hepatic toxicity, cardiac side effects, or idiosyncratic reactions remains a concern. The specific ingredients of the herbs also remain to be elucidated, and some preparations have been found to be contaminated with corticosteroids. At present, Chinese herbal therapy for AD is considered investigational.

ANTIMETABOLITES Mycophenolate mofetil is a purine biosynthesis inhibitor used as an immunosuppressant in organ transplantation that has been used for treatment of refractory AD. Aside from immunosuppression, herpes retinitis and dose-related bone marrow suppression have been reported with its use. Of note, not all patients benefit from treatment. Therefore, the medication should be discontinued if the disease does not respond within 4-8 wk. Methotrexate is an antimetabolite with potent inhibitory effects on inflammatory cytokine synthesis and cell chemotaxis. Methotrexate has been used for patients with recalcitrant AD. In AD, dosing is more frequent than the weekly dosing used for psoriasis. Azathioprine is a purine analogue with anti-inflammatory and antiproliferative effects that has been used for severe AD. Myelosuppression is a significant adverse effect, and thiopurine methyl transferase levels may identify individuals at risk for it. Before any of these drugs is used, patients should be referred to an AD specialist who is familiar with treatment of severe AD, because well-controlled clinical trials of the use of antimetabolites in AD are lacking.

AVOIDING TRIGGERS

It is essential to identify and eliminate triggering factors, both during the period of acute symptoms and on a long-term basis to prevent recurrences.

Irritants

Patients with AD have a low threshold response to irritants that trigger their itch-scratch cycle. Soaps or detergents, chemicals, smoke, abrasive clothing, and exposure to extremes of temperature and humidity are common triggers. Patients with AD should use soaps with minimal defatting properties and a neutral pH. New clothing should be laundered before wearing to decrease levels of formaldehyde and other chemicals. Residual laundry detergent in clothing may trigger the itch-scratch cycle; using a liquid rather than powder detergent and adding a 2nd rinse cycle facilitates removal of the detergent.

Every attempt should be made to allow children with AD to be as normally active as possible. A sport such as swimming may be better tolerated than others that involve intense perspiration, physical contact, or heavy clothing and equipment. Rinsing off chlorine immediately and lubricating the skin after swimming are important. Although ultraviolet light may be beneficial to some patients with AD, high–sun protection factor (SPF) sunscreens should be used to avoid sunburn.

Foods

Food allergy is co-morbid in approximately 40% of infants and young children with moderate to severe AD (Chapter 145). Undiagnosed food allergies in patients with AD may induce eczematous dermatitis in some patients and urticarial reactions, wheezing, or nasal congestion in others. Increased severity of AD symptoms and younger age correlate directly with the presence of food allergy. Removal of food allergens from the diet leads to significant clinical improvement but requires a great deal of education, because most common allergens (egg, milk, peanut, wheat, soy) contaminate many foods and are difficult to avoid.

Potential allergens can be identified by a careful history and performing selective skin prick tests or in vitro blood testing for allergen-specific IgE. Negative skin and blood test results for allergen-specific IgE have a high predictive value for excluding suspected allergens. Positive results of skin or blood tests using foods often do not correlate with clinical symptoms and should be confirmed with controlled food challenges and elimination diets. Extensive elimination diets, which can be nutritionally deficient, are rarely required. Even with multiple positive skin test results, the majority of patients react to fewer than 3 foods under controlled challenge conditions.

Aeroallergens

In older children, AD flares can occur after intranasal or epicutaneous exposure to aeroallergens such as fungi, animal dander, grass, and ragweed pollen. Avoiding aeroallergens, particularly dust mites, can result in clinical improvement of AD. Avoidance measures for dust mite–allergic patients include using dust mite–proof encasings on pillows, mattresses, and box springs; washing bedding in hot water weekly; removing bedroom carpeting; and decreasing indoor humidity levels with air conditioning.

Infections

Patients with AD have increased susceptibility to bacterial, viral, and fungal skin infections. Antistaphylococcal antibiotics are very helpful for treating patients who are heavily colonized or infected with *Staphylococcus aureus*. Erythromycin and azithromycin are usually beneficial for patients who are not colonized with a resistant *S. aureus* strain; however, a first-generation cephalosporin (cephalexin) is recommended for macrolide-resistant *S. aureus*. Topical mupirocin is useful in the treatment of localized impetiginous lesions, with systemic antibiotic for widespread infections. Cytokine-mediated skin inflammation contributes to skin colonization with *S. aureus;* this fact indicates the importance of combining effective anti-inflammatory therapy with antibiotics for treating moderate to severe AD to avoid the need for repeated courses of antibiotics, which can lead to the emergence of antibiotic-resistant strains of *S. aureus*.

Herpes simplex virus (HSV) can provoke recurrent dermatitis and may be misdiagnosed as *S. aureus* infection. The presence of punched-out erosions, vesicles, and infected skin lesions that fail to respond to oral antibiotics suggests HSV infection, which can be diagnosed by a Giemsa-stained Tzanck smear of cells scraped from the vesicle base or by viral polymerase chain reaction or culture. Topical corticosteroids should be temporarily discontinued if HSV infection is suspected. Reports of life-threatening dissemination of HSV infections in patients with AD who have widespread disease mandate antiviral treatment. Dermatophyte infections also can contribute to exacerbation of AD disease activity. Patients with dermatophyte infection or IgE antibodies to *Malassezia furfur* (formerly known as *Pityrosporum ovale*) may benefit from a trial of topical or systemic antifungal therapy.

COMPLICATIONS

Staphylococcus aureus is found in >90% of AD skin lesions. Antibiotic therapy is required if honey-colored crusting, folliculitis, impetigo, and pyoderma are present. Regional lymphadenopathy is common in such cases. The importance of *S. aureus* in AD is supported by the observation that patients with severe AD, even those without overt infection, may show clinical response to combined treatment with antistaphylococcal antibiotics and topical corticosteroids.

AD is associated with recurrent viral skin infections. The most serious viral infection is **Kaposi varicelliform eruption,** or **eczema herpeticum,** which is caused by HSV and affects patients of all ages. The incubation period of 5-12 days is followed by disseminated eruption of multiple, itchy, vesiculopustular lesions. The vesicular lesions are umbilicated, tend to crop, and often become hemorrhagic and crusted. Persons with AD are susceptible to **eczema vaccinatum,** which is similar in appearance to eczema herpeticum and historically follows smallpox (vaccinia virus) vaccination. Cutaneous warts and molluscum contagiosum are additional viral infections affecting children with AD.

Patients with AD have been found to have a greater susceptibility to *Trichophyton rubrum* fungal infections than nonatopic control subjects. There has been particular interest in the role of *M. furfur* in AD because it is a lipophilic yeast commonly present in the seborrheic areas of the skin. IgE antibodies against *M. furfur* have been found in patients with head and neck dermatitis. A reduction of AD severity has been observed in those patients after treatment with antifungal agents.

Exfoliative dermatitis may develop in patients with extensive skin involvement. It is associated with generalized redness, scaling, weeping, crusting, systemic toxicity, lymphadenopathy, and fever and is usually caused by superinfection (e.g., with toxin-producing *S. aureus* or HSV infection) or inappropriate therapy. In some cases, the withdrawal of systemic glucocorticoids used to control severe AD precipitates exfoliative erythroderma.

Eyelid dermatitis and chronic blepharitis may result in visual impairment from corneal scarring. **Atopic keratoconjunctivitis** is usually bilateral and can have disabling symptoms that include itching, burning, tearing, and copious mucoid discharge. Vernal conjunctivitis is associated with papillary hypertrophy or cobblestoning of the upper eyelid conjunctiva. It typically occurs in younger patients and has a marked seasonal incidence with spring exacerbations. **Keratoconus** is a conical deformity of the cornea believed to result from chronic rubbing of the eyes in patients with AD. Cataracts may be a primary manifestation of AD or from extensive use of systemic and topical glucocorticoids, particularly around the eyes.

PROGNOSIS

AD generally tends to be more severe and persistent in young children, particularly if they have null mutations in their filaggrin genes. Periods of remission occur more frequently as patients grow older. Spontaneous resolution of AD has been reported to occur after age 5 yr in 40-60% of patients affected during infancy, particularly for mild disease. Earlier studies suggested that approximately 84% of children outgrow their AD by adolescence; however, later studies reported that AD resolves in approximately 20% of children monitored from infancy until adolescence and becomes less severe in 65%. Of those adolescents treated for mild dermatitis, >50% may experience a relapse of disease as adults, which frequently manifests as hand dermatitis, especially if daily activities require repeated hand wetting. Predictive factors of a poor prognosis for AD include widespread AD in childhood, filaggrin gene null mutations, concomitant allergic rhinitis and asthma, family history of AD in parents or siblings, early age at onset of AD, being an only child, and very high serum IgE levels.

PREVENTION

Breast-feeding or a feeding with a hypoallergenic hydrolyzed formula may be beneficial. Probiotics may also reduce the incidence or severity of AD, but this possibility is unproven. If an infant with AD is diagnosed with food allergy, the breast = feeding mother will need to eliminate the implicated food allergen from her diet. Identification and elimination of triggering factors is the mainstay for prevention of flares as well as for the long-term treatment of AD.

BIBLIOGRAPHY

Please visit the Nelson Textbook of Pediatrics *website at www.expertconsult.com for the complete bibliography.*

Chapter 140
Insect Allergy

Scott H. Sicherer and Donald Y.M. Leung

Allergic responses to stinging or, more rarely, biting insects vary from localized cutaneous reactions to systemic anaphylaxis. Allergic reactions that are caused by inhalation of airborne particles of insect origin result in acute and chronic respiratory symptoms of seasonal or perennial rhinitis, conjunctivitis, and asthma.

ETIOLOGY

Most reactions to biting and stinging insects, such as those induced by mosquitoes, flies, and fleas, are limited to a primary lesion isolated to the area of the bite and do not represent an allergic response. Occasionally, insect bites or stings induce pronounced localized reactions or systemic reactions that may be based on immediate or delayed hypersensitivity reactions. Systemic allergic responses to insects are attributed most typically to immunoglobulin (Ig) E antibody–mediated responses, which are caused primarily by stings from venomous insects of the order Hymenoptera and more rarely from ticks, spiders, scorpions, and *Triatoma* (kissing bug). Members of the order Hymenoptera include apids (honeybee, bumblebee), vespids (yellow jacket, wasp, hornet), and formicids (fire and harvester ants) (Fig. 140-1). Among winged stinging insects, yellow jackets are the most notorious for stinging because they are aggressive and ground dwelling, and they linger near activities involving food. Hornets nest in trees, whereas wasps build honeycomb nests in dark areas such as under porches; both are aggressive if disturbed. Honeybees are less aggressive, nest in tree hollows, and, unlike the stings of other flying Hymenoptera, honeybee stings almost always leave a barbed stinger with venom sac.

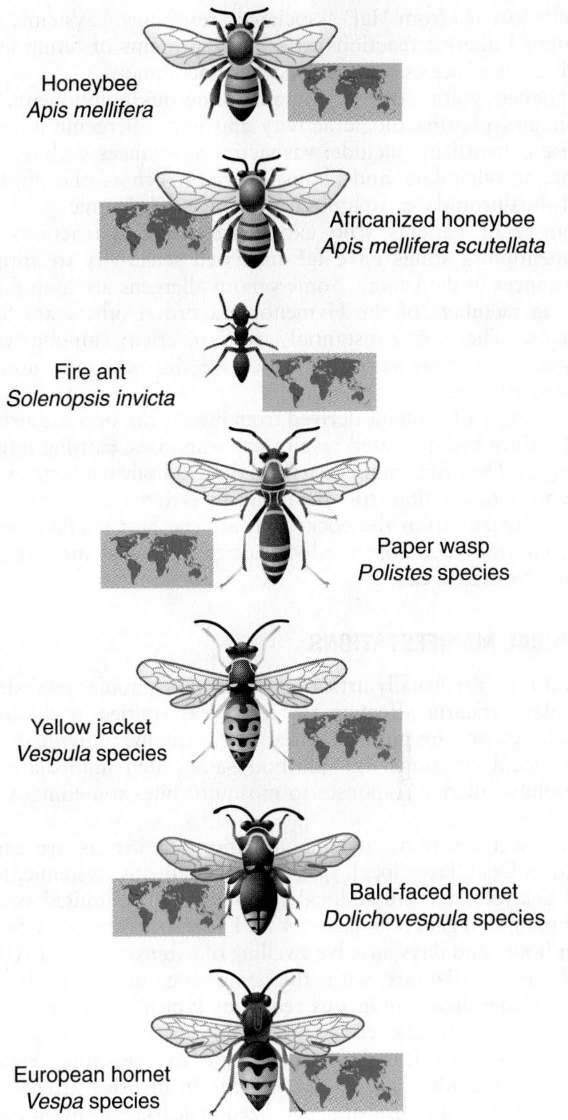

Figure 140-1 Species of Hymenoptera and their geographical distribution. (From Freeman TM: Hypersensitivity to *Hymenoptera* stings, *N Engl J Med* 351:1978–1984, 2004.)

In the USA, fire ants are found increasingly in the Southeast, living in large mounds of soil. When disturbed, the ants attack in large numbers, anchor themselves to the skin by their mandibles, and sting multiple times in a semicircular pattern. Sterile pustules form at the sting sites. Systemic reactions to stinging insects occur in 0.4-0.8% of children and 3% of adults and account for ≈40 deaths each year in the USA.

IgE antibody–mediated allergic responses to airborne particulate matter carrying insect emanations contribute to seasonal and perennial symptoms affecting the upper and lower airways. Seasonal allergy is attributed to exposures to a variety of insects, particularly aquatic insects such as the caddis fly and midge, or lake fly, at a time when larvae pupate and adult flies are airborne. Perennial allergy is attributed to sensitization to insects such as cockroaches and ladybugs as well as house dust mite, which is phylogenetically related to spiders rather than insects and has eight rather than six legs.

PATHOGENESIS

Localized skin responses to biting insects are caused primarily by vasoactive or irritant materials derived from insect saliva, and rarely occur from IgE-associated responses. Systemic IgE-mediated allergic reactions to salivary proteins of biting insects such as mosquitoes are reported but uncommon.

Hymenoptera venoms contain numerous components with toxic and pharmacologic activity and with allergenic potential. These constituents include: vasoactive substances such as histamine, acetylcholine, and kinins; enzymes such as phospholipase and hyaluronidase; apamin; melittin; and formic acid. The majority of patients who experience systemic reactions after Hymenoptera stings have IgE-mediated sensitivity to antigenic substances in the venom. Some venom allergens are homologous among members of the Hymenoptera order; others are family specific. There is substantial cross reactivity among vespid venoms, but these venom allergies are distinct from honeybee venom allergies.

A variety of proteins derived from insects can become airborne and induce IgE-mediated respiratory responses, causing inhalant allergies. The primary allergen from the caddis fly is a hemocyanin-like protein, and that from the midge fly is derived from hemoglobin. Allergens from the cockroach are the best studied and are derived from cockroach saliva, secretions, fecal material, and debris from skin casts.

CLINICAL MANIFESTATIONS

Insect bites are usually urticarial but may be papular or vesicular. Papular urticaria affecting the lower extremities in children is usually caused by multiple bites. Occasionally, individuals have large local reactions. IgE antibody–associated immediate- and late-phase allergic responses to mosquito bites sometimes mimic cellulitis.

Clinical reactions to stinging venomous insects are categorized as local, large local, generalized cutaneous, systemic, toxic, and delayed/late. Simple **local reactions** involve limited swelling and pain, and generally last <24 hr. **Large local reactions** develop over hours and days, involve swelling of extensive areas (>10 cm) that are contiguous with the sting site, and may last for days. **Generalized cutaneous reactions** typically progress within minutes and include cutaneous symptoms of urticaria, angioedema, and pruritus beyond the site of the sting. **Systemic reactions** are identical to anaphylaxis from other triggers and may include symptoms of generalized urticaria, laryngeal edema, bronchospasm, and hypotension. Stings from a large number of insects at once may result in **toxic reactions** of fever, malaise, emesis, and nausea owing to the chemical properties of the venom in large doses. Serum sickness, nephrotic syndrome, vasculitis, neuritis, or encephalopathy may occur as **delayed/late reactions** to stinging insects.

Inhalant allergy caused by insects results in clinical disease similar to that induced by other inhalant allergens such as pollens. Depending on individual sensitivity and exposure, reactions may result in seasonal or perennial rhinitis, conjunctivitis, and asthma.

DIAGNOSIS

The diagnosis of allergy from biting and stinging insects is generally evident from the history of exposure, typical symptoms, and physical findings. The diagnosis of Hymenoptera allergy rests in part on the identification of venom-specific IgE by prick skin testing. The primary reasons to pursue testing are to confirm reactivity when venom immunotherapy (VIT) is being considered or when it is clinically necessary to confirm venom hypersensitivity as a cause of a reaction. Venoms of five Hymenoptera (honeybee, yellow jacket, yellow hornet, white-faced hornet, and wasp) as well as the jack jumper ant in Australia and whole-body extract of fire ant are available for skin testing. Although skin tests are considered to be the most sensitive modality for detection of venom-specific IgE, additional evaluation with an in vitro serum assay for venom-specific IgE is recommended if skin test results are negative in the presence of a convincing history of a severe systemic reaction. With in vitro tests, there is a 20% incidence of both false-positive and false-negative results, so it is not appropriate to exclude venom hypersensitivity based on this test alone. If initial skin prick and in vitro test results are negative in the context of a convincing history of a severe reaction, repeat testing is recommended before one concludes that allergy is unlikely. Skin tests are usually accurate within 1 wk of a sting reaction, but occasionally a refractory period is observed that warrants retesting after 4-6 wk if the initial results are negative. As many as 40% of skin test–positive subjects may not experience anaphylaxis on sting challenge, so testing without an appropriate clinical history is potentially misleading.

The diagnosis of inhalant insect allergy may be evident from a history of typical symptoms induced seasonally in specific geographic regions. A chronic respiratory symptom during long-term exposure, as may occur with cockroach allergy, is less amenable to identification by history alone. Skin prick or in vitro immunoassay tests for specific IgE to the insect are used to confirm inhalant insect allergy. Allergy tests may be particularly warranted for potential cockroach allergy in patients with persistent asthma and known cockroach exposure.

TREATMENT

For local cutaneous reactions caused by insect bites and stings, treatment with cold compresses, topical medications to relieve itching, and, occasionally, the use of a systemic antihistamine and oral analgesic are appropriate. Stingers should be removed promptly by scraping, with caution not to squeeze the venom sac because doing so could inject more venom. Sting sites rarely become infected, possibly owing to the antibacterial actions of venom constituents. Vesicles left by fire ant stings that are scratched open should be cleansed to prevent secondary infection.

Anaphylactic reactions after a Hymenoptera sting are treated exactly like anaphylaxis from any cause. Therapies may include oxygen, epinephrine, intravenous saline, steroids, antihistamines, and other treatments (Chapter 143). Referral to an allergist-immunologist should be considered for patients who have experienced a generalized cutaneous or systemic reaction to an insect sting, need education about avoidance and emergency treatment, may be candidates for VIT, or have a condition that may complicate management of anaphylaxis (use of β-blockers).

Venom Immunotherapy

Hymenoptera VIT is highly effective (95-97%) in decreasing the risk for severe anaphylaxis. The selection of patients for VIT depends on several factors (Table 140-1). Individuals with local reactions regardless of age are not at increased risk for severe systemic reactions on a subsequent sting and are not candidates for VIT. The risk of a systemic reaction for those who experienced a large local reaction is no more than 4-10%; testing or VIT is usually not recommended, and prescription of self-injectable epinephrine is considered optional but usually not necessary. Those who experience severe systemic reactions, with airway involvement or hypotension, and have a positive skin test result should receive immunotherapy. Immunotherapy against winged Hymenoptera is not usually indicated for children ≤16 yr of age in whom stings have caused only generalized urticaria or angioedema, because their risk for a reaction after a subsequent sting is <10%, with isolated skin reactions the most likely event. The risk could be reduced to 1% after treatment with VIT, so it is an option to consider if multiple future stings are anticipated. Immunotherapy against Hymenoptera is indicated in those ≥17 yr of age if venom skin test results are positive and there is a history of generalized urticaria or a systemic reaction, because their risk for future systemic reactions is ≈60-70%. VIT is

Table 140-1 INDICATIONS FOR VENOM IMMUNOTHERAPY AGAINST WINGED HYMENOPTERA

SYMPTOMS	AGE	SKIN TEST/IN VITRO TEST	RISK OF SYSTEMIC REACTION IF UNTREATED (%)*	VIT RECOMMENDED
Large local reaction	Any	Usually not indicated	4-10	Usually not indicated
Generalized cutaneous reaction	≤16 yr	Usually not indicated	9-10	Usually not indicated
	≥17 yr	Positive result	20	Yes
		Negative result	—	No
Systemic reaction	Any	Positive result	Child: 40 Adult: 60-70	Yes
		Negative result	—	Usually no

*Risks generally decrease after 10 yr.

usually not indicated if there is no evidence of IgE to venom. The incidence of adverse effects in the course of treatment is not trivial in adults, as 50% experience large local reactions and about 7% experience systemic reactions. The incidence of both local and systemic reactions is much lower in children. It is uncertain how long immunotherapy with Hymenoptera venom should continue; lifelong treatment has been advocated for patients with very severe reactions. Consideration to discontinue therapy after 3-5 yr has been suggested, however, because >80% of adults who have received 5 yr of therapy tolerate challenge stings without systemic reactions for 5-10 yr after completion of treatment. Long-term responses to treatment are even better for children. Follow-up over a mean of 18 yr of children with moderate to severe insect sting reactions who received VIT for a mean treatment period of 3.5 yr and were stung again showed a reaction rate of only 5%; untreated children experienced a reaction rate of 32%. Whereas duration of therapy with VIT may be individualized, it is clear that a significant number of untreated children retain their allergy.

Less is known about the natural history of fire ant hypersensitivity and efficacy of immunotherapy for this allergy. The criteria for starting immunotherapy are similar to those for hypersensitivities to other Hymenoptera, but there is stronger consideration to treat children ≤16 yr of age with VIT if they have experienced only generalized urticaria. Only whole-body fire ant extract is commercially available for diagnostic skin testing and immunotherapy.

Inhalant Allergy

The symptoms of inhalant allergy caused by insects are managed as for other causes of seasonal or perennial rhinitis (Chapter 137), conjunctivitis (Chapter 141), and asthma (Chapter 138).

PREVENTION

Avoidance of stings and bites is essential. To reduce the risk of stings, sensitized individuals should avoid attractants such as perfumes and bright-colored clothing outdoors, wear gloves when gardening, and wear long pants and shoes with socks when walking in the grass or through fields. Typical insect repellents do not guard against Hymenoptera. Nests of these insects should be removed if they are close to the home.

Individuals who have had generalized cutaneous or systemic reactions to Hymenoptera stings should have immediate access to **self-injectable epinephrine.** Adults responsible for allergic children, and older patients who can self-treat, must be carefully taught the indications for and technique of administration of this medication. Particular attention is necessary for children in out-of-home daycare centers, at school, or attending camps, to ensure that an emergency action plan is in place. The individual at risk for anaphylaxis from an insect sting should also wear an identification bracelet indicating the allergy.

Avoidance of the insect is the preferred management of inhalant allergy. This can prove difficult, particularly, for instance, for those living in multiple-dwelling apartments, where eradication of cockroaches is problematic. Immunotherapy is occasionally undertaken in such cases, but beneficial results have not been thoroughly documented.

BIBLIOGRAPHY

Please visit the Nelson Textbook of Pediatrics *website at www.expertconsult.com for the complete bibliography.*

Chapter 141
Ocular Allergies

Mark Boguniewicz and Donald Y.M. Leung

The eye is a common target of allergic disorders because of its marked vascularity and direct contact with allergens in the environment. The conjunctiva is the most immunologically active tissue of the external eye. Ocular allergies can occur as isolated target organ disease or more commonly in conjunction with nasal allergies. Ocular symptoms can significantly affect quality of life.

CLINICAL MANIFESTATIONS

There are a few distinct entities that constitute allergic eye disease, all of which have bilateral involvement. Sensitization is necessary for all of these except for giant papillary conjunctivitis. Vernal keratoconjunctivitis and atopic keratoconjunctivitis are potentially sight-threatening.

Allergic Conjunctivitis

Allergic conjunctivitis is the most common hypersensitivity response of the eye, affecting approximately 25% of the general population and 30% of children with atopy. It is caused by direct exposure of the mucosal surfaces of the eye to environmental allergens. Patients complain of variable ocular itching, rather than pain, with increased tearing. Clinical signs include bilateral injected conjunctivae with vascular congestion that may progress to chemosis, or conjunctival swelling, and a watery discharge (Fig. 141-1). Allergic conjunctivitis occurs in a seasonal or, less commonly, perennial form. **Seasonal allergic conjunctivitis** is typically associated with allergic rhinitis (Chapter 137) and is most commonly triggered by pollens. Major pollen groups in the temperate zones include trees (late winter to early spring), grasses (late spring to early summer), and weeds (late summer to early fall), but seasons can vary significantly in different parts of the country. Mold spores can also cause seasonal allergy symptoms, principally in the summer and fall. Seasonal allergy symptoms may be aggravated by coincident exposure to perennial allergens. **Perennial allergic conjunctivitis** is triggered by allergens such as animal danders or dust mites that are present throughout the year. Symptoms are usually less severe than with seasonal allergic conjunctivitis. Since pollens and soil molds may be present year round while exposure to perennial allergens such as furred animals may be intermittent, classification as intermittent (i.e.,

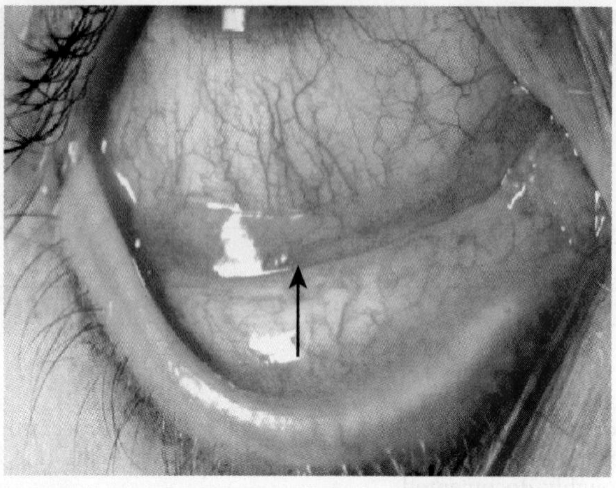

Figure 141-1 Allergic conjunctivitis. Arrow indicates area of chemosis in the conjunctivitis. (From Adkinson NF Jr, Bochner BS, Busse WW, et al, editors: *Middleton's allergy principles and practice*, ed 7, vol 2, Philadelphia, Mosby/Elsevier, p 1221.)

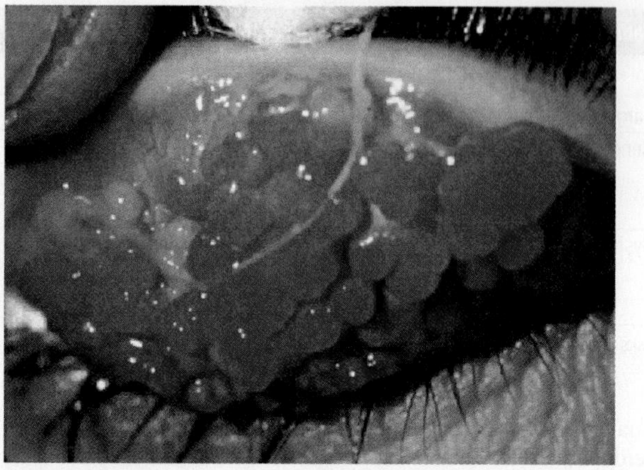

Figure 141-2 Vernal keratoconjunctivitis. Cobblestone papillae and ropey discharge are seen on the underside (tarsal conjunctiva) of the upper eyelid. (From Adkinson NF Jr, Bochner BS, Busse WW, et al, editors: *Middleton's allergy principles and practice*, ed 7, vol 2, Philadelphia, Mosby/Elsevier, p 1224.)

symptoms present <4 days a week or for <4 weeks) and persistent (symptoms present >4 days a week and for >4 weeks) has been proposed.

Vernal Keratoconjunctivitis

Vernal keratoconjunctivitis is a severe bilateral chronic inflammatory process of the upper tarsal conjunctival surface that occurs in a limbal or palpebral form. It may threaten eyesight if there is corneal involvement. Although vernal keratoconjunctivitis is not IgE mediated, it occurs most frequently in children with seasonal allergies, asthma, or atopic dermatitis. Vernal keratoconjunctivitis affects boys twice as often as girls and is more common in persons of Asian and African origin. It affects primarily children in temperate areas, with exacerbations in the spring and summer. Symptoms include severe ocular itching exacerbated by exposure to irritants, light, or perspiration. In addition, patients may complain of severe photophobia, foreign-body sensation, and lacrimation. Giant papillae occur predominantly on the upper tarsal plate and are typically described as **cobblestoning** (Fig. 141-2). Other signs include a stringy or thick, ropey discharge, cobblestone papillae, transient yellow-white points in the limbus (Trantas dots) and conjunctiva (Horner points), corneal "shield" ulcers, and Dennie lines (Dennie-Morgan folds), which are prominent symmetric skinfolds that extend in an arc from the inner canthus beneath and parallel to the lower lid margin. Children with vernal keratoconjunctivitis have measurably longer eyelashes, which may represent a reaction to ocular inflammation.

Atopic Keratoconjunctivitis

Atopic keratoconjunctivitis is a **chronic** inflammatory ocular disorder most commonly involving the lower tarsal conjunctiva. It may threaten eyesight if there is corneal involvement. Almost all patients have **atopic dermatitis,** and a significant number have asthma. Atopic keratoconjunctivitis rarely presents before late adolescence. Symptoms include severe bilateral ocular itching, burning, photophobia, and tearing with a mucoid discharge that are much more severe than in allergic conjunctivitis and persist through-out the year. The bulbar conjunctiva is injected and chemotic; cataracts may occur. Eyelid eczema can extend to the periorbital skin and cheeks with erythema and thick, dry scaling. Secondary staphylococcal blepharitis is common because of eyelid induration and maceration.

Giant Papillary Conjunctivitis

Giant papillary conjunctivitis has been linked to chronic exposure to foreign bodies, such as contact lenses, both hard and soft, ocular prostheses, and sutures. Symptoms and signs include mild bilateral ocular itching, tearing, a foreign body sensation, and excessive ocular discomfort with mild mucoid discharge with white or clear exudate on awakening, which may become thick and stringy. Trantas dots, limbal infiltration, bulbar conjunctival hyperemia, and edema may develop.

Contact Allergy

Contact allergy typically involves the eyelids but can also involve the conjunctivae. It is being recognized more frequently in association with increased exposure to topical medications, contact lens solutions, and preservatives.

DIAGNOSIS

Non-allergic conjunctivitis can be viral, bacterial, or chlamydial in origin. It is typically unilateral but can be bilateral with symptoms initially developing in one eye (Chapter 618). Symptoms include stinging or burning rather than itching and often a foreign body sensation. Ocular discharge can be watery, mucoid, or purulent. Masqueraders of ocular allergy also include nasolacrimal duct obstruction, foreign body, blepharoconjunctivitis, dry eye, uveitis, and trauma.

TREATMENT

Primary treatment of ocular allergies includes avoidance of allergens, cold compresses, and lubrication. Secondary treatment regimens include the use of oral or topical antihistamines (see Table 142-1) and, if necessary, topical decongestants, mast cell stabilizers, and anti-inflammatory agents (Table 141-1). Drugs with dual antihistamine and mast cell blocking activities provide the most advantageous approach in treating allergic conjunctivitis, with both fast-acting symptomatic relief and disease-modifying action. Children often complain of stinging or burning with use of topical ophthalmic preparations and usually prefer oral antihistamines for allergic conjunctivitis. It is important not to contaminate topical ocular medications by allowing the applicator tip to contact the eye or eyelid. Using refrigerated medications may decrease some of the discomfort associated with their use. Topical decongestants act as vasoconstrictors, reducing erythema, vascular congestion, and eyelid edema, but do not diminish the allergic response. Adverse effects of topical vasoconstrictors include burning or stinging and rebound hyperemia or conjunctivitis medicamentosa with chronic use. Combined use of an antihistamine and a vasoconstrictive agent is more effective than use of either agent alone. Use of topical nasal corticosteroids for allergic

Table 141-1 TOPICAL OPHTHALMIC MEDICATIONS FOR ALLERGIC CONJUNCTIVITIS

DRUG AND TRADE NAMES	MECHANISM OF ACTION AND DOSING	CAUTIONS AND ADVERSE EVENTS
Azelastine hydrochloride 0.05% Optivar	Antihistamine Children ≥3 yr: 1 gtt bid	Not for treatment of contact lens–related irritation; the preservative may be absorbed by soft contact lenses. Wait at least 10 min after administration before inserting soft contact lenses.
Emedastine difumarate 0.05% Emadine	Antihistamine Children ≥3 yr: 1 gtt qid	Soft contact lenses should not be worn if the eye is red. Wait at least 10 min after administration before inserting soft contact lenses.
Levocabastine hydrochloride 0.05% Livostin	Antihistamine Children ≥12 yr: 1 gtt bid-qid up to 2 wk	Not for use in patients wearing soft contact lenses during treatment.
Pheniramine maleate 0.3%/naphazoline hydrochloride 0.025% Naphcon-A, Opcon-A	Antihistamine/vasoconstrictor Children >6 yr: 1-2 gtt qid	Avoid prolonged use (>3-4 days) to avoid rebound symptoms. Not for use with contact lenses.
Cromolyn sodium 4% Crolom, Opticrom	Mast cell stabilizer Children >4 yr 1-2 gtt q4-6h	Can be used to treat giant papillary conjunctivitis and vernal keratitis. Not for use with contact lenses.
Lodoxamide tromethamine 0.1% Alomide	Mast cell stabilizer Children ≥2 yr: 1-2 gtt qid up to 3 mo	Can be used to treat vernal keratoconjunctivitis. Not for use in patients wearing soft contact lenses during treatment.
Nedocromil sodium 2% Alocril	Mast cell stabilizer Children ≥3 yr 1-2 gtt bid	Avoid wearing contact lenses while exhibiting the signs and symptoms of allergic conjunctivitis.
Pemirolast potassium 0.1% Alamast	Mast cell stabilizer Children >3 yr: 1-2 gtt qid	Not for treatment of contact lens related irritation; the preservative may be absorbed by soft contact lenses. Wait at least 10 min after administration before inserting soft contact lenses.
Epinastine hydrochloride 0.05% Elestat	Antihistamine/mast cell stabilizer Children ≥3 yr 1 gtt bid	Contact lenses should be removed prior to use. Wait at least 15 min after administration before inserting soft contact lenses. Not for the treatment of contact lens irritation.
Ketotifen fumarate 0.025% Zaditor	Antihistamine/mast cell stabilizer Children ≥3 yr 1 gtt bid q8-12h	Not for treatment of contact lens related irritation; the preservative may be absorbed by soft contact lenses. Wait at least 10 min after administration before inserting soft contact lenses.
Olopatadine hydrochloride 0.1%, 0.2% Patanol Pataday	Antihistamine/mast cell stabilizer Children ≥3 yr: 1 gtt bid (8 hr apart) 1 gtt q day	Not for treatment of contact lens related irritation; the preservative may be absorbed by soft contact lenses. Wait at least 10 min after administration before inserting soft contact lenses.
Ketorolac tromethamine 0.5% Acular	NSAID Children ≥3 yr: 1 gtt qid	Avoid with aspirin or NSAID sensitivity. Use ocular product with caution in patients with complicated ocular surgeries, corneal denervation or epithelial defects, ocular surface diseases (e.g., dry eye syndrome), repeated ocular surgeries within a short period of time, diabetes mellitus, or rheumatoid arthritis; these patients may be at risk for corneal adverse events that may be sight-threatening. Do not use while wearing contact lenses.

NSAID, nonsteroidal anti-inflammatory drug.

rhinoconjunctivitis decreases ocular symptoms, presumably through a naso-ocular reflex.

Tertiary treatment of ocular allergy includes topical or, rarely, oral corticosteroids and should be conducted in conjunction with an ophthalmologist. Local administration of topical corticosteroids may be associated with increased intraocular pressure, viral infections, and cataract formation. Allergen immunotherapy can be very effective in seasonal and perennial allergic conjunctivitis, especially when associated with rhinitis, and can decrease the need for oral or topical medications to control allergy symptoms.

BIBLIOGRAPHY

Please visit the Nelson Textbook of Pediatrics *website at* *www.expertconsult.com* *for the complete bibliography.*

Chapter 142
Urticaria (Hives) and Angioedema

Dan Atkins, Michael M. Frank, Stephen C. Dreskin, and Donald Y.M. Leung

Urticaria and angioedema affect 20% of individuals at some point in their lives. Episodes of hives that last for <6 wk are considered acute, whereas those that occur at least twice a week for >6 wk are designated chronic. The distinction is important, because the causes and mechanisms of urticaria formation and the therapeutic approaches are different in each instance.

ETIOLOGY AND PATHOGENESIS

Acute urticaria and angioedema are often caused by an allergic immunoglobulin (Ig) E–mediated reaction (Table 142-1). This form of urticaria is a self-limited process that occurs when an allergen activates mast cells in the skin. Systemically absorbed allergens that can induce generalized urticaria include foods, drugs (particularly antibiotics), and stinging insect venoms. If an allergen (latex, animal dander) penetrates the skin locally, hives can develop at the site of exposure. Acute urticaria can also result from non–IgE-mediated stimulation of mast cells, caused by radiocontrast agents, viral agents including hepatitis B and Epstein-Barr virus, opiates, and nonsteroidal anti-inflammatory agents. The diagnosis of chronic urticaria is established when lesions recur at least twice a week for > 6 wk and are not physical urticaria or recurrent acute urticaria with repeated exposures to a specific agent (Table 142-2). Often, chronic urticaria is accompanied by angioedema. Rarely, angioedema occurs without urticaria.

Urticaria can also be classified according to the temporal relationship with a stimulus and the duration of a typical hive. Lesions that last 1-2 hr are typical of the physical urticarias, in which an inciting stimulus is only briefly encountered. There is prompt mast cell degranulation, and biopsy of these lesions reveals little or no cellular infiltrate. A second form of urticaria

Table 142-1 ETIOLOGY OF ACUTE URTICARIA

Foods	Egg, milk, wheat, peanuts, tree nuts, soy, shellfish, fish, strawberries (direct mast cell degranulation)
Medications	Suspect all medications, even over-the-counter or homeopathic
Insect stings	Hymenoptera (honeybee, yellow jacket, hornets, wasp, fire ants), biting insects (papular urticaria)
Infections	Bacterial (streptococcal pharyngitis, *Mycoplasma*, sinusitis); viral (hepatitis, mononucleosis [Epstein-Barr virus], coxsackievirus A and B); parasitic *(Ascaris, Ancylostoma, Echinococcus, Fasciola, Filaria, Schistosoma, Strongyloides, Toxocara, Trichinella)*; fungal (dermatophytes, *Candida*)
Contact allergy	Latex, pollen, animal saliva, nettle plants, caterpillars
Transfusion reactions	Blood, blood products, or IV immunoglobulin administration

From Lasley MV, Kennedy MS, Altman LC: Urticaria and angioedema. In Altman LC, Becker JW, Williams PV, editors: *Allergy in primary care,* Philadelphia, 2000, WB Saunders, p 232.

Table 142-2 ETIOLOGY OF CHRONIC URTICARIA

Idiopathic	75-90% of chronic urticaria cases are idiopathic, and 35-40% have immunoglobulin (Ig) G, anti-IgE, and anti-FcεRI (high-affinity IgE receptor α chain) autoantibodies
Physical	Dermatographism
	Cholinergic urticaria
	Cold urticaria
	Delayed pressure urticaria
	Solar urticaria
	Vibratory urticaria
	Aquagenic urticaria
Rheumatologic	Systemic lupus erythematosus
	Juvenile rheumatoid arthritis
Endocrine	Hyperthyroidism
	Hypothyroidism
Neoplastic	Lymphoma
	Mastocytosis
	Leukemia
Angioedema	Hereditary angioedema (autosomal dominant inherited deficiency of C1-esterase inhibitor)
	Acquired angioedema
	Angiotensin-converting enzyme inhibitors

From Lasley MV, Kennedy MS, Altman LC: Urticaria and angioedema. In Altman LC, Becker JW, Williams PV, editors: *Allergy in primary care,* Philadelphia, 2000, WB Saunders, p 234.

can occur spontaneously and last 6-36 hr. These lesions typically have a prominent cellular infiltrate and can be found with food or drug reactions, chronic idiopathic urticaria, chronic autoimmune urticaria, and delayed pressure urticaria. Serum sickness reactions can be seen as a manifestation of drug reactions, and biopsy reveals a small-vessel cutaneous vasculitis. Urticaria in association with systemic lupus erythematosus or other vasculitides appears similar.

Atypical aspects of the gross appearance of the hives or associated symptoms should heighten concern that the urticaria or angioedema may be the manifestation of a systemic disease process. Lesions that burn more than itch, last >24 hr, do not blanch, or are associated with bleeding into the skin (purpura) suggest urticarial vasculitis.

PHYSICAL URTICARIA

Physically induced urticaria and angioedema share the common property of being induced by environmental factors, such as a change in temperature or direct stimulation of the skin with pressure, stroking, vibration, or light (Table 142-3).

Table 142-3 DIAGNOSTIC TESTING FOR URTICARIA AND ANGIOEDEMA

DIAGNOSIS	DIAGNOSTIC TESTING
Food and drug reactions	Elimination of offending agent, skin testing, and challenge with suspected foods
Autoimmune urticaria	Autologous serum skin test; anti-thyroid antibodies
Thyroiditis	Thyroid-stimulating hormone; anti-thyroid antibodies
Infections	Appropriate cultures or serology
Collagen vascular diseases and cutaneous vasculitis	Skin biopsy, CH_{50}, C1q, C4, C3, factor B, immunofluorescence of tissues, antinuclear antibodies, cryoglobulins
Malignancy with angioedema	CH_{50}, C1q, C4, C1-INH determinations
Cold urticaria	Ice cube test
Solar urticaria	Exposure to defined wavelengths of light, red blood cell protoporphyrin, fecal protoporphyrin, and coproporphyrin
Dermatographism	Stroking with narrow object (e.g., tongue blade, fingernail)
Pressure urticaria	Application of pressure for defined time and intensity
Vibratory urticaria	Vibration for 4 min
Aquagenic urticaria	Challenge with tap water at various temperatures
Urticaria pigmentosa	Skin biopsy, test for dermographism
Hereditary angioedema	C4, C2, CH_{50}, C1-INH testing by protein and function
Familial cold urticaria	Challenge by cold exposure, measurement of temperature, white blood cell count, erythrocyte sedimentation rate, and skin biopsy
C3b inactivator deficiency	C3, factor B, C3b inactivator determinations
Chronic idiopathic urticaria	Skin biopsy, immunofluorescence (negative result), autologous skin test

Cold-Dependent Disorders

Cold urticaria is characterized by the rapid onset of localized pruritus, erythema, and urticaria/angioedema after exposure to a cold stimulus. Total-body exposure as seen with swimming in cold water can cause massive release of vasoactive mediators, resulting in hypotension, loss of consciousness and even death if not promptly treated. The diagnosis is confirmed by challenge testing for an isomorphic cold reaction by holding an ice cube in place on the patient's skin for 4 min. In patients with cold urticaria, an urticarial lesion develops about 10 minutes after removal of the ice cube and upon rewarming of the chilled skin. Cold urticaria can be associated with the presence of **cryoproteins** such as cold agglutinins, cryoglobulins, cryofibrinogen, and the Donath-Landsteiner antibody seen in secondary syphilis (paroxysmal cold hemoglobinuria). In patients with cryoglobulins, the isolated proteins appear to transfer cold sensitivity and activate the complement cascade upon in vitro incubation with normal plasma. The term **idiopathic cold urticaria** generally applies to patients without abnormal circulating plasma proteins such as cryoglobulins. Cold urticaria has also been reported after viral infections. Cold urticaria must be distinguished from the **familial cold autoinflammatory syndrome** (see later).

Cholinergic Urticaria

Cholinergic urticaria is characterized by the onset of small punctate wheals surrounded by a prominent erythematous flare associated with exercise, hot showers, and sweating. Once the patient cools down, the rash usually subsides in 30-60 min. Occasionally, symptoms of more generalized cholinergic stimulation, such as lacrimation, wheezing, salivation, and syncope, are observed. These symptoms are mediated by cholinergic nerve fibers that innervate the musculature via parasympathetic neurons and innervate the sweat glands by cholinergic fibers that travel with the sympathetic nerves. Elevated plasma histamine values parallel the onset of urticaria triggered by changes in body temperature.

Dermatographism

The ability to write on skin, termed dermatographism (also called dermographism or urticaria factitia), occurs as an isolated disorder or accompanies chronic urticaria or other physical urticaria such as cholinergic and cold urticaria. It can be diagnosed by observing the skin after stroking it with a tongue depressor or fingernail. In patients with dermatographism, a linear response occurs secondary to reflex vasoconstriction, followed by pruritus, erythema, and a linear wheal.

Pressure-Induced Urticaria and Angioedema

Pressure-induced urticaria differs from most types of urticaria or angioedema in that symptoms typically occur 4-6 hr after pressure has been applied. The disorder is clinically heterogeneous. Some patients may complain of swelling secondary to pressure with normal-appearing skin (no urticaria), so the term *angioedema* is more appropriate. Other lesions are predominantly urticarial and may or may not be associated with significant swelling. When urticaria is present, an infiltrative skin lesion is seen, characterized by a perivascular mononuclear cell infiltrate and dermal edema similar to that seen in chronic idiopathic urticaria. Symptoms occur at sites of tight clothing; foot swelling is common after walking; and buttock swelling may be prominent after sitting for a few hours. This condition can coexist with chronic idiopathic urticaria or can occur separately. The diagnosis is confirmed by challenge testing in which pressure is applied perpendicular to the skin.

Solar Urticaria

Solar urticaria is a rare disorder in which urticaria develops within 1-3 min of sun exposure. Typically, pruritus occurs 1st, in about 30 sec, followed by edema confined to the light-exposed area and surrounded by a prominent erythematous zone caused by an axon reflex. The lesions usually disappear within 1-3 hr after cessation of sun exposure. When large areas of the body are exposed, systemic symptoms may occur, including hypotension and wheezing. Solar urticaria has been classified into 6 types, depending on (1) the wavelength of light that induces skin lesions and (2) the ability or inability to transfer the disorder passively with serum IgE. The rare inborn error of metabolism erythropoietic protoporphyria can be confused with solar urticaria because of the development of itching and burning of exposed skin immediately after sun exposure. In erythropoietic protoporphyria, fluorescence of ultraviolet-irradiated red blood cells can be demonstrated.

Aquagenic Urticaria

Patients with aquagenic urticaria demonstrate small wheals after contact with water, regardless of its temperature, and are thereby distinguishable from patients with cold urticaria or cholinergic urticaria. Direct application of a compress of water to the skin is used to test for the presence of aquagenic urticaria.

CHRONIC IDIOPATHIC URTICARIA AND ANGIOEDEMA

A common disorder of unknown origin, chronic idiopathic urticaria and angioedema is often associated with normal routine laboratory values and no evidence of systemic disease. Chronic urticaria does not appear to result from an allergic reaction. It differs from allergen-induced skin reactions or from physically induced urticaria in that histologic studies reveal a cellular infiltrate predominantly around small venules. Skin examination reveals infiltrative hives with palpably elevated borders, sometimes varying greatly in size and/or shape but generally being rounded.

Biopsy of the typical lesion reveals non-necrotizing, perivascular, mononuclear cellular infiltration. Many types of histopathologic processes can occur in the skin and manifest as urticaria. Patients with **hypocomplementemia** and **cutaneous vasculitis** can have urticaria and/or angioedema. Biopsy of these lesions in patients with urticaria, arthralgias, myalgias, and an elevated erythrocyte sedimentation rate (ESR) as manifestations of necrotizing venulitis can reveal fibrinoid necrosis with a predominantly neutrophilic infiltrate. Yet the urticarial lesions may be clinically indistinguishable from those seen in the more typical, nonvasculitis cases.

There is an increased association of chronic urticaria with the presence of antithyroid antibodies. Affected patients generally have antibodies to thyroglobulin or a microsomally derived antigen (peroxidase) even if they are euthyroid. The incidence of elevated thyroid antibodies in patients with chronic urticaria is ≈12%, compared with 3-6% in the general population. Although some patients show clinical reduction of the urticaria with thyroid replacement therapy, others do not. Therefore, many investigators believe that these are associated, parallel, autoimmune events, although some believe that thyroid autoimmunity is driving the urticaria. There is currently no strong evidence to support the latter hypothesis.

Thirty-five percent to 40% of patients with chronic urticaria have a positive **autologous skin test** (ASST) result: If serum from these patients is intradermally injected into their skin, a significant wheal and flare reaction develops. Such patients frequently have a complement-activating IgG antibody directed against the α subunit of the IgE receptor that can cross link the IgE receptor (α subunit) and degranulate mast cells and basophils. An additional 5-10% of patients with chronic urticaria have anti-IgE antibodies rather than an anti–IgE receptor antibody. These patients, classified as having autoimmune urticaria, tend to have a more severe clinical course than patients without evidence of autoantibodies, but the difference is not dramatic.

DIAGNOSIS

The diagnosis of both acute and chronic urticaria is primarily clinical and requires that the physician be aware of the various forms of urticaria.

Urticaria is transient, pruritic, erythematous, raised wheals, with flat tops and edema that may become tense and painful. The lesions may coalesce and form polycyclic, serpiginous, or annular lesions (Figs. 142-1 and 142-2). Individual lesions usually last 20 min to 3 hr, and rarely more than 24 hr. The lesions often disappear only to reappear at another site. **Angioedema** involves the deeper subcutaneous tissues in locations such as the eyelids, lips, tongue, genitals, and dorsum of the hands or feet.

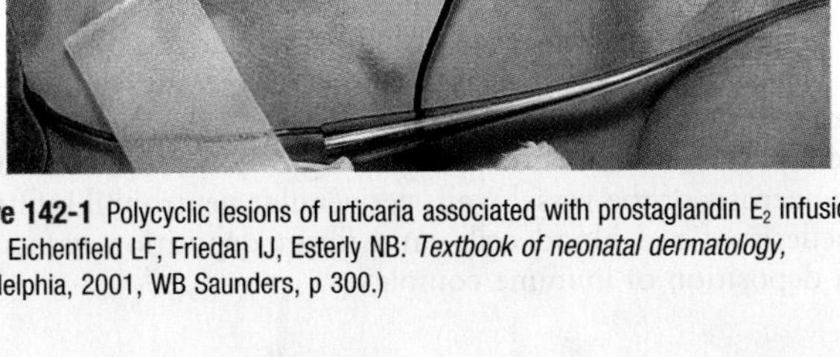

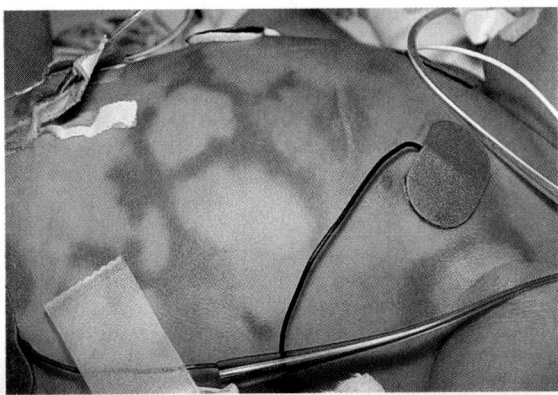

Figure 142-1 Polycyclic lesions of urticaria associated with prostaglandin E_2 infusion. (From Eichenfield LF, Friedan IJ, Esterly NB: *Textbook of neonatal dermatology,* Philadelphia, 2001, WB Saunders, p 300.)

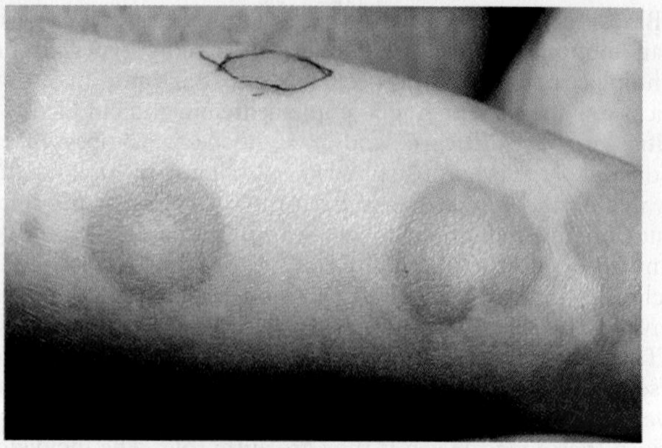

Figure 142-2 Annular urticaria of unknown etiology. (From Eichenfield LF, Friedan IJ, Esterly NB: *Textbook of neonatal dermatology,* Philadelphia, 2001, WB Saunders, p 301.)

Drugs and foods are the most common causes of acute urticaria. Allergy skin testing for foods can be helpful in sorting out causes of acute urticaria, especially when supported by historical evidence. The role of an offending food can then be proven by elimination and careful challenge in a controlled setting. In the absence of information implicating an ingestant cause, skin testing for foods and implementation of elimination diets are generally not useful for either acute or chronic urticaria. Skin testing for aeroallergens is not indicated unless there is a concern about contact urticaria (animal dander or grass pollen). Dermatographism is frequent in patients with urticaria and can complicate allergy skin testing by causing false-positive reactions, but this distinction is usually discernable.

An exogenous cause of chronic urticaria is rarely identified, reflecting an autoimmune or idiopathic etiology. An ASST is useful in establishing the diagnosis of autoimmune urticaria. In vitro testing for serum-derived activity that activates basophils involves detection of the expression of the surface marker CD63 or CD203c by donor basophils after incubation with patient serum. The clinical applicability and significance of these tests remains debated. The **differential diagnosis** of chronic urticaria includes cutaneous or systemic mastocytosis, complement-mediated disorders, malignancies, mixed connective tissue diseases, and cutaneous blistering disorders (e.g., bullous pemphigoid) (see Table 142-2). In general, laboratory testing should be limited to a complete blood cell count with differential, ESR determination, urinalysis, thyroid autoantibody testing, and liver function tests. Further studies are warranted if the patient has fever, arthralgias, or elevated ESR (see Table 142-3). Hereditary angioedema, a potentially life-threatening form of angioedema associated with deficient C1 inhibitor activity, is the most important familial form of angioedema (Chapter 128.3), but is not associated with typical urticaria. In patients with eosinophilia, stools should be obtained for ova and parasite testing, because infection with helminthic parasites has been associated with urticaria. A syndrome of episodic angioedema/urticaria and fever with associated eosinophilia has been described in both adults and children. In contrast to other hypereosinophilic syndromes, this entity has a benign course.

Skin biopsy for diagnosis of possible **urticarial vasculitis** is recommended for urticarial lesions that persist at the same location for >24 hr, those with pigmented or purpuric components, and those that burn more than itch. Collagen vascular diseases such as systemic lupus may manifest urticarial vasculitis as a presenting feature. The skin biopsy in urticarial vasculitis typically shows endothelial cell swelling of postcapillary venules with necrosis of the vessel wall, perivenular neutrophil infiltrate, diapedesis of red blood cells, and fibrin deposition associated with deposition of immune complexes.

Mastocytosis is characterized by mast cell hyperplasia in the bone marrow, liver, spleen, lymph nodes, and skin. Clinical effects of mast cell activation are common, including pruritus, flushing, urtication, abdominal pain, nausea, and vomiting. The diagnosis is confirmed by a bone marrow biopsy showing increased numbers of spindle-shaped mast cells that express CD2 and CD25. **Urticaria pigmentosa** is the most common skin manifestation of mastocytosis and may occur as an isolated skin finding. It appears as small, yellow-tan to reddish brown macules or raised papules that urticate on scratching **(Darier sign).** This sign can be masked by antihistamines. The diagnosis is confirmed by a skin biopsy that shows increased numbers of dermal mast cells.

Physical urticaria should be considered in any patient with chronic urticaria and a suggestive history (see Table 142-3). Papular urticaria commonly occurs in small children, generally on the extremities. It manifests as grouped or linear, highly pruritic wheals or papules mainly on exposed skin at the sites of insect bites.

Exercise-induced anaphylaxis manifests as varying combinations of pruritus, urticaria, angioedema, wheezing, laryngeal obstruction, or hypotension after exercise (Chapter 143). Cholinergic urticaria is differentiated by positive results of heat challenge tests and the rare occurrence of anaphylactic shock. The combination of ingestion of various food allergens (shrimp, celery, or wheat) and postprandial exercise has been associated with urticaria/angioedema and anaphylaxis. In patients with this combination disorder, food or exercise alone does not produce the reaction.

Muckle-Wells syndrome and **familial cold autoinflammatory syndrome (FCAS)** are rare, dominantly inherited conditions associated with recurrent urticaria-like lesions. Muckle-Wells syndrome is characterized by arthritis and limb pain that usually appears in adolescence. It is associated with progressive nerve deafness, recurrent fever, elevated ESR, hypergammaglobulinemia, renal amyloidosis, and a poor prognosis. FCAS is characterized by a cold-induced rash that has urticarial features but is rarely pruritic. Cold exposure leads to additional symptoms such as conjunctivitis, sweating, headache, and nausea. Patient longevity is usually normal.

TREATMENT

Acute urticaria is a self-limited illness requiring little treatment other than antihistamines and avoidance of any identified provocateur. Hydroxyzine and diphenhydramine are sedating but are effective and commonly used for treatment of urticaria. Loratadine, fexofenadine, and cetirizine are also effective and are preferable because of reduced frequency of drowsiness and longer duration of action (Table 142-4). Epinephrine 1:1,000, 0.01 mL/kg (maximum: 0.3 mL) usually provides rapid relief of acute, severe urticaria/angioedema but is seldom required. A short course of oral corticosteroids should be given only for very severe episodes of urticaria and angioedema that are unresponsive to antihistamines.

Most forms of physical urticaria respond to avoidance of triggering stimuli in combination with oral antihistamines. The exception is delayed pressure urticaria, which often requires oral corticosteroids. Cyproheptadine in divided doses is the drug of choice for cold-induced urticaria. Treatment of dermatographism consists of local skin care and antihistamines; for severe symptoms, high doses may be needed. The initial objective of therapy is to decrease pruritus so that the stimulation for scratching is diminished. A combination of antihistamines, sunscreens, and avoidance of sunlight is helpful for most patients.

Chronic urticaria only rarely responds favorably to dietary manipulation. Removal of recognized urticarial aggravators such as salicylates and β-blockers should be considered. The mainstay of therapy is the use of nonsedating or low-sedating H_1 antihistamines. In those patients not showing response to standard

Table 142-4 TREATMENT OF UTICARIA AND ANGIOEDEMA

CLASS/DRUG	DOSE	FREQUENCY
ANTIHISTAMINES, TYPE H_1 (2ND GENERATION)		
Fexofenadine	6-11 yr: 30 mg	bid
	>12 yr: 60 mg	
	Adult: 180 mg	Once daily
Loratadine	2-5 yr: 5 mg	Once daily
	>6 yr: 10 mg	
Desloratadine	6-11 mo: 1 mg	Once daily
	1-5 yr: 1.25 mg	
	6-11 yr: 2.5 mg	
	>12 yr: 5 mg	
Cetirizine	6-24 mo: 2.5 mg	6-12 mo: once daily
	2-6 yr: 2.5-5 mg	12-24 mo: 1-2 daily
	>6 yr: 5-10 mg	2-12 yr: once daily
ANTIHISTAMINES, TYPE H_2		
Cimetidine	Infants: 10-20 mg/kg/day	Divided q6-12h
	Children: 20-40 mg/kg/day	
Ranitidine	1 mo-16 yr: 5-10 mg/kg/day	Divided q12h
Famotidine	3-12 mo: 1 mg/kg/day	Divided q12h
	1-16 yr: 1-2 mg/kg/day	
LEUKOTRIENE PATHWAY MODIFIERS		
Montelukast	12 mo-5 yr: 4 mg	Once daily
	6-14 yr: 5 mg	
	>14 yr: 10 mg	
Zafirlukast	5-11 yr: 10 mg	bid
IMMUNOMODULATORY DRUGS		
Cyclosporine	4-6 mg/kg/day	Once daily*
Sulfasalazine	>6 yr: 30 mg/kg/day	Divided q6h†
Intravenous immunoglobulin (IVIG)	400 mg/kg/day	5 consecutive days

*Monitor blood pressure and serum creatinine, potassium, and magnesium levels monthly.
†Monitor complete blood count and liver function tests at baseline, every 2 wk for 3 mo, and then every 1-3 mo.

doses, pushing the H_1 blockade with higher than the usual recommended doses of these agents is a common next approach. The combined use of H_1- and H_2 antihistamines is sometimes helpful to control chronic urticaria when H_1-type antihistamines alone at higher than standard doses do not work (see Table 142-4). Doxepin is an antagonist of both H_1 and H_2 receptors and can be helpful, but its usefulness is limited by adverse effects. H_2-type antihistamines alone may exacerbate urticaria. Antileukotriene agents in combination with antihistamines are occasionally helpful. If hives persist after maximal H_1- and/or H_2-receptor blockade has been achieved, a brief course of oral corticosteroids may be considered, but long-term steroid use is best avoided. Treatment with cyclosporine 4-6 mg/kg/day has been effective in some adults with chronic urticaria but its use is limited by hypertension and/or nephrotoxicity. Immunomodulatory agents that have been used but remain to be formally proven effective include hydroxychloroquine, sulfasalazine, colchicine, dapsone, mycophenylate and omalizumab (anti-IgE), intravenous immunoglobulin, and plasmapheresis have been used to treat autoimmune chronic urticaria refractory to other therapies.

HEREDITARY ANGIOEDEMA

Hereditary angioedema (HAE) is an inherited disease caused by low levels of the plasma protein C1 inhibitor (C1-INH) (Chapter 128). Patients typically report episodic attacks of angioedema or deep localized swelling, most commonly on a hand or foot, that begin during childhood and become much more severe during adolescence. Cutaneous nonpitting and nonpruritic edema not associated with urticaria is the most common symptom. Patients usually have a prodrome, a tightness or tingling in the area that will swell, lasting most frequently for several hours, followed by the development of angioedema. The swelling usually becomes more severe over about 10 days and then resolves over about the same period. In some patients attacks are preceded by the development of a rash that is erythematous, not raised, and not pruritic. The second major symptom complex noted by patients is attacks of severe abdominal pain caused by edema of the mucosa of any portion of the gastrointestinal tract. The intensity of the pain can approximate that of an acute abdomen, often resulting in unnecessary surgery. Either constipation or diarrhea during these attacks can be noted. The gastrointestinal edema generally follows the same time course to resolution as the cutaneous attacks.

Laryngeal edema, the most feared complication of HAE, can cause complete respiratory obstruction. Although life-threatening attacks are infrequent, more than half of patients with HAE experience laryngeal involvement at some time during their lives. Dental work with the injection of procaine HCL (Novocain) into the gums is a common precipitant, but laryngeal edema can be spontaneous. The clinical condition may deteriorate rapidly, progressing through mild discomfort to complete airway obstruction over a period of hours. Soft tissue edema can be readily seen when the disease involves the throat and uvula. If this edema progresses to difficulty swallowing secretions or a change in the tone of the voice, the patient may require emergency intubation or even tracheostomy to ensure an adequate airway. Other presentations are less common.

In most cases the cause of the attack is unknown, but in some patients trauma or emotional stress clearly precipitates attacks. In some females menstruation also regularly induces attacks. The frequency of attacks varies greatly among affected individuals and at different times in the same individual. Some individuals experience weekly episodes, whereas others may go years between attacks. Episodes can start at any age.

C1-INH is a member of the serpin family of proteases, similar to α-antitrypsin, antithrombin III, and angiotensinogen. These proteins stoichiometrically inactivate their target proteases by forming stable, one-to-one complexes with the protein to be inhibited. Synthesized primarily by hepatocytes, C1-INH is also synthesized by monocytes. The regulation of the protein production is not completely understood, but it is believed that androgens may stimulate C1-INH synthesis, because patients with the disorder respond clinically to androgen therapy with raised serum levels of C1-INH. C1-INH deficiency is an autosomal dominant disease, with as many as 25% of patients giving no family history. Because all C1-INH–deficient patients are heterozygous for this gene defect, it is believed that half the normal level of C1-INH is not sufficient to prevent attacks.

Although named for its action on the first component of complement (C1 esterase), C1-INH also inhibits components of the fibrinolytic, clotting, and kinin pathways. Specifically, C1-INH inactivates plasmin-activated Hageman factor (factor XII), activated factor XI, plasma thromboplastin antecedent, and kallikrein. Within the complement system, C1-INH blocks the activation of C1 and the rest of the classic complement pathway by binding to C1r and C1s. Without C1-INH, unchecked activation of C1 causes cleavage of C4 and C2, the following proteins in the complement cascade. Levels of C3 are normal. The major factor responsible for the edema formation is now known to be bradykinin, an important nonapeptide mediator that can induce leakage of post-capillary venules. Bradykinin is derived from cleavage of the circulating protein high molecular weight kininogen by the plasma enzyme kallikrein.

Two genetic types of C1-INH deficiency are described that result in essentially the same phenotypic expression. The C1-INH gene is located on chromosome 11 in the p11-q13 region. The inheritance is autosomal dominant with incomplete penetrance.

Persons inheriting the abnormal gene can have a clinical spectrum ranging from asymptomatic to severely affected. Type 1 HAE is the most common form, accounting for approximately 85% of cases. Synthesis of C1-INH is blocked at the site of the faulty allele but occurs at the normal allele. The result is transcription of the normal protein, yielding quantitative serum concentrations of C1-INH that are approximately 10-40% of normal. Type 2 HAE accounts for approximately 15% of cases. Mutations near the active site of the inhibitor lead to synthesis of nonfunctional C1-INH protein. Patients with type 2 HAE have either normal or increased concentrations of the protein.

A clinical syndrome resembling HAE and termed type 3 HAE has been described that affects mostly women. In this condition, no abnormalities of complement or of C1-INH have been described, but one third of affected patients have been found to have a gain-of-function abnormality of clotting factor XII.

In the USA, 3 treatment regimens are used for prophylaxis of attacks, but no treatment is currently approved by the U.S. Food and Drug Administration (FDA) for treatment of acute attacks. Impeded androgens like the gonadotropin inhibitor danazol have been found to reliably prevent attacks in the vast majority of patients. Impeded or weak androgens have many side affects that preclude their use in some patients. Their use in children is problematic because of the possibility of premature closure of the epiphyses, and these agents are not used in pregnant women. The fibrinolysis inhibitor ε-aminocaproic acid is effective in preventing attacks and is often used in children, but its use is attended by the development of severe fatigue and muscle weakness over time.

Purified C1-INH prepared from human plasma has been approved for prophylaxis of this disease, but the half-life of this protein is short, on the order of 40 hr. In clinical trials it was given IV two to three times a week. Plasma C1 inhibitor, recombinant C1 inhibitor, a kallikrein antagonist called ecallantide, and a bradykinin type 2 receptor antagonist called Firazyr have all been reported to be effective in the treatment of acute attacks in preliminary double blind studies and are in various stages of review by the FDA.

BIBLIOGRAPHY

Please visit the Nelson Textbook of Pediatrics *website at www.expertconsult.com for the complete bibliography.*

Chapter 143
Anaphylaxis

Hugh A. Sampson and Donald Y.M. Leung

Anaphylaxis is defined as a serious allergic reaction that is rapid in onset and may cause death. Anaphylaxis in children, particularly infants, is frequently underdiagnosed. It occurs when there is a sudden release of potent biologically active mediators from mast cells and basophils, leading to cutaneous (urticaria, angioedema, flushing), respiratory (bronchospasm, laryngeal edema), cardiovascular (hypotension, dysrhythmias, myocardial ischemia), and gastrointestinal (nausea, colicky abdominal pain, vomiting, diarrhea) symptoms.

ETIOLOGY

The most common causes of anaphylaxis in children are different for hospital and community settings. Anaphylaxis occurring in the hospital results primarily from allergic reactions to medications and latex. Food allergy is the most common cause of anaphylaxis occurring outside the hospital, accounting for about one half of the anaphylactic reactions reported in pediatric surveys from the USA, Italy, and South Australia (Table 143-1). Peanut allergy is an important cause of food-induced anaphylaxis, accounting for the majority of fatal and near-fatal reactions. In the hospital, latex is a particular problem for children undergoing multiple operations, such as patients with spina bifida and urologic disorders, and has prompted many hospitals to switch to latex-free products. Patients with latex allergy may also experience food-allergic reactions from homologous proteins in foods such as bananas, kiwi, avocado, chestnut, and passion fruit.

Table 143-1 COMMON CAUSES OF ANAPHYLAXIS IN CHILDREN*

Food: peanuts, tree nuts (walnut, hazelnut, cashew, pistachio, Brazil nut), milk, eggs, fish, shellfish (shrimp, crab, lobster, clam, scallop, oyster), seeds (sesame, cottonseed, pine nuts, psyllium), fruits (apples, banana, kiwi, peaches, oranges, melon), grains (wheat)
Drugs: penicillins, cephalosporins, sulfonamides, nonsteroidal anti-inflammatory agents, opiates, muscle relaxants, vancomycin, dextran, thiamine, vitamin B_{12}, insulin, thiopental, local anesthetics
Hymenoptera venom: honeybee, yellow jacket, wasp, hornet, fire ant
Latex
Allergen immunotherapy
Exercise: food-specific exercise, postprandial (non–food-specific) exercise
Vaccinations: tetanus, measles, mumps, influenza
Miscellaneous: radiocontrast media, gamma globulin, cold temperature, chemotherapeutic agents (asparaginase, cyclosporine, methotrexate, vincristine, 5-fluorouracil), blood products, inhalants (dust and storage mites, grass pollen)
Idiopathic

*In order of frequency.
From Leung DYM, Sampson HA, Geha RS, et al: *Pediatric allergy principles and practice*, St Louis, 2003, Mosby, p 644.

EPIDEMIOLOGY

The overall annual incidence of anaphylaxis in the United States is estimated at 50 cases/100,000 persons/yr, totaling >150,000 cases/yr. An Australian parental survey found that 0.59% of children 3-17 yr of age had experienced at least 1 anaphylactic event.

PATHOGENESIS

Principal pathologic features in fatal anaphylaxis include acute pulmonary hyperinflation, pulmonary edema, intra-alveolar hemorrhaging, visceral congestion, laryngeal edema, and urticaria and angioedema. Acute hypotension is attributed to vasomotor dilation and/or cardiac dysrhythmias.

Most cases of anaphylaxis are the result of activation of mast cells and basophils via cell-bound allergen-specific IgE molecules. Patients initially must be exposed to the responsible allergen to generate allergen-specific antibodies. In many cases, the child and the parent are unaware of the initial exposure, which may be due to passage of food proteins in maternal breast milk. When the child is reexposed to the sensitizing allergen, mast cells and basophils and possibly other cells such as macrophages release a variety of mediators (histamine, tryptase) and cytokines that can produce allergic symptoms in any or all target organs. Clinical anaphylaxis may also be caused by mechanisms other than IgE-mediated reactions, sometimes termed **anaphylactoid reactions**, including direct release of mediators from mast cells by medications and physical factors (morphine, exercise, cold), disturbances of leukotriene metabolism (aspirin and nonsteroidal anti-inflammatory drugs), immune aggregates and complement activation (blood products), and probable complement activation (radiocontrast dyes, dialysis membranes).

CLINICAL MANIFESTATIONS AND DIAGNOSIS

The onset of symptoms may vary somewhat depending on the cause of the reaction. Reactions from ingested allergens (foods, medications) are delayed in onset (minutes to 2 hr) compared with those from injected allergens (insect sting, medications) and tend to have more gastrointestinal symptoms. Initial symptoms vary with the etiology and may include any of the following constellation of symptoms: pruritus about the mouth and face; a sensation of warmth, weakness, and apprehension (sense of doom); flushing, urticaria and angioedema, oral or cutaneous pruritus, tightness in the throat, dry staccato cough and hoarseness, periocular pruritus, nasal congestion, sneezing, dyspnea, deep cough and wheezing; nausea, abdominal cramping, and vomiting, especially with ingested allergens; uterine contractions (manifesting as lower back pain; not uncommon); and faintness and loss of consciousness in severe cases. Some degree of obstructive laryngeal edema is typically encountered with severe reactions. Cutaneous symptoms may be absent in up to 20% of cases, and the acute onset of severe bronchospasm in a previously well asthmatic person should suggest the diagnosis of anaphylaxis. Sudden collapse in the absence of cutaneous symptoms should also raise suspicion of vasovagal collapse, myocardial infarction, aspiration, pulmonary embolism, or seizure disorder. Laryngeal edema, especially with abdominal pain, suggests hereditary angioedema (Chapter 142).

LABORATORY FINDINGS

Laboratory studies may indicate the presence of IgE antibodies to a suspected causative agent, but this result is not definitive. Plasma histamine is elevated for a brief period but is unstable and difficult to measure in a clinical setting. **Plasma β-tryptase** is more stable and remains elevated for several hours but often is not elevated, especially in food-induced anaphylactic reactions.

DIAGNOSIS

A National Institutes of Health (NIH)–sponsored expert panel has recommended an approach to the diagnosis of anaphylaxis (Table 143-2). The differential diagnosis includes other forms of shock (hemorrhagic, cardiogenic, septic), vasopressor reactions including flush syndromes such as carcinoid syndrome, excess histamine syndromes (systemic mastocytosis), and ingestion of monosodium glutamate (MSG), scombroidosis, and heriditary angioedema. In addition, panic attack, vocal cord dysfunction, pheochromocytoma, and red man syndrome (due to vancomycin) should be considered.

Table 143-2 DIAGNOSIS OF ANAPHYLAXIS

Anaphylaxis is highly likely when any *one* of the following three criteria is fulfilled:

1. Acute onset of an illness (minutes to several hours) with involvement of the skin and/or mucosal tissue (e.g., *generalized* hives, pruritus or flushing, swollen lips/tongue/uvula)

   AND AT LEAST ONE OF THE FOLLOWING:

   a. Respiratory compromise (e.g., dyspnea, wheeze/bronchospasm, stridor, reduced peak PEF, hypoxemia)
   b. Reduced BP or associated symptoms of end-organ dysfunction (e.g., hypotonia [collapse], syncope, incontinence)
2. Two or more of the following that occur rapidly after exposure *to a* ***likely*** *allergen for that patient* (minutes to several hours):
   a. Involvement of the skin/mucosal tissue (e.g., *generalized* hives, itch/flush, swollen lips/tongue/uvula)
   b. Respiratory compromise (e.g., dyspnea, wheeze/bronchospasm, stridor, reduced PEF, hypoxemia)
   c. Reduced BP or associated symptoms (e.g., hypotonia [collapse], syncope, incontinence)
   d. *Persistent* gastrointestinal symptoms (e.g., crampy abdominal pain, vomiting)
3. Reduced BP following exposure to ***known*** *allergen for that patient* (minutes to several hours):
   a. Infants and children: low systolic BP (age-specific) or >30% drop in systolic BP
   b. Adults: systolic BP <90 mm Hg or >30% drop from patient's baseline

BP, blood pressure; PEF, peak expiratory flow.
Modified from Sampson HA, Muñoz-Furlong A, Campbell RL, et al: Second symposium on the definition and management of anaphylaxis: summary report. Second National Institute of Allergy and Infectious Disease/Food Allergy and Anaphylaxis Network symposium, *J Allergy Clin Immunol* 117:391–397, 2006.

TREATMENT

Anaphylaxis is a medical emergency requiring aggressive management with **intramuscular** or intravenous epinephrine, intramuscular or intravenous H_1 and H_2 antihistamine antagonists, oxygen, intravenous fluids, inhaled β-agonists, and corticosteroids (Table 143-3). The initial assessment should ensure an adequate airway with effective respiration, circulation, and perfusion. Epinephrine is the most important medication, and there should be no delay in its administration. If an intravenous line is not available, epinephrine should be given by the intramuscular route (0.01 mg/kg; max 0.3-0.5 mg). For children ≥12 yr, many recommend the 0.5-mg intramuscular dose. The intramuscular dose can be repeated 2 or 3 times at intervals of 5 to 15 minutes if an intravenous continuous epinephrine infusion has not yet been started and symptoms persist. Intraosseous infusion is an alternative if an intravenous line is not available (this is an uncommon route). Fluids are also important in patients with shock. Other drugs (antihistamines, glucocorticosteroids) have a secondary role in the management of anaphylaxis. Patients may experience **biphasic anaphylaxis,** which occurs when anaphylactic symptoms recur after apparent resolution. The mechanism of this phenomenon is unknown, but it appears to be more common when therapy is initiated late and symptoms at presentation are more severe. It does not appear to be affected by the administration of corticosteroids during the initial therapy. More than 90% of biphasic responses occur within 4 hr, so patients should be observed for at least 4 hr before being discharged from the emergency department.

PREVENTION

Patients experiencing anaphylactic reactions to foods must be educated in allergen avoidance, including actively reading food labels and acquiring knowledge of potential contamination and high-risk situations, as well as in the early recognition of anaphylactic symptoms and ready administration of emergency medications. Any child with food allergy and a history of asthma, peanut or tree nut allergy, or a previous severe anaphylactic reaction should be given an epinephrine autoinjector (EpiPen, Twinject), liquid cetirizine (or alternatively, diphenhydramine), and a written emergency plan in case of accidental ingestion. A form can be downloaded from the Food Allergy and Anaphylaxis Network at www.foodallergy.org. Patients with egg allergy should be tested before receiving the influenza or yellow fever vaccine, which contain egg protein.

Children experiencing a systemic anaphylactic reaction including respiratory symptoms to an insect sting should be evaluated and treated with immunotherapy, which is more than 90% protective. In cases of food-associated exercise-induced anaphylaxis, children must not exercise within 2-3 hr of ingesting the triggering food and, like children with exercise-induced anaphylaxis, should exercise with a friend, learn to recognize the early signs of anaphylaxis (sensation of warmth and facial pruritus), stop exercising, and seek help immediately if symptoms develop. Any child who is at risk for anaphylaxis should receive emergency medications, education, and a written emergency plan in case of accidental ingestion.

Reactions to medications can be reduced and minimized by using oral medications in preference to injected forms. Hypo-osmolar radiocontrast dyes can be used in patients in

Table 143-3 MANAGEMENT OF A PATIENT WITH ANAPHYLAXIS

DRUG CLASSIFICATION	INDICATION(S) AND DOSAGE(S)	COMMENTS; ADVERSE REACTIONS
PATIENT EMERGENCY MANAGEMENT (DEPENDENT ON SEVERITY OF SYMPTOMS)		
Epinephrine (adrenaline)	Rx of anaphylaxis, bronchospasm, cardiac arrest	Tachycardia, hypertension, nervousness, headache, nausea, irritability, and tremor
0.01 mg/kg up to 0.3 mg	EpiPen Jr (0.15 mg) IM 8-25 kg Twinject Jr (0.15 mg) IM	
	EpiPen (0.3 mg) IM >25 kg Twinject (0.3 mg)	
Cetirizine (liquid)	Antihistamine (competitive of H_1 receptor)	Hypotension, tachycardia, and somnolence
(Zyrtec—5 mg/5 mL)	0.25 mg/kg up to 10 mg PO	
Alt: Diphenhydramine	Antihistamine (competitive of H_1 receptor)	Hypotension, tachycardia, somnolence, and paradoxical excitement
(Benadryl—12.5mg/5mL)	1.25 mg/kg up to 50 mg PO	
Transport **to an Emergency Facility**		
EMERGENCY PERSONNEL MANAGEMENT (DEPENDENT ON SEVERITY OF SYMPTOMS)		
Supplemental oxygen and airway management		
Epinephrine (adrenaline)	Rx of anaphylaxis, bronchospasm, cardiac arrest	Tachycardia, hypertension, nervousness, headache, nausea, irritability, and tremor
0.01 mg/kg up to 0.3 mg	EpiPen Jr (0.15 mg) IM 8-25 kg	May repeat every 10-15 min
	EpiPen (0.3 mg) IM >25 kg	
	0.01 mL/kg/dose of 1:1,000 solution up to 0.3 mL IM	
	0.01 mL/kg/dose of 1:10,000 slow IV push	For severe hypotension
Volume expanders		
Crystalloids (normal saline or Ringer lactate)	30 mL/kg in 1st hour	Rate titrated against blood pressure response
Colloids (hydroxyethyl starch)	10 mL/kg rapidly followed by slow infusion	Rate titrated against blood pressure response
Diphenhydramine (Benadryl—12.5 mg/5 mL)	Antihistamine (competitive of H_1 receptor)	Hypotension, tachycardia, somnolence, and paradoxical excitement
	1.25 mg/kg up to 50 mg IM	
Alt: Cetirizine [liquid] (Zyrtec—5 mg/5 mL)	Antihistamine (competitive of H_1 receptor)	Hypotension, tachycardia, and somnolence
Nebulized albuterol	β-Agonist	Palpitations, nervousness, central nervous system stimulation, tachycardia; use to supplement epinephrine when bronchospasm appears unresponsive; may repeat
	(0.83 mg/mL [3 mL]) via mask with O_2	
Corticosteroids:		
Methylprednisolone	Anti-inflammatory	Hypertension, edema, nervousness, and agitation
Solu-Medrol (IV)	1-2 mg/kg up to 125 mg IV	
Depo-Medrol (IM)	1 mg/kg up to 80 mg IM	
Prednisone	Anti-inflammatory	Hypertension, edema, nervousness, and agitation
For oral use	1 mg/kg up to 75 mg PO	
Ranitidine (Zantac—25 mg/mL)	Antihistamine (competitive of H_2 receptor)	Headache, mental confusion
	1 mg/kg up to 50 mg IV	Should be administered slowly
Alt: Cimetidine (Tagamet—25 mg/mL)	Antihistamine (competitive of H_2 receptor) 4 mg/kg up to 200 mg IV	Headache, mental confusion Should be administered slowly
POST-EMERGENCY MANAGEMENT		
H_1-antagonist	Cetirizine (5-10 mg qd) or loratidine (5-10 mg qd) for 3 days	
Corticosteroids	Oral prednisone (1 mg/kg up to 75 mg) daily for 3 days	
Preventive Treatment		
Follow-up evaluation to determine/confirm etiology		
Immunotherapy for insect sting allergy		
Prescription for EpiPen and antihistamine		
Provide written plan outlining patient emergency management (may download form from *www.foodallergy.org*)		
Patient Education		
Instruction on avoidance of causative agent		
Information on recognizing early signs of anaphylaxis		
Stress early treatment of allergic symptoms to avoid systemic anaphylaxis		

IM, intramuscularly; IV, intravenously; PO, by mouth.

whom previous reactions are suspected. The use of powder-free, low-allergen latex gloves or non-latex gloves and materials should be used in children undergoing multiple operations.

BIBLIOGRAPHY

Please visit the Nelson Textbook of Pediatrics *website at* *www.expertconsult.com* *for the complete bibliography.*

Chapter 144
Serum Sickness

Scott H. Sicherer and Donald Y.M. Leung

Serum sickness is a systemic, immune complex–mediated hypersensitivity vasculitis classically attributed to the therapeutic administration of foreign serum proteins.

ETIOLOGY

Immune complexes involving heterologous (animal) serum proteins and complement activation are important pathogenic mechanisms in serum sickness. Antibody therapies derived from the horse are available for treatment of envenomation by the black widow spider and a variety of snakes, for treatment of botulism, and for immunosuppression (antithymocyte globulin). The availability of alternative medical therapies, modified or bioengineered antibodies, and biologics of human origin have supplanted the use of nonhuman antisera, reducing the risk of serum sickness. Reactions described as "serum sickness–like" are often attributed to drug allergy, triggered in particular by antibiotics (e.g., cefaclor). In contrast to a true immunologic reaction, serum sickness–like reactions do not exhibit the immune complexes, hypocomplementemia, vasculitis, and renal lesions that are seen in serum sickness reactions.

PATHOGENESIS

Serum sickness is a classic example of a type III hypersensitivity reaction caused by antigen-antibody complexes. In the rabbit model using bovine serum albumin as the antigen, symptoms develop with the appearance of antibody against the injected antigen. As free antigen concentration falls and antibody production increases over days, antigen-antibody complexes of various sizes develop in a manner analogous to a precipitin curve. Whereas small complexes usually circulate harmlessly and large complexes are cleared by the reticuloendothelial system, intermediate-sized complexes that develop at the point of slight antigen excess may deposit in blood vessel walls and tissues. There the immune microprecipitates induce vascular and tissue damage through activation of complement and granulocytes.

Complement activation (C3a, C5a) promotes chemotaxis and adherence of neutrophils to the site of immune complex deposition. The processes of immune complex deposition and of neutrophil accumulation may be facilitated by increased vascular permeability, owing to the release of vasoactive amines from tissue mast cells. Mast cells may be activated by binding of antigen to immunoglobulin (Ig) E or through contact with anaphylatoxins (C3a). Tissue injury results from the liberation of proteolytic enzymes and oxygen radicals from the neutrophils.

CLINICAL MANIFESTATIONS

The symptoms of serum sickness generally begin 7-12 days after injection of the foreign material but may appear as late as 3 wk afterward. The onset of symptoms may be accelerated if there has been earlier exposure or previous allergic reaction to the same antigen. A few days before the onset of generalized symptoms, the site of injection may become edematous and erythematous. Symptoms usually include fever, malaise, and rashes (Chapter 637.1). Urticaria and morbilliform rashes are the predominant types of skin eruptions, and pruritus is common. In a prospective study of serum sickness induced by administration of equine antithymocyte globulin, an initial rash was noted in most patients. It began as a thin serpiginous band of erythema along the sides of the hands, fingers, feet, and toes at the junction of the palmar or plantar skin with the skin of the dorsolateral surface. In most patients, the band of erythema was replaced by petechiae or purpura, presumably because of low platelet counts or local damage to small blood vessels. Additional symptoms include edema, myalgia, lymphadenopathy, arthralgia or arthritis involving multiple joints, and gastrointestinal complaints, including pain, nausea, diarrhea, and melena. The disease generally runs a self-limited course, with recovery in 1-2 wk. Carditis, glomerulonephritis, Guillain-Barré syndrome, and peripheral neuritis are rare complications. Serum sickness–like reactions from drugs are characterized by fever, pruritus, urticaria, and arthralgias that usually begin 1-3 wk after drug exposure. The urticarial skin eruption becomes increasingly erythematous as the reaction progresses and can evolve into dusky centers with round plaques.

DIAGNOSIS

Circulating immune complexes are usually detectable, with peak levels at 10-12 days. Serum complement levels (C3 and C4) are generally decreased and reach a nadir at about day 10. C3a anaphylatoxin may be increased. The erythrocyte sedimentation rate (ESR) is usually elevated, and thrombocytopenia is often present. Mild proteinuria, hemoglobinuria, and microscopic hematuria may be seen. Direct immunofluorescence studies of skin lesions often reveal immune deposits of IgM, IgA, IgE, or C3.

TREATMENT

Treatment is primarily supportive, consisting of antihistamines and analgesics. When the symptoms are especially severe, systemic corticosteroids can be used. High doses are given and rapidly reduced as the patient improves. The utility of extracorporeal removal of circulating immune complexes via plasmapheresis requires further study.

PREVENTION

The primary mode of prevention of serum sickness is to seek alternative therapies. In some cases, non–equine-derived formulations may be available (human-derived botulinum immune globulin). Other emerging alternatives are partially digested antibodies of animal origin and engineered (humanized) antibodies. The potential of these therapies to elicit serum sickness–like disease appears low. When only equine antitoxin/antivenom is available, skin tests should be performed before administration of serum, but this procedure indicates the risk only of anaphylaxis, not of serum sickness. Testing generally begins with prick-puncture using a 1:100 dilution of the serum with positive (histamine) and negative (saline) controls and proceeds through increasingly higher doses until a positive response is seen or a top dose of 0.02 mL of a 1:100 dilution injected intracutaneously is reached. A negative response to the strongest solution indicates that anaphylactic sensitivity to horse serum is unlikely.

For patients who have evidence of anaphylactic sensitivity to horse serum, a risk-to-benefit assessment must be made to determine the need to proceed with treatment. If needed, the serum can usually be successfully administered by a process of rapid desensitization using protocols of gradual administration outlined by the manufacturers. Desensitization is transient, and the patient may regain the previous anaphylactic sensitivity. Serum sickness is not prevented by desensitization or by pretreatment with corticosteroids.

BIBLIOGRAPHY
Please visit the Nelson Textbook of Pediatrics *website at www.expertconsult.com for the complete bibliography.*

Chapter 145
Adverse Reactions to Foods

Hugh A. Sampson and Donald Y.M. Leung

Adverse reactions to foods consist of any untoward reaction following the ingestion of a food or food additive and are classically divided into **food intolerances,** which are adverse physiologic responses, and **food hypersensitivities,** which include adverse immunologic responses and allergies (Tables 145-1 to 145-3). Like other atopic disorders, food allergies have increased over the past 3 decades, primarily in "Westernized" countries, and now affect an estimated 3.5% of the U.S. population. Up to 6% of children experience food allergic reactions in the 1st 3 yr of life, including about 2.5% with cow's milk allergy, 1.5% with egg allergy, and 1% with peanut allergy. Most children "outgrow" milk and egg allergies, with about 50% doing so within 3-5 yr. In contrast, about 80-90% of children with peanut, nut, or seafood allergy retain their allergy for life.

Table 145-1 ADVERSE FOOD REACTIONS

FOOD INTOLERANCE
Host Factors
Enzyme deficiencies—lactase (primary or secondary), fructase (maturational delay)
Gastrointestinal disorders—inflammatory bowel disease, irritable bowel syndrome
Idiosyncratic reactions—caffeine in soft drinks ("hyperactivity")
Psychologic—food phobias
Migraines (rare)
Food Factors
Infectious organisms—*Escherichia coli, Staphylococcus aureus, Clostridium*
Toxins—histamine (scombroid poisoning), saxitoxin (shellfish)
Pharmacologic agents—caffeine, theobromine (chocolate, tea), tryptamine (tomatoes), tyramine (cheese)
Contaminants—heavy metals, pesticides, antibiotics
FOOD HYPERSENSITIVITIES
IgE-Mediated
Cutaneous—urticaria, angioedema, morbilliform rashes, flushing, contact urticaria
Gastrointestinal—oral allergy syndrome, gastrointestinal anaphylaxis
Respiratory—acute rhinoconjunctivitis, bronchospasm
Generalized—anaphylactic shock, exercise induced anaphylaxis
Mixed IgE- and Cell-Mediated
Cutaneous—atopic dermatitis, contact dermatitis
Gastrointestinal—allergic eosinophilic esophagitis and gastroenteritis
Respiratory—asthma
Cell Mediated
Cutaneous—contact dermatitis, dermatitis herpetiformis
Gastrointestinal—food protein–induced enterocolitis, proctocolitis, and enteropathy syndromes, celiac disease
Respiratory—food-induced pulmonary hemosiderosis (Heiner syndrome)
Unclassified
Cow's milk–induced anemia

IgE, immunoglobulin E.

ETIOLOGY

Adverse reactions to foods may result from intolerances, which are based on functional properties of foods, or from physiologic responses of the host, including hypersensitivities and adverse immunologic responses (see Table 145-1). Although food represents the largest antigenic load confronting the body, the gut-associated lymphoid tissue (GALT) is able to readily discriminate between "harmless" foods and pathogenic organisms. Ingestion of food normally leads to **oral tolerance,** which is the induction of T-cell anergy and T regulatory cells that enable the systemic immune system to "ignore" the roughly 2% of antigenic protein normally entering the systemic circulation at each meal. In young infants, functional barriers (stomach acidity, intestinal enzymes, glycocalyx) and immunologic barriers (secretory immunoglobulin [Ig] A) are immature, allowing increased penetration of food antigens, and the GALT appears less capable of "tolerizing" than the mature system. Consequently, food hypersensitivity reactions most commonly develop at this susceptible age.

PATHOGENESIS

Food intolerances are the result of a variety of mechanisms, whereas food hypersensitivities are predominantly due to IgE-mediated and/or cell-mediated mechanisms. In susceptible individuals exposed to certain allergens, food-specific IgE antibodies are formed that bind to Fcε receptors on mast cells, basophils, macrophages, and dendritic cells. When food allergens penetrate mucosal barriers and reach cell-bound IgE antibodies, mediators are released that induce vasodilatation, smooth muscle contraction, and mucus secretion, which result in symptoms of immediate hypersensitivity. Activated mast cells and macrophages may release several cytokines that attract and activate other cells, such as eosinophils and lymphocytes, leading to prolonged inflammation. Symptoms elicited during acute IgE-mediated reactions can affect the **skin** (urticaria, angioedema, flushing), **gastrointestinal tract** (oral pruritus, angioedema, nausea, abdominal pain,

Table 145-2 DIFFERENTIAL DIAGNOSIS OF ADVERSE FOOD REACTIONS

GASTROINTESTINAL DISORDERS (WITH VOMITING AND/OR DIARRHEA)
Structural abnormalities (pyloric stenosis, Hirschsprung disease)
Enzyme deficiencies (primary or secondary):
Disaccharidase deficiency—lactase, fructase, sucrase-isomaltase
Galactosemia
Malignancy with obstruction
Other: pancreatic insufficiency (cystic fibrosis), peptic disease
CONTAMINANTS AND ADDITIVES
Flavorings and preservatives—rarely cause symptoms:
Sodium metabisulfite, monosodium glutamate, nitrites
Dyes and colorings—very rarely cause symptoms (urticaria, eczema):
Tartrazine
Toxins:
Bacterial, fungal (aflatoxin), fish-related (scombroid, ciguatera)
Infectious organisms:
Bacteria *(Salmonella, Escherichia coli, Shigella)*
Virus (rotavirus, enterovirus)
Parasites (*Giardia, Akis simplex* [in fish])
Accidental contaminants:
Heavy metals, pesticides
Pharmacologic agents:
Caffeine, glycosidal alkaloid solanine (potato spuds), histamine (fish), serotonin (banana, tomato), tryptamine (tomato), tyramine (cheese)
PSYCHOLOGIC REACTIONS
Food phobias

Table 145-3 NATURAL HISTORY OF FOOD ALLERGY AND CROSS-REACTIVITY BETWEEN COMMON FOOD ALLERGIES

FOOD	USUAL AGE AT ONSET OF ALLERGY	CROSS REACTIVITY	USUAL AGE AT RESOLUTION
Hen's egg white	6-24 mo	Other avian eggs	7 yr (75% of cases resolve)*
Cow's milk	6-12 mo	Goat's milk, sheep's milk, buffalo milk	5 yr (76% of cases resolve)*
Peanuts	6-24 mo	Other legumes, peas, lentils; co-reactivity with tree nuts	Persistent (20% of cases resolve by 5 yr)
Tree nuts	1-2 yr; in adults, onset occurs after cross reactivity to birch pollen	Other tree nuts; co-reactivity with peanuts	Persistent (20% of cases resolve by 7 yr)
Fish	Late childhood and adulthood	Other fish (low cross reactivity with tuna and swordfish)	Persistent†
Shellfish	Adulthood (in 60% of patients with this allergy)	Other shellfish	Persistent
Wheat‡	6-24 mo	Other grains containing gluten	5 yr (80% of cases resolve)
Soybeans‡	6-24 mo	Other legumes	2 yr (67% of cases resolve)
Kiwi	Any age	Banana, avocado, latex	Unknown
Apples, carrots, and peaches§	Late childhood and adulthood	Birch pollen, other fruits, nuts	Unknown

*Recent studies suggest that resolution may occur at a later age.
†Fish allergy that is acquired in childhood can resolve.
‡Although IgE-mediated allergies to wheat and soybeans are frequently suspected food allergies, in practice these diagnoses are rarely confirmed after evaluation by a specialist.
§Allergy to apples, carrots, and peaches (oral allergy syndrome) is commonly caused by heat-labile proteins. Fresh fruit causes oral pruritus, but cooked fruit is tolerated. There is generally no risk of anaphylaxis, although in rare cases, allergies to cross-reactive lipid protein can cause anaphylaxis after ingestion of fruits and vegetables.
From Lack G: Food allergy, *N Engl J Med* 359:1252–1260, 2008, Table 1.

vomiting, diarrhea), **respiratory tract** (nasal congestion, rhinorrhea, nasal pruritus, sneezing, laryngeal edema, dyspnea, wheezing), and **cardiovascular system** (dysrhythmias, hypotension, loss of consciousness). In the other major form of food hypersensitivities, lymphocytes, primarily food allergen–specific T cells, secrete excessive amounts of various cytokines that lead to a "delayed," more chronic inflammatory process affecting the **skin** (pruritus, erythematous rash), **gastrointestinal tract** (cachexia, early satiety, abdominal pain, vomiting, diarrhea), or **respiratory tract** (food-induced pulmonary hemosiderosis). Mixed IgE and cellular responses to food allergens can also lead to chronic disorders such as atopic dermatitis, asthma, and allergic eosinophilic gastroenteritis.

Children in whom IgE-mediated food allergies develop may be sensitized by food allergens penetrating the gastrointestinal barrier, which are **class 1 food allergens,** or by partially homologous allergens such as plant pollens penetrating the respiratory tract, which are **class 2 food allergens.** Any food may serve as a class 1 food allergen, but **egg, milk, peanuts, tree nuts, fish, soy, and wheat** account for 90% of food allergies during childhood. Many of the major allergenic proteins of these foods have been characterized. There is variable but significant cross reactivity with other proteins within an individual food group. Exposure and sensitization to these proteins often occur very early in life, because intact food proteins are passed to the infant through maternal breast milk, and after introduction of solid foods, many parents strive to provide their infants with a highly varied diet. Virtually all milk allergies develop by 12 mo of age and all egg allergies by 18 mo of age, and the median age of 1st peanut allergic reactions is 14 mo. Class 2 food allergens are typically plant or fruit proteins that are partially homologous with pollen proteins (see Table 145-3). With the development of seasonal allergic rhinitis from birch, grass, or ragweed pollens, subsequent ingestion of certain uncooked fruits or vegetables provokes the **oral allergy syndrome.** Intermittent ingestion of allergenic foods may lead to acute symptoms, whereas prolonged exposure may lead to chronic disorders such as atopic dermatitis and asthma. Cell-mediated sensitivity typically develops to class 1 allergens.

CLINICAL MANIFESTATIONS

From a clinical and diagnostic standpoint, it is most useful to subdivide food hypersensitivity disorders according to the predominant target organ and immune mechanism (see Table 145-1).

Gastrointestinal Manifestations

Gastrointestinal food allergies are often the 1st form of allergy to affect infants and young children and typically manifest as irritability, vomiting or "spitting-up," diarrhea, and poor weight gain. Cell-mediated hypersensitivities predominate, making standard allergy tests such as prick skin tests and in vitro tests for food-specific IgE antibodies (e.g., ImmunoCAP) of little diagnostic value.

Food protein–induced enterocolitis syndrome typically manifests in the 1st several months of life as irritability and protracted vomiting and diarrhea and may result in dehydration. Vomiting generally occurs 1-3 hr after feeding, and continued exposure may result in abdominal distention, bloody diarrhea, anemia, and failure to thrive. Symptoms are most commonly provoked by cow's milk or soy protein–based formulas. A similar enterocolitis syndrome occurs in older infants and children from rice, oat, wheat, egg, peanut, nut, chicken, turkey, or fish sensitivity. Hypotension occurs in about 15% of cases after allergen ingestion.

Food protein–induced proctocolitis presents in the 1st few months of life as blood-streaked stools in otherwise healthy infants. About 60% of cases occur among breast-fed infants, with the remainder largely among infants fed cow's milk or soy protein–based formula. Blood loss is typically modest but can occasionally produce anemia.

Food protein–induced enteropathy often manifests in the 1st several months of life as diarrhea, not infrequently steatorrhea, and poor weight gain. Symptoms include protracted diarrhea, vomiting in up to 65% of cases, failure to thrive, abdominal distention, early satiety, and malabsorption. Anemia, edema, and hypoproteinemia occur occasionally. **Cow's milk sensitivity** is the most common cause of this food protein–induced enteropathy in young infants, but it has also been associated with sensitivity to soy, egg, wheat, rice, chicken, and fish in older children. **Celiac disease,** the most severe form of protein-induced enteropathy, occurs in 1:100-1:250 of the U.S. population, although it may be "silent" in many patients (Chapter 330.2). The full-blown form is characterized by extensive loss of absorptive villi and hyperplasia of the crypts, leading to malabsorption, chronic diarrhea, steatorrhea, abdominal distention, flatulence, and weight loss or failure to thrive. Oral ulcers and other extra-intestinal symptoms secondary to malabsorption are not uncommon. Genetically susceptible individuals (HLA-DQ2 or DQ8) demonstrate a cell-mediated response to tissue transglutaminase (tTGase) deamidated gliadin, which is found in wheat, rye, and barley.

Allergic eosinophilic esophagitis may appear from infancy through adolescence, more frequently in boys. In young children, it is primarily cell mediated and manifests as chronic gastroesophageal reflux (GER), intermittent emesis, food refusal, abdominal pain, dysphagia, irritability, sleep disturbance, and failure to respond to conventional reflux medications. Of children <1 yr of age presenting with GER, 40% have cow's milk–induced reflux. **Allergic eosinophilic gastroenteritis** occurs at any age and causes symptoms similar to those of esophagitis as well as prominent weight loss or failure to thrive, both of which are the hallmarks of this disorder. More than 50% of patients with this disorder are atopic, and food-induced IgE-mediated reactions have been implicated in a minority of patients. Generalized edema secondary to hypoalbuminemia may occur in some infants with marked protein-losing enteropathy.

Oral allergy syndrome (pollen-food syndrome) is an IgE-mediated hypersensitivity that occurs in many older children with birch pollen– and ragweed-induced allergic rhinitis. Symptoms are usually confined to the oropharynx and consist of the rapid onset of oral pruritus, tingling and angioedema of the lips, tongue, palate, and throat, and occasionally a sensation of pruritus in the ears and tightness in the throat. Symptoms are generally short lived and are caused by local mast cell activation by fresh fruit and vegetable proteins that cross react with birch pollen (apple, carrot, potato, celery, hazel nuts, kiwi) and ragweed pollen (banana, melons such as watermelon and cantaloupe).

Acute gastrointestinal allergy generally manifests as acute abdominal pain and vomiting that accompany IgE-mediated allergic symptoms in other target organs.

Skin Manifestations

Cutaneous food allergies are also common in infants and young children.

Atopic dermatitis is a form of eczema that generally begins in early infancy and is characterized by pruritus, a chronically relapsing course, and association with asthma and allergic rhinitis (Chapter 139). Although not often apparent from history, at least 30% of children with moderate to severe atopic dermatitis have food allergies. The younger the child and the more severe the eczema, the more likely food allergy is playing a pathogenic role in the disorder.

Acute urticaria and angioedema are among the most common symptoms of food allergic reactions (Chapter 142). The onset of symptoms may be very rapid, within minutes after ingestion of the responsible allergen. Symptoms result from activation of IgE-bearing mast cells by circulating food allergens that are absorbed and circulated rapidly throughout the body. Foods most commonly incriminated in children include egg, milk, peanuts, and nuts, although reactions to various seeds (sesame, poppy) and fruits (kiwi) are becoming more common. Chronic urticaria and angioedema are rarely due to food allergies.

Respiratory Manifestations

Respiratory food allergies are uncommon as isolated symptoms. Although many parents believe that nasal congestion in infants is often caused by milk allergy, many studies show this not to be the case. **Food-induced rhinoconjunctivitis** symptoms typically accompany allergic symptoms in other target organs, such as skin, and consist of typical allergic rhinitis symptoms (periocular pruritus and tearing, nasal congestion and pruritus, sneezing, rhinorrhea). Wheezing occurs in about 25% of IgE-mediated food allergic reactions, but only about 10% of asthmatic patients have food-induced respiratory symptoms.

Food allergic reactions are the single most common cause of anaphylaxis seen in hospital emergency departments. In addition to the rapid onset of cutaneous, respiratory, and gastrointestinal symptoms, patients may demonstrate cardiovascular symptoms, including hypotension, vascular collapse, and cardiac dysrhythmias, which are presumably caused by massive mast cell–mediator release. **Food-associated exercise-induced anaphylaxis** occurs more frequently among teenage athletes, especially females (Chapter 143).

DIAGNOSIS

A thorough medical history is necessary to determine whether a patient's symptomatology represents an adverse reaction (see Table 145-2), whether the adverse food reaction is an intolerance or hypersensitivity reaction, and if the latter, whether it is likely to be an IgE-mediated or a cell-mediated response (Fig. 145-1). The following facts should be established: (1) the food suspected of provoking the reaction and the quantity ingested, (2) the interval between ingestion and the development of symptoms, (3) the types of symptoms elicited by the ingestion, (4) whether ingesting the suspected food produced similar symptoms on other occasions, (5) whether other inciting factors, such as exercise, are necessary, and (6) the interval from the last reaction to the food.

Prick skin tests and in vitro laboratory tests are useful for demonstrating IgE sensitization. Many fruits and vegetables require testing with fresh produce because labile proteins are destroyed during commercial preparation. A negative skin test result virtually excludes an IgE-mediated form of food allergy. Conversely, the majority of children with positive skin test responses to a food do not react when the food is ingested, so more definitive tests, such as quantitative IgE tests or food elimination and challenge, are often necessary to establish a diagnosis of food allergy. Serum food-specific IgE levels ≥15 kU_A/L for milk (≥5 kU_A/L for children ≤1 yr), ≥7 kU_A/L for egg (≥2 kU_A/L for children <3 yr), and ≥14 kU_A/L for peanut are associated with a >95% likelihood of clinical reactivity to these foods in children with suspected reactivity. In the absence of a clear history of reactivity to a food and evidence of food-specific IgE antibodies, definitive studies must be performed before recommendations are made for avoidance or the use of highly restrictive diets that may be nutritionally deficient, logistically impractical, disruptive to the family, and a potential source of future feeding disorders. IgE-mediated food allergic reactions are generally very food specific, so the use of broad exclusionary diets, such as avoidance of all legumes, cereal grains, or animal products, is not warranted (Tables 145-3 and 145-4).

Unfortunately, there are no laboratory studies to help identify foods responsible for cell-mediated reactions. Consequently, **elimination diets followed by food challenges** are the only way to establish the diagnosis. Allergists experienced in dealing with food allergic reactions and able to treat anaphylaxis should perform food challenges. Before a food challenge is initiated, the suspected food should be eliminated from the diet for 10-14 days for IgE-mediated food allergy and up to 8 wk for some cell-mediated disorders, such as allergic eosinophilic esophagitis. Many children with cell-mediated reactions to cow's milk do not tolerate hydrolysate formulas and must receive amino acid–derived formulas (EleCare or Neocate). If symptoms remain unchanged and appropriate elimination diets have been utilized, it is unlikely that food allergy is responsible for the child's disorder.

TREATMENT

Appropriate identification and elimination of foods responsible for food hypersensitivity reactions are the only validated treatments for food allergies. Complete elimination of common foods (milk, egg, soy, wheat, rice, chicken, fish, peanut, nuts) is very difficult because of their widespread use in a variety of processed foods. The Food Allergy and Anaphylaxis Network (www.foodallergy.org or 800-929-4040) provides excellent information to help parents deal with both the practical and emotional issues surrounding these diets. Children with asthma and IgE-mediated food allergy, peanut or nut allergy, or a history of a previous

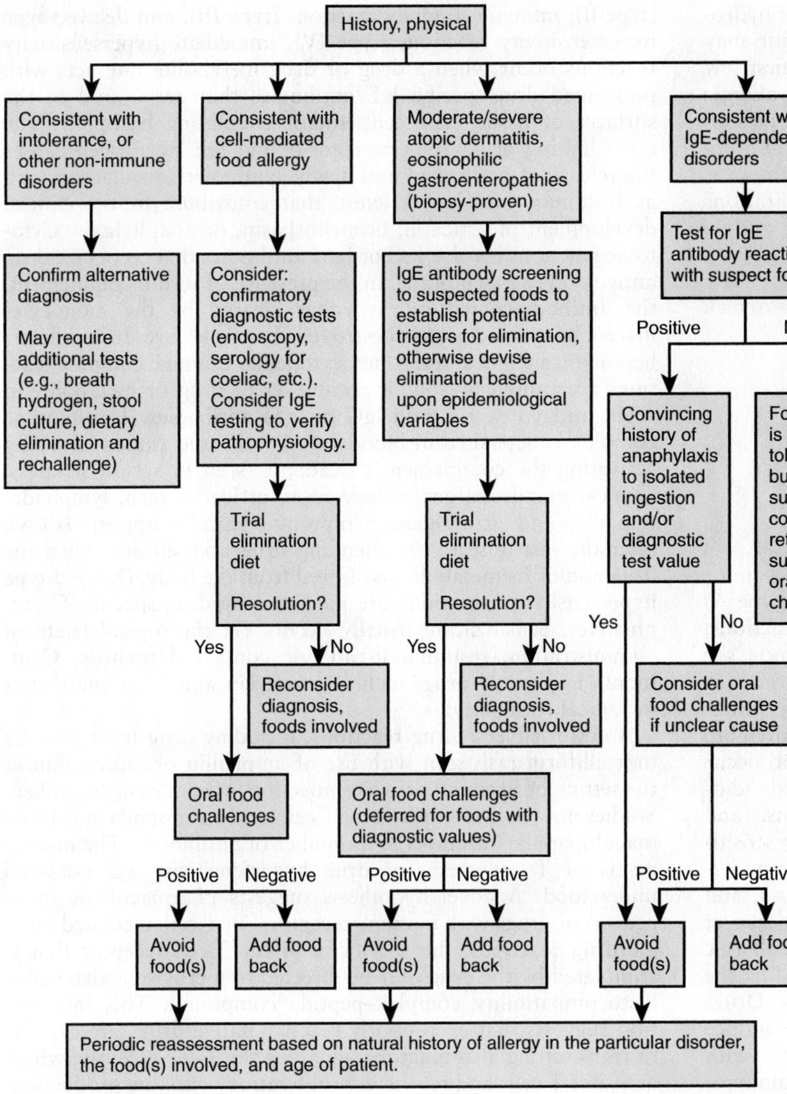

Figure 145-1 General scheme for diagnosis of food allergy. (From Sicherer SH: Food allergy, *Lancet* 360:701–710, 2002.)

Table 145-4 CLINICAL IMPLICATIONS OF CROSS-REACTIVE PROTEINS IN IMMUNOGLOBULIN E–MEDIATED ALLERGY

FOOD FAMILY	RISK OF ALLERGY TO ≥ 1 MEMBER (%; APPROXIMATE)	FEATURE(S)
Legumes	5	Main causes of reactions are peanut, soya, lentil, lupine, and garbanzo
Tree nuts (e.g., hazel, walnut, brazil)	35	Reactions are often severe
Fish	50	Reactions can be severe
Shellfish	75	Reactions can be severe
Grains	20	
Mammalian milks	90	Cow's milk is highly cross reactive with goat's or sheep's milk (92%) but not with mare's milk (4%)
Rosaceae (rock) fruits	55	Risk of reactions to more than three related foods is very low (<10%)
Latex-food	35	For individuals allergic to latex, banana, kiwi, and avocado are the main causes of reactions

From Sicherer SH: Food allergy, *Lancet* 360:701–710, 2002.

severe reaction should be given self-injectable epinephrine (EpiPen) and a written emergency plan in case of accidental ingestion (Chapter 143). Because many food allergies are outgrown, arrangements should be made to have children reevaluated periodically by an allergist to determine whether they have lost their clinical reactivity. A number of clinical trials are under way, evaluating the use of oral immunotherapy and sublingual immunotherapy for the treatment of IgE-mediated food allergies (milk, egg, peanut). In addition, other forms of therapy, such as anti-IgE immunoglobulin therapy, engineered recombinant food protein vaccines, and herbal formulations, are being evaluated and may provide more definitive means of treating food allergies or at least raising the threshold for adverse reactions. In addition, tolerance may be generated by heating (cooking) the food (milk).

PREVENTION

There is no consensus as to whether food allergies can be prevented. At present there is insufficient evidence to support the practice of restricting the maternal diet during pregnancy or breast-feeding or of delaying introduction of various allergenic foods to infants from atopic families. Studies suggest that exclusive breast-feeding and/or supplementation or use of hydrolyzed milk-based formulas for the first 4-6 months of life may reduce allergic disorders (e.g., atopic dermatitis) in the first few years of life in infants at high risk for development of allergic disease. However, the value of further restrictions cannot be supported by the current medical literature. Because some skin preparations contain peanut oil, which may sensitize young infants, especially those with cutaneous inflammation, such preparations should be avoided.

BIBLIOGRAPHY

Please visit the Nelson Textbook of Pediatrics *website at www.expertconsult.com for the complete bibliography.*

Chapter 146
Adverse Reactions to Drugs

Mark Boguniewicz and Donald Y.M. Leung

Adverse drug reactions can be divided into predictable (type A) and unpredictable reactions (type B). **Predictable drug reactions,** including drug toxicity, drug interactions, and adverse effects, are dose dependent, can be related to known pharmacologic actions of the drug, and occur in patients without any unique susceptibility. **Unpredictable drug reactions** are dose independent, often are not related to the pharmacologic actions of the drug, and occur in patients who are genetically predisposed. These include idiosyncratic reactions, allergic (hypersensitivity) reactions, and pseudoallergic reactions. Allergic reactions require prior sensitization, manifest as signs or symptoms characteristic of an underlying allergic mechanism such as anaphylaxis or urticaria, and occur in genetically susceptible individuals. They can occur at doses significantly below the therapeutic range. **Pseudoallergic reactions** resemble allergic reactions but are distinguished by the fact that an immunologic mechanism is not involved. Drug-independent cross-reactive antigens have been shown to induce sensitization manifesting as drug allergy. Patients with cetuximab-induced anaphylaxis were found to have immunoglobulin (Ig) E antibodies in pretreatment samples specific for galactose-α-l,3-galactose. The latter is present on the antigen-binding portion of the cetuximab heavy chain and is similar to structures in the ABO blood group.

EPIDEMIOLOGY

The incidence of adverse drug reactions in the general as well as pediatric populations remains unknown, although data from hospitalized patients show it to be 6.7%, with a 0.32% incidence of fatal adverse drug reactions. Databases such as the FDA MedWatch program (*www.fda.gov/medwatch/index.html*) likely suffer from underreporting. Cutaneous reactions are the most common form of adverse drug reactions, with ampicillin, amoxicillin, penicillin, and trimethoprim-sulfamethoxazole being the most commonly implicated drugs. Although the majority of adverse drug reactions do not appear to be allergic in nature, 6-10% can be attributed to an allergic or immunologic mechanism. Importantly, given the high probability of recurrence of allergic reactions, these reactions should be preventable, and information technology–based interventions may be especially useful to reduce risk of reexposure.

PATHOGENESIS AND CLINICAL MANIFESTATIONS

Immunologically mediated adverse drug reactions have been classified according to the **Gell and Coombs classification:** immediate hypersensitivity reactions (type I), cytotoxic antibody reactions (type II), immune complex reactions (type III), and delayed-type hypersensitivity reactions (type IV). Immediate hypersensitivity reactions occur when a drug or drug metabolite interacts with preformed drug-specific IgE antibodies that are bound to the surfaces of tissue mast cells and/or circulating basophils. The cross linking of adjacent receptor-bound IgE by antigen causes the release of preformed and newly synthesized mediators, such as histamine and leukotrienes, that contribute to the clinical development of urticaria, bronchospasm, or anaphylaxis. Cytotoxic reactions involve IgG or IgM antibodies that recognize drug antigen on cell membrane. In the presence of serum complement, the antibody-coated cell is either cleared by the monocyte-macrophage system or is destroyed. Examples are drug-induced hemolytic anemia and thrombocytopenia. Immune complex reactions are caused by soluble complexes of drug or metabolite in slight antigen excess with IgG or IgM antibodies. The immune complex is deposited in blood vessel walls and causes injury by activating the complement cascade, as seen in serum sickness. Clinical manifestations include fever, urticaria, rash, lymphadenopathy, and arthralgias. Symptoms typically appear 1-3 wk after the last dose of an offending drug and subside when the drug and/or its metabolite is cleared from the body. Delayed-type hypersensitivity reactions are mediated by drug-specific T lymphocytes. Sensitization usually occurs via the topical route of administration, resulting in allergic contact dermatitis. Commonly implicated drugs include neomycin and local anesthetics in topical formulations.

Certain adverse drug reactions, including drug fever and the morbilliform rash seen with use of ampicillin or amoxicillin in the setting of Epstein-Barr virus infection, are not easily classified. Studies now point to the role of T cells and eosinophils in delayed maculopapular reactions to a number of antibiotics. The mechanisms of T cell–mediated drug hypersensitivity are not well understood. A novel hypothesis suggests pharmacologic interactions of drugs with immune receptors. In T cell–mediated allergic drug reactions, the specificity of the T-cell receptor that is stimulated by the drug may be directed to a cross-reactive major histocompatibility complex–peptide compound. This information suggests that even poorly reactive native drugs are capable of transmitting a stimulatory signal via the T-cell receptor, which activates T cells and results in proliferation, cytokine production, and cytotoxicity. Previous contact with the causative drug is not obligatory, and an immune mechanism should be considered as the cause of hypersensitivity, even in reactions that occur with first exposure. Such reactions have been described for radiocontrast media and neuromuscular blocking agents.

Drug Metabolism and Adverse Reactions

Most drugs and their metabolites are not immunologically detectable until they have become covalently attached to a macromolecule. This multivalent hapten-protein complex forms a new immunogenic epitope that can elicit T- and B-lymphocyte responses. The penicillins and related β-lactam antibiotics are highly reactive with proteins and can directly haptenate protein carriers, possibly accounting for the frequency of immune-mediated hypersensitivity reactions with this class of antibiotics.

Incomplete or delayed metabolism of some drugs can give rise to toxic metabolites. Hydroxylamine, a reactive metabolite produced by cytochrome P450 oxidative metabolism, may mediate adverse reactions to sulfonamides. Patients who are slow acetylators appear to be at increased risk (Chapter 56). In addition, cutaneous reactions in patients with AIDS treated with trimethoprim-sulfamethoxazole, rifampin, or other drugs may be due to glutathione deficiency resulting in toxic metabolites. Serum sickness–like reactions in which immune complexes have not been documented, which occur most commonly with cefaclor, may result from an inherited propensity for hepatic biotransformation of drugs into toxic or immunogenic metabolites.

Risk Factors for Hypersensitivity Reactions

Risk factors for adverse drug reactions include prior exposure, previous reactions, age (20-49 yr), route of administration (parenteral or topical), dose (high), and dosing schedule (intermittent) as well as genetic predisposition (slow acetylators). Atopy does not appear to predispose patients to allergic reactions to low molecular weight compounds, but atopic patients in whom an allergic reaction develops have a significantly increased risk of serious reaction. Atopic patients also appear to be at greater risk for pseudoallergic reactions induced by radiocontrast media. Pharmacogenomics has an important role in identifying individuals at risk for certain drug reactions (Chapter 56).

DIAGNOSIS

An accurate medical history is an important first step in evaluating a patient with a possible adverse drug reaction. Suspected drugs need to be identified along with dosages, route of administration, previous exposures, and dates of administration. In addition, underlying hepatic or renal disease may influence drug metabolism. A detailed description of past reactions may yield clues to the nature of the adverse drug reaction. The propensity for a particular drug to cause the suspected reaction can be checked with information in *Physicians' Desk Reference, Drug Eruption Reference Manual,* or directly from the drug manufacturer. It is important to remember, however, that the history may be unreliable, and many patients are inappropriately labeled as being drug allergic. This label can result in inappropriate withholding of a needed drug or class of drugs. In addition, relying solely on the history can lead to overuse of drugs reserved for special indications, such as vancomycin in patients in whom penicillin allergy is suspected. Approximately 80% of patients with a history of penicillin allergy do not have evidence of penicillin-specific IgE antibodies on testing.

Skin testing is the most rapid and sensitive method of demonstrating the presence of IgE antibodies to a specific allergen. It can be performed with high molecular weight compounds such as foreign antisera, hormones, enzymes, and toxoids. Reliable skin testing can also be performed with penicillin but not with most other antibiotics. Most immunologically mediated adverse drug reactions are due to metabolites rather than to parent compounds, and the metabolites for most drugs other than penicillin have not been defined. In addition, many metabolites are unstable or must combine with larger proteins to be useful for diagnosis. Testing with nonstandardized reagents requires caution in interpretation of both positive and negative results, because some drugs can induce nonspecific irritant reactions. Whereas a wheal-and-flare reaction is suggestive of drug-specific IgE antibodies, a negative skin test result does not exclude the presence of such antibodies because the relevant immunogen may not have been used as the testing reagent.

A positive skin test response to the major or minor determinants of penicillin has a 60% positive predictive value for an immediate hypersensitivity reaction to penicillin. In patients in whom skin test responses to the major and minor determinants of penicillin are negative, 97-99% (depending on the reagents used) tolerate the drug without an immediate reaction. At present, the major determinant of penicillin testing reagent PrePen (penicyloyl-polylisne) in the USA is available, but the minor determinant mixture has not been approved by the U.S. Food and Drug Administration (FDA) as a testing reagent. The positive and negative predictive values of skin testing for antibiotics other than penicillin are not well established. Nevertheless, positive immediate hypersensitivity skin test responses to nonirritant concentrations of nonpenicillin antibiotics may be interpreted as a presumptive risk of an immediate reaction to such agents.

Results of direct and indirect Coombs tests are often positive in drug-induced hemolytic anemia. Assays for specific IgG and IgM have been shown to correlate with a drug reaction in immune cytopenia, but, in most other reactions, such assays are not diagnostic. In general, many more patients express humoral or T-cell immune responses to drug determinants than express clinical disease. Serum tryptase is elevated with systemic mast cell degranulation and can be seen with drug-associated mast cell activation, although it is not pathognomonic for drug hypersensitivity, and nonelevated tryptase values can be seen in well-defined anaphylaxis.

TREATMENT

Specific **desensitization,** which involves the progressive administration of an allergen to render effector cells less reactive, is reserved for patients with IgE antibodies to a particular drug for whom an alternative drug is not available or appropriate. Specific protocols for many different drugs have been developed. Desensitization should be performed in a hospital setting, usually in consultation with an allergist and with resuscitation equipment available at all times. Although mild complications, such as pruritus and rash, are fairly common and often respond to adjustments in the drug dose or dosing intervals and medications to relieve symptoms, more severe systemic reactions can occur. Oral desensitization may be less likely to induce anaphylaxis than parenteral administration. Pretreatment with antihistamines or corticosteroids is not usually recommended. It is important to recognize that desensitization to a drug is effective only while the drug continues to be administered and that after a period of interruption or discontinuation, hypersensitivity can recur.

Graded challenges based on the administration of a drug in an incremental fashion until a therapeutic dose is achieved can be attempted with drugs causing non–IgE-mediated reactions, including trimethoprim-sulfamethoxazole. Graded challenges in aspirin- or nonsteroidal anti-inflammatory drug (NSAID)–intolerant patients, particularly those with respiratory reactions, can also be performed. Gradual introduction of a drug may reveal systemic intolerance early enough to prevent progression to a serious or even life-threatening reaction such as Stevens-Johnson syndrome (SJS) or toxic epidermal necrolysis (TEN).

β-Lactam Hypersensitivity

Penicillin is a frequent cause of anaphylaxis and is responsible for the majority of all drug-mediated anaphylactic deaths in the United States. Although IgE-mediated reactions may occur after administration of penicillin by any route, parenteral administration is more likely to cause anaphylaxis. If a patient requires penicillin and has a previous history suggestive of penicillin allergy, it is necessary perform skin tests on the patient for the presence of penicillin-specific IgE with both the major and minor determinants of penicillin. Skin tests for both major and minor determinants of penicillin are necessary because about 20% of patients with documented anaphylaxis do not demonstrate skin reactivity to the major determinant. Unfortunately, as mentioned earlier, the major determinant testing reagent, PrePen, was withdrawn from the market in the USA in 2004 owing to problems with manufacturing. The manufacturer, AllerQuest, LLC (West Hartford, CT), received approval from the FDA in January 2008 to manufacture Pre-Pen (*www.allerquest.com/availability.html*). The minor determinant mixture is currently not licensed and is synthesized as a nonstandardized testing reagent at select academic centers. Although penicillin G is often used as a substitute for the minor determinant mixture, there is a small but significant risk of false-negative skin test results with this approach. Thus, patients should be referred to an allergist capable of performing appropriate testing. If the skin test response is positive to either major or minor determinants of penicillin, the patient should receive an alternative non–cross reacting antibiotic. If administration of penicillin is deemed necessary, desensitization can be performed by an allergist in an appropriate medical setting. Skin testing for penicillin-specific IgE is not predictive for delayed-onset cutaneous, bullous, or immune complex reactions. In addition, penicillin skin testing does not appear to resensitize the patient.

Other β-lactam antibiotics, including semisynthetic penicillins, cephalosporins, carbacephems, and carbapenems, share the β-lactam ring structure. Patients with late-onset morbilliform rashes with amoxicillin are not considered to be at risk for IgE-mediated reactions to penicillin and do not require skin testing before penicillin administration. Up to 100% of patients with Epstein-Barr virus infections treated with ampicillin or amoxicillin can experience a nonpruritic rash. Similar reactions occur in patients who receive allopurinol as treatment for elevated uric acid or have chronic lymphocytic leukemia. If the rash to ampicillin or amoxicillin is urticarial or systemic or the history is unclear, the patient should undergo penicillin skin testing if a penicillin is needed. There have been reports of antibodies specific for semisynthetic penicillin side chains in the absence of β-lactam ring–specific antibodies, although the clinical significance of such side chain–specific antibodies is unclear.

Varying degrees of in vitro cross reactivity have been documented between cephalosporins and penicillins. Although the risk of allergic reactions to cephalosporins in patients with positive skin test responses to penicillin appears to be low (<2%), anaphylactic reactions have occurred after administration of cephalosporins in patients with a history of penicillin anaphylaxis. If a patient has a history of penicillin allergy and requires a cephalosporin, skin testing for major and minor determinants of penicillin should preferably be performed to determine whether the patient has penicillin-specific IgE antibodies. If skin test results are negative, the patient can receive a cephalosporin with no greater risk than found in the general population. If skin test results are positive for penicillin, recommendations may include: administration of an alternative antibiotic; cautious graded challenge with appropriate monitoring, with the recognition that there is a 2% chance of inducing an anaphylactic reaction; and desensitization to the required cephalosporin.

Conversely, patients who require penicillin and have a history of an IgE-mediated reaction to a cephalosporin should also undergo penicillin skin testing. Patients with a negative result can receive penicillin. Patients with a positive result should either receive an alternative medication or undergo desensitization to penicillin. In patients with a history of allergic reaction to one cephalosporin who require another cephalosporin, skin testing with the required cephalosporin can be performed, with the recognition that the negative predictive value of such testing is unknown. If the skin test response to the cephalosporin is positive, the significance of the test should be checked further in control subjects to determine whether the positive response is IgE mediated or an irritant response. The drug can then be administered by graded challenge or desensitization.

Carbapenems (imipenem, meropenem) represent another class of β-lactam antibiotics with a bicyclic nucleus that demonstrate a high degree of cross reactivity with penicillins, although prospective studies now suggest incidence of cross reactivity on skin testing of approximately 1%. In contrast to β-lactam antibiotics, monobactams (aztreonam) have a monocyclic ring structure. Aztreonam-specific antibodies have been shown to be predominantly side chain-specific; data suggest that aztreonam can be safely administered to most penicillin-allergic subjects. On the other hand, administration of aztreonam to a patient with ceftazidime allergy may be associated with increased risk of allergic reaction owing to similarity of side chains.

Sulfonamides

The most common type of reaction to sulfonamides is a maculopapular eruption often associated with fever that occurs after 7-12 days of therapy. Immediate reactions, including anaphylaxis as well as other immunologic reactions, have also been suggested. Hypersensitivity reactions to sulfonamides occur with much greater frequency in HIV-infected individuals. For patients in whom maculopapular rashes develop after sulfonamide administration, both graded challenge and desensitization protocols have been shown to be effective. These regimens should not be used in individuals with a history of SJS or TEN. Hypersensitivity reactions to sulfasalazine used for treatment of inflammatory bowel disease appear to result from the sulfapyridine moiety. Slow desensitization over ≈1 mo permits tolerance of the drug in many patients. In addition, oral and enema forms of 5-aminosalicylic acid (5-ASA), thought to be the pharmacologically active agent in sulfasalazine, are effective alternative therapies.

Stevens-Johnson Syndrome and Toxic Epidermal Necrolysis

Blistering mucocutaneous disorders induced by drugs encompass a spectrum of reactions, including SJS and TEN (Chapter 646). Epidermal detachment of less than 10% is suggestive of SJS, 30% detachment suggests TEN, and 10-30% detachment suggests overlap of the two syndromes. The features of SJS include confluent purpuric macules on face and trunk and severe, explosive mucosal erosions, usually at more than one mucosal surface, accompanied by fever and constitutional symptoms. Ocular involvement may be particularly severe, and the liver, kidneys, and lungs may also be involved. TEN, which appears to be related to keratinocyte apoptosis, manifests as widespread areas of confluent erythema followed by epidermal necrosis and detachment with severe mucosal involvement. The risk of infection and mortality are high. Skin biopsy differentiates subepidermal cleavage characteristic of TEN from intraepidermal cleavage characteristic of the scalded-skin syndrome induced by staphylococcal toxins. TEN must be treated in a burn unit. Corticosteroids are contraindicated because they can significantly increase the risk of infection. High intravenous doses of immunoglobulin have been shown to be beneficial in patients with TEN, likely because of inhibition of Fas-mediated keratinocyte cell death by naturally occurring Fas-blocking antibodies in the intravenous immunoglobulin preparation.

Hypersensitivity to Antiretroviral Agents

A growing number of adverse drug reactions have been observed with antiretroviral agents, including reverse transcriptase inhibitors, protease inhibitors, and fusion inhibitors. Hypersensitivity to abacavir is a well-recognized, multiorgan, potentially life-threatening reaction that occurs in HIV-infected children. The reaction is independent of dose, with onset generally within 9-11 days of initiation of drug therapy. Rechallenge can be accompanied by significant hypotension and potential mortality (rate of 0.03%), and thus hypersensitivity to abacavir is an absolute contraindication for any subsequent use. Prophylaxis with prednisolone does not appear to prevent hypersensitivity reactions to abacavir. Importantly, genetic susceptibility appears to be conferred by the HLA-B*5701 allele, with a positive predictive value of >70% and a negative predictive value of 95-98%. Genetic screening would be cost-effective in white populations but not in African or Asian populations, in which HLA-B*5701 allele frequency is <1%.

Chemotherapeutic Agents

Hypersensitivity reactions to chemotherapeutic drugs have been described, including to monoclonal antibodies. Data now suggest that rapid desensitization to a variety of unrelated agents, including carboplatin, paclitaxel, and rituximab, can be safely achieved in a 12-step protocol. Of note, this approach appears to be successful in both IgE-mediated and non–IgE-mediated reactions.

Biologics

An increasing number of biologic agents has become available for the treatment of autoimmune, allergic, cardiovascular, infectious, and neoplastic diseases. Their use may be associated with a variety of adverse reactions, including hypersensitivity reactions. Given the occurrence of anaphylaxis, including cases with delayed onset and protracted progression in spontaneous postmarketing adverse event reports, the FDA issued a boxed warning regarding risk of anaphylaxis and need for patient monitoring with use of omalizumab (Chapter 138).

Vaccines

Measles-mumps-rubella (MMR) vaccine has been shown to be safe in egg-allergic patients (although rare reactions to gelatin or neomycin can occur). The ovalbumin content in influenza vaccine is variable, and skin testing with the specific vaccine lot is warranted in patients with egg allergy. Patients with positive skin test responses can usually tolerate the vaccine when administered in 1/10 the full dose, followed 15-20 minutes later by 9/10 of the dose and then an observation period of 30 minutes. Of note, some patients who tolerate cooked egg (denatured egg protein) may still react to the vaccine. In addition, the newly introduced live intranasal influenza vaccine is contraindicated in egg-allergic children.

Perioperative Agents

Anaphylactoid reactions occurring during general anesthesia may be caused by induction agents (thiopental) or muscle-relaxing agents (succinylcholine, pancuronium). Quaternary ammonium muscle relaxants (succinylcholine) can act as bivalent antigens in IgE-mediated reactions. Negative skin test results do not necessarily predict that a drug will be tolerated. Latex allergy should always be considered in the differential diagnosis of a perioperative reaction.

Local Anesthetics

Adverse drug reactions associated with local anesthetic agents are primarily toxic reactions resulting from rapid drug absorption, inadvertent intravenous injection, or overdose. Local anesthetics are classified as esters of benzoic acid (group I) or amides (group II). Group I includes benzocaine and procaine; group II includes lidocaine, bupivacaine, and mepivacaine. In suspected local anesthetic allergy, skin testing followed by a graded challenge can be performed or an anesthetic agent from a different group can be used.

Insulin

Insulin use has been associated with a spectrum of adverse drug reactions, including local and systemic IgE-mediated reactions, hemolytic anemia, serum sickness reactions, and delayed-type hypersensitivity. In general, human insulin is less allergenic than porcine insulin, which is less allergenic than bovine insulin, but for individual patients, porcine or bovine insulin may be the least allergenic. Patients treated with nonhuman insulin have had systemic reactions to recombinant human insulin even on the first exposure. More than 50% of patients who receive insulin develop antibodies against the insulin preparation, although there may not be any clinical manifestations. Local cutaneous reactions usually do not require treatment and resolve with continued insulin administration, possibly owing to IgG-blocking antibodies. More severe local reactions can be treated with antihistamines or by splitting the insulin dose between separate administration sites. Local reactions to the protamine component of neutral protamine Hagedorn (NPH) insulin may be avoided by switching to Lente insulin. Immediate-type reactions to insulin, including urticaria and anaphylactic shock, are unusual and almost always occur after re-institution of insulin therapy in sensitized patients. Insulin therapy should not be interrupted if a systemic reaction to insulin occurs and continued insulin therapy is essential. Skin testing may identify a less antigenic insulin preparation. The dose following a systemic reaction is usually reduced to one third, and successive doses are increased in 2-5 unit increments until the dose resulting in glucose control is attained. Insulin skin testing and desensitization are required if insulin treatment is subsequently interrupted for more than 24-48 hr. Immunologic resistance usually occurs when high titers of predominantly IgG antibodies to insulin develop. A rare form of insulin resistance caused by circulating antibodies to tissue insulin receptors is associated with acanthosis nigricans and lipodystrophy. Coexisting insulin allergy may be present in up to a third of patients with insulin resistance. Approximately half of affected patients benefit from substitution with a less reactive insulin preparation, based on skin testing.

Drug-induced Hypersensitivity Syndrome

Drug-induced hypersensitivity syndrome, also referred to as DRESS (drug rash with eosinophilia and systemic symptoms) syndrome, is a potentially life-threatening syndrome that has been described primarily with anticonvulsants (Table 146-1). It is characterized by fever, maculopapular rash, generalized lymphadenopathy, and potentially life-threatening damage of one or more organs, including visceral organ involvement that resolves with discontinuation of the anticonvulsant. Drug-induced hypersensitivity syndrome/DRESS has also been described with minocycline, sulfonamides, aspirin, chlorambucil, and dapsone.

Table 146-1 SERIOUS DRUG ERUPTIONS

DIAGNOSIS	MUCOSAL LESIONS	TYPICAL SKIN LESIONS	PRODROMAL/SIGNS AND SYMPTOMS	DRUG ASSOCIATED (%)	DRUGS MOST OFTEN IMPLICATED	TYPICAL TIME TO ONSET (WK)	ALTERNATIVE CAUSES NOT RELATED TO DRUGS
Drug hypersensitivity syndrome (DHS)	Infrequent	Severe exanthematous rash (could become edematous, pustular, purpuric), exfoliative dermatitis	30-50% involve fever, lymphadenopathy, hepatitis, nephritis, carditis, eosinophilia, atypical lymphocytes	≥90	Phenytoin, carbamazepine, phenobarbital, sulfonamides, allopurinol, minocycline, nitrofurantoin, terbinafine	1-6	Cutaneous lymphoma
Stevens-Johnson syndrome (SJS)	Erosions at ≥2 sites	Crops of lesions on skin, conjunctivae, mouth, and genitalia; detachment of ≤10% of body surface area	High fever, sore throat, rhinorrhea, cough	48-64	Sulfonamides, phenytoin, carbamazepine, barbiturates, allopurinol, aminopenicillins, nonsteroidal anti-inflammatory drugs	1-3	
Toxic epidermal necrolysis (TEN)	Erosions at ≥2 sites	Lesions similar to those with SJS; confluent epidermis separates readily with lateral pressure; detachment of ≥30% of body surface area	Fever, headache, sore throat; nearly all cases involve fever, "acute skin failure," leukopenia, lesions of the respiratory and/or gastrointestinal tracts	43-65	Sulfonamides, phenytoin, carbamazepine, barbiturates, allopurinol, aminopenicillins, nonsteroidal anti-inflammatory drugs	1-3	Exanthematous stage of Kawasaki disease; staphylococcal scalded-skin syndrome

From Segal AR, Doherty KM, Leggott J, et al: Cutaneous reactions to drugs in children, *Pediatrics* 120:e1082–e1096, 2007.

Reactions are treated with discontinuation of the offending agent, systemic steroids, and supportive care.

Red Man Syndrome

Red man syndrome is caused by nonspecific histamine release and is most commonly described with administration of intravenous vancomycin. It can be prevented by slowing the vancomycin infusion rate or by preadministration of H_1-blockers.

Radiocontrast Media

Anaphylactoid reactions to radiocontrast media or dye can occur after intravascular administration and during myelograms or retrograde pyelograms. No single pathogenic mechanism has been defined, but it is likely that mast cell activation accounts for the majority of these reactions. Complement activation has also been described. There is no evidence that sensitivity to seafood or iodine predisposes to radiocontrast media reactions. Predictive tests are not available. Patients who have atopic profiles, who are using β-blockers, and who have had prior anaphylactoid reactions are at increased risk. Other diagnostic alternatives should be considered, or patients can be given low-osmolality radiocontrast media with a pretreatment regimen including oral prednisone, diphenhydramine, and albuterol, with or without cimetidine or ranitidine.

Narcotic Analgesics

Opiates such as morphine and related narcotics can induce direct mast cell degranulation. Patients may experience generalized pruritus, urticaria, and, occasionally, wheezing. If there is a suggestive history and analgesia is required, a nonnarcotic medication should be considered. If this intervention does not control pain, graded challenge with an alternative opiate is an option.

Aspirin and Nonsteroidal Anti-Inflammatory Drugs

Aspirin and nonsteroidal anti-inflammatory drugs (NSAIDs) can cause anaphylactoid reactions or urticaria and/or angioedema in children and, rarely, asthma with or without rhinoconjunctivitis in adolescents. There is no skin or in vitro test to identify patients who may react to aspirin or other NSAIDs. Once aspirin or NSAID intolerance has been established, options include (1) avoidance and (2) pharmacologic desensitization and subsequent continued treatment with aspirin or NSAIDs if indicated. A number of studies suggest that cyclo-oxygenase-2 inhibitors are tolerated by the majority of patients with NSAID-induced adverse reactions.

BIBLIOGRAPHY

Please visit the Nelson Textbook of Pediatrics *website at www.expertconsult.com for the complete bibliography.*

PART XVI Rheumatic Diseases of Childhood

Chapter 147
Evaluation of Suspected Rheumatic Disease

C. Egla Rabinovich

Rheumatic diseases are defined by the constellation of results of the physical examination, autoimmune marker and other serologic tests, tissue pathology, and imaging. Defined diagnostic criteria exist for most rheumatic diseases. Recognition of clinical patterns remains essential for diagnosis because there is no single diagnostic test and results may be positive in the absence of disease. Further clouding diagnosis, children sometimes present with partial criteria that evolve over time or with features of more than one rheumatic disease (**overlap syndromes**). The primary mimics of rheumatic diseases are infection and malignancy but also include metabolic, orthopedic, and chronic pain conditions. Exclusion of possible mimicking disorders is essential before initiation of treatment for a presumptive diagnosis, especially corticosteroids. After careful evaluation has excluded nonrheumatic causes, referral to a pediatric rheumatologist for confirmation of the diagnosis and treatment should be considered.

For the full continuation of this chapter, please visit the Nelson Textbook of Pediatrics *website at www.expertconsult.com.*

Chapter 148
Treatment of Rheumatic Diseases

Esi Morgan DeWitt, Laura E. Schanberg, and C. Egla Rabinovich

The rheumatic diseases of childhood are complex chronic illnesses that present management challenges to both primary care and subspecialty providers. Optimal disease management requires family-centered care delivered by a multidisciplinary team of health care professionals providing medical, psychologic, social, and school support. Rheumatologic conditions, such as juvenile idiopathic arthritis (JIA) and systemic lupus erythematosus (SLE), most often follow a disease course marked by flares and periods of remission, but some children have unremitting disease. Treatment is aimed at achieving and maintaining clinical remission while minimizing medication toxicities. Disease management includes surveillance for potential complications of disease, such as inflammatory eye disease in JIA and early nephritis in SLE.

For the full continuation of this chapter, please visit the Nelson Textbook of Pediatrics *website at www.expertconsult.com.*

Chapter 149
Juvenile Idiopathic Arthritis

Eveline Y. Wu, Heather A. Van Mater, and C. Egla Rabinovich

Juvenile idiopathic arthritis (JIA) (formerly juvenile rheumatoid arthritis) is the most common rheumatic disease in children and one of the more common chronic illnesses of childhood. JIA represents a heterogeneous group of disorders all sharing the clinical manifestation of arthritis. The etiology and pathogenesis of JIA are largely unknown, and the genetic component is complex, making clear distinction among various subtypes difficult. As a result, several classification schemas exist, each with its own limitations. In the Classification Criteria of the American College of Rheumatology (ACR), the term *juvenile rheumatoid arthritis* (JRA) is utilized and categorizes disease into 3 onset types (Table 149-1). Attempting to standardize nomenclature, The International League of Associations for Rheumatology (ILAR) proposed use of a different classification using the term **juvenile idiopathic arthritis (JIA)** (Table 149-2), which is inclusive of all subtypes of chronic juvenile arthritis. We refer to the ILAR classification criteria; enthesitis-related arthritis and psoriatic JIA are covered in Chapter 150 (Tables 149-3 and 149-4).

EPIDEMIOLOGY

The worldwide incidence of JIA ranges from 0.8 to 22.6/100,000 children per year, with prevalence ranges from 7 to 401/ 100,000. These wide-ranging numbers are attributable to population differences, particularly environmental exposure and immunogenetic susceptibility, along with difficulty in case ascertainment and lack of population-based data. It is estimated that 300,000 children in the USA have arthritis, including 100,000 with a form of JIA. Pauciarticular JIA (oligoarthritis) is the most common subtype (50-60%), followed by polyarticular (30-35%) and systemic-onset (10-20%). There is no sex predominance in systemic-onset JIA (SoJIA), but more girls than boys are affected in both pauciarticular (3 : 1) and polyarticular (5 : 1) JIA. The peak age at onset is between 2 and 4 yr for pauciarticular disease. Age of onset has a bimodal distribution in polyarthritis, with peaks at 2-4 yr and 10-14 yr. SoJIA occurs throughout childhood without a peak.

ETIOLOGY

The etiology and pathogenesis of JIA is not completely understood. At least 2 components are considered necessary: immunogenetic susceptibility and an external trigger. JIA is a complex genetic trait in which multiple genes may affect disease susceptibility. Various major histocompatibility complex regions (HLA) class I and class II alleles have been associated with different JIA subtypes. Several non-HLA candidate loci are also associated with JIA, including polymorphisms in the genes encoding tumor necrosis factor (TNF)-α, macrophage inhibitory factor (MIF),

Table 149-1 CRITERIA FOR THE CLASSIFICATION OF JUVENILE RHEUMATOID ARTHRITIS

Age at onset: <16 yr
Arthritis (swelling or effusion, or the presence of 2 or more of the following signs: limitation of range of motion, tenderness or pain on motion, increased heat) in ≥1 joints
Duration of disease: ≥6 wk
Onset type defined by type of articular involvement in the 1st 6 mo after onset:
Polyarthritis: ≥5 inflamed joints
Oligoarthritis: ≤4 inflamed joints
Systemic disease: arthritis with rash and a characteristic quotidian fever
Exclusion of other forms of juvenile arthritis

Modified from Cassidy JT, Levison JE, Bass JC, et al: A study of classification criteria for a diagnosis of juvenile rheumatoid arthritis, *Arthritis Rheum* 29;174–181, 1986.

Table 149-2 CHARACTERISTICS OF THE AMERICAN COLLEGE OF RHEUMATOLOGY (ACR) AND INTERNATIONAL LEAGUE OF ASSOCIATIONS FOR RHEUMATOLOGY (ILAR) CLASSIFICATIONS OF CHILDHOOD CHRONIC ARTHRITIS

PARAMETER	ACR (1977)	ILAR (1997)
Term	Juvenile rheumatoid arthritis (JRA)	Juvenile idiopathic arthritis (JIA)
Minimum duration	≥6 wk	≥6 wk
Age at onset	<16 yr	<16 yr
≤4 joints in 1st 6 mo after presentation	• Pauciarticular	• Oligoarthritis: A. Persistent: <4 joints for course of disease B. Extended: >4 joints after 6 mo
>4 joints in 1st 6 mo after presentation	• Polyarticular	• Polyarticular rheumatoid factor–negative • Polyarticular rheumatoid factor–positive
Fever, rash, arthritis	• Systemic	• Systemic
Other categories included	Exclusion of other forms	• Psoriatic arthritis • Enthesitis-related arthritis • Undifferentiated: A. Fits no other category B. Fits more than one category
Inclusion of psoriatic arthritis, inflammatory bowel disease, ankylosing spondylitis	No (Chapter 150)	Yes

Table 149-3 INTERNATIONAL LEAGUE OF ASSOCIATIONS FOR RHEUMATOLOGY CLASSIFICATION OF JUVENILE IDIOPATHIC ARTHRITIS (JIA)

CATEGORY	DEFINITION	EXCLUSIONS
Systemic-onset JIA	Arthritis in ≥1 joints with, or preceded by, fever of at least 2 wk in duration that is documented to be daily ("quotidian"*) for at least 3 days and accompanied by ≥1 of the following: 1. Evanescent (nonfixed) erythematous rash. 2. Generalized lymph node enlargement. 3. Hepatomegaly or splenomegaly or both. 4. Serositis.†	a. Psoriasis or a history of psoriasis in the patient or a 1st-degree relative. b. Arthritis in an HLA-B27–positive boy beginning after the 6th birthday. c. Ankylosing spondylitis, enthesitis-related arthritis, sacroiliitis with inflammatory bowel disease, Reiter syndrome, or acute anterior uveitis, or a history of one of these disorders in a 1st-degree relative. d. Presence of immunoglobulin M RF on at least 2 occasions at least 3 mo apart.
Oligoarticular JIA	Arthritis affecting 1-4 joints during the 1st 6 mo of disease. Two subcategories are recognized: 1. Persistent oligoarthritis—affecting ≤4 joints throughout the disease course. 2. Extended oligoarthritis—affecting >4 joints after the 1st 6 mo of disease.	a, b, c, d (above) *plus* e. Presence of systemic JIA in the patient.
Polyarthritis (RF-negative)	Arthritis affecting ≥5 joints during the 1st 6 mo of disease; a test for RF is negative.	a, b, c, d, e
Polyarthritis (RF-positive)	Arthritis affecting ≥5 joints during the 1st 6 mo of disease; ≥2 tests for RF at least 3 mo apart during the 1st 6 mo of disease are positive.	a, b, c ,e
Psoriatic arthritis	Arthritis and psoriasis, or arthritis and at least 2 of the following: 1. Dactylitis.‡ 2. Nail pitting§ and onycholysis. 3. Psoriasis in a 1st-degree relative.	b, c, d, e
Enthesitis-related arthritis	Arthritis and enthesitis,ǀ or arthritis or enthesitis with at least 2 of the following: 1. Presence of or a history of sacroiliac joint tenderness or inflammatory lumbosacral pain or both.¶ 2. Presence of HLA-B27 antigen. 3. Onset of arthritis in a male > 6 yr old. 4. Acute (symptomatic) anterior uveitis. 5. History of ankylosing spondylitis, enthesitis-related arthritis, sacroiliitis with inflammatory bowel disease, Reiter syndrome, or acute anterior uveitis in a 1st-degree relative.	a, d, e
Undifferentiated arthritis	Arthritis that fulfills criteria in no category or in ≥2 of the above categories.	

*Quotidian fever is defined as a fever that rises to 39°C once a day and returns to 37°C between fever peaks.
†*Serositis* refers to pericarditis, pleuritis, or peritonitis, or some combination of the three.
‡Dactylitis is swelling of ≥1 digits, usually in an asymmetric distribution, that extends beyond the joint margin.
§A minimum of 2 pits on any one or more nails at any time.
ǀ*Enthesitis* is defined as tenderness at the insertion of a tendon, ligament, joint capsule, or fascia to bone.
¶*Inflammatory lumbosacral pain* refers to lumbosacral pain at rest with morning stiffness that improves on movement.
RF, rheumatoid factor.
From Firestein GS, Budd RC, Harris ED Jr, et al, editors: *Kelley's textbook of rheumatology*, ed 8, Philadelphia, 2009, Saunders/Elsevier.

Table 149-4 OVERVIEW OF THE MAIN FEATURES OF THE SUBTYPES OF JUVENILE IDIOPATHIC ARTHRITIS

INTERNATIONAL LEAGUE OF ASSOCIATIONS FOR RHEUMATOLOGY SUBTYPE	PEAK AGE OF ONSET (YR)	FEMALE: MALE RATIO	PERCENTAGE OF ALL JIA CASES	ARTHRITIS PATTERN	EXTRA-ARTICULAR FEATURES	LABORATORY INVESTIGATIONS	NOTES ON THERAPY
Systemic arthritis	2-4	1:1	<10	Polyarticular, often affecting knees, wrists, and ankles; also fingers, neck, and hips	Daily fever; evanescent rash; pericarditis; pleuritis	Anemia; WBC ↑↑; ESR ↑↑; CRP ↑↑; ferritin ↑; platelets ↑↑ (normal or ↓ in MAS)	Less responsive to standard treatment with MTX and anti-TNF agents; consider interleukin-1 receptor antagonist in resistant cases
Oligoarthritis	<6	4:1	50-60 (but ethnic variation)	Knees ++; ankles, fingers +	Uveitis in ≈30% of cases	ANA positive in ≈60%; other test results usually normal; may have mildly ↑ ESR/CRP	NSAIDS and intra-articular steroids; MTX occasionally required
Polyarthritis: RF-negative	6-7	3:1	30	Symmetric or asymmetric; small and large joints; cervical spine; temporomandibular joint	Uveitis in ≈10%	ANA positive in 40%; RF negative; ESR ↑ or ↑↑; CRP ↑/normal; mild anemia	Standard therapy with MTX and NSAIDs; then, if nonresponsive, anti-TNF agents or other biologics
RF-positive	9-12	9:1	<10	Aggressive symmetric polyarthritis	Rheumatoid nodules in 10%; low-grade fever	RF positive; ESR ↑↑; CRP ↑/normal; mild anemia	Long-term remission unlikely; early aggressive therapy is warranted
Psoriatic arthritis	7-10	2:1	<10	Asymmetric arthritis of small or medium-sized joints	Uveitis in 10%; psoriasis in 50%	ANA positive in 50%; ESR ↑; CRP ↑/ normal; mild anemia	NSAIDs and intra-articular steroids; second-line agents used less commonly
Enthesitis-related arthritis	9-12	1:7	10	Predominantly lower limb joints affected; sometimes axial skeleton (but less than in adult, ankylosing spondylitis)	Acute anterior uveitis; association with reactive arthritis and inflammatory bowel disease	80% of patients positive for HLA-B27	NSAIDs and intra-articular steroids; consider sulfasalazine as alternative to MTX

ANA, antinuclear antibody; CRP, C-reactive protein; ESR, erythrocyte sedimentation rate; JIA, juvenile idiopathic arthritis; MAS, macrophage activation syndrome; MTX, methotrexate; NSAID, nonsteroidal anti-inflammatory drug; RF, rheumatoid factor; TNF, tumor necrosis factor; WBC, white blood cell count.
From Firestein GS, Budd RC, Harris ED Jr, et al, editors: *Kelley's textbook of rheumatology,* ed 8, Philadelphia, 2009, Saunders/Elsevier.

interleukin-6 (IL-6), and IL-1α. Possible nongenetic triggers include bacterial and viral infections (parvovirus B19, rubella, Epstein-Barr virus), enhanced immune responses to bacterial or mycobacterial heat shock proteins, abnormal reproductive hormone levels, and joint trauma.

PATHOGENESIS

JIA is an autoimmune disease associated with alterations in both humoral and cell-mediated immunity. T lymphocytes have a central role, releasing proinflammatory cytokines (e.g., TNF-α, IL-6, and IL-1). The cytokine profile favors type 1 helper T-lymphocyte response. Studies of T-cell receptor expression confirm recruitment of T lymphocytes specific for synovial non-self antigens. Complement consumption, immune complex formation, and B-cell activation also promote inflammation. Inheritance of specific cytokine alleles may predispose to upregulation of inflammatory networks, resulting in systemic-onset disease or more severe articular disease.

Systemic-onset JIA may be more accurately classified as an autoinflammatory disorder, more like familial Mediterranean fever (FMF), than the other subtypes of JIA. This theory is supported by work demonstrating similar expression patterns of a phagocytic protein (S100A12) in SoJIA and FMF, as well as the same marked responsiveness to IL-1 receptor antagonists.

All these immunologic abnormalities cause inflammatory synovitis, characterized pathologically by villous hypertrophy and hyperplasia with hyperemia and edema of the synovial tissue. Vascular endothelial hyperplasia is prominent and is characterized by infiltration of mononuclear and plasma cells with a predominance of T lymphocytes (Fig. 149-1). Advanced and uncontrolled disease leads to pannus formation and progressive erosion of articular cartilage and contiguous bone (Figs. 149-2 and 149-3).

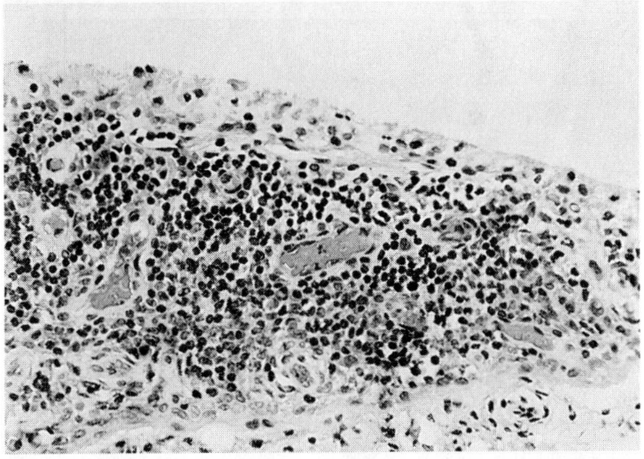

Figure 149-1 Synovial biopsy specimen from a 10 yr old child with oligoarticular juvenile idiopathic arthritis. There is a dense infiltration of lymphocytes and plasma cells in the synovium.

CLINICAL MANIFESTATIONS

Arthritis must be present for a diagnosis of any subtype of JIA to be made. Arthritis is defined by intra-articular swelling or the presence of 2 or more of the following signs: limitation in range of motion, tenderness or pain on motion, and increased heat or erythema. Initial symptoms may be subtle or acute and often include morning stiffness with a limp or gelling after inactivity. Easy fatigability and poor sleep quality may be associated.

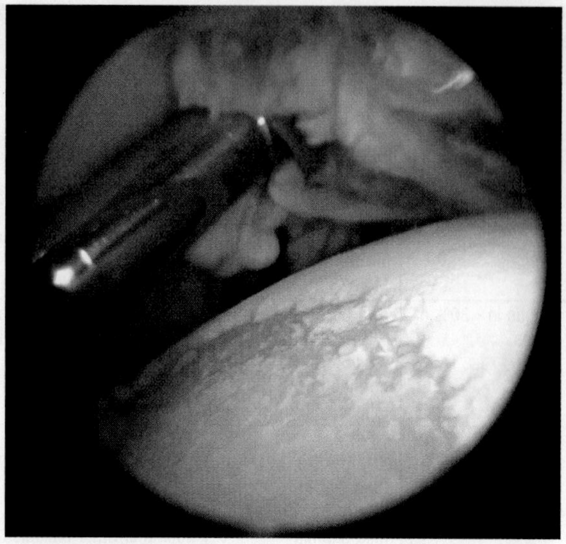

Figure 149-2 Arthroscopy in the shoulder of a child with juvenile idiopathic arthritis showing pannus formation and cartilage erosions. (Courtesy of Dr. Alison Toth.)

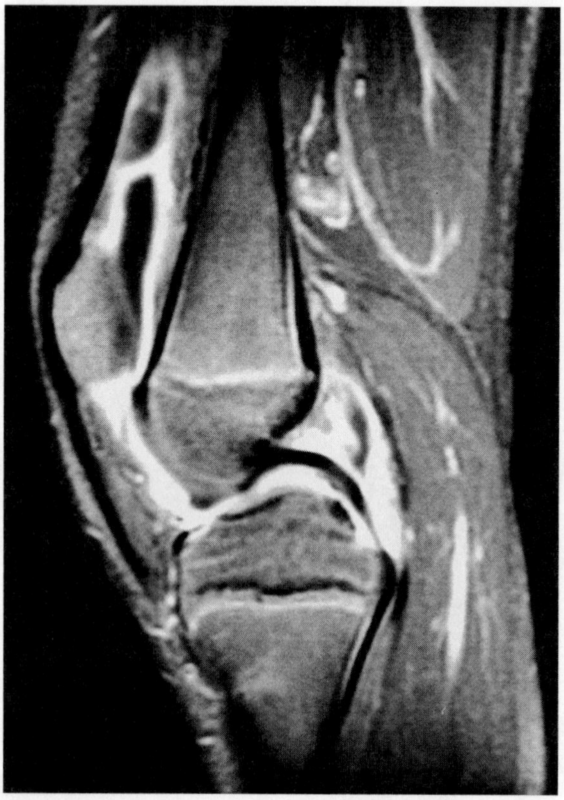

Figure 149-3 MRI with gadolinium of a 10 yr old child with juvenile rheumatoid arthritis (same patient as in Fig. 149-1). The dense white signal in the synovium near the distal femur, proximal tibia, and patella reflects inflammation. MRI of the knee is useful to exclude ligamentous injury, chondromalacia of the patella, and tumor.

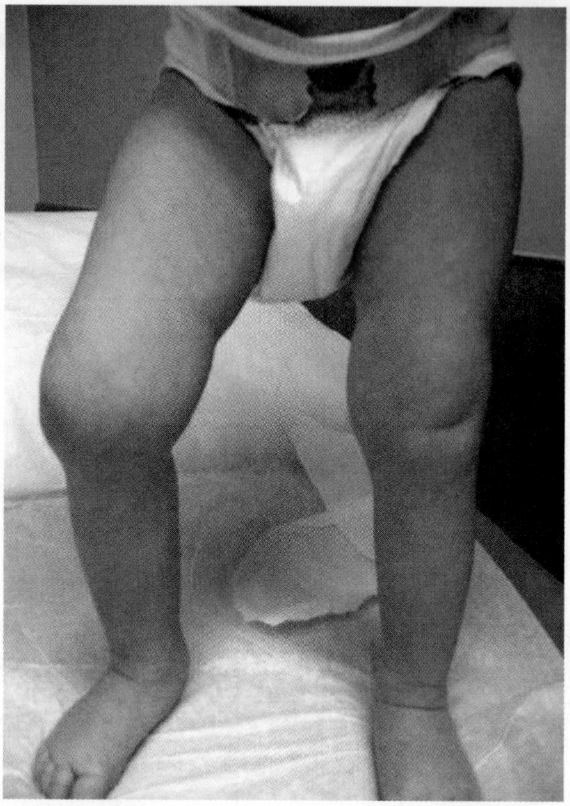

Figure 149-4 Oligoarticular juvenile idiopathic arthritis with swelling and flexion contracture of the right knee.

Involved joints are often swollen, warm to touch, and painful on movement or palpation with reduced range of motion but usually are not erythematous. Arthritis in large joints, especially knees, initially accelerates linear growth, causing the affected limb to be longer and resulting in a discrepancy in limb lengths. Continued inflammation stimulates rapid and premature closure of the growth plate, resulting in shortened bones.

Oligoarthritis is defined as involving ≤4 joints within the first 6 mo of disease onset, predominantly affecting the large joints of the lower extremities, such as the knees and ankles (Fig. 149-4). Often only a single joint is involved. Isolated involvement of upper extremity large joints is less common. Those in whom disease never develops in more than 4 joints are regarded as having **persistent oligoarticular JIA**, whereas evolution of disease in more than 4 joints over time changes the classification to **extended oligoarticular JIA**. The latter often portends a worse prognosis. Involvement of the hip is almost never a presenting sign and suggests a spondyloarthropathy (Chapter 150) or nonrheumatologic cause. The presence of a positive antinuclear antibody (ANA) test result confers increased risk for asymptomatic anterior uveitis, requiring periodic slit-lamp examination (Table 149-5).

Polyarthritis (polyarticular disease) is characterized by inflammation of ≥5 joints in both upper and lower extremities (Figs. 149-5 and 149-6). When rheumatoid factor (RF) is present, polyarticular disease resembles the characteristic symmetric presentation of adult rheumatoid arthritis. **Rheumatoid nodules** on the extensor surfaces of the elbows and over the Achilles tendons, although unusual, are associated with a more severe course and almost exclusively occur in RF-positive individuals. **Micrognathia** reflects chronic temporomandibular joint (TMJ) disease (Fig. 149-7). Cervical spine involvement (Fig. 149-8), manifesting as decreased neck extension, occurs with a risk of atlantoaxial subluxation and neurologic sequelae. Hip disease may be subtle, with findings of decreased or painful range of motion on exam (Fig. 149-9).

Systemic-onset disease (SoJIA) is characterized by arthritis, fever, and prominent visceral involvement, including hepatosplenomegaly, lymphadenopathy, and serositis (pericarditis). The characteristic fever, defined as spiking temperatures to ≥39°C, occurs on a daily or twice-daily basis for at least 2 wk, with a rapid return to normal or subnormal temperatures (Fig. 149-10). The fever is often present in the evening and is frequently accompanied by a characteristic faint, erythematous, macular rash. The

Table 149-5 FREQUENCY OF OPHTHALMOLOGIC EXAMINATION IN PATIENTS WITH JUVENILE IDIOPATHIC ARTHRITIS

TYPE	ANTI-NUCLEAR ANTIBODY TEST RESULT	AGE AT ONSET (YR)	DURATION OF DISEASE (YR)	RISK CATEGORY	EYE EXAMINATION FREQUENCY (MO)
Oligoarthritis or polyarthritis	+	≤6	≤4	High	3
	+	≤6	>4	Moderate	6
	+	≤6	>7	Low	12
	+	>6	≤4	Moderate	6
	+	>6	>4	Low	12
	–	≤6	≤4	Moderate	6
	–	≤6	>4	Low	12
	–	>6	NA	Low	12
Systemic disease	NA	NA	NA	Low	12

From Cassidy J, Kivlin J, Lindsley C, et al; Section on Rheumatology; Section on Ophthalmology: Ophthalmologic examinations in children with juvenile rheumatoid arthritis, *Pediatrics* 117:1843–1845, 2006.

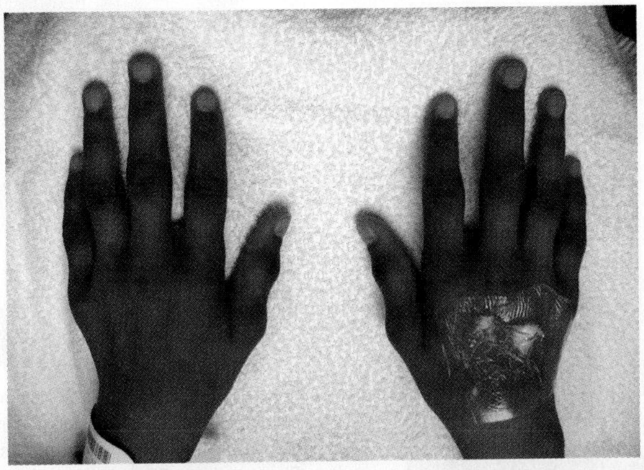

Figure 149-5 Hands and wrists of a girl with polyarticular juvenile idiopathic arthritis that is rheumatoid factor–negative. Notice the symmetric involvement of the wrists, metacarpophalangeal joints, and proximal and distal interphalangeal joints. In this photograph, there is cream with occlusive dressing on the patient's right hand in preparation for placement of an intravenous line for administration of a biologic agent.

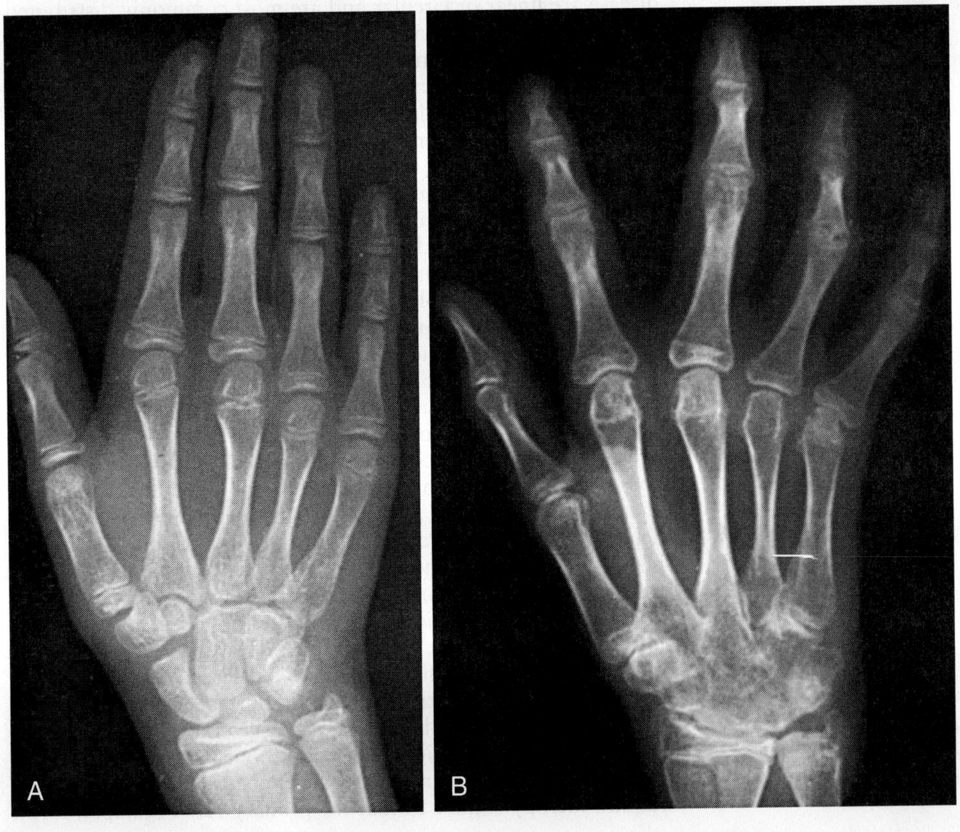

Figure 149-6 Progression of joint destruction in a girl with polyarticular juvenile idiopathic arthritis that is rheumatoid factor–positive, despite doses of corticosteroids sufficient to suppress symptoms in the interval between the radiographs shown in *A* and *B*. *A*, Radiograph of the hand at onset. *B*, Radiograph taken 4 yr later, showing a loss of articular cartilage and destructive changes in the distal and proximal interphalangeal and metacarpophalangeal joints as well as destruction and fusion of wrist bones.

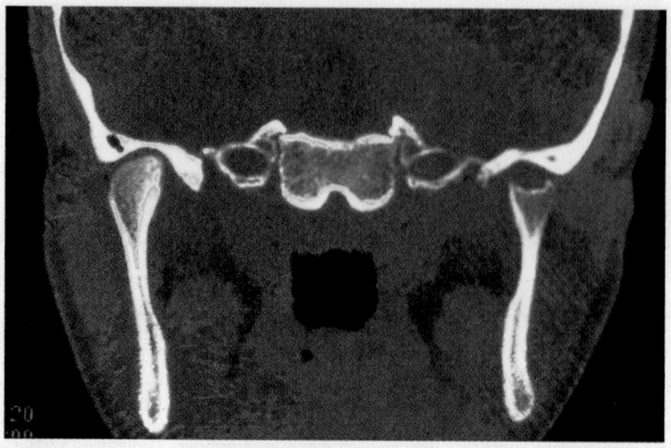

Figure 149-7 CT scan of the temporomandibular joint of a patient with juvenile idiopathic arthritis exhibiting destruction on the right.

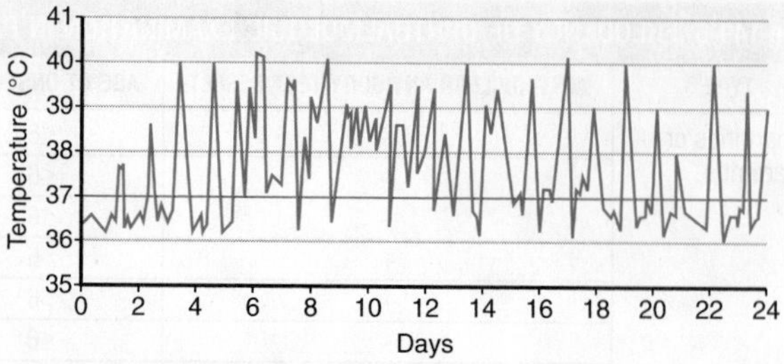

Figure 149-10 High-spiking intermittent fever in a 3 yr old patient with systemic juvenile idiopathic arthritis. (From Ravelli A, Martini A: Juvenile idiopathic arthritis, *Lancet* 369:767–778, 2007.)

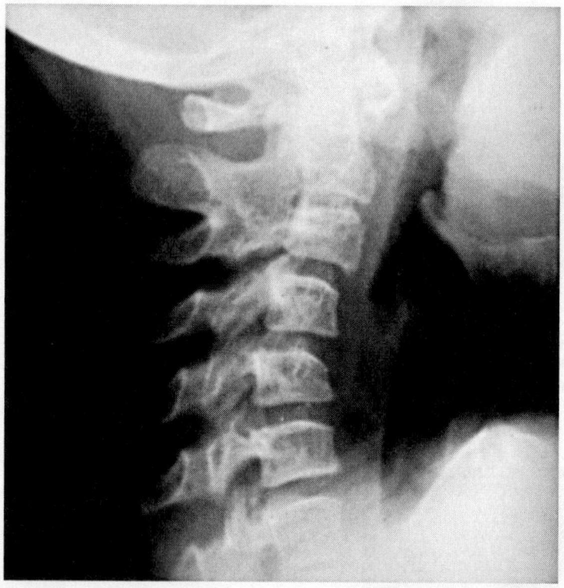

Figure 149-8 Radiograph of the cervical spine of a patient with active juvenile idiopathic arthritis, showing fusion of the neural arch between joints C2 and C3, narrowing and erosion of the remaining neural arch joints, obliteration of the apophyseal space, and loss of the normal lordosis.

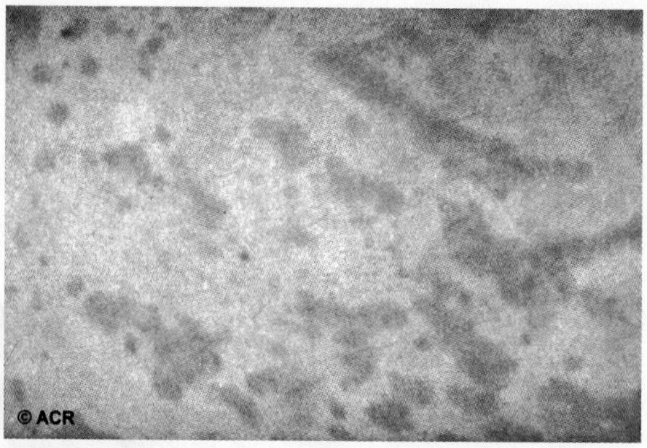

Figure 149-11 The rash of systemic-onset juvenile idiopathic arthritis. The rash is salmon-colored, macular, and nonpruritic. Individual lesions are transient and occur in crops over the trunk and extremities. (Reprinted from the American College of Rheumatology*: Clinical slide collection on the rheumatic diseases*, Atlanta, copyright 1991, 1995, 1997, ACR. Used by permission of the American College of Rheumatology.)

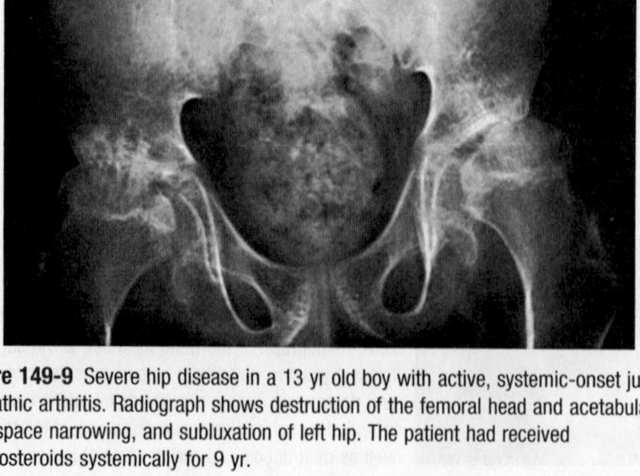

Figure 149-9 Severe hip disease in a 13 yr old boy with active, systemic-onset juvenile idiopathic arthritis. Radiograph shows destruction of the femoral head and acetabula, joint space narrowing, and subluxation of left hip. The patient had received corticosteroids systemically for 9 yr.

evanescent **salmon-colored lesions** classic for systemic-onset disease are linear or circular and are most commonly distributed over the trunk and proximal extremities (Fig. 149-11). The classic rash is nonpruritic and migratory with lesions lasting <1 hr. Fever, rash, hepatosplenomegaly, and lymphadenopathy are present in >70% of affected children. **Koebner phenomenon,** a cutaneous hypersensitivity to superficial trauma, is often present. Heat, such as from a warm bath, also evokes rash. Without arthritis, the differential diagnosis includes the episodic fever syndromes and a fever of unknown origin. Some children initially present with only systemic features, but definitive diagnosis requires presence of arthritis. Arthritis may affect any number of joints, but the course is classically polyarticular, may be very destructive, and includes hip, cervical spine, and TMJ involvement.

Macrophage activation syndrome (MAS) is a rare but potentially fatal complication of SoJIA that can occur at anytime during the disease course. It is also referred to as secondary hemophagocytic syndrome or hemophagocytic lymphohistiocytosis (HLH) (Chapter 501). MAS classically manifests as acute onset of profound anemia associated with thrombocytopenia or leukopenia with high, spiking fevers, lymphadenopathy, and hepatosplenomegaly. Patients may have purpura and mucosal bleeding, as well as elevated fibrin split product values and prolonged prothrombin and partial prothromboplastin times. The erythrocyte sedimentation rate (ESR) falls because of hypofibrinogenemia and hepatic dysfunction, a feature useful in distinguishing MAS from a flare of systemic disease. The diagnosis is suggested by clinical criteria and is confirmed by bone marrow biopsy demonstrating hemophagocytosis (Table 149-6). Emergency treatment with high-dose intravenous methylprednisolone, cyclosporine, or anakinra may be effective. Severe cases may require therapy similar to that for primary HLH (Chapter 501).

Table 149-6 PRELIMINARY DIAGNOSTIC GUIDELINES FOR MACROPHAGE ACTIVATION SYSTEM (MAS) COMPLICATING SYSTEMIC JUVENILE IDIOPATHIC ARTHRITIS (JIA)

LABORATORY CRITERIA
1. Decreased platelet count (≤262 × 10^9/L). 2. Elevations of aspartate aminotransferase (>59 U/L). 3. Decreased white blood cell count (≤4.0 × 10^9/L). 4. Hypofibrinogenemia (≤2.5 g/L).
CLINICAL CRITERIA
1. Central nervous system dysfunction (irritability, disorientation, lethargy, headache, seizures, coma). 2. Hemorrhages (purpura, easy bruising, mucosal bleeding). 3. Hepatomegaly (edge of liver ≥3 cm below the costal arch).
HISTOPATHOLOGIC CRITERION
• Evidence of macrophage hemophagocytosis in the bone marrow aspirate
DIAGNOSTIC RULE
• The diagnosis of MAS requires the presence of any 2 or more laboratory criteria or of any 2 or 3 or more clinical and/or laboratory criteria. A bone marrow aspirate for the demonstration of hemophagocytosis may be required only in doubtful cases.
RECOMMENDATIONS
• The aforementioned criteria are of value only in patients with active systemic JIA. The thresholds of laboratory criteria are provided by way of example only.
COMMENTS
1. The clinical criteria are probably more useful as classification criteria than as diagnostic criteria because they often occur late in the course of MAS and may be, therefore, of limited value for the early suspicion of the syndrome. 2. Other abnormal clinical features in systemic JIA–associated MAS not previously mentioned are: nonremitting high fever, splenomegaly, generalized lymphadenopathy, and paradoxic improvement of signs and symptoms of arthritis. 3. Other abnormal laboratory findings in systemic JIA–associated MAS not previously mentioned are: anemia, erythrocyte sedimentation rate fall, elevated alanine aminotransferase, increased bilirubin, presence of fibrin degradation products, elevated lactate dehydrogenase, hypertriglyceridemia, low sodium levels, decreased albumin, and hyperferritinemia.

From Ravelli A, Magni-Manzoni S, Pistorio A, et al: Preliminary diagnostic guidelines for macrophage activation syndrome complicating systemic juvenile idiopathic arthritis, *J Pediatr* 146:598–604, 2005.

Bone mineral metabolism and skeletal maturation are adversely affected in children with JIA, regardless of subtype. Children with JIA have decreased bone mass (osteopenia), which appears to be associated with increased disease activity. Increased levels of cytokines such as TNF-α and IL-6, both key regulators in bone metabolism, have deleterious effects on bone within the joint as well as systemically in the axial and appendicular bones. Osteoblast and osteoclast development and function have a central role in these negative bone changes. Abnormalities of skeletal maturation become most prominent during the pubertal growth spurt.

DIAGNOSIS

JIA is a clinical diagnosis of exclusion with many mimics and without diagnostic laboratory tests. The meticulous clinical exclusion of other diseases is therefore essential. See Tables 149-1 to 149-4 for classification criteria. Laboratory studies, including tests for ANA and RF, are only supportive and their results may be normal in patients with JIA.

DIFFERENTIAL DIAGNOSIS

The differential diagnosis for arthritis is broad and a careful, thorough investigation for other underlying etiology is imperative. Findings of the history, physical exam, laboratory tests, and radiography help exclude other possible causes. Arthritis can be a presenting manifestation for any of the multisystem rheumatic diseases of childhood, including systemic lupus erythematosus (Chapter 152), juvenile dermatomyositis (Chapter 153), sarcoidosis (Chapter 159), and the vasculitic syndromes (Chapter 161) (Table 149-7). In scleroderma (Chapter 154), limited range of motion due to sclerotic skin overlying a joint may be confused with sequelae from chronic inflammatory arthritis. **Acute rheumatic fever** is characterized by exquisite joint pain and tenderness, a remittent fever, and a migratory polyarthritis. **Autoimmune hepatitis** can also be associated with an acute arthritis.

Many infections are associated with arthritis, and a recent history of infectious symptoms may help make a distinction. Viruses, including parvovirus B19, rubella, Epstein-Barr virus, hepatitis B virus, and HIV, can induce a transient arthritis. Arthritis may follow enteric infections (Chapter 151). **Lyme disease** (Chapter 214) should be considered in children with oligoarthritis living in or visiting endemic areas. Although a history of tick exposure, preceding flu-like illness, and subsequent rash should be sought, they are not always present. Monoarticular arthritis unresponsive to anti-inflammatory treatment may be the result of chronic mycobacterial or other infection such as *Kingella kingae*, and the diagnosis is established by synovial fluid analysis or biopsy. Acute onset of fever and a painful, erythematous, hot joint suggests septic arthritis. Isolated hip pain with limited motion raises the possibility of suppurative arthritis (Chapter 677), osteomyelitis, toxic synovitis, Legg-Calvé-Perthes disease, slipped capital femoral epiphysis, and chondrolysis of the hip (Chapter 670).

Tenderness over insertion of ligaments and tendons and lower extremity arthritis, especially in a boy, raises the possibility of a spondyloarthropathy (Chapter 150). **Psoriatic arthritis** can manifest as limited joint involvement in an unusual distribution (e.g., small joints of the hand and ankle) years prior to onset of cutaneous disease. **Inflammatory bowel disease** may manifest as oligoarthritis, usually affecting joints in the lower extremities, as well as gastrointestinal symptoms, elevations in ESR, and microcytic anemia.

Many conditions present solely with arthralgias (i.e., joint pain). Hypermobility may cause joint pain, especially in the lower extremities. Growing pains should be suspected in a child between the ages of 4 to 12 yr complaining of leg pain in the evenings with normal investigative studies and no morning symptoms. Nocturnal pain also alerts to the possibility of a malignancy. An adolescent with missed school days may suggest a diagnosis of fibromyalgia (Chapter 162).

Children with **leukemia** or **neuroblastoma** may have joint or bone pain resulting from malignant infiltration of the bone, synovium, or, more often, the bone marrow, sometimes months before demonstrating lymphoblasts on peripheral blood smear. Physical examination may reveal no tenderness or a deeper pain to palpation of the bone or pain out of proportion to exam findings. Malignant pain often awakens the child from sleep and may cause cytopenias. Because platelets are an acute-phase reactant, a high ESR with leukopenia and a low normal platelet count may also be a clue to underlying leukemia. In addition, the characteristic quotidian fever of JIA is absent in malignancy. Bone marrow examination is necessary for diagnosis. Some diseases, such as cystic fibrosis, diabetes mellitus, and the glycogen storage diseases, have associated arthropathies (Chapter 163). Swelling that extends beyond the joint can be a sign of lymphedema or Henoch-Schönlein purpura. A peripheral arthritis indistinguishable from JIA occurs in the humoral immunodeficiencies, such as common variable immunodeficiency and X-linked agammaglobulinemia. Skeletal dysplasias associated with a degenerative arthropathy are diagnosed from their characteristic radiologic abnormalities.

LABORATORY FINDINGS

Hematologic abnormalities often reflect the degree of systemic or articular inflammation, with elevated white blood cell and platelet counts and a microcytic anemia. Inflammation may also cause

Table 149-7 CONDITIONS CAUSING ARTHRITIS OR EXTREMITY PAIN

RHEUMATIC AND INFLAMMATORY DISEASES
Juvenile idiopathic arthritis
Systemic lupus erythematosus
Juvenile dermatomyositis
Polyarteritis
Vasculitis
Scleroderma
Sjögren syndrome
Behçet disease
Overlap syndromes
Wegener granulomatosis
Sarcoidosis
Kawasaki syndrome
Henoch-Schönlein purpura
Chronic recurrent multifocal osteomyelitis
SERONEGATIVE SPONDYLOARTHROPATHIES
Juvenile ankylosing spondylitis
Inflammatory bowel disease
Psoriatic arthritis
Reactive arthritis associated with urethritis, iridocyclitis, and mucocutaneous lesions
INFECTIOUS ILLNESSES
Bacterial arthritis (septic arthritis, *Staphylococcus aureus*, pneumococcus, gonococcus, *Haemophilus influenzae*)
Lyme disease
Viral illness (parvovirus, rubella, mumps, Epstein-Barr virus, hepatitis B)
Fungal arthritis
Mycobacterial infection
Spirochetal infection
Endocarditis
REACTIVE ARTHRITIS
Acute rheumatic fever
Reactive arthritis (post-infectious due to *Shigella, Salmonella, Yersinia, Chlamydia,* or meningococcus)
Serum sickness
Toxic synovitis of the hip
Postimmunization
IMMUNODEFICIENCIES
Hypogammaglobulinemia
Immunoglobulin A deficiency
Human immunodeficiency virus
CONGENITAL AND METABOLIC DISORDERS
Gout
Pseudogout
Mucopolysaccharidoses
Thyroid disease (hypothyroidism, hyperthyroidism)
Hyperparathyroidism
Vitamin C deficiency (scurvy)
Hereditary connective tissue disease (Marfan syndrome, Ehlers-Danlos syndrome)
Fabry disease
Farber disease
Amyloidosis (familial Mediterranean fever)
BONE AND CARTILAGE DISORDERS
Trauma
Patellofemoral syndrome
Hypermobility syndrome
Osteochondritis dissecans
Avascular necrosis (including Legg-Calvé-Perthes disease)
Hypertrophic osteoarthropathy
Slipped capital femoral epiphysis
Osteolysis
Benign bone tumors (including osteoid osteoma)
Histiocytosis
Rickets
NEUROPATHIC DISORDERS
Peripheral neuropathies
Carpal tunnel syndrome
Charcot joints
NEOPLASTIC DISORDERS
Leukemia
Neuroblastoma
Lymphoma
Bone tumors (osteosarcoma, Ewing sarcoma)
Histiocytic syndromes
Synovial tumors
HEMATOLOGIC DISORDERS
Hemophilia
Hemoglobinopathies (including sickle cell disease)
MISCELLANEOUS DISORDERS
Pigmented villonodular synovitis
Plant-thorn synovitis (foreign body arthritis)
Myositis ossificans
Eosinophilic fasciitis
Tendinitis (overuse injury)
Raynaud phenomenon
PAIN SYNDROMES
Fibromyalgia
Growing pains
Depression (with somatization)
Reflex sympathetic dystrophy
Regional myofascial pain syndromes

elevations in ESR and C-reactive protein (CRP), though it is not unusual for both to be normal in children with JIA.

Elevated ANA titers are present in 40-85% of children with oligoarticular or polyarticular JIA but are rare with SoJIA. ANA seropositivity is associated with increased risk of **chronic uveitis** in JIA. Approximately 5-10% of patients with polyarticular JIA are seropositive for RF. Anti–cyclic citrullinated peptide (CCP) antibody, like RF, is a marker of more aggressive disease. Both ANA and RF seropositivity can occur in association with transient events, such as viral infection.

Children with SoJIA usually have striking elevations in inflammatory markers and white blood cell and platelet counts. Hemoglobin levels are low, typically in the range of 7 to 10 g/dL, with indices consistent with anemia of chronic disease. The ESR is usually high, except in MAS. Although immunoglobulin levels tend to be high, ANA and RF are uncommon. **Ferritin values** are typically elevated and can be markedly increased in MAS (>10,000 ng/mL). In the setting of MAS, all cell lines have the potential to decline precipitously owing to the consumptive process. A low white blood cell count and/or platelet count in a child with active SoJIA should raise concerns for MAS.

Early radiographic changes of arthritis include soft tissue swelling, periarticular osteoporosis, and periosteal new-bone apposition around affected joints (Fig. 149-12). Continued active disease may lead to subchondral erosions and loss of cartilage, with varying degrees of bony destruction and, potentially, fusion. Characteristic radiographic changes in cervical spine, most frequently in the neural arch joints at C2-C3 (see Fig. 149-8) may progress to atlantoaxial subluxation. MRI is more sensitive than radiography to early changes (Fig. 149-13).

TREATMENT

The goals of treatment are to achieve disease remission, prevent or halt joint damage, and foster normal growth and development. All children with JIA need individualized treatment plans, and management is tailored according to disease subtype and severity, presence of poor prognostic indicators, and response to medications. Disease management also requires monitoring for potential medication toxicities. Please see Chapter 148 for a detailed discussion of the medications used in the treatment of rheumatic diseases.

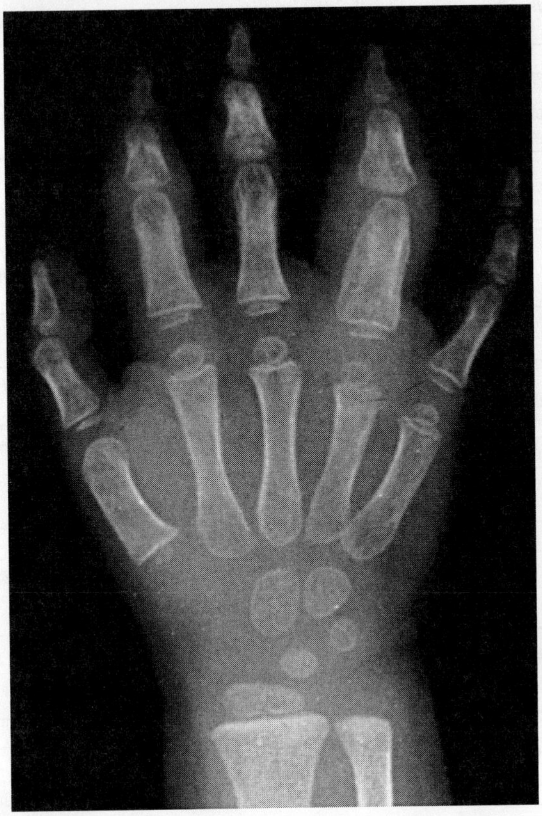

Figure 149-12 Early (6-mo duration) radiographic changes of juvenile idiopathic arthritis: Soft tissue swelling and periosteal new bone formation appear adjacent to the 2nd and 4th proximal interphalangeal joints.

Children with oligoarthritis often show at least partial response to nonsteroidal anti-inflammatory drugs (NSAIDs), with improvement in inflammation and pain (Table 149-8). Those who have no response after 4-6 wk of treatment with NSAIDS or who have functional limitations, such as joint contracture or leg length discrepancy, benefit from injection of intra-articular corticosteroids. Triamcinolone hexacetonide is a long-lasting preparation that provides a prolonged response. A minority of patients with oligoarthritis show no response to NSAIDs and injections, so require treatment with disease-modifying antirheumatic drugs (DMARDs), like patients with polyarticular disease.

NSAIDs alone rarely induce remission in children with polyarticular disease or SoJIA. Methotrexate is the oldest and least toxic of the DMARDs currently available for adjunctive therapy. It may take 6-12 wk to see the effects of methotrexate. Failure of methotrexate monotherapy may warrant the addition of a biologic DMARD. Biologic medications that inhibit proinflammatory cytokines, such as TNF-α and IL-1, have demonstrated excellent disease control. TNF-α antagonists (e.g., etanercept, adalimumab, infliximab) are used to treat children with an inadequate response to methotrexate, with poor prognostic factors, or with severe disease onset. Trials, however, are currently underway to evaluate the role of early and aggressive treatment in the management of JIA. Combination of TNF-α blockade and methotrexate may also be used in children with SoJIA and milder systemic symptoms. When systemic symptoms dominate, initiation of IL-1 receptor antagonist therapy often induces a dramatic and rapid response.

With the advent of newer DMARDs, the use of systemic corticosteroids can often be avoided. Systemic steroids are recommended only for management of severe systemic illness, for bridge therapy during the wait for therapeutic response to a DMARD, and for control of uveitis. Steroids should be avoided, as they impose risks of severe toxicities, including Cushing syndrome, growth retardation, and osteopenia, and they may not prevent joint destruction.

Management of JIA must include periodic slit-lamp ophthalmologic examinations to monitor for asymptomatic uveitis (see Table 149-5). Optimal treatment of uveitis requires collaboration

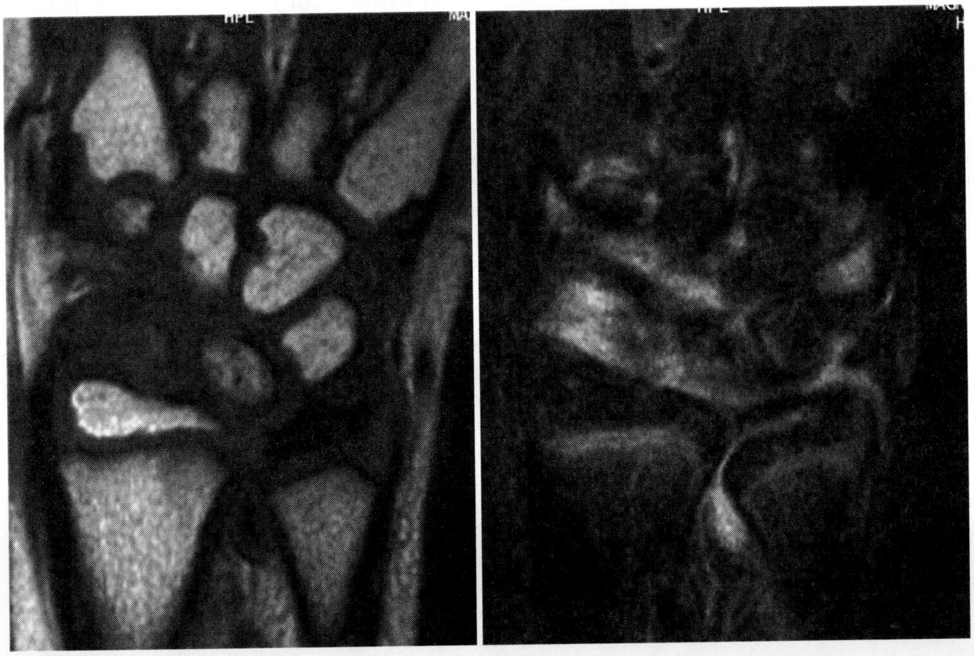

Figure 149-13 MRI of the wrist in a child with wrist arthritis. Image on the *left* shows multiple erosions of carpal bones. Image on the *right,* obtained after administration of gadolinium contrast agent, reveals uptake consistent with active synovitis.

Table 149-8 PHARMACOLOGIC TREATMENT OF JUVENILE IDIOPATHIC ARTHRITIS (JIA)

TYPICAL MEDICATIONS	TYPICAL DOSES	JIA SUBTYPE	SIDE EFFECT(S)
NONSTEROIDAL ANTI-INFLAMMATORY DRUGS			
Naproxen	15 mg/kg/day PO divided bid (maximum dose 500 mg bid)	Polyarticular Systemic onset Oligoarticular	Gastritis, renal toxicity, liver toxicity, pseudoporphyria
Ibuprofen	40 mg/kg/day PO divided tid (maximum dose 800 tid)	Same as above	Same as above
Meloxicam	0.125 mg/kg PO once daily (maximum dose 15 mg daily)	Same as above	Same as above
DISEASE-MODIFYING ANTIRHEUMATIC DRUGS			
Methotrexate	0.5-1 mg/kg PO or SC weekly (maximum dose 25 mg/week)	Polyarticular Systemic onset Extended or refractory oligoarticular	Nausea, vomiting, oral ulcerations, hepatitis, blood count dyscrasias, immunosuppression, teratogenicity
Sulfasalazine	Initial 12.5 mg/kg PO daily; increase by 10 mg/kg/day Maintenance: 40-50 mg/kg divided bid (maximum dose 2 g/day)	Polyarticular	GI upset, allergic reaction, pancytopenia, renal and hepatic toxicity
Leflunomide*	10-20 mg PO daily	Polyarticular	GI upset, hepatic toxicity, allergic rash, alopecia (reversible), teratogenicity (needs washout with cholestyramine)
BIOLOGIC AGENTS **Anti–Tumor Necrosis Factor-α**			
Etanercept	0.8 mg/kg SC weekly or 0.4 mg/kg SC twice weekly (maximum dose 50 mg/wk)	Polyarticular Systemic onset Extended or refractory oligoarticular	Immunosuppressant, concern for malignancy
Infliximab*	3-10 mg/kg IV q 4-8 wk	Same as above	Same as above
Adalimumab	<30 kg: 20 mg SC every other week >30 kg: 40 mg SC every other week	Same as above	Same as above
Anti-Cytotoxic T Lymphocyte–Associated Antigen-4 Immunoglobulin			
Abatacept	<75 kg: 10 mg/kg/dose IV q 4 wk 75-100 kg: 750 mg/dose IV q 4 wk >100 kg: 1,000 mg/dose IV q 4 wk	Polyarticular	Immunosuppressant; concern for malignancy
Anti-CD20			
Rituximab*	750 mg/m^2 IV 2 wk × 2 (maximum dose 1000 mg)	Polyarticular	Immunosuppressant
Interleukin-1 Receptor Antagonist			
Anakinra*	1-2 mg/kg SC daily	Systemic onset	Immunosuppressant

*Not indicated by the U.S. Food and Drug Administration for use in JIA.
bid, twice daily; GI, gastrointestinal; IV, intravenous; PO, oral; SC, subcutaneous; tid, three times daily.

between the ophthalmologist and rheumatologist. Initial management of uveitis may include mydriatics and corticosteroids used topically, systemically, or through periocular injection. DMARDs allow for a decrease in exposure to steroids, and methotrexate and monoclonal antibodies to TNF-α (adalimumab and infliximab) are effective in treating severe uveitis.

Dietary evaluation and counseling to ensure appropriate calcium, vitamin D, protein, and caloric intake are important for children with JIA. Physical therapy and occupational therapy are invaluable adjuncts to any treatment program. A social worker and nurse clinician can be important resources for families, to recognize stresses imposed by a chronic illness, to identify appropriate community resources, and to aid compliance with the treatment protocol.

PROGNOSIS

Although the course of JIA in an individual child is unpredictable, some prognostic generalizations can be made on the basis of disease type and course. Studies analyzing management of JIA in the pre-TNF-α era indicate that up to 50% of patients with JIA have active disease persisting into early adulthood, often with severe limitations of physical function.

Children with persistent oligoarticular disease fare well, with a majority achieving disease remission. Those in whom more extensive disease develops have a poorer prognosis. Children with oligoarthritis, particularly girls who are ANA positive and with onset of arthritis earlier than 6 yr of age are at risk for development of chronic uveitis. There is no association between the activity or severity of the arthritis and the chronic uveitis. Persistent, uncontrolled anterior uveitis (Fig. 149-14) can cause posterior synechiae, cataracts, and band keratopathy, and can result in blindness. Many of these children do well with early diagnosis and implementation of therapy.

The child with polyarticular JIA often has a more prolonged course of active joint inflammation and requires early and aggressive therapy. Predictors of severe and persistent disease include young age at onset, RF seropositivity or rheumatoid nodules, the presence of anti-CCP antibodies, and large numbers of affected joints. Disease involving the hip and hand and wrist is also associated with a poorer prognosis and may lead to significant functional impairment.

SoJIA in children is often the most difficult to control in terms of both articular inflammation and systemic manifestations. Poorer prognosis is related to polyarticular distribution of arthritis, fever lasting >3 mo, and increased inflammatory markers, such as platelet count and ESR, for >6 mo. Newer agents, such as the IL-1 and IL-6 receptor antagonists, hold promise for improving the outcomes for children with severe and prolonged systemic-onset disease.

Orthopedic complications include leg length discrepancy and flexion contractures, particularly of the knees, hips, and wrists.

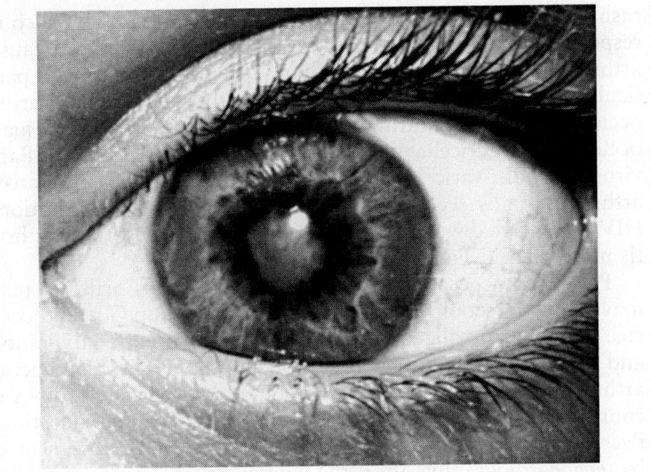

Figure 149-14 Chronic anterior uveitis, or iridocyclitis, of juvenile idiopathic arthritis. Extensive posterior synechiae have resulted in a small, irregular pupil. A well-developed cataract and early band keratopathy can be seen at the medial and lateral margins of the cornea.

Discrepancies in leg length can be managed with a shoe lift on the shorter side to prevent secondary scoliosis. Joint contractures require aggressive medical control of arthritis, often in conjunction with intra-articular corticosteroid injections, appropriate splinting, and stretching of the affected tendons. Popliteal cysts may require no treatment if they are small or intra-articular injection with corticosteroids if they are more problematic.

Psychosocial adaptation may be affected by JIA. Studies indicate that, compared with control subjects, a significant number of children with JIA have problems with lifetime adjustment and employment. Disability not directly associated with arthritis may continue into young adulthood in as many as 20% of patients, together with continuing chronic pain syndromes at a similar frequency. Psychologic complications, including problems with school attendance and socialization, may respond to counseling by mental health professionals.

BIBLIOGRAPHY

Please visit the Nelson Textbook of Pediatrics *website at www.expertconsult.com for the complete bibliography.*

Chapter 150
Ankylosing Spondylitis and Other Spondyloarthritides

James Birmingham and Robert A. Colbert

The diseases collectively referred to as **spondyloarthritides** include ankylosing spondylitis (AS), arthritis associated with inflammatory bowel disease (IBD) and psoriasis, and reactive arthritis following gastrointestinal or genitourinary infections (see Table 150-1 on the *Nelson Textbook of Pediatrics* website at www.expertconsult.com). Pediatric rheumatologists have adopted the International League of Associations for Rheumatology (ILAR) classification scheme for juvenile idiopathic arthritis (JIA) and use the term **enthesitis-related arthritis (ERA)** to encompass most forms of spondyloarthritis in children, except those with co-existing psoriasis.

For the full continuation of this chapter, please visit the Nelson Textbook of Pediatrics *website at www.expertconsult.com.*

Chapter 151
Reactive and Postinfectious Arthritis

James Birmingham and Robert A. Colbert

The role of infectious agents in the pathophysiology of arthritis is a topic of intense study. In addition to causing arthritis by means of direct infection (i.e., septic arthritis; Chapter 677), infection can lead to the generation and deposition of immune complexes as well as antibody or T cell–mediated cross-reactivity with self. Evidence continues to grow that microorganisms also play a role in the development of classic autoimmune diseases, such as systemic lupus erythematosus and juvenile idiopathic arthritis. **Reactive and postinfectious arthritis** are defined as joint inflammation due to a sterile inflammatory reaction following a recent infection. For historical reasons, we use *reactive arthritis* to refer to arthritis that occurs following enteropathic or urogenital infections and *postinfectious arthritis* to describe arthritis that occurs after infectious illnesses not classically considered in the reactive arthritis group, such as infection with group A streptococcus or viruses. In some cases, nonviable components of the initiating organism have been demonstrated in affected joints, and the presence of viable, yet nonculturable, bacteria within the joint remains an area of investigation.

The course of **reactive arthritis** is variable and may remit or progress to a chronic spondyloarthritis including ankylosing spondylitis (Chapter 150). In **postinfectious arthritis**, the pain or joint swelling is usually transient, lasting less than 6 wk, and does not share the typical spondyloarthritis pattern. The distinction between postinfectious arthritis and reactive arthritis is not always clear, either clinically or in terms of pathophysiology.

PATHOGENESIS

Reactive arthritis typically follows enteric infection with *Salmonella, Shigella, Yersinia enterocolitica, Campylobacter jejuni, Cryptosporidium parvum,* or *Giardia intestinalis*, or genitourinary tract infection with *Chlamydia trachomatis* or *Ureaplasma.* Though similar in some respects to reactive arthritis, acute rheumatic fever caused by group A streptococcus (Chapter 176.1), arthritis associated with infective endocarditis (Chapter 431), and the tenosynovitis associated with *Neisseria gonorrhoeae* are considered later.

Approximately 75% of patients with reactive arthritis are HLA-B27 positive. This association has led to the idea that reactive arthritis represents an autoimmune response involving molecular mimicry, whereby autoreactive T lymphocytes cross react with antigens (synovial, cartilaginous, glycosaminoglycan) in the joints presented by HLA-B27; however, this hypothesis remains unproven. Incomplete elimination of bacteria and bacterial products, such as DNA, has also been proposed. A relationship with clinical characteristics of specific infectious disorders is not present. In postinfectious arthritis, several viruses (rubella, varicella-zoster, herpes simplex, cytomegalovirus) have been isolated from the joints of patients. Antigens from other viruses (hepatitis B, adenovirus 7) have been identified in immune complexes from joint tissue.

Patients with reactive arthritis who are HLA-B27 positive have an increased frequency of uveitis and other extra-articular features. In addition, HLA-B27 is a risk factor for persistent gut inflammation following enteric infections, even after resolution of the gastrointestinal infection, and significantly increases the risk that the individual will eventually develop a chronic spondyloarthritis. Nevertheless, reactive arthritis does occur in HLA-B27–negative patients, indicating that other genes play a role in disease susceptibility.

CLINICAL MANIFESTATIONS AND DIFFERENTIAL DIAGNOSIS

Symptoms of reactive arthritis present approximately 2-4 wk following infection. The classic triad of arthritis, urethritis, and conjunctivitis (formerly referred to as Reiter syndrome) is relatively uncommon in children. The arthritis is typically oligoarticular, with a lower extremity predilection. Dactylitis may occur, and enthesitis (Fig. 151-1) is common (Chapter 150). Cutaneous manifestations can occur and may include circinate balanitis, ulcerative vulvitis, oral lesions, and keratoderma blennorrhagica, which is similar in appearance to pustular psoriasis (Fig. 151-2). Systemic symptoms may include fever, malaise, and fatigue. Early in the disease course, markers of inflammation—erythrocyte sedimentation rate (ESR), C-reactive protein (CRP), and platelets—may be markedly elevated.

Familiarity with other causes of postinfectious arthritis is vital when a diagnosis of reactive arthritis is being considered. Numerous viruses are associated with postinfectious arthritis (Table 151-1) and may result in particular patterns of joint involvement. Rubella and hepatitis B virus typically affect the small joints, whereas mumps and varicella often involve large joints, especially the knees. The **hepatitis B arthritis–dermatitis syndrome** is characterized by urticarial rash and a symmetric migratory polyarthritis resembling that of serum sickness. Rubella-associated arthropathy may follow natural rubella infection and, infrequently, rubella immunization. It typically occurs in young women, with an increased frequency with advancing age, and is uncommon in preadolescent children and in males. Arthralgia of the knees and hands usually begins within 7 days of onset of the rash or 10-28 days after immunization. Parvovirus B19, which is responsible for erythema infectiosum (fifth disease), can cause arthralgia, symmetric joint swelling, and morning stiffness, particularly in adult women and less frequently in children. Arthritis occurs occasionally during cytomegalovirus infection and may occur during varicella infections but is rare after Epstein-Barr virus infection. Varicella may also be complicated by suppurative arthritis, usually secondary to group A streptococcus infection. HIV is associated with an arthritis that resembles psoriatic arthritis more than juvenile idiopathic arthritis (JIA).

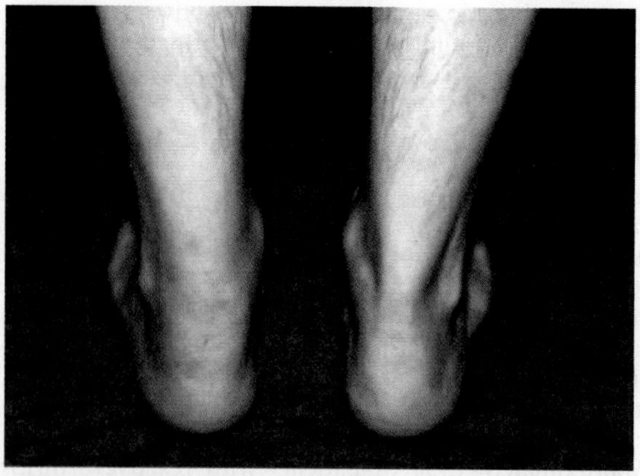

Figure 151-1 Enthesitis—swelling of the posterior aspect of the left heel and lateral aspect of the ankle. (Courtesy of Nora Singer, Case Western Reserve University and Rainbow Babies' Hospital.)

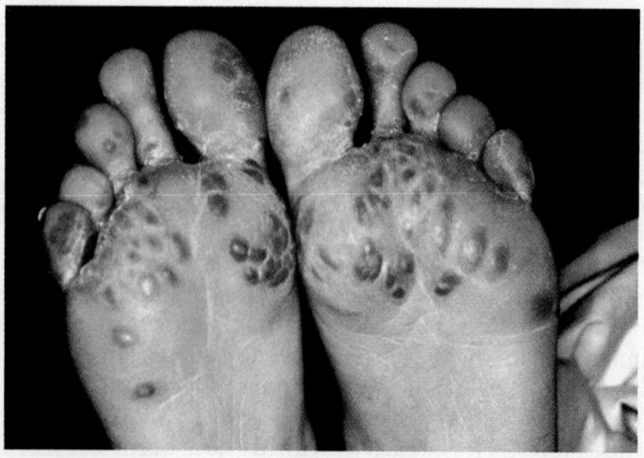

Figure 151-2 Keratoderma blennorrhagica. (Courtesy of Dr. M.F. Rein and The Centers for Disease Control and Prevention Public Health Image Library, 1976. Image #6950.)

Post-streptococcal arthritis is a postinfectious arthritis that may follow infection with either group A or group G streptococcus. It is typically oligoarticular, affecting lower extremity joints, and mild symptoms can persists for months. Post-streptococcal arthritis differs from rheumatic fever, which typically follows a course with painful migratory polyarthritis of brief duration. Because valvular lesions have occasionally been documented by echocardiography after the acute illness, some clinicians consider post-streptococcal arthritis to be an incomplete form of acute rheumatic fever (Chapter 176.1). Certain HLA-DRB1 types may predispose children to development of either post-streptococcal arthritis (HLA-DRB1*01) or acute rheumatic fever (HLA-DRB1*16).

Transient synovitis (toxic synovitis), another form of postinfectious arthritis, typically affects the hip, often after an upper respiratory tract infection (Chapter 670.2). Boys from 3 to 10 yr of age are most commonly affected and have acute onset of severe pain in the hip, with referred pain to the thigh or knee, lasting approximately 1 wk. The ESR and white blood cell count are usually normal. Radiologic or ultrasound examination may confirm widening of the joint space secondary to effusion. Aspiration of joint fluid is often necessary to exclude septic arthritis and results in dramatic clinical improvement. The trigger is presumed to be viral, although responsible microbes have not been identified.

Nonsuppurative arthritis has been reported in children, usually adolescent boys, in association with **severe truncal acne**. Patients

Table 151-1 VIRUSES ASSOCIATED WITH ARTHRITIS

Togaviruses:
Rubivirus:
Rubella
Alphaviruses:
Ross River
Chikungunya
O'nyong-nyong
Mayaro
Sindbis
Ockelbo
Pogosta
Orthopoxviruses:
Variola virus (smallpox)
Vaccinia virus
Parvoviruses
Adenoviruses:
Adenovirus 7
Herpesviruses:
Epstein-Barr
Cytomegalovirus
Varicella-zoster
Herpes simplex
Paramyxoviruses:
Mumps
Hepadnavirus:
Hepatitis B
Enteroviruses:
Echovirus
Coxsackievirus B

Adapted from Cassidy JT, Petty RE: Infectious arthritis and osteomyelitis. In *Textbook of pediatric rheumatology*, ed 5, Philadelphia, 2005, WB Saunders.

often have fever and persistent infection of the pustular lesions. Recurrent episodes may also be associated with a sterile myopathy and may last for several months. Infective endocarditis can be associated with arthralgia, arthritis, or signs suggestive of vasculitis, such as Osler nodes, Janeway lesions, and Roth spots. Post-infectious arthritis, perhaps because of immune complexes, also occurs in children with *N. gonorrhoeae, Neisseria meningitidis, H. influenzae* type b, and *Mycoplasma pneumoniae* infections.

DIAGNOSIS

A recent genitourinary or gastrointestinal infection may suggest the diagnosis of reactive arthritis, but there is no diagnostic test. Although stool or urogenital tract cultures can be performed in an attempt to isolate the triggering organism, the offending agent is not typically identified by the time arthritis is present. Imaging findings are nonspecific or normal. Similarly, documenting previous streptococcal infection may help to diagnose post-infectious arthritis.

Because the preceding infection can be remote or mild and often not recalled by the patient, it is also important to rule out other causes of arthritis. Acute arthritis affecting a single joint suggests septic arthritis, mandating joint aspiration; osteomyelitis may cause pain and an effusion in an adjacent joint but is more often associated with focal bone pain over the site of infection. The diagnosis of postinfectious arthritis is often established by exclusion, after the arthritis has resolved. Arthritis associated with gastrointestinal symptoms or abnormal liver function test results may be triggered by infectious or autoimmune hepatitis. Arthritis or spondyloarthritis may occur in children with inflammatory bowel disease, such as Crohn's disease or ulcerative colitis (Chapter 328). When two or more blood cell lines progressively decrease in concentration in a child with arthritis, parvovirus infection, macrophage activation (hemophagocytic) syndrome, and leukemia should be strongly considered. Persistent arthritis (>6 wk) suggests the possibility of a chronic rheumatic disease, including JIA (Chapters 149 and 150) and systemic lupus erythematosus.

TREATMENT

Specific treatment is unnecessary for most cases of reactive or postinfectious arthritis. Nonsteroidal anti-inflammatory agents are often needed for management of pain and functional limitation. Unless ongoing *Chlamydia* infection is suspected, attempts to treat the offending organism are not warranted. If swelling or arthralgia recurs, further evaluation may be necessary to exclude active infection or evolving rheumatic disease. Intra-articular steroid injections may be utilized for refractory or severely involved joints once acute infection has been ruled out. Systemic steroids or disease-modifying antirheumatic drugs (DMARDs) are rarely indicated but may be considered for chronic disease. Participation in physical activity should be encouraged, and physical therapy may be needed to maintain normal function and prevent muscle atrophy. For post-infectious arthritis due to streptococcal disease, current recommendations include penicillin prophylaxis for at least 1 yr; duration of prophylaxis is controversial.

COMPLICATIONS AND PROGNOSIS

Postinfectious arthritis following viral infections usually resolves without complications unless it is associated with involvement of other organs, such as encephalomyelitis. Children with reactive arthritis after enteric infections occasionally experience inflammatory bowel disease months to years after onset. Both uveitis and carditis have been reported in children diagnosed with reactive arthritis. Reactive arthritis, especially after bacterial enteric infection or genitourinary tract infection with *Chlamydia trachomatis,* has the potential for evolving to chronic arthritis, particularly spondyloarthritis (Chapter 150). The presence of HLA-B27 or significant systemic features increases the risk of chronic disease.

BIBLIOGRAPHY

Please visit the Nelson Textbook of Pediatrics *website at* *www.expertconsult.com* *for the complete bibliography.*

Chapter 152
Systemic Lupus Erythematosus

Stacy P. Ardoin and Laura E. Schanberg

Systemic lupus erythematosus (SLE) is a chronic autoimmune disease characterized by multisystem inflammation and the presence of circulating autoantibodies directed against self-antigens. SLE occurs in children and adults, disproportionately affecting women of reproductive age. Although nearly every organ may be affected, the most commonly involved are the skin, joints, kidneys, blood-forming cells, blood vessels, and central nervous system. Compared with adults, children and adolescents with SLE have more severe disease and more widespread organ involvement.

ETIOLOGY

The pathogenesis of SLE remains unknown, but several factors likely influence risk and severity of disease, including genetics, hormonal milieu, and environmental exposures.

A genetic predisposition to SLE is suggested by the association with **specific genetic abnormalities,** including congenital deficiencies of C1q, C2, and C4 and the finding that individuals with SLE frequently have a family history of SLE or other autoimmune disease. In addition, certain HLA types (including HLA-B8, HLA-DR2, and HLA-DR3) occur with increased frequency in SLE. Although SLE has a clear genetic component, its occurrence is sporadic in families and concordance is incomplete, even among identical twins, suggesting that multiple genes are involved and that nongenetic factors are also important in disease expression.

Because SLE preferentially affects women, especially during their reproductive years, it is suspected that hormonal factors are important in pathogenesis. Ninety percent of individuals with SLE are female, making gender the strongest risk factor for SLE. Estrogens are likely to play a role in SLE, and in vitro and animal model studies suggest that estrogen exposure promotes B-cell autoreactivity. Results of studies on the impact of exogenous estrogen on women with SLE are conflicting. Estrogen-containing oral contraceptives do not appear to induce flares in quiescent SLE, but the risk of flares may be increased in postmenopausal women receiving hormone replacement.

The **environmental exposures** that may trigger the development of SLE remain unknown; however, certain viral infections (including Epstein-Barr virus) may play a role in susceptible individuals, and ultraviolet light exposure is known to aggravate SLE disease activity. Environmental influences also may induce epigenetic modifications to DNA, which increase the risk of SLE and drug-induced lupus. For example, in mouse models, drugs such as procainamide and hydralazine can promote lymphocyte hypomethylation and a lupus-like syndrome.

EPIDEMIOLOGY

The reported prevalence of SLE in children and adolescents (1-6/100,000) is lower than that in adults (20-70/100,000). Prevalence of SLE is highest among African-Americans, Asians, Hispanics, Native Americans, and Pacific Islanders. SLE predominantly affects females, with reported 5:1 ratio prior to puberty, a 9:1 ratio during reproductive years, and near prepubertal ratios in the postmenopausal period. Childhood SLE is rare before 5 yr of age and is usually diagnosed in adolescence. Up to 20% of all individuals with SLE are diagnosed prior to age 16 yr.

PATHOLOGY

Histologic features most suggestive of SLE include findings in the kidney and skin, especially the discoid rash. Renal manifestations of SLE are classified histologically according to the criteria of the International Society of Nephrology (Chapter 508). The finding of diffuse proliferative glomerulonephritis (class IV) significantly increases risk for renal morbidity. Renal biopsies are very helpful to establish the diagnosis of SLE and to stage disease. Immune complexes are commonly found with "full house" deposition of immunoglobulin and complement. The characteristic **discoid rash** depicted in Figure 152-1*D* is characterized on biopsy by hyperkeratosis, follicular plugging, and infiltration of mononuclear cells into the dermal-epidermal junction. The histopathology of photosensitive rashes can be nonspecific, but immunofluorescence examination of both affected and nonaffected skin may reveal deposition of immune complexes within the dermal-epidermal junction. This finding is called the **lupus band test**, which is specific for SLE.

PATHOGENESIS

Developing a model of SLE pathogenesis is challenging, given the need to account for tremendous heterogeneity in disease expression and fluctuations of disease activity over time. It is clear that autoantibodies, cytokines, and aberrant lymphocyte function have important roles in SLE pathogenesis.

A hallmark of SLE is the generation of **autoantibodies** directed against self-antigens, particularly nucleic acids. These intracellular antigens are ubiquitously expressed but are usually inaccessible and cloistered within the cell. During cell necrosis or **apoptosis**, the antigens are released. SLE skin cells are highly susceptible to damage from ultraviolet light, and the resulting cell demise results in release of cell contents, including nucleic antigens. Individuals with SLE may have markedly increased levels of apoptosis or significantly impaired ability to clear cell debris, causing prolonged exposure to these nucleic antigens in the bloodstream and ample opportunity for their recognition by immune cells, leading to production of autoantibodies by B cells. Circulating autoantibodies may form immune complexes and deposit in tissues, leading to local complement activation, initiation of a proinflammatory cascade, and, ultimately, tissue damage. Antibodies to double-stranded DNA can form immune complexes, deposit in glomeruli, and initiate inflammation leading to glomerulonephritis. Many individuals with SLE have circulating

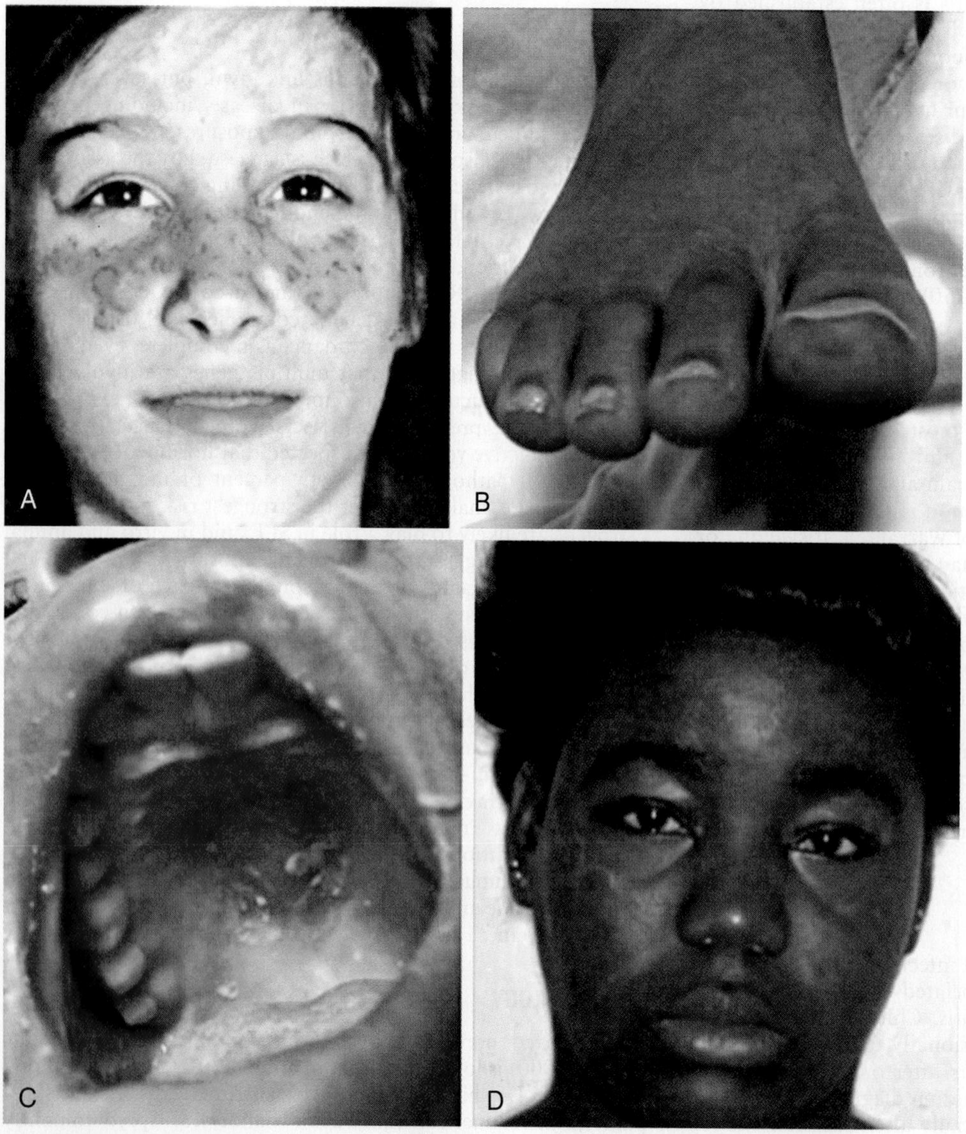

Figure 152-1 Mucocutaneous manifestations of SLE. *A*, Malar rash; *B*, vasculitic rash on toes; *C*, oral mucosal ulcers; *D*, discoid rash in malar distribution.

antibodies to double-stranded DNA yet do not have nephritis, suggesting that autoantibodies alone are not sufficient to cause disease.

Individuals with SLE frequently demonstrate abnormal cytokine levels. In particular, peripheral blood mononuclear cells from patients with SLE exhibit patterns of gene expression suggestive of stimulation by interferon-α (IFN-α). IFN-α production by dendritic cells can be stimulated in vivo by immune complexes. Excess levels of interferon can promote expression of other proinflammatory cytokines and chemokines, maturation of monocytes into dendritic dells, promotion of autoreactive B and T cells, and loss of self-tolerance. Many, but not all, patients with SLE exhibit this **interferon signature.** Other cytokines with increased expression in SLE include interleukin-2 (IL)-2, IL-6, IL-10, IL-12, B-lymphocyte stimulator (BlyS), and anti–tumor necrosis factor-α (TNF-α).

Both B and T cells demonstrate functional impairments in SLE. In active SLE, B-cell populations have impaired tolerance and increased autoreactivity, enhancing B cells' ability to produce autoantibodies following exposure to self-antigen. In addition, cytokines such as BlyS may promote abnormal B-cell number and function. T-cell abnormalities in SLE include increased numbers of memory T cells and decreased number and function of T-regulatory cells. SLE T cells display aberrant signaling and increased autoreactivity. As a result, they are resistant to attrition by normal apoptosis pathways.

CLINICAL MANIFESTATIONS

Any organ system can be involved in SLE, so the potential clinical manifestations are protean (Table 152-1). The presentation of SLE in childhood or adolescence differs from that in adults. The most common presenting complaints of children with SLE include fever, fatigue, hematologic abnormalities, arthralgia, and arthritis. Renal disease in SLE is often asymptomatic; thus careful monitoring of blood pressure and urinalyses is critical. SLE is often characterized by periods of flare and disease quiescence or may follow a more smoldering disease course. The neuropsychiatric complications of SLE may occur with or without apparently active SLE and are particularly difficult to detect in adolescents, who are already at high risk for mood disorders. Long-term complications of SLE and its therapy, including accelerated atherosclerosis and osteoporosis, become clinically evident in young to middle adulthood. SLE is a disease that evolves over time in each affected individual, and new manifestations may arise even many years after diagnosis.

DIAGNOSIS

The diagnosis of SLE requires a comprehensive clinical and laboratory assessment revealing characteristic multisystem disease and excluding other etiologies, including infection and malignancy. Presence of 4 of the 11 American College of Rheumatology 1997 Revised Classification Criteria for SLE (Table 152-2) simultaneously or cumulatively establishes the diagnosis of SLE. Of note, although a positive antinuclear antibody (ANA) test result is not required for the diagnosis of SLE, ANA-negative lupus is extremely rare. Hypocomplementemia, although common in SLE, is not represented among the classification criteria.

DIFFERENTIAL DIAGNOSIS

Multiorgan disease is the hallmark of SLE, and given its wide array of potential clinical manifestations, SLE can be considered in the differential diagnosis of many clinical scenarios, including unexplained fevers, joint pain, arthritis, rash, cytopenias, neurologic or cardiopulmonary abnormalities, and nephritis.

Drug-induced lupus refers to the presence of SLE manifestations triggered by exposure to certain medications, including minocycline, many anticonvulsants, sulfonamides, antiarrhythmic agents, and other drugs (Table 152-3). In individuals prone to SLE, these agents may act as a trigger for true SLE. In others, these agents provoke a reversible lupus-like syndrome. Unlike SLE, drug-induced lupus affects males and females equally. An inherited predisposition toward slow acetylation may increase the risk of drug-induced lupus. Circulating antihistone antibodies are often present in drug-induced SLE, and these antibodies are detected in up to 20% of individuals with SLE. Hepatitis, which

Table 152-1 POTENTIAL CLINICAL MANIFESTATIONS OF SYSTEMIC LUPUS ERYTHEMATOSUS

TARGET ORGAN	POTENTIAL CLINICAL MANIFESTATIONS
Constitutional	Fatigue, anorexia, weight loss, fever, lymphadenopathy
Musculoskeletal	Arthritis, myositis, tendonitis, arthralgias, myalgias, avascular necrosis, osteoporosis
Skin	Malar rash, discoid rash, photosensitive rash, cutaneous vasculitis, livedo reticularis, periungual capillary abnormalities, Raynaud's phenomenon, alopecia, oral and nasal ulcers
Renal	Hypertension, proteinuria, hematuria, edema, nephrotic syndrome, renal failure
Cardiovascular	Pericarditis, myocarditis, conduction system abnormalities, Libman-Sacks endocarditis
Neurologic	Seizures, psychosis, cerebritis, stroke, transverse myelitis, depression, cognitive impairment, headaches, pseudotumor, peripheral neuropathy, chorea, optic neuritis, cranial nerve palsies
Pulmonary	Pleuritis, interstitial lung disease, pulmonary hemorrhage, pulmonary hypertension, pulmonary embolism
Hematologic	Immune-mediated cytopenias (hemolytic anemia, thrombocytopenia or leukopenia), anemia of chronic inflammation, hypercoaguability, thrombocytopenic thrombotic microangiopathy
Gastroenterology	Hepatosplenomegaly, pancreatitis, vasculitis affecting bowel, protein-losing enteropathy
Ocular	Retinal vasculitis, scleritis, episcleritis, papilledema

Table 152-2 AMERICAN COLLEGE OF RHEUMATOLOGY 1997 REVISED CLASSIFICATION CRITERIA FOR SYSTEMIC LUPUS ERYTHEMATOSUS*

Malar rash
Discoid rash
Photosensitivity
Oral or nasal ulcers
Arthritis:
  Nonerosive, affecting 2 or more joints
Serositis:
  Pleuritis, pericarditis, peritonitis
Renal manifestations:
  Persistent proteinuria or cellular casts
  Consistent renal biopsy
Seizure or psychosis
Hematologic manifestations:
  Hemolytic anemia
  Leukopenia (<4,000 leukocytes/mm^3)
  Lymphopenia (<1,500 leukocytes/mm^3)
  Thrombocytopenia (<100,000 thrombocytes/mm^3)
Immunologic abnormalities:
  Positive anti–double-stranded DNA or anti-Smith antibody test result
  False-positive rapid plasma regain RPR test result, positive lupus anticoagulant test result, or elevated anticardiolipin immunoglobulin (Ig) G or IgM antibody
  Positive antinuclear antibody test result

*The presence of 4/11 criteria establishes the diagnosis of SLE. These criteria were developed for classification in clinical trials and not for clinical diagnosis.

Adapted from Hochberg MC: Updating the American College of Rheumatology revised criteria for the classification of systemic lupus erythematosus, *Arthritis Rheum* 40:1725, 1997.

Table 152-3 MEDICATIONS ASSOCIATED WITH DRUG-INDUCED LUPUS

DEFINITE ASSOCIATION
Minocycline, procainamide, hydralazine, isoniazid, penicillamine, diltiazem, interferon-α, methyldopa, chlorpromazine, etanercept, infliximab, adalimumab
PROBABLE ASSOCIATION
Phenytoin, ethosuximide, carbamazepine, sulfasalazine, amiodarone, quinidine, rifampin, nitrofurantoin, beta blockers, lithium, captopril, interferon-gamma, hydrochlorothiazide, glyburide, docetaxel, penicillin, tetracycline, statins, gold, valproate, griseofulvin, gemfibrozil, propylthiouracil

is rare in SLE, is more common in drug-induced lupus. Individuals with drug-induced lupus are less likely to demonstrate antibodies to double-stranded DNA, hypocomplementemia, and significant renal or neurologic disease. In contrast to SLE, manifestations of drug-induced lupus resolve after withdrawal of the offending medication; complete recovery may take several months to years.

LABORATORY FINDINGS

A positive ANA test result is present in 95-99% of individuals with SLE. This test has poor specificity for SLE, as up to 20% of healthy individuals also have a positive ANA test result, making the ANA a poor screening test for SLE. ANA titers are not reflective of disease activity; therefore, repeating ANA titers is not helpful in disease management. Antibodies to double-stranded DNA are more specific for SLE, and in some individuals, anti-dsDNA levels correlate with disease activity, particularly nephritis. Anti-Smith antibody, although found specifically in patients with SLE, does not correlate with disease activity. Serum levels of total hemolytic complement (CH_{50}), C3, and C4 are typically decreased in active disease and often improve with treatment. Table 152-4 lists several autoantibodies found in SLE and their clinical associations. Hypergammaglobulinemia is a common but nonspecific finding. Inflammatory markers, particularly erythrocyte sedimentation rate, are often elevated in active disease. C-reactive protein (CRP) correlates less well with disease activity, and elevated CRP values may reflect infection.

Antiphospholipid antibodies, which increase clotting risk, can be found in up to 66% of children and adolescents with SLE. Antiphospholipid antibodies can be detected by several means, and laboratory features that point to the presence of these antibodies include the presence of anticardiolipin antibodies, prolonged phospholipid-dependent coagulation test results (partial thromboplastin time, dilute Russell viper-venom time), and a circulating **lupus anticoagulant** (which confirms that a prolonged partial thromboplastin time is not corrected with mixing studies). When an arterial or venous clotting event occurs in the presence of an antiphospholipid antibody, **antiphospholipid antibody syndrome** is diagnosed. Antiphospholipid antibody syndrome can occur in the context of SLE or independent of SLE (Chapter 473).

TREATMENT

Treatment of SLE is tailored to the individual, being based on specific disease manifestations and tolerability. For all patients, sunscreen and avoidance of prolonged direct sun exposure and other ultraviolet light may help control disease. Hydroxychloroquine (5-7 mg/kg/day) is recommended for all individuals with SLE if tolerated. In addition to treating mild SLE manifestations such as rash and mild arthritis, hydroxychloroquine prevents SLE flares, improves lipid profiles, and may have a beneficial impact on mortality and renal outcomes. Potential toxicities include retinal pigmentation, impairing color vision; therefore, ophthalmology exams every 6-12 mo are recommended. Nonsteroidal anti-inflammatory agents (NSAIDs) can be useful for management of arthralgias and arthritis; it is important to keep in mind their potential hepatic, renal, and cardiovascular toxicities.

Table 152-4 AUTOANTIBODIES COMMONLY ASSOCIATED WITH SYSTEMIC LUPUS ERYTHEMATOSUS (SLE)

ANTIBODY	CLINICAL ASSOCIATION
Anti–double-stranded DNA	Correlates with disease activity, especially nephritis, in some with SLE
Anti-Smith antibody	Specific for the diagnosis of SLE
Anti-ribonucleoprotein antibody	Increased risk for Raynaud phenomenon and pulmonary hypertension High titer may suggest diagnosis of mixed connective tissue disorder
Anti-Ro antibody (anti-SSA antibody) Anti-La antibody (anti-SSB antibody)	Associated with sicca syndrome May suggest diagnosis of Sjögren syndrome Increased risk of neonatal lupus in offspring (congenital heart block) May be associated with cutaneous and pulmonary manifestations of SLE May be associated with isolated discoid lupus
Antiphospholipid antibodies (including anticardiolipin antibodies)	Increased risk for venous and arterial thrombotic events
Antihistone antibodies	Present in a majority of patients with drug-induced lupus May be present in SLE

Corticosteroids are a mainstay for treatment of significant manifestations of SLE; side effects often limit patient compliance, especially in adolescence, and potential toxicities are worrisome. It is important to limit dose and length of exposure to corticosteroids whenever possible. Potential consequences of corticosteroid therapy include growth disturbance, weight gain, striae, acne, hyperglycemia, hypertension, cataracts, avascular necrosis, and osteoporosis. The optimal dosing of corticosteroids in children and adolescents with SLE remains unknown; severe disease is often treated with high doses of intravenous methylprednisolone (e.g., 30 mg/kg/day for 3 days) or high doses of oral prednisone (1-2 mg/kg/day). As disease manifestations improve, corticosteroid dosages are gradually tapered, along with monitoring for evidence of adrenal insufficiency. It often becomes necessary to introduce steroid-sparing immunosuppressive medications in order to limit cumulative steroid exposure.

Steroid-sparing immunosuppressive agents often used in the treatment of pediatric SLE include methotrexate, leflunomide, azathioprine, mycophenolate mofetil, and cyclophosphamide. Methotrexate, leflunomide, and azathioprine are often used to treat persistent moderate disease, including arthritis, significant cutaneous or hematologic involvement, and pleural disease. In general, intravenous or oral cyclophosphamide is reserved for the most severe, potentially life-threatening SLE manifestations, such as renal, neurologic, and cardiopulmonary disease. Although cyclophosphamide is highly effective in controlling disease, the potential toxicities are significant, including cytopenias, infection, hemorrhagic cystitis, premature gonadal failure, and increased risk of future malignancy. Attention to adequate hydration can attenuate the risk of hemorrhagic cystitis. Fortunately, young girls are at much lower risk of gonadal failure than older women, and the use of gonadotropin-releasing hormone agonists, such as leuprolide acetate, may help prevent gonadal failure. Treatment of significant glomerulonephritis usually involves use of azathioprine, mycophenolate mofetil, or cyclophosphamide. Clinical trials with long-term follow-up are needed to determine optimal approaches to treatment of SLE nephritis. While a randomized, controlled, double-blind trial did not suggest that rituximab is an effective treatment for significant glomerulonephritis, this agent has not been studied in children or in refractory disease. Clinical trials are in progress to assess the safety and efficacy of several biologic agents in SLE, including monoclonal antibodies targeting

Table 152-5 MORBIDITY IN CHILDHOOD LUPUS

Renal	Hypertension, dialysis, transplantation
Central nervous system	Organic brain syndrome, seizures, psychosis, neurocognitive dysfunction
Cardiovascular	Atherosclerosis, myocardial infarction, cardiomyopathy, valvular disease
Immune	Recurrent infection, functional asplenia, malignancy
Musculoskeletal	Osteopenia, compression fractures, osteonecrosis
Ocular	Cataracts, glaucoma
Endocrine	Diabetes, obesity, growth failure, infertility, fetal wastage

From Cassidy JT, Petty RE: *Textbook of pediatric rheumatology*, ed 5, Philadelphia, 2005, Elsevier/Saunders.

CD22, BlyS, IL-10, TNF-α, and IFN-α. Individuals with antiphospholipid antibody syndrome are treated with long-term anticoagulation to prevent future thrombotic events.

Given the lifelong nature of SLE, care of children and adolescents with this disease also involves preventive practices. Owing to the enhanced risk of atherosclerosis in SLE, attention to cholesterol levels, smoking status, body mass index, blood pressure, and other cardiovascular risk factors is warranted. Adequate intake of calcium and vitamin D is necessary to prevent future osteoporosis. Infections commonly complicate SLE, so routine immunization is recommended, including annual influenza vaccination and administration of the 23-valent pneumococcal vaccine. Pregnancy can worsen SLE, and obstetric complications are more common in SLE. In addition, many of the medications used to treat SLE are teratogenic. As a consequence, it is important to counsel adolescent girls about these risks and appropriate contraceptive options.

COMPLICATIONS

Within the first several years of diagnosis, the most common causes of death in individuals with SLE include infection and complications of glomerulonephritis and neuropsychiatric disease (Table 152-5). Over the long term, the most common causes of mortality include complications of atherosclerosis and malignancy. The increased risk of premature atherosclerosis in SLE is not explained by traditional risk factors and is due in part to the chronic immune dysregulation and inflammation associated with SLE. Increased malignancy rates may be caused by immune dysregulation and exposure to medications with carcinogenic potential.

PROGNOSIS

Owing to advances in the diagnosis and treatment of SLE, survival has improved dramatically over the past 50 years. Currently, the 5-year survival rate for pediatric SLE is >90%. However, given their long burden of disease, children and adolescents with SLE face a high risk of future morbidity and mortality from the disease and its complications, especially atherosclerosis and malignancy (see Table 152-5). Given the complex and chronic nature of SLE, it is optimal for children and adolescents with SLE to be treated by pediatric rheumatologists in a multidisciplinary clinic.

BIBLIOGRAPHY

Please visit the Nelson Textbook of Pediatrics *website at* *www.expertconsult.com* *for the complete bibliography.*

152.1 Neonatal Lupus

Stacy P. Ardoin and Laura E. Schanberg

Neonatal lupus, an entity distinct from SLE, is one of the few rheumatic disorders manifesting in the neonate. Clinical manifestations of neonatal lupus include a characteristic annular or macular rash typically affecting the face (especially the periorbital area), trunk, and scalp (Fig. 152-2). Infants may also have cytopenias and hepatitis, but the most feared complication is congenital heart block. Conduction system abnormalities range from prolongation of the PR interval to complete heart block, rarely resulting in progressive cardiomyopathy. The noncardiac manifestations of neonatal lupus are usually reversible, but congenital heart block is permanent. The rash typically appears within the first 6 wk of life after exposure to ultraviolet light and lasts 3-4 mo; however, it can be present at birth. Conduction system abnormalities can be detected in utero beginning at 16 wk of gestational age.

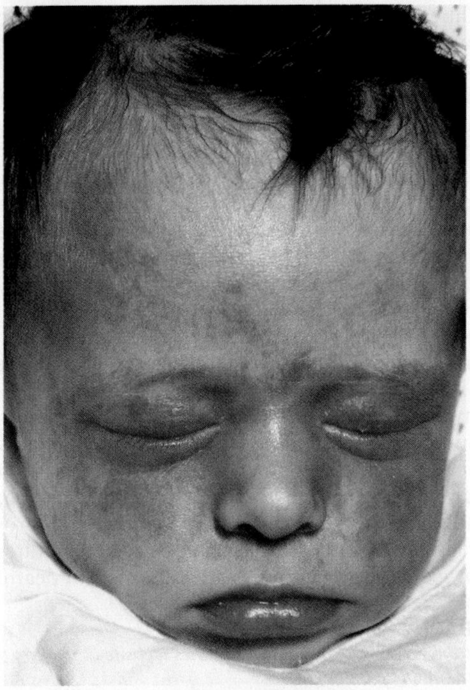

Figure 152-2 Neonatal lupus syndrome. Typical rash, often photosensitive with a malar distribution, appearing as annular plaques with erythema and scaling. (Reproduced, with written parental permission, from Pain C, Beresford MW: Neonatal lupus syndrome, *Paediatr Child Health* 17:223–227, 2007.)

Neonatal lupus results from the passive transfer of maternal immunoglobulin (Ig) G autoantibodies to the fetus. The vast majority of neonatal lupus cases are associated with maternal anti-Ro (also known as SSA) and anti-La antibodies (also known as SSB); however other autoantibodies, including anti-ribonucleoprotein (anti-RNP), have also been reported to cause neonatal lupus. Despite the clear association with maternal autoantibodies, their presence alone is not sufficient to cause disease, as <3% of offspring born to mothers with anti-Ro and anti-La antibodies experience congenital heart block.

In vitro studies suggest that during cardiac development, Ro and La antigens may be exposed on the surface of cardiac cells in the proximity of the atrioventricular node, thus making these antigens accessible to maternal autoantibodies. Binding incites a local immune response, resulting in fibrosis within the conduction system. In the skin, exposure to ultraviolet light results in cell damage and the exposure of Ro and La antigens, inducing a similar local inflammatory response that produces the characteristic rash.

Although the scant clinical trial data have been mixed, both fluorinated corticosteroids and intravenous immunoglobulin have been used in pregnant women with anti-Ro or anti-La antibodies to prevent occurrence or progression of fetal cardiac conduction abnormalities. Significant conduction system abnormalities after birth are treated with cardiac pacing, and severe cardiomyopathy may require cardiac transplantation. Transient, noncardiac manifestations are conservatively managed, with topical steroids used occasionally to treat the rash.

Because maternal autoantibodies gain access to the fetus via the placenta at the 16th wk of gestation, all pregnant women with circulating anti-Ro or anti-La antibody (or those with a history of offspring with neonatal lupus or congenital heart block) are monitored by a pediatric cardiologist with regular fetal electrocardiography from 16 wk of gestation until delivery. If fetal bradycardia is found unexpectedly during in utero monitoring, screening for maternal anti-Ro and anti-La antibodies is warranted.

In contrast to SLE, neonatal lupus is not characterized by ongoing immune dysregulation, although infants with neonatal lupus may be at some increased risk for development of future autoimmune disease. A mother who has borne a child with congenital heart block due to neonatal lupus has a 15% risk of recurrence with future pregnancies. With cardiac pacing, children with conduction system disease have an excellent prognosis. If the conduction defect is not corrected, affected children may be at risk for exercise intolerance, arrhythmias, and death.

BIBLIOGRAPHY

Please visit the Nelson Textbook of Pediatrics *website at* www.expertconsult.com *for the complete bibliography.*

Chapter 153
Juvenile Dermatomyositis

Angela Byun Robinson and Ann M. Reed

Juvenile dermatomyositis (JDM) is the most common inflammatory myositis in children, distinguished by proximal muscle weakness and a characteristic rash. Inflammatory cell infiltrates result in vascular inflammation, the underlying pathology in this disorder.

ETIOLOGY

Evidence suggests that the etiology of JDM is multifactorial, based on genetic predisposition and an unknown environmental trigger. HLA alleles such as B8, DRB1*0301, DQA1*0501, and DQA1*0301 have been associated with increased susceptibility to JDM in selected populations. Maternal microchimerism may play a part in the etiology of JDM by causing graft versus host disease or autoimmune phenomena. Persistent maternal cells have been found in blood and tissue samples of children with JDM. An increased number of these maternal cells are positive for HLA-DQA1*0501, which may assist with transfer or persistence of chimeric cells. Specific cytokine polymorphisms in tumor necrosis factor-α (TNF-α) promoter and variable number tandem repeats of the interleukin-1 receptor antagonist (IL-1Ra) also may increase genetic susceptibility. These polymorphisms are common in the general population. A history of infection in the 3 mo prior to disease onset is commonly reported; multiple studies have failed to produce a causative organism. Constitutional signs and upper respiratory symptoms predominate, but one third of patients report preceding gastrointestinal (GI) symptoms. Group A streptococcus, upper respiratory infections, GI infections, coxsackievirus B, toxoplasma, enteroviruses, parvovirus B19, and multiple other organisms have been postulated as possible pathogens in the etiology of JDM. Despite these concerns, results of serum antibody testing and polymerase chain reaction amplification of the blood and muscle tissue for multiple infectious diseases have not been revealing. Environmental factors may also play a contributing role, with geographic and seasonal clustering reported; however, no clear theory of etiology has emerged.

EPIDEMIOLOGY

The incidence of JDM is approximately 3 cases/1 million children/yr without racial predilection. Peak age of onset is between 4 and 10 yr. There is a second peak of dermatomyositis onset in late adulthood (45-64 yr), but adult-onset dermatomyositis appears to be a distinctly separate entity in prognosis and etiology. In the USA, the ratio of girls to boys with JDM is 2:1. Multiple cases of myositis in a single family are rare, but familial autoimmune disease may be increased in families with children who have JDM than in families of healthy children. Reports of seasonal association have not been confirmed, although clusters of cases may occur.

PATHOGENESIS

Type I interferons may be important in the pathogenesis of juvenile dermatomyositis. Interferon upregulates genes critical in immunoregulation and major histocompatibility class (MHC) class I expression, activates natural killer (NK) cells, and supports dendritic cell maturation. Upregulation of gene products controlled by type I interferons occurs in patients with dermatomyositis, potentially correlating with disease activity and holding promise as clinical biomarkers.

It appears that children with genetic susceptibility to JDM (HLA-DQA1*0501, HLA-DRB*0301) may have prolonged exposure to maternal chimeric cells and/or an unknown environmental trigger. Once triggered, an inflammatory cascade with type I interferon response leads to upregulation of MHC class I expression and maturation of dendritic cells. Overexpression of MHC class I upregulates adhesion molecules, which influence migration of lymphocytes, leading to inflammatory infiltration of muscle. In an autoregulatory feedback loop, muscle inflammation increases the type I interferon response, regenerating the cycle of inflammation. Cells involved in the inflammatory cascade include NK cells (CD56), T-cell subsets (CD4, CD8, Th17), monocytes/macrophages (CD14), and plasmacytoid dendritic cells. Neopterin, interferon-inducible protein 10 (IP-10), monocyte chemoattractant protein (MCP), myxovirus resistance protein (MxA), and von Willebrand factor products as well as other markers of vascular inflammation may be elevated in patients with JDM who have active inflammation.

CLINICAL MANIFESTATIONS

Children with JDM present with either rash, insidious onset of weakness, or both. Fevers, dysphagia or dysphonia, arthritis, muscle tenderness, and fatigue are also commonly reported at diagnosis.

Rash develops as the first symptom in 50% of cases and appears concomitant with weakness only 25% of the time. Children often exhibit extreme photosensitivity to ultraviolet light exposure with generalized erythema in sun-exposed areas. If seen over the chest and neck, this erythema is known as the "**shawl sign.**" Erythema is also commonly seen over the knees and elbows. The characteristic **heliotrope rash** (Fig. 153-1) is a blue-violet discoloration of the eyelids that may be associated with periorbital edema. Facial erythema crossing the nasolabial folds is also common, in contrast to the malar rash without nasolabial involvement typical of systemic lupus erythematosus. Classic **Gottron papules** (Fig. 153-2) are bright pink or pale, shiny, thickened or atrophic plaques over the proximal interphalangeal joints and distal interphalangeal joints and occasionally on the knees, elbows, small joints of the toes, and ankle malleoli. The rash of JDM is sometimes mistaken for eczema or psoriasis. Rarely, a thickened erythematous and scaly rash develops in children over the palms (known as **mechanic's hands**) and soles along the flexor tendons, which is associated with anti-Jo-1 antibodies.

Evidence of small vessel inflammation is often visible in the nail folds and gums as individual capillary loops that are thickened, tortuous, or absent (Fig. 153-3). Telangiectasias may be visible to the naked eye but are more easily visualized under capillaroscopy or with use a magnifier such as an ophthalmoscope. Severe vascular inflammation causes cutaneous ulcers on toes, fingers, axillae, or epicanthal folds.

Weakness associated with JDM is often insidious and difficult to differentiate from fatigue at onset. It is typically symmetric, affecting proximal muscles such as the neck flexors, shoulder girdle, and hip flexors. Parents may report difficulty climbing stairs, combing hair, and getting out of bed. Examination reveals inability to perform a sit-up, head lag in a child after infancy, and **Gower sign** (use of hands on thighs to stand from a sitting position). Patients with JDM may roll to the side rather than sit straight up from lying to compensate for truncal weakness. Approximately half of children exhibit muscle tenderness as a result of muscle inflammation.

Esophageal and respiratory muscles are also affected, resulting in aspiration or respiratory failure. It is essential to assess for dysphonia or nasal speech, palatal elevation with gag, dysphagia, and gastroesophageal reflux by means of history, physical exam, and swallow study, if symptoms are present. Respiratory muscle weakness can be a medical emergency and lead to respiratory failure. Children with respiratory muscle weakness do not manifest typical symptoms of impending respiratory failure with increased work of breathing, instead demonstrating hypercarbia rather than hypoxemia.

Lipodystrophy and **calcinosis** (Fig. 153-4) are thought to be associated with longstanding or undertreated disease. Dystrophic deposition of calcium phosphate, hydroxyapatite, or fluoroapatite crystals occurs in subcutaneous plaques or nodules, resulting in painful ulceration of the skin with extrusion of crystals or calcific liquid. Calcinosis is reported in up to 40% of children with JDM, but the prevalence is thought to be lower in children who are treated early and aggressively. In rare instances, an "exoskeleton" of calcium deposition forms, greatly limiting mobility. Lipodystrophy results in progressive loss of subcutaneous and visceral fat, typically over the face and upper body, and may be associated with a metabolic syndrome similar to polycystic ovarian syndrome with insulin resistance, hirsutism, acanthosis, hypertriglyceridemia, and abnormal glucose tolerance. Lipodystrophy may be generalized or localized.

Rarely, vasculitis of the GI tract develops in children with severe JDM, with crampy abdominal pain, pancreatitis, GI bleeding, and potential for intestinal perforation or infarction. Involvement of the cardiac muscle with pericarditis, myocarditis, and conduction defects has been reported. An association with malignancy at disease onset is observed in adults with dermatomyositis but very rarely in children.

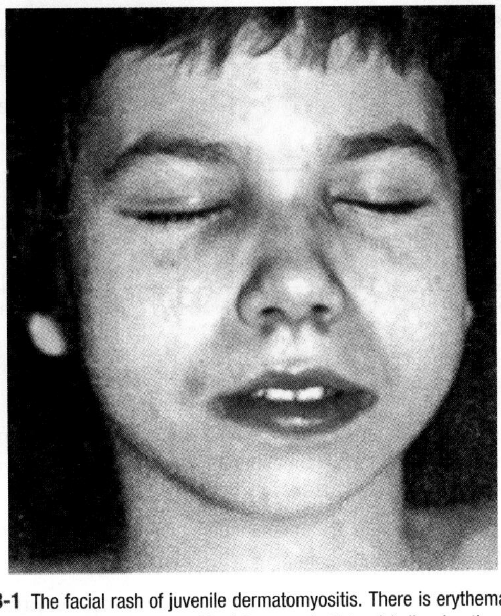

Figure 153-1 The facial rash of juvenile dermatomyositis. There is erythema over the bridge of the nose and malar areas with violaceous (heliotropic) discolorations of the upper eyelids.

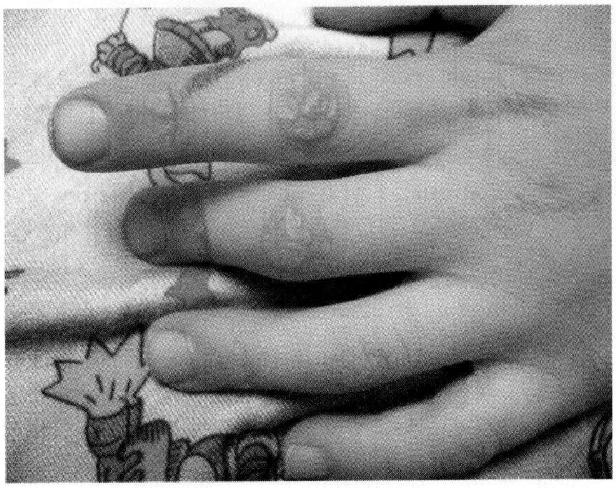

Figure 153-2 The rash of juvenile dermatomyositis. The skin over the metacarpal and proximal interphalangeal joints may be hypertrophic and pale red (Gottron papules).

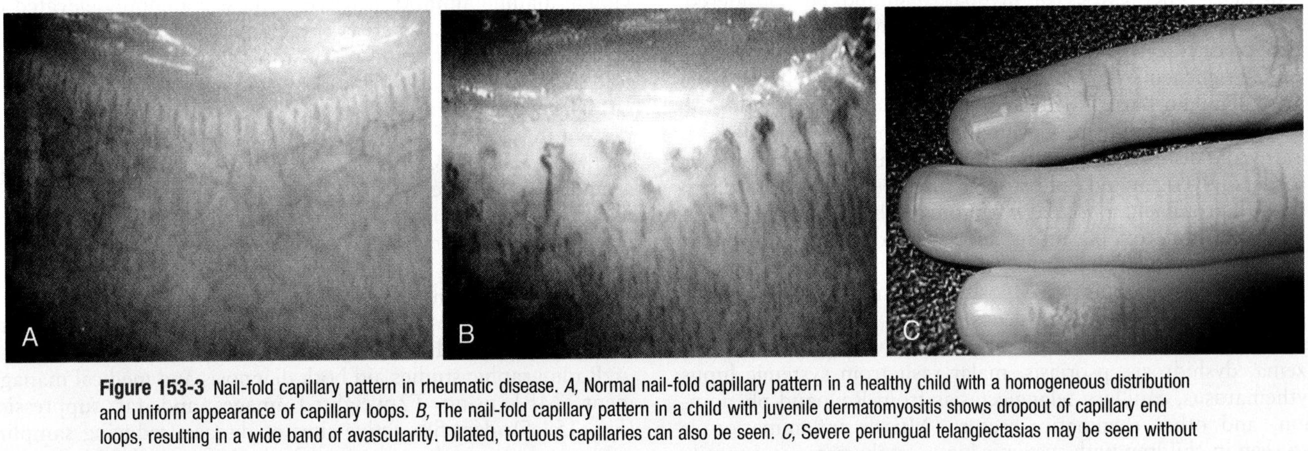

Figure 153-3 Nail-fold capillary pattern in rheumatic disease. *A,* Normal nail-fold capillary pattern in a healthy child with a homogeneous distribution and uniform appearance of capillary loops. *B,* The nail-fold capillary pattern in a child with juvenile dermatomyositis shows dropout of capillary end loops, resulting in a wide band of avascularity. Dilated, tortuous capillaries can also be seen. *C,* Severe periungual telangiectasias may be seen without microscopy.

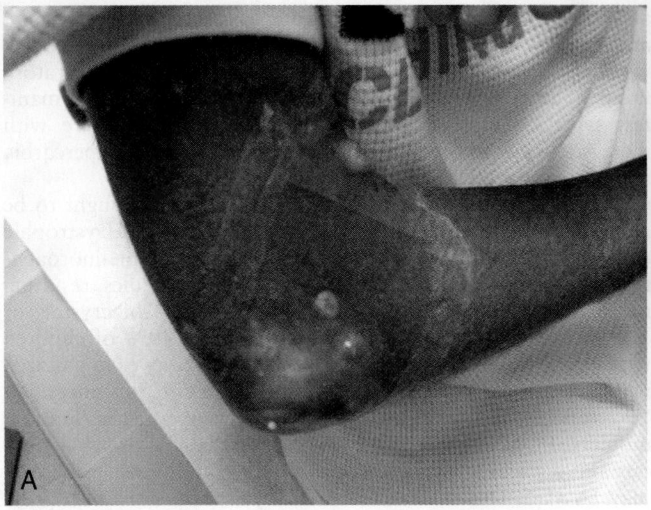

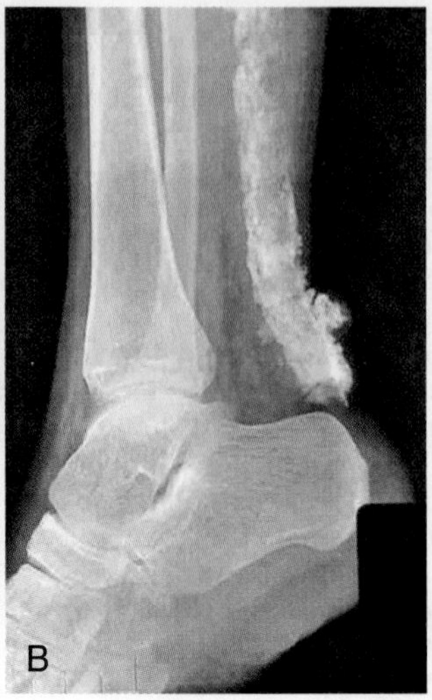

Figure 153-4 Rash and calcifications in dermatomyositis. *A,* Skin effects of calcification. *B,* Radiographic evidence of calcification.

DIAGNOSIS

Diagnosis of dermatomyositis requires the presence of characteristic rash as well as at least three signs of muscle inflammation and weakness (Table 153-1). Diagnostic criteria developed in 1975 predate the use of MRI and have not been validated in children. Diagnosis is often delayed because of the insidious nature of disease onset.

Electromyography shows signs of myopathy and denervation (increased insertional activity, fibrillations, and sharp waves) as well as muscle fiber necrosis (decreased action potential amplitude and duration). Nerve conduction studies are typically normal unless severe muscle necrosis and atrophy are present. It is important that electromyography (EMG) be performed in a center with experience in pediatric EMG and its interpretation. Muscle biopsy is typically indicated when diagnosis is in doubt or for grading disease severity. Biopsy of involved muscle reveals focal necrosis and phagocytosis of muscle fibers, fiber regeneration, endomysial proliferation, inflammatory cell infiltrates and vasculitis, and tubuloreticular inclusion bodies within endothelial cells. Findings of lymphoid structures and vasculopathy may portend more severe disease.

Some children present with classic rash but no apparent muscle weakness or inflammation; this variation is called **amyopathic JDM**. It is unclear whether these children have isolated skin disease or mild undetected muscle inflammation, risking progression to more severe muscle involvement with long-term sequelae such as calcinosis and lipodystrophy if untreated.

Differential diagnosis depends on the presenting symptoms. If the presenting complaint is solely weakness without rash or atypical disease, other causes of myopathy should be considered, including polymyositis, infection-related myositis (influenza A and B, coxsackievirus B, and other viral illnesses), muscular dystrophies (Duchenne and Becker as well as others), myasthenia gravis, Guillain-Barré syndrome, endocrinopathies (hyperthyroidism, hypothyroidism, Cushing syndrome, Addison disease, parathyroid disorders), mitochondrial myopathies, and metabolic disorders (glycogen and lipid storage diseases). Infections associated with prominent muscular symptoms include trichinosis, *Bartonella* infection, toxoplasmosis, and staphylococcal pyomyositis. Blunt trauma and crush injuries may lead to transient rhabdomyolysis with myoglobinuria. Myositis in children may also be associated with vaccinations, drugs, growth hormone, and graft versus host disease. The rash of JDM may be confused with eczema, dyshidrosis, psoriasis, malar rash from systemic lupus erythematosus, capillary telangiectasias from Raynaud phenomenon, and other rheumatic diseases. Muscle inflammation is also seen in children with systemic lupus erythematosus, juvenile idiopathic arthritis, mixed connective tissue disease, inflammatory bowel disease, and anti-neutrophil cytoplasmic antibody (ANCA)–positive vasculitides.

Table 153-1 DIAGNOSTIC CRITERIA FOR JUVENILE DERMATOMYOSITIS

Classic rash	Heliotrope rash of the eyelids Gottron papules
Plus three of the following:	
Weakness	Symmetric Proximal
Muscle enzyme elevation (≥1)	Creatine kinase Aspartate aminotransferase Lactate dehydrogenase Aldolase
Electromyographic changes	Myopathy Denervation
Muscle biopsy	Necrosis Inflammation

Data from Bohan A, Peter JB: Polymyositis and dermatomyositis (second of two parts), *N Engl J Med* 292:403–407, 1975.

LABORATORY FINDINGS

Elevated serum levels of **muscle-derived enzymes** (creatine kinase [CK], aldolase, aspartate aminotransferase, alanine aminotransferase, and lactate dehydrogenase) reflect muscle inflammation. Not all enzyme levels rise with inflammation in a specific individual; alanine aminotransferase is most commonly elevated on initial presentation, whereas the CK level may be normal. The erythrocyte sedimentation rate is often normal, and the rheumatoid factor test result is typically negative. There may be anemia consistent with chronic disease. Antinuclear antibody (ANA) is present in >80% of children with JDM. Results of tests for antibodies to SSA, SSB, Sm, ribonucleoprotein (RNP), and double-stranded DNA are generally negative. Antibodies to Pm/Scl identify a small, distinct subgroup of myopathies with a protracted disease course, often complicated by pulmonary interstitial fibrosis and/or cardiac involvement. Unlike in adults with JDM, presence of myositis-specific autoantibodies (MSAs) is rare in children; positive test results for anti-Jo-1, anti-Mi-2, and other MSAs may portend more significant disease.

Radiographic studies aid both diagnosis and medical management. MRI using T2-weighted images and fat suppression (Fig. 153-5) identifies active sites of disease, reducing sampling error and increasing the sensitivity of muscle biopsy and

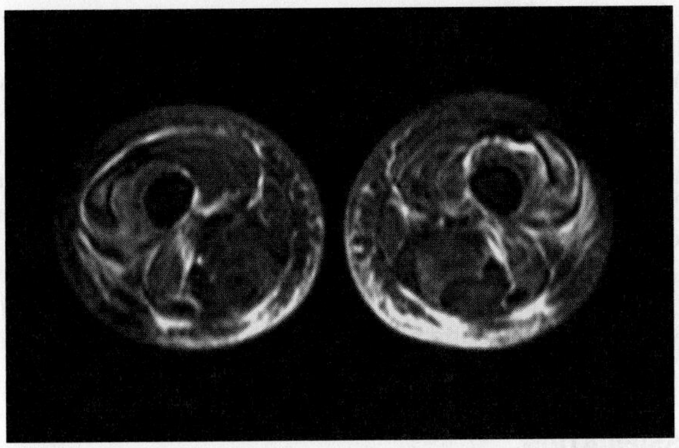

Figure 153-5 MRI using T2-weighting and fat suppression of the proximal muscle of the lower extremities of a child with juvenile dermatomyositis with normal muscle enzyme levels. There is focal inflammatory myopathy. The bright areas reflect the inflammatory response in involved muscle. The darker areas are more normal. Identification of involved areas by MRI directs the location of the muscle biopsy or electromyography.

electromyography, results of which are nondiagnostic in 20% of instances if the procedures are not directed by MRI. Extensive rash and abnormal MRI findings may be found despite normal serum levels of muscle-derived enzymes. Muscle biopsy often demonstrates evidence of disease activity and chronicity that is not suspected from the levels of the serum enzymes alone.

A contrast swallow study may document palatal dysfunction and risk of aspiration. Pulmonary function testing detects a restrictive defect consistent with respiratory weakness and reduced diffusion capacity of carbon monoxide (DLCO) from alveolar fibrosis associated with other connective tissue diseases. Serial measurement of vital capacity or negative inspiratory force can document changes in respiratory weakness, especially in an inpatient setting. Calcinosis is seen easily on radiographs, along the fascial planes and within muscles.

TREATMENT

The aid of an experienced pediatric rheumatologist is invaluable in outlining an appropriate course of treatment for a child with JDM. Prior to the advent of corticosteroids, one third of patients spontaneously improved, one third had a chronic, lingering course, and one third died from the disease. Corticosteroids have altered the course of disease, lowering morbidity and mortality. Methotrexate decreases the length of treatment with corticosteroids, thereby reducing morbidity from steroid toxicity. Intravenous gammaglobulin is frequently used as an adjunct for treatment of severe disease. No evidence-based guidelines for optimal treatment of JDM currently exist.

Corticosteroids are still the mainstay of treatment. In a clinically stable child without debilitating weakness, oral prednisone at 2 mg/kg/day is usually started. Children with GI involvement have decreased absorption of oral steroids and require intravenous administration. In more severe cases with respiratory or oropharyngeal weakness, high-dose pulse methylprednisolone is used (30 mg/kg/day for 3 days, maximum dose 1 g/day) with ongoing weekly or monthly IV dosing along with daily oral corticosteroids as needed. Corticosteroid dosage is slowly tapered over a period of 12-24 mo, after indicators of inflammation (muscle enzymes) normalize and strength improves.

Weekly oral, intravenous, or subcutaneous methotrexate (0.5-1 mg/kg or 15-20 mg/m^2, max 25 mg) is commonly used as a steroid-sparing agent in JDM. The concomitant use of methotrexate halves the cumulative dosage of steroids needed for disease control. Risks of methotrexate include immunosuppression, blood count dyscrasias, chemical hepatitis, pulmonary toxicity, nausea/vomiting, and teratogenicity. Folic acid is typically given with methotrexate starting at a dose of 1 mg daily to reduce toxicity and side effects of folate inhibition (oral ulcers, nausea, and anemia). Children who are taking immunosuppressive medications such as methotrexate should avoid live-virus vaccination, although inactivated influenza vaccination is recommended yearly.

Hydroxychloroquine has little toxicity risk and is used as a secondary disease-modifying agent to reduce rash and maintain remission. Typically, it is administered at doses between 4 and 6 mg/kg/day orally in either tablet or liquid form. Ophthalmologic follow-up 1 to 2 times per year to monitor for rare retinal toxicity due is recommended. Other side effects include hemolysis in patients with glucose-6-phosphate deficiency, GI intolerance, and skin/hair discoloration.

Other medications for severe unresponsive disease include intravenous immunoglobulin, mycophenolate mofetil, cyclosporine, and cyclophosphamide. Children with pharyngeal weakness may need nasogastric or gastrostomy feedings to avoid aspiration, whereas those with GI vasculitis require full bowel rest. Rarely, children with severe respiratory weakness require ventilator therapy and even tracheostomy until the respiratory weakness improves.

Physical therapy and occupational therapy are integral parts of the treatment program, initially for passive stretching early in the disease course and then for direct reconditioning of muscles to regain strength and range of motion once active inflammation has resolved. Bed rest is not indicated, because weight bearing improves bone density and prevents contractures. Social work and psychology services may facilitate adjustment to the frustration of physical impairment in a previously active child.

All children with JDM should avoid sun exposure and apply high–sun protection factor (SPF) sunscreen daily, even in winter and on cloudy days. Vitamin D and calcium supplements are indicated for all children undergoing long-term corticosteroid therapy, in an attempt to reduce osteopenia and osteoporosis from medication.

COMPLICATIONS

Most complications from JDM are related to prolonged and severe weakness, including muscle atrophy, to cutaneous calcifications and scarring or atrophy, and to lipodystrophy. Secondary complications from medical treatments are also common. Children with acute and severe weakness are at risk for aspiration pneumonia and respiratory failure and occasionally require nasogastric feeding and mechanical ventilation until weakness improves. Crampy abdominal pain and occult GI bleeding may indicate bowel wall vasculitis and lead to ischemia, GI bleeding, and perforation if not treated with complete bowel rest and aggressive treatment for the underlying inflammation. Surgery should be avoided if possible, because the GI vasculitis is diffuse and not easily amenable to surgical intervention. Contrast-enhanced CT may show dilation or thickening of the bowel wall, intraluminal air, or evidence of bowel necrosis. Cardiac involvement by JDM is rare but includes arrhythmias.

Pathologic calcifications may be related to severity of disease and prolonged delay to treatment and potentially to genetic polymorphisms of TNF-α-308. Calcium deposits tend to form in subcutaneous tissue and along muscle. Some ulcerate through the skin and drain a soft calcific liquid, and others manifest as hard nodules along extensor surfaces or embedded along muscle. Draining lesions serve as a nidus for cellulitis or osteomyelitis. Nodules cause skin inflammation that may mimic cellulitis. Spontaneous regression of calcium deposits may occur, but there is no evidence-based recommendation for treatment of calcinosis.

Lipodystrophy manifests in 10-40% of patients with JDM and can be difficult to recognize. Fat atrophy may be generalized, partial, or local. Lipodystrophy has been associated with insulin resistance, acanthosis nigricans, dyslipidemia, hypertension, and menstrual irregularity, similar to features seen in polycystic ovarian disease or metabolic syndrome X.

Children receiving prolonged corticosteroid therapy are prone to complications such as cessation of linear growth, weight gain, hirsutism, adrenal suppression, immunosuppression, striae, cushingoid fat deposition, mood changes, osteoporosis, cataracts, avascular necrosis, and steroid myopathy. Families should be counseled on the effects of corticosteroids and advised to use medical alert identification and to consult a nutritionist regarding a low-salt, low-fat diet with adequate vitamin D and calcium supplementation.

PROGNOSIS

The mortality rate in JDM has decreased since the advent of corticosteroids, from 33% to currently about 1%; little is known about the long-term consequences of persistent vascular inflammation. The period of active symptoms has decreased from about 3.5 years to <1.5 years with more aggressive immunosuppressive therapy; the vascular, skin, and muscle symptoms of children with JDM generally respond well to therapy. At 7 years of follow-up, 75% of patients have little to no residual disability, but 25% continue to have chronic weakness and 40% have chronic rash. Up to one third may need long-term medications to control their disease. Children with JDM appear able to repair inflammatory damage to vasculature and muscle.

BIBLIOGRAPHY

Please visit the Nelson Textbook of Pediatrics *website at www.expertconsult.com for the complete bibliography.*

Chapter 154
Scleroderma and Raynaud Phenomenon

Heather A. Van Mater and C. Egla Rabinovich

Juvenile scleroderma encompasses a range of conditions unified by the presence of fibrosis of the skin. Juvenile scleroderma is divided into 2 major categories, **localized scleroderma** (**LS**, also known as **morphea**), which is largely limited to the skin, and **systemic sclerosis** (**SSc**), with organ involvement. Although localized disease is the predominant type seen in pediatric populations, systemic sclerosis is associated with severe morbidity and mortality.

ETIOLOGY AND PATHOGENESIS

The etiology of scleroderma is unknown, but the mechanism of disease appears to be a combination of a vasculopathy, autoimmunity, immune activation, and fibrosis. Triggers, including trauma, infection, and, possibly, subclinical graft versus host reaction from persistent maternal cells (microchimerism), injure vascular endothelial cells, resulting in increased expression of adhesion molecules. These molecules entrap platelets and inflammatory cells, resulting in vascular changes with manifestations such as Raynaud phenomenon and pulmonary hypertension. Inflammatory cells infiltrate the area of initial vascular damage, causing further vascular damage and resulting in thickened artery walls and reduction in capillary numbers. Macrophages and other inflammatory cells then migrate into affected tissues and secrete cytokines that induce fibroblasts to reproduce and synthesize excessive amounts of collagen, resulting in fibrosis and subsequent lipoatrophy, dermal fibrosis, and loss of sweat glands and hair follicles. In late stages, the entire dermis may be replaced by compact collagen fibers.

Autoimmunity is believed to be a key process in the pathogenesis of both localized and systemic scleroderma, given the high percentage of affected children with autoantibodies. Children with localized disease often have a positive ANA test result (42%), and 47% of this subgroup have antihistone antibodies. Other autoantibodies seen include rheumatoid factor (RF) (16%) and antiphospholipid antibodies (12%). The relationship between specific autoantibodies and the various forms of scleroderma is not well understood, and all antibody test results may be negative in a child, especially one who has LS.

CLASSIFICATION

Localized scleroderma is distinct from systemic scleroderma and rarely progresses to systemic disease. Within the category of LS there are several subtypes that are differentiated by both the distribution of the lesions and the depth of involvement (Table 154-1). Up to 15% of children have a combination of 2 or more subtypes.

EPIDEMIOLOGY

Juvenile scleroderma is rare, with an estimated prevalence of 1/100,000. Localized scleroderma is far more common than SSc in children, by a 10:1 ratio, with **plaque morphea** and **linear scleroderma** being the most common subtypes. Linear scleroderma is predominantly a pediatric condition, with 65% of patients diagnosed before age 18. After age 8 yr the female:male ratio for both LS and SSc is approximately 3:1, whereas in patients younger than 8 yr there is no sex predilection.

CLINICAL MANIFESTATIONS

Localized Scleroderma

The onset of scleroderma is generally insidious, and manifestations vary according to disease subtype. The initial skin manifestations of localized disease usually include erythema or a bluish hue seen around an area of waxy induration; subtle erythema may be the only presenting sign (Fig. 154-1). Early edema and erythema are followed by indurated, hypopigmented or hyperpigmented, atrophic lesions (Fig. 154-2). **Linear scleroderma** varies in size from a few centimeters to the entire length of the extremity, with varying depth. Patients sometimes present with arthralgias, synovitis, or flexion contractures (Fig. 154-3). Children also experience limb length discrepancies as a result of growth impairment due to involvement of muscle and bone. Children with **en coup de sabre** (Fig. 154-4) may have symptoms unique to central nervous system (CNS) involvement, such as seizures, hemifacial atrophy, ipsilateral uveitis, and learning/behavioral changes.

Up to 25% of children with LS have extracutaneous manifestations, most commonly arthritis (47%) and neurologic symptoms (17%) associated with en coup de sabre.

Systemic Scleroderma

Systemic scleroderma also has an insidious onset with a prolonged course characterized by periods of remission and exacerbation, ending in either remission or, more commonly, chronic disability and death.

The skin manifestations of SSc include an early phase of edema that spreads proximally from the dorsum of the hands and fingers and includes the face. An eventual decrease in edema is followed by induration and fibrosis of skin, ultimately resulting in loss of subcutaneous fat, sweat glands, and hair follicles. Later, atrophic skin becomes shiny and waxy in appearance. As lesions spread proximally, flexion contractures develop at the elbows, hips, and knees associated with secondary muscle weakness and atrophy. In the face, this process results in a small oral stoma with decreased mouth aperture. Skin ulceration over pressure points, such as the elbows, may be associated with subcutaneous calcifications. Severe Raynaud phenomenon causes ulceration of the fingertips with subsequent loss of tissue pulp and tapered fingers (**sclerodactyly**) (Fig. 154-5). Resorption of the distal tufts of the distal phalanges may occur (**acro-osteolysis**). Hyperpigmented postinflammatory changes surrounded by atrophic depigmentation gives a salt-and-pepper appearance. Over a period of years, remodeling of lesions sometimes results in focal improvement in skin thickening.

Pulmonary disease is the most common visceral manifestation of SSc and includes both arterial and interstitial involvement (alveolitis). Symptoms range from asymptomatic disease to exercise intolerance, dyspnea at rest, and right-sided heart failure.

Table 154-1 CLASSIFICATION OF PEDIATRIC SCLERODERMA (MORPHEA)

LOCALIZED SCLERODERMA
Plaque Morphea
Confined to dermis, occasionally superficial panniculus Well-circumscribed circular area of induration, often a central waxy, ivory-colored area surrounded by a violaceous halo; unilateral
Generalized Morphea
Involves dermis primarily, occasionally panniculus Defined as confluence of individual morphea plaques or lesions in 3 or more anatomic sites; more likely to be bilateral
Bullous Morphea
Bullous lesions that can occur with any of the subtypes of morphea
Linear Scleroderma
Linear lesions can extend through the dermis, subcutaneous tissue, and muscle to underlying bone; more likely unilateral **Limbs/trunk:** One or more linear streaks of the extremities or trunk Flexion contracture occurs when lesion extends over a joint; limb length discrepancies **En coup de sabre:** Involves the scalp and/or face; lesions can extend into the central nervous system, resulting in neurologic sequelae, most commonly seizures and headaches **Parry Romberg syndrome:** Hemifacial atrophy without a clearly definable en coup de sabre lesion; can also have neurologic involvement
Deep Morphea
Involves deeper layers, including panniculus, fascia, and muscle; more likely to be bilateral **Subcutaneous morphea:** Primarily involves the panniculus or subcutaneous tissue Plaques are hyperpigmented and symmetric **Eosinophilic fasciitis:** Fasciitis with marked blood eosinophilia Fascia is the primary site of involvement; typically involves extremities Classic description is "peau d'orange" or orange peel texture, but early disease manifests as edema (see Fig. 154-2) **Morphea profunda:** Deep lesion extending to fascia and sometimes muscle, but may be limited to a single plaque, often on trunk **Disabling pansclerotic morphea of childhood:** Generalized full-thickness involvement of skin on the trunk, face and extremities, sparing finger tips and toes
SYSTEMIC SCLEROSIS
Diffuse
Most common type in childhood Symmetric thickening and hardening of the skin (sclerosis) with fibrous and degenerative changes of viscera
Limited
Rare in childhood Previously known as CREST (calcinosis cutis, Raynaud phenomenon, esophageal dysfunction, sclerodactyly, and telangiectasia) syndrome

Pulmonary arterial hypertension (PAH) is a poor prognostic sign, developing either as a consequence of lung disease or independently as part of the vasculopathy. Clinical manifestations of PAH in children appear late in the course, are subtle, and include cough and dyspnea on exertion. Pulmonary evaluation should include pulmonary function testing (PFT), bronchioalveolar lavage, and high resolution chest CT. PFTs reveal decreased vital capacity and decreased diffusion of carbon monoxide capacity (DLCO), while neutrophilia and/or eosinophilia on bronchioalveolar lavage suggest active alveolitis. Chest CT is much more sensitive than chest radiographs, which are often normal, showing typical basilar ground-glass abnormalities, reticular linear opacities, nodules, honey combing, and mediastinal adenopathy.

Other organ systems are involved in SSc. Gastrointestinal tract disease is seen in 25% of children with the disease. Common manifestations include esophageal and intestinal dysmotility resulting in dysphagia, reflux, dyspepsia, gastroparesis, bacterial overgrowth, dilated bowel loops and pseudo-obstruction, dental caries, as well as malabsorption and failure to thrive. Renal arterial disease can cause chronic or severe episodic hypertension;

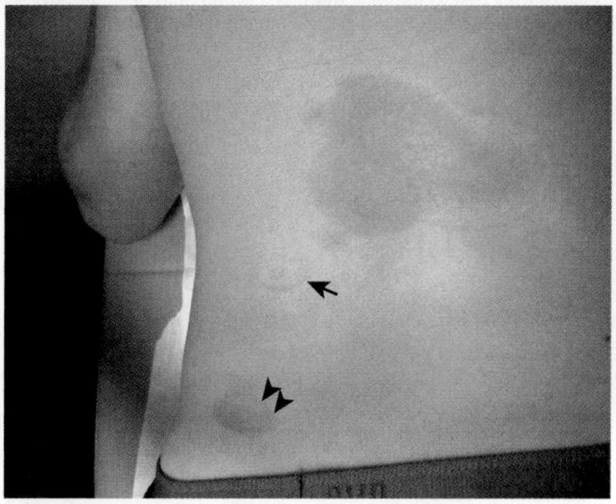

Figure 154-1 Boy with generalized morphea. Note the active circular lesion (*arrowheads*) with a surrounding rim of erythema. The largest lesion has areas of postinflammatory hyperpigmentation and depression with an area of erythema on the right. The small lesion (*arrow*) demonstrates depression due to lipoatrophy.

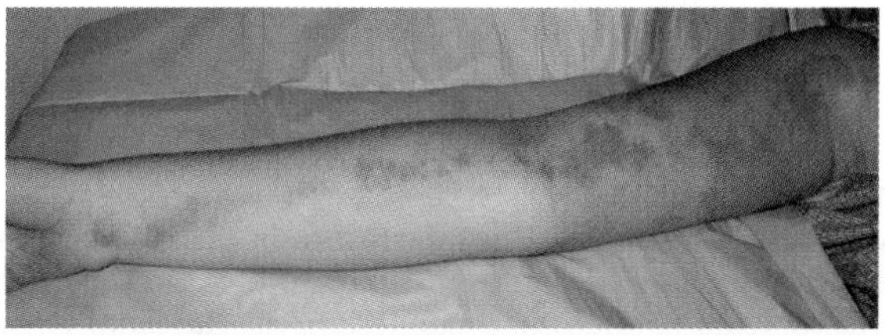

Figure 154-2 Inactive linear scleroderma demonstrating hyperpigmented lesion with areas of normal skin (skip lesions).

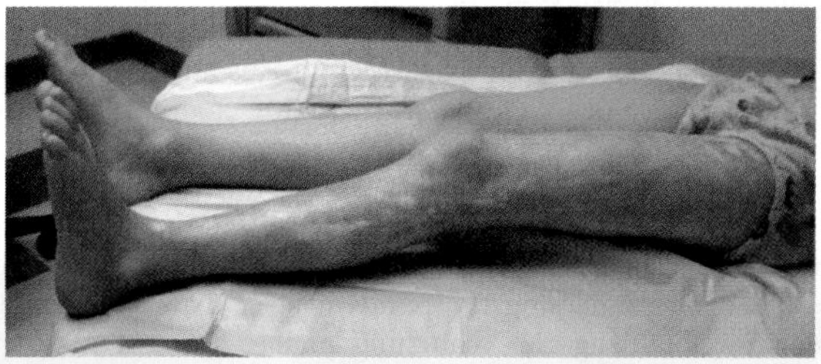

Figure 154-3 Child with untreated linear scleroderma resulting in knee contracture, immobility of ankle, chronic skin breakdown of scar on the lateral knee, and areas of hypopigmentation and hyperpigmentation. The affected leg is 1 cm shorter.

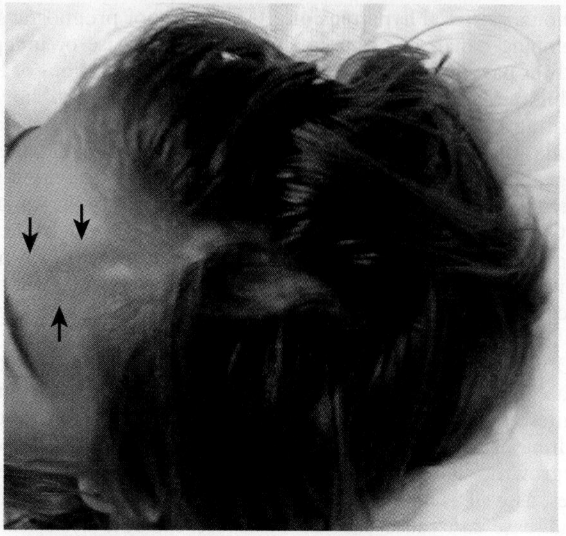

Figure 154-4 Child with en coup de sabre lesion on scalp extending down to forehead. Prior to treatment the skin on the scalp was bound down with chronic skin breakdown. Note the area of hypopigmentation extending down the forehead (*arrows*).

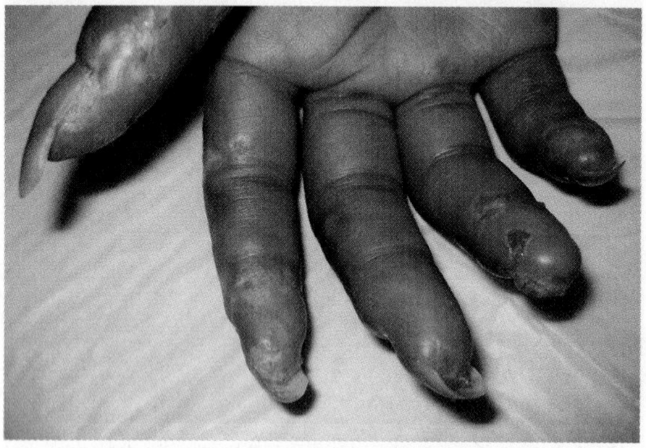

Figure 154-5 Sclerodactyly and finger ulcerations in a patient with systemic sclerosis who is poorly compliant with treatment.

unlike in adult disease, renal crisis is rare. Cardiac fibrosis is associated with arrhythmias, ventricular hypertrophy, and decreased cardiac function. Mortality from juvenile systemic sclerosis is most commonly a result of cardiopulmonary disease.

Raynaud Phenomenon

Raynaud phenomenon (RP) is the most frequent initial symptom in pediatric systemic sclerosis, present in 70% of affected children months to years before other manifestations. *Raynaud phenomenon* refers to the classic triphasic sequence of blanching, cyanosis, and erythema of the digits induced by cold exposure and/or emotional stress. Raynaud phenomenon is most commonly independent of an underlying rheumatic disease (**Raynaud disease**), but it can be a consequence of other diseases as well as scleroderma, such as systemic lupus erythematosus and mixed connective tissue disease (Table 154-2). The color changes are brought about by (1) initial arterial vasoconstriction, resulting in hypoperfusion and pallor (blanching), (2) venous stasis (cyanosis), and (3) reflex vasodilatation caused by the factors released from the ischemic phase (erythema). The color change is classically reproduced by immersing the hands in iced water and reversed by warming. During the blanching phase, there is inadequate tissue perfusion in the affected area, associated with pain and paresthesias and resulting in ischemic damage only when associated with a rheumatic disease. The blanching usually affects the distal fingers but may also involve thumbs, toes, ears, and tip of the nose. The affected area is usually well demarcated and uniformly white.

Table 154-2 CLASSIFICATION OF RAYNAUD PHENOMENON

- Isolated Raynaud phenomenon
- Occupational Raynaud phenomenon:
  - Cold injury
  - Vibrating tools
  - Polyvinyl chloride exposure
- Secondary Raynaud phenomenon:
  - Systemic sclerosis
  - Mixed connective tissue disease
  - Sjögren syndrome
  - Systemic lupus erythematosus
  - Polymyositis/dermatomyositis
  - Rheumatoid arthritis
  - Arteritis
  - Antiphospholipid antibody syndrome
  - Primary biliary cirrhosis
  - Carpal tunnel syndrome
  - Cryoglobulinemia
  - Vasospastic disorders (migraine, Prinzmetal angina)
  - Infection:
    - Hepatitis C
    - Cytomegalovirus (?)
  - Obstructive vascular disease:
    - Atherosclerosis
    - Thromboangiitis obliterans
    - Thoracic outlet syndrome (cervical rib)
  - Metabolic syndrome:
    - Hypothyroid
  - Carcinoid syndrome
  - Drug-induced:
    - Antimigraine
    - β-blocker
    - Bleomycin
    - Interferons
    - Ergotamine derivatives

From Firestein GS, Budd RC, Harris ED Jr, et al, editors: *Kelley's textbook of rheumatology*, ed 8, vol II, Philadelphia, 2009, Saunders/Elsevier.

Raynaud phenomenon often begins in adolescence and is characterized by symmetric occurrence, the absence of tissue necrosis and gangrene, and the lack of manifestations of an underlying rheumatic disease. Children have normal nail-fold capillaries (absence of periungual telangiectasias). Raynaud phenomenon should be distinguished from **acrocyanosis** and **chilblains.** Acrocyanosis is a vasospastic disorder resulting in cool, painless, bluish discoloration in the hands and sometimes feet despite normal tissue perfusion. It may be exacerbated by stimulant medications used to treat attention deficit disorder. Chilblains is a condition with episodic color changes and the development of nodules related to severe cold exposure and spasm-induced vessel and tissue damage; this condition has been associated with systemic lupus erythematosus.

DIAGNOSIS

The diagnosis of localized scleroderma is based on the distribution and depth of characteristic lesions. Biopsy is helpful to confirm the diagnosis. Classification criteria for juvenile systemic sclerosis were recently devised, reflecting differences in presentation and course compared with adult onset disease. The new classification requires proximal sclerosis/induration of the skin as well as the presence of 2 of 20 minor criteria (Table 154-3).

DIFFERENTIAL DIAGNOSIS

The most important condition to differentiate from LS is SSc. Contractures and synovitis from juvenile arthritis can be

Table 154-3 PROVISIONAL CRITERIA FOR THE CLASSIFICATION OF JUVENILE SYSTEMIC SCLEROSIS (SSC)

MAJOR CRITERION (REQUIRED)
Proximal skin sclerosis/induration of the skin
MINOR CRITERIA (AT LEAST 2 REQUIRED)
Cutaneous: sclerodactyly
Peripheral vascular: Raynaud phenomenon, nailfold capillary abnormalities (telangiectasias), digital tip ulcers
Gastrointestinal: dysphagia, gastroesophageal reflux
Cardiac: Arrhythmias, heart failure
Renal: Renal crisis, new-onset arterial hypertension
Respiratory: pulmonary fibrosis (high-resolution computed tomography/radiography), decreased diffusing capacity for carbon monoxide (DLCO), pulmonary arterial hypertension
Neurologic: neuropathy, carpal tunnel syndrome
Musculoskeletal: tendon friction rubs, arthritis, myositis
Serologic: antinuclear antibodies—SSc-selective autoantibodies (anticentromere, anti-topoisomerase I [Scl-70], antifibrillarin, anti-PM/Scl, antifibrillin or anti-RNA polymerase I or III)

From Zulian F, Woo P, Athreya BH, et al: The Pediatric Rheumatology European Society/American College of Rheumatology/European League against Rheumatism provisional classification criteria for juvenile systemic sclerosis, *Arthritis Rheum* 57:203–212, 2007.

differentiated from those due to linear scleroderma by the absence or presence of skin changes. Other conditions to consider include chemically induced scleroderma-like disease, **diabetic cheiroarthropathy, pseudoscleroderma**, and **scleredema.** Pseudoscleroderma is composed of a group of unrelated diseases characterized by patchy or diffuse cutaneous fibrosis without the other manifestations of scleroderma. These include phenylketonuria, syndromes of premature aging, and localized idiopathic fibrosis. **Scleredema** is a transient, self-limited disease of both children and adults that has sudden onset after a febrile illness (especially streptococcal infections) and is characterized by patchy sclerodermatous lesions on the neck and shoulders and extending to the face, trunk, and arms.

LABORATORY FINDINGS

There are no laboratory studies diagnostic of either localized or systemic scleroderma. Although the results of complete blood counts, serum chemistry analyses, and urinalysis are normal, children may have elevated erythrocyte sedimentation rate, eosinophilia, or hypergammaglobulinemia, all of which normalize with treatment. Elevations of muscle enzymes, particularly aldolase, can be seen with muscle involvement. Patients with SSc may have anemia, leukocytosis, and eosinophilia and are more likely to have a high-titer positive ANA test result and to test positive for anti-Scl 70 antibody (anti-topoisomerase I). Imaging studies delineate the affected area and can be used to follow disease progression. MRI is useful in en coup de sabre and Parry Romberg syndrome for determination of CNS or orbital involvement. Infrared thermography utilizes the temperature variation between areas of active and inactive cutaneous disease to help differentiate active disease from damage. The role of ultrasound to look at lesion activity is evolving. High-resolution CT, pulmonary function tests, echocardiography, and manometry are useful tools for diagnosing and monitoring visceral involvement in SSc.

TREATMENT

Treatment for scleroderma varies according to the subtype and severity. Superficial morphea may benefit from topical corticosteroids or ultraviolet (UV) therapy. For lesions involving deeper structures, systemic therapy is recommended. A combination of methotrexate and corticosteroids is effective in treating LS by preventing lesion extension and resulting in significant skin softening and improved range of motion of affected joints. Treatment regimens include 3 months of either monthly high-dose intravenous corticosteroids (30 mg/kg, max dose 1000 mg) for 3 consecutive days a month, or high daily oral corticosteroids (0.5-2 mg/kg/day). In addition, methotrexate is given at 1-mg/kg weekly (max dose 25 mg), usually via subcutaneous administration to optimize bioavailability in doses over 0.5 mg/kg or 20 mg weekly. Physical and occupational therapy are important adjuncts to pharmacologic treatment. Eosinophilic fasciitis often responds well to corticosteroids but may also benefit from methotrexate.

Treatments for juvenile systemic sclerosis target specific disease manifestations. Raynaud phenomenon is treated with cold avoidance. Pharmacologic interventions are generally reserved for more severe disease. Calcium channel blockers (nifedipine 30-60 mg of sustained-release form daily, amlodipine 2.5-10 mg daily) are the most common pharmacologic interventions. Additional potential therapies for Raynaud phenomenon include losartan, prazosin, bosentan, and sildenafil. Angiotensin-converting enzyme inhibitors (captopril, enalapril) are recommended for hypertension associated with renal disease. Methotrexate or mycophenolate mofetil may be beneficial for skin manifestations. Cyclophosphamide is used to treat pulmonary alveolitis and prevent fibrosis. Corticosteroids should be used cautiously in systemic sclerosis due to an association with renal crisis.

PROGNOSIS

Localized scleroderma is usually self-limited, with the initial inflammatory stage followed by a period of stabilization and then softening for an average disease duration of 3-5 yr; there are reports of active disease lasting up to 20 yr. Prolonged disease activity is associated primarily with linear and deep disease subtypes. Localized scleroderma can result in significant morbidity, disfigurement, and disability, especially with the linear and deep subtypes.

Juvenile systemic sclerosis has a more variable prognosis. Although many children have a slow, insidious course, others demonstrate a rapidly progressive form with early organ failure and death. Skin manifestations reportedly soften years after disease onset. Overall, the prognosis of juvenile systemic sclerosis is better than that of the adult form, with 5-, 10-, and 15-year survival rates, respectively, in children of 89%, 80-87%, and 74-87%. The most common cause of death is heart failure due to myocardial and pulmonary fibrosis.

BIBLIOGRAPHY

Please visit the Nelson Textbook of Pediatrics *website at www.expertconsult.com for the complete bibliography.*

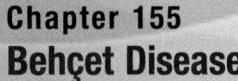

Chapter 155
Behçet Disease

Abraham Gedalia

Behçet disease is an autoinflammatory, multisystem disorder originally described as recurrent oral and genital ulceration associated with relapsing iritis or uveitis and is often characterized by cutaneous, arthritic, neurologic, vascular, and gastrointestinal manifestations.

EPIDEMIOLOGY

The disease is reported commonly in the Mediterranean basin and Asia along the trading route, the so-called Silk Road, and is relatively rare in Europe and the USA. Among the populations of these areas, the estimated prevalence in adults ranges between 20 and 421/ 100,000, although in Europe the prevalence range is 0.6-6.4/100,000. The condition is uncommon in children, who account for an estimated 5% of cases. Most of the pediatric cases are diagnosed in late childhood, although disease symptoms may begin much earlier. On the basis of case reports and the later few series in children, the mean age of onset is 7.5 yr, and the mean age at which patients meet the diagnostic criteria for the diagnosis is 12 yr. The male:female ratio ranges from 1:1.2 to 1:1.4. No sex predominance is seen in adult-onset Behçet disease.

ETIOLOGY AND PATHOGENESIS

The etiology of Behçet disease is unknown, although both genetic and environmental factors may play a significant role in triggering the inflammatory process. Excessive T helper type 1 (Th1) cell activity and increased expression of heat shock proteins (especially HSP60) occur in patients with Behçet disease.

In areas of the world with a high prevalence of disease (along the old Silk Road), HLA-B51 allele located on chromosome 6p has been the most strongly associated risk factor. HLA-B51 may serve as an immunogenetic marker for a subgroup of patients with enhanced neutrophil function and eye involvement. A few cases of transient neonatal Behçet disease in offspring of mothers with the disease have been reported, suggesting that an antibody-mediated immune process may also have a role in the pathogenesis. The basic pathologic lesion is vasculitis of small and medium-sized arteries, with cellular infiltration leading to fibrinoid necrosis and narrowing and obliteration of the vessel lumens. Necrotizing and granulomatous inflammation of large vessels such as the aorta and pulmonary artery may also occur. There is speculation that Behçet disease is an autoinflammatory disease similar to sarcoidosis and inflammatory bowel disease and is caused by dysregulation of the innate immune system.

CLINICAL MANIFESTATIONS

The clinical course is highly variable, with recurrent exacerbations and disease-free intervals of uncertain duration. The most consistent symptom is painful, shallow oral ulcers, usually 2-10 mm in diameter with surrounding erythema, that develop on the buccal mucosa, gingiva, lips, and tongue, persist for days to weeks, and then heal without scarring in 1-3 wk. These oral necrotic ulcers may occur singly or in crops, with a mean of 13 attacks per year. Genital (labia, scrotum, penis) ulcers occur in most patients and follow a parallel course but may heal with scars. Skin manifestations occur in most patients and include erythema nodosum, papulopustular lesions, pseudofolliculitis, and acneiform nodules. **Cutaneous pathergy** is often present, manifesting as an erythematous sterile pustule that develops 24-48 hr after a needle prick. **Ocular manifestations**, including anterior or posterior uveitis and retinal vasculitis, occur less frequently in children than in adults but are more severe in the pediatric population and may progress to blindness. **Arthritis** is common and is usually acute, recurrent, asymmetric, and polyarticular, involving the large joints. Gastrointestinal involvement is variable in different populations and is seen more frequently in Japan. Clinical features include abdominal pain, dyspepsia, and intestinal mucosal ulcerations, especially in the ileocecal region. Central nervous system abnormalities, such as meningoencephalitis, cranial nerve palsies, and psychosis, usually occur later in the course of the disease and indicate a poor prognosis. Fever, orchitis, myositis, pericarditis, nephritis, splenomegaly, and amyloidosis are rare manifestations. There is an increased risk for thrombophlebitis and large vessel thrombosis, including involvement of the superior or inferior vena cava and hepatic veins (**Budd-Chiari syndrome**).

DIAGNOSIS

The diagnosis of Behçet disease is not usually confirmed until the patient is 20-30 yr of age. The International Study Group criteria for diagnosis of Behçet disease are oral aphthae that recur at least 3 times within 12 mo accompanied by 2 of the following: recurrent genital ulcerations, eye lesions (anterior or posterior uveitis, or retinal vasculitis), skin lesions (erythema nodosum, pseudofolliculitis, or acneiforme nodules), and a positive pathergy test result. These criteria have 91% sensitivity and 96% specificity in adults. Laboratory tests are not diagnostic, although the finding of HLA-B51 supports the diagnosis.

DIFFERENTIAL DIAGNOSIS

The differential diagnosis of Behçet disease includes herpes simplex virus infection, inflammatory bowel disease, recurrent aphthous stomatitis, and complex aphthosis (recurrent oral and genital aphthous ulcers or ≥3 persistent oral aphthae). In addition, Stevens-Johnson syndrome and familial Mediterranean fever (in some areas) need to be considered.

TREATMENT

Treatment is based on anecdotal reports. Many drugs, including corticosteroids, colchicine, chlorambucil, azathioprine, cyclosporine, and tacrolimus, have been used. Colchicine is effective against of Behçet disease and shows higher efficacy in children than in adults, especially for oral ulcers, skin rash, joint symptoms, and, occasionally, eye disease. Thalidomide has been reported to be a highly effective and useful therapeutic option for severe oral, genital, and intestinal ulcerations that are unresponsive to other therapies. The successful use of anti–tumor necrosis factor-α (TNF-α) therapy in severe or intractable cases of Behçet disease suggests that these agents may also have a role in its management. The most commonly used anti–TNF-α agent has been infliximab, especially in childhood cases associated with refractory uveitis. In the only placebo-controlled trial, etanercept significantly decreased the mean number of oral ulcers and nodular and papulopustular lesions. Interferon alpha-2a has been used successfully to treat adult patients with Behçet disease. This agent is efficacious and safe in children with corticosteroid-dependent uveitis, allowing tapering of corticosteroid doses. Symptomatic treatment of oral ulcerations may include oral rinses with solutions containing tetracycline, topical anesthetics, and chlorhexidine gluconate.

COMPLICATIONS AND PROGNOSIS

Behçet disease has a variable clinical course with exacerbations and remissions, with the serious complications occurring many years after diagnosis. Blindness may result from posterior uveitis. Gastrointestinal lesions resembling orogenital aphthae occur most commonly in the ileocecal region and rarely lead to perforation. Central nervous system complications include venous sinus thrombosis and parenchymal involvement. Mortality is low and is usually attributable to bowel perforation, thrombosis, or central nervous system involvement.

BIBLIOGRAPHY

Please visit the Nelson Textbook of Pediatrics *website at www.expertconsult.com for the complete bibliography.*

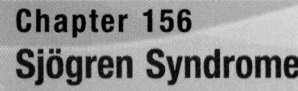

Chapter 156
Sjögren Syndrome

Abraham Gedalia

Sjögren syndrome is a chronic, inflammatory, autoimmune disease characterized by progressive lymphocytic and plasma cell infiltration of the salivary and lacrimal glands. It is rare in children and predominantly affects middle-aged women.

For the full continuation of this chapter, please visit the Nelson Textbook of Pediatrics *website at* *www.expertconsult.com.*

Chapter 157
Hereditary Periodic Fever Syndromes

Abraham Gedalia

Hereditary periodic fever syndromes are a group of **autoinflammatory diseases** caused by an inborn error in the **innate immune system.** They are characterized by recurrent short episodes of fever that are self-limited and occur in the absence of infection or autoimmune reaction, such as high titer autoantibodies or autoreactive T cells. The innate immune system provides the first immunologic line of defense against many microbes and uses **pattern recognition receptors (PRRs)** such as **Toll-like receptors (TLRs)** to recognize a limited number of widely expressed viral and bacterial molecular structures known as **pathogen-associated molecular patterns (PAMPs)**. These pattern recognition receptors stimulate inflammation by activating intracellular proteins (also known as intracellular sensors), which mediate the regulation of nuclear factor-κB (NF-κB), cell apoptosis, and interleukin-1β (IL-1β) through cross-regulated and common signaling pathways. Mutations in these intracellular proteins lead to increased production and secretion of IL-1β, resulting in clinical signs and symptoms.

The most common hereditary periodic fever disorders are familial Mediterranean fever (FMF), tumor necrosis factor (TNF) receptor–associated periodic syndrome (TRAPS), and hyperimmunoglobulinemia D syndrome (HIDS) (Table 157-1). The cryopyrin-associated periodic syndromes (CAPS) include Muckle-Wells syndrome (MWS), familial cold autoinflammatory syndrome (FCAS) (also known as familial cold urticaria [FCU]), and chronic infantile neurologic cutaneous and articular (CINCA) disease (also known as neonatal-onset multisystem inflammatory disease [NOMID]). A syndrome called pyogenic arthritis, pyoderma gangrenosum, and acne (PAPA) and Blau syndrome (known also as familial juvenile systemic granulomatosis) have now been added to this group. Secondary amyloidosis (AA amyloidosis) is a complication in all of these periodic fever disorders, although it is less commonly reported with HIDS. FMF and HIDS are autosomal recessive diseases, whereas TRAPS, PAPA, and Blau syndrome are autosomal dominant conditions. The diagnosis of each of these entities depends on the clinical features and the genetic confirmation (see Table 157-1). Another periodic fever syndrome is periodic fever, aphthous stomatitis, pharyngitis, and cervical adenitis (PFAPA), but it is not clear yet whether PFAPA is an autoinflammatory syndrome (see Table 157-1). Among the conditions that are not in the category of periodic fever and that have been classified as autoinflammatory diseases are Crohn disease, Behçet diseases, early-onset childhood sarcoidosis, systemic juvenile idiopathic arthritis (JIA), and chronic recurrent multifocal osteomyelitis (known also as Majeed syndrome) (Table 157-2).

Table 157-1 SUMMARY OF CLINICAL FINDINGS ASSOCIATED WITH HEREDITARY PERIODIC FEVERS

CLINICAL MANIFESTATIONS	FMF	FCAS	MWS	CINCA/NOMID	TRAPS	HIDS
Duration of attacks	12-72 hr	Minutes-24 hr	1-3 days	Continuous	Often >7 days	3-7 days
Cutaneous manifestations	Erysipeloid erythema	Cold-induced urticaria-like rash	Urticaria-like rash	Urticaria-like rash	Migratory macular rash, underlying myalgia	Nonmigratory maculopapular rash on trunk, limbs, urticaria
Abdominal manifestations	Peritonitis, constipation > diarrhea	Nausea	Sometimes abdominal pain	Uncommon	Peritonitis, diarrhea, or constipation	Severe pain, vomiting, diarrhea > constipation, rarely peritonitis
Pleural, pericardial manifestations	Frequent pleurisy	Not seen	Rare	Rare	Pleurisy, pericarditis	Rare
Arthritis	Monoarthritis, occasionally protracted in the knee or hip	Polyarthralgia	Polyarthralgia, oligoarthritis, large joints	Epiphyseal overgrowth, contractures, intermittent or chronic arthritis	Arthralgia monoarthritis or pauci arthritis in large joints	Systemic polyarthritis, arthralgia
Ocular manifestations	Rare	Conjunctivitis	Conjunctivitis, episcleritis	Conjunctivitis uveitis, vision loss	Conjunctivitis, periorbital edema	Rare
Neurologic manifestations	Headache, aseptic meningitis	Headache	Sensorineural deafness	Headache, deafness, aseptic meningitis, mental retardation	Rare	Headache
Lymph/spleen	Splenomegaly > lymphadenopathy	Not seen	Rare	Adenopathy, hepatosplenomegaly	Splenomegaly > lymphadenopathy	Cervical adenopathy
Vasculitis	Henoch-Schönlein purpura, polyarteritis nodosa	Not seen	Not seen	Occasional	Henoch-Schönlein purpura, lymphocytic vasculitis	Cutaneous vasculitis, rarely HSP
Amyloidosis	Variable risk depending on *MEFV, SAA* genotypes, family history, gender, compliance with treatment	Rare	Occurs in ~25%	May develop in a portion of patients reaching adulthood	Occurs in ≈10%	Rare
Protein	Pyrin	Cryopyrin	Cryopyrin	Cryopyrin	Tumor necrosis factor receptor 1a	Mevalonate kinase
Inheritance	Autosomal recessive	Autosomal dominant	Autosomal dominant	Autosomal dominant	Autosomal dominant	Autosomal recessive

CINCA/NOMID, chronic infantile neurologic cutaneous and articular syndrome, also called neonatal onset multisystem inflammatory disease; FCAS, familial cold autoinflammatory syndrome; FMF, familial Mediterranean fever; HIDS, hyperimmunoglobulinemia D with periodic fever syndrome; HSP, Henoch-Schönlein purpura; MWS, Muckle-Wells syndrome; TRAPS, tumor necrosis factor receptor–associated periodic syndrome.
Modified from Cassidy JT, Petty RE: *Textbook of pediatric rheumatology*, ed 5, Philadelphia, 2005, Elsevier/Saunders.

Table 157-2 RECURRENT OR PERIODIC FEVER SYNDROMES IN CHILDREN

INFECTIOUS DISEASES
Brucellosis Rat-bite fever Relapsing fever
RHEUMATIC DISEASES
Juvenile idiopathic arthritis (systemic onset) Behçet disease Systemic lupus erythematosus Relapsing polychondritis Crohn disease
HEREDITARY AUTOINFLAMMATORY SYNDROMES
Familial Mediterranean fever (FMF) Cryopyrinopathies: Familial cold autoinflammatory syndrome (FCAS) Muckle-Wells syndrome (MWS) Chronic infantile neurologic cutaneous and articular (CINCA) syndrome, also called neonatal onset multisystem inflammatory disease (NOMID) Tumor necrosis factor receptor–associated periodic syndrome (TRAPS) Hyperimmunoglobulinemia D with periodic fever syndrome (HIDS)
CYCLIC HEMATOPOIESIS
Hereditary form Acquired form
IDIOPATHIC CONDITIONS
Periodic fever with aphthous stomatitis, pharyngitis, and adenitis (PFAPA)

From Cassidy JT, Petty RE: *Textbook of pediatric rheumatology*, ed 5, Philadelphia, 2005, Elsevier/Saunders.

FAMILIAL MEDITERRANEAN FEVER

FMF is an autosomal recessive disorder characterized by brief, acute, self-limited episodes of fever and polyserositis that recur at irregular intervals and are associated with development of AA amyloidosis (Chapter 158).

Etiology

The gene responsible for FMF is mapped to a small interval on the short arm of chromosome 16p13.3. It is designated *MEFV* (*ME* for Mediterranean and *FV* for fever) and is a member of the *RoRet* gene family. It has 10 exons that express a 15-kb transcript encoding a 781–amino acid protein known as **pyrin** (from *pyrus*, the Greek word for "fever"), or **marenostrin** (Latin word for "our sea"), which is expressed in myeloid cells. Exon 10 and exon 2 carry most FMF-associated mutations. To date, more than 70 mutations have been discovered, mostly missense mutations. It is unclear whether all are truly disease-related mutations. The 5 most common mutations (M694V, V726A, M694I, M680I, E148Q) are found in more than two thirds of Mediterranean patients with FMF. Haplotypes and mutational analyses show ancestral relationships among carrier chromosomes that have been separated for centuries.

Approximately 70% of patients with clinical manifestations of FMF are heterozygous and have one of the two mutations that are identifiable by genetic analysis. The most common missense mutation is M694V (substitution of methionine with valine at codon 694), which occurs in 20-67% of cases and is associated with full penetrance. Homozygosity for M694V is associated with a greater disease severity and a higher incidence of amyloidosis. It is also associated with increased risk for onset at an early age. The V726A mutation occurs in 7-35% of cases and is associated with milder disease and a lower incidence of amyloidosis. The E148Q mutation is associated with low penetrance and very mild phenotype. These findings suggest that phenotypic differences may reflect different mutations. As with other recessive diseases, it is likely that some heterozygous patients may show attenuated clinical symptoms, with or without increased levels of acute phase reactants.

Epidemiology

FMF occurs primarily among ethnic groups of Mediterranean origin, mainly Sephardic Jews, Turks, Armenians, and individuals of Arab descent. In these populations, the carrier frequency is estimated to be as high as 1 in 5 persons, suggesting a carrier advantage for heterozygotes. Greeks, Hispanics, and Italians are less commonly affected. In addition, cases of FMF are found among non-Mediterranean persons. It is seen rarely among Ashkenazi Jews, Germans, and Anglo-Saxons.

Pathogenesis

The exact pathogenesis of the acute episodes of FMF is unknown. Between episodes, patients with FMF have increased serum levels of interferon-γ and enhanced production of other proinflammatory cytokines, such as TNF-α, IL-1β, IL-6, and IL-8, in circulating leukocytes. Pyrin/marenostrin is a member of the death domain superfamily and consists of 4 different functional domains that interact with other proteins. Of particular interest is the domain known as the **pyrin domain (PYD)**, a 92–amino acid N-terminal domain shared by several proteins that are involved in the regulation of the inflammatory response and apoptosis. Pyrin acts as an anti-inflammatory factor by inhibiting processing of pro–IL-1β cytokine to the active form. This inhibition normally takes place through interactions with a caspase recruitment domain (ASC) and NF-κB. It has been suggested that normally pyrin inhibits the binding of ASC to caspase-1 in a competitive manner. The C-terminal domain of the pyrin molecule interacts with caspase-1, leading to inhibition of IL-1β production. It is speculated that the defective (or mutated) pyrin found in patients with FMF is functionally inactive, allowing binding of ASC to caspase-1 to take place. As a consequence, stimulation of IL-1β processing and secretion occur, resulting in increased IL-1β levels that are responsible for the uncontrolled inflammation (Fig. 157-1). Another possibility that was previously more popular is based on the finding of C5a inhibitor (inactivating enzyme) deficiency in peritoneal and synovial fluids of patients with FMF. C5a is a fragment of complement, an anaphylatoxin, and a potent chemotactic agent (Chapter 127). Normally, C5a inhibitor neutralizes the small amounts of C5a released into serosal cavities before they precipitate overt inflammation. The hypothesis is that a deficiency of C5a inhibitor, which is a consequence of pyrin/marenostrin dysfunction in patients with FMF, allows further accumulation of C5a, leading to the acute attack. Further understanding of pyrin/marenostrin functions will shed light on aspects of FMF pathogenesis that are not yet fully understood.

Clinical Manifestations

The onset of clinical manifestations occurs before 5 yr of age in 65% of cases and before 20 yr of age in 90% of cases. Onset may be as early as 6 mo of age. Exercise, emotional stress, infection, menses, and surgery may precipitate acute episodes. The typical acute episode lasts 1-4 days and includes fever and 1 or more symptoms of sterile peritonitis, manifested as abdominal pain (90%), arthritis or arthralgia (85%), or pleuritis manifested by chest pain (20%). Other serosal tissues, such as the pericardium and tunica vaginalis testis (acute scrotum), are rarely affected. Some patients experience prolonged and protracted episodes of fever and myalgia in upper and lower extremities that may last up to 6 wk. Erysipelas-like rash, myalgia, splenomegaly, scrotal involvement in boys, neurologic involvement, Henoch-Schönlein purpura, and hypothyroidism are other, less common clinical manifestations.

Diagnosis

Genetic testing for the FMF gene confirms the diagnosis of FMF, which is especially important in areas where the disease is rare and less familiar to physicians. Genetic screening using polymerase chain reaction (PCR) and restriction analysis is available in some commercial clinical genetics laboratories. However,

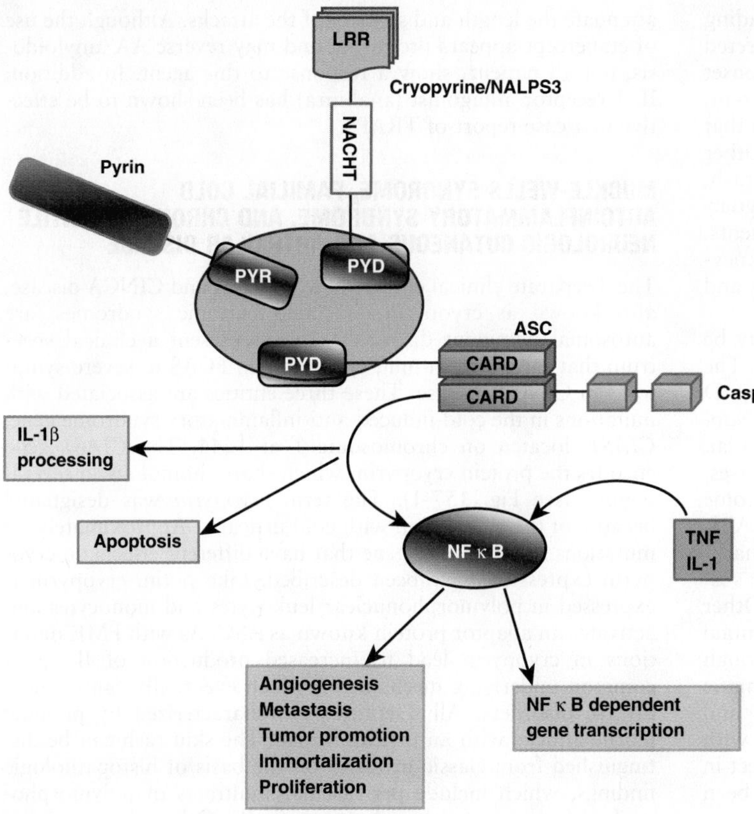

Figure 157-1 Proteins containing pyrin domain (PYD) regulate inflammation through their interaction with apoptotic speck protein (ASC). The assembly of cryopyrin and ASC induces interleukin-1 (IL-1) processing through caspase-1, whereas pyrin may act as an inhibitor. Loss of function by mutations in the pyrin could potentially lead to autoinflammation by reducing the pyrin inhibitory role. Alternatively, gain-of-function mutations in cryopyrin, as found in patients with Muckle-Wells syndrome/familial cold urticaria/neonatal-onset multisystem inflammatory disease, could activate this pathway. ASC participates in apoptosis and activation of nuclear factor–κB (NF-κB), a transcription factor involved in both initiation and resolution of the inflammatory response. LRR, leucine-rich repeat(s); TNF, tumor necrosis factor. (From Padeh S: Periodic fever syndromes, *Pediatr Clin North Am* 52:577–609, 2005.)

genetics laboratories usually screen for only the 10 to 15 most common mutations, and thus, rare mutations will be missed. Therefore, the diagnosis of FMF is still based on clinical manifestations, with genetic testing used as a confirmatory test.

Treatment

Attacks of FMF can be prevented by prophylactic colchicine (0.02-0.03 mg/kg/day; maximum 2 mg/day) in 1 to 2 divided doses. In general, the initial dose should be 0.5 mg/day for children <5 yr of age, 1 mg/day for children 5-10 yr, and 1.5 mg/day for those >10 yr. Approximately 65% of patients experience remission of attacks, 20-30% experience improvement with significant reduction in the number and severity of the episodes, and 5-10% show no response. Colchicine therapy reduces the frequency of acute attacks and also greatly decreases the probability of development of amyloidosis; it may produce partial regression of existing amyloidosis. Poor compliance is common, owing to gastrointestinal side effects and may contribute to treatment failure. Toxic effects (acute myopathy and bone marrow hypoplasia) can be seen with doses >0.1 mg/kg, resulting in lethality at a dose ≥0.8 mg/kg. Colchicine therapy for FMF during pregnancy has not been reported to harm either the mother or her fetus. Prolonged colchicine use seems to have no effects on male or female fertility, pregnancy, fetal development, or development after birth. It has also been shown that biologic treatments, especially the IL-1 inhibitor anakinra, produce a beneficial response in cases of FMF that do not respond to colchicine.

Complications and Prognosis

In 30-50% of untreated children and in 75% of adults with FMF, a form of renal amyloidosis develops in which the amyloid derives from a normal serum protein and an acute-phase reactant, serum amyloid A (SAA), resulting in **AA amyloidosis.** Renal disease manifests as proteinuria that progresses to nephrotic syndrome and renal failure over a period of months to several years. Transplantation may be required for renal failure. Amyloidosis is common among Sephardic Jews and Turks and less common in Armenians. Homozygosity for M694V is associated with a greater disease severity and a higher incidence of amyloidosis. Armenians living in Armenia are reported to have a significantly higher incidence of amyloidosis than their counterparts in North America, suggesting that environmental factors may also play a role. The country of residence rather than the *MEFV* genotype has been playing the major role in the development of amyloidosis. Mortality from FMF usually results from complications of renal failure and amyloidosis, such as infection, thromboembolism, and uremia. Other rare complications are joint contractures, abdominal adhesions, and impairment in social development, although patients are capable of physical activity with some limitations due to their illness.

HYPERIMMUNOGLOBULINEMIA D SYNDROME

HIDS, known also as Dutch fever, is an inherited periodic fever syndrome with an autosomal recessive mode of transmission. This condition is reported primarily among families of European descent, especially Dutch and French, and is caused by mutations in the mevalonate kinase *(MVK)* gene found on chromosome 12 at 12q24. Mevalonate kinase is an enzyme that enhances the metabolism of mevalonic acid, an intermediary product of cholesterol and isoprenoid synthesis pathways (Chapter 80). Cells from patients with HIDS still contain residual *MVK* enzyme activity (1-8%). A complete deficiency of this enzyme causes a distinct disorder known as mevalonic aciduria, which is associated with severe mental retardation, ataxia, myopathy, cataracts, and failure to thrive. In these patients, *MVK* enzyme activity is below the detection level. It is speculated that shortage of isoprenoid end products contributes to increased secretion of IL-1β, which subsequently leads to overt inflammation and fever.

More than 100 different mutations in the *MVK* gene have been reported so far. Some variants are strongly associated with a severe mevalonic aciduria phenotype. The most common mutation is V377I, likely of Dutch origin, which is exclusively associated with a mild phenotype. These mutations are associated with decreased activity of mevalonate kinase in lymphocytes, leading to increased plasma levels of mevalonic acid, which is excreted in large amounts in the urine. The majority of patients have onset within the 1st yr of life. The manifestations include recurrent, short episodes of fever lasting 3-7 days, with abdominal pain that is often accompanied by diarrhea, nausea, and vomiting. Other clinical manifestations include cervical lymphadenopathy, rash, aphthous ulcers, symmetric polyarthritis/arthralgia or oligoarthralgia/arthritis, and occasional splenomegaly. In some patients, the attacks may last several weeks. During the attacks, leukocytosis and increased serum levels of acute-phase reactants and proinflammatory cytokines are commonly present.

HIDS is a difficult diagnosis to make, and diagnosis may be delayed by as long as 10 yr from the onset of symptoms. The finding of elevated serum values of immunoglobulin (Ig) D (>100 mU/mL) is present in ≈80% of patients and strongly supports the diagnosis of HIDS, but it is not diagnostic. In particular, IgD levels may be increased in other autoinflammatory diseases. The symptoms of HIDS may persist for years but tend to become less prominent with time. Unlike in patients with FMF or TRAPS, the incidence of AA amyloidosis in patients with HIDS is remarkably low (3 out of 103 in an international study). The low susceptibility to amyloidosis in HIDS is not fully understood. Other rare complications include joint contractures and abdominal adhesions. There is no known therapy for this condition, although treatment with glucocorticoids may be associated with dramatic or partial relief. Antagonists of IL-1 receptor (anakinra) and TNF-α (etanercept) are effective in case reports of patients with HIDS. A trial of simvastatin showed a beneficial clinical effect in 5 of 6 patients with HIDS. Bone marrow transplantation has been effective in one reported patient.

TUMOR NECROSIS FACTOR RECEPTOR–ASSOCIATED PERIODIC SYNDROME

TRAPS is an autosomal-dominant periodic fever syndrome caused by mutation of the soluble TNF receptor superfamily 1A gene, *TNFRSF1A*. This syndrome was previously known by other names, including **familial Hibernian fever, familial periodic fever,** and **autosomal dominant recurrent fever.** TRAPS is a rare disorder that was initially reported in a few families of Irish and Scottish ancestry, although other ethnic groups, including African-Americans, Japanese, Puerto Rican, and Finnish, may be affected. The *TNFRSF1A* gene is on chromosome 12 at 12p13 and encodes the type 1A TNF receptor protein (TNFR1). In TRAPS a mutation in the *TNFRSF1A* gene leads to a defective TNFR1 molecule on the cell surface that is unable to neutralize TNF-α. More than 50 different disease-associated mutations in *TNFRSF1A* have been reported. Phenotype-genotype correlations have demonstrated that mutations at cysteine residues have a higher penetrance and are associated with a severe disease course and an increased risk of secondary AA amyloidosis.

Patients with TRAPS usually have brief, intermittent febrile episodes, typically lasting 4-6 days and associated with severe abdominal pain, nausea, and vomiting. Oligoarthritis, myalgias, rash, conjunctivitis, and unilateral periorbital edema are universally present in patients with TRAPS (Fig. 157-2). Arthralgias are less common. The acute attacks of TRAPS are slightly longer than the episodes of FMF and may persist for up to 3 wk. AA amyloidosis develops in up to 25% of patients with TRAPS, depending on the specific gene mutation and the duration of attacks. Amyloidosis may affect various organs but commonly involves the kidneys and liver, leading to renal and/or hepatic failure. Increased levels of acute-phase reactants may be seen, with the most specific findings being low serum levels of soluble type 1A TNF receptor and increased serum levels of TNF.

Colchicine has no effect on the acute attacks or on the development of amyloidosis in patients with TRAPS. Prednisone (1 mg/kg; maximum dose 20 mg) may be helpful and can attenuate the length and severity of the attacks. Although the use of etanercept appears promising and may reverse AA amyloidosis, not all patients show a response to this agent. In addition, IL-1 receptor antagonist (anakinra) has been shown to be effective in a case report of TRAPS.

MUCKLE-WELLS SYNDROME, FAMILIAL COLD AUTOINFLAMMATORY SYNDROME, AND CHRONIC INFANTILE NEUROLOGIC CUTANEOUS AND ARTICULAR DISEASE

The 3 separate clinical entities NWS, FCAS, and CINCA disease, also known as cryopyrin-associated periodic syndromes, are autosomal dominant disorders. They represent a clinical spectrum that ranges from mild symptoms in FCAS to severe symptoms in CINCA disease. These three entities are associated with mutations in the cold-induced anti-inflammatory syndrome gene, *CIAS1,* located on chromosome 1 at 1q44. The *CIAS1* gene encodes the protein **cryopyrin,** which shares homology in several regions (see Fig. 157-1). The term *cryopyrin* was designated because of the association with cold urticaria. Approximately 50 mutations in the *CIAS1* gene that have different effects on cryopyrin expression have been described. Like pyrin, cryopyrin is expressed in polymorphonuclear leukocytes and monocytes and activates an adaptor protein known as ASC. As with FMF, mutations in cryopyrin lead to increased production of IL-1β (a common underlying mechanism), which eventually causes these diverse disorders. All 3 entities are characterized by periodic febrile attacks with an urticarial rash. The skin rash can be distinguished from classic urticaria on the basis of histopathologic findings, which include perivascular infiltrates of polymorphonuclear leucocytes rather than mast cells. Other characteristics include arthralgia and arthritis, ocular involvement, and the development of AA amyloidosis. In FCAS, autoinflammatory attacks start within 8 hours of generalized cold exposure. Typically, localized cold exposure does not trigger the episodes. The joint symptoms consist of polyarthralgias (hands, knees, and ankles) in more than 90% of patients. Both MWS and CINCA disease are typically associated with progressive sensorineural hearing loss, optic nerve involvement, and chronic aseptic meningitis. CINCA disease is a more severe entity, typically having a neonatal onset and being associated with dysmorphic features, rash, neurologic disease with mental retardation, and destructive arthropathy, mainly of the knees, which may lead to major malformation and disability (Fig. 157-3). No definitive therapy exists for these conditions, although treatment with colchicine, nonsteroidal anti-inflammatory drugs (NSAIDs), and glucocorticoids may provide some relief. Remarkable responses to anakinra (IL-1 receptor antagonist) in 3 family members with MWS and 18 patients with CINCA disease have been reported. Anakinra seems to improve visual and hearing impairment and in some cases induces amelioration of amyloidosis within 6 mo of treatment. Treatment with rilonacept, an IL-1 trap given by weekly subcutaneous injections, can markedly reduce symptoms and inflammatory markers. In addition, canakinumab, an anti-interleukin-1β monoclonal antibody, has demonstrated efficacy in cryopyrin associated periodic fever syndromes.

Deficiency of the interleukin-1 receptor antagonist produces an autoinflammatory syndrome characterized by inflammation and a pustulosis rash, sterile multifocal osteomyelitis, widened ribs, periosteal elevation, osteopenia, and onset before 1 yr of age. Anakinra is the treatment of choice.

PYOGENIC ARTHRITIS, PYODERMA GANGRENOSUM, AND ACNE AND BLAU SYNDROME

Further understanding of pyrin functions, especially the interactions with other proteins, has led to the discovery of two other entities, PAPA and Blau syndromes. PAPA syndrome is an autosomal dominant disorder with mutations in the gene encoding

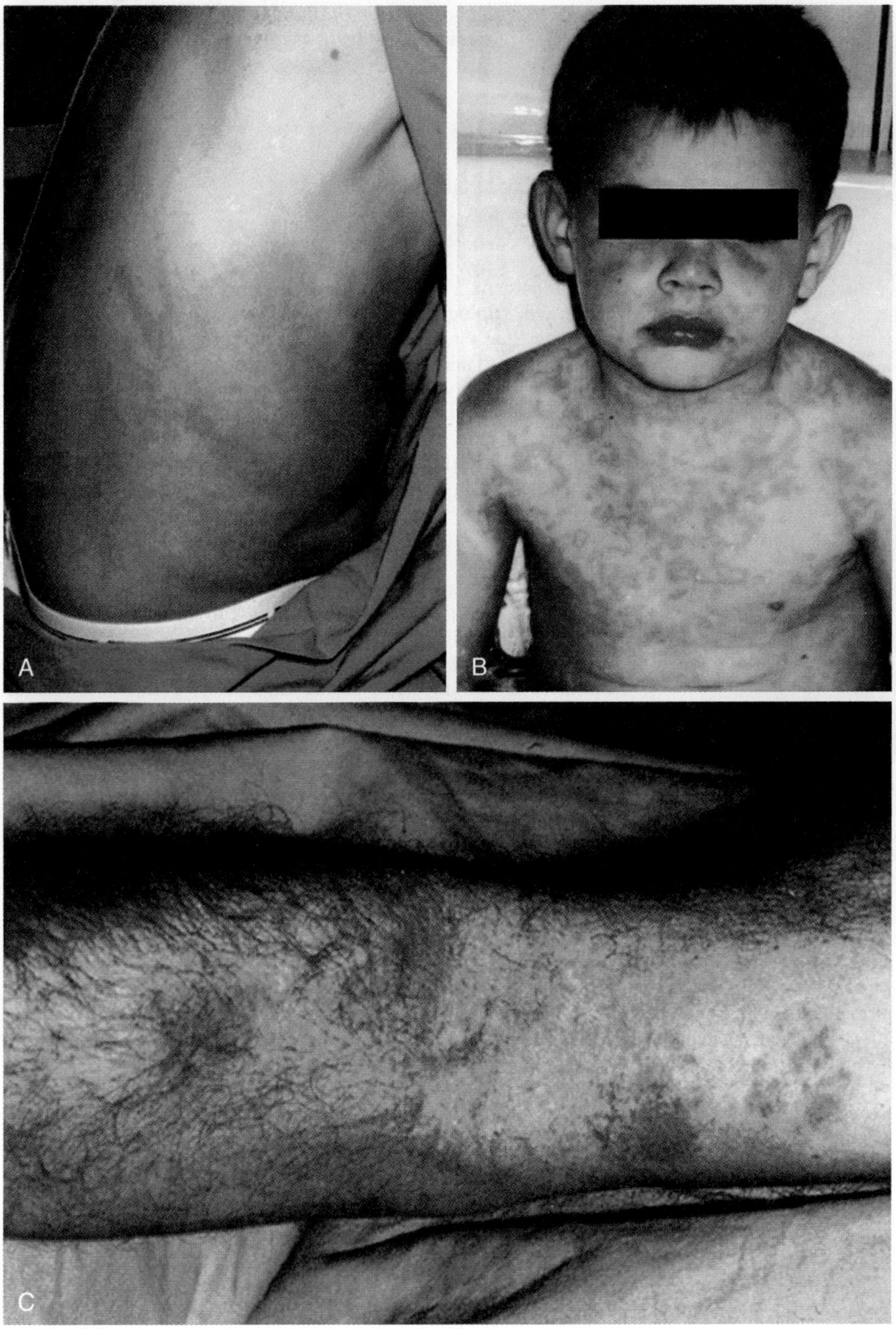

Figure 157-2 Cutaneous manifestations of tumor necrosis factor receptor–associated periodic syndrome. *A,* Right flank of a patient with the T50M mutation. *B,* Serpiginous rash involving the face, neck, torso, and upper extremities of a child with the C30S mutation. *C,* Erythematous, macular patches with crusting on the flexor surface of the right arm of a patient with the T50M mutation.

the adaptor protein proline serine threonine phosphatase–interacting protein (PSTPIP1) located on chromosome 15 at 15q24. Pyoderma gangrenosum and severe cystic acne associated with skin ulcerations are usually seen on the extremities and are triggered by trauma. Typically, the arthritis is sterile and the synovial fluid is rich in neutrophils. **Blau syndrome** is a rare autosomal dominant disorder that manifests as early-onset granulomatous arthritis, uveitis, rash, and flexion contractures at the fingers associated with mutations in the gene encoding CARD15 (caspase recruitment domain 15 protein), also known as NOD2 (nucleotide-binding oligomerization domain 2 protein), located on chromosome 16 at 16q12. Although fever is not a major symptom in PAPA and Blau syndromes, these conditions represent additional rare members of the hereditary periodic fever syndromes family.

PERIODIC FEVER, APHTHOUS STOMATITIS, PHARYNGITIS, AND ADENITIS

Another distinct periodic fever syndrome, PFAPA, also known as **Marshall syndrome,** manifests as episodes of periodic fever, aphthous stomatitis, pharyngitis, and adenitis. PFAPA occurs sporadically and has no ethnic predilection. Symptoms begin around 2-5 yr of age and include recurring fever, malaise, exudative-appearing tonsillitis with negative throat culture results, cervical lymphadenopathy, oral aphthae ulceration, and, less commonly, headache, abdominal pain, and arthralgia. The episodes last 4-6 days, regardless of antipyretic or antibiotic treatment, and occur at a frequency of 8-12 episodes/yr. Findings during the episodes may include mild hepatosplenomegaly, mild

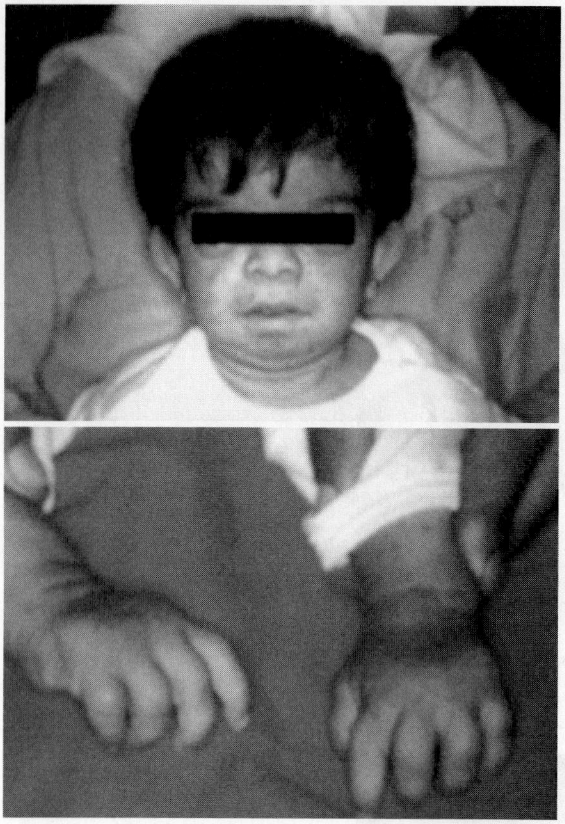

Figure 157-3 A 3 yr old girl with neonatal-onset multisystem inflammatory disease (NOMID)/chronic infantile neurologic cutaneous and articular (CINCA) disease. Note the markedly deformed hands, rash, frontal bossing, and large head. (From Padeh S: Periodic fever syndromes, *Pediatr Clin North Am* 52:577–560, 2005.)

leukocytosis, and elevated acute-phase reactants. Both the frequency and intensity of the episodes diminish over time.

The etiology and the pathogenesis of PFAPA remain unknown. It is not clear whether this syndrome represents an infectious or immunogenetic dysregulation entity. Clinical experience suggests that NSAIDs and antipyretics such as acetaminophen are ineffective in controlling the clinical manifestations of PFAPA. The majority of patients show dramatic response to a single dose of prednisone (1-2 mg/kg) or betamethasone (0.3 mg/kg) with prompt resolution of symptoms within 24 hr. In addition, cimetidine in 3-4 divided doses of 20 mg to 40 mg/kg/day has been reported to be effective in inducing sustained remission after 6 mo of therapy. Complete resolution has also been reported after tonsillectomy in some but not all patients with this disorder. Affected children grow normally and have spontaneous resolution within 4-8 yr with no long-term sequelae. One patient with PFAPA demonstrated TRAPS at age 22 yr.

BIBLIOGRAPHY

Please visit the Nelson Textbook of Pediatrics *website at www.expertconsult.com for the complete bibliography.*

Chapter 158
Amyloidosis
Abraham Gedalia

Amyloidosis comprises a group of diseases characterized by extracellular deposition of insoluble, fibrous amyloid proteins in various body tissues.

For the full continuation of this chapter, please visit the Nelson Textbook of Pediatrics *website at www.expertconsult.com.*

Chapter 159
Sarcoidosis
Eveline Y. Wu and Esi Morgan DeWitt

Sarcoidosis is a rare multisystem granulomatous disease of unknown etiology. The name is derived from a Greek word meaning "fleshlike condition," in reference to the characteristic skin lesions. There appears to be 2 distinct patterns of disease among children with sarcoidosis. The clinical features in older children are similar to those in adults, with frequent pulmonary involvement and lymphadenopathy. In contrast, early-onset sarcoidosis manifesting in children <4 yr of age is characterized by the triad of rash, uveitis, and arthritis.

ETIOLOGY

The etiology of sarcoidosis remains obscure but is likely the result of exposure of a genetically susceptible individual to one or more unidentified antigens. This exposure initiates an exaggerated immune response that ultimately leads to the formation of granulomas. The human major histocompatibility complex is located on chromosome 6, and specific human leukocyte antigen class I and class II alleles are associated with disease phenotype. Genetic polymorphisms involving various cytokines and chemokines may also have a role in development of sarcoidosis. Familial clustering supports the contribution of genetic factors to sarcoidosis susceptibility. Environmental and occupational exposures are also associated with disease risk. There are positive associations between sarcoidosis and agricultural employment, occupational exposure to insecticides, and moldy environments typically associated with microbial bioaerosols.

An autosomal dominant familial form of the disease typified by early onset of skin, eye, and joint involvement is described as **Blau syndrome**. Mutations in the *CARD15/NOD2* gene on chromosome 16 have been found in affected family members and appear to be associated with development of sarcoidosis. Similar genetic mutations also have been found in individuals with early-onset sarcoidosis (rash, uveitis, arthritis) but without a family history of disease, suggesting that this nonfamilial disease and Blau syndrome are genetically and phenotypically identical (Chapter 157).

EPIDEMIOLOGY

Sarcoidosis is rare in childhood, and thus the incidence and prevalence are difficult to determine. A nationwide patient registry of childhood sarcoidosis in Denmark estimated the annual incidence to be 0.22 to 0.27 per 100,000 children. The incidence increases with age, and peak onset occurs at 20-39 yr. The most common age of reported childhood cases is 13-15 yr. Annual incidence is about 11/100,000 in adult white Americans and is three times higher in African Americans. There is no clear sex predominance. Within the USA, the majority of childhood sarcoidosis cases are reported in the Southeastern and South Central states.

PATHOLOGY AND PATHOGENESIS

Noncaseating, epithelioid granulomatous lesions are a cardinal feature of sarcoidosis. Activated macrophages, epithelioid cells, and multinucleated giant cells as well as CD4+ T lymphocytes accumulate and become tightly packed in the center of the granuloma. The causative agent that initiates this inflammatory process is not known. The periphery of the granuloma contains a loose collection of monocytes, CD4+ and CD8+ T lymphocytes, and fibroblasts. The interaction between the macrophages and CD4+ T lymphocytes is important in the formation and maintenance of the granuloma. The activated macrophages secrete high levels of tumor necrosis factor-α (TNF-α) and other proinflammatory mediators. The CD4+ T lymphocytes differentiate into type 1 helper T cells and release interleukin-2 (IL-2) and interferon-γ (IFN-γ), promoting proliferation of lymphocytes. Granulomas may heal or resolve with complete preservation of the parenchyma. In approximately 20% of the lesions, the fibroblasts in the periphery proliferate and produce fibrotic scar tissue, leading to significant and irreversible organ dysfunction.

The sarcoid macrophage is able to produce and secrete 1,25-$(OH)_2$-vitamin D or calcitriol, an active form of vitamin D typically produced in the kidneys. The hormone's natural functions are to increase intestinal absorption of calcium and bone resorption and to decrease renal excretion of calcium and phosphate. An excess in vitamin D may result in hypercalcemia and hypercalciuria in patients with sarcoidosis.

CLINICAL MANIFESTATIONS

Sarcoidosis is a multisystem disease, and granulomatous lesions may occur in any organ of the body. The clinical manifestations depend on the extent and degree of granulomatous inflammation and are extremely variable. Children may present with nonspecific symptoms, such as fever, weight loss, and general malaise. In adults and older children, pulmonary involvement is most frequent, with infiltration of the thoracic lymph nodes and lung parenchyma. Isolated bilateral hilar adenopathy on chest radiograph is the most common finding, but parenchymal infiltrates and miliary nodules may also be seen (Fig. 159-1). Patients with lung involvement are commonly found to have restrictive changes on pulmonary function testing. Symptoms of pulmonary disease are seldom severe and generally consist of a dry, persistent cough.

Extrathoracic lymphadenopathy and infiltration of the liver, spleen, and bone marrow also occur often. Infiltration of the liver and spleen typically leads to isolated hepatomegaly and splenomegaly, respectively, but actual organ dysfunction is rare.

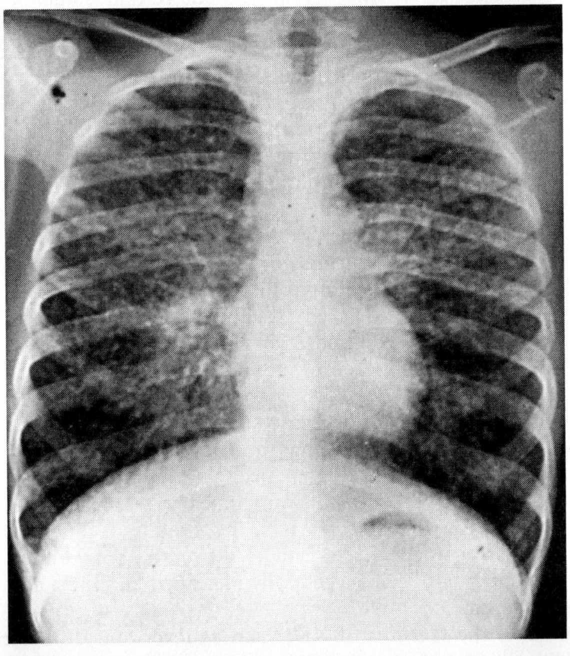

Figure 159-1 Chest radiograph of a 10 yr old girl with sarcoidosis showing widely disseminated peribronchial infiltrates, multiple small nodular densities, hyperaeration of the lungs, and hilar lymphadenopathy.

Cutaneous disease, such as plaques, nodules, erythema nodosum in acute disease, or lupus pernio in chronic sarcoidosis, appears in one quarter of cases and is usually present at onset. Red-brown to purple maculopapular lesions <1 cm on the face, neck, upper back, and extremities are the most common skin finding (Fig. 159-2). Ocular involvement is frequent and has variable manifestations, including anterior or posterior uveitis, conjunctival granulomas, eyelid inflammation, and orbital or lacrimal gland infiltration. The arthritis in sarcoidosis can be confused with juvenile rheumatoid arthritis. Central nervous system (CNS) involvement is rare in childhood but may manifest as seizures, cranial nerve involvement, intracranial mass lesions, and hypothalamic dysfunction. Kidney disease also occurs infrequently in children but typically manifests as renal insufficiency, proteinuria, transient pyuria, or microscopic hematuria as a result of either early monocellular infiltration or granuloma formation in kidney tissue. Only a small fraction of children have hypercalcemia or hypercalciuria, which is therefore an infrequent cause of kidney disease. Sarcoid granulomas can also infiltrate the heart and lead to cardiac arrhythmias and, rarely, sudden death. Other rare sites of disease involvement include blood vessels of any size, the gastrointestinal tract, muscles, bones, and testes.

In contrast to the variable clinical presentation of sarcoidosis in older children, early-onset sarcoidosis classically manifests as the triad uveitis, arthritis, and rash. Pulmonary disease and lymphadenopathy are less common. The arthritis is polyarticular and symmetric, with large boggy effusions. The rash is diffuse, erythematous, papular, and somewhat scaly. Noncaseating granulomas are demonstrated with biopsy of the skin or joint synovium.

LABORATORY FINDINGS

There is no single laboratory test diagnostic of sarcoidosis. Anemia, leukopenia, and eosinophilia may be seen. Other nonspecific findings include hypergammaglobulinemia and elevations in acute-phase reactants, including erythrocyte sedimentation rate and C-reactive protein value. Hypercalcemia and/or hypercalciuria occur in only a small proportion of children with sarcoidosis. Angiotensin-converting enzyme (ACE) is produced by the epithelioid cells of the granuloma, and its serum value may be elevated, but this finding lacks diagnostic sensitivity and specificity. In addition, ACE values may be difficult to interpret because reference values for serum ACE are age dependent. Fluorodeoxyglucose F18 positron emission tomography (^{18}FDG PET) can help identify nonpulmonary sites for a diagnostic biopsy.

DIAGNOSIS

Definitive diagnosis ultimately requires demonstration of the characteristic noncaseating granulomatous lesions in a biopsy

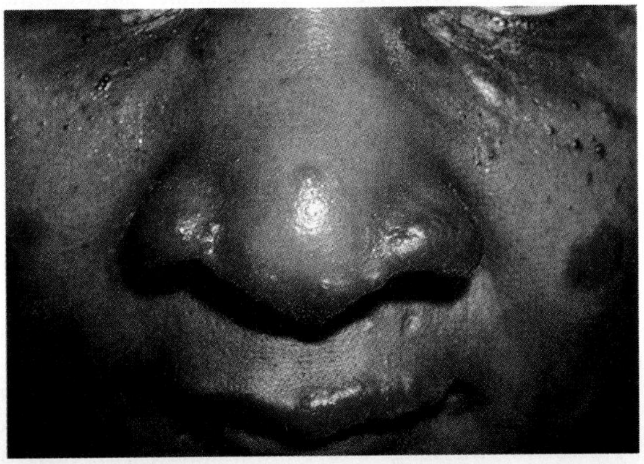

Figure 159-2 Sarcoidosis nodules on the face. (From Shah BR, Laude TA: *Atlas of pediatric clinical diagnosis,* Philadelphia, 2000, WB Saunders.)

specimen (usually taken from the most readily available affected organ) and exclusion of other known causes of granulomatous inflammation. Skin and transbronchial lung biopsies have higher yield, greater specificity, and fewer associated adverse events than biopsy of mediastinal lymph nodes or liver. Additional diagnostic testing should include chest radiography, pulmonary function testing with measurement of diffusion capacity, hepatic enzyme measurements, and renal function asssessment. Ophthalmologic slit-lamp examination is essential, as ocular findings are frequent in sarcoidosis and vision loss is a sequela of untreated disease.

Bronchoalveolar lavage may be used to assess for disease activity, and the fluid typically reveals an excess of lymphocytes with an increased CD4+:CD8+ ratio, 2:1- 13:1. The **Kveim-Siltzbach test** consists of an intradermal injection of homogenated human sarcoid tissue extract followed by observation for the formation of a granuloma several weeks later. This test is rarely used, owing to lack of available validated standardized test materials and safety concerns.

DIFFERENTIAL DIAGNOSIS

Because of its protean manifestations, the differential diagnosis of sarcoidosis is extremely broad and depends largely on the initial clinical manifestations. Granulomatous infections, including tuberculosis, cryptococcosis, pulmonary mycoses (histoplasmosis, blastomycosis, and coccidioidomycosis), brucellosis, tularemia, and toxoplasmosis, must be excluded. Other causes of granulomatous inflammation are Wegener granulomatosis, hypersensitivity pneumonia, chronic berylliosis, and other occupational exposures to metals. Combined variable immunodeficiency may also manifest as granulomatous lesions. Lymphoma should be ruled out in cases of hilar or other lymphadenopathy. Sarcoid arthritis may mimic juvenile rheumatoid arthritis. Evaluation for endocrine disorders is needed in the setting of hypercalcemia or hypercalciuria.

TREATMENT

There are no consensus guidelines for the treatment of childhood sarcoidosis. Treatment should be based on disease severity as well as the number and type of organs involved. Corticosteroids are the mainstay of treatment for most acute and chronic disease manifestations. The optimal dose and duration of corticosteroid therapy in children have not been established. Induction treatment typically begins with oral prednisone or prednisolone (1-2 mg/kg/day up to 40 mg daily) for 8-12 wk until manifestations improve. Corticosteroid dosage is then gradually decreased over 6-12 mo to the minimal effective dose that controls symptoms. Methotrexate may be effective as a corticosteroid-sparing agent. On the basis of the role of TNF-α in the formation of granulomas, there is rationale for use of TNF-α antagonists, and results of a small randomized trial in adults showed modest effect. Other therapeutics used for sarcoidosis manifestations include inhaled corticosteroids (lung), azathioprine (CNS), hydroxychloroquine (skin), thalidomide or its analogs (skin), topical corticosteroids (eye), and nonsteroidal anti-inflammatory drugs (NSAIDs).

PROGNOSIS

The prognosis of childhood sarcoidosis is not well defined. The disease may be self-limited with complete recovery or may persist with a progressive or relapsing course. Outcome is worse in the setting of multiorgan or CNS involvement. Most children requiring treatment experience considerable improvement with corticosteroids, though a significant number have morbid sequelae, mainly involving the lungs and eyes. Children with early-onset sarcoidosis have a poorer prognosis and generally experience a more chronic disease course. The greatest morbidity is associated with ocular involvement, including cataract formation, development of synechiae, and loss of visual acuity or blindness. Progressive polyarthritis may result in joint destruction. The overall mortality rate in childhood sarcoidosis is low.

Serial pulmonary function tests and chest radiographs are useful in following the course of lung involvement. Monitoring for other organ involvement should also include electrocardiogram with consideration of an echocardiogram, urinalysis, renal function tests, and measurements of hepatic enzymes and serum calcium. Other potential indicators of disease activity include inflammatory markers and serum ACE, although changes in ACE level do not always correlate with other indicators of disease status. Given the frequency of asymptomatic eye disease and the ocular morbidity associated with pediatric sarcoidosis, all patients should have an ophthalmologic examination at presentation with monitoring at regular intervals, perhaps every 3-6 mo as recommended in children with juvenile rheumatoid arthritis.

BIBLIOGRAPHY

Please visit the Nelson Textbook of Pediatrics *website at www.expertconsult.com for the complete bibliography.*

Chapter 160
Kawasaki Disease

Mary Beth F. Son and Jane W. Newburger

Kawasaki disease (KD), formerly known as **mucocutaneous lymph node syndrome** and **infantile polyarteritis nodosa,** is an acute febrile illness of childhood seen worldwide in all populations, with the highest incidence occurring in children of Asian background. KD is a vasculitis with a predilection for the coronary arteries, and approximately 20-25% of untreated patients experience coronary artery abnormalities, including aneurysms. KD is the leading cause of acquired heart disease in children in most developed countries, including the USA and Japan.

ETIOLOGY

The cause of KD remains unknown, but certain epidemiologic and clinical features support an infectious origin. These features include the young age group affected, epidemics with wavelike geographic spread of illness, the self-limited nature of the acute febrile illness, and the combination of clinical features fever, rash, enanthem, conjunctival injection, and cervical lymphadenopathy. Further evidence of an infectious trigger includes the infrequent occurrence of the illness in infants younger than 3 mo, likely the result of maternal antibodies, and the virtual absence of cases in adults, likely the result of prior exposures with subsequent immunity. Nonetheless, it is unusual to have multiple cases present at the same time within a family or daycare center. A genetic role in the pathogenesis of KD seems likely, as evidenced by the higher risk of KD in Asian children regardless of country of residence and in siblings and children of individuals with a history of KD. Furthermore, genome-wide association studies, including sibling pair analyses, have identified susceptibility loci.

A KD-associated antigen has been described in cytoplasmic inclusion bodies within ciliated bronchial epithelial cells from acute fatal cases. These inclusions appear consistent with viral protein aggregates and support the hypothesis of a respiratory portal of entry of the KD agent. However, no single infectious etiologic agent has been successfully identified, despite a comprehensive search.

Some of the features of KD, such as fever and diffuse rash, suggest superantigen activity, similar to that seen in toxin-mediated diseases like staphylococcal toxic shock syndrome. Studies of polyclonal activation of T cells, characteristic of superantigen-mediated processes, have yielded conflicting results in patients with KD. Similarly, the role of regulatory T cells, chemokines, and Toll-like receptors in KD has been studied, with inconclusive results. During the subacute phase of illness, levels of all immunoglobulins (Igs) are elevated, suggesting that a vigorous antibody response occurs. As in other forms of vasculitis, it is likely that a common environmental trigger leads to the phenotype of KD in genetically predisposed individuals.

EPIDEMIOLOGY

In 2000, the hospitalization rate for KD in the Kids Inpatient Database was reported to be 17.1/100,000 in children <5 yr of age. Asian and Pacific Islander children are at higher risk for KD; the same database yielded a hospitalization rate for KD of 39/100,000 children of Asian and Pacific Islander background, compared with 19.7/100,000 black, non-Hispanic children, 13.6/100,000 Hispanic children, and 11.4/100,000 white, non-Hispanic children. Between 2001 and 2006, the number of hospitalizations for KD in free-standing children's hospitals participating in the Pediatric Health Information System increased by more than 30%. In Japan, >200,000 cases of KD have been reported since the 1960s. KD is an illness of early childhood, as the median age of illness is 2-3 yr and 80% of children are <5 yr old. KD may occur in adolescents.

Several risk stratification models have been constructed to determine which patients with KD are at highest risk for coronary artery abnormalities. Predictors of poor outcome include young age, male gender, and laboratory abnormalities including neutrophilia, thrombocytopenia, hepatic transaminase elevation, hyponatremia, hypoalbuminemia, and elevated C-reactive protein levels. Asian and Pacific Islander race and Hispanic ethnicity are also risk factors for coronary artery abnormalities. Prolonged fever is associated with the development of coronary artery disease.

PATHOLOGY

KD is a vasculitis that predominantly affects the medium-sized arteries, with a striking predilection for the coronary arteries. Pathologic examination of fatal cases in the acute or subacute stages reveals edema of endothelial and smooth muscle cells with intense inflammatory infiltration of the vascular wall, initially by polymorphonuclear cells but rapidly thereafter by macrophages, lymphocytes (primarily CD8+ T cells), and plasma cells. IgA plasma cells are particularly prominent in the inflammatory infiltrate. In the most severely affected vessels, inflammation involves all three layers of the vascular wall, with destruction of the internal elastic lamina. Loss of structural integrity weakens the vessel wall and results in dilation (ectasia) or saccular or fusiform aneurysm formation. Thrombi may form in the lumen and obstruct blood flow. Over time, the vascular wall can become progressively fibrotic with marked intimal proliferation, producing arterial stenosis or occlusion.

CLINICAL MANIFESTATIONS

Fever is characteristically high (≥101°F), unremitting, and unresponsive to antibiotics. The duration of fever without treatment is generally 1-2 wk but may persist for 3-4 wk. In addition to fever, the **five principal clinical criteria** of KD are: bilateral nonexudative bulbar conjunctival injection with limbal sparing; erythema of the oral and pharyngeal mucosa with strawberry tongue and dry, cracked lips; edema and erythema of the hands and feet; rash of various forms (maculopapular, erythema multiforme, or scarlatiniform) with accentuation in the groin area; and nonsuppurative cervical lymphadenopathy, usually unilateral, with node size >1.5 cm (Table 160-1; Figs. 160-1 to 160-4). Perineal desquamation is common in the acute phase. Periungual desquamation of the fingers and toes begins 1-3 wk after the onset of illness and may progress to involve the entire hand and foot (Fig. 160-5).

Associated symptoms other than the clinical criteria are common in the 10 days prior to diagnosis of KD. Gastrointestinal symptoms (vomiting, diarrhea, or abdominal pain) occur in almost 65% of patients, and respiratory symptoms (interstitial infiltrates, effusions) occur in 30%. Other clinical findings include significant irritability that is especially prominent in infants and likely due to aseptic meningitis, mild hepatitis, hydrops of the gallbladder, urethritis and meatitis with sterile pyuria, and arthritis. Arthritis may occur early in the illness or may develop in the

Table 160-1 CLINICAL AND LABORATORY FEATURES OF KAWASAKI DISEASE

EPIDEMIOLOGIC CASE DEFINITION (CLASSIC CLINICAL CRITERIA)*
Fever persisting at least 5 days†
Presence of at least 4 principal features:
Changes in extremities:
Acute: Erythema of palms, soles; edema of hands, feet
Subacute: Periungual peeling of fingers, toes in weeks 2 and 3
Polymorphous exanthem
Bilateral bulbar conjunctival injection without exudate
Changes in lips and oral cavity: Erythema, lip cracking, strawberry tongue, diffuse injection of oral and pharyngeal mucosa
Cervical lymphadenopathy (>1.5 cm diameter), usually unilateral
Exclusion of other diseases with similar findings‡
OTHER CLINICAL AND LABORATORY FINDINGS
Cardiovascular findings:
Congestive heart failure, myocarditis, pericarditis, valvular regurgitation
Coronary artery abnormalities
Aneurysms of medium-sized noncoronary arteries
Raynaud phenomenon
Peripheral gangrene
Musculoskeletal system:
Arthritis, arthralgias
Gastrointestinal tract:
Diarrhea, vomiting, abdominal pain
Hepatic dysfunction
Hydrops of gallbladder
Central nervous system:
Extreme irritability
Aseptic meningitis
Sensorineural hearing loss
Genitourinary system:
Urethritis/meatitis
Other findings:
Erythema, induration at bacille Calmette-Guérin inoculation site
Anterior uveitis (mild)
Desquamating rash in groin
LABORATORY FINDINGS IN ACUTE KAWASAKI DISEASE
Leukocytosis with neutrophilia and immature forms
Elevated erythrocyte sedimentation rate (ESR)
Elevated C-reactive protein (CRP)
Anemia
Abnormal plasma lipids
Hypoalbuminemia
Hyponatremia
Thrombocytosis after week 1§
Sterile pyuria
Elevated serum transaminases
Elevated serum gamma glutamyl transpeptidase
Pleocytosis of cerebrospinal fluid
Leukocytosis in synovial fluid

*Patients with fever at least 5 days and <4 principal criteria can be diagnosed with Kawasaki disease when coronary artery abnormalities are detected by two-dimensional echocardiography or angiography.

†In the presence of ≥4 principal criteria, Kawasaki disease diagnosis can be made on day 4 of illness. Experienced clinicians who have treated many patients with Kawasaki disease may establish diagnosis before day 4.

‡See differential diagnosis (Table 160-2).

§Some infants present with thrombocytopenia and disseminated intravascular coagulation.

From Newburger JW, Takahashi M, Gerber MA, et al: Diagnosis, treatment, and long-term management of Kawasaki disease, *Pediatrics* 114:1708–1733, 2004.

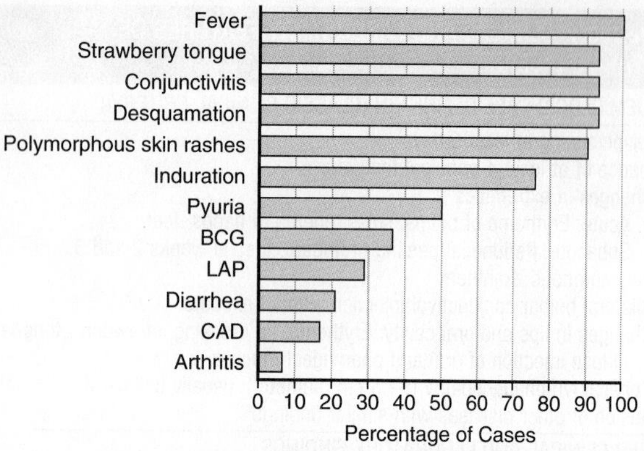

Figure 160-1 Clinical symptoms and signs of Kawasaki disease. A summary of the clinical features from 110 cases of Kawasaki disease seen in Kaohsiung, Taiwan. LAP, lymphadenopathy in head and neck area; BCG, reactivation of bacille Calmette-Guérin inoculation site; CAD, coronary artery dilatation, defined by an internal diameter > 3 mm. (From Wang CL, Wu YT, Liu CA, et al: Kawasaki disease: infection, immunity and genetics, *Pediatr Infect Dis J* 24:998–1004, 2005.)

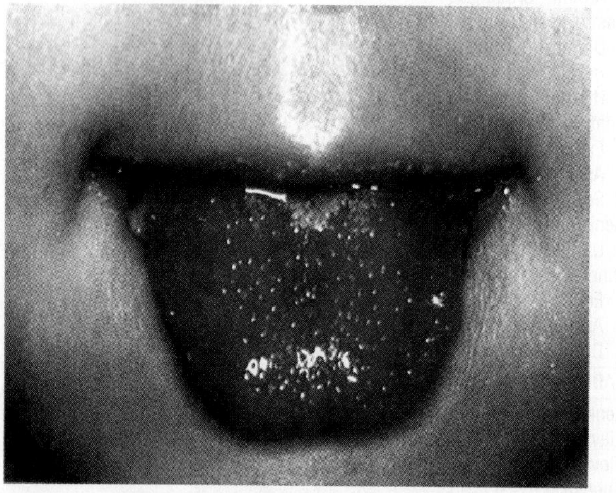

Figure 160-2 Strawberry tongue in mucocutaneous lymph node syndrome (Kawasaki disease). (Courtesy of Tomisaku Kawasaki, MD.) (From Hurwitz S: *Clinical pediatric dermatology*, ed 2, Philadelphia, 1993, WB Saunders.)

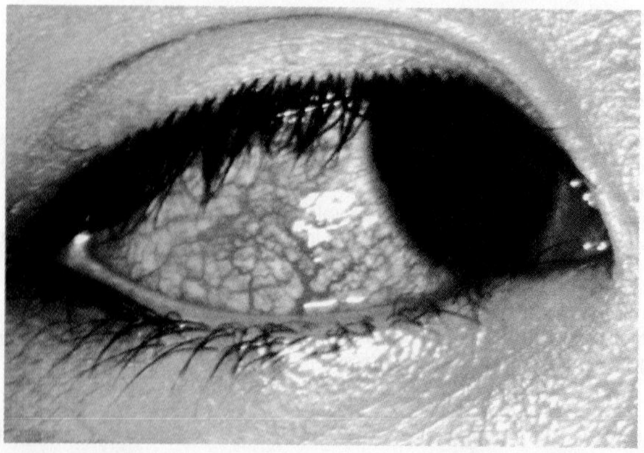

Figure 160-3 Congestion of bulbar conjunctiva in a patient with mucocutaneous lymph node syndrome (Kawasaki disease). (Courtesy of Tomisaku Kawasaki, MD.) (From Hurwitz S: *Clinical pediatric dermatology*, ed 2, Philadelphia, 1993, WB Saunders.)

second or third week. Small or large joints may be affected, and the arthralgias may persist for several weeks. Clinical features that are less consistent with KD include exudative conjunctivitis, exudative pharyngitis, generalized lymphadenopathy, discrete oral lesions, and bullous, pustular, or vesicular rashes.

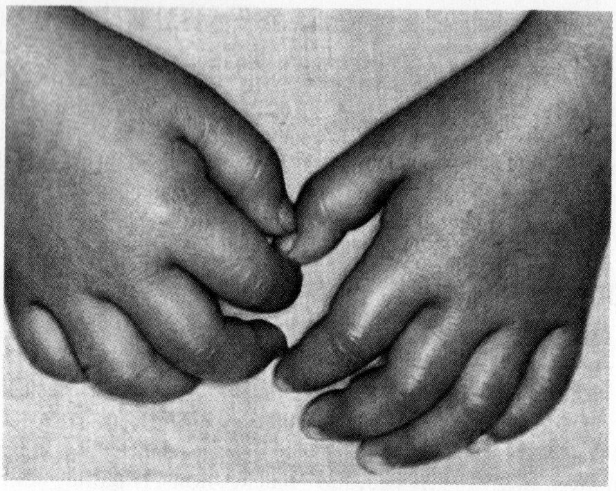

Figure 160-4 Indurative edema of the hands in mucocutaneous lymph node syndrome (Kawasaki disease). (Courtesy of Tomisaku Kawasaki, MD.) (From Hurwitz S: *Clinical pediatric dermatology*, ed 2, Philadelphia, 1993, WB Saunders.)

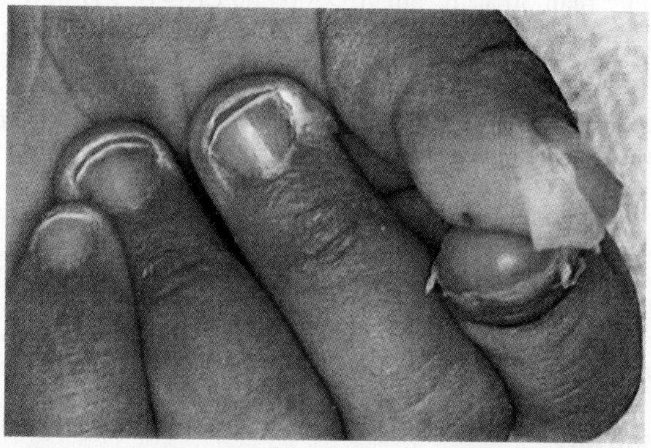

Figure 160-5 Desquamation of the fingers in a patient with mucocutaneous lymph node syndrome (Kawasaki disease). (Courtesy of Tomisaku Kawasaki, MD.) (From Hurwitz S: *Clinical pediatric dermatology*, ed 2, Philadelphia, 1993, WB Saunders.)

Cardiac involvement is the most important manifestation of KD. Myocarditis occurs in most patients with acute KD and manifests as tachycardia out of proportion to fever along with diminished left ventricular systolic function. Occasionally, patients with KD present in shock, with markedly diminished left ventricular function. Pericarditis with a small pericardial effusion can also occur during the acute illness. Mitral regurgitation of at least mild severity is evident on echocardiography in approximately one quarter of patients at presentation but diminishes over time, except among rare patients with coronary aneurysms and ischemic heart disease. Coronary artery aneurysms develop in up to 25% of untreated patients in the second to third week of illness and are best detected by two-dimensional echocardiography. Giant coronary artery aneurysms (≥8 mm internal diameter) pose the greatest risk for rupture, thrombosis or stenosis, and myocardial infarction (Fig. 160-6). Axillary, popliteal, iliac, or other arteries may also be involved by aneurysm, which manifests as a localized pulsating mass.

In the absence of treatment, KD can be divided into 3 clinical phases. The **acute febrile phase** is characterized by fever and the other acute signs of illness and usually lasts 1-2 wk. The **subacute phase** is associated with desquamation, thrombocytosis, the development of coronary aneurysms, and the highest risk of sudden death in patients in whom aneurysms have developed, and generally lasts about 2 wk. The **convalescent phase** begins when all clinical signs of illness have disappeared and continues until the erythrocyte sedimentation rate (ESR) returns to normal, typically about 6-8 wk after the onset of illness.

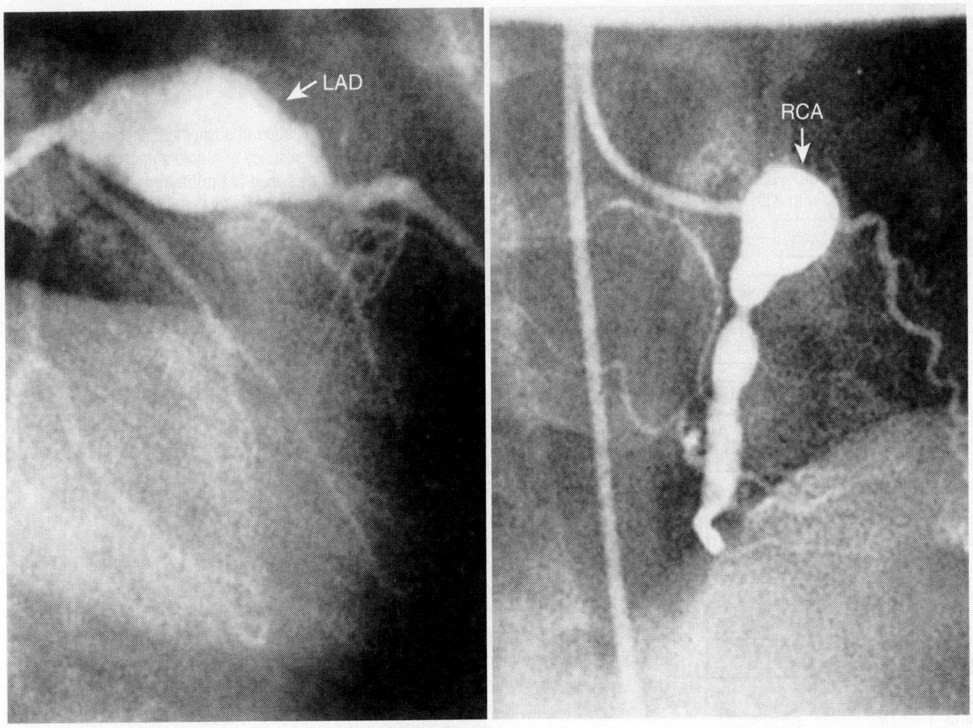

Figure 160-6 Coronary angiogram demonstrating giant aneurysm of the left anterior descending coronary artery (LAD) with obstruction and giant aneurysm of the right coronary artery (RCA) with an area of severe narrowing in 6 yr old boy. (From Newburger JW, Takahashi M, Gerber MA, et al: Diagnosis, treatment, and long-term management of Kawasaki disease, *Pediatrics* 114:1708–1733, 2004.)

LABORATORY FINDINGS

There is no diagnostic test for KD, but patients usually have characteristic laboratory findings. The leukocyte count is normal to elevated, with a predominance of neutrophils and immature forms. Normocytic, normochromic anemia is common. The platelet count is generally normal in the first week of illness and rapidly increases by the second to third week of illness, sometimes exceeding 1,000,000/mm^3. An elevated sedimentation rate and/or C-reactive protein value is universally present in the acute phase of illness. The ESR may remain elevated for weeks. Sterile pyuria, mild elevations of the hepatic transaminases, hyperbilirubinemia, and cerebrospinal fluid pleocytosis may also be present.

Two-dimensional echocardiography is the most useful test to monitor for development of coronary artery abnormalities and should be performed by a pediatric cardiologist. Although frank aneurysms are rarely detected early in the illness, brightness of the arterial walls and lack of normal tapering of the vessels are typical. Moreover, coronary artery dimensions, adjusted for body surface area (BSA), are significantly increased in the first 5 wk after presentation. BSA-adjusted coronary artery dimensions on baseline echocardiography in the first 10 days of illness appear to be good predictors of involvement during early follow-up. Aneurysms have been defined with use of absolute dimensions by the Japanese Ministry of Health and are classified as small (<5 mm internal diameter), medium (5-8 mm internal diameter), or giant (>8 mm internal diameter).

Echocardiography should be performed at diagnosis and again after 2-3 wk of illness. If the results are normal, a repeat study should be performed 6-8 wk after onset of illness. If results of either of the initial studies are abnormal or the patient has recurrent symptoms, more frequent echocardiography or other studies may be necessary. In patients without coronary abnormalities at any time during the illness, performance of echocardiography and a lipid profile is recommended 1 year later. After this time, periodic evaluation for preventive cardiology counseling is warranted, and some experts recommend cardiologic follow-up every 5 yr. For patients with coronary abnormalities, the type of testing and the frequency of cardiology follow-up visits are tailored to the patients' coronary status.

DIAGNOSIS

The diagnosis of KD is based on the presence of characteristic clinical signs. For **classic KD**, the diagnostic criteria require the presence of fever for at least 4 days and at least four of five of the other principal characteristics of the illness (see Table 160-1). In **atypical or incomplete KD**, patients have persistent fever but fewer than four of the five characteristics. In these patients, laboratory and echocardiographic data can assist in the diagnosis (Fig. 160-7). Incomplete cases are most frequent in infants, who, unfortunately, also have the highest likelihood of development of coronary artery abnormalities. Ambiguous cases should be referred to a center with experience in the diagnosis of KD. Establishing the diagnosis with prompt institution of treatment is essential to prevent potentially devastating coronary artery disease.

DIFFERENTIAL DIAGNOSIS

Adenovirus, measles, and scarlet fever lead the list of common childhood infections that mimic KD (Table 160-2). Children with adenovirus typically have exudative pharyngitis and exudative conjunctivitis, allowing differentiation from KD. A common clinical problem is the differentiation of scarlet fever from KD in a child who is a group A streptococcal carrier. Patients with scarlet fever typically have a rapid clinical response to appropriate antibiotic therapy. Such treatment for 24-48 hr with clinical reassessment generally clarifies the diagnosis. Furthermore, ocular findings are quite rare in group A streptococcal pharyngitis and may assist in the diagnosis of KD. Streptococcal and staphylococcal toxin–mediated illnesses must also be considered, especially the toxic shock syndromes.

Measles must also be considered; features of measles that distinguish it from KD include exudative conjunctivitis, Koplik spots, rash that begins on the face and hairline and behind the ears, as well as leukopenia. Cervical lymphadenitis can be the initial diagnosis in children who are ultimately recognized to have KD. Less common infections such as Rocky Mountain spotted fever and leptospirosis are occasionally confused with KD. Rocky Mountain spotted fever is a potentially lethal bacterial infection.

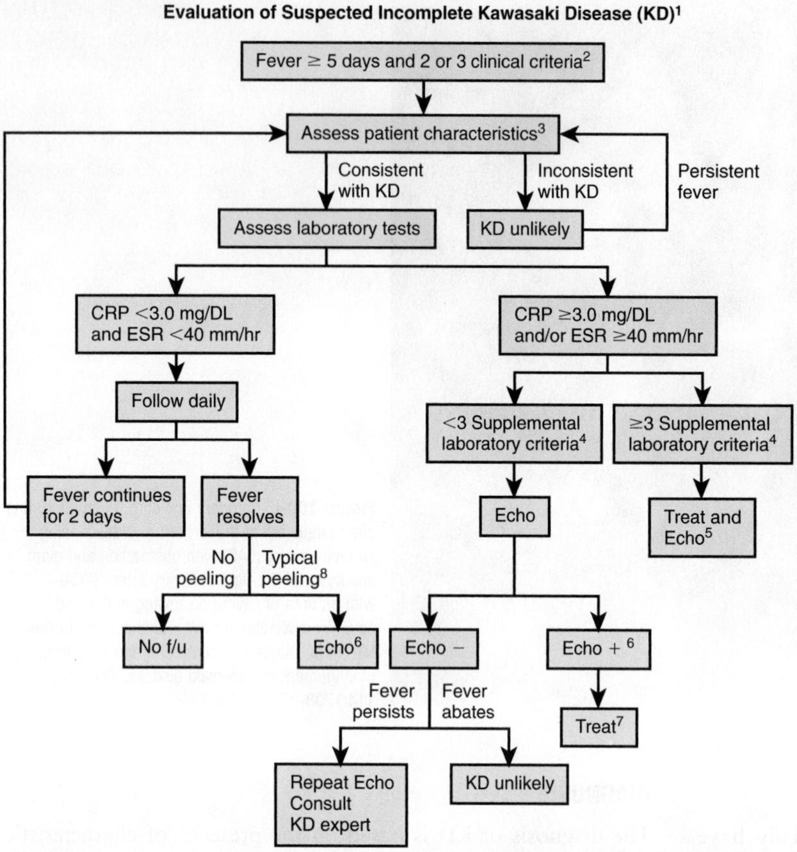

Figure 160-7 Algorithm for evaluation of suspected incomplete Kawasaki disease (KD). *1,* In the absence of a gold standard for diagnosis, this algorithm cannot be evidence based but rather represents the informed opinion of the expert committee. Consultation with an expert should be sought anytime assistance is needed. *2,* Infants ≤6 mo old on day ≥7 of fever or later without other explanation should undergo laboratory testing and, if evidence of systemic inflammation is found, an echocardiogram (Echo), even if they have no clinical criteria. *3,* Patient characteristics suggesting KD are listed in Table 160-1. Characteristics suggesting disease other than KD include exudative conjunctivitis, exudative pharyngitis, discrete intraoral lesions, bullous or vesicular rash, and generalized adenopathy. Consider alternative diagnoses (see Table 160-2). *4,* Supplemental laboratory criteria include albumin ≤3.0 g/dL, anemia for age, elevation of alanine aminotransferase, platelet count after 7 days ≥450,000/mm^3, white blood cell count ≥15,000/mm^3, and urine white blood cell count ≥10 /high-power field. *5,* Can treat before performing echocardiogram. *6,* Echocardiogram findings are considered positive (Echo +) for purposes of this algorithm if any of 3 conditions are met: *z* score of left anterior descending coronary artery (LAD) or right coronary artery (RCA) ≥2.5; coronary arteries meet Japanese Ministry of Health criteria for aneurysms; ≥3 other suggestive features exist, including perivascular brightness, lack of tapering, decreased left ventricle (LV) function, mitral regurgitation, pericardial effusion, or *z* scores in LAD or RCA of 2-2.5. *7,* If echocardiogram findings are positive, treatment should be given to children within 10 days of fever onset and to those beyond day 10 with clinical and laboratory signs (C-reactive protein [CRP], erythrocyte sedimentation rate [ESR]) of ongoing inflammation. *8,* Typical peeling begins under nail beds of fingers and then toes. Echo –, negative echocardiogram findings; f/u, follow-up. (From Newburger JW, Takahashi M, Gerber MA, et al: Diagnosis, treatment, and long-term management of Kawasaki disease, *Pediatrics* 114:1708–1733, 2004.)

Table 160-2 DIFFERENTIAL DIAGNOSIS OF KAWASAKI DISEASE
VIRAL INFECTIONS
• Adenovirus • Enterovirus • Measles • Epstein-Barr virus
BACTERIAL INFECTIONS
• Scarlet fever • Rocky Mountain spotted fever • Leptospirosis • Bacterial cervical lymphadenitis
RHEUMATOLOGIC DISEASE
• Systemic-onset juvenile idiopathic arthritis
OTHER
• Toxic shock syndrome • Staphylococcal scalded skin syndrome • Drug hypersensitivity reactions • Stevens-Johnson syndrome

Its distinguishing features include pronounced myalgias and headache at onset, centripedal rash, and petechiae on the palms and soles. Leptospirosis can also be an illness of considerable severity. Risk factors include exposure to water contaminated with urine from infected animals. The classic description of leptospirosis is of a biphasic illness with a few asymptomatic days between an initial period of fever and headache and a late phase with renal and hepatic failure. In contrast, patients with KD have consecutive days of fever at diagnosis and rarely have renal or hepatic failure.

Children with KD and pronounced myocarditis may demonstrate hypotension with a clinical picture similar to that of toxic shock syndrome. Features of toxic shock syndrome that are not commonly seen in KD include renal insufficiency, coagulopathy, pancytopenia, and myositis. Drug hypersensitivity reactions, including Stevens-Johnson syndrome, share some characteristics with KD. Drug reaction features such as the presence of periorbital edema, oral ulcerations, and a normal or minimally elevated ESR are not seen in KD. Systemic-onset juvenile idiopathic arthritis (systemic juvenile rheumatoid arthritis) is also characterized by fever and rash, but physical findings include diffuse lymphadenopathy and hepatosplenomegaly. Additionally, arthritis develops at some point in the disease course. Laboratory findings may include coagulopathy, elevated fibrin degradation product values, and hyperferritinemia. Interestingly, there are reports of children with systemic-onset juvenile idiopathic arthritis who have echocardiographic evidence of abnormal coronary arteries.

TREATMENT

Patients with acute KD should be treated with 2 g/kg of intravenous gammaglobulin (IVIG) and high-dose aspirin (80-100 mg/kg/day divided q6h) as soon as possible after diagnosis and, ideally, within 10 days of disease onset (Table 160-3). The mechanism of action of IVIG in KD is unknown, but treatment results in rapid defervescence and resolution of clinical signs of illness in 85-90% of patients. The prevalence of coronary disease, which is 20-25% in children treated with aspirin alone, is only 2-4% in those treated with IVIG and aspirin within the first 10 days of illness. Strong consideration should be given to treating patients with persistent fever who are diagnosed after the 10th day of fever. The dose of aspirin is usually decreased from anti-inflammatory to antithrombotic doses (3-5 mg/kg/day as a single dose) after the patient has been afebrile for 48 hr, although some experts prescribe high-dose aspirin until the 14th day of illness. Aspirin is continued for its antithrombotic effect until 6 to 8 wk after illness onset and is then discontinued in patients who have had normal echocardiography findings throughout the course of their illness. Patients with coronary artery abnormalities continue

Table 160-3 TREATMENT OF KAWASAKI DISEASE

ACUTE STAGE
• Intravenous immunoglobulin 2 g/kg over 10-12 hr *AND* • Aspirin 80-100 mg/kg/day divided every 6 hr orally until patient is afebrile for at least 48 hr
CONVALESCENT STAGE
• Aspirin 3-5 mg/kg once daily orally until 6-8 wk after illness onset
LONG-TERM THERAPY FOR PATIENTS WITH CORONARY ABNORMALITIES
• Aspirin 3-5 mg/kg once daily orally • Clopidogrel 1 mg/kg/day (max 75 mg/day) • Most experts add warfarin or low-molecular-weight heparin for those patients at particularly high risk of thrombosis
ACUTE CORONARY THROMBOSIS
• Prompt fibrinolytic therapy with tissue plasminogen activator or other thrombolytic agent under supervision of a pediatric cardiologist

with aspirin therapy and may require anticoagulation, depending on the degree of coronary dilation (see later).

IVIG-resistant KD occurs in approximately 15% of patients and is defined by persistent or recrudescent fever 36 hr after completion of the initial IVIG infusion. Patients with IVIG resistance are at increased risk for coronary artery abnormalities. Typically, another dose of IVIG at 2 g/kg is administered to patients with IVIG resistance. Other therapies that have been used to date include intravenous methylprednisolone and, less often, cyclophosphamide and plasmapheresis. A tumor necrosis factor inhibitor, infliximab, has also been given for the treatment of IVIG-resistant disease, usually if a second dose of IVIG or corticosteroids are ineffective.

COMPLICATIONS

The patient with KD who has had a small solitary aneurysm should continue aspirin indefinitely. Patients with larger or numerous aneurysms may require the addition of other antiplatelet agents or anticoagulation; such decisions should be made in consultation with a pediatric cardiologist. Acute thrombosis may occasionally occur in an aneurysmal or stenotic coronary artery; thrombolytic therapy may be lifesaving in this circumstance.

Long-term follow-up of patients with coronary artery aneurysms should include periodic echocardiography with stress testing and possibly angiography if large aneurysms are present. Catheter intervention with percutaneous transluminal coronary rotational ablation, directional coronary atherectomy, and stent implantation have been used for the management of coronary stenosis due to KD, with some patients requiring coronary artery bypass grafting.

Patients undergoing long-term aspirin therapy should receive annual influenza vaccination to reduce the risk of Reye syndrome. Continuation of aspirin therapy after varicella vaccination can be considered, because the risk of Reye syndrome in children who take salicylates and receive the varicella vaccine is likely to be lower than in those exposed to wild-type varicella without previous vaccination. Alternatively, a different antiplatelet agent can be substituted for aspirin during the 6 wk after varicella vaccination. Because IVIG may interfere with the immune response to live virus vaccines because of specific antiviral antibody, the measles-mumps-rubella and varicella vaccinations should generally be deferred until 11 months after IVIG administration. Other vaccinations do not need to be delayed.

PROGNOSIS

The vast majority of patients with KD return to normal health, as timely treatment reduces the risk of coronary aneurysms to less than 5%. Acute KD recurs in 1-3% of cases. The prognosis for patients with coronary abnormalities depends on the severity of coronary disease; therefore, recommendations for follow-up and management are stratified according to coronary artery status. Published fatality rates are very low, generally <1.0%. Overall, 50% of coronary artery aneurysms regress to normal lumen diameter by 1 to 2 yr after the illness, with smaller aneurysms being more likely to regress. Intravascular ultrasonography has demonstrated that regressed aneurysms are associated with marked myointimal thickening and abnormal functional behavior of the vessel wall. Giant aneurysms are unlikely to resolve and are most likely to lead to thrombosis or stenosis. Coronary artery bypass grafting may be required if myocardial perfusion is significantly impaired; it is best accomplished with the use of arterial grafts, which grow with the child and are more likely than venous grafts to remain patent over the long term. Heart transplantation has been required in rare cases in which revascularization is not feasible because of distal coronary stenoses, distal aneurysms, or severe ischemic cardiomyopathy.

Whether children who have had KD and normal echocardiography findings are at higher risk for the development of atherosclerotic heart disease in adulthood is unclear. Studies of endothelial dysfunction in children with a history of KD and normal coronary dimensions have produced conflicting results. Practical advice in regards to a heart-healthy diet, adequate amounts of exercise, tobacco avoidance, and intermittent lipid monitoring is appropriate for all children with a history of KD.

BIBLIOGRAPHY

Please visit the Nelson Textbook of Pediatrics *website at www.expertconsult.com for the complete bibliography.*

Chapter 161
Vasculitis Syndromes

Stacy P. Ardoin and Edward Fels

Childhood vasculitis encompasses a broad spectrum of diseases that share a common denominator, inflammation of the blood vessels. The pathogenesis of the vasculitides is generally idiopathic; some forms of vasculitis are associated with infectious agents and medications, and others may occur in the setting of preexisting autoimmune disease. The pattern of vessel injury provides insight into the form of vasculitis and serves as a framework to delineate the different vasculitic syndromes. The distribution of vascular injury includes small vessels (capillaries, arterioles, and postcapillary venules), medium vessels (renal arteries, mesenteric vasculature, and coronary arteries), and large vessels (the aorta and its proximal branches). Additionally, some forms of small vessel vasculitis are characterized by the presence of antineutrophil cytoplasmic antibodies (ANCAs), whereas others are associated with immune complex deposition in affected tissues. A combination of clinical features, histologic appearance of involved vessels, and laboratory data is utilized to classify vasculitis (Tables 161-1 to 161-3).

Childhood vasculitis varies from a relatively benign and self-limited disease such as Henoch-Schönlein purpura to catastrophic disease with end-organ damage as seen in Wegener granulomatosis. Vasculitis generally manifests as a heterogeneous multisystem disease. Although some features, such as purpura, are easily identifiable, others, such as hypertension secondary to renal artery occlusion or glomerulonephritis, can be more subtle. Ultimately, the key to recognizing vasculitis relies heavily on pattern recognition. Demonstration of vessel injury and inflammation on biopsy or vascular imaging is required to confirm a diagnosis of vasculitis.

BIBLIOGRAPHY
Please visit the Nelson Textbook of Pediatrics *website at www.expertconsult.com for the complete bibliography.*

161.1 Henoch-Schönlein Purpura

Stacy P. Ardoin and Edward Fels

Henoch-Schönlein purpura (HSP) is the most common vasculitis of childhood and is characterized by leukocytoclastic vasculitis and immunoglobulin (Ig) A deposition in the small vessels in the skin, joints, gastrointestinal tract, and kidney.

Table 161-1 CLASSIFICATION OF CHILDHOOD VASCULITIS

I. PREDOMINANTLY LARGE VESSEL VASCULITIS
• Takayasu arteritis
II. PREDOMINANTLY MEDIUM VESSEL VASCULITIS
• Childhood polyarteritis nodosa • Cutaneous polyarteritis nodosa • Kawasaki disease
III. PREDOMINANTLY SMALL VESSEL VASCULITIS
A. Granulomatous: • Wegener granulomatosis* • Churg-Strauss syndrome* B. Nongranulomatous: • Microscopic polyangiitis* • Henoch-Schönlein purpura • Isolated cutaneous leukocytoclastic vasculitis • Hypocomplementemic urticarial vasculitis
IV. OTHER VASCULITIDES
• Behçet disease • Vasculitis secondary to infection (including hepatitis B–associated polyarteritis nodosa), malignancies, and drugs, including hypersensitivity vasculitis • Vasculitis associated with connective tissue disease • Isolated vasculitis of the central nervous system • Cogan syndrome • Unclassified

*Associated with antineutrophil cytoplasmic antibody.
Adapted from Ozen S, Ruperto N, Dillon MJ, et al: EULAR/PReS endorsed consensus criteria for the classification of childhood vasculitides, *Ann Rheum Dis* 65:936–941, 2006.

EPIDEMIOLOGY

HSP occurs worldwide and affects all ethnic groups. The incidence of HSP is estimated at 14-20/100,000 children per year and affects males more than females, with a 1.2-1.8 : 1 male: female ratio. Approximately 90% of HSP cases occur in children, usually between the ages of 3 and 10 yr. HSP is distinctly less common in adults, in whom severe and chronic complications are often encountered. HSP is more common in the fall, winter, or spring and is unusual in summer months. Many cases of HSP follow a documented upper respiratory infection.

PATHOLOGY

Skin biopsies demonstrate vasculitis of the dermal capillaries and postcapillary venules. The inflammatory infiltrate includes neutrophils and monocytes. Renal histopathology typically shows endocapillary proliferative glomerulonephritis, ranging from a

Table 161-2 FEATURES THAT SUGGEST A VASCULITIC SYNDROME

CLINICAL FEATURES
Fever, weight loss, fatigue of unknown origin Skin lesions (palpable purpura, vasculitic urticaria, livedo reticularis, nodules, ulcers) Neurologic lesions (headache, mononeuritis multiplex, focal central nervous system lesions) Arthralgia or arthritis, myalgia, or myositis Serositis Hypertension Pulmonary infiltrates or hemorrhage
LABORATORY FEATURES
Increased erythrocytes sedimentation rate or C-reactive protein level Leukocytosis, anemia Eosinophilia Antineutrophil cytoplasmic antibodies Elevated factor VIII–related antigen (von Willebrand factor) Cryoglobulins Circulating immune complexes Hematuria, proteinuria, elevated serum creatinine

From Cassidy JT, Petty RE: *Textbook of pediatric rheumatology*, ed 5, Philadelphia, 2005, Elsevier/Saunders.

Table 161-3 CLINICAL AND PATHOLOGIC CHARACTERISTICS OF SOME VASCULITIDES IN CHILDHOOD

SYNDROME	FREQUENCY	VESSELS AFFECTED	CHARACTERISTIC PATHOLOGY
POLYARTERITIS			
Polyarteritis nodosa	Rare	Medium-sized and small muscular arteries and sometimes arterioles	Focal segmental (often near bifurcations); fibrinoid necrosis; gastrointestinal, renal microaneurysms; lesions at various stages of evolution
Kawasaki disease	Common	Coronary and other muscular arteries	Thrombosis, fibrosis, aneurysms, especially of coronary vessels
LEUKOCYTOCLASTIC VASCULITIS			
Henoch-Schönlein purpura	Common	Arterioles and venules, often small arteries and veins	Leukocytoclasis; mixed cells, eosinophils, immunoglobulin A deposits in affected vessels
Hypersensitivity angitis	Rare	Arterioles and venules	Leukocytoclastic or lymphocytic, varying eosinophils, occasionally granulomatous; widespread lesions at same stage of evolution
GRANULOMATOUS VASCULITIS			
Wegener granulomatosis	Rare	Small arteries and veins, occasionally larger vessels	Upper and lower respiratory tract, necrotizing granulomata glomerulonephritis
Churg-Strauss syndrome	Rare	Small arteries and veins, often arterioles and venules	Necrotizing extravascular granulomata; lung involvement; eosinophilia
GIANT CELL ARTERITIS			
Takayasu arteries	Uncommon	Large arteries	Granulomatous inflammation, giant cells; aneurysms, dissection
Temporal arteritis	Rare	Medium-sized and large arteries	Granulomatous inflammation, giant cell arteries

From Cassidy JT, Petty RE: *Textbook of pediatric rheumatology*, ed 5, 2005, Philadelphia, Elsevier/Saunders.

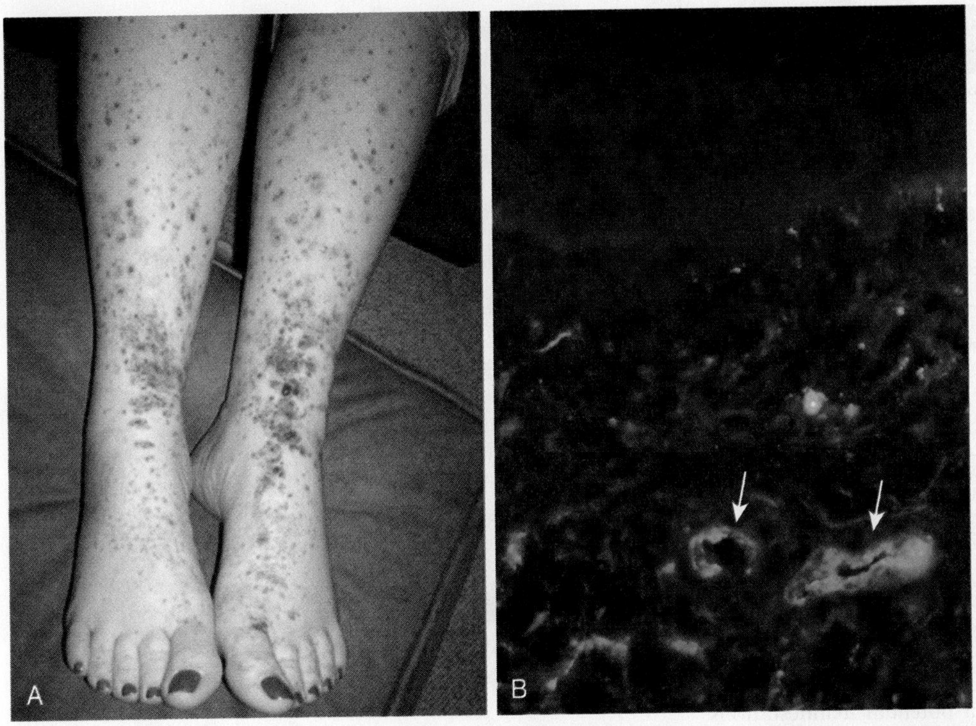

Figure 161-1 *A,* Typical palpable purpura in the lower extremities of a girl with Henoch-Schönlein purpura. *B,* Skin biopsy of lesion from the same patient, showing direct immunofluorescence of immunoglobulin A within the walls of dermal capillaries.

focal segmental process to extensive crescentic involvement. In all tissues, immunofluorescence identifies IgA deposition in walls of small vessels (see Fig. 161-1), accompanied to a lesser extent by deposition of C3, fibrin, and IgM.

PATHOGENESIS

The exact pathogenesis of HSP remains unknown. Given the frequency of preceding upper respiratory infections, including group A streptococcal infections, an infectious trigger is suspected. The common finding of deposition of IgA, specifically IgA_1, suggests that HSP is a disease mediated by IgA and IgA immune complexes. HSP occasionally clusters in families, suggesting a genetic component. HLA-B34 and HLA-DRB1*01 alleles have been linked to HSP nephritis.

CLINICAL MANIFESTATIONS

The hallmark of HSP is its rash: palpable purpura starting as pink macules or wheals and developing into petechiae, raised purpura, or larger ecchymoses. Occasionally, bullae and ulcerations develop. The skin lesions are usually symmetric and occur in gravity-dependent areas (lower extremities) or on pressure points (buttocks) (Figs. 161-1 and 161-2). The skin lesions often evolve in groups, typically lasting 3-10 days, and may recur up to 4 mo after initial presentation. Subcutaneous edema localized to the dorsa of hands and feet, periorbital area, lips, scrotum, or scalp is also common.

Musculoskeletal involvement, including arthritis and arthralgias, is common, occurring in up to 75% of children with HSP. The arthritis tends to be self-limited and oligoarticular, with a predilection for the lower extremities, and does not lead to deformities. The arthritis usually resolves within 2 wk but can recur.

Gastrointestinal manifestations of HSP occur in up to 80% of children with HSP. They include abdominal pain, vomiting, diarrhea, paralytic ileus, melena, intussusception, and mesenteric ischemia or perforation. Endoscopic evaluation is usually not needed but may identify purpura of the intestinal tract.

Renal involvement occurs in up to 50% of children with HSP, manifesting as hematuria, proteinuria, hypertension, frank nephritis, nephrotic syndrome, and acute or chronic renal failure. Progression to end-stage renal disease is uncommon in children (1-2%) (see Chapter 509 for more detailed discussion of HSP renal disease).

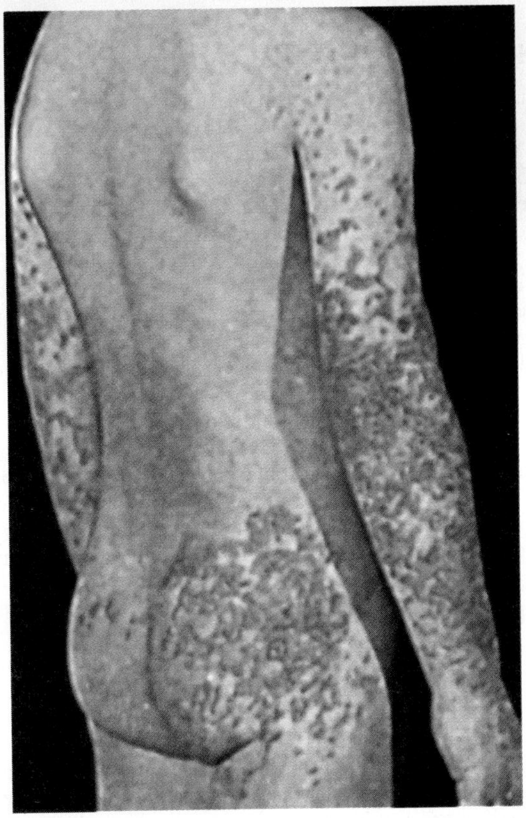

Figure 161-2 Henoch-Schönlein purpura. (From Korting GW: Hautkrankheiten bei Kindern und Jungendlichen, ed 3, Stuttgart, 1982, FK Schattaur Verlag.)

Neurologic manifestations of HSP, due to hypertension or central nervous system (CNS) vasculitis, may also occur. They

Table 161-4 CLASSIFICATION CRITERIA FOR HENOCH-SCHÖNLEIN PURPURA*
AMERICAN COLLEGE OF RHEUMATOLOGY CLASSIFICATION CRITERIA†
Two of the following criteria must be present: • Palpable purpura • Age at onset ≤20 yr • Bowel angina (postprandial abdominal pain, bloody diarrhea) • Biopsy demonstrating intramural granulocytes in small arterioles and/or venules
EUROPEAN LEAGUE AGAINST RHEUMATISM/PEDIATRIC RHEUMATOLOGY EUROPEAN SOCIETY CRITERIA‡
Palpable purpura (in absence of coagulopathy or thrombocytopenia) and one or more of the following criteria must be present: • Diffuse abdominal pain • Arthritis or arthralgia • Biopsy of affected tissue demonstrating predominant immunoglobulin A deposition

*Classification criteria are developed for use in research and not validated for clinical diagnosis.
†Developed for use in adult and pediatric populations. Adapted from Mills JA, Michel BA, Bloch DA, et al: The American College of Rheumatology 1990 criteria for classification of Henoch-Schonlein purpura, *Arthritis Rheum* 33:1114–1121, 1990.
‡Developed for use in pediatric populations only.
Adapted from Ozen S, Ruperto N, Dillon MJ et al: EULAR/PReS endorsed consensus criteria for the classification of childhood vasculitides, *Ann Rheum Dis* 65:936–941, 2006.

include intracerebral hemorrhage, seizures, headaches, and behavior changes. Other less common potential manifestations of HSP are orchitis, carditis, inflammatory eye disease, testicular torsion, and pulmonary hemorrhage.

DIAGNOSIS

The diagnosis of HSP is a clinical one and is often straightforward when the typical rash is present. However, in at least 25% of cases, the rash appears after other manifestations, making early diagnosis challenging. Classification criteria for HSP are summarized in Table 161-4. The differential diagnosis for HSP depends on specific organ involvement but usually includes other small vessel vasculitides, infections, coagulopathies, and other acute intra-abdominal processes.

Acute hemorrhagic edema (AHE), an isolated cutaneous leukocytoclastic vasculitis that affects infants <2 yr of age, resembles HSP clinically. AHE manifests as fever; tender edema of the face, scrotum, hands, and feet; and ecchymosis (usually larger than the purpura of HSP) on the face and extremities (Fig. 161-3). The trunk is spared, but petechiae may be seen in mucous membranes. The patient usually appears well except for the rash. The platelet count is normal or elevated, and the urinalysis results are normal. The younger age, the nature of the lesions, absence of other organ involvement, and a biopsy may help distinguish AHE from HSP.

LABORATORY FINDINGS

No laboratory finding is diagnostic of HSP. Common but nonspecific findings include leukocytosis, thrombocytosis, mild anemia, and elevations of erythrocyte sedimentation rate (ESR) and C-reactive protein (CRP). Occult blood is frequently found in stool specimens. Autoantibody testing is not useful diagnostically except to exclude other diseases. Serum IgA values are often elevated but are not routinely measured. Assessment of renal involvement with blood pressure, urinalysis, and serum creatinine is necessary.

Ultrasound is often used in the setting of gastrointestinal complaints to look for bowel wall edema or the rare occurrence of an associated intussusception. Barium enema can also be used to both diagnose and treat intussusception. Although often unnecessary in typical HSP, biopsies of skin and kidney can provide important diagnostic information, particularly in atypical or severe cases, and characteristically show IgA deposition in affected tissues.

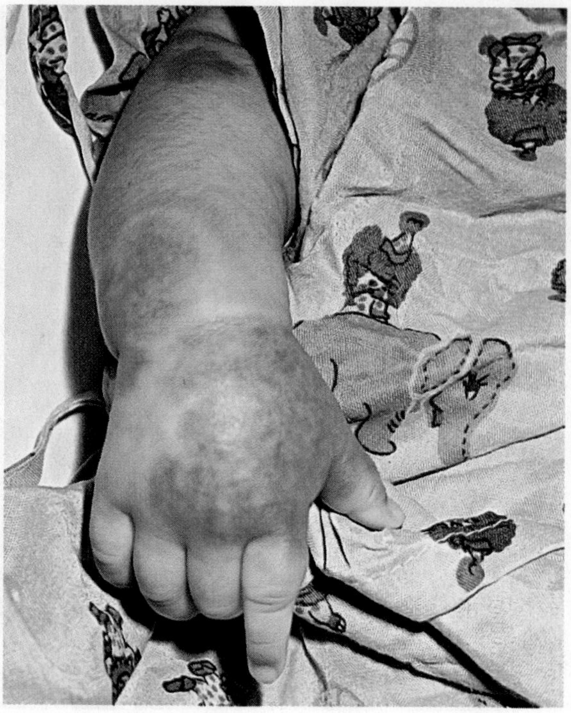

Figure 161-3 Typical lesions of acute hemorrhagic edema on the arm of an infant. (From Eichenfield LF, Frieden IJ, Esterly NB: *Textbook of neonatal dermatology*, Philadelphia, 2001, WB Saunders.)

TREATMENT

Treatment of HSP is supportive, with an emphasis on assuring adequate hydration, nutrition, and analgesia. Controversy continues concerning the appropriate use of glucocorticoids in the management of HSP, but steroids are most often used to treat significant gastrointestinal involvement or other life-threatening manifestations. Empiric use of prednisone (1 mg/kg/day for 1 to 2 wk, followed by taper) reduces abdominal and joint pain but does not alter overall prognosis nor prevent renal disease. Although few data are available to demonstrate efficacy, intravenous immune globulin and plasma exchange are sometimes used in the setting of severe disease. In some cases, chronic HSP renal disease is managed with a variety of immunosuppressants, including azathioprine, cyclophosphamide, and mycophenolate mofetil. End-stage renal disease develops in up to 8% of children with HSP nephritis.

COMPLICATIONS

Acutely, serious gastrointestinal involvement such as intestinal perforation imparts significant morbidity and mortality. Renal disease is the major long-term complication, occurring in 1-2% of children with HSP. Renal disease can develop up to 6 mo after diagnosis but rarely does so if the initial urinalyses findings are normal. It is recommended that children with HSP undergo serial monitoring of blood pressure and urinalyses for 6 mo after diagnosis, especially those who presented with hypertension or urinary abnormalities.

PROGNOSIS

Overall, the prognosis for childhood HSP is excellent, and most children experience an acute, self-limited course. About 30% of children with HSP experience one or more recurrences, typically within 4-6 mo of diagnosis. With each relapse, symptoms are usually milder than at presentation. Children with a more severe initial course are at higher risk for relapse. Chronic renal disease develops in 1-2% of children with HSP, and approximately 8% of those with HSP nephritis go on to have end-stage renal disease.

BIBLIOGRAPHY
Please visit the Nelson Textbook of Pediatrics *website at www.expertconsult.com for the complete bibliography.*

161.2 Takayasu Arteritis

Stacy P. Ardoin and Edward Fels

Takayasu arteritis (TA), also known as "**pulseless disease,**" is a chronic large vessel vasculitis of unknown etiology that predominantly involves the aorta and its major branches.

EPIDEMIOLOGY

Although TA occurs worldwide and can affect all ethnic groups, the disease is most common in Asians. Age of onset is typically between 10 and 40 yr. Up to 20% of individuals with TA are diagnosed prior to age 19 yr. Younger children may be affected but diagnosis in infancy is rare. TA preferentially affects females with a reported 2-4 : 1 female : male ratio in children and adolescents and a 9 : 1 ratio among adults. Occlusive complications are more common in the USA, Western Europe, and Japan, whereas aneurysms predominate in Southeast Asia and Africa.

PATHOLOGY

TA is characterized by inflammation of the vessel wall, starting in the vas vasorum. Involved vessels are infiltrated by T cells, natural killer cells, plasma cells, and macrophages. Giant cells and granulomatous inflammation develop in the media. Persistent inflammation damages the elastic lamina and muscular media, leading to blood vessel dilation and the formation of aneurysms. Progressive scarring and intimal proliferation can result in stenotic or occluded vessels. The subclavian, renal, and carotid arteries are the most commonly involved aortic branches; pulmonary, coronary, and vertebral arteries may also be affected.

PATHOGENESIS

The etiology of TA remains unknown. The presence of abundant T cells with a restricted repertoire of T-cell receptors in TA vascular lesions points to the importance of cellular immunity and suggests the existence of a specific but unknown aortic tissue antigen. Expression of interleukin-1 (IL)-1, IL-6, and tumor necrosis factor-α (TNF-α) is reported to be higher in patients with active TA than in patients with inactive TA and in healthy controls. In addition, some individuals with TA have elevated serum values of anti-endothelial antibodies. A link between TA and tuberculosis infection has been proposed but not proven. The increased prevalence of TA in certain ethnic populations and its occasional occurrence in monozygotic twins and families suggest a genetic predisposition to the disease.

CLINICAL MANIFESTATIONS

The diagnosis of TA is challenging, because early disease manifestations are often nonspecific. As a result, diagnosis can be delayed for several months, and the time to diagnosis is usually longer in children than in adults. Fever, malaise, weight loss, headache, hypertension, myalgias, arthralgias, dizziness, and abdominal pain are common early complaints in the "pre-pulseless" phase of the disease. Among children, hypertension and headache are particularly common presenting manifestations and should prompt consideration of TA when present without alternative explanation. Some individuals with TA report no systemic symptoms and instead present with vascular complications. It is only after substantial vascular injury that evidence of hypoperfusion becomes clinically evident. Later manifestations of disease include diminished pulses, asymmetric blood pressures, claudication, Raynaud phenomenon, renal failure, and symptoms of pulmonary or cardiac ischemia. Inflammation can extend to the aortic valve, resulting in valvular insufficiency. Other findings may include pericardial effusion, pericarditis, pleuritis, splenomegaly, and arthritis.

DIAGNOSIS

Specific pediatric criteria for TA have been proposed, as summarized in Tables 161-5 and 161-6. Radiographic demonstration of large vessel vasculitis is necessary. A thorough physical examination is required to detect an aortic murmur, diminished or asymmetric pulses, and vascular bruits. Four extremity blood pressures should be measured >10 mm Hg; asymmetry in systolic pressure is indicative of disease.

DIFFERENTIAL DIAGNOSIS

In the early phase of TA, when nonspecific symptoms predominate, the differential diagnosis includes a wide array of systemic infections, autoimmune conditions, and malignancies. Although giant cell arteritis, also known as "temporal arteritis," is a common large vessel vasculitis in older adults, this entity is exceedingly rare in childhood. Non-inflammatory conditions that can cause large vessel compromise include fibromuscular dysplasia, Marfan syndrome, and Ehlers-Danlos syndrome.

LABORATORY FINDINGS

The laboratory findings in TA are nonspecific, and there is no specific diagnostic laboratory test. ESR and CRP value are typically elevated, and other nonspecific markers of chronic inflammation may include leukocytosis, thrombocytosis, anemia of chronic inflammation, and hypergammaglobulinemia. Autoantibodies are not useful in diagnosing TA except to help exclude other autoimmune diseases.

Table 161-5 PROPOSED CLASSIFICATION CRITERIA FOR PEDIATRIC-ONSET TAKAYASU ARTERITIS

Angiographic abnormalities (conventional, CT, or magnetic resonance angiography) of the aorta or its main branches and at least one of the following criteria:
- Decreased peripheral artery pulse(s) and/or claudication of extremities
- Blood pressure difference between arms or legs of > 10 mm Hg
- Bruits over the aorta and/or its major branches
- Hypertension (defined by childhood normative data)

Adapted from Ozen S, Ruperton N, Dillon MJ, et al: EULAR/PReS endorsed consensus criteria for the classification of childhood vasculitides, *Ann Rheum Dis* 65:936–941, 2006.

Table 161-6 PATTERNS OF ARTERIAL INVOLVEMENT IN TAKAYASU ARTERITIS

TYPE	INVOLVED ARTERIES
I	Aortic arch only Aortic arch and descending thoracic aorta Aortic arch, thoracic and abdominal aorta Aortic arch and abdominal aorta
II	Descending thoracic aorta only Descending thoracic and abdominal aorta
III	Diffuse aortic involvement
IV	Diffuse aortic and pulmonary artery involvement

Adapted from Hata A, Noda M, Moriwaki R, et al: Angiographic findings of Takayasu arteritis: new classification, *Int J Cardiol* 54(Suppl):S155–S163, 1996.

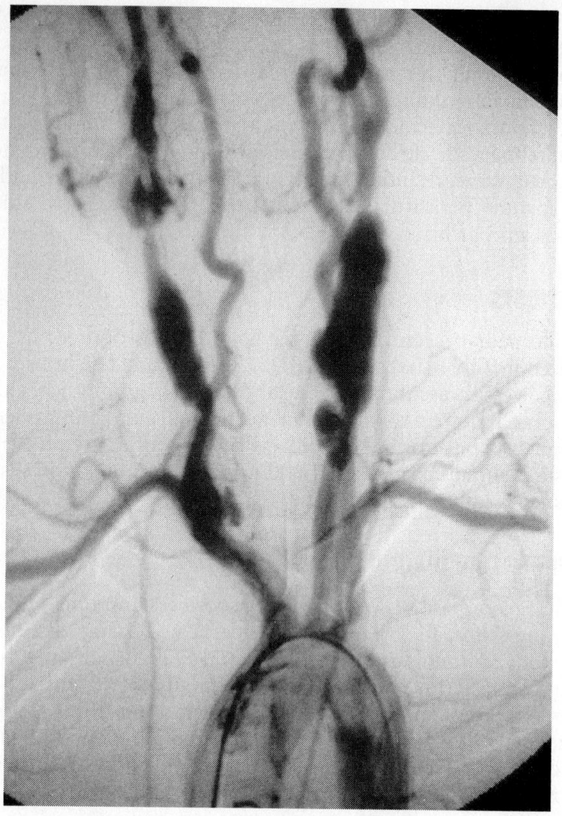

Figure 161-4 Conventional angiogram in a child with Takayasu arteritis showing massive bilateral carotid dilatation, stenosis, and post-stenotic dilatation.

Radiographic assessment is essential to establish large vessel arterial involvement. The gold standard remains conventional arteriography of the aorta and major branches, including carotid, subclavian, pulmonary, renal, and mesenteric branches. Conventional arteriography can identify luminal defects, including dilation, aneurysms, and stenoses, even in smaller vessels such as the mesenteric arteries. Figure 161-4 shows a conventional arteriogram in a child with TA. Although not yet thoroughly validated in TA, magnetic resonance angiography (MRA) and CT angiography (CTA) are gaining acceptance and provide important information about vessel wall thickness and enhancement, although they may not image smaller vessels as well as conventional angiography. Positron emission tomography (PET) may detect vessel wall inflammation but has not been studied extensively. Ultrasound with duplex color-flow Doppler imaging also identifies vessel wall thickening and assesses arterial flow. Echocardiography is recommended to assess for aortic valvular involvement. Serial vascular imaging is usually necessary to assess response to treatment and to detect progressive vascular damage.

TREATMENT

Owing to the rarity of the disease, there is limited evidence to guide therapy. Glucocorticoids are the mainstay of therapy, typically starting with high doses (1 to 2 mg/kg/day of prednisone) followed by gradual dosage tapering. When TA progresses or recurs, steroid-sparing therapy is often required, usually involving methotrexate or azathioprine. Cyclophosphamide is reserved for severe or refractory disease. Results of small case series also suggest that mycophenolate mofetil and anti–TNF-α therapy may be beneficial in select patients. Antihypertensive medications are often necessary to control blood pressure due to renovascular disease.

COMPLICATIONS

Progressive vascular damage can result in arterial stenoses, aneurysms, and occlusions, which produce ischemic symptoms and can be organ- or life-threatening. Potential ischemic complications include stroke, renal impairment or failure, myocardial infarction, mesenteric ischemia, and limb-threatening arterial disease. When these complications occur or are imminent, intervention with surgical vascular grafting or catheter-based angioplasty and stent placement may be necessary to restore adequate blood flow. A high rate of recurrent stenosis has been reported following angioplasty and stent placement. Aortic valve replacement may be required if significant aortic insufficiency develops.

PROGNOSIS

Although up to 20% of individuals with TA have a monophasic course and achieve sustained remission, most suffer relapses. Survival for individuals with TA has improved considerably over the decades, although higher mortality rates are reported in children and adolescents. The overall estimated survival for individuals with TA is 93% at 5 yr and 87% at 10 yr. However, morbidity from vascular complications remains high. Given the chronic endothelial insult and inflammation, children and adolescents with TA are probably at high risk for accelerated atherosclerosis. Early detection and treatment are critical to optimizing outcome in TA.

BIBLIOGRAPHY

Please visit the Nelson Textbook of Pediatrics *website at www.expertconsult.com for the complete bibliography.*

161.3 Polyarteritis Nodosa and Cutaneous Polyarteritis Nodosa

Stacy P. Ardoin and Edward Fels

Polyarteritis nodosa (PAN) is a systemic necrotizing vasculitis affecting small and medium-sized arteries. Aneurysms and stenoses form at irregular intervals throughout affected arteries. Cutaneous PAN is limited to the skin.

EPIDEMIOLOGY

PAN is rare in childhood. Boys and girls are equally affected, and the mean age at presentation is 9 yr. The cause is unknown, but the development of PAN following infections, including group A streptococcus and chronic hepatitis B, suggests that PAN represents a postinfectious autoimmune response. Infections with other organisms, including Epstein-Barr virus, *Mycobacterium tuberculosis*, cytomegalovirus, parvovirus B19, and hepatitis C virus, have also been associated with PAN.

PATHOLOGY

Biopsies show necrotizing vasculitis with granulocytes and monocytes infiltrating the walls of small and medium-sized arteries (Fig. 161-5). Involvement is usually segmental and tends to occur at vessel bifurcations. Granulomatous inflammation is not present, and deposition of complement and immune complexes is rarely observed. Different stages of inflammation are found, ranging from mild inflammatory changes to panmural fibrinoid necrosis associated with aneurysm formation, thrombosis, and vascular occlusion.

PATHOGENESIS

Immune complexes are believed to be pathogenic, but the mechanism is poorly understood. There is no clear genetic association

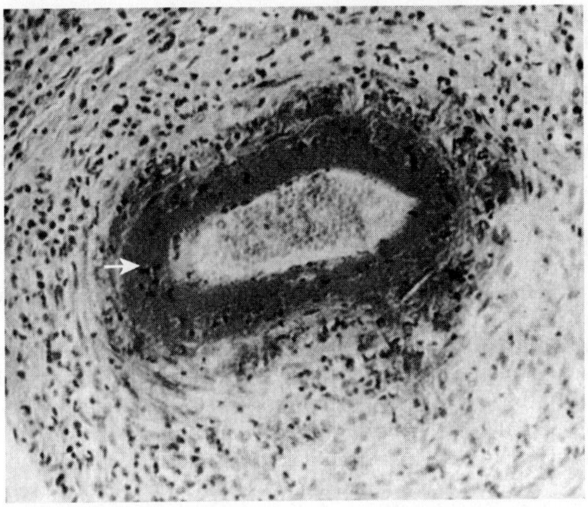

Figure 161-5 Biopsy specimen from a medium-size muscular artery that exhibits marked fibrinoid necrosis of the vessel wall *(arrow).* (From Cassidy JT, Petty RE: Polyarteritis and related vasculitides. In *Textbook of pediatric rheumatology,* ed 5, Philadelphia, 2005, Elsevier/Saunders.)

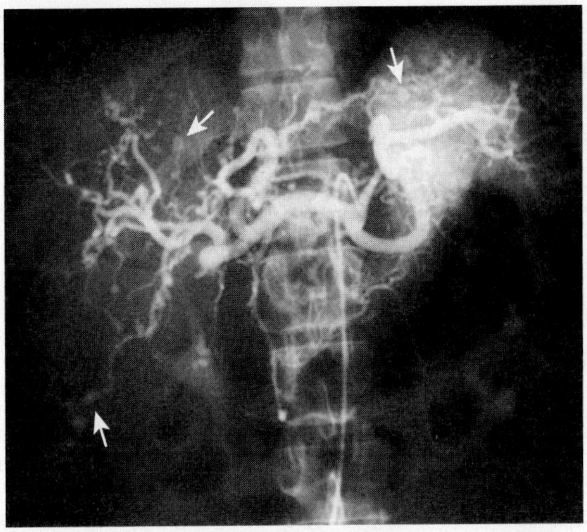

Figure 161-6 Celiac angiography in an 18 yr old boy showing aneurysms in multiple vessels. (From Cassidy JT, Petty RE: Polyarteritis and related vasculitides. In *Textbook of pediatric rheumatology,* ed 5, Philadelphia, 2005, Elsevier/Saunders.)

with PAN, and it is not known why PAN has a predilection for small- and medium-size blood vessels. The inflamed vessel wall becomes thickened and narrowed, impeding blood flow and contributing to end-organ damage characteristic of this disease.

CLINICAL MANIFESTATIONS

The clinical presentation of PAN is variable but generally reflects the distribution of inflamed vessels. Constitutional symptoms are present in most children at disease onset. Weight loss and severe abdominal pain suggest mesenteric arterial inflammation and ischemia. Renovascular arteritis can cause hypertension, hematuria, or proteinuria, although glomerular involvement is not typical. Cutaneous manifestations include purpura, livedo reticularis, ulcerations, and painful nodules. Arteritis affecting the nervous system results in cerebrovascular accidents, transient ischemic attacks, psychosis, and ischemic peripheral neuropathy (mononeuritis multiplex). Myocarditis or coronary arteritis can lead to heart failure and myocardial ischemia; pericarditis and arrhythmias have also been reported. Arthralgias, arthritis, or myalgias are frequently present. Less common symptoms include testicular pain that mimics testicular torsion, bone pain, and vision loss due to retinal arteritis.

DIAGNOSIS

The diagnosis of PAN requires demonstration of vessel involvement on biopsy or angiography. Biopsy of cutaneous lesions shows small or medium vessel vasculitis (see Fig. 161-5). Kidney biopsy in patients with renal manifestations may show necrotizing arteritis. Electromyography in children with peripheral neuropathy identifies affected nerves, and sural nerve biopsy may reveal vasculitis. Conventional arteriography is the gold standard diagnostic imaging study for PAN and reveals areas of aneurysmal dilatation and segmental stenosis, the classic "beads on a string" appearance (Fig. 161-6). MRA and CTA, less invasive imaging alternatives, are gaining acceptance but may not be as effective in identifying small vessel disease or in younger children.

DIFFERENTIAL DIAGNOSIS

Early skin lesions may resemble those of HSP, although the finding of nodular lesions and presence of systemic features help distinguish PAN. Pulmonary lesions suggest ANCA-associated vasculitis or Goodpasture disease. Other rheumatic diseases, including systemic lupus erythematosus, have characteristic target organ involvement and associated autoantibodies distinguishing them from PAN. Prolonged fever and weight loss should also prompt consideration of inflammatory bowel disease or malignancy.

LABORATORY FINDINGS

Nonspecific laboratory findings include elevations of ESR and CRP, anemia, leukocytosis, and hypergammaglobulinemia. Abnormal urine sediment, proteinuria, and hematuria indicate renal disease. Laboratory findings may be normal in cutaneous PAN or similar to those of systemic PAN. Elevated hepatic enzyme values may suggest hepatitis B or C infection. Serologic tests for hepatitis (hepatitis B surface antigen and hepatitis C antibody) should be performed in all patients.

TREATMENT

Oral (1-2 mg/kg/day) and intravenous pulse (30 mg/kg/day) corticosteroids are typically used, frequently in combination with oral or intravenous cyclophosphamide. If hepatitis B is identified, appropriate antiviral therapy should be initiated (Chapter 350). Most cases of cutaneous PAN can be treated with corticosteroids alone at doses of 1-2 mg/kg/day. If an infectious trigger for PAN is identified, antibiotic prophylaxis should be considered. Efficacy data are limited for the treatment of relapsing or refractory cutaneous disease, but dapsone, methotrexate, azathioprine, thalidomide, cyclosporine, and anti-TNF agents have been used successfully.

COMPLICATIONS

Cutaneous nodules may ulcerate and become infected. Hypertension and chronic renal disease may develop from renovascular involvement in PAN. Cardiac involvement may lead to decreased cardiac function or coronary artery disease. Mesenteric vasculitis can predispose to bowel infarction, rupture, and malabsorption. Stroke and rupture of hepatic arterial aneurysm are uncommon complications of this disorder.

PROGNOSIS

The course of PAN varies from mild disease with few complications to a severe, multiorgan disease with high morbidity and mortality. Early and aggressive immunosuppressive therapy increases the likelihood of clinical remission. Compared with disease in adults, childhood PAN is associated with less mortality. Cutaneous PAN is unlikely to transition to systemic disease. Early recognition and treatment of the disease are important to minimizing potential long-term vascular complications.

BIBLIOGRAPHY

Please visit the Nelson Textbook of Pediatrics *website at www.expertconsult.com for the complete bibliography.*

161.4 ANCA-Associated Vasculitis

Stacy P. Ardoin and Edward Fels

The ANCA-associated vasculitides are characterized by small vessel involvement, circulating antineutrophil cytoplasmic antibodies (ANCA), and pauci-immune complex deposition in affected tissues. ANCA-associated vasculitis is categorized into three distinct forms: **Wegener granulomatosis (WG), microscopic polyangiitis (MPA)**, and **Churg-Strauss syndrome (CSS)**.

EPIDEMIOLOGY

WG is a necrotizing granulomatous small vessel vasculitis that occurs at all ages and targets the respiratory tract and the kidneys. Although most cases of WG occur in adults, it does develop in children, with a mean age at diagnosis of 14 yr. There is a female predominance of 3-4:1, and pediatric WG is most prevalent in white persons.

MPA is a small vessel necrotizing vasculitis with clinical features similar to those of WG. CSS is a small vessel necrotizing granulomatous vasculitis associated with a history of refractory asthma and peripheral eosinophilia. MPA and CSS are rare in children, and there does not appear to be a gender predilection in either disease.

PATHOLOGY

Necrotizing vasculitis is the cardinal histologic feature in WG and MPA. Kidney biopsies typically demonstrate crescentic glomerulonephritis with little or no immune complex deposition ("pauci-immune"), in contrast to biopsies from patients with SLE. Although granulomatous inflammation is common in WG and CSS, it is typically not present in MPA. Biopsies showing perivascular eosinophilic infiltrates distinguish CSS syndrome from both MPA and WG (Table 161-7).

PATHOGENESIS

The etiology of ANCA-associated vasculitis remains unknown, although neutrophils, monocytes, and endothelial cells are involved in disease pathogenesis. Neutrophils and monocytes are activated by ANCAs, specifically by the ANCA-associated antigens proteinase-3 (PR3) and myeloperoxidase (MPO), and release proinflammatory cytokines such as TNF-α and IL-8. Localization of these inflammatory cells to the endothelium results in vascular damage characteristic of the ANCA vasculitides. Why the respiratory tract and kidneys are preferential targets in WG and MPA is unknown. Infectious agents and genetic factors have been implicated in disease susceptibility.

CLINICAL MANIFESTATIONS

Early disease course is characterized by nonspecific constitutional symptoms, including fever, malaise, weight loss, myalgias, and arthralgias. In WG, upper airway involvement can manifest as sinusitis, nasal ulceration, epistaxis, otitis media, and hearing loss. Lower respiratory tract symptoms include cough, wheezing, dyspnea, and hemoptysis. Pulmonary hemorrhage can cause rapid respiratory failure. Compared with WG in adults, childhood WG is more frequently complicated by subglottic stenosis (see Fig. 161-5). Inflammation-induced damage to the nasal cartilage can produce a saddle nose deformity (Fig. 161-7). Ophthalmic involvement includes conjunctivitis, scleritis, uveitis, optic neuritis, and invasive orbital pseudotumor (causing proptosis). Perineural vasculitis or direct compression on nerves by granulomatous lesions can cause cranial and peripheral neuropathies. Hematuria, proteinuria, and hypertension signal renal disease. Cutaneous lesions include palpable purpura and ulcers. Venous thromboembolism is a rare but potentially fatal complication of WG. The frequencies of organ system involvement throughout the disease course in WG are: respiratory tract, 84%; kidneys, 88%; joints, 44%; eyes, 60%; skin, 48%; sinuses, 56%; and nervous system, 12%.

The clinical presentation of MPA closely resembles that of WG, although sinus disease is less common. Like WG, CSS frequently causes inflammation of the upper and lower respiratory tract, but cartilage destruction is rare. Unlike in WG, renal involvement in CSS is uncommon, and CSS tends to involve nerves, gastrointestinal tract, pericardium, and skin.

DIAGNOSIS

WG should be considered in children who have recalcitrant sinusitis, pulmonary infiltrates, and evidence of nephritis. Chest radiography often fails to detect pulmonary lesions, and chest CT may show nodules, ground-glass opacities, mediastinal lymphadenopathy, and cavitary lesions (Fig. 161-8). The diagnosis is confirmed by the presence of anti–proteinase 3 (anti-PR3)–specific ANCAs (PR3-ANCAs) and the finding of necrotizing granulomatous vasculitis on pulmonary, sinus, or renal biopsy. The ANCA test result is positive in approximately 90% of children with WG, and the presence of anti-PR3 increases the specificity of the test.

In MPA, ANCAs are also frequently present but have reactivity to myeloperoxidase (MPO-ANCAs). MPA can be distinguished from polyarteritis nodosa (PAN) by the presence of ANCAs and the tendency for small vessel involvement. The

Table 161-7 DIFFERENTIAL DIAGNOSTIC FEATURES OF SMALL VESSEL VASCULITIS

FEATURE	HENOCH-SCHÖNLEIN PURPURA	WEGENER GRANULOMATOSIS	CHURG-STRAUSS SYNDROME	MICROSCOPIC POLYANGIITIS
Signs and symptoms of small vessel vasculitis*	+	+	+	+
Immunoglobulin A–dominant immune deposits	+	−	−	−
Circulating anti-neutrophil cytoplasmic antibodies	−	+ (PR3)	+ (MPO > PR3)	+ (MPO)
Necrotizing vasculitis	−	+	+	+
Granulomatous inflammation	−	+	+	−
Asthma and eosinophilia	−	−	+	−

*Signs and symptoms of small vessel vasculitis include purpura, other rash, arthralgias, arthritis, and constitutional symptoms.
MPO, myeloperoxidase-reactive antibodies; PR3, proteinase 3–reactive antibodies; +, presence; −, absent.
Adapted from Jeannett JC, Falk RJ: Small-vessel vasculitis, *N Engl J Med* 337:1512–1523, 1997.

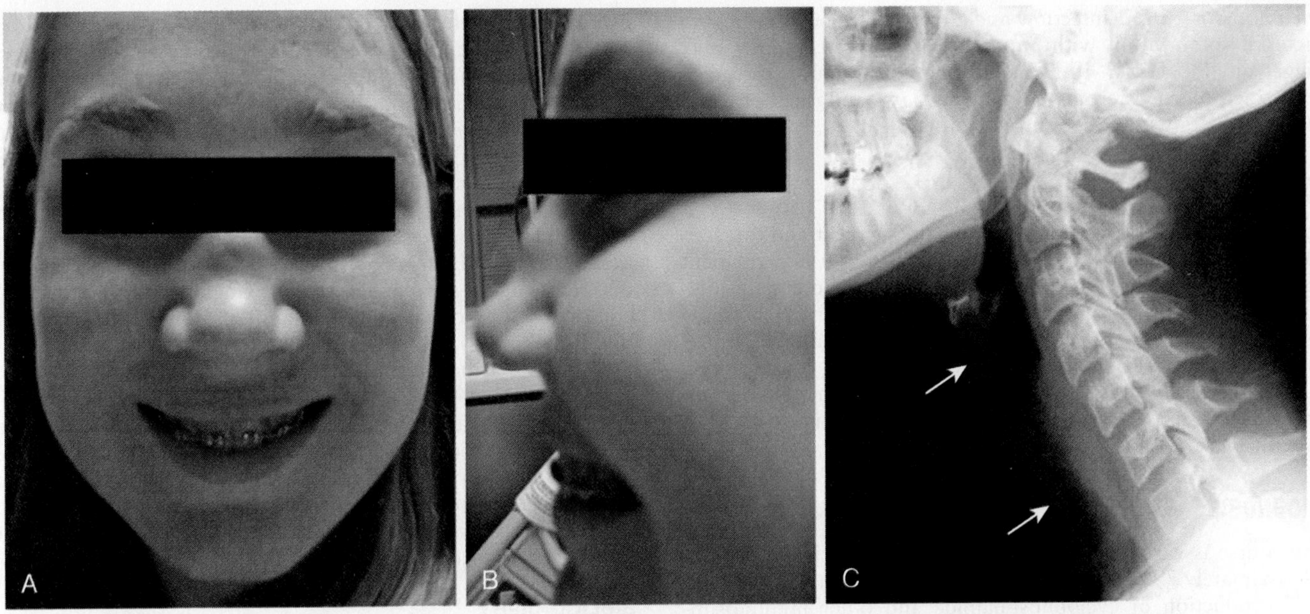

Figure 161-7 *A* and *B,* Anterior and lateral views of saddle nose deformity in an adolescent girl with Wegener granulomatosis. *C,* Segment of subglottic posterior tracheal irregularity (between *arrows*) on lateral neck radiograph in the same patient.

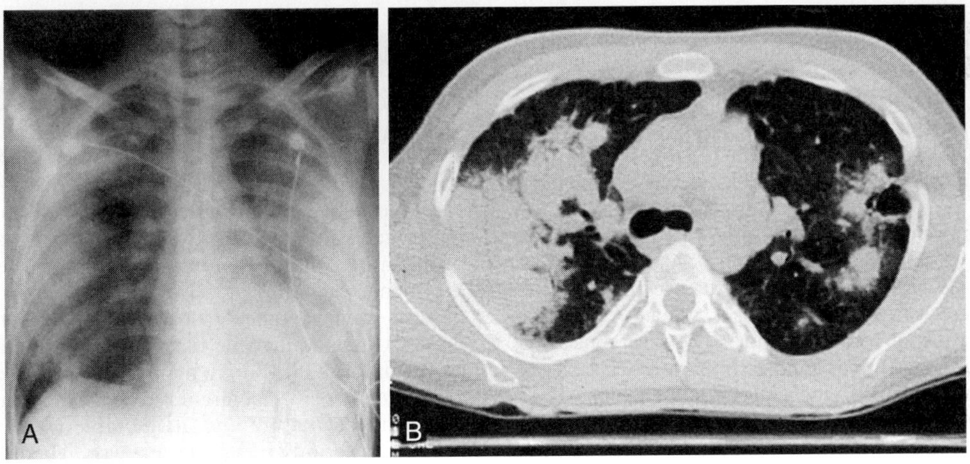

Figure 161-8 Radiographs of lower respiratory tract disease in Wegener granulomatosis. *A,* A chest radiograph of a 14 yr old girl with Wegener granulomatosis and pulmonary hemorrhage. Extensive bilateral, fluffy infiltrates are visualized. (From Cassidy JT, Petty RE: Granulomatous vasculitis, giant cell arteritis and sarcoidosis. In *Textbook of pediatric rheumatology,* ed 3, Philadelphia, 1995, WB Saunders.) *B,* CT scan of the chest in a 17 yr old boy with Wegener granulomatosis. Air space consolidation, septal thickening, and a single cavitary lesion are present. (From Kuhn JP, Slovis TL, Haller JO: *Caffey's pediatric diagnostic imaging,* ed 10, vol 1, Philadelphia, 2004, Mosby.)

ANCA test result is positive in approximately 70% of cases of CSS, and MPO-ANCAs are more common than PR3-ANCAs. The presence of chronic asthma and peripheral eosinophilia suggests the diagnosis of CSS.

DIFFERENTIAL DIAGNOSIS

ANCAs are absent in other granulomatous diseases, such as sarcoidosis and tuberculosis. Goodpasture disease is characterized by antibodies to glomerular basement membrane. Medications such as propylthiouracil, hydralazine, and minocycline are associated with drug-induced ANCA vasculitis. Systemic lupus erythematosus can manifest as pulmonary hemorrhage and nephritis.

LABORATORY FINDINGS

Elevated ESR and CRP values, leukocytosis, and thrombocytosis are present in most patients with an ANCA-associated vasculitis but are nonspecific. Anemia may be due to chronic inflammation or pulmonary hemorrhage. ANCA antibodies show two distinct immunofluorescence patterns: perinuclear (p-ANCAs) and cytoplasmic (c-ANCAs). In addition, ANCAs can also be defined by their specificity for PR3 or MPO antigen. As summarized in Table 161-4, WG is strongly associated with c-ANCAs/anti-PR3 antibodies.

TREATMENT

When the lower respiratory tract or kidneys are significantly involved, initial therapy usually consists of corticosteroids (2 mg/kg/day oral or 30 mg/kg/day × 3 days given intravenously) in conjunction with daily oral cyclophosphamide (2 mg/kg/day). Patients are transitioned to a less toxic medication (usually methotrexate or azathioprine) within 3 to 6 mo once remission is achieved. Trimethoprim-sulfamethoxazole (one 180 mg/800 mg tablet 3 days/wk) is often prescribed both for prophylaxis against

Pneumocystis carinii infection and to reduce upper respiratory bacterial colonization with *Staphylococcus aureus,* which may trigger disease activity. If disease is limited to the upper respiratory tract, corticosteroids (1-2 mg/kg/day) and methotrexate (0.5-1.0 mg/kg/wk) may be first-line treatment.

COMPLICATIONS

Upper respiratory tract lesions can invade the orbit and threaten the optic nerve, and lesions in the ear can cause permanent hearing loss. Respiratory complications include potentially life-threatening pulmonary hemorrhage and upper airway obstruction due to subglottic stenosis. Chronic lung disease secondary to granulomatous inflammation, cavitary lesions, and scarring can predispose to infectious complications. Chronic glomerulonephritis may progress to end-stage renal disease in a subset of patients with advanced or undertreated disease.

PROGNOSIS

The course is variable but is accompanied by disease relapse in approximately 75% of patients. Mortality has been reduced with the introduction of cyclophosphamide and other immunosuppressive agents. Compared with adults, children with ANCA-associated vasculitis have fewer treatment-associated morbidities and malignancies.

BIBLIOGRAPHY

Please visit the Nelson Textbook of Pediatrics *website at* *www.expertconsult.com* *for the complete bibliography.*

161.5 Other Vasculitis Syndromes

Stacy P. Ardoin and Edward Fels

In addition to the more common vasculitides discussed earlier in this chapter, other vasculitic conditions can occur in childhood, the most common of which is Kawasaki disease (discussed in Chapter 160). **Hypersensitivity vasculitis** is a cutaneous vasculitis triggered by medication or toxin exposure. The rash consists of palpable purpura or other nonspecific rash. Skin biopsies reveal characteristic changes of **leukocytoclastic vasculitis** (small vessels with neutrophilic perivascular or extravascular neutrophilic infiltration). **Hypocomplementemic urticarial vasculitis** involves small vessels and manifests as recurrent urticaria that resolves over several days but leaves residual hyperpigmentation. This condition is associated with low levels of complement component C1q and systemic findings that include fever, gastrointestinal symptoms, arthritis, and glomerulonephritis. **Cryoglobulinemic vasculitis** can complicate mixed essential cryoglobulinemia and is a small vessel vasculitis affecting skin, joints, kidneys, and lungs. **Primary angiitis of the central nervous system (PACNS)** represents vasculitis confined to the CNS and requires exclusion of other systemic vasculitides. **Benign angiitis of the central nervous system (BACNS), also known as transient CNS angiopathy,** represents a self-limited variant. **Cogan syndrome** is rare in children; its potential clinical manifestations include constitutional symptoms, inflammatory eye disease, vestibuloauditory dysfunction, arthritis, and aortitis.

Identification of these vasculitis syndromes requires a comprehensive history and physical exam. Other diagnostic considerations are outlined in Table 161-8. Although treatment is tailored to disease severity, treatment generally includes prednisone (up to 2 mg/kg/day) plus steroid-sparing immunosuppressive medications if necessary. For hypersensitivity vasculitis, withdrawal of the triggering medication or toxin is indicated if possible.

Table 161-8 DIAGNOSTIC CONSIDERATIONS FOR OTHER VASCULITIS SYNDROMES

VASCULITIS SYNDROME	APPROACH TO DIAGNOSIS
Hypersensitivity vasculitis	Skin biopsy demonstrating leukocytoclastic vasculitis
Hypocomplementemic urticarial vasculitis	Biopsy of affected tissue demonstrating small vessel vasculitis Low levels of circulating C1q
Cryoglobulinemic vasculitis	Biopsy of affected tissue demonstrating small vessel vasculitis Measurement of serum cryoglobulins Exclusion of hepatitis B and C infections
Primary angiitis of the CNS	Conventional, CT, or MR angiographic evidence of CNS vasculitis Consideration of dura or brain biopsy
Benign angiitis of the CNS	Conventional, CT, or MR angiographic evidence of CNS vasculitis
Cogan syndrome	Ophthalmology and audiology evaluations Conventional, CT, or MR angiographic evidence of CNS or aortic vasculitis

CNS, central nervous system; CT, computed tomography; MR, magnetic resonance.

BIBLIOGRAPHY

Please visit the Nelson Textbook of Pediatrics *website at* *www.expertconsult.com* *for the complete bibliography.*

Chapter 162
Musculoskeletal Pain Syndromes

Kelly K. Anthony and Laura E. Schanberg

Musculoskeletal pain is a frequent complaint of children presenting to general pediatricians and is the most common presenting problem of children referred to pediatric rheumatology clinics. Prevalence estimates of persistent musculoskeletal pain in community samples range from roughly 10% to 30%. Although diseases such as juvenile idiopathic arthritis and systemic lupus erythematosus (SLE) may manifest as persistent musculoskeletal pain, the majority of musculoskeletal pain complaints in children are benign in nature and attributable to trauma, overuse, and normal variations in skeletal growth. There is a subset of children in whom chronic pain complaints develop that persist in the absence of physical and laboratory abnormalities. Children with idiopathic musculoskeletal pain syndromes also typically have marked subjective distress and functional impairment. The treatment of children with musculoskeletal pain syndromes optimally includes both pharmacologic and nonpharmacologic interventions.

CLINICAL MANIFESTATIONS

All chronic musculoskeletal pain syndromes involve pain complaints of at least 3 mo in duration in the absence of objective abnormalities on physical examination and laboratory screening. Additionally, children and adolescents with musculoskeletal pain syndromes often complain of persistent pain despite previous treatment with nonsteroidal anti-inflammatory drugs and analgesic agents. The location varies, with pain complaints either localized to a single extremity or more diffuse and involving multiple extremities. The prevalence of musculoskeletal pain syndromes increases with age and is higher in females, thus rendering adolescent girls at highest risk.

The pain complaints of children and adolescents with musculoskeletal pain syndromes are commonly accompanied by psychologic distress, sleep difficulties, and functional impairment throughout home, school, and peer domains. Psychologic distress can include symptoms of anxiety and depression, such as frequent crying spells, fatigue, sleep disturbance, feelings of worthlessness, poor concentration, and frequent worry. Indeed, a substantial number of children with musculoskeletal pain syndromes display the full range of psychologic symptoms, warranting an additional diagnosis of a comorbid mood or anxiety disorder (e.g., major depressive episode, generalized anxiety disorder). **Sleep disturbance** in children with musculoskeletal pain syndromes may include difficulty falling asleep, multiple night awakenings, disrupted sleep-wake cycles with increased daytime sleeping, nonrestorative sleep, and fatigue.

For children and adolescents with musculoskeletal pain syndromes, the constellation of pain, psychologic distress, and sleep disturbance often leads to a high degree of functional impairment. Poor school attendance is common, and children may struggle to complete other daily activities relating to self-care and participation in household chores. Peer relationships may also be disrupted because of decreased opportunities for social interaction due to pain. Therefore, children and adolescents with musculoskeletal pain syndromes often report loneliness and social isolation, characterized by having few friends and lack of participation in extracurricular activities.

DIAGNOSIS AND DIFFERENTIAL DIAGNOSIS

The diagnosis of a musculoskeletal pain syndrome is typically one of exclusion when careful, repeated physical examinations and laboratory testing do not reveal an etiology. At initial presentation, all children with pain complaints require a thorough clinical history and a complete physical examination to look for an obvious etiology (e.g., sprains, strains, or fractures), characteristics of the pain (localized or diffuse), and evidence of systemic involvement. A comprehensive history can be particularly useful in providing clues to the possibility of underlying illness or systemic disease. The presence of current or recent fever can be indicative of an inflammatory or neoplastic process if the pain is also accompanied by worsening symptoms over time or weight loss.

Subsequent, repeated physical examinations of children with musculoskeletal pain complaints may reveal eventual development and manifestations of rheumatic or other diseases. The need for additional testing should be individualized, depending on the specific symptoms and physical findings. Laboratory screening and/or radiographs should be pursued if there is suspicion of certain underlying disease processes. Possible indicators of a serious, as opposed to a benign, cause of musculoskeletal pain include pain present at rest and relieved by activity, objective evidence of joint swelling on physical examination, stiffness or limited range of motion in joints, bony tenderness, muscle weakness, poor growth and/or weight loss, and constitutional symptoms (e.g., fever, malaise) (Table 162-1). Results of complete blood count and erythrocyte sedimentation rate (ESR) measurement are likely to be abnormal in children whose pain is secondary to a bone or joint infection, SLE, or a malignancy. Bone tumors, fractures, and other focal pathology resulting from infection, malignancy, or trauma can often be indentified through imaging studies, including plain radiographs, MRI, and technetium Tc 99m bone scans.

The presence of persistent pain accompanied by psychologic distress, sleep disturbances, and/or functional impairment and in the absence of objective abnormal laboratory or physical findings suggests the diagnosis of a musculoskeletal pain syndrome. All pediatric musculoskeletal pain syndromes share this general constellation of symptoms at presentation. Several more specific pain syndromes routinely seen by pediatric practitioners can be differentiated by anatomic region and associated symptoms. A comprehensive list of pediatric musculoskeletal pain syndromes is provided in Table 162-2; they include growing pains (Chapter 147), fibromyalgia (Chapter 162.1), complex regional pain syndrome (Chapter 162.2), localized pain syndromes, low back

Table 162-1 POTENTIAL INDICATORS OF BENIGN VS SERIOUS CAUSES OF MUSCULOSKELETAL PAIN

CLINICAL FINDING	BENIGN CAUSE	SERIOUS CAUSE
Effects of rest vs activity on pain	Relieved by rest and worsened by activity	Relieved by activity and present at rest
Time of day pain occurs	End of the day and nights	Morning*
Objective joint swelling	No	Yes
Joint characteristics	Hypermobile/normal	Stiffness, limited range of motion
Bony tenderness	No	Yes
Muscle strength	Normal	Diminished
Growth	Normal growth pattern or weight gain	Poor growth and/or weight loss
Constitutional symptoms (e.g., fever, malaise)	Fatigue without other constitutional symptoms	Yes
Laboratory findings	Normal CBC, ESR, CRP	Abnormal CBC, raised ESR and CRP
Radiographic findings	Normal	Effusion, osteopenia, radiolucent metaphyseal lines, joint space loss, bony destruction

*Cancer pain is often severe and worst at night.
CBC, complete blood count; CRP, C-reactive protein level; ESR, erythrocyte sedimentation rate.
Adapted from Malleson PN, Beauchamp RD: Diagnosing musculoskeletal pain in children, *Can Med Assoc J* 165:183–188, 2001.

Table 162-2 COMMON MUSCULOSKELETAL PAIN SYNDROMES IN CHILDREN BY ANATOMIC REGION

ANATOMIC REGION	PAIN SYNDROME(S)
Shoulder	Impingement syndrome
Elbow	Little League elbow Avulsion fractures Osteochondritis dissecans Tennis elbow Panner disease
Arm	Localized hypermobility syndrome Complex regional pain syndrome
Pelvis and hip	Avulsion injuries Congenital hip dysplasia Legg-Calve-Perthes disease Slipped capital femoral epiphysis
Knee	Osteochondritis dissecans Osgood-Schlatter disease Sinding-Larsen syndrome Patellofemoral syndrome Malalignment syndromes
Leg	Growing pains Complex regional pain syndrome Localized hypermobility syndrome Shin splints Stress fractures Compartment syndromes
Foot	Plantar fasciitis Tarsal coalition Stress fractures Achilles tendinitis Juvenile bunion
Spine	Musculoskeletal strain Spondylolisthesis Spondylolysis Scoliosis Scheuermann disease (kyphosis) Low back pain
Generalized	Hypermobility syndrome Juvenile fibromyalgia Generalized pain syndrome

Adapted from Anthony KK, Schanberg LE: Assessment and management of pain syndromes and arthritis pain in children and adolescents, *Rheum Dis Clin N Am* 33:625–660, 2007.

pain, and chronic sports-related pain syndromes (e.g., Osgood-Schlatter disease).

TREATMENT

The primary goal of treatment for pediatric musculoskeletal pain syndromes is to improve function, and the secondary goal is to relieve pain, although these two desirable outcomes may not occur simultaneously. Indeed, it is common for children with musculoskeletal pain syndromes to continue complaining of pain even as they resume normal function (e.g., increased school attendance and participation in extracurricular activities). For all children and adolescents with pediatric musculoskeletal pain syndromes, regular school attendance is crucial, because school attendance is a hallmark of normal functioning in this age group. The dual nature of treatment targeting both function and pain needs to be clearly explained to children and their families to better define the goals by which treatment successes will be measured.

Recommended treatment modalities typically include physical and/or occupational therapy, pharmacologic interventions, and cognitive-behavioral and/or other psychotherapeutic interventions. The overarching goal of physical therapy is to improve children's physical function and should emphasize participation in aggressive, but graduated aerobic exercise. Pharmacologic interventions should be used judiciously. Low-dose tricyclic antidepressants (amitriptyline 10-50 mg orally 30 min before bedtime) are indicated for treatment of sleep disturbance, whereas the use of selective serotonin reuptake inhibitors (sertraline 10-20 mg daily) may prove useful in treating depression and anxiety if present. Referral for psychologic evaluation is warranted if these symptoms do not resolve with initial treatment efforts or if suicidal ideation is present. Cognitive-behavioral and/or other psychotherapeutic interventions are typically designed to teach children and adolescents coping skills for controlling the behavioral, cognitive, and physiologic responses to pain. Specific components often include cognitive restructuring, relaxation, distraction, and problem-solving skills; additional targets of therapy include sleep hygiene and activity scheduling, all with the goal of restoring normal sleep patterns and activities of daily living. Family-based approaches may be necessary if barriers to treatment success are identified at the family level. Examples of such barriers are parenting strategies or family dynamics that serve to maintain children's pain complaints and maladaptive models for pain coping in the family.

COMPLICATIONS AND PROGNOSIS

Musculoskeletal pain syndromes can negatively affect both child development and future role functioning. Worsening pain and the associated symptoms of depression and anxiety can lead to substantial school absences, peer isolation, and developmental delays later in adolescence and early adulthood. Specifically, adolescents with musculoskeletal pain syndromes may fail to achieve the level of autonomy and independence necessary for age-appropriate activities such as attending college, living away from home, and maintaining a job. Fortunately, not all children and adolescents with musculoskeletal pain syndromes experience this degree of impairment, and the likelihood of positive health outcomes is increased with multidisciplinary treatment.

GROWING PAINS

Also known as benign nocturnal pains of childhood, growing pains affect 10-20% of children, with a peak age incidence between 4 and 8 yr. The most common cause of recurrent musculoskeletal pain in children, growing pains are intermittent and bilateral, predominantly affecting the anterior thigh and calf but not joints. Children most commonly describe cramping or aching that occurs in the late afternoon or evening. Pain often wakes the child from sleep but resolves quickly with massage or analgesics; pain is never present the following morning (Table 162-3). Physical findings are normal, and gait is not impaired. Growing pains are generally considered a benign, time-limited condition; however, there is increasing evidence suggesting that growing pains represent a pain amplification syndrome. Indeed, growing pains persist in a significant percentage of children, with some children developing other pain syndromes such as abdominal pain and headaches. Recent studies suggest that growing pains are more likely to persist in children with a parent who has a history of a pain syndrome and in children who have lower pain thresholds. Treatment focuses on reassurance, education, and healthy sleep hygiene.

Table 162-3 DEFINITION OF "GROWING PAINS"

	INCLUSIONS	EXCLUSIONS
Nature of pain	Intermittent; some pain-free days and nights	Persistent; increasing intensity
Unilateral or bilateral	Bilateral	Unilateral
Location of pain	Anterior thigh, calf, posterior knee—in muscles	Join pain
Onset of pain	Late afternoon or evening	Pain still present next morning
Physical findings	Normal	Swelling, erythema, tenderness; local trauma or infection; reduced joint range of motion; limping
Laboratory findings	Normal	Objective evidence of abnormalities, e.g., from erythrocyte sedimentation rate, radiography, bone scanning

From Evans AM, Scutter SD: Prevalence of "growing pains" in young children, *J Pediatr* 145:255–258, 2004.

BIBLIOGRAPHY

Please visit the Nelson Textbook of Pediatrics *website at www.expertconsult.com for the complete bibliography.*

162.1 Fibromyalgia

Kelly K. Anthony and Laura E. Schanberg

Juvenile primary fibromyalgia syndrome (JPFS) is a common pediatric musculoskeletal pain syndrome. Approximately 25-40% of children with chronic pain syndromes can be diagnosed with JPFS. Although specific diagnostic criteria for JPFS have not been determined, all children and adolescents with JPFS have diffuse musculoskeletal pain in at least 3 areas of the body that persists for at least 3 mo in the absence of an underlying condition. Results of laboratory tests are normal, and physical examination reveals at least 5 well-defined tender points (Fig. 162-1). Children and adolescents with JPFS also present with many associated symptoms, including nonrestorative sleep, fatigue, chronic anxiety or tension, chronic headaches, subjective soft tissue swelling, and pain modulated by physical activity, weather, and anxiety or stress. There is considerable overlap among the symptoms associated with JPFS and the complaints associated with other **functional disorders** (e.g., irritable bowel disease, migraines, temporomandibular joint disorder, premenstrual syndrome, mood and anxiety disorders, and chronic fatigue syndrome), raising speculation that these disorders may be part of a larger spectrum of related syndromes.

Although the precise cause of JPFS is unknown, there is an emerging understanding that the development and maintenance of JPFS are related both to biologic and psychologic factors. JPFS

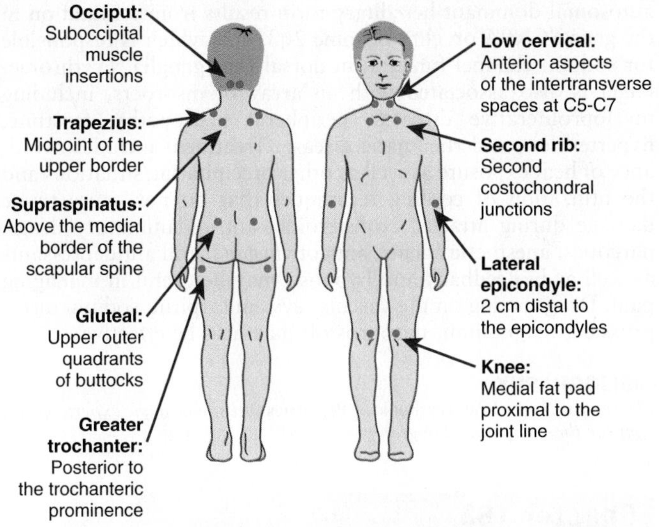

Figure 162-1 Fibromyalgia tender points.

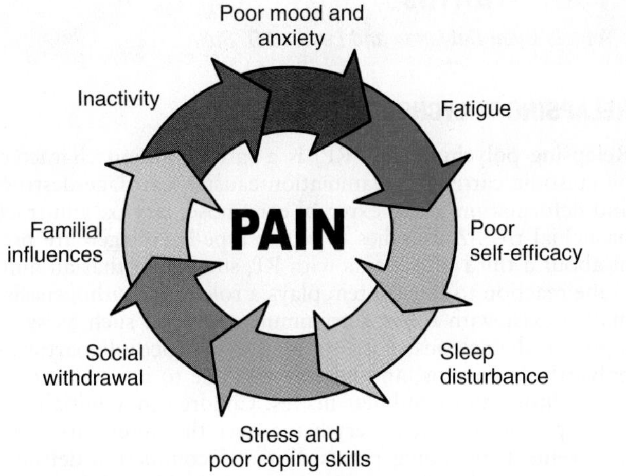

Figure 162-2 Cycle promoting juvenile primary fibromyalgia syndrome symptoms and their maintenance. (Adapted from Anthony KK, Schanberg LE: Juvenile primary fibromyalgia syndrome, *Curr Rheumatol Rep* 3:162–171, 2001.)

is an abnormality of pain processing characterized by disordered sleep physiology, enhanced pain perception with abnormal levels of substance P in cerebrospinal fluid, disordered mood, and dysregulation of hypothalamic-pituitary-adrenal and other neuroendocrine axes resulting in lower tender point pain thresholds and increased pain sensitivity. Children and adolescents with fibromyalgia also often find themselves in a vicious cycle of pain, whereby symptoms build on one another and contribute to the onset and maintenance of new symptoms (Fig. 162-2).

JPFS has a chronic course that can detrimentally affect child health and development. Adolescents with JPFS who do not receive treatment or are inadequately treated may withdraw from school and the social milieu, complicating their transition to adulthood. Treatment of JPFS generally follows consensus statements of the American Pain Society. The major goals are to restore function and to alleviate pain, and treatment should address comorbid mood and sleep disorders. Treatment strategies include parent/child education, pharmacologic interventions, exercise-based interventions, and psychologic interventions. Graduated aerobic exercise is the recommended exercise-based intervention, whereas psychologic interventions should include training in pain coping skills, stress management skills, and sleep hygiene. Drug therapies, although partially unsuccessful in isolation, may include tricyclic antidepressants (amitriptyline 10-50 mg orally 30 minutes before bedtime), selective serotonin reuptake inhibitors (sertraline 10-20 mg daily), and anticonvulsants. Pregabalin was approved by the U.S. Food and Drug Administration (FDA) for treatment of fibromyalgia in adults but has not yet been studied in children. Muscle relaxants are generally not used in children, because they often adversely affect school performance.

Table 162-4 DIAGNOSTIC CRITERIA FOR COMPLEX REGIONAL PAIN SYNDROME

A diagnosis of complex regional pain syndrome (CRPS) requires regional pain, sensory symptoms, *plus* two neuropathic pain descriptors and two physical signs of autonomic dysfunction:
NEUROPATHIC DESCRIPTORS
Burning
Dysesthesia
Paresthesia
Allodynia
Cold hyperalgesia
AUTONOMIC DYSFUNCTION
Cyanosis
Mottling
Hyperhidrosis
Coolness (≥3°F)
Edema

Data from Wilder RT, Berde CB, Wolohan, M, et al: Reflex sympathetic dystrophy in children: clinical characteristics and follow-up of seventy patients, *J Bone Joint Surg Am* 74:910–919, 1992.

BIBLIOGRAPHY

Please visit the Nelson Textbook of Pediatrics *website at www.expertconsult.com for the complete bibliography.*

162.2 Complex Regional Pain Syndrome

Kelly K. Anthony and Laura E. Schanberg

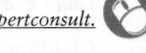

Complex regional pain syndrome (CRPS) is characterized by ongoing burning limb pain that is subsequent to an injury, immobilization, or another noxious event affecting the extremity. CRPS1, formerly called reflex sympathetic dystrophy, has no evidence of nerve injury, whereas CRPS2, formerly called causalgia, follows a prior nerve injury. Key associated features are pain disproportionate to the inciting event, persisting **allodynia** (a heightened pain response to normally non-noxious stimuli), **hyperalgesia** (exaggerated pain reactivity to noxious stimuli), swelling of distal extremities, and indicators of **autonomic dysfunction** (i.e., cyanosis, mottling, and hyperhidrosis) (Table 162-4).

The diagnosis requires the following: an initiating noxious event or immobilization; continued pain, allodynia, hyperalgesia out of proportion to the inciting event; evidence of edema, skin blood flow abnormalities, or sudomotor activity; and exclusion of other disorders. Associated features include atrophy of hair or nails; altered hair growth; loss of joint mobility; weakness, tremor, dystonia; and sympathetically maintained pain.

Although the majority of pediatric patients with CRPS present with a history of immobilization or minor trauma or repeated stress injury (e.g., caused by competitive sports), a sizeable proportion are unable to identify a precipitating event. Usual age of onset is between 9 and 15 yr, and girls with the disease outnumber boys with the disease by as much as 6:1. Childhood CRPS differs from the adult form in that lower extremities rather than upper extremities are most commonly affected. The incidence of CRPS in children is unknown, largely because it is often undiagnosed or diagnosed late, with the diagnosis frequently delayed by nearly a year. Left untreated, CRPS can have severe consequences for children, including bone demineralization, muscle wasting, and joint contractures.

The treatment of CRPS involves a multistage treatment approach. Aggressive physical therapy should be initiated as soon as the diagnosis is made, and cognitive-behavioral therapy (CBT) should be added as needed. Physical therapy is recommended 3 or 4 times/wk, and children may need analgesic premedication at the onset. Physical therapy is initially limited to desensitization and then moves to weight-bearing, range-of-motion, and other functional activities. CBT used as an adjunctive therapy targets psychosocial obstacles to fully participating in physical therapy and provides pain coping skills training. Sympathetic and epidural nerve blocks should be attempted only in refractory cases and only under the auspices of a pediatric pain specialist. The intent of both pharmacologic and adjunctive treatments for CRPS is to provide sufficient pain relief to allow the child to participate in aggressive physical rehabilitation. If CRPS is identified and treated early, the majority of children and adolescents with the disease can be treated successfully with low-dose amitriptyline (10-50 mg orally 30 minutes prior to bedtime), aggressive physical therapy, and CBT. Opioids and anticonvulsants such as gabapentin can also be helpful. Notably, multiple studies have shown that noninvasive treatments, particularly physical therapy and CBT, are at least as efficacious as nerve blocks in children with CRPS.

BIBLIOGRAPHY

Please visit the Nelson Textbook of Pediatrics *website at* *www.expertconsult.com* *for the complete bibliography.*

162.3 Erythromelalgia

Laura E. Schanberg

Children with **erythromelalgia** experience episodes of intense pain, erythema, and heat in their hands and feet (Fig. 162-3) and less commonly in their face, ears, or knees. Symptoms may be triggered by exercise and exposure to heat, and they last for hours and occasionally for days. Although most cases are sporadic, an autosomal dominant hereditary form results from a mutation in the gene *SCN9A* on chromosome 2q31-32, which is responsible for sodium channel function in dorsal root ganglia. Erythromelalgia is also associated with an array of disorders, including myeloproliferative diseases, peripheral neuropathy, frostbite, hypertension, and rheumatic disease. Treatment includes avoidance of heat exposure as well as other precipitating situations and the utilization of cooling techniques that do not cause tissue damage during attacks. Nonsteroidal anti-inflammatory drugs, narcotics, anesthetic agents, anticonvulsants, and antidepressants as well as biofeedback and hypnosis may be useful in managing pain. Drugs acting on the vascular system (aspirin, sodium nitroprusside, magnesium, misoprostol) may also be effective.

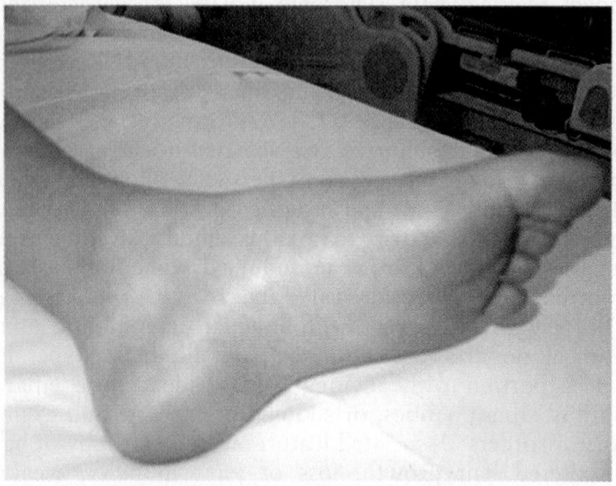

Figure 162-3 Typical redness and edema of the foot in erythromelalgia. (From Pfund Z, Stankovics J, Decsi T, et al: Childhood steroid-responsive acute erythromelalgia with axonal neuropathy of large myelinated fibers: a dysimmune neuropathy? *Neuromusc Disord* 19:49–52, 2009.)

BIBLIOGRAPHY

Please visit the Nelson Textbook of Pediatrics *website at* *www.expertconsult.com* *for the complete bibliography.*

Chapter 163
Miscellaneous Conditions Associated with Arthritis

Angela Byun Robinson and Leonard D. Stein

RELAPSING POLYCHONDRITIS

Relapsing polychondritis (RP) is a rare condition characterized by episodic cartilage inflammation causing cartilage destruction and deformation in the external ears, nose, larynx, and tracheobronchial tree. Antibodies to native type II collagen are present in about a third of patients with RP, suggesting that an autoimmune reaction to this protein plays a role in its pathogenesis. RP may coexist with other autoimmune diseases, such as systemic lupus erythematosus. Patients may experience oligoarthritis or polyarthritis, uveitis, and hearing loss due to inflammation near the auditory and vestibular nerves. Children may initially relate only episodes of intense erythema over the outer ears. Cardiac involvement, including pericarditis and conduction defects, has been reported. Diagnostic criteria established for adults are useful guidelines for evaluating children with suggestive symptoms (see Table 163-1 on the *Nelson Textbook of Pediatrics* website at www.expertconsult.com). The differential diagnosis includes Wegener granulomatosis (Chapter 161.4) and Cogan syndrome, which is characterized by auditory nerve inflammation and keratitis but not chondritis. The clinical course of RP is variable, and flares may remit spontaneously. Flares of disease are often associated with elevations of erythrocyte sedimentation rate (ESR). Many cases respond to nonsteroidal anti-inflammatory drugs, but some require corticosteroids or other immunosuppressive agents (azathioprine, methotrexate, hydroxychloroquine, colchicine, cyclophosphamide, cyclosporine, and anti–tumor necrosis factor [TNF] agents), as reported in small series and case reports. Severe, progressive, and potentially fatal disease resulting from destruction of the tracheobronchial tree and airway obstruction is unusual in childhood.

For the full continuation of this chapter, please visit the Nelson Textbook of Pediatrics *website at* *www.expertconsult.com.*

PART XVII Infectious Diseases

Section 1 GENERAL CONSIDERATIONS

Chapter 164
Diagnostic Microbiology

Anita K.M. Zaidi and Donald A. Goldmann

Laboratory diagnosis of infectious diseases is based on one or more of the following: direct examination of specimens by microscopic or antigenic techniques, isolation of microorganisms in culture, serologic testing for development of antibodies **(serodiagnosis)**, and molecular detection of the pathogen's genome (DNA, RNA). Clinicians must select the appropriate tests and specimens and, when possible, suggest the suspected etiologic agents to the microbiologist, because this information facilitates selection of the most cost-effective diagnostic approach. Additional roles of the microbiology laboratory include testing for antimicrobial drug susceptibility and assisting the hospital epidemiologist in detecting and clarifying the epidemiology of nosocomial infections.

For the full continuation of this chapter, please visit the Nelson Textbook of Pediatrics *website at www.expertconsult.com.*

Section 2 PREVENTIVE MEASURES

Chapter 165
Immunization Practices

Walter A. Orenstein and Larry K. Pickering

Immunization is one of the most beneficial and cost-effective disease-prevention measures. As a result of effective and safe vaccines, smallpox has been eradicated, polio is close to worldwide eradication, and measles and rubella are no longer endemic in the USA. The incidence of most other vaccine-preventable diseases of childhood has been reduced by ≥99% from the annual morbidity prior to development of the corresponding vaccine (Table 165-1). An analysis of effective prevention measures recommended for widespread use by the U.S. Preventive Services Task Force reported that childhood immunization received a perfect score, based on clinically preventable disease burden and cost-effectiveness.

Immunization is the process of inducing immunity against a specific disease. Immunity can be induced either **passively** through administration of antibody-containing preparations or **actively** by administering a vaccine or toxoid to stimulate the immune system to produce a prolonged humoral and/or cellular immune response. As of 2011, infants, children, and adolescents routinely are vaccinated against 16 diseases in the USA: diphtheria, tetanus, pertussis, poliomyelitis, *Haemophilus influenzae* type b (Hib) disease, hepatitis A (HepA), hepatitis B (HepB), measles, mumps, rubella, rotavirus, varicella, pneumococcal disease, meningococcal disease, and influenza. Human papillomavirus (HPV) vaccine has been recommended routinely for girls 11-12 yr of age, with catch-up for females through 26 yr of age. One of the HPV vaccines, HPV4, is recommended for permissive use in males age 11 through 18 yr for prevention of genital warts.

PASSIVE IMMUNITY

Passive immunity is achieved by administration of preformed antibodies to induce transient protection against an infectious agent. Products used include immunoglobulin (IG) administered intramuscularly (IM); specific or hyperimmune IG preparations administered IM; intravenous IG (IVIG); specific or hyperimmunoglobulin preparations administered IV; antibodies of

Table 165-1 REPRESENTATIVE 20TH CENTURY MORBIDITY, CASES IN 2009, AND CHANGE

DISEASE	20TH CENTURY ANNUAL CASES PRECEDING VACCINE DEVELOPMENT	2009 CASES	DECREASE (%)	HEALTHY PEOPLE 2010 COVERAGE GOAL FOR 19-35 MO OLD CHILDREN	COVERAGE JULY 2009
Smallpox	29,005	0	100*	—	—
Diphtheria	21,053	0	100*	4 doses, ≥90%	84%
Measles	503,217	71	>99	1 dose ≥90%	90%
Mumps	162,344	1,991	>99	1 dose, ≥90%	90%
Pertussis	200,752	16,858	92	4 doses, ≥90%	84%
Polio (paralytic)	19,794	1	>99	3 doses, ≥90%	93%
Rubella	47,745	3	>99	1 dose, ≥90%	90%
Congenital rubella syndrome	152	2	99	1 dose, ≥90%	90%
Tetanus	580	18	97	4 doses, ≥90%	84%
H. influenzae type b and unknown (<5 yr)	20,000	213	99	≥3 doses, ≥90%	84%

*Record lows.
Adapted from Roush SW, Murphy TV; Vaccine-Preventable Disease Table Working Group: Historical comparisons of morbidity and mortality for vaccine-preventable diseases in the United States, *JAMA* 298:2155–2163, 2007; and Hinman AR, et al: Vaccine preventable diseases and immunizations, *MMWR Morbid Mortal Wkly Rep* 60:2011 (in press).

animal origin; monoclonal antibodies; and subcutaneous (SC) human IG, which has been licensed to treat patients with primary immunodeficiencies. Passive immunity also can be induced naturally through transplacental transfer of maternal antibodies (IgG) during gestation. Maternally derived transplacental antibodies can provide protection during an infant's first month of life and longer during breast-feeding. Protection for some diseases can persist for as long as a year after birth.

The major indications for passive immunity are to provide protection to immunodeficient children with B-lymphocyte defects who have difficulties making antibodies, persons exposed to infectious diseases or who are at imminent risk of exposure where there is not adequate time for them to develop an active immune response to a vaccine, and persons with an infectious disease as part of specific therapy for that disease (Table 165-2).

Intramuscular Immunoglobulin

IG is a sterile antibody-containing solution, usually derived through cold ethanol fractionation of large pools of human plasma from adults. Antibody concentrations reflect the infectious disease exposure and immunization experience of plasma donors. IG contains 15-18% protein, is predominantly IgG, and is administered intramuscularly. Intravenous use of human intramuscular IG is contraindicated. IG is not known to transmit infectious agents, including viral hepatitis and HIV. The major indications for IG are replacement therapy for children with antibody deficiency disorders, and for passive immunization for measles and hepatitis A.

For replacement therapy, the usual dose of IG is 100 mg/kg or 0.66 mL/kg monthly. The usual interval between doses is 2-4 wk depending on trough IgG concentrations. In practice, **IVIG** has replaced IMIG for this indication. IG can be used to prevent or modify measles if administered to susceptible children within 6 days of exposure (usual dose, 0.25 mL/kg for immunocompetent children, 0.5 mL/kg for immunocompromised children; maximum dose 15 mL) and to prevent or modify HepA if administered to children within 14 days of exposure (usual dose, 0.02 mL/kg). IG also may be administered for prophylaxis of HepA for persons traveling internationally to HepA-endemic areas (0.06 mL/kg) and for children too young for HepA vaccination (<1 yr of age). In children <12 mo of age, adults >40 yr of age, and susceptible children and adults with underlying immunodeficiencies or chronic liver disease, IG is preferred over hepatitis A immunization. In people 12 mo-40 yr of age, HepA immunization is preferred over IG for postexposure prophylaxis and for protection of people traveling to areas where HepA is endemic.

The most common adverse reaction to IG is pain and discomfort at the injection site and, less commonly, flushing, headache, chills, and nausea. More-serious adverse events are rare and have included chest pain, dyspnea, anaphylaxis, and systemic collapse. Patients with selective IgA deficiency can produce antibodies against the trace amounts of IgA in IG preparations and develop reactions after repeat doses. These reactions can include fever, chills, and a shocklike syndrome. Because these reactions are rare, testing for selective IgA deficiencies is not recommended.

Table 165-2 IMMUNE GLOBULIN AND ANIMAL ANTISERA PREPARATIONS

PRODUCT	MAJOR INDICATIONS
Immune globulin for intramuscular injection	Replacement therapy in primary immunodeficiency disorders
	Hepatitis A prophylaxis
	Measles prophylaxis
Intravenous mmunoglobulin (IVIG)	Replacement therapy in primary immune-deficiency disorders
	Kawasaki disease
	Immune-mediated thrombocytopenia
	Pediatric HIV infection
	Hypogammaglobulinemia in chronic B-cell lymphocytic leukemia
	Hematopoietic cell transplantation in adults to prevent graft-versus host disease and infection
	May be useful in a variety of other conditions
Hepatitis B immune globulin (IM)	Postexposure prophylaxis
	Prevention of perinatal infection in infants born to $HBsAg^+$ mothers
Rabies immune globulin (IM)	Postexposure prophylaxis
Tetanus immune globulin (IM)	Wound prophylaxis
	Treatment of tetanus
Varicella-zoster immune globulin (VZIG) (IM) or IVIG	Postexposure prophylaxis of susceptible people at high risk for complications from varicella
Cytomegalovirus IVIG	Prophylaxis of disease in seronegative transplant recipients
Palivizumab (monoclonal antibody) (IM)	Prophylaxis for infants against respiratory syncytial virus (RSV) (Chapter 252)
Vaccinia immune globulin (IV)	Prevent or modify serious adverse events following smallpox vaccination due to vaccinia replication
Botulism IVIG human	Treatment of infant botulism
Diphtheria antitoxin, equine	Treatment of diphtheria
Trivalent botulinum (A,B,E) and bivalent (A,B) botulinum antitoxin, equine	Treatment of food and wound botulism

From Passive immunization. In Pickering LK, Baker CJ, Kimberlin DW, et al, editors: *Red book 2006: report of the Committee on Infectious Diseases*, ed 28, Elk Grove Village, IL, 2009, American Academy of Pediatrics.

Intravenous Immunoglobulin

IVIG is prepared from adult plasma donors using alcohol fractionation and is modified to allow IV use. IVIG is predominantly IgG and is tested to ensure minimum antibody titers to diphtheria, HepB, measles, and polio. Liquid and powder preparations are available. The major **recommended indications** for IVIG are replacement therapy for immunodeficiency disorders; treatment of Kawasaki disease to prevent coronary artery abnormalities and shorten the clinical course; prevention of serious bacterial infections in children with HIV; prevention of serious bacterial infections in persons with hypogammaglobulinemia in chronic B-cell leukemia; immune-mediated thrombocytopenia; and prophylaxis of infection following bone marrow transplantation. IVIG may be helpful for patients with severe toxic shock syndrome, Guillain-Barré syndrome, and anemia caused by parvovirus B19. IVIG is used for many other conditions based on clinical experience. It may be used for varicella postexposure if varicella-zoster immune globulin is not available.

Reactions to IVIG range from 1 to 15%. Some of these reactions appear to be related to the rate of infusion and can be mitigated by decreasing the rate. Such reactions include fever, headache, myalgia, chills, nausea, and vomiting. More serious reactions rarely have been reported, including anaphylactoid events, thromboembolic disorders, aseptic meningitis, and renal insufficiency.

Specific Immune Globulin Preparations

Hyperimmune globulin preparations are derived from donors with high titers of antibodies to specific agents and designed to provide protection against those agents (see Table 165-2).

Hyperimmune Animal Antisera Preparations

Animal antisera preparations are derived from horses. The IG fraction is concentrated using ammonium sulfate, and some products are further treated with enzymes to decrease reactions to foreign proteins. As of 2011, 2 horse antisera preparations are available for humans: diphtheria antitoxin, which is used to treat diphtheria, and botulinum antitoxin, which is available for use in adults with botulism but is not used in infants for whom botulism IVIG (Baby-BIG), a human-derived antitoxin, is licensed. Great care must be exercised before administering animal-derived antisera because of the potential for severe allergic reactions. This includes testing for sensitivity before administration; desensitization, if necessary; and treating potential reactions, including febrile events, serum sickness, and anaphylaxis.

Monoclonal Antibodies

Monoclonal antibodies are antibody preparations produced against a single antigen. They are mass-produced from a hybridoma, created by fusing an antibody-producing B cell with a fast-growing immortal cell such as a cancer cell. A major monoclonal antibody used in infectious diseases is palivizumab, which can prevent severe disease from respiratory syncytial virus (RSV) among children ≤24 mo of age with chronic lung disease (CLD, also called bronchopulmonary dysplasia), with a history of premature birth or with congenital heart lesions or with neuromuscular diseases. The American Academy of Pediatrics (AAP) has developed specific recommendations for use of palivizumab (Chapter 252). RSV-IVIG, a hyperimmune globulin formulated for intravenous administration, is no longer produced in the USA. Monoclonal antibodies also are used to prevent transplant rejection and to treat some types of cancer and autoimmune diseases. Monoclonal antibodies against interleukin 2 (IL-2) and tumor necrosis factor-α (TNF-α) are being used as part of the therapeutic approach to patients with a variety of malignant and autoimmune diseases.

Serious adverse events associated with palivizumab primarily are rare cases of anaphylaxis and hypersensitivity reactions. Adverse reactions to monoclonal antibodies directed at modifying the immune response, such as antibodies against IL-2 or TNF, can be more serious, such as cytokine release syndrome, fever, chills, tremors, chest pain, immunosuppression, and infection with various organisms, including mycobacteria.

ACTIVE IMMUNIZATION

Vaccines are defined as whole or parts of microorganisms administered to prevent an infectious disease. Vaccines can consist of whole inactivated microorganisms (e.g., polio and HepA), parts of the organism (e.g., acellular pertussis, HPV, and HepB), polysaccharide capsules (e.g., pneumococcal and meningococcal polysaccharide vaccines), polysaccharide capsules conjugated to protein carriers (e.g., Hib, pneumococcal, and meningococcal conjugate vaccines), live-attenuated microorganisms (measles, mumps, rubella, varicella, rotavirus, and live-attenuated influenza vaccines), and toxoids (tetanus and diphtheria) (Table 165-3). A **toxoid** is a modified bacterial toxin that is made nontoxic but is still able to induce an active immune response against the toxin.

Immunizing agents can contain a variety of other constituents besides the immunizing antigen. **Suspending fluids** may be sterile water or saline but could be a complex fluid containing small amounts of proteins or other constituents derived from the biologic system used to grow the immunobiologic. **Preservatives, stabilizers,** and **antimicrobial agents** are used to inhibit bacterial growth and to prevent degradation of the antigen. Such components can include gelatin, 2-phenoxyethanol, and specific antimicrobial agents. Preservatives are added to multidose vials of vaccines, primarily to prevent bacterial contamination on repeated entry of the vial. In the past, many vaccines for children contained thimerosal, a preservative containing ethyl mercury. Beginning in 1999, removal of thimerosal as a preservative from vaccines for children was begun as a precautionary measure in the absence of any data on harm from the preservative. This objective was accomplished by switching to single-dose packaging. The only vaccines in the recommended schedule for young children that contain thimerosal as a preservative are some preparations of influenza vaccine. **Adjuvants** are used in some vaccines to enhance the immune response. In the USA, the only adjuvants currently licensed by the Food and Drug Administration (FDA) to be part of vaccines are aluminum salts and ASO4, an adjuvant that contains aluminum hydroxide and monophosphoryl lipid A. Vaccines with adjuvants should be injected deep into muscle masses to avoid local irritation, granuloma formation, and necrosis associated with SC or intracutaneous administration.

Vaccines can induce immunity by stimulating antibody formation, cellular immunity, or both. Protection induced by most vaccines is thought to be mediated primarily by B lymphocytes, which produce antibody. Such antibodies can inactivate toxins, neutralize viruses, and prevent their attachment to cellular receptors, facilitate phagocytosis and killing of bacteria, interact with complement to lyse bacteria, and prevent adhesion to mucosal surfaces by interacting with the bacterial cell surface.

Most B-lymphocyte responses require the assistance of CD4 helper T lymphocytes. These T lymphocyte–dependent responses tend to induce high levels of functional antibody with high avidity, mature over time from primarily an IgM response to long-term persistent IgG, and induce immunologic memory that leads to enhanced responses upon boosting. **T lymphocyte–dependent vaccines,** which include protein moieties, induce good immune responses even in young infants. In contrast, polysaccharide antigens induce B-lymphocyte responses in the absence of T-lymphocyte help. These **T lymphocyte–independent vaccines** are associated with poor immune responses in children <2 yr of age, short-term immunity, and absence of an enhanced or booster response on repeat exposure to the antigen. To overcome problems of plain polysaccharide vaccines, polysaccharides have been **conjugated,** or covalently linked, to protein carriers, converting the vaccine to a T lymphocyte–dependent vaccine. In contrast to plain polysaccharide vaccines, conjugate vaccines induce higher avidity antibody, immunologic memory leading to booster responses on repeat exposure to the antigen, long-term immunity, and herd immunity by decreasing carriage of the organism. As of 2009 in the USA, there were licensed conjugate vaccines to prevent Hib and pneumococcal and meningococcal diseases.

Serum antibodies may be detected as soon as 7-10 days after injection of antigen. Early antibodies are usually of the IgM class that can fix complement. IgM antibodies tend to decline as IgG antibodies increase. The IgG antibodies tend to peak approximately 1 mo after vaccination and with most vaccines persist for some time after a primary vaccine course. Secondary or booster responses occur more rapidly and result from rapid proliferation of memory B and T lymphocytes.

Assessment of the immune response to most vaccines is performed by measuring serum antibodies. Although detection of serum antibody at levels considered protective after vaccination can indicate immunity, loss of detectable antibody over time does not necessarily mean susceptibility to disease. Some vaccines induce immunologic memory, leading to a booster or anamnestic response on exposure to the microorganism, leading to protection from disease. In some instances, cellular immune response is used to evaluate immune status. For some vaccines (e.g., acellular pertussis), there is no accepted serologic correlate of protection.

Live-attenuated vaccines routinely recommended for children and adolescents include measles, mumps, and rubella (MMR); rotavirus; and varicella. In addition, a cold-adapted live-attenuated influenza vaccine (LAIV) is available as an alternative to the trivalent inactivated influenza vaccine (TIV) for children 2-18 yr of age who do not have conditions that place them at high risk for complications from influenza. Live-attenuated vaccines tend to induce long-term immune responses. They replicate,

Table 165-3 CURRENTLY AVAILABLE VACCINES IN THE USA BY TYPE

PRODUCT	TYPE
Anthrax vaccine adsorbed	Cell free filtrate of components including protective antigen
Bacille Calmette-Guérin (BCG) vaccine	Live-attenuated mycobacterial strain used prevent tuberculosis in very limited circumstances
Diphtheria and tetanus toxoids and acellular pertussis (DTaP) vaccine	Toxoids of diphtheria and tetanus and purified and detoxified components from *Bordetella pertussis*
DTaP with *Haemophilus influenzae* type b (DTaP/Hib)	DTaP and Hib polysaccharide conjugated to tetanus toxoid
DTaP–hepatitis B–inactivated polio vaccine (DTaP-HepB-IPV)	DTaP with hepatitis B surface antigen produced through recombinant techniques in yeast with inactivated whole polioviruses
DTaP with IPV and Hib (DTaP-IPV/Hib)	DTaP with inactivated whole polio viruses and Hib polysaccharide conjugated to tetanus toxoid
DTaP and inactivated polio vaccine (DTaP-IPV)	DTaP with inactivated whole polio viruses
Hib conjugate vaccine (Hib)	Polysaccharide conjugated to either tetanus toxoid or meningococcal group B outer membrane protein
Hepatitis A vaccine (HepA)	Inactivated whole virus
Hepatitis A-hepatitis B vaccine (HepA-HepB)	Combined hepatitis A and B vaccine
Hepatitis B vaccine (HepB)	HBsAg produced through recombinant techniques in yeast
Hepatitis B-Hib vaccine (Hib-HepB)	Combined hepatitis B–Hib vaccine; the Hib component is polysaccharide conjugated to meningococcal group B outer membrane protein
Human papillomavirus vaccine (bivalent) (HPV2) and (quadrivalent) (HPV4)	The L1 capsid proteins of HPV types 6, 11, 16, 18 and to prevent cervical cancer and genital warts (HPV4) and types 16 and 18 to prevent cervical cancer (HPV2)
Influenza virus vaccine inactivated (TIV)	Trivalent (A/H_3N_2, A/H_1N_1, and B) split and purified inactivated vaccine containing the hemagglutinin (H) and neuraminidase (N) of each type and other components
Influenza virus vaccine live, intranasal (LAIV)	Live-attenuated, temperature-sensitive, cold-adapted trivalent vaccine containing the H and N genes from the wild strains reassorted to have the 6 other genes from the cold-adapted parent
Japanese encephalitis vaccine	Inactivated whole virus that is purified
Measles, mumps, rubella (MMR) vaccine	Live-attenuated viruses
Measles, mumps, rubella, varicella (MMRV) vaccine	Live-attenuated viruses
Meningococcal conjugate vaccine against serogroups A, C, W135, and Y (MCV4)	Polysaccharide from each serogroup conjugated to diphtheria toxoid or CRM 197
Meningococcal polysaccharide vaccine against serogroups A, C, W135, and Y (MPSV4)	Polysaccharides from each of the serogroups
Pneumococcal conjugate vaccine (13 valent) (PCV13)	Pneumococcal polysaccharides conjugated to a nontoxic form of diphtheria toxin CRM197 Contains 13 serotypes that accounted for >80% of invasive disease in young children prior to vaccine licensure.
Pneumococcal polysaccharide vaccine (23 valent) (PPSV23)	Pneumococcal polysaccharides of 23 serotypes responsible for 85-90% of bacteremic disease in the USA
Poliomyelitis (inactivated, enhanced potency) (IPV)	Inactivated whole virus
Rabies vaccines (human diploid and purified chick embryo cell)	Inactivated whole virus
Rotavirus vaccines (RV5 and RV1)	Bovine rotavirus pentavalent vaccine (RV-5) live reassortment attenuated virus, and human live-attenuated virus (RV1)
Smallpox vaccine	Vaccinia virus, an attenuated pox virus that provides cross-protection against smallpox
Tetanus and diphtheria toxoids, adsorbed (Td, adult use)	Tetanus toxoid plus a reduced quantity of diphtheria toxoid compared to diphtheria toxoid used for children <7 yr of age
Tetanus and diphtheria toxoids adsorbed plus acellular pertussis (Tdap) vaccine	Tetanus toxoid plus a reduced quantity of diphtheria toxoid plus acellular pertussis vaccine to be used in adolescents and adults and in children 7 through 9 yr of age who have not been appropriately immunized with DTaP
Typhoid vaccine (polysaccharide)	Vi capsular polysaccharide of *Salmonella typhi*
Typhoid vaccine (oral)	Live-attenuated Ty21a strain of *Salmonella typhi*
Varicella vaccine	Live-attenuated Oka strain
Yellow fever vaccine	Live-attenuated 17D strain

Data from Centers for Disease Control and Prevention: *U.S. vaccine names* (website). www.cdc.gov/vaccines/about/terms/USvaccines.html. Accessed March 4, 2011.

often similar to natural infections, until an immune response shuts down reproduction. Most live vaccines are administered in 1- or 2-dose schedules. The purpose of repeat doses, such as a second dose of the MMR vaccine, is to induce an initial immune response in persons who failed to respond to the first dose.

The remaining vaccines in the recommended schedule for children and adolescents are inactivated vaccines. Inactivated vaccines tend to require multiple doses to induce an adequate immune response and are more likely to need booster doses to maintain that immunity than live-attenuated vaccines. However, some inactivated vaccines appear to induce long-term immunity, perhaps life-long immunity, after a primary series, including HepB vaccine and inactivated polio vaccine (IPV).

VACCINATION SYSTEM IN THE USA

Vaccine Development

Basic scientific knowledge about an organism, its pathogenesis, and the immune responses thought to be associated with protection are financed primarily through government sponsorship of academic research, although private industry plays a major role (Fig. 165-1). Private industry usually assumes the lead role for guiding potential vaccine candidates through preclinical testing in humans into human clinical trials. There are three phases of prelicensure clinical trials: **phase I,** involving generally <100 participants to gauge safety and dosing; **phase II,** involving several hundred or more participants to refine safety and dosing; and

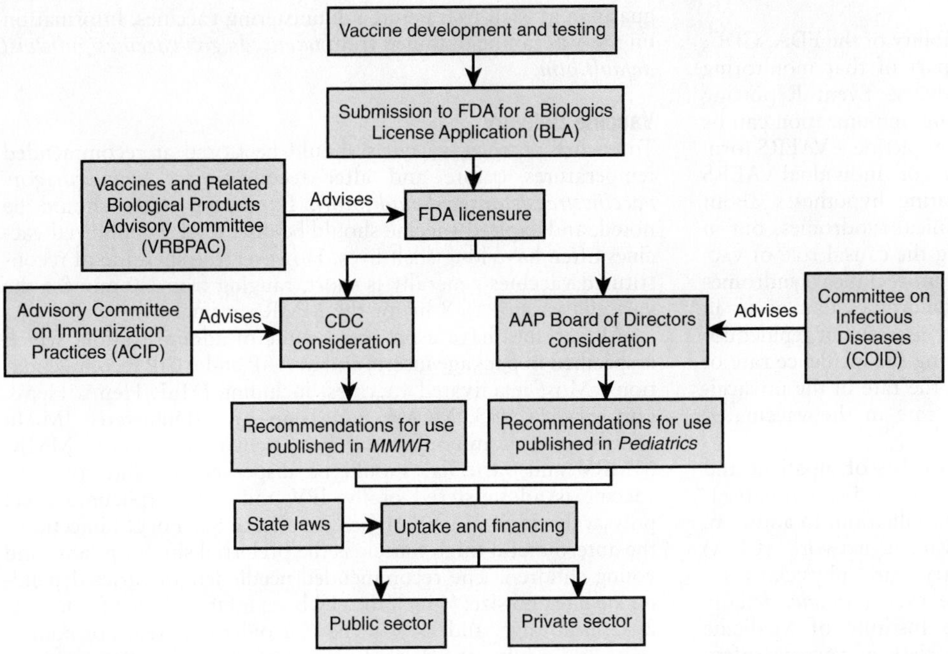

Figure 165-1 Vaccine development and testing. (Modified from Pickering LK, Orenstein WE: Development of pediatric vaccine recommendations and policies. *Semin Pediatr Infect Dis* 13[3]:148–154, 2002.)

phase III or pivotal trials that can involve thousands or tens of thousands of participants. Phase III trials are the major basis for licensure. Following successful clinical development, the sponsor applies to the FDA for vaccine licensure. Estimates for the cost of development for each vaccine range to $800 million or more. Following licensure by the FDA, postlicensure monitoring is performed on hundreds of thousands to millions of people to monitor safety and effectiveness.

Vaccine Production

Vaccine production is primarily a responsibility of private industry. Most of the vaccines recommended routinely for children are produced by only one of the vaccine manufacturers. Only Hib, HepB, HPV, rotavirus, MCV4, diphtheria and tetanus toxoids and acellular pertussis (DTaP), and tetanus and diphtheria toxoids and acellular pertussis (Tdap) vaccines for adolescents and adults have multiple manufacturers. IPV as an IPV-only vaccine has only 1 manufacturer, but IPV also is available in combination products DTaP-HepB-IPV, and DTaP-IPV from another manufacturer. Influenza vaccine for children ≤2 yr of age is produced by 2 manufacturers. MMR, MMRV, varicella, PCV13, and Td vaccines also are produced by manufacturers.

Vaccine Policy

There are 2 major committees that make vaccine policy recommendations for children: the Committee on Infectious Diseases (COID) of the AAP (the Red Book Committee) and the Advisory Committee on Immunization Practices (ACIP) of the Centers for Disease Control and Prevention (CDC). At least annually, the AAP, the ACIP, and the American Academy of Family Physicians (AAFP) issue a **harmonized** childhood and adolescent immunization schedule (*www.cdc.gov/vaccines/recs/schedules/default.htm*). The COID consists primarily of academic pediatric infectious disease specialists with liaisons from practicing pediatricians, professional organizations, and government agencies including the FDA, CDC, and National Institutes of Health (NIH). Recommendations of the COID must be approved by the AAP Board of Directors. The ACIP consists of 15 members who are academic infectious disease experts (for both children and adults), family physicians, state and local public health officials, nurses, and consumers. The ACIP also has extensive liaison representation from major medical societies, government agencies, managed care, and others. The AAP recommendations are published in the *Red Book* and in issues of *Pediatrics*. The ACIP recommendations, available at *www.cdc.gov/vaccines/pubs/ACIP-list.htm,* are official only after approval by the CDC director, which leads to publication in the *Morbidity and Mortality Weekly Report (MMWR)*.

Vaccine Financing

Between 55 and 60% of vaccines routinely administered to children and adolescents <19 yr of age are purchased thorough a contract negotiated by the federal government with licensed vaccine manufacturers. There are 3 major sources of funds that can purchase vaccines through this contract.

The greatest portion comes from the Vaccines for Children (VFC) program, a federal entitlement program. The VFC program covers children on Medicaid, children without any insurance (uninsured), and Native Americans and Alaska Natives. In addition, children who have insurance but whose insurance does not cover immunization (underinsured) can be covered through VFC, but only if they go to a federally qualified health center (FQHC) (*http://www.cms.gov/center/fqhc.asp*). In contrast to other public funding sources that require approval of discretionary funding by legislative bodies, VFC funds are immediately available for new recommendations provided the ACIP votes the vaccine and the recommendation for its use into the VFC program, the federal government negotiates a contract, and the Office of Management and Budget (OMB) apportions funds. The VFC program can provide free vaccines to participating private providers.

The second major federal funding source is the 317 Discretionary Federal Grant Program to states and selected localities. These funds must be appropriated annually by Congress, but in contrast to VFC, they have not had eligibility requirements for use. The third major public source of funds is state appropriations. The VFC program itself does not cover vaccine administration costs. Medicaid covers the administration fees for children enrolled in that program. Parents of other children eligible for VFC must pay administration fees out of pocket, although there is a stipulation in the law that no one eligible for the program can be denied vaccines because of inability to pay the administration fee. The Affordalde Care Act may lead to changes in financing.

Vaccine Safety Monitoring

Monitoring vaccine safety is the responsibility of the FDA, CDC, and vaccine manufacturers. A critical part of that monitoring depends on reports to the Vaccine Adverse Event Reporting System (VAERS). Adverse events following immunization can be reported by calling 1-800-822-7967 or completing a VAERS form that can be obtained from *www.vaers.hhs.gov*. Individual VAERS case reports may be helpful in generating hypotheses about whether vaccines are causing certain clinical syndromes, but in general they are not helpful in evaluating the causal role of vaccines in the adverse event. This is because most clinical syndromes that follow vaccination are similar to syndromes that occur in the absence of vaccination. For causality assessment, epidemiologic studies are often necessary, comparing the incidence rate of the adverse event after vaccination with the rate in the unvaccinated. A statistically significant higher rate in the vaccinated would be consistent with causation.

The Vaccine Safety Datalink (VSD) consists of inpatient and outpatient records of some of the largest managed-care organizations in the USA and facilitates causality evaluation. In addition, the clinical immunization safety assessment network (CISA) has been established to advise primary care physicians on evaluation and management of adverse events (*www.cdc.gov/vaccinesafety/Activities/CISA.html*). The Institute of Medicine (IOM) has reviewed independently a variety of vaccine safety concerns (available at *www.iom.edu/imsafety* and Table 165-4). In no instance did the IOM find that evidence favored acceptance of a causal link between the postulated adverse event and vaccines.

The National Vaccine Injury Compensation Program (NVICP), established in 1988, is designed to compensate persons injured by vaccines in the childhood and adolescent immunization schedule. The program is funded through an excise tax of $0.75 per disease prevented per dose. As of 2010, all of the routinely recommended vaccines that protect children against 16 diseases are covered by this program. The NVICP was established to provide a no-fault system. There is a table of related injuries and time frames. All persons alleging injury from covered vaccines must first file with the program. If the injury meets the requirements of the table, compensation is automatic. If not, the claimant has the responsibility to prove causality. If compensation is accepted, the claimant cannot sue the manufacturer or physician administering the vaccine. If the claimant rejects the judgment of the compensation system, he or she can enter the tort system, but this has only occurred rarely. Information on the NVICP is available at 1-800-338-2382 and *www.hrsa.gov/vaccinecompensation/*. All physicians administering a vaccine covered by the program are required by law to give the approved Vaccine Information Statement (VIS) to the child's parent or guardian at each visit before administering vaccines. Information on the VIS can be obtained from *www.cdc.gov/vaccines/pubs/vis/default.htm*.

Table 165-4 INSTITUTE OF MEDICINE IMMUNIZATION SAFETY REVIEW COMMITTEE REPORTS, 2001-2004

REPORT	DATE OF RELEASE
Measles-mumps-rubella vaccine and autism	April 2001
Thimerosal-containing vaccines and neurodevelopmental disorders	October 2001
Multiple immunizations and immune dysfunction	February 2002*
Hepatitis B vaccine and demyelinating neurologic disorders	May 2002
SV40 contamination of polio vaccine and cancer	October 2002
Vaccinations and sudden unexpected death in infancy	March 2003
Influenza vaccines and neurologic complications	October 2003
Vaccines and autism	May 2004

*Reviews relationship of vaccines to asthma, diabetes, and heterologous infections.
Data from http://www.iom.edu/imsafety.
From Cohn AC et al: Immunizations in the US: a rite of passage, *Pediatr Clin North Am* 52:669–693, 2005.

Vaccine Delivery

To ensure potency, vaccines should be stored at recommended temperatures before and after reconstitution (*www.cdc.gov/vaccines/recs/storage/default.htm*). Expiration dates should be noted, and expired vaccine should be discarded. Lyophilized vaccines often have long shelf lives. However, the shelf life of reconstituted vaccines generally is short, ranging from 30 min for the varicella vaccine to 8 hr for the MMR vaccine.

All vaccines have a preferred route of administration, which is specified in package inserts and in AAP and ACIP recommendations. Most inactivated vaccines, including DTaP, HepA, HepB, Hib, TIV, PCV13, MCV4, and Tdap, are administered IM. In contrast, the commonly used live-attenuated vaccines, MMR, MMRV and varicella, should be dispensed SC and rotavirus vaccine is administered orally. IPV and PPS23 (pneumococcal polysaccharide vaccine) can be given IM or SC. For IM injections, the anterolateral thigh muscle is the preferred site for infants and young children. The recommended needle length varies depending on age and size: ⅝ inch for newborn infants, 1 inch for infants 2-12 mo of age, and 1-1¼ inches for older children. For adolescents and adults, the deltoid muscle of the arm is the preferred site for IM administration with needle lengths of 1-1¼ inches depending on the size of the patient. Most IM injections can be made with 23-25 gauge needles. For SC injections, needle lengths generally range from ⅝ to ¾ inches with 23-25 gauge needles.

RECOMMENDED IMMUNIZATION SCHEDULE

All children in the USA should be vaccinated against 15 diseases (Figs. 165-2 and 165-3) (annually updated schedule available at *http://www.cdc.gov/vaccines/recs/acip/default.htm*). Girls 11-12 yr old should also receive HPV. Boys may receive HPV4 to prevent genital warts, but this is a permissive recommendation.

HepB vaccine is recommended in a 3-dose schedule starting at birth. The birth dose is critical for children born to mothers who are hepatitis B surface antigen positive (HBsAg) or whose immune status is unknown.

The DTaP series consists of 5 doses. The 4th dose of DTaP may be administered as early as 12 mo of age, provided 6 mo has elapsed since the 3rd dose and the child is unlikely to return at 15-18 mo of age. A booster, consisting of an adult preparation of Tdap, is recommended at 11-12 yr of age. Adolescents 13-18 yr of age who missed the 11-12 year old Tdap booster dose should receive a single dose of Tdap if they have completed the diphtheria, tetanus, and pertussis (DTP)/DTaP series. Tdap may be given at any interval following the last Td.

There are 3 licensed preparations of single antigen Hib vaccines. The vaccine conjugated to tetanus toxoid (PRP-T) is given in a 4-dose series, and the Hib vaccine conjugated to meningococcal outer membrane protein (PRP-OMP) is recommended in a 3-dose series. The third Hib vaccine is licensed as a booster for children 15 mo through 4 yr of age.

TIV is recommended for all 6 mo-18 yr old children. Children <9 yr being vaccinated for the 1st time require 2 doses at least 4 wk apart. If such children only received a single dose of TIV the prior season, they need the full 2 doses the following season. However, if 2 doses were received in the prior influenza season, only 1 dose is needed in each subsequent season. TIV usually is given in October or November, although there may be benefits even when administered as late as February or March because influenza seasons most commonly peak in February.

IPV should be given at 2, 4, 6-18 mo and 4-6 yr of age. PCV13 is recommended at 2, 4, 6, and 12-15 mo of age. The final dose in the IPV series should be administered at ≥4 yr of age regardless of the number of previous doses, and the minimal interval from

Recommended Immunization Schedule for Persons Aged 0 Through 6 Years—United States • 2011

For those who fall behind or start late, see the catch-up schedule

Vaccine ▼ Age ►	Birth	1 month	2 months	4 months	6 months	12 months	15 months	18 months	19–23 months	2–3 years	4–6 years
Hepatitis B[1]	HepB	HepB	HepB		HepB	HepB	HepB	HepB			
Rotavirus[2]			RV	RV	RV[2]						
Diphtheria, Tetanus, Pertussis[3]			DTaP	DTaP	DTaP	see footnote[3]	DTaP	DTaP			DTaP
Haemophilus influenzae type b[4]			Hib	Hib	Hib[4]	Hib	Hib				
Pneumococcal[5]			PCV	PCV	PCV	PCV	PCV			PPSV	PPSV
Inactivated Poliovirus[6]			IPV	IPV	IPV	IPV	IPV	IPV			IPV
Influenza[7]					Influenza (Yearly)	Influenza (Yearly)	Influenza (Yearly)	Influenza (Yearly)	Influenza (Yearly)	Influenza (Yearly)	Influenza (Yearly)
Measles, Mumps, Rubella[8]						MMR	MMR	see footnote[8]	see footnote[8]		MMR
Varicella[9]						Varicella	Varicella	see footnote[9]	see footnote[9]		Varicella
Hepatitis A[10]						HepA (2 doses)	HepA (2 doses)	HepA (2 doses)	HepA (2 doses)	HepA Series	HepA Series
Meningococcal[11]										MCV4	MCV4

Gray shading: Range of recommended ages for all children

Black shading: Range of recommended ages for certain high-risk groups (PPSV, HepA Series, MCV4)

This schedule includes recommendations in effect as of December 21, 2010. Any dose not administered at the recommended age should be administered at a subsequent visit, when indicated and feasible. The use of a combination vaccine generally is preferred over separate injections of its equivalent component vaccines. Considerations should include provider assessment, patient preference, and the potential for adverse events. Providers should consult the relevant Advisory Committee on Immunization Practices statement for detailed recommendations: **http://www.cdc.gov/vaccines/pubs/acip-list.htm.** Clinically significant adverse events that follow immunization should be reported to the Vaccine Adverse Event Reporting System (VAERS) at **http://www.vaers.hhs.gov** or by telephone, **800-822-7967**. Use of trade names and commercial sources is for identification only and does not imply endorsement by the U.S. Department of Health and Human Services.

1. **Hepatitis B vaccine (HepB).** (Minimum age: birth)
   At birth:
   - Administer monovalent HepB to all newborns before hospital discharge.
   - If mother is hepatitis B surface antigen (HBsAg)-positive, administer HepB and 0.5 mL of hepatitis B immune globulin (HBIG) within 12 hours of birth.
   - If mother's HBsAg status is unknown, administer HepB within 12 hours of birth. Determine mother's HBsAg status as soon as possible and, if HBsAg-positive, administer HBIG (no later than age 1 week).

   Doses following the birth dose:
   - The second dose should be administered at age 1 or 2 months. Monovalent HepB should be used for doses administered before age 6 weeks.
   - Infants born to HBsAg-positive mothers should be tested for HBsAg and antibody to HBsAg 1 to 2 months after completion of at least 3 doses of the HepB series, at age 9 through 18 months (generally at the next well-child visit).
   - Administration of 4 doses of HepB to infants is permissible when a combination vaccine containing HepB is administered after the birth dose.
   - Infants who did not receive a birth dose should receive 3 doses of HepB on a schedule of 0, 1, and 6 months.
   - The final (3rd or 4th) dose in the HepB series should be administered no earlier than age 24 weeks.
2. **Rotavirus vaccine (RV).** (Minimum age: 6 weeks)
   - Administer the first dose at age 6 through 14 weeks (maximum age: 14 weeks 6 days). Vaccination should not be initiated for infants aged 15 weeks 0 days or older.
   - The maximum age for the final dose in the series is 8 months 0 days
   - If Rotarix is administered at ages 2 and 4 months, a dose at 6 months is not indicated.
3. **Diphtheria and tetanus toxoids and acellular pertussis vaccine (DTaP).** (Minimum age: 6 weeks)
   - The fourth dose may be administered as early as age 12 months, provided at least 6 months have elapsed since the third dose.
4. ***Haemophilus influenzae* type b conjugate vaccine (Hib).** (Minimum age: 6 weeks)
   - If PRP-OMP (PedvaxHIB or Comvax [HepB-Hib]) is administered at ages 2 and 4 months, a dose at age 6 months is not indicated.
   - Hiberix should not be used for doses at ages 2, 4, or 6 months for the primary series but can be used as the final dose in children aged 12 months through 4 years.
5. **Pneumococcal vaccine.** (Minimum age: 6 weeks for pneumococcal conjugate vaccine [PCV]; 2 years for pneumococcal polysaccharide vaccine [PPSV])
   - PCV is recommended for all children aged younger than 5 years. Administer 1 dose of PCV to all healthy children aged 24 through 59 months who are not completely vaccinated for their age.
   - A PCV series begun with 7-valent PCV (PCV7) should be completed with 13-valent PCV (PCV13).
   - A single supplemental dose of PCV13 is recommended for all children aged 14 through 59 months who have received an age-appropriate series of PCV7.
   - A single supplemental dose of PCV13 is recommended for all children aged 60 through 71 months with underlying medical conditions who have received an age-appropriate series of PCV7.
   - The supplemental dose of PCV13 should be administered at least 8 weeks after the previous dose of PCV7. See *MMWR* 2010:59(No. RR-11).
   - Administer PPSV at least 8 weeks after last dose of PCV to children aged 2 years or older with certain underlying medical conditions, including a cochlear implant.
6. **Inactivated poliovirus vaccine (IPV).** (Minimum age: 6 weeks)
   - If 4 or more doses are administered prior to age 4 years an additional dose should be administered at age 4 through 6 years.
   - The final dose in the series should be administered on or after the fourth birthday and at least 6 months following the previous dose.
7. **Influenza vaccine (seasonal).** (Minimum age: 6 months for trivalent inactivated influenza vaccine [TIV]; 2 years for live, attenuated influenza vaccine [LAIV])
   - For healthy children aged 2 years and older (i.e., those who do not have underlying medical conditions that predispose them to influenza complications), either LAIV or TIV may be used, except LAIV should not be given to children aged 2 through 4 years who have had wheezing in the past 12 months.
   - Administer 2 doses (separated by at least 4 weeks) to children aged 6 months through 8 years who are receiving seasonal influenza vaccine for the first time or who were vaccinated for the first time during the previous influenza season but only received 1 dose.
   - Children aged 6 months through 8 years who received no doses of monovalent 2009 H1N1 vaccine should receive 2 doses of 2010–2011 seasonal influenza vaccine. See *MMWR* 2010;59(No. RR-8):33–34.
8. **Measles, mumps, and rubella vaccine (MMR).** (Minimum age: 12 months)
   - The second dose may be administered before age 4 years, provided at least 4 weeks have elapsed since the first dose.
9. **Varicella vaccine.** (Minimum age: 12 months)
   - The second dose may be administered before age 4 years, provided at least 3 months have elapsed since the first dose.
   - For children aged 12 months through 12 years the recommended minimum interval between doses is 3 months. However, if the second dose was administered at least 4 weeks after the first dose, it can be accepted as valid.
10. **Hepatitis A vaccine (HepA).** (Minimum age: 12 months)
    - Administer 2 doses at least 6 months apart.
    - HepA is recommended for children aged older than 23 months who live in areas where vaccination programs target older children, who are at increased risk for infection, or for whom immunity against hepatitis A is desired.
11. **Meningococcal conjugate vaccine, quadrivalent (MCV4).** (Minimum age: 2 years)
    - Administer 2 doses of MCV4 at least 8 weeks apart to children aged 2 through 10 years with persistent complement component deficiency and anatomic or functional asplenia, and 1 dose every 5 years thereafter.
    - Persons with human immunodeficiency virus (HIV) infection who are vaccinated with MCV4 should receive 2 doses at least 8 weeks apart.
    - Administer 1 dose of MCV4 to children aged 2 through 10 years who travel to countries with highly endemic or epidemic disease and during outbreaks caused by a vaccine serogroup.
    - Administer MCV4 to children at continued risk for meningococcal disease who were previously vaccinated with MCV4 or meningococcal polysaccharide vaccine after 3 years if the first dose was administered at age 2 through 6 years.

The Recommended Immunization Schedules for Persons Aged 0 Through 18 Years are approved by the Advisory Committee on Immunization Practices (**http://www.cdc.gov/vaccines/recs/acip**), the American Academy of Pediatrics (**http://www.aap.org**), and the American Academy of Family Physicians (**http://www.aafp.org**).

Department of Health and Human Services • Centers for Disease **Control and Prevention**

Figure 165-2 Recommended immunization schedule for persons aged 0 through 6 years—USA, 2011. (From www.cdc.gov/vaccines/recs/schedules/child-schedule.htm. Accessed February 14, 2011.)

Recommended Immunization Schedule for Persons Aged 7 Through 18 Years—United States • 2011

For those who fall behind or start late, see the schedule below and the catch-up schedule

Vaccine ▼ Age ►	7–10 years	11–12 years	13–18 years
Tetanus, Diphtheria, Pertussis[1]		Tdap	Tdap
Human Papillomavirus[2]	see footnote 2	HPV (3 doses)(females)	HPV Series
Meningococcal[3]	MCV4	MCV4	MCV4
Influenza[4]	Influenza (Yearly)		
Pneumococcal[5]	Pneumococcal		
Hepatitis A[6]	HepA Series		
Hepatitis B[7]	Hep B Series		
Inactivated Poliovirus[8]	IPV Series		
Measles, Mumps, Rubella[9]	MMR Series		
Varicella[10]	Varicella Series		

Range of recommended ages for all children

Range of recommended ages for catch-up immunization

Range of recommended ages for certain high-risk groups

This schedule includes recommendations in effect as of December 21, 2010. Any dose not administered at the recommended age should be administered at a subsequent visit, when indicated and feasible. The use of a combination vaccine generally is preferred over separate injections of its equivalent component vaccines. Considerations should include provider assessment, patient preference, and the potential for adverse events. Providers should consult the relevant Advisory Committee on Immunization Practices statement for detailed recommendations: **http://www.cdc.gov/vaccines/pubs/acip-list.htm.** Clinically significant adverse events that follow immunization should be reported to the Vaccine Adverse Event Reporting System (VAERS) at **http://www.vaers.hhs.gov** or by telephone, **800-822-7967.**

1. **Tetanus and diphtheria toxoids and acellular pertussis vaccine (Tdap).** (Minimum age: 10 years for Boostrix and 11 years for Adacel)
   - Persons aged 11 through 18 years who have not received Tdap should receive a dose followed by Td booster doses every 10 years thereafter.
   - Persons aged 7 through 10 years who are not fully immunized against pertussis (including those never vaccinated or with unknown pertussis vaccination status) should receive a single dose of Tdap. Refer to the catch-up schedule if additional doses of tetanus and diphtheria toxoid–containing vaccine are needed.
   - Tdap can be administered regardless of the interval since the last tetanus and diphtheria toxoid–containing vaccine.
2. **Human papillomavirus vaccine (HPV).** (Minimum age: 9 years)
   - Quadrivalent HPV vaccine (HPV4) or bivalent HPV vaccine (HPV2) is recommended for the prevention of cervical precancers and cancers in females.
   - HPV4 is recommended for prevention of cervical precancers, cancers, and genital warts in females.
   - HPV4 may be administered in a 3-dose series to males aged 9 through 18 years to reduce their likelihood of genital warts.
   - Administer the second dose 1 to 2 months after the first dose and the third dose 6 months after the first dose (at least 24 weeks after the first dose).
3. **Meningococcal conjugate vaccine, quadrivalent (MCV4).** (Minimum age: 2 years)
   - Administer MCV4 at age 11 through 12 years with a booster dose at age 16 years.
   - Administer 1 dose at age 13 through 18 years if not previously vaccinated.
   - Persons who received their first dose at age 13 through 15 years should receive a booster dose at age 16 through 18 years.
   - Administer 1 dose to previously unvaccinated college freshmen living in a dormitory.
   - Administer 2 doses at least 8 weeks apart to children aged 2 through 10 years with persistent complement component deficiency and anatomic or functional asplenia, and 1 dose every 5 years thereafter.
   - Persons with HIV infection who are vaccinated with MCV4 should receive 2 doses at least 8 weeks apart.
   - Administer 1 dose of MCV4 to children aged 2 through 10 years who travel to countries with highly endemic or epidemic disease and during outbreaks caused by a vaccine serogroup.
   - Administer MCV4 to children at continued risk for meningococcal disease who were previously vaccinated with MCV4 or meningococcal polysaccharide vaccine after 3 years (if first dose administered at age 2 through 6 years) or after 5 years (if first dose administered at age 7 years or older).
4. **Influenza vaccine (seasonal).**
   - For healthy nonpregnant persons aged 7 through 18 years (i.e., those who do not have underlying medical conditions that predispose them to influenza complications), either LAIV or TIV may be used.
   - Administer 2 doses (separated by at least 4 weeks) to children aged 6 months through 8 years who are receiving seasonal influenza vaccine for the first time or who were vaccinated for the first time during the previous influenza season but only received 1 dose.
   - Children 6 months through 8 years of age who received no doses of monovalent 2009 H1N1 vaccine should receive 2 doses of 2010-2011 seasonal influenza vaccine. See *MMWR* 2010;59(No. RR-8):33–34.
5. **Pneumococcal vaccines.**
   - A single dose of 13-valent pneumococcal conjugate vaccine (PCV13) may be administered to children aged 6 through 18 years who have functional or anatomic asplenia, HIV infection or other immunocompromising condition, cochlear implant or CSF leak. See *MMWR* 2010;59(No. RR-11).
   - The dose of PCV13 should be administered at least 8 weeks after the previous dose of PCV7.
   - Administer pneumococcal polysaccharide vaccine at least 8 weeks after the last dose of PCV to children aged 2 years or older with certain underlying medical conditions, including a cochlear implant. A single revaccination should be administered after 5 years to children with functional or anatomic asplenia or an immunocompromising condition.
6. **Hepatitis A vaccine (HepA).**
   - Administer 2 doses at least 6 months apart.
   - HepA is recommended for children aged older than 23 months who live in areas where vaccination programs target older children, or who are at increased risk for infection, or for whom immunity against hepatitis A is desired.
7. **Hepatitis B vaccine (HepB).**
   - Administer the 3-dose series to those not previously vaccinated. For those with incomplete vaccination, follow the catch-up schedule.
   - A 2-dose series (separated by at least 4 months) of adult formulation Recombivax HB is licensed for children aged 11 through 15 years.
8. **Inactivated poliovirus vaccine (IPV).**
   - The final dose in the series should be administered on or after the fourth birthday and at least 6 months following the previous dose.
   - If both OPV and IPV were administered as part of a series, a total of 4 doses should be administered, regardless of the child's current age.
9. **Measles, mumps, and rubella vaccine (MMR).**
   - The minimum interval between the 2 doses of MMR is 4 weeks.
10. **Varicella vaccine.**
    - For persons aged 7 through 18 years without evidence of immunity (see *MMWR* 2007;56[No. RR-4]), administer 2 doses if not previously vaccinated or the second dose if only 1 dose has been administered.
    - For persons aged 7 through 12 years, the recommended minimum interval between doses is 3 months. However, if the second dose was administered at least 4 weeks after the first dose, it can be accepted as valid.
    - For persons aged 13 years and older, the minimum interval between doses is 4 weeks.

The Recommended Immunization Schedules for Persons Aged 0 Through 18 Years are approved by the Advisory Committee on Immunization Practices (**http://www.cdc.gov/vaccines/recs/acip**), the American Academy of Pediatrics (**http://www.aap.org**), and the American Academy of Family Physicians (**http://www.aafp.org**).

Department of Health and Human Services • Centers for Disease Control and Prevention

Figure 165-3 Recommended immunization schedule for persons aged 7 through 18 years—USA, 2011. (From www.cdc.gov/vaccines/recs/schedules/child-schedule.htm. Accessed February 14, 2011.)

dose 3 to dose 4 is 6 mo. MMR should be administered at 12-15 mo of age followed by a 2nd dose at 4-6 yr of age. Varicella vaccine should be given at 12-18 mo of age and at 4-6 yr of age.

The quadrivalent measles, mumps, rubella, and varicella (MMRV) vaccine is preferred in place of separate MMR and varicella vaccines at the 4-6 yr old visit. Because of increased febrile seizures associated with combined MMRV vaccine compared to the separate products, use of MMRV is not preferred over use of separate MMR and varicella vaccines for the initial dose at 12-15 mo of age.

Hepatitis A vaccine, licensed for administration to children ≥12 mo of age, is recommended for universal administration to all children at 12-23 mo of age and for certain high-risk groups. The 2 doses in the series should be separated by at least 6 mo.

A 2-dose series of MCV4 is recommended for all adolescents at 11-12 yr and at 16 yr of age. In addition, MCV4 should be administered to people 2 through 55 yr of age with underlying conditions that place them at high risk of meningococcal disease. People with high-risk conditions should receive 2 doses of MCV4 at 0 and 2 mo followed by booster doses.

HPV4 or HPV2 is recommended in a 3-dose series for prevention of cervical precancers and cancers in females. HPV4 may be administered in a 3-dose series to females and males 9 through 18 yr of age to reduce their likelihood of acquiring genital warts. The second dose should be given 1-2 mo after the first; the third is given 6 mo after the first.

Two rotavirus vaccines are available, RotaTeq (RV5) and Rotarix (RV1). With both vaccines, the first dose can be administered as early as 6 wk of age and must be administered by 14 wk 6 days. The final dose in the series must be administered no later than 8 mo of age. The RV5 vaccine is administered in 3 doses at least 4 wk apart. The RV1 vaccine is administered in 2 doses at least 4 wk apart.

The present schedule, excluding influenza vaccine, can require as many as 31 injections, including 22 injections prior to 2 yr of age. Influenza vaccination, starting at 6 mo of age can add an additional 20 injections through 18 yr of age. To reduce the injection burdens, several combination vaccines are available: DTaP-IPV/Hib (Pentacel, Sanofi Pasteur, Swiftwater, PA), DTaP-IPV-HepB (Pediarix, GlaxoSmithKline, Research Triangle Park, NC), Hib (PRP-OMP)-HepB (Comvax, Merck, West Point, PA) MMRV (ProQuad, Merck, West Point, PA), DTaP-IPV (Kinrix, GlaxoSmithKline), and DTaP/Hib (TriHIBit, Sanofi Pasteur). Pentacel is indicated for the first 4 doses of DTaP and Hib vaccine, usually administered at 2, 4, 6, and 15-18 mo of age. Pentacel reduces the number of injections required from 11 to 4. IPV can be administered as part of Pentacel, but a dose of IPV is still indicated on or after the 4th birthday. Pediarix can be used for the first 3 doses of the 3 vaccines, reducing the number of injections from 9 to 3. Comvax can be used as a 3 dose series at 2, 4, and 12-15 mo and potentially reduces the number of injections from 6 (or 8 if another Hib preparation is used) to 3. Kinrix is licensed as a booster for the 5th dose of DTaP and 4th dose of IPV; and TriHIBit is licensed as the 4th dose of the Hib and DTaP series. Because a birth dose of single antigen HepB vaccine is recommended when using combinations, which cannot be administered before 6 wk of age, a 4-dose series for HepB, counting the birth dose, may be used.

The recommended childhood and adolescent immunization schedule establishes a routine adolescent visit at 11-12 yr of age. MCV4 and a Tdap booster should be administered during this visit and HPV can be started. Influenza vaccine should be administered annually. In addition, the 11-12 yr old visit is also an opportune time to review all of the immunizations the child has received previously, to provide any doses that were missed, and to review other age-appropriate preventive services. The 11-12 year old visit establishes an important platform for incorporating other vaccines. Information on the current status of new vaccine licensure and recommendations for use can be obtained at *aapredbook.aappublications.org/news/vaccstatus.shtml* and *www.fda.gov/BiologicsBloodVaccines/Vaccines/ApprovedProducts/UCM093833*.

For children who are at least 1 mo behind in their immunizations, catch-up immunization schedules are available for children 4 mo to 18 yr of age (Fig. 165-4); also available for children <6 yr of age at *www.cdc.gov/vaccines/recs/schedules/child-schedule.htm#catchup*) is an interactive immunization scheduler.

VACCINES RECOMMENDED IN SPECIAL CIRCUMSTANCES

Several vaccines are recommended for children at increased risk for complications from vaccine-preventable diseases or children who have an increased risk for exposure to these diseases.

PCV13 is recommended for all children <5 yr of age who have conditions that place them at high risk for pneumococcal disease. This recommendation includes children with sickle cell disease (SCD) and other sickle cell hemoglobinopathies, including hemoglobin SS, hemoglobin S-C, or hemoglobin S–β-thalassemia, or children who are functionally or anatomically asplenic; children with HIV infection; children who have chronic disease, including chronic cardiac and pulmonary disease (excluding asthma), diabetes mellitus, or CSF leak. Also included are children with immunocompromising conditions, including malignancies (e.g., leukemia, lymphoma, Hodgkin disease); chronic renal failure or nephrotic syndrome; children receiving immunosuppressive chemotherapy, including long-term systemic corticosteroids; and children who have received a solid organ transplant. In addition, children with cochlear implants should be vaccinated. Children at high risk for pneumococcal disease also should receive PPS23 to provide immunity to serotypes not contained in the 13-valent conjugate vaccine. PPS23 should be administered on or after the 2nd birthday and should follow completion of the PCV13 series by at least 6-8 wk. Two doses of PPS23 are recommended, with an interval of 5 yr between doses. Immunization of previously unvaccinated children with high-risk conditions >5 yr of age can be performed with either a dose of PCV13 or a dose of PPS23.

MCV4 is recommended for people with HIV, children with functional or anatomic asplenia, persistent complement component or properdin deficiencies, and as part of outbreak-control programs. MCV4 is preferred and is licensed for children 2-10 yr of age with underlying high-risk conditions.

A variety of vaccines are available for children who will be **traveling** to areas of the world where certain infectious diseases are common in addition to vaccines in the recommended childhood and adolescent schedule (Table 165-5). Vaccines for travelers include typhoid fever, HepA, HepB, Japanese encephalitis, MCV4 or MPS4, rabies, and yellow fever, depending on the location and circumstances of travel. Measles is endemic in many parts of the world. Children 6-11 mo of age may receive a dose of MMR before travel. However, doses of measles vaccine received before the 1st birthday should not be counted in determining compliance with the recommended 2-dose MMR schedule. Additional information on vaccines for international travel can be found at *www.cdc.gov/travel/content/vaccinations.aspx*.

Vaccine recommendations for children with **immunocompromise**, either primary (inherited) or secondary (acquired), vary according to the underlying condition, the degree of immune deficit, the risk for exposure to disease, and the vaccine (Table 165-6). Immunization of children with immunocompromise poses the following potential concerns: the incidence or severity of some vaccine-preventable diseases is higher, and therefore certain vaccines are recommended specifically for certain conditions; vaccines may be less effective during the period of altered immunocompetence and may need to be repeated when immune competence is restored; and because of altered immunocompetence, some children and adolescents may be at increased risk

Catch-up Immunization Schedule for Persons Aged 4 Months Through 18 Years Who Start Late or Who Are More Than 1 Month Behind—United States • 2011

The table below provides catch-up schedules and minimum intervals between doses for children whose vaccinations have been delayed. A vaccine series does not need to be restarted, regardless of the time that has elapsed between doses. Use the section appropriate for the child's age

PERSONS AGED 4 MONTHS THROUGH 6 YEARS

Vaccine	Minimum Age for Dose 1	Minimum Interval Between Doses: Dose 1 to Dose 2	Dose 2 to Dose 3	Dose 3 to Dose 4	Dose 4 to Dose 5
Hepatitis B[1]	Birth	**4 weeks**	**8 weeks** (and at least 16 weeks after first dose)		
Rotavirus[2]	6 wks	**4 weeks**	**4 weeks**[2]		
Diphtheria, Tetanus, Pertussis[3]	6 wks	**4 weeks**	**4 weeks**	**6 months**	**6 months**[3]
Haemophilus influenzae type b[4]	6 wks	**4 weeks** if first dose administered at younger than age 12 months **8 weeks (as final dose)** if first dose administered at age 12–14 months **No further doses needed** if first dose administered at age 15 months or older	**4 weeks**[4] if current age is younger than 12 months **8 weeks (as final dose)**[4] if current age is 12 months or older and first dose administered at younger than age 12 months and second dose administered at younger than 15 months **No further doses needed** if previous dose administered at age 15 months or older	**8 weeks (as final dose)** This dose only necessary for children aged 12 months through 59 months who received 3 doses before age 12 months	
Pneumococcal[5]	6 wks	**4 weeks** if first dose administered at younger than age 12 months **8 weeks (as final dose for healthy children)** if first dose administered at age 12 months or older or current age 24 through 59 months **No further doses needed** for healthy children if first dose administered at age 24 months or older	**4 weeks** if current age is younger than 12 months **8 weeks (as final dose for healthy children)** if current age is 12 months or older **No further doses needed** for healthy children if previous dose administered at age 24 months or older	**8 weeks (as final dose)** This dose only necessary for children aged 12 months through 59 months who received 3 doses before age 12 months or for children at high risk who received 3 doses at any age	
Inactivated Poliovirus[6]	6 wks	**4 weeks**	**4 weeks**	**6 months**[6]	
Measles, Mumps, Rubella[7]	12 mos	**4 weeks**			
Varicella[8]	12 mos	**3 months**			
Hepatitis A[9]	12 mos	**6 months**			

PERSONS AGED 7 THROUGH 18 YEARS

Vaccine	Minimum Age for Dose 1	Dose 1 to Dose 2	Dose 2 to Dose 3	Dose 3 to Dose 4	Dose 4 to Dose 5
Tetanus, Diphtheria/ Tetanus, Diphtheria, Pertussis[10]	7 yrs[10]	**4 weeks**	**4 weeks** if first dose administered at younger than age 12 months **6 months** if first dose administered at 12 months or older	**6 months** if first dose administered at younger than age 12 months	
Human Papillomavirus[11]	9 yrs	**Routine dosing intervals are recommended (females)**[11]			
Hepatitis A[9]	12 mos	**6 months**			
Hepatitis B[1]	Birth	**4 weeks**	**8 weeks** (and at least 16 weeks after first dose)		
Inactivated Poliovirus[6]	6 wks	**4 weeks**	**4 weeks**[6]	**6 months**[6]	
Measles, Mumps, Rubella[7]	12 mos	**4 weeks**			
Varicella[8]	12 mos	**3 months** if person is younger than age 13 years **4 weeks** if person is aged 13 years or older			

1. **Hepatitis B vaccine (HepB).**
   - Administer the 3-dose series to those not previously vaccinated.
   - The minimum age for the third dose of HepB is 24 weeks.
   - A 2-dose series (separated by at least 4 months) of adult formulation Recombivax HB is licensed for children aged 11 through 15 years.
2. **Rotavirus vaccine (RV).**
   - The maximum age for the first dose is 14 weeks 6 days. Vaccination should not be initiated for infants aged 15 weeks 0 days or older.
   - The maximum age for the final dose in the series is 8 months 0 days.
   - If Rotarix was administered for the first and second doses, a third dose is not indicated.
3. **Diphtheria and tetanus toxoids and acellular pertussis vaccine (DTaP).**
   - The fifth dose is not necessary if the fourth dose was administered at age 4 years or older.
4. ***Haemophilus influenzae* type b conjugate vaccine (Hib).**
   - 1 dose of Hib vaccine should be considered for unvaccinated persons aged 5 years or older who have sickle cell disease, leukemia, or HIV infection, or who have had a splenectomy.
   - If the first 2 doses were PRP-OMP (PedvaxHIB or Comvax), and administered at age 11 months or younger, the third (and final) dose should be administered at age 12 through 15 months and at least 8 weeks after the second dose.
   - If the first dose was administered at age 7 through 11 months, administer the second dose at least 4 weeks later and a final dose at age 12 through 15 months.
5. **Pneumococcal vaccine.**
   - Administer 1 dose of 13-valent pneumococcal conjugate vaccine (PCV13) to all healthy children aged 24 through 59 months with any incomplete PCV schedule (PCV7 or PCV13).
   - For children aged 24 through 71 months with underlying medical conditions, administer 1 dose of PCV13 if 3 doses of PCV were received previously or administer 2 doses of PCV13 at least 8 weeks apart if fewer than 3 doses of PCV were received previously.
   - A single dose of PCV13 is recommended for certain children with underlying medical conditions through 18 years of age. See age-specific schedules for details.
   - Administer pneumococcal polysaccharide vaccine (PPSV) to children aged 2 years or older with certain underlying medical conditions, including a cochlear implant, at least 8 weeks after the last dose of PCV. A single revaccination should be administered after 5 years to children with functional or anatomic asplenia or an immunocompromising condition. See *MMWR* 2010;59(No. RR-11).
6. **Inactivated poliovirus vaccine (IPV).**
   - The final dose in the series should be administered on or after the fourth birthday and at least 6 months following the previous dose.
   - A fourth dose is not necessary if the third dose was administered at age 4 years or older and at least 6 months following the previous dose.
   - In the first 6 months of life, minimum age and minimum intervals are only recommended if the person is at risk for imminent exposure to circulating poliovirus (i.e., travel to a polio-endemic region or during an outbreak).
7. **Measles, mumps, and rubella vaccine (MMR).**
   - Administer the second dose routinely at age 4 through 6 years. The minimum interval between the 2 doses of MMR is 4 weeks.
8. **Varicella vaccine.**
   - Administer the second dose routinely at age 4 through 6 years.
   - If the second dose was administered at least 4 weeks after the first dose, it can be accepted as valid.
9. **Hepatitis A vaccine (HepA).**
   - HepA is recommended for children aged older than age 23 months who live in areas where vaccination programs target older children, or who are at increased risk for infection, or for whom immunity against hepatitis A is desired.
10. **Tetanus and diphtheria toxoids (Td) and tetanus and diphtheria toxoids and acellular pertussis vaccine (Tdap).**
    - Doses of DTaP are counted as part of the Td/Tdap series.
    - Tdap should be substituted for a single dose of Td in the catch-up series for children aged 7 through 10 years or as a booster for children aged 11 through 18 years; use Td for other doses.
11. **Human papillomavirus vaccine (HPV).**
    - Administer the series to females at age 13 through 18 years if not previously vaccinated or have not completed the vaccine series.
    - Quadrivalent HPV vaccine (HPV4) may be administered in a 3-dose series to males aged 9 through 18 years to reduce their likelihood of genital warts.
    - Use recommended routine dosing intervals for series catch-up (i.e., the second and third doses should be administered at 1 to 2 and 6 months after the first dose). The minimum interval between the first and second doses is 4 weeks. The minimum interval between the second and third doses is 12 weeks, and the third dose should be administered at least 24 weeks after the first dose.

Information about reporting reactions after immunization is available online at **http://www.vaers.hhs.gov** or by telephone, **800-822-7967**. Suspected cases of vaccine-preventable diseases should be reported to the state or local health department. Additional information, including precautions and contraindications for immunization, is available from the National Center for Immunization and Respiratory Diseases at **http://www.cdc.gov/vaccines** or telephone, **800-CDC-INFO** (800-232-4636).

Department of Health and Human Services • Centers for Disease Control and Prevention

Figure 165-4 Catch-up immunization schedule for persons age 4 mo through 18 yr who start late or who are more than 1 mo behind—USA, 2011. (From www.cdc.gov/vaccines/recs/schedules/child-schedule.htm. Accessed February 14, 2011.)

Table 165-5 RECOMMENDED IMMUNIZATIONS FOR TRAVELERS TO DEVELOPING COUNTRIES*

IMMUNIZATIONS	LENGTH OF TRAVEL		
	Brief, <2 wk	Intermediate, 2 wk-3 mo	Long-term Residential, >3 mo
Review and complete age-appropriate childhood and adolescent schedule (see text for details)	+	+	+
• DTaP, poliovirus, pneumococcal, and *Haemophilus influenzae* type b vaccines may be given at 4-wk intervals if necessary to complete the recommended schedule before departure • Measles: 2 additional doses given if <12 mo of age at 1st dose • Rotavirus • Varicella • HPV • Hepatitis B[†] • Tdap • MCV4			
Yellow fever[‡]	+	+	+
Hepatitis A[§]	+	+	+
Typhoid fever[‖]	±	+	+
Meningococcal disease[¶]	±	±	±
Rabies[#]	±	+	+
Japanese encephalitis**	±	±	+

*See disease-specific chapters for details. For further sources of information, see text.
[†]If there is insufficient time to complete 6 mo primary series, accelerated series can be given (see text for details).
[‡]For regions with endemic infection, see Health Information for International Travel.
[§]Indicated for travelers to areas with intermediate or high endemic rates of hepatitis A virus infection.
[‖]Indicated for travelers who will consume food and liquids in areas of poor sanitation.
[¶]Recommended for regions of Africa with endemic infection and during local epidemics, and required for travel to Saudi Arabia for the Hajj.
[#]Indicated for people with high risk for animal exposure (especially to dogs) and for travelers to countries with endemic infection.
**For regions with endemic infection (see Health Information for International Travel). For high-risk activities in areas experiencing outbreaks, vaccine is recommended, even for brief travel.
DTaP, diphtheria and tetanus toxoids and acellular pertussis; +, recommended; ±, consider.
Modified from Pickering LK, Baker CJ, Kimberlin DW, et al, editors: *Red book 2009: report of the Committee on Infectious Diseases*, ed 28, Elk Grove Village, IL, 2009, American Academy of Pediatrics, p 101.

for an adverse event following receipt of a live viral vaccine. Live-attenuated vaccines generally are contraindicated in immunocompromised people. The exceptions include MMR, which may be given to a child with HIV infection provided the child is asymptomatic or symptomatic without evidence of severe immunosuppression, and varicella vaccine, which may be given to HIV-infected children if the $CD4^+$ lymphocyte count is at least 15%. MMRV is not recommended in these situations.

Altered immunocompetence is considered a precaution for rotavirus; however, the vaccine is contraindicated in children with severe combined immunodeficiency disease. Inactivated vaccines may be administered to immunocompromised children, although, depending on the immune deficit, their effectiveness might not be optimal. Children with complement deficiency disorders may receive all vaccines, including live-attenuated vaccines. In contrast, children with phagocytic disorders may receive both inactivated and live-attenuated viral vaccines but not live-attenuated bacterial vaccines.

Corticosteroids can suppress the immune system. Children receiving corticosteroids (≥2 mg/kg/day or ≥20 mg/day of prednisone or equivalent) for 14 or more days should not receive live vaccines until therapy has been discontinued for at least 1 month. Children on the same dose levels but for <2 wk may receive live viral vaccines as soon as therapy is discontinued, although some experts would wait 2 wk post-therapy. Children receiving lower doses of steroids may be vaccinated while on therapy.

Children and adolescents with malignancy, and those who have undergone solid organ or hematopoietic stem cell transplantation and immunosuppressive or radiation therapy, should not receive live virus and live bacterial vaccines depending on their immune status. Children who have undergone chemotherapy for leukemia may need to be reimmunized with age appropriate single doses of previously administered vaccines.

Preterm infants generally can be vaccinated at the same chronologic age as full-term infants according to the recommended childhood immunization schedule. An exception is the birth dose of HepB vaccine. Infants weighing ≥2 kg and who are stable may receive a birth dose. However, HepB vaccination should be deferred in infants weighing <2 kg at birth until 30 days of age, if born to an HBsAg-negative mother. All preterm, low birth weight infants born to HBsAg-positive mothers should receive HepB IG and HepB vaccine within 12 hr of birth. However, such infants should receive an additional 3 doses of vaccine starting at 30 days of age (see Fig. 165-2).

Some children have situations that are not addressed directly in current immunization schedules. There are general rules that physicians can use to guide immunization decisions in some of these instances. In general, vaccines may be given simultaneously on the same day, whether inactivated or live. Different inactivated vaccines can be administered at any interval between doses. However, because of theoretical concerns about viral interference, different live-attenuated vaccines (MMR, varicella, LAIV) if not administered on the same day, should be given at least 1 mo apart. An inactivated and a live vaccine may be spaced at any interval from each other.

IG does not interfere with killed vaccines. However, IG can interfere with the immune response to measles vaccine and by inference to varicella vaccine. In general, IG, if needed, should be administered at least 2 wk after measles vaccine. Depending on the dose of IG received, MMR should be deferred for as long as 3-11 mo. IG is not expected to interfere with the immune response to LAIV or rotavirus vaccines.

Many agents have been considered for potential use as weapons of bioterrorism. For most of these agents, licensed vaccines are not available in the USA, although vaccines are being developed for some organisms, including botulinum toxoid, Ebola virus, plague, and others. Anthrax vaccine and smallpox (vaccinia) vaccine are available, but they are not recommended for children. Both are indicated in a pre-exposure setting only for selected adults with potential occupational risks of exposure (*www.bt.cdc.gov/* provides details on which groups are recommended for vaccination).

Table 165-6 VACCINATION OF PERSONS WITH PRIMARY AND SECONDARY IMMUNE DEFICIENCIES

PRIMARY				
CATEGORY	SPECIFIC IMMUNODEFICIENCY	CONTRAINDICATED VACCINES*	RISK-SPECIFIC RECOMMENDED VACCINES*	EFFECTIVENESS AND COMMENTS
B lymphocyte (humoral)	Severe antibody deficiencies (e.g., X-linked agammaglobulinemia and common variable immunodeficiency)	OPV† Smallpox LAIV BCG Ty21a (live typhoid) YF	Pneumococcal Consider measles and varicella vaccination	The effectiveness of any vaccine will be uncertain if it depends only on the humoral response (e.g., PPSV, MPSV) IGIV interferes with the immune response to measles vaccine and possibly varicella vaccine.
	Less severe antibody deficiencies (e.g., selective IgA deficiency and IgG subclass deficiency)	OPV† BCG YF Other live vaccines appear to be safe	Pneumococcal	All vaccines probably effective Immune response may be attenuated
T lymphocyte (cell-mediated and humoral)	Complete defects (e.g., SCID disease, complete DiGeorge syndrome)	All live vaccines‡§‖	Pneumococcal	Vaccines may be ineffective
	Partial defects (e.g., most patients with DiGeorge syndrome, Wiskott-Aldrich syndrome, ataxia-telangiectasia)	All live vaccines‡§‖	Pneumococcal Meningococcal Hib (if not administered in infancy)	Effectiveness of any vaccine depends on degree of immune suppression
Complement	Persistent complement, properdin, or factor B deficiency	None	Pneumococcal Meningococcal	All routine vaccines probably effective
Phagocytic function	Chronic granulomatous disease, leukocyte adhesion defect, and myeloperoxidase deficiency	Live bacterial vaccines‡	Pneumococcal¶	All inactivated vaccines safe and probably effective Live viral vaccines probably safe and effective

SECONDARY			
SPECIFIC IMMUNODEFICIENCY	CONTRAINDICATED VACCINES*	RISK-SPECIFIC RECOMMENDED VACCINES*	EFFECTIVENESS AND COMMENTS
HIV/AIDS	OPV† Smallpox BCG LAIV Withhold MMR and varicella in severely immunocompromised persons	Pneumococcal Consider Hib (if not administered in infancy) and meningococcal vaccination	MMR, varicella, rotavirus, and all inactivated vaccines, including inactivated influenza, may be effective#
Malignant neoplasm, transplantation, immunosuppressive or radiation therapy	Live viral and bacterial, depending on immune status‡§	Pneumococcal	Effectiveness of any vaccine depends on degree of immune suppression
Asplenia	None	Pneumococcal Meningococcal Hib (if not administered in infancy)	All routine vaccines probably effective
Chronic renal disease	LAIV	Pneumococcal Hepatitis B**	All routine vaccines probably effective

*Other vaccines that are universally or routinely recommended should be given if not contraindicated.
†OPV is no longer recommended for routine use in the USA.
‡Live bacterial vaccines: BCG and oral Ty21a *Salmonella typhi* vaccine.
§Live viral vaccines: MMR, MMRV, OPV, LAIV, YF, zoster, rotavirus, and vaccinia (smallpox). Smallpox vaccine is not recommended for children or the general public.
‖Regarding T-lymphocyte immunodeficiency as a contraindication for rotavirus vaccine, data exist only for SCID.
¶Pneumococcal vaccine is not indicated for children with chronic granulomatous disease beyond age-based universal recommendations for PCV. Children with chronic granulomatous disease are not at increased risk for pneumococcal disease.
#HIV-infected children should receive immunoglobulin after exposure to measles and may receive varicella, measles, and YF vaccine if CD4+ lymphocyte count is greater than 15%. (For YF vaccine, CD4+ T-lymphocyte count between 15% and 24% is a precaution.)
**Indicated based on the risk from dialysis-based bloodborne transmission.
HIV/AIDS, human immunodeficiency virus/acquired immunodeficiency syndrome; BCG, bacille Calmette-Guérin vaccine; Hib, *Haemophilus influenzae* type b vaccine; IGIV, immune globulin intravenous; LAIV, live, attenuated influenza vaccine; MMR, measles, mumps, rubella vaccine; MPSV, quadrivalent meningococcal polysaccharide vaccine; OPV, oral poliovirus vaccine (live); PPSV, pneumococcal polysaccharide vaccine; SCID, severe combined immunodeficiency disease; TIV, trivalent (inactivated) influenza vaccine; YF, yellow fever.
Adapted from American Academy of Pediatrics: Passive immunization. In Pickering LK, Baker CJ, Kimberlin DW, et al, editors: *Red book: 2009 report of the Committee on Infectious Diseases,* ed 28, Elk Grove Village, IL, 2009, American Academy of Pediatrics, pp 74–75.

PRECAUTIONS AND CONTRAINDICATIONS

Observation of valid precautions and contraindications is critical to ensure that vaccines are used in the safest manner possible and to obtain optimal immunogenicity. When a child presents for immunization with a clinical condition considered a precaution, the physician must weigh benefits and risks to that individual child. If benefits are judged to outweigh risks, then the vaccine or vaccines in question may be administered. A contraindication means the vaccine should not be administered under any circumstances.

A general contraindication for all vaccines is anaphylactic reaction to a prior dose. Anaphylactic hypersensitivity to vaccine constituents is also a contraindication. However, if a vaccine is essential, there are desensitizing protocols for some vaccines. The major constituents of concern are egg proteins for vaccines grown in eggs; gelatin, a stabilizer in many vaccines; and antimicrobial agents. The measles and mumps components of MMR are grown in chick embryo fibroblast tissue culture. However, the amount of egg protein in MMR is so small as not to require any special procedures before administering vaccine to someone with a history of anaphylaxis following egg ingestion.

Vaccines usually should be deferred in children with moderate to severe acute illnesses, regardless of the presence of fever, until the child recovers. However, children with mild illnesses may be vaccinated. Studies of undervaccinated children have documented opportunities that were missed because mild illness was used as an invalid contraindication. Complete tables of contraindications and contraindication misperceptions can be found at *www.cdc.gov/vaccines/recs/vac-admin/contraindications.htm*.

IMPROVING IMMUNIZATION COVERAGE

Standards for child and adolescent immunization practices have been developed to support achievement of high levels of immunization coverage while providing vaccines in a safe and effective manner and educating parents about risks and benefits of vaccines (Table 165-7).

Despite the benefits that vaccines have to offer, many children are underimmunized as a result of not receiving recommended vaccines or not receiving them at the recommended ages. Much of the underimmunization problem can be solved through physician actions. Most children have a regular source of health care. However, missed opportunities to provide immunizations at health care visits include failure to provide all recommended vaccines that could be administered at a single visit during that visit, failure to provide immunizations to children outside of well child care when the conditions children may have are not contraindications to immunizations, and referral of children to public health clinics because of inability to pay for vaccines. Simultaneous administration of multiple vaccines generally is safe and effective. When the benefits of simultaneous vaccination are explained, many parents prefer such immunization rather than needing to make an extra visit. Providing all needed vaccines simultaneously should be the standard of practice.

Only valid contraindications and precautions to vaccine administration should be observed. Ideally immunizations should be provided during well child visits, but using other visits to administer vaccines if there are no contraindications, particularly if a child is behind in the schedule, is important. There is no good evidence that providing immunizations outside of well child care ultimately decreases well child visits.

Financial barriers to immunization should be minimized. Participation in the VFC program allows physicians to receive free vaccines for their eligible patients, which helps such patients be immunized in their medical home.

Several interventions have been shown to help physicians increase immunization coverage in their practices. Reminder systems for children before an appointment or recall systems for children who fail to keep appointments have repeatedly been demonstrated to improve coverage. Assessment and feedback is also an important intervention. Many physicians overestimate the immunization coverage among patients they serve and thus are not motivated to make any changes in their practices to improve performance. Assessing the immunization coverage of patients served by an individual physician and feedback of results can be a major motivator for improvement. Often public health departments can be contacted to provide the assessments and feedback. Alternatively, physicians can perform some self-assessments. Review of approximately 60 consecutive charts of 2 yr old children may provide a reasonable estimate of practice coverage. Another help is to have a staff member review the chart of every patient coming in for a visit and placing immunization needs reminders on the chart for the physician.

Some parents refuse immunization for their child. Pediatricians should try to open a dialogue with such parents to understand the reasons for refusal and try to work with them to overcome their concerns over time during the course of visits. Discussion should be based on the reason for refusal and the knowledge of the parent. Pediatricians should refer patients to reputable sources for vaccine information (Table 165-8) and discuss risks and benefits of vaccines. Physician concerns about liability should be addressed by appropriate documentation of discussions in the chart. The Committee on Bioethics of the AAP has published guidelines for dealing with parents' refusal of immunization. Physicians also might wish to consider having parents sign a refusal waiver. A sample of a refusal to vaccinate waiver can be found at *www.aap.org/immunization/pediatricians/pdf/ReducingVaccineLiability.pdf*.

Table 165-7 STANDARDS FOR CHILD AND ADOLESCENT IMMUNIZATION PRACTICES

AVAILABILITY OF VACCINES
Vaccination services are readily available. Vaccinations are coordinated with other health care services and provided in a medical home when possible. Barriers to vaccination are identified and minimized. Patient costs are minimized.
ASSESSMENT OF VACCINATION STATUS
Health care professionals review the vaccination and health status of patients at every encounter to determine which vaccines are indicated. Health care professionals assess for and follow only medically accepted contraindications.
EFFECTIVE COMMUNICATION ABOUT VACCINE BENEFITS AND RISKS
Parents or guardians and patients are educated about the benefits and risks of vaccination in a culturally appropriate manner and in easy-to-understand language.
PROPER STORAGE AND ADMINISTRATION OF VACCINES AND DOCUMENTATION OF VACCINATIONS
Health care professionals follow appropriate procedures for vaccine storage and handling. Up-to-date, written vaccination protocols are accessible at all locations where vaccines are administered. Persons who administer vaccines and staff who manage or support vaccine administration are knowledgeable and receive ongoing education. Health care professionals simultaneously administer as many indicated vaccine doses as possible. Vaccination records for patients are accurate, complete, and easily accessible. Health care professionals report adverse events following vaccination promptly and accurately to the Vaccine Adverse Event Reporting System (VAERS) and are aware of a separate program, the National Vaccine Injury Compensation Program (VICP). All personnel who have contact with patients are appropriately vaccinated.
IMPLEMENTATION OF STRATEGIES TO IMPROVE VACCINATION COVERAGE
Systems are used to remind parents or guardians, patients, and health care professionals when vaccinations are due and to recall those who are overdue. Office- or clinic-based patient record reviews and vaccination coverage assessments are performed annually. Health care professionals practice community-based approaches.

From the National Vaccine Advisory Committee: Standards for child and adolescent immunization practices. *Pediatrics* 112:958–963, 2003.

BIBLIOGRAPHY

Please visit the Nelson Textbook of Pediatrics *website at www.expertconsult.com for the complete bibliography.*

165.1 International Immunization Practices

Jean-Marie Okwo-Bele and John David Clemens

Vaccines are used to prevent infectious diseases around the world. However, the types of vaccines in use, the indications and contraindications, and the immunization schedules vary substantially. Most developing countries follow the immunization schedules promulgated by the World Health Organization's Immunization Programme; the latest update is available at *www.who.int/immunization/policy/Immunization_routine_table2.pdf*.

Table 165-8 VACCINE WEBSITES AND RESOURCES

ORGANIZATION	WEBSITE
HEALTH PROFESSIONAL ASSOCIATIONS	
American Academy of Family Physicians (AAFP)	*www.familydoctor.org/online/famdocen/home.html*
American Academy of Pediatrics (AAP)	*www.aap.org/*
AAP Childhood Immunization Support Program	*www.aap.org/immunization/*
American Medical Association (AMA)	*www.ama-assn.org/*
American Nurses Association (ANA)	*www.nursingworld.org/*
Association of State and Territorial Health Officials (ASTHO)	*www.astho.org/*
Association of Teachers of Preventive Medicine (ATPM)	*www.atpm.org/*
National Medical Association (NMA)	*www.nmanet.org/*
NONPROFIT GROUPS AND UNIVERSITIES	
Albert B. Sabin Vaccine Institute	*www.sabin.org/*
Allied Vaccine Group (AVG)	*www.vaccine.org/*
Children's Vaccine Program	*www.path.org/vaccineresources/*
Every Child By Two (ECBT)	*www.ecbt.org/*
Global Alliance for Vaccines and Immunization (GAVI)	*www.gavialliance.org/*
Health on the Net Foundation (HON)	*www.hon.ch/*
National Healthy Mothers, Healthy Babies Coalition (HMHB)	*www.hmhb.org/*
Immunization Action Coalition (IAC)	*www.immunize.org/*
Institute for Vaccine Safety (IVS), Johns Hopkins University	*www.vaccinesafety.edu/*
Institute of Medicine	*www.iom.edu/Activities/PublicHealth/ImmunizationSafety.aspx*
National Alliance for Hispanic Health	*www.hispanichealth.org/*
National Network for Immunization Information (NNii)	*www.immunizationinfo.org/*
Parents of Kids with Infectious Diseases (PKIDS)	*www.pkids.org/*
The Vaccine Education Center at the Children's Hospital of Philadelphia	*www.chop.edu/service/vaccine-education-center/home.html*
The Vaccine Place	*www.vaccineplace.com/?fa=home*
GOVERNMENT ORGANIZATIONS	
Centers for Disease Control and Prevention (CDC)	
Public Health Image Library	*www.phil.cdc.gov/phil/home.asp*
Travelers' Health	*www.cdc.gov/travel/*
Vaccines and Immunizations	*www.cdc.gov/vaccines/*
Vaccine Safety	*www.cdc.gov/vaccinesafety/index.html*
Department of Health and Human Services (HHS)	
National Vaccine Program Office (NVPO)	*www.hhs.gov/nvpo/*
Health Resources and Services Administration	
National Vaccine Injury Compensation Program	*www.hrsa.gov/vaccinecompensation/*
National Institute of Allergy and Infectious Diseases (NIAID)	
Vaccines	*www.niaid.nih.gov/topics/vaccines/Pages/Default.aspx*
World Health Organization (WHO)	
Immunization, Vaccines, and Biologicals	*www.who.int/immunization/en/*

According to this schedule, all children should be vaccinated at birth against tuberculosis with bacille Calmette-Guérin (BCG) vaccine. Many children also receive a dose of the live-attenuated oral polio vaccine (OPV) at this time. Immunization visits are scheduled for 6, 10, and 14 wk of age when DTP vaccine and OPV are administered. Measles vaccine is given at 9 mo of age. Nearly all developing countries have implemented HepB vaccination. Three schedule options may be used depending on epidemiologic and programmatic considerations. HepB vaccine can be given at the same time as DTP vaccine doses at 6, 9, and 14 wk of age, often in combination vaccines. To prevent perinatal transmission, the first dose should be administered as soon as possible after birth (<24 hr) and at 6 and 14 wk of age. Yellow fever and Japanese encephalitis vaccines are recommended for infants 9 mo of age living in endemic areas. Substantial efforts have been made to incorporate Hib vaccines into all but 10 developing countries that are eligible for support by the GAVI Alliance (Global Alliance for Vaccines and Immunisation), often within a DPT-based combination vaccine.

In the next few yr, the support from the GAVI Alliance will facilitate the adoption of rotavirus and pneumococcal conjugate vaccines into developing country immunization programs. The increased coverage with these additional vaccines will considerably reduce the global childhood morbidity and mortality due to pneumonia, meningitis, and diarrheal diseases.

In 1988, the World Health Assembly endorsed the goal of eradicating polio from the world by the end of 2000. While that goal has not been reached, endemic polio transmission has been curtailed to three countries in south Asia (India, Pakistan, and Afghanistan) and one country in Africa. Other countries have had outbreaks from imported cases. The principal strategy has been use of OPV both for routine immunization as well as in mass campaigns, at least twice per year, during which all children <5 yr of age are targeted for immunization, regardless of prior immunization status. Once termination of wild polio virus transmission is achieved, the eventual goal is to stop use of OPV, which can rarely cause vaccine-associated polio and which is capable of mutating and taking on the phenotypic characteristics of the wild viruses.

The countries in Latin America have maintained the elimination of indigenous circulation of measles since 2002. The strategy called for attainment of high routine immunization coverage of infants with a dose at 9 mo of age, a 1-time mass campaign targeting all persons 9 mo-14 yr of age regardless of prior immunization status, and follow-up campaigns of children born since the prior campaign, generally every 3-5 yr. Meanwhile, global measles mortality in all ages has been reduced by nearly 70%, from an estimated 757,000 deaths in 2000 to 242,000 in 2006. The largest percentage in mortality reduction, 91%, was achieved in Africa, which has scaled up the implementation of the successful elimination strategy initiated in the Americas. Latin American countries have now embarked on efforts to eliminate indigenous rubella with strategies consisting of both routine immunization and mass campaigns.

Immunization schedules in the industrialized world are substantially more variable than in the developing world. Immunization recommendations for Canada are developed by the Canadian National Advisory Committee on Immunization (NACI) but are implemented somewhat differently by each province. The Canadian schedule is similar to the U.S. immunization schedule (*http://www.phac-aspc.gc.ca/im/is-cv/index-eng.php*). Conjugate meningococcal serogroup C vaccine (MCV-C) is recommended in a 3-dose series at 2, 4, and 6 mo of age. A single dose is recommended after 12 mo of age if the child has never been immunized or has received <3 doses in infancy. The province of Ontario, Canada, has a recommendation for annual vaccination of all persons 6 mo and older with trivalent influenza vaccine.

There is tremendous variation in vaccines used and the immunization schedules recommended in Europe. European immunization schedules can be reviewed at *www.who.int/vaccines/globalsummary/immunization/ScheduleSelect.cfm*. As an example, the UK developed an immunization schedule during the late 1980s that includes visits at 2, 3, and 4 mo of age where a combination DTaP-Hib-IPV vaccine is administered. Following evidence that a three-dose series of Hib vaccine at these ages was insufficient to ensure long-term, high-grade protection, a booster dose was added at 12 mo of age. MMR is recommended in a 2-dose schedule at 13 mo and 3-5 yr of age. During the 2nd MMR visit, a booster of DTaP and IPV is provided. A Td/IPV booster is recommended between 13 and 18 yr of age. PCV7 is recommended at 2, 4, and 13 mo of age. The UK was the first country to use MCV-C vaccine during a massive catch-up campaign for children, adolescents, and young adults. The effectiveness of the vaccine in the 1st year was 88% or greater, and herd immunity was induced with an approximate two-thirds reduction in the incidence among unvaccinated children. MCV-C is administered at 3, 4, and 12 mo of age. In September 2008, HPV vaccine was recommended for girls 12-13 yr old. As of July 2009, the UK schedule did not include HepB vaccine, varicella vaccine, or influenza vaccine for universal childhood immunization (see *www.immunisation.nhs.uk/*).

The Japanese immunization schedule in 2009 is substantially different from that in the USA. The Japanese do not use MMR and rely on individual vaccines for measles and rubella or combined MR. Japanese children also are vaccinated routinely against polio with OPV; against diphtheria, tetanus, and pertussis with DTaP; against Japanese encephalitis; and against tuberculosis with BCG. Adults 65 yr of age and older receive annual influenza vaccinations. The Japanese schedule does not include any vaccines against encapsulated bacteria.

Some children come to the USA having started or completed international immunization schedules with vaccines produced outside of the USA. In general, doses administered in other countries should be considered valid if administered at the same ages as recommended in the USA. For missing doses, age-inappropriate doses, lost immunization records, or other concerns, pediatricians have 2 options: Administer or repeat missing or inappropriate doses or perform serologic tests, and if they are negative, administer vaccines.

BIBLIOGRAPHY

Please visit the Nelson Textbook of Pediatrics *website at www.expertconsult.com for the complete bibliography.*

Chapter 166
Infection Prevention and Control

Michael J. Chusid and Mary M. Rotar

Infection prevention and control (IPC) is playing an ever more important role in pediatric medicine. To be fully effective, such programs require a functional infrastructure that addresses collaboration with the public health system, widespread immunizations, and use of appropriate techniques to prevent transmission of infection within the general population and within health care institutions. The increased focus upon preventing nosocomial infection is emphasized by the fact that 5 of the 16 elements of the Joint Commission's 2009 National Patient Safety Goals relate to prevention of health care–associated infection (HAI): hand hygiene, unanticipated death or major permanent loss of function associated with a health care-associated infection, central line–associated bloodstream infections, surgical site infections, and infections with multidrug-resistant organisms. Additionally, governmental agencies and insurance providers have reduced or eliminated payment to institutions for expenses associated with certain HAIs.

For the full continuation of this chapter, please visit the Nelson Textbook of Pediatrics *website at www.expertconsult.com.*

Chapter 167
Child Care and Communicable Diseases

Linda A. Waggoner-Fountain

More than 23.7 million children <5 yr of age attend a child care facility. These facilities can include some type of out-of-home care on a routine basis such as nursery school, preschool, or a full-day program based either in a child care center or in another person's home. Regardless of the age at entry, children entering day care are more prone to infections. Exposure to larger groups of children increases a child's probability of getting sick. Child-care facilities can be classified on the basis of size of enrollment, ages of attendees, health status of the children enrolled, and type of setting. As defined in the USA, **child-care facilities** consist of child-care centers, small and large family child-care homes, and facilities for ill children or for children with special needs. Centers are licensed and regulated by state governments and care for a larger number of children than are cared for in family homes. In contrast, **family child-care homes** are designated as small (1-6 children) or large (7-12 children), may be full day or part day, and may be designed for either daily or sporadic attendance. Family child-care homes generally are not licensed or registered, depending on state requirements.

For the full continuation of this chapter, please visit the Nelson Textbook of Pediatrics *website at www.expertconsult.com.*

Chapter 168
Health Advice for Children Traveling Internationally

Jessica K. Fairley and Chandy C. John

The health risks and pretravel requirements for children traveling internationally, particularly those <2 yr of age, differ from those for adults. In the USA, recommendations and vaccine requirements for travel to different countries are provided by the Centers for Disease Control and Prevention (CDC) and are available online at *www.cdc.gov/travel/content/vaccinations.aspx*.

For the full continuation of this chapter, please visit the Nelson Textbook of Pediatrics *website at www.expertconsult.com.*

Chapter 169
Fever

Linda S. Nield and Deepak Kamat

DEFINITION

Fever is defined as a rectal temperature ≥38°C, and a value >40°C is called hyperpyrexia. Body temperature fluctuates in a defined normal range (36.6°C-37.9°C rectally), so that the highest point is reached in early evening and the lowest point is reached in the morning. Any abnormal rise in body temperature should be considered a symptom of an underlying condition.

For the full continuation of this chapter, please visit the Nelson Textbook of Pediatrics *website at www.expertconsult.com.*

Chapter 170
Fever without a Focus

Linda S. Nield and Deepak Kamat

Fever without a focus refers to a rectal temperature of 38°C or higher as the sole presenting feature. The terms "fever without localizing signs" and "fever of unknown origin" (FUO) are subcategories of fever without a focus.

FEVER WITHOUT LOCALIZING SIGNS

Fever of acute onset, with duration of <1 wk and without localizing signs, is a common diagnostic dilemma in children <36 mo of age. The etiology and evaluation of fever without localizing signs depends on the age of the child. Traditionally, 3 age groups are considered: neonates or infants to 1 mo of age, infants >1 mo to 3 mo of age, and children >3 mo to 3 yr of age. In 1993, practice guidelines were published to aid the clinician in evaluating the otherwise healthy 0 to 36 mo old with fever without a source. However, with the advent and extensive use of the conjugate *Haemophilus influenzae* type b (Hib) and *Streptococcus pneumoniae* vaccines, the rates of infections with these 2 pathogens have decreased substantially. As a consequence, modifications to the 1993 guidelines have been advocated as described later. Children in high-risk groups (Table 170-1) require a more-aggressive approach and consideration of a broader differential diagnosis.

Neonates

Neonates who experience fever without focus are a challenge to evaluate because they display limited signs of infection, making it difficult to clinically distinguish between a serious bacterial infection and self-limited viral illness. Immature immune responses in the first few months of life also increase the significance of fever in the young infant. In general, neonates who have a fever and do not appear ill have a 7% risk of having a serious bacterial infection. Serious bacterial infections include occult bacteremia, meningitis, pneumonia, osteomyelitis, septic arthritis, enteritis, and urinary tract infections. Although neonates with serious infection can acquire community pathogens, they are mainly at risk for late-onset neonatal bacterial diseases (group B streptococci, *Escherichia coli*, and *Listeria monocytogenes*) and perinatally acquired herpes simplex virus (HSV) infection.

Practice guidelines recommend that if a neonate has had a fever recorded at home by a reliable parent, the patient should be treated as a febrile neonate. If excessive clothing and blankets encasing the infant are suspected of falsely elevating the body temperature, then the excessive coverings should be removed and the temperature retaken in 15 to 30 minutes. If body temperature is normal after the covers are removed, then the infant is considered afebrile.

Owing to the unreliability of physical findings and the presence of an immature immune system, all febrile neonates should be hospitalized; blood, urine, and cerebrospinal fluid (CSF) should be cultured, and the child should receive empirical intravenous antibiotics. CSF studies should include cell counts, glucose and protein levels, Gram stain, and culture; HSV and enterovirus polymerase chain reaction should be considered. Stool culture

Table 170-1 FEBRILE PATIENTS AT INCREASED RISK FOR SERIOUS BACTERIAL INFECTIONS

RISK GROUP	DIAGNOSTIC CONSIDERATIONS
IMMUNOCOMPETENT PATIENTS	
Neonates (<28 days)	Sepsis and meningitis caused by group B streptococcus, *Escherichia coli, Listeria monocytogenes*; neonatal herpes simplex virus infection, enteroviruses
Infants 1-3 mo	Serious bacterial disease in 10-15%, including bacteremia in 5%; urinary tract infection
Infants and children 3-36 mo	Occult bacteremia in <0.5% of children immunized with both *Haemophilus influenzae* type b and pneumococcal conjugate vaccines; urinary tract infections
Hyperpyrexia (>40°C)	Meningitis, bacteremia, pneumonia, heatstroke, hemorrhagic shock-encephalopathy syndrome
Fever with petechiae	Bacteremia and meningitis caused by *Neisseria meningitidis, H. influenzae* type b, and *Streptococcus pneumoniae*
IMMUNOCOMPROMISED PATIENTS	
Sickle cell disease	Sepsis, pneumonia, and meningitis caused by *S. pneumoniae*, osteomyelitis caused by *Salmonella* and *Staphylococcus aureus*
Asplenia	Bacteremia and meningitis caused by *N. meningitidis, H. influenzae* type b, and *S. pneumoniae*
Complement or properdin deficiency	Sepsis caused by *N. meningitidis*
Agammaglobulinemia	Bacteremia, sinopulmonary infections
AIDS	*S. pneumoniae, H. influenzae* type b, and *Salmonella* infections
Congenital heart disease	Infective endocarditis; brain abscess with right-to-left shunting
Central venous line	*Staphylococcus aureus*, coagulase-negative staphylococci, *Candida*
Malignancy	Bacteremia with gram-negative enteric bacteria, *S. aureus*, and coagulase-negative staphylococci; fungemia with *Candida* and *Aspergillus*

and chest radiograph may also be part of the evaluation. Combination antibiotics such as ampicillin and cefotaxime are recommended. Acyclovir should be included if HSV infection is suspected owing to the presence of CSF pleocytosis or known maternal history of genital HSV, especially at the time of delivery.

1 Month to 3 Months

The large majority of children with fever without localizing signs in the 1-3 mo age group likely have a viral syndrome. In contrast to bacterial infections, most viral diseases have a distinct seasonal pattern: respiratory syncytial virus and influenza A virus infections are more common during the winter, whereas enterovirus infections usually occur in the summer and fall. Although a viral infection is the most likely etiology, fever in this age group should always suggest the possibility of serious bacterial disease. Organisms to consider include group B streptococcus, *L. monocytogenes*, *Salmonella enteritis*, *E. coli*, *Neisseria meningitidis*, *S. pneumoniae*, Hib, and *Staphylococcus aureus*. Pyelonephritis is more common in uncircumcised infant boys and infants with urinary tract anomalies. Other potential bacterial diseases in this age group include otitis media, pneumonia, omphalitis, mastitis, and other skin and soft tissue infections.

Ill-appearing (toxic) febrile infants ≤3 mo of age require prompt hospitalization and immediate parenteral antimicrobial therapy after cultures of blood, urine, and CSF are obtained. Ampicillin (to cover *L. monocytogenes* and enterococcus) plus either ceftriaxone or cefotaxime is an effective initial antimicrobial regimen for ill-appearing infants without focal findings. This regimen is effective against the usual bacterial pathogens causing sepsis, urinary tract infection, and enteritis in young infants. However, if meningitis is suspected because of CSF abnormalities, vancomycin should be included to treat possible penicillin-resistant *S. pneumoniae* until the results of culture and susceptibility tests are known.

Many academic institutions have investigated the optimal management of low-risk patients in this age group with fever without a focus (Table 170-2). The use of viral diagnostic studies (enteroviruses, respiratory viruses, rotavirus, and herpesvirus) in combination with the Rochester Criteria or similar criteria can enhance the ability to determine which infants are at high risk for serious bacterial infections (see Table 170-2). Febrile infants in whom a virus has been detected are at low or no risk of a serious bacterial infection. Well-appearing infants 1-3 mo of age can be managed safely using low-risk laboratory and clinical criteria as indicated in Table 170-2 if reliable parents are involved and close follow-up is assured.

Infants 1-3 mo of age with fever who appear generally well; who have been previously healthy; who have no evidence of skin, soft tissue, bone, joint, or ear infection; and who have a peripheral white blood cell (WBC) count of 5,000-15,000 cells/μL, an absolute band count of <1,500 cells/μL, and normal urinalysis and negative culture (blood and urine) results are unlikely to have a serious bacterial infection. The negative predictive value with 95% confidence of these criteria for any serious bacterial infection is >98% and for bacteremia is >99%. Among serious bacterial infections, pyelonephritis is the most common and may be seen in well-appearing infants who have fever without a focus or in those who appear ill. Urinalysis may be negative in infants <2 mo of age with pyelonephritis. Bacteremia is present in <30% of infants with pyelonephritis.

The decision to obtain CSF studies in the well-appearing 1-3 mo old infant depends on the decision to administer empirical antibiotics. If close observation without antibiotics is planned, a lumbar puncture may be deferred. If the child deteriorates clinically, a full sepsis evaluation should be performed, and intravenous antibiotics should be administered. If empirical antibiotics are initiated, CSF studies should be obtained, preferably before administering antibiotics.

Table 170-2 LOW RISK CRITERIA IN 1-3 MONTHS OLD WITH FEVER

BOSTON CRITERIA
Infants are at low risk if they appear well, have normal physical examination, have a caretaker reachable by telephone, and laboratory tests are as follows: • CBC: <20,000 WBC/mm³ • Urine: negative leukocyte esterase • CSF: leukocyte count less than 10 × 10⁶/L,
PHILADELPHIA PROTOCOL
Infants are at low risk if they appear well, have a normal physical examination, and laboratory tests are as follows: • CBC: <15,000 WBC/mm³; band: total neutrophil ratio <0.2 • Urine: <10 WBC/HPF; no bacteria on Gram stain • CSF: <8 WBC/mm³; no bacteria on Gram stain • Chest radiograph: no infiltrate • Stool: no RBC; few to no WBC
PITTSBURGH GUIDELINES
Infants are at low risk if they appear well, have a normal physical examination, and laboratory tests are as follows: • CBC: 5,000-15,000 WBC; peripheral absolute band count <1500/mm³ • Urine (enhanced urinalysis): 9 WBC/mm³ and no bacteria on Gram stain • CSF: 5 WBC/mm³ and negative Gram stain; if bloody tap, then WBC : RBC ≤ 1 : 500 • Chest radiograph: no infiltrate • Stool: 5 WBC/HPF with diarrhea
ROCHESTER CRITERIA
Infants are at low risk if they appear well, have a normal physical examination, and laboratory findings are as follows: • CBC: 5,000-15,000 WBC/mm3; absolute band count ≤1500/mm³ • Urine: <10 WBC/HPF at 40× • Stool: <5 WBC/HPF if diarrhea

CBC, complete blood count; CSF, cerebrospinal fluid; HPF, high-powered field; RBC, red blood cell; WBC: white blood cell.

3 Months to 36 Months of Age

Approximately 30% of febrile children in the 3-36 mo age group have no localizing signs of infection. Viral infections are the cause of the vast majority of fevers in this population, but serious bacterial infections do occur and are caused by the same pathogens listed for patients 1-3 mo of age, except for the perinatally acquired infections. *S. pneumoniae*, *N. meningitidis*, and *Salmonella* account for most cases of occult bacteremia. Hib was an important cause of occult bacteremia in young children before universal immunization with conjugate Hib vaccines and remains common in underdeveloped countries that have not implemented these vaccines.

Risk factors indicating increased probability of occult bacteremia include temperature ≥39°C, WBC count ≥15,000/μL, and elevated absolute neutrophil count, band count, erythrocyte sedimentation rate, or C-reactive protein. The incidence of bacteremia and/or pneumonia or pyelonephritis, among infants 3-36 mo of age increases as the temperature (especially >40°C) and WBC count (especially >25,000) increase. However, no combination of laboratory tests or clinical assessment is completely accurate in predicting the presence of occult bacteremia. Socioeconomic status, race, sex, and age (within the range of 3-36 mo) do not appear to affect the risk for occult bacteremia.

Without therapy, occult bacteremia due to pneumococcus can resolve spontaneously without sequelae, can persist, or can lead to localized infections such as meningitis, pneumonia, cellulitis, pericarditis, osteomyelitis, or suppurative arthritis. The pattern of sequelae may be related to host factors and the offending organism. In some children, the occult bacteremic illness can represent the early signs of serious localized infection rather than a transient disease state. Hib bacteremia is characteristically associated with a higher risk for localized serious infection than is bacteremia due to *S. pneumoniae*. Hospitalized children with Hib bacteremia often develop focal infections, such as meningitis, epiglottitis, cellulitis, pericarditis, or osteoarticular infection, and spontaneous resolution of bacteremia is rare. Among patients with pneumococcal bacteremia (occult or focal), spontaneous resolution occurs in 30-40%, with a higher rate of spontaneous resolution among well-appearing children.

Important bacterial infections among children 3-36 mo of age with localizing signs include otitis media, sinusitis, pneumonia (not always evident without a chest x-ray), enteritis, urinary tract infection, osteomyelitis, and meningitis.

Treatment of toxic-appearing febrile children 3-36 mo of age who do not have focal signs of infection includes hospitalization and prompt institution of antimicrobial therapy after specimens of blood, urine, and CSF are obtained for culture. Consensus practice guidelines published in 1993 recommended that children 3-36 mo of age who have a temperature of <39°C and do not appear toxic be observed as outpatients without performing diagnostic tests or administering antimicrobial agents. For nontoxic-appearing infants with a rectal temperature of ≥39°C, options include obtaining a blood culture and administering empirical antibiotic therapy (ceftriaxone, a single dose of 50 mg/kg, not to exceed 1 g); if the WBC count is >15,000/µL, obtaining a blood culture and beginning empirical antibiotic therapy; or obtaining a blood culture and observing as outpatients without empirical antibiotic therapy, with return for re-evaluation within 24 hr. Guidelines for managing febrile children 3-36 mo of age who have received both Hib and *S. pneumoniae* conjugate vaccines have not been established, but careful observation without empirical administration of antibiotic therapy is generally prudent. Because fully vaccinated young children are at a much lower risk of occult bacteremia and meningitis as the cause of acute fever without localizing signs, some advocate that the only laboratory tests needed in this age group when temperature is >39°C are a urinalysis and urine culture for circumcised boys <6 mo of age and uncircumcised boys and all girls <24 mo of age. Regardless of the management option (Table 170-3), the family should be instructed to return immediately if the child's condition deteriorates or new symptoms develop.

Empirical antibiotic therapy for well-appearing children <36 mo of age who have not received Hib and *S. pneumoniae* conjugate vaccines and who have a rectal temperature of >39°C and a WBC count of >15,000/µL is strongly recommended. If blood cultures are obtained and *S. pneumoniae* is isolated from the blood, the child should return to the physician as soon as possible after the culture results are known. If the child appears well, is afebrile, and has a normal physical exam, a second blood culture should be obtained and the child should be treated with 7-10 days of oral antimicrobial therapy. If the child appears ill and continues to have fever with no identifiable focus of infection at the time of follow-up, or if *H. influenzae*, or *N. meningitidis* is present in the initial blood culture, the child should have a repeat blood culture, be evaluated for meningitis (including lumbar puncture), and receive treatment in the hospital with appropriate intravenous antimicrobial agents. If the child develops a localized infection, therapy should be directed toward the likely pathogens.

FEVER OF UNKNOWN ORIGIN

The classification of FUO is best reserved for children with fever documented by a health care provider and for which the cause could not be identified after 3 wk of evaluation as an outpatient or after 1 wk of evaluation in the hospital (Table 170-4).

Etiology

The many causes of FUO in children are infections and rheumatologic (connective tissue or autoimmune) diseases (Table 170-5). Neoplastic disorders should also be seriously considered, although most children with malignancies do not have fever alone. The possibility of drug fever should be considered if the patient is receiving any drug. Drug fever is usually sustained and not

Table 170-3 MANAGEMENT OF FEVER WITHOUT LOCALIZING SIGNS

GROUP	MANAGEMENT
Any toxic-appearing child 0-36 mo and temperature ≥38°C	Hospitalize, broad cultures plus other tests,* parenteral antibiotics
Child <1 mo and temperature ≥38°C	Hospitalize, broad cultures plus other tests,* parenteral antibiotics
Child 1-3 mo and temperature ≥38°C	Two-step process 1. Determine risk based on history, physical examination, and laboratory studies. Low risk: • Uncomplicated medical history • Normal physical examination • Normal laboratory studies • Urine: negative leukocyte esterase, nitrite and <10 WBC/HPF • Peripheral blood: 5,000-15,000 WBC/mm³; <1,500 bands or band : total neutrophil ratio <0.2 • Stool studies if diarrhea (no RBC and <5 WBC/HPF) • CSF cell count (<8 WBC/mm³) and negative Gram stain • Chest radiograph without infiltrate 2. If child fulfills all low-risk criteria, administer no antibiotics, ensure follow-up in 24 hr and access to emergency care if child deteriorates. Daily follow-up should occur until blood, urine, and CSF cultures are final. If any cultures are positive, child returns for further evaluation and treatment. If child does not fulfill all low-risk criteria, hospitalize and administer parenteral antibiotics until all cultures are final and definitive diagnosis determined and treated.
Child 3-36 mo and temperature 38-39°C	Reassurance that diagnosis is likely self-limiting viral infection, but advise return with persistence of fever, temperatures >39°C, and new signs and symptoms
Child 3-36 mo and temperature >39°C	Two-step process: 1. Determine immunization status 2. If received conjugate pneumococcal and *H. influenzae* type b vaccines, obtain urine studies (urine WBC, leukocyte esterase, nitrite, and culture) for all girls, all boys <6 mo old, all uncircumcised boys <2 yr, all children with recurrent urinary tract infections If did not receive conjugate pneumococcal and *H. influenzae* type b vaccines, manage according to the 1993 Guidelines (see Baraff et al. *Pediatrics* 1993;92:1-12)

*Other tests may include chest radiograph, stool studies, herpes simplex polymerase chain reaction.
CSF, cerebrospinal fluid; HPF, high-powered field; RBC, red blood cell; WBC, white blood cell.

Table 170-4 SUMMARY OF DEFINITIONS AND MAJOR FEATURES OF THE FOUR SUBTYPES OF FEVER OF UNKNOWN ORIGIN

FEATURE	CLASSIC FUO	HEALTH CARE–ASSOCIATED FUO	IMMUNE-DEFICIENT FUO	HIV-RELATED FUO
Definition	>38.0°C, >3 wk, >2 visits or 1 wk in hospital	≥38.0°C, >1 wk, not present or incubating on admission	≥38.0°C, >1 wk, negative cultures after 48 hr	≥38.0°C, >3 wk for outpatients, >1 wk for inpatients, HIV infection confirmed
Patient location	Community, clinic, or hospital	Acute care hospital	Hospital or clinic	Community, clinic, or hospital
Leading causes	Cancer, infections, inflammatory conditions, undiagnosed, habitual hyperthermia	Health care–associated infections, postoperative complications, drug fever	Majority due to infections, but cause documented in only 40-60%	HIV (primary infection), typical and atypical mycobacteria, CMV, lymphomas, toxoplasmosis, cryptococcosis, immune reconstitution inflammatory syndrome (IRIS)
History emphasis	Travel, contacts, animal and insect exposure, medications, immunizations, family history, cardiac valve disorder	Operations and procedures, devices, anatomic considerations, drug treatment	Stage of chemotherapy, drugs administered, underlying immunosuppressive disorder	Drugs, exposures, risk factors, travel, contacts, stage of HIV infection
Examination emphasis	Fundi, oropharynx, temporal artery, abdomen, lymph nodes, spleen, joints, skin, nails, genitalia, rectum or prostate, lower limb deep veins	Wounds, drains, devices, sinuses, urine	Skin folds, IV sites, lungs, perianal area	Mouth, sinuses, skin, lymph nodes, eyes, lungs, perianal area
Investigation emphasis	Imaging, biopsies, sedimentation rate, skin tests	Imaging, bacterial cultures	CXR, bacterial cultures	Blood and lymphocyte count; serologic tests; CXR; stool examination; biopsies of lung, bone marrow, and liver for cultures and cytologic tests; brain imaging
Management	Observation, outpatient temperature chart, investigations, avoidance of empirical drug treatments	Depends on situation	Antimicrobial treatment protocols	Antiviral and antimicrobial protocols, vaccines, revision of treatment regimens, good nutrition
Time course of disease	Months	Weeks	Days	Weeks to months
Tempo of investigation	Weeks	Days	Hours	Days to weeks

CMV, cytomegalovirus; CXR, chest radiograph; FUO, fever of unknown origin.
Adapted from Mandell GL, Bennett, JE, Dolin R, editors: *Mandell, Douglas, and Bennett's principles and practice of infectious diseases*, ed 7, Philadelphia, 2010, Churchill Livingstone/Elsevier, 2010, p 780, Table 51-1.

associated with other symptoms. Discontinuation of the drug is associated with resolution of the fever, generally within 72 hr, although certain drugs, such as iodides, are excreted for a prolonged period with fever that can persist for as long as 1 mo after drug withdrawal.

Most fevers of unknown or unrecognized origin result from atypical presentations of common diseases. In some cases, the presentation as an FUO is characteristic of the disease, such as juvenile idiopathic arthritis, but the definitive diagnosis can be established only after prolonged observation because initially there are no associated or specific findings on physical examination and all laboratory results are negative or normal.

In the USA, the systemic infectious diseases most commonly implicated in children with FUO are salmonellosis, tuberculosis, rickettsial diseases, syphilis, Lyme disease, cat-scratch disease, atypical prolonged presentations of common viral diseases, infectious mononucleosis, cytomegalovirus (CMV) infection, viral hepatitis, coccidioidomycosis, histoplasmosis, malaria, and toxoplasmosis. Less common infectious causes of FUO include tularemia, brucellosis, leptospirosis, and rat-bite fever. AIDS alone is not usually responsible for FUO, although febrile illnesses often occur in patients with AIDS as a result of opportunistic infections (see Table 170-4).

Juvenile idiopathic arthritis (JIA) and systemic lupus erythematosus (SLE) are the connective tissue diseases associated most commonly with FUO. Inflammatory bowel disease, rheumatic fever, and Kawasaki disease are also commonly reported as causes of FUO. If factitious fever (inoculation of pyogenic material or manipulation of the thermometer by the patient or parent) is suspected, the presence and pattern of fever should be documented in the hospital. Prolonged and continuous observation, which can include electronic or video surveillance, of patients is imperative. FUO lasting >6 mo is uncommon in children and suggests granulomatous or autoimmune disease. Repeat interval evaluation, including history, physical examination, laboratory evaluation, and roentgenographic studies is required.

Diagnosis

The evaluation of FUO requires a thorough history and physical examination supplemented by a few screening laboratory tests and additional laboratory and radiographic tests as indicated by the history or abnormalities on examination or initial screening (see Table 170-5).

HISTORY The age of the patient is helpful in evaluating FUO. Children >6 yr of age often have a respiratory or genitourinary tract infection, localized infection (abscess, osteomyelitis), JIA, or, rarely, leukemia. Adolescent patients are more likely to have tuberculosis, inflammatory bowel disease, autoimmune processes, or lymphoma, in addition to the causes of FUO found in younger children.

A history of exposure to wild or domestic animals should be solicited. Zoonotic infections in the USA are increasing in incidence and are often acquired from pets that are not overtly ill. Immunization of dogs against specific disorders such as leptospirosis can prevent canine disease but does not always prevent the animal from carrying and shedding leptospires, which may be transmitted to household contacts. A history of ingestion of rabbit or squirrel meat might provide a clue to the diagnosis of oropharyngeal, glandular, or typhoidal tularemia. A history of tick bite or travel to tick- or parasite-infested areas should be obtained.

Any history of pica should be elicited. Ingestion of dirt is a particularly important clue to infection with *Toxocara canis* (visceral larva migrans) or *Toxoplasma gondii* (toxoplasmosis).

A history of unusual dietary habits or travel as early as the birth of the child should be sought. Malaria, histoplasmosis, and coccidioidomycosis can re-emerge years after visiting or living in an endemic area. It is important to identify prophylactic immunizations and precautions taken by the patient against ingestion of contaminated water or food during foreign travel. Rocks, dirt, and artifacts from geographically distant regions that have been collected and brought into the home as souvenirs can serve as vectors of disease.

Table 170-5 DIAGNOSTIC CONSIDERATIONS OF FEVER OF UNKNOWN ORIGIN IN CHILDREN

ABSCESSES
Abdominal Brain Dental Hepatic Pelvic Perinephric Rectal Subphrenic Psoas
BACTERIAL DISEASES
Actinomycosis *Bartonella henselae* (cat-scratch disease) Brucellosis *Campylobacter* *Francisella tularensis* (tularemia) *Listeria monocytogenes* (listeriosis) Meningococcemia (chronic) *Mycoplasma pneumoniae* Rat-bite fever (*Streptobacillus moniliformis*; streptobacillary form of rat-bite fever) *Salmonella* Tuberculosis Whipple disease Yersiniosis
LOCALIZED INFECTIONS
Cholangitis Infective endocarditis Mastoiditis Osteomyelitis Pneumonia Pyelonephritis Sinusitis Spirochetes *Borrelia burgdorferi* (Lyme disease) Relapsing fever (*Borrelia recurrentis*) Leptospirosis Rat-bite fever (*Spirillum minus*; spirillary form of rat-bite fever) Syphilis
FUNGAL DISEASES
Blastomycosis (extrapulmonary) Coccidiodomycosis (disseminated) Histoplasmosis (disseminated) *Chlamydia* Lymphogranuloma venereum Psittacosis *Rickettsia* *Ehrlichia canis* Q fever Rocky Mountain spotted fever Tick-borne typhus
VIRUSES
Cytomegalovirus Hepatitis viruses HIV Infectious mononucleosis (Epstein-Barr virus)
PARASITIC DISEASES
Amebiasis Babesiosis Giardiasis Malaria Toxoplasmosis Trichinosis Trypanosomiasis Visceral larva migrans (*Toxocara*)
RHEUMATOLOGIC DISEASES
Behçet disease Juvenile dermatomyositis Juvenile rheumatoid arthritis Rheumatic fever Systemic lupus erythematosus
HYPERSENSITIVITY DISEASES
Drug fever Hypersensitivity pneumonitis Serum sickness Weber-Christian disease
NEOPLASMS
Atrial myxoma Cholesterol granuloma Hodgkin disease Inflammatory pseudotumor Leukemia Lymphoma Pheochromocytoma Neuroblastoma Wilms tumor
GRANULOMATOUS DISEASES
Crohn disease Granulomatous hepatitis Sarcoidosis
FAMILIAL AND HEREDITARY DISEASES
Anhidrotic ectodermal dysplasia Fabry disease Familial dysautonomia Familial Hiberian fever Familial Mediterranean fever Hypertriglyceridemia Ichthyosis Sickle cell crisis
MISCELLANEOUS
Addison disease Castleman disease Chronic active hepatitis Cyclic neutropenia Diabetes insipidus (non-nephrogenic and nephrogenic) Factitious fever Hemophagocytic syndromes Hypothalamic-central fever Infantile cortical hyperostosis Inflammatory bowel disease Kawasaki disease Kikuchi-Fujimoto disease Metal fume fever Pancreatitis Periodic fevers Poisoning Pulmonary embolism Thrombophlebitis Thyrotoxicosis, thyroiditis

A medication history should be pursued rigorously. This history should elicit information about over-the-counter preparations and topical agents, including eye drops, that may be associated with atropine-induced fever.

The genetic background of a patient also is important. Descendants of the Ulster Scots may have FUO because they are afflicted with nephrogenic diabetes insipidus. Familial dysautonomia (Riley-Day syndrome), a disorder in which hyperthermia is recurrent, is more common among Jews than other population groups. Ancestry from the Mediterranean should suggest the possibility of familial Mediterranean fever (FMF). Both FMF and hyperimmunoglobulin D syndrome are inherited as autosomal-recessive

Table 170-6 EXAMPLES OF SUBTLE PHYSICAL FINDINGS HAVING SPECIAL SIGNIFICANCE IN PATIENTS WITH FEVER OF UNKNOWN ORIGIN

BODY SITE	PHYSICAL FINDING	DIAGNOSIS
Head	Sinus tenderness	Sinusitis
Temporal artery	Nodules, reduced pulsations	Temporal arteritis
Oropharynx	Ulceration	Disseminated histoplasmosis
	Tender tooth	Periapical abscess
Fundi or conjunctivae	Choroid tubercle	Disseminated granulomatosis*
	Petechiae, Roth's spot	Endocarditis
Thyroid	Enlargement, tenderness	Thyroiditis
Heart	Murmur	Infective or marantic endocarditis
Abdomen	Enlarged iliac crest lymph nodes, splenomegaly	Lymphoma, endocarditis, disseminated granulomatosis*
Rectum	Perirectal fluctuance, tenderness	Abscess
	Prostatic tenderness, fluctuance	Abscess
Genitalia	Testicular nodule	Periarteritis nodosa
	Epididymal nodule	Disseminated granulomatosis
Lower extremities	Deep venous tenderness	Thrombosis or thrombophlebitis
Skin and nails	Petechiae, splinter hemorrhages, subcutaneous nodules, clubbing	Vasculitis, endocarditis

*Includes tuberculosis, histoplasmosis, coccidioidomycosis, sarcoidosis, and syphilis.
From Mandell GL, Bennett, JE, Dolin R, editors: *Mandell, Douglas, and Bennett's principles and practice of infectious diseases*, ed 7, Philadelphia, 2010, Churchill Livingstone/Elsevier, 2010, p 785, Table 51-8.

disorders. Tumor necrosis factor receptor–associated periodic syndrome (TRAPS) and Muckle-Wells syndrome are inherited as autosomal dominant traits.

PHYSICAL EXAMINATION A complete physical examination is essential to find any physical clues to the underlying diagnosis (Table 170-6). The child's general appearance, including sweating during fever, should be noted. The continuing absence of sweat in the presence of an elevated or changing body temperature suggests dehydration due to vomiting, diarrhea, or central or nephrogenic diabetes insipidus. It also should suggest anhidrotic ectodermal dysplasia, familial dysautonomia, or exposure to atropine.

A careful ophthalmic examination is important. Red, weeping eyes may be a sign of connective tissue disease, particularly polyarteritis nodosa. Palpebral conjunctivitis in a febrile patient may be a clue to measles, coxsackievirus infection, tuberculosis, infectious mononucleosis, lymphogranuloma venereum, and cat-scratch disease. In contrast, bulbar conjunctivitis in a child with FUO suggests Kawasaki disease or leptospirosis. Petechial conjunctival hemorrhages suggest infective endocarditis. Uveitis suggests sarcoidosis, JIA, SLE, Kawasaki disease, Behçet disease, and vasculitis. Chorioretinitis suggests CMV, toxoplasmosis, and syphilis. Proptosis suggests an orbital tumor, thyrotoxicosis, metastasis (neuroblastoma), orbital infection, Wegener granulomatosis, or pseudotumor.

The ophthalmoscope should also be used to examine nailfold capillary abnormalities that are associated with connective tissue diseases such as juvenile dermatomyositis and systemic scleroderma. Immersion oil or lubricating jelly is placed on the skin adjacent to the nailbed, and the capillary pattern is observed with the ophthalmoscope set on +40.

FUO is sometimes caused by hypothalamic dysfunction. A clue to this disorder is failure of pupillary constriction due to absence of the sphincter constrictor muscle of the eye. This muscle develops embryologically when hypothalamic structure and function also are undergoing differentiation.

Fever resulting from familial dysautonomia may be suggested by lack of tears, an absent corneal reflex, or a smooth tongue with absence of fungiform papillae. Tenderness to tapping over the sinuses or the upper teeth suggests sinusitis. Recurrent oral candidiasis may be a clue to various disorders of the immune system.

Fever blisters are common findings in patients with pneumococcal, streptococcal, malarial, and rickettsial infection. These lesions also are common in children with meningococcal meningitis (which usually does not manifest as FUO) but rarely are seen in children with meningococcemia. Fever blisters also are occasionally seen with *Salmonella* or staphylococcal infections.

Hyperemia of the pharynx, with or without exudate, suggests infectious mononucleosis, CMV infection, toxoplasmosis, salmonellosis, tularemia, Kawasaki disease, or leptospirosis.

The muscles and bones should be palpated carefully. Point tenderness over a bone can suggest occult osteomyelitis or bone marrow invasion from neoplastic disease. Tenderness over the trapezius muscle may be a clue to subdiaphragmatic abscess. Generalized muscle tenderness suggests dermatomyositis, trichinosis, polyarteritis, Kawasaki disease, or mycoplasmal or arboviral infection.

Rectal examination can reveal perirectal lymphadenopathy or tenderness, which suggests a deep pelvic abscess, iliac adenitis, or pelvic osteomyelitis. A guaiac test should be obtained; occult blood loss can suggest granulomatous colitis or ulcerative colitis as the cause of FUO.

Repetitive chills and temperature spikes are common in children with septicemia (regardless of cause), particularly when associated with kidney disease, liver or biliary disease, infective endocarditis, malaria, brucellosis, rat-bite fever, or a loculated collection of pus. The general activity of the patient and the presence or absence of rashes should be noted. Hyperactive deep tendon reflexes can suggest thyrotoxicosis as the cause of FUO.

LABORATORY EVALUATION The laboratory evaluation of the child with FUO and whether the evaluation will occur in the inpatient or outpatient realm are determined on a case-by-case basis. Hospitalization may be required for laboratory or radiographic studies that are unavailable or impractical in an ambulatory setting, for more-careful observation, or for temporary relief of parents' anxiety. The tempo of diagnostic evaluation should be adjusted to the tempo of the illness; haste may be imperative in a critically ill patient, but if the illness is more chronic, the evaluation can proceed in systematic fashion and can be carried out in an outpatient setting. If there are no clues in the patient's history or on physical examination that suggest a specific infection or area of suspicion, it is unlikely that diagnostic studies will be helpful. In that common scenario, continued surveillance and repeated re-evaluations of the child should be employed to detect any new clinical findings.

Although ordering a large number of diagnostic tests in every child with FUO according to a predetermined list is discouraged, certain studies should be considered in the evaluation. A complete blood cell count with a differential white blood cell count and a urinalysis should be part of the initial laboratory evaluation. An absolute neutrophil count of <5,000/μL is evidence against indolent bacterial infection other than typhoid fever. Conversely, in patients with a polymorphonuclear leukocyte count of >10,000/μL or a nonsegmented polymorphonuclear leukocyte count of >500/μL a severe bacterial infection is highly likely. Direct examination of the blood smear with Giemsa or Wright stain can reveal organisms of malaria, trypanosomiasis, babesiosis, or relapsing fever.

An erythrocyte sedimentation rate (ESR) of >30 mm/hr indicates inflammation and the need for further evaluation for infectious, autoimmune, or malignant diseases. An ESR of >100 mm/hr suggests tuberculosis, Kawasaki disease, malignancy, or autoimmune disease. A low ESR does not eliminate the possibility of infection or JIA. C-reactive protein is another acute-phase reactant that becomes elevated and returns to normal more rapidly than the ESR. Experts may prefer to check 1 of the 2 because there is no evidence that measuring both the ESR and C-reactive protein in the same patient with FUO is clinically useful.

Blood cultures should be obtained aerobically. Anaerobic blood cultures have an extremely low yield and should be obtained only if there are specific reasons to suspect anaerobic infection. Multiple or repeated blood cultures may be required to detect bacteremia associated with infective endocarditis, osteomyelitis, or deep-seated abscesses. Polymicrobial bacteremia suggests factitious self-induced infection or gastrointestinal (GI) pathology. The isolation of leptospires, *Francisella,* or *Yersinia* can require selective media or specific conditions not routinely used. Urine culture should be obtained routinely.

Tuberculin skin testing (TST) should be performed with intradermal placement of 5 units of purified protein derivative (PPD) that has been kept appropriately refrigerated.

Radiographic examination of the chest, sinuses, mastoids, or GI tract may be indicated by specific historical or physical findings. Radiographic evaluation of the GI tract for inflammatory bowel disease may be helpful in evaluating selected children with FUO and no other localizing signs or symptoms.

Examination of the bone marrow can reveal leukemia; metastatic neoplasm; mycobacterial, fungal, or parasitic diseases; and histiocytosis, hemophagocytosis, or storage diseases. If a bone marrow aspirate is performed, cultures for bacteria, mycobacteria, and fungi should be obtained.

Serologic tests can aid in the diagnosis of infectious mononucleosis, CMV infection, toxoplasmosis, salmonellosis, tularemia, brucellosis, leptospirosis, cat-scratch disease, Lyme disease, rickettsial disease, and, on some occasions, JIA. The clinician should be aware that the reliability and sensitivity and specificity of these tests vary; for instance, serologic tests for Lyme disease outside of reference laboratories have been generally unreliable.

Radionuclide scans may be helpful in detecting abdominal abscesses as well as osteomyelitis, especially if the focus cannot be localized to a specific limb or multifocal disease is suspected. Gallium citrate (^{67}Ga) localizes inflammatory tissues (leukocytes) associated with tumors or abscesses. ^{99m}Tc phosphate is useful for detecting osteomyelitis before plain roentgenograms demonstrate bone lesions. Granulocytes tagged with indium (^{111}In) or iodinated IgG may be useful in detecting localized pyogenic processes. ^{18}F-fluorodeoxyglucose positron emission tomography (FDG-PET) is a helpful imaging modality in adults with an FUO and can contribute to an ultimate diagnosis in 30-60% of patients. Echocardiograms can demonstrate the presence of a vegetation on the leaflets of heart valves, suggesting infective endocarditis. Ultrasonography can identify intra-abdominal abscesses of the liver, subphrenic space, pelvis, or spleen.

Total body CT or MRI (both with contrast) permits detection of neoplasms and collections of purulent material without the use of surgical exploration or radioisotopes. CT and MRI are helpful in identifying lesions of the head, neck, chest, retroperitoneal spaces, liver, spleen, intra-abdominal and intrathoracic lymph nodes, kidneys, pelvis, and mediastinum. CT or ultrasound-guided aspiration or biopsy of suspicious lesions has reduced the need for exploratory laparotomy or thoracotomy. MRI is particularly useful for detecting osteomyelitis if there is concern about a specific limb. Diagnostic imaging can be very helpful in confirming or evaluating a suspected diagnosis but rarely leads to an unsuspected cause, and in the case of CT scans, the child is exposed to large amounts of radiation.

Biopsy is occasionally helpful in establishing a diagnosis of FUO. Bronchoscopy, laparoscopy, mediastinoscopy, and GI endoscopy can provide direct visualization and biopsy material when organ-specific manifestations are present. When employing any of the more-invasive testing, the risk:benefit ratio for the patient must always be taken into consideration before proceeding further.

Treatment

The ultimate treatment of FUO is tailored to the underlying diagnosis. Fever and infection in children are not synonymous; antimicrobial agents should not be used as antipyretics, and empirical trials of medication should generally be avoided. An exception may be the use of antituberculous treatment in critically ill children with suspected disseminated tuberculosis. Empirical trials of other antimicrobial agents may be dangerous and can obscure the diagnosis of infective endocarditis, meningitis, parameningeal infection, or osteomyelitis. After a complete evaluation, antipyretics may be indicated to control fever and relieve symptoms.

Prognosis

Children with FUO have a better prognosis than do adults. The outcome in a child depends on the primary disease process, which is usually an atypical presentation of a common childhood illness. In many cases, no diagnosis can be established and fever abates spontaneously. In as many as 25% of cases in whom fever persists, the cause of the fever remains unclear, even after thorough evaluation.

BIBLIOGRAPHY

Please visit the Nelson Textbook of Pediatrics *website at www.expertconsult.com for the complete bibliography.*

Chapter 171
Infections in Immunocompromised Persons

Marian G. Michaels and Michael Green

Infection and disease develop when the host immune system fails to adequately protect against potential pathogens. In persons with an intact immune system, infection occurs in the setting of naiveté to the microbe and no pre-existing microbe-specific immunity or when protective barriers of the body such as the skin have been breached. Healthy children are able to meet the challenge of most infectious agents with an immunologic armamentarium capable of preventing significant disease. Once an infection begins to develop, an array of immune responses is set into action to control the disease and prevent it from reappearing. In contrast, immunocompromised children might not have this same capability. Depending on the level and type of immune defect, the affected child might not be able to contain the pathogen or to develop an appropriate immune response to prevent recurrence (Chapter 116).

For the full continuation of this chapter, please visit the Nelson Textbook of Pediatrics *website at www.expertconsult.com.*

171.1 Infections Occurring with Primary Immunodeficiencies

Marian G. Michaels and Michael Green

As the field of genetics and molecular biology has exploded, so has the identification and recognition of primary immunodeficiencies. More than 120 genes have been identified to account for >150 different primary immunodeficiencies. This section highlights the infectious disease problems associated with the major forms of deficiency.

For the full continuation of this chapter, please visit the Nelson Textbook of Pediatrics *website at www.expertconsult.com.*

171.2 Infections Occurring with Acquired Immunodeficiencies

Marian G. Michaels and Michael Green

Immunodeficiencies can be secondarily acquired as a result of infections or as a consequence of other underlying disorders such as malignancy, cystic fibrosis, diabetes mellitus, sickle cell disease, or malnutrition. Immunosuppressive medications used to prevent rejection after organ transplantation, to prevent graft versus host disease (GVHD) after stem cell transplantation (Chapter 131), or to treat malignancies can also leave the host vulnerable to infections. Similarly, medications used to control collagen vascular or other autoimmune diseases may be associated with an increased risk for developing infection. Any process that disrupts the normal mucosal and skin barriers (e.g., burns, surgery, indwelling catheters) can lead to an increased risk for infection.

For the full continuation of this chapter, please visit the Nelson Textbook of Pediatrics *website at* *www.expertconsult.com*.

171.3 Prevention of Infection in Immunocompromised Persons

Marian G. Michaels and Michael Green

Infections cannot be completely prevented in children who have defects in 1 or more arms of their immune system, although some measures can decrease the risks for infection. Replacement immunoglobulin is a benefit to children with primary B-cell deficiencies. Interferon-γ, trimethoprim-sulfamethoxazole, and oral antifungal agents reduce the number of infections occurring in children with chronic granulomatous disease. Children who have depressed cellular immunity from primary diseases, who have advanced HIV infection, or who take immunosuppressive medications benefit from prophylaxis against *P. jiroveci*. Immunizations prevent many infections and are particularly important for children with compromised immune systems. When possible, immunizations should be administered before any treatment that would compromise the child's immune system.

For the full continuation of this chapter, please visit the Nelson Textbook of Pediatrics *website at* *www.expertconsult.com*.

Chapter 172 Infection Associated with Medical Devices

Patricia M. Flynn

Despite the therapeutic successes and convenience of the many synthetic devices used in pediatric patients, infectious complications are problematic. The pathogenesis of device-related infection is not completely defined, but many factors are important, including the susceptibility of the host, the composition of the device, the ability of microorganisms to adhere to the device itself or to the biofilm that quickly forms on it, and environmental factors that include the insertion technique and maintenance of the device.

For the full continuation of this chapter, please visit the Nelson Textbook of Pediatrics *website at* *www.expertconsult.com*.

Section 3 ANTIBIOTIC THERAPY

Chapter 173 Principles of Antibacterial Therapy

Mark R. Schleiss

Antibacterial therapy in infants and children presents many challenges. A daunting problem is the paucity of pediatric data regarding pharmacokinetics and optimal dosages; pediatric recommendations are therefore (unfortunately) extrapolated from studies in adults. A 2nd challenge is the need for the clinician to consider important differences among various age groups with respect to the pathogenic species responsible for pediatric bacterial infections. Age-appropriate antibiotic dosing and toxicities must also be considered, taking into account the developmental status and physiology of infants and children. Finally, the style of usage of antibiotics has some important differences compared with usage in adult patients. Specific antibiotic therapy is optimally driven by a **microbiologic diagnosis,** predicated on isolation of the pathogenic organism from a sterile body site, and supported by antimicrobial susceptibility testing. Given the inherent difficulties that can arise in collecting specimens from pediatric patients, and given the increased risk of serious bacterial infection in young infants, much of pediatric infectious diseases practice is based on a **clinical diagnosis** with **empirical** use of antibacterial agents before or even without eventual identification of the specific pathogen.

For the full continuation of this chapter, please visit the Nelson Textbook of Pediatrics *website at* *www.expertconsult.com*.

Section 4 GRAM-POSITIVE BACTERIAL INFECTIONS

Chapter 174 *Staphylococcus*

James K. Todd

Staphylococci are hardy, aerobic, gram-positive bacteria that grow in pairs and clusters and are ubiquitous as normal flora of humans and present on fomites and in dust. They are resistant to heat and drying and may be recovered from nonbiologic environments weeks to months after contamination. Strains are classified as *Staphylococcus aureus* if they are coagulase positive or as 1 of the many species of **coagulase-negative staphylococci** (e.g., *Staphylococcus epidermidis, Staphylococcus saprophyticus, Staphylococcus haemolyticus,* etc). Often, *S. aureus* produces a yellow or orange pigment and β-hemolysis on blood agar and *S.*

epidermidis produces a white pigment with variable hemolysis results, although definitive species confirmation requires further testing. *S. aureus* has many virulence factors that mediate various serious diseases, whereas coagulase-negative staphylococci tend to be less pathogenic unless an indwelling foreign body (e.g., intravascular catheter) is present. Emerging antimicrobial resistance has become important, especially to the β-lactam antibiotics and less often to vancomycin.

174.1 *Staphylococcus aureus*

James K. Todd

S. aureus is the most common cause of pyogenic infection of the skin and soft tissue, causing impetigo, furuncles (boils), cellulitis, abscess, lymphadenitis, paronychia, omphalitis, and wound infection. Bacteremia (primary and secondary) is common and can be associated with or result in osteomyelitis, suppurative arthritis, deep abscesses, pneumonia, empyema, endocarditis, pyomyositis, pericarditis, and rarely meningitis. Toxin-mediated diseases, including food poisoning, staphylococcal scarlet fever, scalded skin syndrome, and toxic shock syndrome (TSS), are caused by certain *S. aureus* strains. Methicillin resistance is a global problem.

ETIOLOGY

Disease may result from tissue invasion or injury caused by various toxins and enzymes produced by the organism. Strains of *S. aureus* can be identified by the virulence factors they produce and can be classified by various molecular techniques.

Adhesion of *S. aureus* to mucosal cells is mediated by **teichoic acid** in the cell wall; exposure to the submucosa or subcutaneous sites increases adhesion to fibrinogen, fibronectin, collagen, and other proteins. Different strains of *S. aureus* produce many different virulence factors that have 1 or more of 4 different roles: protect the organism from host defenses, localize infection, cause local tissue damage, and act as toxins affecting noninfected tissue sites.

Most strains of *S. aureus* possess factors that protect the organism from host defenses. Many staphylococci produce a loose polysaccharide capsule, or **slime layer,** which may interfere with opsonophagocytosis. Production of **coagulase** and/or clumping factor differentiates *S. aureus* from *S. epidermidis* and other coagulase-negative staphylococci. Clumping factor interacts with fibrinogen to cause large clumps of organisms, interfering with effective phagocytosis. Coagulase causes plasma to clot by interacting with fibrinogen and this may have an important role in localization of infection (abscess formation). **Protein A** is present in most strains of *S. aureus* but not coagulase-negative staphylococci and reacts specifically with immunoglobulin G1 (IgG1), IgG2, and IgG4. It is located on the outermost coat of the cell wall and can absorb serum immunoglobulins, preventing antibacterial antibodies from acting as opsonins and thus inhibiting phagocytosis. Other enzymes elaborated by staphylococci include **catalase** (inactivates hydrogen peroxide, promoting intracellular survival), **penicillinase** or **β-lactamase** (inactivates penicillin at the molecular level), and lipase (associated with skin infection).

Many strains of *S. aureus* produce substances that cause local tissue destruction. A number of immunologically distinct hemolysins that act on cell membranes and cause tissue necrosis have been identified (α-toxin, β-hemolysin, δ-hemolysin). **Panton-Valentine leukocidin (PVL)**, which is produced by many current strains of *S. aureus* and has been associated with invasive skin disease, combines with the phospholipid of the phagocytic cell membrane, producing increased permeability, leakage of protein, and eventual death of the cell.

Many strains of *S. aureus* release 1 or more exotoxins. **Exfoliatins A and B** are serologically distinct proteins that produce localized (bullous impetigo) or generalized (scalded skin syndrome, staphylococcal scarlet fever) dermatologic complications (Chapter 651). Exfoliatins produce skin separation by splitting the desmosome and altering the intracellular matrix in the stratum granulosum.

One or more staphylococcal **enterotoxins (types A, B, C_1, C_2, D, E)** are elaborated by most strains of *S. aureus*. Ingestion of preformed enterotoxin A or B is associated with **food poisoning,** resulting in vomiting and diarrhea and, in some cases, profound hypotension. By 10 yr of age, almost all individuals have antibodies to at least 1 enterotoxin.

Toxic shock syndrome toxin-1 (TSST-1) is associated with TSS related to menstruation and focal staphylococcal infection. TSST-1 is a superantigen that induces production of interleukin-1 and tumor necrosis factor, resulting in hypotension, fever, and multisystem involvement. Enterotoxin A and enterotoxin B also may be associated with nonmenstrual TSS.

EPIDEMIOLOGY

Many neonates are colonized within the 1st wk of life, and 20-40% of normal individuals carry at least 1 strain of *S. aureus* in the anterior nares at any given time.

The organisms may be transmitted from the nose to the skin, where colonization seems to be more transient. Persistent umbilical, vaginal, and perianal carriage may occur.

Heavily colonized nasal carriers (often aggravated by a viral upper respiratory tract infection) are particularly effective disseminators. Exposure to *S. aureus* generally occurs by autoinoculation or direct contact with the hands of other colonized individuals. Handwashing between patient contacts is essential to decrease the nosocomial spread of staphylococci. Spread via fomites is rare.

Invasive disease may follow colonization. Antibiotic therapy with a drug to which *S. aureus* is resistant favors colonization and the development of infection. Other factors that increase the likelihood of infection include wounds, skin disease, ventriculoperitoneal shunts, intravenous or intrathecal catheterization, corticosteroid treatment, malnutrition, and azotemia. Viral infections of the respiratory tract, especially influenza virus, may predispose to secondary bacterial infection with staphylococci.

PATHOGENESIS

The development of staphylococcal disease is related to resistance of the host to infection and to virulence of the organism (Fig. 174-1). The intact skin and mucous membranes serve as barriers to invasion by staphylococci. Defects in the mucocutaneous barriers produced by trauma, surgery, foreign surfaces (sutures, shunts, intravascular catheters), and burns increase the risk for infection.

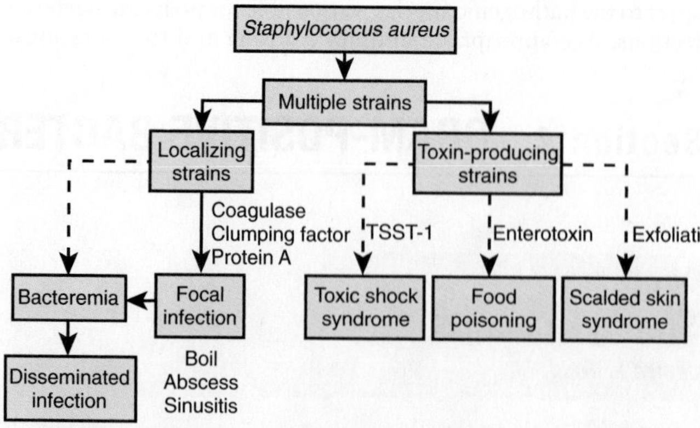

Figure 174-1 Relationship of virulence factors and diseases associated with *Staphylococcus aureus*. TSST-1, toxic shock syndrome toxin-1.

Infants may acquire type-specific humoral immunity to staphylococci transplacentally. Older children and adults develop antibodies to staphylococci as a result of colonization or minor infections. Antibody to the various *S. aureus* toxins appears to protect against those specific toxin-mediated diseases, but humoral immunity does not necessarily protect against focal or disseminated *S. aureus* infection with the same organisms.

Congenital defects in chemotaxis (Job syndrome, Chédiak-Higashi syndrome, Wiskott-Aldrich syndrome) and defective phagocytosis and killing (neutropenia, chronic granulomatous disease) increase the risk for staphylococcal infections. Patients with HIV infection have neutrophils that are defective in their ability to kill *S. aureus* in vitro. Patients with recurrent staphylococcal infection should be evaluated for immune defects, especially those involving neutrophil dysfunction.

CLINICAL MANIFESTATIONS

The signs and symptoms vary with the location of the infection, which is most commonly the skin but may be any tissue. Disease states of various degrees of severity are generally a result of local suppuration, systemic dissemination with metastatic infection, or systemic effects of toxin production. Although the nasopharynx and skin of many persons may be colonized with *S. aureus*, disease due to this organism is relatively uncommon. Skin infections due to *S. aureus* are considerably more prevalent among persons living in low socioeconomic circumstances and particularly among those in tropical climates.

Newborn

S. aureus is an important cause of neonatal infections (Chapter 103).

Skin

S. aureus is an important cause of pyogenic skin infections, including impetigo contagiosa, ecthyma, bullous impetigo, folliculitis, hydradenitis, furuncles, carbuncles, staphylococcal scalded skin syndrome, and staphylococcal scarlet fever. Infection may also complicate wounds or occur as superinfection of other noninfectious skin disease (eczema). Recurrent furunculosis is associated with repeated episodes of pyoderma over months to years. Recurrent skin and soft tissue infections are commonly noted with community-associated methicillin-resistant *S. aureus* (MRSA) and often affect the lower extremities and buttocks. *S. aureus* is also an important cause of wound infections and can cause deep soft tissue involvement, including cellulitis and rarely necrotizing fasciitis.

Respiratory Tract

Infections of the upper respiratory tract due to *S. aureus* are rare, in particular considering the frequency with which the anterior nares are colonized. In normal hosts, otitis media (Chapter 632) and sinusitis (Chapter 372) are rarely caused by *S. aureus*. *S. aureus* sinusitis is relatively common in children with cystic fibrosis or defects in leukocyte function and may be the only focus of infection in some children with toxic shock syndrome. Suppurative parotitis is a rare infection, but *S. aureus* is a common cause. A membranous **tracheitis** that complicates viral croup may be due to infection with *S. aureus*, but other organisms are also possible. Patients typically have high fever, leukocytosis, and evidence of severe upper airway obstruction. Direct laryngoscopy or bronchoscopy shows a normal epiglottis with subglottic narrowing and thick, purulent secretions within the trachea. Treatment requires careful airway management and appropriate antibiotic therapy.

Pneumonia (Chapter 392) due to *S. aureus* may be primary (hematogenous) or secondary after a viral infection such as influenza. Hematogenous pneumonia may be secondary to septic emboli from right-sided endocarditis or septic thrombophlebitis, with or without the presence of intravascular devices. Inhalation pneumonia is caused by alteration of mucociliary clearance (see cystic fibrosis, Chapter 395), leukocyte dysfunction, or bacterial adherence initiated by a viral infection. Common symptoms and signs include high fever, abdominal pain, tachypnea, dyspnea, and localized or diffuse bronchopneumonia or lobar disease. *S. aureus* often causes a **necrotizing pneumonitis** that may be associated with development of empyema, pneumatoceles, pyopneumothorax, and bronchopleural fistulas.

Sepsis

S. aureus bacteremia and sepsis may be primary or associated with any localized infection. The onset may be acute and marked by nausea, vomiting, myalgia, fever, and chills. Organisms may localize subsequently at any site (usually a single deep focus) but are found especially in the heart valves, lungs, joints, bones, and abscesses.

In some instances, especially in young adolescent males, disseminated *S. aureus* disease occurs, characterized by fever, persistent bacteremia despite antibiotics, and focal involvement of 2 or more separate tissue sites (skin, bone, joint, kidney, lung, liver, heart).

In these cases, endocarditis and septic thrombophlebitis must be ruled out.

Muscle

Localized staphylococcal abscesses in muscle associated with elevation of muscle enzymes sometimes without septicemia have been called **pyomyositis.** This disorder has been reported most frequently from tropical areas but also occurs in the USA in otherwise healthy children. Multiple abscesses occur in 30-40% of cases. History may include prior trauma at the site of the abscess. Surgical drainage and appropriate antibiotic therapy are essential.

Bones and Joints

S. aureus is the most common cause of osteomyelitis and suppurative arthritis in children (Chapters 676 and 677).

Central Nervous System

Meningitis (Chapter 595.1) caused by *S. aureus* is not common; it is associated with penetrating cranial trauma and neurosurgical procedures (craniotomy, cerebrospinal fluid [CSF] shunt placement) and less frequently with endocarditis, parameningeal foci (epidural or brain abscess), diabetes mellitus, or malignancy. The CSF profile of *S. aureus* meningitis is indistinguishable from that in other forms of bacterial meningitis.

Heart

S. aureus is a common cause of acute endocarditis (Chapter 431) on native valves. Perforation of heart valves, myocardial abscesses, heart failure, conduction disturbances, acute hemopericardium, purulent pericarditis, and sudden death may ensue.

Kidney

S. aureus is a common cause of renal and perinephric abscess (Chapter 532), usually of hematogenous origin. Pyelonephritis and cystitis due to *S. aureus* are unusual.

Toxic Shock Syndrome (TSS)

S. aureus is the principal cause of TSS (Chapter 174.2), which should be suspected in anyone with fever, shock, and/or a scarlet fever-like rash.

Intestinal Tract

Staphylococcal enterocolitis rarely follows overgrowth of normal bowel flora by *S. aureus*, which can occur as a result of broad-spectrum oral antibiotic therapy. Diarrhea is associated with blood and mucus. Peritonitis associated with *S. aureus* in patients receiving long-term ambulatory peritoneal dialysis usually involves the catheter tunnel. Removal of the catheter is required to achieve a bacteriologic cure.

Food poisoning (Chapter 332) may be caused by ingestion of **preformed** enterotoxins produced by staphylococci in contaminated foods. Approximately 2-7 hr after ingestion of the toxin, sudden, severe vomiting begins. Watery diarrhea may develop, but fever is absent or low. Symptoms rarely persist longer than 12-24 hr. Rarely, shock and death may occur.

DIAGNOSIS

The diagnosis of *S. aureus* infection depends on isolation of the organism from nonpermissive sites such as cellulitis aspirates, abscess cavities, blood, bone or joint aspirates, or other sites of infection. Swab cultures of surfaces are not as useful, as they may reflect surface contamination rather than the true cause of infection. Tissue samples or fluid aspirates in a syringe provide the best culture material. Isolation from the nose or skin does not necessarily imply causation because these sites may be normally colonized sites. Because of the high prevalence of MRSA, the increasing severity of *S. aureus* infections, and the fact that bacteremia is not universally present even in severe *S. aureus* infections, it is usually important to obtain a nonpermissive culture of any potential focus of infection as well as a blood culture prior to starting antibiotic treatment. The organism can be grown readily in liquid and on solid media. After isolation, identification is made on the basis of Gram stain and coagulase, clumping factor, and protein A reactivity. Patterns of susceptibility to antibiotics should be assessed in serious cases, as antimicrobial resistance is increasingly common.

Diagnosis of *S. aureus* food poisoning is made on the basis of epidemiologic and clinical findings. Food suspected of contamination should be cultured and can be tested for enterotoxin.

Differential Diagnosis

Skin lesions due to *S. aureus* may be indistinguishable from those due to group A streptococci; the former usually expand slowly, while the latter are more prone to spread rapidly. *S. aureus* pneumonia can be suspected on the basis of chest roentgenograms that reveal pneumatoceles, pyopneumothorax, or lung abscess (Fig. 174-2). Fluctuant skin and soft tissue lesions also can be caused by other organisms, including *Mycobacterium tuberculosis*, atypical mycobacteria, *Bartonella henselae* (cat-scratch disease), *Francisella tularensis*, and various fungi, among others.

Treatment

Antibiotic therapy alone is rarely effective in individuals with undrained abscesses or with infected foreign bodies. Loculated collections of purulent material should be relieved by incision and drainage. Foreign bodies should be removed, if possible. Therapy always should be initiated with an antibiotic consistent with the local staphylococcal susceptibility patterns as well as the severity of infection. Penicillin and amoxicillin are not appropriate, because more than 90% of all staphylococci isolated, regardless of source, are resistant to these agents. For serious infections, parenteral treatment is indicated, at least at the outset, until symptoms are controlled. Serious *S. aureus* infections, with or without abscesses, tend to persist and recur, necessitating prolonged therapy.

The antibiotic used as well as the dose, route, and duration of treatment depend on the site of infection, the response of the patient to treatment, and the susceptibility of the organisms recovered from blood or from local sites of infection. For most patients with serious *S. aureus* infection, intravenous treatment is recommended until the patient has become afebrile and other signs of infection have improved. Oral therapy is often continued for a period of time, especially in patients with chronic infection or underlying host defense problems. Treatment of *S. aureus* osteomyelitis (Chapter 676), meningitis (Chapter 595.1), and endocarditis (Chapter 431) are discussed in their respective chapters.

Initial treatment for serious infections thought to be due to methicillin-susceptible *S. aureus* (MSSA) should include semisynthetic penicillin (e.g., nafcillin, oxacillin) or less often a 1st generation cephalosporin (e.g., cefazolin). MRSA is both an important hospital and community-acquired pathogen. Community-associated MRSA infections are common throughout the USA, even in children without pre-existing risk factors. Resistance to semisynthetic penicillins and cephalosporins is related to a novel penicillin-binding protein (PB2A) that is relatively insensitive to antibiotics containing a β-lactam ring. MRSA strains appear to be at least as virulent as their methicillin-sensitive counterparts. Vancomycin (40-60 mg/kg/24 hr divided every 6 hr IV) can be used as the initial treatment for penicillin-allergic individuals and those with suspected serious *S. aureus* infections that might be due to MRSA. Serum levels of vancomycin should be

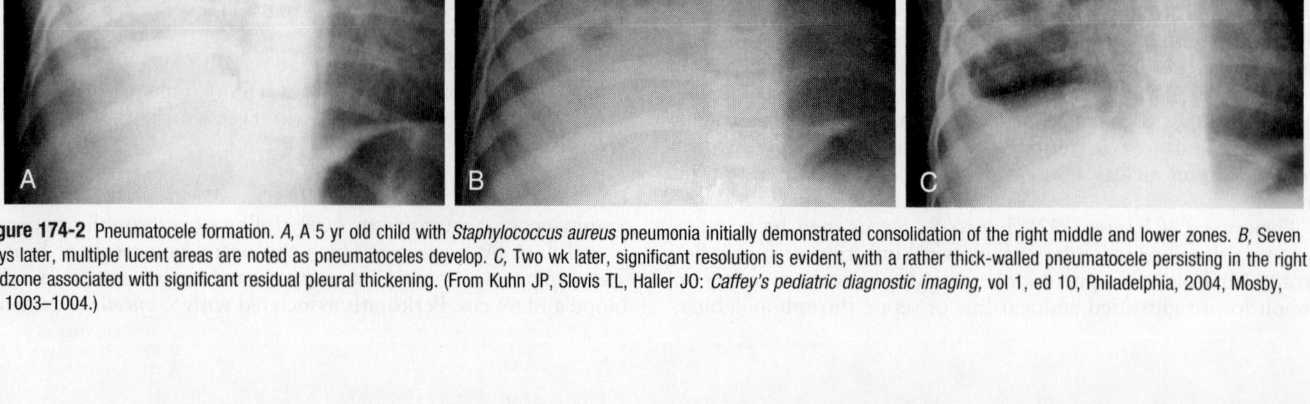

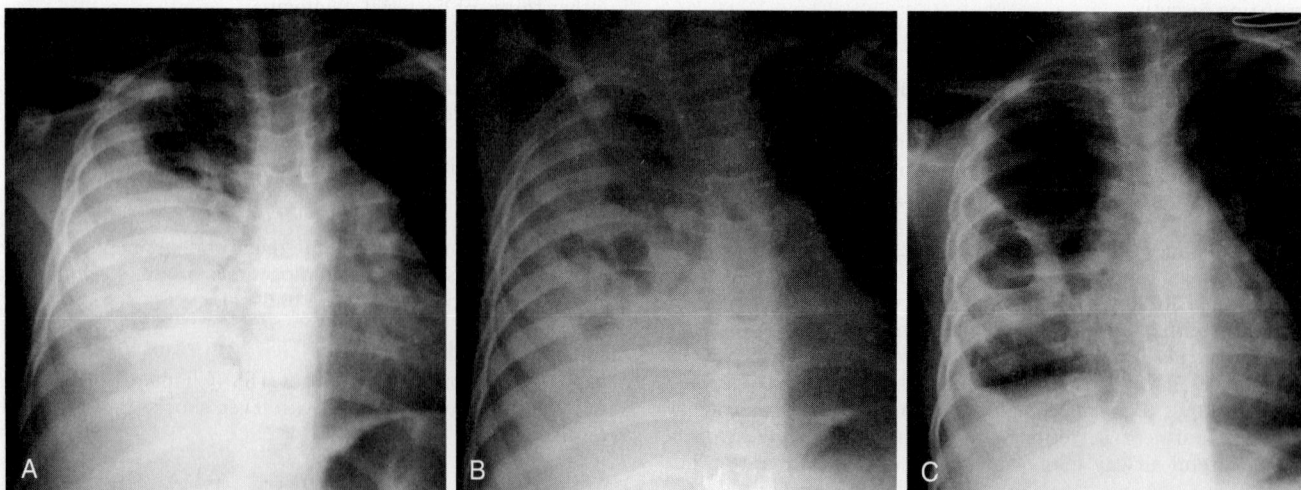

Figure 174-2 Pneumatocele formation. *A,* A 5 yr old child with *Staphylococcus aureus* pneumonia initially demonstrated consolidation of the right middle and lower zones. *B,* Seven days later, multiple lucent areas are noted as pneumatoceles develop. *C,* Two wk later, significant resolution is evident, with a rather thick-walled pneumatocele persisting in the right midzone associated with significant residual pleural thickening. (From Kuhn JP, Slovis TL, Haller JO: *Caffey's pediatric diagnostic imaging,* vol 1, ed 10, Philadelphia, 2004, Mosby, pp 1003–1004.)

monitored, with trough concentrations of 10-20 µg/mL, depending on the case. MRSA is also resistant to cephalosporins and carbapenems and is unreliably susceptible to the quinolones. Linezolid, daptomycin, quinupristin-dalfopristin, vancomycin with linezolid and gentamicin, and vancomycin with trimethoprim-sulfamethoxazole may be useful for serious *S. aureus* infections highly resistant to other antibiotics (Table 174-1).

Rare vancomycin intermediate and vancomycin-resistant strains have also been reported, mostly in patients being treated with vancomycin, emphasizing the need for restricting the prescription of unnecessary antibiotics and the importance of isolation of the causative organism and susceptibility testing in serious infections.

Serious *S. aureus* infections (septicemia, endocarditis, central nervous system infections, TSS) should be treated initially with intravenous vancomycin or methicillin, nafcillin, or oxacillin depending on the local staphylococcal resistance pattern until the causative organism is isolated and its susceptibility determined. Rifampin or gentamicin may be added for synergy in serious infections (endocarditis).

In many of these infections, oral antimicrobials may be substituted to complete the course of treatment after an initial period of parenteral therapy and determination of antimicrobial susceptibilities. Despite in vitro susceptibility of *S. aureus* to ciprofloxacin and other quinolone antibiotics, these agents should not be used in serious staphylococcal infections, because their use has been associated with rapid development of resistance. Trimethoprim-sulfamethoxazole may be an effective oral antibiotic for many strains of both methicillin-susceptible *S. aureus* (MSSA) and MRSA.

Dicloxacillin (50-100 mg/kg/24 hr divided 4 times per day PO) and cephalexin (25-100 mg/kg/24 hr divided 3 to 4 times

Table 174-1 PARENTERAL ANTIMICROBIAL AGENT(S) FOR TREATMENT OF BACTEREMIA AND OTHER SERIOUS *STAPHYLOCOCCUS AUREUS* INFECTIONS

SUSCEPTIBILITY	ANTIMICROBIAL AGENTS	COMMENTS
I. INITIAL EMPIRIC THERAPY (ORGANISM OF UNKNOWN SUSCEPTIBILITY)		
Drugs of choice:	Vancomycin ± gentamicin or rifampin	For life-threatening infections (i.e., septicemia, endocarditis, CNS infection); linezolid could be substituted if the patient has received several recent courses of vancomycin
	Nafcillin or oxacillin*	For non–life-threatening infection without signs of sepsis (e.g., skin infection, cellulitis, osteomyelitis, pyarthrosis) when rates of MRSA colonization and infection in the community are low
	Clindamycin	For non–life-threatening infection without signs of sepsis when rates of MRSA colonization and infection in the community are substantial and prevalence of clindamycin resistance is low
	Vancomycin	For non–life-threatening, hospital-acquired infections
II. METHICILLIN-SUSCEPTIBLE, PENICILLIN-RESISTANT *S. AUREUS* (MSSA)		
Drugs of choice:	Nafcillin or oxacillin*,†	
Alternatives (depending on susceptibility results):	Cefazolin*	
	Clindamycin	
	Vancomycin	Only for penicillin- and cephalosporin-allergic patients
	Ampicillin + sulbactam	
III. MRSA		
A. Health Care–Associated (Multidrug-Resistant)		
Drugs of choice:	Vancomycin ± gentamicin or ± rifampin†	
Alternatives: susceptibility testing results available before alternative drugs are used		
	Trimethoprim-sulfamethoxazole	
	Linezolid‡	
	Quinupristin-dalfopristin‡	
	Fluoroquinolones	Not recommended for people younger than 18 yr of age or as monotherapy
B. Community (Not Multidrug-Resistant)		
Drugs of choice:	Vancomycin†	For life-threatening infections
	Vancomycin ± gentamicin (or ± rifampin†)	For pneumonia, septic arthritis, osteomyelitis, skin or soft tissue infections
		For skin or soft tissue infections
Alternatives:	Clindamycin (if strain susceptible by "D test)	
	Trimethoprim-sulfamethoxazole	
IV. VANCOMYCIN INTERMEDIATELY SUSCEPTIBLE OR VANCOMYCIN-RESISTANT *S. AUREUS*†		
Drugs of choice:	Optimal therapy is not known	Dependent on in vitro susceptibility test results
	Linezolid‡	
	Daptomycin§	
	Quinupristin-dalfopristin‡	
Alternatives:	Vancomycin + linezolid ± gentamicin	
	Vancomycin + trimethoprim-sulfamethoxazole†	

*Penicillin- and cephalosporin-allergic patients should receive vancomycin as initial therapy for serious infections.
†One of the adjunctive agents, gentamicin or rifampin, should be added to the therapeutic regimen for life-threatening infections such as endocarditis or CNS infection or infections with a vancomycin-intermediate or vancomycin-resistant *S. aureus* strain. Consultation with an infectious diseases specialist should be considered to determine which agent to use and duration of use.
‡Linezolid and quinupristin-dalfopristin are 2 agents with activity in vitro and efficacy in adults with multidrug-resistant, gram-positive organisms, including *S. aureus*. Because experience with these agents in children is limited, consultation with an infectious diseases specialist should be considered before use.
§Daptomycin is active in vitro against multidrug-resistant, gram-positive organisms, including *S. aureus*, but has not been used often in children. Daptomycin is approved by the U.S. Food and Drug Administration only for the treatment of complicated skin and skin structure infections in patients 18 yr of age and older.
CNS, central nervous system; MRSA, methicillin-resistant *S. aureus*.
From the American Academy of Pediatrics: *Red book: 2009 report of the Committee on Infectious Diseases*, ed 28, Elk Grove Village, IL, 2009, American Academy of Pediatrics, pp 610–611.

per day PO) are absorbed well orally and are effective for MSSA. Amoxicillin-clavulanate (40-80 mg amoxicillin/kg/24 hr divided 3 times per day PO) is also effective. Clindamycin (30-40 mg/kg/24 hr divided 3 to 4 times per day PO) has proved effective for the treatment of skin, soft tissue, bone, and joint infections due to susceptible *S. aureus* strains confirmed by a clinical microbiology laboratory using the "D-test." Clindamycin is bacteriostatic and should not be used to treat endocarditis, brain abscess, or meningitis due to *S. aureus*. Given that the mechanism of action of clindamycin involves inhibition or protein synthesis, many experts use clindamycin to treat *S. aureus* toxin–mediated illnesses (TSS) to inhibit toxin production. The duration of oral therapy depends on the response as determined by the clinical response and roentgenographic and laboratory findings.

Skin and soft tissue infection and respiratory tract infection may often be managed by oral therapy or by an initial brief course of parenteral antibiotics followed by oral medication. Ceftaroline (IV) is approved for MRSA skin infections in adults.

PROGNOSIS

Untreated *S. aureus* septicemia is associated with a high fatality rate, which have been reduced significantly by appropriate antibiotic treatment. *S. aureus* pneumonia can be fatal at any age but is more likely to be associated with high morbidity and mortality in young infants or in patients whose therapy has been delayed. Prognosis also may be influenced by numerous host factors, including nutrition, immunologic competence, and the presence or absence of other debilitating diseases. In most cases with abscess formation, surgical drainage is necessary.

PREVENTION

S. aureus infection is transmitted primarily by direct contact. Strict attention to handwashing techniques is the most effective measure for preventing the spread of staphylococci from one individual to another (Chapter 166). Use of a hand wash containing chlorhexidine or alcohol is recommended. In hospitals or other institutional settings, all persons with acute *S. aureus* infections should be isolated until they have been treated adequately. There should be constant surveillance for nosocomial *S. aureus* infections within hospitals. When MRSA is recovered, strict isolation of affected patients has been shown to be the most effective method for preventing nosocomial spread of infection. Thereafter, control measures should be directed toward identification of new isolates and strict isolation of newly colonized or infected patients. Clusters of cases may be defined by molecular typing. If associated with a singular molecular strain, it may also be necessary to identify colonized hospital personnel and eradicate carriage in affected individuals.

Patients with recurrent *S. aureus* skin infection may be treated with hypochlorite baths (1 teaspoon common bleach solution per gallon of water), an appropriate oral antibiotic, and nasal mupirocin in an attempt to prevent recurrences.

Food poisoning (Chapter 332) may be prevented by excluding individuals with *S. aureus* infections of the skin from the preparation and handling of food. Prepared foods should be eaten immediately or refrigerated appropriately to prevent multiplication of *S. aureus* with which the food may have been contaminated.

BIBLIOGRAPHY

Please visit the Nelson Textbook of Pediatrics *website at* *www.expertconsult.com* *for the complete bibliography.*

174.2 Toxic Shock Syndrome

James K. Todd

TSS is an acute multisystem disease characterized by fever, hypotension, an erythematous rash with subsequent desquamation on the hands and feet, and multisystem involvement including vomiting, diarrhea, myalgias, nonfocal neurologic abnormalities, conjunctival hyperemia, and strawberry tongue.

ETIOLOGY

TSS is caused by TSST-1–producing and some enterotoxin-producing strains of *S. aureus*, which may colonize the vagina or cause focal sites of staphylococcal infection.

EPIDEMIOLOGY

Many cases occur in menstruating women 15-25 yr of age and who use tampons or other vaginal devices (diaphragm, contraceptive sponge). TSS also occurs in children, nonmenstruating women, and men usually associated with an identifiable focus of *S. aureus* infection. **Nonmenstrual TSS** has occurred with *S. aureus* infection of nasal packing or infections including wound infections, sinusitis, tracheitis, pneumonia, empyema, abscesses, burns, osteomyelitis, and primary bacteremia. Without antimicrobial therapy, menstrual TSS has a 30% recurrence rate if tampons are used, with secondary cases being milder and occurring within 5 mo of the original episode. The overall mortality rate of treated patients is 3-5%. Most strains of *S. aureus* associated with TSS have been susceptible to the semi-synthetic β-lactam antibiotics, including 1st generation cephalosporins, but some methicillin/cephalosporin–resistant cases have been reported.

PATHOGENESIS

The primary toxin associated with TSS is TSST-1, which acts as a superantigen causing massive loss of fluid from the intravascular space. TSST-1–negative *S. aureus* strains have been isolated from patients with TSS, suggesting that other toxins (primarily the enterotoxins) have a role in TSS (especially nonmenstrual). Epidemiologic and in vitro studies suggest that these toxins are selectively produced in a clinical environment consisting of a neutral pH, a high P_{CO_2}, and an "aerobic" P_{O_2}, which are the conditions found in the vagina with tampon use during menstruation. Approximately 90% of adults have antibody to TSST-1 without a history of clinical TSS, suggesting that most individuals are colonized at some point with a toxin-producing organism at a site (anterior nares) where low-grade or inactive toxin exposure results in an immune response without disease. The risk factors for symptomatic disease include a nonimmune host colonized with a toxin-producing organism, which is exposed to focal growth conditions (menstruation plus tampon use or abscess) that induce toxin production. It appears that some hosts may have a varied cytokine response to exposure to TSST-1, helping to explain a spectrum of severity of TSS that may include staphylococcal scarlet fever.

CLINICAL MANIFESTATIONS

The diagnosis of TSS is based on clinical manifestations (Table 174-2). The onset is abrupt, with high fever, vomiting, and diarrhea, and is accompanied by sore throat, headache, and myalgias. A diffuse erythematous macular rash (sunburn-like or scarlatiniform) appears within 24 hr and may be associated with hyperemia of pharyngeal, conjunctival, and vaginal mucous membranes. A strawberry tongue is common. Symptoms often include alterations in the level of consciousness, oliguria, and hypotension, which in severe cases may progress to shock and disseminated intravascular coagulation. Complications, including acute respiratory distress syndrome, myocardial dysfunction, and renal failure, are commensurate with the degree of shock. Recovery occurs within 7-10 days and is associated with desquamation, particularly of palms and soles; hair and nail loss have also been observed after 1-2 mo. Many cases of apparent scarlet fever

Table 174-2 DIAGNOSTIC CRITERIA OF STAPHYLOCOCCAL TOXIC SHOCK SYNDROME

MAJOR CRITERIA (ALL REQUIRED)
Acute fever; temperature >38.8°C Hypotension (orthostatic, shock; below age-appropriate norms) Rash (erythroderma with convalescent desquamation)
MINOR CRITERIA (ANY 3 OR MORE)
Mucous membrane inflammation (vaginal, oropharyngeal or conjuctival hyperemia, strawberry tongue) Vomiting, diarrhea Liver abnormalities (bilirubin or transaminase greater than twice upper limit of normal) Renal abnormalities (urea nitrogen or creatinine greater than twice upper limit of normal, or greater than 5 white blood cells per high power field) Muscle abnormalities (myalgia or creatinine phosphokinase greater than twice upper limit of normal) Central nervous system abnormalities (alteration in consciousness without focal neurological signs) Thrombocytopenia (100,000/mm^3 or less)
EXCLUSIONARY CRITERIA
Absence of another explanation Negative blood cultures (except occasionally for *Staphylococcus aureus*)

From the American Academy of Pediatrics *Red book: 2009 report of the Committee on Infectious Diseases*, ed 28, Elk Grove Village, IL, 2009, American Academy of Pediatrics, p 602.

without shock may be caused by TSST-1-producing *S. aureus* strains.

DIAGNOSIS

There is no specific laboratory test; appropriate selective tests reveal involvement of multiple organ systems, including the hepatic, renal, muscular, gastrointestinal, cardiopulmonary, and central nervous systems. Bacterial cultures of the associated focus (vagina, abscess) before administration of antibiotics usually yield *S. aureus,* although this is not a required element of the definition.

Differential Diagnosis

Group A streptococcus can cause a similar TSS-like illness, termed **streptococcal TSS** (Chapter 176), which is often associated with severe streptococcal sepsis or a focal streptococcal infection such as cellulitis, necrotizing fasciitis, or pneumonia.

Kawasaki disease closely resembles TSS clinically but is usually not as severe or rapidly progressive. Both conditions are associated with fever unresponsive to antibiotics, hyperemia of mucous membranes, and an erythematous rash with subsequent desquamation. However, many of the clinical features of TSS are usually absent or rare in Kawasaki disease, including diffuse myalgia, vomiting, abdominal pain, diarrhea, azotemia, hypotension, acute respiratory distress syndrome, and shock (Chapter 160). Kawasaki disease typically occurs in children younger than 5 yr. Scarlet fever, Rocky Mountain spotted fever, leptospirosis, toxic epidermal necrolysis, sepsis, and measles must also be considered in the differential diagnosis.

TREATMENT

Parenteral administration of a β-lactamase–resistant antistaphylococcal antibiotic (nafcillin, oxacillin, or a 1st generation cephalosporin) or vancomycin in areas where MRSA is common is recommended after appropriate cultures have been obtained. The addition of clindamycin is recommended to reduce toxin production. Drainage of the vagina by removal of any retained tampons in menstrual TSS and of focally infected sites in nonmenstrual TSS is important for successful treatment. Antistaphylococcal therapy may also reduce the risk for recurrence in menstrual TSS.

Fluid replacement should be aggressive to prevent or treat hypotension, renal failure, and cardiovascular collapse. Inotropic agents may be needed to treat shock; corticosteroids and intravenous immunoglobulin may be helpful in severe cases.

PREVENTION

The risk for acquiring menstrual TSS (1-2 cases/100,000 menstruating women) is low. Changing tampons at least every 8 hr is recommended. If a fever, rash, or dizziness develops during menstruation, any tampon should be removed immediately and medical attention should be sought.

BIBLIOGRAPHY

Please visit the Nelson Textbook of Pediatrics *website at www.expertconsult.com for the complete bibliography.*

174.3 Coagulase-Negative Staphylococci

James K. Todd

S. epidermidis is just 1 of many recognized species of coagulase-negative staphylococci (CONS) affecting or colonizing humans. Originally thought to be avirulent commensal bacteria, CONS is now recognized to cause infections in patients with indwelling foreign devices, including intravenous catheters, hemodialysis shunts and grafts, CSF shunts (meningitis), peritoneal dialysis catheters (peritonitis), pacemaker wires and electrodes (local infection), prosthetic cardiac valves (endocarditis), and prosthetic joints (arthritis). CONS is a common cause of nosocomial neonatal infection. *S. haemolyticus,* another CONS species, is an important cause of invasive infection and may develop resistance to vancomycin and teicoplanin.

EPIDEMIOLOGY

CONS consist of normal inhabitants of the human skin, throat, mouth, vagina, and urethra. *S. epidermidis* is the most common and persistent species, representing 65-90% of staphylococci present on the skin and mucous membranes. Colonization, sometimes with strains acquired from hospital staff, precedes infection; alternatively, direct inoculation during surgery may initiate infection of CSF shunts, prosthetic valves, or indwelling vascular lines. For epidemiologic purposes, CONS can be identified on the basis of molecular DNA methods.

PATHOGENESIS

CONS produce an **exopolysaccharide** protective biofilm, or **slime layer,** that surrounds the organism and may enhance adhesion to foreign surfaces, resist phagocytosis, and impair penetration of antibiotics.

CLINICAL MANIFESTATIONS

The low virulence of CONS usually requires the presence of another factor, such as immune compromise or a foreign body, for development of clinical disease.

Bacteremia

CONS, specifically *S. epidermidis,* are the most common cause of nosocomial bacteremia, usually in association with central vascular catheters. In neonates, CONS bacteremia, with or without a central venous catheter, may be manifested as apnea, bradycardia, temperature instability, abdominal distention, hematochezia, meningitis in the absence of CSF pleocytosis, cutaneous abscesses, and persistence of positive blood cultures despite adequate antimicrobial therapy. In most circumstances, CONS bacteremia is indolent and is not usually associated with overwhelming septic shock.

Endocarditis
Infection of native heart valves or the right atrial wall secondary to an infected thrombosis at the end of a central line may produce endocarditis. *S. epidermidis* and other CONS may rarely produce native valve subacute indolent endocarditis in previously normal patients without a central venous catheter. CONS is a common cause of prosthetic valve endocarditis, presumably due to inoculation at the time of surgery. Infection of the valve sewing ring, with abscess formation and dissection, produces valve dysfunction, dehiscence, arrhythmias, or valve obstruction (Chapter 431).

Central Venous Catheter Infection
Central venous catheters become infected through the exit site and subcutaneous tunnel, which provide a direct path to the bloodstream. *S. epidermidis* is the most common CONS, owing in part to its high rate of cutaneous colonization. **Line sepsis** is usually manifested as fever and leukocytosis; tenderness and erythema may be present at the exit site or along the subcutaneous tunnel. Catheter thrombosis may complicate line sepsis.

Cerebrospinal Fluid Shunts
CONS, introduced at the time of surgery, is the most common pathogen associated with CSF shunt meningitis. Most (70-80%) infections occur within 2 mo of the operation and are manifested by signs of meningeal irritation, fever, increased intracranial pressure (headache), and peritonitis due to the intra-abdominal position of the distal end of the shunt tubing.

Urinary Tract Infection
S. saprophyticus is a common cause of primary urinary tract infections in sexually active females. Manifestations are similar to those characteristics of urinary tract infection due to *Escherichia coli* (Chapter 532). CONS also causes asymptomatic urinary tract infection in hospitalized patients with urinary catheters and after urinary tract surgery or transplantation.

DIAGNOSIS
Because *S. epidermidis* is a common skin inhabitant and may contaminate poorly collected blood cultures, differentiating bacteremia from contamination is often difficult. True bacteremia should be suspected if blood cultures grow rapidly (within 24 hr), ≥2 blood cultures are positive with the same CONS, and clinical and laboratory signs and symptoms compatible with CONS sepsis are present and subsequently resolve with appropriate therapy. No blood culture that is positive for CONS in a neonate or patient with intravascular catheter should be considered contaminated without careful assessment of the foregoing criteria and examination of the patient. Before initiating presumptive antimicrobial therapy in such patients, it is always prudent to draw 2 separate blood cultures to facilitate subsequent interpretation if CONS is grown.

TREATMENT
Most CONS strains are resistant to methicillin. Vancomycin is the drug of choice for methicillin-resistant strains. The addition of rifampin to vancomycin may increase antimicrobial efficacy. In many cases of CONS infection associated with foreign bodies, the catheter, valve, or shunt must be removed to ensure a cure. Prosthetic heart valves and CSF shunts usually have to be removed to treat the infection adequately.

Antibiotic therapy given through an infected central venous catheter (through each lumen) may effectively cure CONS line sepsis. If the catheter or reservoir is no longer needed, it should be removed. Unfortunately, removal is not always possible owing to the therapeutic requirements of the underlying disease (nutrition for short bowel syndrome, chemotherapy for malignancy). A trial of intravenous vancomycin is indicated to attempt to preserve the use of the central line as long as systemic manifestations of infection are not severe.

Peritonitis caused by *S. epidermidis* in patients on continuous ambulatory peritoneal dialysis is an infection that may be treated with intravenous or intraperitoneal antibiotics without removing the dialysis catheter. If the organism is resistant to methicillin, vancomycin adjusted for renal function is appropriate therapy.

PROGNOSIS
Most episodes of CONS bacteremia respond successfully to antibiotics and removal of any foreign body that is present. Poor prognosis is associated with malignancy, neutropenia, and infected prosthetic or native heart valves. CONS increases morbidity, the duration of hospitalization, and mortality rates among patients with underlying complicated illnesses.

BIBLIOGRAPHY
Please visit the Nelson Textbook of Pediatrics *website at www.expertconsult.com for the complete bibliography.*

Chapter 175
Streptococcus pneumoniae (Pneumococcus)

Timothy R. Peters and Jon S. Abramson

Streptococcus pneumoniae (pneumococcus) is a very important pathogen that kills more than 1 million children each year worldwide. Childhood pneumococcal disease is prevalent and commonly severe, causes numerous clinical syndromes, and is a major cause of life-threatening pneumonia, bacteremia, and meningitis. Antimicrobial resistance in pneumococcus is a major public health problem, with 15-30% of isolates worldwide classified as multidrug-resistant (MDR, resistant to ≥3 classes of antibiotics). Pneumococcal polysaccharide-protein conjugate vaccines (PCVs) developed for infants have been highly successful in the control of disease caused by virulent vaccine-specific serotypes. Epidemiologic surveillance reveals a dynamic pneumococcal ecology with emergence of highly virulent, MDR serotypes. Ongoing vaccine development and distribution efforts remain our best approach to control of this threat to childhood health.

ETIOLOGY
S. pneumoniae is a gram-positive, lancet-shaped, polysaccharide encapsulated diplococcus, occurring occasionally as individual cocci or in chains. More than 90 serotypes have been identified by type-specific capsular polysaccharides. Antisera to some pneumococcal polysaccharides cross react with other pneumococcal types, defining serogroups (e.g., 6A and 6B). Encapsulated strains cause most serious disease in humans. Capsular polysaccharides impede phagocytosis. Virulence is related in part to capsular size, but pneumococcal types with capsules of the same size can vary widely in virulence.

On solid media, *S. pneumoniae* forms unpigmented, umbilicated colonies surrounded by a zone of incomplete (α) hemolysis. *S. pneumoniae* is bile soluble (i.e., 10% deoxycholate) and optochin-sensitive. *S. pneumoniae* is closely related to the viridans groups of *Streptococcus mitis*, which typically overlap phenotypically with pneumococci. The conventional laboratory definition of pneumococci continues to rely on bile and optochin sensitivity, although considerable confusion occurs in distinguishing pneumococci and other α-hemolytic streptococci. Pneumococcal capsules can be microscopically visualized and typed by exposing organisms to type-specific antisera that combine with their unique capsular polysaccharide, rendering the capsule refractile (Quellung reaction). Specific antibodies to capsular polysaccharides confer protection on the host, promoting opsonization and phagocytosis. Additionally, $CD4^+$ T cells have a direct role in antibody-independent immunity to pneumococcal nasopharyngeal colonization. Conjugated PCVs promote T-cell immunity and protect against pneumococcal colonization, in contrast to the pneumococcal polysaccharide vaccine (PPSV23) used primarily in adults that does not affect nasopharyngeal colonization.

EPIDEMIOLOGY

Most healthy individuals carry various *S. pneumoniae* serotypes in their upper respiratory tract; >90% of children between 6 mo and 5 yr of age harbor *S. pneumoniae* in the nasopharynx at some time. A single serotype usually is carried by a given individual for an extended period (45 days to 6 mo). Carriage does not consistently induce local or systemic immunity sufficient to prevent later reacquisition of the same serotype. Rates of pneumococcal carriage peak during the 1st and 2nd yr of life and decline gradually thereafter. Carriage rates are highest in institutional settings and during the winter, and rates are lowest in summer. Nasopharyngeal carriage of pneumococci is common among young children attending out-of-home care, with rates of 21-59% in point prevalence studies and 65% in longitudinal studies. During the past 4 decades, serotypes 4, 6B, 9V, 14, 18C, 19F, and 23F have constituted the majority of invasive isolates in children in the U.S. and other developed countries; strains belonging to serotypes 6B, 9V, 14, and 19F frequently have reduced susceptibility to penicillin. Since licensure of the PCVs, the prevalence of carriage and infection with vaccine serotypes has substantially declined and a shift to increased carriage or infections with nonvaccine serotypes has occurred (Fig. 175-1). Indirect protection of unvaccinated persons has occurred since PCV introduction, and this herd protection is likely due to decreases in nasopharyngeal carriage of virulent pneumococcal vaccine serotypes.

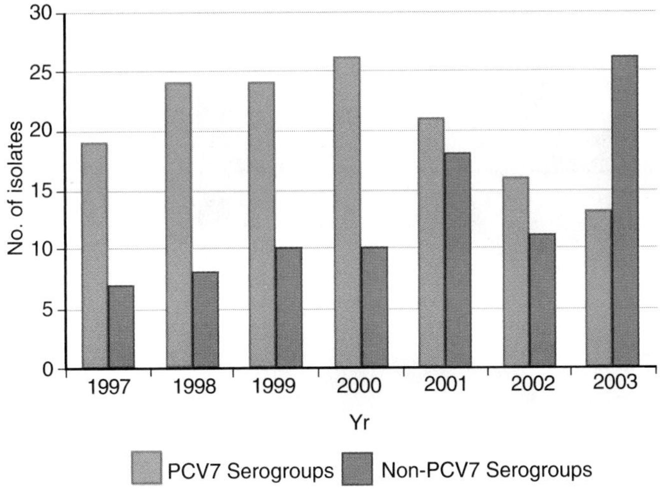

Figure 175-1 Number of isolates from *Streptococcus pneumoniae* serogroups included in the heptavalent pneumococcal conjugate vaccine (PCV7 [Prevnar; Wyeth Lederle Vaccines]) and from nonvaccine serogroups recovered from children treated at Primary Children's Medical Center (Salt Lake City, UT), by year. (From Byington CL, Samore MH, Stoddard GJ, et al: Temporal trends of invasive disease due to *Streptococcus pneumoniae* among children in the intermountain west: emergence of nonvaccine serogroups, *Clin Infect Dis* 41:21–29, 2005.)

S. pneumoniae is the most frequent cause of bacteremia, bacterial pneumonia, and otitis media and the second most common cause of meningitis in children, next to *Neisseria meningitidis*. The decreased ability in children <2 yr of age to produce antibody against the T-cell independent polysaccharide antigens and the high prevalence of colonization may explain an increased susceptibility to pneumococcal infection and the decreased effectiveness of polysaccharide vaccines. Males are more commonly affected than females. Native American and African-American children have rates of invasive disease that are 2- to 10-fold higher than other healthy children. Prior to the introduction of PCVs into routine childhood immunization schedules, rates of invasive pneumococcal disease in the USA peaked at 6-11 mo of age, with attack rates of >540/100,000 in healthy children. Following the universal use of PCVs, rates of infection have fallen in both high-risk and healthy children. In Tennessee, peak rates of infection have fallen from 235/100,000 to 46/100,000 in children <2 yr of age and the proportion of penicillin-resistant strains in invasive disease have fallen from 59.8% to 30.4%.

Pneumococcal disease usually occurs sporadically but can be spread from person to person by respiratory droplet transmission. The frequency and severity of pneumococcal disease are increased in patients with sickle cell disease, asplenia, deficiencies in humoral (B cell) and complement-mediated immunity, HIV infection, certain malignancies (e.g., leukemia, lymphoma), chronic heart, lung, or renal disease (particularly the nephrotic syndrome), cerebrospinal fluid (CSF) leak, and cochlear implants. Other high-risk groups are noted in Table 175-1. *S. pneumoniae* is an important cause of secondary bacterial pneumonia in patients with influenza. During influenza epidemics and pandemics, most deaths result from bacterial pneumonia, and pneumococcus is the predominant bacterial pathogen isolated in this setting. Pneumococcal co-pathogenicity may be important in disease caused by other respiratory viruses as well.

Table 175-1 CHILDREN AT HIGH OR MODERATE RISK OF INVASIVE PNEUMOCOCCAL INFECTION

HIGH RISK (INCIDENCE OF INVASIVE PNEUMOCOCCAL DISEASE = 150 CASES/100,000 PEOPLE PER YEAR)
Children with: • Sickle cell disease, congenital or acquired asplenia, or splenic dysfunction • Human immunodeficiency virus infection • Cochlear implants
PRESUMED HIGH RISK (INSUFFICIENT DATA TO CALCULATE RATES)
Children with: • Congenital immune deficiency; some B- (humoral) or T-lymphocyte deficiencies, complement deficiencies (particularly C1, C2, C3, and C4), or phagocytic disorders (excluding chronic granulomatous disease) • Chronic cardiac disease (particularly cyanotic congenital heart disease and cardiac failure) • Chronic pulmonary disease (including asthma treated with high-dose oral corticosteroid therapy) • Cerebrospinal leaks from a congenital malformation, skull fracture, or neurologic procedure • Chronic renal insufficiency, including nephrotic syndrome • Diseases associated with immunosuppressive therapy or radiation therapy (including malignant neoplasms, leukemias, lymphomas, and Hodgkin disease) and solid organ transplantation • Diabetes mellitus
MODERATE RISK (INCIDENCE OF INVASIVE PNEUMOCOCCAL DISEASE = 20 CASES/100,000 PEOPLE PER YEAR)
• All children 24-35 mo of age • Children 36-59 mo of age attending out-of-home child care • Children 36-59 mo of age who are black or of American Indian/Alaska Native descent

From American Academy of Pediatrics: *Red book: 2006 report of the Committee on Infectious Diseases*, ed 27, Elk Grove Village, IL, 2006, American Academy of Pediatrics, p 527.

PATHOGENESIS

Invasion of the host is affected by a number of factors. Nonspecific defense mechanisms, including the presence of other bacteria in the nasopharynx, may limit multiplication of pneumococci. Aspiration of secretions containing pneumococci is hindered by the epiglottic reflex and by respiratory epithelial cilia, which move infected mucus toward the pharynx. Similarly, normal ciliary flow of fluid from the middle ear through the eustachian tube and sinuses to the nasopharynx usually prevents infection with nasopharyngeal flora, including pneumococci. Interference with these normal clearance mechanisms by allergy, viral infection, or irritants (e.g., smoke) may allow colonization and subsequent infection with these organisms in otherwise normally sterile sites.

Virulent pneumococci are intrinsically resistant to phagocytosis by alveolar macrophages. Pneumococcal disease frequently is facilitated by viral respiratory tract infection, which may produce mucosal injury, diminish epithelial ciliary activity, and depress the function of alveolar macrophages and neutrophils. Phagocytosis may be impeded by respiratory secretions and alveolar exudate. In the lungs and other tissues, the spread of infection is facilitated by the antiphagocytic properties of the pneumococcal capsule. Surface fluids of the respiratory tract contain only small amounts of IgG and are deficient in complement. During inflammation, there is limited influx of IgG, complement, and neutrophils. Phagocytosis of bacteria by neutrophils may occur, but normal human serum may not opsonize pneumococci and facilitate phagocytosis by alveolar macrophages. In tissues, pneumococci multiply and spread through the lymphatics or bloodstream or, less commonly, by direct extension from a local site of infection (e.g., sinuses). In bacteremia, the severity of disease is related to the number of organisms in the bloodstream and to the integrity of specific host defenses. A poor prognosis correlates with very large numbers of pneumococci and high concentrations of capsular polysaccharide in the blood and CSF.

Invasive pneumococcal disease is 30- to 100-fold more prevalent in children with sickle cell disease and other hemoglobinopathies and in children with congenital or surgical asplenia than in the general population. This risk is greatest in infants <2 yr of age since at that age antibody production to most serotypes is poor. The increased frequency of pneumococcal disease in asplenic persons is related to both deficient opsonization of pneumococci as well as absence of clearance by the spleen of circulating bacteria. Children with sickle cell disease also have deficits in the antibody-independent properdin (alternative) pathway of complement activation, in addition to functional asplenia. Both complement pathways contribute to antibody-independent and antibody-dependent opsonophagocytosis of pneumococci. With advancing age (e.g., >5 yr), children with sickle cell disease produce anticapsular antibody, augmenting antibody-dependent opsonophagocytosis and greatly reducing, but not eliminating, the risk of severe pneumococcal disease. Deficiency of many of the complement components (e.g., C2 and C3) is associated with recurrent pyogenic infection, including *S. pneumonia* infection. The efficacy of phagocytosis also is diminished in patients with B- and T-cell immunodeficiency syndromes (e.g., agammaglobulinemia, severe combined immune deficiency) or loss of immune globulin (e.g., nephrotic syndrome) and is largely caused by a deficiency of opsonic anticapsular antibody. These observations suggest that opsonization of pneumococci depends on the alternative complement pathway in antibody-deficient persons and that recovery from pneumococcal disease depends on the development of anticapsular antibodies that act as opsonins, enhancing phagocytosis and killing of pneumococci. Children with HIV infection also have high rates of invasive pneumococcal infection similar to or greater than that of children with sickle cell disease, although rates of invasive pneumococcal disease decreased after the introduction of highly active antiretroviral therapy (HAART).

CLINICAL MANIFESTATIONS

The signs and symptoms of pneumococcal infection are related to the anatomic site of disease. Common clinical syndromes include otitis media (Chapter 632), sinusitis (Chapter 372), pneumonia (Fig. 175-2) (Chapter 392), and sepsis (Chapter 64). Before routine use of PCVs, pneumococci caused >80% of bacteremia episodes in infants 3-36 mo of age with fever without an identifiable source (i.e., occult bacteremia). Bacteremia may be followed by meningitis (Chapter 595), osteomyelitis (Chapter 676), suppurative arthritis (Chapter 677), endocarditis (Chapter 431), and rarely, brain abscess (Chapter 596). Primary peritonitis (Chapter 363) may occur in children with peritoneal effusions due to nephrotic syndrome and other conditions. Local complications of infection may occur, causing empyema, pericarditis, mastoiditis, epidural abscess, or meningitis. Hemolytic-uremic syndrome (Chapter 478.4) and disseminated intravascular

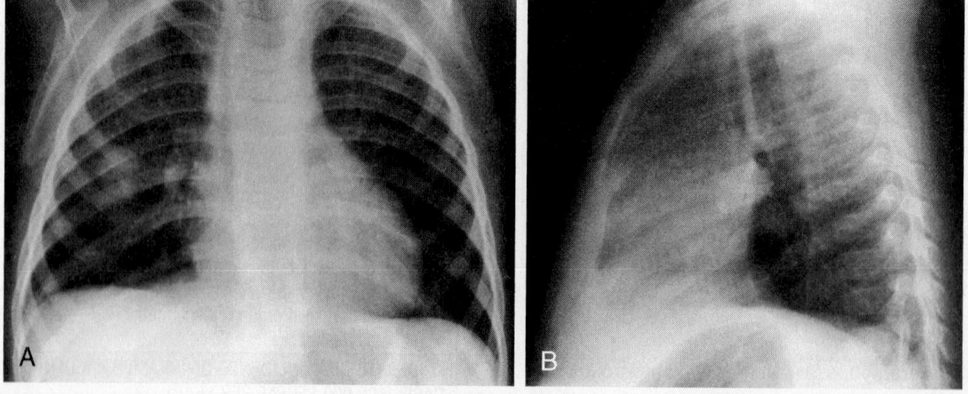

Figure 175-2 Bacterial pneumonia: "round" pneumonia *(Streptococcus pneumoniae)* in an 11 mo old girl with a 2 day history of cough and spiking fever. There was leukocytosis with a shift to the left. *A,* The anteroposterior view shows a round, nodular area of consolidation in the right midlung. *B,* On the lateral projection, the nodule lying in the right middle lobe appears somewhat triangular. Such round pneumonias are usually caused by one of the common bacterial pathogens and are most commonly located in the superior segment of a lower lobe. Confusion with a metastatic lesion is possible, but the clinical findings are those of pneumonia. An important radiographic clue is that the consolidation typically appears round on the frontal projection, a shape that does not persist on the lateral view (here the infiltrate appears triangular). (From Hilton SVW, Edwards DK, editors: *Practical pediatric radiology,* ed 3, Philadelphia, 2006, Elsevier, p 329.)

coagulation also occur as rare complications of pneumococcal infections. Epidemic conjunctivitis caused by nonencapsulated or encapsulated pneumococci occurs as well.

DIAGNOSIS

The diagnosis of pneumococcal infection is established by recovery of *S. pneumoniae* from the site of infection or the blood. Although pneumococci may be found in the nose or throat of patients with otitis media, pneumonia, septicemia, or meningitis, cultures of these locations are generally not helpful for diagnosis as they are not indicative of causation. Blood cultures should be obtained in children with pneumonia, meningitis, arthritis, osteomyelitis, peritonitis, pericarditis, or gangrenous skin lesions. Due to the implementation of universal vaccination with PCVs, there has been a substantial decrease in the incidence of occult bacteremia, but blood cultures should still be considered in febrile patients with clinical toxicity or significant leukocytosis. Leukocytosis often is pronounced, with total white blood cell counts frequently >15,000/mm^3. In severe cases of pneumococcal disease, white blood cell count may be low.

Pneumococci can be identified in body fluids as gram-positive, lancet-shaped diplococci. Early in the course of pneumococcal meningitis, many bacteria may be seen in relatively acellular cerebrospinal fluid. With current methods of continuously monitored blood culture systems, the average time to isolation of pneumococcal organisms is 14-15 hr. Pneumococcal latex agglutination tests for urine or other body fluids suffer from poor sensitivity and add little to Gram-stained fluids and standard cultures.

TREATMENT

The incidence of high-level β-lactam resistance and MDR strains have expanded dramatically during the past several decades. Spread of pneumococcal β-lactam and macrolide resistance is largely due to global spread of worldwide clones primarily of serotypes 6A, 6B, 9V, 14, 19F, and 23F, and introduction of PCVs appears to have decreased the overall incidence of pneumococcal resistance. In contrast, fluoroquinolone resistance is more commonly due to spontaneous mutation than clonal spread. Widespread use of antibiotics contributes to the spread of resistant strains. Some serotypes can undergo capsule switching (i.e., change from one serotype to another) in association with the development of antibiotic resistance.

Resistance in pneumococcal organisms to penicillin and the extended spectrum cephalosporins cefotaxime and ceftriaxone is defined by the minimum inhibitory concentration (MIC) as well as clinical syndrome. Pneumococci are considered susceptible, intermediate, or resistant to various antibacterial agents based on specific MIC breakpoints. For patients with pneumococcal meningitis, penicillin-susceptible strains have an MIC ≤0.06 µg/mL and penicillin resistant strains have an MIC ≥0.12 µg/mL. For patients with pneumococcal pneumonia, breakpoints are higher; in particular, penicillin susceptible strains have an MIC ≤2 µg/mL, and penicillin resistant strains have an MIC ≥8 µg/mL. For patients with meningitis, cefotaxime and ceftriaxone susceptible strains have an MIC ≤0.5 µg/mL and resistant strains have an MIC ≥2.0 µg/mL. For patients with nonmeningeal pneumococcal disease, breakpoints are higher, and cefotaxime- and ceftriaxone-susceptible strains have an MIC ≤1.0 µg/mL and resistant strains have an MIC ≥2 µg/mL. In cases where the pneumococcus is resistant to erythromycin but sensitive to clindamycin, **a D-test should be performed** to determine whether clindamycin resistance can be induced; if the D-test is positive, clindamycin should not be used to complete treatment of the patient. More than 30% of pneumococcal isolates are resistant to trimethoprim-sulfamethoxazole; levofloxacin resistance has also been reported. All isolates from children with severe infections should be tested for antibiotic susceptibility given widespread pneumococcal MDR strains. Resistance to vancomycin has not been seen to date, but vancomycin-tolerant pneumococci that are killed at a slower rate have been reported, and these tolerant pneumococci may be associated with a worse clinical outcome. Linezolid is an oxazolidinone antibacterial with activity against MDR gram-positive organisms including pneumococcus and has been used in the treatment of MDR pneumococcal pneumonia, meningitis, and severe otitis. Despite early favorable studies, use of this drug is limited by myelosuppression and high cost, and linezolid resistance in pneumococcus has been reported.

Children 1 mo of age or older with suspected pneumococcal meningitis should be treated with combination therapy using vancomycin (60 mg/kg/24 hr divided q 6 hr IV), and high-dose cefotaxime (300 mg/kg/24 hr divided q 8 hr IV) or ceftriaxone (100 mg/kg/24 hr divided q 12 hr IV). Proven pneumococcal meningitis can be treated with penicillin alone, or cefotaxime or ceftriaxone alone, if the isolate is penicillin-susceptible. If the organism is nonsusceptible (i.e., intermediate or full resistance) to penicillin but susceptible to cefotaxime and ceftriaxone, pneumococcal meningitis can be treated with cefotaxime or ceftriaxone alone. However, if the organism is nonsusceptible to penicillin and to cefotaxime or ceftriaxone, pneumococcal meningitis should be treated with combination vancomycin plus cefotaxime or ceftriaxone, not with vancomycin alone, and consideration should be given to the addition of rifampin.

For invasive infections outside the central nervous system (e.g., lobar pneumonia with or without bacteremia), high-dose cefotaxime and ceftriaxone are effective, even for those infections caused by cephalosporin-intermediate or -resistant strains. For individuals who are allergic to penicillin, clindamycin, erythromycin (or related macrolides, e.g., azithromycin or clarithromycin), cephalosporins (standard dosing), and trimethoprim-sulfamethoxazole may provide effective alternative therapy for susceptible strains, depending on the site of infection (e.g., clindamycin may be effective for pneumococcal infections other than meningitis). Higher doses of amoxicillin (80-100 mg/kg/24 hr) have been successful in the treatment of otitis media caused by penicillin-nonsusceptible strains. Empirical treatment of pneumococcal disease should be based on knowledge of susceptibility patterns in specific communities.

PROGNOSIS

Prognosis depends on the integrity of host defenses, virulence and numbers of the infecting organism, the age of the host, the site and extent of the infection, and the adequacy of treatment. The mortality rate for pneumococcal meningitis is approximately 10% in most studies. Pneumococcal meningitis results in sensorineural hearing loss in 20-30% of patients and can cause other serious neurologic sequelae including paralysis, epilepsy, blindness, and intellectual deficits.

PREVENTION

Immunologic responsiveness and efficacy following administration of pneumococcal polysaccharide vaccines is unpredictable in children <2 yr of age. PPSV23 contains purified polysaccharide of 23 pneumococcal serotypes responsible for >95% of cases of invasive disease. The clinical efficacy of these vaccines is controversial and studies have yielded conflicting results. In contrast, PCVs (see Table 175-2) provoke "protective" antibody responses in 90% of infants given these vaccines at 2, 4, and 6 mo of age, and greatly enhanced responses (e.g., immunologic memory) are apparent after "booster" doses given at 12-15 mo of age. In addition, PCVs reduce nasopharyngeal carriage of vaccine serotypes by up to 60-70%. In efficacy trials in the USA, infant immunization with PCV7 decreased invasive infections from pneumococcal vaccine serotypes by >93% and lobar pneumonias

Table 175-2 COMPARISON OF PNEUMOCOCCAL VACCINES LICENSED IN USA OR IN ADVANCED DEVELOPMENT (PCV7 SEROTYPES IN BOLD)

CARRIER PROTEIN	PNEUMOCOCCAL CAPSULAR POLYSACCHARIDES	MANUFACTURER
Diphtheria CRM_{197} protein	**4,6B, 9V, 14, 18C, 19F, 23F**	Wyeth Lederle (PCV7, Prevnar)
Diphtheria CRM_{197} protein	1, 3, **4**, 5, 6A, **6B**, 7F, **9V**, **14**, **18C**, 19A, **19F**, **23F**	Wyeth Lederle (PCV13, Prevnar 13)
Haemophilus influenzae protein D Tetanus and diphtheria toxoids	1, **4**, 5, **6B**, 7F, **9V**, **14**, **18C**, **19F**, **23F**	GlaxoSmithKline (PCV10, Synflorix)
None	1, 2, 3, **4**, 5, **6B**, 7F, 8, 9N, **9V**, 10A, 11A, 12F, **14**, 15B, 17F, **18C**, 19A, **19F**, 20, 22F, **23F**, 33F	Sanofi Pasteur MSD (PPSV23, Pneumovax II)

by >73%. Its administration was associated with a 6-7% decrease in otitis media, but greater reduction in complications of otitis media such as tympanostomy tube placement. From 2000 (PCV7 introduction) to 2005, invasive pneumococcal disease in U.S. children <5 yr of age decreased by 94%. PCV7 has significantly decreased rates of invasive pneumococcal disease in children with sickle cell disease, and preliminary studies suggest substantial protection for HIV-infected children and splenectomized adults. Adverse events after the administration of PCV7 have included local swelling and redness and slightly increased rates of fever, when used in conjunction with other childhood vaccines. There have been multiple reports of increases of empyema due to serotypes 1, 3, and 19A; necrotizing pneumonia due to serotype 3 and serogroup 19; bacteremia due to serotypes 3 and 8; and mastoiditis and recalcitrant acute otitis media due to MDR serotype 19A. These observations inform the serotype composition of new PCVs (Table 175-2).

Immunization with PVC13 is recommended for all infants on a schedule for primary immunization, in previously unvaccinated infants, and for transition for those partially vaccinated with PCV7 (Tables 175-3 and 175-4). High-risk children ≥2 yr of age, such as those with asplenia, sickle cell disease, some types of immune deficiency (e.g., antibody deficiencies), HIV infection, cochlear implant, CSF leak, diabetes mellitus, and chronic lung, heart, or kidney disease (including nephrotic syndrome), may benefit also from PPSV23 administered after 2 yr of age following priming with the scheduled doses of PCV13. Thus, it is recommended that children ≥2 yr of age with these underlying conditions receive supplemental vaccination with PPSV23. A second dose of PPSV23 is recommended 5 yr after the first dose of PPSV23 for persons aged ≥2 yr who are immunocompromised, have sickle cell disease, or functional or anatomic asplenia.

Immunization with pneumococcal vaccines also may prevent pneumococcal disease caused by nonvaccine serotypes that are serotypically related to a vaccine strain (e.g., 6A and 6B). However, because current vaccines do not eliminate all pneumococcal invasive infections, penicillin prophylaxis is recommended for children at high risk of invasive pneumococcal disease, including children with asplenia or sickle cell disease. Oral penicillin V potassium (125 mg bid for children <3 yr; 250 mg bid for children ≥3 yr) decreases the incidence of pneumococcal sepsis in children with sickle cell disease. Once monthly intramuscular benzathine penicillin G (600,000 U q 3-4 wk for children <60 lb; 1,200,000 U q 3-4 wk for children ≥60 lb) may also provide prophylaxis. Erythromycin may be used in children with penicillin allergy, but its efficacy is unproved. Prophylaxis in sickle cell disease has been safely discontinued after the 5th birthday in children who have received all recommended pneumococcal vaccine doses and who had not experienced invasive

Table 175-3 RECOMMENDED ROUTINE VACCINATION SCHEDULE FOR 13-VALENT PNEUMOCOCCAL CONJUGATE VACCINE (PCV13) AMONG INFANTS AND CHILDREN WHO HAVE NOT RECEIVED PREVIOUS DOSES OF 7-VALENT VACCINE (PCV7) OR PCV13, BY AGE AT FIRST DOSE—ADVISORY COMMITTEE ON IMMUNIZATION PRACTICES (ACIP), USA, 2010

AGE AT FIRST DOSE (MO)	PRIMARY PCV13 SERIES*	PCV13 BOOSTER DOSE†
2-6	3 doses	1 dose at age 12-15 mo
7-11	2 doses	1 dose at age 12-15 mo
12-23	2 doses	—
24-59 (healthy children)	1 dose	—
24-71 (children with certain chronic diseases or immunocompromising conditions)	2 doses	—

*Minimum interval between doses is 8 weeks except for children vaccinated at age <12 months for whom minimum interval between doses is 4 weeks. Minimum age for administration of first dose is 6 weeks.
†Given at least 8 weeks after the previous dose.
From Centers for Disease Control and Prevention: Licensure of a 13-valent pneumococcal conjugate vaccine (PCV13) and recommendations for use among children—Advisory Committee on Immunization Practices (ACEP), 2010, *MMWR Morb Mortal Wkly Rep* 59:258–261, 2010, p 260, Table 3.

Table 175-4 RECOMMENDED TRANSITION SCHEDULE FROM 7-VALENT PNEUMOCOCCAL CONJUGATE VACCINE (PCV7) TO 13-VALENT VACCINE (PCV13) VACCINATION AMONG INFANTS AND CHILDREN, ACCORDING TO NUMBER OF PREVIOUS PCV7 DOSES RECEIVED—ADVISORY COMMITTEE ON IMMUNIZATION PRACTICES (ACIP), USA, 2010

INFANT SERIES 2 mo	INFANT SERIES 4 mo	INFANT SERIES 6 mo	BOOSTER DOSE ≥12 mo*	SUPPLEMENTAL PCV13 DOSE 14-59 mo†
PCV7	PCV13	PCV13	PCV13	—
PCV7	PCV7	PCV13	PCV13	—
PCV7	PCV7	PCV7	PCV13	—
PCV7	PCV7	PCV7	PCV7	PCV13

*No additional PCV13 doses are indicated for children age 12-23 months who have received 2 or 3 doses of PCV before age 12 months and at least 1 dose of PCV13 at age ≥12 months.
†For children with underlying medical conditions (see Table 175-1), a single supplemental PCV13 dose is recommended through age 71 months.
From Centers for Disease Control and Prevention: Licensure of a 13-valent pneumococcal conjugate vaccine (PCV13) and recommendations for use among children—Advisory Committee on Immunization Practices (ACEP), 2010, *MMWR Morb Mortal Wkly Rep* 59:258–261, 2010, p 260, Table 3.

pneumococcal disease. Prophylaxis is often administered for at least 2 yr after splenectomy or up to 5 yr of age. Efficacy in children >5 yr of age and adolescents is unproved. If oral antibiotic prophylaxis is used, strict compliance must be encouraged. Given the rapid emergence of penicillin-resistant pneumococci, especially in children receiving long-term, low-dose therapy, prophylaxis cannot be relied on to prevent disease. High-risk children with fever should be promptly evaluated and treated regardless of vaccination or penicillin prophylaxis history.

BIBLIOGRAPHY

Please visit the Nelson Textbook of Pediatrics *website at www.expertconsult.com for the complete bibliography.*

Chapter 176
Group A Streptococcus

Michael A. Gerber

Group A streptococcus (GAS), also known as *Streptococcus pyogenes,* is a common cause of infections of the upper respiratory tract (pharyngitis) and the skin (impetigo, pyoderma) in children and is a less common cause of perianal cellulitis, vaginitis, septicemia, pneumonia, endocarditis, pericarditis, osteomyelitis, suppurative arthritis, myositis, cellulitis, and omphalitis. These microorganisms also cause distinct clinical entities (scarlet fever and erysipelas), as well as a toxic shock syndrome and necrotizing fasciitis. GAS is also the cause of 2 potentially serious nonsuppurative complications: rheumatic fever (Chapters 176.1 and 432) and acute glomerulonephritis (Chapter 505.1).

ETIOLOGY

Group A streptococci are gram-positive coccoid-shaped bacteria that tend to grow in chains. They are broadly classified by their reactions on mammalian red blood cells. The zone of complete hemolysis that surrounds colonies grown on blood agar distinguishes β-hemolytic (complete hemolysis) from α-hemolytic (green or partial hemolysis) and γ (nonhemolytic) species. The β-hemolytic streptococci can be divided into groups by a group-specific polysaccharide (**Lancefield carbohydrate C**) located in the cell wall. More than 20 serologic groups are identified, designated by the letters A through V. Serologic grouping by the Lancefield method is precise, but group A organisms can be identified more readily by any one of a number of latex agglutination, coagglutination, or enzyme immunoassay procedures. Group A strains can also be distinguished from other groups by differences in sensitivity to bacitracin. A disk containing 0.04 U of bacitracin inhibits the growth of most group A strains, whereas other groups are generally resistant to this antibiotic. GAS can be subdivided into >100 serotypes on the basis of the **M protein** antigen, which is located on the cell surface and in fimbriae that project from the outer edge of the cell. M typing has traditionally relied primarily on the serologic typing of the surface M protein using available polyclonal sera. However, it is frequently difficult to detect M proteins in this way; a molecular approach to M typing GAS isolates using the polymerase chain reaction is based on sequencing the *emm* gene of GAS that encodes the M protein. More than 180 distinct M types have been identified using *emm* typing, and there has been a good correlation between the known serotypes and the *emm* types.

M serotyping has been valuable for epidemiologic studies; particular GAS diseases tend to be associated with certain M types. Types 1, 12, 28, 4, 3, and 2 (in that order) are the most common causes of uncomplicated streptococcal pharyngitis in the USA. The M types commonly associated with pharyngitis rarely cause skin infections, and the M types commonly associated with skin infections rarely cause pharyngitis. A few of the **pharyngeal** strains (M type 12) have been associated with glomerulonephritis, but far more of the **skin** strains (M types 49, 55, 57, and 60) have been considered nephritogenic. A few of the pharyngeal serotypes, but none of the skin strains, have been associated with acute rheumatic fever. Rheumatogenic potential is not solely dependent on the serotype but is a characteristic of specific strains within several serotypes.

EPIDEMIOLOGY

Humans are the natural reservoir for GAS. These bacteria are highly communicable and can cause disease in normal individuals of all ages who do not have type-specific immunity against the particular serotype involved. Disease in neonates is uncommon, probably because of maternally acquired antibody. The incidence of pharyngeal infections is highest in children 5-15 yr of age, especially in young school-aged children. These infections are most common in the northern regions of the USA, especially during winter and early spring. Children with untreated acute pharyngitis spread GAS by airborne salivary droplets and nasal discharge. Transmission is favored by close proximity; therefore, schools, military barracks, and homes are important environments for spread. The incubation period for pharyngitis is usually 2-5 days. GAS has the potential to be an important upper respiratory tract pathogen and to produce outbreaks of disease in the daycare setting. Foods containing GAS occasionally cause explosive outbreaks of pharyngotonsillitis. Children are usually not infectious 24 hr after appropriate antibiotic therapy has been started. Chronic pharyngeal carriers of GAS rarely transmit this organism to others.

Streptococcal pyoderma (impetigo, pyoderma) occurs most frequently during the summer in temperate climates, or year round in warmer climates, when the skin is exposed and abrasions and insect bites are more likely to occur (Chapter 657). Colonization of healthy skin by GAS usually precedes the development of impetigo. Because GAS cannot penetrate intact skin, impetigo usually occurs at the site of open lesions (insect bites, traumatic wounds, burns). Although impetigo serotypes may colonize the throat, spread is usually from skin to skin, not via the respiratory tract. Fingernails and the perianal region can harbor GAS and play a role in disseminating impetigo. Multiple cases of impetigo in the same family are common. Both impetigo and pharyngitis are more likely to occur among children living in crowded homes and in poor hygienic circumstances.

The incidence of **severe invasive** GAS infections, including bacteremia, streptococcal toxic shock syndrome, and necrotizing fasciitis, has increased in recent years. The incidence appears to be highest in the very young and in older persons. Prior to the routine use of varicella vaccine, varicella was the most commonly identified risk factor in children. Other risk factors include diabetes mellitus, HIV infection, intravenous drug use, and chronic pulmonary or chronic cardiac disease. The portal of entry is unknown in almost 50% of the cases of severe invasive GAS infection; in most cases, it is believed to be skin or mucous membrane. Severe invasive disease rarely follows GAS pharyngitis.

PATHOGENESIS

Virulence of GAS depends primarily on the M protein, and strains rich in M protein resist phagocytosis in fresh human blood, whereas M-negative strains do not. GAS isolated from chronic pharyngeal carriers contains little or no M protein and are relatively avirulent. The M protein antigen stimulates the production of protective antibodies. These antibodies are type specific. They protect against infection with a homologous M type but confer no immunity against other M types. Therefore, multiple GAS infections attributable to different M types are common during childhood and adolescence. By adult life, individuals are probably immune to many of the common M types in the environment, but because of the large number of serotypes it is doubtful that total immunity is ever achieved.

GAS produces a large variety of enzymes and toxins, including erythrogenic toxins (known as *streptococcal pyrogenic exotoxins*). Streptococcal **pyrogenic exotoxins** A, B, and C are responsible for the **rash of scarlet fever** and are elaborated by streptococci that are infected with a particular bacteriophage. These exotoxins stimulate the formation of specific antitoxin antibodies that provide immunity against the scarlatiniform rash but not against other streptococcal infections. Because GAS can produce 3 different rash-producing pyrogenic exotoxins (A, B, or C), a 2nd attack of scarlet fever may sometimes occur. Streptococcal pyrogenic exotoxins A, B, and C, as well as several newly discovered exotoxins, appear to be involved in the pathogenesis of invasive GAS disease, including the **streptococcal toxic shock syndrome.**

The roles of most of the other streptococcal toxins and enzymes in human disease have yet to be established. Many of these extracellular substances are antigenic and stimulate antibody production after an infection. However, these antibodies bear no relationship to immunity. Their measurement is useful for evidence of a recent streptococcal infection. The test for antibodies against streptolysin O (antistreptolysin O) is the most commonly used antibody determination. Because the immune response to extracellular antigens varies among individuals as well as with the site of infection, it is sometimes necessary to measure other streptococcal antibodies, such as anti-deoxyribonuclease (anti-DNase).

CLINICAL MANIFESTATIONS

The most common infections caused by GAS involve the respiratory tract and the skin and soft tissues.

Respiratory Tract Infections

GAS is an important cause of acute pharyngitis (Chapter 373) and pneumonia (Chapter 392).

Scarlet Fever

Scarlet fever is an upper respiratory tract infection associated with a characteristic rash, which is caused by an infection with **pyrogenic exotoxin (erythrogenic toxin)**-producing GAS in individuals who do not have antitoxin antibodies. It is now encountered less commonly and is less virulent than in the past, but the incidence is cyclic, depending on the prevalence of toxin-producing strains and the immune status of the population. The modes of transmission, age distribution, and other epidemiologic features are otherwise similar to those for GAS pharyngitis.

The rash appears within 24-48 hours after onset of symptoms, although it may appear with the first signs of illness (Fig. 176-1*A*). It often begins around the neck and spreads over the trunk and extremities. It is a diffuse, finely papular, erythematous eruption producing a bright red discoloration of the skin, which blanches on pressure. It is often more intense along the creases of the elbows, axillae, and groin. The skin has a goose-pimple appearance and feels rough. The face is usually spared, although the cheeks may be erythematous with pallor around the mouth. After 3-4 days, the rash begins to fade and is followed by desquamation, 1st on the face, progressing downward, and often resembling a mild sunburn. Occasionally, sheetlike desquamation may occur around the free margins of the fingernails, the palms, and the soles. Examination of the pharynx of a patient with scarlet fever reveals essentially the same findings as with GAS pharyngitis. In addition, the tongue is usually coated and the papillae are swollen (Fig. 176-1*B*). After desquamation, the reddened papillae are prominent, giving the tongue a strawberry appearance (Fig. 176-1*C*).

Typical scarlet fever is not difficult to diagnose; the milder form with equivocal pharyngeal findings can be confused with viral exanthems, Kawasaki disease, and drug eruptions. Staphylococcal infections are occasionally associated with a scarlatiniform rash. A history of recent exposure to a GAS infection is helpful. Identification of GAS in the pharynx confirms the diagnosis, if uncertain.

Impetigo

Impetigo (or pyoderma) has traditionally been classified into 2 clinical forms: bullous and nonbullous (Chapter 657). Nonbullous impetigo is the more common form and is a superficial infection of the skin that appears first as a discrete papulovesicular lesion surrounded by a localized area of redness. The vesicles rapidly become purulent and covered with a thick, confluent, amber-colored crust that gives the appearance of having been stuck on the skin. The lesions may occur anywhere but are more common on the face and extremities. If untreated, nonbullous impetigo is a mild but chronic illness, often spreading to other parts of the body, but occasionally is self-limited. Regional **lymphadenitis** is common. Nonbullous impetigo is generally not

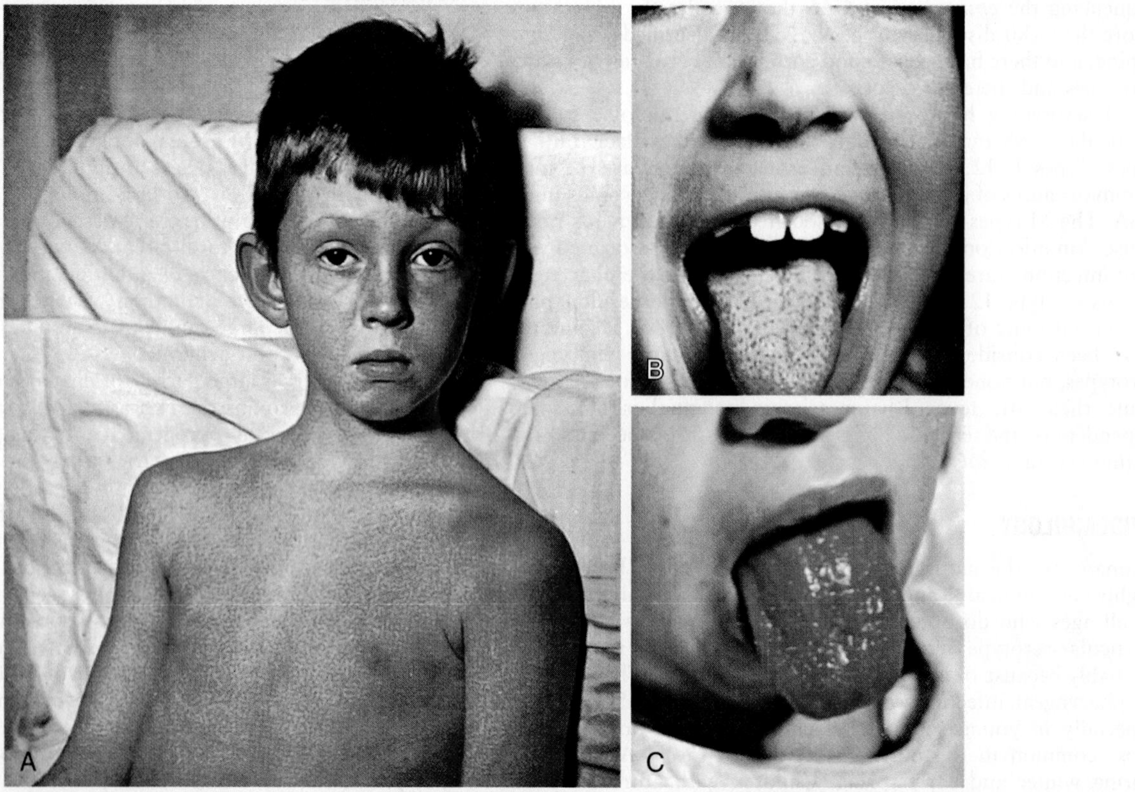

Figure 176-1 Scarlet fever. *A,* Punctate, erythematous rash (2nd day). *B,* White strawberry tongue (1st day). *C,* Red strawberry tongue (3rd day). (Courtesy Dr. Franklin H. Top, Professor and Head of the Department of Hygiene and Preventive Medicine, State University of Iowa, College of Medicine, Iowa City, IA; and Parke, Davis & Company's *Therapeutic Notes.* From Gershon AA, Hotez PJ, Katz SL: *Krugman's infectious diseases of children,* ed 11, Philadelphia, 2004, Mosby, plate 53.)

accompanied by fever or other systemic signs or symptoms. Impetiginized excoriations around the nares are seen with active GAS infections of the nasopharynx particularly in young children. However, impetigo is not usually associated with an overt streptococcal infection of the upper respiratory tract.

Bullous impetigo is less common and occurs most often in neonates and young infants. It is characterized by flaccid, transparent bullae usually <3 cm in diameter on previously untraumatized skin. The usual distribution involves the face, buttocks, trunk, and perineum. Although *Staphylococcus aureus* has traditionally been accepted as the sole pathogen responsible for bullous impetigo, there has been confusion about the organisms responsible for nonbullous impetigo. In most episodes of nonbullous impetigo, either GAS or *S. aureus,* or a combination of these 2 organisms, is isolated. Earlier investigations suggested that GAS was the causative agent in most cases of nonbullous impetigo and that *S. aureus* was only a secondary invader. However, studies have demonstrated the recent emergence of *S. aureus* as the causative agent in most cases of nonbullous impetigo. Culture of the lesions is the only way to distinguish nonbullous impetigo caused by *S. aureus* from that caused by GAS.

Erysipelas

Erysipelas is a relatively rare acute GAS infection involving the deeper layers of the skin and the underlying connective tissue. The skin in the affected area is swollen, red, and very tender. Superficial blebs may be present. The most characteristic finding is the sharply defined, slightly elevated border. At times, reddish streaks of lymphangitis project out from the margins of the lesion. The onset is abrupt, and signs and symptoms of a systemic infection, such as high fever, are often present. Cultures obtained by needle aspirate of the inflamed area often reveal the causative agent.

Perianal Dermatitis

Perianal dermatitis, also called **perianal streptococcal disease,** is a distinct clinical entity characterized by well-demarcated, perianal erythema associated with anal pruritus, painful defecation, and blood-streaked stools. Physical examination reveals flat, pink to beefy-red perianal erythema with sharp margins extending as far as 2 cm from the anus. Erythema may involve the vulva and vagina. Lesions may be very tender and, particularly when chronic, may fissure and bleed. Systemic symptoms and fever are unusual.

Vaginitis

GAS is a common cause of vaginitis in prepubertal girls (Chapter 543). Patients usually have a serous discharge with marked erythema and irritation of the vulvar area, accompanied by discomfort in walking and in urination.

Severe Invasive Disease

Invasive GAS infection is defined by isolation of GAS from a normally sterile body site and includes 3 overlapping clinical syndromes. The 1st is GAS toxic shock syndrome, which is differentiated from other types of invasive GAS infections by the presence of shock and multiorgan system failure early in the course of the infection (Table 176-1). The second is GAS necrotizing fasciitis characterized by extensive local necrosis of subcutaneous soft tissues and skin. The third is the group of focal and systemic infections that do not meet the criteria for toxic shock syndrome or necrotizing fasciitis and includes bacteremia with no identified focus, meningitis, pneumonia, peritonitis, puerperal sepsis, osteomyelitis, suppurative arthritis, myositis, and surgical wound infections.

The pathogenic mechanisms responsible for severe, invasive GAS infections, including streptococcal toxic shock syndrome and necrotizing fasciitis, have yet to be defined completely, but an association with streptococcal pyrogenic exotoxins has been suggested. The three original streptococcal pyrogenic exotoxins (A, B, C), the newly discovered streptococcal pyrogenic exotoxins, and potentially other, as yet unidentified toxins produced by GAS act as superantigens, which stimulate an intense activation and proliferation of T lymphocytes and macrophages resulting in the production of large quantities of cytokines. These cytokines are capable of producing shock and tissue injury, and are believed to be responsible for many of the clinical manifestations of severe, invasive GAS infections.

Table 176-1 DEFINITION OF STREPTOCOCCAL TOXIC SHOCK SYNDROME

Clinical criteria
Hypotension plus 2 or more of the following:
Renal impairment
Coagulopathy
Hepatic involvement
Adult respiratory distress syndrome
Generalized erythematous macular rash
Soft tissue necrosis
Definite case
Clinical criteria plus group A streptococcus from a normally sterile site
Probable case
Clinical criteria plus group A streptococcus from a nonsterile site

DIAGNOSIS

When attempting to decide whether to perform a microbiologic test on a patient presenting with acute pharyngitis, consideration of the clinical and epidemiologic findings should take place before the test is performed. A history of close contact with a well-documented case of GAS pharyngitis is helpful, as is an awareness of a high prevalence of GAS infections in the community. The signs and symptoms of streptococcal and nonstreptococcal pharyngitis overlap too broadly to allow the requisite diagnostic precision on clinical grounds alone. The clinical diagnosis of GAS pharyngitis cannot be made with certainty even by the most experienced physicians, and bacteriologic confirmation is required.

Culture of a throat swab on a sheep blood agar plate remains the standard for the documentation of the presence of GAS in the upper respiratory tract and for the confirmation of the clinical diagnosis of acute GAS pharyngitis. If performed correctly, a single throat swab cultured on a blood-agar plate has a sensitivity of 90-95% for detecting the presence of GAS in the pharynx.

A disadvantage of culturing a throat swab on a blood-agar plate is the delay (overnight or longer) in obtaining the culture result. **Rapid antigen detection** tests have been developed for the identification of GAS directly from throat swabs. Although these rapid tests are more expensive than the blood-agar culture, the advantage they offer over the traditional procedure is the speed with which they can provide results. Rapid identification and treatment of patients with streptococcal pharyngitis can reduce the risk for the spread of GAS, allowing the patient to return to school or work sooner, and can reduce the acute morbidity of this illness.

The great majority of the rapid antigen detection tests that are currently available have an excellent specificity of >95% when compared with blood-agar plate cultures. False-positive test results are unusual, and, therefore, therapeutic decisions can be made on the basis of a positive test result with confidence. Unfortunately, the sensitivity of most of these tests is 80-90%, possibly lower, when compared with the blood-agar plate culture. Therefore, a negative test does not exclude the presence of GAS, and a confirmatory throat culture should be performed. Newer tests may be more sensitive than other rapid antigen detection tests and perhaps may even be as sensitive as blood-agar plate cultures. However, the definitive studies to determine whether some rapid antigen detection tests are significantly more sensitive than others, and, whether any of these tests are sensitive enough to be used routinely without throat culture confirmation of negative test results, have not been performed. Some experts believe that physicians who use a rapid antigen detection test without culture backup should compare the results with that specific test to those of throat cultures to confirm adequate sensitivity in their practice.

GAS infection can also be diagnosed retrospectively on the basis of an elevated or increasing streptococcal antibody titer. The antistreptolysin O assay is the streptococcal antibody test most commonly used. Because streptolysin O also is produced by group C and G streptococcus, the test is not specific for group A infection. The antistreptolysin O response can be feeble in patients with streptococcal impetigo, and its usefulness for this condition is limited. In contrast, the anti-DNase B responses are present after both skin and throat infections. A significant antibody increase is usually defined as an increase in titer of 2 or more dilution increments between the acute phase and convalescent phase specimens, regardless of the actual height of the antibody titer. Physicians frequently misinterpret streptococcal antibody titers because of a failure to appreciate that the normal levels of these antibodies are higher among school-aged children compared to adults. Both the traditional ASO and anti-DNase B tests are neutralization assays. Newer tests use latex agglutination or nephelometric assays. Unfortunately, these newer tests have not been well-standardized against the traditional neutralization assays. Physicians need to be aware of these potential problems when interpreting the results of streptococcal serologic testing performed on their patients.

A commercially available slide agglutination test for the detection of antibodies to several streptococcal antigens is the Streptozyme test (Wampole Laboratories, Stamford, CT). This test is less well standardized and less reproducible than other antibody tests, and it should not be used as a test for evidence of a preceding GAS infection.

Differential Diagnosis

Viruses are the most common cause of acute pharyngitis in children. Respiratory viruses such as influenza virus, parainfluenza virus, rhinovirus, coronavirus, adenovirus, and respiratory syncytial virus are frequent causes of acute pharyngitis. Other viral causes of acute pharyngitis include enteroviruses and herpes simplex virus (HSV). Epstein-Barr virus (EBV) is a frequent cause of acute pharyngitis that is often accompanied by other clinical findings of infectious mononucleosis (e.g., splenomegaly, generalized lymphadenopathy). Systemic infections with other viral agents including cytomegalovirus, rubella virus, measles virus, and HIV may be associated with acute pharyngitis.

GAS is the most common cause of bacterial pharyngitis, accounting for 15-30% of the cases of acute pharyngitis in children. Groups C and G β-hemolytic streptococcus (Chapter 178) also produce acute pharyngitis in children. *Arcanobacterium haemolyticum* and *Fusobacterium necrophorum* are additional less common causes. *Neisseria gonorrhoeae* can occasionally cause acute pharyngitis in sexually active adolescents. Other bacteria such as *Francisella tularensis* and *Yersinia enterocolitica* as well as mixed infections with anaerobic bacteria (Vincent angina) are rare causes of acute pharyngitis. *Chlamydia pneumoniae* and *Mycoplasma pneumoniae* have been implicated as causes of acute pharyngitis, particularly in adults. *Corynebacterium diphtheriae* (Chapter 180) can cause pharyngitis but is rare because of universal immunization. Although other bacteria such as *Staphylococcus aureus, Haemophilus influenzae,* and *Streptococcus pneumoniae* are frequently cultured from the throats of children with acute pharyngitis, their etiologic role in pharyngitis has not been established.

GAS pharyngitis is the only common cause of acute pharyngitis for which antibiotic therapy is definitely indicated. Therefore, when confronted with a patient with acute pharyngitis, the clinical decision that usually needs to be made is whether the pharyngitis is attributable to GAS.

TREATMENT

Antibiotic therapy for patients with GAS pharyngitis can prevent acute rheumatic fever, shorten the clinical course of the illness, reduce transmission of the infection to others, and prevent suppurative complications. For the patient with classic scarlet fever, antibiotic therapy should be started immediately, but for the vast majority of patients who present with much less distinctive findings, treatment should be withheld until there is some form of bacteriologic confirmation either by throat culture or rapid antigen detection test. Rapid antigen detection tests, because of their high degree of specificity, have made it possible to initiate antibiotic therapy immediately for someone with a positive test result.

GAS is exquisitely sensitive to penicillin, and resistant strains have never been encountered. Penicillin is, therefore, the drug of choice (except in patients who are allergic to penicillin) for pharyngeal infections as well as for suppurative complications. Treatment with oral penicillin V (250 mg/dose bid-tid for ≤60 lb and 500 mg/dose bid-tid for >60 lb PO) is recommended but it must be taken for a full 10 days even though there is symptomatic improvement in 3-4 days. Penicillin V (phenoxyethylpenicillin) is preferred over penicillin G because it may be given without regard to mealtime. The major problem with all forms of oral therapy is the risk that the drug will be discontinued before the 10-day course has been completed. Therefore, when oral treatment is prescribed, the necessity of completing a full course of therapy must be emphasized. If the parents seem unlikely to comply with oral therapy because of family disorganization, difficulties in comprehension, or other reasons, parenteral therapy with a single intramuscular injection of benzathine penicillin G (600,000 IU for ≤60 lb, 1.2 million IU for >60 lb, IM) is the most efficacious and often the most practical method of treatment. Disadvantages include soreness around the site of injection, which may last for several days, and potential for injection into nerves or blood vessels if not administered correctly. The local reaction is diminished when benzathine penicillin G is combined in a single injection with procaine penicillin G, although precautions are necessary to ensure that an adequate amount of benzathine penicillin G is administered.

In several comparative clinical trials, once daily amoxicillin (50 mg/kg, maximum 1,000 mg) for 10 days has been shown to be effective in treating GAS pharyngitis. This somewhat broader-spectrum agent has the advantage of once-daily dosing, which may enhance adherence. In addition, amoxicillin is relatively inexpensive and is considerably more palatable than penicillin V suspension.

A 10-day course of a narrow spectrum oral cephalosporin is recommended for most penicillin-allergic individuals. Several reports indicate that a 10-day course with an oral cephalosporin is superior to 10 days of oral penicillin in eradicating GAS from the pharynx. Analysis of these data suggests that the difference in eradication is due mainly to a higher rate of eradication of carriers included unintentionally in these clinical trials. Some penicillin-allergic persons (up to 10%) are also allergic to cephalosporins, and these agents should not be used in patients with immediate (anaphylactic-type) hypersensitivity to penicillin. Most oral broad-spectrum cephalosporins are considerably more expensive than penicillin or amoxicillin, and the former agents are more likely to select for antibiotic-resistant flora.

Oral clindamycin is an appropriate agent for treating penicillin-allergic patients and resistance to clindamycin among GAS isolates in the USA is currently only about 1%. An oral macrolide (erythromycin or clarithromycin) or azalide (azithromycin) is also an appropriate agent for patients allergic to penicillins. Ten days of therapy is indicated except for azithromycin, which is given for 5 days. Erythromycin is associated with substantially higher rates of gastrointestinal side effects than the other agents. In recent years, macrolide resistance rates among pharyngeal isolates of GAS in most areas of the USA have been around 5-8%. Sulfonamides and the tetracyclines are not indicated for treatment of GAS infections.

Most oral antibiotics must be administered for the conventional 10 days to achieve maximal pharyngeal eradication rates of GAS, but certain newer agents have been reported to achieve comparable bacteriologic and clinical cure rates when given for 5 days or less. However, definitive results from comprehensive studies are not available to allow final evaluation of these proposed shorter courses of oral antibiotic therapy. Therefore, they cannot be recommended at this time. In addition, these antibiotics have a much broader spectrum than penicillin and are generally more expensive, even when administered for short courses.

The majority of patients with GAS pharyngitis respond clinically to antimicrobial therapy, and GAS is eradicated from the pharynx. Post-treatment throat cultures are indicated only in the relatively few patients who remain symptomatic, whose symptoms recur, or who have had rheumatic fever and are, therefore, at unusually high risk for recurrence.

Antibiotic therapy for a patient with nonbullous impetigo can prevent local extension of the lesions, spread to distant infectious foci, and transmission of the infection to others. However, the ability of antibiotic therapy to prevent poststreptococcal glomerulonephritis has not been demonstrated. Patients with a few superficial, isolated lesions and no systemic signs can be treated with topical antibiotics. Mupirocin is a safe and effective agent that has become the topical treatment of choice. If there are widespread lesions or systemic signs, oral therapy with coverage for both GAS and *S. aureus* is needed. With the rapid emergence of methicillin-resistant *S. aureus* in many communities, consideration should be given to using clindamycin alone or a combination of trimethoprim-sulfamethoxazole and amoxicillin as first-line therapy. Oral cefuroxime is an effective treatment of perianal streptococcal disease.

Theoretical considerations and experimental data suggest that intravenous clindamycin is a more effective agent for the treatment of severe, invasive GAS infections than intravenous penicillin. However, because a small proportion of the GAS isolates in the USA are resistant to clindamycin, clindamycin should be used in combination with penicillin for these infections until susceptibility to clindamycin has been established. If **necrotizing fasciitis** is suspected, immediate surgical exploration or biopsy is required to identify a deep soft tissue infection that should be debrided immediately. Patients with **streptococcal toxic shock syndrome** require rapid and aggressive fluid replacement, management of respiratory or cardiac failure, if present, and anticipatory management of multiorgan system failure. Limited data suggest that intravenous gamma globulin may be effective in the management of streptococcal toxic shock syndrome. Intravenous immunoglobulin should be reserved for those patients who do not respond to other therapeutic measures.

COMPLICATIONS

Suppurative complications from the spread of GAS to adjacent structures were common before antibiotics became available. Cervical lymphadenitis, peritonsillar abscess, retropharyngeal abscess, otitis media, mastoiditis, and sinusitis still occur in children in whom the primary illness has gone unnoticed or in whom treatment of the pharyngitis has been inadequate. GAS pneumonia can also occur.

Acute rheumatic fever (Chapter 176.1) and acute poststreptococcal glomerulonephritis (Chapter 505.1) are both nonsuppurative sequelae of infections with GAS that occur after an asymptomatic latent period. They are both characterized by lesions remote from the site of the GAS infection. Acute rheumatic fever and acute glomerulonephritis differ in their clinical manifestations, epidemiology, and potential morbidity. In addition, acute glomerulonephritis can occur after a GAS infection of either the upper respiratory tract or the skin, but acute rheumatic fever can occur only after an infection of the upper respiratory tract.

Poststreptococcal Reactive Arthritis

Poststreptococcal reactive arthritis has been used to describe a syndrome characterized by the onset of acute arthritis following an episode of GAS pharyngitis in a patient whose illness does not otherwise fulfill the Jones criteria for the diagnosis of acute rheumatic fever. There is still considerable debate about whether this entity represents a distinct syndrome or is a manifestation of acute rheumatic fever. Although poststreptococcal reactive arthritis usually involves the large joints, in contrast to the arthritis of acute rheumatic fever, it may involve small peripheral joints as well as the axial skeleton and is typically nonmigratory. The latent period between the antecedent episode of GAS pharyngitis and the poststreptococcal reactive arthritis may be considerably shorter (usually <10 days) than that typically seen with acute rheumatic fever. In contrast to the arthritis of acute rheumatic fever, poststreptococcal reactive arthritis does not respond dramatically to therapy with aspirin or other nonsteroidal antiinflammatory agents. In addition, the reactive arthritis is usually not migratory, and fewer patients have a fever >38°C. Even though no more than half of the patients with poststreptococcal reactive arthritis who have a throat culture performed have GAS isolated, all have serologic evidence of a recent GAS infection. Because a small proportion of patients with poststreptococcal reactive arthritis have been reported to subsequently develop valvular heart disease, these patients should be carefully observed for several months for clinical evidence of carditis. Some experts recommend that these patients receive secondary prophylaxis for up to 1 yr; however, the effectiveness of this approach is not well established. If clinical evidence of carditis is not observed, the prophylaxis can then be discontinued. If valvular disease is detected, the patient should be classified as having had acute rheumatic fever and should continue to receive secondary prophylaxis.

Pediatric Autoimmune Neuropsychiatric Disorders Associated with *Streptococcus pyogenes* (PANDAS)

PANDAS describes a group of neuropsychiatric disorders (particularly obsessive-compulsive disorders, tic disorders, and Tourette syndrome) for which a possible relationship with GAS infections has been suggested (Chapter 22). It has been demonstrated that patients with Sydenham chorea (a manifestation of acute rheumatic fever) frequently have obsessive-compulsive symptoms and that a subset of patients with obsessive-compulsive and tic disorders will have chorea as well as acute exacerbations following GAS infections. Therefore, it has been proposed that this subset of patients with obsessive-compulsive and tic disorders produce autoimmune antibodies in response to a GAS infection that cross react with brain tissue similar to the autoimmune response believed to be responsible for the manifestations of Sydenham chorea. It has also been suggested that secondary prophylaxis that prevents recurrences of Sydenham chorea might also be effective in preventing recurrences of obsessive-compulsive and tic disorders in these patients. Because of the proposed autoimmune mechanism, it has also been suggested that these patients may benefit from immunoregulatory therapy such as plasma exchange or intravenous immunoglobulin therapy. The possibility that PANDAS could represent an extension of the spectrum of acute rheumatic fever is intriguing, but it should be considered only as a yet-unproven hypothesis. Until carefully designed and well-controlled studies have established a causal relationship between PANDAS and GAS infections, routine laboratory testing for GAS to diagnose, long-term antistreptococcal prophylaxis to prevent, or immunoregulatory therapy (e.g., intravenous immunoglobulin, plasma exchange) to treat exacerbations of this disorder are not recommended (Chapter 22).

PROGNOSIS

The prognosis for appropriately treated GAS pharyngitis is excellent, and complete recovery is the rule. When therapy is provided within 9 days of onset, acute rheumatic fever is prevented. There is no evidence that acute poststreptococcal glomerulonephritis can be prevented once pharyngitis or pyoderma with a nephritogenic strain of GAS has occurred. In rare instances, particularly in neonates or in children whose response to infection is compromised, fulminant pneumonia, septicemia, and death may occur despite usually adequate therapy.

PREVENTION

The only specific indication for long-term use of antibiotics to prevent GAS infections is for patients with a history of acute rheumatic fever or rheumatic heart disease. Mass prophylaxis is generally not feasible except to reduce the number of infections during epidemics of impetigo and to control epidemics of pharyngitis in military populations and in schools. Because the ability of antimicrobial agents to prevent GAS infections is limited, a streptococcal vaccine offers the possibility of a more effective approach.

Results of phase 1 and phase 2 studies in adults of a 26-valent plus streptococcal protective antigen (Spa) M protein-based recombinant vaccine demonstrated that the vaccine was well tolerated with no evidence of induction of human tissue-reactive antibodies. The vaccine was also immunogenic and produced opsonizing bactericidal antibodies. Published data suggest that immunization with this candidate vaccine could produce protection against approximately 85% of the isolates causing pharyngitis, 93% of the isolates associated with acute rheumatic fever, and 88% of the isolates associated with invasive GAS disease in the USA and could have significant impact on the overall burden of GAS disease. However, matching a multivalent M type specific vaccine to current circulating strains is likely to be less complete in Asia and other developing areas of the world. In addition, emergence of new *emm* types and the possibility that nonvaccine serotypes or genotypes of clinical importance may replace those contained in the vaccine is a concern. Other current candidate GAS vaccines such as a C5a peptidase, cysteine protease, fibronectin-binding protein, and group A carbohydrate vaccine are based on common protective antigens and would result in increased strain coverage and reduced concerns for serotype replacement.

BIBLIOGRAPHY

Please visit the Nelson Textbook of Pediatrics *website at www.expertconsult.com for the complete bibliography.*

176.1 Rheumatic Fever

Michael A. Gerber

ETIOLOGY

There is considerable evidence to support the link between GAS upper pharyngitis tract infections and acute rheumatic fever and rheumatic heart disease. As many as 66% of the patients with an acute episode of rheumatic fever have a history of an upper respiratory tract infection several weeks before, and the peak age and seasonal incidence of acute rheumatic fever closely parallel those of GAS infections. Patients with acute rheumatic fever almost always have serologic evidence of a recent GAS infection. Their antibody titers are usually considerably higher than those seen in patients with GAS infections without acute rheumatic fever. Outbreaks of GAS pharyngitis in closed communities, such as boarding schools or military bases, may be followed by outbreaks of acute rheumatic fever. Antimicrobial therapy that eliminates GAS from the pharynx also prevents initial episodes of acute rheumatic fever, and long-term, continuous prophylaxis that prevents GAS pharyngitis also prevents recurrences of acute rheumatic fever.

Not all of the serotypes of GAS can cause rheumatic fever. When some strains (M type 4) were present in a very susceptible rheumatic population, no recurrences of rheumatic fever occurred. In contrast, episodes of pharyngitis with other serotypes prevalent in the same population were associated with frequent recurrences. The concept of rheumatogenicity is further supported by the observation that although serotypes of GAS frequently associated with skin infection are often isolated from the upper respiratory tract, they rarely cause recurrences of rheumatic fever in individuals with a previous history of rheumatic fever. In addition, certain serotypes of GAS (M types 1, 3, 5, 6, 18, 24) are more frequently isolated from patients with acute rheumatic fever than are other serotypes.

EPIDEMIOLOGY

The incidence of acute rheumatic fever in some developing countries exceeds 50 per 100,000 children. Worldwide, rheumatic heart disease remains the most common form of acquired heart disease in all age groups, accounting for as much as 50% of all cardiovascular disease and as much as 50% of all cardiac admissions in many developing countries. Striking differences are evident in the incidence of acute rheumatic fever and rheumatic heart disease among different ethnic groups within the same country; many, but not all, of these differences appear to be related to differences in socioeconomic status.

In the USA, at the beginning of the 20th century, acute rheumatic fever was a leading cause of death among children and adolescents, with annual incidence rates of 100-200/100,000 population. In addition, rheumatic heart disease was a leading cause of heart disease among adults <40 yr of age. At that time, as many as ¼ of the hospital beds in the USA were occupied by patients with acute rheumatic fever or its complications. By the 1940s, the annual incidence of acute rheumatic fever had decreased to 50/100,000, and over the next 4 decades, the decline in incidence accelerated rapidly. By the early 1980s, the annual incidence in some areas of the USA was as low as 0.5/100,000 population. This sharp decline in the incidence of acute rheumatic fever has been observed in other industrialized countries as well.

The explanation for this dramatic decline in the incidence of acute rheumatic fever and rheumatic heart disease in the USA and other industrialized countries is not clear. Historically, acute rheumatic fever has been associated with poverty, particularly in urban areas. Much of the decline in the incidence of acute rheumatic fever in industrialized countries during the preantibiotic era can probably be attributed to improvements in living conditions. A number of studies have suggested that, of the various manifestations of poverty, crowding, which contributes to the spread of GAS infections, is the one most closely associated with the incidence of acute rheumatic fever. The decline in incidence of acute rheumatic fever in industrialized countries over the past 4 decades has also been attributable in large measure to the greater availability of medical care and to the widespread use of antibiotics. Antibiotic therapy of GAS pharyngitis has been important in preventing initial attacks and, particularly, recurrences of the disease. In addition, the decline can be attributed, at least in part, to a shift in the prevalent strains of GAS from rheumatogenic to nonrheumatogenic strains.

A dramatic outbreak of acute rheumatic fever in the Salt Lake City area began in early 1985, and 198 cases were reported by the end of 1989. Other outbreaks were reported between 1984 and 1988 in Columbus and Akron, OH; Pittsburgh, PA; Nashville and Memphis, TN; New York, NY; Kansas City, MO; Dallas, TX; and among recruits at the San Diego Naval Training

Center in California and at the Fort Leonard Wood Army Training Base in Missouri. Evidence suggests that this resurgence of acute rheumatic fever was focal and not nationwide.

Certain rheumatogenic serotypes (types 1, 3, 5, 6, and 18) that were isolated infrequently during the 1970s and early 1980s dramatically reappeared during these focal outbreaks. The appearance of these rheumatogenic strains in selected communities was probably a major factor in these outbreaks of acute rheumatic fever. Another property of GAS that has been associated with rheumatogenicity is the formation of highly mucoid colonies. Mucoid strains of GAS had only rarely been isolated from throat cultures in recent years. However, during these focal outbreaks of acute rheumatic fever, mucoid strains of GAS were commonly isolated from patients, family members, and members of the surrounding community.

In addition to the specific characteristics of the infecting GAS, the risk of a particular person developing acute rheumatic fever is also dependent on various host factors. The incidence of both initial attacks and recurrences of acute rheumatic fever peaks in children 5-15 yr of age, the age of greatest risk for GAS pharyngitis. Patients who have had one attack of acute rheumatic fever tend to have recurrences, and the clinical features of the recurrences tend to mimic those of the initial attack. In addition, there appears to be a genetic predisposition to acute rheumatic fever. Studies in twins have shown a higher concordance rate of acute rheumatic fever in monozygotic than in dizygotic twin pairs. Some investigators have also demonstrated an association between the presence of both specific human leukocyte antigen (HLA) markers and a specific B-cell alloantigen (D8/17) and susceptibility to acute rheumatic fever; others have been unable to confirm these associations.

PATHOGENESIS

The pathogenic link between a GAS infection of the upper respiratory tract and an attack of acute rheumatic fever, characterized by organ and tissue involvement far removed from the pharynx, is still not clear. One of the major obstacles to understanding the pathogenesis of acute rheumatic fever and rheumatic heart disease has been the inability to establish an animal model. Several theories of the pathogenesis of acute rheumatic fever and rheumatic heart disease have been proposed, but only 2 are seriously considered: the cytotoxicity theory and the immunologic theory.

The cytotoxicity theory suggests that a GAS toxin may be involved in the pathogenesis of acute rheumatic fever and rheumatic heart disease. GAS produces several enzymes that are cytotoxic for mammalian cardiac cells, such as streptolysin O, which has a direct cytotoxic effect on mammalian cells in tissue culture. Most of the proponents of the cytotoxicity theory have focused on this enzyme. However, one of the major problems with the cytotoxicity hypothesis is its inability to explain the latent period between GAS pharyngitis and the onset of acute rheumatic fever.

An immune-mediated pathogenesis for acute rheumatic fever and rheumatic heart disease has been suggested by the clinical similarity of acute rheumatic fever to other illnesses produced by immunopathogenic processes and by the latent period between the GAS infection and acute rheumatic fever. The antigenicity of a large variety of GAS products and constituents and the immunologic cross reactivity between GAS components and mammalian tissues also lends support to this hypothesis. Common antigenic determinants are shared between certain components of GAS (M protein, protoplast membrane, cell wall group A carbohydrate, capsular hyaluronate) and specific mammalian tissues (e.g., heart, brain, joint). For example, certain M proteins (M1, M5, M6, and M19) share epitopes with human tropomyosin and myosin. Additionally, the involvement of GAS superantigens such as pyrogenic exotoxins in the pathogenesis of acute rheumatic fever has been proposed.

Table 176-2 GUIDELINES FOR THE DIAGNOSIS OF INITIAL ATTACK OF RHEUMATIC FEVER (JONES CRITERIA, UPDATED 1992)

MAJOR MANIFESTATIONS*	MINOR MANIFESTATIONS	SUPPORTING EVIDENCE OF ANTECEDENT GROUP A STREPTOCOCCAL INFECTION
Carditis Polyarthritis Erythema marginatum Subcutaneous nodules Chorea	**Clinical features:** Arthralgia Fever	Positive throat culture or rapid streptococcal antigen test Elevated or increasing streptococcal antibody titer
	Laboratory features: Elevated acute phase reactants: Erythrocyte sedimentation rate C-reactive protein Prolonged PR interval	

*The presence of 2 major or of 1 major and 2 minor manifestations indicates a high probability of acute rheumatic fever if supported by evidence of preceding group A streptococcal infection.
From Jones criteria, updated 1992. *JAMA* 268:2069–2073, 1992. Copyright American Medical Association.

CLINICAL MANIFESTATIONS AND DIAGNOSIS

Because no clinical or laboratory finding is pathognomonic for acute rheumatic fever, T. Duckett Jones in 1944 proposed guidelines to aid in diagnosis and to limit overdiagnosis. The **Jones criteria,** as revised in 1992 by the American Heart Association (AHA) (Table 176-2) are intended only for the diagnosis of the initial attack of acute rheumatic fever and not for recurrences. There are **5 major** and **4 minor criteria** and an absolute requirement for evidence (microbiologic or serologic) of recent GAS infection. The diagnosis of acute rheumatic fever can be established by the Jones criteria when a patient fulfills 2 major criteria or 1 major and 2 minor criteria and meets the absolute requirement. Even with strict application of the Jones criteria, overdiagnosis as well as underdiagnosis of acute rheumatic fever may occur. There are 3 circumstances in which the diagnosis of acute rheumatic fever can be made without strict adherence to the Jones criteria. Chorea may occur as the only manifestation of acute rheumatic fever. Similarly, indolent carditis may be the only manifestation in patients who 1st come to medical attention months after the onset of acute rheumatic fever. Finally, although most patients with recurrences of acute rheumatic fever fulfill the Jones criteria, some may not.

Major Manifestations

There are 5 major criteria.

MIGRATORY POLYARTHRITIS Arthritis occurs in about 75% of patients with acute rheumatic fever and typically involves larger joints, particularly the knees, ankles, wrists, and elbows. Involvement of the spine, small joints of the hands and feet, or hips is uncommon. Rheumatic joints are generally hot, red, swollen, and exquisitely tender; even the friction of bedclothes is uncomfortable. The pain can precede and can appear to be disproportionate to the other findings. The joint involvement is characteristically migratory in nature; a severely inflamed joint can become normal within 1-3 days without treatment, as 1 or more other large joints become involved. Severe arthritis can persist for several weeks in untreated patients. Monoarticular arthritis is unusual unless anti-inflammatory therapy is initiated prematurely, aborting the progression of the migratory polyarthritis. If a child with fever and arthritis is suspected of having acute rheumatic fever, it frequently is useful to withhold salicylates and observe for migratory progression. A dramatic response to even small doses of salicylates is another characteristic feature of the arthritis, and the absence of such a response should suggest an alternative diagnosis.

Rheumatic arthritis is typically not deforming. Synovial fluid in acute rheumatic fever usually has 10,000-100,000 white blood cells/mm^3 with a predominance of neutrophils, a protein level of about 4 g/dL, a normal glucose level, and forms a good mucin clot. Frequently, arthritis is the earliest manifestation of acute rheumatic fever and may correlate temporally with peak anti-streptococcal antibody titers. *There is often an inverse relationship between the severity of arthritis and the severity of cardiac involvement.*

CARDITIS Carditis and resultant chronic rheumatic heart disease are the most serious manifestations of acute rheumatic fever and account for essentially all of the associated morbidity and mortality. Rheumatic carditis is characterized by pancarditis, with active inflammation of myocardium, pericardium, and endocardium (Chapter 432). Cardiac involvement during acute rheumatic fever varies in severity from fulminant, potentially fatal exudative pancarditis to mild, transient cardiac involvement. Endocarditis (valvulitis) is a universal finding in rheumatic carditis, whereas the presence of pericarditis or myocarditis is variable. Myocarditis and/or pericarditis without evidence of endocarditis is rarely due to rheumatic heart disease. Most cases consist of either isolated mitral valvular disease or combined aortic and mitral valvular disease. Isolated aortic or right-sided valvular involvement is uncommon. Serious and long-term illness is related entirely to valvular heart disease as a consequence of a single attack or recurrent attacks of acute rheumatic fever. Valvular insufficiency is characteristic of both acute and convalescent stages of acute rheumatic fever, whereas valvular stenosis usually appears several years or even decades after the acute illness. However, in developing countries where acute rheumatic fever often occurs at a younger age, mitral stenosis and aortic stenosis may develop sooner after acute rheumatic fever than in developed countries and can occur in young children.

Acute rheumatic carditis usually presents as tachycardia and cardiac murmurs, with or without evidence of myocardial or pericardial involvement. Moderate to severe rheumatic carditis can result in cardiomegaly and congestive heart failure with hepatomegaly and peripheral and pulmonary edema. Echocardiographic findings include pericardial effusion, decreased ventricular contractility, and aortic and/or mitral regurgitation. Mitral regurgitation is characterized by a high-pitched apical holosystolic murmur radiating to the axilla. In patients with significant mitral regurgitation, this may be associated with an apical mid-diastolic murmur of relative mitral stenosis. Aortic insufficiency is characterized by a high-pitched decrescendo diastolic murmur at the upper left sternal border.

Clinically, rheumatic carditis is almost always associated with a murmur of valvulitis. Several investigators and advisory groups have suggested that subclinical valvular regurgitation be accepted as evidence of rheumatic carditis. Subclinical valvular regurgitation is echocardiographically identified pathological mitral or aortic regurgitation inaudible to skilled auscultation. Although controversial, subclinical valvular regurgitation is not currently accepted as either a major or minor Jones criterion by the AHA in the guidelines for the diagnosis of acute rheumatic fever (Chapter 432).

Carditis occurs in about 50-60% of all cases of acute rheumatic fever. Recurrent attacks of acute rheumatic fever in patients who had carditis with the initial attack are associated with high rates of carditis. The major consequence of acute rheumatic carditis is chronic, progressive valvular disease, particularly valvular stenosis, which can require valve replacement.

CHOREA Sydenham chorea occurs in about 10-15% of patients with acute rheumatic fever and usually presents as an isolated, frequently subtle, neurologic behavior disorder. Emotional lability, incoordination, poor school performance, uncontrollable movements, and facial grimacing, exacerbated by stress and disappearing with sleep, are characteristic. Chorea occasionally is unilateral. The latent period from acute GAS infection to chorea is usually longer than for arthritis or carditis and can be months. Onset can be insidious, with symptoms being present for several months before recognition. Clinical maneuvers to elicit features of chorea include (1) demonstration of **milkmaid's grip** (irregular contractions of the muscles of the hands while squeezing the examiner's fingers), (2) spooning and pronation of the hands when the patient's arms are extended, (3) wormian darting movements of the tongue upon protrusion, and (4) examination of handwriting to evaluate fine motor movements. Diagnosis is based on clinical findings with supportive evidence of GAS antibodies. However, in patients with a long latent period from the inciting streptococcal infection, antibody levels may have declined to normal. Although the acute illness is distressing, chorea rarely, if ever, leads to permanent neurologic sequelae.

ERYTHEMA MARGINATUM Erythema marginatum is a rare (<3% of patients with acute rheumatic fever) but characteristic rash of acute rheumatic fever. It consists of erythematous, serpiginous, macular lesions with pale centers that are not pruritic (Fig. 176-2). It occurs primarily on the trunk and extremities, but not on the face, and it can be accentuated by warming the skin.

SUBCUTANEOUS NODULES Subcutaneous nodules are a rare (≤1% of patients with acute rheumatic fever) finding and consist of firm nodules approximately 1 cm in diameter along the extensor surfaces of tendons near bony prominences. There is a correlation between the presence of these nodules and significant rheumatic heart disease.

Minor Manifestations

The 2 clinical minor manifestations are arthralgia (in the absence of polyarthritis as a major criterion) and fever (typically temperature ≥102°F and occurring early in the course of illness). The 2 laboratory minor manifestations are elevated acute-phase reactants (e.g., C-reactive protein, erythrocyte sedimentation rate) and prolonged PR interval on electrocardiogram (1st degree heart block). However, a prolonged P-R interval alone does not constitute evidence of carditis or predict long-term cardiac sequelae.

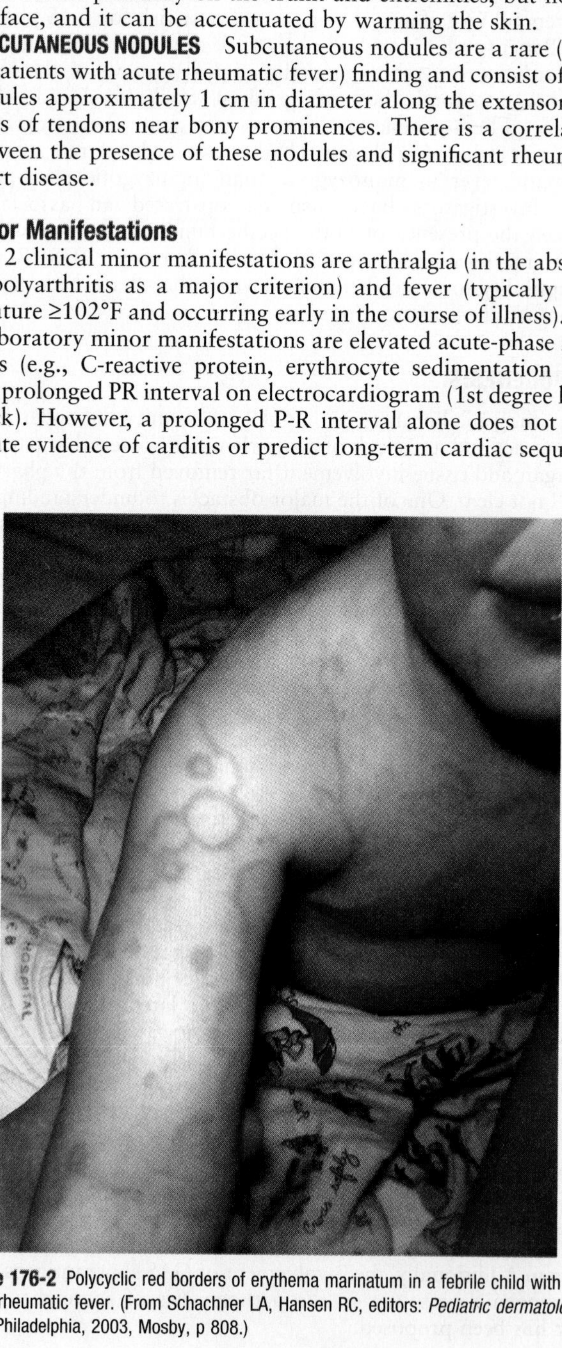

Figure 176-2 Polycyclic red borders of erythema marinatum in a febrile child with acute rheumatic fever. (From Schachner LA, Hansen RC, editors: *Pediatric dermatology,* ed 3, Philadelphia, 2003, Mosby, p 808.)

Recent Group A Streptococcus Infection

An absolute requirement for the diagnosis of acute rheumatic fever is supporting evidence of a recent GAS infection. Acute rheumatic fever typically develops 2-4 wk after an acute episode of GAS pharyngitis at a time when clinical findings of pharyngitis are no longer present and when only 10-20% of the throat culture or rapid streptococcal antigen test results are positive. One third of patients with acute rheumatic fever have no history of an antecedent pharyngitis. Therefore, evidence of an antecedent GAS infection is usually based on elevated or increasing serum antistreptococcal antibody titers. A slide agglutination test (Streptozyme) has been introduced, and it is purported to detect antibodies against 5 different GAS antigens. Although this test is rapid, relatively simple to perform, and widely available, it is less standardized and less reproducible than other tests and should not be used as a diagnostic test for evidence of an antecedent GAS infection. If only a single antibody is measured (usually antistreptolysin O), only 80-85% of patients with acute rheumatic fever have an elevated titer; however, 95-100% have an elevation if 3 different antibodies (antistreptolysin O, anti-DNase B, antihyaluronidase) are measured. Therefore, when acute rheumatic fever is suspected clinically, multiple antibody tests should be performed. Except for patients with chorea, clinical findings of acute rheumatic fever generally coincide with peak antistreptococcal antibody responses. Most patients with chorea have elevation of antibodies to 1 or more GAS antigens. However, in patients in whom there is a long latent period from the inciting GAS infection, antibody levels may have declined to within the normal range. The diagnosis of acute rheumatic fever should not be made in patients with elevated or increasing streptococcal antibody titers who do not fulfill the Jones criteria because such titer changes may be coincidental. This is most often true in younger, school-aged children, many of whom have GAS pyoderma in the summer or unrelated GAS pharyngitis during the winter and spring months.

Differential Diagnosis

The differential diagnoses of rheumatic fever include many infectious as well as noninfectious illnesses (Table 176-3). When children present with arthritis, a collagen vascular disease must be considered. Rheumatoid arthritis in particular must be distinguished from acute rheumatic fever. Children with rheumatoid arthritis tend to be younger and usually have less joint pain relative to their other clinical findings than those with acute rheumatic fever. Spiking fevers, lymphadenopathy, and splenomegaly are more suggestive of rheumatoid arthritis than acute rheumatic fever. The response to salicylate therapy is also much less dramatic with rheumatoid arthritis than with acute rheumatic fever. Systemic lupus erythematosus can usually be distinguished from acute rheumatic fever on the basis of the presence of antinuclear antibodies with systemic lupus erythematosus. Other causes of arthritis such as gonococcal arthritis, malignancies, serum sickness, Lyme disease, sickle cell disease, and reactive arthritis related to gastrointestinal infections (e.g., *Shigella, Salmonella, Yersinia*) should also be considered.

When carditis is the sole major manifestation of suspected acute rheumatic fever, viral myocarditis, viral pericarditis, Kawasaki disease, and infective endocarditis should also be considered. Patients with infective endocarditis may present with both joint and cardiac manifestations. These patients can usually be distinguished from patients with acute rheumatic fever by blood cultures and the presence of associated findings (e.g., hematuria, splenomegaly, splinter hemorrhages). When chorea is the sole major manifestation of suspected acute rheumatic fever, Huntington chorea, Wilson disease, systemic lupus erythematosus, and various encephalitides should also be considered. These other diseases are usually identified by the history, laboratory studies, and clinical findings.

Table 176-3 DIFFERENTIAL DIAGNOSIS OF ACUTE RHEUMATIC FEVER

ARTHRITIS	CARDITIS	CHOREA
Rheumatoid arthritis	Viral myocarditis	Huntington chorea
Reactive arthritis (e.g., *Shigella, Salmonella, Yersinia*)	Viral pericarditis	Wilson disease
Serum sickness	Infective endocarditis	Systemic lupus erythematosus
Sickle cell disease	Kawasaki disease	Cerebral palsy
Malignancy	Congenital heart disease	Tics
Systemic lupus erythematosus	Mitral valve prolapse	Hyperactivity
Lyme disease (*Borrelia burgdorferi*)	Innocent murmurs	
Gonococcal infection (*Neisseria gonorrhoeae*)		

TREATMENT

All patients with acute rheumatic fever should be placed on bed rest and monitored closely for evidence of carditis. They can be allowed to ambulate as soon as the signs of acute inflammation have subsided. However, patients with carditis require longer periods of bed rest.

Antibiotic Therapy

Once the diagnosis of acute rheumatic fever has been established and regardless of the throat culture results, the patient should receive 10 days of orally administered penicillin or erythromycin or a single intramuscular injection of benzathine penicillin to eradicate GAS from the upper respiratory tract. After this initial course of antibiotic therapy, the patient should be started on long-term antibiotic prophylaxis.

Anti-inflammatory Therapy

Anti-inflammatory agents (e.g., salicylates, corticosteroids) should be withheld if arthralgia or atypical arthritis is the only clinical manifestation of presumed acute rheumatic fever. Premature treatment with one of these agents may interfere with the development of the characteristic migratory polyarthritis and thus obscure the diagnosis of acute rheumatic fever. Agents such as acetaminophen can be used to control pain and fever while the patient is being observed for more definite signs of acute rheumatic fever or for evidence of another disease.

Patients with typical migratory polyarthritis and those with carditis without cardiomegaly or congestive heart failure should be treated with oral salicylates. The usual dose of aspirin is 100 mg/kg/day in 4 divided doses PO for 3-5 days, followed by 75 mg/kg/day in 4 divided doses PO for 4 wk. Determination of the serum salicylate level is not necessary unless the arthritis does not respond or signs of salicylate toxicity (tinnitus, hyperventilation) develop. There is no evidence that nonsteroidal antiinflammatory agents are any more effective than salicylates.

Patients with carditis and cardiomegaly or congestive heart failure should receive corticosteroids. The usual dose of prednisone is 2 mg/kg/day in 4 divided doses for 2-3 wk followed by a tapering of the dose that reduces the dose by 5 mg/24 hr every 2-3 days. At the beginning of the tapering of the prednisone dose, aspirin should be started at 75 mg/kg/day in 4 divided doses for 6 wk. Supportive therapies for patients with moderate to severe carditis include digoxin, fluid and salt restriction, diuretics, and oxygen. The cardiac toxicity of digoxin is enhanced with myocarditis.

Termination of the antiinflammatory therapy may be followed by the reappearance of clinical manifestations or of laboratory abnormalities. These "rebounds" are best left untreated unless the clinical manifestations are severe; salicylates or steroids should be reinstated in such cases.

Sydenham Chorea

Because chorea often occurs as an isolated manifestation after the resolution of the acute phase of the disease, anti-inflammatory agents are usually not indicated. Sedatives may be helpful early in the course of chorea; phenobarbital (16-32 mg every 6-8 hr PO) is the drug of choice. If phenobarbital is ineffective, then haloperidol (0.01-0.03 mg/kg/24 hr divided bid PO) or chlorpromazine (0.5 mg/kg every 4-6 hr PO) should be initiated.

COMPLICATIONS

The arthritis and chorea of acute rheumatic fever resolve completely without sequelae. Therefore, the long-term sequelae of rheumatic fever are usually limited to the heart (Chapter 432).

The AHA has published updated recommendations regarding the use of prophylactic antibiotics to prevent infective endocarditis (Chapter 431). The AHA recommendations do not suggest routine prophylaxis any longer for patients with rheumatic heart disease. However, the maintenance of optimal oral health care remains an important component of an overall health care program. For the relatively few patients with rheumatic heart disease in whom IE prophylaxis remains recommended, such as those with prosthetic valves or prosthetic material used in valve repair, the current AHA recommendations should be followed (Chapter 431). These recommendations advise using an agent other than a penicillin to prevent IE in those receiving penicillin prophylaxis for rheumatic fever because oral α-hemolytic streptococci are likely to have developed resistance to penicillin.

PROGNOSIS

The prognosis for patients with acute rheumatic fever depends on the clinical manifestations present at the time of the initial episode, the severity of the initial episode, and the presence of recurrences. Approximately 70% of patients with carditis during the initial episode of acute rheumatic fever recover with no residual heart disease; the more severe the initial cardiac involvement, the greater the risk is for residual heart disease. Patients without carditis during the initial episode are unlikely to have carditis with recurrences. In contrast, patients with carditis during the initial episode are likely to have carditis with recurrences, and the risk for permanent heart damage increases with each recurrence. Patients who have had acute rheumatic fever are susceptible to recurrent attacks following reinfection of the upper respiratory tract with GAS. Therefore, these patients require long-term continuous chemoprophylaxis.

Before antibiotic prophylaxis was available, 75% of patients who had an initial episode of acute rheumatic fever had one or more recurrences during their lifetimes. These recurrences were a major source of morbidity and mortality. The risk of recurrence is highest immediately after the initial episode and decreases with time.

Approximately 20% of patients who present with "pure" chorea who are not given secondary prophylaxis develop rheumatic heart disease within 20 yr. Therefore, patients with chorea, even in the absence of other manifestations of rheumatic fever, require long-term antibiotic prophylaxis.

PREVENTION

Prevention of both initial and recurrent episodes of acute rheumatic fever depends on controlling GAS infections of the upper respiratory tract. Prevention of initial attacks (primary prevention) depends on identification and eradication of the GAS that produces episodes of acute pharyngitis. Individuals who have already suffered an attack of acute rheumatic fever are particularly susceptible to recurrences of rheumatic fever with any subsequent GAS upper respiratory tract infection, whether or not they are symptomatic. Therefore, these patients should receive continuous antibiotic prophylaxis to prevent recurrences (secondary prevention).

Primary Prevention

Appropriate antibiotic therapy instituted before the 9th day of symptoms of acute GAS pharyngitis is highly effective in preventing 1st attacks of acute rheumatic fever from that episode. However, about 30% of patients with acute rheumatic fever do not recall a preceding episode of pharyngitis.

Secondary Prevention

Secondary prevention is directed at preventing acute GAS pharyngitis in patients at substantial risk of recurrent acute rheumatic fever. Secondary prevention requires continuous antibiotic prophylaxis, which should begin as soon as the diagnosis of acute rheumatic fever has been made and immediately after a full course of antibiotic therapy has been completed. Because patients who have had carditis with their initial episode of acute rheumatic fever are at a relatively high risk for having carditis with recurrences and for sustaining additional cardiac damage, they should receive long-term antibiotic prophylaxis well into adulthood and perhaps for life.

Patients who did not have carditis with their initial episode of acute rheumatic fever have a relatively low risk for carditis with recurrences. Antibiotic prophylaxis should continue in these patients until the patient reaches 21 yr of age or until 5 yr have elapsed since the last rheumatic fever attack, whichever is longer. The decision to discontinue prophylactic antibiotics should be made only after careful consideration of potential risks and benefits and of epidemiologic factors such as the risk for exposure to GAS infections.

The regimen of choice for secondary prevention is a single intramuscular injection of benzathine penicillin G (600,000 IU for children ≤60 lb and 1.2 million IU for those >60 lb) every 4 wk (Table 176-4). In certain high-risk patients, and in certain areas of the world where the incidence of rheumatic fever is particularly high, use of benzathine penicillin G every 3 wk may be necessary because levels of penicillin may decrease to marginally effective amounts after 3 wk. In the USA, the administration of benzathine penicillin G every 3 wk is recommended only for those who have recurrent acute rheumatic fever despite adherence to a 4-wk regimen. In compliant patients, continuous oral antimicrobial prophylaxis can be used. Penicillin V given twice daily and sulfadiazine given once daily are equally effective when used in such patients. For the exceptional patient who is allergic to both penicillin and sulfonamides, a macrolide (erythromycin or

Table 176-4 CHEMOPROPHYLAXIS FOR RECURRENCES OF ACUTE RHEUMATIC FEVER

DRUG	DOSE	ROUTE
Penicillin G benzathine	600,000 U for children, ≤60 lb 1.2 million U for children >60 lb, every 4 wk*	Intramuscular
OR		
Penicillin V	250 mg, twice a day	Oral
OR		
Sulfadiazine or sulfisoxazole	0.5 g, once a day for patients ≤60 lb	Oral
	1.0 g, once a day for patients >60 lb	
FOR PEOPLE WHO ARE ALLERGIC TO PENICILLIN AND SULFONAMIDE DRUGS		
Macrolide or azalide	Variable	Oral

*In high-risk situations, administration every 3 weeks is recommended.
From Gerber MA, Baltimore RS, Eaton CB, et al: Prevention of rheumatic fever and diagnosis and treatment of acute streptococcal pharyngitis: a scientific statement from the American Heart Association Rheumatic Fever, Endocarditis, and Kawasaki Disease Committee of the Council on Cardiovascular Disease in the Young, *Circulation* 119:1541–1551, 2009.

Table 176-5 DURATION OF PROPHYLAXIS FOR PEOPLE WHO HAVE HAD ACUTE RHEUMATIC FEVER: RECOMMENDATIONS OF THE AMERICAN HEART ASSOCIATION

CATEGORY	DURATION
Rheumatic fever without carditis	5 yr or until 21 yr of age, whichever is longer
Rheumatic fever with carditis but without residual heart disease (no valvular disease*)	10 yr or until 21 yr of age, whichever is longer
Rheumatic fever with carditis and residual heart disease (persistent valvular disease*)	10 yr or until 40 yr of age, whichever is longer, sometimes lifelong prophylaxis

*Clinical or echocardiographic evidence.
From Gerber MA, Baltimore RS, Eaton CB, et al: Prevention of rheumatic fever and diagnosis and treatment of acute streptococcal pharyngitis: a scientific statement from the American Heart Association Rheumatic Fever, Endocarditis, and Kawasaki Disease Committee of the Council on Cardiovascular Disease in the Young, *Circulation* 119:1541–1551, 2009.

clarithromycin) or azalide (azithromycin) may be used. The duration of secondary prophylaxis is noted in Table 176-5.

BIBLIOGRAPHY

Please visit the Nelson Textbook of Pediatrics *website at www.expertconsult.com for the complete bibliography.*

Chapter 177
Group B Streptococcus

Catherine S. Lachenauer and Michael R. Wessels

Group B streptococcus (GBS), or *Streptococcus agalactiae,* is a major cause of neonatal bacterial sepsis in the USA. While advances in prevention strategies have led to a decline in the incidence of neonatal disease, GBS remains a major pathogen for neonates, pregnant women, and nonpregnant adults.

ETIOLOGY

Group B streptococci are facultative anaerobic gram-positive cocci that form chains or diplococci in broth and small gray-white colonies on solid medium. GBS is definitively identified by demonstration of the Lancefield group B carbohydrate antigen, such as with latex agglutination techniques widely used in clinical laboratories. Presumptive identification can be established on the basis of a narrow zone of β-hemolysis on blood agar, resistance to bacitracin and trimethoprim-sulfamethoxazole, lack of hydrolysis of bile esculin, and elaboration of CAMP factor (named for the discoverers, Christie, Atkins, and Munch-Petersen), an extracellular protein that, in the presence of the β toxin of *Staphylococcus aureus,* produces a zone of enhanced hemolysis on sheep's blood agar. Individual GBS strains are serologically classified according to the presence of one of the structurally distinct capsular polysaccharides, which are important virulence factors and stimulators of antibody-associated immunity. Ten GBS capsular types have been identified: types Ia, Ib, II, III, IV, V, VI, VII, VIII, and IX.

EPIDEMIOLOGY

GBS emerged as a prominent neonatal pathogen in the late 1960s. For the next 2 decades, the incidence of neonatal GBS disease remained fairly constant, affecting 1.0-5.4/1,000 liveborn infants in the USA. Two patterns of disease were seen: **early-onset disease,** which presents at <7 days of age, and **late-onset disease,** which presents at 7 days of age or later. In the 1990s, widespread implementation of maternal chemoprophylaxis led to a striking 65%

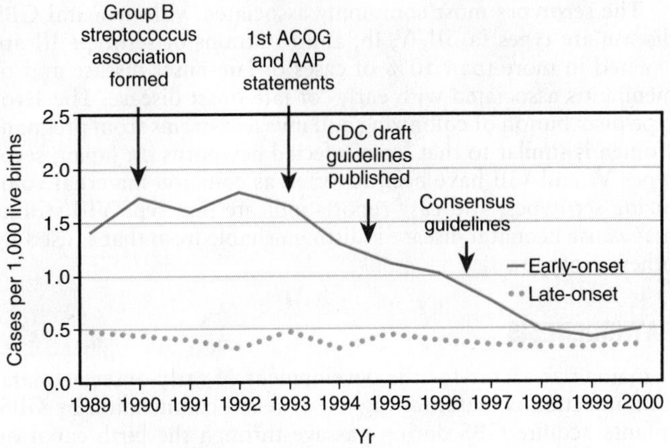

Figure 177-1 Incidence of early-onset and late-onset invasive group B streptococcus disease in three active surveillance areas (California, Georgia, and Tennessee), 1989 through 2000, and activities for the prevention of group B streptococcus disease. Arrows designate the dates when prevention activities occurred. ACOG, American College of Obstetricians and Gynecologists; AAP, American Academy of Pediatrics; CDC, Centers for Disease Control and Prevention. (Adapted from Centers for Disease Control and Prevention: Early-onset group B streptococcal disease—United States, 1998-1999, *MMWR* 49:793–796, 2000; Schrag SJ, Zywicki S, Farley MM, et al: Group B streptococcal disease in the era of intrapartum antibiotic prophylaxis, *N Engl J Med* 342:15–20, 2000.)

decrease in the incidence of early-onset neonatal GBS disease in the USA, from 1.7/1,000 live births to 0.6/1,000 live births, whereas the incidence of late-onset disease remained essentially stable at approximately 0.4/1,000 (Fig. 177-1). Release of revised guidelines in 2002 coincided with a further reduction in the incidence of early-onset neonatal disease. In other developed countries, rates of neonatal GBS disease are similar to those in the USA prior to use of GBS chemoprophylaxis. In the developing world, GBS is not a major cause of neonatal sepsis, even though the prevalence of maternal vaginal colonization with GBS (a major risk factor for neonatal disease) among women from developing countries is similar to that reported among women living in the USA. The incidence of neonatal GBS disease is higher in premature and low birthweight infants, although most cases occur in full-term infants.

Colonization by GBS in healthy adults is common. Vaginal or rectal colonization occurs in up to approximately 30% of pregnant women and is the usual source for GBS transmission to newborn infants. In the absence of maternal chemoprophylaxis, approximately 50% of infants born to colonized women acquire GBS colonization, and 1-2% of these infants develop invasive disease. Heavy maternal colonization increases the risk for infant colonization and development of early-onset disease. Additional risk factors for early-onset disease include prolonged rupture of membranes, intrapartum fever, prematurity, maternal bacteriuria during pregnancy, or previous delivery of an infant who developed GBS disease. Risk factors for late-onset disease are less well defined. Whereas late-onset disease may follow vertical transmission, horizontal acquisition from nursery or other community sources has also been described.

GBS is also an important cause of invasive disease in adults. GBS may cause urinary tract infections, bacteremia, endometritis, chorioamnionitis, and wound infection in pregnant and parturient women. In nonpregnant adults, especially those with underlying medical conditions such as diabetes mellitus, cirrhosis, or malignancy, GBS may cause serious infections such as bacteremia, skin and soft tissue infections, endocarditis, pneumonia, and meningitis. In the era of maternal chemoprophylaxis, most invasive GBS infections occur in nonpregnant adults. Unlike neonatal disease, the incidence of invasive GBS disease in adults has increased substantially, doubling between 1990 and 2007.

The serotypes most commonly associated with neonatal GBS disease are types Ia, III, V, Ib, and II. Strains of serotype III are isolated in more than 50% of cases of late-onset disease and of meningitis associated with early- or late-onset disease. The serotype distribution of colonizing and invasive strains from pregnant women is similar to that from infected newborns. In Japan, serotypes VI and VIII have been reported as common maternal colonizing serotypes, and case reports indicate that type VIII strains may cause neonatal disease indistinguishable from that caused by other serotypes.

PATHOGENESIS

A major risk factor for the development of early-onset neonatal GBS infection is maternal vaginal or rectal colonization by GBS. Infants acquire GBS during passage through the birth canal or, in some cases, via ascending infection. Fetal aspiration of infected amniotic fluid may occur. The incidence of early-onset GBS infection increases with the length of rupture of membranes. Infection may also occur through seemingly intact membranes. In cases of late-onset infection, GBS may be vertically transmitted or acquired later from maternal or nonmaternal sources.

Several bacterial factors are implicated in the pathophysiology of invasive GBS disease. Foremost among these is the type-specific capsular polysaccharide. Strains that are associated with invasive disease in humans elaborate more capsular polysaccharide than do colonizing isolates. All GBS capsular polysaccharides are high molecular weight polymers and contain a short side chain terminating in *N*-acetylneuraminic acid (sialic acid). Studies in type III GBS show that the sialic acid component of the capsular polysaccharide prevents activation of the alternative complement pathway in the absence of type-specific antibody. Thus, the capsular polysaccharide appears to exert a virulence effect by protecting the organism from opsonophagocytosis in the nonimmune host. In addition, type-specific virulence attributes are suggested by the fact that type III strains are implicated in most cases of late-onset neonatal GBS disease and meningitis. Type III strains are taken up by brain endothelial cells more efficiently in vitro than are strains of other serotypes, although studies using acapsular mutant strains demonstrate that it is not the capsule itself that facilitates cellular invasion. Other putative GBS virulence factors include GBS surface proteins, which may play a role in adhesion to host cells; C5a peptidase, which is postulated to inhibit the recruitment of polymorphonuclear cells into sites of infection; β-hemolysin, which has been associated with cell injury in vitro studies; and hyaluronidase, which has been postulated to act as a spreading factor in host tissues.

In a classic study, among pregnant women colonized with type III GBS, those who gave birth to healthy infants had higher levels of capsular polysaccharide-specific antibody than those who gave birth to infants who developed invasive disease. In addition, there is a high correlation of antibody to GBS type III in mother-infant paired sera. These observations indicate that transplacental transfer of maternal antibody is critically involved in neonatal immunity to GBS. Optimal immunity to GBS also requires an intact complement system. The classic complement pathway is an important component of GBS immunity in the absence of specific antibody; antibody-mediated opsonophagocytosis may also proceed via the alternative complement pathway. These and other results indicate that anticapsular antibody can overcome the prevention of C3 deposition on the bacterial surface by the sialic acid component of the type III capsule.

The precise steps between GBS colonization and invasive disease remain unclear. In vitro studies showing GBS entry of alveolar epithelium and pulmonary vasculature endothelial cells suggest that GBS may gain access to the bloodstream via invasion from the alveolar space, perhaps following intrapartum aspiration of infected fluid. β-Hemolysin/cytolysin may facilitate GBS entry into the bloodstream following inoculation into the lungs. However, highly encapsulated GBS strains enter eukaryotic cells poorly in vitro compared with capsule-deficient organisms, yet are associated with virulence clinically and in experimental infection models.

GBS induces the release of proinflammatory cytokines. The group B antigen and the peptidoglycan component of the GBS cell wall are potent inducers of tumor necrosis factor-α release in vitro, whereas purified type III capsular polysaccharide is not. Even though the capsule plays a central role in virulence through avoidance of immune clearance, the capsule does not directly contribute to cytokine release and the resultant inflammatory response.

The complete genome sequences of type III, V, and Ia GBS strains have been reported, emphasizing a genomic approach to better understanding GBS. Analysis of these sequences shows that GBS is closely related to *Streptococcus pyogenes* and *Streptococcus pneumoniae.* Many known and putative GBS virulence genes are clustered in **pathogenicity islands** that also contain mobile genetic elements, suggesting that interspecies acquisition of genetic material plays an important role in genetic diversity.

CLINICAL MANIFESTATIONS

Two syndromes of neonatal GBS disease are distinguishable on the basis of age at presentation, epidemiologic characteristics, and clinical features (Table 177-1). **Early-onset neonatal GBS disease** presents within the 1st 6 days of life and is often associated with maternal obstetric complications, including chorioamnionitis, prolonged rupture of membranes, and premature labor. Infants may appear ill at the time of delivery, and most infants become ill within the 1st 24 hr of birth. In utero infection may result in septic abortion. The most common manifestations of early-onset GBS disease are sepsis (50%), pneumonia (30%), and meningitis (15%). Asymptomatic bacteremia is uncommon but can occur. In symptomatic patients, nonspecific signs such as hypothermia or fever, irritability, lethargy, apnea, and bradycardia may be present. Respiratory signs are prominent regardless of the presence of pneumonia and include cyanosis, apnea, tachypnea, grunting, flaring, and retractions. A fulminant course with hemodynamic abnormalities, including tachycardia, acidosis, and shock, may ensue. Persistent fetal circulation may develop. Clinically and radiographically, pneumonia associated with early-onset GBS disease is difficult to distinguish from respiratory distress syndrome. Patients with meningitis often present with nonspecific findings, as described for sepsis or pneumonia, with more specific signs of central nervous system (CNS) involvement initially being absent.

Late-onset neonatal GBS disease occurs on or after 7 days of life and most commonly manifests as bacteremia (45-60%) and meningitis (25-35%). Focal infections involving bone and joints, skin and soft tissue, the urinary tract, or lungs have been reported in approximately 20% of patients with late-onset disease. Cellulitis and adenitis are often localized to the submandibular or

Table 177-1 CHARACTERISTICS OF EARLY- AND LATE-ONSET GBS DISEASE

	EARLY-ONSET DISEASE	LATE-ONSET DISEASE
Age at onset	0-6 days	7-90 days
Increased risk after obstetric complications	Yes	No
Common clinical manifestations	Sepsis, pneumonia, meningitis	Bacteremia, meningitis, other focal infections
Common serotypes	Ia, III, V, II, Ib	III predominates
Case fatality rate	4.7%	2.8%

Adapted from Schrag SJ, Zywicki S, Farley MM, et al: Group B streptococcal disease in the era of intrapartum antibiotic prophylaxis, *N Engl J Med* 342:15–20, 2000.

parotid regions. In contrast to early-onset disease, maternal obstetric complications are not risk factors for the development of late-onset GBS disease. Infants with late-onset disease are often less severely ill on presentation than infants with early-onset disease and the disease is often less fulminant.

Invasive GBS disease in children beyond early infancy is uncommon. In a multistate surveillance study in the 1990s, 2% of all cases of invasive GBS disease were identified in children age 90 days to 14 yr. Two of the more common syndromes associated with childhood GBS disease beyond early infancy are bacteremia and endocarditis. HIV infection should be considered in children with invasive GBS disease beyond the neonatal period.

DIAGNOSIS

A major challenge is distinguishing between respiratory distress syndrome and invasive neonatal GBS infection in preterm infants because the 2 illnesses share clinical and radiographic features. Severe apnea, early onset of shock, abnormalities in the peripheral leukocyte count, and greater lung compliance may be more likely in infants with GBS disease. Other neonatal pathogens, including *Escherichia coli* and *Listeria monocytogenes,* may cause illness that is clinically indistinguishable from that due to GBS.

The diagnosis of invasive GBS disease is established by isolation and identification of the organism from a normally sterile site, such as blood, urine, or cerebrospinal fluid (CSF). Isolation of GBS from gastric or tracheal aspirates or from skin or mucous membranes indicates colonization and is not diagnostic of invasive disease. CSF should be examined in all neonates suspected of having sepsis, because specific CNS signs are often absent in the presence of meningitis, especially in early-onset disease. Antigen detection methods that use group B polysaccharide-specific antiserum, such as latex particle agglutination, are available for testing of urine, blood, and CSF, but these tests are less sensitive than culture. Moreover, antigen is often detected in urine samples collected by bag from otherwise healthy neonates who are colonized with GBS on the perineum or rectum.

LABORATORY FINDINGS

Frequently present are abnormalities in the peripheral white blood cell count, including an increased or decreased absolute neutrophil count, an elevated band count, an elevated ratio of bands to total neutrophils, or leukopenia. Elevations in the C-reactive protein level have been investigated as a potential early marker of GBS sepsis but are unreliable. Findings on chest radiograph are often indistinguishable from those of respiratory distress syndrome and may include reticulogranular patterns, patchy infiltrates, generalized opacification, pleural effusions, or increased interstitial markings.

TREATMENT

Penicillin G is the treatment of choice of confirmed GBS infection. Initial empirical therapy of neonatal sepsis should include ampicillin and an aminoglycoside (or cefotaxime), both for the need for broad coverage pending organism identification and for synergistic bactericidal activity. Once GBS has been definitively identified and a good clinical response has occurred, therapy may be completed with penicillin alone. Especially in cases of meningitis, high doses of penicillin (450,000-500,000 U/kg/day) or ampicillin (300 mg/kg/day) are recommended because of the relatively high mean inhibitory concentration of penicillin for GBS as well as the potential for a high initial CSF inoculum. The duration of therapy varies according to the site of infection (Table 177-2) and should be guided by clinical circumstances. Extremely ill near-term patients with respiratory failure have been successfully treated with extracorporeal membrane oxygenation.

Table 177-2 RECOMMENDED DURATION OF THERAPY FOR MANIFESTATIONS OF GBS DISEASE

TREATMENT	DURATION
Bacteremia without a focus	10 days
Meningitis	2-3 wk
Ventriculitis	4 wk
Osteomyelitis	4 wk

Adapted from the American Academy of Pediatrics: Group B streptococcal infections. In Pickering LK, editor: *Red book: 2000 report of the Committee on Infectious Diseases*, ed 25, Elk Grove Village, IL, 2000, American Academy of Pediatrics, pp 537–544.

In cases of GBS meningitis, some experts recommend that additional CSF be sampled at 24-48 hr to determine whether sterility has been achieved. Persistent GBS growth may indicate an unsuspected intracranial focus or an insufficient antibiotic dose.

For **recurrent neonatal GBS** disease, standard intravenous antibiotic therapy followed by attempted eradication of GBS mucosal colonization has been suggested. This suggestion is based on the findings in several studies that invasive isolates from recurrent episodes are often identical to each other and to colonizing strains from the affected infant. Rifampin has most frequently been used for this purpose, but one report demonstrates that eradication of GBS colonization in infants is not reliably achieved by rifampin therapy. Optimal management of this uncommon situation remains unclear.

PROGNOSIS

Studies from the 1970s and 1980s showed that up to 30% of infants surviving GBS meningitis had major long-term neurologic sequelae, including developmental delay, spastic quadriplegia, microcephaly, seizure disorder, cortical blindness, or deafness; less severe neurologic complications may be present in other survivors. Periventricular leukomalacia and severe developmental delay may result from GBS disease and accompanying shock in premature infants, even in the absence of meningitis. The outcome of focal GBS infections outside of the CNS, such as bone or soft tissue infections, is generally favorable.

In the 1990s, the case fatality rates associated with early- and late-onset neonatal GBS disease were 4.7% and 2.8%, respectively. Mortality is higher in premature infants; 1 study reported a case fatality rate of 30% in infants whose gestational age was <33 wk and 2% in infants whose gestational age was 37 wk or older. The case fatality rate in children aged 3 mo to 14 yr was 9%, and in nonpregnant adults was 11.5%.

PREVENTION

Persistent morbidity and mortality from perinatal GBS disease despite advances in neonatal care has spurred intense investigation into modes of prevention. Two basic approaches to GBS prevention have been investigated: (1) elimination of colonization from the mother or infant (chemoprophylaxis), and (2) induction of protective immunity (immunoprophylaxis).

Chemoprophylaxis

Administration of antibiotics to pregnant women **before** the onset of labor does not reliably eradicate maternal GBS colonization and is not an effective means of preventing neonatal GBS disease. Interruption of neonatal colonization is achievable through administration of antibiotics to the mother during labor (Chapter 103). Infants born to GBS-colonized women with premature labor or prolonged rupture of membranes who were given intrapartum chemoprophylaxis had a substantially lower rate of GBS colonization (9% vs 51%) and early-onset disease (0% vs 6%) than did the infants born to women who were not treated. Maternal postpartum febrile illness was also decreased in the treatment group.

In the mid-1990s, guidelines for chemoprophylaxis were issued that specified administration of intrapartum antibiotics to women identified as high-risk by either culture-based or risk factor–based criteria. These guidelines were revised in 2002 after epidemiologic data indicated the superior protective effect of the culture-based approach in the prevention of neonatal GBS disease (Chapter 103). According to current recommendations, vaginorectal GBS screening cultures should be performed for all pregnant women at 35-37 wk gestation. Any woman with a positive prenatal screening culture, GBS bacteriuria during pregnancy, or a previous infant with invasive GBS disease should receive intrapartum antibiotics. Women whose culture status is unknown (culture not done, incomplete, or results unknown) and who deliver prematurely (<37 wk gestation) or experience prolonged rupture of membranes (≥18 hr) or intrapartum fever (≥38.0°C) should also receive intrapartum chemoprophylaxis. If amnionitis is suspected, broad-spectrum antibiotic therapy that includes an agent active against GBS should replace GBS prophylaxis. Routine intrapartum prophylaxis is not recommended for women with GBS colonization undergoing planned cesarean delivery who have not begun labor or had rupture of membranes.

These guidelines also suggest an approach for the management of infants born to mothers who received intrapartum chemoprophylaxis (Chapter 103). Data from a large epidemiologic study indicate that the administration of maternal intrapartum antibiotics does not change the clinical spectrum or delay the onset of clinical signs in infants who developed GBS disease despite maternal prophylaxis. Thus, the Centers for Disease Control and Prevention guidelines reserve a full diagnostic evaluation for those infants who appear clinically ill or whose mothers are suspected of having chorioamnionitis.

A significant concern with maternal intrapartum prophylaxis has been that large-scale antibiotic use among parturient women might lead to increased rates of antimicrobial resistance or infection in infants with organisms other than GBS. To date, an increase in the incidence of non-GBS early-onset neonatal infections has been seen only in premature, low birthweight, and very low birthweight infants, in whom risk factors other than maternal chemoprophylaxis may play a role. At present, the substantial decline in early-onset neonatal GBS disease favors continued broad-scale intrapartum chemoprophylaxis, but continued surveillance is required. Penicillin remains the preferred agent for chemoprophylaxis, because of its narrow spectrum and the universal penicillin susceptibility of GBS isolates associated with human infection. Occasional GBS isolates have demonstrated reduced in vitro susceptibility to penicillin and other β-lactam antibiotics in association with mutations in penicillin-binding proteins. However, such strains have not been reported in invasive infection. Because of recent reports indicating frequent resistance of GBS to erythromycin (up to 32%) and clindamycin (up to 15%), cefazolin should be used in most cases of intrapartum chemoprophylaxis for penicillin-intolerant women. For penicillin-allergic women at high risk for anaphylaxis, clindamycin or erythromycin should be used, if isolates are demonstrated to be susceptible. Vancomycin should be used if isolates are resistant to clindamycin and erythromycin or if susceptibility to these agents is unknown.

A limitation of the maternal chemoprophylaxis strategy is that intrapartum antibiotic use is unlikely to have an impact on late-onset neonatal disease, miscarriages or stillbirths attributed to GBS, or adult GBS disease. In addition, with wider implementation of maternal chemoprophylaxis, an increasing percentage of early-onset neonatal disease has been in patients born to women with negative cultures, that is, false-negative screens.

Maternal Immunization

Human studies demonstrate that transplacental transfer of naturally acquired maternal antibody to the GBS capsular polysaccharide protects newborns from invasive GBS infection and that efficient transplacental passage of vaccine-induced GBS antibodies occurs. Conjugate vaccines composed of the GBS capsular polysaccharides coupled to carrier proteins have been produced for human use. In early clinical trials, conjugate GBS vaccines were well tolerated and induced levels of functional antibodies well above the range believed to be protective in greater than 90% of recipients. A vaccine containing type III polysaccharide coupled to tetanus toxoid was safely administered to pregnant women and elicited functionally active type-specific antibody that was efficiently transported to the fetus. Administration of a multivalent polysaccharide-protein vaccine before or during pregnancy should lead to transplacental passage of vaccine-induced antibody that protects the fetus and newborn against infection by several GBS serotypes. Such a vaccine would eliminate the need for cumbersome cultures during pregnancy, would circumvent the various risks associated with large-scale antibiotic prophylaxis, and would likely have an impact on both early- and late-onset disease. Intrapartum chemoprophylaxis will likely remain an important aspect of prevention, particularly for women in whom opportunities for GBS immunization are missed and for infants born so early that levels of transplacentally acquired antibodies may not be high enough to be protective.

BIBLIOGRAPHY

Please visit the Nelson Textbook of Pediatrics *website at www.expertconsult.com for the complete bibliography.*

Chapter 178
Non–Group A or B Streptococci

Michael A. Gerber

The genus *Streptococcus* comprises >30 species. *Streptococcus pneumoniae* (Chapter 175), group A streptococcus (Chapter 176), and group B streptococcus (Chapter 177) are the most common causes of human streptococcal infections. The β-hemolytic streptococci of Lancefield groups C to H and K to V and the α-hemolytic streptococci that cannot be classified within a Lancefield group (the viridans streptococci) commonly colonize intact body surfaces (the pharynx, skin, gastrointestinal tract, genitourinary tract) and also cause infections in humans (see Table 178-1 on the *Nelson Textbook of Pediatrics* website at www.expertconsult.com). Of the non–group A β-hemolytic streptococci, groups C and G streptococcus are the most frequent cause of human disease. The enterococci were once classified among the group D streptococci but are now a separate genus, *Enterococcus* (Chapter 179).

For the full continuation of this chapter, please visit the Nelson Textbook of Pediatrics *website at www.expertconsult.com.*

Chapter 179
Enterococcus

David B. Haslam

Enterococcus has long been recognized as a pathogen in select populations and over the past 2 decades has become a common and particularly troublesome cause of hospital-acquired infection. Enterococci were formerly classified with *Streptococcus bovis* and *Streptococcus equinus* as the Lancefield group D streptococci and are now placed in a separate genus. These organisms are notorious for their frequent resistance to antibiotics.

For the full continuation of this chapter, please visit the Nelson Textbook of Pediatrics *website at www.expertconsult.com.*

Chapter 180
Diphtheria (*Corynebacterium diphtheriae*)
E. Stephen Buescher

Diphtheria is an acute toxic infection caused by *Corynebacterium* species, typically *Corynebacterium diphtheriae* and rarely toxigenic strains of *Corynebacterium ulcerans.* Although diphtheria was reduced from a major cause of childhood death to a medical rarity in the Western hemisphere in the early 20th century, current reminders of the fragility of this success emphasize the necessity to continue vigorous promotion of those same principles across the global community.

For the full continuation of this chapter, please visit the Nelson Textbook of Pediatrics *website at www.expertconsult.com.*

Chapter 181
Listeria monocytogenes
Robert S. Baltimore

Listeriosis in humans is caused principally by *Listeria monocytogenes,* 1 of 6 species of the genus *Listeria* that are widely distributed in the environment and throughout the food chain. Human infections can usually be traced to an animal reservoir. Infection occurs most commonly at the extremes of age. In the pediatric population, perinatal infections predominate and usually occur secondary to maternal infection or colonization. Outside the newborn period, disease is most commonly encountered in immunosuppressed (T-cell deficiencies) children and adults and in the elderly. In the USA, food-borne outbreaks are caused by improperly processed dairy products and contaminated vegetables, and principally affect the same individuals at risk for sporadic disease.

For the full continuation of this chapter, please visit the Nelson Textbook of Pediatrics *website at www.expertconsult.com.*

Chapter 182
Actinomyces
Richard F. Jacobs and Gordon E. Schutze

Actinomyces organisms are slow-growing, gram-positive bacteria that are part of the endogenous oral flora in humans. Their filamentous structure gives them a fungus-like appearance. Infection caused by these bacteria is termed **actinomycosis,** which is a chronic, granulomatous, suppurative disease characterized by direct extension to contiguous tissue across natural anatomic barriers with the formation of numerous draining fistulas and sinus tracts. These infections usually involve the cervicofacial, thoracic, abdominal, or pelvic regions.

For the full continuation of this chapter, please visit the Nelson Textbook of Pediatrics *website at www.expertconsult.com.*

Chapter 183
Nocardia
Richard F. Jacobs and Gordon E. Schutze

Nocardia organisms cause localized and disseminated disease in children and adults. These organisms are primarily opportunistic pathogens infecting immunocompromised persons. Infection caused by these bacteria is termed **nocardiosis,** which consists of acute, subacute, or chronic suppurative infections with a tendency for remissions and exacerbations.

For the full continuation of this chapter, please visit the Nelson Textbook of Pediatrics *website at www.expertconsult.com.*

Section 5 GRAM-NEGATIVE BACTERIAL INFECTIONS

Chapter 184
Neisseria meningitidis (Meningococcus)
Dan M. Granoff and Janet R. Gilsdorf

Neisseria meningitidis (also referred to as *meningococcus*) lives as a commensal in the nasopharynx of humans and is typically carried by 10% or more of the population at any one time. Relatively rarely the organism enters the bloodstream and may cause devastating disease. Why invasive meningococcal disease develops in a small proportion of exposed individuals is still largely not understood. Paradoxically, *N. meningitidis* also is unique for its ability to cause epidemic bacterial meningitis and sepsis. Although the last major meningococcal epidemic in the USA was in the 1940s, the organism remains an important cause of serious endemic disease in the country and of epidemic disease throughout the world. Despite advances in critical care medicine, previously healthy children and adolescents continue to succumb to fulminant meningococcal disease.

ETIOLOGY

N. meningitidis is a fastidious encapsulated, oxidase-positive, aerobic diplococcus. In gram-stained specimens, the microbes appear as gram-negative, kidney-shaped pairs. There are 13 chemically and serologically distinct meningococcal capsular groups, of which five, designated A, B, C, W-135 and Y, are responsible for almost all cases of human disease. Meningococcal strains also are subclassified on the basis of antigenic variation in two porin molecules, PorB (serotype) and PorA (serosubtype). The PorA serologic classification is gradually being replaced by a parallel classification system, called *variable region (VR) sequence types,* which are based on amino acid variation at two surface-accessible loops on the PorA molecule. Genetic lineages of strains can be inferred from multilocus sequence typing (MLST), which is based on polymorphisms in seven housekeeping genes.

The meningococcus readily exchanges genes encoding key antigens. The characterization of strains based on the product of one or two genetic loci therefore does not provide a reliable reflection of the underlying genetic or epidemiologic relationships between isolates. In practice, a combination of MLST, capsular group, and sequence variation in several protein antigens is used to determine epidemiologic relatedness of strains. These techniques have established that endemic meningococcal disease is caused by genetically heterogeneous strains and that outbreaks are usually caused by single strains.

EPIDEMIOLOGY

Meningococci are transmitted by aerosol droplets or through contact with respiratory secretions, such as through kissing or sharing a drinking glass. The organism is not thought to survive for long periods in the environment, and transmission is decreased during periods of high ambient ultraviolet B radiation. Viral respiratory infections (influenza), exposure to tobacco smoke, marijuana use, bar patronage, binge drinking, attendance at nightclubs, and freshmen college students living in dormitories are all associated with increased rates of meningococcal carriage or disease. Respiratory viruses and/or exposure to smoke may alter the mucosal surface and enhance bacterial binding and/or decrease clearance of the organism from the nasopharynx.

Meningococcal disease is a global problem. Disease incidence rates are highly cyclic. After a decade of relatively high incidence in the 1990s, rates in the USA have steadily decreased. Over the last 10 years, the annual incidence averaged ≈1- 2/100,000 population, resulting in ≈2000 to 3500 culture-confirmed cases per year. The actual number of cases likely was higher, because in countries such as the United Kingdom, where polymerase chain reaction (PCR) methods are used routinely for diagnosis of suspected cases, only 50% of PCR-confirmed cases are culture-confirmed. In the USA, most cases of meningococcal disease are sporadic. Small outbreaks in elementary or secondary schools or colleges account for <2% of all cases.

The highest age-incidence of meningococcal disease occurs in infants <1 yr old (average annual rates of 5-9/100,000 population). The high rate in this age group is not entirely understood. It may be attributable to immature alternative and lectin complement pathways and to lack of acquired serum antibodies. In the absence of immunization, incidence rates decline by age 2-4 yr (1-2/100,000), with a further decline after age 4 yr (0.5/100,000). A secondary peak in incidence occurs among adolescents (1-3/100,000), which may be related to increased exposure from social activities.

In the USA, the majority of cases of disease in the first year of life is caused by capsular group B strains. After age 1 yr, disease is roughly equally distributed among group B, C, and Y strains. In most other industrialized countries group B strains predominate at all ages, in part because of introduction of routine group C meningococcal conjugate vaccination in infants and/or toddlers. For reasons not understood, disease in children caused by group Y strains was uncommon in the USA before the 1990s and remains relatively uncommon outside the country.

Since World War II, disease from group A strains has been largely confined to developing countries. The highest incidence of group A disease is in sub-Saharan Africa, with annual endemic rates of 10-25/ 100,000. Every 7 to 10 yr this region experiences large group A pandemics with annual rates as high as 1000/100,000. The onset of cases in the sub-Saharan region typically begins during the dry season and subsides with the rainy season, and may reemerge the following dry season. Endemic and epidemic meningococcal disease in this region has also been caused by group W-135 and X strains. These strains are infrequent causes of disease in other areas of the world, although W-135 isolates have been associated with outbreaks among pilgrims returning from the Hajj.

PATHOGENESIS

After exposure to meningococci, attachment of an organism to nasopharyngeal mucosal cells is mediated by specific bacterial adhesins. Multiple adhesins have been identified, but among the most important are pili and two opacity-associated proteins, Opa and Opc. CD46 and other, unidentified host cell receptors mediate pilus attachment. Opa and Opc interact with heparin sulfate proteoglycans and extracellular matrix proteins such as fibronectin and vitronectin. There are also specific receptor interactions, the most important being carcino-embryonic antigen cell adhesion molecule (CEACAM) proteins. Contact between the bacteria and host cells initiates internalization of the bacteria within membrane-bound vesicles. These molecular events lead to replication of the organism and establishment of an asymptomatic carrier state.

Although carriage can persist for weeks to months, onset of invasive meningococcal disease usually occurs within a few days to a week after acquisition of the organism. Development of disease depends on the virulence of the organism, innate susceptibility of the host, and presence or absence of serum antibodies capable of activating complement-mediated bacteriolysis and/or opsonophagocytosis. The strains responsible for invasive disease are always encapsulated and are usually derived from a limited number of so-called hypervirulent genetic lineages. Although these strains can be found in asymptomatic carriers, the majority of carrier strains either are nonencapsulated or are encapsulated organisms derived from diverse genetic lineages, many of which rarely cause disease.

The most important virulence determinant is the presence of a capsular polysaccharide, which enhances resistance of the organism to killing by normal human serum and helps resist opsonophagocytic killing. Additionally, endotoxin (lipopolysaccharide) has an essential role in stimulating cytokines and activating coagulation and bleeding, which are the clinical hallmarks of severe meningococcal sepsis. The ability of the organism to scavenge iron from human transferrin and lactoferrin and to bind human factor H (fH), a downregulating molecule in the complement cascade, are additional important mechanisms that allow meningococci to evade innate host defenses and to survive and grow in human serum or blood.

The severity of meningococcal disease is related to the circulating level of endotoxin in the bloodstream. During bacterial growth, outer membrane blebs, which are rich in endotoxin, are released. Meningococcal endotoxin is composed of lipopolysaccharide—also referred to as lipo-oligosaccharide (LOS) because of the presence of repeating short saccharides instead of long-chain saccharides characteristic of endotoxins of many other gram-negative bacteria. The lipid A portion of meningococcal LOS is responsible for the toxicity of the molecule, which is sensed by host cells through Toll-like receptors (TLRs), most notably TLR4 in association with an accessory protein, MD-2. Stimulation of TLR4 activates genes via pathways related to nuclear factor-κB (NF-κB), which leads to production of multiple proinflammatory cytokines including tumor necrosis factor-α (TNF-α), interleukin-1β (IL-1β), IL-6, and IL-8. Subsequently both the extrinsic (by way of induction of tissue factor expression on endothelial cells and monocytes) and intrinsic pathways of coagulation are activated. Progression of capillary leak and disseminated intravascular coagulopathy (DIC) can lead to multiple organ system failure, septic shock, and death. Following initiation of antibiotic therapy, circulating LOS and TNF-α levels can increase transiently as a result of rapid bacterial lysis, which then decreases with clearance of viable microbes. Activation of the complement and clotting cascades can continue well beyond this point, especially in fulminant cases.

Diffuse vasculitis and DIC are common with meningococcemia. Leukocyte-rich fibrin clots are seen in small vessels, including arterioles and capillaries. The resulting focal hemorrhage and necrosis that initially manifest as purpura in the skin may occur in any organ. The heart, central nervous system, skin, mucous and serous membranes, and adrenal glands are affected in most fatal cases, and microbes are often present in these lesions. Myocarditis is present in >50% of patients who die of meningococcal disease. Diffuse adrenal hemorrhage without vasculitis, the **Waterhouse-Friderichsen syndrome,** is common during fulminant meningococcemia. Meningitis is characterized by acute inflammatory cells in the leptomeninges and perivascular spaces. Focal cerebritis is uncommon.

About 10% of cases of meningococcal meningitis are caused by naturally occurring LOS mutants with penta-acylated instead of hexa-acylated lipid A. The penta-acylated mutant is poorly recognized by human TLR4 and, as a result, has attenuated endotoxin activity. Patients with meningitis caused by penta-acylated mutant strains are reported to have milder clinical syndromes, including decreased coagulopathy, than patients infected by strains that have the more common form of LOS with hexa-acylated lipid A.

Immunity

Naturally acquired serum antibodies to meningococci are elicited by asymptomatic carriage of pathogenic and nonpathogenic strains as well as by carriage of antigenically related species such as *Neisseria lactamica.* Bactericidal antibodies are produced against capsular polysaccharide and outer membrane proteins. Immunoglobulin M (IgM), IgG, and IgA responses are induced within a few weeks after nasopharyngeal colonization. Ongoing natural exposures may help maintain immunity.

The role of complement-mediated serum bactericidal antibodies is protective in military recruits exposed to epidemic group C meningococcal disease. Recruits with serum bactericidal titers of 1:4 or greater were protected from disease. The importance of serum bactericidal antibody also is underscored by a greatly increased risk of acquiring meningococcal disease in persons with inherited late complement component deficiencies (C5-C9), who lack bactericidal activity because of an inability to form a complement membrane attack complex. However, vaccine-induced antibodies in patients with late complement component deficiencies have opsonic activity, and in one study, meningococcal polysaccharide vaccination decreased the incidence of meningococcal disease among C5-C9 deficient individuals. These observations support an independent contribution of opsonophagocytic activity to protection against meningococcal disease and provide the rationale for the recommendation to immunize complement-deficient patients with meningococcal vaccines.

Host Factors

Persons with inherited deficiencies of properdin, factor D, or terminal complement components have up to a 1000-fold higher risk for development of meningococcal disease than complement-sufficient persons. The risk of meningococcal disease is also increased in patients with acquired complement deficiencies associated with diseases such as nephrotic syndrome, systemic lupus erythematosus, and hepatic failure.

Among persons with complement deficiencies, meningococcal disease is more prevalent during late childhood and adolescence, when carriage rates are higher than in children <10 yr; meningococcal infections may be recurrent. Although meningococcal disease can occasionally be overwhelming in patients with late complement component deficiency, cases are more typically described as being less severe than in complement-sufficient persons, perhaps reflecting the fact that these cases are often caused by unusual capsular groups such as W-135 and X. Although protective against early infection, extensive complement activation and bacteriolysis may contribute to the pathogenesis of severe disease once bacterial invasion has occurred.

A large number of host genetic factors appear to affect the risk and/or severity of meningococcal disease. The molecules implicated involved polymorphisms at epithelial surfaces, the complement cascade, pattern recognition receptors, clotting factors, or inflammatory mediators. To date, the strongest associations implicate genetic variation in complement regulators, particularly genes encoding mannose-binding protein (MBL), which is part of the lectin complement pathway, or in factor H, which is a down-regulator in the complement cascade. Factor H binds specifically to the surface of *N. meningitidis,* which enhances resistance to complement-killing of the bacteria and is critical for evasion of host defenses. Most other studies to identify susceptibility genes enrolled relatively small numbers of patients, and the results have not yet been confirmed or validated. Children with the IgG receptor allotype, FcγRIIa R/R131 (i.e., homozygous for arginine at position 131) are reported to have increased severity of meningococcal disease. One reason may be that neutrophils with this Fc receptor allotype exhibit less effective opsonophagocytosis than those with allotypes containing histidine at this position. Plasminogen activator converts plasminogen into its active form, plasmin, which elicits fibrinolysis. Functional polymorphisms in the promoter region of the gene for plasminogen-activator-inhibitor-1, which result in higher inhibitor levels and decreased fibrinolysis, have been associated with increased severity of meningococcal disease. The presence of factor V Leiden, which is known to increase the risk of thrombosis, also may exacerbate meningococcal purpura fulminans.

CLINICAL MANIFESTATIONS

The spectrum of meningococcal disease varies widely, and recognized patterns include bacteremia without sepsis, meningococcemia without meningitis, meningitis with or without meningococcemia, and chronic infection. At least 80% of cases have overt clinical signs. Occult meningococcal bacteremia often manifests as fever with or without associated symptoms that suggest minor viral infections. Resolution of bacteremia may occur without antibiotics, but sustained bacteremia leads to meningitis in ≈60% of cases and to distant infection of other tissues. *N. meningitidis* is isolated from blood in about 65% of patients with meningococcal infections, from cerebrospinal fluid (CSF) in about 50% of patients, and from joint fluid in 1% of patients.

Acute meningococcemia may initially mimic illnesses caused by viruses or other bacteria, causing pharyngitis, fever, myalgias, weakness, vomiting, diarrhea, and/or headache. A fine maculopapular rash is evident in about 7% of cases, with onset typically early in the course of infection. Limb pain, myalgias, or refusal to walk occurs often and is the primary complaint in 7% of otherwise clinically unsuspected cases. Cold hands or feet and abnormal skin color are also early signs. In fulminant meningococcemia, the disease progresses rapidly over several hours from fever without other signs to septic shock characterized by prominent petechiae and purpura (**purpura fulminans**), hypotension, DIC, acidosis, adrenal hemorrhage, renal failure, myocardial failure, and coma (Fig. 184-1). Meningitis may or may not be present.

Meningococcal meningitis is indistinguishable from meningitis due to other bacteria. Headache, photophobia, lethargy, vomiting, nuchal rigidity, and other signs of meningeal irritation are typically present. Seizures and focal neurologic signs occur less frequently than in patients with meningitis due to *Streptococcus pneumoniae* or *Haemophilus influenzae* type b. A meningoencephalitis-like picture can occur that may be associated with rapidly progressive cerebral edema, which may be more common with capsular group A infection.

Among 402 patients <21 yr old reported in three case series of all types of invasive meningococcal disease during the 1980s to early 2000s, about 80% presented with fever, 40% had hypotension or decreased peripheral perfusion, and 50% had petechiae and/or purpura. Purpura fulminans developed in 16%. Other presenting symptoms and signs included emesis (34%), lethargy (30%), irritability (21%), diarrhea (6%), rhinorrhea (10%), seizure (6%), and septic arthritis (8%). Radiographic evidence of pneumonia was present initially in 8% of patients in one series. Pleural effusion or empyema occurred in 15% of cases with meningococcal pneumonia and mechanical ventilation was required in 26% and vasopressor support in 35%.

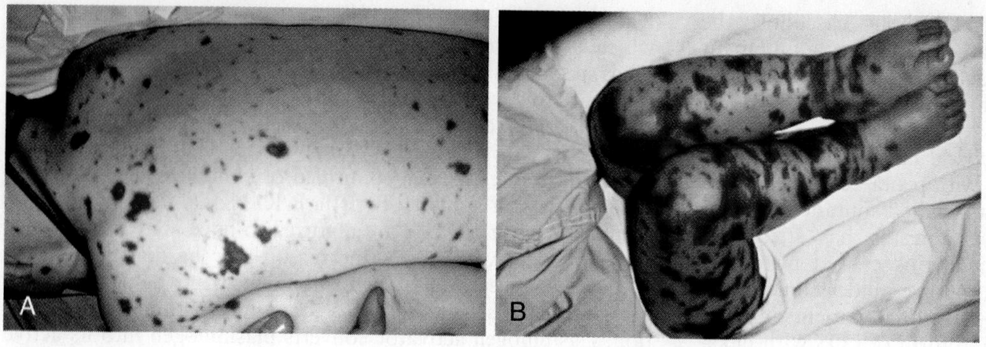

Figure 184-1 *A,* Purpuric rash in a 3 yr old with meningococcemia. *B,* Purpura fulminans in an 11 mo old with meningococcemia. (From Thompson ED, Herzog KD: Fever and rash. In Zaoutis L, Chiang V, editors: *Comprehensive pediatric hospital medicine,* Philadelphia, 2007, Mosby, p 332, Figs. 62-6 and 62-7.)

Nonsuppurative (presumed immune complex) arthritis developed in 4-6%. Uncommon manifestations of meningococcal disease include endocarditis, purulent pericarditis, pneumonia, endophthalmitis, mesenteric lymphadenitis, osteomyelitis, sinusitis, otitis media, and periorbital cellulitis. Primary purulent conjunctivitis can lead to invasive disease. *N. meningitidis* infections of the genitourinary tract are rare, but urethritis, cervicitis, vulvovaginitis, orchitis, and proctitis may occur.

Chronic meningococcemia, which occurs rarely, is characterized by fever, nontoxic appearance, arthralgias, headache, and a maculopapular to pustular rash, often with a hemorrhagic component. Symptoms are intermittent, with a mean duration of illness of 6-8 wk. Blood culture results are usually positive but cultures may initially be sterile. Chronic meningococcemia may spontaneously resolve, but meningitis can develop in untreated cases.

DIAGNOSIS

Definitive diagnosis of meningococcal disease is established by isolation of *N. meningitidis* from a normally sterile body fluid such as blood, CSF, or synovial fluid. Meningococci are sometimes identified in Gram stain preparation and/or culture of petechial or purpuric skin lesions and occasionally are seen on Gram stain of the buffy coat layer of a spun blood sample. Culture results often are negative if the patient has been treated with antibiotics prior to collection of the culture specimen. Isolation of the organism from the nasopharynx is not diagnostic for invasive disease.

In patients with meningococcal meningitis, the cellular and chemical characteristics of the CSF are those of acute bacterial meningitis, showing gram-negative diplococci on Gram stain in 75% of cases. CSF culture results may be positive in patients with meningococcemia in the absence of CSF pleocytosis or clinical evidence of meningitis; conversely, positive CSF specimens that are positive for Gram stain are sometimes culture negative. Overdecolorized pneumococci in Gram stain preparations can be mistaken for meningococci, and, therefore, empirical therapy should not be narrowed to *N. meningitidis* infection on the basis of Gram stain findings alone.

Detection of capsular polysaccharide antigens by rapid latex agglutination tests in CSF can support the diagnosis in cases clinically consistent with meningococcal disease and is found in 53-90% of cases. Because false-positive results are reported and results do not significantly affect clinical practice, latex agglutination tests are not routinely recommended. These tests are most useful when their results are positive in the setting of partially treated infections in which Gram stain and culture results are negative. On the other hand, latex agglutination tests of serum or urine are not clinically useful. Capsular antigen tests are not reliable for group B strains because of cross reactions with other bacterial species (*Escherichia coli* K1 antigen). PCR-based assays for detection of meningococci in blood and CSF have been developed, and multiplex PCR assays that detect several bacterial species associated with meningitis, including the meningococcus, are under development.

Other laboratory findings include leukocytopenia or leukocytosis, often with increased percentages of neutrophils and band forms, thrombocytopenia, proteinuria, and hematuria. Elevations of erythrocyte sedimentation rate (ESR) and C-reactive protein, hypoalbuminemia, hypocalcemia, and metabolic acidosis, often with increased lactate levels, are common. Patients with DIC have decreased serum concentrations of prothrombin and fibrinogen and prolonged coagulation times.

DIFFERENTIAL DIAGNOSIS

Meningococcal disease can appear similar to sepsis or meningitis caused by many other gram-negative bacteria, *S. pneumoniae, Staphylococcus aureus,* or group A streptococcus; to Rocky Mountain spotted fever, ehrlichiosis, or epidemic typhus; and to bacterial endocarditis. Viral and other infectious etiologies of meningoencephalitis should be considered in some cases. Autoimmune vasculitides (especially Henoch-Schönlein purpura), serum sickness, hemolytic-uremic syndrome, Kawasaki disease, idiopathic thrombocytopenic purpura, drug eruptions, and ingestion of various poisons can have features that overlap with those of meningococcal infection.

Benign petechial rashes are common in viral and group A streptococcal infections. The nonpetechial, blanching maculopapular rash observed in some cases of meningococcal disease may initially be confused with a viral exanthem.

TREATMENT

Empirical therapy should be initiated immediately for possible invasive meningococcal infections. β-Lactam antibiotics are the drugs of choice. Because of concerns about penicillin- or cephalosporin-resistant *S. pneumoniae,* intravenous (IV) vancomycin (60 mg/kg/day, divided in four doses, each dose given every 6 hr) should be added empirically as a second drug as part of initial empiric regimens for bacterial meningitis of unknown cause (Chapter 595.1). More specific therapy for meningococcal disease may be initiated when culture and antibiotic susceptibility results become available (Table 184-1). Although ciprofloxacin may be an alternative to cephalosporins for treatment of meningococcal infection, ciprofloxacin-resistant meningococci have been identified. Therapy in children is generally continued for 5-7 days.

Early treatment of meningococcal infections may prevent serious sequelae, but timely early diagnosis is often difficult in the absence of petechial or purpuric skin findings. High fever and leukocytosis with increased neutrophil and band counts are common in older children and adolescents with otherwise unsuspected meningococcal infection. Empiric outpatient treatment with careful follow-up of selected patients during meningococcal outbreaks and of nontoxic children with petechial rashes can be considered after blood culture specimens are obtained. Most of the latter do not have meningococcal infection.

Table 184-1 TREATMENT OF *NEISSERIA MENINGITIDIS* INVASIVE INFECTIONS

DRUG	ROUTE OF ADMINISTRATION	DOSE	DOSING INTERVAL (hr)	MAXIMUM DAILY DOSE
Penicillin G	IM or IV	250,000-300,000 U/kg/day	4 to 6	24 million U
Ampicillin	IM or IV	200-400 mg/kg/day	6	6-12 g
Cefotaxime	IM or IV	200-300 mg/kg/day	6-8	8-10 g
Ceftriaxone	IM or IV	100 mg/kg/day	12-24	4 g
Alternative therapy in the face of life-threatening β-lactam allergy:				
Chloramphenicol*	IV	50-100 mg/kg/day	6	2-4 g
Ciprofloxacin†	IV	18-30 mg/kg/day	8-12	800-1600 mg
Meropenem	IV	60-120 mg/kg/day	8	4-6 g

*Monitor blood levels to avoid toxicity.
†Licensed for individuals > age 18 yr.
IM, intramuscular; IV, intravenous.

Isolates of *N. meningitidis* with decreased susceptibility to penicillin (minimal inhibitory concentration of penicillin of 0.1-1.0 mg/mL) have been reported from Europe, Africa, Canada, and the USA. Decreased susceptibility is caused, at least in part, by altered penicillin-binding protein 2 and does not appear to adversely affect the response to therapy. In 2006 such strains represented ≈4% of isolates in the USA. Routine susceptibility testing of meningococcal isolates is not performed by many U.S. clinical microbiology laboratories.

Optimal supportive care is essential. Many adjunctive therapies have been attempted, but to date, none has shown clear benefit in children. Dexamethasone therapy for 2 to 4 days, with the first dose given before or during the initiation of antibiotic therapy, has decreased mortality in adults with *S. pneumoniae* meningitis; the benefit in patients with meningococcal meningitis has not been firmly established. Anticoagulant or fibrinolytic agents and vasodilators have been used with variable success in anecdotal reports. Activated protein C therapy is not recommended for infants with severe sepsis and purpura fulminans because of the increased risk of intracranial hemorrhage associated with its use.

Most children with meningococcal disease who do not require intubation or vasopressor support show ready response to antibiotics plus supportive care and demonstrate clinical improvement within 24-72 hr. Those requiring mechanical ventilation and other critical care interventions often have prolonged and complicated courses that may require hospitalization for weeks. Children with severe disease who show poor response to aggressive fluid and inotropic therapies may have adrenal insufficiency and may benefit from hydrocortisone supplementation. Extracorporeal membrane oxygenation, plasmapheresis, and hyperbaric oxygen have been described anecdotally as having limited success.

COMPLICATIONS

Acute complications of severe meningococcal disease are related to the vasculitis, DIC, and hypotension. Focal skin infarctions usually heal but can become secondarily infected, resulting in significant scarring and requiring skin grafting. The dry gangrene of extremities often seen with purpura fulminans may necessitate amputations. Adrenal hemorrhage, endophthalmitis, arthritis, endocarditis, pericarditis, myocarditis, pneumonia, lung abscess, peritonitis, and renal infarcts can occur during acute infection. Avascular necrosis of epiphyses and epiphyseal-metaphyseal defects can result from the generalized DIC and may lead to growth disturbances and late skeletal deformities.

Deafness is the most frequent neurologic sequela of meningitis, occurring in 5-10% of children. Cerebral arterial or venous thrombosis with resultant cerebral infarction can occur in severe cases. Meningococcal meningitis is rarely complicated by subdural effusion or empyema or by brain abscess. Other rare neurologic sequelae include ataxia, seizures, blindness, cranial nerve palsies, hemiparesis or quadriparesis, and obstructive hydrocephalus. The last often manifests 3-4 wk after onset of illness.

Nonsuppurative complications of meningococcal disease appear to be **immune complex mediated** and become apparent 4-9 days after the onset of illness. Arthritis and cutaneous vasculitis (erythema nodosum) are most common. The **arthritis** usually is monoarticular or oligoarticular, involves large joints, and is associated with sterile effusions that respond to nonsteroidal anti-inflammatory agents. Long-term sequelae are uncommon. Because most patients with meningococcal meningitis become afebrile by the 7th hospital day, persistence or recrudescence of fever after 5 days of antibiotics warrants evaluation for immune complex–mediated complications.

Reactivation of latent herpes simplex virus infections (primarily herpes labialis) is common during meningococcal infection.

PROGNOSIS

The mortality rate for invasive meningococcal disease remains about 10% in the USA despite modern medical interventions. Most deaths occur within 48 hr of hospitalization in children with meningococcemia. Poor prognostic factors on presentation include hypothermia or extreme hyperpyrexia, hypotension or shock, purpura fulminans, seizures, leukopenia, thrombocytopenia (including DIC), acidosis, and high circulating levels of endotoxin and TNF-α. The presence of petechiae for <12 hr before admission, absence of meningitis, and low or normal ESR indicate rapid, fulminant progression and poorer prognosis.

Screening for complement deficiency after resolution of the acute infection should be performed in older children, adolescents, and adults with meningococcal infection and in young children with recurrent infection or with first episodes caused by strains with unusual capsular groups such as W-135 or X.

PREVENTION

Close contacts of patients with meningococcal disease are at increased risk for infection. Antibiotic prophylaxis is indicated for household, daycare, and nursery school contacts and for anyone who has had contact with the patient's oral secretions during the 7 days before onset of illness. Prophylaxis of contacts should be offered as soon as possible (Table 184-2), ideally within 24 hr of diagnosis of the patient. Because prophylaxis is not 100% effective, close contacts should be carefully monitored and brought to medical attention if they experience fever. Prophylaxis is not routinely recommended for medical personnel except those with intimate exposure, such as through mouth-to-mouth resuscitation, intubation, or suctioning before antibiotic therapy was begun.

Neither penicillin nor ampicillin treatment eradicates nasopharyngeal carriage; patients with meningococcal infection treated with penicillin or ampicillin should receive prophylaxis before hospital discharge. Droplet precautions should be observed for hospitalized patients for 24 hr after initiation of effective therapy. All confirmed or probable cases of meningococcal infection must be reported to the local public health department.

Vaccination

As of October 2010, three quadrivalent meningococcal vaccines containing capsular groups A, C, W-135, and Y are licensed in the USA. MPSV4 (Menomune, Sanfi Pasteur) contains only purified polysaccharides. The other two are conjugates of either purified polysaccharides coupled with diphtheria toxoid (MCV4-DT, Menactra, Sanofi Pasteur), or oligosaccharides coupled with a mutant, nontoxic diphtheria toxin, CRM_{197} (MenACWY-CRM, Menveo, Novartis Vaccines). All three vaccines are safe and effective. The conjugate vaccines more frequently cause transient fever and local redness, pain, or swelling at the injection site than MPSV4, which is attributed to the presence of the carrier proteins in the conjugate vaccines.

Following a single dose in otherwise healthy adolescents, all three vaccines elicit serum bactericidal antibody titers that peak at about 4-6 wk. These titers reflect the ability of the sera to kill the bacteria in the presence of complement. By 3 yr, half of vaccinated adolescents have serum titers <1:4 when measured with human complement. Titers of 1:4 or greater with human complement are considered protective.

Both meningococcal conjugate vaccines are more immunogenic in children than MPSV4 and, at all ages, the conjugate vaccines elicit serum bactericidal antibodies of superior quality (avidity) and persistence. The conjugate vaccines also prime for immunologic memory, which results in booster responses to a second injection. Vaccination also has the potential to decrease meningococcal carriage. In contrast, MPSV4 vaccination induces immunologic hyporesponsiveness to a subsequent injection of MPSV4 or conjugate vaccine. There is no evidence that MPSV4 vaccination decreases carriage. For all of these reasons, use of either conjugate vaccine is preferred over MPSV4.

In the USA, routine meningococcal vaccination is recommended for all children beginning at age 11 yr. In this age group, about 75% of meningococcal disease is caused by strains with capsular groups C, Y, or W-135 and therefore is potentially vaccine preventable. On the basis of reviews of age-related immunogenicity, disease burden, and cost effectiveness, the Advisory Committee on Immunization Practices (ACIP) and the American Academy of Pediatrics (AAP) do not recommend routine meningococcal vaccination for children < 11 yr. Beginning at age 2 yr, vaccination should be given to children with underlying conditions associated with increased risk of meningococcal disease (Table 184-3). As of October 2010, MPSV4 and MCV4-DT are the only vaccines approved by the FDA for use in this age group. MenACWY-CRM, however, is reported to be safe and immunogenic in children 2-10 yr, and regulatory approval by the FDA for this age group is under consideration.

The majority of otherwise healthy adolescents who were immunized at age 11-12 yr will have undetectable serum bactericidal titers by age 16 yr. Those engaging in social activities common to this age group, such as intimate kissing, smoking, or nightclub attendance, are at increased risk of exposure to *N. meningitidis*. At the October 2010 ACIP meeting, the Committee voted in favor of a booster dose of meningococcal conjugate vaccine for all adolescents aged 16 yr who received a first dose at age 11-12 yr (see later).

In the United Kingdom, the combination of a mass catch-up group C conjugate immunization campaign in 1999 and introduction of routine infant group C conjugate immunization resulted in a 95% decrease in group C disease. Similar results have been reported in other European countries and in Canada. Decreased nasopharyngeal carriage of group C strains among both vaccinees and nonvaccinees (herd immunity) also has been documented in the United Kingdom. In the USA, MenACWY-CRM and a new combination conjugate vaccine, meningococcal C,Y and *Haemophilus influenzae* type b, are likely to receive regulatory approval for use in infants and toddlers, the age groups with the highest incidence of meningococcal disease. In the meantime, the U.S. strategy targets adolescents. Immunization at this age may decrease carriage and have an indirect effect on lowering the incidence of disease in younger age groups that are not currently targeted for routine meningococcal immunization.

Table 184-2 ANTIBIOTIC PROPHYLAXIS TO PREVENT *NEISSERIA MENINGITIDIS* INFECTION

DRUG	DOSE	DURATION
Rifampin:		2 days (4 doses)
Infants <1 mo	5 mg/kg PO every 12 hr	
Children >1 mo	10mg/kg PO every 12hr	
Adults	600 mg PO every 12 hr	
Ceftriaxone:		
Children <15 yr	125 mg IM	1 dose
Children >15 yr	250 mg IM	1 dose
Ciprofloxacin, persons >18 yr	500 mg PO	1 dose

IM, intramuscular; PO, by mouth.

Table 184-3 RECOMMENDATIONS FOR MENINGOCOCCAL VACCINATION

POPULATION GROUP	<2 YR	2-10 YR	11-19 YR	20-55 YR
General population	Not recommended	Not recommended	A single dose of MCV4 or MenACWY-CRM at age 11-12 yr (at preadolescent assessment visit) or at high school entry (at approximately age 15 yr). A booster dose 5 yr later (see text).*	Not recommended
GROUPS AT INCREASED RISK				
Anatomic or immune compromised†	Not usually recommended	Two doses of MCV4-DT, separated by 8 wk with a booster dose 3-5 yr later‡	Two doses of MCV4-DT or MenACYW-CRM, separated by 8 wk with a booster dose at 5 yr	Two doses of MCV4-DT or MenACYW-CRM, separated by 8 wk with a booster dose at 5 yr
Increased exposure§	Not usually recommended	A single dose of MCV4-DT with a booster dose 3-5 yr later‡	A single dose of MCV4-DT or MenACYW-CRM with a booster dose 5 yr later	A single dose of MCV4-DT or MenACYW-CRM with a booster dose at 5 yr

Adapted from recommendations of the ACIP and AAP (see Bibliography), and updated to reflect recommendations adopted at the ACIP meeting of October 27, 2010.

*Otherwise healthy adolescents who received a first dose at age 11-12 yr should receive a booster dose of a meningococcal conjugate vaccine at 16 yr of age. For those given a first dose at age 13-15 yr, and who have not yet reached their 21st birthday, the booster dose should be given 5 yr after the first dose.

†Includes persons who have complement component deficiencies, anatomic or functional asplenia, and children infected with HIV.

‡Persons previously vaccinated at 7 yr of age or older and are at prolonged increased risk should be revaccinated 5 yr after their previous meningococcal vaccine. Persons previously vaccinated at ages 2-6 yr and are at prolonged increased risk should be revaccinated 3 yr after their previous meningococcal vaccination.

§Military personnel, microbiologists and persons traveling to areas where *Neisseria meningitidis* is hyperendemic or epidemic, for example, visitors to the "meningitis belt" of sub-Saharan Africa during the dry season (December-June). Vaccination also is required by the government of Saudi Arabia for all travelers to Mecca during the annual Hajj.

The group B polysaccharide capsule cross-reacts with glycosylated protein antigens present in brain, heart, and kidney and therefore is not a safe vaccine antigen. Several counties (Cuba, Norway, and New Zealand) successfully controlled group B epidemics by immunizing with tailor-made outer membrane vesicle (OMV) vaccines prepared from the respective epidemic strains. The principal limitation of OMV vaccines is that the bactericidal antibody responses are directed against PorA, which is antigenically variable. OMV vaccines are not available in the USA, where group B organisms demonstrate considerable PorA diversity. Promising alternative approaches for prevention of group B disease include two recombinant protein vaccines. Both vaccines are based on a novel antigen called factor H-binding protein (fHbp), given either alone (two antigenic variants) or in combination with two other recombinant proteins and an OMV vaccine. These vaccines are currently undergoing evaluation of safety and immunogenicity in infants, toddlers, and adolescents.

Recommendations for meningococcal vaccination can be found in Table 184-3. **MCV4-DT or MenACWY-CRM as a single dose is routinely recommended for all adolescents at 11-12 yr at the preadolescent visit, and adolescents at age 15 yr or high school entry if not previously vaccinated.** MPSV4 remains an acceptable alternative for this age group when conjugate vaccines are unavailable. MCV4-DT or MenACWY-CRM and the Tdap (tetanus and diphtheria toxoids and acellular pertussis booster) vaccine should be administered at separate injection sites to adolescents during the same visit if both vaccines are indicated. If this is not feasible, the meningococcal conjugate vaccines and Tdap can be administered in either sequence with a minimum interval of 1 mo between vaccines. MenACWY-CRM also can be administered at separate injection sites with Tdap and HPV vaccines. Either conjugate vaccine is also recommended for all incoming college freshmen living in dormitories who have not been previously immunized with a meningococcal vaccine. Many colleges and universities, and some states, have mandated meningococcal immunization of all matriculating freshmen. Because of waning immunity, otherwise healthy adolescents who received a first dose at age 11-12 yr should receive a booster dose of a meningococcal conjugate vaccine at 16 yr of age. For those given a first dose at age 13-15 yr, and who have not yet reached their 21st birthday, the booster dose should be given 5 yr after the first dose.

Two doses of MCV4-DT separated by 8 wk are recommended for children beginning at age 2 yr who are at increased risk of meningococcal disease because of immune or anatomic defects. These include children with anatomic or functional asplenia, complement component deficiencies, and those infected with HIV. Persons with immune or anatomic defects who have previously been vaccinated with a single dose should receive a booster dose at the earliest opportunity and then continue to receive boosters. For those immunized at 2-6 yr of age, a booster dose can be given after 3 yr. For those initially vaccinated at 7 yr of age or older, the booster dose can be given after 5 yr.

A single dose of MCV4-DT is recommended beginning at age 2 yr for otherwise healthy children traveling to areas of the world with high endemic or epidemic meningococcal disease rates such as sub-Saharan Africa. For children who continue to be at increased risk of exposure, a booster dose can be given after 3-5 yr (see above).

Cases of Guillain-Barré syndrome (GBS) with onset temporally associated with the administration of MCV4-DT had been reported to the Vaccine Adverse Events Reporting System. The data do not permit exclusion of a small increase in risk for GBS over what would be expected in the absence of a meningococcal conjugate vaccination program. A possible risk of GBS should be discussed during the informed consent process. Except in children at high risk for development of meningococcal disease, MCV4 vaccination should be avoided when there is a past medical history of GBS.

BIBLIOGRAPHY

Please visit the Nelson Textbook of Pediatrics *website at www.expertconsult.com for the complete bibliography.*

Chapter 185
Neisseria gonorrhoeae (Gonococcus)

Toni Darville

Neisseria gonorrhoeae produces several forms of **gonorrhea,** an infection of the genitourinary tract mucous membranes and rarely of the mucosa of the rectum, oropharynx, and conjunctiva. Gonorrhea transmitted by sexual contact or perinatally is 2nd only to chlamydial infections in the number of cases reported to the Centers for Disease Control and Prevention (CDC) in the USA. This high prevalence and the development of antibiotic-resistant strains have produced significant morbidity in adolescents.

ETIOLOGY

N. gonorrhoeae is a nonmotile, aerobic, non–spore-forming, gram-negative intracellular diplococcus with flattened adjacent surfaces. Optimal growth occurs at 35-37°C and at pH 7.2-7.6 in an atmosphere of 3-5% carbon dioxide. The specimen should be inoculated immediately onto fresh, moist, modified Thayer-Martin or specialized transport media because gonococci do not tolerate drying. Thayer-Martin medium contains antimicrobial agents that inhibit hardier normal flora present in clinical specimens that may otherwise overgrow gonococci. Presumptive identification may be based on colony appearance, Gram stain appearance, and production of cytochrome oxidase. Gonococci are differentiated from other *Neisseria* species by the fermentation of glucose but not maltose, sucrose, or lactose. Gram-negative diplococci are seen in infected material, often within polymorphonuclear leukocytes.

Like all gram-negative bacteria, *N. gonorrhoeae* possesses a cell envelope composed of an inner cytoplasmic membrane, a middle layer of peptidoglycan, and an outer membrane. The outer membrane contains lipo-oligosaccharides (endotoxin), phospholipid, and a variety of proteins that contribute to cell adherence, tissue invasion, and resistance to host defenses. The 2 systems primarily used to characterize gonococcal strains are auxotyping and serotyping. Auxotyping is based on genetically stable requirements of strains for specific nutrients or cofactors as defined by an isolate's ability to grow on chemically defined media. The most widely used serotyping system is based on a porin called PorI, a trimeric outer membrane protein that makes up a substantial part of the gonococcal envelope structure. Antibodies generated to *PorI* have been used to serotype gonococci (e.g., PorIA-4 and PorIB-12), and changes in PorI proteins present in a community are believed to occur, at least in part, as a result of selective immune pressure.

EPIDEMIOLOGY

N. gonorrhoeae infection occurs only in humans. The organism is shed in the exudate and secretions of infected mucosal surfaces and is transmitted through intimate contact, such as sexual contact or parturition, and rarely by contact with fomites. Gonococcal infections in the newborn period are generally acquired during delivery. Gonorrhea is the most common sexually transmitted infection found in sexually abused children. Rarely, *N. gonorrhoeae* may be spread by sexual play among children, but the index patient is likely to be a victim of sexual abuse. Gonococcal infections in children are acquired rarely through household exposure to infected caretakers. In such cases, the possibility of sexual abuse should be seriously considered.

The number of reported cases of gonorrhea increased steadily in the USA from 1964 to 1977, fluctuated through the early 1980s, and increased until 1987, when reported rates were 323/100,000. Rates decreased annually from 1987 to 1996, when reported rates were 123/100,000 population. Since 1996, rates declined or were stable, although in 2005 the national rate (116/100,000 population) increased for the first time since 1999. The decline in gonorrhea prevalence may be attributed to recommendations by the CDC that only highly effective antimicrobial agents be used to treat gonorrhea. The incidence of gonorrhea is highest in high-density urban areas among persons < 24 yr of age who have multiple sex partners and engage in unprotected sexual intercourse. Increases in gonorrhea prevalence have been noted among men who have sex with men (MSM). Risk factors include nonwhite race, homosexuality, increased number of sexual partners, prostitution, presence of other sexually transmitted infections, unmarried status, poverty, and failure to use condoms. Auxotyping and serotyping techniques and, more recently, molecular typing methods have been used to analyze the spread of individual strains of *N. gonorrhoeae* within a community.

Maintenance and subsequent spread of gonococcal infections in a community require a hyperendemic, high-risk core group such as prostitutes or adolescents with multiple sexual partners. This observation reflects the fact that most persons who have gonorrhea cease sexual activity and seek care, unless economic need or other factors (e.g., drug addiction) drive persistent sexual activity. Thus, many core transmitters belong to a subset of infected persons who lack or ignore symptoms and continue to be sexually active, underscoring the importance of seeking out and treating the sexual contacts of infected persons who present for treatment.

Gonococcal infection of **neonates** usually results from peripartum exposure to infected exudate from the cervix of the mother. An acute infection begins 2-5 days after birth. The incidence of neonatal infection depends on the prevalence of gonococcal infection among pregnant women, prenatal screening for gonorrhea, and neonatal ophthalmic prophylaxis.

PATHOGENESIS AND PATHOLOGY

N. gonorrhoeae infects primarily columnar epithelium, because stratified squamous epithelium is relatively resistant to invasion. Mucosal invasion by gonococci results in a local inflammatory response that produces a purulent exudate consisting of polymorphonuclear leukocytes, serum, and desquamated epithelium. The gonococcal lipo-oligosaccharide (endotoxin) exhibits direct cytotoxicity, causing ciliostasis and sloughing of ciliated epithelial cells. Once the gonococcus traverses the mucosal barrier, the lipo-oligosaccharide binds bactericidal immunoglobulin M (IgM) antibody and serum complement, causing an acute inflammatory response in the subepithelial space. Tumor necrosis factor and other cytokines are thought to mediate the cytotoxicity of gonococcal infections.

Gonococci may ascend the urogenital tract, causing urethritis or epididymitis in postpubertal males and acute endometritis, salpingitis, and peritonitis (collectively termed **acute pelvic inflammatory disease** or **PID**) in postpubertal females. Dissemination from the fallopian tubes through the peritoneum to the liver capsule results in **perihepatitis (Fitz-Hugh–Curtis syndrome)**. Gonococci that invade the lymphatics and blood vessels may cause inguinal lymphadenopathy; perineal, perianal, ischiorectal, and periprostatic abscesses; and disseminated gonococcal infection (DGI).

A number of gonococcal virulence and host immune factors are involved in the penetration of the mucosal barrier and subsequent manifestations of local and systemic infection. Selective pressure from different mucosal environments probably leads to changes in the outer membrane of the organism, including expression of variants of pili, opacity or Opa proteins (formerly protein II), and lipo-oligosaccharides. These changes may enhance gonococcal attachment, invasion, replication, and evasion of the host's immune response.

For infection to occur, the gonococcus must first attach to host cells. A gonococcal IgA protease inactivates IgA1 by cleaving the molecule in the hinge region and may be an important factor in colonization or invasion of host mucosal surfaces. Gonococci adhere to the microvilli of nonciliated epithelial cells by hairlike protein structures (pili) that extend from the cell wall. Pili are thought to protect the gonococcus from phagocytosis and complement-mediated killing. Pili undergo high-frequency antigenic variation that may aid in the organism's escape from the host immune response and may provide specific ligands for different cell receptors. Opacity proteins, most of which confer an opaque appearance to colonies, are also thought to function as ligands to facilitate binding to human cells. Gonococci that express certain Opa proteins adhere to and are phagocytosed by human neutrophils in the absence of serum.

Other phenotypic changes that occur in response to environmental stresses allow gonococci to establish infection. Examples include iron-repressible proteins for binding transferrin or lactoferrin, anaerobically expressed proteins, and proteins that are synthesized in response to contact with epithelial cells. Gonococci may grow in vivo under anaerobic conditions or in an environment with a relative lack of iron.

Approximately 24 hr after attachment, the epithelial cell surface invaginates and surrounds the gonococcus in a phagocytic vacuole. This phenomenon is thought to be mediated by the insertion of gonococcal outer membrane protein I into the host cell, causing alterations in membrane permeability. Subsequently, phagocytic vacuoles begin releasing gonococci into the subepithelial space by means of exocytosis. Viable organisms may then cause local disease (i.e., salpingitis) or disseminate through the bloodstream or lymphatics.

Serum IgG and IgM directed against gonococcal proteins and lipo-oligosaccharides lead to complement-mediated bacterial lysis. Stable serum resistance to this bactericidal antibody probably results from a particular type of porin protein expressed in gonococci (most contain PorIA), predisposing to disseminated disease. *N. gonorrhoeae* differentially subverts the effectiveness of complement and alters the inflammatory responses elicited in human infection. Isolates from cases of DGI typically resist killing by normal serum (i.e., are serum resistant), inactivate more C3b, generate less C5a, and result in less inflammation at local sites. PID isolates are serum sensitive, inactivate less C3b, generate more C5a, and result in more inflammation at local sites. IgG antibody directed against gonococcal reduction-modifiable protein (Rmp) blocks complement-mediated killing of *N. gonorrhoeae*. Anti-Rmp blocking antibodies may harbor specificity for outer membrane protein sequences shared with other neisserial species or Enterobacteriaceae, may be directed against unique Rmp upstream cysteine loop–specific sequences, or both. Preexisting antibodies directed against Rmp facilitate transmission of gonococcal infection to exposed women; Rmp is highly conserved in *N. gonorrhoeae,* and the blocking of mucosal defenses may be one of its functions. Gonococcal adaptation also appears to be important in the evasion of killing by neutrophils. Examples include sialylation of lipo-oligosaccharides, increases in catalase production, and changes in the expression of surface proteins.

Host factors may influence the incidence and manifestations of gonococcal infection. Prepubertal girls are susceptible to vulvovaginitis and, rarely, experience salpingitis. *N. gonorrhoeae* infects noncornified epithelium, and the thin noncornified vaginal epithelium and alkaline pH of the vaginal mucin predispose this age group to infection of the lower genital tract. Estrogen-induced cornification of the vaginal epithelium in neonates and mature females resists infection. Postpubertal females are more susceptible to salpingitis, especially during menses, when diminished bactericidal activity of the cervical mucus and reflux of blood from the uterine cavity into the fallopian tubes facilitate passage of gonococci into the upper reproductive tract.

Populations at risk for DGI include asymptomatic carriers; neonates; menstruating, pregnant, and postpartum women; homosexuals; and immunocompromised hosts. The asymptomatic carrier state implies failure of the host immune system to recognize the gonococcus as a pathogen, the capacity of the gonococcus to avoid being killed, or both. Pharyngeal colonization has been proposed as a risk factor for DGI. The high rate of asymptomatic infection in pharyngeal gonorrhea may account for this phenomenon. Women are at greater risk for development of DGI during menstruation, pregnancy, and the postpartum period, presumably because of the maximal endocervical shedding and decreased peroxidase bactericidal activity of the cervical mucus during these periods. A lack of neonatal bactericidal IgM antibody is thought to account for the increased susceptibility of neonates to DGI. Persons with terminal complement component deficiencies (C5-C9) are at considerable risk for development of recurrent episodes of DGI.

CLINICAL MANIFESTATIONS

Gonorrhea is manifested by a spectrum of clinical presentations from asymptomatic carriage, to the characteristic localized urogenital infections, to disseminated systemic infection (Chapter 114).

Asymptomatic Gonorrhea

The incidence of asymptomatic gonorrhea in children has not been ascertained. Gonococci have been isolated from the oropharynx of young children who have been abused sexually by male contacts; oropharyngeal symptoms are usually absent. Most genital tract infections produce symptoms in children. However, as many as 80% of sexually mature females with urogenital gonorrhea infections are asymptomatic in settings in which most infections are detected through screening or other case-finding efforts. This situation is in contrast to that in men, who are asymptomatic only 10% of the time. Asymptomatic rectal carriage of *N. gonorrhoeae* has been documented in 40-60% of females with urogenital infection. Most persons with positive rectal culture results are asymptomatic. Most pharyngeal gonococcal infections are asymptomatic. The importance of documenting pharyngeal infection is debated. Most cases resolve spontaneously, transmission from the pharynx to other patients is uncommon, and the pharynx is rarely the only site of infection. Nevertheless, asymptomatic pharyngeal infection may lead to systemic infection and is occasionally the source of transmission to sexual partners.

Uncomplicated Gonorrhea

Genital gonorrhea has an incubation period of 2-5 days in men and 5-10 days in women. Primary infection develops in the urethra of males, the vulva and vagina of prepubertal females, and the cervix of postpubertal females. Neonatal ophthalmitis occurs in both sexes.

Urethritis is usually characterized by a purulent discharge and by dysuria without urgency or frequency. Untreated urethritis in males resolves spontaneously in several weeks or may be complicated by epididymitis, penile edema, lymphangitis, prostatitis, or seminal vesiculitis. Gram-negative intracellular diplococci are found in the discharge.

In prepubertal females, **vulvovaginitis** is usually characterized by a purulent vaginal discharge with a swollen, erythematous, tender, and excoriated vulva. Dysuria may occur. In postpubertal females, symptomatic gonococcal cervicitis and urethritis are characterized by purulent discharge, suprapubic pain, dysuria, intermenstrual bleeding, and dyspareunia. The cervix may be inflamed and tender. In urogenital gonorrhea limited to the lower genital tract, pain is not enhanced by moving the cervix, and the adnexa are not tender to palpation. Purulent material may be expressed from the urethra or ducts of the Bartholin gland. Rectal gonorrhea is often asymptomatic but may cause proctitis with symptoms of anal discharge, pruritus, bleeding, pain, tenesmus, and constipation. Asymptomatic rectal gonorrhea may not be due to anal intercourse but may represent colonization from vaginal infection.

Gonococcal **ophthalmitis** may be unilateral or bilateral and may occur in any age group after inoculation of the eye with infected secretions. Ophthalmia neonatorum due to *N. gonorrhoeae* usually appears from 1 to 4 days after birth (Chapter 618). Ocular infection in older patients results from inoculation or autoinoculation from a genital site. The infection begins with mild inflammation and a serosanguineous discharge. Within 24 hr, the discharge becomes thick and purulent, and tense edema of the eyelids with marked chemosis occurs. If the disease is not treated promptly, corneal ulceration, rupture, and blindness may follow.

Disseminated Gonococcal Infection

Hematogenous dissemination occurs in 1-3% of all gonococcal infections, more frequently after asymptomatic primary infections than symptomatic infections. Women account for the majority of cases, with symptoms beginning 7-30 days after infection and within 7 days of menstruation. The most common manifestations are asymmetric arthralgia, petechial or pustular acral skin lesions, tenosynovitis, suppurative arthritis, and, rarely, carditis, meningitis, and osteomyelitis. The most common initial symptom is acute onset of polyarthralgia with fever. Only 25% of patients complain of skin lesions. Most deny genitourinary symptoms; however, primary mucosal infection is documented by genitourinary cultures. Results of approximately 80-90% of cervical cultures are positive in women with DGI. In males, urethral culture results are positive in 50-60%, pharyngeal culture results are positive in 10-20%, and rectal culture results are positive in 15% of cases.

DGI has been classified into 2 clinical syndromes that have some overlapping features. The 1st and more common is the **tenosynovitis-dermatitis syndrome,** which is characterized by fever, chills, skin lesions, and polyarthralgia predominantly involving the wrists, hands, and fingers. Blood culture results are positive in approximately 30-40% of cases, and results of synovial fluid cultures are almost uniformly negative. The 2nd syndrome is the **suppurative arthritis syndrome,** in which systemic symptoms and signs are less prominent and monarticular arthritis, often involving the knee, is more common. A polyarthralgia phase may precede the monarticular infection. In cases of monarticular involvement, synovial fluid culture results are positive in approximately 45-55%, and synovial fluid findings are consistent with septic arthritis. Blood culture results are usually negative. DGI in neonates usually occurs as a polyarticular suppurative arthritis.

Dermatologic lesions usually begin as painful, discrete, 1- to 20-mm pink or red macules that progress to maculopapular, vesicular, bullous, pustular, or petechial lesions. The typical necrotic pustule on an erythematous base is distributed unevenly over the extremities, including the palmar and plantar surfaces, usually sparing the face and scalp. The lesions number between 5 and 40, and 20-30% may contain gonococci. Although immune complexes may be present in DGI, complement levels are normal, and the role of the immune complexes in pathogenesis is uncertain.

Acute endocarditis is an uncommon (1-2%) but often fatal manifestation of DGI that usually leads to rapid destruction of the aortic valve. Acute pericarditis is a rarely described entity in patients with disseminated gonorrhea. Meningitis with *N. gonorrhoeae* has been documented. Signs and symptoms are similar to those of any acute bacterial meningitis.

DIAGNOSIS

It is not possible to distinguish gonococcal from nongonococcal urethritis on the basis of symptoms and signs alone. Gonococcal urethritis and vulvovaginitis must be distinguished from other infections that produce a purulent discharge, including β-hemolytic streptococci, *Chlamydia trachomatis, Mycoplasma hominis, Trichomonas vaginalis,* and *Candida albicans.* Rarely, infection with human herpes simplex virus type 2 may produce symptoms similar to those of gonorrhea.

In males with symptomatic urethritis, a presumptive diagnosis of gonorrhea can be made by identification of gram-negative intracellular diplococci (within leukocytes) in the urethral discharge. A similar finding in females is not sufficient because *Mima polymorpha* and *Moraxella,* which are normal vaginal flora, have a similar appearance. The sensitivity of the Gram stain for diagnosing gonococcal cervicitis and asymptomatic infections is also low. The presence of commensal *Neisseria* species in the oropharynx prevents the use of the Gram stain for diagnosis of pharyngeal gonorrhea. Nonpathogenic *Neisseria* organisms are not found intracellularly.

Specific testing for *N. gonorrhoeae* is recommended because a specific diagnosis might enhance partner notification. Highly sensitive and specific testing methods are available. Culture, nucleic acid hybridization tests, and nucleic acid amplification tests (NAATs) are available for the detection of genitourinary infection. Culture and nucleic acid hybridization tests require female endocervical or male urethral swab specimens. NAATs offer the widest range of testing specimen types; they are cleared by the U.S. Food and Drug Administration (FDA) for use with endocervical swabs, vaginal swabs, male urethral swabs, and female and male urine. However, product inserts for each NAAT vendor must be carefully examined to assess current indications. Nonculture tests are not FDA cleared for use with specimens from the rectum and pharynx or for use with specimens obtained from the oropharynx, rectum, or genital tract of children. Nonculture gonococcal tests for gonococci (e.g., gram-stained smear, nucleic acid hybridization tests, and NAATs) should not be used without standard culture in children because of the legal implications of a diagnosis of *N. gonorrhoeae* infection in a child. Nonculture tests cannot provide antimicrobial susceptibility results, so in cases of persistent gonococcal infection after treatment, clinicians should perform both culture and antimicrobial susceptibility testing.

Material for cervical cultures is obtained as follows: After the exocervix is wiped, a swab is placed in the cervical os and rotated gently for several seconds. Male urethral specimens are obtained by placement of a small swab 2-3 cm into the urethra. Rectal swabs are best obtained by passing of a swab 2-4 cm into the anal canal; specimens that are heavily contaminated by feces should be discarded. For optimal culture results, specimens should be obtained with noncotton swabs (e.g., a urethrogenital calcium alginate–tipped swab [Calgiswab, Puritan Medical Products, Guilford, ME]), inoculated directly onto culture plates, and incubated immediately. The choice of anatomic sites to culture depends on the sites exposed and the clinical manifestations. Samples from the urethra should be cultured for heterosexual men, and samples from the endocervix and rectum should be cultured for all females, regardless of a history of anal intercourse. A pharyngeal culture specimen should be obtained from both men and women if symptoms of pharyngitis are present or in the case of oral exposure to a person known to have genital gonorrhea. In a suspected case of child sexual abuse, rectal, pharyngeal, and urethral (males) or vaginal (females) swabs should be cultured. Culture of the endocervix should not be attempted until after puberty.

Specimens from sites that are normally colonized by other organisms (e.g., cervix, rectum, pharynx) should be inoculated on a selective culture medium, such as modified Thayer-Martin medium (fortified with vancomycin, colistin, nystatin, and trimethoprim to inhibit growth of indigenous flora). Specimens from sites that are normally sterile or minimally contaminated (i.e., synovial fluid, blood, cerebrospinal fluid) should be inoculated on a nonselective chocolate agar medium. If DGI is suspected, blood, pharynx, rectum, urethra, cervix, and synovial fluid (if involved) should be cultured. Cultured specimens should be incubated promptly at 35-37°C in 3-5% carbon dioxide. When specimens must be transported to a central laboratory for culture plating, a reduced, non-nutrient holding medium (i.e., Amies modified Stuart medium) preserves specimens with minimal loss of viability for up to 6 hr. When transport may delay culture plating by more than 6 hr, it is preferable to inoculate the sample directly onto a culture medium and transport it at an ambient temperature in a candle jar. The Transgrow and JEMBEC (John E. Martin Biological Environmental Chamber) systems of modified Thayer-Martin medium are alternative transport systems.

Gonococcal arthritis must be distinguished from other forms of septic arthritis as well as from rheumatic fever, rheumatoid arthritis, inflammatory bowel disease, and arthritis secondary to rubella or rubella immunization. Gonococcal conjunctivitis in the newborn period must be differentiated from chemical conjunctivitis caused by silver nitrate drops as well as from conjunctivitis caused by *C. trachomatis, Staphylococcus aureus,* group A or B streptococcus, *Pseudomonas aeruginosa, Streptococcus pneumoniae,* or human herpes simplex virus type 2.

TREATMENT

All patients who are presumed or proven to have gonorrhea should be evaluated for concurrent syphilis, hepatitis B, HIV, and *C. trachomatis* infection. The incidence of *Chlamydia* co-infection is 15-25% among males and 35-50% among females. Patients beyond the neonatal period should be treated presumptively for *C. trachomatis* infection unless a negative chlamydial NAAT result is documented at the time treatment is initiated for gonorrhea. However, if chlamydial test results are not available or if a non-NAAT result is negative for *Chlamydia,* patients should be treated for both gonorrhea and *Chlamydia* infection (Chapter 218.2). Sexual partners exposed in the preceding 60 days should be examined, culture specimens should be collected, and presumptive treatment should be started.

Because of the prevalence of penicillin-resistant *N. gonorrhoeae,* ceftriaxone (a 3rd-generation cephalosporin) is recommended as initial therapy for all ages. Antimicrobial resistance in *N. gonorrhoeae* occurs as plasmid-mediated resistance to penicillin and tetracycline and chromosomally mediated resistance to penicillins, tetracyclines, spectinomycin, and fluoroquinolones. As a consequence of widespread fluoroquinolone-resistant gonorrhea in the USA, this class of antibiotics is no longer recommended for the treatment of gonorrhea in this country.

Adolescent and Adult Infections

A single dose of ceftriaxone (125 mg intramuscularly [IM]) eradicates pharyngeal and uncomplicated urogenital gonococcal infections. Ceftriaxone is safe and effective in pregnant women and probably aborts incubating syphilis. Alternative regimens include cefixime (400 mg by mouth [PO]) in a single dose. The efficacy of cefixime against incubating syphilis is uncertain. Other single-dose cephalosporin therapies that are considered alternative treatment regimens for uncomplicated urogenital and anorectal gonococcal infections include ceftizoxime 500 mg IM; cefoxitin 2 g IM, administered with probenecid 1 g PO; and cefotaxime 500 mg IM. Some evidence indicates that cefpodoxime 400 mg and cefuroxime axetil 1 g might be oral alternatives. Spectinomycin (40 mg/kg, maximum dose 2 g) in a single IM dose remains highly effective for genital and rectal gonorrhea in the USA but is ineffective for pharyngeal infection and does not inhibit *Treponema pallidum.* Regardless of the regimen chosen, treatment should be followed by a regimen active against *C. trachomatis* unless *Chlamydia* infection is ruled out by a negative chlamydial NAAT result. The recommended regimen is doxycycline (100 mg PO twice daily for 7 days) or azithromycin (1g PO in a single dose). Adolescents and adults who are asymptomatic after treatment need not under culture for confirmation of cure.

Pregnant women should not be treated with quinolones or tetracyclines. Those infected with *N. gonorrhoeae* should be treated with a recommended or alternate cephalosporin. Either azithromycin or amoxicillin is recommended for treatment of presumptive or proven *C. trachomatis* infection during pregnancy.

The initial management of DGI includes hospitalization and parenteral administration of ceftriaxone (1 g/day). Alternative cephalosporins include cefotaxime (1 g intravenously [IV] every 8 hr) and ceftizoxime (1g IV every 8 hr). Patients should be examined for clinical evidence of endocarditis and meningitis. Treatment may be switched to oral regimens after 24-48 hr and as clinical improvement is obvious. Oral regimens include cefixime (400 mg PO bid) and cefpodoxime (400 mg PO bid) to complete 7 days of therapy. Fluoroquinolones may be an alternative treatment option if antimicrobial susceptibility to these agents can be documented by culture.

Gonococcal conjunctivitis should be treated with ceftriaxone (1g IM in a single dose) with lavage of the infected eye with saline. Meningitis is treated with ceftriaxone (1-2 g IV every 12 hr) for 10-14 days. Endocarditis is treated for >4 wk with ceftriaxone (1-2 g IV every 12 hr). Concurrent therapy for treatment of genital *Chlamydia* infection is important.

Infant and Pediatric Infections

Uncomplicated gonococcal infections in children should be treated with ceftriaxone in a single dose (50 mg/kg IM, not to exceed 125 mg). Children who have bacteremia or arthritis should be treated with ceftriaxone (50 mg/kg/day, maximum 1 g/day if <45 kg) for a minimum of 7 days. Meningitis should be treated for 10-14 days, and endocarditis for a minimum of 28 days, with ceftriaxone (50 mg/kg/dose every 12 hr with maximum of 1-2 g IV every 12 hr). Neonatal gonococcal ophthalmia is treated effectively with a single dose of ceftriaxone (50 mg/kg IM, not to exceed 125 mg); a single dose of cefotaxime (100 mg/kg IM) is an acceptable alternative. The conjunctivae should be irrigated frequently with physiologic saline solution. Infants born to mothers who have gonococcal infection should also receive a single dose of ceftriaxone (50 mg/kg IM, not to exceed 125 mg). Neonatal sepsis should be treated parenterally for a minimum of 7 days, and meningitis for a minimum of 10 days. Cefotaxime is recommended for infants with hyperbilirubinemia, because ceftriaxone competes for bilirubin binding sites on albumin. Neonates with gonococcal ophthalmitis must be hospitalized and evaluated for DGI.

Pelvic Inflammatory Disease

PID encompasses a spectrum of infectious diseases of the upper genital tract due to *N. gonorrhoeae*, *C. trachomatis*, and endogenous flora (streptococci, anaerobes, gram-negative bacilli). For women with more severe symptoms, parenteral therapy should be initiated in the hospital. A commonly recommended therapeutic regimen is cefoxitin (2g IV every 6 hr) or cefotetan (2g IV every 12 hr) plus doxycycline (100 mg PO or IV every 12 hr). Alternative regimens include clindamycin (900 mg IV every 8 hr) plus a loading dose of gentamicin (2 mg/kg IV) followed by maintenance gentamicin (1.5 mg/kg every 8 hr), and ampicillin/sulbactam (3 g IV every 6 hr) plus doxycycline (100 mg PO or IV every 12 hr). Clinical experience should guide transition to oral therapy, which usually can be initiated within 24 hr of improvement. Thereafter, oral doxycycline is given to complete 14 days of total therapy.

Parenteral therapy and oral therapy appear to be similar in clinical efficacy for women with PID of mild to moderate severity. Clinical response to outpatient treatment is similar among younger and older women. The decision to hospitalize adolescents with acute PID should be based on clinical criteria used for older women. Those who do not show response to oral therapy within 72 hr should be reevaluated to confirm the diagnosis and then should receive parenteral therapy. Recommended oral regimens are as follows: a single dose of ceftriaxone (250 mg IM) plus doxycycline (100 mg PO bid) with or without metronidazole (500 mg PO bid) for 14 days; and single doses of cefoxitin (2 g IM) and probenecid (1 g PO) plus doxycycline (100 mg PO bid) with or without metronidazole (500 mg PO bid) for 14 days. If the patient has an intrauterine device, it must be removed and an alternative form of birth control used. Sexual partners should be examined and treated for uncomplicated gonorrhea. Follow-up culture (test of cure) after cephalosporin-doxycycline therapy of gonococcal infection is not recommended owing to the low treatment failure rate. A follow-up examination and culture are recommended in 1-2 mo to evaluate the possibility of re-infection or, rarely, treatment failure.

COMPLICATIONS

Complications of gonorrhea result from the spread of gonococci from a local site of invasion. The interval between primary infection and development of a complication is usually days to weeks. In postpubertal females, endometritis may occur, especially during menses, and may progress to salpingitis and peritonitis (PID). Manifestations of PID include signs of lower genital tract infection (e.g., vaginal discharge, suprapubic pain, cervical tenderness) and upper genital tract infection (e.g., fever, leukocytosis, elevated erythrocyte sedimentation rate, and adnexal tenderness or mass). The differential diagnosis includes gynecologic diseases (ovarian cyst, ovarian tumor, ectopic pregnancy) and intra-abdominal disorders (appendicitis, urinary tract infection, inflammatory bowel disease).

Once inside the peritoneum, gonococci may seed the liver capsule, causing a perihepatitis with right upper quadrant pain (Fitz-Hugh–Curtis syndrome), with or without signs of salpingitis. Perihepatitis may also be caused by *C. trachomatis*. Progression to PID occurs in about 20% of cases of gonococcal cervicitis, and *N. gonorrhoeae* is isolated in approximately 40% of cases of PID in the USA. Untreated cases may lead to hydrosalpinx, pyosalpinx, tubo-ovarian abscess, and eventual sterility. Even with adequate treatment of PID, the risk for sterility due to bilateral tubal occlusion approaches 20% after 1 episode of salpingitis and exceeds 60% after 3 or more episodes. The risk for ectopic pregnancy is increased approximately sevenfold after 1 or more episodes of salpingitis. Additional sequelae of PID include chronic pain, dyspareunia, and increased risk for recurrent PID.

Urogenital gonococcal infection acquired during the 1st trimester of pregnancy carries a high risk for septic abortion. After 16 wk, infection leads to chorioamnionitis, a major cause of premature rupture of the membranes and premature delivery.

PROGNOSIS

Prompt diagnosis and correct therapy ensure complete recovery from uncomplicated gonococcal disease. Complications and permanent sequelae may be associated with delayed treatment, recurrent infection, metastatic sites of infection (meninges, aortic valve), and delayed or topical therapy of gonococcal ophthalmia.

PREVENTION

Efforts to develop a gonococcal pilus vaccine have been unsuccessful thus far. The high degree of interstrain and intrastrain antigenic variability of pili poses a formidable deterrent to the development of a single effective pilus vaccine. Other gonococcal surface structures, such as the porin protein, stress proteins, and lipo-oligosaccharides, may prove more promising as vaccine candidates. In the absence of a vaccine, prevention of gonorrhea can be achieved through education, use of barrier contraceptives (especially condoms and spermicides), intensive epidemiologic and bacteriologic surveillance (screening sexual contacts), and early identification and treatment of infected contacts.

Gonococcal ophthalmia neonatorum can be prevented by instilling 2 drops of a 1% solution of silver nitrate into each conjunctival sac shortly after birth (Chapter 618). Erythromycin (0.5%) or tetracycline (1%) ophthalmic ointment may also be used.

BIBLIOGRAPHY

Please visit the Nelson Textbook of Pediatrics *website at www.expertconsult.com for the complete bibliography.*

Chapter 186
Haemophilus influenzae

Robert S. Daum

An effective vaccine to prevent *Haemophilus influenzae* type b disease introduced in the USA and many other countries has resulted in a dramatic decrease in the incidence of infections caused by this organism. However, mortality and morbidity from *H. influenzae* type b infection remain a problem worldwide, primarily in developing countries. Occasional cases of invasive disease caused by non–type b organisms continue to occur but infrequently. Nontypable members of the species are important causes of otitis media and sinusitis.

ETIOLOGY

H. influenzae is a fastidious, gram-negative, pleomorphic coccobacillus that requires factor X (hematin) and factor V (phosphopyridine nucleotide) for growth. Some *H. influenzae* isolates are surrounded by a polysaccharide capsule and can be serotyped into 6 antigenically and biochemically distinct types designated by letters a-f.

EPIDEMIOLOGY

Before the advent of an effective type b conjugate vaccine in 1988, *H. influenzae* type b was a major cause of serious disease among children in all countries. There was a striking age distribution of cases, with >90% in children <5 yr of age and the majority in children <2 yr of age. The annual attack rate of invasive disease was 64-129 cases/100,000 children <5 yr of age per year. Invasive disease caused by other capsular serotypes has been much less frequent but continues to occur. The incidence of invasive disease caused by b and non–type b serotypes has been estimated at about 0.08 and 1.02 cases/100,000 children <5 yr of age per year, respectively, in the USA. Nonencapsulated (nontypable) *H. influenzae* organisms also occasionally cause invasive disease, especially in neonates, immunocompromised children, and children in developing countries. The estimated rate of invasive disease due to nontypable *H. influenzae* in the USA is 1.88/100,000 children <5 yr of age per year. Nontypable isolates are common etiologic agents in otitis media, sinusitis, and chronic bronchitis.

Humans are the only natural hosts for *H. influenzae*, which is part of the normal respiratory flora in 60-90% of healthy children. Most isolates are nontypable. Before the advent of conjugate vaccine immunization, *H. influenzae* type b could be isolated from the pharynx of 2-5% of healthy preschool and school-aged children, with lower rates among infants and adults. Asymptomatic colonization with *H. influenzae* type b occurs at a much lower rate in immunized populations.

The continued circulation of the type b organism despite current vaccine coverage levels suggests that elimination of type b disease may be a formidable task. The few cases of type b invasive disease in the USA now occur in both unvaccinated and fully vaccinated children. Approximately one half of cases occur in young infants too young to have received a complete primary vaccine series. Among the cases in patients who are old enough to have received a complete vaccine series, the majority are underimmunized. To highlight this point, during a recent shortage of *H. influenzae* type b vaccine, invasive disease developed in five children in Minnesota, all of whom were incompletely immunized. Continued efforts will be necessary to provide currently available conjugate vaccines to children in developing countries, where affordability remains an important issue.

In the pre-vaccine era, certain groups and individuals had an increased incidence of invasive type b disease, including Alaskan Eskimos, Apaches, Navajos, and African-Americans. Persons with certain chronic medical conditions were also known to be at increased risk for invasive disease, including those with sickle cell disease, asplenia, congenital and acquired immunodeficiencies, and malignancies. Unvaccinated infants with invasive *H. influenzae* type b infection are also at increased risk for recurrence, reflecting the fact that they typically do not develop a protective immune response to *H. influenzae*.

Socioeconomic risk factors for invasive *H. influenzae* type b disease included child care outside the home, the presence of siblings of elementary school age or younger, short duration of breastfeeding, and parental smoking. A history of otitis media was associated with an increased risk for invasive disease. Much less is known about the epidemiology of invasive disease due to non–type b strains, and it is not clear whether the epidemiologic features of type b disease apply to disease caused by non–type b isolates.

Among age-susceptible household contacts who have been exposed to a case of invasive *H. influenzae* type b disease, there is increased risk for secondary cases of invasive disease in the first 30 days, especially in susceptible children <24 mo of age. Whether a similar increased risk occurs for contacts of individuals with non–type b disease is unknown.

The mode of transmission is most commonly direct contact or inhalation of respiratory tract droplets containing *H. influenzae*. The incubation period for invasive disease is variable, and the exact period of communicability is unknown. Most children with invasive *H. influenzae* type b disease are colonized in the nasopharynx before initiation of antimicrobial therapy; 25-40% may remain colonized during the first 24 hr of therapy.

With the decline of disease caused by type b organisms, disease caused by other serotypes (a, c-f) and nontypable organisms has been recognized more clearly. There is no evidence that these non–type b infections have increased in frequency. However, clusters of type a and, less often, type f and type e infections have occurred.

PATHOGENESIS

The pathogenesis of disease begins with adherence to respiratory epithelium and colonization of the nasopharynx, which is mediated by pilus and non-pilus adherence factors. The mechanism of entry into the intravascular compartment is unclear but appears to be influenced by cytotoxic factors. Once in the bloodstream, *H. influenzae* type b and perhaps other encapsulated strains resist intravascular clearance mechanisms at least in part via the presence of a polysaccharide capsule. In the case of *H. influenzae* type b, the magnitude and duration of bacteremia influence the likelihood of dissemination of bacteria to sites such as the meninges and joints.

Noninvasive *H. influenzae* infections such as otitis media, sinusitis, and bronchitis are usually caused by nontypable strains. These organisms gain access to sites such as the middle ear and sinus cavities by direct extension from the nasopharynx. Factors facilitating spread from the pharynx include eustachian tube dysfunction and antecedent viral infections of the upper respiratory tract.

Antibiotic Resistance

Most *H. influenzae* isolates are susceptible to ampicillin or amoxicillin, but about a third produce a β-lactamase and are therefore resistant. β-Lactamase–negative ampicillin-resistant (BLNAR) isolates have been identified that manifest resistance by production of a β-lactam–insensitive cell wall synthesis enzyme called PBP3.

Amoxicillin-clavulanate is uniformly active against *H. influenzae* clinical isolates except for the rare BLNAR isolates. Among macrolides, azithromycin is active against about 99% of *H. influenzae* isolates; in contrast, the activity of erythromycin and clarithromycin against *H. influenzae* clinical isolates is poor. *H. influenzae* resistance to 3rd-generation cephalosporins has not been documented. Resistance to trimethoprim-sulfamethoxazole is infrequent (≈10%), and resistance to quinolones is believed to be rare.

Immunity

In the pre-vaccine era, the most important known element of host defense was antibody directed against the type b capsular polysaccharide polyribosylribitol phosphate (PRP). Anti-PRP antibody is acquired in an age-related fashion and facilitates clearance of *H. influenzae* type b from blood, in part related to opsonic activity. Antibodies directed against antigens such as outer membrane proteins or lipopolysaccharides may also have a role in opsonization. Both the classic and alternative complement pathways are important in defense against *H. influenzae* type b.

Before the introduction of vaccination, protection from *H. influenzae* type b infection was presumed to correlate with the concentration of circulating anti-PRP antibody at the time of exposure. A serum antibody concentration of 0.15-1.0 µg/mL was considered protective against invasive infection. Unimmunized infants >6 mo of age and young children usually lacked an anti-PRP antibody concentration of this magnitude and were susceptible to disease after encountering *H. influenzae* type b. This lack of antibody in infants and young children may have reflected a maturational delay in the immunologic response to thymus-independent type 2 (TI-2) antigens such as unconjugated PRP, presumably explaining the high incidence of type b infections in infants and young children in the pre-vaccine era.

The conjugate vaccines (Table 186-1) act as thymus-dependent antigens and elicit serum antibody responses in infants and young children. These vaccines are believed to prime memory antibody responses on subsequent encounters with PRP. The concentration of circulating anti-PRP antibody in a child primed by a conjugate vaccine may not correlate precisely with protection, presumably because a memory response may occur rapidly on exposure to PRP and provide protection.

Much less is known about immunity to other *H. influenzae* serotypes or to nontypable isolates. For nontypable isolates, evidence suggests that antibodies directed against 1 or more outer membrane proteins are bactericidal and protect against experimental challenge. A variety of antigens have been evaluated in an attempt to identify vaccine candidates for nontypable *H. influenzae,* including outer membrane proteins (P1, P2, P4, P5, P6, D15, and Tbp A/B), lipopolysaccharide, various adhesins, and lipoprotein D.

Table 186-1 *HAEMOPHILUS INFLUENZAE* TYPE B CONJUGATE VACCINES AVAILABLE IN THE USA

ABBREVIATION	TRADE NAME	MANUFACTURER	PROTEIN CARRIER	AVAILABLE COMBINATION VACCINES
PRP-OMP	PedvaxHIB	Merck & Co., Inc., Whitehouse Station, NJ	OMP	COMVAX* (PRP-OMP and hepatitis B vaccine)
PRP-T	ActHIB (PRP-T)	Sanofi Pasteur Inc., Swiftwater, PA	Tetanus toxoid	Pentacel (PRP-T, DTaP, and IPV vaccines)

*COMVAX should not be used for hepatitis B immunization at birth.
DTaP, diphtheria and tetanus toxoids and acellular pertussis; HIB, *Haemophilus influenzae* type B; IPV, trivalent, inactivated polio vaccine; OMP, outer membrane protein complex of *Neisseria meningitidis*; PRP, polyribosylribitol phosphate.

DIAGNOSIS

Presumptive identification of *H. influenzae* is established by direct examination of the collected specimen after staining with Gram reagents. Because of its small size, pleomorphism, and occasional poor uptake of stain as well as the tendency for proteinaceous fluids to have a red background, *H. influenzae* is sometimes difficult to visualize. Furthermore, given that identification of microorganisms on smear by either technique requires at least 10^5 bacteria/mL, failure to visualize them does not preclude their presence.

Culture of *H. influenzae* requires prompt transport and processing of specimens because the organism is fastidious. Specimens should not be exposed to drying or temperature extremes. Primary isolation of *H. influenzae* can be accomplished on chocolate agar or on blood agar plates using the staphylococcus streak technique.

Serotyping of *H. influenzae* is accomplished by slide agglutination with type-specific antisera. Accurate serotyping is essential to monitor progress toward elimination of type b invasive disease. Timely reporting of cases to public health authorities should be ensured.

CLINICAL MANIFESTATIONS AND TREATMENT

The initial antibiotic therapy of invasive infections possibly due to *H. influenzae* should be a parenterally administered antimicrobial agent effective in sterilizing all foci of infection and effective against ampicillin-resistant strains, usually an extended-spectrum cephalosporin such as cefotaxime or ceftriaxone. These antibiotics have achieved popularity because of their relative lack of serious adverse effects and ease of administration. After the antimicrobial susceptibility of the isolate has been determined, an appropriate agent can be selected to complete the therapy. Ampicillin remains the drug of choice for the therapy of infections due to susceptible isolates. If the isolate is resistant to ampicillin, ceftriaxone can be administered once daily in selected circumstances for outpatient therapy.

Oral antimicrobial agents are sometimes used to complete a course of therapy initiated by the parenteral route and are typically initial therapy for noninvasive infections such as otitis media and sinusitis. If the organism is susceptible, amoxicillin is the drug of choice. An oral 3rd-generation cephalosporin (e.g., cefixime, cefdinir) or amoxicillin-clavulanate may be used when the isolate is resistant to ampicillin.

Meningitis

In the pre-vaccine era, meningitis accounted for more than half of invasive *H. influenzae* disease. Clinically, meningitis caused by *H. influenzae* type b cannot be differentiated from meningitis caused by *Neisseria meningitidis* or *Streptococcus pneumoniae* (Chapter 595.1). It may be complicated by other foci of infection such as the lungs, joints, bones, and pericardium.

Antimicrobial therapy should be administered intravenously for 7-14 days for uncomplicated cases. Cefotaxime, ceftriaxone, and ampicillin cross the blood-brain barrier during acute inflammation in concentrations adequate to treat *H. influenzae* meningitis. Intramuscular therapy with ceftriaxone is an alternative in patients with normal organ perfusion.

The prognosis of *H. influenzae* type b meningitis depends on the age at presentation, duration of illness before appropriate antimicrobial therapy, cerebrospinal fluid (CSF) capsular polysaccharide concentration, and rapidity with which organisms are cleared from CSF, blood, and urine. Clinically manifested inappropriate secretion of antidiuretic hormone and evidence of focal neurologic deficits at presentation are poor prognostic features. About 6% of patients with *H. influenzae* type b meningitis are left with some hearing impairment, probably because of inflammation of the cochlea and the labyrinth. Dexamethasone (0.6 mg/kg/day divided every 6 hours for 2 days), particularly when given shortly before or concurrent with the initiation of antimicrobial therapy, decreases the incidence of hearing loss. Major neurologic sequelae of *H. influenzae* type b meningitis include behavior problems, language disorders, delayed development of language, impaired vision, mental retardation, motor abnormalities, ataxia, seizures, and hydrocephalus.

Cellulitis

Children with *H. influenzae* cellulitis often have an antecedent upper respiratory tract infection. They usually have no prior history of trauma, and the infection is thought to represent seeding of the organism to the involved soft tissues during bacteremia. The head and neck, particularly the cheek and preseptal region of the eye, are the most common sites of involvement. The involved region generally has indistinct margins and is tender and indurated. Buccal cellulitis is classically erythematous with a violaceous hue, although this sign may be absent. *H. influenzae* may often be recovered directly from an aspirate of the leading edge, although this procedure is seldom performed. The blood culture may also reveal the causative organism. Other foci of infection may be present concomitantly, particularly in children <18 mo of age. A diagnostic lumbar puncture should be considered at the time of diagnosis in these children.

Parenteral antimicrobial therapy is indicated until patients become afebrile, after which an appropriate orally administered antimicrobial agent may be substituted. A 7- to 10-day course is customary.

Preseptal Cellulitis

Infection involving the superficial tissue layers anterior to the orbital septum is termed preseptal cellulitis, which may be caused by *H. influenzae*. Uncomplicated preseptal cellulitis does not imply a risk for visual impairment or direct central nervous system extension. However, concurrent bacteremia may be associated with the development of meningitis. *H. influenzae* preseptal cellulitis is characterized by fever, edema, tenderness, warmth of the lid, and, occasionally, purple discoloration. Evidence of interruption of the integument is usually absent. Conjunctival drainage may be associated. *S. pneumoniae, Staphylococcus aureus,* and group A streptococcus cause clinically indistinguishable preseptal cellulitis. The latter two pathogens are more likely when fever is absent and the integument is interrupted (e.g., an insect bite or trauma).

Children with preseptal cellulitis in whom *H. influenzae* and *S. pneumoniae* are etiologic considerations (young age, high fever, intact integument) should undergo blood culture, and a diagnostic lumbar puncture should be considered.

Parenteral antibiotics are indicated for preseptal cellulitis. Because methicillin-susceptible and methicillin-resistant *S. aureus, S. pneumoniae,* and group A β-hemolytic streptococci are other causes, empirical therapy should include agents active against these pathogens. Patients with preseptal cellulitis without concurrent meningitis should receive parenteral therapy for about 5 days, until fever and erythema have abated. In uncomplicated cases, antimicrobial therapy should be given for 10 days.

Orbital Cellulitis

Infections of the orbit are infrequent and usually develop as complications of acute ethmoid or sphenoid sinusitis. Orbital cellulitis may manifest as lid edema but is distinguished by the presence of proptosis, chemosis, impaired vision, limitation of the extraocular movements, decreased mobility of the globe, or pain on movement of the globe. The distinction between preseptal and orbital cellulitis may be difficult and is best delineated by CT.

Orbital infections are treated with parenteral therapy for at least 14 days. Underlying sinusitis or orbital abscess may require surgical drainage and more prolonged antimicrobial therapy.

Supraglottitis or Acute Epiglottitis

Supraglottitis is a cellulitis of the tissues comprising the laryngeal inlet (Chapter 377). It has become exceedingly rare since the introduction of conjugate type b vaccines. Direct bacterial invasion of the involved tissues is probably the initiating pathophysiologic event. This dramatic, potentially lethal condition can occur at any age. Because of the risk of sudden, unpredictable airway obstruction, supraglottitis is a medical emergency. Other foci of infection, such as meningitis, are rare. Antimicrobial therapy directed against *H. influenzae* and other etiologic agents should be administered parenterally but only after the airway is secured, and therapy should be continued until patients are able to take fluids by mouth. The duration of antimicrobial therapy is typically 7 days.

Pneumonia

The true incidence of *H. influenzae* pneumonia in children is unknown because invasive procedures required to obtain culture specimens are seldom performed (Chapter 392). In the prevaccine era, type b bacteria were believed to be the usual cause. The signs and symptoms of pneumonia due to *H. influenzae* cannot be differentiated from those of pneumonia due to many other microorganisms. Other foci of infection may be present concomitantly.

Children < 12 mo of age in whom *H. influenzae* pneumonia is suspected should receive parenteral antimicrobial therapy initially because of their increased risk for bacteremia and its complications. Older children who do not appear severely ill may be managed with an orally administered antimicrobial. Therapy is continued for 7-10 days. Uncomplicated pleural effusion associated with *H. influenzae* pneumonia requires no special intervention. However, if empyema develops, surgical drainage is indicated.

Suppurative Arthritis

Large joints, such as the knee, hip, ankle, and elbow, are affected most commonly (Chapter 677). Other foci of infection may be present concomitantly. Although single joint involvement is the rule, multiple joint involvement occurs in about 6% of cases. The signs and symptoms of septic arthritis caused by *H. influenzae* are indistinguishable from those of arthritis caused by other bacteria.

Uncomplicated septic arthritis should be treated with an appropriate antimicrobial administered parenterally for at least 5-7 days. If the clinical response is satisfactory, the remainder of the course of antimicrobial treatment may be given orally. Therapy is typically given for 3 wk for uncomplicated septic arthritis, but it may be continued beyond 3 wk, until the C-reactive protein concentration is normal.

Pericarditis

H. influenzae is a rare cause of pericarditis (Chapter 434). Affected children often have had an antecedent upper respiratory tract infection. Fever, respiratory distress, and tachycardia are consistent findings. Other foci of infection may be present concomitantly.

The diagnosis may be established by recovery of the organism from blood or pericardial fluid. Gram stain or detection of PRP in pericardial fluid, blood, or urine (when type b organisms are the cause) may aid the diagnosis. Antimicrobials should be provided parenterally in a regimen similar to that used for meningitis (Chapter 595.1). Pericardiectomy is useful for draining the purulent material effectively and preventing tamponade and constrictive pericarditis.

Bacteremia without an Associated Focus

Bacteremia due to *H. influenzae* may be associated with fever without any apparent focus of infection (Chapter 170). In this situation, risk factors for "occult" bacteremia include the magnitude of fever (≥39°C) and the presence of leukocytosis (≥15,000 cells/µL). In the pre-vaccine era, meningitis developed in about 25% of children with occult *H. influenzae* type b bacteremia if left untreated. In the vaccine era, this *H. influenzae* infection has become exceedingly rare. When it does occur, the child should be re-evaluated for a focus of infection and a second blood culture performed. In general, the child should be hospitalized and given parenteral antimicrobial therapy after a diagnostic lumbar puncture and chest radiograph are obtained.

Miscellaneous Infections

Urinary tract infection, epididymo-orchitis, cervical adenitis, acute glossitis, infected thyroglossal duct cysts, uvulitis, endocarditis, endophthalmitis, primary peritonitis, osteomyelitis, and periappendiceal abscess are rarely caused by *H. influenzae.*

Invasive Disease in Neonates

Neonates rarely have invasive *H. influenzae* infection. In the infant with illness within the first 24 hr of life, especially in association with maternal chorioamnionitis or prolonged rupture of membranes, transmission of the organism to the infant is likely to have occurred through the maternal genital tract, which may be (<1%) colonized with nontypable *H. influenzae.* Manifestations of neonatal invasive infection include bacteremia with sepsis, pneumonia, respiratory distress syndrome with shock, conjunctivitis, scalp abscess or cellulitis, and meningitis. Less commonly, mastoiditis, septic arthritis, and congenital vesicular eruption may occur.

Otitis Media

Acute otitis media is one of the most common infectious diseases of childhood (Chapter 632). It results from the spread of bacteria from the nasopharynx through the eustachian tube into the middle ear cavity. Usually because of a preceding viral upper respiratory tract infection, the mucosa in the area becomes hyperemic and swollen, resulting in obstruction and an opportunity for bacterial multiplication in the middle ear.

The most common bacterial pathogens are *S. pneumoniae, H. influenzae,* and *Moraxella catarrhalis.* Most *H. influenzae* isolates causing otitis media are nontypable. Ipsilateral conjunctivitis may also be present. Amoxicillin (80-90 mg/kg/day) is a suitable first-line oral antimicrobial agent, because the probability that the causative isolate is resistant to amoxicillin and the risk for invasive potential are sufficiently low to justify this approach. Alternatively, in certain cases, a single dose of ceftriaxone constitutes adequate therapy.

In the case of treatment failure or if a β-lactamase–producing isolate is obtained by tympanocentesis or from drainage fluid, amoxicillin-clavulanate (Augmentin) and erythromycin-sulfisoxazole (Pediazole) are among the available alternatives. Erythromycin-sulfisoxazole is useful for patients allergic to β-lactam antibiotics.

Conjunctivitis

Acute infection of the conjunctivae is common in childhood (Chapter 618). In neonates, *H. influenzae* is an infrequent cause. However, it is an important pathogen in older children, as are *S. pneumoniae* and *S. aureus.* Most *H. influenzae* isolates associated with conjunctivitis are nontypable, although type b isolates and other serotypes are occasionally found. Empirical treatment of conjunctivitis beyond the neonatal period usually consists of topical antimicrobial therapy with sulfacetamide. Topical fluoroquinolone therapy is to be avoided because of its broad spectrum, high cost, and high rate of emerging resistance among many bacterial species. Ipsilateral otitis media caused by the same organism may be present and requires oral antibiotic therapy.

Sinusitis

H. influenzae is an important cause of acute sinusitis in children, second in frequency only to *S. pneumoniae* (Chapter 372). Chronic sinusitis lasting >1 yr or severe sinusitis requiring hospitalization is often caused by *S. aureus* or anaerobes such as *Peptococcus, Peptostreptococcus,* and *Bacteroides.* Nontypable *H. influenzae* and viridans group streptococci are also frequently recovered.

For uncomplicated sinusitis, amoxicillin is acceptable initial therapy. However, if clinical improvement does not occur, a broader-spectrum agent, such as amoxicillin-clavulanate, may be appropriate. A 10-day course is sufficient for uncomplicated sinusitis. Hospitalization for parenteral therapy is rarely required; the usual reason is suspicion of progression to orbital cellulitis.

PREVENTION

Universal immunization with *H. influenzae* type b conjugate vaccine is recommended for all infants. Prophylaxis is indicated if close contacts of an index patient with type b disease are unvaccinated. The contagiousness of non–type b *H. influenzae* infections is not known, and prophylaxis is not recommended.

Vaccine

Two *H. influenzae* type b conjugate vaccines are currently marketed in the USA, PRP–outer membrane protein (PRP-OMP) and PRP–tetanus toxoid (PRP-T), which differ in the carrier protein used and the method of conjugating the polysaccharide to the protein (see Table 186-1 and Chapter 165). They are often sold in combination with other vaccines. One combination vaccine, which consists of PRP-OMP combined with hepatitis B vaccine (COMVAX, Merck & Co., Inc., Whitehouse Station, NJ), can be used for doses recommended at 2, 4, and 12-15 mo of age. Another consists of DTaP vaccine (diphtheria and tetanus toxoids and acellular pertussis), IPV vaccine (trivalent, inactivated polio vaccine) and PRP-T, (Pentacel, Sanofi Pasteur Inc., Swiftwater, PA) that can be used for doses recommended at 2, 4, 6, and 12-15 mo of age.

Prophylaxis

Unvaccinated children <48 mo of age who are in close contact with an index case of invasive *H. influenzae* type b infection are at increased risk for invasive infection. The risk for secondary disease for children >3 mo of age is inversely related to age. About half of the secondary cases among susceptible household contacts occur in the first week after hospitalization of the patient with the index case. Because many children are now protected against *H. influenzae* type b by prior immunization, the need for prophylaxis has greatly decreased. When prophylaxis is used, rifampin is indicated for all members of the household or close contact group, including the index patient, if the group includes ≥1 child <48 mo of age who is not fully immunized.

Parents of children hospitalized for invasive *H. influenzae* type b disease should be informed of the increased risk for secondary infection in other young children in the same household if they are not fully immunized. Parents of children exposed to a single case of invasive *H. influenzae* type b disease in a child-care center or nursery school should be similarly informed, although there is disagreement about the need for rifampin prophylaxis for these children.

For prophylaxis, children should be given rifampin orally (0-1 mo of age, 10 mg/kg/dose; >1 mo of age, 20 mg/kg/dose, not to exceed 600 mg/dose) once a day for 4 consecutive days. The adult dose is 600mg once daily. Rifampin prophylaxis is not recommended for pregnant women.

BIBLIOGRAPHY

Please visit the Nelson Textbook of Pediatrics *website at www.expertconsult.com for the complete bibliography.*

Chapter 187
Chancroid (*Haemophilus ducreyi*)

H. Dele Davies and Parvin H. Azimi

Chancroid is a sexually transmitted disease characterized by painful genital ulceration and inguinal lymphadenopathy.

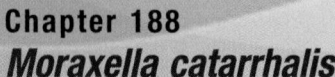

For the full continuation of this chapter, please visit the Nelson Textbook of Pediatrics *website at www.expertconsult.com.*

Chapter 188
Moraxella catarrhalis

Timothy F. Murphy

Moraxella catarrhalis, an unencapsulated gram-negative diplococcus, is a human-specific pathogen that colonizes the respiratory tract beginning in infancy. Colonization and infection with *M. catarrhalis* are increasing in countries in which pneumococcal conjugate vaccines are used widely. The most important clinical manifestation of *M. catarrhalis* infection in children is otitis media.

For the full continuation of this chapter, please visit the Nelson Textbook of Pediatrics *website at www.expertconsult.com.*

Chapter 189
Pertussis (*Bordetella pertussis* and *Bordetella parapertussis*)

Sarah S. Long

Pertussis is an acute respiratory tract infection that was well described initially in the 1500s. Sydenham first used the term *pertussis,* meaning intense cough, in 1670; it is preferable to **whooping cough** because most infected individuals do not "whoop."

ETIOLOGY

Bordetella pertussis is the sole cause of epidemic pertussis and the usual cause of sporadic pertussis. *Bordetella parapertussis* is an occasional cause of sporadic pertussis that contributes significantly to total cases of pertussis in Eastern and Western Europe but accounts for <5% of *Bordetella* isolates in the USA. *B. pertussis* and *B. parapertussis* are exclusive pathogens of humans and some primates.

B. bronchiseptica is a common animal pathogen. Occasional case reports in humans may involve any body site and typically occur in immunocompromised persons or young children with intense exposure to animals. Protracted coughing (which in some cases is paroxysmal) can be caused by *Mycoplasma,* parainfluenza viruses, influenza viruses, enteroviruses, respiratory syncytial viruses, or adenoviruses.

EPIDEMIOLOGY

There are 60 million cases of pertussis each year worldwide, resulting in >500,000 deaths. Before vaccination was available, pertussis was the leading cause of death due to communicable disease among children <14 yr of age in the USA, with 10,000 deaths annually. Widespread use of pertussis vaccine led to a >99% decline in cases. The pivotal role of vaccination in disease control is reflected in the continued high incidence of pertussis in developing countries and the resurgence in other countries where vaccine coverage is low or where less potent vaccine may have been used.

After the low number of 1,010 cases in the USA reported in 1976, there was an increase in annual pertussis incidence to 1.2 cases/100,000 population from 1980 through 1989, with epidemic pertussis in many states in 1989-1990, 1993, and 1996. Since then pertussis has become increasingly endemic, with less cycling or seasonality and with shifting burden of disease to young infants, adolescents, and adults. By 2004, the incidence of reported pertussis in the USA was 8.9 cases/100,000 population, and the number of cases (25,827) was the highest reported since 1959. Of these cases, 10% occurred among infants <6 mo of age (incidence of 136.5/100,000 population). A total of 40 pertussis-related deaths were reported in 2005, and 16 in 2006; >90% occurred among young infants. Approximately 60% of cases currently are in adolescents and adults. Pertussis is the only vaccine-preventable disease for which universal immunization in the USA is recommended that continues to be endemic. Prospective and serologic studies suggest that pertussis is underrecognized, especially among adolescents and adults, in whom the actual number of cases is estimated to be 600,000 annually. A number of studies have documented pertussis in 13-32% of adolescents and adults with cough illness for >7 days.

Pertussis is extremely contagious, with attack rates as high as 100% in susceptible individuals exposed to aerosol droplets at close range. *B. pertussis* does not survive for prolonged periods in the environment. Chronic carriage by humans is not documented. After intense exposure as in households, the rate of subclinical infection is as high as 80% in fully immunized or previously infected individuals. When carefully sought, a symptomatic source case can be found for most patients.

Neither natural disease nor vaccination provides complete or lifelong immunity against pertussis re-infection or disease. Protection against typical disease begins to wane 3-5 yr after vaccination and is unmeasurable after 12 yr. Subclinical re-infection undoubtedly has contributed significantly to immunity against disease ascribed previously to both vaccine and prior infection. Despite history of disease or complete immunization, outbreaks of pertussis have occurred in the elderly, in nursing homes, in residential facilities with limited exposures, in highly immunized suburbia, and in preadolescents, adolescents, and adults with significant time since immunization. Possible explanations for change in epidemiology include waning immunity post immunization, an aging cohort who received less effective vaccine, and increased awareness and diagnosis. Without natural re-infection with *B. pertussis* or repeated booster vaccinations, adolescents and adults are susceptible to clinical disease if exposed, and mothers provide little if any passive protection to young infants. Coughing adolescents and adults (usually not recognized as having pertussis) are the major reservoir for *B. pertussis* and are the usual sources of infection for infants and children.

PATHOGENESIS

Bordetella organisms are tiny, fastidious, gram-negative coccobacilli that colonize only ciliated epithelium. The exact mechanism of disease symptomatology remains unknown. *Bordetella* species share a high degree of DNA homology among virulence genes. Only *B. pertussis* expresses **pertussis toxin** (PT), the major virulence protein. PT has numerous proven biologic activities (e.g., histamine sensitivity, insulin secretion, leukocyte dysfunction), some of which may account for systemic manifestations of disease. PT causes lymphocytosis immediately in experimental animals by rerouting lymphocytes to remain in the circulating blood pool. PT appears to have a central but not a singular role in pathogenesis. *B. pertussis* produces an array of other biologically active substances, many of which are postulated to have a role in disease and immunity. After aerosol acquisition, **filamentous hemagglutinin** (FHA), some **agglutinogens** (especially fimbriae [Fim] types 2 and 3), and a 69-kd nonfimbrial surface protein called **pertactin** (Pn) are important for attachment to ciliated respiratory epithelial cells. **Tracheal cytotoxin,** adenylate cyclase, and PT appear to inhibit clearance of organisms. Tracheal cytotoxin, dermonecrotic factor, and adenylate cyclase are postulated to be predominantly responsible for the local epithelial damage that produces respiratory symptoms and facilitates absorption of PT.

CLINICAL MANIFESTATIONS

Classically, pertussis is a prolonged disease, divided into catarrhal, paroxysmal, and convalescent stages. The **catarrhal stage** (1-2 wk) begins insidiously after an incubation period ranging from 3-12 days with nondistinctive symptoms of congestion and rhinorrhea variably accompanied by low-grade fever, sneezing, lacrimation, and conjunctival suffusion. As initial symptoms wane, coughing marks the onset of the **paroxysmal stage** (2-6 wk). The cough begins as a dry, intermittent, irritative hack and evolves into the inexorable paroxysms that are the hallmark of pertussis. A well-appearing, playful toddler with insignificant provocation suddenly expresses an anxious aura and may clutch a parent or comforting adult before beginning a machine-gun burst of uninterrupted cough on a single exhalation, chin and chest held forward, tongue protruding maximally, eyes bulging and watering, face purple, until coughing ceases and a loud whoop follows as inspired air traverses the still partially closed airway. *Post-tussive emesis* is common, and exhaustion is universal. The number and severity of paroxysms escalate over days to a week and remain at that plateau for days to weeks. At the peak of the paroxysmal stage, patients may have more than 1 episode hourly. As the paroxysmal stage fades into the **convalescent stage** (≥2 wk), the number, severity, and duration of episodes diminish.

Infants <3 mo of age do not display the classic stages. The catarrhal phase lasts only a few days or is unnoticed, and then, after the most insignificant startle from a draft, light, sound, sucking, or stretching, a well-appearing young infant begins to choke, gasp, gag, and flail the extremities, with face reddened. Cough may not be prominent, especially in the early phase. Whoop infrequently occurs in infants <3 mo of age who at the end of a paroxysm lack stature or muscular strength to create sudden negative intrathoracic pressure. Apnea and cyanosis can follow a coughing paroxysm, or apnea can occur without a cough. Apnea may be the only symptom. Apnea and cyanosis both are more common with pertussis than with neonatal viral infections, including respiratory syncytial virus (RSV). The paroxysmal and convalescent stages in young infants are lengthy. Paradoxically, in infants, cough and whooping may become louder and more classic in convalescence. Convalescence includes intermittent paroxysmal coughing throughout the 1st yr of life, including "exacerbations" with subsequent respiratory illnesses; these are not due to recurrent infection or reactivation of *B. pertussis.*

Adolescents and previously immunized children have foreshortening of all stages of pertussis. Adults have no distinct stages. Classically, adolescents and adults describe a sudden feeling of strangulation followed by uninterrupted coughs, feeling of suffocation, bursting headache, diminished awareness, and then a gasping breath, usually without a whoop. Post-tussive emesis and intermittency of paroxysms separated by hours of well-being are specific clues to the diagnosis in adolescents and adults. At least 30% of older individuals with pertussis have nonspecific cough illness, distinguished only by duration, which is usually >21 days.

Findings on physical examination generally are uninformative. Signs of lower respiratory tract disease are not expected unless complicating secondary bacterial pneumonia is present. Conjunctival hemorrhages and petechiae on the upper body are common.

DIAGNOSIS

Pertussis should be suspected in any individual who has pure or predominant complaint of cough, especially if the following features are absent: fever, malaise or myalgia, exanthem or enanthem, sore throat, hoarseness, tachypnea, wheezes, and rales. For sporadic cases, a clinical case definition of cough of ≥14 days' duration with at least 1 associated symptom of paroxysms, whoop, or post-tussive vomiting has a sensitivity of 81% and a specificity of 58% for culture confirmation. Pertussis should be suspected in older children whose cough illness is escalating at 7-10 days and whose coughing episodes are not continuous. Pertussis should be suspected in infants <3 mo of age with gagging, gasping, apnea, cyanosis, or an apparent life-threatening event (ALTE). Sudden infant death is occasionally caused by *B. pertussis.*

Adenoviral infections are usually distinguishable by associated features, such as fever, sore throat, and conjunctivitis. *Mycoplasma* causes protracted episodic coughing, but patients usually have a history of fever, headache, and systemic symptoms at the onset of disease as well as more continuous cough and frequent finding of rales on auscultation of the chest. Epidemics of *Mycoplasma* and *B. pertussis* in young adults can be difficult to distinguish on clinical grounds. Although pertussis is often included in the laboratory evaluation of young infants with afebrile pneumonia, *B. pertussis* is not associated with staccato cough (breath with every cough), purulent conjunctivitis, tachypnea, rales or wheezes that typify infection due to *Chlamydia trachomatis,* or predominant lower respiratory tract signs that typify infection due to RSV. Unless an infant with pertussis has secondary pneumonia (and then appears ill), the findings on examination between paroxysms are entirely normal, including respiratory rate.

Leukocytosis (15,000-100,000 cells/mm^3) due to absolute lymphocytosis is characteristic in the catarrhal stage. Lymphocytes are of T- and B-cell origin and are normal small cells, rather than the large atypical lymphocytes seen with viral infections. Adults, partially immune children, and, occasionally, young infants have less impressive lymphocytosis. Absolute increase in neutrophils suggests a different diagnosis or secondary bacterial infection. Eosinophilia is not a manifestation of pertussis. A severe course and death are correlated with extreme leukocytosis (median peak white blood cell count in fatal vs nonfatal cases, 94 vs 18 × 10^9 cells/L, respectively) and thrombocytosis (median peak platelet count in fatal vs nonfatal cases, 782 vs 556 × 10^9/L, respectively). Mild hyperinsulinemia and reduced glycemic response to epinephrine have been demonstrated, although hypoglycemia is reported only occasionally. Chest radiographic findings are only mildly abnormal in the majority of hospitalized infants, showing perihilar infiltrate or edema (sometimes with a butterfly appearance) and variable atelectasis. Parenchymal consolidation suggests secondary bacterial infection. Pneumothorax, pneumomediastinum, and subcutaneous emphysema can be seen occasionally.

All current methods for confirmation of infection due to *B. pertussis* have limitations in sensitivity, specificity, or practicality. Isolation of *B. pertussis* in culture remains the gold standard for diagnosis. Careful attention must be directed to specimen collection, transport, and isolation technique. The specimen is obtained with deep nasopharyngeal aspiration or with the use of a flexible swab, preferably a Dacron or calcium alginate–tipped swab, held in the posterior nasopharynx for 15-30 sec (or until cough occurs). A 1.0% casamino acid liquid is acceptable for holding a specimen up to 2 hr; Stainer-Scholte broth or Regan-Lowe semisolid transport medium is used for longer transport periods, up to 4 days. The preferred isolation media are Regan-Lowe charcoal agar with 10% horse blood and 5-40 μg/mL cephalexin and Stainer-Scholte media with cyclodextrin resins. Cultures are incubated at 35-37°F in a humid environment and examined daily for 7 days for slow-growing, tiny, glistening colonies. Direct fluorescent antibody (DFA) testing of potential isolates using specific antibody for *B. pertussis* and *B. parapertussis* maximizes recovery rates. Direct testing of nasopharyngeal secretions by DFA is a rapid test but is reliable only in laboratories with continuous experience. Polymerase chain reaction (PCR) analysis to test nasopharyngeal wash specimens has a sensitivity similar to that of culture and averts difficulties of isolation, but a standardized validated test is not yet available universally. Results of DFA, culture, and PCR are all expected to be positive in unimmunized, untreated children during the catarrhal and early paroxysmal stages of disease. Less than 10% of any of these test results are positive in partially or remotely immunized individuals tested in the paroxysmal stage. Serologic tests for detection of antibodies to *B. pertussis* antigens in acute and convalescent samples are the most sensitive tests in immunized individuals and are useful epidemiologically. A single serum sample showing immunoglobulin G (IgG) antibody to pertussis toxin elevated >2 standard deviations above the mean of the immunized population (≈100 EU/mL) indicates recent infection. Standardization of tests and cut point for a positive result are currently being investigated. Tests for IgA and IgM pertussis antibody, or antibody to antigens other than PT, are not reliable methods for diagnosis of pertussis.

TREATMENT

Goals of therapy are to limit the number of paroxysms, to observe the severity of the cough, to provide assistance when necessary, and to maximize nutrition, rest, and recovery without sequelae (Table 189-1). Infants <3 mo of age with suspected pertussis are always admitted to hospital, as are those between 3 and 6 mo of age unless witnessed paroxysms are not severe, and patients of any age if significant complications occur. Prematurely born young infants and children with underlying cardiac, pulmonary, muscular, or neurologic disorders have a high risk for severe, potentially fatal disease.

The specific, limited goals of hospitalization are to: (1) assess progression of disease and likelihood of life-threatening events at peak of disease; (2) prevent or treat complications; and (3) educate parents in the natural history of the disease and in care that will be given at home. Heart rate, respiratory rate, and pulse oximetry are monitored continuously with alarm settings so that paroxysms can be witnessed and recorded by health care personnel. Detailed cough records and documentation of feeding, vomiting, and weight change provide data to assess severity. Typical paroxysms that are not life threatening have the following features: duration <45 sec; red but not blue color change; tachycardia, bradycardia (not <60 beats/min in infants), or oxygen desaturation that spontaneously resolves at the end of the paroxysm; whooping or strength for self-rescue at the end of the paroxysm; self-expectorated mucus plug; and post-tussive exhaustion but not unresponsiveness. Assessing the need to provide oxygen, stimulation, or suctioning requires skilled personnel who can document an infant's ability for self-rescue but who will intervene rapidly and expertly when necessary. The benefit of a quiet, dimly lighted, undisturbed, comforting environment cannot be overestimated or forfeited in a desire to monitor and intervene. Feeding children with pertussis is challenging. The risk of precipitating cough by nipple feeding does not warrant nasogastric, nasojejunal, or parenteral alimentation in most infants. The composition or thickness of formula does not affect the quality of secretions, cough, or retention. Large-volume feedings are avoided.

Table 189-1 CAVEATS IN ASSESSMENT AND CARE OF INFANTS WITH PERTUSSIS

Infants with potentially fatal pertussis may appear well between episodes.
A paroxysm must be witnessed before a decision is made between hospital and home care.
Only analysis of carefully compiled cough record permits assessment of severity and progression of illness.
Suctioning of nose, oropharynx, or trachea should not be performed on a "preventive" schedule.
Feeding in the period following a paroxysm may be more successful than after napping.
Family support begins at the time of hospitalization with empathy for the child's and family's experience to date, transfer of the burden of responsibility for the child's safety to the health care team, and delineation of assessments and treatments to be performed.
Family education, recruitment as part of the team, and continued support after discharge are essential.

Within 48-72 hr, the direction and severity of disease are obvious, usually from analysis of recorded information. Many infants have marked improvement upon hospitalization and antibiotic therapy, especially if they are hospitalized early in the course of disease or have been removed from aggravating environmental smoke, excessive stimulation, or a dry or polluting heat source. Hospital discharge is appropriate if over a 48-hr period disease severity is unchanged or diminished, no intervention is required during paroxysms, nutrition is adequate, no complication has occurred, and parents are adequately prepared for care at home. Apnea and seizures occur in the incremental phase of illness and in patients with complicated disease. Portable oxygen, monitoring, or suction apparatus should not be needed at home.

Infants who have apnea, paroxysms that repeatedly lead to life-threatening events despite passive delivery of oxygen, or respiratory failure require intubation, pharmaceutically induced paralysis, and ventilation.

Antibiotics

An antimicrobial agent is always given when pertussis is suspected or confirmed, primarily to limit the spread of infection and secondarily for possible clinical benefit. Macrolides are preferred agents and are similar to one another in terms of in vitro activity (Table 189-2). Resistance has been reported rarely. A 7- to 10-fold relative risk for infantile hypertrophic pyloric stenosis (IHPS) has been reported in neonates treated with orally administered erythromycin. Azithromycin is the preferred agent for most patients and particularly in neonates, although cases of IHPS have followed its use. All infants <1 mo of age treated with any macrolide should be monitored for symptoms of pyloric stenosis. Benefits of post-exposure prophylaxis for infants far outweigh risk of IHPS.

Adjunct Therapies

No rigorous clinical trial has demonstrated a beneficial effect of β_2-adrenergic stimulants such as salbutamol and albuterol. Fussing associated with aerosol treatment triggers paroxysms. No randomized, blinded clinical trial of sufficient size has been performed to evaluate the usefulness of corticosteroids in the management of pertussis; their clinical use is not warranted.

Isolation

Patients with suspected pertussis are placed in respiratory isolation with use of masks by all health care personnel entering the room. Screening for cough should be performed upon entrance of patients to emergency departments, offices, and clinics to begin isolation immediately and until 5 days after initiation of macrolide therapy. Children and staff with pertussis in child-care facilities or schools should be excluded until macrolide prophylaxis has been taken for 5 days.

Care of Household and Other Close Contacts

A macrolide agent should be given promptly to all household contacts and other close contacts, such as those in daycare,

Table 189-2 RECOMMENDED ANTIMICROBIAL TREATMENT AND POSTEXPOSURE PROPHYLAXIS FOR PERTUSSIS, BY AGE GROUP

AGE GROUP	PRIMARY AGENTS		ALTERNATE AGENT*	
	Azithromycin	Erythromycin	Clarithromycin	TMP-SMZ
<1 mo	Recommended agent. 10 mg/kg/day in a single dose for 5 days (only limited safety data available)	Not preferred Erythromycin is substantially associated with infantile hypertrophic pyloric stenosis Use if azithromycin is unavailable; 40-50 mg/kg/day in 4 divided doses for 14 days	Not recommended (safety data unavailable)	Contraindicated for infants aged <2 mo (risk for kernicterus)
1-5 mo	10 mg/kg/day in a single dose for 5 days	40-50 mg/kg/day in 4 divided doses for 14 days	15 mg/kg/day in 2 divided doses for 7 days	Contraindicated at age <2 mo For infants aged ≥2 mo: TMP 8mg/kg/day plus SMZ 40 mg/kg/day in 2 divided doses for 14 days
Infants aged ≥6 mo and children	10 mg/kg in a single dose on day 1 (maximum 500 mg), then 5 mg/kg/day (maximum 250 mg) on days 2-5	40-50 mg/kg/day (maximum 2 g/day) in 4 divided doses for 14 days	15 mg/kg/day in 2 divided doses (maximum 1 g/day) for 7 days	TMP 8 mg/kg/day plus SMZ 40 mg/kg/day in 2 divided doses for 14 days
Adults	500 mg in a single dose on day 1 then 250 mg/day on days 2-5	2 g/day in 4 divided doses for 14 days	1 g/day in 2 divided doses for 7 days	TMP 320mg/day, SMZ 1,600mg/day in 2 divided doses for 14 days

*Trimethoprim-sulfamethoxazole (TMP-SMZ) can be used as an alternative agent to macrolides in patients aged ≥2 mo who are allergic to macrolides, who cannot tolerate macrolides, or who are infected with a rare macrolide-resistant strain of *Bordetella pertussis.*

From Centers for Disease Control and Prevention: Recommended antimicrobial agents for treatment and postexposure prophylaxis of pertussis: 2005 CDC guidelines, *MMWR Morbid Mortal Wkly Rep* 54:1–16, 2005.

regardless of age, history of immunization, and symptoms (see Table 189-2). The same age-related drugs and doses used for prophylaxis are used for treatment. Visitation and movement of coughing family members in the hospital must be assiduously controlled until erythromycin has been taken for 5 days. In close contacts <7 yr of age who have received fewer than 4 doses of pertussis-containing vaccines, vaccination should be initiated or continued to complete the recommended series. Children <7 yr of age who received a 3rd dose >6 mo before exposure or a 4th dose ≥3 yr before exposure should receive a booster dose. Individuals ≥9 yr of age should be given a Tdap (adolescent/adult formulation of tetanus and diphtheria toxoids and acellular pertussis) booster if they have not previously received Tdap. Unmasked health care personnel (HCP) exposed to untreated cases should be evaluated for post-exposure prophylaxis and follow-up. Coughing HCP with or without known exposure to pertussis should be promptly evaluated for pertussis.

COMPLICATIONS

Infants <6 mo of age have excessive mortality and morbidity; infants <2 mo of age have the highest reported rates of pertussis-associated hospitalization (82%), pneumonia (25%), seizures (4%), encephalopathy (1%), and death (1%). Infants <4 mo of age account for 90% of cases of fatal pertussis. Preterm birth and young maternal age are significantly associated with fatal pertussis. Neonates with pertussis have substantially longer hospitalizations, greater need for oxygen, and greater need for mechanical ventilation than neonates with viral respiratory infection.

The principal complications of pertussis are apnea, secondary infections (such as otitis media and pneumonia), and physical sequelae of forceful coughing. Fever, tachypnea or respiratory distress between paroxysms, and absolute neutrophilia are clues to pneumonia. Expected pathogens include *Staphylococcus aureus, Streptococcus pneumoniae,* and bacteria of oropharyngeal flora. Increased intrathoracic and intra-abdominal pressure during coughing can result in conjunctival and scleral hemorrhages, petechiae on the upper body, epistaxis, hemorrhage in the central nervous system (CNS) and retina, pneumothorax and subcutaneous emphysema, and umbilical and inguinal hernias. Laceration of the lingual frenulum occurs occasionally.

The need for intensive care and mechanical ventilation is usually limited to infants <3 mo of age and infants with underlying conditions. Respiratory failure due to apnea may precipitate need for intubation and ventilation through the days when disease peaks; prognosis is good. Progressive pulmonary hypertension in very young infants and secondary bacterial pneumonia are severe complications of pertussis and are the usual causes of death. Pulmonary hypertension and cardiogenic shock with fatal outcome are associated with extreme elevations of lymphocyte and platelet counts. Autopsies in fatal cases show luminal aggregates of leukocytes in the pulmonary vasculature. Extracorporeal membrane oxygenation of infants with pertussis in whom mechanical ventilation failed has been associated with >80% fatality (questioning the advisability of this procedure). Exchange transfusion or leukopheresis, however, has been associated with drop in lymphocyte and platelet counts, with recovery in several reported cases.

CNS abnormalities occur at a relatively high frequency in pertussis and are almost always a result of hypoxemia or hemorrhage associated with coughing or apnea in young infants. Apnea or bradycardia or both may result from apparent laryngospasm or vagal stimulation just before a coughing episode, from obstruction during an episode, or from hypoxemia following an episode. Lack of associated respiratory signs in some young infants with apnea raises the possibility of a primary effect of PT on the CNS. Seizures are usually a result of hypoxemia, but hyponatremia from excessive secretion of antidiuretic hormone during pneumonia can occur. The only neuropathology documented in humans is parenchymal hemorrhage and ischemic necrosis.

Bronchiectasis has been reported rarely after pertussis. Children who have pertussis before the age of 2 yr may have abnormal pulmonary function into adulthood.

PREVENTION

Universal immunization of children with pertussis vaccine, beginning in infancy with periodic reinforcing doses through adolescence and adulthood, is central to the control of pertussis (Chapter 165). There is no serologic correlate of protection from *B. pertussis.*

DTaP Vaccines

Several diphtheria and tetanus toxoids combined with acellular pertussis (DTaP) vaccines or combination products currently are licensed in the USA for children <7 yr of age. DTaP vaccines have fewer adverse effects than the vaccines containing whole-cell pertussis (DTP), which continue to be given to infants and children in many other countries. Acellular pertussis vaccines all contain inactivated PT and 2 or more other bacterial components (FHA, Pn, and Fim 2 and 3). Clinical efficacy against severe pertussis, defined as paroxysmal cough >21 days, is 80-85%. Mild local and systemic adverse events as well as more serious events (including high fever, persistent crying of ≥3 hr in duration, hypotonic hyporesponsive episodes, and seizures) occur significantly less frequently among infants who receive DTaP than in those who receive DTP vaccine. DTaP-containing vaccines can be administered simultaneously with any other vaccines used in standard schedules for children.

Four doses of DTaP should be administered during the 1st 2 years of life, generally at ages 2, 4, 6, and 15-18 mo of age. The 4th dose may be administered as early as 12 mo of age, provided that 6 mo have elapsed since the 3rd dose. The 5th dose of DTaP is recommended for children at 4-6 yr of age; a 5th dose is not necessary if the 4th dose in the series is administered on or after the 4th birthday. A birth dose of DTaP is not effective, but commencement of vaccination at 6 wk of age, with monthly doses through the 3rd dose, can be considered in high-risk settings.

When feasible, the same DTaP product is recommended for all doses of the primary vaccination series. Local reactions increase in rate and severity with successive doses of DTaP, although never reaching the magnitude of reactions following similar doses of DTP. Swelling of the entire thigh or upper arm has been reported in 2-3% of vaccinees after the 4th or 5th doses of a variety of DTaP products. Swelling may be accompanied by pain, erythema, and fever. Limitation of activity is less than might be expected. Swelling subsides spontaneously without sequelae. The pathogenesis is unknown. Extensive limb swelling after the 4th dose of DTaP usually is not associated with a similar reaction to the 5th dose and is not a contraindication to subsequent dose(s).

Exempting children from pertussis immunization should be considered only in the narrow limits as recommended. Exemptors have been shown to have significantly increased risk for pertussis and to play a role in outbreaks of pertussis among immunized populations. Although well-documented pertussis confers short-term protection, the duration of protection is unknown; immunization should be completed on schedule in children diagnosed with pertussis. Improper vaccine storage reduces immunity.

Tdap Vaccines

Two tetanus toxoid, reduced diphtheria toxoid, and acellular pertussis vaccine, adsorbed (Tdap) products were licensed in 2005 and were recommended universally in 2006 for use in individuals 11-18 years of age and in older individuals as a single-dose booster vaccine to provide protection against tetanus, diphtheria, and pertussis. Because of heightened risk in adolescents for pertussis and the evidence of association of pertussis with young infants of adolescent mothers, the American Academy of Pediatrics (AAP) includes pregnant adolescents who are in their second or third trimester in Tdap recommendations. The preferred age for Tdap vaccination is 11-12 yr. All adolescents 11-18 yr of age who received Td, but not Tdap, should receive a single dose of Tdap to provide protection against pertussis. There is no minimum interval required between vaccines containing tetanus or diphtheria toxoid and Tdap. There is no contraindication to concurrent administration of any other indicated vaccine. In 2010, Tdap was recommended for children 7-10 yr old with incomplete pertussis vaccination prior to age 7 yr as well as for those ≥65 yr who have contact with infants. An important objective of administering Tdap is to protect adolescents and adults against pertussis in order to control endemic and epidemic spread to young infants who have not completed primary immunization and are at high risk for pertussis and its complications. In provinces and territories in Canada where Tdap was administered to 14 to 16 yr old adolescents, marked reduction in pertussis has been documented in adolescents and younger age groups, possibly as a result of herd protection. In 2008 and pending further data, the CDC recommendations for pregnant adult women showed preference for the cocoon strategy (immediate postpartum Tdap immunization of mother and all household and other contacts of the infant) over maternal immunization during pregnancy.

BIBLIOGRAPHY

Please visit the Nelson Textbook of Pediatrics *website at www.expertconsult.com for the complete bibliography.*

Chapter 190 *Salmonella*

Zulfiqar Ahmed Bhutta

Salmonellosis is a common and widely distributed food-borne disease that is a global major public health problem that affects millions of individuals and results in significant mortality. Salmonellae live in the intestinal tracts of warm- and cold-blooded animals. Some species are ubiquitous, whereas others are specifically adapted to a particular host.

The sequencing of the *Salmonella enterica* serovar Typhi (previously called *Salmonella typhi*) and *Salmonella typhimurium* genomes has indicated an almost 95% genetic homology between the organisms. However, the clinical diseases caused by the 2 organisms differ considerably. Orally ingested salmonellae survive at the low pH of the stomach and evade the multiple defenses of the small intestine in order to gain access to the epithelium. Salmonellae preferentially enter M cells, which transport them to the lymphoid cells (T and B) in the underlying Peyer patches. Once across the epithelium, *Salmonella* serotypes that are associated with systemic illness enter intestinal macrophages and disseminate throughout the reticuloendothelial system. By contrast, non-typhoidal *Salmonella* (NTS) serovars induce an early local inflammatory response, which results in the infiltration of polymorphonuclear leukocytes into the intestinal lumen and diarrhea. The NTS serovars cause a gastroenteritis of rapid onset and brief duration, in contrast to typhoid, which has a considerably longer incubation period and duration of illness and in which systemic illness predominates and only a small proportion of children get diarrhea. These differences in the manifestations of infection by the two groups of pathogens, one predominantly causing intestinal inflammation and the other leading to systemic disease, may be related to specific genetic pathogenicity islands on the organisms. NTS serovars are unable to overcome defense mechanisms that limit bacterial dissemination from the intestine to systemic circulation in immunocompetent individuals and produce a self-limiting gastroenteritis. In contrast, *S. typhi* may possess unique virulence traits that allow it to overcome mucosal barrier functions in immunocompetent hosts, resulting in a severe systemic illness. Interestingly, the frequencies of typhoid in immunocompetent and immunocompromised individuals do not differ.

The nomenclature of *Salmonella* reflects the species name *Salmonella enterica* with a number of serovars. *Salmonella* nomenclature has undergone considerable alterations. The original taxonomy was based on clinical syndromes *(S. typhi, S. cholerAesuis, S. paratyphi).* With adoption of serologic analysis, a *Salmonella* species was defined subsequently as "a group of related fermentation phage-type," with the result that each *Salmonella* serovar was regarded as a species in itself. Although this classification is simplistic, its use until 2004 resulted in identification of 2,501 serovars of *Salmonella,* which led to the need for further categorization to aid communication among scientists, public health officials, and the public.

All *Salmonella* serovars form a single DNA hybridization group, a single species called *S. enterica* composed of several subspecies (Table 190-1). Each subspecies contains various serotypes defined by the O and H antigens. To further simplify the

Table 190-1 SALMONELLA NOMENCLATURE

TRADITIONAL USAGE	FORMAL NAME	CDC DESIGNATION
S. typhi	*S. enterica** subsp. enterica ser. Typhi	*S.* ser. Typhi
S. dublin	*S. enterica* subsp. enterica ser. Dublin	*S.* ser. Dublin
S. typhimurium	*S. enterica* subsp. enterica ser. Typhimurium	*S.* ser. Typhimurium
S. choleraesuis	*S. enterica* subsp. enterica ser. Choleraesuis	*S.* ser. Choleraesuis
S. marina	*S. enterica* subsp. houtenae ser. Marina	*S.* ser. Marina

CDC, U.S. Centers for Disease Control and Prevention; subsp, subspecies; ser., serovar.
*Some authorities prefer *S. choleraesuis* or *S. enteritidis* rather than *S. enterica* to describe the species.

nomenclature for physicians and epidemiologists, the names for the common serovars are kept for subspecies I strains, which represent >99.5% of the *Salmonella* strains isolated from humans and other warm-blooded animals.

190.1 Nontyphoidal Salmonellosis

Zulfiqar Ahmed Bhutta

ETIOLOGY

Salmonellae are motile, nonsporulating, nonencapsulated, gram-negative rods that grow aerobically and are capable of facultative anaerobic growth. They are resistant to many physical agents but can be killed by heating to 130°F (54.4°C) for 1 hr or 140°F (60°C) for 15 min. They remain viable at ambient or reduced temperatures for days and may survive for weeks in sewage, dried foodstuffs, pharmaceutical agents, and fecal material. Like other members of the family Enterobacteriaceae, *Salmonella* possesses somatic O antigens and flagellar H antigens.

With the exception of a few serotypes that affect only 1 or a few animal species, such as *Salmonella dublin* in cattle and *S. choleraesuis* in pigs, most serotypes have a broad host spectrum. Typically, such strains cause gastroenteritis that is often uncomplicated and does not need treatment but can be severe in the young, the elderly, and patients with weakened immunity. The causes are typically *Salmonella* Enteritidis (*Salmonella enterica* serotype Enteritidis) and *Salmonella* Typhimurium (*S. enterica* serotype Typhimurium), the 2 most important serotypes for salmonellosis transmitted from animals to humans. Nontyphoidal salmonellae have emerged as a major cause of bacteremia in Africa, especially among populations with high incidence of HIV infection.

EPIDEMIOLOGY

Salmonellosis constitutes a major public health burden and represents a significant cost to society in many countries. It is estimated that in the USA alone an estimated 1.4 million nontyphoidal *Salmonella* infections occurred in 2007, with an estimated $2.5 billion cost due to lost productivity and medical treatment. Although there is little information on the epidemiology and the burden of *Salmonella* gastroenteritis from developing countries, *Salmonella* infections are recognized as major causes of childhood diarrheal illness. With the growing burden of HIV infections and malnutrition in Africa, nontyphoidal *Salmonella* bacteremic infections have emerged as a major cause of morbidity and mortality among children and adults.

Nontyphoidal *Salmonella* infections have a worldwide distribution, with an incidence proportional to the standards of hygiene, sanitation, availability of safe water, and food preparation practices. In the developed world, the incidence of *Salmonella* infections and outbreaks has increased several-fold over the past few decades, which may be related to modern practices of mass food production that increase the potential for epidemics. *Salmonella* gastroenteritis accounts for over half of all episodes of bacterial diarrhea in the USA, with incidence peaks at the extremes of ages, among young infants and the elderly. Most human infections have been caused by *S.* Enteritidis; the prevalence of this organism has decreased over the past decade, with *S.* Typhimurium overtaking it in some countries.

The rise in *Salmonella* infections in many parts of the world over the past 3 decades may also be related to intensive animal husbandry practices, which selectively promote the rise of certain strains, especially drug-resistant varieties that emerge in response to the use of antimicrobials in food animals. Poultry products were traditionally regarded as a common source of salmonellosis, but consumption of a range of foods has now been associated with outbreaks, including fruits and vegetables. Although this change in epidemiology may be related to selective pressure from the use of antimicrobials, there may be other factors, such as the rise of strains with a selective propensity to develop resistance and virulence. It appears that multidrug-resistant strains of *Salmonella* are more virulent than susceptible strains and that poorer outcome does not simply relate to the delay in treatment response due to empirical choice of an ineffective antibiotic. Strains of multidrug-resistant *Salmonella* such as *S.* Typhimurium phage type DT104 harbor a genomic island that contains many of the drug resistance genes. It is possible that these integrons also contain genes that express virulence factors. The global spread of multidrug-resistant *S.* Typhimurium phage type DT104 in animals and humans may be related to the growing use of antimicrobials and may be facilitated by international and national trade of infected animals.

Several risk factors are associated with outbreaks of *Salmonella* infections. Animals constitute the principal source of human nontyphoidal *Salmonella* disease, and cases have occurred in which individuals have had contact with infected animals, including domestic animals such as cats, dogs, reptiles, pet rodents, and amphibians. Specific serotypes may be associated with particular animal hosts; children with *S. enterica* serovar Marina typically have exposure to pet lizards. In 1996 more than 50,000 cases of salmonellosis related to domestic lizards were reported to the U.S. Centers for Disease Control and Prevention (CDC). Domestic animals probably acquire the infection in the same way that humans do, through consumption of contaminated raw meat, poultry, or poultry-derived products. Animal feeds containing fishmeal or bone meal contaminated with *Salmonella* are an important source of infection for animals. Moreover, subtherapeutic concentrations of antibiotics are often added to animal feed to promote growth. Such practices promote the emergence of antibiotic-resistant bacteria, including *Salmonella,* in the gut flora of the animals, with subsequent contamination of their meat. There is strong evidence to link resistance of *S.* Typhimurium to fluoroquinolones with the use of this group of antimicrobials in animal feeds. Animal-to-animal transmission can occur, but most infected animals are asymptomatic.

An increasing number of produce-associated foodborne outbreaks in the USA associated with bacterial contamination are primarily from *Salmonella.* Although almost 80% of *Salmonella* infections are discrete, outbreaks can pose an inordinate burden on public health systems. In an evaluation of 604 outbreaks of foodborne disease in schools in the USA, *Salmonella* was the most commonly identified pathogen, accounting for 36% of outbreak reports with a known etiology. *Salmonella* infections in chickens increase the risk for contamination of eggs, and both poultry and eggs have been regarded as a dominant cause of common-source outbreaks. However, a growing proportion of *Salmonella* outbreaks are also associated with other food sources. The CDC reports that between 2002 and 2003, 31 food produce–associated

Salmonella outbreaks were reported, compared with only 29 poultry-related outbreaks. The food sources included many fruits and vegetables, such as tomatoes, sprouts, watermelon, cantaloupe, lettuce, and mangoes.

In addition to the effect of antibiotic use in animal feeds, the relationship of *Salmonella* infections to prior antibiotic use among children in the previous month is well recognized. This increased risk for infection in people who have received antibiotics for an unrelated reason may be related to alterations in gut microbial ecology, which predispose them to colonization and infection with antibiotic-resistant *Salmonella* isolates. These resistant strains of *Salmonella* are also more virulent. It is estimated that antimicrobial resistance in *Salmonella* may result in about 30,000 additional *Salmonella* infections annually, leading to about 300 hospitalizations and 10 deaths.

Given the ubiquitous nature of the organism, nosocomial infections with nontyphoidal *Salmonella* strains can also occur through contaminated equipment and diagnostic or pharmacologic preparations, particularly those of animal origin (pancreatic extracts, pituitary extracts, bile salts). Hospitalized children are at increased risk for severe and complicated *Salmonella* infections, especially with drug-resistant organisms.

PATHOGENESIS

The estimated number of bacteria that must be ingested to cause symptomatic disease in healthy adults is 10^6 to 10^8 *Salmonella* organisms. The gastric acidity inhibits multiplication of the salmonellae, and most organisms are rapidly killed at gastric pH ≤2.0. Achlorhydria, buffering medications, rapid gastric emptying after gastrectomy or gastroenterostomy, and a large inoculum enable viable organisms to reach the small intestine. Neonates and young infants have hypochlorhydria and rapid gastric emptying, which contribute to their increased vulnerability to symptomatic salmonellosis. In infants who typically take fluids, the inoculum size required to produce disease is also comparatively smaller because of faster transit through the stomach.

Once they reach the small and large intestines, the ability of *Salmonella* organisms to multiply and cause infection depends on the infecting dose as well as competition with normal flora. Prior antibiotic therapy may alter this relationship, as might factors such as co-administration of antimotility agents. The typical intestinal mucosal response to nontyphoidal *Salmonella* infection is an enterocolitis with diffuse mucosal inflammation and edema, sometimes with erosions and microabscesses. *Salmonella* organisms are capable of penetrating the intestinal mucosa, although destruction of epithelial cells and ulcers are usually not found. Intestinal inflammation with polymorphonuclear leukocytes and macrophages usually involves the lamina propria. Underlying intestinal lymphoid tissue and mesenteric lymph nodes enlarge and may demonstrate small areas of necrosis. Such lymphoid hypertrophy may cause interference with the blood supply to the gut mucosa. Hyperplasia of the reticuloendothelial system (RES) is also found within the liver and spleen. If bacteremia develops, it may lead to localized infection and suppuration in almost any organ.

Although *S.* Typhimurium can cause systemic disease in humans, intestinal infection usually results in a localized enteritis that is associated with a secretory response in the intestinal epithelium. Intestinal infection also induces secretion of interleukin-8 (IL-8) from the basolateral surface and other chemoattractants from the apical surface, directing recruitment and transmigration of neutrophils into the gut lumen and thus preventing the systemic spread of the bacteria (Fig. 190-1).

Interestingly, virulence traits that contribute to the host response are common to all nontyphoidal *Salmonella* serovars. These include (1) the type III secretion system (TTSS-1) encoded on *Salmonella* pathogenicity island-1 (SP1), which mediates invasion of the intestinal epithelium; (2) the TTSS encoded on SP2 (TTSS-2), which is required for survival within macrophages; and (3) expression of strong agonists of innate pattern recognition receptors (lipopolysaccharide and flagellin), which are important for triggering an TLR-mediated inflammatory response mediated by Toll-like receptors (TLRs). These observations suggest that *S.* Typhimurium must have acquired additional factors that further modulate the host response during infection.

Salmonella species invade epithelial cells in vitro by a process of bacteria-mediated endocytosis involving cytoskeletal rearrangement, disruption of the epithelial cell brush border, and the subsequent formation of membrane ruffles (Fig. 190-2). An adherent and invasive phenotype of *S. enterica* is activated under conditions similar to those found in the human small intestine (high osmolarity, low oxygen). The invasive phenotype is mediated in part by *Salmonella* pathogenicity island 1, a 40-kb region that encodes regulator proteins such as HilA, the type 3 secretory system involved in invasion of epithelial cells, and a variety of other products. In humans the TLR-dependent interleukin-12/interferon-λ (IL-12/IFN-λ) is a major immunoregulatory system that bridges innate and adaptive immunity and is responsible for restricting the systemic spread of nontyphoidal *Salmonella*.

Shortly following invasion of the gut epithelium, invasive *Salmonella* organisms encounter macrophages within the gut-associated lymphoid tissue. The interaction between *Salmonella* and macrophages results in alteration in the expression of a number of host genes, including those encoding proinflammatory mediators (inducible nitric oxide synthase [iNOS], chemokines, IL-1β), receptors or adhesion molecules (tumor necrosis factor-α receptor [TNF-αR], CD40, intercellular adhesion molecule 1 [ICAM-1]), and anti-inflammatory mediators (transforming growth factor-β1 and -β2 [TGF-β1] and TGF-β2). Other upregulated genes include those involved in cell death or apoptosis (intestinal epithelial cell protease, TNF-R1, Fas) and transcription factors (early growth response 1[Egr-1], IFN regulatory factor 1 [IRF-1]). *S.* Typhimurium can induce rapid macrophage death in vitro, which depends on the host cell protein caspase-1 and is mediated by the effector protein SipB (*Salmonella* invasion protein B). Intracellular *S.* Typhimurium is found within specialized *Salmonella* organisms containing vacuoles that have diverged from the normal endocytic pathway. This ability to survive within monocytes/macrophages is essential for *S.* Typhimurium to establish a systemic infection in the mouse. The mucosal proinflammatory response to *S.* Typhimurium infection and the subsequent recruitment of phagocytic cells to the site may also facilitate systemic spread of the bacteria.

Some virulence traits are shared by all salmonellae, but others are serotype restricted. These virulence traits have been defined in tissue culture and murine models, and it is likely that clinical features of human *Salmonella* infection will eventually be related to specific DNA sequences. With most diarrhea-associated nontyphoidal salmonelloses, the infection does not extend beyond the lamina propria and the local lymphatics. Specific virulence genes are related to the ability to cause bacteremia. These genes are found significantly more often in strains of *S.* Typhimurium isolated from the blood than in strains recovered from stool. Although both *S. dublin* and *S. choleraesuis* have a greater propensity to rapidly invade the bloodstream with little or no intestinal involvement, the development of disease after infection with *Salmonella* depends on the number of infecting organisms, their virulence traits, and several host defense factors. Various host factors may also affect the development of specific complications or clinical syndromes (Table 190-2) and of these, HIV infections are assuming greater importance in Africa in all age groups.

Bacteremia is possible with any *Salmonella* serotype, especially in individuals with reduced host defenses and especially in those with altered reticuloendothelial or cellular immune function. Thus, children with HIV infection, chronic granulomatous disease, and leukemia are more likely to demonstrate bacteremia after *Salmonella* infection, although the majority of children with

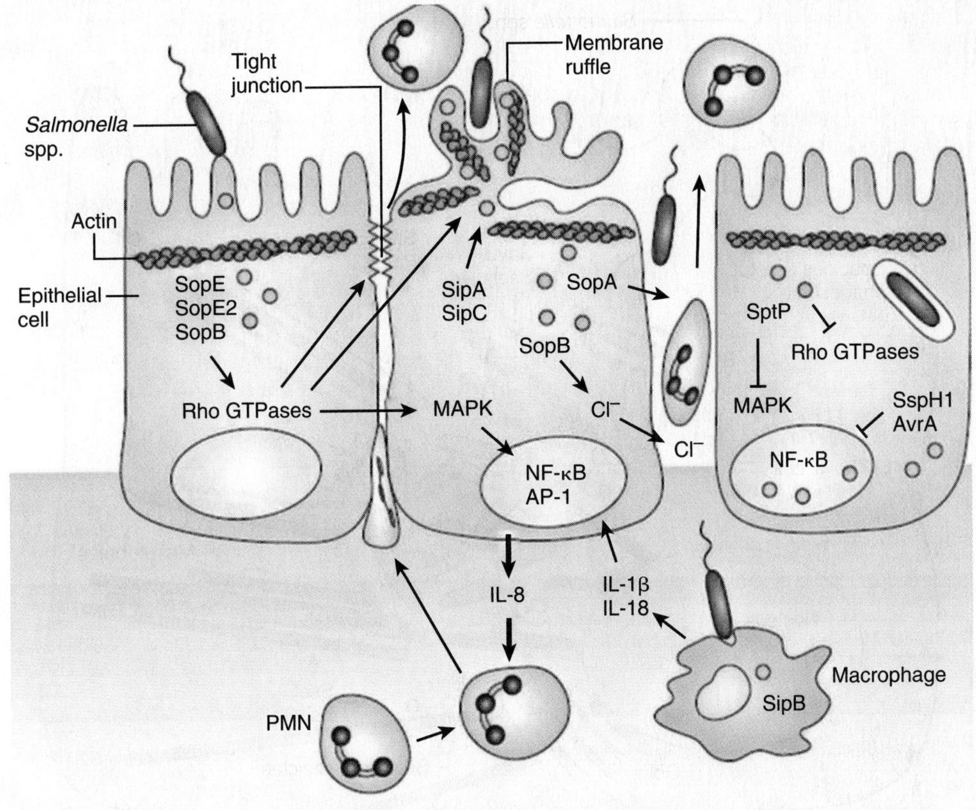

Figure 190-1 On contact with the epithelial cell, salmonellae assemble the *Salmonella* pathogenicity island 1–encoded type III secretion system (TTSS-1) and translocate effectors (*yellow spheres*) into the eukaryotic cytoplasm. Effectors such as SopE, SopE2 and SopB then activate host Rho guanosine triphosphatase (GTPases), resulting in the rearrangement of the actin cytoskeleton into membrane ruffles, induction of mitogen-activated protein kinase (MAPK) pathways, and destabilization of tight junctions. Changes in the actin cytoskeleton, which are further modulated by the actin-binding proteins SipA and SipC, lead to bacterial uptake. MAPK signaling activates the transcription factors activator protein-1 (AP-1) and nuclear factor-κB (NF-κB), which turn on production of the proinflammatory polymorphonuclear leukocyte (PMN) chemokine interleukin (IL)-8. SipB induces caspase-1 activation in macrophages, with the release of IL-1β and IL-18, so augmenting the inflammatory response. In addition, SopB stimulates Cl^- secretion by its inositol phosphatase activity. The destabilization of tight junctions allows the transmigration of PMNs from the basolateral to the apical surface, paracellular fluid leakage, and access of bacteria to the basolateral surface. However, the transmigration of PMNs also occurs in the absence of tight-junction disruption and is further promoted by SopA. The actin cytoskeleton is restored, and MAPK signaling is turned off by the enzymatic activities of SptP. This also results in the down-modulation of inflammatory responses, to which SspH1 and AvrA also contribute by inhibiting activation of NF-κB. (From Haraga A, Ohlson MB, Miller SI: Salmonellae interplay with host cells, *Nat Rev Microbiol* 6:53–66, 2008.)

Salmonella bacteremia in Africa are HIV negative. Children with *Schistosoma mansoni* infection and hepatosplenic involvement as well as chronic malarial anemia are also at a greater risk for development of chronic salmonellosis. Children with sickle cell disease are at increased risk for *Salmonella* septicemia and osteomyelitis. This risk may be related to the presence of numerous infarcted areas in the gastrointestinal tract, bones, and RES as well as reduced phagocytic and opsonizing capacity of patients, which allow the organism to flourish.

Some inherited defects, such as IL-12 deficiency (IL-12 β1 chain deficiency, IL-12 p40 subunit deletion) are associated with increased risk for *Salmonella* infections, suggesting a key role for IL-12 in the clearance of *Salmonella*. IL-12 is produced by activated macrophages and is a potent inducer of IFN-γ by natural killer cells and T lymphocytes. Given the putative protective role of IL-12 against malarial infection, *Salmonella* infection of phagocytes may secondarily affect IL-12 production and thus produce a vicious circle of chronic malaria and salmonella co-infection.

CLINICAL MANIFESTATIONS

Acute Enteritis

The most common clinical presentation of salmonellosis is acute enteritis. After an incubation period of 6-72 hr (mean 24 hr), there is an abrupt onset of nausea, vomiting, and crampy abdominal pain, located primarily in the periumbilical area and right lower quadrant, followed by mild to severe watery diarrhea and sometimes by diarrhea containing blood and mucus. A large proportion of children with acute enteritis are febrile, although younger infants may exhibit a normal or subnormal temperature. Symptoms usually subside within 2-7 days in healthy children, and fatalities are rare. However, some children experience severe disease with a septicemia-like picture (high fever, headache, drowsiness, confusion, meningismus, seizures, abdominal distention). The stool typically contains a moderate number of polymorphonuclear leukocytes and occult blood. Mild leukocytosis may be detected.

Bacteremia

Although the precise incidence of bacteremia following *Salmonella* gastroenteritis is unclear, transient bacteremia can occur in 1-5% of children with *Salmonella* diarrhea. Bacteremia can occur with minimal associated symptoms in newborns and very young infants, but in older infants it typically follows gastroenteritis and can be associated with fever, chills, and septic shock. In patients with AIDS, recurrent septicemia appears despite antibiotic therapy, often with a negative stool culture result for *Salmonella* and sometimes with no identifiable focus of infection.

Nontyphoidal *Salmonella* gastrointestinal infections commonly cause bacteremia in developing countries. High rates of invasive disease with *S.* Typhimurium and *S.* Enteritidis reported

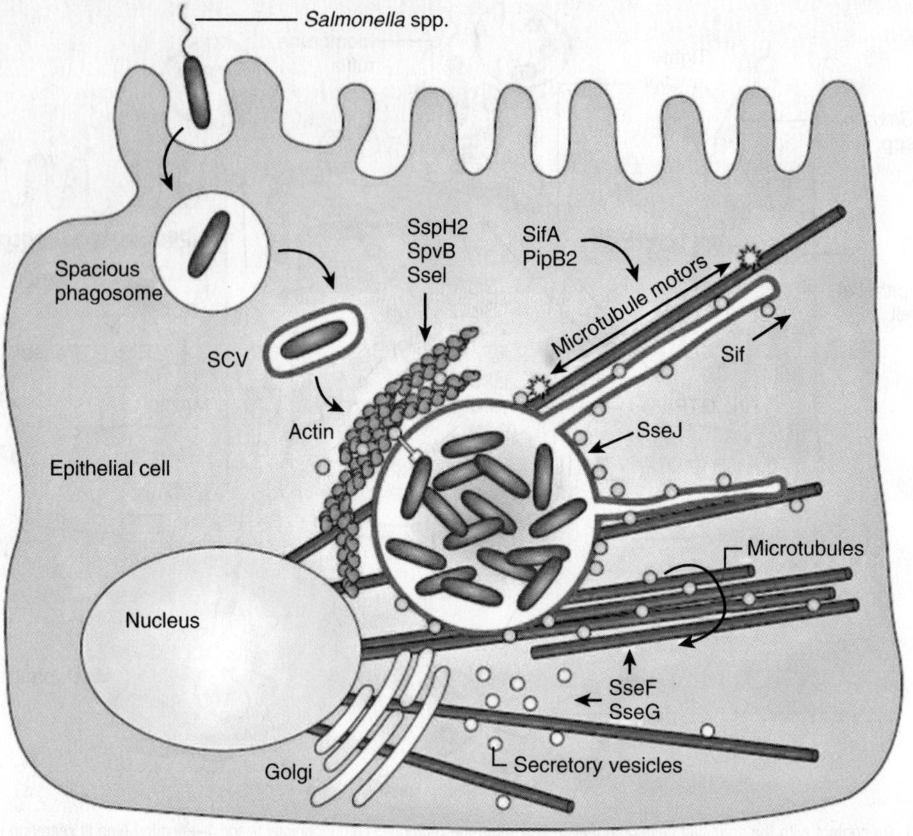

Figure 190-2 Formation of the *Salmonella*-containing vacuole (SCV) and induction of the Salmonella pathogenicity island 12 (SPI2) type III secretion system (TTSS) within the host cell. Shortly after internalization by macropinocytosis, salmonellae are enclosed in a spacious phagosome that is formed by membrane ruffles. Later, the phagosome fuses with lysosomes, acidifies, and shrinks to become adherent around the bacterium, and so is called the SCV. It contains the endocytic marker lysosomal associated membrane protein 1 (LAMP-1; *purple*). The *Salmonella* pathogenicity island 2 TTSS (TTSS-2) is induced within the SCV and translocates effector proteins (*yellow spheres*) across the phagosomal membrane several hours after phagocytosis. The TTSS-2 effectors SifA and PipB2 contribute to formation of *Salmonella*-induced filament along microtubules (*green*) and regulate microtubule-motor (*yellow star shape*) accumulation on the Sif and the SCV. SseJ is a deacylase that is active on the phagosome membrane. SseF and SseG cause microtubule bundling adjacent to the SCV and direct Golgi-derived vesicle traffic toward the SCV. Actin accumulates around the SCV in a TTSS-2–dependent manner, in which SspH2, SpvB, and SseI are thought to have a role. (From Haraga A, Ohlson MB, Miller SI: Salmonellae interplay with host cells, *Nat Rev Microbiol* 6:53–66, 2008.)

Table 190-2 HOST FACTORS AND CONDITIONS PREDISPOSING TO THE DEVELOPMENT OF SYSTEMIC DISEASE WITH NONTYPHOIDAL *SALMONELLA* STRAINS

Neonates and young infants (≤3 mo of age)
HIV/AIDS
Other immunodeficiencies and chronic granulomatous disease
Immunosuppressive and corticosteroid therapies
Malignancies, especially leukemia and lymphoma
Hemolytic anemia, including sickle cell disease, malaria, and bartonellosis
Collagen vascular disease
Inflammatory bowel disease
Achlorhydria or use of antacid medications
Impaired intestinal motility
Schistosomiasis, malaria
Malnutrition

from Africa (38-70% of isolates) suggest an association with HIV infections and malaria.

Extraintestinal Focal Infections

Following bacteremia, salmonellae have the propensity to seed and cause focal suppurative infection of many organs. The most common focal infections involve the skeletal system, meninges, intravascular sites, and sites of preexisting abnormalities. The peak incidence of ***Salmonella* meningitis** is in infancy, and the infection may be associated with a florid clinical course, high mortality, and neurologic sequelae in survivors.

COMPLICATIONS

Salmonella gastroenteritis can be associated with acute dehydration and complications that result from delayed presentation and inadequate treatment. Bacteremia in younger infants and immunocompromised individuals can have serious consequences and potentially fatal outcomes. *Salmonella* organisms can seed many organ systems, leading to osteomyelitis in children with sickle cell disease, among other infections. Reactive arthritis may follow *Salmonella* gastroenteritis, usually in adolescents with the HLA-B27 antigen.

In certain high-risk groups, especially those with impaired immunity, the course of *Salmonella* gastroenteritis may be more complicated. Neonates, infants younger than 6 mo, and children with primary or secondary immunodeficiency may have symptoms that persist for several weeks. The course of illness and complications may also be affected by coexisting pathologies. In children with AIDS, *Salmonella* infection frequently becomes widespread and overwhelming, causing multisystem involvement, septic shock, and death. In patients with inflammatory bowel disease, especially active ulcerative colitis, *Salmonella* gastroenteritis may lead to rapid development of toxic megacolon, bacterial translocation, and sepsis. In children with schistosomiasis, the *Salmonella* may persist and multiply within schistosomes, leading to chronic infection unless the schistosomiasis is effectively treated. Prolonged or intermittent bacteremia is associated with low-grade fever, anorexia, weight loss, diaphoresis, and myalgias and may occur in children with underlying problems and an RES dysfunction such as hemolytic anemia or malaria.

DIAGNOSIS

Clinical features that are specific to *Salmonella* gastroenteritis and thus would allow differentiation from other bacterial causes of diarrhea are few. Definitive diagnosis of *Salmonella* infection is based on clinical correlation of the presentation and culture of and subsequent identification of *Salmonella* organisms from feces or other body fluids. In children with gastroenteritis, cultures of stools have higher yields than rectal swabs. In children with nontyphoidal *Salmonella* gastroenteritis, prolonged fever lasting ≥5 days and young age should be recognized as risk factors closely associated with development of bacteremia. In patients with sites of local suppuration, aspirated specimens should be gram-stained and cultured. *Salmonella* organisms grow well on nonselective or enriched media, such as blood agar, chocolate agar, and nutrient broth, but stool specimens containing mixed bacterial flora require a selective medium, such as MacConkey, xylose-lysine-deoxycholate (XLD), bismuth sulfite (BBL), or *Salmonella-Shigella* (SS) agar for isolation.

Although other rapid diagnostic methods, such as latex agglutination and immunofluorescence, have been developed for rapid diagnosis of *Salmonella* in cultures, there are few comparable tests for rapid serologic detection. Polymerase chain reaction (PCR) techniques may offer a rapid alternative to classic cultures but are as yet not in widespread use in clinical settings.

TREATMENT

Appropriate therapy relates to the specific clinical presentation of *Salmonella* infection. In children with gastroenteritis, rapid clinical assessment, correction of dehydration and electrolyte disturbances, and supportive care, are key (Chapter 332). Antibiotics are not generally recommended for the treatment of isolated uncomplicated *Salmonella* gastroenteritis because they may suppress normal intestinal flora and prolong both the excretion of *Salmonella* and the remote risk for creating the chronic carrier state (usually in adults). However, given the risk for bacteremia in infants (<3 mo of age) and that of disseminated infection in high-risk groups with immune compromise (HIV, malignancies, immunosuppressive therapy, sickle cell anemia, immunodeficiency states), these children must receive an appropriate empirically chosen antibiotic until culture results are available (Table 190-3). The *S.* Typhimurium phage type DT104 strain is usually resistant to the following 5 drugs: ampicillin, chloramphenicol, streptomycin, sulfonamides, and tetracycline. An increasing proportion of *S.* Typhimurium phage type DT104 isolates also have reduced susceptibility to fluoroquinolones. Given the higher mortality associated with multidrug-resistant *Salmonella* infections, it is necessary to perform susceptibility tests on all human isolates. Infections with suspected drug-resistant *Salmonella* should be closely monitored and treated with appropriate antimicrobial therapy.

PROGNOSIS

Most healthy children with *Salmonella* gastroenteritis recover fully. However, malnourished children and children who do not receive optimal supportive treatment (Chapters 55 and 332) are at risk for development of prolonged diarrhea and complications.

Table 190-3 TREATMENT OF *SALMONELLA* GASTROENTERITIS

ORGANISM AND INDICATION	DOSE AND DURATION OF TREATMENT
Salmonella infections in infants <3 mo of age or immunocompromised persons (in addition to appropriate treatment for underlying disorder)	Cefotaxime 100-200 mg/kg/day every 6 hr for 5-14 days
	or
	Ceftriaxone 75 mg/kg/day once daily for 7 days
	or
	Ampicillin 100 mg/kg/day every 6 hr for 7 days
	or
	Cefixime 15 mg/kg/day for 7-10 days

Table 190-4 RECOMMENDATIONS FOR PREVENTING TRANSMISSION OF *SALMONELLA* FROM REPTILES AND AMPHIBIANS TO HUMANS

Pet store owners, health care providers, and veterinarians should provide information to owners and potential purchasers of reptiles and amphibians about the risks for and prevention of salmonellosis from these pets.
Persons at increased risk for infection or serious complications from salmonellosis (e.g., children aged <5 yr and immunocompromised persons) should avoid contact with reptiles and amphibians and any items that have been in contact with reptiles and amphibians.
Reptiles and amphibians should be kept out of households that include children aged <5 yr or immunocompromised persons. A family expecting a child should remove any pet reptile or amphibian from the home before the infant arrives.
Reptiles and amphibians should not be allowed in child-care centers.
Persons should always wash their hands thoroughly with soap and water after handling reptiles and amphibians or their cages.
Reptiles and amphibians should not be allowed to roam freely throughout a home or living area.
Pet reptiles and amphibians should be kept out of kitchens and other food preparation areas. Kitchen sinks should not be used to bathe reptiles and amphibians or to wash their dishes, cages, or aquariums. If bathtubs are used for these purposes, they should be cleaned thoroughly and disinfected with bleach.
Reptiles and amphibians in public settings (e.g., zoos and exhibits) should be kept from direct or indirect contact with patrons except in designated animal contact areas equipped with adequate handwashing facilities. Food and drink should not be allowed in animal contact areas.

From the Centers for Disease Control and Prevention: Reptile-associated salmonellosis—selected states, 1998-2002, *MMWR Morbid Mortal Wkly Rep* 52:1206–1210, 2003.

Young infants and immunocompromised patients often have systemic involvement, a prolonged course, and extraintestinal foci. In particular, children with HIV infection and *Salmonella* infections can have a florid course.

After infection, nontyphoidal salmonellae are excreted in feces for a median of 5 wk.

A prolonged carrier state after nontyphoidal salmonellosis is rare (<1%) but may be seen in children with biliary tract disease and cholelithiasis after chronic hemolysis. Prolonged carriage of *Salmonella* organisms is rare in healthy children but has been reported in those with underlying immune deficiency. During the period of *Salmonella* excretion, the individual may infect others, directly by the fecal-oral route or indirectly by contaminating foods.

PREVENTION

Control of the transmission of *Salmonella* infections to humans requires control of the infection in the animal reservoir, judicious use of antibiotics in dairy and livestock farming, prevention of contamination of foodstuffs prepared from animals, and use of appropriate standards in food processing in commercial and private kitchens (Table 190-4). Because large outbreaks are often related to mass food production, it should be recognized that contamination of just one piece of machinery used in food processing may cause an outbreak; meticulous cleaning of equipment is essential. Clean water supply and education in handwashing and food preparation and storage are critical to reducing person-to-person transmission. *Salmonella* may remain viable when cooking practices prevent food from reaching a temperature greater than 150°F (65.5°C) for >12 min. Parents should be advised of the risk of reptiles as pets in households with young infants.

In contrast to developed countries, relatively little is known about the transmission of nontyphoidal *Salmonella* infections in developing countries, and it is likely that person-to-person transmission may be relatively more important in some settings. Although some vaccines have been used in animals, no human vaccine against nontyphoidal *Salmonella* infections is currently available. Infections should be reported to public health authorities so that outbreaks can be recognized and investigated. Given the rapid rise of antimicrobial resistance among *Salmonella* isolates, it is imperative that there is rigorous regulation of the use of antimicrobials in animal feeds.

BIBLIOGRAPHY

Please visit the Nelson Textbook of Pediatrics *website at www.expertconsult.com for the complete bibliography.*

190.2 Enteric Fever (Typhoid Fever)

Zulfiqar Ahmed Bhutta

Enteric fever (more commonly termed *typhoid fever*) remains endemic in many developing countries. Given the ease of modern travel, cases are regularly reported from most developed countries, usually from returning travelers.

ETIOLOGY

Typhoid fever is caused by *Salmonella enterica* serovar Typhi (*S.* Typhi), a gram-negative bacterium. A very similar but often less severe disease is caused by *S.* Paratyphi A and rarely by *S.* Paratyphi B (Schotmulleri) and *S.* Paratyphi C (Hirschfeldii). The ratio of disease caused by *S.* Typhi to that caused by *S.* Paratyphi is about 10 to 1, although the proportion of *S.* Paratyphi A infections is increasing in some parts of the world for reasons that are unclear. Although *S.* Typhi shares many genes with *Escherichia coli* and at least 95% with *S.* Typhimurium, several unique gene clusters known as *pathogenicity islands* and other genes have been acquired during evolution. The inactivation of single genes as well as the acquisition or loss of single genes or large islands of DNA may have contributed to host adaptation and restriction of *S.* Typhi.

One of the most specific gene products is the polysaccharide capsule Vi (virulence), which is present in about 90% of all freshly isolated *S.* Typhi and has a protective effect against the bactericidal action of the serum of infected patients.

EPIDEMIOLOGY

It is estimated that more than 21.7 million typhoid cases and more than 200,000 deaths occur annually, the vast majority in Asia. Additionally, an estimated 5.4 million cases due to paratyphoid occur each year. Given the paucity of microbiologic facilities in developing countries, these figures may be more representative of the clinical syndrome rather than of culture-proven disease. In most developed countries, the incidence of typhoid fever is <15 cases/100,000 population, with most cases occurring in travelers. In contrast, the incidence may vary considerably in the developing world, with estimated rates ranging from 100 to 1,000 cases/100,000 population. There are significant differences in the age distribution and population at risk. Population-based studies from South Asia also indicate that the age-specific incidence of typhoid may be highest in children <5 yr of age, in association with comparatively higher rates of complications and hospitalization.

Typhoid fever has been notable for the emergence of drug resistance. Following sporadic outbreaks of chloramphenicol-resistant typhoid, many strains of *S.* Typhi have developed plasmid-mediated multidrug resistance to all 3 of the primary antimicrobials: ampicillin, chloramphenicol, and trimethoprim-sulfamethoxazole. There has also been considerable increase in nalidixic acid–resistant isolates of *S.* Typhi as well as the emergence of fluoroquinolone-resistant isolates. Nalidixic acid–resistant isolates first emerged in Southeast Asia and India and now account for the majority of travel-associated cases of typhoid fever in the USA.

S. Typhi is highly adapted to infection of humans to the point that it has lost the ability to cause transmissible disease in other animals. The discovery of the large number of pseudogenes in *S.* Typhi suggests that the genome of this pathogen has undergone degeneration to facilitate a specialized association with the human host. Thus, direct or indirect contact with an infected person (sick or chronic carrier) is a prerequisite for infection. Ingestion of foods or water contaminated with *S.* Typhi from human feces is the most common mode of transmission, although water-borne outbreaks due to poor sanitation or contamination have been described in developing countries. In other parts of the world, oysters and other shellfish cultivated in water contaminated by sewage and the use of night soil as fertilizer may also cause infection.

PATHOGENESIS

Enteric fever occurs through the ingestion of the organism, and a variety of sources of fecal contamination have been reported, including street foods and contamination of water reservoirs.

Human volunteer experiments established an infecting dose of about 10^5-10^9 organisms, with an incubation period ranging from 4 to 14 days, depending on the inoculating dose of viable bacteria. After ingestion, *S.* Typhi organisms are thought to invade the body through the gut mucosa in the terminal ileum, possibly through specialized antigen-sampling cells known as *M cells* that overlie gut-associated lymphoid tissues, through enterocytes, or via a paracellular route. *S.* Typhi crosses the intestinal mucosal barrier after attachment to the microvilli by an intricate mechanism involving membrane ruffling, actin rearrangement, and internalization in an intracellular vacuole. In contrast to nontyphoidal *Salmonella*, *S.* Typhi expresses virulence factors that allow it to downregulate the pathogen recognition receptor–mediated host inflammatory response. Within the Peyer patches in the terminal ileum, *S.* Typhi can traverse the intestinal barrier through several mechanisms, including the M cells in the follicle-associated epithelium, epithelial cells, and dendritic cells. At the villi, *Salmonella* can enter through the M cells or by passage through or between compromised epithelial cells.

On contact with the epithelial cell, S. typhi assembles TTSS-1 and translocates effectors into the cytoplasm. These effectors activate host Rho guanosine triphosphatases (GTPases), resulting in the rearrangement of the actin cytoskeleton into membrane ruffles, induction of mitogen-activated protein kinase (MAPK) pathways, and destabilization of tight junctions. Changes in the actin cytoskeleton are further modulated by the actin-binding proteins SipA and SipC and lead to bacterial uptake. MAPK signaling activates the transcription factors activator protein-1 (AP-1) and nuclear factor-κB (NF-κB), which turn on production of IL-8. The destabilization of tight junctions allows the transmigration of polymorphonuclear leukocytes (PMNs) from the basolateral surface to the apical surface, paracellular fluid leakage, and access of bacteria to the basolateral surface. Shortly after internalization of *S.* Typhi by macropinocytosis, salmonellae are enclosed in a spacious phagosome that is formed by membrane ruffles. Later, the phagosome fuses with lysosomes, acidifies, and shrinks to become adherent around the bacterium, forming the

Salmonella-containing vacuole (SCV). TTSS-2 is induced within the SCV and translocates effector proteins SifA and PipB2, which contribute to *Salmonella*-induced filament (Sif) formation along microtubules (see Fig. 190-2).

After passing through the intestinal mucosa, *S.* Typhi organisms enter the mesenteric lymphoid system and then pass into the bloodstream via the lymphatics. This primary bacteremia is usually asymptomatic, and blood culture results are frequently negative at this stage of the disease. The blood-borne bacteria are disseminated throughout the body and are thought to colonize the organs of the RES, where they may replicate within macrophages. After a period of bacterial replication, *S.* Typhi organisms are shed back into the blood, causing a secondary bacteremia that coincides with the onset of clinical symptoms and marks the end of the incubation period (Fig. 190-3).

In vitro studies with human cell lines have shown qualitative and quantitative differences in the epithelial cell response to *S.* Typhi and *S.* Typhimurium with regard to cytokine and chemokine secretion. Thus, by avoiding the triggering of an early inflammatory response in the gut, *S.* Typhi could instead colonize deeper tissues and organ systems. Infection with *S.* Typhi produces an inflammatory response in the deeper mucosal layers and underlying lymphoid tissue, with hyperplasia of Peyer patches and subsequent necrosis and sloughing of overlying epithelium. The resulting ulcers can bleed but usually heal without scarring or stricture formation. The inflammatory lesion may occasionally penetrate the muscularis and serosa of the intestine and produce perforation. The mesenteric lymph nodes, liver, and spleen are hyperemic and generally have areas of focal necrosis as well. A mononuclear response may be seen in the bone marrow in association with areas of focal necrosis. The morphologic changes of *S.* Typhi infection are less prominent in infants than in older children and adults.

It is thought that several virulence factors, including TTSS-2, may be necessary for the virulence properties and ability to cause systemic infection. The surface Vi polysaccharide capsular antigen found in *S.* Typhi interferes with phagocytosis by preventing the binding of C3 to the surface of the bacterium. The ability of organisms to survive within macrophages after phagocytosis is an important virulence trait encoded by the PhoP regulon and may be related to metabolic effects on host cells. The occasional occurrence of diarrhea may be explained by the presence of a toxin related to cholera toxin and *E. coli* heat-labile enterotoxin. The clinical syndrome of fever and systemic symptoms is produced by a release of proinflammatory cytokines (IL-6, IL-1β, and TNF-α) from the infected cells.

In addition to the virulence of the infecting organisms, host factors and immunity may also play an important role in predisposition to infection. There is an association between susceptibility to typhoid fever and human genes within the major histocompatibility complex class II and class III loci. Patients who are infected with HIV are at significantly higher risk for clinical infection with *S.* Typhi and *S.* Paratyphi. Similarly, patients with *Helicobacter pylori* infection have an increased risk of acquiring typhoid fever.

CLINICAL FEATURES

The incubation period of typhoid fever is usually 7-14 days but depends on the infecting dose and ranges between 3 and 30 days. The clinical presentation varies from a mild illness with low-grade fever, malaise, and slight, dry cough to a severe clinical picture with abdominal discomfort and multiple complications.

Many factors influence the severity and overall clinical outcome of the infection. They include the duration of illness before the initiation of appropriate therapy, choice of antimicrobial treatment, age, previous exposure or vaccination history, virulence of the bacterial strain, quantity of inoculum ingested, and several host factors affecting immune status.

The presentation of typhoid fever may also differ according to age. Although data from South America and other parts of Africa suggest that typhoid may manifest as a mild illness in young children, presentation may vary in different parts of the world. There is emerging evidence from south Asia that the presentation of typhoid may be more dramatic in children <5 yr of age, with comparatively higher rates of complications and hospitalization. Diarrhea, toxicity, and complications such as disseminated intravascular coagulopathy (DIC) are also more common in infancy, resulting in higher case fatality rates. However, some of the other features and complications of typhoid fever seen in adults, such as relative bradycardia, neurologic manifestations, and gastrointestinal bleeding, are rare in children.

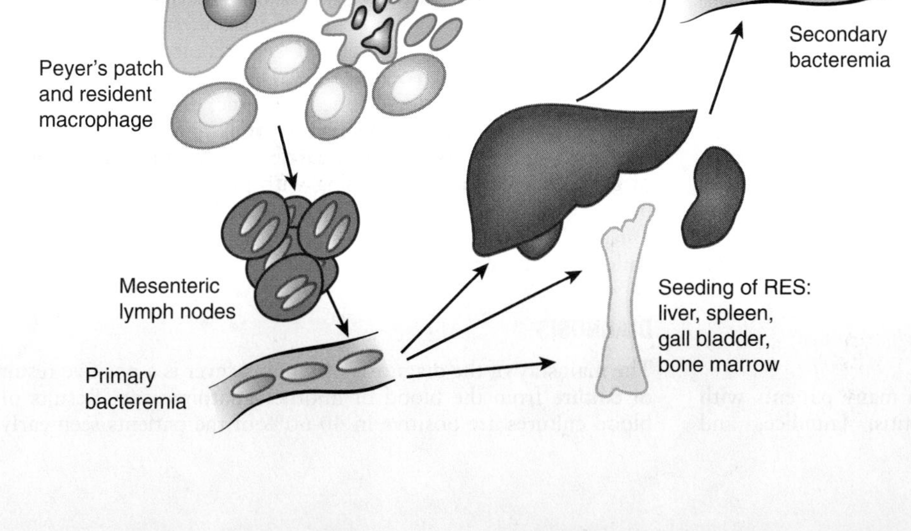

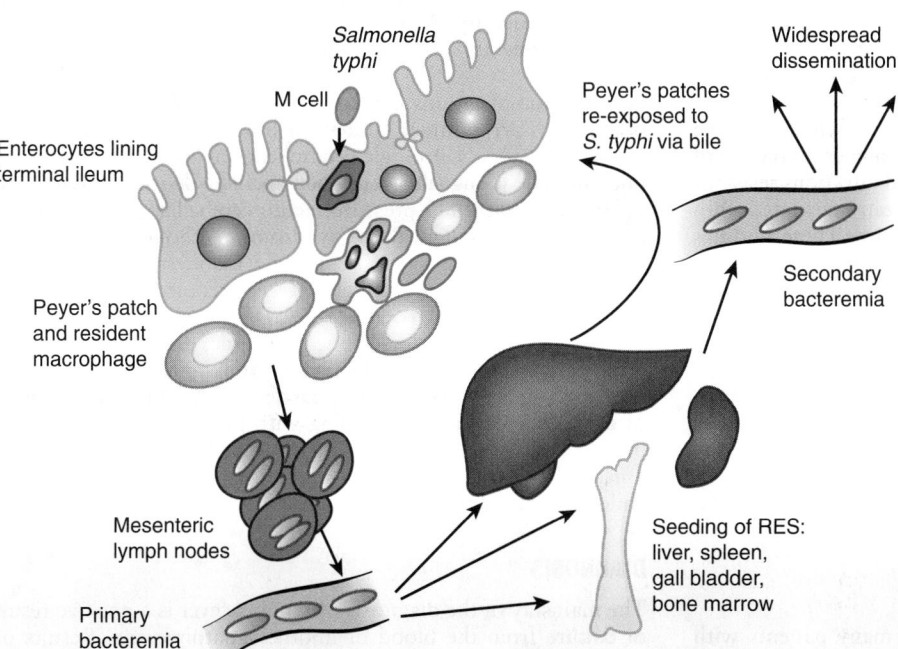

Figure 190-3 Pathogenesis of typhoid fever. RES, reticuloendothelial system. (Adapted from Richens J: Typhoid fever. In Cohen J, Powderly WG, Opal SM, editors: *Infectious diseases,* ed 2, London, 2004, Mosby, pp 1561–1566.)

Table 190-5 COMMON CLINICAL FEATURES OF TYPHOID FEVER IN CHILDREN*

FEATURE	RATE (%)
High-grade fever	95
Coated tongue	76
Anorexia	70
Vomiting	39
Hepatomegaly	37
Diarrhea	36
Toxicity	29
Abdominal pain	21
Pallor	20
Splenomegaly	17
Constipation	7
Headache	4
Jaundice	2
Obtundation	2
Ileus	1
Intestinal perforation	0.5

*Data collected in Karachi, Pakistan, from 2,000 children.

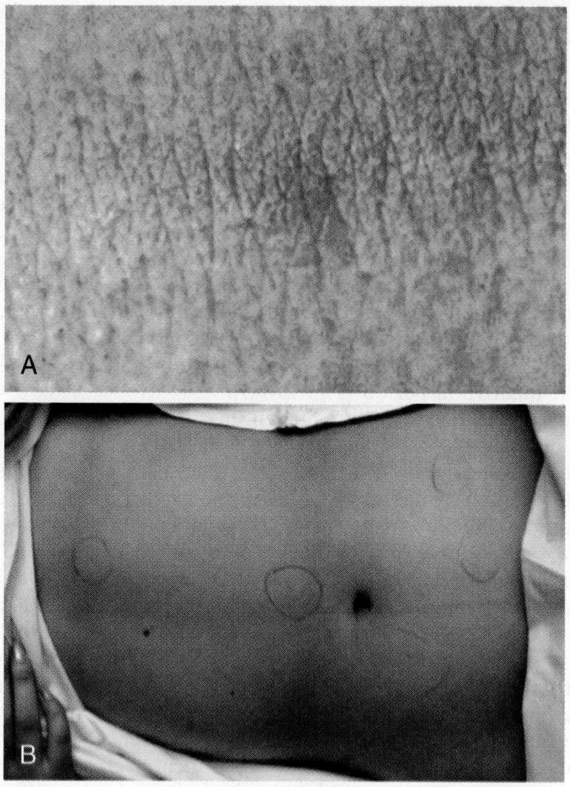

Figure 190-4 *A,* A rose spot in a volunteer with experimental typhoid fever. *B,* A small cluster of rose spots is usually located on the abdomen. These lesions may be difficult to identify, especially in dark-skinned people. (From Huang DB, DuPont HL: Problem pathogens: Extra-intestinal complications of *Salmonella enterica* serotype Typhi infection, *Lancet Infect Dis* 5:341–348, 2005.)

Typhoid fever usually manifests as high-grade fever with a wide variety of associated features, such as generalized myalgia, abdominal pain, hepatosplenomegaly, abdominal pain, and anorexia (Table 190-5). In children, diarrhea may occur in the earlier stages of the illness and may be followed by constipation. In the absence of localizing signs, the early stage of the disease may be difficult to differentiate from other endemic diseases such as malaria and dengue fever. The fever may rise gradually, but the classic stepladder rise of fever is relatively rare. In about 25% of cases, a macular or maculopapular rash (rose spots) may be visible around the 7th-10th day of the illness, and lesions may appear in crops of 10-15 on the lower chest and abdomen and last 2-3 days (Fig. 190-4). These lesions may be difficult to see in dark-skinned children. Patients managed as outpatients present with fever (99%) but have less emesis, diarrhea, hepatomegaly, splenomegaly, and myalgias than patients who require admission to the hospital.

The presentation of typhoid fever may be tempered by coexisting morbidities and early diagnosis and administration of antibiotics. In malaria-endemic areas and in parts of the world where schistosomiasis is common, the presentation of typhoid may also be atypical. It is also recognized that multidrug-resistant *S.* Typhi infection is a more severe clinical illness with higher rates of toxicity, complications, and case fatality rates, which may be related to the greater virulence as well as higher numbers of circulating bacteria. The emergence of typhoid infections resistant to nalidixic acid and fluorquinolones has been associated with higher rates of morbidity and treatment failure. These findings may have implications for treatment algorithms, especially in endemic areas with high rates of multidrug-resistant and nalidixic acid– or fluoroquinolone-resistant typhoid.

If no complications occur, the symptoms and physical findings gradually resolve within 2-4 wk; however, the illness may be associated with malnutrition in a number of affected children. Although enteric fever caused by *S.* Paratyphi organisms has been classically regarded as a milder illness, there have been several outbreaks of infection with drug-resistant *S.* Paratyphi A, suggesting that paratyphoid fever may also be severe, with significant morbidity and complications.

COMPLICATIONS

Although altered liver function is found in many patients with enteric fever, clinically significant hepatitis, jaundice, and cholecystitis are relatively rare and may be associated with higher rates of adverse outcome. Intestinal hemorrhage (<1%) and perforation (0.5-1%) are infrequent among children. Intestinal perforation may be preceded by a marked increase in abdominal pain (usually in the right lower quadrant), tenderness, vomiting, and features of peritonitis. Intestinal perforation and peritonitis may be accompanied by a sudden rise in pulse rate, hypotension, marked abdominal tenderness and guarding, and subsequent abdominal rigidity. A rising white blood cell count with a left shift and free air on abdominal radiographs may be seen in such cases.

Rare complications include toxic myocarditis, which may manifest as arrhythmias, sinoatrial block, or cardiogenic shock (Table 190-6). Neurologic complications are also relatively uncommon among children; they include delirium, psychosis, increased intracranial pressure, acute cerebellar ataxia, chorea, deafness, and Guillain-Barré syndrome. Although case fatality rates may be higher with neurologic manifestations, recovery usually occurs with no sequelae. Other reported complications include fatal bone marrow necrosis, DIC, hemolytic-uremic syndrome, pyelonephritis, nephrotic syndrome, meningitis, endocarditis, parotitis, orchitis, and suppurative lymphadenitis.

The propensity to become a carrier follows the epidemiology of gallbladder disease, increasing with patient age and the antibiotic resistance of the prevalent strains. Although limited data are available, rates of chronic carriage are generally lower in children than adults.

DIAGNOSIS

The mainstay of the diagnosis of typhoid fever is a positive result of culture from the blood or another anatomic site. Results of blood cultures are positive in 40-60% of the patients seen early

Table 190-6 EXTRAINTESTINAL INFECTIOUS COMPLICATIONS OF TYPHOID FEVER CAUSED BY *SALMONELLA ENTERICA* SEROTYPE TYPHI

ORGAN SYSTEM INVOLVED	PREVALENCE (%)	RISK FACTORS	COMPLICATIONS
Central nervous system	3-35	Residence in endemic region, malignancy, endocarditis, congenital heart disease, paranasal sinus infections, pulmonary infections, meningitis, trauma, surgery, and osteomyelitis of the skull	Encephalopathy, cerebral edema, subdural empyema, cerebral abscess, meningitis, ventriculitis, transient parkinsonism, motor neuron disorders, ataxia, seizures, Guillain-Barré syndrome, psychosis
Cardiovascular system	1-5	Cardiac abnormalities—e.g., existing valvular abnormalities, rheumatic heart disease, or congenital heart defects	Endocarditis, myocarditis, pericarditis, arteritis, congestive heart failure
Pulmonary system	1-6	Residence in endemic region, past pulmonary infection, sickle cell anaemia, alcohol abuse, diabetes, HIV infection	Pneumonia, empyema, bronchopleural fistula
Bone and joint	<1	Sickle cell anemia, diabetes, systemic lupus erythematosus, lymphoma, liver disease, previous surgery or trauma, extremes of age, and steroid use	Osteomyelitis, septic arthritis
Hepatobiliary system	1-26	Residence in endemic region, pyogenic infections, intravenous drug use, splenic trauma, HIV, hemoglobinopathy	Cholecystitis, hepatitis, hepatic abscesses, splenic abscess, peritonitis, paralytic ileus
Genitourinary system	<1	Urinary tract, pelvic pathology, and systemic abnormalities	Urinary tract infection, renal abscess, pelvic infections, testicular abscess, prostatitis, epididymitis
Soft tissue infections	At least 17 cases reported in the English language literature	Diabetes	Psoas abscess, gluteal abscess, cutaneous vasculitis
Hematologic	At least 5 cases reported in the English language literature		Hemophagocytosis syndrome

From Huang DB, DuPont HL: Problem pathogens: extra-intestinal complications of *Salmonella enterica* serotype Typhi infection, *Lancet Infect Dis* 5:341–348, 2005.

in the course of the disease, and stool and urine culture results become positive after the 1st wk. The stool culture result is also occasionally positive during the incubation period. However, the sensitivity of blood cultures in diagnosing typhoid fever in many parts of the developing world is limited because widespread liberal antibiotic use may render bacteriologic confirmation difficult. Although bone marrow cultures may increase the likelihood of bacteriologic confirmation of typhoid, collection of the specimens is difficult and relatively invasive.

Results of other laboratory investigations are nonspecific. Although blood leukocyte counts are frequently low in relation to the fever and toxicity, there is a wide range in counts; in younger children leukocytosis is common and may reach 20,000-25,000 cells/mm^3. Thrombocytopenia may be a marker of severe illness and may accompany DIC. Liver function test results may be deranged, but significant hepatic dysfunction is rare.

The classic Widal test measures antibodies against O and H antigens of *S.* Typhi but lacks sensitivity and specificity in endemic areas. Because many false-positive and false-negative results occur, diagnosis of typhoid fever by Widal test alone is prone to error. Other relatively newer diagnostic tests using monoclonal antibodies have been developed that directly detect *S.* Typhi–specific antigens in the serum or *S.* Typhi Vi antigen in the urine. However, few have proved sufficiently robust in large-scale evaluations. A nested polymerase chain reaction analysis using *H1-d* primers has been used to amplify specific genes of *S.* Typhi in the blood of patients; it is a promising means of making a rapid diagnosis, especially given the low level of bacteremia in enteric fever. Despite these innovations, the mainstay of diagnosis of typhoid remains clinical in much of the developing world, and several diagnostic algorithms have been evaluated in endemic areas.

DIFFERENTIAL DIAGNOSIS

In endemic areas, typhoid fever may mimic many common febrile illnesses without localizing signs. In children with multisystem features and no localizing signs, the early stages of enteric fever may be confused with alternative conditions, such as acute gastroenteritis, bronchitis, and bronchopneumonia. Subsequently, the differential diagnosis includes malaria; sepsis with other bacterial pathogens; infections caused by intracellular microorganisms, such as tuberculosis, brucellosis, tularemia, leptospirosis, and rickettsial diseases; and viral infections such as Dengue fever, acute hepatitis, and infectious mononucleosis.

TREATMENT

An early diagnosis of typhoid fever and institution of appropriate treatment are essential. The vast majority of children with typhoid can be managed at home with oral antibiotics and close medical follow-up for complications or failure of response to therapy. Patients with persistent vomiting, severe diarrhea, and abdominal distention may require hospitalization and parenteral antibiotic therapy.

There are general principles of management of typhoid. Adequate rest, hydration, and attention are important to correct fluid and electrolyte imbalance. Antipyretic therapy (acetaminophen 10-15 mg/kg every 4-6 hr by mouth [PO]) should be provided as required. A soft, easily digestible diet should be continued unless the patient has abdominal distention or ileus. Antibiotic therapy is critical to minimize complications (Table 190-7). It has been suggested that traditional therapy with either chloramphenicol or amoxicillin is associated with relapse rates of 5-15% and 4-8%, respectively, whereas use of the quinolones and third-generation cephalosporins is associated with higher cure rates. The antibiotic treatment of typhoid fever in children is also influenced by the prevalence of antimicrobial resistance. Over the past 2 decades, emergence of multidrug-resistant strains of *S.* Typhi (i.e., isolates fully resistant to amoxicillin, trimethoprim-sulfamethoxazole, and chloramphenicol) has necessitated treatment with fluoroquinolones, which are the antimicrobial drug of choice for treatment of salmonellosis in adults, or cephalosporins. The emergence of resistance to quinolones has placed tremendous pressure on public health systems because alternative therapeutic options are limited.

Although some investigators have suggested that children with typhoid should be treated with fluoroquinolones like adults, others have questioned this approach on the basis of the potential development of further resistance to fluoroquinolones and the fact that quinolones are still not approved for widespread use in

Table 190-7 TREATMENT OF TYPHOID FEVER IN CHILDREN

SUSCEPTIBILITY	OPTIMAL THERAPY Antibiotic	Daily Dose (mg/kg/day)	Days	ALTERNATIVE EFFECTIVE DRUGS Antibiotic	Daily Dose (mg/kg/day)	Days
UNCOMPLICATED TYPHOID FEVER						
Fully sensitive	Chloramphenicol	50-75	14-21	Fluoroquinolone, e.g., ofloxacin or ciprofloxacin	15	5-7*
	Amoxicillin	75-100	14			
Multidrug-resistant	Fluoroquinolone	15	5-7	Azithromycin	20	7
	or					
	Cefixime	15-20	7-14	Cefixime	15-20	7-14
Quinolone-resistant†	Azithromycin	8-10	7	Cefixime	20	7-14
	or					
	Ceftriaxone	75	10-14			
SEVERE TYPHOID FEVER						
Fully sensitive	Ampicillin	100	14	Fluoroquinolone, e.g., ofloxacin or ciprofloxacin	15	10-14
	or					
	Ceftriaxone	60-75	10-14			
Multidrug-resistant	Fluoroquinolone	15	10-14	Ceftriaxone	60	10-14
				or		
				Cefotaxime	80	10-14
Quinolone-resistant	Ceftriaxone	60-75	10-14	Azithromycin	20	7
				Gatifloxacin	10	7

*A 3-day course is also effective, particularly for epidemic containment.

†The optimum treatment for quinolone-resistant typhoid fever has not been determined. Azithromycin, 3rd-generation cephalosporins, or high-dose fluoroquinolones for 10-14 days is effective.

Modified from World Health Organization: Treatment of typhoid fever. Background document: the diagnosis, prevention and treatment of typhoid fever. In: *Communicable disease surveillance and response: vaccines and biologicals,* Geneva, 2003, World Health Organization, pp 19–23. http://whqlibdoc.who.int/hq/2003/WHO_V&B_03.07.pdf.

children. A Cochrane systematic review of the treatment of typhoid fever also indicates that there is little evidence to support the carte blanche administration of fluoroquinolones in all cases of typhoid.

In addition to antibiotics, the importance of supportive treatment and maintenance of appropriate fluid and electrolyte balance must be underscored. Although additional treatment with dexamethasone (3 mg/kg for the initial dose, followed by 1 mg/kg every 6 hr for 48 hr) has been recommended for severely ill patients with shock, obtundation, stupor, or coma, corticosteroids should be administered only under strict controlled conditions and supervision, because their use may mask signs of abdominal complications.

PROGNOSIS

The prognosis for a patient with enteric fever depends on the rapidity of diagnosis and institution of appropriate antibiotic therapy. Other factors are the patient's, age, general state of health, and nutrition, the causative *Salmonella* serotype, and the appearance of complications. Infants and children with underlying malnutrition and patients infected with multidrug-resistant isolates are at higher risk for adverse outcomes.

Despite appropriate therapy, 2-4% of infected children may experience relapse after initial clinical response to treatment. Individuals who excrete *S.* Typhi for ≥3 mo after infection are regarded as chronic carriers. The risk for becoming a carrier is low in children (<2% for all infected children) and increases with age. A chronic urinary carrier state can develop in children with schistosomiasis.

PREVENTION

Of the major risk factors for outbreaks of typhoid, contamination of water supplies with sewage is the most important. Other risk factors for development of typhoid fever are congestion, contact with another patient or a febrile individual, and lack of water and sanitation services. During outbreaks, central chlorination as well as domestic water purification is important. In endemic situations, consumption of street foods, especially ice cream and cut fruit, has been recognized as an important risk factor. The human-to-human spread by chronic carriers is also important, and attempts should therefore be made to target food handlers and high-risk groups for *S.* Typhi carriage screening. Once identified, chronic carriers must be counseled as to the risk for disease transmission and the importance of handwashing.

The classic heat-inactivated whole-cell vaccine for typhoid is associated with an unacceptably high rate of side effects and has been largely withdrawn from public health use. Globally, 2 vaccines are currently available for potential use in children. An oral, live-attenuated preparation of the Ty21a strain of *S.* Typhi has been shown to have good efficacy (67-82%) for up to 5 yr. Significant adverse effects are rare. The Vi capsular polysaccharide can be used in people ≥2 yr of age. It is given as a single intramuscular dose, with a booster every 2 yr, and has a protective efficacy of 70-80%. The vaccines are currently recommended for anyone traveling into endemic areas, but a few countries have introduced large-scale vaccination strategies. Previous studies in South America have demonstrated protection against typhoid among schoolchildren with the use of an oral attenuated Ty21 strain vaccine.

Several large-scale demonstration projects using the Vi polysaccharide vaccine in Asia have demonstrated protective efficacy against typhoid fever across all age groups, but the data on protection among young children (<5 yr) showed important differences between studies. The recent Vi-conjugate vaccine has been shown to have a protective efficacy exceeding 90% in younger children and may offer protection in parts of the world where a large proportion of preschool children are at risk for the disease enteric or typhoid fever.

BIBLIOGRAPHY

Please visit the Nelson Textbook of Pediatrics *website at www.expertconsult.com for the complete bibliography.*

Chapter 191
Shigella

Theresa J. Ochoa and Thomas G. Cleary

Shigella causes an acute invasive enteric infection clinically manifested by diarrhea that is often bloody. The term *dysentery* is used to describe the syndrome of bloody diarrhea with fever, abdominal cramps, rectal pain, and mucoid stools. Bacillary dysentery is a term often used to distinguish dysentery caused by *Shigella* from amoebic dysentery caused by *Entamoeba histolytica*.

ETIOLOGY

Four species of *Shigella* are responsible for bacillary dysentery: *S. dysenteriae* (serogroup A), *S. flexneri* (serogroup B), *S. boydii* (serogroup C), and *S. sonnei* (serogroup D). There are 13 serotypes in group A, six serotypes and 15 subserotypes in group B, 18 serotypes in group C, and one serotype in group D. Species classification has important therapeutic implications because the species differ in both geographic distribution and antimicrobial susceptibility.

EPIDEMIOLOGY

It is estimated that there are approximately 165 million cases of shigellosis each year, resulting in >1 million deaths; most of these cases and deaths occur in developing countries. In the USA, approximately 14,000 cases per year are documented. Although infection can occur at any age, it is most common in the 2nd and 3rd years of life. Approximately 70% of all episodes and 60% of all *Shigella*-related deaths involve children <5 years old. Infection in the first 6 mo of life is rare for reasons that are not clear. Breast milk contains antibodies to both virulence plasmid-coded antigens and lipopolysaccharides in endemic areas, and breast-feeding might partially explain the age-related incidence.

Asymptomatic infection of children and adults occurs commonly in endemic areas. Infection with *Shigella* occurs most often during the warm months in temperate climates and during the rainy season in tropical climates. Both sexes are affected equally. In industrialized societies, *S. sonnei* is the most common cause of bacillary dysentery, with *S. flexneri* second in frequency; in preindustrial societies, *S. flexneri* is most common, with *S. sonnei* second in frequency. *S. boydii* is found primarily in India. *S. dysenteriae* serotype 1 tends to occur in massive epidemics, although it is also endemic in Asia and Africa, where it is associated with high mortality rates (5-15%).

Contaminated food (often a salad or other item requiring extensive handling of the ingredients) and water are important vectors. Exposure to both fresh and saltwater is a risk factor for infection. Rapid spread within families, custodial institutions, and child-care centers demonstrates the ability of shigellae to be transmitted from one individual to the next and the requirement for ingestion of very few organisms to cause illness. As few as 10 *S. dysenteriae* serotype 1 organisms can cause dysentery. In contrast, ingestion of 10^8-10^{10} *Vibrio cholerae* is necessary to cause cholera.

PATHOGENESIS

The basic virulence trait shared by all shigellae is the ability to invade intestinal epithelial cells. This characteristic is encoded on a large (220 Kb) plasmid that is responsible for synthesis of a group of polypeptides involved in cell invasion and killing. Shigellae that lose the virulence plasmid are no longer pathogenic. *Escherichia coli* that harbor a closely related plasmid containing these invasion genes (enteroinvasive *E. coli*) behave clinically like shigellae. The virulence plasmid encodes a type III secretion system (TTSS) required to trigger entry into epithelial cells and apoptosis in macrophages. This secretion system translocates effector molecules from the bacterial cytoplasm to the membrane and cytoplasm of target host cells. The TTSS is composed of approximately 50 proteins, including Mxi and Spa proteins involved in assembly and regulation of the TTSS, chaperones (IpgA, IpgC, IpgE, and Spa15), transcription activators (VirF, VirB, and MxiE), translocators (IpaB, IpaC, and IpaD), and approximately 25 effector proteins. In addition to the major plasmid-encoded virulence traits, chromosomally encoded factors are also required for full virulence.

Shigella passes the epithelial cell barrier by transcytosis through M cells and encounters resident macrophages. The bacteria evade degradation in macrophages by inducing apoptosis, which is accompanied by proinflammatory signaling. Free bacteria invade the epithelial cells from the basolateral side, move into the cytoplasm by actin polymerization, and spread to adjacent cells. Proinflammatory signaling by macrophages and epithelial cells further activates the innate immune response involving NK cells and attracts polymorphonuclear leukocytes (PMNs). The influx of PMNs disintegrates the epithelial cell lining, which initially exacerbates the infection and tissue destruction by facilitating the invasion of more bacteria. Ultimately, PMNs phagocytose and kill *Shigella*, thus contributing to the resolution of the infection.

Some shigellae make toxins including Shiga toxin and enterotoxins. Shiga toxin is a potent exotoxin that inhibits protein synthesis and is produced in significant amounts by *S. dysenteriae* serotype 1, by a subset of *E. coli*, which are known as Shiga toxin–producing *E. coli* (STEC), and occasionally by other organisms. This toxin mediates the severe complication of hemolytic-uremic syndrome (HUS). It is unclear whether the watery diarrhea phase of shigellosis is caused by one of the other enterotoxins. Targeted deletion of the genes for enterotoxins *(ShET1* and *ShET2)* decreased the incidence of fever and dysentery in volunteers during vaccine-development studies. Lipopolysaccharides are virulence factors for all shigellae; other traits are important for only a few serotypes (e.g., Shigatoxin synthesis by *S. dysenteriae* serotype 1 and ShET1 by *S. flexneri* 2a).

The pathologic changes of shigellosis take place primarily in the colon, the target organ for *Shigella*. The changes are most intense in the distal colon, although pancolitis can occur. Shigellae cross the colonic epithelium through M cells in the follicle-associated epithelium overlying the Peyer patches. Grossly, localized or diffuse mucosal edema, ulcerations, friable mucosa, bleeding, and exudate may be seen. Microscopically, ulcerations, pseudomembranes, epithelial cell death, infiltration extending from the mucosa to the muscularis mucosae by PMNs and mononuclear cells, and submucosal edema occur.

IMMUNITY

Innate immunity to *Shigella* infection is characterized by the induction of acute inflammation with massive recruitment of PMNs and subsequently massive tissue destruction. In humans, analysis of cytokine expression in rectal biopsies of infected patients at the acute phase of the disease has revealed upregulation of proinflammatory genes, such as those encoding interleukin (IL)-1β, IL-6, IL-8, tumor necrosis factor (TNF)-α, and TNF-β, although antiinflammatory genes encoding IL-10 and TGF-β are also upregulated. Control of *Shigella* invasion in intestinal epithelial cells depends on interferon (IFN)-γ. *Shigella*-specific immunity elicited upon natural infection is characterized by the induction of a humoral response. Local secretory IgA and serum IgG are produced against LPS and some protein effectors (Ipas). Natural protective immunity arises only after several episodes of infection, is of short duration, and seems to be effective in limiting reinfection, particularly in young children.

CLINICAL MANIFESTATIONS AND COMPLICATIONS

Bacillary dysentery is clinically similar regardless of infecting serotype. There are some clinical differences, particularly relating to the greater severity and risk of complications with *S. dysenteriae* serotype 1 infection. Ingestion of shigellae is followed by an incubation period of 12 hr to several days before symptoms ensue. Severe abdominal pain, high fever, emesis, anorexia, generalized toxicity, urgency, and painful defecation characteristically occur. The diarrhea may be watery and of large volume initially, evolving into frequent, small-volume, bloody mucoid stools. Most children never progress to the stage of bloody diarrhea, but some have bloody stools from the outset. Significant dehydration is related to the fluid and electrolyte losses in feces and emesis. Untreated diarrhea can last 1-2 wk; only about 10% of patients have diarrhea persisting for >10 days. Persistent diarrhea occurs in malnourished infants, children with AIDS, and occasionally previously normal children. Even nondysenteric disease can be complicated by persistent illness.

Physical examination initially shows abdominal distention and tenderness, hyperactive bowel sounds, and a tender rectum on digital examination. Neurologic findings are among the most common extraintestinal manifestations of bacillary dysentery, occurring in as many as 40% of hospitalized children. Enteroinvasive *E. coli* can cause similar neurologic toxicity. Convulsions, headache, lethargy, confusion, nuchal rigidity, or hallucinations may be present before or after the onset of diarrhea. The cause of these neurologic findings is not understood. In the past, these symptoms were attributed to the neurotoxicity of Shiga toxin, but it is now clear that this explanation is wrong because the organisms isolated from children with *Shigella*-related seizures are usually not Shiga toxin producers. Seizures sometimes occur when little fever is present, suggesting that simple febrile convulsions do not explain their appearance. Hypocalcemia or hyponatremia may be associated with seizures in a small number of patients. Although symptoms often suggest central nervous system infection and cerebrospinal fluid pleocytosis with minimally elevated protein levels can occur, meningitis due to shigellae is rare. Based on animal studies, it has been suggested that proinflammatory mediators, including TNF-α and interleukin-1β, nitric oxide, and corticotropin-releasing hormone, all play a role in the enhanced susceptibility to seizures caused by *S. dysenteriae*.

The most common complication of shigellosis is dehydration. Inappropriate secretion of antidiuretic hormone with profound hyponatremia can complicate dysentery, particularly when *S. dysenteriae* is the etiologic agent. Hypoglycemia and protein-losing enteropathy are common. Other major complications include sepsis and disseminated intravascular coagulation, particularly in very young, malnourished children. Given that shigellae penetrate the intestinal mucosal barrier, these events are surprisingly uncommon.

Shigella and sometimes other gram-negative enteric bacilli are recovered from blood cultures in 1-5% of patients in whom blood cultures are taken; because patients selected for blood cultures represent a biased sample, the risk of bacteremia in unselected cases of shigellosis is presumably lower. Bacteremia is more common with *S. dysenteriae* serotype 1 than with other shigellae; the mortality rate is high (~20%) when sepsis occurs.

Neonatal shigellosis is rare. Neonates might have only low-grade fever with mild, nonbloody diarrhea. However, complications occur more commonly than in older children and include septicemia, meningitis, dehydration, colonic perforation, and toxic megacolon.

S. dysenteriae serotype 1 infection is commonly complicated by hemolysis, anemia, and HUS. This syndrome is caused by Shiga toxin–mediated vascular endothelial injury. *E. coli* that produce Shiga toxins (e.g., *E. coli* O157:H7, *E. coli* O111:NM, *E. coli* O26:H11) also cause HUS (Chapter 512).

Rectal prolapse, toxic megacolon or pseudomembranous colitis (usually associated with *S. dysenteriae*), cholestatic hepatitis, conjunctivitis, iritis, corneal ulcers, pneumonia, arthritis (usually 2-5 wk after enteritis), reactive arthritis, cystitis, myocarditis, and vaginitis (typically with a blood-tinged discharge associated with *S. flexneri*) are uncommon events. Although rare, surgical complications of shigellosis can be severe; the most common are intestinal obstruction and appendicitis with and without perforation.

On average, severity of illness and risk of death are least with disease caused by *S. sonnei* and greatest with infection by *S. dysenteriae* type 1. Risk groups for severe illness and poor outcomes include infants; adults >50 yr; children who are not breastfed; children recovering from measles; malnourished children and adults; and patients who develop dehydration, unconsciousness, or hypo- or hyperthermia or have a history of convulsion when first seen. Death is a rare outcome in well-nourished older children. Multiple factors contribute to death in malnourished children with shigellosis, including illness in the first year of life, altered consciousness, dehydration, hypothermia, thrombocytopenia, anemia, hyponatremia, renal failure, hyperkalemia hypoglycemia, bronchopneumonia, and bacteremia.

The rare syndrome of severe toxicity, convulsions, extreme hyperpyrexia, and headache followed by brain edema and a rapidly fatal outcome without sepsis or significant dehydration (Ekiri syndrome or "lethal toxic encephalopathy") is not well understood.

DIFFERENTIAL DIAGNOSIS

Although clinical features suggest shigellosis, they are insufficiently specific to allow confident diagnosis. Infection by *Campylobacter jejuni*, *Salmonella* spp, enteroinvasive *E. coli*, Shiga toxin–producing *E. coli* (e.g. *E. coli* O157:H7), *Yersinia enterocolitica*, *Clostridium difficile*, and *Entamoeba histolytica* as well as inflammatory bowel disease can cause confusion.

DIAGNOSIS

Presumptive data supporting a diagnosis of bacillary dysentery include the finding of fecal leukocytes (usually >50 or 100 PMNs per high power field, confirming the presence of colitis), fecal blood, and demonstration in peripheral blood of leukocytosis with a dramatic left shift (often with more bands than segmented neutrophils). The total peripheral white blood cell count is usually 5,000-15,000 cells/mm^3, although leukopenia and leukemoid reactions occur.

Culture of both stool and rectal swab specimens optimizes the chance of diagnosing *Shigella* infection. Culture media should include MacConkey agar as well as selective media such as xylose-lysine deoxycholate (XLD) and SS agar. Transport media should be used if specimens cannot be cultured promptly. Appropriate media should be used to exclude *Campylobacter* spp and other agents. Studies of outbreaks and illness in volunteers show that the laboratory is often not able to confirm the clinical suspicion of shigellosis even when the pathogen is present. Multiple fecal cultures improve the yield of *Shigella*. The diagnostic inadequacy of cultures makes it incumbent on the clinician to use judgment in the management of clinical syndromes consistent with shigellosis. Use of polymerase chain reaction (PCR) analysis of stool for specific genes such as *ipaH*, *virF*, or *virA* can detect cases not diagnosed by culture, but it is usually available only in research laboratories. In children who appear to be toxic, blood cultures should be obtained, especially in very young or malnourished infants because of their increased risk of bacteremia.

TREATMENT

As with gastroenteritis from other causes, the first concern in a child with suspected shigellosis should be for fluid and electrolyte correction and maintenance (Chapter 332). Drugs that retard intestinal motility (e.g., diphenoxylate hydrochloride with atropine [Lomotil] or loperamide [Imodium]) should not be used because of the risk of prolonging the illness.

Nutrition is a key concern in areas where malnutrition is common. A high-protein diet during convalescence enhances growth in the following 6 mo. A single large dose of vitamin A (200,000 IU) lessens severity of shigellosis in settings where vitamin A deficiency is common. Zinc supplementation (20 mg elemental zinc for 14 days) has been shown to significantly decrease the duration of diarrhea, improve weight gain during recovery and immune response to the *Shigella*, and decrease diarrheal disease in the subsequent 6 mo in malnourished children.

The next concern is a decision about the use of antibiotics. Although some authorities recommend withholding antibacterial therapy because of the self-limited nature of the infection, the cost of drugs, and the risk of emergence of resistant organisms, there is a persuasive logic in favor of empirical treatment of all children in whom shigellosis is strongly suspected. Even if not fatal, the untreated illness can cause a child to be quite ill for weeks; chronic or recurrent diarrhea can ensue. Malnutrition can develop or worsen during prolonged illness, particularly in children in developing countries. The risk of continued excretion and subsequent infection of family contacts further argues against the strategy of withholding antibiotics.

Shigella species have variable antimicrobial susceptibility. In general, *S. flexneri* tends to be more resistant than *S. boydii*. There are major geographic variations in antibiotic susceptibility of shigellae. In most developing countries and in some industrialized countries such as the USA, *Shigella* strains are often resistant to ampicillin and trimethoprim-sulfamethoxazole (TMP-SMX). Therefore, these drugs should usually not be used for empirical treatment of suspected shigellosis. Oral ampicillin (100 mg/kg/24 hr orally, divided 4 times/day) or TMP-SMX (10 mg/kg/24 hr orally of the TMP component in 2 divided doses) may be used if the strain is known to be susceptible (e.g., in an outbreak due to a defined strain). Amoxicillin is less effective than ampicillin for treatment of ampicillin-sensitive strains. Ceftriaxone (50 mg/kg/24 hr as a single daily dose IV or IM) can be used for empirical therapy, especially for small infants.

The oral 3rd-generation cephalosporin cefixime can also be used. Oral 1st and 2nd-generation cephalosporins are inadequate as alternative drugs despite in vitro susceptibility. Nalidixic acid (55 mg/kg/24 hr orally divided 4 times/day) is also an acceptable alternative drug when available. Azithromycin (12 mg/kg/24 hr orally for the first day, followed by 6 mg/kg/24 hr for the next 4 days) has proven to be an effective alternative drug for shigellosis. Ciprofloxacin (30 mg/kg/24 hr divided into 2 doses) used to be a back-up drug to treat shigellosis but is now the drug of choice recommended by WHO for all patients with bloody diarrhea, irrespective of their ages.

Although quinolones have been reported to cause arthropathy in immature animals, the risk of joint damage in children appears to be minimal and is outweighed by the value of these drugs for treatment of this potentially life-threatening disease. However, some experts recommend that these agents be reserved for seriously ill children with bacillary dysentery due to an organism that is suspected or known to be resistant to other agents, because overuse of quinolones promotes development of resistance to these drugs. Treatment in general is for a 5-day course.

Treatment of patients in whom *Shigella* infection is suspected on clinical grounds of should be initiated when they are first evaluated. Stool culture is obtained to exclude other pathogens and to assist in antibiotic changes should a child fail to respond to empirical therapy. A child who has typical dysentery and who responds to initial empirical antibiotic treatment should be continued on that drug for a full 5-day course even if the stool culture is negative. The logic of this recommendation is based on the proven difficulty of culturing *Shigella* from stools of ill patients during adult volunteer infection studies. In a child who fails to respond to therapy of a dysenteric syndrome in the presence of initially negative stool culture results, additional cultures should be obtained and the child should be re-evaluated for other possible diagnoses.

PREVENTION

Numerous measures have been recommended to decrease the risk of *Shigella* transmission to children. Mothers should be encouraged to prolong breast-feeding of infants. Families and day care personnel should be educated in proper handwashing techniques and encouraged to wash hands after using the toilet, changing diapers, or engaging in preparation of foods. They should be taught how to manage potentially contaminated materials such as raw vegetables, soiled diapers, and diaper-changing areas. Children with diarrhea should be excluded from child care facilities. Children should be supervised when handwashing after they use the toilet. Caretakers should be informed of the risk of transmission if they prepare food when they are ill with diarrhea. Families should be educated regarding the risk of swallowing contaminated water from ponds, lakes, or untreated pools.

There is not yet a vaccine that is effective for preventing infection by *Shigella*. Several candidate vaccines are under development, mostly against *S. flexneri*. Measles immunization can substantially reduce the incidence and severity of diarrheal diseases, including shigellosis. Every infant should be immunized against measles at the recommended age.

BIBLIOGRAPHY

Please visit the Nelson Textbook of Pediatrics *website at www.expertconsult.com for the complete bibliography.*

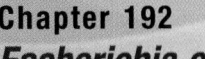

Chapter 192 Escherichia coli

Theresa J. Ochoa and Thomas G. Cleary

Escherichia coli are important causes of enteric infections as well as urinary tract infections (Chapter 532), sepsis and meningitis in the newborn (Chapter 103), and bacteremia and sepsis in immunocompromised patients (Chapter 171) and in patients with intravascular devices (Chapter 172).

E. coli species are members of the Enterobacteriaceae family. They are facultatively anaerobic, gram-negative bacilli that usually ferment lactose. Most fecal *E. coli* do not cause diarrhea. Six major groups of diarrheagenic *E. coli* have been characterized on the basis of clinical, biochemical, and molecular-genetic criteria: enterotoxigenic *E. coli* (ETEC); enteroinvasive *E. coli* (EIEC); enteropathogenic *E. coli* (EPEC); Shiga toxin–producing *E. coli* (STEC), also known as enterohemorrhagic *E. coli* (EHEC) or verotoxin producing *E. coli* (VTEC); enteroaggregative *E. coli* (EAEC or EggEC); and diffusely adherent *E. coli* (DAEC).

Because *E. coli* are normal fecal flora, pathogenicity is defined by demonstration of virulence characteristics and association of those traits with illness (Table 192-1). The mechanism by which *E. coli* produces diarrhea typically involves adherence of organisms to a glycoprotein or glycolipid receptor, followed by production of some noxious substance that injures or disturbs the function of intestinal cells. The genes for virulence properties and for antibiotic resistance are often carried on transferable plasmids, pathogenicity islands, or bacteriophages. In the developing world, the various diarrheagenic *E. coli* cause frequent infections in the first few years of life. They occur with increased frequency during the warm months in temperate climates and during rainy season months in tropical climates. Most diarrheagenic *E. coli* strains (except STEC) require a large inoculum of organisms to

Table 192-1 CLINICAL CHARACTERISTICS, PATHOGENESIS, AND DIAGNOSIS OF DIARRHEAGENIC *ESCHERICHIA COLI*

PATHOGEN	POPULATIONS AT RISK	CHARACTERISTICS OF DIARRHEA		MAIN VIRULENCE FACTORS			DIAGNOSIS
		Watery	Bloody	Duration	Adherence Factors	Toxins	Target Genes for PCR
ETEC	>1 yr old and travelers	+++	—	Acute	Colonization factor antigens (CFs or CFAs); ECP	Heat-labile enterotoxin (LT) Heat-stable enterotoxin (ST)	LT, ST
EIEC	>1 yr old	+	++	Acute	Invasion plasmid antigen (IpaABCD)		IpaH or ial
EPEC	<2 yr old, especially infants <6 mo	+++	—	Acute or persistent	A/E lesion, intimin/Tir, EspABD Bfp	EspF, Map, EAST1	eae, bfpA
STEC	6 mo–10 yr and the elderly	+	+++	Acute	A/E lesion, intimin/Tir Esp ABD	Shiga toxins (Stx1, Stx2, and variants of Stx2)	eae, Stx1, Stx2
EAEC	<2 yr old and travelers	+++	—	Acute or persistent	Aggregative adherence Fimbriae (AAF)	ShET1, EAST1, Pet	AggR or AA plasmid
DAEC	>1 yr old and travelers	++	—	Acute or persistent	Afa/Dr, AIDA-I	Not fully defined	daaC or daaD

AA, aggregative adherence; AggR, EAEC transcriptional activator; AIE lesion, attaching and effacing lesion; Bfp bundle forming pilus; daaC/D genes defining DAEC virulence; DAEC diffusely adherent *E. coli*; *eae*, intimin gene; EAEC, enteroaggregative *E. coli*; EAST1, Enteroaggregative heat stable toxin; ECP, *Escherichia coli* common pilus; EIEC, enteroinvasive *E. coli*; EPEC, enteropathogenic *E. coli*; EspABD, *E. coli* secreted proteins A, B, and D; ETEC, enterotoxigenic *E. coli*; ialL, invasiveness plasmid of EIEC; Pet, Autotransporter toxin; ShET1, Shigella enterotoxin 1; STEC, shigatoxin-producing *E. coli*; Tir, translocated intimin receptor.
+, present; ++, common; +++, very common.

induce disease. Infection is most likely when food-handling or sewage-disposal practices are suboptimal. The diarrheagenic *E. coli* are also important in North America and Europe, although their epidemiology is less well defined in these areas than in the developing world. Recent data in North America suggest that the various diarrheagenic *E. coli* could be the etiology of as much as 30% of infectious diarrhea in children <5 yr of age.

ENTEROTOXIGENIC *ESCHERICHIA COLI*

ETEC account for a sizeable fraction of dehydrating infantile diarrhea in the developing world (10-30%) and of traveler's diarrhea (20-60% of cases). ETEC are also responsible for 3-39% of overall diarrhea episodes in children in the developing world. The typical signs and symptoms include explosive watery, nonmucoid, nonbloody diarrhea, abdominal pain, nausea, vomiting, and little or no fever. The illness is usually self-limited and resolves in 3-5 days, but occasionally lasts >1 wk.

ETEC cause few or no structural alterations in the gut mucosa. Diarrhea is caused by colonization of the small intestine and subsequent elaboration of enterotoxins. ETEC strains secrete a heat-labile enterotoxin (LT) and/or a heat-stable enterotoxin (ST). LT, a large molecule consisting of five receptor-binding subunits and one enzymatically active subunit, is structurally, functionally, and immunologically related to cholera toxin produced by *Vibrio cholerae*. LT stimulates adenylate cyclase, resulting in increased cyclic adenosine monophosphate (cAMP). ST is a small molecule not related to LT or cholera toxin. ST stimulates guanylate cyclase, resulting in increased cyclic guanosine monophosphate (cGMP). The genes carrying these toxins are encoded on plasmids.

Colonization of the intestine requires fimbrial colonization factor antigens (CFs or CFAs), which promote adhesion to the intestinal epithelium. CFs are antigenic fimbriae that are currently targets for vaccine development. There are at least 25 CF types; these antigens are composed of coli surface (CS) antigens and can be expressed alone or in combination. Prevalent colonization factors include CFA/I, CS1-CS7, CS14, and CS17. However, CFs have not been detected on all ETEC strains. A large proportion of strains produce a type IV pilus called *longus*, which functions as a colonization factor and is found among several other gram-negative bacterial pathogens. ETEC strains also have the common pilus, produced by commensal and pathogenic *E. coli* strains. Among the nonfimbrial adhesions, TibA is a potent bacterial adhesin that mediates bacterial attachment and invasion of cells.

For many years, the O serogroup was used to distinguish pathogenic from commensal *E. coli*. Because the pathogenic *E. coli* are now defined and classified by using probes or primers for specific virulence genes, determining the O serogroup has become less important. Of the >180 *E. coli* serogroups, only a relatively small number typically are ETEC. The most common O groups are O6, O8, O128 and O153, and these serogroups only account for half of the ETEC strains based on some large retrospective studies.

ENTEROINVASIVE *ESCHERICHIA COLI*

Clinically, EIEC infections present either with watery diarrhea or a dysentery syndrome with blood, mucus, and leukocytes in the stools, as well as fever, systemic toxicity, crampy abdominal pain, tenesmus, and urgency. The illness resembles bacillary dysentery, because EIEC share virulence genes with *Shigella* spp. EIEC are mostly described in outbreaks; however, endemic disease occurs in developing countries where these bacteria can be isolated. In some areas of the developing world as many as 5% of sporadic diarrhea episodes and 20% of bloody diarrhea cases are caused by EIEC strains.

EIEC cause colonic lesions with ulcerations, hemorrhage, mucosal and submucosal edema, and infiltration by polymorphonuclear leukocytes. EIEC strains behave like *Shigella* in their capacity to invade gut epithelium and produce a dysentery-like illness. The invasive process involves initial entry into cells, intracellular multiplication, intracellular and intercellular spread, and host-cell death. All bacterial genes necessary for entry into the host cell are clustered within a 30-kb region of a large virulence plasmid; these genes are closely related to those found on the invasion plasmid of *Shigella* spp. This region carries genes encoding the entry-mediating proteins, which code for proteins forming a type III secretion apparatus required for secreting the invasins (IpaA-D and IpgD). IpaB and IpaC have been identified as the primary effector proteins of epithelial cell invasion. The type III secretion apparatus is a system triggered by contact with host cells; bacteria use it to transport proteins into the host cell plasma membrane and inject toxins into the cytoplasm.

EIEC encompass a small number of serogroups (O28ac, O29, O112ac, O124, O136, O143, O144, O152, O159, O164, O167, and some untypable strains). These serogroups have lipopolysaccharide (LPS) antigens related to *Shigella* LPS, and, like shigellae, are nonmotile (they lack H or flagellar antigens) and are usually not lactose fermenting.

ENTEROPATHOGENIC *ESCHERICHIA COLI*

EPEC are a major cause of acute and persistent diarrhea in children <2 yr of age in developing countries (20-30% of infant diarrhea). In developed countries, EPEC are responsible for occasional outbreaks in daycare centers and pediatric wards. Profuse watery, nonbloody diarrhea with mucus, vomiting, and low-grade fever are common symptoms. Persistent diarrhea (>14 days) can lead to malnutrition, a potentially serious outcome of EPEC infection in infants in the developing world. Studies have shown that breast-feeding is protective against diarrhea due to EPEC.

EPEC colonization causes blunting of villi, inflammatory changes, and sloughing of superficial mucosal cells; these lesions can be found from the duodenum through the colon. EPEC induce a characteristic attaching and effacing (A/E) histopathologic lesion, which is defined by the intimate attachment of bacteria to the epithelial surface and effacement of host cell microvilli. Factors responsible for the A/E lesion formation are encoded by the locus of enterocyte effacement (LEE), which is a pathogenicity island that contains the genes for a type III secretion system, the translocated intimin receptor (Tir) and intimin, and multiple effector proteins such as the *E. coli*–secreted proteins (EspA-B-D). Some strains adhere to the host's intestinal epithelium in a pattern known as *localized adherence* (LA); this trait is mediated in part by the type IV bundle forming pilus (Bfp) encoded on a plasmid (the EAF plasmid). After initial contact, proteins are translocated through filamentous appendages forming a physical bridge between the bacteria and the host cell; bacterial effectors (EspB, EspD, Tir) are translocated through these conduits. Tir moves to the surface of host cells, where it is bound by a bacterial outer membrane protein intimin (encoded by the *eae* gene). Intimin-Tir binding triggers polymerization of actin and other cytoskeletal components at the site of attachment. The result of these cytoskeletal changes is intimate bacterial attachment to the host cell, enterocyte effacement, and pedestal formation.

Other LEE-encoded effectors include Map, EspF, EspG, EspH, and SepZ. Various other effector proteins are encoded outside the LEE and secreted by the type III secretion system (the non–LEE-encoded proteins or Nle). The contribution of these putative effectors (NleA/EspI, NleB, NleC, NleD, etc.) to virulence is still under investigation. There is variability in presence and expression of virulence genes among EPEC strains.

The *eae* (intimin) and *bfp*A (bundle-forming pilus) genes are use for identifying EPEC and for subdividing this group of bacteria into typical and atypical strains. *E. coli* strains that are $eae^+/bfpA^+$ are classified as typical EPEC; most of these strains belong to classic O:H serotypes. On the other hand, *E. coli* strains that are $eae^+/bfpA^-$ are classified as atypical EPEC. Typical EPEC have been considered for many years to be the leading cause of infantile diarrhea in developing countries and were considered rare in industrialized countries where atypical EPEC seemed to be a more important cause of diarrhea. However, current data suggest that atypical EPEC are more prevalent than typical EPEC in both developed and developing countries, even in persistent diarrhea cases.

The classic EPEC serogroups include strains of 12 O serogroups: O26, O55, O86, O111, O114, O119, O125, O126, O127, O128, O142, and O158. However, various *E. coli* strains defined as EPEC based on presence of the intimin gene, belong to nonclassic EPEC serogroups, especially the atypical strains.

SHIGA TOXIN–PRODUCING *ESCHERICHIA COLI*

STEC have been shown to cause a wide spectrum of diseases. STEC infections may be asymptomatic. Patients who develop intestinal symptoms can have mild diarrhea or severe hemorrhagic colitis. The gastrointestinal illness is characterized by abdominal pain with diarrhea that is initially watery but within a few days can become blood-streaked or grossly bloody. Although this pattern resembles that of shigellosis or EIEC disease, it differs in that fever is an uncommon manifestation. Most persons infected with STEC recover from the infection without further complication. However, 5-10% of children with STEC hemorrhagic colitis go on within a few days to develop systemic complications such as hemolytic-uremic syndrome (HUS), characterized by acute kidney failure, thrombocytopenia, and microangiopathic hemolytic anemia (Chapter 512). Severe illness occurs most often among children from 6 months to 10 years of age. The elderly can also develop HUS or thrombotic thrombocytopenic purpura.

STEC are transmitted person to person (e.g., in families and day care centers) as well as by food and water; ingestion of a small number is sufficient to cause disease with some strains. Poorly cooked hamburger is a common cause of food-borne outbreaks, although many other foods (apple cider, lettuce, spinach, mayonnaise, salami, dry fermented sausage, and unpasteurized dairy products) have also been incriminated.

STEC affect the colon most severely. These organisms adhere to intestinal cells, and most strains that affect humans produce attaching-effacing lesions like those seen with EPEC. The attachment mechanism has genes (*intimin, tir, EspA-D*, etc.) very closely related to those of EPEC. However, in addition to enterocyte attachment, these bacteria produce toxins that kill cells. These toxins (Shiga toxins [Stx]) are the key virulence factors of STEC. In the past these toxins were also called verotoxins or Shiga-like toxins. There are two major Shiga toxin families, Stx1 and Stx2, with multiple subtypes. Some STEC produce only Stx1 and others produce only Stx2, but many STEC have genes for several toxins. Stx1 is essentially identical to Shiga toxin, the protein synthesis–inhibiting exotoxin of *Shigella dysenteriae* serotype 1, whereas Stx2 and variants of Stx2 are more distantly related to Shiga toxin.

These toxins are composed of a single A subunit noncovalently associated with a pentamer composed of identical B subunits. The B subunits bind to globotriaosylceramide (Gb_3), a glycosphingolipid receptor on host cells. The A subunit is taken up by endocytosis. The toxin target is the 28S rRNA, which is depurinated by the toxin at a specific adenine residue, causing protein synthesis to cease and affected cells to die. These toxins are carried on lambdoid bacteriophages that are normally inactive when inserted into the bacterial chromosome; when the phages are induced to replicate (e.g., by the stress induced by many antibiotics), they cause lysis of the bacteria and release of large amounts of toxin. It is generally thought that the toxins enter the systemic circulation after translocation across the intestinal epithelium and damage vascular endothelial cells, resulting in activation of the coagulation cascade, formation of microthrombi, intravascular hemolysis, and ischemia.

Clinical outcome of STEC infection depends on both epithelial attachment and the toxin(s) produced by the infecting strain. The Stx2 family of toxins is associated with a higher risk of causing HUS. Strains that make only Stx1 often cause only watery diarrhea and are uncommonly associated with HUS.

The most common STEC serotypes are *E. coli* O157:H7, *E. coli* O111:NM, and *E. coli* O26:H11, although several hundred other STEC serotypes have also been described.

ENTEROAGGREGATIVE *ESCHERICHIA COLI*

EAEC are associated with acute and persistent pediatric diarrhea in developing countries, most prominently in children <2 yr of age. EAEC are also etiologic agents in AIDS-associated chronic diarrhea and acute traveler's diarrhea. Typical EAEC illness is manifested by watery, mucoid, secretory diarrhea with low-grade fever and little or no vomiting. The watery diarrhea can persist ≥14 days. In some studies many patients have grossly bloody stools. EAEC have been associated with growth retardation and malnutrition in infants in the developing world.

EAEC form a characteristic biofilm on the intestinal mucosa and induce shortening of the villi, hemorrhagic necrosis, and inflammatory responses. The proposed model of pathogenesis of EAEC involves three phases: adherence to the intestinal mucosa by way of the aggregative adherence fimbriae or related adhesins; enhanced production of mucus; and production of toxins and inflammation that results in damage of the mucosa and intestinal secretion. Diarrhea caused by EAEC is predominantly secretory. The intestinal inflammatory response (elevated fecal lactoferrin, interleukin [IL]-8 and IL-1β) may be related to growth impairment and malnutrition.

EAEC are recognized by adherence to HEp-2 cells in an aggregative, stacked-brick–like pattern, called *aggregative adherence* (AA). EAEC virulence factors include the aggregative adherence fimbriae (AAF-I and AAF-II) that confers the AA phenotype. Some strains produce toxins including the plasmid-encoded enterotoxin EAST1, homolog of the ETEC heat-stable toxin; an autotransporter toxin called *Pet*; and the chromosomally encoded enterotoxin ShET1. Other virulence factors include outer membrane and secreted proteins such as dispersin.

Strains of *E. coli* categorized as EAEC belong to multiple serogroups, including O3, O7, O15, O44, O77, O86, O126, and O127. EAEC is a heterogeneous group of *E.coli*. The original diagnostic criteria (HEp-2 cell adherence pattern) identified many strains that are probably not true pathogens; genetic criteria appear to more reliably identify true pathogens. A transcriptional activator called *AggR* controls expression of plasmid-borne and chromosomal virulence factors. Identification of AggR or members of the AggR regulator appears to reliably identify illness-associated pathogenic EAEC strains.

DIFFUSELY ADHERENT *ESCHERICHIA COLI*

Although the status of DAEC as true pathogens has been in doubt, multiple studies in both developed and developing countries have associated these organisms with diarrhea, particularly in children after the first year or two of life. Discrepancies among epidemiologic studies may be explained by age-dependent susceptibility to diarrhea or by the use of inappropriate detection methods. Data suggest that these organisms also cause traveler's diarrhea in adults. DAEC produces acute watery diarrhea that is usually not dysenteric but is often prolonged.

DAEC strains have been identified on the basis of their diffuse adherence pattern (DA) on cultured epithelial cells. Two putative adherence factors have been described for DAEC strains. One of the adherence factors is the surface fimbriae (designated F1845) that are responsible for the diffuse adherence phenotype in a prototype strain. These fimbriae are homologous with members of the Afa/Dr family of adhesins, which are identified by hybridization with a specific probe, *daaC*, common to operons encoding Afa/Dr adhesions. A second putative adhesin associated with the DA phenotype is an outer membrane protein, designated AIDA-I. The contribution of other putative effectors (*icuA, fimH, afa, agg-3A, pap, astA, shET1)* to virulence is still under investigation.

Bacteria expressing Afa/Dr adhesins interact with membrane-bound receptors, including the recognition of decay-accelerating factor. The structural and functional lesions induced by DAEC include loss of microvilli and decrease in the expression and enzyme activities of functional brush border–associated proteins. Afa/Dr DAEC isolates produce a secreted autotransporter toxin that induces marked fluid accumulation in the intestine.

Serogroups associated with DAEC strains are less well defined than are those of other diarrheagenic *E. coli*.

DIAGNOSIS

The clinical features of illness are seldom distinctive enough to allow confident diagnosis, and routine laboratory studies are of very limited value. Diagnosis currently depends heavily on laboratory studies that are not readily available to practitioners. Practical, non–DNA-dependent, methods for routine diagnosis of diarrheagenic *E. coli* have been developed primarily for the STEC. Serotype O157:H7 is suggested by isolation of an *E. coli* that fails to ferment sorbitol on MacConkey sorbitol medium; latex agglutination confirms that the organism contains O157 LPS. Other STEC can be detected in routine hospital laboratories using commercially available enzyme immunoassay or latex agglutination to detect Shiga toxins, although variable sensitivity of commercial immunoassays has limited their value.

The diagnosis of other diarrheagenic *E. coli* infection is typically made based on tissue culture assays (e.g., HEp-2-cells assay for EPEC, EAEC, DAEC) or identification of specific virulence factors of the bacteria by phenotype (e.g., toxins) or genotype. DNA probes for genes encoding the various virulence traits are the best diagnostic tests but are currently available only as a research tool. Multiplex, real-time, or conventional polymerase chain reaction (PCR) can be used for presumptive diagnosis of isolated *E. coli* colonies. The genes commonly used for diagnostic PCR are LT and ST for ETEC, *IpaH* or *iaL* for EIEC, *eae* and *bfp*A for EPEC, *eae, Stx1* and *Stx2* for STEC, *AggR* or the AA plasmid for EAEC, and *daa*C or *daa*D for DAEC. Suspected organisms can be forwarded to reference or research laboratories for definitive evaluation, although such effort is seldom necessary.

Other laboratory data are at best nonspecific indicators of etiology. Fecal leukocyte examination of the stool is often positive with EIEC or mildly elevated with other diarrheagenic *E. coli*. With EIEC and STEC there may be an elevated peripheral blood polymorphonuclear leukocyte count with a left shift. Fecal lactoferrin, IL-8, and IL-1β can be used as inflammatory markers. Electrolyte changes are nonspecific, reflecting only fluid loss.

TREATMENT

The cornerstone of management is appropriate fluid and electrolyte therapy. In general, this therapy should include oral replacement and maintenance with rehydration solutions such as those specified by the World Health Organization. Pedialyte and other readily available oral rehydration solutions are acceptable alternatives. After refeeding, continued supplementation with oral rehydration fluids is appropriate to prevent recurrence of dehydration. Early refeeding (within 6-8 hr of initiating rehydration) with breast milk or infant formula or solid foods should be encouraged. Prolonged withholding of feeding can lead to chronic diarrhea and malnutrition. If the child is malnourished, oral zinc should be given to speed recovery and decrease the risk of future diarrheal episodes.

Specific antimicrobial therapy of diarrheagenic *E. coli* is problematic because of the difficulty of making an accurate rapid diagnosis of these pathogens and the unpredictability of antibiotic susceptibilities. Treatment is complicated by the fact that these organisms are often multiply resistant to antibiotics due to their previous exposure to inappropriate antibiotic therapy. Multiple studies in developing countries have found diarrheagenic *E. coli* strains to be commonly resistant to antibiotics such as trimethoprim-sulfamethoxazole (TMP-SMX) and ampicillin (60-70%). There are no randomized controlled studies of antibiotics for the treatment of diarrheagenic *E. coli* diarrhea in children; most data come from case series or clinical trials in traveler's diarrhea. ETEC respond to antimicrobial agents such as TMP-SMX when the *E. coli* strains are susceptible. ETEC cases from traveler's diarrhea trials respond to ciprofloxacin, azithromycin, and rifaximin. However, other than for a child recently returning from travel in the developing world, empirical treatment of severe *watery diarrhea* with antibiotics is seldom appropriate.

EIEC infections may be treated before the availability of culture results because the clinician suspects shigellosis and has begun empirical therapy. If the organisms prove to be susceptible, TMP-SMX is an appropriate choice. Although treatment of EPEC infection with TMP-SMX intravenously or orally for 5 days may be effective in speeding resolution, the lack of a rapid diagnostic test makes treatment decisions difficult. Ciprofloxacin or rifaximin are useful for EAEC traveler's diarrhea, but pediatric data are sparse. Specific therapy for DAEC has not been defined.

The STEC represent a particularly difficult therapeutic dilemma; many antibiotics can induce toxin production and phage-mediated bacterial lysis with toxin release. Antibiotics should not be given for STEC infection because they can increase the risk of hemolytic-uremic syndrome (Chapter 512).

PREVENTION OF ILLNESS

In the developing world, prevention of disease caused by diarrheagenic *E. coli* is probably best done by maintaining prolonged breast-feeding, paying careful attention to personal hygiene, and following proper food- and water-handling procedures. People traveling to these places can be best protected by handwashing, consuming only processed water, bottled beverages, breads, fruit juices, fruits that can be peeled, or foods that are served steaming hot.

Prophylactic antibiotic therapy is effective in adult travelers but has not been studied in children and is not recommended. Public health measures, including sewage disposal and food-handling practices, have made pathogens that require large inocula to produce illness relatively uncommon in industrialized countries. Foodborne outbreaks of STEC are a problem for which no adequate solution has been found. During the occasional hospital outbreak of EPEC disease, attention to enteric isolation precautions and cohorting may be critical.

The nature of protective immunity against diarrheagenic *E. coli* is not fully understood, and no vaccines are available for clinical use in children. There are several vaccine candidates based on bacterial toxins or colonization factors that have shown promise for prevention of ETEC in adult travelers.

BIBLIOGRAPHY

Please visit the Nelson Textbook of Pediatrics *website at www.expertconsult.com for the complete bibliography.*

Chapter 193
Cholera

Anna Lena Lopez

Cholera is a rapidly dehydrating diarrheal disease that can lead to death, if appropriate treatment is not provided immediately. Although rare in industrialized countries, cholera has a propensity to cause outbreaks in areas with poor hygiene and inadequate sanitation and water facilities. These outbreaks may be explosive, especially when they occur in populations residing in crowded conditions, such as refugee camps. Reports from the World Health Organization (WHO) indicate that cholera is on the rise, with more cases being reported annually from 2006 and 2007 compared to the annual average of 2002-2005. In 2007, there were 177,963 cholera cases reported, with 4,031 deaths; actual figures may be higher.

ETIOLOGY

The disease is caused by *Vibrio cholerae*, a gram-negative comma-shaped bacillus, subdivided into serogroups by its somatic O antigen. Of the more than 200 serogroups, only serogroups O1 and O139 have been associated with epidemics, although some non-O1, non-O139 *V. cholerae* strains (e.g., O75 and O141) are pathogenic and can cause small outbreaks. A flagellar H antigen is present but is not used for species identification. The O1 serogroup is further divided into classical and the El Tor biotypes based on its biochemical characteristics. Since the turn of the century, only O1 El Tor has been reported; hybrids and variants of *V. cholerae* O1 El Tor possessing classical genes have been reported in Asia and Africa. Each biotype may be further subdivided into Inaba, Ogawa, and Hikojima serotypes based on the antigenic determinants on the O antigen. Inaba strains have A and C antigenic determinants, whereas Ogawa strains have A and B antigenic determinants. Hikojima strains produce all 3 antigenic determinants but are unstable and rare.

EPIDEMIOLOGY

The first 6 cholera pandemics originated in the Indian subcontinent and were caused by classical O1 *V. cholerae*. The seventh pandemic is the most extensive of all and is caused by *V. cholerae* O1 El Tor. It began in 1961 in Sulawesi, Indonesia, and has spread to the Indian subcontinent, Southeast Asia, Africa, Oceania, Southern Europe, and the Americas. In 1991, *V. cholerae* O1 El Tor first appeared in Peru before rapidly spreading in the Americas. Cholera becomes endemic in areas following outbreaks when a large segment of the population develops immunity to the disease after recurrent exposure. The disease is now endemic in parts of East, Southern, and Northwest Africa, as well as in South and Southeast Asia (Fig. 193-1).

In 1992, the first non-O1 *V. cholerae* that resulted in epidemics was identified in India and Bangladesh and was designated *V. cholerae* O139. From 1992 to 1994, this organism replaced O1 as the predominant cause of cholera in South Asia but has since been an uncommon etiologic agent.

The hybrid El Tor strains were first identified sporadically in Bangladesh. In 2004, during routine surveillance in Mozambique, isolates of *V. cholerae* O1 El Tor carrying classical genes were identified. Since then, hybrid and variant El Tor strains have been reported in other parts of Asia and Africa and have caused outbreaks in India and Vietnam. Although the classical biotype has virtually disappeared, its genes remain within the El Tor biotype.

Humans are the only known hosts, but free-living and plankton-associated *V. cholerae* exist in the marine environment. The organism thrives best in moderately salty water but can survive in rivers and freshwater if nutrient levels are high, as occurs when there is organic pollution such as human feces. The formation of a biofilm on abiotic surfaces and the ability to enter a viable but nonculturable state has been hypothesized as factors that allow *V. cholerae* to persist in the environment. Surface sea temperature, pH, chlorophyll content, the presence of iron compounds and chitin, and climatic conditions such as amount of rainfall and sea level rise are all important environmental factors that influence the survival of *V. cholerae* in the environment and the expression of cholera toxin, an important virulence determinant.

Consumption of contaminated water and ingestion of undercooked shellfish are the main modes of transmission, with the latter more often seen in developed countries. Previous studies in Bangladesh revealed that children aged 2-4 yr have the highest incidence of the disease; data from two endemic areas in Jakarta, Indonesia, and Kolkata, India, revealed that the incidence of disease was highest among infants and children <2 yr of age. On the other hand, all age groups were commonly affected in areas where the disease has not gained a foothold. In epidemic and endemic settings, the disease usually first appears in men. Persons with blood group O, decreased gastric acidity, malnutrition, immunocompromised state, and absence of local intestinal immunity (prior exposure by infection or vaccination) are at increased risk for developing severe disease. Household contacts of cholera-infected patients are at high risk for the disease, because the stools of infected patients contain high concentrations of *V. cholerae* (up to 10^8/gof stool).

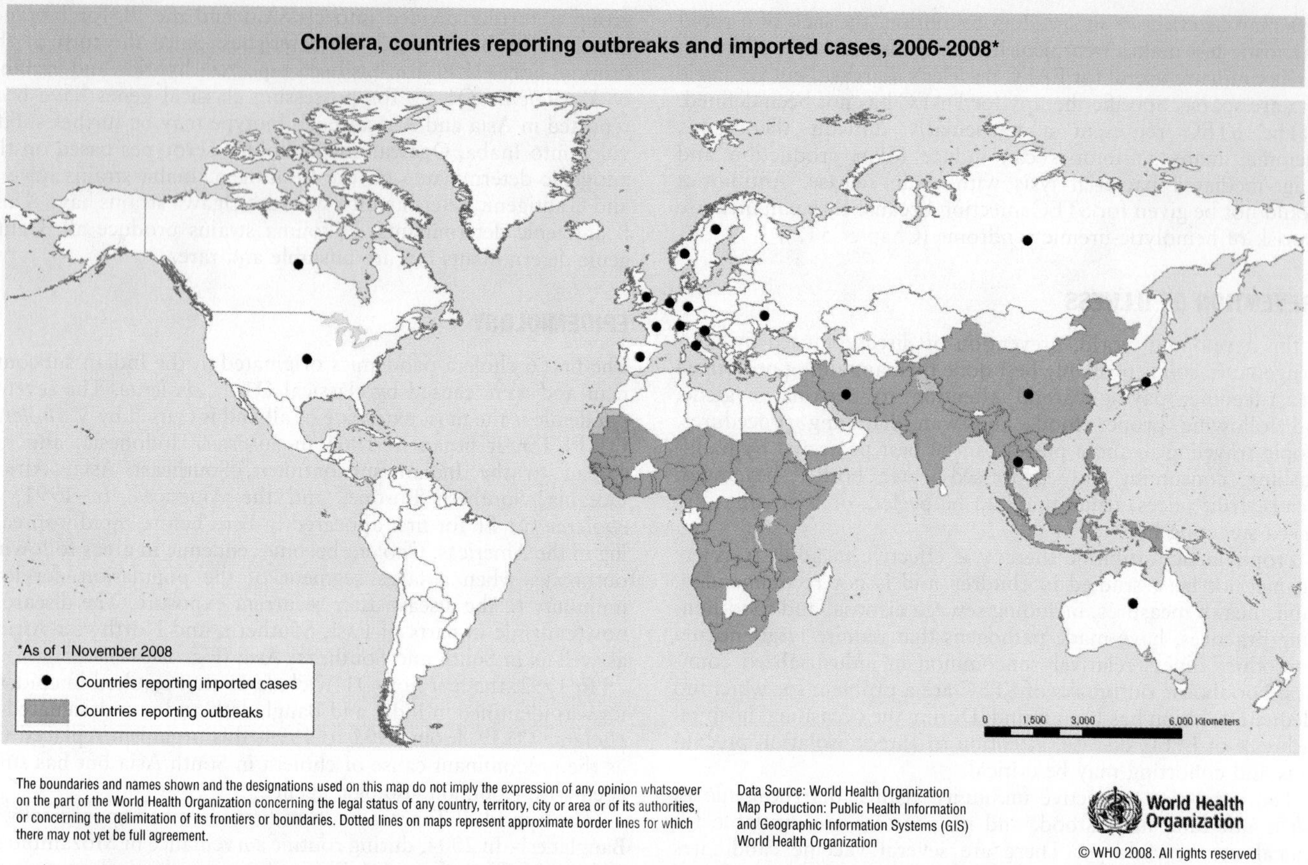
Cholera, countries reporting outbreaks and imported cases, 2006-2008*
*As of 1 November 2008
Countries reporting imported cases
Countries reporting outbreaks
0 1,500 3,000 6,000 Kilometers
The boundaries and names shown and the designations used on this map do not imply the expression of any opinion whatsoever on the part of the World Health Organization concerning the legal status of any country, territory, city or area or of its authorities, or concerning the delimitation of its frontiers or boundaries. Dotted lines on maps represent approximate border lines for which there may not yet be full agreement.
Data Source: World Health Organization
Map Production: Public Health Information and Geographic Information Systems (GIS) World Health Organization
World Health Organization
© WHO 2008. All rights reserved

Figure 193-1 Countries reporting cholera outbreaks and imported cholera cases to WHO from 2006-2008. (From World Health Organization: *Cholera, areas reporting outbreaks, 2007-2009* (website). gamapserver.who.int/mapLibrary/Files/Maps/Global_ChoeraCases_ITHRiskMap.png. Accessed August 9, 2010.)

PATHOGENESIS

Following ingestion of *V. cholerae* from the environment, several changes occur in the vibrios while they traverse the human intestine: increased expression of genes required for nutrient acquisition, downregulation of chemotactic response, and expression of motility. Together these changes allow the vibrios to reach a hyperinfectious state, leading to lower infectious doses in secondarily infected persons.

Large inocula of bacteria (>10^8) are required for severe cholera to occur; however, for persons whose gastric barrier is disrupted, a much lower dose (10^5) is required. If the vibrios survive gastric acidity, they then colonize the small intestine through various factors such as toxin coregulated pili (TCP) and motility, leading to efficient delivery of cholera toxin. The cholera toxin consists of five binding B subunits and one active A subunit. The B subunits are responsible for binding to the GM1 ganglioside receptors located in the small intestinal epithelial cells. After binding, the A subunit is then released into the cell, where it stimulates adenylate cyclase and initiates a cascade of events. An increase in cyclic adenosine monophosphate (cAMP) leads to an increase in chloride secretion by the crypt cells, which in turn leads to inhibition of absorption of sodium and chloride by the microvilli. These events eventually lead to massive purging of electrolyte rich isotonic fluid in the small intestine that exceeds the absorptive capacity of the colon, resulting in rapid dehydration and depletion of electrolytes, including sodium, chloride, bicarbonate, and potassium. Metabolic acidosis and hypokalemia then ensues.

CLINICAL MANIFESTATIONS

Most cases of cholera are mild or inapparent. Among symptomatic cases, around 20% develop severe dehydration that can rapidly lead to death. Following an incubation period of 1 to 3 days (range, several hours to 5 days), acute watery diarrhea and vomiting ensues. The onset may be sudden, with profuse watery diarrhea, but some patients have a prodrome of anorexia and abdominal discomfort and the stool may initially be brown. Diarrhea can progress to painless purging of profuse rice-water stools (suspended flecks of mucus) with a fishy smell, which is the hallmark of the disease. Vomiting with clear watery fluid is usually present at the onset of the disease.

Cholera gravis, the most severe form of the disease, results when purging rates of 500-1000 mL/hr occur. This purging leads to dehydration manifested by decreased urine output, sunken fontanels (in infants), sunken eyes, absence of tears, dry oral mucosa, shriveled hands and feet (washerwoman's hands), poor skin turgor, thready pulse, tachycardia, hypotension, and vascular collapse (Fig. 193-2). Patients with metabolic acidosis can present with typical Kussmaul breathing. Although patients may be initially thirsty and awake, they rapidly progress to obtundation and coma. If fluid losses are not rapidly corrected, death can occur within hours.

LABORATORY FINDINGS

Findings associated with dehydration such as elevated urine specific gravity and hemoconcentration are evident. Hypoglycemia is a common finding due to decreased food intake during the acute illness. Serum potassium may be initially normal or even high in the presence of metabolic acidosis; however, as the acidosis is corrected, hypokalemia can become evident. Metabolic acidosis due to bicarbonate loss is a prominent finding in severe cholera. Serum sodium and chloride levels may be normal or decreased, depending on the severity of the disease.

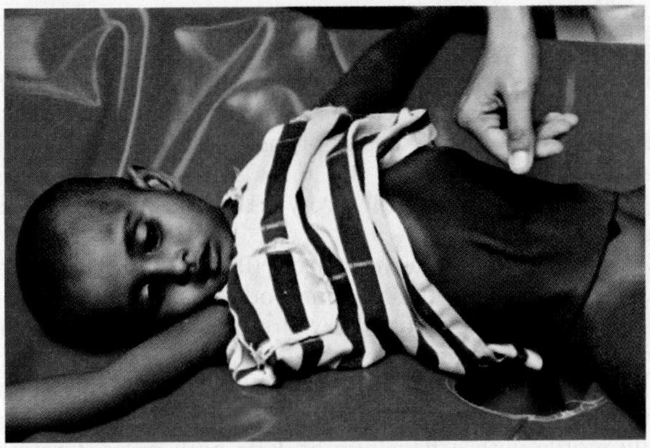

Figure 193-2 A child, lying on a cholera cot, showing typical signs of severe dehydration from cholera. The patient has sunken eyes, lethargic appearance, and poor skin turgor, but within 2 hr was sitting up, alert, and eating normally. (From Sack DA, Sack RB, Nair GB, et al: Cholera, *Lancet* 363:223–233, 2004.)

DIAGNOSIS AND DIFFERENTIAL DIAGNOSIS

In children who have acute watery diarrhea with severe dehydration and have recently traveled to an area known to have cholera, the disease may be suspected pending laboratory confirmation. Cholera differs from other diarrheal disease in that it often occurs in large outbreaks affecting both adults and children.

Treatment of dehydration should begin as soon as possible. Diarrhea due to other etiologic causes (e.g., enterotoxigenic *Escherichia coli* or rotavirus) may be difficult to distinguish from cholera clinically. Microbiologic isolation of *V. cholerae* remains the gold standard for diagnosis. Although definitive diagnosis is not required for treatment to be initiated, laboratory confirmation is necessary for epidemiologic surveillance. *V. cholerae* may be isolated from stools, vomitus, or rectal swabs. Specimens may be transported on Cary-Blair media, if they cannot be processed immediately. Selective media such as thiosulfate citrate bile salts sucrose (TCBS) agar that inhibit normal flora should be used. Because most laboratories in industrialized countries do not routinely culture for *V. cholerae*, clinicians should request appropriate cultures for clinically suspected cases.

Stool examination reveals few fecal leukocytes and erythrocytes because cholera does not cause inflammation. Dark-field microscopy may be used for rapid identification of typical "darting motility" in wet mounts of rice-water stools, which disappears once specific antibodies against *V. cholerae* O1 or O139 are added. Rapid diagnostic tests are currently being evaluated that will allow use at the bedside. Molecular identification with the use of polymerase chain reaction (PCR) and DNA probes are available but often not used in areas where cholera exists.

COMPLICATIONS

Delayed initiation of rehydration therapy or inadequate rehydration often lead to complications. Renal failure due to prolonged hypotension can occur. Unless potassium supplementation is provided, hypokalemia can lead to nephropathy and focal myocardial necrosis. Hypoglycemia is common among children and can lead to seizures unless it is appropriately corrected.

TREATMENT

Rehydration is the mainstay of therapy (Chapter 332). Effective and timely case management considerably decreases mortality. Children with mild or moderate dehydration may be treated with oral rehydration solution (ORS) unless the patient is in shock, is obtunded, or has intestinal ileus. Vomiting is not a contraindication to ORS. Severely dehydrated patients require intravenous fluid, ideally with lactated Ringer solution. When available, rice-based ORS should be used during rehydration, because this fluid has been shown to be superior to standard ORS in children and adults with cholera. Close monitoring is necessary, especially during the first 24 hr of illness, when large amounts of stool may be passed. After rehydration, patients have to be reassessed every 1-2 hr, or more frequently if profuse diarrhea is ongoing. Feeding should not be withheld during diarrhea. Frequent, small feedings are better tolerated than less frequent, large feedings.

Table 193-1 SUGGESTED ANTIMICROBIALS FOR SUSPECTED CHOLERA CASES WITH SEVERE DEHYDRATION

ANTIBIOTIC OF CHOICE*	ALTERNATIVE
Doxycycline (adults and older children): 300 mg given as a single dose *or* Tetracycline 12.5 mg/kg/dose 4 times/day × 3 days (up to 500 mg per dose × 3 days)	Erythromycin 12.5 mg/kg/dose 4 times a day × 3 days (up to 250 mg 4 times a day × 3 days)

*Selection of an antimicrobial should be based on sensitivity patterns of strains of *Vibrio cholerae* 01 or 0139 in the area.

Adapted from World Health Organization: *The treatment of diarrhea: a manual for physicians and other senior health workers—4th revision,* Geneva, 2005, World Health Organization.

As soon as vomiting stops (usually within 4-6 hr after initiation of rehydration therapy), an antibiotic to which local *V. cholerae* strains are sensitive must be administered. Antibiotics (Table 193-1) shorten the duration of illness, decrease fecal excretion of vibrios, decrease the volume of diarrhea, and reduce the fluid requirement during rehydration. Single-dose doxycycline increases compliance; there have been increasing reports of resistance to tetracyclines. Ciprofloxacin, azithromycin, and trimethoprim-sulfamethoxazole are also effective against cholera. Cephalosporins and aminoglycosides are not clinically effective against cholera and therefore should not be used, even if in vitro tests show strains to be sensitive.

Zinc should be given as soon as vomiting stops. Zinc deficiency is common among children in many developing countries. Zinc supplementation among children <5 yr of age has been shown to shorten the duration of diarrhea and reduce subsequent diarrhea episodes when given daily for 14 days at the time of the illness. For children <6 mo of age, 10 mg of oral zinc may be given daily for 2 wk, and for children aged 6 mo to 12 yr, 20 mg of oral zinc may be given daily for 2 wk.

PREVENTION

Improved personal hygiene, access to clean water, and sanitation are the mainstays of cholera control. Appropriate case management substantially decreases case fatalities to <1%. Travelers from developed countries often have no prior exposure to cholera and are therefore at risk of developing the disease. Children travelling to cholera-affected areas should avoid drinking potentially contaminated water and eating high-risk foods such as raw or undercooked fish and shellfish.

No country or territory requires vaccination against cholera as a condition for entry. There is no cholera vaccine licensed in the USA. An internationally licensed killed whole-cell oral cholera vaccine with recombinant B subunit (Dukoral, SBL/Crucell) has been available in more than 60 countries, including the European Union, and provides protection against cholera in endemic areas as well as cross-protection against certain strains of enterotoxigenic *E. coli* (ETEC). Older-generation parenteral cholera vaccines have not been recommended by WHO, due to the limited protection they confer and their high reactogenicity. Oral cholera vaccines (OCVs) have been available for >2 decades and are mostly used by travelers from industrialized countries going to cholera-affected areas. Although WHO has recommended the use of OCV in the control of cholera in certain endemic and epidemic situations since 2001, these vaccines have not been extensively adopted. Table 193-2 shows currently licensed vaccines and

Table 193-2 INTERNATIONALLY LICENSED ORAL CHOLERA VACCINES

VACCINE TRADE NAME	CONTENTS	DOSING SCHEDULE FOR CHOLERA
Dukoral (SBL/Crucell)	1 mg of recombinant B subunit of cholera toxin plus 2.5×10^{10} of the following strains of *V. cholerae*: Formalin-killed El Tor Inaba (Phil 6973) Heat-killed classical Inaba (Cairo 48) Heat-killed classical Ogawa (Cairo 50) Formalin-killed classical Ogawa (Cairo 50)	Children 2-6 yr: 3 doses, 1-6 wk apart Adults and children >6 yr: 2 doses, 1-6 wk apart
Orochol (Berna Biotech/Crucell)	Live-attenuated classical *V. cholerae* 01 CVD 103- HgR	One dose for children and adults aged ≥2 yr of age

dosing schedules. Live-attenuated oral cholera vaccine (Orochol, Berna Biotech/Crucell) has not been shown to be protective against cholera in a clinical trial in an endemic area and is no longer manufactured.

BIBLIOGRAPHY

Please visit the Nelson Textbook of Pediatrics *website at* *www.expertconsult.com* *for the complete bibliography.*

Chapter 194
Campylobacter

Gloria P. Heresi, Shahida Baqar, and James R. Murphy

Campylobacter jejuni and *Campylobacter coli* are global zoonoses and are among the most common causes of human intestinal infections. Infection with these organisms may be followed by severe immunoreactive diseases and possibly immunoproliferative disorders.

ETIOLOGY

The family Campylobacteriaceae includes >20 species. Those known or considered pathogenic for humans include *C. jejuni*, *C. fetus*, *C. coli*, *C. hyointestinalis*, *C. lari*, *C. upsaliensis*, *C. concisus*, *C. sputorum*, *C. rectus*, *C. mucosalis*, *C. jejuni* subspecies *doylei*, *C. curvus*, *C. gracilis*, and *C. cryaerophila*. Additional *Campylobacter* species have been isolated from clinical specimens, but their roles as pathogens have not been established. *C. jejuni* and *C. coli* are the most important pathogens of the genus. More than 100 serotypes of *C. jejuni* have been identified.

Campylobacter organisms are thin (0.2-0.4 µm wide), curved, gram-negative, non–spore-forming rods (1.5-3.5 µm long) that usually have tapered ends. They are smaller than most other enteric bacterial pathogens and have variable morphology, including short comma- or S-shaped organisms and long, multispiraled, filamentous, seagull-shaped organisms. Individual organisms are usually motile with a flagellum at 1 or both poles. Growth on solid media results in small (0.5-1 mm), slightly raised, smooth colonies. Visible growth in blood cultures is often not apparent until 5-14 days after inoculation. Most *Campylobacter* organisms are microaerophilic and do not oxidize or ferment carbohydrates. Selective culture media developed to enhance isolation of *C. jejuni* may inhibit the growth of other *Campylobacter* species. *C. jejuni* has a circular chromosome of 1.64 million base pairs (30.6% G+C) that is predicted to encode 1,654 proteins and 54 stable RNA species. The genome is unusual in that there are virtually no insertion sequences or phage-associated sequences and very few repeat sequences.

Clinical presentations differ, in part, by species (Table 194-1). Intestinal disease is usually associated with *C. jejuni* and *C. coli*, and extraintestinal and systemic infections are most often associated with *C. fetus*. *C. jejuni* septicemia is increasingly recognized and can occur without gastrointestinal signs or symptoms. Less commonly, enteritis is recognized in association with isolation of *C. lari*, *C. fetus*, and other *Campylobacter* species.

EPIDEMIOLOGY

Human campylobacterioses most commonly result from ingestion of contaminated poultry (chicken, turkey) or raw milk and less commonly from drinking water, pets (cats, dogs, hamsters), and farm animals. Infections are more common in resource-limited settings, are prevalent year-round in tropical areas, and can exhibit seasonal peaks in temperate regions (late summer and early fall in most of the USA). In industrialized countries, *Campylobacter* infections peak in early childhood and in persons 15-44 yr of age. Each year in the USA there are an estimated 2.4 million cases of *Campylobacter* infections, resulting in >100

Table 194-1 *CAMPYLOBACTER* SPECIES ASSOCIATED WITH HUMAN DISEASE

SPECIES	DISEASES IN HUMANS	COMMON SOURCES
C. jejuni	Gastroenteritis, bacteremia, Guillain-Barré syndrome	Poultry, raw milk, cats, dogs, cattle, swine, monkeys, water
C. coli	Gastroenteritis, bacteremia	Poultry, raw milk, cats, dogs, cattle, swine, monkeys, oysters, water
C. fetus	Bacteremia, meningitis, endocarditis, mycotic aneurysm, diarrhea	Sheep, cattle, birds
C. hyointestinalis	Diarrhea, bacteremia, proctitis	Swine, cattle, deer, hamsters, raw milk, oysters
C. lari	Diarrhea, colitis, appendicitis, bacteremia, urinary tract infection	Seagulls, water, poultry, cattle, dogs, cats, monkeys, oysters, mussels
C. upsaliensis	Diarrhea, bacteremia, abscesses, enteritis, colitis, hemolyticuremic	Cats, other domestic pets
C. concisus	Diarrhea, gastritis, enteritis, periodontitis	Human oral cavity
C. sputorum	Diarrhea, bedsores, abscesses, periodontitis	Human oral cavity, cattle, swine
C. rectus	Periodontitis	
C. mucosalis	Enteritis	Swine
C. jejuni subspecies doylei	Diarrhea, colitis, appendicitis, bacteremia, urinary tract infection	Swine
C. curvus	Gingivitis, alveolar abscess	Poultry, raw milk, cats, dogs, cattle, swine, monkeys, water, human oral cavity
C. gracilis	Head and neck abscess, abdominal abscess, empyema	
C. cryaerophila	Diarrhea	Swine

deaths. Medical record keeping in the Netherlands has allowed analyses showing that each resident acquires asymptomatic *Campylobacter* infection every 2 years and that asymptomatic infection progresses to symptomatic infection in approximately 1% of colonized persons.

Although chickens are a classic source of *Campylobacter,* many animal sources of human food can harbor *Campylobacter,* including seafood. Additionally, many animals kept as pets carry *Campylobacter,* and insects inhabiting contaminated environments can acquire the organism. Direct or indirect exposure to this plethora of environmental sources is the origin of most human infections. Airborne transmission of *Campylobacter* can occur in farm workers. There is increasing evidence that the use of antimicrobials in animal foods increases the prevalence of antibiotic-resistant *Campylobacter* isolated from humans.

Human infection can result from exposure to as few as a few hundred colony-forming units. At times, *C. jejuni* and *C. coli* spread person to person, perinatally, and at child care centers where diapered toddlers are present. Persons infected with *C. jejuni* usually shed the organism for weeks but can shed for months.

PATHOGENESIS

The conceptual model for the pathogenesis of *C. jejuni* enteritis includes mechanisms to transit the stomach, adhere to intestinal mucosal cells, and initiate intestinal lumen fluid accumulation. Most *Campylobacter* isolates are acid sensitive. Host conditions associated with reduced gastric acidity and foods capable of shielding organisms in transit through the stomach are postulated to be factors that allow *Campylobacter* to reach the intestine. Subsequently, bacterial motility, surface proteins, and surface glycans facilitate adhesion to intestinal mucosal cells. Lumen fluid accumulation is associated with direct damage to mucosal cells resulting from bacterial invasion and potentially from a cholera-like toxin and other cytotoxins. Additionally, *C. jejuni* can have mechanisms that enable transit away from the mucosal surface. This armamentarium appears to be differentially deployed by various *C. jejuni* organisms.

Campylobacter differ from other enteric bacterial pathogens in that they have both N- and O-linked glycosylation capacities. N-linked glycosylation is associated with molecules expressed on the bacterial surface, and O-linked glycosylation appears limited to flagella. Slipped-strand mispairing in glycosylation loci results in modified, antigenically distinct surface structures. It is hypothesized that antigenic variation provides a mechanism for immune evasion.

C. fetus possesses a high molecular weight S layer protein that mediates high-level resistance to serum-mediated killing and phagocytosis and is thus thought to be responsible for the propensity to produce bacteremia. *C. jejuni* and *C. coli* are generally sensitive to serum-mediated killing, but serum-resistant variants exist. It has been suggested that these serum-resistant variants may be more capable of systemic dissemination.

There is a strong association between **Guillain-Barré syndrome** and preceding infection with some serotypes of *C. jejuni* (Chapter 608). Molecular mimicry between nerve tissue and *Campylobacter* surface antigens may be the triggering factor in *Campylobacter*-associated Guillain-Barré syndrome, including the Miller-Fisher variant, which is characterized by ataxia, areflexia, and ophthalmoplegia. Reactive arthritis and erythema nodosum can also occur. Most *Campylobacter* infections are not followed by immunoreactive complications, indicating that factors in addition to molecular mimicry are required for these complications.

There is increasing evidence of an association between *Campylobacter* infection and irritable bowel syndrome. It is proposed that low-grade inflammation caused by *Campylobacter,* below the threshold that can be detected by endoscopy, results in cross-talk with gut nerves, leading to symptoms.

CLINICAL MANIFESTATIONS

The varied clinical presentations of *Campylobacter* infections link to the species involved and to host factors such as age, immunocompetence, and underlying conditions. The most common presentation is acute enteritis.

Acute Gastroenteritis

Diarrhea is usually caused by *C. jejuni* (90-95%) or *C. coli* and rarely by *C. lari, C. hyointestinalis,* or *C. upsaliensis.* The incubation period is 1-7 days. Patients typically have a prodrome comprising fever, headache, and myalgia and within a day develop loose, watery stools or, less commonly, bloody, mucus-containing stools that are characteristic of dysentery. In severe cases, blood appears in the stools 2-4 days after the onset of symptoms. Fever may be the only manifestation initially, but 60-90% of older children also complain of abdominal pain. The abdominal pain is periumbilical and may be cramping, sometimes persisting after the stools return to normal. The abdominal pain can mimic appendicitis or intussusception.

Mild disease lasts 1-2 days and resembles viral gastroenteritis. Most patients recover in <1 wk, although 20-30% of patients remain ill for 2 wks and 5-10% are symptomatic for >2 wks. Fatalities are rare. Persistent or recurrent *Campylobacter* gastroenteritis and emergence of erythromycin resistance during therapy have been reported in immunocompetent persons, patients with hypogammaglobulinemia (congenital or acquired), and patients with AIDS. Persistent infection can mimic chronic inflammatory bowel disease, and thus *Campylobacter* infection should be ruled out when considering a diagnosis of inflammatory bowel disease. Fecal shedding of the organisms in untreated patients usually lasts for 2-3 wk, with a range from a few days to several months. Shedding tends to be relatively longer in young children. Acute appendicitis, mesenteric lymphadenitis, and ileocolitis have been reported in patients who have had appendectomies during *C. jejuni* infection.

Bacteremia

With the exception of bacteremia due to *C. fetus,* bacteremia with *Campylobacter* occurs most often among malnourished children, patients with chronic illnesses or immunodeficiency (HIV, others), and at the extremes of age and is usually asymptomatic. *C. fetus* causes bacteremia in adults with or without identifiable focal infection, usually in the setting of underlying conditions such as malignancy or diabetes mellitus. When symptomatic, *C. jejuni* bacteremia is associated with fever, headache, malaise, and abdominal pain. Relapsing or intermittent fever is associated with night sweats, chills, and weight loss when the illness is prolonged. Lethargy and confusion can occur, but focal neurologic signs are unusual without cerebrovascular disease or meningitis. A cough is present occasionally, usually without pulmonary parenchymal involvement. Diarrhea, jaundice, and hepatomegaly are uncommon. Moderate leukocytosis may be found. Transient asymptomatic bacteremia, rapidly fatal septicemia, and prolonged bacteremia of 8-13 wk have been described. Occasional reports describe bacteremia with *C. upsaliensis.*

Focal Extraintestinal Infections

Focal infections caused by *C. jejuni* are rare and occur mainly among neonates and immunocompromised patients, with examples including meningitis, pneumonia, thrombophlebitis, pancreatitis, cholecystitis, ileocecitis with right lower quadrant pain mimicking appendicitis, urinary tract infection, arthritis, peritonitis, myocarditis, pericarditis, and endocarditis. *C. fetus* shows a predilection for vascular endothelium, causing endocarditis, pericarditis, thrombophlebitis, and mycotic aneurysms, and can also cause meningitis, septic arthritis, osteomyelitis, urinary tract infection, lung abscess, and cholangitis. *C. hyointestinalis* has

been associated with proctitis, *C. upsaliensis* with breast abscesses, and *C. rectus* with periodontitis.

Perinatal Infections

Severe perinatal infections are uncommon and are caused most often by *C. fetus* and rarely by *C. jejuni*. Maternal *C. fetus* and *C. jejuni* infections may be asymptomatic and can result in abortion, stillbirth, premature delivery, or neonatal infection with sepsis and meningitis. Neonatal infection with *C. jejuni* is associated with diarrhea that may be bloody.

DIAGNOSIS

The clinical presentation of *Campylobacter* enteritis can be similar to that of enteritis caused by other bacterial enteropathogens. The differential diagnosis includes *Shigella, Salmonella,* invasive *Escherichia coli, E. coli* O157:H7, *Yersinia enterocolitica, Aeromonas, Vibrio parahaemolyticus,* and amebiasis. Fecal leukocytes are found in as many as 75% of cases, and fecal blood is present in 50% of cases. The presence of bloody stools, fever, and abdominal pain should result in an evaluation for *Campylobacter.*

The diagnosis of *Campylobacter* enteritis is usually confirmed by identification of the organism in cultures of stool or rectal swabs. Selective media such as Skirrow or Butzler media and microaerophilic conditions (5-10% oxygen) are commonly used. Some *C. jejuni* grow best at 42°C. Filtration methods are available and can preferentially enrich for *Campylobacter* by selecting for their small size. These methods allow subsequent culture of the enriched sample on antibiotic free media, enhancing rates of isolation of *Campylobacter* organisms inhibited by the antibiotics included in standard selective media. Isolation of Campylobacter from normally sterile sites does not require enhancement procedures.

For rapid diagnosis of *Campylobacter* enteritis, direct carbol fuchsin stain of fecal smear, indirect fluorescence antibody test, dark-field microscopy, or latex agglutination can be used. Antigen detection by enzyme immunoassay is nearly as sensitive and specific as culture. Species-specific DNA probes and specific gene amplification by polymerase chain reaction (PCR) have been described. Serologic diagnosis is also possible.

COMPLICATIONS

Severe, prolonged *C. jejuni* infection can occur in patients with immunodeficiencies, including hypogammaglobulinemia and malnutrition. In patients with AIDS, an increased frequency and severity of *C. jejuni* infection have been reported; severity correlates inversely with CD4 count.

Reactive Arthritis

Reactive arthritis can accompany *Campylobacter* enteritis in adolescents and adults, especially patients who are positive for HLA-B27. This manifestation appears 5-40 days after the onset of diarrhea, involves mainly large joints, and resolves without sequelae. The arthritis is typically migratory and occurs without fever. Synovial fluid lacks bacteria. Reactive arthritis with conjunctivitis, urethritis, and rash (including erythema nodosum) also occurs but is less common.

Guillain-Barré Syndrome

Guillain-Barré syndrome (GBS) is an acute demyelinating disease of the peripheral nervous system characterized clinically by acute flaccid paralysis and is the most common cause of neuromuscular paralysis worldwide (Chapter 608). GBS carries a mortality rate of ~2%, and ~20% of patients with this disease develop major neurologic sequelae. *C. jejuni* is an important causal factor for GBS, which has been reported 1-12 wk after culture-proven *C. jejuni* gastroenteritis in 1 of every 3,000 *C. jejuni* infections. Stool cultures obtained from patients with GBS at the onset of neurologic symptoms have yielded *C. jejuni* in >25% of the cases. Serologic studies suggest that 20-45% of patients with GBS have evidence of recent *C. jejuni* infection. The management of GBS includes supportive care, intravenous immunoglobulin, and plasma exchange.

Other Complications

IgA nephropathy and immune complex glomerulonephritis with *C. jejuni* antigens in the kidneys have been reported. *Campylobacter* infection has also been associated with hemolytic anemia.

TREATMENT

Fluid replacement, correction of electrolyte imbalance, and supportive care are the mainstays of treatment of children with *Campylobacter* gastroenteritis (Chapter 332). Antimotility agents can cause prolonged or fatal disease and should not be used.

The need for antibiotic therapy in patients with uncomplicated gastroenteritis is controversial. Data suggest a shortened duration of symptoms and intestinal shedding of organisms if erythromycin ethylsuccinate or azithromycin is initiated early in the disease in patients with the dysenteric form of *Campylobacter* enteritis.

Most *Campylobacter* isolates are susceptible to macrolides, aminoglycosides, chloramphenicol, imipenem, and clindamycin and are resistant to cephalosporins, tetracyclines, rifampin, penicillins, trimethoprim, and vancomycin. Antibiotic resistance among *C. jejuni* has become a serious worldwide problem. Quinolone resistance has developed and is related to the use of quinolones in veterinary medicine. Erythromycin-resistant *Campylobacter* isolates remain uncommon, and erythromycin or azithromycin is the drug of choice if therapy is required. Antibiotics are recommended for patients with the dysenteric form of the disease, high fever, or a severe course and for children who are immunosuppressed or have underlying diseases. Sepsis is treated with parenteral antibiotics such as an aminoglycoside, meropenem, or imipenem.

For extraintestinal infection caused by *C. fetus*, prolonged therapy is advised. *C. fetus* isolates resistant to erythromycin have been reported.

PROGNOSIS

Although *Campylobacter* gastroenteritis is usually self-limited, immunosuppressed children (including children with AIDS) can experience a protracted or severe course. Septicemia in newborns and immunocompromised hosts has a poor prognosis, with an estimated mortality rate of 30-40%.

PREVENTION

Most human campylobacterioses are sporadic and are acquired from infected animals or contaminated foods. Interventions to minimize transmission include preparing food under conditions that kill *Campylobacter* and that prevent recontamination after cooking (not using the same surfaces, utensils, or containers for both uncooked and cooked food), ensuring that water sources are not contaminated and that water is kept in clean containers, and taking steps to prevent direct transmission from infected persons or infected domestic pets. Breast-feeding appears to decrease symptomatic *Campylobacter* disease but does not reduce colonization.

Several approaches at immunization are being studied, including the use of live-attenuated organisms, subunit vaccines, and killed whole-cell vaccines.

BIBLIOGRAPHY

Please visit the Nelson Textbook of Pediatrics *website at* *www.expertconsult.com* *for the complete bibliography.*

Chapter 195
Yersinia

Anupama Kalaskar, Gloria P. Heresi, and James R. Murphy

The genus *Yersinia* is a member of the family Enterobacteriaceae and comprises >14 named species, 3 of which are established as human pathogens. *Yersinia enterocolitica* is by far the most common *Yersinia* species causing human disease and produces fever, abdominal pain that can mimic appendicitis, and diarrhea. *Yersinia pseudotuberculosis* is most often associated with mesenteric lymphadenitis. *Yersinia pestis* is the agent of plague and most commonly causes an acute febrile lymphadenitis (bubonic plague) and less commonly occurs as septicemic, pneumonic, or meningeal plague. Untreated and delayed treated plague has significant mortality. Other *Yersinia* organisms are uncommon causes of infections of humans, and their identification is often an indicator of immunodeficiency. *Yersinia* is enzootic and can colonize pets. Infection of humans most often results from contact with infected animals or their tissues; ingestion of contaminated water, milk, or meat; or, for *Y. pestis,* the bite of infected fleas. Association with human disease is less clear for *Y. frederiksenii, Y. intermedia, Y. kristensenii, Y. aldovae, Y. bercovieri, Y. mollaretii, Y. rohdei,* and *Y. ruckeri.* Some *Yersinia* isolates replicate at low temperatures (1-4°C) or survive at high temperatures (50-60°C). Thus, common food preparation and storage and common pasteurization methods might not limit the number of bacteria. Most are sensitive to oxidizing agents.

195.1 *Yersinia enterocolitica*

Anupama Kalaskar, Gloria P. Heresi, and James R. Murphy

ETIOLOGY

Y. enterocolitica is a large, gram-negative coccobacillus that exhibits little or no bipolarity when stained with methylene blue and carbol fuchsin. These facultative anaerobes grow well on common culture media and are motile at 22°C but not at 37°C. *Y. enterocolitica* includes pathogenic and nonpathogenic members.

EPIDEMIOLOGY

This agent is transmitted to humans through food, water, animal contact, and contaminated blood products. Transmission can occur from mother to newborn. *Y. enterocolitica* appears to have a global distribution but is seldom a cause of tropical diarrhea. There is approximately 1 culture- confirmed *Y. enterocolitica* infection per 100,000 population/yr in the USA, and infection may be more common in Northern Europe. Cases are more common in colder months and among younger persons and boys. Most infections in children are among those <7 yr of age, with the majority among children <1 yr of age.

Natural reservoirs of *Y. enterocolitica* include pigs, rodents, rabbits, sheep, cattle, horses, dogs, and cats, with pigs being the major animal reservoir. Contact with feral animals or a colonized pet is a common source of human infections. Culture and molecular techniques have found the organism in a variety of foods, including vegetable juice, pasteurized milk, and carrots and in water. A source of sporadic *Y. enterocolitica* infections is pig offal (chitterlings). In one study, 71% of human isolates were indistinguishable from the strains isolated from pigs. *Y. enterocolitica* is an occupational threat to butchers. In part because of its capacity to multiply at refrigerator temperatures, *Y. enterocolitica* is transmitted at times by intravenous injection of contaminated fluids, including blood products.

Y. enterocolitica infections have increased, and *Y. pseudotuberculosis* infections have declined, leading to the suggestion that the former organism is replacing the latter in an ecologic niche. In part, the mass production of animals, development of meat factories based on chains of cold storage, and international trade of meat products and animals are believed to be the reasons for the increasing prevalence of yersiniosis in humans. There is evidence that under farm conditions pigs can be raised free of *Y. enterocolitica.*

PATHOGENESIS

The organisms most often enter by the alimentary tract and cause mucosal ulcerations in the ileum. Necrotic lesions of Peyer patches and mesenteric lymphadenitis occur. If septicemia develops, suppurative lesions can be found in infected organs. Infection can trigger reactive arthritis and erythema nodosum.

Adherence, invasion, and toxin production are established as essential mechanisms of pathogenesis. Bacterial components, some associated with the bacterial type III secretion apparatus, can actively suppress immunologic capacities, suggesting that immunosuppression can contribute to pathogenesis. Motility appears to be required for *Y. enterocolitica* pathogenesis. Serogroups that predominate in human illness are O:3, O:8, O:9, and O:5,27. Virulence traits are both chromosomal and plasmid encoded. Possibly because pathogenic strains require iron, patients with **iron overload** as in hemochromatosis, thalassemia, and sickle cell disease are at high risk for infection.

CLINICAL MANIFESTATIONS

Disease occurs most often as enterocolitis with diarrhea, fever, and abdominal pain. Acute enteritis is more common among younger children, and mesenteric lymphadenitis that can mimic appendicitis may be found in older children and adolescents. Stools may be watery or contain leukocytes and, less commonly, frank blood and mucus. *Y. enterocolitica* is excreted in stool for 1-4 wk. Family contacts of a patient are often found to be asymptomatically colonized with *Y. enterocolitica. Y. enterocolitica* septicemia is less common and is most often found in very young children (<3 mo of age) and immunocompromised persons. Systemic infection is associated with splenic and hepatic abscesses, osteomyelitis, meningitis, endocarditis, and mycotic aneurysms. Exudative pharyngitis, pneumonia, empyema, lung abscess, and acute respiratory distress syndrome uncommonly occur. *Y. enterocolitica* infection in immunocompromised persons can manifest with physical and CT findings suggesting colon cancer with liver metastases.

Reactive complications include erythema nodosum, arthritis, and the uveitis rash syndrome. These manifestations may be more common in selected populations (northern Europeans), in association with HLA-B27, and in girls. *Y. enterocolitica* has been associated with Kawasaki disease.

DIAGNOSIS

Y. enterocolitica is easily cultured from normally sterile sites but requires special procedures for isolation from stool, where other bacteria can outgrow it. Cold enrichment, where a sample is held in buffered saline, can result in preferential growth of *Yersinia,* but the procedure takes weeks. Polymerase chain reaction (PCR) and DNA microarray are more sensitive than culture with DNA microarray more sensitive and accurate than multiplex PCR. Many laboratories do not routinely perform the procedures required to detect *Y. enterocolitica.* Procedures targeted to this organism must be specifically requested. A history indicating contact with environmental sources of *Yersinia* and detection of fecal leukocytes are helpful indicators of a need to test for *Y. enterocolitica.* The isolation of a *Yersinia* from stool should be followed by tests to confirm that the isolate is a pathogen. Serodiagnosis is possible but not readily available.

DIFFERENTIAL DIAGNOSIS

The clinical presentation is similar to other forms of bacterial enterocolitis. The most common considerations include *Shigella, Salmonella, Campylobacter, Clostridium difficile*, enteroinvasive *Escherichia coli, Y. pseudotuberculosis*, and occasionally *Vibrio* diarrheal disease (Chapter 332). Amebiasis, appendicitis, Crohn disease, ulcerative colitis, diverticulitis, and pseudomembranous colitis should also be considered.

TREATMENT

Enterocolitis in an immunocompetent patient is a self-limiting disease, and no benefit from antibiotic therapy is established. Patients with systemic infection and very young children (in whom septicemia is common) should be treated. Many *Yersinia* organisms are susceptible to trimethoprim-sulfamethoxazole (TMP-SMX), aminoglycosides, 3rd-generation cephalosporins, and quinolones. TMP-SMX is the recommended empirical treatment in children, because it has activity against most strains and is well tolerated. In severe infections such as bacteremia, 3rd-generation cephalosporins with or without aminoglycosides are effective. *Y. enterocolitica* produces β-lactamases, which are responsible for resistance to penicillins and 1st-generation cephalosporins. Patients on deferoxamine should discontinue iron chelation therapy during treatment for *Y. enterocolitica*, especially if they have complicated gastrointestinal infection or extraintestinal infection.

COMPLICATIONS

Reactive arthritis, erythema nodosum, erythema multiforme, hemolytic anemia, thrombocytopenia, and systemic dissemination of bacteria have been reported in association with *Y. enterocolitica* infection. Septicemia is more common in younger children, and reactive arthritis is more common in older patients. Arthritis appears to be mediated by immune complexes, and viable organisms are not present in involved joints.

PREVENTION

Prevention centers on reducing contact with environmental sources of *Yersinia*. Breaking or sterilization of the chain from animal reservoirs to humans holds the greatest potential to reduce infections, and the techniques applied must be tailored to the reservoirs in each geographic area. There is no licensed vaccine.

BIBLIOGRAPHY

Please visit the Nelson Textbook of Pediatrics *website at www.expertconsult.com for the complete bibliography.*

195.2 *Yersinia pseudotuberculosis*

Anupama Kalaskar, Gloria P. Heresi, and James R. Murphy

Y. pseudotuberculosis has a worldwide distribution; *Y. pseudotuberculosis* disease is less common than *Y. enterocolitica* disease. The most common form of disease is a mesenteric lymphadenitis that produces an appendicitis-like syndrome. *Y. pseudotuberculosis* is associated with a Kawasaki disease–like illness in about 8% of cases (Chapter 160).

ETIOLOGY

Y. pseudotuberculosis is a gram-negative aerobic and facultative anaerobic coccobacillus that does not ferment lactose; is oxidase negative, catalase producing, and urea splitting; and shares many morphologic and culture characteristics with *Y. enterocolitica*. It is differentiated biochemically from *Y. enterocolitica* on the basis of ornithine decarboxylase activity and on fermentation of sucrose, sorbitol, cellobiose, and other tests, although some overlap between species occurs. Antisera to somatic O antigens and sensitivity to *Yersinia* phages can also be used to differentiate the 2 species. Subspecies-specific DNA sequences that allow direct probe- and primer-specific differentiation of *Y. pestis, Y. pseudotuberculosis*, and *Y. enterocolitica* have been described. *Y. pseudotuberculosis* is more closely related to *Y. pestis* than to *Y. enterocolitica*.

EPIDEMIOLOGY

Y. pseudotuberculosis is zoonotic, with reservoirs in wild rodents, rabbits, deer, farm animals, various birds, and domestic animals, including cats and canaries. Transmission to humans is by consumption of or contact with contaminated animals or contact with an environmental source contaminated by animals (often water). Infections are more commonly reported from Europe, in boys, and in the winter. Direct evidence of transmission of *Y. pseudotuberculosis* to humans by consumption of lettuce and raw carrots has been published. *Y. pseudotuberculosis* bacteremia is an increasingly recognized problem in HIV-infected patients.

PATHOGENESIS

Ileal and colonic mucosal ulceration and mesenteric lymphadenitis are hallmarks of the infection. Necrotizing epithelioid granulomas may be seen in the mesenteric lymph nodes, but the appendix is often grossly and microscopically normal. The mesenteric nodes are often the only source of isolation of the organisms. *Y. pseudotuberculosis* antigens bind directly to HLA class II molecules and can function as superantigens, which might account for the clinical illness resembling Kawasaki disease.

CLINICAL MANIFESTATIONS

Pseudoappendicitis with abdominal pain, right lower quadrant tenderness, fever, and leukocytosis is the most common clinical presentation. Enterocolitis and extraintestinal spread are uncommon. Iron overload, diabetes mellitus, and chronic liver disease are often found concomitantly with extraintestinal *Y. pseudotuberculosis* infection. Renal involvement with tubulointerstitial nephritis, azotemia, pyuria, and glucosuria can occur.

DIAGNOSIS

PCR of involved tissue can be used to identify the organism; isolation by culture can require an extended interval. Involved mesenteric lymph nodes removed at appendectomy can yield the organism by culture. Ultrasound examination of children with unexplained fever and abdominal pain can reveal a characteristic picture of enlarged mesenteric lymph nodes, thickening of the terminal ileum, and no image of the appendix. *Y. pseudotuberculosis* is rarely recovered from stool. Serologic procedures are available but not in most routine laboratories.

DIFFERENTIAL DIAGNOSIS

Appendicitis (most commonly), inflammatory bowel disease, and other intra-abdominal infections should be considered. Kawasaki disease, staphylococcal or streptococcal disease, leptospirosis, Stevens-Johnson syndrome, and collagen vascular diseases, including acute-onset juvenile rheumatoid arthritis, can mimic the syndrome with prolonged fever and rash. *Clostridium difficile* colitis, meningitis, encephalitis, enteropathic arthropathies, acute pancreatitis, sarcoidosis, toxic shock syndrome, typhoid fever, and ulcerative colitis may also be considered.

TREATMENT

Uncomplicated mesenteric lymphadenitis due to *Y. pseudotuberculosis* is a self-limited disease, and antimicrobial therapy is not required. Culture-confirmed bacteremia should be treated with an aminoglycoside, ampicillin, TMP-SMX, a 3rd-generation cephalosporin, or chloramphenicol.

COMPLICATIONS

An illness with presentation similar to Kawasaki disease can occur. There may be fever of 1-2 days' duration; strawberry tongue; pharyngeal erythema; a scarlatiniform rash; cracked, red, swollen lips; conjunctivitis; sterile pyuria; periungual desquamation; and thrombocytosis. Coronary aneurysm formation has been described. Erythema nodosum and reactive arthritis can follow infection.

PREVENTION

Avoiding exposure to potentially infected animals and good food-handling practices can prevent infection. The sporadic nature of the disease makes application of targeted prevention measures difficult.

BIBLIOGRAPHY
Please visit the Nelson Textbook of Pediatrics *website at www.expertconsult.com for the complete bibliography.*

195.3 Plague *(Yersinia pestis)*

Anupama Kalaskar, Gloria P. Heresi, and James R. Murphy

ETIOLOGY

Y. pestis is a gram-negative, facultative anaerobe that is a pleomorphic nonmotile, non-spore-forming coccobacillus and is a potential agent of bioterrorism (Chapter 704). The bacterium has several chromosomal and plasmid-associated factors that are essential to virulence and to survival in mammalian hosts and fleas. *Y. pestis* shares bipolar staining appearance with *Y. pseudotuberculosis* and can be differentiated by biochemical reactions, serology, phage sensitivity, and molecular techniques. The *Y. pestis* genome has been determined and is ~4,600,000 base pairs in size.

EPIDEMIOLOGY

Plague is endemic in at least 24 countries. About 3,000 cases are reported worldwide per year, with 100-200 deaths (2004). Plague is uncommon in the USA (0-40 reported cases/yr); most of these cases occur west of a line from east Texas to east Montana, with 80% of cases in New Mexico, Arizona, and Colorado. Transmission to humans is most commonly from wild animal sources, although most cases of inhalation plague reported to the Centers for Disease Control and Prevention (CDC) were associated with exposure to infected free-roaming domestic cats. The epidemic form of disease killed about 25% of the population of Europe in the Middle Ages in one of a number of epidemics and pandemics. The epidemiology of epidemic plague involves extension of infection from the zoonotic reservoirs to urban rats, *Rattus rattus* and *Rattus norvegicus,* and from fleas of urban rats to humans. Epidemics are no longer seen. Selective pressure exerted by plague pandemics in medieval Europe is hypothesized for enrichment of a deletion mutation in the gene encoding CCR5 (CCR5-Δ32). The enhanced frequency of this mutation in European populations endows about 10% of European descendants with resistance to HIV-1.

The most common mode of transmission of *Y. pestis* to humans is by the bite of infected fleas. Historically, most human infections are thought to have resulted from bites of fleas that acquired infection from feeding on infected urban rats. Less commonly, infection is caused by contact with infectious body fluids or tissues or inhaling infectious droplets. Sylvatic plague can exist as a stable enzootic infection or as an epizootic disease with high host mortality. Ground squirrels, rock squirrels, prairie dogs, rats, mice, bobcats, cats, rabbits, and chipmunks may be infected. Transmission among animals is usually by flea bite or by ingestion of contaminated tissue. *Xenopsylla cheopis* is the flea most commonly associated with transmission to humans, but >30 species of fleas have been demonstrated as vector competent, and *Pulex irritans,* the human flea, can transmit plague and might have been an important vector in some historical epidemics. Both sexes are similarly affected by plague, and transmission is more common in colder regions and seasons, possibly because of temperature effects on *Y. pestis* infections in vector fleas.

PATHOGENESIS

In the most common form of plague, infected fleas regurgitate organisms into a patient's skin during feeding. The bacteria translocate to regional lymph nodes, where *Y. pestis* replicates, resulting in bubonic plague. In the absence of rapidly implemented specific therapy, bacteremia can occur, resulting in purulent, necrotic, and hemorrhagic lesions in many organs. Both plasmid and chromosomal genes are required for full virulence. Pneumonic plague occurs when infected material is inhaled. The organism is highly transmissible from persons with pneumonic plague and from domestic cats with pneumonic infection. This high transmissibility and high morbidity and mortality have provided an impetus for attempts to use *Y. pestis* as a biological weapon.

CLINICAL MANIFESTATIONS

Y. pestis infection can manifest as several clinical syndromes; infection can also be subclinical. The 3 principal clinical presentations of plague are bubonic, septicemic, and pneumonic. **Bubonic plague** is the most common form and accounts for 80-90% of cases in the USA. From 2-8 days after a flea bite, lymphadenitis develops in lymph nodes closest to the inoculation site, including the inguinal (most common), axillary, or cervical region. These buboes are remarkable for tenderness. Fever, chills, weakness, prostration, headache, and the development of septicemia are common. The skin might show insect bites or scratch marks. Purpura and gangrene of the extremities can develop as a result of disseminated intravascular coagulation. These lesions may be the origin of the name Black Death. Untreated plague results in death in >50% of symptomatic patients. Death can occur within 2-4 days after onset of symptoms.

Occasionally, *Y. pestis* establishes systemic infection and induces the systemic symptoms seen with bubonic plague without causing a bubo (**primary septicemic plague**). Because of the delay in diagnosis linked to the lack of the bubo, septicemic plague carries a higher case fatality rate than bubonic plague. In some regions, bubo-free septicemic plague accounts for 25% of cases.

Pneumonic plague is the least common but most dangerous and lethal form of the disease. Pneumonic plague can result from hematogenous dissemination, or rarely as primary pneumonic plague after inhalation of the organism from a human or animal with plague pneumonia or potentially from a biological attack. Signs of pneumonic plague include severe pneumonia with high fever, dyspnea, and hemoptysis.

Plague meningitis, tonsillitis, or gastroenteritis can occur. Meningitis tends to be a late complication following inadequate treatment. Tonsillitis and gastroenteritis can occur with or without apparent bubo formation or lymphadenopathy.

DIAGNOSIS

Plague should be suspected in patients with fever and history of exposure to small animals in endemic areas. Thus, bubonic plague is suspected in a patient with a painful swollen lymph node, fever, and prostration who has been exposed to fleas or rodents in the western USA. A history of camping or the presence of flea bites increases the index of suspicion.

Y. pestis is readily transmitted to humans by some routine laboratory manipulations. Thus, *it is imperative to clearly notify a laboratory* when submitting a sample suspected of containing *Y. pestis.* Laboratory diagnosis is based on bacteriologic culture or direct visualization using Gram, Giemsa, or Wayson stains of lymph node aspirates, blood, sputum, or exudates. *Y. pestis* grows slowly under routine culture conditions and best at temperatures that differ from those used for routine cultures in many clinical laboratories. ELISA and PCR are available but are not in routine clinical use. A rapid antigen test is under development. Suspected isolates of *Y. pestis* should be forwarded to a reference laboratory for confirmation. Special containment shipping precautions are required. Cases of plague should be reported to local and state health departments and the CDC.

DIFFERENTIAL DIAGNOSIS

The Gram stain of *Y. pestis* may be confused with *Enterobacter agglomerans.* Mild and subacute forms of bubonic plague may be confused with other disorders causing localized lymphadenitis and lymphadenopathy. Septicemic plague may be indistinguishable from other forms of overwhelming bacterial sepsis like tularemia and cat-scratch disease.

Pulmonary manifestations of plague are similar to those of anthrax, Q fever, and tularemia, all agents with bioterrorism and biological warfare potential. Thus, the presentation of a suspected case, and especially any cluster of cases, requires immediate reporting. Additional information on this aspect of plague and procedures can be found at *www.bt.cdc.gov/agent/plague/*.

TREATMENT

Patients in whom bubonic plague is suspected should be placed in isolation until 2 days after starting antibiotic treatment to prevent the potential spread of the disease if the patient develops pneumonia. The treatment of choice for bubonic plague historically has been streptomycin (30 mg/kg/day, maximum 2 g/day, divided every 12 hr IM for 10 days). Intramuscular streptomycin is inappropriate for septicemia because absorption may be erratic when perfusion is poor. The poor central nervous system penetration of streptomycin makes this an inappropriate drug for meningitis. Streptomycin might not be widely and immediately available. Gentamicin (children, 7.5 mg/kg IM or IV divided every 8 hr; adults, 5 mg/kg IM or IV once daily) has been shown to be as efficacious as streptomycin. Alternative treatments include doxycycline (<45 kg, 2-5 mg/kg/day every 12 hr IV, maximum 200 mg/day; not recommended for children <8 yr of age; ≥45 kg, 100 mg every 12 hr PO), ciprofloxacin (30 mg/kg/day divided every 12 hr, maximum 400 mg every 12 hr IV), and chloramphenicol (50-100 mg/kg/day IV divided every 6 hr). Meningitis is usually treated with chloramphenicol. Resistance to these agents and relapses are rare. *Y. pestis* is susceptible to fluoroquinolones in vitro, which is effective in treating experimental plague in animals. *Y. pestis* is susceptible to penicillin in vitro, but this is ineffective in treatment of human disease. Mild disease may be treated with oral chloramphenicol or tetracycline in children >8 yr of age. Clinical improvement is noted within 48 hr of initiating treatment.

Postexposure prophylaxis should be given to close contacts of patients with pneumonic plague. Antimicrobial prophylaxis is recommended within 7 days of exposure for persons with direct, close contact with a pneumonic plague patient or those exposed to an accidental or terrorist-induced aerosol. Recommended regimens include a 7-day course of tetracycline, doxycycline, or TMP-SMX. Contacts of cases of uncomplicated bubonic plague do not require prophylaxis. *Y. pestis* is a potential agent of bioterrorism that can require mass casualty prophylaxis (Chapter 704).

PREVENTION

Avoidance of exposure to infected animals and fleas is the best method of prevention of infection. In the USA, special care is required in environments inhabited by rodent reservoirs of *Y. pestis* and their ectoparasites. Patients with plague should be isolated if they have pulmonary symptoms, and infected materials should be handled with extreme care.

BIBLIOGRAPHY

Please visit the Nelson Textbook of Pediatrics *website at* www.expertconsult.com *for the complete bibliography.*

Chapter 196
Aeromonas and *Plesiomonas*

Guenet H. Degaffe, Gloria P. Heresi, and James R. Murphy

Aeromonas and *Plesiomonas* are pathogenic gram-negative bacilli that commonly cause enteritis and less frequently cause skin and soft tissue infections and septicemia. They are common in fresh and brackish water and colonize animals and plants in these niches.

196.1 *Aeromonas*

Guenet H. Degaffe, Gloria P. Heresi, and James R. Murphy

ETIOLOGY

Aeromonas is a member of the family Aeromonadaceae. These organisms are oxidase-positive, facultatively anaerobic, gram-negative bacilli that ferment glucose. At least 17 phenotypic species are known, including 8 that are recognized as human pathogens. *A. hydrophila, A. veronii* biotype sobria, and *A. caviae* are the species most often associated with human infection. *A. trota* is being isolated with increasing frequency from human stool.

For the full continuation of this chapter, please visit the Nelson Textbook of Pediatrics *website at* www.expertconsult.com.

196.2 *Plesiomonas shigelloides*

Guenet H. Degaffe, Gloria P. Heresi, and James R. Murphy

ETIOLOGY

Plesiomonas shigelloides is most commonly associated with acute enteritis and rarely with extraintestinal infections. The organism is a facultative, anaerobic, gram-negative non–spore forming bacillus with over 100 serotypes (100 somatic [O] and 50 flagellar [H] antigens). It is catalase and oxidase positive, able to ferment xylose, and motile, with 2-5 polar flagella.

For the full continuation of this chapter, please visit the Nelson Textbook of Pediatrics *website at* www.expertconsult.com.

Chapter 197 *Pseudomonas, Burkholderia,* and *Stenotrophomonas*

197.1 *Pseudomonas aeruginosa*

Thomas S. Murray and Robert S. Baltimore

ETIOLOGY

Pseudomonas aeruginosa is a gram-negative rod and is a strict aerobe. It can multiply in a great variety of environments that contain minimal amounts of organic compounds. Strains from clinical specimens do not ferment lactose, are oxidase positive, and may produce β-hemolysis on blood agar. Many produce pigments including pyocyanin, pyoverdin, and pyorubrin that diffuse into and color the surrounding medium. Strains of *Pseudomonas* can be differentiated for epidemiologic purposes by serologic, phage, and pyocin typing and by genome restriction fragment length polymorphisms using pulsed-field gel electrophoresis.

EPIDEMIOLOGY

P. aeruginosa is a classic opportunist. It rarely causes disease in people who do not have a predisposing risk factor. Compromised host defense mechanisms owing to trauma, neutropenia, mucositis, immunosuppression, or impaired mucociliary transport explain the predominant role of this organism in producing opportunistic infections. The rate of *P. aeruginosa* bacteremia in children is 3.8/1,000 patients over 10 yr, with a 20% mortality rate; rates vary according to the prevalent underlying diseases. *P. aeruginosa* and other pseudomonads frequently enter the hospital environment on the clothes, skin, or shoes of patients or hospital personnel, with plants or vegetables brought into the hospital, and in the gastrointestinal tracts of patients. Colonization of any moist or liquid substance may ensue; the organisms may be found growing in any water reservoir, including distilled water, and in hospital kitchens and laundries, some antiseptic solutions, and equipment used for respiratory therapy. Colonization of skin, throat, stool, and nasal mucosa of patients is low at admission to the hospital but increases to as high as 50-70% with prolonged hospitalization and with the use of broad-spectrum antibiotics, chemotherapy, mechanical ventilation, and urinary catheters. Patients' intestinal microbial flora may be altered by the use of broad-spectrum antibiotics, which reduces resistance to colonization and permits *P. aeruginosa* in the environment to populate the gastrointestinal tract. Intestinal mucosal breakdown associated with medications, especially cytotoxic agents, and nosocomial enteritis may provide a pathway by which *P. aeruginosa* spreads to the lymphatics or bloodstream.

PATHOLOGY

The pathologic manifestations of *Pseudomonas* infections depend on the site and type of infection. Due to its elaboration of toxins and invasive factors, the organism can often be seen invading blood vessels and causing vascular necrosis. In some infections there is spread through tissues with necrosis and microabscess formation. In patients with cystic fibrosis, focal and diffuse bronchitis/bronchiolitis leading to bronchiolitis obliterans has been reported.

PATHOGENESIS

Invasiveness of *P. aeruginosa* is mediated by a host of virulence factors. Bacterial attachment is facilitated by pili that adhere to epithelium damaged by prior injury or infection. Extracellular proteins, proteases, elastases, and cytotoxin disrupt cell membranes, and in response, host-produced cytokines cause capillary vascular permeability and induce an inflammatory response. Dissemination and bloodstream invasion follow extension of local tissue damage and are facilitated by the antiphagocytic properties of endotoxin, the exopolysaccharide, and protease cleavage of immunoglobulin G. *P. aeruginosa* also produces numerous exotoxins, including **exotoxin A,** which causes local necrosis and facilitates systemic bacterial invasion. *P. aeruginosa* possesses a type III secretion system (TTSS) that is important for virulence in multiple animal models. This needle structure inserts into host cell membranes and allows secretion of exotoxins directly into host cells. *P. aeruginosa* strains with the gene encoding the TTSS dependent phospholipase ExoU have been associated with increased mortality compared with ExoU-negative strains in retrospective studies of patients with *P. aeruginosa* ventilator-associated pneumonia. The host responds to infection by producing antibodies to *Pseudomonas* exotoxin A and endotoxin.

In addition to acute infection, *P. aeruginosa* is also capable of chronic persistence thought to be due in part to the formation of biofilms, organized communities of bacteria encased in an extracellular matrix that protects the organisms from the host immune response and the effects of antibiotics. Biofilm formation requires pilus-mediated attachment to a surface, proliferation of the organism, and production of exopolysaccharide as the main component of the extracellular matrix. A mature biofilm is resistant to many antimicrobials and difficult to eradicate with current therapies.

CLINICAL MANIFESTATIONS

Most clinical patterns (Table 197-1) are related to opportunistic infections (Chapter 171) or are associated with shunts and indwelling catheters (Chapter 172). *P. aeruginosa* may be introduced into a minor wound of a healthy person as a secondary invader, and cellulitis and a localized abscess that exudes green or blue pus may follow. The characteristic skin lesions of *Pseudomonas,* **ecthyma gangrenosum,** whether caused by direct inoculation or metastatic secondary to septicemia, begin as pink macules and progress to hemorrhagic nodules and eventually to ulcers with ecchymotic and gangrenous centers with eschar formation, surrounded by an intense red areola.

Outbreaks of dermatitis and urinary tract infections caused by *P. aeruginosa* have been reported in healthy persons after use of pools or hot tubs. Skin lesions of folliculitis develop several hours to 2 days after contact with these water sources. Skin lesions may be erythematous, macular, papular, or pustular. Illness may vary from a few scattered lesions to extensive truncal involvement. In some children, malaise, fever, vomiting, sore throat, conjunctivitis, rhinitis, and swollen breasts may be associated with dermal lesions.

Pseudomonads other than *P. aeruginosa* rarely cause disease in healthy children, but pneumonia and abscesses due to *Burkholderia cepacia,* otitis media due to *P. putrefaciens* or *P. stutzeri,* abscesses due to *P. fluorescens,* and cellulitis and septicemia and osteomyelitis due to *S. maltophilia* have been reported. Septicemia and endocarditis due to *S. maltophilia* have also been associated with abuse of intravenous drugs.

Burns and Wound Infection

The surfaces of burns or wounds are frequently populated by *Pseudomonas* and other gram-negative organisms; this initial colonization with a low number of adherent organisms is a necessary prerequisite to invasive disease. *P. aeruginosa* colonization of a burn site may develop into burn wound sepsis, which has a high mortality rate when the density of organisms reaches a critical concentration. Administration of antibiotics may diminish the susceptible microbiologic flora, permitting strains of relatively resistant *Pseudomonas* to flourish. Multiplication of organisms

Table 197-1 *PSEUDOMONAS AERUGINOSA* INFECTIONS

INFECTION	COMMON CLINICAL CHARACTERISTICS
Endocarditis	Native right-sided (tricuspid) valve disease with intravenous drug abuse
Pneumonia	Compromised local (lung) or systemic host defense mechanisms; nosocomial (respiratory), bacteremic (malignancy), or abnormal mucociliary clearance (cystic fibrosis) may be pathogenetic; cystic fibrosis is associated with mucoid *Pseudomonas aeruginosa* organisms producing capsular slime
Central nervous system infection	Meningitis, brain abscess; contiguous spread (mastoiditis, dermal sinus tracts, sinusitis); bacteremia or direct inoculation (trauma, surgery)
External otitis	Swimmer's ear; humid warm climates, swimming pool contamination
Malignant otitis externa	Invasive, indolent, febrile toxic, destructive necrotizing lesion in young infants, immunosuppressed neutropenic patients, or diabetic patients; associated with 7th nerve palsy and mastoiditis
Chronic mastoiditis	Ear drainage, swelling, erythema; perforated tympanic membrane
Keratitis	Corneal ulceration; contact lens keratitis
Endophthalmitis	Penetrating trauma, surgery, penetrating corneal ulceration; fulminant progression
Osteomyelitis/septic arthritis	Puncture wounds of foot and osteochondritis; intravenous drug abuse; fibrocartilaginous joints, sternum, vertebrae, pelvis; open fracture osteomyelitis; indolent pyelonephritis and vertebral osteomyelitis
Urinary tract infection	Iatrogenic, nosocomial; recurrent urinary tract infections in children, instrumented patients, and those with obstruction or stones
Intestinal tract infection	Immunocompromised, neutropenia, typhlitis, rectal abscess, ulceration, rarely diarrhea; peritonitis in peritoneal dialysis
Ecthyma gangrenosum	Metastatic dissemination; hemorrhage, necrosis, erythema, eschar, discrete lesions with bacterial invasion of blood vessels; also subcutaneous nodules, cellulitis, pustules, deep abscesses
Primary and secondary skin infections	Local infection; burns, trauma, decubitus ulcers, toe web infection, green nail (paronychia); whirlpool dermatitis; diffuse, pruritic, folliculitis, vesiculopustular or maculopapular, erythematous lesions

in devitalized tissues or associated with prolonged use of intravenous or urinary catheters increases the risk for septicemia with *P. aeruginosa*, a major problem in burned patients (Chapter 68).

Cystic Fibrosis
P. aeruginosa is common in children with cystic fibrosis, with a prevalence that increases with increasing age and severity of pulmonary disease (Chapter 395). Initial infection may be caused by nonmucoid strains of *P. aeruginosa*, but after a variable period of time, mucoid strains of *P. aeruginosa* that produce the antiphagocytic exopolysaccharide alginate, which are rarely encountered in other conditions predominate. Repeated isolation of mucoid *P. aeruginosa* from the sputum is associated with increased morbidity and mortality. The infection begins insidiously or even asymptomatically, and the progression has a highly variable pace. In children with cystic fibrosis, antibody does not eradicate the organism and antibiotics are only partially effective; thus, after infection becomes chronic it cannot be completely eradicated. Repeated courses of antibiotics select for *P. aeruginosa* strains that are highly antibiotic resistant.

Immunocompromised Persons
Children with leukemia or other debilitating malignancies, particularly those who are receiving immunosuppressive therapy and who are neutropenic, are extremely susceptible to septicemia due to invasion of the bloodstream by *Pseudomonas* that is colonizing the respiratory or gastrointestinal tract. Signs of sepsis are often accompanied by a generalized vasculitis, and hemorrhagic necrotic lesions may be found in all organs, including the skin (ecthyma gangrenosum). Hemorrhagic or gangrenous perirectal cellulitis or abscesses may occur, associated with ileus and profound hypotension.

Nosocomial Pneumonia
Although not a frequent cause of community-acquired pneumonia in children, *P. aeruginosa* is an increasingly important cause of community-acquired pneumonia in adults and of nosocomial pneumonia, especially ventilator-associated pneumonia, in patients of all ages. *P. aeruginosa* has historically been found to contaminate ventilators, tubing, and humidifiers. Such contamination is uncommon because of disinfection practices and routine changing of equipment. Nevertheless, colonization of the upper respiratory tract and the gastrointestinal tract may be followed by aspiration of *P. aeruginosa*-contaminated secretions, resulting in severe pneumonia. Prior use of broad-spectrum antibiotics is a risk factor for colonization with antibiotic-resistant strains of *P. aeruginosa*. One of the most challenging situations is distinguishing between colonization and pneumonia in intubated patients. This distinction can often only be resolved by using invasive culture techniques such as bronchoscopy with bronchial brushing or quantitative bronchoalveolar lavage.

Infants
P. aeruginosa is an occasional cause of nosocomial bacteremia in newborns and accounts for 2-5% of positive blood culture results in neonatal intensive care units. A frequent focus preceding bacteremia is **conjunctivitis.** Older infants may occasionally present with community-acquired sepsis due to *P. aeruginosa*, but this circumstance is uncommon. In the few reports describing community-acquired sepsis, preceding conditions included ecthyma-like skin lesions, virus-associated transient neutropenia, and prolonged contact with contaminated bath water or a hot tub.

DIAGNOSIS

P. aeruginosa infection is rarely clinically distinctive. Diagnosis depends on recovery of the organism from the blood, cerebrospinal fluid, urine, or needle aspirate of the lung, or from purulent material obtained by aspiration of subcutaneous abscesses or areas of cellulitis. Rarely, skin lesions that resemble *P. aeruginosa* infection may follow septicemia due to *Aeromonas hydrophila*, other gram-negative bacilli, and *Aspergillus*. When *P. aeruginosa* is recovered from nonsterile sites such as skin, mucous membranes, voided urine, and the upper respiratory tract, quantitative cultures are useful to differentiate colonization from invasive infection. In general, ≥100,000 colony forming units/mL of fluid or gram of tissue is evidence suggestive of invasive infection.

TREATMENT

Systemic infections with *Pseudomonas* should be treated promptly with an antibiotic to which the organism is susceptible in vitro. Response to treatment may be limited, and prolonged treatment may be necessary for systemic infection in immunocompromised hosts.

Septicemia and other aggressive infections should be treated with either 1 or 2 bactericidal agents. While the number of agents required is controversial, little evidence shows that more than 1 agent is needed for individuals with normal immunity or when treating urinary tract infections, but *dual therapy* is often used for a synergistic effect in immunocompromised patients or when the susceptibility of the organism is in doubt. Whether the use of 2 agents delays the development of resistance is also controversial, with evidence both for and against. Appropriate antibiotics for single-agent therapy include ceftazidime, cefepime, ticarcillin-clavulanate, and piperacillin-tazobactam. Gentamicin or another aminoglycoside may be used concomitantly for synergistic effect.

Ceftazidime has proved to be extremely effective in patients with cystic fibrosis (150-250 mg/kg/day divided every 6-8 hr IV to a maximum of 6 g/day). Piperacillin or piperacillin-tazobactam (300-450 mg/kg/day divided every 6-8 hr IV to a maximum of 12 g/day) also has proved to be effective therapy for susceptible strains of *P. aeruginosa* when combined with an aminoglycoside. Additional effective antibiotics include imipenem-cilastatin, meropenem, and aztreonam. Ciprofloxacin is effective but is not approved in the USA for persons <18 yr of age except for oral treatment of urinary tract infections or when there are not other agents to which the organism is susceptible. It is important to base continued treatment on the results of susceptibility tests because antibiotic resistance of *P. aeruginosa* to 1 or more antibiotics is increasing.

P. aeruginosa displays intrinsic and acquired resistance to antibiotics. It has many mechanisms for resistance to multiple classes of antibiotics including but not limited to genetic mutation, production of β-lactamases, and drug efflux pumps. Critical care units throughout the USA have documented a rising rate of resistance of *P. aeruginosa* to all of the major classes of antibiotics.

Meningitis can occur from spread from a contiguous focus, as a secondary focus when there is bacteremia, or after invasive procedures. *Pseudomonas* meningitis is best treated with ceftazidime in combination with an aminoglycoside such as gentamicin, both given intravenously. Concomitant intraventricular or intrathecal treatment with gentamicin may be required when intravenous therapy fails but is not recommended for routine use.

SUPPORTIVE CARE

Pseudomonas infections vary in severity from superficial to intense septic presentations. With severe infections there is often multisystem involvement and systemic inflammatory response. Supportive care is similar to severe sepsis caused by other gram-negative bacilli and requires support of blood pressure, oxygenation, and appropriate fluid management.

PROGNOSIS

The prognosis is dependent primarily on the nature of the underlying factors that predisposed the patient to *Pseudomonas* infection. In severely immunocompromised patients, the prognosis for patients with *P. aeruginosa* sepsis is poor unless susceptibility factors such as neutropenia or hypogammaglobulinemia can be reversed. Resistance of the organism to 1st line antibiotics also decreases the chance of survival. The outcome may be improved by combined antimicrobial therapy and is improved when there is a urinary tract portal of entry, absence of neutropenia or recovery from neutropenia, and drainage of local sites of infection. *Pseudomonas* is recovered from the lungs of most children who die of cystic fibrosis and adds to the slow deterioration of these patients. The prognosis for normal development is poor in the few infants who survive *Pseudomonas* meningitis.

PREVENTION

Prevention of infections is dependent on limiting contamination of the health care environment and preventing transmission to patients. Effective hospital infection control programs are necessary to identify and eradicate sources of the organism as quickly as possible. In hospitals, infection can be transmitted to children by the hands of personnel, from washbasin surfaces, from catheters, and from solutions used to rinse suction catheters.

Strict attention to hand hygiene, before and between contacts with patients may prevent or interdict epidemic disease. Meticulous care and sterile procedures in suctioning of endotracheal tubes, insertion and maintenance of indwelling catheters, and removal of catheters as soon as medically reasonable greatly reduce the hazard of extrinsic contamination by *Pseudomonas* and other gram-negative organisms.

Prevention of follicular dermatitis caused by *Pseudomonas* contamination of whirlpools or hot tubs is possible by maintaining pool water at a pH of 7.2-7.8.

Infections in burned patients may be minimized by protective isolation, debridement of devitalized tissue, and topical applications of bactericidal cream. Administration of intravenous immunoglobulin may be used. Approaches under investigation to prevent infection include development of a *Pseudomonas* vaccine and development of hyperimmune globulin against *Pseudomonas*. No vaccine is currently licensed in the USA.

Pseudomonas infection of dermal sinuses communicating with the cerebrospinal space can be prevented by early identification and surgical repair. *Pseudomonas* infection of the urinary tract is often associated with the presence of an indwelling catheter. Urinary tract infections may be minimized or prevented by prompt removal of the catheter and by early identification and corrective surgery of obstructive lesions when present.

BIBLIOGRAPHY

Please visit the Nelson Textbook of Pediatrics *website at www.expertconsult.com for the complete bibliography.*

197.2 *Burkholderia*

Thomas S. Murray and Robert S. Baltimore

BURKHOLDERIA CEPACIA

Burkholderia cepacia is a filamentous gram-negative rod. It is ubiquitous in the environment but may be difficult to isolate from respiratory specimens in the laboratory, requiring an enriched, selective media oxidation fermentation base supplemented with polymyxin B–bacitracin-lactose agar (OFPBL) and as long as 3 days of incubation.

For the full continuation of this chapter, please visit the Nelson Textbook of Pediatrics *website at www.expertconsult.com.*

197.3 *Stenotrophomonas*

Thomas S. Murray and Robert S. Baltimore

Stenotrophomonas maltophilia (formerly *Xanthomonas maltophilia* or *Pseudomonas maltophilia*) is a short to medium-sized straight gram-negative bacillus. It is ubiquitous in nature and can be found in the hospital environment, especially in tap water, standing water, and nebulizers. Strains isolated in the laboratory may be contaminants, may be a commensal from the colonized surface of a patient, or may represent an invasive pathogen. The species is an opportunist and is frequently recovered from patients with cystic fibrosis after multiple courses of antimicrobial therapy. Serious infections usually occur among those requiring intensive care, including neonatal intensive care, typically patients with ventilator-associated pneumonia or catheter-associated infections. Prolonged antibiotic exposure appears to be a frequent factor in nosocomial *S. maltophilia* infections, probably due to its endogenous antibiotic resistance pattern. Common types of infection include pneumonia following airway colonization and aspiration, urinary tract infection, endocarditis, and osteomyelitis. Strains vary as to antibiotic susceptibility.

For the full continuation of this chapter, please visit the Nelson Textbook of Pediatrics *website at www.expertconsult.com.*

Chapter 198
Tularemia *(Francisella tularensis)*

Gordon E. Schutze and Richard F. Jacobs

Tularemia is a zoonotic infection caused by the gram-negative bacterium *Francisella tularensis*. Tularemia is primarily a disease of wild animals; human disease is incidental and usually results from contact with blood-sucking insects or live or dead wild animals. The illness caused by *F. tularensis* is manifested by different clinical syndromes, the most common of which consists of an ulcerative lesion at the site of inoculation with regional lymphadenopathy or lymphadenitis. It is also a potential agent of bioterrorism (Chapter 704).

ETIOLOGY

F. tularensis, the causative agent of tularemia, is a small, nonmotile, pleomorphic, gram-negative coccobacillus that can be classified into 4 main subspecies (*F. tularensis tularensis* [type A], *F. tularensis holarctica* [type B], *F. tularensis mediasiatica*, and *F. tularensis novicida*). Type A can be further subdivided into 4 distinct genotypes (A1a, A1b, A2a, A2b) with A1b appearing to produce more serious disease in humans. Type A is found exclusively in North America and is associated with wild rabbits, ticks, and tabanid flies (e.g., deer flies), whereas type B may be found in North America, Europe, and Asia and is associated with semiaquatic rodents, hares, mosquitoes, ticks, tabanid flies, water (e.g., ponds, rivers), and marine animals. Human infections with type B are usually milder and have lower mortality rates compared to infections with type A.

EPIDEMIOLOGY

During 1990-2000, a total of 1,368 cases of tularemia were reported in the USA from 44 states, averaging 124 cases (range 86-193) per year (Fig. 198-1). Four states accounted for 56% of all reported tularemia cases: Arkansas, 315 cases (23%); Missouri, 265 cases (19%); South Dakota, 96 cases (7%); and Oklahoma, 90 cases (7%).

Transmission

Of all the zoonotic diseases, tularemia is unusual because of the different modes of transmission of disease. A large number of animals serve as a reservoir for this organism, which can penetrate both intact skin and mucous membranes. Transmission can occur through the bite of infected ticks or other biting insects, by contact with infected animals or their carcasses, by consumption of contaminated foods or water, or through inhalation, as might occur in a laboratory setting. This organism is not, however, transmitted from person to person. In the USA, rabbits and ticks are the principal reservoirs. Most disease due to rabbit exposure occurs in the winter, and disease due to tick exposure occurs in the warmer months (April-September). *Amblyomma americanum* (Lone Star tick), *Dermacentor variabilis* (dog tick), and *Dermacentor andersoni* (wood tick) are the most common tick vectors. These ticks usually feed on infected small rodents and later feed on humans. Taking that blood meal through a fecally contaminated field transmits the infection.

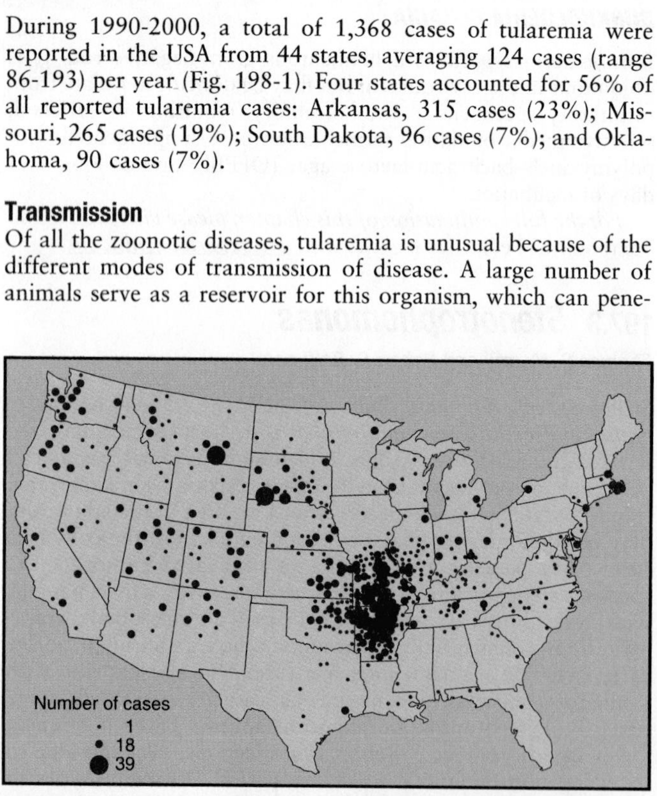

Figure 198-1 Reported cases of tularemia in the USA from 1990-2000, based on 1,347 patients reporting county of residence in the continental USA. Alaska reported 10 cases in 4 counties during 1990-2000. The circle size is proportional to the number of cases, ranging from 1 to 39 cases. (From the Centers for Disease Control and Prevention: Tularemia—United States, 1990-2000, *MMWR Morb Mortal Wkly Rep* 51:181–184, 2002.)

PATHOGENESIS

The most common portal of entry for human infection is through the skin or mucous membrane. This may occur through the bite of an infected insect or by way of unapparent abrasions. Inhalation or ingestion of *F. tularensis* can also result in infection. Usually $>10^8$ organisms are required to produce infection if they are ingested, but as few as 10 organisms may cause disease if they are inhaled or injected into the skin. Within 48-72 hr after injection into the skin, an erythematous, tender, or pruritic papule may appear at the portal of entry. This papule may enlarge and form an ulcer with a black base, followed by regional lymphadenopathy. Once *F. tularensis* reaches the lymph nodes, the organism may multiply and form granulomas. Bacteremia may also be present, and although any organ of the body may be involved, the reticuloendothelial system is the most commonly affected.

Conjunctival inoculation may result in infection of the eye with preauricular lymphadenopathy. Inhalation, aerosolization, or hematogenous spread of the organisms can result in pneumonia. Chest roentgenograms of such patients may reveal patchy infiltrates rather than areas of consolidation. Pleural effusions may also be present and may contain blood. In pulmonary infections, mediastinal adenopathy may be present; in oropharyngeal disease, patients may develop cervical lymphadenopathy. Typhoidal tularemia may be used to describe severe bacteremic disease, regardless of the mode of transmission or portal of entry.

Infection with tularemia stimulates the host to produce antibodies. This antibody response, however, has only a minor role in fighting this infection. The body is dependent on cell-mediated immunity to contain and eradicate this infection. Infection is usually followed by specific protection; thus, chronic infection or reinfection is unlikely.

CLINICAL MANIFESTATIONS

Although it may vary, the average incubation period from infection until clinical symptoms appear is 3 days (range, 1-21 days). A sudden onset of fever with other associated symptoms is common (Table 198-1). Physical examination may include lymph-

Table 198-1 COMMON CLINICAL MANIFESTATIONS OF TULAREMIA IN CHILDREN

SIGN OR SYMPTOM	FREQUENCY (%)
Lymphadenopathy	96
Fever (>38.3°C)	87
Ulcer/eschar/papule	45
Pharyngitis	43
Myalgias/arthralgias	39
Nausea/vomiting	35
Hepatosplenomegaly	35

Table 198-2 CLINICAL SYNDROMES OF TULAREMIA IN CHILDREN

CLINICAL SYNDROME	FREQUENCY (%)
Ulceroglandular	45
Glandular	25
Pneumonia	14
Oropharyngeal	4
Oculoglandular	2
Typhoidal	2
Other*	6

*Includes meningitis, pericarditis, hepatitis, peritonitis, endocarditis, and osteomyelitis.

adenopathy, hepatosplenomegaly, or skin lesions. Various skin lesions have been described, including erythema multiforme and erythema nodosum. Approximately 20% of patients may develop a generalized maculopapular rash that occasionally becomes pustular. These clinical manifestations of tularemia have been divided into various syndromes (Table 198-2).

Ulceroglandular and glandular disease are the 2 most common forms of tularemia diagnosed in children. The most common glands involved are usually the cervical or posterior auricular nodes owing to a tick bite on the head or neck. If an ulcer is present, it is erythematous and painful and may last from 1 to 3 wk. The ulcer is located at the portal of entry. After the ulcer develops, regional lymphadenopathy ensues. These nodes may vary in size from 0.5 to 10 cm and may appear singly or in clusters. These affected nodes may become fluctuant and drain spontaneously, but most usually resolve with treatment. Late suppuration of the involved nodes has been described in 25-30% of patients despite effective therapy. Examination of this material from such lymph nodes usually reveals sterile necrotic material.

Pneumonia caused by *F. tularensis* usually presents as variable parenchymal infiltrates that are unresponsive to β-lactam antimicrobial agents. Inhalation-related infection has been described in laboratory workers who are working with the organism; it results in a relatively high mortality rate. Aerosols from farming activities involving rodent contamination (haying, threshing) or animal carcass destruction with lawn mowers have been reported to cause pneumonia as well. Patchy parenchymal infiltrates can also be demonstrated in other forms of tularemia. Patchy segmental infiltrates, hilar adenopathy, and pleural effusions are the most common abnormalities demonstrated on chest roentgenograms. Patients may also complain of a nonproductive cough, dyspnea, or pleuritic chest pain.

Oropharyngeal tularemia results from consumption of poorly cooked meats or contaminated water. This syndrome is characterized by acute pharyngitis, with or without tonsillitis, and cervical lymphadenitis. Infected tonsils may become large and develop a yellowish-white membrane that may resemble the membranes associated with diphtheria. Gastrointestinal disease may also occur and usually presents with mild, unexplained diarrhea but may progress to rapidly fulminant and fatal disease.

Oculoglandular tularemia is uncommon, but when it does occur, the portal of entry is the conjunctiva. Contact with contaminated fingers or debris from crushed insects is the most common way of applying the organisms to the conjunctiva. The conjunctiva is painful and inflamed, with yellowish nodules and pinpoint ulcerations. Purulent conjunctivitis with ipsilateral preauricular or submandibular lymphadenopathy is referred to as **Parinaud oculoglandular syndrome.**

Typhoidal tularemia is usually associated with a large inoculum of organisms and usually presents with fever, headaches, and signs or symptoms of endotoxemia. Patients typically are critically ill, and symptoms mimic those with other forms of sepsis. Clinicians practicing in tularemia-endemic regions must always consider this diagnosis in critically ill children.

DIAGNOSIS

The history and physical examination of the patient may suggest the diagnosis of tularemia, especially if the patient lives in or has visited an endemic region. A history of animal or tick exposure may be especially helpful. Hematologic blood tests are nondiagnostic. Results of routine cultures and smears are positive in only approximately 10% of cases. *F. tularensis* can be cultured in the microbiology laboratory on cysteine–glucose–blood agar, but care should be taken to alert the personnel in the laboratory if this is attempted so that they can take the proper precautions to protect themselves from acquiring infection.

The diagnosis of tularemia is most commonly established through the use of a standard and highly reliable serum agglutination test. In the standard tube agglutination test, a single titer of ≥1:160 in a patient with a compatible history and physical findings can establish the diagnosis. A 4-fold increase in titer from paired serum samples collected 2-3 wk apart is also diagnostic. False-negative serologic responses can be obtained early in the infection, and as many as 30% of individuals require longer than 3 wk before testing positive. Once infected, patients may have a positive agglutination test result (1:20 to 1:80) that may persist for life.

Other testing techniques available include a microagglutination test, enzyme-linked immunosorbent assay, analysis of urine for tularemia antigen, and polymerase chain reaction. These techniques may become more popular in the future but at this time have a limited role in establishing the diagnosis of tularemia.

Differential Diagnosis

The differential diagnosis of ulceroglandular or glandular tularemia includes cat scratch disease *(Bartonella henselae);* infectious mononucleosis; Kawasaki syndrome; lymphadenopathy caused by *Staphylococcus aureus,* group A streptococcus, *Mycobacterium tuberculosis, Toxoplasma gondii,* nontuberculous mycobacteria, and *Sporothrix schenckii;* plague; anthrax; melioidosis; and rat-bite fever. Oculoglandular disease may also occur with other infectious agents, such as *B. henselae, Treponema pallidum, Coccidioides immitis,* herpes simplex virus, adenoviruses, and the bacterial agents responsible for purulent conjunctivitis. Oropharyngeal tularemia must be differentiated from the same diseases that cause ulceroglandular/glandular disease and from cytomegalovirus, herpes simplex, adenovirus, and other viral or bacterial etiologies. Pneumonic tularemia must be differentiated from the other non–β-lactam-responsive organisms such as *Mycoplasma, Chlamydia,* mycobacteria, fungi, and rickettsia. Typhoidal tularemia must be differentiated from other forms of sepsis as well as from enteric fever (typhoid and paratyphoid fever) and brucellosis.

TREATMENT

All strains of *F. tularensis* are susceptible to gentamicin and streptomycin. Gentamicin (5 mg/kg/day divided bid or tid IV or IM) is the drug of choice for the treatment of tularemia in children because of the limited availability of streptomycin (30-40 mg/kg/day divided bid IM) and the fewer adverse effects of gentamicin. Therapy is typically continued for 7-10 days, but in mild cases, 5-7 days may be sufficient. Chloramphenicol and tetracyclines have been used, but the high relapse rate has limited their use in children. Early data suggested that *F. tularensis* is susceptible to the 3rd generation cephalosporins (cefotaxime, ceftriaxone), but clinical case reports demonstrate a nearly universal failure rate with these agents. Quinolones are active against *F. tularensis* and have been used for treatment of disease due to the type B subspecies *holarctica.* Further data are required before quinolone therapy can be routinely recommended for human disease caused by the type A subspecies *tularensis* encountered in North America.

Patients typically have defervescence within 24-48 hr after starting therapy, and relapses are uncommon if gentamicin or streptomycin is used. Patients who have not started on appropriate therapy early may respond more slowly to antimicrobial therapy. Late suppuration of involved lymph nodes may occur despite adequate therapy but usually contain sterile material.

PROGNOSIS

Poor outcomes are associated with a delay in recognition and treatment, but with rapid recognition and treatment, fatalities are exceedingly rare. The mortality rate for severe untreated disease (e.g., pneumonia, typhoidal disease) can be as high as 30% in these situations, but in general, the overall mortality rate is <1%.

PREVENTION

Prevention of tularemia is based on avoiding exposure. Children living in tick-endemic regions should be taught to avoid tick-infested areas, and families should have a tick control plan for their immediate environment and for their pets. Protective clothing should be worn when entering a tick-infested area, but more importantly, children should undergo frequent tick checks during and after their time in these areas. Skin repellents such as *N,N*-diethyl-3-methylbenzamide (DEET) can be used safely in infants and children to 2 mo of age. Avoiding taking young infants into tick-endemic regions is the most prudent approach. If DEET-containing compounds are used, they should be used sparingly on the exposed skin, avoiding the hands and face on children <1 yr of age. The repellent should be washed off completely after leaving the high-risk region. Clothing repellents that use permethrin have been demonstrated to be an effective addition to the use of protective clothing. If ticks are found on the child, forceps should be used to pull the tick straight out. The skin should be cleansed before and after this procedure.

Children should also be taught to avoid sick and dead animals. Dogs and cats are most likely to bring these animals to a child's attention. Children should be encouraged to wear gloves while cleaning wild game. A vaccine is available for adults with high-risk vocations (e.g., veterinarians), but there are no recommendations for use in children. Prophylactic antimicrobial agents are not effective in preventing tularemia and should not be used after exposure.

BIBLIOGRAPHY

Please visit the Nelson Textbook of Pediatrics *website at www.expertconsult.com for the complete bibliography.*

Chapter 199
Brucella

Gordon E. Schutze and Richard F. Jacobs

Human brucellosis, caused by organisms of the genus *Brucella*, continues to be a major public health problem worldwide. Humans are accidental hosts and acquire this zoonotic disease from direct contact with an infected animal or consumption of products of an infected animal. Although brucellosis is widely recognized as an occupational risk among adults working with livestock, much of the brucellosis in children is food-borne and is associated with consumption of unpasteurized milk products. It is also a potential agent of bioterrorism (Chapter 704).

ETIOLOGY

Brucella abortus (cattle), *B. melitensis* (goat/sheep), *B. suis* (swine), and *B. canis* (dog) are the most common organisms responsible for human disease. These organisms are small, aerobic, non–spore-forming, nonmotile, gram-negative coccobacillary bacteria that are fastidious in their growth but can be grown on various laboratory media including blood and chocolate agars.

EPIDEMIOLOGY

Because of improved sanitation, brucellosis has become rare in industrialized countries. Brucellosis exists worldwide and is especially prevalent in the Mediterranean basin, Arabian Gulf, Indian subcontinent, and parts of Mexico and Central and South America. In industrialized countries, recreational or occupational exposure to infected animals is a major risk factor for the development of disease. In the USA, 50% of cases occur in California and Texas. Among children, geographic locations that are endemic for *B. melitensis* remain areas of increased risk for the development of infection. In such locations, unpasteurized milk from goats or camels may be used to feed children, thus leading to the development of brucellosis. A history of travel to endemic regions or consumption of exotic food or unpasteurized dairy or dairy products may be an important clue to the diagnosis of human brucellosis.

PATHOGENESIS

Routes of infection for these organisms include inoculation through cuts or abrasions in the skin, inoculation of the conjunctival sac of the eye, inhalation of infectious aerosols, or ingestion of contaminated meat or dairy products. The risk for infection depends on the nutritional and immune status of the host, the route of inoculum, and the species of *Brucella*. For reasons that remain unclear, *B. melitensis* and *B. suis* tend to be more virulent than *B. abortus* or *B. canis*.

The major virulence factor for *Brucella* appears to be its cell wall lipopolysaccharide. Strains containing smooth lipopolysaccharide have been demonstrated to have greater virulence and are more resistant to killing by polymorphonuclear leukocytes. These organisms are facultative intracellular pathogens that can survive and replicate within the mononuclear phagocytic cells (monocytes, macrophages) of the reticuloendothelial system. Even though *Brucella* are chemotactic for entry of leukocytes into the body, the leukocytes are less efficient at killing these organisms than other bacteria despite the assistance of serum factors such as complement.

Organisms that are not phagocytosed by the leukocytes are ingested by the macrophages and become localized within the reticuloendothelial system. Specifically, they reside within the liver, spleen, lymph nodes, and bone marrow and result in **granuloma** formation. Antibodies are produced against the lipopolysaccharide and other cell wall antigens. This provides a means of diagnosis and probably has a role in long-term immunity. The major factor in recovery from infection appears to be development of a cell-mediated response resulting in macrophage activation and enhanced intracellular killing. Specifically, sensitized T lymphocytes release cytokines (e.g., interferon-γ and tumor necrosis factor-α), which activate the macrophages and enhance their intracellular killing capacity.

CLINICAL MANIFESTATIONS

Brucellosis is a systemic illness that can be very difficult to diagnose in children without a history of animal or food exposure. Symptoms can be acute or insidious in nature and are usually nonspecific, beginning 2-4 wk after inoculation. Although the clinical manifestations do vary, the classic triad of fever, arthralgia/arthritis, and hepatosplenomegaly can be demonstrated in most patients. Some present as a fever of unknown origin. Other associated symptoms include abdominal pain, headache, diarrhea, rash, night sweats, weakness/fatigue, vomiting, cough, and pharyngitis. A common constellation of symptoms in children is refusal to eat, lassitude, refusal to bear weight, and failure to thrive. Besides hepatosplenomegaly, the physical findings on examination are usually few, with the exception of arthritis. The fever pattern can vary widely, and virtually any organ or tissue can be involved.

If abnormalities are demonstrated on physical examination, monoarticular arthritis of the knees and hips in children and of the sacroiliac joint in adolescents and adults can be found. Although headache, mental inattention, and depression may be demonstrated in patients with brucellosis, invasion of the nervous system occurs in only about 1% of cases. Neonatal and congenital infections with these organisms have also been described. These have been transmitted transplacentally, from breast milk, and through blood transfusions. The signs and symptoms associated with brucellosis are vague and not pathognomonic.

DIAGNOSIS

Routine laboratory examinations of the blood are not helpful; thrombocytopenia, neutropenia, anemia, or pancytopenia may occur. A history of exposure to animals or ingestion of unpasteurized dairy products may be more helpful. A definitive diagnosis is established by recovering the organisms in the blood, bone marrow, or other tissues. Although automated culture systems and the use of the lysis-centrifugation method have shortened the isolation time from weeks to days, it is prudent to alert the clinical microbiology laboratory that brucellosis is suspected. Isolation of the organism still may require as long as 4 wk from a blood culture sample unless the laboratory is using an automated culture system such as the lysis centrifugation method where the organism can be recovered in <5 days. Bone marrow cultures may be superior to blood cultures when evaluating patients with previous antimicrobial therapy. Caution is advised when using automated bacterial identification systems, because isolates have been misidentified as other gram-negative organisms (*Haemophilus influenzae* type b).

In the absence of positive culture results, various serologic tests have been applied to the diagnosis of brucellosis. The serum agglutination test (SAT) is the most widely used and detects antibodies against *B. abortus, B. melitensis,* and *B. suis.* This method does not detect antibodies against *B. canis* because this organism lacks the smooth lipopolysaccharide. No single titer is ever diagnostic, but most patients with acute infections have titers of ≥1:160. Low titers may be found early in the course of the illness, requiring the use of acute and convalescent sera testing to confirm the diagnosis. Because patients with active infection have both an immunoglobulin M (IgM) and an IgG response and the SAT measures the total quantity of agglutinating antibodies, the total quantity of IgG is measured by treatment of the serum with 2-mercaptoethanol. This fractionation is important in determining the significance of the antibody titer because low levels of IgM can remain in the serum for weeks to months after the infection has been treated. It is important to remember that all titers must be interpreted in light of a patient's history and physical examination. False-positive results due to cross-reacting antibodies to other gram-negative organisms such as *Yersinia enterocolitica, Francisella tularensis,* and *Vibrio cholerae* can occur. In addition, the prozone effect can give false-negative results in the presence of high titers of antibody. To avoid this issue, serum that is being tested should be diluted to ≥1:320.

Among newer tests, the enzyme immunoassay appears to be the most sensitive method for detecting *Brucella* antibodies but less specific as compared to agglutination tests. Polymerase chain reaction assays are also becoming available but at this time are mostly limited to research facilities but could be particularly useful in patients with complications (e.g., neurobrucellosis) where serologic testing often fails.

Differential Diagnosis

Brucellosis may be confused with other infections such as tularemia, cat scratch disease, typhoid fever, and fungal infections due to histoplasmosis, blastomycosis, or coccidioidomycosis. Infections caused by *Mycobacterium tuberculosis,* atypical mycobacteria, rickettsiae, and *Yersinia* can present in a similar fashion to brucellosis.

TREATMENT

Many antimicrobial agents are active in vitro against the *Brucella* species, but the clinical effectiveness does not always correlate with these results. Doxycycline is the most useful antimicrobial agent and, when combined with an aminoglycoside, is associated with the fewest relapses (Table 199-1). Treatment failures with β-lactam antimicrobial agents, including the 3rd generation cephalosporins, may be due to the intracellular nature of the organism. Agents that provide intracellular killing are required for eradication of this

Table 199-1 RECOMMENDED THERAPY FOR THE TREATMENT OF BRUCELLOSIS

AGE AND CONDITION	ANTIMICROBIAL AGENT	DOSE	ROUTE	DURATION
≥8 yr	Doxycycline	2-4 mg/kg/day; maximum 200 mg/day	PO	6 wk
	+			
	Rifampin	15-20 mg/kg/day; maximum 600-900 mg/day	PO	6 wk
	Alternative:			
	Doxycycline	2-4 mg/kg/day; maximum 200 mg/day	PO	6 wk
	+			
	Streptomycin	15-30 mg/kg/day; maximum 1 g/day	IM	2 wk
	or			
	Gentamicin	3-5 mg/kg/day	IM/IV	2 wk
<8 yr	Trimethoprim-sulfamethoxazole (TMP-SMZ)	TMP (10 mg/kg/day; maximum 480 mg/day) and SMZ (50 mg/kg/day; maximum 2.4 g/day)	PO	4-8 wk
	+			
	Rifampin	15-20 mg/kg/day	PO	6 wk
Meningitis, osteomyelitis, endocarditis				
	Doxycycline	2-4 mg/kg/day; maximum 200 mg/day	PO	4-6 mo
	+			
	Gentamicin	3-5 mg/kg/day	IV	2 wk
	±			
	Rifampin	15-20 mg/kg/day; maximum 600-900 mg/day	PO	4-6 mo

infection. Similarly, it is apparent that prolonged treatment is the key to preventing disease relapse. Relapse is confirmed by isolation of *Brucella* within weeks to months after therapy has ended and is usually not associated with antimicrobial resistance.

The onset of initial antimicrobial therapy may precipitate a Jarisch-Herxheimer–like reaction, presumably due to a large antigen load. It is rarely severe enough to require corticosteroid therapy.

PROGNOSIS

Before the use of antimicrobial agents, the course of brucellosis was often prolonged and may have led to death. Since the institution of specific therapy, most deaths are due to specific organ system involvement (e.g., endocarditis) in complicated cases. The prognosis after specific therapy is excellent if patients are compliant with the prolonged therapy (see Table 199-1).

PREVENTION

Prevention of brucellosis is dependent on effective eradication of the organism from cattle, goats, and swineherds as well as from other animals. Pasteurization of milk and dairy products for human consumption remains an important aspect of prevention. No vaccine currently exists for use in children and, therefore, education of the public continues to have a prominent role in prevention of this disease.

BIBLIOGRAPHY

Please visit the Nelson Textbook of Pediatrics *website at www.expertconsult.com for the complete bibliography.*

Chapter 200
Legionella

Lucy S. Tompkins

Legionellosis comprises **Legionnaires disease** (*Legionella* pneumonia), other invasive extrapulmonary *Legionella* infections, and an acute flulike illness known as **Pontiac fever.** In contrast to the syndromes associated with invasive disease, Pontiac fever is a self-limiting illness that develops after aerosol exposure and may represent a toxic or hypersensitivity response to *Legionella*.

For the full continuation of this chapter, please visit the Nelson Textbook of Pediatrics *website at www.expertconsult.com.*

Chapter 201
Bartonella

Barbara W. Stechenberg

The spectrum of disease resulting from human infection with *Bartonella* species includes the association of bacillary angiomatosis and cat-scratch disease (CSD) with *Bartonella henselae*. Six major *Bartonella* species are pathogenic for humans: *B. henselae, Bartonella quintana, Bartonella bacilliformis, Bartonella elizabethae, Bartonella vinsonii,* and *Bartonella clarridgeiae* (Table 201-1). Several other *Bartonella* species have been found in animals, particularly rodents and moles.

Members of the genus *Bartonella* are gram-negative, oxidase-negative, fastidious aerobic rods that ferment no carbohydrates. *B. bacilliformis* is the only species that is motile, achieving motility by means of polar flagella. Optimal growth is obtained on fresh media containing 5% or more sheep or horse blood in the presence of 5% carbon dioxide. The use of lysis centrifugation for specimens from blood on chocolate agar for extended periods (2-6 wk) enhances recovery.

BIBLIOGRAPHY

Please visit the Nelson Textbook of Pediatrics *website at www.expertconsult.com for the complete bibliography.*

201.1 Bartonellosis *(Bartonella bacilliformis)*

Barbara W. Stechenberg

The 1st human *Bartonella* infection described was bartonellosis, a geographically distinct disease caused by *B. bacilliformis*. There are 2 predominant forms of illness due to *B. bacilliformis*: **Oroya fever,** a severe, febrile hemolytic anemia, and **verruca peruana** (verruga peruana), an eruption of hemangioma-like lesions. *B. bacilliformis* also causes asymptomatic infection. Bartonellosis is also called **Carrión disease** in honor of the Peruvian medical student who inoculated himself with blood from a verruca and 21 days later had Oroya fever. He died 39 days after the inoculation, thus proving the unitary etiology of the 2 clinical illnesses.

ETIOLOGY

B. bacilliformis is a small, motile, gram-negative organism with a brush of 10 or more unipolar flagella, which appear to be important components for invasiveness. An obligate aerobe, it grows best at 28°C in semisolid nutrient agar containing rabbit serum and hemoglobin.

EPIDEMIOLOGY

Bartonellosis is a zoonosis found only in mountain valleys of the Andes Mountains in Peru, Ecuador, Colombia, Chile, and Bolivia at altitudes and environmental conditions favorable for the vector, which is the sandfly, *Lutzomyia verrucarum*.

PATHOGENESIS

After the sandfly bite, *Bartonella* organisms enter the endothelial cells of blood vessels, where they proliferate. Found throughout the reticuloendothelial system, they then re-enter the bloodstream and parasitize erythrocytes. They bind on the cells, deform the membranes, and then enter intracellular vacuoles. The resultant **hemolytic anemia** may involve as many as 90% of circulating erythrocytes. Patients who survive this acute phase may or may not experience the cutaneous manifestations, which are nodular hemangiomatous lesions or verrucae ranging in size from a few millimeters to several centimeters.

CLINICAL MANIFESTATIONS

The incubation period is 2-14 wk. Patients may be totally asymptomatic or may have nonspecific symptoms such as headache and malaise without anemia.

Oroya fever is characterized by fever with rapid development of anemia. Clouding of the sensorium and delirium are common symptoms and may progress to overt psychosis. Physical examination demonstrates signs of severe hemolytic anemia, including icterus and pallor, sometimes in association with generalized lymphadenopathy.

In the pre-eruptive stage of **verruca peruana** (Fig. 201-1), patients may complain of arthralgias, myalgias, and paresthesias. Inflammatory reactions such as phlebitis, pleuritis, erythema nodosum, and encephalitis may develop. The appearance of verrucae is pathognomonic of the eruptive phase. Lesions vary greatly in size and number.

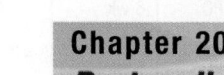

Table 201-1 *BARTONELLA* SPECIES CAUSING HUMAN DISEASE

DISEASE	ORGANISM	VECTOR	PRIMARY RISK FACTOR
Bartonellosis	*B. bacilliformis*	Sandfly (*Lutzomyia verrucarum*)	Living in endemic areas (Andes Mountains)
Cat-scratch disease	*B. henselae*	Cat	Cat scratch or bite
	B. clarridgeiae (1 case)		
Trench fever	*B. quintana*	Human body louse	Body louse infestation during outbreak
Bacteremia, endocarditis	*B. henselae* *B. quintana*	Cat for *B. henselae* Human body louse for *B. quintana*	Severe immunosuppression
	B. elizabethae, B. vinsonii		
Bacillary angiomatosis	*B. henselae*	Cat for *B. henselae*	Severe immunosuppression
	B. quintana	Human body louse for *B. quintana*	
Peliosis hepatis	*B. henselae*	Cat for *B. henselae*	Severe immunosuppression
	B. quintana	Human body louse for *B. quintana*	

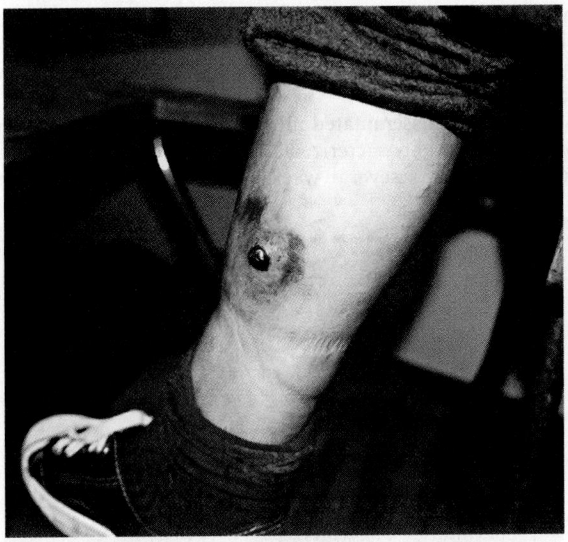

Figure 201-1 A single large lesion of verruca peruana on the leg of an inhabitant of the Peruvian Andes. Such lesions are prone to superficial ulceration, and their vascular nature may lead to copious bleeding. Ecchymosis of the skin surrounding the lesion is also evident. (Courtesy of Dr. J.M. Crutcher, Oklahoma State Department of Health, Oklahoma City.)

DIAGNOSIS

The diagnosis is established on clinical grounds in conjunction with a blood smear demonstrating organisms or with blood culture. The anemia is macrocytic and hypochromic, with reticulocyte counts as high as 50%. *B. bacilliformis* may be seen on Giemsa stain preparation as red-violet rods in the erythrocytes. In the recovery phase, organisms change to a more coccoid form and disappear from the blood. In the absence of anemia, the diagnosis depends on blood cultures. In the eruptive phase, the typical verruca confirms the diagnosis. Antibody testing has been used to document infection.

TREATMENT

B. bacilliformis is sensitive to many antibiotics, including rifampin, tetracycline, and chloramphenicol. Treatment is very effective in rapidly diminishing fever and eradicating the organism from the blood. Chloramphenicol (50-75 mg/kg/day) has been considered the drug of choice, because it is also useful in the treatment of concomitant infections such as *Salmonella*. Fluoroquinolones have been used successfully as well. Blood transfusions and supportive care are critical in patients with severe anemia. Antimicrobial treatment for verruca peruana is considered when there are >10 cutaneous lesions, if the lesions are erythematous or violaceous, or if the onset of the lesions was <1 mo before presentation. Oral rifampin is effective in the healing of lesions. Surgical excision may be needed for lesions that are large and disfiguring or that interfere with function.

PREVENTION

Prevention depends on avoidance of the vector, particularly at night, by the use of protective clothing and insect repellents (Chapter 168).

BIBLIOGRAPHY

Please visit the Nelson Textbook of Pediatrics *website at* *www.expertconsult.com* *for the complete bibliography.*

201.2 Cat-Scratch Disease (*Bartonella henselae*)

Barbara W. Stechenberg

The most common presentation of *Bartonella* infection is CSD, which is a subacute, regional lymphadenitis caused by *B. henselae*. It is the most common cause of chronic lymphadenitis that persists for >3 wk.

ETIOLOGY

B. henselae can be cultured from the blood of healthy cats. *B. henselae* organisms are the small pleomorphic gram-negative bacilli visualized with Warthin-Starry stain in affected lymph nodes from patients with CSD. Development of serologic tests that showed prevalence of antibodies in 84-100% of cases of CSD, culturing of *B. henselae* from CSD nodes, and detection of *B. henselae* by polymerase chain reaction (PCR) in the majority of lymph node samples and pus from patients with CSD confirmed the organism as the cause of CSD. Occasional cases of CSD may be caused by other organisms; 1 report described a veterinarian with CSD caused by *B. clarridgeiae*.

EPIDEMIOLOGY

CSD is common, with more than 24,000 estimated cases per year in the USA. It is transmitted by cutaneous inoculation. Most (87-99%) patients have had contact with cats, many of which are kittens <6 mo of age, and >50% have a definite history of a cat scratch or bite. Cats have high-level *Bartonella* bacteremia for months without any clinical symptoms; kittens are more frequently bacteremic than adult cats. Transmission between cats occurs via the cat flea, *Ctenocephalides felis*. In temperate zones, the majority of cases occur between September and March, perhaps in relation to the seasonal breeding of domestic cats or to the close proximity of family pets in the fall and winter. In tropical zones, there is no seasonal prevalence. Distribution is worldwide, and infection occurs in all races.

Cat scratches appear to be more common among children, and boys are affected more often than girls. CSD is a sporadic illness; usually only 1 family member is affected, even though many siblings play with the same kitten. However, clusters do occur, with family cases within weeks of one another. Anecdotal reports have implicated other sources, such as dog scratches, wood splinters, fishhooks, cactus spines, and porcupine quills.

PATHOGENESIS

The pathologic findings in the primary inoculation **papule** and affected lymph nodes are similar. Both show a central avascular necrotic area with surrounding lymphocytes, giant cells, and histiocytes. Three stages of involvement occur in affected nodes, sometimes simultaneously in the same node. The first stage consists of generalized enlargement with thickening of the cortex and hypertrophy of the germinal center and with a predominance of lymphocytes. Epithelioid granulomas with Langhans giant cells are scattered throughout the node. The middle stage is characterized by granulomas that increase in density, fuse, and become infiltrated with polymorphonuclear leukocytes, with beginning central necrosis. In the final stage, necrosis progresses with formation of large pus-filled sinuses. This purulent material may rupture into surrounding tissue. Similar granulomas have been found in the liver, spleen, and osteolytic lesions of bone when those organs are involved.

CLINICAL MANIFESTATIONS

After an incubation period of 7-12 days (range 3-30 days), 1 or more 3- to 5-mm red papules develop at the site of cutaneous inoculation, often reflecting a linear cat scratch. These lesions are often overlooked because of their small size but are found in at least 65% of patients when careful examination is performed (Fig. 201-2). Lymphadenopathy is generally evident within a period of 1-4 wk (Fig. 201-3). Chronic regional lymphadenitis is the hallmark, affecting the 1st or 2nd set of nodes draining the entry site. Affected lymph nodes in order of frequency include the axillary, cervical, submandibular, preauricular, epitrochlear, femoral, and inguinal nodes. Involvement of more than 1 group of nodes occurs in 10-20% of patients, although at a given site, half the cases involve several nodes.

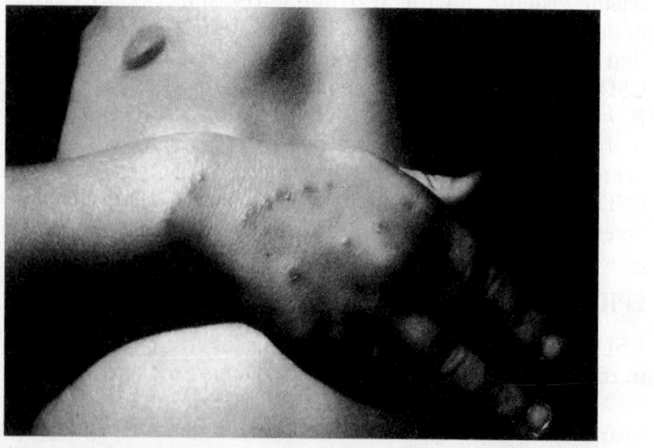

Figure 201-2 A child with typical cat-scratch disease demonstrating the original scratch injuries and the primary papule that soon thereafter developed proximal to the middle finger. (Courtesy of Dr. V.H. San Joaquin, University of Oklahoma Health Sciences Center, Oklahoma City.)

Nodes involved are usually tender and have overlying erythema but without cellulitis. They usually range between 1 and 5 cm in size, although they can become much larger. Between 10% and 40% eventually suppurate. The duration of enlargement is usually 1-2 mo, with persistence up to 1 yr in rare cases. Fever occurs in about 30% of patients, usually 38-39°C. Other nonspecific symptoms, including malaise, anorexia, fatigue, and headache, affect less than a third of patients. Transient rashes, which may occur in about 5% of patients, are mainly truncal maculopapular rashes. Erythema nodosum, erythema multiforme, and erythema annulare are also reported.

CSD is usually a self-limited infection that spontaneous resolves within a few weeks to months. The most common atypical presentation is **Parinaud oculoglandular syndrome,** which is unilateral conjunctivitis followed by preauricular lymphadenopathy and occurs in 2-17% of patients with CSD (Fig. 201-4). Direct eye inoculation as a result of rubbing with the hands after cat contact is the presumed mode of spread. A conjunctival granuloma may be found at the inoculation site. The involved eye is usually not painful and has little or no discharge but may be quite red and swollen. Submandibular or cervical lymphadenopathy may also occur.

More severe, disseminated illness occurs in a small percentage of patients and is characterized by presentation with high fever, often persisting for several weeks. Other prominent symptoms

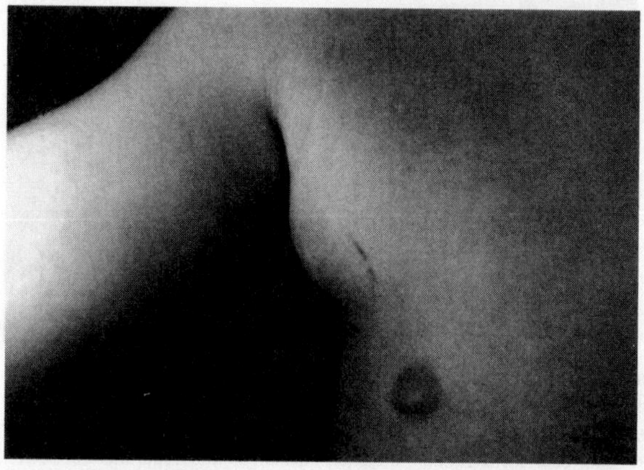

Figure 201-3 Right axillary lymphadenopathy followed the scratches and development of a primary papule in this child with typical cat-scratch disease. (From Mandell GL, Bennett JE, Dolin R, editors: *Principles and practice of infectious diseases,* ed 6, vol 2, Philadelphia, 2006, Elsevier, p 2737.)

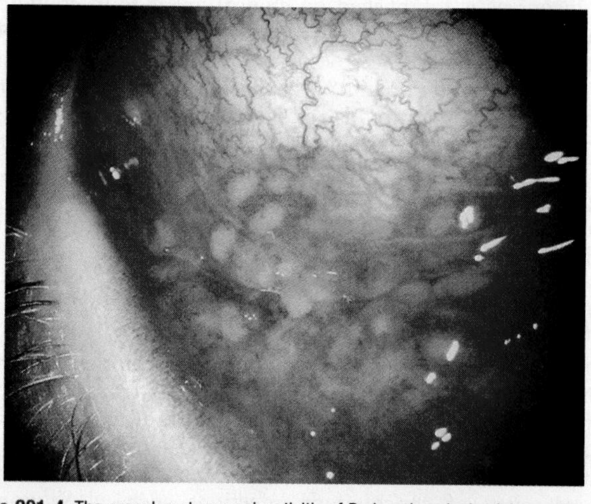

Figure 201-4 The granulomatous conjunctivitis of Parinaud oculoglandular syndrome is associated with ipsilateral local lymphadenopathy, usually preauricular and less commonly submandibular. (From Mandell GL, Bennett JE, Dolin R, editors: *Principles and practice of infectious diseases,* ed 6, vol 2, Philadelphia, 2006, Elsevier, p 2739.)

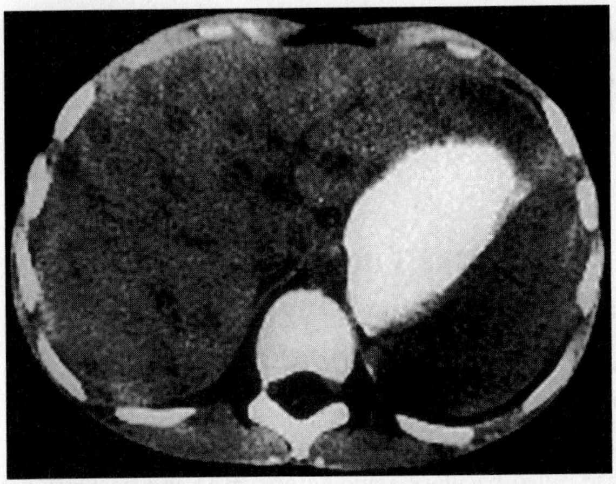

Figure 201-5 In this CT scan of a patient with hepatic involvement of cat-scratch disease, the absence of enhancement of the multiple lesions after contrast infusion is consistent with the granulomatous inflammation of this entity. Treated empirically with various antibiotics without improvement before establishment of this diagnosis, the patient subsequently recovered fully with no further antimicrobial therapy. (Courtesy of Dr. V.H. San Joaquin, University of Oklahoma Health Sciences Center, Oklahoma City.)

include significant abdominal pain and weight loss. **Hepatosplenomegaly** may occur, although hepatic dysfunction is rare (Fig. 201-5). Granulomatous changes may be seen in the liver and spleen. Another common site of dissemination is bone, with the development of **granulomatous osteolytic lesions,** associated with localized pain but without erythema, tenderness, or swelling. Other uncommon manifestations are neuroretinitis with papilledema and stellate macular exudates, encephalitis, fever of unknown origin, and atypical pneumonia.

DIAGNOSIS

In most cases, the diagnosis can be strongly suspected on clinical grounds in a patient with history of exposure to a cat. The U.S. Centers for Disease Control and Prevention (CDC) has developed an indirect immunofluorescent assay (IFA) that has shown good correlation with disease. Other IFA and enzyme-linked immunoassay tests are commercially available, although little comparative data are available. Most patients have elevated antibody titers at presentation; however, the timing of immunoglobulin G (IgG) and IgM response to *B. henselae* can be quite variable. There is cross reactivity among *Bartonella* species, particularly *B. henselae* and *B. quintana*.

If tissue specimens are obtained, bacilli may be visualized with Warthin-Starry and Brown-Hopps tissue stains. *Bartonella* DNA can be identified through PCR analysis of tissue specimens. Culturing of the organism is not generally practical for clinical diagnosis.

Differential Diagnosis

The differential diagnosis of CSD includes virtually all causes of lymphadenopathy (Chapter 490). The more common entities include pyogenic lymphadenitis, primarily from staphylococcal or streptococcal infections, atypical mycobacterial infections, and malignancy. Less common entities are tularemia, brucellosis, and sporotrichosis. Epstein-Barr virus, cytomegalovirus, and *Toxoplasma gondii* infections usually cause more generalized lymphadenopathy.

LABORATORY FINDINGS

Routine laboratory tests are not helpful. The erythrocyte sedimentation rate is often elevated. The white blood cell count may be normal or mildly elevated. Hepatic transaminases may be elevated in systemic disease. Ultrasonography or CT may reveal many granulomatous nodules in the liver and spleen; the nodules appear as hypodense round irregular lesions.

TREATMENT

Antibiotic treatment of CSD is not always needed and is not clearly beneficial. For most patients, treatment consists of conservative symptomatic care and observation. Studies show a significant discordance between in vitro activity of antibiotics and clinical effectiveness. For many patients, diagnosis is considered in the context of failure to respond to β-lactam antibiotic treatment of presumed staphylococcal lymphadenitis.

A small prospective study of oral azithromycin (500 mg on day 1, and then 250 mg on days 2-5; for smaller children, 10 mg/kg/24hr on day 1 and 5 mg/kg/24hr on days 2-5) showed a decrease in initial lymph node volume in 50% of patients during the 1st 30 days, but after 30 days there was no difference in lymph node volume. No other clinical benefit was found. For the majority of patients, CSD is self-limited, and resolution occurs over weeks to months without antibiotic treatment. Azithromycin, clarithromycin, trimethoprim-sulfamethoxazole, rifampin, ciprofloxacin, and gentamicin appear to be the best agents if treatment is considered.

Suppurative lymph nodes that become tense and extremely painful should be drained by needle aspiration, which may need to be repeated. Incision and drainage of nonsuppurative nodes should be avoided because chronic draining sinuses may result. Surgical excision of the node is rarely necessary.

Children with hepatosplenic CSD appear to respond well to rifampin at a dose of 20 mg/kg for 14 days, either alone or in combination with trimethoprim-sulfamethoxazole.

COMPLICATIONS

Encephalopathy, which can occur in as many as 5% of patients with CSD, typically manifests 1-3 wk after the onset of lymphadenitis as the sudden onset of neurologic symptoms, which often include seizures, combative or bizarre behavior, and altered level of consciousness. Imaging studies are generally normal. The cerebrospinal fluid is normal or shows minimal pleocytosis and protein elevation. Recovery occurs without sequelae in nearly all patients but may take place slowly over many months.

Other neurologic manifestations include peripheral facial nerve paralysis, myelitis, radiculitis, compression neuropathy, and cerebellar ataxia. One patient has been reported to have encephalopathy with persistent cognitive impairment and memory loss.

Stellate macular retinopathy has been associated with several infections, including CSD. Children and young adults present with unilateral or rarely bilateral loss of vision with central scotoma, optic disc swelling, and macular star formation from exudates radiating out from the macula. The findings usually resolve completely, with recovery of vision, generally within 2-3 mo. The optimal treatment for the neuroretinitis is unknown, although treatment of adults with doxycycline and rifampin for 4-6 wk has had good results.

Hematologic manifestations include hemolytic anemia, thrombocytopenic purpura, nonthrombocytopenic purpura, and eosinophilia. **Leukocytoclastic vasculitis** similar to Henoch-Schönlein purpura has been reported in association with CSD in 1 child. A systemic presentation of CSD with pleurisy, arthralgia or arthritis, mediastinal masses, enlarged nodes at the head of the pancreas, and atypical pneumonia also has been reported.

PROGNOSIS

The prognosis for CSD in a normal host is generally excellent, with resolution of clinical findings over weeks to months. Recovery is occasionally slower and may take as long as a year.

PREVENTION

Person-to-person spread of *Bartonella* infections is not known. Isolation of the affected patient is not necessary. Prevention would require elimination of cats from households, which is not practical or necessarily desirable. Awareness of the risk of cat (and particularly kitten) scratches should be emphasized to parents.

BIBLIOGRAPHY

Please visit the Nelson Textbook of Pediatrics *website at www.expertconsult.com for the complete bibliography.*

201.3 Trench Fever *(Bartonella quintana)*

Barbara W. Stechenberg

ETIOLOGY

The causative agent of trench fever was first designated *Rickettsia quintana,* was then assigned to the genus *Rochalimaea,* and now has been reassigned as *B. quintana.*

EPIDEMIOLOGY

Trench fever was first recognized as a distinct clinical entity during World War I, when more than a million troops in the trenches were infected. The disease became quiescent until World War II, when it again was epidemic. It is extremely rare in the USA.

Humans are the only known reservoir. No other animal is naturally infected, and usual laboratory animals are not susceptible. The human **body louse,** *Pediculus humanus* var. *corporis,* is the vector and is capable of transmission to a new host 5-6 days after feeding on an infected person. Lice excrete the organism for life; transovarian passage does not occur. Humans may have prolonged asymptomatic bacteremia for years.

CLINICAL MANIFESTATIONS

The incubation period for trench fever averages about 22 days (range 4-35 days). The clinical presentation is highly variable. Symptoms can be very mild and brief. About half of infected persons have a single febrile illness with abrupt onset lasting 3-6 days. In other patients, prolonged, sustained fever may occur. More commonly, patients have periodic febrile illness with 3 to 8 episodes lasting 4-5 days each, sometimes occurring over a period of a year or more. This form is reminiscent of malaria or relapsing fever *(Borrelia recurrentis).* Afebrile bacteremia can occur.

Clinical findings usually consist of fever (typically with a temperature of 38.5-40°C), malaise, chills, sweats, anorexia, and severe headache. Common findings include marked conjunctival injection, tachycardia, myalgias, arthralgias, and severe pain in the neck, back, and legs. **Crops of erythematous macules** or **papules** may occur on the trunk in as many as 80% of patients. Splenomegaly and mild liver enlargement may be noted.

DIAGNOSIS

In non-epidemic situations, it is impossible to establish a diagnosis of trench fever on clinical grounds, because the findings are not distinctive. A history of body louse infection or having been in an area of epidemic disease should heighten suspicions. *B. quintana* can be cultured from the blood with modification to include culture on epithelial cells. Serologic tests for *B. quintana* are available, but there is cross reaction with *B. henselae.*

TREATMENT

There are no controlled trials of treatment, but patients with trench fever typically show dramatic response to tetracycline or chloramphenicol, with rapid defervescence.

201.4 Bacillary Angiomatosis and Bacillary Peliosis Hepatis *(Bartonella henselae* and *Bartonella quintana)*

Barbara W. Stechenberg

Both *B. henselae* and *B. quintana* cause vascular proliferative disease called **bacillary angiomatosis** (BA) and **bacillary peliosis** in severely immunocompromised persons, primarily adult patients with AIDS or cancer and organ transplant recipients. Subcutaneous and lytic bone lesions are strongly associated with *B. quintana,* whereas peliosis hepatis is associated exclusively with *B. henselae.*

BACILLARY ANGIOMATOSIS

Lesions of cutaneous BA, also known as *epithelioid angiomatosis,* are the most easily identified and recognized form of *Bartonella* infection in immunocompromised hosts. They are found primarily in patients with AIDS who have very low CD4 counts. The clinical appearance can be quite diverse. The vasoproliferative lesions of BA may be cutaneous or subcutaneous and may resemble the vascular lesions (verruca peruana) of *B. bacilliformis* in immunocompetent persons, characterized by erythematous papules on an erythematous base with a collarette of scale. They may enlarge to form large pedunculated lesions and may ulcerate. Trauma may result in profuse bleeding.

BA may be clinically indistinguishable from Kaposi sarcoma. Other considerations in the differential diagnosis are pyogenic granuloma and verruca peruana *(B. bacilliformis).* Deep soft tissue masses caused by BA may mimic a malignancy.

Osseous BA lesions commonly involve the long bones. These lytic lesions are very painful and highly vascular and are occasionally associated with an overlying erythematous plaque. The high degree of vascularity produces a very positive result on a technetium-Tc 99m methylene diphosphonate bone scan, resembling that of a malignant lesion.

Lesions can be found in virtually any organ, producing similar vascular proliferative lesions. They may appear raised, nodular, or ulcerative when seen on endoscopy or bronchoscopy. They may be associated with enlarged lymph nodes with or without an obvious local cutaneous lesion. Brain parenchymal lesions have been described.

BACILLARY PELIOSIS

Bacillary peliosis affects the reticuloendothelial system, primarily the liver (**peliosis hepatis**) and less frequently the spleen and lymph nodes. It is a vasoproliferative disorder characterized by random proliferation of venous lakes surrounded by fibromyxoid stroma harboring numerous bacillary organisms. Clinical findings include fever and abdominal pain in association with abnormal results of liver function tests, particularly a markedly increased alkaline phosphatase level. Cutaneous BA or splenomegaly may be associated, with or without thrombocytopenia or pancytopenia. The vascular proliferative lesions in the liver and spleen appear on CT scan as hypodense lesions scattered throughout the parenchyma. The differential diagnosis includes hepatic Kaposi sarcoma, lymphoma, and disseminated infection with *Pneumocystis carinii* or *Mycobacterium avium* complex.

BACTEREMIA AND ENDOCARDITIS

B. henselae, B. quintana, B. vinsonii, and *B. elizabethae* all have been reported to cause bacteremia or endocarditis. They are associated with symptoms such as prolonged fevers, night sweats, and profound weight loss. A cluster of cases in Seattle in 1993 occurred in a homeless population with chronic alcoholism. These patients with high fever or hypothermia were thought to represent "urban trench fever," but no body louse infestation was associated. Some cases of culture-negative endocarditis may represent *Bartonella* endocarditis. One report described central nervous system involvement with *B. quintana* infection in 2 children.

DIAGNOSIS

Diagnosis of BA is made initially by biopsy. The characteristic small vessel proliferation with mixed inflammatory response and the staining of bacilli by Warthin-Starry silver staining distinguish BA from pyogenic granuloma or Kaposi sarcoma (Chapter 254). Travel history can usually preclude verruca peruana.

Culture is impractical for CSD but is the diagnostic procedure for suspected bacteremia or endocarditis. Use of the lysis centrifugation technique or fresh chocolate or heart infusion agar with 5% rabbit blood with prolonged incubation may increase the yield of culture. PCR can also be a useful tool.

TREATMENT

Bartonella infections in immunocompromised hosts caused by both *B. henselae* and *B. quintana* have been treated successfully with antimicrobial agents. BA responds rapidly to erythromycin, azithromycin, and clarithromycin, which are the drugs of choice. Alternative choices are doxycycline or tetracycline. Severely ill patients with peliosis hepatis, endocarditis, or osteomyelitis may be treated initially with intravenous erythromycin or doxycycline and the addition of rifampin or gentamicin. The use of an aminoglycoside for a minimum of 2 wk is associated with improved prognosis in endocarditis. A Jarisch-Herxheimer reaction may occur. Relapses may follow, and prolonged treatment for several months may be necessary.

PREVENTION

Immunocompromised persons should consider the potential risks of cat ownership because of the risks for *Bartonella* infections as well as toxoplasmosis and enteric infections. Those who elect to obtain a cat should adopt or purchase a cat >1 yr of age and in good health. Prompt washing of any wounds from cat bites or scratches is essential.

BIBLIOGRAPHY

Please visit the Nelson Textbook of Pediatrics *website at www.expertconsult.com for the complete bibliography.*

Section 6 ANAEROBIC BACTERIAL INFECTIONS

Chapter 202
Botulism (*Clostridium botulinum*)

Stephen S. Arnon

Three naturally occurring forms of human botulism are known: infant (intestinal toxemia) botulism (the most common in the USA), food-borne (classic) botulism, and wound botulism. Two other forms, both human-made, also occur: inhalational botulism from inhaling accidentally aerosolized toxin and iatrogenic botulism from overdosage of therapeutic or cosmetic use of botulinum toxin.

ETIOLOGY

Botulism is the acute, flaccid paralysis caused by the neurotoxin produced by *Clostridium botulinum* or, infrequently, an equivalent neurotoxin produced by rare strains of *Clostridium butyricum* and *Clostridium baratii. C. botulinum* is a gram-positive, spore-forming, obligate anaerobe whose natural habitat worldwide is soil, dust, and marine sediments. The organism is found in a wide variety of fresh and cooked agricultural products. Spores of some *C. botulinum* strains endure boiling for several hours, enabling the organism to survive efforts at food preservation. In contrast, botulinum toxin is heat labile and easily destroyed by heating at ≥85°C for 5 min. Neurotoxigenic *C. butyricum* has been isolated from a soybean food and from soils near Lake Weishan in China, the site of food-borne botulism outbreaks associated with this organism. Little is known about the ecology of neurotoxigenic *C. baratii.*

Botulinum toxin is a simple dichain protein consisting of a 100-kd heavy chain that contains the neuronal attachment sites and a 50-kd light chain that is taken into the cell after binding. Botulinum toxin is the most poisonous substance known, the parenteral human lethal dose being estimated at 10^{-6} mg/kg. The toxin blocks neuromuscular transmission and causes death through airway and respiratory muscle paralysis. Seven antigenic toxin types, designated by letters A-G, are distinguished by the inability of neutralizing antibody against 1 toxin type to protect against a different toxin type. Toxin types are further differentiated into subtypes by differences in the nucleotide sequences of their toxin genes. Like the gene for tetanus toxin, the gene for botulinum toxin for some toxin types and subtypes resides on a plasmid.

The 7 toxin types serve as convenient clinical and epidemiologic markers. Toxin types A, B, E, and F are well-established causes of human botulism, whereas types C and D cause illness in other animals. Neurotoxigenic *C. butyricum* strains produce a type E toxin, whereas neurotoxigenic *C. baratii* strains produce a type F toxin. Type G has not been established as a cause of either human or animal disease. The phenomenal potency of botulinum toxin occurs because its 7 light chains are zinc-endopeptidases whose substrates are 1 or 2 proteins of the docking complex by which synaptic vesicles fuse with the terminal neuronal cell membrane and release acetylcholine into the synaptic cleft.

EPIDEMIOLOGY

Infant botulism has been reported from all inhabited continents except Africa. Notably, the infant is the only family member who is ill. The most striking epidemiologic feature of infant botulism is its age distribution, in which in 95% of cases the infants are between 3 wk and 6 mo of age, with a broad peak from 2 to 4 mo of age. Cases have been recognized in infants as young as

1.5 days or as old as 382 days at onset. The male : female ratio of hospitalized cases is approximately 1 : 1, and cases have occurred in most racial and ethnic groups.

Infant botulism is an uncommon and often unrecognized illness. In the USA, about 80-100 hospitalized cases are diagnosed annually; more than 2,500 cases were reported from 1976 to 2010. The full clinical spectrum of infant botulism includes mild outpatient cases and fulminant sudden death cases. Approximately 40% of U.S. hospitalized cases have been reported from California. Consistent with the known asymmetric soil distribution of *C. botulinum* toxin types, most cases west of the Mississippi River have been caused by type A strains, whereas most cases east of the Mississippi River have been caused by type B strains. One case each in New Mexico, Washington, Ohio, California, Iowa, and Colorado has been caused by *C. baratii* and type F toxin. Four cases in Italy have resulted from *C. butyricum* and type E toxin. Identified risk factors for the illness include breast-feeding, the ingestion of honey, and a slow intestinal transit time (<1 stool/day). Breast-feeding may provide protection against fulminant sudden death from infant botulism. Under rare circumstances of altered intestinal anatomy, physiology, and microflora, older children and adults may contract infant-type botulism.

Food-borne botulism results from the ingestion of a food in which *C. botulinum* has multiplied and produced its toxin. Outbreaks in North America have been associated with baked potatoes, sautéed onions, and chopped garlic served in restaurants, revising the traditional view of food-borne botulism as resulting mainly from home-canned foods. Other outbreaks in the USA have occurred from commercial foods sealed in plastic pouches that relied solely on refrigeration to prevent outgrowth of *C. botulinum* spores. Uncanned foods responsible for food-borne botulism cases include peyote tea, the hazelnut flavoring added to yogurt, sweet cream cheese, sautéed onions in "patty melt" sandwiches, potato salad, and fresh and dried fish. A trend toward a single case per outbreak or of cases manifesting separately in different cities or hospitals portends that physicians cannot rely on the temporal and geographic clustering of cases to suggest the diagnosis.

Most types of preserved foods have been implicated in food-borne botulism, but the usual offenders in the USA are the "low-acid" (pH ≥ 6.0) home-canned foods such as jalapeño peppers, asparagus, olives, and beans. The potential for food-borne botulism exists throughout the world, but outbreaks occur most commonly in the temperate zones rather than the tropics, where preservation of fruits, vegetables, and other foods is less common.

Approximately 5-10 outbreaks and 20-25 cases of food-borne botulism have occurred annually in the USA. Most of the continental U.S. outbreaks resulted from proteolytic type A or type B strains, which produce a strongly putrefactive odor in the food that some people find necessary to verify by tasting. In contrast, in Alaska and Canada, most food-borne outbreaks have resulted from nonproteolytic type E strains in Native American foods, such as fermented salmon eggs and seal flippers, which do not exhibit signs of spoilage. A further hazard of type E strains is their ability to grow at the temperatures maintained by household refrigerators (5°C).

Wound botulism is an exceptionally rare disease, with <400 cases reported worldwide, but it is important to pediatrics because adolescents and children may be affected. Although many cases have occurred in young, physically active males at greatest risk for traumatic injury, wound botulism also occurs with crush injuries in which no break in the skin is evident. In the past 15 yr, wound botulism from injection has become increasingly common in adult heroin abusers in the western USA and in Europe, not always with evident abscess formation or cellulitis.

A single outbreak of **inhalational botulism** was reported in 1962 in which 3 laboratory workers in Germany were exposed unintentionally to aerosolized botulinum toxin. Some patients in the USA have been hospitalized by accidental overdose of therapeutic or cosmetic botulinum toxin.

PATHOGENESIS

All forms of botulism produce disease through a final common pathway. Botulinum toxin is carried by the bloodstream to peripheral cholinergic synapses, where it binds irreversibly, blocking acetylcholine release and causing impaired neuromuscular and autonomic transmission. **Infant botulism** is an infectious disease that results from ingesting the spores of any of the 3 botulinum toxin-producing clostridial strains, with subsequent spore germination, multiplication, and production of botulinum toxin in the large intestine. **Food-borne botulism** is an intoxication that results when preformed botulinum toxin contained in an improperly preserved or inadequately cooked food is swallowed. **Wound botulism** results from spore germination and colonization of traumatized tissue by *C. botulinum;* it is the analog of tetanus. **Inhalational botulism** occurs when aerosolized botulinum toxin is inhaled. A bioterrorist attack could result in large or small outbreaks of inhalational or food-borne botulism (Chapter 704).

Botulinum toxin is not a cytotoxin and does not causes overt macroscopic or microscopic pathology. Secondary pathologic changes (pneumonia, petechiae on intrathoracic organs) may be found at autopsy. No diagnostic technique is available to identify botulinum toxin bound at the neuromuscular junction. The healing process in botulism consists of sprouting of new terminal unmyelinated motor neurons. Movement resumes when these new twigs locate noncontracting muscle fibers and reinnervate them by inducing formation of a new motor end plate. In experimental animals, this process takes about 4 wk.

CLINICAL MANIFESTATIONS

Botulinum toxin is distributed hematogenously. Because relative blood flow and density of innervation are greatest in the bulbar musculature, all forms of botulism manifest neurologically as a symmetric, descending, flaccid paralysis beginning with the cranial nerve musculature. It is not possible to have botulism without having multiple bulbar palsies, yet in infants, such symptoms as poor feeding, weak suck, feeble cry, drooling, and even obstructive apnea are often not recognized as bulbar in origin (Fig. 202-1). Patients with evolving illness may already have generalized weakness and hypotonia in addition to bulbar palsies when first examined. In contrast to botulism caused by *C. botulinum,* a majority of the rare cases caused by intestinal colonization with *C. butyricum* are associated with a Meckel diverticulum accompanying abdominal distention, often leading to misdiagnosis as an acute abdomen. The also rare *C. baratii* type F infant botulism cases have been characterized by very young age at onset, rapidity of onset, and greater severity of paralysis.

In older children with **food-borne** or **wound botulism,** the onset of neurologic symptoms follows a characteristic pattern of diplopia, blurred vision, ptosis, dry mouth, dysphagia, dysphonia, and dysarthria, with decreased gag and corneal reflexes. Importantly, because the toxin acts only on motor nerves, paresthesias are not seen in botulism, except when a patient hyperventilates from anxiety. The sensorium remains clear, but this fact may be difficult to ascertain because of the slurred speech.

Food-borne botulism begins with gastrointestinal symptoms of nausea, vomiting, or diarrhea in about 30% of cases. These symptoms are thought to result from metabolic by-products of growth of *C. botulinum* or from the presence of other toxic contaminants in the food because gastrointestinal distress is rarely observed in wound botulism. Constipation may occur in food-borne botulism once flaccid paralysis becomes evident. Illness usually begins 12-36 hr after ingestion of the contaminated food but can range from as little as 2 hr to as long as 8

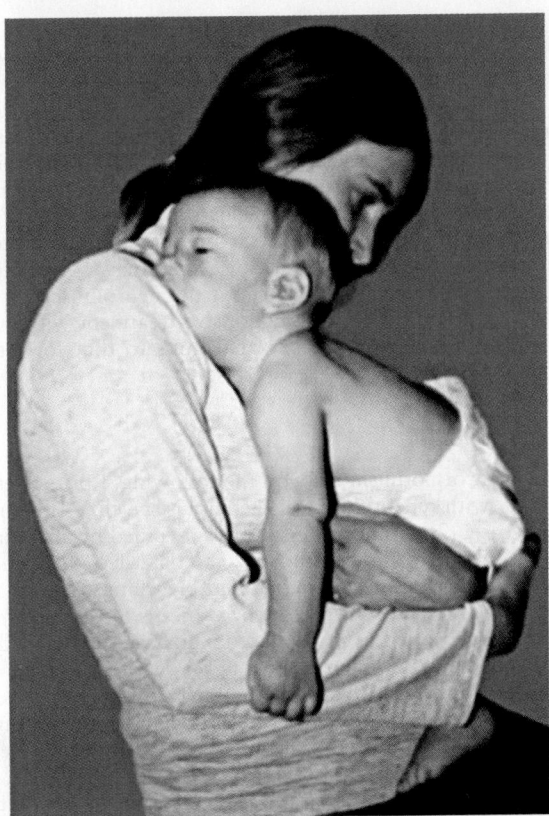

Figure 202-1 A 3 mo old infant with mild infant botulism showing signs of ptosis, an expressionless face, and hypotonia of the neck, trunk, and limbs. The additional bulbar palsies—ophthalmoplegia, weak cry, weak sucking, and dysphagia (drooling)—are not apparent in the photograph. (From Arnon SS, Schechter R, Maslanka SE, et al: Human botulism immune globulin for the treatment of infant botulism, *N Engl J Med* 354: 462–471, 2006.)

days. The incubation period in **wound botulism** is 4-14 days. Fever may be present in wound botulism but is absent in food-borne botulism unless a secondary infection (often pneumonia) is present. All forms of botulism display a wide spectrum of clinical severity, from the very mild, with minimal ptosis, flattened facial expression, minor dysphagia, and dysphonia, to the fulminant, with rapid onset of extensive paralysis, frank apnea, and fixed, dilated pupils. Fatigability with repetitive muscle activity is the clinical hallmark of botulism.

Infant botulism differs in apparent initial symptoms of illness only because the infant cannot verbalize them. Usually, the 1st indication of illness is a decreased frequency or even absence of defecation, although this sign is frequently overlooked. Parents typically notice inability to feed, lethargy, weak cry, and diminished spontaneous movement. Dysphagia may be evident as secretions drooling from the mouth. Gag, suck, and corneal reflexes diminish as the paralysis advances. Oculomotor palsies may be evident only with sustained observation. Paradoxically, the pupillary light reflex may be unaffected until the child is severely paralyzed, or it may be initially sluggish. Loss of head control is typically a prominent sign. Respiratory arrest may occur suddenly from airway occlusion by unswallowed secretions or from obstructive flaccid pharyngeal musculature. Occasionally, the diagnosis of infant botulism is suggested by a respiratory arrest that occurs after the infant is curled into position for lumbar puncture.

In mild cases or in the early stages of illness, the physical signs of infant botulism may be subtle and easily missed. Eliciting cranial nerve palsies and fatigability of muscular function requires careful examination. Ptosis may not be seen unless the head of the child is kept erect.

Table 202-1 DIAGNOSES CONSIDERED IN SUBSEQUENTLY LABORATORY-CONFIRMED CASES OF INFANT BOTULISM

ADMISSION DIAGNOSIS	SUBSEQUENTLY CONSIDERED DIAGNOSES
Suspected sepsis, meningitis	Guillain-Barré syndrome
Pneumonia	Myasthenia gravis
Dehydration	Disorders of amino acid metabolism
Viral syndrome	Hypothyroidism
Hypotonia of unknown etiology	Drug ingestion
	Organophosphate poisoning
Constipation	Brainstem encephalitis
Failure to thrive	Heavy metal poisoning (Pb, Mg, As)
Spinal muscular atrophy (Werdnig-Hoffmann disease)	Poliomyelitis
	Viral polyneuritis
	Hirschsprung disease
	Metabolic encephalopathy
	Medium chain acetyl–CoA dehydrogenase (MCAD) deficiency

DIAGNOSIS

Clinical diagnosis of botulism is confirmed by specialized laboratory testing that requires hours to days to complete. Therefore, clinical diagnosis is the foundation for early recognition of and response to all forms of botulism. Routine laboratory studies, including those of the cerebrospinal fluid (CSF), are normal in botulism unless dehydration, undernourishment (metabolic acidosis and ketosis), or secondary infection is present.

The **classic triad of botulism** is the acute onset of a symmetric flaccid descending paralysis with clear sensorium, no fever, and no paresthesias. Suspected botulism represents a medical and public health emergency that is immediately reportable by telephone in most U.S. health jurisdictions. State health departments (1st call) and the U.S. Centers for Disease Control and Prevention (CDC; telephone 770-488-7100 at any time) can arrange for diagnostic testing, epidemiologic investigation, and provision of equine antitoxin.

The diagnosis of botulism is unequivocally established by demonstration of the presence of botulinum toxin in serum or of *C. botulinum* toxin or organisms in wound material, enema fluid, or feces. *C. botulinum* is not part of the normal resident intestinal flora of humans, and its presence in the setting of acute flaccid paralysis is diagnostic. An epidemiologic diagnosis of food-borne botulism can be established when *C. botulinum* organisms and toxin are found in food eaten by patients.

Electromyography (EMG) can sometimes distinguish between causes of acute flaccid paralysis, although results may be variable, including normal, in patients with botulism. The distinctive EMG finding in botulism is facilitation (potentiation) of the evoked muscle action potential at high-frequency (50-Hz) stimulation. In infant botulism, a characteristic pattern, known by the acronym **BSAP** (brief, small, abundant motor unit action potentials), is present only in clinically weak muscles. Nerve conduction velocity and sensory nerve function are normal in botulism.

Infant botulism requires a high index of suspicion for early diagnosis (Table 202-1). "Rule out sepsis" remains the most common admission diagnosis. If a previously healthy infant (commonly 2-4 mo of age) demonstrates weakness with difficulty in sucking, swallowing, crying, or breathing, infant botulism should be considered a likely diagnosis. A careful cranial nerve examination is then very helpful.

Differential Diagnosis

Botulism is frequently misdiagnosed, most often as a polyradiculoneuropathy (Guillain-Barré or Miller Fisher syndrome), myasthenia gravis, or a disease of the central nervous system (Tables 202-1 and 202-2). In the USA, botulism is more likely than

Table 202-2 DIAGNOSES CONSIDERED IN FOOD-BORNE AND WOUND BOTULISM

Acute gastroenteritis
Myasthenia gravis
Guillain-Barré syndrome
Organophosphate poisoning
Meningitis
Encephalitis
Psychiatric illness
Cerebrovascular accident
Poliomyelitis
Hypothyroidism
Aminoglycoside-associated paralysis
Tick paralysis
Hypocalcemia
Hypermagnesemia
Carbon monoxide poisoning
Hyperemesis gravidarum
Laryngeal trauma
Diabetic complications
Inflammatory myopathy
Overexertion

Guillain-Barré syndrome, intoxication, or poliomyelitis to cause a cluster of cases of acute flaccid paralysis. Botulism differs from other flaccid paralyses in its prominent cranial nerve palsies disproportionate to milder weakness and hypotonia below the neck, in its symmetry, and in its absence of sensory nerve damage. Spinal muscular atrophy may closely mimic infant botulism at presentation.

Additional diagnostic procedures may be useful in rapidly excluding botulism as the cause of paralysis. The CSF is unchanged in botulism but is abnormal in many central nervous system diseases. Although the CSF protein concentration is eventually elevated in Guillain-Barré syndrome, it may be normal early in illness. Imaging of the brain, spine, and chest may reveal hemorrhage, inflammation, or neoplasm. A test dose of edrophonium chloride briefly reverses paralytic symptoms in many patients with myasthenia gravis and, reportedly, in some with botulism. A close inspection of the skin, especially the scalp, may reveal an attached tick that is causing paralysis. Possible organophosphate intoxication should be pursued aggressively because specific antidotes (oximes) are available and because the patient may be part of a commonly exposed group, some of whom have yet to demonstrate illness. Other tests that require days for results include stool culture for *Campylobacter jejuni* as a precipitant of Guillain-Barré syndrome, spinal muscular atrophy and other genetic (including mitochondrial) disorders, and assays for the autoantibodies that cause myasthenia gravis, Lambert-Eaton syndrome, and Guillain-Barré syndrome.

TREATMENT

Human botulism immune globulin, given intravenously (BIG-IV), is licensed for the treatment of infant botulism caused by type A or B botulinum toxin. Treatment with BIG-IV consists of a single intravenous infusion of 50-100 mg/kg (see package insert) that should be given as soon as possible after infant botulism is suspected in order to immediately end the toxemia that is the cause of the illness. Treatment should not be delayed for laboratory confirmation. In the USA, BIG-IV may be obtained from the California Department of Health Services (24-hr telephone 510-231-7600; www.infantbotulism.org). The use of BIG-IV shortens mean hospital stay from ≈6 wks to 2 wks. Most of the decrease in length of hospital stay results from the reduced time that the patient requires ventilation and in intensive care. Hospital costs are reduced by >$100,000 per case (in 2004 dollars).

Older patients with suspected food, wound, or inhalational botulism may be treated with 1 vial of investigational equine heptavalent botulinum antitoxin (H-BAT), available in the USA through the CDC by way of state and local health departments.

Antibiotic therapy is not part of the treatment of uncomplicated infant or food-borne botulism, because the toxin is primarily an intracellular molecule that is released into the intestinal lumen with vegetative bacterial cell death and lysis. Antibiotics are reserved for the treatment of secondary infections, and in the absence of antitoxin therapy, a nonclostridiocidal antibiotic such as trimethoprim-sulfamethoxazole is preferred. Aminoglycoside antibiotics should be avoided because they may potentiate the blocking action of botulinum toxin at the neuromuscular junction. Wound botulism requires aggressive treatment with antibiotics and antitoxin in a manner analogous to that for tetanus (Chapter 203).

SUPPORTIVE CARE

Management of botulism rests on the following 3 principles: (1) fatigability with repetitive muscle activity is the clinical hallmark of the disease; (2) complications are best avoided by anticipating them; and (3) meticulous supportive care is a necessity. The 1st principle applies mainly to feeding and breathing. *Correct positioning is imperative to protect the airway and improve respiratory mechanics.* The patient is placed face up on a rigid-bottomed crib (or bed), the head of which is tilted at 30 degrees. A small cloth roll is placed under the cervical vertebrae to tilt the head back so that secretions drain to the posterior pharynx and away from the airway. In this tilted position, the abdominal viscera pull the diaphragm down, thereby improving respiratory mechanics. The patient's head and torso should not be elevated by bending the middle of the bed; in such a position, the hypotonic thorax would slump into the abdomen and breathing would be compromised.

About half of patients with infant botulism require endotracheal intubation, which is best done prophylactically. The indications include diminished gag and cough reflexes and progressive airway obstruction by secretions. With meticulous management techniques (especially proper tube diameter), monitoring, and positioning, patients have tolerated months of intubation without subglottic stenosis or need for tracheostomy.

Feeding should be done by a nasogastric or nasojejunal tube until sufficient oropharyngeal strength and coordination enable feeding by breast or bottle. Expressed breast milk is the most desirable food for infants, in part because of its immunologic components (e.g., secretory immunoglobulin A [sIgA], lactoferrin, leukocytes). Tube feeding also assists in the restoration of peristalsis, a nonspecific but probably essential part of eliminating *C. botulinum* from the intestinal flora. Intravenous feeding (hyperalimentation) is discouraged because of the potential for infection and the advantages of tube feeding.

Because sensation remains intact, providing auditory, tactile, and visual stimuli is beneficial. Maintaining strong central respiratory drive is essential, so sedatives and central nervous system depressants are best avoided. Full hydration and stool softeners such as lactulose may mitigate the protracted constipation. Cathartics are not recommended. Patients with food-borne and infant botulism excrete *C. botulinum* toxin and organisms in their feces, often for weeks, and care should be taken in handling their excreta. When bladder palsy occurs in severe cases, gentle suprapubic pressure with the patient in the sitting position with the head supported may help attain complete voiding and reduce the risk for urinary tract infection. Families of affected patients may require emotional and financial support, especially when the paralysis of botulism is prolonged.

COMPLICATIONS

Almost all of the complications of botulism are nosocomial, and a few are iatrogenic (Table 202-3). Some critically ill, pharmacologically paralyzed patients who must spend weeks or months on

Table 202-3 COMPLICATIONS OF INFANT BOTULISM

Acute respiratory distress syndrome
Aspiration
Clostridium difficile enterocolitis
Hypotension
Inappropriate antidiuretic hormone secretion
Long bone fractures
Misplaced or plugged endotracheal tube
Nosocomial anemia
Otitis media
Pneumonia
Pneumothorax
Recurrent atelectasis
Seizures secondary to hyponatremia
Sepsis
Subglottic stenosis
Tracheal granuloma
Tracheitis
Transfusion reaction
Urinary tract infection

ventilators in intensive care units inevitably experience some of these complications. Suspected "relapses" of infant botulism usually reflect premature hospital discharge or an inapparent underlying complication such as pneumonia, urinary tract infection, or otitis media.

PROGNOSIS

When the regenerating nerve endings have induced formation of a new motor end plate, neuromuscular transmission is restored. In the absence of complications, particularly those related to hypoxia, the prognosis in infant botulism is for full and complete recovery. Hospital stay in untreated infant botulism averages 5.7 wk but differs significantly by toxin type, with patients with untreated type B disease being hospitalized a mean of 4.2 wk and those with untreated type A disease 6.7 wk.

In the USA, the case fatality ratio for hospitalized cases of infant botulism is <1%. Patients with untreated infant botulism appear after recovery to have an increased incidence of strabismus that requires timely screening and treatment.

The case fatality ratio in food-borne and wound botulism varies by age, with younger patients having the best prognosis. Some adults with botulism have reported chronic weakness and fatigue for more than 1 yr as sequelae.

PREVENTION

Food-borne botulism is best prevented by adherence to safe methods of home canning (pressure cooker and acidification), by avoiding suspicious foods, and by heating all home canned foods to 85°C for ≥5 min. Wound botulism is best prevented by not using illicit drugs and by treatment of contaminated wounds with thorough cleansing, surgical debridement, and provision of appropriate antibiotics.

Most patients with infant botulism probably inhaled and then swallowed airborne clostridial spores; these cases cannot be prevented. The one identified, avoidable source of botulinum spores for infants is honey. *Honey is an unsafe food for any child younger than 1 yr.* Corn syrups were once thought to be a possible source of botulinum spores, but evidence indicates otherwise. Breast-feeding appears to slow the onset of infant botulism and to diminish the risk for sudden death in infants in whom the disease develops.

BIBLIOGRAPHY

Please visit the Nelson Textbook of Pediatrics *website at www.expertconsult.com for the complete bibliography.*

Chapter 203
Tetanus (*Clostridium tetani*)

Stephen S. Arnon

ETIOLOGY

Tetanus is an acute, spastic paralytic illness historically called **lockjaw** that is caused by the neurotoxin produced by *Clostridium tetani,* a motile, gram-positive, spore-forming obligate anaerobe whose natural habitat worldwide is soil, dust, and the alimentary tracts of various animals. *C. tetani* forms spores terminally, producing a drumstick or tennis racket appearance microscopically. Tetanus spores can survive boiling but not autoclaving, whereas the vegetative cells are killed by antibiotics, heat, and standard disinfectants. Unlike many clostridia, *C. tetani* is not a tissue-invasive organism and instead causes illness through the effects of a single toxin, **tetanospasmin,** more commonly referred to as **tetanus toxin.** Tetanospasmin is the 2nd most poisonous substance known, surpassed in potency only by botulinum toxin. The human lethal dose of tetanus toxin is estimated to be 10^{-5} mg/kg.

EPIDEMIOLOGY

Tetanus occurs worldwide and is endemic in approximately 90 developing countries, although its incidence varies considerably. The most common form, **neonatal (or umbilical) tetanus,** kills approximately 500,000 infants each year, with about 80% of deaths in just 12 tropical Asian and African countries. It occurs in infants whose mothers are not immunized. In addition, an estimated 15,000-30,000 unimmunized women worldwide die each year of **maternal tetanus,** which results from postpartum, postabortal, or postsurgical wound infection with *C. tetani.* Approximately 50 cases of tetanus are reported each year in the USA, mostly in persons >60 yr of age, although cases also occur in toddlers and neonates. Approximately 20% of children in the USA 10-16 yr of age lack a protective antibody level. The majority of childhood cases of tetanus in the USA have occurred in unimmunized children whose parents objected to vaccination.

Most non-neonatal cases of tetanus are associated with a traumatic injury, often a penetrating wound inflicted by a dirty object such as a nail, splinter, fragment of glass, or unsterile injection. Tetanus occurring after illicit drug injection is becoming more common. The disease also occurs after the use of contaminated suture material and after intramuscular injection of medicines, most notably quinine for chloroquine-resistant falciparum malaria. The disease may also occur in association with animal bites, abscesses (including dental abscesses), ear and other body piercing, chronic skin ulceration, burns, compound fractures, frostbite, gangrene, intestinal surgery, ritual scarification, infected insect bites, and female circumcision. Rare cases have no history of trauma.

PATHOGENESIS

Tetanus occurs after introduced spores germinate, multiply, and produce tetanus toxin in the low oxidation-reduction potential (E_h) of an infected injury site. A plasmid carries the toxin gene. Toxin is released after vegetative bacterial cell death and lysis. Tetanus toxin (and the botulinum toxins) is a 150-kd simple protein consisting of a heavy chain (100 kd) and a light (50 kd) chain joined by a single disulfide bond. Tetanus toxin binds at the neuromuscular junction and enters the motor nerve by endocytosis, after which it undergoes retrograde axonal transport to the cytoplasm of the α-motoneuron. In the sciatic nerve, the transport rate was found to be 3.4 mm/hr. The toxin exits the motoneuron in the spinal cord and next enters adjacent spinal inhibitory interneurons, where it prevents release of the neurotransmitters glycine and γ-aminobutyric acid (GABA). Tetanus toxin thus blocks the normal inhibition of antagonistic muscles on which voluntary coordinated movement depends; in consequence, affected muscles sustain maximal contraction and cannot relax. The autonomic nervous system is also rendered unstable in tetanus.

The phenomenal potency of tetanus toxin is enzymatic in nature. The light chain of tetanus toxin (and of several botulinum toxins) is a zinc-containing endoprotease whose substrate is synaptobrevin, a constituent protein of the docking complex that enables the synaptic vesicle to fuse with the terminal neuronal cell membrane. The heavy chain of the toxin contains its binding and internalization domains.

Because *C. tetani* is not an invasive organism, its toxin-producing vegetative cells remain where introduced into the wound, which may display local inflammatory changes and a mixed bacterial flora.

CLINICAL MANIFESTATIONS

Tetanus is most often generalized but may also be localized. The incubation period typically is 2-14 days but may be as long as months after the injury. In **generalized tetanus,** the presenting symptom in about half of cases is **trismus** (masseter muscle spasm, or lockjaw). Headache, restlessness, and irritability are early symptoms, often followed by stiffness, difficulty chewing, dysphagia, and neck muscle spasm. The so-called **sardonic smile of tetanus (risus sardonicus)** results from intractable spasms of facial and buccal muscles. When the paralysis extends to abdominal, lumbar, hip, and thigh muscles, the patient may assume an arched posture of extreme hyperextension of the body, or **opisthotonos,** with the head and the heels bent backward and the body bowed forward with only the back of the head and the heels touching the supporting surface. Opisthotonos is an equilibrium position that results from unrelenting total contraction of opposing muscles, all of which display the typical boardlike rigidity of tetanus. Laryngeal and respiratory muscle spasm can lead to airway obstruction and asphyxiation. Because tetanus toxin does not affect sensory nerves or cortical function, the patient unfortunately remains conscious, in extreme pain, and in fearful anticipation of the next tetanic seizure. The seizures are characterized by sudden, severe tonic contractions of the muscles, with fist clenching, flexion, and adduction of the arms and hyperextension of the legs. Without treatment, the seizures range from a few seconds to a few minutes in length with intervening respite periods, but as the illness progresses, the spasms become sustained and exhausting. The smallest disturbance by sight, sound, or touch may trigger a tetanic spasm. Dysuria and urinary retention result from bladder sphincter spasm; forced defecation may occur. Fever, occasionally as high as 40°C, is common because of the substantial metabolic energy consumed by spastic muscles. Notable autonomic effects include tachycardia, dysrhythmias, labile hypertension, diaphoresis, and cutaneous vasoconstriction. The tetanic paralysis usually becomes more severe in the 1st wk after onset, stabilizes in the 2nd wk, and ameliorates gradually over the ensuing 1-4 wk.

Neonatal tetanus, the infantile form of generalized tetanus, typically manifests within 3-12 days of birth as progressive difficulty in feeding (sucking and swallowing), associated hunger, and crying. Paralysis or diminished movement, stiffness and rigidity to the touch, and spasms, with or without opisthotonos, are characteristic. The umbilical stump may hold remnants of dirt, dung, clotted blood, or serum, or it may appear relatively benign.

Localized tetanus results in painful spasms of the muscles adjacent to the wound site and may precede generalized tetanus. **Cephalic tetanus** is a rare form of localized tetanus involving the bulbar musculature that occurs with wounds or foreign bodies in the head, nostrils, or face. It also occurs in association with chronic otitis media. Cephalic tetanus is characterized by retracted eyelids, deviated gaze, trismus, risus sardonicus, and spastic paralysis of the tongue and pharyngeal musculature.

DIAGNOSIS

The picture of tetanus is one of the most dramatic in medicine, and the diagnosis may be established clinically. The typical setting is an unimmunized patient (and/or mother) who was injured or born within the preceding 2 wk, who presents with trismus, other rigid muscles, and a clear sensorium.

Results of routine laboratory studies are usually normal. A peripheral leukocytosis may result from a secondary bacterial infection of the wound or may be stress induced from the sustained tetanic spasms. The cerebrospinal fluid is normal, although the intense muscle contractions may raise intracranial pressure. Neither the electroencephalogram nor the electromyogram shows a characteristic pattern. *C. tetani* is not always visible on Gram stain of wound material and is isolated in only about 30% of cases.

DIFFERENTIAL DIAGNOSIS

Fully developed, generalized tetanus cannot be mistaken for any other disease. However, trismus may result from parapharyngeal, retropharyngeal, or dental abscesses or, rarely, from acute encephalitis involving the brainstem. Either rabies or tetanus may follow an animal bite, and rabies may manifest as trismus with seizures. Rabies may be distinguished from tetanus by hydrophobia, marked dysphagia, predominantly clonic seizures, and pleocytosis (Chapter 266). Although strychnine poisoning may result in tonic muscle spasms and generalized seizure activity, it seldom produces trismus, and unlike in tetanus, general relaxation usually occurs between spasms. Hypocalcemia may produce tetany that is characterized by laryngeal and carpopedal spasms, but trismus is absent. Occasionally, epileptic seizures, narcotic withdrawal, or other drug reactions may suggest tetanus.

TREATMENT

Management of tetanus requires eradication of *C. tetani* and the wound environment conducive to its anaerobic multiplication, neutralization of all accessible tetanus toxin, control of seizures and respiration, palliation, provision of meticulous supportive care, and, finally, prevention of recurrences.

Surgical wound excision and debridement are often needed to remove the foreign body or devitalized tissue that created anaerobic growth conditions. Surgery should be performed promptly after administration of **human tetanus immunoglobulin** (TIG) and antibiotics. Excision of the umbilical stump in the neonate with tetanus is no longer recommended.

Tetanus toxin cannot be neutralized by TIG after it has begun its axonal ascent to the spinal cord. TIG should be given as soon as possible in order to neutralize toxin that diffuses from the wound into the circulation before the toxin can bind at distant muscle groups. The optimal dose of TIG has not been determined. A single intramuscular injection of 500 U of TIG is sufficient to neutralize systemic tetanus toxin, but total doses as high as 3,000-6,000 U are also recommended. Infiltration of TIG into the wound is now considered unnecessary. If TIG is unavailable, use of human intravenous immunoglobulin (IVIG) may be necessary. IVIG contains 4-90 U/mL of TIG; the optimal dosage of

IVIG for treating tetanus is not known, and its use is not approved for this indication. Another alternative is equine- or bovine-derived tetanus antitoxin (TAT). The usual dose of TAT is 50,000-100,000 U, with half given intramuscularly and half intravenously, but as little as 10,000 U may be sufficient. TAT is not available in the USA. Approximately 15% of patients given the usual dose of TAT experience serum sickness. When TAT is used, it is essential to check for possible sensitivity to horse serum; desensitization may be needed. The human-derived immunoglobulins are much preferred because of their longer half-lives (30 days) and the virtual absence of allergic and serum sickness adverse effects. Intrathecal TIG, given to neutralize tetanus toxin in the spinal cord, is not effective.

Penicillin G (100,000 U/kg/day divided every 4-6 hr IV for 10-14 days) remains the antibiotic of choice because of its effective clostridiocidal action and its diffusibility, which is an important consideration because blood flow to injured tissue may be compromised. Metronidazole (500 mg every 8hr IV for adults) appears to be equally effective. Erythromycin and tetracycline (for persons >8 yr of age) are alternatives for penicillin-allergic patients.

All patients with generalized tetanus need muscle relaxants. Diazepam provides both relaxation and seizure control. The initial dose of 0.1-0.2 mg/kg every 3-6 hr given intravenously is subsequently titrated to control the tetanic spasms, after which the effective dose is sustained for 2-6 wk before a tapered withdrawal. Magnesium sulfate, other benzodiazepines (midazolam), chlorpromazine, dantrolene, and baclofen are also used. Intrathecal baclofen produces such complete muscle relaxation that apnea often ensues; like most other agents listed, baclofen should be used only in an intensive care unit setting. The highest survival rates in generalized tetanus are achieved with neuromuscular blocking agents such as vecuronium and pancuronium, which produce a general flaccid paralysis that is then managed by mechanical ventilation. Autonomic instability is regulated with standard α- or β- (or both) blocking agents; morphine has also proved useful.

SUPPORTIVE CARE

Meticulous supportive care in a quiet, dark, secluded setting is most desirable. Because tetanic spasms may be triggered by minor stimuli, the patient should be sedated and protected from all unnecessary sounds, sights, and touch, and all therapeutic and other manipulations must be carefully scheduled and coordinated. Endotracheal intubation may not be required, but it should be done to prevent aspiration of secretions before laryngospasm develops. A tracheostomy kit should be immediately at hand for unintubated patients. Endotracheal intubation and suctioning easily provoke reflex tetanic seizures and spasms, so early tracheostomy should be considered in severe cases not managed by pharmacologically induced flaccid paralysis. Therapeutic botulinum toxin has been used for this purpose, that is, to overcome trismus.

Cardiorespiratory monitoring, frequent suctioning, and maintenance of the patient's substantial fluid, electrolyte, and caloric needs are fundamental. Careful nursing attention to mouth, skin, bladder, and bowel function is needed to avoid ulceration, infection, and obstipation. Prophylactic subcutaneous heparin may be of value but must be balanced with the risk for hemorrhage.

COMPLICATIONS

The seizures and the severe, sustained rigid paralysis of tetanus predispose the patient to many complications. Aspiration of secretions and pneumonia may have begun before the first medical attention was received. Maintaining airway patency often mandates endotracheal intubation and mechanical ventilation with their attendant hazards, including pneumothorax and mediastinal emphysema. The seizures may result in lacerations of the mouth or tongue, in intramuscular hematomas or rhabdomyolysis with myoglobinuria and renal failure, or in long bone or spinal fractures. Venous thrombosis, pulmonary embolism, gastric ulceration with or without hemorrhage, paralytic ileus, and decubitus ulceration are constant hazards. Excessive use of muscle relaxants, which are an integral part of care, may produce iatrogenic apnea. Cardiac arrhythmias, including asystole, unstable blood pressure, and labile temperature regulation reflect disordered autonomic nervous system control that may be aggravated by inattention to maintenance of intravascular volume needs.

PROGNOSIS

Recovery in tetanus occurs through regeneration of synapses within the spinal cord and thereby the restoration of muscle relaxation. However, because an episode of tetanus does not result in the production of toxin-neutralizing antibodies, active immunization with tetanus toxoid at discharge with provision for completion of the primary series is mandatory.

The most important factor that influences outcome is the quality of supportive care. Mortality is highest in the very young and the very old. A favorable prognosis is associated with a long incubation period, absence of fever, and localized disease. An unfavorable prognosis is associated with onset of trismus <7 days after injury and with onset of generalized tetanic spasms <3 days after onset of trismus. Sequelae of hypoxic brain injury, especially in infants, include cerebral palsy, diminished mental abilities, and behavioral difficulties. Most fatalities occur within the 1st wk of illness. Reported case fatality rates for generalized tetanus are 5-35%, and for neonatal tetanus they extend from <10% with intensive care treatment to >75% without it. Cephalic tetanus has an especially poor prognosis because of breathing and feeding difficulties.

PREVENTION

Tetanus is an entirely preventable disease. A serum antibody titer of ≥0.01 U/mL is considered protective. Active immunization should begin in early infancy with combined diphtheria toxoid–tetanus toxoid–acellular pertussis (DTaP) vaccine at 2, 4, and 6 mo of age, with a booster at 4-6 yr of age and at 10-yr intervals thereafter throughout adult life (tetanus and reduced diphtheria toxoid [Td] or tetanus, and reduced diphtheria and pertussis toxoids [Tdap]). Immunization of women with tetanus toxoid prevents neonatal tetanus, and the World Health Organization is currently engaged in a global campaign for elimination of neonatal tetanus through maternal immunization with at least 2 doses of tetanus toxoid. For unimmunized persons >7 yr of age, the primary immunization series consists of 3 doses of Td toxoid given intramuscularly, with the 2nd given 4-6 wk after the 1st and the 3rd given 6-12 mo after the 2nd.

Arthus reactions (type III hypersensitivity reactions), a localized vasculitis associated with deposition of immune complexes and activation of complement, are reported rarely after tetanus vaccination. Mass immunization campaigns in developing countries have occasionally provoked a widespread hysterical reaction.

Wound Management

Tetanus prevention measures after trauma consist of inducing active immunity to tetanus toxin and of passively providing antitoxic antibody (Table 203-1). Tetanus prophylaxis is an essential part of all wound management, but specific measures depend on

Table 203-1 TETANUS PROPHYLAXIS IN ROUTINE WOUND MANAGEMENT

HISTORY OF ABSORBED TETANUS TOXOID	CLEAN, MINOR WOUNDS Tdap or Td†	TIG‡	OTHER WOUNDS* Tdap or Td†	TIG‡
Uncertain, or <3 doses	Yes	No	Yes	Yes
3 or more doses	No§	No	No‖	No

*Such as, but not limited to, wounds contaminated with dirt, feces, and saliva; puncture wounds; avulsions; wounds resulting from missiles, crushing, burns, and frostbite.
†For children <7 yr of age, DTaP is preferred to tetanus toxoid alone if <3 doses of DTaP have been previously given. If pertussis vaccine is contraindicated, DT is given. For persons ≥7 yr of age, Td (or Tdap for adolescents 11-18 yr of age) is preferred to tetanus toxoid alone. Tdap is preferred to Td for adolescents 11-18 yr of age who have never received Tdap. Td is preferred to tetanus toxoid for adolescents who received Tdap previously or when Tdap is not available.
‡TIG should be administered for tetanus-prone wounds in HIV-infected patients regardless of the history of tetanus immunizations.
§Yes, if ≥10 yr since the last tetanus toxoid–containing vaccine dose.
‖Yes, if ≥5 yr since the last tetanus toxoid–containing vaccine dose. (More frequent boosters are not needed and can accentuate adverse events.)
DT, diphtheria and tetanus toxoid vaccine; DTaP, combined diphtheria toxoid–tetanus toxoid–acellular pertussis vaccine; Td, tetanus toxoid and reduced diphtheria toxoid vaccine; Tdap, tetanus toxoid, reduced diphtheria toxoid, and acellular pertussis vaccine; TIG, tetanus immune globulin.
Adapted from the Centers for Disease Control and Prevention: Preventing tetanus, diphtheria, and pertussis among adolescents: use of tetanus toxoid, reduced diphtheria toxoid and acellular pertussis vaccines. Recommendations of the Advisory Committee on Immunization Practices (ACIP), *MMWR Morbid Mortal Wkly Rep* 55:1–43, 2006.

the nature of the injury and the immunization status of the patient. Regrettably, prevention of tetanus must now be included in planning for the consequences of bombings and other possible civilian mass-casualty events.

Tetanus toxoid should always be given after a dog or other animal bite, even though *C. tetani* is infrequently found in canine mouth flora. All non-minor wounds require human TIG except those in a fully immunized patient. In any other circumstance (e.g., patients with an unknown or incomplete immunization history; crush, puncture, or projectile wounds; wounds contaminated with saliva, soil, or feces; avulsion injuries; compound fractures; or frostbite), TIG 250 U should be given intramuscularly, with 500 U for highly tetanus-prone wounds (i.e., unable to be debrided, with substantial bacterial contamination, or >24 hr since injury). If TIG is unavailable, use of human IGIV may be considered. If neither of these products is available, then 3,000-5,000U of equine- or bovine-derived TAT may be given intramuscularly after testing for hypersensitivity. Even at this dose, serum sickness may occur.

The wound should undergo immediate, thorough surgical cleansing and debridement to remove foreign bodies and any necrotic tissue in which anaerobic conditions might develop. Tetanus toxoid should be given to stimulate active immunity and may be administered concurrently with TIG (or TAT) if given in separate syringes at widely separated sites. A tetanus toxoid booster (preferably Td or Tdap) is administered to all persons with any wound if the tetanus immunization status is unknown or incomplete. A booster is administered to injured persons who have completed the primary immunization series if (1) the wound is clean and minor but ≥10 yr have passed since the last booster or (2) the wound is more serious and ≥5 yr have passed since the last booster. Persons who experienced an Arthus reaction after a dose of tetanus toxoid–containing vaccine should not receive Td more frequently than every 10 yr, even for tetanus prophylaxis as part of wound management. In a situation of delayed wound care, active immunization should be started at once. Although fluid tetanus toxoid produces a more rapid immune response than the absorbed or precipitated toxoids, the absorbed toxoid results in a more durable titer.

BIBLIOGRAPHY

Please visit the Nelson Textbook of Pediatrics *website at www.expertconsult.com for the complete bibliography.*

Chapter 204
Clostridium difficile Infection

Ethan A. Mezoff and Mitchell B. Cohen

Clostridium difficile **infection** (CDI), also known as *pseudomembranous colitis, antibiotic-associated diarrhea,* or *C. difficile–*associated diarrhea, refers to gastrointestinal colonization with *C. difficile* resulting in a diarrheal illness. Reports have indicated an increase in both incidence and severity of CDI.

ETIOLOGY

C. difficile is a gram-positive, anaerobic bacillus capable of forming a spore that is resistant to killing by alcohol. Organisms causing symptomatic disease produce one or both of the following: **toxin A** and **toxin B.** These toxins affect intracellular signaling pathways, resulting in inflammation and cell death. The cytotoxic **Binary toxin**, an AB toxin, is not present in the majority of strains but has been detected in recent epidemic strains.

EPIDEMIOLOGY

The incidence of CDI increased 48%, from 2.5 to 3.7 cases/1000 pediatric admissions, between 2001 and 2006. The age group most affected was 1 to 5 yr old children, with an 85% increase in CDI rates. Concurrent with this rise in incidence, disease severity has also increased, as evidenced by changes in colectomy and mortality rates in adults (thus far increases in colectomy and mortality rates have not been observed in the pediatric population).

A hypervirulent strain, denoted NAP1/BI/027, has acquired fluoroquinolone resistance, leading to outbreaks throughout North American and European hospitals. This strain produces binary toxin and exhibits 16- and 23-fold increases in the production of toxins A and B production, respectively. The specific role of this hypervirulent strain in the changing epidemiology of CDI is not yet completely understood.

Asymptomatic carriage occurs with non–toxin-producing strains as well as in neonates, who may lack the toxin receptor. Carrier frequency rates of 50% may occur in children younger than 1 yr but decline to 3% by age 2. Carriers can infect other susceptible individuals.

Risk factors for CDI include use of broad-spectrum antibiotics, hospitalization, gastrointestinal surgery, inflammatory bowel disease, chemotherapy, enteral feeding, proton pump–inhibiting agents, and chronic illness. Once thought to be exclusively a nosocomial, iatrogenic disease, CDI is increasingly recognized in the community. Half of all community-acquired cases occur in the pediatric population, and 35% of these infections occur with no history of antibiotic exposure.

PATHOGENESIS

Disease is caused by gastrointestinal infection with a toxin-producing strain. Any process that disrupts normal flora, impairs the normal gastrointestinal immune response (e.g., inflammatory bowel disease [IBD]), or inhibits intestinal motility may lead to infection. Normal bowel flora appears to be protective, conferring "colonization resistance."

By affecting intracellular signaling pathways and cytoskeletal organization, toxins induce an inflammatory response and cell death, leading to diarrhea and pseudomembrane formation. Antibodies against toxin A have been shown to confer protection from symptomatic disease, and failure of antibody production has been shown to occur in patients with recurrent disease.

CLINICAL MANIFESTATIONS

Infection with toxin-producing strains of *C. difficile* leads to a spectrum of disease ranging from mild, self-limited diarrhea to explosive, watery diarrhea with occult blood or mucous, to pseudomembranous colitis, and even death. **Pseudomembranous colitis** describes a bloody diarrhea with accompanying fever, abdominal pain/cramps, nausea, and vomiting. Rarely, small gut involvement, bacteremia, abscess formation, toxic megacolon, and even death can occur.

Symptoms of CDI generally begin less than a week after colonization and may develop during or weeks after antibiotic exposure. They are generally more severe in certain populations, including patients receiving chemotherapy, patients with chronic gastrointestinal disease (e.g., IBD), and some patients with cystic fibrosis.

DIAGNOSIS

CDI is diagnosed by the detection of a *C. difficile* **toxin** in the stool of a symptomatic patient. Most patients present with a history of recent antibiotic use, but the absence of antibiotic exposure should not dissuade the astute clinician from considering this diagnosis and ordering the appropriate test.

The standard for toxin detection is the tissue culture cytotoxicity assay. This assay detects only toxin B and requires 24-48 hr. It has been supplanted in most clinical laboratories by the enzyme immunoassay, which requires less time, a lower level of expertise, and less expense. The enzyme immunoassay is a same-day test for one or both toxins with sufficient specificity (94-100%) but less than ideal sensitivity (88-93%). Toxin detection rates shift by age group, from predominantly toxin A in neonates to predominantly toxin B in adolescence. Accordingly, testing for both toxins is recommended in pediatric populations to reduce the rate of false-negative results.

Stool culture is a sensitive test, but it is not specific, as it does not differentiate between toxin-producing and non–toxin-producing strains. Pseudomembranous nodules and characteristic plaques may be seen on colonoscopy or sigmoidoscopy.

TREATMENT

Initial treatment of CDI involves discontinuation of any nonvital antibiotic therapy and administration of fluid/electrolyte replacement. For mild cases, this treatment may be curative. Persistent symptoms or moderate to severe disease warrants antimicrobial therapy directed against *C. difficile*.

Oral metronidazole (20-40 mg/kg/day by mouth [PO] divided every 6-8 hr for 7-10 days) works well in mild to moderate infection. It is the least expensive approach, though studies comparing it to vancomycin have shown a significantly longer time to symptom resolution as well as a higher failure rate when metronidazole is use to treat severe disease. Vancomycin (25-40 mg/kg/day PO divided every 6 hrs for 7-10 days) is the only therapy approved by the U.S. Food and Drug Administration for use against infection with *C. difficile*. Vancomycin exhibits ideal pharmacologic properties for treatment of this enteric pathogen, as it is not absorbed in the gut. This agent is suggested as a first-line agent for severe disease as manifested by hypotension, peripheral leukocytosis, or severe pseudomembranous colitis. A concern about using it as first line therapy in all cases is the potential for emergence of vancomycin-resistant enterococci (VRE). Nitazoxanide and fidaxomicin are other agents that are effective in treating CDI in adults.

PROGNOSIS

The response rate to initial treatment of CDI is greater than 95%; however, both the treatment failure rate and recurrence rate have increased over the last two decades. Additionally, the risk of subsequent reappearance increases with each recurrence.

Initial recurrence rates are between 5% and 30%, and CDIs generally recur within 4 wk of treatment. Some recurrences are due to incomplete eradication of the original strain, and others to reinfection with a different strain. Treatment for the initial recurrence involves retreatment with the original antibiotic course.

Multiple recurrences of CDI may be due to a suboptimal immune response, failure to kill organisms that have sporulated, or failure of delivery of antibiotic to the site of infection in the case of ileus or toxic megacolon. In the case of the first two causes, treatment with pulsed or tapered vancomycin has been shown to decrease recurrence rates. In addition to this approach, other antibiotics (rifaximin or nitazoxanide), toxin-binding polymers (Tolevamer), fecal transplantation, and probiotics (*Saccharomyces boulardii* or *Lactobacillus* GG) have been used. Though not well studied in children, *S. boulardii* has been shown to significantly decrease recurrence rates when used as an adjunct to vancomycin therapy in adults. Because failure to manifest an adequate antitoxin immune response is associated with a higher frequency of recurrent CDI, intravenous immune globulin (IVIG) has been used to treat recurrent disease. In the case of ileus or toxic megacolon, an enema of vancomycin may be used to directly place the antibiotic at the site of infection, although most often intravenous therapy is first attempted in this circumstance.

It is important to recognize that postinfectious diarrhea may be due to other causes. Examples are post-infectious irritable bowel syndrome, microscopic colitis, and IBD. A test of cure is not recommended in the asymptomatic patient.

PREVENTION

Strategies for prevention of CDI include the following: recognition of common sites of acquisition (hospitals, childcare settings, extended care facilities), effective environmental cleaning (i.e., use of chlorinated cleaning solutions), appropriate antibiotic prescription practices, cohorting of infected patients, and proper handwashing with soap and water.

BIBLIOGRAPHY

Please visit the Nelson Textbook of Pediatrics *website at www.expertconsult.com for the complete bibliography.*

Chapter 205
Other Anaerobic Infections

Michael J. Chusid

Anaerobic bacteria are among the most numerous organisms colonizing humans. Anaerobes are present in soil and are normal inhabitants of all living animals, but infections caused by anaerobes are relatively uncommon. Anaerobes are relatively or entirely intolerant of exposure to oxygen. Most are **facultative anaerobes**, being able to survive in the presence of oxygen but growing better in reduced oxygen tensions. **Obligate anaerobes** cannot survive any exposure to oxygen.

For the full continuation of this chapter, please visit the Nelson Textbook of Pediatrics *website at www.expertconsult.com.*

Section 7 MYCOBACTERIAL INFECTIONS

Chapter 206
Principles of Antimycobacterial Therapy

Stacene R. Maroushek

The treatment of mycobacterial infection and disease can be challenging. Patients require therapy with multiple agents, the offending pathogens commonly exhibit complex drug resistance patterns, and patients often have underlying conditions that affect drug choice and monitoring. Several of the drugs have not been well studied in children, and current recommendations are extrapolated from the experience in adults.

For the full continuation of this chapter, please visit the Nelson Textbook of Pediatrics *website at www.expertconsult.com.*

Chapter 207
Tuberculosis (*Mycobacterium tuberculosis*)

Jeffrey R. Starke

During the last decade of the 20th century the number of new cases of tuberculosis increased worldwide. Currently, 95% of tuberculosis cases occur in developing countries where HIV/AIDS epidemics have had the greatest impact and where resources are often unavailable for proper identification and treatment of these diseases (Figs. 207-1 and 207-2). In many industrialized countries, most cases of tuberculosis occur in foreign-born populations (Figs. 207-3 and 207-4). The World Health Organization (WHO) estimates that >8 million new cases of tuberculosis occur and that approximately 2 million people die of tuberculosis worldwide each year. Almost 1.3 million cases and 450,000 deaths occur in children each year. More than 30% of the world's population is infected with *Mycobacterium tuberculosis*. If present trends continue, 10 million new cases are expected to occur annually by 2010, with Africa having more cases than any other region of the world (see Fig. 207-1). In the USA, after a resurgence in the late 1980s, the total number of cases of tuberculosis began to decrease in 1992, but tuberculosis continues to be a public health concern (see Fig. 207-3).

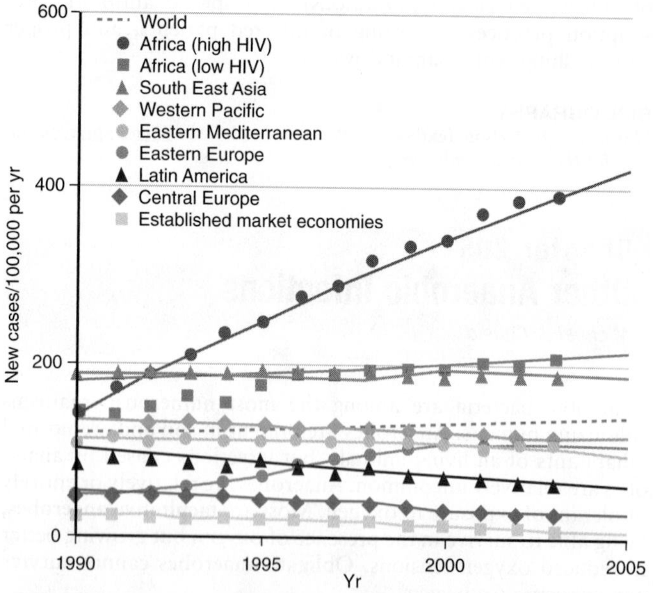

Figure 207-1 Trajectories of tuberculosis epidemic for 9 epidemiologically different regions of the world. Points mark trends in estimated incidence rates, derived from case notifications for 1990-2003. Groupings of countries based on WHO regions. High HIV = incidence >4% in adults aged 15-49 yr in 2003; low HIV = <4%. Established market economies = all 30 OECD (Organization for Economic Co-operation and Development) countries, except Mexico, Slovakia, and Turkey, plus Singapore. Countries in each region are listed in full elsewhere. (From Dye C: Global epidemiology of tuberculosis, *Lancet* 367:938–940, 2006.)

ETIOLOGY

There are 5 closely related mycobacteria in the *M. tuberculosis* complex: *M. tuberculosis, M. bovis, M. africanum, M. microti,* and *M. canetti. M. tuberculosis* is the most important cause of tuberculosis disease in humans. The tubercle bacilli are non–spore-forming, nonmotile, pleomorphic, weakly gram-positive curved rods 2-4 µm long. They can appear beaded or clumped in stained clinical specimens or culture media. They are obligate aerobes that grow in synthetic media containing glycerol as the carbon source and ammonium salts as the nitrogen source (Loewenstein-Jensen culture media). These mycobacteria grow best at 37-41°C, produce niacin, and lack pigmentation. A lipid-rich cell wall accounts for resistance to the bactericidal actions of antibody and complement. A hallmark of all mycobacteria is **acid fastness**—the capacity to form stable mycolate complexes with arylmethane dyes such as crystal violet, carbolfuchsin, auramine, and rhodamine. Once stained, they resist decoloration with ethanol and hydrochloric or other acids.

Mycobacteria grow slowly, with a generation time of 12-24 hr. Isolation from clinical specimens on solid synthetic media usually takes 3-6 wk, and drug susceptibility testing requires an additional 4 wk. Growth can be detected in 1-3 wk in selective liquid medium using radiolabeled nutrients (e.g., the BACTEC radiometric system), and drug susceptibilities can be determined in an additional 3-5 days. Once mycobacterial growth is detected, the species of mycobacteria present can be determined within hours using high-pressure liquid chromatography analysis (based on the fact that each species has a unique fingerprint of mycolic acids) or DNA probes. The presence of *M. tuberculosis* in clinical specimens sometimes can be detected directly within hours using **nucleic acid amplification** (**NAA**) tests (including polymerase chain reaction) that employ a DNA probe complementary to mycobacterial DNA or RNA. Data from children are limited, but the sensitivity of some NAA techniques is similar to that for culture for pulmonary tuberculosis and is better than culture for extrapulmonary disease. Restriction fragment length polymorphism (RFLP) profiling of mycobacteria is a helpful tool to study the epidemiology of tuberculosis.

EPIDEMIOLOGY

Latent tuberculosis infection (**LTBI**) occurs after the inhalation of infective droplet nuclei containing *M. tuberculosis*. A reactive tuberculin skin test (TST) and the absence of clinical and radiographic manifestations are the hallmark of this stage. The word *tuberculosis* refers to disease that occurs when signs and symptoms or radiographic changes become apparent. Untreated infants with LTBI have up to a 40% likelihood of developing tuberculosis, with the risk for progression decreasing gradually

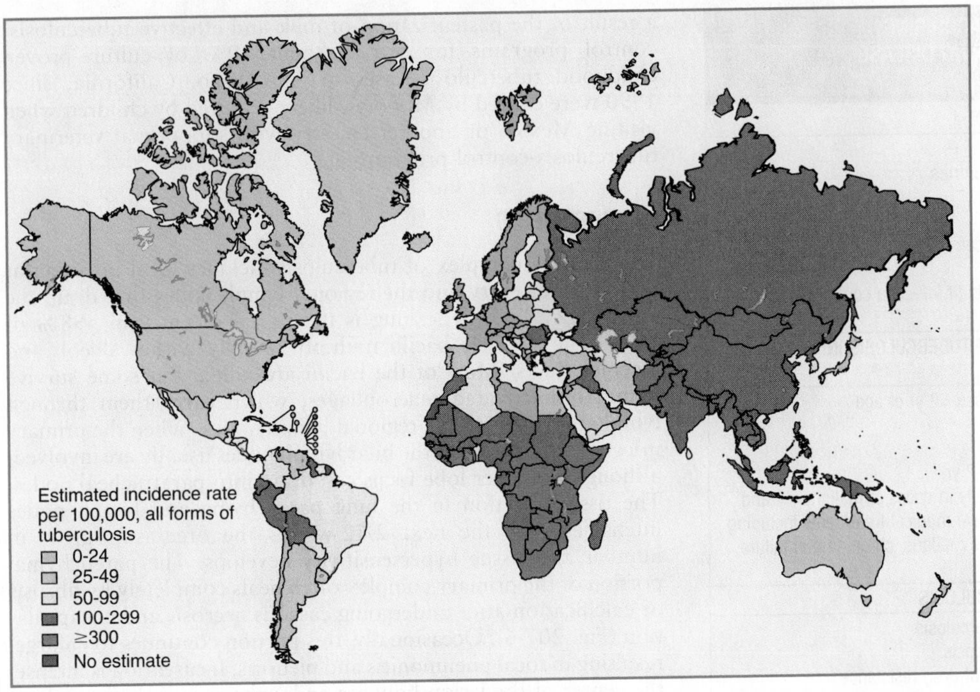

Figure 207-2 Distribution of tuberculosis in the world in 2003. (From Dye C: Global epidemiology of tuberculosis, *Lancet* 367:938–940, 2006.)

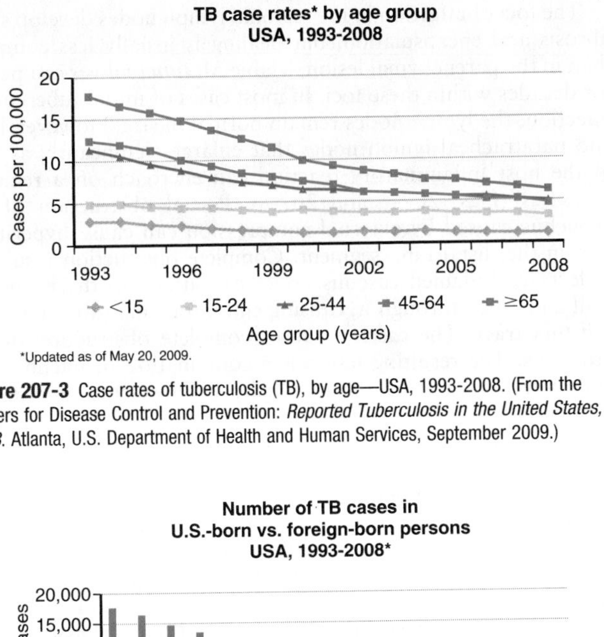

Figure 207-3 Case rates of tuberculosis (TB), by age—USA, 1993-2008. (From the Centers for Disease Control and Prevention: *Reported Tuberculosis in the United States, 2008.* Atlanta, U.S. Department of Health and Human Services, September 2009.)

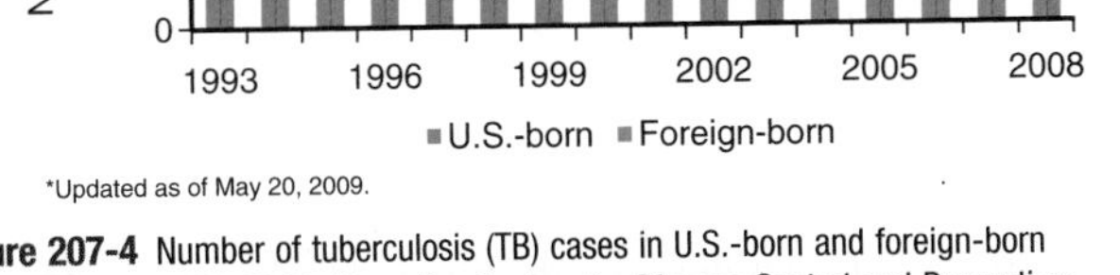

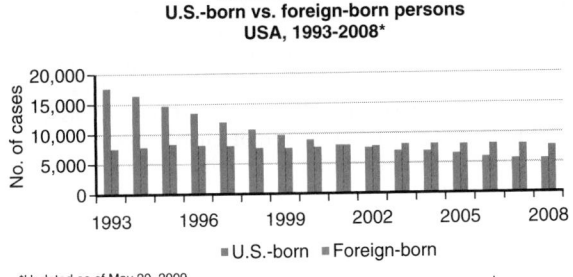

Figure 207-4 Number of tuberculosis (TB) cases in U.S.-born and foreign-born persons—USA, 1993-2008. (From the Centers for Disease Control and Prevention: *Reported Tuberculosis in the United States, 2008.* Atlanta, U.S. Department of Health and Human Services, September 2009.)

through childhood to adult lifetime rates of 5-10%. The greatest risk for progression occurs in the first 2 yr after infection.

The World Health Organization estimates that 30% of the world's population (2 billion people) are infected with *M. tuberculosis.* Infection rates are highest in Africa, Asia, and Latin America (see Fig. 207-2). The global burden of tuberculosis continues to grow owing to several factors, including the impact of HIV epidemics, population migration patterns, increasing poverty, social upheaval and crowded living conditions in developing countries and in inner city populations in developed countries, inadequate health coverage and poor access to health services, and inefficient tuberculosis control programs.

Tuberculosis case rates decreased steadily in the USA during the 1st half of the 20th century, long before the advent of antituberculosis drugs, as a result of improved living conditions and, likely, genetic selection favoring persons resistant to developing disease. A resurgence of tuberculosis in the late 1980s was associated primarily with the HIV epidemic and transmission of the organism in congregate settings, adding to increased immigration and poor tuberculosis control (see Fig. 207-3). Since 1992, the number of reported cases of tuberculosis has decreased each year, reaching a record low of 12,904 cases (rate of 4.2/100,000 population) in the year 2008. Of these, 786 (6.1%) cases occurred in children <15 yr of age (rate 1.3/100,000 population). The decline in overall incidence was mostly due to a substantial decrease in cases in persons born in the USA. About 59% of all cases were among foreign-born persons. The total number of cases among foreign-born persons increased 5% between 1992 and 2005 (see Fig. 207-4). In all age groups, the proportion of reported cases was strikingly higher in foreign-born and nonwhite persons, even though the number of cases among foreign-born children <15 yr of age has declined. In white populations in the USA, tuberculosis rates are highest among the elderly who acquired the infection decades ago. In contrast, among nonwhite populations, tuberculosis is most common in young adults and children <5 yr of age. The age range of 5-14 yr is often called the "favored age," because in all human populations this group has the lowest rate of tuberculosis disease. Among adults two thirds of cases occur in men, but in children there is no significant difference in sex distribution.

In the USA, most children are infected with *M. tuberculosis* in their home by someone close to them, but outbreaks of childhood tuberculosis also occur in elementary and high schools, nursery schools, daycare centers and homes, churches, school buses, and sports teams. HIV-infected adults with tuberculosis can transmit *M. tuberculosis* to children, and children with HIV infection are at increased risk for developing tuberculosis after infection. Specific groups are at high risk for acquiring tuber-

Table 207-1 GROUPS AT HIGH RISK FOR ACQUIRING TUBERCULOSIS INFECTION AND DEVELOPING DISEASE IN COUNTRIES WITH LOW INCIDENCE
RISK FACTORS FOR TUBERCULOSIS INFECTION
Children exposed to high-risk adults Foreign-born persons from high-prevalence countries Homeless persons Persons who inject drugs Present and former residents or employees of correctional institutions, homeless shelters, and nursing homes Health care workers caring for high-risk patients (if infection control is not adequate)
RISK FACTORS FOR PROGRESSION OF LATENT TUBERCULOSIS INFECTION TO TUBERCULOSIS DISEASE
Infants and children ≤4 yr of age, especially those <2 yr of age Adolescents and young adults Persons co-infected with HIV Persons with skin test conversion in the past 1-2 yr Persons who are immunocompromised, especially in cases of malignancy and solid organ transplantation, immunosuppressive medical treatments including anti–tumor necrosis factor therapies, diabetes mellitus, chronic renal failure, silicosis, and malnutrition
RISK FACTORS FOR DRUG-RESISTANT TUBERCULOSIS
Personal or contact history of treatment for tuberculosis Contacts of patients with drug-resistant tuberculosis Birth or residence in a country with a high rate of drug resistance Poor response to standard therapy Positive sputum smears (acid-fast bacilli) or culture ≥2 month after initiating appropriate therapy

culosis infection and progressing from LTBI to tuberculosis (Table 207-1).

The incidence of **drug-resistant** tuberculosis has increased dramatically throughout the world. In the USA, about 8% of *M. tuberculosis* isolates are resistant to at least isoniazid, whereas 1% are resistant to both isoniazid and rifampin. Resistance to isoniazid remained relatively stable between 1992 and 2008, as did the proportion of cases that were multidrug resistant (about 1%). In some countries, drug resistance rates range from 20% to 50%. The major reasons for the development of drug resistance are the patient's poor adherence to treatment and provision of inadequate drug regimens by the physician or national tuberculosis program.

TRANSMISSION

Transmission of *M. tuberculosis* is person to person, usually by airborne mucus droplet nuclei, particles 1-5 µm in diameter that contain *M. tuberculosis*. Transmission rarely occurs by direct contact with an infected discharge or a contaminated fomite. The chance of transmission increases when the patient has a positive acid-fast smear of sputum, an extensive upper lobe infiltrate or cavity, copious production of thin sputum, and severe and forceful cough. Environmental factors such as poor air circulation enhance transmission. Most adults no longer transmit the organism within several days to 2 weeks after beginning adequate chemotherapy, but some patients remain infectious for many weeks. Young children with tuberculosis rarely infect other children or adults. Tubercle bacilli are sparse in the endobronchial secretions of children with pulmonary tuberculosis, and cough is often absent or lacks the tussive force required to suspend infectious particles of the correct size. Children and adolescents with adult-type cavitary or endobronchial pulmonary tuberculosis can transmit the organism. Airborne transmission of *M. bovis* and *M. africanum* can also occur. *M. bovis* can penetrate the gastrointestinal (GI) mucosa or invade the lymphatic tissue of the oropharynx when large numbers of the organism are ingested. Human infection with *M. bovis* is rare in developed countries as a result of the pasteurization of milk and effective tuberculosis-control programs for cattle. About 30% of culture-proven childhood tuberculosis cases in San Diego, California, since 1990 were caused by *M. bovis,* likely acquired by children when visiting Mexico or another country with suboptimal veterinary tuberculosis-control programs.

PATHOGENESIS

The primary complex of tuberculosis includes local infection at the portal of entry and the regional lymph nodes that drain the area (Fig. 207-5). The lung is the portal of entry in >98% of cases. The tubercle bacilli multiply initially within alveoli and alveolar ducts. Most of the bacilli are killed, but some survive within nonactivated macrophages, which carry them through lymphatic vessels to the regional lymph nodes. When the primary infection is in the lung, the hilar lymph nodes usually are involved, although an upper lobe focus can drain into paratracheal nodes. The tissue reaction in the lung parenchyma and lymph nodes intensifies over the next 2-12 wk as the organisms grow in number and tissue **hypersensitivity** develops. The parenchymal portion of the primary complex often heals completely by fibrosis or calcification after undergoing caseous necrosis and encapsulation (Fig. 207-6). Occasionally, this portion continues to enlarge, resulting in focal pneumonitis and pleuritis. If caseation is intense, the center of the lesion liquefies and empties into the associated bronchus, leaving a residual cavity.

The foci of infection in the regional lymph nodes develop some fibrosis and encapsulation, but healing is usually less complete than in the parenchymal lesion. Viable *M. tuberculosis* can persist for decades within these foci. In most cases of initial tuberculosis infection, the lymph nodes remain normal in size. However, hilar and paratracheal lymph nodes that enlarge significantly as part of the host inflammatory reaction can encroach on a regional bronchus (Figs. 207-7 and 207-8). Partial obstruction of the bronchus caused by external compression can cause hyperinflation in the distal lung segment. Complete obstruction results in atelectasis. Inflamed caseous nodes can attach to the bronchial wall and erode through it, causing endobronchial tuberculosis or a fistula tract. The caseum causes complete obstruction of the bronchus. The resulting lesion is a combination of pneumonitis and atelectasis and has been called a **collapse-consolidation** or **segmental lesion** (Fig. 207-9).

During the development of the **primary complex (Ghon complex)**, which is the combination of a parenchymal pulmonary lesion and a corresponding lymph node site, tubercle bacilli are often carried to most tissues of the body through the blood and lymphatic vessels. Although seeding of the organs of the reticuloendothelial system is common, bacterial replication is more likely to occur in organs with conditions that favor their growth, such as the lung apices, brain, kidneys, and bones. **Disseminated tuberculosis** occurs if the number of circulating bacilli is large and the host's cellular immune response is inadequate. More often the number of bacilli is small, leading to clinically inapparent metastatic foci in many organs. These remote foci usually become encapsulated, but they may be the origin of both extrapulmonary tuberculosis and reactivation tuberculosis in some persons.

The time between initial infection and clinically apparent disease is variable. Disseminated and meningeal tuberculosis are early manifestations, often occurring within 2-6 mo of acquisition. Significant lymph node or endobronchial tuberculosis usually appears within 3-9 mo. Lesions of the bones and joints take several years to develop, whereas renal lesions become evident decades after infection. Extrapulmonary manifestations develop in 25-35% of children with tuberculosis, compared with about 10% of immunocompetent adults with tuberculosis.

Pulmonary tuberculosis that occurs >1 yr after the primary infection is usually caused by endogenous regrowth of bacilli

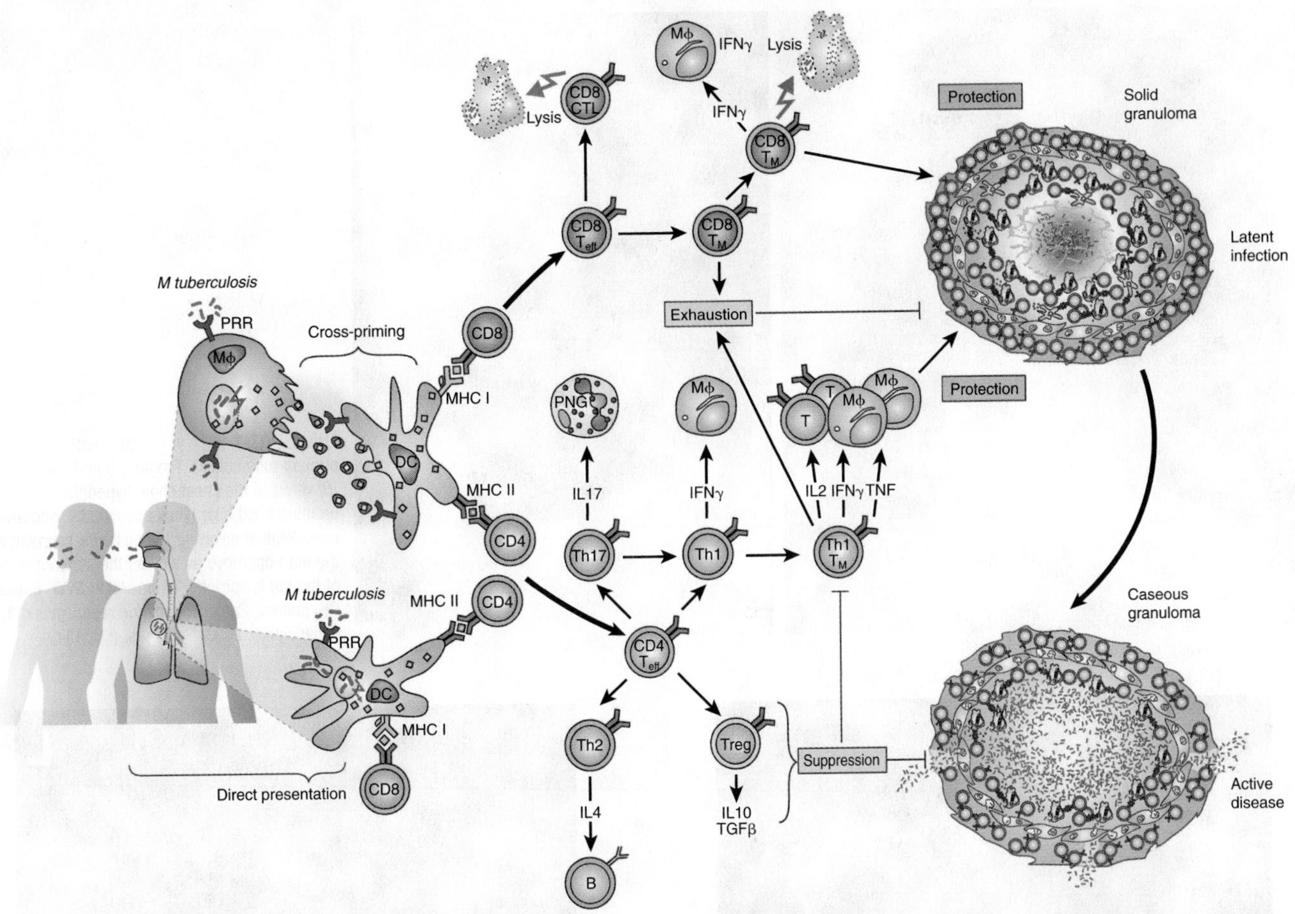

Figure 207-5 Overview of the immune response in tuberculosis. Control of *Mycobacterium tuberculosis* is mainly the result of productive teamwork between T-cell populations and macrophages (Mφ). *M. tuberculosis* survives within macrophages and dendritic cells (DCs) inside the phagosomal compartment. Gene products of MHC class II are loaded with mycobacterial peptides that are presented to CD4 T cells. CD8 T-cell stimulation requires loading of MHC I molecules by mycobacterial peptides in the cytosol, either by egression of mycobacterial antigens into the cytosol or cross-priming, by which macrophages release apoptotic bodies carrying mycobacterial peptides. These vesicles are taken up by DCs and peptides presented. The CD4 T-helper (Th) cells polarize into different subsets. DCs and macrophages express pattern recognition receptors (PRRs), which sense molecular patterns on pathogens. Th1 cells produce IL-2 for T-cell activation, interferon-γ (IFN-γ), or tumor necrosis factor (TNF) for macrophage activation. Th17 cells, which activate polymorphonuclear granulocytes (PNGs), contribute to the early formation of protective immunity in the lung after vaccination. Th2 cells and regulatory T cells (Treg) counter-regulate Th1-mediated protection via IL4, transforming growth factor β (TGF-β), or IL10. CD8 T cells produce IFN-γ and TNF, which activate macrophages. They also act as cytolytic T lymphocytes (CTL) by secreting perforin and granulysin, which lyse host cells and directly attack *M. tuberculosis.* These effector T cells (T_{eff}) are succeeded by memory T cells T_M). T_M cells produce multiple cytokines, notably IL2, IFN-γ, and TNF. During active containment in solid granuloma, *M. tuberculosis* recesses into a dormant stage and is immune to attack. Exhaustion of T cells is mediated by interactions between T cells and DCs through members of the programmed death 1 system. Treg cells secrete IL10 and TGF-β, which suppress Th1. This process allows resuscitation of *M. tuberculosis*, which leads to granuloma caseation and active disease. B, B cell. (From Kaufman SHE, Hussey G, Lambert PH: New vaccines for tuberculosis. *Lancet* 375:2110–2118, 2010.)

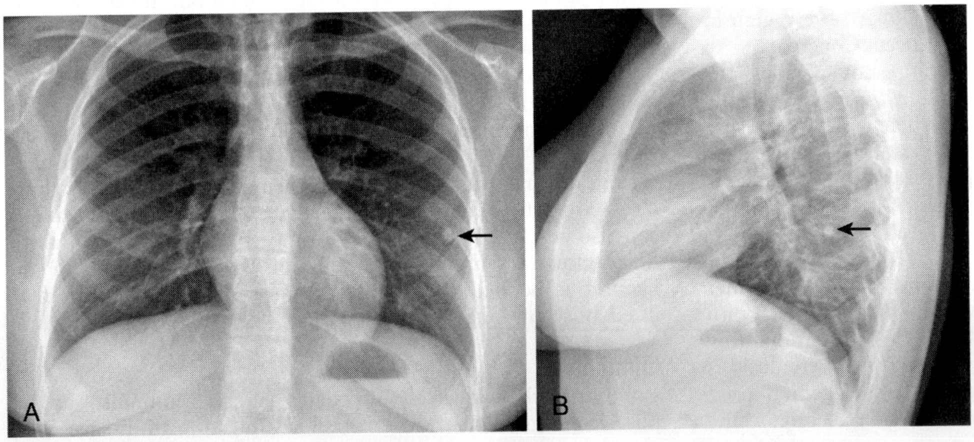

Figure 207-6 *A* and *B*, Posteroanterior and lateral chest radiograph images of an adolescent showing a 7-mm calcified granuloma in the left lower lobe *(arrows).* (From Lighter J, Rigaud M: Diagnosing childhood tuberculosis: traditional and innovative modalities, *Curr Prob Pediatr Adolesc Health Care* 39:55–88, 2009.)

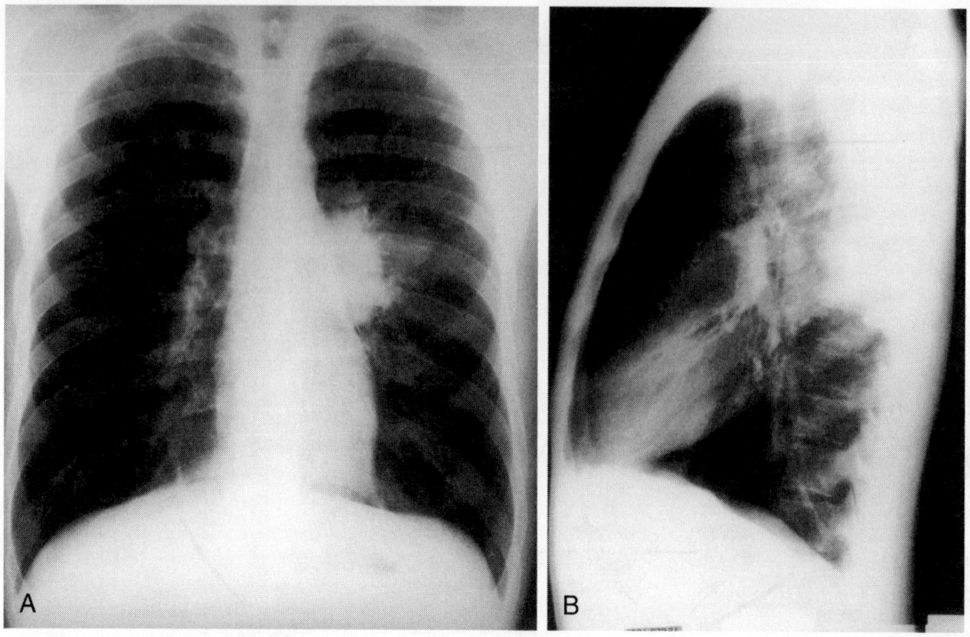

Figure 207-7 A 14 yr old child with proven primary tuberculosis. Frontal *(A)* and lateral *(B)* views of the chest show hyperinflation, prominent left hilar lymphadenopathy, and alveolar consolidation involving the posterior segment of the left upper love as well as the superior segment of the left lower lobe. (From Hilton SVW, Edwards DK, editors: *Practical pediatric radiology,* ed 3, Philadelphia, 2003, Saunders, p 334.)

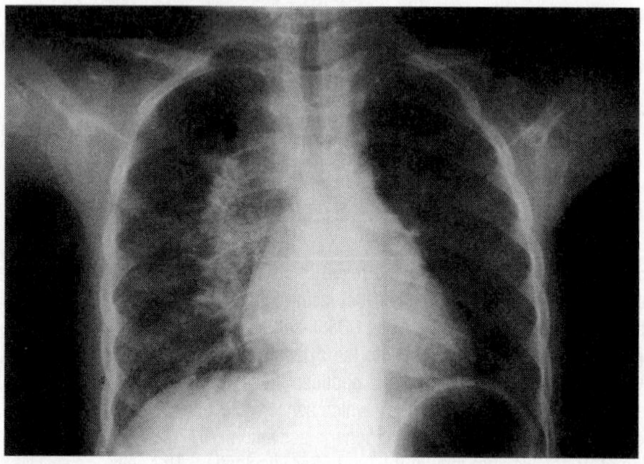

Figure 207-8 An 8 yr old child with a history of cough. A single frontal view of the chest shows marked right hilar and paratracheal lymphadenopathy with alveolar disease involving the right middle and lower lung fields. This was also a case of primary tuberculosis. (From Hilton SVW, Edwards DK, editors: *Practical pediatric radiology,* ed 3, Philadelphia, 2003, Saunders, p 335.)

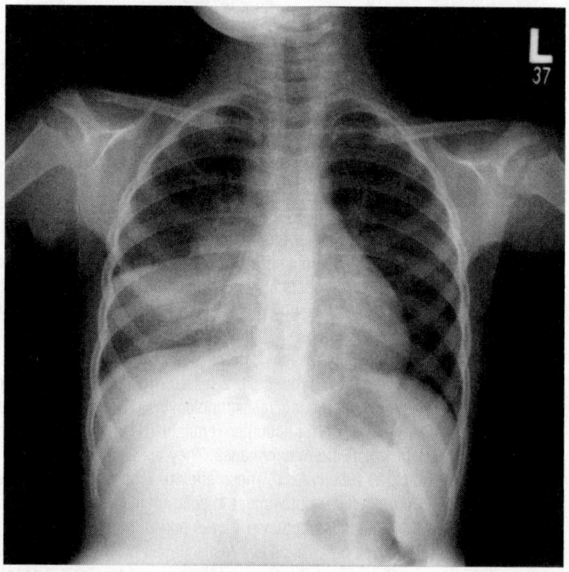

Figure 207-9 Right-sided hilar lymphadenopathy and collapse-consolidation lesions of primary tuberculosis in a 4 yr old child.

persisting in partially encapsulated lesions. This **reactivation tuberculosis** is rare in children but is common among adolescents and young adults. The most common form is an infiltrate or cavity in the apex of the upper lobes, where oxygen tension and blood flow are great.

The risk for dissemination of *M. tuberculosis* is very high in HIV-infected persons. Reinfection also can occur in persons with advanced HIV or AIDS. In immunocompetent persons the response to the initial infection with *M. tuberculosis* usually provides protection against reinfection when a new exposure occurs. However, exogenous reinfection has been reported to occur in adults without immune compromise in highly endemic areas.

Pregnancy and the Newborn

Pulmonary and particularly extrapulmonary tuberculosis other than lymphadenitis in a pregnant woman is associated with increased risk for prematurity, fetal growth retardation, low birthweight, and perinatal mortality. Congenital tuberculosis is rare because the most common result of female genital tract tuberculosis is infertility. Congenital transmission usually occurs from a lesion in the placenta through the umbilical vein. Primary infection in the mother just before or during pregnancy is more likely to cause congenital infection than is reactivation of a previous infection. The tubercle bacilli first reach the fetal liver, where a primary focus with periportal lymph node involvement can occur. Organisms pass through the liver into the main fetal circulation and infect many organs. The bacilli in the lung usually remain dormant until after birth, when oxygenation and pulmonary circulation increase significantly. Congenital tuberculosis can also be caused by aspiration or ingestion of infected amniotic fluid. However, the most common route of infection for the neonate is postnatal airborne transmission from an adult with infectious pulmonary tuberculosis.

Immunity

Conditions that adversely affect cell-mediated immunity predispose to progression from tuberculosis infection to disease. Rare specific genetic defects associated with deficient cell-mediated immunity in response to mycobacteria include interleukin (IL)-12 receptor B1 deficiency and complete and partial interferon-γ (IFN-γ) receptor 1 chain deficiencies. Tuberculosis infection is associated with a humoral antibody response, which appears to play little role in host defense. Shortly after infection, tubercle bacilli replicate in both free alveolar spaces and within inactivated alveolar macrophages. Sulfatides in the mycobacterial cell wall inhibit fusion of the macrophage phagosome and lysosomes, allowing the organisms to escape destruction by intracellular enzymes. **Cell-mediated immunity** develops 2-12 wk after infection, along with tissue hypersensitivity (see Fig. 207-6). After bacilli enter macrophages, lymphocytes that recognize mycobacterial antigens proliferate and secrete lymphokines and other mediators that attract other lymphocytes and macrophages to the area. Certain lymphokines activate macrophages, causing them to develop high concentrations of lytic enzymes that enhance their mycobactericidal capacity. A discrete subset of regulator helper and suppressor lymphocytes modulates the immune response. Development of specific cellular immunity prevents progression of the initial infection in most persons.

The pathologic events in the initial tuberculosis infection seem to depend on the balance among the mycobacterial antigen load; cell-mediated immunity, which enhances intracellular killing; and tissue hypersensitivity, which promotes extracellular killing. When the antigen load is small and the degree of tissue sensitivity is high, granuloma formation results from the organization of lymphocytes, macrophages, and fibroblasts. When both antigen load and the degree of sensitivity are high, granuloma formation is less organized. Tissue necrosis is incomplete, resulting in formation of caseous material. When the degree of tissue sensitivity is low, as is often the case in infants or immunocompromised persons, the reaction is diffuse and the infection is not well contained, leading to dissemination and local tissue destruction. Tumor necrosis factor (TNF) and other cytokines released by specific lymphocytes promote cellular destruction and tissue damage in susceptible persons.

Tuberculin Skin Testing

The development of delayed-type hypersensitivity (DTH) in most persons infected with the tubercle bacillus makes the TST a useful diagnostic tool. The **Mantoux TST** is the intradermal injection of 0.1 mL purified protein derivative (PPD) stabilized with Tween 80. T cells sensitized by prior infection are recruited to the skin, where they release lymphokines that induce induration through local vasodilatation, edema, fibrin deposition, and recruitment of other inflammatory cells to the area. The amount of induration in response to the test should be measured by a trained person 48-72 hr after administration. In some patients the onset of induration is >72 hr after placement; this is also a positive result. Immediate hypersensitivity reactions to tuberculin or other constituents of the preparation are short lived (<24 hr) and not considered a positive result. Tuberculin sensitivity develops 3 wk to 3 mo (most often in 4-8 wk) after inhalation of organisms.

Host-related factors can depress the skin test reaction in a child infected with *M. tuberculosis,* including very young age, malnutrition, immunosuppression by disease or drugs, viral infections (measles, mumps, varicella, influenza), vaccination with live-virus vaccines, and overwhelming tuberculosis. Corticosteroid therapy can decrease the reaction to tuberculin, but the effect is variable. TST done at the time of initiating corticosteroid therapy is usually reliable. Approximately 10% of immunocompetent children with tuberculosis disease (up to 50% of those with meningitis or disseminated disease) do not react initially to PPD; most become reactive after several months of antituberculosis therapy. Nonreactivity may be specific to tuberculin or more global to a variety of antigens, so positive "control" skin tests with a negative tuberculin test never rule out tuberculosis. The other common reasons for a false-negative skin test are poor technique and misreading of the results.

False-positive reactions to tuberculin can be caused by cross sensitization to antigens of nontuberculous mycobacteria (NTM), which generally are more prevalent in the environment as one approaches the equator. These cross reactions are usually transient over months to years and produce less than 10-12 mm of induration. Previous vaccination with bacille Calmette-Guérin (BCG) also can cause a reaction to a TST, especially if 2 or more BCG vaccinations have been given. Approximately 50% of the infants who receive a BCG vaccine never develop a reactive TST, and the reactivity usually wanes in 2-3 yr in those with initially positive skin test results. Older children and adults who receive a BCG vaccine are more likely to develop tuberculin reactivity, but most lose the reactivity by 5-10 yr after vaccination. When skin test reactivity is present, it usually causes <10 mm of induration, although larger reactions occur in some persons. In general in the USA, a tuberculin skin reaction of ≥10 mm in a BCG-vaccinated child or adult is considered positive and necessitates further diagnostic evaluation and treatment, although many such patients do not have LTBI. Prior vaccination with BCG is never a contraindication to tuberculin testing.

The appropriate size of induration indicating a positive Mantoux TST result varies with related epidemiologic and risk factors. In children with no risk factors for tuberculosis, skin test reactions are usually false-positive results. The American Academy of Pediatrics (AAP) and Centers for Disease Control and Prevention (CDC) discourage routine testing of children and recommend targeted tuberculin testing of children at risk identified through periodic screening surveys conducted by the primary care provider (Table 207-2). Possible exposure to an adult with or at high risk for infectious pulmonary tuberculosis is the most crucial risk factor for children. Reaction size limits for determining a positive tuberculin test result vary with the person's risk for infection (Table 207-3). For adults and children at the highest risk for having infection progress to disease (those with recent contact with infectious persons, clinical illnesses consistent with tuberculosis, or HIV infection or other immunosuppression), a reactive area of ≥5 mm is classified as a positive result, indicating infection with *M. tuberculosis.* For other high-risk groups, a reactive area of ≥10 mm is considered positive. For low-risk persons, especially those residing in communities where the prevalence of tuberculosis is low, the cutoff point for a positive reaction is ≥15 mm. An increase of induration of ≥10 mm within a 2-yr period is considered a TST conversion at any age.

Interferon-γ Release Assays

Two blood tests (T-SPOT.TB and QuantiFERON-TB) detect IFN-γ generation by the patient's T cells in response to specific *M. tuberculosis* antigens (ESAT-6, CFP-10, and TB7.7). The QuantiFERON-TB test measures whole blood concentrations of IFN-γ, and the T-SPOT.TB test measures the number of lymphocytes producing IFN-γ. The test antigens are not present on *M. bovis*–BCG and *M. avium* complex, the major groups of environmental mycobacteria, so one would expect fewer false-positive results. Both tests have internal positive and negative controls. These tests have several theoretical and practical advantages over the TST, including the need for only one patient encounter, lack of cross reaction with BCG vaccination and most other mycobacteria, and absence of boosting (increasing reaction to the TST with serial testing).

When specificity is important, such as in persons who received a BCG vaccination, the IFN-γ release assays (IGRAs) are the preferred test. However, IGRAs should be interpreted with caution when used for children <5 yr of age and immunocompromised patients owing to the relative lack of data and the increased propensity for indeterminate results (mostly owing to failure of the positive control) in these groups.

Table 207-2 TUBERCULIN SKIN TEST (TST) OR INTERFERON-γ RELEASE ASSAY (IGRA) RECOMMENDATIONS FOR INFANTS, CHILDREN, AND ADOLESCENTS*

Children for whom immediate TST or IGRA is indicated[†]: • Contacts of people with confirmed or suspected contagious tuberculosis (contact investigation) • Children with radiographic or clinical findings suggesting tuberculosis disease • Children immigrating from countries with endemic infection (e.g., Asia, Middle East, Africa, Latin America, countries of the former Soviet Union) including international adoptees • Children with travel histories to countries with endemic infection and substantial contact with indigenous people from such countries[‡]
Children who should have annual TST or IGRA: • Children infected with HIV • Incarcerated adolescents
CHILDREN AT INCREASED RISK FOR PROGRESSION OF LTBI TO TUBERCULOSIS DISEASE
Children with other medical conditions, including diabetes mellitus, chronic renal failure, malnutrition, and congenital or acquired immunodeficiencies deserve special consideration. Without recent exposure, these children are not at increased risk of acquiring tuberculosis infection. Underlying immunodeficiencies associated with these conditions theoretically would enhance the possibility for progression to severe disease. Initial histories of potential exposure to tuberculosis should be included for all of these patients. If these histories or local epidemiologic factors suggest a possibility of exposure, immediate and periodic TST should be considered. **An initial TST or IGRA should be performed before initiation of immunosuppressive therapy, including prolonged steroid administration, use of tumor necrosis factor-alpha antagonists, or immunosuppressive therapy in any child requiring these treatments.**

*Bacille Calmette-Guérin immunization is not a contraindication to a TST.
[†]Beginning as early as 3 mo of age.
[‡]If the child is well, the TST should be delayed for up to 10 wk after return.
LTBI, latent tuberculosis infection.
From American Academy of Pediatrics: *Red book: 2009 report of the Committee on Infectious Diseases*, ed 28, Elk Grove Village, IL, 2009, American Academy of Pediatrics, p 684.

Table 207-3 DEFINITIONS OF POSITIVE TUBERCULIN SKIN TEST (TST) RESULTS IN INFANTS, CHILDREN, AND ADOLESCENTS*

INDURATION ≥5 mm
Children in close contact with known or suspected contagious people with tuberculosis disease
Children suspected to have tuberculosis disease: • Findings on chest radiograph consistent with active or previously tuberculosis disease • Clinical evidence of tuberculosis disease[†] • Children receiving immunosuppressive therapy[‡] or with immunosuppressive conditions, including HIV infection
INDURATION ≥10 mm
Children at increased risk of disseminated tuberculosis disease: • Children younger than 4 yr of age • Children with other medical conditions, including Hodgkin disease, lymphoma, diabetes mellitus, chronic renal failure, or malnutrition (see Table 207-2)
Children with increased exposure to tuberculosis disease: • Children born in high-prevalence regions of the world • Children often exposed to adults who are HIV infected, homeless, users of illicit drugs, residents of nursing homes, incarcerated or institutionalized, or migrant farm workers • Children who travel to high-prevalence regions of the world
INDURATION ≥15 mm
Children ≥4 yr of age without any risk factors

*These definitions apply regardless of previous bacille Calmette-Guérin (BCG) immunization; erythema at TST site does not indicate a positive test result. Tests should be read at 48 to 72 hr after placement.
[†]Evidence by physical examination or laboratory assessment that would include tuberculosis in the working differential diagnosis (e.g., meningitis).
[‡]Including immunosuppressive doses of corticosteroids.
From American Academy of Pediatrics: *Red book: 2009 report of the Committee on Infectious Diseases*, ed 28, Elk Grove Village, IL, 2009, American Academy of Pediatrics, p 681.

CLINICAL MANIFESTATIONS AND DIAGNOSIS

The majority of children with tuberculosis infection develop no signs or symptoms at any time. Occasionally, infection is marked by low-grade fever and mild cough, and it is rarely marked by high fever, cough, malaise, and flulike symptoms that resolve within 1 wk. The proportion of extrapulmonary tuberculosis cases has increased since 1990 in the USA. About 15% of tuberculosis cases in adults are extrapulmonary, and 25-30% of children with tuberculosis have an extrapulmonary presentation.

Primary Pulmonary Disease

The **primary complex** includes the parenchymal pulmonary focus and the regional lymph nodes. About 70% of lung foci are subpleural, and localized pleurisy is common. The initial parenchymal inflammation usually is not visible on chest radiograph, but a localized, nonspecific infiltrate may be seen before the development of tissue hypersensitivity. All lobar segments of the lung are at equal risk for initial infection. Two or more primary foci are present in 25% of cases. The hallmark of primary tuberculosis in the lung is the relatively large size of the regional lymphadenitis compared with the relatively small size of the initial lung focus (see Figs. 207-6 to 207-9). As DTH develops, the hilar lymph nodes continue to enlarge in some children, especially infants, compressing the regional bronchus and causing obstruction. The usual sequence is hilar lymphadenopathy, focal hyperinflation, and then atelectasis. The resulting radiographic shadows have been called collapse-consolidation or segmental tuberculosis (see Fig. 207-9). Rarely, inflamed caseous nodes attach to the endobronchial wall and erode through it, causing endobronchial tuberculosis or a fistula tract. The caseum causes complete obstruction of the bronchus, resulting in extensive infiltrate and collapse. Enlargement of the subcarinal lymph nodes can cause compression of the esophagus and, rarely, a bronchoesophageal fistula.

Most cases of tuberculous bronchial obstruction in children resolve fully with appropriate treatment. Occasionally, there is residual calcification of the primary focus or regional lymph nodes. The appearance of calcification implies that the lesion has been present for at least 6-12 mo. Healing of the segment can be complicated by scarring or contraction associated with cylindrical bronchiectasis, but this is rare.

Children can have lobar pneumonia without impressive hilar lymphadenopathy. If the primary infection is progressively destructive, liquefaction of the lung parenchyma can lead to formation of a thin-walled primary tuberculosis cavity. Rarely, bullous tuberculous lesions occur in the lungs and lead to pneumothorax if they rupture. Erosion of a parenchymal focus of tuberculosis into a blood or lymphatic vessel can result in dissemination of the bacilli and a **miliary pattern,** with small nodules evenly distributed on the chest radiograph (Fig. 207-10).

The symptoms and physical signs of primary pulmonary tuberculosis in children are surprisingly meager considering the degree of radiographic changes often seen. When active case finding is performed, up to 50% of infants and children with radiographically moderate to severe pulmonary tuberculosis have no physical findings. Infants are more likely to experience signs and symptoms. Nonproductive cough and mild dyspnea are the most common symptoms. Systemic complaints such as fever, night sweats, anorexia, and decreased activity occur less often. Some infants have difficulty gaining weight or develop a true failure-to-thrive syndrome that often does not improve significantly until several months of effective treatment have been taken. Pulmonary signs are even less common. Some infants and young children with bronchial obstruction have localized wheezing or decreased breath sounds that may be accompanied by tachypnea or, rarely, respiratory distress. These pulmonary symptoms and signs are occasionally alleviated by antibiotics, suggesting bacterial superinfection.

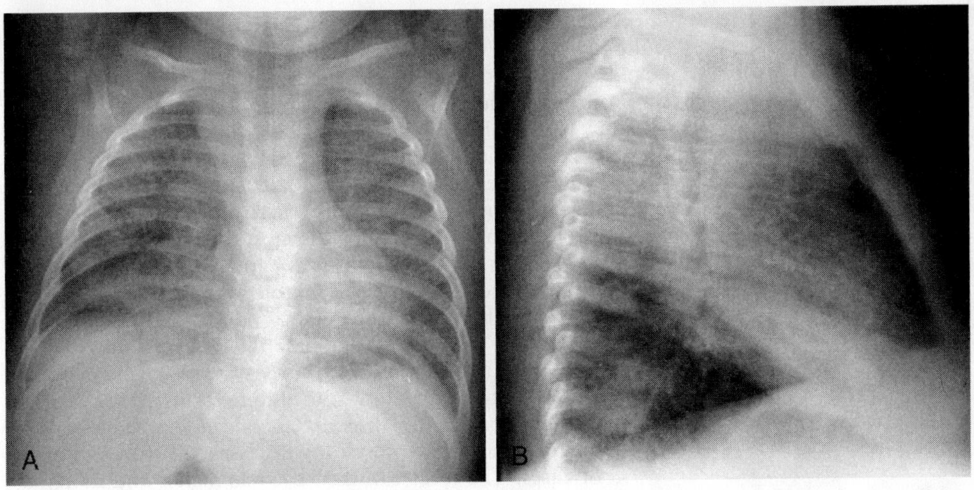

Figure 207-10 Posteroanterior *(A)* and lateral *(B)* chest radiographs of an infant with miliary tuberculosis. The child's mother had failed to complete treatment for pulmonary tuberculosis twice within 3 yr of this child's birth.

The most specific confirmation of pulmonary tuberculosis is isolation of *M. tuberculosis*. Sputum specimens for culture should be collected from adolescents and older children who are able to expectorate. Induced sputum with a jet nebulizer and chest percussion followed by nasopharyngeal suctioning is effective in children as young as 1 mo. Sputum induction provides samples for both culture and smear staining, whereas gastric aspirates are usually cultured. The traditional culture specimen in young children is the early morning gastric acid obtained before the child has arisen and peristalsis has emptied the stomach of the pooled secretions that have been swallowed overnight. However, even under optimal conditions, 3 consecutive morning gastric aspirates yield the organisms in <50% of cases. The culture yield from bronchoscopy is even lower, but this procedure can demonstrate the presence of endobronchial disease or a fistula. Negative cultures never exclude the diagnosis of tuberculosis in a child. The presence of a positive TST or IGRA, an abnormal chest radiograph consistent with tuberculosis, and history of exposure to an adult with infectious tuberculosis is adequate proof that the disease is present. Drug susceptibility test results of the isolate from the adult source can be used to determine the best therapeutic regimen for the child. Cultures should be obtained from the child whenever the source case is unknown or the source case has possible drug-resistant tuberculosis.

Progressive Primary Pulmonary Disease

A rare but serious complication of tuberculosis in a child occurs when the primary focus enlarges steadily and develops a large caseous center. Liquefaction can cause formation of a primary cavity associated with large numbers of tubercle bacilli. The enlarging focus can slough necrotic debris into the adjacent bronchus, leading to further intrapulmonary dissemination. Significant signs or symptoms are common in locally progressive disease in children. High fever, severe cough with sputum production, weight loss, and night sweats are common. Physical signs include diminished breath sounds, rales, and dullness or egophony over the cavity. The prognosis for full but usually slow recovery is excellent with appropriate therapy.

Reactivation Tuberculosis

Pulmonary tuberculosis in adults usually represents endogenous reactivation of a site of tuberculosis infection established previously in the body. This form of tuberculosis is rare in childhood but can occur in adolescence. Children with a healed tuberculosis infection acquired at <2 yr of age rarely develop chronic reactivation pulmonary disease, which is more common in those who acquire the initial infection at >7 yr of age. The most common pulmonary sites are the original parenchymal focus, lymph nodes, or the apical seedings (**Simon foci**) established during the hematogenous phase of the early infection. This form of disease usually remains localized to the lungs, because the established immune response prevents further extrapulmonary spread. The most common radiographic presentations of this type of tuberculosis are extensive infiltrates or thick-walled cavities in the upper lobes.

Older children and adolescents with reactivation tuberculosis are more likely to experience fever, anorexia, malaise, weight loss, night sweats, productive cough, hemoptysis, and chest pain than children with primary pulmonary tuberculosis. However, physical examination findings usually are minor or absent, even when cavities or large infiltrates are present. Most signs and symptoms improve within several weeks of starting effective treatment, although the cough can last for several months. This form of tuberculosis may be highly contagious if there is significant sputum production and cough. The prognosis for full recovery is excellent when patients are given appropriate therapy.

Pleural Effusion

Tuberculous pleural effusions, which can be local or general, originate in the discharge of bacilli into the pleural space from a subpleural pulmonary focus or caseated lymph node. Asymptomatic local pleural effusion is so common in primary tuberculosis that it is basically a component of the primary complex. Larger and clinically significant effusions occur months to years after the primary infection. Tuberculous pleural effusion is uncommon in children <6 yr of age and rare in children <2 yr of age. Effusions are usually unilateral but can be bilateral. They are rarely associated with a segmental pulmonary lesion and are uncommon in disseminated tuberculosis. Often the radiographic abnormality is more extensive than would be suggested by physical findings or symptoms (Fig. 207-11).

Clinical onset of tuberculous pleurisy is often sudden, characterized by low to high fever, shortness of breath, chest pain on deep inspiration, and diminished breath sounds. The fever and other symptoms can last for several weeks after the start of antituberculosis chemotherapy. The TST is positive in only 70-80% of cases. The prognosis is excellent, but radiographic resolution often takes months. Scoliosis is a rare complication from a long-standing effusion.

Examination of pleural fluid and the pleural membrane is important to establish the diagnosis of tuberculous pleurisy. The pleural fluid is usually yellow and only occasionally tinged with blood. The specific gravity is usually 1.012-1.025, the protein level is usually 2-4 g/dL, and the glucose concentration may be low, although it is usually in the low-normal range (20-40 mg/dL). Typically there are several hundred to several thousand white blood cells per cubic millimeter, with an early predominance of polymorphonuclear cells followed by a high percentage of lymphocytes. Acid-fast smears of the pleural fluid are rarely

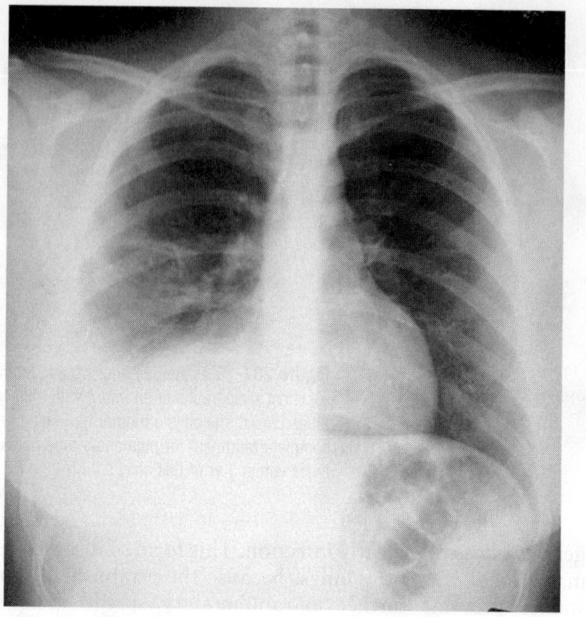

Figure 207-11 Pleural tuberculosis in a 16 yr old girl.

positive. Cultures of the fluid are positive in <30% of cases. Biopsy of the pleural membrane is more likely to yield a positive acid-fast stain or culture, and granuloma formation usually can be demonstrated.

Pericardial Disease

The most common form of cardiac tuberculosis is pericarditis. It is rare, occurring in 0.5-4% of tuberculosis cases in children. Pericarditis usually arises from direct invasion or lymphatic drainage from subcarinal lymph nodes. The presenting symptoms are nonspecific, including low-grade fever, malaise, and weight loss. Chest pain is unusual in children. A pericardial friction rub or distant heart sounds with pulsus paradoxus may be present. The pericardial fluid is typically serofibrinous or hemorrhagic. Acid-fast smear of the fluid rarely reveals the organism, but cultures are positive in 30-70% of cases. The culture yield from pericardial biopsy may be higher, and the presence of granulomas often suggests the diagnosis. Partial or complete pericardiectomy may be required when constrictive pericarditis develops.

Lymphohematogenous (Disseminated) Disease

Tubercle bacilli are disseminated to distant sites, including liver, spleen, skin, and lung apices, in all cases of tuberculosis infection. The clinical picture produced by lymphohematogenous dissemination depends on the quantity of organisms released from the primary focus and the adequacy of the host's immune response. Lymphohematogenous spread is usually asymptomatic. Rare patients experience protracted hematogenous tuberculosis caused by the intermittent release of tubercle bacilli as a caseous focus erodes through the wall of a blood vessel in the lung. Although the clinical picture may be acute, more often it is indolent and prolonged, with spiking fever accompanying the release of organisms into the bloodstream. Multiple organ involvement is common, leading to hepatomegaly, splenomegaly, lymphadenitis in superficial or deep nodes, and papulonecrotic tuberculids appearing on the skin. Bones and joints or kidneys also can become involved. Meningitis occurs only late in the course of the disease. Early pulmonary involvement is surprisingly mild, but diffuse involvement becomes apparent with prolonged infection.

The most clinically significant form of disseminated tuberculosis is **miliary disease,** which occurs when massive numbers of tubercle bacilli are released into the bloodstream, causing disease in 2 or more organs. Miliary tuberculosis usually complicates the primary infection, occurring within 2-6 mo of the initial infection. Although this form of disease is most common in infants and young children, it is also found in adolescents and older adults, resulting from the breakdown of a previously healed primary pulmonary lesion. The clinical manifestations of miliary tuberculosis are protean, depending on the load of organisms that disseminate and where they lodge. Lesions are often larger and more numerous in the lungs, spleen, liver, and bone marrow than other tissues. Because this form of tuberculosis is most common in infants and malnourished or immunosuppressed patients, the host's immune incompetence probably also plays a role in pathogenesis.

The onset of miliary tuberculosis is sometimes explosive, and the patient can become gravely ill in several days. More often, the onset is insidious, with early systemic signs, including anorexia, weight loss, and low-grade fever. At this time, abnormal physical signs are usually absent. Generalized lymphadenopathy and hepatosplenomegaly develop within several weeks in about 50% of cases. The fever can then become higher and more sustained, although the chest radiograph usually is normal and respiratory symptoms are minor or absent. Within several more weeks, the lungs can become filled with tubercles, and dyspnea, cough, rales, or wheezing occur. The lesions of miliary tuberculosis are usually smaller than 2-3 mm in diameter when first visible on chest radiograph (see Fig. 207-10). The smaller lesions coalesce to form larger lesions and sometimes extensive infiltrates. As the pulmonary disease progresses, an alveolar-air block syndrome can result in frank respiratory distress, hypoxia, and pneumothorax, or pneumomediastinum. Signs or symptoms of meningitis or peritonitis are found in 20-40% of patients with advanced disease. Chronic or recurrent headache in a patient with miliary tuberculosis usually indicates the presence of meningitis, whereas the onset of abdominal pain or tenderness is a sign of tuberculous peritonitis. **Cutaneous lesions** include papulonecrotic tuberculids, nodules, or purpura. Choroid tubercles occur in 13-87% of patients and are highly specific for the diagnosis of miliary tuberculosis. Unfortunately, the TST is nonreactive in up to 40% of patients with disseminated tuberculosis.

Diagnosis of disseminated tuberculosis can be difficult, and a high index of suspicion by the clinician is required. Often the patient presents with fever of unknown origin. Early sputum or gastric aspirate cultures have a low sensitivity. Biopsy of the liver or bone marrow with appropriate bacteriologic and histologic examinations more often yields an early diagnosis. The most important clue is usually history of recent exposure to an adult with infectious tuberculosis.

The resolution of miliary tuberculosis is slow, even with proper therapy. Fever usually declines within 2-3 wk of starting chemotherapy, but the chest radiographic abnormalities might not resolve for many months. Occasionally, corticosteroids hasten symptomatic relief, especially when air block, peritonitis, or meningitis is present. The prognosis is excellent if the diagnosis is made early and adequate chemotherapy is given.

Upper Respiratory Tract Disease

Tuberculosis of the upper respiratory tract is rare in developed countries but is still observed in developing countries. Children with laryngeal tuberculosis have a croup-like cough, sore throat, hoarseness, and dysphagia. Most children with laryngeal tuberculosis have extensive upper lobe pulmonary disease, but occasional patients have primary laryngeal disease with a normal chest radiograph. Tuberculosis of the middle ear results from aspiration of infected pulmonary secretions into the middle ear or from hematogenous dissemination in older children. The most common signs and symptoms are painless unilateral otorrhea, tinnitus, decreased hearing, facial paralysis, and a perforated tympanic membrane. Enlargement of lymph nodes in the preauricular or anterior cervical chains can accompany this infection. Diagnosis is difficult, because stains and cultures of ear fluid are often negative, and histology of the affected tissue often shows a

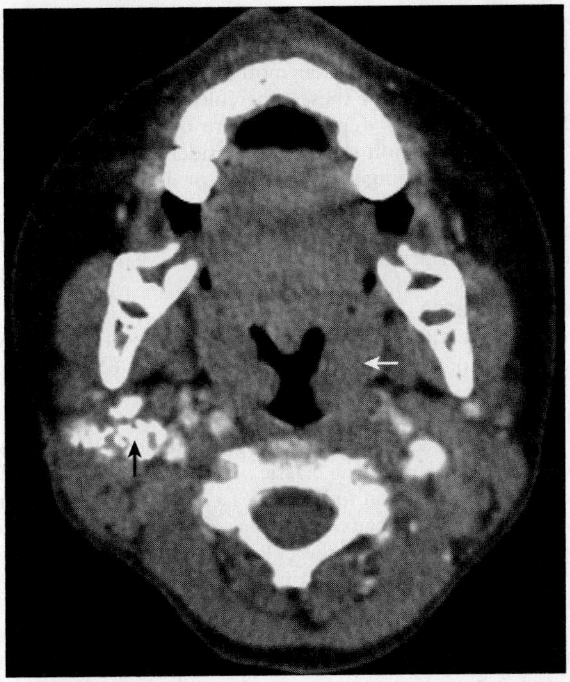

Figure 207-12 Axial CT image of the neck in an 8 yr old boy shows calcified right cervical lymphadenopathy *(black arrow)* with tonsillar swelling *(white arrow)*. (From Lighter J, Rigaud M: Diagnosing childhood tuberculosis: traditional and innovative modalities, *Curr Prob Pediatr Adolesc Health Care* 39:55–88, 2009.)

nonspecific acute and chronic inflammation without granuloma formation.

Lymph Node Disease

Tuberculosis of the superficial lymph nodes, often referred to as **scrofula,** is the most common form of extrapulmonary tuberculosis in children (Fig. 207-12). Historically, scrofula was usually caused by drinking unpasteurized cow's milk laden with *M. bovis.* Most current cases occur within 6-9 mo of initial infection by *M. tuberculosis,* although some cases appear years later. The tonsillar, anterior cervical, submandibular, and supraclavicular nodes become involved secondary to extension of a primary lesion of the upper lung fields or abdomen. Infected nodes in the inguinal, epitrochlear, or axillary regions result from regional lymphadenitis associated with tuberculosis of the skin or skeletal system. The nodes usually enlarge gradually in the early stages of lymph node disease. They are discrete, nontender, and firm but not hard. The nodes often feel fixed to underlying or overlying tissue. Disease is most often **unilateral,** but bilateral involvement can occur because of the crossover drainage patterns of lymphatic vessels in the chest and lower neck. As infection progresses, multiple nodes are infected, resulting in a mass of matted nodes. Systemic signs and symptoms other than a low-grade fever are usually absent. The TST is usually reactive, but the chest radiograph is normal in 70% of cases. The onset of illness is occasionally more acute, with rapid enlargement, tenderness, and fluctuance of lymph nodes and with high fever. The initial presentation is rarely a fluctuant mass with overlying cellulitis or skin discoloration.

Lymph node tuberculosis can resolve if left untreated but more often progresses to caseation and necrosis. The capsule of the node breaks down, resulting in the spread of infection to adjacent nodes. Rupture of the node usually results in a draining sinus tract that can require surgical removal. Tuberculous lymphadenitis can usually be diagnosed by fine-needle aspiration of the node and responds well to antituberculosis therapy, although the lymph nodes do not return to normal size for months or even years. Surgical removal is not usually necessary and must be combined with antituberculous medication because the lymph node disease is only one part of a systemic infection.

A definitive diagnosis of tuberculous adenitis usually requires histologic or bacteriologic confirmation, which is best accomplished by fine-needle aspiration for culture, stain, and histology. If fine-needle aspiration is not successful in establishing a diagnosis, excisional biopsy of the involved node is indicated. Culture of lymph node tissue yields the organism in only about 50% of cases. Many other conditions can be confused with tuberculous adenitis, including infection due to NTM, cat scratch disease *(Bartonella henselae),* tularemia, brucellosis, toxoplasmosis, tumor, branchial cleft cyst, cystic hygroma, and pyogenic infection. The most common problem is distinguishing infection due to *M. tuberculosis* from lymphadenitis caused by NTM in geographic areas where NTM are common. Both conditions are usually associated with a normal chest radiograph and a reactive TST. An important clue to the diagnosis of tuberculous adenitis is an epidemiologic link to an adult with infectious tuberculosis. In areas where both diseases are common, the only way to distinguish them may be culture of the involved tissue.

Central Nervous System Disease

Tuberculosis of the central nervous system (CNS) is the most serious complication in children and is fatal without prompt and appropriate treatment. Tuberculous meningitis usually arises from the formation of a metastatic caseous lesion in the cerebral cortex or meninges that develops during the lymphohematogenous dissemination of the primary infection. This initial lesion increases in size and discharges small numbers of tubercle bacilli into the subarachnoid space. The resulting gelatinous exudate infiltrates the corticomeningeal blood vessels, producing inflammation, obstruction, and subsequent infarction of cerebral cortex. The brain stem is often the site of greatest involvement, which accounts for the commonly associated dysfunction of cranial nerves III, VI, and VII. The exudate also interferes with the normal flow of cerebrospinal fluid (CSF) in and out of the ventricular system at the level of the basilar cisterns, leading to a communicating hydrocephalus. The combination of vasculitis, infarction, cerebral edema, and hydrocephalus results in the severe damage that can occur gradually or rapidly. Profound abnormalities in electrolyte metabolism due to salt wasting or the syndrome of inappropriate antidiuretic hormone secretion also contribute to the pathophysiology of tuberculous meningitis.

Tuberculous meningitis complicates about 0.3% of untreated tuberculosis infections in children. It is most common in children between 6 mo and 4 yr of age. Occasionally, tuberculous meningitis occurs many years after the infection, when rupture of 1 or more of the subependymal tubercles discharges tubercle bacilli into the subarachnoid space. The clinical progression of tuberculous meningitis may be rapid or gradual. Rapid progression tends to occur more often in infants and young children, who can experience symptoms for only several days before the onset of acute hydrocephalus, seizures, and cerebral edema. More commonly, the signs and symptoms progress slowly over several weeks and can be divided into 3 stages.

The **1st stage** typically lasts 1-2 wk and is characterized by nonspecific symptoms such as fever, headache, irritability, drowsiness, and malaise. Focal neurologic signs are absent, but infants can experience a stagnation or loss of developmental milestones. The **2nd stage** usually begins more abruptly. The most common features are lethargy, nuchal rigidity, seizures, positive Kernig and Brudzinski signs, hypertonia, vomiting, cranial nerve palsies, and other focal neurologic signs. The accelerating clinical illness usually correlates with the development of hydrocephalus, increased intracranial pressure, and vasculitis. Some children have no evidence of meningeal irritation but can have signs of encephalitis, such as disorientation, movement disorders, or speech impairment. The **3rd stage** is marked by coma, hemiplegia or paraplegia, hypertension, decerebrate posturing, deterioration of vital signs, and eventually death.

The prognosis of tuberculous meningitis correlates most closely with the clinical stage of illness at the time treatment is initiated. The majority of patients in the 1st stage have an excellent outcome, whereas most patients in the 3rd stage who survive have permanent disabilities, including blindness, deafness, paraplegia, diabetes insipidus, or mental retardation. The prognosis for young infants is generally worse than for older children. It is imperative that antituberculosis treatment be considered for any child who develops basilar meningitis and hydrocephalus, cranial nerve palsy, or stroke with no other apparent etiology. Often the key to the correct diagnosis is identifying an adult who has infectious tuberculosis and is in contact with the child. Because of the short incubation period of tuberculous meningitis, the illness has not yet been diagnosed in the adult in many cases.

The diagnosis of tuberculous meningitis can be difficult early in its course, requiring a high degree of suspicion on the part of the clinician. The TST is nonreactive in up to 50% of cases, and 20-50% of children have a normal chest radiograph. The most important laboratory test for the diagnosis of tuberculous meningitis is examination and culture of the lumbar CSF. The CSF leukocyte count usually ranges from 10 to 500 cells/mm^3. Polymorphonuclear leukocytes may be present initially, but lymphocytes predominate in the majority of cases. The CSF glucose is typically <40mg/dL but rarely <20mg/dL. The protein level is elevated and may be markedly high (400-5,000mg/dL) secondary to hydrocephalus and spinal block. Although the lumbar CSF is grossly abnormal, ventricular CSF can have normal chemistries and cell counts because this fluid is obtained from a site proximal to the inflammation and obstruction. During early stage I, the CSF can resemble that of viral aseptic meningitis only to progress to the more-severe CSF profile over several weeks. The success of the microscopic examination of acid-fast-stained CSF and mycobacterial culture is related directly to the volume of the CSF sample. Examinations or culture of small amounts of CSF are unlikely to demonstrate *M. tuberculosis*. When 5-10 mL of lumbar CSF can be obtained, the acid-fast stain of the CSF sediment is positive in up to 30% of cases and the culture is positive in 50-70% of cases. Cultures of other fluids, such as gastric aspirates or urine, can help confirm the diagnosis.

Radiographic studies can aid in the diagnosis of tuberculous meningitis. CT or MRI of the brain of patients with tuberculous meningitis may be normal during early stages of the disease. As disease progresses, basilar enhancement and communicating hydrocephalus with signs of cerebral edema or early focal ischemia are the most common findings. Some small children with tuberculous meningitis can have one or several clinically silent tuberculomas, occurring most often in the cerebral cortex or thalamic regions.

Another manifestation of CNS tuberculosis is the **tuberculoma,** a tumor-like mass resulting from aggregation of caseous tubercles that usually manifests clinically as a brain tumor. Tuberculomas account for up to 40% of brain tumors in some areas of the world but are rare in North America. In adults tuberculomas are most often supratentorial, but in children they are often infratentorial, located at the base of the brain near the cerebellum. Lesions are most often singular but may be multiple. The most common symptoms are headache, fever, and convulsions. The TST is usually reactive, but the chest radiograph is usually normal. Surgical excision is sometimes necessary to distinguish tuberculoma from other causes of brain tumor. However, surgical removal is not necessary because most tuberculomas resolve with medical management. Corticosteroids are usually administered during the 1st few weeks of treatment or in the immediate postoperative period to decrease cerebral edema. On CT or MRI of the brain, tuberculomas usually appear as discrete lesions with a significant amount of surrounding edema. Contrast medium enhancement is often impressive and can result in a ring-like lesion. Since the advent of CT, the paradoxical development of tuberculomas in patients with tuberculous meningitis who are receiving ultimately effective chemotherapy has been recognized. The cause and nature of these tuberculomas are poorly understood, but they do not represent failure of antimicrobial treatment. This phenomenon should be considered whenever a child with tuberculous meningitis deteriorates or develops focal neurologic findings while on treatment. Corticosteroids can help alleviate the occasionally severe clinical signs and symptoms that occur. These lesions can persist for months or even years.

Cutaneous Disease

Cutaneous tuberculosis is rare in the USA but occurs worldwide and accounts for 1-2% of tuberculosis (Chapter 657).

Bone and Joint Disease

Bone and joint infection complicating tuberculosis is most likely to involve the vertebrae. The classic manifestation of tuberculous spondylitis is progression to Pott disease, in which destruction of the vertebral bodies leads to gibbus deformity and kyphosis (Chapter 671.4). Skeletal tuberculosis is a late complication of tuberculosis and has become a rare entity since the availability of antituberculosis therapy but is more likely to occur in children than in adults. Tuberculous bone lesions can resemble pyogenic and fungal infections or bone tumors. Multifocal bone involvement can occur. A bone biopsy is essential to confirm the diagnosis.

Abdominal and Gastrointestinal Disease

Tuberculosis of the oral cavity or pharynx is quite unusual. The most common lesion is a painless ulcer on the mucosa, palate, or tonsil with enlargement of the regional lymph nodes. Tuberculosis of the parotid gland has been reported rarely in endemic countries. Tuberculosis of the esophagus is rare in children but may be associated with a tracheoesophageal fistula in infants. These forms of tuberculosis are usually associated with extensive pulmonary disease and swallowing of infectious respiratory secretions. However, they can occur in the absence of pulmonary disease, presumably by spread from mediastinal or peritoneal lymph nodes.

Tuberculous peritonitis occurs most often in young men and is uncommon in adolescents and rare in children. Generalized peritonitis can arise from subclinical or miliary hematogenous dissemination. Localized peritonitis is caused by direct extension from an abdominal lymph node, intestinal focus, or genitourinary tuberculosis. Rarely, the lymph nodes, omentum, and peritoneum become matted and can be palpated as a doughy irregular nontender mass. Abdominal pain or tenderness, ascites, anorexia, and low-grade fever are typical manifestations. The TST is usually reactive. The diagnosis can be confirmed by paracentesis with appropriate stains and cultures, but this procedure must be performed carefully to avoid entering a bowel that is intertwined with the matted omentum.

Tuberculous enteritis is caused by hematogenous dissemination or by swallowing tubercle bacilli discharged from the patient's own lungs. The jejunum and ileum near Peyer patches and the appendix are the most common sites of involvement. The typical findings are shallow ulcers that cause pain, diarrhea or constipation, weight loss, and low-grade fever. Mesenteric adenitis usually complicates the infection. The enlarged nodes can cause intestinal obstruction or erode through the omentum to cause generalized peritonitis. The clinical presentation of tuberculous enteritis is nonspecific, mimicking other infections and conditions that cause diarrhea. The disease should be suspected in any child with chronic GI complaints and a reactive TST or positive IGRA. Biopsy, acid-fast stain, and culture of the lesions are usually necessary to confirm the diagnosis.

Genitourinary Disease

Renal tuberculosis is rare in children, because the incubation period is several years or longer. Tubercle bacilli usually reach the kidney during lymphohematogenous dissemination. The organisms often can be recovered from the urine in cases of miliary tuberculosis and in some patients with pulmonary tuberculosis in the absence of renal parenchymal disease. In true renal tuberculosis, small caseous foci develop in the renal parenchyma and release *M. tuberculosis* into the tubules. A large mass develops near the renal cortex that discharges bacteria through a fistula into the renal pelvis. Infection then spreads locally to the ureters, prostate, or epididymis. Renal tuberculosis is often clinically silent in its early stages, marked only by sterile pyuria and microscopic hematuria. Dysuria, flank or abdominal pain, and gross hematuria develop as the disease progresses. Superinfection by other bacteria is common and can delay recognition of the underlying tuberculosis. Hydronephrosis or ureteral strictures can complicate the disease. Urine cultures for *M. tuberculosis* are positive in 80-90% of cases, and acid-fast stains of large volumes of urine sediment are positive in 50-70% of cases. The TST is nonreactive in up to 20% of patients. An intravenous pyelogram or CT scan often reveals mass lesions, dilatation of the proximal ureters, multiple small filling defects, and hydronephrosis if ureteral stricture is present. Disease is most often unilateral.

Tuberculosis of the genital tract is uncommon in both boys and girls before puberty. This condition usually originates from lymphohematogenous spread, although it can be caused by direct spread from the intestinal tract or bone. Adolescent girls can develop genital tract tuberculosis during the primary infection. The fallopian tubes are most often involved (90-100% of cases), followed by the endometrium (50%), ovaries (25%), and cervix (5%). The most common symptoms are lower abdominal pain and dysmenorrhea or amenorrhea. Systemic manifestations are usually absent, and the chest radiograph is normal in the majority of cases. The TST is usually reactive. Genital tuberculosis in adolescent boys causes epididymitis or orchitis. The condition usually manifests as a unilateral nodular painless swelling of the scrotum. Involvement of the glans penis is extremely rare. Genital abnormalities and a positive TST in an adolescent boy or girl suggests genital tract tuberculosis.

Disease in HIV-Infected Children

Most cases of tuberculosis in HIV-infected children are seen in developing countries. The rate of tuberculosis disease in HIV-infected children is 30 times higher than in non–HIV-infected children in the USA. Establishing the diagnosis of tuberculosis in an HIV-infected child may be difficult, because skin test reactivity can be absent (with a negative IGRA), culture confirmation is difficult, and the clinical features of tuberculosis are similar to many other HIV-related infections and conditions. Tuberculosis in HIV-infected children is often more severe, progressive, and likely to occur in extrapulmonary sites. Radiographic findings are similar to those in children with normal immune systems, but lobar disease and lung cavitation are more common. Nonspecific respiratory symptoms, fever, and weight loss are the most common complaints. Rates of drug-resistant tuberculosis tend to be higher in HIV-infected adults and probably are also higher in HIV-infected children.

The mortality rate of HIV-infected children with tuberculosis is high, especially as the CD4 lymphocyte numbers decrease. In adults, the host immune response to tuberculosis infection appears to enhance HIV replication and accelerate the immune suppression caused by HIV. Increased mortality rates are attributed to progressive HIV infection rather than tuberculosis. Therefore, HIV-infected children with potential exposures and/or recent infection should be promptly evaluated and treated for tuberculosis. Conversely, all children with tuberculosis disease should be tested for HIV co-infection, because of the potential benefits of early diagnosis and treatment of HIV infection and because the presence of HIV can necessitate a longer duration of treatment.

Perinatal Disease

Symptoms of congenital tuberculosis may be present at birth but more commonly begin by the 2nd or 3rd wk of life. The most common signs and symptoms are respiratory distress, fever, hepatic or splenic enlargement, poor feeding, lethargy or irritability, lymphadenopathy, abdominal distention, failure to thrive, ear drainage, and skin lesions. The clinical manifestations vary in relation to the site and size of the caseous lesions. Many infants have an abnormal chest radiograph, most often with a miliary pattern. Some infants with no pulmonary findings early in the course of the disease later develop profound radiographic and clinical abnormalities. Hilar and mediastinal lymphadenopathy and lung infiltrates are common. Generalized lymphadenopathy and meningitis occur in 30-50% of patients.

The clinical presentation of tuberculosis in newborns is similar to that caused by bacterial sepsis and other congenital infections, such as syphilis, toxoplasmosis, and cytomegalovirus. The diagnosis should be suspected in an infant with signs and symptoms of bacterial or congenital infection whose response to antibiotic and supportive therapy is poor and in whom evaluation for other infections is unrevealing. The most important clue for rapid diagnosis of congenital tuberculosis is a maternal or family history of tuberculosis. Often, the mother's disease is discovered only after the neonate's diagnosis is suspected. The infant's TST is negative initially but can become positive in 1-3 mo. A positive acid-fast stain of an early morning gastric aspirate from a newborn usually indicates tuberculosis. Direct acid-fast stains on middle-ear discharge, bone marrow, tracheal aspirate, or biopsy tissue (especially liver) can be useful. The CSF should be examined and cultured, although the yield for isolating *M. tuberculosis* is low. The mortality rate of congenital tuberculosis remains very high because of delayed diagnosis; many children have a complete recovery if the diagnosis is made promptly and adequate chemotherapy is started.

TREATMENT

The basic principles of management of tuberculosis disease in children and adolescents are the same as those in adults. Several drugs are used to effect a relatively rapid cure and prevent the emergence of secondary drug resistance during therapy (Tables 207-4 and 207-5). The choice of regimen depends on the extent of tuberculosis disease, the host, and the likelihood of drug resistance (Chapter 206 and Table 206-1). The standard therapy of intrathoracic tuberculosis (pulmonary disease and/or hilar lymphadenopathy) in children recommended by the CDC and AAP is a 6 mo regimen of isoniazid and rifampin supplemented in the 1st 2 mo of treatment by pyrazinamide and ethambutol. Several clinical trials have shown that this regimen yields a success rate approaching 100%, with an incidence of clinically significant adverse reactions of <2%. Nine month regimens of only isoniazid and rifampin are also highly effective for drug-susceptible tuberculosis, but the necessary length of treatment, the need for good adherence by the patient, and the relative lack of protection against possible initial drug resistance have led to the use of shorter regimens with additional medications. Most experts recommend that all drug administration be directly observed, meaning that a health care worker is physically present when the medications are administered to the patients. When **directly observed therapy** is used, intermittent (twice weekly) administration of drugs after an initial period as short as 2 wk of daily therapy is as effective in children as daily therapy for the entire course.

Extrapulmonary tuberculosis is usually caused by small numbers of mycobacteria. In general, the treatment for most forms of extrapulmonary tuberculosis in children, including cervical lymphadenopathy, is the same as for pulmonary tuberculosis. Exceptions are bone and joint, disseminated, and CNS tuberculosis, for which there are inadequate data to recommend

Table 207-4 COMMONLY USED DRUGS FOR THE TREATMENT OF TUBERCULOSIS IN INFANTS, CHILDREN, AND ADOLESCENTS

DRUG	DOSAGE FORMS	DAILY DOSAGE, mg/kg	TWICE A WEEK DOSAGE, mg/kg PER DOSE	MAXIMUM DOSE	ADVERSE REACTIONS
Ethambutol	Tablets: 100 mg 400 mg	20	50	2.5 g	Optic neuritis (usually reversible), decreased red-green color discrimination, gastrointestinal tract disturbances, hypersensitivity
Isoniazid*	Scored tablets: 100 mg 300 mg Syrup: 10 mg/ mL	10-15†	20-30	Daily, 300 mg Twice a week, 900 mg	Mild hepatic enzyme elevation, hepatitis,† peripheral neuritis, hypersensitivity
Pyrazinamide*	Scored tablets: 500 mg	20-40	50	2 g	Hepatotoxic effects, hyperuricemia, arthralgias, gastrointestinal tract upset
Rifampin*	Capsules: 150 mg 300 mg Syrup formulated in syrup from capsules	10-20	10-20	600 mg	Orange discoloration of secretions or urine, staining of contact lenses, vomiting, hepatitis, influenza-like reaction, thrombocytopenia, pruritus; oral contraceptives may be ineffective

*Rifamate is a capsule containing 150 mg of isoniazid and 300 mg of rifampin. Two capsules provide the usual adult (>50 kg) daily doses of each drug. Rifater is a capsule containing 50 mg of isoniazid, 120 mg of rifampin, and 300 mg of pyrazinamide. Isoniazid and rifampin also are available for parenteral administration.
†When isoniazid in a dosage exceeding 10 mg/kg per day is used in combination with rifampin, the incidence of hepatotoxic effects may be increased.
From American Academy of Pediatrics: *Red book: 2009 report of the Committee on Infectious Diseases*, ed 28, Elk Grove Village, IL, 2009, American Academy of Pediatrics, p 689.

Table 207-5 LESS COMMONLY USED DRUGS FOR TREATING DRUG-RESISTANT TUBERCULOSIS IN INFANTS, CHILDREN, AND ADOLESCENTS*

DRUGS	DOSAGE, FORMS	DAILY DOSAGE, mg/kg	MAXIMUM DOSE	ADVERSE REACTIONS
Amikacin†	Vials, 500 mg, 1 g	15-30 (IV or IM administration)	1 g	Auditory and vestibular toxic effects, nephrotoxic effects
Capreomycin†	Vials, 1 g	15-30 (IM administration)	1 g	Auditory and vestibular toxicity and nephrotoxic effects
Cycloserine	Capsules, 250 mg	10-20, given in 2 divided doses	1 g	Psychosis, personality changes, seizures, rash
Ethionamide	Tablets, 250 mg	15-20, given in 2-3 divided doses	1 g	Gastrointestinal tract disturbances, hepatotoxic effects, hypersensitivity reactions, hypothyroidism
Kanamycin	Vials: 75 mg/2 mL 500 mg/2 mL 1 g/3 mL	15-30 (IM or IV administration)	1 g	Auditory and vestibular toxic effects, nephrotoxic effects
Levofloxacin‡	Tablets: 250 mg 500 mg Vials, 25 mg/ mL	Adults: 500-1000 mg (once daily) Children: not recommended	1 g	Theoretic effect on growing cartilage, gastrointestinal tract disturbances, rash, headache, restlessness, confusion
para-Aminosalicylic acid (PAS)	Packets, 3 g	200-300 (bid-qid)	10 g	Gastrointestinal tract disturbances, hypersensitivity, hepatotoxic effects
Streptomycin†	Vials: 1 g 4 g	20-40 (IM administration)	1 g	Auditory and vestibular toxic effects, nephrotoxic effects, rash

*These drugs should be used in consultation with a specialist in tuberculosis.
†Dose adjustment in renal insufficiency.
‡Levofloxacin currently is not approved for use in children younger than 18 yr of age; its use in younger children necessitates assessment of the potential risks and benefits.
From American Academy of Pediatrics: *Red book: 2009 report of the Committee on Infectious Diseases*, ed 28, Elk Grove Village, IL, 2009, American Academy of Pediatrics, p 692.

6 mo therapy. These infections are treated for 9-12 mo. Surgical débridement in bone and joint disease and ventriculoperitoneal shunting in CNS disease are often necessary.

The optimal treatment of tuberculosis in HIV-infected children has not been established. HIV-seropositive adults with tuberculosis can be treated successfully with standard regimens that include isoniazid, rifampin, pyrazinamide, and ethambutol. The total duration of therapy should be 6-9 mo, or 6 mo after culture of sputum becomes sterile, whichever is longer. Data for children are limited to isolated case reports and small series. Most experts believe that HIV-seropositive children with drug-susceptible tuberculosis should receive the standard 4-drug regimen for the 1st 2 mo followed by isoniazid and rifampin for a total duration of at least 9 mo. Children with HIV infection appear to have more frequent adverse reactions to antituberculosis drugs and must be monitored closely during therapy. Co-administration of rifampin and some antiretroviral agents results in subtherapeutic blood levels of protease inhibitors and non-nucleoside reverse transcriptase inhibitors and toxic levels of rifampin. Concomitant administration of these drugs is not recommended. Treatment of HIV-infected children is often empirical based on epidemiologic and radiographic information, because the radiographic appearance of other pulmonary complications of HIV in children, such as lymphoid interstitial pneumonitis and bacterial pneumonia, may be similar to that of tuberculosis. Therapy should be considered when tuberculosis cannot be excluded.

Drug-Resistant Tuberculosis

The incidence of drug-resistant tuberculosis is increasing in many areas of the world, including North America. There are two major types of drug resistance. **Primary resistance** occurs when a person is infected with *M. tuberculosis* that is already resistant to a particular drug. **Secondary resistance** occurs when drug-resistant organisms emerge as the dominant population during treatment. The major causes of secondary drug resistance are poor adherence to the medication by the patient or inadequate treatment regimens prescribed by the physician. Nonadherence to one drug is more likely to lead to secondary resistance than is failure to take all drugs. Secondary resistance is rare in children because of the small size of their mycobacterial population. Therefore, most drug resistance in children is primary, and patterns of drug resistance among children tend to mirror those found among adults in the same population. The main predictors of drug-resistant tuberculosis among adults are history of previous antituberculosis treatment, co-infection with HIV, and exposure to another adult with infectious drug-resistant tuberculosis.

Treatment of drug-resistant tuberculosis is successful only when at least 2 bactericidal drugs are given to which the infecting strain of *M. tuberculosis* is susceptible. When a child has possible drug-resistant tuberculosis, usually 4 or 5 drugs should be administered initially until the susceptibility pattern is determined and a more-specific regimen can be designed. The specific treatment plan must be individualized for each patient according to the results of susceptibility testing on the isolates from the child or the adult source case. Treatment duration of 9 mo with rifampin, pyrazinamide, and ethambutol is usually adequate for isoniazid-resistant tuberculosis in children. When resistance to isoniazid and rifampin is present, the total duration of therapy often must be extended to 12-18 mo, and twice-a-week regimens should not be used. The prognosis of single- or multidrug-resistant tuberculosis in children is usually good if the drug resistance is identified early in the treatment, appropriate drugs are administered under directly observed therapy, adverse reactions from the drugs do not occur, and the child and family are in a supportive environment. The treatment of drug-resistant tuberculosis in children always should be undertaken by a clinician with specific expertise in the treatment of tuberculosis.

Extensively drug resistant (XDR) TB with resistance to isoniazid, rifampicin, any fluoroquinolone, and any one of capreomycin, kanamycin, or amikacin is a growing problem, particularly in developing countries and patients with HIV.

Corticosteroids

Corticosteroids are useful in treating some children with tuberculosis disease. They are most beneficial when the host inflammatory reaction contributes significantly to tissue damage or impairment of organ function. There is convincing evidence that corticosteroids decrease mortality rates and long-term neurologic sequelae in some patients with **tuberculous meningitis** by reducing vasculitis, inflammation, and, ultimately, intracranial pressure. Lowering the intracranial pressure limits tissue damage and favors circulation of antituberculosis drugs through the brain and meninges. Short courses of corticosteroids also may be effective for children with **endobronchial tuberculosis** that causes respiratory distress, localized emphysema, or segmental pulmonary lesions. Several randomized clinical trials have shown that corticosteroids can help relieve symptoms and constriction associated with acute tuberculous **pericardial effusion.** Corticosteroids can cause dramatic improvement in symptoms in some patients with tuberculous pleural effusion and shift of the mediastinum. However, the long-term course of disease is probably unaffected. Some children with severe **miliary tuberculosis** have dramatic improvement with corticosteroid therapy if the inflammatory reaction is so severe that alveolocapillary block is present. There is no convincing evidence that 1 corticosteroid preparation is better than another. The most commonly prescribed regimen is prednisone, 1-2 mg/kg/day in 1-2 divided doses orally for 4-6 wk, followed by gradual tapering.

Supportive Care

Children receiving treatment should be followed carefully to promote adherence to therapy, to monitor for toxic reactions to medications, and to ensure that the tuberculosis is being adequately treated. Adequate nutrition is important. Patients should be seen at monthly intervals and should be given just enough medication to last until the next visit. Anticipatory guidance with regard to the administration of medications to children is crucial. The physician should foresee difficulties that the family might have in introducing several new medications in inconvenient dosage forms to a young child. The clinician must report all cases of suspected tuberculosis in a child to the local health department to be sure that the child and family receive appropriate care and evaluation.

Nonadherence to treatment is the major problem in tuberculosis therapy. The patient and family must know what is expected of them through verbal and written instructions in their primary language. About 30-50% of patients taking long-term treatment are significantly nonadherent with self-administered medications, and clinicians are usually not able to determine in advance which patients will be nonadherent. Preferably, directly observed therapy should be instituted with the help of the local health department.

Latent *Mycobacterium tuberculosis* Infection (LTBI)

The following aspects of the natural history and treatment of LTBI in children must be considered in the formulation of recommendations about therapy: (1) infants and children <5 yr of age with LTBI have been infected recently; (2) the risk for progression to disease is high; (3) untreated infants with LTBI have up to a 40% chance of development of tuberculosis disease; (4) the risk for progression decreases gradually through childhood; (5) infants and young children are more likely to have life-threatening forms of tuberculosis, including meningitis and disseminated disease; and (6) children with LTBI have more years at risk for development of disease than adults. Because of these factors, and the excellent safety profile of isoniazid in children, there is a tendency to err on the side of overtreatment in infants and young children.

Isoniazid therapy for LTBI appears to be more effective for children than adults, with several large clinical trials demonstrating risk reduction of 70-90%. The risk of isoniazid-related hepatitis is minimal in infants, children, and adolescents, who generally tolerate the drug better than adults.

The recommended regimen for treatment of LTBI in children is a 9-mo course of isoniazid as self-administered daily therapy or by twice-weekly directly observed therapy (DOT). Analysis of data from several studies has demonstrated that the efficacy decreased significantly if isoniazid was taken for <9 mo. Isoniazid given twice weekly has been used extensively to treat LTBI in children, especially schoolchildren and close contacts of case patients. DOT should be considered when it is unlikely that the child and family will adhere to daily self-administration, or if the child is at increased risk for rapid development of disease (newborns and infants, recent contacts, immunocompromised children). For healthy children taking isoniazid but no other potentially hepatotoxic drugs, routine biochemical monitoring and supplementation with pyridoxine are not necessary. A 3-mo regimen of rifampin and isoniazid has been used in England, with programmatic data suggesting that the regimen is effective, but this regimen is not recommended in the USA. Rifampin alone for 6 mo has been used for the treatment of LTBI in infants, children, and adolescents when isoniazid could not be tolerated or the child has had contact with a case patient infected with an isoniazid-resistant but rifamycin-susceptible organism. However, no controlled clinical trials have been conducted. For children with multidrug-resistant tuberculosis infection, the regimen will depend on the drug susceptibility profile of the contract case's organism; usually an expert in tuberculosis should be consulted in such cases.

No controlled studies have been published regarding the efficacy of any form of treatment for LTBI in HIV-infected children. A 9-mo course of daily isoniazid is recommended. Most experts recommend that routine monitoring of serum hepatic enzyme concentrations be performed and pyridoxine be given when HIV-infected children are treated with isoniazid. The optimal duration of rifampin therapy in children with LTBI is not known, but many experts recommend at least a 6-mo course.

Isoniazid should be given to young children who have negative skin test or IGRA results but who have known recent exposure to an adult with contagious tuberculosis disease. This practice is often referred to as window prophylaxis. By the time delayed hypersensitivity develops (2-3 mo), an untreated child already may have developed severe tuberculosis. For these children, tuberculin skin or IGRA testing is repeated 3 mo after contact with the source case for tuberculosis has been broken (*broken contact* is defined as physical separation or adequate initial treatment of the source case). If the second test result is positive, isoniazid therapy is continued for the full 9-mo duration, but if the result of the second test is negative, treatment can be stopped.

PREVENTION

The highest priority of any tuberculosis control program should be case finding and treatment, which interrupts transmission of infection between close contacts. All children and adults with symptoms suggestive of tuberculosis disease and those in close contact with an adult with suspected infectious pulmonary tuberculosis should be tested for tuberculosis infection (by TST or IGRA) and examined as soon as possible. On average, 30-50% of household contacts to infectious cases are infected, and 1% of contacts already have overt disease. This scheme relies on effective and adequate public health response and resources. Children, particularly young infants, should receive high priority during contact investigations, because their risk for infection is high and they are more likely to rapidly develop severe forms of tuberculosis.

Mass testing of large groups of children for tuberculosis infection is an inefficient process. When large groups of children at low risk for tuberculosis are tested, the vast majority of skin test reactions are actually false-positive reactions due to biologic variability or cross sensitization with NTM. However, testing of high-risk groups of adults or children should be encouraged, because most of these persons with positive TST or IGRA results have tuberculosis infection. Testing should take place only if effective mechanisms are in place to ensure adequate evaluation and treatment of the persons who test positive.

Bacille Calmette-Guérin Vaccination

The only available vaccine against tuberculosis is the BCG, named for the 2 French investigators responsible for its development. The original vaccine organism was a strain of *M. bovis* attenuated by subculture every 3 wk for 13 yr. This strain was distributed to dozens of laboratories that continued to subculture the organism on different media under various conditions. The result has been production of many BCG vaccines that differ widely in morphology, growth characteristics, sensitizing potency, and animal virulence.

The administration route and dosing schedule for the BCG vaccines are important variables for efficacy. The preferred route of administration is intradermal injection with a syringe and needle, because it is the only method that permits accurate measurement of an individual dose.

The BCG vaccines are extremely safe in immunocompetent hosts. Local ulceration and regional suppurative adenitis occur in 0.1-1% of vaccine recipients. Local lesions do not suggest underlying host immune defects and do not affect the level of protection afforded by the vaccine. Most reactions are mild and usually resolve spontaneously, but chemotherapy is needed occasionally. Surgical excision of a suppurative draining node is rarely necessary and should be avoided if possible. Osteitis is a rare complication of BCG vaccination that appears to be related to certain strains of the vaccine that are no longer in wide use. Systemic complaints such as fever, convulsions, loss of appetite, and irritability are extraordinarily rare after BCG vaccination. Profoundly immunocompromised patients can develop disseminated BCG infection after vaccination. Children with HIV infection appear to have rates of local adverse reactions to BCG vaccines that are comparable with rates in immunocompetent children. However, the incidence in these children of disseminated infection months to years after vaccination is currently unknown.

Recommended vaccine schedules vary widely among countries. The official recommendation of the World Heath Organization is a single dose administered during infancy, in populations where the risk for tuberculosis is high. However, infants with known HIV infection should not receive a BCG vaccination. In some countries repeat vaccination is universal, though no clinical trials support this practice. In others it is based on either TST or the absence of a typical scar. The optimal age for administration and dosing schedule are unknown because adequate comparative trials have not been performed.

Although dozens of BCG trials have been reported in various human populations, the most useful data have come from several controlled trials. The results of these studies have been disparate. Some demonstrated a great deal of protection from BCG vaccines, but others showed no efficacy at all. A recent meta-analysis of published BCG vaccination trials suggested that BCG is 50% effective in preventing pulmonary tuberculosis in adults and children. The protective effect for disseminated and meningeal tuberculosis appears to be slightly higher, with BCG preventing 50-80% of cases. A variety of explanations for the varied responses to BCG vaccines have been proposed, including methodologic and statistical variations within the trials, interaction with NTM that either enhances or decreases the protection afforded by BCG, different potencies among the various BCG vaccines, and genetic factors for BCG response within the study populations. BCG vaccination administered during infancy has little effect on the ultimate incidence of tuberculosis in adults, suggesting that the effect of the vaccine is time limited.

BCG vaccination has worked well in some situations but poorly in others. Clearly, BCG vaccination has had little effect on the ultimate control of tuberculosis throughout the world, because more than 5 billion doses have been administered but tuberculosis remains epidemic in most regions. BCG vaccination does not substantially influence the chain of transmission, because cases of contagious pulmonary tuberculosis in adults that can be prevented by BCG vaccination constitute a small fraction of the sources of infection in a population. The best use of BCG vaccination appears to be prevention of life-threatening forms of tuberculosis in infants and young children.

BCG vaccination has never been adopted as part of the strategy for the control of tuberculosis in the USA. Widespread use of the vaccine would render subsequent TST less useful. However, BCG vaccination can contribute to tuberculosis control in selected population groups. BCG is recommended for TST-negative infants and children who are at high risk for intimate and prolonged exposure to persistently untreated or ineffectively treated adults with infectious pulmonary tuberculosis and cannot be removed from the source of infection or placed on long-term preventive therapy, and it is recommended for those who are continuously exposed to persons with tuberculosis who have bacilli that are resistant to isoniazid and rifampin. Any child receiving BCG vaccination should have a documented negative TST before receiving the vaccine. After receiving the vaccine, the child should be separated from the possible sources of infection until it can be demonstrated that the child has had a vaccine response, demonstrated by tuberculin reactivity, which usually develops within 1-3 mo.

Active research to develop new tuberculosis vaccines has led to the creation and preliminary testing of several vaccine candidates based on attenuated strains of mycobacteria, subunit proteins, or DNA. The genome of *M. tuberculosis* has been sequenced, allowing researchers to further study and better understand the pathogenesis and host immune responses to tuberculosis.

Perinatal Tuberculosis

The most effective way of preventing tuberculosis infection and disease in the neonate or young infant is through appropriate testing and treatment of the mother and other family members. High-risk pregnant women should be tested with a TST or IGRA, and those with a positive test result should receive a chest radiograph with appropriate abdominal shielding. If the mother has a negative chest radiograph and is clinically well, no separation of the infant and mother is needed after delivery. The child needs no special evaluation or treatment if he or she remains asymptomatic. Other household members should undergo testing for tuberculosis infection and further evaluation as indicated.

If the mother has suspected tuberculosis at the time of delivery, the newborn should be separated from the mother until the chest radiograph is obtained. If the mother's chest radiograph is abnormal, separation should be maintained until the mother has been evaluated thoroughly, including examination of the sputum. If the mother's chest radiograph is abnormal but the history, physical examination, sputum examination, and evaluation of the radiograph show no evidence of current active tuberculosis, it is reasonable to assume that the infant is at low risk for infection. The mother should receive appropriate treatment, and she and her infant should receive careful follow-up care. In addition, all household members should be evaluated for tuberculosis.

If the mother's chest radiograph or acid-fast sputum smear shows evidence of current tuberculosis disease, additional steps are necessary to protect the infant. Isoniazid therapy for newborns has been so effective that separation of the mother and infant is no longer considered mandatory. Separation should occur only if the mother is ill enough to require hospitalization, has been or is expected to become nonadherent to treatment, or has suspected drug-resistant tuberculosis. Isoniazid treatment for the infant should be continued until the mother has been shown to be sputum culture negative for ≥3 mo. At that time, a Mantoux TST should be placed on the child. If the test is positive, isoniazid is continued for a total duration of 9-12 mo; if the test is negative, isoniazid can be discontinued. If isoniazid resistance is suspected or the mother's adherence to medication is in question, separation of the infant from the mother should be considered. The duration of separation must be at least as long as is necessary to render the mother noninfectious. An expert in tuberculosis should be consulted if the young infant has potential exposure to the mother or another adult with tuberculosis disease caused by an isoniazid-resistant strain of *M. tuberculosis*.

Although isoniazid is not thought to be teratogenic, the treatment of pregnant women who have asymptomatic tuberculosis infection is often deferred until after delivery. However, symptomatic pregnant women or those with radiographic evidence of tuberculosis disease should be appropriately evaluated. Because pulmonary tuberculosis is harmful to both the mother and the fetus and represents a great danger to the infant after delivery, tuberculosis in pregnant women always should be treated. The most common regimen for drug-susceptible tuberculosis is isoniazid, rifampin, and ethambutol. The aminoglycosides and ethionamide should be avoided because of their teratogenic effect. The safety of pyrazinamide in pregnancy has not been established.

BIBLIOGRAPHY

Please visit the Nelson Textbook of Pediatrics *website at* *www.expertconsult.com* *for the complete bibliography.*

Chapter 208
Hansen Disease (*Mycobacterium leprae*)

Dwight A. Powell and Vijay Pannikar

Hansen disease (**leprosy**) is a chronic disease resulting from infection with *Mycobacterium leprae* and moderated by the ensuing host response. The respiratory mucosa, skin, and peripheral nervous system are most prominently affected, with occasional testicular and ocular involvement. Humans were long believed to be the sole host of *M. leprae,* but naturally acquired infection has been documented in armadillos in the southeastern USA, and experimental infection has been established in primates, nude mice, and armadillos.

For the full continuation of this chapter, please visit the Nelson Textbook of Pediatrics *website at* *www.expertconsult.com.*

Chapter 209
Nontuberculous Mycobacteria

Jakko van Ingen and Dick van Soolingen

Nontuberculous mycobacteria (NTM), also referred to as **atypical mycobacteria** or **mycobacteria other than tuberculosis (MOTT)**, are members of the family Mycobacteriaceae and the genus *Mycobacterium*. Genetically, NTM constitute a highly diverse group of bacteria that differ from *Mycobacterium tuberculosis* complex bacteria in their pathogenicity, nutritional requirements, ability to produce pigments, enzymatic activity, and drug-susceptibility patterns. In contrast to the *M. tuberculosis* complex, NTM are acquired from environmental sources and not by person-to-person spread. Their omnipresence in our environment implies that the clinical relevance of NTM isolation from clinical specimens is often unclear; a positive culture might reflect contamination rather than true NTM disease. NTM are associated with pediatric lymphadenitis, otomastoiditis, serious lung infections, and, albeit rarely, disseminated disease. Treatment is long-term and cumbersome and often requires adjunctive surgical treatment. Guidelines on diagnosis and treatment are provided by the American and British Thoracic Societies.

ETIOLOGY

NTM are ubiquitous in the environment all over the world, existing as saprophytes in soil and water but also as opportunistic pathogens in animals, including swine, birds, and cattle. Many of the 130 validly published NTM species have been isolated from environmental and animal samples, implying that humans are constantly exposed to NTM from the environment, for instance during showering. Owing to the introduction of molecular identification tools such as 16S rDNA gene sequencing, the number of identified NTM species has grown to more than 130; the clinical relevance (i.e., the percentage of isolates that are causative agents of true NTM disease, rather than contamination) differs significantly by species.

In the USA, *M. avium-intracellulare* complex (MAC) and *M. kansasii* are most often isolated from clinical samples, yet the isolation frequency of these species differs significantly by geographical area. MAC bacteria have been commonly isolated from natural and synthetic environments in the USA, and cases of MAC disease have been successfully linked to home exposure to shower and tap water. Although the designation *M. avium* suggests that *M. avium* infections are derived from birds (*avium* being Latin for "of birds"), molecular typing has pointed out that *M. avium* strains that cause pediatric lymphadenitis and adult pulmonary disease represent the *M. avium hominissuis* subgrouping that is mainly found in humans and pigs and not in birds.

Some NTM have well-defined ecologic niches that help explain infection patterns. The natural reservoir for *M. marinum* is fish and other cold-blooded animals, and hence infections due to *M. marinum* follow skin injury in an aquatic environment. *M. fortuitum* complex bacteria and *M. chelonae* are ubiquitous in water and have caused clusters of nosocomial surgical wound and venous catheter–related infections. *M. ulcerans* is associated with severe, chronic skin infections (**Buruli ulcer disease**) and is endemic mainly in West Africa and Australia, although other foci exist. Its incidence is highest in children <15 yr old. *Mycobacterium ulcerans* had been commonly detected in environmental samples by polymerase chain reaction (PCR) but was only recently recovered by culture from a Water Strider (*Gerris* sp.) from Benin.

EPIDEMIOLOGY

Humans are exposed to NTM very commonly. In rural counties in the USA, where *M. avium* is prevalent in swamps, the **prevalence** of asymptomatic infections with *M. avium* complex as measured by skin test sensitization approaches 70% by adulthood. Still, the incidence and prevalence of the various NTM disease types remain largely unknown, especially for pediatric NTM disease. In Australian children, the overall **incidence** of NTM infection was found to be 0.84 per 100,000, with lymphadenitis accounting for two thirds of cases. The incidence of pediatric NTM disease in the Netherlands has been estimated at 0.77 infections per 100,000 children per year, with lymphadenitis making up 92% of all infections.

In comparison, estimations of the prevalence of NTM from respiratory samples in adults are 5-14.1/100,000 persons per year, with important differences between countries or regions. Because pulmonary NTM disease progresses slowly, over years rather than months, and usually takes several years to cure, the prevalence of pulmonary NTM disease is much higher than incidence rates would suggest.

The paradigm that NTM disease is a rare entity limited to developed countries is changing. In recent studies in African countries with a high prevalence of HIV infection, it has been found that NTM might play a much larger role as a cause of tuberculosis-like disease of children and adults than previously assumed.

PATHOGENESIS

The histologic appearances of lesions caused by *M. tuberculosis* and NTM are often indistinguishable. The classic pathologic lesion consists of **caseating granulomas.** Compared with *M. tuberculosis* infections, NTM infections are more likely to result in granulomas that are **noncaseating,** ill defined (nonpalisading), and irregular or serpiginous. Granuloma formation during NTM disease might even be absent, with only chronic inflammatory changes observed.

In patients with AIDS and disseminated NTM infection, the inflammatory reaction is usually scant and tissues are filled with large numbers of histiocytes packed with acid-fast bacilli. These disseminated NTM infections typically occur only after the number of CD4 T-lymphocytes has fallen below 50/μL, suggesting that specific T-cell products or activities are required for immunity to mycobacteria.

The pivotal roles of interferon-γ (IFN-γ), interleukin (IL)-12 and tumor necrosis factor (TNF)-α in pathogenesis are demonstrated by the high incidence of (mostly disseminated) NTM disease in children with interferon-γ and IL-12 pathway deficiencies and in persons treated with agents that neutralize TNF-α.

Observed differences in pathogenicity, clinical relevance, and spectrum of clinical disease associated with the various NTM species emphasize the importance of bacterial factors in the pathogenesis of NTM disease, though exact virulence factors remain unknown.

CLINICAL MANIFESTATIONS

Lymphadenitis of the superior anterior cervical or submandibular lymph nodes is the most common manifestation of NTM infection in children (Table 209-1). Preauricular, posterior cervical, axillary, and inguinal nodes are involved occasionally. Lymphadenitis is most common in children 1-5 yr of age and has been related to their tendency to put objects contaminated with soil, dust, or standing water into their mouths. Given the constant environmental exposure to NTM, the occurrence of these infections might also reflect an atypical immune response of a subset of the infected children during or after their first contact with NTM.

Affected children usually lack constitutional symptoms and present with a unilateral subacute and slowly enlarging lymph node or group of closely approximated nodes >1.5 cm that are firm, painless, freely movable, and not erythematous (Fig. 209-1).

Table 209-1 DISEASES CAUSED BY NONTUBERCULOUS MYCOBACTERIAL SPECIES

CLINICAL DISEASE	COMMON SPECIES	LESS-COMMON SPECIES
Cutaneous infection	*M. chelonae, M. fortuitum, M. abscessus, M. marinum*	*M. ulcerans**
Lymphadenitis	MAC	*M. kansasii, M. haemophilum, M. malmoense*†
Otologic infection	*M. abscessus*, MAC	*M. fortuitum*
Pulmonary infection	MAC, *M. kansasii, M. abscessus*	*M. xenopi, M. malmoense,*† *M. szulgai, M. fortuitum, M. simiae*
Catheter-associated infection	*M. chelonae, M. fortuitum*	*M. abscessus*
Skeletal infection	MAC, *M. kansasii, M. fortuitum*	*M. chelonae, M. marinum, M. abscessus, M. ulcerans**
Disseminated	MAC	*M. kansasii, M. genavense, M. haemophilum, M. chelonae*

*Not endemic in the USA.
†Found primarily in Northern Europe.
MAC, *Mycobacterium avium* complex.
From American Academy of Pediatrics: *Red book: 2009 report of the Committee on Infectious Diseases*, ed 28, Elk Grove Village, IL, 2009, American Academy of Pediatrics, p 703.

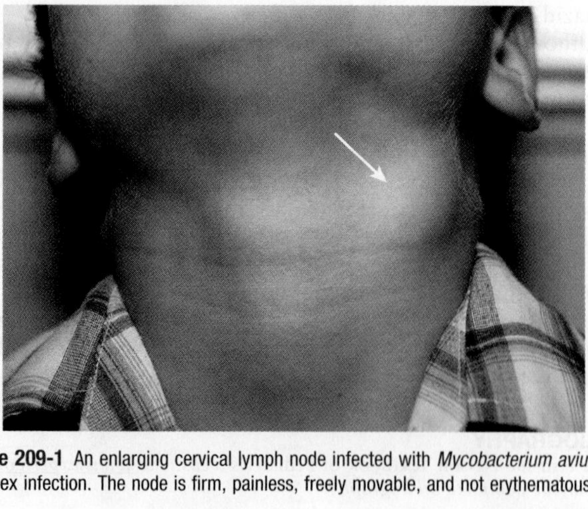

Figure 209-1 An enlarging cervical lymph node infected with *Mycobacterium avium* complex infection. The node is firm, painless, freely movable, and not erythematous.

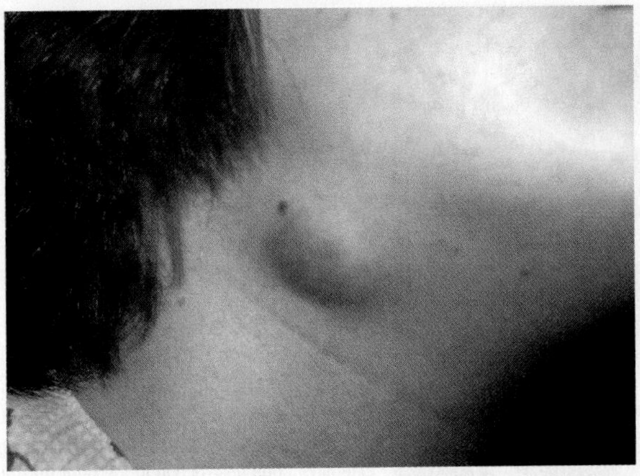

Figure 209-2 A suppurating cervical lymph node infected with *Mycobacterium avium* complex.

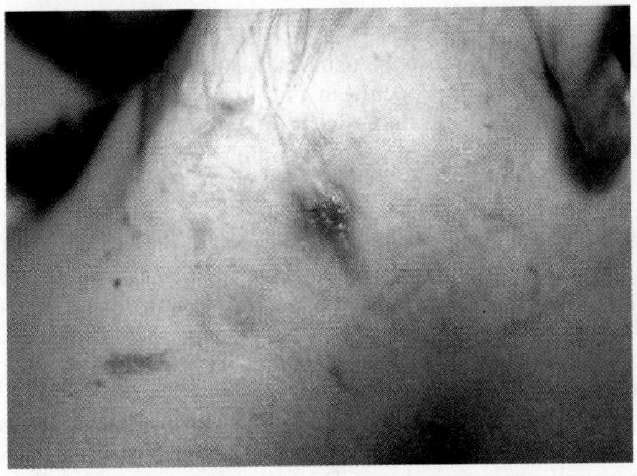

Figure 209-3 A ruptured cervical lymph node infected with *Mycobacterium avium* complex, which resembles the classic scrofula of tuberculosis.

The involved nodes occasionally resolve without treatment, but most undergo rapid suppuration after several weeks (Fig. 209-2). The center of the node becomes fluctuant, and the overlying skin becomes erythematous and thin. Eventually, the nodes rupture and form cutaneous sinus tracts that drain for months or years, resembling the classic scrofula of tuberculosis (Fig. 209-3).

In the USA, *M. avium* complex accounts for approximately 80% of NTM lymphadenitis in children. Birds are an unlikely source of these *M. avium* complex infections, as molecular typing has shown that the lymphadenitis-associated *M. avium* bacteria are of the human or porcine subtype rather than the bird type. *M. kansasii* accounts for most other cases of lymphadenitis in the USA. *M. malmoense* and *M. haemophilum* are described. The former is only common in northwestern Europe; for the latter, underestimation is likely because the bacteria require specific culture conditions (hemin-enriched media, low incubation temperatures). On the basis of PCR analysis of lymph node samples from lymphadenitis cases in the Netherlands, *M. haemophilum* was the second most common cause of this infection after *M. avium* complex.

Cutaneous disease caused by NTM is rare in children (see Table 209-1). Infection usually follows percutaneous inoculation with fresh or salt water contaminated by *M. marinum*. Within 2-6 wk after exposure, an erythematous papule develops at the site of minor abrasions on the elbows, knees, or feet (**swimming pool granuloma**) and on the hands and fingers of fish tank owners, mostly inflicted during tank cleaning (**fish tank granuloma**). These lesions are usually nontender and enlarge over 3-5 wk to form violaceous plaques. Nodules or pustules can develop, and occasionally these lesions ulcerate, resulting in a serosanguineous discharge. The lesions sometimes resemble sporotrichosis, with satellite lesions near the site of entry, extending along the superficial lymphatics. Lymphadenopathy is usually absent. Although most infections remain localized to skin, penetrating *M. marinum* infections can result in tenosynovitis, bursitis, osteomyelitis, or arthritis.

M. ulcerans infection is the third most common mycobacterial infection in immunocompetent patients, after *M. tuberculosis* and *M. leprae* infection, and causes cutaneous disease in children living in tropical regions of Africa, South America, Asia, and parts of Australia. In some communities in West Africa, up to 16% of people have been affected. Infection follows percutaneous inoculation from minor trauma, such as pricks and cuts from plants or insect bites. After an incubation period of approximately 3 mo, lesions appear as an erythematous nodule, most commonly on legs or arms. The lesion undergoes central necrosis and ulceration. The lesion, often called a **Buruli ulcer** after the region in Uganda where a large number of cases was reported, has a characteristic undermined edge, expands over several weeks, and can result in extensive, deep soft tissue destruction or bone involvement. Lesions are typically painless, and constitutional symptoms are unusual. Lesions might heal slowly over 6-9 mo or might continue to spread, leading to deformities and contractures.

Skin and soft tissue infections caused by rapidly growing mycobacteria such as *M. fortuitum, M. chelonae,* or *M. abscessus* are rare in children and usually follow percutaneous inoculation from puncture or surgical wounds and minor abrasions. Clinical disease usually arises after a 4-6 wk incubation period and manifests as localized cellulitis, painful nodules, or a draining abscess. *M. haemophilum* can cause painful subcutaneous nodules, which often ulcerate and suppurate in immunocompromised patients, particularly after kidney transplantation.

NTM are an uncommon cause of **catheter-associated infections** but are becoming increasingly recognized in this respect. Infections caused by *M. fortuitum, M. chelonae,* or *M. abscessus* can manifest as bacteremia or localized catheter tunnel infections.

Otomastoiditis, or chronic otitis media, is a rare extrapulmonary NTM disease type that specifically affects children with tympanostomy tubes and a history of topical antibiotic or steroid use. *M. abscessus* is the most common causative agent, followed by *M. avium* complex (see Table 209-1). Patients present with painless, chronic otorrhea resistant to antibiotic therapy. CT imaging can reveal destruction of the mastoid bone with mucosal swelling (Fig. 209-4). Delayed or unsuccessful treatment can result in permanent hearing loss. In unusual circumstances, NTM causes other **bone** and **joint infections** that are indistinguishable from those produced by *M. tuberculosis* or other bacterial agents. Such infections usually result from operative incision or accidental puncture wounds. *M. fortuitum* infections from puncture wounds of the foot resemble infections caused by *Pseudomonas aeruginosa* and *Staphylococcus aureus*.

Pulmonary infections are the most common form of NTM illness in adults but are rare in children. *M. avium* complex bacteria, the most commonly identified organisms (see Table 209-1), are capable of causing acute pneumonitis, chronic cough, or wheezing associated with paratracheal or peribronchial lymphadenitis and airway compression in normal children. Associated constitutional symptoms such as fever, anorexia, and weight loss occur in 60% of these children. Chest radiographic findings are very similar to those for primary tuberculosis, with unilateral infiltrates and hilar lymphadenopathy (Fig. 209-5). Pleural effusion is uncommon. Rare cases of progression to endobronchial granulation tissue have been reported.

Pulmonary infections usually occur in adults with underlying chronic lung disease. The onset is insidious and consists of cough and fatigue, progressing to weight loss, night sweats, low-grade fever, and generalized malaise in severe cases. Thin-walled cavities

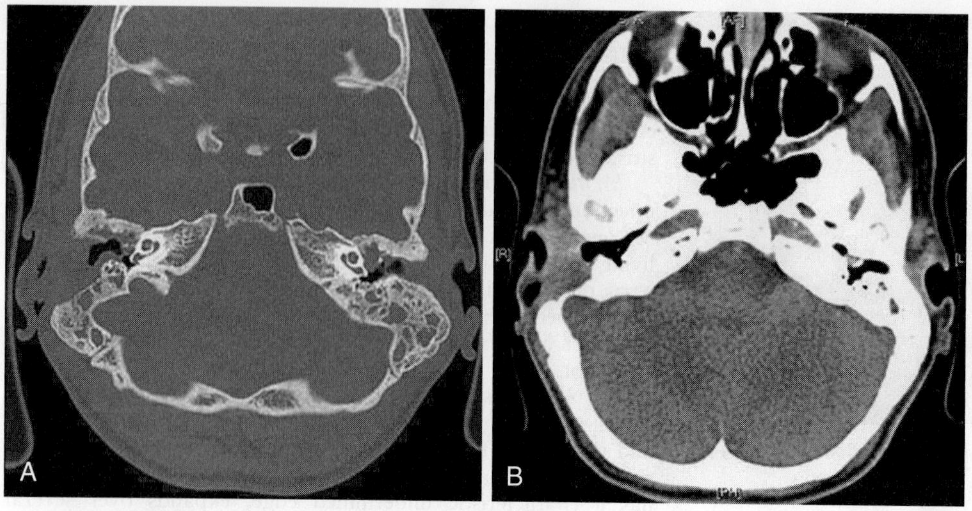

Figure 209-4 Computed tomography images of the middle ear of a 6 yr old child infected with *Mycobacterium abscessus* demonstrating extensive bone destruction in the right mastoid and associated right-sided mucosal swelling. *A*, Bone tissue window setting. *B*, Soft tissue window setting.

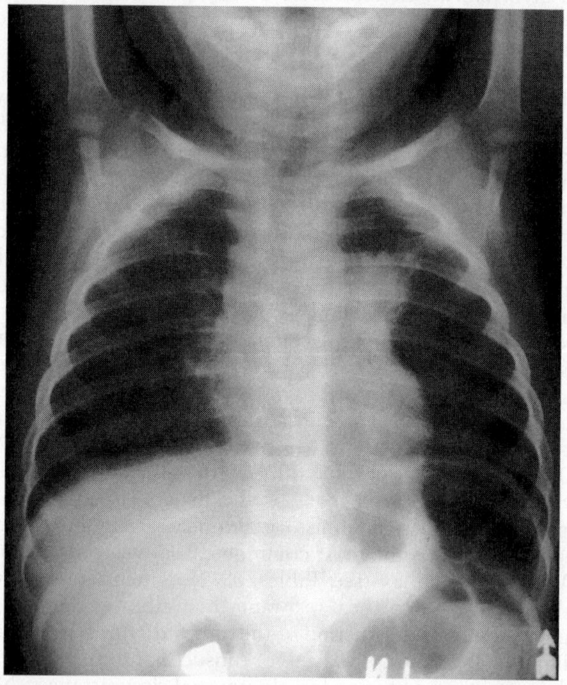

Figure 209-5 Chest radiograph of a 2 yr old child infected with *Mycobacterium avium* complex demonstrating a left upper lobe infiltrate and left hilar lymphadenopathy.

with minimal surrounding parenchymal infiltrates are characteristic, but radiographic findings can resemble those of tuberculosis. A separate disease manifestation occurs in postmenopausal women and is radiologically characterized by bronchiectasis and nodular lesions, often affecting the middle lobe and lingula.

Chronic pulmonary infections specifically affect children with **cystic fibrosis** and are generally caused by *M. abscessus* and *M. avium* complex. *M. abscessus* primarily affects children, and *M. avium* complex is most common among adults. The percentage of patients with cystic fibrosis with at least one sputum culture positive for NTM is 6-8.1% overall and increases with age; in cystic fibrosis patients <12 yr of age, a prevalence of 3.9% has been reported. The strong representation of *M. abscessus* in these patients is remarkable, because this bacterium is an uncommon isolate in other categories of patients. There are indications that NTM infections in patients with cystic fibrosis further accelerate the decline in lung function; antimycobacterial therapy can result in weight gain and improved lung function in affected patients.

Disseminated disease is usually associated with *M. avium* complex infection and occurs in immunocompromised children. The first category of patients with disseminated disease includes persons with mutations in genes coding for the IFN-γ receptor (IFNGR) or the IL-12 receptor, or for IL-12 production. Patients with complete **IFNGR deficiency** have severe disease that is difficult to treat. Those with partial IFNGR deficiency or IL-12 pathway mutations have milder disease that can respond to interferon-γ and antimycobacterial therapy. **Multifocal osteomyelitis** is particularly prevalent in persons with the IFNGR1 818del4 mutation. Recurrences, even years after a course of treatment, and multiple infections have been well documented. The second category of patients affected by **disseminated disease** is patients with **AIDS**. Disseminated NTM disease in patients with AIDS usually appears when CD4 cell counts are <50 cells/mm^3; in younger children (especially those <2 yr of age) these infections occur at higher CD4 cell counts. The most recent estimate of its incidence is 0.14-0.2 episodes per 100 person-years, a 10-fold decrease from its incidence before highly active antiretroviral therapy (HAART) was available.

Colonization of the respiratory or gastrointestinal tract probably precedes disseminated *M. avium* complex infections, but screening studies of respiratory secretions or stool samples are not useful to predict dissemination. Continuous high-grade bacteremia is common, and multiple organs are infected, most commonly including lymph nodes, liver, spleen, bone marrow, and gastrointestinal tract. Thyroid, pancreas, adrenal gland, kidney, muscle, and brain can also be involved. The most common signs and symptoms of disseminated *M. avium* complex infections in AIDS patients are fever, night sweats, chills, anorexia, marked weight loss, wasting, weakness, generalized lymphadenopathy, and hepatosplenomegaly. Jaundice, elevated alkaline phosphatase or lactate dehydrogenase levels, anemia, and neutropenia can occur. Imaging studies usually demonstrate massive lymphadenopathy of hilar, mediastinal, mesenteric, or retroperitoneal nodes. The survival in children with AIDS has improved considerably with the availability of HAART therapy.

Disseminated disease in children without any apparent immunodeficiency is exceedingly rare.

DIAGNOSIS

For infections of lymph nodes, skin, bone, and soft tissues, isolation of the causative NTM bacteria by *Mycobacterium* **culture**, preferably with histologic confirmation of granulomatous inflammation, normally suffices for diagnosis. The differential diagnosis of NTM lymphadenitis includes acute bacterial lymphadenitis, tuberculosis, cat scratch disease (*Bartonella henselae*), mononucleosis, toxoplasmosis, brucellosis, tularemia, and malignancies, especially lymphomas. Differentiation between NTM and *M. tuberculosis* may be difficult, but children with NTM lymphadenitis usually have a Mantoux tuberculin skin test reaction of <15 mm induration, unilateral anterior cervical node involvement, a normal chest x-ray, and no history of exposure to adult tuberculosis. Definitive diagnosis requires excision of the involved nodes for culture and histology. Fine needle aspiration for **PCR** and culture can enable earlier diagnosis, before excisional biopsy.

The diagnosis of **pulmonary NTM infection** in children is difficult because many species of NTM, including *M. avium* complex, are omnipresent in our environment and can contaminate, or occasionally be present in, clinical samples. As a result, isolation of these bacteria from nonsterile specimens (respiratory and digestive tract) does not necessarily reflect true infection. To determine the clinical relevance of isolation of NTM, the diagnostic criteria of the American and British Thoracic Societies are an important support. These criteria take into consideration clinical features and radiologic, pathologic, and microbiologic findings. The hallmark of these criteria is the need for **multiple positive cultures** yielding the same NTM species to make a definitive diagnosis of pulmonary NTM disease. In children, definitive diagnosis often requires invasive procedures such as bronchoscopy and pulmonary or endobronchial biopsy; in cystic fibrosis patients, more-aggressive sample pretreatment is necessary to prevent overgrowth by other species, especially *Pseudomonas* spp. The chance that isolation of NTM is clinically relevant differs significantly by species; some species are more likely causative agents of true pulmonary disease (*M. avium, M. kansasii, M. abscessus, M. malmoense*), whereas others are most likely contaminants (*M. gordonae, M. fortuitum, M. chelonae*).

Blood cultures are 90-95% sensitive in AIDS patients with disseminated infection. *M. avium* complex may be detected within 7-10 days of inoculation in nearly all patients by radiometric or continuously monitored automated blood culture systems. Commercially available DNA probes differentiate NTM from *M. tuberculosis*. If DNA probes cannot identify the causative mycobacteria, DNA sequencing of bacterial housekeeping genes will always yield a clue to the identity of these NTM. Identification of histiocytes containing numerous acid-fast bacilli from bone marrow and other biopsy tissues provides a rapid presumptive diagnosis of disseminated mycobacterial infection.

TREATMENT

Therapy for NTM infections is long-term and cumbersome; **expert consultation** is advised. Therapy involves medical, surgical, or combined treatment (Chapter 206 and Table 206-3). Isolation of the infecting strain followed by **drug susceptibility testing** is ideal, because it provides a baseline for drug susceptibility. Important discrepancies exist between in vitro drug susceptibility and in vivo response to treatment, explained in part by synergism, mainly among first-line antituberculosis drugs. In vitro, slow growers (*M. kansasii, M. marinum, M. xenopi, M. ulcerans,* and *M. malmoense*) are usually susceptible to the first-line antituberculosis drugs rifampicin and ethambutol; *M. avium* complex bacteria are often resistant to these drugs alone but susceptible to the combination and have variable susceptibility to other antibiotics, most importantly the macrolides. Rapid growers (*M. fortuitum, M. chelonae, M. abscessus*) are highly resistant to antituberculosis drugs and often have inducible macrolide resistance mechanisms. Susceptibility to macrolides, aminoglycosides, carbapenems, tetracyclines, and glycylcyclines are most relevant for therapy guidance. In all NTM infections, multiple-drug therapy is essential to avoid development of resistance.

The preferred treatment of NTM lymphadenitis is complete **surgical excision** (Table 206-3). Nodes should be removed while still firm and encapsulated. Excision is more difficult if extensive caseation with extension to surrounding tissue has occurred, and complications of facial nerve damage or recurrent infection are more likely in such cases. Incomplete surgical excision is not advised, because chronic drainage can develop. If there is concern for possible *M. tuberculosis* infection, therapy with isoniazid, rifampin, ethambutol, and pyrazinamide should be administered until cultures confirm the cause to be NTM (Chapter 207). If for some reason surgery of NTM lymphadenitis cannot be performed, removal of infected tissue is incomplete, or recurrence or chronic drainage develops, a 3-6 mo trial of chemotherapy is warranted. Although there are no published controlled trials, several case reports and small series have reported successful treatment with chemotherapy alone or combined with surgical excision. Clarithromycin or azithromycin combined with rifabutin or ethambutol are the most commonly reported therapy regimens (Table 206-3).

Post-traumatic cutaneous NTM lesions in immunocompetent patients usually heal spontaneously after incision and drainage without other therapy (Table 206-3). ***M. marinum*** is susceptible to rifampin, amikacin, ethambutol, sulfonamides, trimethoprim-sulfamethoxazole, and tetracycline. Therapy with a combination of these drugs, particularly rifampin and ethambutol, may be given for 3-4 mo. Corticosteroid injections should not be used. Superficial infections with *M. fortuitum* or *M. chelonae* usually resolve after surgical incision and open drainage, but deep-seated or catheter-related infections require removal of infected central lines and therapy with parenteral amikacin plus cefoxitin or clarithromycin.

Some localized forms of *M. ulcerans* skin disease (**Buruli ulcer**) can heal spontaneously; for most forms, excisional surgery with primary closure or skin grafting is recommended. Provisional guidelines by the World Health Organization (WHO) recommend treatment with rifampin and streptomycin, with or without surgery. In clinical experience, a drug treatment duration of 8 wk generally leads to low recurrence levels. Physiotherapy after surgery is essential to prevent contractures and functional disabilities.

Pulmonary infections should be treated initially with isoniazid, rifampin, ethambutol, and pyrazinamide pending culture identification and drug susceptibility testing. For slow-growing NTM, a combination of rifampin or rifabutin, ethambutol, and clarithromycin is recommended; after culture conversion, treatment should be continued for at least 1 yr. In adult patients with pre-existing pulmonary disease, the role of the macrolides is still debated. For pulmonary disease caused by rapidly growing NTM, a combination of macrolides, fluoroquinolones, aminoglycosides, cefoxitin, and carbapenems is the optimal therapy; three or four-drug regimens are selected on the basis of drug susceptibility testing results. In cystic fibrosis patients, there may be a role for inhaled antibiotics.

Patients with disseminated *M. avium* complex and IL-12 pathway defects or IFNGR deficiency should be treated for at least 12 mo with clarithromycin or azithromycin combined with rifampin or rifabutin and ethambutol. Fluoroquinolones have some in vitro activity, though clinical studies have not settled their role in treatment regimens. In vitro susceptibility testing for clarithromycin and the fluoroquinolones is important to guide therapy. Once the clinical illness has resolved, lifelong daily prophylaxis with azithromycin or clarithromycin is advisable to prevent recurrent disease. The use of interferon adjunctive therapy is determined by the specific genetic defect.

In children with **AIDS, prophylaxis** with azithromycin or clarithromycin is indicated to prevent infection with *M. avium* complex. Although few pediatric studies exist, the U.S. Public Health Service recommends either azithromycin (20 mg/kg once weekly PO, maximum 1,200 mg/dose) or clarithromycin (7.5 mg/kg/dose twice daily PO, maximum 500 mg/dose) for HIV-infected children with significant immune deficiency as defined by the CD4 count (children ≥6 yr, CD4 count <50/µL; 2-6 yr, CD4 count <75/ µL; 1-2 yr, CD4 count <500/µL; <1 yr, CD4 count <750/µL). Prophylaxis may be safely discontinued in children aged >2 yr receiving stable HAART for >6 mo and experiencing sustained (>3 mo) CD4 cell recovery well above the age-specific target for initiation of prophylaxis: >100 cells/µL for children aged ≥6 yr and >200 cells/µL for children aged 2-5 yr. For children <2 yr of age, no specific recommendations for discontinuing MAC prophylaxis exist.

BIBLIOGRAPHY

Please visit the Nelson Textbook of Pediatrics *website at www.expertconsult.com for the complete bibliography.*

Section 8 SPIROCHETAL INFECTIONS

Chapter 210 Syphilis *(Treponema pallidum)*

Maria Jevitz Patterson and H. Dele Davies

Syphilis is a chronic systemic sexually transmitted infection that can be easily treated if detected early but manifests with protean clinical symptoms and significant morbidity if left unchecked.

ETIOLOGY

Syphilis is caused by *Treponema pallidum,* a long, motile spirochete with finely tapered ends belonging to the family *Spirochaetaceae*. The pathogenic members of this genus include *T. pallidum* subspecies *pallidum* (venereal syphilis), *T. pallidum* subspecies *pertenue* (yaws), *T. pallidum* subspecies *endemicum* (bejel or endemic syphilis), and *T. pallidum* subspecies *carateum* (pinta). Because these microorganisms stain poorly and are below the detection limits of conventional light microscopy, detection in clinical specimens requires dark-field or phase contrast microscopy or direct immunofluorescent staining. *T. pallidum* cannot be cultured in vitro.

EPIDEMIOLOGY

In addition to presentation at sexually transmitted disease clinics, patients with syphilis are increasingly seen by primary care providers in private practice settings. Two forms of syphilis occur in children. **Acquired syphilis** is transmitted almost exclusively by sexual contact, including oral sexual exposure. Less common modes of transmission include transfusion of contaminated blood or direct contact with infected tissues. After an epidemic resurgence of primary and secondary syphilis in the USA that peaked in 1989, the annual rate declined 90% by 2000. The total number of cases of primary and secondary syphilis has subsequently increased since 2000, particularly among men who have sex with men. Despite a decrease among women for almost a decade, their rates have also increased every year since 2004. By 2007, U.S. reported cases of syphilis had risen for the 7th straight year, a 15% increase from 2006 among men and women. Cases of congenital syphilis rose by 13% in the same time period (Fig. 210-1). Rates in the southern USA and among non-Hispanic blacks are disproportionately high.

Congenital syphilis results from transplacental transmission of spirochetes. Women with primary and secondary syphilis and spirochetemia are more likely to transmit infection to the fetus than are women with latent infection. Transmission can occur at any stage of pregnancy. The incidence of congenital infection in offspring of untreated or poorly treated infected women remains highest during the first 4 yr after acquisition of primary infection, secondary infection, and early latent disease. Risk factors most commonly associated with congenital syphilis are lack of prenatal care and cocaine drug abuse, unprotected sexual contact, trading of sex for drugs, and poor treatment of syphilis during pregnancy (Fig. 210-2). Confirmed cases of acquired or congenital syphilis should be reported to the local health department.

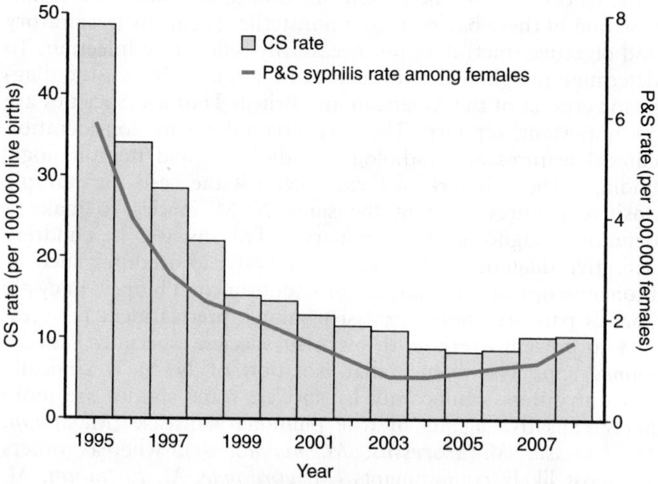

Figure 210-1 Congenital syphilis (CS) rate among infants aged <1 yr and rate of primary and secondary syphilis (P&S) among girls and women aged ≥10 yr: National Electronic Telecommunication System for Surveillance, USA, 1995-2008. CS rates from 1995 to 2006 were calculated using yearly live birth data as denominators. Rates for 2007 and 2008 were calculated using live birth data for 2006. (From Centers for Disease Control and Prevention: *National vital statistics system: birth data* [website]. http://www.cdc.gov/nchs/births.htm. Accessed August 25, 2010.) P&S syphilis rates were calculated using bridged race population estimates for 2000-2007 based on 2000 U.S. Census counts. (From CDC Wonder: *Bridged-race resident population estimates, United States, state and county, for the years 1990-2008* (website). http://wonder.cdc.gov/wonder/help/bridged-race.html. Accessed August 25, 2010.) (From Centers for Disease Control and Prevention: Congenital syphilis—United States, 2003-2008, *MMWR Morb Mortal Wkly Rep* 59:413–417, 2010.)

CLINICAL MANIFESTATIONS AND LABORATORY FINDINGS

Many persons infected with syphilis are asymptomatic for years or do not recognize the early signs of disease. **Primary syphilis** is characterized by a chancre and regional lymphadenitis. A **painless papule** appears at the site of entry (usually the genitals) 2-6 wk after inoculation that develops into a clean, painless, but highly contagious ulcer with raised borders (**chancre**) containing abundant *T. pallidum*. Extragenital chancres can occur at other sites of primary entry. Oral lesions can be mistaken for aphthous ulcers or herpes. Adjacent lymph nodes are generally enlarged and nontender. The chancre heals spontaneously within 4-6 wk, leaving a thin scar.

Untreated patients develop manifestations of **secondary syphilis** related to spirochetemia 2-10 wk after the chancre heals. Manifestations of secondary syphilis include a generalized nonpruritic maculopapular rash, notably involving the palms and soles (Fig. 210-3). Pustular lesions can also develop. **Condylomata lata,** gray-white to erythematous wartlike plaques, can occur in moist areas around the anus and vagina, and white

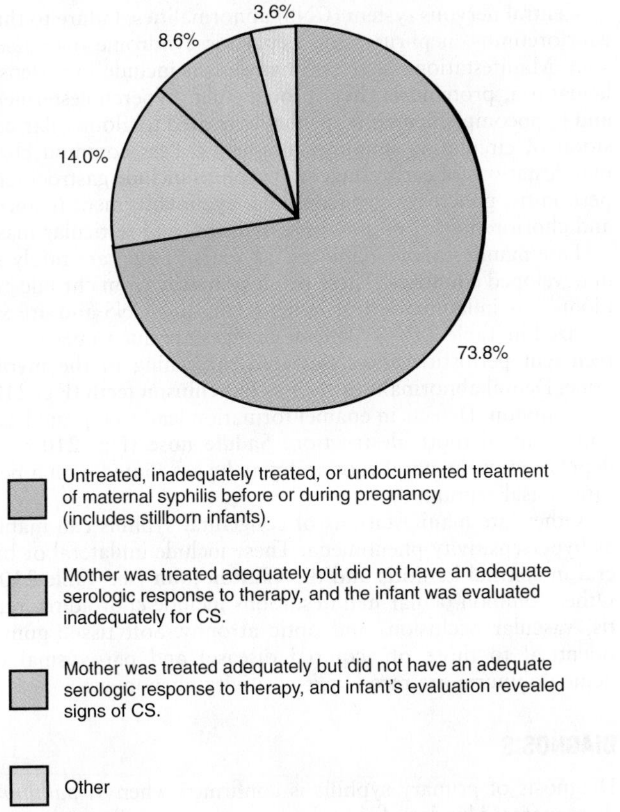

3.6%
8.6%
14.0%
73.8%
Untreated, inadequately treated, or undocumented treatment of maternal syphilis before or during pregnancy (includes stillborn infants).
Mother was treated adequately but did not have an adequate serologic response to therapy, and the infant was evaluated inadequately for CS.
Mother was treated adequately but did not have an adequate serologic response to therapy, and infant's evaluation revealed signs of CS.
Other

Figure 210-2 Diagnoses of congenital syphilis (CS) in the USA, 2002. (From Centers for Disease Control and Prevention: Primary and secondary syphilis—United States, 2002, *MMWR Morb Mortal Wkly Rep* 52:1117–1120, 2003.)

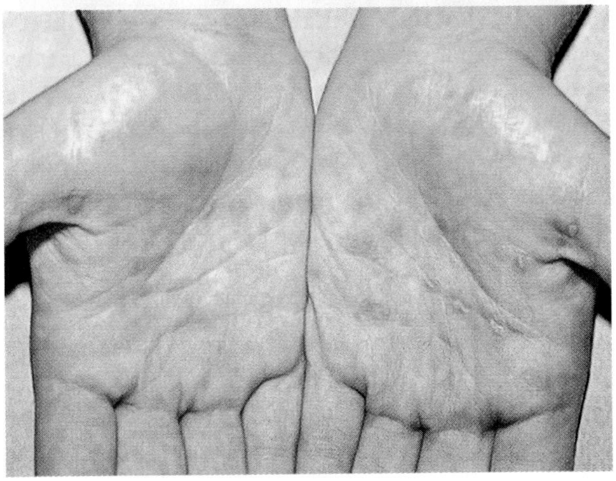

Figure 210-3 Secondary syphilis. Ham-colored palmar macules on an adolescent with secondary syphilis. (From Weston WL, Lane AT, Morelli JG: *Color textbook of pediatric dermatology*, ed 3, St Louis, Mosby, 2002.)

plaques (**mucous patches**) may be found in mucous membranes. A **flulike illness** with low-grade fever, headache, malaise, anorexia, weight loss, sore throat, myalgias, arthralgias, and generalized lymphadenopathy is often present. Renal, hepatic, and ophthalmologic manifestations may be present. Meningitis occurs in 30% of patients with secondary syphilis and is characterized by cerebrospinal fluid (CSF) pleocytosis and elevated protein level. Patients with meningitis might not show neurologic symptoms. Secondary infection becomes **latent** within 1-2 mo after onset of rash. Relapses with secondary manifestations can occur during the first year of latency (the **early latent period**). **Late syphilis**

Table 210-1 LATE MANIFESTATIONS OF CONGENITAL SYPHILIS

SYMPTOM/SIGN	DESCRIPTION/COMMENTS
Olympian brow	Bony prominence of the forehead due to persistent or recurrent periostitis
Clavicular or Higouménaki sign	Unilateral or bilateral thickening of the sternoclavicular third of the clavicle
Saber shins	Anterior bowing of the midportion of the tibia
Scaphoid scapula	Convexity along the medial border of the scapula
Hutchinson teeth	Peg-shaped upper central incisors; they erupt during 6th yr of life with abnormal enamel, resulting in a notch along the biting surface
Mulberry molars	Abnormal 1st lower (6 yr) molars characterized by small biting surface and excessive number of cusps
Saddle nose*	Depression of the nasal root, a result of syphilitic rhinitis destroying adjacent bone and cartilage
Rhagades	Linear scars that extend in a spoke-like pattern from previous mucocutaneous fissures of the mouth, anus, and genitalia
Juvenile paresis	Latent meningovascular infection; it is rare and typically occurs during adolescence with behavioral changes, focal seizures, or loss of intellectual function
Juvenile tabes	Rare spinal cord involvement and cardiovascular involvement with aortitis
Hutchinson triad	Hutchinson teeth, interstitial keratitis, and 8th nerve deafness
Clutton joint	Unilateral or bilateral painless joint swelling (usually involving knees) due to synovitis with sterile synovial fluid; spontaneous remission usually occurs after several wk
Interstitial keratitis	Manifests with intense photophobia and lacrimation, followed within weeks or months by corneal opacification and complete blindness.
Eighth nerve deafness	May be unilateral or bilateral, appears at any age, manifests initially as vertigo and high-tone hearing loss, and progresses to permanent deafness

*A perforated nasal septum may be an associated abnormality.

follows and may be either asymptomatic (**late latent**) or symptomatic (**tertiary**). Tertiary disease is marked by neurologic, cardiovascular, and **gummatous lesions** (nonsuppurative granulomas of the skin and musculoskeletal system resulting from the host's hypersensitivity reaction).

Congenital Infection

Untreated syphilis during pregnancy has a vertical transmission rate approaching 100%, with profound effects on pregnancy outcome. Fetal or perinatal death occurs in 40% of affected infants. Premature delivery can also occur. Neonates can also be infected at delivery by contact with an active genital lesion.

Most infected infants are asymptomatic at birth and are identified only by routine prenatal screening. In the absence of treatment, symptoms develop within weeks or months. Among infants symptomatic at birth or in the first months of life, manifestations have traditionally been divided into early and late stages. All stages of congenital syphilis are characterized by a vasculitis, with progression to necrosis and fibrosis. The **early signs** appear during the first 2 yr of life, and the **late signs** appear gradually during the first 2 decades. Early manifestations vary and involve multiple organ systems, resulting from transplacental spirochetemia and are analogous to the secondary stage of acquired syphilis (Table 210-1). Hepatosplenomegaly, jaundice, and elevated liver enzymes are common. Histologically, liver involvement includes bile stasis, fibrosis, and extramedullary hematopoiesis. Lymphadenopathy tends to be diffuse and resolve spontaneously, although shotty nodes can persist.

Coombs-negative hemolytic anemia is characteristic. Thrombocytopenia is often associated with platelet trapping in an enlarged spleen. Characteristic osteochondritis and periostitis (Fig. 210-4) and a mucocutaneous rash (Fig. 210-5*A*, *B*) manifesting with erythematous maculopapular or vesiculobullous lesions followed by desquamation involving hands and feet (see Fig. 210-5C) are common. Mucous patches, persistent rhinitis (**snuffles**), and condylomatous lesions (Fig. 210-6) are highly characteristic features of mucous membrane involvement and contain abundant spirochetes. Blood and moist open lesions from infants with congenital syphilis and children with acquired primary or secondary syphilis are infectious until 24 hours of appropriate treatment.

Bone involvement is common. Roentgenographic abnormalities include **Wimberger's lines** (metaphyseal demineralization of the medial aspect of the proximal tibia), multiple sites of osteochondritis at the wrists, elbows, ankles, and knees, and periostitis of the long bones and rarely the skull. The osteochondritis is painful, often resulting in irritability and refusal to move the involved extremity (**pseudoparalysis of Parrot**).

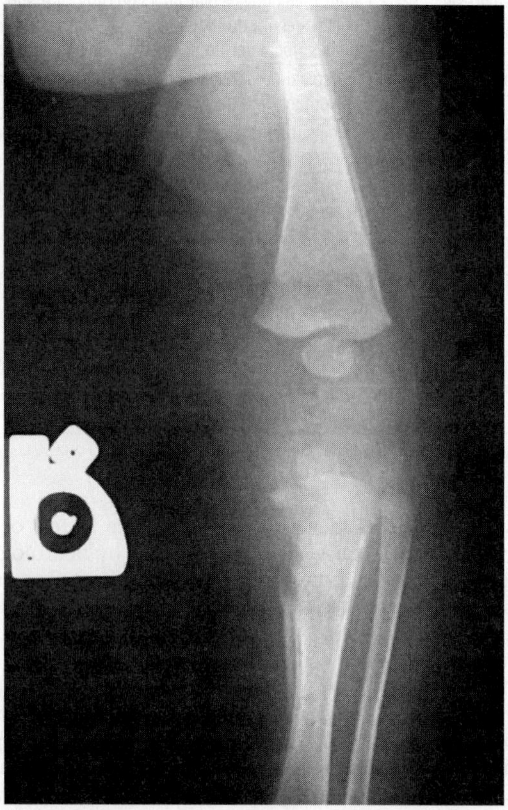

Figure 210-4 Osteochondritis and periostitis in a newborn with congenital syphilis.

Central nervous system (CNS) abnormalities, failure to thrive, chorioretinitis, nephritis, and nephrotic syndrome may also be seen. Manifestations of renal involvement include hypertension, hematuria, proteinuria, hypoproteinemia, hypercholesterolemia, and hypocomplementemia, probably related to glomerular deposition of circulating immune complexes. Less common clinical manifestations of early congenital syphilis include gastroenteritis, peritonitis, pancreatitis, pneumonia, eye involvement (glaucoma and chorioretinitis), nonimmune hydrops, and testicular masses.

Late manifestations (children >2 years of age) are rarely seen in developed countries. These result primarily from chronic granulomatous inflammation of bone, teeth, and CNS and are summarized in Table 210-1. Skeletal changes are due to persistent or recurrent periostitis and associated thickening of the involved bone. Dental abnormalities such as **Hutchinson teeth** (Fig. 210-7) are common. Defects in enamel formation lead to repeated caries and eventual tooth destruction. **Saddle nose** (Fig. 210-8) is a depression of the nasal root and may be associated with a perforated nasal septum.

Other late manifestations of congenital syphilis can manifest as hypersensitivity phenomena. These include unilateral or bilateral interstitial keratitis and the **Clutton joint** (see Table 210-1). Other common ocular manifestations include choroiditis, retinitis, vascular occlusion, and optic atrophy. Soft tissue gummas (identical to those of acquired disease) and paroxysmal cold hemoglobinuria are rare hypersensitivity phenomena.

DIAGNOSIS

Diagnosis of primary syphilis is confirmed when *T. pallidum* is demonstrated by dark-field microscopy or direct fluorescent antibody testing on specimens from skin lesions, placenta, or

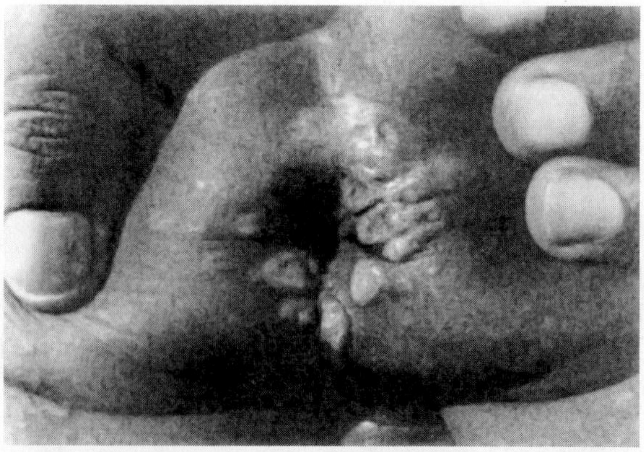

Figure 210-6 Perianal condylomata lata. (From Karthikeyan K, Thappa DM: Early congenital syphilis in the new millennium, *Pediatr Dermatol* 19:275–276, 2002.)

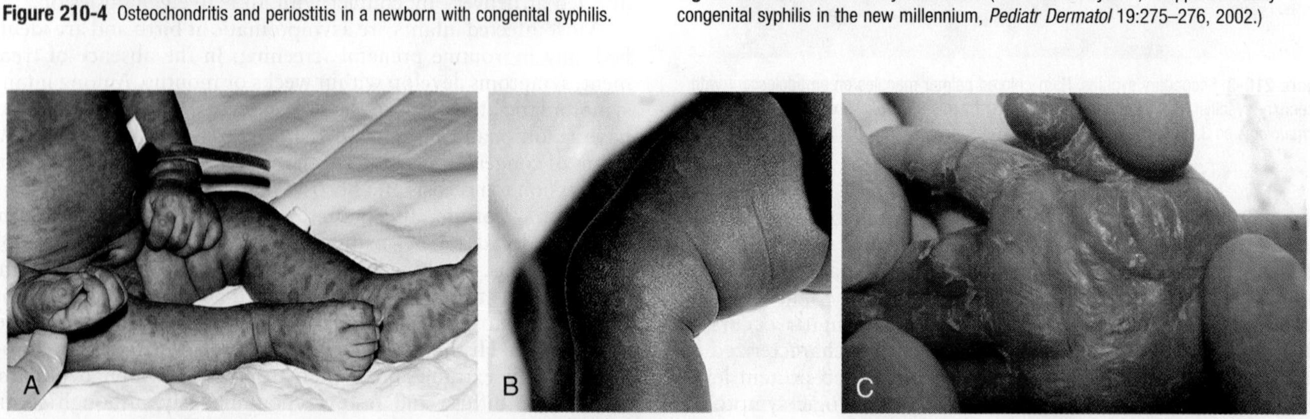

Figure 210-5 *A* and *B*, Papulosquamous plaques in 2 infants with syphilis. *C*, Desquamation on the palm of a newborn's hand. (*A* and *B*, From Eichenfeld LF, Frieden IJ, Esterly NB, editors: *Textbook of neonatal dermatology*, Philadelphia, 2001, WB Saunders, p 196. *C*, Courtesy of Dr. Patricia Treadwell.)

umbilical cord. Nucleic acid–based amplification assays such as polymerase chain reaction (PCR) are not commercially available. Serologic testing for syphilis remains the principal means for diagnosis and typically involves screening with a nontreponemal test followed by a confirmatory treponemal test.

The **Venereal Disease Research Laboratory (VDRL)** and **rapid plasma reagin (RPR)** tests are sensitive **nontreponemal tests** that detect antibodies against phospholipid antigens on the treponeme surface that cross react with mammalian cardiolipin-lecithin-cholesterol antigens. The quantitative results of these tests are helpful in screening and in monitoring therapy. Titers increase with active disease, including treatment failure or reinfection, and decline with adequate treatment (Fig. 210-9). Nontreponemal tests usually become nonreactive within 1 yr of adequate therapy for primary syphilis and within 2 yr of adequate treatment for secondary disease. Uncommonly some patients become **serofast** (nontreponemal titers persisting at low levels for long periods). In congenital infection, these tests become nonreactive within a few months after adequate treatment. Certain conditions such as infectious mononucleosis and other infections, connective tissue diseases, and pregnancy can give false-positive VDRL results. False-positive results are less common with the use of purified cardiolipin-lecithin-cholesterol antigen. All positive maternal serologic tests for syphilis, regardless of titer, necessitate thorough investigation. Antibody excess can give a false-negative reading unless the serum is diluted (**prozone effect**). False-negative results can also occur in early primary syphilis, in latent syphilis of long duration, and in late congenital syphilis.

Treponemal tests traditionally are used to confirm diagnosis and measure specific *T. pallidum* antibody and include the *T. pallidum* hemagglutination assay (TPHA), the fluorescent

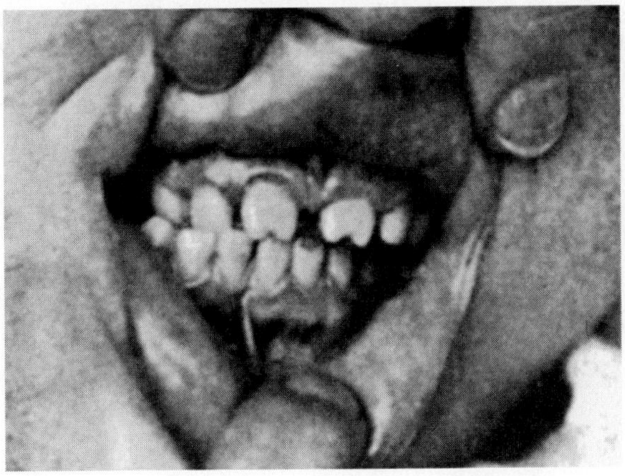

Figure 210-7 Hutchinson teeth as a late manifestation of congenital syphilis.

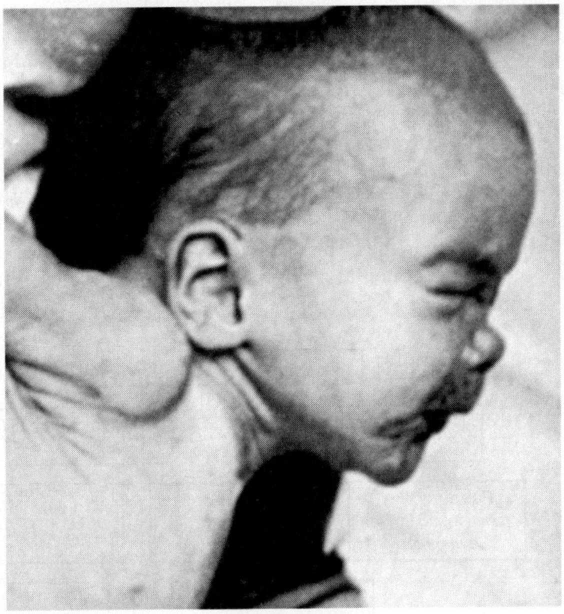

Figure 210-8 Saddle nose in a newborn with congenital syphilis.

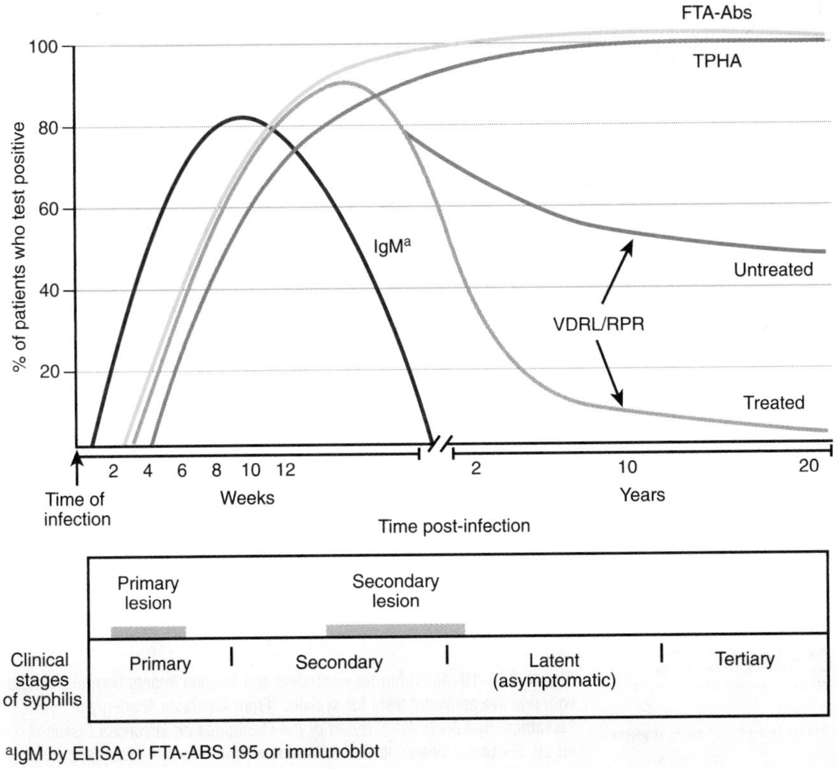

Figure 210-9 Common patterns of serologic reactivity in syphilis patients. FTA-Abs, fluorescent treponemal antibody absorption (test); RPR, rapid plasma reagin (test); TPHA, *Treponema pallidum* hemagglutination assay; VDRL, Venereal Disease Research Laboratory (test). (From Peeling RW, Ye H: Diagnostic tools for preventing and managing maternal and congenital syphilis: an overview, *Bull World Health Organ* 82:439–446, 2004.)

treponemal antibody absorption (FTA-ABS) test, and the *T. pallidum* particle agglutination (TPPA) test. Treponemal antibody titers become positive soon after initial infection and usually remain positive for life, even with adequate therapy (see Fig. 210-9). These antibody titers do not correlate with disease activity. Traditionally they are useful for diagnosis of a 1st episode of syphilis and for distinguishing false-positive results of nontreponemal antibody tests but cannot accurately identify length of time of infection, response to therapy, or reinfection.

There is limited cross reactivity of treponemal antibody tests with other spirochetes, including the causative organisms of Lyme disease (*Borrelia burgdorferi*), yaws, endemic syphilis, and pinta. Only venereal syphilis and Lyme disease are found in the USA. Nontreponemal tests (VDRL, RPR) are uniformly nonreactive in Lyme disease.

Enzyme-linked immunosorbent assays (ELISAs) to detect treponemal immunoglobulin G (IgG) and immunoglobulin M (IgM) have been developed. Such assays should allow developing countries quality screening programs at the point-of-service because WHO currently relies on syndromic management of sexually transmitted infections, where patients are treated for all likely causes of their constellation of signs and symptoms. In the USA use of ELISAs has confounded screening because it switches the traditional algorithm: the treponemal-specific testing is done before the nontreponemal testing. Because the former remain positive for life, clinical and epidemiologic data are required to provide clear guidelines to distinguish cured disease, latent but potentially active disease, and true false-positive tests. Interim CDC guidelines suggest that persons with reactive treponemal but nonreactive nontreponemal testing who have not been previously treated for syphilis should be offered treatment for late latent syphilis. Interpretation of nontreponemal and treponemal serologic tests in the newborn may be confounded by maternal IgG antibodies transferred to the fetus. Passively acquired antibody is suggested by neonatal titer at least 4-fold (i.e., a 2-tube dilution) less than the maternal titer. This conclusion can be verified by gradual decline in antibody in the infant, usually becoming undetectable by 3-6 mo of age.

The diagnosis of neurosyphilis remains difficult but is often established by demonstrating pleocytosis and increased protein in the CSF and a positive CSF VDRL test along with neurologic symptoms. The CSF VDRL test is specific but relatively insensitive (22-69%) for neurosyphilis. CSF PCR and IgM Western immunoblot tests are under development to assist in diagnosis of neurosyphilis.

Dark-field microscopy of scrapings from primary lesions or congenital or secondary lesions can reveal *T. pallidum,* often before serology becomes positive, but this technique is usually not available in clinical practice. Placental examination by gross and microscopic techniques can be useful in the diagnosis of congenital

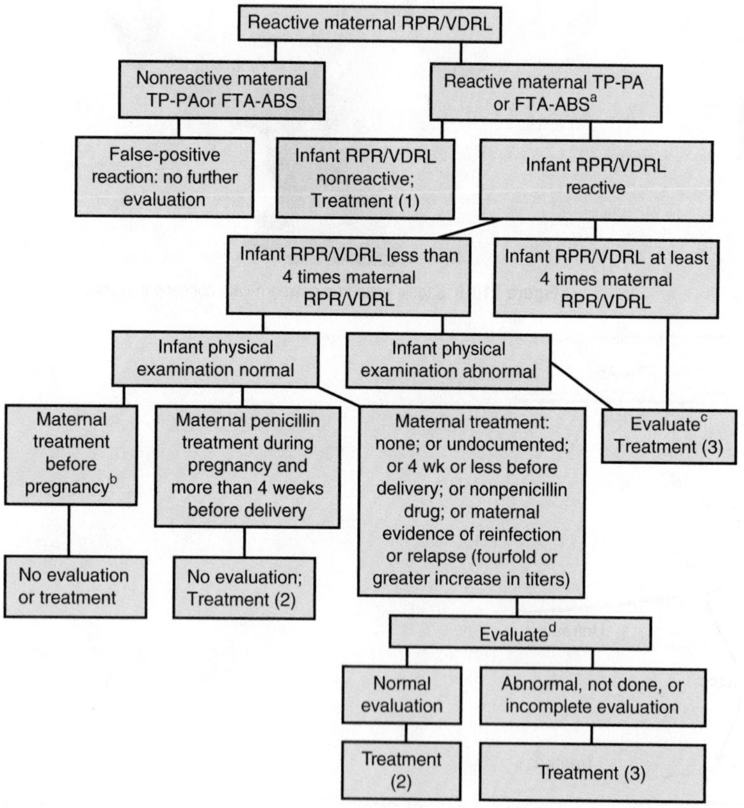

RPR indicates rapid plasma reagin (test); VDRL, Venereal Disease Research Laboratory (test); TP-PA, *Treponema pallidum* particle agglutination (test); FTA-ABS, fluorescent treponema antibody absorption (test).

a Test for human immunodeficiency virus (HIV) antibody. Infants of HIV-infected mothers do not require different evaluation or treatment.

b Women who maintain a VDRL titer 1:2 or less (RPR 1:4 or less) beyond 1 year after successful treatment are considered serofast.

c Evaluation consists of complete blood cell (CBC) and platelet count; cerebrospinal fluid (CSF) examination for cell count, protein, and quantitative VDRL. Other tests as clinically indicated: long-bone and chest radiographs, neuroimaging, auditory brainstem response, eye examination, liver function tests.

d CBC, platelet count; CSF examination for cell count, protein, and quantitative VDRL; long-bone radiography.

TREATMENT:

(1) If the mother has had no treatment, undocumented treatment, treatment 4 weeks or less before delivery or evidence of reinfection or relapse (fourfold or greater increase in titers) AND the infant's physical examination is normal, THEN treat infant with a single intramuscular (IM) injection of benzathine penicillin (50 000 U/kg). If these criteria are not met, no treatment is required. In both scenarios, no additional evaluation is needed.

(2) Benzathine penicillin G, 50 000 U/kg, IM, x 1 dose.

(3) Aqueous penicillin G, 50 000 U/kg, IV, every 12 hours (1 week of age or younger), every 8 hours (older than 1 week), or procaine penicillin G, 50 000 U/kg, IM, single daily dose, x 10 days.

Figure 210-10 Algorithm for evaluating and treating infants born to mothers with reactive serologic tests for syphilis. (From American Academy of Pediatrics: *Red book: 2009 report of the Committee on Infectious Diseases,* ed 28, Elk Grove Village, IL, 2009, American Academy of Pediatrics, p 645.)

syphilis. The disproportionately large placentas are characterized histologically by focal proliferative villitis, endovascular and perivascular arteritis, and focal or diffuse immaturity of placental villi.

Congenital Syphilis

Diagnosis of congenital syphilis requires thorough review of maternal testing, treatment, and the dynamics of response. Proactive evaluation and treatment of exposed neonates is critical (Fig. 210-10 and Table 210-2). Symptomatic infants should be thoroughly evaluated and treated. Guidelines for evaluating and managing asymptomatic infants considered at risk for congenital syphilis because the maternal nontreponemal and treponemal serology is positive are shown in Table 210-3.

Diagnosis of neurosyphilis in the newborn with syphilitic infection is confounded by poor sensitivity of the CSF VDRL test in this age group and lack of CSF abnormalities. A positive CSF VDRL test in a newborn warrants treatment for neurosyphilis, even though it might reflect passive transfer of antibodies from serum to CSF. It is now accepted that all infants with a presumptive diagnosis of congenital syphilis should be treated with regimens effective for neurosyphilis because CNS involvement cannot be reliably excluded. Diagnosis of syphilis beyond early infancy should lead to consideration of possible child abuse.

For infants with proven or highly probable disease or abnormal physical findings, complete evaluation including serologic tests (RPR or VDRL), complete blood count with differential and platelet count, liver function tests, long-bone radiographs, ophthalmology examination, auditory brainstem response, and other tests as indicated should be performed. For infants with a positive VDRL or RPR test result and normal physical examination whose mothers were inadequately treated, further evaluation is not necessary if 10 days of parenteral therapy is administered.

Table 210-2 CLUES THAT SUGGEST A DIAGNOSIS OF CONGENITAL SYPHILIS*

EPIDEMIOLOGIC BACKGROUND	CLINICAL FINDINGS
Untreated early syphilis in the mother	Osteochondritis, periostitis
Untreated latent syphilis in the mother	Snuffles, hemorrhagic rhinitis
An untreated mother who has contact with a known syphilitic during pregnancy	Condylomata lata
Mother treated for syphilis during pregnancy with a drug other than penicillin	Bullous lesions, palmar or plantar rash
Mother treated for syphilis during pregnancy without follow-up to demonstrate 4-fold change in titer	Mucous patches
Mother co-infected with HIV	Hepatomegaly, splenomegaly
	Jaundice
	Nonimmune hydrops fetalis
	Generalized lymphadenopathy
	Central nervous system signs; elevated cell count or protein in cerebrospinal fluid
	Hemolytic anemia, diffuse intravascular coagulation, thrombocytopenia
	Pneumonitis
	Nephrotic syndrome
	Placental villitis or vasculitis (unexplained enlarged placenta)
	Intrauterine growth restriction

*Arranged in decreasing order of confidence of diagnosis.
Modified from Remington JS, Klein JO, Wilson CB, et al, editors: *Infectious diseases of the fetus and newborn infant,* ed 6, Philadelphia, 2006, Saunders, p 556.

TREATMENT

T. pallidum remains extremely sensitive to penicillin, with no evidence of emerging penicillin resistance, and thus penicillin remains the treatment drug of choice (Tables 210-3 and 210-4). Parenteral penicillin G is the only documented effective treatment for congenital syphilis, syphilis during pregnancy, and neurosyphilis. Aqueous crystalline penicillin G is preferred over procaine penicillin, because it better achieves and sustains the minimum concentration of 0.018 µg/mL (0.03 U/mL) needed for 7-10 days to achieve treponemicidal levels. Although nonpenicillin regimens are available to the penicillin-allergic patient, desensitization followed by standard penicillin therapy is the most reliable strategy. An acute systemic febrile reaction called the **Jarisch-Herxheimer reaction** (due to massive release of endotoxin-like antigens during

Table 210-3 RECOMMENDED MANAGEMENT OF NEONATES (≤1 MO OF AGE) BORN TO MOTHERS WITH SEROLOGIC TESTS FOR SYPHILIS

CLINICAL STATUS	EVALUATION (IN ADDITION TO PHYSICAL EXAMINATION AND QUANTITATIVE NONTREPONEMAL TESTING)	ANTIMICROBIAL THERAPY*
Proven or highly probable disease†	CSF analysis for VDRL, cell count, and protein CBC and platelet count Other tests as clinically indicated (e.g., long-bone radiography, liver function tests, ophthalmologic examination)	Aqueous crystalline penicillin G, 100 000-150 000 U/kg/day, administered as 50,000 U/kg/dose IV q12hr during the first 7 days of life and 18hr thereafter for a total of 10 days *or* Penicillin G procaine, 50,000 U/kg/day IM in a single dose × 10 days
Normal physical examination and serum quantitative nontreponemal titer ≤4 times the maternal titer:		
a) (i) Mother was not treated or inadequately treated or has no documented treatment; (ii) mother was treated with erythromycin or other nonpenicillin regimen; (iii) mother received treatment ≤4 wk before delivery; (iv) maternal evidence of reinfection or relapse (<4-fold decrease in titers)	CSF analysis for VDRL, cell count, and protein§ CBC and platelet count§ Long-bone radiography§	Aqueous crystalline penicillin G IV × 10 days§ *or* Penicillin G procaine‡ 50,000 U/kg IM in a single dose × 10 days§ *or* Penicillin G benzathine‡ 50,000 U/kg IM in a single dose§
b) (i) Adequate maternal therapy given >4 wk before delivery; (ii) mother has no evidence of reinfection or relapse	None	Clinical, serologic follow-up, and penicillin G benzathine 50,000 U/kg IM in a single dose‖
c) Adequate therapy before pregnancy and mother's nontreponemal serologic titer remained low and stable during pregnancy and at delivery	None	None¶

*If >1 day of therapy is missed, the entire course should be restarted.
†Abnormal physical examination, serum quantitative nontreponemal titer that is fourfold greater than the mother's titer, or positive result of dark-field or fluorescent antibody test of body fluid(s).
‡Penicillin G benzathine and penicillin G procaine are approved for IM administration only.
§A complete evaluation (CSF analysis, bone radiography, CBC) is not necessary if 10 days of parenteral therapy is administered, but it may be useful to support a diagnosis of congenital syphilis. If a single dose of penicillin G benzathine is used, then the infant must be evaluated fully, results of the full evaluation must be normal, and follow-up must be certain. If any part of the infant's evaluation is abnormal or not performed or if the CSF analysis is uninterpretable, the 10-day course of penicillin is required.
‖Some experts would not treat the infant but would provide close serologic follow-up.
¶Some experts would treat with penicillin G benzathine, 50,000 U/kg, as a single IM injection, if follow-up is uncertain.
CBC, complete blood cell count; CSF, cerebrospinal fluid; VDRL, Venereal Disease Research Laboratory.
From American Academy of Pediatrics: *Red book: 2009 report of the Committee on Infectious Diseases*, ed 28, Elk Grove Village, IL, 2009, American Academy of Pediatrics, p 645.

Table 210-4 RECOMMENDED TREATMENT FOR SYPHILIS IN PATIENTS >1 MONTH OF AGE

STATUS	CHILDREN	ADULTS
Congenital syphilis	Aqueous crystalline penicillin G 200 000-300 000 U/kg/day IV administered as 50,000 U/kg 14-6hr × 10 days*	
Primary, secondary, and early latent syphilis†	Penicillin G benzathine,‡ 50,000 U/kg, IM, up to the adult dose of 2.4 million U in a single dose	Penicillin G benzathine,‡ 2.4 million U IM in a single dose *or* *If allergic to penicillin and not pregnant,* doxycycline 100 mg PO bid × 14 days *or* Tetracycline 500 mg PO qid × 14 days
Late latent syphilis§ or syphilis of unknown duration	Penicillin G benzathine,‡ 50,000 U/kg IM up to the adult dose of 2.4 million U, administered as 3 single doses at 1-wk intervals (total 150,000 U/kg, up to the adult dose of 7.2 million U)	Penicillin G benzathine‡ 7.2 million U total administered as 3 doses of 2.4 million U IM, each at 1-wk intervals *or* *If allergic to penicillin and not pregnant,* doxycycline 100 mg PO bid × 4 wk *or* Tetracycline 500 mg PO qid × 4 wk
Tertiary syphilis		Penicillin G benzathine‡ 7.2 million U total, administered as 3 doses of 2.4 million U IM at 1-wk intervals *If allergic to penicillin and not pregnant, same as for late latent syphilis*
Neurosyphilis‖	Aqueous crystalline penicillin G 200,000-300,000 U/kg/day q4-6hr × 10-14 days in doses not to exceed the adult dose	Aqueous crystalline penicillin G 18-24 million U/day administered as 3-4 million U IV q4hr × 10-14 days¶ *or* Penicillin G procaine,‡ 2.4 million U IM once daily *plus* probenecid 500 mg PO qid, both × 10-14 days¶

*If the patient has no clinical manifestations of disease, the CSF examination is normal, and the CSF VDRL result is negative, some experts would treat with up to 3 weekly doses of penicillin G benzathine 50,000 U/kg IM. Some experts also suggest giving these patients a single dose of penicillin G benzathine 50,000 U/kg IM after the 10-day course of IV aqueous penicillin.
†Early latent syphilis is defined as being acquired within the preceding year.
‡Penicillin G benzathine and penicillin G procaine are approved for IM administration only.
§Late latent syphilis is defined as syphilis beyond 1 year's duration.
‖Patients who are allergic to penicillin should be desensitized.
¶Some experts administer penicillin G benzathine 2.4 million U IM, once per week for up to 3 weeks after completion of these neurosyphilis treatment regimens.
CSF, cerebrospinal fluid; VDRL, Venereal Disease Research Laboratory.
From American Academy of Pediatrics: *Red book: 2009 report of the Committee on Infectious Diseases,* ed 28, Elk Grove Village, IL, 2009, American Academy of Pediatrics, p 647, Table 3.76.

bacterial lysis) occurs in 15-20% of patients with acquired or congenital syphilis treated with penicillin. It is not an indication for discontinuing penicillin therapy.

Acquired Syphilis

Primary, secondary, and early latent disease is treated with a single dose of benzathine penicillin G (50,000 units/kg IM, maximum 2.4 million units). Nonpregnant penicillin-allergic patients without neurosyphilis may be treated with either doxycycline (100 mg PO twice daily for 2 wk) or tetracycline (500 mg PO four times daily for 2 wk). Azalide and macrolide resistance has been documented in several US cities, compromising the effective use of the class of antibiotics.

Patients co-infected with HIV are at increased risk for neurologic complications and higher rates of treatment failure. CDC guidelines recommend the same treatment of primary and secondary syphilis as for patients who are not infected with HIV, but some experts recommend 3 weekly doses of benzathine penicillin G. HIV-infected patients with late latent syphilis or latent syphilis of unknown duration should have a CSF evaluation for neurosyphilis before treatment.

Sex partners of infected persons of any stage should be evaluated and treated. Persons exposed ≤90 days preceding diagnosis in a sex partner should be treated presumptively even if seronegative. Persons exposed >90 days before the diagnosis in a sex partner should be treated if seropositive or if serologic tests are not available. Follow-up serology should be performed on treated patients to establish adequacy of therapy, and all patients should be tested for other sexually transmitted diseases, including HIV.

Syphilis in Pregnancy

When clinical or serologic findings suggest active infection or when diagnosis of active syphilis cannot be excluded with certainty, treatment is indicated. Patients should be treated with the penicillin regimen appropriate for the woman's stage of syphilis. Women who have been adequately treated in the past do not require additional therapy unless quantitative serology suggests evidence of reinfection (**4-fold elevation in titer**). Doxycycline and tetracycline should not be administered during pregnancy, and macrolides do not effectively prevent fetal infection. Pregnant patients who are allergic to penicillin should be desensitized and treated with penicillin.

Congenital Syphilis

Adequate maternal therapy should eliminate the risk for congenital syphilis. All infants born to mothers with syphilis should be followed until nontreponemal serology is negative. The infant should be treated if there is any uncertainty about the adequacy of maternal treatment.

Congenital syphilis is treated with aqueous penicillin G (100,000-150,000 U/kg/24 hr divided every 12 hr IV for the 1st wk of life, and every 8 hr thereafter) or procaine penicillin G (50,000 U/kg IM once daily) given for 10 days. Both penicillin regimens are recognized as adequate therapy for congenital syphilis, but higher concentrations of penicillin are achieved in the CSF of infants treated with intravenous aqueous penicillin G than in those treated with intramuscular procaine penicillin. Treated infants should be followed every 2-3 months to confirm at least a 4-fold decrease in nontreponemal titers. Treated infants with congenital neurosyphilis should undergo clinical and CSF evaluation at 6-mo intervals until CSF is normal. In a very low risk neonate who is asymptomatic and whose mother was treated appropriately, without evidence of relapse or reinfection, but with a low and stable VDRL titer (serofast), no evaluation is necessary. Some specialists would treat such an infant with a single dose of benzathine penicillin G 50,000 U/kg IM.

PREVENTION

Testing is indicated at any time for persons with suspicious lesions, a history of recent sexual exposure to a person with syphilis, or diagnosis of another sexually transmitted infection, including HIV infection. Timely treatment lessens risk of community spread. Vaccine prevention remains elusive, confounded by the treponeme's ability to evade the immune system.

Congenital Syphilis

Routine prenatal screening for syphilis remains the most important factor in identifying infants at risk for developing congenital syphilis and is legally required at the beginning of prenatal care in all states. In pregnant women without optimal prenatal care, serologic screening for syphilis should be performed at the time pregnancy is diagnosed. Any woman who is delivered of a stillborn infant ≥20 wk of gestation should be tested for syphilis. In communities and populations with a high prevalence of syphilis and in patients at high risk, testing should be performed at least 2 additional times: at the beginning of the 3rd trimester (28 wk) and at delivery. Some states mandate repeat testing at delivery for all women, underscoring the importance of preventive screening. Women at high risk for syphilis should be screened even more frequently, either monthly or pragmatically in the case of inconsistent prenatal care, at every medical encounter because they can have repeat infections during pregnancy or reinfection late in pregnancy.

No newborn should leave the hospital without the maternal serologic status having been determined at least once during pregnancy. In states conducting newborn screening for syphilis, both the mother's and infant's serologic results should be known before discharge. In addition, all previously uninvestigated infants of an infected mother should be screened.

BIBLIOGRAPHY

Please visit the Nelson Textbook of Pediatrics *website at* *www.expertconsult.com* *for the complete bibliography.*

Chapter 211 Nonvenereal Treponemal Infections

Stephen K. Obaro and H. Dele Davies

Nonvenereal treponemal infections—yaws, bejel (endemic syphilis), and pinta—are caused by different subspecies of *Treponema pallidum* and occur in tropical and subtropical areas. The causative agents of nonvenereal treponematoses—*T. pertenue, T. pallidum* subspecies *endemicum,* and *T. carateum*—cannot be distinguished from *T. pallidum* by morphologic or serologic tests. These diseases are characterized by a relapsing clinical course and prominent skin involvement. Penicillin remains the treatment of choice for syphilis and nonvenereal treponemal infections.

211.1 Yaws *(Treponema pertenue)*

Stephen K. Obaro and H. Dele Davies

Yaws is the most prevalent nonveneral treponematosis. It is a contagious, chronic, relapsing infection involving the skin and bony structures caused by the spirochete *T. pertenue,* which is identical to *T. pallidum* microscopically and serologically. It occurs in tropical regions with heavy rainfall and annual temperatures ≥27°C (80°F). Almost all cases occur in children in tropical and subtropical countries. It is also referred to as "framboesia," "pian," "parangi," and "bouba." A high percentage of the population is infected in endemic areas.

For the full continuation of this chapter, please visit the Nelson Textbook of Pediatrics *website at* *www.expertconsult.com.*

211.2 Bejel (Endemic Syphilis; *Treponema pallidum* subspecies *endemicum*)

Stephen K. Obaro and H. Dele Davies

Bejel, or endemic syphilis, affects children in remote rural communities living in poor hygienic conditions. Bejel, unlike yaws, can occur in temperate as well as dry, hot climates. Infection with *T. pallidum* subspecies *endemicum* follows penetration of the spirochete through traumatized skin or mucous membranes. In experimental infections, a primary papule forms at the inoculation site after an incubation period of 3 wk. A primary lesion is almost never visualized in human infections; however, primary ulcers have been described surrounding the nipples of nursing mothers with infected children.

For the full continuation of this chapter, please visit the Nelson Textbook of Pediatrics *website at* *www.expertconsult.com.*

211.3 Pinta *(Treponema carateum)*

Stephen K. Obaro and H. Dele Davies

Pinta is a chronic, nonvenereally transmitted infection caused by *Treponema pallidum subspecies carateum,* a spirochete morphologically and serologically indistinguishable from other human treponemes. This is perhaps the mildest of the nonvenereal treponematoses. The disease is endemic in Mexico, Central America, South America, and parts of the West Indies and largely affects children <15 yr of age.

For the full continuation of this chapter, please visit the Nelson Textbook of Pediatrics *website at* *www.expertconsult.com.*

Chapter 212 *Leptospira*

H. Dele Davies and Melissa Beth Rosenberg

Leptospirosis is a common and widespread zoonosis in the world and is caused by spirochetes of the genus *Leptospira.*

ETIOLOGY

Leptospira are aerobic spiral bacteria with a terminal hook at 1 or both ends. Pathogenic leptospires belong to a single species, *Leptospira interrogans,* which includes >200 distinct serovars. A single serovar can produce a variety of distinct syndromes, and a single clinical manifestation may be caused by multiple serotypes. Nonpathogenic leptospires are classified as *Leptospira biflexa,* with >60 serovars.

EPIDEMIOLOGY

Most human cases of leptospirosis occur in tropical and subtropical countries, but the distribution is worldwide. The rat is the principal source of human infection, but leptospires infect many species of domestic and feral animals, including livestock, birds, fish, dogs, cats, and wild animals, including reptiles. Infected animals excrete spirochetes in their urine for prolonged periods. Most human cases result from occupational exposure to water or soil contaminated with rat urine. Groups with a high incidence of leptospirosis include persons exposed occupationally or recreationally to contaminated soil or water, agricultural workers, veterinarians, abattoir workers, meat inspectors, rodent control workers, laboratory workers, and workers in other occupations that require contact with animals. The major animal reservoir in the USA is the dog. Transmission via animal bites and directly from person to person has been rarely reported.

PATHOLOGY AND PATHOGENESIS

Leptospires enter humans through abrasions and cuts in the skin or through mucous membranes. After penetration, they circulate in the bloodstream to all body organs, causing endothelial lining damage of small blood vessels with secondary ischemic damage to the end organs.

CLINICAL MANIFESTATIONS

The spectrum of human leptospirosis ranges from asymptomatic infection (most cases) to severe disease with multiorgan dysfunction and death. The onset is usually abrupt, and the illness tends to follow a biphasic course (Fig. 212-1). After an incubation period of 7-12 days, there is an **initial** or **septicemic phase** lasting 2-7 days, during which leptospires can be isolated from the blood, cerebrospinal fluid (CSF), and other tissues. This phase may be followed by a brief period of well-being before onset of a second symptomatic **immune** or **leptospiruric phase**. This phase is associated with the appearance of circulating antibody, disappearance of organisms from the blood and CSF, and appearance of signs and symptoms associated with localization of leptospires in the tissues. Despite the presence of circulating antibody, leptospires can persist in the kidney, urine, and aqueous humor. The immune phase can last for several weeks. Symptomatic infection may be anicteric or icteric.

Anicteric Leptospirosis

The **septicemic phase** of anicteric leptospirosis has an abrupt onset with flulike signs of fever, shaking chills, lethargy, severe headache, malaise, nausea, vomiting, and severe debilitating myalgia most prominent in the lower extremities, lumbosacral spine, and abdomen. Bradycardia and hypotension can occur, but circulatory collapse is uncommon. Conjunctival suffusion with photophobia and orbital pain (in the absence of chemosis and purulent exudate), generalized lymphadenopathy, and hepatosplenomegaly may also be present. A transient (<24 hr) erythematous maculopapular, urticarial, petechial, purpuric, or desquamating rash occurs in 10% of cases. Rarer manifestations include pharyngitis, pneumonitis, arthritis, carditis, cholecystitis, and orchitis. The **second** or **immune phase** can follow a brief asymptomatic interlude and is characterized by recurrence of fever and aseptic meningitis. CSF abnormalities include a modest elevation in pressure, pleocytosis with early polymorphonuclear leukocytosis followed by mononuclear predominance rarely exceeding 500 cells/mm^3, normal or slightly elevated protein levels, and normal glucose values. Although 80% of infected children have abnormal CSF profiles, only 50% have meningeal manifestations. Encephalitis, cranial and peripheral neuropathies, papilledema, and paralysis are uncommon. A self-limited unilateral or bilateral uveitis can occur during this phase, rarely resulting in permanent visual impairment. Central nervous system symptoms usually resolve spontaneously within 1 wk, with almost no mortality.

Icteric Leptospirosis (Weil Syndrome)

Weil syndrome is a rare (<10% of cases) severe form of leptospirosis seen more commonly in adults (>30 yr) than in children. The initial manifestations are similar to those described for anicteric leptospirosis. The immune phase, however, is characterized by jaundice, renal failure, thrombocytopenia, and, in fulminant cases, hemorrhage and cardiovascular collapse. Hepatic involvement leads to right upper quadrant pain, hepatomegaly, direct and indirect hyperbilirubinemia, and modestly elevated serum levels of hepatic enzymes. Liver function usually returns to normal after recovery. All patients have abnormal findings on urinalysis (hematuria, proteinuria, and casts), and azotemia is common, often associated with oliguria or anuria. Acute kidney failure occurs in 16-40% of cases and is the principal cause of death. Abnormal electrocardiograms are present in 90% of cases, but congestive heart failure is uncommon. Transient thrombocytopenia occurs in >50% of cases. Rarely, hemorrhagic manifestations occur, including epistaxis, hemoptysis, and pulmonary, gastrointestinal, and adrenal hemorrhage. The mortality rate is 5-15%.

DIAGNOSIS

Leptospirosis should be considered in the differential diagnosis of acute flulike febrile illnesses with a history of direct contact with animals or with soil or water contaminated with animal urine. This disease may be difficult to distinguish clinically from dengue or malaria.

Use of Warthin-Starry silver staining, polymerase chain reaction, and immunofluorescent and immunohistochemical methods permits diagnosis of leptospirosis from infected tissue or body fluids. The diagnosis is most often made by serologic testing and less often by isolation of the infecting organism from clinical specimens. Serologic tests for *Leptospira* include genus-specific and serogroup-specific tests. The reference method is the **microscopic agglutination test**, a serogroup-specific assay using live antigen suspension of leptospiral serovars and dark-field microscopy for agglutination. A 4-fold or greater increase in titer in paired sera confirms the diagnosis. Agglutinins usually appear by the 12th day of illness and reach a maximum titer by the 3rd wk. Low titers can persist for years. Approximately 10% of infected persons do not have detectable agglutinins, presumably because

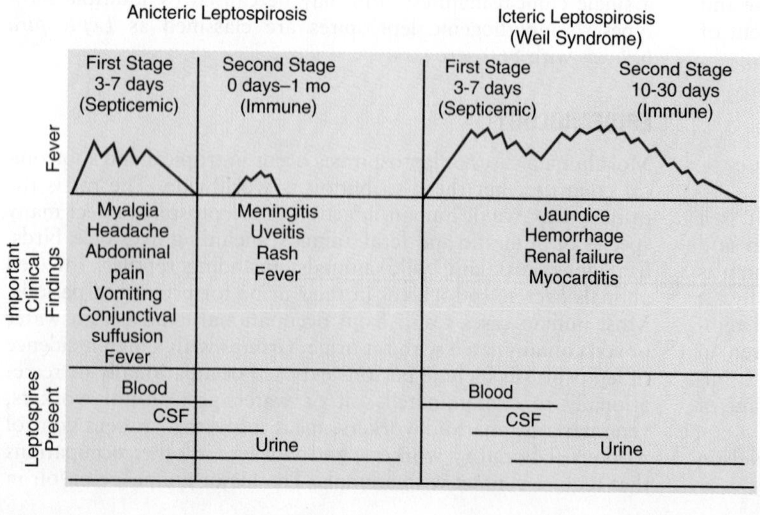

Figure 212-1 Stages of anicteric and icteric leptospirosis. Correlation between clinical findings and presence of leptospires in body fluids, CSF, cerebrospinal fluid. (Reprinted with permission from Feigin RD, Anderson DC: Human leptospirosis, *CRC Crit Rev Clin Lab Sci* 5:413–467, 1975. Copyright CRC Press, Inc, Boca Raton, FL.)

available antisera do not identify all *Leptospira* serotypes. Enzyme-linked immunosorbent assay (ELISA) methods, including an immunoglobulin M-specific dot-ELISA test, are also available. Phase-contrast and dark-field microscopy are insensitive for spirochete detection.

Unlike other pathogenic spirochetes, leptospires can be recovered from the blood or CSF during the first 10 days of illness and from urine after the 2nd week by repeated culture of small inoculum (i.e., 1 drop of blood or CSF in 5 mL of medium) on commercially available media-containing rabbit serum or bovine serum albumin and long-chain fatty acids. However, the inoculum in clinical specimens is small, and growth can take up to 13 wk.

TREATMENT

Despite in vitro sensitivity of *Leptospira* to penicillin and tetracycline, the effectiveness of these antibiotics in treating human leptospirosis is unclear due to the naturally high spontaneous recovery rates. Some studies suggest that initiation of treatment before the 7th day shortens the clinical course and decreases the severity of the infection; thus treatment with penicillin or tetracycline (in children ≥9 yr of age) should be instituted early when the diagnosis is suspected. Parenteral penicillin G (6-8 million U/m^2/day divided every 4 hr IV for 7 days) is recommended, with tetracycline (10-20 mg/kg/day divided every 6 hr PO or IV for 7 days) as an alternative for patients allergic to penicillin. Oral amoxicillin is an alternative therapy for children <9 yr of age.

PREVENTION

Prevention of human leptospirosis infection is facilitated by instituting rodent control measures and avoiding contaminated water and soil. Immunization of livestock and family pets is recommended as a means of eliminating animal reservoirs. Attempts at a human vaccine have been challenging. Protective clothing should be worn by persons at risk for occupational exposure. Leptospirosis has been prevented in American soldiers stationed in the tropics by administering doxycycline (200 mg PO once a week) as prophylaxis. This approach may be similarly effective for travelers to highly endemic areas for short periods.

BIBLIOGRAPHY

Please visit the Nelson Textbook of Pediatrics *website at* *www.expertconsult.com* *for the complete bibliography.*

Chapter 213
Relapsing Fever (*Borrelia*)

H. Dele Davies and Stephen K. Obaro

Relapsing fever is characterized by recurring fevers and flulike symptoms such as headaches, myalgia, arthralgia, and rigors.

ETIOLOGY

Relapsing fever is an infection transmitted by arthropods (lice or ticks) and caused by spirochetes of the genus *Borrelia*.

For the full continuation of this chapter, please visit the Nelson Textbook of Pediatrics *website at* *www.expertconsult.com*.

Chapter 214
Lyme Disease (*Borrelia burgdorferi*)

Stephen C. Eppes

Lyme disease is the most common vector-borne disease in the USA and has become an important public health problem.

ETIOLOGY

Lyme disease is caused by the spirochete *Borrelia burgdorferi* sensu lato (broad sense). In North America, *B. burgdorferi* sensu stricto (strict sense) causes virtually all cases, and in Europe, the species *B. afzelii* and *B. garinii* also cause disease. The 3 major outer-surface proteins called OspA, OspB, and OspC (which are highly charged basic proteins of molecular weights of about 31, 34, and 23 kd, respectively) and the 41 kd flagellar protein are important targets for the immune response. Differences in the molecular structure of the different species are associated with differences in the clinical manifestations of Lyme borreliosis in Europe and the USA. These differences include the greater incidence of radiculoneuritis in Europe.

EPIDEMIOLOGY

Lyme disease has been reported from >50 countries. In the USA approximately 20,000 cases were reported in 2006; however, because of incomplete reporting of cases, it is estimated that the actual number of cases is much higher. From 1992 through 2006, 93% of cases occurred in 10 states: Connecticut, Delaware, Maryland, Massachusetts, Minnesota, New Jersey, New York, Pennsylvania, Rhode Island, and Wisconsin (Fig. 214-1). In endemic areas, the reported annual incidence ranges from 20 to 100 cases/100,000 population, although this figure may be as high as 600 cases/100,000 population in hyperendemic areas. In Europe, most cases occur in the Scandinavian countries and in central Europe, especially Germany, Austria, and Switzerland. The reported incidence is highest among children 5-9 yr of age, with a second peak of disease activity in middle-aged adults. In the USA, Lyme disease is diagnosed in boys slightly more often than in girls, and 94% of patients are of European descent. Early Lyme disease (described later) usually occurs from spring to early fall, corresponding to deer tick activity. Late disease (chiefly arthritis) occurs year round. Among adults, outdoor occupation and leisure activities are risk factors; for children, location of residence in an endemic area is the most important risk for infection.

TRANSMISSION

Lyme disease is a zoonosis caused by the transmission of *B. burgdorferi* to humans through the bite of an infected tick of the

Reported Cases of Lyme Disease - USA, 2009

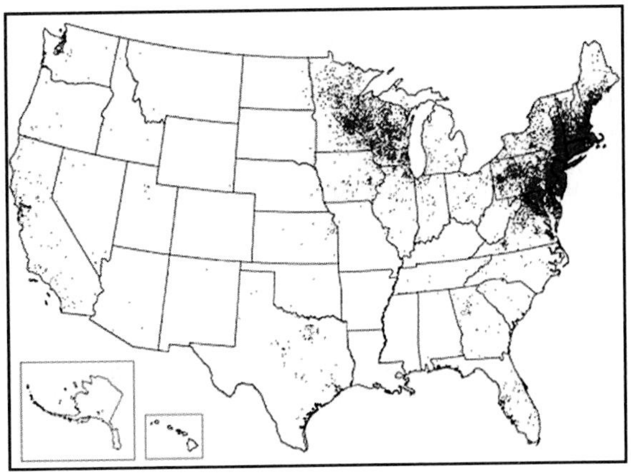

1 dot placed randomly within county of residence for each confirmed case

Figure 214-1 The approximate distribution of predicted risk for Lyme disease in the USA. The risk varies by the distribution of *Ixodes scapularis* and *Ixodes pacificus*, the proportion of ticks that are infected at each stage of the tick's life cycle, and the presence of grassy or wooded locations favored by white-tailed deer. (From the Centers for Disease Control and Prevention: *Reported cases of Lyme disease—United States, 2009* [website]. http://www.cdc.gov/ncidod/dvbid/lyme/ld_Incidence.htm. Accessed November 11, 2010.)

Ixodes genus. In the eastern and midwestern USA, the vector is *Ixodes scapularis,* the black-legged tick that is commonly known as the deer tick, which is responsible for most cases of Lyme disease in the USA. The vector on the Pacific Coast is *Ixodes pacificus,* the western black-legged tick. *Ixodes* ticks have a 2-yr, 3-stage life cycle. The larvae hatch in the early summer and are usually uninfected with *B. burgdorferi.* The tick can become infected at any stage of its life cycle by feeding on a host, usually a small mammal such as the white-footed mouse (*Peromyscus leucopus*), which is a natural reservoir for *B. burgdorferi.* The larvae overwinter and emerge the following spring in the nymphal stage, which is the stage of the tick most likely to transmit the infection. The nymphs molt to adults in the fall and then adults spend the second winter attached to white tailed deer (*Odocoileus virginianus*). The females lay their eggs the following spring before they die, and the 2-yr life cycle begins again.

Several factors are associated with increased risk for transmission of *B. burgdorferi* from ticks to humans. The proportion of infected ticks varies by geographic area and by stage of the tick's life cycle. In endemic areas in the northeastern and midwestern USA, 15-25% of nymphal ticks and 35-50% of adult ticks are infected with *B. burgdorferi.* By contrast, *I. pacificus* often feeds on lizards, which are not a competent reservoir for *B. burgdorferi,* reducing the chance that these ticks will be infected. The risk for transmission of *B. burgdorferi* from infected *Ixodes* ticks is related to the duration of feeding. Experiments in animals have shown that infected nymphal ticks must feed for 36-48 hr, and infected adults must feed for 48-72 hr, before the risk for transmission of *B. burgdorferi* becomes substantial. If the tick is recognized and removed promptly, transmission of *B. burgdorferi* will not occur.

Ixodes scapularis also transmits other microorganisms, namely *Anaplasma phagocytophilum* and *Babesia microti.* Simultaneous transmission can result in co-infections with these organisms and *B. burgdorferi.*

PATHOLOGY AND PATHOGENESIS

Similar to other spirochetal infections, untreated Lyme disease is characterized by asymptomatic infection, clinical disease that can occur in stages, and a propensity for cutaneous and neurologic manifestations.

The skin is the initial site of infection by *B. burgdorferi.* Inflammation induced by *B. burgdorferi* leads to the development of the characteristic rash, **erythema migrans**. Early disseminated Lyme disease results from the spread of spirochetes through the bloodstream to tissues throughout the body. The spirochete adheres to the surfaces of a wide variety of different types of cells, but the principal target organs are skin, central and peripheral nervous system, joints, heart, and eyes. Because the organism can persist in tissues for prolonged periods, symptoms can appear very late after initial infection.

The symptoms of early disseminated and late Lyme disease are due to inflammation mediated by interleukin 1 and other lymphokines in response to the presence of the organism. It is likely that relatively few organisms actually invade the host, but cytokines serve to amplify the inflammatory response and lead to much of the tissue damage. Lyme disease is characterized by inflammatory lesions that contain both T and B lymphocytes, macrophages, plasma cells, and mast cells. The refractory symptoms of late Lyme disease can have an immunogenetic basis. Persons with certain HLA-DR allotypes may be genetically predisposed to develop chronic Lyme arthritis. An autoinflammatory response in the synovium can result in clinical symptoms long after the bacteria have been killed.

CLINICAL MANIFESTATIONS

The clinical manifestations of Lyme disease are divided into early and late stages (Table 214-1). Early Lyme disease is further classified as early localized or early disseminated disease. Untreated patients can progressively develop clinical symptoms of each stage of the disease, or they can present with early disseminated or with late disease without apparently having had any symptoms of the earlier stages of Lyme disease.

Table 214-1 CLINICAL STAGES OF LYME DISEASE

DISEASE STAGE	TIMING AFTER TICK BITE	TYPICAL CLINICAL MANIFESTATIONS
Early localized	3-30 days	EM (single), variable constitutional symptoms (headache, fever, myalgia, arthralgia, fatigue)
Early disseminated	3-12 wk	EM (single or multiple), worse constitutional symptoms, cranial neuritis, meningitis, carditis, ocular disease
Late	>2 mo	Arthritis

EM, erythema migrans.

Early Localized Disease

The first clinical manifestation of Lyme disease in most patients is erythema migrans (Fig. 214-2). Although it usually occurs 7-14 days after the bite, the onset of the rash has been reported from 3 to 30 days later. The initial lesion occurs at the site of the bite. The rash is generally either uniformly erythematous or a target lesion with central clearing; rarely, there are vesicular or necrotic areas in the center of the rash. Occasionally the rash is itchy or painful, though usually it is asymptomatic. The lesion can occur anywhere on the body, although the most common locations are the axilla, periumbilical area, thigh, and groin. It is not unusual for the rash to occur on the neck or face, especially in young children. Without treatment, the rash gradually expands (hence the name *migrans*) to an average diameter of 15 cm and typically remains present for 1-2 wk. Erythema migrans may be associated with systemic features, including fever, myalgia, headache, or malaise. Co-infection with *Babesia microti* or *Anaplasma phagocytophilum* during early infection with *B. burgdorferi* is associated with more severe systemic symptoms.

Early Disseminated Disease

In the USA, about 20% of patients with acute *B. burgdorferi* infection develop secondary erythema migrans lesions, a common manifestation of early disseminated Lyme disease, caused by hematogenous spread of the organisms to multiple skin sites (Fig. 214-3). The secondary lesions, which can develop several days or weeks after the first lesion, are usually smaller than the primary lesion and are often accompanied by more severe constitutional symptoms. The most common early neurologic manifestations are peripheral facial nerve palsy and meningitis. Lyme meningitis usually has an indolent onset with days to weeks of symptoms that can include headache, neck pain and stiffness, and fatigue. Fever is variably present.

The clinical findings of papilledema, cranial neuropathy (especially cranial nerve VII), and erythema migrans, which are present individually or together in 90% of cases, help differentiate Lyme from viral meningitis, in which these findings are rarely present. Lyme aseptic meningitis can be accompanied by significant elevations of intracranial pressure, which can sometimes last weeks or even months. All of the cranial nerves except the olfactory have been reported to be involved with Lyme disease, but the most common are VI and especially VII. In endemic areas, Lyme disease is the leading cause of peripheral facial nerve palsy. It is often the initial or the only manifestation of Lyme disease and is occasionally bilateral. Laboratory findings indicating meningitis are present in more than half of the cases of peripheral facial nerve palsy. The facial paralysis usually lasts 2-8 wk and resolves completely in most cases. Radiculoneuritis and other peripheral neuropathies can occur but are more common in Europe.

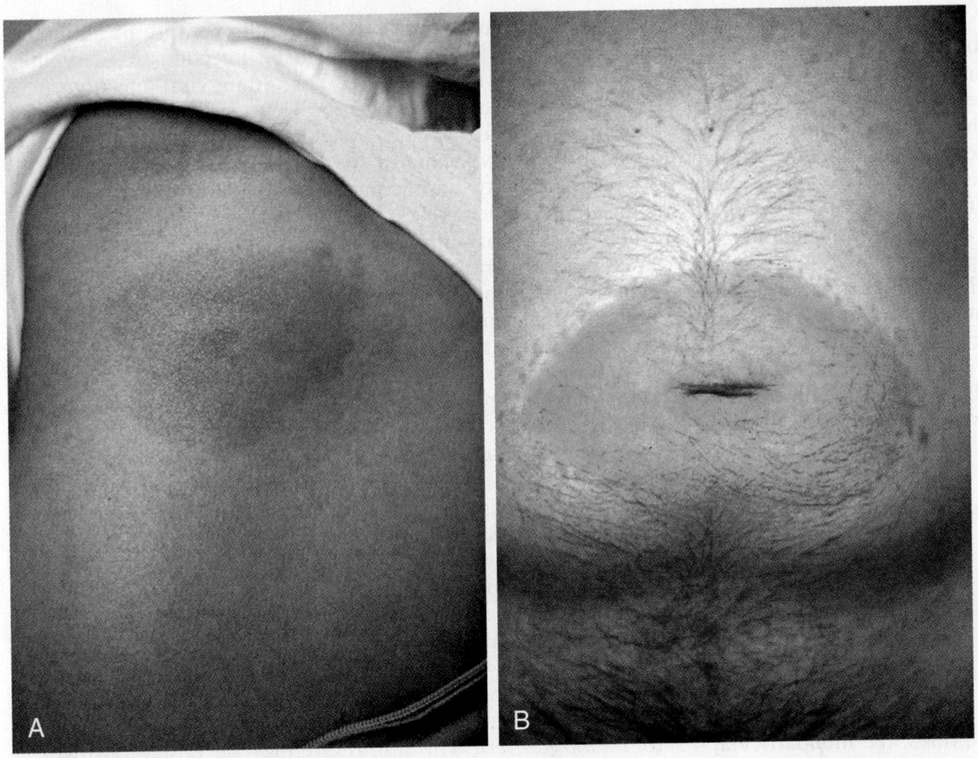

Figure 214-2 Skin manifestations of Lyme borreliosis. *A,* Erythema migrans on the upper leg, showing central clearing. *B,* Erythema migrans expanding around the umbilicus; note central clearing. (From Stanek G, Strle F: Lyme borreliosis, *Lancet* 362:1639–1647, 2003.)

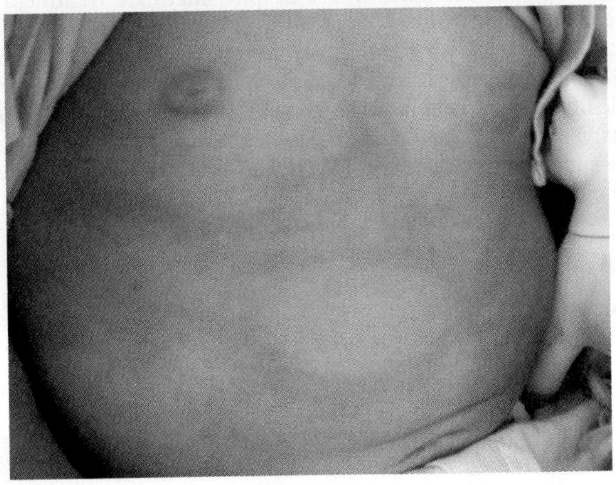

Figure 214-3 Multiple erythema migrans in a boy with early disseminated Lyme disease.

Cardiac involvement occurs in 5-15% of early disseminated Lyme disease and usually takes the form of heart block, which can be 1st, 2nd, or 3rd degree, and the rhythm can fluctuate rapidly. Rarely, myocardial dysfunction can occur. Patients presenting with suspected or proven early disseminated Lyme disease should have a careful cardiac examination and might need electrocardiography. Lyme carditis is a treatable condition and is the only manifestation of Lyme disease that has been fatal.

Of the ocular conditions reported in Lyme disease, papilledema and uveitis are most common.

Late Disease

Arthritis is the usual manifestation of late Lyme disease and begins weeks to months after the initial infection. Arthritis typically involves the large joints, especially the knee, which is affected in 90% of cases; involvement is usually monoarticular. The hallmark of Lyme arthritis is joint swelling, which is due to synovial effusion and sometimes synovial hypertrophy. The swollen joint may be only mildly symptomatic or it may be painful and tender, though patients usually do not experience the severe pain and systemic toxicity that are common in pyogenic arthritis. If untreated, the arthritis can last several weeks, resolve, and then be followed by recurrent attacks in the same or other joints.

Late manifestations of Lyme disease involving the central nervous system, sometimes termed *late neuroborreliosis*, are rarely reported in children. In adults, chronic encephalitis and polyneuritis have been attributed to Lyme disease. The term *Lyme encephalopathy* has been used to describe chronic encephalitis (demonstrable by objective measures), but other literature has also used this term in reference to memory loss and other cognitive sequelae after Lyme disease has been treated. At times, the vague term *chronic Lyme disease* has been used to describe symptomatology in persons who might have never had well-documented infection with *B. burgdorferi* at all, have serologic evidence of prior infection but current symptoms not consistent with Lyme disease, or have persistent symptoms after having received appropriate antibiotic therapy. Post–Lyme disease syndrome is now the preferred term for this last group.

Congenital Lyme Disease

In endemic areas, infection can occur during pregnancy, although congenital infection appears to be a rare event. *B. burgdorferi* has been identified from several abortuses and from a few liveborn children with congenital anomalies; however, the tissues in which the spirochete has been identified usually have not shown histologic evidence of inflammation. Severe skin and cardiac manifestations have been described in a few cases, but no consistent pattern of fetal damage has been identified to suggest a clinical syndrome of congenital infection. Furthermore, studies conducted in endemic areas have indicated that there is no difference in the prevalence of congenital malformations among the offspring of women with serum antibodies against *B. burgdorferi* and the offspring of those without such antibodies.

Laboratory Findings

Standard laboratory tests rarely are helpful in diagnosing Lyme disease because any associated laboratory abnormalities usually are nonspecific. The peripheral white blood cell count may be either normal or elevated. The erythrocyte sedimentation rate may be elevated. Liver transaminases are occasionally mildly elevated. In Lyme arthritis, the white blood cell count in joint fluid can range from 25,000 to 100,000/mL, often with a preponderance of polymorphonuclear cells. When meningitis is present, there usually is a low-grade pleocytosis with a lymphocytic and monocytic predominance. The CSF protein level may be elevated, but the glucose concentration usually is normal. Gram stain and routine bacterial cultures are negative. Imaging of the CNS (e.g., magnetic resonance imaging and single photon emission computed tomography [SPECT]) occasionally reveals abnormalities, but there is no definitive pattern in Lyme disease. The main role of imaging is to exclude other diagnoses.

DIAGNOSIS

In the appropriate epidemiologic setting, typical erythema migrans is virtually pathognomonic. The diagnosis of erythema migrans may be difficult because the rash initially can be confused with nummular eczema, tinea corporis, granuloma annulare, an insect bite, or cellulitis. The relatively rapid expansion of erythema migrans helps distinguish it from these other skin lesions. The other clinical manifestations of Lyme disease are less specific and may be confused with other conditions; the monoarticular or pauciarticular arthritis sometimes is confused with a septic joint or other causes of arthritis in children, such as juvenile rheumatoid arthritis or rheumatic fever; the facial nerve palsy due to Lyme disease is clinically indistinguishable from idiopathic Bell palsy, although bilateral involvement is much more common with Lyme disease; Lyme meningitis generally occurs in the warmer months, the same period that enteroviral disease is prevalent. Therefore, for all disease manifestations other than erythema migrans, it is recommended to have laboratory confirmation of infection with *B. burgdorferi.*

Although *B. burgdorferi* has been isolated from blood, skin, CSF, myocardium, and the synovium of patients with Lyme disease, the organism is difficult to isolate in culture (cultivation is largely relegated to research laboratories). Infection is usually identified by the detection of antibody in serum. Although some laboratories offer polymerase chain reaction (PCR) as a diagnostic test for Lyme disease, its sensitivity may be poor because of the low concentrations of bacteria in many sites, especially cerebrospinal fluid (CSF). Other antigen-based tests, including a test for *B. burgdorferi* antigens in urine, have been unreliable. Clinicians should be aware that some laboratories use alternative diagnostic tests and/or alternative interpretive criteria that are not evidence based, leading to a false diagnosis of Lyme disease.

Serology

Following the transmission of *B. burgdorferi* from a tick bite, specific immunoglobulin M (IgM) antibodies appear first, usually at 3-4 wk, peak at 6-8 wk, and subsequently decline. Sometimes a prolonged elevation of IgM antibodies occurs despite effective antimicrobial treatment. (For that reason, the results of tests for specific IgM antibodies alone should not be used as a reliable indicator of either active or recent infection.) Specific IgG antibodies usually appear at 4-8 wk, peak after 4-6 mo, and can remain elevated for years, particularly in patients with arthritis. The antibody response to *B. burgdorferi* may be blunted in patients with early Lyme disease who are treated promptly with an effective antimicrobial agent.

By far the most common method used to detect IgG and IgM antibodies is the **enzyme-linked immunosorbent assay (ELISA)**. This method is sensitive but not optimally specific. The ELISA sometimes produces false-positive results because of antibodies that cross-react with other spirochetal infections (e.g., syphilis, leptospirosis, or relapsing fever), or certain viral infections (e.g., Epstein-Barr virus or parvovirus B19) or that occur in certain autoimmune diseases (e.g., systemic lupus erythematosus). The positive predictive value of the ELISA result depends primarily on the plausibility that the patient has Lyme disease based on the clinical and epidemiologic history and the physical examination (**the pretest probability**). For patients who have been in endemic areas with opportunities for *Ixodes* tick exposure and who have typical clinical manifestations of Lyme disease, the pretest probability is high and positive ELISA results are usually true positives. For patients who are from nonendemic areas and/or who have little risk for *Ixodes* tick exposures and/or have nonspecific symptoms (low pretest probability), rates of false-positive results are high.

Western immunoblotting is well standardized, and there are accepted criteria for interpretation. Five of 10 IgG bands and 2 of 3 IgM bands is considered positive. The Western blot is not as sensitive as ELISA, especially in early infection, but it is highly specific. Any positive or equivocal ELISA should be confirmed with Western blotting. This two-tier testing is the recommended laboratory evaluation of most cases of Lyme disease and is associated with a high degree of sensitivity and specificity when used appropriately.

Clinicians should be aware that Lyme disease might not be the cause of a patient's symptoms despite the presence of antibodies to *B. burgdorferi*. The test result may be falsely positive (as described for ELISA), or the patient might have been infected previously. Antibodies to *B. burgdorferi* that develop with infection can persist for many years despite adequate treatment and clinical cure of the disease. In addition, because some people who become infected with *B. burgdorferi* are asymptomatic, the background rate of seropositivity among patients who have never had clinically apparent Lyme disease may be substantial in endemic areas. Finally, because antibodies against *B. burgdorferi* persist after successful treatment, there is no reason to obtain follow-up serologic tests.

TREATMENT

Treatment recommendations are given in Table 214-2. These have been developed by the Infectious Diseases Society of America

Table 214-2 RECOMMENDED TREATMENT OF LYME DISEASE

DRUG	PEDIATRIC DOSING
Amoxicillin	50 mg/kg/day in 3 divided doses (max 1,500 mg/day)
Doxycycline	4 mg/kg/day in 2 divided doses (max 200 mg/day) (see text regarding doxycycline use in children)
Cefuroxime axetil	30 mg/kg/day in 2 divided doses (max 1,000 mg/day)
Ceftriaxone (IV)*†	50-75 mg/kg/day once daily (max 2,000 mg/day)
RECOMMENDED THERAPY BASED ON CLINICAL MANIFESTATION	
Erythema migrans	Oral regimen, 14-21 days
Meningitis	Ceftriaxone, 10-28 days
Cranial nerve palsy	Oral regimen, 14-21 days (see text regarding possible need for lumbar puncture)
Cardiac disease	Oral regimen or ceftriaxone, 14-21 days (see text for specifics)
Arthritis‡	Oral regimen, 28 days
Late neurologic disease	Ceftriaxone, 14-28 days

*Cefotaxime and penicillin G are alternative parenteral agents
†Doses of 100 mg/kg/day can be used for meningitis
‡Persistent arthritis can be treated with a second oral regimen or ceftriaxone.
From Wormser GP, Dattwyler RJ, Shapiro ED, et al: The clinical assessment, treatment, and prevention of Lyme disease, human granulocytic anaplasmosis, and babesiosis: clinical practice guidelines by the Infectious Diseases Society of America, *Clin Infect Dis* 43:1089–1134, 2006.

(IDSA) and are based on the best available evidence. There have been more clinical trials involving adults than children, so some of the pediatric recommendations derive from results of studies in adults.

Most patients can be treated with an oral regimen of antibiotic therapy. Young children are generally treated with amoxicillin. Doxycycline has the advantages of good CNS penetration and is active against *Anaplasma phagocytophilum*, which may be transmitted at the same time as *B. burgdorferi* in certain geographic areas. In general, children <8 yr of age should not be treated with doxycycline because of the risk of permanent staining of the teeth (although courses of ≤2 wk are usually safe in this regard). Patients who are treated with doxycycline should be alerted to the risk for developing photosensitivity in sun-exposed areas while taking the medication; long sleeves, long pants, and hat are recommended for activities in direct sunlight. The only oral cephalosporin proved to be effective for the treatment of Lyme disease is cefuroxime axetil, which is an alternative for persons who cannot take doxycycline and who are allergic to penicillin (it is also more expensive). Results with macrolide antibiotics, including azithromycin, have been disappointing.

Parenteral therapy is recommended for patients with central nervous system infection and higher degrees of heart block. Patients with arthritis that fails to resolve after an initial course of oral therapy can be re-treated with an oral regimen or can receive intravenous antibiotic therapy. Ceftriaxone is usually favored because of its excellent anti-borrelial activity, tolerability, and once-daily dosing regimen, which can usually be done on an outpatient basis.

Peripheral facial nerve palsy can be treated using an oral antibiotic. However, many of these patients have concomitant meningitis. Patients with meningitis should receive a parenteral antibiotic. Experts are divided on whether every patient with Lyme-associated facial palsy should have a CSF analysis, but clinicians should consider lumbar puncture for patients with significant headache, neck pain or stiffness, or papilledema.

Patients with symptomatic cardiac disease, second- or third-degree heart block, or significantly prolonged PR interval should be hospitalized and monitored closely. These patients should receive a parenteral antibiotic. Patients with mild first-degree heart block can be treated with an oral antibiotic.

Some patients develop a **Jarisch-Herxheimer reaction** soon after treatment is initiated; this results from lysis of the borrelia. The manifestations of this reaction are fever, diaphoresis, and myalgia. These symptoms resolve spontaneously within 24-48 hr, although administration of nonsteroidal anti-inflammatory drugs (NSAIDs) often is beneficial. NSAIDs also may be useful in treating symptoms of early Lyme disease and of Lyme arthritis. Co-infections with other pathogens transmitted by *Ixodes* ticks should be treated according to standard recommendations.

Criteria for the post–Lyme disease syndrome have been proposed by the IDSA. There is no clear evidence that this condition is related to persistence of the organism. Studies in adults have shown little benefit associated with prolonged or repeated treatment with oral or parenteral antibiotics.

PROGNOSIS

There is a widespread misconception that Lyme disease is difficult to cure and that chronic symptoms and clinical recurrences are common. The most likely reason for apparent treatment failure is an incorrect diagnosis of Lyme disease.

The prognosis for children treated for Lyme disease is excellent. Children treated for erythema migrans rarely progress to late Lyme disease. The long-term prognosis for patients who are treated beginning in the late phase of Lyme disease also is excellent. Although chronic and recurrent arthritis does occur rarely, especially among patients with certain HLA allotypes (an autoimmune process), most children who are treated for Lyme arthritis are cured and have no sequelae. Although there are rare reports of adults who have developed late neuroborreliosis, usually among persons with Lyme disease in whom treatment was delayed for months or years, similar cases in children are rare.

PREVENTION

The best way to avoid Lyme disease is to avoid tick-infested areas. Children should be examined for deer ticks after known or potential exposure. If a deer tick attachment is noted, the tick should be grasped at the mouthparts with a forceps or tweezers; if these are not available, the tick should be covered with a tissue. The recommended method of tick removal is to pull directly outward without twisting; infection is usually preventable if the tick is removed before 48 hours of attachment. The overall risk for acquiring Lyme disease after a tick bite is low (1-3%) in most endemic areas. Patients and families can be advised to watch the area for development of erythema migrans and to seek medical attention if the rash or constitutional symptoms occur. If infection develops, early treatment of the infection is highly effective. A study of prophylaxis after a tick bite found that a single dose of doxycycline in adults (200 mg PO) was 87% effective in preventing Lyme disease; data in children using this strategy are lacking. Most people are not able to identify the species or the stage of the tick (in some instances reported "tick" bites prove not to be from ticks), and therefore administration of antimicrobial **prophylaxis is not recommended** routinely. The routine testing of ticks that have been removed from humans for evidence of *B. burgdorferi* is not recommended, because the value of a positive test result for predicting infection in the human host is unknown.

Personal protective measures that may be effective in reducing the chance of tick bites include wearing protective clothing (long pants tucked into socks, long-sleeved shirts) when entering tick-infested areas, checking for and promptly removing ticks, and using tick repellents such as DEET. This chemical can safely be used on pants, socks and shoes; care must be used with heavy or repeated application on skin, particularly in infants, because of the risk of systemic absorption and toxicity.

BIBLIOGRAPHY

Please visit the Nelson Textbook of Pediatrics *website at www.expertconsult.com for the complete bibliography.*

Section 9 MYCOPLASMAL INFECTIONS

Chapter 215
Mycoplasma pneumoniae

Dwight A. Powell

Among the 5 *Mycoplasma* species isolated from the human respiratory tract, *Mycoplasma pneumoniae* is the only recognized human pathogen and is a major cause of respiratory infections in school-aged children and young adults.

ETIOLOGY

Mycoplasmas are the smallest self-replicating biologic system and are dependent on attachment to host cells for obtaining essential precursors such as nucleotides, fatty acids, sterols, and amino acids. They are distinguished by the complete absence of a cell wall, double-stranded DNA, and small genomes ranging from 577 to 1,380 kb. *M. pneumoniae* is fastidious, and growth in commercially available culture systems is too slow to be of practical clinical use.

EPIDEMIOLOGY

M. pneumoniae infections occur worldwide and throughout the year. In contrast to the acute, short-lived epidemics of some respiratory viral agents, *M. pneumoniae* infection is endemic in larger communities, with epidemic outbreaks occurring every 4-7 yr. In smaller communities, infections are sporadic, with long-lasting and smoldering outbreaks occurring at irregular intervals. Community outbreaks can spread largely through school contacts, but up to 40% of household members of an infected student also develop mycoplasma infection.

The occurrence of mycoplasmal illness is related, in part, to age and pre-exposure immunity. Overt illness is unusual before 3 yr of age. Children <5 yr of age appear to have mild illness associated with upper respiratory tract involvement, vomiting, and diarrhea. The peak incidence of lower respiratory illness occurs in school-aged children. *M. pneumoniae* accounts for 7-40% of all community-acquired pneumonias among children 3-15 yr of age. Recurrent infections occur infrequently but are well documented to occur in adults at intervals of 4-7 yr.

TRANSMISSION

Infection occurs through the respiratory route by large droplet spread. The incubation period is 1-3 wk. High transmission rates have been documented within families, with a high percentage of secondary cases developing lower respiratory tract infections. Outbreaks can occur in closed settings (military recruits, institutions, summer camps for children) or can occur as community-wide epidemics.

PATHOLOGY AND PATHOGENESIS

Cells of the ciliated respiratory epithelium are the target cells of *M. pneumoniae* infection. The organism is an elongated snakelike structure with an attachment tip characterized by an electron-dense core and a trilaminar outer membrane. Attachment to the ciliary membrane is mediated by a complex network of interactive adhesion and adherence-accessory proteins localized to this specialized attachment tip (P1/B/C, P30, P65, P24, and P41). These proteins cooperate structurally and functionally to mobilize and concentrate adhesion proteins at the tip and permit mycoplasmal colonization of mucous membranes. Avirulent phenotypes that arise through spontaneous mutations at high frequency cannot synthesize specific cytoadherence-related proteins or are unable to stabilize them at the tip organelle.

Virulent organisms attach to ciliated respiratory epithelial cell surfaces through sialated glycoprotein or sulfated glycolipid receptors and burrow down between cells, resulting in ciliostasis and eventual sloughing of the cells. Mechanisms of cytopathology have not been determined completely; one possibility is the transmission to cells of various cytotoxins such as hydrogen peroxide. *M. pneumoniae* can also produce a protein similar to the S1 subunit of pertussis toxin. Intracellular organisms have not been found in vivo, and *M. pneumoniae* rarely invades beyond the respiratory tract basement membrane. However, *M. pneumoniae* can invade certain cell lines in vitro and survive in the cytoplasm or perinuclear regions for prolonged periods. *M. pneumoniae* has been detected by polymerase chain reaction (PCR) in many nonrespiratory sites. These observations suggest that *M. pneumoniae* causes more extrapulmonary infections and chronic disease than appreciated.

A possible mechanism of *M. pneumoniae* disease is the release of various proinflammatory and anti-inflammatory cytokines. *M. pneumoniae* infection may induce numerous interleukins, interferons, tumor necrosis factor-α, and other cytokines. The disease produced by *M. pneumoniae* is complex; the immunologic response of the host may be responsible for the manifestations of disease itself as well as for protection against infection, depending on the qualitative and quantitative balance of humoral and cellular immunity. Although it is well documented that specific cell-mediated immunity and antibody titers against *M. pneumoniae* increase with age (and therefore probably follow repeated infections), the immune mechanisms that protect against or clear infection are not defined. Patients with immunodeficiencies such as hypogammaglobulinemia and sickle cell disease can have more-severe mycoplasmal pneumonia than do immunocompetent hosts. *M. pneumoniae* can persist for years in the respiratory tract of patients with hypogammaglobulinemia despite multiple courses of antibiotics. *M. pneumoniae* is a common infectious cause of acute chest syndrome in sickle cell disease, but it is not prevalent in patients with AIDS.

CLINICAL MANIFESTATIONS

Tracheobronchitis and bronchopneumonia are the most commonly recognized clinical syndromes associated with *M. pneumoniae* infection. Although the onset of illness may be abrupt, it is usually characterized by gradual onset of headache, malaise, fever, and sore throat, followed by progression of lower respiratory symptoms, including hoarseness and cough. Coryza is unusual with *M. pneumoniae* pneumonia and usually suggests a viral etiology. Although the clinical course in untreated patients is variable, coughing usually worsens during the 1st wk of illness, with all symptoms usually resolving within 2 wk. The cough is initially nonproductive, but older children and adolescents might produce frothy, white sputum. The symptoms are usually more severe than the physical signs, which appear later in the disease. Crackles are fine and are the most prominent signs. With progression of the disease, the fever intensifies, the cough becomes more troublesome, and the patient can become dyspneic.

Radiographic findings are not specific. Pneumonia is usually described as interstitial or bronchopneumonic, and involvement is most common in the lower lobes, with unilateral, centrally dense infiltrates present in 75% of cases. Lobar pneumonia is seen infrequently. Hilar lymphadenopathy occurs in up to one third of patients. Significant amounts of pleural fluid are unusual, but patients with large pleural effusions due to *M. pneumoniae* have been described as having severe disease associated with lobar infiltrates and necrotizing pneumonia. The white blood cell and differential counts are usually normal, whereas the erythrocyte sedimentation rate is often elevated.

Additional respiratory illnesses caused occasionally by *M. pneumoniae* include undifferentiated upper respiratory tract infections, pharyngitis, sinusitis, croup, and bronchiolitis. *M. pneumoniae* may be a common trigger of wheezing in asthmatic children or can cause chronic colonization and resulting lung dysfunction in adolescent and adult asthma patients. Otitis media and bullous myringitis have been described but are rarely seen without associated lower respiratory tract infection. Encephalitis and postinfectious demyelination occur but are less common than respiratory tract infections.

DIAGNOSIS

No specific clinical, epidemiologic, or laboratory observations permit a definite diagnosis of mycoplasmal infection early in the clinical course. However, certain observations are suggestive and can be helpful. Pneumonia in school-aged children and young adults always suggests *M. pneumoniae* disease, especially if cough is a prominent finding. Cultures on special media of the throat or sputum might demonstrate *M. pneumoniae*, but growth generally requires incubation for >1 wk, and few commercial laboratories maintain the capability of culturing *M. pneumoniae*. Positive *M. pneumoniae* immunoglobulin M (IgM) antibody identified by indirect fluorescence or enzyme-linked immune assay (EIA) more specifically supports the diagnosis. IgM antibodies may be positive for 6-12 mo after infection. A 4-fold increase in IgG *M. pneumoniae* antibody titer by complement fixation or EIA between acute and convalescent sera obtained 10 days to 3 wk after the onset of illness is diagnostic. PCR of a nasopharyngeal or throat swab (doing both can increase sensitivity) for *M. pneumoniae* DNA is very specific (>97%) in many studies but has a sensitivity of only 50-70% when compared to 4-fold rise in antibody titer. Combined use of PCR and IgM antibody may be the most reliable approach to diagnose the acute illness. When *M. pneumoniae* is confirmed in the community in a few patients, the probability of the existence of more widespread mycoplasmal illness is greatly increased.

TREATMENT

M. pneumoniae illness is usually mild, and hospitalization is generally unnecessary. *M. pneumoniae* is typically sensitive to erythromycin, clarithromycin, azithromycin, and the tetracyclines in vitro, although macrolide resistant strains have been reported from Asia, Europe, and the USA. Macrolides are effective in shortening the course of mycoplasmal illnesses, although they do not have bactericidal activity. Hence, there may be delay in eradicating the organism from the respiratory tract. Two multicenter studies of pediatric community-acquired pneumonia demonstrated equal efficacy between erythromycin and clarithromycin or azithromycin. These newer macrolides were better tolerated and more effective at eradication of *M. pneumoniae* from the respiratory tract. The recommended treatment is clarithromycin (15 mg/kg/day divided bid PO for 10 days) or azithromycin (10 mg/kg once PO on day 1 and 5 mg/kg once daily PO on days 2-5), which eradicate *M. pneumoniae* in 100% of patients studied. Prophylaxis with azithromycin has been shown to substantially reduce the secondary attack rate in institutional outbreaks.

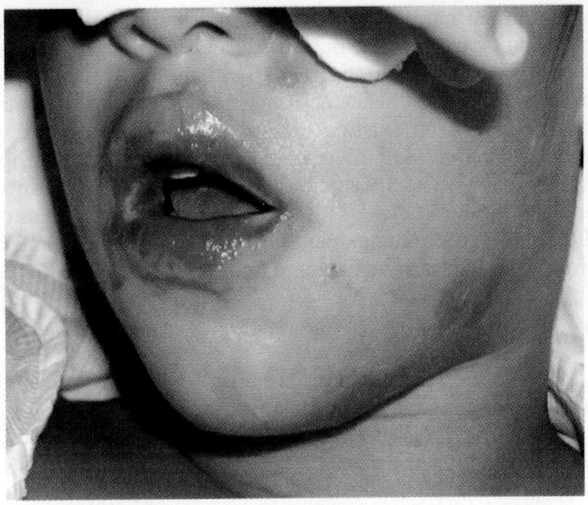

Figure 215-1 Lip changes found in Stevens-Johnson syndrome associated with *Mycoplasma pneumoniae* infection.

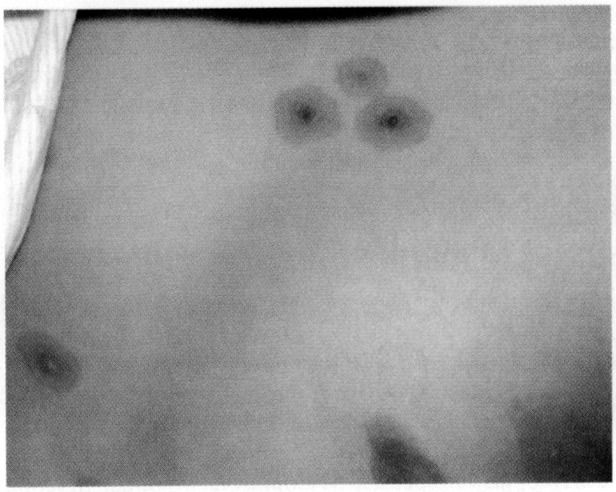

Figure 215-2 Classic erythema multiforme skin lesions found in Stevens-Johnson syndrome associated with *Mycoplasma pneumoniae* infection.

COMPLICATIONS

Complications are unusual. Despite the reportedly rare isolation of *M. pneumoniae* from nonrespiratory sites such as joints, pleural fluid, and cerebrospinal fluid (CSF), the availability of PCR to detect specific segments of *M. pneumoniae* DNA has led to increasing identification of *M. pneumoniae* in nonrespiratory sites, particularly the central nervous system (CNS). Nonrespiratory illness can therefore involve direct invasion with *M. pneumoniae* or can involve autoimmune mechanisms, which is reflected by the frequency with which human antigens cross react with *M. pneumoniae*. Patients with or without respiratory symptoms can manifest illness involving the skin, CNS, blood, heart, gastrointestinal tract, and joints. Skin lesions include a variety of exanthemas, most notably maculopapular rashes, erythema multiforme, and Stevens-Johnson syndrome (SJS). *M. pneumoniae* is the most common infectious agent identified as a cause of SJS, which usually develops 3-21 days after initial respiratory symptoms, lasts <14 days, and is rarely associated with severe complications (Figs. 215-1 and 215-2). *M. pneumoniae* has been linked to an atypical SJS with oral mucositis but absence of rash.

Neurologic complications include meningoencephalitis, transverse myelitis, aseptic meningitis, cerebellar ataxia, Bell palsy, deafness, brainstem syndrome, acute demyelinating encephalitis, and Guillain-Barré syndrome. Neurologic complications occur 3-28 days (mean, 10 days) after respiratory illness but may not be preceded by respiratory illness in 20% of cases. Encephalitis occurring within 5 days of the onset of prodromal symptoms may be caused by direct *M. pneumoniae* infection of the CNS, although CSF PCR is positive in <5% of cases. Encephalitis occurring >7 days after onset of prodromal symptoms is more likely to be due to an autoimmune response. *M. pneumoniae* accounts for 5-15% of all forms of childhood encephalitis and most commonly manifests as fever, lethargy, and impaired consciousness. Seizures, focal motor deficit, ataxia, or meningeal signs are less common. Concomitant infection with viral agents such as herpes simplex virus, human herpesvirus 6, enteroviruses, or respiratory viruses is found in about one third of patients. Involvement of the brainstem can result in severe dystonia and movement disorders. The CSF may be normal or have a mild mononuclear pleocytosis. Diagnosis is confirmed with positive CSF PCR, positive PCR from a throat swab, or the presence of definitive serum antibody titers. Findings on MRI include focal ischemic changes, ventriculomegaly, diffuse edema, or multifocal white matter inflammatory lesions consistent with postinfectious demyelinating encephalomyelitis.

Common **hematologic complications** include mild degrees of hemolysis with a positive Coombs test and minor reticulocytosis 2-3 wk after the onset of illness. Severe hemolysis is associated with high titers of cold hemagglutinins (≥1:512) and occurs rarely. Thrombocytopenia and coagulation defects occur occasionally. Mild hepatitis, pancreatitis, and protein-losing hypertrophic gastropathy are rarely reported gastrointestinal complications. Myocarditis, pericarditis, and a rheumatic fever–like syndrome are uncommon manifestations, but arrhythmias, ST- and T-wave changes, and cardiac dilation with heart failure can accompany *M. pneumoniae* infection, particularly in adults. Transient monoarticular arthritis has been reported in up to 1% of patients.

It is unclear from existing literature whether antibiotic treatment of *M. pneumoniae* infection decreases the risk for complications. There is also no specific established therapy for most of the complications. Corticosteroids have been the most commonly used agents in the management of severe *M. pneumoniae* complications, particularly neurologic complications.

PROGNOSIS

Fatal *M. pneumoniae* infections are rare. Anatomic abnormalities such as altered lung perfusion, mild bronchiectasis, and bronchial wall thickening have been detected by high-resolution CT in approximately one third of children 1-2 yr following *M. pneumoniae* pneumonia. Abnormalities in pulmonary gas diffusion have been reported in nearly half of children 6 mo after recovery from *M. pneumoniae*. Patients generally recover without complications, although sequelae of encephalitis may be severe and permanent.

BIBLIOGRAPHY

Please visit the Nelson Textbook of Pediatrics *website at* www.expertconsult.com *for the complete bibliography.*

Chapter 216
Genital Mycoplasmas *(Mycoplasma hominis, Mycoplasma genitalium, and Ureaplasma urealyticum)*

Dwight A. Powell

Three *Mycoplasma* species, *Mycoplasma hominis, Mycoplasma genitalium,* and *Ureaplasma urealyticum,* are human urogenital pathogens. They are often associated with sexually transmitted infections such as nongonococcal urethritis (NGU) or puerperal infections such as endometritis. *M. hominis* and *U. urealyticum* commonly colonize the female genital tract and can cause chorioamnionitis, colonization of neonates, and perinatal infections. Two other genital *Mycoplasma* species, *M. fermentans* and *M. penetrans,* are identified in respiratory or genitourinary secretions more in HIV-infected patients.

ETIOLOGY

M. hominis and *U. urealyticum* require sterols for growth, can grow in cell-free media, and produce characteristic colonies on agar. Colonies of *M. hominis* are 200-300 µm in diameter with a "fried-egg" appearance, and colonies of *U. urealyticum* are 16-60 µm in diameter. These organisms are resistant to β-lactams because they lack a cell wall and are resistant to sulfonamides and trimethoprim because they do not produce folic acid. *M. hominis* is susceptible to clindamycin and quinolones but resistant to macrolides and rifampin. Increasing numbers of tetracycline-resistant strains are being reported. Using 16s ribosomal RNA sequencing, *U. urealyticum* has been subdivided into two species: *U. urealyticum* and *U. parvum.* Most are susceptible to macrolides and advanced generation quinolones but resistant to ciprofloxacin and clindamycin. Susceptibility to aminoglycosides and tetracyclines is variable. *M. genitalium* can be isolated only in cell culture systems and with difficulty. Identification in most studies has required polymerase chain reaction (PCR).

EPIDEMIOLOGY

M. hominis and *U. urealyticum* colonize the genital and urinary tracts of postpubertal women and men. Female colonization is maximal in the vagina and less in the endocervix, urethra, and endometrium. Male colonization occurs primarily in the urethra. Colonization rates are directly related to sexual activity and are highest among persons with multiple sexual partners. Colonization rates are <10% among prepubertal children and sexually inactive adults and vary from 40% to 90% among pregnant women.

TRANSMISSION

Genital mycoplasmas are transmitted by sexual contact. *M. genitalium* has been identified predominantly in the male urethra and is capable of attaching to human spermatozoa, suggesting a mechanism for sexual transmissibility.

Vertical transmission rates among neonates born to colonized women are 25-60%. The usual route of neonatal acquisition is contamination from colonized amniotic fluid or during vaginal delivery. However, neonatal colonization can occur in the presence of intact amniotic fluid membranes and with delivery by cesarean section. Neonatal colonization rates are higher among infants who weigh <1,500 g, are born in the presence of chorioamnionitis, and are born to mothers of lower socioeconomic status. Organisms are recovered from the newborn's throat, vagina, rectum, and, occasionally, eyes for as long as 3 mo after birth.

PATHOLOGY AND PATHOGENESIS

Genital mycoplasmas can produce chronic inflammation of the genitourinary tract and amniotic fluid membranes. *U. urealyticum* can infect the amniotic sac early in gestation without rupturing the amniotic membranes, resulting in a clinically silent, chronic chorioamnionitis characterized by an intense inflammatory response. Attachment to fetal human tracheal epithelium can cause ciliary disarray, clumping, and loss of epithelial cells. *U. urealyticum* induces macrophages in vitro to increase production of interleukin 6 (IL-6) and tumor necrosis factor 2. Very low birthweight infants colonized with *U. urealyticum* have increased levels of monocyte chemoattractant protein and IL-8, which are proinflammatory agents possibly associated with development of chronic lung disease of prematurity (CLD). Immunity appears to require serotype-specific antibody. Thus, a lack of maternal antibody might account for a higher risk for disease in premature newborns.

CLINICAL MANIFESTATIONS

In adults and sexually active adolescents, genital mycoplasmas are associated with sexually transmitted diseases and are uncommonly associated with focal infections outside the genital tract. *M. hominis* has been described causing septicemia, endocarditis, wound infection, osteomyelitis, lymphadenitis, pneumonia, meningitis, brain abscess, arthritis, amnionitis, and postpartum fever. Life-threatening mediastinitis, sternal wound infections, pleuritis, peritonitis, and pericarditis have been reported with high mortality rates in patients following organ transplantation. Extragenital *U. urealyticum* infections are rarely described but include osteomyelitis, arthritis, meningitis, mediastinitis, infection of aortic grafts, and postcesarean wound infections. Patients with hypogammaglobulinemia appear to be at high risk for chronic arthritis caused by various *Mycoplasma* spp.

U. urealyticum and *M. genitalium* are recognized pathogens of NGU. Approximately 30% of NGU in male patients may be caused by these organisms either alone or with *Chlamydia trachomatis* (Chapter 516.1). Disease is most common in young adults but is also prevalent in sexually active adolescents. The average incubation period is 2-3 wk, with symptoms typically consisting of scant mucoid-white urethral discharge, dysuria, and penile discomfort. The discharge is often evident only in the morning or after the urethra is stripped. Rare complications of NGU are epididymitis and proctitis. Approximately 20-60% of patients with *M. genitalium* NGU develop recurrent or chronic urethritis despite 1-2 wk of treatment with doxycycline alone.

Neonates

Genital mycoplasmas are associated with a variety of fetal and neonatal infections. *U. urealyticum* can cause clinically inapparent chorioamnionitis resulting in an increase in fetal death or premature delivery. Up to 50% of infants <34 wk of gestational age may have *U. urealyticum* recovered from tracheal, blood, cerebrospinal fluid (CSF), or lung biopsy specimens. In a study of 351 preterm infants between 23-32 wk of gestational age, isolation of *U. urealyticum* or *M. hominis* from cord blood correlated with the development of systemic inflammatory response syndrome. The role of these organisms causing severe respiratory insufficiency, the need for assisted ventilation, the development of CLD, or death remains controversial. Two meta-analyses of published studies showed a relative risk of 1.72 and 2.83 for the relationship between respiratory colonization with *U. urealyticum* and development of CLD. However, 2 small randomized, controlled trials of erythromycin therapy in high-risk preterm infants with tracheobronchial colonization of *U. urealyticum* failed to show any difference in treated vs nontreated infants in the development of CLD.

M. hominis and *U. urealyticum* have been isolated from the CSF of premature and, in a few cases, full-term infants. Simultaneous isolation of other pathogens is unusual, and most infants have no overt signs of central nervous system (CNS) infection. CSF pleocytosis is not a consistent observation, and spontaneous clearance of mycoplasmas has been documented without specific therapy. *U. urealyticum* meningitis has been associated with intraventricular hemorrhage and hydrocephalus. Meningitis caused by *M. hominis* was thought to be benign but in a review of 29 reported cases, 8 (28%) died and 8 (28%) were left with neurologic sequelae. The onset of meningitis varies from 1 to 196 days of life; organisms can persist in the CSF without therapy for days to weeks. *M. hominis* and *U. urealyticum* have also been described to cause neonatal conjunctivitis, lymphadenitis, pharyngitis, pneumonitis, osteomyelitis, brain abscess, pericarditis, meningoencephalitis, and scalp abscess.

DIAGNOSIS

Confirmation of genital tract infection is difficult because of high colonization rates in the vagina and urethra. NGU is confirmed by Gram stain of urethral discharge showing ≥3 polymorphonuclear leukocytes per oil-immersion field and the absence of gram-negative diplococci (i.e., *Neisseria gonorrhoeae*). A urethral swab or exudate should be cultured for *C. trachomatis* and *U. urealyticum*. *M. genitalium* can only be identified by PCR testing.

Neonates

U. urealyticum and *M. hominis* have been isolated from urine, blood, CSF, tracheal aspirates, pleural fluid, abscesses, and lung tissue. Premature neonates who are clinically ill with pneumonitis, focal abscesses, or CNS disease (particularly progressive hydrocephalus with or without pleocytosis) for whom bacterial cultures are negative or in whom there is no improvement with standard antibiotic therapy warrant cultures for genital mycoplasmas. Isolation requires special media, and clinical specimens must be cultured immediately or be frozen at −80°C to prevent loss of organisms. When inoculated into broth containing arginine (for *M. hominis*) or urea (for *U. urealyticum*), growth is indicated by an alkaline pH. Identification of *U. urealyticum* on agar requires 1-2 days of growth and visualization with the dissecting microscope, whereas *M. hominis* is apparent to the eye but can require 1 wk to grow. Cultures from the upper respiratory tract are probably meaningless owing to high colonization rates. Cultures of the lower respiratory tract through endotracheal aspirate or biopsy are essential.

TREATMENT

Recommended treatment for NGU in boys is azithromycin (1 g PO as a single dose) and doxycycline (100 mg PO twice daily for 7 days). Recurrent NGU after completion of treatment suggests the presence of azithromycin-resistant *M. genitalium*. Retreatment with moxifloxicin may be most effective. Sexual partners should also be treated to avoid recurrent disease in the index case. Nongenital mycoplasmal infections can require surgical drainage and prolonged antibiotic therapy.

Neonates

Therapy for neonatal genital mycoplasma infections is indicated in infections associated with a pure growth of the organism and evidence that the disease manifestations are compatible with an infectious process rather than merely colonization. The role of therapy in preventing CLD in very low birthweight infants awaits results of further studies. Treatment is based on predictable antimicrobial sensitivities, because susceptibility testing is not readily available for individual isolates. For symptomatic CNS infections, cures have been described with chloramphenicol, doxycycline, and moxifloxacin. The long-term consequences of asymptomatic CNS infection with genital mycoplasmas, especially in the absence of pleocytosis, are unknown. Because mycoplasmas can spontaneously clear from the CSF, therapy should involve minimal risks.

BIBLIOGRAPHY

Please visit the Nelson Textbook of Pediatrics *website at* *www.expertconsult.com* *for the complete bibliography.*

Section 10 CHLAMYDIAL INFECTIONS

Chapter 217
Chlamydophila pneumoniae

Stephan A. Kohlhoff and Margaret R. Hammerschlag

Chlamydophila (Chlamydia) pneumoniae is a common cause of lower respiratory tract diseases, including pneumonia in children and bronchitis and pneumonia in adults.

ETIOLOGY

Chlamydiae are obligate intracellular pathogens that have established a unique niche in host cells. Chlamydiae cause a variety of diseases in animal species at virtually all phylogenic levels. The most significant human pathogens are *C. pneumoniae* and *C. trachomatis* (Chapter 218). *C. psittaci* is the cause of psittacosis, an important zoonosis (Chapter 219).

Chlamydiae have a gram-negative envelope without detectable peptidoglycan, although recent genomic analysis has revealed that both *C. pneumoniae* and *C. trachomatis* encode proteins forming a nearly complete pathway for synthesis of peptidoglycan, including penicillin-binding proteins. Chlamydiae also share a group-specific lipopolysaccharide antigen and use host adenosine triphosphate (ATP) for the synthesis of chlamydial proteins. Although chlamydiae are auxotrophic for 3 of 4 nucleoside triphosphates, they encode functional glucose-catabolizing enzymes that can be used to generate ATP. As with peptidoglycan synthesis, for some reason these genes are turned off. All chlamydiae also encode an abundant surface exposed protein called the *major outer membrane protein* (MOMP, or OmpA). The MOMP is the major determinant of the serologic classification of *C. trachomatis* and *C. psittaci* isolates.

EPIDEMIOLOGY

C. pneumoniae is primarily a human respiratory pathogen. The organism has also been isolated from nonhuman species, including horses, koalas, reptiles, and amphibians, where it also causes respiratory infection, although the role that these infections might play in transmission to humans is unknown. *C. pneumoniae* appears to affect individuals of all ages. The proportion of community-acquired pneumonias associated with *C. pneumoniae* infection is 2-19%, varying with geographic location, the age group examined, and the diagnostic methods used. Several studies of the role of *C. pneumoniae* in lower respiratory tract infection in pediatric populations have found evidence of infection in 0-18% of patients based on serology or culture for diagnosis. In one study, almost 20% of the children with *C. pneumoniae* infection were co-infected with *M. pneumonia. C. pneumoniae* may also be responsible for 10-20% of episodes of acute chest syndrome in children with sickle cell disease, up to 10% of asthma exacerbations, 10% of episodes of bronchitis, and 5-10% episodes of pharyngitis in children. Asymptomatic infection appears to be common based on epidemiologic studies.

Transmission probably occurs from person to person through respiratory droplets. Spread of the infection appears to be enhanced by close proximity, as is evident from localized outbreaks in enclosed populations, such as military recruits and in nursing homes.

PATHOGENESIS

Chlamydiae are characterized by a unique developmental cycle (Fig. 217-1) with morphologically distinct infectious and reproductive forms: the elementary body (EB) and reticulate body (RB). Following infection, the infectious EBs, which are 200-400 µm in diameter, attach to the host cell by a process of electrostatic binding and are taken into the cell by endocytosis that does not depend on the microtubule system. Within the host cell, the EB remains within a membrane-lined phagosome. The phagosome does not fuse with the host cell lysosome. The inclusion membrane is devoid of host cell markers, but lipid markers traffic to the inclusion, which suggests a functional interaction with the Golgi apparatus. The EBs then differentiate into RBs that undergo binary fission. After ~36 hr, the RBs differentiate into EBs. At ~48 hr, release can occur by cytolysis or by a process of exocytosis or extrusion of the whole inclusion, leaving the host cell intact. Chlamydiae can also enter a persistent state after treatment with certain cytokines such as interferon-γ, treatment with antibiotics, or restriction of certain nutrients. While chlamydiae are in the persistent state, metabolic activity is reduced. The ability to cause prolonged, often subclinical, infection is one of the major characteristics of chlamydiae.

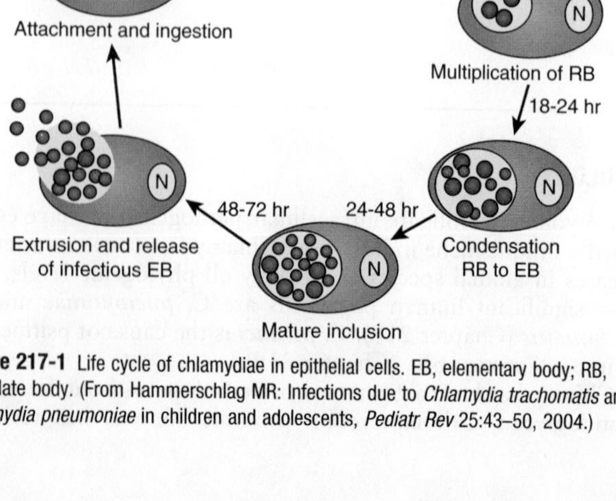

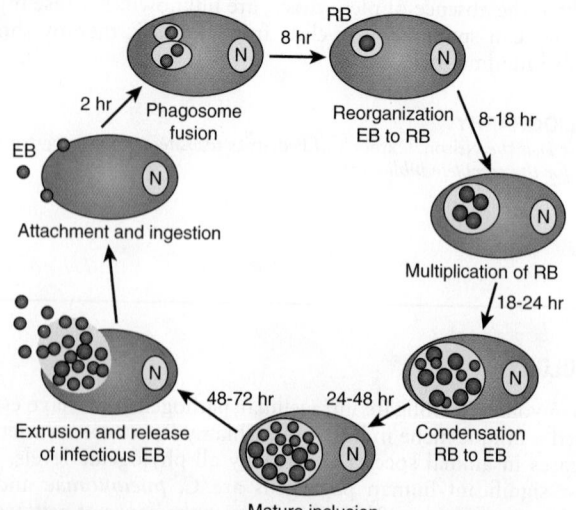

Figure 217-1 Life cycle of chlamydiae in epithelial cells. EB, elementary body; RB, reticulate body. (From Hammerschlag MR: Infections due to *Chlamydia trachomatis* and *Chlamydia pneumoniae* in children and adolescents, *Pediatr Rev* 25:43–50, 2004.)

CLINICAL MANIFESTATIONS

Infections caused by *C. pneumoniae* cannot be readily differentiated from those caused by other respiratory pathogens, especially *M. pneumoniae*. The pneumonia usually occurs as a classic atypical (or nonbacterial) pneumonia characterized by mild to moderate constitutional symptoms, including fever, malaise, headache, cough, and often pharyngitis. Severe pneumonia with pleural effusions and empyema has been described. Milder respiratory infections have been described, which can manifest as a pertussis-like illness.

C. pneumoniae can serve as an infectious trigger for asthma, can cause pulmonary exacerbations in patients with cystic fibrosis, and produce acute chest syndrome in patients with sickle cell anemia. *C. pneumoniae* has been isolated from middle ear aspirates of children with acute otitis media, most of the time as co-infection with other bacteria. Asymptomatic respiratory infection has been documented in 2-5% of adults and children and can persist for ≥1 yr.

DIAGNOSIS

It is not possible to differentiate *C. pneumoniae* from other causes of atypical pneumonia on the basis of clinical findings. Auscultation reveals the presence of rales and often wheezing. The chest radiograph often appears worse than the patient's clinical status would indicate and can show mild, diffuse involvement or lobar infiltrates with small pleural effusions. The complete blood count may be elevated with a left shift but is usually unremarkable.

Specific diagnosis of *C. pneumoniae* infection is based on isolation of the organism in tissue culture. *C. pneumoniae* grows best in cycloheximide-treated HEp-2 and HL cells. The optimum site for culture is the posterior nasopharynx; the specimen is collected with wire-shafted swabs in the same manner as that used for *C. trachomatis*. The organism can be isolated from sputum, throat cultures, bronchoalveolar lavage fluid, and pleural fluid, but few laboratories perform such cultures because of technical difficulties. Polymerase chain reaction (PCR) testing is the most promising technology in the development of a rapid, nonculture method for detection of *C. pneumoniae*.

Serologic diagnosis can be accomplished using the microimmunofluorescence (MIF) or the complement fixation (CF) tests. The CF test is genus specific and is also used for diagnosis of lymphogranuloma venereum (Chapter 218.4) and psittacosis (Chapter 219). Its sensitivity in hospitalized patients with *C. pneumoniae* infection and children is variable. The Centers for Disease Control and Prevention (CDC) has proposed modifications in the serologic criteria for diagnosis. Although the MIF test was considered to be the only currently acceptable serologic test, the criteria were made significantly more stringent. Acute infection, using the MIF test, was defined by a 4-fold increase in immunoglobulin G (IgG) titer or an IgM titer of ≥16; use of a single elevated IgG titer was discouraged. An IgG titer of ≥16 was thought to indicate past exposure, but neither elevated IgA titers nor any other serologic marker was thought to be a valid indicator of persistent or chronic infection. Because diagnosis would require paired sera, this would be a retrospective diagnosis. The CDC did not recommend the use of any enzyme-linked immune assay for detection of antibody to *C. pneumoniae*, because there is concern about the inconsistent correlation of these results with culture results. Studies of *C. pneumoniae* infection in children with pneumonia and asthma show that >50% of children with culture-documented infection have no detectable MIF antibody.

TREATMENT

The optimum dose and duration of antimicrobial therapy for *C. pneumoniae* infections remain uncertain. Most treatment studies have used only serology for diagnosis, and thus microbiologic efficacy cannot be assessed. Prolonged therapy for ≥2 wk is required for some patients, because recrudescent symptoms and persistent positive cultures have been described following 2 wk of erythromycin and 30 days of tetracycline or doxycycline.

Tetracyclines, erythromycin, the macrolides (azithromycin and clarithromycin), and quinolones show in vitro activity. The ketolides also have promising in vitro activity. Like *C. psittaci*, *C. pneumoniae* is resistant to sulfonamides. The results of treatment studies have shown that erythromycin (40 mg/kg/day PO divided twice a day for 10 days), clarithromycin (15 mg/kg/day PO divided twice a day for 10 days), and azithromycin (10 mg/kg PO on day 1, and then 5 mg/kg/day PO on days 2-5) are effective for eradication of *C. pneumoniae* from the nasopharynx of children with pneumonia in approximately 80% of cases.

PROGNOSIS

Clinical response to antibiotic therapy varies. Coughing often persists for several weeks even after therapy.

BIBLIOGRAPHY

Please visit the Nelson Textbook of Pediatrics *website at* www.expertconsult.com *for the complete bibliography.*

Chapter 218
Chlamydia trachomatis

Margaret R. Hammerschlag

Chlamydia trachomatis is subdivided into 2 biovars: lymphogranuloma venereum (LGV) and trachoma, which is the agent of human oculogenital diseases other than LGV. Although the strains of both biovars have almost complete DNA homology, they differ in growth characteristics and virulence in tissue culture and animals. In developed countries, *C. trachomatis* is the most prevalent sexually transmitted disease, causing urethritis in men, cervicitis and salpingitis in women, and conjunctivitis and pneumonia in infants.

218.1 Trachoma

Margaret R. Hammerschlag

Trachoma is the most important preventable cause of **blindness** in the world. It is caused primarily by the A, B, Ba, and C serotypes of *C. trachomatis*. It is endemic in the Middle East and Southeast Asia and among Navajo Indians in the southwestern USA. In areas that are endemic for trachoma, such as Egypt, genital chlamydial infection is caused by the serotypes responsible for oculogenital disease: D, E, F, G, H, I, J, and K. The disease is spread from eye to eye. Flies are a common vector.

Trachoma begins as a **follicular conjunctivitis**, usually in early childhood. The follicles heal, leading to conjunctival scarring that can result in an entropion, with the eyelid turning inward so that the lashes abrade the cornea. It is the corneal ulceration secondary to the constant trauma that leads to scarring and blindness. Bacterial superinfection can also contribute to scarring. Blindness occurs years after the active disease.

Trachoma can be diagnosed clinically. The World Health Organization (WHO) suggests that at least 2 of 4 criteria must be present for a diagnosis of trachoma: lymphoid follicles on the upper tarsal conjunctivae, typical conjunctival scarring, vascular pannus, and limbal follicles. The diagnosis is confirmed by culture or staining tests for *C. trachomatis* performed during the active stage of disease. Serologic tests are not helpful clinically because of the long duration of the disease and the high seroprevalence in endemic populations.

Poverty and lack of sanitation are important factors in the spread of trachoma. As socioeconomic conditions improve, the incidence of the disease decreases substantially. Endemic trachoma has been controlled in most instances by administering topical tetracyclines (or, rarely, erythromycin ointment) daily for periods of 6-10 wk or intermittently over a 6-mo period. Oral doxycycline is effective but is contraindicated in children <8 yr of age. Oral erythromycin requires frequent dosing, which is impractical in the control of endemic trachoma. Several studies have reported that 1-6 doses of oral azithromycin are equivalent to 30 days of treatment with topical oxytetracycline/polymyxin ointment. The WHO recommends single-dose azithromycin (20 mg/kg, maximum 1g) for the treatment of trachoma in children. A study from Tanzania demonstrated that mass treatment with a single dose of azithromycin to all the residents of a village dramatically reduced the prevalence and intensity of infection. This effect continued for 2 years after treatment, probably by interrupting the transmission of ocular *C. trachomatis* infection.

BIBLIOGRAPHY

Please visit the Nelson Textbook of Pediatrics *website at* www.expertconsult.com *for the complete bibliography.*

218.2 Genital Tract Infections

Margaret R. Hammerschlag

EPIDEMIOLOGY

There are an estimated 3 million new cases of chlamydial sexually transmitted infections each year in the USA. *C. trachomatis* is a major cause of epididymitis and is the cause of 23-55% of all cases of nongonococcal urethritis, although the proportion of chlamydial nongonococcal urethritis has been gradually declining. As many as 50% of men with gonorrhea may be co-infected with *C. trachomatis*. The prevalence of chlamydial cervicitis among sexually active women is 2-35%. Rates of infection among girls 15-19 yr of age exceed 20% in many urban populations but can be as high as 15% in suburban populations as well.

Children who have been sexually abused can acquire anogenital *C. trachomatis* infection, which is usually asymptomatic. Culture is the only method that should be used for diagnosis of *C. trachomatis* from these sites when a prepubertal child is being tested for suspected sexual abuse. However, because perinatally acquired rectal and vaginal *C. trachomatis* infections can persist for ≥3 years, the detection of *C. trachomatis* in the vagina or rectum of a young child is not absolute evidence of sexual abuse.

CLINICAL MANIFESTATIONS

The trachoma biovar of *C. trachomatis* causes a spectrum of disease in sexually active adolescents and adults. Up to 75% of women with *C. trachomatis* have no symptoms of infection. *C. trachomatis* can cause urethritis (acute urethral syndrome), epididymitis, cervicitis, salpingitis, proctitis, and pelvic inflammatory disease. The symptoms of chlamydial genital tract infections are less acute than those of gonorrhea, consisting of a discharge that is usually mucoid rather than purulent. Asymptomatic urethral infection is common in sexually active men. Autoinoculation from the genital tract to the eyes can lead to concomitant inclusion conjunctivitis.

DIAGNOSIS

Definitive diagnosis of genital chlamydial infection is accomplished by isolation of the organism in tissue culture and confirmed by microscopic identification of the characteristic inclusions using fluorescent antibody staining in culture specimens obtained from the urethra in men and the endocervix in women. Care should be taken to obtain epithelial cells, not only discharge. *C. trachomatis* can be cultured in cycloheximide-treated HeLa, McCoy, and HEp-2 cells. Chlamydia culture has been further defined by the Centers for Disease Control and Prevention (CDC) as isolation of the organism in tissue culture and as confirmation of the characteristic intracytoplasmic inclusions by fluorescent antibody staining.

Alternatively, a nonculture method, specifically a nucleic acid amplification test (NAAT) can be used. These tests have high sensitivity, perhaps even detecting 10-20% greater than culture, while retaining high specificity. Three Food and Drug Administration (FDA)-approved NAATs are comercially available for detecting *C. trachomatis*: polymerase chain reaction (PCR; Amplicor Chlamydia test, Roche Molecular Diagnostics, Nutley, NJ), strand displacement amplification (SDA; ProbeTec, BD Diagnostic Systems, Sparks, MD), and transcription-mediated amplification (TMA; Amp CT, Gen-Probe, San Diego, CA). PCR and SDA are DNA amplification tests that use primers that target gene sequences on the cryptogenic *C. trachomatis* plasmid that are present at approximately 10 copies in each infected cell. TMA is a ribosomal RNA amplification assay. All 3 assays are also available as co-amplification tests for simultaneously detecting *C. trachomatis* and *Neisseria gonorrhoeae.*

The currently available commercial NAATs are FDA approved for cervical swabs from adolescent girls and women, urethral swabs from adolescent boys and men, and urine from adolescents and adults. The latest version of TMA was recently approved for use with vaginal swabs in adolescents and adults. Use of urine avoids the necessity for a clinical pelvic examination and can greatly facilitate screening in certain populations, especially adolescents, although several studies have now demonstrated that endocervical specimens and vaginal swabs are superior to urine for NAAT. Self-collected vaginal specimens appear to be as reliable as specimens obtained by a health care professional.

Data on use of NAATs for vaginal specimens or urine from children are very limited and insufficient to allow making a recommendation for their use. The CDC recommends that NAATs may be used as an alternative to culture only if confirmation is available. Confirmation tests should consist of a 2nd FDA-approved NAAT that targets a different gene sequence from the initial test.

The etiology of most cases of nonchlamydial nongonococcal urethritis is unknown, although *Ureaplasma urealyticum* and possibly *Mycoplasma genitalium* are implicated in up to one third of cases (Chapter 216). Proctocolitis may develop in individuals who have a rectal infection with an LGV strain (see Chapter 218.4, later).

TREATMENT

The 1st-line treatment regimens recommended by the CDC for uncomplicated *C. trachomatis* genital infection in men and nonpregnant women include azithromycin (1 g PO as a single dose) and doxycycline (100 mg PO twice a day for 7 days). Alternative regimens are erythromycin base (500 mg PO 4 times a day for 7 days), erythromycin ethylsuccinate (800 mg PO 4 times a day for 7 days), ofloxacin (300 mg PO twice a day for 7 days), and levofloxacin (500 mg PO once daily for 7 days). The high erythromycin dosages might not be well tolerated. Doxycycline and quinolones are contraindicated in pregnant women, and quinolones are contraindicated in persons younger than 18 yr. For pregnant women, the recommended treatment regimen is erythromycin base (500 mg PO twice a day for 7 days) or amoxicillin (500 mg PO 3 times a day for 7 days). Alternative regimens for pregnant women are erythromycin base (250 mg PO 4 times a day for 14 days), erythromycin ethylsuccinate (800 mg PO 4 times a day for 7 days or 400 mg PO 4 times a day for 14 days), and azithromycin (1 g PO in a single dose). Amoxicillin at a dosage of 500 mg PO 3 times a day for 7 days is as effective as any of the erythromycin regimens and is much better tolerated. However, experience with all these regimens is still limited.

Empirical treatment without microbiologic diagnosis is recommended only for patients at high risk for infection who are unlikely to return for follow-up evaluation, including adolescents with multiple sex partners. These patients should be treated empirically for both *C. trachomatis* and gonorrhea.

Sex partners of patients with nongonococcal urethritis should be treated if they have had sexual contact with the patient during the 60 days preceding the onset of symptoms. The most recent sexual partner should be treated even if the last sexual contact was more than 60 days from onset of symptoms.

COMPLICATIONS

Complications of genital chlamydial infections in women include perihepatitis (Fitz-Hugh-Curtis syndrome) and salpingitis. Of women with untreated chlamydial infection who develop pelvic inflammatory disease, up to 40% will have significant sequelae; approximately 17% will suffer from chronic pelvic pain, approximately 17% will become infertile, and approximately 9% will have an ectopic (tubal) pregnancy. Adolescent girls may be at higher risk for developing complications, especially salpingitis, than older women. Salpingitis in adolescent girls is also more likely to lead to tubal scarring, subsequent obstruction with secondary infertility, and increased risk for ectopic pregnancy. Approximately 50% of neonates born to pregnant women with untreated chlamydial infection will acquire *C. trachomatis* infection (see Chapter 218.3, next). Women with *C. trachomatis* infection have a 3-5-fold increased risk for acquiring HIV infection.

PREVENTION

Timely treatment of sex partners is essential for decreasing risk for reinfection. Sex partners should be evaluated and treated if they had sexual contact during the 60 days preceding onset of symptoms in the patient. The most recent sex partner should be treated even if the last sexual contact was >60 days. Patients and their sex partners should abstain from sexual intercourse until 7 days after a single-dose regimen or after completion of a 7-day regimen.

Annual routine screening for *C. trachomatis* is recommended for all sexually active female adolescents, for all women 20-25 years of age, and for older women with risk factors such as new or multiple partners or inconsistent use of barrier contraceptives. Sexual risk assessment might indicate more frequent screening of some women.

BIBLIOGRAPHY
Please visit the Nelson Textbook of Pediatrics *website at www.expertconsult.com for the complete bibliography.*

218.3 Conjunctivitis and Pneumonia in Newborns

Margaret R. Hammerschlag

EPIDEMIOLOGY

Chlamydial genital infection is reported in 5-30% of pregnant women, with a risk for vertical transmission at parturition to newborn infants of about 50%. The infant may become infected at 1 or more sites, including the conjunctivae, nasopharynx, rectum, and vagina. Transmission is rare following cesarean section with intact membranes. The introduction of systematic prenatal screening for *C. trachomatis* infection and treatment of pregnant women has resulted in a dramatic decrease in the incidence of neonatal chlamydial infection in the USA. However, in countries where prenatal screening is not done, such as the Netherlands, *C. trachomatis* remains an important cause of neonatal infection, accounting for >60% of neonatal conjunctivitis.

Inclusion Conjunctivitis

Approximately 30-50% of infants born to mothers with active, untreated chlamydial infection develop clinical conjunctivitis. Symptoms usually develop 5-14 days after delivery, or earlier in infants born after prolonged rupture of membranes. The presentation is extremely variable and ranges from mild conjunctival injection with scant mucoid discharge to severe conjunctivitis with copious purulent discharge, chemosis, and pseudomembrane formation. The conjunctiva may be very friable and miight bleed when stroked with a swab. Chlamydial conjunctivitis must be differentiated from gonococcal ophthalmia, which is sight threatening. At least 50% of infants with chlamydial conjunctivitis also have nasopharyngeal infection.

Pneumonia

Pneumonia due to *C. trachomatis* can develop in 10-20% of infants born to women with active, untreated chlamydial infection. Only about 25% of infants with nasopharyngeal chlamydial infection develop pneumonia. *C. trachomatis* pneumonia of infancy has a very characteristic presentation. Onset usually occurs between 1 and 3 mo of age and is often insidious, with persistent cough, tachypnea, and absence of fever. Auscultation reveals rales; wheezing is uncommon. The absence of fever and wheezing helps to distinguish *C. trachomatis* pneumonia from respiratory syncytial virus pneumonia. A distinctive laboratory finding is the presence of peripheral eosinophilia (>400 cells/mm^3). The most consistent finding on chest radiograph is hyperinflation accompanied by minimal interstitial or alveolar infiltrates.

Infections at Other Sites

Infants born to mothers with *C. trachomatis* can develop infection in the rectum or vagina. Although infection in these sites appears to be totally asymptomatic, it can cause confusion if it is identified at a later date. Perinatally acquired rectal, vaginal, and nasopharyngeal infections can persist for ≥3 years. *C. pneumoniae* can also be confused with *C. trachomatis* infection in nasopharyngeal cultures if a genus-specific monoclonal antibody is used to confirm the culture.

DIAGNOSIS

Definitive diagnosis is achieved by isolation of *C. trachomatis* in cultures of specimens obtained from the conjunctiva or nasopharynx. Nonculture methods including direct fluorescent antibody (DFA) and NAATs are available, but only the DFA is currently approved for diagnosis of chlamydial conjunctivitis with sensitivities of ≥90% and specificities of ≥95% for conjunctival specimens compared with culture. Accuracy for nasopharyngeal specimens is not as good. Data on use of NAATs for diagnosis of *C. trachomatis* in children are limited. Limited data suggest that PCR may be equivalent to culture for detecting *C. trachomatis* in the conjunctiva of infants with conjunctivitis.

TREATMENT

The recommended treatment regimen for *C. trachomatis* conjunctivitis or pneumonia in infants is erythromycin (base or ethylsuccinate, 50 mg/kg/day divided 4 times a day PO for 14 days). The rationale for using oral therapy for conjunctivitis is that 50% or more of these infants have concomitant nasopharyngeal infection or disease at other sites, and studies have demonstrated that topical therapy with sulfonamide drops and erythromycin ointment is not effective. The failure rate with oral erythromycin remains 10-20%, and some infants require a 2nd course of treatment. The results of 1 small study suggest that a short course of azithromycin (20 mg/kg/day once daily PO for 3 days) is as effective as 14 days of erythromycin. Mothers (and their sexual contacts) of infants with *C. trachomatis* infections should be empirically treated for genital infection. An association between treatment with oral erythromycin and infantile hypertrophic pyloric stenosis has been reported in infants <6 wk of age who were given the drug for prophylaxis after nursery exposure to pertussis.

PREVENTION

Neonatal gonococcal prophylaxis with topical erythromycin or tetracycline ointment, or silver nitrate, does not appear to prevent chlamydial ophthalmia or nasopharyngeal colonization with *C. trachomatis* or chlamydial pneumonia. The most effective method of controlling perinatal chlamydial infection is screening and treatment of pregnant women. For treatment of *C. trachomatis* infection in pregnant women, the CDC currently recommends either azithromycin (1 g PO as a single dose) or amoxicillin (500 mg PO 3 times a day for 7 days) as 1st-line regimens. Erythromycin base (250 mg PO 4 times a day for 14 days) and erythromycin ethylsuccinate (800 mg 4 times a day for 7 days, or 400 mg PO 4 times a day for 14 days) are listed as alternative regimens. Reasons for failure of maternal treatment to prevent infantile chlamydial infection include poor compliance and reinfection from an untreated sexual partner.

BIBLIOGRAPHY
Please visit the Nelson Textbook of Pediatrics *website at www.expertconsult.com for the complete bibliography.*

218.4 Lymphogranuloma Venereum

Margaret R. Hammerschlag

LGV is a systemic sexually transmitted disease caused by the L_1, L_2, and L_3 serotypes of the LGV biovar of *C. trachomatis*. Unlike strains of the trachoma biovar, LGV strains have a predilection for lymphoid tissue. About 20 cases of LGV have been reported in children, and <1,000 cases are reported in adults in the USA annually. There has been a resurgence of LGV infections among men who have sex with men in Europe and the USA. Many of the men were HIV infected and used illicit drugs, specifically methamphetamines.

CLINICAL MANIFESTATIONS

The 1st stage of LGV is characterized by the appearance of the primary lesion, a painless, usually transient papule on the genitals. The 2nd stage is characterized by usually unilateral femoral or inguinal lymphadenitis with enlarging, painful buboes. The nodes may break down and drain, especially in men. In women, the vulvar lymph drains to the retroperitoneal nodes. Fever, myalgia, and headache are common. The 3rd stage is a genitoanorectal syndrome with rectovaginal fistulas, rectal strictures, and urethral destruction. Among men who have sex with men, rectal infection with LGV can produce a severe, acute proctocolitis, which can be confused with inflammatory bowel disease or malignancy.

DIAGNOSIS

LGV can be diagnosed by serologic testing or by culture of *C. trachomatis* or molecular testing for *C. trachomatis* from a specimen aspirated from a bubo. Most patients with LGV have complement-fixing antibody titers of >1:16. Chancroid and herpes simplex virus can be distinguished clinically from LGV by the concurrent presence of painful genital ulcers. Syphilis can be differentiated by serologic tests. However, co-infections can occur.

TREATMENT

Doxycycline (100 mg PO bid for 21 days) is the recommended treatment. The alternative regimen is erythromycin base (500 mg PO 4 times/day for 21 days). Azithromycin (1 g PO once weekly for 3 wk) may also be effective but clinical data are lacking. Sex partners of patients with LGV should be treated if they have had sexual contact with the patient during the 30 days preceding the onset of symptoms.

BIBLIOGRAPHY

Please visit the Nelson Textbook of Pediatrics *website at www.expertconsult.com for the complete bibliography.*

Chapter 219
Psittacosis *(Chlamydophila psittaci)*

Stephan A. Kohlhoff and Margaret R. Hammerschlag

Chlamydophila psittaci, the agent of psittacosis (also known as **parrot fever** and **ornithosis**), is primarily an animal pathogen and causes human disease oncommonly. In birds, *C. psittaci* infection is known as *avian chlamydiosis.*

For the full continuation of this chapter, please visit the Nelson Textbook of Pediatrics *website at www.expertconsult.com.*

Section 11 RICKETTSIAL INFECTIONS

Chapter 220
Spotted Fever and Transitional Group Rickettsioses

Megan E. Reller and J. Stephen Dumler

Rickettsia species were classically divided into "spotted fever" and "typhus" groups based on serologic reactions. The outer membrane protein A (*ompA*) gene is present in spotted fever but not typhus group organisms. Complete genome sequences have further refined distinctions, and several species that possess *ompA,* but are genetically distinct from others in the spotted fever group, have been reassigned to a "transitional" group. Many members of the spotted fever group of rickettsiae are pathogenic for humans (Table 220-1). These include the tick-borne agents *Rickettsia rickettsii,* the cause of Rocky Mountain spotted fever (RMSF); *R. conorii,* the cause of Mediterranean spotted fever (MSF) or boutonneuse fever; *R. sibirica,* the cause of North Asian tick typhus; *R. japonica,* the cause of Oriental spotted fever; *R. honei,* the cause of Flinders Island spotted fever or Thai tick typhus; *R. africae,* the cause of African tick bite fever; and unnamed Israeli spotted fever rickettsia, and possibly others. Members of the transitional group include *R. akari,* the cause of mite-transmitted rickettsialpox; *R. felis,* the cause of cat flea–transmitted typhus; and *R. australis,* the cause of tick-transmitted Queensland tick typhus.

Infections with other members of the spotted fever and transitional groups are clinically similar to MSF, with fever, maculopapular rash, and eschar at the site of the tick bite. Israeli spotted fever is generally associated with a more severe course, including death in children. African tick bite fever is relatively mild, can include a vesicular rash, and often manifests with multiple eschars. New potentially pathogenic rickettsial species have been identified, including *R. slovaca,* the cause of TIBOLA (tick-borne lymphadenopathy), and *R. parkeri,* a cause of eschars in patients bitten by *Amblyomma maculatum* ticks in North America. *R. rickettsii, R. parkeri, R. felis,* and *R. akari* are the only members of the spotted fever and transitional groups that cause autochthonous disease in the USA.

220.1 Rocky Mountain Spotted Fever *(Rickettsia rickettsii)*

Megan E. Reller and J. Stephen Dumler

Rocky Mountain spotted fever (RMSF) is the most frequently identified and most severe rickettsial disease in the USA. It is also the most common vector-borne disease in the USA after Lyme disease. Although considered uncommon, RMSF is greatly underdiagnosed and underreported. RMSF should be considered in the differential diagnosis of fever, headache, and rash in the summer months, especially after tick exposure. Because fulminant disease and death are associated with delays in treatment, patients in whom the illness is clinically suspected should be treated promptly.

ETIOLOGY

RMSF results from systemic infection of endothelial cells by the obligate intracellular bacterium *R. rickettsii.*

EPIDEMIOLOGY

The term **Rocky Mountain spotted fever** is historical, because the agent was discovered in the Bitterroot Range of the Rocky Mountains of Montana. Few cases are now reported from this region.

Table 220-1 SUMMARY OF RICKETTSIAL DISEASES OF HUMANS, INCLUDING *RICKETTSIA, ORIENTIA, EHRLICHIA, ANAPLASMA, NEORICKETTSIA,* AND *COXIELLA*

GROUP OR DISEASE AGENT		ARTHROPOD VECTOR, TRANSMISSION HOSTS		GEOGRAPHIC DISTRIBUTION	PRESENTING CLINICAL FEATURES*	COMMON LAB ABNORMALITIES	DIAGNOSTIC TESTS	TREATMENT†
SPOTTED FEVER GROUP								
Rocky Mountain spotted fever	*Rickettsia rickettsii*	Tick bite: *Dermacentor* species (wood tick, dog tick) *Rhipicephalus sanguineus* (brown dog tick)	Dogs Rodents	Western hemisphere	Fever, headache, rash,* emesis, diarrhea, tender calf muscles	AST, ALT ↓Na (mild) ↓Platelets ±Leukopenia Left shift	Early: IH, DFA, PCR After 1st wk: IFA	**Doxycycline** Tetracycline Chloramphenicol
Mediterranean spotted fever (Boutonneuse fever)	*Rickettsia conorii*	Tick bite: *R. sanguineus* (brown dog tick)	Dogs Rodents	Africa, Mediterranean, India, Middle East	Painless eschar (tache noir) with regional lymphadenopathy, fever, headache, rash,* myalgias	AST, ALT ↓Na (mild) ↓Platelets ±Leukopenia Left shift	Early: IH, DFA, PCR After 1st wk: IFA	**Doxycycline** Tetracycline Chloramphenicol Azithromycin Clarithromycin Fluoroquinolones
African tick-bite fever	*Rickettsia africae*	Tick bite	Cattle Goats?	Sub-Saharan Africa, Caribbean	Fever, single or multiple eschars, regional lymphadenopathy, rash* (can be vesicular)	AST, ALT ↓Platelets	Early: IH, DFA After 1st wk: IFA	**Doxycycline**
Tick-borne lymphadenopathy (TIBOLA)	*Rickettsia slovaca*	Tick bite: *Dermacentor*	?	Europe	Eschar (scalp), painful lymphadenopathy	?	PCR	**Doxycycline**
TRANSITIONAL GROUP								
Rickettsialpox	*Rickettsia akari*	Mite bite	Mice	North America, Russia, Ukraine, Adriatic, Korea, South Africa	Painless eschar, ulcer or papule; tender regional lymphadenopathy, fever, headache, rash*(can be vesicular)	↓WBC	Early: IH, DFA After 1st wk: IFA	**Doxycycline** Chloramphenicol
Cat flea typhus	*Rickettsia felis*	Flea bite	Opossums Cats Dogs	Western hemisphere, Europe	Fever, rash,* headache	?	Early: PCR After 1st wk: IFA	**Doxycycline**
TYPHUS GROUP								
Murine typhus	*Rickettsia typhi*	Flea feces	Rats Opossums	Worldwide	Fever, headache, rash,* myalgias, emesis, lymphadenopathy, hepatosplenomegaly	AST, ALT ↓Na (mild) ↓WBC ↓ Platelets	Early: DFA After 1st wk: IFA	**Doxycycline** Chloramphenicol
Epidemic (louse-borne) typhus (Recrudescent form: Brill-Zinsser disease)	*Rickettsia prowazekii*	Louse feces	Humans	South America, Central America, Mexico, Africa, Asia, Eastern Europe	Fever, headache, abdominal pain, rash,* CNS involvement	AST, ALT ↓Platelets	Early: None After 1st wk: IgG/IgM, IFA	**Doxycycline** Tetracycline Chloramphenicol
Flying squirrel (sylvatic) typhus	*Rickettsia prowazekii*	Louse feces? Flea feces or bite?	Flying squirrels	Eastern USA	Same as above (often milder)	AST, ALT ↓Platelets	Early: None After 1st wk: IFA	**Doxycycline** Tetracycline Chloramphenicol

Continued

Table 220-1 SUMMARY OF RICKETTSIAL DISEASES OF HUMANS, INCLUDING *RICKETTSIA, ORIENTIA, EHRLICHIA, ANAPLASMA, NEORICKETTSIA,* AND *COXIELLA*—cont'd

GROUP OR DISEASE AGENT		ARTHROPOD VECTOR, TRANSMISSION HOSTS		GEOGRAPHIC DISTRIBUTION	PRESENTING CLINICAL FEATURES*	COMMON LAB ABNORMALITIES	DIAGNOSTIC TESTS	TREATMENT†
SCRUB TYPHUS								
Scrub typhus	*Orientia tsutsugamushi*	Chigger bite: *Leptotrombidium*	Rodents?	South Asia, Japan, Indonesia, Korea, China, Russia, Australia	Fever, rash,* headache, painless eschar, hepatosplenomegaly, gastrointestinal symptoms	↓Platelets AST, ALT	Early: None After 1st wk: IFA	**Doxycycline** Tetracycline Chloramphenicol ***If Doxycycline resistant:*** **Rifampicin** Azithromycin
EHRLICHIOSIS AND ANAPLASMOSIS								
Human monocytic ehrlichiosis	*Ehrlichia chaffeensis*	Tick bite: *Amblyomma americanum* (lone star tick)	Deer Dogs	USA Europe? Africa? Asia?	Fever, headache, malaise, myalgias, rash*‡, hepatosplenomegaly,‡ swollen hands/feet‡	AST, ALT ↓WBC ↓Platelets ↓Na (mild)	Early: PCR After 1st wk: IFA	**Doxycycline** Tetracycline
Human granulocytic anaplasmosis	*Anaplasma phagocytophilum*	Tick bite: *Ixodes* species	Rodents Deer Ruminants	USA, Europe, Asia	Fever, headache, malaise, myalgias	AST, ALT ↓WBC, ↓ANC ↓Platelets ↓Na (mild)	Early: PCR, blood smear After 1st wk: IFA	**Doxycycline** Tetracycline Rifampin
Ewingii ehrlichiosis	*Ehrlichia ewingii*	Tick bite: *Amblyomma americanum* (lone star tick)	Dogs Deer	USA (south-central southeast)	Fever, headache, malaise, myalgias	AST, ALT, ↓WBC ↓Platelets ↓Na (mild)	Early: PCR After 1st wk: IFA	**Doxycycline** Tetracycline
Sennetsu ehrlichiosis	*Neorickettsia sennetsu*	Ingestion of fish helminth?	Unknown	Japan Malaysia	Fever, "mononucleosis" symptoms, postauricular and posterior cervical lymphadenopathy	Atypical lymphocytosis	Early: None After 1st wk: IFA	**Doxycycline** Tetracycline
Q FEVER								
Q Fever: acute (for chronic, see text)	*Coxiella burnetti*	Inhale infected aerosols: contact with parturient animals, abattoir, contaminated cheese and milk, ?ticks	Cattle Sheep Goats Cats Rabbits	Worldwide	Fever, headache, arthralgias, myalgias, gastrointestinal symptoms, cough, pneumonia, rash (children)	AST, ALT WBC ↓ Platelets Interstitial infiltrate	Early: PCR After 1st wk: IFA	**Doxycycline** Tetracycline Fluoroquinolones Trimethoprim-sulfamethoxazole

*Rash is infrequently present at initial presentation but appears during the first week of illness.
†Preferred treatment is in **bold**.
‡Often present in children but not adults.
ALT, alanine aminotransferase; ANC, absolute neutrophil count; AST, aspartate aminotransferase; CNS, central nervous system; DFA, direct fluorescent antibody; IFA, indirect fluorescent antibody; IgG, immunoglobulin G; IgM, immunoglobulin M; IH, immunohistochemistry; PCR, polymerase chain reaction; WBC, white blood cell count.

Cases have been reported throughout the continental USA (except Vermont and Maine), southwestern Canada, Mexico, Central America, and South America, but not from outside of the Western Hemisphere. In 2006, most cases were reported from North Carolina, Tennessee, Missouri, Oklahoma, Virginia, Arkansas, Alabama, Maryland, Georgia, and South Carolina. Human incursion into previously uninhabited areas has resulted in cases being described in new areas, such as the Northeast USA. The incidence of RMSF has been cyclical but has generally increased over the past decades. The mean number of cases reported each year to the Centers for Disease Control and Prevention (CDC) has steadily increased (515 during 1993-1998, 1,071 during 2001-2004, and 2,000 cases in 2006-2008). Habitats favored by ticks, including wooded areas or coastal grassland and salt marshes, are associated with disease. Foci of intense infection are found both in rural and urban areas. Clustering of cases within families likely reflects shared environmental exposures. In the USA, 90% of cases occur between April and September, months in which humans spend the most time outdoors. The highest age-specific incidence of RMSF among children is seen in those >5 yr of age, with boys outnumbering girls.

TRANSMISSION

Ticks are the natural hosts, reservoirs, and vectors of *R. rickettsii.* Ticks maintain the infection in nature by transovarial transmission (passage of the organism from infected ticks to their progeny). Ticks harboring rickettsiae are substantially less fecund than uninfected ticks; thus, horizontal transmission (acquisition of rickettsiae by taking a blood meal from transiently rickettsemic animal hosts such as small mammals or dogs) significantly contributes to maintenance of rickettsial infections in ticks. Ticks transmit the infectious agent to mammalian hosts (including humans) via infected saliva during feeding. The pathogen *R. rickettsii* in ticks becomes virulent after exposure to blood or increased temperature; thus, the longer the tick is attached, the greater the risk of transmission. The principal tick hosts of *R. rickettsii* are *Dermacentor variabilis* (the American dog tick) in the eastern USA and Canada, *Dermacentor andersoni* (the wood tick) in the western USA and Canada, *Rhipicephalus sanguineus* (the common brown dog tick) in the southwestern USA and in Mexico, and *Amblyomma cajennense* in Central and South America (Fig. 220-1).

Dogs can serve as reservoir hosts for *R. rickettsii,* can develop RMSF themselves, and can bring infected ticks into contact with humans. Serologic studies suggest that many patients with RMSF likely acquired the illness from ticks carried by the family dog.

Humans can also become infected when trying to remove an attached tick, because *R. rickettsii*–containing tick fluids or feces can be rubbed into the open wound at the bite site or into the conjunctivae by contaminated fingers. Finally, inhalation of aerosolized rickettsiae has caused severe infections and deaths in laboratory workers.

PATHOLOGY AND PATHOGENESIS

Systemic infection is most obvious on the skin (rash), but nearly all organs and tissues are affected. Following inoculation of tick saliva into the dermis, the rickettsiae attach to the vascular endothelium via protein ligands and initiate rickettsia-mediated injury to host cell membranes. Damage to the membranes induces endocytosis, and the internalized rickettsiae then gain access to the cytosol by continued lysis of vacuolar membranes. Members of the spotted fever group actively initiate intracellular actin polymerization to achieve directional movement, and rickettsiae can easily invade neighboring cells despite minimal initial damage to host cells. The rickettsiae proliferate and damage the host cells by peroxidative membrane alterations, protease activation, or continued phospholipase activity.

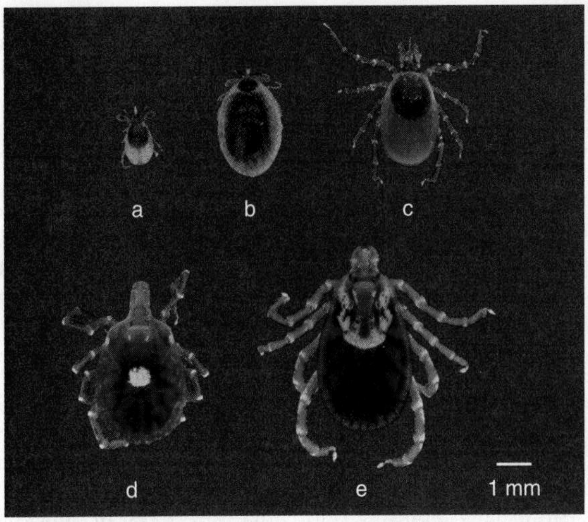

Figure 220-1 Tick vectors of agents of human rickettsial diseases. An unengaged nymph (a), engorged nymph (b), and adult female (c) of *Ixodes scapularis* (deer tick), the vector of *Anaplasma phagocytophilum,* the cause of human granulocytic anaplasmosis. An adult female (d) of *Amblyomma americanum* (lone star tick), the vector of *Ehrlichia chaffeensis* and *Ehrlichia ewingii,* the causes of human monocytic ehrlichiosis and ewingii ehrlichiosis, respectively. An adult female (e) of *Dermacentor variabilis* (American dog tick), the vector of *Rickettsia rickettsii,* the cause of Rocky Mountain spotted fever.

The histologic correlate of the initial macular or maculopapular rash is perivascular infiltrates of lymphoid and histiocytic cells with edema but without significant endothelial damage. Proliferation of rickettsiae within the cytoplasm of infected endothelial cells leads to lymphohistiocytic or leukocytoclastic vasculitis of small venules and capillaries, which manifests as a petechial rash. This process ultimately results in microvascular leakage, tissue hypoperfusion, and possibly end-organ ischemic injury. Rickettsiae are contained within endothelial cells of inflamed vessels that may be eccentrically involved. Infrequently, inflammation leads to nonocclusive thrombi. Very rarely, small and large vessels become completely obliterated by thrombosis, which leads to tissue infarction or hemorrhagic necrosis. Interstitial pneumonitis and vascular leakage in the lungs can lead to noncardiogenic pulmonary edema, and meningoencephalitis can cause significant cerebral edema.

The presence of the infectious agent initiates an inflammatory cascade, including release of cytokines such as tumor necrosis factor-α (TNF-α), interleukin 1β, and interferon-γ (IFN-γ). Infection of endothelial cells by *R. rickettsii* induces surface E-selectin expression and procoagulant activity. Release of chemokines and expression of vascular selectin results in infiltration of the damaged endothelial cells by lymphocytes, macrophages, and occasionally neutrophils. Local inflammatory and immune responses have been suspected to contribute to the vascular injury characteristic of rickettsioses; however, the benefits of effective inflammation and immunity are greater. Blockade of TNF-α and IFN-γ action in animal models diminishes survival and increases the morbidity of spotted fever group infections, probably by abrogating upregulation of nitric oxide synthase and arginine-dependent intracellular killing. Direct contact of infected endothelial cells with perforin-producing CD8 T lymphocytes and IFN-γ–producing natural killer cells helps control the infection. Infection of endothelial cells with *Rickettsia* leads to upregulated expression of procoagulant molecules and consumption of coagulation factors, platelet adhesion, dissolution of endothelium junctional proteins, and emigration of leukocytes and can lead to disseminated intravascular coagulation (DIC).

CLINICAL MANIFESTATIONS

The incubation period of RMSF in children varies from 2 to 14 days, with a median of 7 days. In 60% of cases, patients or their parents report a history of removing an attached tick, although the site of the tick bite is usually unapparent. Epidemiologic clues include living in or visiting an endemic area, playing or hiking in the woods, typical season, similar illness in family members, and close contact with a dog (especially one that is sick). Inapparent or mild illness probably occurs infrequently, but the illness might not be reported. In patients presenting for care, the illness is initially nonspecific, with symptoms including headache, anorexia, myalgias, and restlessness. *Pain and tenderness of calf muscles are particularly common in children.* Gastrointestinal symptoms including nausea, vomiting, diarrhea, and abdominal pain occur commonly (39-63%) early in the disease.

The typical **clinical triad of fever, headache, and rash** is observed in 44% of patients overall but is present in only 3% at presentation. Fever and headache persist if the illness is untreated. Fever can exceed 40°C and may be persistently elevated or can fluctuate dramatically. Headache is severe, unremitting, and unresponsive to analgesics.

Rash usually appears only after 2-4 days of illness, and approximately 5% of children and up to 20% of adults never develop a rash that is recognized. Rash occurs more reliably in children than in adults. Initially, discrete, pale, rose-red blanching macules or maculopapules appear, characteristically on the extremities, including the ankles, wrists, or lower legs (Fig. 220-2). The rash then spreads rapidly to involve the entire body, including the soles and palms. After several days, the rash becomes more petechial or hemorrhagic, sometimes with palpable purpura. In severe disease, the petechiae can enlarge into ecchymosis, which can become necrotic. Severe vascular obstruction secondary to the rickettsial vasculitis and thrombosis is uncommon but can result in gangrene of the digits, earlobes, scrotum, nose, or an entire limb.

Central nervous system infection usually manifests as meningismus and changes in sensorium. In addition, patients can manifest ataxia, seizures, coma, or auditory deficits. CSF parameters are usually normal, but one third have mononuclear pleocytosis (<10-300 cells/μL) and 20% have elevated protein (<200 mg/dL). Neuroimaging studies generally reveal only subtle abnormalities that do not alter treatment. Cerebral edema, meningeal enhancement, and prominent perivascular spaces have been observed in patients with severe disease.

Other pulmonary disease occurs more commonly in adults than in children and can manifest clinically as rales, infiltrates, and noncardiogenic pulmonary edema. Other findings can include conjunctival suffusion, periorbital edema, dorsal hand and foot edema, and hepatosplenomegaly. Severe disease can include myocarditis, acute renal failure, and vascular collapse.

Persons with **glucose-6-phosphate dehydrogenase (G6PD) deficiency** are at increased risk for fulminant RMSF, defined as death from *R. rickettsii* infection within 5 days. The clinical course of fulminant RMSF is characterized by profound coagulopathy and extensive thrombosis leading to kidney, liver, and respiratory failure. Clinical features associated with a fatal outcome include stupor, respiratory distress, acute renal failure, hepatomegaly, jaundice, and a DIC-like syndrome.

Occasionally, infection of vessels with rickettsiae appear to be a local process, such as appendicitis or cholecystitis. Thorough evaluation usually reveals evidence of a systemic process, and unnecessary surgical interventions are avoided.

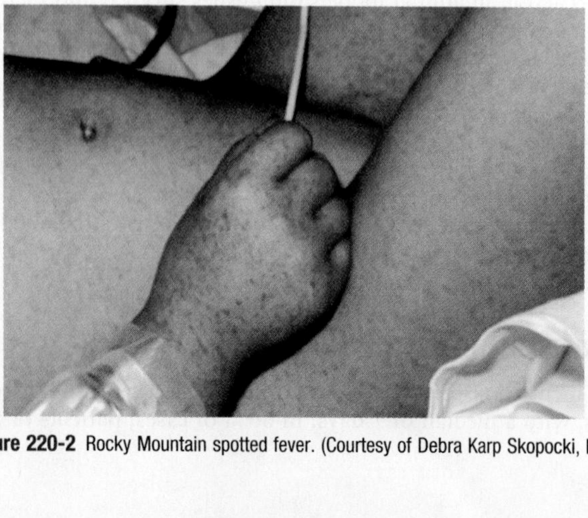

Figure 220-2 Rocky Mountain spotted fever. (Courtesy of Debra Karp Skopocki, MD.)

LABORATORY FINDINGS

Laboratory abnormalities are common but nonspecific. Often, the total white blood cell count is initially normal or low, but leukocytosis can develop as the illness progresses. Other characteristic abnormalities include a left-shifted leukocyte differential, anemia (33%), thrombocytopenia (<150,000 platelets/μL in 33%), hyponatremia (<130 mEq/mL in 20%), and elevated serum aminotransferase levels (50%).

DIAGNOSIS

Delays in diagnosis and treatment are associated with severe disease and death. Because no reliable diagnostic test is available to confirm RMSF acutely, the decision to treat must be based on compatible epidemiologic, clinical, and laboratory features. RMSF should be considered in patients presenting spring through fall with an acute febrile illness accompanied by headache and myalgia (particularly if they report exposure to ticks or contact with a dog or have been in forested or tick-infested rural areas). A history of tick exposure, a rash (especially if on the palms or soles), a normal or low leukocyte count with a marked left shift, a relatively low or decreasing platelet count, and a low serum sodium concentration are all clues that can support a diagnosis of RMSF. In patients without a rash or in dark-skinned patients in whom a rash can be difficult to appreciate, the diagnosis can be exceptionally elusive and delayed. One half of pediatric deaths occur within 9 days of onset of symptoms. Thus, treatment should not be withheld pending definitive laboratory results for a patient with clinically suspected illness. Further, prompt response to early treatment is diagnostically helpful.

If a rash is present, a vasculotropic rickettsial infection can be diagnosed as early as day 3 of illness with biopsy of a petechial lesion and immunohistochemical or immunofluorescent demonstration of specific rickettsial antigen in the endothelium. Although very specific, the sensitivity of this method is probably 70% at most. Further, it can be adversely influenced by prior antimicrobial therapy, suboptimal selection of skin lesions for biopsy, and examination of insufficient tissue because the infection is very focal. Tissue or blood can also be evaluated for *R. rickettsii* nucleic acids by polymerase chain reaction (PCR) at the CDC and selected public health or reference laboratories; however, PCR on blood is less sensitive than PCR on tissue and of similar sensitivity to tissue immunohistology, probably because the level of rickettsemia is generally very low (<6 rickettsiae/mL).

Definitive diagnosis is most often accomplished by serology, which is retrospective, because a rise in titer is not seen until after the 1st week of illness. The gold standard for the diagnosis of RMSF is a 4-fold increase in IgG antibody titer by indirect fluorescent antibody assay (IFA) between acute and convalescent (at 2-4 wk) sera or demonstration of seroconversion. A single titer is neither sensitive (patients can die before seroconversion) nor specific (an elevated titer can represent prior infection). With current serologic methods, RMSF cannot be reliably distinguished from other spotted fever group rickettsiae infections. Cross reactions with typhus group rickettsiae also occur, but titers may be lower for the typhus group. Cross reactions are not seen with *Ehrlichia* or *Anaplasma* infections. Weil-Felix antibody testing should not be performed, because it lacks both sensitivity and specificity. *RMSF is a reportable disease in the USA.*

DIFFERENTIAL DIAGNOSIS

Other rickettsial infections are easily confused with RMSF, especially all forms of human ehrlichiosis and murine typhus. RMSF can also mimic a variety of other pathogens, such as meningococcemia and enteroviruses. Negative blood cultures can exclude meningococcemia. PCR can differentiate enterovirus from *R. rickettsii* in patients with aseptic meningitis and a lymphocytic pleocytosis in the CSF. Other diseases in the differential diagnosis are typhoid fever, secondary syphilis, Lyme disease, leptospirosis, rat-bite fever, scarlet fever, toxic shock syndrome, rheumatic fever, rubella, parvovirus infection, Kawasaki disease, idiopathic thrombocytopenic purpura, thrombotic thrombocytopenic purpura, Henoch-Schönlein purpura, hemolytic uremic syndrome, aseptic meningitis, acute gastrointestinal illness, acute abdomen, hepatitis, infectious mononucleosis, hemophagocytic syndromes, dengue fever, and drug reactions.

TREATMENT

The time-proven effective therapies for RMSF are tetracyclines and chloramphenicol. The treatment of choice for suspected RMSF in patients of all ages, including for young children, is doxycycline (4 mg/kg/day divided every 12 hr PO or IV, maximum 200 mg/day). Tetracycline (25-50 mg/kg/day divided every 6 hr PO, maximum 2 g/day) is an alternative. Chloramphenicol (50-100 mg/kg/day divided every 6 hr IV, maximum 4 g/day) should be reserved for patients with doxycycline allergy and for pregnant women, because chloramphenicol has been shown to be an independent risk factor for increased mortality vs. tetracycline. If used, chloramphenicol should be monitored to maintain serum concentrations of 10-30 µg/mL. Chloramphenicol is preferred for pregnant women because of doxycycline's potential adverse effects on the fetus's teeth and bone and the mother's liver. Although tetracycline and doxycycline may be associated with tooth discoloration in children <8 yr of age, RMSF is a life-threatening illness for which prompt therapy is imperative. Tooth discoloration is dose dependent and it is unlikely that children with RMSF will require multiple courses. Chloramphenicol has rarely been associated with aplastic anemia and is no longer available as an oral preparation in the USA. An additional benefit of doxycycline over chloramphenicol is its effectiveness against potential concomitant ehrlichial infection. Sulfonamides should not be used, because they are associated with greater morbidity and mortality with RMSF. Other antibiotics, including penicillins, cephalosporins, and aminoglycosides, are not effective. The use of alternative antimicrobial agents, such as fluoroquinolones and the macrolides (azithromycin and clarithromycin), has not been evaluated.

Therapy should be continued for a minimum of 5-7 days and until the patient has been afebrile for at least 3 days to avoid relapse, especially in patients treated early. Treated patients usually defervesce within 48 hr, so the duration of therapy is usually <10 days.

SUPPORTIVE CARE

Most infections resolve rapidly with appropriate antimicrobial therapy and do not require hospitalization or other supportive care. On occasion, severe infections require intensive care. Particular attention to hemodynamic status is required in severely ill children, because iatrogenic pulmonary or cerebral edema is easy to precipitate owing to diffuse microvascular injury of the lungs, meninges, and brain. Judicious use of corticosteroids for meningoencephalitis has been advocated by some, but no controlled trials have been conducted.

COMPLICATIONS

Complications of RMSF include noncardiogenic pulmonary edema from pulmonary microvascular leakage, cerebral edema from meningoencephalitis, and multiorgan damage (hepatitis, pancreatitis, cholecystitis, epidermal necrosis, and gangrene) mediated by rickettsial vasculitis and/or the accumulated effects of hypoperfusion and ischemia (acute renal failure). Long-term neurologic sequelae are more likely to occur in patients who have been hospitalized for ≥2 wk and include paraparesis; hearing loss; peripheral neuropathy; bladder and bowel incontinence; cerebellar, vestibular, and motor dysfunction; and language disorders. Learning disabilities and behavioral problems are the most common neurologic sequelae among children who have survived severe disease.

PROGNOSIS

Delays in diagnosis and therapy are significant factors associated with death or severe illness. Before the advent of effective antimicrobial therapy for RMSF, the case fatality rate was 10% for children and 30% for adults. A case fatality rate of 8.5% was documented in Texas from 1986 through 1996. The overall mortality rate is now 2-7%. Diagnosis based on serology alone underestimates the true mortality of RMSF, because patients often die before developing a serologic response. Deaths occur despite the availability of effective therapeutic agents, indicating the need for clinical vigilance and a low threshold for early empiric therapy. Even with administration of appropriate antimicrobials, delayed therapy can lead to irreversible vascular or end-organ damage and long-term sequelae or death. Early therapy in uncomplicated cases usually leads to rapid defervescence within 1-3 days and recovery within 7-10 days. A slower response may be seen if therapy is delayed. In those who survive despite no treatment, fever subsides in 2-3 wks.

PREVENTION

No vaccines are available. Prevention of RMSF is best accomplished by preventing or treating tick-infestation in dogs, avoiding wooded or grassy areas where ticks reside, using insect repellents containing DEET, wearing protective clothing, and carefully inspecting children who have been playing in the woods or fields for ticks. Recovery from infection yields lifelong immunity.

Prompt and complete **removal of attached ticks** helps reduce the risk for transmission because rickettsiae in the ticks need to be reactivated to become virulent, and this requires at least several hours to days of exposure to body heat or blood. Contrary to popular belief, the application of petroleum jelly, 70% isopropyl alcohol, fingernail polish, or a hot match are not effective in removing ticks. A tick can be safely removed by grasping the mouth parts with a pair of forceps at the site of attachment to the skin and applying gentle and steady pressure to achieve retraction without twisting, thereby removing the entire tick and its mouth parts. The site of attachment should then be disinfected. Ticks should not be squeezed or crushed, because their fluids may be infectious. The removed tick should be soaked in alcohol or flushed down the toilet, and hands should be washed to avoid accidental inoculation into conjunctivae, mucous membranes, or breaks in skin. Prophylactic antimicrobial therapy should not be administered, because tetracyclines and chloramphenicol are only rickettsiastatic, simply delaying the onset of illness and confusing the clinical picture by prolonging the incubation period.

220.2 Mediterranean Spotted Fever or Boutonneuse Fever *(Rickettsia conorii)*

Megan E. Reller and J. Stephen Dumler

Boutonneuse fever is caused by *R. conorii* and its related subspecies and was first described in Tunisia in 1909. It is also called

Mediterranean spotted fever (MSF), Kenya tick typhus, Indian tick typhus, Israeli spotted fever, and Astrakhan fever. It is a moderately severe vasculotropic rickettsiosis that is often initially associated with an eschar at the site of the tick bite. Minor differences in clinical presentation could be associated with genetic diversity of the rickettsial subspecies.

ETIOLOGY

MSF is caused by systemic endothelial cell infection by the obligate intracellular bacterium *R. conorii.* Similar species are distributed globally, such as *R. sibirica* in Russia, China, Mongolia, and Pakistan; *R. australis* and *R. honei* in Australia; *R. japonica* in Japan; and *R. africae* in South Africa (see Table 220-1). Analysis of antigens and related DNA sequences show that all are closely related to *R. rickettsii*, the cause of Rocky Mountain Spotted Fever (RMSF).

EPIDEMIOLOGY

R. conorii is distributed over a large geographic region, including India, Pakistan, Russia, Ukraine, Georgia, Israel, Morocco, southern Europe, Ethiopia, Kenya, and South Africa. Reported cases of MSF in southern Europe have steadily increased since 1980, and the seroprevalence is 11-26% in some areas. The peak in reported cases occurs during July and August in the Mediterranean basin; in other regions it occurs during warm months when ticks are active.

TRANSMISSION

Transmission occurs after the bite of the brown dog tick, *R. sanguineus,* or other tick species such as *Dermacentor, Haemaphysalis, Amblyomma, Hyalomma,* and *Ixodes.* Clustering of human cases of boutonneuse fever, infected ticks, and infected dogs implicate the household dog as a potential vehicle for transmission.

PATHOLOGY AND PATHOGENESIS

The underlying pathology seen with MSF is nearly identical to that of RMSF, except that eschars are often present at the site of tick bite where inoculation of rickettsiae occurs. The histopathology of the resultant lesion includes necrosis of dermal and epidermal tissues with a superficial crust; a dermis densely infiltrated by lymphocytes, histiocytes, and scattered neutrophils; and damaged capillaries and venules in the dermis. Immunohistochemical stains confirm that the lesions contain rickettsia-infected endothelial cells, but the vasculature structure might not be apparent owing to extensive inflammation and necrosis. The necrosis results from both direct rickettsia-mediated vasculitis and resultant extensive local inflammation. Rickettsiae thus have ready access to lymphatics and venous blood and disseminate to cause systemic disease.

CLINICAL MANIFESTATIONS AND LABORATORY FINDINGS

Typical findings include fever, headache, myalgias, and a maculopapular rash that appears 3-5 days after onset of fever. In about 70% of patients, a painless eschar or **tache noire** appears at the site of the tick bite with accompanying regional lymphadenopathy. Although previously considered self-limited, this infection can be severe, mimicking RMSF. Findings can include purpuric skin lesions, neurologic deficits, respiratory and/or acute renal failure, severe thrombocytopenia, and death in 1.4-5.6% of cases. As with RMSF, a particularly severe form occurs in patients with G6PD deficiency and in patients with underlying conditions such as alcoholic liver disease or diabetes mellitus. Fortunately, disease is generally milder in children.

DIAGNOSIS

Laboratory diagnosis of MSF and related spotted fever group rickettsioses is the same as that for RMSF. Cases may be confirmed by immunohistologic or immunofluorescent demonstration of rickettsiae in skin biopsies, in vitro cultivation via centrifugation-assisted shell vial tissue culture, or demonstration of seroconversion or a 4-fold rise in serum antibody titer to spotted fever group rickettsiae between acute and convalescent sera. Antibodies to spotted fever group antigens cross react, so RMSF in the USA or MSF in Europe, Africa, and Asia cannot be distinguished by these methods.

DIFFERENTIAL DIAGNOSIS

The differential diagnosis includes conditions also associated with single eschars, such as anthrax, bacterial ecthyma, brown recluse spider bite, rat-bite fever (caused by *Spirillum minus*), and other rickettsioses (such as rickettsialpox, African tick-bite fever, and scrub typhus). The spotted fever group rickettsia *R. africae* causes African tick typhus, a milder illness than MSF that is often associated with multiple eschars and occasionally a vesicular rash. African tick typhus can be contracted in North Africa, where MSF also occurs and is a common infection of travelers to sub-Saharan Africa who encounter bush or high grasslands on safari.

TREATMENT AND SUPPORTIVE CARE

MSF is effectively treated with tetracycline, doxycycline, chloramphenicol, ciprofloxacin, ofloxacin, levofloxacin, azithromycin, or clarithromycin. The treatment of choice is doxycycline (4 mg/kg/day divided every 12 hr PO or IV, maximum 200 mg/day). Tetracycline and chloramphenicol are alternatives, as for RMSF. Azithromycin (10 mg/kg/day once daily PO for 3 days) and clarithromycin (15 mg/kg/day divided twice daily PO for 7 days) are also used. Specific fluoroquinolone regimens effective for children have not been established. Intensive care may be required.

COMPLICATIONS

The complications of MSF are similar to those of RMSF. The case fatality rate is approximately 2%. Particularly severe infections have been noted in patients with underlying medical conditions, including G6PD deficiency and diabetes mellitus.

PREVENTION

MSF is transmitted by tick bites, and prevention is the same as recommended for RMSF. No vaccine is currently available.

220.3 Rickettsialpox *(Rickettsia akari)*

Megan E. Reller and J. Stephen Dumler

Rickettsialpox is caused by *Rickettsia akari,* a transitional group *Rickettsia* species that is transmitted by the **mouse mite,** *Allodermanyssus sanguineus.* The mouse host for this mite is widely distributed in cities in the USA, Europe, and Asia. Seroepidemiologic studies suggest a high prevalence of this infection in urban settings. The disease is uncommon and is usually mild. Unlike the situation with most forms of rickettsiosis, the macrophage is an important target cell for *R. akari.*

Rickettsialpox is best known because of its association with a varicelliform rash. In fact, this rash is a modified form of an antecedent typical macular or maculopapular rash like those seen in other vasculotropic rickettsioses. At presentation, most patients have fever, headache, and chills. In up to 90% of cases, there is a painless papular or ulcerative lesion or eschar at the initial site of inoculation, which may be associated with regional lymphadenopathy that is often tender. In some patients, the maculopapular rash becomes vesicular, involving the trunk, head, and extremities. The infection generally resolves spontaneously and does not require therapy. However, a short course of doxycycline hastens resolution and is sometimes used in patients >8 yr of age and in young children with relatively severe illness. Complications and fatalities are rare.

BIBLIOGRAPHY

Please visit the Nelson Textbook of Pediatrics *website at* www.expertconsult.com *for the complete bibliography.*

Chapter 221
Scrub Typhus (*Orientia tsutsugamushi*)

Megan E. Reller and J. Stephen Dumler

Scrub typhus is an important cause of acute febrile illness in South and East Asia and the Pacific. Recent reports suggest the emergence of doxycycline-resistant strains. Concurrent scrub typhus can inhibit the replication of HIV virus.

ETIOLOGY

The causative agent of scrub typhus, or tsutsugamushi fever, is *Orientia tsutsugamushi,* which is distinct from other spotted fever and typhus group rickettsiae (see Table 220-1). *O. tsutsugamushi* lacks both lipopolysaccharide and peptidoglycan in its cell wall. Like other vasculotropic rickettsiae, *O. tsutsugamushi* infects endothelial cells and causes vasculitis, the predominant clinicopathologic feature of the disease. However, the organism also infects cardiac myocytes and macrophages.

EPIDEMIOLOGY

Approximately 1 million infections occur each year, and it is estimated that more than 1 billion people are at risk. Scrub typhus occurs mostly in Asia, including areas delimited by Korea, Pakistan, and northern Australia. Outside these tropical and subtropical regions, the disease occurs in Japan, the Primorye of far eastern Russia, Tajikistan, Nepal, and nontropical China, including Tibet. Cases imported to the USA and other parts of the world are reported. Most infections in children are acquired in rural areas. In Thailand, scrub typhus is the cause of 1-8% of acute fevers of unknown origin. Infections are most common during rainy months, usually June through November. Reported cases in boys are higher than in girls.

TRANSMISSION

O. tsutsugamushi is transmitted via the bite of the larval stage (chigger) of a trombiculid mite (*Leptotrombidium*), which serves as both vector and reservoir. Transovarial transmission (passage of the organism from infected ticks to their progeny) and transmission of the organism from infected animals to mites both occur. Because only the larval stage takes blood meals, a role for horizontal transmission from infected rodent hosts to uninfected mites has not been proved. Multiple serotypes of *O. tsutsugamushi* are recognized, and some share antigenic cross reactivity; however, they do not stimulate protective cross immunity.

PATHOLOGY AND PATHOGENESIS

The pathogenesis of scrub typhus is uncertain. Recent studies suggest that the process is stimulated by widespread infection of vascular endothelial cells, which corresponds to the distribution of disseminated vasculitic and perivascular inflammatory lesions observed in histopathologic examinations. In autopsy series, the major result of the vascular injury appears to be hemorrhage. However, it is very likely that the vascular injury initiated by the infection is sustained by immune-mediated inflammation that together cause significant vascular leakage. The net result is significant vascular compromise and ensuing end-organ injury, most often manifested in the brain and lungs, as with other vasculotropic rickettsioses.

CLINICAL MANIFESTATIONS AND LABORATORY FINDINGS

Scrub typhus can be mild or severe in children. Most patients present with fever for 9-11 days (range, 1-30 days) before seeking medical care. Regional or generalized lymphadenopathy is reported in 23-93% of patients, hepatomegaly in about two thirds, and splenomegaly in about one third of children with scrub typhus. Gastrointestinal symptoms, including abdominal pain, vomiting, and diarrhea, occur in up to 40% of children at presentation. A single painless eschar with an erythematous rim at the site of the chigger bite is seen in 7-68% of cases, and a maculopapular rash is present in <30%. Leukocyte and platelet counts are most commonly within normal ranges, although thrombocytopenia occurs in one quarter to one third of children, and leukocytosis is observed in about 40%.

DIAGNOSIS AND DIFFERENTIAL DIAGNOSIS

Owing to the potential for severe complications, diagnosis and decision to initiate treatment should be based on clinical suspicion and confirmed by *O. tsutsugamushi* serologic tests such as indirect fluorescent antibody (IFA) or immunoperoxidase assays. The IFA assay is 92% sensitive with ≥11 days of fever. Although the rickettsiae can be cultivated using tissue culture methods, and polymerase chain reaction tests appear highly sensitive, these diagnostic methods are not widely available. The differential diagnosis includes fever of unknown origin, enteric fever, typhoid fever, dengue hemorrhagic fever, other rickettsioses, tularemia, anthrax, dengue, leptospirosis, malaria, and infectious mononucleosis.

TREATMENT AND SUPPORTIVE CARE

The recommended treatment regimen for scrub typhus is doxycycline (4 mg/kg/day PO or IV divided every 12 hr, maximum 200 mg/day). Alternative regimens include tetracycline (25-50 mg/kg/day PO divided every 6 hr, maximum 2 g/day) or chloramphenicol (50-100 mg/kg/day divided every 6 hr IV, maximum 4 g/24 hr). If used, chloramphenicol should be monitored to maintain serum concentrations of 10-30 µg/mL. Therapy should be continued for a minimum of 5 days and until the patient has been afebrile for ≥3 days to avoid relapse. However, a single dose of oral doxycycline was reported effective for all 38 children treated with this regimen in a large series of children with scrub typhus from Thailand. Most children respond rapidly to doxycycline or chloramphenicol within 1-2 days (range, 1-5 days). Highly virulent or potentially doxycycline-resistant *O. tsutsugamushi* strains have emerged in some regions of Thailand. Clinical trials showed that azithromycin may be as effective and that rifampicin is superior to doxycycline in such cases. Likewise, a retrospective analysis in Korean children with scrub typhus showed that roxithromycin was as effective as either doxycycline or chloramphenicol, suggesting a role as an alternative therapy for children or pregnant women. The use of ciprofloxacin in pregnant women resulted in an adverse outcome in 5 of 5 pregnancies among Indian women. Intensive care may be required for hemodynamic management of severely affected patients.

COMPLICATIONS

Serious complications include pneumonitis in 20-35% and meningoencephalitis in approximately 10% of children. Acute renal failure, myocarditis, and a septic shock–like syndrome occur much less often. Cerebrospinal fluid examination shows a mild mononuclear pleocytosis with normal glucose levels. Chest x-rays reveal transient perihilar or peribronchial interstitial infiltrates in most children who are examined. The case fatality rate in untreated patients may be as high as 30% if left untreated, although deaths in children are uncommon.

PREVENTION

Prevention is based on avoidance of the chiggers that transmit *O. tsutsugamushi*. Protective clothing is the next most useful mode of prevention. Infection provides immunity to reinfection by homologous but not heterologous strains; however, because natural strains are highly heterogeneous, infection does not always provide complete protection against reinfection.

BIBLIOGRAPHY

Please visit the Nelson Textbook of Pediatrics *website at www.expertconsult.com for the complete bibliography.*

Chapter 222
Typhus Group Rickettsioses

Megan E. Reller and J. Stephen Dumler

Members of the typhus group of rickettsiae (see Table 220-1) include *Rickettsia typhi*, the cause of murine typhus, and *Rickettsia prowazekii*, the cause of louse-borne or epidemic typhus. *R. typhi* is transmitted to humans by fleas, and *R. prowazekii* is transmitted in the feces of body lice. Louse-borne or epidemic typhus is widely considered to be the most virulent of rickettsial diseases, with a high case fatality rate even with treatment. Murine typhus is moderately severe and likely under-reported worldwide. The genomes of both *R. typhi* and *R. prowazekii* are genetically similar.

222.1 Murine Typhus *(Rickettsia typhi)*

Megan E. Reller and J. Stephen Dumler

ETIOLOGY

Murine typhus is caused by *R. typhi*, a rickettsia transmitted from infected fleas to rats, other rodents, or opossums and back to fleas. Transovarial transmission (passage of the organism from infected fleas to their progeny) in fleas is inefficient. Transmission depends on distribution by the flea to uninfected mammals that become transiently rickettsemic and transmit the organism to uninfected fleas.

Rickettsia felis is a novel agent species identified as a cause of a murine typhus-like illness worldwide. This new rickettsia is genetically a member of a transitional *Rickettsia* group and is capable of highly efficient transovarial transmission in cat fleas. This organism is found in cat fleas obtained from areas endemic for murine typhus in the USA and increasingly worldwide.

EPIDEMIOLOGY

Murine typhus has a worldwide distribution and occurs especially in warm coastal ports, where it is maintained in a cycle involving rat fleas (*Xenopsylla cheopis*) and rats (*Rattus* species). Peak incidence occurs when rat populations are highest during spring, summer, and fall. In the USA, the disease is most prevalent in south Texas and southern California, although seroprevalence studies among children indicate a higher than anticipated rate of infection broadly across the southeast and south-central USA, expanding the endemic areas in which pediatricians must be alert for this infection. In the coastal areas of south Texas, the disease is seen predominantly from March through June and is associated with opossums, cats, and cat fleas (*Ctenocephalides felis*).

TRANSMISSION

R. typhi normally cycles between rodents or mid-size animals such as opossums and their fleas. Human acquisition of murine typhus occurs when rickettsiae-infected flea feces contaminate flea bite wounds.

PATHOLOGY AND PATHOGENESIS

R. typhi is a vasculotropic rickettsia that causes disease in a manner similar to *R. rickettsii* (Chapter 220.1). *R. typhi* organisms in flea feces deposited on the skin as part of the flea feeding reflex are inoculated into the pruritic flea bite wound. After an interval for local proliferation, the rickettsiae spread systemically to infect the endothelium in many tissues. As with spotted fever group rickettsiae, typhus group rickettsiae infect endothelial cells, but unlike the spotted fever group rickettsiae, they polymerize intracellular actin poorly, have limited intracellular mobility, and probably cause cellular injury by mechanical lysis after accumulating in large numbers within the endothelial cell cytoplasm. Intracellular infection leads to endothelial cell damage, recruitment of inflammatory cells, and vasculitis. The inflammatory cell infiltrates bring in a number of effector cells, including macrophages that produce proinflammatory cytokines, and CD4, CD8, and natural killer lymphocytes, which can produce immune cytokines such as interferon-γ or participate in cell-mediated cytotoxic responses. Intracellular rickettsial proliferation of typhus group rickettsiae is inhibited by cytokine-mediated mechanisms and nitric oxide–dependent and –independent mechanisms.

Pathologic findings include systemic vasculitis in response to rickettsiae within endothelial cells. This manifests as interstitial pneumonitis, meningoencephalitis, interstitial nephritis, myocarditis, and mild hepatitis with periportal lymphohistiocytic infiltrates. As vasculitis and inflammatory damage accumulate, multiorgan damage can ensue.

CLINICAL MANIFESTATIONS

Murine typhus is a moderately severe infection that is similar to other vasculotropic rickettsioses. The incubation period varies from 1 to 2 wk. The initial presentation is often nonspecific, and fever of undetermined origin is the most common presentation. Pediatric patients exhibit the typically important clues for murine typhus somewhat less often than for the other vasculotropic rickettsioses, including rash (48-80%), myalgias (29-57%), vomiting (29-45%), cough (15-40%), headache (19-77%), and diarrhea or abdominal pain (10-40%). Lymphadenopathy and hepatosplenomegaly are reported often among children with murine typhus in Europe. Although neurologic involvement is a common finding in adults with murine typhus, photophobia, confusion, stupor, coma, seizures, meningismus, and ataxia are seen in <17% of hospitalized children and <6% of infected children treated as outpatients. A petechial rash is observed only in ≤13% of children, and the usual appearance is that of macules or maculopapules distributed on the trunk and extremities. The rash can involve both the soles and palms.

LABORATORY FINDINGS

Although nonspecific, laboratory findings that may be helpful include mild leukopenia (36-40%) with a moderate left shift, mild to marked thrombocytopenia (43-60%), hyponatremia (20-66%), hypoalbuminemia (46-87%), and elevated aspartate aminotransferase (82%) and alanine aminotransferase (38%). Elevations in serum urea nitrogen are usually due to prerenal mechanisms.

DIAGNOSIS AND DIFFERENTIAL DIAGNOSIS

As for other vasculotropic rickettsioses, delays in diagnosis and therapy are associated with increased morbidity and mortality; thus, diagnosis must be based on clinical suspicion. Occasionally, patients present with findings suggesting pharyngitis, bronchitis, hepatitis, gastroenteritis, or sepsis; thus, the differential diagnosis may be extensive.

Confirmation of the diagnosis is usually accomplished by comparing acute and convalescent-phase antibody titers obtained with the indirect fluorescent antibody assay. Research tools now being evaluated include polymerase chain reaction amplification of rickettsial nucleic acids in acute-phase blood, rickettsial culture by the centrifugation-assisted shell vial assay, and immunohistology on skin biopsy.

TREATMENT

Therapy for murine typhus includes tetracyclines or chloramphenicol, similar to treatment for Rocky Mountain spotted fever. No controlled trials of other antimicrobial agents have been performed. Ciprofloxacin has been used effectively to treat murine typhus, but treatment failures have been reported. In vitro experiments suggest that minimal inhibitory concentrations of azithromycin and clarithromycin for *R. typhi* should be easily achieved.

The time-honored recommended treatment for murine typhus is doxycycline (4 mg/kg/day divided every 12 hr PO or IV, maximum 200 mg/day). Alternative regimens include tetracycline (25-50 mg/kg/day divided every 6 hr PO, maximum 2 g/day) or chloramphenicol (50-100 mg/kg/day divided every 6 hr IV, maximum 4 g/day). Therapy should be continued for a minimum of 5 days and until the patient has been afebrile for at least 3 days to avoid relapse, especially in patients treated early.

SUPPORTIVE CARE

Although disease is usually mild, 7% of children with murine typhus require intensive care to manage complications such as meningoencephalitis or a disseminated intravascular coagulation–like condition. As for other rickettsial infections with significant systemic vascular injury, careful hemodynamic management is mandatory to avoid pulmonary or cerebral edema.

COMPLICATIONS

Complications of murine typhus in pediatric patients are uncommon; however, relapse, stupor, facial edema, dehydration, splenic rupture, and meningoencephalitis are reported. Predominance of abdominal pain has led to surgical exploration to exclude a perforated viscus.

PREVENTION

Control of murine typhus was dependent on elimination of the flea reservoir and control of flea hosts, and this remains important. However, with the recognition of cat fleas as potentially significant reservoirs and vectors, the presence of these flea vectors and their mammalian hosts in suburban and urban areas where close human exposures occur will probably pose increasingly difficult control problems. It is not known with certainty if infection confers protective immunity; reinfection appears to be rare.

222.2 Epidemic Typhus *(Rickettsia prowazekii)*

Megan E. Reller and J. Stephen Dumler

ETIOLOGY

Humans are considered the principal or only reservoir of *R. prowazekii,* the causative agent of epidemic or louse-borne typhus and its recrudescent form, Brill-Zinsser disease. Another reservoir exists in flying squirrels and their ectoparasites in a sylvatic cycle with small rodents. *R. prowazekii* is the most pathogenic member of the genus *Rickettsia* and multiplies to very large intracellular quantities before rupture of infected endothelial cells.

EPIDEMIOLOGY

The infection is characteristically seen in winter or spring and especially during times of poor hygienic practices associated with crowding, war, famine, extreme poverty, and civil strife. A cause of some sporadic cases of a mild, typhus-like illness in the USA has been confirmed as *R. prowazekii;* such cases are associated with exposure to flying squirrels harboring infected lice or fleas. *R. prowazekii* organisms isolated from these squirrels appear to be genetically similar to isolates obtained during typical outbreaks.

Most cases of louse-borne typhus in the developed world are sporadic, but outbreaks have been identified in Africa (Ethiopia, Nigeria, and Burundi), Mexico, Central America, South America, Eastern Europe, Afghanistan, Russia, northern India, and China within the past 25 years. Following the Burundi Civil War in 1993, 35,000-100,000 cases of epidemic typhus were diagnosed in displaced refugees, resulting in an estimated 6,000 deaths.

TRANSMISSION

Human body lice (*Pediculus humanus corporis*) become infected by feeding on rickettsemic persons. The ingested rickettsiae infect the midgut epithelial cells of the lice and are passed into the feces, which in turn is introduced into a susceptible human host through abrasions or perforations in the skin, through the conjunctivae, or rarely through inhalation after drying in clothing, bedding, or furniture.

CLINICAL MANIFESTATIONS

Louse-borne typhus can be mild or severe in children. The incubation period is usually <14 days. The typical clinical manifestations include fever, severe headache, abdominal tenderness, and rash in most patients, as well as chills (82%), myalgias (70%), arthralgias (70%), anorexia (48%), nonproductive cough (38%), dizziness (35%), photophobia (33%), nausea (32%), abdominal pain (30%), tinnitus (23%), constipation (23%) meningismus (17%), visual disturbances (15%), vomiting (10%), and diarrhea (7%). However, investigation of recent African outbreaks has shown a lower incidence of rash (25%) and a high incidence of delirium (81%) and cough associated with pneumonitis (70%). The rash is initially pink or erythematous and blanches. In 1/3 of patients, red, nonblanching macules and petechiae appear predominantly on the trunk. Infections identified during the pre-antibiotic era typically produced a variety of central nervous system findings, including delirium (48%), coma (6%), and seizures (1%). Estimates of case fatality rates range between 3.8% and 20% in outbreaks.

Brill-Zinsser disease is an unusual form of typhus that becomes recrudescent months to years after the primary infection, thus rarely affecting children. When rickettsemic, these infected patients can transmit the agent to lice, potentially providing the initial event that triggers an outbreak if hygienic conditions permit.

TREATMENT

Recommended treatment regimens for louse-borne or sylvatic typhus are identical to those used for murine typhus. The treatment of choice is doxycycline (4 mg/kg/day divided every 12 hr PO or IV, maximum 200 mg/day). Alternative treatments include tetracycline (25-50 mg/kg/day divided every 6 hr PO, maximum 2 g/day) or chloramphenicol (50-100 mg/kg/day divided every 6 hr IV, maximum 4 g/day). Therapy should be continued for a minimum of 5 days and until the patient has been afebrile for at least 3 days to avoid relapse, especially in patients treated early. Good evidence exists that doxycycline as a single 200 mg oral dose (4.4 mg/kg if <45 kg) is also efficacious.

PREVENTION

Immediate destruction of vectors with an insecticide is important in the control of an epidemic. Lice live in clothing rather than on the skin; thus, searches for ectoparasties should include examination of clothes. For epidemic typhus, antibiotic therapy and delousing measures interrupt transmission, reduce the prevalence of infection in the human reservoir, and diminish the impact of an outbreak. Dust containing excreta from infected lice is stable and capable of transmitting typhus, and care must be taken to prevent its inhalation. Infection confers solid protective immunity. However, recrudescence can occur years later with Brill-Zinsser disease, implying that immunity is nonsterile.

BIBLIOGRAPHY

Please visit the Nelson Textbook of Pediatrics *website at* www.expertconsult.com *for the complete bibliography.*

Chapter 223
Ehrlichioses and Anaplasmosis

Megan E. Reller and J. Stephen Dumler

ETIOLOGY

In 1987, clusters of bacteria confined within cytoplasmic vacuoles of circulating leukocytes (morulae), particularly mononuclear leukocytes, were detected in the peripheral blood of a severely ill patient with suspected Rocky Mountain spotted fever (RMSF). The etiologic agent of this case and other similar cases was found to resemble a canine pathogen in the genus *Ehrlichia*. In 1990, *Ehrlichia chaffeensis* was cultivated and identified as the predominant cause of "human ehrlichiosis." Seroepidemiologic investigations showed that *E. chaffeensis* infections are transmitted by ticks and occur more often than RMSF in some geographic areas.

In 1994, the observation of other cases in which morulae were found only within circulating neutrophils and serology for *E. chaffeensis* was negative led to the recognition of another species. In these cases, serologic reactions were strongest to *Ehrlichia phagocytophila* and *Ehrlichia equi*, pathogens of ruminant and horse granulocytes, respectively. DNA of these bacteria was also found in the blood of infected persons. In 1996, the agent was cultivated in vitro; in 2001, the human agent and the 2 veterinary pathogens were unified into a single species and placed into the genus *Anaplasma* under the name *Anaplasma phagocytophilum* on the basis of genetic studies.

In 1996, a veterinary pathogen of canine neutrophils, *Ehrlichia ewingii*, was identified as the causative agent of some human infections initially thought to be due to *E. chaffeensis* because of the presence of morulae within circulating neutrophils. The infection is generally milder, but it can cause severe disease in children and adults with pre-existing immunosuppression, including organ transplant recipients or persons with HIV infection. Although not yet cultivated in vitro, it is serologically cross reactive with *E. chaffeensis*.

Although these infections are caused by bacteria assigned to various genera, the name ehrlichiosis has been applied to all. **Human monocytic ehrlichiosis (HME)** is used to describe disease characterized by infection of predominantly monocytes caused by *E. chaffeensis*, **human granulocytic anaplasmosis (HGA)** to describe disease of circulating neutrophils caused by *Anaplasma phagocytophilum*, and **ewingii ehrlichiosis** caused by *E. ewingii* (see Table 220-1).

All are tick-transmitted, small, obligate intracellular bacteria with gram-negative–type cell walls and are now classified in the Anaplasmataceae family. *Neorickettsia* (formerly *Ehrlichia*) *sennetsu* is another related bacterium that rarely causes human disease and is not transmitted by ticks. *E. chaffeensis* alters host signaling and transcription to cause the endosome to enter a receptor recycling pathway that avoids phagosome-lysosome fusion and allows the growth of a **morula,** an intravacuolar aggregate of bacteria. Little is known about the vacuoles in which *A. phagocytophilum* and *E. ewingii* grow. These bacteria are pathogens of phagocytic cells in mammals, and characteristically each species has a specific host cell affinity: *E. chaffeensis* and *N. sennetsu* infect mononuclear phagocytes, and *A. phagocytophilum* and *E. ewingii* infect neutrophils. Infection leads to direct modifications in function of the host cell that protect the bacterium from host defenses; yet, host immune and inflammatory reactions might in part account for many of the clinical manifestations seen in all forms of ehrlichiosis.

EPIDEMIOLOGY

Infections with *E. chaffeensis* occur across the southeastern, south central, and mid-Atlantic states in a distribution that parallels that of RMSF; cases have also been reported in northern California. Suspected cases with appropriate serologic and occasionally molecular evidence have been reported in Europe, Africa, and the Far East, including China and Korea. Human infections with *E. ewingii* have only been identified in the USA in areas where *E. chaffeensis* also exists, perhaps owing to a shared tick vector. Canine infections are documented in both sub-Saharan Africa and in South America.

Although the median age of patients with ehrlichiosis and anaplasmosis is generally older (>42 yr), many infected children have been identified. Little is known about the epidemiology of *E. ewingii* infections, although many patients have also been children. All infections are strongly associated with tick exposure and tick bites and are identified predominantly during May through September. Although both nymphal and adult ticks can transmit infection, nymphs are more likely to transmit disease, because they are most active during the summer.

TRANSMISSION

The predominant tick species that harbors *E. chaffeensis* and *E. ewingii* is *Amblyomma americanum*, the Lone Star tick. Additional vectors such as *Dermacentor variabilis*, the American dog tick, have not been proved but might explain the presence of HME outside the known range of *A. americanum* (see Fig. 220-1). The tick vectors of *A. phagocytophilum* are *Ixodes*, including *I. scapularis* (black-legged or deer tick) in the eastern USA (Fig. 220-1), *I. pacificus* (western black-legged tick) in the western USA, *I. ricinus* (sheep tick) in Europe, and *I. persulcatus* in Eurasia. *Ixodes* species ticks also transmit *Borrelia burgdorferi, Babesia microti,* and, in Europe, tick-borne encephalitis-associated flaviviruses. Co-infections with these agents and *A. phagocytophilum* have been documented in children and adults.

Ehrlichia and *Anaplasma* species are maintained in nature predominantly by horizontal transmission (tick to mammal to tick), because the organisms are not transmitted to the progeny of infected adult female ticks (transovarial transmission). The major reservoir host for *E. chaffeensis* is the white-tailed deer (*Odocoileus virginianus*), which is found abundantly in many parts of the USA. A reservoir for *A. phagocytophilum* in the eastern USA appears to be the white-footed mouse, *Peromyscus leucopus.* Deer or domestic ruminants may also have persistent asymptomatic infections, but the genetic variants in these reservoirs might not be infectious for humans. Efficient transmission requires persistent infections of mammals, long recognized in dogs with *Ehrlichia canis,* ruminants with *A. phagocytophilum,* and other hosts of various ehrlichial species. Although *E. chaffeensis* and *A. phagocytophilum* can cause persistent infections in animals, documentation of chronic infections in humans is exceedingly rare. Transmission of *Ehrlichia* can occur within hours of tick attachment, in contrast to the 1-2 days of attachment required for transmission of *B. burgdorferi* to occur. Transmission of *A. phagocytophilum* is via the bite of the small nymphal stage of *Ixodes* spp., including *I. scapularis* (see Fig. 220-1), which is very active during late spring and early summer in the eastern USA.

PATHOLOGY AND PATHOGENESIS

Although human monocytic ehrlichiosis and anaplasmosis often clinically mimics RMSF or typhus, vasculitis is rare. Pathologic findings include mild, diffuse perivascular lymphohistiocytic infiltrates; Kupffer cell hyperplasia; mild lobular hepatitis with infrequent apoptotic hepatocytes; infiltrates of mononuclear phagocytes in the spleen, lymph nodes, and bone marrow with occasional erythrophagocytosis; granulomas of the liver and bone marrow in patients with *E. chaffeensis* infections; and hyperplasia of one or more bone marrow hematopoietic lineages.

The exact pathogenetic mechanisms are poorly understood, but histopathologic examinations suggest diffuse mononuclear phagocyte activation and poorly regulated host immune and inflammatory reactions. This activation results in moderate to profound leukopenia and thrombocytopenia despite a hypercellular bone marrow, and deaths often are related to severe hemorrhage or secondary opportunistic infections. Hepatic and other organ-specific injury occurs by an unknown mechanism that appears to be unrelated to direct infection. Meningoencephalitis with a mononuclear cell pleocytosis in the cerebrospinal fluid (CSF) occurs with HME but is rare with HGA.

CLINICAL MANIFESTATIONS

The clinical manifestations of HME, HGA, and ewingii ehrlichiosis are similar. Many well-characterized infections of HME and HGA of variable severity have been reported in children, including 1 death each from HME and HGA. Children with ehrlichiosis are often ill for 4-12 days, shorter than in adults. In series of children with HME, most required hospitalization and many (25%) required intensive care; this might represent preferential reporting of severe cases. Population-based studies have documented that seroconversion often occurs in children who are well or who have only a mild illness.

Fewer pediatric cases of *E. ewingii* infection are reported, so the clinical manifestations related to this infection are less well characterized. However, in adults *E. ewingii* and monocytic ehrlichiosis are clinically similar. The incubation period (time from last tick bite or exposure) appears to range from 2 days to 3 wks. Nearly 25% of patients do not report a tick bite. Clinically, the ehrlichioses are nonspecific illnesses. Fever (~100%) and headache (~75%) are most common, but many patients also report myalgias, anorexia, nausea, and vomiting. With HME, rash is more common in children (nearly 66%) than in adults (33%). The rash is usually macular or maculopapular, but petechial lesions can occur. Photophobia, conjunctivitis, pharyngitis, arthralgias, and lymphadenopathy are less consistent features. Hepatomegaly and splenomegaly are detected in nearly 50% of children with ehrlichiosis. Edema of the face, hands, and feet occurs more commonly in children than in adults, but arthritis is uncommon in both groups.

Meningoencephalitis with a lymphocyte-predominant CSF pleocytosis is an uncommon but potentially severe complication of HME that appears to be rare with HGA. CSF protein may be elevated and glucose may be mildly depressed in adults with HME meningoencephalitis, but CSF protein and glucose in affected children are typically normal. In 1 series, 19% of adult patients with CNS symptoms and abnormal CSF died despite normal CTs of the brain.

LABORATORY FINDINGS

Characteristically, most children with monocytic ehrlichiosis present with leukopenia (58-72%), lymphopenia (75-78%), and thrombocytopenia (80-92%); cytopenias reach a nadir several days into the illness. Lymphopenia is common in both HME and HGA, and neutropenia is reported in adults with HGA. Leukocytosis can also occur. Despite the presence of pancytopenia, examination usually reveals a cellular or reactive bone marrow in adults. Interestingly, granulomas and granulomatous inflammation are identified in nearly 75% of bone marrow specimens examined from patients with proven cases of *E. chaffeensis* infection, but this finding is not present in patients with HGA. Mild to severe hepatic injury is documented by the common (83-91%) finding of elevated serum transaminase levels. Hyponatremia (<135 mEq/L) is present in most cases. Kidney involvement in children manifests as elevated levels of serum creatinine and blood urea nitrogen. A clinical picture similar to disseminated intravascular coagulopathy has also been reported.

DIAGNOSIS

A delay in diagnosis or treatment can contribute to increased morbidity or mortality; thus, treatment must be begun early based on clinical suspicion. Because both HME and anaplasmosis can cause death, therapy should not be withheld while waiting for the results of confirmatory testing. In fact, prompt response to therapy supports the diagnosis.

The 1st patient and several subsequent pediatric patients with *E. chaffeensis* infection were identified presumptively on the basis of typical *Ehrlichia* morulae in peripheral blood leukocytes (Fig. 223-1*A*). This finding has been too infrequent to be considered a useful diagnostic tool. In contrast, HGA presents with a small but significant percentage (1-40%) of circulating neutrophils (Fig. 223-1*B*) containing typical morulae in 20-60% of patients. The distinction between the 2 infections relies on polymerase chain reaction (PCR) amplification of species-specific DNA sequences or on the demonstration of specific antibodies to *E. chaffeensis* or *A. phagocytophilum* with low titer or absent antibodies to the other agent.

Diagnostic criteria can **confirm** or **suggest ehrlichioses** in a clinically compatible case. *E. chaffeensis* and *A. phagocytophilum* infections can be confirmed by demonstrating a fourfold change in IgG titer by indirect immunofluorescence assay (IFA) between paired sera *or* detection of specific DNA by PCR *or* demonstration of ehrlichial antigen in a tissue sample by immunohistochemistry *or* isolation of the organism in cell culture. A single specific titer of ≥64 or identification of morulae in

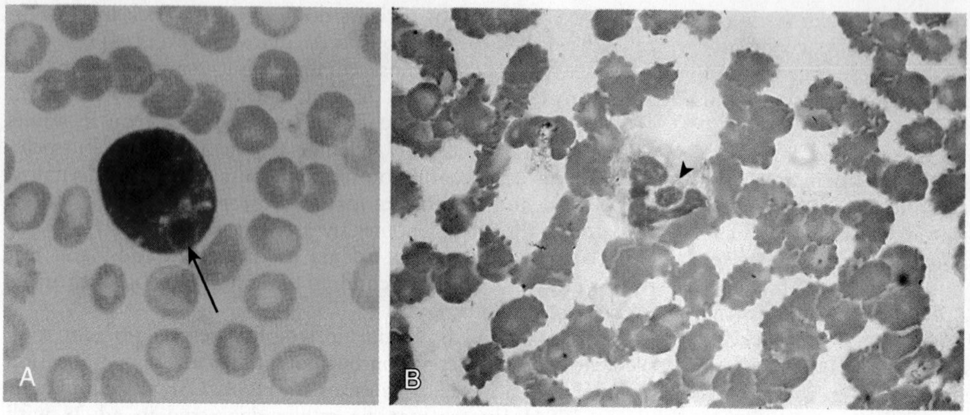

Figure 223-1 Morulae in peripheral blood leukocytes in patients with human monocytic ehrlichiosis and human granulocytic anaplasmosis. *A,* A morula *(arrow)* containing *Ehrlichia chaffeensis* in a monocyte. *B,* A morula *(arrowhead)* containing *Anaplasma phagocytophilum* in a neutrophil. Wright stains, original magnifications ×1,200. *E. chaffeensis* and *A. phagocytophilum* have similar morphologies but are serologically and genetically distinct.

monocytes or macrophages for *E. chaffeensis* or in neutrophils or eosinophils for *A. phagocytophilum* by microscopy is suggestive. *Ehrlichia ewingii* can only be confirmed by PCR, because it has not been cultured and antigens are not available. *E. ewingii* infection induces antibodies that cross react with *E. chaffeensis* in routine serologic tests and can only be differentiated by identification of specific nucleic acids. Patients with HGA have serologic reactions to *E. chaffeensis* in up to 15% of cases, and thus serodiagnosis depends on testing with both *E. chaffeensis* and *A. phagocytophilum* antigens and demonstrating a 4-fold or higher difference between titers. During the acute phase of illness when antibodies might not be detected, PCR amplification of specific *E. chaffeensis* or *A. phagocytophilum* DNA sequences is sensitive in 50-86% of cases. Although *E. chaffeensis* and *A. phagocytophilum* have both been cultivated in tissue culture, this method does not provide a timely result.

DIFFERENTIAL DIAGNOSIS

Because of the nonspecific presentation, ehrlichiosis mimics other arthropod-borne infections such as RMSF, tularemia, babesiosis, Lyme disease, murine typhus, relapsing fever, and Colorado tick fever. Other potential diagnoses often considered include otitis media, streptococcal pharyngitis, infectious mononucleosis, Kawasaki disease, endocarditis, respiratory or gastrointestinal viral syndromes, hepatitis, leptospirosis, Q fever, collagen-vascular diseases, and leukemia. If rash and disseminated intravascular coagulopathy predominate, meningococcemia, bacterial sepsis, and toxic shock syndrome are also suspected. Meningoencephalitis might suggest aseptic meningitis due to enterovirus or herpes simplex virus, bacterial meningitis, or RMSF. Severe respiratory disease may be confused with bacterial, viral, and fungal causes of pneumonia.

TREATMENT

Both HME and HGA are effectively treated with tetracyclines, especially doxycycline, and the majority of patients usually improve within 48 hr. In vitro tests document that both *E. chaffeensis* and *A. phagocytophilum* have minimal inhibitory concentrations to chloramphenicol above blood levels that can be safely achieved. Therefore, a short course of doxycycline is the recommended regimen. Doxycycline can be used safely in children <8 yr of age because tooth discoloration is dose dependent and the need for multiple courses is unlikely. Few data exist to recommend alternative therapies; however, both *E. chaffeensis* and *A. phagocytophilum* are susceptible in vitro to rifampin, which has been used successfully to treat HGA in pregnant women and children.

The recommended regimen for patients of all ages with severe or complicated HME and HGA is doxycycline (4 mg/kg/day PO or IV divided every 12 hr, maximum dose 200 mg/day). An alternative regimen is tetracycline 25-50 mg/kg/day divided every 6 hr PO, maximum 2 g/day. Therapy should be continued for ≥5 days and until the patient has been afebrile for ≥2-4 days.

Other broad-spectrum antibiotics, including penicillins, cephalosporins, aminoglycosides, and macrolides, are not effective. In vitro studies suggest that fluoroquinolones are active against *A. phagocytophilum*, although at least one patient relapsed when levofloxacin was discontinued. *E. chaffeensis* is naturally resistant to fluoroquinolones owing to a single nucleotide change in *gyrA,* which suggests that *A. phagocytophilum* could also become resistant to fluoroquinolones rapidly.

COMPLICATIONS AND PROGNOSIS

Fatal monocytic ehrlichiosis has been reported in 1 pediatric patient where the findings were initially dominated by pulmonary involvement with respiratory failure complicated by nosocomial bacterial pneumonia. The pattern of severe pulmonary involvement culminating in diffuse alveolar damage and acute respiratory distress syndrome (ARDS) and secondary nosocomial or opportunistic infections is now well documented with HME and HGA in adults. One child with HGA died after 3 wk of fever, thrombocytopenia, and lymphadenopathy suspected to be a hematologic malignancy. Other severe complications include a toxic shock–like illness, meningoencephalitis with long-term neurologic sequelae, brachial plexopathy, demyelinating polyneuropathy, myocarditis, rhabdomyolysis, and renal failure. Patients who are immunocompromised (e.g., HIV infection, high-dose corticosteroid therapy, cancer chemotherapy, immunosuppression for organ transplantation) are at high risk for fulminant *E. chaffeensis* infection.

PREVENTION

HME, HGA, and ewingii ehrlichiosis are tick-borne diseases, and any activity that increases exposure to ticks increases risk. Avoiding tick-infested areas, wearing appropriate light-colored clothing, spraying tick repellents on clothing, carefully inspecting for ticks after exposure, and promptly removing any attached ticks diminish the risk of HME and HGA. The interval between tick attachment and transmission of the agents may be as short as 4 hr; thus, any attached tick should be removed promptly. The role of prophylactic therapy for ehrlichiosis and anaplasmosis after tick bites has not been investigated. It is not known if infection confers protective immunity; however, reinfection appears to be exceedingly rare.

BIBLIOGRAPHY

Please visit the Nelson Textbook of Pediatrics *website at www.expertconsult.com for the complete bibliography.*

Chapter 224
Q Fever (*Coxiella burnetii*)

Megan E. Reller and J. Stephen Dumler

Q fever (for **query fever,** the name given following an outbreak of febrile illness in an abattoir in Queensland, Australia) is rarely reported in children but is probably underdiagnosed. Symptomatic patients can have acute or chronic disease.

ETIOLOGY

Although previously classified within the order Rickettsiales, *Coxiella burnetii* (the causative agent of Q fever) is genetically distinct from the genera *Rickettsia, Orientia, Ehrlichia,* and *Anaplasma.* Hence, based on small subunit rRNA gene sequencing, it has been reassigned to the order Legionellales, family Coxiellaceae. *C. burnetii* is highly infectious for both humans and animals; even a single organism can cause infection. The agent has been nationally notifiable since 1999 and is listed as a Category B agent of bioterrorism by the Centers for Disease Control and Prevention. Unlike *Rickettsia,* the organism can enter a sporogenic differentiation cycle, which renders it highly resistant to chemical and physical treatments.

C. burnetii resides intracellularly within macrophages. The organism undergoes a lipopolysaccharide phase variation similar to that described for smooth and rough strains of Enterobacteriaceae. Unlike *Ehrlichia, Anaplasma,* and *Chlamydia, C. burnetii* that express phase I lipopolysaccharide can survive and proliferate within acidified phagosomes to form aggregates of >100 bacteria. In contrast, organisms that express phase II lipopolysaccharide are killed in the phagolysosome.

EPIDEMIOLOGY

The disease is reported worldwide, except in New Zealand. Although seroepidemiologic studies suggest that infection occurs just as often in children as in adults, children less often present with clinical disease than do adults. Approximately 60% of infections are asymptomatic, and only 5% of symptomatic patients require hospitalization. Seroprevalence surveys show that 6-70% of children in endemic European and African communities have evidence of past infection, and in France the overall incidence of Q fever is estimated to be 50 cases per 100,000 persons. Cases in Africa are likely misdiagnosed as malaria. Reported cases of Q fever in the USA have increased by 6.5-fold from 26 cases in 2001 to 171 cases in 2007, which might reflect an increase in incidence, increased reporting after September 11, 2001, improved diagnostic tools, or a combination of factors. Reported cases in Asia and Australia have also increased. Most infections in children are identified during the lamb birthing season in Europe (January through June), following farm visits, or after exposure to placentas of dogs, cats, and rabbits. The largest community outbreak ever described occurred in the southeastern part of the Netherlands in 2008 and was associated with intensive goat farming. More than 20% of cases of clinically recognized acute or chronic Q fever occur in immunosuppressed hosts or in persons with prosthetic valves or damaged native valves or vessels. Although infections are recognized more often in men than in women, reported cases in boys and girls are equal.

TRANSMISSION

In contrast to other rickettsial infections, humans usually acquire *C. burnetii* by inhaling infectious aerosols (e.g., contaminated barnyard dust) or ingesting (and likely aspirating) contaminated foods. Ticks are rarely implicated. Cattle, sheep, and goats are the primary reservoirs, but infection in other livestock and domestic pets has also been described. Organisms are excreted in milk, urine, and feces of infected animals, but especially in amniotic fluids and the placenta. An increase in incidence has been associated with the seasonal mistral winds in France that coincide with lamb birthing season and with consumption of cheese among children in Greece. In Nova Scotia and Maine, exposure to newborn animals, especially kittens, has been associated with small outbreaks of Q fever in families. Exposure to domestic ruminants is the major risk in Europe and Australia, although many urban dwellers in France also acquire Q fever without such an exposure. Clinical Q fever during pregnancy can result from primary infection or reactivation of latent infection and has been associated with miscarriage, intrauterine growth retardation, and premature births. Obstetricians and other related health care workers are at risk for acquiring infection because of the quantity of *C. burnetii* sequestered in the placenta.

PATHOLOGY AND PATHOGENESIS

The pathology of Q fever depends on the mode of transmission, route of dissemination, specific tissues involved, and course of the infection. When acquired via inhalation, a mild interstitial lymphocytic pneumonitis and macrophage- and organism-rich intra-alveolar exudates are often seen. When the liver is involved, a mild to moderate lymphocytic lobular hepatitis may be seen. Inflammatory pseudotumors can develop in the pulmonary parenchyma or other tissues. Classic fibrin-ring ("doughnut") granulomas, generally associated with acute, self-limited infections, occasionally are identified in liver, bone marrow, meninges, and other organs. Typically, infected tissues are also infiltrated by lymphocytes and histiocytes.

Recovery from symptomatic or asymptomatic acute infection can result in persistent subclinical infection and may be maintained by dysregulated cytokine responses. The persistence of *C. burnetii* in tissue macrophages at sites of pre-existing tissue damage elicits low-grade chronic inflammation and, depending on the site of involvement, can result in irreversible cardiac valve damage, persistent vascular injury, or osteomyelitis. Endocarditis of native or prosthetic valves is characterized by infiltrates of macrophages and lymphocytes in necrotic fibrinous valvular vegetations and an absence of granulomas.

CLINICAL MANIFESTATIONS AND COMPLICATIONS

Only about 40-50% of people infected with *C. burnetii* develop symptoms. Two forms of symptomatic disease occur. **Acute Q fever** is more common and usually manifests as self-limited undifferentiated fever or an influenza-like illness with interstitial pneumonitis. **Chronic Q fever** in adults usually involves native heart valves, prosthetic valves, or other endovascular prostheses. Q fever osteomyelitis is less common but proportionally more common in children.

Acute Q Fever

Acute Q fever develops about 3 wk (range, 14-39 days) after exposure to the causative agent. The severity of illness in children ranges from subclinical infection to a systemic illness of sudden onset characterized by high fever, severe frontal headache, nonproductive cough, chest pain, vomiting, diarrhea, abdominal pain, arthralgias, and myalgias. About 40% of children with acute Q fever present with fever, 25% with pneumonia or an influenza-like illness, >10% with meningoencephalitis, and >10% with myocarditis. Other manifestations include pericarditis, hepatitis, hemophagocytosis, rhabdomyolysis, and hemolytic uremic syndrome. Rash, ranging from maculopapular to purpuric lesions, is an unusual finding in adults with Q fever but is observed in ~50% of pediatric patients. Rigors and night sweats are common in adults with Q fever and occur less often in children. Prominent clinical findings that can create diagnostic confusion include fatigue, vomiting, abdominal pain, and meningismus. Hepatomegaly and splenomegaly may be detected in some patients.

Routine laboratory investigations in pediatric acute Q fever are usually normal but can reveal mild leukocytosis and thrombocytopenia. Up to 85% of children have modestly elevated serum hepatic transaminase levels that usually normalize within 10 days. Hyperbilirubinemia is uncommon in the absence of complications. C-reactive protein is uniformly elevated in pediatric Q fever. Chest x-ray films are abnormal in 27% of all patients; in children, the most common findings include single or multiple bilateral infiltrates with reticular markings in the lower lobes.

Acute Q fever in children is usually a self-limited illness, with fever persisting for only 7-10 days compared with 2-3 wk in adults. However, severe infections, such as myocarditis requiring cardiac transplantation, meningoencephalitis, pericarditis, and hemophagocytosis, have been reported.

Chronic Q Fever

The risk for developing chronic Q fever is strongly correlated with advancing age and underlying conditions such as cardiac valve damage or immunosuppression. Thus, chronic Q fever is rarely diagnosed in children. A review identified only 5 cases of chronic Q fever endocarditis and 6 cases of osteomyelitis among children, none of whom had known predisposing immune deficiencies. Four of the 5 cases of endocarditis occurred in children with underlying congenital heart abnormalities and involved the aortic, pulmonary, and tricuspid valves. Four of the 6 children with Q fever osteomyelitis had a prior diagnosis or clinical courses consistent with idiopathic chronic recurrent multifocal osteomyelitis. A long interval before diagnosis and lack of high fever are common in pediatric cases of chronic Q fever. Although Q fever endocarditis often results in death (23-65% of cases) in adults, mortality has not been reported for children. Endocarditis associated with chronic Q fever can occur months to years after acute infection and can occur in the absence of recognized acute Q fever.

LABORATORY FINDINGS

Laboratory features in children with chronic Q fever are poorly documented; adult patients often have an erythrocyte sedimentation rate of >20 mm/hr (80% of cases), hypergammaglobulinemia (54%), and hyperfibrinogenemia (67%). In children, the presence of rheumatoid factor in >50% of cases and circulating immune complexes in nearly 90% suggest an autoimmune process, as do anti-platelet antibodies, anti–smooth muscle antibodies, antimitochondrial antibodies, circulating anticoagulants, and positive direct Coombs tests.

DIAGNOSIS AND DIFFERENTIAL DIAGNOSIS

Although uncommonly diagnosed, Q fever should be considered in children who have fever of unknown origin, atypical pneumonia, myocarditis, meningoencephalitis, culture-negative endocarditis, or recurrent osteomyelitis and who live in rural areas or who are in close contact with domestic livestock, cats, or animal products.

The diagnosis of Q fever is most easily and commonly confirmed by testing acute and convalescent sera (2-4 wk apart), which show a 4-fold increase in indirect fluorescent antibody titers to phase I and phase II *C. burnetii* antigens. Predominant, elevated, or increasing titers of phase II antibody are characteristic of acute Q fever, and the appearance and persistence of titers of phase II antibody greater than phase I indicate chronic Q fever. Elevated titers of phase I immunoglobulin A (IgA) antibody are reported to be diagnostic for Q fever endocarditis; however, 1 evaluation showed that a phase I IgG titer of <800 is inconsistent with chronic Q fever. Cross reaction with antibodies to *Legionella* and *Bartonella* can occur.

Although culture has been considered the gold standard, sensitivity (compared with a composite standard including serology and PCR) is low. *C. burnetii* has been cultivated in tissue culture cells, which can become positive within 48 hr, but isolation and antimicrobial susceptibility testing of *C. burnetii* should be attempted only in specialized biohazard facilities. Testing by polymerase chain reaction (PCR) can be performed on blood, serum, and tissue samples and is available in some public health, reference, or research laboratories. Although PCR has been helpful in patients with equivocal titers; sensitivity has been improved by real-time methods and use of repeated sequences as targets. Immunohistochemical staining has also been used, but suffers from simila problems similar to PCR's.

The differential diagnosis depends on the clinical presentation. In patients with respiratory disease, *Mycoplasma pneumoniae, Chlamydophila pneumoniae,* legionellosis, psittacosis, and Epstein-Barr virus infection should be considered. In patients with granulomatous hepatitis, tuberculous and nontuberculous mycobacterial infections, salmonellosis, visceral leishmaniasis, toxoplasmosis, Hodgkin disease, monocytic ehrlichiosis, granulocytic anaplasmosis, brucellosis, cat scratch disease (*Bartonella henselae*), or autoimmune disorders such as sarcoidosis should be considered. Culture-negative endocarditis suggests infection with *Brucella, Bartonella,* or HACEK organisms *(Haemophilus, Aggregatibacter, Cardiobacterium hominis, Eikenella corrodens, Kingella)*, partially treated bacterial endocarditis, or nonbacterial endocarditis.

TREATMENT

Selection of an appropriate antimicrobial regimen for children is difficult owing to the lack of rigorous studies, the limited therapeutic window for drugs that are known to be efficacious, and the potential length of therapy required to preclude relapse.

Most pediatric patients with Q fever have a self-limited illness that is identified only on retrospective serologic evaluation. However, to prevent potential complications, patients with acute Q fever should be treated within 3 days of onset of symptoms, because therapy started >3 days after onset of illness has little effect on the course of acute Q fever. Because early confirmatory testing is not possible now, empirical therapy is warranted in clinically suspected cases. Doxycycline (4 mg/kg/day PO or IV divided every 12 hr, maximum 200 mg/day) is the drug of choice. Tetracycline and doxycycline may be associated with tooth discoloration in children <9 yr of age; however, most experts consider the benefits of treatment with doxycycline to be greater than the risks. Tooth discoloration is dose and duration dependent, and it is unlikely that children will require multiple courses. During pregnancy, Q fever is best treated with trimethoprim-sulfamethoxazole. The fluoroquinolones have also proved effective, and success with a combination of a fluoroquinolone and rifampin has also been achieved with prolonged therapy (16-21 days). Macrolides, including erythromycin and clarithromycin, are less effective alternatives.

For chronic Q fever, especially endocarditis, therapy for 18-36 mo is mandatory. The current recommended regimen for chronic Q fever endocarditis is a combination of doxycycline and hydroxychloroquine for ≥18 mo. For patients with heart failure, valve replacement may be necessary. Interferon-γ therapy has been used as adjunct therapy for intractable Q fever.

PREVENTION

Recognition of the disease in livestock or other domestic animals should alert communities to the risk for human infection. Milk from infected herds must be pasteurized at temperatures sufficient to destroy *C. burnetii*. *C. burnetii* is resistant to significant environmental conditions but may be inactivated with a solution of

1% Lysol, 1% formaldehyde, or 5% hydrogen peroxide. Special isolation measures are not required because person-to-person transmission is rare, except when others are exposed to the placenta of an infected patient. A vaccine preparation is available and provides protection against Q fever for at least 5 yr in abattoir workers. Because the vaccine is strongly reactogenic and no trials in children have been conducted, it should only be used when extreme risk is judged to exist. Clusters of cases resulting from intense natural exposures, such as in slaughterhouses or on farms, are well documented. Clusters of cases that occur in the absence of such an exposure should be investigated as potential sentinel events for bioterrorism.

BIBLIOGRAPHY

Please visit the Nelson Textbook of Pediatrics *website at www.expertconsult.com for the complete bibliography.*

Section 12 FUNGAL INFECTIONS

Chapter 225
Principles of Antifungal Therapy

William J. Steinbach, Michael Cohen-Wolkowiez, and Daniel K. Benjamin, Jr.

Due to advances in aggressive antineoplastic agents and organ transplantation, invasive fungal infections are a major cause of morbidity and mortality in children. Fortunately, the therapeutic armamentarium for invasive fungal infections has markedly increased since the turn of the century (See Table 225-1 on the *Nelson Textbook of Pediatrics* website at www.expertconsult.com).

For the full continuation of this chapter, please visit the Nelson Textbook of Pediatrics *website at www.expertconsult.com.*

Chapter 226
Candida

P. Brian Smith and Daniel K. Benjamin, Jr.

Candidiasis encompasses many clinical syndromes that may be caused by several species of *Candida*. Invasive candidiasis (*Candida* infections of the blood and other sterile body fluids) is a leading cause of infection-related mortality in hospitalized immunocompromised patients.

Candida exists in 3 morphologic forms: oval to round **blastospores or yeast cells** (3-6 mm in diameter); double-walled **chlamydospores** (7-17 mm in diameter), which are usually at the terminal end of a pseudohypha; and **pseudomycelium,** which is a mass of pseudohyphae and represents the tissue phase of *Candida*. **Pseudohyphae** are filamentous processes that elongate from the yeast cell without the cytoplasmic connection of a true hypha. *Candida* grows aerobically on routine laboratory media but can require several days of incubation.

C. albicans accounts for most human infections, but *C. parapsilosis, C. tropicalis, C. krusei, C. lusitaniae, C. glabrata,* and several other species are commonly isolated from hospitalized children. *C. albicans* forms a germ tube when suspended in rabbit or human serum and incubated for 1-2 hr; a rapid **germ tube test** should therefore be performed before further identification tests are conducted. Thereafter, differentiation and susceptibility testing are important owing to increasing frequency of fluconazole resistance. The other clinically important *Candida* species can be identified within 48 hr on the basis of biochemical test results.

Treatment of invasive *Candida* infections is complicated by the emergence of non-albicans strains. Amphotericin B deoxycholate is inactive against approximately 20% of strains of *C. lusitaniae*. Fluconazole is useful for many *Candida* infections but is inactive against all strains of *C. krusei* and 5-25% of strains of *C. glabrata*. Susceptibility testing of these clinical isolates is recommended.

226.1 Neonatal Infections

P. Brian Smith and Daniel K. Benjamin, Jr.

Candida is a common cause of oral mucous membrane infections (**thrush**) and perineal skin infections (***Candida* diaper dermatitis**) in newborn infants (Chapter 658). Rare presentations include **congenital cutaneous candidiasis,** caused by an ascending infection into the uterus during gestation, and **invasive fungal dermatitis,** a postnatal infection skin infection resulting in positive blood cultures. Invasive candidiasis is a common infectious complication in the neonatal intensive care unit (NICU) because of improved survival of the extremely preterm infants.

EPIDEMIOLOGY

Candida species are the third most common cause of bloodstream infection in premature infants. The cumulative incidence is <0.3% among infants >2,500 g birthweight admitted to the NICU. The cumulative incidence increases to 12% for infants <750 g birthweight. In addition the incidence varies greatly by individual NICU. In the National Institutes of Health–sponsored Neonatal Research Network, the cumulative incidence of candidiasis among infants <1,000 g birthweight is 2.4-20.4%.

Up to 10% of full-term infants are colonized as the result of vertical transmission from the mother at birth, with slightly higher rates of colonization in preterm infants. Colonization rates increase to >50% among infants admitted to the NICU by 1 mo of age. H_2 blockers and broad-spectrum antibiotics facilitate *Candida* colonization and overgrowth.

Significant risk factors for neonatal invasive candidiasis include prematurity, low birthweight, exposure to broad-spectrum antibiotic administration, abdominal surgery, and presence of a central venous catheter.

PATHOGENESIS

The immune system of premature infants has deficiencies in chemotaxis, cytokine production, phagocytosis, and production of type-specific antibodies. These immune defects combined with an underdeveloped layer of skin, need for invasive measures (endotracheal tubes, central venous catheters), and exposure to broad-spectrum antibiotics place preterm infants at great risk for invasive candidiasis. Preterm infants are also at high risk for spontaneous intestinal perforations and necrotizing enterocolitis. Both conditions require abdominal surgery, prolonged exposure to broad-spectrum antibiotics, and total parenteral administration requiring placement of central venous catheters. Each of these factors increases the risk of invasive candidiasis.

CLINICAL MANIFESTATIONS

The manifestations of neonatal candidiasis vary in severity from oral thrush and *Candida* diaper dermatitis (Chapter 226.2) to invasive candidiasis that can manifest with overwhelming sepsis (Chapter 226.3). Signs of invasive candidiasis among preterm neonates are often nonspecific and include temperature instability, lethargy, apnea, hypotension, respiratory distress, abdominal distention, and hyperglycemia or hypoglycemia.

Central nervous system (CNS) involvement is common and is more accurately described as meningoencephalitis. *Candida* infections involving the CNS often result in abscesses leading to unremarkable cerebrospinal fluid parameters (white blood cell count, glucose, protein) in the presence of CNS infection. **Endophthalmitis** is an uncommon complication affecting <5% of neonates with invasive candidiasis. In addition, candidemia is associated with an increased risk of severe retinopathy of prematurity. Renal involvement commonly complicates neonatal invasive candidiasis. Renal involvement may be limited to candiduria or can manifest with diffuse infiltration of *Candida* throughout the renal parenchyma or the presence of *Candida* and debris within the collecting system. Other affected organs include the heart, bones, joints, liver, and spleen.

DIAGNOSIS

Mucocutaneous infections are most often diagnosed by direct clinical exam. Scrapings of skin lesions may be examined with a microscope after Gram staining or suspension in KOH. Definitive diagnosis of invasive disease requires histologic demonstration of the fungus in tissue specimens or recovery of the fungus from normally sterile body fluids. Hematologic parameters are sensitive but not specific. Although thrombocytopenia occurs in >80% of preterm infants with invasive candidiasis, thrombocytopenia also occurs in 75% of preterm infants with gram-negative bacterial sepsis and nearly 50% of infants with gram-positive bacterial sepsis. Blood cultures have very low sensitivity for invasive candidiasis. In a study of autopsy-proven candidiasis in adult patients, the sensitivity of multiple blood cultures for detecting single-organ disease was 28%. Blood culture volumes in neonates are typically only 0.5-1 mL, making the sensitivity in this population almost certainly lower.

Assessment of neonates in the presence of documented candidemia should include ultrasound or computerized tomography of the head to evaluate for abscesses; ultrasound of the liver, kidney, and spleen; cardiac echocardiography; ophthalmologic exam; lumbar puncture; and urine culture.

TREATMENT

In the absence of systemic manifestations, topical antifungal therapy is the treatment of choice for congenital cutaneous candidiasis in full-term infants. Congenital cutaneous candidiasis in preterm infants can progress to systemic disease, and therefore systemic therapy is warranted.

Every attempt should be made to remove or replace central venous catheters once the diagnosis of candidemia is confirmed. Delayed removal has been consistently associated with increased mortality and morbidity including poor neurodevelopmental outcomes. No well-powered randomized, controlled trials exist to guide length and type of therapy.

Systemic antifungal therapy should be administered for 21 days from the last positive *Candida* culture. Amphotericin B deoxycholate has been the mainstay of therapy for systemic candidiasis and is active against both yeast and mycelial forms. Nephrotoxicity, hypokalemia, and hypomagnesemia are common, but amphotericin B deoxycholate is better tolerated in neonates than in adult patients. *C. lusitaniae*, an uncommon pathogen in neonates, is resistant to amphotericin B deoxycholate. Fluconazole is very useful for treatment of invasive neonatal *Candida* infections, especially urinary tract infections. Fluconazole is inactive against all strains of *C. krusei* and some isolates of *C. glabrata*. The echinocandins have excellent activity against most *Candida* species and have been used successfully in patients with resistant organisms or in whom other therapies have failed. Several studies have described the pharmacokinetics of antifungals in infants (Table 226-1).

Table 226-1 DOSING OF ANTIFUNGAL AGENTS IN INFANTS* AND NUMBER OF SUBJECTS <1 YR OF AGE STUDIED WITH REPORTED PHARMACOKINETIC PARAMETERS

DRUG	INFANTS STUDIED	SUGGESTED DOSE
Amphotericin B deoxycholate	15	1 mg/kg/day
Amphotericin B lipid complex	28	5 mg/kg/day
Liposomal amphotericin B	17	5 mg/kg/day
Amphotericin B colloidal dispersion	0	5 mg/kg/day
Fluconazole	55	12 mg/kg/day
Micafungin†	48	10 mg/kg/day
Caspofungin‡	22	50 mg/m²/day
Anidulafungin‡,§	0	1.5 mg/kg/day

*Voriconazole dosing has not been investigated in the nursery.
†Micafungin has been studied in infants <120 days of life at this dosage. Dosing for older infants should be 4-8 mg/kg.
‡Caspofungin and anidulafungin should generally be avoided, because dosing sufficient to penetrate brain tissue has not been studied.
§The formulation for anidulafungin contains alcohol and should generally be avoided in premature infants; an alcohol-free formulation is undergoing clinical investigation in 2009-2011.

PROGNOSIS

Mortality following invasive candidiasis in premature infants has been consistently reported to be around 20% in large studies. Candidiasis is also associated with poor neurodevelopmental outcomes, chronic lung disease, and severe retinopathy of prematurity.

BIBLIOGRAPHY

Please visit the Nelson Textbook of Pediatrics *website at www.expertconsult.com for the complete bibliography.*

226.2 Infections in Immunocompetent Children and Adolescents

P. Brian Smith and Daniel K. Benjamin, Jr.

ORAL CANDIDIASIS

Oral thrush is a superficial mucous membrane infection that affects approximately 2-5% of normal newborns. *C. albicans* is the most commonly isolated species. Oral thrush can develop as early as 7-10 days of age. The use of antibiotics, especially in the 1st year of life, can lead to recurrent or persistent thrush. It is characterized by pearly white, curdish material visible on the tongue, palate, and buccal mucosa. Oral thrush may be asymptomatic or can cause pain, fussiness, and decreased feeding, leading to inadequate nutritional intake and dehydration. It is uncommon after 1 yr of age but can occur in older children treated with antibiotics. Persistent or recurrent thrush with no obvious predisposing reason, such as recent antibiotic treatment, warrants investigation of an underlying immunodeficiency, especially vertically transmitted HIV infection.

Treatment of mild cases might not be necessary. When treatment is warranted, the most commonly prescribed antifungal agent is nystatin. For recalcitrant or recurrent infections, a single dose of fluconazole may be useful. In breast-fed infants, simultaneous treatment of infant and mother with topical nystatin or oral fluconazole may be indicated.

DIAPER DERMATITIS

Diaper dermatitis is the most common infection caused by *Candida* (Chapter 658) and is characterized by a confluent erythematous rash with satellite pustules. *Candida* diaper dermatitis often complicates other noninfectious diaper dermatitides and often occurs following a course of oral antibiotics.

A common practice is to presumptively treat any diaper rash that has been present for >3 days with topical antifungal therapy such as nystatin, clotrimazole, or miconazole. If significant inflammation is present, the addition of hydrocortisone 1% may be useful for the 1st 1-2 days, but topical corticosteroids should be used cautiously in infants because the relatively potent topical corticosteroid can lead to adverse effects. Frequent diaper changes and short periods without diapers are important adjunctive treatments.

UNGUAL AND PERIUNGUAL INFECTIONS

Paronychia and onychomycosis may be caused by *Candida,* although *Trichophyton* and *Epidermophyton* are much more common causes (Chapter 655). *Candida* onychomycosis differs from tinea infections by its propensity to involve the fingernails and not the toenails, and by the associated paronychia. *Candida* paronychia often respond to treatment consisting of keeping the hands dry and using a topical antifungal agent. For ungual infections, a short course of systemic azole therapy may be necessary.

VULVOVAGINITIS

Vulvovaginitis is a common *Candida* infection of pubertal and postpubertal female patients (Chapter 543). Predisposing factors include pregnancy, use of oral contraceptive, and use of oral antibiotics. Prepubertal girls with *Candida* vulvovaginitis usually have a predisposing factor such as diabetes mellitus or prolonged antibiotic treatment. Clinical manifestations can include pain or itching, dysuria, vulvar or vaginal erythema, and an opaque white or cheesy exudate. More than 80% of cases are caused by *C. albicans.*

Candida vulvovaginitis can be effectively treated with either vaginal creams or troches of nystatin, clotrimazole, or miconazole. Oral therapy with a single dose of fluconazole is also effective.

226.3 Infections in Immunocompromised Children and Adolescents

P. Brian Smith and Daniel K. Benjamin, Jr.

ETIOLOGY

C. albicans is the most common cause of invasive candidiasis among immunocompromised pediatric patients and is associated with higher rates of mortality and end-organ involvement than are non-*albicans* species.

CLINICAL MANIFESTATIONS

HIV-Infected Children

Oral thrush and diaper dermatitis are the most common *Candida* infections in HIV-infected children. Besides oral thrush, 3 other types of oral *Candida* infections can occur in HIV-infected children: atrophic candidiasis, which manifests as a fiery erythema of the mucosa or loss of papillae of the tongue; chronic hyperplastic candidiasis, which presents with oral symmetric white plaques; and angular cheilitis, in which there is erythema and fissuring of the angles of the mouth. Topical antifungal therapy may be effective, but systemic treatment with fluconazole or itraconazole is usually necessary. Symptoms of dysphagia or poor oral intake can indicate progression to *Candida* **esophagitis,** requiring systemic antifungal therapy. In HIV patients, esophagitis can also be caused by cytomegalovirus, HSV, reflux, or lymphoma; *Candida* is the most common cause, and *Candida* esophagitis can occur in the absence of thrush.

Candida dermatitis and onychomycosis are more common in HIV-infected children. These infections are generally more severe than they are in immunocompetent children and can require systemic antifungal therapy.

Cancer and Transplant Patients

Fungal infections, especially *Candida* and *Aspergillus* infections, are a significant problem in oncology patients with chemotherapy-associated neutropenia (Chapter 171); the risk of these infections increases after 5 days of neutropenia and fever. Accordingly, empirical antifungal therapy is usually added to the antimicrobial regimen, if fever and neutropenia persist for ≥5 days. The triazoles and echinocandins have similar efficacy and improved safety profiles compared with either amphotericin B deoxycholate or lipid-complex formulations of amphotericin.

Bone marrow transplant recipients have a much higher risk of fungal infections because of the dramatically prolonged duration of neutropenia. Fluconazole prophylaxis decreases the incidence of candidemia in bone marrow transplant recipients. The echinocandins (anidulafungin, caspofungin, micafungin) and voriconazole have been successfully used as monotherapy or in combination with each other and amphotericin B deoxycholate. The use of myelopoietic colony-stimulating factor affects the duration of neutropenia after chemotherapy and is associated with decreased risk for candidemia. When *Candida* infection occurs in this population, the lung, spleen, kidney, and liver are involved in >50% of cases.

Solid organ transplant recipients are also at increased risk for superficial and invasive *Candida* infections. Studies in liver transplant recipients demonstrate the utility of antifungal prophylaxis with amphotericin B deoxycholate, fluconazole, voriconazole, or caspofungin.

Catheter-Associated Infections

Central venous catheter infections occur most often in oncology patients but can affect any patient with a central catheter (Chapter 172). Neutropenia, use of broad-spectrum antibiotics, and parenteral alimentation are associated with increased risk for *Candida* central catheter infection. Treatment requires removing or replacing the catheter and a 2-3 wk course of systemic antifungal therapy.

DIAGNOSIS

The diagnosis is often presumptive in neutropenic patients with prolonged fever because positive blood fungal cultures occur only in a minority of patients who are later found to have disseminated infection. If isolated, *Candida* grows readily on routine blood culture media, with ≥90% of positive cultures identified within 72 hr.

TREATMENT

Echinocandins are favored for moderately or severely ill children; fluconazole is acceptable for those infected with susceptible organism and less critically ill; amphotericin B products are also acceptable. Fluconazole is not effective against *C. krusei* and

Table 226-2 DOSING OF ANTIFUNGAL AGENTS IN CHILDREN >1 YEAR OF AGE FOR TREATMENT OF INVASIVE DISEASE

DRUG	SUGGESTED DOSAGE
Amphotericin B deoxycholate	1 mg/kg/day
Amphotericin B lipid complex	5 mg/kg/day
Liposomal amphotericin B	5 mg/kg/day
Amphotericin B colloidal dispersion	5 mg/kg/day
Fluconazole	12 mg/kg/day
Voriconazole	7 mg/kg every 12 hr
Micafungin*	4-8 mg/kg/day
Caspofungin†	50 mg/m²/day
Anidulafungin	1.5 mg/kg/day

*Use adult dosages in children >8 yr of age.
†Loading doses should be used for caspofungin and anidulafungin: 70 mg/m² and 3.0 mg/kg, respectively.

some isolates of *C. glabrata*. Amphotericin B deoxycholate is inactive against approximately 20% of strains of *C. lusitaniae*, and therefore susceptibility testing should be performed for all strains (Table 226-2).

BIBLIOGRAPHY

Please visit the Nelson Textbook of Pediatrics *website at* www.expertconsult.com *for the complete bibliography.*

226.4 Chronic Mucocutaneous Candidiasis

P. Brian Smith and Daniel K. Benjamin, Jr.

Chronic mucocutaneous candidiasis is a group of heterogeneous immune disorders with a primary defect of T-lymphocyte responsiveness to *Candida*. Endocrinopathies (hypoparathyroidism, Addison disease), hyperimmunoglobulin E syndrome (Job syndrome), autoimmune disorders, HIV, and inhaled corticosteroid use are associated with chronic mucocutaneous candidiasis (Chapter 119). Although the underlying immune disorders are varied, the presentations of chronic mucocutaneous candidiasis are usually similar. Symptoms can begin in the 1st few months of life or as late as the 2nd decade of life. The disorder is characterized by chronic and severe *Candida* skin and mucous membrane infections. Patients rarely develop systemic *Candida* disease. Topical antifungal therapy can provide limited improvement early in the course of the disease, but systemic courses of azoles are usually necessary. The infection usually responds temporarily to treatment but is not eradicated and recurs.

Chapter 227
Cryptococcus neoformans

Jane M. Gould and Stephen C. Aronoff

ETIOLOGY

Cryptococcosis is an invasive fungal disease caused by a monomorphic, encapsulated yeast. *Cryptococcus neoformans* var. *neoformans* is the most common etiologic agent worldwide and is the predominant pathogenic fungal infection among persons infected with HIV.

EPIDEMIOLOGY

C. neoformans var. *neoformans* (serotypes A, D, and AD) is distributed in temperate climates predominantly in soil contaminated with droppings from certain avian species, including pigeons, canaries, and cockatoos. It may also be found on fruits and vegetables and may be carried by cockroaches. *C. neoformans* var. *gattii* (serotypes B and C) is found in the tropics and subtropics and has been associated with several species of eucalyptus trees. This species causes endemic disease primarily in immunologically competent hosts living in the tropics and is associated with the formation of large granulomas known as **cryptococcomas.** The distribution and ecology of *C. gattii* seem to be changing, and this organism can now be found in association with a wide range of trees, including firs and oaks. *C. gattii* has caused disease in 19 patients residing in Oregon and Washington, most occurring since 2006. Pulmonary disease with or without meningoencephalitis was the most common manifestation. It is critical to distinguish between the two cryptococcal species because *C. gattii* is less susceptible to fluconazole. *Cryptococcus laurentii* has been occasionally reported as a cause of invasive fungal disease, usually in immunocompromised patients and most recently in the premature neonatal population.

C. neoformans exposure is much more common than previously thought. Seroprevalence studies in temperate urban environments have shown that most children >2 yr of age and nearly all adults have been exposed to this organism. Despite this high prevalence, clinical disease is unusual in immunocompetent persons and is rare in children. Pigeon breeders and laboratory personnel who work with *Cryptococcus* are at greatest risk. Cryptococcosis is also rare (<1%) among HIV-infected children but occurs in 5-10% of HIV-infected adults, with higher rates of infection reported from developing countries. Pediatric cases of cryptococcosis are evenly divided among immunocompetent and immunocompromised persons. Cryptococcosis is the third most common invasive fungal infection after candidiasis and aspergillosis in solid organ transplant patients. Other risk factors for cryptococcal infection include diabetes mellitus, renal failure, cirrhosis, and use of corticosteroids, chemotherapy agents, and monoclonal antibodies such as etanercept, infliximab, and alemtuzumab. Interestingly organ transplant recipients who are receiving calcineurin-inhibitor based immunosuppression are less likely to have cryptococcal CNS infection and more likely to have disease limited to the lung, because these agents have antifungal activity in vivo.

PATHOGENESIS

In most cases *C. neoformans* is acquired by inhalation of fungal spores (<5-10 µm), which are engulfed by alveolar macrophages. Local inoculation leads to cutaneous or ophthalmic infection rarely. An additional portal of entry can be seen with organ transplantation of infected tissue. Direct entry through the gastrointestinal tract can also occur. After entry into the body, either latent infection or acute disease is produced. Cell-mediated immunity is the most important host defense for producing granulomatous inflammation and thus containing cryptococcal infection. Patients with compromised cell-mediated immunity have the highest risk for developing cryptococcal disease. In most immunocompetent persons, infection is limited to the lung. When the immune system fails to contain the infection, dissemination follows, with potential involvement of the brain, meninges, skin, eyes, prostate, and skeletal system.

In immunocompetent patients, *C. neoformans* can produce both a suppurative and granulomatous tissue reaction or a granulomatous reaction alone with varying degrees of necrosis. Healing is characterized by fibrosis usually without calcification. In immunocompromised patients tissue reactions may be minimal or absent, leading to the proliferation of yeast and the development of mucoid cystic lesions. Pulmonary cryptococcosis produces granulomas that are often subpleural in location and contain yeast forms. Cystic cryptococcomas occur in the CNS of

20% of non–HIV-infected patients with disseminated disease and may be found in the absence of overt meningitis. Granulomas and microabscesses containing yeast occur in patients with skin and bone infection.

CLINICAL MANIFESTATIONS

The manifestations of cryptococcal infection reflect the route of inoculation and the immunocompetence of the host. Sites of infection include lung, CNS, blood, skin, bone, and mucous membranes.

Pneumonia

Pneumonia is the most common form of cryptococcosis. Asymptomatic pulmonary infections occur often, especially among pigeon breeders, bird fanciers, and laboratory workers. Asymptomatic carriage can occur in persons with underlying chronic lung disease. Progressive pulmonary disease is symptomatic with fever, cough, pleuritic chest pain, and constitutional symptoms. In a 2006 review of 24 patients with pulmonary cryptococcosis, cough was the most common symptom. Pulmonary disease often precedes disseminated infection in immunocompromised persons. Chest radiographs can demonstrate a poorly localized bronchopneumonia, nodular changes, or lobar consolidations; cavities and pleural effusions are rare. Immunocompromised patients can have alveolar and interstitial infiltrates that can mimic pneumocystis pneumonia. In adults with HIV infection, cryptococcal pneumonia is usually asymptomatic, although >90% of patients have concomitant CNS infection.

Disseminated Infection

Disseminated infection usually follows primary pulmonary disease, especially among immunocompromised persons. Advanced HIV infection is the most common predisposing factor for disseminated cryptococcosis. Other major predisposing conditions include lymphoproliferative disorders, corticosteroid therapy, primary immunodeficiencies affecting both T- and B-cell lineages, and immunosuppressive therapy for rheumatic disorders, celiac disease, and organ transplantation.

Meningitis

Subacute or chronic meningitis is the most common clinical manifestation of disseminated cryptococcal infection. The clinical presentation is variable and prognostic. Good outcomes are associated with headache as the initial symptom, normal mental status, absence of a predisposing condition, normal cerebrospinal fluid (CSF) opening pressure, normal CSF glucose, negative India ink stain, absence of extraneural infection by culture, and cryptococcal antigen titers in CSF and serum of <1:32. Overt symptoms of meningitis and HIV infection predict a poor outcome. HIV-infected patients typically present with unexplained fevers, headache, and malaise; cryptococcal antigen titers in these patients are often >1:1,024. CT of the brain identifies cryptococcomas in as many as 30% of patients with disseminated infection, even with no clinical signs of CNS involvement. The mortality rate for cryptococcal meningitis is 15-30%, and most deaths occur within several weeks of diagnosis. The fatality rates are higher among HIV-infected patients, who had relapse rates of >50% before the use of lifelong maintenance highly active antiretroviral therapy (HAART). In adults, relapse rates have decreased to <5% with daily fluconazole therapy. Relapse is unusual in adequately treated immunocompetent persons. Postinfectious sequelae are common and include hydrocephalus, decreased visual acuity, deafness, cranial nerve palsies, seizures, and ataxia.

Sepsis Syndrome

Sepsis syndrome is a rare manifestation of cryptococcosis and occurs almost exclusively among HIV-infected patients. Fever is followed by respiratory distress and multiorgan system disease that is often fatal.

Cutaneous Infection

Cutaneous disease most commonly follows disseminated cryptococcosis and rarely local inoculation. Early lesions are erythematous, may be single or multiple, and are variably indurated and tender. Lesions often become ulcerated with central necrosis and raised borders. Cutaneous cryptococcosis in immunocompromised patients can resemble molluscum contagiosum.

Skeletal Infection

Skeletal infection occurs in approximately 5% of patients with disseminated infection but rarely in HIV-infected patients. The onset of symptoms is insidious and chronic. Bone involvement is typified by soft tissue swelling and tenderness, and arthritis is characterized by effusion, erythema, and pain on motion. Skeletal disease is unifocal in approximately 75% of cases. The vertebrae are the most common sites of infection, followed by the tibia, ileum, rib, femur, and humerus. Concomitant bone and joint disease results from contiguous spread.

Ocular Infection

Chorioretinitis is rare, occurs primarily in adults, and is usually a manifestation of disseminated disease, although direct inoculation of the eye has been described. Eye infection is characterized by the acute loss of visual acuity, eye pain, visual floaters, and photophobia. Examination usually reveals choroiditis with or without retinitis. Retinal and vitreal masses and anterior uveitis are seen less commonly. Eye disease is often a manifestation of disseminated infection and is associated with a mortality rate of >20%. Only 15% of survivors recover full vision.

Lymph Nodes

Lymphonodular disease has been reported in 2 children, 1 of whom had an underlying immunodeficiency. Lymphonodular cryptococcosis is characterized by disseminated lymphadenopathy including thoracic and abdominal nodes, subcutaneous lesions, liver granulomas, and concomitant pulmonary disease.

DIAGNOSIS

Recovery of the fungus by culture or demonstration of the fungus in histologic sections of infected tissue is definitive. A latex agglutination test, which detects cryptococcal antigen in serum and CSF, is the most useful diagnostic test. Titers of >1:4 in bodily fluid strongly suggest infection, and titers of >1:1,024 reflect high burden of yeast, poor host immune response, and greater likelihood of therapeutic failure. India ink preparations of CSF are useful prognostically but are less sensitive than culture and antigen detection. Skin test antigens are poorly characterized, and the sensitivity and specificity of this test are unknown. Serum cryptococcal antibody tests have poor sensitivity and specificity and are generally not helpful in diagnosing cryptococcosis. Cryptococci can grow easily on standard fungal and bacterial culture media. Colonies can be seen within 48 to 72 hours when grown aerobically at standard temperatures.

TREATMENT

The choice of treatment depends on the sites of involvement and the host immune status. The immunocompetent patient with asymptomatic or mild disease limited to the lungs may be closely observed without therapy or, alternatively, treated with oral fluconazole (pediatric dose 6-12 mg/kg/day and adult dose 200-400 mg/day) or itraconazole (pediatric dose 5-10 mg/kg/day divided every 12 hours and adult dose 200-400 mg/day) for 3-12 mo, with the duration dependent on clinical response.

Patients with cryptococcemia or severe symptoms and non–HIV-immunocompromised hosts with lung disease with cryptococcal antigen titers of >1:8 or with CNS, urinary tract, or cutaneous disease should be treated in a staged approach, because these factors suggest disseminated disease. In general, these patients receive induction therapy with amphotericin B (0.7-1 mg/kg/day) plus flucytosine (100-150 mg/kg/day divided every 6 hours assuming normal kidney function) for a minimum of 2 wi, keeping serum flucytosine concentrations between 40 and 60 µg/mL. Depending on the clinical response, induction therapy may be continued as long as 6-10 wk.

Induction is followed by a consolidation phase with oral fluconazole or itraconazole for 6-12 mo. Itraconazole does not penetrate well into CSF, so consolidation therapy for CNS disease should be accomplished with fluconazole. Lifelong maintenance therapy may be required for children who remain immunocompromised. Lipid-complex amphotericin B (3-6 mg/kg/day) is recommended for patients intolerant of the deoxycholate amphotericin, although experience with this agent in children with cryptococcosis is limited. The current echinocandins do not have clinical activity against cryptococcal infections. Effectiveness of anticryptococcal therapy is monitored by serial cryptococcal antigen testing. Serum or CSF values of ≥1:8 predict relapse. Ventriculoperitoneal shunts may be required for patients with hydrocephalus, and aggressive medical management of increased intracranial pressure might also be required.

Because of the high rate of relapse, pulmonary, CNS, or disseminated cryptococcal infections in HIV-infected patients require induction, consolidation, and maintenance therapy. Patients with pulmonary disease most often require lifelong therapy with fluconazole or itraconazole. For those with CNS disease, the most commonly used regimen is amphotericin B (0.7 mg/kg/day) and flucytosine (100 mg/kg/day) for a minimum of 2 wk and as long as 6-10 wk (induction), followed by fluconazole for a minimum of 8-10 wk (consolidation). Fluconazole should be continued for life (maintenance therapy) after the completion of consolidation therapy. Itraconazole should be used only in cases where the patient is intolerant or has failed fluconazole therapy due to the higher relapse rates with itraconazole. Cessation of maintenance therapy in children whose HIV infection is well controlled on HAART has not been well studied to date.

Cutaneous infections are usually treated medically, although surgical biopsy may be required for diagnosis. Skeletal infections generally require surgical débridement in addition to systemic antifungal therapy. Chorioretinitis also requires systemic antifungal therapy with amphotericin B and either fluconazole or flucytosine, both of which achieve high drug concentrations in the vitreous.

PREVENTION

Persons at high risk should avoid exposures such as bird droppings. Effective HAART for persons with HIV infection reduces the risk of cryptococcal disease. Fluconazole prophylaxis is effective for preventing cryptococcosis in patients with AIDS and $CD4^+$ lymphocyte counts <100/µL. A cryptococcal glucuronoxylomannan (GXM)–tetanus toxoid conjugate vaccine has been developed that elicits protective antibodies in mice but awaits clinical trials in children. Passive immunization with protective monoclonal antibodies has yet to be studied in children.

BIBLIOGRAPHY

Please visit the Nelson Textbook of Pediatrics *website at www.expertconsult.com for the complete bibliography.*

Chapter 228
Malassezia

Martin E. Weisse and Ashley M. Maranich

Members of the genus *Malassezia* include the causative agents of **tinea versicolor** and have been associated with other dermatologic conditions and with fungemia in patients with indwelling catheters. *Malassezia* are commensal lipophilic yeasts with a predilection for the sebum-rich areas of the skin. They are considered a part of the normal skin flora, with presence established by 3-6 mo of age.

For the full continuation of this chapter, please visit the Nelson Textbook of Pediatrics *website at www.expertconsult.com.*

Chapter 229
Aspergillus

Luise E. Rogg and William J. Steinbach

The aspergilli are ubiquitous fungi whose normal ecological niche is that of a soil saprophyte that recycles carbon and nitrogen. The genus *Aspergillus* contains approximately 185 species, but most human disease is caused by *A. fumigatus*, *A. flavus*, *A. niger*, *A. terreus*, and *A. nidulans*. Invasive disease is most commonly caused by *A. fumigatus*. *Aspergillus* reproduces asexually via production of sporelike conidia. Most cases of *Aspergillus* disease (**aspergillosis**) are due to inhalation of airborne conidia that subsequently germinate into fungal hyphae and invade host tissue. People are likely exposed to conidia on a daily basis. When inhaled by an immunocompetent person, conidia are rarely deleterious, presumably because they are efficiently cleared by phagocytic cells. Macrophage- and neutrophil-mediated host defenses are required for resistance to invasive disease. Disease can develop in hosts with neutropenia or suppressed macrophage function or after exposure to unusually high doses of conidia.

Aspergillus is a relatively unusual pathogen in that it can create very different disease states depending on the host characteristics, including allergic (hypersensitivity), saprophytic (noninvasive), or invasive disease. Immunodeficient hosts are at risk for invasive disease, whereas immunocompetent hosts tend to develop allergic disease. Disease manifestations include primary allergic reactions; colonization of the lungs or sinuses; localized infection of the lung or skin; invasive pulmonary disease; or widely disseminated disease of the lungs, brain, skin, eye, bone, heart, and other organs. Clinically, these syndromes often manifest with mild, nonspecific, and late-onset symptoms, particularly in the immunosuppressed host, complicating accurate diagnosis and timely treatment.

229.1 Allergic Disease (Hypersensitivity Syndromes)

Luise E. Rogg and William J. Steinbach

ASTHMA

Attacks of atopic asthma can be triggered by inhalation of *Aspergillus* spores, producing allergic responses and subsequent bronchospasm. Exposure to fungi, especially *Aspergillus*, needs to be considered as a trigger in a patient with an asthma flare.

EXTRINSIC ALVEOLAR ALVEOLITIS

Extrinsic alveolar alveolitis is a hypersensitivity pneumonitis that occurs due to repetitive inhalational exposure to inciting materials, including *Aspergillus* conidia. Symptoms typically occur shortly after exposure and include fever, cough, and dyspnea. Neither blood nor sputum eosinophilia is present. Chronic exposure to the triggering material can lead to pulmonary fibrosis.

ALLERGIC BRONCHOPULMONARY ASPERGILLOSIS

Allergic bronchopulmonary aspergillosis (ABPA) is a hypersensitivity disease resulting from immunologic sensitization to *Aspergillus* antigens. It is primarily seen in patients with asthma or cystic fibrosis. Inhalation of conidia produces noninvasive colonization of the bronchial airways, resulting in persistent inflammation and development of hypersensitivity inflammatory responses. Disease manifestations are due to abnormal immunologic responses to *A. fumigatus* antigens and include wheezing, pulmonary infiltrates, bronchiectasis, and even fibrosis.

There are 7 primary diagnostic criteria for ABPA: episodic bronchial obstruction, peripheral eosinophilia, immediate cutaneous reactivity to *Aspergillus* antigens, precipitating antibodies to *Aspergillus* antigen, elevated IgE, pulmonary infiltrates, and central bronchietasis. Secondary diagnostic criteria include repeated detection of *Aspergillus* from sputum by identification of morphologically consistent fungal elements or direct culture, coughing up brown plugs or specks, elevated *Aspergillus* antigen–specific immunoglobulin E (IgE) antibodies, and late skin reaction to *Aspergillus* antigen. Radiologically, bronchial wall thickening, pulmonary infiltrates, and central bronchiectasis can be seen.

Treatment depends on relieving inflammation via an extended course of systemic corticosteroids. Addition of the antifungal agent itraconazole is used to decrease the fungal burden and diminish the inciting stimulus for inflammation. Because disease activity is correlated with serum IgE levels, these levels are used as one marker to define duration of therapy. An area of research interest is the utility of anti-IgE antibody therapy in the management of ABPA.

ALLERGIC *ASPERGILLUS* SINUSITIS

Allergic *Aspergillus* sinusitis is thought to be similar in etiology to ABPA. It has been primarily described in young adult patients with asthma and may or may not be seen in combination with ABPA. Patients often present with symptoms of chronic sinusitis or recurrent acute sinusitis, such as congestion, headaches, and rhinitis, and are found to have nasal polyps and opacification of multiple sinuses on imaging. Laboratory findings can include elevated IgE levels, precipitating antibodies to *Aspergillus* antigen, and immediate cutaneous reactivity to *Aspergillus* antigens. Sinus tissue specimens might contain eosinophils, Charcot-Leyden crystals, and fungal elements consistent with *Aspergillus* species. Surgical drainage is an important aspect of treatment, often accompanied by courses of either systemic or inhaled steroids. Use of an antifungal agent may also be considered.

BIBLIOGRAPHY

Please visit the Nelson Textbook of Pediatrics *website at* *www.expertconsult.com* *for the complete bibliography.*

229.2 Saprophytic (Noninvasive) Syndromes

Luise E. Rogg and William J. Steinbach

PULMONARY ASPERGILLOMA

Aspergillomas are masses of fungal hyphae, cellular debris, and inflammatory cells that proliferate without vascular invasion, generally in the setting of pre-existing cavitary lesions or ectatic bronchi. These cavitary lesions can occur as a result of infections such as tuberculosis, histoplasmosis, or resolved abscesses or secondary to congenital or acquired defects such as pulmonary cysts or bullous emphysema. Patients may be asymptomatic, with diagnosis made through imaging for other reasons, or they might present with hemoptysis, cough, or fever. On imaging, there may be thickening of the walls of a cavity initially, or later, a solid round mass separated from the cavity wall, as the fungal ball develops. Detection of *Aspergillus* antibody in the serum suggests this diagnosis. Treatment is indicated for control of complications, such as hemoptysis. Surgical resection is the definitive treatment but has been associated with significant risks. Systemic antifungal treatment with azole-class agents may be indicated in certain patients.

CHRONIC PULMONARY ASPERGILLOSIS

Chronic aspergillosis can occur in patients with normal immune systems or mild degrees of immunosuppression. Three categories have been proposed to describe different manifestations of chronic aspergillosis. The first is chronic cavitary pulmonary aspergillosis (CCPA), which is similar to aspergilloma, except that multiple cavities form and expand with occupying fungal balls. The second is chronic fibrosing pulmonary aspergillosis, where the multiple individual lesions progress to significant pulmonary fibrosis. The final is chronic necrotizing pulmonary aspergillosis (CNPA), also known as *subacute invasive* or *semi-invasive pulmonary aspergillosis*, a slowly progressive subset found in patients with mild to moderate immune impairment.

Management of CCPA can sometimes be via surgical resection, though long-term antifungal therapy, as for invasive aspergillosis, is indicated. Management of CNPA is similar to that of invasive pulmonary aspergillosis; however, the disease is more indolent, and thus there is a greater emphasis on oral therapy. Direct instillation of antifungals into the lesion cavity has been employed with some success.

SINUSITIS

Sinus aspergillosis typically manifests with chronic sinus symptoms that are refractory to antibacterial treatment. Imaging can demonstrate mucosal thickening in the case of *Aspergillus* sinusitis or a single mass within the maxillary or ethmoid sinus in the case of sinus aspergilloma. If untreated, sinusitis can progress and extend into the ethmoid sinuses and orbits. Therapy of sinusitis depends on surgical débridement and drainage, including surgical removal of the fungal mass in cases of sinus aspergilloma.

OTOMYCOSIS

Aspergillus can colonize the external auditory canal, with possible extension to the middle ear and mastoid air spaces if the tympanic membrane is disrupted by concurrent bacterial infection. Symptoms include pain, itching, decreased unilateral hearing, or otorrhea. Otomycosis is more often seen in patients with impaired mucosal immunity, such as patients with hypogammaglobulinemia, diabetes mellitus, chronic eczema, or HIV and those using chronic steroids. Treatments have not been well studied, but topical treatment with acetic or boric acid instillations or azole creams as well as oral azoles such as voriconazole, itraconazole, and posaconazole have been described.

BIBLIOGRAPHY

Please visit the Nelson Textbook of Pediatrics *website at www.expertconsult.com for the complete bibliography.*

229.3 Invasive Disease

Luise E. Rogg and William J. Steinbach

Invasive aspergillosis (IA) occurs after conidia enter the body, escape immunologic control mechanisms, and germinate into fungal hyphae that subsequently invade tissue parenchyma and vasculature. The invasion of the vasculature can result in thrombosis and localized necrosis and facilitates hematogenous dissemination. The incidence of IA appears to be increasing, possibly due to better management of other infections found in the at-risk populations and more use of severely immunosuppressive therapies for a widening array of diseases. The most common site of primary infection is the lung, but primary infection is also seen in the sinuses and skin and rarely elsewhere. Secondary infection can be seen after hematogenous spread, often to the skin, CNS, eye, bone, and heart.

IA is primarily a disease of immunocompromised hosts, and risk factors include cancer or chemotherapy-induced neutropenia, particularly if severe and/or prolonged, stem cell transplantation, especially during the initial pre-engraftment phase or if complicated by graft vs host disease, neutrophil or macrophage dysfunction such as occur in severe combined immunodeficiency (SCID) or chronic granulomatous disease (CGD), prolonged high-dose steroid use, HIV, or solid organ transplantation. There have only been a few studies in the pediatric age group to identify risk factors for IA, but allogeneic bone marrow transplantation and acute myelogenous leukemia have been suggested. Well-defined incidence of IA among pediatric patients has not been determined to date.

INVASIVE PULMONARY ASPERGILLOSIS

Invasive pulmonary aspergillosis is the most common form of aspergillosis. It plays a significant role in morbidity and mortality in the patient populations at increased risk for IA, namely stem cell and solid organ transplant recipients, cancer patients, patients with primary immunodeficiencies, and patients receiving immunomodulatory therapy. Presenting symptoms can include fever despite initiation of empirical broad-spectrum antibacterial therapy, cough, chest pain, hemoptysis, and pulmonary infiltrates. Patients on high-dose steroids are less likely to present with fever. Symptoms in these immunocompromised patients can be very vague, and thus maintaining a high index of suspicion when confronted with a high-risk patient is essential.

Diagnosis

Imaging can be helpful, although no finding is pathognomonic for invasive pulmonary disease. Characteristically, multiple, ill-defined nodules can be seen, though lobar or diffuse consolidation is not uncommon and normal chest X-rays can be seen even late in the disease evolution. Classic radiologic signs on CT include the **halo sign,** when angioinvasion produces a hemorrhagic nodule surrounded by ischemia. Early on there is a rim of ground-glass opacification surrounding a nodule. Over time, these lesions evolve into cavitary lesions or lesions with an **air crescent** when the lung necroses around the fungal mass, often seen during recovery from neutropenia. Unfortunately, these findings are not specific to invasive pulmonary aspergillosis and can also be seen in other pulmonary fungal infections, as well as pulmonary hemorrhage and organizing pneumonia. In addition, several reviews of imaging results of pediatric aspergillosis cases suggest that cavitation and air crescent formation are less common among these patients than among adult patients. On MRI, the typical finding for pulmonary disease is the **target sign,** a nodule with lower central signal compared to the rim-enhancing periphery.

Diagnosis of IA can be complicated for a number of reasons. Conclusive diagnosis requires culture of *Aspergillus* from a normally sterile site and histologic identification of tissue invasion by fungal hyphae consistent with *Aspergillus* morphology. However, obtaining tissue specimens is often practically impossible in critically ill patients. In addition, depending on the specimen type, a positive result from culture can represent colonization rather than infection. Isolation of *Aspergillus* from blood cultures is uncommon, likely because fungemia is low-level and intermittent.

Serology can be useful in the diagnosis of allergic *Aspergillus* syndromes as well as aspergilloma but is low yield for invasive disease, likely because of deficient immune responses in the high-risk immunocompromised population. Bronchoalveolar lavage (BAL) can be useful, but negative results cannot be used to rule out disease, owing to inadequate sensitivity. Addition of molecular biologic assays such as antigen detection and polymerase chain reaction (PCR) can improve the diagnostic yield of BAL for aspergillosis. An enzyme-linked immunosorbent assay (ELISA)-based assay for galactomannan, one of the components of the *Aspergillus* cell wall, has been developed to aid the diagnosis of invasive aspergillosis. This newer molecular test is useful when used in serial monitoring for development of infection and has been shown to be the most sensitive in detecting disease in cancer patients or hematopoietic stem cell transplant recipients. Earlier reports of increased false-positive reactions in children versus adults have been refuted. This test appears to have high rates of false negativity in patients with congenital immunodeficiency (e.g., CGD) and invasive *Aspergillus* infections. An ongoing area of research involves the use of serial monitoring of galactomannan levels to provide guidance for duration of therapy. PCR-based assays are in development for the diagnosis of aspergillosis but are still being optimized and are not yet commercially available.

Treatment

Successful treatment of IA hinges on the ability to reconstitute normal immune function and use of effective antifungal agents until immune recovery can be achieved. Therefore, lowering overall immunosuppression via cessation of corticosteroid use is vital to improve the ultimate outcome. In 2008, new treatment guidelines for *Aspergillus* infections were published by the Infectious Diseases Society of America, marking a major shift in management recommendations. In the past, first-line therapy was amphotericin B, notable for low response rates and significant infusion reactions and drug toxicity. Liposomal formulations of amphotericin B have been developed, which are associated with decreased toxicity and may still have a role as first-line therapy for invasive infection in certain patients.

Primary therapy is now the azole-class antifungal voriconazole, based on multiple studies showing both improved response rates and survival in patients receiving voriconazole when compared to amphotericin B. In addition, voriconazole is better tolerated than amphotericin B and can be given orally as well as intravenously. Azoles are metabolized through the cytochrome P-450 system, and thus medication interactions can be a significant complication. Other triazole antifungals are also available, including posaconazole, which is approved for antifungal prophylaxis and may be an alternative agent for first-line treatment of IA. Although the dosing of itraconazole and voriconazole have been established for pediatric patients, the pharmacokinetic studies for posaconazole have not yet been done.

The echinocandin class of antifungals may also a play a role in treatment of IA, but to date, these agents are generally employed as second-line medications, particularly for salvage therapy. There have been insufficient studies to permit any recommendations for combination antifungal therapy. Unfortunately, even with the new classes of antifungals, complete or partial response rates for treatment of IA are only approximately 50%. To augment antifungal therapies, patients have been treated with growth factors to increase neutrophil counts, granulocyte transfusions, interferon-γ, and surgery.

Special Populations

Patients with CGD represent a pediatric population at particular risk for pulmonary aspergillosis. Invasive pulmonary aspergillosis can be the first serious infection identified in these patients, and the lifetime risk of development is estimated to be 33%. The onset of symptoms is often gradual, with slow development of fever, fatigue, pneumonia, and elevated sedimentation rate. The neutrophils of patients with CGD surround the collections of fungal elements but cannot kill them, thereby permitting local invasion with extension of disease to the pleura, ribs, and vertebrae, though angioinvasion is not seen. Imaging in these patients is much less likely to reveal the halo sign, infarcts, or cavitary lesions and instead generally shows areas of tissue destruction due to the ongoing inflammatory processes.

CUTANEOUS ASPERGILLOSIS

Cutaneous aspergillosis can occur as a primary disease or as a consequence of hematogenous dissemination or spread from underlying structures. Primary cutaneous disease classically occurs at sites of skin disruption, such as intravenous access device locations, adhesive dressings, or sites of injury or surgery. Premature infants are particularly at risk, given their immature skin and need for multiple access devices. Cutaneous disease in transplant recipients tends to reflect hematogenous distribution from a primary site of infection, often the lungs. Lesions are erythematous indurated papules that progress to painful, ulcerated, necrotic lesions. Treatment depends on the combination of surgical débridement and antifungal therapy, with systemic voriconazole recommended as primary therapy.

INVASIVE SINONASAL DISEASE

Invasive *Aspergillus* sinusitis represents a difficult diagnosis because the clinical presentation tends to be highly variable. Patients can present with congestion, rhinorrhea, epistaxis, headache, facial pain or swelling, orbital swelling, fever, or abnormal appearance of the nasal turbinates. Because noninvasive imaging can be normal, diagnosis rests on direct visualization via endoscopy and biopsy. Sinus mucosa may be pale, discolored, granulating, or necrotic depending on the stage and extent of disease. The infection can invade adjacent structures, including the eye and brain. This syndrome is difficult to distinguish clinically from other types of invasive fungal disease of the sinuses such as zygomycosis, rendering obtaining specimens for culture and histology extremely important. If the diagnosis is confirmed, treatment should be with voriconazole. Because voriconazole is not active against the Zygomycetes, amphotericin B formulations should be considered pending definitive diagnosis.

CENTRAL NERVOUS SYSTEM

The primary site of *Aspergillus* infection tends to be the lungs, but as the hyphae invade into the vasculature, fungal elements can dislodge and travel through the bloodstream, permitting establishment of secondary infection sites. One of the sites commonly involved in disseminated disease is the central nervous system (CNS). Cerebral aspergillosis can also arise secondary to local extension of sinus disease. The presentation of cerebral aspergillosis is highly variable but can include changes in mental status, seizures, paralysis, coma, and ophthalmoplegia. As the hyphae invade the CNS vasculature, hemorrhagic infarcts develop that convert to abscesses. Biopsy is required for definitive diagnosis, but patients are often too ill to tolerate surgery. Imaging can be helpful for diagnosis, and MRI is preferred. Lesions tend to be multiple, located in the basal ganglia, have intermediate intensity with no enhancement, and have no mass effect. CT shows hypodense, well-demarcated lesions, sometimes with ring enhancement and edema. Diagnosis often depends on characteristic imaging findings in a patient with known aspergillosis at other sites. Galactomannan assay testing of CSF has been studied and may become a future methodology to confirm the diagnosis. In general, the prognosis for CNS aspergillosis is extremely poor, likely owing to the late onset at presentation. Reversal of immunosuppression is extremely important. Surgical resection of lesions may be useful. Voriconazole is thought to be the best therapy, and itraconazole, posaconazole, and liposomal formulations of amphotericin B are alternative options.

EYE

Fungal endophthalmitis and keratitis may be seen in patients with disseminated *Aspergillus* infection. Pain, photophobia, and decreased visual acuity may be present, though many patients are asymptomatic. Emergent ophthalmologic evaluation is important when these entities are suspected. Endophthalmitis is treated with intravitreal injection of either amphotericin B or voriconazole along with surgical intervention and systemic antifungal therapy with amphotericin B or voriconazole. Keratitis requires topical and systemic antifungal therapy.

BONE

Aspergillus osteomyelitis can occur, most commonly in the vertebrae. Rib involvement occurs owing to extension of disease in patients with CGD and is most often caused by *A. nidulans*. Treatment depends on the combination of surgical débridement and systemic antifungals. Arthritis can develop owing to hematogenous dissemination or local extension, and treatment depends on joint drainage combined with antifungal therapy. Amphotericin B has been the most commonly employed agent in the past, although voriconazole is the preferred first-line therapy now.

HEART

Cardiac infection can occur as a result of surgical contamination, secondary to disseminated infection, or as a result of direct extension from a contiguous focus of infection and includes endocarditis, myocarditis, and pericarditis. Treatment requires surgical intervention in the case of endocarditis and pericarditis, along with systemic antifungals, sometimes lifelong due to possibility of recurrent infection.

EMPIRICAL ANTIFUNGAL THERAPY

Because the diagnosis of invasive *Aspergillus* infections is often complicated and delayed, empirical initiation of antifungal therapy is often considered in high-risk patients. At present, antifungal coverage with amphotericin B (conventional or liposomal), voriconazole, itraconazole, or the echinocandin caspofungin should be considered in patients at risk for prolonged neutropenia or with findings suggesting invasive fungal infections. At this time, our ability to diagnose and treat infections due to *Aspergillus* remains suboptimal, particularly among pediatric patients. Additional study of antigen detection assays based on galactomannan and other *Aspergillus* cell wall components as well as standardization of PCR-based assays will facilitate diagnosis. The optimal treatment remains another challenging question, because current therapeutic regimens tend to produce complete or partial response only about half of the time. In the future, we may have additional information on multiagent regimens that combine different antifungal classes as well as novel antifungal agents in our armamentarium.

BIBLIOGRAPHY

Please visit the Nelson Textbook of Pediatrics *website at* *www.expertconsult.com* *for the complete bibliography.*

Chapter 230
Histoplasmosis (*Histoplasma capsulatum*)

Jane M. Gould and Stephen C. Aronoff

ETIOLOGY

Histoplasmosis is caused by *Histoplasma capsulatum*, a dimorphic fungus found in the environment as a saprophyte in the mycelial (mold) form and in tissues in the parasitic form as yeast.

EPIDEMIOLOGY

The saprophytic form is found in soil throughout the midwestern USA, primarily along the Ohio and Mississippi rivers. Sporadic cases of human and animal histoplasmosis have been reported from 31 of the 48 contiguous states. In parts of Kentucky and Tennessee, almost 90% of the population >20 yr of age have positive skin test results for histoplasmin. *Histoplasma* is endemic to parts of the Caribbean islands, Central and South America, certain areas of Southeast Asia, and the Mediterranean. *H. capsulatum* thrives in soil rich in nitrates such as areas that are heavily contaminated with bird or bat droppings or decayed wood. Fungal spores are often carried on the wings of birds. Focal outbreaks of histoplasmosis have been reported after aerosolization of microconidia resulting from construction in areas previously occupied by starling roosts or chicken coops or by chopping decayed wood. Unlike birds, bats are actively infected with *Histoplasma*. Focal outbreaks of histoplasmosis have also been reported after intense exposure to bat guano in caves and along bridges frequented by bats. Person-to-person transmission does not occur.

PATHOGENESIS

Inhalation of microconidia (fungal spores) is the initial stage of human infection. The conidia reach the alveoli, germinate, and proliferate as yeast. Alternatively, spores can remain as mold with the potential for activation. Most infections are asymptomatic or self-limited. When disseminated disease occurs, any organ system can be involved. The initial infection is a bronchopneumonia. As the initial pulmonary lesion ages, giant cells form, followed by formation of caseating or noncaseating granulomas and central necrosis. Granulomas contain viable yeast, and disease can relapse. At the time of spore germination, yeast cells are phagocytosed by alveolar macrophages, where they replicate and gain access to the reticuloendothelial system via the pulmonary lymphatic system and hilar lymph nodes. Dissemination with splenic involvement typically follows the primary pulmonary infection. In normal hosts, specific cell-mediated immunity follows in approximately 2 weeks, enabling sensitized T-cells to activate macrophages and kill the organism. The initial pulmonary lesion resolves within 2-4 mo but may undergo calcification resembling the Ghon complex of tuberculosis. Alternatively, "buckshot" calcifications involving the lung and spleen may be seen. Unlike tuberculosis, reinfection with *H. capsulatum* occurs and can lead to exaggerated host responses in some cases.

CLINICAL MANIFESTATIONS

There are 3 forms of human histoplasmosis: acute pulmonary infection, chronic pulmonary histoplasmosis, and progressive disseminated histoplasmosis.

Acute pulmonary histoplasmosis follows initial or recurrent respiratory exposure to microconidia. The majority of patients are asymptomatic. Symptomatic disease occurs more often in young children; in older patients, symptoms follow exposure to large inocula in closed spaces (e.g., chicken coops or caves) or prolonged exposure (e.g., camping on contaminated soil, chopping decayed wood). The median incubation time is 14 days. The prodrome is not specific and usually consists of flulike symptoms including headache, fever, chest pain, cough, and myalgias. Hepatosplenomegaly occurs more often in infants and young children. Symptomatic infections may be associated with significant respiratory distress and hypoxia and can require intubation, ventilation, and steroid therapy. Acute pulmonary disease can also manifest with a prolonged illness (10 days to 3 wk) consisting of weight loss, dyspnea, high fever, asthenia, and fatigue. In 10% of patients, infection is a sarcoid-like disease with arthritis or arthralgia, erythema nodosum, keratoconjunctivitis, iridocyclitis, and pericarditis. Pericarditis, with effusions both pericardial and pleural, is a self-limited benign condition that develops as a result of an inflammatory reaction to adjacent mediastinal disease. The effusions are exudative, and the organism is rarely culturable from fluid. Most children with acute pulmonary disease have normal chest radiographs. Patients with symptomatic disease typically have a patchy bronchopneumonia; hilar lymphadenopathy is variably present. In young children, the pneumonia can coalesce. Focal or buckshot calcifications are convalescent findings in patients with acute pulmonary infection.

Exaggerated host responses to fungal antigens within the lung parenchyma or hilar lymph nodes produce thoracic complications of acute pulmonary histoplasmosis. Histoplasmomas are of parenchymal origin and are usually asymptomatic. These fibroma-like lesions are often concentrically calcified and single. Rarely, these lesions produce broncholithiasis associated with "stone spitting," wheezing, and hemoptysis. In endemic regions, these lesions can mimic parenchymal tumors and are occasionally diagnosed at lung biopsy. Mediastinal granulomas form when reactive hilar lymph nodes coalesce and mat together. Although these lesions are usually asymptomatic, huge granulomas can compress the mediastinal structures, producing symptoms of esophageal, bronchial, or vena caval obstruction. Local extension and necrosis can produce pericarditis or pleural effusions. Mediastinal fibrosis is a rare complication of mediastinal granulomas and represents an uncontrolled fibrotic reaction arising from the hilar nodes. Structures within the mediastinum become encased within a fibrotic mass, producing obstructive symptomatology. Superior vena cava syndrome, pulmonary venous obstruction with a mitral stenosis–like syndrome, and pulmonary artery obstruction with congestive heart failure have been described. Dysphagia accompanies esophageal entrapment, and a syndrome of cough, wheeze, hemoptysis, and dyspnea accompanies bronchial obstruction.

Chronic pulmonary histoplasmosis is an opportunistic infection in adult patients with centrilobular emphysema. This entity is rare in children.

Progressive disseminated histoplasmosis accounts for 10% of histoplasmosis cases and affects infants and immunocompromised patients. Disseminated disease of childhood occurs almost exclusively in children <2 yr of age because of a relative immature cellular immune system and follows primary pulmonary infection. The mortality of progressive disseminated histoplasmosis without therapy is 100%. Fever is the most common finding and can persist for weeks to months before the condition is diagnosed.

The majority of patients have hepatosplenomegaly, lymphadenopathy, anemia, and thrombocytopenia. Pneumonia and pancytopenia are variably present. Some patients develop mucous membrane ulcerations and skin findings such as nodules, ulcers, or molluscum-like papules. Half of the infected infants have transient T-cell deficiencies, and many experience transient hyperglobulinemia. Elevated acute phase reactants and hypercalcemia are typically seen but are not specific for disseminated histoplasmosis. Although chest radiographs are normal in more than half of these children, the yeast can often be identified on bone marrow examination.

Children who are immunosuppressed (cancer patients, organ transplant recipients, patients with HIV infection) are at increased risk for disseminated histoplasmosis. In children who are not infected with HIV, disseminated disease manifests with unexplained fevers, weight loss, lymphadenopathy, and interstitial pulmonary disease. Extrapulmonary infection is a characteristic of disseminated disease and can include destructive bony lesions, oropharyngeal ulcers, Addison disease, meningitis, multifocal chorioretinitis, cutaneous infection, and endocarditis. Elevated liver function test results and high serum concentrations of angiotensin-converting enzyme may be observed.

Disseminated histoplasmosis in an HIV-infected patient is an AIDS-defining illness. Disseminated disease is often preceded or followed by another opportunistic infection in this patient population. HIV-infected patients at greatest risk for acquiring disseminated histoplasmosis are those with a history of exposure to avian excreta or bat guano, no prior history of antiretroviral therapy, or no history of previous antifungal prophylaxis. Fever and weight loss occur in most patients. In the majority of patients, pulmonary disease develops; hepatosplenomegaly, lymphadenopathy, skin rashes, and meningoencephalitis are variably present. A sepsis-like syndrome has been identified in a small number of HIV-infected patients with disseminated histoplasmosis and is characterized by the rapid onset of shock, multiorgan failure, and coagulopathy. Reactive hemophagocytic syndrome has been described in immunocompromised patients with severe disseminated histoplasmosis. Transplacental transmission of *H. capsulatum* has been reported in immunocompromised mothers.

DIAGNOSIS

Histoplasma typically grows within 6 wk on Sabouraud agar at 25 °C. Identification of tuberculate macroconidia allow for only a presumptive diagnosis, because *Sepedonium* also form similar structures. A confirmatory test using a chemiluminescent DNA probe for *H. capsulatum* is necessary to establish a definitive identification. Recovery of *H. capsulatum* by culture differs with the form of infection. In normal hosts with symptomatic or asymptomatic acute pulmonary histoplasmosis, sputum cultures are rarely obtained and are variably positive; cultures of bronchoalveolar lavage fluid appear to have a slightly higher yield than sputum cultures. Sputum cultures are positive in 60% of adults with chronic pulmonary histoplasmosis. The yeast can be recovered from blood or bone marrow in >90% of patients with progressive disseminated histoplasmosis. Blood cultures are sterile in patients with acute pulmonary histoplasmosis, and cultures from any source are typically sterile in patients with the sarcoid form of the disease. Yeast forms may be demonstrated histologically in tissue from patients with complicated forms of acute pulmonary disease (histoplasmoma, mediastinal granuloma, and mediastinal fibrosis). Tissue should be stained with methenamine silver or periodic acid–Schiff stains, and yeast can be found within or outside of macrophages. Wright stain of peripheral blood can demonstrate fungal elements within leukocytes. Polymerase chain reaction assay enables more accurate and early diagnosis but is not widely available.

Detection of fungal polysaccharide antigen by radioimmunoassay is the most widely available diagnostic study for patients with suspected progressive disseminated histoplasmosis. In HIV-infected patients as well as others at risk for disseminated disease, histoplasma-associated antigen can be demonstrated in the urine, blood, or bronchoalveolar lavage fluid in >90% of cases. False-positive results on urinary antigen testing can occur in patients with *Blastomyces dermatitidis, Coccidioides immitis* and *posadasii, Paracoccidioides brasiliensis,* and *Penicillium marneffei.* False-positive results on serum antigen testing can occur with rheumatoid factor and treatment with rabbit antithymocyte globulin. Antigen detection by enzyme immunoassay (EIA) has comparable sensitivity, improved specificity, but limited availability; however, both the radioimmunoassay and the EIA are more sensitive when urine is tested rather than serum. Serum, urine, and bronchoalveolar lavage fluid from patients with acute or chronic pulmonary infections are variably antigen positive. Sequential measurement of antigen in patients with disseminated disease is useful for monitoring response to therapy.

Seroconversion continues to be useful for the diagnosis of acute pulmonary histoplasmosis, its complications, and chronic pulmonary disease. Serum antibody to yeast and mycelium-associated antigens is classically measured by complement fixation. Although titers of >1:8 are found in >80% of patients with histoplasmosis, titers of ≥1:32 are most significant for the diagnosis of recent infection. Complement-fixation antibody titers are often not significant early in the infection and do not become positive until 4-6 wk after exposure. A 4-fold increase in either yeast or mycelial-phase titers or a single titer of ≥1:32 is presumptive evidence of active infection. Complement fixation titers may be falsely positive in patients with other systemic mycoses such as *Blastomyces dermatitidis* and *Coccidioides immitis* and may be falsely negative in immunocompromised patients. Antibody detection by immunodiffusion is less sensitive but more specific than complement fixation and is used to confirm questionably positive complement fixation titers. Skin testing is useful only for epidemiologic studies because cutaneous reactivity is lifelong, and intradermal injection can elicit an immune response in otherwise seronegative persons.

TREATMENT

Antifungal therapy is not warranted for persons with asymptomatic or mildly symptomatic acute pulmonary histoplasmosis. Oral itraconazole or fluconazole should be considered in patients with acute pulmonary infections who fail to improve clinically within 1 mo. Itraconazole is superior to fluconazole in treatment of histoplasmosis in adults. Patients with primary or re-exposure pulmonary histoplasmosis who become hypoxemic or require ventilatory support should receive amphotericin B (0.7-1.0 mg/kg/day) or amphotericin B lipid complex (3-5 mg/kg/day) until improved; continued therapy with oral itraconazole (5.0-10.0 mg/kg/day in 2 divided doses not to exceed 400 mg daily) for a minimum of 12 weeks is also recommended. The lipid preparations of amphotericin are not preferred. Patients with severe obstructive symptoms caused by granulomatous mediastinal disease may be treated sequentially with amphotericin B followed by itraconazole for 6-12 mo. Patients with milder mediastinal disease may be treated with oral itraconazole alone. Some experts recommend that surgery be reserved for patients who fail to improve after 1 mo of intensive amphotericin B therapy. Sarcoid-like disease with or without pericarditis may be treated with nonsteroidal anti-inflammatory agents for 2-12 wk.

Amphotericin B continues to be the cornerstone of therapy for infants with progressive disseminated histoplasmosis. In one study, sequential therapy with amphotericin B and oral ketoconazole for 3 mo was curative in 88% of patients. Alternatively, amphotericin B (1.0 mg/kg/day) or its lipid complex may be given acutely for 4-6 wk or amphotericin B (1.0 mg/kg/day) may be given for 2-4 wk followed by oral itraconazole (5.0-10.0 mg/kg/day in 2 divided doses) as maintenance therapy for 3 months, depending on histoplasma antigen status. Longer therapy may be needed in patients with severe disease, immunosuppression or primary immunodeficiency syndromes. It is recommended to monitor blood levels of itraconazole during treatment, aiming for a concentration of ≥1.0 µg/mL but <10 µg/mL to avoid potential drug toxicity. It is also recommended to monitor urine antigen levels during therapy and for 12 mo after therapy has ended to ensure cure. In general, amphotericin B lipid complex may be substituted in severely ill children who are intolerant of the classic drug preparation. The newer azoles (voriconzaole and posaconazole) have not been well studied in the treatment of histoplasmosis and are currently not recommended.

Relapses in HIV-infected patients with progressive disseminated histoplasmosis are common. Currently, induction therapy with amphotericin B or lipid complex amphotericin B is recommended. Lifelong suppressive therapy with daily itraconazole (5.0 mg/kg/day up to adult dose of 200 mg/day) is also required. For severely immunocompromised HIV-infected children living in endemic regions, itraconazole (2-5 mg/kg every 12-24 hr) may be used prophylactically. Care must be taken to avoid interactions between antifungal azoles and protease inhibitors.

BIBLIOGRAPHY

Please visit the Nelson Textbook of Pediatrics *website at www.expertconsult.com for the complete bibliography.*

Chapter 231
Blastomycosis (*Blastomyces dermatitidis*)

Gregory M. Gauthier and Bruce S. Klein

ETIOLOGY

Blastomyces dermatitidis belongs to a group of fungi that exhibit thermal dimorphism. In the soil, these fungi grow as mold and produce spores, which are the infectious particles. When inhaled into the lungs, the spores convert into pathogenic yeast and cause infection.

EPIDEMIOLOGY

B. dermatitidis causes disease in immunocompetent and immunocompromised children. Only 2-13% of blastomycosis cases occur in patients <18 yr of age. Neonatal blastomycosis is rare and can be transmitted through the placenta to the fetus. In North America, the geographic distribution of blastomycosis cases is restricted to the Midwest, south-central, and southeastern USA and parts of Canada bordering the Great Lakes and Saint Lawrence River Valley. Infections have also been reported from Africa, India, the Middle East, and Central and South America. *B. dermatitidis* grows in sandy soils that have decaying vegetation and are near water. Most infections with *B. dermatitidis* are sporadic; however, outbreaks have been well described. The severity of infection is influenced by the size of the inhaled inoculum and the integrity of the patient's immune system.

PATHOGENESIS

The ability to convert from spores to yeast in the lung is a crucial event in the pathogenesis of infection with *B. dermatitidis* and other dimorphic fungi. This phase transition enables *B. dermatitidis* to evade the host immune system and establish infection. In the yeast form, *B. dermatitidis* produces BAD-1 (*Blastomyces* adhesin-1; formerly WI-1), an essential virulence factor that is displayed on the cell wall and secreted. BAD-1 promotes binding of yeast to macrophages in lung alveoli, blocks the deposition of complement on the yeast surface, binds calcium, and suppresses the production of pro-inflammatory cytokines in the host.

The phase transition from mold to yeast is a complex event that involves alteration in cell wall composition, metabolism, intracellular signaling, and gene expression. In *B. dermatitidis*, this transition is regulated, in part, by a histidine kinase known as *DRK1* (dimorphism regulating kinase-1). This sensor kinase controls not only the conversion of mold to yeast but also spore production, cell wall composition, and *BAD-1* expression; the loss of *DRK1* expression through gene disruption renders *B. dermatitidis* avirulent in a murine model of blastomycosis.

CLINICAL MANIFESTATIONS

The clinical manifestations of blastomycosis are heterogeneous and include subclinical infection, symptomatic pneumonia, and disseminated disease. Clinical disease develops 3 wk to 3 mo following exposure to *B. dermatitidis*. Asymptomatic or subclinical infections are estimated to occur in 50% of patients.

The most common clinical manifestation of blastomycosis is acute pneumonia. Symptoms include fever, dyspnea, cough, and malaise. Respiratory failure can occur in patients with severe pulmonary disease. Chest imaging typically demonstrates airspace consolidation, which can involve the upper or lower lobes. Other radiographic features include nodular, reticulonodular, and miliary patterns. Hilar adenopathy and pleural effusions are uncommon. Because the clinical and radiographic features can mimic bacterial pneumonia, patients can be mistakenly treated with antibiotics, resulting in disease progression. Patients with chronic pneumonia present with fevers, chills, night sweats, cough, weight loss, hemoptysis, dyspnea, and chest pain. Airspace consolidation, masslike lesions, or cavitary disease can be present on chest roetenography. These features can mimic tuberculosis or malignancy.

Extrapulmonary blastomycosis most often affects the skin or bone, but can involve almost any organ. The incidence of extrapulmonary disease in children is not well defined; the rate of disseminated disease is thought to be similar to the rate in adults (25-40%). The skin is the most common site for extrapulmonary blastomycosis, which is usually the result of hematogenous dissemination. Direct inoculation of *B. dermatitidis* into the skin from trauma or a laboratory accident can result in primary cutaneous blastomycosis. Skin manifestations include plaques, papules, ulcers, nodules, and verrucous lesions. The bone is the second most common site of extrapulmonary involvement, including the ribs, skull, spine, and long bones. Clinical symptoms of bone involvement include bone pain, soft tissue swelling, sinus formation, and ulceration. Patients with osteomyelitis often have pulmonary or cutaneous manifestations of blastomycosis. Complications include paraspinal abscess, vertebral collapse, and septic arthritis. Genitourinary blastomycosis occurs in 10-30% of adults but is rare in children.

Blastomycosis of the central nervous system (CNS) occurs in <5-10% of immunocompetent patients and can result in brain abscess or meningitis. Some patients with CNS blastomycosis have widely disseminated disease. Symptoms include headache, altered mental status, memory loss, seizure, cranial nerve deficits, and focal neurologic deficits. Lumbar puncture demonstrates leukocytosis with a lymphocyte predominance, elevated protein, and low glucose. Growth of *B. dermatitidis* in culture from cerebral spinal fluid is uncommon.

DIAGNOSIS

The diagnosis of blastomycosis requires a high index of suspicion, because the clinical and radiographic manifestations can mimic other diseases. Blastomycosis should be included in the differential diagnosis for patients with pneumonia who live in or visit areas in which this pathogen is endemic, fail to respond to antibiotics, or have chronic skin lesions or osteomyelitis. Growth of

B. dermatitidis in culture from sputum, skin, bone, or other clinical specimens provides a definitive diagnosis. Sputum specimens should be stained with 10% potassium hydroxide or calcofluor white. Histopathology shows neutrophilic infiltration with noncaseating granulomas (pyogranulomas). *B. dermatitidis* yeast in tissue samples can be visualized using Gomori methenamine silver (GMS) or periodic acid–Schiff (PAS) stains. Yeast are 8-20 µm in size, have a double refractile cell wall, and display broad-based budding.

Serologic methods including complement fixation and immunodiffusion suffer from poor sensitivity. In contrast, the *Blastomyces* urine antigen test has a sensitivity of 92.9%; however, it cross-reacts upon infection with other dimorphic fungi, reducing its specificity.

TREATMENT

Antifungal therapy is influenced by the severity of the infection, involvement of the central nervous system, and the integrity of the host's immune system. Newborns with blastomycosis should be treated with amphotericin B deoxycholate 1 mg/kg/day. Children with mild to moderately severe infection can be treated with itraconazole 10 mg/kg/day (maximum 400 mg/day) for 6-12 mo. Children with severe disease or underlying immunocompromise should be treated with amphotericin B deoxycholate 0.7-1.0 mg/kg/day, or lipid formulation 3-5 mg/kg/day, until there is clinical improvement, generally 7-14 days, and then itraconazole 10 mg/kg/day (maximum 400 mg/day) for a total of 12 mo. CNS blastomycosis requires therapy with a lipid formulation of amphotericin B at 5 mg/kg/day for 4-6 wk followed by itraconazole, fluconazole, or voriconazole for ≥12 mo.

For patients receiving itraconazole, the oral antifungal of choice, serum drug levels need to be measured 14 days into therapy (goal ≥1 µg/mL) and liver function tests should be monitored periodically. The newest azole antifungal drugs, voriconazole and posaconazole, have activity against *B. dermatitidis*; however, clinical experience with these drugs remains limited. The echinocandins (caspofungin, micafungin, and anidulofungin) should not be used to treat blastomycosis. Serial measurement of urine antigen levels to assess response to therapy appears promising, but the clinical usefulness of this strategy remains to be determined.

BIBLIOGRAPHY

Please visit the Nelson Textbook of Pediatrics *website at www.expertconsult.com for the complete bibliography.*

Chapter 232 Coccidioidomycosis (*Coccidioides* Species)

Martin B. Kleiman

ETIOLOGY

Coccidioidomycosis (valley fever, San Joaquin fever, desert rheumatism, coccidioidal granuloma) is caused by *Coccidioides* spp., soil-dwelling dimorphic fungi. *Coccidioides* spp. grow in the environment as spore-bearing (arthroconidia-bearing) mycelial forms. In their parasitic form, they appear as unique, endosporulating spherules in infected tissue. The 2 recognized species, *C. immitis* and *C. posadasii,* cause similar illnesses.

EPIDEMIOLOGY

Coccidioides spp. inhabit soil in arid regions. *C. immitis* is primarily found in California's San Joaquin Valley. *C. posadasii* is endemic to southern regions of Arizona, Utah, Nevada, New Mexico, western Texas, and regions of Mexico and Central and South America.

Population migrations into endemic areas and increasing numbers of immunosuppressed persons have caused coccidioidomycosis to become an important health problem. Infection rates increased from 2000 to 2007. About 150,000 newly reported infections occur annually in the USA. Coccidioidin skin test positivity in 5-7 yr old students in a highly endemic area demonstrated a decline from 10% to 2% in a 58-yr period ending in 2000. During 2002, 153 children required hospitalization for coccidioidomycosis, and infection was fatal in 9% of cases.

Infection results from inhalation of spores. Incidence increases during windy, dry periods that follow rainy seasons. Seismic events, archaeological excavations, and other activities that disturb contaminated sites have caused outbreaks. Person-to-person transmission does not occur. Rarely, infections result from spores that contaminate fomites or grow beneath casts or wound dressings of infected patients. Infection has also resulted from transplantation of organs from infected donors and from mother to fetus or newborn. Visitors to endemic areas can acquire infections, and diagnosis may be delayed when they are evaluated in nonendemic areas. Spores are highly virulent, and *Coccidioides* spp. are potential agents of bioterrorism (Chapter 704).

PATHOGENESIS

Inhaled spores reach terminal bronchioles where they transform into septated spherules that resist phagocytosis and within which many endospores develop. Released endospores transform into new spherules, and the process results in an acute focus of infection. Endospores can also disseminate lymphohematogenously. Eventually, a granulomatous reaction predominates. Both recovery and protection upon re-exposure depend on effective cellular immunity.

CLINICAL MANIFESTATIONS

The clinical spectrum (Fig. 232-1) encompasses pulmonary and extrapulmonary disease. Pulmonary infection occurs in 95% of cases and can be divided into primary, complicated, and residual infections. About 60% of infections are asymptomatic. Symptoms in children are milder than those in adults. The incidence of extrapulmonary dissemination in children approaches that of adults.

Primary Coccidioidomycosis

The incubation period is 1-4 wk, with an average of 10-16 days. Early symptoms include malaise, chills, fever, and night sweats. Chest discomfort occurs in 50-70% of patients and varies from mild tightness to severe pain. Headache and/or backache are sometimes reported. An evanescent, generalized, fine macular erythematous or urticarial eruption may be seen within the first few days of infection. Erythema nodosum can occur (more often in women) and is sometimes accompanied by an erythema multiforme rash, usually 3-21 days after the onset of symptoms. The

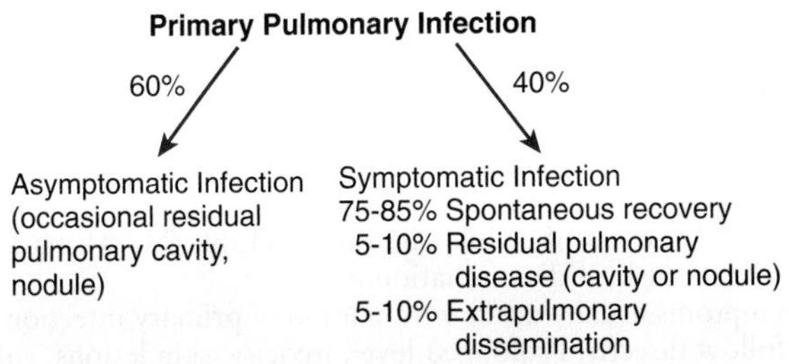

Figure 232-1 Natural history of coccidioidomycosis.

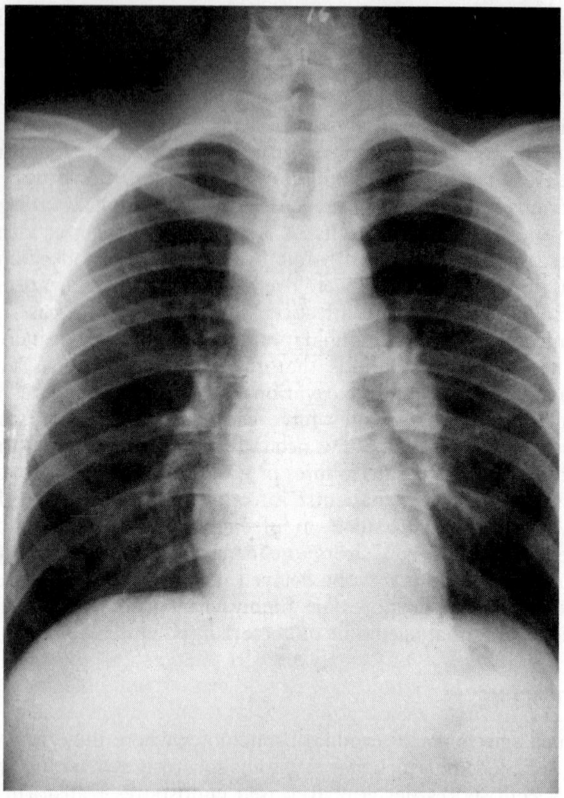

Figure 232-2 Chest radiograph of a 19 yr old man with acute primary coccidioidomycosis. There is prominent hilar lymphadenopathy and mediastinal widening.

clinical constellation of erythema nodosum, fever, chest pain, and arthralgias (especially knees and ankles) has been termed *desert rheumatism* and *valley fever*. The chest examination is often normal even if radiographic findings are present. Dullness to percussion, friction rub, or fine rales may be present. Pleural effusions can occur and can become large enough to compromise respiratory status. Hilar and mediastinal lymphadenopathy are common (Fig. 232-2).

Complicated Pulmonary Infection

Complicated infections include severe and persistent pneumonia, progressive primary coccidioidomycosis, progressive fibrocavitary disease, transient cavities that develop in areas of pulmonary consolidation, and empyema that follows rupture of a cavity into the pleural space. Some cavities persist, are thin-walled, peripheral, and cause no symptoms; occasionally there is mild hemoptysis, and rarely there is serious hemorrhage. Rarely, acute respiratory insufficiency occurs following intense exposure; this is associated with high mortality.

Residual Pulmonary Coccidioidomycosis

Residual pulmonary coccidioidomycosis includes fibrosis as well as persisting pulmonary nodules. Nodules are present in 5-7% of infections and sometimes require differentiation from malignancy.

Dissseminated (Extrapulmonary) Infection

Clinically apparent dissemination occurs in 0.5% of patients. Its incidence is increased in infants; men; persons of Filipino, African, and Latin American ancestry; and in other Asians. Primary or acquired disorders of cellular immunity (Table 232-1) markedly increase the risk of dissemination.

Symptoms usually occur within 6 mo of primary infection and can follow directly. Prolonged fever, toxicity, skin lesions, subcutaneous and/or osseous cold abscesses, and laryngeal lesions can herald onset. Organism-specific skin lesions have a predilection for the nasolabial area and appear initially as papules, which evolve to form pustules, plaques, abscesses, and verrucous plaques. Biopsy of these lesions demonstrates spherules. Basilar meningitis is the most common manifestation and may be accompanied by ventriculitis, ependymitis, cerebral vasculitis, abscess, and syringomyelia. Headache, vomiting, meningismus, and cranial nerve dysfunction are often present. Untreated meningitis is almost invariably fatal. Bone infections account for 20-50% of extrapulmonary manifestations, are often multifocal, and can affect adjacent structures. Miliary dissemination and peritonitis can mimic tuberculosis.

Table 232-1 RISK FACTORS FOR POOR OUTCOME IN PATIENTS WITH ACTIVE COCCIDIOIDOMYCOSIS

PRIMARY INFECTIONS
Severe, prolonged (≥6 wk), or progressive infection
RISK FACTORS FOR EXTRAPULMONARY DISSEMINATION
Primary or acquired cellular immune dysfunction (including patients receiving tumor necrosis factor inhibitors)
Neonates, infants, the elderly
Male sex (adult)
Filipino, African, Native American, or Latin American ethnicity
Late-stage pregnancy and early postpartum period
Standardized complement fixation antibody titer >1:16 or increasing titer with persisting symptoms
Blood group B
HLA class II allele-DRBI*1301

DIAGNOSIS

Nonspecific tests have limited usefulness. The complete blood count might show an elevated eosinophil count, and marked eosinophilia can accompany dissemination.

Culture, Histopathologic Findings, and Antigen Detection

Although diagnostic, culture is positive in only 8.3% of respiratory tract specimens and in only 3.2% of all other sites. *Coccidioides* is isolated from clinical specimens as the spore-bearing mold form, and thus the laboratory should be informed and use special precautions when the diagnosis is suspected. The observation of endosporulating spherules in histopathologic specimens is also diagnostic.

A quantitative enzyme immunoassay (EIA) (MiraVista Diagnostics) that detects coccidioidal galactomannan in urine has excellent specificity and is positive in 70% of patients with severe infections. Although the EIA can cross-react with other endemic mycoses, interpretation is often straightforward because there is negligible geographic overlap with areas endemic for other mycoses.

Cerebrospinal fluid (CSF) analysis should be performed in patients with suspected dissemination. The findings in meningitis are similar to those seen with tuberculous meningitis (Chapter 207). Eosinophilic pleocytosis may be present. Fungal stains and culture are usually negative. Volumes of 10 mL in adults have improved the yield of culture.

Serology

Serologic tests provide valuable diagnostic information but may be falsely negative early in self-limited infections and in immunocompromised patients. Three major methods are used, including EIA, complement fixation (CF), and immunodiffusion (ID). EIA and CF tests are best done in experienced reference laboratories.

Immunoglobulin M (IgM) specific antibody becomes measurable in 50% of infected patients 1 wk after onset and in 90%

of infected patients by 3 wk. EIA is sensitive and can detect IgM and IgG antibody; it is less specific than other methods, and confirmation with ID or CF may be needed. IgG antibodies measured by CF appear between the 2nd and 3rd wk but can take several months; follow-up testing is needed if tests are negative and clinical suspicion persists. In the presence of CF titers of 1:2 or 1:4, a positive IDF test can help corroborate significance. IgG-specific antibody can persist for months, with titers elevated in proportion to the severity of illness. CF titers >1:16 are suggestive of dissemination. Direct comparison of the results of CF (IgG) antibody tests measured by different methodologies should be interpreted with caution. IgG antibody titers used to monitor disease activity should be tested concurrently with serum samples taken earlier in the illness using the same methodology.

C. immitis antibody is present in CSF in 95% of patients with meningitis and is usually diagnostic. Rarely, "spillover" in patients without meningitis but with high IgG titers in serum can be present in CSF. Isolation of *Coccidioides* from CSF culture of patients with meningitis is uncommon, although culture of large volumes of CSF may improve sensitivity.

Imaging Procedures
During primary infection, chest radiography may be normal or demonstrate consolidation, single or multiple circumscribed lesions, or soft pulmonary densities. Hilar and subcarinal lymphadenopathy is often present (see Fig. 232-2). Cavities tend to be thin-walled (Fig. 232-3). Pleural effusions vary in size. The presence of miliary or reticulonodular lesions is prognostically unfavorable. Isolated or multiple osseous lesions are usually lytic and often affect cancellous bone. Lesions can affect adjacent structures, and vertebral lesions can impact the spinal cord.

TREATMENT
Based on the few rigorous clinical trials performed in adults and the opinions of experts in the management of coccidioidomycosis, consensus treatment guidelines have been developed (Table 232-2). Consultation with experts in an area of endemicity should be considered when formulating a plan of management.

Patients should be followed closely because late relapse can occur, especially in patients who are immunosuppressed or have severe manifestations. Treatment is recommended for all HIV-infected patients with active coccidioidomycosis and CD4 counts <250/μL. Following successful treatment, antifungals may be stopped if the CD4 count exceeds 250/μL. Treatment should be continued if the CD4 count remains less than 250/μL and should be given indefinitely in all HIV-infected patients with coccidioidal meningitis.

First-line agents include oral and intravenous preparations of fluconazole (6-12 mg/kg/day IV or PO) and itraconazole (5-10 mg/kg/day). Serum levels of itraconazole should be monitored.

Amphotericin B is preferred for initial treatment of severe infections. Amphotericin B deoxycholate is less costly than lipid formulations and is often well tolerated in children. Once a daily dose of amphotericin B deoxycholate of 1-1.5 mg/kg/day is achieved, the frequency of administration can be reduced to 3 times weekly. The recommended total dosage ranges from 15 mg/kg to 45 mg/kg and is determined by the clinical response. Lipid formulations of amphotericin are recommended for patients with impaired renal function, patients receiving other nephrotoxic agents, or if amphotericin B deoxycholate is not tolerated. Some experts prefer liposomal amphotericin to treat CNS infections because it achieves higher levels in brain parenchyma. Amphotericin B preparations do not cross the blood-brain barrier to effectively treat *Coccidioides* spp., but they can mask the signs of meningitis. Infections during pregnancy should be treated with amphotericin B, because the azoles are potentially teratogenic.

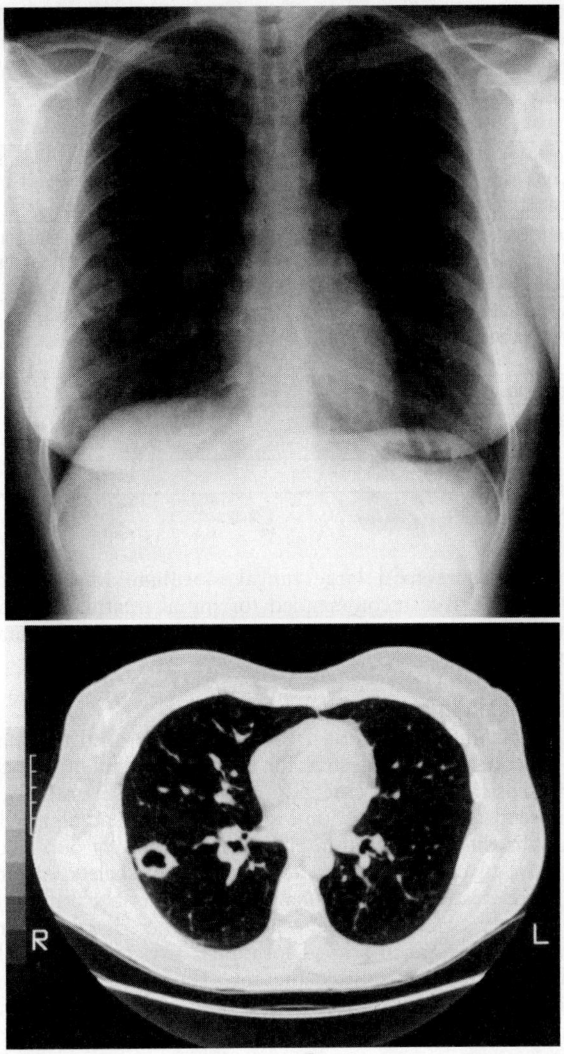

Figure 232-3 *Top*, Chest radiograph revealing a chronic cavitary lesion in the right lung of a woman with coccidioidomycosis. *Bottoml*, CT showing the same cavity in the right lung.

Voriconazole and posaconazole have been used successfully as salvage therapy in infections failing the standard agents.

Primary Pulmonary Infection
Primary pulmonary coccidioidomycosis resolves in 95% of patients without risk factors for dissemination; antifungal therapy does not lessen the frequency of dissemination or pulmonary residua. When it is elected to defer antifungal therapy, visits are recommended as needed and at 3-6 mo intervals for 2 yr and as needed.

Patients with significant or prolonged symptoms are more likely to incur benefit from antifungal agents, but there are no established criteria upon which to base the decision. Commonly used indicators in adults are summarized in Table 232-2. A treatment trial in adults with primary respiratory infections examined outcomes of antifungal therapy prescribed on the basis of severity and compared them to an untreated group with less severe symptoms; complications occurred only in patients in the treatment group and only in those in whom treatment was stopped. If treatment is elected, a 3-6 mo course of fluconazole (6-12 mg/kg/day) or itraconazole (5-10 mg/kg/day) is recommended.

Diffuse Pneumonia
Diffuse reticulonodular densities or miliary infiltrates, sometimes accompanied by severe illness, can occur in dissemination or

Table 232-2 INDICATIONS FOR TREATMENT OF COCCIDIOIDOMYCOSIS IN ADULTS

INDICATION	TREATMENT
Acute pneumonia, mild	Observe without antifungal treatment at 1-3 mo intervals for ≥1 yr; some experts recommend antifungal treatment
Weight loss >10%; sweats >3 wk; infiltrates at least half of one lung or parts of both lungs; prominent or persistent hilar lymphadenopathy; CF titers >1:16; inability to work, symptoms >2 mo	Treat with an azole daily for 3-6 mo, with follow up at 1-3 mo intervals for ≥1 yr
Uncomplicated acute pneumonia, special circumstances: immunosuppression, late pregnancy, Filipino or African ancestry, age >55 yr, other chronic diseases (diabetes, cardiopulmonary disease), symptoms >2 mo	Treat with an azole daily for 3-6 mo, with follow up at 1-3 mo intervals for ≥1 yr Treat with amphotericin B if in late pregnancy
Diffuse pneumonia: reticulonodular or miliary infiltrates suggest underlying immunodeficiency and possible fungemia, pain	Treat initially with amphotericin B if significant hypoxia or rapid deterioration, followed by an azole for ≥1 yr In mild cases, an azole for ≥1 yr
Chronic pneumonia	Treat with an azole for ≥1 yr
Disseminated disease, nonmeningeal	Treat with an azole for ≥1 yr except in severe or rapidly worsening cases for which amphotericin B is recommended
Disseminated disease, meningeal	Treat with fluconazole (some add intrathecal amphotericin B) and treat indefinitely

CF, complement fixation.

follow exposure to a large fungal inoculum. In this setting, amphotericin B is recommended for initial treatment followed thereafter by extended treatment with high-dose fluconazole (Table 232-2).

Disseminated Infection (Extrapulmonary)

For **nonmeningeal infection** (see Table 232-2), oral fluconazole and itraconazole are effective for treating disseminated coccidioidomycosis that is not extensive, is not progressing rapidly, and has not affected the CNS. Some experts recommend higher doses for adults than were used in clinical trials. A subgroup analysis showed a tendency for improved response of skeletal infections that were treated with itraconazole. Amphotericin B deoxycholate is used as an alternative, especially if there is rapid worsening and lesions are in critical locations. Voriconazole has been used successfully as salvage therapy. The optimal duration of therapy with the azoles has not been clearly defined. Late relapses have occurred after lengthy treatment and favorable clinical response.

Meningitis

Therapy with oral fluconazole is currently preferred for coccidioidal meningitis. In adults, a dosage >400 mg/day is recommended by some experts. Itraconazole at a dosage of 400-600 mg/day in adults has been reported to have a comparable effect. Some experts use intrathecal, intraventricular, or intracisternally administered amphotericin B in addition to an azole, believing that the clinical response may be faster. Patients who respond to the azole should continue treatment indefinitely. Hydrocephalus is a common occurrence and is not necessarily a marker of treatment failure. In the event of treatment failure with azoles, intrathecal therapy with amphotericn B deoxycholate is indicated, with or without the azole treatment. Cerebral vasculitis can occur and can predispose to cerebral ischemia, infarction, or hemorrhage. The efficacy of steroids in high dosage is unresolved. Salvage therapy with voriconazole has been found to be effective.

Surgical Management

If a cavity is located peripherally or there is recurrent bleeding or pleural extension, excision may be needed. Infrequently, bronchopleural fistula or recurrent cavitation occur as surgical complications; rarely, dissemination can result. Perioperative intravenous therapy with amphotericin B may be considered. Drainage of cold abscesses, synovectomy, and curettage or excision of osseous lesions are sometimes needed. Local and systemic administration of amphotericin B can be used to treat coccidioidal articular disease.

PREVENTION

Prevention relies on education about ways to reduce exposure. Physicians practicing in nonendemic regions should incorporate careful travel histories when evaluating patients with symptoms compatible with coccidioidomycosis.

BIBLIOGRAPHY

Please visit the Nelson Textbook of Pediatrics *website at www.expertconsult.com for the complete bibliography.*

Chapter 233
Paracoccidioides brasiliensis

Jane M. Gould and Stephen C. Aronoff

ETIOLOGY

Paracoccidioidomycosis (South American or Brazilian blastomycosis, Lutz-Splendore-Almeida disease) is an uncommon fungal infection endemic in South America, with cases reported in Central America and Mexico. The etiologic agent, *Paracoccidioides brasiliensis*, is a thermally dimorphic fungus found in the environment in the mycelial (mold) form and in tissues as yeast.

For the full continuation of this chapter, please visit the Nelson Textbook of Pediatrics *website at www.expertconsult.com.*

Chapter 234
Sporotrichosis *(Sporothrix schenckii)*

David M. Fleece and Stephen C. Aronoff

ETIOLOGY

Sporotrichosis is a rare fungal infection that occurs worldwide both sporadically and in outbreaks. The etiologic agent, *Sporothrix schenckii*, exhibits temperature dimorphism, existing as a mold at environmental temperatures (25°C-30°C) and as a yeast in vivo (37°C).

For the full continuation of this chapter, please visit the Nelson Textbook of Pediatrics *website at www.expertconsult.com.*

Chapter 235
Zygomycosis (Mucormycosis)
Jane M. Gould and Stephen C. Aronoff

ETIOLOGY

Zygomycosis refers to a group of opportunistic fungal infections caused by dimorphic fungi of the class Zygomycetes, which are primitive, fast-growing fungi that are largely saprophytic and ubiquitous. These organisms are found commonly in soil, in decaying plant and animal matter, and on moldy cheese, fruit, and bread.

For the full continuation of this chapter, please visit the Nelson Textbook of Pediatrics *website at www.expertconsult.com.*

Chapter 236
Pneumocystis jirovecii
Francis Gigliotti and Terry W. Wright

Pneumocystis jirovecii pneumonia (interstitial plasma cell pneumonitis) in an immunocompromised person is a life-threatening infection. Primary infection in the immunocompetent person is usually subclinical and goes unrecognized. The disease most likely results from new or repeat acquisition of the organism rather than reactivation of latent organisms. Even in the most severe cases, with rare exceptions, the organisms remain localized to the lungs.

For the full continuation of this chapter, please visit the Nelson Textbook of Pediatrics *website at www.expertconsult.com.*

Section 13 VIRAL INFECTIONS

Chapter 237
Principles of Antiviral Therapy
Mark R. Schleiss

Antiviral chemotherapy typically involves a delicate interplay between host cellular functions and viral targets of action. Many antiviral agents exert significant host cellular toxicity, a limitation that has hindered antiviral drug development. In spite of this limitation, a number of agents are licensed for use against viruses, particularly herpesviruses, respiratory viruses, and hepatitis viruses. In addition to licensed antivirals and recommended regimens (see Table 237-1 on the *Nelson Textbook of Pediatrics* website at www.expertconsult.com), several studies are actively enrolling children for evaluation of novel antiviral therapeutic approaches. These studies are funded by the National Institutes of Health and administered through the Collaborative Antiviral Study Group (CASG), and up-to-date information is available about active clinical protocols at the CASG web page (*http://medicine.uab.edu/Peds/CASG/*).

For the full continuation of this chapter, please visit the Nelson Textbook of Pediatrics *website at www.expertconsult.com.*

Chapter 238
Measles
Wilbert H. Mason

Measles is highly contagious and was once an inevitable experience during childhood. Owing to widespread vaccination, endemic transmission has been interrupted in the USA; indigenous or imported cases (in children or adults) have occasionally resulted in epidemics in the USA in unimmunized or partially immunized American or foreign-born children. In some areas of the world, measles remains a serious threat to children.

ETIOLOGY

Measles virus is a single-stranded, lipid-enveloped RNA virus in the family Paramyxoviridae and genus *Morbillivirus*. Other members of the genus *Morbillivirus* affect a variety of mammals, such as rinderpest virus in cattle and distemper virus in dogs, but humans are the only host of measles virus. Of the 6 major structural proteins of measles virus, the 2 most important in terms of induction of immunity are the hemagglutinin (H) protein and the fusion (F) protein. The neutralizing antibodies are directed against the H protein, and antibodies to the F protein limit proliferation of the virus during infection. Small variations in genetic composition have also been identified that result in no effect on protective immunity but provide molecular markers that can distinguish between viral types. These markers have been useful in the evaluation of endemic spread of measles.

EPIDEMIOLOGY

The measles vaccine has changed the epidemiology of measles dramatically. Once worldwide in distribution, endemic transmission of measles has been interrupted in many countries where there is widespread vaccine coverage. Historically, measles caused universal infection in childhood in the USA, with 90% of children acquiring the infection before 15 yr of age. Morbidity and mortality associated with measles decreased prior to the introduction of the vaccine as a result of improvements in health care and nutrition. However, the incidence declined dramatically following the introduction of the measles vaccine in 1963. The attack rate fell from 313 cases/100,000 population in 1956-1960 to 1.3 cases/100,000 in 1982-1988.

A nationwide indigenous measles outbreak occurred in 1989-1991, resulting in >55,000 cases, 11,000 hospitalizations, and 123 deaths, demonstrating that the infection had not yet been conquered. This resurgence was attributed to vaccine failure in a small number of school-aged children, low coverage of preschool-aged children, and more rapid waning of maternal antibodies in infants born to mothers who had never experienced wild-type measles infection. Implementation of the 2-dose vaccine policy and more intensive immunization strategies resulted in interruption of endemic transmission in the USA in 1993. The current rate is <1 case/1,000,000 population.

Measles continues to be imported into the USA from abroad; therefore, continued maintenance of >90% immunity through vaccination is necessary to prevent widespread outbreaks from occurring (Fig. 238-1).

In 2008, 131 cases of measles were reported to the U.S. Centers for Disease Control and Prevention (CDC) in the first 7 months of the year, the highest year-to-date number of cases since 1996. Seven outbreaks accounted for 106 (81%) of the cases. Of the total, 17 patients (13%) had acquired the infection abroad

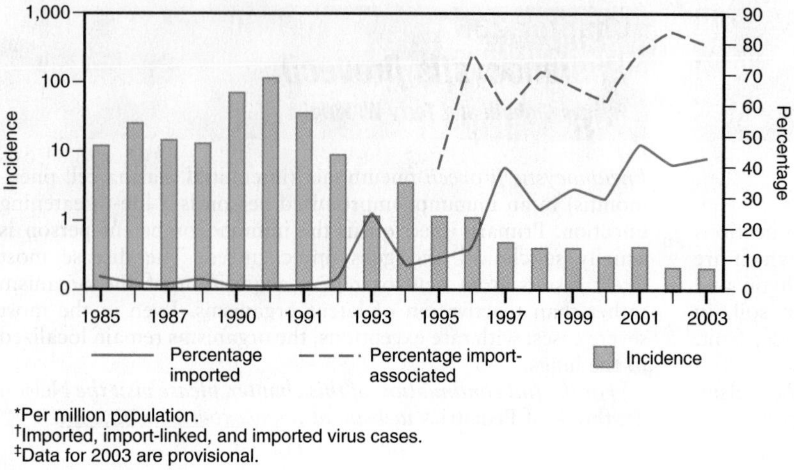

Figure 238-1 Incidence* and percentage of import-associated† measles cases, by year in the USA, 1985–2003‡. (From the Centers for Disease Control and Prevention: Epidemiology of measles—United States, 2001–2003, *MMWR Morb Mortal Wkly Rep* 53:713–716, 2004.)

and 99 cases (76%) were linked epidemiologically with the importations. These importation-associated cases occurred primarily among unvaccinated school-aged children whose parents had religious or philosophical objections to vaccination. Measles continues to be imported from abroad, and outbreaks will continue to occur in communities with low vaccination rates.

TRANSMISSION

The portal of entry of measles virus is through the respiratory tract or conjunctivae following contact with large droplets or small-droplet aerosols in which the virus is suspended. Patients are infectious from 3 days before to up to 4-6 days after the onset of rash. Approximately 90% of exposed susceptible individuals experience measles. Face-to-face contact is not necessary, because viable virus may be suspended in air for as long as 1 hr after the patient with the source case leaves a room. Secondary cases due to spread of aerosolized virus have been reported in physicians' offices and in hospitals.

PATHOLOGY

Measles infection causes necrosis of the respiratory tract epithelium and an accompanying lymphocytic infiltrate. Measles produces a small vessel vasculitis on the skin and on the oral mucous membranes. Histology of the rash and exanthem reveals intracellular edema and dyskeratosis associated with formation of epidermal syncytial giant cells with up to 26 nuclei. Viral particles have been identified within these giant cells. In lymphoreticular tissue, lymphoid hyperplasia is prominent. Fusion of infected cells results in multinucleated giant cells, the **Warthin-Finkeldey giant cells** that are pathognomonic for measles, with up to 100 nuclei and intracytoplasmic and intranuclear inclusions.

PATHOGENESIS

Measles consists of 4 phases: incubation period, prodromal illness, exanthematous phase, and recovery. During incubation, measles virus migrates to regional lymph nodes. A primary viremia ensues that disseminates the virus to the reticuloendothelial system. A secondary viremia spreads virus to body surfaces. The prodromal illness begins after the secondary viremia and is associated with epithelial necrosis and giant cell formation in body tissues. Cells are killed by cell-to-cell plasma membrane fusion associated with viral replication that occurs in many body tissues, including cells of the central nervous system (CNS). Virus shedding begins in the prodromal phase. With onset of the rash, antibody production begins, and viral replication and symptoms begin to subside. Measles virus also infects CD4+ T cells, resulting in suppression of the Th1 immune response and a multitude of other immunosuppressive effects.

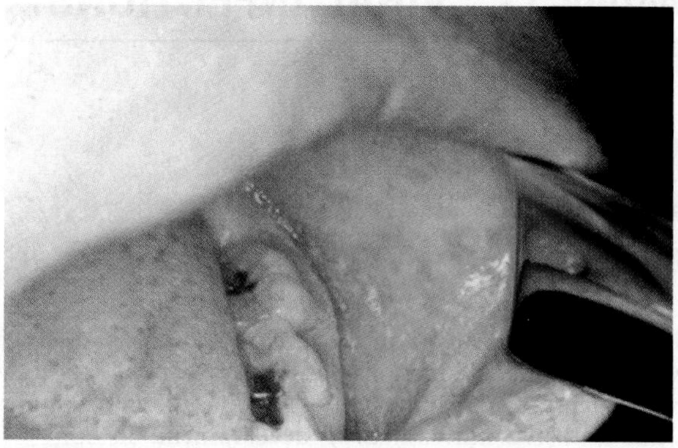

Figure 238-2 Koplik spots on the buccal mucosa during the 3rd day of rash. (From Centers for Disease Control and Prevention: *Public health image library, image #4500* [website]. http://phil.cdc.gov/phil/details.asp.)

CLINICAL MANIFESTATIONS

Measles is a serious infection characterized by high fever, an enanthem, cough, coryza, conjunctivitis, and a prominent exanthem. After an incubation period of 8-12 days, the prodromal phase begins with a mild fever followed by the onset of conjunctivitis with photophobia, coryza, a prominent cough, and increasing fever. **Koplik spots** represent the enanthem and are the pathognomonic sign of measles, appearing 1 to 4 days prior to the onset of the rash (Fig. 238-2). They first appear as discrete red lesions with bluish white spots in the center on the inner aspects of the cheeks at the level of the premolars. They may spread to involve the lips, hard palate, and gingiva. They also may occur in conjunctival folds and in the vaginal mucosa. Koplik spots have been reported in 50-70% of measles cases but probably occur in the great majority.

Symptoms increase in intensity for 2-4 days until the 1st day of the rash. The rash begins on the forehead (around the hairline), behind the ears, and on the upper neck as a red maculopapular eruption. It then spreads downward to the torso and extremities, reaching the palms and soles in up to 50% of cases. The exanthem frequently becomes confluent on the face and upper trunk (Fig. 238-3).

With the onset of the rash, symptoms begin to subside. The rash fades over about 7 days in the same progression as it evolved, often leaving a fine desquamation of skin in its wake. Of the major symptoms of measles, the cough lasts the longest, often up

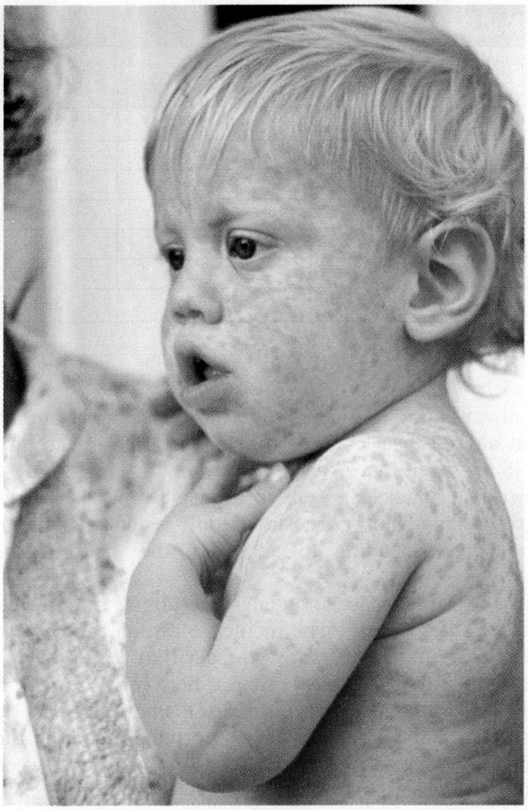

Figure 238-3 A child with measles displaying the characteristic red blotchy pattern on his face and body. (From Kremer JR, Muller CP: Measles in Europe—there is room for improvement, *Lancet* 373:356–358, 2009.)

to 10 days. In more severe cases, generalized lymphadenopathy may be present, with cervical and occipital lymph nodes especially prominent.

INAPPARENT MEASLES INFECTION

In individuals with passively acquired antibody, such as infants and recipients of blood products, a subclinical form of measles may occur. The rash may be indistinct, brief, or, rarely, entirely absent. Likewise, some individuals who have received vaccine, when exposed to measles, may have a rash but few other symptoms. Persons with inapparent or subclinical measles do not shed measles virus and do not transmit infection to household contacts.

Children who had received the original formalin-inactivated measles vaccine at times demonstrated a more severe form of disease called **atypical measles.** Such patients had onset of high fever and headache followed by the appearance of a maculopapular rash on the extremities that become petechial and purpuric and progressed in a centripetal direction. The illness was frequently complicated by pneumonia and pleural effusions. It is thought that atypical measles was caused by development of circulating immune complexes that formed as a result of an abnormal immune response to the vaccine.

LABORATORY FINDINGS

The diagnosis of measles is almost always based on clinical and epidemiologic findings. Laboratory findings in the acute phase include reduction in the total white blood cell count, with lymphocytes decreased more than neutrophils. Absolute neutropenia has been known to occur, however. In measles not complicated by bacterial infection, the erythrocyte sedimentation rate and C-reactive protein level are normal.

DIAGNOSIS

In the absence of a recognized measles outbreak, confirmation of the clinical diagnosis is often recommended. Serologic confirmation is most conveniently made by identification of immunoglobulin M (IgM) antibody in serum. IgM antibody appears 1-2 days after the onset of the rash and remains detectable for about 1 mo. If a serum specimen is collected <72 hr after onset of rash and is negative for measles antibody, a second specimen should be obtained. Serologic confirmation may also be made by demonstration of a fourfold rise in IgG antibodies in acute and convalescent specimens collected 2-4 wk later. Viral isolation from blood, urine, or respiratory secretions can be accomplished by culture at the CDC or local or state laboratories. Molecular detection by polymerase chain reaction (PCR) is possible but is a research tool.

DIFFERENTIAL DIAGNOSIS

Typical measles is unlikely to be confused with other illnesses, especially if Koplik spots are observed. Measles in the later stages or inapparent or subclinical infections may be confused with a number of other exanthematous immune-mediated illnesses and infections, including rubella, adenoviruses, enteroviruses, and Epstein-Barr virus. Exanthem subitum (in infants) and erythema infectiosum (in older children) may also be confused with measles. *Mycoplasma pneumoniae* and group A streptococcus may also produce rashes similar to that of measles. Kawasaki syndrome can cause many of the same findings as measles but lacks discrete intraoral lesions (Koplik spots) and a severe prodromal cough, and typically leads to elevations of neutrophils and acute-phase reactants. In addition, the characteristic thrombocytosis of Kawasaki syndrome is absent in measles (Chapter 160). Drug eruptions may occasionally be mistaken for measles.

COMPLICATIONS

Complications of measles are largely attributable to the pathogenic effects of the virus on the respiratory tract and immune system (Table 238-1). Several factors make complications more likely. Morbidity and mortality from measles are greatest in patients <5 yr of age (especially <1 yr of age) and >20 yr of age. In developing countries, higher case fatality rates have been associated with crowding, which are possibly attributable to larger inoculum doses after household exposure. Severe malnutrition in children results in suboptimal immune response and higher morbidity and mortality with measles infection. Low serum retinol levels in children with measles have been shown to be associated with higher measles morbidity and mortality in developing countries and in the USA. Measles infection lowers serum retinol concentrations, so subclinical cases of hyporetinolemia may be made symptomatic during measles. Measles infection in immunocompromised persons is associated with increased morbidity and mortality. Among patients with malignancy in whom measles develops, pneumonitis occurs in 58% and encephalitis in 20%.

Pneumonia is the most common cause of death in measles. It may manifest as **giant cell pneumonia** caused directly by the viral infection or as superimposed bacterial infection. The most common bacterial pathogens are *Streptococcus pneumoniae, Haemophilus influenzae,* and *Staphylococcus aureus.* Following severe measles pneumonia, the final common pathway to a fatal outcome is often the development of bronchiolitis obliterans.

Croup, tracheitis, and bronchiolitis are common complications in infants and toddlers with measles. The clinical severity of these complications frequently requires intubation and ventilatory support until the infection resolves.

Acute otitis media is the most common complication of measles and was of particularly high incidence during the epi-

Table 238-1 COMPLICATIONS BY AGE FOR REPORTED MEASLES CASES, USA, 1987-2000

COMPLICATION	OVERALL (67,032 CASES WITH AGE INFORMATION)	NO. (%) OF PERSONS WITH COMPLICATION BY AGE GROUP				
		<5 yr (n = 28,730)	5-9 yr (n = 6,492)	10-19 yr (n = 18,580)	20-29 yr (n = 9,161)	<30 yr (n = 4,069)
Any	19,480 (29.1)	11,883 (41.4)	1,173 (18.1)	2,369 (12.8)	2,656 (29.0)	1,399 (34.4)
Death	177 (0.3)	97 (0.3)	9 (0.1)	18 (0.1)	26 (0.3)	27 (0.7)
Diarrhea	5,482 (8.2)	3,294 (11.5)	408 (6.3)	627 (3.4)	767 (8.4)	386 (9.5)
Encephalitis	97 (0.1)	43 (0.2)	9 (0.1)	13 (0.1)	21 (0.2)	11 (0.3)
Hospitalization	12,876 (19.2)	7,470 (26.0)	612 (9.4)	1,612 (8.7)	2,075 (22.7)	1,107 (27.2)
Otitis media	4,879 (7.3)	4,009 (14.0)	305 (4.7)	338 (1.8)	157 (1.7)	70 (1.7)
Pneumonia	3,959 (5.9)	2,480 (8.6)	183 (2.8)	363 (2.0)	554 (6.1)	379 (9.3)

From Perry RT, Halsey NA: The clinical significance of measles: a review, *Clin Infect Dis* 189(Suppl 1):S4–S16, 2004.

demic of the late 1980s and early 1990s because of the relatively young age of affected children. Sinusitis and mastoiditis also occur as complications. Viral and/or bacterial tracheitis is seen and can be life threatening. Retropharyngeal abscess has also been reported.

Measles infection is known to suppress skin test responsiveness to purified tuberculin antigen. There may be a higher rate of activation of pulmonary tuberculoses in populations of individuals infected with *Mycobacterium tuberculosis* who are then exposed to measles.

Diarrhea and vomiting are common symptoms associated with acute measles, and diffuse giant cell formation is found in the epithelium the gastrointestinal tract. Dehydration is a common consequence, especially in young infants and children. Appendicitis may occur from obstruction of the appendiceal lumen by lymphoid hyperplasia.

Febrile seizures occur in <3% of children with measles. Encephalitis following measles has been a long-associated complication, often with an unfavorable outcome. Rates of 1-3/1,000 cases of measles have been reported, with greater numbers occurring in adolescents and adults than in preschool or school-aged children. Encephalitis is a postinfectious, immunologically mediated process and is not due to a direct effect by the virus. Clinical onset begins during the exanthem and manifests as seizures (56%), lethargy (46%), coma (28%), and irritability (26%). Findings in cerebrospinal fluid (CSF) include lymphocytic pleocytosis in 85% of cases and elevated protein concentration. Approximately 15% of patients with measles encephalitis die, and 20-40% suffer long-term sequelae, including mental retardation, motor disabilities, and deafness.

Measles encephalitis in immunocompromised patients results from direct damage to the brain by the virus. Subacute measles encephalitis manifests 1-10 mo after measles in immunocompromised patients, particularly those with AIDS, lymphoreticular malignancies, and immunosuppression. Signs and symptoms include seizures, myoclonus, stupor, and coma. In addition to intracellular inclusions, abundant viral nucleocapsids and viral antigen are seen in brain tissue. Progressive disease and death almost always occur.

A severe form of measles rarely seen now is **hemorrhagic measles** or **"black measles."** It manifested as a hemorrhagic skin eruption and was often fatal. Keratitis, appearing as multiple punctate epithelial foci, resolved with recovery from the infection. Thrombocytopenia sometimes occurred following measles.

Myocarditis is a rare complication of measles. Miscellaneous bacterial infections have been reported, including bacteremia, cellulitis, and toxic shock syndrome. Measles during pregnancy has been associated with high maternal morbidity, fetal wastage and stillbirths, and congenital malformations in 3% of live born infants.

Subacute Sclerosing Panencephalitis

Subacute sclerosing panencephalitis (SSPE) is a chronic complication of measles with a delayed onset and an outcome that is nearly always fatal. It appears to result from a persistent infection with an altered measles virus that is harbored intracellularly in the CNS for several yr. After 7-10 yr the virus apparently regains virulence and attacks the cells in the CNS that offered the virus protection. This "slow virus infection" results in inflammation and cell death, leading to an inexorable neurodegenerative process.

SSPE is a rare disease and generally follows the prevalence of measles in a population. The incidence rate in the USA in 1960 was 0.61 cases/million persons younger than 20 yr. By 1980 the rate had fallen to 0.06 cases/ million. Between 1956 and 1982 a total of 634 cases had been reported to the national SSPE registry. After 1982 about 5 cases/ yr were reported annually in the USA, and only 2-3 cases/ yr in the early 1990s. However, between 1995 and 2000, reported cases in the USA increased and 13 cases were reported in 2000. Nine of the 13 cases occurred in foreign-born individuals. This "resurgence" may be the result of an increased incidence of measles between 1989 and 1991. Although the age of onset ranges from <1 to <30 yr, the illness is primarily one of children and adolescents. Measles at an early age favors the development of SSPE: 50% of patients with SSPE had primary measles before 2 yr of age, and 75% before 4 yr of age. Males are affected twice as often as females, and there appear to be more cases reported from rural rather than urban populations. Recent observations from the registry indicate a higher prevalence among children of Hispanic origin.

The pathogenesis of SSPE remains enigmatic. Factors that seem to be involved include defective measles virus and interaction with a defective or immature immune system. The virus isolated from brain tissue of patients with SSPE is missing 1 of the 6 structural proteins, the matrix or M protein. This protein is responsible for assembly, orientation, and alignment of the virus in preparation for budding during viral replication. Immature virus may be able to reside, and possibly propagate, within neuronal cells for long periods. The fact that most patients with SSPE were exposed at a young age suggests that immune immaturity is involved in pathogenesis. In addition, the intracellular location of the virus sequesters it from the immune system, especially from humoral immunity.

Clinical manifestations of SSPE begin insidiously 7-13 yr after primary measles infection. Subtle changes in behavior or school performance appear, including irritability, reduced attention span, and temper outbursts. This initial phase (stage I) may at times be missed because of brevity or mildness of the symptoms. Fever, headache, and other signs of encephalitis are absent. The hallmark of the second stage is massive myoclonus, which coincides with extension of the inflammatory process site to deeper structures in the brain, including the basal ganglia. Involuntary movements and repetitive myoclonic jerks begin in single muscle groups but give way to massive spasms and jerks involving both axial and appendicular muscles. Consciousness is maintained. In the third stage, involuntary movements disappear and are replaced by choreoathetosis, immobility, dystonia, and lead pipe rigidity that result from destruction of deeper centers in the basal ganglia.

Sensorium deteriorates into dementia, stupor, and then coma. The fourth stage is characterized by loss of critical centers that support breathing, heart rate, and blood pressure. Death soon ensues. Progression through the clinical stages may follow courses characterized as acute, subacute, or chronic progressive.

The diagnosis of SSPE can be established through documentation of a compatible clinical course and at least 1 of the following supporting findings: (1) measles antibody detected in CSF, (2) characteristic electroencephalographic findings, and (3) typical histologic findings in and/or isolation of virus or viral antigen from brain tissue obtained by biopsy or postmortem examination.

CSF analysis reveals normal cells but elevated IgG and IgM antibody titers in dilutions >1:8. Electroencephalographic patterns are normal in stage I, but in the myoclonic phase, suppression-burst episodes are seen that are characteristic of but not pathognomonic for SSPE. Brain biopsy is no longer routinely indicated for diagnosis of SSPE.

Management of SSPE is primarily supportive and similar to care provided to patients with other neurodegenerative diseases. A large randomized clinical trial compared the use of oral inosine pranobex (isoprinosine) alone to oral inosine pranobex and intraventricular interferon-α2b. The treatment courses for both groups were 6 months. Although there were no differences in the rates of stabilization or improvement at 6 months (34% vs 35%), the investigators concluded that these rates were substantially better than historically reported spontaneous improvement rates, which are 5-10%.

Virtually all patients eventually succumb to SSPE. Most die within 1-3 yr of onset from infection or loss of autonomic control mechanisms. Prevention of SSPE depends on prevention of primary measles infection through vaccination. SSPE has been described in patients who have no history of measles infection and only exposure to the vaccine virus. However, wild-type virus, not vaccine virus, has been found in brain tissue of at least some of these patients, suggesting that they had had subclinical measles previously.

TREATMENT

Management of measles is supportive. Antiviral therapy is not effective in the treatment of measles in otherwise normal patients. Maintenance of hydration, oxygenation, and comfort are goals of therapy. Antipyretics for comfort and fever control are useful. For patients with respiratory tract involvement, airway humidification and supplemental oxygen may be of benefit. Respiratory failure due to croup or pneumonia may require ventilatory support. Oral rehydration is effective in most cases, but severe dehydration may require intravenous therapy. Prophylactic antimicrobial therapy to prevent bacterial infection is not indicated.

Measles infection in immunocompromised patients is highly lethal. Ribavirin is active in vitro against measles virus. Anecdotal reports of ribavirin therapy with or without intravenous gamma globulin suggest some benefit in individual patients. However, no controlled trials have been performed, and ribavirin is not licensed in the USA for treatment of measles.

Vitamin A

Vitamin A deficiency in children in developing countries has long been known to be associated with increased mortality from a variety of infectious diseases, including measles. In the USA, studies in the early 1990s documented that 22-72% of children with measles had low retinol levels. In addition, one study demonstrated an inverse correlation between the level of retinol and severity of illness. Several randomized controlled trials of vitamin A therapy in the developing world and the USA have demonstrated reduced morbidity and mortality from measles. The American Academy of Pediatrics suggests vitamin A therapy for selected patients with measles (Table 238-2).

Table 238-2 RECOMMENDATIONS FOR VITAMIN A TREATMENT OF CHILDREN WITH MEASLES

INDICATIONS
Children 6 mo-2 yr of age hospitalized with measles and its complications (e.g., croup, pneumonia, and diarrhea). (Limited data are available about the safety of and need for vitamin A supplementation for infants <6 mo of age).
Children >6 mo of age with measles who are not already receiving vitamin A supplementation and who have any of the following risk factors: • Immunodeficiency • Clinical evidence of vitamin A deficiency • Impaired intestinal absorption • Moderate to severe malnutrition • Recent immigration from areas where high mortality rates attributed to measles have been observed
REGIMEN
Parenteral and oral formulations of vitamin A are available in the USA. The recommended dosage, administered as a capsule, is: • Single dose of 200,000 IU orally for children ≥1 yr of age (100,000 IU for children 6 mo–1 yr of age and 50,000 IU for infants <6 mo of age)
The dose should be repeated the next day and again 4 wk later for children with ophthalmologic evidence of vitamin A deficiency

Data from the American Academy of Pediatrics: *Red book: 2009 report of the Committee on Infectious Diseases*, ed 28, Elk Grove Village, IL, 2009, American Academy of Pediatrics, p 446.

PROGNOSIS

In the early 20th century, deaths due to measles varied between 2,000 and 10,000, or about 10 deaths per 1,000 cases of measles. With improvements in health care and antimicrobial therapy, better nutrition, and decreased crowding, the death-to-case ratio fell to 1/1,000 cases. Between 1982 and 2002, the CDC estimated that there were 259 deaths caused by measles in the USA, with a death-to-case ratio of 2.5-2.8/1,000 cases of measles. Pneumonia and encephalitis were complications in most of the fatal cases, and immunodeficiency conditions were identified in 14-16% of deaths.

PREVENTION

Patients shed measles virus from 7 days after exposure to 4-6 days after the onset of rash. Exposure of susceptible individuals to patients with measles should be avoided during this period. In hospitals, standard and airborne precautions should be observed for this period. Immunocompromised patients with measles will shed virus for the duration of the illness, so isolation should be maintained throughout the disease.

Vaccine

Measles vaccine in the USA is available as a monovalent preparation or combined with the rubella (MR) or measles-mumps-rubella (MMR) vaccine, the last of which is the recommended form in most circumstances (Table 238-3). Following the measles resurgence of 1989-1991, a second dose of measles vaccine was added to the schedule. The current recommendations include a first dose at 12-15 mo followed by a second dose at 4-6 yr of age. Seroconversion is slightly lower in children who receive the first dose before or at 12 mo of age (87% at 9 mo, 95% at 12 mo, and 98% at 15 mo) because of persisting maternal antibody. For children who have not received 2 doses by 11-12 yr of age, a second dose should be provided. Infants who receive a dose before 12 mo of age should be given 2 additional doses at 12-15 mo and 4-6 yr of age.

Adverse events from the MMR vaccine include fever (usually 6-12 days following vaccination), rash in about 5% of vaccines, and, rarely, transient thrombocytopenia. Children prone to febrile seizures may experience an event following vaccination, so the risks and benefits of vaccination should be discussed with parents. Encephalopathy and autism have not been shown to

Table 238-3 RECOMMENDATIONS FOR MEASLES IMMUNIZATION

CATEGORY	RECOMMENDATIONS
Unimmunized, no history of measles (12-15 mo of age)	A 2-dose schedule (with MMR) is recommended The first dose is recommended at 12-15 mo of age; the 2nd is recommended at 4-6 yr of age
Children 6-11 mo of age in epidemic situations or prior to international travel	Immunize (with monovalent measles vaccine, or if not available, MMR); reimmunization (with MMR) at 12-15 mo of age is necessary, and a 3rd dose is indicated at 4-6 yr of age
Children 4-12 yr of age who have received 1 dose of measles vaccine at ≥12 mo of age	Reimmunize (1 dose)
Students in college and other post–high school institutions who have received 1 dose of measles vaccine at ≥12 mo of age	Reimmunize (1 dose)
History of immunization before the 1st birthday	Consider susceptible and immunize (2 doses)
History of receipt of inactivated measles vaccine or unknown type of vaccine, 1963-1967	Consider susceptible and immunize (2 doses)
Further attenuated or unknown vaccine given with IG	Consider susceptible and immunize (2 doses)
Allergy to eggs	Immunize; no reactions likely
Neomycin allergy, nonanaphylactic	Immunize; no reactions likely
Severe hypersensitivity (anaphylaxis) to neomycin or gelatin	Avoid immunization
Tuberculosis	Immunize; if patient has untreated tuberculosis disease, start antituberculosis therapy before immunizing
Measles exposure	Immunize and/or give IG, depending on circumstances
HIV-infected	Immunize (2 doses) unless severely immunocompromised
Personal or family history of seizures	Immunize; advise parents of slightly increased risk of seizures
IG or blood recipient	Immunize at the appropriate interval (see Table 238-4)

IG, immunoglobulin; MMR, measles-mumps-rubella vaccine.
From American Academy of Pediatrics: *Red book: 2009 report of the Committee on Infectious Diseases,* ed 28, Elk Grove Village, IL, 2009, American Academy of Pediatrics, p 450.

Table 238-4 SUGGESTED INTERVALS BETWEEN IMMUNOGLOBULIN ADMINISTRATION AND MEASLES IMMUNIZATION*

INDICATION FOR IMMUNOGLOBULIN	DOSE			
	Route	Units (U) or Milliliters (mL)	mg IgG/kg	Interval (mo)†
Tetanus (as tetanus IG)	IM	250 U	10	3
Hepatitis A prophylaxis (as IG):				
Contact prophylaxis	IM	0.02 mL/kg	3.3	3
International travel	IM	0.06 mL/kg	10	3
Hepatitis B prophylaxis (as hepatitis B IG)	IM	0.06 mL/kg	10	3
Rabies prophylaxis (as rabies IG)	IM	20 IU/kg	22	4
Varicella prophylaxis (as VariZIG)	IM	125 U/10 kg (maximum 625 U)	20-40	5
Measles prophylaxis (as IG):				
Standard	IM	0.25 mL/kg	40	5
Immunocompromised host	IM	0.50 mL/kg	80	6
Respiratory syncytial virus prophylaxis (palivizumab monoclonal antibody)	IM	—	15 mg/kg (monoclonal)	None
Cytomegalovirus immune globulin	IV	3 mL/kg	150	6
Blood transfusion:				
Washed RBCs	IV	10 mL/kg	Negligible	0
RBCs, adenine-saline added	IV	10 mL/kg	10	3
Packed RBCs	IV	10 mL/kg	20-60	5
Whole blood	IV	10 mL/kg	80-100	6
Plasma or platelet products	IV	10 mL/kg	160	7
Replacement (or therapy) of immune deficiencies (as IGIV)	IV	—	300-400	8
ITP (as IGIV)	IV	—	400	8
ITP	IV	—	1,000	10
ITP or Kawasaki disease	IV	—	1,600-2,000	11

*Immunization in the form of measles-mumps-rubella (MMR), measles-mumps-rubella-varicella (MMRV), or monovalent measles vaccine.
†These intervals should provide sufficient time for decreases in passive antibodies in all children to follow for an adequate response to measles vaccine. Physicians should not assume that children are fully protected against measles during these intervals. Additional doses of IG or measles vaccine may be indicated after exposure to measles (see text).
IG, immunoglobulin; IgG, immunoglobulin G; IGIV, intravenous IG; ITP, immune (formerly termed "idiopathic") thrombocytopenic purpura; RBCs, red blood cells.
Modified from American Academy of Pediatrics: *Red book: 2009 report of the committee on infectious disease,* ed 28, Elk Grove Village, IL, 2009, American Academy of Pediatrics, p 448.

be causally associated with the MMR vaccine nor vaccine constituents.

A review of the effect of measles vaccination on the epidemiology of SSPE has demonstrated that measles vaccination protects against SSPE and does not accelerate the course of SSPE or trigger the disease in those already infected with wild measles virus.

Passively administered immune globulin may inhibit the immune response to live measles vaccine, and administration should be delayed for variable amounts of time based on the dose of immune globulin (Table 238-4).

Live vaccines should not be administered to pregnant women or to immunodeficient or immunosuppressed patients. However, patients with HIV who are not severely immunocompromised should be immunized. Because measles virus may suppress the cutaneous response to tuberculous antigen, skin testing for tuberculosis should be performed before or at the same time as administration of the vaccine. Individuals infected with *M. tuberculosis* should be receiving appropriate treatment at the time of administration of measles vaccine.

Postexposure Prophylaxis

Susceptible individuals exposed to measles may be protected from infection by either vaccine administration or immunization with immune globulin. The vaccine is effective in prevention or modification of measles if given within 72 hr of exposure. Immune globulin may be given up to 6 days after exposure to prevent or modify infection. Immunocompetent children should receive 0.25 mL/kg intramuscularly, and immunocompromised children should receive 0.5 mL/kg (maximum dose in both cases is 15 mL/kg). Immune globulin is indicated for susceptible household contacts of measles patients, especially infants <6 mo of age, pregnant women, and immunocompromised persons.

BIBLIOGRAPHY

Please visit the Nelson Textbook of Pediatrics *website at www.expertconsult.com for the complete bibliography.*

Chapter 239 Rubella

Wilbert H. Mason

Rubella (**German measles** or **3-day measles**) is a mild, often exanthematous disease of infants and children that is typically more severe and associated with more complications in adults. Its major clinical significance is transplacental infection and fetal damage as part of the **congenital rubella syndrome (CRS)**.

ETIOLOGY

Rubella virus is a member of the family Togaviridae and is the only species of the genus *Rubivirus*. It is a single-stranded RNA virus with a lipid envelope and 3 structural proteins, including a nucleocapsid protein that is associated with the nucleus and 2 glycoproteins, E1 and E2, that are associated with the envelope. The virus is sensitive to heat, ultraviolet light, and extremes of pH but is relatively stable at cold temperatures. Humans are the only known host.

EPIDEMIOLOGY

In the prevaccine era, rubella appeared to occur in major epidemics every 6-9 yr, with smaller peaks interspersed every 3-4 yr, and was most common in preschool and school-aged children. Following introduction of the rubella vaccine, the incidence fell by >99%, with a relatively higher percentage of infections reported among persons >19 yr of age. After years of decline, a resurgence of rubella and CRS occurred during 1989-1991 (Fig. 239-1). Subsequently, a 2-dose recommendation for rubella vaccine was implemented and resulted in a decrease in incidence of rubella from 0.45/100,000 in 1990 to 0.1/100,000 in 1999 and a corresponding decrease of CRS, with an average of 6 infants with CRS reported annually from 1992 to 2004. Mothers of these infants tended to be young, Hispanic, or foreign born. The number of reported cases of rubella continued to decline in the early part of this decade.

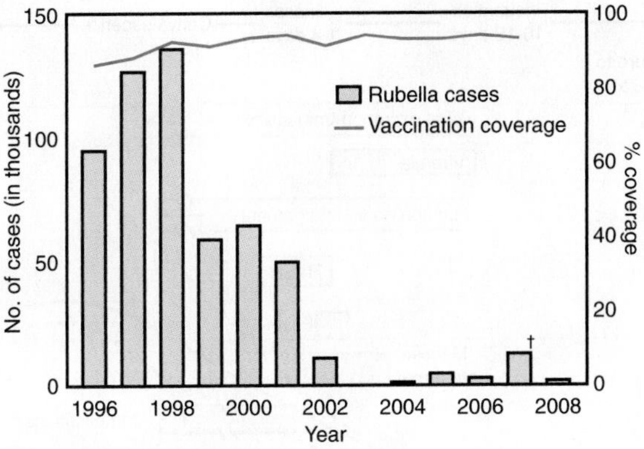

*Includes rubella cases reported to Pan American Health Organization as of September 20, 2008.

†Increase in cases in 2007, mainly attributed to outbreaks in Argentina, Brazil, and Chile.

Figure 239-1 Number of confirmed rubella cases and percentage coverage with first dose of measles-containing vaccine—the Americas, 1996–2008.* (From Centers for Disease Control and Prevention: Progress toward elimination of rubella and congenital rubella syndrome—the Americas, 2003–2008, *MMWR Morb Mortal Wkly Rep* 2008;57:1176–1179, 2008.)

PATHOLOGY

Little information is available on the pathologic findings in rubella occurring postnatally. The few reported studies of biopsy or autopsy material from cases of rubella revealed only nonspecific findings of lymphoreticular inflammation and mononuclear perivascular and meningeal infiltration. The pathologic findings for CRS are often severe and may involve nearly every organ system (Table 239-1).

PATHOGENESIS

The viral mechanisms for cell injury and death in rubella are not well understood for either postnatal or congenital infection. Following infection, the virus replicates in the respiratory epithelium, then spreads to regional lymph nodes (Fig. 239-2). Viremia ensues and is most intense from 10 to 17 days after infection. Viral shedding from the nasopharynx begins about 10 days after infection and may be detected up to 2 wk following onset of the rash. The period of highest communicability is from 5 days before to 6 days after the appearance of the rash.

The most important risk factor for severe congenital defects is the stage of gestation at the time of infection. Maternal infection during the 1st 8 wk of gestation results in the most severe and widespread defects. The risk for congenital defects has been estimated at 90% for maternal infection before 11 wk of gestation, 33% at 11-12 wk, 11% at 13-14 wk, and 24% at 15-16 wk. Defects occurring after 16 wk of gestation are uncommon, even if fetal infection occurs.

Causes of cellular and tissue damage in the infected fetus may include tissue necrosis due to vascular insufficiency, reduced cellular multiplication time, chromosomal breaks, and production of a protein inhibitor causing mitotic arrests in certain cell types. The most distinctive feature of congenital rubella is chronicity. Once the fetus is infected early in gestation, the virus persists in fetal tissue until well beyond delivery. Persistence suggests the possibility of ongoing tissue damage and reactivation, most notably in the brain.

CLINICAL MANIFESTATIONS

Postnatal infection with rubella is a mild disease not easily discernible from other viral infections, especially in children. Following an incubation period of 14-21 days, a prodrome consisting

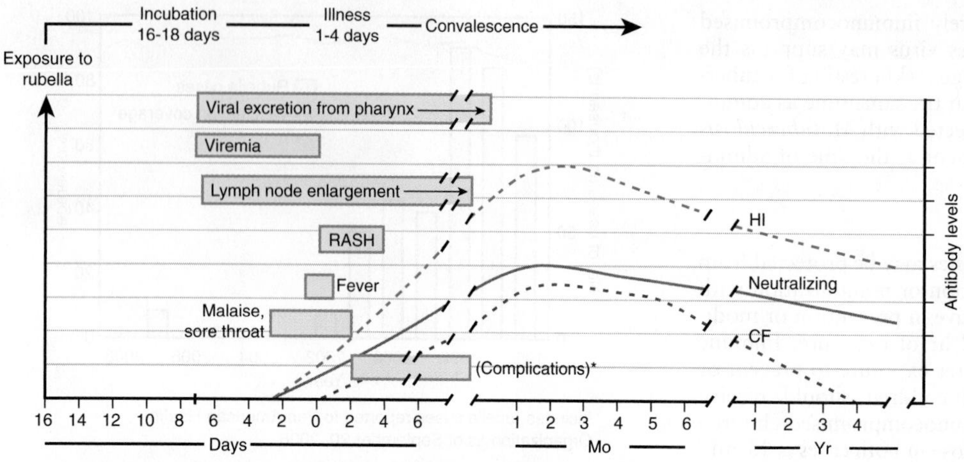

Figure 239-2 Pathophysiologic events in postnatally acquired rubella virus infection. *Possible complications include arthralgia and/or arthritis, thrombocytopenic purpura, and encephalitis. (From Lamprecht CL: Rubella virus. In Beshe RB, editor: *Textbook of human virology,* ed 2, Littleton, MA, 1990, PSG Publishing, p 685.)

Table 239-1 PATHOLOGIC FINDINGS IN CONGENITAL RUBELLA SYNDROME

SYSTEM	PATHOLOGIC FINDINGS
Cardiovascular	Patent ductus arteriosus
	Pulmonary artery stenosis
	Ventriculoseptal defect
	Myocarditis
Central nervous system	Chronic meningitis
	Parenchymal necrosis
	Vasculitis with calcification
Eye	Microphthalmia
	Cataract
	Iridocyclitis
	Ciliary body necrosis
	Glaucoma
	Retinopathy
Ear	Cochlear hemorrhage
	Endothelial necrosis
Lung	Chronic mononuclear interstitial pneumonitis
Liver	Hepatic giant cell transformation
	Fibrosis
	Lobular disarray
	Bile stasis
Kidney	Interstitial nephritis
Adrenal gland	Cortical cytomegaly
Bone	Malformed osteoid
	Poor mineralization of osteoid
	Thinning cartilage
Spleen, lymph node	Extramedullary hematopoiesis
Thymus	Histiocytic reaction
	Absence of germinal centers
Skin	Erythropoiesis in dermis

of low-grade fever, sore throat, red eyes with or without eye pain, headache, malaise, anorexia, and lymphadenopathy begins. Suboccipital, postauricular, and anterior cervical lymph nodes are most prominent. In children, the 1st manifestation of rubella is usually the rash, which is variable and not distinctive. It begins on the face and neck as small, irregular pink macules that coalesce, and it spreads centrifugally to involve the torso and extremities, where it tends to occur as discrete macules (Fig. 239-3). About the time of onset of the rash, examination of the oropharynx may reveal tiny, rose-colored lesions (**Forchheimer spots**) or petechial hemorrhages on the soft palate. The rash fades

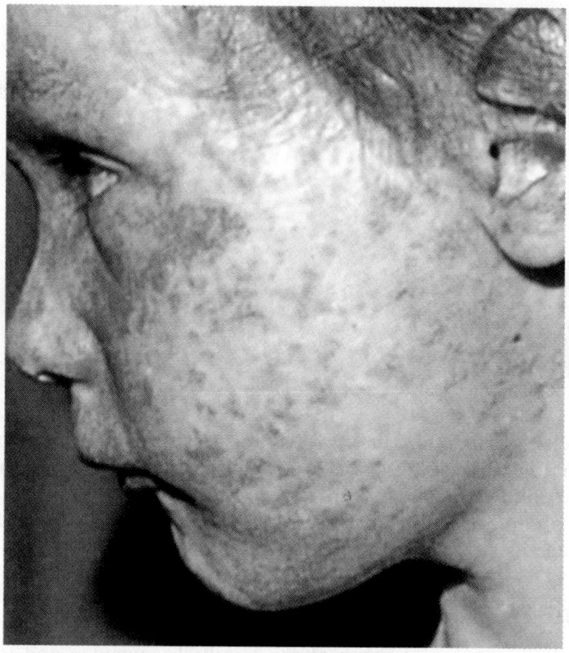

Figure 239-3 Rash of rubella.

from the face as it extends to the rest of the body so that the whole body may not be involved at any 1 time. The duration of the rash is generally 3 days, and it usually resolves without desquamation. Subclinical infections are common, and 25-40% of children may not have a rash.

LABORATORY FINDINGS

Leukopenia, neutropenia, and mild thrombocytopenia have been described during postnatal rubella.

DIAGNOSES

Specific diagnosis of rubella is important for epidemiologic reasons, for diagnosis of infection in pregnant women, and for confirmation of the diagnosis of congenital rubella. The most common diagnostic test is rubella immunoglobulin M (IgM) enzyme immunosorbent assay. As with any serologic test, the positive predictive value of testing decreases in populations with low prevalence of disease. Tests should be performed in the context of a supportive history of exposure or consistent clinical findings. The relative sensitivity and specificity of commercial kits used in most laboratories range from 96% to 99% and 86% to 97%, respectively. A caveat for testing of congenitally infected infants early in infancy is that false-negative results may occur owing to competing immunoglobulin (Ig) G antibodies circulating in these patients. In such patients, an IgM capture assay, reverse transcriptase polymerase chain reaction (PCR) test, or viral culture should be performed for confirmation.

DIFFERENTIAL DIAGNOSES

Rubella may manifest as distinctive features suggesting the diagnosis. It is frequently confused with other infections because it is uncommon, similar to other viral exanthematous diseases, and demonstrates variability in the presence of typical findings. In severe cases it may resemble measles. The absence of Koplik spots and a severe prodrome as well as a shorter course allow for differentiation from measles. Other diseases frequently confused with rubella include infections caused by adenoviruses, parvovirus B19 (erythema infectiosum), Epstein-Barr virus, enteroviruses, and *Mycoplasma pneumoniae*.

COMPLICATIONS

Complications following postnatal infection with rubella are infrequent and generally not life threatening.

Postinfectious **thrombocytopenia** occurs in about 1/3,000 cases of rubella and occurs more frequently among children and in girls. It manifests about 2 wk following the onset of the rash as petechiae, epistaxis, gastrointestinal bleeding, and hematuria. It is usually self-limited.

Arthritis following rubella occurs more commonly among adults, especially women. It begins within 1 wk of onset of the exanthem and classically involves the small joints of the hands. It also is self-limited and resolves within weeks without sequelae. There are anecdotal reports and some serologic evidence linking rubella with rheumatoid arthritis, but a true causal association remains speculative.

Encephalitis is the most serious complication of postnatal rubella. It occurs in 2 forms: a postinfectious syndrome following acute rubella and a rare progressive panencephalitis manifesting as a neurodegenerative disorder years following rubella.

Postinfectious encephalitis is uncommon, occurring in 1/5,000 cases of rubella. It appears within 7 days after onset of the rash, consisting of headache, seizures, confusion, coma, focal neurologic signs, and ataxia. Fever may recrudesce with the onset of neurologic symptoms. Cerebrospinal fluid (CSF) may be normal or have a mild mononuclear pleocytosis and/or elevated protein concentration. Virus is rarely, if ever, isolated from CSF or brain, suggesting a noninfectious pathogenesis. Most patients recover completely, but mortality rates of 20% and long-term neurologic sequelae have been reported.

Progressive rubella panencephalitis (PRP) is an extremely rare complication of either acquired rubella or CRS. It has an onset and course similar to those of the subacute sclerosing panencephalitis (SSPE) associated with measles (Chapter 238). Unlike in the postinfectious form of rubella encephalitis, however, rubella virus may be isolated from brain tissue of the patient with PRP, suggesting an infectious pathogenesis, albeit a "slow" one. The clinical findings and course are undistinguishable from those of SSPE and transmissible spongiform encephalopathies (Chapter 270). Death occurs 2-5 yr after onset.

Other neurologic syndromes rarely reported with rubella include Guillain-Barré syndrome and peripheral neuritis. Myocarditis is a rare complication.

Congenital Rubella Syndrome

In 1941 an ophthalmologist first described a syndrome of cataracts and congenital heart disease that he correctly associated with rubella infections in the mothers during early pregnancy (Table 239-2). Shortly after the first description, hearing loss was recognized as a common finding often associated with microcephaly. In 1964-1965 a pandemic of rubella occurred, with 20,000 cases reported in the USA leading to >11,000 spontaneous or therapeutic abortions and 2,100 neonatal deaths. From this experience emerged the expanded definition of CRS that included numerous other transient or permanent abnormalities.

Nerve deafness is the single most common finding among infants with CRS. Most infants have some degree of intrauterine growth restriction. Retinal findings described as **salt-and-pepper retinopathy** are the most common ocular abnormality but have little early effect on vision. Unilateral or bilateral cataracts are the most serious eye finding, occurring in about a third of infants (Fig. 239-4). Cardiac abnormalities occur in half of the children infected during the 1st 8 wk of gestation. Patent ductus arteriosus is the most frequently reported cardiac defect, followed by lesions of the pulmonary arteries and valvular disease. Interstitial pneumonitis leading to death in some cases has been reported. Neurologic abnormalities are common and may progress following birth. Meningoencephalitis is present in 10-20% of infants with CRS and may persist for up to 12 mo. Longitudinal follow-up through 9-12 yr of infants without initial retardation revealed progressive development of additional sensory, motor, and behavioral abnormalities, including hearing loss and autism. PRP has also been recognized rarely after CRS. Subsequent postnatal growth retardation and ultimate short stature have been reported

Table 239-2 CLINICAL MANIFESTATIONS OF CONGENITAL RUBELLA SYNDROME IN 376 CHILDREN FOLLOWING MATERNAL RUBELLA*

MANIFESTATION	RATE (%)
Deafness	67
Ocular	71
Cataracts	29
Retinopathy	39
Heart disease†	48
Patent ductus arteriosus	78
Right pulmonary artery stenosis	70
Left pulmonary artery stenosis	56
Valvular pulmonic stenosis	40
Low birthweight	60
Psychomotor retardation	45
Neonatal purpura	23
Death	35

*Other findings: hepatitis, linear streaking of bone, hazy cornea, congenital glaucoma, delayed growth.
†Findings in 87 patients with congenital rubella syndrome and heart disease who underwent cardiac angiography.
From Cooper LZ, Ziring PR, Ockerse AB, et al: Rubella: clinical manifestations and management, *Am J Dis Child* 118:18–29, 1969.

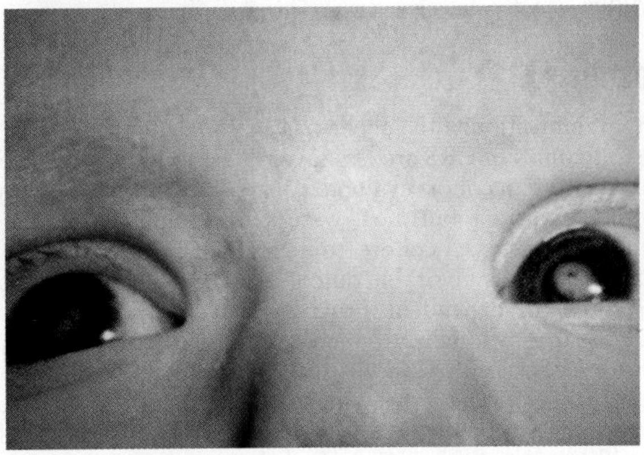

Figure 239-4 Bilateral cataracts in infant with congenital rubella syndrome.

in a minority of cases. Rare reports of immunologic deficiency syndromes have also been described.

A variety of late-onset manifestations of CRS have been recognized. In addition to PRP, they include diabetes mellitus (20%), thyroid dysfunction (5%), and glaucoma and visual abnormalities associated with the retinopathy, which had previously been considered benign.

TREATMENT

There is no specific treatment available for either acquired rubella or CRS.

SUPPORTIVE CARE

Postnatal rubella is generally a mild illness that requires no care beyond antipyretics and analgesics. Intravenous immunoglobulin or corticosteroids can be considered for severe, nonremitting thrombocytopenia.

Management of children with CRS is more complex and requires pediatric, cardiac, audiologic, ophthalmologic, and neurologic evaluation and follow-up because many manifestations may not be readily apparent initially or may worsen with time. Hearing screening is of special importance, because early intervention may improve outcomes in children with hearing problems due to CRS.

PROGNOSIS

Postnatal infection with rubella has an excellent prognosis. Long-term outcomes of CRS are less favorable and somewhat variable. In an Australian cohort evaluated 50 yr after infection, many had chronic conditions but most were married and had made good social adjustments. A cohort from New York from the mid-1960s epidemic had less favorable outcomes, with 30% leading normal lives, 30% in dependent situations but functional, and 30% requiring institutionalization and continuous care.

Re-infection with wild virus occurs postnatally in both individuals who were previously infected with wild-virus rubella and in vaccinated individuals. Re-infection is defined serologically as a significant increase in IgG antibody level and/or an IgM response in an individual who has a documented preexisting rubella-specific IgG above an accepted cutoff. Re-infection may result in an anamnestic IgG response, an IgM and IgG response, or clinical rubella. There have been 29 reports of CRS following maternal re-infection in the literature. Re-infection with serious adverse outcomes to adults or children is rare and of unknown significance.

PREVENTION

Patients with postnatal infection should be isolated from susceptible individuals for 7 days after onset of the rash. Standard plus droplet precautions are recommended for hospitalized patients. Children with CRS may excrete the virus in respiratory secretions up to 1 yr of age, so contact precautions should be maintained for them until then, unless repeated cultures of urine and pharyngeal secretions have negative results. Similar precautions apply to patients with CRS with regard to attendance in school and out-of-home child care.

Exposure of susceptible pregnant women poses a potential risk to the fetus. For pregnant women exposed to rubella, a blood specimen should be obtained as soon as possible for rubella IgG–specific antibody testing; a frozen aliquot also should be saved for later testing. If the rubella antibody test result is positive, the mother is likely immune. If the rubella antibody test is negative, a 2nd specimen should be obtained 2-3 wk later and tested concurrently with the saved specimen. If both of these test negative, a 3rd specimen should be obtained 6 wk after exposure and tested concurrently with the saved specimen. If both the 2nd and 3rd specimens test negative, infection has not occurred. A negative 1st specimen and a positive test result in either the 2nd or 3rd specimen indicate that seroconversion has occurred in the mother, , suggesting recent infection. Counseling should be provided about the risks and benefits of termination of pregnancy. The routine use of immune globulin for susceptible pregnant women exposed to rubella is not recommended and is considered only if termination of pregnancy is not an option because of maternal preferences. In such circumstances, immune globulin 0.55 mL/kg IM may be given with the understanding that prophylaxis may reduce the risk for clinically apparent infection but does not guarantee prevention of fetal infection.

VACCINATION

Rubella vaccine in the USA consists of the attenuated RA 27/3 strain that is usually administered in combination with measles and mumps (MMR) or also with varicella (MMRV) in a 2-dose regimen at 12-15 mo and 4-6 yr of age. It theoretically may be effective as postexposure prophylaxis if administered within 3 days of exposure. Vaccine should not be administered to severely immunocompromised patients (e.g., transplant recipients). Patients with HIV infection who are not severely immunocompromised may benefit from vaccination. Fever is not a contraindication, but if a more serious illness is suspected, immunization should be delayed. Immune globulin preparations may inhibit the serologic response to the vaccine (Chapter 165). Vaccine should not be administered during pregnancy. If pregnancy occurs within 28 days of immunization, the patient should be counseled on the theoretical risks to the fetus. Studies of >200 women who had been inadvertently immunized with rubella vaccine during pregnancy showed that none of their offspring developed CRS. Therefore, interruption of pregnancy is probably not warranted.

Adverse reactions to rubella vaccination are uncommon in children. MMR administration is associated with fever in 5-15% of vaccines and rash in about 5%. Arthralgia and arthritis are more common following rubella vaccination in adults. Approximately 25% of postpubertal women experience arthralgia, and 10% experience arthritis. Peripheral neuropathies and transient thrombocytopenia may also occur.

As part of the worldwide effort to eliminate endemic rubella virus transmission and occurrence of CRS, maintaining high population immunity through vaccination coverage and high-quality integrated measles-rubella surveillance have been emphasized as being vital to its success.

BIBLIOGRAPHY

Please visit the Nelson Textbook of Pediatrics *website at www.expertconsult.com for the complete bibliography.*

Chapter 240
Mumps

Wilbert H. Mason

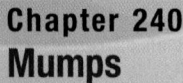

Mumps is an acute self-limited infection, once commonplace but now unusual in developed countries because of widespread use of vaccination. It is characterized by fever, bilateral or unilateral parotid swelling and tenderness, and the frequent occurrence of meningoencephalitis and orchitis. Although no longer common in countries with extensive vaccination programs, mumps remains endemic in the rest of the world, warranting continued vaccine protection.

ETIOLOGY

Mumps virus is in the family Paramyxoviridae and the genus *Rubulavirus*. It is a single-stranded pleomorphic RNA virus encapsulated in a lipoprotein envelope and possessing 7 structural proteins. Two surface glycoproteins, HN (hemagglutinin-neuraminidase) and F (fusion), mediate absorption of the virus to host cells and penetration into cells, respectively. Both of these proteins stimulate production of protective antibodies. Mumps virus exists as a single immunotype, and humans are the only natural host.

EPIDEMIOLOGY

In the prevaccine era, mumps occurred primarily in young children between the ages of 5 and 9 yr and in epidemics about every 4 yr. Mumps infection occurred more often in the winter and spring months. In 1968, just after the introduction of the mumps vaccine, 185,691 cases were reported in the USA. Following the recommendation for routine use of mumps vaccine in 1977, the incidence of mumps in young children fell dramatically (Fig. 240-1), the disease occurring instead in older children, adolescents, and young adults. Outbreaks continued to occur *even in highly vaccinated* populations as a result of to vaccine failure and also of undervaccination of susceptible persons. After implementation of the 2-dose recommendation for the measles-mumps-rubella (MMR) vaccine for measles control in 1989, the number of mumps cases declined further. During 2001-2003, <300 mumps cases were reported each year. In 2006, the largest mumps epidemic in the last 20 years occurred in the USA. A total of 6584 cases occurred, 85% of them in 8 Midwestern states. Twenty-nine percent of the cases occurred in patients 18-24 yr old, most of whom were attending college. An analysis of 4039 patients with mumps seen in the first 7 months of the epidemic indicated that 63% had received >2 doses of the MMR vaccine.

Mumps is spread from person to person by respiratory droplets. Virus appears in the saliva from up to 7 days before to as long as 7 days after onset of parotid swelling. The period of maximum infectiousness is 1-2 days before to 5 days after onset of parotid swelling. Viral shedding before onset of symptoms and in asymptomatic infected individuals impairs efforts to contain the infection in susceptible populations. The U.S. Centers for Disease Control and Prevention (CDC), the American Academy of Pediatrics, and the Health Infection Control Practices Advisory Committee recommend an isolation period of 5 days after onset of parotitis for patients with mumps in both community and health care settings.

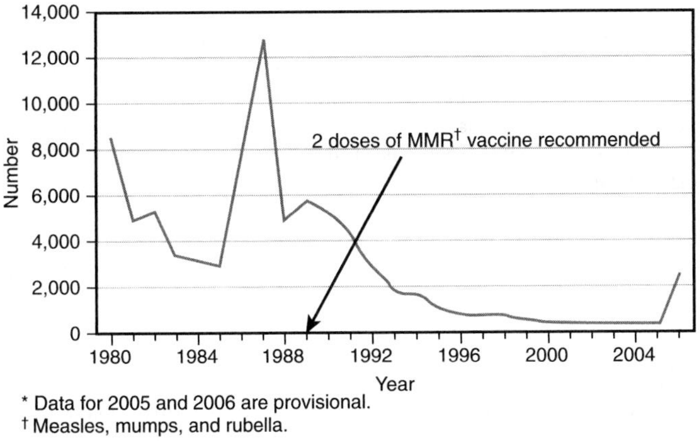

Figure 240-1 Number of reported mumps cases by year in the USA from 1980 to 2006 (data for 2005 and 2006 are provisional). Mumps vaccine was first licensed in 1967 and recommended for routine use in 1977. After expanded recommendation for 2 doses of measles-mumps-rubella (MMR) vaccine in 1989 for measles control, mumps incidence further declined. During 2001–2003 there were <300 mumps cases each year, a 99% decline from the 185,691 cases reported in 1968. More than 2,500 cases were reported in the 1st half of 2006 as part of a multistate outbreak, the largest number of cases in the USA since 1991. (From the Centers for Disease Control and Prevention: Summary of notifiable diseases—United States, 2004, *MMWR Morb Mortal Wkly Rep* 53:1–79, 2006.).

PATHOLOGY AND PATHOGENESIS

Mumps virus targets the salivary glands, central nervous system (CNS), pancreas, testes, and, to a lesser extent, thyroid, ovaries, heart, kidneys, liver, and joint synovia.

Following infection, initial viral replication occurs in the epithelium of the upper respiratory tract. Infection spreads to the adjacent lymph nodes by the lymphatic drainage, and viremia ensues, spreading the virus to targeted tissues. Mumps virus causes necrosis of infected cells and is associated with a lymphocytic inflammatory infiltrate. Salivary gland ducts are lined with necrotic epithelium, and the interstitium is infiltrated with lymphocytes. Swelling of tissue within the testes may result in focal ischemic infarcts. The cerebrospinal fluid (CSF) frequently contains mononuclear pleocytosis, even in individuals without clinical signs of meningitis.

CLINICAL MANIFESTATIONS

The incubation period for mumps ranges from 12 to 25 days but is usually 16-18 days. Mumps virus infection may result in clinical presentation ranging from asymptomatic or nonspecific symptoms to the typical illness associated with parotitis with or without complications involving several body systems. The typical patient presents with a prodrome lasting 1-2 days and consisting of fever, headache, vomiting, and achiness. Parotitis then appears and may be unilateral initially but becomes bilateral in about 70% of cases (Fig. 240-2). The parotid gland is tender, and parotitis may be preceded or accompanied by ear pain on the ipsilateral side. Ingestion of sour or acidic foods or liquids may enhance pain in the parotid area. As swelling progresses, the angle of the jaw is obscured and the ear lobe may be lifted upward and outward (Figs. 240-2 and 240-3). The opening of Stensen duct may be red and edematous. The parotid swelling peaks in approximately 3 days, then gradually subsides over 7 days. Fever and the other systemic symptoms resolve in 3-5 days. A morbilliform rash is rarely seen. Submandibular salivary glands may also be involved or may be enlarged without parotid swelling. Edema over the sternum due to lymphatic obstruction may also occur.

DIAGNOSIS

When mumps was highly prevalent, the diagnosis could be made on the basis of a history of exposure to mumps infection, an appropriate incubation period, and development of typical clini-

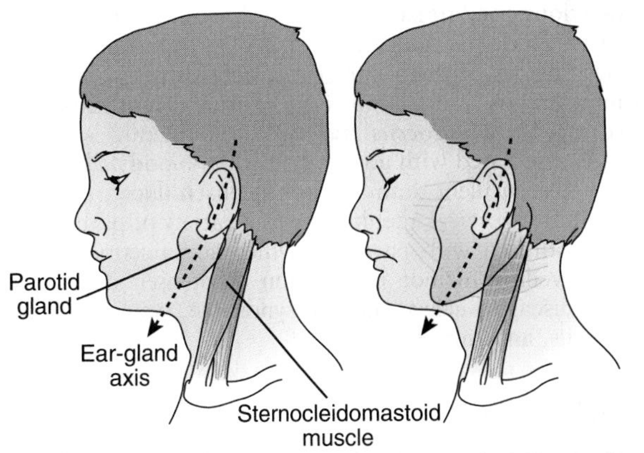

Figure 240-2 Schematic drawing of a parotid gland infected with mumps (*right*) compared with a normal gland (*left*). An imaginary line bisecting the long axis of the ear divides the parotid gland into 2 equal parts. These anatomic relationships are not altered in the enlarged gland. An enlarged cervical lymph node is usually posterior to the imaginary line. (From Mumps [epidemic parotitis]. In Krugman S, Ward R, Katz SL, editors: *Infectious diseases in children,* ed 6, St Louis, 1977, Mosby, p 182.)

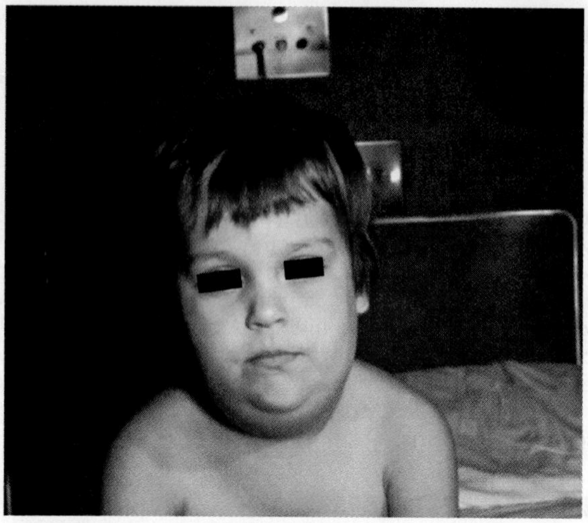

Figure 240-3 A child with mumps showing parotid swelling. (From the Centers for Disease Control and Prevention: *Public health image library [PHIL]* [website]. http://phil.cdc.gov/phil/home.asp. Accessed March 8, 2011.)

cal findings. Confirmation of the presence of parotitis could be made with demonstration of an elevated serum amylase value. Leukopenia with a relative lymphocytosis was a common finding. Today, in patients with parotitis lasting >2 days and of unknown cause, a specific diagnosis of mumps should be confirmed or ruled out by virologic or serologic means. This step may be accomplished by isolation of the virus in cell culture, detection of viral antigen by direct immunofluorescence, or identification of nucleic acid by reverse transcriptase polymerase chain reaction. Virus can be isolated from upper respiratory tract secretions, CSF, or urine during the acute illness. Serologic testing is usually a more convenient and available mode of diagnosis. A significant increase in serum mumps immunoglobulin G (IgG) antibody between acute and convalescent serum specimens as detected by complement fixation, neutralization hemagglutination, or enzyme immunoassay (EIA) tests establishes the diagnosis. Mumps IgG antibodies may cross react with antibodies to parainfluenza virus in serologic testing. More commonly, an EIA for mumps IgM antibody is used to identify recent infection. Skin testing for mumps is neither sensitive nor specific and should not be used.

DIFFERENTIAL DIAGNOSIS

Parotid swelling may be caused by many other infectious and noninfectious conditions. Viruses that have been shown to cause parotitis include parainfluenza 1 and 3 virus, influenza A virus, cytomegalovirus, Epstein-Barr virus, enteroviruses, lymphocytic choriomeningitis virus, and HIV. Purulent parotitis, usually caused by *Staphylococcus aureus,* is unilateral, is extremely tender, is associated with an elevated white blood cell count, and may involve purulent drainage from Stensen duct. Submandibular or anterior cervical adenitis due to a variety of pathogens may also be confused with parotitis. Other noninfectious causes of parotid swelling include obstruction of Stensen duct, collagen vascular diseases such as Sjögren syndrome, systemic lupus erythematosus, and tumor.

COMPLICATIONS

The most common complications of mumps are meningitis, with or without encephalitis, and gonadal involvement. Uncommon complications include conjunctivitis, optic neuritis, pneumonia, nephritis, pancreatitis, and thrombocytopenia.

Maternal infection with mumps during the 1st trimester of pregnancy results in increased fetal wastage. No fetal malformations have been associated with intrauterine mumps infection. However, perinatal mumps disease has been reported in infants born to mothers who acquired mumps late in gestation.

Meningitis and Meningoencephalitis

Mumps virus is neurotropic and is thought to enter the CNS via the choroid plexus and infect the choroidal epithelium and ependymal cells, both of which can be found in CSF along with mononuclear leukocytes. Symptomatic CNS involvement occurs in 10-30% of infected individuals, but CSF pleocytosis has been found in 40-60% of patients with mumps parotitis. The meningoencephalitis may occur before, along with, or following the parotitis. It most commonly manifests 5 days after the parotitis. Clinical findings vary with age. Infants and young children have fever, malaise, and lethargy, whereas older children, adolescents, and adults complain of headache and demonstrate meningeal signs. In 1 series of children with mumps and meningeal involvement, findings were fever in 94%, vomiting in 84%, headache in 47%, parotitis in 47%, neck stiffness in 71%, lethargy in 69%, and seizures in 18%. In typical cases, symptoms resolve in 7-10 days. CSF in mumps meningitis has a white blood cell pleocytosis of 200-600/mm^3 with a predominance of lymphocytes. The CSF glucose content is normal in most patients, but a moderate hypoglycorrhachia (glucose content 20-40 mg/dL) may be seen in 10-20% of patients. The CSF protein content is normal or mildly elevated.

Less common CNS complications of mumps include transverse myelitis, aqueductal stenosis, and facial palsy. Sensorineural hearing loss is rare but has been estimated to occur in 0.5-5.0/100,000 cases of mumps. There is some evidence that this sequela is more likely in patients with meningoencephalitis.

Orchitis and Oophoritis

In adolescent and adult males, orchitis is 2nd only to parotitis as a common finding in mumps. Involvement in prepubescent boys is extremely rare, but after puberty, orchitis occurs in 30-40% of males. It begins within days following onset of parotitis in the majority of cases and is associated with moderate to high fever, chills, and exquisite pain and swelling of the testes. In ≤30% of cases the orchitis is bilateral. Atrophy of the testes may occur, but sterility is rare even with bilateral involvement.

Oophoritis is uncommon in postpubertal females but may cause severe pain and may be confused with appendicitis when located on the right side.

Pancreatitis

Pancreatitis may occur in mumps with or without parotid involvement. Severe disease is rare, but fever, epigastric pain, and vomiting are suggestive. Epidemiologic studies have suggested that mumps may be associated with the subsequent development of diabetes mellitus, but a causal link has not been established.

Cardiac Involvement

Myocarditis has been reported in mumps, and molecular studies have identified mumps virus in heart tissue taken from patients with endocardial fibroelastosis.

Arthritis

Arthralgia, monoarthritis, and migratory polyarthritis have been reported in mumps. Arthritis is seen with or without parotitis and usually occurs within 3 wk of onset of parotid swelling. It is generally mild and self-limited.

Thyroiditis

Thyroiditis is rare following mumps. It has not been reported without parotitis and may occur weeks after the acute infection. Most cases resolve, but some become relapsing and result in hypothyroidism.

TREATMENT

No specific antiviral therapy is available for mumps. Management should be aimed at reducing the pain associated with meningitis or orchitis and maintaining adequate hydration. Antipyretics may be given for fever.

PROGNOSIS

The outcome of mumps is nearly always excellent, even when the disease is complicated by encephalitis, although fatal cases due to CNS involvement or myocarditis have been reported.

PREVENTION

Immunization with the live mumps vaccine is the primary mode of prevention used in the USA. It is given as part of the MMR 2-dose vaccine schedule, at 12-15 mo of age for the 1st dose and 4-6 yr of age for the 2nd dose. If not given at 4-6 yr, the 2nd dose should be given before children enter puberty. Antibody develops in 95% of vaccinees after 1 dose. One study showed vaccine effectiveness of 88% for 2 doses of MMR vaccine, compared with 64% for a single dose. Immunity appears to be long lasting. However, studies from the United Kingdom and the recent epidemic in the USA suggest that both antibody levels and vaccine effectiveness may decline, contributing to mumps outbreaks in older vaccinated populations.

As a live-virus vaccine, MMR should not be administered to pregnant women or to severely immunodeficient or immunosuppressed individuals. HIV-infected patients who are not severely immunocompromised may receive the vaccine, because the risk for severe infection with mumps outweighs the risk for serious reaction to the vaccine. Individuals with anaphylactoid reactions to egg or neomycin may be at risk for immediate-type hypersensitivity reactions to the vaccine. Persons with other types of reactions to egg or reactions to other components of the vaccine are not restricted from receiving the vaccine.

In 2006, in response to the multistate outbreak in the USA, evidence of immunity to mumps through vaccination was redefined. Acceptable presumptive evidence of immunity to mumps now consists of 1 of the following: (1) documentation of adequate vaccination, (2) laboratory evidence of immunity, (3) birth before 1957, and (4) documentation of physician-diagnosed mumps. Evidence of immunity through documentation of adequate vaccination is now defined as 1 dose of a live mumps virus vaccine for preschool-aged children and adults not at high risk and 2 doses for school-aged children (i.e., grades K-12) and for adults at high risk (i.e., health care workers, international travelers, and students at post–high school educational institutions).

All persons who work in health care facilities should be immune to mumps. Adequate mumps vaccination for health care workers born during or after 1957 consists of 2 doses of a live mumps virus vaccine. Health care workers with no history of mumps vaccination and no other evidence of immunity should receive 2 doses, with >28 days between doses. Health care workers who have received only 1 dose previously should receive a 2nd dose. Because birth before 1957 is only presumptive evidence of immunity, health care facilities should consider recommending 1 dose of a live mumps virus vaccine for unvaccinated workers born before 1957 who do not have a history of physician-diagnosed mumps or laboratory evidence of mumps immunity. During an outbreak, health care facilities should strongly consider recommending 2 doses of a live mumps virus vaccine to unvaccinated workers born before 1957 who do not have evidence of mumps immunity.

Adverse reactions to mumps virus vaccine are rare. Parotitis and orchitis have been reported rarely. Other reactions such as febrile seizures, deafness, rash, purpura, encephalitis, and meningitis may not be causally related to the strain of mumps vaccine virus used for immunization in the USA. Higher rates of aseptic meningitis following vaccination for mumps have been associated with vaccine strains used elsewhere in the world, including the Leningrad 3 and Urabe Am 9 strains. Transient suppression of reactivity to tuberculin skin testing has been reported after mumps vaccination.

BIBLIOGRAPHY

Please visit the Nelson Textbook of Pediatrics *website at www.expertconsult.com for the complete bibliography.*

Chapter 241
Polioviruses

Eric A.F. Simões

ETIOLOGY

The polioviruses are nonenveloped, positive-stranded RNA viruses belonging to the Picornaviridae family, in the genus *Enterovirus,* and consist of 3 antigenically distinct serotypes (types 1, 2, and 3). Polioviruses spread from the intestinal tract to the central nervous system (CNS), where they cause aseptic meningitis and poliomyelitis, or polio. The polioviruses are extremely hardy and can retain infectivity for several days at room temperature.

EPIDEMIOLOGY

The most devastating result of poliovirus infection is paralysis, although 90-95% of infections are inapparent but induce protective immunity. Clinically apparent but nonparalytic illness occurs in about 5% of all infections, with paralytic polio occurring in about 1/1,000 infections among infants to about 1/100 infections among adolescents. In developed countries prior to universal vaccination, epidemics of paralytic poliomyelitis occurred primarily in adolescents. Conversely, in developing countries with poor sanitation, infection early in life results in infantile paralysis. Improved sanitation explains the virtual eradication of polio from the USA in the early 1960s, when only about 65% of the population was immunized with the Salk vaccine, which contributed to the disappearance of circulating wild-type poliovirus in the USA and Europe. Poor sanitation and crowding have permitted the continued transmission of poliovirus in certain poor countries in Africa and Asia, despite massive global efforts to eradicate polio, which in some areas involve an average of 12-13 doses of polio vaccine administered to children in the 1st 5 yr of life (Fig. 241-1).

TRANSMISSION

Humans are the only known reservoir for the polioviruses, which are spread by the fecal-oral route. Poliovirus has been isolated from feces for >2 wk before paralysis to several weeks after the onset of symptoms.

PATHOGENESIS

Polioviruses infect cells by adsorbing to the genetically determined **poliovirus receptor.** The virus penetrates the cell, is uncoated, and releases viral RNA. The RNA is translated to produce proteins responsible for replication of the RNA, shutoff of host cell protein synthesis, and synthesis of structural elements that compose the capsid. Mature virus particles are produced in 6-8 hr and are released into the environment by disruption of the cell.

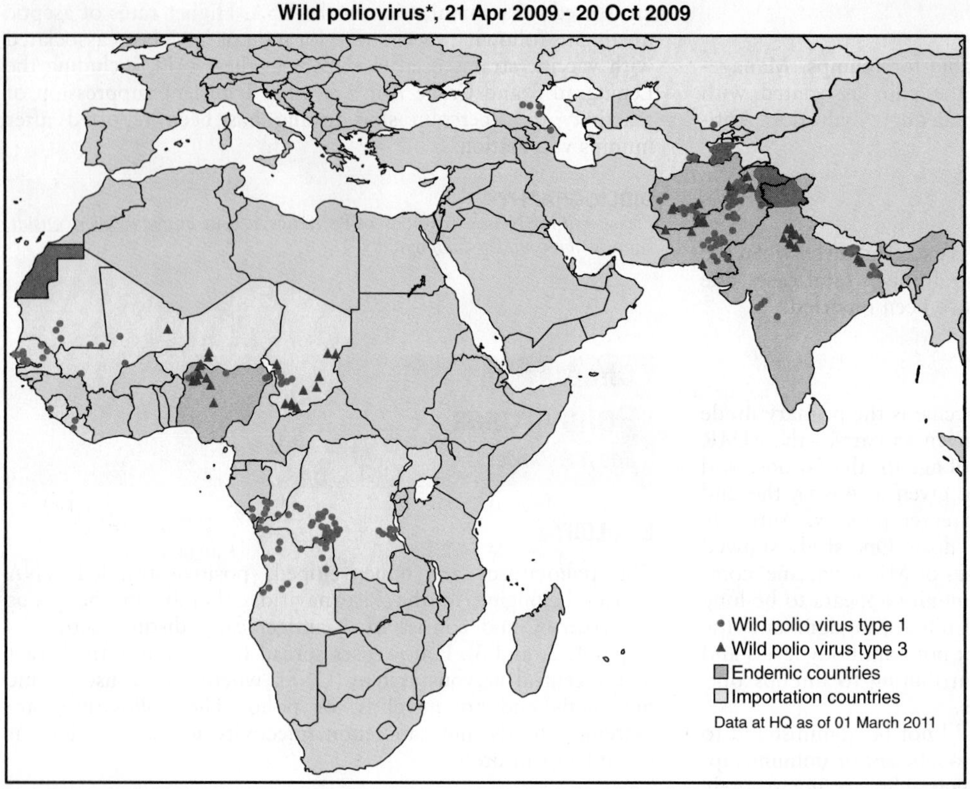

Figure 241-1 Wild poliovirus cases in 2010 worldwide. (From World Health Organization: *Global polio eradication initiative* [website]. http://www.polioeradication.org/Portals/0/Image/Data&Monitoring/yearmap.jpg. Accessed March 8, 2011.)

In the contact host, wild-type and vaccine strains of polioviruses gain host entry via the gastrointestinal tract. The primary site of replication is in the M cells lining the mucosa of the small intestine. Regional lymph nodes are infected, and primary viremia occurs after 2-3 days. The virus seeds multiple sites, including the reticuloendothelial system, brown fat deposits, and skeletal muscle. Wild-type poliovirus probably accesses the CNS along peripheral nerves. Vaccine strains of polioviruses do not replicate in the CNS, a feature that accounts for the safety of the live-attenuated vaccine. Occasional **revertants** (by nucleotide substitution) of these vaccine strains develop a neurovirulent phenotype and cause **vaccine-associated paralytic poliomyelitis (VAPP)**. Reversion occurs in the small intestine and probably accesses the CNS via the peripheral nerves. Because poliovirus replicates in endothelial cells, the theory of viremic spread to the CNS was favored; however, poliovirus has almost never been cultured from the cerebrospinal fluid (CSF) of patients with paralytic disease, and patients with aseptic meningitis due to poliovirus never have paralytic disease. With the 1st appearance of non-CNS symptoms, a secondary viremia probably occurs as a result of enormous viral replication in the reticuloendothelial system.

The exact mechanism of entry into the CNS is not known. Once entry is gained, however, the virus may traverse neural pathways, and multiple sites within the CNS are often affected. The effect on motor and vegetative neurons is most striking and correlates with the clinical manifestations. Perineuronal inflammation, a mixed inflammatory reaction with both polymorphonuclear leukocytes and lymphocytes, is associated with extensive neuronal destruction. Petechial hemorrhages and considerable inflammatory edema also occurs in areas of poliovirus infection. The poliovirus primarily infects motor neuron cells in the spinal cord (**the anterior horn cells**) and the medulla oblongata (the cranial nerve nuclei). Because of the overlap in muscle innervation by 2-3 adjacent segments of the spinal cord, clinical signs of weakness in the limbs develop when more than 50% of motor neurons are destroyed. In the medulla, less extensive lesions cause paralysis, and involvement of the reticular formation that contains the vital centers controlling respiration and circulation may have a catastrophic outcome. Involvement of the intermediate and dorsal areas of the horn and the dorsal root ganglia in the spinal cord results in hyperesthesia and myalgias that are typical of acute poliomyelitis. Other neurons affected are the nuclei in the roof and vermis of the cerebellum, the substantia nigra, and, occasionally, the red nucleus in the pons; there may be variable involvement of thalamic, hypothalamic, and pallidal nuclei and the motor cortex.

Apart from the histopathology of the CNS, inflammatory changes occur generally in the reticuloendothelial system. Inflammatory edema and sparse lymphocytic infiltration are prominently associated with hyperplastic lymphocytic follicles.

Infants acquire immunity transplacentally from their mothers. Transplacental immunity disappears at a variable rate during the 1st 4-6 mo of life. Active immunity after natural infection is probably lifelong but protects against the infecting serotype only; infections with other serotypes are possible. Poliovirus neutralizing antibodies develop within several days after exposure as a result of replication of the virus in the M cells in the intestinal tract and deep lymphatic tissues. This early production of circulating immunoglobulin (Ig) G antibodies protects against CNS invasion. Local (mucosal) immunity, conferred mainly by secretory IgA, is an important defense against subsequent re-infection of the gastrointestinal tract.

CLINICAL MANIFESTATIONS

The incubation period of poliovirus from contact to initial clinical symptoms is usually considered to be 8-12 days, with a range of 5-35 days. Poliovirus infections with wild-type virus may follow 1 of several courses: **inapparent infection,** which occurs in 90-95% of cases and causes no disease and no sequelae; abortive poliomyelitis; nonparalytic poliomyelitis; or paralytic poliomyelitis. Paralysis, if it occurs, appears 3-8 days after the initial symptoms. The clinical manifestations of paralytic polio caused by wild or vaccine strains are comparable, although the incidence of abortive and nonparalytic paralysis with vaccine-associated poliomyelitis is unknown.

Abortive Poliomyelitis

In about 5% of patients, a nonspecific influenza-like syndrome occurs 1-2 wk after infection, which is termed abortive poliomyelitis. Fever, malaise, anorexia, and headache are prominent features, and there may be sore throat and abdominal or muscular pain. Vomiting occurs irregularly. The illness is short-lived, lasting up to 2-3 days. The **physical examination** may be normal or may reveal nonspecific pharyngitis, abdominal or muscular tenderness, and weakness. Recovery is complete, and no neurologic signs or sequelae develop.

Nonparalytic Poliomyelitis

In about 1% of patients infected with wild-type poliovirus, signs of abortive poliomyelitis are present, as are more intense headache, nausea, and vomiting, as well as soreness and stiffness of the posterior muscles of the neck, trunk, and limbs. Fleeting paralysis of the bladder and constipation are frequent. Approximately two thirds of these children have a short symptom-free interlude between the 1st phase (**minor illness**) and the 2nd phase (CNS disease or **major illness**). Nuchal rigidity and spinal rigidity are the basis for the diagnosis of nonparalytic poliomyelitis during the 2nd phase.

Physical examination reveals nuchal-spinal signs and changes in superficial and deep reflexes. Gentle forward flexion of the occiput and neck elicits nuchal rigidity. The examiner can demonstrate head drop by placing the hands under the patient's shoulders and raising the patient's trunk. Although normally the head follows the plane of the trunk, in poliomyelitis it often falls backward limply, but this response is not due to true paresis of the neck flexors. In struggling infants it may be difficult to distinguish voluntary resistance from clinically important true nuchal rigidity. The examiner may place the infant's shoulders flush with the edge of the table, support the weight of the occiput in the hand, and then flex the head anteriorly. True nuchal rigidity persists during this maneuver. When open, the anterior fontanel may be tense or bulging.

In the early stages the reflexes are normally active and remain so unless paralysis supervenes. Changes in reflexes, either increased or decreased, may precede weakness by 12-24 hr. The superficial reflexes, the cremasteric and abdominal reflexes, and the reflexes of the spinal and gluteal muscles are usually the 1st to diminish. The spinal and gluteal reflexes may disappear before the abdominal and cremasteric reflexes. Changes in the deep tendon reflexes generally occur 8-24 hr after the superficial reflexes are depressed and indicate impending paresis of the extremities. Tendon reflexes are absent with paralysis. Sensory defects do not occur in poliomyelitis.

Paralytic Poliomyelitis

Paralytic poliomyelitis develops in about 0.1% of persons infected with poliovirus, causing 3 clinically recognizable syndromes that represent a continuum of infection differentiated only by the portions of the CNS most severely affected. These are (1) spinal paralytic poliomyelitis, (2) bulbar poliomyelitis, and (3) polioencephalitis.

Spinal paralytic poliomyelitis may occur as the 2nd phase of a biphasic illness, the 1st phase of which corresponds to abortive poliomyelitis. The patient then appears to recover and feels better for 2-5 days, after which severe headache and fever occur with exacerbation of the previous systemic symptoms. Severe muscle pain is present, and sensory and motor phenomena (e.g., paresthesia, hyperesthesia, fasciculations, and spasms) may develop. On physical examination the distribution of paralysis is characteristically spotty. Single muscles, multiple muscles, or groups of muscles may be involved in any pattern. Within 1-2 days, asymmetric flaccid paralysis or paresis occurs. Involvement of 1 leg is most common, followed by involvement of 1 arm. The proximal areas of the extremities tend to be involved to a greater extent than the distal areas. To detect mild muscular weakness, it is often necessary to apply gentle resistance in opposition to the muscle group being tested. Examination at this point may reveal nuchal stiffness or rigidity, muscle tenderness, initially hyperactive deep tendon reflexes (for a short period) followed by absence or diminution of reflexes, and paresis or flaccid paralysis. In the spinal form there is weakness of some of the muscles of the neck, abdomen, trunk, diaphragm, thorax, or extremities. Sensation is intact; sensory disturbances, if present, suggest a disease other than poliomyelitis.

The paralytic phase of poliomyelitis is extremely variable; some patients progress during observation from paresis to paralysis, whereas others recover, either slowly or rapidly. The extent of paresis or paralysis is directly related to the extent of neuronal involvement; paralysis occurs if >50% of the neurons supplying the muscles are destroyed. The extent of involvement is usually obvious within 2-3 days; only rarely does progression occur beyond this interval. Paralysis of the lower limbs is often accompanied by bowel and bladder dysfunction ranging from transient incontinence to paralysis with constipation and urinary retention.

The onset and course of paralysis are variable in developing countries. The biphasic course is rare; typically the disease manifests in a single phase in which prodromal symptoms and paralysis occur in a continuous fashion. In developing countries, where a history of intramuscular injections precedes paralytic poliomyelitis in about 50-60% of patients, patients may present initially with fever and paralysis (**provocation paralysis**). The degree and duration of muscle pain are also variable, ranging from a few days usually to a week. Occasionally spasm and increased muscle tone with a transient increase in deep tendon reflexes occur in some patients, whereas in most patients, flaccid paralysis occurs abruptly. Once the temperature returns to normal, progression of paralytic manifestations stops. Little recovery from paralysis is noted in the 1st days or weeks, but, if it is to occur, is usually evident within 6 mo. The return of strength and reflexes is slow and may continue to improve as long as 18 mo after the acute disease. Lack of improvement from paralysis within the 1st several weeks or months after onset is usually evidence of permanent paralysis. Atrophy of the limb, failure of growth, and deformity are common and are especially evident in the growing child.

Bulbar poliomyelitis may occur as a clinical entity without apparent involvement of the spinal cord. Infection is a continuum, and designation of the disease as bulbar implies only dominance of the clinical manifestations by dysfunctions of the cranial nerves and medullary centers. The clinical findings seen with bulbar poliomyelitis with respiratory difficulty (other than paralysis of extraocular, facial, and masticatory muscles) include (1) nasal twang to the voice or cry caused by palatal and pharyngeal weakness (hard-consonant words such as "cookie" and "candy" bring this feature out best); (2) inability to swallow smoothly, resulting in accumulation of saliva in the pharynx, indicating partial immobility (holding the larynx lightly and asking the patient to swallow will confirm such immobility); (3) accumulated pharyngeal secretions, which may cause irregular respirations that appear interrupted and abnormal even to the point of falsely simulating intercostal or diaphragmatic weakness; (4) absence of effective coughing, shown by constant fatiguing efforts to clear the throat; (5) nasal regurgitation of saliva and fluids as a result of palatal paralysis, with inability to separate the oropharynx from the nasopharynx during swallowing; (6) deviation of the palate, uvula, or tongue; (7) involvement of vital centers in the medulla, which manifest as irregularities in rate, depth, and rhythm of respiration; as cardiovascular alterations, including blood pressure changes (especially increased blood pressure), alternate flushing and mottling of the skin, and cardiac arrhythmias; and as rapid changes in body temperature; (8) paralysis of 1 or both vocal cords, causing hoarseness, aphonia, and ultimately asphyxia unless the problem is recognized on laryngoscopy and managed by immediate tracheostomy; and (9) the **rope sign,** an acute angulation between the chin and larynx caused by weakness of the hyoid muscles (the hyoid bone is pulled posteriorly, narrowing the hypopharyngeal inlet).

Uncommonly, bulbar disease may culminate in an ascending paralysis (Landry type), in which there is progression cephalad from initial involvement of the lower extremities. Hypertension and other autonomic disturbances are common in bulbar involvement and may persist for a week or more or may be transient. Occasionally, hypertension is followed by hypotension and shock and is associated with irregular or failed respiratory effort, delirium, or coma. This kind of bulbar disease may be rapidly fatal.

The course of bulbar disease is variable; some patients die as a result of extensive, severe involvement of the various centers in the medulla; others recover partially but require ongoing respiratory support, and others recover completely. Cranial nerve involvement is seldom permanent. Atrophy of muscles may be evident, patients immobilized for long periods may experience pneumonia, and renal stones may form as a result of hypercalcemia and hypercalciuria secondary to bone resorption.

Polioencephalitis is a rare form of the disease in which higher centers of the brain are severely involved. Seizures, coma, and spastic paralysis with increased reflexes may be observed. Irritability, disorientation, drowsiness, and coarse tremors are often present with peripheral or cranial nerve paralysis that coexists or ensues. Hypoxia and hypercapnia caused by inadequate ventilation due to respiratory insufficiency may produce disorientation without true encephalitis. The manifestations are common to encephalitis of any cause and can be attributed to polioviruses only with specific viral diagnosis or if accompanied by flaccid paralysis.

Paralytic poliomyelitis with ventilatory insufficiency results from several components acting together to produce ventilatory insufficiency resulting in hypoxia and hypercapnia. It may have profound effects on many other systems. Because respiratory insufficiency may develop rapidly, close continued clinical evaluation is essential. Despite weakness of the respiratory muscles, the patient may respond with so much respiratory effort associated with anxiety and fear that overventilation may occur at the outset, resulting in respiratory alkalosis. Such effort is fatiguing and contributes to respiratory failure.

There are certain characteristic patterns of disease. Pure spinal poliomyelitis with respiratory insufficiency involves tightness, weakness, or paralysis of the respiratory muscles (chiefly the diaphragm and intercostals) without discernible clinical involvement of the cranial nerves or vital centers that control respiration, circulation, and body temperature. The cervical and thoracic spinal cord segments are chiefly affected. Pure bulbar poliomyelitis involves paralysis of the motor cranial nerve nuclei with or without involvement of the vital centers. Involvement of the 9th, 10th, and 12th cranial nerves results in paralysis of the pharynx, tongue, and larynx with consequent airway obstruction. Bulbospinal poliomyelitis with respiratory insufficiency affects the respiratory muscles and results in coexisting bulbar paralysis.

The clinical findings associated with involvement of the respiratory muscles include (1) anxious expression; (2) inability to speak without frequent pauses, resulting in short, jerky, "breathless" sentences; (3) increased respiratory rate; (4) movement of the ala nasi and of the accessory muscles of respiration; (5) inability to cough or sniff with full depth; (6) paradoxical abdominal movements caused by diaphragmatic immobility due to spasm or weakness of 1 or both leaves; and (7) relative immobility of the intercostal spaces, which may be segmental, unilateral, or bilateral. When the arms are weak, and especially when deltoid paralysis occurs, there may be impending respiratory paralysis because the phrenic nerve nuclei are in adjacent areas of the spinal cord. Observation of the patient's capacity for thoracic breathing while the abdominal muscles are splinted manually indicates minor degrees of paresis. Light manual splinting of the thoracic cage helps assess the effectiveness of diaphragmatic movement.

DIAGNOSIS

Poliomyelitis should be considered in any unimmunized or incompletely immunized child with paralytic disease. VAPP should be considered in any child with paralytic disease occurring 7-14 days after receiving the orally administered polio vaccine (OPV). VAPP can occur at later times after administration and should be considered in any child with paralytic disease in countries or regions where wild-type poliovirus has been eradicated and the OPV has been administered to the child or a contact. The combination of fever, headache, neck and back pain, asymmetric flaccid paralysis without sensory loss, and pleocytosis does not regularly occur in any other illness.

The World Health Organization (WHO) recommends that the laboratory diagnosis of poliomyelitis be confirmed by isolation and identification of poliovirus in the stool, with specific identification of wild-type and vaccine-type strains. In suspected cases of acute flaccid paralysis, 2 stool specimens should be collected 24-48 hr apart as soon as possible after the diagnosis of poliomyelitis is suspected. Poliovirus concentrations are high in the stool in the 1st week after the onset of paralysis, which is the optimal time for collection of stool specimens. Polioviruses may be isolated from 80-90% of specimens from acutely ill patients, whereas <20% of specimens from such patients may yield virus within 3-4 wk after onset of paralysis. Because most children with spinal or bulbospinal poliomyelitis have constipation, rectal straws may be used to obtain specimens; ideally a minimum of 8-10 g of stool should be collected. In laboratories that can isolate poliovirus, isolates should be sent to either the U.S. Centers for Disease Control and Prevention (CDC) or to one of the WHO-certified poliomyelitis laboratories where DNA sequence analysis can be performed to distinguish between wild poliovirus and neurovirulent, revertant OPV strains. With the current WHO plan for global eradication of poliomyelitis, most regions of the world (the Americas, Europe, Australia) have been certified wild-poliovirus free; in these areas, poliomyelitis is most often caused by vaccine strains. Hence it is critical to differentiate between wild-type and revertant vaccine-type strains.

The CSF is often normal during the minor illness and typically contains a pleocytosis with 20-300 cells/mm^3 with CNS involvement. The cells in the CSF may be polymorphonuclear early during the course of the disease but shift to mononuclear cells soon afterward. By the 2nd week of major illness, the CSF cell count falls to near-normal values. In contrast, the CSF protein content is normal or only slightly elevated at the outset of CNS disease but usually rises to 50-100 mg/dL by the 2nd week of illness. In polioencephalitis, the CSF may remain normal or show minor changes. Serologic testing demonstrates seroconversion or a fourfold or greater increase in antibody titers from the acute phase of illness to 3-6 wk later.

DIFFERENTIAL DIAGNOSIS

Poliomyelitis should be considered in the differential diagnosis of any case of paralysis, and is only 1 of many causes of acute flaccid paralysis in children and adults. There are numerous other causes of acute flaccid paralysis (Table 241-1). In most conditions, the clinical features are sufficient to differentiate between these various causes, but in some cases nerve conduction studies and electromyograms in addition to muscle biopsies may be required.

The possibility of polio should be considered in any case of acute flaccid paralysis even in countries where polio has been eradicated. The diagnoses most often confused with polio are VAPP, West Nile virus and other enteroviruses, as well as

Table 241-1 DIFFERENTIAL DIAGNOSIS OF ACUTE FLACCID PARALYSIS

SITE, CONDITION, FACTOR, OR AGENT	CLINICAL FINDINGS	ONSET OF PARALYSIS	PROGRESSION OF PARALYSIS	SENSORY SIGNS AND SYMPTOMS	REDUCTION OR ABSENCE of DEEP TENDON REFLEXES	RESIDUAL PARALYSIS	PLEOCYTOSIS
ANTERIOR HORN CELLS OF SPINAL CORD							
Poliomyelitis (wild and vaccine-associated paralytic poliomyelitis)	Paralysis	Incubation period 7-14 days (4-35 days)	24-48 hr to onset of full paralysis; proximal → distal, asymmetric	No	Yes	Yes	Aseptic meningitis (moderate polymorphonuclear leukocytes at 2-3 days)
Nonpolio enterovirus	Hand-foot-and-mouth disease, aseptic meningitis, acute hemorrhagic conjunctivitis	As in poliomyelitis	As in poliomyelitis	No	Yes	Yes	As in poliomyelitis
West Nile virus	Meningitis encephalitis	As in poliomyelitis	As in poliomyelitis	No	Yes	Yes	Yes
OTHER NEUROTROPIC VIRUSES							
Rabies virus		Mo- yr	Acute, symmetric, ascending	Yes	Yes	No	±
Varicella-zoster virus	Exanthematous vesicular eruptions	Incubation period 10-21 days	Acute, symmetric, ascending	Yes	±	±	Yes
Japanese encephalitis virus		Incubation period 5-15 days	Acute, proximal, asymmetric	±	±	±	Yes
GUILLAIN-BARRÉ SYNDROME							
Acute inflammatory polyradiculoneuropathy	Preceding infection, bilateral facial weakness	Hours to 10 days	Acute, symmetric, ascending (days to 4 wk)	Yes	Yes	±	No
Acute motor axonal neuropathy	Fulminant, widespread paralysis, bilateral facial weakness, tongue involvement	Hours to 10 days	1-6 days	No	Yes	±	No
ACUTE TRAUMATIC SCIATIC NEURITIS							
Intramuscular gluteal injection	Acute, asymmetric	Hours to 4 days	Complete, affected limb	Yes	Yes	±	No
Acute transverse myelitis	Preceding *Mycoplasma pneumoniae Schistosoma*, other parasitic or viral infection	Acute, symmetric hypotonia of lower limbs	Hours to days	Yes	Yes, early	Yes	Yes
Epidural abscess	Headache, back pain, local spinal tenderness, meningismus	Complete		Yes	Yes	±	Yes
Spinal cord compression; trauma		Complete	Hours to days	Yes	Yes	±	±
NEUROPATHIES							
Exotoxin of *Corynebacterium diphtheriae*	In severe cases, palatal paralysis, blurred vision	Incubation period 1-8 wk (paralysis 8-12 wk after onset of illness)		Yes	Yes		±
Toxin of *Clostridium botulinum*	Abdominal pain, diplopia, loss of accommodation, mydriasis	Incubation period 18-36 hr	Rapid, descending, symmetric	±	No		No
Tick bite paralysis	Ocular symptoms	Latency period 5-10 days	Acute, symmetric, ascending	No	Yes		No
DISEASES OF THE NEUROMUSCULAR JUNCTION							
Myasthenia gravis	Weakness, fatigability, diplopia, ptosis, dysarthria		Multifocal	No	No	No	No
DISORDERS OF MUSCLE							
Polymyositis	Neoplasm, autoimmune disease	Subacute, proximal → distal	Weeks to months	No	Yes		No
Viral myositis		Pseudoparalysis	Hours to days	No	No		No
METABOLIC DISORDERS							
Hypokalemic periodic paralysis		Proximal limb, respiratory muscles	Sudden postprandial	No	Yes	±	No
INTENSIVE CARE UNIT WEAKNESS							
Critical illness polyneuropathy	Flaccid limbs and respiratory weakness	Acute, following systemic inflammatory response syndrome/sepsis	Hours to days	±	Yes	±	No

Modified from Marx A, Glass JD, Sutter RW: Differential diagnosis of acute flaccid paralysis and its role in poliomyelitis surveillance, *Epidemiol Rev* 22:298–316, 2000.

Guillain-Barré syndrome, transverse myelitis, and traumatic paralysis. In Guillain-Barré syndrome, which is the most difficult to distinguish from poliomyelitis, the paralysis is characteristically symmetric, and sensory changes and pyramidal tract signs are common; these are absent in poliomyelitis. Fever, headache, and meningeal signs are less notable, and the CSF has few cells but an elevated protein content. Transverse myelitis progresses rapidly over hours to days, causing an acute symmetric paralysis of the lower limbs with concomitant anesthesia and diminished sensory perception. Autonomic signs of hypothermia in the affected limbs are common, and there is bladder dysfunction. The CSF is usually normal. Traumatic neuritis occurs from a few hours to a few days after the traumatic event, is asymmetric, acute, and affects only 1 limb. Muscle tone and deep tendon reflexes are reduced or absent in the affected limb with pain in the gluteus. The CSF is normal.

Conditions causing pseudoparalysis do not present with nuchal-spinal rigidity or pleocytosis. These causes include unrecognized trauma, transient (toxic) synovitis, acute osteomyelitis, acute rheumatic fever, scurvy, and congenital syphilis (pseudoparalysis of Parrot).

TREATMENT

There is no specific antiviral treatment for poliomyelitis. The management is supportive and aimed at limiting progression of disease, preventing ensuing skeletal deformities, and preparing the child and family for the prolonged treatment required and for permanent disability if this seems likely. Patients with the nonparalytic and mildly paralytic forms of poliomyelitis may be treated at home. All intramuscular injections and surgical procedures are contraindicated during the acute phase of the illness, especially in the 1st week of illness, because they might result in progression of disease.

Abortive Poliomyelitis

Supportive treatment with analgesics, sedatives, an attractive diet, and bed rest until the child's temperature is normal for several days is usually sufficient. Avoidance of exertion for the ensuing 2 wk is desirable, and careful neurologic and musculoskeletal examinations should be performed 2 mo later to detect any minor involvement.

Nonparalytic Poliomyelitis

Treatment for the nonparalytic form is similar to that for the abortive form; in particular, relief is indicated for the discomfort of muscle tightness and spasm of the neck, trunk, and extremities. Analgesics are more effective when they are combined with the application of hot packs for 15-30 min every 2-4 hr. Hot tub baths are sometimes useful. A firm bed is desirable and can be improvised at home by placing table leaves or a sheet of plywood beneath the mattress. A footboard or splint should be used to keep the feet at a right angle to the legs. Because muscular discomfort and spasm may continue for some weeks, even in the nonparalytic form, hot packs and gentle physical therapy may be necessary. Patients with nonparalytic poliomyelitis should also be carefully examined 2 mo after apparent recovery to detect minor residual effects that might cause postural problems in later years.

Paralytic Poliomyelitis

Most patients with the paralytic form of poliomyelitis require hospitalization with complete physical rest in a calm atmosphere for the 1st 2-3 weeks. Suitable body alignment is necessary for comfort and to avoid excessive skeletal deformity. A neutral position with the feet at right angles to the legs, the knees slightly flexed, and the hips and spine straight is achieved by use of boards, sandbags, and, occasionally, light splint shells. The position should be changed every 3-6 hr. Active and passive movements are indicated as soon as the pain has disappeared. Moist hot packs may relieve muscle pain and spasm. Opiates and sedatives are permissible only if no impairment of ventilation is present or impending. Constipation is common, and fecal impaction should be prevented. When bladder paralysis occurs, a parasympathetic stimulant such as bethanechol may induce voiding in 15-30 min; some patients show no response to this agent, and others respond with nausea, vomiting, and palpitations. Bladder paresis rarely lasts more than a few days. If bethanechol fails, manual compression of the bladder and the psychologic effect of running water should be tried. If catheterization must be performed, care must be taken to prevent urinary tract infections. An appealing diet and a relatively high fluid intake should be started at once unless the patient is vomiting. Additional salt should be provided if the environmental temperature is high or if the application of hot packs induces sweating. Anorexia is common initially. Adequate dietary and fluid intake can be maintained by placement of a central venous catheter. An orthopedist and a physiatrist should see patients as early in the course of the illness as possible and should assume responsibility for their care before fixed deformities develop.

The management of pure bulbar poliomyelitis consists of maintaining the airway and avoiding all risk of inhalation of saliva, food, and vomitus. Gravity drainage of accumulated secretions is favored by using the head-low (foot of bed elevated 20-25 degrees) prone position with the face to one side. Patients with weakness of the muscles of respiration or swallowing should be nursed in a lateral or semiprone position. Aspirators with rigid or semirigid tips are preferred for direct oral and pharyngeal aspiration, and soft, flexible catheters may be used for nasopharyngeal aspiration. Fluid and electrolyte equilibrium is best maintained by intravenous infusion because tube or oral feeding in the 1st few days may incite vomiting. In addition to close observation for respiratory insufficiency, the blood pressure should be measured at least twice daily because hypertension is not uncommon and occasionally leads to hypertensive encephalopathy. Patients with pure bulbar poliomyelitis may require tracheostomy because of vocal cord paralysis or constriction of the hypopharynx; most patients who recover have little residual impairment, although some exhibit mild dysphagia and occasional vocal fatigue with slurring of speech.

Impaired ventilation must be recognized early; mounting anxiety, restlessness, and fatigue are early indications for preemptive intervention. Tracheostomy is indicated for some patients with pure bulbar poliomyelitis, spinal respiratory muscle paralysis, or bulbospinal paralysis because such patients are generally unable to cough, sometimes for many months. Mechanical respirators are often needed.

COMPLICATIONS

Paralytic poliomyelitis may be associated with numerous complications. Acute gastric dilatation may occur abruptly during the acute or convalescent stage, causing further respiratory embarrassment; immediate gastric aspiration and external application of ice bags are indicated. Melena severe enough to require transfusion may result from single or multiple superficial intestinal erosions; perforation is rare. Mild hypertension for days or weeks is common in the acute stage and probably related to lesions of the vasoregulatory centers in the medulla and especially to underventilation. In the later stages, because of immobilization, hypertension may occur along with hypercalcemia, nephrocalcinosis, and vascular lesions. Dimness of vision, headache, and a lightheaded feeling associated with hypertension should be regarded as premonitory of a frank convulsion. Cardiac irregularities are uncommon, but electrocardiographic abnormalities suggesting myocarditis are not rare. Acute pulmonary edema occurs occasionally, particularly in patients with arterial hypertension. Hypercalcemia occurs because of skeletal decalcification that begins soon after immobilization and results in hypercalciuria, which in turn predisposes the patient to urinary calculi, especially when urinary stasis and infection are present. High fluid intake is the only effective prophylactic measure.

PROGNOSIS

The outcome of inapparent, abortive poliomyelitis and aseptic meningitis syndromes is uniformly good, with death being exceedingly rare and with no long-term sequelae. The outcome of paralytic disease is determined primarily by degree and severity of CNS involvement. In severe bulbar poliomyelitis, the mortality rate may be as high as 60%, whereas in less severe bulbar involvement and/or spinal poliomyelitis, the mortality rate varies from 5% to 10%, death generally occurring from causes other than the poliovirus infection.

Maximum paralysis usually occurs 2-3 days after the onset of the paralytic phase of the illness, with stabilization followed by gradual return of muscle function. The recovery phase lasts usually about 6 mo, beyond which persisting paralysis is permanent. Generally, paralysis is more likely to develop in male children but female adults. Mortality and the degree of disability are greater after the age of puberty. Pregnancy is associated with an increased risk for paralytic disease. Tonsillectomy and intramuscular injections may enhance the risk for acquisition of bulbar and localized disease, respectively. Increased physical activity, exercise, and fatigue during the early phase of illness have been cited as factors leading to a higher risk for paralytic disease. Finally, it has been clearly demonstrated that type 1 poliovirus has the greatest propensity for natural poliomyelitis, and type 3 for VAPP.

Postpolio Syndrome

After an interval of 30-40 yr, as many as 30-40% of persons who survived paralytic poliomyelitis in childhood may experience muscle pain and exacerbation of existing weakness or development of new weakness or paralysis. This entity, referred to as postpolio syndrome, has been reported only in persons who were infected in the era of wild-type poliovirus circulation. Risk factors for postpolio syndrome include increasing length of time since acute poliovirus infection, presence of permanent residual impairment after recovery from acute illness, and female sex.

PREVENTION

Vaccination is the only effective method of preventing poliomyelitis. Hygienic measures help limit the spread of the infection among young children, but immunization is necessary to control transmission among all age groups. Both the inactivated polio vaccine (IPV), which is currently produced with the use of better methods than those for the original vaccine and is sometimes referred to as enhanced IPV, and the live-attenuated OPV have established efficacy in preventing poliovirus infection and paralytic poliomyelitis. Both vaccines induce production of antibodies against the 3 strains of poliovirus. IPV elicits higher serum IgG antibody titers, but the OPV also induces significantly greater mucosal IgA immunity in the oropharynx and gastrointestinal tract, which limits replication of the wild poliovirus at these sites. Transmission of wild poliovirus by fecal spread is limited in OPV recipients. The immunogenicity of IPV is not affected by the presence of maternal antibodies, and IPV has no adverse effects. Live vaccine may undergo reversion to neurovirulence as it multiplies in the human intestinal tract and may cause VAPP in vaccinees or in their contacts. The overall risk for recipients is 1 case/6.2 million doses. As of January 2000, the IPV-only schedule is recommended for routine polio vaccination in the USA. All children should receive 4 doses of IPV, at 2 mo, 4 mo, 6-18 mo, and 4-6 yr of age.

In 1988, the World Health Assembly resolved to eradicate poliomyelitis globally by 2000, and remarkable progress had been made toward reaching this target. To achieve it, the WHO used 4 basic strategies: routine immunization, National Immunization Days (NIDs), acute flaccid paralysis surveillance, and "mop-up" immunization. The OPV is the only vaccine recommended by the WHO for eradication of the disease. By the end of 1999, at least 1 set of NIDs had been conducted in every polio-endemic country in the world. This strategy has resulted in a >99% decline in poliomyelitis cases; and in early 2002, there were only 10 countries in the world endemic for poliomyelitis. Globally there were 496 cases of polio, of which 483 were confirmed as wild virus in 2001. As of November 30, 2010, 821 confirmed WPV1 cases, 77 WPV3 cases, and 41 vaccine-associated cases had been reported worldwide since the beginning of the year. This figure is double that in 2001. As long as the OPV is being used, there is the potential that circulating vaccine-derived poliovirus (VDPV) will acquire the neurovirulent phenotype and transmission characteristics of the wild-type polioviruses. VDPV emerges from the OPV because of continuous replication in immunodeficient persons (iVDPVs) or by circulation in populations with low vaccine coverage (cVDPVs). The risk appears to be highest with the type 2 strain. Outbreaks of cVDPV2 occurred in Hispaniola, the Philippines, and Madagascar in 2001, and endemic cVDPV2 circulation occurred in Egypt from 1983 to 1993. A cVDPV2 outbreak in Nigeria, which involved 292 cases from 2005 to 2009, is ongoing. The independent lineages in Nigeria and unrelated cVDPV2 outbreaks in the Democratic Republic of Congo and Ethiopia that emerged with cVDPV2 in countries incompletely protected with OPV suggest that the main risk factor for cVDPV circulation is low levels of vaccine coverage. The rate of VAPP in the USA was 1 case of paralytic disease per 760,000 1st doses of OPV distributed, with 93% of recipient cases and 76% of VAPP occurring after administration of the 1st or 2nd dose of OPV. The risk for paralysis in the immunodeficient recipient may be as much as 6,800 times that in normal subjects. HIV has not been found to be a cause for long-term excretion of virus.

Several countries are global priorities because they face challenges in eradication of the disease (see Fig. 241-1). Polioviruses are endemic in India, Pakistan, Afghanistan, and Nigeria. The Global Polio Eradication Initiative began in 1988. By 2006, transmission of virulent polio virus type 2 had been interrupted globally and transmission of indigenous type 1 and type 3 (WPV1 and WPV3) had been interrupted in all but four countries world wide (Afghanistan, India, Nigeria and Pakistan). During 2002-2006, 20 previously polio-free countries were infected by importations of WPV1 originating from Nigeria, and 3 polio-free African countries by WPV1 imported from India. Relatively few importations occurred in 2007, but during 2008-2009 additional WPV1 and WPV3 occurred in 15 countries in Africa, including 5 that had interrupted outbreaks resulting from earlier outbreaks (see Fig. 241-1). In April 2010, Tajikistan reported an outbreak of poliomyelitis in 20 districts with 458 cases. This strain (WPV1 from northern India) has spread to other central Asian countries and to the Russian Federation.

For the 4 countries with uninterrupted outbreaks, there are 3 main reasons for the failure to eradicate polio. In India, the suboptimal efficacy of OPV in key areas in Northern India, the suboptimal campaign quality in Nigeria, parts of Pakistan and southern Afghanistan and the 5 countries with prolonged transmission of imported virus as well as security-compromised areas in parts of Afghanistan and Pakistan were the main difficulties faced in 2009. In India, massive campaigns with monovalent OPV1 (mOPV1) that has been shown to have higher immunogenicity than trivalent OPV has resulted in a decrease in transmission of WPV1. In Nigeria, a similar strategy has resulted in higher community-based immunity, and successive campaigns using mOPV1 and mOPV3 are being used currently. In India, where suboptimal immunogenicity is an issue, injectable IPV is being considered as part of that strategy.

Global synchronous cessation of the OPV may need to be coordinated by the WHO after coordinated mass campaigns. Transition to IPV in developed countries with high rates of immunization coverage is encouraged. In countries where the risk for VAPP is higher than the risk for transmission of poliomyelitis, the injectable poliovirus vaccines continue to confer immunity and are being used routinely, and in other countries that either cannot afford IPV or in which transmission is endemic, the OPV will continue to be used both in routine immunization and in the NID strategy.

BIBLIOGRAPHY
Please visit the Nelson Textbook of Pediatrics *website at* *www.expertconsult.com* *for the complete bibliography.*

Chapter 242
Nonpolio Enteroviruses

Mark J. Abzug

The genus *Enterovirus* contains a large number of agents that produce a broad range of illnesses. The genus name reflects the importance of the gastrointestinal tract as the primary site of invasion and replication and the source for transmission. Viremic spread to distant sites accounts for the majority of clinical manifestations.

ETIOLOGY

Enteroviruses are non-enveloped, single-stranded, positive-sense viruses in the Picornaviridae ("small RNA virus") family, which also includes the genera *Rhinovirus, Hepatovirus* (hepatitis A virus), and *Parechovirus* and genera containing related animal viruses. The original human enterovirus subgroups—polioviruses (Chapter 241), coxsackieviruses (named after Coxsackie, New York, where they were discovered), and echoviruses (named from the acronym *e*nteric *c*ytopathic *h*uman *o*rphan *viruses*, applied before disease associations were identified)—were differentiated by their replication patterns in tissue culture and animals (Table 242-1). The human enteroviruses have been reclassified on the basis of nucleotide and amino acid sequences into 5 species, polioviruses and human enteroviruses A-D. Enterovirus types are distinguished by antigenic and genetic sequence differences; newer enteroviruses are classified by numbering. Although 100 or more types have been described, 10-15 account for the majority of disease. No disease is uniquely associated with any specific serotype, although certain manifestations are preferentially associated with specific serotypes.

Table 242-1 CLASSIFICATION OF HUMAN ENTEROVIRUSES

Family	Picornaviridae
Genus	*Enterovirus*
Subgroups*	Poliovirus serotypes 1-3
	Coxsackie A virus serotypes 1-22, 24 (23 **reclassified** as echovirus 9)
	Coxsackie B virus serotypes 1-6
	Echovirus serotypes 1-9, 11-27, 29-33 (echoviruses 10 and 28 **reclassified** as non-enteroviruses; echovirus 34 **reclassified** as coxsackie A virus 24; echoviruses 22 and 23 **reclassified** within the genus *Parechovirus*)
	Numbered enterovirus serotypes (enterovirus 72 **reclassified** as hepatitis A virus)

*The human enteroviruses have been alternatively classified on the basis of nucleotide and amino acid sequences into 5 species (polioviruses and human enteroviruses A-D).

EPIDEMIOLOGY

Enterovirus infections are common and have a worldwide distribution. In temperate climates there is an annual epidemic peak in summer/fall, although some transmission occurs year-round. Enteroviruses are responsible for 33-65% of acute febrile illnesses and 55-65% of hospitalizations for suspected sepsis in infants during the summer and fall in the USA, and 25% year-round. In tropical and semitropical areas, enteroviruses circulate year-round. In general, only a few serotypes circulate simultaneously. Infections by different serotypes can occur within the same season. Factors associated with increased incidence and/or severity include young age, male sex, poor hygiene, overcrowding, and low socioeconomic status; >25% of symptomatic infections occur in children <1 yr of age. Breast-feeding reduces the risk for infection, likely via enterovirus-specific antibodies.

Humans are the only known reservoir for human enteroviruses. Virus is primarily spread person to person, by the fecal-oral and respiratory routes, and vertically, from mother to neonate, prenatally or in the peripartum period, or, possibly, via breast-feeding. Enteroviruses can survive on environmental surfaces, permitting transmission via fomites. Enteroviruses also can frequently be isolated from water sources and sewage and can survive for months in wet soil. Although environmental contamination (of drinking water, swimming pools and ponds, and hospital water reservoirs) may occasionally be responsible for transmission, it is often considered the result, rather than the cause, of human infection. Transmission occurs within families (if a member of a household is infected, there is ≥50% risk of spread to nonimmune household contacts), daycare centers, playgrounds, summer camps, orphanages, and hospital nurseries; severe secondary infections may occur in nursery outbreaks. Diaper changing is a risk factor for spread, whereas handwashing decreases transmission. Tick-borne transmission has been suggested.

Large outbreaks of enterovirus infections have included epidemics of echovirus meningitis in numerous countries (echoviruses 4, 6, 9, 13, and 30 commonly); epidemics of hand-foot-and-mouth disease with severe central nervous system (CNS) and/or cardiopulmonary disease in young children due to enterovirus 71 in Asia and Australia; outbreaks of acute hemorrhagic conjunctivitis due to enterovirus 70, coxsackievirus A24, and coxsackievirus A24 variant in tropical and temperate regions; and community outbreaks of uveitis. Reverse transcription polymerase chain reaction (RT-PCR), restriction fragment length polymorphism (RFLP) analysis, single-strand conformation polymorphism analysis, heteroduplex mobility analysis, and genomic sequencing help identify outbreaks and allow phylogenetic analyses that demonstrate, depending on the outbreak, commonality of outbreak strains, differences among epidemic strains and older prototype strains, changes in circulating viral subgroups over time, co-circulation of multiple genetic lineages, and associations between specific genogroups and epidemiologic and clinical characteristics. Genetic analyses have demonstrated recombination and genetic drift that lead to evolutionary changes in genomic sequence and antigenicity and extensive genetic diversity. Recombination events associated with emergence of new subgenotypes of enterovirus 71 may contribute to sequential outbreaks.

The incubation period is typically 3-6 days, except for a 1- to 3-day incubation period for acute hemorrhagic conjunctivitis. Infected children, both symptomatic and asymptomatic, frequently shed cultivable enteroviruses from the respiratory tract for <1-3 wk, whereas fecal shedding continues up to 7-11 wk. Enterovirus RNA appears to be shed from mucosal sites for longer periods.

PATHOGENESIS

Following acquisition by the oral or respiratory route, initial replication occurs in the pharynx and intestine, possibly within mucosal M cells. The absence of an envelope favors survival in the gastrointestinal tract. Cell surface macromolecules, including poliovirus receptor, integrin very late activation antigen VLA-2, decay accelerating factor/complement regulatory protein (DAF/CD55), intercellular adhesion molecule-1 (ICAM-1), and coxsackievirus-adenovirus receptor, serve as receptors, as does sialic acid for enterovirus 70 and coxsackievirus A24 variants infecting the eye. Two or more enteroviruses may invade and replicate in the gastrointestinal tract simultaneously, but replication of 1 type often hinders growth of the heterologous type (**interference**).

After the virus attaches to a cell surface receptor, a conformational change in surface capsid proteins facilitates penetration and uncoating with release of viral RNA in the cytoplasm. Translation of the positive-sense RNA results in synthesis of a polyprotein that undergoes cleavage by proteinases encoded in the polyprotein. Several proteins produced guide synthesis of negative-sense RNA that serves as a template for replication of new positive-sense RNA. The genome is approximately 7,500 nucleotides long and includes a highly conserved 5′ noncoding region important for replication efficiency and a highly conserved 3′ polyA region, which flank a continuous region encoding viral proteins. The 5 end is covalently linked to a small viral protein (VPg) necessary for initiation of RNA synthesis. There is significant variation within genomic regions encoding the structural proteins (with corresponding variability in antigenicity). Replication is followed by further cleavage of proteins and assembly into 30-nm icosahedral virions. Of the 4 structural proteins (VP1-VP4) in the capsid (additional regulatory proteins such as an RNA-dependent RNA polymerase and proteases are also present in the virion), VP1 is the most important determinant of serotype specificity. Approximately 10^4-10^5 virions are released from an infected cell by lysis within 5-10 hr of infection.

Initial replication in the pharynx and intestine is followed within days by multiplication in lymphoid tissue such as tonsils, Peyer patches, and regional lymph nodes. A primary, transient viremia (**minor viremia**) results in spread to distant parts of the reticuloendothelial system, including the liver, spleen, bone marrow, and distant lymph nodes. Host immune responses may limit replication and progression beyond the reticuloendothelial system, resulting in subclinical infection. Clinical infection occurs if replication proceeds in the reticuloendothelial system and virus spreads via a secondary, sustained viremia (**major viremia**) to target organs such as the CNS, heart, and skin. Tropism to target organs is determined in part by the infecting serotype.

Enteroviruses can damage a wide variety of organs and systems, including the CNS, heart, liver, lungs, pancreas, kidneys, muscle, and skin. Damage is mediated by necrosis and the inflammatory response. CNS infections are often associated with mononuclear pleocytosis of the cerebrospinal fluid (CSF), composed of macrophages and activated T lymphocytes, and a mixed meningeal inflammatory response. Parenchymal involvement may affect the cerebral white and gray matter, cerebellum, basal ganglia, brainstem, and spinal cord with perivascular and parenchymal mixed or lymphocytic inflammation, gliosis, cellular degeneration, and neuronophagocytosis. Encephalitis during epidemics of enterovirus 71 has been characterized by severe involvement of the brainstem, spinal cord gray matter, hypothalamus, and subthalamic and dentate nuclei, and frequently complicated by pulmonary edema and/or interstitial pneumonitis and cardiopulmonary failure, presumed to be secondary to brainstem damage, sympathetic hyperactivity, and CNS and systemic inflammatory responses (including cytokine and chemokine overexpression), and, only occasionally, myocarditis.

Enterovirus myocarditis is characterized by perivascular and interstitial mixed inflammatory infiltrates and myocyte damage, possibly mediated by viral cytolytic (e.g., cleavage of dystrophin) and innate and adaptive immune-mediated mechanisms. Chronic inflammation may persist after viral clearance. The potential for enteroviruses to cause persistent infection is controversial. Persistent infection has been implicated in dilated cardiomyopathy and in myocardial infarction, with enteroviral RNA sequences and/or antigens demonstrated in cardiac tissues in some, but not other, series. Infections with enteroviruses such as coxsackievirus B4 have been implicated as a trigger for type 1 diabetes in genetically susceptible hosts, and persistent infection in the pancreas or intestine has been suggested. Similarly, persistent infection has been implicated in amyotrophic lateral sclerosis and Sjögren syndrome, and evidence of chronic infection has been described in some studies of chronic fatigue syndrome but not in others.

Severe **neonatal infections** can manifest as hepatic necrosis, hemorrhage, inflammation, endotheliitis, and veno-occlusive disease; myocardial mixed inflammatory infiltrates, edema, and necrosis; meningeal and brain inflammation, hemorrhage, gliosis, necrosis, and white matter damage; inflammation, hemorrhage, thrombosis, and necrosis in the lungs, pancreas, and adrenal glands; and disseminated intravascular coagulation. In utero infections are characterized by placentitis and infection of multiple fetal organs such as heart, lung, and brain.

Development of circulating type-specific neutralizing antibodies appears to be the most important immune defense, mediating prevention against and recovery from infection. Immunoglobulin M (IgM) antibodies, followed by long-lasting IgA and IgG antibodies, and secretory IgA, mediating mucosal immunity, are produced. Although local re-infection of the gastrointestinal tract can occur, replication is usually limited and not associated with disease. In vitro and animal experiments suggest that heterotypic antibody may enhance disease caused by a different serotype. Innate and cellular defenses (macrophages and cytotoxic T lymphocytes) may also play important roles in recovery from infection. Altered cellular responses to enterovirus 71, including T lymphocyte depletion, were associated with severe meningoencephalitis ± pulmonary edema during recent epidemics.

Hypogammaglobulinemia and agammaglobulinemia predispose to severe, often chronic enterovirus infections. Similarly, perinatally infected neonates lacking maternal type-specific antibody to the infecting virus are at risk for severe disease. Other risk factors for significant illness include young age, immune suppression (post-transplantation and lymphoid malignancy), and, according to animal models and/or epidemiologic observations, exercise, cold exposure, malnutrition, and pregnancy. Specific HLA genes have been linked to enterovirus 71 susceptibility and severe disease.

CLINICAL MANIFESTATIONS

Manifestations are protean, ranging from asymptomatic infection or undifferentiated febrile or respiratory illnesses in the majority, to, less frequently, severe diseases such as meningoencephalitis, myocarditis, and neonatal sepsis. A majority of individuals are asymptomatic or have very mild illness, yet may serve as significant sources for spread of infection. Symptomatic disease is generally more common in young children.

Nonspecific Febrile Illness

Nonspecific febrile illnesses are the most common symptomatic manifestations, especially in infants and young children. These are difficult to clinically differentiate from serious infections such as bacteremia and bacterial meningitis, necessitating diagnostic testing, presumptive therapy, and hospitalizations for suspected bacterial infection in young infants.

Illness usually begins abruptly with fever of 38.5-40°C (101-104°F), malaise, and irritability. Other symptoms are lethargy, anorexia, diarrhea, nausea, vomiting, abdominal discomfort, rash, sore throat, and respiratory symptoms, and, in older children, headache and myalgia. Findings are generally nonspecific and may include mild conjunctivitis pharyngeal injection and cervical lymphadenopathy. Meningitis may be present, but, in infants, specific clinical features distinguishing those with meningitis are often lacking. Fever lasts a mean of 3 days and, occasionally, is biphasic. Duration of illness is usually 4-7 days but can range from 1 day to >1 wk. White blood cell (WBC) count and results of routine laboratory tests are generally normal. Concomitant enterovirus and bacterial infection has been observed in a small number of infants.

Enterovirus illnesses may be associated with a wide variety of skin manifestations, including macular, maculopapular, urticarial, vesicular, and petechial eruptions. Rare cases of idiopathic thrombocytopenic purpura have been reported. Enteroviruses have also been implicated in pityriasis rosea. In general, the frequency of cutaneous manifestations is inversely related to age. Serotypes commonly associated with rashes are echoviruses 9, 11, 16, and 25; coxsackie A viruses 2, 4, 9, and 16; and coxsackie B viruses 3-5. Virus can occasionally be recovered from vesicular skin lesions.

Hand-Foot-and-Mouth Disease

Hand-foot-and-mouth disease, one of the more distinctive rash syndromes, is most frequently caused by coxsackievirus A16, sometimes in large outbreaks, and can also be caused by enterovirus 71; coxsackie A viruses 5, 7, 9, and 10; coxsackie B viruses 2 and 5; and some echoviruses. It is usually a mild illness, with or without low-grade fever. The oropharynx is inflamed and contains scattered vesicles on the tongue, buccal mucosa, posterior pharynx, palate, gingiva, and/or lips (Fig. 242-1). These may ulcerate, leaving 4- to 8-mm shallow lesions with surrounding erythema. Maculopapular, vesicular, and/or pustular lesions may occur on the hands and fingers, feet, and buttocks and groin; the hands are more commonly involved than the feet (see Fig. 242-1). Lesions on the hands and feet are usually tender, 3- to 7-mm vesicles that occur more commonly on dorsal surfaces but frequently also on palms and soles. Vesicles resolve in about 1 wk. Buttock lesions do not usually progress to vesiculation. Disseminated vesicular rashes may complicate preexisting eczema. Hand-foot-and-mouth disease caused by enterovirus 71 is frequently more severe than coxsackievirus A16 disease, with high rates of neurologic and cardiopulmonary involvement, including brainstem encephalomyelitis, neurogenic pulmonary edema, pulmonary hemorrhage, shock, and rapid death, especially in young children. Coxsackievirus A16 also can occasionally be associated with complications such as myocarditis, pericarditis, and shock.

Herpangina

Herpangina is characterized by sudden onset of fever, sore throat, dysphagia, and lesions in the posterior pharynx. Temperatures range from normal to 41°C (106°F); fever tends to be greater in younger patients. Headache and backache may occur in older children, and vomiting and abdominal pain occur in 25% of cases. Characteristic lesions, present on the anterior tonsillar pillars, soft palate, uvula, tonsils, posterior pharyngeal wall, and, occasionally, the posterior buccal surfaces, are discrete 1- to 2-mm vesicles and ulcers that enlarge over 2-3 days to 3-4 mm and are surrounded by erythematous rings that vary in size up to 10 mm. Typically about 5 lesions are present, with a range of 1 to >15. The remainder of the pharynx appears normal or minimally erythematous. Most cases are mild and have no complications; however, some are associated with meningitis or more severe illness. Fever generally lasts 1-4 days, and resolution of symptoms occurs in 3-7 days. A variety of enteroviruses cause herpangina, including enterovirus 71, although coxsackie A viruses are implicated most often.

Respiratory Manifestations

Symptoms such as sore throat and coryza frequently accompany and sometimes dominate enterovirus illnesses. Findings include upper respiratory symptoms, wheezing, exacerbation of asthma, apnea, respiratory distress, pneumonia, otitis media, bronchiolitis, croup, parotitis, and pharyngotonsillitis, which may occasionally be exudative. Lower respiratory tract infection may be significant in immunocompromised patients.

Pleurodynia (**Bornholm disease**), caused most frequently by coxsackie B viruses 3, 5, 1, and 2 and echoviruses 1 and 6, is an epidemic or sporadic illness characterized by paroxysmal thoracic pain, due to myositis involving chest and abdominal wall muscles. In epidemics, children and adults are affected, but most cases occur in persons younger than 30 yr. Malaise, myalgias, and headache are followed by sudden onset of fever and spasmodic, pleuritic pain in the chest or upper abdomen aggravated by coughing, sneezing, deep breathing, or other movement. During spasms, which last from a few minutes to several hours, pain may be severe and respirations are usually rapid, shallow, and grunting, suggesting pneumonia or pleural inflammation. A pleural friction rub may be noted during pain episodes, although chest radiographs are generally normal. Pain localized to the abdomen is frequently crampy, suggesting colic in the younger child. A pale, sweaty, shocklike appearance may suggest intestinal obstruction; tenderness and guarding may suggest appendicitis and peritonitis. Illness usually lasts 3-6 days, and, occasionally, up to 2 wk. It is frequently biphasic and is rarely associated with recurrent episodes over a few weeks, with less prominent fever during recurrences. Pleurodynia may be associated with meningitis, orchitis, myocarditis, or pericarditis.

Life-threatening pulmonary edema, hemorrhage, and/or interstitial pneumonitis may occur in patients with enterovirus 71 encephalitis.

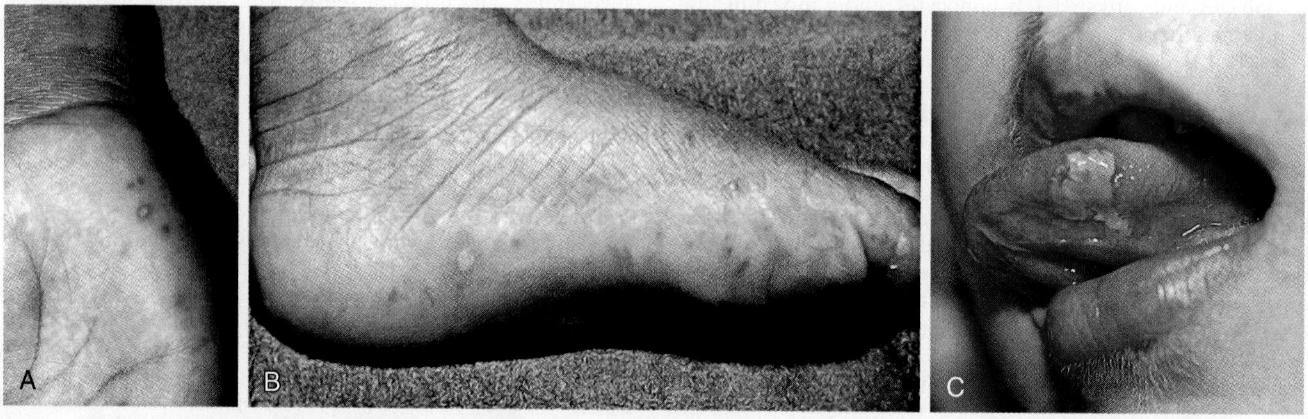

Figure 242-1 *A,* Oval blisters of the palms in a child with hand-foot-and-mouth disease (coxsackievirus A16 infection). *B,* Oval blisters on the feet of a child with hand-foot-and-mouth disease. *C,* Erosion of the tongue in a child with hand-foot-and-mouth disease. (From Weston WL, Lane AT, Morelli JG: *Color textbook of pediatric dermatology,* ed 3, St Louis, 2002, Mosby, p 109.)

Ocular Manifestations

Epidemics of **acute hemorrhagic conjunctivitis,** primarily caused by enterovirus 70 and coxsackievirus A24/A24 variant, are explosive, spreading mainly via eye-hand-fomite-eye transmission. School-aged children, teenagers, and adults 20-50 yr of age have the highest attack rates. Sudden onset of severe eye pain is associated with photophobia, blurred vision, lacrimation, conjunctival erythema and congestion, lid edema, preauricular lymphadenopathy, and, in some cases, subconjunctival hemorrhages and superficial punctate keratitis. Eye discharge is initially serous but becomes mucopurulent with secondary bacterial infection. Systemic symptoms including fever are rare, although manifestations suggestive of pharyngoconjunctival fever occasionally occur. Recovery is usually complete within 1-2 wk. Polyradiculoneuropathy or paralytic disease following enterovirus 70 disease occurs occasionally. Other enteroviruses have occasionally been implicated as causes of keratoconjunctivitis.

Epidemic and sporadic uveitis in infants caused by subtypes of enteroviruses 11 and 19 can be associated with severe complications, including destruction of the iris, cataracts, and glaucoma. Enteroviruses have been implicated in cases of chorioretinitis, uveoretinitis, optic neuritis, and unilateral acute idiopathic maculopathy.

Myocarditis and Pericarditis

Enteroviruses account for approximately 25-35% of cases of myocarditis and pericarditis with proven cause (Chapters 433 and 434). Coxsackie B viruses are most commonly implicated, although coxsackie A viruses and echoviruses also may be causative. Adolescents and young adults, especially males, are disproportionately affected. Myopericarditis may be the dominant feature or it may be part of disseminated disease, as in neonates. Disease ranges from relatively mild to severe. Upper respiratory symptoms frequently precede fatigue, dyspnea, chest pain, congestive heart failure, and dysrhythmias. Presentations may mimic myocardial infarction; sudden death may also occur (including apparent sudden infant death syndrome). A pericardial friction rub indicates pericardial involvement. Chest radiography often demonstrates cardiac enlargement. Electrocardiography frequently reveals ST segment, T wave, and/or rhythm abnormalities, and echocardiography may confirm cardiac dilatation, reduced contractility, and/or pericardial effusion. Myocardial enzyme serum concentrations may be elevated. The acute mortality of enterovirus myocarditis is 0-4%. Recovery is complete without residual disability in the majority. Occasionally, chronic cardiomyopathy, inflammatory ventricular microaneurysms, or constrictive pericarditis may result. The role of persistent infection in chronic dilated cardiomyopathy is controversial. Enteroviruses have also been implicated in late adverse cardiac events following heart transplantation and acute coronary events, and in peripartum cardiomyopathy. Myocardial dysfunction observed in enterovirus 71 epidemics most commonly has occurred without evidence of myocarditis and may be of neurogenic origin; however, true myocarditis has also been described.

Gastrointestinal and Genitourinary Manifestations

Symptoms such as emesis (especially with meningitis), diarrhea (rarely severe), and abdominal pain are frequent but generally not dominant. Diarrhea, hematochezia, pneumatosis intestinalis, and necrotizing enterocolitis have occurred in premature infants during nursery outbreaks. Enterovirus infection has been implicated in chronic intestinal inflammation in hypogammaglobulinemic patients, sporadic hepatitis in normal children, severe hepatitis in neonates, and pancreatitis, which may result in transient exocrine pancreatic insufficiency.

Coxsackie B viruses are 2nd only to mumps as causes of orchitis. The illness is frequently biphasic; fever and pleurodynia or meningitis are followed, in about 2 wk, by orchitis, often with epididymitis. Enteroviruses have also been implicated in cases of nephritis and IgA nephropathy.

Neurologic Manifestations

Enteroviruses are the most common cause of viral meningitis in mumps-immunized populations, accounting for up to 90% or more of cases in which a cause is identified. Meningitis is particularly common in infants, especially those <3 mo of age, often in community epidemics. Frequently implicated serotypes include coxsackie B viruses 2-5; echoviruses 4, 6, 7, 9, 11, 13, 16, and 30; parechoviruses 1-6; and enteroviruses 70 and 71. Most cases in infants and young children are mild and lack specific signs and symptoms. Fever is present in 50-100%, accompanied by irritability, malaise, headache, photophobia, nausea, emesis, anorexia, lethargy, hypotonia, rash, cough, rhinorrhea, pharyngitis, diarrhea, and/or myalgia. Nuchal rigidity is apparent in more than half of children >1-2 yr of age. Some cases are biphasic, with fever and nonspecific symptoms for a few days followed by return of fever with meningeal signs several days later. Fever usually resolves in 3-5 days, and other symptoms in infants and young children usually resolve within 1 wk. Symptoms tend to be more severe and longer lasting in adults. CSF findings include pleocytosis (generally <500 but occasionally as high as 1,000-8,000 WBCs/mm^3; often predominantly polymorphonuclear cells in the 1st 48 hr before becoming mostly mononuclear); normal or slightly low glucose content (10% <40 mg/dL); and normal or mildly increased protein content (generally <100 mg/dL). CSF occasionally has normal parameters despite positive viral culture or PCR results, particularly in the 1st few months of life. Complications occur in approximately 10% of young children, including simple and complex seizures, obtundation, increased intracranial pressure, syndrome of inappropriate antidiuretic hormone secretion, ventriculitis, transient cerebral arteriopathy, and coma. The prognosis for most children is good.

Enteroviruses are also responsible for ≥10-20% of cases of encephalitis with an identified cause. Frequently implicated serotypes include echoviruses 3, 4, 6, 9, and 11; coxsackie B viruses 2, 4, and 5; coxsackie A virus 9; and enterovirus 71. After initial nonspecific symptoms, there is progression to confusion, weakness, lethargy, and/or irritability. Depression is usually generalized, although focal findings, including focal motor seizures, hemichorea, acute cerebellar ataxia, aphasia, extrapyramidal symptoms, and/or focal imaging abnormalities, may occur. Manifestations range from altered mental status to coma to decerebrate status. Long-term sequelae, including epilepsy, weakness, cranial nerve palsy, spasticity, psychomotor retardation, and hearing loss, or death may follow severe disease. Persistent or recurrent cases have been observed rarely.

Neurologic disorders have been prominent in recent epidemics of enterovirus 71 disease. The majority of affected children had hand-foot-and-mouth disease, some had herpangina, and others had no mucocutaneous manifestations. Neurologic syndromes in a fraction of children included meningitis, meningoencephalomyelitis, poliomyelitis-like acute flaccid paralysis, Guillain-Barré syndrome, transverse myelitis, cerebellar ataxia, opsoclonus-myoclonus syndrome, benign intracranial hypertension, and brainstem encephalitis (**rhombencephalitis** involving the midbrain, pons, and medulla). The last is characterized by myoclonus, vomiting, ataxia, nystagmus, tremor, cranial nerve abnormalities, autonomic dysfunction, and MRI demonstration of brainstem lesions. Although the disease was mild and reversible in some children, others had rapid progression to neurogenic pulmonary edema and hemorrhage, cardiopulmonary failure, shock, and coma. High mortality rates have been reported, especially in children <5 yr of age. Deficits such as central hypoventilation, bulbar dysfunction, neurodevelopmental delay, cerebellar defects, attention deficit/hyperactivity–related symptoms, and limb weakness and atrophy have been observed among survivors, especially those who experienced cardiopulmonary failure during their acute illness. Similar clinical pictures have been produced by other enterovirus serotypes (e.g., echovirus 7).

Patients with **antibody deficiencies** and **combined immunodeficiencies** (including human immunodeficiency virus infection and acute lymphocytic leukemia) are at risk for acute or, more commonly, **chronic meningoencephalitis.** The latter is characterized by persistent CSF abnormalities, viral detection by culture or PCR for years, and recurrent encephalitis and/or progressive neurologic deterioration, including insidious intellectual or personality deterioration, altered mental status, seizures, motor weakness, and increased intracranial pressure. Although disease may wax and wane, deficits generally become progressive and ultimately are frequently fatal or lead to long-term sequelae. A **dermatomyositis-like syndrome,** hepatitis, arthritis, myocarditis, or disseminated infection may also occur. Chronic enterovirus meningoencephalitis has become less common now that treatment with antibody replacement with high-dose intravenous immunoglobulin is available.

A variety of nonpoliovirus enteroviruses, including enteroviruses 70 and 71, coxsackie A viruses 7 and 24, coxsackie B viruses, and several echoviruses, can cause poliomyelitis-like acute flaccid paralysis with motor weakness due to anterior horn cell involvement. Disease tends to be milder than that caused by poliovirus, with less bulbar involvement and less persistent weakness. Other neurologic syndromes include cerebellar ataxia, transverse myelitis, Guillain-Barré syndrome, acute disseminated encephalomyelitis, peripheral neuritis, optic neuritis, other cranial neuropathies, sudden hearing loss, tinnitus, and inner ear disorders such as vestibular neuritis.

Myositis and Arthritis

Although myalgia is common, direct evidence of muscle involvement, including rhabdomyolysis, muscle swelling, focal myositis, and polymyositis, has uncommonly been reported. A dermatomyositis-like syndrome and arthritis can be seen in enterovirus-infected hypogammaglobulinemic patients. Enteroviruses are a rare cause of arthritis in normal hosts.

Neonatal Infections

Neonatal infections are relatively common, with a disease incidence comparable to or greater than that of neonatal herpes simplex virus, cytomegalovirus, and group B streptococcus disease. Infection frequently is caused by coxsackie B viruses 2-5 and echoviruses 6, 9, 11, and 19, although many serotypes have been implicated, including, in later years, coxsackie B virus 1 and echovirus 30. Enteroviruses may be acquired vertically before, during, or after delivery, including possible transmission via breast milk; horizontally from family members; or by sporadic or epidemic transmission in nurseries. In utero infection can lead to fetal demise, nonimmune hydrops fetalis, or neonatal illness; additionally, intrauterine infection has been speculatively linked to congenital anomalies, intrauterine growth retardation, neurodevelopmental sequelae, unexplained neonatal illness and death, and increased risk of type 1 diabetes.

Neonatal infection may range from asymptomatic (the majority) to benign febrile illness to severe multisystem disease. Most affected newborns are full term and previously well; maternal history often reveals a recent viral illness, including fever and, frequently, abdominal pain. Neonatal symptoms may occur as early as day 1 of life, with onset of severe disease generally within the 1st 2 wk of life. Frequent findings include fever or hypothermia, irritability, lethargy, anorexia, rash (usually maculopapular, occasionally petechial or papulovesicular), jaundice, respiratory symptoms, apnea, hepatomegaly, abdominal distention, emesis, diarrhea, and decreased perfusion. Most patients have benign courses, with resolution of fever in an average of 3 days and of other symptoms in about 1 wk. A biphasic course may occur occasionally. A minority have severe disease dominated by any combination of sepsis, meningoencephalitis, myocarditis, hepatitis, coagulopathy, and pneumonitis. Meningoencephalitis may be manifested by focal or complex seizures, bulging fontanelle, nuchal rigidity, or reduced level of consciousness. Myocarditis, most often associated with coxsackie B virus infection, may be suggested by tachycardia, dyspnea, cyanosis, and cardiomegaly. Hepatitis and pneumonitis are associated with echovirus infection, although they may occur with coxsackie B viruses. Gastrointestinal manifestations may predominate in premature neonates. Laboratory and radiographic evaluation may reveal leukocytosis, thrombocytopenia, CSF pleocytosis, CNS white matter damage, elevations of serum transaminases and bilirubin, coagulopathy, pulmonary infiltrates, and electrocardiographic changes.

Complications of severe neonatal disease include CNS necrosis and generalized or focal neurologic compromise; arrhythmias, congestive heart failure, myocardial infarction, and pericarditis; hepatic necrosis and failure; intracranial or other bleeding; adrenal necrosis and hemorrhage; and rapidly progressive pneumonitis and pulmonary hypertension. Myositis, arthritis, necrotizing enterocolitis, inappropriate antidiuretic hormone secretion, hemophagocytic syndrome, bone marrow failure, and sudden death are rare events. Mortality with severe disease is significant and most often associated with hepatitis and bleeding complications, myocarditis, or pneumonitis.

The majority of survivors of severe neonatal disease have gradual resolution of hepatic and cardiac dysfunction, although chronic calcific myocarditis and ventricular aneurysm can occur. Meningoencephalitis may be associated with speech and language impairment; cognitive deficits; spasticity, hypotonicity, or weakness; seizure disorders; microcephaly or hydrocephaly; and ocular abnormalities. However, most survivors appear not to have long-term sequelae. Risk factors for severe disease include illness onset in the first few days of life, maternal illness just prior to or at delivery, prematurity, male sex, infection by echovirus 11 or a coxsackie B virus, positive serum viral culture result, absence of neutralizing antibody to the infecting virus, and evidence of severe hepatitis and/or multisystem disease.

Stem Cell Transplant Recipients and Patients with Malignancies

Severe and/or prolonged enterovirus infections in stem cell transplant recipients include progressive pneumonia, severe diarrhea, pericarditis, heart failure, meningoencephalitis, and disseminated disease. Enterovirus-associated hemophagocytic syndrome, meningitis, encephalitis, and myocarditis have been reported in children with malignancies. Infections in both groups are associated with high fatality rates.

DIAGNOSIS

Clues to enterovirus infection include characteristic findings such as hand-foot-and-mouth disease or herpangina lesions, consistent seasonality, known community outbreak, and exposure to enterovirus-compatible disease. In the neonate, history of maternal fever, malaise, and/or abdominal pain near delivery during enterovirus season is suggestive.

Viral culture using a combination of cell lines is the gold standard for confirmation. Sensitivity ranges from 50% to 75% and can be increased by sampling of multiple sites. In children with meningitis, yield of culture is enhanced by sampling CSF plus the throat and rectum. In neonates, yields of 30-70% are achieved when blood, urine, CSF, and mucosal swabs are cultured. A major limitation is the inability of most coxsackie A viruses to grow in culture. Yield may also be limited by neutralizing antibody in patient specimens, improper specimen handling, or insensitivity of the cell lines. Culture is relatively slow, with 3-8 days usually required to detect growth. Centrifugation-enhanced antigen detection coupled with culture (shell vial

Table 242-2 DIFFERENTIAL DIAGNOSIS OF ENTEROVIRUS INFECTIONS

CLINICAL MANIFESTATION	BACTERIAL PATHOGENS	VIRAL PATHOGENS
Nonspecific febrile illness	*Streptococcus pneumoniae, Haemophilus influenzae* type b, *Neisseria meningitidis*	Influenza viruses, human herpesviruses 6 and 7
Exanthems/enanthems	Group A streptococcus, *Staphylococcus aureus, N. meningitidis*	Herpes simplex virus, adenoviruses, varicella-zoster virus, Epstein-Barr virus, measles virus, rubella virus, human herpesviruses 6 and 7
Respiratory illness/ conjunctivitis	*S. pneumoniae, H. influenzae* (nontypable and type b), *N. meningitidis, Mycoplasma pneumoniae, Chlamydia pneumoniae*	Adenoviruses, influenza viruses, respiratory syncytial virus, parainfluenza viruses, rhinovirus, human metapneumovirus
Myocarditis/pericarditis	*S. aureus, H. influenzae* type b, *M. pneumoniae*	Adenoviruses, influenza virus, parvovirus, cytomegalovirus
Meningitis/encephalitis	*S. pneumoniae, H. influenzae* type b, *N. meningitidis, Mycobacterium tuberculosis, Borrelia burgdorferi, M. pneumoniae, Bartonella henselae, Listeria monocytogenes*	Herpes simplex virus, West Nile virus, influenza viruses, adenovirus, Epstein-Barr virus, mumps virus, lymphocytic choriomeningitis virus, arboviruses
Neonatal infections	Group B streptococcus, gram-negative enteric bacilli, *L. monocytogenes, Enterococcus*	Herpes simplex virus, adenoviruses, cytomegalovirus, rubella virus

techniques) can shorten the time to detection, but the sensitivity of this method has been limiting. Although cultivation of an enterovirus from any site can generally be considered evidence of recent infection, isolation from the rectum or stool can reflect more remote shedding. Similarly, recovery from a mucosal site may suggest an association with an illness, whereas recovery from a normally sterile site (e.g., CSF, blood, or tissue) is more conclusive evidence of causation. Serotype identification is generally required only for investigation of an outbreak or an unusual disease manifestation or to distinguish nonpoliovirus enteroviruses from vaccine or wild-type polioviruses.

Direct testing for nucleic acid overcomes the imperfect sensitivity and delayed results of culture. RT-PCR detection of highly conserved areas of the enterovirus genome can detect the majority of enteroviruses, including coxsackie A viruses (but frequently not the parechoviruses) in CSF; serum; urine; conjunctival, nasopharyngeal, throat, tracheal, rectal, stool, and dried blood spot specimens; and tissues such as myocardium, liver, and brain. Sensitivity and specificity of RT-PCR are high, with results in as short as 2-3 hr. Real-time, quantitative PCR assays and nested PCR assays with enhanced sensitivity have been developed, as have enterovirus-containing multiplex PCR assays, nucleic acid sequence–based amplification (NASBA) assays, culture-enhanced PCR assays, and PCR-based microarray assays. Results of PCR testing of CSF from children with meningitis and from hypogammaglobulinemic patients with chronic meningoencephalitis are frequently positive despite negative culture results. PCR testing of tracheal aspirates of children with myocarditis has good concordance with testing of myocardial specimens. In ill neonates and young infants, PCR testing of serum and urine has higher yields than culture, and viral load in blood is correlated with severity. Routine application of CSF PCR for infants and young children with suspected meningitis decreases the number of diagnostic tests, duration of hospital stay, antibiotic use, and overall costs. Sequence analysis of amplified nucleic acid can be used for serotype identification and phylogenetic analysis. Serotype-specific (e.g., enterovirus 71 and coxsackie A virus 16) PCR assays have also been developed. For enterovirus 71, the yield of specimens other than CSF (throat, nasopharyngeal, rectal, and vesicle swabs and CNS tissue) is greater (by PCR or culture) than the yield of CSF specimens, which are infrequently virus-positive.

Enterovirus infections can be detected serologically by a rise, in serum or CSF, of neutralizing, complement fixation, enzyme-linked immunosorbent assay (ELISA), or other type-specific antibody or by serotype-specific IgM antibody. However, serologic testing requires presumptive knowledge of the infecting serotype or an assay with sufficiently broad cross reactivity. Sensitivity may be limited. Except for epidemiologic studies or severe cases characteristic of specific serotypes (e.g., enterovirus 71), serology is generally less useful than culture or nucleic acid detection.

DIFFERENTIAL DIAGNOSIS

The differential diagnosis of enterovirus infections varies with the clinical presentation (Table 242-2).

TREATMENT

In the absence of a proven antiviral agent for enterovirus infections, supportive care is the mainstay of treatment. Newborns and young infants with nonspecific febrile illnesses and children with meningitis frequently require diagnostic evaluations for bacterial and herpes simplex virus infection and hospitalization for presumptive treatment until tests rule out these diagnoses. Neonates with severe disease and infants and children with myocarditis or concerning neurologic diseases (e.g., enterovirus 71 neurologic and/or cardiopulmonary disease) may require intensive supportive care, including cardiorespiratory support and blood products. Milrinone has been suggested as a useful agent in severe enterovirus 71 cardiopulmonary disease. Liver and cardiac transplantation have been performed for neonates with progressive end-organ failure.

Use of immune globulin to treat enterovirus infections is predicated on two assumptions: that the humoral immune response is a key defense against enterovirus infection and lack of neutralizing antibody is a risk factor for symptomatic infection. Immune globulin products contain neutralizing antibodies to many commonly circulating serotypes, although titers vary with serotype and among products. Anecdotal, uncontrolled use of intravenous immune globulin or infusion of maternal convalescent plasma to treat newborns with severe disease has been reported. The one randomized, controlled trial was too small to demonstrate significant clinical benefits, although neonates who received immune globulin containing high neutralizing titers to their own isolates had shorter periods of viremia and viruria. Immune globulin has been administered intravenously and intraventricularly to treat hypogammaglobulinemic patients with chronic enterovirus meningoencephalitis, and intravenously in oncology patients with severe infections, with variable success. Intravenous immune globulin and corticosteroids have been used for patients with neurologic disease caused by enterovirus 71 and other enteroviruses; modulation of cytokine profiles after administration of intravenous immune globulin for enterovirus 71–associated brainstem encephalitis has been demonstrated. A retrospective study suggested that treatment of presumed viral myocarditis with immune globulin was associated with improved outcome; however, virologic diagnoses were not made. Evaluation of corticosteroids and cyclosporine and other immunosuppressive therapy for myocarditis has been inconclusive. Successful treatment of enterovirus myocarditis with interferon-α has been reported anecdotally, and interferon-β treatment was associated with viral clearance and improved cardiac function in chronic cardiomyopathy associated with persistence of enterovirus or adenovirus genome. Activity of interferon-α against enterovirus 71 has been demonstrated in animal models.

Antiviral agents that act at several steps in the enterovirus life cycle—attachment, penetration, uncoating, translation, polyprotein processing, protease activity, and replication—are being evaluated. Candidates include pharmacologically active chemical compounds, small interfering RNAs and DNA-like antisense agents, purine nucleoside analogues, enzyme inhibitors of signal transduction pathways, interferon-inducing oligodeoxynucleotides, and herbal compounds. The investigational agent that advanced furthest, pleconaril, inhibits attachment and uncoating of picornaviruses (enteroviruses and rhinoviruses). This oral medication was associated with modest acceleration of symptom resolution in some pediatric and adult studies of enterovirus meningitis and slightly faster resolution of picornavirus upper respiratory tract infections. Uncontrolled experience suggested possible benefits in high-risk infections, such as neonatal disease, myocarditis, encephalitis, paralytic disease, and infections in immunodeficient patients (including chronic meningoencephalitis). Viral resistance was observed in a minority of patients. Application for licensure was denied owing to concern about potential medication interactions. A randomized trial in neonates with severe hepatitis, coagulopathy, and/or myocarditis is in progress. Design and evaluation of candidate agents active against enterovirus 71 is a current priority. Of currently available agents, lactoferrin and ribavirin have demonstrated activity in vitro and/or in animal models.

COMPLICATIONS AND PROGNOSIS

The prognosis in the majority of enterovirus infections is excellent. Morbidity and mortality are associated primarily with myocarditis, neurologic disease, severe neonatal infections, and infections in immune compromised hosts.

PREVENTION

The 1st line of defense is hygiene, such as handwashing to prevent fecal-oral and respiratory spread within families, schools, and institutional settings; avoidance of sharing utensils and drinking containers and other potential fomites; and disinfection of contaminated surfaces. Treatment of drinking water and swimming pools may be important. Infection control techniques such as cohorting have proven effective in limiting nursery outbreaks. Prophylactic administration of immune globulin or convalescent plasma has been used in nursery epidemics; simultaneous use of infection control interventions makes it difficult to determine efficacy.

Pregnant women near term should avoid contact with individuals ill with possible enterovirus infections. If a pregnant woman experiences a suggestive illness, it is advisable not to proceed with emergency delivery unless there is concern for fetal compromise or obstetric emergencies cannot be excluded. Rather, it may be advantageous to extend pregnancy, allowing the fetus to passively acquire protective antibodies. A strategy of prophylactically administering immune globulin to neonates born to mothers with enterovirus infections is untested.

Maintenance antibody replacement with high-dose intravenous immune globulin for patients with hypogammaglobulinemia has reduced the incidence of chronic enterovirus meningoencephalitis. Vaccines for non-poliovirus enteroviruses are not available, but candidates for virulent serotypes are being investigated. Approaches being evaluated include enterovirus 71 virus–like particle vaccines, enterovirus 71 and coxsackie B virus 3 VP1 capsid protein gene-containing vaccines, breast milk enriched in enterovirus 71 VP1 capsid protein or lactoferrin, and interferon-γ–expressing recombinant viral vectors.

BIBLIOGRAPHY

Please visit the Nelson Textbook of Pediatrics *website at* *www.expertconsult.com* *for the complete bibliography.*

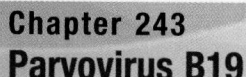

Chapter 243
Parvovirus B19

William C. Koch

Parvovirus B19 is the cause of **erythema infectiosum** or **fifth disease.**

ETIOLOGY

Parvovirus B19 (B19) is a member of the genus *Erythrovirus* in the family Parvoviridae. Parvoviruses are small DNA viruses that infect a variety of animal species. As a group, parvoviruses include a number of important animal pathogens, such as canine parvovirus and feline panleukopenia virus; B19 does not infect other animals, and animal parvoviruses do not infect humans. B19 is one of only two parvoviruses that are pathogenic in humans. The other such virus is the newly described human bocavirus. Although the clinical significance of human bocavirus is not yet fully defined, this virus may be associated with upper and lower respiratory tract infection in young children and will not be further discussed in this chapter.

B19 is composed of an icosahedral protein capsid without an envelope and contains a single-stranded DNA genome of approximately 5.5 kb. It is relatively heat and solvent resistant. It is antigenically distinct from other mammalian parvoviruses and has only one known serotype. Parvoviruses replicate in mitotically active cells and require host cell factors present in late S phase to replicate. B19 can be propagated in vitro only in erythropoietin-stimulated erythropoietic cells derived from human bone marrow, umbilical cord blood, or primary fetal liver culture.

EPIDEMIOLOGY

Infections with parvovirus B19 are common and occur worldwide. Clinically apparent infections, such as the rash illness of erythema infectiosum and transient aplastic crisis, are most prevalent in school-aged children, 70% of cases occurring in patients between 5 and 15 yr of age. Seasonal peaks occur in the late winter and spring, with sporadic infections throughout the year. Seroprevalence increases with age, 40-60% of adults having evidence of prior infection.

Transmission of B19 is by the respiratory route, presumably via large droplet spread from nasopharyngeal viral shedding. The transmission rate is 15-30% among susceptible household contacts, and mothers are more commonly infected than fathers. In outbreaks of erythema infectiosum in elementary schools, the secondary attack rates range from 10% to 60%. Nosocomial outbreaks also occur, with secondary attack rates of 30% among susceptible health care workers.

Although respiratory spread is the primary mode of transmission, B19 is also transmissible in blood and blood products, as documented among children with hemophilia receiving pooled-donor clotting factor. Given the resistance of the virus to solvents, fomite transmission could be important in child-care centers and other group settings, but this mode of transmission has not been established.

PATHOGENESIS

The primary target of B19 infection is the erythroid cell line, specifically erythroid precursors near the pronormoblast stage.

Viral infection produces cell lysis leading to a progressive depletion of erythroid precursors and a transient arrest of erythropoiesis. The virus has no apparent effect on the myeloid cell line. The tropism for erythroid cells is related to the erythrocyte P blood group antigen, which is the primary cell receptor for the virus and is also found on endothelial cells, placental cells, and fetal myocardial cells. Thrombocytopenia and neutropenia are often observed clinically, but the pathogenesis of these abnormalities is unexplained.

Experimental infection of normal volunteers with B19 revealed a biphasic illness. From 7 to 11 days after inoculation, subjects had viremia and nasopharyngeal viral shedding with fever, malaise, and rhinorrhea. Reticulocyte counts dropped to undetectable levels but resulted in only a mild, clinically insignificant fall in serum hemoglobin. With the appearance of specific antibodies, symptoms resolved and serum hemoglobin returned to normal. Several subjects experienced a rash associated with arthralgia 17-18 days after inoculation. Some manifestations of B19 infection, such as transient aplastic crisis, appear to be a direct result of viral infection, whereas others, including the exanthem and arthritis, appear to be **postinfectious phenomena** related to the immune response. Skin biopsy of patients with erythema infectiosum reveals edema in the epidermis and a perivascular mononuclear infiltrate compatible with an immune-mediated process.

Individuals with **chronic hemolytic anemia** and increased red blood cell (RBC) turnover are very sensitive to minor perturbations in erythropoiesis. Infection with B19 leads to a transient arrest in RBC production and a precipitous fall in serum hemoglobin, often requiring transfusion. The reticulocyte count drops to undetectable levels, reflecting the lysis of infected erythroid precursors. Humoral immunity is crucial in controlling infection. Specific immunoglobulin M (IgM) appears within 1-2 days of infection and is followed by anti-B19 IgG, which leads to control of the infection, restoration of reticulocytosis, and a rise in serum hemoglobin.

Individuals with **impaired humoral immunity** are at increased risk for more serious or persistent infection with B19, which usually manifests as chronic RBC aplasia, although neutropenia, thrombocytopenia, and marrow failure are also described. Children undergoing chemotherapy for leukemia or other forms of cancer, transplant recipients, and patients with congenital or acquired immunodeficiency states (including AIDS) are at risk for chronic B19 infections.

Infections in the **fetus** and **neonate** are somewhat analogous to infections in immunocompromised persons. B19 is associated with nonimmune fetal hydrops and stillbirth in women experiencing a primary infection but does not appear to be teratogenic. Like most mammalian parvoviruses, B19 can cross the placenta and cause fetal infection during primary maternal infection. Parvovirus cytopathic effects are seen primarily in erythroblasts of the bone marrow and sites of extramedullary hematopoiesis in the liver and spleen. Fetal infection can presumably occur as early as 6 wk of gestation, when erythroblasts are first found in the fetal liver; after the 4th mo of gestation, hematopoiesis switches to the bone marrow. In some cases, fetal infection leads to profound fetal anemia and subsequent high-output cardiac failure (Chapter 97). **Fetal hydrops** ensues and is often associated with fetal death. There may also be a direct effect of the virus on myocardial tissue that contributes to the cardiac failure. However, most infections during pregnancy result in normal deliveries at term. Some of the asymptomatic infants from these deliveries have been reported to have chronic postnatal infection with B19 that is of unknown significance.

CLINICAL MANIFESTATIONS

Many infections are clinically inapparent. Infected children characteristically demonstrate the rash illness of erythema infectiosum. Adults, especially women, frequently experience acute polyarthropathy with or without a rash.

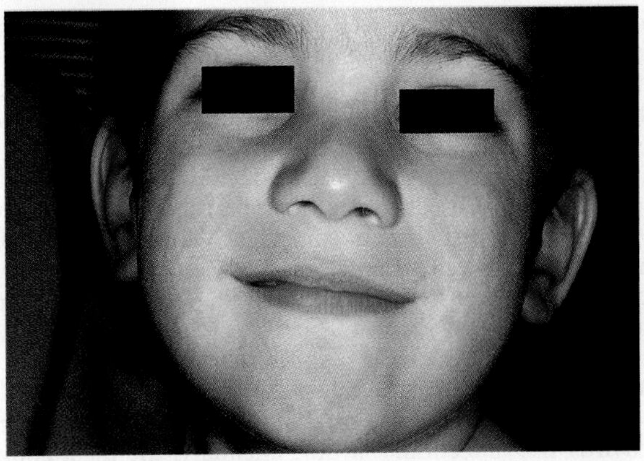

Figure 243-1 Erythema infectiosum. Erythema of the bilateral cheeks, which has been likened to a "slapped cheek" appearance. (From Paller AS, Macini AJ: *Hurwitz clinical pediatric dermatology,* ed 3, Philadelphia, 2006, Elsevier Saunders, p 431.)

Erythema Infectiosum (Fifth Disease)

The most common manifestation of parvovirus B19 is erythema infectiosum, also known as *fifth disease*, which is a benign, self-limited exanthematous illness of childhood.

The incubation period for erythema infectiosum is 4-28 days (average 16-17 days). The prodromal phase is mild and consists of low-grade fever in 15-30% of cases, headache, and symptoms of mild upper respiratory tract infection. The hallmark of erythema infectiosum is the characteristic rash, which occurs in 3 stages that are not always distinguishable. The initial stage is an erythematous facial flushing, often described as a **"slapped-cheek" appearance** (Fig. 243-1). The rash spreads rapidly or concurrently to the trunk and proximal extremities as a diffuse macular erythema in the 2nd stage. Central clearing of macular lesions occurs promptly, giving the rash a **lacy, reticulated appearance** (Fig. 243-2). The rash tends to be more prominent on extensor surfaces, sparing the palms and soles. Affected children are afebrile and do not appear ill. Some have petechiae. Older children and adults often complain of mild pruritus. The rash resolves spontaneously without desquamation but tends to wax and wane over 1-3 wk. It can recur with exposure to sunlight, heat, exercise, and stress. Lymphadenopathy and atypical papular, purpuric, vesicular rashes are also described.

Arthropathy

Arthritis and arthralgia may occur in isolation or with other symptoms. Joint symptoms are much more common among adults and older adolescents with B19 infection. Females are affected more frequently than males. In one large outbreak of fifth disease, 60% of adults and 80% of adult women reported joint symptoms. Joint symptoms range from diffuse polyarthralgia with morning stiffness to frank arthritis. The joints most often affected are the hands, wrists, knees, and ankles, but practically any joint may be affected. The joint symptoms are self-limited and, in the majority of patients, resolve within 2-4 wk. Some patients may have a prolonged course of many months, suggesting rheumatoid arthritis. Transient rheumatoid factor positivity is reported in some of these patients but with no joint destruction.

Transient Aplastic Crisis

The transient arrest of erythropoiesis and absolute reticulocytopenia induced by B19 infection leads to a sudden fall in serum hemoglobin in individuals with chronic hemolytic conditions. This B19-induced RBC aplasia or transient aplastic crisis occurs in patients with all types of chronic hemolysis and/or rapid RBC turnover, including sickle cell disease, thalassemia, hereditary spherocytosis, and pyruvate kinase deficiency. In contrast to children with erythema infectiosum only, patients with aplastic crisis are ill with fever, malaise, and lethargy and have signs and symptoms of profound anemia, including pallor, tachycardia, and tachypnea. Rash is rarely present. The incubation period for transient aplastic crisis is shorter than that for erythema infectiosum because the crisis occurs coincident with the viremia. Children with sickle cell hemoglobinopathies may also have a concurrent vasoocclusive pain crisis, further confusing the clinical presentation.

Immunocompromised Persons

Persons with impaired humoral immunity are at risk for chronic parvovirus B19 infection. Chronic anemia is the most common manifestation, sometimes accompanied by neutropenia, thrombocytopenia, or complete marrow suppression. Chronic infections occur in persons receiving cancer chemotherapy or immunosuppressive therapy for transplantation and persons with congenital immunodeficiencies, AIDS, and functional defects in IgG production who are thereby unable to generate neutralizing antibodies.

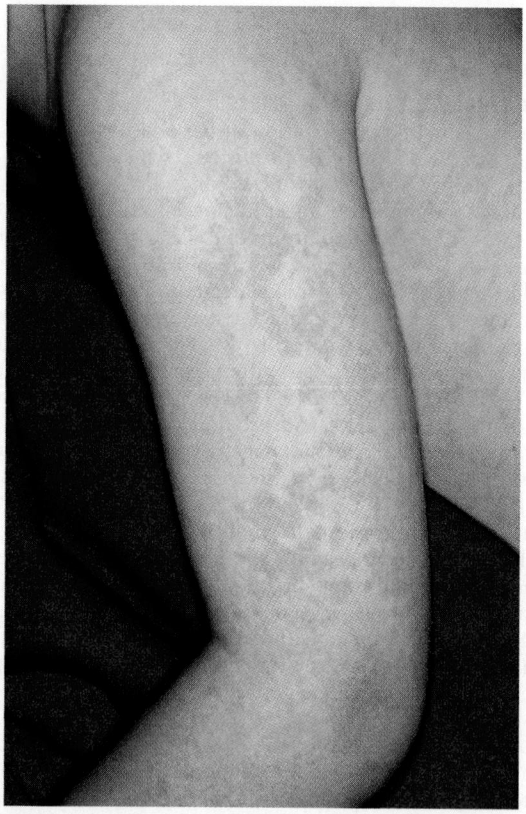

Figure 243-2 Erythema infectiosum. Reticulate erythema on the upper arm of a patient with erythema infectiosum. (From Paller AS, Macini AJ: *Hurwitz clinical pediatric dermatology,* ed 3, Philadelphia, 2006, Elsevier Saunders, p 431.)

Fetal Infection

Primary maternal infection is associated with nonimmune fetal hydrops and intrauterine fetal demise, with the risk for fetal loss after infection estimated at <5%. The mechanism of fetal disease appears to be a viral-induced RBC aplasia at a time when the fetal erythroid fraction is rapidly expanding, leading to profound anemia, high-output cardiac failure, and fetal hydrops. Viral DNA has been detected in infected abortuses. The second trimester seems to be the most sensitive period, but fetal losses are reported at every stage of gestation. If maternal B19 infection is suspected, fetal ultrasonography and measurement of the peak systolic flow velocity of the middle cerebral artery are sensitive, noninvasive procedures to diagnose fetal anemia and hydrops. Most infants infected in utero are born normally at term, including some who have had ultrasonographic evidence of hydrops. A small subset of infants infected in utero may acquire a chronic or persistent postnatal infection with B19 that is of unknown significance. Congenital anemia associated with intrauterine B19 infection has been reported in a few cases, sometimes following intrauterine hydrops. This process may mimic other forms of congenital hypoplastic anemia (e.g., Diamond-Blackfan syndrome). Fetal infection with B19 has not been associated with other birth defects. B19 is only one of many causes of hydrops fetalis (Chapter 97.2).

Myocarditis

B19 infection has been associated with myocarditis in fetuses, infants, children, and a few adults. Diagnosis has often been based on serologic findings suggestive of a concurrent B19 infection, but in many cases B19 DNA has been demonstrated in cardiac tissue. B19-related myocarditis is plausible because fetal myocardial cells are known to express P antigen, the cell receptor for the virus. In the few cases in which histology is reported, a predominantly lymphocytic infiltrate is described. Outcomes have varied from complete recovery to chronic cardiomyopathy to fatal cardiac arrest. Although B19-associated myocarditis seems to be a rare occurrence, there appears to be enough evidence to consider B19 as a potential cause of lymphocytic myocarditis, especially in infants and immunocompromised persons.

Other Cutaneous Manifestations

A variety of atypical skin eruptions have been reported with B19 infection. Most of these are petechial or purpuric in nature, often with evidence of vasculitis on biopsy. Among these rashes, the **papular-purpuric "gloves and socks" syndrome (PPGSS)** is well established in the dermatologic literature as distinctly associated with B19 infection (Fig. 243-3). PPGSS is characterized by fever, pruritus, and painful edema and erythema localized to the distal

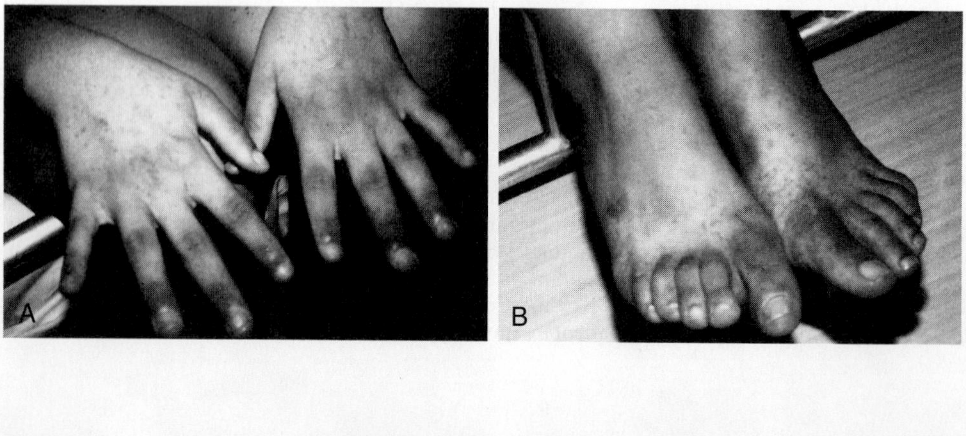

Figure 243-3 Papular-purpuric acrodermatitis with glove-and-sock–like distribution and edema of the fingers (*A*) and toes (*B*). (From Messina MF, Ruggeri C, Rosano M, et al: Purpuric gloves and socks syndrome caused by parvovirus B19 infection, *Pediatr Infect Dis J* 22:755–756, 2003.)

extremities in a distinct "gloves and socks" distribution, followed by acral petechiae and oral lesions. The syndrome is self-limited and resolves within a few weeks. Although PPGSS was initially described in young adults, a number of reports of the disease in children have since been published. In those cases linked to B19 infection, the eruption is accompanied by serologic evidence of acute infection.

DIAGNOSIS

The diagnosis of erythema infectiosum is usually based on clinical presentation of the typical rash and rarely requires virologic confirmation. Similarly, the diagnosis of a typical transient aplastic crisis in a child with sickle cell disease is generally made on clinical grounds without specific virologic testing.

Serologic tests for the diagnosis of B19 infection are available. B19-specific IgM develops rapidly after infection and persists for 6-8 weeks. Anti-B19 IgG serves as a marker of past infection or immunity. Determination of anti-B19 IgM is the best marker of recent/acute infection on a single serum sample; seroconversion of anti-B19 IgG antibodies in paired sera can also be used to confirm recent infection. Demonstration of anti-B19 IgG in the absence of IgM, even in high titer, is not diagnostic of recent infection.

Serologic diagnosis is unreliable in immunocompromised persons; diagnosis in these patients requires methods to detect viral DNA. Because the virus cannot be isolated by standard cell culture, methods to detect viral particles or viral DNA, such as polymerase chain reaction and nucleic acid hybridization, are necessary to establish the diagnosis. These tests are not widely available outside of research centers or reference laboratories. Prenatal diagnosis of B19-induced fetal hydrops can be accomplished by detection of viral DNA in fetal blood or amniotic fluid by these methods.

DIFFERENTIAL DIAGNOSIS

The rash of erythema infectiosum must be differentiated from rubella, measles, enteroviral infections, and drug reactions. Rash and arthritis in older children should prompt consideration of juvenile rheumatoid arthritis, systemic lupus erythematosus, serum sickness, and other connective tissue disorders.

TREATMENT

There is no specific antiviral therapy for B19 infection. Commercial lots of intravenous immune globulin (IVIG) have been used with some success to treat B19-related episodes of anemia and bone marrow failure in immunocompromised children. Specific antibody may facilitate clearance of the virus; it is not always necessary, however, because cessation of cytotoxic chemotherapy with subsequent restoration of immune function often suffices. In patients whose immune status is not likely to improve, such as patients with AIDS, administration of IVIG may give only a temporary remission, and periodic re-infusions may be required. In patients with AIDS, clearance of B19 infection has been reported after initiation of highly active antiretroviral therapy (HAART) without the use of IVIG.

No controlled studies have been published regarding dosing of IVIG for B19-induced RBC aplasia. Doses reported with good results in a limited number of cases include 200 mg/kg/day for 5-10 days and 1g/kg/day for 3 days. IVIG should not be used for treatment of B19-induced arthropathy.

B19-infected fetuses with anemia and hydrops have been managed successfully with intrauterine RBC transfusions, but this procedure has significant attendant risks. Once fetal hydrops is diagnosed, regardless of the suspected cause, the mother should be referred to a fetal therapy center for further evaluation because of the high risk for serious complications (Chapter 97.2).

COMPLICATIONS

Erythema infectiosum is often accompanied by arthralgias or arthritis in adolescents and adults that may persist after resolution of the rash. B19 may rarely cause thrombocytopenic purpura. Neurologic conditions, including aseptic meningitis, encephalitis, and peripheral neuropathy, have been reported in both immunocompromised and healthy individuals in association with B19 infection. The incidence of stroke may be increased in children with sickle cell disease following B19-induced transient aplastic crisis. B19 is also a cause of infection-associated hemophagocytic syndrome, usually in immunocompromised persons.

PREVENTION

Children with erythema infectiosum are not likely to be infectious at presentation because the rash and arthropathy represent immune-mediated, postinfectious phenomena. Isolation and exclusion from school or child care are unnecessary and ineffective after diagnosis.

Children with B19-induced RBC aplasia, including the transient aplastic crisis, are infectious upon presentation and demonstrate a more intense viremia. Most of these children require transfusions and supportive care until their hematologic status stabilizes. They should be isolated in the hospital to prevent spread to susceptible patients and staff. Isolation should continue for at least 1 wk and until after resolution of fever. Pregnant caregivers should not be assigned to these patients. Exclusion of pregnant women from workplaces where children with erythema infectiosum may be present (e.g., primary and secondary schools) is not recommended as a general policy because it is unlikely to reduce their risk. There are no data to support the use of IVIG for postexposure prophylaxis in pregnant caregivers or immunocompromised children. No vaccine is currently available.

BIBLIOGRAPHY

Please visit the Nelson Textbook of Pediatrics *website at www.expertconsult.com for the complete bibliography.*

Chapter 244
Herpes Simplex Virus

Lawrence R. Stanberry

The 2 closely related herpes simplex viruses (HSVs), HSV type 1 (HSV-1) and HSV type 2 (HSV-2), cause a variety of illnesses, depending on the anatomic site where the infection is initiated, the immune state of the host, and whether the symptoms reflect primary or recurrent infection. Common infections involve the skin, eye, oral cavity, and genital tract. Infections tend to be mild and self-limiting, except in the immunocompromised patient and newborn infant, in whom they may be severe and life threatening.

Primary infection occurs in individuals who have not been infected previously with either HSV-1 or HSV-2. Because these individuals are HSV seronegative and have no pre-existing immunity to HSV, primary infections can be severe. **Nonprimary 1st infection** occurs in individuals previously infected with 1 type of HSV (e.g., HSV-1) who have become infected for the 1st time with the other HSV type (in this case, HSV-2). Because immunity to one HSV type provides some cross protection against disease caused by the other HSV type, nonprimary 1st infections tend to be less severe than true primary infections. During primary and nonprimary initial infections, HSV establishes latent infection in regional sensory ganglion neurons. Virus is maintained in this latent state for the life of the host but periodically can reactivate and cause **recurrent infection.** Symptomatic recurrent infections tend to be less severe and of shorter duration than 1st infections. Asymptomatic recurrent infections are extremely common. They cause no physical distress, although patients with recurrent infections are contagious and can transmit the virus to susceptible individuals. Re-infection with a new strain of either HSV-1 or HSV-2 at a previously infected anatomic site (e.g., the genital tract) can occur but is relatively uncommon, suggesting that host immunity, perhaps site-specific local immunity, resulting from the initial infection affords protection against exogenous re-infection. This observation suggests that it might be feasible to develop effective HSV vaccines.

ETIOLOGY

HSVs contain a double-stranded DNA genome of approximately 152 kb that encodes at least 84 proteins. The DNA is contained within an icosadeltahedral capsid, which is surrounded by an outer envelope composed of a lipid bilayer containing at least 12 viral glycoproteins. These glycoproteins are the major targets for humoral immunity, whereas other nonstructural proteins are important targets for cellular immunity. Two encoded proteins, viral DNA polymerase and thymidine kinase, are targets for antiviral drugs. HSV-1 and HSV-2 have a similar genetic composition with extensive DNA and protein homology. One important difference in the 2 viruses is their glycoprotein G genes, which have been exploited to develop a new generation of commercially available, accurate, type-specific serologic tests that can be used to discriminate whether a patient has been infected with HSV-1, HSV-2, or both.

EPIDEMIOLOGY

HSV infections are ubiquitous, and there are no seasonal variations in risk for infection. The only natural host is humans, and the mode of transmission is direct contact between mucocutaneous surfaces. There are no documented incidental transmissions from inanimate objects such as toilet seats.

All infected individuals harbor latent infection and experience recurrent infections, which may be symptomatic or may go unrecognized, and thus are periodically contagious. This information helps explain the widespread prevalence of HSV.

HSV-1 and HSV-2 are equally capable of causing initial infection at any anatomic site but differ in their capacity to cause recurrent infections. HSV-1 has a greater propensity to cause recurrent oral infections, whereas HSV-2 has a greater proclivity to cause recurrent genital infections. For this reason, HSV-1 infection typically results from contact with contaminated oral secretions, whereas HSV-2 infection most commonly results from anogenital contact.

HSV seroprevalence rates are highest in developing countries and among lower socioeconomic groups, although high rates of HSV-1 and HSV-2 infections are found in developed nations and among persons of the highest socioeconomic strata. Incident HSV-1 infections are more common during childhood and adolescence but are also found throughout later life. Data from the U.S. population–based National Health and Nutrition Examination Survey (NHANES) conducted between 1999 and 2004 showed a consistent increase of HSV-1 prevalence with age, which rose from 39% in adolescents 14-19-yr of age to 65% among those 40-49 yr of age. HSV-1 seroprevalence was not influenced by gender but rates were highest in Mexican-Americans (80.8%), intermediate in non-Hispanic blacks (68.3%), and lowest in non-Hispanic whites (50.1%), The NHANES study found an overall HSV-2 prevalence of 17% with a steady increased with age from 1.6% in the 14-19 yr age group to 26.4% in the 40-49-yr group. The rate was higher among females than males (22.8% and 11.2%, respectively) and varied by race and ethnic group, with an overall seroprevalence of 41.7% in blacks, 13.6% in Mexican-Americans, and 13.0% in whites. Modifiable factors that predicted HSV-2 seropositivity included less education, poverty, cocaine use, and a greater lifetime number of sexual partners. Studies show that only about 10% of HSV-2–seropositive subjects report a history of genital herpes, emphasizing the asymptomatic nature of most HSV infections.

A 3-yr longitudinal study of Midwestern adolescent girls 12-15 yr of age found that 44% were seropositive for HSV-1 and 7% for HSV-2 at enrollment. At the end of the study, 49% were seropositive for HSV-1 and 14% for HSV-2. The attack rates, based on the number of cases per 100 person-years, were 3.2 for HSV-1 infection among all girls and 4.4 for HSV-2 infection among girls who reported being sexually experienced. Findings of this study indicate that sexually active young women have a high attack rate for genital herpes and suggest that genital herpes should be considered in the differential diagnosis of any young woman who reports recurrent genitourinary complaints. In this study, participants with pre-existing HSV-1 antibodies had a significantly lower attack rate for HSV-2 infection, and those who became infected were less likely to have symptomatic disease than girls who were HSV seronegative when they entered the study. Prior HSV-1 infection appears to afford adolescent girls some protection against becoming infected with HSV-2; in adolescent girls infected with HSV-2, the pre-existing HSV-1 immunity appears to protect against development of symptomatic genital herpes.

Neonatal herpes is an uncommon but potentially fatal infection of the fetus or more likely the newborn. It is not a reportable disease in most states, and therefore there are no solid epidemiologic data regarding its frequency in the general population. In King County, Washington, the estimated incidence of neonatal herpes per was 2.6 cases/100,000 live births in the late 1960s, 11.9 from 1978 to 1981, and 31 from 1982 to 1999. This increase in neonatal herpes cases parallels the increase in cases of genital herpes. The estimated rate of neonatal herpes is 1/3,000-5,000 live births, which is higher than reported for the reportable perinatally acquired sexually transmitted infections such as congenital syphilis and gonococcal ophthalmia. More than 90% of the cases are the result of maternal-fetal transmission. The risk for transmission is greatest during a primary or nonprimary 1st infection (30-50%) and much lower when the exposure is during a recurrent infection (<2%). Infants born to mothers dually infected with HIV and HSV-2 are also at higher risk for acquiring HIV than infants born to HIV-positive mothers who are not HSV-2 infected. It is estimated that approximately 25% of pregnant women are HSV-2 infected and that approximately 2% of pregnant women acquire HSV-2 infection during pregnancy.

HSV is a leading cause of sporadic, fatal encephalitis in children and adults. In the USA it is estimated that there are 1,250 cases annually of HSV encephalitis.

PATHOGENESIS

In the immunocompetent host the pathogenesis of HSV infection involves viral replication in skin and mucous membranes followed by replication and spread in neural tissue. Viral infection typically begins at a cutaneous **portal of entry** such as the oral cavity, genital mucosa, ocular conjunctiva, or breaks in keratinized epithelia. Virus replicates locally, resulting in the death of the cell, and sometimes produces clinically apparent inflammatory responses that facilitate the development of characteristic herpetic vesicles and ulcers. Virus also enters nerve endings and spreads beyond the portal of entry to sensory ganglia by intraneuronal transport. Virus replicates in some sensory neurons, and the progeny virions are sent via intraneuronal transport mechanisms back to the periphery, where they are released from nerve endings and replicate further in skin or mucosal surfaces. It is virus moving through this neural arc that is primarily responsible for the development of characteristic herpetic lesions, although most HSV infections do not reach a threshold necessary to cause clinically recognizable disease. Although many sensory neurons become productively infected during the initial infection, some infected neurons do not initially support viral replication. It is in these neurons that the virus establishes a **latent infection,** a condition in which the viral genome persists within the neuronal nucleus in a largely metabolically inactive state. Intermittently throughout the life of the host, undefined changes can occur in latently infected neurons that trigger the virus to begin to replicate. This replication occurs despite the host's having established a variety of humoral and cellular immune responses that successfully controlled the initial infection. With reactivation of the latent neuron, progeny virions are produced and transported within nerve fibers back to cutaneous sites somewhere in the vicinity of the initial infection, where further replication occurs and causes recurrent infections. Recurrent infections may be symptomatic (with typical or atypical herpetic lesions) or asymptomatic. In either case, virus is shed at the site where cutaneous replication occurs and can be transmitted to susceptible individuals who come in contact with the site or with contaminated secretions. Latency and reactivation are the mechanisms by which the virus is successfully maintained in the human population.

Viremia, or hematogenous spread of the virus, does not appear to play an important role in HSV infections in the immunocompetent host but can occur in neonates, individuals with eczema, and severely malnourished children. It is also seen in patients with depressed or defective cell-mediated immunity, such as occurs with HIV infection or some immunosuppressive therapies. Viremia can result in dissemination of the virus to visceral organs, including the liver and adrenals. Hematogenous dissemination of virus to the central nervous system appears to only occur in neonates.

The pathogenesis of HSV infection in newborns is complicated by their relative immunologic immaturity. The source of virus in neonatal infections is typically but not exclusively the mother. Transmission generally occurs during delivery, although it is well documented to occur even with cesarean delivery with intact fetal membranes. The most common portals of entry are the conjunctiva, mucosal epithelium of the nose and mouth, and breaks or abrasions in the skin that occur with scalp electrode use or forceps delivery. With prompt antiviral therapy, virus replication may be restricted to the site of inoculation (the skin, eye, or mouth). However, virus may also extend from the nose to the respiratory tract to cause pneumonia, move via intraneuronal transport to the central nervous system to cause encephalitis, or spread by hematogenous dissemination to visceral organs and the brain. Factors that may influence neonatal HSV infection include the virus type, portal of entry, inoculum of virus to which the infant is exposed, gestational age of the infant, and presence of maternally derived antibodies specific to the virus causing infection. Latent infection is established during neonatal infection, and survivors may experience recurrent cutaneous and neural infections.

CLINICAL MANIFESTATIONS

The hallmarks of common HSV infections are skin vesicles and shallow ulcers. Classic infections manifest as small, 2- to 4-mm vesicles that may be surrounded by an erythematous base. These may persist for a few days before evolving into shallow, minimally erythematous ulcers. The vesicular phase tends to persist longer when keratinized epithelia is involved and be brief, sometimes fleeting, when moist mucous membranes are the site of infection. Because HSV infections are common and their natural history is influenced by many factors, including portal of entry, immune status of the host, and whether it is an initial or recurrent infection, the typical manifestations are seldom classic. Most infections are asymptomatic or unrecognized, and nonclassic presentations such as small skin fissures and small erythematous nonvesicular lesions are common.

Acute Oropharyngeal Infections

Herpes gingivostomatitis most often affects children 6 mo to 5 yr of age but is seen across the age spectrum. It is an extremely painful condition with sudden onset, pain in the mouth, drooling, refusal to eat or drink, and fever of up to 40.0-40.6°C. The gums become markedly swollen, and vesicles may develop throughout the oral cavity, including the gums, lips, tongue, palate, tonsils, pharynx, and perioral skin (Fig. 244-1). The vesicles may be more extensively distributed than typically seen with enteroviral herpangina. During the initial phase of the illness there may be tonsillar exudates suggestive of bacterial pharyngitis. The vesicles are generally present only a few days before progressing to form shallow indurated ulcers that may be covered with a yellow-gray membrane. Tender submandibular, submaxillary, and cervical lymphadenopathy is common. The breath may be foul as a result of overgrowth of anaerobic oral bacteria. Untreated, the illness resolves in 7-14 days, although the lymphadenopathy may persist for several weeks.

In older children, adolescents, and college students, the initial HSV oral infection may manifest as pharyngitis and tonsillitis rather than gingivostomatitis. The vesicular phase is often over by the time the patient presents to a health care provider, and signs and symptoms may be indistinguishable from those of streptococcal pharyngitis, consisting of fever, malaise, headache, sore throat, and white plaques on the tonsils. The course of illness is typically longer than for untreated streptococcal pharyngitis.

Herpes Labialis

Fever blisters, or **cold sores,** are the most common manifestation of recurrent HSV-1 infections. The most common site of herpes labialis is the vermilion border of the lip, although lesions sometimes occur on the nose, chin, cheek, or oral mucosa. Older patients report experiencing burning, tingling, itching, or pain

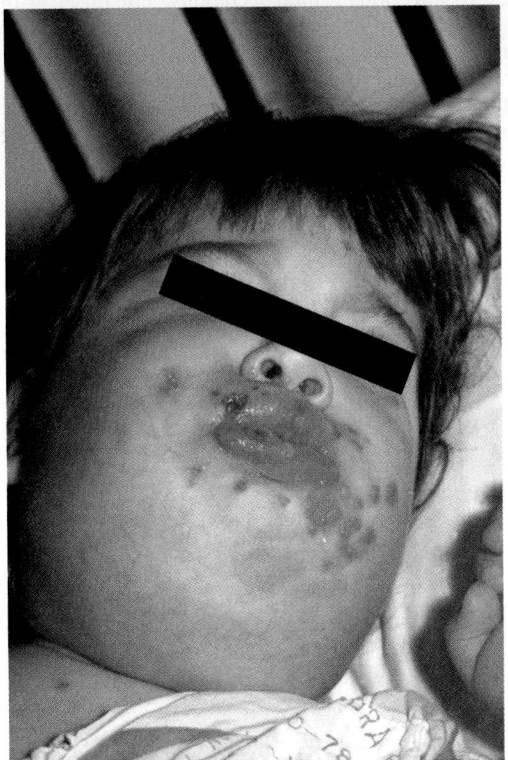

Figure 244-1 Clustered perioral vesicles and erosions in an infant with primary herpetic gingivostomatitis. (From Schachner LA, Hansen RC, editors: *Pediatric dermatology,* ed 3, Philadelphia, 1988, Mosby, p 1078.)

3-6 hr (rarely as long as 24-48 hr) before the development of the herpes lesion. The lesion generally begins as a small grouping of erythematous papules that over a few hours progress to create a small, thin-walled vesicle. The vesicles may form shallow ulcers or become pustular. The short-lived ulcer dries and develops a crusted scab. Complete healing without scarring occurs with re-epithelialization of the ulcerated skin, usually within 6-10 days. Some patients experience local lymphadenopathy but no constitutional symptoms.

Cutaneous Infections

In the healthy child or adolescent, cutaneous HSV infections are generally the result of skin trauma with macro- or micro-abrasions and exposure to infectious secretions. This situation most often occurs in play or contact sports such as wrestling (**herpes gladiatorum**) and rugby (**scrumpox**). As with other HSV infections, an initial cutaneous infection establishes a latent infection that can subsequently result in recurrent infections at or near the site of the initial infection. Pain, burning, itching, or tingling often precedes the herpetic eruption by a few hours to a few days. Like herpes labialis, lesions begin as grouped, erythematous papules that progress to vesicles, pustules, ulcers, and crusts and then healing without scarring in 6-10 days. Although herpes labialis typically results in a single lesion, a cutaneous HSV infection results in multiple discrete lesions and involves a larger surface area. Regional lymphadenopathy may occur but systemic symptoms seldom do. Recurrences are sometimes associated with local edema and lymphangitis or local neuralgia.

Herpes whitlow is a term generally applied to HSV infection of fingers or toes, although strictly speaking it refers to HSV infection of the paronychia. Among children, this condition is most commonly seen in infants and toddlers who suck the thumb or fingers and who are experiencing either a symptomatic or a subclinical oral HSV-1 infection (Fig. 244-2). An HSV-2 herpes whitlow occasionally develops in an adolescent as a result of exposure to infectious genital secretions. The onset of the infection is heralded by itching, pain, and erythema 2-7 days after exposure. The cuticle becomes erythematous and tender and may appear to contain pus, although if it is incised, little fluid is present. Incising the lesion is discouraged, as this maneuver typically prolongs recovery and increases the risk for secondary bacterial infection. Lesions and associated pain typically persist for about 10 days, followed by rapid improvement and complete recovery in 18-20 days. Regional lymphadenopathy is common, and lymphangitis and neuralgia may occur. Unlike other recurrent herpes infections, recurrent herpetic whitlows are often as painful as the primary infection but are generally shorter in duration.

Cutaneous HSV infections can be severe or life threatening in patients with disorders of the skin such as eczema (eczema herpeticum), pemphigus, burns, and Darier disease, and following laser skin resurfacing. The lesions are frequently ulcerative and nonspecific in appearance, although typical vesicles may be seen in adjacent normal skin (Fig. 244-3). If untreated, these lesions can progress to disseminated infection and death. Recurrent infections are common but generally less severe than the initial infection.

Genital Herpes

Genital HSV infection is common in sexually experienced adolescents and young adults, but up to 90% of infected individuals are unaware they are infected. Infection may result from genital-genital transmission (usually HSV-2) or oral-genital transmission (usually HSV-1). Symptomatic and asymptomatic individuals periodically shed virus from anogenital sites and hence can transmit the infection to sexual partners or, in the case of pregnant women, to their newborns. Classic primary genital herpes may be preceded by a short period of local burning and tenderness before vesicles develop on genital mucosal surfaces or keratinized skin and sometimes around the anus or on the buttocks and thighs. Vesicles on mucosal surfaces are short lived and rupture to produce shallow, tender ulcers covered with a yellowish gray exudate and surrounded by an erythematous border. Vesicles on keratinized epithelium persist for a few days before progressing to the pustular stage and then crusting.

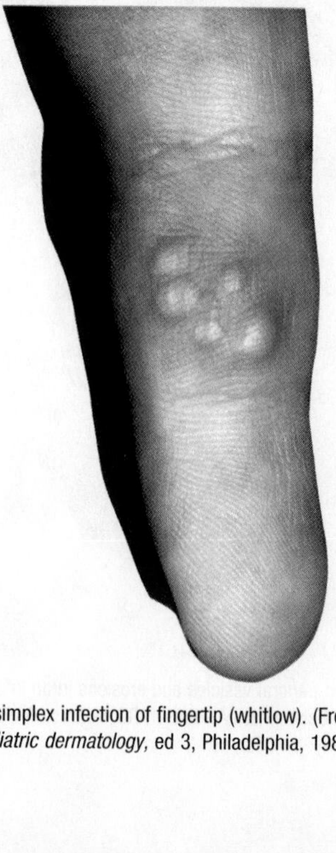

Figure 244-2 Herpes simplex infection of fingertip (whitlow). (From Schachner LA, Hansen RC, editors: *Pediatric dermatology,* ed 3, Philadelphia, 1988, Mosby, p 1079.)

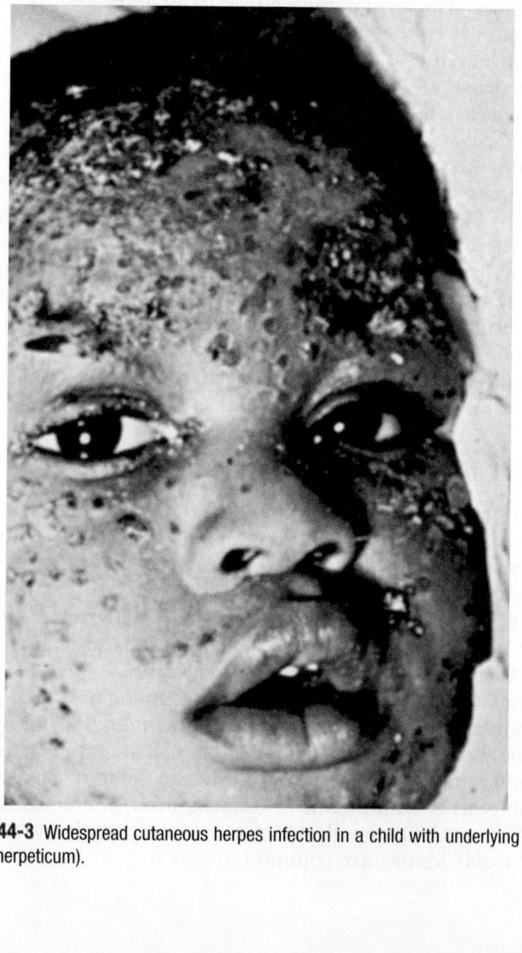

Figure 244-3 Widespread cutaneous herpes infection in a child with underlying eczema (eczema herpeticum).

Patients may experience urethritis and dysuria severe enough to cause urinary retention and bilateral, tender inguinal and pelvic lymphadenopathy. Women may experience a watery vaginal discharge, and men may have a clear mucoid urethral discharge. Significant local pain and systemic symptoms such as fever, headache, and myalgia are common. Aseptic meningitis develops in an estimated 15% of cases. The course of classic primary genital herpes from onset to complete healing is 2-3 wk.

Most patients with symptomatic primary genital herpes experience at least 1 recurrent infection in the following year. Recurrent genital herpes is usually less severe and of shorter duration than the primary infection. Some patients experience a sensory prodrome with pain, burning, and tingling at the site where vesicles subsequently develop. Asymptomatic recurrent anogenital HSV infections are common, and all HSV-2–seropositive individuals appear to periodically shed virus from anogenital sites. Most sexual transmissions and maternal-neonatal transmissions of virus result from asymptomatic shedding episodes.

Genital infections caused by HSV-1 and HSV-2 are indistinguishable, but HSV-1 causes significantly fewer subsequent episodes of recurrent infection; hence, knowing which virus is causing the infection has important prognostic value. Genital HSV infection increases the risk for acquiring HIV infection.

Rarely, genital HSV infections are identified in young children and preadolescents. Although genital disease in children should raise concerns about possible sexual abuse, there are documented cases of autoinoculation, in which a child has inadvertently transmitted virus from contaminated oral secretions to his or her own genitalia.

Ocular Infections

HSV ocular infections may involve the conjunctiva, cornea, or retina and may be primary or recurrent. Conjunctivitis or keratoconjunctivitis is usually unilateral and is often associated with blepharitis and tender preauricular lymphadenopathy. The conjunctiva appears edematous but there is rarely purulent discharge. Vesicular lesions may be seen on the lid margins and periorbital skin. Patients typically have fever. Untreated infection generally resolves in 2-3 wk. Obvious corneal involvement is rare, but when it occurs it can produce ulcers that are described as appearing dendritic or geographic. Extension to the stroma is uncommon although more likely to occur in patients inadvertently treated with corticosteroids. When it occurs it may be associated with corneal edema, scarring, and corneal perforation. Recurrent infections tend to involve the underlying stroma, and repeated recurrences can cause progressive corneal scarring and injury that can lead to blindness.

Retinal infections are rare and are more likely among infants with neonatal herpes and immunocompromised persons with disseminated HSV infections.

Central Nervous System Infections

HSV encephalitis is the leading cause of sporadic, nonepidemic encephalitis in children and adults in the USA. It is an acute necrotizing infection generally involving the frontal and/or temporal cortex and the limbic system and, beyond the neonatal period, is almost always caused by HSV-1. The infection may manifest as nonspecific findings, including fever, headache, nuchal rigidity, nausea, vomiting, generalized seizures, and alteration of consciousness. Injury to the frontal or temporal cortex or limbic system may produce findings more indicative of HSV encephalitis, including anosmia, memory loss, peculiar behavior, expressive aphasia and other changes in speech, hallucinations, and focal seizures. The untreated infection progresses to coma and death in 75% of cases. Examination of the cerebrospinal fluid (CSF) typically shows a moderate number of mononuclear cells and polymorphonuclear leukocytes, a mildly elevated protein concentration, a normal or slightly decreased glucose concentration, and often a moderate number of erythrocytes.

HSV is also a cause of aseptic meningitis and is the most common cause of recurrent aseptic meningitis (**Mollaret meningitis**).

Infections in Immunocompromised Persons

Severe, life-threatening HSV infections can occur in patients with compromised immune functions, including neonates, the severely malnourished, those with primary and secondary immunodeficiencies diseases including AIDS, and those on some immunosuppressive regimens, particularly for cancer and organ transplantation. Mucocutaneous infections, including mucositis and esophagitis, are most common, although their presentations may be atypical and can result in lesions that slowly enlarge, ulcerate, become necrotic, and extend to deeper tissues. Other HSV infections include tracheobronchitis, pneumonitis, and anogenital infections. Disseminated infection can result in a sepsis-like presentation, with liver and adrenal involvement, disseminated intravascular coagulopathy, and shock.

Perinatal Infections

HSV infection may be acquired in utero, during the birth process, or during the neonatal period. Intrauterine and postpartum infections are well described but occur infrequently. Postpartum transmission may be from the mother or another adult with a nongenital (typically HSV-1) infection such as herpes labialis. Most cases of neonatal herpes result from maternal infection and transmission, usually during passage through a contaminated infected birth canal of a mother with asymptomatic genital herpes. Transmission is well documented in infants delivered by cesarean section. Fewer than 30% of mothers of an infant with neonatal herpes have a history of genital herpes. The risk for infection is higher in infants born to mothers with primary genital infection (>30%) than with recurrent genital infection (<2%). Use of scalp electrodes may also increase risk.

Neonatal HSV infection is thought to never be asymptomatic. Its clinical presentation reflects timing of infection, portal of entry, and extent of spread. Infants with intrauterine infection typically have skin vesicles or scarring, eye findings including chorioretinitis and keratoconjunctivitis, and microcephaly or hydranencephaly that are present at delivery. Few infants survive without therapy, and those who do generally have severe sequelae. Infants infected during delivery or postpartum present with 1 of the following 3 patterns of disease: (1) disease localized to the skin, eyes, or mouth; (2) encephalitis with or without skin, eye, and mouth **(SEM) disease**; and (3) disseminated infection involving multiple organs, including the brain, lungs, liver, heart, adrenals, and skin.

Infants with SEM disease generally present at 5-11 days of life and typically demonstrate a few small vesicles, particularly on the presenting part or at sites of trauma such as with scalp electrode placement. If untreated, SEM disease in infants may progress to encephalitis or disseminated disease.

Infants with encephalitis typically present at 8-17 days of life with clinical findings suggestive of bacterial meningitis, including irritability, lethargy, poor feeding, poor tone, and seizures. Fever is relatively uncommon, and skin vesicles occur in only about 60% of cases (Fig. 244-4). If untreated, 50% of infants with HSV encephalitis die and most survivors have severe neurologic sequelae.

Infants with disseminated HSV infections generally become ill at 5-11 days of life. Their clinical picture is similar to that of infants with bacterial sepsis, consisting of hyperthermia or hypothermia, irritability, poor feeding, and vomiting. They may also exhibit respiratory distress, cyanosis, apneic spells, jaundice, purpuric rash, and evidence of central nervous system infection; seizures are common. Skin vesicles are seen in about 75% of cases. If untreated, the infection causes shock and disseminated intravascular coagulation; approximately 90% of these infants die, and most survivors have severe neurologic sequelae.

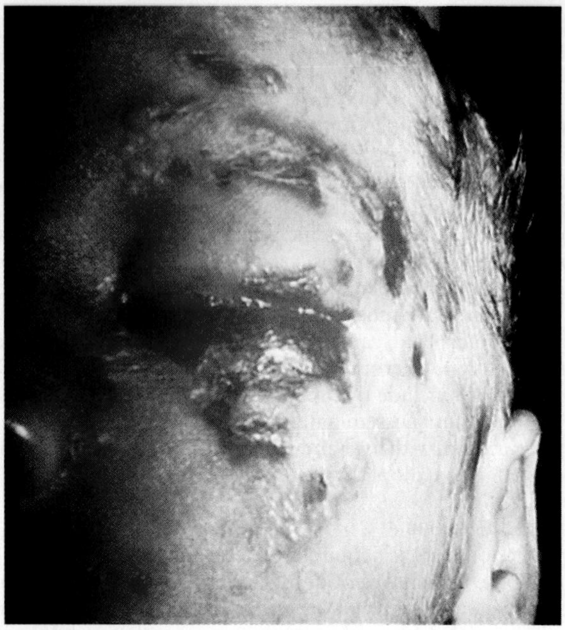

Figure 244-4 Vesicular-pustular lesions on the face of a neonate with herpes simplex virus infection. (From Kohl S: Neonatal herpes simplex virus infection, *Clin Perinatol* 24:129–150, 1997.)

DIAGNOSIS

The clinical diagnosis of HSV infections, particularly life-threatening infections and genital herpes, should be confirmed by laboratory test, preferably isolation of virus or viral DNA detection by polymerase chain reaction (PCR). Histologic findings or imaging studies may support the diagnosis but should not substitute for virus-specific tests. HSV immunoglobulin M (IgM) tests are notoriously unreliable, and the demonstration of a four-fold or greater rise in HSV-specific IgG titers between acute and convalescent serum samples is useful only in retrospect.

Virus culture remains the gold standard for diagnosing HSV infections. The highest yield comes from rupturing a suspected herpetic vesicle and vigorously rubbing the base of the lesion to collect fluid and cells. Culturing dried, crusted lesions is generally of low yield. Although not as sensitive as viral culture, direct detection of HSV antigens in clinical specimens can be done rapidly and has very good specificity. The use of PCR for detection of HSV DNA is highly sensitive and specific and in some instances can be performed rapidly. It is the test of choice in examining CSF in cases of suspected HSV encephalitis.

Evaluation of the neonate with suspected HSV infection should include cultures of suspicious lesions as well as eye and mouth swabs and PCR of CSF. Culture or antigen detection should be used in evaluating lesions associated with suspected acute genital herpes. HSV-2 type-specific antibody tests are useful for evaluating sexually experienced adolescents or young adults who have a history of unexplained recurrent nonspecific urogenital signs and symptoms, but these tests are less useful for general screening in populations in which HSV-2 infections are of low prevalence.

Because most HSV diagnostic tests take at least a few days to complete, treatment should not be withheld but rather initiated promptly in order to ensure the maximum therapeutic benefit.

LABORATORY FINDINGS

Most self-limited HSV infections cause few changes in routine laboratory parameters. Mucocutaneous infections may cause a moderate polymorphonuclear leukocytosis. In HSV meningoencephalitis there can be an increase in mononuclear cells and protein in CSF, the glucose content may be normal or reduced, and red blood cells may be present. The electroencephalogram and MRI of the brain may show temporal lobe abnormalities in HSV encephalitis beyond the neonatal period. Encephalitis in the neonatal period tends to be more global and not limited to the temporal lobe. Disseminated infection may cause elevated liver enzymes, thrombocytopenia, and abnormal coagulation.

TREATMENT (CHAPTER 237)

Three antiviral drugs are available in the USA for the management of HSV infections, namely acyclovir, valacyclovir, and famciclovir. All 3 are available in oral form, but only acyclovir is available in a suspension form. Acyclovir has the poorest bioavailability and hence requires more frequent dosing. Valacyclovir, a prodrug of acyclovir, and famciclovir, a prodrug of penciclovir, both have very good oral bioavailability and are dosed once or twice daily. Acyclovir and penciclovir are also available in a topical form but these provide limited or no benefit to patients with recurrent mucocutaneous HSV infections. Only acyclovir has an intravenous formulation. Early initiation of therapy results in the maximal therapeutic benefit. All 3 drugs have exceptional safety profiles and are safe to use in pediatric patients. Doses should be modified in patients with renal impairment.

Resistance to acyclovir and penciclovir is rare in immunocompetent persons but does occur in immunocompromised persons. Virus isolates from immunocompromised persons whose HSV infection is not responding or is worsening with acyclovir therapy should be tested for drug sensitivities. Foscarnet and cidofovir have been used in the treatment of HSV infections caused by acyclovir-resistant mutants.

Topical trifluorothymidine, vidarabine, and idoxuridine are used in the treatment of herpes keratitis.

Patients with genital herpes also require counseling to address psychosocial issues, including possible stigma, and to help them understand the natural history and management of this chronic infection.

Acute Mucocutaneous Infections

For gingivostomatitis, oral acyclovir (15 mg/kg/dose 5 times a day PO for 7 days, maximum 1 g/day) started within 72 hr of onset reduces the severity and duration of the illness. Pain associated with swallowing may limit oral intake of infants and children, putting them at risk for dehydration. Intake should be encouraged through the use of cold beverages, ice cream, and yogurt.

For **herpes labialis**, oral treatment is superior to topical antiviral therapy. For treatment of a recurrence in adolescents, oral valacyclovir (2,000 mg bid PO for 1 day), acyclovir (200-400 mg 5 times daily PO for 5 days), or famciclovir (1,500 mg once daily PO for 1 day) shortens the duration of the episode. Long-term daily use of oral acyclovir (400 mg bid PO) or valacyclovir (500 mg once daily PO) has been used to prevent recurrences in individuals with frequent or severe recurrences.

Anecdotal reports suggest that treatment of adolescents with **herpes gladiatorum** with oral acyclovir (200 mg 5 times daily PO for 7-10 days) or valacyclovir (500 mg bid PO for 7-10 days) at the first signs of the outbreak can shorten the course of the recurrence. For patients with a history of recurrent herpes gladiatorum, chronic daily prophylaxis with valacyclovir (500-1,000 mg daily) has been reported to prevent recurrences.

There are no clinical trials assessing the benefit of antiviral treatment for **herpetic whitlow.** High-dose oral acyclovir (1,600-2,000 mg/day divided in 2-3 doses PO for 10 days) started at the 1st signs of illness has been reported to abort some recurrences and reduce the duration of others in adults.

A clinical trial in adults has established the effectiveness of oral acyclovir (200 mg 5 times a day PO for 5 days) in the treatment of **eczema herpeticum**; however, serious infections should be treated with intravenous acyclovir. Oral-facial HSV infections can reactivate after cosmetic facial laser resurfacing, causing extensive disease and scarring. Treatment of adults beginning the day before the procedure with either valacyclovir (500 mg twice daily PO for 10-14 days) or famciclovir (250-500 mg bid PO for 10 days) has been reported to be effective in preventing the infections. HSV infections in **burn patients** can be severe or life threatening and have been treated with intravenous acyclovir (10-20 mg/kg/day divided every 8 hr IV).

Antiviral drugs are not effective in the treatment of HSV-associated **erythema multiforme,** but their daily use as for herpes labialis prophylaxis has been shown to prevent recurrences of erythema multiforme.

Genital Herpes

Pediatric patients, usually adolescents or young adults, with suspected first-episode genital herpes should be treated with antiviral therapy. Treatment of the initial infection reduces the severity and duration of the illness but has no effect on the frequency of subsequent recurrent infections. Treatment options for adolescents include acyclovir (400 mg tid PO for 7-10 days), famciclovir (750 mg tid PO for 7-10 days), or valacyclovir (1000 mg bid PO for 7-10 days). The twice-daily valacyclovir option avoids treatment during school hours. For smaller children, acyclovir suspension can be used at a dose of 10-20 mg/kg/dose 4 times daily not to exceed the adult dose. The first episode of genital herpes can be extremely painful, and use of analgesics is generally indicated. All patients with genital herpes should be offered counseling to help them deal with psychosocial issues and understand the chronic nature of the illness.

There are 3 strategic options regarding the management of recurrent infections. The choice should be guided by several factors, including the frequency and severity of the recurrent infections, the psychologic impact of the illness on the patient, and concerns regarding transmission to a susceptible sexual partner. Option 1 is no therapy; option 2 is episodic therapy; and option 3 is long-term suppressive therapy. For **episodic therapy,** treatment should be initiated at the 1st signs of an outbreak. Recommended choices for episodic therapy in adolescents include famciclovir (1,000 mg bid PO for 1 day), acyclovir (800 mg tid PO for 2 days), or valacyclovir (500 mg bid PO for 3 days). Long-term suppressive therapy offers the advantage that it prevents most outbreaks, improves patient quality of life in terms of the psychosocial impact of genital herpes, and, with daily valacyclovir therapy, also reduces (but does not eliminate) the risk for sexual transmission to a susceptible sexual partner. Options for **long-term suppressive therapy** are acyclovir (400 mg bid PO), famciclovir (250 mg bid PO), and valacyclovir (500-1,000 mg qd PO).

Ocular Infections

HSV ocular infections can result in blindness. Management should involve consultation with an ophthalmologist.

Central Nervous System Infections

Patients older than neonates who have herpes encephalitis should be promptly treated with intravenous acyclovir (10 mg/kg every 8 hr given as a 1-hr infusion for 14-21 days). Treatment for increased intracranial pressure, management of seizures, and respiratory compromise may be required.

Infections in Immunocompromised Persons

Severe mucocutaneous and disseminated HSV infections in immunocompromised patients should be treated with intravenous acyclovir (5-10 mg/kg or 250 mg/m^2 every 8 hr) until there is evidence of resolution of the infection. Oral antiviral therapy with acyclovir, famciclovir, or valacyclovir has been used for treatment of less severe HSV infections and for suppression of recurrences during periods of significant immunosuppression. Drug resistance does occur occasionally in immunocompromised patients, and in individuals whose HSV infection does not respond to antiviral drug therapy, viral isolates should be tested to determine sensitivity. Acyclovir-resistant viruses are often also resistant to famciclovir but may be sensitive to foscarnet or cidofovir.

Perinatal Infections

All infants with proven or suspected neonatal HSV infection should be begun promptly on high-dose intravenous acyclovir (60 mg/kg/day divided every 8 hr IV). Treatment may be discontinued in infants shown by laboratory testing not to be infected. Infants with HSV disease limited to skin, eyes, and mouth should be treated for 14 days, whereas those with disseminated or central nervous system disease should receive 21 days of therapy. Patients receiving high-dose therapy should be monitored for neutropenia.

PROGNOSIS

Most HSV infections are self-limiting, last from a few days (for recurrent infections) to 2-3 wk (for primary infections), and heal without scarring. Recurrent oral-facial herpes in a patient who has undergone dermabrasion or laser resurfacing can be severe and lead to scarring. Because genital herpes is a sexually transmitted infection, it can be stigmatizing, and its psychologic consequences may be much greater than its physiologic effects. Some HSV infections can be severe and without prompt antiviral therapy may have grave consequences. Life-threatening conditions include neonatal herpes, herpes encephalitis, and HSV infections in immunocompromised patients, burn patients, and severely malnourished infants and children. Recurrent ocular herpes can lead to corneal scarring and blindness.

PREVENTION

Transmission of infection occurs through exposure to virus either as the result of skin-to-skin contact or from contact with contaminated secretions. Good handwashing and, when appropriate, the use of gloves provide health care workers with excellent protection against HSV infection in the workplace. Health care workers with active oral-facial herpes or herpes whitlow should take precautions, particularly when caring for high-risk patients such as newborns, immunocompromised individuals, and patients with chronic skin conditions. Patients and parents should be advised about good hygienic practices, including handwashing and avoiding contact with lesions and secretions, during active herpes outbreaks. Schools and daycare centers should clean shared toys and athletic equipment such as wrestling mats at least daily after use. Athletes with active herpes infections who participate in contact sports such as wrestling and rugby should be excluded from practice or games until the lesions are completely healed. Genital herpes can be prevented by avoiding genital-genital and oral-genital contact. The risk for acquiring genital herpes can be reduced but not eliminated through the correct and consistent use of condoms. Male circumcision is associated with a reduced risk of acquiring genital HSV infection. The risk for transmitting genital HSV-2 infection to a susceptible sexual partner can be reduced but not eliminated by the daily use of oral valacyclovir by the infected partner. No vaccine is currently available, but a subunit vaccine intended for the prevention of genital herpes is in advanced clinical development.

For **pregnant women** with **active genital herpes** at the time of delivery, the risk for mother-to-baby transmission can be reduced but not eliminated by delivering the baby via a cesarean section (within 4-6 hr of rupture of membranes). The risk for recurrent genital herpes and therefore the need for cesarean delivery can be reduced but not eliminated in pregnant women with a history of genital herpes by the daily use of oral acyclovir, valacyclovir, or famciclovir during the last 4 wk of gestation, which is recommended by the American College of Obstetrics and Gynecology.

Infants delivered vaginally to women with first-episode genital herpes are at very high risk for acquiring HSV infection. The nasopharynx and umbilicus should be cultured at delivery and on day 2 of life. Some authorities recommend that these infants receive anticipatory acyclovir therapy for at least 2 wk, and others treat such infants if signs develop or if the 48-hr cultures have positive results. Infants delivered to women with a history of recurrent genital herpes are at low risk for development of neonatal herpes. In this setting parents should be educated about the signs and symptoms of neonatal HSV infection and should be instructed to seek care without delay at the first suggestion of infection. When the situation is in doubt, infants should be evaluated and the nasopharynx and umbilicus cultured for neonatal herpes and intravenous acyclovir begun until culture results are negative or until another explanation can be found for the signs and symptoms.

Recurrent genital HSV infections can be prevented by the daily use of oral acyclovir, valacyclovir, or famciclovir, and these drugs have been used to prevent recurrences of oral-facial (labialis) and cutaneous (gladiatorum) herpes. Oral and intravenous acyclovir has also been used to prevent recurrent HSV infections in immunocompromised patients. Use of sun blockers has also been reported to be effective in preventing recurrent oral-facial herpes in patients with a history of sun-induced recurrent disease.

BIBLIOGRAPHY

Please visit the Nelson Textbook of Pediatrics *website at www.expertconsult.com for the complete bibliography.*

Chapter 245
Varicella-Zoster Virus Infections

Philip S. LaRussa and Mona Marin

Varicella-zoster virus (VZV) causes primary, latent, and recurrent infections. The primary infection is manifested as varicella (**chickenpox**) and results in establishment of a lifelong latent infection of sensory ganglion neurons. Reactivation of the latent infection causes herpes zoster (**shingles**). Although often a mild illness of childhood, chickenpox can cause substantial morbidity and mortality in otherwise healthy children; it increases morbidity and mortality in immunocompetent infants, adolescents, adults, as well as in immunocompromised persons; it predisposes to severe group A streptococcus and *Staphylococcus aureus* infections. Varicella and herpes zoster can be treated with antiviral drugs. Primary clinical disease can be prevented by immunization with live-attenuated VZV vaccine (varicella vaccine). Herpes zoster vaccine (zoster vaccine), which contains the same VZV strain used in the varicella vaccine but with a higher potency, is recommended for persons ≥60 yr of age to boost their immunity to VZV in order to reduce the rates of herpes zoster and its major complication, painful postherpetic neuralgia.

ETIOLOGY

VZV is a neurotropic human herpesvirus with similarities to herpes simplex virus, which is also α-herpesvirus. These viruses are enveloped with double-stranded DNA genomes that encode more than 70 proteins, including proteins that are targets of cellular and humoral immunity.

EPIDEMIOLOGY

Before the introduction of varicella vaccine in 1995, varicella was an almost universal communicable infection of childhood in the USA. Most children were infected by 15 yr of age, with fewer than 5% of adults remaining susceptible. This pattern of infection at younger ages is characteristic in all countries in temperate climates. In tropical areas, varicella occurs among older persons, with many cases occurring among adults. In the USA, annual varicella epidemics occurred in winter and spring, accounting for about 4 million cases, 11,000-15,000 hospitalizations, and 100-150 deaths every year. Varicella is a more serious disease in young infants, adults, and immunocompromised persons, in whom there are higher rates of complications and deaths than in healthy children. Within households, transmission of VZV to susceptible individuals occurs at a rate of 65-86%; more casual contact, such as occurs in a school classroom, is associated with lower attack rates among susceptible children. Patients with varicella are contagious 24-48 hr before the rash is evident and until vesicles are crusted, usually 3-7 days after onset of rash. Susceptible persons may also acquire varicella after close, direct contact with adults or children who have herpes zoster.

Since implementation of the 1-dose varicella vaccination program in 1995, there have been substantial declines in varicella morbidity and mortality in the USA. By 2005, vaccination coverage had increased to 90% and varicella cases had declined 90-91% from those in 1995 in sites where active surveillance was being conducted. By 2002, varicella-related hospitalizations had declined 88% from 1994 and 1995. Deaths had decreased by 87% overall from 1990-1994 to 2003-2005; in persons age <20 yr there was a 96% decline in deaths. Declines in morbidity and mortality were seen in all age groups, including infants <12 mo of age who were not eligible for vaccination, indicating protection from exposure by indirect vaccination effects. Although the age-specific incidence has declined in all age groups, the median age at infection has increased, and cases now are occurring predominantly in children in upper elementary school rather than in the preschool years. This change in varicella epidemiology highlights the importance of offering vaccine to every susceptible child, adolescent, and adult.

The continued occurrence of breakthrough infections, though most commonly mild, and of outbreaks in settings with high 1-dose varicella vaccine coverage prompted adoption in 2006 of a routine 2-dose childhood varicella vaccination program for all individuals without evidence of immunity, regardless of age.

Herpes zoster is due to the reactivation of latent VZV. It is uncommon in childhood and shows no seasonal variation in incidence. Zoster is not caused by exposure to a patient with varicella; exposures to varicella boost the cell-mediated immune response to VZV in individuals with prior infection, decreasing the likelihood of reactivation of latent virus. The lifetime risk for herpes zoster for individuals with a history of varicella is 10-20%, with 75% of cases occurring after 45 yr of age. Herpes zoster is very rare in healthy children <10 yr of age, with the exception of infants who were infected in utero or in the 1st year of life, who have an increased risk for development of zoster in the first years of life. Herpes zoster in children tends to be milder than disease in adults and is less frequently associated with postherpetic neuralgia. Herpes zoster occurs more frequently, occasionally multiple times, and may be severe in children receiving immunosuppressive therapy for malignancy or other diseases and in those who have HIV infection. The zoster vaccine, recommended for adults 60 yr of age and older, reduces both the frequency of herpes zoster and its most frequent complication, postherpetic neuralgia.

The attenuated VZV in the varicella vaccine can establish latent infection and reactivate as herpes zoster. However, the risk for development of subsequent herpes zoster is lower after vaccine

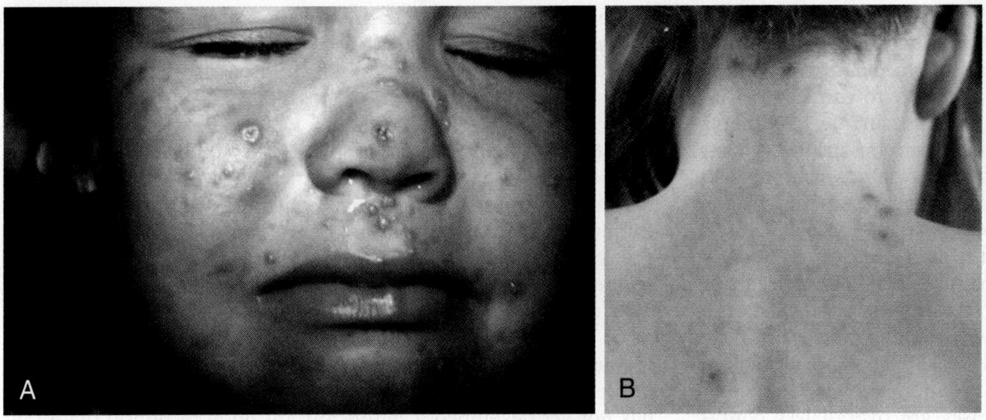

Figure 245-1 *A,* Varicella lesions in unvaccinated persons display the characteristic "cropping" distribution, or manifest themselves in clusters; the simultaneous presence of lesions in various stages of evolution is characteristic. *B,* Breakthrough varicella lesions are predominantly maculopapular, and vesicles are less common; the illness is most commonly mild with <50 lesions. (*A,* Courtesy of the Centers for Disease Control and Prevention [CDC]; *B,* Courtesy of the CDC and Dr. John Noble, Jr.)

than after natural VZV infection among immunocompromised children. Post-licensure data also suggest the same trend in healthy vaccinees.

PATHOGENESIS

VZV is transmitted in oropharyngeal secretions and in the fluid of skin lesions either by airborne spread or through direct contact. Primary infection (varicella) results from inoculation of the virus onto the mucosa of the upper respiratory tract and tonsillar lymphoid tissue. During the early part of the 10- to 21-day incubation period, virus replicates in the local lymphoid tissue, and then a brief subclinical viremia spreads the virus to the reticuloendothelial system. Widespread cutaneous lesions occur during a second viremic phase that lasts 3-7 days. Peripheral blood mononuclear cells carry infectious virus, generating new crops of vesicles during this period of viremia. VZV is also transported back to the mucosa of the upper respiratory tract and oropharynx during the late incubation period, permitting spread to susceptible contacts 1-2 days before the appearance of rash. Host immune responses limit viral replication and facilitate recovery from infection. In the immunocompromised child, the failure of immune responses, especially cell-mediated immune responses, results in continued viral replication that may lead to disseminated infection with resultant complications in the lungs, liver, brain, and other organs. Virus is transported in a retrograde manner through sensory axons to the dorsal root ganglia throughout the spinal cord, where the virus establishes latent infection in the neurons and satellite cells associated with these axons. Subsequent **reactivation** of latent virus causes **herpes zoster,** a vesicular rash that usually is dermatomal in distribution. During herpes zoster, necrotic changes may be produced in the associated ganglia. The skin lesions of varicella and herpes zoster have identical histopathology, and infectious VZV is present in both. Varicella elicits humoral and cell-mediated immunity that is highly protective against symptomatic reinfection. Suppression of cell-mediated immunity to VZV correlates with an increased risk for VZV reactivation as herpes zoster.

CLINICAL MANIFESTATIONS

Varicella is an acute febrile rash illness that was common in children in the USA before the universal childhood vaccination program. It has variable severity but is usually self limited. It may be associated with severe complications, including staphylococcal and streptococcal superinfection, pneumonia, encephalitis, bleeding disorders, congenital infection, and life-threatening perinatal infection. Herpes zoster, uncommon in children, causes localized cutaneous symptoms but may disseminate in immunocompromised patients.

Varicella

The illness usually begins 14-16 days after exposure, although the incubation period can range from 10 to 21 days. Subclinical varicella is rare; almost all exposed, susceptible persons experience a rash. Prodromal symptoms may be present, particularly in older children and adults. Fever, malaise, anorexia, headache, and occasionally mild abdominal pain may occur 24-48 hours before the rash appears. Temperature elevation is usually moderate, usually 100-102°F, but may be as high as 106°F; fever and other systemic symptoms usually resolve within 2-4 days after the onset of the rash.

Varicella lesions often appear first on the scalp, face, or trunk. The initial exanthem consists of intensely pruritic erythematous macules that evolve through the papular stage to form clear, fluid-filled vesicles. Clouding and umbilication of the lesions begin in 24-48 hr. While the initial lesions are crusting, new crops form on the trunk and then the extremities; the simultaneous presence of lesions in various stages of evolution is characteristic of varicella (Fig. 245-1). The distribution of the rash is predominantly central or centripetal, in contrast to that in smallpox, which is more prominent on the face and distal extremities. Ulcerative lesions involving the mucosa of oropharynx and vagina are also common; many children have vesicular lesions on the eyelids and conjunctivae, but corneal involvement and serious ocular disease are rare. The average number of varicella lesions is about 300, but healthy children may have fewer than 10 to more than 1,500 lesions. In cases resulting from secondary household spread and in older children, more lesions usually occur, and new crops of lesions may continue to develop for a longer time. The exanthem may be much more extensive in children with skin disorders, such as eczema or recent sunburn. Hypopigmentation or hyperpigmentation of lesion sites persists for days to weeks in some children, but severe scarring is unusual unless the lesions were secondarily infected.

The **differential diagnosis** of varicella includes vesicular rashes caused by other infectious agents, such as herpes simplex virus, enterovirus, monkey pox, rickettsial pox, and *S. aureus;* drug reactions; disseminated herpes zoster; contact dermatitis; and insect bites. Severe varicella was the most common illness confused with smallpox before the eradication of smallpox.

Varicella in Vaccinated Individuals ("Breakthrough Varicella")

One dose of varicella vaccine is >97% effective in preventing severe varicella and is 85% (median; range 44-100%) effective in preventing all disease after exposure to wild-type VZV. This means that after close exposure to VZV, as may occur in a household or an outbreak setting in a school or daycare center, about 1 of every 5 children receiving 1-dose vaccination children may experience breakthrough varicella. Exposure to VZV may also result in asymptomatic infection in the previously immunized child. **Breakthrough disease** is varicella that occurs in a person vaccinated >42 days before rash onset and is caused by **wild-type VZV.** In the early stages of the varicella vaccination program, rash occurring within the 1st 2 weeks after vaccination was most commonly wild-type VZV, reflecting exposure to varicella before vaccination could provide protection. Rash occurring 14-42 days after vaccination was due to either wild or vaccine strains, reflecting breakthrough varicella or vaccine-associated rash, respectively. As varicella disease continues to decline, rashes in the interval 0-42 days after vaccination will be less commonly caused by wild-type VZV. The rash in breakthrough disease is frequently atypical and predominantly maculopapular, vesicles are seen less commonly, and the illness is most commonly mild with <50 lesions, shorter duration of rash, fewer complications, and little or no fever. However, approximately 25-30% of breakthrough cases are not mild, with clinical features more similar to those of wild-type infection. Breakthrough cases are overall **less contagious** than wild-type infections within household settings, but contagiousness varies proportionally with the number of lesions: typical breakthrough cases (<50 lesions) are about a third as contagious as unvaccinated cases, whereas breakthrough cases with ≥50 lesions are as contagious as wild-type cases. Therefore, children with breakthrough disease should be considered potentially infectious and excluded from school until lesions have crusted or, if there are no vesicles present, until no new lesions are occurring. Transmission has been documented to occur from breakthrough cases in household, child-care, and school settings.

Fewer studies have evaluated the performance of the 2-dose varicella vaccine regimen. One clinical trial estimated the 2-dose vaccine effectiveness for preventing all disease at 98%. Breakthrough cases have been reported among 2-dose vaccinees, although recipients of 2 doses of varicella vaccine are less likely to have breakthrough disease than those receiving one dose.

Progressive Varicella

Progressive varicella, with visceral organ involvement, coagulopathy, severe hemorrhage, and continued vesicular lesion development, is a severe complication of primary VZV infection. Severe abdominal pain, which may reflect involvement of mesenteric lymph nodes or the liver, or the appearance of hemorrhagic vesicles in otherwise healthy adolescents and adults, immunocompromised children, pregnant women, and newborns, may herald severe disease. Although rare in healthy children, the risk for progressive varicella is highest in children with congenital cellular immune deficiency disorders and those with malignancy, particularly if chemotherapy was given during the incubation period and the absolute lymphocyte count is <500 cells/mm^3. The mortality rate for children who acquired varicella while undergoing treatment for malignancy and who were not treated with antiviral therapy approaches 7%; varicella-related deaths usually occur within 3 days after the diagnosis of varicella **pneumonia.** Children who acquire varicella after organ transplantation are also at risk for progressive VZV infection. Children undergoing long-term, low-dose systemic corticosteroid therapy are not considered to be at higher risk for severe varicella, but progressive varicella does occur in patients receiving high-dose corticosteroids and has been reported in patients receiving inhaled corticosteroids as well as in asthmatic persons receiving multiple short courses of systemic corticosteroid therapy. Unusual clinical findings of varicella, including lesions that develop a unique hyperkeratotic appearance and continued new lesion formation for weeks or months, have been described in children with untreated, late stage **HIV infection.** Immunization of HIV-infected children who have a CD4+ T-lymphocyte value ≥15% as well as children with leukemia and solid organ tumors who are in remission and whose chemotherapy can be interrupted for 2 wk around the time of immunization or has been terminated has reduced this problem. Since the advent of the universal immunization program, many children who would become immunocompromised later in life because of disease or treatment are protected before the immunosuppression occurs; also, due to reductions in varicella incidence, immunocompromised children are less likely to be exposed to varicella.

Neonatal Varicella

Mortality is particularly high in neonates born to susceptible mothers who contracted varicella around the time of delivery. Infants whose mothers demonstrate varicella in the period from 5 days prior to delivery to 2 days afterward are at high risk for severe varicella. The infant acquires the infection transplacentally as a result of maternal viremia, which may occur up to 48 hr prior to onset of maternal rash. The infant's rash usually occurs toward the end of the 1st week to the early part of the 2nd week of life (although it may be as soon as 2 days). Because the mother has not yet developed a significant antibody response, the infant receives a large dose of virus without the moderating effect of maternal anti-VZV antibody. If the mother demonstrates varicella >5 days prior to delivery, she still may pass virus to the soon-to-be-born child, but infection is attenuated because of transmission of maternal VZV-specific antibody across the placenta. This moderating effect of maternal antibody is present if delivery occurs after 30 wk of gestation, when maternal immunoglobulin G (IgG) is able to cross the placenta. The recommendations for human varicella zoster immune globulin (VariZIG) reflect the differing risks to the exposed infant. Newborns whose mothers demonstrate varicella 5 days before to 2 days after delivery should receive 1 vial of VariZIG as soon as possible. Although neonatal varicella may occur in about half of these infants despite administration of VariZIG, it is usually mild. All premature infants born <28 wk gestation to a mother with active varicella at delivery (even if the maternal rash has been present for >1 wk) should receive VariZIG. If VariZIG is not available, intravenous immune globulin (IGIV) may provide some protection, although varicella-specific antibody titers may vary from lot to lot. Because perinatally acquired varicella may be life threatening, the infant should be treated with acyclovir (10 mg/kg every 8 hr IV) when lesions develop. Neonatal varicella can also follow a postpartum exposure of an infant delivered to a mother who was susceptible to VZV, although the frequency of complications declines rapidly in the weeks after birth. Infants with community-acquired varicella who experience severe varicella, especially those who have a complication such as pneumonia, hepatitis, or encephalitis, should also receive treatment with IV acyclovir (10 mg/kg every 8 hr IV). Infants with neonatal varicella who receive prompt antiviral therapy have an excellent prognosis.

Congenital Varicella Syndrome

In utero transmission of VZV can occur; however, because most adults in temperate climates are immune, varicella complicating pregnancy is unusual. When pregnant women do contract varicella early in pregnancy, experts estimate that as many as 25% of the fetuses may become infected. Fortunately, clinically apparent disease in the infant is uncommon: the congenital varicella syndrome occurs in approximately 0.4% of infants born to women who have varicella during pregnancy before 13 wk of gestation and approximately 2% of infants born to women with varicella between 13 and 20 wk of gestation. Before availability of varicella vaccine in the USA, 44 cases of congenital varicella syndrome were estimated to occur each year. The congenital varicella syndrome is characterized by cicatricial skin scarring in a zoster-like distribution, limb hypoplasia, and neurologic (e.g., microcephaly, cortical atrophy, seizures, and mental retardation), eye (e.g., chorioretinitis, microphthalmia, and cataracts), renal (e.g., hydroureter and hydronephrosis) and autonomic nervous system abnormalities (neurogenic bladder, swallowing dysfunction, and aspiration pneumonia). Most of the stigmata can be attributed to virus-induced injury to the nervous system, although there is no obvious explanation why certain regions of the

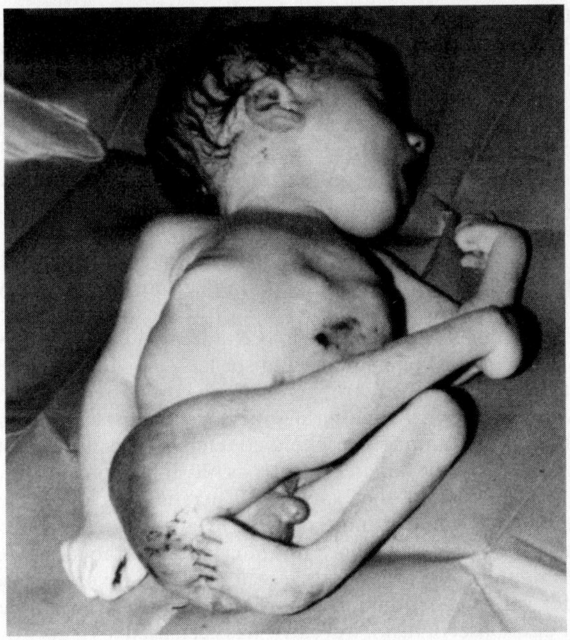

Figure 245-2 Newborn with congenital varicella syndrome. The infant had severe malformations of both lower extremities and cicatricial scarring over his left abdomen.

body are preferentially infected during fetal VZV infection. The characteristic cutaneous lesion has been called a cicatrix, a zigzag scarring, in a **dermatomal** distribution, often associated with atrophy of the affected limb (Fig. 245-2). Many infants with severe manifestations of congenital varicella syndrome (atrophy and scarring of a limb) have significant neurologic deficiencies.

There are rare case reports of fetal abnormalities following the development of herpes zoster in the mother; whether or not these cases truly represent the congenital varicella syndrome is unclear. If it does occur, the congenital syndrome acquired as a result of maternal herpes zoster is exceedingly rare.

The diagnosis of VZV fetopathy is based mainly on the history of gestational varicella combined with the presence of characteristic abnormalities in the newborn infant. Virus cannot be cultured from the affected newborn, but viral DNA may be detected in tissue samples by polymerase chain reaction (PCR). VZV-specific IgM antibody is detectable in the cord blood sample in some infants, although the IgM titer drops quickly postpartum and can be nonspecifically positive. Chorionic villus sampling and fetal blood collection for the detection of viral DNA, virus, or antibody have been used in an attempt to diagnose fetal infection and embryopathy. The usefulness of these tests for patient management and counseling has not been defined. Because these tests may not distinguish between infection and disease, their utility may primarily be that of reassurance when the result is negative. A persistently positive VZV IgG antibody titer at 12-18 mo of age is a reliable indicator of prenatal infection in the asymptomatic child, as is the development of zoster in the 1st year of life without evidence of postnatal infection.

Varicella immune globulin has often been administered to the susceptible mother exposed to varicella, but whether this step modifies infection in the fetus is uncertain. Similarly, acyclovir treatment may be given to the mother with severe varicella. A prospective registry of acyclovir use in the 1st trimester demonstrated that the occurrence of birth defects approximates that found in the general population. Acyclovir is a class B drug for pregnancy and should be considered only when the benefit to the mother outweighs the potential risk to the fetus. The efficacy of acyclovir treatment of the pregnant woman in preventing or modifying the severity of congenital varicella is not known, but its use should be considered to protect the mother from severe disease. Finally, because the damage caused by fetal VZV infection does not progress in the postpartum period, antiviral treatment of infants with congenital VZV syndrome is not indicated.

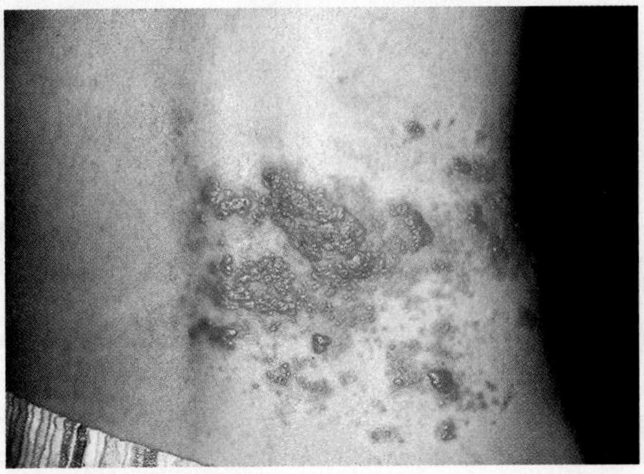

Figure 245-3 Herpes zoster involving the lumbar dermatome. (From Mandell GL, Bennett JE, Dolin R, editors: *Principles and practice of infectious diseases,* ed 6, vol 2, Philadelphia, 2005, Elsevier, p 1783.)

Herpes Zoster

Herpes zoster manifests as vesicular lesions clustered within 1 or, less commonly, 2 adjacent dermatomes (Fig. 245-3). In the elderly, herpes zoster typically begins with burning pain followed by clusters of skin lesions in a dermatomal pattern. Almost half of the elderly with herpes zoster experience complications; the most frequent complication is postherpetic neuralgia, a painful condition that affects the nerves despite resolution of the shingles skin lesions. Unlike herpes zoster in adults, zoster in children is infrequently associated with localized pain, hyperesthesia, pruritus, and low-grade fever. In children, the rash is mild, with new lesions appearing for a few days; symptoms of acute neuritis are minimal; and complete resolution usually occurs within 1-2 wk. Unlike in adults, postherpetic neuralgia is very unusual in children. Approximately 4% of patients suffer a 2nd episode of herpes zoster; 3 or more episodes are rare. Transverse myelitis with transient paralysis is a rare complication of herpes zoster. An increased risk for herpes zoster early in childhood has been described in children who acquire infection with VZV in utero or in the 1st year of life (Fig. 245-4).

Immunocompromised children may have more severe herpes zoster, which is similar to that in adults, including postherpetic neuralgia. Immunocompromised patients may also experience disseminated cutaneous disease that mimics varicella as well as visceral dissemination with pneumonia, hepatitis, encephalitis, and disseminated intravascular coagulopathy. Severely immunocompromised children, particularly those with advanced HIV infection, may have unusual, chronic or relapsing cutaneous disease, retinitis, or central nervous system (CNS) disease without rash. The finding of a lower risk for herpes zoster among vaccinated children with leukemia than in those who have had varicella disease suggests that varicella vaccine virus reactivates less commonly than wild-type VZV. The risk for herpes zoster in healthy vaccinated children may be lower than in children who had wild-type varicella disease, although many more years of follow-up will be needed to determine that this is the case.

DIAGNOSIS

Laboratory evaluation has not been considered necessary for the diagnosis or management of healthy children with varicella or herpes zoster. However, as disease declines to low levels, laboratory confirmation of all varicella cases may be necessary. The atypical nature of breakthrough varicella, with a higher

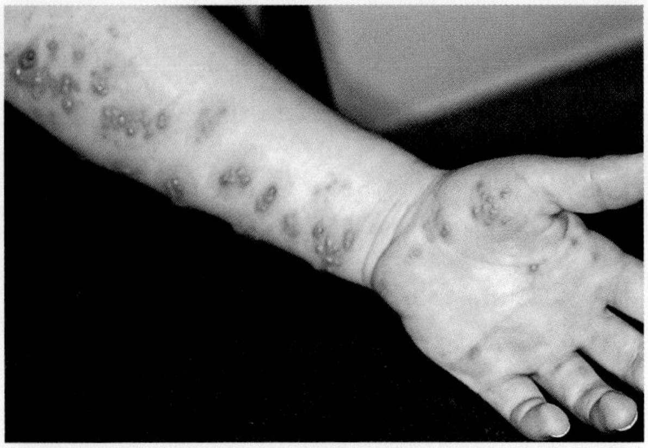

Figure 245-4 Many groups of blisters occurring over the arm in a child with herpes zoster. (From Weston WL, Lane AT, Morelli JG: *Color textbook of pediatric dermatology,* ed 3, Philadelphia, 2002, Mosby, Fig. 8-28.)

proportion of rashes being papular rather than vesicular, will pose diagnostic challenges. In addition, severe cases of varicella may need virologic confirmation to distinguish them from pox virus infections.

Leukopenia is typical during the 1st 72 hours after onset of rash; it is followed by a relative and absolute lymphocytosis. Results of liver function tests are also usually (75%) mildly elevated. Patients with neurologic complications of varicella or uncomplicated herpes zoster have a mild lymphocytic pleocytosis and a slight to moderate increase in protein content of the cerebrospinal fluid; the cerebrospinal fluid glucose concentration is usually normal.

Rapid laboratory diagnosis of VZV is often important in high-risk patients and can be important for infection control. Confirmation of varicella (or herpes simplex virus) can be accomplished by most referral hospital laboratories and all state health laboratories. VZV can be identified quickly by direct fluorescence assay (DFA) of cells from cutaneous lesions (vesicular fluid) in 15-20 min, by rapid culture with specific immunofluorescence staining (shell vial technique) in 48-72 hr, and by PCR amplification testing (vesicular fluid, crusts) in 2 hr to days, depending on availability. Although multinucleated giant cells can be detected with nonspecific stains (**Tzanck smear**), they have poor sensitivity and do not differentiate VZV from herpes simplex virus infections. Infectious virus may be recovered by means of tissue culture methods; such methods require specific expertise, and virus may take days to weeks to grow. VZV IgG antibodies can be detected by several methods, and a fourfold or greater rise in IgG antibodies is confirmatory of acute infection. VZV IgG antibody tests can also be valuable to determine the immune status of individuals whose clinical history of varicella is unknown or equivocal. Testing for VZV IgM antibodies is not useful for clinical diagnosis because commercially available methods are unreliable and the kinetics of the IgM response is not well defined. Reliable VZV-specific IgM assays are available in certain reference laboratories, including a capture-IgM assay available at the national VZV laboratory at the Centers for Disease Control and Prevention. Strain identification (genotyping) can distinguish wild-type VZV from the vaccine strain; however, genotyping is available only at highly specialized reference laboratories.

TREATMENT

Antiviral treatment modifies the course of both varicella and herpes zoster. Antiviral drug resistance is rare but has occurred in children with HIV infection who have been treated with acyclovir for extended periods; foscarnet is the only drug available for the treatment of acyclovir-resistant VZV infections.

Varicella

The only antiviral drug available in liquid formulation that is licensed for pediatric use is acyclovir. Given the safety profile of acyclovir and its demonstrated efficacy in the treatment of varicella, treatment of all children, adolescents, and adults with varicella is acceptable. However, acyclovir therapy is not recommended routinely by the American Academy of Pediatrics for treatment of uncomplicated varicella in the otherwise healthy child because of the marginal benefit, the cost of the drug, and the low risk for complications of varicella. Oral therapy with acyclovir (20 mg/kg/dose, maximum 800 mg/dose) given as 4 doses/day for 5 days can be used to treat uncomplicated varicella in: nonpregnant individuals >13 yr of age and children >12 mo of age with chronic cutaneous or pulmonary disorders, individuals receiving short-term, intermittent, or aerosolized corticosteroid therapy, individuals receiving long-term salicylate therapy, and possibly secondary cases among household contacts. To be most effective, treatment should be initiated as early as possible, preferably within 24 hr of the onset of the exanthem. There is less clinical benefit if treatment is initiated more than 72 hr after onset of the exanthem. Acyclovir therapy does not interfere with the induction of VZV immunity. **Intravenous therapy** is indicated for severe disease and for varicella in immunocompromised patients (even if begun 72 hr after onset of rash). Acyclovir has been used to treat varicella in pregnant women; its safety for the fetus has not been established. Some experts recommend the use of famciclovir or valacyclovir in older children who can swallow tablets. Although these drugs do not have specific U.S. Food and Drug Administration–approved indications for treatment of varicella, they are highly active against VZV by the same mechanism as acyclovir and are better absorbed by the oral route than acyclovir.

Any patient who has signs of disseminated VZV, including pneumonia, severe hepatitis, thrombocytopenia, or encephalitis, should receive immediate treatment. IV acyclovir (500 mg/m^2 every 8 hr IV) therapy initiated within 72 hr of development of initial symptoms decreases the likelihood of progressive varicella and visceral dissemination in high-risk patients. Treatment is continued for 7–10 days or until no new lesions have appeared for 48 hr. Delaying antiviral treatment in high-risk individuals until it is obvious that prolonged new lesion formation is occurring is not advisable because visceral dissemination occurs during the same period.

Acyclovir-resistant VZV has been identified in children infected with HIV. These children may be treated with intravenous foscarnet, 120 mg/kg/day divided every 8 hr for up to 3 wk. The dose should be modified in the presence of renal insufficiency. Resistance to foscarnet has been reported with prolonged use.

Herpes Zoster

Antiviral drugs are effective for treatment of herpes zoster. In healthy adults, acyclovir (800 mg 5 times a day PO for 5 days), famciclovir (500 mg tid PO for 7 days), and valacyclovir (1,000 mg tid PO for 7 days) reduce the duration of the illness and the risk for development of postherpetic neuralgia; concomitant corticosteroid use improves the quality of life in the elderly. In otherwise healthy children, herpes zoster is a less severe disease, and postherpetic neuralgia is rare. Therefore, treatment of uncomplicated herpes zoster in the child with an antiviral agent may not always be necessary, although some experts would treat with oral acyclovir (20 mg/kg/dose, maximum 800 mg/dose) to shorten the duration of the illness. It is important to start antiviral therapy as soon as possible. Delay beyond 72 hr from onset of rash limits its effectiveness.

In contrast, herpes zoster in **immunocompromised** children can be severe, and disseminated disease may be life threatening. Patients at high risk for disseminated disease should receive acyclovir (500 mg/m^2 or 10 mg/kg every 8 hr IV). Oral acyclovir, famciclovir, or valacyclovir are options for immunocompromised patients with uncomplicated herpes zoster and who are considered at low risk for visceral dissemination.

Use of corticosteroids in the treatment of herpes zoster in children is not recommended.

COMPLICATIONS

The complications of VZV infection occur with varicella or with reactivation of infection, more commonly in immunocompromised patients. In the otherwise healthy child, mild varicella hepatitis is relatively common but rarely clinically symptomatic. Mild thrombocytopenia occurs in 1-2% of children with varicella and may be associated with transient petechiae. Purpura, hemorrhagic vesicles, hematuria, and gastrointestinal bleeding are rare complications that may have serious consequences. Other complications of varicella, some of them rare, include cerebellar ataxia, encephalitis, pneumonia, nephritis, nephrotic syndrome, hemolytic-uremic syndrome, arthritis, myocarditis, pericarditis, pancreatitis, and orchitis. A reduction in the number and rates of varicella-related complications is expected in the vaccine era. Serious varicella-related complications in vaccinated persons have been reported rarely. In addition, declines in varicella-related hospitalizations and deaths in the USA since implementation of the varicella vaccination program provide supporting evidence that varicella vaccine reduces severe complications from varicella.

Bacterial Infections

Secondary bacterial infections of the skin, usually caused by group A streptococci and *S. aureus,* may occur in up to 5% of children with varicella. These range from impetigo to cellulitis, lymphadenitis, and subcutaneous abscesses. An early manifestation of secondary bacterial infection is erythema of the base of a new vesicle. Recrudescence of fever 3-4 days after the initial exanthem may also herald a secondary bacterial infection. Varicella is a well-described risk factor for serious invasive infections caused by group A streptococcus, which can have a fatal outcome. The more invasive infections, such as varicella gangrenosa, bacterial sepsis, pneumonia, arthritis, osteomyelitis, cellulitis, and necrotizing fasciitis, account for much of the morbidity and mortality of varicella in otherwise healthy children. Bacterial toxin–mediated diseases (toxic shock syndrome) also may complicate varicella. A substantial decline in varicella-related invasive bacterial infections has been associated with the use of the varicella vaccine.

Encephalitis and Cerebellar Ataxia

Encephalitis (1/50,000 cases of varicella in unvaccinated children) and acute cerebellar ataxia (1/4,000 cases of varicella in unvaccinated children) are well-described neurologic complications of varicella; morbidity from CNS complications is highest among patients younger than 5 yr or older than 20 yr. Nuchal rigidity, altered consciousness, and seizures characterize meningoencephalitis. Patients with cerebellar ataxia have a gradual onset of gait disturbance, nystagmus, and slurred speech. Neurologic symptoms usually begin 2-6 days after the onset of the rash but may occur during the incubation period or after resolution of the rash. Clinical recovery is typically rapid, occurring within 24-72 hr, and is usually complete. Although severe hemorrhagic encephalitis, analogous to that caused by herpes simplex virus, is very rare in children with varicella, the consequences are similar to those of herpes encephalitis. Reye syndrome (hepatic dysfunction with hypoglycemia and encephalopathy) associated with varicella and other viral illnesses such as influenza has become rare now that salicylates are no longer used as antipyretics in these situations (Chapter 353).

Pneumonia

Varicella pneumonia is a severe complication that accounts for most of the increased morbidity and mortality in adults and other high-risk populations, but pneumonia may also complicate varicella in young children. Respiratory symptoms, which may include cough, dyspnea, cyanosis, pleuritic chest pain, and hemoptysis, usually begin within 1-6 days after the onset of the rash. Smoking has been described as a risk factor for severe pneumonia complicating varicella. The frequency of varicella pneumonia may be greater in the parturient.

PROGNOSIS

Primary varicella has a mortality rate of 2-3/100,000 cases, with the lowest case fatality rates among children 1-9 yr of age (~1 death per 100,000 cases). Compared with these age groups, infants have a 4 times greater risk of dying and adults have a 25 times greater risk of dying. Approximately 100 deaths occurred in the USA annually before the introduction of the varicella vaccine; the most common complications among people who died from varicella were pneumonia, CNS complications, secondary infections, and hemorrhagic conditions. The mortality rate of untreated primary infection is 7-14% in immunocompromised children and may approach 50% in untreated adults with pneumonia.

Neuritis with herpes zoster should be managed with appropriate analgesics. Postherpetic neuralgia can be a severe problem in adults and may persist for months, requiring care by a specialist in pain management.

PREVENTION

VZV transmission is difficult to prevent because an infected person is contagious for 24-48 hr before the rash appears. Infection control practices, including caring for infected patients in isolation rooms with filtered air systems, are essential. All health care workers should have evidence of varicella immunity (Table 245-1). Unvaccinated health care workers without other evidence of immunity who have had a close exposure to VZV should be furloughed for days 8-21 after exposure because they are potentially infectious during this period.

Vaccine

Varicella is a vaccine-preventable disease. Varicella vaccine contains live, attenuated VZV (Oka strain) and is indicated for subcutaneous administration. Varicella vaccine is recommended for routine administration as a 2-dose regimen to healthy children at ages 12-15 mo and 4-6 yr. Catch-up vaccination with the

Table 245-1 EVIDENCE OF IMMUNITY TO VARICELLA

Evidence of immunity to varicella consists of *any* of the following:

- Documentation of age-appropriate vaccination with a varicella vaccine:
  - Preschool-aged children (i.e., aged >12 mo): 1 dose
  - School-aged children, adolescents, and adults: 2 doses*
- Laboratory evidence of immunity† or laboratory confirmation of disease
- Birth in the USA before 1980§
- Diagnosis or verification of a history of varicella disease by a health-care provider¶
- Diagnosis or verification of a history of herpes zoster by a health-care provider

*For children who received their first dose at age <13 yr and for whom the interval between the 2 doses was ≥28 days, the second dose is considered valid.

†Commercial assays can be used to assess disease-induced immunity, but they lack sensitivity to always detect vaccine-induced immunity (i.e., they might yield false-negative results).

§For health-care personnel, pregnant women, and immunocompromised persons, birth before 1980 should not be considered evidence of immunity.

¶Verification of history or diagnosis of typical disease can be provided by any health care provider (e.g., school or occupational clinic nurse, nurse practitioner, physician assistant, or physician). For persons reporting a history of, or reporting with, atypical or mild cases, assessment by a physician or his/her designee is recommended, and one of the following should be sought: (1) an epidemiologic link to a typical varicella case or to a laboratory-confirmed case or (2) evidence of laboratory confirmation if it was performed at the time of acute disease. When such documentation is lacking, persons should not be considered as having a valid history of disease, because other diseases might mimic mild atypical varicella.

second dose is recommended for children and adolescents who received only 1 dose. Vaccination with 2 doses is recommended for all persons without evidence of immunity. The minimum recommended interval between the two doses is 3 mo for persons ≤12 yr of age and 4 wk for older children, adolescents, and adults. Administration of varicella vaccine within 4 wk of measles-mumps-rubella (MMR) vaccine has been associated with a higher risk for breakthrough disease; therefore, it is recommended that the vaccines either be administered simultaneously at different sites or be given at least 4 wk apart.

Varicella vaccine is contraindicated for pregnant women and persons with cell-mediated immune deficiencies, including those with leukemia, lymphoma, and other malignant neoplasms affecting the bone marrow or lymphatic systems. Compassionate-use protocols are available for immunization of children with leukemia in remission. The vaccine should be considered for HIV-infected children with a CD4+ T-lymphocyte percentage ≥15%. These children should receive 2 doses of vaccine, 3 mo apart. Specific guidelines for immunizing these children should be reviewed before vaccination. Children with isolated humoral immunodeficiencies may receive varicella vaccine.

Zoster vaccine was licensed in 2006 for use as a single immunization of individuals ≥60 yr of age for prevention of herpes zoster and to decrease the frequency of postherpetic neuralgia. It is not indicated for the treatment of zoster or postherpetic neuralgia.

Vaccine-associated Adverse Events

Varicella vaccine is safe and well tolerated. The incidence of injection site complaints observed ≤3 days after vaccination was slightly higher after dose 2 (25%) than after dose 1 (22%). A mild vaccine-associated varicelliform rash was reported in approximately 1-3% of healthy vaccinees, consisting of 6-10 papular-vesicular, erythematous lesions with peak occurrence 8-21 days after vaccination. Transmission of vaccine virus to susceptible contacts is a very rare occurrence.

Postexposure Prophylaxis

Vaccine given to healthy children within 3-5 days after exposure (as soon as possible is preferred) is effective in preventing or modifying varicella, especially in a household setting where exposure is very likely to result in infection. Varicella vaccine is now recommended for postexposure use and for outbreak control. Oral acyclovir administered late in the incubation period may modify subsequent varicella in the healthy child; however, its use in this manner is not recommended until it can be further evaluated.

High-titer anti-VZV immune globulin as postexposure prophylaxis is recommended for immunocompromised children, pregnant women, and newborns exposed to varicella. Human varicella-zoster immune globulin (VariZIG) is distributed in the USA by FFF Enterprises, California (1-800-843-7477). The recommended dose is 1 vial (125 units) for each 10-kg increment of body weight (maximum 625 units) given intramuscularly as soon as possible but within 96 hr after exposure.

Although licensed pooled immune globulin intravenous (IGIV) preparations contain antivaricella antibodies, the titer varies from lot to lot. The recommended dose of IGIV for postexposure prophylaxis (in situations in which administration of VariZIG does not appear possible within 96 hr of exposure) is 400 mg/kg administered once within 96 hr of exposure. Immunocompromised patients who have received high-dose IGIV (100-400 mg/kg) for other indications within 2-3 wk before VZV exposure can be expected to have serum antibodies to VZV.

Newborns whose mothers demonstrate varicella 5 days before to 2 days after delivery should receive 1 vial of VariZIG. VariZIG is also indicated for: pregnant women without evidence of immunity; premature infants born at <28 wks of gestation (or weight <1,000 g) who were exposed to varicella during the neonatal period, regardless of maternal immunity; and premature infants born at >28 wks of gestation who were exposed to varicella and whose mothers have no evidence of varicella immunity. If possible, adults should be tested for VZV IgG antibodies before VariZIG administration, because many adults with no clinical history of varicella are immune. Anti-VZV antibody prophylaxis may ameliorate disease but does not eliminate the possibility of progressive disease, nor does it ensure that varicella is not transmitted to close susceptible contacts; patients should be monitored and treated with acyclovir if necessary once lesions develop.

Close contact between a susceptible high-risk patient and a patient with herpes zoster is also an indication for VariZIG prophylaxis. Passive antibody administration or treatment does not reduce the risk for herpes zoster or alter the clinical course of varicella or herpes zoster when given after the onset of symptoms.

BIBLIOGRAPHY

Please visit the Nelson Textbook of Pediatrics *website at www.expertconsult.com for the complete bibliography.*

Chapter 246
Epstein-Barr Virus

Hal B. Jenson

Infectious mononucleosis is the best-known clinical syndrome caused by Epstein-Barr virus (EBV). It is characterized by systemic somatic complaints consisting primarily of fatigue, malaise, fever, sore throat, and generalized lymphadenopathy. Originally described as **glandular fever,** it derives its name from the mononuclear lymphocytosis with atypical-appearing lymphocytes that accompany the illness. Other pathogens may cause a mononucleosis-like illness.

ETIOLOGY

EBV, a member of the γ-herpesviruses, causes >90% of cases of infectious mononucleosis. Two distinct types of EBV, **type 1 and type 2 (also called type A and type B),** have been characterized and have 70-85% sequence homology. EBV-1 is more prevalent worldwide, although EBV-2 is more common in Africa than in the USA and Europe. Both types lead to persistent, lifelong, latent infection. Dual infections with both types have been documented among immunocompromised persons. EBV-1 induces in vitro growth transformation of B cells more efficiently then EBV-2, but no type-specific disease manifestations or clinical differences have been identified. Co-acquisition of multiple EBV genotypes has been shown by heteroduplex tracking assays to occur commonly in otherwise healthy patients with infectious mononucleosis. Only a single genotype tends to be cultured.

As many as 5-10% of **infectious mononucleosis–like illnesses** are caused by primary infection with cytomegalovirus, *Toxoplasma gondii,* adenovirus, viral hepatitis, HIV, and possibly rubella virus. In the majority of EBV-negative infectious mononucleosis–like illnesses, the exact cause remains unknown.

EPIDEMIOLOGY

The epidemiology of infectious mononucleosis is related to the epidemiology and age of acquisition of EBV infection. EBV infects >95% of the world's population. It is transmitted via penetrative sexual intercourse and in oral secretions such as "deep kissing" and sharing water bottles. Among children, transmission may occur by exchange of saliva from child to child, such as occurs between children in out-of-home child care. Nonintimate contact, environmental sources, and fomites do not contribute to spread of EBV.

EBV is shed in oral secretions consistently for >6 mo after acute infection and then intermittently for life. As many as 20-30% of healthy EBV-infected persons excrete virus at any particular time. Immunosuppression permits reactivation of latent EBV; 60-90% of EBV-infected immunosuppressed patients shed the virus. EBV is also found in male and female genital secretions and, especially type 2, is spread through sexual contact.

Infection with EBV in developing countries and among socioeconomically disadvantaged populations of developed countries usually occurs during infancy and early childhood. In central Africa, almost all children are infected by 3 yr of age. Primary infection with EBV during childhood is usually inapparent or indistinguishable from other infections of childhood; the clinical syndrome of infectious mononucleosis is practically unknown in undeveloped regions of the world. Among more affluent populations in industrialized countries, infection during childhood is also common but occurs less frequently, presumably because of high standards of hygiene, with approximately 30% of infections during adolescence and young adulthood. Primary EBV infection in adolescents and adults manifests in >50% of cases as the **classic triad** fatigue, pharyngitis, and generalized lymphadenopathy, which constitute the major clinical manifestations of infectious mononucleosis. This syndrome may be seen at all ages but is rarely apparent in children <4 yr of age, when most EBV infections are asymptomatic, or in adults >40 yr of age, of whom most individuals have already been infected by EBV. The true incidence of the syndrome of infectious mononucleosis is unknown but is estimated to occur in 20-70/100,000 persons/year; in young adults, the incidence increases to about 1/1,000 persons/year. The prevalence of serologic evidence of past EBV infection increases with age; almost all adults in the USA are seropositive.

PATHOGENESIS

After acquisition in the oral cavity, EBV initially infects oral epithelial cells, possibly contributing to the symptoms of pharyngitis. After intracellular viral replication and cell lysis with release of new virions, virus spreads to contiguous structures such as the salivary glands, with eventual viremia and infection of B lymphocytes in the peripheral blood and the entire lymphoreticular system, including the liver and spleen. The atypical lymphocytes that are characteristic of infectious mononucleosis are CD8+ T lymphocytes, which exhibit both suppressor and cytotoxic functions that develop in response to the infected B lymphocytes. This relative as well as absolute increase in CD8+ lymphocytes results in a transient reversal of the normal 2:1 CD4+/CD8+ (helper/suppressor) T-lymphocyte ratio. Many of the clinical manifestations of infectious mononucleosis may result, at least in part, from cytokine release from the host immune response, which is effective in reducing the EBV load to <1 copy/10^5 circulating B lymphocytes, equivalent to <10 copies/µg of DNA from whole blood. The EBV load is more variable among immunocompromised persons and can be >4,000 copies/µg of DNA.

Epithelial cells of the uterine cervix may become infected by sexual transmission of the virus, although local symptoms have not been described after sexual transmission. EBV is consistently found intracellularly in smooth muscle cells of leiomyosarcomas of immunocompromised persons but not in leiomyosarcomas of immunocompetent persons.

EBV, like the other herpesviruses, establishes lifelong latent infection after the primary illness. The latent virus is carried in oropharyngeal epithelial cells and systemically in memory B lymphocytes as multiple episomes in the nucleus. The viral episomes replicate with cell division and are distributed to both daughter cells. Viral integration into the cell genome is not typical. Only a few viral proteins, including the EBV-determined nuclear antigens (EBNAs), are produced during latency. These proteins are important in maintaining the viral episome during the latent state. Progression to viral replication begins with production of EBV early antigens (EAs), proceeds to viral DNA replication, is followed by production of viral capsid antigen (VCA), and culminates in cell death and release of mature virions. Reactivation with viral replication occurs at a low rate in populations of latently infected cells and is responsible for intermittent viral shedding in oropharyngeal secretions of infected individuals. Reactivation is apparently asymptomatic and is not recognized to be accompanied by distinctive clinical symptoms.

ONCOGENESIS

EBV was the first human virus to be associated with malignancy. EBV infection may result in a spectrum of proliferative disorders ranging from self-limited, usually benign disease such as infectious mononucleosis to aggressive, nonmalignant proliferations such as the virus-associated hemophagocytic syndrome to lymphoid and epithelial cell malignancies. Benign EBV-associated proliferations include oral hairy leukoplakia, primarily in adults with AIDS, and lymphoid interstitial pneumonitis, primarily in children with AIDS. Malignant EBV-associated proliferations include nasopharyngeal carcinoma, Burkitt lymphoma, Hodgkin disease, lymphoproliferative disorders, and leiomyosarcoma in immunodeficient states, including AIDS. There is no firm evidence of development of EBV quasispecies that would contribute to the pathogenesis of EBV-positive malignancies.

Nasopharyngeal carcinoma occurs worldwide but is 10 times more common in persons in southern China, where it is the most common malignant tumor among adult men. It is also common among whites in North Africa and Inuit in North America. Patients usually present with cervical lymphadenopathy, eustachian tube blockage, and nasal obstruction with epistaxis. All malignant cells of undifferentiated nasopharyngeal carcinoma contain a high copy number of EBV episomes. Persons with undifferentiated and partially differentiated, nonkeratinizing nasopharyngeal carcinomas have elevated EBV antibody titers that are both diagnostic and prognostic. High levels of immunoglobulin A (IgA) antibody to EA and VCA may be detected in asymptomatic individuals and can be used to follow response to tumor therapy (Table 246-1). Cells of well-differentiated, keratinizing nasopharyngeal carcinoma contain a low number of or no EBV genomes; people with this disease have EBV serologic patterns similar to those of the general population.

CT and MRI are helpful in both identifying and defining masses in the head and neck. The diagnosis is established by biopsy of the mass or of a suspicious cervical lymph node. Surgery is important for staging and diagnosis. Radiation therapy is effective for control of the primary tumor and regional nodal metastases. Chemotherapy with 5-fluorouracil, cisplatin, and methotrexate is effective but not always curative. The prognosis is good if the tumor is localized.

Endemic (African) Burkitt lymphoma, often found in the jaw, is the most common childhood cancer in equatorial East Africa and New Guinea (Chapter 490.2). The median age at onset is 5 yr. These regions are holoendemic for *Plasmodium falciparum* malaria and have a high rate of EBV infection early in life. The constant malarial exposure acts as a B-lymphocyte mitogen that contributes to the polyclonal B-lymphocyte proliferation with EBV infection, impairs T-lymphocyte surveillance of EBV-infected B lymphocytes, and increases the risk for development of Burkitt lymphoma. Approximately 98% of cases of endemic Burkitt lymphoma contain the EBV genome, compared with only 20% of cases of nonendemic (sporadic or American) Burkitt lymphoma. Individuals with Burkitt lymphoma have unusually and characteristically high levels of antibody to VCA and EA that correlate with the risk for developing tumor (see Table 246-1).

All cases of Burkitt lymphoma, including those that are EBV negative, are monoclonal and demonstrate chromosomal translocation of the *c-myc* proto-oncogene to the constant region of

Table 246-1 CORRELATION OF CLINICAL STATUS AND SEROLOGIC RESPONSES TO EPSTEIN-BARR VIRUS INFECTION*

CLINICAL STATUS	SEROLOGIC RESPONSE					
	Heterophile Antibodies (Qualitative Test)	EBV-Specific Antibody				
		IgM-VCA	IgG-VCA	EA-D	EA-R	EBNA
Negative reaction	–	<1:8[†]	<1:10[†]	<1:10[†]	<1:10[†]	<1:2.5[†]
Susceptible	–	–	–	–	–[§]	–
Acute primary infection: infectious mononucleosis	+	1:32-1:256	1:160-1:640	1:40-1:160	–[§]	– to 1:2.5
Recent primary infection: infectious mononucleosis	±	– to 1:32	1:320-1:1,280	1:40-1:160	–[‡]	1:5-1:10
Remote infection	–	–	1:40-1:160	–[§]	– to 1:40	1:10-1:40
Reactivation: immunosuppressed or immunocompromised	–	–	1:320-1:1,280	–[§]	1:80-1:320	– to 1:160
Burkitt lymphoma	–	–	1:320-1:1,280	–[§]	1:80-1:320	1:10-1:80
Nasopharyngeal carcinoma	–	–	1:320-1:1,280	1:40-1:160	–[‖]	1:20-1:160

*The data were obtained from numerous studies. Individual responses outside the characteristic range may occur.
[†]Or the lowest test dilution.
[‡]In young children and adults with asymptomatic seroconversion, the anti–early antigen response may be mainly to the EA-R component.
[§]A minority of individuals have the anti–early antigen response mainly to the EA-D component.
[‖]A minority of individuals have the anti–early antigen response mainly to the EA-R component.
EA-D, diffuse staining component of early antigen; EA-R, cytoplasmic restricted component of early antigen; EBNA, EBV-determined nuclear antigens; EBV, Epstein-Barr virus; Ig, immunoglobulin; VCA, viral capsid antigen; –, negative; +, positive.
Reprinted with permission from Jenson HB: Epstein-Barr virus. In Detrick B, Hamilton RG, Folds JD, editors: *Manual of molecular and clinical laboratory immunology,* ed 7, Washington, DC, 2006, American Society for Microbiology.

the immunoglobulin heavy-chain locus, t(8;14), to the κ constant light-chain locus, t(2;8), or to the λ constant light-chain locus, t(8;22). This translocation results in the deregulation and constitutive transcription of the *c-myc* gene with overproduction of a normal *c-myc* product that autosuppresses *c-myc* production on the untranslocated chromosome.

The incidence of **Hodgkin disease** peaks in childhood in developing countries and in young adulthood in developed countries. Levels of EBV antibodies are consistently elevated preceding development of Hodgkin disease; only a small minority of patients with the disease is seronegative for EBV. Infection with EBV appears to increase the risk for Hodgkin disease by a factor of 2-4. EBV is associated with more than 50% of cases of mixed cellularity Hodgkin disease and approximately 25% of cases of the nodular sclerosing subtype and is rarely associated with lymphocyte-predominant Hodgkin disease. Immunohistochemical studies have localized EBV to the Reed-Sternberg cells and their variants, the pathognomonic malignant cells of Hodgkin disease.

Failure to control EBV infection may result from host immunologic deficits. The prototype is the **X-linked lymphoproliferative syndrome (Duncan syndrome)**, an X chromosome–linked recessive disorder of the immune system associated with severe, persistent, and sometimes fatal EBV infection (Chapter 118). Approximately two thirds of affected patients, who are male, die of disseminated and fulminating lymphoproliferation involving multiple organs at the time of primary EBV infection. Surviving patients acquire hypogammaglobulinemia, B-cell lymphoma, or both; most of these patients die within 10 yr.

Numerous congenital and acquired immunodeficiency syndromes are associated with an increased incidence of EBV-associated B-lymphocyte lymphoma, especially central nervous system lymphoma, and leiomyosarcoma. The incidence of lymphoproliferative syndromes parallels the degree of immunosuppression. A decline in T-cell function evidently permits EBV to escape from immune surveillance. Congenital immunodeficiencies predisposing to EBV-associated lymphoproliferation include the X-linked lymphoproliferative syndrome, common-variable immunodeficiency, ataxia-telangiectasia, Wiskott-Aldrich syndrome, and Chédiak-Higashi syndrome. Individuals with acquired immunodeficiencies resulting from anticancer chemotherapy, immunosuppression after solid organ or bone marrow transplantation, or HIV infection have a significantly increased risk for EBV-associated lymphoproliferation. The lymphomas may be focal or diffuse, and they are usually histologically polyclonal but may become monoclonal. Their growth is not reversed upon cessation of immunosuppression.

EBV is found intracellularly in all of the smooth muscle cells of leiomyosarcomas occurring in immunocompromised persons, including HIV-infected patients and transplant recipients, but not in leiomyosarcomas occurring in immunocompetent persons.

EBV is also associated with carcinoma of the salivary glands. Other tumors putatively associated with EBV include some T-lymphocyte lymphomas (including lethal midline), angioimmunoblastic lymphadenopathy-like lymphoma, thymomas and thymic carcinomas derived from thymic epithelial cells, supraglottic laryngeal carcinomas, lymphoepithelial tumors of the respiratory tract and gastrointestinal tract, and gastric adenocarcinoma. The precise contribution of EBV to these various malignancies is not well defined.

CLINICAL MANIFESTATIONS

The incubation period of infectious mononucleosis in adolescents is 30-50 days. In children, it may be shorter. The majority of cases of primary EBV infection in infants and young children are clinically silent. In older patients, the onset of illness is usually insidious and vague. Patients may complain of malaise, fatigue, acute or prolonged (>1 wk) fever, headache, sore throat, nausea, abdominal pain, and myalgia. This prodromal period may last 1-2 wk. The sore throat and fever gradually worsen until patients seek medical care. Splenic enlargement may be rapid enough to cause left upper quadrant abdominal discomfort and tenderness, which may be the presenting complaint.

The classic physical examination findings are generalized lymphadenopathy (90% of cases), splenomegaly (50% of cases), and hepatomegaly (10% of cases). Lymphadenopathy occurs most commonly in the anterior and posterior cervical nodes and the submandibular lymph nodes and less commonly in the axillary and inguinal lymph nodes. Epitrochlear lymphadenopathy is particularly suggestive of infectious mononucleosis. Symptomatic hepatitis or jaundice is uncommon, but elevated liver enzyme values are common. Splenomegaly to 2-3 cm below the costal margin is typical; massive enlargement is uncommon.

The sore throat is often accompanied by moderate to severe pharyngitis with marked tonsillar enlargement, occasionally with exudates (Fig. 246-1). Petechiae at the junction of the hard and soft palate are frequently seen. The pharyngitis resembles that caused by streptococcal infection. Other clinical findings may include rashes and edema of the eyelids.

Rashes are usually maculopapular and have been reported in 3-15% of patients. Up to 80% of patients with infectious mononucleosis experience **"ampicillin rash"** if treated with ampicillin

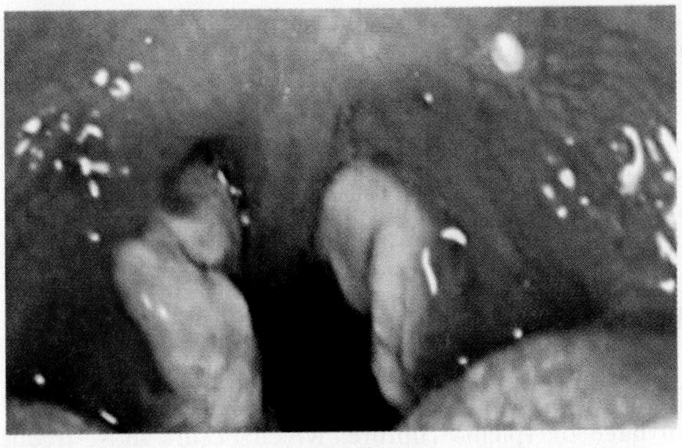

Figure 246-1 Tonsillitis with membrane formation in infectious mononucleosis. (Courtesy of Alex J. Steigman, MD.)

or amoxicillin. This vasculitic rash is probably immune mediated and resolves without specific treatment. EBV is also associated with **Gianotti-Crosti syndrome,** a symmetric rash on the cheeks with multiple erythematous papules, which may coalesce into plaques, and persists for 15-50 days. The rash has the appearance of atopic dermatitis and may appear on the extremities and buttocks.

DIAGNOSIS

The diagnosis of infectious mononucleosis implies primary EBV infection. A presumptive diagnosis may be made from the presence of typical clinical symptoms with atypical lymphocytosis in the peripheral blood. The diagnosis is usually confirmed by serologic testing, for either heterophile antibody or specific EBV antibodies.

Culture of EBV is tedious and requires 4-6 wk. The culture method is the **transformation assay,** which is performed by co-cultivation of oropharyngeal or genital secretions, peripheral blood (10-30 mL), or tumor with human umbilical cord lymphocytes. The cultures are observed for 6 wk for signs of **cell transformation:** proliferation and rapid growth, mitotic figures, large vacuoles, granular morphology, and cell aggregation. EBV **immortalizes** the umbilical cord cells, resulting in cell lines that harbor the EBV strain isolated from the patient and that can be maintained in vitro in perpetuity.

Differential Diagnosis

Infectious mononucleosis–like illnesses may be caused by primary infection with cytomegalovirus, *T. gondii,* adenovirus, viral hepatitis, HIV, or possibly rubella virus. Cytomegalovirus infection is a particularly common cause in adults. Streptococcal pharyngitis may cause sore throat and cervical lymphadenopathy indistinguishable from that of infectious mononucleosis but is not associated with hepatosplenomegaly. In approximately 5% of patients with EBV-associated infectious mononucleosis, throat cultures are positive for group A streptococcus, representing pharyngeal streptococcal carriage. Failure of a patient with streptococcal pharyngitis to improve within 48-72 hr should evoke suspicion of infectious mononucleosis. The most serious problem in the diagnosis of acute illness arises in the occasional patient with extremely high or low white blood cell counts, moderate thrombocytopenia, and even hemolytic anemia. In these patients, bone marrow examination and hematologic consultation are warranted to exclude the possibility of leukemia.

LABORATORY TESTS

In >90% of cases of EBV infection there is leukocytosis at 10,000-20,000 cells/mm^3, of which at least two thirds are lymphocytes; atypical lymphocytes usually account for 20-40% of the total number. The atypical cells are mature T lymphocytes that have been antigenically activated. When compared with regular lymphocytes microscopically, atypical lymphocytes are larger overall, with larger, eccentrically placed indented and folded nuclei with a lower nucleus-to-cytoplasm ratio. Although atypical lymphocytosis may be seen with many of the infections usually causing lymphocytosis, the highest degree of atypical lymphocytes is classically seen with EBV infection. Other syndromes associated with atypical lymphocytosis include acquired cytomegalovirus infection (in contrast to congenital cytomegalovirus infection), toxoplasmosis, viral hepatitis, rubella, roseola, mumps, tuberculosis, typhoid, *Mycoplasma* infection, and malaria, as well as some drug reactions. Mild thrombocytopenia to 50,000-200,000 platelets/mm^3 occurs in >50% of patients but only rarely is associated with purpura. Mild elevation of hepatic transaminase values occurs in approximately 50% of uncomplicated cases but is usually asymptomatic and not associated with jaundice.

Heterophile Antibody Test

Heterophile antibodies agglutinate cells from species different from those in the source serum. The transient heterophile antibodies seen in infectious mononucleosis, also known as *Paul-Bunnell antibodies,* are IgM antibodies detected by the Paul-Bunnell-Davidsohn test for sheep red blood cell (RBC) agglutination. The heterophile antibodies of infectious mononucleosis agglutinate sheep or, for greater sensitivity, horse RBCs but not guinea pig kidney cells. This adsorption property differentiates this response from the heterophile response found in patients with serum sickness, rheumatic diseases, and some normal individuals. Titers >1:28 or >1:40, depending on the dilution system used, after absorption with guinea pig kidney cells are considered positive.

Results of the sheep RBC agglutination test are often positive for several months after infectious mononucleosis; those of the horse RBC agglutination test may be positive for as long as 2 yr. The most widely used method is the qualitative rapid slide test using horse erythrocytes. It detects heterophile antibody in 90% of cases of EBV-associated infectious mononucleosis in older children and adults but in only up to 50% of cases in children <4 yr of age because they typically have a lower titer. From 5% to 10% of cases of infectious mononucleosis are not caused by EBV and are not uniformly associated with a heterophile antibody response. The false-positive rate is <10%, usually resulting from erroneous interpretation. If the heterophile test result is negative and an EBV infection is suspected, EBV-specific antibody testing is indicated.

Specific Epstein-Barr Virus Antibodies

EBV-specific antibody testing is useful to confirm acute EBV infection, especially in heterophile-negative cases, or to confirm past infection and determine susceptibility to future infection. Several distinct EBV antigen systems have been characterized for diagnostic purposes (Fig. 246-2 and Table 246-1). The EBNA, EA, and VCA systems are most useful for diagnostic purposes. The acute phase of infectious mononucleosis is characterized by rapid IgM and IgG antibody responses to VCA in all cases and an IgG response to EA in most cases. The IgM response to VCA is transient but can be detected for at least 4 wk and occasionally for up to 3 mo. The laboratory must take steps to remove rheumatoid factor from the specimen, which may otherwise cause a false-positive IgM VCA result. The IgG response to VCA usually peaks late in the acute phase, declines slightly over the next several weeks to months, and then persists at a relatively stable level for life.

Anti-EA antibodies are usually detectable for several months but may persist or may be detected intermittently at low levels for many years. Antibodies to the diffuse-staining component of EA, EA-D, are found transiently in 80% of patients during the

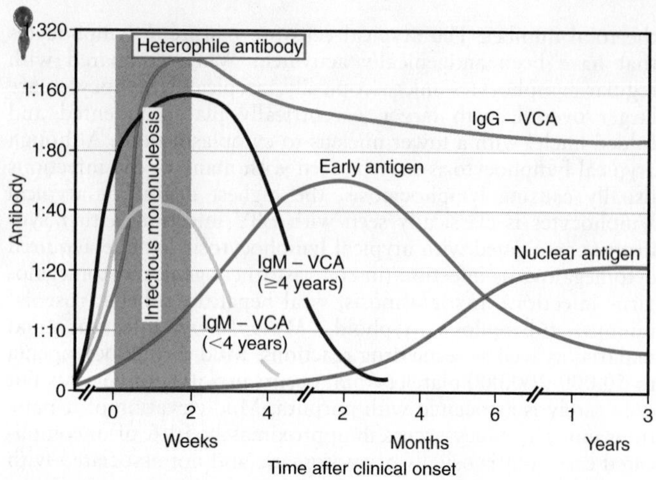

Figure 246-2 Schematic representation of the development of antibodies to various Epstein-Barr virus antigens in patients with infectious mononucleosis. Antibody titers are calculated as geometric mean values expressed as reciprocals of the serum dilution. The immunoglobulin M (IgM) response to viral capsid antigen (VCA) is divided because of the significant differences noted according to age of the patient. IgG, immunoglobulin G. (Reprinted with permission from Jenson HB: Epstein-Barr virus. In Detrick B, Hamilton RG, Folds JD, editors: *Manual of molecular and clinical laboratory immunology,* ed 7, Washington, DC, 2006, American Society for Microbiology.)

acute phase of infectious mononucleosis and reach high titers in patients with nasopharyngeal carcinoma. Antibodies to the cytoplasmic-restricted component of EA, EA-R, emerge transiently in the convalescence from infectious mononucleosis and often attain high titers in patients with EBV-associated Burkitt lymphoma, which in the terminal stage of the disease may be exceeded by antibodies to EA-D. High levels of antibodies to EA-D or EA-R may be found also in immunocompromised patients with persistent EBV infections and active EBV replication. Anti-EBNA antibodies are the last to develop in infectious mononucleosis, gradually appearing 3-4 mo after the onset of illness and remaining at low levels for life. Absence of anti-EBNA when other antibodies are present implies recent infection, whereas the presence of anti-EBNA implies infection occurring more than 3-4 mo previously. The wide range of individual antibody responses and the various laboratory methods used can occasionally make interpretation of an antibody profile difficult. The detection of IgM antibody to VCA is the most valuable and specific serologic test for the diagnosis of acute EBV infection and is generally sufficient to confirm the diagnosis.

TREATMENT

There is no specific treatment for infectious mononucleosis. Therapy with high doses of acyclovir, with or without corticosteroids, decreases viral replication and oropharyngeal shedding during the period of administration but does not reduce the severity or duration of symptoms or alter the eventual outcome. Rest and symptomatic treatments are the mainstays of management. Bed rest is necessary only when the patient has debilitating fatigue. As soon as there is definite symptomatic improvement, the patient should be allowed to begin to resume normal activities. Because blunt abdominal trauma may predispose patients to splenic rupture, it is customary and prudent to advise against participation in contact sports and strenuous athletic activities during the first 2-3 wk of illness or while splenomegaly is present.

Short courses of corticosteroids (<2 wk) may be helpful for complications of infectious mononucleosis, but this use has not been evaluated critically. Some appropriate indications include incipient airway obstruction, thrombocytopenia with hemorrhaging, autoimmune hemolytic anemia, seizures, and meningitis. A recommended regimen is prednisone 1 mg/kg/day (maximum: 60 mg/day) or equivalent for 7 days followed by a dosage taper over another 7 days. There are no controlled data showing efficacy of corticosteroids in any of these conditions. In view of the potential and unknown hazards of immunosuppression for a virus infection with oncogenic complications, corticosteroids should not be used in uncomplicated cases of infectious mononucleosis.

COMPLICATIONS

Very few patients with infectious mononucleosis experience complications. The most feared complication is subcapsular splenic hemorrhage or splenic rupture, which occurs most frequently during the second week of the disease at a rate of <0.5% of cases in adults; the rate in children is unknown but is probably much lower. Rupture is commonly related to trauma, which often may be mild and is rarely fatal. Swelling of the tonsils and oropharyngeal lymphoid tissue may be substantial and may cause airway obstruction that manifests as drooling, stridor, and interference with breathing. Airway compromise with progressive symptoms occurs in <5% of cases and is a common indication for hospitalization with infectious mononucleosis. It may be managed by elevation of the head of the bed and administration of intravenous hydration, humidified air, and systemic corticosteroids. Respiratory distress with incipient or actual airway occlusion should be managed by tonsilloadenoidectomy followed by endotracheal intubation for 12-24 hr in an intensive care setting.

Many uncommon and unusual neurologic conditions have been reported to be associated with EBV infectious mononucleosis. Headache is present in about half of cases, with severe neurologic manifestations, such as seizures and ataxia, in 1-5% of cases. Perceptual distortions of sizes, shapes, and spatial relationships, known as the **Alice in Wonderland syndrome (metamorphopsia)**, may be a presenting symptom. There may be meningitis with nuchal rigidity and mononuclear cells in the cerebrospinal fluid, facial nerve palsy, transverse myelitis, and encephalitis. Most patients with confirmed EBV encephalitis, however, do not demonstrate the typical symptoms of infectious mononucleosis.

Guillain-Barré syndrome or Reye syndrome may follow acute illness. Hemolytic anemia, often with a positive Coombs test result and with cold agglutinins specific for RBC i antigen, occurs in 3% of cases. The onset is typically in the first 2 wk of illness and lasts <1 mo. Aplastic anemia is a rare complication that usually manifests 3-4 wk after the onset of illness, usually with recovery in 4-8 days, but some cases do require bone marrow transplantation. Mild thrombocytopenia and neutropenia are common, but severe thrombocytopenia (<20,000 platelets/μL) or severe neutropenia (<1,000 neutrophils/μL) is rare. Myocarditis or interstitial pneumonia may occur, and both resolve in 3-4 wk. Other rare complications are pancreatitis, parotitis, and orchitis.

PROGNOSIS

The prognosis for complete recovery is excellent. The major symptoms typically last 2-4 wk followed by gradual recovery. Individuals often harbor multiple strains of EBV, and second infections with a different type of EBV (type 1 or type 2) have been demonstrated in immunocompromised persons, but symptoms or second clinical episodes of infectious mononucleosis have not been documented. Prolonged and debilitating fatigue, malaise, and some disability that may wax and wane for several weeks to 6 mo are common complaints even in otherwise unremarkable cases. Occasional persistence of fatigue for a few years after infectious mononucleosis is well recognized. There is no convincing evidence linking EBV infection or EBV reactivation to chronic fatigue syndrome (Chapter 115).

PREVENTION

It is impractical to try to prevent EBV infection because the virus is ubiquitous and often acquired by oral contact early in life. A recombinant EBV subunit glycoprotein 350 (gp350) candidate vaccine in a 3-dose regimen shows promise for preventing infectious mononucleosis and potentially EBV-associated malignancies as well.

BIBLIOGRAPHY

Please visit the Nelson Textbook of Pediatrics *website at* *www.expertconsult.com* *for the complete bibliography.*

Chapter 247 Cytomegalovirus

Sergio Stagno

Human cytomegalovirus (CMV) is widely distributed. Most CMV infections are inapparent, but the virus can cause a variety of clinical illnesses that range in severity from mild to fatal. CMV is the most common cause of congenital infection, which occasionally causes the syndrome of cytomegalic inclusion disease (hepatosplenomegaly, jaundice, petechia, purpura, and microcephaly) in neonates. In immunocompetent adults, CMV infection is occasionally characterized by a mononucleosis-like syndrome. In immunosuppressed persons, including transplant recipients and patients with AIDS, CMV pneumonitis, retinitis, and gastrointestinal disease are common and can be fatal.

Primary infection occurs in a seronegative, susceptible host. Recurrent infection represents reactivation of latent infection or reinfection of a seropositive immune host. Disease may result from primary or recurrent CMV infection, but the former is more commonly associated with severe disease.

ETIOLOGY

CMV is the largest of the herpesviruses and has a diameter of 200 nm with a double-stranded DNA viral genome of 240 kb in a 64-nm core enclosed by an icosahedral capsid composed of 162 capsomers. The core is assembled in the nucleus of the host cells. The capsid is surrounded by a poorly defined amorphous tegument, which is itself surrounded by a loosely applied, lipid-containing envelope. The tegument contains the most immunogenic proteins of the virion, including targets of T-lymphocyte and antibody responses. The envelope is acquired during the budding process through the nuclear membrane into a cytoplasmic vacuole, which contains the protein components of the envelope. The envelope glycoproteins induce strong antibody responses, including neutralizing antibodies in the infected host. Mature viruses exit the cells by cell lysis (fibroblasts) or by poorly defined exocytic pathways. Routine serologic tests do not define specific serotypes. In contrast, restriction endonuclease analysis of CMV DNA shows that human strains are not genetically identical unless obtained from epidemiologically related cases.

EPIDEMIOLOGY

Seroepidemiologic surveys demonstrate CMV infection in every population examined worldwide. The prevalence of infection increases with age and is higher in developing countries and among lower socioeconomic strata of the more developed nations.

Transmission sources of CMV include saliva, breast milk, cervical and vaginal secretions, urine, semen, tears, blood products, and organ allographs. The spread of CMV requires very close or intimate contact because it is very labile. Transmission occurs by direct person-to-person contact, but indirect transmission is possible via contaminated fomites.

The incidence of congenital CMV infection ranges from 0.2% to 2.2% (average 1%) of all live births, with the higher rates among populations with a lower economic standard of living. The risk for fetal infection is greatest with maternal primary CMV infection (30%) and much less likely with recurrent infection (<1%). In the USA, 1-4% of pregnant women acquire primary CMV infection, and as many as 8,000 newborns have neurodevelopmental sequelae associated with congenital CMV infection.

Perinatal transmission is common, accounting for an incidence of 10-60% through the 1st 6 mo of life. The most important perinatal sources of virus are genital tract secretions at delivery and breast milk. Among CMV-seropositive mothers, virus is detectable in breast milk in 96%, with postnatal transmission occurring in approximately 38% of infants, resulting in symptomatic infection in nearly half of very low birthweight infants. Infected infants may excrete virus for years in saliva and urine.

After the 1st year of life, the prevalence of infection depends on group activities, with child-care centers contributing to rapid spread of CMV among children. Infection rates of 50-80% during childhood are common. For children who are not exposed to other toddlers, the rate of infection increases very slowly throughout the 1st decade of life. A 2nd peak occurs in adolescence as a result of sexual transmission. Seronegative child-care workers and parents of young children shedding CMV have a 10-20% annual risk of acquiring CMV, in contrast to the risk of 1-3% per year for the general population.

Hospital workers are not at increased risk for acquiring CMV infection from patients. With the implementation of universal precautions, the risk of nosocomial transmission of CMV to health care workers is expected to be lower than the risk of acquiring the infection in the community.

CMV infection may be transmitted in transplanted organs (kidney, heart, bone marrow). Following transplantation, many patients excrete CMV as a result of infection acquired from the donor organ or from reactivation of latent infection caused by immunosuppression. Seronegative transplant recipients of organs from seropositive donors are at greatest risk for severe disease.

Nosocomial infection is a hazard of transfusion of blood and blood products. In a population with a 50% prevalence of CMV infection, the risk has been estimated at 2.7% per unit of whole blood. Leukocyte transfusions pose a much greater risk. Infection is usually asymptomatic, but even in well children and adults there is a risk for disease if the recipient is seronegative and receives multiple units. Immunocompromised patients and seronegative premature infants have a much higher (10-30%) risk for disease.

PATHOGENESIS

Clinical CMV disease generally results from a combination of altered cellular immunity, uncontrolled viral replication with increased virus burden, multiorgan involvement, and end-organ disease secondary to direct viral cytopathic effects. Increased levels of virus replication, as ascertained by genome copy numbers, are useful in identifying patients at risk for invasive disease and dissemination of infection. The presence of CMV in areas of inflammation increases the expression of soluble mediators such as cytokines and chemokines, leading to recruitment of inflammatory cells. The interactions between the virus and host inflammatory response seem to lead to persistent viral replication, viral gene expression, and dissemination.

CLINICAL MANIFESTATIONS

The signs and symptoms of CMV infection vary with age, route of transmission, and immunocompetence of the patient. The infection is subclinical in most patients. In infants and young children, primary CMV infection occasionally causes pneumonitis, hepatomegaly, hepatitis, and petechial rashes. In older children, adolescents, and adults, CMV may cause a mononucleosis-like syndrome characterized by fatigue, malaise, myalgia, headache, fever, hepatosplenomegaly, elevated liver enzyme values, and atypical lymphocytosis. The course of CMV mononucleosis is generally mild, lasting 2-3 wk. Clinical presentations include occasionally persistent fever, overt hepatitis, and a morbilliform rash. Recurrent infections are asymptomatic in the immunocompetent host.

Immunocompromised Persons

The risk of CMV disease is increased in immunocompromised persons, with both primary and recurrent infections (Chapter 171). Illness with a primary infection includes pneumonitis (most common), hepatitis, chorioretinitis, gastrointestinal disease, or fever with leukopenia as an isolated entity or as a manifestation of generalized disease, which may be fatal. The risk is greatest in bone marrow transplant recipients and in patients with AIDS. Pneumonia, retinitis, and involvement of the central nervous system and gastrointestinal tract are usually severe and progressive. Submucosal ulcerations can occur anywhere in the gastrointestinal tract and may lead to hemorrhage and perforation. Pancreatitis and cholecystitis may also occur.

Congenital Infection

Symptomatic congenital CMV infection was originally termed **cytomegalic inclusion disease**. Only 5% of all congenitally infected infants have severe cytomegalic inclusion disease, another 5% have mild involvement, and 90% are born with subclinical, but still chronic, CMV infection. The characteristic signs and symptoms of clinically manifested infections include intrauterine growth restriction, prematurity, hepatosplenomegaly and jaundice, blueberry muffin–like rash, thrombocytopenia and purpura, and microcephaly and intracranial calcifications. Other neurologic problems include chorioretinitis, sensorineural hearing loss, and mild increases in cerebrospinal fluid protein. Symptomatic newborns are usually easy to identify. Congenital infections that are symptomatic and most severe and those resulting in sequelae are more likely to be caused by primary rather than reactivated infections in pregnant women. Re-infection with a different strain of CMV can lead to symptomatic congenital infection. Asymptomatic congenital CMV infection is likely a leading cause of sensorineural hearing loss, which occurs in approximately 7-10% of all infants with congenital CMV infection, whether symptomatic at birth or not.

Perinatal Infection

Infections resulting from exposure to CMV in the maternal genital tract at delivery or in breast milk occur despite the presence of maternally derived, passively acquired antibody. Approximately 6-12% of seropositive mothers transmit CMV by contaminated cervical-vaginal secretions and 40% by breast milk to their infants, who usually remain asymptomatic and do not exhibit sequelae. Occasionally, perinatally acquired CMV infection is associated with pneumonitis and a sepsis-like syndrome. Premature and ill full-term infants may have neurologic sequelae and psychomotor retardation. However, the risk for hearing loss, chorioretinitis, and microcephaly does not appear to be increased. Very low birthweight infants with transfusion-acquired or breast milk–acquired CMV infection have a much greater risk of morbidity.

DIAGNOSIS

Active CMV infection is best confirmed by virus isolation from urine, saliva, bronchoalveolar washings, breast milk, cervical secretions, buffy coat, and tissues obtained by biopsy. Rapid identification (within 24 hr) is routinely available with the centrifugation-enhanced rapid culture system based on the detection of CMV early antigens using monoclonal antibodies. Several methods are used for rapid quantitative detection of CMV antigens, and quantitative polymerase chain reaction (PCR) assays are also available. The presence of viral shedding and active infection does not distinguish between primary and recurrent infections. A primary infection is confirmed by seroconversion or the simultaneous detection of immunoglobulin (Ig) M and IgG antibodies with low functional avidity. A simple increase in antibody titers in initially seropositive patients must be interpreted with caution, because such an increase is occasionally observed years after primary infection. IgG antibodies persist for life. For the first weeks after primary infection, the functional avidity of IgG class antibodies is very low, rising to a peak in 4-5 mo. IgM antibodies can be demonstrated transiently in both symptomatic and asymptomatic infection at 4-16 wk, which is during the acute phase of symptomatic disease. IgM antibodies are occasionally found with these assays (0.2-1%) in patients with recurrent infection.

Recurrent infection is defined by the reappearance of viral excretion in a patient known to have been seropositive in the past. The distinction between reactivation of endogenous virus and re-infection with a different strain of CMV requires CMV-DNA analysis or the measurement of antibodies against strain-specific epitopes of CMV, such as glycoprotein H epitopes.

In immunocompromised persons, excretion of CMV, increases in IgG titers, and even the presence of IgM antibodies are common, greatly confounding the ability to distinguish primary and recurrent infections. Demonstrating viremia by buffy coat culture, detection of CMV antigenemia, or detection of CMV DNA by PCR implies active disease and worse prognosis regardless of whether the type of infection is primary, recurrent, or uncertain.

Congenital Infection

The definitive method for diagnosis of congenital CMV infection is virus isolation or demonstration of CMV DNA by PCR, which must be performed during the 1st 2 weeks of life because viral excretion afterwards may represent infection acquired at birth or shortly thereafter. Urine and saliva are the best specimens for culture and saliva, and cord blood is best for PCR. Infants with congenital CMV infection may excrete CMV in the urine for several years. An IgG antibody test is of little diagnostic value because a positive result also reflects maternal antibodies, although a negative result excludes the diagnosis of congenital CMV infection. Demonstration of stable or rising titers in serial specimens during the 1st year of life does not help, because acquired infection in the first few months of life is common. IgM tests lack sensitivity and specificity and are unreliable for diagnosis of congenital CMV infection.

IgM antibody tests and the measurement of CMV IgG avidity can identify women at high risk for transmitting CMV in utero. Fetal infection can be confirmed by viral isolation from amniotic fluid. The sensitivity of this method is excellent after the 22nd wk of gestation. The detection of viral genome by PCR in amniotic fluid is equally sensitive and specific; quantitative PCR demonstrating 10^5 genome equivalents per mL of amniotic fluid is a predictor of symptomatic congenital infection.

TREATMENT

Ganciclovir, foscarnet, and cidofovir are inhibitors of viral DNA polymerase shown to be effective in CMV disease and are approved for use in the USA. Treatment is seldom indicated for immunocompetent persons but is recommended for immunocompromised persons and remains controversial for infants with symptomatic congenital infection.

Immunocompromised Persons

The more severe the immunosuppression, such as that required after bone marrow transplantation, the more severe is the CMV disease. Ganciclovir combined with immune globulin, either standard intravenous immunoglobulin (IVIG) or hyperimmune CMV IVIG, has been used to treat life-threatening CMV infections in immunocompromised hosts (bone marrow, heart, and kidney transplant recipients and patients with AIDS). Two published regimens are: ganciclovir (7.5 mg/kg/day divided every 8 hr IV for 14 days) with CMV IVIG (400 mg/kg on days 1, 2, and 7, and 200 mg/kg on day 14); and ganciclovir (7.5 mg/kg/day divided every 8 hr IV for 20 days with IVIG 500 mg/kg every other day for 10 doses).

CMV retinitis and gastrointestinal disease appear to be clinically responsive to therapy but, like viral excretion, often recur on cessation. Toxicity with ganciclovir is frequent and often severe and includes neutropenia, thrombocytopenia, liver dysfunction, reduction in spermatogenesis, and gastrointestinal and renal abnormalities. Oral valganciclovir, the orally bioavailable prodrug of ganciclovir, causes less toxicity and appears to be as effective as IV ganciclovir. Foscarnet is an alternative antiviral agent, although there is limited information on its use in children. CMV prophylaxis with ganciclovir or acyclovir reduces the risk of morbidity in solid organ transplantation. Prophylactic treatment with valacyclovir in adults (900 mg PO once daily for 90 days) is a safe and effective regimen to prevent CMV disease in kidney and pancreas transplant recipients.

Patients with CMV mononucleosis usually recover fully, although some have protracted symptoms. Most immunocompromised patients also recover uneventfully, but many experience severe pneumonitis, with a high fatality rate if hypoxemia develops. CMV infection and disease may be fatal in individuals with increased susceptibility to infections, such as patients with AIDS.

Congenital Infection

A randomized controlled study with ganciclovir (6 mg/kg/dose every 12 hr IV for the 1st 6 wk of life) concluded that treatment both prevents hearing deterioration and improves or maintains normal hearing function at 6 mo of age, and may prevent hearing deterioration that occurs after 1 yr of age. Drug-related toxicity was common, with significant neutropenia developing in 63% of ganciclovir-treated patients, compared with 21% in the untreated group. The logistic obstacles of intravenous therapy for the 1st 6 wk of life, limited benefit, and adverse effects have limited enthusiasm for this regimen. A randomized study of oral valganciclovir, is under way to compare the efficiency of 42 days of treatment with 6 mo of treatment.

PREVENTION

The use of CMV-free blood products, especially for premature newborns, and, whenever possible, the use of organs from CMV-free donors for transplantation represent important measures to prevent CMV infection and disease in patients at high risk.

Pregnant women who are CMV seropositive are at low risk of delivering a symptomatic newborn. If possible, pregnant women should undergo CMV serologic testing, especially if they provide care for young children who are potential CMV excreters. Pregnant women who are CMV seronegative should be counseled regarding good handwashing and other hygienic measures and avoidance of contact with oral secretions of others. Those with suspected recent CMV infection may undergo additional diagnostic evaluations to ascertain in utero transmission and fetal disease. An uncontrolled trial has shown that the use of CMV hyperimmune globulin in pregnant women with primary CMV can lessen the risk of transmission to the unborn baby and can even reduce the risk of disease in the infected fetus.

Passive Immunoprophylaxis

The use of IVIG or CMV IVIG for prophylaxis of infection in solid organ and bone marrow transplant recipients reduces the risk of symptomatic disease but does not prevent infection. The efficacy of prophylaxis is more striking when the hazard of primary CMV infection is greatest, such as in bone marrow transplantation. There is no consensus for a uniform prophylaxis regimen for CMV infection. Recommended regimens include either IVIG (1,000 mg/kg) or CMV IVIG (500 mg/kg) given as a single intravenous dose beginning within 72 hr of transplantation and once weekly thereafter until 90-120 days after transplantation.

Active Immunization

The beneficial role of immunity is substantial, as illustrated by the fact that most cases of severe disease follow primary infection, especially with congenital infection, transfusion-acquired infection, and infection in transplant recipients.

The 1st vaccine tested in humans was developed from the live attenuated Towne strain of CMV, which proved immunogenic but did not prevent infection in renal transplant recipients or normal adult women. However, in renal transplant recipients the vaccine reduced the virulence of primary infection. Promising results have been obtained with a CMV vaccine consisting of recombinant envelope glycoprotein B (gB) combined with the adjuvant MF59. In a double-blind placebo-controlled trial of seronegative adult women results showed that after 3 doses this vaccine induced antibodies to gB, neutralizing antibodies, and cell-mediated immunity. A later study of 464 women randomly assigned to receive either this gB subunit vaccine or placebo showed prevention of maternal infection as measured by seroconversion to CMV proteins other than gB in about 50% of vaccines. One congenital infection occurred among infants of this immunized group, whereas 3 infections occurred in the placebo group.

BIBLIOGRAPHY

Please visit the Nelson Textbook of Pediatrics *website at* *www.expertconsult.com* *for the complete bibliography.*

Chapter 248
Roseola (Human Herpes Viruses 6 and 7)

Mary T. Caserta

Human herpesvirus 6 (HHV-6) and human herpesvirus 7 (HHV-7) cause ubiquitous infection in infancy and early childhood. HHV-6 is responsible for the majority of cases of **roseola infantum (exanthema subitum** or **sixth disease**) and has been associated with other diseases, including encephalitis, especially in immunocompromised hosts. A small percentage of children with roseola have primary infection with HHV-7.

ETIOLOGY

HHV-6 and HHV-7 are the sole members of the *Roseolovirus* genus in the Betaherpesvirinae subfamily of human herpesviruses. Human cytomegalovirus (CMV), the only other β-herpesvirus, shares limited sequence homology with HHV-6 and HHV-7. Morphologically all human herpesviruses are composed of an icosahedral nucleocapsid, protein-dense tegument, and lipid envelope. Within the nucleocapsid, HHV-6 and HHV-7 each contain large, linear, double-stranded DNA genomes that encode >80 unique proteins.

Two strain groups of HHV-6 have been recognized, HHV-6 variant A and variant B. The genomes of HHV-6 A and B are highly conserved, with approximately 90% sequence identity. However, they can be distinguished by restriction fragment length polymorphisms, reactivity with monoclonal antibodies, differential growth in tissue culture cell lines, and epidemiology. Accordingly, some researchers propose that they should be separate viruses. Although the frequency of detection of HHV-6 variant A DNA differs among studies, variant B is the overwhelmingly predominant strain found in both normal and immunocompromised hosts by both culture and polymerase chain reaction (PCR). Primary infection with HHV-6 variant A has been detected in children in Africa. It is not clear whether the differences in the detection of HHV-6 variant A DNA and variant B DNA relate to different tissue tropism, differences in mode or age of acquisition, differences in the ability to cause human disease, or the geographical location of the population studied.

EPIDEMIOLOGY

Primary infection with HHV-6 is acquired rapidly by essentially all children following the loss of maternal antibodies in the first few months of infancy, 95% of children being infected with HHV-6 by 2 yr of age. The peak age of primary HHV-6 infection is 6-9 mo of life, with infections occurring sporadically and without seasonal predilection. Infection with HHV-7 is also widespread but occurs later in childhood and at a slower rate; only 50% of children have evidence of prior infection with HHV-7 by 3 yr of age. Seroprevalence reaches 75% at 3-6 yr of age. In a small study of children with primary HHV-7 infection, the mean age of the patients was 26 mo, significantly older than that of children with acute HHV-6 infection.

Although it is presumed that children acquire primary infection with HHV-6 and HHV-7 from the saliva of asymptomatic adults, congenital infection with HHV-6 occurs in 1% of newborns. Two mechanisms of vertical transmission of HHV-6 have been identified, transplacental infection and chromosomal integration (CI-HHV6). HHV-6 is unique among the human herpesviruses in that it is integrated at the telomere end of human chromosomes at a frequency of 0.2-2.2% of the population and is passed from parent to child via the germline. Chromosomal integration has been identified as the major mechanism by which HHV-6 is vertically transmitted, accounting for 86% of congenital infections, with one third due to HHV-6 variant A. The clinical consequences of chromosomal integration or transplacental infection with HHV-6 have yet to be determined. In one series of infants identified with HHV-6 congenital infection, no evidence of disease was present in the early neonatal period. Congenital infection with HHV-7 has not been demonstrated. DNA of both HHV-6 and HHV-7 has been identified in the cervical secretions of pregnant women, suggesting an additional role for sexual or perinatal transmission of these viruses. Breast milk does not appear to play a role in transmission of either HHV-6 or HHV-7.

PATHOLOGY/PATHOGENESIS

Primary HHV-6 infection causes a viremia that can be demonstrated by co-culture of the patient's peripheral blood mononuclear cells (PBMCs) with mitogen-stimulated cord blood mononuclear cells. HHV-6 has a recognizable cytopathic effect, consisting of the appearance of large refractile mononucleated or multinucleated cells with intracytoplasmic and/or intranuclear inclusions. Infected cells exhibit a slightly prolonged life span in cultures; however, lytic infection predominates. HHV-6 infection also induces apoptosis of T cells and may lead to cell expiration via loss of mitochondrial membrane potential as well as alteration of interferon and retinoic acid-induced cell death signals. In vitro, HHV-6 can infect a broad range of cell types, including primary T cells, monocytes, natural killer (NK) cells, dendritic cells, and astrocytes. HHV-6 has also been documented to infect B-cell, megakaryocytic, endothelial, and epithelial cell lines. Human astrocytes, oligodendrocytes, and microglia have been infected with HHV-6 ex-vivo. The broad tropism of HHV-6 is consistent with the recognition that CD46, a complement regulatory protein present on the surface of all nucleated cells, is a cellular receptor for HHV-6. The CD4 molecule has been identified as a receptor for HHV-7. HHV-7 has been demonstrated to reactivate HHV-6 from latency in vitro. Whether this phenomenon occurs in vivo remains unknown.

Primary infection with HHV-6 and HHV-7 is followed by lifelong latency or persistence of virus at multiple sites. HHV-6 exists in a true state of viral latency in monocytes and macrophages. The detection of replicating HHV-6 in cultures of primary CD34+ hematopoietic stem cells has also been described, suggesting that cellular differentiation is a trigger of viral reactivation. This observation may be clinically significant because of the possibility that HHV-6 may cause either primary or reactivated infection during hematopoietic stem cell transplantation. Additionally, HHV-6 and HHV-7 infection may be persistent in salivary glands, and DNA for both HHV-6 and HHV-7 can be routinely detected in the saliva of both adults and children. HHV-7 can also be isolated in tissue culture from saliva, but HHV-6 cannot. HHV-6 DNA has been identified in the cerebrospinal fluid (CSF) of children both during and subsequent to primary infection as well as in brain tissue from immunocompetent adults at autopsy, implicating the central nervous system (CNS) as an additional important site of either viral latency or persistence. HHV-7 DNA has also been found in adult brain tissue but at a significantly lower frequency.

CLINICAL MANIFESTATIONS

Roseola infantum (**exanthem subitum**, or **sixth disease**) is an acute, self-limited disease of infancy and early childhood. It is characterized by the abrupt onset of high fever, which may be accompanied by fussiness. The fever usually resolves acutely after 72 hr ("crisis") but may gradually fade over a day ("lysis") coincident with the appearance of a faint pink or rose-colored, nonpruritic, 2- to 3-mm morbilliform rash on the trunk (Fig. 248-1). The rash usually lasts 1-3 days but is often described as evanescent and may be visible only for hours, spreading from the trunk to the face and extremities. Because the rash is variable in appearance, location, and duration, it is not distinctive. Associated signs are sparse but can include mild injection of the pharynx, palpebral conjunctivae, or tympanic membranes and enlarged suboccipital nodes. In Asian countries, ulcers at the uvulopalatoglassal junction (**Nagayama spots**) are commonly reported in infants with roseola.

High fever (mean 39.7°C) is the most consistent finding associated with primary HHV-6 infection. Rash detected either during the illness or following defervescence has been reported in approximately 20% of infected children in the USA. Additional symptoms and signs include irritability, inflamed tympanic membranes, rhinorrhea and congestion, gastrointestinal complaints, and encephalopathy. Symptoms of lower respiratory tract involvement such as cough are identified significantly less frequently in children with primary HHV-6 infection than in children with other febrile illnesses. The mean duration of illness due to primary HHV-6 infection is 6 days, with 15% of children having fever for 6 or more days. Primary infection with HHV-6 accounts for a significant burden of illness on the health care system; one study found that 24% of visits to emergency departments by infants between 6 and 9 mo of age were due to primary HHV-6 infection. A population-based study of primary HHV-6 infection has confirmed that 93% of infants had symptoms and were more likely to visit a physician than non-infected infants. Fever was less likely to be present with HHV-6 infection in children <6 mo of age but was significantly more common in older infants and children.

Much less is known about the clinical manifestations of HHV-7 infection. Primary infection with HHV-7 has been identified in a small number of children with roseola in whom the

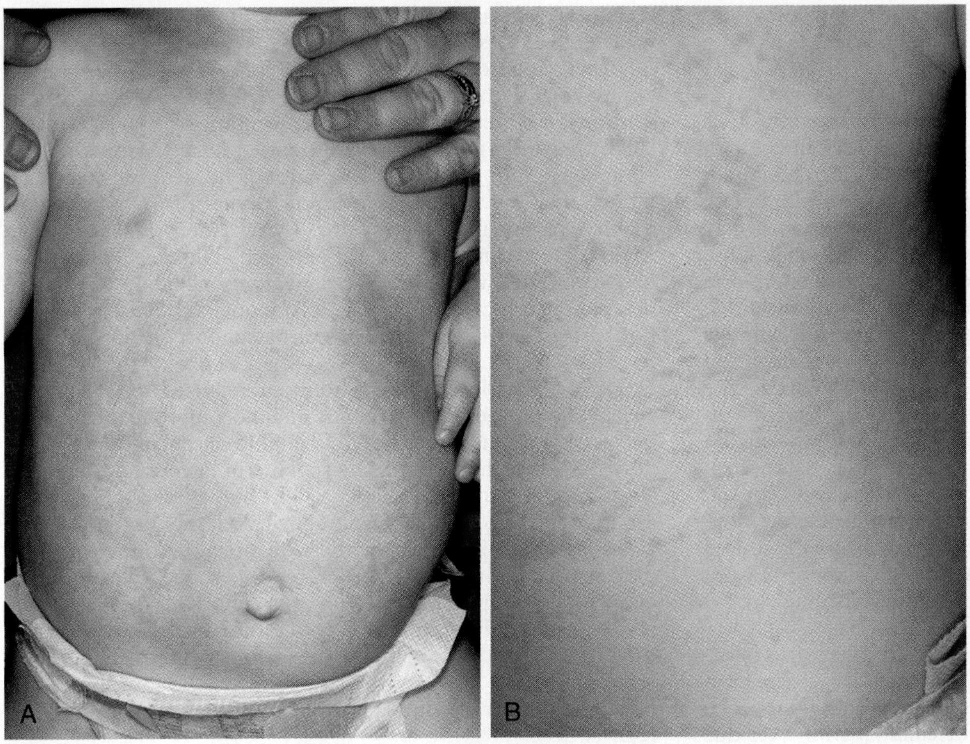

Figure 248-1 Roseola infantum. Erythematous, blanching macules and papules (*A*) in an infant who had high fever for 3 days preceding development of the rash. On closer inspection (*B*), some lesions reveal a subtle peripheral halo of vasoconstriction. (From Paller AS, Mancinin AJ, editors: *Hurwitz clinical pediatric dermatology*, ed 3, Philadelphia, 2006, Elsevier, p 434.)

illness is indistinguishable from that due to HHV-6. Secondary cases of roseola due to infection with HHV-7 have also been reported. Additionally, primary infection with HHV-7 may be asymptomatic or may cause a nonspecific febrile illness lasting approximately 3 days.

LABORATORY FINDINGS

The most characteristic laboratory findings noted in children with primary HHV-6 infection are lower mean numbers of total white blood cells (8900/mm^3), lymphocytes (3400/mm^3), and neutrophils (4500/mm^3), than in febrile children without primary HHV-6 infection. Similar hematologic findings have been reported during primary infection with HHV-7. Thrombocytopenia, elevated serum transaminase values, and atypical lymphocytes have also been noted sporadically in children with primary HHV-6 infection.

Results of CSF analyses reported in patients with encephalitis thought to be due to HHV-6 have been normal or demonstrated only mild CSF pleocytosis with slight elevations of protein. Areas of hyperintense signal on T2-weighted and FLAIR (fluid attenuation inversion recovery) images of the hippocampus, uncus, and amygdale have been found on MRI, as well as increased metabolism within the hippocampus on positron emission tomography (PET) scanning.

DIAGNOSIS

Although roseola is generally a benign self-limited disease, its diagnosis can exclude other, more serious disorders that cause fever and rash. A history of 3 days of high fever in an otherwise nontoxic 10 mo old infant with a blanching maculopapular rash on the trunk suggests a diagnosis of roseola. Likewise, a specific diagnosis of HHV-6 is not usually necessary except in situations in which the manifestations of the infection are severe or unusual and might benefit from antiviral therapy.

The diagnosis of primary infection with either HHV-6 or HHV-7 is confirmed by demonstrating the presence of actively replicating virus in the patient's blood sample coupled with seroconversion. Viral culture is the gold standard method to document active viral replication. Unfortunately, culture is expensive, time consuming, and available only in research laboratories. Two other methods used to identify active HHV-6 replication are the detection of viral DNA by PCR on acellular fluids such as plasma and reverse transcriptase PCR (RT-PCR) on PBMC samples designed to detect viral transcription and protein production. Quantitative PCR for HHV-6 genome copy numbers on various specimens is also frequently reported and is commercially available. However, the role of this methodology is not clear, as a specific value of DNA that can discriminate between patients with viremia and those who are culture negative has not been determined. Complicating the use of molecular assays for the detection of active replication of HHV-6 is the recognition that individuals with chromosomally integrated HHV-6 have persistently high viral loads of HHV-6 DNA in plasma, PBMCs, and CSF in the absence of disease and viremia.

Serologic methods including indirect immunofluorescence assays, enzyme-linked immunosorbent assay (ELISA), neutralization assays, and immunoblot have been described for the measurement of concentrations of antibodies to HHV-6 and HHV-7 in serum or plasma and are commercially available. Although IgM antibody is produced early in infection with HHV-6, assays designed to measure this response have not proved useful in the diagnosis of primary or reactivated infection. The absence of IgG antibody in an infant >6 mo of age combined with the presence of replicating virus is strong evidence of primary infection with either HHV-6 or HHV-7. Alternatively, the demonstration of seroconversion between acute and convalescent samples also confirms primary infection but is not clinically useful in the acute care setting. Unfortunately, serologic assays have not been found reliable in the detection of HHV-6 reactivation and cannot be used to differentiate between infection with HHV-6 variants A and B. Additionally, limited antibody cross reactivity has been demonstrated between HHV-6 and HHV-7, complicating the interpretation of serologic assays, especially if low titers are reported.

Differential Diagnosis

Primary infection with either HHV-6 or HHV-7 usually causes an undifferentiated febrile illness that may be very difficult to distinguish from other common viral infections of childhood. This difficulty also applies to the early stages of roseola, before the development of rash. Once the rash is present, roseola may be confused with other exanthematous diseases of childhood, especially measles and rubella. Children with **rubella** often have a prodrome characterized by mild illness with low-grade fever, sore throat, arthralgia, and gastrointestinal complaints, unlike those with roseola. On physical examination, suboccipital and posterior auricular lymph nodes are prominent up to 1 wk before the rash of rubella is evident and persist during the exanthematous phase. Additionally, the rash of rubella usually begins on the face and spreads to the chest, like that in measles. The associated symptoms of **measles** virus infection include cough, coryza, and conjunctivitis, with high fever coincident with the development of rash, unlike in roseola. Roseola may also be confused with scarlet fever, though the latter is rare in children <2 yr of age and causes a characteristic sandpaper-like rash concurrent with fever.

Roseola may be confused with illness due to enterovirus infections, especially in the summer and fall months. Drug hypersensitivity reactions may also be difficult to distinguish from roseola. Antibiotics are frequently prescribed for children with fever due to roseola before the appearance of rash. A child who then demonstrates rash after the resolution of fever may erroneously be labeled as being drug allergic.

COMPLICATIONS

Convulsions are the most common complication of roseola and are recognized in up to one third of patients. Seizures are also the most common complication of children with primary HHV-6 infection, occurring in approximately 15%, with a peak age at 12-15 mo. Children with primary HHV-6 infection have also been reported to have a higher frequency of partial seizures, prolonged seizures, post-ictal paralysis, and repeated seizures than children with febrile seizures not associated with HHV-6. In a study limited to children with primary HHV-6 infection and seizures, 30% of patients had prolonged seizures, 29% had focal seizures, and 38% had repeated seizures.

A prospective study of children 2-35 mo of age with suspected encephalitis or severe illness with convulsions and fever found that 17% had primary infection with either HHV-6 or HHV-7, and status epilepticus was the most common presentation. Despite the reported severity of seizures during primary infection with HHV-6 and HHV-7, limited data suggest that there may be a decreased risk of recurrent seizures after primary infection with HHV-6 than of febrile seizures due to other causes.

Case reports and small patient series have described additional complications in children with primary HHV-6 infection, including encephalitis, acute disseminated demyelination, acute cerebellitis, hepatitis, and myocarditis. Late-developing long-term sequelae, including developmental disabilities and autistic-like features, have been reported rarely in children who have CNS symptoms during primary HHV-6 infection.

An association between recurrent seizures and reactivated or persistent infection of the CNS by HHV-6 has been suggested. Studies evaluating brain tissue specimens have implicated HHV-6 in as many as 35% of patients with temporal lobe epilepsy, high viral loads being found in the hippocampus or lateral temporal lobe regions. HHV-6 protein production has also been identified in a small number of resected tissue specimens. Primary astrocytes obtained from these samples had undetectable levels of a glutamate transporter, suggesting the loss of ability to control glutamate levels as a possible mechanism for the development of recurrent seizures.

Reactivation of HHV-6 has been reported in several different populations with and without disease with the use of various methods of detection. The best documentation of HHV-6 reactivation has been in immunocompromised hosts, especially those patients who have undergone hematopoietic stem cell transplantation (HSCT). Such reactivation occurs in approximately 35-50% of patients, typically at 2-4 weeks after transplantation. Many of the clinical complications seen following HSCT have been associated with HHV-6 reactivation, including fever, rash, delayed engraftment of platelets or monocytes, and graft versus host disease with variable degrees of support in the literature for each.

HHV-6 reactivation has also been reported as a cause of encephalitis in both normal and immunocompromised hosts. A distinct syndrome of post-HSCT limbic encephalitis has been described; it is characterized by short-term memory dysfunction, confusion, and insomnia with seizures noted either clinically or on prolonged electroencephalography (EEG) monitoring. HHV-6 DNA has been identified in the CSF in the majority of these patients. Additionally, HHV-6 proteins were identified in astrocytes of the hippocampus in one post mortem specimen, suggesting active HHV-6 infection at the time of death. Because of the variability in sensitivity of PCR methods and the high prevalence of HHV-6 DNA in multiple body sites following primary infection, it is very difficult to evaluate the validity of these reports.

TREATMENT

Supportive care is usually all that is needed for infants with roseola. Parents should be advised to maintain hydration and may use antipyretics if the child is especially uncomfortable with the fever. Specific antiviral therapy is not recommended for routine cases of primary HHV-6 or HHV-7 infection. Unusual or severe manifestations of primary or presumed reactivated HHV-6 infection such as encephalitis, especially in immunocompromised patients, may benefit from treatment. Ganciclovir, foscarnet, and cidofovir all demonstrate inhibitory activity against HHV-6 in vitro similar to their activity against CMV. Case reports suggest that all three drugs, alone or in combination, can decrease HHV-6 viral replication, as evidenced by decreased viral loads in plasma and CSF. However, clinical data regarding efficacy are sparse and contradictory, with no randomized trials to guide use. Additionally, in vitro resistance of HHV-6 to ganciclovir has been described. Foscarnet appears to be most likely to have activity against HHV-7 on the basis of in vitro testing, but no clinical data are available.

PROGNOSIS

Roseola is generally a self-limited illness associated with complete recovery. The majority of children with primary infections with HHV-6 and HHV-7 also recover uneventfully without sequelae. Although seizures are a common complication of primary infection with HHV-6 and HHV-7, the risk of recurrent seizures does not appear to be higher than that associated with other causes of febrile seizures.

PREVENTION

Primary infections with HHV-6 and HHV-7 are widespread throughout the human population with no current means of interrupting transmission.

BIBLIOGRAPHY

Please visit the Nelson Textbook of Pediatrics *website at* *www.expertconsult.com* *for the complete bibliography.*

Chapter 249
Human Herpesvirus 8

Mary T. Caserta

Human herpesvirus 8 (HHV-8) was first identified in tissue specimens from patients with **Kaposi sarcoma (KS)**. Because of this association it is also known as **Kaposi sarcoma–associated herpesvirus** (KSHV). HHV-8 has since been recognized as the etiologic agent of two additional lymphoproliferative disorders: **primary effusion based lymphoma** (PEL) and **multicentric Castleman disease.**

ETIOLOGY

HHV-8 is a γ-2-human herpesvirus genetically most similar to Epstein-Barr virus. The virus contains a large DNA genome encoding for 85-95 unique proteins. Infection is followed by both lytic and latent viral states with different degrees of viral replication associated with distinct disease manifestations.

EPIDEMIOLOGY

The prevalence of infection with HHV-8 varies both geographically and by population and roughly matches the epidemiology of KS. HHV-8 is endemic in Africa and parts of South America, with infection rates of up to 30-60% by adolescence. Seroprevalence >20% has also been found in regions bordering the Mediterranean. In contrast, infection rates <5% are noted in North America, central Europe, and Asia. However, within geographical regions, the prevalence of infection varies with risk behaviors, rates of 30-75% being found among men who have sex with men in North America and Europe. HHV-8 DNA can be detected in saliva and genital tract secretions. Taken together, these findings lead to the recognition that saliva is the major mode of transmission to children in areas where HHV-8 infection is endemic, whereas sexual contact is a source of infection among adults in low-prevalence areas. Other less common routes of HHV-8 transmission include blood transfusion, bone marrow transplantation, and solid organ transplantation. Vertical transmission may occur in regions where HHV-8 is highly endemic, but the risk appears low.

PATHOLOGY/PATHOGENESIS

HHV-8 contains multiple genes that impact cell cycle regulation and the host immune response. Viral proteins interfere with the function of the tumor suppressor molecules p53 and retinoblastoma protein, induce the expression of pro-angiogenesis factors vascular endothelial growth factor (VEGF) A and VEGF receptor-2, and lead to upregulation of the human mammalian target of rapamycin (mTOR) pathway, which is instrumental in the control of cell growth and metabolism. HHV-8 also encodes a homolog of human interleukin-6 (IL-6), which can bind and activate cytokine receptors and serve as a host cell autocrine growth factor. Additionally, viral proteins are associated with the constitutive expression of the transcription factor nuclear factor-κB (NF-κB). All of these proteins may be potential targets for therapeutic intervention.

CLINICAL MANIFESTATIONS

Although subclinical infection appears to be common, symptomatic primary HHV-8 infection has been described in immunocompetent children. Patients commonly had fever and a maculopapular rash or a mononucleosis-like syndrome, with full recovery the rule.

KS has several different clinical forms; each includes multifocal, angiogenic lesions arising from vascular endothelial cells infected with HHV-8. Classic KS is an indolent disorder seen in elderly men with limited involvement of the skin of the lower extremities. Endemic KS is more aggressive, occurring in children and young people, primarily in Africa, and can include visceral involvement as well as widespread cutaneous lesions (patches, plaques, or nodules). Post-transplantation KS and AIDS-related KS are the most severe forms, with disseminated lesions often in the gastrointestinal tract and lungs in addition to the skin.

Primary effusion–based lymphoma is a rare disease caused by HHV-8 that is seen most commonly in HIV-infected individuals. It consists of lymphomatous invasion of the serosal surfaces of the pleura, pericardium, and peritoneum. Similarly, **multicentric Castleman disease** is an unusual lymphoproliferative disorder characterized by anemia, thrombocytopenia, generalized lymphadenopathy, and constitutional symptoms and frequently associated with HHV-8 infection and a high degree of viral replication.

DIAGNOSIS

Serologic assays, including immunofluorescence, enzyme-linked immunosorbent assay (ELISA), and Western blot, are the primary methods of diagnosing infection with HHV-8. However, testing has limited sensitivity, specificity, and reproducibility and is primarily a research tool. Additionally, the loss of antibodies over time, referred to as *seroreversion,* has been described, further complicating serodiagnosis. Immunohistochemistry and molecular methods are available for the detection of the HHV-8 genome in tissue samples.

TREATMENT

Treatment for KS, PEL, and multicentric Castleman disease is multifaceted and includes attempts to control malignant proliferations with traditional radiotherapy and chemotherapeutic regimens as well as agents aimed at specific cellular pathways targeted by HHV-8 proteins. Therapies such as rapamycin to block the mTOR pathway, proteosome inhibitors aimed at decreasing the activation of NF-κB, and monoclonal antibodies to block the IL-6 receptor or CD20 are under investigation. Additionally, in patients with HIV infection, highly active antiretroviral treatment (HAART) is a mainstay of therapy for the treatment of HHV-8–related disease. Oral valganciclovir decreases both the quantity and frequency of detection of HHV-8 in saliva, suggesting that specific antiviral therapy might also play a role in treatment or prevention of diseases due to HHV-8.

BIBLIOGRAPHY

Please visit the Nelson Textbook of Pediatrics *website at www.expertconsult.com for the complete bibliography.*

Chapter 250
Influenza Viruses

Peter F. Wright

Influenza viral infections cause a broad array of respiratory illnesses that are responsible for significant morbidity and mortality in children on a yearly basis. Influenza viruses have the potential for causing periodic global pandemics with even higher penetrance of illness, as witnessed by the pandemic 2009 novel H1N1 strain.

ETIOLOGY

Influenza viruses are members of the family Orthomyxoviridae. They are large, single-stranded RNA viruses with a segmented genome encased in a lipid-containing envelope. The 2 major surface proteins that determine the serotype of influenza, hemagglutinin (HA) and neuraminidase (NA), project as spikes through the envelope. Influenza viruses are divided into three types: A, B, and C. Influenza virus types A and B are the primary human pathogens and cause epidemic disease. Influenza virus type C is a sporadic cause of predominantly upper respiratory tract disease. Influenza virus types A and B are further divided into serotypically distinct strains that circulate on a yearly basis through the population.

EPIDEMIOLOGY

Influenza A viruses have a complex epidemiology involving avian and mammalian hosts that serve as reservoirs for diverse strains with the potential for infecting the human population. The segmented nature of the influenza genome allows reassortment to occur between an animal virus and a human virus when co-infection occurs. Thus, potentially any of 15 HAs and 9 NAs residing in animal reservoirs may be introduced into humans; these influenza A viruses behave epidemiologically as though they were immunologically distinct serotypes without apparent cross-protection. Minor changes within a serotype are termed *antigenic drift*; major changes in serotype are termed *antigenic shift*. Migratory birds can spread disease, as illustrated by H5N1 avian influenza. The introduction of novel HA strains has occurred in the Far East with H5N1 and H9N2 viruses, in the Netherlands with H7N7 virus, and in Mexico with the 2009 novel swine-origin H1N1 virus.

The highly virulent avian H5N1 influenza virus remains a potential threat to spread more broadly in the human population. By mid 2009, >400 cases had been documented. It has demonstrated major virulence, with mortality consistently >50% in humans in direct contact with infected poultry, although it has not yet acquired the ability to spread readily from person to person.

The novel H1N1 virus emerged in Mexico in the spring of 2009 and circulated widely enough that by June of 2009 it was declared a global pandemic. In the fall of 2009 it circulated throughout the USA, generally producing mild disease but occasionally resulting in death, especially in pregnant women and in patients with underlying disease. Influenza B virus has much less capacity for major antigenic change and no identified animal reservoir.

The worldwide epidemiology of influenza viruses demonstrates annual spread between the Northern and Southern hemispheres, with the origins of new strains often traced to Asia. When a virus identified by a novel and serologically distinct HA or NA enters the population, there is potential for a pandemic of influenza with excess morbidity and mortality on a global scale in a largely nonimmune population. The most dramatic pandemic in recorded history occurred in 1918, when influenza was estimated to have killed >20 million people. More common is the almost yearly variation in the antigenic composition of the surface proteins, conferring a selective advantage to a new strain and resulting in localized epidemics of disease with hospitalization and mortality greatest in infants, the elderly, and patients with underlying cardiopulmonary disease. Each year's strain is novel for infants, because they have no pre-existing antibody except for maternally transferred antibody in the first few months of life.

The attack rate and frequency of isolation of influenza are highest in young children. In a typical year as many as 30-50% of children have serologic evidence of infection. Influenza is marked by increased school absenteeism and a yearly peak in sick visits to the pediatrician. Children undergoing primary exposure to an influenza strain have higher levels and more prolonged shedding of the virus than adults, making the former extremely effective transmitters of infection. Influenza is a disease of the colder months of the year in temperate climates. Spread of influenza appears to occur by small-particle aerosol, and transmission through a community is rapid, with the highest incidence of illness occurring within 2-3 wk of introduction. Influenza has been implicated in hospital spread of infection and may complicate the original illness that required hospitalization.

On a country or global basis, 1 or 2 predominant strains spread to create the annual epidemic. Until 2009, influenza type A strains with the H1N1 and H3N2 serotypes and type B strains were co-circulating, and either type could predominate in a given year, making predictions about the serotype and severity of the upcoming influenza season difficult. It is not clear whether the novel H1N1 strain will alter this pattern.

Strain variants are identified by their HA and NA serotypes, by the geographic area from which they were originally isolated, by their isolate number, and by year of isolation. Thus, the seasonal influenza vaccine for 2009-2010 was trivalent, containing A/Brisbane/59/2007 (H1N1)–like, A/Brisbane/10/2007 (H3N2)–like, and B/Brisbane 60/2008–like antigens.

PATHOGENESIS

Influenza virus attaches to sialic acid residues on cells via the HA and, by endocytosis, makes its way into vacuoles, where with progressive acidification there is fusion to the endosomal membrane and release of the viral RNA into the cytoplasm. The RNA is transported to the nucleus and transcribed. Newly synthesized RNA is returned to the cytoplasm and translated into proteins, which are transported to the cell membrane. Subsequently, viral assembly and budding through the cell membrane take place. In a manner that is not well understood, the packaging usually incorporates the appropriate 10 segments of the genome. A host cell–mediated proteolytic cleavage of the HA occurs at some point in the assembly or release of the virus, which is essential for successful fusion and release from the endosome and amplification of virus titer. In humans, the influenza virus replicative cycle is confined to the respiratory epithelium. With primary infection, virus replication continues for 10-14 days.

Influenza virus causes a lytic infection of the respiratory epithelium with loss of ciliary function, decreased mucus production, and desquamation of the epithelial layer. These changes permit secondary bacterial invasion, either directly through the epithelium or, in the case of the middle ear space, through obstruction of the normal drainage through the eustachian tube. Influenza types A and B have been reported to cause myocarditis, and influenza type B can cause myositis. Reye syndrome can result with the use of salicylates during influenza type B infection (Chapter 353).

The exact immune mechanisms involved in termination of primary infection and protection against re-infection are not well understood but may correspond to the induction of cytokines that inhibit viral replication, such as interferon and tumor necrosis factor. The incubation period of influenza can be as short as 48-72 hr. The extremely short incubation period of influenza and the growth of influenza virus on the mucosal surface pose particular problems for invoking an adaptive immune response. Antigen presentation occurs primarily at mucosal sites acting through the bronchial tract–associated lymphoid tract. The most easily detected humoral response is directed against the HA. High serum antibody levels inhibiting HA activity are generated by inactivated vaccine and correlate with protection. Mucosally produced immunoglobulin A (IgA) antibodies are thought to be the most effective and immediate protective response generated during influenza infection. Unfortunately, detectable IgA antibodies against influenza virus persist for a relatively short period. Because of the short duration of

Table 250-1 RELATIVE FREQUENCY OF SYMPTOMS AND SIGNS DURING CLASSIC INFLUENZA IN OLDER CHILDREN AND ADOLESCENTS

VARIABLE	OCCURRENCE
SYMPTOMS	
Chilly sensation	++++
Cough	+++
Headache	+++
Sore throat	+++
Prostration	++
Nasal stuffiness	++
Diarrhea	++
Dizziness	+
Eye irritation or pain	+
Vomiting	+
Myalgia	+
SIGNS	
Fever	++++
Pharyngitis	+++
Conjunctivitis (mild)	++
Rhinitis	++
Cervical lymphadenopathy	+
Pulmonary rales, wheezes, or rhonchi	+

++++, 76-100%; +++, 51-75%; ++, 26-50%; +, 1-25%.

appreciable IgA as well as strain variation, symptomatic re-infection with influenza virus can be seen at intervals of 3-4 yr. Although heterotypic immunity can be demonstrated in the mouse through cell-mediated immune mechanisms directed toward common internal proteins, heterotypic immunity has been more difficult to show in humans.

CLINICAL MANIFESTATIONS

Influenza types A and B cause predominantly respiratory illness. The onset of illness is abrupt and is dominated by fever, myalgias, chills, headache, malaise, and anorexia; coryza, pharyngitis, and dry cough are associated features overshadowed by the other systemic signs (Table 250-1). The predominant symptoms may localize anywhere in the respiratory tract, producing an isolated upper respiratory tract illness, croup, bronchiolitis, or pneumonia. More than any other respiratory virus, influenza virus causes systemic signs such as high temperature, myalgia, malaise, and headache. Many of these signs and symptoms may be mediated through cytokine production by the respiratory tract epithelium, because there is no systemic spread of the virus. The typical duration of the febrile illness is 2-4 days. Cough may persist for longer periods, and evidence of small airway dysfunction is often found weeks later.

Owing to the high transmissibility of influenza, other family members or close contacts of an infected person often experience a similar illness. Influenza is a less distinct illness in younger children and infants. The infected young infant or child may be highly febrile and toxic in appearance, prompting a full diagnostic work-up. Despite some distinctive features of influenza, the illness it causes is often indistinguishable from that caused by other respiratory viruses, such as respiratory syncytial virus, parainfluenza virus, and adenovirus.

LABORATORY FINDINGS

The clinical laboratory abnormalities associated with influenza are nonspecific. Relative leukopenia is frequently seen. Chest radiographs show evidence of atelectasis or infiltrate in about 10% of children.

Table 250-2 ANTIVIRAL MEDICATION DOSING RECOMMENDATIONS FOR TREATMENT OR CHEMOPROPHYLAXIS OF 2009 H1N1 INFECTION*

MEDICATION	TREATMENT (5 DAYS)	CHEMOPROPHYLAXIS (10 DAYS)
OSELTAMIVIR		
Adults	75-mg capsule twice per day	75-mg capsule once per day
Children ≥ 12 months:		
≤15 kg (≤33 lbs)	30 mg twice daily	30 mg once per day
>15-23 kg (>33-51 lbs)	45 mg twice daily	45 mg once per day
>23-40 kg (>51-88 lbs)	60 mg twice daily	60 mg once per day
>40 kg (>88 lbs)	75 mg twice daily	75 mg once per day
ZANAMIVIR		
Adults	10 mg (two 5-mg inhalations) twice daily	10 mg (two 5-mg inhalations) once daily
Children (≥7 yr or older for treatment, ≥5 yr for chemoprophylaxis)	10 mg (two 5-mg inhalations) twice daily	10 mg (two 5-mg inhalations) once daily

*Published as Updated interim recommendations for the use of antiviral medications in the treatment and prevention of influenza for the 2009-2010 season October 16, 2009; available at www.cdc.gov/h1n1flu/recommendations.htm. For current details, consult annually updated recommendations from the Advisory Committee on Immunization Practices of the Centers for Disease Control and Prevention, at www.cdc.gov/flu/.

DIAGNOSIS AND DIFFERENTIAL DIAGNOSIS

The diagnosis of influenza depends on epidemiologic, clinical, and laboratory considerations. In the context of an epidemic, the clinical diagnosis of influenza in a young child who has fever without a focus, malaise, and respiratory symptoms can be made with some certainty. The laboratory confirmation of influenza can be made in the following 4 ways:

- If seen early in the illness, virus can be isolated from the nasopharynx by inoculation of the specimen into embryonated eggs or selective cell lines that support the growth of influenza. The presence of influenza in the culture is confirmed by hemadsorption, which depends on the capacity of the HA to bind red cells.
- Reliable diagnostic tests for influenza types A and B are available that use variations of polymerase chain reaction viral genome detection technology.
- Rapid virus detection can be achieved by direct fluorescence on exfoliated cells or antigen capture in an enzyme-linked immunosorbent assay.
- The diagnosis can be confirmed serologically with use of acute and convalescent sera collected around the time of the illness and tested by hemagglutination inhibition.

TREATMENT

Two classes of antiviral drugs may be effective in the treatment of influenza. Guidelines for the use of the neuraminidase inhibitors zanamivir and oseltamivir against the novel H1N1 virus include use for children from the ages of 7 yr and 1 yr, respectively (Table 250-2). These drugs are given either as an inhalation (zanamivir) or orally (oseltamivir). Their effectiveness can be strain specific, as exemplified by the current seasonal H1N1 virus, which is resistant to oseltamivir but sensitive to zanamivir. Oseltamivir is not approved for use in children younger than 1 yr. Limited safety data on oseltamivir treatment of seasonal influenza in children younger than 1 yr suggest that severe adverse events are rare. Oseltamivir is authorized for emergency use in children younger than 1 yr by the U.S. Food and Drug Administration (Table 250-3).

The 2nd class of drugs includes amantadine and rimantadine, which can be used in influenza type A outbreaks. These 2

Table 250-3 OSELTAMIVIR DOSING RECOMMENDATIONS FOR ANTIVIRAL TREATMENT OR CHEMOPROPHYLAXIS IN CHILDREN <1 YR*

AGE	RECOMMENDED TREATMENT DOSE FOR 5 DAYS	RECOMMENDED PROPHYLAXIS DOSE FOR 10 DAYS
<3 mo	12 mg twice daily	Not recommended unless situation judged critical, because of limited data on use in this age group
3-5 mo	20 mg twice daily	20 mg once daily
6-11 mo	25 mg twice daily	25 mg once daily

*Published as Updated interim recommendations for the use of antiviral medications in the treatment and prevention of influenza for the 2009-2010 season October 16, 2009; available at www.cdc.gov/h1n1flu/recommendations.htm. For current details, consult annually updated recommendations from the Advisory Committee on Immunization Practices of the Centers for Disease Control and Prevention, at www.cdc.gov/flu/.

antivirals are not effective against influenza type B strains and are not approved for use in children <1 yr of age. The H5 avian influenza virus is often resistant to amantadine and rimantadine. The novel H1N1 strain and the current seasonal H3N2 viruses are also resistant. It is important to review annual recommendations and updates published by the Centers for Disease Control and Prevention (CDC) before prescribing influenza antivirals.

Each class of drug must be given within the 1st 48 hr of symptoms to decrease the severity and duration of influenza. Confusion and inability to concentrate or sleep are seen in some patients given amantadine. Drug resistance can develop fairly quickly during a course of amantadine or rimantadine therapy. All of these drugs are only an adjunct to a strong vaccination program. The family setting and schoolroom may be appropriate places to try to prevent secondary illness by drug treatment, particularly when exposed individuals have underlying conditions that predispose them to severe or complicated influenza infection.

SUPPORTIVE CARE

Adequate fluid intake and rest are important components in the management of influenza. Acetaminophen or ibuprofen (but not salicylates because of the risk for Reye syndrome; Chapter 353) should be used as antipyretics to control fever. The most difficult question for parents is the appropriate timing of consultation with a health care provider. Bacterial superinfections are relatively common, and when they occur, antibiotic therapy should be administered. Bacterial superinfections should be suspected with recrudescence of fever, prolonged fever, or deterioration in clinical status. With uncomplicated influenza, children should feel better after the 1st 48-72 hr of symptoms.

COMPLICATIONS

Otitis media and pneumonia are common complications of influenza in young children. Acute otitis media may be seen in up to 25% of cases of documented influenza. Pneumonia accompanying influenza may be a primary viral process. An acute hemorrhagic pneumonia may be seen in the most severe cases, as was frequent with the highly virulent strain seen in 1918 and as has been seen in patients with the current H5 avian influenza. The more common cause of pneumonia is probably secondary bacterial infection through the damaged epithelial layer. Unusual clinical manifestations of influenza include acute myositis seen with influenza type B, which follows the acute respiratory illness by 5-7 days and is marked by muscle weakness and pain, particularly in the calf muscles, and myoglobinuria. Myocarditis also follows influenza, and toxic shock syndrome can be associated with toxin-producing staphylococcal colonization. Influenza is particularly severe in children with underlying cardiopulmonary disease, including congenital and acquired valvular disease, cardiomyopathy, bronchopulmonary dysplasia, asthma, cystic fibrosis, and neuromuscular diseases affecting the accessory muscles of breathing. Pregnant women are at special risk for severe influenza. Virus is shed for longer periods in children receiving cancer chemotherapy and children with immunodeficiency.

Table 250-4 SUMMARY OF SEASONAL INFLUENZA VACCINATION RECOMMENDATIONS, 2009: CHILDREN AND ADOLESCENTS AGED 6 MO-18 YR*

All children aged 6 mo-18 yr should be vaccinated annually.

Children and adolescents at higher risk for influenza complications should continue to be a focus of vaccination efforts as providers and programs transition to routinely vaccinating all children and adolescents, including those who:
- Are aged 6 mo–4 yr (59 mo)
- Have chronic pulmonary (including asthma), cardiovascular (except hypertension), renal, hepatic, cognitive, neurologic/neuromuscular, hematologic, or metabolic disorders (including diabetes mellitus)
- Are immunosuppressed (including immunosuppression caused by medications or by human immunodeficiency virus)
- Are receiving long-term aspirin therapy and therefore might be at risk for experiencing Reye syndrome after influenza virus infection
- Are residents of long-term care facilities
- Will be pregnant during the influenza season.

*Children aged <6 mo cannot receive influenza vaccination. Household and other close contacts (e.g., daycare providers) of children aged <6 mo, including older children and adolescents, should be vaccinated.

PROGNOSIS

The prognosis for recovery from influenza is excellent, although full return to normal levels of activity and freedom from cough usually require weeks rather than days.

PREVENTION

Influenza vaccination of targeted populations is the best means of preventing severe disease due to influenza. Recommendations for use of influenza vaccine have become progressively broader as the impact of influenza is appreciated in such groups as pregnant women and young children. Chemoprophylaxis with the drugs discussed in the treatment section is a secondary means of prevention.

Vaccines

Inactivated and live-attenuated seasonal influenza vaccines with H3, H1, and B strains become available each summer, their formulations having incorporated changes to reflect the strains anticipated to circulate in the coming winter. The Advisory Committee on Immunization Practices publishes guidelines for their use each year when the vaccines are formulated and released. These guidelines are widely publicized but appear initially in the *Morbidity and Mortality Weekly Report* published by the CDC. Anyone who wants to reduce his or her chances of acquiring influenza can be vaccinated. It is recommended that all children are at special risk of influenza receive vaccination (Table 250-4). Nevertheless, certain high-risk groups should be prioritized, particularly when vaccine is in short supply or is made late in the year in response to an emerging epidemic. Guidelines are sufficiently complicated and differ enough from year to year that only the following broad recommendations can be given:

- In addition to the universal recommendation for pediatric patients older than 6 mo, household contacts and out-of-home caregivers of children 0-6 mo of age are a targeted group.
- Because of the decreased potential for causing febrile reactions, only split-virus vaccines are recommended for children <12 yr of age.

- Two doses of vaccine (0.25 mL for 6-36 mo of age; 0.5 mL for 3-8 yr of age) at least 1 mo apart are recommended for primary immunization of children <9 yr of age.
- Live-attenuated vaccines that are administered intranasally are not recommended for children <2 yr of age or for children 2-4 yr old who have asthma. Trials in children have consistently shown a very high efficacy, in the range of 90%. Ease of administration, response to a single dose, and high efficacy of these vaccines could serve to increase effective influenza vaccination among children.

CHEMOPROPHYLAXIS

Amantadine, oseltamivir, and zanamivir are licensed for prophylaxis of influenza A infections (see Table 250-2). These agents are recommended as a 10-day course for prophylaxis for vaccinated and unvaccinated high-risk patients and their unvaccinated health care providers during influenza A outbreaks in closed settings, for unvaccinated persons and health care providers during community influenza A outbreaks, and for immunodeficient persons and those for whom the influenza vaccine is contraindicated during the period of peak influenza A activity.

BIBLIOGRAPHY

Please visit the Nelson Textbook of Pediatrics *website at www.expertconsult.com for the complete bibliography.*

Chapter 251
Parainfluenza Viruses

Angela Jean Peck Campbell and Peter F. Wright

Parainfluenza viruses (PIVs) are common causes of respiratory illness in infants and children and are second only to respiratory syncytial virus as an important viral cause of lower respiratory tract infections in young children and immunocompromised patients. These viruses cause a spectrum of upper and lower respiratory tract illnesses but are particularly associated with croup (laryngotracheitis or laryngotracheobronchitis), bronchiolitis, and pneumonia.

ETIOLOGY

The PIVs are members of the Paramyxoviridae family. Four PIVs cause illness in humans, classified as types 1-4, with diverse manifestations of infection. Type 4 is divided into 2 antigenic subgroups, A and B. PIVs have a nonsegmented, single-stranded RNA genome with a lipid-containing envelope derived from budding through the cell membrane. The major antigenic moieties are the HN and F envelope spike glycoproteins, which exhibit hemagglutinin-neuraminidase and fusion functions, respectively.

EPIDEMIOLOGY

By 5 yr of age, most children have experienced primary infection with PIV types 1, 2, and 3 (Table 251-1). PIV-3 infections often occur in the first 6 mo of life, whereas PIV-1 and PIV-2 are more common after infancy. In the USA and temperate climates, PIV-1 and PIV-2 have biennial epidemics in the fall, usually alternating years in which their serotype is most prevalent. PIV-3 is endemic throughout the year but typically peaks in late spring. In years with less PIV-1 activity, the PIV-3 season may extend longer or have a second peak in the fall. The epidemiology of PIV-4 is less well defined, because it is difficult to grow in tissue culture and was often excluded from early studies.

PIVs are spread primarily from the respiratory tract by inhalation of large respiratory droplets or contact with infected secretions. PIVs are notable for causing outbreaks of respiratory infections in hospital wards, clinics, neonatal nurseries, and other institutional settings. The incubation period from exposure to symptom onset is 2-6 days. Children are likely to excrete virus from the oropharynx for 2-3 wk, but excretion can be more prolonged even in immunocompetent children; in immunocompromised patients, excretion may persist for months. Primary infection does not confer permanent immunity, and re-infections are common throughout life. Re-infections are generally mild and self limited.

PATHOGENESIS

PIVs replicate in the respiratory epithelium. The propensity to cause illness in the upper large airways is presumably related to preferential replication in the larynx, trachea, and bronchi in comparison with other viruses. Some PIVs induce cell-to-cell fusion. During the budding process, cell membrane integrity is lost, and viruses can induce cell death through the process of apoptosis. In children, the most severe illness coincides with the time of maximal viral shedding. However, disease severity is likely related to the inflammatory response as much as to direct cytopathic effects of the virus.

Table 251-1 CHARACTERISTICS OF PARAINFLUENZA VIRUS (PIV) INFECTIONS IN CHILDREN

	PIV-1	PIV-2	PIV-3	PIV-4
Seasonality	Biennial epidemics in fall, often alternating with PIV-2	Annual epidemics in fall, often alternating with PIV-1	Endemic throughout year, peaks in spring (higher activity when less PIV-1 circulating)	Insufficient data
Age groups	≈75% infected by age 5 yr, peak incidence age 2-3 yr	≈60% infected by age 5 yr, peak incidence age 1-2 yr	90-100% infected by age 5 yr, ≈50% by age 1 yr; children <6 mo at high risk	≈50% infec yr
Clinical syndromes (manifestations of virus types, relative to one another):				
Common cold	+++	+++	+++	+++
Acute otitis media	++	++	+++	+
Croup	++++	+++	++	+
Bronchiolitis	++	++	++++	+
Pneumonia	++	++	++++	+
Diagnostic methods (reliability of method for diagnosis):				
Culture	++	++	++	Not reliable
Rapid detection/immunofluorescence	++	++	+++	+
Polymerase chain reaction	++++	++++	++++	++++

++++, 76-100%; +++, 51-75%; ++, 26-50%; +, 1-25%.

Virus-specific immunoglobulin (Ig) A antibody levels correlate with protection from PIV infection. Circulating serum antibody is also likely to play a role in protection against PIV acquisition and progression to severe infection. Patients with compromised cellular immunity have severe, prolonged disease, suggesting that T cells are critical to controlling and terminating PIV infection.

CLINICAL MANIFESTATIONS

Most PIV infections manifest themselves primarily in the upper respiratory tract (see Table 251-1). The most common types of illness consist of some combination of low-grade fever, rhinorrhea, cough, pharyngitis, and hoarseness and may be associated with vomiting or diarrhea. Rarely, PIV infection has been associated with parotitis. The illnesses usually last 4-5 days. The generally mild illness pattern is belied by a spectrum of rarer but more serious illnesses that result in hospitalization. PIVs account for 50% of hospitalizations for croup and at least 15% of cases of bronchiolitis and pneumonia. PIV-1 and to a lesser extent PIV-2 cause more cases of croup, whereas PIV-3 is more likely to infect the small air passages and cause pneumonia, bronchiolitis, or bronchitis. Any PIV can cause lower respiratory tract disease, particularly during primary infection or in immunosuppressed patients.

LABORATORY FINDINGS

Conventional laboratory diagnosis of infection is accomplished by PIV isolation in tissue culture. Direct immunofluorescent (IF) staining is available in some centers for rapid identification of virus antigen in respiratory secretions. Many laboratories perform polymerase chain reaction (PCR) viral genomic testing, which greatly increases sensitivity of PIV detection (see Table 251-1). For viral culture or IF, a nasal wash or aspirate provides the best sample, but for PCR, nasal swabs are also appropriate.

DIAGNOSIS AND DIFFERENTIAL DIAGNOSIS

The diagnosis of PIV infection in children is often based only on clinical and epidemiologic criteria. Croup is a clinical diagnosis and must be distinguished from foreign body aspiration, epiglottitis, pharyngeal abscess, and subglottic hemangioma. Although the radiographic "steeple sign," consisting of progressive narrowing of the subglottic region, is characteristic of croup, differential considerations include acute epiglottitis, thermal injury, angioedema, and bacterial tracheitis. Manifestation of PIV lower respiratory tract disease may be similar to that of a number of other respiratory viral infections; therefore, identification of virus should be specifically sought by the most sensitive diagnostic means available for certain severe illnesses, such as pneumonia in immunocompromised children.

TREATMENT

There are no approved treatments for PIV infections with the exception of croup. For croup, the possibility of rapid respiratory compromise should influence the acuity of care given (Chapter 377). Humidified air has not been shown to be effective. Generally a single dose of oral, intramuscular, or intravenous dexamethasone (0.6 mg/kg) should be part of the management of croup in the office or emergency room setting. This dose may be repeated, but there are no guidelines to compare outcomes of single- and multiple-dose treatment schedules. Nebulized epinephrine (either racemic epinephrine 2.25%, 0.5 mL in 2.5 mL of saline, or L-epinephrine, 1:1000 dilution in 5 mL of saline) may also provide temporary symptomatic improvement. Children should be observed for at least 2 hr after receiving epinephrine treatment for return of obstructive symptoms. Repeated treatments may obviate the need for intubation. Oxygen should be administered for hypoxia, and supportive care with analgesics and antipyretics is reasonable for fever and discomfort associated with PIV infections. The indications for antibiotics are limited to well-documented secondary bacterial infections of the middle ear(s) or lower respiratory tract.

Ribavirin has some antiviral activity against PIVs in vitro and in animal models. Inhaled ribavirin should be considered for severely immunocompromised children with PIV pneumonia. Promising strategies for drug development include hemagglutinin-neuraminidase inhibitors and synthetic small interfering RNAs.

COMPLICATIONS

Eustachian tube obstruction can lead to secondary bacterial invasion of the middle ear space and acute otitis media in 30-50% of PIV infections. Similarly, obstruction of the paranasal sinuses can lead to sinusitis. The destruction of cells in the upper airways can lead to secondary bacterial invasion and resultant bacterial tracheitis, and antecedent PIV infection of lower airways may predispose to bacterial pneumonia. Non-respiratory complications of PIV are rare but include aseptic meningitis, encephalitis, acute disseminated encephalomyelitis, rhabdomyolysis, myocarditis, and pericarditis.

PROGNOSIS

The prognosis for full recovery from PIV infection in the normal child is excellent, with no long-term pulmonary sequelae.

PREVENTION

Vaccine development is focused on live intranasal PIV-3 vaccines. The candidates include a cold-adapted virus of human origin, an attenuated bovine PIV-3, and a newer construct using the bovine PIV-3 vaccine with insertion of human PIV-3 HN and F genes and the F protein of respiratory syncytial virus. The measure of protection afforded by vaccines will be difficult to assess, because symptomatic re-infection is seen and the frequency of serious infection in the general population is low. Nonetheless, it is clear that prevention of acute respiratory illness caused by PIVs, particularly lower respiratory tract infections among infants and young children, is a worthwhile goal.

BIBLIOGRAPHY

Please visit the Nelson Textbook of Pediatrics *website at www.expertconsult.com for the complete bibliography.*

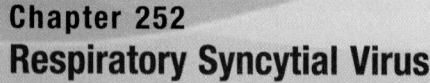

Chapter 252
Respiratory Syncytial Virus

James E. Crowe, Jr.

Respiratory syncytial virus (RSV) is the major cause of bronchiolitis (Chapter 383) and viral pneumonia in children <1 yr of age and is the most important respiratory tract pathogen of early childhood.

ETIOLOGY

RSV is an enveloped RNA virus with a single-stranded negative-sense genome that replicates entirely in the cytoplasm of infected cells and matures by budding from the apical surface of the cell membrane. Because this virus has a nonsegmented genome, it cannot undergo antigenic shift by reassortment like the influenza viruses do. The virus belongs to the family Paramyxoviridae, along with parainfluenza and measles viruses, and is in the subfamily Pneumovirinae, which also contains the human metapneumovirus (Chapter 253). It is the only member of the genus *Pneumovirus* that infects humans. There are 2 antigenic subgroups of RSV, their differentiation based primarily on variation in 1 of the 2 surface proteins, the G glycoprotein that is responsible for attachment. This antigenic variation caused by point mutations due to infidelity of the virus RNA polymerase may to some degree contribute to the frequency with which RSV re-infects children and adults.

RSV replicates in a wide variety of cell line monolayer cultures in vitro, and in HeLa or HEp-2 cells produces characteristic syncytial cytopathology, from which the virus derives its name. Interestingly, it is now known that the virus does not cause large syncytia in polarized epithelial cells in vitro, and it is not clear that syncytium formation occurs to any significant degree in vivo.

EPIDEMIOLOGY

RSV is distributed worldwide and appears in yearly epidemics. In temperate climates, these epidemics occur each winter over 4-5 mo. During the remainder of the year, infections are sporadic and much less common. In the Northern hemisphere, epidemics usually peak in January, February, or March, but peaks have been recognized as early as December and as late as June. Some areas in the USA, such as Florida, report a moderate incidence year-round. In the Southern hemisphere, outbreaks also occur during winter months in that hemisphere. RSV outbreaks often overlap with outbreaks of influenza and human metapneumovirus but are generally more consistent from year to year and result in more disease overall, especially among infants <6 mo of age. In the tropics, the epidemic pattern is less clear. This pattern of widespread annual outbreaks and the high incidence of infection during the 1st 3-4 mo of life are unique among human viruses.

Transplacentally acquired anti-RSV maternal immunoglobulin (Ig) G serum antibodies, if present in high concentration, appear to provide partial but incomplete protection. These IgGs may account for the lower severity of RSV infections during the 1st 4-6 wk of life, except among infants born prematurely, who receive less maternal immunoglobulin. Breast-feeding provides substantial protection against severe disease to female infants but not to male infants. RSV is one of the most contagious viruses that affect humans. Infection is nearly universal among children by their 2nd birthdays. Re-infection occurs at a rate of 10-20% per epidemic throughout childhood, with a lower frequency among adults. In situations of high exposure, such as daycare centers, attack rates are nearly 100% among previously uninfected infants and 60-80% for 2nd and subsequent infections.

Re-infection may occur as early as a few weeks after recovery but usually takes place during subsequent annual outbreaks. Antigenic variation is not required for re-infection, as shown by the fact that a proportion of adults inoculated repeatedly with the same experimental preparation of wild-type virus can be re-infected multiple times. The immune response of infants is poor in quality, magnitude, and durability. The severity of illness during re-infection in childhood is usually lower and appears to be a function of both partial immunity and increased age.

Asymptomatic RSV infection is rare in young children. Most infants experience coryza and pharyngitis, often with fever and frequently with otitis media due to virus in the middle ear or bacterial superinfection following eustachian tube dysfunction. The lower respiratory tract is involved to a varying degree with bronchiolitis and bronchopneumonia in about a third of children. The hospitalization rate for RSV infection in otherwise healthy infants is typically 0.5-4%, depending on region, gender, socioeconomic status, exposure to cigarette smoke, gestational age, and family history of atopy. The admitting diagnosis is usually bronchiolitis with hypoxia, although this condition is often indistinguishable from RSV pneumonia in infants, and, indeed, the 2 processes frequently coexist. All RSV diseases of the lower respiratory tract (excluding croup) have their highest incidence at 6 wk-7 mo of age and decrease in frequency thereafter. The syndrome of bronchiolitis is much less common after the 1st birthday. The terminology used for diagnosis of virus-associated wheezing illnesses in toddlers is confusing, as these illnesses are variably termed wheezing associated respiratory infection (WARI), "wheezy bronchitis," exacerbation of reactive airways disease, or asthma attack. Because many toddlers wheeze during RSV infection but do not go on to have lifelong asthma, it is best to use this diagnostic term only later in life. Viral pneumonia is a persistent problem throughout childhood, although RSV becomes less prominent as the etiologic agent after the 1st year. RSV plays a causative role in an estimated 40-75% of cases of hospitalized bronchiolitis, 15-40% of cases of childhood pneumonia, and 6-15% of cases of croup.

Bronchiolitis and pneumonia resulting from RSV are more common in boys than in girls by a ratio of about 1.5:1. Other risk factors with similar impact include ≥1 sibling in the home, white race, rural residence, maternal smoking, and maternal education <12 yr. The medical factors in infants associated with highest risk are bronchopulmonary dysplasia, congenital heart disease, immunodeficiency, and prematurity. Still, most infants admitted to hospital because of RSV infection do not have strong easily identifiable risk factors. Therefore, any strategy for prophylaxis only of individuals with strong risk factors probably could prevent only about 10% of hospitalizations, even if it was 100% effective in treated high-risk individuals.

The incubation period from exposure to 1st symptoms is about 3-5 days. The virus is excreted for variable periods, probably depending on severity of illness and immunologic status. Most infants with lower respiratory tract illness shed infectious virus for 1-2 wk after hospital admission. Excretion for 3 wk and even longer has been documented. Spread of infection occurs when large, infected droplets, either airborne or conveyed on hands or other fomites, are inoculated in the nasopharynx of a susceptible subject. RSV is probably introduced into most families by young schoolchildren undergoing re-infection. Typically, in the space of a few days, 25-50% of older siblings and one or both parents acquire upper respiratory tract infections, but infants becomes more severely ill with fever, otitis media, or lower respiratory tract disease.

Nosocomial infection during RSV epidemics is an important concern. Virus is usually spread from child to child on the hands of caregivers. Adults undergoing re-infection also have been implicated in spread of the virus. Contact precautions are sufficient to prevent spread when compliance is meticulous, as the virus is not usually spread by small particle aerosol. Adherence to isolation procedures by caregivers often is not complete, however.

PATHOGENESIS

Bronchiolitis is caused by obstruction and collapse of the small airways during expiration. Infants are particularly apt to experience small airway obstruction because of the small size of their normal bronchioles; airway resistance is proportional to $1/\text{radius}^4$. There has been relatively little pathologic examination of RSV disease in the lower airways of otherwise healthy subjects. Airway narrowing likely is caused by virus-induced necrosis of the bronchiolar epithelium, hypersecretion of mucus, and round cell infiltration and edema of the surrounding submucosa. These changes result in formation of mucus plugs obstructing bronchioles, with consequent hyperinflation or collapse of the distal lung tissue. In interstitial pneumonia, the infiltration is more generalized, and epithelial shedding may extend to both the bronchi and the alveoli. In older subjects, smooth muscle hyperreactivity may contribute to airway narrowing, but the airways of young infants typically do not exhibit a high degree of reversible smooth muscle hyperreactivity during RSV infection.

Several facts suggest that elements of the host response may cause inflammation and contribute to tissue damage. The immune response required to eliminate virus-infected cells is a double-edged sword, reducing the cells producing virus but causing host cell death in the process. A large number of soluble factors, such as cytokines, chemokines, and leukotrienes, are released in the process, and skewing of the patterns of these responses may predispose some individuals to more severe disease. There is also evidence that genetic factors may predispose to more severe bronchiolitis.

Children who received a formalin-inactivated, parenterally administered RSV vaccine in the 1960s experienced more severe and more frequent bronchiolitis upon subsequent natural exposure to wild-type RSV than did their age-matched controls. Several children died during naturally acquired RSV infection after vaccination. This event has greatly inhibited progress in RSV vaccine development, because of both an incomplete understanding of the mechanism and a reluctance to test new experimental vaccines that might induce the same type of response.

Some studies have identified the presence of both RSV and human metapneumovirus viral RNA in airway secretions in a significant proportion of infants requiring assisted ventilation and intensive care. It may be that **co-infection** is associated with more severe disease; positive results of polymerase chain reaction (PCR) analysis must be interpreted carefully because this positivity can remain for prolonged periods after infection, even when infectious virus is no longer detectable.

It is not clear how often superimposed bacterial infection plays a pathogenic role in RSV lower respiratory tract disease. RSV bronchiolitis in infants is probably exclusively a viral disease, although there is evidence that bacterial pneumonia can be triggered by respiratory viral infection, including with RSV. A large clinical study of pneumococcal vaccine showed that childhood vaccination reduced the incidence of viral pneumonia by about 30%, suggesting viral-bacterial interactions that we currently do not fully understand.

CLINICAL MANIFESTATIONS

Typically, the first sign of infection in infants with RSV is rhinorrhea. Cough may appear simultaneously but more often does so after an interval of 1-3 days, at which time there may also be sneezing and a low-grade fever. Soon after the cough develops, the child who experiences bronchiolitis begins to wheeze audibly. If the disease is mild, the symptoms may not progress beyond this stage. Auscultation often reveals diffuse fine inspiratory crackles and expiratory wheezes. Rhinorrhea usually persists throughout the illness, with intermittent fever. Chest radiograph findings at this stage are frequently normal.

If the illness progresses, cough and wheezing worsen and air hunger ensues, with increased respiratory rate, intercostal and subcostal retractions, hyperexpansion of the chest, restlessness, and peripheral cyanosis. Signs of severe, life-threatening illness are central cyanosis, tachypnea of >70 breaths/min, listlessness, and apneic spells. At this stage, the chest may be significantly hyperexpanded and almost silent to auscultation because of poor air movement.

Chest radiographs of infants hospitalized with RSV bronchiolitis have normal findings in about 30% of cases, with the other 70% showing hyperexpansion of the chest, peribronchial thickening, and interstitial infiltrates. Segmental or lobar consolidation is unusual and pleural effusion is rare.

In some infants, the course of the illness may resemble that of pneumonia, the prodromal rhinorrhea and cough being followed by dyspnea, poor feeding, and listlessness, with a minimum of wheezing and hyperexpansion. Although the clinical diagnosis is pneumonia, wheezing is often present intermittently and the chest radiographs may show air trapping.

Fever is an inconstant sign in RSV infection. In young infants, particularly those who were born prematurely, periodic breathing and apneic spells have been distressingly frequent signs, even with relatively mild bronchiolitis. Apnea is not necessarily caused by respiratory exhaustion, but rather appears to be a consequence of alterations in central control of breathing.

RSV infections in profoundly immunocompromised hosts may be severe at any age of life. The mortality associated with RSV pneumonia in the first few weeks after hematopoietic stem cell or solid organ transplantation in both children and adults is high. RSV infection does not seem to be more severe in HIV-infected patients with reasonable control of HIV disease, although these patients may shed virus for prolonged periods.

DIAGNOSIS

Bronchiolitis is a clinical diagnosis. RSV can be suspected with varying degrees of certainty on the basis of the season of the year and the presence of the virus in the community. Other epidemiologic features that may be helpful are the presence of colds in older household contacts and the age of the child. The other respiratory viruses that attack infants frequently during the first few months of life are parainfluenza virus type 3, human metapneumovirus, and influenza. Rhinovirus is frequently found in the respiratory tract of children, and there is growing evidence that this virus may contribute to lower respiratory tract disease.

Routine laboratory tests are of minimal diagnostic use in most cases of bronchiolitis or pneumonia caused by RSV. The white blood cell count is normal or elevated, and the differential cell count may be normal with either a neutrophilic or mononuclear predominance. Hypoxemia as measured by pulse oximetry or arterial blood gas analysis is frequent and tends to be more marked than anticipated from the clinical findings. A normal or elevated blood CO_2 value in a patient with a markedly elevated respiratory rate is a sign of respiratory failure.

The most important diagnostic concern is to identify bacterial or chlamydial involvement. When bronchiolitis is not accompanied by infiltrates on chest radiographs, there is little likelihood of a bacterial component. In infants 1-4 mo of age, interstitial pneumonitis may be caused by *Chlamydia trachomatis* (Chapter 218). With *C. trachomatis* pneumonia there may be a history of conjunctivitis, and the illness tends to be of subacute onset. Coughing and inspiratory crackles may be prominent; wheezing is not. Fever is usually absent.

Lobar consolidation without other signs or with pleural effusion should be considered of bacterial etiology until proved otherwise. Other signs suggesting bacterial pneumonia are neutrophilia, neutropenia in the presence of severe disease, ileus or other abdominal signs, high temperature, and circulatory collapse. In such instances, antibiotics should be initiated.

Definitive diagnosis of RSV infection is based on the detection in respiratory secretions of live virus by cell culture. The presence of viral RNA (detected by a molecular diagnostic test using reverse transcription PCR [RT-PCR]) or viral antigens (detected by a rapid diagnostic test, usually a membrane blotting test incorporating antibody detection of viral proteins) is strongly supportive in the right clinical setting. The antigen test is less sensitive than culture, and RT-PCR analysis is more sensitive. An aspirate of mucus or a nasopharyngeal wash from the child's posterior nasal cavity is the optimal specimen. Nasopharyngeal or throat swabs are less preferable but acceptable. A tracheal aspirate is unnecessary, but endotracheal tube lavage fluid from patients intubated for mechanical ventilation can be tested. The specimen should be placed on ice, taken directly to the laboratory, and processed immediately for culture, antigen detection, or PCR analysis.

TREATMENT

The treatment of uncomplicated cases of bronchiolitis is symptomatic. Humidified oxygen and suctioning are usually indicated for hospitalized infants who are hypoxic. Many infants are slightly to moderately dehydrated, and therefore fluids should be carefully administered in amounts somewhat greater than those for maintenance. Often intravenous or tube feeding is helpful when sucking is difficult because of tachypnea.

There is disagreement among experts regarding the usefulness of epinephrine or β_2-agonists in RSV bronchiolitis. Most patients do not receive lasting benefit from prolonged therapy, which is associated with a relatively high frequency of side effects. Corticosteroid therapy is not indicated except in older children with an established diagnosis of asthma, because its use is associated with prolonged virus shedding and is of no proven clinical benefit.

In nearly all instances of bronchiolitis, antibiotics are not useful, and their inappropriate use contributes to development of antibiotic resistance. Interstitial pneumonia in infants 1-4 mo old may be caused by *C. trachomatis,* and macrolide therapy may be indicated for that infection.

Ribavirin is an antiviral agent delivered through an oxygen hood, face mask, or endotracheal tube with use of a small particle aerosol generator most of the day for 3-5 days. Early small trials of its use suggested a modest beneficial effect on the course of RSV pneumonia, with some reduction in the duration of both mechanical ventilation and hospitalization. Subsequent studies failed to document a clear beneficial effect of ribavirin. Most medical centers do not use ribavirin currently for RSV infection. The monoclonal antibody palivizumab is licensed for prophylaxis in high-risk infants, but small clinical trials using the antibody as a therapy during established infection have not shown benefit to date.

PROGNOSIS

The mortality rate of hospitalized infants with RSV infection of the lower respiratory tract is low in the developed world. Almost all deaths occur among young, premature infants or infants with underlying disease of the neuromuscular, pulmonary, cardiovascular, or immunologic system. It is estimated, however, that hundreds of thousands of children worldwide in resource-poor settings die each year from RSV.

Many children with asthma have a history of bronchiolitis in infancy. There is recurrent wheezing in 30-50% of children with severe RSV bronchiolitis in infancy. The likelihood of recurrence is increased in the presence of an allergic diathesis (e.g., eczema, hay fever, or a family history of asthma). With a clinical presentation of bronchiolitis in a patient >1 yr of age, there is an increasing probability that, although the episode may be virus induced, this is likely the first of multiple wheezing attacks that will later be diagnosed as hyperreactive airways disease or asthma. Asthma is difficult to diagnose in the first years of life. It is not clear at this time whether early, severe RSV wheezing disease causes some cases of asthma or whether subjects destined to suffer asthma present with symptoms first when provoked by RSV infection during infancy.

PREVENTION

In the hospital, the most important preventive measures are aimed at blocking nosocomial spread. During RSV season, high-risk infants should be separated from all infants with respiratory symptoms. Gowns, gloves, and careful handwashing should be used for the care of all infants with suspected or established RSV infection. A high level of compliance with contact isolation is essential. Viral laboratory tests are adequate for diagnosis in the setting of acute disease, but they are not designed to detect low levels of virus. Therefore, contact precaution isolation should be observed for most patients admitted for acute disease assigned for the duration of hospitalization; rapid antigen tests should not be used to determine whether or not a patient still requires isolation. Ideally, patients with RSV or metapneumovirus infections are housed separately, because co-infection may be associated with more severe disease.

Passive Immunoprophylaxis

Administration of palivizumab (15 mg/kg IM once a month), a neutralizing humanized murine monoclonal antibody against RSV, is recommended for protecting high-risk children against serious complications from RSV disease. Immunoprophylaxis reduces the frequency and total days of hospitalization for RSV infections in high-risk infants in about half of cases. Palivizumab is administered monthly from the beginning to the end of the RSV season (usually October-December and March-May, respectively, in temperate Northern hemisphere regions).

Candidates for immunoprophylaxis include children who have lung disease or were born very prematurely. Children <2 yr of age with chronic lung disease requiring supplemental oxygen or other medical therapy currently or within the 6 mo before the RSV season should receive prophylaxis for the 1st 2 RSV seasons if they have severe lung disease, and only for the 1st RSV season for less severe lung disease. Children <2 yr of age with hemodynamically significant congenital heart disease (heart failure, cyanosis, pulmonary hypertension) are also candidates for this therapy. Infants should receive seasonal RSV prophylaxis up to 12 mo of age if they were born at <28 wk of gestation, and up to 6 mo of age if they were born at 29-32 wk of gestation. Infants born between 32 and 35 wk of gestation should receive prophylaxis only if they have other risk factors. Adverse events with palivizumab are uncommon. An enhanced-affinity version of the antibody is in late-stage development as a second-generation drug.

Vaccine

There is no licensed vaccine against RSV. The challenge for development of live agents has been to produce attenuated vaccine strains that infect infants in the nasopharynx after topical inoculation without producing unacceptable symptoms, that remain genetically stable during shedding, and that induce protection against severe disease following re-infection. The most promising live-attenuated virus candidates have been engineered in the laboratory from cold-passaged strains of RSV, according to a basic strategy that yielded the live poliovirus and influenza virus vaccine strains.

BIBLIOGRAPHY

Please visit the Nelson Textbook of Pediatrics *website at www.expertconsult.com for the complete bibliography.*

Chapter 253
Human Metapneumovirus

James E. Crowe, Jr.

Human metapneumovirus (HMPV), a respiratory virus identified in 2001, is emerging as one of the most common causes of serious lower respiratory tract illness in children throughout the world.

ETIOLOGY

HMPV is an enveloped, single-stranded nonsegmented negative-sense RNA genome of the Paramyxoviridae family, which is divided into 2 subfamilies, Pneumovirinae and Paramyxovirinae. The Pneumovirinae subfamily includes the 2 genera *Metapneumovirus* and *Pneumovirus,* which includes respiratory syncytial virus (RSV). HMPV and the avian pneumoviruses (APVs) are highly related and are separated into the separate genus *Metapneumovirus* because the gene order in the nonsegmented genome is slightly altered and APVs/HMPVs lack the genes for 2 nonstructural proteins, NS1 and NS2, that are encoded at the 3′ end of RSV genomes. These proteins are thought to counteract host type I interferons. The absence of NS1/NS2 in the metapneumoviruses may contribute to decreased pathogenicity of HMPV relative to wild-type RSV strains.

Full-length sequences of a number of HMPV genomes have been determined. The genome is predicted to encode 9 proteins in the order 3′-N-P-M-F-M2-(orf1 and 2)-SH-G-L-5′. The genome also contains noncoding 3′ leader, 5′ trailer, and intergenic regions, consistent with the organization of most paramyxoviruses, with a viral promoter contained in the 3′ end of the genome. The F (fusion), G (glycosylated), and SH (short hydrophobic) proteins are integral membrane proteins on the surfaces of infected cells and virion particles. The F protein is a classic type I integral membrane viral fusion protein that contains 2 heptad repeats in the extracellular domain that facilitate membrane fusion. There is a predicted protein cleavage site near a hydrophobic fusion peptide that likely is cleaved by an extracellular protease, activating the F protein for fusion. The predicted attachment (G) protein of HMPV exhibits the basic features of a glycosylated type II mucin-like protein. The HMPV G protein differs from the RSV G protein in that it lacks a cysteine noose structure. This protein may inhibit innate immune responses. The internal proteins of the virus appear similar in function to those of other paramyxoviruses.

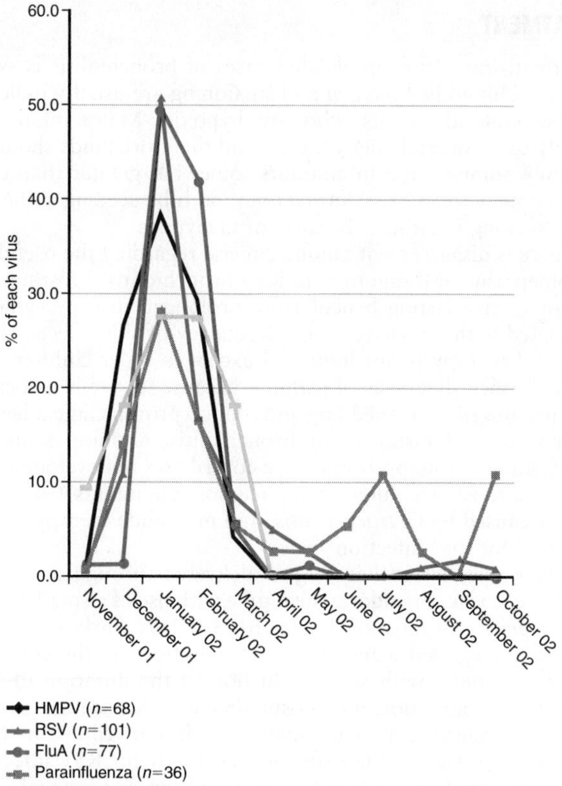

Figure 253-1 Temporal distribution of respiratory viruses among children hospitalized with lower respiratory tract infections from November 2001 through October 2002. Data are displayed as the proportion of each virus detected monthly. FluA, influenza A; HMPV, human metapneumovirus; RSV, respiratory syncytial virus. (From Wolf DG, Greenberg D, Kalkstein D, et al: Comparison of human metapneumovirus, respiratory syncytial virus and influenza A virus lower reparatory tract infections in hospitalized young children, *Pediatr Infect Dis J* 25:320–324, 2006.)

EPIDEMIOLOGY

HMPV outbreaks occur in annual epidemics during late winter and early spring in temperate climates, often overlapping with the second half of the annual RSV epidemic (Fig. 253-1). Sporadic infection does occur year round. The usual period of viral shedding is likely to be several weeks after primary infection in infants. The incubation period is 3-5 days. Humans are the only source of virus. Transmission is thought to occur by close or direct contact with contaminated secretions involving large-particle aerosols, droplets, or contaminated surfaces. Nosocomial infections have been reported, and contact isolation with excellent handwashing for health care providers is indicated in medical settings. This virus affects the elderly, immunocompromised patients, and patients with reactive airways disease more severely than otherwise healthy individuals.

PATHOLOGY

Infection is usually limited to the superficial layer of airway epithelial cells. Infection is associated with a local inflammatory infiltrate consisting of lymphocytes and macrophages. Immunocompromised individuals have evidence of both acute and organizing injuries during prolonged infection.

PATHOGENESIS

Infection occurs via inoculation of the upper respiratory tract. Infection can spread rapidly to the lower respiratory tract, but it is not clear whether the spread is mediated by cell-to-cell spread or aspiration of infected materials from the upper tract. Severe lower respiratory tract illness, especially wheezing, occurs mainly during the 1st 6 mo of life, at a time when the airways are of a small diameter and high resistance. Maternal serum neutralizing antibodies that cross the placenta may afford a relative protection against severe disease for several weeks or months after birth. Once infection is established, it is suspected that cytotoxic T cells recognize and eliminate virus-infected cells, thus terminating the infection but also causing some cytopathology. Individuals with an underlying predisposition to reactive airways disease (including adults) are susceptible to severe wheezing during re-infection later in life, suggesting that HMPV may cause smooth muscle hyperactivity, inflammation, or increased mucus production in such individuals. Infection in otherwise healthy individuals resolves without apparent long-term consequences in most cases.

CLINICAL MANIFESTATIONS

HMPV is associated with the common cold (complicated by otitis media in about 30% of cases) and with lower respiratory tract illnesses such as bronchiolitis, pneumonia, croup, and exacerbation of reactive airways disease. The profile of signs and symptoms caused by HMPV is very similar to that caused by RSV (Table 253-1). Approximately 5-10% of outpatient lower respiratory tract illnesses in otherwise healthy young children is associated with HMPV infection, which is 2nd in incidence only to RSV. Children with RSV or HMPV infection require supplemental oxygen and medical intensive care at similar frequencies.

About 50% of the cases of lower respiratory tract illness in children occur in the 1st 6 mo of life, suggesting that young age is a major risk factor for severe disease. Both young adults and the elderly can have HMPV infection that requires medical care including hospitalization, but severe disease occurs at much lower frequencies in adults than in young children. Severe disease in older subjects is most common in immunocompromised patients and can be fatal. A significant number of both adult and pediatric patients with asthma exacerbations have HMPV infection; it is not clear whether the virus causes long-term wheezing. RSV and

Table 253-1 CLINICAL MANIFESTATIONS OF HUMAN METAPNEUMOVIRUS IN CHILDREN

COMMON (>50%)
Fever >38°C Cough Rhinitis, coryza Wheezing Tachypnea, retractions Hypoxia (O_2 saturation <94%) Chest radiograph demonstration of infiltrates or hyperinflation
LESS COMMON
Otitis media Pharyngitis Rales
RARE
Conjunctivitis Hoarseness Encephalitis Fatal respiratory failure in immunocompromised children

HMPV co-infections have been reported; coinfections may be more severe, resulting in pediatric intensive care unit admissions. It is difficult to define true co-infections because the viral genome can be detected by reverse transcriptase polymerase chain reaction (RT-PCR) in respiratory secretions for at least several weeks after illness, even when virus shedding has terminated.

LABORATORY FINDINGS

The virus can be seen only with electron microscopy. The virus grows in primary monkey kidney cells or LLC-MK2 cell or Vero cell line monolayer cultures, but its efficient isolation requires an experienced laboratory technician. Conventional bright-field microscopy of infected cell monolayer cultures often reveals cytopathic effect only after multiple passages in cell culture. The characteristics of the cytopathic effect are not sufficiently distinct to allow identification of the virus on this basis alone, even by a trained observer. Direct antigen tests for identification of HMPV antigens in nasopharyngeal secretions are available. Some laboratories have success with the use of immunofluorescence staining with monoclonal or polyclonal antibodies to detect HMPV in nasopharyngeal secretions and shell vial cultures or in monolayer cultures in which virus has been cultivated. The most sensitive test for identification of HMPV in clinical samples is RT-PCR, usually performed with primers directed to internal genes such as the nucleoprotein gene. Detection by this modality is also available in some multiplex PCR tests for panels of respiratory viruses. Real-time RT-PCR tests offer enhanced sensitivity and specificity, including assays designed to detect viruses from the 4 known genetic lineages.

DIAGNOSIS AND DIFFERENTIAL DIAGNOSIS

In temperate areas, the diagnosis should be suspected during the late winter in infants or young children with wheezing or pneumonia and a negative RSV diagnostic test result. The diseases caused by RSV and HMPV cannot be distinguished clinically. Many other common respiratory viruses, such as parainfluenza viruses, influenza viruses, adenoviruses, rhinoviruses, and coronaviruses, can cause similar disease in young children. Some of these viruses can be identified by PCR genetic testing or conventional cell culture means.

COMPLICATIONS

Co-infection with bacteria is not common in HMPV infection, except for the local complication of otitis media.

TREATMENT

There is no specific treatment at this time for HMPV infection. Management consists of supportive care. The rate of bacterial lung infection or bacteremia associated with HMPV infection is not fully defined but is suspected to be very low. Antibiotics are usually not indicated in treatment of infants hospitalized for HMPV bronchiolitis or pneumonia.

SUPPORTIVE CARE

Treatment is supportive and includes careful attention to hydration, monitoring of respiratory status by physical examination and measurement of oxygen saturation, use of supplemental oxygen, and, if necessary, mechanical ventilation.

PROGNOSIS

Most infants and children recover from acute HMPV infection without apparent long-term consequences. Many experts believe an association exists between severe HMPV infections in infancy and risk for recurrent wheezing or the development of asthma; however, it is not clear whether the virus causes these conditions or precipitates their 1st manifestations.

PREVENTION

The only method of prevention of HMPV infection is reduction of exposure. Contact precautions are recommended for the duration of HMPV-associated illness among hospitalized infants and young children. Patients known to have HMPV infection should be housed in single rooms or with a cohort of HMPV-infected patients. It may be wise to care for patients with RSV infection in a separate cohort from HMPV-infected patients to prevent co-infection. Preventive measures include limiting, where feasible, exposure to contagious settings during annual epidemics (daycare centers) and emphasis on hand hygiene in all settings, including the home, especially during periods when the contacts of high-risk children have respiratory infections. However, providers should keep in mind that infection is universal in the first several years of life. Therefore, reduction of exposure makes most sense during the 1st 6 mo of life, when infants are at highest risk for severe disease.

BIBLIOGRAPHY

Please visit the Nelson Textbook of Pediatrics *website at www.expertconsult.com for the complete bibliography.*

Chapter 254
Adenoviruses

John V. Williams

Adenoviruses (AdVs) are a common cause of human disease. Conjunctivitis is a familiar illness associated with AdVs, but these viruses also cause upper and lower respiratory disease, pharyngitis, gastroenteritis, and hemorrhagic cystitis. AdVs can cause severe disease in immunocompromised hosts. Outbreaks of AdV occur in communities and close populations, notably the military. No specific antivirals that are highly effective against AdVs are available. Vaccines are available for serotypes 4 and 7 but are used only for military populations.

ETIOLOGY

Adenoviruses were first isolated from human adenoidal surgical specimens in 1953. They are nonenveloped viruses with an

Table 254-1 ADENOVIRUS SEROTYPES WITH ASSOCIATED INFECTIONS

SPECIES	SEROTYPE	PREFERRED SITE OF INFECTION
A	12, 18, 31	Gastrointestinal
B1	3, 7, 16, 21, 50	Respiratory
B2	11, 14, 34, 35	Renal/urinary tract epithelium
C	1, 2, 5, 6	Respiratory
D	8, 9, 10, 13, 15, 17, 19a, 19p, 20, 22-30, 32, 33, 36, 37, 38, 39, 42-48, 49, 51	Ocular
E	4	Respiratory
F	40, 41	Gastrointestinal

icosahedral protein capsid. The double-stranded DNA genome is contained within the particle complexed with several viral proteins. Antigenic variability in surface proteins of the virion defines >50 serotypes grouped into seven species. Species differ in their tissue tropism and target organs, causing distinct clinical infections (Table 254-1). AdV can be shed from the gastrointestinal tract for prolonged periods and can establish chronic low-level infection of the tonsils and adenoids.

EPIDEMIOLOGY

AdVs circulate worldwide and cause endemic infections year-round in immunocompetent hosts. Asymptomatic infections are also common. Only about one third of all known human AdV serotypes are associated with clinically apparent disease. The most prevalent types in recent surveillance studies are AdVs 3, 2, 1, and 5. Epidemics of conjunctivitis (often severe), pharyngitis, and respiratory disease occur, especially in schools and military settings. Outbreaks of febrile respiratory illness caused by AdV 4 and AdV 7 are a major source of morbidity in military barracks, with attack rates ranging from 25% to >90%. Spread of AdV occurs by respiratory and fecal-oral routes. An important factor in AdV transmission, especially in epidemics, is the ability of the nonenveloped particle to survive on inanimate objects in the environment. Nosocomial outbreaks have been reported.

PATHOGENESIS

AdVs bind to cell surface receptors and trigger internalization by endocytosis. Acidification of the endosome induces conformational changes in the capsid, leading to eventual translocation of the genome to the cell nucleus. Viral messenger RNA transcription and genomic replication occur in the nucleus. Progeny virion particles assemble in the nucleus. Lysis of the cell releases new infectious particles and causes damage to epithelial mucosa, sloughing of cell debris, and inflammation. AdVs recruit neutrophils, macrophages, and natural killer cells to the site of infection and induce these cells to elaborate a number of cytokines and chemokines. Host immune response thus contributes to the symptoms of AdV infection, but specific mechanisms of pathogenesis are poorly understood.

CLINICAL MANIFESTATIONS

AdVs cause a variety of common clinical syndromes in both immunocompetent and immunocompromised hosts. These syndromes are difficult to distinguish reliably from similar illnesses caused by other pathogens, such as respiratory syncytial virus (RSV), human metapneumovirus (HMPV), human rhinovirus (HRV), rotavirus, group A streptococcus, and other common viral and bacterial pathogens.

Acute Respiratory Disease

Respiratory tract infections are common manifestations of AdV infections in children and adults. AdV cause an estimated 5-10% of all childhood respiratory disease. Primary infections in infants may manifest as bronchiolitis or pneumonia. AdV pneumonia may manifest as features more typical of bacterial disease (lobar infiltrates, high fever, parapneumonic effusions). Pharyngitis due to AdV typically includes symptoms of coryza, sore throat, and fever. The virus can be identified in 15-20% of children with isolated pharyngitis, mostly in preschool children and infants.

Ocular Infections

Common follicular conjunctivitis due to AdV is self-limiting and requires no specific treatment. A more severe form, called *epidemic keratoconjunctivitis*, involves the cornea and conjunctiva. Pharyngoconjunctival fever is a distinct syndrome that includes a high temperature, pharyngitis, nonpurulent conjunctivitis, and preauricular and cervical lymphadenopathy.

Gastrointestinal Infections

AdVs can be detected in the stools of 5-10% of children with acute diarrhea. Most cases of acute diarrhea are self-limiting, though severe disease can occur. Enteric infection with AdV is often asymptomatic, so the causative role in these episodes is frequently uncertain. AdV may also cause mesenteric adenitis.

Hemorrhagic Cystitis

Hemorrhage cystitis consists of a sudden onset of hematuria, dysuria, frequency, and urgency with negative urine bacterial culture results. Urinalysis may show sterile pyuria in addition to red blood cells; the illness resolves on its own in 1-2 wk.

Other Complications

Rarely, AdVs are associated with myocarditis, hepatitis, or meningoencephalitis in immunocompetent individuals.

Adenoviruses in Immunocompromised Patients

Immunocompromised persons are at high risk for severe disease due to AdVs, particularly recipients of hematopoietic stem cell transplants (HSCTs) and solid organ transplants. Organ failure due to pneumonia, hepatitis, gastroenteritis, and disseminated infection occurs primarily in these patients. AdV infection in HSCT recipients commonly manifests as pulmonary or disseminated disease and is most likely to occur in the first 100 days after transplantation. Infections due to AdV in solid organ transplant recipients usually involve the transplanted organ. Immunocompromised children are at greater risk than immunocompromised adults for complicated AdV infection, presumably because of a lack of pre-existing immunity. Additional risk factors are T cell–depleted grafts, high-level immunosuppression, and presence of graft versus host disease. Some experts advocate a preemptive screening approach to detect and treat AdV infection early in immunocompromised patients, with the intent to prevent dissemination and severe illness in this vulnerable population.

DIAGNOSIS

AdV may be suspected as the etiology of an illness on the basis of epidemiologic or clinical features; neither of these categories is specific enough to firmly establish the diagnosis. Rapid tests for AdV are not commercially available. Most AdV serotypes grow well in culture, although this method requires 2-7 days and thus is not helpful for early identification. Molecular techniques such as polymerase chain reaction (PCR) offer rapid, sensitive, and specific diagnosis of AdV infections and are most useful clinically for the management of suspected AdV infections in immunocompromised hosts. The frequency of asymptomatic shedding of AdV makes assigning causality to this pathogen difficult at times. Serology is generally useful only in epidemiologic investigations.

COMPLICATIONS

AdV pneumonia can lead to respiratory failure requiring mechanical ventilation, especially in the immunocompromised patient. Secondary bacterial pneumonias do not appear to be as common following AdV infection as they are after influenza infection, but data for this issue are limited. Severe AdV pneumonia has been linked to chronic lung disease and bronchiolitis obliterans in a minority of cases. Epidemic keratoconjunctivitis is a sight-threatening form of AdV infection. Nearly any form of AdV infection can be fatal in an HSCT or solid organ transplant recipient. Refractory severe anemia requiring repeated blood transfusions can develop in HSCT recipients with hemorrhagic cystitis. . Mortality rates of up to 60-80% have been reported in transplant recipients with disseminated AdV or AdV pneumonia.

TREATMENT

Supportive care is the mainstay of AdV treatment in most cases. Patients with severe AdV conjunctivitis should be referred for ophthalmologic consultation. No specific antiviral therapy has been shown to produce a definite clinical benefit against AdV infection. The nucleoside analogue cidofovir has in vitro activity against most AdV serotypes. Cidofovir is used topically to treat epidemic keratoconjunctivitis, although topical steroids are often prescribed later in the disease course to limit the inflammatory component. Cidofovir may be used intravenously for AdV infections in immunocompromised patients. Cidofovir is highly nephrotoxic; however, prehydration, concomitant administration of probenecid, and weekly dosing may alleviate renal toxicity. Clinical studies suggest benefit from cidofovir, but there are no prospective, randomized controlled trials of cidofovir for AdV. In addition, no formal guidelines or recommendations for treatment exist. Anecdotal descriptions of benefit from intravenous immunoglobulin (IVIG) and donor lymphocyte infusion have also been reported.

PREVENTION

Environmental and fomite transmission of AdVs occurs readily; therefore, simple measures such as handwashing and cleaning reduce spread. Live attenuated AdV 4 and AdV 7 vaccines were used effectively in the USA military from the 1970s until 1999. Cessation of their use led to widespread outbreaks in barracks, and these vaccines have been re-introduced into military use. AdVs are highly immunogenic and have been used as gene therapy vectors and vaccine vectors for other pathogens, including malaria and HIV, but no AdV-specific vaccines are commercially available.

BIBLIOGRAPHY

Please visit the Nelson Textbook of Pediatrics *website at* *www.expertconsult.com* *for the complete bibliography.*

Chapter 255
Rhinoviruses

E. Kathryn Miller and John V. Williams

Human rhinoviruses (HRVs) are the most frequent cause of the **common cold** in both adults and children. Although rhinoviruses were once thought to cause only the common cold, it is now known that they are associated with lower respiratory infections in adults and children. Many HRVs do not grow in culture; studies using molecular diagnostic tools such as polymerase chain reaction (PCR) have revealed that HRVs are leading causes of both mild and serious respiratory illnesses in children.

ETIOLOGY

Human rhinoviruses are members of the Picornaviridae family ("pico" = small; "rna" = RNA genome). Traditional methods of virus typing using immune antiserum have identified ≈ 100 serotypes, classified into HRVA and HRVB species on the basis of genetic sequence similarity. A novel group of HRVs designated HRVC has been detected by reverse transcriptase PCR (RT-PCR) but has not yet been cultivated. Virus gene sequence analysis demonstrates that HRVC are a genetically distinct species. The increased proportions of HRV reported in recent PCR-based studies may partly be due to detection of these previously unknown HRVC viruses in addition to improved detection of known HRVA and HRVB strains.

EPIDEMIOLOGY

Rhinoviruses are distributed worldwide, and there is no proven correlation between serotypes and epidemiologic or clinical characteristics. Multiple serotypes may circulate in a community simultaneously, and particular HRV strains may be isolated during consecutive epidemic seasons, suggesting persistence in a community over an extended period. In temperate climates the incidence of HRV infection peaks in fall, with another peak in spring, but HRV infections occur year-round. Rhinoviruses are the major infectious trigger for asthma among young children, and numerous studies have described a sharp increase in asthmatic attacks in this age group when school opens in the fall. Peak HRV incidence in the tropics occurs during the rainy season, from June to October.

Rhinoviruses are present in high concentrations in nasal secretions and can be detected in the lower airways. Rhinovirus particles are nonenveloped and quite hardy, persisting for several hours in secretions on hands or other surfaces such as telephones, light switches, doorknobs, and stethoscopes. Transmission occurs when infected secretions carried on contaminated fingers are rubbed onto nasal or conjunctival mucosa. Rhinoviruses are present in aerosols produced by talking, coughing, and sneezing. Children are the most important reservoir of the virus.

PATHOGENESIS

The majority of HRVs infect respiratory epithelial cells via intercellular adhesion molecule-1 (ICAM-1), but some HRV strains utilize the LDL (low-density lipoprotein) receptor. Infection begins in the nasopharynx and spreads to the nasal mucosa and in some cases to bronchial epithelial cells in the lower airway. Rhinoviruses do not appear to cause significant direct cellular damage, so it is thought that many of the pathogenic effects are produced by the host immune response. Rhinovirus infection of bronchial epithelial cells in vitro induces the secretion of many inflammatory chemokines and cytokines. Both innate and adaptive immune mechanisms are important in HRV pathogenesis and clearance. HRV-specific nasal immunoglobulin (Ig) A can be detected on day 3 after infection, followed by the production of serum IgM and IgG after 7-8 days. Neutralizing IgG to HRV may prevent or limit the severity of illness following re-infection. Cross protection between antibodies to different HRV serotypes is limited in breadth and duration. Both allergen exposure and elevated IgE values predispose patients with asthma to more severe respiratory symptoms in response to HRV infection. Abnormalities in the host cellular response to HRV infection that result in impaired apoptosis and increased viral replication may be responsible for the severe and prolonged symptoms in individuals with asthma.

CLINICAL MANIFESTATIONS

Most HRV infections produce clinical symptoms, but approximately 15% are asymptomatic. Typical symptoms of sneezing, nasal congestion, rhinorrhea, and sore throat develop following an incubation period of 1-4 days. Cough and hoarseness are present in one third of cases. Fever is less common with HRV than with other common respiratory viruses, including influenza virus, RSV, and HMPV. Symptoms are frequently more severe and last longer in children, with 70% of children still reporting symptoms by day 10, compared with 20% of adults. Virus can be shed for as long as 3 wk.

HRVs are the most prevalent agents associated with acute wheezing, otitis media, and hospitalization for respiratory illness in children and are an important cause of severe pneumonia and exacerbation of asthma or chronic obstructive pulmonary disease (COPD) in adults. HRV-associated hospitalizations are more frequent in young infants than in older children and in children with a history of wheezing or asthma. HRV infection in immunocompromised hosts may be life threatening.

DIAGNOSIS

Culturing HRV is labor intensive and relatively low yield. Sensitive and specific diagnostic methods based on RT-PCR are commercially available. An important caveat of HRV detection is the fact that HRV infection can be asymptomatic, and thus the presence of the virus does not prove causality in all cases. Serology is impractical owing to the great number of HRV serotypes. Presumptive clinical diagnosis based on symptoms and seasonality is not specific, because many other viruses cause similar clinical illnesses. Bacterial culture or antigen testing may exclude streptococcal pharyngitis. Rapid detection techniques for HRV might lessen the use of unnecessary antibiotics or procedures.

COMPLICATIONS

Possible complications of HRV infection include sinusitis, otitis media, asthma exacerbation, bronchiolitis, pneumonia, and, rarely, death. HRV-associated wheezing during infancy is a significant risk factor for the development of childhood asthma. This effect appears to remain until adulthood, but the mechanisms have not been elucidated.

TREATMENT

Supportive care is the mainstay of HRV treatment. The symptoms of HRV infection are commonly treated with analgesics, decongestants, antihistamines, or antitussives. *Data are limited on the effectiveness of such over-the-counter cold medications for children.* If bacterial superinfections are highly suspected or diagnosed, antibiotics may be appropriate. *Antibiotics are not indicated for uncomplicated viral upper respiratory infection.* Vaccines have not been successfully developed because of the numerous HRV serotypes and limited cross protection between serotypes.

PREVENTION

Good handwashing remains the mainstay of prevention of HRV infection and should be reinforced frequently, especially in young children, the predominant "vectors" for disease.

BIBLIOGRAPHY
Please visit the Nelson Textbook of Pediatrics *website at www.expertconsult.com for the complete bibliography.*

Chapter 256
Coronaviruses
Mark R. Denison

Coronaviruses are increasingly recognized as important pathogens of humans. They cause up to 15% of common colds and are implicated as causes of croup, asthma exacerbations, and lower respiratory tract infections, including bronchiolitis and pneumonia. In addition there is evidence that coronaviruses may be causes of enteritis or colitis in neonates and infants and may be underappreciated as agents of meningitis or encephalitis. The discovery that **severe acute respiratory syndrome (SARS)** is caused by a novel human coronavirus (**SARS-CoV**) has led to increased surveillance and the recognition of additional human coronaviruses, revealing that new coronaviruses enter human populations from zoonotic vectors such as bats.

For the full continuation of this chapter, please visit the Nelson Textbook of Pediatrics *website at www.expertconsult.com.*

256.1 Severe Acute Respiratory Syndrome–Associated Coronavirus
Mark R. Denison

The SARS outbreak of 2003 was contained and ultimately halted through a remarkable cooperative effort among countries around the world; the occurrence of several laboratory-acquired cases as well as sporadic cases likely associated with animal-to-human transmission in 2004 demonstrates the potential threat posed by trans-species transmission of coronaviruses. The identification of bats as likely reservoirs of SARS-like coronaviruses as well as large numbers of coronaviruses related to all other mammalian groups suggests mechanisms for ongoing introduction into human populations.

For the full continuation of this chapter, please visit the Nelson Textbook of Pediatrics *website at www.expertconsult.com.*

Chapter 257
Rotaviruses, Caliciviruses, and Astroviruses
Dorsey M. Bass

Diarrhea is a leading cause of childhood mortality in the world, accounting for 5-10 million deaths/yr. In early childhood, the single most important cause of severe dehydrating diarrhea is rotavirus infection. Rotavirus and other gastroenteritis viruses not only are major causes of pediatric mortality but also lead to significant morbidity. Children in the USA have been estimated to have a risk of hospitalization for rotavirus diarrhea of 1:43, corresponding to 80,000 hospitalizations annually.

ETIOLOGY

Rotavirus, astrovirus, caliciviruses such as the **Norwalk agent,** and enteric adenovirus are the medically important pathogens of human viral gastroenteritis (Chapter 332).

Rotaviruses are in the Reoviridae family and cause disease in virtually all mammals and birds. These viruses are a wheel-like, triple-shelled icosahedron containing 11 segments of double-stranded RNA. The diameter of the particles on electron microscopy is approximately 80 nm. Rotaviruses are classified by serogroup (A, B, C, D, E, F, and G) and subgroup (I or II). Rotavirus strains are species specific and do not cause disease in heterologous hosts. Group A includes the common human pathogens as well as a variety of animal viruses. Group B rotavirus is reported as a cause of severe disease in infants and adults in China only. Occasional human outbreaks of group C rotavirus are reported. The other serogroups infect only nonhumans.

Subgrouping of rotaviruses is determined by the antigenic structure of the inner capsid protein, VP6. Serotyping of rotaviruses, described for group A only, is determined by classic cross-neutralization testing and depends on the outer capsid glycoproteins, VP7 and VP4. The VP7 serotype is referred to as the *G type* (for glycoprotein). There are 10 G serotypes, of which 4 cause most illness and vary in occurrence from year to year and region to region. The VP4 serotype is referred to as the P type. There are 11 P serotypes. Although both VP4 and VP7 elicit neutralizing immunoglobulin (Ig) G antibodies, the relative role of these systemic antibodies compared with that of mucosal IgA antibodies and cellular responses in protective immunity remains unclear.

Caliciviruses, which constitute the Caliciviridae family, are small 27- to 35-nm viruses that are the most common cause of gastroenteritis outbreaks in older children and adults. Caliciviruses also cause a rotavirus-like illness in young infants. They are positive-sense, single-stranded RNA viruses with a single structural protein. Human caliciviruses are divided into 2 genera, the noroviruses and sapoviruses. Caliciviruses have been named for locations of initial outbreaks: Norwalk, Snow Mountain, Montgomery County, Sapporo, and others. Caliciviruses and astroviruses are sometimes referred to as **small, round viruses** on the basis of appearance on electron microscopy.

Astroviruses, which constitute the Astroviridae family, are important agents of viral gastroenteritis in young children, with a high incidence in both the developing and developed worlds. Astroviruses are positive-sense, single-stranded RNA viruses. They are small particles, approximately 30 nm in diameter, with a characteristic central 5- or 6-pointed star when viewed on electron microscopy. The capsid consists of 3 structural proteins. There are 8 known human serotypes.

Enteric adenoviruses are a common cause of viral gastroenteritis in infants and children. Although many adenovirus serotypes exist and are found in human stool, especially during and after typical upper respiratory tract infections (Chapter 254), only serotypes 40 and 41 cause gastroenteritis. These strains are very difficult to grow in tissue culture. The virus consists of an 80-nm-diameter icosahedral particle with a relatively complex double-stranded DNA genome.

Aichi virus is a picornavirus that has been associated with gastroenteritis and was initially described in Asia. Several other viruses that may cause diarrheal disease in animals have been postulated but not well established as human gastroenteritis viruses. These include coronaviruses, toroviruses, and pestiviruses. The **picobirnaviruses** are an unclassified group of small (30 nm), single-stranded RNA viruses that have been found in 10% of patients with HIV-associated diarrhea.

EPIDEMIOLOGY

Worldwide, rotavirus is estimated to cause >111 million cases of diarrhea annually in children younger than 5 yr. Of these, 18 million cases are considered at least moderately severe, with approximately 500,000 deaths per year. Rotavirus causes 3 million cases of diarrhea, 80,000 hospitalizations, and 20-40 deaths annually in the USA.

Rotavirus infection is most common in winter months in temperate climates. In the USA, the annual winter peak spreads from west to east (Fig. 257-1). Unlike the spread of other winter viruses, such as influenza, this wave of increased incidence is not due to a single prevalent strain or serotype. Typically, several serotypes predominate in a given community for 1 or 2 seasons, while nearby locations may harbor unrelated strains. Disease tends to be most severe in patients 3-24 mo of age, although 25% of the cases of severe disease occur in children >2 yr of age, with serologic evidence of infection developing in virtually all children by 4-5 yr of age. Infants younger than 3 mo are relatively protected by transplacental antibody and possibly breast-feeding. Infections in neonates and in adults in close contact with infected children are generally asymptomatic. Some rotavirus strains have stably colonized newborn nurseries for years, infecting virtually all newborns without causing any overt illness.

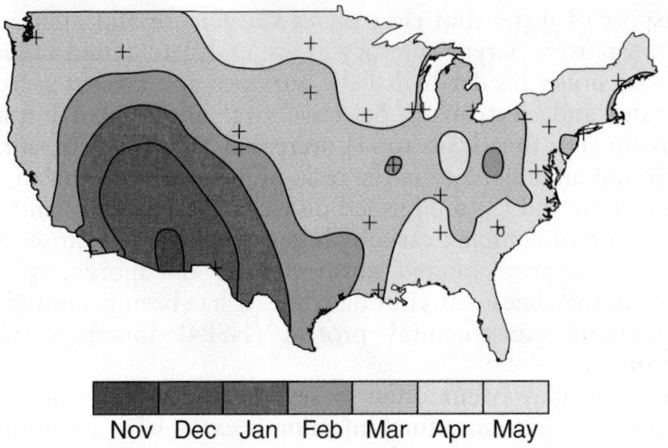

Figure 257-1 Peak rotavirus activity by month in the USA for July 1996–June 1997. This pattern is typical of the annual rotavirus activity each year. (From the Centers for Disease Control and Prevention: Laboratory-based surveillance for rotavirus—United States, July 1996-June 1997, *MMWR Morb Mortal Wkly Rep* 46:1092–1094, 1997.)

Rotavirus and the other gastrointestinal viruses spread efficiently via a fecal-oral route, and outbreaks are common in children's hospitals and child-care centers. The virus is shed in stool at very high concentration before and for days after the clinical illness. Very few infectious virions are needed to cause disease in a susceptible host.

The epidemiology of **astroviruses** is not as thoroughly studied as that of rotavirus, but they are a common cause of mild to moderate watery winter diarrhea in children and infants and an uncommon pathogen in adults. Hospital outbreaks are common. **Enteric adenovirus** gastroenteritis occurs year-round, mostly in children younger than 2 yr. Nosocomial outbreaks occur but are less common than with rotavirus and astrovirus. **Calicivirus** is best known for causing large, explosive outbreaks among older children and adults, particularly in settings such as schools, cruise ships, and hospitals. Often a single food, such as shellfish or water used in food preparation, is identified as a source. Like astrovirus and rotavirus, caliciviruses are also commonly found in winter infantile gastroenteritis.

PATHOGENESIS

Viruses that cause human diarrhea selectively infect and destroy villus tip cells in the small intestine. Biopsies of the small intestines show variable degrees of villus blunting and round cell infiltrate in the lamina propria. Pathologic changes may not correlate with the severity of clinical symptoms and usually resolve before the clinical resolution of diarrhea. The gastric mucosa is not affected despite the commonly used term *gastroenteritis,* although delayed gastric emptying has been documented during Norwalk virus infection.

In the small intestine, the upper villus enterocytes are differentiated cells, which have both digestive functions, such as hydrolysis of disaccharides, and absorptive functions, such as the transport of water and electrolytes via glucose and amino acid co-transporters. Crypt enterocytes are undifferentiated cells that lack the brush border hydrolytic enzymes and are net secretors of water and electrolytes. Selective viral infection of intestinal villus tip cells thus leads to (1) decreased absorption of salt and water and an imbalance in the ratio of intestinal fluid absorption to secretion and (2) diminished disaccharidase activity and malabsorption of complex carbohydrates, particularly lactose. Most evidence supports altered absorption as the more important factor in the genesis of viral diarrhea. It has been proposed that a rotavirus nonstructural protein (NSP4) functions as an enterotoxin.

Viremia may occur often in severe, primary infections, but symptomatic **extraintestinal infection** is extremely rare in immunocompetent persons—although immunocompromised patients may rarely experience hepatic and renal involvement. The increased vulnerability of infants (compared with older children and adults) to severe morbidity and mortality from gastroenteritis viruses may relate to a number of factors, including decreased intestinal reserve function, lack of specific immunity, and decreased nonspecific host defense mechanisms such as gastric acid and mucus. Viral enteritis greatly enhances intestinal permeability to luminal macromolecules and has been postulated to increase the risk for food allergies.

CLINICAL MANIFESTATIONS

Rotavirus infection typically begins after an incubation period of <48 hr (range 1-7 days) with mild to moderate fever as well as vomiting, followed by the onset of frequent, watery stools. All 3 symptoms are present in about 50-60% of cases. Vomiting and fever typically abate during the 2nd day of illness, but diarrhea often continues for 5-7 days. The stool is without gross blood or white blood cells (WBCs). Dehydration may develop and progress rapidly, particularly in infants. The most severe disease typically occurs among children 4-36 mo of age. Malnourished children and children with underlying intestinal disease such as short-bowel syndrome are particularly likely to acquire severe rotavirus diarrhea. Rarely, immunodeficient children experience severe and prolonged illness. Although most newborns infected with rotavirus are asymptomatic, some outbreaks of necrotizing enterocolitis have been associated with the appearance of a new rotavirus strain in the affected nurseries.

The clinical course of **astrovirus** appears to be similar to that of rotavirus, with the notable exception that the disease tends to be milder, with less significant dehydration. **Adenovirus enteritis** tends to cause diarrhea of longer duration, often 10-14 days. The **Norwalk virus** has a short (12-hr) incubation period. Vomiting and nausea tend to predominate in illness associated with the Norwalk virus, and the duration is brief, usually consisting of 1-3 days of symptoms. The clinical and epidemiologic picture of Norwalk virus often closely resembles so-called food poisoning from preformed toxins such as *Staphylococcus aureus* and *Bacillus cereus.*

DIAGNOSIS

In most cases, a satisfactory diagnosis can be made on the basis of the clinical and epidemiologic features. Enzyme-linked immunosorbent assays (ELISAs), which offer >90% specificity and sensitivity, are available for detection of group A rotavirus, caliciviruses, and enteric adenovirus in stool samples. Latex agglutination assays are also available for group A rotavirus and are less sensitive than ELISA. Research tools include electron microscopy of stools, RNA polymerase chain reaction analysis to identify G and P antigens, and culture. The diagnosis of viral gastroenteritis should always be questioned in patients with persistent or high fever, blood or WBCs in the stool, or persistent severe or bilious vomiting, especially in the absence of diarrhea.

LABORATORY FINDINGS

Isotonic dehydration with acidosis is the most common finding in children with severe viral enteritis. The stools are free of blood and leukocytes. Although the WBC count may be moderately elevated secondary to stress, the marked left shift seen with invasive bacterial enteritis is absent.

DIFFERENTIAL DIAGNOSIS

The differential diagnosis includes other infectious causes of enteritis, such as bacteria and protozoa. Occasionally, surgical conditions such as appendicitis, bowel obstruction, and intussusception may initially mimic viral gastroenteritis.

TREATMENT

Avoiding and treating dehydration are the main goals in treatment of viral enteritis. A secondary goal is maintenance of the nutritional status of the patient (Chapters 55 and 332).

There is no routine role for antiviral drug treatment of viral gastroenteritis. Controlled studies have shown no benefit from antiemetics or antidiarrheal drugs, and there is a significant risk for serious side effects with both types of agents. Antibiotics are similarly of no benefit. Immunoglobulins have been administered orally to both normal and immunodeficient patients with severe rotavirus gastroenteritis, but this treatment is currently considered experimental. Therapy with probiotic organisms such as *Lactobacillus* species has been shown to be helpful only in mild cases and not in dehydrating disease.

Supportive Treatment

Rehydration via the oral route can be accomplished in most patients with mild to moderate dehydration (Chapters 55 and 332). Severe rehydration requires immediate intravenous therapy followed by oral rehydration. Modern oral rehydration solutions containing appropriate quantities of sodium and glucose promote optimum absorption of fluid from the intestine. There is no evidence that a particular carbohydrate source (rice) or addition of amino acids improves the efficacy of these solutions for children with viral enteritis. Other clear liquids, such as flat soda, fruit juice, and sports drinks, are inappropriate for rehydration of young children with significant stool loss. Rehydration via the oral (or nasogastric) route should be done over 6-8 hr, and feedings begun immediately thereafter. Providing the rehydration fluid at a slow, steady rate, typically 5 mL/min, reduces vomiting and improves the success of oral therapy. Rehydration solution should be continued as a supplement to make up for ongoing excessive stool loss. Initial intravenous fluids are required for the infant in shock or the occasional child with intractable vomiting.

After rehydration has been achieved, resumption of a normal diet for age has been shown to result in a more rapid recovery from viral gastroenteritis. Prolonged (>12 hr) administration of exclusive clear liquids or dilute formula is without clinical benefit and actually prolongs the duration of diarrhea. Breastfeeding should be continued even during rehydration. Selected infants may benefit from lactose-free feedings (such as soy formula and lactose-free cow's milk) for several days, although this step is not necessary for most children. Hypocaloric diets low in protein and fat such as **BRAT** (*b*ananas, *r*ice, cereal, *a*pplesauce, and *t*oast) have not been shown to be superior to a regular diet.

PROGNOSIS

Most fatalities occur in infants with poor access to medical care and are attributed to dehydration. Children may be infected with rotavirus each year during the 1st 5yr of life, but each subsequent infection decreases in severity. Primary infection results in a predominantly serotype-specific immune response, whereas re-infection, which is usually with a different serotype, induces a broad immune response with cross-reactive heterotypic antibody. After the initial natural infection, children have limited protection against subsequent asymptomatic infection (38%) and greater protection against mild diarrhea (73%) and moderate to severe diarrhea (87%). After the 2nd natural infection, protection increases against subsequent asymptomatic infection (62%) and mild diarrhea (75%) and is complete (100%) against moderate to severe diarrhea. After the 3rd natural infection, there is even higher protection against subsequent asymptomatic infection (74%) and near-complete protection against even mild diarrhea (99%).

PREVENTION

Good hygiene reduces the transmission of viral gastroenteritis, but even in the most hygienic societies, virtually all children become infected as a result of the efficiency of infection of the gastroenteritis viruses. Good handwashing and isolation procedures can help control nosocomial outbreaks. The role of breastfeeding in prevention or amelioration of rotavirus infection may be small, given the variable protection observed in a number of studies. Vaccines offer the best hope for control of these ubiquitous infections.

Vaccines

A trivalent rotavirus vaccine was licensed in the USA in 1998 and was subsequently linked to an increased risk for intussusception, especially during the 3- to 14-day period after the 1st dose and the 3- to 7-day period after the 2nd dose. The vaccine was withdrawn from the market in 1999. Subsequently 2 new live, oral rotavirus vaccines have been approved in the USA after extensive safety and efficacy testing.

A live, oral, pentavalent rotavirus vaccine was approved in 2006 for use in the USA. The vaccine contains 5 reassortant rotaviruses isolated from human and bovine hosts. Four of the reassortant rotaviruses express 1 serotype of the outer protein VP7 (G1, G2, G3, or G4), and the 5th expresses the protein P1A (genotype P[8]) from the human rotavirus parent strain. The pentavalent vaccine protects against rotavirus gastroenteritis when administered as a 3-dose series at 2, 4, and 6 mo of age. The 1st dose should be administered between 6 and 12 wk of age, with all 3 doses completed by 32 wk of age. The vaccine provides substantial protection against rotavirus gastroenteritis, with primary efficacy of 98% against severe rotavirus gastroenteritis caused by G1-G4 serotypes and 74% efficacy against rotavirus gastroenteritis of any severity through the 1st rotavirus season after vaccination. It provides a 96% reduction in hospitalizations for rotavirus gastroenteritis through the 1st 2yr after the 3rd dose. In a study of >70,000 infants, the pentavalent vaccine did not increase the risk for intussusception.

Another new monovalent rotavirus vaccine was licensed in the USA and also appears to be safe and effective. It is an attenuated monovalent human rotavirus and is administered as 2 oral doses at 2 and 4 mo of age. The vaccine has 85% efficacy against severe gastroenteritis and was found to reduce hospital admissions for all diarrhea by 42%. Despite being monovalent, the vaccine is effective in prevention of all 4 common serotypes of human rotavirus.

Preliminary surveillance data on rotavirus incidence from the U.S. Centers for Disease Control and Prevention (CDC) suggest that rotavirus vaccination greatly reduced the disease burden in the USA during the 2007-2008 rotavirus season. Given the incomplete vaccine coverage during this period, the results suggest a degree of "herd immunity" from rotavirus immunization. Vaccine-associated disease has been reported in vaccine recipients who have severe combined immunodeficiency disease (a contraindication). In addition, vaccine-derived virus may undergo reassortment and become more virulent, producing diarrhea in unvaccinated siblings.

BIBLIOGRAPHY

Please visit the Nelson Textbook of Pediatrics *website at* *www.expertconsult.com* *for the complete bibliography.*

Chapter 258
Human Papillomaviruses

Anna-Barbara Moscicki

Human papillomaviruses (HPVs) cause a variety of proliferative cutaneous and mucosal lesions, including common skin warts, benign and malignant anogenital tract lesions, and life-threatening respiratory papillomas. Most HPV-related infections in children and adolescents are benign.

ETIOLOGY

The papillomaviruses are small (55-nm), DNA-containing viruses that are ubiquitous in nature, infecting most mammalian and many nonmammalian animal species. Strains are almost always species-specific. More than 100 different types of HPVs have been identified through comparison of sequence homologies. The different HPV types typically cause disease in specific anatomic sites; >30 HPV types have been identified from genital tract specimens.

EPIDEMIOLOGY

HPV infections of the skin are common, and most individuals are probably infected with one or more HPV types at some time. There are no animal reservoirs for HPV; all transmission is presumably person-to-person. There is little evidence to suggest that HPV is transmitted by fomites. Common warts, including palmar and plantar warts, are frequently seen in children and adolescents, in whom they infect the hands and feet, common areas of frequent minor trauma.

Human papillomavirus is the most prevalent viral sexually transmitted infection in the USA. Up to 70% of sexually active women eventually acquire HPV through sexual transmission; most have their first infection within 3 yr of beginning sexual intercourse. The greatest risk for HPV in sexually active adolescents is exposure to new non–condom-using sexual partners, underscoring the ease of transmission of this virus through sexual contact. As with many other genital pathogens, perinatal transmission to newborns also occurs, but infections appear transient. Detection of HPV in older preadolescent children is rare. If lesions are detected in a child >3 yr of age, the possibility of sexual abuse should be raised.

The most common manifestation of HPV is latent infection, defined by the detection of HPV DNA in the absence of any detectable HPV-associated lesion. Approximately 20% of sexually active adolescents have detectable HPV at any given time and have normal cytologic findings and no detectable lesions. External genital warts are much less common, occurring in <1% of adolescents. The most common clinically detected lesion in adolescent women is the cervical lesion termed **low-grade squamous intraepithelial lesion (LSIL)** (Table 258-1). This lesion appears to occur in 25-30% of adolescents infected with HPV. LSILs are considered benign cellular changes associated with HPV infection. As with HPV DNA detection, most LSILs regress spontaneously in young women and do not require any intervention or therapy. Less commonly, HPV can induce more severe cellular

Table 258-1 BETHESDA SYSTEM FOR REPORTING CERVICAL/VAGINAL CYTOLOGY

DESCRIPTIVE DIAGNOSIS OF EPITHELIAL CELL ABNORMALITIES	EQUIVALENT TERMINOLOGY
SQUAMOUS CELL	
Atypical squamous cells of undetermined significance (ASC-US)	Squamous atypia
Atypical squamous cells, cannot exclude HSIL (ASC-H)	
Low-grade squamous intraepithelial lesion (LSIL)	Mild dysplasia, condylomatous atypia, HPV-related changes, koilocytic atypia, cervical intraepithelial neoplasia (CIN) 1
High-grade squamous intraepithelial lesion (HSIL)	Moderate dysplasia, CIN 2, severe dysplasia, CIN 3, carcinoma in situ
GLANDULAR CELL	
Endometrial cells, cytologically benign, in a postmenopausal woman	
Atypical glandular cells of undetermined significance	
Endocervical adenocarcinoma	
Endometrial adenocarcinoma	
Extrauterine adenocarcinoma	
Adenocarcinoma, not otherwise specified	

changes, termed **high-grade squamous intraepithelial lesions (HSILs)** (Chapter 547).

Although HSILs are considered precancerous lesions, they rarely progress to invasive cancer. HSILs occur in approximately 0.4-3% of sexually active women, whereas invasive cervical cancer occurs in 8 cases/100,000 adult women. In true virginal populations, including children who are not sexually abused, rates of both clinical disease and HPV detection are very low to zero. In the USA, there are approximately 12,000 new cases and 3,700 deaths from cervical cancer each year. Worldwide, cervical cancer is the 2nd most common cause of cancer deaths among women.

Some infants may acquire papillomaviruses during passage through an infected birth canal, leading to recurrent **respiratory papillomatosis.** Cases also have been reported after cesarean section. The maximum incubation period for emergence of clinically apparent lesions (genital warts or laryngeal papillomas) after perinatally acquired infection is unknown but appears to be 6 mo (Chapter 382.2).

Genital warts appearing in later childhood may result from sexual abuse with HPV transmission during the abusive contact. Genital warts may represent a sexually transmitted infection even in some very young children. Their presence is cause to suspect that possibility. A child with genital warts should therefore be provided with a complete evaluation for evidence of possible abuse (Chapter 37.1), including the presence of other sexually transmitted infections (Chapter 114). Presence of genital warts in a child does not confirm sexual abuse, because perinatally transmitted genital warts may go undetected until the child is older. Typing for specific genital HPV types in children is not helpful in diagnosis or to confirm sexual abuse status, because the same genital types occur in both perinatal transmission and abuse. Nonetheless, the type detected in the infant is not always the same as the mother's type, suggesting other sources of HPV acquisition.

PATHOGENESIS

Initial HPV infection of the cervix is thought to begin by viral invasion of the basal cells of the epithelium, a process that is enhanced by disruption of the epithelium caused by trauma or inflammation. It is thought that the virus initially remains relatively dormant because virus is present without any evidence of clinical disease. The life cycle of HPV depends on the differentiation program of keratinocytes. The pattern of HPV transcription varies throughout the epithelial layer as well as through different stages of disease (LSIL, HSIL, invasive cancer). Understanding of HPV transcription enhances understanding of its ability to behave as an oncovirus. Early region proteins, E6 and E7, function as trans-activating factors that regulate cellular transformation. Complex interactions between E6- and E7-transcribed proteins and host proteins result in the perturbation of normal processes that regulate cellular DNA synthesis. The perturbations caused by E6 and E7 are primarily disruption of the anti-oncoproteins p53 and retinoblastoma protein (Rb), respectively, contributing to the development of anogenital cancers. Disruption of these proteins results in continued cell proliferation, even under the circumstances of DNA damage, which leads to basal cell proliferation, chromosomal abnormalities, and aneuploidy, hallmarks of SIL development.

Evidence of productive viral infection occurs in benign lesions such as external genital warts and LSILs, with the abundant expression of viral capsid proteins in the superficial keratinocytes. The appearance of the HPV-associated koilocyte is due to the expression of E4, a structural protein that causes collapse of the cytoskeleton. Low level expression of E6 and E7 proteins results in cell proliferation seen in the basal cell layer of LSILs. LSILs are a manifestation of active viral replication and protein expression. However, as the lesions advance in grade, expression of those products important in the process of cell transformation, such as E6 and E7, now predominate, rather than structural proteins, resulting in the chromosomal abnormalities and aneuploidy characteristic of the higher-grade lesions.

Cutaneous lesions (common and genital warts) are not associated with malignant HPV types and do not have any malignant potential except in the rare skin disorder **epidermodysplasia verruciformis.** Genital lesions caused by HPV may be broadly grouped into those with little to no malignant potential (low risk) and those with greater malignant potential (high risk). **Low-risk HPV types,** 6 and 11, are most commonly found in genital warts and are rarely if ever found isolated in malignant lesions. **High-risk HPV types,** specifically types 16 and 18, which cause about 70% of cervical cancer, are commonly found in SILs and invasive anogenital cancers. Other HPV types found in invasive cancers but at much lower frequencies include types 31, 33, 35, 39, 45, 51, 52, 56, 58, 59, 68, 73, and 82. HPV 16 is also most commonly found in women without lesions, making the connection with cancer confusing. Lesions may also be infected simultaneously with multiple HPV types. Almost all latent infections with low-risk types spontaneously resolve over time. Genital and common warts in general resolve without therapy but may take years to do so. Although 85-90% of high-risk type infections resolve as well, they are more likely than low-risk types to persist. This observation seems to be particularly true for HPV 16, which has a slower rate of regression than some of the other high-risk types. Persistent high-risk–type infections are associated with increased risk for development of HSILs and invasive cancer. LSILs have similar regression patterns as latent infection in young women: 92-95% of LSILs in young women spontaneously regress within 3 yr. Although HSILs are less likely to regress than latent infections or LSILs, progression to invasive cancer is still rare, with only 5-15% showing progression.

Most infants with recognized genital warts are infected with the low-risk types. In contrast, children with a history of sexual abuse have a clinical picture more like that of adult genital warts, consisting of mixed low- and high-risk types. There are rare reports of HPV-associated genital malignancies occurring in preadolescent children and adolescents. On the other hand, HSILs do occur in sexually active adolescents. There is also a concern that younger age of sexual debut has contributed to the increase

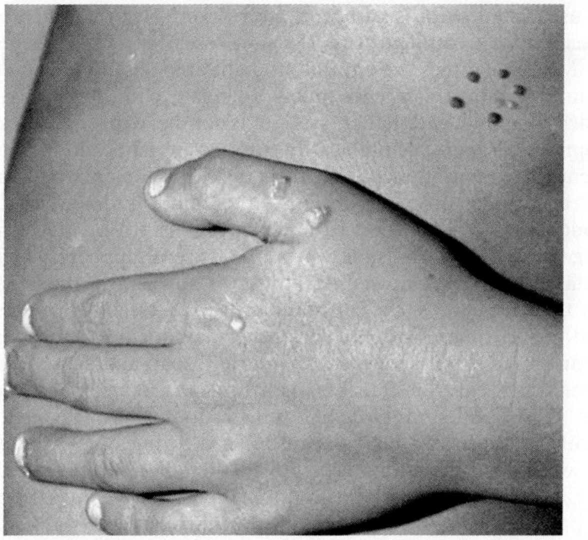

Figure 258-1 Common warts of the left hand and the chest wall. (From Meneghini CL, Bonifaz E: *An atlas of pediatric dermatology,* Chicago, 1986, Year Book Medical Publishers, p 45.)

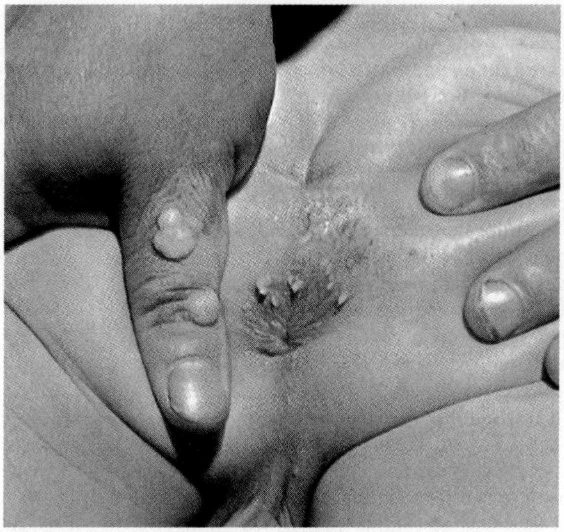

Figure 258-2 Common warts of the hand in a mother and perianal condylomata acuminata in her son. (From Meneghini CL, Bonifaz E: *An atlas of pediatric dermatology,* Chicago, 1986, Year Book Medical Publishers, p 44.)

in invasive cervical cancer seen in women <50 yr of age in the USA. HPV is considered necessary but not sufficient for the development of invasive cancers. Other risk factors for which there is relatively strong suggestive evidence of association include smoking, prolonged oral contraceptive use, *Chlamydia trachomatis* and herpes simplex virus infections, and greater parity.

CLINICAL MANIFESTATIONS

The clinical findings in HPV infection depend on the site of epithelial infection.

Skin Lesions

The typical HPV-induced lesions of the skin are proliferative, papular, and hyperkeratotic. Common warts are raised circinate lesions with a keratinized surface (Fig. 258-1). Plantar and palmar warts are practically flat. Multiple warts are common and may create a mosaic pattern. Flat warts appear as small (1-5 mm), flat, flesh-colored papules.

Genital Warts

Genital warts may be found throughout the perineum around the anus, vagina, and urethra, as well as in the cervical, intravaginal, and intra-anal areas (Fig. 258-2). Intra-anal warts occur predominantly in patients who have had receptive anal intercourse, in contrast with perianal warts, which may occur in men and women without a history of anal sex. Although rare, lesions caused by genital genotypes can also be found on other mucosal surfaces, such as conjunctivae, gingiva, and nasal mucosa. They may be single or multiple lesions and are frequently found in multiple anatomic sites. External genital warts can be flat, dome-shaped, keratotic, pedunculated, and cauliflower-shaped and may occur singly, in clusters, or as plaques. On mucosal epithelium, the lesions are softer. Depending on the size and anatomic location, lesions may be pruritic and painful, may cause burning with urination, may be friable and bleed, or may become superinfected. Adolescents are frequently disturbed by the development of genital lesions. Other rarer lesions caused by HPV of the external genital area include Bowen disease, bowenoid papulosis, squamous cell carcinomas, Buschke-Löwenstein tumors, and vulvar intraepithelial neoplasias (VINs).

Squamous intraepithelial lesions detected with cytology are usually invisible to the naked eye and require the aid of colposcopic magnification and acetic acid. With aid, the lesions appear white and show evidence of neovascularity. SILs can occur on the cervix, vagina, vulva, and intra-anus. Invasive cancers tend to be more exophytic, with aberrant-appearing vasculature. These lesions are rarely found in non–sexually active individuals.

Laryngeal Papillomatosis

The median age at onset of recurrent laryngeal papillomatosis is 3 yr. Children present with hoarseness, an altered cry, and sometimes stridor. Rapid growth of respiratory papillomas can occlude the upper airway, causing respiratory compromise. These lesions may recur within weeks of removal, requiring frequent surgery. The lesions do not become malignant unless treated with irradiation.

DIAGNOSIS

The diagnosis of external genital warts and common warts may be reliably determined by visual inspection of a lesion by an experienced observer and does not require additional tests for confirmation. A biopsy should be considered if the diagnosis is uncertain, the lesions do not respond to therapy, or the lesions worsen during therapy.

Screening for cervical cancer begins with cytology, which is either performed by Papanicolaou (Pap) smear or liquid-based cytology. Screening guidelines, which were updated in 2009 by the American Society for Colposcopy and Cervical Pathology (ASCCP) and American College of Obstetrics and Gynecology, recommend to start screening at age 21 yr. Screening earlier is more likely to result in unnecessary referrals for colposcopy, because most lesions in this group are likely to be LSILs and therefore to regress. Annual cytology is recommended until at least 3 normal cytology results are obtained. After this, the recommended frequency interval varies between 1-3 yr. The recommended terminology used for cytologic evaluation is based on the Bethesda system (see Table 258-1). Terminology used for histology is based on the World Health Organization recommendation using cervical intraepithelial neoplasia (CIN) 1, 2, and 3 (see Table 258-1). Although the purpose of screening is to identify CIN 3+ lesions, the majority of these lesions are found in women who were referred for **atypical squamous cells of undetermined significance (ASCUS)** or LSILs on cytology. On the other hand, few CIN 3 or cancers exist in adolescent populations. Cytologic evaluation of cervical cells is a screening test and not confirmatory. New guidelines often take years before their uptake. If cytology is obtained in an adolescent, the 2006 ASCCP guidelines for management of abnormal cytology and histology should be followed. For adolescents, ASCUS and LSIL are treated the same. The current recommendation for adolescents with ASCUS or LSIL is to repeat cytology every 12 mo for up to 24 mo. For persistent ASCUS or LSILs at 2 yr or 24 mo of follow-up, referral for colposcopy is recommended. Adolescents with HSIL at any visit should be referred for colposcopy and biopsy. In adult women, HSIL can be treated without histologic confirmation. However, this approach should be avoided in adolescents because HSIL is often misdiagnosed in this group.

In adult women older than 21 yr, high-risk HPV testing can be used to assist in ASCUS triage. The latter recommendation was based on the observations that adult women with ASCUS and a positive HPV test result for high-risk types are more likely to have CIN 2/3 than women with a negative HPV test result. HPV testing in adolescents, whether used for ASCUS triage or follow-up, is not recommended because of the high prevalence of HPV. If HPV testing is performed inadvertently, it is recommended to ignore the HPV test result. Once the LSIL is confirmed by histology (i.e., CIN 1), treatment of CIN 1 is not recommended; women can be followed with cytology at 12-mo intervals. An adolescent in whom histology confirms CIN 2/3 or CIN 2 can be followed by colposcopy and cytology at 6-mo intervals if the patient is compliant. If CIN 2/3 continues to persistent at 2 yr of follow-up, treatment is recommended. CIN 3 in adolescents is recommended to be treated as in adults. These guidelines and updates can be found at www.asccp.org.

Very sensitive tests for the presence of HPV DNA, RNA, and proteins are becoming generally available, although they are not required for the diagnosis of external genital warts or related conditions. There are no indications for HPV DNA testing in adolescents or children.

DIFFERENTIAL DIAGNOSIS

A number of other conditions should be considered, including condyloma latum, seborrheic keratoses, dysplastic and benign nevi, molluscum contagiosum, pearly penile papules, and neoplasms. Condyloma latum is due to secondary syphilis and can be diagnosed with dark-field microscopy and standard serologic tests for syphilis. Seborrheic keratoses are common, localized, hyperpigmented lesions that are rarely associated with malignancy. Molluscum contagiosum is caused by a poxvirus, is highly infectious, and is often umbilicated. Pearly penile papules occur at the penile corona and are normal variants that require no treatment.

TREATMENT

Most common (plantar, palmar, skin) warts eventually resolve spontaneously (Chapter 659). Symptomatic lesions should be removed. Removal includes a variety of self-applied therapies, including salicylic acid preparations and provider-applied therapies (cryotherapy, laser therapy, electrosurgery). Genital warts in children and adolescents are benign and usually remit, but only over an extended period. It is recommended that genital lesions be treated if the patient or the parent requests therapy. As for common warts, treatment is categorized into self-applied and provider-applied. No one therapy has been shown to be more efficacious than any other. Provider-applied therapies include surgical treatments (electrosurgery, surgical excision, laser surgery) and office-based treatment (cryotherapy with liquid nitrogen or a cryoprobe, podophyllin resin 10-25%, and bi- or tri-chloroacetic acid). Office-based treatments are usually applied once a week for 3-6 wk. Podophyllin resins have lost favor to other methods because of the variability in preparations. Intralesional interferon is no more effective than other therapies and is associated with significant adverse effects; this therapy is reserved for treatment of recalcitrant cases.

Many therapies are painful, and children should not undergo painful genital treatments unless adequate pain control is provided. Parents and patients should not be expected to apply painful therapies themselves. In adolescents and adults, recommended patient-applied treatment regimens for external genital warts include topical podofilox, imiquimod, and sinecatechins. Podofilox 0.5% solution (using a cotton swab) or gel (using a finger) is applied to visible warts in a cycle of applications twice a day for 3 days followed by 4 days of no therapy, repeated for up to a total of 4 cycles. Imiquimod 5% cream is applied at bedtime, 3 times a week, every other day, for up to 16 wk; the treated area should be washed with mild soap and water 6-10 hr after treatment. Sinecatechins is a topical product approved by the U.S. Food and Drug Administration (FDA) for external genital wart treatment that can be used 3 times daily for up to 16 wk. None of the patient-applied therapies are approved for use during pregnancy, and podophyllin resin is contraindicated in pregnancy. For any of the nonsurgical treatments, prescription is contraindicated in a patient with any history of hypersensitivity to any product constituents.

If HPV exposure as a result of sexual abuse is suspected or known, the clinician should ensure that the child's safety has been achieved and is maintained.

When indicated, the most common treatments for CIN 2/3 are ablative treatments, including cryotherapy and loop electrosurgical excisional procedure. Because laser therapy is expensive and requires anesthesia, its use has fallen from favor in relatively straightforward cases. Once confirmed by histology with CIN 1, LSILs can be observed indefinitely. Decision to treat a persistent CIN 1 rests between the provider and patient. Risks of treatment, including premature delivery in a pregnant patient, should be discussed prior to any treatment decision.

COMPLICATIONS

The presence of HPV lesions in the genital area may be a cause of profound embarrassment to a child or parent. Complications of therapy are uncommon; chronic pain (vulvodynia) or hypoesthesia may occur at the treatment site. Lesions may heal with hypopigmentation or hyperpigmentation and less commonly with depressed or hypertrophic scars. Surgical therapies can lead to infection and scarring. Premature delivery and low birthweight in future pregnancies are complications of excisional therapy for CIN.

It is estimated that 5-15% of untreated CIN 3 lesions will progress to cervical cancer. Most cancer is prevented by early detection and treatment of these lesions. Despite screening, cervical cancer develops rapidly in a few adolescents and young women. The reason for the rapid development of cancer in these rare cases remains unknown, but host genetic defects are likely underlying causes. Respiratory papillomas rarely become malignant, unless they have been treated with irradiation. Vulvar condylomas rarely become cancerous. HPV-associated cancers of the vagina, vulva, anus, penis, and oral cavity are much rarer than cervical tumors, and therefore screening for them is not currently recommended. However, these tumors are more common in women with cervical cancer; hence, it is recommended to screen women with cervical cancer for these tumors with visual inspection.

PROGNOSIS

With all forms of therapy, genital warts commonly recur, and approximately half of children and adolescents require a 2nd or 3rd treatment. Recurrence is also evident in patients with respiratory papillomatosis. Patients and parents should be warned of this likelihood. Combination therapy for genital warts (imiquimod and podofilox) does not improve response and may increase complications. Prognosis of cervical disease is better, with 85-90% cure rates after a single treatment with loop electrosurgical excision procedure (LEEP). Cryotherapy has a slight less cure rate. Recalcitrant disease should prompt an evaluation and is common in immunocompromised individuals, specifically men and women infected with HIV.

PREVENTION

The only means of preventing HPV infection is to avoid direct contact with lesions. Condoms may reduce the risk for HPV transmission; condoms also prevent other sexually transmitted infections, which are risk factors associated with SIL development. In addition, condoms appear to hasten the regression of LSILs in women. Avoiding smoking cigarettes is important in preventing cervical cancer. Prolonged oral contraceptive use and parity have been shown to be risks for cervical cancer. However, the mechanisms associated with these factors have not been identified, and consequently no change in counseling is recommended.

HPV vaccines show efficacy against type-specific persistence and development of type-specific disease. A quadrivalent HPV vaccine containing types 6, 11, 16, and 18 was licensed in the USA 2006, and a bivalent HPV vaccine containing types 16 and 18 in 2009. The efficacy of these vaccines is mediated by the development of neutralizing antibodies. Vaccination is recommended routinely for all girls at 11-12 yr of age and is administered intramuscularly in the deltoid region in a 3-dose series at 0, 1, 2, and 6 mo. It is important that vaccination take place in children before they become sexually active, because the rate of HPV acquisition is high shortly after the onset of sexual activity. Vaccine can be given to girls as young as 9 yr of age, and a catch-up vaccination is recommended in girls 13-26 yr. Individuals who are already infected with 1 or more vaccine-related HPV types prior to vaccination are protected from clinical disease caused by the remaining vaccine HPV types. However, the vaccines are not therapeutic. The quadrivalent vaccine is also licensed to be administered in a 3-dose series to males aged 9 through 26 years to reduce their likelihood of acquiring genital warts and developing anal dysplasia and cancer.

BIBLIOGRAPHY
Please visit the Nelson Textbook of Pediatrics *website at www.expertconsult.com for the complete bibliography.*

Chapter 259
Arboviral Encephalitis in North America

Scott B. Halstead

The arthropod-borne (arbovirus) viral encephalitides are a group of clinically similar severe neurologic infections caused by several different viruses. They are transmitted by mosquitoes during outdoor exposure in warmer weather in overlapping regions across most of the USA and much of southern Canada.

ETIOLOGY

The principal causes of the arthropod-borne encephalitides of North America are West Nile encephalitis (WNE), the St. Louis encephalitis (SLE), a complex of viruses included in the California encephalitis (CE) group of viruses, and, less frequently, western equine encephalitis (WEE), eastern equine encephalitis (EEE), and Colorado tick fever. The etiologic agents belong to different viral taxa: alphaviruses of the family Togaviridae (EEE and WEE), Flaviviridae (WNE, SLE), the California complex of the family Bunyaviridae (CE), and Reoviridae (Colorado tick fever virus). Alphaviruses are 69-nm, enveloped, positive-sense RNA viruses that evolved from a common Venezuelan equine encephalitis–like viral ancestor in the Western hemisphere. Flaviviruses are 40- to 50-nm, enveloped, positive-sense RNA viruses that evolved from a common ancestor. They are globally distributed and responsible for many important human viral diseases. The California serogroup, 1 of 16 Bunyavirus groups, are 75- to 115-nm enveloped viruses possessing a 3-segment, negative-sense RNA genome. Reoviruses are 60- to 80-nm double-stranded RNA viruses.

EPIDEMIOLOGY

Eastern Equine Encephalitis

In the USA, EEE is a very low incidence disease, with a median of 8 cases occurring annually in the Atlantic and Gulf States from 1964-2007 (Fig. 259-1). Transmission occurs often in focal endemic areas of the coast of Massachusetts, the 6 southern counties of New Jersey, and northeastern Florida. In North America, the virus is maintained in freshwater swamps in a zoonotic cycle involving *Culiseta melanura* and birds. Various other mosquito species obtain viremic meals from birds and transmit the virus to horses and humans. Virus activity varies markedly from year to year in response to still unknown ecologic factors. Most infections in birds are silent, but infections in pheasants are often fatal, and epizootics in these species are used as sentinels for periods of increased viral activity. Cases have been recognized on Caribbean islands. The case : infection ratio is lowest in children (1 : 8) and somewhat higher in adults (1 : 29).

Western Equine Encephalitis

WEE infections occur principally in the USA and Canada west of the Mississippi River (see Fig. 259-1), mainly in rural areas where water impoundments, irrigated farmland, and naturally flooded land provide breeding sites for *Culex tarsalis*. The virus is transmitted in a cycle involving mosquitoes, birds, and other vertebrate hosts. Humans and horses are susceptible to encephalitis. The case : infection ratio varies by age, having been estimated at 1 : 58 in children younger than 4 yr and 1 : 1,150 in adults. Infections are most severe at the extremes of life; a third of cases occur in children younger than 1 yr. Recurrent human epidemics have been reported from the Yakima Valley in Washington State and the Central Valley of California; the largest outbreak on record resulted in 3,400 cases and occurred in Minnesota, North and South Dakota, Nebraska, and Montana as well as Alberta, Manitoba, and Saskatchewan, Canada. Epizootics in horses precede human epidemics by several weeks. For the past 20 yr, only 3 cases of WEE have been reported, presumably reflecting successful mosquito abatement.

St. Louis Encephalitis

Cases of SLE are reported from nearly all states; the highest attack rates occur in the Gulf and central states (see Fig. 259-1). Epidemics frequently occur in urban and suburban areas; the largest, in 1975, involved 1,800 persons living in Houston, Chicago, Memphis, and Denver. Cases often cluster in areas where there is ground water or septic systems, which support mosquito breeding. The principal vectors are *Culex pipiens* and *Culex quinquefasciatus* in the central Gulf States, *Culex nigripalpus* in Florida, and *Culex tarsalis* in California. SLE virus is maintained in nature in a bird-mosquito cycle. Viral amplification occurs in bird species abundant in residential areas (e.g., sparrows, blue jays, and doves). Virus is transmitted in the late summer and early fall. The case : infection ratio may be as high as 1 : 300. Age-specific attack rates are lowest in children and highest in individuals older than 60 yr. The most recent small outbreaks were in Florida in 1990 and Louisiana in 2001. For the past 15 years there have been a mean of 18 cases annually.

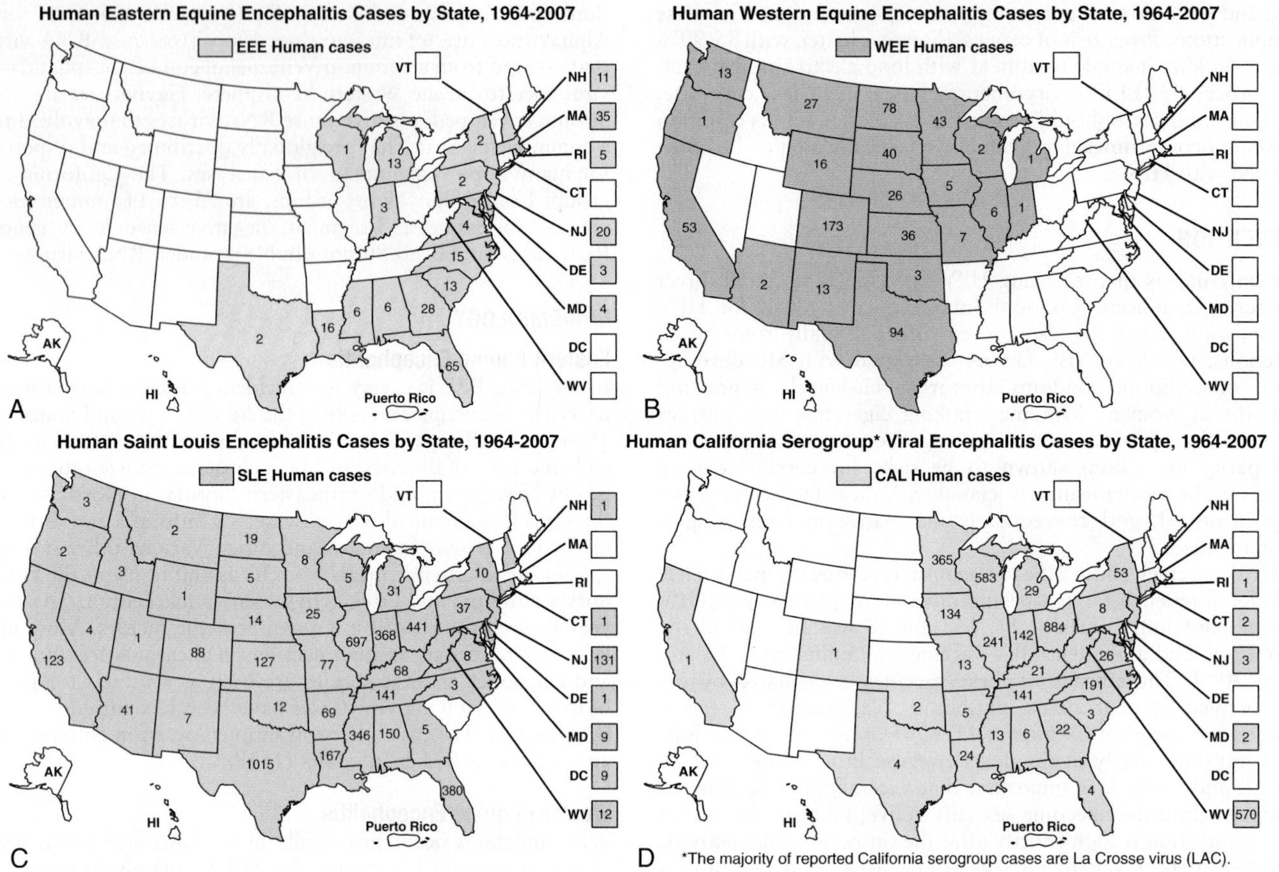

Figure 259-1 The distribution and incidence of reported cases of eastern equine encephalitis *(A)*, western equine encephalitis *(B)*, St. Louis encephalitis *(C)*, and California serogroup encephalitis *(D)* reported by state to the Centers for Disease Control and Prevention, 1964–2007.

West Nile Encephalitis

WNE virus has been implicated as the cause of sporadic summertime cases of human encephalitis and meningitis in Israel, India, Pakistan, Romania, Russia, and the USA. All American WNE viruses are genetically similar and are related to a virus recovered from a goose in Israel in 1998. WNE virus survives in a broad enzootic cycle in the USA and within 4 yr had spread to most states east of the Rocky Mountains plus California (Fig. 259-2). Every state in the continental USA plus 9 provinces in Canada have reported mosquito, bird, mammalian, or human West Nile infection. Through the end of 2008 28,813 total cases had been reported, 30-40% of which were encephalitis, with 1064 deaths. Summer/fall epidemics are common (Fig. 259-3). West Nile virus has entered the blood supply through asymptomatic viremic blood donors. Blood banks screen for West Nile virus RNA (Fig. 259-4). West Nile virus has also been transmitted to humans via the placenta, breast milk, and organ transplantation. Throughout its range, the virus is maintained in nature by transmission between mosquitoes of the *Culex* genus and various species of birds. In the USA, human infections are largely acquired from *Culex pipiens*. Horses are the non-avian vertebrates most likely to exhibit disease with WNE infection. During the 2002 transmission season, 14,000 equine cases were reported, with a mortality rate of 30%. Disease occurs predominantly in individuals >50 yr of age.

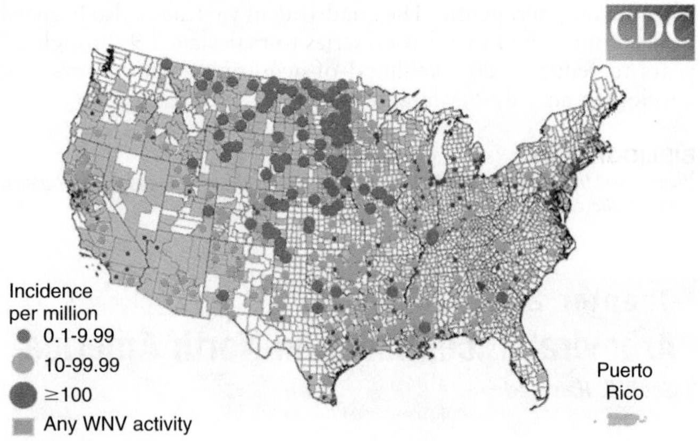

Figure 259-2 Incidence of West Nile virus neuroinvasive disease in humans—USA, 2008. (From the Centers for Disease Control and Prevention: West Nile virus activity—United States, January 1-December 31, 2008 as reported to CDC's ArboNET system.)

La Crosse/California Encephalitis

La Crosse viral infections are endemic in the USA, occurring annually from July to September, principally in the north-central and central states (See Fig. 259-1). Infections occur in peridomestic environments as the result of bites from *Aedes triseriatus* mosquitoes, which often breed in tree holes. The virus is maintained vertically in nature by transovarial transmission and can be spread between mosquitoes by copulation and amplified in mosquito populations by viremic infections in various vertebrate hosts. Amplifying hosts include chipmunks, squirrels, foxes, and woodchucks. A case:infection ratio of 1:22-300 has been surmised. La Crosse encephalitis is principally a disease of children, who may account for to 75% of cases. A mean of 100 cases have been reported annually for the past 10 years.

Colorado Tick Fever

Colorado tick fever virus is transmitted by the wood tick *Dermacentor andersoni*, which inhabits high-elevation areas of states

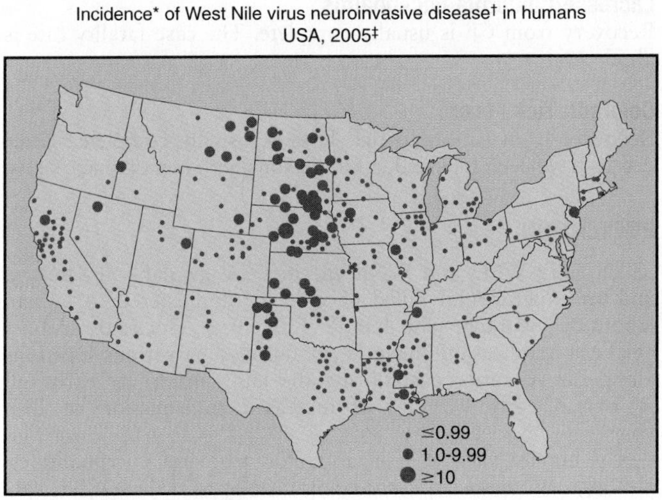

*Per 100,000 county residents.
†Meningitis, encephalitis, or acute flaccid paralysis.
‡Provisional data as of December 1, 2005.

Figure 259-3 Number of reported West Nile virus neuroinvasive disease† cases in humans, by week of illness onset—USA, 2005.‡ (From the Centers for Disease Control and Prevention: West Nile virus activity—United States, January 1-December 1, 2005, *MMWR Morbid Mortal Wkly Rep* 54:1253–1256, 2005.)

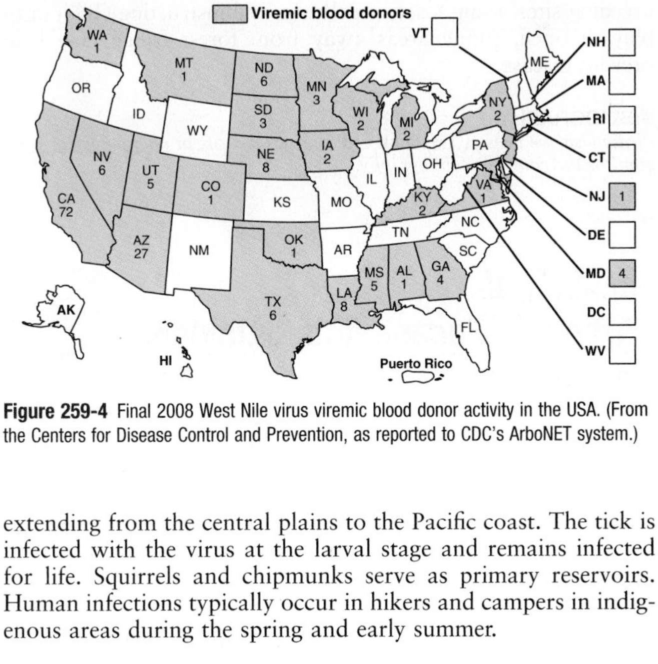

Figure 259-4 Final 2008 West Nile virus viremic blood donor activity in the USA. (From the Centers for Disease Control and Prevention, as reported to CDC's ArboNET system.)

extending from the central plains to the Pacific coast. The tick is infected with the virus at the larval stage and remains infected for life. Squirrels and chipmunks serve as primary reservoirs. Human infections typically occur in hikers and campers in indigenous areas during the spring and early summer.

CLINICAL MANIFESTATIONS

The arboviruses produce symptoms of encephalitis, except West Nile virus and Colorado tick fever virus, which most commonly manifest as flulike illnesses and only occasionally cause encephalitis.

Eastern Equine Encephalitis

EEE virus Infections result in fulminant encephalitis with a rapid progression to coma and death in one third of cases. In infants and children, abrupt onset of fever, irritability, and headache are followed by lethargy, confusion, seizures, and coma. High temperature, bulging fontanel, stiff neck, and generalized flaccid or spastic paralysis are observed. There may be a brief prodrome of fever, headache, and dizziness. Unlike most other viral encephalitides, the peripheral white blood cell count usually demonstrates a marked leukocytosis, and the cerebrospinal fluid (CSF) may show marked pleocytosis. Pathologic changes are found in the cortical and gray matter, with viral antigens localized to neurons. There is necrosis of neurons, neutrophilic infiltration, and perivascular cuffing by lymphocytes.

Western Equine Encephalitis

In WEE, there may be a prodrome with symptoms of an upper respiratory tract infection. The onset is usually sudden with chills, fever, dizziness, drowsiness, increasing headache, malaise, nausea and vomiting, stiff neck, and disorientation. Infants typically present with the sudden cessation of feeding, fussiness, fever, and protracted vomiting. Convulsions and lethargy develop rapidly. On physical examination, patients are somnolent, exhibit meningeal signs, and have generalized motor weakness and reduced deep tendon reflexes. In infants, a bulging fontanel, spastic paralysis, and generalized convulsions may be observed. On pathologic examination, disseminated small focal abscesses, small focal hemorrhages, and patchy areas of demyelination are distinctive.

St. Louis Encephalitis

Clinical manifestations of SLE vary from a mild flulike illness to fatal encephalitis. There may be a prodrome of nonspecific symptoms with subtle changes in coordination or mentation of several days to 1wk in duration. Early signs and symptoms include fever, photophobia, headache, malaise, nausea, vomiting, and neck stiffness. About half of patients exhibit abrupt onset of weakness, incoordination, disturbed sensorium, restlessness, confusion, lethargy, and delirium or coma. The peripheral white blood cell count is modestly elevated, with 100-200 cells/mm^3 found in the CSF. On autopsy, the brain shows scattered foci of neuronal damage and perivascular inflammation.

West Nile Encephalitis

WNE may be asymptomatic, but when clinical features appear, they include an abrupt onset of high fever, headache, myalgias, and nonspecific signs of emesis, rash, abdominal pain, or diarrhea. Most infections manifest as a flulike febrile illness, whereas a minority of patients demonstrate meningitis or encephalitis or both. Rarely there may be cardiac dysrhythmias, myocarditis, rhabdomyolysis, optic neuritis, uveitis, retinitis, orchitis, pancreatitis, or hepatitis. WNE disease in the USA has been accompanied by prolonged lymphopenia and an acute asymmetric polio-like paralytic illness with CSF pleocytosis involving the anterior horn cells of the spinal cord. A striking but uncommon feature has been Parkinsonism and movement disorders (with tremor and myoclonus).

Lacrosse/California Encephalitis

The clinical spectrum includes a mild febrile illness, aseptic meningitis, and fatal encephalitis. Children typically present with a prodrome of 2-3 days with fever, headache, malaise, and vomiting. The disease evolves with clouding of the sensorium, lethargy, and, in severe cases, focal or generalized seizures. On physical examination, children are lethargic but not disoriented. Focal neurologic signs, including weakness, aphasia, and focal or generalized seizures, have been reported in 16-25% of cases. CSF shows low to moderate leukocyte counts. On autopsy, the brain shows focal areas of neuronal degeneration, inflammation, and perivascular cuffing.

Colorado Tick Fever

Colorado tick fever begins with the abrupt onset of a flulike illness, including high temperature, malaise, arthralgias and myalgia, vomiting, headache, and decreased sensorium. Rash is uncommon. The symptoms rapidly disappear after 3 days of illness. However, in approximately half of patients, a 2nd identical episode recurs 24-72 hr after the 1st, producing the typical "saddleback" temperature curve of Colorado tick fever.

Complications, including encephalitis, meningoencephalitis, and a bleeding diathesis, develop in 3-7% of infected persons and may be more common in children younger than 12 yr.

DIAGNOSIS

The etiologic diagnosis of a specific arboviral infection is established by testing an acute-phase serum ≥5 days after onset of illness for the presence of virus-specific immunoglobulin (Ig) M antibodies using an indirect immunofluorescence test or an enzyme-linked immunosorbent assay (ELISA) IgM capture test. Alternatively, acute and convalescent sera can be tested for a fourfold or greater increase in ELISA, hemagglutination inhibition, or neutralizing IgG antibody titers. Commercial serologic diagnostic kits are marketed, especially for West Nile viral infections. Serum and CSF should be tested for West Nile virus–specific IgM. However, IgM may reflect past infection, because it may be present up to 12 mo after infection. The diagnosis may also be established by isolation in cell cultures of virus in brain tissue, obtained by brain biopsy or at autopsy, or by identification of viral RNA reverse transcriptase polymerase chain reactions.

The diagnosis of encephalitis may be aided by CT or MRI and by electroencephalography. Focal seizures or focal findings on CT or MRI or electroencephalography should suggest the possibility of herpes simplex encephalitis, which should be treated with acyclovir (Chapter 244).

TREATMENT

There is no specific treatment for arboviral encephalitides, although oral ribavirin may have been of benefit in a case of La Crosse encephalitis. The treatment of acute arboviral encephalitis is intensive supportive care (Chapter 62), including control of seizures (Chapter 586).

PROGNOSIS

Fatalities occur with all arboviral encephalitides. With the exception of EEE, most resolve without residua.

Eastern Equine Encephalitis

The prognosis in EEE is better for patients with a prolonged prodrome; the occurrence of convulsions conveys a poor prognosis. Patient fatality rates are 33-75% and are highest in the elderly. Residual neurologic defects are common, especially in children.

Western Equine Encephalitis

Patient fatality rates in WEE are 3-9% and highest in the elderly. Major neurologic sequelae have been reported in up to 13% of cases and may be as high as 30% in infants. Parkinsonian syndrome has been reported as a residual in adult survivors.

St. Louis Encephalitis

The principal risk factor for fatal outcome of SLE is advanced age, with patient fatality rates being as high as 80% in early outbreaks. In children, mortality rates are 2-5%. In adults, underlying hypertensive cardiovascular disease has been a risk factor for fatal outcome. Recovery from SLE is usually complete, but the rate of serious neurologic sequelae has been reported to be as high as 10% in children.

West Nile Encephalitis

Cases of and deaths due to WNE occur mainly in the elderly, although many serologic surveys show that persons of all ages are infected. During 2002-2004, there were 648 deaths among 16,557 cases, a 3.8% mortality rate. Paralysis may result in permanent weakness.

Lacrosse/California Encephalitis

Recovery from CE is usually complete. The case fatality rate is about 1%.

Colorado Tick Fever

Recovery from Colorado tick fever is usually complete. Three deaths have been reported, all in persons with hemorrhagic signs.

PREVENTION

Killed EEE, WEE, and WNE vaccines are available for horses, and an experimental killed vaccine is administered to human laboratory workers who handle EEE virus. Flocks of sentinel chickens or pheasants have been stationed at various locations along the Atlantic coast during the late summer or early fall to obtain early warning of increased transmission of EEE virus.

No human vaccine is licensed for arboviral encephalitides, although WNE vaccines are being developed. Killed WNE vaccines are licensed for veterinary use. Extensive water management and mosquito abatement programs in California have reduced transmission of WEE and the incidence of human infections. Urban WNE and SLE outbreaks in the eastern USA, Texas, and the Midwest have been controlled by the application of ultra-low-volume adulticide chemicals applied from trucks or low-flying aircraft.

Because infections in children may occur as a result of summer daytime mosquito biting in residential areas, sealing mosquito breeding sites, using insect repellents, and instructing children to play in open, sunny areas away from forest fringe may help prevent disease.

BIBLIOGRAPHY

Please visit the Nelson Textbook of Pediatrics *website at* *www.expertconsult.com* *for the complete bibliography.*

Chapter 260
Arboviral Encephalitis outside North America

Scott B. Halstead

The principal causes of arboviral encephalitis outside North America are Venezuelan equine encephalitis (VEE) virus, Japanese encephalitis (JE) virus, tick-borne encephalitis (TBE), and West Nile (WN) virus (Table 260-1).

260.1 Venezuelan Equine Encephalitis

Scott B. Halstead

The VEE virus was isolated from an epizootic in Venezuelan horses in 1938. Human cases were first identified in 1943. Hundreds of thousands of equine and human cases have occurred over the past 70 yr. During 1971, epizootics moved through Central America and Mexico to southern Texas. After 2 decades of quiescence, epizootic disease emerged again in Venezuela and Colombia in 1995.

ETIOLOGY

VEE is an alphavirus of the family Togaviridae. VEE circulates in nature in 6 subtypes. Virus types I and III have multiple antigenic variants. Types IAB and IC have caused epizootics and human epidemics.

Table 260-1 VECTORS AND GEOGRAPHIC DISTRIBUTION OF ARBOVIRAL ENCEPHALITIS OUTSIDE NORTH AMERICA

GENUS	VIRUS AND DISEASE	VECTOR	GEOGRAPHIC DISTRIBUTION
Flavivirus	Japanese encephalitis	*Culex tritaeniorhynchus*	Asia/Japan to Sri Lanka
	Murray Valley encephalitis	*Culex annulirostris*	Eastern Australia
	Rocio	*Psorophora* or *Aedes*	Sao Paulo, Brazil
	West Nile	*Culex* and others	Europe to Australia
	Tick-borne encephalitis	*Ixodes ricinus*	Europe
		Ixodes persulcatus	Russia
Togavirus	Venezuelan equine encephalitis	*Culex* and others	Northern South America

EPIDEMIOLOGY

The majority of epizootics resulting from types IAB and IC have occurred in Venezuela and Colombia. The virus resides in ill-defined sylvatic reservoirs in the South American rain forests. Known hosts include rodents and aquatic birds with transmission by *Culex melaconion* species. Vectors for horse-to-horse and horse-to-human transmission include *Aedes taeniorhynchus* and *Psorophora confinnis.* Epizootics move rapidly, up to several miles per day. Human cases are proportional to and follow epizootic occurrences. Viremia levels in human blood are high enough to infect mosquitoes. Because virus can be recovered from human pharyngeal swabs, and household attack rates are often as high as 50%, it is widely believed that person-to-person transmission occurs, although direct evidence is lacking. Virus types II-VI are restricted to relatively small foci; each has a unique vector-host relationship and rarely results in human infections.

CLINICAL MANIFESTATIONS

The incubation period is 2-5 days, followed by the abrupt onset of fever, chills, headache, sore throat, myalgia, malaise, prostration, photophobia, nausea, vomiting, and diarrhea. In 5-10% of cases, there is a biphasic illness; the 2nd phase is heralded by seizures, projectile vomiting, ataxia, confusion, agitation, and mild disturbances in consciousness. There is cervical lymphadenopathy and conjunctival suffusion. Cases of meningoencephalitis may demonstrate **cranial nerve palsy,** motor weakness, paralysis, seizures, and coma. Microscopic examination of tissues reveals inflammatory infiltrates in lymph nodes, spleen, lung, liver, and brain. Lymph nodes show cellular depletion, necrosis of germinal centers, and lymphophagocytosis. The liver shows patchy hepatocellular degeneration, the lungs demonstrate a diffuse interstitial pneumonia with intra-alveolar hemorrhages, and the brain shows patchy cellular infiltrates.

DIAGNOSIS

The etiologic diagnosis of VEE is established by testing an acute-phase serum collected early in the illness for the presence of virus-specific immunoglobulin (Ig) M antibodies or, alternatively, demonstrating a fourfold or greater increase in IgG antibody titers by testing paired acute and convalescent sera. The virus can also be identified by polymerase chain reaction (PCR).

TREATMENT

There is no specific treatment for VEE. The treatment is intensive supportive care (Chapter 62), including control of seizures (Chapter 586).

PROGNOSIS

In patients with VE meningoencephalitis, the fatality rate ranges from 10% to 25%. Sequelae include nervousness, forgetfulness, recurrent headache, and easy fatigability.

PREVENTION

Several veterinary vaccines are available to protect equines. VEE virus is highly infectious in laboratory settings, and biosafety level 3 containment should be used. An experimental vaccine is available for use in laboratory workers.

BIBLIOGRAPHY

Please visit the Nelson Textbook of Pediatrics *website at* *www.expertconsult.com* *for the complete bibliography.*

260.2 Japanese Encephalitis

Scott B. Halstead

Epidemics of encephalitis were reported in Japan from the late 1800s.

ETIOLOGY

JE virus is a positive-sense, single-stranded RNA virus of the family Flaviviridae.

EPIDEMIOLOGY

JE is a mosquito-borne viral disease of humans as well as horses, swine, and other domestic animals that causes human infections and acute disease in a vast area of Asia, northern Japan, Korea, China, Taiwan, Philippines, and the Indonesian archipelago and from Indochina through the Indian subcontinent. *Culex tritaeniorhynchus summarosus,* a night-biting mosquito that feeds preferentially on large domestic animals and birds but only infrequently on humans, is the principal vector of zoonotic and human JE in northern Asia. A more complex ecology prevails in southern Asia. From Taiwan to India, *C. tritaeniorhynchus* and members of the closely related *Culex vishnui* group are vectors. Before the introduction of JE vaccine, summer outbreaks of JE occurred regularly in Japan, Korea, China, Okinawa, and Taiwan. Over the past decade, there has been a pattern of steadily enlarging recurrent seasonal outbreaks in Vietnam, Thailand, Nepal, and India, with small outbreaks in the Philippines, Indonesia, and the northern tip of Queensland, Australia. Seasonal rains are accompanied by increases in mosquito populations and JE transmission. Pigs serve as amplifying host.

The annual incidence in endemic areas ranges from 1-10/10,000 population. Children <15 yr of age are principally affected, with nearly universal exposure by adulthood. The case : infection ratio for JE virus has been variously estimated at 1:25 to 1:1,000. Higher ratios have been estimated for populations indigenous to enzootic areas. JE occurs in travelers visiting Asia; therefore, a travel history in the diagnosis of encephalitis is critical.

CLINICAL MANIFESTATIONS

After a 4- to 14-day incubation period, cases typically progress through the following 4 stages: prodromal illness (2-3 days), acute stage (3-4 days), subacute stage (7-10 days), and convalescence (4-7 wk). Onset may be characterized by abrupt onset of fever, headache, respiratory symptoms, anorexia, nausea, abdominal pain, vomiting, and sensory changes, including psychotic episodes. Grand mal seizures are seen in 10-24% of children with JE; parkinsonian-like nonintention tremor and cogwheel rigidity are seen less frequently. Particularly characteristic are **rapidly** changing central nervous system signs (e.g., hyperreflexia followed by hyporeflexia or plantar responses that change). The sensory status of the patient may vary from confusion through disorientation and delirium to somnolence, progressing to coma. There is usually a mild pleocytosis (100-1,000 leukocytes/mm^3) in the cerebrospinal fluid, initially polymorphonuclear but in a few days predominantly lymphocytic. Albuminuria is common. Fatal cases usually progress rapidly to coma, and the patient dies within 10 days.

DIAGNOSIS

JE should be suspected in patients reporting exposure to night-biting mosquitoes in endemic areas during the transmission season. The etiologic diagnosis of JE is established by testing an acute-phase serum collected early in the illness for the presence of virus-specific IgM antibodies or, alternatively, demonstrating a fourfold or greater increase in IgG antibody titers by testing paired acute and convalescent sera. The virus can also be identified by PCR.

TREATMENT

There is no specific treatment for JE. The treatment is intensive supportive care (Chapter 62), including control of seizures (Chapter 586).

PROGNOSIS

Patient fatality rates for JE are 24-42% and are highest in children 5-9 yr of age and in adults older than 65 yr. The frequency of sequelae is 5-70% and is directly related to the age of the patient and severity of disease. Sequelae are most common in patients younger than 10 yr at the onset of disease. The more common sequelae are mental deterioration, severe emotional instability, personality changes, motor abnormalities, and speech disturbances.

PREVENTION

Travelers to endemic countries who plan to be in rural areas of the endemic region during the expected period of seasonal transmission and travelers in rural areas experiencing endemic transmission should receive JE vaccine. An inactivated vaccine manufactured in Japan by intracerebral injection of young mice and available throughout the world has been taken off the market owing to a high incidence of adverse events. In 2008-2009, tissue culture–based JE vaccine (IXIARO) was licensed in Europe, Australia, and the USA. In the USA, this vaccine (also called IC51) is licensed for use in older children and adults and is distributed by Novartis (Basel). For this vaccine, JE virus is grown in Vero cells, then formalin inactivated and administered intramuscularly as two 0.5-mL doses, 28 days apart. The final dose should be completed at least 1 wk prior to the patient's expected arrival in a JE endemic area. This vaccine contains alum and protamine sulfate and has exhibited only mild adverse events. A highly efficacious live-attenuated single-dose JE vaccine developed in China for children is licensed and marketed in some Asian countries. This vaccine can be co-administered with live-attenuated measles vaccine without altering the immune responses to either vaccine. In humans, prior dengue virus infection provides partial protection from clinical JE.

Personal measures should be taken to reduce exposure to mosquito bites, especially for short-term residents in endemic areas. They consist of avoiding evening outdoor exposure, using insect repellents, covering the body with clothing, and using bed nets or house screening.

Commercial pesticides, widely used by rice farmers in Asia, are effective in reducing populations of *C. tritaeniorhynchus*. Fenthion, fenitrothion, and phenthoate are effectively adulticidal and larvicidal. Insecticides may be applied from portable sprayers or from helicopters or light aircraft.

BIBLIOGRAPHY

Please visit the Nelson Textbook of Pediatrics *website at* *www.expertconsult.com* *for the complete bibliography.*

260.3 Tick-Borne Encephalitis

Scott B. Halstead

TBE was identified by Russian scientists in 1937 and was subsequently shown to be widespread in Europe, where it was identified as the cause of milk-borne encephalitis.

ETIOLOGY

TBE virus is a positive-sense, single-stranded RNA virus of the family Flaviviridae.

EPIDEMIOLOGY

TBE refers to neurotropic tick-transmitted flaviviral infections occurring across the Eurasian land mass. In the Far East, the disease is called *Russian spring-summer encephalitis*; the milder, often biphasic form in Europe is simply called tick-borne encephalitis. TBE is found in all countries of Europe except Portugal and the Benelux countries. The incidence is particularly high in Austria, Poland, Hungary, Czech Republic, Slovakia, former Yugoslavia, and Russia. The incidence tends to be very focal. Seroprevalence is as high as 50% in farm and forestry workers. The majority of cases occur in adults, but even young children may be infected while playing in the woods or on picnics or camping trips. The seasonal distribution of cases is midsummer in southern Europe, with a longer season in Scandinavia and the Russian Far East. TBE can be excreted from the milk of goats, sheep, or cows. Before World War II, when milk was consumed unpasteurized, milk-borne cases of TBE were common.

Viruses are transmitted principally by hard ticks of *Ixodes ricinus* in Europe and *Ixodes persulcatus* in the Far East. Viral circulation is maintained by a combination of transmission from ticks to birds, rodents, and larger mammals and transtadial transmission from larval to nymphal and adult stages. In some parts of Europe and Russia, ticks feed actively during the spring and early fall, giving rise to the name "spring-summer encephalitis."

CLINICAL MANIFESTATIONS

After an incubation period of 7-14 days, the European form begins as an acute nonspecific febrile illness that is followed in 5-30% of cases by meningoencephalitis. The Far Eastern variety more often results in encephalitis with higher case fatality and sequelae rates. The 1st phase of illness is characterized by fever, headache, myalgia, malaise, nausea, and vomiting for 2-7 days. Fever disappears and after 2-8 days may return accompanied by vomiting, photophobia, and signs of meningeal irritation in children and more severe encephalitic signs in adults. This phase rarely lasts more than 1 wk.

DIAGNOSIS

The diagnosis of TBE should be suspected in any patient reporting a tick bite in an endemic area during the transmission season. The etiologic diagnosis of TBE is established by testing an acute-phase serum collected early in the illness for the presence of virus-specific IgM antibodies or, alternatively, demonstrating a fourfold or greater increase in IgG antibody titers by testing paired acute and convalescent sera. The virus can also be identified by PCR.

TREATMENT

There is no specific treatment for TBE. The treatment is intensive supportive care (Chapter 62), including control of seizures (Chapter 586).

PROGNOSIS

The main risk for fatal outcome is advanced age; the fatality rate in adults is about 1%, but sequelae in children are rare. Transient unilateral paralysis of an upper extremity is a common finding in adults. Common sequelae include chronic fatigue, headache, sleep disorders, and emotional disturbances.

PREVENTION

Specific Ig has been given to persons with seasonal tick bite exposure, although efficacy of this preventive therapy is not well studied. Effective inactivated vaccines for human use, made from virus grown in tissue culture, are licensed in Russia and Europe. They are administered in a 3-dose series.

BIBLIOGRAPHY
Please visit the Nelson Textbook of Pediatrics *website at* *www.expertconsult.com* *for the complete bibliography.*

Chapter 261
Dengue Fever and Dengue Hemorrhagic Fever

Scott B. Halstead

Dengue fever, a benign syndrome caused by several arthropod-borne viruses, is characterized by biphasic fever, myalgia or arthralgia, rash, leukopenia, and lymphadenopathy. **Dengue hemorrhagic fever** (Philippine, Thai, or Singapore hemorrhagic fever; hemorrhagic dengue; acute infectious thrombocytopenic purpura) is a severe, often fatal, febrile disease caused by dengue viruses. It is characterized by capillary permeability, abnormalities of hemostasis, and, in severe cases, a protein-losing shock syndrome (**dengue shock syndrome**), which is thought to have an immunopathologic basis.

ETIOLOGY

There are at least 4 distinct antigenic types of dengue virus, which is a member of the family Flaviviridae. In addition, 3 other arthropod-borne viruses (arboviruses) cause similar or identical febrile diseases with rash (Table 261-1).

Table 261-1 VECTORS AND GEOGRAPHIC DISTRIBUTION OF DENGUE-LIKE DISEASES

VIRUS	GEOGRAPHIC GENUS AND DISEASE	VECTOR	DISTRIBUTION
Togavirus	Chikungunya	*Aedes aegypti* *Aedes africanus*	Africa, India, Southeast Asia
Togavirus	O'nyong-nyong	*Anopheles funestus*	East Africa
Flavivirus	West Nile fever	*Culex molestus* *Culex univittatus*	Europe, Africa, Middle East, India

EPIDEMIOLOGY

Dengue viruses are transmitted by mosquitoes of the Stegomyia family. *Aedes aegypti*, a daytime biting mosquito, is the principal vector, and all 4 virus types have been recovered from it. In most tropical areas, *A. aegypti* is highly urbanized, breeding in water stored for drinking or bathing and in rainwater collected in any container. Dengue viruses have also been recovered from *Aedes albopictus*, as in the 2001 Hawaiian epidemic, whereas outbreaks in the Pacific area have been attributed to several other *Aedes* species. These species breed in water trapped in vegetation. In Southeast Asia and West Africa, dengue virus may be maintained in a cycle involving canopy-feeding jungle monkeys and *Aedes* species, which feed on monkeys.

Epidemics were common in temperate areas of the Americas, Europe, Australia, and Asia until early in the 20th century. Dengue fever and dengue-like disease are now endemic in tropical Asia, the South Pacific Islands, northern Australia, tropical Africa, the Caribbean, and Central and South America. Dengue fever occurs frequently among travelers to these areas. Locally acquired disease has been reported in Florida and Texas, and imported cases in the USA occur in travelers to endemic areas.

Dengue outbreaks in urban areas infested with *A. aegypti* may be explosive; up to 70-80% of the population may be involved. Most disease occurs in older children and adults. Because *A. aegypti* has a limited flight range, spread of an epidemic occurs mainly through viremic human beings and follows the main lines of transportation. Sentinel cases may infect household mosquitoes; a large number of nearly simultaneous secondary infections give the appearance of a contagious disease. Where dengue is endemic, children and susceptible foreigners may be the only persons to acquire overt disease, adults having become immune.

Dengue-Like Diseases

Dengue-like diseases may also occur in epidemics. Epidemiologic features depend on the vectors and their geographic distribution (see Table 261-1). Chikungunya virus is widespread in the most populous areas of the world. In Asia, *A. aegypti* is the principal vector; in Africa, other Stegomyia species may be important vectors. In Southeast Asia, dengue and chikungunya outbreaks occur concurrently. Outbreaks of o'nyong-nyong and West Nile fever usually involve villages or small towns, in contrast to the urban outbreaks of dengue and chikungunya.

Dengue Hemorrhagic Fever

Dengue hemorrhagic fever occurs where multiple types of dengue virus are simultaneously or sequentially transmitted. It is endemic in all of tropical America and Asia, where warm temperatures and the practices of water storage in homes plus outdoor breeding sites result in large, permanent populations of *A. aegypti*. Under these conditions, infections with dengue viruses of all types are common, and 2nd infections with heterologous types are frequent.

Second dengue infections are relatively mild in the majority of instances, ranging from an inapparent infection through an undifferentiated upper respiratory tract or dengue-like disease, but may also progress to dengue hemorrhagic fever. Nonimmune foreigners, both adults and children, who are exposed to dengue virus during outbreaks of hemorrhagic fever have classic dengue fever or even milder disease. The differences in clinical manifestations of dengue infections between natives and foreigners in Southeast Asia are related more to immunologic status than to racial susceptibility. Dengue hemorrhagic fever can occur during primary dengue infections, most frequently in infants whose mothers are immune to dengue.

Dengue 3 virus strains circulating in mainland Southeast Asia since 1983 are associated with a particularly severe clinical syndrome, characterized by encephalopathy, hypoglycemia, markedly elevated liver enzyme values, and, occasionally, jaundice.

PATHOGENESIS

Fatalities with chikungunya and West Nile fever infections have been ascribed to hemorrhage or viral encephalitis.

The pathogenesis of dengue hemorrhagic fever is incompletely understood, but epidemiologic studies suggest that it is usually associated with 2nd infections with dengue types 1-4. Retrospective studies of sera from human mothers whose infants acquired dengue hemorrhagic fever and prospective studies in children acquiring sequential dengue infections have shown that the circulation of infection-enhancing antibodies at the time of infection is the strongest risk factor for development of severe disease. Absence of cross-reactive neutralizing antibodies and presence of enhancing antibodies from passive transfer or active production are the best correlates of risk for dengue hemorrhagic fever. Monkeys that are infected sequentially or are receiving small quantities of enhancing antibodies have enhanced viremias. In humans studied early during the course of secondary dengue infections, viremia levels directly predicted disease severity. When dengue virus immune complexes attach to macrophage Fc receptors, a signal is sent that suppresses innate immunity, resulting in enhanced viral production. In the Americas, dengue hemorrhagic fever and dengue shock syndrome have been associated with dengue types 1-4 strains of recent Southeast Asian origin. Recent occurrences of sizable dengue hemorrhagic fever outbreaks in India, Pakistan, and Bangladesh also appear to be related to imported dengue strains.

Early in the acute stage of secondary dengue infections, there is rapid activation of the complement system. Shortly before or during shock, blood levels of soluble tumor necrosis factor receptor, interferon-γ, and interleukin-2 are elevated. C1q, C3, C4, C5-C8, and C3 proactivators are depressed, and C3 catabolic rates are elevated. These factors or virus itself may interact with endothelial cells to produce increased vascular permeability through the nitric oxide final pathway. The blood clotting and fibrinolytic systems are activated, and levels of factor XII (Hageman factor) are depressed. The mechanism of bleeding in dengue hemorrhagic fever is not known, but a mild degree of disseminated intravascular coagulopathy, liver damage, and thrombocytopenia may operate synergistically. Capillary damage allows fluid, electrolytes, small proteins, and, in some instances, red blood cells to leak into extravascular spaces. This internal redistribution of fluid, together with deficits caused by fasting, thirsting, and vomiting, results in hemoconcentration, hypovolemia, increased cardiac work, tissue hypoxia, metabolic acidosis, and hyponatremia.

Usually no pathologic lesions are found to account for death. In rare instances, death may be due to gastrointestinal or intracranial hemorrhages. Minimal to moderate hemorrhages are seen in the upper gastrointestinal tract, and petechial hemorrhages are common in the interventricular septum of the heart, on the pericardium, and on the subserosal surfaces of major viscera. Focal hemorrhages are occasionally seen in the lungs, liver, adrenals, and subarachnoid space. The liver is usually enlarged, often with fatty changes. Yellow, watery, and at times blood-tinged effusions are present in serous cavities in about 75% of patients.

Dengue virus is frequently absent in tissues at the time of death; viral antigens or RNA have been localized to macrophages in liver, spleen, lung, and lymphatic tissues.

CLINICAL MANIFESTATIONS

The incubation period is 1-7 days. The clinical manifestations are variable and are influenced by the age of the patient. In infants and young children, the disease may be undifferentiated or characterized by fever for 1-5 days, pharyngeal inflammation, rhinitis, and mild cough. A majority of infected older children and adults experience sudden onset of fever, with temperature rapidly increasing to 39.4-41.1°C (103-106°F), usually accompanied by frontal or retro-orbital pain, particularly when pressure is applied to the eyes. Occasionally, severe back pain precedes the fever (back-break fever). A transient, macular, generalized rash that blanches under pressure may be seen during the 1st 24-48 hr of fever. The pulse rate may be slow relative to the degree of fever. Myalgia and arthralgia occur soon after the onset and increase in severity. Joint symptoms may be particularly severe in patients with chikungunya or o'nyong-nyong infection. From the 2nd to 6th day of fever, nausea and vomiting are apt to occur, and generalized lymphadenopathy, cutaneous hyperesthesia or hyperalgesia, taste aberrations, and pronounced anorexia may develop.

About 1-2 days after defervescence, a generalized, morbilliform, maculopapular rash appears that spares the palms and soles. It disappears in 1-5 days; desquamation may occur. Rarely there is edema of the palms and soles. About the time this 2nd rash appears, the body temperature, which has previously decreased to normal, may become slightly elevated and demonstrate the characteristic biphasic temperature pattern.

Dengue Hemorrhagic Fever

Differentiation between dengue fever and dengue hemorrhagic fever is difficult early in the course of illness. A relatively mild 1st phase with abrupt onset of fever, malaise, vomiting, headache, anorexia, and cough is followed after 2-5 days by rapid clinical deterioration and collapse. In this 2nd phase, the patient usually has cold, clammy extremities, a warm trunk, flushed face, diaphoresis, restlessness, irritability, mid-epigastric pain, and decreased urinary output. Frequently, there are scattered petechiae on the forehead and extremities; spontaneous ecchymoses may appear, and easy bruising and bleeding at sites of venipuncture are common. A macular or maculopapular rash may appear, and there may be circumoral and peripheral cyanosis. Respirations are rapid and often labored. The pulse is weak, rapid, and thready, and the heart sounds are faint. The liver may enlarge to 4-6 cm below the costal margin and is usually firm and somewhat tender. Approximately 20-30% of cases of dengue hemorrhagic fever are complicated by shock (dengue shock syndrome). Fewer than 10% of patients have gross ecchymosis or gastrointestinal bleeding, usually after a period of uncorrected shock. After a 24- to 36-hr period of crisis, convalescence is fairly rapid in the children who recover. The temperature may return to normal before or during the stage of shock. Bradycardia and ventricular extrasystoles are common during convalescence.

DIAGNOSIS

A clinical diagnosis of dengue fever derives from a high index of suspicion and knowledge of the geographic distribution and environmental cycles of causal viruses. Because clinical findings vary and there are many possible causative agents, the term *dengue-like disease* should be used until a specific diagnosis is established. A case is confirmed by isolation of the virus, virus antigen, or genome by polymerase chain reaction (PCR) analysis as well as demonstration of a fourfold or greater increase in antibody titers. A probable case is a typical acute febrile illness with supportive serology and occurrence at a location where there are confirmed cases.

The World Health Organization criteria for **dengue hemorrhagic fever** are fever (2-7 days in duration or biphasic), minor or major hemorrhagic manifestations, thrombocytopenia (≤100,000/mm^3), and objective evidence of increased capillary permeability (hematocrit increased by ≥20%), pleural effusion or ascites (by chest radiography or ultrasonography), or hypoalbuminemia. **Dengue shock syndrome** criteria include those for dengue hemorrhagic fever as well as hypotension, tachycardia, narrow pulse pressure (≤20 mm Hg), and signs of poor perfusion (cold extremities).

Virologic diagnosis can be established by serologic tests, by detection of viral proteins or viral RNA or the isolation of the virus from blood leukocytes or acute phase serum. Following primary and secondary dengue infections, there is a relatively transient appearance of anti-dengue immunoglobulin (Ig) M antibodies. These disappear after 6-12 wk, a feature that can be used to time a dengue infection. In 2nd primary dengue infections, most antibody is of the IgG class. Serologic diagnosis depends on a fourfold or greater increase in IgG antibody titer in paired sera by hemagglutination inhibition, complement fixation, enzyme immunoassay, or neutralization test. Carefully standardized IgM and IgG capture enzyme immunoassays are now widely used to identify acute-phase antibodies from patients with primary or secondary dengue infections in single-serum samples. Usually such samples should be collected not earlier than 5 days nor later than 6 wk after onset. It may not be possible to distinguish the infecting virus by serologic methods alone, particularly when there has been prior infection with another member of the same arbovirus group. Virus can be recovered from acute-phase serum after inoculating tissue culture or living mosquitoes. Viral RNA can be detected in blood or tissues by specific complementary RNA probes or amplified first by = PCR or by real-time PCR. A viral nonstructural protein, NS1, is released by infected cells into the circulation and can be detected using monoclonal or polyclonal antibodies. The detection of NS1 is the basis of commercial tests, including rapid lateral flow tests. These tests offer reliable point of care diagnosis of acute dengue infection.

DIFFERENTIAL DIAGNOSIS

The differential diagnosis of dengue fever includes dengue-like diseases, viral respiratory and influenza-like diseases, the early stages of malaria, mild yellow fever, scrub typhus, viral hepatitis, and leptospirosis.

Four arboviral diseases have dengue-like courses but without rash: Colorado tick fever, sandfly fever, Rift Valley fever, and Ross River fever. Colorado tick fever occurs sporadically among campers and hunters in the western USA; sandfly fever in the Mediterranean region, the Middle East, southern Russia, and parts of the Indian subcontinent; and Rift Valley fever in North, East, Central, and South Africa. Ross River fever is endemic in much of eastern Australia, with epidemic extension to Fiji. In adults, Ross River fever often produces protracted and crippling arthralgia involving weight-bearing joints.

Because meningococcemia, yellow fever (Chapter 262), other viral hemorrhagic fevers (Chapter 263), many rickettsial diseases, and other severe illnesses caused by a variety of agents may produce a clinical picture similar to dengue hemorrhagic fever, the etiologic diagnosis should be made only when epidemiologic or serologic evidence suggests the possibility of a dengue infection.

LABORATORY FINDINGS

In dengue fever, pancytopenia may occur after the 3-4 days of illness. Neutropenia may persist or reappear during the latter stage of the disease and may continue into convalescence with white blood cell counts <2,000/mm^3. Platelet counts rarely fall below 100,000/mm^3. Venous clotting, bleeding and prothrombin times, and plasma fibrinogen values are within normal ranges. The tourniquet test result may be positive. Mild acidosis, hemoconcentration, increased transaminase values, and hypoproteinemia may occur during some primary dengue virus infections. The electrocardiogram may show sinus bradycardia, ectopic ventricular foci, flattened T waves, and prolongation of the P-R interval.

The most common hematologic abnormalities during dengue hemorrhagic fever and dengue shock syndrome are hemoconcentration with an increase of >20% in hematocrit, thrombocytopenia, prolonged bleeding time, and moderately decreased prothrombin level that is seldom <40% of control. Fibrinogen levels may be subnormal, and fibrin split product values are elevated. Other abnormalities include moderate elevations of serum transaminase levels, consumption of complement, mild metabolic acidosis with hyponatremia, occasionally hypochloremia, slight elevation of serum urea nitrogen, and hypoalbuminemia. Roentgenograms of the chest reveal pleural effusions (right > left) in nearly all patients with dengue shock syndrome.

TREATMENT

Treatment of uncomplicated dengue fever is supportive. Bed rest is advised during the febrile period. Antipyretics should be used to keep body temperature <40°C (104°F). Analgesics or mild sedation may be required to control pain. Aspirin is contraindicated and should not be used because of its effects on hemostasis. Fluid and electrolyte replacement is required for deficits caused by sweating, fasting, thirsting, vomiting, and diarrhea.

Dengue Hemorrhagic Fever and Dengue Shock Syndrome

Management of dengue hemorrhagic fever and dengue shock syndrome includes immediate evaluation of vital signs and degrees of hemoconcentration, dehydration, and electrolyte imbalance. Close monitoring is essential for at least 48 hr, because shock may occur or recur precipitously early in the disease. Patients who are cyanotic or have labored breathing should be given oxygen. Rapid intravenous replacement of fluids and electrolytes can frequently sustain patients until spontaneous recovery occurs. Normal saline is more effective in treating shock than the more expensive Ringer lactated saline. When pulse pressure is ≤10 mm Hg or when elevation of the hematocrit persists after replacement of fluids, plasma or colloid preparations are indicated.

Care must be taken to avoid overhydration, which may contribute to cardiac failure. Transfusions of fresh blood or platelets suspended in plasma may be required to control bleeding; they should not be given during hemoconcentration, but only after evaluation of hemoglobin or hematocrit values. Salicylates are contraindicated because of their effect on blood clotting.

Sedation may be required for children who are markedly agitated. Use of vasopressors has not resulted in a significant reduction of mortality over that observed with simple supportive therapy. Disseminated intravascular coagulation may require treatment (Chapter 477). Corticosteroids do not shorten the duration of disease or improve prognosis in children receiving careful supportive therapy.

Hypervolemia during the fluid reabsorptive phase may be life threatening and is heralded by a decrease in hematocrit with wide pulse pressure. Diuretics and digitalization may be necessary.

COMPLICATIONS

Primary infections with dengue fever and dengue-like diseases are usually self-limited and benign. Fluid and electrolyte losses, hyperpyrexia, and febrile convulsions are the most frequent complications in infants and young children. Epistaxis, petechiae, and purpuric lesions are uncommon but may occur at any stage. Swallowed blood from epistaxis, vomited or passed by rectum, may be erroneously interpreted as gastrointestinal bleeding. In adults and possibly in children, underlying conditions may lead to clinically significant bleeding. Convulsions may occur during high temperature, especially with chikungunya fever. Infrequently, after the febrile stage, prolonged asthenia, mental depression, bradycardia, and ventricular extrasystoles may occur in children.

In endemic areas, dengue hemorrhagic fever should be suspected in children with a febrile illness suggestive of dengue fever who experience hemoconcentration and thrombocytopenia.

PROGNOSIS

The prognosis of dengue fever may be adversely affected by passively acquired antibody or by prior infection with a closely related virus that predisposes to development of dengue hemorrhagic fever.

Dengue Hemorrhagic Fever

Death has occurred in 40-50% of patients with shock, but with adequate intensive care deaths should occur in <1% of cases. Survival is directly related to early and intense supportive treatment. Infrequently, there is residual brain damage due to prolonged shock or occasionally to intracranial hemorrhage.

PREVENTION

Several types of dengue type 1-4 vaccines are under development, and a killed vaccine for chikungunya is efficacious but not licensed. Prophylaxis consists of avoiding **mosquito bites** through the use of insecticides, repellents, body covering with clothing, screening of houses, and destruction of *A. aegypti* breeding sites. If water storage is mandatory, a tight-fitting lid or a thin layer of oil may prevent egg laying or hatching. A larvicide, such as Abate [O,O′-(thiodi-p-phenylene) O,O,O,O′-tetramethyl phosphorothioate], available as a 1% sand-granule formation and effective at a concentration of 1 ppm, may be added safely to drinking water. Ultra-low-volume spray equipment effectively dispenses the adulticide malathion from truck or airplane for rapid intervention during an epidemic. Only personal anti-mosquito measures are effective against mosquitoes in the field, forest, or jungle.

The possibility exists that incomplete dengue vaccination may sensitize a recipient so that ensuing dengue infection could result in hemorrhagic fever. Vaccination with yellow fever 17D strain has no effect on the severity of dengue illness, although seroconversion rates to a dengue type 2 vaccine was enhanced in persons immune to yellow fever.

BIBLIOGRAPHY

Please visit the Nelson Textbook of Pediatrics *website at www.expertconsult.com for the complete bibliography.*

Chapter 262
Yellow Fever

Scott B. Halstead

Yellow fever is an acute infection characterized in its most severe form by fever, jaundice, proteinuria, and hemorrhage. The virus is mosquito-borne and occurs in epidemic or endemic form in South America and Africa. Seasonal epidemics occurred in cities located in temperate areas of Europe and the Americas until 1900, and epidemics continue in West, Central, and East Africa.

For the full continuation of this chapter, please visit the Nelson Textbook of Pediatrics *website at www.expertconsult.com.*

Chapter 263
Other Viral Hemorrhagic Fevers

Scott B. Halstead

Viral hemorrhagic fevers are a loosely defined group of clinical syndromes in which hemorrhagic manifestations are either common or especially notable in severe illness. Both the etiologic agents and clinical features of the syndromes differ, but disseminated intravascular coagulopathy may be a common pathogenetic feature.

Table 263-1 VIRAL HEMORRHAGE FEVERS (HFs)

MODE OF TRANSMISSION	DISEASE	VIRUS
Tick-borne	Crimean-Congo HF*	Congo
	Kyasanur Forest disease	Kyasanur Forest disease
	Omsk HF	Omsk
Mosquito-borne†	Dengue HF	Dengue (four types)
	Rift Valley fever	Rift Valley fever
	Yellow fever	Yellow fever
Infected animals or materials to humans	Argentine HF	Junin
	Bolivian HF	Machupo
	Lassa fever*	Lassa
	Marburg disease*	Marburg
	Ebola HF*	Ebola
	Hemorrhagic fever with renal syndrome	Hantaan

*Patients may be contagious; nosocomial infections are common.
†Chikungunya virus is associated infrequently with petechiae and epistaxis. Severe hemorrhagic manifestations have been reported in some cases.

ETIOLOGY

Six of the viral hemorrhagic fevers are caused by arthropod-borne viruses (arboviruses) (Table 263-1). Four are togaviruses of the family Flaviviridae: Kyasanur Forest disease, Omsk, dengue (Chapter 261), and yellow fever (Chapter 262) viruses. Three are of the family Bunyaviridae: Congo, Hantaan, and Rift Valley fever (RVF) viruses. Four are of the family Arenaviridae: Junin, Machupo, Guanarito, and Lassa viruses. Two are of the family Filoviridae: Ebola and Marburg viruses. The Filoviridae are enveloped, filamentous RNA viruses that are sometimes branched, unlike any other known virus.

EPIDEMIOLOGY AND CLINICAL MANIFESTATIONS

With some exceptions, the viruses causing viral hemorrhagic fevers are transmitted to humans via a nonhuman entity. The specific ecosystem required for viral survival determines the geographic distribution of disease. Although it is commonly thought that all viral hemorrhagic fevers are arthropod borne, 7 may be contracted from environmental contamination caused by animals or animal cells or from infected humans (see Table 263-1). Laboratory and hospital infections have occurred with many of these agents. Lassa fever and Argentine and Bolivian hemorrhagic fevers are reportedly milder in children than in adults.

Crimean-Congo Hemorrhagic Fever

Sporadic human infection with Crimean-Congo hemorrhage fever in Africa provided the original virus isolation. Natural foci are recognized in Bulgaria, western Crimea, and the Rostov-on-Don and Astrakhan regions; a somewhat similar disease occurs in Kazakhstan and Uzbekistan. Index cases were followed by nosocomial transmission in Pakistan and Afghanistan in 1976, in the Arabian Peninsula in 1983, and in South Africa in 1984. Outbreaks have been reported from Pakistan, Oman, and southern Russia. In the Russian Federation, the vectors are *Hyalomma marginatum* and *Hyalomma anatolicum,* which, along with hares and birds, may serve as viral reservoirs. Disease occurs from June to September, largely among farmers and dairy workers.

Kyasanur Forest Disease

Human cases of Kyasanur Forest disease occur chiefly in adults in an area of Mysore State, India. The main vectors are 2 Ixodidae ticks, *Haemaphysalis turturis* and *Haemaphysalis spinigera.* Monkeys and forest rodents may be amplifying hosts. Laboratory infections are common.

Omsk Hemorrhagic Fever

Omsk hemorrhagic fever occurs throughout south-central Russia and northern Romania. Vectors may include *Dermacentor pictus* and *Dermacentor marginatus,* but direct transmission from moles and muskrats to humans seems well established. Human disease occurs in a spring-summer-autumn pattern, paralleling the activity of vectors. This infection occurs most frequently in persons with outdoor occupational exposure. Laboratory infections are common.

Rift Valley Fever

The virus causing RVF is responsible for epizootics involving sheep, cattle, buffalo, certain antelopes, and rodents in North, Central, East, and South Africa. The virus is transmitted to domestic animals by *Culex theileri* and several *Aedes* species. Mosquitoes may serve as reservoirs by transovarial transmission. An epizootic in Egypt in 1977-1978 was accompanied by thousands of human infections, principally among veterinarians, farmers, and farm laborers. Smaller outbreaks occurred in Senegal in 1987, Madagascar in 1990, and Saudi Arabia and Yemen in 2000-2001. Humans are most often infected during the slaughter or skinning of sick or dead animals. Laboratory infection is common.

Argentine Hemorrhagic Fever

Before introduction of vaccine, hundreds to thousands of cases of Argentine hemorrhage fever occurred annually from April through July in the maize-producing area northwest of Buenos Aires that reaches to the eastern margin of the Province of Cordoba. Junin virus has been isolated from the rodents *Mus musculus, Akodon arenicola,* and *Calomys laucha laucha.* It infects migrant laborers who harvest the maize and who inhabit rodent-contaminated shelters.

Bolivian Hemorrhagic Fever

The recognized endemic area of Bolivian hemorrhagic fever consists of the sparsely populated province of Beni in Amazonian Bolivia. Sporadic cases occur in farm families who raise maize, rice, yucca, and beans. In the town of San Joaquin, a disturbance in the domestic rodent ecosystem may have led to an outbreak of household infection caused by Machupo virus transmitted by chronically infected *Calomys callosus,* ordinarily a field rodent. Mortality rates are high in young children.

Venezuelan Hemorrhagic Fever

In 1989, an outbreak of hemorrhagic illness occurred in the farming community of Guanarito, Venezuela, 200 miles south of Caracas. Subsequently, in 1990-1991, there were 104 cases reported with 26 deaths due to Guanarito virus. Cotton rats *(Sigmodon alstoni)* and cane rats *(Zygodontomys brevicauda)* have been implicated as likely reservoirs of Venezuelan hemorrhage fever.

Lassa Fever

Lassa virus has an unusual potential for human-to-human spread, which has resulted in many small epidemics in Nigeria, Sierra Leone, and Liberia. Medical workers in Africa and the USA have also contracted the disease. Patients with acute Lassa fever have been transported by international aircraft, necessitating extensive surveillance among passengers and crews. The virus is probably maintained in nature in a species of African peridomestic rodent, *Mastomys natalensis.* Rodent-to-rodent transmission and infection of humans probably operate via mechanisms established for other arenaviruses.

Marburg Disease

Until recently, the world experience of Marburg disease had been limited to 26 primary and 5 secondary cases in Germany and Yugoslavia in 1967, and to small outbreaks in Zimbabwe in 1975, Kenya in 1980 and 1988, and South Africa in 1983. But, in 1999 a large outbreak occurred in Congo Republic and a still larger outbreak in Uige Province, Angola, with 351 cases and 312 deaths in 2005. In laboratory and clinical settings, transmission occurs by direct contact with tissues of the African green monkey or with infected human blood or semen. A reservoir in bats has been demonstrated. It appears that the virus is transmitted by close contact between fructivorous bats and from bats by aerosol to humans.

Ebola Hemorrhagic Fever

Ebola virus was isolated in 1976 from a devastating epidemic involving small villages in northern Zaire and southern Sudan; smaller outbreaks have occurred subsequently. Outbreaks have initially been nosocomial. Attack rates have been highest in the birth- 1 yr old and 15-50 yr old age groups. The virus is closely related to Marburg virus. Ebola virus has been particularly active recently, with an outbreak in Kikwit, Zaire, in 1995, followed recently by scattered outbreaks in Uganda and Central and West Africa. The virus has been recovered from chimpanzees, and antibodies have been found in other subhuman primates, which apparently acquire infection from a zoonotic reservoir in bats. The mode of transmission to humans is unknown. Reston virus, related to Ebola, has been recovered from Philippine monkeys and pigs and has caused subclinical infections in workers in monkey colonies in the USA.

Hemorrhagic Fever with Renal Syndrome

The endemic area of hemorrhage fever with renal syndrome (HFRS), also known as *epidemic hemorrhagic fever* and *Korean hemorrhagic fever*, includes Japan, Korea, far eastern Siberia, north and central China, European and Asian Russia, Scandinavia, Czechoslovakia, Romania, Bulgaria, Yugoslavia, and Greece. Although the incidence and severity of hemorrhagic manifestations and the mortality are lower in Europe than in northeastern Asia, the renal lesions are the same. Disease in Scandinavia, **nephropathia epidemica,** is caused by a different although antigenically related virus, Puumala virus, associated with the bank vole, *Clethrionomys glareolus.* Cases occur predominantly in the spring and summer. There appears to be no age factor in susceptibility, but because of occupational hazards, young adult men are most frequently attacked. Rodent plagues and evidence of rodent infestation have accompanied endemic and epidemic occurrences. Hantaan virus has been detected in lung tissue and excreta of *Apodemus agrarius coreae.* Antigenically related agents have been detected in laboratory rats and in urban rat populations around the world, including Prospect Hill virus in the wild rodent *Microtus pennsylvanicus* in North America and Sin Nombre virus in the deer mouse in the southern and southwestern USA; these viruses are causes of hantavirus pulmonary syndrome (Chapter 265). Rodent-to-rodent and rodent-to-human transmission presumably occurs via the respiratory route.

CLINICAL MANIFESTATIONS

Dengue hemorrhagic fever (Chapter 261) and yellow fever (Chapter 262) cause similar syndromes in children in endemic areas.

Crimean-Congo Hemorrhagic Fever

The incubation period of 3-12 days is followed by a febrile period of 5-12 days and a prolonged convalescence. Illness begins suddenly with fever, severe headache, myalgia, abdominal pain, anorexia, nausea, and vomiting. After 1-2 days, fever may subside until the patient experiences an erythematous facial or truncal flush and injected conjunctivae. A 2nd febrile period of 2-6 days then develops, with a hemorrhagic enanthem on the soft palate and a fine petechial rash on the chest and abdomen. Less frequently, there are large areas of purpura and bleeding from the gums, nose, intestines, lungs, or uterus. Hematuria and proteinuria are relatively rare. During the hemorrhagic stage, there is usually tachycardia with diminished heart sounds and occasionally hypotension. The liver is usually enlarged, but there is no icterus. In protracted cases, central nervous system signs include delirium, somnolence, and progressive clouding of consciousness. Early in the disease, leukopenia with relative lymphocytosis, progressively worsening thrombocytopenia, and gradually increasing anemia occur. In convalescence there may be hearing and memory loss. The mortality rate is 2-50%.

Kyasanur Forest Disease and Omsk Hemorrhagic Fever

After an incubation period of 3-8 days, both Kyasanur Forest disease and Omsk hemorrhagic fever begin with sudden onset of fever and headache. Kyasanur Forest disease is characterized by severe myalgia, prostration, and bronchiolar involvement; it often manifests without hemorrhage but occasionally with severe gastrointestinal bleeding. In Omsk hemorrhagic fever, there is moderate epistaxis, hematemesis, and a hemorrhagic enanthem but no profuse hemorrhage; bronchopneumonia is common. In both diseases, severe leukopenia and thrombocytopenia, vascular dilatation, increased vascular permeability, gastrointestinal hemorrhages, and subserosal and interstitial petechial hemorrhages occur. Kyasanur Forest disease may be complicated by acute degeneration of renal tubules and focal liver damage. In many patients, recurrent febrile illness may follow an afebrile period of 7-15 days. This 2nd phase takes the form of a meningoencephalitis.

Rift Valley Fever

Most Rift Valley fever infections have occurred in adults with signs and symptoms resembling those of dengue fever (Chapter 261). Onset is acute, with fever, headache, prostration, myalgia, anorexia, nausea, vomiting, conjunctivitis, and lymphadenopathy. The fever lasts 3-6 days and is often biphasic. Convalescence is often prolonged. In the 1977-1978 outbreak many patients died after showing signs that included purpura, epistaxis, hematemesis, and melena. RVF affects the uvea and posterior chorioretina; macular scarring, vascular occlusion, and optic atrophy occur, resulting in permanent visual loss in a high proportion of patients with mild to severe RVF. At autopsy in one report, extensive eosinophilic degeneration of the parenchymal cells of the liver were observed.

Argentine, Venezuelan, and Bolivian Hemorrhagic Fevers and Lassa Fever

The incubation period in Argentine, Venezuelan, and Bolivian hemorrhagic fevers and Lassa fever is commonly 7-14 days; the acute illness lasts for 2-4 wk. Clinical illnesses range from undifferentiated fever to the characteristic severe illness. **Lassa fever** is most often clinically severe in white persons. Onset is usually gradual, with increasing fever, headache, diffuse myalgia, and anorexia (Table 263-2). During the 1st wk, signs frequently include a sore throat, dysphagia, cough, oropharyngeal ulcers, nausea, vomiting, diarrhea, and pains in the chest and abdomen. Pleuritic chest pain may persist for 2-3 wk. In Argentine and Bolivian hemorrhagic fevers, and less frequently in Lassa fever, a petechial enanthem appears on the soft palate 3-5 days after onset and at about the same time on the trunk. The tourniquet test result may be positive. The clinical course of Venezuelan hemorrhagic fever has not been well described.

Table 263-2 CLINICAL STAGES OF LASSA FEVER

STAGE	SYMPTOMS
1 (days 1-3)	General weakness and malaise. High fever, >39°C, constant with peaks of 40-41°C
2 (days 4-7)	Sore throat (with white exudative patches) very common; headache; back, chest, side, or abdominal pain; conjunctivitis; nausea and vomiting; diarrhea; productive cough; proteinuria; low blood pressure (systolic <100 mm Hg); anemia
3 (after 7 days)	Facial edema; convulsions; mucosal bleeding (mouth, nose, eyes); internal bleeding; confusion or disorientation
4 (after 14 days)	Coma and death

From Richmond JK, Baglole DJ: Lassa fever: epidemiology, clinical features, and social consequences, *Br Med J* 327: 1271–1275, 2003.

In 35-50% of all patients, these diseases may become severe, with persistent high temperature, increasing toxicity, swelling of the face or neck, microscopic hematuria, and frank hemorrhages from the stomach, intestines, nose, gums, and uterus. A syndrome of **hypovolemic shock** is accompanied by pleural effusion and renal failure. **Respiratory distress** resulting from airway obstruction, pleural effusion, or congestive heart failure may occur. A total of 10-20% of patients experience late neurologic involvement, characterized by intention tremor of the tongue and associated speech abnormalities. In severe cases, there may be intention tremors of the extremities, seizures, and delirium. The cerebrospinal fluid is normal. In Lassa fever, nerve deafness occurs in early convalescence in 25% of cases. Prolonged convalescence is accompanied by alopecia and, in Argentine and Bolivian hemorrhagic fevers, by signs of autonomic nervous system lability, such as postural hypotension, spontaneous flushing or blanching of the skin, and intermittent diaphoresis.

Laboratory studies reveal marked leukopenia, mild to moderate thrombocytopenia, proteinuria, and, in Argentine hemorrhagic fever, moderate abnormalities in blood clotting, decreased fibrinogen, increased fibrinogen split products, and elevated serum transaminases. There is focal, often extensive eosinophilic necrosis of liver parenchyma, focal interstitial pneumonitis, focal necrosis of the distal and collecting tubules, and partial replacement of splenic follicles by amorphous eosinophilic material. Usually bleeding occurs by diapedesis with little inflammatory reaction. The mortality rate is 10-40%.

Marburg Disease and Ebola Hemorrhagic Fever

After an incubation period of 4-7 days, illness begins abruptly with severe frontal headache, malaise, drowsiness, lumbar myalgia, vomiting, nausea, and diarrhea. A **maculopapular** eruption begins 5-7 days later on the trunk and upper arms. It becomes generalized and often hemorrhagic and exfoliates during convalescence. The exanthem is accompanied by a dark red enanthem on the hard palate, conjunctivitis, and scrotal or labial edema. Gastrointestinal hemorrhage occurs as the severity of illness increases. Late in the illness, the patient may become tearfully depressed with marked hyperalgesia to tactile stimuli. In fatal cases, patients become hypotensive, restless, and confused and lapse into coma. Convalescent patients may experience alopecia and may have paresthesias of the back and trunk. There is a marked leukopenia with necrosis of granulocytes. **Disseminated intravascular coagulopathy** and thrombocytopenia are universal and correlate with severity of disease; there are moderate abnormalities in concentrations of clotting proteins and elevations of serum transaminases and amylase. The mortality rate of Marburg disease is 25-85%, and that of Ebola hemorrhagic fever 50-90%. High viral loads in acute-phase blood samples convey a poor prognosis.

Hemorrhagic Fever with Renal Syndrome

In most cases, HFRS is characterized by fever, petechiae, mild hemorrhagic phenomena, and mild proteinuria, followed by relatively uneventful recovery. In 20% of recognized cases, the disease may progress through 4 distinct phases. The febrile phase is ushered in with fever, malaise, and facial and truncal flushing. It lasts 3-8 days and ends with thrombocytopenia, petechiae, and proteinuria. The hypotensive phase, of 1-3 days, follows defervescence. Loss of fluid from the intravascular compartment may result in marked hemoconcentration. Proteinuria and ecchymoses increase. The oliguric phase, usually 3-5 days in duration, is characterized by a low output of protein-rich urine, increasing nitrogen retention, nausea, vomiting, and dehydration. Confusion, extreme restlessness, and hypertension are common. The diuretic phase, which may last for days or weeks, usually initiates clinical improvement. The kidneys show little concentrating ability, and rapid loss of fluid may result in severe dehydration and shock. Potassium and sodium depletion may be severe. Fatal cases manifest as abundant protein-rich retroperitoneal edema and marked hemorrhagic necrosis of the renal medulla. The mortality rate is 5-10%.

DIAGNOSIS

Diagnosis of these viral hemorrhagic fevers depends on a high index of suspicion in endemic areas. In nonendemic areas, histories of recent travel, recent laboratory exposure, or exposure to an earlier case should evoke suspicion of a viral hemorrhagic fever.

In all viral hemorrhagic fevers, the viral agent circulates in the blood at least transiently during the early febrile stage. Togaviruses and bunyaviruses can be recovered from acute-phase serum samples by inoculation into tissue culture or living mosquitoes. Argentine, Bolivian, and Venezuelan hemorrhagic fever viruses can be isolated from acute-phase blood or throat washings by intracerebral inoculation into guinea pigs, infant hamsters, or infant mice. Lassa virus may be isolated from acute-phase blood or throat washings by inoculation into tissue cultures. For Marburg disease and Ebola hemorrhagic fever, acute-phase throat washings, blood, and urine may be inoculated into tissue culture, guinea pigs, or monkeys. The viruses are readily identified on electron microscopy, with a filamentous structure differentiating them from all other known agents. Specific complement-fixing and immunofluorescent antibodies appear during convalescence. The virus of HFRS is recovered from acute-phase serum or urine by inoculation into tissue culture. A variety of antibody tests using viral subunits is becoming available. Serologic diagnosis depends on demonstration of seroconversion or a fourfold or greater increase in immunoglobulin G antibody titer in acute and convalescent serum specimens collected 3-4 wk apart. Viral RNA may also be detected in blood or tissues with use of reverse transcriptase polymerase chain reaction analysis.

Handling blood and other biologic specimens is hazardous and must be performed by specially trained personnel. Blood and autopsy specimens should be placed in tightly sealed metal containers, wrapped in absorbent material inside a sealed plastic bag, and shipped on dry ice to laboratories with biocontainment safety level 4 facilities. Even routine hematologic and biochemical tests should be done with extreme caution.

Differential Diagnosis

Mild cases of hemorrhagic fever may be confused with almost any self-limited systemic bacterial or viral infection. More severe cases may suggest typhoid fever; epidemic, murine, or scrub typhus; leptospirosis; or a rickettsial spotted fever, for which effective chemotherapeutic agents are available. Many of these disorders may be acquired in geographic or ecologic locations endemic for a viral hemorrhagic fever.

TREATMENT

Ribavirin administered intravenously is effective in reducing mortality in Lassa fever and HFRS. Further information and advice about management, control measures, diagnosis, and collection of biohazardous specimens can be obtained from Centers for Disease Control and Prevention, National Center for Infectious Diseases, Special Pathogens Branch, Atlanta, Georgia 30333 (404-639-1115).

The therapeutic principle involved in all of these diseases, especially HFRS, is the reversal of dehydration, hemoconcentration, renal failure, and protein, electrolyte, or blood losses. The contribution of disseminated intravascular coagulopathy to the hemorrhagic manifestations is unknown, and the management of hemorrhage should be individualized. Transfusions of fresh blood and platelets are frequently given. Good results have been reported in a few patients after the administration of clotting factor concentrates. The efficacy of corticosteroids, ε-aminocaproic acid, pressor amines, and α-adrenergic blocking agents has not been established. Sedatives should be selected with regard to the possibility of kidney or liver damage. The successful management of HFRS may require renal dialysis.

Although whole blood transfusions from Ebola virus–immune donors are thought to be therapeutic, studies in a monkey model were unable to confirm this outcome.

PREVENTION

A live-attenuated vaccine (Candid-I) for Argentine hemorrhagic fever (Junin virus) is highly efficacious. A form of inactivated mouse brain vaccine is reported to be effective in preventing Omsk hemorrhagic fever. Inactivated RVF vaccines are widely used to protect domestic animals and laboratory workers. HFRS inactivated vaccine is licensed in Korea, and killed and live-attenuated vaccines are widely used in China. A vaccinia-vector glycoprotein vaccine provides protection against Lassa fever in monkeys. A single dose of a recombinant vesicular stomatitis virus vaccine containing surface glycoproteins from Ebola and Marburg viruses is effective in preventing virus hemorrhagic fevers due to several strains of filovirus in a monkey model.

Prevention of **mosquito-borne** and **tick-borne infections** includes use of repellents, wearing of tight-fitting clothing that fully covers the extremities, and careful examination of the skin after exposure with removal of any vectors found. Diseases transmitted from a rodent-infected environment can be prevented through methods of rodent control; elimination of refuse and breeding sites is particularly successful in urban and suburban areas.

Crimean-Congo hemorrhagic fever, Lassa fever, Marburg disease, and Ebola hemorrhagic fever may be **transmitted in hospital settings.** Patients should be isolated until they are virus-free or for 3 wk after illness. Patients' urine, sputum, blood, clothing, and bedding should be disinfected. Disposable syringes and needles should be used. Prompt and strict enforcement of barrier nursing may be lifesaving. The mortality rate among medical workers contracting these diseases is 50%. A few entirely asymptomatic Ebola infections result in strong antibody production.

BIBLIOGRAPHY

Please visit the Nelson Textbook of Pediatrics *website at www.expertconsult.com for the complete bibliography.*

Chapter 264
Lymphocytic Choriomeningitis Virus

Daniel J. Bonthius

Lymphocytic choriomeningitis virus (LCMV) is a prevalent human pathogen and an important cause of meningitis in children and adults. This virus is capable of crossing the placenta and infecting the fetus and is also an important cause of neurologic birth defects and encephalopathy in the newborn.

For the full continuation of this chapter, please visit the Nelson Textbook of Pediatrics *website at www.expertconsult.com.*

Chapter 265
Hantavirus Pulmonary Syndrome

Scott B. Halstead

The Hantavirus pulmonary syndrome (HPS) is caused by multiple closely related hantaviruses that have been identified from the western USA, with sporadic cases reported from the eastern USA (see Fig. 265-1 on the *Nelson Textbook of Pediatrics* website at www.expertconsult.com) and Canada and important foci of disease in several countries in South America. HPS is characterized by a febrile prodrome followed by the rapid onset of noncardiogenic pulmonary edema and hypotension or shock. Sporadic cases in the USA caused by related viruses may manifest with renal involvement. Cases in Argentina and Chile sometimes include severe gastrointestinal hemorrhaging; nosocomial transmission has been documented in this geographic region only.

For the full continuation of this chapter, please visit the Nelson Textbook of Pediatrics *website at www.expertconsult.com.*

Chapter 266
Rabies

Rodney E. Willoughby, Jr.

Rabies virus is a bullet-shaped, negative-sense, single-stranded, enveloped RNA virus from the family Rhabdoviridae, genus *Lyssavirus*. There currently are 7 known genotypes of *Lyssavirus*; more are under taxonomic consideration. The classic rabies virus (genotype 1) is distributed worldwide and naturally infects a large variety of animals. The other 6 genotypes are more geographically confined, with none found in the Americas. All 7 *Lyssavirus* genotypes have been associated with rabies in humans, although type 1 accounts for the great majority of cases. Within genotype 1, a number of genetic variants have been defined. Each variant is specific to a particular animal reservoir, although cross-species transmission can occur.

EPIDEMIOLOGY

Rabies is present on all continents except Antarctica. Rabies predominantly afflicts under-aged, poor, and geographically isolated populations. Approximately 50,000 cases of human rabies occur in Africa and Asia annually. Theoretically, rabies virus can infect any mammal (which then can transmit disease to humans), but true animal reservoirs that maintain the presence of rabies virus in the population are limited to terrestrial carnivores and bats. Worldwide, transmission from dogs accounts for >90% of human cases. In Africa and Asia, other animals serve as prominent reservoirs, such as jackals, mongooses, and raccoon dogs. In industrialized nations canine rabies has been largely controlled through the routine immunization of pets. In the USA, raccoons are the most commonly infected wild animal along the eastern seaboard. Three phylogenies of skunk rabies are endemic in the Midwest (north and south) and California, and gray foxes harbor rabies in Arizona and Texas and mongooses in Puerto Rico. Rabies occurs infrequently in livestock. Among American domestic pets, infected cats outnumber infected dogs, probably because cats frequently prowl unsupervised and are not uniformly subject to vaccine laws. Rabies is rare in small mammals, including mice, squirrels, and rabbits; to date, no animal-to-human transmission from these animals has been documented.

The epidemiology of human rabies in the USA is dominated by cryptogenic bat rabies. Bats are migratory in the spring and fall; rabid bats are identified in every state of the union except Hawaii. In one study, the largest proportion of cases of human rabies were infected with a bat variant, and in almost all cases of bat-associated human rabies there was no history of a bat bite.

In the USA, 30,000 episodes of rabies postexposure prophylaxis (PEP) occur annually. Between 1 and 3 human cases are diagnosed annually, half postmortem. There have been two outbreaks of rabies associated with solid organ and corneal transplantations.

TRANSMISSION

Rabies virus is found in large quantities in the saliva of infected animals, and transmission occurs almost exclusively through inoculation of the infected saliva through a bite or scratch from a rabid mammal. Approximately 35-50% of people bitten by a known rabies-infected animal and receiving no PEP experience rabies. The transmission rate is increased if the victim has suffered multiple bites and if the inoculation occurs in highly innervated parts of the body such as the face and the hands. Infection does not occur after exposure of intact skin to infected secretions, but virus may enter the body through intact mucous membranes. Claims that spelunkers may experience rabies after inhaling bat excreta have come under doubt, although inhalational exposure can occur during laboratory accidents.

No case of nosocomial transmission to a health care worker has been documented to date, but caregivers of a patient with rabies are advised to use full barrier precautions. The virus is rapidly inactivated in the environment, and contamination of fomites is not a mechanism of spread.

PATHOGENESIS

After inoculation, rabies virus replicates slowly and at low levels in muscle or skin. This slow initial step likely accounts for the disease's long incubation period. Virus then enters the peripheral motor nerve, utilizing the nicotinic acetylcholine receptor and possibly several other receptors for entry. Once in the nerve, the virus travels by fast axonal transport, crossing synapses roughly every 12 hr. Rapid dissemination occurs throughout the brain and spinal cord before symptoms appear. Infection of the dorsal root ganglia is apparently futile but causes the characteristic radiculitis. Infection concentrates in the brainstem, accounting for autonomic dysfunction and relative sparing of cognition. Despite severe neurologic dysfunction with rabies, histopathology reveals limited damage, inflammation, or apoptosis. The pathologic hallmark of rabies, the Negri body, is composed of clumped viral nucleocapsids that create cytoplasmic inclusions on routine histology. Negri bodies can be absent in documented rabies virus infection. Rabies may be a metabolic disorder of neurotransmission; tetrahydrobiopterin (BH_4) deficiency in human rabies causes severe deficiencies in dopamine, norepinephrine, and serotonin metabolism.

After infection of the central nervous system, the virus travels anterograde through the peripheral nervous system to virtually all innervated organs. It is through this route that the virus infects the salivary glands. Many victims of rabies die from uncontrolled cardiac dysrhythmia.

Deficiency of BH_4, an essential cofactor for neuronal nitric oxide synthase, is predicted to lead to spasm of the basilar arteries. Onset of vasospasm has been confirmed in a few patients within 5-8 days of first hospitalization, at about the time coma supervenes in the natural history.

CLINICAL MANIFESTATIONS

The incubation period for rabies is 1-3 mo but is variable. In severe wounds to the head, symptoms may occur within 5 days after exposure, and occasionally the incubation period can extend to >6 mo. Rabies has 2 principal clinical forms. **Encephalitic** or **"furious" rabies** begins with nonspecific symptoms, including fever, sore throat, malaise, headache, nausea and vomiting, and weakness. These symptoms are often accompanied by paresthesias and pruritus at or near the site of the bite that then extend along the affected limb. Soon thereafter the patient begins to demonstrate typical symptoms of severe encephalitis, with agitation, depressed mentation, and occasionally seizures. Characteristically patients with rabies encephalitis initially have periods of lucidity intermittent with periods of profound encephalopathy. Hydrophobia and aerophobia are the cardinal signs of rabies; they are unique to humans and are not universal. Phobic spasms are manifested by agitation and fear created by being offered a drink or fanning of air in the face, which in turn produce choking and aspiration through spasms of the pharynx, neck, and diaphragm. The illness is relentlessly progressive. There is a dissociation of electrophysiologic or encephalographic activity with findings of brainstem coma caused by anterograde denervation. Death almost always occurs within 1-2 days of hospitalization in developing countries and by 18 days of hospitalization with intensive care.

A 2nd form of rabies known as **paralytic** or **"dumb" rabies** is seen much less frequently and is characterized principally by fevers and ascending motor weakness affecting both the limbs and the cranial nerves. Most patients with paralytic rabies also have some element of encephalopathy as the disease progresses subacutely.

DIFFERENTIAL DIAGNOSIS

The differential diagnosis of rabies encephalitis includes all forms of severe cerebral infections, tetanus, and some intoxications and envenomations. Rabies can be confused with psychiatric illness, drug abuse, and conversion disorders. Paralytic rabies is most frequently confused with Guillain-Barré syndrome. The diagnosis of rabies is frequently delayed in Western countries because of its rarity and the unfamiliarity of the medical staff with the infection. These considerations highlight the need to pursue a history of contact with an animal belonging to one of the known reservoirs for rabies or to establish a travel history to a rabies-endemic region.

DIAGNOSIS

The Centers for Disease Control and Prevention (CDC) require a number of tests to confirm a clinically suspected case of rabies. The virus can be grown both in cell culture and after animal injection, but identification of rabies by these methods is prolonged. Rabies antigen is detected through immunofluorescence of saliva or biopsies of hairy skin or brain. Corneal impressions are not recommended. Rabies virus RNA has been detected in saliva, skin, and brain by the reverse transcription polymerase chain reaction (RT-PCR). RT-PCR is the most sensitive available assay for the diagnosis of rabies when done iteratively. Rabies-specific antibody can be detected in serum or cerebrospinal fluid (CSF) samples, but most patients die while seronegative. Antirabies antibodies are present in the sera of patients who have received an incomplete course of the rabies vaccine, precluding a meaningful interpretation in this setting. Antibody in CSF is rarely detected after vaccination and is considered diagnostic of rabies regardless of immunization status. CSF abnormalities in cell count, glucose, and protein content are minimal and are not diagnostic. MRI findings in the brain are late.

TREATMENT AND PROGNOSIS

Rabies is generally fatal. There are 3 survivors from rabies infection through the use of the Milwaukee Protocol (www.mcw.edu/rabies). Deep sedation is induced to avoid dysautonomia while the immune response develops. Survival is estimated at 20%; neurologic outcome can be very good. Among 6 survivors of rabies after failure of vaccine prophylaxis, only 2 had a satisfactory neurologic outcome. Neither rabies immune globulin (RIG) nor rabies vaccine alters the course of disease once symptoms have appeared. Antiviral treatments have not been effective. Ribavirin, which delays the immune response, is to be avoided during early management. In contrast, appearance of the normal antibody response at 7-10 days is associated with clearance of salivary viral load. Nimodipine is recommended as prophylaxis against cerebrovascular spasm.

PREVENTION

Primary prevention of rabies infection includes vaccination of domestic animals and education to avoid wild animals, stray animals, and animals with unusual behavior.

Immunization and Fertility Control of Animal Reservoirs

The introduction of routine rabies immunization for domestic pets in the USA and Europe during the middle of the 20th century virtually eliminated infection in dogs, which prior to that time had been the principal transmitter of rabies to humans in developed as well as nonindustrialized countries. Since the 1990s, efforts in Europe and North America have shifted to immunization of wildlife reservoirs of rabies, where rabies is newly emerging. These programs have employed bait laced with either an attenuated rabies vaccine or a recombinant rabies surface glycoprotein inserted into vaccinia, distributed by air or hand into areas inhabited by rabid animals. Human contact with vaccine-laden bait has occurred infrequently. Adverse events after such contact have been rare, but the vaccinia vector poses a threat to the same population at risk for vaccinia itself, namely, pregnant women, immunocompromised persons, and people with chronic dermatologic conditions. Mass culling of endemic reservoirs has never worked; vaccination and fertility control abort outbreaks. Bats are ubiquitous and very important for insect control. Less than 1% of free-flying bats but >8% of downed bats and bats found in dwellings are rabid.

Postexposure Prophylaxis

The relevance of rabies for most pediatricians centers on evaluating whether an animal exposure warrants PEP (Table 266-1). No case of rabies has been documented in a person receiving the fully recommended schedule of PEP since introduction of modern cellular vaccines in the 1970s.

Given the incubation period for rabies, PEP is a medical urgency, not emergency. Algorithms have been devised to aid practitioners in deciding when to initiate rabies PEP (Fig. 266-1). The decision to proceed ultimately depends on the local epidemiology of animal rabies as determined by active surveillance programs, information that can be obtained from local and state health departments. In general, bats, raccoons, skunks, coyotes, and foxes should be considered rabid unless proven otherwise through euthanasia and testing of brain tissue, whereas bites from small herbivorous animals (squirrels, hamsters, gerbils, chipmunks, rats, mice, and rabbits) can be discounted. The response to bites from a pet, particularly a dog, cat, or ferret, depends on local surveillance statistics and on whether the animal is available for observation.

The approach to nonbite bat exposures is controversial. In response to the observation that most cases of rabies in the USA have been caused by bat variants and that the majority of affected patients had no recollection of a bat bite, the CDC has recommended that rabies PEP be considered after any physical contact with bats and when a bat is found in the same room as persons who may not be able to accurately report a bite, assuming that the animal is unavailable for testing. Such people include young children, the mentally disabled, and intoxicated individuals. Other nonbite contacts (e.g., handling a carcass, exposure to an animal playing with a carcass, or coming into contact with blood or excreta from a potentially rabid animal) usually do not require PEP.

In all instances of a legitimate exposure, effort should be made to recover the animal for quarantine and observation or brain examination after euthanasia. Testing obviates the need for PEP over half the time. In most instances PEP can be deferred until the results of observation or brain histology are known. In dogs, cats, and ferrets, symptoms of rabies always occur within several days of viral shedding; therefore, in these animals a 10-day observation period is sufficient to eliminate the possibility of rabies.

No duration of time between exposure and onset of symptoms should preclude rabies prophylaxis. Rabies PEP is most effective when applied expeditiously. Nevertheless, the series should be begun in the asymptomatic person as soon as possible, regardless of the length of time since the bite. *The vaccine and RIG are contraindicated once symptoms develop.*

Table 266-1 RABIES POSTEXPOSURE PROPHYLAXIS GUIDE

ANIMAL TYPE	EVALUATION AND DISPOSITION OF ANIMAL	POSTEXPOSURE PROPHYLAXIS RECOMMENDATIONS
Dogs, cats, and ferrets	Healthy and available for 10 days of observation	Prophylaxis only if animal shows signs of rabies*
	Rabid or suspected of being rabid†	Immediate immunization and RIG
	Unknown (escaped)	Consult public health officials for advice
Bats, skunks, raccoons, foxes, and most other carnivores; woodchucks	Regarded as rabid unless geographic area is known to be free of rabies or until animal proven negative by laboratory tests†	Immediate immunization and RIG
Livestock, rodents, and lagomorphs (rabbits, hares, and pikas)	Consider individually	Consult public health officials. Bites of squirrels, hamsters, guinea pigs, gerbils, chipmunks, rats, mice and other rodents, rabbits, hares, and pikas almost never require antirabies treatment.

*During the 10-day observation period, at the first sign of rabies in the biting dog, cat, or ferret, treatment of the exposed person with RIG (human) and vaccine should be initiated. The animal should be euthanized immediately and tested.

†The animal should be euthanized and tested as soon as possible. Holding for observation is not recommended. Immunization is discontinued if immunofluorescent test result for the animal is negative.

RIG, rabies immune globulin.

From American Academy of Pediatrics: *Red book 2009: report of the Committee on Infectious Diseases*, ed 28, Elk Grove Village, IL, 2009, American Academy of Pediatrics.

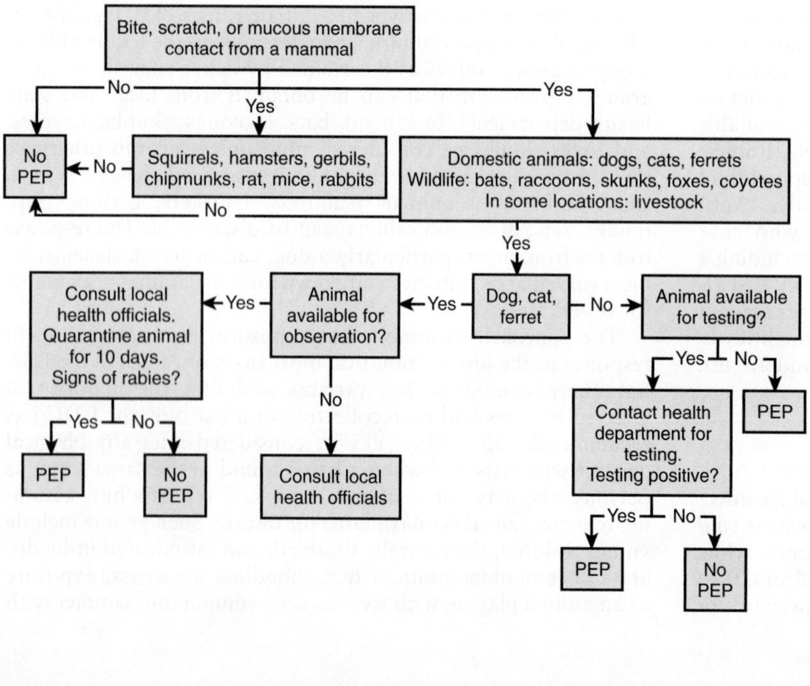

Figure 266-1 Algorithm for evaluating a child for rabies postexposure prophylaxis (PEP). This and any other algorithm should be used in concert with local epidemiologic information regarding the incidence of animal rabies in any given location.

The 1st step in rabies PEP is to cleanse the wound thoroughly. Soapy water is sufficient for an enveloped virus, and its effectiveness is supported by broad experience. Other commonly used disinfectants, such as iodine-containing preparations, are virucidal and should be used in addition to soap when available. Probably the most important aspect of this component is that the wound is cleansed with copious volumes of disinfectant and primary closure is avoided. Antibiotics and tetanus prophylaxis (Chapter 203) should be applied with the use of usual wound care criteria.

The 2nd component of rabies PEP consists of passive immunization with RIG. Most failures of PEP are attributed to not using RIG. Human RIG, the formulation used in industrialized countries, is administered at a dose of 20 IU/kg. As much of the dose is infused around the wound as possible, and the remainder is injected intramuscularly in a limb distant from the one injected with the killed vaccine. Like other immune globulin preparations, RIG interferes with the take of live viral vaccines for at least 4 mo after administration of the RIG dose. Human RIG is not available in many parts of the developing world. Equine RIG serves as a substitute for the human immune globulin preparation in some areas. Modern preparations of equine RIG are associated with fewer side effects than prior products composed of crude horse serum. Regrettably, for a large segment of the world's population, no passive immunization product is available at all. Monoclonal antibody products are in clinical trials and may alleviate this deficiency.

The 3rd component of rabies PEP is immunization with inactivated vaccine. In the developed world, cell-based vaccines have replaced previous preparations. Two formulations currently are available in the USA, namely, RabAvert (Chiron Behring Vaccines, Maharashtra, India), a purified chick-embryo cell cultivated vaccine, and Imovax Rabies (Aventis Pasteur, Bridgewater, NJ), cultivated in human diploid cell cultures. In both children and adults, both vaccines are administered intramuscularly in a 1-mL volume in the deltoid or anterolateral thigh on days 0, 3, 7, and 14 after presentation. Injection into the gluteal area has been associated with a blunted antibody response, so this area should not be used. The rabies vaccines can be safely administered during pregnancy. In most persons the vaccine is well tolerated; most adverse effects are related to booster doses. Pain and erythema at the injection site occur commonly, and local adenopathy, headache, and myalgias occur in 10-20% of patients. Approximately 5% of patients who receive the human diploid cell vaccine experience an immune complex–mediated allergic reaction, including rash, edema, and arthralgias, several days after a booster dose. The World Health Organization (WHO) has approved schedules using smaller amounts of vaccine, administered intradermally, that are immunogenic and protective (*www.who.int/rabies/human/postexp/en/*), but none is approved for use in the USA. Other cell culture–derived rabies virus vaccines are available in the developing world. A few countries still produce nerve tissue–derived vaccines; these preparations are poorly immunogenic, and cross reactivity with human nervous tissue may occur with their use, producing severe neurologic symptoms even in the absence of rabies infection.

Pre-Exposure Prophylaxis

The killed rabies vaccine can be given to prevent rabies in persons at high risk for exposure to wild-type virus, including laboratory personnel working with rabies virus, veterinarians, and others likely to be exposed to rabid animals as part of their occupation. Pre-exposure prophylaxis should be considered for persons traveling to a rabies-endemic region where there is a credible risk for a bite or scratch from a rabies-infected animal, particularly if there is likely to be a shortage of RIG or cell culture–based vaccine (Chapter 168). Rabies vaccine as part of the routine vaccine series is under investigation in some countries. The schedule for pre-exposure prophylaxis consists of 3 intramuscular injections on days 0, 7, and 21 or 28. PEP in the patient who has received pre-exposure prophylaxis or a prior full schedule of PEP consists of 2 doses of vaccine (1 each on days 0 and 3) and does not require RIG. Immunity from pre-exposure prophylaxis wanes after several years and requires boosting if the potential for exposure to rabid animals recurs.

BIBLIOGRAPHY

Please visit the Nelson Textbook of Pediatrics *website at* *www.expertconsult.com* *for the complete bibliography.*

Chapter 267
Polyomaviruses

Gregory A. Storch

The polyomaviruses are small (45-nm), nonenveloped, double-stranded circular DNA viruses with genomes of approximately 5,000 bp. JC virus and BK viruses infect humans and cause disease. Two other polyomaviruses, designated KI virus and WU virus, can be detected in respiratory samples from children; the role of these viruses as pathogens is still under investigation. A fifth polyomavirus, called *Merkel cell polyomavirus*, can be detected in tumor tissue from individuals with Merkel cell carcinoma, an unusual neuroectodermal tumor of the skin that occurs primarily in elderly and immunocompromised individuals. A sixth human polyomavirus has been isolated from patients with the dermatologic condition trichodysplasia granulosa. The new virus has been provisionally named Trichodysplasia spinulosa virus. Trichodysplasia granulosa is a condition of the skin that occurs in immunocompromised individuals and involves the development of follicular papules and keratin spines, usually involving the face. JC and BK viruses are closely related to each other, with about 75% genome homology. KI and WU have a similar relationship to each other but are distinct from other human and animal polyomaviruses. Merkel cell polyomavirus is also distinct from the other human polyomaviruses.

For the full continuation of this chapter, please visit the Nelson Textbook of Pediatrics *website at* *www.expertconsult.com*.

Chapter 268
Acquired Immunodeficiency Syndrome (Human Immunodeficiency Virus)

Ram Yogev and Ellen Gould Chadwick

Advances in research and major improvements in the treatment and management of HIV infection have brought about a substantial decrease in the incidence of new HIV infections and AIDS in children born in the USA and Western Europe. However, worldwide, HIV infection rates continue to rise with an estimated 1,000 children were newly infected with HIV each day in 2009, most of whom were from resource-limited countries. Increasing numbers of children have lost 1 or both parents to AIDS, resulting in more than 1.5 million AIDS orphans reported thus far in the epidemic. HIV infection in children progresses more rapidly than in adults, and up to half of untreated children die within the 1st 2 yr of life. This rapid progression is correlated with higher viral burden and faster depletion of infected CD4 lymphocytes in infants and children than in adults. Accurate diagnostic tests and the availability of potent drugs to inhibit HIV replication have dramatically increased the ability to prevent and control this devastating disease.

ETIOLOGY

HIV-1 and HIV-2 are members of the Retroviridae family and belong to the *Lentivirus* genus, which includes cytopathic viruses causing diverse diseases in several animal species. The HIV-1 genome contains 2 copies of single-stranded RNA that is 9.2 kb in size. At both ends of the genome there are identical regions, called **long terminal repeats,** which contain the regulation and expression genes of HIV. The remainder of the genome includes 3 major sections: the **GAG** region, which encodes the viral core proteins (p24, p17, p9, and p6, which are derived from the precursor p55); the **POL** region, which encodes the viral enzymes (i.e., reverse transcriptase [p51], protease [p10], and integrase [p32]); and the **ENV** region, which encodes the viral envelope proteins (gp120 and gp41, which are derived from the precursor gp160). Other regulatory proteins, such as tat (p14), rev (p19), nef (p27), vpr (p15), vif (p23), vpu in HIV-1 (P16), and vpx in HIV-2 (P15) are involved in transactivation, viral messenger RNA expression, viral replication, induction of cell cycle arrest, promotion of nuclear import of viral reverse transcription complexes, downregulation of CD4 receptors and class I major histocompatibility complex, proviral DNA synthesis, and virus release and infectivity (Fig. 268-1).

The major external viral protein of HIV-1 is a heavily glycosylated gp120 protein that is associated with the transmembrane glycoprotein gp41; gp41 is very immunogenic and is used to detect HIV-1 antibodies in diagnostic assays; gp120 is a complex molecule that includes the highly variable **V3 loop.** This region is immunodominant for neutralizing antibodies. The heterogeneity of gp120 presents major obstacles in establishing an effective HIV vaccine. The gp120 glycoprotein also carries the binding site for the CD4 molecule, the most common host cell surface receptor of T lymphocytes. This tropism for $CD4^+$ T cells is beneficial to the virus because of the resulting reduction in the effectiveness of the host immune system. Other CD4-bearing cells include macrophages and microglial cells. The observations that $CD4^-$ cells are also infected by HIV and that some $CD4^+$ T cells are resistant to such infections suggests that other cellular attachment sites are needed for the interaction between HIV and human cells. Several chemokines serve as co-receptors for the envelope glycoproteins, permitting membrane fusion and entry into the cell. Most HIV strains have a specific tropism for 1 of the chemokines, including the fusion-inducing molecule **CXCR-4,** which has been

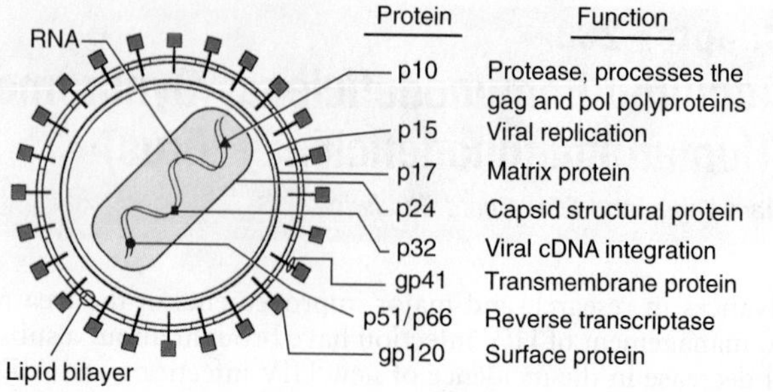

Figure 268-1 The human immunodeficiency virus and associated proteins and their functions.

shown to act as a co-receptor for HIV attachment to lymphocytes, and **CCR-5**, a β chemokine receptor that facilitates HIV entry into macrophages. Several other chemokine receptors (CCR-3) have also been shown in vitro to serve as virus co-receptors. Other mechanisms of attachment of HIV to cells use non-neutralizing antiviral antibodies and complement receptors. The Fab portion of these antibodies attaches to the virus surface, and the Fc portion binds to cells that express Fc receptors (macrophages, fibroblasts), thus facilitating virus transfer into the cell. Other cell surface receptors, such as mannose-binding protein on macrophages or DC-specific C-type lectin (DC-SIGN) on dendritic cells, also bind to the HIV-1 envelope glycoprotein and increase the efficiency of viral infectivity. Cell-to-cell transfer of HIV without formation of fully formed particles is a more rapid mechanism of spreading the infection to new cells than direct infection by the virus.

Following viral attachment, gp120 and the CD4 molecule undergo conformational changes, and gp41 interacts with the fusion receptor on the cell surface. Viral fusion with the cell membrane allows entry of viral RNA into the cell cytoplasm. This process involves accessory viral proteins (nef, vif) and binding of cyclophilin A (a host cellular protein) to p24. Viral DNA copies are then transcribed from the virion RNA through viral reverse transcriptase enzyme activity, and duplication of the DNA copies produces double-stranded circular DNA. The HIV-1 reverse transcriptase is error prone and lacks error-correcting mechanisms. Thus, many mutations arise, creating wide genetic variation in HIV-1 isolates even within an individual patient. The circular DNA is transported into the cell nucleus, where it is integrated into chromosomal DNA and referred to as the *provirus*. The provirus has the advantage of latency, as it can remain dormant for extended periods. Integration usually occurs near active genes, which allow a high level of viral production in response to various external factors such as an increase in inflammatory cytokines (by infection with other pathogens) and cellular activation. Depending on the relative expression of the viral regulatory genes (tat, rev, nef), the proviral DNA may encode production of the viral RNA genome, which in turn leads to production of viral proteins necessary for viral assembly.

HIV-1 transcription is followed by translation. A capsid polyprotein is cleaved to produce, among others, the virus-specific protease (p10). This enzyme is critical for HIV-1 assembly. Several HIV-1 antiprotease drugs have been developed, targeting the increased sensitivity of the viral protease, which differs from the cellular proteases. The RNA genome is then incorporated into the newly formed viral capsid that requires zinc finger domains (p7) and the matrix protein (p17). As new virus is formed, it buds through specialized membrane areas, known as *lipid rafts*, and is released.

Full length sequencing of the HIV-1 genome demonstrated 3 different groups (M [main], O [outlier], N [non-M, non-O]) probably occurring from multiple zoonotic infections from primates in different geographic regions. The same technique identified 8 groups with HIV-2 isolates. Group M diversified to 9 subtypes (or clades A to D, F to H, J and K) In each region of the world, certain clades predominate, for example, clade A in Central Africa, clade B in the USA and South America, clade C in South Africa, clade E in Thailand, and clade F in Brazil. While some subtypes have been identified for Group O, none was found with any of the HIV-2 groups. Clades are mixed in some patients due to HIV recombination, and some crossing between groups (i.e., M and O) has been reported.

HIV-2 has a similar life cycle to HIV-1 and is known to cause infection in several monkey species. Subtypes A and B are the major causes of infection in humans but rarely cause infection in children. HIV-2 differs from HIV-1 in its accessory genes (for example, it has no *vpu* gene but contains the *vpx* gene, which is not found in HIV-1). It is most prevalent in Western Africa, but increasing numbers of cases are reported from Europe and Southern Asia. The diagnosis of HIV-2 infection is more difficult because of major differences in the genetic sequences between HIV-1 and HIV-2. Thus, several of the standard confirmatory assays (immunoblot), which are HIV-1 specific, may give indeterminate results with HIV-2 infection. If HIV-2 infection is suspected, a combination screening test that detects antibody to HIV-1 and HIV-2 peptides should be used. In addition, the rapid HIV detection tests have been less reliable in patients suspected to be dually infected with HIV-1 and HIV-2, because of lower antibody concentrations against HIV-2.

EPIDEMIOLOGY

The World Health Organization (WHO) estimated that in 2009, 2.5 million children worldwide were living with HIV-1 infection, 90% of who were from Sub-Saharan Africa. While between 2004 and 2009 the global number of children born with HIV decreased by 24% and deaths from AIDS-related illnesses among children <15 yr of age declined by 19%, still 370,000 children (<15 yr) were newly infected with HIV in 2009 alone. These trends reflect the slow but steady expansion of services to prevent transmission of HIV to infants and an increase in access to treatment for children. Worldwide, 50% of HIV-infected individuals are women, most of who have become infected through heterosexual contact in their child-bearing years. Through 2009, an estimated 16.6 million children have been orphaned by AIDS, which is defined as having one or both parents die from AIDS.

There have been 9,600 American children <13 yr of age diagnosed with AIDS from the beginning of the epidemic through 2007. The number of U.S. children with AIDS diagnosed each year increased from 1984 to 1992 but then declined by more than 95% to <100 cases annually by 2003, largely due to the success of prenatal screening and perinatal antiretroviral treatment of HIV-infected mothers and infants. There are now ~8,500 children and adolescents living with HIV or AIDS in the USA. Virtually all HIV infections in children <13 yr of age in the USA are the result of **vertical transmission** from an HIV-infected mother. Children of racial and ethnic minority groups are disproportionately over-represented, particularly non-Hispanic African-Americans and Hispanics. Race and ethnicity is not a risk factor for HIV infection but more likely reflects other factors that may be predictive of increased risk for HIV infection, such as lack of educational and economic opportunities and higher rates of intravenous drug use. New York, Florida, and California account for most cases of HIV in children in the USA.

Although adolescents (13-24 yr of age) represent a minority of U.S. AIDS cases (approximately 5%), they constitute a growing population of newly infected individuals, with 15% of all new cases of HIV diagnosed in 2006 occurring between the ages of 13 and 24 yr. The highest incidence of new adolescent infections has been among African-American males who have sex with males, and more than 50% report being unaware of their diagnosis. Considering the long latency period between the time of infection and the development of clinical symptoms, reliance on

AIDS case definition surveillance data significantly under-represents the impact of the disease in adolescents. Based on a median incubation period of 8-12 yr, it has been estimated that 15-20% of all AIDS cases were acquired between 13 and 19 yr of age.

Risk factors for HIV infection vary by gender in adolescents. More than 87% of males between the ages of 13 and 19 yr with HIV/AIDS acquire infection through sex with males (MSM). In contrast, 88% of adolescent females with AIDS are infected through heterosexual contact. As in the pediatric population, adolescent racial and ethnic minority populations are over-represented, especially among females. A greater proportion of female adolescents have AIDS (male : female ratio 1.5 : 1) than do female adults >25 yr of age (male : female ratio 2.9 : 1).

Transmission

Transmission of HIV-1 occurs via sexual contact, parenteral exposure to blood, or vertical transmission from mother to child. The primary route of infection in the pediatric population is vertical transmission, accounting for almost all new cases. Rates of transmission of HIV from mother to child have varied in different parts of the USA and among countries. The USA and Europe have documented transmission rates in untreated women between 12-30%. Transmission rates in Africa and Haiti are higher (range is 25-52%). Perinatal treatment of HIV-infected mothers with antiretroviral drugs has dramatically decreased these rates to <2% in pregnant women on effective therapy.

Vertical transmission of HIV can occur before (**intrauterine**), during (**intrapartum**), or after delivery (through **breast-feeding**). Intrauterine transmission has been suggested by identification of HIV by culture or polymerase chain reaction (PCR) in fetal tissue as early as 10 wk. First trimester placental tissue from HIV-infected women has been demonstrated to contain HIV by in situ hybridization and immunocytochemistry. It is generally accepted that 30-40% of infected newborns are infected in utero, because this percentage of infants has laboratory evidence of infection (positive viral culture or PCR) within the 1st wk of life. Some studies have found that viral detection soon after birth also correlates with early onset of symptoms and rapid progression to AIDS, consistent with more long-standing infection during gestation.

The highest percentage of HIV-infected children acquires the virus intrapartum, evidenced by the fact that 60-70% of infected infants do not demonstrate detectable virus until after 1 wk of age. The mechanism of transmission appears to be exposure to infected blood and cervicovaginal secretions in the birth canal, where HIV is found in high titers during late gestation and delivery. An international registry of HIV-exposed twins found that first-born twins were 3 times more likely to be infected, reflecting the longer time that twin A is exposed to the birth canal.

Breast-feeding is the least common route of vertical transmission in industrialized nations but responsible for as many as 40% of perinatal infections in resource-limited countries. Both free and cell-associated viruses have been detected in breast milk from HIV-infected mothers. The risk for transmission through breast-feeding in chronically infected women is approximately 9-16% but 29-53% in women who acquire HIV postnatally, suggesting that the viremia experienced by the mother during primary infection at least triples the risk for transmission. It seems reasonable for women to substitute infant formula for breast milk if they are known to be HIV-infected or are at risk for ongoing sexual or parenteral exposure to HIV. However, the WHO recommends that in developing countries where other diseases (diarrhea, pneumonia, malnutrition) substantially contribute to a high infant mortality rate, the benefit of breast-feeding outweighs the risk for HIV transmission, and HIV-infected women in developing countries should breast-feed their infants for at least the 1st 6 mo of life (see later section on prevention).

Several risk factors influence the rate of vertical transmission: preterm delivery (<34 wk gestation), a low maternal antenatal CD4 count, and use of recreational drugs during pregnancy. The most important variables appear to be >4 hr duration of ruptured membranes and birthweight <2,500 g, each of which doubles the transmission rate. Elective cesarean delivery decreases transmission by 87% if used in conjunction with zidovudine therapy in the mother and infant. Because these data predated the advent of **highly active antiretroviral therapy (HAART)**, the additional benefit of cesarean section is probably negligible if the mother's viral load is <1,000 copies/mL. Although several studies have shown an increased rate of transmission in women with advanced disease (i.e., AIDS) or high viral load (>50,000 copies/mL), some transmitting mothers in each group were asymptomatic or had a low, but detectable, viral load. Thus, in the USA it is recommended to consider cesarean section if the viral load is >1,000 copies/mL.

Transfusions of infected blood or blood products has accounted for 3-6% of all pediatric AIDS cases. The period of highest risk was between 1978 and 1985, before the availability of HIV antibody-screened blood products. Whereas the prevalence of HIV infection in individuals with hemophilia treated before 1985 was as high as 70%, heat treatment of factor VIII concentrate and HIV antibody screening of donors has virtually eliminated HIV transmission in this population. Donor screening has dramatically reduced, but not eliminated, the risk for blood transfusion–associated HIV infection: nucleic acid amplification testing of "minipools" (pools of 16-24 donations) performed on antibody-nonreactive blood donations (to identify donations made during the window period before seroconversion) reduced the residual risk of transfusion-transmitted HIV-1 to approximately 1 in 2 million blood units. However, in many resource-limited countries, screening of blood is not uniform, and the risk for transmitting HIV infection via transfusion is substantial.

Although HIV can be isolated rarely from saliva, it is in very low titers (<1 infectious particle/mL) and has not been implicated as a transmission vehicle. Studies of hundreds of household contacts of HIV-infected individuals have found that the risk for household HIV transmission is practically nonexistent. Only a few cases have been reported in which urine or feces (possibly devoid of visible blood) have been proposed as a possible vehicle of HIV transmission.

In the pediatric population, sexual transmission is infrequent, but a small number of cases resulting from sexual abuse have been reported. Sexual contact is a major route of transmission in the adolescent population, accounting for most of the cases.

PATHOGENESIS

HIV infection affects most of the immune system and disrupts its homeostasis (Fig. 268-2). In most cases, the initial infection is caused by low amounts of a single virus. Therefore, disease may be prevented by prophylactic drug(s) or vaccine. When the mucosa serves as the portal of entry for HIV, the 1st cells to be affected are the dendritic cells. These cells collect and process antigens introduced from the periphery and transport them to the lymphoid tissue. HIV does not infect the dendritic cell but binds to its DC-SIGN surface molecule, allowing the virus to survive until it reaches the lymphatic tissue. In the lymphatic tissue (e.g., lamina propria, lymph nodes), the virus selectively binds to cells expressing CD4 molecules on their surface, primarily helper T lymphocytes ($CD4^+$ T cells) and cells of the monocyte-macrophage lineage. Other cells bearing CD4, such as microglia, astrocytes, oligodendroglia, and placental tissue containing villous Hofbauer cells, may also be infected by HIV. Additional factors (co-receptors) are necessary for HIV fusion and entry into cells. These factors include the chemokines CXCR4 (fusion) and CCR5. Other chemokines (CCR1, CCR3) may be necessary for the fusion of certain HIV strains. Several host genetic determinants affect the susceptibility to HIV infection, the progression of disease, and the response to treatment. These genetic variants vary in different populations. A deletion in the CCR5 gene that is protective

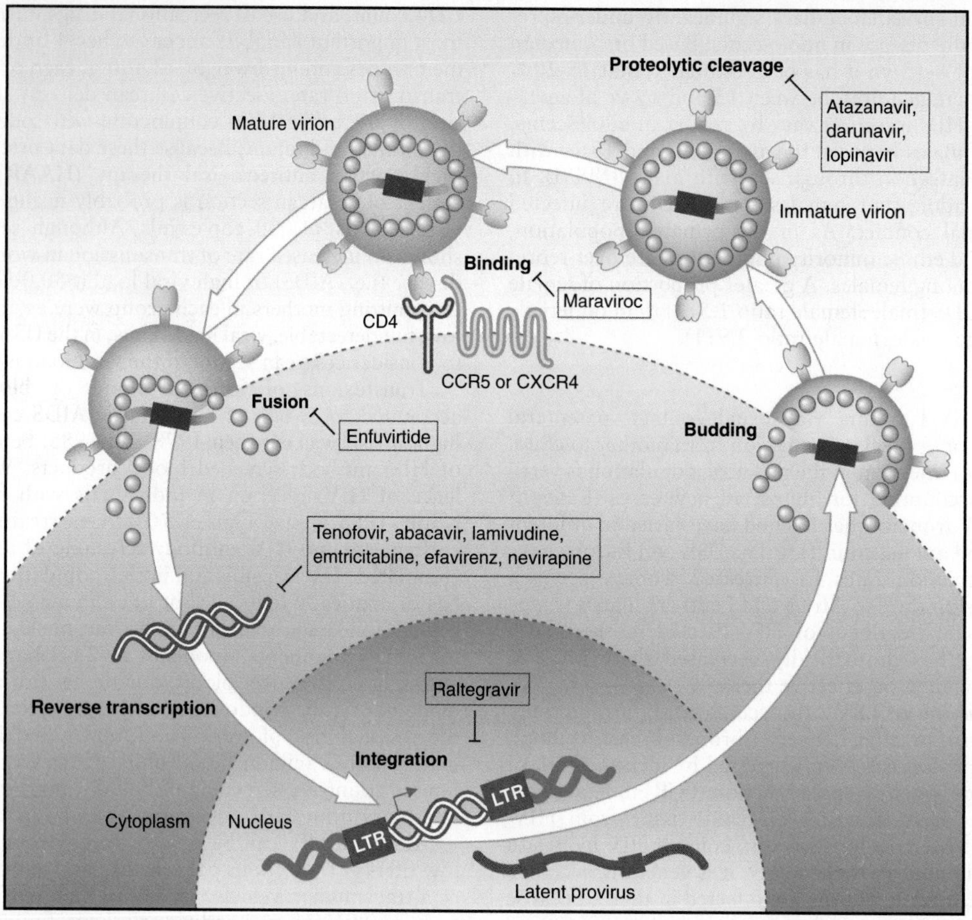

Figure 268-2 HIV life cycle and antiretroviral drug targets. Present antiretroviral drugs span 6 classes that target 5 unique steps in the HIV life cycle (binding, fusion, reverse transcription, integration, and proteolytic cleavage). The most common drugs used in resource-rich regions to target each step are shown. Extracellular virions enter their target cell through a complex 3-step process, which is (1) attachment to the CD4 receptor, (2) binding to the CCR5 or CXCR4 co-receptors, or both, and (3) membrane fusion. Maraviroc blocks CCR5 binding and enfuvirtide blocks fusion. The HIV reverse transcriptase enzyme catalyses transcription of HIV RNA into double-stranded HIV DNA, a step inhibited by nucleoside analogues and non-nucleoside reverse transcriptase inhibitors (NNRTIs). The HIV integrase enzyme facilitates incorporation of HIV DNA into host chromosomes and this step is inhibited by raltegravir and other integrase inhibitors. After transcription and translation of the HIV genome, immature virions are produced and bud from the cell surface. The HIV protease enzyme cleaves polypeptide chains, allowing the virus to mature. This last step is inhibited by HIV protease inhibitors. (From Volberding PA, Deeks SG: Antiretroviral therapy and management of HIV infection, *Lancet* 376:49–60, 2010, Fig 1, p 50.)

against HIV infection (CCR5Δ32) is relatively common in whites but is rare in blacks. Several other genes that regulate chemokine receptors, ligands, histocompatibility complex, and cytokines have also been found to influence the outcome of HIV infection. Usually, $CD4^+$ lymphocytes migrate to the lymphatic tissue in response to viral antigens and then become activated and proliferate, making them highly susceptible to HIV infection. This antigen-driven migration and accumulation of CD4 cells within the lymphoid tissue may contribute to the generalized lymphadenopathy characteristic of the acute retroviral syndrome in adults and adolescents. HIV preferentially infects the very cells that respond to it (HIV-specific memory CD4 cells), accounting for the progressive loss of these cells and the subsequent loss of control of HIV replication. The continued destruction of memory CD4+ cells in the gastrointestinal tract leads to reduced integrity of the gastrointestinal epithelium followed by leakage of bacterial particles into the blood and increased inflammatory response, which cause further CD4+ cell loss. When HIV replication reaches a threshold (usually within 3-6 wk from the time of infection), a burst of plasma viremia occurs. This intense viremia causes **flu or mononucleosis-like symptoms** (fever, rash, lymphadenopathy, arthralgia) in 50-70% of infected adults. With establishment of a cellular and humoral immune response within 2-4 mo, the viral load in the blood declines substantially, and patients enter a phase characterized by a lack of symptoms and a return of CD4 cells to only moderately decreased levels.

Early HIV-1 replication in children has no apparent clinical manifestations. Whether tested by virus isolation or by PCR for viral nucleic acid sequences, fewer than 40% of HIV-1–infected infants demonstrate evidence of the virus at birth. The virus load increases by 1-4 mo, and almost all HIV-infected infants have detectable HIV-1 in peripheral blood by 4 mo of age.

In adults, the long period of clinical latency (up to 8-12 yr) is not indicative of viral latency. In fact, there is a very high turnover of virus and CD4 lymphocytes (more than a billion cells per day), gradually causing deterioration of the immune system, marked by depletion of CD4 cells. Several mechanisms for the depletion of CD4 cells in adults and children have been suggested, including HIV-mediated single cell killing, formation of multinucleated giant cells of infected and uninfected CD4 cells (**syncytia formation**), virus-specific immune responses (natural killer cells, antibody-dependent cellular cytotoxicity), superantigen-mediated activation of T cells (rendering them more susceptible to infection with HIV), autoimmunity, and programmed cell death (apoptosis). The viral burden is greater in the lymphoid organs than in the peripheral blood during the asymptomatic period. As HIV virions and their immune complexes migrate through the lymph nodes, they are trapped in the network of dendritic follicular cells. Because the ability of HIV to replicate in T cells depends on the state of activation of the cells, the immune activation that takes place within the microenvironment of the lymph nodes in HIV disease serves to promote infection of new CD4 cells as well as subsequent viral replication within these cells. Monocytes can be productively infected by HIV yet resist killing, explaining their role as reservoirs of HIV and as effectors of tissue damage in organs such as the brain.

Cell-mediated and humoral responses occur early in the infection. CD8 T cells play an important role in containing the infection. These cells produce various ligands (MIP-1α, MIP-1β, RANTES), which suppress HIV replication by blocking the binding of the virus to the co-receptors (CCR5). HIV-specific cytotoxic T lymphocytes (CTLs) develop against both the structural (ENV, POL, GAG) and regulatory (tat) viral proteins. The CTLs appear at the end of the acute infection, as viral replication is controlled by killing HIV-infected cells before new viruses are produced and by secreting potent antiviral factors that compete with the virus for its receptors (CCR5). Neutralizing antibodies appear later in the infection and seem to help in the continued suppression of viral replication during clinical latency. There are at least 2 possible mechanisms that control the steady-state viral load level during the chronic clinical latency. One mechanism may be the limited availability of activated CD4 cells, which prevent further increase in viral load. The other mechanism is development of an active immune response, which is influenced by the amount of viral antigen and limits viral replication at a steady state. There is no general consensus about which of these 2 mechanisms is more important. The CD4 cell limitation mechanism accounts for the effect of antiretroviral therapy, whereas the immune response mechanism emphasizes the importance of immune modulation treatment (cytokines, vaccines) to increase the efficiency of immune-mediated control. A group of cytokines that includes tumor necrosis factor-α (TNF-α), TNF-β, interleukin 1 (IL-1), IL-2, IL-3, IL-6, IL-8, IL-12, IL-15, granulocyte-macrophage colony-stimulating factor, and macrophage colony-stimulating factor plays an integral role in upregulating HIV expression from a state of quiescent infection to active viral replication. Other cytokines such as interferon-γ (IFN-γ), IFN-β, and IL-13 exert a suppressive effect on HIV replication. Certain cytokines (IL-4, IL-10, IFN-γ, TGF-β) reduce or enhance viral replication depending on the infected cell type. The interactions among these cytokines influence the concentration of viral particles in the tissues. Plasma concentrations of cytokines need not be elevated for them to exert their effect, because they are produced and act locally in the tissues. Thus, even during states of apparent immunologic quiescence, the complex interaction of cytokines sustains a constant level of viral expression, particularly in the lymph nodes.

Commonly HIV isolated during the clinical latency period grows slowly in culture and produces low titers of reverse transcriptase. These isolates use CCR5 as their co-receptor. By the late stages of clinical latency, the isolated virus is phenotypically different. It grows rapidly and to high titers in culture and uses CXCR4 as its co-receptor. The switch from CCR5-receptor to CXCR4 receptor increases the capacity of the virus to replicate, to infect a broader range of target cells (CXCR4 is more widely expressed on resting and activated immune cells), and to kill T cells more rapidly and efficiently. As a result, the clinical latency phase is over and progression toward AIDS is noted. The **progression of disease** is related temporally to the gradual disruption of lymph node architecture and degeneration of the follicular dendritic cell network with loss of its ability to trap HIV particles. The virus is freed to recirculate, producing high levels of viremia and an increased disappearance of CD4 T cells during the later stages of disease.

Before HAART was available, **3 distinct patterns of disease** were described in children. Approximately 15-25% of HIV-infected newborns in developed countries present with a **rapid disease course**, with onset of AIDS and symptoms during the 1st few months of life and a median survival time of 6-9 mo if untreated. In resource-poor countries, the majority of HIV-infected newborns will have this rapidly progressing disease. It has been suggested that if intrauterine infection coincides with the period of rapid expansion of CD4 cells in the fetus, the virus could effectively infect the majority of the body's immunocompetent cells. The normal migration of these cells to the marrow, spleen, and thymus would result in efficient systemic delivery of HIV, unchecked by the immature immune system of the fetus. Thus, infection would be established before the normal ontogenic development of the immune system, causing more severe impairment of immunity. Most children in this group have a positive HIV-1 culture and/or detectable virus in the plasma (median level 11,000 copies/mL) in the 1st 48 hr of life. This early evidence of viral presence suggests that the newborn was infected in utero. The viral load rapidly increases, peaking by 2-3 mo of age (median 750,000 copies/mL) and staying high for at least the 1st 2 yr of life.

The majority of perinatally infected newborns (60-80%) in developed countries present with a much **slower progression** of disease, with a median survival time of 6 yr representing the 2nd pattern of disease. Many patients in this group have a negative viral culture or PCR in the 1st wk of life and are therefore considered to be infected intrapartum. In a typical patient, the viral load rapidly increases, peaking by 2-3 mo of age (median 100,000 copies/mL) and then slowly declines over a period of 24 mo. The slow decline in viral load is in sharp contrast to the rapid decline after primary infection seen in adults. This observation can be explained only partially by the immaturity of the immune system in newborns and infants.

The 3rd pattern of disease occurs in a small percentage (<5%) of perinatally infected children referred to as **long-term survivors (LTS)**, who have minimal or no progression of disease with relatively normal CD4 counts and very low viral loads for longer than 8 yr. Mechanisms for the delay in disease progression include effective humoral immunity and/or CTL responses, host genetic factors (e.g., HLA profile), and infection with attenuated (defective gene) virus. A subgroup of the LTS called "elite survivors" has no detectable viruses in the blood and may reflect different or greater mechanisms of protection from disease progression.

HIV-infected children have changes in the immune system that are similar to those in HIV-infected adults. CD4 cell depletion may be less dramatic because infants normally have a relative lymphocytosis. A value of 1,500 CD4 cells/mm^3 in children <1 yr of age is indicative of severe CD4 depletion and is comparable to <200 CD4 cells/mm^3 in adults. Lymphopenia is relatively rare in perinatally infected children and is usually only seen in older children or those with end-stage disease. Although cutaneous anergy is common during HIV infection, it is also frequent in healthy children <1 yr of age, and thus its interpretation is difficult to interpret in infected infants. The depletion of CD4 cells also decreases the response to soluble antigens such as in vitro mitogens phytohemagglutinin and concanavalin A.

Polyclonal activation of B cells occurs in most children early in the infection, as evidenced by elevation of IgA, IgM, IgE, and particularly IgG (**hypergammaglobulinemia**), with high levels of anti–HIV-1 antibody. This response may reflect both dysregulation of T-cell suppression of B-cell antibody synthesis and active CD4 enhancement of B-lymphocyte humoral response. As a result, antibody response to routine childhood vaccinations may be abnormal. The B-cell dysregulation precedes the CD4 depletion in many children, and may serve as a surrogate marker of HIV infection in symptomatic children in whom specific diagnostic tests (PCR, culture) are not available or are too expensive. Despite the increased levels of immunoglobulins, some children lack specific antibodies or protective antibodies. Hypogammaglobulinemia is very rare (<1%).

Table 268-1 PEDIATRIC HIV CLASSIFICATION FOR CHILDREN YOUNGER THAN 13 YEARS

IMMUNOLOGIC DEFINITIONS	IMMUNOLOGIC CATEGORIES: AGE-SPECIFIC CD4⁺ T-LYMPHOCYTE COUNT AND PERCENTAGE OF TOTAL LYMPHOCYTES*						CLINICAL CLASSIFICATIONS†			
	<12 mo		1-5 yr		6-12 yr					
	µL	%	µL	%	µL	%	N: No Signs or Symptoms	A: Mild Signs and Symptoms	B: Moderate Signs and Symptoms‡	C: Severe Signs and Symptoms‡
1: No evidence of suppression	≥1500	≥25	≥1000	≥25	≥500	≥25	N1	A1	B1	C1
2: Evidence of moderate suppression	750-1499	15-24	500-999	15-24	200-499	15-24	N2	A2	B1	C2
3: Severe suppression	<750	<15	<500	<15	<200	<15	N3	A3	B3	C3

*To convert values in µL to Système International units (× 10^9/L), multiply by 0.001.
†Children whose HIV infection status is not confirmed are classified by using this grid with a letter E (for perinatally exposed) placed before the appropriate classification code (e.g., EN2).
‡Lymphoid interstitial pneumonitis in category B or any condition in category C is reportable to state and local health departments as acquired immunodeficiency syndrome (AIDS-defining conditions) (see Table 273-2 for further definition of clinical categories).
Modified from the Centers for Disease Control and Prevention: 1994 revised classification system for human immunodeficiency virus infection in children less than 13 years of age. Official authorized addenda: human immunodeficiency virus infection codes and official guidelines for coding and reporting ICD-9-CM, *MMWR Recomm Rep* 43(RR-12):1–19, 1994.
From *Red book: 2009 report of the Committee on Infectious Diseases*, ed 28, Elk Grove Village, IL, 2009, American Academy of Pediatrics, p 384.

Central nervous system (CNS) involvement is more common in pediatric patients than in adults. Macrophages and microglia play an important role in HIV neuropathogenesis, and data suggest that astrocytes may also be involved. Although the specific mechanisms for encephalopathy in children are not yet clear, the developing brain in young infants is affected by at least 2 mechanisms. The virus itself may directly infect various brain cells or cause indirect damage to the nervous system by the release of cytokines (IL-1α, IL-1β, TNF-α, IL-2) or reactive oxygen from HIV-infected lymphocytes or macrophages.

Appropriate therapy with antiretroviral agents may result in **immune reconstitution inflammatory syndrome (IRIS)**, which is characterized by an increased inflammatory response from the recovered immune system to subclinical opportunistic infections (e.g., tuberculosis, herpes simplex virus (HSV) infection, toxoplasmosis, CMV infection, cryptococcal infection). This condition is more commonly observed in patients with progressive disease and severe CD4⁺ T-lymphocyte depletion. Patients with IRIS develop fever and worsening of the clinical manifestations of the opportunistic infection or new manifestations (e.g., enlargement of lymph nodes, pulmonary infiltrates, etc.), typically within the 1st few weeks after initiation of antiretroviral therapy. Determining whether the symptoms represent IRIS, worsening of a current infection, a new opportunistic infection, or drug toxicity is often very difficult. If the syndrome does represent IRIS, adding nonsteroidal anti-inflammatory agents or corticosteroids may alleviate the inflammatory reaction, although the use of corticosteroids is controversial. The inflammation may take weeks or months to subside. In most cases, continuation of anti-HIV treatment while treating the opportunistic infection (with or without antiinflamatory agents) is sufficient. If opportunistic infection is suspected prior to initiation of antiretroviral therapy, appropriate antimicrobial treatment should be given first.

CLINICAL MANIFESTATIONS

The clinical manifestations of HIV infection vary widely among infants, children, and adolescents. In most infants, physical examination at birth is normal. Initial symptoms may be subtle, such as lymphadenopathy and hepatosplenomegaly, or nonspecific, such as failure to thrive, chronic or recurrent diarrhea, respiratory symptoms, or oral thrush, and may be distinguishable only by their persistence. Whereas systemic and pulmonary findings are common in the USA and Europe, chronic diarrhea, wasting, and severe malnutrition predominate in Africa. Clinical manifestations found more commonly in children than adults with HIV infection include recurrent bacterial infections, chronic parotid swelling, lymphocytic interstitial pneumonitis (LIP), and early onset of progressive neurologic deterioration.

The HIV classification system is used to categorize the stage of pediatric disease by using 2 parameters: clinical status and degree of immunologic impairment (Table 268-1). Among the clinical categories, **category A (mild symptoms)** includes children with at least 2 mild symptoms such as lymphadenopathy, parotitis, hepatomegaly, splenomegaly, dermatitis, and recurrent or persistent sinusitis or otitis media (Table 268-2). **Category B (moderate symptoms)** includes children with LIP, oropharyngeal thrush persisting for >2 mo, recurrent or chronic diarrhea, persistent fever for >1 mo, hepatitis, recurrent (HSV) stomatitis, HSV esophagitis, HSV pneumonitis, disseminated varicella (i.e., with visceral involvement), cardiomegaly, or nephropathy (see Table 268-2). **Category C (severe symptoms)** includes children with opportunistic infections (e.g. esophageal or lower respiratory tract candidiasis, cryptosporidiosis (>1 mo), disseminated mycobacterial or cytomegalovirus infection, *Pneumocystis* pneumonia, or cerebral toxoplasmosis [onset >1 mo of age]), recurrent bacterial infections (sepsis, meningitis, pneumonia), encephalopathy, malignancies, and severe weight loss.

The immune classification is based on the absolute CD4 lymphocyte count or the percentage of CD4 cells (see Table 268-1). Age adjustment of the absolute CD4 count is necessary because counts that are relatively high in normal infants decline steadily until 6 yr of age, when they reach adult norms. If there is a discrepancy between the CD4 count and percentage, the disease is classified into the more severe category.

Infections

Approximately 20% of AIDS-defining illnesses in children are recurrent bacterial infections caused primarily by encapsulated organisms such as *Streptococcus pneumoniae* and *Salmonella* (Table 268-3) due to disturbances in humoral immunity. Other pathogens, including *Staphylococcus, Enterococcus, Pseudomonas aeruginosa, Haemophilus influenzae,* and other gram-positive and gram-negative organisms, may also be seen. The most common serious infections in HIV-infected children are bacteremia, sepsis, and bacterial pneumonia, accounting for >50% of infections in these patients. Meningitis, urinary tract infections, deep-seated abscesses, and bone/joint infections occur less frequently. Milder recurrent infections, such as otitis media, sinusitis, and skin and soft tissue infections, are very common and may be chronic with atypical presentations.

Opportunistic infections (OIs) are generally seen in children with severe depression of the CD4 count. In adults, these infections usually represent reactivation of a latent infection acquired early in life. In contrast, young children generally have primary infection and often have a more fulminant course of disease reflecting the lack of prior immunity. This principle is best illustrated by *Pneumocystis jirovecii* (formerly *Pneumocystis carinii*) pneumonia, the most common opportunistic infection in the pediatric population (Chapter 236). The peak incidence of *Pneumocystis* pneumonia occurs at age 3-6 mo in the setting of undiagnosed perinatally acquired disease, with the highest mortality rate in children <1 yr

Table 268-2 CLINICAL CATEGORIES FOR CHILDREN YOUNGER THAN 13 YEARS OF AGE WITH HIV INFECTION

CATEGORY N: NOT SYMPTOMATIC

Children who have no signs or symptoms considered to be the result of HIV infection or have only 1 of the conditions listed in category A.

CATEGORY A: MILDLY SYMPTOMATIC

Children with 2 or more of the conditions listed but none of the conditions listed in categories B and C.

- Lymphadenopathy (≥0.5 cm at more than 2 sites; bilateral at 1 site)
- Hepatomegaly
- Splenomegaly
- Dermatitis
- Parotitis
- Recurrent or persistent upper respiratory tract infection, sinusitis, or otitis media

CATEGORY B: MODERATELY SYMPTOMATIC

Children who have symptomatic conditions other than those listed for category A or C that are attributed to HIV infection.

- Anemia (hemoglobin <8 g/dL [<80 g/L]), neutropenia (white blood cell count <1,000/µL [$<1.0 \times 10^9$/L]), and/or thrombocytopenia (platelet count $<100 \times 10^3$/µL [$<100 \times 10^9$/L]) persisting for ≥30 days
- Bacterial meningitis, pneumonia, or sepsis (single episode)
- Candidiasis, oropharyngeal (thrush), persisting (>2 mo) in children older than 6 mo of age
- Cardiomyopathy
- Cytomegalovirus infection, with onset before 1 mo of age
- Diarrhea, recurrent or chronic
- Hepatitis
- Herpes simplex virus (HSV) stomatitis, recurrent (>2 episodes within 1 yr)
- HSV bronchitis, pneumonitis, or esophagitis with onset before 1 mo of age
- Herpes zoster (shingles) involving at least 2 distinct episodes or more than 1 dermatome
- Leiomyosarcoma
- Lymphoid interstitial pneumonia or pulmonary lymphoid hyperplasia complex
- Nephropathy
- Nocardiosis
- Persistent fever (lasting >1 mo)
- Toxoplasmosis, onset before 1 mo of age
- Varicella, disseminated (complicated chickenpox)

CATEGORY C: SEVERELY SYMPTOMATIC

- Serious bacterial infections, multiple or recurrent (i.e., any combination of at least 2 culture-confirmed infections within a 2 yr period), of the following types: septicemia, pneumonia, meningitis, bone or joint infection, or abscess of an internal organ or body cavity (excluding otitis media, superficial skin or mucosal abscesses, and indwelling catheter-related infections)
- Candidiasis, esophageal or pulmonary (bronchi, trachea, lungs)
- Coccidioidomycosis, disseminated (at site other than or in addition to lungs or cervical or hilar lymph nodes); cryptococcosis, extrapulmonary
- Cryptosporidiosis or isosporiasis with diarrhea persisting >1 mo
- Cytomegalovirus disease with onset of symptoms after 1 mo of age (at a site other than liver, spleen, or lymph nodes)
- Encephalopathy (at least 1 of the following progressive findings present for at least 2 mo in the absence of a concurrent illness other than HIV infection that could explain the findings): (1) failure to attain or loss of developmental milestones or loss of intellectual ability, verified by standard developmental scale or neuropsychologic tests; (2) impaired brain growth or acquired microcephaly demonstrated by head circumference measurements or brain atrophy demonstrated by CT or MRI (serial imaging required for children younger than 2 yr of age); or (3) acquired symmetric motor deficit manifested by 2 or more of the following: paresis, pathologic reflexes, ataxia, or gait disturbance
- HSV infection causing a mucocutaneous ulcer that persists for greater than 1 mo or bronchitis, pneumonitis, or esophagitis for any duration affecting a child older than 1 mo of age
- Histoplasmosis, disseminated (at a site other than or in addition to lungs or cervical or hilar lymph nodes)
- Kaposi sarcoma
- Lymphoma, primary, in brain
- Lymphoma, small, noncleaved cell (Burkitt), or immunoblastic; or large-cell lymphoma of B-lymphocyte or unknown immunologic phenotype
- *Mycobacterium tuberculosis* infection, disseminated or extrapulmonary
- *Mycobacterium,* other species or unidentified species infection, disseminated (at a site other than or in addition to lungs, skin, or cervical or hilar lymph nodes)
- *Pneumocystis jiroveci* pneumonia
- Progressive multifocal leukoencephalopathy
- *Salmonella* (nontyphoid) septicemia, recurrent
- Toxoplasmosis of the brain with onset after 1 mo of age
- Wasting syndrome in the absence of a concurrent illness other than HIV infection that could explain the following findings: (1) persistent weight loss >10% of baseline; (2) downward crossing of at least 2 of the following percentile lines on the weight-for-age chart (e.g., 95th, 75th, 50th, 25th, 5th) in a child 1 yr of age or older; OR (3) <5th percentile on weight-for-height chart on 2 consecutive measurements, ≥30 days apart; PLUS (1) chronic diarrhea (i.e., at least 2 loose stools per day for >30 days); OR (2) documented fever (for >30 days, intermittent or constant)

Modified from the Centers for Disease Control and Prevention: 1994 revised classification system for human immunodeficiency virus infection in children less than 13 years of age. Official authorized addenda: human immunodeficiency virus infection codes and official guidelines for coding and reporting ICD-9-CM, *MMWR Recomm Rep* 43(RR-12):1–19, 1994.

of age. Aggressive approaches to treatment have improved the outcome substantially. While the overall incidence of opportunistic infections has markedly declined since the era of combination antiretroviral therapy (ART), OIs still occur in patients with severe immunodepletion as the result of unchecked viral replication, which often accompanies poor ART adherence.

The classic clinical presentation of *Pneumocystis* pneumonia includes acute onset of fever, tachypnea, dyspnea, and marked hypoxemia; in some children, more indolent development of hypoxemia may precede other clinical or x-ray manifestations. Chest x-ray findings most commonly consist of interstitial infiltrates or diffuse alveolar disease, which rapidly progresses. Nodular lesions, streaky or lobar infiltrates, or pleural effusions may occasionally be seen. Diagnosis is established by demonstration of *P. jirovecii* with appropriate staining of bronchoalveolar fluid lavage; rarely, an open lung biopsy is necessary.

The 1st line therapy for *Pneumocystis* pneumonia is intravenous trimethoprim-sulfamethoxazole (TMP-SMZ) (15-20 mg/kg/day of the TMP component every 6 hr IV) with adjunctive corticosteroids if the $Pa{O_2}$ is <70 mm Hg while breathing room air. When the patient has improved, therapy with oral TMP-SMZ should be continued for a total of 21 days while the corticosteroids are weaned. Alternative therapy for *Pneumocystis* pneumonia includes intravenous administration of pentamidine (4 mg/kg/day). Other regimens such as TMP plus dapsone, clindamycin plus primaquine, or atovaquone are used as alternatives in adults but have not been widely used in children to date.

Atypical mycobacterial infection, particularly with *Mycobacterium avium-intracellulare* complex (MAC), may cause disseminated disease in HIV-infected children who are severely immunosuppressed. The incidence of MAC infection in ART-naïve children with <100 CD4 cells/mm^3 has been estimated to be as high as 10%, but effective combination ART that results in viral suppression has made MAC infections rare. Disseminated MAC infection is characterized by fever, malaise, weight loss, and night sweats; diarrhea, abdominal pain, and rarely intestinal perforation or jaundice (due to biliary tract obstruction by lymphadenopathy) may also be present. Diagnosis is made by isolation of MAC from blood, bone marrow, or tissue; the isolated presence of MAC in the stool does not confirm a diagnosis of disseminated MAC. Treatment can reduce symptoms and prolong life but is at best only capable of suppressing the infection if severe CD4 depletion persists. Therapy should include at least 2 drugs: clarithromycin or azithromycin and ethambutol. A 3rd

Table 268-3 1993 REVISED CASE DEFINITION OF AIDS-DEFINING CONDITIONS FOR ADULTS AND ADOLESCENTS 13 YEARS OF AGE AND OLDER

Candidiasis of bronchi, trachea, or lungs
Candidiasis, esophageal
Cervical cancer, invasive
Coccidioidomycosis, disseminated or extrapulmonary
Cryptococcosis, extrapulmonary
Cryptosporidiosis, chronic intestinal (>1 mo duration)
Cytomegalovirus disease (other than liver, spleen, or nodes)
Cytomegalovirus retinitis (with loss of vision)
Encephalopathy, HIV related
Herpes simplex: chronic ulcer(s) (>1 mo duration) or bronchitis, pneumonitis, or esophagitis
Histoplasmosis, disseminated or extrapulmonary
Isosporiasis, chronic intestinal (>1 mo duration)
Kaposi sarcoma
Lymphoma, Burkitt (or equivalent term)
Lymphoma, immunoblastic (or equivalent term)
Lymphoma, primary or brain
Mycobacterium avium complex or *Mycobacterium kansasii* infection, disseminated or extrapulmonary
Mycobacterium tuberculosis infection, any site, pulmonary or extrapulmonary
Mycobacterium, other species or unidentified species infection, disseminated or extrapulmonary
Pneumocystis jiroveci pneumonia
Pneumonia, recurrent
Progressive multifocal leukoencephalopathy
Salmonella septicemia, recurrent
Toxoplasmosis of brain
Wasting syndrome attributable to HIV
$CD4^+$ T-lymphocyte count <200/µL (0.20×10^9/L) or $CD4^+$ lymphocyte percentage <15%

Modified from the Centers for Disease Control and Prevention: 1993 revised classification system for HIV infection and expanded surveillance case definition for AIDS among adolescents and adults, *MMWR Recomm Rep* 41(RR-17):1–19, 1992.

drug (rifabutin, rifampin, ciprofloxacin, levofloxacin, or amikacin) is generally added to decrease the emergence of drug-resistant isolates. Careful consideration of possible drug interactions with antiretroviral agents is necessary before initiation of disseminated MAC therapy. Drug susceptibilities should be ascertained, and the treatment regimen should be adjusted accordingly in the event of inadequate clinical response to therapy. Because of the great potential for toxicity with most of these medications, surveillance for adverse effects should be ongoing.

Oral candidiasis is the most common fungal infection seen in HIV-infected children. Oral nystatin suspension (2-5 mL qid) is often effective. Clotrimazole troches or fluconazole (3-6 mg/kg PO QD) are an effective alternative. Oral thrush progresses to involve the esophagus in as many as 20% of children with severe CD4 depletion, presenting with symptoms such as anorexia, dysphagia, vomiting, and fever. Treatment with oral fluconazole for 7-14 days generally results in rapid improvement in symptoms. Fungemia rarely occurs, usually in the setting of indwelling venous catheters, and up to 50% of cases may be caused by non-albicans species. Disseminated histoplasmosis, coccidioidomycosis, and cryptococcosis are rare in pediatric patients but may occur in endemic areas. Parasitic infections such as intestinal cryptosporidiosis and microsporidiosis and rarely isosporiasis or giardiasis are other opportunistic infections that cause significant morbidity. Although these intestinal infections are usually self-limiting in healthy hosts, they cause severe chronic diarrhea in HIV-infected children with low CD4 counts, often leading to malnutrition. Nitazoxanide therapy has been found to be partially effective at improving cryptosporidia diarrhea, but immune reconstitution with HAART is the most important factor for clearance of the infection. Albendazole has been reported to be effective against some microsporidia, and TMP-SMZ appears to be effective for isosporiasis.

Viral infections, especially with the herpesvirus group, pose significant problems for HIV-infected children. HSV causes recurrent gingivostomatitis, which may be complicated by local and distant cutaneous dissemination. Primary varicella-zoster virus (VZV) infection (chickenpox) may be prolonged and complicated by bacterial infections or visceral dissemination, including pneumonitis. Recurrent, atypical, or chronic episodes of herpes zoster are often debilitating and require prolonged therapy with acyclovir; in rare instances, VZV has developed resistance to acyclovir, requiring the use of foscarnet. Disseminated cytomegalovirus (CMV) infection occurs in the setting of severe CD4 depletion (<50 CD4 cells/mm³) and may involve single or multiple organs. Retinitis, pneumonitis, esophagitis, gastritis with pyloric obstruction, hepatitis, colitis, and encephalitis have been reported, but these complications are rarely seen if HAART is given. Ganciclovir (6 mg/kg bid IV) and foscarnet (60 mg/kg tid IV) are the drugs of choice and are often given together in children with sight-threatening CMV retinitis. An intraocular ganciclovir implant plus oral valganciclovir has also been efficacious in adults and older children with CMV retinitis. Measles may occur despite immunization and may present without the typical rash. It often disseminates to the lung or brain with a high mortality rate.

Respiratory viruses such as respiratory syncytial virus (RSV) and adenovirus may present with prolonged symptoms and persistent viral shedding. In parallel with the increased prevalence of genital tract human papillomavirus (HPV) infection, cervical intraepithelial neoplasia (CIN) and anal intraepithelial neoplasia (AIN) also occur with increased frequency among HIV-1–infected adult women compared with HIV-seronegative women. The relative risk for CIN is 5-10 times higher for HIV-1 seropositive women. Multiple modalities are used to treat HPV infection (Chapter 258), although none is uniformly effective and the recurrence rate is high among HIV-1–infected persons.

Central Nervous System

The incidence of CNS involvement in perinatally infected children is 50-90% in resource-limited countries but significantly lower in developed countries, with a median onset at 19 mo of age. Manifestations may range from subtle developmental delay to progressive encephalopathy with loss or plateau of developmental milestones, cognitive deterioration, impaired brain growth resulting in acquired microcephaly, and symmetric motor dysfunction. **Encephalopathy** may be the initial manifestation of the disease or may present much later when severe immune suppression occurs. With progression, marked apathy, spasticity, hyperreflexia, and gait disturbance may occur, as well as loss of language and oral, fine, and/or gross motor skills. The encephalopathy may progress intermittently, with periods of deterioration followed by transiently stable plateaus. Older children may exhibit behavioral problems and learning disabilities. Associated abnormalities identified by neuroimaging techniques include cerebral atrophy in up to 85% of children with neurologic symptoms, increased ventricular size, basal ganglia calcifications, and, less frequently, leukomalacia.

Fortunately, since the advent of HAART, the incident rate of encephalopathy has dramatically declined to as low as 0.08% in 2006. However, as HIV-infected children progress through adolescence and young adulthood, other subtle manifestations of CNS disease are evident, such as cognitive deficits, attention problems, and psychiatric disorders. Living with a chronic, often stigmatizing, disease, parental loss, and the requirement for lifelong pristine medication adherence compounds these issues, making it challenging for these youth as they inherit responsibility for managing their disease as adults.

Focal neurologic signs and seizures are unusual and may imply a co-morbid pathologic process such as a CNS tumor, opportunistic infection, or stroke. **CNS lymphoma** may present with new onset focal neurologic findings, headache, seizures, and mental status changes. Characteristic findings on neuroimaging studies include a hyperdense or isodense mass with variable contrast enhancement or a diffusely infiltrating contrast-enhancing mass. **CNS toxoplasmosis** is exceedingly rare in young infants, but may occur in HIV-infected adolescents and is typically associated with serum antitoxoplasma IgG as a marker of infection. Other opportunistic infections of the CNS are rare and include infection with CMV, JC virus (**progressive *multifocal leukoencephalopathy***), HSV, *Cryptococcus neoformans*, and *Coccidioides immitis*. Although the true incidence of cerebrovascular disorders (both hemorrhagic and nonhemorrhagic strokes) is unclear, 6-10% of children from large clinical series have been affected.

Respiratory Tract

Recurrent upper respiratory tract infections such as otitis media and sinusitis are very common. Although the typical pathogens (*S. pneumoniae, H. influenzae, Moraxella catarrhalis*) are most common, but unusual pathogens such as *P. aeruginosa*, yeast, and anaerobes may be present in chronic infections and result in complications such as invasive sinusitis and mastoiditis.

LIP is the most common chronic lower respiratory tract abnormality reported to the Centers for Disease Control and Prevention (CDC); historically this occurred in approximately 25% of HIV-infected children, although the incidence has declined in the combination ART era. LIP is a chronic process with nodular lymphoid hyperplasia in the bronchial and bronchiolar epithelium, often leading to progressive alveolar capillary block over months to years. It has a characteristic chronic diffuse reticulonodular pattern on chest radiography rarely accompanied by hilar lymphadenopathy, allowing a presumptive diagnosis to be made radiographically before the onset of symptoms. There is an insidious onset of tachypnea, cough, and mild to moderate hypoxemia with normal auscultatory findings or minimal rales. Progressive disease presents with symptomatic hypoxemia, which usually resolves with oral corticosteroid therapy, accompanied by digital clubbing. Several studies suggest that LIP is a lymphyproliferative response to a primary Epstein-Barr virus infection in the setting of HIV infection.

Most symptomatic HIV-infected children experience at least 1 episode of pneumonia during the course of their disease. *S. pneumoniae* is the most common bacterial pathogen, but *P. aeruginosa* and other Gram-negative pneumonias may occur in end-stage disease and are often associated with acute respiratory failure and death. Rarely, severe recurrent bacterial pneumonia results in bronchiectasis. *Pneumocystis* pneumonia is the most common opportunistic infection, but other pathogens, including CMV, *Aspergillus, Histoplasma,* and *Cryptococcus* can cause pulmonary disease. Infection with common respiratory viruses, including respiratory syncytial virus, parainfluenza, influenza, and adenovirus, may occur simultaneously and have a protracted course and period of viral shedding from the respiratory tract. Pulmonary and extrapulmonary tuberculosis (TB) has been reported with increasing frequency in HIV-infected children in low-resource countries, although it is considerably more common in HIV-infected adults. Due to drug interactions between rifampin and ritonavir-based ART and poor tolerability of the combination of multiple drugs required, treatment of TB/HIV co-infection is particularly challenging in children.

Cardiovascular System

Subclinical cardiac abnormalities in HIV-infected children are common, persistent, and often progressive. Young children with symptomatic HIV infection often have dilated cardiomyopathy and left ventricular hypertrophy; the 2 yr cumulative incidence of congestive heart failure is almost 5%. Children with encephalopathy or other AIDS-defining conditions have the highest rate of adverse cardiac outcomes. Resting sinus tachycardia has been reported in up to 64% and marked sinus arrhythmia in 17% of HIV-infected children. Hemodynamic instability occurs more frequently with advanced HIV disease. Gallop rhythm with tachypnea and hepatosplenomegaly appear to be the best clinical indicators of congestive heart failure in HIV-infected children; anticongestive therapy is generally very effective, especially when initiated early. Electrocardiography and echocardiography are helpful in assessing cardiac function before the onset of clinical symptoms. There is increasing concern that premature cardiovascular disease will be seen in children who have disease- or treatment-related hyperlipidemia, and prospective studies will be needed to assess this risk.

Gastrointestinal and Hepatobiliary Tract

Oral manifestations of HIV disease include erythematous or pseudomembranous candidiasis, periodontal disease (e.g., ulcerative gingivitis or periodontitis), salivary gland disease (i.e., swelling, xerostomia), and rarely ulcerations or oral hairy leukoplakia. Gastrointestinal tract involvement is common in HIV-infected children. A variety of pathogens can cause gastrointestinal disease, including bacteria (*Salmonella, Campylobacter,* MAC), protozoa (*Giardia, Cryptosporidium, Isospora,* microsporidia), viruses (CMV, HSV, rotavirus), and fungi (*Candida*). MAC and the protozoal infections are most severe and protracted in patients with severe CD4 cell depletion. Infections may be localized or disseminated and affect any part of the gastrointestinal tract from the oropharynx to the rectum. Oral or esophageal ulcerations, either viral in origin or idiopathic, are painful and often interfere with eating. AIDS enteropathy, a syndrome of malabsorption with partial villous atrophy not associated with a specific pathogen, has been postulated to be a result of direct HIV infection of the gut. Disaccharide intolerance is common in HIV-infected children with chronic diarrhea.

The most common symptoms of gastrointestinal disease are chronic or recurrent diarrhea with malabsorption, abdominal pain, dysphagia, and failure to thrive (FTT). Prompt recognition of weight loss or poor growth velocity in the absence of diarrhea is critical. Linear growth impairment often correlates with the level of HIV viremia. Supplemental enteral feedings should be instituted, either by mouth or with nighttime nasogastric tube feedings in cases associated with more severe chronic growth problems; placement of a gastrostomy tube for nutritional supplementation may be necessary. The wasting syndrome, defined as a loss of >10% of body weight, is not as common as FTT in pediatric patients, but the resulting malnutrition is associated with a grave prognosis. Chronic liver inflammation evidenced by fluctuating serum levels of transaminases with or without cholestasis is relatively common, often without identification of an etiologic agent. Cryptosporidial cholecystitis is associated with abdominal pain, jaundice, and elevated gamma GT. In some patients, chronic hepatitis caused by CMV, hepatitis B, hepatitis C, or MAC may lead to portal hypertension and liver failure. Several of the antiretroviral drugs or other drugs such as didanosine, protease inhibitors, nevirapine, and dapsone may also cause reversible elevation of transaminases.

Pancreatitis with increased pancreatic enzymes with or without abdominal pain, vomiting, and fever may be the result of drug therapy (e.g., with pentamidine, didanosine, or lamivudine) or, rarely, opportunistic infections such as MAC or CMV.

Renal Disease

Nephropathy is an unusual presenting symptom of HIV infection, more commonly occurring in older symptomatic children. A direct effect of HIV on renal epithelial cells has been suggested as the cause, but immune complexes, hyperviscosity of the blood (secondary to hyperglobulinemia), and nephrotoxic drugs are other possible factors. A wide range of histologic abnormalities has been reported, including focal glomerulosclerosis, mesangial hyperplasia, segmental necrotizing glomerulonephritis, and minimal change disease. Focal glomerulosclerosis generally progresses to renal failure within 6-12 mo, but other histologic abnormalities in children may remain stable without significant renal insufficiency for prolonged periods. Nephrotic syndrome is the most common manifestation of pediatric renal disease, with edema, hypoalbuminemia, proteinuria, and azotemia with normal blood pressure. Cases resistant to steroid therapy may benefit from cyclosporine therapy. Polyuria, oliguria, and hematuria have also been observed in some patients.

Skin Manifestations

Many cutaneous manifestations seen in HIV-infected children are inflammatory or infectious disorders that are not unique to HIV infection. These disorders tend to be more disseminated and respond less consistently to conventional therapy than in the uninfected child. Seborrheic dermatitis or eczema that is severe and unresponsive to treatment may be an early nonspecific sign of HIV infection. Recurrent or chronic episodes of HSV, herpes zoster, molluscum contagiosum, flat warts, anogenital warts, and candidal infections are common and may be difficult to control.

Allergic drug eruptions are also common, in particular related to non-nucleoside reverse transcription inhibitors, and generally respond to withdrawal of the drug but also may resolve spontaneously without drug interruption: rarely, progression to Stevens-Johnson syndrome has been reported. Epidermal hyperkeratosis with dry, scaling skin is frequently observed, and sparse hair or hair loss may be seen in the later stages of the disease.

Hematologic and Malignant Diseases

Anemia occurs in 20-70% of HIV-infected children, more commonly in children with AIDS. The anemia may be due to chronic infection, poor nutrition, autoimmune factors, virus-associated conditions (hemophagocytic syndrome, parvovirus B19 red cell aplasia), or the adverse effect of drugs (zidovudine). In children with low erythropoietin levels, subcutaneous recombinant erythropoietin has been successful in treating the anemia.

Leukopenia occurs in almost 30% of untreated HIV-infected children, and neutropenia often occurs. Multiple drugs used for treatment or prophylaxis for opportunistic infections, such as *Pneumocystis* pneumonia, MAC, and CMV, or antiretroviral drugs (zidovudine) may also cause leukopenia and/or neutropenia. In cases in which therapy cannot be changed, treatment with subcutaneous granulocyte colony-stimulating factor may be necessary.

Thrombocytopenia has been reported in 10-20% of patients. The etiology may be immunologic (i.e., circulating immune complexes or antiplatelet antibodies) or less commonly due to drug toxicity, or the cause may be unknown. Antiretroviral therapy may also reverse thrombocytopenia in ARV-naïve patients. Treatment with intravenous immunoglobulin (IVIG) or anti-D offers temporary improvement in most patients already taking ARVs. If ineffective, a course of steroids may be an alternative, but consultation with a hematologist should be sought. Deficiency of clotting factors (factors II, VII, IX) is not rare in children with advanced HIV disease and is often easy to correct with vitamin K. A novel disease of the thymus has been observed in a few HIV-infected children. These patients were found to have characteristic anterior mediastinal multilocular thymic cysts without clinical symptoms. Histologic examination shows focal cystic changes, follicular hyperplasia, and diffuse plasmocytosis and multinucleated giant cells. Spontaneous involution occurs in some cases.

In contrast to the more frequent occurrence in adults, malignant diseases have been reported infrequently in HIV-infected children, representing only 2% of AIDS-defining illnesses. Non-Hodgkin lymphoma, primary CNS lymphoma, and leiomyosarcoma are the most commonly reported neoplasms among HIV-infected children. Epstein-Barr virus is associated with most lymphomas and with all leiomyosarcomas (Chapter 246). Kaposi sarcoma, which is caused by human herpesvirus 8, occurs frequently among HIV-infected adults but is exceedingly uncommon among HIV-infected children in resource rich countries (Chapter 249).

DIAGNOSIS

All infants born to HIV-infected mothers test antibody-positive at birth because of passive transfer of maternal HIV antibody across the placenta during gestation. Most uninfected infants without ongoing exposure (i.e., who are not breast-fed) lose maternal antibody between 6 and 12 mo of age and are known as **seroreverters.** Because a small proportion of uninfected infants continue to test HIV antibody positive for up to 18 mo of age, positive IgG antibody tests, including the rapid tests, cannot be used to make a definitive diagnosis of HIV infection in infants younger than this age. The presence of IgA or IgM anti-HIV in the infant's circulation can indicate HIV infection, because these immunoglobulin classes do not cross the placenta; however, IgA and IgM anti-HIV assays have been both insensitive and nonspecific and therefore are not valuable for clinical use. In any child >18 mo of age, demonstration of IgG antibody to HIV by a repeatedly reactive enzyme immunoassay (EIA) and confirmatory Western blot test establishes the diagnosis of HIV infection. Breast-fed infants should have antibody testing performed 12 wk following cessation of breast-feeding to identify those who became infected at the end of lactation by the HIV-infected mother. Certain diseases (e.g., syphilis, autoimmune diseases) may cause false-positive or indeterminate results. In such cases specific viral diagnostic tests (see later) have to be done.

Several rapid HIV tests are currently available with sensitivity and specificity better than those of the standard EIA. Many of these new tests require only a single step that allows test results to be reported within less than half an hour. Incorporating rapid HIV testing during delivery or immediately after birth is crucial for the care of HIV-exposed newborns whose HIV status was unknown during pregnancy. A positive rapid test has to be confirmed by Western blot testing. However, if 2 different rapid tests (testing different HIV-associated antibodies) are positive, there is no need for further verification with Western blot testing.

Viral diagnostic assays, such as HIV DNA or RNA PCR or HIV culture, are considerably more useful in young infants, allowing a definitive diagnosis in most infected infants by 1-6 mo of age (Table 268-4). By 3-4 mo of age, the HIV culture and/or PCR identifies all infected infants. HIV DNA PCR is the preferred virologic assay in developed countries. Almost 40% of infected newborns have positive test results in the 1st 2 days of life, with >90% testing positive by 2 wk of age. Plasma HIV RNA assays, which detect viral replication, are as sensitive as the DNA PCR for early diagnosis. HIV culture has similar sensitivity to HIV DNA PCR; it is more technically complex and expensive, and results are often not available for several weeks compared with 2-3 days for PCR.

Table 268-4 LABORATORY DIAGNOSIS OF HIV INFECTION

TEST	COMMENT
HIV DNA PCR	Preferred test to diagnose HIV-1 subtype B infection in infants and children younger than 18 mo of age; highly sensitive and specific by 2 wk of age and available; performed on peripheral blood mononuclear cells. False negatives can occur in non-B subtype HIV-1 infections
HIV culture	Expensive, not easily available, requires up to 4 wk to do test; not recommended
HIV RNA PCR	Less sensitive than DNA PCR for routine testing of infants, because a negative result cannot be used to exclude HIV infection definitively. Some assays preferred test to identify non-B subtype HIV-1 infections.

Ag, antigen; ICD, immune complex dissociated; PCR, polymerase chain reaction.
From *Red book: 2009 report of the Committee on Infectious Diseases,* ed 28, Elk Grove Village, IL, 2009, American Academy of Pediatrics, p 386.

Viral diagnostic testing should be performed within the 1st 12-24 hr of life. Almost 40% of HIV-infected children can be identified at this time. It seems that many of these children have a more rapid progression of their disease and deserve more aggressive therapy. In exposed children with negative virologic testing at 1-2 days of life, additional testing should be done at 1-2 mo of age and at 4-6 mo of age; some also favor testing at age 14 days as almost 90% of the infected infants can be identified and earlier initiation of antiretroviral therapy can be initiated. A positive virologic assay (i.e., detection of HIV by PCR, culture, or p24 antigen) suggests HIV infection and should be confirmed by a repeat test on a 2nd specimen as soon as possible. A diagnosis of HIV infection can be made with 2 positive virologic test results obtained from different blood samples.

Although the perinatal use of prophylactic zidovudine to prevent vertical transmission has not affected the predictive value of viral diagnostic testing, the more intensive antiviral combinations (protease inhibitors) in pregnant women do not affect the DNA PCR but the effect on the RNA PCR is unknown. HIV infection can be reasonably excluded if an infant has had at least 2 negative virologic test results with at least 1 test performed at ≥4 mo of age. In some parts of the world where non–subtype B are common (i.e., outside of the USA), interpretation of a negative PCR test result should be done with caution because the assay may not detect the particular subtype (e.g., group O). Close clinical monitoring with serologic testing (by 18 mo of age) or culture (if possible) is recommended. In older infants, 2 or more negative HIV antibody tests performed at least 1 mo apart past 6 mo of age in the absence of hypogammaglobulinemia or clinical evidence of HIV disease can reasonably exclude HIV infection. The infection can be excluded definitively if the same parameters are met when the infant is at least 18 mo of age.

TREATMENT

The currently available therapy does not eradicate the virus and cure the patient and instead suppresses the virus for extended periods of time and changes the course of the disease to a chronic process. Decisions about antiretroviral therapy for pediatric HIV-infected patients are based on the magnitude of viral replication (viral load), CD4 lymphocyte count or percentage, and clinical condition. Because antiretroviral therapy changes as new drugs become available, decisions regarding therapy should be made in consultation with an expert in pediatric HIV infection. Plasma viral load monitoring and measurement of CD4 values have made it possible to implement rational treatment strategies for viral suppression as well as to assess the efficacy of a particular drug combination. The following principles form the basis for antiretroviral treatment: (1) uninterrupted HIV replication causes destruction of the immune system and progression to AIDS; (2) the magnitude of the viral load predicts the rate of disease progression, and the CD4 cell count reflects the risk of opportunistic infections and HIV infection complications; (3) combinations of HAART, which include at least 3 drugs, should be the initial treatment. Potent combination therapy that suppresses HIV replication to an undetectable level restricts the selection of antiretroviral-resistant mutants; drug-resistant strains are the major factor limiting successful viral suppression and delay of disease progression; (4) the goal of sustainable suppression of HIV replication is best achieved by the simultaneous initiation of combinations of antiretroviral agents to which the patient has not been exposed previously and that are not cross-resistant to drugs with which the patient has been treated previously; and (5) adherence to the complex drug regimens is crucial for a successful outcome.

Combination Therapy

Antiretroviral drugs licensed as of 2010 are categorized by their mechanism of action, such as preventing viral entrance into $CD4^+$ T cells, inhibiting the HIV reverse transcriptase or protease enzymes, or inhibiting integration of the virus into the human DNA. Within the reverse transcriptase inhibitors, a further subdivision can be made: **nucleoside (or nucleotide) reverse transcriptase inhibitors (NRTIs)** and **non-nucleoside reverse transcriptase inhibitors (NNRTIs)** (see Fig. 268-2). The NRTIs have a similar structure to the building blocks of DNA (e.g., thymidine, cytosine). When incorporated into DNA, they act like chain terminators and block further incorporation of nucleosides, preventing viral DNA synthesis. As of 2010, 7 NRTIs were licensed in the USA (Table 268-5). Among the NRTIs, thymidine analogs (e.g., stavudine [d4T], zidovudine [ZDV]) are found in higher concentrations in activated or dividing cells, and nonthymidine analogs (e.g., didanosine [ddI], lamivudine [3TC]) have more activity in resting cells. Activated cells are thought to produce >99% of the population of HIV virions. In contrast, resting cells account for <1% of the population but may serve as a reservoir for HIV. Suppression of replication in both populations is thought to be an important component of long-term viral control. NNRTIs (i.e., nevirapine, efavirenz, etravirine) act differently than the NRTIs. They attach to the reverse transcriptase and restrict its motility, reducing the activity of the enzyme. The **protease inhibitors** (PIs) are potent agents that act farther along the viral replicative cycle. As of 2010, 9 PIs were licensed in the USA, but only 5 of these agents (ritonavir, nelfinavir, fosamprenavir, tipranavir, and lopinavir) have pediatric formulations (e.g., liquid or powder) (see Table 268-5). The PIs bind to the site where the viral long polypeptides are cut to individual, mature, and functional core proteins that produce the infectious virions before they leave the cell. The virus entry into the cell is a complex process that involves cellular receptors and fusion. Several drugs have been developed to prevent this process. The **fusion inhibitor,** enfuvirtide, which binds to viral gp41, causes conformational changes that prevent fusion of the virus with the $CD4^+$ cell and entry into the cell. Maraviroc is an example of a selective CCR5 co-receptor antagonist that blocks the attachment of the virus to this chemokine (an essential process in the viral binding and fusion to the $CD4^+$ cells). **Integrase inhibitors** like raltegravir block the enzyme that catalyzes the incorporation of the viral genome into the host's DNA.

While the principal site of viral replication is lymphoid tissue, sanctuary sites such as the CNS may harbor residual virions with the potential to be a source of local or persistent disease. Impaired penetration of drugs to these compartments could result in development of resistance. Although data on CNS penetration of antiviral agents are presently limited, ZDV, d4T, and 3TC appear to achieve inhibitory concentrations in the CNS. Nevirapine also penetrates the CSF, but protease inhibitors are actively transported out of the CNS, thereby limiting their potential efficacy at this site.

By targeting different points in the viral life cycle and stages of cell activation and by delivering drug to all tissue sites, maximal viral suppression may be feasible. Combinations of 3 drugs, a thymidine analog NRTI (ZDV) and a nonthymidine analog NRTI (3TC) to suppress replication in both active and resting cells and a protease inhibitor (lopinavir/ritonavir or nelfinavir) or an NNRTI (efavirenz) have been shown to produce prolonged viral suppression. Less potent combinations such as triple NRTIs (abacavir, zidovudine, lamivudine) may be considered in special situations when there are concerns about significant drug interactions or adherence to a complex drug regimen. Combination treatment increases the rate of toxicities (see Table 268-5), and complex drug-drug interactions exist among many of the antiretroviral drugs. Many protease inhibitor drugs are inducers or inhibitors of the cytochrome P450 system and are therefore likely to have serious interactions with multiple drug classes, including nonsedating antihistamines and psychotropic, vasoconstrictor, antimycobacterial, cardiovascular, analgesic, and gastrointestinal drugs (cisapride). Whenever new

Text continued on page 1172.

Table 268-5 SUMMARY OF ANTIRETROVIRAL THERAPIES AVAILABLE IN 2009

DRUG (TRADE NAMES, FORMULATIONS)	DOSING	SIDE EFFECTS	COMMENTS
NUCLEOSIDE/NUCLEOTIDE REVERSE TRANSCRIPTASE INHIBITORS (NRTIs)		Class adverse effects: Lactic acidosis with hepatic steatosis	
Abacavir Ziagen, ABC Tablet: 300 mg Oral solution: 20 mg/mL Trizivir: combination of ZDV, 3TC, ABC (300, 150, 300 mg) Epzicom: combination of 3TC, ABC (300, 600 mg)	Children: ≥3 mo to 13 yr: 8 mg/kg bid (maximum dose 300 mg bid) 13 yr and older: 300 mg bid Adults: 600 mg once daily (no such data for <16 yr) Trizavir (>40 kg): 1 tablet bid Epzicom (>16 yr of age): 1 tablet bid	Common: Nausea, vomiting, anorexia, fever, headache, diarrhea, rash Less common: Hypersensitivity, lactic acidosis with hepatic steatosis, pancreatitis, elevated triglycerides, myocardial infarction	Can be given with food. Genetic screening for HLAB*5701 is recommended prior to initiation of ABC-containing treatment. If test is positive avoid ABC. Do not restart ABC in patients who had hypersensitivity-like symptoms (e.g., flu-like symptoms).
Didanosine Videx, ddI Powder for oral solution (prepared with solution containing antacid): 10 mg/mL	2 wk to <3 mo: 50 mg/m^2 bid 3-8 mo: 100 mg/m^2 bid >8 mo: 120 mg/m^2 (range 90-150 g/m^2) bid Adolescents (>13 yr) and adults <60 kg: 250 mg once daily (to increase adherence) >60 kg: 400 mg once daily (to increase adherence)	Common: Diarrhea, abdominal pain, nausea, vomiting Less common: Pancreatitis, peripheral neuropathy, electrolyte abnormalities, lactic acidosis with hepatic steatosis, hepatomegaly, retinal depigmentation	Food decreases bioavailability up to 50%. Take 30 min before or 2 hr after meal. Tablets dissolved in water are stable for 1 hr (4 hr in buffered solution). Drug interactions: Antacids/gastric acid antagonists may increase bioavailability; possible decreased absorption of fluoroquinolones, ganciclovir, ketoconazole, itraconazole, dapsone. Combination with d4T enhances toxicity, also common if combined with tenofavir.
Videx EC Capsule, delayed release: 125, 200, 250, 400 mg Generic: 200, 250, 400 mg	Children: Not established 20-25 kg: 200 mg once daily 25-60 kg: 250 mg once daily ≥60 kg: 400 mg once daily	Same as for ddI	Same as ddI
Emtricitabine Emtriva, FTC Capsules: 200 mg Oral solution: 10 mg/mL Truvada: Combination FTC, TDF (200, 300 mg) Atripla: Combination FTC, TDF, EFV (200, 300, 600 mg)	Infants: 0-3 mo: 3 mg/kg once daily Children ≥3 mo to 17 yr: 6 mg/kg (maximum 240 mg) once daily >33 kg: 200 mg capsule or solution once daily Truvada or Atripla adult dose: 1 tablet once daily	Common: Headache, insomnia, diarrhea, nausea, skin discoloration Less common: Lactic acidosis with hepatic steatosis, neutropenia	Closely monitor patients with hepatitis B co-infection. Can be given without regard to food. Oral solution should be refrigerated.
Lamivudine Epivir, Epivir HBV, 3TC Tablet: 150 (scored), 300 mg (Epivir) 100 mg (Epivir HBV) Solution: 5 mg/mL (Epivir HBV), 10 mg/mL (Epivir) Combavir: combination of ZDV, 3TC (300, 150 mg) Trizivir and Epzicon combination (see ABC)	Neonates (<30 days): 2 mg/kg bid >1 mo: 4 mg/kg bid (maximum 150 mg bid) ≥50 kg: 150 mg bid or 300 mg once daily Combavir (>30 kg): 1 tablet bid	Common: Headache, nausea, Less common: Pancreatitis, peripheral neuropathy, lactic acidosis with hepatic steatosis, lipodystrophy	No food restrictions. Drug interactions: Trimethoprim/sulfamethoxazole increases 3TC levels. Combination with ZDV may prevent ZDV resistance. Patient should be screened for HBV and if positive watched for HBV exacerbation when 3TC is discontinued.
Stavudine Zerit, d4T Capsule: 15, 20, 30, 40 mg Solution: 1 mg/mL	Neonates (0-13 days): 0.5 mg/kg bid 14 days to 30 kg: 1 mg/kg bid. 30-60 kg: 30 mg bid >60 kg: 40 mg bid	Common: Headache, nausea, hyperlipidemia, fat maldistribution Less common: Peripheral neuropathy, pancreatitis, lactic acidosis with hepatic steatosis.	No food restrictions. Should not be administered with ZDV due to virologic antagonism. Higher incidence of lactic acidosis than other NRTIs. Increased toxicity if combined with ddI.
Tenofovir Viread, TDF Tablet: 300 mg Truvada: combination of FTC, TDF (200, 300 mg) Atripla: Combination of FTC, TDF, EFV (200, 300, 600 mg)	<12 yr: 8 mg/kg once daily >12 yr and 35 kg: 300 mg once daily adults: 300 mg once daily Truvada and atripla (see FTC)	Common: Nausea, vomiting, diarrhea Less common: Lactic acidosis with hepatic steatosis, hepatomegaly, reduced bone density, renal toxicity	High-fat meal increases absorption; co-administration with ddI may increase ddI toxicity, decrease ATV levels (therefore boosting ATV with ritonavir (RTV) is required). ATV and LPV increase TDF levels and potential toxicity. Screen for HBV before TDF given, as exacerbation of hepatitis may occur when TDF is discontinued.
Zidovudine Retrovir, AZT, ZDV Capsule: 100 mg Tablet: 300 mg Syrup: 10 mg/mL Injection: 10 mg/mL Combavir: combination of ZDV, 3TC (300, 150 mg) Trizavir: Combination of ZDV, 3TC, ABC (300, 150, 300 mg)	**Prophylaxis and treatment:** 0- 6 wk: Premature infants: 1.5 mg/kg IV every 12 hr OR 2 mg/kg orally every 12 hr for age 0-4 wk, then increase to every 8 hr at 2 wk (for gestational age >30 wk) or at 4 wk (for gestational age <30 wk) Neonate/infant: 2.7 mg/kg orally every 8 hr OR 4 mg/kg orally every 12 hr OR 1.5 mg/kg/dose IV every 6 hr (infuse over 30 min)	Common: Bone marrow suppression (e.g., macrocytic anemia, leukopenia) headache, nausea, vomiting, anorexia Less common: Liver toxicity, lactic acidosis with hepatic steatosis, myopathy, fat redistribution	No food restrictions. Drug interactions: should not be given with d4T Rifampin may increase metabolism Cimetidine, fluconazole, valproic acid may decrease metabolism Gancyclovir, ribovirin increase ZDV toxicity Dose adjustment required in renal and/or liver impairment.

Table 268-5 SUMMARY OF ANTIRETROVIRAL THERAPIES AVAILABLE IN 2009—cont'd			
DRUG (TRADE NAMES, FORMULATIONS)	DOSING	SIDE EFFECTS	COMMENTS
	Treatment: 6 wk to 18 yr: 180-240 mg/m^2 every 12 hr or 4 kg to < 9 kg: 12 mg/kg bid 9 kg to <30 kg: 9 mg/kg bid >30 kg: 300 mg bid Adolescents and adults: 200 mg tid or 300 mg bid Combavir (see 3TC) Trizavir (see ABC)		
NON-NUCLEOSIDE REVERSE TRANSCRIPTASE INHIBITORS (NNRTIs)		Class adverse effects: Rash-mild to severe, usually within 1st 6 wk. Discontinue the drug if severe rash (with blistering, desquamation, muscle involvement, or fever).	
Efavirenz Sustiva, EFV Capsule: 50, 200 mg Tablet: 600 mg Atripla combination of EFV, FTC, TDF (600, 200, 300 mg)	Children <3 yr: Not established Children ≥3 yr and weight >10 kg: Given once daily Weight 10 to <15 kg: 200 mg; 15 to <20 kg: 250 mg; 20 to <25 kg: 300 mg; 25 to <32.5 kg: 350 mg; 32.5 to <40 kg: 400 mg; ≥40 kg: 600 mg Atripla (see FTC)	Common: Skin rashes, CNS abnormalities (e.g., abnormal dreams, impaired concentration, insomnia, depression, hallucination) Less common: Increased liver enzymes; potentially teratogenic	Capsules can be opened for mixing in food. Can be given without regard to food except fatty foods (because absorption is increased 50%). Drug interactions: Efavirenz induces/inhibits CYP 3A4 enzymes. Increase clearance of drugs metabolized by this pathway (e.g., antihistamines, sedatives and hypnotics, cisapride, ergot derivatives, warfarin, ethinyl estradiol) and several other ARVs (i.e., protease inhibitors). Drugs that induce CYP 3A4 (e.g., phenobarbital, rifampin, rifabutin) decrease efavirenz levels. Clarithromycin levels decrease with EFV and azithromycin should be considered.
Etravirine Intelence, ETR, TMC 125 Tablet: 100 mg	Pediatric: Not established Adolescents and adults: 200 mg bid	Common: Nausea, skin rashes, diarrhea Less common: Hypersensitivity reactions	Given only with food. Inducer of CYP 3A4 enzymes and inhibitor of CYP 2C9 and CYP 2C19 causing multiple interactions which should be checked before initiating ETR. Should not be given in combination with TPV, Fos-APV, RTV or other NNRTIs.
Nevirapine Viramune, NVP Tablet: 200 mg Suspension: 10 mg/mL	15 days to 8 yr: 200 mg/m^2 once daily for 14 days then same dose bid (maximum 200 mg per dose) > 8 yr: 120-150 mg/m^2 once daily for 14 days then bid (maximum 200 mg per dose) Adolescents and adults: 200 mg once daily for 14 days then 200 mg bid	Common: Skin rash, headache, fever, nausea, abnormal liver function tests Less common: Hepatotoxicity (rarely life threatening), hypersensitivity reactions	No food restrictions. Drug interactions: Induces hepatic CYP 450A enzymes (including CYP 3A and CYP 2B6) activity and decreases protease inhibitors concentrations (e.g., IND, SQV, LPV). Should not be given with ATV. Reduces ketoconazole concentrations (fluconazole should be used as an alternative). Rifampin decreases nevirapine serum levels. Anticonvulsants and psychotropic drugs using same metabolic pathways as NVP should be monitored. Oral contraceptives may also be affected.
PROTEASE INHIBITORS		Class adverse effects: Hyperglycemia, hyperlipidemia (except atazanavir), lipodystrophy, increased transaminases, increased bleeding disorders in hemophiliacs. Can induce metabolism of ethinyl estradiol; use alternate contraception (other than estrogen-containing oral contraceptives). All undergo hepatic metabolism, mostly by CYP 3A4, with many drug interactions!	
Atazanavir Reyataz, ATV Capsules: 100, 150, 200, 300 mg	<6 yr: Not established 6-18 yr: 15 to <25 kg: 150 mg + 80 RTV once daily 25 to <32 kg: 200 mg + 100 RTV once daily 32 to <39 kg: 250 mg + 100 RTV once daily >39 kg: 300 mg + 100 RTV once daily If given with EFV (600 mg): 400 mg + 100 RTV once daily 13 yr and NOT tolerating RTV once daily: 620 mg/m^2 once daily with food	Common: Elevation of indirect bilirubin; headache, arthralgia, depression, insomnia, nausea, vomiting, diarrhea, paresthesias Less common: Prolongation of PR interval on ECG; rash, rarely Stevens-Johnson syndrome, diabetes mellitus, nephrolithiasis	Administer with food to increase absorption. Review drug interactions before initiating because ATV inhibits CYP 3A4, CYP 1A2,CYP 2C9 and UGT1A1 enzymes. Use with caution with cardiac conduction disease or liver impairment. Combination with EFV should not be used in treatment-experienced patients because it decreases ATV levels. TDF, antacids, H_2-receptor antagonists and proton-pump inhibitors decreases ATN concentrations. Patients taking buffered ddI should take it at least 2 hr before ATV.
Darunavir Prezista, DRV, Tablets: 75, 150, 400, 600 mg	<6 yr: Not established >6 yr: 20 to <30 kg: 375 mg DRV + 50 mg RTV bid 30 to <40 kg: 450 DRV mg + 60 mg RTV bid >40 kg: 600 mg DRV + 100 mg RTV Adults: 600 mg DRV + 100 mg RTV, bid or 800 mg DRV + 100 mg RTV once daily (with food)	Common: Diarrhea, nausea, vomiting, abdominal pain, fatigue, headache Less common: Skin rashes (including Stevens-Johnson syndrome), lipid and liver enzyme elevations, hyperglycemia, fat maldistribution	DRV should not be given without food and without RTV. Contraindicated for concurrent therapy with cisapride, ergot alkaloids, benzodiazepines, pimozide or any major CYP 3A4 substrates. Use with caution in patients taking anticonvulsants, strong CYP 3A4 inhibitors, or moderate/strong CYP 3A4 inducers. Adjust dose with concurrent rifamycin therapy. Contains sulfa moiety: potential for cross-sensitivity with sulfonamide class.

Continued

Table 268-5 SUMMARY OF ANTIRETROVIRAL THERAPIES AVAILABLE IN 2009—cont'd

DRUG (TRADE NAMES, FORMULATIONS)	DOSING	SIDE EFFECTS	COMMENTS
Fosamprenavir Lexiva, FPV Tablets: 700 mg Suspension: 50 mg/mL	≥2 yr: ARV naïve: 30 mg/kg (maximum 1400 mg) bid or 18 mg/kg FPV (maximum 700 mg) + 3 mg/kg RTV (maximum 100 mg) bid >6 yr (ARV experienced): 18 mg/kg FPV (maximum 700 mg) + 3 mg/kg RTV (maximum 100 mg) bid Adolescent >47 kg and adults: FPV 1,400 mg bid OR FPV 1,400 mg + RTV 200 mg once daily For PI-experienced, the once daily dose is not recommended	Common: Nausea, vomiting, perioral paresthesias, headache, rash, lipid abnormalities Less common: Stevens-Johnson syndrome, fat redistribution, neutropenia, elevated creatine kinase, hyperglycemia, diabetes mellitus, elevated liver enzymes, angioedema, nephrolithiasis	Tablet no food restrictions but suspension should be given with food. FPV is an inhibitor of the CYP 450 system and an inducer, inhibitor and substrate of CYP 3A4 which can cause multiple drug interactions. Use with caution in sulfa-allergic individuals.
Indinavir Crixivan, IDV Capsule: 100, 200, 400 mg	Infants: Not approved Children: 500 mg/m^2 every 8 hr (max dose: 800 mg per dose) Adolescents and adults: 800 mg IDV every 8 hr or 800 mg IDV + 100 or 200 mg RTV every 12 hr Dosing with EFV: IDV 1,000 mg every 8 hr + EFV 600 mg once daily	Common: Nausea, abdominal pain, hyperbilirubinemia, headache, dizziness, lipid abnormalities, nephrolithiasis, metallic taste Less common: fat redistribution, hyperglycemia, diabetes mellitus, hepatitis, acute hemolytic anemia	Administer on empty stomach. When co-administered with boosting dose of ritonavir, no food restrictions. Reduce dose (600 mg IDV q8h) with mild to moderate liver dysfunction. Adequate hydration (48 oz fluid/day in adults) necessary to minimize risk of nephrolithiasis. IDV is cytochrome P450 3A4 inhibitor and substrate, which can cause multiple drug interactions: rifampin reduces levels; ketoconazole, ritonavir, and other protease inhibitors increase IDV levels. Do not co-administer with astemizole cisapride, terfenadine.
Lopinavir/Ritonavir Kaletra, LPV/r, Tablets: 200/50 mg, 100/25 mg Solution: 80/20 mg per/mL (contains 42% alcohol)	14 days to 6 mo: 300 mg/m^2 LPV/75 mg/m^2 RTV bid OR 16 mg/kg LPV/4 mg/kg RTV bid Children:<15 kg: 12 mg/kg LPV/3 mg/kg RTV bid 15-40 kg: 10 mg/kg LPV/2.5 mg/kg RTV bid >40 kg: 400 mg LPV/100 mg RTV bid Adolescents (>18 yr) and adults: 400 mg LPV/100 mg RTV bid or 800 mg LPV/200 mg RTV once daily	More common: Diarrhea, headache, nausea and vomiting, lipid elevation Less common: Fat redistribution, hyperglycemia, diabetes mellitus, pancreatitis, hepatitis, PR interval prolongation	No food restrictions. High-fat meal is recommended if oral solution is used. Adjust dose when used with NNRTIs (e.g., NVP, EFV) and other protease inhibitors (e.g., FAPV, NFV); interacts with drugs using CYP 3A4, which can cause multiple drug interactions.
Nelfinavir Viracept, NFV Tablet: 250, 625 mg Powder for suspension: 50 mg/1 level scoop, 200 mg/teaspoon	<2 yr: Not recommended Children 2-13 yr: 45-55 mg/kg bid or 25-35 mg/kg tid Adolescents and adults: 750 mg tid or 1,250 mg bid	Common: Diarrhea asthenia, abdominal pain, skin rashes, lipid abnormalities Less common: Exacerbation of liver disease, fat redistribution, hyperglycemia diabetes mellitus, elevation of liver enzymes	Administer with a meal to optimize absorption; avoid acidic food or drink (e.g., orange juice). Tablet can be crushed or dissolved in water to administer as a solution. Drug interactions: Nelfinavir inhibits CYP 3A4 activity, which may cause multiple drug interactions. Rifampin, phenobarbital, and carbamazepine reduce levels. Ketoconazole, ritonavir, indinavir, and other protease inhibitors increase levels. Do not co-administer astemizole, cisapride, terfenadine.
Ritonavir Norvir, RTV Capsule: 100 mg Tablet: 100 mg Solution: 80 mg/mL (contains 43% alcohol)	The major use is to enhance other PIs; dose varies (see information for specific PI)	Common: Nausea, headache, vomiting, abdominal pain, diarrhea, taste aversion, lipids abnormalities, perioral paresthesias Less common: Fat redistribution, hyperglycemia, diabetes mellitus pancreatitis, hepatitis, PR interval prolongation	Administration with food enhances bioavailability and reduces GI symptoms. RTV solution should not be refrigerated. RTV is potent inhibitor of CYP 3A4 and CYP2D6 and inducer of CYP3A4 and CYP1A2 that leads to many drug interactions (e.g., protease inhibitors, antiarrhythmics, antidepressants, cisapride).

Table 268-5 SUMMARY OF ANTIRETROVIRAL THERAPIES AVAILABLE IN 2009—cont'd

DRUG (TRADE NAMES, FORMULATIONS)	DOSING	SIDE EFFECTS	COMMENTS
Saquinavir Invirase, SQV Hard gelatin: 200 mg Film-coated tablets: 500 mg	Infants and children <2 yr: Not established SQV must be boosted with RTV >2 yr: 5-<15 kg: 50 mg/kg + 3 mg/kg RTV bid 15-40 kg: 50 mg/kg + 2.5 mg/kg RTV bid >40: 50 mg/kg + 100 RTV bid Adolescent and adults: 1,000 mg + 100 mg RTV bid	Common: Diarrhea, abdominal pain, headache, nausea, skin rashes, lipid abnormalities Less common: Fat distribution, diabetes mellitus, pancreatitis, elevated liver transaminases, fat maldistribution	Administration with a high-fat meal or grapefruit juice enhances bioavailability. Use only in combination with ritonavir boosting dose. SQV is metabolized by CYP 3A4 which may cause many drug interactions: Rifampin, phenobarbital, and carbamazepine decrease serum levels; saquinavir may decrease metabolism of calcium channel antagonists; azoles (e.g., ketoconazole), macrolides.
Tipranavir Aptivus, TPV Capsule: 250 mg solution 100 mg/mL (contains 116 IU vitamin E/mL)	<2yr: Not established. TPV must be boosted with RTV 2-18 yr: 375 mg/m^2 TPV + 150 mg/ m^2 RTV (maximum 500 mg TPV + 200 mg RTV) bid or 14 mg TPV + 6 mg RTV per kg (maximum-same) bid Adults: 500 mg TPV +200 mg RTV, bid	Common: Diarrhea, nausea, fatigue, vomiting, headache, skin rashes, elevated liver enzymes, lipid abnormalities Less common: Fat redistribution, hepatitis, hyperglycemia, diabetes mellitus: intracranial hemorrhage	No food restrictions. Better tolerated with meal. Can inhibit human platelet aggregation: use with caution in patients at risk for increased bleeding (trauma, surgery, etc.) or in patients receiving concurrent medications that may increase the risk of bleeding. TPV is metabolized by CYP 3A4 which may cause many drug interactions. Contraindicated in patients with hepatic insufficiency or receiving concurrent therapy with amiodarone, cisapride, ergot alkaloids, benzodiazepines, pimozide. TPV contains sulfonamide moiety and caution should be taken in patients with sulfonamide allergy.
FUSION INHIBITORS			
Enfuvirtide Fuzeon, T-20, ENF Injection: Lyophilized powder of 108 mg reconstituted in 1.1 mL of sterile water delivers 90 mg/mL	<6 yr: Not established Children >6 yr to 16 yr: 2 mg/kg (maximum 90 mg) bid >16 yr and adult: 90 mg bid	Common: Local injection site reactions in 98% (e.g., erythema, induration nodules, cysts, ecchymoses) Less common: Increased incidence of bacterial pneumonia, hypersensitivity including fever, nausea, vomiting, chills, elevated liver enzymes, hypotension, immune-mediated reactions (e.g., glomerulonephritis, Guillain-Barré syndrome, respiratory distress)	Must be given subcutaneously. Severity of reactions increased if given intramuscularly. Apply ice after injection and massage the area to reduce local reactions. Injection sites should be rotated.
ENTRY INHIBITORS			
Maraviroc Selzentry, MVC Tablets: 150, 300 mg	Not approved for children or adolescents <16 yr Adolescents >16 yr and adults: 150 mg bid if given together with another PI (except TPV) 300 mg bid if given with CYP 3A4 inhibitors (e.g., NRTI, TPV, NVP, ENF, RAL) 600 mg bid if given with drugs that are not potent CYP 3A4 inducers (e.g., EFV, ETR, rifampin, phenobarbital)	Common: Fever, URI symptoms, skin rashes, abdominal pain, musculoskeletal symptoms, dizziness Less common: Cardiovascular abnormalities, cholestatic jaundice, rhabdomyolysis, myositis	No food restrictions. MVC is a CYP 3A4 and P-glycoprotein (Pgp) substrate which may cause many drug interactions. Tropism assay to exclude the presence of CXCR4 HIV is required before using MVC. Caution should be used when given to patients with hepatic impairment, cardiac disease receiving CYP 3A4 or Pgp modulating drugs.
INTEGRASE INHIBITORS			
Raltegravir Isentress, RAL, Tablets: 400 mg	<16 yr: Not established >16 yr and adults: 400 mg bid	Common: Nausea, headache, dizziness, diarrhea, fatigue Less common: Abdominal pain, vomiting, itching, CPK elevation, myopathy, rhabdomyolysis	No food restrictions. RGV is metabolized by UGT1A1 glucuronidation and inducers of this system (e.g., rifampin, TPV) will reduce RGV levels; whereas inhibitors (e.g., ATV) will increase it.

Antiretroviral drugs often have significant drug-drug interactions, with each other and with other classes of medicines, which should be reviewed before initiating any new medication.
The information in this table is not all-inclusive. Updated and additional information on dosing, drug-drug interactions, and toxicities is available on the AIDSinfo website at *www.aidsinfo.nih.gov*.
Modified from the Panel on Antiretroviral Therapy and Medical Management of HIV-Infected Children: *Guidelines for use of antiretroviral agents in pediatric HIV infection. August 16, 2010* (PDF file). aidsinfo.nih.gov/contentFiles/PediatricGuidelines.pdf. Accessed January 4, 2011.

medications are added to an antiretroviral treatment regimen, especially a protease inhibitor–containing regimen, a pharmacist and/or HIV specialist should be consulted to address possible drug interactions. The inhibitory effect of ritonavir (a protease inhibitor) on the cytochrome P450 system has been exploited, and small doses of the drug are added to several other protease inhibitors (lopinavir, tipranavir, atazanavir) to slow their metabolism by the P450 system and to improve their pharmacokinetic profile. This strategy provides more effective drug levels with less toxicity and less frequent dosing.

Adherence

Adherence to the medications schedules and dosages is fundamental to antiretroviral therapy success. Therefore, assessment of the likelihood of adherence to treatment is an important factor in deciding whether and when to initiate therapy. Numerous studies have shown that compliance of <90% results in less successful suppression of the viral load. In addition, several studies have documented that almost half of the pediatric patients surveyed were nonadherent to their regimen. Poor adherence to prescribed medication regimens results in subtherapeutic drug concentrations and enhances development of resistance. Several barriers to adherence are unique to children with HIV infection. Combination antiretroviral regimens are often unpalatable and require extreme dedication on the part of the caregiver and child; a reluctance to disclose the child's disease to others reduces social support; there may be a tendency to skip doses if the caregiver is not around or when the child is in school. Adolescents have other issues that reduce adherence. Denial of their infection, unstructured lifestyle, wishing to be the same as their peers, depression, anxiety, and alcohol and substance abuse are just a few of the barriers for a long-term adherence in this growing population. These and other barriers make participation of the family in the decision to initiate therapy essential. Intensive education on the relationship of drug adherence to viral suppression, training on drug administration, frequent follow-up visits, peer support, pager messaging, and commitment of the caregiver and the patient (despite the inconvenience of adverse effects, dosing schedule, and so on) are critical for successful antiviral treatment.

Initiation of Therapy

HIV-infected children with symptoms (clinical category A, B, or C) or with evidence of immune dysfunction (immune category 2 or 3) should be treated with antiretroviral therapy, regardless of age or viral load (see Tables 268-1 and 268-2). Children <1 yr of age are at high risk for disease progression, and immunologic and virologic tests to identify those likely to develop rapidly progressive disease are less predictive than in older children. Therefore, such infants should be treated with antiretroviral agents as soon as the diagnosis of HIV infection has been confirmed, regardless of clinical or immunologic status or viral load. Data suggest that HIV-infected infants who are treated before the age of 3 mo control their HIV infection better than infants whose antiretroviral therapy started later than 3 mo of age. Some of these infants even become HIV seronegative and lose their HIV specific immune response.

There is still a debate on when to start therapy in children older than 1 yr of age. Most guidelines recommend deferring treatment if the CD4 is ≥25% in children 1-5 yr of age or the CD4 count is above 350-500 cells/mm^3 in children >5 yr of age, with a viral load of <100,000 copies/mm^3 because there are concerns regarding drug adherence, safety, and durability of antiretroviral response. These children should be monitored regularly for evidence of virologic, immunologic, or clinical progression, at which point therapy should be initiated as long as potential adherence issues are addressed. Some clinicians advocate treating such children to prevent the inevitable immunologic deterioration that will otherwise occur.

Dosing

Data on antiretroviral drug dosages for neonates are often limited. Because of the immaturity of the neonatal liver, premature infants and newborns often require an increase in the dosing interval of drugs primarily cleared through hepatic glucuronidation. Children are usually treated with higher doses (per kg weight) than adults due to reduced absorption or increased elimination.

Adolescents should have antiretroviral dosages prescribed on the basis of Tanner staging of puberty rather than on the basis of age. Pediatric dosing ranges should be used during early puberty (Tanner stages I, II, and III), whereas adult dosing schedules should be followed in adolescents in late puberty (Tanner stages IV and V).

Changing Antiretroviral Therapy

Therapy should be changed when the current regimen is judged ineffective as evidenced by increase in viral load, deterioration of the CD4 cell count, or clinical progression. Development of toxicity or intolerance to drugs is another reason to consider a change in therapy. When a change is considered, the patient and family should be reassessed for adherence problems. Because adherence is a major issue in this population, resistance testing (while on antiretroviral medications) is important in identifying adherence issues (e.g., detectable virus sensitive to current drugs) or development of resistance (e.g., evidence of resistance mutations to given drugs). In both situations, other contributing factors such as poor absorption, incorrect dose, or drug-drug interactions should be carefully reviewed. While considering possible new drug choices, potential cross-resistance should be addressed. In addition, few patients who have virologic failure may still demonstrate improved CD4 cell counts (discordant response). Impaired replication ability of the resistant virus and enhanced cytotoxic T lymphocyte (CTL) effects are some of the reasons for this discordant response. In these patients, delay in changing therapy may be considered as long as the immunologic benefit is evident. Ideally, when a decision is made to change the antiretroviral therapy, all drugs should be changed. However, in many situations (previous antiretroviral experience, intolerance, toxicity) this is not possible, and, therefore, at least 2 drugs should be changed based on the resistance mutation genotype (if available) or previous regimen used.

Monitoring Antiretroviral Therapy

Children need to be seen within 1 to 2 wk after initiation of new antiretroviral therapy to assure compliance and to screen for potential side effects. Virologic and immunologic surveillance (using HIV RNA copy number and CD4 lymphocyte count or percentage) as well as clinical assessment should be performed regularly during antiretroviral therapy. Initial virologic response (i.e., at least a 5-fold [0.7 $\log_{10}$] reduction in viral load) should be achieved within 4-8 wk of initiating antiretroviral therapy. The maximum response to therapy usually occurs within 12-16 wk but may be later (24 wk) in very young infants. Thus, HIV RNA levels should be measured at 4 wk and 3-4 mo after therapy initiation. Once an optimal response has occurred, viral load should then be measured at least every 3-6 mo. If the response is unsatisfactory, another viral load should be performed as soon as possible to verify the results before a change in therapy is considered. The CD4 cells respond more slowly to successful treatment and, therefore, can be monitored less frequently. Potential toxicity should be monitored closely for the 1st 8-12 wk, and if no clinical or laboratory toxicity is documented, a follow-up visit every 3-4 mo is adequate. Monitoring for potential toxicity should be tailored to the drugs taken. These toxicities include hematologic complications (e.g., ZDV); hypersensitivity rash (e.g., EFV); lipodystrophy (e.g., redistribution of body fat seen with NRTIs, protease inhibitors); hyperlipidemia (elevation of cholesterol and triglyceride concentrations), hyperglycemia and insulin resistance, and mitochondrial toxicity leading to severe lactic acidosis (e.g., D4T, ddI), ECG abnormalities (e.g., atazanavir, lopinavir), abnormal bone mineral metabolism (e.g., tenofavir), and hepatic toxicity including severe hepatomegaly with steatosis.

Resistance to Antiretroviral Therapy

Young children are at greater risk than adults for developing resistance because they have higher viral loads than adults and are more limited by which ARV options are available. The high mutation rate of HIV (mainly due to the absence of error-correcting mechanisms) severely impairs the success of antiretroviral therapy. Failure to reduce the viral load to <50 copies/mL increases the risk for developing resistance. Even effectively treated patients do not completely suppress viral replication, and persistence of HIV transcription and evolution of envelope sequences continues in the latent cellular reservoirs. The accumulation of resistance mutations progressively diminishes the potency of the antiretroviral therapy and challenges the physician to find new regimens. For some drugs (e.g., nevirapine, 3TC) a single mutation is associated with resistance, while for other drugs (e.g., ZDV, lopinavir) several mutations are needed before resistance develops. Testing for drug resistance, especially when devising a new regimen, is becoming the standard of care. Two types of tests are available. The **phenotypic assay** measures the virus susceptibility in various concentrations of the drug, and the **genotypic assay** predicts the virus susceptibility from mutations identified in the HIV genome isolated from the patient. Several studies have shown that treatment success was higher in patients whose antiretroviral therapy was guided by genotype or phenotype testing.

Supportive Care

Even before antiretroviral drugs were available, a significant impact on the quality of life and survival of HIV-infected children was achieved when supportive care was given. A multidisciplinary team approach is desirable for successful management. Close attention should be paid to nutritional status, which is often delicately balanced and may require aggressive enteral supplementation; Painful oropharyngeal lesions and dental caries may interfere with eating, and thus routine dental evaluations and careful attention to oral hygiene should be encouraged. Paradoxically, an increasing number of adolescents with perinatally-acquired or behavioral risk-acquired disease are obese. Some teens experience ARV-related central lipo-accumulation, but others have poor dietary habits and inactivity as the cause of their obesity, in parallel to epidemic obesity in the USA. Development should be evaluated regularly with provision of necessary physical, occupational, and/or speech therapy. Recognition of pain in the young child may be difficult, and effective nonpharmacologic and pharmacologic protocols for pain management should be instituted.

Infants born to HIV-infected mothers should receive ZDV prophylaxis for 4-6 weeks +/− additional ART to prevent transmission. Guidelines for such prophylaxis are updated at least yearly and can be accessed at *http://www.aidsinfo.nih.gov/default.aspx*. A complete blood count, differential leukocyte count, and platelet count should be performed at 4 wk of age to monitor ZDV toxicity. If the child is found to be HIV-infected or if the HIV status is not clear, these tests should be continued every 1-3 mo to assess the hematologic effect of the disease or its treatment (prophylactic TMP-SMZ and antiretroviral therapy). If the child is found to be HIV infected, baseline laboratory assessment (e.g., CD4 count, HIV RNA, CBC, chemistries) should be done. Viral load and CD4 lymphocyte counts should be performed at 1 and 3 mo of age and should be repeated every 3 mo. The frequency of the test should be increased (every 4-6 wk) if the CD4 lymphocyte count or percentage declines rapidly.

All HIV-exposed and infected children should receive standard pediatric immunizations. In general, live oral polio vaccine should not be given (Fig. 268-3). The risk and benefits of rotavirus vaccination should be considered in infants born to HIV-infected mothers. Because <1% of these infants in developed countries will develop HIV infection, the vaccine should be given. In other situations, the considerable attenuation of the vaccine's strains should be taken into account and unless the infant has clinical symptoms of AIDS or CD4 <15%, vaccination seems to be appropriate. Other live bacterial vaccines (e.g., bacillus Calmette-Guérin [BCG]) should be avoided due to the high incidence of BCG-related disease in HIV-infected infants. Varicella and measles-mumps-rubella (MMR) vaccines are recommended for children who are not severely immunosuppressed (i.e., CD4 cell percentage ≥15%), but neither varicella nor MMR vaccines should be given to severely immunocompromised children (i.e., CD4 cell <15%). Of note, prior immunizations do not always provide protection, as evidenced by outbreaks of measles and pertussis in immunized HIV-infected children. Durability of vaccine-induced titers is often short, especially if vaccines are administered when the child's CD4 cell is <15%, and re-immunization when the CD4 count has increased (i.e., >15%) may be indicated.

Prophylactic regimens are integral for the care of HIV-infected children. All infants between 4-6 wk and 1 yr of age who are proven to be HIV-infected should receive prophylaxis to prevent *Pneumocystis jiroveci* infection regardless of the CD4 count or percentage (see Tables 268-6 and 268-7). Infants exposed to

Vaccine	Birth	1 mo	2 mo	4 mo	6 mo	12 mo	15 mo	18 mo	24 mo	4-6 yr	11-12 yr	14-16 yr
Hepatitis B	Hep B	Hep B			Hep B							
Measles, Mumps, Rubella*						MMR†	MMR†					
Influenza					Influenza‡							
Pneumococcal Conjugate and Hemophilus b			PCV Hib	PCV Hib	PCV Hib	PCV Hib					Pneumococcal§	
Diphtheria, Tetanus, Pertussis			DTap	DTap	DTap		DTap					
Polio (inactivated)			Polio	Polio	Polio							
Varicella						Varicella						
Hepatitis A						Hep A‖						
Rotavirus*			RV¶	RV	RV							

* See text.
† Contraindicated in children with AIDS or CD4+ <15%. Give two doses 1-3 mo apart.
‡ Revaccination is recommended every year. Attenuated vaccine can be used >2 yr of age only if CD4+ >15%.
§ Revaccination with pneumococcal polysaccharide vaccine (PPV) every 5 yr.
‖ Two doses at least 6 mo apart.
¶ First dose 6 through 14 wk of age and final dose no later than 8 mo 0 d of age. If using Rotarix only 2 doses (2 and 4 mo) are needed.

Figure 268-3 Routine childhood immunization schedule for HIV-infected children.

Table 268-6 RECOMMENDATIONS FOR PCP PROPHYLAXIS AND CD4 MONITORING FOR HIV-EXPOSED INFANTS AND HIV-INFECTED CHILDREN, BY AGE AND HIV INFECTION STATUS

AGE/HIV INFECTION STATUS	PCP PROPHYLAXIS	CD4 MONITORING
Birth to 4-6 wk, HIV exposed	No prophylaxis	None
HIV infection reasonably excluded*	No prophylaxis	None
4-6 wk to 4 mo, HIV exposed	Prophylaxis	3 mo
6 wk to 1 yr HIV-infected or indeterminate	Prophylaxis	6, 9, and 12 mo
1-5 yr, HIV infected	Prophylaxis if:	Every 3-4 mo†
	CD4 <500 cells/µL or <15%	
> 6 yr, HIV infected	Prophylaxis if:	Every 3-4 mo†
	CD4 <200 cells/µL or <15%‡	

The National Perinatal HIV Hotline (1-888-448-8765) provides consultation on all aspects of perinatal HIV care.

PCP, *Pneumocystis carinii* (some suggest *jirovecii*) pneumonia.

*See text.

†More frequent monitoring (e.g., monthly) is recommended for children whose CD4 counts or percentages are approaching the threshold at which prophylaxis is recommended.

‡Prophylaxis should be considered on a case-by-case basis for children who might otherwise be at risk for PCP, such as children with rapidly declining CD4 counts or percentages or children with category C conditions. Children who have had PCP should receive lifelong PCP prophylaxis.

HIV-infected mothers should receive the same prophylaxis until they are proven to be noninfected; however, prophylaxis does not have to be initiated if there is strong presumptive evidence of noninfection (i.e., non–breast-fed infant with 2 negative HIV PCR tests at >14 days and 4 wk of age, respectively). When the HIV-infected child is >1 yr of age, prophylaxis should be given according to the CD4 lymphocyte count (Table 268-6). The best prophylactic regimen is 150 mg/m^2/day of trimethoprim component of TMP/SMZ given as 1-2 daily doses 3 days per wk. For severe adverse reactions to TMP/SMZ, alternative therapies include dapsone, atovaquone, or aerosolized pentamidine.

Prophylaxis against MAC should be offered to HIV-infected children with advanced immunosuppression (i.e., CD4 lymphocyte count <750 cells/mm^3 in children <1 yr of age, <500 for children 1-2 yr of age, <75 cells/mm^3 in children 2-5 yr of age, and <50 cells/mm^3 in children >6 yr of age) (Table 268-7). The drugs of choice are azithromycin (20 mg/kg [maximum 1200 mg] once a week PO or 5 mg/kg [maximum 250 mg] once daily PO) or clarithromycin (7.5 mg/kg bid PO).

Based on adult data, primary prophylaxis against opportunistic infections may be discontinued if patients have experienced sustained (>6 mo duration) immune reconstitution with HAART. Even if patients have had opportunistic infections such as *Pneumocystis* pneumonia or disseminated MAC, it may also be possible to discontinue prophylaxis if immune reconstitution has been sustained.

All HIV-infected children should have tuberculin skin testing (5 tuberculin units purified protein derivation [PPD]) for TB at least once per year. If the child is living in close contact with a person with tuberculosis, he or she should be tested more frequently. Recently, assays that determine IFN-γ release from lymphocytes following stimulation by specific *M. tuberculosis* antigens were found to be more specific than the skin testing in adults. Limited data suggest that they are less sensitive in diagnosing TB in children, and therefore caution should be used in interpreting negative results of such tests in children. To reduce the incidence of other potential infections, parents should be counseled about (1) the importance of good handwashing, (2) avoiding raw or undercooked food *(Salmonella)*, (3) avoiding drinking or swimming in lake or river water or being in contact with young farm animals *(Cryptosporidium)*, and (4) the risk of playing with pets (*Toxoplasma* and *Bartonella* from cats, *Salmonella* from reptiles).

Because of the frequent changes in these guidelines, physicians providing care to few HIV-exposed or infected children should periodically consult physicians with expertise in pediatric HIV infection as well as the U.S. Pediatric Guidelines for treatment of HI- infected children found at *http://www.aidsinfo.nih.gov*.

PROGNOSIS

The improved understanding of the pathogenesis of HIV infection in children and the availability of more effective antiretroviral drugs has changed the prognosis considerably. In settings with ready access to early diagnosis and antiretroviral therapy, progression of the disease to AIDS has significantly diminished. Since the advent of HAART in the mid-1990s, mortality in perinatally infected children has declined >90% and the mean age at death has doubled from ~9 yr of age in the pre-HAART era to >18 yr of age by 2006. Even with only partial reduction of viral load, children may have both significant immunologic and clinical benefits. In general, the best prognostic indicators are the sustained suppression of plasma viral load and restoration of a normal CD4$^+$ lymphocyte count. If determinations of viral load and CD4 lymphocytes are available, the results can be used to evaluate prognosis. It is unusual to see rapid progression in an infant with a viral load <100,000 copies/mL. In contrast, a high viral load (>100,000 copies/mL) over time is associated with greater risk for disease progression and death. CD4 lymphocyte percentage is another prognostic indicator, and the mortality rate is higher in patients with a CD4 lymphocyte percentage <15%. To define prognosis more accurately, the use of changes in both markers (CD4 lymphocyte percentage and plasma viral load) is recommended.

In resource-limited countries where antiretroviral therapy and molecular diagnostic tests are less available, a clinical staging system has been used to predict progression of disease and when to initiate antiretroviral therapy. The suggested clinical staging is similar to the classification recommended in the revised 1994 CDC classification. Unfortunately, this system has a low sensitivity for diagnosing HIV-infected children. Children with opportunistic infections (*Pneumocystis* pneumonia, MAC), encephalopathy, or wasting syndrome have the worst prognosis, with 75% dying before 3 yr of age. Persistent fever and/or oral thrush, serious bacterial infections (meningitis, pneumonia, sepsis), hepatitis, persistent anemia (<8.0 g/dL), and/or thrombocytopenia (<100,000/mm^3) also suggest a poor outcome, with >30% of such children dying before age 3 yr of age. In contrast, lymphadenopathy, splenomegaly, hepatomegaly, lymphoid interstitial pneumonitis, and parotitis are indicators of a better prognosis.

PREVENTION

Use of antiretroviral therapy for interruption of perinatal transmission from mother-to-child has been one of the greatest achievements of HIV research. In the landmark Pediatric Clinical Trials Protocol 076, ZDV chemoprophylaxis was administered to pregnant women as early as 4 wk of gestation, during labor and delivery, and to the newborn for the 1st 6 wk of life and reduced vertical transmission by 75% when compared with placebo treated mother-infant pairs. Maternal HAART has been documented to decrease the rate of perinatal HIV-1 transmission to <2% and <1% if the mother's viral RNA level is <1000 copies/mL at delivery. Therefore, the CDC recommends that women be treated with a HAART regimen irrespective of viral load or CD4 count during pregnancy, with collaboration between the HIV-specialist and the obstetrician. Cesarean section (C-section) as a prevention strategy was examined in a multinational meta-analysis, which showed that the combination of elective C-section and maternal ZDV

Table 268-7 PROPHYLAXIS TO PREVENT FIRST EPISODE OF OPPORTUNISTIC INFECTIONS AMONG HIV-EXPOSED AND HIV-INFECTED INFANTS AND CHILDREN, USA*

PATHOGEN	PREVENTIVE REGIMEN Indication	First Choice	Alternative
STRONGLY RECOMMENDED AS STANDARD OF CARE			
Pneumocystis pneumonia†	HIV-infected or HIV-indeterminate infants aged 1-12 mo; HIV-infected children aged 1-5 yr with CD4 count of <500 cells/mm³ or CD4 percentage of <15%; HIV-infected children aged 6-12 yr with CD4 count of <200 cells/mm³ or CD4 percentage of <15%	TMP-SMX, 150/750 mg/m² body surface area per day (max: 320/1600 mg) orally divided into 2 doses daily and administered 3 times weekly on consecutive days. Acceptable alternative dosage schedules for same dose: single dose orally 3 times weekly on consecutive days; 2 divided doses orally daily; or 2 divided doses orally 3 times weekly on alternate days	Dapsone: children aged ≥1 mo, 2 mg/kg body weight (max 100 mg) orally daily; or 4 mg/kg body weight (max 200 mg) orally weekly. Atovaquone: children aged 1-3 mo and >24 mo, 30 mg/kg body weight orally daily; children aged 4-24 mo, 45 mg/kg body weight orally daily. Aerosolized pentamidine: children aged ≥5 yr, 300 mg every mo by Respirgard II (Marquest, Englewood, CO) nebulizer.
Malaria	Living or traveling to area in which malaria is endemic	Recommendations are the same for HIV-infected and HIV-uninfected children. Refer to *http://www.cdc.gov/malaria/* for the most recent recommendations based on region and drug susceptibility. Mefloquine, 5 mg/kg body weight orally 1 time weekly (max 250 mg) Atovaquone/proguanil (Malarone) 1 time daily 11-20 kg = 1 pediatric tablet (62.5 mg/25 mg) 21-30 kg = 2 pediatric tablets (125 mg/50 mg) 31-40 kg = 3 pediatric tablets (187.5 mg/75 mg) >40 kg = 1 adult tablet (250 mg/100 mg)	Doxycycline, 100 mg orally daily for children >8 yr (2.2 mg/kg/day). Chloroquine 5 mg/kg base (equal 7.5 mg/kg chloroquine phosphate) orally up to 300 mg weekly (only for regions where the parasite is sensitive).
Mycobacterium tuberculosis			
Isoniazid-sensitive	TST reaction ≥5 mm or prior positive TST result without treatment; or regardless of current TST result and previous treatment, close contact with any person who has contagious TB. TB disease must be excluded before start of treatment.	Isoniazid, 10-15 mg/kg body weight (max 300 mg) orally daily for 9 mo; or 20-30 mg/kg body weight (max 900 mg) orally 2 times weekly for 9 mo	Rifampin, 10-20 mg/kg body weight (max 600 mg) orally daily for 4-6 mo
Isoniazid-resistant	Same as previous pathogen; increased probability of exposure to isoniazid-resistant TB	Rifampin, 10-20 mg/kg body weight (max 600 mg) orally daily for 4-6 mo	Uncertain
Multidrug-resistant (isoniazid and rifampin)	Same as previous pathogen; increased probability of exposure to multidrug-resistant TB	Choice of drugs requires consultation with public health authorities and depends on susceptibility of isolate from source patient	
Mycobacterium avium complex‡	For children aged ≥6 yr with CD4 count of <50 cells/mm³; aged 2-5 yr with CD4 count of <75 cells/mm³; aged 1-2 yr with CD4 count of <500 cells/mm³; aged <1 yr with CD4 count of <750 cells/mm³	Clarithromycin, 7.5 mg/kg body weight (max 500 mg) orally 2 times daily, or azithromycin, 20 mg/kg body weight (max 1,200 mg) orally weekly	Azithromycin, 5 mg/kg body weight (max 250 mg) orally daily; children aged ≥6 yr, rifabutin, 300 mg orally daily
Varicella-zoster virus§	Substantial exposure to varicella or shingles with no history of varicella or zoster or seronegative status for VZV by a sensitive, specific antibody assay or lack of evidence for age-appropriate vaccination	Varicella-zoster immune globulin (VariZIG), 125 IU per 10 kg (max 625 IU) IM, administered within 96 hr after exposure‖	If VariZIG is not available or <96 hr have passed since exposures, some experts recommend prophylaxis with acyclovir 20 mg/kg body weight (max 800 mg) per dose orally 4 times a day for 5-7 days. Another alternative to VariZIG is intravenous immune globulin (IVIG), 400 mg/kg, administered once. IVIG should be administered within 96 hr after exposure
Vaccine-preventable pathogens	Standard recommendations for HIV-exposed and HIV-infected children	Routine vaccinations (see Fig. 268-3)	

Continued

Table 268-7 PROPHYLAXIS TO PREVENT FIRST EPISODE OF OPPORTUNISTIC INFECTIONS AMONG HIV-EXPOSED AND HIV-INFECTED INFANTS AND CHILDREN, USA—cont'd

PATHOGEN	PREVENTIVE REGIMEN Indication	First Choice	Alternative
USUALLY RECOMMENDED			
Toxoplasma gondii¶	Immunoglobulin G (IgG) antibody to *Toxoplasma* and severe immunosuppression: HIV-infected children aged <6 yr with CD4 <15%; HIV-infected children aged ≥6 yr with CD4 <100 cells/mm^3	TMP-SMX, 150/750 mg/m^2 body surface area daily orally in 2 divided doses Acceptable alternative dosage schedules for same dosage: single dose orally 3 times weekly on consecutive days; or 2 divided doses orally 3 times weekly on alternate days	Dapsone (children aged ≥1 mo), 2 mg/kg body weight or 15 mg/m^2 body surface area (max 25 mg) orally daily, PLUS pyrimethamine, 1 mg/kg body weight (max 25 mg) orally daily; PLUS leucovorin, 5 mg orally every 3 days Atovaquone (children aged 1-3 mo and >24 mo, 30 mg/kg body weight orally daily; children aged 4-24 mo, 45 mg/kg body weight orally daily) with or without pyrimethamine, 1 mg/kg body weight or 15 mg/m^2 body surface area (max 25 mg) orally daily; PLUS leucovorin, 5 mg orally every 3 days
NOT RECOMMENDED FOR MOST CHILDREN—INDICATED FOR USE ONLY IN UNUSUAL CIRCUMSTANCES			
Invasive bacterial infections	Hypogammaglobulinemia (i.e., IgG <400 mg/dL)	IVIG (400 mg/kg body weight every 2-4 wk)	
Cytomegalovirus	CMV antibody positivity and severe immunosuppression (CD4 <50 cells/mm^3)	Valganciclovir, 900 mg orally 1 time daily with food for older children who can receive adult dosing	

*Information in these guidelines might not represent FDA approval or FDA-approved labeling for products or indications. Specifically, the terms "safe" and "effective" might not be synonymous with the FDA-defined legal standards for product approval.
†Daily trimethoprim-sulfamethoxazole (TMP-SMX) reduces the frequency of certain bacterial infections. TMP-SMX, dapsone-pyrimethamine, and possibly atovaquone (with or without pyrimethamine) protect against toxoplasmosis; however, data have not been prospectively collected. Compared with weekly dapsone, daily dapsone is associated with lower incidence of PCP but higher hematologic toxicity and mortality. Patients receiving therapy for toxoplasmosis with sulfadiazine-pyrimethamine are protected against PCP and do not need TMP-SMX.
‡Substantial drug interactions can occur between rifamycins (i.e., rifampin and rifabutin) and protease inhibitors and non-nucleoside reverse transcriptase inhibitors. A specialist should be consulted.
§Children routinely being administered intravenous immunoglobulin (IVIG) should receive VariZIG if the last dose of IVIG was administered >21 days before exposure.
||As of 2007, VariZIG can be obtained only under a treatment Investigational New Drug protocol (1-800-843-7477, FFF Enterprises, Temecula, CA).
¶Protection against toxoplasmosis is provided by the preferred anti-*Pneumocystis* regimens and possibly by atovaquone.
HIV, human immunodeficiency virus; PCP, *Pneumocystis* pneumonia; TMP-SMX, trimethoprim-sulfamethoxazole; TST, tuberculin skin test; TB, tuberculosis; IM, intramuscularly; IVIG, intravenous immunoglobulin; IgG, immunoglobulin G; CMV, cytomegalovirus; VZV, varicella-zoster virus; FDA, U.S. Food and Drug Administration.
From Centers for Disease Control and Prevention: Guidelines for the prevention and treatment of opportunistic infections among HIV-exposed and HIV-infected children, *MMWR Recomm Rep* 58(RR-11):127–128, 2009, Table 1.

treatment reduced transmission by 87%. However, these data were obtained prior to the advent of HAART, and the additional benefit of elective C-section to the HAART-treated mother is not clear. In women whose viral load at the time of delivery is >1,000 copies/mL, the potential benefit of C-section should be considered to further reduce the risk for vertical transmission.

Retrospective data suggest that even if a mother has received no antiretroviral therapy during gestation or delivery, the 6-wk component of the ZDV prophylactic regimen instituted for the newborn as soon as possible after delivery (preferably within 12-24 hr of birth) results in a significant reduction of transmission rate. Full-term infants and preterm infants should be treated with oral ZDV (see Table 268-5).

Oral nevirapine, a non-nucleoside reverse transcriptase inhibitor, given once to women in labor and once to the infant during the 1st 48-72 hr of life, capitalizes on the prolonged half-life of this drug. In Africa, single dose nevirapine (SD NVP) has been shown to reduce perinatal transmission by almost 50%, providing a simple and highly cost-effective regimen for resource-poor countries. However, women and infants who have received SD NVP and subsequently require ART within 6 mo of delivery have a significantly higher rate of virologic failure if a NVP-based regimen is used. Therefore, the WHO has also recommended that pregnant women be treated with a HAART regimen appropriate for their own health, if possible. For those who do not meet indications for therapy, a regimen known to prevent vertical HIV-1 transmission should be offered, such as ZDV from 14 weeks of pregnancy plus/minus a single dose of nevirapine (SD NVP) during labor and oral ZDV + 3TC during labor and for 1 week postpartum; their non–breast-feeding infants should also receive ZDV or NVP for 6 weeks. Studies in non–breast-feeding mothers in Thailand have shown that 3rd trimester ZDV with SD NVP in labor with 7 days of ZDV ± SD NVP to the infant is associated with a transmission rate of <2%. These regimens offer simpler, less expensive, effective approaches to preventing perinatal transmission when longer-term regimens are difficult to implement.

Although the most effective way to prevent postpartum transmission of HIV is to eliminate breast-feeding altogether and substitute replacement feeding, there is increasing evidence that early weaning may not be safe in very resource constrained settings, due to the high risk of malnutrition and diarrhea in formula-fed infants without a consistent source of clean water. The WHO has recommended exclusive breast-feeding (no additional solids or fluids other than water) for at least 6 mo in resource-limited settings, unless there is an acceptable, feasible, affordable, sustainable, and safe (AFASS) replacement feeding option. Multiple international studies have shown that there are 2 efficacious approaches to interrupt breast-feeding transmission. One option is to treat mothers with triple ART for the duration of breast-feeding and their infants with daily nevirapine from birth to 6 weeks of age; this is critical for mothers who require ART for their own health. The other option, only for women with relatively strong CD4 counts who do not require ART for their own health, is to discontinue maternal ART 1 wk after delivery and treat the infant with daily nevirapine from birth until all exposure to breast milk has ended. As more data become available, guidelines for prevention of mother to child transmission will be regularly updated at *http://www.aidsinfo.nih.gov/default.aspx* and the WHO website (*http://www.who.int/en/index.html*).

Now that it is clear that perinatal transmission can be reduced dramatically by treating pregnant mothers, a compelling argument can be made for prenatal identification of HIV-1 infection in the mother. The benefit of therapy both for the mother's health and to prevent transmission to the infant cannot be overemphasized. The recommended universal prenatal HIV-1 counseling and HIV-1 testing with consent for all pregnant women has reduced the number of new infections dramatically in many areas of the USA and Europe. For women not tested during pregnancy, the use of rapid HIV antibody testing during labor or on the 1st day of life for the infant is a way to provide perinatal prophylaxis to an additional group of at-risk infants.

Prevention of sexual transmission involves avoiding the exchange of bodily fluids. In sexually active adolescents, condoms should be an integral part of programs to reduce sexually transmitted diseases, including HIV-1. Unprotected sex with older partners or with multiple partners and use of recreational drugs is common among HIV-1–infected adolescents, increasing their risk. Educational efforts about avoidance of risk factors are essential for older school-aged children and adolescents and should begin before the onset of sexual activity. In addition, promising new research for sexually active adults may translate to increased prevention for adolescents. Three African trials have demonstrated that male circumcision was associated with a 50-60% reduction in risk of HIV acquisition in young men. For women, use of a 1% vaginal gel formulation of tenofovir during intercourse was found to reduce HIV acquisition by nearly 40%. Other topical microbicides are being investigated. Recently, a double-blind study of pre-exposure prophylaxis in males having sex with men using once daily dosing of co-formulated tenofovir and emtricitabine resulted in a 44% reduction in the incidence of HIV (95% confidence interval, 15 to 63; P=0.005). Of interest, the incidence of HIV transmission was reduced by 73% when participants took the drug on 90% or more days.

Despite prolonged suppression of viremia, it is obvious that HAART will not fully restore health and is associated with long term toxicity. In addition, adherence is a major challenge and resources will not be available to expand HAART to all patients who need it. Thus, recent discoveries of new antiretroviral drugs, new vaccines, and advances in our understanding of HIV latency are encouraging developments on the long road to a cure.

BIBLIOGRAPHY

Please visit the Nelson Textbook of Pediatrics *website at www.expertconsult.com for the complete bibliography.*

Chapter 269 Human T-Lymphotropic Viruses (1 and 2)

Hal B. Jenson

ETIOLOGY

Human T-lymphotropic viruses 1 (HTLV-1) and 2 (HTLV-2) are members of the *Deltaretrovirus* genus of the Retroviridae family, which are single-stranded RNA viruses that encode reverse transcriptase, an RNA-dependent DNA polymerase that transcribes the single-stranded viral RNA into a double-stranded DNA copy. HTLV-1 and -2 share approximately 65% genome homology and infect T cells, B cells, and synovial cells via the ubiquitous glucose transporter type 1 (GLUT1), which serves as the virus receptor. Circular viral DNA is transported into the nucleus where it is integrated into chromosomal DNA (provirus), evading the typical mechanisms of immune surveillance and resulting in lifelong infection. The host response is mediated by cytotoxic T lymphocytes resulting in lysis of infected cells. An exuberant inflammatory response with overproduction of cytokines contributes to developing nonmalignant disease. In addition, HTLV-1 was the first human retrovirus to be associated with cancer, as the cause of adult T-cell leukemia/lymphoma (ATL).

For the full continuation of this chapter, please visit the Nelson Textbook of Pediatrics *website at www.expertconsult.com.*

Chapter 270 Transmissible Spongiform Encephalopathies

David M. Asher

The transmissible spongiform encephalopathies (TSEs) are slow infections of the human nervous system, consisting of at least 4 diseases of humans (see Table 270-1 on the *Nelson Textbook of Pediatrics* website at www.expertconsult.com): kuru; Creutzfeldt-Jakob disease (CJD) with its variants—sporadic CJD (sCJD), familial CJD (fCJD), iatrogenic CJD (iCJD), and new-variant or variant CJD (vCJD); Gerstmann-Sträussler-Scheinker syndrome (GSS); and fatal familial insomnia (FFI), or the even more rare sporadic fatal insomnia syndrome. TSEs also affect animals; the most common and best-known TSEs of animals are scrapie in sheep, bovine spongiform encephalopathy (BSE or mad cow disease) in cattle, and a chronic wasting disease (CWD) of deer, elk, and moose found in parts of the USA and Canada. All TSEs have similar clinical manifestations and histopathology, and all are “slow” infections with very long asymptomatic incubation periods (often years), durations of several months or more, and overt disease affecting only the nervous system. The most striking neuropathologic change that occurs in each TSE, to a greater or lesser extent, is spongy degeneration of the cerebral cortical gray matter.

For the full continuation of this chapter, please visit the Nelson Textbook of Pediatrics *website at www.expertconsult.com.*

Section 14 ANTIPARASITIC THERAPY

Chapter 271 Principles of Antiparasitic Therapy

Mark R. Schleiss and Sharon F. Chen

Parasites are divided into 2 main groups taxonomically: **protozoans,** which are unicellular, and **helminths,** which are multicellular. Chemotherapeutic agents appropriate for 1 group may not be appropriate for the other, and not all drugs are readily available. Some drugs are available only from the manufacturer, some are not available in the USA, and some are available through the Centers for Disease Control and Prevention Drug Service (telephone: 404-639-3670, weekdays; 404-639-2888, evenings, weekends, and holidays) (see Tables 271-1 and 271-2 on the *Nelson Textbook of Pediatrics* website at www.expertconsult.com).

For the full continuation of this chapter, please visit the Nelson Textbook of Pediatrics *website at www.expertconsult.com.*

Section 15 PROTOZOAN DISEASES

Chapter 272
Primary Amebic Meningoencephalitis

Martin E. Weisse and Stephen C. Aronoff

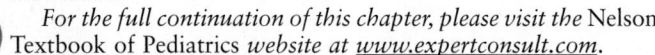

Naegleria, Acanthamoeba, and *Balamuthia* are small, free-living amebae that cause human amebic meningoencephalitis, which has 2 distinct clinical presentations. The more common is an acute, usually fatal **amebic meningitis** that is caused by *Naegleria* and occurs in previously healthy children and young adults. **Granulomatous amebic meningoencephalitis** is caused by *Acanthamoeba, Balamuthia,* and *Sappinia* and is a more indolent infection that is more likely to occur in immunocompromised individuals.

For the full continuation of this chapter, please visit the Nelson Textbook of Pediatrics *website at www.expertconsult.com.*

Chapter 273
Amebiasis

Edsel Maurice T. Salvana and Robert A. Salata

Entamoeba histolytica infects up to 10% of the world's population; endemic foci are particularly common in the tropics, especially in areas with low socioeconomic and sanitary standards. In most infected individuals, *E. histolytica* parasitizes the lumen of the gastrointestinal tract and causes few symptoms or sequelae. The 2 most common forms of disease caused by *E. histolytica* are **amebic colitis** with parasitic invasion of the intestinal mucosa and **amebic liver abscess** with dissemination of the parasite to the liver.

ETIOLOGY

Two morphologically identical but genetically distinct species of *Entamoeba* commonly infect humans. *Entamoeba dispar,* the more prevalent species, does not cause symptomatic disease. *E. histolytica,* the pathogenic species, causes a spectrum of disease and can become invasive. Patients previously described as asymptomatic carriers of *E. histolytica* based on microscopy findings were likely harboring *E. dispar.* Five other species of nonpathogenic *Entamoeba* can colonize the human gastrointestinal tract: *E. coli, E. hartmanni, E. gingivalis, E. moshkovskii,* and *E. polecki.*

Infection is acquired through the ingestion of parasite cysts, which measure 10-18 mm in diameter and contain 4 nuclei. Cysts are resistant to harsh environmental conditions including the concentrations of chlorine commonly used in water purification but can be killed by heating to 55°C. After ingestion, cysts are resistant to gastric acidity and digestive enzymes and germinate in the small intestine to form trophozoites. These large, actively motile organisms colonize the lumen of the large intestine and may invade the mucosal lining. Infection is not transmitted by trophozoites, as these rapidly degenerate outside the body and are unable to survive the low pH of the stomach if swallowed.

EPIDEMIOLOGY

Prevalence of infection with *E. histolytica* varies greatly depending on region and socioeconomic status. Most prevalence studies have not distinguished between *E. histolytica* and *E. dispar,* and thus the true prevalence of *E. histolytica* infection is not known. It is estimated that infection with *E. histolytica* leads to 50 million cases of symptomatic disease and 40,000-110,000 deaths annually. Amebiasis is the 3rd leading parasitic cause of death worldwide. Prospective studies have shown that 4-10% of individuals infected with *E. histolytica* develop amebic colitis and that <1% of infected individuals develop disseminated disease, including amebic liver abscess. These numbers vary by region; for example, in South Africa and Vietnam, liver abscesses form a disproportionately large number of the cases of invasive disease due to *E. histolytica.* Amebic liver abscesses are rare in children and occur equally in male and female children; in adults, amebic liver abscesses occur predominantly in men.

Amebiasis is endemic to Africa, Latin America, India, and Southeast Asia. In the USA, amebiasis is seen most frequently in immigrants from and in travelers to developing countries. Residents of mental health institutions and men who have sex with men are also at increased risk for invasive amebiasis. Food or drink contaminated with *Entamoeba* cysts and direct fecal-oral contact are the most common means of infection. Untreated water and night soil (human feces used as fertilizer) are important sources of infection. Food handlers shedding amebic cysts play a role in spreading infection. Direct contact with infected feces also results in person-to-person transmission.

PATHOGENESIS

Trophozoites are responsible for tissue invasion and destruction. These attach to colonic epithelial cells by a galactose and *N*-acetyl-D-galactosamine (Gal/GalNac)-specific lectin. This lectin is also thought to be responsible for resistance to complement-mediated lysis. Once attached to the colonic mucosa, amebae release proteinases that allow for penetration through the epithelial layer. Host cells are destroyed by cytolysis and apoptosis. Cytolysis is mediated by trophozoite release of **amoebapores** (pore-forming proteins), phospholipases, and hemolysins. Amoebapores may also be partially responsible for the induction of apoptosis that occurs in mice with amebic liver disease and colitis. Early invasive amebiasis produces significant inflammation, due in part to parasite-mediated activation of nuclear factor-κB (NF-κB). Once *E. histolytica* trophozoites invade the intestinal mucosa, the organisms multiply and spread laterally underneath the intestinal epithelium to produce the characteristic **flask-shaped ulcers.** Amebae produce similar lytic lesions if they reach the liver. These lesions are commonly called *abscesses,* although they contain no granulocytes. Well-established ulcers and amebic liver abscesses demonstrate little local inflammatory response.

Immunity to infection is associated with a mucosal secretory IgA response against the Gal/GalNac lectin. Neutrophils appear to be important in initial host defense, but *E. histolytica*–induced epithelial cell damage releases neutrophil chemoattractants, and *E. histolytica* is able to kill neutrophils, which then release mediators that further damage epithelial cells. The disparity between the extent of tissue destruction by amebae and the absence of a local host inflammatory response in the presence of systemic humoral (antibody) and cell-mediated responses may reflect both parasite-mediated apoptosis and the ability of the trophozoite to kill not only epithelial cells but neutrophils, monocytes, and macrophages.

The sequencing of the *E. histolytica* genome has led to further insights into the pathogenesis of *E. histolytica* disease. The genome is functionally tetraploid, and there is evidence of lateral gene transfer from bacteria. It has been demonstrated that the **amoebapore-A** (Ap-A) gene along with other important genes can be epigenetically silenced using plasmids with specifically engineered sequences or short hairpin RNAs. Transcriptional profiling using proteomics and microarrays have likewise identified several candidate virulence factors. Several classes of proteases that may be associated pathogenesis have been identified, including a novel *E. histolytica* **rhomboid protease 1** (EhROM1), which may be involved in immune evasion.

CLINICAL MANIFESTATIONS

Clinical presentations range from asymptomatic cyst passage to amebic colitis, amebic dysentery, ameboma, and extraintestinal disease. *E. histolytica* infection is asymptomatic in about 90% of persons but has the potential to become invasive and should be treated. Severe disease is more common in young children, pregnant women, malnourished individuals, and persons taking corticosteroids. Extraintestinal disease usually involves the liver, but less common extraintestinal manifestations include amebic brain abscess, pleuropulmonary disease, ulcerative skin, and genitourinary lesions.

Amebic Colitis

Amebic colitis may occur within 2 wk of infection or may be delayed for months. The onset is usually gradual, with colicky abdominal pains and frequent bowel movements (6-8/day). Diarrhea is frequently associated with tenesmus. Almost all stool is heme-positive, but most patients do not present with grossly bloody stools. Generalized constitutional symptoms and signs are characteristically absent, with fever documented in only one third of patients. Amebic colitis affects all age groups, but its incidence is strikingly high in children 1-5 yr of age. Severe amebic colitis in infants and young children tends to be rapidly progressive with more frequent extraintestinal involvement and high mortality rates, particularly in tropical countries. Amebic dysentery can result in dehydration and electrolyte disturbances.

Amebic Liver Abscess

Amebic liver abscess, a serious manifestation of disseminated infection, is uncommon in children. Although diffuse liver enlargement has been associated with intestinal amebiasis, liver abscesses occur in <1% of infected individuals and may appear in patients with no clear history of intestinal disease. Amebic liver abscess may occur months to years after exposure, so obtaining a careful travel history is critical. In children, fever is the hallmark of amebic liver abscess and is frequently associated with abdominal pain, distention, and enlargement and tenderness of the liver. Changes at the base of the right lung, such as elevation of the diaphragm and atelectasis or effusion, may also occur.

HIV Co-Infection

Though some studies have shown higher rates of amebic colonization in HIV-positive men in East Asia compared to HIV-uninfected men, this association was not found in other areas of the world. While cellular immune dysfunction associated with HIV infection may, in turn affect humoral immunity, the higher prevalence of amebiasis in this group of patients is more likely due to higher intestinal colonization rates rather than a true association with immunodeficiency.

LABORATORY FINDINGS

Laboratory examination findings are often unremarkable in uncomplicated amebic colitis, although mild anemia may be seen. Laboratory findings in amebic liver abscess are a slight leukocytosis, moderate anemia, high erythrocyte sedimentation rate, and elevations of hepatic enzyme (particularly alkaline phosphatase) levels. Stool examination for amebae is negative in more than half of patients with documented amebic liver abscess. Ultrasonography, CT, or MRI can localize and delineate the size of the abscess cavity (Fig. 273-1). The most common finding is a single abscess in the right hepatic lobe in about a half of these cases. Higher resolution ultrasound and CT studies have shown that left lobe abscess and multiple abscesses occur more often than previously recognized.

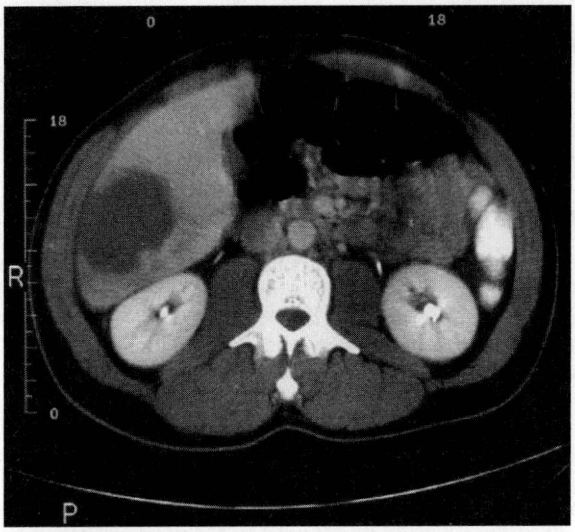

Figure 273-1 Abdominal CT scan of a patient with an amebic liver abscess. (From Miller Q, Kenney JM, Cotlar AM: Amebic abscess of the liver presenting as acute cholecystitis, *Curr Surg* 57:476–479, 2000, Fig 1, p 477.)

DIAGNOSIS AND DIFFERENTIAL DIAGNOSIS

A diagnosis of amebic colitis is made in the presence of compatible symptoms with detection of *E. histolytica* antigens in stool. This approach has a greater than 95% sensitivity and specificity and coupled with a positive serology test is the most accurate means of diagnosis in developed countries. The *E. histolytica* II stool antigen detection test (TechLab, Blacksburg, VA) is able to distinguish *E. histolytica* from *E. dispar* infection. Microscopic examination of stool samples has a sensitivity of 60%. Sensitivity can be increased to 85-95% by examining 3 stools, since excretion of cysts can be intermittent. However, microscopy cannot differentiate between *E. histolytica* and *E. dispar* unless phagocytosed erythrocytes (specific for *E. histolytica*) are seen. In highly endemic areas, trophozoites without phagocytosed erythrocytes may reflect co-infection with *E. dispar* in a patient with another cause of colitis, such as shigellosis. Endoscopy and biopsies of suspicious areas should be performed when stool sample results are negative and suspicion for amebiasis remains high.

Various serum antiamebic antibody tests are available. Serologic results are positive in 70-80% of patients with invasive disease (colitis or liver abscess) at presentation and in >90% of patients after 7 days of disease symptoms. The most sensitive serologic test, indirect hemagglutination, yields a positive result even years after invasive infection. Therefore, many uninfected adults and children in highly endemic areas demonstrate antibodies to *E. histolytica*. Polymerase chain reaction (PCR) detection in stool of *E. histolytica* is also able to distinguish *E. histolytica* from *E. dispar* but is less sensitive (72%) than the stool antigen test. Rapid antigen and antibody tests for bedside diagnosis in the developing world have been developed and are currently being tested. In addition, a loop-mediated isothermal amplification assay (LAMP) that can be optimized for field use is under development.

The **differential diagnosis** for amebic colitis includes colitis due to bacterial (*Shigella, Salmonella,* enteropathogenic *Escherichia coli, Campylobacter, Yersinia, Clostridium difficile*), mycobacterial (tuberculosis and atypical mycobacteria), and viral (cytomegalovirus) pathogens, as well as noninfectious causes such as inflammatory bowel disease (IBD). Pyogenic liver abscess due to bacterial infection, hepatoma, and echinococcal cysts are in the differential for amebic liver abscess. However, echinococcal cysts are rarely associated with systemic symptoms such as fever unless there is cyst rupture or leakage.

COMPLICATIONS

Complications of amebic colitis include acute necrotizing colitis, ameboma, toxic megacolon, extraintestinal extension, or local perforation and peritonitis. Less commonly, a chronic form of amebic colitis develops, often recurring over several years. Amebomas are nodular foci of proliferative inflammation that sometimes develops in the wall of the colon. Chronic amebiasis should be excluded before initiating corticosteroid treatment for IBD, as corticosteroid therapy given during active amebic colitis is associated with high mortality rates.

An amebic liver abscess may rupture into the peritoneum, pleural cavity, skin, and pericardium. Cases of amebic abscesses in extrahepatic sites, including the lung and brain, have been reported.

TREATMENT

Invasive amebiasis is treated with a nitroimidazole such as **metronidazole** or **tinidazole** and then a **luminal amebicide** (Table 273-1). Tinidazole has similar efficacy to metronidazole with shorter and simpler dosing and less frequent adverse effects. These adverse effects include nausea, abdominal discomfort, and a metallic taste that disappears after completion of therapy. Therapy with a nitroimidazole should be followed by treatment with a luminal agent, such as paromomycin (which is preferred) or iodoquinol. Diloxanide furoate can also be used in children >2 yr of age, but it is no longer available in the USA. Paromomycin should not be given concurrently with metronidazole or tinidazole, because diarrhea is a common side effect of paromomycin and may confuse the clinical picture. Asymptomatic intestinal infection with *E. histolytica* should be treated preferably with paromomycin or alternatively with either iodoquinol or diloxanide furoate. For fulminant cases of amebic colitis, some experts suggest adding dehydroemetine (1 mg/kg/day subcutaneously or IM, never IV), available only through the Centers for Disease Control and Prevention. Patients should be hospitalized for monitoring if dehydroemetine is administered. Dehydroemetine should be discontinued if tachycardia, T-wave depression, arrhythmia, or proteinuria develops.

Broad-spectrum antibiotic therapy may be indicated in fulminant colitis to cover possible spillage of intestinal bacteria into the peritoneum and translocation into the bloodstream. Intestinal perforation and toxic megacolon are indications for surgery. In amebic liver abscess, image-guided aspiration of large lesions or left lobe abscesses may be necessary if rupture is imminent or if the patient shows a poor clinical response 4-6 days after administration of amebicidal drugs. A Cochrane meta-analysis comparing metronidazole and metronidazole plus aspiration in uncomplicated amebic liver abscess showed that there is insufficient evidence to make any recommendation for or against this approach. Chloroquine, which concentrates in the liver, may also be a useful adjunct to nitroimidazoles in the treatment of amebic liver abscess. To confirm cure, stool examination should be repeated every 2 wk following completion of therapy until clear.

Table 273-1 DRUG TREATMENT FOR AMEBIASIS

MEDICATION	ADULT DOSAGE (ORAL)	PEDIATRIC DOSAGE (ORAL)*
INVASIVE DISEASE		
Metronidazole	Colitis or liver abscess: 750 mg tid for 7-10 days	Colitis or liver abscess: 35-50 mg/kg/day in 3 divided doses for 7-10 days
or		
Tinidazole	Colitis: 2 g once daily for 3 days	Colitis: 50 mg/kg/day once daily for 3 days
	Liver abscess: 2 g once daily for 3-5 days	Liver abscess: 50 mg/kg/day once daily for 3-5 days
Followed by:		
Paromomycin (preferred)	500 mg tid for 7 days	25-35 mg/kg/day in 3 divided doses for 7 days
or		
Diloxanide furoate† *or*	500 mg tid for 10 days	20 mg/kg/day in 3 divided doses for 7 days
Iodoquinol	650 mg tid for 20 days	30-40 mg/kg/day in 3 divided doses for 20 days
ASYMPTOMATIC INTESTINAL COLONIZATION		
Paromomycin (preferred)	As for invasive disease	As for invasive disease
or		
Diloxanide furoate†		
or		
Iodoquinol		

*All pediatric dosages are up to a maximum of the adult dose.
†Not available in the USA.

PROGNOSIS

Most infections evolve to either an asymptomatic carrier state or eradication. Extraintestinal infection carries about a 5% mortality rate.

PREVENTION

Control of amebiasis can be achieved by exercising proper sanitation and avoiding fecal-oral transmission. Regular examination of food handlers and thorough investigation of diarrheal episodes may help identify the source of infection No prophylactic drug or vaccine is currently available for amebiasis. Immunization with a combination of Gal/GalNAc lectin and CpG oligodeoxynucleotides has been shown to be protective to amebic trophozoite challenge in animals.

BIBLIOGRAPHY

Please visit the Nelson Textbook of Pediatrics *website at www.expertconsult.com for the complete bibliography.*

Chapter 274
Giardiasis and Balantidiasis

274.1 *Giardia lamblia*

Chandy C. John

Giardia lamblia is a flagellated protozoan that infects the duodenum and small intestine. Infection results in clinical manifestations that range from asymptomatic colonization to acute or chronic diarrhea and malabsorption. Infection is more prevalent in children than in adults. *Giardia* is endemic in areas of the world with poor levels of sanitation. It is also an important cause of morbidity in developed countries, where it is associated with urban child-care centers, residential institutions for the developmentally delayed, and water-borne and food-borne outbreaks. *Giardia* is a particularly significant pathogen in people with malnutrition, certain immunodeficiencies, and cystic fibrosis.

ETIOLOGY

The life cycle of *G. lamblia* (also known as *Giardia intestinalis* or *Giardia duodenalis*) is composed of 2 stages: trophozoites and cysts. *Giardia* infects humans after ingestion of as few as 10-100 cysts (which measure 8-10 mm in diameter). Each ingested cyst produces 2 trophozoites in the duodenum. After excystation, trophozoites colonize the lumen of the duodenum and proximal jejunum, where they attach to the brush border of the intestinal epithelial cells and multiply by binary fission. The body of the trophozoite is teardrop shaped, measuring 10-20 mm in length and 5-15 mm in width. *Giardia* trophozoites contain 2 oval nuclei anteriorly, a large ventral disk, a curved median body posteriorly, and 4 pairs of flagella. As detached trophozoites pass down the intestinal tract, they encyst to form oval cysts that contain 4 nuclei. Cysts are passed in stools of infected individuals and may remain viable in water for as long as 2 mo. Their viability often is not affected by the usual concentrations of chlorine used to purify water for drinking.

Giardia strains that infect humans are diverse biologically, as shown by differences in antigens, restriction endonuclease patterns, DNA fingerprinting, isoenzyme patterns, and pulsed-field gel electrophoresis. Studies suggest that different *Giardia* genotypes may cause unique clinical manifestations, but these findings appear to vary according to the geographic region tested.

EPIDEMIOLOGY

Giardia occurs worldwide and is the most common intestinal parasite identified in public health laboratories in the USA, where it is estimated that up to 2 million cases of giardiasis occur annually. *Giardia* infection usually occurs sporadically but is a frequently identified etiologic agent of outbreaks associated with drinking water. The age-specific prevalence of giardiasis is high during childhood and begins to decline after adolescence. The asymptomatic carrier rate of *G. lamblia* in the USA is as high as 20-30% in children younger than 36 mo of age attending child-care centers. Asymptomatic carriage may persist for several months.

Transmission of *Giardia* is common in certain high-risk groups, including children and employees in child-care centers, consumers of contaminated water, travelers to certain areas of the world, men who have sex with men, and persons exposed to certain animals. The major reservoir and vehicle for spread of *Giardia* appears to be water contaminated with *Giardia* cysts, but food-borne transmission occurs. The seasonal peak in age-specific case reports coincides with the summer recreational water season and might be a result of the extensive use of communal swimming venues by young children, the low infectious dose, and the extended periods of cyst shedding that can occur. In addition, *Giardia* cysts are relatively resistant to chlorination and to ultraviolet light irradiation. Boiling is effective for inactivating cysts.

Person-to-person spread also occurs, particularly in areas of low hygiene standards, frequent fecal-oral contact, and crowding. Individual susceptibility, lack of toilet training, crowding, and fecal contamination of the environment all predispose to transmission of enteropathogens, including *Giardia,* in child-care centers. Child-care centers play an important role in transmission of urban giardiasis, with secondary attack rates in families as high as 17-30%. Children in child-care centers may pass cysts for several months. Campers who drink untreated stream or river water, particularly in the western USA, and residents of institutions for the developmentally delayed are also at increased risk for infection.

Humoral immunodeficiencies, including common variable hypogammaglobulinemia and X-linked agammaglobulinemia, predispose humans to chronic symptomatic *Giardia* infection, suggesting the importance of humoral immunity in controlling giardiasis. Selective immunoglobulin A (IgA) deficiency is also associated with *Giardia* infection. Although many individuals with AIDS have relatively mild *Giardia* infections, some reports suggest that severe *Giardia* infection, often refractory to treatment, may occur in a subset of individuals with AIDS. There is a higher incidence of *Giardia* infection in patients with cystic fibrosis, probably owing to local factors such as the increased amount of mucus, which may protect the organism against host factors in the duodenum. Human milk contains glycoconjugates and secretory IgA antibodies that may provide protection to nursing infants.

CLINICAL MANIFESTATIONS

The incubation period of *Giardia* infection usually is 1-2 wk but may be longer. A broad spectrum of clinical manifestations occurs, depending on the interaction between *G. lamblia* and the host. Children who are exposed to *G. lamblia* may experience asymptomatic excretion of the organism, acute infectious diarrhea, or chronic diarrhea with persistent gastrointestinal tract signs and symptoms, including failure to thrive and abdominal pain or cramping. Giardia was the cause of 15% of nondysenteric diarrhea in children examined in U.S. outpatient clinics in 1 study. Most infections in both children and adults are asymptomatic. There usually is no extraintestinal spread, but occasionally trophozoites may migrate into bile or pancreatic ducts.

Symptomatic infections occur more frequently in children than in adults. Most symptomatic patients usually have a limited period of acute diarrheal disease with or without low-grade fever, nausea, and anorexia; in a small proportion of patients, an intermittent or more protracted course characterized by diarrhea, abdominal distention and cramps, bloating, malaise, flatulence, nausea, anorexia, and weight loss develops (Table 274-1). Stools initially may be profuse and watery and later become greasy and foul smelling and may float. Stools do not contain blood, mucus, or fecal leukocytes. Varying degrees of malabsorption may occur. Abnormal stool patterns may alternate with periods of constipation and normal bowel movements. Malabsorption of sugars, fats, and fat-soluble vitamins has been well documented and may be responsible for substantial weight loss. *Giardia* has been associated with iron deficiency in internationally adopted children. Giardiasis has been associated with growth stunting and repeated *Giardia* infections with a decrease in cognitive function in children in endemic areas.

DIAGNOSIS

Giardiasis should be considered in children who have acute nondysenteric diarrhea, persistent diarrhea, intermittent diarrhea and

Table 274-1 CLINICAL SIGNS AND SYMPTOMS OF GIARDIASIS

SYMPTOM	FREQUENCY (%)
Diarrhea	64-100
Malaise, weakness	72-97
Abdominal distention	42-97
Flatulence	35-97
Abdominal cramps	44-81
Nausea	14-79
Foul-smelling, greasy stools	15-79
Anorexia	41-73
Weight loss	53-73
Vomiting	14-35
Fever	0-28
Constipation	0-27

constipation, malabsorption, chronic crampy abdominal pain and bloating, failure to thrive, or weight loss. It should be particularly high in the differential diagnosis of children in child care, children in contact with an index case, children with a history of recent travel to an endemic area, and children with humoral immunodeficiencies. Testing for giardiasis should be standard for internationally adopted children from *Giardia*-endemic areas, and screening for iron deficiency should be considered in internationally adopted children with giardiasis.

Stool enzyme immunoassay (EIA) or direct fluorescent antibody tests for *Giardia* antigens are now the tests of choice for giardiasis in most situations. EIA is less reader dependent and more sensitive for detection of *Giardia* than microscopy. Some studies have reported that a single stool is sufficiently sensitive for detection of *Giardia* by EIA, while others suggest that sensitivity is increased with testing of 2 samples. Traditionally, a diagnosis of giardiasis has been established by microscopy documentation of trophozoites or cysts in stool specimens, but 3 stool specimens are required to achieve a sensitivity of >90%. In patients in whom other parasitic intestinal infections are in the differential diagnosis, microscopy examination of stool allows evaluation for these infections in addition to *Giardia*. Laboratories can reduce reagent and personnel costs by pooling specimens submitted for detection of *Giardia* before evaluation by microscopy or EIA. Polymerase chain reaction (PCR) and gene probe–based detection systems specific for *Giardia* have been used in environmental monitoring but at present remain research tools. Multiplex PCR testing for multiple parasitic pathogens may become a viable option for testing in the future.

In patients with chronic symptoms in whom giardiasis is suspected but in whom testing of stool specimens for *Giardia* yields a negative result, aspiration or biopsy of the duodenum or upper jejunum should be considered. In a fresh specimen, trophozoites usually can be visualized by direct wet mount. An alternate method of directly obtaining duodenal fluid is the commercially available Entero-Test (Hedeco Corp, Mountain View, CA), but this method is less sensitive than aspiration or biopsy. The biopsy can be used to make touch preparations and tissue sections for identification of *Giardia* and other enteric pathogens and also to visualize changes in histology. Biopsy of the small intestine should be considered in patients with characteristic clinical symptoms, negative stool and duodenal fluid specimen findings, and 1 or more of the following: abnormal radiographic findings (such as edema and segmentation in the small intestine); abnormal lactose tolerance test result; absent secretory IgA level; hypogammaglobulinemia; or achlorhydria. Duodenal biopsy may show findings consistent with chronic inflammation, including eosinophilic infiltration of the lamina propria.

Radiographic contrast studies of the small intestine may show nonspecific findings such as irregular thickening of the mucosal folds. Blood cell counts usually are normal. Giardiasis is not tissue invasive and is not associated with peripheral blood eosinophilia.

TREATMENT

Children with acute diarrhea in whom *Giardia* organisms are identified should receive therapy. In addition, children who manifest failure to thrive or exhibit malabsorption or gastrointestinal tract symptoms such as chronic diarrhea should be treated.

Asymptomatic excreters generally are not treated except in specific instances such as in outbreak control, for prevention of household transmission by toddlers to pregnant women and patients with hypogammaglobulinemia or cystic fibrosis, and in situations requiring oral antibiotic treatment where *Giardia* may have produced malabsorption of the antibiotic.

The U.S. Food and Drug Administration (FDA) has approved tinidazole and nitazoxanide for the treatment of *Giardia* in the USA. Both medications have been used to treat *Giardia* in thousands of patients in other countries and have excellent safety and efficacy against *Giardia* (Table 274-2). Tinidazole has the advantage of single-dose treatment and very high efficacy (>90%), while nitazoxanide has the advantage of a suspension form, high efficacy (80-90%), and very few adverse effects. Metronidazole, though never approved by the FDA for treatment of *Giardia,* is also highly effective (80-90% cure rate), and the generic form is considerably less expensive than tinidazole or nitazoxanide. Frequent adverse effects are seen with metronidazole therapy, and it requires 3 times a day dosing for 5-7 days. Suspension forms of tinidazole and metronidazole must be compounded by a pharmacy; neither drug is sold in suspension form.

Table 274-2 DRUG TREATMENT FOR GIARDIASIS

MEDICATION	ADULT DOSAGE (ORAL)	PEDIATRIC DOSAGE (ORAL)*
RECOMMENDED		
Tinidazole	2 g once	>3 yr: 50 mg/kg once
Nitazoxanide	500 mg bid for 3 days	1-3 yr: 100 mg (5 mL) bid for 3 days
		4-11 yr: 200 mg (10 mL) bid for 3 days
		>12 yr: 500 mg bid for 3 days
Metronidazole	250 mg tid for 5-7 days	15 mg/kg/day in 3 divided doses for 5-7 days
ALTERNATIVE		
Albendazole	400 mg once a day for 5 days	>6 yr: 400 mg once a day for 5 days
Furazolidone	100 mg qid for 10 days	6 mg/kg/day in 4 divided doses for 10 days
Paromomycin	25-35 mg/kg/day in 3 divided doses for 5-10 days	Not recommended
Quinacrine†	100 mg tid for 5-7 days	6 mg/kg/day in 3 divided doses for 5 days

*All pediatric dosages are up to a maximum of the adult dose.
†Not commercially available. Can be compounded by Medical Center Pharmacy in New Haven, CT (203-785-6818) or Panorama Compounding Pharmacy in Van Nuys, CA (800-247-9767).

Second line alternatives for the treatment of patients with giardiasis include furazolidone, albendazole, paromomycin, and quinacrine (see Table 274-2). Furazolidone, albendazole, and paromomycin are less effective than tinidazole, nitazoxanide, and metronidazole. Furazolidone has been prescribed for children because it is available in liquid form. Albendazole has few adverse effects and is effective against many helminths, making it useful for treatment when multiple intestinal parasites are identified or suspected. Paromomycin is a nonabsorbable aminoglycoside and is less effective than other agents but is recommended for treatment of pregnant women with giardiasis because of potential teratogenic effects of other agents. Quinacrine is effective and inexpensive but is not available commercially and must be obtained from compounding pharmacies (see Table 274-2). Refractory cases of giardiasis have been successfully treated with nitazoxanide, prolonged courses of tinidazole, or a 3-week course of metronidazole and quinacrine.

PROGNOSIS

Symptoms recur in some patients in whom reinfection cannot be documented and in whom an immune deficiency such as an immunoglobulin abnormality is not present, despite use of appropriate therapy. Several studies have demonstrated that variability in antimicrobial susceptibility exists among strains of *Giardia,* and in some instances resistant strains have been demonstrated. Combined therapy may be useful for infection that persists after single-drug therapy, assuming reinfection has not occurred and the medication was taken as prescribed.

PREVENTION

Infected persons and persons at risk should practice strict handwashing after any contact with feces. This point is especially important for caregivers of diapered infants in child-care centers, where diarrhea is common and *Giardia* organism carriage rates are high.

Methods to purify public water supplies adequately include chlorination, sedimentation, and filtration. Inactivation of *Giardia* cysts by chlorine requires the coordination of multiple variables such as chlorine concentration, water pH, turbidity, temperature, and contact time. These variables cannot be appropriately controlled in all municipalities and are difficult to control in swimming pools. Individuals, especially children in diapers, should avoid swimming if they have diarrhea. Individuals should also avoid swallowing recreational water and drinking untreated water from shallow wells, lakes, springs, ponds, streams, and rivers.

Travelers to endemic areas are advised to avoid uncooked foods that might have been grown, washed, or prepared with water that was potentially contaminated. Purification of drinking water can be achieved by a filter with a pore size of <1 mm or that has been National Sanitation Foundation rated for cyst removal, or by brisk boiling of water for at least 1 min. Treatment of water with chlorine or iodine is less effective but may be used as an alternate method when boiling or filtration is not possible.

BIBLIOGRAPHY

Please visit the Nelson Textbook of Pediatrics *website at* www.expertconsult.com *for the complete bibliography.*

274.2 Balantidiasis

Chandy C. John

Balantidium coli is a ciliated protozoan and is the largest protozoan that parasitizes humans. Both trophozoites and cysts may be identified in feces. Disease caused by this organism is uncommon in the USA and generally is reported where there is a close association of humans with pigs, which are the natural hosts of *B. coli.* Because the organism infects the large intestine, symptoms are consistent with large bowel disease, similar to those associated with amebiasis and trichuriasis, and include nausea, vomiting, lower abdominal pain, tenesmus, and bloody diarrhea. Symptoms associated with chronic infection include abdominal cramps, watery diarrhea with mucus, occasionally bloody diarrhea, and colonic ulcers similar to those associated with *Entamoeba histolytica.* Extraintestinal spread of *B. coli* is rare and usually occurs only in immunocompromised patients. Most infections are asymptomatic.

Diagnosis using direct saline mounts is established by identification of trophozoites (50-100 mm long) or spherical or oval cysts (50-70 mm in diameter) in stool specimens. Trophozoites usually are more numerous than cysts. The recommended treatment regimen is metronidazole (45 mg/kg/day divided tid PO, maximum 750 mg/dose) for 5 days, or tetracycline (40 mg/kg/day divided qid PO, maximum 500 mg/dose) for 10 days for persons >8 yr of age. An alternative is iodoquinol (40 mg/kg/day divided tid PO, maximum 650 mg/dose) for 20 days. Prevention of contamination of the environment by pig feces is the most important means for control.

BIBLIOGRAPHY

Please visit the Nelson Textbook of Pediatrics *website at* www.expertconsult.com *for the complete bibliography.*

Chapter 275
Cryptosporidium, Isospora, Cyclospora, and Microsporidia

Patricia M. Flynn

The spore-forming intestinal protozoa *Cryptosporidium, Isospora,* and *Cyclospora* are important intestinal pathogens in both immunocompetent and immunocompromised hosts. *Cryptosporidium, Isospora,* and *Cyclospora* are coccidian parasites that predominantly infect the epithelial cells lining the digestive tract. Microsporidia were formerly considered spore-forming protozoa and have recently been reclassified as fungi. Microsporidia are ubiquitous, obligate intracellular parasites that infect many other organ systems in addition to the gastrointestinal tract and cause a broader spectrum of disease.

CRYPTOSPORIDIUM

Cryptosporidium is recognized as a leading protozoal cause of diarrhea in children worldwide and is a common cause of outbreaks in child-care centers; it is also a significant pathogen in immunocompromised patients.

Etiology

Cryptosporidium hominis and *Cryptosporidium parvum* cause most cases of cryptosporidiosis in humans. Disease is initiated by ingestion of infectious oocysts that release 4 sporozoites that invade enterocytes, primarily in the small intestine. The infection progresses through 2 stages: the asexual stage, which allows autoinfection at the luminal surface of the epithelium, and the sexual stage, which results in production of oocysts that are shed in the stools. The cysts are immediately infectious to other hosts or can reinfect the same host.

Epidemiology

Cryptosporidiosis is associated with diarrheal illness worldwide and is more prevalent in developing countries and among children <2 yr of age. It has been implicated as an etiologic agent of persistent diarrhea in the developing world and as a cause of significant morbidity and mortality from malnutrition, including permanent effects on growth.

Transmission of *Cryptosporidium* to humans can occur by close association with infected animals, via person-to-person transmission, or from environmentally contaminated water. Although zoonotic transmission, especially from cows, occurs in persons in close association with animals, person-to-person transmission is probably responsible for cryptosporidiosis outbreaks within hospitals and child-care centers where rates as high as 67% have been reported. Recommendations to prevent outbreaks in child-care centers include strict handwashing, use of protective clothes or diapers capable of retaining liquid diarrhea, and separation of diapering and food-handling areas and responsibilities.

Outbreaks of cryptosporidial infection have been associated with contaminated community water supplies and recreational waters in several states in the USA and the U.K. Wastewater in the form of raw sewage and runoff from dairies and grazing lands can contaminate both drinking and recreational water sources. It is estimated that *Cryptosporidium* oocysts are present in 65-97% of the surface water in the USA. The organism's small size (4-6 μm in diameter), resistance to chlorination, and ability to survive for long periods outside a host create problems in public water supplies.

Clinical Manifestations

The incubation period is 2-14 days. Infection with *Cryptosporidium* is associated with profuse, watery, nonbloody diarrhea that can be accompanied by diffuse crampy abdominal pain, nausea, vomiting, and anorexia. Although less common in adults, vomiting occurs in >80% of children with cryptosporidiosis. Nonspecific symptoms such as myalgia, weakness, and headache also may occur. Fever occurs in 30-50% of cases. Malabsorption, lactose intolerance, dehydration, weight loss, and malnutrition often occur in severe cases. Recently, the clinical spectrum and disease severity has been linked with both the infecting species and host HLA class I and II alleles.

In immunocompetent persons, the disease is usually self-limiting, although diarrhea may persist for several weeks and oocyst shedding may persist many weeks after symptoms resolve. Chronic diarrhea is common in individuals with immunodeficiency, such as congenital hypogammaglobulinemia or HIV infection. Symptoms and oocyst shedding can continue indefinitely and may lead to severe malnutrition, wasting, anorexia, and even death.

Cryptosporidiosis in **immunocompromised hosts** is often associated with biliary tract disease, characterized by fever, right upper quadrant pain, nausea, vomiting, and diarrhea. It also has been associated with pancreatitis. Respiratory tract disease, with symptoms of cough, shortness of breath, wheezing, croup, and hoarseness, is very rare.

Diagnosis

Infection can be diagnosed by microscopy using modified acid-fast stain or polymerase chain reaction (PCR), but enzyme-linked immunoassays are the diagnostic method of choice. In stool, oocysts appear as small, spherical bodies (2-6 µm) and stain red with modified acid-fast staining. Because *Cryptosporidium* does not invade below the epithelial layer of the mucosa, fecal leukocytes are not found in stool specimens. Oocyst shedding in feces can be intermittent, and several fecal specimens (at least 3 for an immunocompetent host) should be collected for microscopic examination. Serologic diagnosis is not helpful in acute cryptosporidiosis.

In tissue sections, *Cryptosporidium* organisms can be found along the microvillus region of the epithelia that line the gastrointestinal tract. The highest concentration usually is detected in the jejunum. Histologic section results reveal villus atrophy and blunting, epithelial flattening, and inflammation of the lamina propria.

Treatment

Often the diarrheal illness due to cryptosporidiosis is self-limited in immunocompetent patients and requires no specific antimicrobial therapy. Treatment should focus on supportive care, including rehydration orally or, if fluid losses are severe, intravenously. Nitazoxanide (100 mg bid PO for 3 days for children 1-3 yr of age, 200 mg bid PO for children 4-11 yr of age; 500 mg bid PO for children ≥12 yr of age) has been approved for treatment of diarrhea caused by *Cryptosporidium*. Clinical studies have not demonstrated that nitazoxanide is superior to placebo in trials of HIV-infected or immunocompromised patients. In adult patients with AIDS, combination therapy with paromomycin (1 g bid PO) and azithromycin (600 mg/day PO) for 4 wk followed by paromomycin monotherapy for 8 wk has been used with limited success. Treatment with orally administered human serum immunoglobulin or bovine colostrum has been successful in several anecdotal reports.

ISOSPORA

Like *Cryptosporidium, Isospora belli* has been implicated as a cause of diarrhea in institutional outbreaks and in travelers and has also been linked with contaminated water and food. *Isospora* appears to be more common in tropical and subtropical climates and in developing areas, including South America, Africa, and Southeast Asia. *Isospora* has not been associated with animal contact. It is also an infrequent cause of diarrhea in patients with AIDS in the USA but may infect up to 15% of AIDS patients in Haiti.

The life cycle and pathogenesis of infection with *Isospora* species are similar to those of *Cryptosporidium* organisms except that oocysts excreted in the stool are not immediately infectious and must undergo further maturation below 37°C. Histologic appearance of gastrointestinal epithelium reveals blunting and atrophy of the villi, acute and chronic inflammation, and crypt hyperplasia.

The **clinical manifestations** are indistinguishable from those of cryptosporidiosis, although fever may be a more common finding. Eosinophilia may be present, contrasting with other enteric protozoan infections. The diagnosis is established by detecting the oval, 22-33 µm long by 10-19 µm wide, oocysts by using modified acid-fast staining of the stool. Each oocyst contains 2 sporocysts with 4 sporozoites in each. Fecal leukocytes are not detected.

Isosporiasis responds promptly to **treatment** with oral trimethoprim-sulfamethoxazole (TMP-SMZ) (5 mg TMP and 25 mg SMZ/kg/dose; maximum 160 mg TMP and 800 mg SMZ/dose qid for 10 days, and then bid for 3 wk). In patients with AIDS, relapses are common and often necessitate maintenance therapy. Ciprofloxacin, nitazoxanide, or a regimen of pyrimethamine alone or with folinic acid is effective in patients intolerant of sulfonamide drugs.

CYCLOSPORA

Cyclospora cayetanensis is a coccidian parasite similar to but larger than *Cryptosporidium*. The organism infects both immunocompromised and immunocompetent individuals and is more common in children <18 mo of age. The pathogenesis and pathologic findings of cyclosporiasis are similar to those of isosporiasis. Asymptomatic carriage of the organism has been found, but travelers who harbor the organism almost always have diarrhea. Outbreaks of cyclosporiasis have been linked with contaminated food and water. Implicated foods include raspberries, lettuce, snow peas, basil, and other fresh food items. After fecal excretion, the oocysts must sporulate to become infectious. This finding explains the lack of person-to-person transmission.

The **clinical manifestations** of cyclosporiasis are similar to those of cryptosporidiosis and isosporiasis and follow an incubation period of approximately 7 days. Moderate *Cyclospora* illness is characterized by a median of 6 stools/day with a median duration of 10 days (range 3-25 days). The duration of diarrhea in immunocompetent persons is characteristically longer in cyclosporiasis than in the other intestinal protozoan illnesses. Associated symptoms frequently include fatigue; abdominal bloating or gas; abdominal cramps or pain; nausea; muscle, joint, or body aches; fever; chills; headache; and weight loss. Vomiting may occur. Bloody stools are uncommon. Biliary disease has been reported. Intestinal pathology includes inflammation with villus blunting.

The diagnosis is established by identification of oocysts in the stool. Oocysts are wrinkled spheres, measure 8-10 µm in diameter, and resemble large *Cryptosporidium* organisms. Each oocyst contains 2 sporocysts, each with 2 sporozoites. The organisms can be seen by using modified acid-fast, auramine-phenol, or modified trichrome staining but stain less consistently than *Cryptosporidium*. They can also be detected with phenosafranin stain and by autofluorescence using strong green or intense blue under ultraviolet epifluorescence. New molecular diagnostic testing, including real-time PCR, is currently under investigation. Fecal leukocytes are not present.

The **treatment** of choice for cyclosporiasis is TMP-SMZ (5 mg TMP and 25 mg SMZ/kg/dose bid PO for 7 days, maximum 160 mg TMP and 800 mg SMZ/dose). Ciprofloxacin or nitazoxanide is effective in patients intolerant of sulfonamide drugs.

MICROSPORIDIA

Microsporidia are ubiquitous and infect most animal groups, including humans. At least 14 species of the phylum Microsporidia have been linked with human disease in both immunocompetent and immunocompromised hosts. The species most commonly associated with gastrointestinal disease are *Enterocytozoon bieneusi* and *Encephalitozoon intestinalis.*

Although still not definitive, the source of human infections is likely zoonotic. Like *Cryptosporidium,* there is concern for water-borne transmission through occupational and recreational contact with contaminated water sources. There is also the potential for food-borne outbreaks; the organisms have been identified on vegetables as a consequence of contaminated irrigation water. Vector-borne transmission is hypothesized because one species, *Brachiola algerae,* typically infects mosquitoes. Finally, transplacental transmission has been reported in animals but not in humans. Once infected, intracellular division produces new spores that can spread to nearby cells, disseminate to other host tissues, or be passed into the environment via feces. Spores also have been detected in urine and respiratory epithelium, suggesting that some body fluids may also be infectious. Once in the environment, microsporidial spores remain infectious for up to 4 mo.

Initially, microsporidial intestinal infection had been almost exclusively reported in patients with AIDS, but there is increasing evidence that immunocompetent individuals are also commonly infected. Microsporidia-associated diarrhea is intermittent, copious, watery, and nonbloody. Abdominal cramping and weight loss may be present; fever is unusual. Disseminated disease involving most organs, involving liver, heart, kidney, bladder, biliary tract, lung, bone, skeletal muscle, and sinuses, has been reported.

Microsporidia stain with hematoxylin-eosin, Giemsa, Gram, periodic acid–Schiff, and acid-fast stains but are often overlooked because of their small size (1-2 µm) and the absence of associated inflammation in surrounding tissues. Electron microscopy remains the reference method of detection. Multiple research laboratories report success with PCR technology in detecting microsporidia, both in human and environmental samples.

There is no proven **therapy** for microsporidial intestinal infections. *E. intestinalis* infection usually responds to albendazole (adult dose 400 mg bid PO for 3 wk). Fumagillin (adult dose 20 mg tid PO for 2 wk) was effective in a small controlled study. Atovaquone and nitazoxanide have also been reported to decrease symptoms, but controlled clinical trials have not been performed. Improvement in underlying HIV infection with aggressive antiviral therapy also improves microsporidiosis symptoms.

BIBLIOGRAPHY

Please visit the Nelson Textbook of Pediatrics *website at* www.expertconsult.com *for the complete bibliography.*

Chapter 276
Trichomoniasis *(Trichomonas vaginalis)*

Edsel Maurice T. Salvana and Robert A. Salata

Trichomoniasis, caused by the protozoan parasite *Trichomonas vaginalis,* is the most common nonviral sexually transmitted disease worldwide. It primarily causes vulvovaginitis in women but has been implicated in pelvic inflammatory disease, adverse outcomes in pregnancy, chronic prostatitis, and an increased risk of transmission of HIV.

EPIDEMIOLOGY

Over 170 million new cases of trichomoniasis occur yearly, the majority in resource-limited settings. Prevalence and incidence rates are likely underestimated, as most men and up to 30% of women are asymptomatic. Diagnostic accuracy using wet mount microscopy, the mainstay of diagnosis, is less sensitive than previously assumed. While the disease is easily treated, sequelae of untreated infection remain a significant cause of morbidity due to high reinfection rates from untreated partners, underrecognition of asymptomatic cases, and insensitive diagnostics.

From 5 to 8 million cases of trichomoniasis occur each year in the USA. A population-based study conducted in 2005 showed a prevalence of 2.8% in women, 1.7% in men, and an overall prevalence of 2.3%. The incidence of trichomoniasis is highest among females with multiple sexual partners and in groups with the highest rates of other sexually transmitted infections. *T. vaginalis* is recovered from >60% of female partners of infected men and 70% of male sexual partners of infected women. Vaginal trichomoniasis is rare until menarche. Its presence in a younger child should raise the possibility of **sexual abuse.**

Trichomoniasis may be transmitted to neonates during passage through an infected birth canal. Infection in this setting is usually self-limited, but rare cases of neonatal vaginitis and respiratory infection have been reported.

PATHOGENESIS

T. vaginalis is an anaerobic, flagellated protozoan parasite. Infected vaginal secretions contain 10^1 to 10^5 or more protozoa/mL. *T. vaginalis* is pear shaped and exhibits characteristic twitching motility in wet mount (Fig. 276-1). Reproduction is by binary fission. It exists only as **vegetative cells;** cyst forms have not been described. *T. vaginalis* damages host cells and tissues by a number of mechanisms. Adhesion molecules allow attachment of *T. vaginalis* to host cells, and hydrolases, proteases, and cytotoxic molecules act to destroy or impair the integrity of host cells. Parasite-specific antibodies and lymphocyte priming occur in response to infection, but durable protective immunity does not occur.

CLINICAL MANIFESTATIONS

The **incubation period** in females is 5-28 days. Symptoms may begin or exacerbate with menses. Most infected women eventually develop symptoms, although up to one third remain asymptomatic. Common signs and symptoms include a copious malodorous gray, frothy vaginal discharge, vulvovaginal irritation, dysuria, and dyspareunia. Physical examination may reveal a frothy discharge with vaginal erythema and cervical hemorrhages ("strawberry cervix"). The discharge usually has a pH of

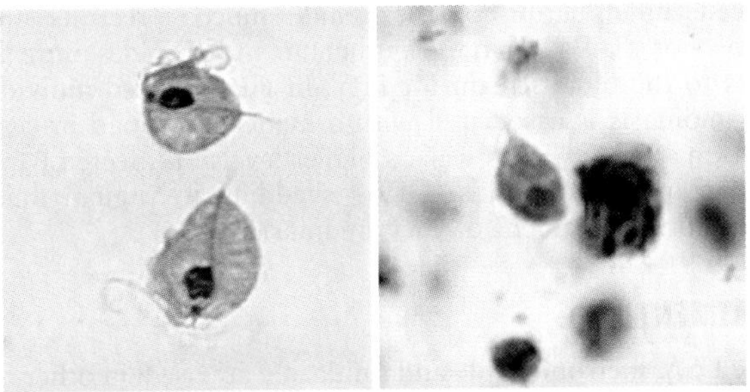

Figure 276-1 *Trichomonas vaginalis* trophozoites stained with Giemsa *(left)* and iron hematoxylin *(right).* (From the Centers for Disease Control and Prevention: *Laboratory identification of parasites of public health concern. Trichomoniasis* (website). www.dpd.cdc.gov/dpdx/HTML/ImageLibrary/Trichomoniasis_il.htm. Accessed August 30, 2010.)

>4.5. Abdominal discomfort is unusual and should prompt evaluation for pelvic inflammatory disease (Chapter 114).

Most infections in males are asymptomatic. Symptomatic males usually have dysuria and scant urethral discharge. Trichomonads occasionally cause epididymitis, prostatic involvement, and superficial penile ulceration. Infection is often self-limited, spontaneously resolving in 36% of men. *Trichomonas* has been implicated as a cause of recurrent or relapsing urethritis and can be isolated in 3-20% of men with **nongonococcal urethritis.** Treatment failures with standard therapy for gonorrhea and *Chlamydia* are frequently treated with antitrichomonal therapy.

DIAGNOSIS

Trichomonads may be recognized in vaginal secretions by using the wet mount technique. This technique has been estimated to have a sensitivity of 60-70%; studies using more sensitive assays with nucleic acid probes and polymerase chain reaction (PCR) have suggested that this is closer to 35-60%. Although *Trichomonas* is sometimes seen on Pap smears and urine, these methods are not considered reliable tests for disease. Wet mount examination of material obtained by platinum loop from the anterior urethra may reveal the organism in 50-90% of infected men. Microscopic examination of urine sediment after prostatic massage is also useful in infected men. Culture of the organism is the gold standard for detection, and commercial culture media are available. Enzyme-linked immunosorbent assay and direct fluorescent antigen testing of vaginal secretions are more sensitive than wet mount testing but less sensitive than culture for detection of *T. vaginalis* infection. In women, DNA immunoblot and PCR testing of vaginal secretions have similar sensitivity and specificity to culture. In men, these methods appear to be more sensitive at detection of infection than culture. Nucleic acid amplification testing (NAAT) and immunologic diagnostic kits for diagnosis of *Trichomonas* alone and in combination with other gynecologic diseases such as *Candida* and *Gardnerella* have been evaluated by multiple studies and have been found to be accurate and easy to use. At least 2 point-of-care kits for rapid testing, Affirm VP III (BD Diagnostic Systems, Sparks, MD) and OSOM *Trichomonas* Rapid Test (Genzyme Diagnostics, Cambridge, MA), have received approval by the U.S. Food and Drug Administration (FDA). Conventional and multiplex PCR assays for clinical use have been developed, and preliminary testing results are promising. Patients with *T. vaginalis* should be screened for other sexually transmitted infections, including *Chlamydia* and gonorrhea.

COMPLICATIONS

Untreated trichomoniasis has been associated with pelvic inflammatory disease, premature delivery, low birthweight, tubal infertility, and vaginal cuff cellulitis. *T. vaginalis* infection increases the risk of acquisition and transmission of HIV. *Trichomonas*-induced inflammation of the genital mucosa recruits greater numbers of $CD4^+$ cells in the epithelium and provides more direct access to the bloodstream for HIV. In HIV-infected individuals, trichomoniasis is associated with a higher viral load in cervical secretions and semen as well as higher levels of infected lymphocytes in urogenital fluids. HIV-1 shedding in vaginal fluids is decreased by treatment of trichomoniasis.

TREATMENT

In the USA, **metronidazole** and **tinidazole** are used; in other countries ornidazole is also used. Both metronidazole (single-dose regimen of 2 g orally as a single dose for adolescent and adults; alternative regimen, 500 mg orally bid for 7 days) and tinidazole (single 2 g dose orally in adolescents and adults) are used as first-line treatment. For children infected prior to adolescence, the recommended regimen is metronidazole 15 mg/kg/day divided in 3 doses orally for 7 days; tinidazole is not approved for dosing in younger children. Topical metronidazole gel is not efficacious when used as the sole therapy for *T. vaginalis* infection, but it may decrease symptoms in individuals with severe infection when used in conjunction with oral therapy. Sexual partners should be treated simultaneously to prevent reinfection. Multiple head-to-head trials comparing the efficacy between single-dose/short courses of metronidazole and single-dose tinidazole have shown either non-inferiority or superior efficacy for tinidazole. A Cochrane meta-analysis demonstrated that single dose tinidazole was superior compared to short-course metronidazole in clinical efficacy and parasitologic cure rates and had significantly fewer side effects. Tinidazole is more expensive than metronidazole and is generally reserved for treatment failures or metronidazole intolerance.

Treatment failures have been reported with metronidazole, although poor response can usually be overcome by higher doses of drugs. Second-line treatment recommendations include either a 7-day course of metronidazole 500 mg twice daily or a single dose of tinidazole. If this treatment fails, either metronidazole or tinidazole at 2 g daily for 5 days is recommended. Further treatment failure should be referred to an infectious diseases specialist and may require susceptibility testing, which is available from the Centers for Disease Control and Prevention. Metronidazole has not been shown to be teratogenic during pregnancy in humans but is currently classified as a category C drug. At least 2 prospective studies showed an association between premature births or low birth weight with metronidazole treatment of asymptomatic *T. vaginalis* infection in pregnancy. Further studies are needed to confirm these findings. Treatment of symptomatic trichomoniasis in pregnancy should be weighed against possible risks, while treatment of asymptomatic disease should be delayed as much as possible to near term.

PREVENTION

Prevention of *T. vaginalis* infection is best accomplished by treatment of all sexual partners of an infected person and by programs aimed at prevention of all sexually transmitted infections (Chapter 114). No vaccine is available, and drug prophylaxis is not recommended.

BIBLIOGRAPHY

Please visit the Nelson Textbook of Pediatrics *website at www.expertconsult.com for the complete bibliography.*

Chapter 277
Leishmaniasis *(Leishmania)*

Peter C. Melby

The leishmaniases are a diverse group of diseases caused by intracellular protozoan parasites of the genus *Leishmania,* which are transmitted by phlebotomine sandflies. Multiple species of *Leishmania* are known to cause human disease involving the skin and mucosal surfaces and the visceral reticuloendothelial organs. Cutaneous disease is generally mild but may cause cosmetic disfigurement. Mucosal and visceral leishmaniasis is associated with significant morbidity and mortality.

ETIOLOGY

Leishmania organisms are members of the Trypanosomatidae family and include 2 subgenera, *Leishmania (Leishmania)* and *Leishmania (Viannia)*. The parasite is dimorphic, existing as a flagellate promastigote in the insect vector and as an aflagellate amastigote that resides and replicates within mononuclear phagocytes of the vertebrate host. Within the sandfly vector the promastigote changes from a noninfective procyclic form to an infective metacyclic stage. Fundamental to this transition are changes that take place in the terminal polysaccharides of the surface lipophosphoglycan (LPG), which allow forward migration of the infective parasites from the sandfly midgut to the mouth parts and inoculation of the host during a blood meal. Metacyclic LPG also plays an important role in the entry and survival of *Leishmania* in the mammalian host by conferring complement resistance and by facilitating entry into the macrophage by way of multiple receptors, including complement receptors 1 and 3. Once within the macrophage, the promastigote transforms to an amastigote and resides and replicates within a phagolysosome. The parasite is resistant to the acidic, hostile environment of the macrophage and eventually ruptures the cell and goes on to infect other macrophages. Infected macrophages have a diminished capacity to initiate and respond to an inflammatory response, thus providing a safe haven for the intracellular parasite.

EPIDEMIOLOGY

The leishmaniases are estimated to affect 10-50 million people in endemic tropical and subtropical regions on all continents except Australia and Antarctica. The different forms of the disease are distinct in their causes, epidemiologic characteristics, transmission, and geographic distribution. The leishmaniases may occur sporadically throughout an endemic region or may occur in epidemic focuses. With only rare exceptions, the *Leishmania* organisms that primarily cause cutaneous disease do not cause visceral disease.

Localized cutaneous leishmaniasis (LCL) in the Old World is caused by *L. (Leishmania) major* and *L. (L.) tropica* in North Africa, the Middle East, central Asia, and the Indian subcontinent. *L. (L.) aethiopica* is a cause of LCL and diffuse cutaneous leishmaniasis (DCL) in Kenya and Ethiopia. **Visceral leishmaniasis** (VL) in the Old World is caused by *L. (L.) donovani* in Kenya, Sudan, India, Pakistan, and China and by *L. (L.) infantum* in the Mediterranean basin, Middle East, and central Asia. *L. infantum* is also a cause of LCL (without visceral disease) in this same geographic distribution. *L. tropica* also has been recognized as an uncommon cause of visceral disease in the Middle East and India. In the New World, *L. (L.) mexicana* causes LCL in a region stretching from southern Texas through Central America. *L. (L.) amazonensis, L. (L.) pifanoi, L. (L.) garnhami,* and *L. (L.) venezuelensis* cause LCL in South America, the Amazon basin, and northward. Members of the *Viannia* subgenus (*L. [V.] braziliensis, L. [V.] panamensis, L. [V.] guyanensis,* and *L. [V.] peruviana*) cause LCL from the northern highlands of Argentina northward to Central America. Members of the *Viannia* subgenus also cause **mucosal leishmaniasis** (ML) in a similar geographic distribution. VL in the New World is caused by *L. (L.) chagasi* (now considered to be the same organism as *L. infantum*), which is distributed from Mexico (rare) through Central and South America. *L. infantum/chagasi* can also cause LCL in the absence of visceral disease.

The maintenance of *Leishmania* in most endemic areas is through a zoonotic transmission cycle. In general, the dermotropic strains in both the Old and New Worlds are maintained in rodent reservoirs, and the domestic dog is the usual reservoir for *L. infantum/chagasi*. The transmission between reservoir and sandfly is highly adapted to the specific ecologic characteristics of the endemic region. Human infections occur when human activities bring them in contact with the zoonotic cycle. Anthroponotic transmission, in which humans are the presumed reservoir, occurs with *L. tropica* in some urban areas of the Middle East and Central Asia, and with *L. donovani* in India and Sudan. Congenital transmission of *L. donovani* or *L. infantum/chagasi* has been reported.

There is a resurgence of leishmaniasis in long-standing endemic areas as well as in new foci. Tens of thousands of cases of LCL occurred in an outbreak in Kabul, Afghanistan, and severe epidemics with >100,000 deaths from VL have occurred in India and Sudan. VL is most prevalent among the poorest of the poor, with substandard housing contributing to the vector-borne transmission and undernutrition leading to increased host susceptibility. The emergence of the leishmaniases in new areas is the result of (1) movement of a susceptible population into existing endemic areas, usually because of agricultural or industrial development or timber harvesting; (2) increase in vector and/or reservoir populations as a result of agriculture development projects; (3) increase in anthroponotic transmission owing to rapid urbanization in some focuses; and (4) increase in sandfly density resulting from a reduction in vector control programs.

PATHOLOGY

Histopathologic analysis of the LCL lesion shows intense chronic granulomatous inflammation involving the epidermis and dermis. Occasionally, neutrophils and even microabscesses can be seen. The lesions of DCL are characterized by dense infiltration with vacuolated macrophages containing abundant amastigotes. ML is characterized by an intense granulomatous reaction with prominent tissue necrosis, which may include adjacent cartilage or bone. In VL there is prominent reticuloendothelial cell hyperplasia in the liver, spleen, bone marrow, and lymph nodes. Amastigotes are abundant in the histiocytes and Kupffer cells. Late in the course of disease, splenic infarcts are common, centrilobular necrosis and fatty infiltration of the liver occur, the normal marrow elements are replaced by parasitized histiocytes, and erythrophagocytosis is present.

PATHOGENESIS

Cellular immune mechanisms determine resistance or susceptibility to infection with *Leishmania*. Resistance is mediated by interleukin 12 (IL-12)–driven generation of a T helper 1 (Th1) cell response, with interferon-γ inducing classical macrophage activation and parasite killing. Susceptibility is associated with expansion of IL-4–producing Th2 cells and/or the production of IL-10 and transforming growth factor-β, which are inhibitors of macrophage-mediated parasite killing, and the generation of regulatory T cells and alternatively activated macrophages. Patients with ML exhibit a hyperresponsive cellular immune reaction that may contribute to the prominent tissue destruction seen in this form of the disease. Patients with DCL or active VL demonstrate minimal or absent *Leishmania*-specific cellular immune responses, but these responses recover after successful therapy.

Within endemic areas, people who have had a subclinical infection can be identified by a positive delayed-type hypersensitivity response to leishmanial antigens (**Montenegro skin test**). Subclinical infection occurs considerably more frequently than does active cutaneous or visceral disease. Host factors (genetic background, concomitant disease, nutritional status), parasite factors (virulence, size of the inoculum), and possibly vector-specific factors (vector genotype, immunomodulatory salivary constituents) influence the expression as either subclinical infection or active disease. Within endemic areas the prevalence of skin test result positivity increases with age and the incidence of clinical disease decreases with age, indicating that immunity is acquired in the population over time. Individuals with prior active disease or subclinical infection are usually immune to a subsequent clinical infection.

CLINICAL MANIFESTATIONS

The different forms of the disease are distinct in their causes, epidemiologic features, transmission, and geographic distribution.

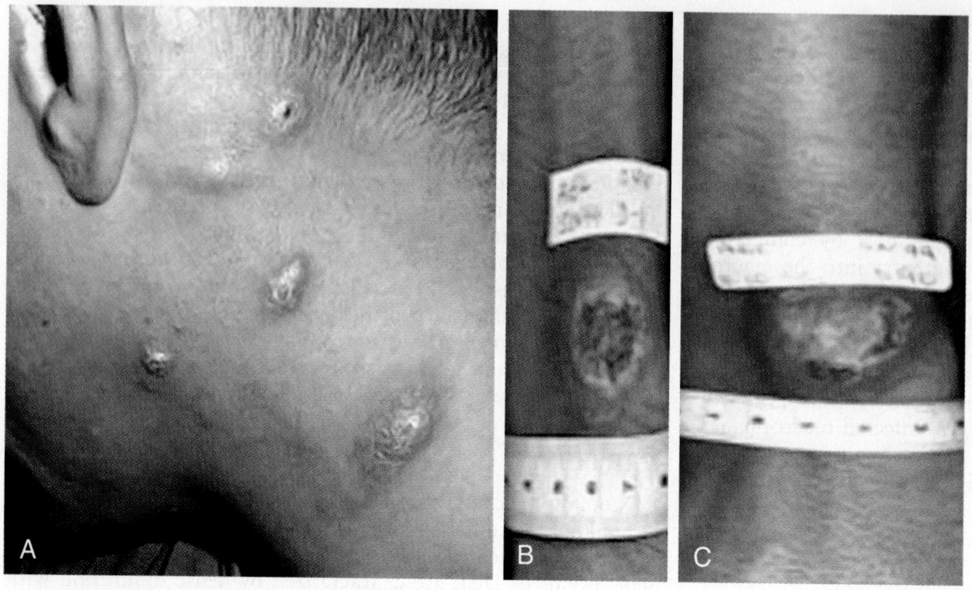

Figure 277-1 Cutaneous and mucosal disease. *A,* Old World infection *(Leishmania major)* acquired in Iraq; note 5 papular and nodular lesions on neck. *B,* New World infection *(Leishmania panamensis)* in Colombia; purely ulcerative lesion is characteristic of New World disease. *C,* Healed infection in patient shown in *B* 70 days after 20 days of meglumine antimoniate treatment; note paper-thin scar tissue over flat re-epithelialized skin. (*A,* Courtesy of P. Weina. *B,* Courtesy of J. Soto. *A-C,* Modified from Murray HW, Berman JD, Davies CR, et al: Advances in leishmaniasis, *Lancet* 366:1561–1577, 2005.)

Localized Cutaneous Leishmaniasis

LCL (**Oriental sore**) can affect individuals of any age, but children are the primary victims in many endemic regions. It may present as 1 or a few papular, nodular, plaquelike, or ulcerative lesions that are usually located on exposed skin, such as the face and extremities (Fig. 277-1). Rarely, >100 lesions have been recorded. The lesions typically begin as a small papule at the site of the sandfly bite, which enlarges to 1-3 cm in diameter and may ulcerate over the course of several weeks to months. The shallow ulcer is usually nontender and surrounded by a sharp, indurated, erythematous margin. There is no drainage unless a bacterial superinfection develops. Lesions caused by *L. major* and *L. mexicana* usually heal spontaneously after 3-6 mo, leaving a depressed scar. Lesions on the ear pinna caused by *L. mexicana,* called **chiclero ulcer** because they were common in chicle harvesters in Mexico and Central America, often follow a chronic, destructive course. In general, lesions caused by *L. (Viannia)* species tend to be larger and more chronic. Regional lymphadenopathy and palpable subcutaneous nodules or lymphatic cords, the so-called sporotrichoid appearance, are also more common when the patient is infected with organisms of the *Viannia* subgenus. If lesions do not become secondarily infected, there are usually no complications aside from the residual cutaneous scar.

Diffuse Cutaneous Leishmaniasis

DCL is a rare form of leishmaniasis caused by organisms of the *L. mexicana* complex in the New World, and *L. aethiopica* in the Old World. DCL manifests as large nonulcerating macules, papules, nodules, or plaques that often involve large areas of skin and may resemble lepromatous leprosy. The face and extremities are most commonly involved. Dissemination from the initial lesion usually takes place over several years. It is thought that an immunologic defect underlies this severe form of cutaneous leishmaniasis.

Mucosal Leishmaniasis

ML (**espundia**) is an uncommon but serious manifestation of leishmanial infection resulting from hematogenous metastases to the nasal or oropharyngeal mucosa from a cutaneous infection. It is usually caused by parasites in the *L. (Viannia)* complex. Approximately half of the patients with mucosal lesions have had active cutaneous lesions within the preceding 2 yr, but ML may not develop until many years after resolution of the primary lesion. ML occurs in <5% of individuals who have, or have had, LCL caused by *L. (V.) braziliensis.* Patients with ML most commonly have nasal mucosal involvement and present with nasal congestion, discharge, and recurrent epistaxis. Oropharyngeal and laryngeal involvement is less common but associated with severe morbidity. Marked soft tissue, cartilage, and even bone destruction occurs late in the course of disease and may lead to visible deformity of the nose or mouth, nasal septal perforation, and tracheal narrowing with airway obstruction.

Visceral Leishmaniasis

VL (**kala-azar**) typically affects children <5 yr of age in the New World and Mediterranean region (*L. infantum/chagasi*) and older children and young adults in Africa and Asia (*L. donovani*). After inoculation of the organism into the skin by the sandfly, the child may have a completely asymptomatic infection or an oligosymptomatic illness that either resolves spontaneously or evolves into active kala-azar. Children with asymptomatic infection are transiently seropositive but show no clinical evidence of disease. Children who are oligosymptomatic have mild constitutional symptoms (malaise, intermittent diarrhea, poor activity tolerance) and intermittent fever; most will have a mildly enlarged liver. In most of these children the illness will resolve without therapy, but in approximately 25% it will evolve to active kala-azar within 2-8 mo. Extreme incubation periods of several years have rarely been described. During the 1st few weeks to months of disease evolution the fever is intermittent, there is weakness and loss of energy, and the spleen begins to enlarge. The classic clinical features of high fever, marked splenomegaly, hepatomegaly, and severe cachexia typically develop approximately 6 mo after the onset of the illness, but a rapid clinical course over 1 mo has been noted in up to 20% of patients in some series (Fig. 277-2). At the terminal stages of kala-azar the hepatosplenomegaly is massive, there is gross wasting, the pancytopenia is profound, and jaundice, edema, and ascites may be present. Anemia may be severe enough to precipitate heart failure. Bleeding episodes, especially epistaxis, are frequent. The late stage of the illness is often complicated by secondary bacterial infections, which frequently are a cause of death. A younger age at the time of infection and underlying malnutrition may be risk factors for the development and more rapid evolution of active VL. Death occurs in >90% of patients without specific antileishmanial treatment.

VL is an opportunistic infection associated with HIV infection. Most cases have occurred in southern Europe and Brazil, often as a result of needle sharing associated with illicit drug use, with the potential for many more cases as the endemic regions for HIV and VL converge. Leishmaniasis may also result from

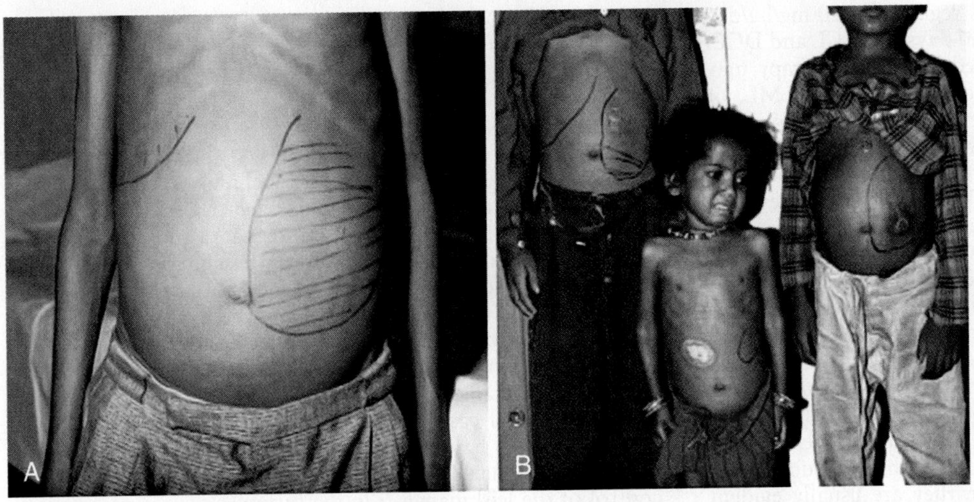

Figure 277-2 Visceral leishmaniasis (*Leishmania donovani*) in Bihar State, India. *A,* Hepatosplenomegaly and wasting in a young man. *B,* Children with burn marks over enlarged spleen or liver—local shaman's unsuccessful remedy. (*A,* Courtesy of D. Sacks. *B,* Courtesy of R. Kenney. *A-B,* Modified from Murray HW, Berman JD, Davies CR, et al: Advances in leishmaniasis, *Lancet* 366:1561–1577, 2005.)

reactivation of a long-standing subclinical infection. Frequently there is an atypical clinical presentation of VL in HIV-infected individuals with prominent involvement of the gastrointestinal tract and absence of the typical hepatosplenomegaly.

A small percentage of patients previously treated for VL develop diffuse skin lesions, a condition known as **post–kala-azar dermal leishmaniasis (PKDL)**. These lesions may appear during or shortly after therapy (Africa) or up to several years later (India). The lesions of PKDL are hypopigmented, erythematous, or nodular and commonly involve the face and torso. They may persist for several months or for many years.

LABORATORY FINDINGS

Patients with cutaneous or mucosal leishmaniasis generally do not have abnormal laboratory results unless the lesions are secondarily infected with bacteria. Laboratory findings associated with classic kala-azar include anemia (hemoglobin 5-8 mg/dL), thrombocytopenia, leukopenia (2,000-3,000 cells/μL), elevated hepatic transaminase levels, and hyperglobulinemia (>5 g/dL) that is mostly immunoglobulin G (IgG).

DIFFERENTIAL DIAGNOSIS

Diseases that should be considered in the differential diagnosis of LCL include sporotrichosis, blastomycosis, chromomycosis, lobomycosis, cutaneous tuberculosis, atypical mycobacterial infection, leprosy, ecthyma, syphilis, yaws, and neoplasms. Infections such as syphilis, tertiary yaws, histoplasmosis, paracoccidioidomycosis, as well as sarcoidosis, Wegener granulomatosis, midline granuloma, and carcinoma may have clinical features similar to those of ML. VL should be strongly suspected in the patient with prolonged fever, weakness, cachexia, marked splenomegaly, hepatomegaly, cytopenias, and hypergammaglobulinemia who has had potential exposure in an endemic area. The clinical picture may also be consistent with that of malaria, typhoid fever, miliary tuberculosis, schistosomiasis, brucellosis, amebic liver abscess, infectious mononucleosis, lymphoma, and leukemia.

DIAGNOSIS

The development of one or several slowly progressive, nontender, nodular, or ulcerative lesions in a patient who had potential exposure in an endemic area should raise suspicion of LCL.

Serologic tests for diagnosis of ML or LCL generally have low sensitivity and specificity and offer little for diagnosis. Serologic testing by enzyme immunoassay, indirect fluorescence assay, or direct agglutination is very useful in VL because of the very high level of antileishmanial antibodies. An enzyme-linked immunosorbent assay using a recombinant antigen (K39) has a sensitivity and specificity for VL that is close to 100%. A negative serologic test result in an immunocompetent individual is strong evidence against a diagnosis of VL. Serodiagnostic tests have positive findings in only about half of the patients who are co-infected with HIV.

Definitive diagnosis of leishmaniasis is established by the demonstration of amastigotes in tissue specimens or isolation of the organism by culture. Amastigotes can be identified in Giemsa-stained tissue sections, aspirates, or impression smears in about half of the cases of LCL but only rarely in the lesions of ML. Culture of a tissue biopsy or aspirate, best performed by using Novy-McNeal-Nicolle (NNN) biphasic blood agar medium, yields a positive finding in only about 65% of cases of CL. Identification of parasites in impression smears, histopathologic sections, or culture medium is more readily accomplished in DCL than in LCL. In patients with VL, smears or cultures of material from splenic, bone marrow, or lymph node aspirations are usually diagnostic. In experienced hands, **splenic aspiration** has a higher diagnostic sensitivity, but it is rarely performed in the USA because of the risk for bleeding complications. A positive culture result allows speciation of the parasite, usually by isoenzyme analysis by a reference laboratory, which may have therapeutic and prognostic significance.

TREATMENT

Specific antileishmanial therapy is not routinely indicated for uncomplicated LCL caused by strains that have a high rate of spontaneous resolution and self-healing *(L. major, L. mexicana)*. Lesions that are extensive, severely inflamed, or located where a scar would result in disability (near a joint) or cosmetic disfigurement (face or ear), that involve the lymphatics, or that do not begin healing within 3-4 mo should be treated. Cutaneous lesions suspected or known to be caused by members of the *Viannia* subgenus (New World) should be treated because of the low rate of spontaneous healing and the potential risk for development of mucosal disease. Similarly, patients with lesions caused by *L. tropica* (Old World), which are typically chronic and nonhealing, should be treated. All patients with VL or ML should receive therapy.

The pentavalent antimony compounds (sodium stibogluconate [Pentostam, GlaxoSmithKline, Uxbridge, UK] and meglumine antimoniate [Glucantime, Aventis, Strasbourg, France]) have been the mainstay of antileishmanial chemotherapy for >40 yr. These drugs have similar efficacies, toxicities, and treatment regimens. Currently, for sodium stibogluconate (available in the USA from the Centers for Disease Control and Prevention,

Atlanta, Georgia), the recommended regimen is 20 mg/kg/day intravenously or intramuscularly for 20 days (for LCL and DCL) or 28 days (for ML and VL). Repeated courses of therapy may be necessary in patients with severe cutaneous lesions, ML, or VL. An initial clinical response to therapy usually occurs in the 1st wk of therapy, but complete clinical healing (re-epithelialization and scarring for LCL and ML, and regression of splenomegaly and normalization of cytopenias for VL) is usually not evident for weeks to a few months after completion of therapy. Cure rates with this regimen of 90-100% for LCL, 50-70% for ML, and 80-100% for VL were common in the 1990s, but clinical resistance to antimony therapy has become common in parts of India, East Africa, and Latin America. Furthermore, a very low cure rate in children <5 yr of age has been reported in Colombia. Relapses are common in patients who do not have an effective antileishmanial cellular immune response, such as those who have DCL or are co-infected with HIV. These patients often require multiple courses of therapy or a chronic suppressive regimen. When clinical relapses occur, they are usually evident within 2 mo after completion of therapy. Adverse effects of antimony therapy are dose and duration dependent and commonly include fatigue, arthralgias and myalgias (50%), abdominal discomfort (30%), elevated hepatic transaminase level (30-80%), elevated amylase and lipase levels (almost 100%), mild hematologic changes (slightly decreased leukocyte count, hemoglobin level, and platelet count) (10-30%), and nonspecific T-wave changes on electrocardiography (30%). Sudden death due to cardiac toxicity is extremely rare and is usually associated with use of very high doses of pentavalent antimony.

Amphotericin B desoxycholate and the amphotericin lipid formulations are very useful in the treatment of VL or ML and in some regions have replaced antimony as first-line therapy. Amphotericin B desoxycholate at doses of 0.5-1.0 mg/kg every day or every other day for 14-20 doses achieved a cure rate for VL of close to 100%, but the renal toxicity commonly associated with amphotericin B was common. The lipid formulations of amphotericin B are especially attractive for treatment of leishmaniasis because the drugs are concentrated in the reticuloendothelial system and are less nephrotoxic. Liposomal amphotericin B is highly effective, with a 90-100% cure rate for VL in immunocompetent children, some of whom were refractory to antimony therapy. Liposomal amphotericin B (Ambisome, Gilead Sciences, Foster City, CA) is approved by the U.S. Food and Drug Administration for treatment of VL at a recommended dose for immunocompetent patients of 3 mg/kg on days 1-5, 14, and 21 and should be considered for first-line therapy in the USA. Therapy for immunocompromised patients may need to be prolonged. Parenteral treatment of VL with the aminoglycoside paromomycin (aminosidine) has efficacy (~95%) similar to that of amphotericin B in India. Recombinant human interferon-γ has been successfully used as an adjunct to antimony therapy in the treatment of refractory cases of ML and VL. It is not effective alone and has the frequent side effects of fever and flulike symptoms. Miltefosine, a membrane-activating alkylphospholipid, has been recently developed as the 1st oral treatment for VL and has a cure rate of 95% in Indian patients with VL when administered orally at 50-100 mg/day for 28 days. Gastrointestinal adverse effects were frequent but did not require discontinuation of the drug. Treatment of LCL with oral drugs has had only modest success. Ketoconazole has been effective in treating adults with LCL caused by L. major, L. mexicana, and L. panamensis but not L. tropica or L. braziliensis. Fluconazole 200 mg orally once daily for 6 wk was demonstrated in adults to modestly increase the rate of healing of CL caused by L. major in Saudi Arabia. Miltefosine 2.5 mg/kg/day orally for 20 days had a 91% efficacy in treating CL in Colombia (L. panamensis) but was significantly less effective in patients from Guatemala (L. braziliensis). Topical treatment of CL with paromomycin plus methylbenzethonium chloride ointment has been effective in selected areas in the both Old and New World. Enhanced drug development efforts and clinical trials of new drugs are clearly needed, especially in children.

PREVENTION

Personal protective measures should include avoidance of exposure to the nocturnal sandflies and, when necessary, the use of insect repellent and permethrin-impregnated mosquito netting. Where peridomiciliary transmission is present, community-based residual insecticide spraying has had some success in reducing the prevalence of leishmaniasis, but long-term effects are difficult to maintain. Control or elimination of infected reservoir hosts (e.g., seropositive domestic dogs) has had limited success. Where anthroponotic transmission is thought to occur, early recognition and treatment of cases are essential. Several vaccines have been demonstrated to have efficacy in experimental models, and vaccination of humans or domestic dogs may have a role in the control of the leishmaniases in the future.

BIBLIOGRAPHY

Please visit the Nelson Textbook of Pediatrics *website at www.expertconsult.com for the complete bibliography.*

Chapter 278
African Trypanosomiasis (Sleeping Sickness; *Trypanosoma brucei* Complex)

Edsel Maurice T. Salvana and Robert A. Salata

Over 60 million people in nearly 40 countries are at risk for infection with *Trypanosoma brucei* complex, the causative agent of sleeping sickness. Also known as *human African trypanosomiasis* (HAT), this disease is restricted to sub-Saharan Africa, the range of the tsetse fly vector, where at least 300,000 people are infected. It is a disease of extreme poverty, with an increasing burden observed in remote rural areas. HAT comes in 2 geographically and clinically distinct forms. *Trypanosoma brucei gambiense* causes a chronic infection lasting years and mostly affects people who live in Western and Central Africa (**West African sleeping sickness, Gambian trypanosomiasis**). *Trypanosoma brucei rhodesiense,* a zoonosis, presents as an acute illness lasting several weeks and usually occurs in residents of eastern and southern Africa (**East African sleeping sickness, Rhodesian trypanosomiasis**).

ETIOLOGY

HAT is a vector-borne disease caused by parasitic, flagellated kinetoplastid protozoans of 2 subspecies of *Trypanosoma brucei.* It is transmitted to humans through the bite of *Glossina*, commonly known as the **tsetse fly.**

The tsetse fly feeds on the blood of humans and wild game animals and penetrates intact mucous membranes and skin. Humans usually contract East African HAT when they venture from towns to rural areas to visit woodlands or livestock, highlighting the importance of zoonotic reservoirs in this disease. West African HAT is contracted closer to settlements. This form only requires a small vector population and thus has been particularly difficult to eradicate. Because of low rates of infection in tsetse flies, the life cycle of this form necessitates close and repeated contact between humans and insects to permit frequent biting. While animal reservoirs occur, these reservoirs are less important than for East African HAT, and the main source of infection remains chronically infected human hosts.

LIFE CYCLE

Trypanosoma brucei undergoes several stages of development in the insect and mammalian host. Upon ingestion with a blood meal, nonproliferative stumpy forms of the parasite, which are optimally adapted to surviving in *Glossina,* transform into procyclic forms in the insect's midgut. These procyclic forms proliferate and undergo further development into epimastigotes, which then become infective metacyclic forms that migrate to the insect's salivary glands. The life cycle within the tsetse fly takes 15-35 days. On inoculation into the mammalian host, the metacyclic stage transforms into proliferative long and slender forms in the bloodstream and the lymphatics, eventually penetrating the central nervous system. These slender forms appear in waves in the peripheral blood, with each wave followed by a febrile crisis and heralding the formation of a new antigenic variant. The slender forms transform into intermediate forms, which become nonproliferative stumpy forms that are ingested by *Glossina* and start the cycle anew.

Direct transmission to humans has been reported, either mechanically through contact with the contaminated mouth parts of tsetse flies with viable slender forms during feeding or vertically to infants by way of the placenta of infected mothers.

EPIDEMIOLOGY

HAT is a major public health problem in sub-Saharan Africa. It occurs in the region between latitudes 15 degrees north and 15 degrees south, corresponding roughly to the area where the annual rainfall creates optimal climatic conditions for *Glossina* flies to thrive.

Thirty-two thousand cases of HAT are reported annually, although an incidence of up to 70,000 cases/yr is estimated to occur; 24,000 deaths per year are attributed to HAT. By far, the bulk of reported cases are made up of *T. brucei gambiense*, with approximately two thirds of the cases coming from the Democratic Republic of the Congo. The incidence of HAT has been dropping in recent years, reflecting more aggressive and cohesive control programs, but these programs need to be sustained before the possibility of elimination can be considered realistic. Over 1.5 million disability-adjusted life years were lost to HAT in 2002, although this number does not take into account morbidity from acute and chronic infection, toxic side effects of treatment, or economic burden from losses of trypanosome-infected livestock.

T. brucei rhodesiense infection is restricted to the eastern third of the endemic area in tropical Africa, stretching from Ethiopia to the northern boundaries of South Africa. *T. brucei gambiense* occurs mainly in the western half of the continent's endemic region. *Glossina* captured in endemic foci show a low rate of infection, usually <5%. Rhodesian HAT, which has an acute and often fatal course, greatly reduces chances of transmission to tsetse flies. The ability of *T. brucei rhodesiense* to multiply rapidly in the bloodstream and infect other species of mammals helps maintain its life cycle. The insect vector is able to transmit disease for up to 6 mo.

PATHOGENESIS

The initial entry site of the organisms develops a hard, painful, red nodule known as a trypanosomal **chancre.** It contains long, thin trypanosomes multiplying beneath the dermis and is surrounded by a lymphocytic cellular infiltrate. Dissemination into the blood and lymphatic systems follows, with subsequent localization to the CNS. Histopathologic findings in the brain are consistent with meningoencephalitis, with lymphocytic infiltration and perivascular cuffing of the membranes. The appearance of **morular** cells (large, strawberry-like cells, supposedly derived from plasma cells) is a characteristic finding in chronic disease.

Antigenic variation of **variant surface glycoproteins (VSG)** on the trypanosome's surface enables evasion of acquired immunity during infection. Both *T. brucei gambiense* and *T. brucei rhodesiense* have acquired resistance to trypanolytic factors in human serum, the most well-studied of which is **apolipoprotein L-1** (APOL1), through the expression of a protein known as *serum resistance-associated protein* (SRA). A frameshift mutation in the APOL1 gene in 1 patient enabled infection with a nonhuman trypanosome, *Trypanosoma evansi*, and treatment with recombinant APOL1 restored trypanolytic activity. Mechanisms underlying virulence in HAT are still incompletely understood, although severity of disease seems to be dependent on the host inflammatory response, particularly IFN-γ production in the central nervous system (CNS) and blood.

CLINICAL MANIFESTATIONS

Clinical presentations vary not only because of the 2 subspecies of organisms but also because of differences in host response in the indigenous population of endemic areas and in newcomers or visitors. Visitors usually suffer more from the acute symptoms, but in untreated cases death is inevitable for natives and visitors alike. Symptoms usually occur within 1-4 wk of infection. The clinical syndromes of HAT are trypanosomal chancre, hemolymphatic stage, and meningoencephalitic stage.

Trypanosomal Chancre

The site of the tsetse fly bite may be the 1st presenting feature. A nodule or chancre develops in 2-3 days and becomes a painful, hard, red nodule surrounded by an area of erythema and swelling within 1 wk. Nodules are commonly seen on the lower limbs and sometimes also on the head. They subside spontaneously in about 2 wk, leaving no permanent scar.

Hemolymphatic Stage (Stage 1)

The most common presenting features of acute HAT occur at the time of invasion of the bloodstream by the parasites, 2-3 wk after infection. Patients usually present with irregular episodes of fever, each lasting up to 7 days, accompanied by headache, sweating, and generalized lymphadenopathy. Attacks may be separated by symptom-free intervals of days or even weeks. Painless, nonmatted lymphadenopathy, most commonly of the posterior cervical and supraclavicular nodes, is 1 of the most constant signs, particularly in the Gambian form. A common feature of trypanosomiasis in Caucasians is the presence of blotchy, irregular, nonpruritic, erythematous macules, which may appear any time after the 1st febrile episode, usually within 6-8 wk. The majority of macules have a normal central area, giving the rash a circinate outline. This rash is seen mainly on the trunk and is evanescent, fading in 1 place only to appear at another site. Examination of the blood during this stage may show anemia, leukopenia with relative monocytosis, and elevated levels of IgM. Cardiac manifestations of HAT have also been reported but are generally limited to nonspecific ST-T wave electrocardiographic abnormalities. Histopathologic characterization shows a lymphomonohistiocytic infiltrate in the interstitium and there is no penetration of the myocardial cells, unlike that for American trypanosomiasis (Chapter 279). Progression of cardiac pathology to congestive heart failure has not been reported, and the perimyocarditis is usually self-limited and/or readily resolves with treatment.

Meningoencephalitic Stage (Stage 2)

Neurologic symptoms and signs are nonspecific, including irritability, insomnia, and irrational and inexplicable anxieties with frequent changes in mood and personality. Neurologic symptoms may precede invasion of the CNS by the organisms. In untreated *T. brucei rhodesiense* infections, CNS invasion occurs within 3-6 wk and is associated with recurrent bouts of headache, fever, weakness, and signs of acute toxemia. Tachycardia may be

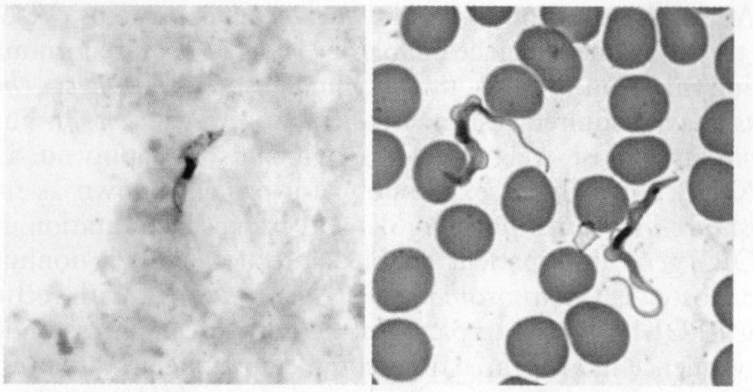

Figure 278-1 *Trypanosoma brucei* sp. trypomastigotes in thick blood smear stained with Giemsa *(left)* and thin blood smear stained with Wright-Giemsa *(right)*. (From the Centers for Disease Control and Prevention: *Laboratory identification of parasites of public health concern. Trypanosomiasis, African* [website]. www.dpd.cdc.gov/dpdx/HTML/ImageLibrary/TrypanosomiasisAfrican_il.htm. Accessed August 30, 2010.)

evidence of myocarditis. Death occurs in 6-9 mo as a result of secondary infection or cardiac failure.

In Gambian HAT, cerebral symptoms appear within 2 yr after the acute symptoms. An increase in drowsiness during the day and insomnia at night reflect the continuous progression of infection and may be accompanied by anemia, leukopenia, and muscle wasting. Patients are also at increased risk for infection.

The chronic, diffuse meningoencephalitis without localizing symptoms is the form referred to as **sleeping sickness.** Drowsiness and an uncontrollable urge to sleep are the major features of this stage of the disease and become almost continuous in the terminal stages. Tremor or rigidity with stiff and ataxic gait, suggest involvement of the basal ganglia. Psychotic changes occur in almost one third of untreated patients. Although untreated disease has been generally regarded to be uniformly fatal, this belief has been challenged recently, and there is some evidence that at least partial immunity and even spontaneous resolution may occur.

DIAGNOSIS

Definitive diagnosis can be established during the early stages by examination of a fresh, thick blood smear, which permits visualization of the motile active forms (Fig. 278-1). HAT can also be detected from blood using a variety of sensitive techniques: quantitative buffy coat smears and mini anion exchange resins are common examples. The **card agglutination trypanosomiasis test** (CATT) is of value for epidemiologic purposes and in screening for *T. brucei gambiense*. Dried, Giemsa-stained smears should be examined for the detailed morphologic features of the organisms. If a thick blood or buffy coat smear is negative, concentration techniques may help.

Aspiration of an enlarged lymph node can also be used to obtain material for parasitologic examination. If positive, cerebrospinal fluid should also be examined for the organisms. Technology based on polymerase chain reaction (PCR) for detection of trypanosomes to the species level has been validated in animal infection but is currently unsuitable for field work and is not yet cost effective for extensive use in human populations. Several PCR methods have been developed, including those that use internal transcribed spacer (ITS) regions of ribosomal RNA and can detect mixed infections.

TREATMENT

The choice of chemotherapeutic agents for treatment is dependent upon the stage of the infection and the causative organisms.

Stage 1 Treatment

Hematogenous forms of both Rhodesian and Gambian HAT can be treated with either suramin or pentamidine, which are better tolerated than drugs for stage 2 or CNS disease but are associated with substantial risks of toxicity. **Suramin** is a polysulphonated symmetrical naphthalene derivative given as a 10% solution for intravenous administration. A **test dose** (10 mg for children; 100-200 mg for adults) is initially administered to detect rare idiosyncratic reactions of shock and collapse. The dose for subsequent IV injections is 20 mg/kg (maximum 1 g) administered on days 1, 3, 7, 14, and 21. Suramin is nephrotoxic, and thus a urinalysis should be performed before each dose. Marked proteinuria, blood, or casts is a contraindication to continuation of suramin. Resistance is rare but has been reported.

Pentamidine isethionate (4 mg/kg/day IM for 7-10 days daily or on alternate days) concentrates to high levels in trypanosomes and is highly trypanocidal. It is better tolerated than suramin but carries significant risk of hypoglycemia, nephrotoxicity, hypotension, leukopenia, and liver enzyme elevation. Because of its potency, long half-life, and toxicity, short course treatment is desirable and is being investigated.

Stage 2 Treatment

If CNS invasion is present, melarsoprol is the drug of choice. **Melarsoprol** is an arsenical compound with trypanosomicidal effects. It is used outside the USA for treatment of late hemolymphatic and CNS HAT. It is the only effective treatment for late *T. brucei rhodesiense* disease and is the most widely used drug for stage 2 HAT. Treatment of children is initiated at 0.36 mg/kg once daily IV, with gradually escalating doses every 1-5 days to 3.6 mg/kg once daily IV; treatment is usually 10 doses (18-25 mg/kg total dose). Treatment of adults is with melarsoprol 2-3.6 mg/kg once daily IV for 3 days; and after 1 wk, 3.6 mg/kg once daily IV for 3 days, which is repeated after 10-21 days. An alternative regimen is 2.2 mg/kg once daily for 10 days. Guidelines recommend 18-25 mg/kg total over 1 mo. Reactions such as fever, abdominal pain, and chest pain are rare but may occur during or shortly after administration. Serious toxic effects include encephalopathy and exfoliative dermatitis.

Eflornithine is used as an alternative to melarsoprol. It is more effective against *T. brucei gambiense* and variably effective against *T. brucei rhodesiense*. It was previously in short supply, although the recent use of eflornithine as a facial hair suppressing agent breathed new life into the compound. Because of an improved supply, emerging melarsopol resistance, and some evidence of lesser toxicity, there has been a push to use the drug as a first-line treatment. It is given at a dose of 100 mg/kg/day every 6 hr IV for 14 days. Major pharmaceutical companies have generously donated large quantities of trypanosomicidal drugs, including eflornithine, pentamidine, suramin, and nifurtimox, to the global eradication effort.

With the recent influx of research funding into neglected tropical diseases, several new candidate therapeutic agents have emerged, including at least 1 oral form. Pafuramidine maleate (DB289) is an O-methyl amidoxime prodrug that is metabolized systemically to diamidine furamidine (DB75). It is only active against stage I disease; side effects have included fever and pruritus but have generally been mild in early phase II trials. It is currently undergoing evaluation in phase III clinical trials. Other drugs in the pipeline include diminazine, which has been used as a veterinary trypanocide, as well as nifurtimox, which is currently being evaluated in trials and for compassionate use in cases of melarsoprol failure. Combination therapy holds substantial promise and may become the preferred mode of treatment, since drugs act synergistically and the improved efficacy allows the doses of each drug to be reduced leading to decreased toxicity.

PREVENTION

A vaccine or consistently effective prophylactic therapy is not available. A single injection of pentamidine (3-4 mg/kg IM) provides protection against Gambian trypanosomiasis for at least 6 months, but the effect against the Rhodesian form is uncertain.

Vaccine development is particularly challenging because of the antigenic variation due to VSGs. Recent work in African lions has shown some trypanosomal cross-species acquired immunity in spite of the VSGs and may suggest novel pathways for vaccine development.

Control of trypanosomiasis in endemic areas of Africa is an ongoing challenge, and even though early successes in reducing disease burden are encouraging, the increasing cost of treatment per case as the overall number of patients decline may lead to premature termination of intensive control efforts. Moreover, underreporting of cases remains a challenge. Vector control programs to control *Glossina* have been essential in controlling disease, coupled with the use of screens, traps, and sanitary measures. Encouraging neutral-colored clothing that is not attractive to the tsetse fly may reduce bites. Using serology and parasitologic methods, mobile medical surveillance of the population at risk by specialized staff is critical. The creation of referral centers for evaluation and treatment is still needed, especially because of the toxic nature of treatment. Ground spraying of insecticides, aerial spraying, and the use of cloth and live animal baits have proven successful. Transgenic techniques to restrict the ability of the tsetse fly to survive and transmit pathogens are also being developed.

The full genome sequencing of the *T. brucei* and *Trypanosoma cruzi* parasites has revealed a conserved core proteome of about 6,200 genes in large gene clusters. This advance has helped identify genes relevant to the disease and its possible prevention, as well as the design of new antitrypanosomal drugs including those that target specific metabolic pathways.

Wigglesworthia glossinidia is an obligate endosymbiont found in the *Glossina* vector and has been shown to be intimately involved in female fly fecundity and overall survival of the fly. This endosymbiont represents a new target for vector control and a possible vehicle to introduce foreign gene products that may affect the development of the parasite.

BIBLIOGRAPHY

Please visit the Nelson Textbook of Pediatrics *website at* www.expertconsult.com *for the complete bibliography.*

Chapter 279
American Trypanosomiasis (Chagas Disease; *Trypanosoma cruzi*)

Edsel Maurice T. Salvana, Laila Woc-Colburn, and Robert A. Salata

American trypanosomiasis or Chagas disease is a vector-borne disease caused by the protozoan *Trypanosoma cruzi*. Its natural vectors are the bloodsucking insects of the family Reduviidae. It can also be transmitted vertically from mother to child and through blood transfusion and organ transplantation. While acute American trypanosomiasis usually manifests as a nonspecific febrile illness, chronic Chagas disease is associated with cardiomyopathy and severe gastrointestinal abnormalities.

ETIOLOGY

American trypanosomiasis is a caused by *Trypanosoma cruzi*, a parasitic, flagellated kinetoplastid protozoan (Fig. 279-1). The main vectors for *T. cruzi* are insects of the order Triatominae, which includes *Triatoma infestans, Rhodnius prolixus,* and *Panstrongylus megistus.*

LIFE CYCLE

T. cruzi has 3 recognizable morphogenetic phases: amastigotes, trypomastigotes, and epimastigotes (Figures 279-1 and 279-2). **Amastigotes** are intracellular forms found in mammalian tissues that are spherical and have a short flagellum but form clusters of oval shapes (pseudocysts) within infected tissues. **Trypomastigotes** are spindle-shaped, extracellular, nondividing forms that are found in blood and are responsible for both transmission of infection to the insect vector and cell-to-cell spread of infection. **Epimastigotes** are found in the midgut of the vector insect and multiply in the midgut and rectum of arthropods, differentiating into **metacyclic trypomastigotes.** Metacyclic trypomastigotes are the infectious form for humans and are released onto the skin of a human when the insect defecates close to the site of a bite, entering via the damaged skin or mucous membranes. Once in the host, these multiply intracellularly as amastigotes and are released into the circulation when the cell dies. Blood-borne trypomastigotes circulate until they enter another host cell or are taken up by the bite of another insect, completing the life cycle.

EPIDEMIOLOGY

Chagas disease is found only in the Western hemisphere, specifically the Americas, particularly in Southern Patagonia (Fig. 279-3). Natural transmission only occurs within this region, but the disease may arise elsewhere due to migration and transmission through contaminated blood. Multilateral efforts coordinated by the World Health Organization (WHO) in large-scale vector control, blood donor screening to prevent transmission through transfusion, and case-finding and treatment of chronically infected mothers and newborn infants have effectively halted transmission in a number of areas of South America. The number of cases has dropped from a peak of 24 million in 1984 to a current estimate of 8-10 million. The lack of international consensus guidelines on case definition, mass screening, and treatment recommendations for the different stages of the disease severely hamper the prospects for elimination of this disease. Moreover, the lack of clear therapeutic endpoints, logistic difficulties in drug procurement, and substantial drug toxicity presents substantial

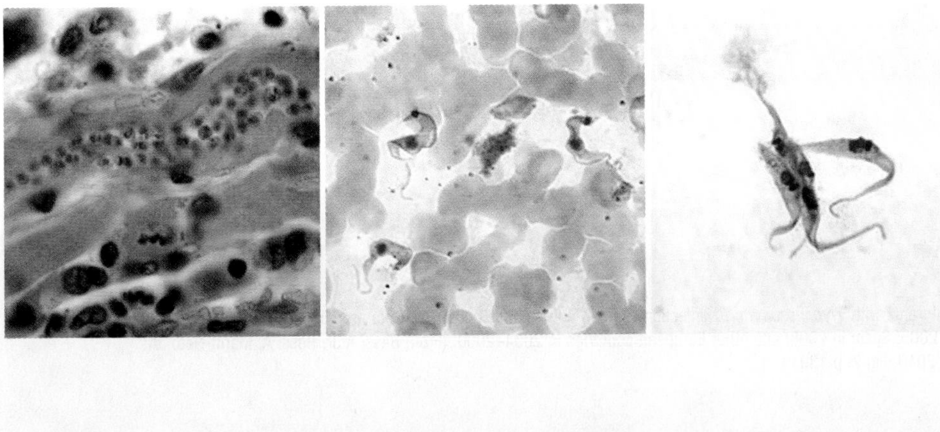

Figure 279-1 Stages of *Trypanosoma cruzi*. *From left to right:* amastigote, trypomastigote, and epimastigote. (From the Centers for Disease Control and Prevention: *Laboratory identification of parasites of public health concern. Trypanosomiasis, American* [website]. www.dpd.cdc.gov/dpdx/HTML/ImageLibrary/TrypanosomiasisAmerican_il.htm. Accessed August 30, 2010.)

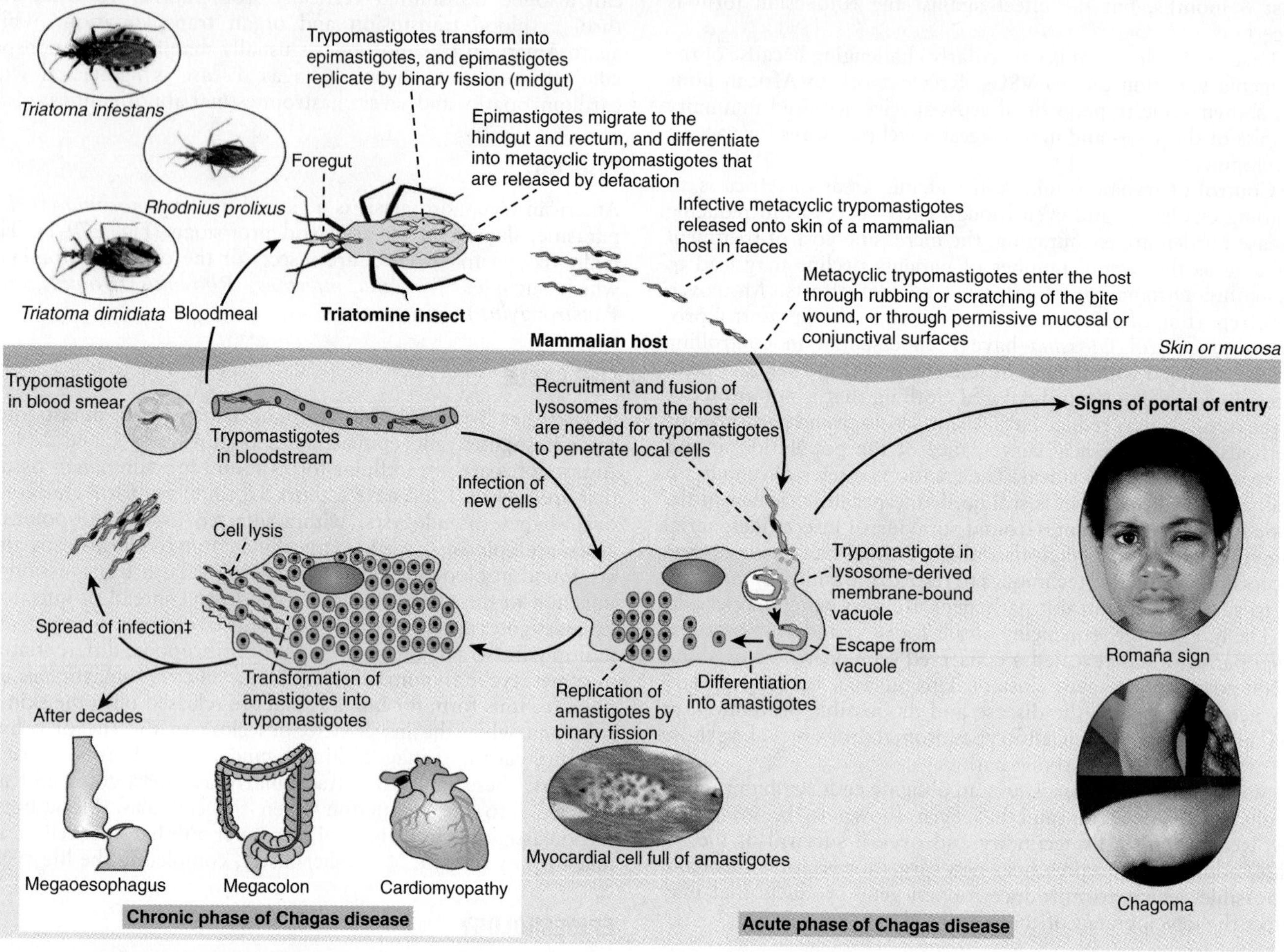

Figure 279-2 Vector-borne transmission and life cycle of *Trypanosoma cruzi*. (From Rassi A Jr, Rassi A, Marin-Neto JA: Chagas disease, *Lancet* 375:1388–1400, 2010, Fig 1, p 1389.)

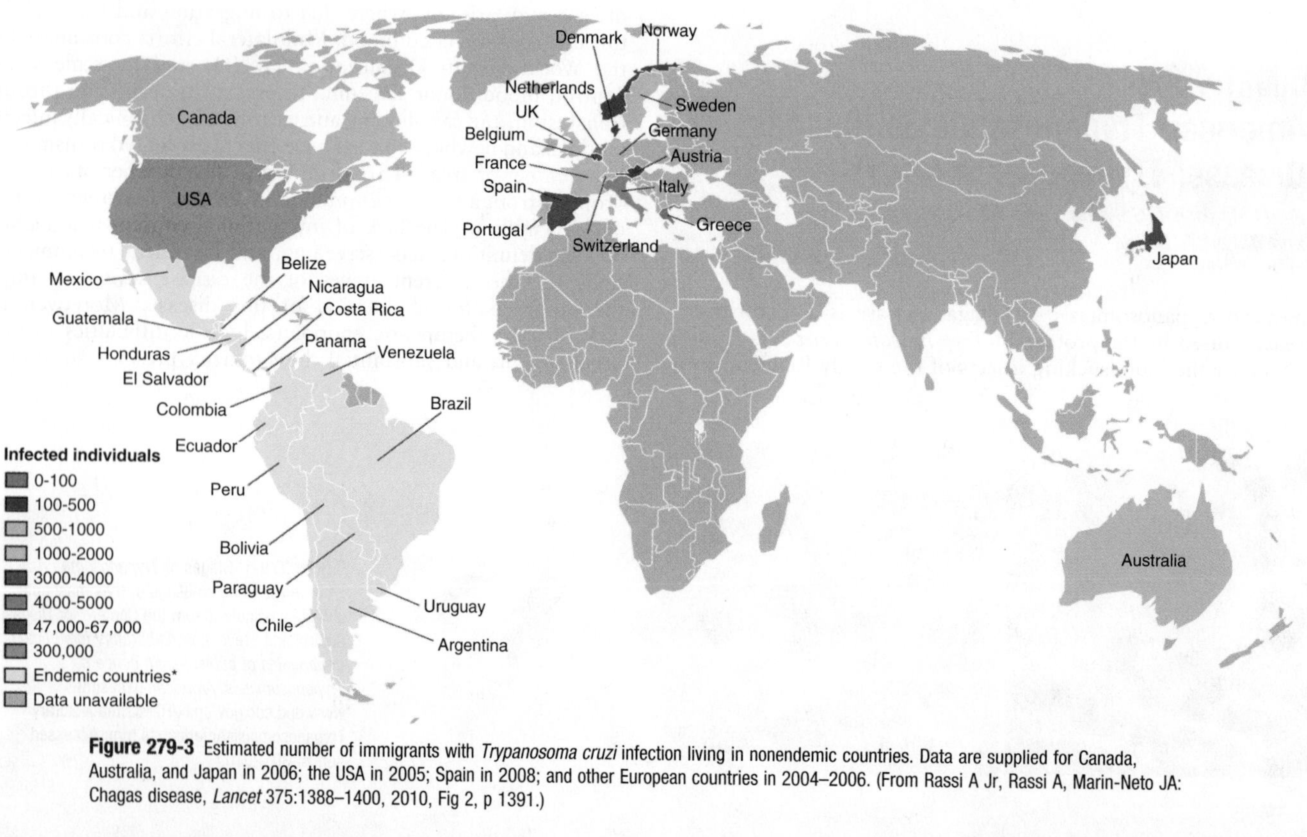

Figure 279-3 Estimated number of immigrants with *Trypanosoma cruzi* infection living in nonendemic countries. Data are supplied for Canada, Australia, and Japan in 2006; the USA in 2005; Spain in 2008; and other European countries in 2004–2006. (From Rassi A Jr, Rassi A, Marin-Neto JA: Chagas disease, *Lancet* 375:1388–1400, 2010, Fig 2, p 1391.)

Table 279-1 VECTOR-BORNE TRANSMISSION AND LIFE CYCLE OF *TRYPANOSOMA CRUZI*

	GEOGRAPHICAL DISTRIBUTION	PREDOMINANT POPULATION	INCUBATION TIME	CLINICAL PRESENTATION	DIAGNOSIS	MORTALITY
Vectorial	Endemic countries	Children and adolescents	1-2 wk	Asymptomatic; fever, malaise, lymphadenopathy, hepatosplenomegaly, subcutaneous edema; signs of portal of entry (Romaña sign, chagoma); myocarditis, meningoencephalitis	Parasite detection by microscopy; fresh blood specimen; stained blood smears; buffy coat preparation (microhematocrit technique); or serum precipitate (Strout technique)	Low (<5-10%*)
Transfusion-based	Endemic and nonendemic countries	Adults	8-120 days	Same as for vectorial but excluding signs of portal of entry	Same as for vectorial	Variable†
Congenital	Endemic and nonendemic countries	Neonates and children younger than 1 yr	Up to a few weeks	Asymptomatic; abortion, neonatal death, prematurity, low birthweight, low Apgar score; hypotonicity, fever, hepatosplenomegaly, respiratory distress, anemia; myocarditis, meningoencephalitis, megaviscera, edema	Microhematocrit with cord blood or peripheral blood from neonate; 2 or more samples in the 1st month of life; IgG serology at 6-9 mo of age is microhematocrit negative or not done	Unknown
Oral	Amazon basin and regional outbreaks	Individuals of any age from the same family or community	3-22 days	Same as for transfusion-based plus headache, myalgia, vomiting, abdominal pain, jaundice, diarrhea, and digestive hemorrhage	Same as for vectorial	High (8-35%)
Reactivation-based	Endemic and nonendemic countries	Patients with associated immunosuppressive states	Variable	Same as for transfusion-based plus panniculitis, subcutaneous parasite-containing nodules, and skin ulcers	Same as for vectorial, and parasites can also be detected in tissues by microscopy or PCR	Variable†

*Refers to symptomatic cases; since 95% of acute infections from vectorial transmission are asymptomatic and 5-10% of patients with acute symptoms die, estimated mortality in this phase of infection is between 1 in 200 and 1 in 400.
†Depends on the underlying disease and the patient's clinical condition.
From Rassi A Jr, Rassi A, Marin-Neto JA: Chagas disease, *Lancet* 375:1388–1400, 2010, Table 2, p 1393.

barriers to the formulation and adoption of universal treatment guidelines.

Infection is divided into 3 main phases: acute (Table 279-1), indeterminate, and chronic. Acute infection is the most amenable to treatment. Indeterminate infection is asymptomatic but associated with a positive antibody titer. Up to 30% of infected persons proceed to chronic *T. cruzi* infection and develop symptoms. While it was initially believed that chronic infection without treatment does not clear, at least 3 well-documented cases of spontaneous resolution without treatment have been reported. It is still unclear how this parasitic protozoan escapes the immune system because, unlike African trypanosomiasis (Chapter 278), antigenic variation is not observed.

T. cruzi infection is primarily a zoonosis, and humans are incidental hosts. *T. cruzi* has a large sylvan reservoir and has been isolated from numerous animal species. The presence of reservoirs and vectors of *T. cruzi,* and the socioeconomic and educational levels of the population are the most important risk factors for vector-borne transmission to humans. The arthropod vectors for *T. cruzi* are the **reduviid insects** or **triatomines,** variably known as **wild bedbugs, assassin bugs,** or **kissing bugs.** Insect vectors are found in rural, wooded areas and acquire infection through ingestion of blood from humans or animals with circulating trypomastigotes.

Housing conditions are very important in the transmission chain. Incidence and prevalence of infection depends on the adaptation of the triatomines to human dwellings as well as the vector capacity of the species. Animal reservoirs of reduviid bugs include dogs, cats, rats, opossum, guinea pigs, monkeys, bats, and raccoons. Humans often become infected when land in enzootic areas is developed for agricultural or commercial purposes. Although reduviid insects can be found in warmer regions of the USA as far north as Maryland, Chagas disease is extremely rare owing to the higher standard of domestic housing. Most acute cases in the USA are associated with laboratory accidents. Approximately 100,000 immigrants from endemic countries living in the USA are likely infected with *T. cruzi,* and several cases have been reported among immigrants in American cities. Chagas disease may be a significant contributor to otherwise diagnosed cases of primary dilated idiopathic cardiomyopathy.

Humans can be infected transplacentally, occurring in 10.5% of infected mothers and causing congenital Chagas disease. Transplacental infection is associated with premature birth, fetal wastage, and placentitis. Previously, up to 1,000 neonates infected with *T. cruzi* were born every year in Argentina; this number has substantially decreased since widespread control programs were initiated. Disease transmission can occur through blood transfusions in endemic areas from asymptomatic blood donors. Seropositivity rates in endemic areas are as high as 20%. The risk for transmission through a single blood transfusion from a chagasic donor is 13-23%. A blood screening test for *T. cruzi* was approved by the U.S. Food and Drug Administration in December of 2006, and the American Red Cross began routinely screening donated blood in January 2007. Since then, nearly 800 cases of Chagas disease have been detected and confirmed in the USA blood supply (*www.aabb.org/Content/Programs_and_Services/Data_Center/Chagas/*). Percutaneous injection as a result of laboratory accidents is also a documented mode of transmission. Oral transmission through contaminated food has been reported. Although breast-feeding is a very uncommon mode of transmission, women with acute infections should not nurse until they have been treated.

PATHOGENESIS

Acute Disease

At the site of entry or puncture site, neutrophils, lymphocytes, macrophages, and monocytes infiltrate. *T. cruzi* organisms are engulfed by macrophages and are sequestered in membrane-bound vacuoles. Trypanosomes lyse the phagosomal membrane, escape into the cytoplasm, and replicate. A local tissue reaction, the **chagoma,** develops, and the process extends to a local lymph node (see Fig. 279-2). Blood forms appear, and the process disseminates. Immune recognition of parasites is incompletely understood but probably involves toll-like receptor (TLR)-independent mechanisms.

Chronic Disease

The pathophysiology of chronic Chagas disease is incompletely understood, and the mechanism remains controversial. Two theories have been proposed, although other factors may come into play. The 1st mechanism involves direct tissue destruction by low level parasite persistence. The 2nd mechanism involves molecular mimicry of host antigens by the parasite, resulting in autoantibodies that produce (1) an inflammatory reaction associated with direct damage to host tissue, and/or (2) direct stimulation of adrenergic and muscarinic cholinergic receptors associated with dysautonomia and increased risk of arrhythmia.

T. cruzi strains demonstrate selective parasitism for certain tissues. Most strains are myotropic and invade smooth, skeletal, and heart muscle cells. Attachment is mediated by specific receptors on the trypomastigotes that attach to complementary glycoconjugates on the host cell surface. Attachment to cardiac muscle results in inflammation of the endocardium and myocardium, edema, focal necrosis in the contractile and conducting systems, periganglionitis, and lymphocytic inflammation. The heart becomes enlarged, and endocardial thrombosis or aneurysm may result. Right bundle branch block is also common. Trypanosome parasites also attach to neural cells and reticuloendothelial cells. In patients with gastrointestinal tract involvement, myenteric plexus destruction leads to pathologic organ dilatation. Immunologic mechanisms for control of parasitism and resistance are not fully understood. Despite strong acquired immunity, parasitologic cure in chronic infection is exceedingly rare. Antigenic variation that is typical of African trypanosomiasis (Chapter 278) is not seen with American trypanosomiasis. Antibodies involved with resistance to *T. cruzi* are related to the phase of infection. Immunoglobulin G antibodies, probably to several major surface antigens, mediate immunophagocytosis of *T. cruzi* by macrophages. Conditions that depress cell-mediated immunity increase the severity of *T. cruzi* infection. Macrophages likely play a major role in protection against *T. cruzi* infection, especially in the acute phase. Interferon-γ stimulates macrophage killing of amastigotes through oxidative mechanisms.

CLINICAL MANIFESTATIONS

Acute Chagas disease in children is usually asymptomatic or is associated with a mild febrile illness characterized by malaise, facial edema, and lymphadenopathy (Table 279-1). Infants often demonstrate local signs of inflammation at the site of parasite entry, which is then referred to as a **chagoma.** Approximately 50% of children come to medical attention with the **Romaña sign** (unilateral, painless eye swelling), conjunctivitis, and preauricular lymphadenitis. Patients complain of fatigue and headache. Fever can persist from 4-5 weeks. More severe systemic presentations can occur in children younger than 2 yr old and may include lymphadenopathy, hepatosplenomegaly, and meningoencephalitis. A cutaneous morbilliform eruption can accompany the acute syndrome. Anemia, lymphocytosis, hepatitis, and thrombocytopenia have also been described.

The heart, central nervous system, peripheral nerve ganglia, and reticuloendothelial system are often heavily parasitized. The heart is the primary target organ. The intense parasitism can result in acute inflammation and in 4-chamber cardiac dilatation. Diffuse myocarditis and inflammation of the conduction system can lead to the development of fibrosis. Histologic examination reveals the characteristic **pseudocysts,** which are the intracellular aggregates of amastigotes.

Intrauterine infection in pregnant women can cause spontaneous abortion or premature birth. In children with congenital infection, severe anemia, hepatosplenomegaly, jaundice, and convulsions can mimic congenital cytomegalovirus infection, toxoplasmosis, and erythroblastosis fetalis. *T. cruzi* can be visualized in the cerebrospinal fluid in meningoencephalitis. Children usually undergo spontaneous remission in 8-12 wk and enter an indeterminate phase with lifelong low-grade parasitemia and development of antibodies to many *T. cruzi* cell surface antigens. The mortality rate is 5-10%, with deaths caused by acute myocarditis with resultant heart failure, or meningoencephalitis. Acute Chagas disease should be differentiated from malaria, schistosomiasis, visceral leishmaniasis, brucellosis, typhoid fever, and infectious mononucleosis.

Autonomic dysfunction and peripheral neuropathy can occur. Central nervous system involvement in Chagas disease is uncommon. If granulomatous encephalitis occurs in the acute infection, it is usually fatal.

Chronic Chagas disease may be asymptomatic or symptomatic. The most common presentation of chronic *T. cruzi* infection is **cardiomyopathy,** manifested by congestive heart failure, arrhythmia, and thromboembolic events. Electrocardiographic abnormalities include partial or complete atrioventricular block and right bundle branch block. Left bundle branch block is unusual. Pathologic examination of infected heart muscle reveals muscle atrophy, myonecrosis, myocytolysis, fibrosis, and lymphocytic infiltration. Myocardial infarction has been reported and may be secondary to left apical aneurysm embolization or necrotizing arteriolitis of the microvasculature. Left ventricular apical aneurysms are pathognomonic of chronic chagasic cardiomyopathy.

T. cruzi–infected human peripheral blood mononuclear and endothelial cells synthesize increased levels of interleukin 1β (IL-1β), IL-6, and tumor necrosis factor (TNF). These cytokines result in increasing leukocyte recruitment and smooth muscle cell proliferation, which may be responsible for some of the manifestations of the disease. Viral myocarditis, rheumatic heart disease, and endomyocardial fibrosis can mimic chronic chagasic cardiomyopathy.

Gastrointestinal manifestations of chronic Chagas disease occur in 8-10% of patients and involve a diminution in the Auerbach plexus and Meissner plexus. There are also preganglionic lesions and a reduction in the number of dorsal motor nuclear cells of the vagus nerve. Characteristically, this involvement presents clinically as **megaesophagus** and **megacolon.** Sigmoid dilatation, volvulus, and fecalomas are often found in megacolon. Loss of ganglia in the esophagus results in abnormal dilatation; the esophagus can reach up to 26 times its normal weight and hold up to 2 L of excess fluid. Megaesophagus presents as dysphagia, odynophagia, and cough. Esophageal body abnormalities occur independently of lower esophageal dysfunction. Megaesophagus can lead to esophagitis and cancer of the esophagus. Aspiration pneumonia and pulmonary tuberculosis are also more common in patients with megaesophagus.

Immunocompromised Persons

T. cruzi infections in immunocompromised persons may be caused by transmission from an asymptomatic donor of blood products or reactivation of prior infection. Organ donation to allograft recipients can result in a devastating form of the illness. Cardiac transplantation for Chagas cardiomyopathy has resulted in reactivation, despite prophylaxis and postoperative treatment with benznidazole. HIV infection also leads to reactivation; cerebral lesions are more common in these patients and can mimic those of toxoplasmic encephalitis. In immunocompromised patients at risk for reactivation, serologic testing and close monitoring are necessary.

DIAGNOSIS

A careful history with attention to geographic origin and travel is important. A **peripheral blood smear** or a Giemsa-stained smear during the acute phase of illness may show motile trypanosomes, which is diagnostic for Chagas disease (see Fig. 279-1). These are only seen in the 1st 6-12 wk of illness. Buffy coat smears may improve yield.

Most persons seek medical attention during the chronic phase of the disease, when parasites are not found in the bloodstream and clinical symptoms are not diagnostic. Serologic testing is used for diagnosis, most commonly enzyme-linked immunosorbent assay (ELISA), indirect hemagglutination and indirect fluorescent antibody testing. No single serology test is sufficiently reliable to make the diagnosis, so repeat or parallel testing using a different method or antigen is required to confirm the result of an initial positive serologic test, and in the case of discordant results a 3rd test may be employed. Confirmatory tests have been proposed, including the radiologic immunoprecipitation assay (RIPA, used as a confirmatory test in blood donors in the USA) and Western blot assays based on trypomastigote excreted-secreted antigens (TESA-WB).

Nonimmunologic methods of diagnosis are also available. Mouse inoculation and xenodiagnosis (allowing uninfected reduviid bugs to feed on a patient's blood and examining the intestinal contents of those bugs 30 days after the meal) are quite sensitive. Polymerase chain reaction (PCR) of nuclear and kinetoplast DNA sequences have been developed and are highly sensitive in acute disease but are less reliable for the detection of chronic disease. Parasites may also be cultured in Novy-MacNeal-Nicolle (NNN) media.

TREATMENT

Biochemical differences between the metabolism of American trypanosomes and that of mammalian hosts have been exploited for chemotherapy. Trypanosomes are very sensitive to oxidative radicals and do not possess catalase or glutathione reductase/glutathione peroxidase, which are key enzymes in scavenging free radicals. All trypanosomes also have an unusual reduced nicotinamide adenine dinucleotide phosphate (NADPH)-dependent disulfide reductase. Drugs that stimulate H_2O_2 generation or prevent its utilization are potential trypanosomicidal agents. Other biochemical pathways that have been targeted include ergosterol synthesis using azole compounds and the hypoxanthine-guanine phosphoribosyltransferase (HGPRT) pathway using allopurinol.

Drug treatment for *T. cruzi* infection is currently limited to nifurtimox and benznidazole. Both are effective against trypomastigotes and amastigotes and have been used to eradicate parasites in the acute stages of infection. Treatment responses vary according to the phase of Chagas disease, duration of treatment, dose, age of the patient, and geographic origin of the patient. Neither drug is safe in pregnancy.

Nifurtimox has been used most extensively and is about 60% percent effective in preventing progression to chronic disease if given in the acute or early stages of infection. Efficacy in chronic disease is variable and has been disappointing for the most part. Nifurtimox generates highly toxic oxygen metabolites through the action of nitroreductases, which produce unstable nitroanion radicals, which in turn react with oxygen to produce peroxide and superoxide free radicals. The treatment regimen for children 1-10 yr of age is 15-20 mg/kg/day divided 4 times a day PO for 90 days; for children 11-16 yr of age, 12.5-15 mg/kg/day divided 4 times a day PO for 90 days; and for children >16 yr of age, 8-10 mg/kg/day divided 3 times a day to 4 times a day PO for 90-120 days. Nifurtimox has been associated with weakness, anorexia, gastrointestinal disturbances, toxic hepatitis, tremors, seizures, and hemolysis in patients with glucose-6-phosphate dehydrogenase deficiency.

Benznidazole is a nitroimidazole derivative that may be slightly more effective than nifurtimox. While benznidazole is capable of inducing the production of free oxide radicals, the dose at which it is given is not effective for this mode of action. Instead, its nitroreduction intermediates may form covalent bonds or interact in other ways with parasitic DNA, lipids, and proteins and cause damage to parasite components. The recommended treatment regimen for children <12 yr of age is 10 mg/kg/day divided twice daily PO for 60 days, and for those >12 yr of age, it is 5-7 mg/kg/day divided twice daily PO for 60 days. This drug is associated with significant toxicity, including rash, photosensitivity, peripheral neuritis, granulocytopenia, and thrombocytopenia. While treatment is generally recommended for acute Chagas disease and is likely effective in the early stages of infection as well, the treatment of asymptomatic (or indeterminate) and symptomatic chronic disease is controversial. Multiple trials with long-term follow-up have yielded mixed results, with an estimated response rate of 10-20% for chronic disease. The definition of response in itself is problematic, and parasitologic cure is nearly impossible to demonstrate given the limitations of the sensitivity and specificity of detection methods. Instead, serologic conversion is seen as an appropriate treatment response, although some patients who achieve this still eventually develop symptoms. Recommendations from authorities have been mixed, with some advocating for treatment regardless of disease phase, and others recommending against treatment due to uncertain benefit and the toxicity of the drugs involved. Proponents of the latter approach instead advocate symptomatic treatment of disease manifestations. Treatment of congestive heart failure is generally in line with recommendations for management of dilated cardiomyopathy due to other causes. Beta-blockers have been validated in the management of these patients. Digitalis toxicity occurs frequently in patients with Chagas cardiomyopathy. Pacemakers may be necessary in cases of severe heart block. Although cardiac transplantation has been used successfully in chagasic patients, it is reserved for those with the most severe disease manifestations. Plasmapheresis to remove antibodies with adrenergic activity has been proposed for refractory patients as this approach has been tried and has worked in patients with dilated cardiomyopathy from other causes. However, its application to Chagas disease is unproven.

A light, balanced diet is recommended for megaesophagus. Surgery or dilation of the lower esophageal sphincter treats megaesophagus; pneumatic dilation is the superior mode of therapy. Nitrates and nifedipine have been used to reduce lower esophageal sphincter pressure in patients with megaesophagus. Treatment of megacolon is surgical and symptomatic. Treatment of meningoencephalitis is also supportive.

In accidental infection when parasitic penetration is certain, treatment should be immediately initiated and continued for 10-15 days. Blood is usually collected and serologic samples tested for seroconversion at 15, 30, and 60 days.

PREVENTION

Massive coordinated vector control programs under the auspices of the WHO and the institution of widespread blood donor screening and targeted surveillance of chronically infected mothers and infants at risk have effectively eliminated or at least drastically reduced transmission in most endemic countries. As Chagas disease remains linked to poverty, improvement of living conditions is likewise essential to successful control and eradication. Education of residents in endemic areas, use of bed nets, use of insecticides, and destruction of adobe houses that harbor reduviid bugs are effective methods to control the bug population. Synthetic pyrethroid insecticides help keep houses free of vectors for up to 2 years and have low toxicity for humans. Paints incorporating insecticides have also been used. Vaccine development thus far has been unsuccessful, as the parasite uses incompletely understood means to evade immune surveillance.

Blood transfusions in endemic areas are a significant risk. Gentian violet, an amphophilic cationic agent that acts photodynamically, has been used to kill the parasite in blood. Photoirradiation of blood containing gentian violet and ascorbate generates free radicals and superoxide anions that are trypanosomicidal. Mepacrine and maprotiline have also been used to eradicate the parasite in blood transfusions.

Because immigrants can carry this disease to nonendemic areas, serologic testing should be performed in blood and organ donors from endemic areas. Potential seropositive donors can be identified by determining whether they have been or have spent extensive time in an endemic area. Questionnaire-based screening of potentially infected blood and organ donors from areas endemic for infection can reduce the risk for transmission. Seropositivity should be considered a contraindication to organ donation.

BIBLIOGRAPHY

Please visit the Nelson Textbook of Pediatrics *website at* *www.expertconsult.com* *for the complete bibliography.*

Chapter 280
Malaria *(Plasmodium)*

Chandy C. John and Peter J. Krause

Malaria is an acute and chronic illness characterized by paroxysms of fever, chills, sweats, fatigue, anemia, and splenomegaly. It has played a major role in human history, causing harm to more people than perhaps any other infectious disease. Malaria is of overwhelming importance in the developing world today, with an estimated 300 to 500 million cases and more than 1 million deaths each year. Most malarial deaths occur among infants and young children. Although malaria is not endemic in the USA, approximately 1,000 imported cases are recognized in the USA each year. Physicians practicing in nonendemic areas should consider the diagnosis of malaria in any febrile child who has returned from a malaria-endemic area within the previous year, because delay in diagnosis and treatment can result in severe illness or death.

ETIOLOGY

Malaria is caused by intracellular *Plasmodium* protozoa transmitted to humans by female *Anopheles* mosquitoes. Prior to 2004, only 4 species of *Plasmodium* were known to cause malaria in humans: *P. falciparum, P. malariae, P. ovale*, and *P. vivax*. In 2004 *P. knowlesi* (a primate malaria species) was also shown to cause human malaria, and cases of *P. knowlesi* infection have been documented in Malaysia, Indonesia, Singapore, and the Philippines. Malaria also can be transmitted through blood transfusion, use of contaminated needles, and from a pregnant woman to her fetus. The risk for blood transmission is small and decreasing in the USA but may occur by way of whole blood, packed red blood cells, platelets, leukocytes, and organ transplantation.

EPIDEMIOLOGY

Malaria is a major worldwide problem, occurring in more than 100 countries with a combined population of over 1.6 billion people (Fig. 280-1). The principal areas of transmission are Africa, Asia, and South America. *P. falciparum* and *P. malariae* are found in most malarious areas. *P. falciparum* is the predominant species in Africa, Haiti, and New Guinea. *P. vivax* predominates in Bangladesh, Central America, India, Pakistan, and Sri Lanka. *P. vivax* and *P. falciparum* predominate in Southeast Asia, South America, and Oceania. *P. ovale* is the least common species and is transmitted primarily in Africa. Transmission of malaria has been eliminated in most of North America (including the USA), Europe, and the Caribbean, as well as Australia, Chile, Israel, Japan, Korea, Lebanon, and Taiwan.

Most cases of malaria in the USA occur among previously infected visitors to the USA from endemic areas and among U.S. citizens who travel to endemic areas without appropriate chemoprophylaxis. The most common regions of acquisition of the 10,100 cases of malaria reported to the Centers for Disease Control and Prevention (CDC) among U.S. citizens between 1985 and 2001 were sub-Saharan Africa (58%), Asia (18%), and the Caribbean and Central or South America (16%). Most of the fatal cases were caused by *P. falciparum* (94% or 66 of the 70 cases), of which 47 (71%) were acquired in sub-Saharan Africa.

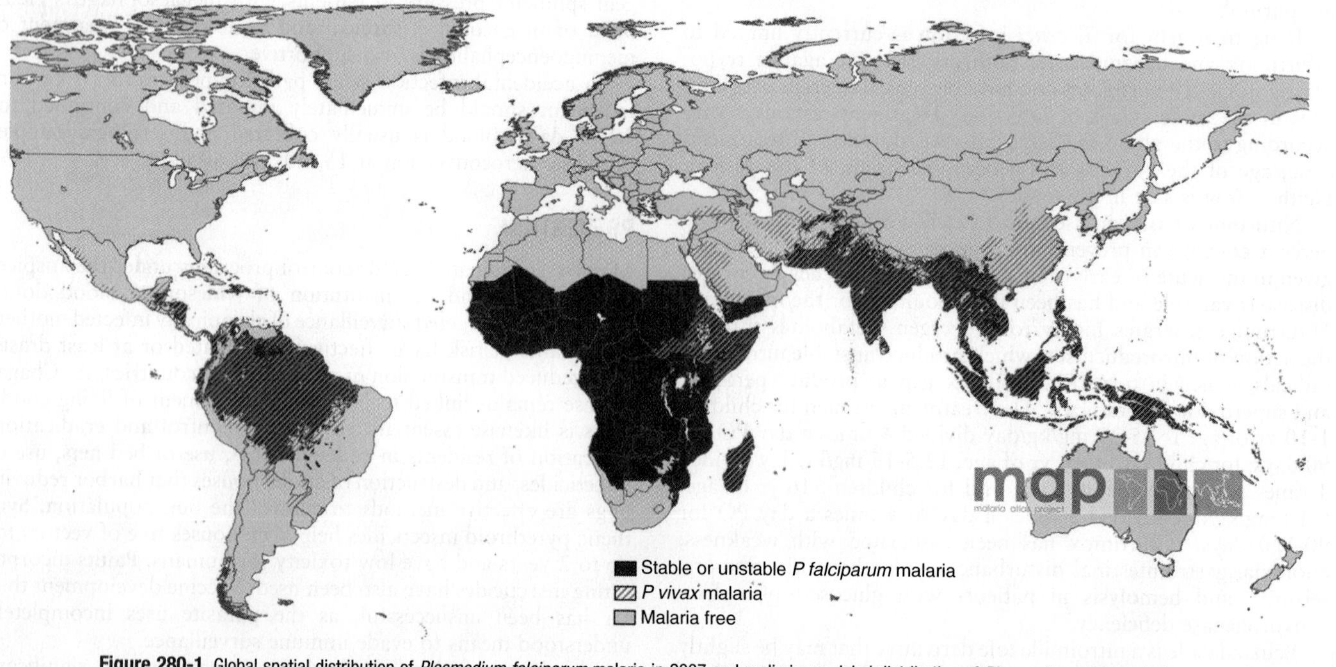

Figure 280-1 Global spatial distribution of *Plasmodium falciparum* malaria in 2007 and preliminary global distribution of *Plasmodium vivax* malaria. (From Crawley J, Chu C, Mtove G, et al: Malaria in children, *Lancet* 375:1468–1478, 2010, Fig 1, p 1469.)

Rare cases of apparent locally transmitted malaria have been reported since the 1950s. These cases are likely due to transmission from untreated and often asymptomatic infected individuals from malaria endemic countries who travel to the USA and infect local mosquitoes or to infected mosquitoes from malaria endemic areas that are transported to the USA on airplanes.

PATHOGENESIS

Plasmodium species exist in a variety of forms and have a complex life cycle that enables them to survive in different cellular environments in the human host (asexual phase) and the mosquito (sexual phase) (Fig. 280-2). A marked amplification of *Plasmodium*, from approximately 10^2 to as many as 10^{14} organisms, occurs during a 2-step process in humans, with the 1st phase in hepatic cells (exoerythrocytic phase) and the 2nd phase in the red cells (erythrocytic phase). The **exoerythrocytic phase** begins with inoculation of sporozoites into the bloodstream by a female *Anopheles* mosquito. Within minutes, the sporozoites enter the hepatocytes of the liver, where they develop and multiply asexually as a schizont. After 1-2 wk, the hepatocytes rupture and release thousands of merozoites into the circulation. The tissue schizonts of *P. falciparum, P. malariae,* and apparently *P. knowlesi* rupture once and do not persist in the liver. There are 2 types of tissue schizonts for *P. ovale* and *P. vivax*. The primary type ruptures in 6-9 days, and the secondary type remains dormant in the liver cell for weeks, months, or as long as 5 yr before releasing merozoites and causing relapse of infection. The **erythrocytic phase** of *Plasmodium* asexual development begins when the merozoites from the liver penetrate erythrocytes. Once inside the erythrocyte, the parasite transforms into the **ring form,** which then enlarges to become a **trophozoite.** These latter 2 forms can be identified with Giemsa stain on blood smear, the primary means of confirming the diagnosis of malaria (Fig. 280-3). The trophozoite multiplies asexually to produce a number of small erythrocytic **merozoites** that are released into the bloodstream when the erythrocyte membrane ruptures, which is associated with fever. Over time, some of the merozoites develop into male and female gametocytes that complete the *Plasmodium* life cycle when they are ingested during a blood meal by the female anopheline mosquito. The male and female gametocytes fuse to form a **zygote** in the stomach cavity of the mosquito. After a series of further transformations, sporozoites enter the salivary gland of the mosquito and are inoculated into a new host with the next blood meal.

Four important pathologic processes have been identified in patients with malaria: fever, anemia, immunopathologic events, and tissue anoxia. Fever occurs when erythrocytes rupture and

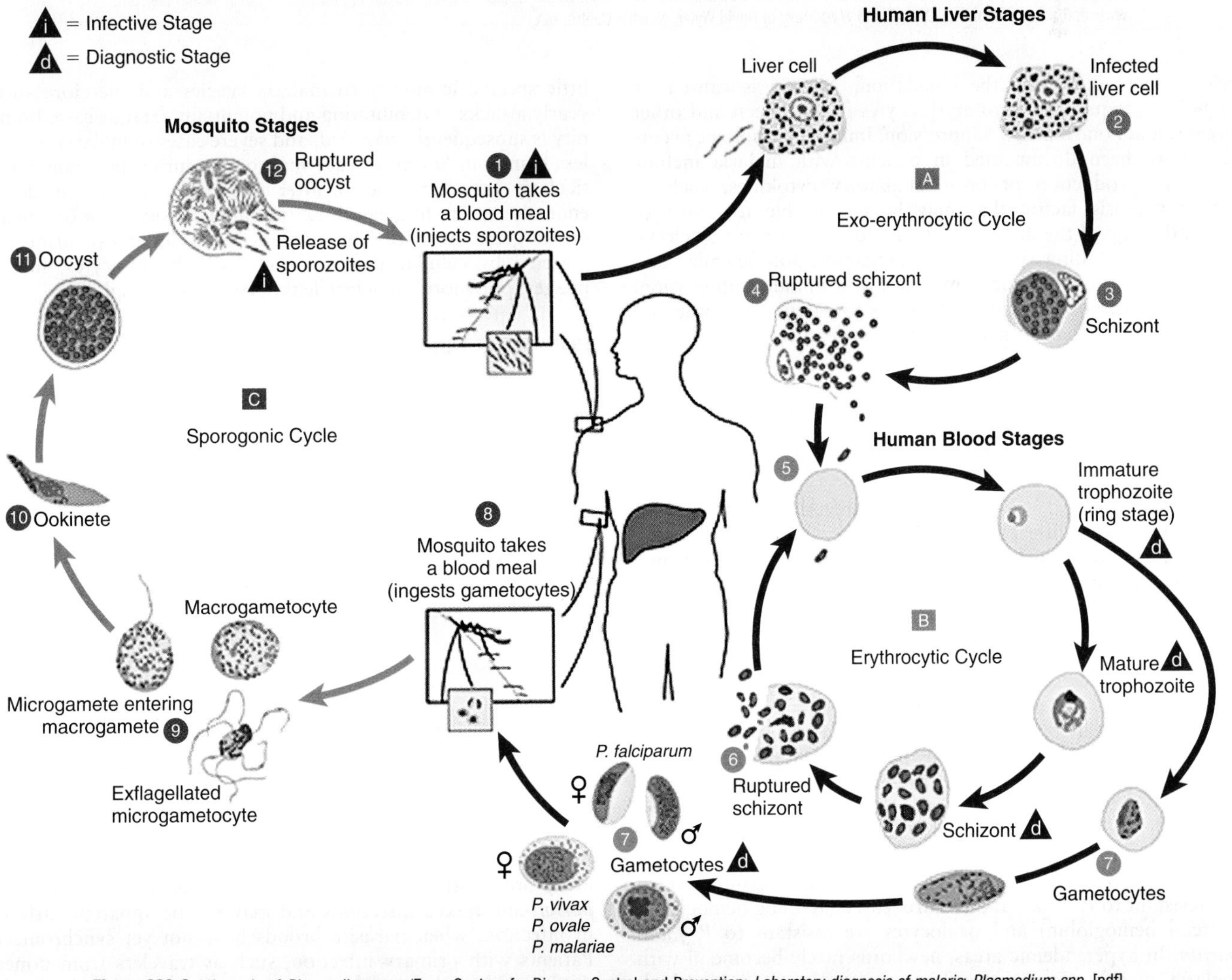

Figure 280-2 Life cycle of *Plasmodium* spp. (From Centers for Disease Control and Prevention: *Laboratory diagnosis of malaria: Plasmodium spp.* [pdf]. www.dpd.cdc.gov/dpdx/HTML/PDF_Files/Parasitemia_and_LifeCycle.pdf. Accessed September 20, 2010.)

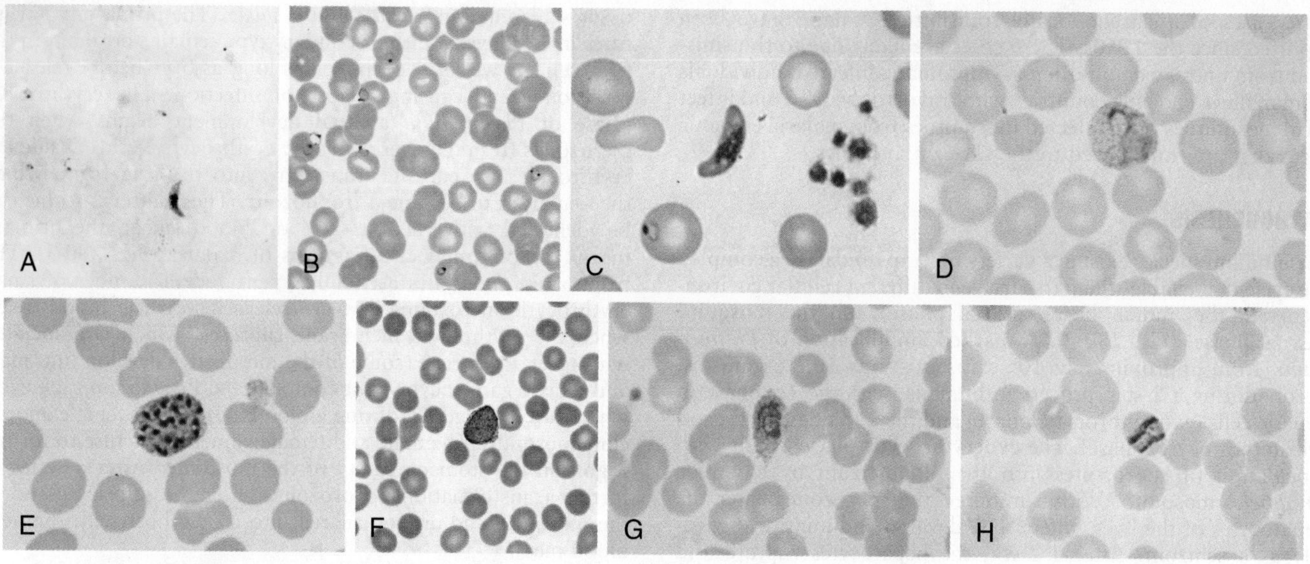

Figure 280-3 Giemsa-stained thick *(A)* and thin *(B-H)* smears used for the diagnosis of malaria and the speciation of *Plasmodium* parasites. *A,* Multiple signet-ring *Plasmodium falciparum* trophozoites, which are visualized outside erythrocytes. *B,* A multiply infected erythrocyte containing signet-ring *P. falciparum* trophozoites, including an accolade form positioned up against the inner surface of the erythrocyte membrane. *C,* Banana-shaped gametocyte unique to *P. falciparum. D,* Ameboid trophozoite characteristic of *Plasmodium vivax.* Both *P. vivax–* and *Plasmodium ovale*–infected erythrocytes exhibit Schuffner dots and tend to be enlarged compared with uninfected erythrocytes. *E, P. vivax* schizont. Mature *P. falciparum* parasites, by contrast, are rarely seen on blood smears because they sequester in the systemic microvasculature. *F, P. vivax* spherical gametocyte. *G, P. ovale* trophozoite. Note Schuffner dots and ovoid shapes of the infected erythrocyte. *H,* Characteristic band form trophozoite of *Plasmodium malariae,* containing intracellular pigment hemozoin. (*A, B,* and *F* from Centers for Disease Control and Prevention: *DPDx: laboratory identification of parasites of public health concern.* www.dpd.cdc.gov/dpdx/. *C, D, E, G,* and *H* courtesy of David Wyler, Newton Centre, MA.)

release merozoites into the circulation. Anemia is caused by hemolysis, sequestration of erythrocytes in the spleen and other organs, and bone marrow suppression. Immunopathologic events that have been documented in patients with malaria include excessive production of proinflammatory cytokines, such as tumor necrosis factor, that may be responsible for most of the pathology of the disease, including tissue anoxia; polyclonal activation resulting in both hypergammaglobulinemia and the formation of immune complexes; and immunosuppression. Cytoadherence of infected erythrocytes to vascular endothelium occurs in *P. falciparum* malaria and may lead to obstruction of blood flow and capillary damage, with resultant vascular leakage of blood, protein, and fluid and tissue anoxia. In addition, hypoglycemia and lactic acidemia are caused by anaerobic metabolism of glucose. The cumulative effects of these pathologic processes may lead to cerebral, cardiac, pulmonary, intestinal, renal, and hepatic failure.

Immunity after *Plasmodium* species infection is incomplete, preventing severe disease but still allowing future infection. In some cases, parasites circulate in small numbers for a long time but are prevented from rapidly multiplying and causing severe illness. Repeated episodes of infection occur because the parasite has developed a number of immune evasive strategies, such as intracellular replication, vascular cytoadherence that prevents infected erythrocytes from circulating through the spleen, rapid antigenic variation, and alteration of the host immune system resulting in partial immune suppression. The human host response to *Plasmodium* infection includes natural immune mechanisms that prevent infection by other *Plasmodium* species, such as those of birds or rodents, as well as several alterations in erythrocyte physiology that prevent or modify malarial infection. Erythrocytes containing hemoglobin S (sickle erythrocytes) resist malaria parasite growth, erythrocytes lacking Duffy blood group antigen are resistant to *P. vivax*, and erythrocytes containing hemoglobin F (fetal hemoglobin) and ovalocytes are resistant to *P. falciparum.* In hyperendemic areas, newborns rarely become ill with malaria, in part because of passive maternal antibody and high levels of fetal hemoglobin. Children 3 mo to 2-5 yr of age have little specific immunity to malaria species and therefore suffer yearly attacks of debilitating and potentially fatal disease. Immunity is subsequently acquired, and severe cases of malaria become less common. Severe disease may occur during pregnancy, particularly 1st pregnancies or after extended residence outside the endemic region. In general, extracellular *Plasmodium* organisms are targeted by antibody, whereas intracellular organisms are targeted by cellular defenses such as T lymphocytes, macrophages, polymorphonuclear leukocytes, and the spleen.

CLINICAL MANIFESTATIONS

Children and adults are asymptomatic during the initial phase of infection, the incubation period of malaria infection. The usual incubation periods are 9-14 days for *P. falciparum*, 12-17 days for *P. vivax*, 16-18 days for *P. ovale,* and 18-40 days for *P. malariae*. The incubation period can be as long as 6-12 mo for *P. vivax* and can also be prolonged for patients with partial immunity or incomplete chemoprophylaxis. A prodrome lasting 2-3 days is noted in some patients before parasites are detected in the blood. Prodromal symptoms include headache, fatigue, anorexia, myalgia, slight fever, and pain in the chest, abdomen, and joints.

The classic presentation of malaria is seldom noted with other infectious diseases and consists of **paroxysms** of fever alternating with periods of fatigue but otherwise relative wellness. Febrile paroxysms are characterized by high fever, sweats, and headache, as well as myalgia, back pain, abdominal pain, nausea, vomiting, diarrhea, pallor, and jaundice. Paroxysms coincide with the rupture of schizonts that occurs every 48 hr with *P. vivax* and *P. ovale,* resulting in fever spikes every other day. Rupture of schizonts occurs every 72 hr with *P. malariae*, resulting in fever spikes every 3rd or 4th day. Periodicity is less apparent with *P. falciparum* and mixed infections and may not be apparent early on in infection, when parasite broods have not yet synchronized. Patients with primary infection, such as travelers from nonendemic regions, also may have irregular symptomatic episodes for 2-3 days before regular paroxysms begin. Children with malaria

Table 280-1 WORLD HEALTH ORGANIZATION CRITERIA FOR SEVERE MALARIA, 2000

Impaired consciousness
Prostration
Respiratory distress
Multiple seizures
Jaundice
Hemoglobinuria
Abnormal bleeding
Severe anemia
Circulatory collapse
Pulmonary edema

often lack typical paroxysms and have nonspecific symptoms, including fever (may be low-grade but is often greater than 104°F), headache, drowsiness, anorexia, nausea, vomiting, and diarrhea. Distinctive physical signs may include splenomegaly (common), hepatomegaly, and pallor due to anemia. Typical laboratory findings include anemia, thrombocytopenia, and a normal or low leukocyte count. The erythrocyte sedimentation rate (ESR) is often elevated.

P. falciparum is the most severe form of malaria and is associated with higher density parasitemia and a number of complications. The most common serious complication is severe anemia, which also is associated with other malaria species. Serious complications that appear unique to *P. falciparum* include cerebral malaria, acute renal failure, respiratory distress from metabolic acidosis, algid malaria and bleeding diatheses (see later section on complications, and Table 280-1). The diagnosis of *P. falciparum* malaria in a nonimmune individual constitutes a medical emergency. Severe complications and death can occur if appropriate therapy is not instituted promptly. In contrast to malaria caused by *P. ovale, P. vivax,* and *P. malariae,* which usually results in parasitemias of less than 2%, malaria caused by *P. falciparum* can be associated with parasitemia levels as high as 60%. The differences in parasitemia reflect the fact that *P. falciparum* infects both immature and mature erythrocytes, while *P. ovale* and *P. vivax* primarily infect immature erythrocytes and *P. malariae* infects only mature erythrocytes. Like *P. falciparum, P. knowlesi* has a 24 hr replication cycle and can also lead to very high density parasitemia.

P. vivax malaria has long been considered less severe than *P. falciparum* malaria, but recent reports suggest that in some areas of Indonesia it is as frequent a cause of severe disease and death as P. *falciparum*. Severe disease and death from *P. vivax* are usually due to severe anemia and sometimes to splenic rupture. *P. ovale* malaria is the least common type of malaria. It is similar to *P. vivax* malaria and commonly is found in conjunction with *P. falciparum* malaria. *P. malariae* is the mildest and most chronic of all malaria infections. Nephrotic syndrome is a rare complication of *P. malariae* infection that is not observed with any other human malaria species. Nephrotic syndrome associated with *P. malariae* infection is poorly responsive to steroids. Low-level, undetected *P. malariae* infection may be present for years and is sometimes unmasked by immunosuppression or physiological stress such as splenectomy or corticosteroid treatment.

Recrudescence after a primary attack may occur from the survival of erythrocyte forms in the bloodstream. Long-term relapse is caused by release of merozoites from an exoerythrocytic source in the liver, which occurs with *P. vivax* and *P. ovale*, or from persistence within the erythrocyte, which occurs with *P. malariae* and rarely with *P. falciparum*. A history of typical symptoms in a person more than 4 wk after return from an endemic area is therefore more likely to be *P. vivax, P. ovale,* or *P. malariae* infection than *P. falciparum* infection. In the most recent survey of malaria in the USA among individuals in whom a malaria species was identified, 48.6% of cases were due to *P. falciparum*, 22. 1% to *P. vivax*, 3.5% to *P. malariae*, and 2.5% to *P. ovale*. Ninety-four percent of *P. falciparum* infections were diagnosed within 30 days of arrival in the USA, and 99% within 90 days of arrival. In contrast, 50.7% of *P. vivax* cases occurred more than 30 days after arrival in the USA.

Congenital malaria is acquired from the mother prenatally or perinatally and is a serious problem in tropical areas but is rarely reported in the USA. In endemic areas, congenital malaria is an important cause of abortions, miscarriages, stillbirths, premature births, intrauterine growth retardation, and neonatal deaths. Congenital malaria usually occurs in the offspring of a nonimmune mother with *P. vivax* or *P. malariae* infection, although it can be observed with any of the human malaria species. The 1st sign or symptom most commonly occurs between 10 and 30 days of age (range 14 hr to several months of age). Signs and symptoms include fever, restlessness, drowsiness, pallor, jaundice, poor feeding, vomiting, diarrhea, cyanosis, and hepatosplenomegaly. Malaria is often severe during pregnancy and may have an adverse effect on the fetus or neonate, resulting in intrauterine growth retardation and low birthweight, even in the absence of transmission from mother to child.

DIAGNOSIS

Any child who presents with fever or unexplained systemic illness and has traveled or resided in a malaria-endemic area within the previous year should be assumed to have life-threatening malaria until proven otherwise. Malaria should be considered regardless of the use of chemoprophylaxis. Important criteria that suggest *P. falciparum* malaria include symptoms occurring less than 1 mo after return from an endemic area, more than 2% parasitemia, ring forms with double chromatin dots, and erythrocytes infected with more than 1 parasite.

The diagnosis of malaria is established by identification of organisms on Giemsa-stained smears of peripheral blood (see Fig. 280-3) or by rapid immunochromatographic assay. Giemsa stain is superior to Wright stain or Leishman stain. Both thick and thin blood smears should be examined. The concentration of erythrocytes on a **thick smear** is 20-40 times that on a thin smear and is used to quickly scan large numbers of erythrocytes. The **thin smear** allows for positive identification of the malaria species and determination of the percentage of infected erythrocytes and is useful in following the response to therapy. Identification of the species is best made by an experienced microscopist and checked against color plates of the various *Plasmodium* species (see Fig. 280-3). Morphologically it is impossible to distinguish *P. knowlesi* from *P. malariae*, so polymerase chain reaction (PCR) detection by a reference lab or the CDC is required. Although *P. falciparum* is most likely to be identified from blood just after a febrile paroxysm, the timing of the smears is less important than their being obtained several times a day over a period of 3 successive days. A single negative blood smear does not exclude malaria. Most symptomatic patients with malaria will have detectable parasites on thick blood smears within 48 hr. For nonimmune persons, symptoms typically occur 1 to 2 days before parasites are detectable on blood smear.

The BinaxNOW Malaria test is approved by the U.S. Food and Drug Administration (FDA) for rapid diagnosis of malaria. This immunochromatographic test for *P. falciparum* histidine rich protein (HRP2) and aldolase is approved for testing for *P. falciparum* and *P. vivax*. Aldolase is present in all 5 of the malaria species that infect humans. Thus, a positive result for *P. vivax* could be due to *P. ovale* or *P. malariae* infection. Sensitivity and specificity for *P. falciparum* (94-99% and 94-99%, respectively) and *P. vivax* (87-93% and 99%, respectively) are good, but sensitivity for *P. ovale* and *P. malariae* are lower. Sensitivity for *P. falciparum* decreases at lower levels of parasitemia, so microscopy is still advised in areas where expert microscopy is available. The test is simple to perform and can be done in the field or laboratory in 10 min. PCR is even more sensitive than microscopy but is technically more complex. It is available in some reference laboratories, but the time delay in availability of results generally precludes its use for acute diagnosis of malaria.

DIFFERENTIAL DIAGNOSIS

The differential diagnosis of malaria is broad and includes viral infections such as influenza and hepatitis, sepsis, pneumonia, meningitis, encephalitis, endocarditis, gastroenteritis, pyelonephritis, babesiosis, brucellosis, leptospirosis, tuberculosis, relapsing fever, typhoid fever, yellow fever, amebic liver abscess, Hodgkin disease, and collagen vascular disease.

TREATMENT

Physicians caring for patients with malaria or traveling to endemic areas need to be aware of current information regarding malaria because the problem of resistance to antimalarial drugs is changing and has greatly complicated therapy and prophylaxis. The best source for such information is the CDC Malaria Hotline, which is available to physicians 24 hr a day (770-488-7788 from 8:00 A.M. to 4:30 P.M. Eastern Standard Time (EST) and 770-488-7100 from 4:30 P.M. to 8:00 A.M. EST on weekends and holidays; ask the operator to page the person on call for the Malaria Epidemiology Branch). **Fever without an obvious cause in any patient who has left a *P. falciparum* endemic area within 30 days and is nonimmune should be considered a medical emergency.** Thick and thin blood smears should be obtained immediately, and all children with symptoms of severe disease should be hospitalized. If blood films are negative, they should be repeated every few hours. If the patient is severely ill, antimalarial therapy should be initiated immediately. Outpatient therapy generally is not given to nonimmune children but may be considered in immune or semi-immune children who have low-level parasitemia (less than 1%), no evidence of complications defined by the World Health Organization (WHO), no vomiting, and a lack of toxic appearance; who are able to contact the physician or emergency department at any time; and in whom follow-up within 24 hr is assured.

P. falciparum Malaria

Malarious regions considered chloroquine-sensitive include Central America west of the Panama Canal, Haiti, the Dominican Republic, and most of the Middle East except Iran, Oman, Saudi Arabia, and Yemen. Individuals traveling from areas with chloroquine-susceptible *P. falciparum* can be treated with chloroquine if they do not have severe malaria. Malaria acquired in *P. falciparum* areas with chloroquine resistance or where there is any doubt about chloroquine sensitivity after conferring with the CDC should be treated with drugs other than chloroquine (Table 280-2). Intravenous quinidine gluconate (or quinine if outside the USA) should be administered for cases of complicated malaria (see Table 280-2) or patients unable to retain oral medications because of vomiting. These patients should be admitted to the intensive care unit for monitoring of complications, plasma quinidine levels, and adverse effects during quinidine administration. During administration of quinidine, blood pressure monitoring for hypotension and cardiac monitoring for widening of the QRS complex or lengthening of the QTc interval should be performed continuously, and blood glucose monitoring for hypoglycemia should be performed periodically. Cardiac adverse events may require temporary discontinuation of the drug or slowing of the intravenous infusion. Parenteral therapy should be continued until the parasitemia is less than 1%, which usually occurs within 48 hr, and the patient can tolerate oral medication. Quinidine gluconate (USA) or quinine sulfate (other countries) is administered for a total of 3 days for malaria acquired in Africa or South America and for 7 days for malaria acquired in Southeast Asia. Doxycycline, tetracycline, or clindamycin is then given orally to complete the therapeutic course (see Table 280-2). Although there are no data to support the use of sequential quinine and atovaquone-proguanil, the difficulty of maintaining compliance with oral quinine has led many clinicians to complete oral therapy after IV quinine with a complete course of atovaquone-proguanil.

Parenterally administered artesunate or artemether can be substituted for quinine for treatment of severe malaria in children and adults (see Table 280-2). Artesunate is now available on special request from the CDC (770-488-7788) for treatment of severe malaria, but empirical therapy should not be delayed while awaiting delivery of artesunate. Oral and rectal administration of these artemisinin-based antimalarial drugs is effective in treatment of malaria, but such formulations are not indicated or approved in the USA.

Patients from areas with chloroquine-resistant *P. falciparum* who have mild to moderate infection, parasitemia less than 1%, no evidence of complications, and no vomiting and who can take oral medication should be given either oral atovaquone-proguanil (Malarone), oral artemether-lumefantrine (Coartem), or oral quinine plus doxycycline, tetracycline, or clindamycin (see Table 280-2). Coartem is approved by the FDA for the treatment of uncomplicated malaria and is an appealing choice because it is highly effective and well-tolerated. Pediatric dosing is well established, but pediatric dispersible tablets, available in some other countries, are not yet available in the USA. Coartem should not be used in children with known QT interval prolongation. Patients who acquire *P. falciparum* in Thailand, Myanmar, or Cambodia should receive 7 days of quinine therapy if they are prescribed quinine. Mefloquine is contraindicated for use in patients with a known hypersensitivity to mefloquine or with a history of epilepsy or severe psychiatric disorders. Mefloquine is not recommended for persons with cardiac conduction abnormalities but may be administered to persons concurrently receiving β-blockers if they have no underlying arrhythmia. Quinidine or quinine may exacerbate the adverse effects of mefloquine and should generally not be given to patients who have received mefloquine unless there are no other alternatives.

Patients with uncomplicated *P. falciparum* malaria acquired in areas without chloroquine resistance should be treated with oral chloroquine phosphate. If the parasite count does not drop rapidly (within 24-48 hr) and become negative after 4 days, chloroquine resistance should be assumed and the patient started on a different antimalarial regimen.

Supportive therapy is very important and includes red blood cell transfusion(s) to maintain the hematocrit at more than 20%, exchange transfusion in *P. falciparum* malaria with parasitemia greater than 10% and evidence of severe complications (e.g., severe malarial anemia, cerebral malaria), supplemental oxygen and ventilatory support for pulmonary edema or cerebral malaria, careful intravenous rehydration for severe malaria, intravenous glucose for hypoglycemia, anticonvulsants for cerebral malaria with seizures, and dialysis for renal failure. Exchange transfusion is thought be useful in severe malaria with high-level parasitemia, but no randomized clinical trial has ever been conducted to assess its utility. Corticosteroids are not recommended for cerebral malaria.

P. vivax, *P. ovale*, *P. malariae*, or *P. knowlesi* Malaria

Uncomplicated infection due to *P. vivax*, *P. ovale*, or *P. malariae* can usually be treated with chloroquine (see Table 280-2). Chloroquine remains the initial drug of choice for *P. vivax* malaria in the absence of good data on drug alternatives. Indications for using alternative therapy are worsening or new symptoms, persistent *P. vivax* parasitemia after 72 hours, and possibly acquisition of infection in Oceania or India. Patients with *P. vivax* or *P. ovale* malaria should also be given primaquine once daily for 14 days to prevent relapse from the hypnozoite forms that remain

Table 280-2 CDC GUIDELINES FOR TREATMENT OF MALARIA IN THE USA

CDC Malaria Hotline: (770) 488-7788 Monday-Friday 8 am to 4:30 pm EST; (770) 488-7100 after hours, weekends, and holidays

CLINICAL DIAGNOSIS/*PLASMODIUM* SPECIES	REGION INFECTION ACQUIRED	RECOMMENDED DRUG AND ADULT DOSE	RECOMMENDED DRUG AND PEDIATRIC DOSE *PEDIATRIC DOSE SHOULD NEVER EXCEED ADULT DOSE*
Uncomplicated malaria/ *P. falciparum* or Species not identified If "species not identified" is subsequently diagnosed as *P. vivax* or *P. ovale:* see *P. vivax* and *P. ovale* (below) re: treatment with primaquine	**Chloroquine-resistant or unknown resistance**[1] (All malarious regions except those specified as chloroquine-sensitive listed in the box below. Middle Eastern countries with chloroquine-resistant *P. falciparum* include Iran, Oman, Saudi Arabia, and Yemen. Of note, infections acquired in the Newly Independent States of the former Soviet Union and Korea to date have been uniformly caused by *P. vivax* and should therefore be treated as chloroquine-sensitive infections.)	**A. Atovaquone-proguanil (Malarone)**[2] **Adult tab = 250 mg atovaquone/100 mg proguanil** 4 adult tabs po qd × 3 days	**A. Atovaquone-proguanil (Malarone)**[2] **Adult tab = 250 mg atovaquone/100 mg proguanil** **Peds tab = 62.5 mg atovaquone/25 mg proguanil** 5-8 kg: 2 peds tabs po qd × 3 days 9-10 kg: 3 peds tabs po qd × 3 days 11-20 kg: 1 adult tab po qd × 3 days 21-30 kg: 2 adult tabs po qd × 3 days 31-40 kg: 3 adult tabs po qd × 3 days >40 kg: 4 adult tabs po qd × 3 days
		B. Artemether-lumefantrine (Coartem)[2] **1 tablet = 20 mg artemether and 120 mg lumefantrine** A 3-day treatment schedule with a total of 6 oral doses is recommended for both adult and pediatric patients based on weight. The patient should receive the initial dose, followed by the second dose 8 hr later, and then 1 dose po bid for the following 2 days. 5 to <15 kg: 1 tablet per dose 15 to <25 kg: 2 tablets per dose 25 to <35 kg: 3 tablets per dose >35 kg: 4 tablets per dose	
		C. Quinine sulfate plus one of the following: doxycycline, tetracycline, or clindamycin **Quinine sulfate:** 542 mg base (=650 mg salt)[3] po tid × 3 or 7 days[4] **Doxycycline:** 100 mg po bid × 7 days **Tetracycline:** 250 mg po qid × 7 days **Clindamycin:** 20 mg base/kg/day po divided tid × 7 days	**C. Quinine sulfate**[3] **plus one of the following: doxycycline,**[5] **tetracycline,**[5] **or clindamycin** **Quinine sulfate:** 8.3 mg base/kg (=10 mg salt/kg) po tid × 3 or 7 days[4] **Doxycycline:** 2.2 mg/kg po every 12 hr × 7 days **Tetracycline:** 25 mg/kg/day po divided qid × 7 days **Clindamycin:** 20 mg base/kg/day po divided tid × 7 days
		D. Mefloquine (Lariam and generics)[6] 684 mg base (=750 mg salt) po as initial dose, followed by 456 mg base (=500 mg salt) po given 6-12 hr after initial dose Total dose =1,250 mg salt	**D. Mefloquine (Lariam and generics)**[6] 13.7 mg base/kg (=15 mg salt/kg) po as initial dose, followed by 9.1 mg base/kg (=10 mg salt/kg) po given 6-12 hr after initial dose Total dose = 25 mg salt/kg
Uncomplicated malaria/ *P. falciparum* or Species not identified	**Chloroquine-sensitive** (Central America west of Panama Canal; Haiti; the Dominican Republic; and most of the Middle East)	**Chloroquine phosphate (Aralen and generics)** 600 mg base (=1,000 mg salt) po immediately, followed by 300 mg base (=500 mg salt) po at 6, 24, and 48 hr Total dose: 1,500 mg base (=2,500 mg salt) **OR** **Hydroxychloroquine (Plaquenil and generics)** 620 mg base (=800 mg salt) po immediately, followed by 310 mg base (=400 mg salt) po at 6, 24, and 48 hr Total dose: 1,550 mg base (=2,000 mg salt)	**Chloroquine phosphate (Aralen and generics)** 10 mg base/kg po immediately, followed by 5 mg base/kg po at 6, 24, and 48 hr Total dose: 25 mg base/kg **OR** **Hydroxychloroquine (Plaquenil and generics)** 10 mg base/kg po immediately, followed by 5 mg base/kg po at 6, 24, and 48 hr Total dose: 25 mg base/kg
Uncomplicated malaria/ *P. malariae* or *P. knowlesi*	**All regions**	**Chloroquine phosphate:** Treatment as above **OR** **Hydroxychloroquine:** Treatment as above	**Chloroquine phosphate:** Treatment as above **OR** **Hydroxychloroquine:** Treatment as above

[1]NOTE: There are 4 options (A, B, C, or D) available for treatment of uncomplicated malaria caused by chloroquine-resistant *P. falciparum*. Options A, B, and C are equally recommended. Because of a higher rate of severe neuropsychiatric reactions seen at treatment doses, we do not recommend option D (mefloquine) unless the other options cannot be used. For option C, because there is more data on the efficacy of quinine in combination with doxycycline or tetracycline, these treatment combinations are generally preferred to quinine in combination with clindamycin.

[2]Take with food or whole milk. If patient vomits within 30 min of taking a dose, then they should repeat the dose.

[3]U.S. manufactured quinine sulfate capsule is in a 324 mg dosage; therefore 2 capsules should be sufficient for adult dosing. Pediatric dosing may be difficult due to unavailability of noncapsule forms of quinine.

[4]For infections acquired in Southeast Asia, quinine treatment should continue for 7 days. For infections acquired elsewhere, quinine treatment should continue for 3 days.

[5]Doxycycline and tetracycline are not indicated for use in children less than 8 yr old. For children less than 8 yr old with chloroquine-resistant *P. falciparum*, atovaquone-proguanil and artemether-lumefantrine are recommended treatment options; mefloquine can be considered if no other options are available. For children less than 8 yr old with chloroquine-resistant *P. vivax*, mefloquine is the recommended treatment. If it is not available or is not being tolerated and if the treatment benefits outweigh the risks, atovaquone-proguanil or artemether-lumefantrine should be used instead.

[6]Treatment with mefloquine is not recommended in persons who have acquired infections from Southeast Asia due to drug resistance.

Continued

Table 280-2 CDC GUIDELINES FOR TREATMENT OF MALARIA IN THE UNITED STATES—cont'd

CLINICAL DIAGNOSIS/*PLASMODIUM* SPECIES	REGION INFECTION ACQUIRED	RECOMMENDED DRUG AND ADULT DOSE	RECOMMENDED DRUG AND PEDIATRIC DOSE *PEDIATRIC DOSE SHOULD NEVER EXCEED ADULT DOSE*
Uncomplicated malaria/*P. vivax* or *P. ovale*	**All regions** Note: For suspected chloroquine-resistant *P. vivax*, see row below	**Chloroquine phosphate plus primaquine phosphate**[7] **Chloroquine phosphate:** Treatment as above **Primaquine phosphate:** 30 mg base po qd × 14 days **OR** **Hydroxychloroquine plus primaquine phosphate**[7] **Hydroxychloroquine:** Treatment as above **Primaquine phosphate:** 30 mg base po qd × 14 days	**Chloroquine phosphate plus primaquine phosphate**[7] **Chloroquine phosphate:** Treatment as above **Primaquine:** 0.5 mg base/kg po qd × 14 days **OR** **Hydroxychloroquine plus primaquine phosphate**[7] **Hydroxychloroquine:** Treatment as above **Primaquine phosphate:** 30 mg base po qd × 14 days
Uncomplicated malaria/*P. vivax*	**Chloroquine-resistant**[8] (Papua New Guinea and Indonesia)	**A. Quinine sulfate plus either doxycycline or tetracycline plus primaquine phosphate**[7] **Quinine sulfate:** Treatment as above **Doxycycline or tetracycline:** Treatment as above **Primaquine phosphate:** Treatment as above	**A. Quinine sulfate plus either doxycycline**[5] **or tetracycline**[5] **plus primaquine phosphate**[7] **Quinine sulfate:** Treatment as above **Doxycycline or tetracycline:** Treatment as above **Primaquine phosphate:** Treatment as above
		B. Atovaquone-proguanil plus primaquine phosphate **Atovaquone-proguanil:** Treatment as above **Primaquine phosphate:** Treatment as above	**B. Atovaquone-proguanil plus primaquine phosphate** **Atovaquone-proguanil:** Treatment as above **Primaquine phosphate:** Treatment as above
		C. Mefloquine plus primaquine phosphate[7] **Mefloquine:** Treatment as above **Primaquine phosphate:** Treatment as above	**C. Mefloquine plus primaquine phosphate**[7] **Mefloquine:** Treatment as above **Primaquine phosphate:** Treatment as above
Uncomplicated malaria: alternatives for pregnant women[9-12]	**Chloroquine-sensitive** (see uncomplicated malaria sections above for chloroquine-sensitive species by region)	**Chloroquine phosphate:** Treatment as above **OR** **Hydroxychloroquine:** Treatment as above	Not applicable
	Chloroquine resistant *P. falciparum*[1] (see sections above for regions with chloroquine resistant ***P. falciparum***)	**Quinine sulfate plus clindamycin** **Quinine sulfate:** Treatment as above **Clindamycin:** Treatment as above	Not applicable
	Chloroquine-resistant *P. vivax* (see uncomplicated malaria sections above for regions with chloroquine-resistant ***P. vivax***)	**Quinine sulfate** **Quinine sulfate:** 650 mg[3] salt po tid × 7 days	Not applicable

[7]Primaquine is used to eradicate any hypnozoites that may remain dormant in the liver, and thus prevent relapses, in *P. vivax* and *P. ovale* infections. Because primaquine can cause hemolytic anemia in G6PD-deficient persons, G6PD screening must occur prior to starting treatment with primaquine. For persons with borderline G6PD deficiency or as an alternate to the above regimen, primaquine may be given 45 mg orally 1 time per wk for 8 wk; consultation with an expert in infectious disease and/or tropical medicine is advised if this alternative regimen is considered in G6PD-deficient persons. Primaquine must not be used during pregnancy.

[8]NOTE: There are three options (A, B, or C) available for treatment of uncomplicated malaria caused by chloroquine-resistant *P. vivax*. High treatment failure rates due to chloroquine-resistant *P. vivax* have been well documented in Papua New Guinea and Indonesia. Rare case reports of chloroquine-resistant *P. vivax* have also been documented in Burma (Myanmar), India, and Central and South America. Persons acquiring *P. vivax* infections outside of Papua New Guinea or Indonesia should be started on chloroquine. If the patient does not respond, the treatment should be changed to a chloroquine-resistant *P. vivax* regimen and CDC should be notified (Malaria Hotline number listed above). For treatment of chloroquine-resistant *P. vivax* infections, options A, B, and C are equally recommended.

[9]For pregnant women diagnosed with uncomplicated malaria caused by chloroquine-resistant *P. falciparum* or chloroquine-resistant *P. vivax* infection, treatment with doxycycline or tetracycline is generally not indicated. However, doxycycline or tetracycline may be used in combination with quinine (as recommended for non-pregnant adults) if other treatment options are not available or are not being tolerated, and the benefit is judged to outweigh the risks.

[10]Atovaquone-proguanil and artemether-lumefantrine are generally not recommended for use in pregnant women, particularly in the 1st trimester due to lack of sufficient safety data. For pregnant women diagnosed with uncomplicated malaria caused by chloroquine-resistant *P. falciparum* infection, atovaquone-proguanil or artemether-lumefantrine may be used if other treatment options are not available or are not being tolerated, and if the potential benefit is judged to outweigh the potential risks.

[11]Because of a possible association with mefloquine treatment during pregnancy and an increase in stillbirths, mefloquine is generally not recommended for treatment in pregnant women. However, mefloquine may be used if it is the only treatment option available and if the potential benefit is judged to outweigh the potential risks.

[12]For *P. vivax* and *P. ovale* infections, primaquine phosphate for radical treatment of hypnozoites should not be given during pregnancy. Pregnant patients with *P. vivax* and *P. ovale* infections should be maintained on chloroquine prophylaxis for the duration of their pregnancy. The chemoprophylactic dose of chloroquine phosphate is 300 mg base (= 500 mg salt) orally once per week. After delivery, pregnant patients who do not have G6PD deficiency should be treated with primaquine.

Table 280-2 CDC GUIDELINES FOR TREATMENT OF MALARIA IN THE UNITED STATES—cont'd

CLINICAL DIAGNOSIS/*PLASMODIUM* SPECIES	REGION INFECTION ACQUIRED	RECOMMENDED DRUG AND ADULT DOSE	RECOMMENDED DRUG AND PEDIATRIC DOSE *PEDIATRIC DOSE SHOULD NEVER EXCEED ADULT DOSE*
Severe malaria[13-16]	**All regions**	**Quinidine gluconate**[14] **plus one of the following: doxycycline, tetracycline, or clindamycin** **Quinidine gluconate:** 6.25 mg base/kg (=10 mg salt/kg) loading dose IV over 1-2 hr, then 0.0125 mg base/kg/min (=0.02 mg salt/kg/min) continuous infusion for at least 24 hr. An alternative regimen is 15 mg base/kg (=24 mg salt/kg) loading dose IV infused over 4 hr, followed by 7.5 mg base/kg (=12 mg salt/kg) infused over 4 hr every 8 hr, starting 8 hr after the loading dose (see package insert). Once parasite density <1% and patient can take oral medication, complete treatment with oral quinine, dose as above. Quinidine/quinine course = 7 days in Southeast Asia; = 3 days in Africa or South America. **Doxycycline:** Treatment as above. If patient not able to take oral medication, give 100 mg IV every 12 hr and then switch to oral doxycycline (as above) as soon as patient can take oral medication. For IV use, avoid rapid administration. Treatment course = 7 days. **Tetracycline:** Treatment as above **Clindamycin:** Treatment as above. If patient not able to take oral medication, give 10 mg base/kg loading dose IV followed by 5 mg base/kg IV every 8 hr. Switch to oral clindamycin (oral dose as above) as soon as patient can take oral medication. For IV use, avoid rapid administration. Treatment course = 7 days. ***Investigational new drug (contact CDC for information):*** **Artesunate followed by one of the following: atovaquone proguanil (Malarone), doxycycline (clindamycin in pregnant women), or mefloquine**	**Quinidine gluconate**[14] **plus one of the following: doxycycline,**[4] **tetracycline,**[4] **or clindamycin** **Quinidine gluconate:** Same mg/kg dosing and recommendations as for adults. **Doxycycline:** Treatment as above. If patient not able to take oral medication, may give IV. For children <45 kg, give 2.2 mg/kg IV every 12 hr and then switch to oral doxycycline (dose as above) as soon as patient can take oral medication. For children >45 kg, use same dosing as for adults. For IV use, avoid rapid administration. Treatment course = 7 days. **Tetracycline:** Treatment as above **Clindamycin:** Treatment as above. If patient not able to take oral medication, give 10 mg base/kg loading dose IV followed by 5 mg base/kg IV every 8 hr. Switch to oral clindamycin (oral dose as above) as soon as patient can take oral medication. For IV use, avoid rapid administration. Treatment course = 7 days. ***Investigational new drug (contact CDC for information):*** **Artesunate followed by one of the following: atovaquone-proguanil (Malarone), clindamycin, or mefloquine**

[13]Persons with a positive blood smear OR history of recent possible exposure and no other recognized pathology who have one or more of the following clinical criteria (impaired consciousness/coma, severe normocytic anemia, renal failure, pulmonary edema, acute respiratory distress syndrome, circulatory shock, disseminated intravascular coagulation, spontaneous bleeding, acidosis, hemoglobinuria, jaundice, repeated generalized convulsions, and/or parasitemia of >5%) are considered to have manifestations of more severe disease. Severe malaria is most often caused by *P. falciparum.*

[14]Patients diagnosed with severe malaria should be treated aggressively with parenteral antimalarial therapy. Treatment with IV quinidine should be initiated as soon as possible after the diagnosis has been made. Patients with severe malaria should be given an intravenous loading dose of quinidine unless they have received more than 40 mg/kg of quinine in the preceding 48 hr or if they have received mefloquine within the preceding 12 hr. Consultation with a cardiologist and a physician with experience treating malaria is advised when treating malaria patients with quinidine. During administration of quinidine, blood pressure monitoring (for hypotension) and cardiac monitoring (for widening of the QRS complex and/or lengthening of the QTc interval) should be monitored continuously and blood glucose (for hypoglycemia) should be monitored periodically. Cardiac complications, if severe, may warrant temporary discontinuation of the drug or slowing of the intravenous infusion.

[15]Consider exchange transfusion if the parasite density (i.e., parasitemia) is >10% OR if the patient has altered mental status, non–volume overload pulmonary edema, or renal complications. The parasite density can be estimated by examining a monolayer of red blood cells (RBCs) on the thin smear under oil immersion magnification. The slide should be examined where the RBCs are more or less touching (approximately 400 RBCs per field). The parasite density can then be estimated from the percentage of infected RBCs and should be monitored every 12 hr. Exchange transfusion should be continued until the parasite density is <1% (usually requires 8-10 units). IV quinidine administration should not be delayed for an exchange transfusion and can be given concurrently throughout the exchange transfusion.

[16]Pregnant women diagnosed with severe malaria should be treated aggressively with parenteral antimalarial therapy.

Adapted from Centers for Disease Control and Prevention: *Guidelines for treatment of malaria in the United States* (pdf). www.cdc.gov/malaria/resources/pdf/treatmenttable73109.pdf. Accessed September 20, 2010.

dormant in the liver. Some strains may require 2 courses of primaquine. Testing for glucose-6-phosphate dehydrogenase deficiency must be performed before initiation of primaquine, because it can cause hemolytic anemia in such patients. Unfortunately, no alternatives to primaquine currently exist for eradication of the hypnozoite forms of *P. vivax* or *P. ovale*. Patients with any type of malaria must be monitored for possible recrudescence with repeat blood smears at the end of therapy because recrudescence may occur more than 90 days after therapy with low-grade resistant organisms. If vomiting precludes oral administration, chloroquine can be given by nasogastric tube. Based on limited evidence, chloroquine plus sulfadoxine-pyrimethamine should be used to treat *P. knowlesi* infections. For cases of severe malaria due to any Plasmodium species, intravenous quinidine or quinine along with a second drug (clindamycin, doxycycline, or tetracycline) should be used, as for P. falciparum. Patients with any type of malaria must be monitored for possible recrudescence with repeat blood smears at the end of therapy, because recrudescence may occur more than 90 days after therapy with low-grade resistant organisms. For children living in endemic areas, mothers should be encouraged to treat fever with an antimalarial drug. If such children are severely ill, they should be given the same therapy as nonimmune children.

COMPLICATIONS OF *P. FALCIPARUM* MALARIA

WHO has identified 10 complications of *P. falciparum* malaria that define severe malaria (see Table 280-1). The most common complications in children are severe anemia, impaired consciousness (including cerebral malaria), respiratory distress (due to metabolic acidosis), multiple seizures, prostration, and jaundice.

Severe malarial anemia (hemoglobin level less than 5 g/dL) is the most common severe complication of malaria in children and is the leading cause of anemia leading to hospital admission in African children. Anemia is associated with hemolysis, but removal of infected erythrocytes by the spleen and impairment of erythropoiesis likely play a greater role than hemolysis in the pathogenesis of severe malarial anemia. The primary treatment for severe malarial anemia is blood transfusion. With appropriate and timely treatment, severe malarial anemia usually has a relatively low mortality (~1%).

Cerebral malaria is defined as the presence of coma in a child with *P. falciparum* parasitemia and an absence of other reasons for coma. Children with altered mental status who are not in coma fall into the larger category of impaired consciousness. Cerebral malaria is most common in children in areas of mid-level transmission and in adolescents or adults in areas of very low transmission. It is less frequently seen in areas of very high transmission. Cerebral malaria often develops after the patient has been ill for several days but may develop precipitously. Cerebral malaria is associated with a fatality rate of 20-40% and is associated with long-term cognitive impairment in children. Repeated seizures are frequent in children with cerebral malaria. Hypoglycemia is common, but children with true cerebral malaria fail to arouse from coma even after receiving a dextrose infusion that normalizes their glucose level. Physical findings may be normal or may include high fever, seizures, muscular twitching, rhythmic movement of the head or extremities, contracted or unequal pupils, retinal hemorrhages, hemiplegia, absent or exaggerated deep tendon reflexes, and a positive Babinski sign. Lumbar puncture reveals increased pressure and cerebrospinal fluid protein with no pleocytosis and normal glucose and protein concentrations. Treatment of cerebral malaria other than antimalarial medications is largely supportive and includes evaluation of and treatment of seizures and hypoglycemia. Although increased intracranial pressure has been documented in some children with cerebral malaria, treatment with mannitol and corticosteroids has not improved outcomes in these children.

Respiratory distress is a poor prognostic indicator in severe malaria and appears to be due to metabolic acidosis rather than intrinsic pulmonary disease. To date, no successful interventions for treatment of metabolic acidosis in children with severe malaria have been described, but trials of dichloroacetate treatment and fluid expansion are ongoing.

Seizures are a common complication of severe malaria, particularly cerebral malaria. Benzodiazepines are first-line therapy for seizures, and intrarectal diazepam has been used successfully in children with malaria and seizures. Many seizures resolve with a single dose of diazepam. For persistent seizures, phenobarbital or phenytoin are the standard medications used. Phenytoin may be preferred for seizure treatment, particularly in hospitals or clinics where ventilatory support is not available. However, no comparative trials of the 2 drugs have been performed, and phenytoin is considerably more expensive than phenobarbital. There are currently no drugs recommended for seizure prophylaxis in children with severe malaria. Phenobarbital prophylaxis decreased seizure activity but increased mortality in 1 major study of children with severe malaria, probably because of the respiratory depression associated with phenobarbital that may have been exacerbated by benzodiazepine therapy.

Hypoglycemia is a complication of malaria that is more common in children, pregnant women, and patients receiving quinine therapy. Patients may have a decreased level of consciousness that can be confused with cerebral malaria. Any child with impaired consciousness and malaria should have a glucose level checked, and if glucometers are not available, an empirical bolus of dextrose should be given. Hypoglycemia is associated with increased mortality and neurologic sequelae.

Circulatory collapse (**algid malaria**) is a rare complication that manifests as hypotension, hypothermia, rapid weak pulse, shallow breathing, pallor, and vascular collapse. Death may occur within hours. Severe malaria is occasionally accompanied by bacteremia, which may have been the cause of some of the cases previously referred to as algid malaria. Any child with severe malaria and hypotension should have a blood culture obtained and be treated empirically for bacterial sepsis.

Long-term cognitive impairment occurs in 25% of children with cerebral malaria and also occurs in children with repeated episodes of uncomplicated disease. Prevention of attacks in these children significantly improves educational attainment.

Tropical splenomegaly syndrome is a chronic complication of *P. falciparum* malaria in which massive splenomegaly persists after treatment of acute infection. The syndrome is characterized by marked splenomegaly, hepatomegaly, anemia, and an elevated IgM level. Tropical splenomegaly syndrome is thought to be caused by an impaired immune response to *P. falciparum* antigens. Prolonged antimalarial prophylaxis (for at least several years) is required to treat this syndrome if the child remains in a malaria endemic area. Spleen size gradually regresses on antimalarial prophylaxis but often increases again if prophylaxis is stopped.

Other complications in children include jaundice, which is associated with a worse outcome, and prostration. Prostration is defined as the inability to sit, stand, or eat without support, in the absence of impaired consciousness. Prostration also has been associated with increased mortality in some studies, but the pathophysiology of this process is not well understood. Uncommon complications include hemoglobinuria, abnormal bleeding, pulmonary edema, and renal failure. These are uncommon complications in children with severe malaria and are more common in adults, particularly pulmonary edema and renal failure.

PREVENTION

Malaria prevention consists of reducing exposure to infected mosquitoes and chemoprophylaxis. The most accurate and current information on areas in the world where malaria risk and drug resistance exist can be obtained by contacting local and state health departments or the CDC or consulting *Health Information for International Travel*, which is published by the U.S. Public Health Service.

Travelers to endemic areas should remain in well-screened areas from dusk to dawn, when the risk for transmission is highest. They should sleep under permethrin-treated mosquito netting and spray insecticides indoors at sundown. During the day the travelers should wear clothing that covers the arms and legs, with trousers tucked into shoes or boots. Mosquito repellent should be applied to thin clothing and exposed areas of the skin, with applications repeated every 1-2 hr. A child should not be taken outside from dusk to dawn, but if at risk for exposure, a solution with 25-35% DEET (not greater than 40%) should be applied to exposed areas except for the eyes, mouth, or hands. Hands are excluded because they are often placed in the mouth. DEET should then be washed off as soon as the child comes back inside. The American Academy of Pediatrics recommends that DEET solutions be avoided in children less than 2 mo of age. Adverse reactions to DEET include rashes, toxic encephalopathy, and seizures, but these reactions occur almost exclusively with inappropriate application of high concentrations of DEET. Even with these precautions, a child should be taken to a physician immediately if he or she develops illness when traveling to a malarious area.

Chemoprophylaxis is necessary for all visitors to and residents of the tropics who have not lived there since infancy, including children of all ages (Table 280-3). Health care providers should consult the latest information on resistance patterns before prescribing prophylaxis for their patients. Chloroquine is given in the few remaining areas of the world free of chloroquine-resistant malaria strains. In areas where chloroquine-resistant *P. falciparum* exists, atovaquone-proguanil, mefloquine, or doxycycline may be given as chemoprophylaxis. Atovaquone-proguanil is generally recommended for shorter trips (up to 2 wk), since it must be taken daily. Pediatric tablets are available and are generally well tolerated, although the taste is sometimes unpleasant to very young children. For longer trips, mefloquine is preferred, as it is given only once a week. Mefloquine does not have a pediatric formulation and has an unpleasant taste that usually requires that the cut tablet be "disguised" in another food, such as chocolate syrup. Mefloquine should not be given to children if they have a known hypersensitivity to mefloquine, are receiving cardiotropic drugs, have a history of convulsive or certain psychiatric disorders, or travel to an area where mefloquine resistance exists (the borders of Thailand with Myanmar and Cambodia, the western provinces of Cambodia, and the eastern states of Myanmar). Atovaqoune-proguanil is started 1-2 days before travel, and mefloquine is started 2 wk before travel. It is important that these doses are given, both to allow therapeutic levels of the drugs to be achieved and also to be sure that the drugs are tolerated. Doxycycline is an alternative for children over 8 yr of age. It must be given daily and should be given with food. Side effects of doxycycline include photosensitivity and vaginal yeast infections. Provision of medication for self-treatment is controversial, but it can be considered in individuals who refuse to take prophylaxis or will be in very remote areas without accessible medical care. Provision of medication for self-treatment of malaria should be done in consultation with a travel medicine specialist, and the medication provided should be different than that used for prophylaxis.

A number of other efforts are currently underway to prevent malaria in malaria endemic countries. Some have been highly successful, leading to a significant decrease in malaria incidence in many countries in Africa, Asia, and South America in the last 5 yr. These interventions include the use of insecticide-treated bed nets (which have decreased all-cause mortality in children under 5 yr of age in several highly malaria endemic areas by ~20%), indoor residual spraying with long-lasting insecticides, and the use of artemisinin-combination therapy for first-line malaria treatment. The 1st malaria vaccine to have any degree of efficacy is the RTS,S vaccine, which is based on the circumsporozoite protein of *P. falciparum*. In various clinical trials, this vaccine has shown an efficacy of 26-56% against uncomplicated malaria and 38-50% against severe malaria in young children in malaria endemic areas in periods as long as 45 mo after vaccination. The vaccine is now in large phase III trials. Given the relatively low efficacy of this vaccine, it will likely be used as part of a multipronged strategy in endemic areas that includes the already successful interventions mentioned. Numerous other vaccines are also in current clinical trials, and it is hoped that future vaccines will improve upon the efficacy of the RTS,S vaccine. There is currently no vaccine with sufficient efficacy to be considered for prevention of malaria in travelers.

Table 280-3 CHEMOPROPHYLAXIS OF MALARIA FOR CHILDREN

AREA	DRUG	DOSAGE (ORAL)
Chloroquine-resistant area	Mefloquine*†	<10 kg: 4.6 mg base (5 mg salt)/kg/wk
		10-19 kg: 1/4 tab/wk
		20-30 kg: 1/2 tab/wk
		31-45 kg: 3/4 tab/wk
		>45 kg: 1 tab/wk (228 mg base)
	Doxycyline‡	2 mg/kg daily (max 100 mg)
	Atovaquone/proguanil§ (Malarone)	Pediatric tabs: 62.5 mg atovaquone/25 mg proguanil Adult tabs: 250 mg proguanil/100 mg proguanil
		5-8 kg: 1/2 pediatric tab once daily (off-label)
		9-10 kg: 3/4 pediatric tab once daily (off-label)
		11-20 kg: 1 pediatric tab once daily
		21-30 kg: 2 pediatric tabs once daily
		31-40 kg: 3 pediatric tabs once daily
		>40 kg: 1 adult tab once daily
Chloroquine-susceptible area	Chloroquine phosphate	5 mg base/kg/wk (max 300 mg base)

*Chloroquine and mefloquine should be started 1-2 wk prior to departure and continued for 4 wk after last exposure.

†Mefloquine resistance exists in western Cambodia and along the Thailand-Cambodia and Thailand-Myanmar borders. Travelers to these areas should take doxycycline or atovaquone-proguanil. See text for precautions about mefloquine use.

‡Doxycycline should be started 1-2 days prior to departure and continued for 4 wk after last exposure. Do not use in children <8 yr of age or in pregnant women.

§Atovaquone/proguanil (Malarone) should be started 1-2 days prior to departure and continued for 7 days after last exposure. Should be taken with food or a milky drink. Not recommended in pregnant women, children <5 kg, and women breast-feeding infants <5 kg. Contraindicated in individuals with severe renal impairment (creatinine clearance <30 mL/min).

BIBLIOGRAPHY

Please visit the Nelson Textbook of Pediatrics *website at* *www.expertconsult.com* *for the complete bibliography.*

Chapter 281
Babesiosis (*Babesia*)

Peter J. Krause

Babesiosis is an emerging malaria-like disease caused by intraerythrocytic protozoa that are transmitted by hard body (ixodid) ticks. The clinical manifestations of babesiosis range from subclinical illness to fulminant disease resulting in death.

For the full continuation of this chapter, please visit the Nelson Textbook of Pediatrics *website at* *www.expertconsult.com*.

Chapter 282
Toxoplasmosis *(Toxoplasma gondii)*

Rima McLeod

Toxoplasma gondii, an obligate intracellular protozoan, is acquired perorally, transplacentally, or, rarely, parenterally in laboratory accidents; by transfusion; or from a transplanted organ. In immunologically normal children, acute acquired infection may be asymptomatic, cause lymphadenopathy, or affect almost any organ. Once acquired, latent encysted organisms persist in the host throughout life. In immunocompromised infants or children, either initial acquisition or recrudescence of latent organisms often causes signs or symptoms related to the central nervous system (CNS). If untreated, congenital infection often causes disease either perinatally or later in life, most frequently chorioretinitis and CNS lesions. Other manifestations such as intrauterine growth retardation, cognitive and motor deficits, fever, lymphadenopathy, rash, hearing loss, pneumonitis, hepatitis, and thrombocytopenia also occur. Congenital toxoplasmosis in infants with HIV infection may be fulminant.

ETIOLOGY

T. gondii is a coccidian protozoan that multiplies only in living cells. The tachyzoites are oval or crescent-like, measuring 2-4 × 4-7 µm. Tissue cysts, which are 10-100 µm in diameter, may contain thousands of parasites and remain in tissues, especially the CNS and skeletal and heart muscle, for the life of the host. *Toxoplasma* can multiply in all tissues of mammals and birds.

Newly infected cats and other Felidae species excrete infectious *Toxoplasma* oocysts in their feces. *Toxoplasma* organisms are transmitted to cats by ingestion of infected meat containing encysted bradyzoites or by ingestion of oocysts excreted by other recently infected cats. The parasites then multiply through schizogonic and gametogonic cycles in the distal ileal epithelium of the cat intestine. Oocysts containing 2 sporocysts are excreted, and, under proper conditions of temperature and moisture, each sporocyst matures into 4 sporozoites. For about 2 wk the cat excretes 10^5-10^7 oocysts/day, which may retain their viability for >1 yr in a suitable environment. Oocysts sporulate 1-5 days after excretion and are then infectious. Oocysts are killed by drying or boiling but not exposure to bleach. Oocysts have been isolated from soil and sand frequented by cats, and outbreaks associated with contaminated water have been reported. Oocysts and tissue cysts are sources of animal and human infections (Fig. 282-1). There are 3 clonal and atypical types of *T. gondii* that have different virulence for mice (and perhaps for humans) and form different numbers of cysts in the brains of outbred mice.

There is one predominant clonal type in France, Austria, and Poland, and nonarchetypal parasites in Brazil, Guyana, French Guiana, and Central America.

EPIDEMIOLOGY

Toxoplasma infection is ubiquitous in animals and is one of the most common latent infections of humans throughout the world. Incidence varies considerably among people and animals in different geographic areas. In many areas of the world, approximately 3-35% of pork, 7-60% of lamb, and 0-9% of beef contain *T. gondii* organisms. Significant antibody titers are detected in 50-80% of residents of some localities such as France, Brazil, and Central America, and in <5% in other areas. There is a higher prevalence of infection in warmer, more humid climates.

Human infection is usually acquired orally by eating undercooked or raw meat that contains cysts or food or other material contaminated with oocysts from acutely infected cats. Freezing meat to −20°C or heating meat to 66°C renders the cysts noninfectious. Outbreaks of acute acquired infection have occurred in families who have consumed the same infected food. *Toxoplasma* organisms are not transmitted from person to person except for transplacental infection from mother to fetus and, rarely, by organ transplantation or transfusion.

Seronegative transplant recipients who receive an organ or bone marrow from seropositive donors have experienced life-threatening illness requiring therapy. Seropositive recipients may have increased serologic titers without associated disease.

Congenital Toxoplasmosis

Transmission to the fetus usually follows acquisition of infection by an immunologically normal mother during gestation. Congenital transmission from mothers infected before pregnancy is extremely rare except for immunocompromised women who are chronically infected. The incidence of congenital infection in the USA ranges from 1/1,000 to 1/8,000 live births. The incidence of infection among pregnant women depends on the general risk for infection in the specific locale and the proportion of the population that has not been infected previously.

PATHOGENESIS

T. gondii is acquired by children and adults from ingesting food that contains cysts or that is contaminated with oocysts usually from acutely infected cats. Oocysts also may be transported to food by flies and cockroaches. When the organism is ingested, bradyzoites are released from cysts or sporozoites from oocysts. The organisms enter gastrointestinal cells where they multiply, rupture cells, infect contiguous cells, enter the lymphatics, and disseminate hematogenously throughout the body. Tachyzoites proliferate, producing necrotic foci surrounded by a cellular reaction. With development of a normal immune response that is both humoral and cell-mediated, tachyzoites disappear from tissues. In immunocompromised persons and also some apparently immunocompetent persons, acute infection progresses and may cause potentially lethal disease, including pneumonitis, myocarditis, or encephalitis.

Alterations of T-lymphocyte populations during acute *T. gondii* infection are common and include lymphocytosis, increased CD8 count, and decreased CD4:CD8 ratio. Depletion of CD4 cells in patients with AIDS may contribute to severe manifestations of toxoplasmosis. Characteristic lymph node changes include reactive follicular hyperplasia with irregular clusters of epithelioid histiocytes that encroach on and blur margins of germinal centers, and focal distention of sinuses with monocytoid cells.

Cysts form as early as 7 days after infection and remain for the life of the host. During latent infection they produce little or no inflammatory response but can cause recrudescent disease in immunocompromised persons. Recrudescent chorioretinitis occurs in children with postnatal infection but more often in older children and adults with congenital infection.

Congenital Toxoplasmosis

When a mother acquires infection during gestation, organisms may disseminate hematogenously to the placenta. Infection may be transmitted to the fetus transplacentally or during vaginal delivery. Of untreated maternal infections acquired in the 1st trimester, approximately 17% of fetuses are infected, usually with severe disease. Of untreated maternal infection acquired in the 3rd trimester, approximately 65% of fetuses are infected, usually with disease that is mild or inapparent at birth. These different rates of transmission and outcomes are most likely related to placental blood flow, virulence, inoculum of *T. gondii,* and immunologic capacity of the mother to limit parasitemia.

Examination of the placenta of infected newborns may reveal chronic inflammation and cysts. Tachyzoites can be seen with Wright or Giemsa stains but are best demonstrated with immu-

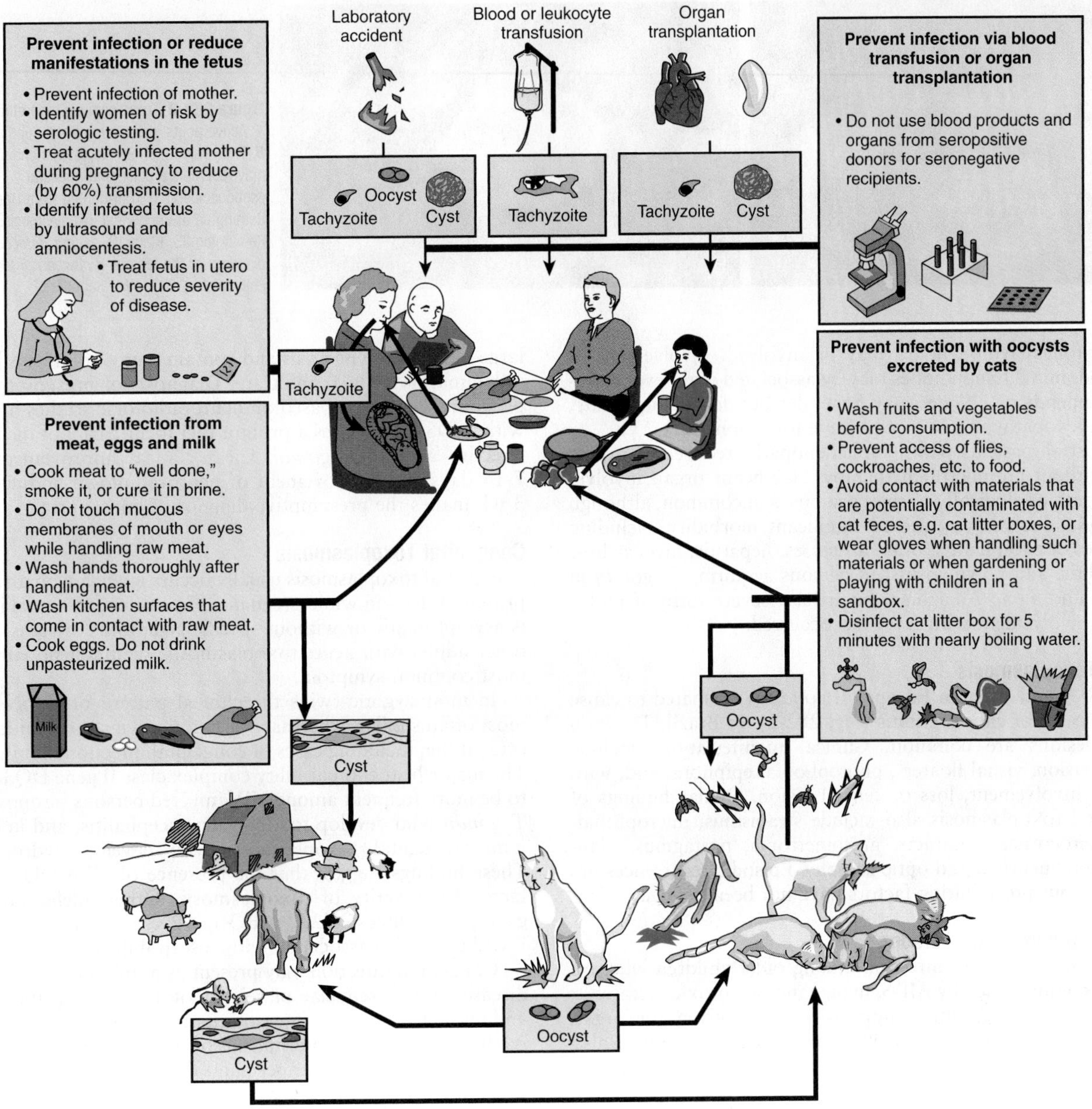
Laboratory accident
Blood or leukocyte transfusion
Organ transplantation
Prevent infection or reduce manifestations in the fetus
• Prevent infection of mother.
• Identify women of risk by serologic testing.
• Treat acutely infected mother during pregnancy to reduce (by 60%) transmission.
• Identify infected fetus by ultrasound and amniocentesis.
• Treat fetus in utero to reduce severity of disease.
Oocyst
Tachyzoite
Cyst
Tachyzoite
Tachyzoite
Cyst
Prevent infection via blood transfusion or organ transplantation
• Do not use blood products and organs from seropositive donors for seronegative recipients.
Tachyzoite
Prevent infection from meat, eggs and milk
• Cook meat to "well done," smoke it, or cure it in brine.
• Do not touch mucous membranes of mouth or eyes while handling raw meat.
• Wash hands thoroughly after handling meat.
• Wash kitchen surfaces that come in contact with raw meat.
• Cook eggs. Do not drink unpasteurized milk.
Milk
Prevent infection with oocysts excreted by cats
• Wash fruits and vegetables before consumption.
• Prevent access of flies, cockroaches, etc. to food.
• Avoid contact with materials that are potentially contaminated with cat feces, e.g. cat litter boxes, or wear gloves when handling such materials or when gardening or playing with children in a sandbox.
• Disinfect cat litter box for 5 minutes with nearly boiling water.
Oocyst
Cyst
Oocyst
Cyst

Figure 282-1 Life cycle of *Toxoplasma gondii* and prevention of toxoplasmosis by interruption of transmission to humans.

noperoxidase technique. Tissue cysts stain well with periodic acid–Schiff and silver stains as well as with the immunoperoxidase technique. Gross or microscopic areas of necrosis may be present in many tissues, especially the CNS, choroid and retina, heart, lungs, skeletal muscle, liver, and spleen. Areas of calcification occur in the brain.

Almost all congenitally infected individuals who are not treated manifest signs or symptoms of infection, such as chorioretinitis, by adolescence. Some severely involved infants with congenital infection appear to have *Toxoplasma* antigen–specific cell-mediated anergy, which may be important in the pathogenesis of disease.

CLINICAL MANIFESTATIONS

Manifestations of primary infection with *T. gondii* are highly variable and are influenced primarily by host immunocompetence. There may be no signs or symptoms or severe disease. Reactivation of previously asymptomatic congenital toxoplasmosis usually manifests as ocular toxoplasmosis.

Acquired Toxoplasmosis

Immunocompetent children who acquire infection postnatally generally do not have clinically recognizable symptoms. When clinical manifestations are apparent, they may include almost any combination of fever, stiff neck, myalgia, arthralgia, maculopapular rash that spares the palms and soles, localized or generalized lymphadenopathy, hepatomegaly, hepatitis, reactive lymphocytosis, meningitis, brain abscess, encephalitis, confusion, malaise, pneumonia, polymyositis, pericarditis, pericardial effusion, and myocarditis. Chorioretinitis is usually unilateral and occurs in approximately 1% of cases in the USA. Half the cases of ocular toxoplasmosis in English children are due to acute acquired infection; the appearance does not distinguish acute vs. congenital infection. Symptoms may be present for a few days only or may persist many months. The most common manifestation is enlargement of 1 or a few cervical lymph nodes. Cases of *Toxoplasma* lymphadenopathy rarely resemble infectious mononucleosis, Hodgkin's disease, or other lymphadenopathies (Chapter 484). In the pectoral area in older girls and women, enlarged nodes may be confused with breast neoplasms. Mediastinal, mesenteric, and

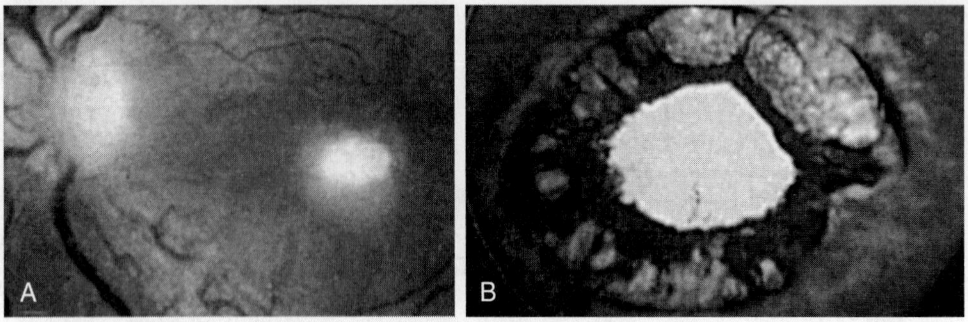

Figure 282-2 Toxoplasmic chorioretinitis. *A,* Active acute lesion by indirect ophthalmoscopy. *B,* The healed foci of toxoplasmic chorioretinitis may resemble a coloboma (macular pseudocoloboma). (*B,* Adapted from Desmonts G, Remington J: Congenital toxoplasmosis. In Remington JS, Klein JO, editors: *Infectious diseases of the fetus and newborn infant,* ed 5, Philadelphia, 2001, WB Saunders.)

retroperitoneal lymph nodes may be involved. Involvement of intra-abdominal lymph nodes may be associated with fever, mimicking appendicitis. Nodes may be tender but do not suppurate. Lymphadenopathy may wax and wane for as long as 1-2 yr.

Almost all patients with lymphadenopathy recover spontaneously without antimicrobial therapy. Significant organ involvement in immunologically normal persons is uncommon, although some individuals have suffered significant morbidity, including rare cases of encephalitis, brain abscesses, hepatitis, myocarditis, pericarditis, and polymyositis. In persons acquiring *T. gondii* in Guyana and along Amazon tributaries, a severe form of multivisceral involvement with fever has occurred.

Ocular Toxoplasmosis

In the USA and Western Europe, *T. gondii* is estimated to cause 35% of cases of chorioretinitis (Fig. 282-2). In Brazil, *T. gondii* retinal lesions are common. Clinical manifestations include blurred vision, visual floaters, photophobia, epiphora, and, with macular involvement, loss of central vision. Ocular findings of congenital toxoplasmosis also include strabismus, microphthalmia, microcornea, cataracts, anisometropia, nystagmus, glaucoma, optic neuritis, and optic atrophy. Episodic recurrences are common, but precipitating factors have not been defined.

Immunocompromised Persons

Disseminated *T. gondii* infection among older children who are immunocompromised by AIDS, malignancy, cytotoxic therapy or corticosteroids, or immunosuppressive drugs given for organ transplantation involves the CNS in 50% of cases and may also involve the heart, lungs, and gastrointestinal tract. Stem cell transplant recipients present a special problem, because active infection is particularly difficult to diagnose. After transplantation, *T. gondii*-specific antibody levels may remain the same, increase, or decrease and can even become undetectable. Most often immunoglobulin G (IgG) antibody is present; thus, toxoplasmosis in these patients almost always results from transplantation from a seropositive individual to a seronegative recipient. Active infection is often fulminant and rapidly fatal.

Congenital *T. gondii* infection in infants with HIV infection is rare and is often a severe and fulminant disease with substantial CNS involvement. Alternatively, it may be more indolent in presentation, with focal neurologic deficits or systemic manifestations such as pneumonitis.

From 25-50% of persons with *T. gondii* antibodies and **HIV infection** without antiretroviral treatment eventually experience toxoplasmic encephalitis, which is fatal if not treated. Highly active antiretroviral therapy and trimethoprim-sulfamethoxazole prophylaxis have diminished the incidence of toxoplasmosis in patients with HIV infection, but toxoplasmic encephalitis remains a presenting manifestation in 20% of adult patients with AIDS. Typical findings include fever, headache, altered mental status, psychosis, cognitive impairment, seizures, and focal neurologic defects, including hemiparesis, aphasia, ataxia, visual field loss, cranial nerve palsies, and dysmetria or movement disorders. In adult patients with AIDS, toxoplasmic retinal lesions are often large with diffuse necrosis and contain many organisms but little inflammatory cellular infiltrate. Diagnosis of presumptive toxoplasmic encephalitis based on neuroradiologic studies in patients with AIDS necessitates a prompt therapeutic trial of medications effective against *T. gondii.* Clear clinical improvement within 7-14 days and improvement of neuroradiologic findings within 3 wk makes the presumptive diagnosis almost certain.

Congenital Toxoplasmosis

Congenital toxoplasmosis usually occurs when a woman acquires primary infection while pregnant. Most often, maternal infection is asymptomatic or without specific symptoms or signs. As with other adults with acute toxoplasmosis, lymphadenopathy is the most common symptom.

In monozygotic twins the clinical pattern of involvement is most often similar, whereas in dizygotic twins the manifestations often differ, including cases of congenital infection in only 1 twin. The major histocompatibility complex class II gene DQ3 appears to be more frequent among HIV-infected persons seropositive for *T. gondii* who develop toxoplasmic encephalitis, and in children with congenital toxoplasmosis who develop hydrocephalus. These findings suggest that the presence of HLA-DQ3 is a risk factor for severity of toxoplasmosis. Other allelic variants of genes, including Col2A, ABC4r, P2X7r, Nalp1, TLR9, and ERAAP are also associated with susceptibility.

Congenital infection may present as a mild or severe neonatal disease or with sequelae or relapse of a previously undiagnosed and untreated infection later in infancy or even later in life. There is a wide variety of manifestations of congenital infection, ranging from hydrops fetalis and perinatal death to small size for gestational age, prematurity, peripheral retinal scars, persistent jaundice, mild thrombocytopenia, cerebrospinal fluid (CSF) pleocytosis, and the characteristic triad of chorioretinitis, hydrocephalus, and cerebral calcifications. More than 50% of congenitally infected infants are considered normal in the perinatal period, but almost all such children develop ocular involvement later in life if they are not treated during infancy. Neurologic signs such as convulsions, setting-sun sign with downward gaze, and hydrocephalus with increased head circumference may be associated with or without substantial cerebral damage or with relatively mild inflammation obstructing the aqueduct of Sylvius. If affected infants are treated promptly, signs and symptoms may resolve and development may be normal.

The spectrum and frequency of neonatal manifestations of 210 newborns with congenital *Toxoplasma* infection identified by a serologic screening program of pregnant women are presented in Table 282-1. In this study, 10% had severe congenital toxoplasmosis with CNS involvement, eye lesions, and general systemic manifestations; 34% had mild involvement with normal clinical examination results other than retinal scars or isolated intracranial calcifications; and 55% had no detectable manifestations. These numbers represent an underestimation of the incidence of severe congenital infection for several reasons: the most severe cases, including most of those individuals who died, were not referred; therapeutic abortion was often performed when acute acquired

Table 282-1 SIGNS AND SYMPTOMS IN 210 INFANTS WITH PROVED CONGENITAL *TOXOPLASMA* INFECTION*

FINDING	NO. EXAMINED	NO. POSITIVE (%)
Prematurity	210	
Birthweight <2,500 g		8 (3.8)
Birthweight 2,500-3,000 g		5 (7.1)
Intrauterine growth retardation		13 (6.2)
Icterus	201	20 (10)
Hepatosplenomegaly	210	9 (4.2)
Thrombocytopenic purpura	210	3 (1.4)
Abnormal blood count (anemia, eosinophilia)	102	9 (4.4)
Microcephaly	210	11 (5.2)
Hydrocephaly	210	8 (3.8)
Hypotonia	210	12 (5.7)
Convulsions	210	8 (3.8)
Psychomotor retardation	210	11 (5.2)
Intracranial calcification x-ray	210	24 (11.4)
Ultrasound	49	5 (10)
Computed tomography	13	11 (84)
Abnormal electroencephalogram	191	16 (8.3)
Abnormal cerebrospinal fluid	163	56 (34.2)
Microphthalmia	210	6 (2.8)
Strabismus	210	111 (5.2)
Chorioretinitis	210	
Unilateral		34 (16.1)
Bilateral		12 (5.7)

*Infants were identified by prospective study of infants born to women who acquired *Toxoplasma gondii* infection during pregnancy.
Data adapted from Couvreur J, Desmonts G, Tournier G, et al: A homogeneous series of 210 cases of congenital toxoplasmosis in 0 to 11-month-old infants detected prospectively, *Ann Pediatr (Paris)* 31:815–819, 1984.

infection of the mother was diagnosed early during pregnancy; in utero spiramycin therapy may have diminished the severity of infection; and only 13 infants had brain CT and 23% did not have a CSF examination. Routine newborn examinations often yield normal findings for congenitally infected infants, but more careful evaluations may reveal significant abnormalities. In 1 study of 28 infants identified by a universal state-mandated serologic screening program for *T. gondii*–specific IgM, 26 had normal findings on routine newborn examination and 14 had significant abnormalities detected with more careful evaluation. The abnormalities included retinal scars (7 infants), active chorioretinitis (3 infants), and CNS abnormalities (8 infants). In Fiocruz, Belo Horizonte, Brazil, infection is common, occurring in 1/600 live births. Half of these infected infants have active chorioretinitis at birth.

There is also a wide spectrum of symptoms of untreated congenital toxoplasmosis that presents later in the 1st yr of life (Table 282-2). More than 80% of these children have IQ scores of <70, and many have convulsions and severely impaired vision.

SYSTEMIC SIGNS

From 25% to >50% of infants with clinically apparent disease at birth are born prematurely. Intrauterine growth retardation, low Apgar scores, and temperature instability are common. Other manifestations may include lymphadenopathy, hepatosplenomegaly, myocarditis, pneumonitis, nephrotic syndrome, vomiting, diarrhea, and feeding problems. Bands of metaphyseal lucency and irregularity of the line of provisional calcification at the epiphyseal plate may occur without periosteal reaction in the ribs, femurs, and vertebrae. Congenital toxoplasmosis may be confused with erythroblastosis fetalis resulting from isosensitization, although the Coombs test result is usually negative with congenital *T. gondii* infection.

Table 282-2 SIGNS AND SYMPTOMS OCCURRING BEFORE DIAGNOSIS OR DURING THE COURSE OF UNTREATED ACUTE CONGENITAL TOXOPLASMOSIS IN 152 INFANTS (A) AND IN 101 OF THESE SAME CHILDREN AFTER THEY HAD BEEN FOLLOWED 4 YR OR MORE (B)

SIGNS AND SYMPTOMS	FREQUENCY OF OCCURRENCE IN PATIENTS WITH	
	"Neurologic" Disease*	"Generalized" Disease†
A. INFANTS	**108 PATIENTS (%)**	**44 PATIENTS (%)**
Chorioretinitis	102 (94)	29 (66)
Abnormal cerebrospinal fluid	59 (55)	37 (84)
Anemia	55 (51)	34 (77)
Convulsions	54 (50)	8 (18)
Intracranial calcification	54 (50)	2 (4)
Jaundice	31 (29)	35 (80)
Hydrocephalus	30 (28)	0 (0)
Fever	27 (25)	34 (77)
Splenomegaly	23 (21)	40 (90)
Lymphadenopathy	18 (17)	30 (68)
Hepatomegaly	18 (17)	34 (77)
Vomiting	17 (16)	21 (48)
Microcephalus	14 (13)	0 (0)
Diarrhea	7 (6)	11 (25)
Cataracts	5 (5)	0 (0)
Eosinophilia	6 (4)	8 (18)
Abnormal bleeding	3 (3)	8 (18)
Hypothermia	2 (2)	9 (20)
Glaucoma	2 (2)	0 (0)
Optic atrophy	2 (2)	0 (0)
Microphthalmia	2 (2)	0 (0)
Rash	1 (1)	11 (25)
Pneumonitis	0 (0)	18 (41)
B. CHILDREN ≥4 YR OF AGE	**70 PATIENTS (%)**	**31 PATIENTS (%)**
Mental retardation	62 (89)	25 (81)
Convulsions	58 (83)	24 (77)
Spasticity and palsies	53 (76)	18 (58)
Severely impaired vision	48 (69)	13 (42)
Hydrocephalus or microcephalus	31 (44)	2 (6)
Deafness	12 (17)	3 (10)
Normal	6 (9)	5 (16)

*Patients with otherwise undiagnosed central nervous system disease in the 1st yr of life.
†Patients with otherwise undiagnosed non-neurologic diseases during the 1st 2 mo of life.
Adapted from Eichenwald H: A study of congenital toxoplasmosis. In Slim JC, editor: *Human toxoplasmosis*, Copenhagen, 1960, Munksgaard, pp 41–49. Study performed in 1947. The most severely involved institutionalized patients were not included in the later study of 101 children.

Skin

Cutaneous manifestations among newborn infants with congenital toxoplasmosis include rashes, petechiae, ecchymoses, and large hemorrhages secondary to thrombocytopenia. Rashes may be fine punctate, diffuse maculopapular, lenticular, deep blue-red, sharply defined macular, or diffuse blue and papular. Macular rashes involving the entire body including the palms and soles, exfoliative dermatitis, and cutaneous calcifications have been described. Jaundice with hepatic involvement and/or hemolysis, cyanosis due to interstitial pneumonitis from congenital infection, and edema secondary to myocarditis or nephrotic syndrome may be present. Jaundice and conjugated hyperbilirubinemia may persist for months.

Endocrine Abnormalities

Endocrine abnormalities may occur secondary to hypothalamic or pituitary involvement or end-organ involvement. Reported endo-

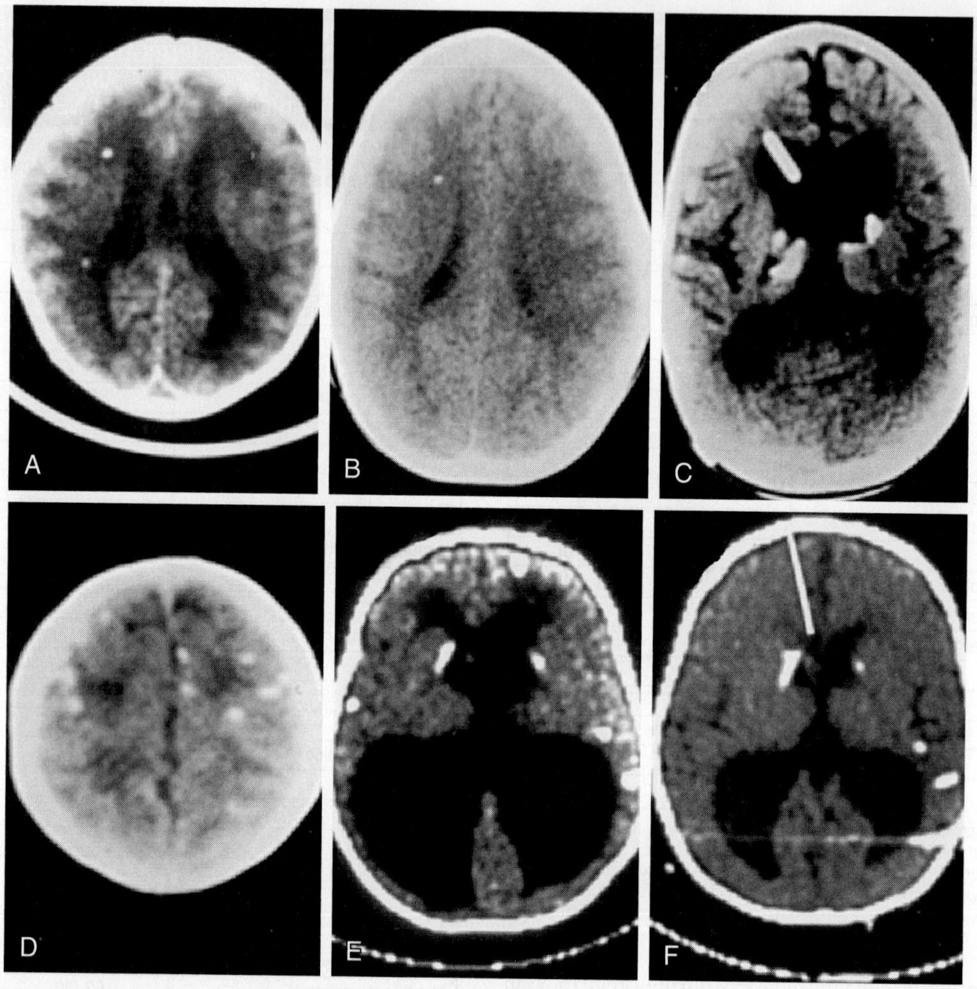

Figure 282-3 Head CT scans of infants with congenital toxoplasmosis. *A,* CT scan at birth that shows areas of hypolucency, mildly dilated ventricles, and small calcifications. *B,* CT scan of the same child at 1 yr of age (after antimicrobial therapy for 1 yr). This scan is normal with the exception of 2 small calcifications. This child's Mental Development Index (MDI) at 1 yr of age was 140 by the Bayley Scale of Infant Development. *C,* CT scan from a 1 yr old infant who was normal at birth. His meningoencephalitis became symptomatic in the 1st weeks of life but was not diagnosed correctly and remained untreated during his 1st 3 mo of life. At 3 mo of age, development of hydrocephalus and bilateral macular chorioretinitis led to the diagnosis of congenital toxoplasmosis, and antimicrobial therapy was initiated. This scan shows significant residual atrophy and calcifications. This child had substantial motor dysfunction, development delays, and visual impairment. *D,* CT scan obtained during the 1st mo of life of a microcephalic child. Note the numerous calcifications. This child's IQ scores using the Stanford-Binet Intelligence Scale for children when she was 3 yr of age and the Wechsler Preschool and Primary Scale Intelligence when she was 5 yr of age were 100 and 102, respectively. She received antimicrobial therapy during her 1st yr of life. *E,* CT scan with hydrocephalus owing to aqueductal stenosis, before shunt. *F,* Scan from the same patient as the scan in *E,* after shunt. This child's IQ scores using the Stanford-Binet Intelligence Scale for children were approximately 100 when she was 3 and 6 yr of age. (Adapted from McAuley J, Boyer K, Patel D, et al: Early and longitudinal evaluations of treated infants and children and untreated historical patients with congenital toxoplasmosis: the Chicago Collaborative Treatment Trial, *Clin Infect Dis* 18:38–72, 1994.)

crinopathies include myxedema, persistent hypernatremia with vasopressin-sensitive diabetes insipidus without polyuria or polydipsia, sexual precocity, and partial anterior hypopituitarism.

Central Nervous System

Neurologic manifestations of congenital toxoplasmosis vary from massive acute encephalopathy to subtle neurologic syndromes. Toxoplasmosis should be considered as a potential cause of any undiagnosed neurologic disease in children <1 yr of age, especially if retinal lesions are present.

Hydrocephalus may be the sole clinical neurologic manifestation of congenital toxoplasmosis and may be compensated but most often requires shunt placement. Hydrocephalus may present prenatally and progress during the perinatal period, or, less commonly, may present later in life. Patterns of seizures are protean and have included focal motor seizures, petit and grand mal seizures, muscular twitching, opisthotonus, and hypsarrhythmia. Spinal or bulbar involvement may be manifested by paralysis of the extremities, difficulty swallowing, and respiratory distress. Microcephaly usually reflects severe brain damage, but some children with microcephaly caused by congenital toxoplasmosis who have been treated have normal or superior cognitive function. Untreated congenital toxoplasmosis that is symptomatic in the 1st yr of life can cause substantial diminution in cognitive function and developmental delay. Intellectual impairment also occurs in some children with subclinical infection without or despite treatment with pyrimethamine and sulfonamides. Seizures and focal motor defects may become apparent after the newborn period, even when infection is subclinical at birth.

CSF abnormalities occur in at least 30% of infants with congenital toxoplasmosis. A CSF protein level of >1 g/dL is characteristic of severe CNS toxoplasmosis and is usually accompanied by hydrocephalus. Local production of *T. gondii*–specific IgG and IgM antibodies may be demonstrated. CT of the brain is useful to detect calcifications, determine ventricular size, and demonstrate porencephalic cystic structures (Fig. 282-3). Calcifications occur throughout the brain, but there is a propensity for development of calcifications in the caudate nucleus and basal ganglia, choroid plexus, and subependyma. MRI and contrast-enhanced CT brain scans are useful for detecting active inflammatory lesions. MRIs that take only a brief time (<45 sec) for imaging or ultrasonography may be useful for following ventricular size. Treatment in utero and in the 1st yr of life results in improved neurologic outcomes.

Eyes

Almost all untreated congenitally infected infants develop chorioretinal lesions by adulthood, and about 50% will have severe visual impairment. *T. gondii* causes a focal necrotizing retinitis in congenitally infected individuals (see Fig. 282-2). Retinal detachment may occur. Any part of the retina may be involved, either unilaterally or bilaterally, including the maculae. The optic nerve may be involved, and toxoplasmic lesions that involve projections of the visual pathways in the brain or the visual cortex also may lead to visual impairment. In association with retinal lesions and vitritis, the anterior uvea may be intensely inflamed, leading to erythema of the external eye. Other ocular findings include cells and protein in the anterior chamber, large keratic precipitates, posterior synechiae, nodules on the iris, and neovascular formation on the surface of the iris, sometimes with increased intraocular pressure and glaucoma. The extraocular musculature may also be involved directly. Other manifestations include strabismus, nystagmus, visual impairment, and microphthalmia. Enucleation has been required for a blind, phthisic, painful eye. The differential diagnosis of ocular toxoplasmosis includes congenital coloboma and inflammatory lesions caused by cytomegalovirus, *Treponema pallidum, Mycobacterium tuberculosis,* or vasculitis. Ocular toxoplasmosis may be a recurrent and progressive disease that requires multiple courses of therapy. Limited data suggest that occurrence of lesions in the early years of life may be prevented by instituting antimicrobial treatment with pyrimethamine and sulfonamides during the 1st yr of life and that treatment of the infected fetus in utero followed by treatment in the 1st yr of life with pyrimethamine, sulfadiazine, and leukovorin reduces the incidence and the severity of the retinal disease.

Ears

Sensorineural hearing loss, both mild and severe, may occur. It is not known whether this is a static or progressive disorder. Treatment in the 1st yr of life is associated with decreased frequency of hearing loss.

DIAGNOSIS

Diagnosis of acute *Toxoplasma* infection can be established by culture of *T. gondii* from blood or body fluids; identification of tachyzoites in sections or preparations of tissues and body fluids, amniotic fluid, or placenta; identification of cysts in the placenta or tissues of a fetus or newborn; and characteristic lymph node histologic features. Serologic tests also are very useful for diagnosis. Polymerase chain reaction (PCR) also is useful to identify *T. gondii* DNA in CSF, amniotic fluid, infant peripheral blood, and urine to definitively establish the diagnosis.

Culture

Organisms are isolated by inoculation of body fluids, leukocytes, or tissue specimens into mice or tissue cultures. Body fluids should be processed and inoculated immediately, but *T. gondii* has been isolated from tissues and blood that have been stored overnight or even for 4-5 days at 4°C. Freezing or treatment of specimens with formalin kills *T. gondii.* From 6 to 10 days after inoculation into mice, or earlier if mice die, peritoneal fluids should be examined for tachyzoites. If inoculated mice survive for 6 wk and seroconvert, definitive diagnosis is made by visualization of *Toxoplasma* cysts in mouse brain. If cysts are not seen, subinoculations of mouse tissue into other mice are performed.

Microscopic examination of tissue culture inoculated with *T. gondii* shows necrotic, heavily infected cells with numerous extracellular tachyzoites. Isolation of *T. gondii* from blood or body fluids reflects acute infection. Except in the fetus or neonate, it is usually not possible to distinguish acute from past infection by isolation of *T. gondii* from tissues such as skeletal muscle, lung, brain, or eye obtained by biopsy or at autopsy.

Diagnosis of acute infection can be established by demonstration of tachyzoites in biopsy tissue sections, bone marrow aspirate, or body fluids such as CSF or amniotic fluid. Immunofluorescent antibody and immunoperoxidase staining techniques may be necessary, because it is often difficult to distinguish the tachyzoite using ordinary stains. Tissue cysts are diagnostic of infection but do not differentiate between acute and chronic infection, although the presence of many cysts suggests recent acute infection. Cysts in the placenta or tissues of the newborn infant establish the diagnosis of congenital infection. Characteristic histologic features strongly suggest the diagnosis of toxoplasmic lymphadenitis.

Serologic Testing

Multiple serologic tests may be necessary to confirm the diagnosis of congenital or acutely acquired *Toxoplasma* infection. Each laboratory that reports serologic test results must have established values for their tests that diagnose infection in specific clinical settings, provide interpretation of their results, and ensure appropriate quality control before therapy is based on serologic test results. Serologic test results used as the basis for therapy should be confirmed in a reference laboratory.

The **Sabin-Feldman dye test** is sensitive and specific. It measures primarily IgG antibodies. Results should be expressed in international units (IU/mL), based on international standard reference sera available from the World Health Organization.

The **IgG indirect fluorescent-antibody (IgG-IFA) test** measures the same antibodies as the dye test, and the titers tend to be parallel. These antibodies usually appear 1-2 wk after infection, reach high titers (≥1 : 1,000) after 6-8 wk, and then decline over months to years. Low titers (1 : 4 to 1 : 64) usually persist for life. Antibody titer does not correlate with severity of illness. Approximately half of the commercially available IFA kits for *T. gondii* have been found to be improperly standardized and may yield significant numbers of false-positive and false-negative results.

An **agglutination test** (Bio-Mérieux, Lyon, France) that is available commercially in Europe uses formalin-preserved whole parasites to detect IgG antibodies. This test is accurate, simple to perform, and inexpensive.

The **IgM-IFA test** is useful for the diagnosis of acute infection with *T. gondii* in the older child because IgM antibodies appear earlier, often by 5 days after infection, and diminish more quickly than IgG antibodies. In most instances, IgM antibodies rise rapidly (1 : 50 to <1 : 1,000) and then fall to low titers (1 : 10 or 1 : 20) or disappear after weeks or months. However, some patients continue to have positive IgM results with low titers for several years. The IgM-IFA test detects *Toxoplasma*-specific IgM in only approximately 25% of congenitally infected infants at birth. IgM antibodies may not be present in sera of immunocompromised patients with acute toxoplasmosis or in patients with reactivation of ocular toxoplasmosis. The IgM-IFA test may yield false-positive results as a result of rheumatoid factor.

The **double-sandwich IgM enzyme-linked immunosorbent assay (IgM-ELISA)** is more sensitive and specific than the IgM-IFA test for detection of *Toxoplasma* IgM antibodies. In the older child, serum IgM-ELISA *Toxoplasma* antibodies of >2.0 (a value of 1 reference laboratory; each laboratory must establish its own value) indicates that *Toxoplasma* infection most likely has been acquired recently. The IgM-ELISA identifies approximately

50-75% of infants with congenital infection. IgM-ELISA avoids both the false-positive results from rheumatoid factor and the false-negative results from high levels of passively transferred maternal IgG antibody in fetal serum, as may occur in the IgM-IFA test. Results obtained with commercial kits must be interpreted with caution, because false-positive reactions are not infrequent. Care must also be taken to determine whether kits have been standardized for diagnosis of infection in specific clinical settings, such as in the newborn infant. The **IgA-ELISA** also is a sensitive test for detection of maternal and congenital infection, and results may be positive when those of the IgM-ELISA are not.

The **immunosorbent agglutination assay (ISAGA)** combines trapping of a patient's IgM, IgA, or IgE to a solid surface and use of formalin-fixed organisms or antigen-coated latex particles. It is read as an agglutination test. There are no false-positive results from rheumatoid factor or antinuclear antibodies. The IgM-ISAGA is more sensitive than the IgM-ELISA and may detect specific IgM antibodies before and for longer periods than the IgM-ELISA.

At present, the IgM-ISAGA, the **IgA-ISAGA,** and the **IgA-ELISA** are the best tests for diagnosis of congenital infection in the newborn. The **IgE-ELISA** and **IgE-ISAGA** are also sometimes useful in establishing the diagnosis of congenital toxoplasmosis or acute acquired *T. gondii* infection. The presence of IgM antibodies in the older child or adult can never be used alone to diagnose acute acquired infection.

The **differential agglutination test** (HS/AC) compares antibody titers obtained with formalin-fixed tachyzoites **(HS antigen)** with titers obtained using acetone- or methanol-fixed tachyzoites **(AC antigen)** to differentiate recent and remote infections in adults and older children. This method may be particularly useful in differentiating remote infection in pregnant women, because levels of IgM and IgA antibodies detectable by ELISA or ISAGA may remain elevated for months to years in adults and older children.

The **avidity test** can be helpful to time infection. A high-avidity test result indicates that infection began >16 wk earlier, which is especially useful in determining time of acquisition of infection in the 1st or final 16 wk of gestation. A low-avidity test result may be present for many months and is not diagnostic of recent acquisition of infection.

A relatively higher level of *Toxoplasma* antibody in the aqueous humor or in CSF demonstrates local production of antibody during active ocular or CNS toxoplasmosis. This comparison is performed, and a coefficient [C] is calculated as follows:

$$C = \frac{\text{Antibody titer in body fluid}}{\text{Antibody titer in serum}} \times \frac{\text{Concentration of IgG in serum}}{\text{Concentration of IgG in body fluid}}$$

Significant coefficients [C] are >8 for ocular infection, >4 for CNS for congenital infection, and >1 for CNS infection in patients with AIDS. If the serum dye test titer is >300 IU/mL, most often it is not possible to demonstrate significant local antibody production using this formula with either the dye test or the IgM-IFA test titer. IgM antibody may be detectable in CSF.

Comparative **Western immunoblot** tests of sera from a mother and infant may detect congenital infection. Infection is suspected when the mother's serum and her infant's serum contain antibodies that react with different *Toxoplasma* antigens.

The **enzyme-linked immunofiltration assay (ELIFA)** using micropore membranes permits simultaneous study of antibody specificity by immunoprecipitation and characterization of antibody isotypes by immunofiltration with enzyme-labeled antibodies. This method is capable of detecting 85% of cases of congenital infection in the 1st few days of life.

PCR is used to amplify the DNA of *T. gondii,* which then can be detected by using a DNA probe. Detection of repetitive *T. gondii* genes, the B1 or 529 bp, 300 copy gene, in amniotic fluid is the PCR target of choice for establishing the diagnosis of congenital *Toxoplasma* infection in the fetus. Sensitivity and specificity of this test in amniotic fluid obtained to diagnose infections acquired between 17 and 21 wk of gestation are approximately 95%. Before and after that time, PCR with the 529 bp, 300 copy repeat gene as the template is 92% sensitive and 100% specific for detection of congenital infection. PCR of vitreous or aqueous fluids also has been used to diagnose ocular toxoplasmosis. PCR of peripheral white blood cells, CSF, and urine has been used to detect congenital infection.

Lymphocyte blastogenesis to *Toxoplasma* antigens has been used to diagnose congenital toxoplasmosis when the diagnosis is uncertain and other test results are negative. However, a negative result does not exclude the diagnosis because many infected newborns do not respond to *T. gondii* antigens.

Acquired Toxoplasmosis

Recent infection is diagnosed by seroconversion from a negative to a positive IgG antibody titer (in the absence of transfusion); a 2 tube increase in *Toxoplasma*-specific IgG titer when serial sera are obtained 3 wk apart and tested in parallel; or the detection of *Toxoplasma*-specific IgM antibody in conjunction with other tests, but never alone.

Ocular Toxoplasmosis

IgG antibody titers of 1:4 to 1:64 are usual in older children with active *Toxoplasma* chorioretinitis. Presence of antibodies measurable only when serum is tested undiluted is helpful in establishing the diagnosis. The diagnosis is likely with characteristic retinal lesions and positive serologic tests. PCR of aqueous or vitreous fluid has been used to diagnose ocular toxoplasmosis but is infrequently performed because of risks associated with obtaining fluid.

Immunocompromised Persons

IgG antibody titers may be low, and *Toxoplasma*-specific IgM is often absent in immunocompromised stem cell transplant recipients, but not kidney or heart transplant recipients with toxoplasmosis. Demonstration of *Toxoplasma* antigens or DNA in serum, blood, and CSF may identify disseminated *Toxoplasma* infection in immunocompromised persons. Resolution of CNS lesions during a therapeutic trial of pyrimethamine and sulfadiazine has been useful to diagnose toxoplasmic encephalitis in patients with AIDS. Brain biopsy has been used to establish the diagnosis if there is no response to a therapeutic trial and to exclude other likely diagnoses such as CNS lymphoma.

Congenital Toxoplasmosis

Fetal ultrasound examination, performed every 2 wk during gestation, beginning at the time acute acquired infection is diagnosed in a pregnant woman, and PCR analysis of amniotic fluid are used for prenatal diagnosis. *T. gondii* may also be isolated from the placenta at delivery.

Serologic tests are also useful in establishing a diagnosis of congenital toxoplasmosis. Either persistent or rising titers in the dye test or IFA test, or a positive IgM-ELISA or IgM-ISAGA result is diagnostic of congenital toxoplasmosis. The half-life of IgM is about 2 days, so if there is a placental leak, the level of IgM antibodies in the infant's serum decreases significantly, usually within 1 wk. Passively transferred maternal IgG antibodies may require many months to a year to disappear from the infant's serum, depending on the magnitude of the original titer. Synthesis of *Toxoplasma* antibody is usually demonstrable by the 3rd mo of life if the infant is untreated. If the infant is treated, synthesis may be delayed for as long as the 9th mo of life and, infrequently, may not occur at all. When an infant begins to synthesize IgG antibody, infection may be documented serologically even without demonstration of IgM antibodies by an increase in the ratio of specific serum IgG antibody titer to the total IgG, whereas the ratio will decrease if the specific IgG antibody has been passively transferred from the mother.

Newborns suspected of having congenital toxoplasmosis should be evaluated by general, ophthalmologic, and neurologic examinations; head CT scan; attempt to isolate *T. gondii* from the placenta and infant's leukocytes from peripheral blood buffy coat; measurement of serum *Toxoplasma*-specific IgG, IgM, IgA, and IgE antibodies, and the levels of total serum IgM and IgG; lumbar puncture including analysis of CSF for cells, glucose, protein, *Toxoplasma*-specific IgG and IgM antibodies, and level of total IgG; and testing of CSF for *T. gondii* by PCR and inoculation into mice. Presence of *Toxoplasma*-specific IgM in CSF that is not contaminated with blood or confirmation of local antibody production of *Toxoplasma*-specific IgG antibody in CSF establishes the diagnosis of congenital *Toxoplasma* infection.

Many manifestations of congenital toxoplasmosis occur in other perinatal infections, especially congenital cytomegalovirus infection. Neither cerebral calcification nor chorioretinitis is pathognomonic. The clinical picture in the newborn infant may also be compatible with sepsis, aseptic meningitis, syphilis, or hemolytic disease. Some children <5 yr of age with chorioretinitis have postnatally acquired *T. gondii* infection.

TREATMENT

Pyrimethamine and sulfadiazine act synergistically against *Toxoplasma,* and combination therapy is indicated for many of the forms of toxoplasmosis. Use of pyrimethamine is contraindicated during the 1st trimester of pregnancy. Spiramycin should be used to attempt to prevent vertical transmission of infection to the fetus of acutely infected pregnant women. Pyrimethamine inhibits the enzyme dihydrofolate reductase (DHFR), and thus the synthesis of folic acid, and therefore produces a dose-related, reversible, and usually gradual depression of the bone marrow. Neutropenia is most common but rarely has treatment been reported to result in thrombocytopenia and anemia. Reversible neutropenia is the most common adverse effect in treated infants. All patients treated with pyrimethamine should have platelet and leukocyte counts twice weekly. Seizures may occur with overdosage of pyrimethamine. Folinic acid, as calcium leukovorin, should always be administered concomitantly and for 1 wk after treatment with pyrimethamine is discontinued to prevent bone marrow suppression. Potential toxic effects of sulfonamides (e.g., crystalluria, hematuria, and rash) should be monitored. Hypersensitivity reactions occur, especially in patients with AIDS.

Acquired Toxoplasmosis

Patients with acquired toxoplasmosis and lymphadenopathy do not need specific treatment unless they have severe and persistent symptoms or evidence of damage to vital organs. If such signs and symptoms occur, treatment with pyrimethamine, sulfadiazine, and leukovorin should be initiated. Patients who appear to be immunocompetent but have severe and persistent symptoms or damage to vital organs (e.g., chorioretinitis, myocarditis) need specific therapy until these specific symptoms resolve, followed by therapy for an additional 2 wk. Therapy is usually administered for at least 4-6 wk. The optimal duration of therapy is unknown. A loading dose of pyrimethamine for older children is 2 mg/kg/day divided bid (maximum 50 mg/day), given for the 1st 2 days of treatment. The maintenance dose is 1 mg/kg/day (maximum 50 mg/day). Sulfadiazine is administered to children >1 yr of age at a dosage of 100 mg/kg/day divided bid (maximum 4 g/day). Leukovorin is administered orally at a dosage of 5-20 mg 3 times a week (or even daily depending on the leukocyte count).

Ocular Toxoplasmosis

Patients with ocular toxoplasmosis are usually treated with pyrimethamine, sulfadiazine, and leukovorin for approximately 1 wk after the lesion develops a quiescent appearance (i.e., sharp borders and associated inflammatory cells in the vitreous resolve), which usually occurs in 2-4 wk. Within 7-10 days the borders of the retinal lesions sharpen, and visual acuity usually returns to that noted before development of the acute lesion. Systemic corticosteroids have been administered concomitantly with antimicrobial treatment when lesions involve the macula, optic nerve head, or papillomacular bundle. Corticosteroids are never given alone and are begun after loading doses of pyrimethamine and sulfadiazine have been administered (2 days). Most new lesions appear contiguous to old ones. Very rarely, vitrectomy and removal of the lens are needed to restore visual acuity. Suppressive treatment has prevented frequent recurrences of vision-threatening lesions.

Immunocompromised Persons

Serologic evidence of acute infection in an immunocompromised patient, regardless of whether signs and symptoms of infection are present or tachyzoites are demonstrated in tissue, are indications for therapy similar to that described for immunocompetent persons with symptoms of organ injury. It is important to establish the diagnosis as rapidly as possible and institute treatment early. In immunocompromised patients other than those with AIDS, therapy should be continued for at least 4-6 wk beyond complete resolution of all signs and symptoms of active disease. Careful follow-up observation of these patients is imperative because relapse may occur, requiring prompt reinstitution of therapy. Relapse is frequent in patients with AIDS, and suppressive therapy with pyrimethamine and sulfonamides, or trimethoprim-sulfamethoxazole, traditionally has been continued for life. It is possible to discontinue maintenance therapy when the CD4 count remains at >200 cells/μL for 4-6 mo and all lesions have resolved. Therapy usually induces a beneficial response clinically, but it does not eradicate cysts. Treatment of *T. gondii*–seropositive patients with AIDS should be continued as long as CD4 counts remain at <200 cells/μL. Prophylactic treatment with trimethoprim-sulfamethoxazole for *Pneumocystis carinii* pneumonia significantly reduces the incidence of toxoplasmosis in patients with AIDS.

Congenital Toxoplasmosis

All newborns infected with *T. gondii* should be treated whether or not they have clinical manifestations of the infection because treatment may be effective in interrupting acute disease that damages vital organs. Infants should be treated for 1 yr with pyrimethamine (2 mg/kg/day divided bid for 2 days, then 1 mg/kg/day for 2 or 6 mo, and then 1 mg/kg given on Monday, Wednesday, and Friday [or more often], PO), sulfadiazine (100 mg/kg/day divided bid PO), and leukovorin (5-10 mg given on Monday, Wednesday, and Friday, or more often depending on neutrophil count, PO). The relative efficacy in reducing sequelae of infection and the safety of treatment with 2 vs 6 mo of the higher dosage of pyrimethamine are being compared in the U.S. National Collaborative Study. Updated information about this study and these regimens is available from Dr. Rima McLeod (773-834-4131). Pyrimethamine and sulfadiazine are available only in tablet form and can be prepared as suspensions. Prednisone (1 mg/kg/day divided bid PO) has been utilized in addition when active chorioretinitis involves the macula or otherwise threatens vision or the CSF protein is >1,000 mg/dL at birth, but the efficacy is not established. Prednisone is continued only for as long as the active inflammatory process in the posterior pole of the eye is vision threatening or CSF protein is >1,000 mg/dL and then tapered rapidly if the duration of treatment has been brief.

Pregnant Women with *T. gondii* Infection

The immunologically normal pregnant woman who acquired *T. gondii* before conception does not need treatment to prevent congenital infection of her fetus. Although data are not available to allow for a definitive time interval, if infection occurs during the 6 mo prior to conception, it is reasonable to evaluate the fetus by use of PCR with amniotic fluid and ultrasonography and treat to prevent congenital infection in the fetus in the same manner as described for the acutely infected pregnant patient.

Treatment of a pregnant woman who acquires infection at any time during pregnancy reduces the chance of congenital infection in her infant. Spiramycin (1 g every 8 hr PO without food) is recommended for prevention of fetal infection if the mother develops acute toxoplasmosis during pregnancy. Spiramycin is available in the USA through the Food and Drug Administration (301-796-1600, attn. Leo Chan) after the diagnosis of acute infection is confirmed in a reference laboratory (650-326-8120). Adverse reactions are infrequent and include paresthesias, rash, nausea, vomiting, and diarrhea. Pyrimethamine (50 mg once daily PO), sulfadiazine (1.5-2 g bid PO), and leukovorin (10 mg once daily PO) are recommended for treatment of the pregnant woman whose fetus has confirmed or probable fetal infection except in the 1st trimester. In the 1st trimester when there is definite infection, sulfadiazine alone is recommended because pyrimethamine is potentially teratogenic at that time. Spiramycin treatment is used early in gestation when it is uncertain whether there is fetal infection. Treatment of the mother of an infected fetus with pyrimethamine and sulfadiazine reduces infection in the placenta and the severity of disease in the newborn. Delay in maternal treatment during gestation results in greater brain and eye disease in the infant. Diagnostic amniocentesis should be performed at >17-18 wk of gestation in pregnancies when there is high suspicion of fetal infection. Overall sensitivity of PCR for amniotic fluid is at 85% between 17 and 21 wk of gestation. The sensitivity of PCR using amniotic fluid for diagnosis of fetal infection is 92% in early and late gestation when amniotic fluid is tested for presence of the 529 bp, 300 copy gene. After 24 weeks gestation, incidence of transmission is high and pregnant women who are infected acutely after that time are often treated with pyrimethamine and sulfadiazine to treat the fetus.

The approach in France to congenital toxoplasmosis includes systematic serologic screening of all women of childbearing age and again intrapartum each month during gestation, at term, and 1 mo after term. Mothers with acute infection are treated with spiramycin, which decreases the transmission from 60-23%. Ultrasonography and amniocentesis for PCR at approximately 18 wk of gestation are used for fetal diagnosis, which have 97% sensitivity and 100% specificity. Confidence intervals for sensitivity are largest early and late in gestation. Fetal infection is treated with pyrimethamine and sulfadiazine. Termination of pregnancy is very rare at present. Treatment with pyrimethamine and sulfadiazine during pregnancy usually has an excellent outcome, with normal development of children. Only 19% have subtle findings of congenital infection, including intracranial calcifications (13%) and chorioretinal scars (6%), although 39% have chorioretinal scars detected at follow-up observation during later childhood. Several studies have demonstrated improved outcomes with shorter times between diagnosis and initiation of treatment.

Chronically infected pregnant women who are immunocompromised have transmitted *T. gondii* to their fetuses. Such women should be treated with spiramycin throughout gestation. The optimal management for prevention of congenital toxoplasmosis in the fetus of a pregnant woman with HIV infection and inactive *T. gondii* infection is unknown. If the pregnancy is not terminated, some investigators suggest that the mother should be treated with spiramycin during the 1st 14 wk of gestation and thereafter with pyrimethamine and sulfadiazine until term. There are no accepted guidelines. In a study of adult patients with AIDS, pyrimethamine (75 mg once daily PO) combined with high dosages of intravenously administered clindamycin (1,200 mg every 6 hr IV) appeared equal in efficacy to sulfadiazine and pyrimethamine in the treatment of toxoplasmic encephalitis. Other experimental agents include the macrolides roxithromycin and azithromycin.

Active choroidal neovasular membranes due to toxoplasmic chorioretinitis have been treated successfully in children with intravitreal injection of antibody to VegF.

PROGNOSIS

Early institution of specific treatment for congenitally infected infants usually cures the active manifestations of toxoplasmosis, including active chorioretinitis, meningitis, encephalitis, hepatitis, splenomegaly, and thrombocytopenia. Rarely, hydrocephalus resulting from aqueductal obstruction may develop or become worse during therapy. Treatment appears to reduce the incidence of some sequelae such as diminished cognitive and abnormal motor function. Without therapy and in some treated patients as well, chorioretinitis often recurs. Children with extensive involvement at birth may function normally later in life or have mild to severe impairment of vision, hearing, cognitive function, and other neurologic functions. Delays in diagnosis and therapy, perinatal hypoglycemia, hypoxia, hypotension, repeated shunt infections, and severe visual impairment are associated with a poorer prognosis. The prognosis is guarded but is not necessarily poor for infected babies. Treatment with pyrimethamine and sulfadiazine does not eradicate encysted parasites.

Studies in Lyon and Paris, France, demonstrated that outcome of treated fetal toxoplasmosis, even when infection is acquired early in gestation, is usually favorable if no hydrocephalus is detected on ultrasound, and treatment with pyrimethamine and sulfadiazine is initiated promptly. The SYROCOT study in Europe indicated that outcome is improved with shorter times between diagnosis and initiation of treatment of fetal toxoplasmosis. Work in Lyon, France, has indicated a low incidence of recurrent eye disease in children with congenital toxoplasmosis who had been treated in utero and in their 1st yr of life. The National Collaborative Chicago-based Congenital Toxoplasmosis Study (NCCCTS) (1981-2004) in the USA found that neurologic, developmental, audiologic, and ophthalmologic outcomes are considerably better for most, but not all, children who were treated in their 1st yr of life with pyrimethamine and sulfadiazine (with leukovorin) when compared to children who had not been treated or were treated for only 1 mo in earlier decades. The mean age of the children in this study is 10.8 yr at the time of this analysis, and most of the children had not yet entered their teenage years, which is a time when recurrent disease may increase.

PREVENTION

Counseling pregnant women about the methods of preventing transmission of *T. gondii* (see Fig. 282-1) during pregnancy can reduce acquisition of infection during gestation. Women who do not have specific antibody to *T. gondii* before pregnancy should only eat well-cooked meat during pregnancy and avoid contact with oocysts excreted by cats. Cats that are kept indoors, maintained on prepared food, and not fed fresh, uncooked meat should not contact encysted *T. gondii* or shed oocysts. Serologic screening, ultrasound monitoring, and treatment of pregnant women during gestation can also reduce the incidence and manifestations of congenital toxoplasmosis. No protective vaccine is available.

BIBLIOGRAPHY

Please visit the Nelson Textbook of Pediatrics *website at* *www.expertconsult.com* *for the complete bibliography.*

Section 16 HELMINTHIC DISEASES

Chapter 283
Ascariasis (*Ascaris lumbricoides*)

Arlene E. Dent and James W. Kazura

ETIOLOGY

Ascariasis is caused by the nematode, or roundworm, *Ascaris lumbricoides*. Adult worms of *A. lumbricoides* inhabit the lumen of the small intestine and have a life span of 10-24 mo. The reproductive potential of *Ascaris* is prodigious; a gravid female worm produces 200,000 eggs/day. The fertile ova are oval in shape with a thick mammillated covering measuring 45-70 µm in length and 35-50 µm in breadth (Fig. 283-1). After passage in the feces, the eggs embryonate and become infective in 5-10 days under favorable environmental conditions. Adult worms can live for 12-18 mo (Fig. 283-2).

EPIDEMIOLOGY

Ascariasis occurs globally and is the most prevalent human helminthiasis in the world. It is most common in tropical areas of the world where environmental conditions are optimal for maturation of ova in the soil. Approximately 1 billion persons are estimated to be infected, with 4 million cases in the USA. Key factors linked with a higher prevalence of infection include poor socioeconomic conditions, use of human feces as fertilizer, and geophagia. Even though infection can occur at any age, the highest rate is in preschool or early school-aged children. Transmission is primarily hand to mouth but may also involve ingestion of contaminated raw fruits and vegetables. Transmission is enhanced by the high output of eggs by fecund female worms and resistance of ova to the outside environment. *Ascaris* eggs can remain viable at 5-10°C for as long as 2 yr.

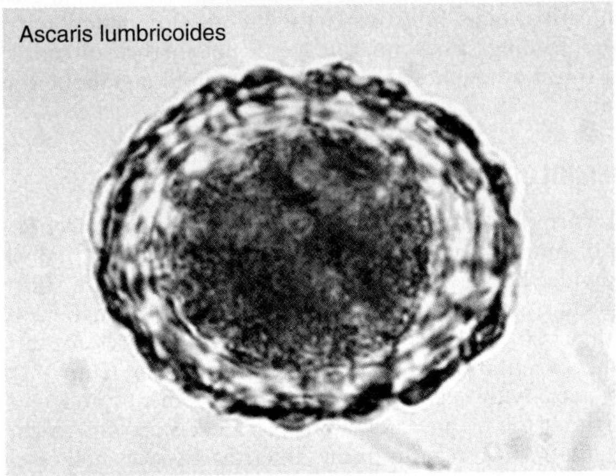

Figure 283-1 Soil-transmitted helminth eggs. (From Bethony J, Brooker S, Albonico M, et al: Soil-transmitted helminth infections: ascariasis, trichuriasis, and hookworm, *Lancet* 367:1521–1532, 2006.)

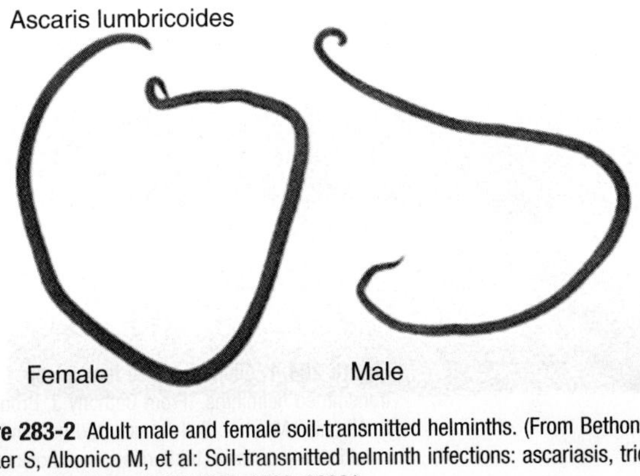

Figure 283-2 Adult male and female soil-transmitted helminths. (From Bethony J, Brooker S, Albonico M, et al: Soil-transmitted helminth infections: ascariasis, trichuriasis, and hookworm, *Lancet* 367:1521–1532, 2006.)

PATHOGENESIS

Ascaris ova hatch in the small intestine after ingestion by the human host. Larvae are released, penetrate the intestinal wall, and migrate to the lungs by way of the venous circulation. The parasites then cause **pulmonary ascariasis** as they enter into the alveoli and migrate through the bronchi and trachea. They are subsequently swallowed and return to the intestines, where they mature into adult worms. Female *Ascaris* begin depositing eggs in 8-10 wk.

CLINICAL MANIFESTATIONS

The clinical presentation depends on the intensity of infection and the organs involved. Most individuals have low to moderate worm burdens and have no symptoms or signs. The most common clinical problems are due to pulmonary disease and obstruction of the intestinal or biliary tract. Larvae migrating through these tissues may cause allergic symptoms, fever, urticaria, and granulomatous disease. The pulmonary manifestations resemble Loeffler syndrome and include transient respiratory symptoms such as cough and dyspnea, pulmonary infiltrates, and blood eosinophilia. Larvae may be observed in the sputum. Vague abdominal complaints have been attributed to the presence of adult worms in the small intestine, although the precise contribution of the parasite to these symptoms is difficult to ascertain. A more serious complication occurs when a large mass of worms leads to acute bowel obstruction. Children with heavy infections may present with vomiting, abdominal distention, and cramps. In some cases, worms may be passed in the vomitus or stools. *Ascaris* worms occasionally migrate into the biliary and pancreatic ducts, where they cause cholecystitis or pancreatitis. Worm migration through the intestinal wall can lead to peritonitis. Dead worms can serve as a nidus for stone formation. Studies show that chronic infection with *A. lumbricoides* (often coincident with other helminth infections) impairs growth, physical fitness, and cognitive development.

DIAGNOSIS

Microscopic examination of fecal smears can be used for diagnosis because of the high number of eggs excreted by adult female worms (see Fig. 283-1). A high index of suspicion in the appropriate clinical context is needed to diagnose pulmonary ascariasis or obstruction of the gastrointestinal tract. Ultrasound examination of the abdomen is capable of visualizing intraluminal adult worms.

TREATMENT

Although several chemotherapeutic agents are effective against ascariasis, none have documented utility during the pulmonary phase of infection. Treatment options for gastrointestinal ascariasis include albendazole (400 mg PO once, for all ages), mebendazole (100 mg bid PO for 3 days or 500 mg PO once for all ages), or pyrantel pamoate (11 mg/kg PO once, maximum 1 g). Piperazine citrate (75 mg/kg/day for 2 days maximum 3.5 g/day), which causes neuromuscular paralysis of the parasite and rapid expulsion of the worms, is the treatment of choice for intestinal or biliary obstruction and is administered as syrup through a nasogastric tube. Surgery may be required for cases with severe obstruction. Nitazoxanide (100 mg bid PO for 3 days for children 1-3 yr of age, 200 mg bid PO for 3 days for children 4-11 yr, and 500 mg bid PO for 3 days for adolescents and adults) produces cure rates comparable with single-dose albendazole.

PREVENTION

Although ascariasis is the most prevalent worm infection in the world, little attention has been given to its control. Anthelmintic chemotherapy programs can be implemented in 1 of 3 ways: (1) offering universal treatment to all individuals in an area of high endemicity; (2) offering treatment targeted to groups with high frequency of infection, such as children attending primary school; or (3) offering individual treatment based on intensity of current or past infection. Improving sanitary conditions and sewage facilities, discontinuing the practice of using human feces as fertilizer, and education are the most effective long-term preventive measures.

BIBLIOGRAPHY

Please visit the Nelson Textbook of Pediatrics *website at www.expertconsult.com for the complete bibliography.*

Chapter 284
Hookworms (*Necator americanus* and *Ancylostoma* spp.)

Peter J. Hotez

ETIOLOGY

Two major genera of hookworms, which are nematodes or roundworms, infect humans. *Necator americanus,* the only representative of its genus, is a major anthropophilic hookworm and is the most common cause of human hookworm infection. Hookworms of the genus *Ancylostoma* includes the major anthropophilic hookworm *Ancylostoma duodenale* that also causes classic hookworm infection and the less common zoonotic species *A. ceylanicum, A. caninum,* and *A. braziliense.* Human zoonotic infection with the dog hookworm *A. caninum* is associated with an eosinophilic enteritis syndrome. The larval stage of *A. braziliense,* whose definitive hosts include dogs and cats, is the principal cause of cutaneous larva migrans.

The infective larval stages of the anthropophilic hookworms live in a developmentally arrested state in warm, moist soil. Larvae infect humans either by penetrating through the skin (*N. americanus* and *A. duodenale*) or when they are ingested (*A. duodenale*). Larvae entering the human host by skin penetration undergo **extraintestinal migration** through the venous circulation and lungs before they are swallowed, whereas orally ingested larvae may undergo extraintestinal migration or remain in the gastrointestinal tract. Larvae returning to the small intestine undergo 2 molts to become adult sexually mature male and female worms ranging in length from 5 to 13 mm. The buccal capsule of the adult hookworm is armed with cutting plates (*N. americanus*) or teeth (*A. duodenale*) to facilitate attachment to the mucosa and submucosa of the small intestine. Hookworms can remain in the intestine for 1-5 yr, where they mate and produce eggs. Although approximately 2 mo is required for the larval stages of hookworms to undergo extraintestinal migration and develop into mature adults, *A. duodenale* larvae may remain developmentally arrested for many months before resuming development in the intestine. Mature *A. duodenale* female worms produce about 30,000 eggs/day; daily egg production by *N. americanus* is <10,000/day (Fig. 284-1). The eggs are thin shelled and ovoid, measuring approximately 40-60 µm. Eggs that are deposited on soil with adequate moisture and shade develop into 1st stage larvae and hatch. Over the ensuing several days and under appropriate conditions, the larvae molt twice to the infective stage. Infective larvae are developmentally arrested and nonfeeding. They migrate vertically in the soil until they either infect a new host or exhaust their lipid metabolic reserves and die.

EPIDEMIOLOGY

Hookworm infection is one of the most prevalent infectious diseases of humans, affecting an estimated 576 million individuals worldwide. Because of the requirement for adequate soil moisture, shade, and warmth, hookworm infection is usually confined to rural areas, especially where human feces are used for fertilizer or where sanitation is inadequate. Hookworm is an infection associated with economic underdevelopment and poverty throughout the tropics and subtropics. Sub-Saharan Africa, East Asia, and tropical regions of the Americas have the highest prevalence of hookworm infection. High rates of infection are often

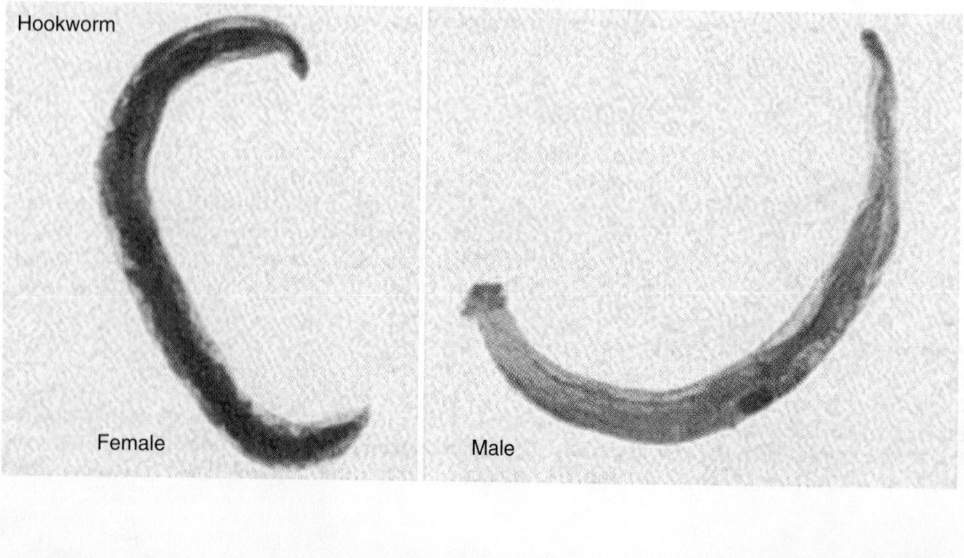

Figure 284-1 Adult male and female soil-transmitted helminths. (From Bethony J, Brooker S, Albonico M, et al: Soil-transmitted helminth infections: ascariasis, trichuriasis, and hookworm, *Lancet* 367:1521–1532, 2006.)

associated with cultivation of certain agricultural products such as tea in India; sweet potato, corn, cotton, and mulberry trees in China; coffee in Central and South America; and rubber in Africa. It is not uncommon to find dual *N. americanus* and *A. duodenale* infections. *N. americanus* predominates in Central and South America as well as in Southern China and southeast Asia, whereas *A. duodenale* predominates in North Africa, in northern India, in China north of the Yangtze River, and among aboriginal people in western Australia. The ability of *A. duodenale* to withstand somewhat harsher environmental and climatic conditions may reflect its ability to undergo arrested development in human tissues. *A. ceylanicum* infection occurs in India and southeast Asia.

Eosinophilic enteritis caused by *A. caninum* was 1st described in Queensland, Australia, with 2 reported cases in the USA. Because of its global distribution in dogs, it was initially anticipated that human *A. caninum* infections would be identified in many locales, but this has not been found.

PATHOGENESIS

The major morbidity of human hookworm infection is a direct result of intestinal blood loss. Adult hookworms adhere tenaciously to the mucosa and submucosa of the proximal small intestine by using their cutting plates or teeth and a muscular esophagus that creates negative pressure in their buccal capsules. At the attachment site, host inflammation is downregulated by the release of antiinflammatory polypeptides by the hookworm. Rupture of capillaries in the lamina propria is followed by blood extravasation, with some of the blood ingested directly by the hookworm. After ingestion, the blood is anticoagulated, the red blood cells are lysed, and the hemoglobin released and digested. Each adult *A. duodenale* hookworm causes loss of an estimated 0.2 mL of blood/day; blood loss is less for *N. americanus*. Individuals with light infections suffer from very little blood loss and, consequently, may have hookworm infection but not hookworm disease. There is a direct correlation between the number of adult hookworms in the gut and the volume of fecal blood loss. Hookworm disease results only when individuals with moderate and heavy infections experience sufficient blood loss to develop iron deficiency and anemia. Hypoalbuminemia and consequent edema and anasarca from the loss of intravascular oncotic pressure can also occur. These features depend heavily on the dietary reserves of the host.

CLINICAL MANIFESTATIONS

Chronically infected children with moderate and heavy hookworm infections suffer from intestinal blood loss that results in **iron deficiency** and can lead to **anemia** as well as protein malnutrition. Prolonged iron deficiency associated with hookworms in childhood can lead to physical growth retardation and cognitive and intellectual deficits.

Anthropophilic hookworm larvae elicit dermatitis sometimes referred to as **ground itch** when they penetrate human skin. The vesiculation and edema of ground itch are exacerbated by repeated infection. Infection with a zoonotic hookworm, especially *A. braziliense,* can result in lateral migration of the larvae to cause the characteristic cutaneous tracts of **cutaneous larva migrans** (Chapter 284.1). Cough subsequently occurs in *A. duodenale* and *N. americanus* hookworm infection when larvae migrate through the lungs to cause laryngotracheobronchitis, usually about 1 wk after exposure. Pharyngitis also can occur.

Intestinal hookworm infection may occur without specific gastrointestinal complaints, although pain, anorexia, and diarrhea have been attributed to the presence of hookworms. Eosinophilia is often 1st noticed in early gastrointestinal infection. The major clinical manifestations are related to intestinal blood loss. Heavily infected children exhibit all of the signs and symptoms of iron deficiency anemia and protein malnutrition. In some cases, children with chronic hookworm disease acquire a yellow-green pallor known as **chlorosis.**

An infantile form of ancylostomiasis resulting from heavy *A. duodenale* infection has been described. Affected infants experience diarrhea, melena, failure to thrive, and profound anemia. Infantile ancylostomiasis has significant mortality.

Eosinophilic enteritis caused by *A. caninum* is associated with colicky abdominal pain that begins in the epigastrium and radiates outward and is usually exacerbated by food. Extreme cases may mimic acute appendicitis.

DIAGNOSIS

Children with hookworm release eggs that can be detected by direct fecal examination (Fig. 284-2). Quantitative methods are available to determine whether a child has a heavy worm burden that can cause hookworm disease. The eggs of *N. americanus* and *A. duodenale* are morphologically indistinguishable. Species identification typically requires egg hatching and differentiation of 3rd stage infective larvae; newer methods using polymerase chain reaction methods are under development.

In contrast, eggs are generally not present in the feces of patients with eosinophilic enteritis caused by *A. caninum*. Eosinophilic enteritis is often diagnosed by demonstrating ileal and colonic ulcerations by colonoscopy in the presence of significant blood eosinophilia. An adult canine hookworm may occasionally be recovered during colonoscopic biopsy. Patients with this syndrome develop IgG and IgE serologic responses.

TREATMENT

The goal of **deworming** is removal of the adult hookworms with an anthelmintic drug. The benzimidazole anthelmintics, mebendazole and albendazole, are effective at eliminating hookworms from the intestine, although multiple doses are sometimes required. Albendazole (400 mg PO once, for all ages) usually achieves high cure rates, although *N. americanus* adult hookworms are sometimes more refractory and require additional doses. Mebendazole (100 mg bid PO for 3 days, for all ages) is also effective. In many developing countries, mebendazole is administered as a single dose of 500 mg; however, the cure rates with this regimen can be as low as 10% or less. According to the World Health Organization, children should be encouraged to chew tablets of albendazole or mebendazole because forcing very young children to swallow large tablets may cause choking or asphyxiation. Mebendazole is recommended for

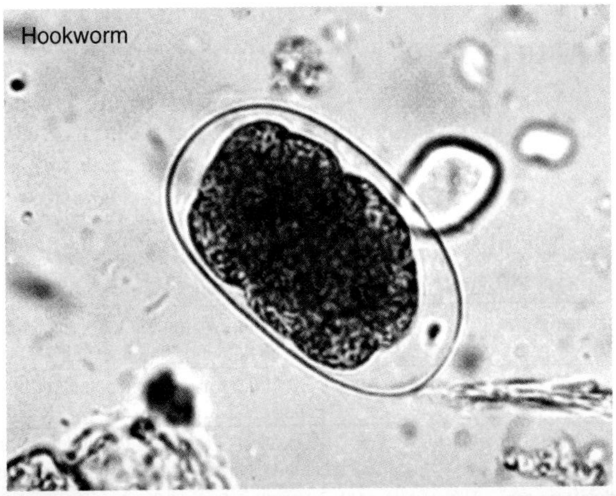

Figure 284-2 Soil-transmitted helminth eggs. (From Bethony J, Brooker S, Albonico M, et al: Soil-transmitted helminth infections: ascariasis, trichuriasis, and hookworm, *Lancet* 367:1521–1532, 2006.)

A. caninum–associated eosinophilic enteritis, although recurrences are common. Because the benzimidazoles have been reported to be embryotoxic and teratogenic in laboratory animals, their safety during pregnancy and in young children is a potential concern and the risks vs benefits must be carefully considered. The World Health Organization currently support the use of benzimidazoles in infected children ≥1 yr of age but at a reduced dose (200 mg for albendazole) in the youngest age group (1-2 yr old). Pyrantel pamoate (11 mg/kg PO once daily for 3 days, maximum dose 1 g) is available in liquid form and is an effective alternative to the benzimidazoles. Replacement therapy with oral iron is not usually required to correct hookworm-associated iron deficiency in children.

PREVENTION

In 2001, the World Health Assembly urged its member states to implement programs of periodic deworming in order to control the morbidity of hookworm and other soil-transmitted helminth infections. Although anthelmintic drugs are effective at eliminating hookworms from the intestine, the high rates of reinfection among children suggest that drug chemotherapy alone is not effective for controlling hookworm in highly endemic areas. Moreover data suggest that the efficacy of mebendazole decreases with frequent, periodic use, leading to concerns about the possible emergence of anthelmintic drug resistance. In order to reduce the reliance exclusively on anthelmintic drugs, a recombinant human hookworm vaccine has been developed and is undergoing clinical testing. Economic development and associated improvements in sanitation, health education, and avoidance of human feces as fertilizer remain critical for reducing hookworm transmission and endemicity.

BIBLIOGRAPHY

Please visit the Nelson Textbook of Pediatrics *website at www.expertconsult.com for the complete bibliography.*

284.1 Cutaneous Larva Migrans

Peter J. Hotez

ETIOLOGY

Cutaneous larva migrans (**creeping eruption**) is caused by the larvae of several nematodes, primarily hookworms, which are not usually parasitic for humans (Table 284-1). *A. braziliense,* a hookworm of dogs and cats, is the most common cause, but other animal hookworms may also produce the disease.

EPIDEMIOLOGY

Cutaneous larva migrans is usually caused by *A. braziliense,* which is endemic to the southeastern USA and Puerto Rico.

CLINICAL MANIFESTATIONS

After penetrating the skin, larvae localize at the epidermal-dermal junction and migrate in this plane, moving at a rate of 1-2 cm/day. The response to the parasite is characterized by raised, erythematous, serpiginous tracks, which occasionally form bullae (Fig. 284-3). These lesions may be single or numerous and are usually localized to an extremity, although any area of the body may be affected. As the organism migrates, new areas of involvement may appear every few days. Intense localized pruritus, without any systemic symptoms, may be associated with the lesions. Bacterial superinfection can occur.

DIAGNOSIS

Cutaneous larva migrans is diagnosed by clinical examination of the skin. Patients are often able to recall the exact time and location of exposure, because the larvae produce intense itching at the site of penetration. Eosinophilia may occur but is uncommon.

TREATMENT

If left untreated, the larvae die, and the syndrome resolves within a few weeks to several months. Treatment with ivermectin

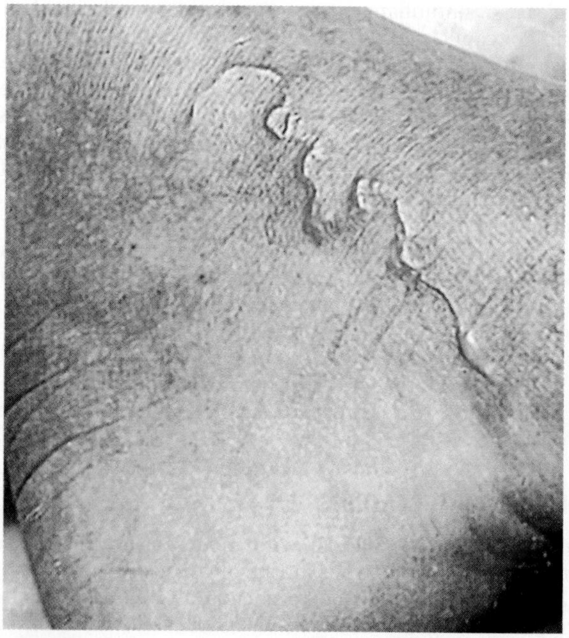

Figure 284-3 Creeping eruption of cutaneous larva migrans. (From Korting GW: *Hautkrankheiten bei kindern und jugendlichen,* Stuttgart, Germany, 1969, FK Schattauer Verlag.)

Table 284-1 ETIOLOGIES OF THE CUTANEOUS LARVA MIGRANS SYNDROME ACCORDING TO CUTANEOUS PRESENTATION

CAUSATIVE AGENT	CUTANEOUS TRACK	OTHER CUTANEOUS SIGNS
Animal hookworm	1-10 burrows, on the feet or buttocks, about 3 mm wide and up to 15-20 cm long, slow-moving (2-5 cm/day), chronic (weeks to months)	Highly pruritic, vesiculobullous lesions, impetiginization, hookworm folliculitis
Pelodera strongyloides	10-100 burrows, on abdomen or buttocks, 1-2 cm long, 2-3 mm wide, may persist for months	Pruritus, follicular papules and pustules
Strongyloides stercoralis	Usually 1 burrow, on the abdomen or buttocks; lasts for hours only, may recur, fast-moving (larva currens)	Pruritus, urticaria
Gnathostoma spp. (*G. hispidum*, etc.)	Usually 1 burrow located anywhere, lasts for days, medium-fast-moving	Cutaneous migratory edema (eosinophilic panniculitis), cellulitis, papules, and nodules

From Caumes E, Danis M: From creeping eruption to hookworm-related cutaneous larva migrans, *Lancet Infect Dis* 4:659–660, 2004.

(200 μg/kg daily PO for 1-2 days), albendazole (400 mg daily PO for 3 days, for all ages), or topical thiabendazole hastens resolution, if symptoms warrant treatment. Nausea and vomiting frequently preclude repeated administration of oral thiabendazole. The safety of ivermectin in young children (<15 kg) and pregnant women remains to be established. Ivermectin should be taken on an empty stomach with water.

BIBLIOGRAPHY

Please visit the Nelson Textbook of Pediatrics *website at* *www.expertconsult.com* *for the complete bibliography.*

Chapter 285
Trichuriasis (*Trichuris trichiura*)

Arlene E. Dent and James W. Kazura

ETIOLOGY

Trichuriasis is caused by the **whipworm**, *Trichuris trichiura*, a nematode, or roundworm, that inhabits the cecum and ascending colon of humans. The principal hosts of *T. trichiura* are humans who acquire infection by ingesting embryonated, barrel-shaped eggs (Fig. 285-1). The larvae escape from the shell in the upper small intestine and penetrate the intestinal villi. The worms slowly move toward the cecum, where the anterior three quarters whiplike portion remains within the superficial mucosa and the short posterior end is free in the lumen (Fig. 285-2). In 1-3 mo, the adult female worm begins producing 5,000-20,000 eggs/day. After excretion in the feces, embryonic development occurs in 2-4 wk with optimal temperature and soil conditions. The adult worm life span is approximately 2 yr.

EPIDEMIOLOGY

Trichuriasis occurs throughout the world and is especially common in poor rural communities with inadequate sanitary facilities and soil contaminated with human or animal feces. Trichuriasis is one of the most prevalent human helminthiases, with an estimated 1 billion infected individuals worldwide. In many parts of the world where protein-energy malnutrition and anemia are common, the prevalence of *T. trichiura* infection can be as high as 95%. It is estimated that 2.2 million people are infected in the rural southeastern USA. The highest rate of infection occurs among children 5-15 yr of age. Infection develops after ingesting embryonated ova by direct contamination of hands, food (raw fruits and vegetables fertilized with human feces), or drink. Transmission can also occur indirectly through flies or other insects.

CLINICAL MANIFESTATIONS

Most persons harbor low worm burdens and do not have symptoms. Some individuals may have a history of right lower quadrant or vague periumbilical pain. Adult *Trichuris* suck approximately 0.005 mL of blood/worm/day. Children, who are most likely to be heavily infected, frequently suffer from disease. Clinical manifestations include chronic dysentery, rectal prolapse, anemia, poor growth, as well as developmental and cognitive deficits. There is no significant eosinophilia, even though a portion of the worm is embedded in the mucosa of the large bowel.

DIAGNOSIS

Because egg output is so high, fecal smears frequently reveal the characteristic barrel-shaped ova of *T. trichiura*.

TREATMENT

Mebendazole (100 mg bid PO for 3 days or 500 mg PO once for all ages) is the drug of choice and is safe and effective, in part because it is poorly absorbed from the gastrointestinal tract. It

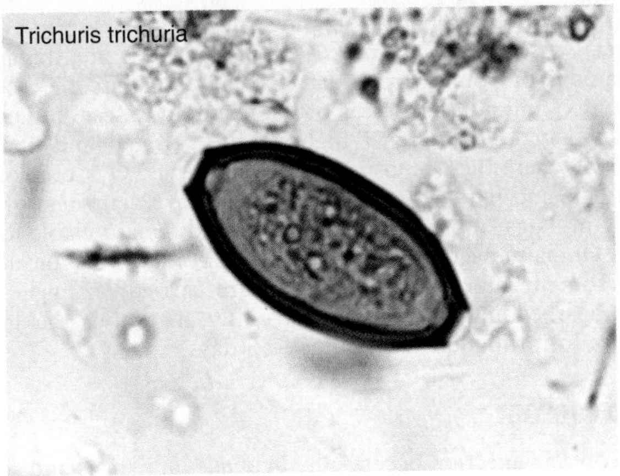

Figure 285-1 Soil-transmitted helminth eggs. (From Bethony J, Brooker S, Albonico M, et al: Soil-transmitted helminth infections: ascariasis, trichuriasis, and hookworm, *Lancet* 367:1521–1532, 2006.)

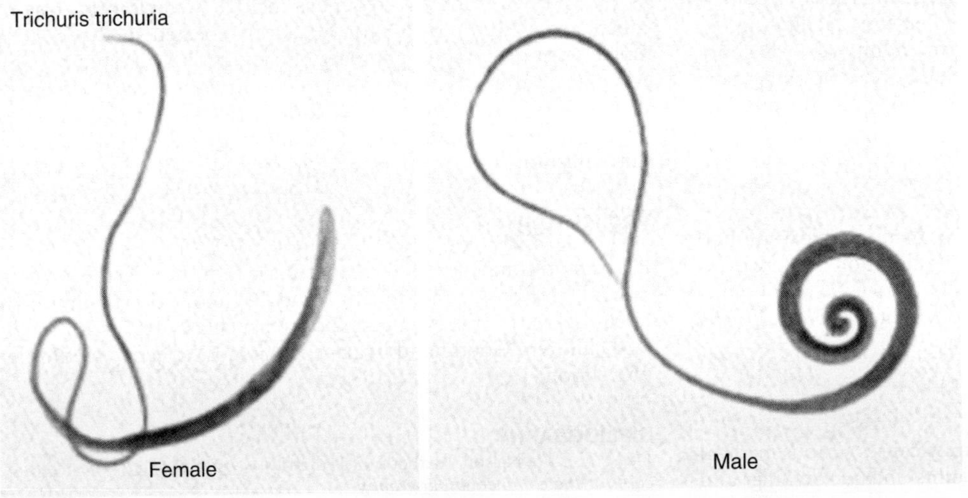

Figure 285-2 Adult male and female soil-transmitted helminths. (From Bethony J, Brooker S, Albonico M, et al: Soil-transmitted helminth infections: ascariasis, trichuriasis, and hookworm, *Lancet* 367:1521–1532, 2006.)

reduces egg output by 90-99% and has cure rates of 70-90%. Albendazole (400 mg PO once for all ages) is an alternative, but with heavy infections the daily dose of albendazole should be administered for 3 days. Recent analysis indicates that currently recommended single-dose oral regimens of mebendazole and albendazole lack efficacy in curing *Trichuris* infections. Nitazoxanide (100 mg bid PO for 3 days for children 1-3 yr of age, 200 mg bid PO for 3 days for children 4-11 yr of age, and 500 mg bid PO for 3 days for adolescents and adults) has been shown to produce higher cure rates than single-dose albendazole.

PREVENTION

Disease can be prevented by personal hygiene, improved sanitary conditions, and eliminating the use of human feces as fertilizer.

BIBLIOGRAPHY

Please visit the Nelson Textbook of Pediatrics *website at* *www.expertconsult.com* *for the complete bibliography.*

Chapter 286
Enterobiasis *(Enterobius vermicularis)*

Arlene E. Dent and James W. Kazura

ETIOLOGY

The cause of enterobiasis, or **pinworm** infection, is *Enterobius vermicularis,* which is a small (1 cm in length), white, threadlike nematode, or roundworm, that typically inhabits the cecum, appendix, and adjacent areas of the ileum and ascending colon. Gravid females migrate at night to the perianal and perineal regions, where they deposit up to 15,000 eggs. Ova are convex on 1 side and flattened on the other and have diameters of ~30 × 60 µm. Eggs embryonate within 6 hr and remain viable for 20 days. Human infection occurs by the fecal-oral route typically by ingestion of embryonated eggs that are carried on fingernails, clothing, bedding, or house dust. After ingestion, the larvae mature to form adult worms in 36-53 days.

EPIDEMIOLOGY

Enterobiasis infection occurs in individuals of all ages and socioeconomic levels. It is prevalent in regions with temperate climates and is the most common helminth infection in the USA. It infects 30% of children worldwide, and humans are the only known host. Infection occurs primarily in institutional or family settings that include children. The prevalence of pinworm infection is highest in children 5-14 yr of age. It is common in areas where children live, play, and sleep close together, thus facilitating egg transmission. Because the life span of the adult worm is short, chronic parasitism is likely due to repeated cycles of reinfection. Autoinoculation can occur in individuals who habitually put their fingers in their mouth.

PATHOGENESIS

Enterobius infection may cause symptoms by mechanical stimulation and irritation, allergic reactions, and migration of the worms to anatomic sites where they become pathogenic. *Enterobius* infection has been associated with concomitant *Dientamoeba fragilis* infection, which causes diarrhea.

CLINICAL MANIFESTATIONS

Pinworm infection is innocuous and rarely causes serious medical problems. The most common complaints include itching and restless sleep secondary to nocturnal **perianal** or **perineal pruritus.** The precise cause and incidence of pruritus are unknown but may be related to the intensity of infection, psychologic profile of the infected individual and his or her family, or allergic reactions to the parasite. Eosinophilia is not observed in most cases, because tissue invasion does not occur. Aberrant migration to ectopic sites occasionally may lead to appendicitis, chronic salpingitis, pelvic inflammatory disease, peritonitis, hepatitis, and ulcerative lesions in the large or small bowel.

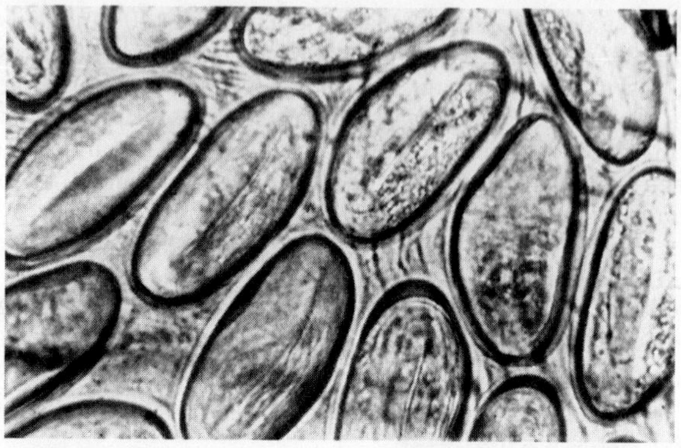

Figure 286-1 Eggs of *Enterobius vermicularis* adherent to cellulose acetate tape. (From Guerrant RL, Walker DH, Weller PF, et al: *Tropical infectious diseases,* Philadelphia, 1999, Churchill Livingstone, p 949.)

DIAGNOSIS

A history of nocturnal perianal pruritus in children strongly suggests enterobiasis. Definitive diagnosis is established by identification of parasite eggs or worms. Microscopic examination of adhesive cellophane tape pressed against the perianal region early in the morning frequently demonstrates eggs (Fig. 286-1). Repeated examinations increase the chance of detecting ova; a single examination detects 50% of infections, 3 examinations 90%, and 5 examinations 99%. Worms seen in the perianal region should be removed and preserved in 75% ethyl alcohol until microscopic examination can be performed. Digital rectal examination may also be used to obtain samples for a wet mount. Routine stool samples rarely demonstrate *Enterobius* ova.

TREATMENT

Anthelmintic drugs should be administered to infected individuals and their family members. A single oral dose of mebendazole (100 mg PO for all ages) repeated in 2 wk results in cure rates of 90-100%. Alternative regimens include a single oral dose of albendazole (400 mg PO for all ages) repeated in 2 wk, or a single dose of pyrantel pamoate (11 mg/kg PO, maximum 1 g). Morning bathing removes a large portion of eggs. Frequent changing of underclothes, bed clothes, and bed sheets decreases environmental egg contamination and may decrease the risk for autoinfection.

PREVENTION

Household contacts can be treated at the same time as the infected individual. Repeated treatments every 3-4 mo may be required in circumstances with repeated exposure, such as with institutionalized children. Good hand hygiene is the most effective method of prevention.

BIBLIOGRAPHY

Please visit the Nelson Textbook of Pediatrics *website at* *www.expertconsult.com* *for the complete bibliography.*

Chapter 287
Strongyloidiasis (*Strongyloides stercoralis*)

Arlene E. Dent and James W. Kazura

ETIOLOGY

Strongyloidiasis is caused by the nematode, or roundworm, *Strongyloides stercoralis.* Only adult female worms inhabit the small intestine. The nematode reproduces in the human host by parthenogenesis and releases eggs containing mature larvae into the intestinal lumen. Rhabditiform larvae immediately emerge from the ova and are passed in feces, where they can be visualized by stool examination. Rhabditiform larvae either differentiate into free-living adult male and female worms or metamorphose into the infectious filariform larvae. Sexual reproduction occurs only in the free-living stage. Humans are usually infected through skin contact with soil contaminated with infectious larvae. Larvae penetrate the skin, enter the venous circulation and then pass to the lungs, break into alveolar spaces, and migrate up the bronchial tree. They are then swallowed and pass through the stomach, and adult female worms develop in the small intestine. Egg deposition begins about 28 days after initial infection.

The **hyperinfection syndrome** occurs when large numbers of larvae transform into infective organisms during their passage in feces and then reinfect (autoinfect) the host by way of the lower gastrointestinal tract or perianal region. This cycle may be accelerated in immunocompromised persons, particularly those with depressed T-cell function.

EPIDEMIOLOGY

S. stercoralis infection is prevalent in tropical and subtropical regions of the world and endemic in several areas of Europe, the southern USA, and Puerto Rico. Transmission requires appropriate environmental conditions, particularly warm, moist soil. Poor sanitation and crowded living conditions are conducive to high levels of transmission. Dogs and cats can act as reservoirs. The highest prevalence of infection in the USA (4% of the general population) is in impoverished rural areas of Kentucky and Tennessee. Infection may be especially common among residents of mental institutions, veterans who were prisoners of war in areas of high endemicity, and refugees and immigrants. Because of internal autoinfection, individuals may remain infected for decades. Individuals with hematologic malignancies, autoimmune diseases, malnutrition, and drug-induced immunosuppression (especially corticosteroids) are at high risk for the hyperinfection syndrome. Patients with AIDS may experience a rapid course of disseminated strongyloidiasis with a fatal outcome.

PATHOGENESIS

The initial host immune response to infection is production of immunoglobulin E (IgE) and eosinophilia in blood and tissues, which presumably prevents dissemination and hyperinfection in the immunocompetent host. Adult female worms in otherwise healthy and asymptomatic individuals may persist in the gastrointestinal tract for years. If infected persons become immunocompromised, the reduction in cellular and humoral immunity may lead to an abrupt and dramatic increase in parasite load with systemic dissemination.

CLINICAL MANIFESTATIONS

Approximately 30% of infected individuals are asymptomatic. The remaining patients have symptoms that correlate with the 3 stages of infection: invasion of the skin, migration of larvae through the lungs, and parasitism of the small intestine by adult worms. **Larva currens** is the manifestation of an allergic reaction to filariform larvae that migrate through the skin, where they leave pruritic, tortuous, urticarial tracks. The lesions may recur and are typically found over the lower abdominal wall, buttocks, or thighs, resulting from larval migration from defecated stool. Pulmonary disease secondary to larval migration through the lung rarely occurs and may resemble **Loeffler syndrome** (cough, wheezing, shortness of breath, transient pulmonary infiltrates accompanied by eosinophilia). Gastrointestinal strongyloidiasis is characterized by indigestion, crampy abdominal pain, vomiting, diarrhea, steatorrhea, protein-losing enteropathy, protein-caloric malnutrition, and weight loss. Edema of the duodenum with irregular mucosal folds, ulcerations, and strictures can be seen radiographically. Infection may be chronic in nature and is associated with **eosinophilia.**

Strongyloidiasis is potentially lethal because of the ability of the parasite to cause overwhelming hyperinfection in immunocompromised persons. The **hyperinfection syndrome** is characterized by an exaggeration of the clinical features that develop in symptomatic immunocompetent individuals. The onset is usually sudden, with generalized abdominal pain, distention, and fever. Multiple organs can be affected as massive numbers of larvae disseminate throughout the body and introduce bowel flora. The latter may result in bacteremia and septicemia. Cutaneous manifestations may include petechiae and purpura. Cough, wheezing, and hemoptysis are indicative of pulmonary involvement. Whereas eosinophilia is a prominent feature of strongyloidiasis in immunocompetent persons, this sign may be absent in immunocompromised persons. Because of the low incidence of strongyloidiasis in industrialized countries, it is often misdiagnosed, resulting in a significant delay in treatment.

DIAGNOSIS

Intestinal strongyloidiasis is diagnosed by examining feces or duodenal fluid for the characteristic larvae (Fig. 287-1). Several stool samples should be examined either by direct smear, Koga agar plate method, or the Baermann test. Alternatively, duodenal

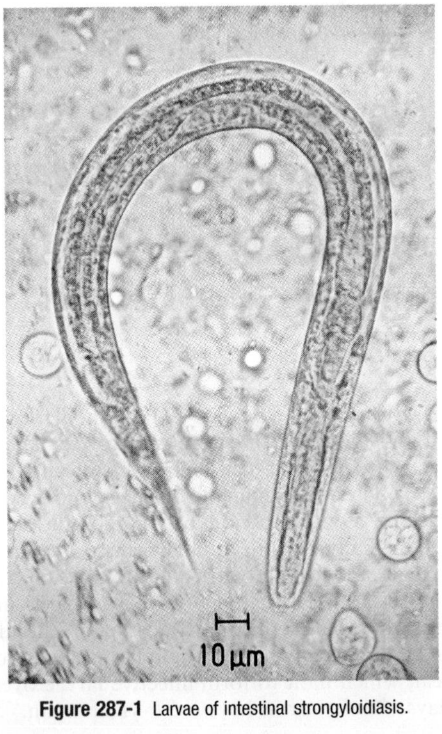

Figure 287-1 Larvae of intestinal strongyloidiasis.

fluid can be sampled by the **enteric string test** (Entero-Test) or aspiration via endoscopy. In children with the hyperinfection syndrome, larvae may be found in sputum, gastric aspirates, and rarely in small intestinal biopsy specimens. An enzyme-linked immunosorbent assay for IgG antibody to *Strongyloides* may be more sensitive than parasitologic methods for diagnosing intestinal infection in the immunocompetent host. The utility of the assay in diagnosing infection in immunocompromised subjects with the hyperinfection syndrome has not been determined. Eosinophilia is common.

TREATMENT

Treatment is directed at eradication of infection. Ivermectin (200 µg/kg/day once daily PO for 1-2 days) is the drug of choice for uncomplicated strongyloidiasis. It is equally effective and associated with fewer adverse effects than thiabendazole (25 mg/kg/dose bid PO for 2 days, maximum 3 g/day), which is the traditional treatment. Patients with the hyperinfection syndrome should be treated with ivermectin for 7-10 days and may require repeated courses. Reducing the dose of immunosuppressive therapy and treatment of concomitant bacterial infections are essential in the management of the hyperinfection syndrome. Close follow-up with repeated stool examination is necessary to ensure complete elimination of the parasite. *Strongyloides* antibodies decrease within 6 mo after successful treatment.

PREVENTION

Sanitary practices designed to prevent soil and person-to-person transmission are the most effective control measures. Wearing shoes is a main preventive strategy. Reduction in transmission in institutional settings can be achieved by decreasing fecal contamination of the environment such as by the use of clean bedding. Because infection is uncommon in most settings, case detection and treatment are advisable. Individuals who will be given prolonged high dose corticosteroids, immunosuppressive drugs before organ transplantation, or cancer chemotherapy should have a screening examination for *S. stercoralis*. If infected, they should be treated before immunosuppression is initiated.

BIBLIOGRAPHY

Please visit the Nelson Textbook of Pediatrics *website at www.expertconsult.com for the complete bibliography.*

Chapter 288
Lymphatic Filariasis (*Brugia malayi*, *Brugia timori*, and *Wuchereria bancrofti*)

Arlene E. Dent and James W. Kazura

ETIOLOGY

The filarial worms *Brugia malayi* (**Malayan filariasis**), *Brugia timori*, and *Wuchereria bancrofti* (**bancroftian filariasis**) are threadlike nematodes that cause similar infections. Infective larvae are introduced into humans during blood feeding by the mosquito vector. Over a period of 4-6 mo, the larval forms develop into sexually mature adult worms. Once an adequate number of male and female worms accumulate in the afferent lymphatic vessels, adult female worms release large numbers of microfilariae that circulate in the bloodstream. The life cycle of the parasite is completed when mosquitoes ingest microfilariae in a blood meal, which molt to form infective larvae over a period of 10-14 days. Adult worms have a 5-7 yr life span.

EPIDEMIOLOGY

More than 120 million people living in tropical Africa, Asia, and Latin America are infected; approximately 10-20% of these individuals have clinically significant morbidity attributable to filariasis. *W. bancrofti* is transmitted in Africa, Asia, and Latin America and accounts for 90% of lymphatic filariasis. *B. malayi* is restricted to the South Pacific and Southeast Asia, and *B. timori* is restricted to several islands of Indonesia. Travelers from nonendemic areas of the world who spend brief periods of time in endemic areas are rarely infected. Global elimination has been targeted for 2020.

CLINICAL MANIFESTATIONS

The clinical manifestations of *B. malayi*, *B. timori*, and *W. bancrofti* infection are similar; manifestations of acute infection include transient, recurrent lymphadenitis and lymphangitis, The early signs and symptoms include episodic fever, lymphangitis of an extremity, lymphadenitis (especially the inguinal and axillary areas), headaches, and myalgias that last a few days to several weeks. These symptoms are caused by an acute inflammatory response triggered by death of adult worms. Initial damage to lymphatic vessels may remain subclinical for years. The syndrome is most frequently observed in young persons 10-20 yr of age. Manifestations of chronic lymphatic filariasis occur mostly in adults 30 yr of age or older and result from anatomic and functional obstruction to lymph flow. This obstruction results in lymphedema of the legs, arms, breasts, and/or genitalia. Male genital involvement such as hydrocele is very common in *W. bancrofti* infection but uncommon in *Brugia* species infection. Chronic lymphedema predisposes affected extremities to bacterial superinfections, sclerosis, and verrucous skin changes, resulting in elephantitis, which may involve 1 or more limbs, the breasts, or genitalia. It is uncommon for children to have overt signs of chronic filariasis.

Tropical Pulmonary Eosinophilia

The presence of microfilariae in the body has no apparent pathologic consequences except in persons with tropical pulmonary eosinophilia, a syndrome of filarial etiology in which microfilariae are found in the lungs and lymph nodes but not the bloodstream. It occurs only in individuals who have lived for years in endemic areas. Men 20-30 yr of age are most likely to be affected, although the syndrome occasionally occurs in children. The presentation includes paroxysmal nocturnal cough with dyspnea, fever, weight loss, and fatigue. Rales and rhonchi are found on auscultation of the chest. The x-ray findings may occasionally be normal, but increased bronchovascular markings, discrete opacities in the middle and basal regions of the lung, or diffuse miliary lesions are usually present (Fig. 288-1). Recurrent episodes may result in interstitial fibrosis and chronic respiratory insufficiency in untreated individuals. Hepatosplenomegaly and generalized lymphadenopathy are often seen in children. The diagnosis is suggested by residence in a filarial endemic area, eosinophilia (>2,000/µL), compatible clinical symptoms, increased serum IgE (>1,000 IU/mL), and high titers of antimicrofilarial antibodies in the absence of microfilaremia. Although microfilariae may be found in sections of lung or lymph node, biopsy of these tissues is unwarranted in most situations. The clinical response to diethylcarbamazine (2 mg/kg/dose tid PO for 12-21 days) is the final criterion for diagnosis; the majority of patients improve with this therapy. If symptoms recur, a 2nd course of the anthelmintic should be administered. Patients with chronic symptoms are less likely to show improvement than those who have been ill for a short time.

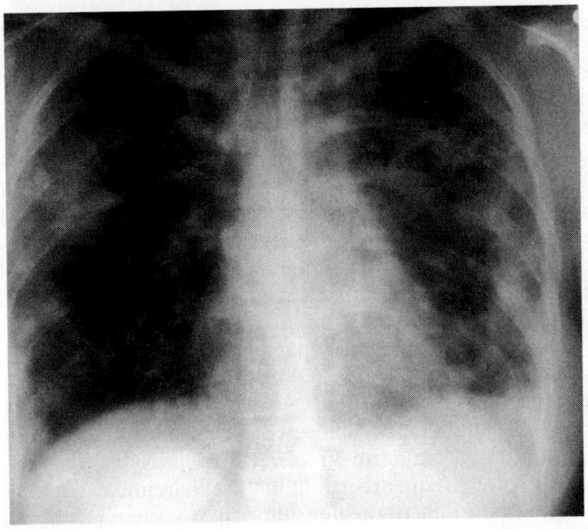

Figure 288-1 Chest radiograph of a woman with tropical pulmonary eosinophilia. Reticulondular opacities are scattered throughout both lungs. (From Mandell GL, Bennett JE, Dolin R, editors: *Principles and practice of infectious diseases,* vol 2, ed 6, Philadelphia, 2006, Elsevier, p 3274.)

DIAGNOSIS

Demonstration of microfilariae in the blood is the primary means for confirming the diagnosis of lymphatic filariasis. Because microfilaremia is **nocturnal** in most cases, blood samples should be obtained between 10 P.M. and 2 A.M. Anticoagulated blood is passed through a Nuclepore filter that is stained and examined microscopically for microfilariae. Adult worms or microfilariae can be identified in tissue specimens obtained at biopsy. Infection with *W. bancrofti* in the absence of blood-borne microfilariae may be diagnosed by detection of parasite antigen in the serum. Adult worms in lymphatic vessels can be visualized by ultrasonography.

TREATMENT

The use of antifilarial drugs in the management of acute lymphadenitis and lymphangitis is controversial. No controlled studies demonstrate that administration of drugs such as diethylcarbamazine modifies the course of acute lymphangitis. Diethylcarbamazine may be given to asymptomatic microfilaremic persons to lower the intensity of parasitemia. The drug also kills a proportion of the adult worms. Because treatment-associated complications such as pruritus, fever, generalized body pain, hypotension, and even death may occur, especially with high microfilarial levels, the dose of diethylcarbamazine should be increased gradually (children, 1 mg/kg PO as a single dose on day 1, 1 mg/kg tid PO on day 2, 1-2 mg/kg tid PO on day 3, and 6 mg/kg/day divided tid PO on days 4-14; adults, 50 mg PO on day 1, 50 mg tid PO on day 2, 100 mg tid PO on day 3, and 6 mg/kg/day divided tid PO on days 4-14). For patients with no microfilaria in the blood, the full dose (6 mg/kg/day divided tid PO) can be given beginning on day 1. Repeat doses may be necessary to further reduce the microfilaremia and kill lymph-dwelling adult parasites. *W. bancrofti* is more sensitive than *B. malayi* to diethylcarbamazine.

Global programs to control and ultimately eradicate lymphatic filariasis currently recommend a single annual dose of diethylcarbamazine (6 mg/kg PO once) in combination with albendazole (400 mg PO once) for 5 yr. In co-endemic areas of filariasis and onchocerciasis, mass drug applications with single-dose ivermectin (150 µg/kg PO once) and albendazole are used because of severe adverse reactions with diethylcarbamazine in onchocerciasis-infected individuals. Five years of annual mass treatment is thought to be necessary to stop transmission. Adjuvant medicines (e.g., doxycycline) that target endosymbiont bacteria (*Wolbachia*) in filarial parasites may accelerate eradication.

BIBLIOGRAPHY

Please visit the Nelson Textbook of Pediatrics *website at* *www.expertconsult.com* *for the complete bibliography.*

Chapter 289
Other Tissue Nematodes

Arlene E. Dent and James W. Kazura

ONCHOCERCIASIS *(ONCHOCERCA VOLVULUS)*

Infection with *Onchocerca volvulus* leads to onchocerciasis or **river blindness.** Onchocerciasis occurs primarily in West Africa but also Central and East Africa and is the world's 2nd leading infectious cause of blindness. There are scattered foci in Central and South America. *O. volvulus* larvae are transmitted to humans by way of the bite of *Simulium* black flies that breed in fast-flowing streams. The larvae penetrate the skin and migrate through the connective tissue and eventually develop into adult worms that can be found tangled in fibrous tissue. Adult worms can live in the human body for up to 14 yr. Female worms produce large numbers of microfilariae that migrate through the skin, connective tissue, and eye. Most infected individuals are asymptomatic. In heavily infected subjects, clinical manifestations are due to localized host inflammatory reactions to dead or dying microfilariae. These reactions produce pruritic dermatitis, punctate keratitis, corneal pannus formation, and chorioretinitis. Adult worms in **subcutaneous nodules** are not painful and tend to occur over bony prominences of the hip. The **diagnosis** can be established by obtaining snips of skin covering the scapulae, iliac crests, buttocks, or calves. The snips are immersed in saline for several hours and examined microscopically for microfilariae that have emerged into the fluid. The diagnosis can also be established by demonstrating microfilariae in the cornea or anterior chamber on slit-lamp examination or finding adult worms on a nodule biopsy specimen. Ophthalmology consultation should be obtained before treatment of eye lesions. A single dose of ivermectin (150 µg/kg PO) is the drug of choice and clears microfilariae from the skin for several months but has no effect on the adult worm. Treatment with ivermectin should be repeated at 3-6 mo intervals if there are continuing symptoms or evidence of eye infection. Adverse effects of ivermectin therapy include fever, urticaria, and pruritus and are more frequent in individuals not born in endemic areas who acquired the infection following periods of intense exposure, such as Peace Corps volunteers. Patients with concurrent loiasis may develop encephalopathy with ivermectin therapy. Doxycycline, which kills endosymbiont bacteria *(Wolbachia)* of *O. volvulus*, may contribute to amicrofilaremia. Personal protection includes avoiding areas where biting flies are numerous, wearing protective clothing, and using insect repellent. Vector control and mass ivermectin distribution programs have been implemented in Africa in a successful effort to reduce the prevalence of onchocerciasis.

LOIASIS *(LOA LOA)*

Loiasis is caused by infection with the tissue nematode *Loa loa.* The parasite is transmitted to humans via diurnally biting flies *(Chrysops)* that live in the rain forests of West and Central Africa. Migration of adult worms through skin, subcutaneous tissue, and subconjunctival area can lead to transient episodes of pruritus, erythema, localized edema known as **Calabar swellings,** which are nonerythematous areas of subcutaneous edema 10-20 cm in

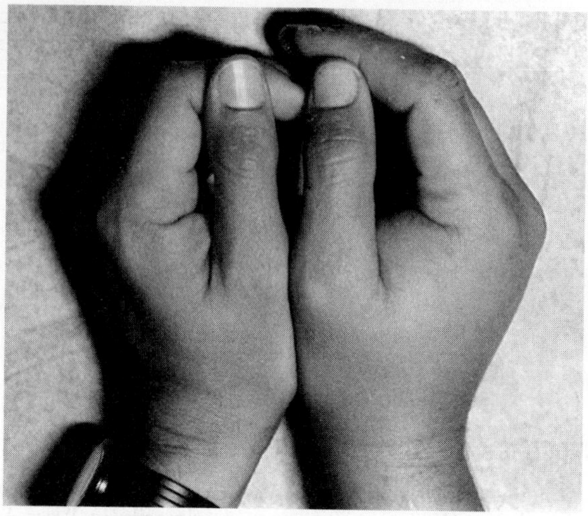

Figure 289-1 Calabar swelling of the right hand. (From Guerrant RL, Walker DH, Weller PF, et al: *Tropical infectious diseases*, Philadelphia, 1999, Churchill Livingstone, p 863.)

diameter typically found around joints such as the wrist or the knee (Fig. 289-1), or eye pain. They resolve over several days to weeks and may recur at the same or different sites. Although lifelong residents of endemic regions may have microfilaremia and eosinophilia, these individuals are often asymptomatic. In contrast, travelers to endemic regions may have a hyperreactive response to *L. loa* infection characterized by frequent recurrences of swelling, high-level eosinophilia, debilitation, and serious complications such as glomerulonephritis and encephalitis. Diagnosis is usually established on clinical grounds, often assisted by the infected individual reporting a worm being seen crossing the conjunctivae. Microfilariae may be detected in blood smears collected between 10 AM and 2 PM. Adult worms should be surgically excised when possible. Diethylcarbamazine is the agent of choice for eradication of microfilaremia, but the drug does not kill adult worms. Because treatment-associated complications such as pruritus, fever, generalized body pain, hypertension, and even death may occur, especially with high microfilarial levels, the dose of diethylcarbamazine should be increased gradually (children, 1 mg/kg PO on day 1, 1 mg/kg tid PO on day 2, 1-2 mg/kg tid PO on day 3, 6 mg/kg/day divided tid PO on days 4-21; adults, 50 mg PO on day 1, 50 mg tid PO on day 2, 100 mg tid PO on day 3, 6 mg/kg/day divided tid PO on days 4-21). Full doses can be instituted on day 1 in persons without microfilaremia. Individuals concurrently infected with *O. volvulus* are at increased risk for developing encephalopathy with ivermectin treatment. A single dose of ivermectin (150 μg/kg) decreases microfilarial densities in the blood in persons with high-density microfilaremia. A 3 wk course of albendazole can also be used to slowly reduce microfilarial levels as a result of embryotoxic effects on the adult worms. Antihistamines or corticosteroids may be used to limit allergic reactions secondary to killing of microfilariae. Personal protective measures include avoiding areas where biting flies are present, wearing protective clothing, and using insect repellents. Diethylcarbamazine (300 mg PO once weekly) prevents infection in travelers who spend prolonged periods of time in endemic areas. *L. loa* do not harbor *Wolbachia* endosymbionts, and therefore doxycycline has no effect on infection.

INFECTION WITH ANIMAL FILARIAE

The most commonly recognized zoonotic filarial infections are caused by members of the genus *Dirofilaria*. The worms are introduced into humans by the bites of mosquitoes containing 3rd stage larvae. The most common filarial zoonosis in the USA is *Dirofilaria tenuis*, a parasite of raccoons. In Europe, Africa, and Southeast Asia, infections are most commonly caused by the dog parasite *Dirofilaria repens*. The **dog heartworm,** *Dirofilaria immitis*, is the 2nd most commonly encountered filarial zoonosis worldwide. Other genera, including *Dipetalonema*-like worms, *Onchocerca*, and *Brugia*, are rare causes of zoonotic filarial infections.

Animal filariae do not undergo normal development in the human host. The clinical manifestations and pathologic findings correspond to the anatomic site of infection and can be categorized into 4 major groups: subcutaneous, lung, eye, and lymphatic. Pathologic examination of affected tissue reveals a localized foreign body reaction around a dead or dying parasite. The lesion consists of granulomas with eosinophils, neutrophils, and tissue necrosis. *D. tenuis* does not leave the subcutaneous tissues, whereas *Brugia beaveri* eventually localizes to superficial lymph nodes. Infections may be present for up to several months. *D. immitis* larvae migrate for several months in subcutaneous tissues and most frequently result in a well-circumscribed coinlike lesion in a single lobe of the lung. The chest x-ray typically reveals a solitary pulmonary nodule 1-3 cm in diameter. Definitive diagnosis and cure depend on surgical excision and identification of the nematode within the surrounding granulomatous response. *D. tenuis* and *B. beaveri* infections present as painful 1-5 cm rubbery nodules in the skin of the trunk, extremities, and around the orbit. Patients often report having been engaged in activities predisposing to exposure to infected mosquitoes, such as working or hunting in swampy areas. Diagnosis and management is by surgical excision.

ANGIOSTRONGYLUS CANTONENSIS

Angiostrongylus cantonensis, the **rat lungworm,** is the most common cause of eosinophilic meningitis worldwide. Rats are the definitive host. Human infection follows ingestion of 3rd stage larvae in raw or undercooked intermediate hosts such as snails and slugs, or transport hosts such as freshwater prawns, frogs, and fish. Most cases are sporadic, but clusters have been reported, including consumption of lettuce contaminated with intermediate or transport hosts. Even though most infections have been described in Southeast Asia, the South Pacific, and Taiwan, shipboard travel of infected rats has spread the parasite to Madagascar, Africa, the Caribbean, and, most recently, Australia and North America. Larvae penetrate the vasculature of the intestinal tract and migrate to the meninges, where they usually die but induce eosinophilic aseptic meningitis. Patients present 2-35 days after ingestion of larvae with severe headache, neck pain or nuchal rigidity, hyperesthesias and paresthesias (often migrating), fatigue, fever, rash, pruritus, nausea, and vomiting. Neurologic involvement varies from asymptomatic to paresthesias, severe pain, weakness, and focal neurologic findings such as cranial nerve palsies. Symptoms can last for several weeks to months, especially headache. Coma and death due to hydrocephalus occur rarely in heavy infections. Peripheral blood eosinophilia is not always present on initial examination but peaks about 5 wk after exposure, often when symptoms are improving. Cerebrospinal fluid (CSF) analysis reveals pleocytosis with >10% eosinophils in more than half of patients, with mildly elevated protein and normal glucose levels, and an elevated opening pressure. Head CT or MRI is usually unremarkable. The diagnosis is established clinically with supporting travel and diet history. A sensitive and specific enzyme-linked immunosorbent assay (ELISA) is available on a limited basis from the Centers for Disease Control and Prevention for testing either CSF or serum. Treatment is primarily supportive because the majority of infections are mild and most patients recover within 2 mo without neurologic sequelae. Analgesics should be given for headache. Careful, repeated lumbar punctures should be performed to relieve hydrocephalus. Anthelmintic drugs have not been shown to influence the outcome and may exacerbate neurologic symptoms. The use of corticosteroids may shorten the duration of persistent and severe headaches. There is a higher incidence of permanent neurologic sequelae and mortality among children than among adults. Infection can be avoided by not eating raw or undercooked crabs, prawns, or snails.

ANGIOSTRONGYLUS COSTARICENSIS

Angiostrongylus costaricensis is a nematode that infects several species of rodents and causes abdominal angiostrongyliasis, which has been described predominantly in Latin America and the Caribbean. The mode of transmission to humans, who are accidental hosts, is unknown. It is speculated that infectious larvae from a molluscan intermediate host, such as the slug *Vaginulus plebeius,* contaminate water or vegetation that are inadvertently consumed (chopped up in salads or on vegetation contaminated with their mucus secretions). Although this slug is not indigenous to the continental USA, it has been found on imported flowers and produce. The incubation period for abdominal angiostrongyliasis is unknown, but limited data suggest it ranges from 2 wk to several months after ingestion of larvae. Third stage larvae migrate from the gastrointestinal tract to the mesenteric arteries, where they mature into adults. These eggs degenerate and elicit an eosinophilic granulomatous reaction. The clinical findings of abdominal angiostrongyliasis **mimic appendicitis,** although the former are typically more indolent. Children can have fever, right lower quadrant pain, a tumor-like mass, abdominal rigidity, and painful rectal examination. Most patients have leukocytosis with eosinophilia. Radiologic examination may show bowel wall edema, spasticity, or filling defects in the ileocecal region and the ascending colon. Examination of stool for ova and parasites is not useful for *A. costaricensis* but is useful for evaluating the presence of other intestinal parasites. An ELISA is available for diagnosis on a limited basis from the Centers for Disease Control and Prevention, but the specificity of the test is low, and it is known to cross react with *Toxocara, Strongyloides,* and *Paragonimus.* Many patients undergo laparotomy for suspected appendicitis and are found to have a mass in the terminal ileum to the ascending colon. No specific treatment is known for abdominal angiostrongyliasis. Even though the use of anthelmintic therapy has not been studied systematically, thiabendazole or diethylcarbamazine has been suggested. The prognosis is generally good. Most cases are self-limited, although surgery may be required in some patients. Cornerstones of prevention include avoidance of slugs and not ingesting raw food and water that may be contaminated with imperceptible slugs or slime from slugs. Rat control is also important in preventing the spread of infection.

DRACUNCULIASIS *(DRACUNCULUS MEDINENSIS)*

Dracunculiasis is caused by the guinea worm, *Dracunculus medinensis.* The World Health Organization has targeted dracunculiasis for eradication. As of 2008, the transmission of the infection was confined to 5 countries (Sudan, Ghana, Mali, Niger, and Nigeria), with Sudan reporting 61% and Ghana reporting 35% of global cases. Humans become infected by **drinking contaminated stagnant water** that contains immature forms of the parasite in the gut of tiny crustaceans (copepods or water fleas). Larvae are released in the stomach, penetrate the mucosa, mature, and mate. About 1 yr later, the adult female worm (1-2 mm in diameter and up to 1 m long) migrates and partially emerges through the human host skin, usually of the legs. Thousands of immature larvae are released when the affected body part is immersed in the water. The cycle is completed when larval forms are ingested by the crustaceans. Infected humans have no symptoms until the worm reaches the subcutaneous tissue, causing a **stinging papule** that may be accompanied by urticaria, nausea, vomiting, diarrhea, and dyspnea. The lesion vesiculates, ruptures, and forms a painful ulcer in which a portion of the worm is visible. Diagnosis is established clinically. Larvae can be identified by microscopic examination of the discharge fluid. **Metronidazole** (25 mg/kg/day tid PO for 10 days, maximum dose 750 mg) decreases local inflammation. Although the drug does not kill the worm, it facilitates its removal. The worm must be physically removed by rolling the slowly emerging 1 m long parasite onto a thin stick over a week. Topical corticosteroids shorten the time to complete healing while topical antibiotics decrease the risk of secondary bacterial infection. Dracunculiasis can be prevented by boiling or chlorinating drinking water or passing the water through a cloth sieve before consumption. Eradication is dependent on behavior modification and education.

GNATHOSTOMA SPINIGERUM

Gnathostoma spinigerum is a dog and cat nematode endemic to Southeast Asia, Japan, China, Bangladesh, and India, but has been identified in Mexico and parts of South America. Infection is acquired by ingesting intermediate hosts containing larvae of the parasite such as raw or undercooked freshwater fish, chickens, pigs, snails, or frogs. Penetration of the skin by larval forms and prenatal transmission has also been described. Nonspecific signs and symptoms such as generalized malaise, fever, urticaria, anorexia, nausea, vomiting, diarrhea, and epigastric pain develop 24-48 hr after ingestion of *G. spinigerum.* Ingested larvae penetrate the gastric wall and migrate through soft tissue for up to 10 yr. Moderate to severe eosinophilia can develop. Cutaneous gnathostomiasis manifests as intermittent episodes of localized, migratory nonpitting edema associated with pain, pruritus, or erythema. Central nervous system involvement in gnathostomiasis is suggested by focal neurologic findings, initially neuralgia followed within a few days by paralysis or changes in mental status. Multiple cranial nerves may be involved, and the cerebrospinal fluid may be xanthochromic but typically shows an eosinophilic pleocytosis. Diagnosis of gnathostomiasis is based on clinical presentation and epidemiologic background. Brain and spinal cord lesions may be seen on CT or MRI. Serologic testing varies in sensitivity and specificity and is available through the Centers for Disease Control and Prevention. There is no well-documented effective chemotherapy, although **albendazole** (400 mg PO bid for 21 days) has been suggested to be useful. Multiple courses may be needed. Corticosteroids have been used to relieve focal neurologic deficits. Surgical resection of the *Gnathostoma* is the major mode of therapy and the treatment of choice. Blind surgical resection of subcutaneous areas of diffuse swelling is not recommended because the worm can rarely be located. Prevention through the avoidance of ingestion of poorly cooked or raw fish, poultry, or pork should be emphasized for individuals living in or visiting endemic areas.

BIBLIOGRAPHY

Please visit the Nelson Textbook of Pediatrics *website at www.expertconsult.com for the complete bibliography.*

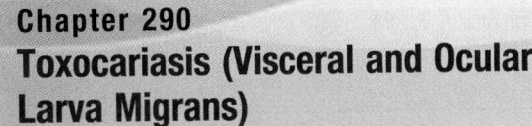

Chapter 290
Toxocariasis (Visceral and Ocular Larva Migrans)

Arlene E. Dent and James W. Kazura

ETIOLOGY

Most cases of human toxocariasis are caused by the **dog roundworm,** *Toxocara canis.* Adult female *T. canis* worms live in the intestinal tracts of young puppies and their lactating mothers. Large numbers of eggs are passed in the feces of dogs and embryonate under optimal soil conditions. *Toxocara* eggs can survive relatively harsh environmental conditions and are resistant to freezing and extremes of moisture and pH. Humans ingest embryonated eggs contaminating soil, hands, or fomites. The larvae hatch and penetrate the intestinal wall and travel via the circulation to the liver, lung, and other tissues. Humans do not excrete *T. canis* eggs because the larvae are unable to complete their maturation to adult worms in the intestine. The **cat roundworm,** *Toxocara cati,* is responsible for far fewer cases of visceral larva migrans (VLM) than *T. canis.* Ingestion of infective larvae of the raccoon ascarid *Baylisascaris procyonis* rarely leads to VLM, but can cause neural larva migrans resulting in fatal eosinophilic meningitis. Ingestion of larvae from the opossum ascarid *Lagochilascaris minor* leads to VLM rarely.

EPIDEMIOLOGY

Human *T. canis* infections have been reported in nearly all parts of the world, primarily in temperate and tropical areas where dogs are popular household pets. Young children are at highest risk because of their unsanitary play habits and tendency to place fingers in the mouth. Other behavioral risk factors include pica, contact with puppy litters, and institutionalization. In North America, the highest prevalences of infection are in the southeastern USA and Puerto Rico, particularly among socially disadvantaged African-American and Hispanic children. In the USA, serosurveys show that 4.6-7.3% of children are infected. Assuming an unrestrained and untreated dog population, toxocariasis is prevalent in settings where other geohelminth infections such as ascariasis, trichuriasis, and hookworm infections are common.

PATHOGENESIS

T. canis larvae secrete large amounts of immunogenic glycosylated proteins. These antigens induce immune responses that lead to eosinophilia and polyclonal and antigen-specific immunoglobulin E (IgE) production. The characteristic histopathologic lesions are granulomas containing eosinophils, multinucleated giant cells (histiocytes), and collagen. Granulomas are typically found in the liver but may also occur in the lungs, central nervous system (CNS), and ocular tissues. Clinical manifestations reflect the intensity and chronicity of infection, anatomic localization of larvae, and host granulomatous responses.

CLINICAL MANIFESTATIONS

There are 3 major clinical syndromes associated with human toxocariasis: VLM, ocular larva migrans (OLM), and covert toxocariasis (Table 290-1). The classic presentation of VLM includes eosinophilia, fever, and hepatomegaly, and occurs most commonly in toddlers with a history of pica and exposure to puppies. The findings include fever, cough, wheezing, bronchopneumonia, anemia, hepatomegaly, leukocytosis, eosinophilia, and positive *Toxocara* serology. Cutaneous manifestations such as pruritis, eczema, and urticaria can be present. OLM tends to occur in older children without signs or symptoms of VLM. Presenting symptoms include unilateral visual loss, eye pain, white pupil, or strabismus that develops over a period of weeks. Granulomas occur on the posterior pole of the retina and may be mistaken for retinoblastoma. Serologic testing for *Toxocara* has allowed the identification of individuals with less obvious or covert symptoms of infection. These children may have nonspecific complaints that do not constitute a recognizable syndrome. Common findings include hepatomegaly, abdominal pain, cough, sleep disturbance, failure to thrive, and headache with elevated *Toxocara* antibody titers. Eosinophilia may be present in only 50-75% of cases. The prevalence of positive *Toxocara* serology in the general population supports the notion that most children with *T. canis* infection are asymptomatic and will not develop overt clinical sequelae over time. A correlation between positive *Toxocara* serology and allergic asthma has also been described.

DIAGNOSIS

A presumptive diagnosis can be established in a young child with **eosinophilia** (>20%), leukocytosis, hepatomegaly, fevers, wheezing, and a history of geophagia and exposure to puppies or unrestrained dogs. Supportive laboratory findings include hypergammaglobulinemia and elevated isohemagglutinin titers to A and B blood group antigens. Most patients with VLM have an absolute eosinophil count of >500/μL. Eosinophilia is less common in subjects with OLM. Biopsy confirms the diagnosis. When biopsies cannot be obtained, an enzyme-linked immunosorbent assay using excretory-secretory proteins harvested from *T. canis* larvae maintained in vitro is the standard serologic test used to confirm toxocariasis. The sensitivity is approximately 78% and specificity 92% at a titer of 1:42. The sensitivity for OLM is significantly less. The diagnosis of OLM can be established in patients with typical clinical findings of a retinal or peripheral pole granuloma or endophthalmitis with elevated antibody titers. Vitreous and aqueous humor fluid anti-*Toxocara* titers are usually greater than serum titers. The diagnosis of covert toxocariasis should be considered in individuals with chronic weakness, abdominal pain, or allergic signs with eosinophilia and increased IgE. In temperate regions of the world, nonparasitic causes of eosinophilia that should be considered in the differential diagnosis include allergies, drug hypersensitivity, lymphoma, vasculitis, and the idiopathic hypereosinophilic syndrome (Chapter 123).

TREATMENT

Most cases do not require treatment because signs and symptoms are mild and subside over a period of weeks to months. Several anthelmintic drugs have been used for symptomatic cases, often with adjunctive corticosteroids to limit inflammatory responses that presumably result from release of *Toxocara* antigens by dying parasites. Albendazole (400 mg bid PO for 5 days for all

Table 290-1 CLINICAL SYNDROMES OF HUMAN TOXOCARIASIS

SYNDROME	CLINICAL FINDINGS	AVERAGE AGE	INFECTIOUS DOSE	INCUBATION PERIOD	LABORATORY FINDINGS	ELISA
Visceral larva migrans	Fevers, hepatomegaly, asthma	5 yr	Moderate to high	Weeks to months	Eosinophilia, leukocytosis, elevated IgE	High (≥1:16)
Ocular larva migrans	Visual disturbances, retinal granulomas, endophthalmitis, peripheral granulomas	12 yr	Low	Months to years	Usually none	Low (<1:512)
Covert toxocariasis	Abdominal pain, gastrointestinal symptoms, weakness, hepatomegaly, pruritus, rash	School age to adult	Low to moderate	Weeks to years	±Eosinophilia, ±elevated IgE	Low to moderate

ELISA, enzyme-linked immunosorbent assay; IgE, immunoglobulin E; ±, with or without.
Adapted from Liu LX: Toxocariasis and larva migrans syndrome. In Guerrant RL, Walker DH, Weller PF, editors: *Tropical infectious diseases: principles, pathogens & practice,* Philadelphia, 1999, Churchill-Livingstone, p 908.

ages) has demonstrated efficacy in both children and adults. Mebendazole (100-200 mg bid PO for 5 days for all ages) is also useful. Anthelmintic treatment of CNS and ocular disease should be extended (3-4 wk). Even though there are no clinical trials regarding therapy of OLM, a course of oral corticosteroids such as prednisone (1 mg/kg/day PO for 2-4 wk) has been recommended to suppress local inflammation while treatment with anthelmintic agents is initiated.

PREVENTION

Transmission can be minimized by public health measures that prevent dog feces from contaminating the environment. These include keeping dogs on leashes and excluding pets from playgrounds and sandboxes that toddlers use. Children should be discouraged from putting dirty fingers in their mouth and eating dirt. Vinyl covering of sandboxes reduces the viability of *T. canis* eggs. Widespread veterinary use of broad-spectrum anthelmintics effective against *Toxocara* may lead to a decline in parasite transmission to humans.

BIBLIOGRAPHY

Please visit the Nelson Textbook of Pediatrics *website at* *www.expertconsult.com* *for the complete bibliography.*

Chapter 291
Trichinosis (*Trichinella spiralis*)

Arlene E. Dent and James W. Kazura

ETIOLOGY

Human trichinosis (trichinellosis) is caused by consumption of meat containing encysted larvae of *Trichinella spiralis,* a tissue-dwelling nematode with a worldwide distribution. After ingestion of raw or inadequately cooked meat containing viable *Trichinella* larvae, the organisms are released from the cyst by acid-pepsin digestion of the cyst walls in the stomach and then pass into the small intestine. The larvae invade the small intestine columnar epithelium at the villi base and develop into adult worms. The adult female produces about 500 larvae over 2 wk and is then expelled in the feces. The larvae enter the bloodstream and seed striated muscle by burrowing into individual muscle fibers. Over a period of 3 wk, they coil as they increase about 10 times in length and become capable of infecting a new host if ingested. The larvae eventually become encysted and can remain viable for years.

EPIDEMIOLOGY

Despite veterinary public health efforts to control and eradicate the parasite, reemergence of the disease has been observed in many areas of the world in the past 10-20 yr. Trichinosis is most common in Asia, Latin America, and Central Europe. Swine fed with garbage may become infected when given uncooked trichinous scraps, usually pig meat, or when the carcasses of infected wild animals such as rats are eaten. Prevalence rates of *T. spiralis* in domestic swine range from 0.001% in the USA to ≥25% in China. The resurgence of this disease can be attributed to translocations of animal populations, human travel, and export of food as well as ingestion of sylvatic *Trichinella* (*T. brivoti, T. nativa, T. pseudospiralis,* and *T. murrelli*) through game meat. In the USA from 1997 to 2001, wild game meat (especially bear meat) was the most common source of infection. Most outbreaks occur from the consumption of *T. spiralis*–infected pork (or horse meat in areas of the world where horse is eaten) obtained from a single source.

PATHOGENESIS

During the 1st 2-3 wk after infection, pathologic reactions to infection are limited to the gastrointestinal tract and include a mild, partial villous atrophy with an inflammatory infiltrate of neutrophils, eosinophils, lymphocytes, and macrophages in the mucosa and submucosa. Larvae are released by female worms and disseminate over the next several weeks. Skeletal muscle fibers show the most striking changes with edema and basophilic degeneration. The muscle fiber may contain the typical coiled worm, the cyst wall derived from the host cell, and the surrounding lymphocytic and eosinophilic infiltrate.

CLINICAL MANIFESTATIONS

The development of symptoms depends on the number of viable larvae ingested. Most infections are asymptomatic or mild, and children often show milder symptoms than adults who consumed the same amount of infected meat. Watery diarrhea is the most common symptom corresponding to maturation of the adult worms in the gastrointestinal tract, which occurs during the 1st 1-2 wk after ingestion. Patients may also complain of abdominal discomfort and vomiting. Fulminant enteritis may develop in individuals with extremely high worm burdens. The classic symptoms of facial and periorbital edema, fever, weakness, malaise, and myalgia peak about 2-3 wk after the infected meat is ingested as the larvae migrate and then encyst in the muscle. Headache, cough, dyspnea, dysphagia, subconjunctival and splinter hemorrhages, and a macular or petechial rash may occur. Patients with high intensity infection may die from myocarditis, encephalitis, or pneumonia. In symptomatic patients, eosinophilia is common and may be dramatic.

DIAGNOSIS

The Centers for Disease Control and Prevention diagnostic criteria for trichinosis require positive serology or muscle biopsy for *Trichinella* with 1 or more compatible clinical symptoms (eosinophilia, fever, myalgia, facial or periorbital edema). To declare a discrete outbreak, at least one person must have positive serology or muscle biopsy. Antibodies to *Trichinella* are detectable about 3 wk after infection. Severe muscle involvement results in elevated serum creatine phosphokinase and lactic dehydrogenase levels. Muscle biopsy is not usually necessary, but if needed, a sample should be obtained from a tender swollen muscle. A history of eating undercooked meat supports the diagnosis. The cysts may calcify and be visible by radiograph.

TREATMENT

Recommended treatment of trichinosis is mebendazole (200-400 mg tid PO for 3 days then 400-500 mg tid PO for 10 days, for all ages) to eradicate the adult worms if a patient has ingested contaminated meat within the previous 1 wk. An alternative regimen is albendazole (400 mg bid PO for 8-14 days, for all ages). There is no consensus for treatment of muscle stage trichinosis. Systemic corticosteroids along with mebendazole may be used, although evidence for efficacy is anecdotal. Thiabendazole (25 mg/kg bid PO for 10 days) and mebendazole (200 mg bid PO for 10 days) are effective against muscle larvae; mebendazole may have been less active but thiabendazole was poorly tolerated.

PREVENTION

Trichinella larvae can be killed by cooking meat (≥55°C) until there is no trace of pink fluid or flesh, or storage in a freezer (−15°C) for ≥3 wk. Freezing to kill larvae should only be applied to pork meat, as larvae in horse, wild boar, or game meat can remain viable even after 4 wk of freezing. Smoking, salting, and drying meat are unreliable methods of killing *Trichinella*. Strict adherence to pubic health measures including garbage feeding regulations, stringent rodent control, prevention of exposure of pigs and other livestock to animal carcasses, constructing barriers between livestock, wild animals, and domestic pets, and proper handling of wild animal carcasses by hunters can reduce infection with *Trichinella*. Current meat inspection for trichinosis is by direct digestion and visualization of encysted larvae in meat samples. Serologic testing does not have a role in meat inspection.

BIBLIOGRAPHY

Please visit the Nelson Textbook of Pediatrics *website at* *www.expertconsult.com* *for the complete bibliography.*

Chapter 292
Schistosomiasis *(Schistosoma)*

Charles H. King and Amaya Lopez Bustinduy

The term schistosomiasis encompasses the acute and chronic inflammatory disorders caused by human infection with *Schistosoma* spp. parasites. Disease is related to both the systemic and focal effects of schistosome infection and its consequent host immune responses, which often result in disabling morbidity for the affected patient.

ETIOLOGY

Schistosoma organisms are the trematodes, or flukes, that parasitize the bloodstream. Five schistosome species infect humans: *Schistosoma haematobium, S. mansoni, S. japonicum, S. intercalatum,* and *S. mekongi*. Humans are infected through contact with water contaminated with **cercariae**, the free-living infective stage of the parasite. These motile, forked-tail organisms emerge from infected snails and are capable of penetrating intact human skin. As they reach maturity, adult worms migrate to specific anatomic sites characteristic of each schistosome species: *S. haematobium* adults are found in the perivesical and periureteral venous plexus, *S. mansoni* in the inferior mesenteric veins, and *S. japonicum* in the superior mesenteric veins. *S. intercalatum* and *S. mekongi* are usually found in the mesenteric vessels. Adult schistosome worms (1-2 cm long) are clearly adapted for an intravascular existence. The female accompanies the male in a groove formed by the lateral edges of its body. On fertilization, female worms begin oviposition in the small venous tributaries. The eggs of the 3 main schistosome species have characteristic morphologic features: *S. haematobium* has a terminal spine, *S. mansoni* has a lateral spine, and *S. japonicum* has a smaller size with a short, curved spine (Fig. 292-1). Parasite eggs provoke significant granulomatous inflammatory response, which allows them to ulcerate through host tissues to reach the lumen of the urinary tract or intestines. They are carried to the outside environment in urine or feces, where they will hatch if deposited in freshwater. Motile **miracidia** emerge, infect specific freshwater snail intermediate hosts, and divide asexually. After 4-12 wk, the infective cercariae are released by the snails into the contaminated water.

EPIDEMIOLOGY

Schistosomiasis infects >207 million people worldwide, primarily children and young adults. Prevalence is increasing in many areas as population density increases and new irrigation projects provide broader habitats for vector snails. Humans are the definitive host for the 5 clinically important species of schistosomes, although *S. japonicum* may infect some animals such as dogs, rats, pigs, and cattle. *S. haematobium* is prevalent in Africa and the Middle East; *S. mansoni* is prevalent in Africa, the Middle East, the Caribbean, and South America; and *S. japonicum* is prevalent in China, the Philippines, and Indonesia, with some sporadic foci in parts of Southeast Asia. The other 2 species are less prevalent. *S. intercalatum* is found in West and Central Africa, and *S. mekongi* is found only along the upper Mekong River in the Far East.

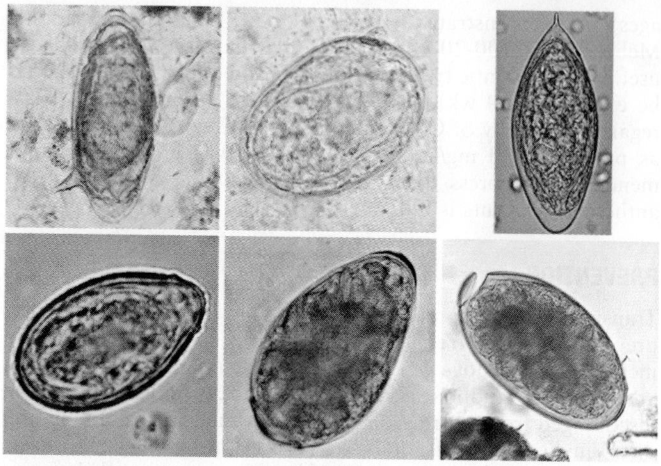

Figure 292-1 Eggs of common human trematodes. Clockwise from upper left: *Schistosoma mansoni, Schistosoma japonicum, Schistosoma haematobium, Clonorchis sinensis, Paragonimus westermani,* and *Fasciola hepatica* (note the partially open operculum). (From Centers for Disease Control and Prevention: *DPDx: laboratory identification of parasites of public health concern.* http://www.dpd.cdc.gov/DPDx/.)

Transmission depends on disposal of excreta, the presence of specific intermediate snail hosts, and the patterns of water contact and social habits of the population (Fig. 292-2). The distribution of infection in endemic areas shows that prevalence increases with age to a peak at 10-20 yr of age. Measuring intensity of infection (by quantitative egg count in urine or feces) demonstrates that the heaviest worm loads are found in the younger age groups. Therefore, schistosomiasis is most prevalent and most severe in children and young adults, who are at maximal risk for suffering from its acute and chronic sequelae.

PATHOGENESIS

Both the early and late manifestations of schistosomiasis are immunologically mediated. Acute schistosomiasis, known as *snail fever* or *Katayama syndrome*, is a febrile illness that represents an immune complex disease associated with early infection and oviposition. The major pathology of infection occurs later, with chronic schistosomiasis, in which retention of eggs in the host tissues is associated with chronic granulomatous injury. Eggs may be trapped at sites of deposition (urinary bladder, ureters, intestine) or be carried by the bloodstream to other organs, most commonly the liver and less often the lungs and central nervous system. The host response to these eggs involves local as well as systemic manifestations. The cell-mediated immune response leads to granulomas composed of lymphocytes, macrophages, and eosinophils that surround the trapped eggs and add significantly to the degree of tissue destruction. Granuloma formation in the bladder wall and at the ureterovesical junction results in the major disease manifestations of schistosomiasis haematobia: hematuria, dysuria, and obstructive uropathy. Intestinal as well as hepatic granulomas underlie the pathologic sequelae of the other schistosome infections: ulcerations and fibrosis of intestinal wall, hepatosplenomegaly, and portal hypertension due to presinusoidal obstruction of blood flow. In terms of systemic disease, antischistosome inflammation increases circulating levels of proinflammatory cytokines

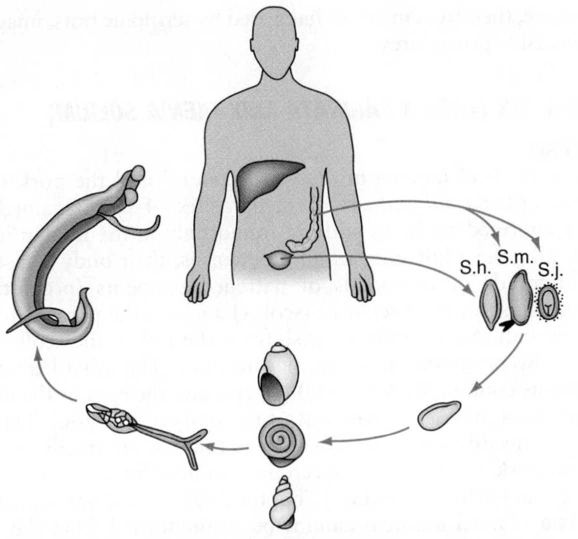

Figure 292-2 Life cycle of schistosomes. Eggs are passed in stools for *Schistosoma mansoni* (S.m.) and *Schistosoma japonicum* (S.j.) and in urine for *Schistosoma haematobium* (S.h.). The eggs hatch in freshwater, miracidia invade specific snail intermediate hosts, and in a few weeks, forked-tail cercariae are liberated. These infective forms penetrate human skin, pass through a migratory phase in the lung and liver, and then pass to their final habitat in the portal venous system (S.m. and S.j.) or the urinary bladder venous plexus (S.h.). Two other species infect humans, although less frequently. *Schistosoma intercalatum* produces terminal spined eggs that may be found in feces, whereas *Schistosoma mekongi* produces eggs similar to but smaller than those of *S. japonicum,* which also may be found in stools. All 5 species of schistosomes have characteristic snail intermediate hosts. (From Mandell GL, Bennett JE, Dolin R, editors: *Principles and practice of infectious diseases,* vol 2, ed 6, Philadelphia, 2006, Elsevier, p 3278.)

such as tumor necrosis factor (TNF)-α and interleukin (IL)-6, associated with elevated levels of C-reactive protein. These responses are associated with hepcidin-mediated inhibition of iron uptake and utilization, leading to anemia of chronic inflammation. Schistosomiasis-related undernutrition may be the result of similar pathways of chronic inflammation. Acquired partial protective immunity against schistosomiasis has been demonstrated in some animal species and may occur in humans.

CLINICAL MANIFESTATIONS

Most chronically infected individuals experience mild symptoms and may not seek medical attention; the more severe symptoms of schistosomiasis occur mainly in those who are heavily infected or who have been infected over longer periods of time. In addition to organ-specific morbidities, infected patients may demonstrate anemia, chronic pain, diarrhea, exercise intolerance, and undernutrition. Cercarial penetration of human skin may result in a papular pruritic rash known as schistosomal dermatitis or **swimmer's itch.** It is more pronounced in previously exposed individuals and is characterized by edema and massive cellular infiltrates in the dermis and epidermis. Acute schistosomiasis, **Katayama syndrome,** may occur, particularly in heavily infected individuals 4-8 wk after exposure; this is a serum sickness–like syndrome manifested by the acute onset of fever, chills, sweating, lymphadenopathy, hepatosplenomegaly, and eosinophilia. Acute schistosomiasis most commonly presents in 1st time visitors to endemic areas who experience primary infection at an older age.

Symptomatic children with chronic schistosomiasis haematobia usually complain of frequency, dysuria, and hematuria. Urine examination shows erythrocytes, parasite eggs, and occasional eosinophiluria. In endemic areas, moderate to severe pathologic lesions have been demonstrated in the urinary tract of >20% of infected children. The extent of disease correlates with the intensity of infection, but significant morbidity can occur even in lightly infected children. The advanced stages of schistosomiasis haematobia are associated with chronic renal failure, secondary infections, and cancer of the bladder.

Children with chronic schistosomiasis mansoni, japonica, intercalatum, or mekongi may have intestinal symptoms; colicky abdominal pain and bloody diarrhea are the most common. However, the intestinal phase may remain subclinical, and the late syndrome of hepatosplenomegaly, portal hypertension, ascites, and hematemesis may then be the 1st clinical presentation. Liver disease is due to granuloma formation and subsequent fibrosis; no appreciable liver cell injury occurs, and hepatic function may be preserved for a long time. Schistosome eggs may escape into the lungs, causing pulmonary hypertension and cor pulmonale. *S. japonicum* worms may migrate to the brain vasculature and produce localized lesions that cause seizures. Transverse myelitis rarely has been reported in children or young adults with either acute or chronic *S. haematobium* or *S. mansoni* infection.

DIAGNOSIS

Schistosome eggs are found in the excreta of infected individuals; quantitative methods should be used to provide an indication of the burden of infection. For diagnosis of schistosomiasis haematobia, a volume of 10 mL of urine should be collected around midday, which is the time of maximal egg excretion, and filtered for microscopic examination. Stool examination by the Kato thick smear procedure is the method of choice for diagnosis and quantification of other schistosome infections.

TREATMENT

Treatment of children with schistosomiasis should be based on an appreciation of the intensity of infection and the extent of disease. The recommended treatment for schistosomiasis is praziquantel (40 mg/kg/day divided bid PO for 1 day for schistosomiasis haematobia, mansoni, and intercalatum; 60 mg/kg/day divided tid PO for 1 day for schistosomiasis japonica and mekongi). For *S. mansoni,* oxamniquine has been effective in some areas where praziquantel has been less effective.

PREVENTION

Transmission in endemic areas may be decreased by reducing the parasite load in the human population. The availability of oral, single-dose, effective chemotherapeutic agents may help achieve this goal. When added to drug-based programs, other measures such as improved sanitation, focal application of molluscicides, and animal vaccination may prove useful in breaking the cycle of transmission. Ultimately, control of schistosomiasis is closely linked to economic and social development.

BIBLIOGRAPHY

Please visit the Nelson Textbook of Pediatrics *website at www.expertconsult.com for the complete bibliography.*

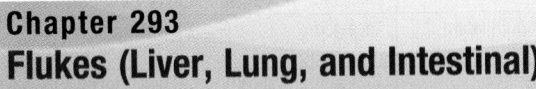

Chapter 293
Flukes (Liver, Lung, and Intestinal)

Charles H. King and Amaya Lopez Bustinduy

Several different trematodes, or flukes, can parasitize humans and cause disease. Flukes are endemic worldwide but are more prevalent in the less developed parts of the world. They include *Schistosoma,* or the blood flukes (Chapter 292), as well as fluke species that cause infection in the human biliary tree, lung tissue, and intestinal tract. These latter trematodes are characterized by complex life cycles. Sexual reproduction of adult worms in the definitive host produces eggs that are passed in the stool. Larvae, called *miracidia*, develop in freshwater. These, in turn, infect certain species of mollusks (snails or clams), in which asexual multiplication by parasite larvae produces cercariae. Cercariae then seek a 2nd intermediate host such as an insect, crustacean, or fish or attach to vegetation to produce infectious metacercariae. Humans acquire liver, lung, and intestinal fluke infections by eating uncooked, lightly cooked, pickled, or smoked foods containing these infectious parasite cysts. The "alternation of generations" requires that flukes parasitize more than 1 host (often 3) to complete their life cycle. Because parasitic flukes are dependent on these nonhuman species for transmission, the distribution of human fluke infection closely matches the ecologic range of the flukes.

For the full continuation of this chapter, please visit the Nelson Textbook of Pediatrics *website at www.expertconsult.com.*

Chapter 294
Adult Tapeworm Infections

Ronald Blanton

Cestodes are segmented flat worms popularly referred to as *tapeworms*. The family is large with a wide range of sizes (8 mm to 10 m) and morbidities. Their life cycle is usually distributed between 2 hosts, although some species, such as *Taenia solium*, can complete development in 1 host and others, such as *Diphyllobothrium latum*, require 3 hosts. A consistent theme in cestode developmental biology is that the adult, sexually replicating stages inhabit the gastrointestinal tract and have low pathogenicity, whereas, the asexually reproducing intermediate stages are tissue invasive and are potentially the cause of very serious morbidity. Depending on the species, humans can be host to either stage or both (Table 294-1). The most important invasive cestodes, *T. solium* (Chapter 295) and *Echinococcus* species (Chapter 296), are presented in subsequent chapters. The differential distribution of adult versus intermediate stages also influences diagnostic approaches. Infection with the adult worm can be easily diagnosed by finding eggs or segments of adult worms in the stool, whereas the invasive stage of the parasite cannot be observed in any easily sampled fluid. Infection with an intermediate stage, therefore, must be diagnosed by serologic tests, imaging, or invasive procedures.

TAENIASIS (*TAENIA SAGINATA* AND *TAENIA SOLIUM*)

Etiology

The adult **beef tapeworm** *(Taenia saginata)* and the **pork tapeworm** *(Taenia solium)* are large parasites (4-10 m) named for their intermediate hosts and are found only in the human intestine. Like the adult stage of all tapeworms, their body is a series of hundreds or thousands of flattened segments (**proglottids**) whose most anterior segment (**scolex**) anchors the parasite to the bowel wall. New segments arise from the tail of the scolex followed by progressively more mature ones. The gravid terminal segments contain 50,000-100,000 eggs, and the eggs or the intact proglottids themselves pass out of the body in the stool. These 2 tapeworms differ most significantly in that the intermediate stage of the pork tapeworm (cysticercus) can also infect humans and cause significant morbidity (Chapter 295). A 3rd species found in Asia *(Taenia asiatica)* cannot be distinguished from the beef tapeworm, but its intermediate stage infects the liver of pigs and may produce invasive disease in humans.

Epidemiology

The pork and beef tapeworms are distributed worldwide, with the highest risk for infection in Central America, Africa, India, Southeast Asia, and China. The prevalence in adults may not reflect the prevalence in young children, because cultural practices may dictate how well meat is cooked and how much is served to children.

Pathogenesis

Uncomplicated infection with the adult beef or pork tapeworm by itself is an infrequent source of symptoms. When children ingest raw or undercooked infected meat, gastric acid and bile facilitate release of the immature scolex that attaches to the lumen of the small intestine. The parasite adds new segments, and after 2-3 mo the terminal segments mature, become gravid, and appear in stool.

Clinical Manifestations

Adult beef and pork tapeworms cause very little overt morbidity apart from nonspecific abdominal symptoms. The proglottids of

Table 294-1 COMMON CESTODE PARASITES OF HUMANS, THEIR TYPICAL VECTORS, AND THEIR USUAL SYMPTOMS

PARASITE SPECIES	DEVELOPMENTAL STAGE FOUND IN HUMANS	COMMON NAME	TRANSMISSION SOURCE	SYMPTOMS ASSOCIATED WITH INFECTION
Taenia saginata	Tapeworm	Beef tapeworm	Cysts in beef	Abdominal discomfort, proglottid migration
Taenia solium	Tapeworm	Pork tapeworm	Cysticerci in pork	Minimal
Taenia solium (cysticercus cellulosae)	Cysticerci	Cysticercosis	Eggs from infected humans	Local inflammation, mass effect; if in central nervous system, seizures, hydrocephalus, arachnoiditis
Taenia asiatica	Tapeworm Cysticerci—uncertain	Asian *Taenia*	Pigs	Unknown; may be invasive for liver or brain
Diphyllobothrium latum	Tapeworm	Fish tapeworm	Plerocercoid cysts in fresh water fish	Usually minimal; with prolonged or heavy infection, vitamin B_{12} deficiency
Hymenolepis nana	Tapeworm, cysticercoids	Dwarf tapeworm	Infected humans	Mild abdominal discomfort
Dipylidium caninum	Tapeworm	None	Domestic dogs and cats	Eosinophilia, anal puritis confused with pinworm
Echinococcus granulosus	Larval cysts	Hydatid cyst disease	Eggs from infected dogs	Mass effect leading to pain, obstruction of adjacent organs; less commonly, secondary bacterial infection, distal spread of daughter cysts
Echinococcus multilocularis	Larval cysts	Alveolar cyst disease	Eggs from infected canines	Local invasion and mass effect leading to organ dysfunction; distal metastasis possible
Taenia multiceps	Larval cysts	Coenurosis, bladder worm	Eggs from infected dogs	Local inflammation and mass effect
Spirometra mansonoides	Larval cysts	Sparganosis	Cysts from infected copepods, frogs, snakes	Local inflammation and mass effect

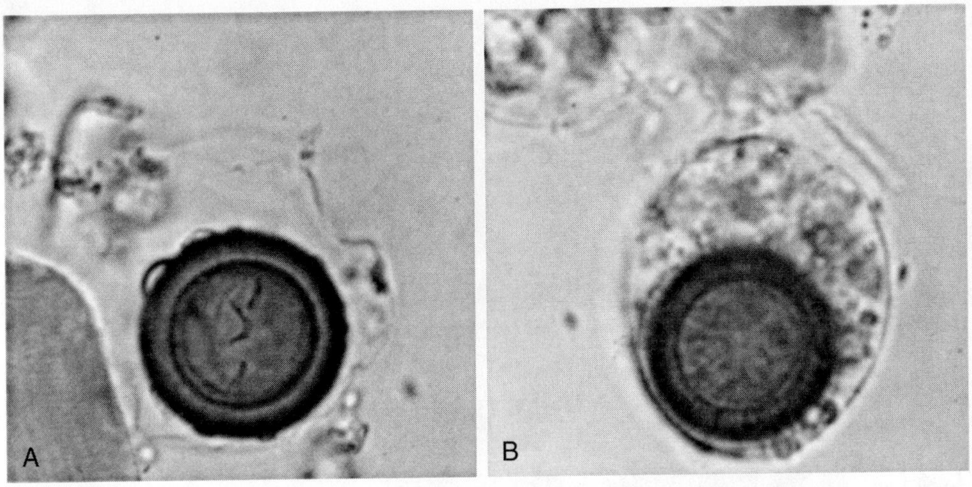

Figure 294-1 *A* and *B*, Eggs of *Taenia saginata* recovered from feces (original magnification ×400). The eggs are generally bile stained, dark, and prismatic. There is occasionally some surrounding cellular material from the proglottid in which the egg develops, which is more evident in *B* than in *A*. The larva within the egg shows 3 pairs of hooklets (*A*), which may occasionally be observed in motion.

these tapeworms can be noticeable in stool or underwear. They are also motile and sometimes produce anal pruritus. The adult beef and pork tapeworms are rare causes of intestinal obstruction, pancreatitis, cholangitis, and appendicitis.

Diagnosis

It is important to identify the infecting species of tapeworm. Carriers of adult pork tapeworms are at increased risk for transmitting eggs with the pathogenic intermediate stage (**cysticercus**) to themselves or others, whereas children infected with the beef tapeworm are a risk only to livestock. Because proglottids are generally passed intact, visual examination for gravid proglottids in the stool is a sensitive test; these segments may be used to identify species. Eggs, by contrast, are often absent from stool and cannot reliably distinguish between *T. saginata* and *T. solium* (Fig. 294-1). If the parasite is completely expelled, the scolex of each species is diagnostic. The scolex of *T. saginata* has only a set of 4 anteriorly oriented suckers, whereas *T. solium* is armed with a double row of hooks in addition to suckers. The proglottids of *T. saginata* have more than 20 branches from a central uterine structure, and those of *T. solium* have 10 or fewer. When in doubt, more proglottids should be obtained or the sample should be referred to a laboratory with parasitologic expertise. Only molecular methods can be used to distinguish *T. saginata* from *T. asiatica*.

Differential Diagnosis

Anal pruritus may mimic symptoms of pinworm *(Enterobius vermicularis)* infection. *D. latum* or even *Ascaris lumbricoides* may be mistaken for *T. saginata* or *T. solium* in stools.

Treatment

Infections with all adult tapeworms respond to praziquantel (25 mg/kg PO once). An alternative treatment for taeniasis is niclosamide (50 mg/kg PO once for children, 2 g PO once for adults). However, this medication is no longer available in the USA. The parasite is usually expelled on the day of administration.

Prevention

Prolonged freezing or thorough cooking of beef and pork kills the parasite. Appropriate human sanitation can interrupt transmission by preventing infection in livestock.

DIPHYLLOBOTHRIASIS *(DIPHYLLOBOTHRIUM LATUM)*

Etiology

The **fish tapeworm,** *Diphyllobothrium latum,* is the longest human tapeworm (>10 m) and has an organization similar to that of other adult cestodes. An elongated scolex equipped with slits (**bothria**) along each side but no suckers or hooks is followed by thousands of segments looped in the small bowel. The terminal gravid proglottid detaches periodically but tends to disintegrate before expulsion, thus releasing its eggs into the feces. In contrast to taeniids, the life cycle of *D. latum* requires 2 intermediate hosts. Small fresh water crustaceans (copepods) take up the larvae that hatch from parasite eggs. The parasite passes up the food chain as small fish eat the copepods and are in turn eaten by larger fish. In this way, the juvenile parasite becomes concentrated in pike, walleye, perch, burbot, and perhaps salmon associated with aquaculture of this species. Consumption of raw or undercooked fish leads to human infection with adult fish tapeworms.

Epidemiology

The fish tapeworm is most prevalent in the temperate climates of Europe, North America, and Asia but may be found in cold lakes at high altitudes in South America and Africa. In North America, the prevalence is highest in Alaska, Canada, and the northern USA. The tapeworm is found in fish from those areas brought to market in the continental USA. Persons who prepare raw fish for home or commercial use or who sample fish before cooking are particularly at risk for infection.

Pathogenesis

The adult worm efficiently scavenges vitamin B_{12} for its own use in the constant production of large numbers of segments and as many as 1 million eggs per day. As a result, diphyllobothriasis causes megaloblastic anemia in 2-9% of infections. Children with other causes of vitamin B_{12} or folate deficiency such as chronic infectious diarrhea, celiac disease, or congenital malabsorption are more likely to develop symptomatic infection.

Clinical Manifestations

Infection is largely asymptomatic, except in those who develop B_{12} or folate deficiency. Megaloblastic anemia with leukopenia, thrombocytopenia, glossitis, and signs of spinal cord posterior column degeneration (loss of vibratory sense, proprioception, and coordination) can be evidence of advanced nutritional deficiency due to diphyllobothriasis. It should be mentioned that an invasive form of infection termed sparganosis results when the intermediate form of this or other members of this group of tapeworm are introduced subcutaneously. Skin, muscle, eye, and brain have been sites of invasion.

Diagnosis

Parasitologic examination of the stool is useful because eggs are abundant in the feces and have morphology distinct from that of all other tapeworms. The eggs are ovoid and have an operculum, which is a cap structure at one end that opens to release the embryo (Fig. 294-2). The worm itself has a distinct scolex and

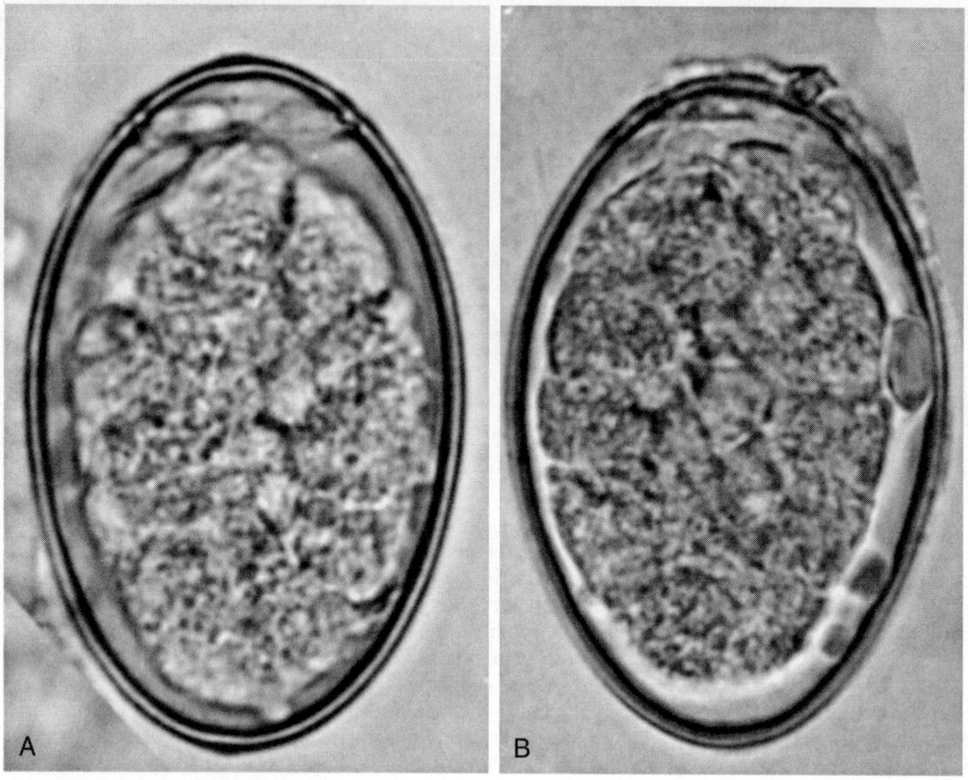

Figure 294-2 *A* and *B*, Eggs of *Diphyllobothrium latum* as seen in feces (original magnification ×400). The caplike operculum is at the upper end of the egg here.

proglottid morphology; however, these are not likely to be passed spontaneously.

Differential Diagnosis
A segment or a whole section of the worm might be confused with *Taenia* or *Ascaris* after it is passed. Pernicious anemia, bone marrow toxins, and dietary restrictions may contribute to or mimic diphyllobothriasis.

Treatment
As with all adult tapeworms, *D. latum* infections respond to praziquantel (5-10 mg/kg PO once).

Prevention
The intermediate stage is easily eliminated by brief cooking or prolonged freezing. Because humans are the major reservoir for adult worms, health education is one of the most important tools for preventing transmission, together with improved human sanitation.

HYMENOLEPIASIS *(HYMENOLEPIS)*
Infection with *Hymenolepis nana,* the **dwarf tapeworm,** is very common in developing countries. It is a major cause of eosinophilia, and although it rarely causes overt disease, the presence of *H. nana* eggs in stool may serve as a marker for exposure to poor hygienic conditions. The intermediate stage develops in various hosts (e.g., rodents, ticks, and fleas), and the entire life cycle can be completed in humans. Therefore, hyperinfection with thousands of small adult worms in a single child may occur. A similar infection may occur less commonly with the species *Hymenolepis diminuta.* Eggs but not segments may be found in the stool. *H. nana* infection responds to praziquantel (25 mg/kg PO once).

DIPYLIDIASIS *(DIPYLIDIUM CANINUM)*
Dipylidium caninum is a common tapeworm of domestic dogs and cats, yet human infection is relatively rare. Direct transmission between pets and humans does not occur; human infection requires ingestion of the parasite's intermediate host, the dog or cat flea. Infants and small children are particularly susceptible because of their level of hygiene, generally more intimate contact with pets, and activities in areas where fleas can be encountered. Anal pruritus, vague abdominal pain, and diarrhea have at times been associated with dipylidiasis, which is thus sometimes confused with pinworm *(E. vermicularis).* Dipylidiasis responds to treatment with praziquantel (5-10 mg/kg PO once). Deworming pets and flea control are the best preventive measures.

BIBLIOGRAPHY
Please visit the Nelson Textbook of Pediatrics *website at www.expertconsult.com for the complete bibliography.*

Chapter 295
Cysticercosis
Ronald Blanton

ETIOLOGY
Humans can be the definitive host (parasite sexual reproduction) as well as the intermediate host (parasite asexual reproduction) of *Taenia solium,* the **pork tapeworm.** Infection with the invasive intermediate stage (**cysticercus**) is called **cysticercosis.** Unlike *Taenia saginata,* the intermediate stage of *T. solium* is invasive with a tropism for the central nervous system (CNS) in humans, causing **neurocysticercosis.** The risk of cysticercosis may be the same for individuals who eat or do not eat pork, since humans acquire the intermediate form by ingestion of food or water contaminated with the eggs of *T. solium.* By contrast, consumption of infected undercooked pork produces intestinal infection with the adult worm (Chapter 294). Individuals harboring an adult worm may infect themselves with the eggs by the fecal-oral route. Reverse peristalsis in the small intestine has also been

implicated as a means of autoinfection. In the small intestine, the egg releases an **oncosphere** that crosses the gut wall and spreads hematogenously to many tissues, primarily brain and muscle. Wherever the eggs lodge, they produce small (0.2-0.5 cm) fluid-filled bladders containing a single **protoscolex**, the juvenile-stage parasite.

EPIDEMIOLOGY

The pork tapeworm is distributed worldwide wherever pigs are raised. Intense transmission occurs in Central and South America, India, Indonesia, Korea, and China as well as some areas of Africa. In these areas, 20-50% of cases of epilepsy may be due to cysticercosis. Most cases of cysticercosis in the USA are imported; transmission is uncommon but occurs.

PATHOGENESIS

Living, intact cystic stages usually do not provoke a strong immunologic response. Intact cysts can be associated with disease when the initial parasite invasion of the brain is massive or when they obstruct the flow of cerebrospinal fluid (CSF). Most cysts remain viable for 5-10 yr and then begin to degenerate, followed by a vigorous host response. The natural history of cysts is to resolve by complete resorption or calcification.

CLINICAL MANIFESTATIONS

Seizures are the presenting finding in ~70% of cases, although any cognitive or neurologic abnormality ranging from psychosis to stroke may be a manifestation of cysticercosis. It is useful to classify neurocysticercosis as parenchymal, intraventricular, meningeal, spinal, or ocular on the basis of anatomic location, clinical presentation, and radiologic appearance. Prognosis and management vary with location.

Parenchymal neurocysticercosis produces seizures as well as focal neurologic deficits. The seizures are generalized in 80% of cases but frequently begin as simple or complex partial seizures. Rarely, cerebral infarction can result from obstruction of small terminal arteries or vasculitis. With extensive frontal lobe disease, symptoms of intellectual deterioration with dementia or parkinsonism may obfuscate diagnosis until focal signs appear. A fulminant encephalitis-like presentation also occurs, most frequently in children who have had a massive initial infection. Intraventricular neurocysticercosis (5-10% of all cases) is associated with hydrocephalus and acute, subacute, or intermittent signs of increased intracranial pressure without localizing signs. The 4th ventricle is the most common site for obstruction and symptoms; cysts in the lateral ventricles are less likely to cause obstruction. Meningeal neurocysticercosis is associated with signs of meningeal irritation and also increased intracranial pressure that results from edema, inflammation, or the presence of a cyst obstructing flow of CSF. Chronic basilar meningitis is associated with many forms of neurocysticercosis, but predominantly meningeal presentations. Racemose neurocysticercosis is a meningeal form of disease in which large, lobulated cysts appear in the basal cisterns. **Spinal neurocysticercosis** presents with evidence of spinal cord compression, nerve root pain, transverse myelitis, or meningitis. Ocular neurocysticercosis causes decreased visual acuity due to cysticerci floating in the vitreous, retinal detachment, iridocyclitis, or orbital mass effect. Outside of the CNS, cysts can sometimes be palpated under the skin, and very heavy infections in skeletal or heart muscle can result in myositis or carditis.

DIAGNOSIS

Neurocysticercosis should be suspected in a child with onset of any neurologic, cognitive, or personality disorder and who also has a history of residence in an endemic area or a care provider from an endemic area. Seizures, hydrocephalus, unilateral visual impairment, or symptoms of encephalitis are particularly suspicious. Proglottids (segments) or eggs are observed in feces from only 25% of cases of neurocysticercosis; therefore, imaging studies and serologic tests are necessary to confirm a clinical suspicion.

The most useful diagnostic study for parenchymal disease is MRI of the head. MRI provides the most information about cyst viability and associated inflammation. The protoscolex is sometimes visible within the cyst, which provides a pathognomonic sign for cysticercosis (Fig. 295-1*A*). The MRI also better detects basilar arachnoiditis (Fig. 295-1*B*), intraventricular cysts (Fig 295-1*C*), as well as those in the spinal cord. CT is best for identifying calcifications. A solitary parenchymal cyst, with or without contrast enhancement, and numerous calcifications are the most common findings in children (Fig. 295-2). Plain films may reveal calcifications in muscle or brain consistent with cysticercosis, but these are often nondiagnostic in children and may also be found in congenital toxoplasmosis.

Serologic diagnosis using the enzyme-linked immunotransfer blot (EITB) is available commercially in the USA and through the Centers for Disease Control and Prevention. Serum antibody testing has ~90% sensitivity and specificity; testing of CSF is not required. Persons with many parenchymal cysts almost always have a positive serum EITB test result. Cases with solitary lesions or old calcified disease may not have detectable antibodies. Neurocysticercosis is the most important and most frequent cause of **eosinophilia** in CSF, but this is not a consistent finding.

DIFFERENTIAL DIAGNOSIS

Neurocysticercosis can be confused clinically with encephalitis, stroke, meningitis, and many other conditions (Table 295-1). Clinical suspicion is based on travel history or a history of contact with an individual who might carry an adult tapeworm. On imaging studies, cysticerci can be difficult to distinguish from tuberculomas, histoplasmosis, blastomycosis, toxoplasmosis, sarcoidosis, vasculitis, and tumor.

TREATMENT

The initial objectives of the management of cysticerosis are to diagnosis and manage hydrocephalus due to ventricular obstruction. The next is to control seizure activity. Most associated seizures can be readily controlled using standard anticonvulsant regimens. If seizures are recurrent or associated with calcified lesions, treatment should be continued for 2-3 yr before attempting weaning from anticonvulsants. The inclusion of antiparasitic drugs is controversial, but evidence appears to increasingly point to benefit in certain cases. Causes other than cysticercosis, especially tuberculoma, must be excluded (see Table 295-1).

The natural history of parenchymal lesions is to resolve spontaneously with or without antiparasitic drugs. Most children present with solitary parenchymal cysts that resolve as readily with as without therapy. Other forms of the disease are less common in children. By contrast, multiple lesions and complex presentations are typical of disease in adults. One double-blind, placebo-controlled study demonstrated a significant decrease in generalized seizures for cysticercosis in adults treated with antiparasitic therapy. Subsequently, meta-analyses of 4-6 randomized, controlled trials suggested an overall 2-fold decrease in recurrence of generalized seizures in patients treated with albendazole compared to those not treated. The benefit to children was significantly less, perhaps since most of these infections were with only 1-2 cysts. There is little evidence that the management of acute symptoms improves with these drugs, and they are not indicated where there are only degenerating or calcified lesions.

Subarachnoid disease has a poor prognosis if untreated, but antiparasitic treatment is associated with a better outcome in

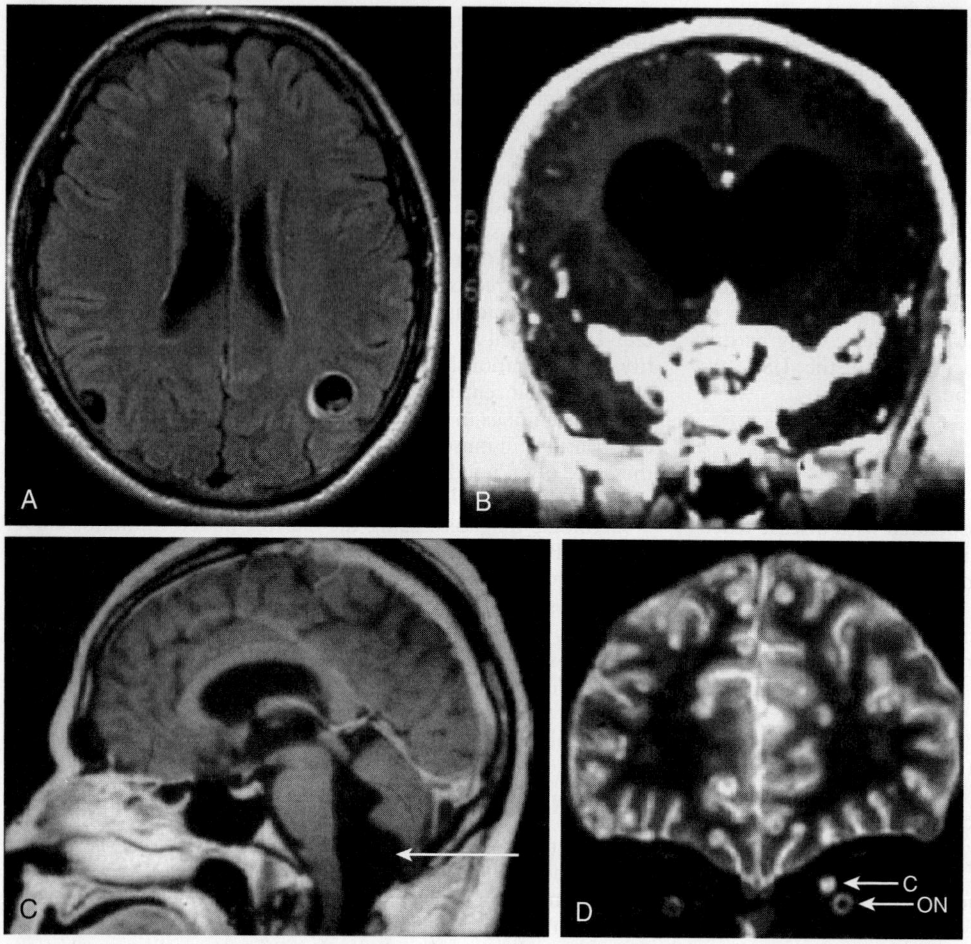

Figure 295-1 *A,* MRI (T1 weighted) demonstrating 2 parenchymal cysts with protoscolices. *B,* MRI (T1 weighted) of cysticercal basilar arachnoiditis. *C,* MRI (T1 weighted) showing a cyst below the 4th ventricle *(arrow). D,* MRI (T2 weighted) showing a cysticercus (C) above the optic nerve (ON).

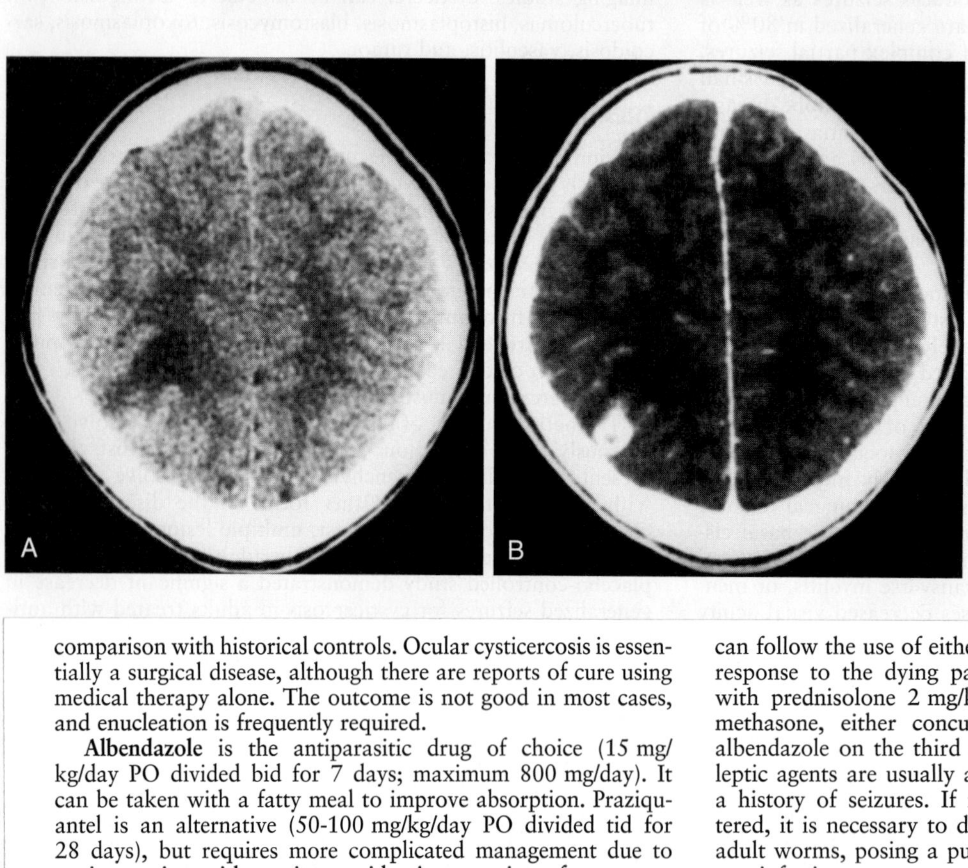

Figure 295-2 CT image of a solitary lesion of neurocysticercosis with *(A)* and without *(B)* contrast, showing contrast enhancement. (Courtesy of Dr. Wendy G. Mitchell and Dr. Marvin D. Nelson, Children's Hospital, Los Angeles.)

comparison with historical controls. Ocular cysticercosis is essentially a surgical disease, although there are reports of cure using medical therapy alone. The outcome is not good in most cases, and enucleation is frequently required.

Albendazole is the antiparasitic drug of choice (15 mg/kg/day PO divided bid for 7 days; maximum 800 mg/day). It can be taken with a fatty meal to improve absorption. Praziquantel is an alternative (50-100 mg/kg/day PO divided tid for 28 days), but requires more complicated management due to an interaction with corticosteroids. A worsening of symptoms can follow the use of either drug due to the host's inflammatory response to the dying parasite. Patients should be medicated with prednisolone 2 mg/kg/day or 0.15 mg/kg/day oral dexamethasone, either concurrent with albendazole, or starting albendazole on the third day of corticosteroids. Single antiepileptic agents are usually administered as well if there has been a history of seizures. If no anticysticercal drugs are administered, it is necessary to determine whether these patients carry adult worms, posing a public health risk and risk of continued autoinfection.

Table 295-1 DIFFERENTIAL DIAGNOSIS OF NEUROCYSTICERCOSIS ON NEUROIMAGING

SINGLE NON-ENHANCING CYSTIC LESION
Hydatid disease Arachnoid cysts Porencephaly Cystic astrocytoma Colloid cyst (third ventricle)
SEVERAL NON-ENHANCING CYSTIC LESIONS
Multiple metastases Hydatid disease (rare)
ENHANCING LESIONS
Tuberculosis Mycosis Toxoplasmosis Abscess Early glioma Metastasis Arteriovenous malformation
CALCIFICATIONS
Tuberous sclerosis Tuberculosis Cytomegalovirus infection Toxoplasmosis

From Garcia HH, Gonzalez AE, Evans CAW, et al: *Taenia solium* cysticercosis, *Lancet* 361:547–556, 2003.

PREVENTION

All family members of index cases of cysticercosis as well as persons handling the food of index cases should be examined for signs of disease or evidence of adult worms. Attention to personal hygiene, proper handwashing by food handlers, and avoidance of fresh fruits and vegetables in areas endemic for *T. solium* help prevent ingestion of eggs. All pork should be cooked thoroughly. Veterinary vaccines for several cestode infections have a high degree of efficacy and have a potential role in decreasing parasite transmission.

BIBLIOGRAPHY
Please visit the Nelson Textbook of Pediatrics *website at www.expertconsult.com for the complete bibliography.*

Chapter 296
Echinococcosis (*Echinococcus granulosus* and *Echinococcus multilocularis*)

Ronald Blanton

ETIOLOGY

Echinococcosis (**hydatid disease** or **hydatidosis**) is the most widespread, serious human cestode infection in the world (Fig. 296-1). Two major *Echinococcus* species are responsible for distinct clinical presentations, *E. granulosus* (**cystic hydatid disease**) and the more malignant *E. multilocularis* (**alveolar hydatid disease**). The adult parasite is a small (2-7 mm) tapeworm with only 2-6 segments that inhabits the intestines of dogs, wolves, dingoes, jackals, coyotes, and foxes. These carnivores pass the eggs in their stool, which contaminates the soil, pasture, and water, as well as their own fur. Domestic animals such as sheep, goats, cattle, and camels ingest *E. granulosus* eggs while grazing. Humans are also infected by consuming food or water contaminated with eggs or by direct contact with infected dogs. The larvae hatch, penetrate the gut, and are carried by the vascular or lymphatic systems to the liver, lungs, and less commonly bones, brain, or heart.

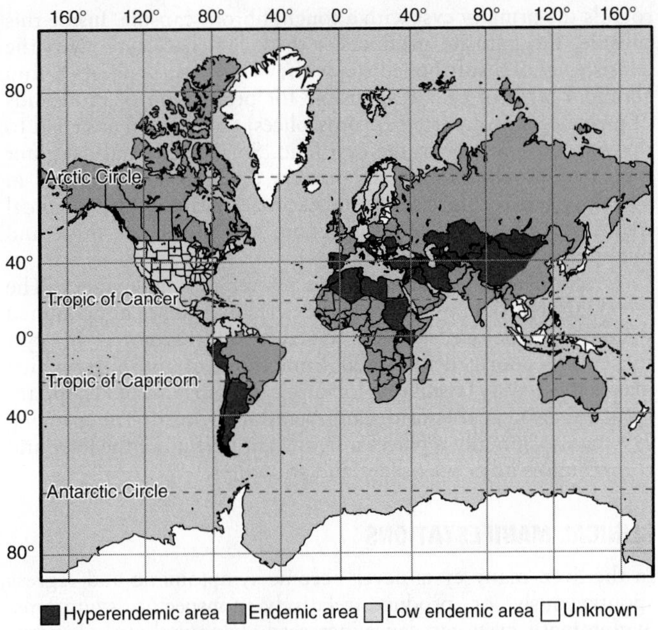

Figure 296-1 Worldwide distribution of cystic echinococcosis. (From McManus DP, Zhang W, Li J, et al: Echinococcosis, *Lancet* 362:1295–1304, 2003.)

E. granulosus shows high intraspecific variation. One distinct variant is found in a sylvatic wolf/moose cycle in North America and Siberia. The transmission cycle of *E. multilocularis* is similar to that of *E. granulosus,* except that this species is mainly sylvatic and uses small rodents as its natural intermediate hosts. The rodents are consumed by foxes, their natural predators, and sometimes by dogs and cats.

EPIDEMIOLOGY

There is potential for transmission of this parasite to humans wherever there are herd animals and dogs. Even in urban areas, dogs may be infected by eating entrails after home slaughter of domestic animals. Cysts have been detected in up to 10% of the human population in northern Kenya and Western China. In South America, the disease is prevalent in sheepherding areas of the Andes, the beef-herding areas of the Brazilian/Argentine Pampas, and Uruguay. Among developed countries, the disease is recognized in Italy, Greece, Portugal, Spain, and Australia, and is reemergent in dogs in Great Britain. In North America, transmission occurs by way of the sylvatic cycle in Alaska, Canada, and Isle Royale on Lake Superior, as well as in foci of the domestic cycle in sheep raising areas of western USA.

Transmission of *E. multilocularis* occurs primarily in temperate climates of Northern Europe, Siberia, Turkey, and China. Transmission is decreasing among native peoples in Alaska and Canada as dogs are replaced by mechanized forms of transportation. A separate species, *Echinococcus vogeli,* causes polycystic disease similar to alveolar hydatidosis in South America.

PATHOGENESIS

In areas endemic for *E. granulosus,* the parasite is often acquired in childhood, but liver cysts require many years to become large enough to detect or cause symptoms. In children, the lung is a common site, whereas in adults 70% of cysts develop in the right lobe of the liver. Cysts can also develop in bone, the genitourinary system, bowels, subcutaneous tissues, and brain. The host surrounds the primary cyst with a tough, fibrous capsule. Inside this capsule, the parasite produces a thick lamellar layer with the consistency of a soft-boiled egg white. This layer supports a thin germinal layer of cells responsible for production of thousands of juvenile-stage parasites (**protoscolices**) that remain attached to the wall or float free in the cyst fluid. Smaller internal daughter cysts may develop within the primary cyst capsule. The fluid in a healthy cyst is colorless, crystal clear, and watery. After medical treatment or with bacterial infection, it may become thick and bile stained.

Infection with *E. multilocularis* resembles a malignancy. The secondary reproductive units bud externally and are not confined within a single well-defined structure. Furthermore, the cyst tissues are poorly demarcated from those of the host, which makes these cysts unsuitable for surgical removal. The secondary cysts are also capable of distant metastatic spread. The growing cyst mass eventually replaces a significant portion of the liver and compromises adjacent tissues and structures.

CLINICAL MANIFESTATIONS

In the liver, many cysts never become symptomatic and regress spontaneously or produce relatively nonspecific symptoms. Symptomatic cysts can cause increased abdominal girth, hepatomegaly, a palpable mass, vomiting, or abdominal pain. However, the more serious complications result from compression of adjacent structures, spillage of cyst contents, and location of cysts in sensitive areas, such as the reproductive tract, brain, and bone. Anaphylaxis can occur with cyst rupture or spontaneous spillage, due to trauma or intraoperatively. Spillage can also be catastrophic long-term, since each protoscolex can form a new cyst. Jaundice due to cystic hydatid disease is rare. In the lung, cysts produce chest pain, cough, or hemoptysis. Bone cysts may cause pathologic fractures, and cysts in the genitourinary system may produce hematuria or infertility.

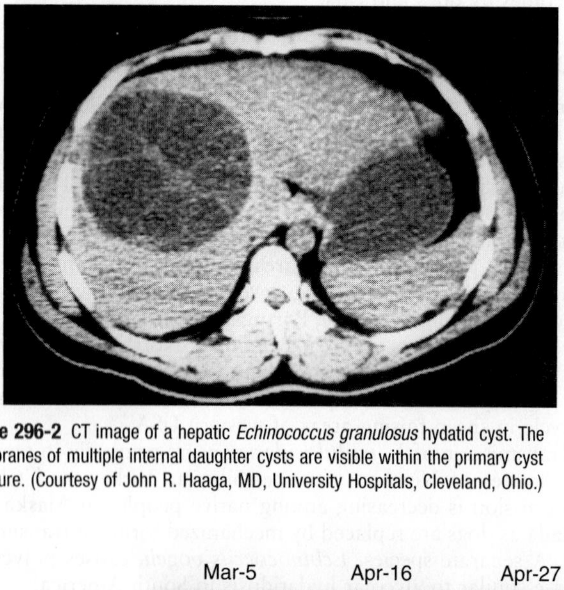

Figure 296-2 CT image of a hepatic *Echinococcus granulosus* hydatid cyst. The membranes of multiple internal daughter cysts are visible within the primary cyst structure. (Courtesy of John R. Haaga, MD, University Hospitals, Cleveland, Ohio.)

In alveolar hydatid disease, cyst tissue continues to proliferate and may separate and metastasize distantly. The proliferating mass compromises hepatic tissue or the biliary system and causes progressive obstructive jaundice and hepatic failure. Symptoms also occur from expansion of extrahepatic foci.

DIAGNOSIS

Subcutaneous nodules, hepatomegaly, or a palpable abdominal mass may be found. The parasite cannot be recovered from any easily accessible body fluid unless a lung cyst ruptures, after which protoscolices or layers of cyst wall may briefly be seen in sputum. Ultrasonography is the most valuable tool for both the diagnosis and treatment of cystic hydatid disease of the liver. The presence of internal membranes and falling echogenic cyst material (**hydatid sand**) observed in real time aid in the diagnosis. Alveolar disease is less cystic in appearance and resembles a diffuse solid tumor. CT findings (Fig. 296-2) are similar to those of ultrasonography and may at times be useful in distinguishing alveolar from cystic hydatid disease in geographic regions where both occur. CT or MRI is also important in planning a surgical intervention. Lung hydatid is usually apparent on chest x-ray (Fig. 296-3).

Serologic studies may be useful in confirming a diagnosis of cystic echinococcosis, but the false-negative rate may be >50%. Most patients with alveolar hydatidosis develop detectable antibody responses. Current tests use crude or partially purified antigens that can cross react in individuals infected with other parasitic infections, such as cysticercosis or schistosomiasis.

DIFFERENTIAL DIAGNOSIS

Benign hepatic cysts are common but can be distinguished by the absence of either internal membranes or hydatid sand. The density of bacterial hepatic abscesses is distinct from the watery cystic fluid characteristic of *E. granulosus* infection, but hydatid cysts may also be complicated by secondary bacterial infection. Alveolar echinococcosis is often confused with hepatoma and cirrhosis and presents features suggestive of pancreatic carcinoma, metastatic liver disease, and cholangitis.

TREATMENT

For simple, accessible cysts surrounded by tissue, ultrasound- or CT-guided Percutaneous Aspiration, Instillation (hypertonic saline or another scolicidal agent) and Re-aspiration (**PAIR**) is the preferred therapy. Compared with surgical treatment alone, PAIR plus albendazole results in similar cyst disappearance with fewer adverse events and fewer days in the hospital. Compared to albendazole alone, PAIR with or without albendazole provides significantly better cyst reduction and symptomatic relief. Spillage with PAIR is surprisingly uncommon, but prophylactic albendazole therapy is routinely administered >1 wk prior to PAIR or surgery and continued for 1 mo thereafter. Albendazole treatment for 4 wk prior to any procedure is probably warranted, but may remove the diagnostic value of aspiration in some cases.

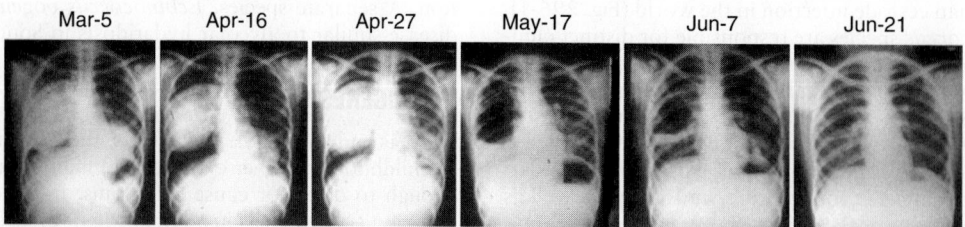

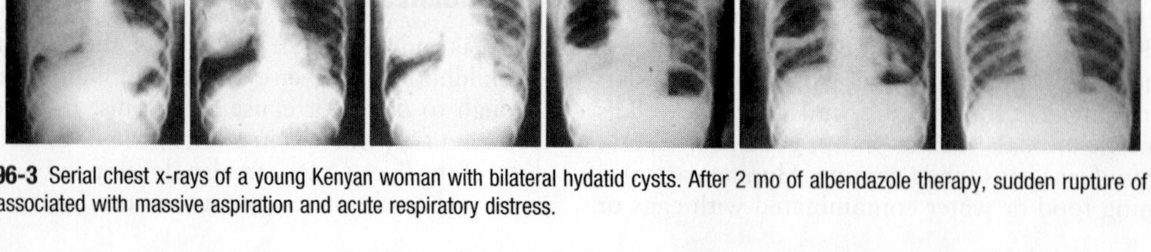

Figure 296-3 Serial chest x-rays of a young Kenyan woman with bilateral hydatid cysts. After 2 mo of albendazole therapy, sudden rupture of the right cyst was associated with massive aspiration and acute respiratory distress.

PAIR is contraindicated in pregnancy and for bile-stained cysts, which should not be injected with a scolicidal agent because of increased risk for biliary complications.

Indications for surgery are the presence of large liver cysts with multiple daughter cysts, single superficially situated liver cysts that may rupture spontaneously or as the result of a trauma, infected cysts, cysts communicating with the biliary tree and/or exerting pressure on adjacent vital organs, and cysts in the lung, brain, kidney, or bones. For conventional surgery, the inner cyst wall (only laminate and germinal layers are of parasite origin) can be easily peeled from the fibrous layer, although some studies suggest that removal of the whole capsule has a better outcome. The cavity should then be topically sterilized and either closed or filled with omentum. Considerable care must be taken to avoid spillage of cyst contents, because cyst fluid contains viable protoscolices, each capable of producing secondary cysts wherever it lodges. An additional risk is anaphylaxis due to spilled cyst fluid, so it is therefore useful to employ a surgeon experienced in this surgery.

Nonpregnant patients with cysts not amenable to PAIR or surgery or with contraindications can be managed with albendazole (15 mg/kg/day divided bid PO for 1-6 mo, maximum 800 mg/day). A favorable response occurs in 40-60% of patients. Adverse effects include occasional alopecia, mild gastrointestinal disturbance, and elevated transaminases on prolonged use. Because of leukopenia, the U.S. Food and Drug Administration recommends that blood counts be monitored at the beginning and every 2 wk during therapy. Corticosteroids are not indicated unless patients show signs of immediate hypersensitivity. Ultrasonographic indications of successful therapy are reduction in diameter, a change in shape from spherical to elliptic or flat, progressive increase in echogenicity and density of cyst fluid, and detachment of membranes from the capsule (**water lily sign**).

Alveolar hydatidosis is frequently incurable by any modality, except by partial hepatectomy, lobectomy, or liver transplantation for limited disease. Medical therapy with albendazole may slow the progression of alveolar hydatidosis, and some patients have been maintained on long-term suppressive therapy, but the infection generally recurs if albendazole is stopped.

PROGNOSIS

Factors predictive of success with chemotherapy are age of the cyst (<2 yr), low internal complexity of the cyst, and small size. The site of the cyst is not important, although cysts in bone respond poorly. For alveolar hydatidosis, if surgical removal is unsuccessful, the average mortality is 92% by 10 yr after diagnosis.

PREVENTION

Important measures to interrupt transmission include, above all, thorough handwashing, avoiding contact with dogs in endemic areas, boiling or filtering water when camping, proper disposal of animal carcasses, and proper meat inspection. Strict procedures for proper disposal of refuse from slaughterhouses must be instituted and followed so that dogs or wild carnivores do not have access to entrails. Other useful measures are control or treatment of the feral dog population and regular praziquantel treatment of pets and working dogs in endemic areas. A vaccine is available.

BIBLIOGRAPHY

Please visit the Nelson Textbook of Pediatrics *website at www.expertconsult.com for the complete bibliography.*

PART XVIII The Digestive System

Section 1 CLINICAL MANIFESTATIONS OF GASTROINTESTINAL DISEASE

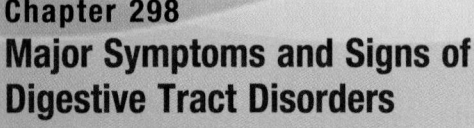

Chapter 297
Normal Digestive Tract Phenomena
Chris A. Liacouras

Gastrointestinal function varies with maturity; what is a physiologic event in a newborn or infant might be a pathologic symptom at an older age. A fetus can swallow amniotic fluid as early as 12 wk of gestation, but nutritive sucking in neonates 1st develops at about 34 wk of gestation. The coordinated oral and pharyngeal movements necessary for swallowing solids develop within the 1st few months of life. Before this time, the tongue thrust is upward and outward to express milk from the nipple, instead of a backward motion, which propels solids toward the esophageal inlet. By 1 mo of age, infants appear to show preferences for sweet and salty foods. Infants' interest in solids increases at about 4 mo of age. The recommendation to begin solids at 6 mo of age is based on nutritional and cultural concepts rather than maturation of the swallowing process (Chapter 42). Infants swallow air during feeding, and burping is encouraged to prevent gaseous distention of the stomach.

For the full continuation of this chapter, please visit the Nelson Textbook of Pediatrics *website at www.expertconsult.com.*

Chapter 298
Major Symptoms and Signs of Digestive Tract Disorders
Raman Sreedharan and Chris A. Liacouras

Disorders of organs outside the gastrointestinal (GI) tract can produce symptoms and signs that mimic digestive tract disorders and should be considered in the differential diagnosis (Table 298-1). In children with normal growth and development, treatment may be initiated without a formal evaluation based on a presumptive diagnosis after taking a history and performing a physical examination. Poor weight gain or weight loss is often associated with a significant pathologic process and usually necessitates a more formal evaluation.

DYSPHAGIA

Difficulty in swallowing is termed *dysphagia*. Painful swallowing is termed **odynophagia. Globus** is the sensation of something stuck in the throat without a clear etiology. Swallowing is a complex process that starts in the mouth with mastication and lubrication of food that is formed into a bolus. The bolus is pushed to the pharynx by the tongue. The pharyngeal phase of swallowing is rapid and involves protective mechanisms to prevent food from entering the airway. The epiglottis is lowered over the larynx while the soft palate is elevated against the nasopharyngeal wall; respiration is temporarily arrested while the upper esophageal sphincter opens to allow the bolus to enter the esophagus. In the esophagus, peristaltic coordinated muscular contractions push the food bolus toward the stomach. The lower esophageal sphincter relaxes shortly after the upper esophageal sphincter, so liquids that rapidly clear the esophagus enter the stomach without resistance.

Dysphagia is classified as oropharyngeal dysphagia and esophageal dysphagia. **Oropharyngeal dysphagia** occurs when the transfer of the food bolus from the mouth to the esophagus is impaired (also termed *transfer dysphagia*). The striated muscles of the mouth, pharynx, and upper esophageal sphincter are affected in oropharyngeal dysphagia. Neurologic and muscular disorders can give rise to oropharyngeal dysphagia (Table 298-2). The most serious complication of oropharyngeal dysphagia is life-threatening aspiration.

A complex sequence of neuromuscular events is involved in the transfer of foods to the upper esophagus. Abnormalities of the muscles involved in the ingestion process and their innervation, strength, or coordination are associated with transfer dysphagia in infants and children. In such cases, an oropharyngeal problem is usually part of a more generalized neurologic or muscular problem (botulism, diphtheria, neuromuscular disease). Painful oral lesions, such as acute viral stomatitis or trauma, occasionally interfere with ingestion. If the nasal air passage is seriously obstructed, the need for respiration causes severe distress when suckling. Although severe structural, dental, and salivary abnormalities would be expected to create difficulties, ingestion proceeds relatively well in most affected children if they are hungry.

Esophageal dysphagia occurs when there is difficulty in transporting the food bolus down the esophagus. Esophageal dysphagia can result from neuromuscular disorders or mechanical obstruction (Table 298-3). Primary motility disorders causing impaired peristaltic function and dysphagia are rare in children. Achalasia is an esophageal motility disorder with associated inability of relaxation of the lower esophageal sphincter, and it rarely occurs in children. Motility of the distal esophagus is disordered after surgical repair of tracheoesophageal fistula or achalasia. Abnormal motility can accompany collagen vascular disorders. Mechanical obstruction can be intrinsic or extrinsic. Intrinsic structural defects cause a fixed impediment to the passage of food bolus due to a narrowing within the esophagus, as in a stricture, web, or tumor. Extrinsic obstruction is due to compression from vascular rings, mediastinal lesions, or vertebral abnormalities. Structural defects typically cause more problems in swallowing solids than liquids. In infants, esophageal web, tracheobronchial remnant, or vascular ring can cause dysphagia. An esophageal stricture secondary to esophagitis (chronic gastroesophageal reflux, eosinophilic esophagitis, chronic infections) occasionally has dysphagia as the first manifestation. An esophageal foreign body or a stricture secondary to a caustic ingestion also causes dysphagia. A Schatzki ring, a thin ring of mucosal tissue near the lower esophageal sphincter, is another mechanical cause of recurrent dysphagia, and again is rare in children.

When dysphagia is associated with a delay in passage through the esophagus, the patient may be able to point to the level of the chest where the delay occurs, but esophageal symptoms are

Table 298-1 SOME NONDIGESTIVE TRACT CAUSES OF GASTROINTESTINAL SYMPTOMS IN CHILDREN

ANOREXIA
Systemic disease: inflammatory, neoplastic
Cardiorespiratory compromise
Iatrogenic: drug therapy, unpalatable therapeutic diets
Depression
Anorexia nervosa
VOMITING
Inborn errors of metabolism
Medications: erythromycin, chemotherapy, nonsteroidal anti-inflammatory drugs
Increased intracranial pressure
Brain tumor
Infection of the urinary tract
Labyrinthitis
Adrenal insufficiency
Pregnancy
Psychogenic
Abdominal migraine
Toxins
Renal disease
DIARRHEA
Infection: otitis media, urinary
Uremia
Medications: antibiotics, cisapride
Tumors: neuroblastoma
Pericarditis
CONSTIPATION
Hypothyroidism
Spina bifida
Psychomotor retardation
Dehydration: diabetes insipidus, renal tubular lesions
Medications: narcotics
Lead poisoning
Infant botulism
ABDOMINAL PAIN
Pyelonephritis, hydronephrosis, renal colic
Pneumonia
Pelvic inflammatory disease
Porphyria
Angioedema
Endocarditis
Abdominal migraine
Familial Mediterranean fever
Sexual or physical abuse
Systemic lupus erythematosus
School phobia
Sickle cell crisis
Vertebral disk inflammation
Psoas abscess
Pelvic osteomyelitis
Medications
ABDOMINAL DISTENTION OR MASS
Ascites: nephrotic syndrome, neoplasm, heart failure
Discrete mass: Wilms tumor, hydronephrosis, neuroblastoma, mesenteric cyst, hepatoblastoma, lymphoma
Pregnancy
JAUNDICE
Hemolytic disease
Urinary tract infection
Sepsis
Hypothyroidism
Panhypopituitarism

Table 298-2 CAUSES OF OROPHARYNGEAL DYSPHAGIA

NEUROMUSCULAR DISORDERS
Cerebral palsy
Brain tumors
Cerebrovascular accidents
Polio and postpolio syndromes
Multiple sclerosis
Myositis
Dermatomyositis
Myasthenia gravis
Muscular dystrophies
METABOLIC AND AUTOIMMUNE DISORDERS
Hyperthyroidism
Systemic lupus erythematosus
Sarcoidosis
Amyloidosis
INFECTIOUS DISEASE
Meningitis
Botulism
Diphtheria
Lyme disease
Neurosyphilis
Viral infection: polio, Coxsackievirus, herpes, cytomegalovirus
STRUCTURAL LESIONS
Inflammatory: abscess, pharyngitis
Congenital web
Cricopharyngeal bar
Dental problems
Bullous skin lesions
Plummer- Vinson syndrome
Zenker diverticulum
Extrinsic compression: osteophytes, lymph nodes, thyroid swelling
OTHER
Corrosive injury
Side effects of medications
After surgery
After radiation therapy

Adapted from Gasiorowska A, Faas R: Current approach to dysphagia, *Gastroenterol Hepatol* 5(4):269–279, 2009.

usually referred to the suprasternal notch. When a patient points to the suprasternal notch, the impaction can be found anywhere in the esophagus.

REGURGITATION

Regurgitation is the effortless movement of stomach contents into the esophagus and mouth. It is not associated with distress, and infants with regurgitation are often hungry immediately after an episode. The lower esophageal sphincter prevents reflux of gastric contents into the esophagus. Regurgitation is a result of gastroesophageal reflux through an incompetent or, in infants, immature lower esophageal sphincter. This is often a developmental process, and regurgitation or “spitting” resolves with maturity. Regurgitation should be differentiated from vomiting, which denotes an active reflex process with an extensive differential diagnosis (Table 298-4).

ANOREXIA

Anorexia means prolonged lack of appetite. Hunger and satiety centers are located in the hypothalamus; it seems likely that afferent nerves from the GI tract to these brain centers are important

Table 298-3 CAUSES OF ESOPHAGEAL DYSPHAGIA

NEUROMUSCULAR DISORDERS
GERD
Achalasia cardia
Diffuse esophageal spasm
Scleroderma
MECHANICAL
Intrinsic Lesions
Foreign bodies
Esophagitis: GERD, eosinophilic esophagitis
Stricture: corrosive injury, pill induced, peptic
Esophageal webs
Esophageal rings
Esophageal diverticula
Neoplasm
Extrinsic Lesions
Vascular compression
Mediastinal lesion
Cervical osteochondritis
Vertebral abnormalities

GERD, gastroesophageal reflux disease.
Adapted from Gasiorowska A, Faas R: Current approach to dysphagia, *Gastroenterol Hepatol* 5(4):269–279, 2009.

Table 298-4 DIFFERENTIAL DIAGNOSIS OF EMESIS DURING CHILDHOOD

INFANT	CHILD	ADOLESCENT
COMMON		
Gastroenteritis Gastroesophageal reflux Overfeeding Anatomic obstruction* Systemic infection Pertussis syndrome Otitis media	Gastroenteritis Systemic infection Gastritis Toxic ingestion Pertussis syndrome Medication Reflux (GERD) Sinusitis Otitis media Anatomic obstruction*	Gastroenteritis GERD Systemic infection Toxic ingestion Gastritis Sinusitis Inflammatory bowel disease Appendicitis Migraine Pregnancy Medication Ipecac abuse, bulimia Concussion
RARE		
Adrenogenital syndrome Inborn error of metabolism Brain tumor (increased intracranial pressure) Subdural hemorrhage Food poisoning Rumination Renal tubular acidosis Ureteropelvic junction obstruction	Reye syndrome Hepatitis Peptic ulcer Pancreatitis Brain tumor Increased intracranial pressure Middle ear disease Chemotherapy Achalasia Cyclic vomiting (migraine) Esophageal stricture Duodenal hematoma Inborn error of metabolism	Reye syndrome Hepatitis Peptic ulcer Pancreatitis Brain tumor Increased intracranial pressure Middle ear disease Chemotherapy Cyclic vomiting (migraine) Biliary colic Renal colic Diabetic ketoacidosis

GERD, gastroesophageal reflux disease.
*Includes malrotation, pyloric stenosis, intussusception.

determinants of the anorexia that characterizes many diseases of the stomach and intestine. Satiety is stimulated by distention of the stomach or upper small bowel, the signal being transmitted by sensory afferents, which are especially dense in the upper gut. Chemoreceptors in the intestine, influenced by the assimilation of nutrients, also affect afferent flow to the appetite centers. Impulses reach the hypothalamus from higher centers, possibly influenced by pain or the emotional disturbance of an intestinal disease. Other regulatory factors include hormones, ghrelin, leptin, and plasma glucose, which, in turn, reflect intestinal function (Chapter 44).

VOMITING

Vomiting is a highly coordinated reflex process that may be preceded by increased salivation and begins with involuntary retching. Violent descent of the diaphragm and constriction of the abdominal muscles with relaxation of the gastric cardia actively force gastric contents back up the esophagus. This process is coordinated in the medullary vomiting center, which is influenced directly by afferent innervation and indirectly by the chemoreceptor trigger zone and higher central nervous system (CNS) centers. Many acute or chronic processes can cause vomiting (see Tables 298-1 and 298-4).

Vomiting caused by obstruction of the GI tract is probably mediated by intestinal visceral afferent nerves stimulating the vomiting center (Table 298-5). If obstruction occurs below the 2nd part of the duodenum, vomitus is usually bile stained. Emesis can also become bile stained with repeated vomiting in the absence of obstruction when duodenal contents are refluxed into the stomach. Nonobstructive lesions of the digestive tract can also cause vomiting; this includes diseases of the upper bowel, pancreas, liver, or biliary tree. CNS or metabolic derangements can lead to severe, persistent emesis.

Cyclic vomiting is a syndrome with numerous episodes of vomiting interspersed with well intervals. The North American Society for Pediatric Gastroenterology, Hepatology and Nutrition consensus statement on the diagnosis and management of cyclic vomiting criteria are listed in Table 298-6. Rome III criteria for Functional GI disorders (FGIDs) have 2 criteria for cyclic vomiting in children, and both these criteria have to be present for a diagnosis of cyclic vomiting: 2 or more periods of intense nausea and unremitting vomiting or retching lasting hours to days and return to usual state of health lasting weeks to months.

The onset of cyclic vomiting is usually between 2 and 5 yr of age but has been observed in infants and adults. The frequency of vomiting episodes is variable (average of 12 episodes per yr) with each episode typically lasting 2-3 days and 4 or more emesis episodes per hour. The episodes usually occur in the early hours of the morning or upon wakening. Patients can have a prodrome of nausea, pallor, intolerance of noise or light, lethargy, and headache. Epigastric pain, abdominal pain, diarrhea, and fever are seen in many patients, making the diagnosis difficult. Precipitants include infection, physical stress, and psychologic stress.

Several theories have been proposed as causative factors including a migraine-related mechanism, mitochondrial disorders, and autonomic dysfunction. More than 80% of affected children have a first-degree relative with migraines; many patients develop migraines later in life. Many children show evidence for sympathetic autonomic dysfunction of sudomotor systems. The differential diagnosis includes GI anomalies (malrotation, duplication cysts, choledochal cysts, recurrent intussusceptions), CNS disorders (neoplasm, epilepsy, vestibular pathology), nephrolithiasis, cholelithiasis, hydronephrosis, metabolic-endocrine disorders (urea cycle, fatty acid metabolism, Addison disease, porphyria, hereditary angioedema, familial Mediterranean fever), chronic appendicitis, and inflammatory bowel disease. Laboratory evaluation is based on a careful history and physical examination and may include, if indicated, endoscopy, contrast GI radiography, brain MRI, and metabolic studies (lactate, organic acids, ammonia). Treatment includes hydration and antiemetics (e.g., ondansetron). Prevention may be possible with

Table 298-5 CAUSES OF GASTROINTESTINAL OBSTRUCTION

ESOPHAGUS
Congenital
Esophageal atresia
Vascular rings
Schatzki ring
Tracheobronchial remnant
Acquired
Esophageal stricture
Foreign body
Achalasia
Chagas disease
Collagen vascular disease
STOMACH
Congenital
Antral webs
Pyloric stenosis
Acquired
Bezoar, foreign body
Pyloric stricture (ulcer)
Chronic granulomatous disease of childhood
Eosinophilic gastroenteritis
Crohn disease
Epidermolysis bullosa
SMALL INTESTINE
Congenital
Duodenal atresia
Annular pancreas
Malrotation/volvulus
Malrotation/Ladd bands
Ileal atresia
Meconium ileus
Meckel diverticulum with volvulus or intussusception
Inguinal hernia
Intestinal duplication
Acquired
Postsurgical adhesions
Crohn disease
Intussusception
Distal ileal obstruction syndrome (cystic fibrosis)
Duodenal hematoma
Superior mesenteric artery syndrome
COLON
Congenital
Meconium plug
Hirschsprung disease
Colonic atresia, stenosis
Imperforate anus
Rectal stenosis
Pseudo-obstruction
Volvulus
Colonic duplication
Acquired
Ulcerative colitis (toxic megacolon)
Chagas disease
Crohn disease
Fibrosing colonopathy (cystic fibrosis)

Table 298-6 CRITERIA FOR CYCLICAL VOMITING SYNDROME

All of the criteria must be met for the consensus definition of cyclical vomiting syndrome:

- At least 5 attacks in any interval, or a minimum of 3 attacks during a 6-month period
- Episodic attacks of intense nausea and vomiting lasting 1 hr to 10 days and occurring at least 1 wk apart
- Stereotypical pattern and symptoms in the individual patient
- Vomiting during attacks occurs ≥4 times/hr for ≥1 hr
- Return to baseline health between episodes
- Not attributed to another disorder

Li, B UK, Lefevre F, Chelimsky GG, et al: North American Society for Pediatric Gastroenterology, Hepatology, and Nutrition Consensus Statement on the Diagnosis and Management of Cyclic Vomiting Syndrome, *J Pediatr Gastroenterol Nutr* 47:379–393, 2008.

Table 298-7 COMPLICATIONS OF VOMITING

COMPLICATION	PATHOPHYSIOLOGY	HISTORY, PHYSICAL EXAMINATION, AND LABORATORY STUDIES
Metabolic	Fluid loss in emesis	Dehydration
	HCl loss in emesis	Alkalosis; hypochloremia
	Na, K loss in emesis	Hyponatremia; hypokalemia
	Alkalosis →	
	• Na into cells	
	• HCO_3 loss in urine	Urine pH 7-8
	• Na and K loss in urine	Urine Na ↑, K ↑
	Hypochloremia → Cl conserved by kidneys	Urine Cl ↓
Nutritional	Emesis of calories and nutrients Anorexia for calories and nutrients	Malnutrition; "failure to thrive"
Mallory-Weiss tear	Retching → tear at lesser curve of gastroesophageal junction	Forceful emesis → hematemesis
Esophagitis	Chronic vomiting → esophageal acid exposure	Heartburn; hemoccult + stool
Aspiration	Aspiration of vomitus, especially in context of obtundation	Pneumonia; neurologic dysfunction
Shock	Severe fluid loss in emesis or in accompanying diarrhea	Dehydration (accompanying diarrhea can explain acidosis?)
	Severe blood loss in hematemesis	Blood volume depletion
Pneumomediastinum, pneumothorax	Increased intrathoracic pressure	Chest x-ray
Petechiae, retinal hemorrhages	Increased intrathoracic pressure	Normal platelet count

From Kliegman RM, Greenbaum LA, Lye PS, editors: *Practical strategies in pediatric diagnosis and therapy,* ed 2, Philadelphia, 2004, Elsevier, p 318.

lifestyle changes and prophylactic medications (cyproheptadine, propranolol, amitriptyline, phenobarbital) based on the patient's age.

Potential complications of emesis are noted in Table 298-7. Broad management strategies for vomiting in general and specific causes of emesis are noted in Tables 298-8 and 298-9.

DIARRHEA

Diarrhea is best defined as excessive loss of fluid and electrolyte in the stool. Acute diarrhea is defined as sudden onset of exces-

Table 298-8 PHARMACOLOGIC THERAPIES FOR VOMITING EPISODES

THERAPEUTIC DRUG CLASS	DRUG	DOSAGE
REFLUX		
Dopamine antagonist	Metoclopramide (Reglan)	0.1-0.2 mg/kg PO or IV qid
GASTROPARESIS		
Dopamine antagonist	Metoclopramide (Reglan)	0.1-0.2 mg/kg PO or IV qid
Motilin agonist	Erythromycin	3-5 mg/kg PO or IV tid-qid
INTESTINAL PSEUDO-OBSTRUCTION		
Stimulation of intestinal migratory myoelectric complexes	Octreotide (Sandostatin)	1 μg/kg SC bid-tid
CHEMOTHERAPY		
Dopamine antagonist	Metoclopramide	0.5-1.0 mg/kg IV qid, with antihistamine prophylaxis of extrapyramidal side effects
Serotoninergic 5-HT$_3$ antagonist	Ondansetron (Zofran)	0.15-0.3 mg/kg IV or PO tid
Phenothiazines (extrapyramidal, hematologic side effects)	Prochlorperazine (Compazine)	≈0.3 mg/kg PO bid-tid
	Chlorpromazine (Thorazine)	>6 mo of age: 0.5 mg/kg PO or IV tid-qid
Steroids	Dexamethasone (Decadron)	0.1 mg/kg PO tid
Cannabinoids	Tetrahydrocannabinol (Nabilone)	0.05-0.1 mg/kg PO bid-tid
POSTOPERATIVE		
	Ondansetron, phenothiazines	See under chemotherapy
MOTION SICKNESS, VESTIBULAR DISORDERS		
Antihistamine	Dimenhydrinate (Dramamine)	1 mg/kg PO tid-qid
Anticholinergic	Scopolamine (Transderm Scop)	Adults: 1 patch/3 days
ADRENAL CRISIS		
Steroids	Cortisol	2 mg/kg IV bolus followed by 0.2-0.4 mg/kg/hr IV (±1 mg/kg IM)
CYCLIC VOMITING SYNDROME		
Supportive		
Analgesic	Meperidine (Demerol)	1-2 mg/kg IV or IM q4-6 hr
Anxiolytic, sedative	Lorazepam (Ativan)	0.05-0.1 mg/kg IV q6hr
Antihistamine, sedative	Diphenhydramine (Benadryl)	1.25 mg/kg IV q6hr
Abortive		
Serotoninergic 5-HT$_3$ antagonist:	Ondansetron	See above
	Granisetron (Kytril)	10 μg/kg IV q4-6 hr
Nonsteroidal anti-inflammatory agent (GI ulceration side effect)	Ketorolac (Toradol)	0.5-1.0 mg/kg IV q6-8 hr
Serotoninergic 5-HT$_{1D}$ agonist	Sumatriptan (Imitres)	>40 kg: 20 mg intranasally or 25 mg PO, one time only
PROPHYLACTIC*		
Antimigraine, β-adrenergic blocker	Propranolol (Inderal)	0.5-2.0 mg/kg PO bid
Antimigraine, antihistamine	Cyproheptadine (Periactin)	0.25-0.5 mg/kg/day PO ÷ bid-tid
Antimigraine, tricyclic antidepressant	amitriptyline (Elavil)	0.33-0.5 mg/kg PO tid, and titrate to maximum of 3.0 mg/kg/day as needed Obtain baseline ECG at start of therapy, and consider monitoring drug levels
Antimigraine antiepileptic	Phenobarbital (Luminal)	2-3 mg/kg qhs
	Erythromycin (see above)	
Low-estrogen oral contraceptives	Consider for catamenial CVS episodes	

*If >1 CVS bout/month or symptoms are extremely disabling; taken daily.
CVS, cyclic vomiting syndrome; ECG, electrocardiogram; GI, gastrointestinal.
From Kliegman RM, Greenbaum LA, Lye PS, editors: *Practical strategies in pediatric diagnosis and therapy,* ed 2, Philadelphia, 2004, Elsevier, p 317.

sively loose stools of >10 mL/kg/day in infants and >200 g/24 hr in older children, which lasts <14 days. When the episode lasts >14 days, it is called *chronic* or *persistent diarrhea.*

Normally, a young infant has approximately 5 mL/kg/day of stool output; the volume increases to 200 g/24 hr in an adult. The greatest volume of intestinal water is absorbed in the small bowel; the colon concentrates intestinal contents against a high osmotic gradient. The small intestine of an adult can absorb 10-11 L/day of a combination of ingested and secreted fluid, whereas the colon absorbs approximately 0.5 L. Disorders that interfere with absorption in the small bowel tend to produce voluminous diarrhea, whereas disorders compromising colonic absorption produce lower-volume diarrhea. Dysentery (small-volume, frequent bloody stools with mucus, tenesmus, and urgency) is the predominant symptom of colitis.

The basis of all diarrheas is disturbed intestinal solute transport and water absorption. Water movement across intestinal membranes is passive and is determined by both active and passive fluxes of solutes, particularly sodium, chloride, and glucose. The pathogenesis of most episodes of diarrhea can be explained by secretory, osmotic, or motility abnormalities or a combination of these (Table 298-10).

Secretory diarrhea occurs when the intestinal epithelial cell solute transport system is in an active state of secretion. It is often caused by a secretagogue, such as cholera toxin, binding to a receptor on the surface epithelium of the bowel and thereby stimulating intracellular accumulation of cyclic adenosine monophosphate (cAMP) or cyclic guanosine monophosphate (cGMP). Some intraluminal fatty acids and bile salts cause the colonic mucosa to secrete through this mechanism. Diarrhea not associated with an exogenous secretagogue can also have a secretory component (congenital microvillus inclusion disease). Secretory diarrhea is usually of large volume and persists even with fasting. The stool osmolality is indicated by the electrolytes and the ion gap is 100 mOsm/kg or less. The ion gap is calculated by subtracting the concentration of electrolytes from total osmolality:

$$\text{Ion gap} = \text{Stool osmolality} - [(\text{stool Na} + \text{stool K}) \times 2]$$

Osmotic diarrhea occurs after ingestion of a poorly absorbed solute. The solute may be one that is normally not well absorbed (magnesium, phosphate, lactulose, or sorbitol) or one that is not well absorbed because of a disorder of the small bowel (lactose with lactase deficiency or glucose with rotavirus diarrhea). Malabsorbed carbohydrate is fermented in the colon, and short-chain fatty acids (SCFAs) are produced. Although SCFAs can be absorbed in the colon and used as an energy source, the net effect is increase in the osmotic solute load. This form of diarrhea is usually of lesser volume than a secretory diarrhea and stops with fasting. The osmolality of the stool will not be explained by the electrolyte content, because another osmotic component is present and the anion gap is >100 mOsm.

Motility disorders can be associated with rapid or delayed transit and are not generally associated with large-volume diarrhea. Slow motility can be associated with bacterial overgrowth leading to diarrhea. The differential diagnosis of common causes of acute and chronic diarrhea is noted in Table 298-11.

Table 298-9 SUPPORTIVE AND NONPHARMACOLOGIC THERAPIES FOR VOMITING EPISODES

DISEASE	THERAPY
All	Treat cause • Obstruction: operate • Allergy: change diet (± steroids) • Metabolic error: Rx defect • Acid peptic disease: H_2RAs, PPIs, etc.
Complications	
Dehydration	IV fluids, electrolytes
Hematemesis	Transfuse, correct coagulopathy
Esophagitis	H_2RAs, PPIs
Malnutrition	NG or NJ drip feeding useful for many chronic conditions
Meconium ileus	Gastrografin enema
DIOS	Gastrografin enema; balanced colonic lavage solution (e.g., GoLytely)
Intussusception	Barium enema; air reduction enema
Hematemesis	Endoscopic: injection sclerotherapy or banding of esophageal varices; injection therapy, fibrin sealant application, or heater probe electrocautery for selected upper GI tract lesions
Sigmoid volvulus	Colonoscopic decompression
Reflux	Positioning; dietary measures (infants: rice cereal, 1 tbs/oz of formula)
Psychogenic components	Psychotherapy; tricyclic antidepressants; anxiolytics (e.g., diazepam: 0.1 mg/kg PO tid-qid)

DIOS, distal intestinal obstruction syndrome; GI, gastrointestinal; H_2RA, H_2-receptor antagonist; NG, nasogastric; NJ, nasojejunal; PPIs, proton pump inhibitors; tbs, tablespoon.
From Kliegman RM, Greenbaum LA, Lye PS, editors: *Practical strategies in pediatric diagnosis and therapy*, ed 2, Philadelphia, 2004, Elsevier, p 319.

CONSTIPATION

Any definition of constipation is relative and depends on stool consistency, stool frequency, and difficulty in passing the stool. A normal child might have a soft stool only every 2nd or 3rd day without difficulty; this is not constipation. A hard stool passed with difficulty every 3rd day should be treated as constipation. Constipation can arise from defects either in filling or emptying the rectum (Table 298-12).

A nursing infant might have very infrequent stools of normal consistency; this is usually a normal pattern. True constipation in the neonatal period is most likely secondary to Hirschsprung disease, intestinal pseudo-obstruction, or hypothyroidism.

Table 298-10 MECHANISMS OF DIARRHEA

PRIMARY MECHANISM	DEFECT	STOOL EXAMINATION	EXAMPLES	COMMENT
Secretory	Decreased absorption, increased secretion, electrolyte transport	Watery, normal osmolality with ion gap <100 mOsm/kg	Cholera, toxigenic *Escherichia coli;* carcinoid, VIP, neuroblastoma, congenital chloride diarrhea, *Clostridium difficile,* cryptosporidiosis (AIDS)	Persists during fasting; bile salt malabsorption can also increase intestinal water secretion; no stool leukocytes
Osmotic	Maldigestion, transport defects ingestion of unabsorbable substances	Watery, acidic, and reducing substances; increased osmolality with ion gap >100 mOsm/kg	Lactase deficiency, glucose-galactose malabsorption, lactulose, laxative abuse	Stops with fasting; increased breath hydrogen with carbohydrate malabsorption; no stool leukocytes
Increased motility	Decreased transit time	Loose to normal-appearing stool, stimulated by gastrocolic reflex	Irritable bowel syndrome, thyrotoxicosis, postvagotomy dumping syndrome	Infection can also contribute to increased motility
Decreased motility	Defect in neuromuscular unit(s) stasis (bacterial overgrowth)	Loose to normal-appearing stool	Pseudo-obstruction, blind loop	Possible bacterial overgrowth
Decreased surface area (osmotic, motility)	Decreased functional capacity	Watery	Short bowel syndrome, celiac disease, rotavirus enteritis	Might require elemental diet plus parenteral alimentation
Mucosal invasion	Inflammation, decreased colonic reabsorption, increased motility	Blood and increased WBCs in stool	*Salmonella, Shigella,* infection; amebiasis; *Yersinia, Campylobacter* infections	Dysentery evident in blood, mucus, and WBCs

VIP, vasoactive intestinal peptide; WBC, white blood cell.
From Kliegman RM, Greenbaum LA, Lye PS, editors: *Practical strategies in pediatric diagnosis and therapy*, ed 2, Philadelphia, 2004, Elsevier, p 274.

Table 298-11 DIFFERENTIAL DIAGNOSIS OF DIARRHEA

INFANT	CHILD	ADOLESCENT
ACUTE		
Common		
Gastroenteritis (viral > bacterial) Systemic infection Antibiotic associated Overfeeding	Gastroenteritis (viral > bacterial) Food poisoning Systemic infection Antibiotic associated	Gastroenteritis (viral > bacterial) Food poisoning Antibiotic associated
Rare		
Primary disaccharidase deficiency Hirschsprung toxic colitis Adrenogenital syndrome Neonatal opiate withdrawal	Toxic ingestion Hemolytic uremic syndrome Intussusception	Hyperthyroidism Appendicitis
CHRONIC		
Common		
Postinfectious secondary lactase deficiency Cow's milk or soy protein intolerance Chronic nonspecific diarrhea of infancy Excessive fruit juice (sorbitol) ingestion Celiac disease Cystic fibrosis AIDS enteropathy	Postinfectious secondary lactase deficiency Irritable bowel syndrome Celiac disease Lactose intolerance Excessive fruit juice (sorbitol) ingestion Giardiasis Inflammatory bowel disease AIDS enteropathy	Irritable bowel syndrome Inflammatory bowel disease Lactose intolerance Giardiasis Laxative abuse (anorexia nervosa) Constipation with encopresis
Rare		
Primary immune defects Glucose-galactose malabsorption Microvillus inclusion disease (microvillus atrophy) Congenital transport defects (chloride, sodium) Primary bile acid malabsorption Factitious syndrome by proxy Hirschsprung disease Shwachman syndrome Secretory tumors Acrodermatitis enteropathica Lymphangiectasia Abetalipoproteinemia Eosinophilic gastroenteritis Short bowel syndrome Intractable diarrhea syndrome Autoimmune enteropathy	Acquired immune defects Secretory tumors Pseudo-obstruction Sucrase-isomaltase deficiency Eosinophilic gastroenteritis	Secretory tumor Primary bowel tumor Parasitic infections and venereal diseases Appendiceal abscess Addison disease

From Kliegman RM, Greenbaum LA, Lye PS, editors: *Practical strategies in pediatric diagnosis and therapy*, ed 2, Philadelphia, 2004, Elsevier, p 272.

Table 298-12 CAUSES OF CONSTIPATION

- Nonorganic (functional)—retentive
- Organic
  - Anatomic
    - Anal stenosis, atresia with fistula
    - Imperforate anus
    - Anteriorly displaced anus
    - Intestinal stricture (post necrotizing enterocolitis)
    - Anal stricture
  - Abnormal musculature
    - Prune-belly syndrome
    - Gastroschisis
    - Down syndrome
    - Muscular dystrophy
  - Intestinal nerve or muscle abnormalities
    - Hirschsprung disease
    - Pseudo-obstruction (visceral myopathy or neuropathy)
    - Intestinal neuronal dysplasia
  - Spinal cord defects
    - Tethered cord
    - Spinal cord trauma
    - Spina bifida
  - Drugs
    - Anticholinergics
    - Narcotics
    - Methylphenidate
    - Phenytoin
    - Antidepressants
    - Chemotherapeutic agents (vincristine)
    - Pancreatic enzymes (fibrosing colonopathy)
    - Lead
    - Vitamin D intoxication
  - Metabolic disorders
    - Hypokalemia
    - Hypercalcemia
    - Hypothyroidism
    - Diabetes mellitus, diabetes insipidus
  - Intestinal disorders
    - Celiac disease
    - Cow's milk protein intolerance
    - Cystic fibrosis (meconium ileus equivalent)
    - Inflammatory bowel disease (stricture)
    - Tumor
  - Connective tissue disorders
    - Systemic lupus erythematosus
    - Scleroderma
  - Psychiatric diagnosis
    - Anorexia nervosa

Defective rectal filling occurs when colonic peristalsis is ineffective (in cases of hypothyroidism or opiate use and when bowel obstruction is caused either by a structural anomaly or by Hirschsprung disease). The resultant colonic stasis leads to excessive drying of stool and a failure to initiate reflexes from the rectum that normally trigger evacuation. Emptying the rectum by spontaneous evacuation depends on a defecation reflex initiated by pressure receptors in the rectal muscle. Stool retention, therefore, can also result from lesions involving these rectal muscles, the sacral spinal cord afferent and efferent fibers, or the muscles of the abdomen and pelvic floor. Disorders of anal sphincter relaxation can also contribute to fecal retention.

Constipation tends to be self-perpetuating, whatever its cause. Hard, large stools in the rectum become difficult and even painful to evacuate; thus, more retention occurs and a vicious circle ensues. Distention of the rectum and colon lessens the sensitivity of the defecation reflex and the effectiveness of peristalsis. Eventually, watery content from the proximal colon might percolate around hard retained stool and pass per rectum unperceived by the child. This involuntary **encopresis** may be mistaken for diarrhea. Constipation itself does not have deleterious systemic organic effects, but urinary tract stasis can accompany severe long-standing cases and constipation can generate anxiety, having a marked emotional impact on the patient and family.

ABDOMINAL PAIN

There is considerable variation among children in their perception and tolerance for abdominal pain. This is one reason the evaluation of chronic abdominal pain is difficult. A child with functional abdominal pain (no identifiable organic cause) may be as uncomfortable as one with an organic cause. It is very important to distinguish between organic and nonorganic (functional) abdominal pain because the approach for the management is based on this. Normal growth and physical examination (including a rectal examination) are reassuring in a child who is suspected of having functional pain.

A specific cause may be difficult to find, but the nature and location of a pain-provoking lesion can usually be determined from the clinical description. Two types of nerve fibers transmit

Table 298-13 CHRONIC ABDOMINAL PAIN IN CHILDREN

DISORDER	CHARACTERISTICS	KEY EVALUATIONS
NONORGANIC		
Functional abdominal pain	Nonspecific pain, often periumbilical	Hx and PE; tests as indicated
Irritable bowel syndrome	Intermittent cramps,diarrhea, and constipation	Hx and PE
Non-ulcer dyspepsia	Peptic ulcer–like symptoms without abnormalities on evaluation of the upper GI tract	Hx; esophagogastroduodenoscopy
GASTROINTESTINAL TRACT		
Chronic constipation	Hx of stool retention, evidence of constipation on examination	Hx and PE; plain x-ray of abdomen
Lactose intolerance	Symptoms may be associated with lactose ingestion; bloating, gas, cramps, and diarrhea	Trial of lactose-free diet; lactose breath hydrogen test
Parasite infection (especially *Giardia*)	Bloating, gas, cramps, and diarrhea	Stool evaluation for O&P; specific immunoassays for *Giardia*
Excess fructose or sorbitol ingestion	Nonspecific abdominal pain, bloating, gas, and diarrhea	Large intake of apples, fruit juice, or candy or chewing gum sweetened with sorbitol
Crohn disease	See Chapter 328	
Peptic ulcer	Burning or gnawing epigastric pain; worse on awakening or before meals; relieved with antacids	Esophagogastroduodenoscopy or upper GI contrast x-rays
Esophagitis	Epigastric pain with substernal burning	Esophagogastroduodenoscopy
Meckel's diverticulum	Periumbilical or lower abdominal pain; may have blood in stool	Meckel scan or enteroclysis
Recurrent intussusception	Paroxysmal severe cramping abdominal pain; blood may be present in stool with episode	Identify intussusception during episode or lead point in intestine between episodes with contrast studies of GI tract
Internal, inguinal, or abdominal wall hernia	Dull abdomen or abdominal wall pain	PE, CT of abdominal wall
Chronic appendicitis or appendiceal mucocele	Recurrent RLQ pain; often incorrectly diagnosed, may be rare cause of abdominal pain	Barium enema, CT
GALLBLADDER AND PANCREAS		
Cholelithiasis	RUQ pain, might worsen with meals	Ultrasound of gallbladder
Choledochal cyst	RUQ pain, mass ± elevated bilirubin	Ultrasound or CT of RUQ
Recurrent pancreatitis	Persistent boring pain, might radiate to back, vomiting	Serum amylase and lipase ± serum trypsinogen; ultrasound or CT of pancreas
GENITOURINARY TRACT		
Urinary tract infection	Dull suprapubic pain, flank pain	Urinalysis and urine culture; renal scan
Hydronephrosis	Unilateral abdominal or flank pain	Ultrasound of kidneys
Urolithiasis	Progressive, severe pain; flank to inguinal region to testicle	Urinalysis, ultrasound, IVP, CT
Other genitourinary disorders	Suprapubic or lower abdominal pain; genitourinary symptoms	Ultrasound of kidneys and pelvis; gynecologic evaluation
MISCELLANEOUS CAUSES		
Abdominal migraine	See text; nausea, family Hx migraine	Hx
Abdominal epilepsy	Might have seizure prodrome	EEG (can require >1 study, including sleep-deprived EEG)
Gilbert syndrome	Mild abdominal pain (causal or coincidental?); slightly elevated unconjugated bilirubin	Serum bilirubin
Familial Mediterranean fever	Paroxysmal episodes of fever, severe abdominal pain, and tenderness with other evidence of polyserositis	Hx and PE during an episode, DNA diagnosis
Sickle cell crisis	Anemia	Hematologic evaluation
Lead poisoning	Vague abdominal pain ± constipation	Serum lead level
Henoch-Schönlein purpura	Recurrent, severe crampy abdominal pain, occult blood in stool, characteristic rash, arthritis	Hx, PE, urinalysis
Angioneurotic edema	Swelling of face or airway, crampy pain	Hx, PE, upper GI contrast x-rays, serum C1 esterase inhibitor
Acute intermittent porphyria	Severe pain precipitated by drugs, fasting, or infections	Spot urine for porphyrins

abd, abdominal; EEG, electroencephalogram; GI, gastrointestinal; Hx, history; IVP, intravenous pyelogrophy; O&P, ova and parasites; PE, physical exam; RLQ, right lower quadrant; RUQ, right upper quadrant.

Table 298-14 DISTINGUISHING FEATURES OF ACUTE GASTROINTESTINAL TRACT PAIN IN CHILDREN

DISEASE	ONSET	LOCATION	REFERRAL	QUALITY	COMMENTS
Pancreatitis	Acute	Epigastric, left upper quadrant	Back	Constant, sharp, boring	Nausea, emesis, tenderness
Intestinal obstruction	Acute or gradual	Periumbilical-lower abdomen	Back	Alternating cramping (colic) and painless periods	Distention, obstipation, emesis, increased bowel sounds
Appendicitis	Acute	Periumbilical, then localized to lower right quadrant; generalized with peritonitis	Back or pelvis if retrocecal	Sharp, steady	Anorexia, nausea, emesis, local tenderness, fever with peritonitis
Intussusception	Acute	Periumbilical-lower abdomen	None	Cramping, with painless periods	Hematochezia, knees in pulled-up position
Urolithiasis	Acute, sudden	Back (unilateral)	Groin	Sharp, intermittent, cramping	Hematuria
Urinary tract infection	Acute	Back	Bladder	Dull to sharp	Fever, costo-vertebral angle tenderness, dysuria, urinary frequency

painful stimuli in the abdomen. In skin and muscle, A fibers mediate sharp localized pain; C fibers from viscera, peritoneum, and muscle transmit poorly localized, dull pain. These afferent fibers have cell bodies in the dorsal root ganglia, and some axons cross the midline and ascend to the medulla, midbrain, and thalamus. Pain is perceived in the cortex of the postcentral gyrus, which can receive impulses arising from both sides of the body. In the gut, the usual stimulus provoking pain is tension or stretching. Inflammatory lesions can lower the pain threshold, but the mechanisms producing pain of inflammation are not clear. Tissue metabolites released near nerve endings probably account for the pain caused by ischemia. Perception of these painful stimuli can be modulated by input from both cerebral and peripheral sources. Psychologic factors are particularly important. Features of abdominal pain are noted in Tables 298-13 and 298-14. Pain that suggests a potentially serious organic etiology is associated with age <5 yr; fever; weight loss; bile or blood-stained emesis; jaundice; hepatosplenomegaly; back or flank pain or pain in a location other than the umbilicus; awakening from sleep in pain; referred pain to shoulder, groin or back; elevated ESR, WBC, or CRP; anemia; edema; or a strong family history of inflammatory bowel disease (IBD) or celiac disease.

Visceral pain tends to be dull and aching and is experienced in the dermatome from which the affected organ receives innervations. So, most often, the pain and tenderness is not felt over the site of the disease process. Painful stimuli originating in the liver, pancreas, biliary tree, stomach, or upper bowel are felt in the epigastrium; pain from the distal small bowel, cecum, appendix, or proximal colon is felt at the umbilicus; and pain from the distal large bowel, urinary tract, or pelvic organs is usually suprapubic. The pain from the cecum, ascending colon, and descending colon sometimes is felt at the site of the lesion due to the short mesocecum and corresponding mesocolon. The pain due to appendicitis is initially felt in the periumbilical region, and pain from the transverse colon is usually felt in the supra pubic region. The shifting (localization) of pain is a pointer toward diagnosis; for example, periumbilical pain of a few hours localizing to the right lower quadrant suggests appendicitis. Radiation of pain can be helpful in diagnosis; for example, in biliary colic the radiation of pain is toward the inferior angle of the right scapula, pancreatic pain radiated to the back, and the renal colic pain is radiated to the inguinal region on the same side.

Somatic pain is intense and is usually well localized. When the inflamed viscus comes in contact with the somatic organ like the parietal peritoneum or the abdominal wall, pain is localized to that site. Peritonitis gives rise to generalized abdominal pain with rigidity, involuntary guarding, rebound tenderness, and cutaneous hyperesthesia on physical examination.

Referred pain from extraintestinal locations, due to shared central projections with the sensory pathway from the abdominal wall, can give rise to abdominal pain, as in pneumonia when the parietal pleural pain is referred to the abdomen.

Table 298-15 DIFFERENTIAL DIAGNOSIS OF GASTROINTESTINAL BLEEDING IN CHILDHOOD

INFANT	CHILD	ADOLESCENT
COMMON		
Bacterial enteritis Milk protein allergy Intussusception Swallowed maternal blood Anal fissure Lymphonodular hyperplasia	Bacterial enteritis Anal fissure Colonic polyps Intussusception Peptic ulcer/gastritis Swallowed epistaxis Prolapse (traumatic) gastropathy secondary to emesis Mallory-Weiss syndrome	Bacterial enteritis Inflammatory bowel disease Peptic ulcer/gastritis Prolapse (traumatic) gastropathy secondary to emesis Mallory-Weiss syndrome Colonic polyps Anal fissure
RARE		
Volvulus Necrotizing enterocolitis Meckel diverticulum Stress ulcer, gastritis Coagulation disorder (hemorrhagic disease of newborn) Esophagitis	Esophageal varices Esophagitis Meckel diverticulum Lymphonodular hyperplasia Henoch-Schönlein purpura Foreign body Hemangioma, arteriovenous malformation Sexual abuse Hemolytic-uremic syndrome Inflammatory bowel disease Coagulopathy Duplication cyst	Hemorrhoids Esophageal varices Esophagitis Pill ulcer Telangiectasia-angiodysplasia Graft versus host disease Duplication cyst

GASTROINTESTINAL HEMORRHAGE

Bleeding can occur anywhere along the GI tract, and identification of the site may be challenging (Table 298-15). Bleeding that originates in the esophagus, stomach, or duodenum can cause **hematemesis.** When exposed to gastric or intestinal juices, blood quickly darkens to resemble coffee grounds; massive bleeding is likely to be red. Red or maroon blood in stools, **hematochezia,** signifies either a distal bleeding site or massive hemorrhage above the distal ileum. Moderate to mild bleeding from sites above the distal ileum tends to cause blackened stools of tarry consistency (**melena**); major hemorrhages in the duodenum or above can also cause melena.

Erosive damage to the mucosa of the GI tract is the most common cause of bleeding, although variceal bleeding secondary to portal hypertension occurs often enough to require consideration. Prolapse gastropathy producing subepithelial hemorrhage and Mallory-Weiss lesions secondary to mucosal tears associated with emesis are causes of upper intestinal bleeds. Vascular malformations are a rare cause in children; they are difficult to identify. Upper intestinal bleeding is evaluated with an EGD (esophagogastroduodenoscopy). Evaluation of the small intestine is facilitated by capsule endoscopy. The capsule-sized imaging device is swallowed in older children or placed endoscopically in younger children. Lower GI bleeding is investigated with a colonoscopy. In brisk intestinal bleeding of unknown location, a tagged red blood cell (RBC) scan is helpful in locating the site of the bleeding. Occult blood in stool is usually detected by using commercially available fecal occult blood testing cards, which are based on a chemical reaction between the chemical guaiac and oxidizing action of a substrate (hemoglobin), giving a blue color. The guaiac test is very sensitive, but random testing can miss chronic blood loss, which can lead to iron-deficiency anemia. GI hemorrhage can produce hypotension and tachycardia but rarely causes GI symptoms; brisk duodenal or gastric bleeding can lead to nausea, vomiting, or diarrhea. The breakdown products of intraluminal blood might tip patients into hepatic coma if liver function is already compromised and can lead to elevation of serum bilirubin.

ABDOMINAL DISTENTION AND ABDOMINAL MASSES

Enlargement of the abdomen can result from diminished tone of the wall musculature or from increased content: fluid, gas, or solid. Ascites, the accumulation of fluid in the peritoneal cavity, distends the abdomen both in the flanks and anteriorly when it is large in volume. This fluid shifts with movement of the patient and conducts a percussion wave. Ascitic fluid is usually a transudate with a low protein concentration resulting from reduced plasma colloid osmotic pressure of hypoalbuminemia and/or from raised portal venous pressure. In cases of portal hypertension, the fluid leak probably occurs from lymphatics on the liver surface and from visceral peritoneal capillaries, but ascites does not usually develop until the serum albumin level falls. Sodium excretion in the urine decreases greatly as the ascitic fluid accumulates and, thus, additional dietary sodium goes directly to the peritoneal space, taking with it more water. When ascitic fluid contains a high protein concentration, it is usually an exudate caused by an inflammatory or neoplastic lesion.

When fluid distends the gut, either obstruction or imbalance between absorption and secretion should be suspected. The factors causing fluid accumulation in the bowel lumen often cause gas to accumulate, too. The result may be audible gurgling noises. The source of gas is usually swallowed air, but endogenous flora can increase considerably in malabsorptive states and produce excessive gas when substrate reaches the lower intestine. Gas in the peritoneal cavity (pneumoperitoneum) is usually due to perforated viscus and can cause abdominal distention depending on the amount of gas leak. A tympanitic percussion note, even over solid organs such as the liver, indicates a large collection of gas in the peritoneum.

An abdominal organ can enlarge diffusely or be affected by a discrete mass. In the digestive tract, such discrete masses can occur in the lumen, wall, omentum, or mesentery. In a constipated child, mobile, nontender fecal masses are often found. Congenital anomalies, cysts, or inflammatory processes can affect the wall of the gut. Gut wall neoplasms are extremely rare in children. The pathologic enlargement of liver, spleen, bladder, and kidneys can give rise to abdominal distention.

JAUNDICE

See Chapters 96.3 and 348.

BIBLIOGRAPHY

Please visit the Nelson Textbook of Pediatrics *website at www.expertconsult.com for the complete bibliography.*

Section 2 THE ORAL CAVITY

Chapter 299 Development and Developmental Anomalies of the Teeth

Norman Tinanoff

INITIATION

The primary teeth form in dental crypts that arise from a band of epithelial cells incorporated into each developing jaw. By 12 wk of fetal life, each of these epithelial bands (**dental laminae**) has 5 areas of rapid growth on each side of the maxilla and the mandible, seen as rounded, budlike enlargements. Organization of adjacent mesenchyme takes place in each area of epithelial growth, and the 2 elements together are the beginning of a tooth.

After the formation of these crypts for the 20 primary teeth, another generation of tooth buds forms lingually (toward the tongue), which will develop into the succeeding permanent incisors, canines, and premolars that eventually replace the primary teeth. This process takes place from ~5 mo of gestation for the central incisors to ~10 mo of age for the 2nd premolars. The permanent 1st, 2nd, and 3rd molars, on the other hand, arise from extension of the dental laminae distal to the 2nd primary molars; buds for these teeth develop at ~4 mo of gestation, 1 yr of age, and 4-5 yr of age, respectively.

HISTODIFFERENTIATION-MORPHODIFFERENTIATION

As the epithelial bud proliferates, the deeper surface invaginates and a mass of mesenchyme becomes partially enclosed. The epithelial cells differentiate into the ameloblasts that lay down an organic matrix that forms enamel; the mesenchyme forms the dentin and dental pulp.

CALCIFICATION

After the organic matrix has been laid down, the deposition of the inorganic mineral crystals takes place from several sites of calcification that later coalesce. The characteristics of the inorganic portions of a tooth can be altered by disturbances in formation of the matrix, decreased availability of minerals, or the

Table 299-1 CALCIFICATION, CROWN COMPLETION, AND ERUPTION

TOOTH	FIRST EVIDENCE OF CALCIFICATION	CROWN COMPLETED	ERUPTION
PRIMARY DENTITION			
Maxillary			
Central incisor	3-4 mo in utero	4 mo	7½ mo
Lateral incisor	4½ mo in utero	5 mo	8 mo
Canine	5½ mo in utero	9 mo	16-20 mo
First molar	5 mo in utero	6 mo	12-16 mo
Second molar	6 mo in utero	10-12 mo	20-30 mo
Mandibular			
Central incisor	4½ mo in utero	4 mo	6½ mo
Lateral incisor	4½ mo in utero	4¼ mo	7 mo
Canine	5 mo in utero	9 mo	16-20 mo
First molar	5 mo in utero	6 mo	12-16 mo
Second molar	6 mo in utero	10-12 mo	20-30 mo
PERMANENT DENTITION			
Maxillary			
Central incisor	3-4 mo	4-5 yr	7-8 yr
Lateral incisor	10 mo	4-5 yr	8-9 yr
Canine	4-5 mo	6-7 yr	11-12 yr
First premolar	1½-1¾ yr	5-6 yr	10-11 yr
Second premolar	2-2¼ yr	6-7 yr	10-12 yr
First molar	At birth	2½-3 yr	6-7 yr
Second molar	2½-3 yr	7-8 yr	12-13 yr
Third molar	7-9 yr	12-16 yr	17-21 yr
Mandibular			
Central incisor	3-4 mo	4-5 yr	6-7 yr
Lateral incisor	3-4 mo	4-5 yr	7-8 yr
Canine	4-5 mo	6-7 yr	9-10 yr
First premolar	1¾-2 yr	5-6 yr	10-12 yr
Second premolar	2¼-2½ yr	6-7 yr	11-12 yr
First molar	At birth	2½-3 yr	6-7 yr
Second molar	2½-3 yr	7-8 yr	11-13 yr
Third molar	8-10 yr	12-16 yr	17-21 yr

Modified from Logan WHG, Kronfeld R: Development of the human jaws and surrounding structures from birth to age 15 years, *J Am Dent Assoc* 20:379, 1993.

incorporation of foreign materials. Such disturbances can affect the color, texture, or thickness of the tooth surface. Calcification of primary teeth begins at 3-4 mo in utero and concludes postnatally at ~12 mo with mineralization of the 2nd primary molars (Table 299-1).

ERUPTION

At the time of tooth bud formation, each tooth begins a continuous movement toward the oral cavity. The times of eruption of the primary and permanent teeth are listed in Table 299-1.

ANOMALIES ASSOCIATED WITH TOOTH DEVELOPMENT

Both failures and excesses of tooth initiation are observed. Developmentally missing teeth can result from environmental insult, a genetic defect involving only teeth, or the manifestation of a syndrome. **Anodontia,** or absence of teeth, occurs when no tooth buds form (ectodermal dysplasia, or familial missing teeth) or when there is a disturbance of a normal site of initiation (the area of a palatal cleft). The teeth that are most commonly absent include the 3rd molars, the maxillary lateral incisors, and the mandibular 2nd premolars.

If the dental lamina produces more than the normal number of buds, supernumerary teeth occur, most often in the area between the maxillary central incisors. Because they tend to disrupt the position and eruption of the adjacent normal teeth, their identification by radiographic examination is important. Supernumerary teeth also occur with cleidocranial dysplasia (Chapter 303) and in the area of cleft palates.

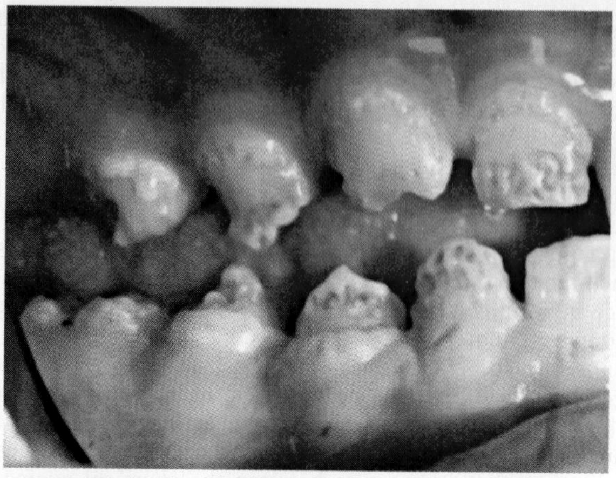

Figure 299-1 Amelogenesis imperfecta, hypoplastic type. The enamel defect results in areas of missing or thin enamel as well as grooves and pits.

Twinning, in which 2 teeth are joined together, is most often observed in the mandibular incisors of the primary dentition. It can result from gemination, fusion, or concrescence. **Gemination** is the result of the division of 1 tooth germ to form a bifid crown on a single root with a common pulp canal; an extra tooth appears to be present in the dental arch. **Fusion** is the joining of incompletely developed teeth that, owing to pressure, trauma, or crowding, continue to develop as 1 tooth. Fused teeth are sometimes joined along their entire length; in other cases, a single wide crown is supported on 2 roots. **Concrescence** is the attachment of the roots of closely approximated adjacent teeth by an excessive deposit of cementum. This type of twinning, unlike the others, is found most often in the maxillary molar region.

Disturbances during differentiation can result in alterations in dental morphology, such as **macrodontia** (large teeth) or **microdontia** (small teeth). The maxillary lateral incisors can assume a slender, tapering shape (**peg-shaped laterals**).

Amelogenesis imperfecta represents a group of hereditary conditions that manifest in enamel defects of the primary and permanent teeth without evidence of systemic disorders (Fig. 299-1). The teeth are covered by only a thin layer of abnormally formed enamel through which the yellow underlying dentin is seen. The primary teeth are generally affected more than the permanent teeth. Susceptibility to caries is low, but the enamel is subject to destruction from abrasion. Complete coverage of the crown may be indicated for dentin protection, to reduce tooth sensitivity, and for improved appearance.

Dentinogenesis imperfecta, or hereditary opalescent dentin, is a condition analogous to amelogenesis imperfecta in which the odontoblasts fail to differentiate normally, resulting in poorly calcified dentin (Fig. 299-2). This autosomal dominant disorder can also occur in patients with **osteogenesis imperfecta.** The enamel-dentin junction is altered, causing enamel to break away. The exposed dentin is then susceptible to abrasion, in some cases worn to the gingiva. The teeth are opaque and pearly, and the pulp chambers are generally obliterated by calcification. Both primary and permanent teeth are usually involved. If there is excessive wear of the teeth, selected complete coverage of the teeth may be indicated to prevent further tooth loss and improve appearance.

Localized disturbances of calcification that correlate with periods of illness, malnutrition, premature birth, or birth trauma are common. **Hypocalcification** appears as opaque white patches

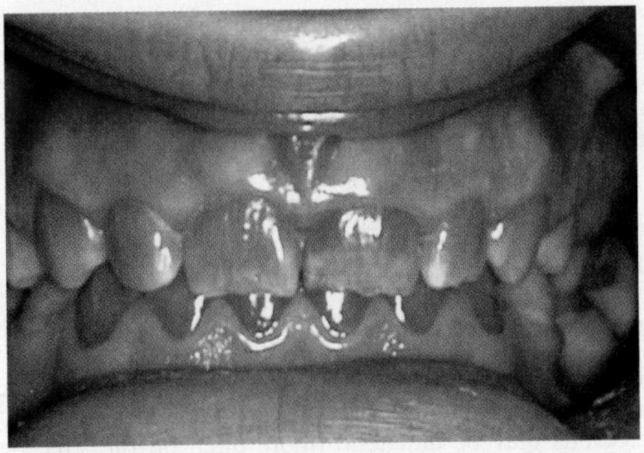

Figure 299-2 Dentinogenesis imperfecta. The bluish, opalescent sheen on several of these teeth results from genetically defective dentin. This condition may be associated with osteogenesis imperfecta. (From Nazif MM, Martin BS, McKibben DH, et al: Oral disorders. In Zitelli BJ, Davis HW, editors: *Atlas of pediatric physical diagnosis*, ed 4, Philadelphia, 2002, Mosby, p 703.)

or horizontal lines on the tooth; **hypoplasia** is more severe and manifests as pitting or areas devoid of enamel. Systemic conditions, such as renal failure and cystic fibrosis, are associated with enamel defects. Local trauma to the primary incisors can also affect calcification of permanent incisors.

Fluorosis (mottled enamel) can result from systemic fluoride consumption >0.05 mg/kg/day during enamel formation. This high fluoride consumption can be caused by residing in an area of high fluoride content of the drinking water (>2.0 ppm), swallowing excessive fluoridated toothpaste, or inappropriate fluoride prescriptions. Excessive fluoride during enamel formation affects ameloblastic function, resulting in inconspicuous white, lacy patches on the enamel to severe brownish discoloration and hypoplasia. The latter changes are usually seen with fluoride concentrations in the drinking water >5.0 ppm.

Discolored teeth can result from incorporation of foreign substances into developing enamel. Neonatal hyperbilirubinemia can produce blue to black discoloration of the primary teeth. Porphyria produces a red-brown discoloration. Tetracyclines are extensively incorporated into bones and teeth and, if administered during the period of formation of enamel, can result in brown-yellow discoloration and hypoplasia of the enamel. Such teeth fluoresce under ultraviolet light. The period at risk extends from ~4 mo of gestation to 7 yr of life. Repeated or prolonged therapy with tetracycline carries the highest risk.

Delayed eruption of the 20 primary teeth can be familial or indicate systemic or nutritional disturbances such as hypopituitarism, hypothyroidism, cleidocranial dysplasia, trisomy 21, and multiple syndromes. Failure of eruption of single or small groups of teeth can arise from local causes such as malpositioned teeth, supernumerary teeth, cysts, or retained primary teeth. Premature loss of primary teeth is most commonly caused by premature eruption of the permanent teeth. If the entire dentition is advanced for age and sex, precocious puberty or hyperthyroidism should be considered.

Natal teeth are observed in ~1/2,000 newborn infants; usually, there are 2 in the position of the mandibular central incisors. Natal teeth are present at birth, whereas **neonatal teeth** erupt in the 1st mo of life. Attachment of natal and neonatal teeth is generally limited to the gingival margin, with little root formation or bony support. They may be a supernumerary or a prematurely erupted primary tooth. A radiograph can easily differentiate between the 2 conditions. Natal teeth are associated with cleft palate, Pierre Robin syndrome, Ellis-van Creveld syndrome, Hallermann-Streiff syndrome, pachyonychia congenita, and other anomalies. A family history of natal teeth or premature eruption is present in 15-20% of affected children.

Natal or neonatal teeth occasionally result in pain and refusal to feed and can produce maternal discomfort because of abrasion or biting of the nipple during nursing. If the tooth is mobile there is a danger of detachment, with aspiration of the tooth. Because the tongue lies between the alveolar processes during birth, it can become lacerated, and, occasionally, the tip is amputated (**Riga-Fede disease**). Decisions regarding extraction of prematurely erupted primary teeth must be made on an individual basis.

Exfoliation failure occurs when a primary tooth is not shed before the eruption of its permanent successor. Most often the primary tooth exfoliates eventually, but in some cases, the primary tooth needs to be extracted. This occurs most commonly in the mandibular incisor region.

BIBLIOGRAPHY

Please visit the Nelson Textbook of Pediatrics *website at* *www.expertconsult.com* *for the complete bibliography.*

Chapter 300
Disorders of the Oral Cavity Associated with Other Conditions

Norman Tinanoff

Disorders of the teeth and surrounding structures can occur in isolation or in combination with other systemic conditions (Table 300-1). Most commonly, medical conditions that occur during tooth development can affect tooth formation or appearance. Damage to teeth during their development is permanent.

Table 300-1 DENTAL PROBLEMS ASSOCIATED WITH SELECTED MEDICAL CONDITIONS

MEDICAL CONDITION	COMMON ASSOCIATED DENTAL OR ORAL FINDINGS
Cleft lip and palate	Missing teeth, extra (supernumerary) teeth, shifting of arch segments, feeding difficulties, speech problems
Kidney failure	Mottled enamel (permanent teeth), facial dysmorphology
Cystic fibrosis	Stained teeth with extensive medication, mottled enamel
Immunosuppression	Oral candidiasis with potential for systemic candidiasis, cyclosporine-induced gingival hyperplasia
Low birth weight	Palatal groove, narrow arch with prolonged oral intubation; enamel defects of primary teeth
Heart defects with susceptibility to bacterial endocarditis	Bacteremia from dental procedures or trauma
Neutrophil chemotactic deficiency	Juvenile periodontitis (loss of supporting bone around teeth)
Juvenile diabetes (uncontrolled)	Juvenile periodontitis
Neuromotor dysfunction	Oral trauma from falling; malocclusion (open bite); gingivitis from lack of hygiene
Prolonged illness (generalized) during tooth formation	Enamel hypoplasia of crown portions forming during illness
Seizures	Gingival enlargement if phenytoin is used
Maternal infections	Syphilis: abnormally shaped teeth
Vitamin D–dependent rickets	Enamel hypoplasia

Chapter 301
Malocclusion
Norman Tinanoff

The oral cavity is essentially a masticatory instrument. The purpose of the anterior teeth is to bite off portions of large amounts of food. The posterior teeth reduce foodstuff to a soft, moist bolus. The cheeks and tongue force the food onto the areas of tooth contact. Establishing a proper relationship between the mandibular and maxillary teeth is important for physiologic and cosmetic reasons.

For the full continuation of this chapter, please visit the Nelson Textbook of Pediatrics *website at www.expertconsult.com.*

Chapter 302
Cleft Lip and Palate
Norman Tinanoff

Clefts of the lip and palate are distinct entities closely related embryologically, functionally, and genetically. Although there are a variety of theories, it is commonly thought that cleft of the lip appears because of hypoplasia of the mesenchymal layer, resulting in a failure of the medial nasal and maxillary processes to join. Cleft of the palate appears to represent failure of the palatal shelves to approximate or fuse.

INCIDENCE AND EPIDEMIOLOGY

The incidence of cleft lip with or without cleft palate is ~1/750 white births; the incidence of cleft palate alone is ~1/2,500 white births. Clefts of the lip are more common in males. Possible causes include maternal drug exposure, a syndrome-malformation complex, or genetic factors. Although both appear to occur sporadically, the presence of susceptibility genes appears important. There are ~400 syndromes associated with cleft lip and palates. There are families in which a cleft lip or palate, or both, is inherited in a dominant fashion (van der Woude syndrome), and careful examination of parents is important to distinguish this type from others, because the recurrence risk is 50%. The *IRF6* gene is responsible for the van der Woude syndrome and some cases of nonsyndromic clefts. The severity of the disease is independent of predisposing genes. Ethnic factors also affect the incidence of cleft lip and palate; the incidence is highest among Asians (~1/500) and Native Americans (~1/300), and lowest among blacks (~1/2500). The incidence of associated congenital malformations (chromosomal aneuploidy, holoprosencephaly) and of impairment in development is increased in children with cleft defects, especially in those with cleft palate alone. The risks of recurrence of cleft defects within families were discussed in Chapters 72 and 75.

CLINICAL MANIFESTATIONS

Cleft lip can vary from a small notch in the vermilion border to a complete separation involving skin, muscle, mucosa, tooth, and bone. Clefts may be unilateral (more often on the left side) or bilateral and can involve the alveolar ridge (Fig. 302-1).

Isolated cleft palate occurs in the midline and might involve only the uvula or can extend into or through the soft and hard palates to the incisive foramen. When associated with cleft lip, the defect can involve the midline of the soft palate and extend into the hard palate on one or both sides, exposing one or both of the nasal cavities as a unilateral or bilateral cleft palate. The palate can also have a submucosal cleft indicated by a bifid uvula, partial separation of muscle with intact mucosa, or a palpable notch at the posterior of the palate.

TREATMENT

A complete program of habilitation for the child with a cleft lip or palate can require years of special treatment by a team consisting of a pediatrician, plastic surgeon, otolaryngologist, oral and maxillofacial surgeon, pediatric dentist, prosthodontist, orthodontist, speech therapist, geneticist, medical social worker, psychologist, and public health nurse. The child's physician should be responsible for seeking the coordinated use of specialists and for parental counseling and guidance.

The immediate problem in an infant born with a cleft lip or palate is feeding. Although some advocate the construction of a plastic obturator to assist in feedings, most believe that with the use of soft artificial nipples with large openings, a squeezable bottle, and proper instruction, feeding of infants with clefts can be achieved with relative ease and effectiveness.

Surgical closure of a cleft lip is usually performed by 3 mo of age, when the infant has shown satisfactory weight gain and is free of any oral, respiratory, or systemic infection. Modification of the Millard rotation-advancement technique is the most commonly used technique; a staggered suture line minimizes notching of the lip from retraction of scar tissue. The initial repair may be revised at 4 or 5 yr of age. Corrective surgery on the nose may be delayed until adolescence. Nasal surgery can also be performed at the time of the lip repair. Cosmetic results depend on

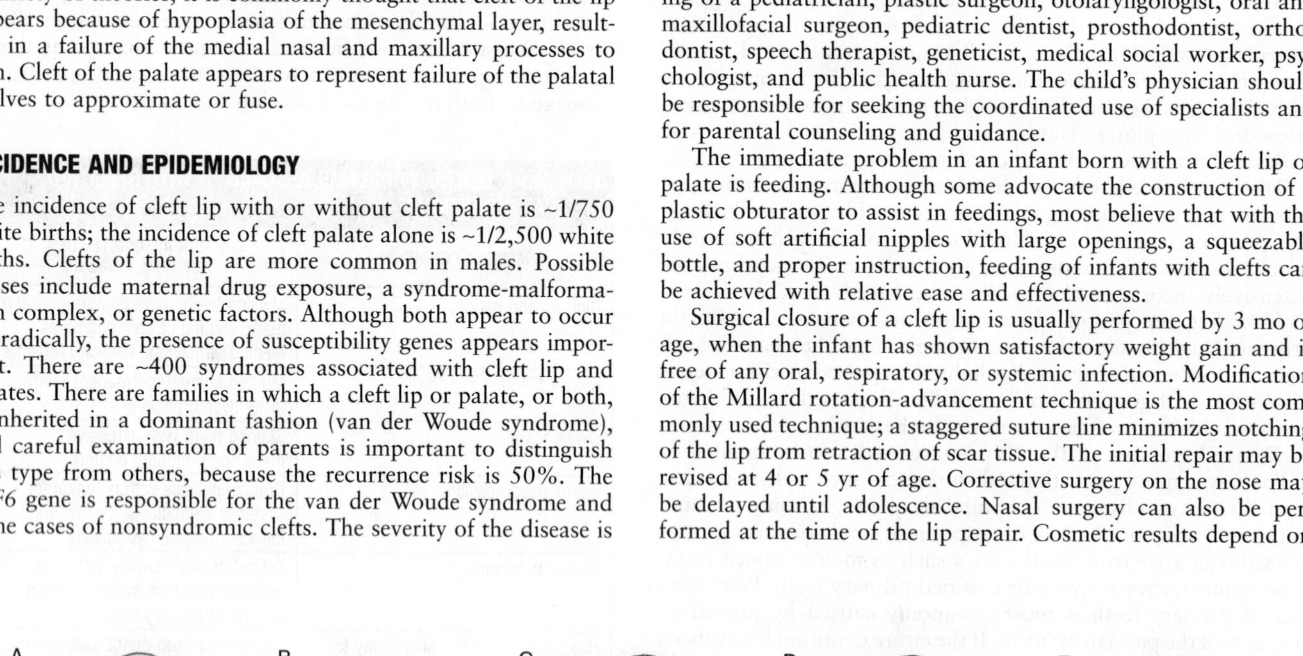

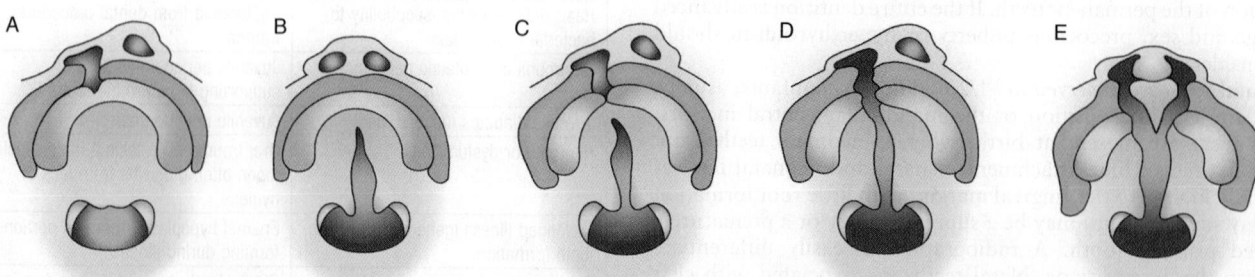

Figure 302-1 Non-syndromic orofacial clefts. *A,* Cleft lip and alveolus. *B,* Cleft palate. *C,* Incomplete unilateral cleft lip and palate. *D,* Complete unilateral cleft lip and palate. *E,* Complete bilateral cleft lip and palate. (From Shaw WC: *Orthodontics and occlusal management,* Oxford, England, 1993, Butterworth-Heinemann.)

the extent of the original deformity, healing potential of the individual patient, absence of infection, and the skill of the surgeon.

Because clefts of the palate vary considerably in size, shape, and degree of deformity, the timing of surgical correction should be individualized. Criteria such as width of the cleft, adequacy of the existing palatal segments, morphology of the surrounding areas (width of the oropharynx), and neuromuscular function of the soft palate and pharyngeal walls affect the decision. The goals of surgery are the union of the cleft segments, intelligible and pleasant speech, reduction of nasal regurgitation, and avoidance of injury to the growing maxilla.

In an otherwise healthy child, closure of the palate is usually done before 1 yr of age to enhance normal speech development. When surgical correction is delayed beyond the 3rd yr, a contoured speech bulb can be attached to the posterior of a maxillary denture so that contraction of the pharyngeal and velopharyngeal muscles can bring tissues into contact with the bulb to accomplish occlusion of the nasopharynx and help the child develop intelligible speech.

A cleft palate usually crosses the alveolar ridge and interferes with the formation of teeth in the maxillary anterior region. Teeth in the cleft area may be displaced, malformed, or missing. Missing teeth or teeth that are nonfunctional are replaced by prosthetic devices.

POSTOPERATIVE MANAGEMENT

During the immediate postoperative period, special nursing care is essential. Gentle aspiration of the nasopharynx minimizes the chances of the common complications of atelectasis or pneumonia. The primary considerations in postoperative care are maintenance of a clean suture line and avoidance of tension on the sutures. The infant is fed with a Mead Johnson bottle and the arms are restrained with elbow cuffs. A fluid or semifluid diet is maintained for 3 wk; feeding is continued with a Mead Johnson bottle or a cup. The patient's hands, toys, and other foreign bodies must be kept away from the surgical site.

SEQUELAE

Recurrent otitis media and subsequent hearing loss are frequent with cleft palate. Displacement of the maxillary arches and malposition of the teeth usually require orthodontic correction. Misarticulations and velopharyngeal dysfunction are often associated with cleft lip and palate and may be present or persist because of physiologic dysfunction, anatomic insufficiency, malocclusion, or inadequate surgical closure of the palate. Such speech is characterized by the emission of air from the nose and by a hypernasal quality with certain sounds or by compensatory misarticulations (glottal stops). Before and sometimes after palatal surgery, the speech defect is caused by inadequacies in function of the palatal and pharyngeal muscles. The muscles of the soft palate and the lateral and posterior walls of the nasopharynx constitute a valve that separates the nasopharynx from the oropharynx during swallowing and in the production of certain sounds. If the valve does not function adequately, it is difficult to build up enough pressure in the mouth to make such explosive sounds as p, b, d, t, h, y, or the sibilants s, sh, and ch, and such words as "cats," "boats," and "sisters" are not intelligible. After operation or the insertion of a speech appliance, speech therapy is necessary.

VELOPHARYNGEAL DYSFUNCTION

The speech disturbance characteristic of the child with a cleft palate can also be produced by other osseous or neuromuscular abnormalities where there is an inability to form an effective seal between oropharynx and nasopharynx during swallowing or phonation. The abnormality may be in the structure of the palate or pharynx or in the muscles attached to these structures. In a child who has the potential for abnormal speech, adenoidectomy can precipitate overt hypernasality. A submucous cleft palate can also cause this problem. In such cases, the adenoid mass might have facilitated velopharyngeal closure when contacted by the elevated soft palate. If the neuromuscular function is adequate, compensation in palatopharyngeal movement might take place and the speech defect might improve, although speech therapy is necessary. In other cases, slow involution of the adenoids can allow gradual compensation in palatal and pharyngeal muscular function. This might explain why a speech defect does not become apparent in some children who have a submucous cleft palate or similar anomaly predisposing to palatopharyngeal incompetence.

Velopharyngeal dysfunction (VPD) can also occur in children with an inherent palatal abnormality (velocardiofacial syndrome). A craniofacial disorders team and a geneticist should evaluate VPD.

Clinical Manifestations

Although clinical signs vary, the symptoms of VPD are similar to those of a cleft palate. There may be hypernasal speech (especially noted in the articulation of pressure consonants such as p, b, d, t, h, v, f, and s); conspicuous constricting movement of the nares during speech; inability to whistle, gargle, blow out a candle, or inflate a balloon; loss of liquid through the nose when drinking with the head down; otitis media; and hearing loss. Oral inspection might reveal a cleft palate or a relatively short palate with a large oropharynx; absent, grossly asymmetric, or minimal muscular activity of the soft palate and pharynx during phonation or gagging; or a submucous cleft. The last is suggested by a bifid uvula, by a translucent membrane in the midline of the soft palate (revealing lack of continuity of muscles), by palpable notching in the posterior border of the hard palate instead of a posterior nasal spinous process, or by forward or V-shaped displacement or grooving on the soft palate during phonation or gagging.

VPD may also be demonstrated radiographically. The head should be carefully positioned to obtain a true lateral view; one film is obtained with the patient at rest and another during continuous phonation of the vowel u as in "boom." The soft palate contacts the posterior pharyngeal wall in normal function, whereas in velopharyngeal dysfunction such contact is absent.

In selected cases of VPD, the palate may be retropositioned or pharyngoplasty may be performed using a flap of tissue from the posterior pharyngeal wall. Dental speech appliances have also been used successfully. The type of surgery used is best tailored to the findings on nasoendoscopy.

BIBLIOGRAPHY
Please visit the Nelson Textbook of Pediatrics *website at www.expertconsult.com for the complete bibliography.*

Chapter 303
Syndromes with Oral Manifestations

Norman Tinanoff

Many syndromes have distinct or accompanying facial, oral, and dental manifestations (Apert syndrome, Chapter 585; Crouzon disease, Chapter 585; Down syndrome, Chapter 76).

Osteogenesis imperfecta is often accompanied by effects on the teeth, termed **dentinogenesis imperfecta** (Chapter 299,

Fig. 299-2). Depending on the severity of presentation, treatment of the dentition varies from routine preventive and restorative monitoring to covering affected posterior teeth with stainless steel crowns, to prevent further tooth loss and improve appearance. Dentinogenesis imperfecta can also occur in isolation without the bony effects.

Another syndrome, **cleidocranial dysplasia,** has orofacial variations such as frontal bossing, mandibular prognathism, and a broad nasal base. Tooth eruption is often delayed. The primary teeth can be abnormally retained and the permanent teeth remain unerupted. Supernumerary teeth are common, especially in the premolar area. Although the erupted teeth are usually free of hypoplasia, variations in the size and shape of the teeth are common. Extensive dental rehabilitation therapy may be needed to maintain effective mastication.

Ectodermal dysplasias (Chapter 641) are a heterogeneous group of conditions in which oral manifestations range from little or no involvement (the dentition is completely normal) to cases in which the teeth can be totally or partially absent or malformed. Because alveolar bone does not develop in the absence of teeth, the alveolar processes can be either totally or partially absent, and the resultant overclosure of the mandible causes the lips to protrude. Facial development is otherwise not disturbed. Teeth, when present, can range from normal to small and conical. If aplasia of the buccal and labial salivary glands is present, dryness and irritation of the oral mucosa can occur. People with ectodermal dysplasia might need partial or full dentures, even at a very young age. The vertical height between the jaws is thus restored, improving the position of the lips and facial contours as well as restoring masticatory function.

Pierre Robin syndrome consists of micrognathia usually accompanied by a high arched or cleft palate (Fig. 303-1). The tongue is usually of normal size, but the floor of the mouth is foreshortened. The air passages can become obstructed, particularly on inspiration, usually requiring treatment to prevent suffocation. The infant should be maintained in a prone or partially prone position so that the tongue falls forward to relieve respiratory obstruction. Some patients require tracheostomy. Mandibular distraction procedures in the neonate can improve mandibular size, enhance respiration, and facilitate oral feedings.

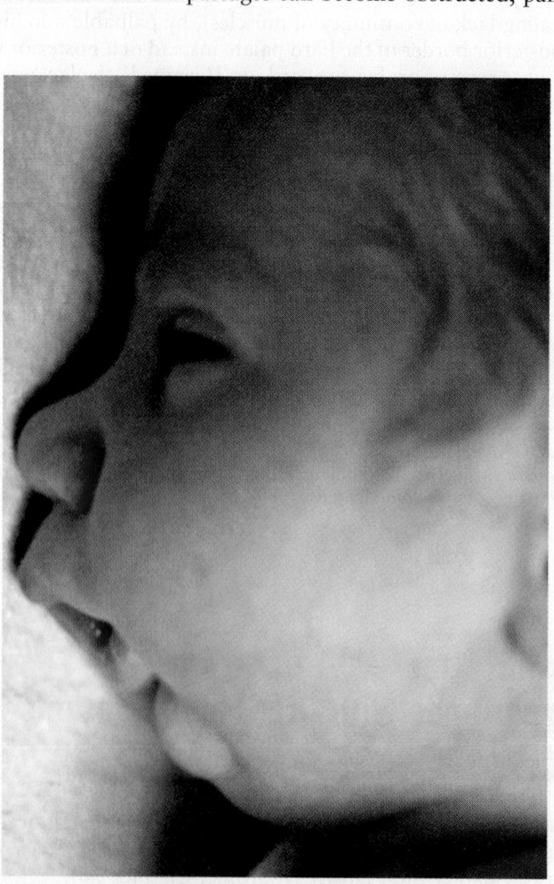

Figure 303-1 Pierre Robin syndrome. (From Clark DA: *Atlas of neonatology,* ed 7, Philadelphia, 2000, WB Saunders, p 144.)

Sufficient spontaneous mandibular growth can take place within a few months to relieve the potential airway obstruction. Often the growth of the mandible achieves a normal profile in 4-6 yr. The feeding of infants with mandibular hypoplasia requires great care and patience but can usually be accomplished without resorting to gavage. Thirty to 50% of children with Pierre Robin syndrome have **Stickler syndrome**, an autosomal dominant condition that includes other findings such as prominent joints, arthritis, hypotonia, hyperextensible joints, mitral valve prolapse, and ocular problems (retinal detachment, myopia, cataracts).

In **mandibulofacial dysostosis** (Treacher Collins syndrome or Franceschetti syndrome), the facial appearance is characterized by downward sloping palpebral fissures, colobomas of the lower eyelids, sunken cheekbones, blind fistulas opening between the angles of the mouth and the ears, deformed pinnae, atypical hair growth extending toward the cheeks, receding chin, and large mouth. Facial clefts, abnormalities of the ears, and deafness are common. The disorder is autosomal dominant, often with incomplete penetrance. The mandible is usually hypoplastic; the ramus may be deficient, and the coronoid and condylar processes are flat or even aplastic. The palatal vault may be either high or cleft. Dental malocclusions are common. The teeth may be widely separated, hypoplastic, or displaced or have an open bite. Orthodontic and routine dental treatments are indicated.

Hemifacial microsomia is usually characterized by unilateral hypoplasia of the mandible and can be associated with partial paralysis of the facial nerve, macrostomia, blind fistulas between the angles of the mouth and the ears, and deformed external ears. Severe facial asymmetry and malocclusion can develop because of the absence or hypoplasia of the mandibular condyle on the affected side. Congenital condylar deformity tends to increase with age. Early craniofacial surgery may be indicated to minimize the deformity. This disorder can be associated with ocular and vertebral anomalies (oculo-auriculo-vertebral spectrum, including Goldenhar syndrome); therefore, radiographs of the vertebrae and ribs should be considered to determine the extent of skeletal involvement.

BIBLIOGRAPHY

Please visit the Nelson Textbook of Pediatrics *website at www.expertconsult.com for the complete bibliography.*

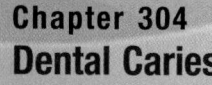

Chapter 304
Dental Caries
Norman Tinanoff

ETIOLOGY

The development of dental caries depends on interrelationships among the tooth surface, dietary carbohydrates, and specific oral bacteria. Organic acids produced by bacterial fermentation of dietary carbohydrates reduce the pH of dental plaque adjacent to the tooth to a point where demineralization occurs. The initial demineralization appears as an opaque **white spot lesion** on the enamel, and with progressive loss of tooth mineral, cavitation of the tooth occurs (Fig. 304-1).

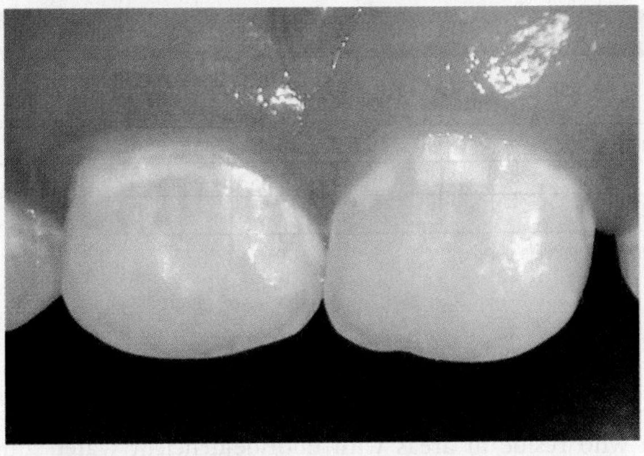

Figure 304-1 Initial carious lesions (white spot lesions) around the necks of the maxillary central incisors.

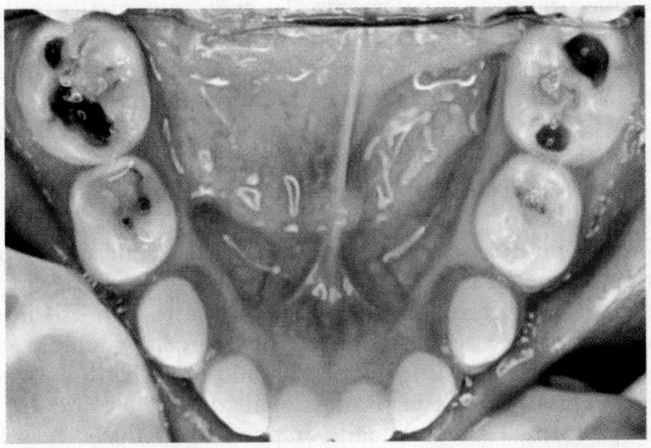

Figure 304-2 Rampant caries in a 3 yr old child. Note darkened and cavitated lesions on the fissure surfaces of mandibular molars.

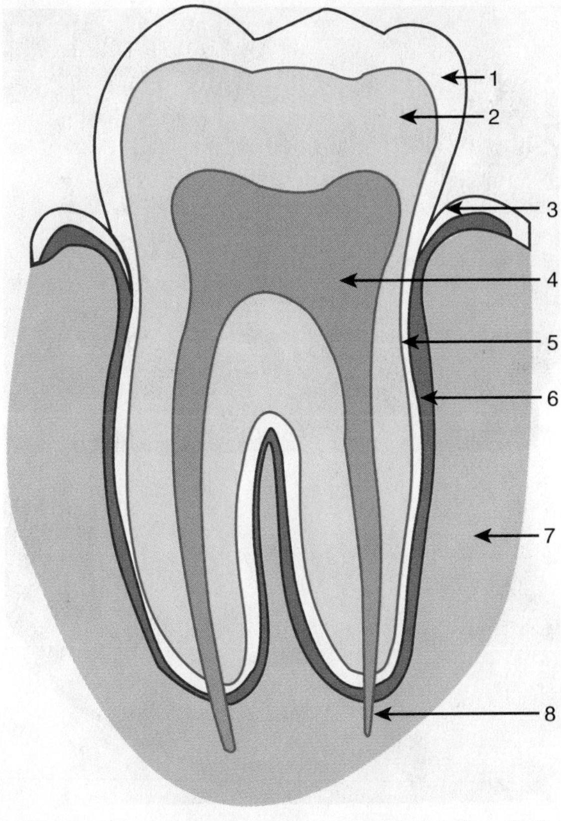

Figure 304-3 Basic dental anatomy: 1, enamel; 2, dentin; 3, gingival margin; 4, pulp; 5, cementum; 6, periodontal ligament; 7, alveolar bone; 8, neurovascular bundle.

The group of microorganisms *Streptococcus mutans* are associated with the development of dental caries. These bacteria have the ability to adhere to enamel, produce abundant acid, and survive at low pH. Once the enamel surface cavitates, other oral bacteria (lactobacilli) can colonize the tooth, produce acid, and foster further tooth demineralization. Demineralization from bacterial acid production is determined by the frequency of carbohydrate consumption and by the type of carbohydrate. Sucrose is the most cariogenic sugar because one of its byproducts during bacterial metabolism is glucan, a polymer that enables bacteria to adhere more readily to tooth structures. Dietary behaviors, such as consuming sweetened beverages in a nursing bottle or frequently consuming sticky candies, increase the cariogenic potential of foods because of the long retention of sugar in the mouth.

EPIDEMIOLOGY

The incidence of dental caries has decreased in developed countries in the past 30 years but has not decreased and remains highly prevalent among low-income children and children from developing countries. More than half of the children in the United States have dental caries, with most of those having caries primarily in the pits and fissures of the occlusal (biting) surfaces of the molar teeth.

CLINICAL MANIFESTATIONS

Dental caries of the primary dentition usually begins in the pits and fissures. Small lesions may be difficult to diagnose by visual inspection, but larger lesions are evident as darkened or cavitated lesions on the tooth surfaces (Fig. 304-2). Rampant dental caries in infants and toddlers, referred to as **early childhood caries** (ECC), is the result of a child colonized early with cariogenic bacteria and the frequent ingestion of sugar, either in the bottle or in solid foods. The carious process in this situation is initiated earlier and consequently can affect the maxillary incisors first and then progress to the molars as they erupt.

The prevalence of ECC is 30-50% in children from low socioeconomic backgrounds and as high as 70% in some Native American groups. Besides high frequency of sugar consumption and colonization with cariogenic bacteria, other enabling factors include low socioeconomic status of the family, other family member with carious teeth, recent immigrant status of the child, and the visual presence of dental plaque on the child's teeth. Children who develop caries at a young age are known to be at high risk for developing further caries as they get older. Therefore, the appropriate prevention of early childhood caries can result in the elimination of major dental problems in toddlers and less decay in later childhood.

COMPLICATIONS

Left untreated, dental caries usually destroy most of the tooth and invade the dental pulp (Fig. 304-3), leading to an inflammation of the pulp (**pulpitis**) and significant pain. Pulpitis can progress to pulp necrosis, with bacterial invasion of the alveolar bone causing a dental abscess (Fig. 304-4). Infection of a primary tooth can disrupt normal development of the successor permanent tooth. In some cases this process leads to sepsis and infection of the facial space.

TREATMENT

The age at which dental caries occurs is important in dental management. Children <3 yr of age lack the developmental

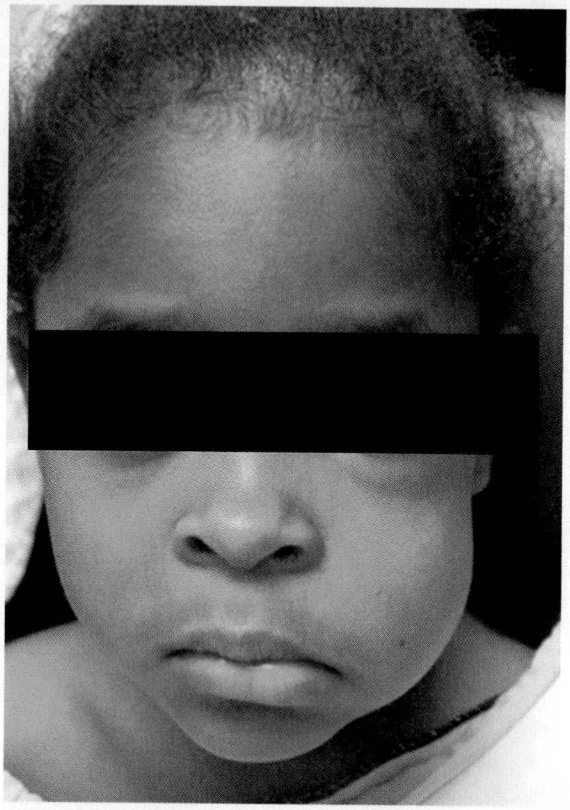

Figure 304-4 Facial swelling from an abscessed primary molar. Resolution of the inflammation can be achieved by a course of antibiotics, followed by either extraction or root canal of the offending tooth.

ability to cooperate with dental treatment and often require restraint, sedation, or general anesthesia to repair carious teeth. After age 4 yr, children can generally cope with dental restorative care with the use of local anesthesia.

Dental treatment, using silver amalgam, plastic composite, or stainless steel crowns, can restore most teeth affected with dental caries. If caries involves the dental pulp, a partial removal of the pulp (pulpotomy) or complete removal of the pulp (pulpectomy) may be required. If a tooth requires extraction, a space maintainer may be indicated to prevent migration of teeth, which subsequently leads to malposition of permanent successor teeth.

Clinical management of the pain and infection associated with untreated dental caries varies with the extent of involvement and the medical status of the patient. Dental infection localized to the dentoalveolar unit can be managed by local measures (extraction, pulpectomy). Oral antibiotics are indicated for dental infections associated with fever, cellulitis, and facial swelling, or if it is difficult to anesthetize the tooth in the presence of inflammation. Penicillin is the antibiotic of choice, except in patients with a history of allergy to this agent. Clindamycin and erythromycin are suitable alternatives. Oral analgesics, such as ibuprofen, are usually adequate for the pain control.

PREVENTION

Because they are seeing infants and toddlers on a periodicity schedule, physicians have an important role in screening children <3 yr of age for dental caries; providing preventive instructions; applying preventive measures, such as fluoride varnish; and referring the child to a dentist if problems exist.

Fluoride

The most effective preventive measure against dental caries is communal water supplies optimized to 1 ppm fluoride. Children who reside in areas with fluoride-deficient water supplies and are at risk for caries benefit from dietary fluoride supplements (Table 304-1). If the patient uses a private water supply, it is necessary to get the water tested for fluoride levels before prescribing fluoride supplements. To avoid potential overdoses, no fluoride prescription should be written for more than a total of 120 mg of fluoride. However, because of confusion regarding fluoride supplements among practitioners and parents, association of supplements with fluorosis, and lack of parent compliance with the daily administration, supplements may no longer be the first-line approach for preventing caries in preschool children.

Table 304-1 SUPPLEMENTAL FLUORIDE DOSAGE SCHEDULE

AGE	FLUORIDE IN HOME WATER (ppm) <0.3	0.3-0.6	>0.6
6 mo-3 yr	0.25*	0	0
3-6 yr	0.50	0.25	0
6-16 yr	1.00	0.50	0

*Milligrams of fluoride per day.

Topical fluoride on a daily basis can be achieved by using fluoridated toothpaste. Supervised use of a "pea-sized" amount of toothpaste (approximately 1/4 g) on the toothbrush in children <6 yr of age reduces the risk of fluorosis. Children <2 yr of age, who are at risk for caries, should brush with a "smear" of fluoridated toothpaste. Professional topical fluoride applications performed semiannually reportedly reduce caries by approximately 30%. Fluoride varnish is ideal for professional applications in preschool children because of ease of use, even with non–dental health providers, and its safety due to single-dose dispensers. Products that are available now come in containers of 0.25, 0.4, or 0.6 mL of varnish, corresponding to 12.5, 20, or 30 mg fluoride, respectively. Fluoride varnish should be administered twice a year for preschool children at moderate caries risk and four times a year for children at high caries risk.

Oral Hygiene

Daily brushing, especially with fluoridated toothpaste, helps prevent dental caries. Most children <8 yr of age do not have the coordination required for adequate tooth brushing. Accordingly, parents should assume responsibility for the child's oral hygiene, with the degree of parental involvement appropriate to the child's changing abilities.

Diet

Frequent consumption of fruit juice is not generally recognized by parents for its high cariogenic potential. Therefore, consuming sweetened beverages in a nursing bottle or sippy cup should be discouraged, and special efforts must be made to instruct parents that their child should only consume juices at meal times and not exceed 6 oz per day.

Dental Sealant

Plastic dental sealants have been shown to be effective in preventing caries on the pit and fissure of the primary and permanent molars. Sealants are most effective when placed soon after teeth erupt and used in children with deep grooves and fissures in the molar teeth.

BIBLIOGRAPHY

Please visit the Nelson Textbook of Pediatrics *website at www.expertconsult.com for the complete bibliography.*

Chapter 305
Periodontal Diseases

Norman Tinanoff

The periodontium includes the gingiva, alveolar bone, cementum, and periodontal ligament (see Fig. 304-3).

GINGIVITIS

Poor oral hygiene results in the accumulation of dental plaque at the tooth-gingival interface that activates an inflammatory response, expressed as localized or generalized reddening and swelling of the gingiva. More than half of American school children experience gingivitis. In severe cases, the gingiva spontaneously bleeds and there is oral malodor. Treatment is proper oral hygiene (careful toothbrushing and flossing); complete resolution can be expected. Fluctuations in hormonal levels during the onset of puberty can increase inflammatory response to plaque. Gingivitis in healthy children is unlikely to progress to periodontitis (inflammation of the periodontal ligament resulting in loss of alveolar bone).

AGGRESSIVE PERIODONTITIS IN CHILDREN (PREPUBERTAL PERIODONTITIS)

Periodontitis in children before puberty is a rare disease that often begins between the time of eruption of the primary teeth and the age of 4 or 5 yr. The disease occurs in localized and generalized forms. There is rapid bone loss, often leading to premature loss of primary teeth. It is often associated with systemic problems, including neutropenia, leukocyte adhesion or migration defects, hypophosphatasia, Papillon-Lefèvre syndrome, leukemia, and histiocytosis X. In many cases, however, there is no apparent underlying medical problem. Nonetheless, diagnostic work-ups are necessary to rule out underlying systemic disease.

Treatment includes aggressive professional teeth cleaning, strategic extraction of affected teeth, and antibiotic therapy. There are few reports of long-term successful treatment to reverse bone loss surrounding primary teeth.

AGGRESSIVE PERIODONTITIS IN ADOLESCENTS (LOCALIZED JUVENILE PERIODONTITIS)

Aggressive periodontitis in adolescents is characterized by rapid alveolar bone loss, especially around the permanent incisors and 1st molars. Overall prevalence in the United States is <1%, but the prevalence among African-Americans is reportedly 2.5%. This form of periodontitis is associated with a strain of *Aggregatibacter (Actinobacillus)* bacteria. In addition, the neutrophils of patients with aggressive periodontitis can have chemotactic or phagocytic defects. If left untreated, affected teeth lose their attachment and can exfoliate. Treatment varies with the degree of involvement. Patients whose disease is diagnosed at onset are usually managed by surgical or nonsurgical debridement in conjunction with antibiotic therapy. Prognosis depends on the degree of initial involvement and compliance with therapy.

TEETHING

Teething can lead to intermittent localized discomfort in the area of erupting primary teeth, irritability, low-grade fevers, and excessive salivation; many children have no apparent difficulties. Treatment of symptoms includes oral analgesics and ice rings for the child to "gum." Similar manifestations can also arise when the 1st permanent molars erupt at about age 6 yr.

CYCLOSPORINE- OR PHENYTOIN-INDUCED GINGIVAL OVERGROWTH

The use of cyclosporine to suppress organ rejection or phenytoin for anticonvulsant therapy, and in some cases calcium channel blockers, is associated with generalized enlargement of the gingiva. Phenytoin and its metabolites have a direct stimulatory action on gingival fibroblasts, resulting in accelerated synthesis of collagen. Phenytoin induces less gingival hyperplasia in patients who maintain meticulous oral hygiene.

Gingival hyperplasia occurs in 10-30% of patients treated with phenytoin. Severe manifestations can include gross enlargement of the gingiva, sometimes covering the teeth; edema and erythema of the gingiva; secondary infection, resulting in abscess formation; migration of teeth; and inhibition of exfoliation of primary teeth and subsequent impaction of permanent teeth. Treatment should be directed toward prevention and, if possible, discontinuation of cyclosporine or phenytoin. Patients undergoing long-term treatment with these drugs should receive frequent dental examinations and oral hygiene care. Severe forms of gingival overgrowth are treated by gingivectomy, but the lesion recurs if drug use is continued.

ACUTE PERICORONITIS

Acute inflammation of the flap of gingiva that partially covers the crown of an incompletely erupted tooth is common in mandibular permanent molars. Accumulation of debris and bacteria between the gingival flap and tooth precipitates the inflammatory response. A variant of this condition is a gingival abscess due to entrapment of bacteria because of orthodontic bands or crowns. Trismus and severe pain may be associated with the inflammation. Untreated cases can result in facial space infections and facial cellulitis.

Treatment includes local debridement and irrigation, warm saline rinses, and antibiotic therapy. When the acute phase has subsided, extraction of the tooth or resection of the gingival flap prevents recurrence. Early recognition of the partial impaction of mandibular 3rd molars and their subsequent extraction prevents these areas from developing pericoronitis.

NECROTIZING PERIODONTAL DISEASE (ACUTE NECROTIZING ULCERATIVE GINGIVITIS)

Necrotizing periodontal disease, in the past sometimes referred to as "trench mouth," is a distinct periodontal disease associated with oral spirochetes and fusobacteria. It is not clear, however, whether bacteria initiate the disease or are secondary. It rarely develops in healthy children in developed countries, with a prevalence in the United States of <1%, but is seen more often in children and adolescents from developing areas of Africa, Asia, and South America. In certain African countries, where affected children usually have protein malnutrition, the lesion can extend into adjacent tissues, causing necrosis of facial structures (cancrum oris, or noma).

Clinical manifestations of necrotizing periodontal disease include necrosis and ulceration of gingiva between the teeth, an adherent grayish pseudomembrane over the affected gingiva, oral malodor, cervical lymphadenopathy, malaise, and fever. The condition may be mistaken for acute herpetic gingivostomatitis. Dark-field microscopy of debris obtained from necrotizing lesions demonstrates dense spirochete populations.

Treatment of necrotizing periodontal disease is divided into an acute management with local debridement, oxygenating agents (direct application of 10% carbamide peroxide in anhydrous glycerol qid), and analgesics. Dramatic resolution usually occurs within 48 hr. If a patient is febrile, antibiotics (penicillin or metronidazole) may be an important adjunctive therapy. A 2nd phase of treatment may be necessary if the acute phase of the disease has caused irreversible morphologic damage to the periodontium. The disease is not contagious.

BIBLIOGRAPHY
Please visit the Nelson Textbook of Pediatrics *website at* *www.expertconsult.com* *for the complete bibliography.*

Chapter 306

Dental Trauma

Norman Tinanoff

Traumatic oral injuries may be categorized into three groups: injuries to teeth, injuries to soft tissue (contusions, abrasions, lacerations, punctures, avulsions, and burns), and injuries to jaw (mandibular and/or maxillary fractures).

INJURIES TO TEETH

Approximately 10% of children between 18 mo and 18 yr of age sustain significant tooth trauma. There appear to be 3 age periods of greatest predilection: toddlers (1-3 yr), usually due to falls or child abuse; school-aged children (7-10 yr), usually from bicycle and playground accidents; and adolescents (16-18 yr), often the result of fights, athletic injuries, and automobile accidents. Injuries to teeth are more common among children with protruding front teeth. Children with craniofacial abnormalities or neuromuscular deficits are also at increased risk for dental injury. Injuries to teeth can involve the hard dental tissues, the dental pulp (nerve), and injuries to the periodontal structure (surrounding bone and attachment apparatus) (Fig. 306-1 and Table 306-1).

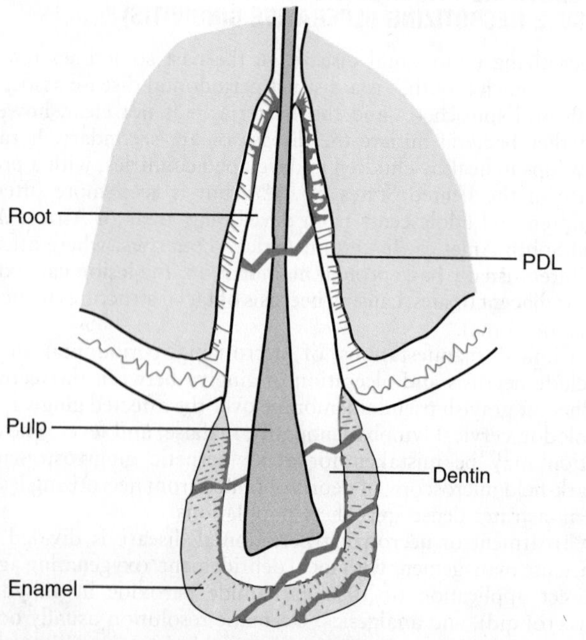

Figure 306-1 Tooth fractures can involve enamel, dentin, or pulp and can occur in the crown or root of a tooth. PDL, periodontal ligament. (From Pinkham JR: *Pediatric dentistry: infancy through adolescence*, Philadelphia, 1988, WB Saunders, p 172.)

Fractures of teeth may be uncomplicated (confined to the hard dental tissues) or complicated (involving the pulp). Exposure of the pulp results in its bacterial contamination, which can lead to infection and pulp necrosis. Such pulp exposure complicates therapy and can lower the likelihood of a favorable outcome.

The teeth most often affected are the maxillary incisors. Uncomplicated crown fractures are treated by covering exposed dentin and by placing an aesthetic restoration. Complicated crown fractures usually require **endodontic therapy** (root canal). Crown-root fractures and root fractures usually require extensive dental therapy. Such injuries in the primary dentition can interfere with normal development of the permanent dentition, and therefore, significant injuries of the primary incisor teeth are usually managed by extraction.

Traumatic oral injuries should be referred to a dentist as soon as possible. Even when the teeth appear intact, a dentist should promptly evaluate the patient. Baseline data (radiographs, mobility patterns, responses to specific stimuli) enable the dentist to assess the likelihood of future complications.

INJURIES TO PERIODONTAL STRUCTURES

Trauma to teeth with associated injury to periodontal structures that hold the teeth usually manifests as mobile or displaced teeth. Such injuries are more common in the primary than in the permanent dentition. Categories of trauma to the periodontium include concussion, subluxation, intrusive luxation, extrusive luxation, and avulsion.

Concussion

Injuries that produce minor damage to the periodontal ligament are termed *concussions.* Teeth sustaining such injuries are not mobile or displaced but react markedly to percussion (gentle hitting of the tooth with an instrument). This type of injury usually requires no therapy and resolves without complication. Primary incisors that sustain concussion can change color, indicating pulpal degeneration, and should be evaluated by a dentist.

Table 306-1 INJURIES TO CROWNS OF TEETH

TYPE OF TRAUMA	DESCRIPTION	TREATMENT AND REFERRAL
Enamel infraction (crazing)	Incomplete fracture of enamel without loss of tooth structure	Initially might not require therapy but should be assessed periodically by dentist
Enamel fractures	Fracture of only the tooth enamel	Tooth may be smoothed or treated to replace fragment
Enamel and dentin fracture	Fracture of enamel and dentinal layer of the tooth. Tooth may be sensitive to cold or air. Pulp may become necrotic, leading to periapical abscess.	Refer as soon as possible. Area should be treated to preserve the integrity of the underlying pulp.
Enamel, dentin fracture involving the pulp	Bacterial contamination can lead to pulpal necrosis and periapical abscess. The tooth might have the appearance of bleeding or might display a small red spot.	Refer immediately. The dental therapy of choice depends on the extent of injury, the condition of the pulp, the development of the tooth, time elapsed from injury, and any other injuries to the supporting structures. Therapy is directed toward minimizing contamination in an effort to improve the prognosis.

From Josell SD, Abrams RG: Managing common dental problems and emergencies, *Pediatr Clin North Am* 38:1325–1342, 1991.

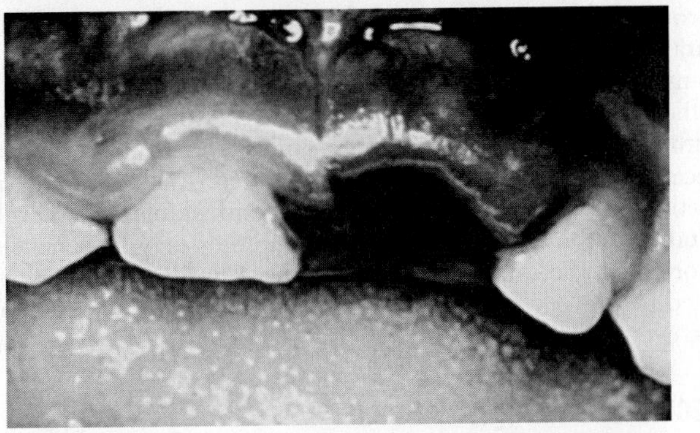

Figure 306-2 Intruded primary incisor that appears avulsed (knocked out).

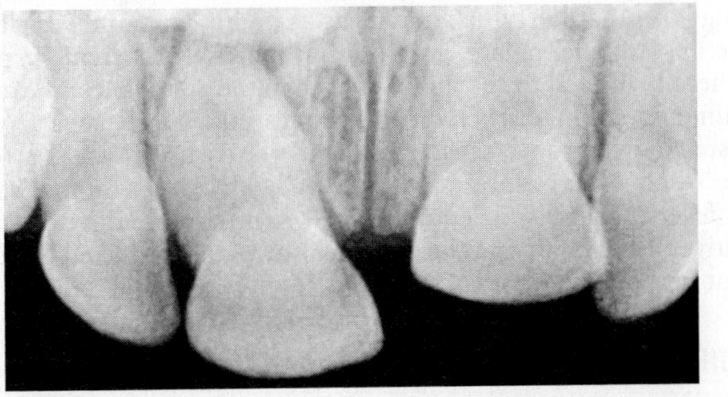

Figure 306-3 Occlusal radiograph documents intrusion of "missing tooth" presented in Figure 306-2.

Subluxation

Subluxated teeth exhibit mild to moderate horizontal mobility and/or vertical mobility. Hemorrhage is usually evident around the neck of the tooth at the gingival margin. There is no displacement of the tooth. Many subluxated teeth need to be immobilized by splints to ensure adequate repair of the periodontal ligament. Some of these teeth develop pulp necrosis.

Intrusion

Intruded teeth are pushed up into their socket, sometimes to the point where they are not clinically visible. Intruded primary incisors can give the false appearance of being avulsed (knocked out). To rule out avulsion, a dental radiograph is indicated (Figs. 306-2 and 306-3).

Extrusion

Extrusion injury is characterized by displacement of the tooth from its socket. The tooth is usually displaced to the lingual (tongue) side, with fracture of the wall of the alveolar socket. These teeth need immediate treatment; the longer the delay, the more likely the tooth will be fixed in its displaced position. Therapy is directed at reduction (repositioning the tooth) and fixation (splinting). The pulp of such teeth often becomes necrotic and requires endodontic therapy. Extrusive luxation in the primary dentition is usually managed by extraction because complications of reduction and fixation can result in problems with development of permanent teeth.

Avulsion

If avulsed permanent teeth are replanted within 20 min after injury, good success may be achieved; if the delay exceeds 2 hr, however, failure (root resorption, ankylosis) is common. The likelihood that normal reattachment will follow replantation of the tooth is related to the viability of the periodontal ligament. Parents confronted with this emergency situation can be instructed to do the following:

- Find the tooth.
- Rinse the tooth. (Do not scrub the tooth. Do not touch the root. After plugging the sink drain, hold the tooth by the crown and rinse it under running tap water.)
- Insert the tooth into the socket. (Gently place it back into its normal position. Do not be concerned if the tooth extrudes slightly. If the parent or child is too apprehensive for replantation of the tooth, the tooth should be placed in cold cow's milk or other cold isotonic solution.)
- Go directly to the dentist. (In transit, the child should hold the tooth in its socket with a finger. The parent should buckle a seatbelt around the child and drive safely.)

After the tooth is replanted, it must be immobilized to facilitate reattachment; endodontic therapy is always required. The initial signs of complications associated with replantation can appear as early as 1 wk after trauma or as late as several years later. Close dental follow-up is indicated for at least 1 yr.

PREVENTION

To minimize the likelihood of dental injuries:

- Every child or adolescent who engages in contact sports should wear a mouth guard, which may be constructed by a dentist or purchased at any athletic goods store.
- Helmets with face guards should be worn by children or adolescents with neuromuscular problems or seizure disorders to protect the head and face during falls.
- Helmets should also be used during biking, skating, and skateboarding.
- All children or adolescents with protruding incisors should be evaluated by a pediatric dentist or orthodontist.

ADDITIONAL CONSIDERATIONS

Children who experience dental trauma might also have sustained head or neck trauma, and therefore neurologic assessment is warranted. Tetanus prophylaxis should be considered with any injury that disrupts the integrity of the oral tissues. The possibility of child abuse should always be considered.

Chapter 307
Common Lesions of the Oral Soft Tissues

Norman Tinanoff

OROPHARYNGEAL CANDIDIASIS

Oropharyngeal infection with *Candida albicans* (thrush, moniliasis) (Chapter 226.1) is common in neonates from contact with the organism in the birth canal or breast. The lesions of oropharyngeal candidiasis (OPC) appears as white plaques covering all or part of the oropharyngeal mucosa. These plaques are removable from the underlying surface, which is characteristically inflamed and has pinpoint hemorrhages. The diagnosis is confirmed by direct microscopic examination on potassium hydroxide smears and culture of scrapings from lesions. OPC is usually self-limited in the healthy newborn infant, but topical application of nystatin to the oral cavity of the baby and to the nipples of breast-feeding mothers will hasten recovery.

OPC is also a major problem during myelosuppressive therapy. **Systemic candidiasis** (SC), a major cause of morbidity and mortality during myelosuppressive therapy, develops almost exclusively in patients who have had prior oropharyngeal, esophageal, or intestinal candidiasis. This observation implies that prevention of OPC should reduce the incidence of SC. The use of oral rinses of 0.2% chlorhexidine solution, plus systemic antifungals may be effective in preventing OPC, SC, or candidal esophagitis.

APHTHOUS ULCERS

The aphthous ulcer (canker sore) is a distinct oral lesion, prone to recurrence. The differential diagnosis is noted in Table 307-1. Aphthous ulcers are reported to develop in 20% of the population. Their etiology is unclear, but allergic or immunologic reactions, emotional stress, genetics, and injury to the soft tissues in the mouth have been implicated. Aphthous-like lesions may be associated with inflammatory bowel disease, Behçet disease, gluten-sensitive enteropathy, periodic fever-aphthae-pharyngitis-adenitis syndrome, Sweet syndrome, HIV infection (especially if ulcers are large and slow to heal), and cyclic neutropenia. Clinically, these ulcers are characterized by well-circumscribed, ulcerative lesions with a white necrotic base surrounded by a red halo. The lesions last 10-14 days and heal without scarring. Over-the-counter palliative therapies, such as benzocaine and topical lidocaine, are effective, as well as topical steroids. Tetracycline has been shown to have benefit with severe outbreaks, but caution is necessary in pregnant women and young children to prevent tetracycline tooth staining during a child's tooth development.

HERPETIC GINGIVOSTOMATITIS

After an initial incubation period of ~1 wk, the initial infection with herpes simplex virus manifests as fever and malaise, usually in a child <5 yr (Chapter 244). The oral cavity can show various expressions, including the gingiva becoming erythematous, mucosal hemorrhages, and clusters of small vesicles erupting throughout the mouth. There is often involvement of the mucocutaneous margin and perioral skin (Fig. 307-1). The oral symptoms generally are accompanied by fever, lymphadenopathy, and difficulty eating and drinking. The symptoms usually regress within 2 wk without scarring. Fluids should be encouraged because the child may become dehydrated. Analgesics and anesthetic rinses can make the child more comfortable. Oral acyclovir if taken within the first 3 days of symptoms may be beneficial in shortening the duration of symptoms. Caution should be exercised to prevent autoinoculation or transmission of infection to the eyes.

Table 307-1 DIFFERENTIAL DIAGNOSIS OF ORAL ULCERATION

CONDITION	COMMENT
COMMON	
Aphthous (canker sore)	Painful, circumscribed lesions; recurrences
Traumatic	Accidents, chronic cheek biter, or after dental local anesthesia
Hand, foot, mouth disease	Painful; lesions on tongue, anterior oral cavity, hands, and feet
Herpangina	Painful; lesions confined to soft palate and oropharynx
Herpetic gingivostomatitis	Vesicles on mucocutaneous borders; painful, febrile
Recurrent herpes labialis	Vesicles on lips; painful
Chemical burns	Alkali, acid, aspirin; painful
Heat burns	Hot food, electrical
UNCOMMON	
Neutrophil defects	Agranulocytosis, leukemia, cyclic neutropenia; painful
Systemic lupus erythematosus	Recurrent, may be painless
Behçet's syndrome	Resembles aphthous lesions; associated with genital ulcers, uveitis
Necrotizing ulcerative gingivostomatitis	Vincent stomatitis; painful
Syphilis	Chancre or gumma; painless
Oral Crohn disease	Aphthous-like; painful
Histoplasmosis	Lingual

RECURRENT HERPES LABIALIS

Approximately 90% of the population develops antibodies to herpes simplex virus. In periods of quiescence, the virus is thought to remain latent in sensory neurons. Unlike primary herpetic gingivostomatitis, which manifests as multiple painful vesicles on the lips, tongue, palate, gingiva, and mucosa, recurrent herpes is generally limited to the lips. Other than the annoyance of causing pain and an unattractive appearance, there are generally no systemic symptoms. Reactivation of the virus is thought to be the result of exposure to ultraviolet light, tissue trauma, stress, or fevers. There is little advantage of antiviral therapy over palliative therapies in an otherwise healthy patient affected by recurrent herpes.

BOHN NODULES

Bohn nodules are small developmental anomalies located along the buccal and lingual aspects of the mandibular and maxillary ridges and in the hard palate of the neonate. These lesions arise from remnants of mucous gland tissue. Treatment is not necessary, because the nodules disappear within a few weeks.

DENTAL LAMINA CYSTS

Dental lamina cysts are small cystic lesions located along the crest of the mandibular and maxillary ridges of the neonate. These lesions arise from epithelial remnants of the dental lamina. Treatment is not necessary; they disappear within a few weeks.

FORDYCE GRANULES

Almost 80% of adults have multiple yellow-white granules in clusters or plaquelike areas on the oral mucosa, most commonly on the buccal mucosa or lips. They are aberrant sebaceous glands. The glands are present at birth, but they can hypertrophy and 1st

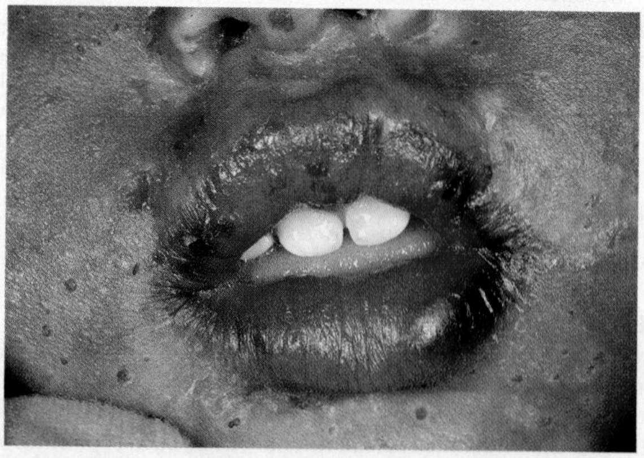

Figure 307-1 Herpetic gingivostomatitis. Lip erosions with multiple perioral herpetic lesions. (From Paller AS, Mancini AJ, editors: *Hurwitz clinical pediatric dermatology*, ed 3, Philadelphia, 2006, Elsevier /Saunders, p 398.)

appear as discrete yellowish papules during the preadolescent period in ~50% of children. No treatment is necessary.

PARULIS

The parulis (gum boil) is a soft reddish papule located adjacent to the root of a chronically abscessed tooth. It occurs at the end-point of a draining dental sinus tract. Treatment consists of diagnosing which tooth is abscessed and extracting it or performing root canal on the offending tooth.

CHEILITIS

This dryness of the lips followed by scaling and cracking and accompanied by a characteristic burning sensation is common in children. Cheilitis may be caused by sensitivity to contact substances, lip licking, vitamin deficiency, weakened immune system, or fungal or bacterial infections. Cheilitis often occurs in association with fever. Treatment may include antifungal or antibacterial agents and frequent application of petroleum jelly.

ANKYLOGLOSSIA

Ankyloglossia or "tongue-tie" is characterized by an abnormally short lingual frenum that can hinder the tongue movement but rarely interferes with feeding or speech. The frenum might spontaneously lengthen as the child gets older. If the extent of the ankyloglossia is severe, speech may be affected and surgical correction may be indicated.

GEOGRAPHIC TONGUE

Geographic tongue (migratory glossitis) is a benign and asymptomatic lesion and is characterized by one or more smooth, bright red patches, often showing a yellow, gray, or white membranous margin on the dorsum of an otherwise normally roughened tongue. The condition has no known cause, and no treatment is indicated (Chapter 656).

FISSURED TONGUE

The fissured tongue (scrotal tongue) is a malformation manifested clinically by numerous small furrows or grooves on the dorsal surface (Chapter 656). If the tongue is painful, brushing the tongue or irrigating with water can reduce the bacteria in the fissures.

Chapter 308
Diseases of the Salivary Glands and Jaws

Norman Tinanoff

With the exception of mumps (Chapter 240), disease of the salivary glands is rare in children. Bilateral enlargement of the submaxillary glands can occur in AIDS, cystic fibrosis, Epstein-Barr virus infection, and malnutrition and, transiently, during acute asthmatic attacks. Chronic vomiting can be accompanied by enlargement of the parotid glands. Benign salivary gland hypertrophy has been associated with endocrinopathies: thyroid disease, diabetes, and disorders of the pituitary-adrenal axis.

For the full continuation of this chapter, please visit the Nelson Textbook of Pediatrics *website at www.expertconsult.com.*

Chapter 309
Diagnostic Radiology in Dental Assessment

Norman Tinanoff

The **panoramic radiograph** provides a single tomographic image of the upper and lower jaw, including all the teeth and supporting structures. The x-ray tube rotates about the patient's head with reciprocal movement of the film or image receptor during the exposure. The panoramic image shows the mandibular bodies, rami, and condyles; maxillary sinuses; and a majority of the facial buttresses. Such images are used to show abnormalities of tooth number, development and eruption pattern, cystic and neoplastic lesions, bone infections, and fracture, as well as dental caries and periodontal disease (see Fig. 309-1 on the *Nelson Textbook of Pediatrics* website at www.expertconsult.com).

For the full continuation of this chapter, please visit the Nelson Textbook of Pediatrics *website at www.expertconsult.com.*

Section 3 THE ESOPHAGUS

Chapter 310
Embryology, Anatomy, and Function of the Esophagus

Seema Khan and Susan R. Orenstein

The esophagus is a hollow muscular tube, separated from the pharynx above and the stomach below by 2 tonically closed sphincters. Its primary function is to convey ingested material from the mouth to the stomach. Largely lacking digestive glands and enzymes, and exposed only briefly to nutrients, it has no active role in digestion.

For the full continuation of this chapter, please visit the Nelson Textbook of Pediatrics *website at www.expertconsult.com.*

310.1 Common Clinical Manifestations and Diagnostic Aids

Seema Khan and Susan R. Orenstein

COMMON CLINICAL MANIFESTATIONS

Manifestations include pain, obstruction or difficulty swallowing, abnormal retrograde movement of gastric contents (reflux, regurgitation, or vomiting), or bleeding; esophageal disease can also engender respiratory symptoms. Pain in the chest unrelated to swallowing (**heartburn**) can be a sign of esophagitis, but similar pain might also represent cardiac, pulmonary, or musculoskeletal disease or visceral hyperalgesia. Pain during swallowing (**odynophagia**) localizes the disease more discretely to the pharynx and esophagus and often represents inflammatory mucosal disease. Complete esophageal obstruction can be produced acutely by esophageal foreign bodies, including food impactions; can be congenital, as in esophageal atresia; or can evolve over time as a peptic stricture occludes the esophagus. Difficulty swallowing (**dysphagia**) can be produced by incompletely occlusive esophageal obstruction (by extrinsic compression, intrinsic narrowing, or foreign bodies) but can also result from dysmotility of the esophagus (whether primary/idiopathic or secondary to systemic disease). Inflammatory lesions of the esophagus without obstruction or dysmotility are a 3rd cause of dysphagia; eosinophilic esophagitis, most often afflicting older boys, is relatively common.

For the full continuation of this chapter, please visit the Nelson Textbook of Pediatrics *website at www.expertconsult.com.*

Chapter 311
Congenital Anomalies

311.1 Esophageal Atresia and Tracheoesophageal Fistula

Seema Khan and Susan R. Orenstein

Esophageal atresia (EA) is the most common congenital anomaly of the esophagus, affecting ~1/4,000 neonates. Of these, >90% have an associated tracheoesophageal fistula (TEF). In the most common form of EA, the upper esophagus ends in a blind pouch and the TEF is connected to the distal esophagus. The types of EA and TEF and their relative frequencies are shown in Figure 311-1. The exact cause is still unknown; associated features include advanced maternal age, European ethnicity, obesity, low socioeconomic status, and tobacco smoking. This defect has survival rates of >90%, owing largely to improved neonatal intensive care, earlier recognition, and appropriate intervention. Infants weighing <1,500 g at birth have the highest risk for mortality. Fifty percent of infants are nonsyndromic without other anomalies, and the rest have associated anomalies, most often associated with the VATER or VACTERL (vertebral, anorectal, [cardiac], tracheal, esophageal, renal, radial, [limb]) syndrome. These syndromes generally are associated with normal intelligence. Despite low concordance among twins and the low incidence of familial cases, genetic factors have a role in the pathogenesis of TEF in some patients as suggested by discrete mutations in syndromic cases: Feingold syndrome *(N-MYC)*, CHARGE syndrome (*c*oloboma of the eye, central nervous system anomalies; *h*eart defects; *a*tresia of the choanae; *r*etardation of growth and/or development; *g*enital and/or urinary defects [hypogonadism]; *e*ar anomalies and/or deafness) *(CHD7)*, and anophthalmia-esophageal-genital syndrome *(SOX2)*.

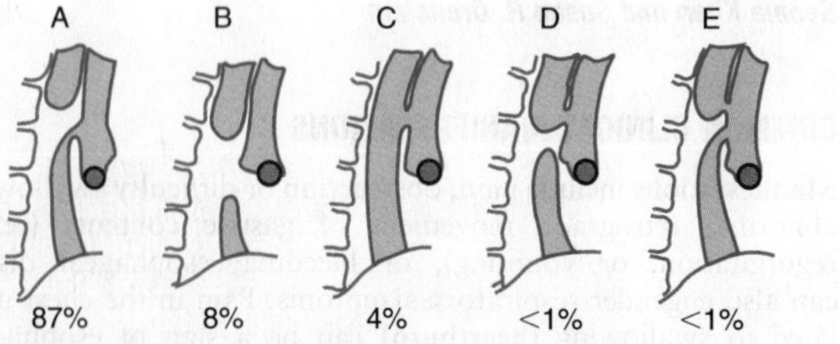

Figure 311-1 *A-E,* Diagrams of the 5 most commonly encountered forms of esophageal atresia and tracheoesophageal fistula, shown in order of frequency.

PRESENTATION

The neonate with EA typically has frothing and bubbling at the mouth and nose after birth as well as episodes of coughing, cyanosis, and respiratory distress. Feeding exacerbates these symptoms, causes regurgitation, and can precipitate aspiration. Aspiration of gastric contents via a distal fistula causes more damaging pneumonitis than aspiration of pharyngeal secretions from the blind upper pouch. The infant with an isolated TEF in the absence of EA ("H-type" fistula) might come to medical attention later in life with chronic respiratory problems, including refractory bronchospasm and recurrent pneumonias.

DIAGNOSIS

In the setting of early-onset respiratory distress, the inability to pass a nasogastric or orogastric tube in the newborn suggests esophageal atresia. Maternal polyhydramnios might alert the physician to EA. Plain radiography in the evaluation of respiratory distress might reveal a coiled feeding tube in the esophageal pouch and/or an air-distended stomach, indicating the presence of a coexisting TEF (Fig. 311-2). Conversely, pure EA can manifest as an airless scaphoid abdomen. In isolated TEF (H type), an esophagogram with contrast medium injected under pressure can

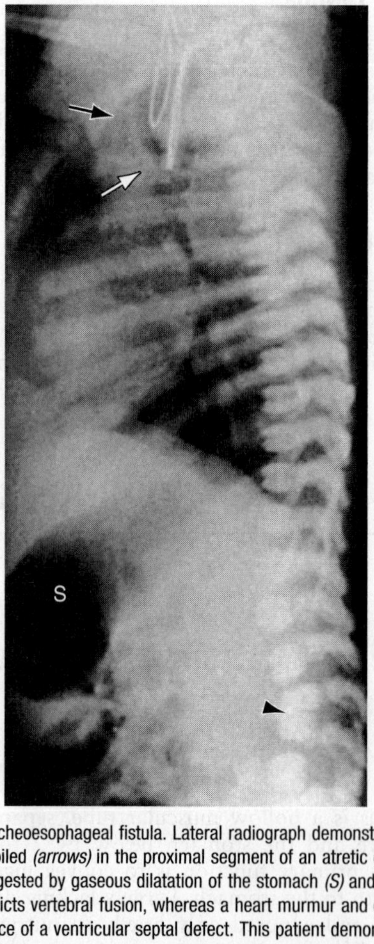

Figure 311-2 Tracheoesophageal fistula. Lateral radiograph demonstrating a nasogastric tube coiled *(arrows)* in the proximal segment of an atretic esophagus. The distal fistula is suggested by gaseous dilatation of the stomach *(S)* and small intestine. The *arrowhead* depicts vertebral fusion, whereas a heart murmur and cardiomegaly suggest the presence of a ventricular septal defect. This patient demonstrated elements of the VATER (vertebral, anorectal, tracheal, esophageal, renal, radial) anomalad. (From Balfe D, Ling D, Siegel M: The esophagus. In Putman CE, Ravin CE, editors: *Textbook of diagnostic imaging,* Philadelphia, 1988, WB Saunders.)

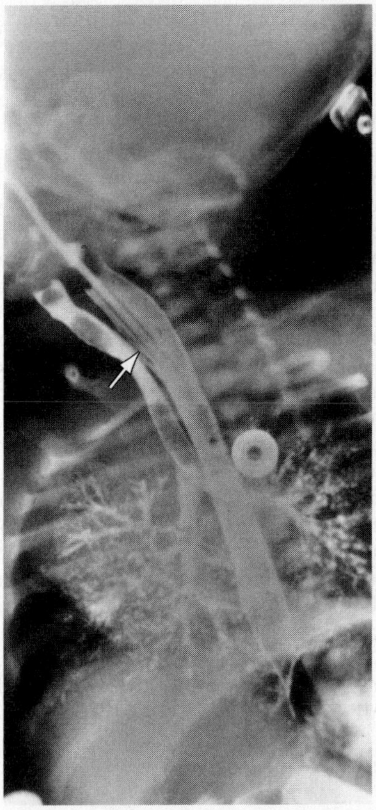

Figure 311-3 H-type fistula *(arrow)* demonstrated in an infant after barium swallow on frontal-oblique chest x-ray. The tracheal aspect of the fistula is characteristically superior to the esophageal aspect. Barium is seen to outline the tracheobronchial tree. (From Wyllie R, Hyams JS, editors: *Pediatric gastrointestinal and liver disease*, ed 3, Philadelphia, 2006, Saunders Elsevier, p 299.)

demonstrate the defect (Fig. 311-3). Alternatively, the orifice may be detected at bronchoscopy or when methylene blue dye injected into the endotracheal tube during endoscopy is observed in the esophagus during forced inspiration.

MANAGEMENT

Initially, maintaining a patent airway and preventing aspiration of secretions are paramount. Prone positioning minimizes movement of gastric secretions into a distal fistula, and esophageal suctioning minimizes aspiration from a blind pouch. Endotracheal intubation with mechanical ventilation is to be avoided if possible because it can worsen distention of abdominal viscera. Surgical ligation of the TEF and primary end-to-end anastomosis of the esophagus are performed when feasible. In the premature or otherwise complicated infant, a primary closure may be delayed by temporizing with fistula ligation and gastrostomy tube placement. If the gap between the atretic ends of the esophagus is >3-4 cm, primary repair cannot be done; options include using gastric, jejunal, or colonic segments interposed as a neo-esophagus. Careful search must be undertaken for the common associated cardiac and other anomalies. Thoracoscopic surgical repair is now considered feasible and associated with favorable long-term outcomes.

OUTCOME

The majority of children with EA and TEF grow up to lead normal lives, but complications are often challenging, particularly during the first 5 yr of life. Complications of surgery include anastomotic leak, refistulization, and anastomotic stricture. Gastroesophageal reflux disease (GERD), resulting from intrinsic abnormalities of esophageal function, often combined with delayed gastric emptying, contributes to management challenges in many cases. GERD contributes significantly to the respiratory disease (**reactive airway disease**) that often complicates EA and TEF and also worsens the frequent anastomotic strictures after repair of EA.

Many patients have an associated tracheomalacia that improves as the child grows.

BIBLIOGRAPHY

Please visit the Nelson Textbook of Pediatrics *website at* *www.expertconsult.com* *for the complete bibliography.*

311.2 Laryngotracheoesophageal Clefts

Seema Khan and Susan R. Orenstein

Laryngotracheoesophageal clefts are uncommon anomalies that result when the septum between the esophagus and trachea fails to develop fully, leading to a common channel defect between the pharyngoesophagus and laryngotracheal lumen, thus making the laryngeal closure incompetent during swallowing or reflux. Other developmental anomalies, such as esophageal atresia and tracheoesophageal fistula, are seen in 20% of patients with clefts. Early in life, the infant presents with stridor, choking, cyanosis, aspiration of feedings, and recurrent chest infections. The diagnosis is difficult and usually requires direct endoscopic visualization of the larynx and esophagus. When contrast radiography is used, material is often seen in the esophagus and trachea. Treatment is surgical repair, which can be complex if the defects are long.

Chapter 312
Obstructing and Motility Disorders of the Esophagus

Seema Khan and Susan R. Orenstein

Obstructing lesions classically produce **dysphagia** to solids earlier and more noticeably than to liquids and can manifest when the infant liquid diet begins to incorporate solids; this is in contrast to **dysphagia** from **dysmotility,** in which swallowing of liquids is affected as early as, or earlier than, solids. In most instances of dysphagia, evaluation begins with fluoroscopy, which may include videofluoroscopic evaluation of swallowing, particularly if aspiration is a primary symptom. Secondary studies are often endoscopic if intrinsic obstruction is suspected or manometric if dysmotility is suspected; other imaging studies may be used in particular cases. Congenital lesions can require surgery, whereas webs and peptic strictures might respond adequately to endoscopic (or bougie) dilation. Peptic strictures, once dilated, should prompt consideration of fundoplication for ongoing prophylaxis.

EXTRINSIC

Esophageal duplication cysts are the most commonly encountered foregut duplications. These cysts are lined by intestinal epithelium, have a well-developed smooth muscle wall, and are attached to the normal gastrointestinal tract. Two thirds occur on the right side of the esophagus. The most common presentation is respiratory distress caused by compression of the adjacent airways. Dysphagia is a common symptom in older children. Upper gastrointestinal bleeding can occur as a result of acid-secreting gastric mucosa in the duplication wall. **Neuroenteric cysts** might contain glial elements and are associated with **vertebral anomalies.** Diagnosis is made on either barium swallow or chest CT. Treatment is surgical; laparoscopic approach to excision is also possible.

Enlarged mediastinal or subcarinal **lymph nodes,** caused by infection (tuberculosis, histoplasmosis) or neoplasm (lymphoma), are the most common external masses that compress the esophagus and produce obstructive symptoms. **Vascular anomalies** can also compress the esophagus; *dysphagia lusoria* is a term denoting the dysphagia produced by a developmental vascular anomaly, which is often an aberrant right subclavian artery or right-sided or double aortic arch (Chapter 426.1).

INTRINSIC

Intrinsic narrowing of the esophageal lumen can be congenital or acquired. The etiology is suggested by the location, the character of the lesion, and the clinical situation. The lower esophagus is the most common location for peptic strictures, which are generally somewhat ragged and several cm long. Thin membranous rings, including the Schatzki ring at the squamocolumnar junction, can also occlude this area. In the mid esophagus, congenital narrowing may be associated with the esophageal atresia–tracheoesophageal fistula complex, in which some of the lesions might incorporate cartilage and might be impossible to dilate safely; alternatively, reflux esophagitis can induce a ragged and extensive narrowing that appears more proximal than the usual peptic stricture, often because of an associated hiatal hernia. Congenital webs or rings can narrow the upper esophagus. The upper esophagus can also be narrowed by an inflammatory stricture occurring after a caustic ingestion or due to epidermolysis bullosa. Cricopharyngeal achalasia can appear radiographically as a cricopharyngeal "bar" posteriorly in the upper esophagus. **Eosinophilic esophagitis** (**EoE**) is currently one of the most common causes for esophageal obstructive symptoms. Although the pathogenesis of obstructive EoE is not yet completely explained and seems to vary among individual patients, endoscopy or radiology demonstrate stricture formation in some children with EoE, and in others a noncompliant esophagus is evident, with thickened wall layers demonstrable by ultrasonography.

BIBLIOGRAPHY

Please visit the Nelson Textbook of Pediatrics *website at* *www.expertconsult.com* *for the complete bibliography.*

Chapter 313
Dysmotility

Seema Khan and Susan R. Orenstein

UPPER ESOPHAGEAL AND UPPER ESOPHAGEAL SPHINCTER DYSMOTILITY (STRIATED MUSCLE)

Cricopharyngeal **achalasia** signifies a failure of complete relaxation of the upper esophageal sphincter (UES), whereas cricopharyngeal **incoordination** implies full relaxation of the UES but incoordination of the relaxation with the pharyngeal contraction. These entities are usually detected on videofluoroscopic evaluation of swallowing (sometimes accompanied by visible cricopharyngeal prominence, termed a *bar*), but often the most precise definition of the dysfunction is obtained with manometry. A self-limited form of cricopharyngeal incoordination occurs in infancy and remits spontaneously in the 1st year of life if nutrition is maintained despite the dysphagia. In older children, idiopathic cricopharyngeal **spasm** is usually treated by myotomy of the UES. It is important, however, to evaluate such children thoroughly, including cranial MRI to detect **Arnold Chiari malformations,** which can manifest in this way but are best treated by cranial decompression, rather than esophageal surgery. Cricopharyngeal spasm may be severe enough to produce posterior pharyngeal (Zenker) **diverticulum** above the obstructive sphincter; this entity occurs rarely in children.

Systemic causes of swallowing dysfunction that can affect the oropharynx, UES, and upper esophagus include cerebral palsy, Arnold Chiari malformations, syringomyelia, bulbar palsy or cranial nerve defects (Möbius syndrome, transient infantile paralysis of the superior laryngeal nerve), transient pharyngeal muscle dysfunction, spinal muscular atrophy (including Werdnig-Hoffmann disease), muscular dystrophy, multiple sclerosis, infections (botulism, tetanus, poliomyelitis, diphtheria), inflammatory and autoimmune diseases (dermatomyositis, myasthenia gravis, polyneuritis, scleroderma), and familial dysautonomia. All of these can produce dysphagia. Medications (nitrazepam, benzodiazepines) and tracheostomy can adversely affect the function of the UES and thereby produce dysphagia.

LOWER ESOPHAGEAL AND LOWER ESOPHAGEAL SPHINCTER DYSFUNCTION (SMOOTH MUSCLE)

Causes of dysphagia due to more distal primary esophageal dysmotility include achalasia, diffuse esophageal spasm, nutcracker esophagus, and hypertensive LES; all but achalasia are rare in children. Secondary causes include Hirschsprung disease, pseudoobstruction, inflammatory myopathies, scleroderma, and diabetes.

Achalasia is a primary esophageal motor disorder of unknown etiology characterized by loss of LES relaxation and loss of esophageal peristalsis, both contributing to a functional obstruction of the distal esophagus. Degenerative, autoimmune (antibodies to Auerbach plexus), and infectious (Chagas disease due to *Trypanosoma cruzi*) factors are possible causes. In rare cases, achalasia is familial or part of the achalasia, alacrima, and corticotropin insensitivity, known as **Allgrove syndrome.** *Pseudoachalsia* refers to achalasia caused by various forms of cancer via obstruction of the gastroesophageal junction, infiltration of the submucosa and muscularis of the LES, or as part of the paraneoplastic syndrome with formation of anti-Hu antibodies. Pathologically, in achalasia, inflammation surrounds ganglion cells, which are decreased in number. There is selective loss of postganglionic inhibitory neurons that normally lead to sphincter relaxation, leaving postganglionic cholinergic neurons unopposed. This imbalance produces high basal LES pressures and insufficient LES relaxation. The loss of esophageal peristalsis can be a secondary phenomenon.

Achalasia manifests with regurgitation and dysphagia for solids and liquids and may be accompanied by undernutrition or respiratory symptoms; retained esophageal food can produce esophagitis. The mean age in children is 8.8 yr, with a mean duration of symptoms before diagnosis of 23 mo; it is uncommon before school age. Chest radiograph shows an air-fluid level in a dilated esophagus. **Barium fluoroscopy** reveals a smooth tapering of the lower esophagus leading to the closed LES, resembling a bird's beak (Fig. 313-1). Loss of primary peristalsis in the distal esophagus with retained food and poor emptying are often

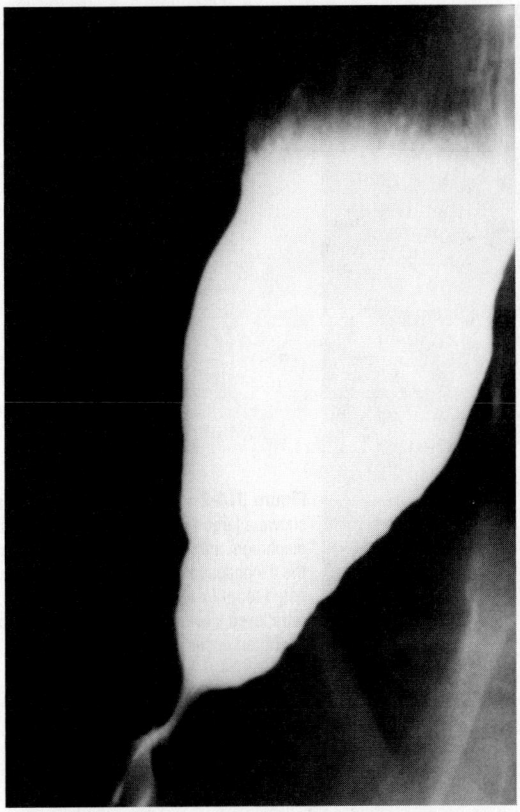

Figure 313-1 Barium esophagogram of a patient with achalasia demonstrating dilated esophagus and narrowing at the lower esophageal sphincter. Note retained secretions layered on top of barium in the esophagus.

present. **Manometry** is the most sensitive diagnostic test; it reveals the defining features of aperistalsis in the distal esophageal body and incomplete or absent LES relaxation, often accompanied by high pressure LES and low-amplitude esophageal body contractions.

The 2 most effective treatment options are pneumatic dilatation and surgical (Heller) myotomy. Pneumatic dilatation is the initial treatment of choice. Surgeons often supplement a myotomy with an antireflux procedure to prevent the gastroesophageal reflux disease that otherwise often ensues when the sphincter is rendered less competent. Calcium channel blockers (nifedipine) and phosphodiesterase inhibitors offer temporary relief of dysphagia. Endoscopic injection of the LES with **botulinum toxin** counterbalances the selective loss of inhibitory neurotransmitters by inhibiting the release of acetylcholine from nerve terminals and may be an effective therapy. Botulinum toxin is effective in 50-65% of patients and is expensive; half the patients might require a repeat injection within 1 yr. Most eventually require dilatation or surgery.

Diffuse esophageal spasm causes chest pain and dysphagia and affects adolescents and adults. It is diagnosed **manometrically** and can be treated with nitrates or calcium channel blocking agents.

Gastroesophageal reflux disease constitutes the most common cause of nonspecific abnormalities of esophageal motor function, probably through the effect of the esophageal inflammation on the musculature.

BIBLIOGRAPHY

Please visit the Nelson Textbook of Pediatrics *website at www.expertconsult.com for the complete bibliography.*

Chapter 314
Hiatal Hernia

Seema Khan and Susan R. Orenstein

Herniation of the stomach through the esophageal hiatus can occur as a common sliding hernia (type 1), in which the gastroesophageal junction slides into the thorax, or it can be paraesophageal (type 2), in which a portion of the stomach (usually the fundus) is insinuated next to the esophagus inside the gastroesophageal junction in the hiatus (Figs. 314-1 and 314-2). A combination of sliding and paraesophageal types (type 3) is present in some patients. Sliding hernias are often associated with gastroesophageal reflux, especially in developmentally delayed children. The relationship to hiatal hernias in adults is unclear. Medical treatment is not directed at the hernia but at the gastroesophageal reflux, unless failure of medical therapy prompts correction of the hernia at the time of fundoplication.

A paraesophageal hernia can be an isolated congenital anomaly or associated with gastric volvulus, or it may be encountered after fundoplication for gastroesophageal reflux, especially if the edges of a dilated esophageal diaphragmatic hiatus have not been approximated. Fullness after eating and upper abdominal pain are the usual symptoms. Infarction of the herniated stomach is rare.

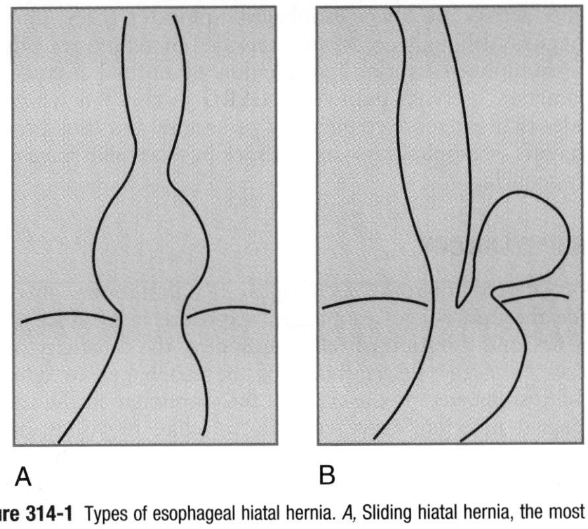

Figure 314-1 Types of esophageal hiatal hernia. *A,* Sliding hiatal hernia, the most common type. *B,* Paraesophageal hiatal hernia.

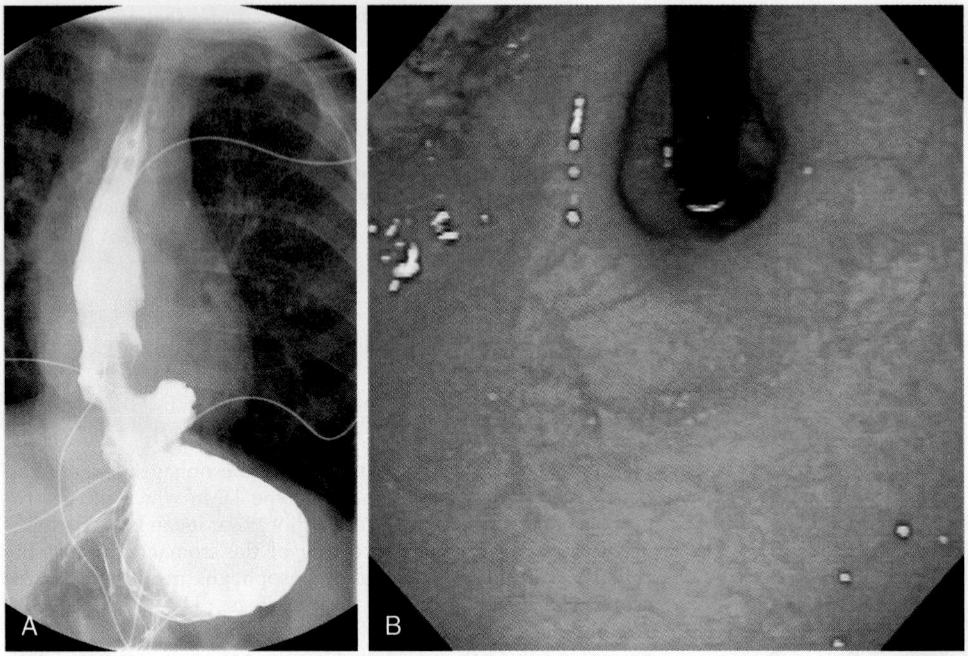

Figure 314-2 *A,* An upper gastrointestinal series shows a large hiatal hernia that extends above the diaphragm and impedes the exit of contrast from the esophagus into the stomach. Contrast is also noted to reflux to the upper esophagus. *B,* A retroflexed view of the hernia from the stomach during an upper endoscopy.

Chapter 315
Gastroesophageal Reflux Disease

Seema Khan and Susan R. Orenstein

Gastroesophageal reflux disease (GERD) is the most common esophageal disorder in children of all ages. Gastroesophageal reflux (GER) signifies the retrograde movement of gastric contents across the lower esophageal sphincter (LES) into the esophagus. Although occasional episodes of reflux are physiologic, exemplified by the regurgitation of normal infants, the phenomenon becomes **pathologic GERD** in children who have episodes that are more frequent or persistent, and thus produce esophagitis or esophageal symptoms, or in those who have respiratory sequelae.

PATHOPHYSIOLOGY

Factors determining the esophageal manifestations of reflux include the duration of esophageal exposure (a product of the frequency and duration of reflux episodes), the causticity of the refluxate, and the susceptibility of the esophagus to damage. The LES, supported by the crura of the diaphragm at the gastroesophageal junction, together with valvelike functions of the esophagogastric junction anatomy, form the antireflux barrier. In the context of even the normal intra-abdominal pressure augmentations that occur during daily life, the frequency of reflux episodes is increased by insufficient LES tone, by abnormal frequency of LES relaxations, and by hiatal herniation that prevents the LES pressure from being proportionately augmented by the crura during abdominal straining. Normal intra-abdominal pressure augmentations may be further exacerbated by straining or respiratory efforts. The duration of reflux episodes is increased by lack of swallowing (e.g., during sleep) and by defective esophageal peristalsis. Vicious cycles ensue because chronic esophagitis produces esophageal peristaltic dysfunction (low-amplitude waves, propagation disturbances), decreased LES tone, and inflammatory esophageal shortening that induces hiatal herniation, all worsening reflux.

Transient LES relaxation (TLESR) is the primary mechanism allowing reflux to occur. TLESRs occur independent of swallowing, reduce LES pressure to 0-2 mm Hg (above gastric), and last >10 sec; they appear by 26 wk of gestation. A vagovagal reflex, composed of afferent mechanoreceptors in the proximal stomach, a brainstem pattern generator, and efferents in the LES, regulates TLESRs. Gastric distention (postprandially, or due to abnormal gastric emptying or air swallowing) is the main stimulus for TLESRs. Whether GERD is caused by a higher frequency of TLESRs or by a greater incidence of reflux during TLESRs is debated; each is likely in different persons. Straining during a TLESR makes reflux more likely, as do positions that place the gastroesophageal junction below the air-fluid interface in the stomach. Other factors influencing gastric pressure-volume dynamics, such as increased movement, straining, obesity, large-volume or hyperosmolar meals, and increased respiratory effort (coughing, wheezing) can have the same effect.

EPIDEMIOLOGY AND NATURAL HISTORY

Infant reflux becomes evident in the 1st few months of life, peaks at ~4 mo, and resolves in up to 88% by 12 mo and nearly all by 24 mo. Symptoms in **older children** tend to be chronic, waxing and waning, but completely resolving in no more than half, which resembles adult patterns. The histologic findings of esophagitis have been shown to persist in infants who have naturally resolving symptoms of reflux. GERD likely has genetic predispositions: family clustering of GERD symptoms, endoscopic esophagitis, hiatal hernia, Barrett esophagus, and adenocarcinoma have been identified. As a continuously variable and common disorder, complex inheritance involving multiple genes and environmental factors is likely. Genetic linkage is indicated by the strong evidence of GERD in studies with monozygotic twins. A pediatric autosomal dominant form with otolaryngologic and respiratory manifestations has been located to chromosome 13q14, and the locus is termed GERD1.

CLINICAL MANIFESTATIONS

Most of the common clinical manifestations of esophageal disease can signify the presence of GERD. **Infantile reflux** manifests more often with regurgitation (especially postprandially), signs of esophagitis (irritability, arching, choking, gagging, feeding aversion), and resulting failure to thrive; symptoms resolve spontaneously in the majority by 12–24 mo. **Older children** can have regurgitation during the preschool years; complaints of abdominal and chest pain supervene in later childhood and adolescence. Occasional children present with neck contortions (arching, turning of head), designated **Sandifer syndrome.** The respiratory presentations are also age dependent: GERD in infants can manifest as obstructive apnea or as stridor or lower airway disease in which reflux complicates primary airway disease such as laryngomalacia or bronchopulmonary dysplasia. Otitis media, sinusitis, lymphoid hyperplasia, hoarseness, vocal cord nodules, and laryngeal edema have all been associated with GERD. Airway manifestations in older children are more commonly related to asthma or to otolaryngologic disease such as laryngitis or sinusitis. Despite the high prevalence of GERD symptoms in asthmatic children, data showing direction of causality are conflicting.

DIAGNOSIS

For most of the typical GERD presentations, particularly in older children, a thorough history and physical examination suffice initially to reach the diagnosis. This initial evaluation aims to identify the pertinent positives in support of GERD and its complications and the negatives that make other diagnoses unlikely. The history may be facilitated and standardized by questionnaires (e.g., the Infant Gastroesophageal Reflux Questionnaire, the I-GERQ, and its derivative, the I-GERQ-R), which also permit quantitative scores to be evaluated for their diagnostic discrimination and for evaluative assessment of improvement or worsening of symptoms. Important other diagnoses to consider in the evaluation of an infant or a child with chronic vomiting are milk and other food allergies, eosinophilic esophagitis, pyloric stenosis, intestinal obstruction (especially malrotation with intermittent volvulus), nonesophageal inflammatory diseases, infections, inborn errors of metabolism, hydronephrosis, increased intracranial pressure, rumination, and bulimia. Focused diagnostic testing, depending on the presentation and the differential diagnosis, can then supplement the initial examination.

Most of the esophageal tests are of some use in particular patients with suspected GERD. **Contrast (usually barium) radiographic** study of the esophagus and upper gastrointestinal tract is performed in children with vomiting and dysphagia to evaluate for achalasia, esophageal strictures and stenosis, hiatal hernia, and gastric outlet or intestinal obstruction (Fig. 315-1). It has poor sensitivity and specificity in the diagnosis of GERD due to its limited duration and the inability to differentiate physiologic GER from GERD.

Extended **esophageal pH monitoring** of the distal esophagus, no longer considered the sine qua non of a GERD diagnosis, provides a quantitative and sensitive documentation of acidic reflux episodes, the most important type of reflux episodes for pathologic reflux. The distal esophageal pH probe is placed at a level corresponding to 87% of the nares-LES distance, based on regression equations using the patient's height, on fluoroscopic visualization, or on manometric identification of the LES. Normal values of distal esophageal acid exposure (pH <4) are generally established as <5-8% of the total monitored time, but these quantitative normals are insufficient to establish or disprove a diagnosis of pathologic GERD. The most important indications for esophageal pH monitoring are for assessing efficacy of acid suppression during treatment, evaluating apneic episodes in conjunction with a pneumogram and perhaps impedance, and evaluating atypical GERD presentations such as chronic cough, stridor, and asthma. Dual pH probes, adding a proximal esophageal probe to the standard distal one, are used in the diagnosis of extraesophageal GERD, identifying upper esophageal acid exposure times of ~1% of the total time as threshold values for abnormality.

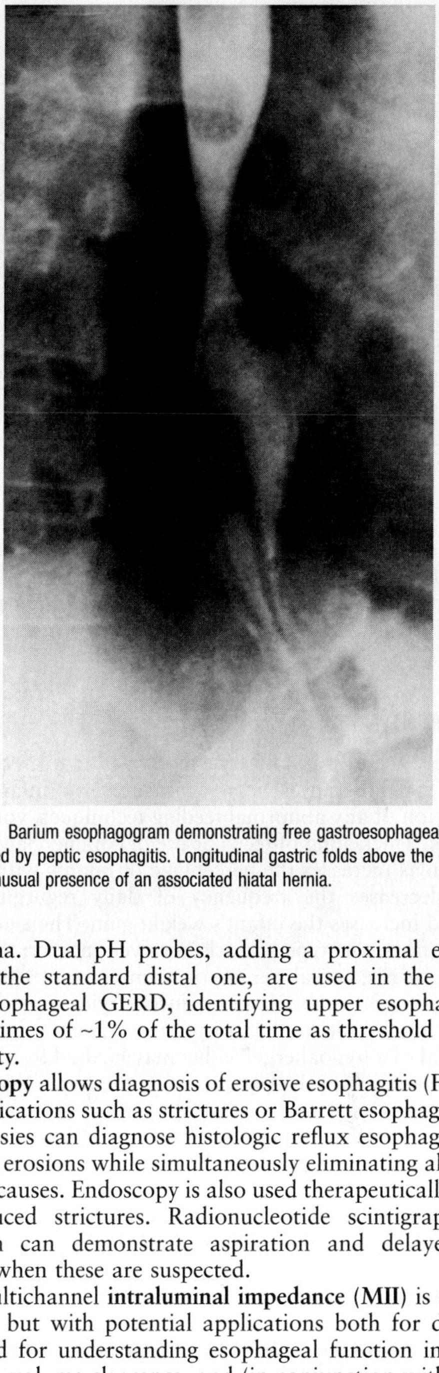

Figure 315-1 Barium esophagogram demonstrating free gastroesophageal reflux. Note stricture caused by peptic esophagitis. Longitudinal gastric folds above the diaphragm indicate the unusual presence of an associated hiatal hernia.

Endoscopy allows diagnosis of erosive esophagitis (Fig. 315-2) and complications such as strictures or Barrett esophagus; esophageal biopsies can diagnose histologic reflux esophagitis in the absence of erosions while simultaneously eliminating allergic and infectious causes. Endoscopy is also used therapeutically to dilate reflux-induced strictures. Radionucleotide scintigraphy using technetium can demonstrate aspiration and delayed gastric emptying when these are suspected.

The multichannel **intraluminal impedance (MII)** is a cumbersome test, but with potential applications both for diagnosing GERD and for understanding esophageal function in terms of bolus flow, volume clearance, and (in conjunction with manometry) motor patterns associated with GERD. Owing to the multiple sensors and a distal pH sensor, it is possible to document acidic reflux, weakly acidic reflux, and weakly alkaline reflux with MII. It is an important tool in those with respiratory symptoms particularly for the determination of nonacid reflux.

Laryngotracheobronchoscopy evaluates for visible airway signs that are associated with extraesophageal GERD, such as posterior laryngeal inflammation and vocal cord nodules; it can permit diagnosis of silent aspiration (during swallowing or during reflux) by bronchoalveolar lavage with subsequent quantification of lipid-laden macrophages in airway secretions. Detection of pepsin in tracheal fluid is a marker of reflux-associated aspiration of gastric contents. Esophageal manometry permits evaluation for dysmotility, particularly in preparation for antireflux surgery.

Empirical antireflux therapy, using a time-limited trial of high-dose proton pump inhibitor (PPI), is a cost-effective strategy for

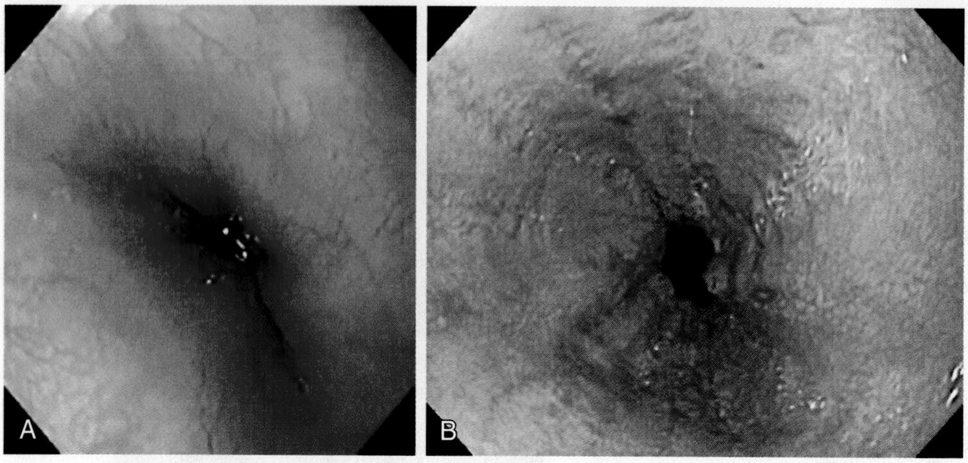

Figure 315-2 Endoscopic image of a normal esophagus *(A)* and erosive peptic esophagitis *(B)*.

diagnosis in adults; although not formally evaluated in older children, it has also been applied to this age group. Failure to respond to such empirical treatment, or a requirement for the treatment for prolonged periods, mandates formal diagnostic evaluation.

MANAGEMENT

Conservative therapy and lifestyle modification form the foundation of GERD therapy. Dietary measures for infants include normalization of any abnormal feeding techniques, volumes, and frequencies. Thickening of feeds or use of commercially prethickened formulas increases the percentage of infants with no regurgitation, decreases the frequency of daily regurgitation and emesis, and increases the infant's weight gain. The evidence does not clearly favor one type of thickener over another; the addition of a Tbsp of rice cereal per oz of formula results in a greater caloric density (30 kcal/oz), and reduced crying time, although it might not modify the number of nonregurgitant reflux episodes. A short trial of a hypoallergenic diet may be used to exclude milk or soy protein allergy before pharmacotherapy. Older children should be counseled to avoid acidic or reflux-inducing foods (tomatoes, chocolate, mint) and beverages (juices, carbonated and caffeinated drinks, alcohol). Weight reduction for obese patients and elimination of smoke exposure are other crucial measures at all ages.

Positioning measures are particularly important for infants, who cannot control their positions independently. Seated position worsens infant reflux and should be avoided in infants with GERD. Esophageal pH monitoring demonstrates more reflux episodes in infants in supine and side positions compared with the prone position, but evidence that the supine position reduces the risk of sudden infant death syndrome has led the American Academy of Pediatrics and the North American Society of Pediatric Gastroenterology and Nutrition to recommend supine positioning during sleep. When the infant is awake and observed, prone position and upright carried position can be used to minimize reflux. The efficacy of positioning for older children is unclear, but some evidence suggests a benefit to left side position and head elevation during sleep. The head should be elevated by elevating the head of the bed, rather than using excess pillows, to avoid abdominal flexion and compression that might worsen reflux.

Pharmacotherapy is directed at ameliorating the acidity of the gastric contents or at promoting their aboral movement. **Antacids** are the most commonly used antireflux therapy and are readily available over the counter. They provide rapid but transient relief of symptoms by acid neutralization. The long-term regular use of antacids cannot be recommended because of side effects of diarrhea (magnesium antacids) and constipation (aluminum antacids) and rare reports of more serious side effects of chronic use.

Histamine-2 receptor antagonists (H2RAs: cimetidine, famotidine, nizatidine, and ranitidine) are widely used antisecretory agents that act by selective inhibition of histamine receptors on gastric parietal cells. There is a definite benefit of H2RAs in treatment of mild-to-moderate reflux esophagitis. H2RAs have been recommended as first-line therapy because of their excellent overall safety profile, but they are being superseded by PPIs in this role, as increased experience with pediatric use and safety, US Food and Drug Administration (FDA) approval, and pediatric formulations and dosing are acquired.

PPIs (omeprazole, lansoprazole, pantoprazole, rabeprazole, and esomeprazole) provide the most potent antireflux effect by blocking the hydrogen-potassium ATPase channels of the final common pathway in gastric acid secretion. PPIs are superior to H2RAs in the treatment of severe and erosive esophagitis. Pharmacodynamic studies have indicated that children require higher doses of PPIs than adults on a per-weight basis. The use of PPIs to treat infants and children deemed to have GERD on the basis of symptoms has considerably increased in recent years. Controlled trials in infants with GERD diagnosed on the basis of symptoms alone have suggested an efficacy similar to placebo and have raised a safety concern.

Prokinetic agents available in the United States include metoclopramide (dopamine-2 and 5-HT_3 antagonist), bethanechol (cholinergic agonist), and erythromycin (motilin receptor agonist). Most of these increase LES pressure; some improve gastric emptying or esophageal clearance. None affects the frequency of TLESRs. The available controlled trials have not demonstrated much efficacy for GERD. In 2009, the FDA announced a black box warning for metoclopramide, linking its chronic use (>3 mo) with tardive dyskinesia, the rarely reversible movement disorder. Baclofen is a centrally acting γ-aminobutyric acid (GABA) agonist that has been shown to decrease reflux by decreasing TLESRs in healthy adults and in a small number of neurologically impaired children with GERD. New agents of great interest include peripherally acting GABA agonists devoid of central side effects, and metabotropic glutamate receptor 5 (mGluR5) antagonists that are reported to reduce TLESRs, but are as yet inadequately studied for this indication in children.

Surgery, usually **fundoplication**, is effective therapy for intractable GERD in children, particularly those with refractory esophagitis or strictures and those at risk for significant morbidity from chronic pulmonary disease. It may be combined with a gastrostomy for feeding or venting. The availability of potent acid-suppressing medication mandates more-rigorous analysis of the relative risks (or costs) and benefits of this relatively irreversible therapy in comparison to long-term pharmacotherapy. Some of the risks of fundoplication include a wrap that is "too tight" (producing dysphagia or gas-bloat) or "too loose" (and thus incompetent). Surgeons may choose to perform a "tight" (360°, Nissen) or variations of a "loose" (<360°, Thal, Toupet, Boix-Ochoa) wrap or to add a gastric drainage procedure (pyloroplasty) to improve gastric emptying, based on their experience and the patient's disease. Preoperative accuracy of diagnosis of GERD and the skill of the surgeon are 2 of the most important predictors of successful outcome. Long-term studies suggest that fundoplications often become incompetent in children, as in adults, with reflux recurrence rates of up to 14% for Nissen and up to 20% for loose wraps; this fact currently combines with the potency of PPI therapy that is now available to shift practice toward long-term pharmacotherapy in many cases. Fundoplication procedures may be performed as open operations, by laparoscopy, or by endoluminal (gastroplication) techniques. Pediatric experience is limited with endoscopic application of radiofrequency therapy (Stretta procedure) to a 2-3 cm area of the LES and cardia to create a high-pressure zone to reduce reflux.

BIBLIOGRAPHY

Please visit the Nelson Textbook of Pediatrics *website at www.expertconsult.com for the complete bibliography.*

315.1 Complications of Gastroesophageal Reflux Disease

Seema Khan and Susan R. Orenstein

ESOPHAGEAL: ESOPHAGITIS AND SEQUELAE—STRICTURE, BARRETT ESOPHAGUS, ADENOCARCINOMA

Esophagitis can manifest as irritability, arching, and feeding aversion in infants; chest or epigastric pain in older children; and, rarely, as hematemesis, anemia, or Sandifer syndrome at any age. Erosive esophagitis is found in approximately 12% of children with GERD symptoms and is more common in boys, older children, neurologically abnormal children, children with severe chronic respiratory disease, and in those with hiatal hernia. Prolonged and severe esophagitis leads to formation of strictures, generally located in the distal esophagus, producing dysphagia, and requiring repeated esophageal dilations and often fundoplication. Long-standing esophagitis predisposes to metaplastic transformation of the normal esophageal squamous epithelium into intestinal columnar epithelium, termed **Barrett esophagus,** a precursor of esophageal adenocarcinoma. Both Barrett esophagus and adenocarcinoma occur more in white males and in those with increased duration, frequency, and severity of reflux symptoms. This transformation increases with age to plateau in the 5th decade; adenocarcinoma is thus rare in childhood. Barrett esophagus, uncommon in children, warrants periodic surveillance biopsies, aggressive pharmacotherapy, and fundoplication for progressive lesions.

NUTRITIONAL

Esophagitis and regurgitation may be severe enough to induce failure to thrive because of caloric deficits. Enteral (nasogastric or nasojejunal, or percutaneous gastric or jejunal) or parenteral feedings are sometimes required to treat such deficits.

EXTRAESOPHAGEAL: RESPIRATORY ("ATYPICAL") PRESENTATIONS

GERD should be included in the differential diagnosis of children with unexplained or refractory otolaryngologic and respiratory complaints. GERD can produce respiratory symptoms by direct contact of the refluxed gastric contents with the respiratory tract (aspiration, laryngeal penetration, or microaspiration) or by reflexive interactions between the esophagus and respiratory tract (inducing laryngeal closure or bronchospasm). Often, GERD and a primary respiratory disorder, such as asthma, interact and a vicious cycle between them worsens both diseases. Many children with these extraesophageal presentations do not have typical GERD symptoms, making the diagnosis difficult. These atypical GERD presentations require a thoughtful approach to the differential diagnosis that considers a multitude of primary otolaryngologic (infections, allergies, postnasal drip, voice overuse) and pulmonary (asthma, cystic fibrosis) disorders. Therapy for the GERD must be more intense (usually incorporating a PPI) and prolonged (usually at least 3-6 mo). Subspecialist assistance from the perspective of the airway disease (otolaryngology, pulmonology) and the reflux disease (gastroenterology) is often warranted for specialized diagnostic testing and for optimizing intensive management.

APNEA AND STRIDOR

These upper airway presentations have been linked with GERD in case reports and epidemiologic studies; temporal relationships between them and reflux episodes have been demonstrated in some patients by esophageal pH-MII studies, and a beneficial response to therapy for GERD provides further support in a number of case series. An evaluation of 1,400 infants with apnea attributed the apnea to GERD in 50%, but other studies have failed to find an association. Apnea and apparent life-threatening event (ALTE) due to reflux is generally obstructive, owing to laryngospasm that may be conceived of as an abnormally intense protective reflex. At the time of such apnea, infants have often been provocatively positioned (supine or flexed seated), have been recently fed, and have shown signs of obstructive apnea, with unproductive respiratory efforts. Thus far, however, the evidence suggests that for the large majority of infants presenting with apnea and ALTE, GERD is not causal. Stridor triggered by reflux generally occurs in infants anatomically predisposed toward stridor (laryngomalacia, micrognathia). Spasmodic croup, an episodic frightening upper airway obstruction, can be an analogous condition in older children. Esophageal pH probe studies might fail to demonstrate linkage of these manifestations with reflux owing to the buffering of gastric contents by infant formula and the episodic nature of the conditions. Pneumograms can fail to identify apnea if they are not designed to identify obstructive apnea by measuring nasal airflow.

Reflux laryngitis and other otolaryngologic manifestations (also known as laryngopharyngeal reflux) can be attributed to GERD. **Hoarseness,** voice fatigue, throat clearing, chronic cough, pharyngitis, sinusitis, otitis media, and a sensation of globus have been cited. Laryngopharyngeal signs of GERD include edema and hyperemia (of the posterior surface), contact ulcers, granulomas, polyps, subglottic stenosis, and interarytenoid edema. The paucity of well-controlled evaluations of the association contributes to the skepticism with which these associations may be considered. Other risk factors irritating the upper respiratory passages can predispose some patients with GERD to present predominantly with these complaints.

Asthma co-occurs with GERD in ~50% of children with asthma, which contrasts to the prevalence of each condition independently in ~10% of children. Many studies have reported a strong association between asthma and reflux as determined by history, pH-MII, endoscopy, and esophageal histology. However, this association does not clarify the direction of causality in individual cases and thus does not indicate which patients with asthma are likely to benefit from anti-GERD therapy. Children with asthma who are particularly likely to have GERD as a provocative factor are those with symptoms of reflux disease, those with refractory or steroid-dependent asthma, and those with nocturnal worsening of asthma. Endoscopic evaluation that discloses esophageal sequelae of GERD provides an impetus to embark on the aggressive (high dose and many months' duration) therapy of GERD.

Dental erosions constitute the most common oral lesion of GERD, the lesions being distinguished by their location on the lingual surface of the teeth. The severity seems to correlate with the presence of reflux symptoms and the presence of an acidic milieu due to reflux in the proximal esophagus and oral cavity. The other common factors that can produce similar dental erosions are juice consumption and bulimia.

BIBLIOGRAPHY

Please visit the Nelson Textbook of Pediatrics *website at* *www.expertconsult.com* *for the complete bibliography.*

Chapter 316

Eosinophilic Esophagitis and Non-GERD Esophagitis

Seema Khan and Susan R. Orenstein

EOSINOPHILIC ESOPHAGITIS

The esophageal epithelium in eosinophilic esophagitis (EoE) is infiltrated by eosinophils, typically in a density exceeding 15 per high-power field (hpf). Presenting symptoms include vomiting, feeding problems, chest or epigastric pain, and dysphagia with occasional food impactions or strictures. Most patients are male. The mean age at diagnosis is 7 yr (range 1-17 yr), and the duration of symptoms is 3 yr. Most patients have other atopic diseases and associated food allergies; laboratory abnormalities can include peripheral eosinophilia and elevated immunoglobulin E (IgE) levels. Endoscopically, the esophagus presents a granular, furrowed, ringed, or exudative appearance (Fig. 316-1); esophageal histology reveals eosinophilia, with cut-points for diagnosis variably chosen at 15-20/hpf. Up to 30% children with EoE have grossly normal esophageal mucosa. EoE is differentiated from gastroesophageal reflux disease (GERD) by its general lack of erosive esophagitis, by its greater eosinophil density, and by its refractoriness to antireflux therapies. Gastroesophageal reflux disease may be an important coexisting diagnosis. Evaluation of EoE should include a thorough search for food and environmental allergies via skin prick (IgE mediated) and patch (non–IgE mediated) tests.

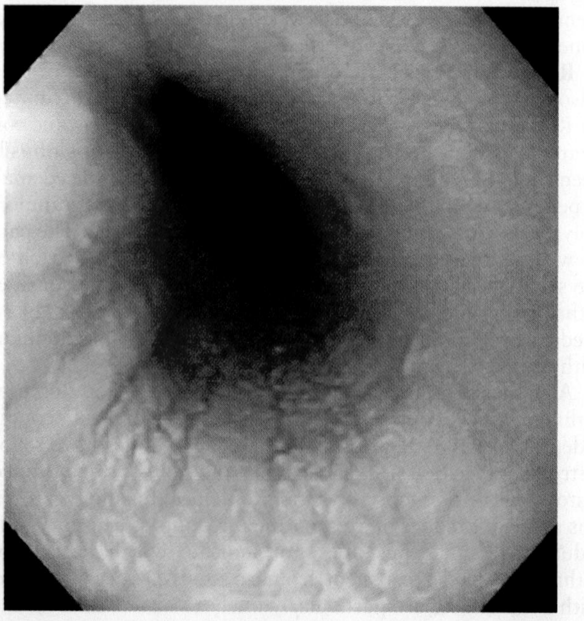

Figure 316-1 Endoscopic image of eosinophilic esophagitis with characteristic mucosal appearance of furrowing and white specks.

Treatment involves dietary restrictions that take one of 3 forms: elimination diets guided by circumstantial evidence and food allergy test results; "six food elimination diet" removing the major food allergens (milk, soy, wheat, egg, peanuts and tree nuts, seafood); and elemental diet composed exclusively of an amino acid–based formula. Successful clinical and histologic remission is observed in 70-98% patients. Topical and systemic corticosteroids have been used successfully for nonresponders and for nonallergic ("primary") EoE, with symptomatic and histologic remission rates reaching 90%. Therapies under investigation include anti–interleukin 5 (anti-IL-5) antibody (mepolizumab, reslizumab). Little is yet known about its natural history, but it seems that EoE is a chronic remitting and relapsing disorder with a potential for complications such as stricture formation.

INFECTIVE ESOPHAGITIS

Uncommon, and most often affecting immunocompromised children, infective esophagitis is caused by fungal agents, such as *Candida* and *Torulopsis glabrata;* viral agents, such as herpes simplex, cytomegalovirus, HIV, and varicella zoster; and, rarely, bacterial infections, including diphtheria and tuberculosis. The typical presenting signs and symptoms are odynophagia, dysphagia, and retrosternal pain; there may also be fever, nausea, and vomiting. Esophageal candidiasis manifests as concurrent oropharyngeal infection in 11% of patients, and it can affect immunocompetent and immunocompromised children. Esophageal viral infections can also manifest in immunocompetent hosts as an acute febrile illness. Infectious esophagitis, like other forms of esophageal inflammation, occasionally progresses to esophageal stricture. Diagnosis of infectious esophagitis is made by endoscopy (ulcerations, exudates) and histopathologic examination; adding polymerase chain reaction, tissue-viral culture, and immunocytochemistry enhances the diagnostic sensitivity and precision. Treatment is with appropriate antimicrobial agents, analgesics, and antacids.

"PILL" ESOPHAGITIS

This acute injury is produced by contact with a damaging agent. Medications implicated in "pill" esophagitis include tetracycline, potassium chloride, ferrous sulfate, nonsteroidal anti-inflammatory medications, and alendronate. Most often the offending tablet is ingested at bedtime with inadequate water. This practice often produces acute discomfort followed by progressive retrosternal pain, odynophagia, and dysphagia. Endoscopy shows a focal lesion often localized to one of the anatomic narrowed regions of the esophagus or to an unsuspected pathologic narrowing. Treatment is supportive; lacking much evidence, antacids, topical anesthetics, and bland or liquid diets are often used.

BIBLIOGRAPHY

Please visit the Nelson Textbook of Pediatrics *website at* *www.expertconsult.com* *for the complete bibliography.*

Chapter 317
Esophageal Perforation
Seema Khan and Susan R. Orenstein

The majority of esophageal perforations in children either are from blunt trauma (automobile injury, gunshot wounds, child abuse) or are iatrogenic. Cardiac massage, the Heimlich maneuver, nasogastric tube placement, traumatic laryngoscopy or endotracheal intubation, excessively vigorous postpartum suctioning of the airway during neonatal resuscitation, difficult upper endoscopy, sclerotherapy of esophageal varices, esophageal compression by a cuffed endotracheal tube, and pneumatic dilatation for therapy of achalasia have all been implicated. Esophageal rupture has followed forceful vomiting in patients with anorexia and has followed esophageal injury due to caustic ingestion, foreign body ingestion, food impactions, pill esophagitis, or eosinophilic esophagitis.

For the full continuation of this chapter, please visit the Nelson Textbook of Pediatrics *website at* *www.expertconsult.com*.

Chapter 318
Esophageal Varices
Seema Khan and Susan R. Orenstein

Portal hypertension is defined as an elevation of portal venous pressure to levels 10-12 mm Hg higher than pressures present in the inferior vena cava (Chapter 359). Decompression of this hypertension through portosystemic collateral circulation via the coronary vein, in conjunction with the left gastric veins, gives rise to esophageal varices. Most esophageal varices are "uphill varices"; less commonly, those that arise in the absence of portal hypertension and with superior vena cava (SVC) obstruction are "downhill varices." Their treatment is directed at the underlying cause of the SVC abnormality. Hemorrhage from esophageal varices is the major cause of morbidity and mortality due to portal hypertension. Presentation is with significant hematemesis and melena; whereas most patients have liver disease, some children with entities such as extrahepatic portal venous thrombosis might have been previously asymptomatic. Any child with hematemesis and splenomegaly should be presumed to have esophageal variceal bleeding until proved otherwise.

For the full continuation of this chapter, please visit the Nelson Textbook of Pediatrics *website at* *www.expertconsult.com*.

Chapter 319
Ingestions

319.1 Foreign Bodies in the Esophagus
Seema Khan and Susan R. Orenstein

The majority (80%) of foreign body ingestions occur in children, most of whom are between 6 mo and 3 yr of age. Youngsters with developmental delays and those with psychiatric disorders are also at increased risk. Coins and small toy items are the most commonly ingested foreign bodies. Food impactions are less common in children than in adults and usually occur in children with an underlying structural anomaly or motility disorder, such as repair of esophageal atresia or eosinophilic esophagitis. Most esophageal foreign bodies lodge at the level of the cricopharyngeus (upper esophageal sphincter [UES]), the aortic arch, or just superior to the diaphragm at the gastroesophageal junction (lower esophageal sphincter [LES]).

At least 30% of children with esophageal foreign bodies may be totally asymptomatic, so any history of foreign body ingestion should be taken seriously and investigated. An initial bout of choking, gagging, and coughing may be followed by excessive salivation, dysphagia, food refusal, emesis, or pain in the neck, throat, or sternal notch regions. Respiratory symptoms such as stridor, wheezing, cyanosis, or dyspnea may be encountered if the esophageal foreign body impinges on the larynx or membranous posterior tracheal wall. Cervical swelling, erythema, or subcutaneous crepitations suggest perforation of the oropharynx or proximal esophagus.

Evaluation of the child with a history of foreign body ingestion starts with plain anteroposterior (AP) radiographs of the neck, chest, and abdomen, along with lateral views of the neck and chest. The flat surface of a coin in the esophagus is seen on the AP view and the edge on the lateral view (Fig. 319-1). The reverse is true for coins lodged in the trachea; here, the edge is seen anteroposteriorly and the flat side is seen laterally. Disk batteries can look like coins (Fig. 319-2) and have a much higher risk of burns and necrosis (Fig. 319-3). Materials such as plastic, wood, glass, aluminum, and bones may be radiolucent; failure to visualize the object with plain films in a symptomatic patient warrants urgent endoscopy. Although barium contrast studies may be helpful in the occasional asymptomatic patient with negative plain films, their use is to be discouraged because of the potential of aspiration as well as making subsequent visualization and object removal more difficult.

Treatment of esophageal foreign bodies usually merits endoscopic visualization of the object and underlying mucosa and removal of the object; therapeutic endoscopy is most conservatively done with an endotracheal tube protecting the airway. Sharp objects in the esophagus, disk button batteries, or foreign bodies associated with respiratory symptoms mandate urgent removal. Button batteries, in particular, must be expediently removed because they can induce mucosal injury in as little as 1 hr of contact time and involve all esophageal layers within 4 hr (see Fig. 319-3). Asymptomatic blunt objects and coins lodged in the esophagus can be observed for up to 24 hr in anticipation of passage into the stomach. If there are no problems in handling secretions, meat impactions can be observed for up to 12 hr. In patients without prior esophageal surgeries, glucagon (0.05 mg/kg IV) can sometimes be useful in facilitating passage of distal esophageal food boluses by decreasing the LES pressure. The use of meat tenderizers or gas-forming agents can lead to perforation and are not recommended. An alternative technique for removing esophageal coins impacted for <24 hr, performed most safely by experienced radiology personnel, consists of passage of a Foley catheter beyond the coin at fluoroscopy, inflating the balloon, and then pulling the catheter and coin back simultaneously with the patient in a prone oblique position. Concerns about the lack of direct mucosal visualization and, when tracheal intubation is not used, the lack of airway protection prompt caution in the use of this technique. Bougienage of esophageal coins toward the stomach in selected uncomplicated pediatric cases has been suggested to be an effective, safe, and economical modality where endoscopy might not be routinely available.

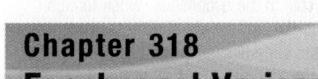

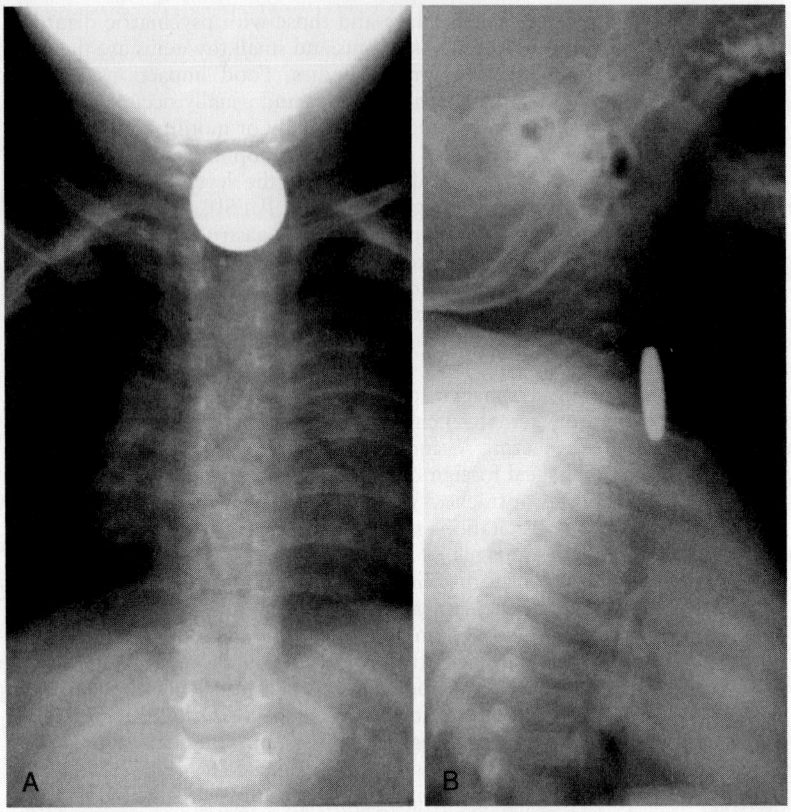

Figure 319-1 Radiographs of a coin in the esophagus. When foreign bodies lodge in the esophagus, the flat surface of the object is seen in the anteroposterior view *(A)* and the edge is seen in the lateral view *(B)*. The reverse is true for objects in the trachea. (Courtesy of Beverley Newman, MD.)

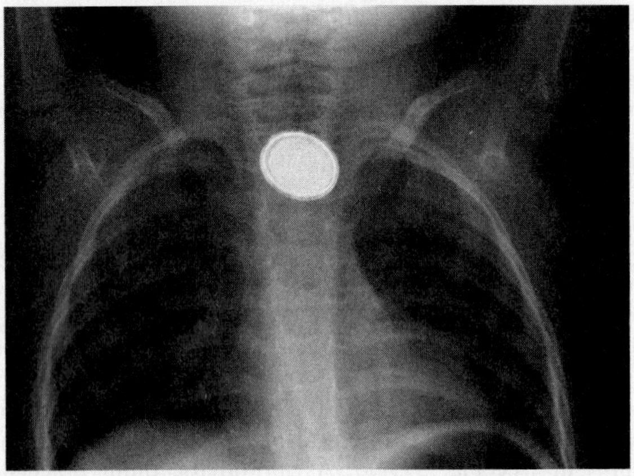

Figure 319-2 Disk battery impacted in esophagus. Note the double rim. (From Wyllie R, Hyams JS, editors: *Pediatric gastrointestinal and liver disease,* ed 3, Philadelphia, 2006, Saunders.)

BIBLIOGRAPHY

Please visit the Nelson Textbook of Pediatrics *website at* *www.expertconsult.com* *for the complete bibliography.*

319.2 Caustic Ingestions

Seema Khan and Susan R. Orenstein

Ingestion of caustic substances can result in esophagitis, necrosis, perforation, and stricture formation (Chapter 58). Most cases (70%) are accidental ingestions of liquid alkali substances that produce severe, deep liquefaction necrosis; drain decloggers are most common, and because they are tasteless, more is ingested (Table 319-1). **Acidic agents** (20% of cases) are bitter, so less may be consumed; they produce coagulation necrosis and a

Table 319-1 INGESTIBLE CAUSTIC MATERIALS AROUND THE HOUSE

CATEGORY	MOST DAMAGING AGENTS	OTHER AGENTS
Alkaline drain cleaners, milking machine pipe cleaners	Sodium or potassium hydroxide	Ammonia Sodium hypochlorite Aluminum particles
Acidic drain openers	Hydrochloric acid Sulfuric acid	
Toilet cleaners	Hydrochloric acid Sulfuric acid Phosphoric acid Other acids	Ammonium chloride Sodium hypochlorite
Oven and grill cleaners	Sodium hydroxide Perborate (borax)	
Denture cleaners	Persulfate (sulfur) Hypochlorite (bleach)	
Dishwasher detergent • Liquid • Powdered	Sodium hydroxide Sodium hypochlorite Sodium carbonate	
Bleach	Sodium hypochlorite	Ammonia salt
Swimming pool chemicals	Acids, alkalis, chlorine	
Battery acid (liquid)	Sulfuric acid	
Disk batteries	Electric current	Zinc or other metal salts
Rust remover	Hydrofluoric, phosphoric, oxalic, and other acids	
Household de-limers	Phosphoric acid Hydroxyacetic acid Hydrochloric acid	
Barbeque cleaners	Sodium and potassium hydroxide	
Glyphosate surfactant (RoundUp) acid	Glyphosate herbicide	Surfactants

Source: National Library of Medicine: *Health and safety information on household products* (website). http://householdproducts.nlm.nih.gov/. Accessed April 28, 2010.
From Wyllie R, Hyams JS, editors: *Pediatric gastrointestinal and liver disease,* ed 3, Philadelphia, 2006, Saunders.

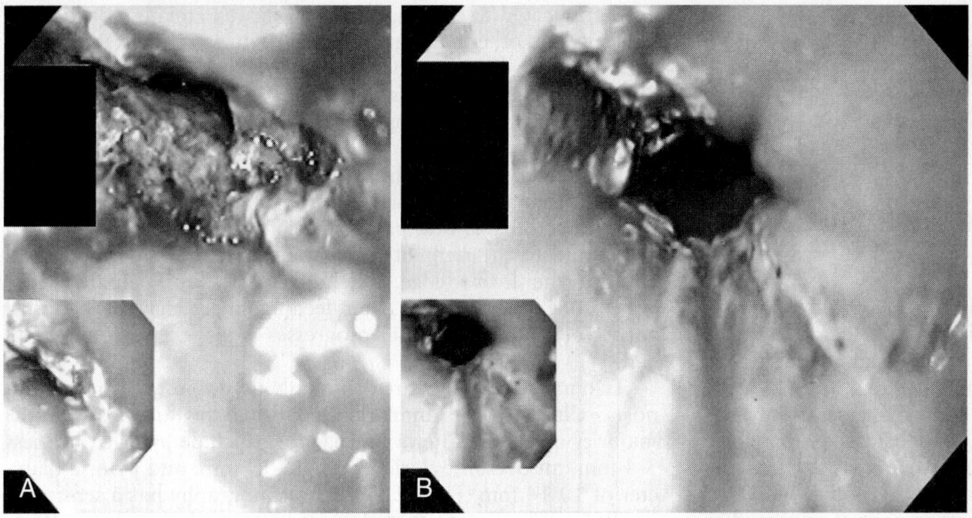

Figure 319-3 *A,* Disk battery in esophagus with necrotic debris at burn sites. *B,* Typical bilateral esophageal burn after removal of disk battery. (From Wyllie R, Hyams JS, editors: *Pediatric gastrointestinal and liver disease,* ed 3, Philadelphia, 2006, Saunders.)

somewhat protective thick eschar. They can produce severe gastritis, and volatile acids can result in respiratory symptoms. Children <5 yr of age account for half of the cases of caustic ingestions, and boys are far more commonly involved than girls.

Caustic ingestions produce signs and symptoms such as vomiting, drooling, refusal to drink, oral burns, dysphagia, dyspnea, abdominal pain, hematemesis, and stridor. Twenty percent of patients develop esophageal strictures. Absence of oropharyngeal lesions does not exclude the possibility of significant esophagogastric injury, which can lead to perforation or stricture. The absence of symptoms is usually associated with no or minimal lesions; hematemesis, respiratory distress, or presence of at least 3 symptoms predicts severe lesions. An upper endoscopy is recommended as the most efficient means of rapid identification of tissue damage and must be undertaken in all symptomatic children.

Dilution by water or milk is recommended as acute treatment, but neutralization, induced emesis, and gastric lavage are contraindicated. Treatment depends on the severity and extent of damage (Table 319-2). Stricture risk is increased by circumferential ulcerations, white plaques, and sloughing of the mucosa. Strictures can require treatment with dilation, and in some severe cases, surgical resection and colon or small bowel interposition are needed. Silicone stents (self-expanding) placed endoscopically after a dilatation procedure can be an alternative and conservative approach to the management of strictures. Rare late cases of superimposed esophageal carcinoma are reported. The role of corticosteroids is controversial; they are not recommended in 1st-degree burns, but they can reduce the risk of strictures in more-advanced caustic esophagitis. Some centers also use antibiotics in the initial treatment of caustic esophagitis on the premise that reducing superinfection in the necrotic tissue bed will in turn lower the risk of stricture formation. However, multiple studies examining the role of antibiotics in caustic esophagitis have not reported a clinically significant benefit even in those with grade 2 or greater severity of esophagitis.

Table 319-2 SEVERITY OF ESOPHAGEAL INJURY FOLLOWING CAUSTIC INGESTION AS GRADED BY ENDOSCOPIC APPEARANCE OF THE ESOPHAGUS

SEVERITY	ENDOSCOPIC APPEARANCE OF ESOPHAGEAL MUCOSA
Grade 0	Normal mucosa
Grade 1	Erythema
Grade 2	Erythema, sloughing, ulceration, and exudates (not circumferential)
Grade 3	Deep mucosal sloughing and ulceration (circumferential)
Grade 4	Eschar, full thickness injury and perforation

BIBLIOGRAPHY

Please visit the Nelson Textbook of Pediatrics *website at www.expertconsult.com for the complete bibliography.*

Section 4 STOMACH AND INTESTINES

Chapter 320
Normal Development, Structure, and Function

Chris A. Liacouras

DEVELOPMENT

The primitive gut is recognizable by the 4th wk of gestation and is composed of the foregut, midgut, and hindgut. The **foregut** gives rise to the upper gastrointestinal (GI) tract including the esophagus, stomach, and duodenum to the level of the insertion of the common bile duct. The **midgut** gives rise to the rest of the small bowel and the large bowel to the level of the mid-transverse colon. The **hindgut** forms the remainder of the colon and upper anal canal. The rapid growth of the midgut causes it to protrude out of the abdominal cavity through the umbilical ring during fetal development. The midgut subsequently returns to the peritoneal cavity and rotates counterclockwise until the cecum lies in the right lower quadrant. The process is normally complete by the 8th wk of gestation.

For the full continuation of this chapter, please visit the Nelson Textbook of Pediatrics *website at www.expertconsult.com.*

Chapter 321
Pyloric Stenosis and Other Congenital Anomalies of the Stomach

321.1 Hypertrophic Pyloric Stenosis

Anna Klaudia Hunter and Chris A. Liacouras

Hypertrophic pyloric stenosis occurs in 1-3/1,000 infants in the United States. It is more common in whites of northern European ancestry, less common in blacks, and rare in Asians. Males (especially first-borns) are affected approximately 4 to 6 times as often as females. The offspring of a mother and, to a lesser extent, the father who had pyloric stenosis are at higher risk for pyloric stenosis. Pyloric stenosis develops in approximately 20% of the male and 10% of the female descendants of a mother who had pyloric stenosis. The incidence of pyloric stenosis is increased in infants with B and O blood groups. Pyloric stenosis is occasionally associated with other congenital defects, including tracheoesophageal fistula and hypoplasia or agenesis of the inferior labial frenulum.

ETIOLOGY

The cause of pyloric stenosis is unknown, but many factors have been implicated. Pyloric stenosis is usually not present at birth and is more concordant in monozygotic than dizygotic twins. It is unusual in stillbirths and probably develops after birth. Pyloric stenosis has been associated with eosinophilic gastroenteritis, Apert syndrome, Zellweger syndrome, trisomy 18, Smith-Lemli-Opitz syndrome, and Cornelia de Lange syndrome. An association has been found with the use of erythromycin in neonates with highest risk if the medication is given within the 1st 2 wk of life. There have also been reports of higher incidence of pyloric stenosis among mostly female infants of mothers treated with macrolide antibiotics during pregnancy and breastfeeding. Abnormal muscle innervation, elevated serum levels of prostaglandins, and infant hypergastrinemia has been implicated. Reduced levels of neuronal nitric oxide synthase (nNOS) have been found with altered expression of the nNOS exon 1c regulatory region, which influences the expression of the nNOS gene. Reduced nitric oxide might contribute to the pathogenesis of pyloric stenosis.

CLINICAL MANIFESTATIONS

Nonbilious vomiting is the initial symptom of pyloric stenosis. The vomiting may or may not be projectile initially but is usually progressive, occurring immediately after a feeding. Emesis might follow each feeding, or it may be intermittent. The vomiting usually starts after 3 wk of age, but symptoms can develop as early as the 1st wk of life and as late as the 5th mo. About 20% have intermittent emesis from birth that then progresses to the classic picture. After vomiting, the infant is hungry and wants to feed again. As vomiting continues, a progressive loss of fluid, hydrogen ion, and chloride leads to hypochloremic metabolic alkalosis. Greater awareness of pyloric stenosis has led to earlier identification of patients with fewer instances of chronic malnutrition and severe dehydration and at times a subclinical self-resolving hypertrophy.

Hyperbilirubinemia is the most common clinical association of pyloric stenosis, also known as *icteropyloric syndrome.* Unconjugated hyperbilirubinemia is more common than conjugated and usually resolves with surgical correction. It may be associated with a decreased level of glucuronyl transferase as seen in ~5% of affected infants; mutations in the bilirubin uridine diphosphate glucuronosyl transferase gene *(UGT1A1)* have also been implicated. If conjugated hyperbilirubinemia is a part of the presentation, other etiologies need to be investigated. Other coexistent clinical diagnoses have been described, including eosinophilic gastroenteritis, hiatal hernia, peptic ulcer, congenital nephrotic syndrome, congenital heart disease, and congenital hypothyroidism.

The diagnosis has traditionally been established by palpating the pyloric mass. The mass is firm, movable, ~2 cm in length, olive shaped, hard, best palpated from the left side, and located above and to the right of the umbilicus in the mid-epigastrium beneath the liver's edge. The olive is easiest palpated after an episode of vomiting. After feeding, there may be a visible gastric peristaltic wave that progresses across the abdomen (Fig. 321-1).

Two imaging studies are commonly used to establish the diagnosis. Ultrasound examination confirms the diagnosis in the majority of cases. Criteria for diagnosis include pyloric thickness 3-4 mm, an overall pyloric length 15-19 mm, and pyloric diameter of 10-14 mm (Fig. 321-2). Ultrasonography has a sensitivity of ~95%. When contrast studies are performed, they demonstrate an elongated pyloric channel (string sign), a bulge of the pyloric muscle into the antrum (shoulder sign), and parallel streaks of barium seen in the narrowed channel, producing a "double tract sign" (Fig. 321-3).

DIFFERENTIAL DIAGNOSIS

Gastric waves are occasionally visible in small, emaciated infants who do not have pyloric stenosis. Infrequently, gastroesophageal reflux, with or without a hiatal hernia, may be confused with pyloric stenosis. Gastroesophageal reflux disease can be differentiated from pyloric stenosis by radiographic studies. Adrenal insufficiency from the adrenogenital syndrome can simulate pyloric stenosis, but the absence of a metabolic acidosis and elevated serum potassium and urinary sodium concentrations of adrenal insufficiency aid in differentiation (Chapter 570). Inborn errors of metabolism can produce recurrent emesis with alkalosis (urea cycle) or acidosis (organic acidemia) and lethargy, coma, or seizures. Vomiting with diarrhea suggests gastroenteritis, but patients with pyloric stenosis occasionally have diarrhea. Rarely, a pyloric membrane or pyloric duplication results in projectile vomiting, visible peristalsis, and, in the case of a duplication, a palpable mass. Duodenal stenosis proximal to the ampulla of Vater results in the clinical features of pyloric stenosis but can be differentiated by the presence of a pyloric mass on physical examination or ultrasonography.

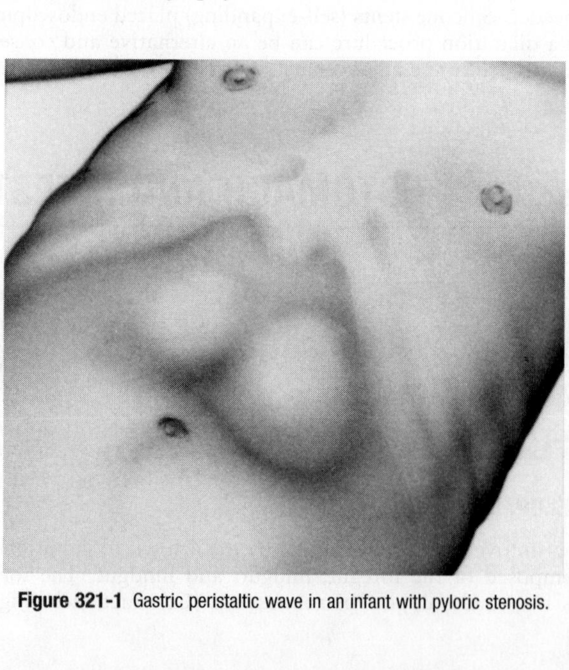

Figure 321-1 Gastric peristaltic wave in an infant with pyloric stenosis.

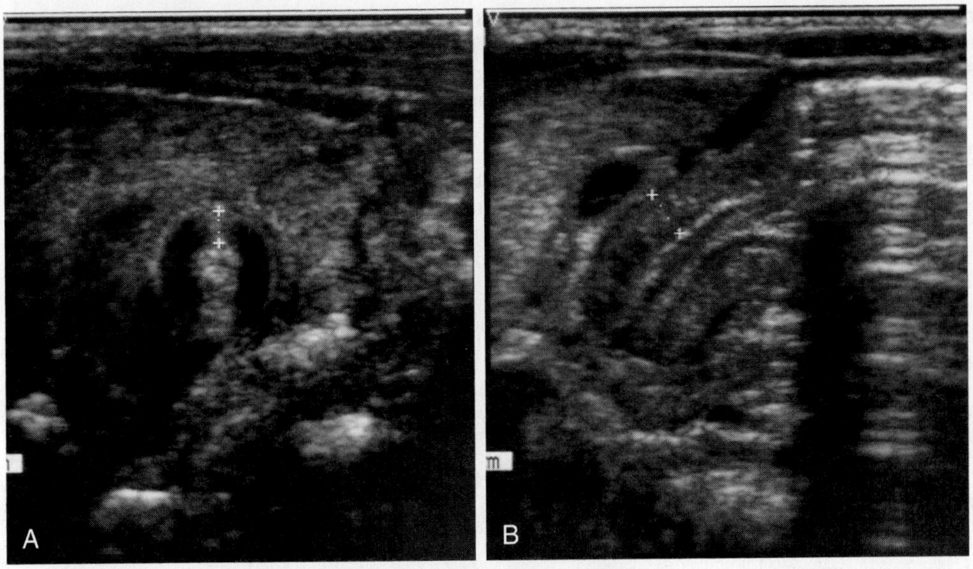

Figure 321-2 *A,* Transverse sonogram demonstrating a pyloric muscle wall thickness of >4 mm (distance between *crosses*). *B,* Horizontal image demonstrating a pyloric channel length >14 mm (wall thickness outlined between *crosses*) in an infant with pyloric stenosis.

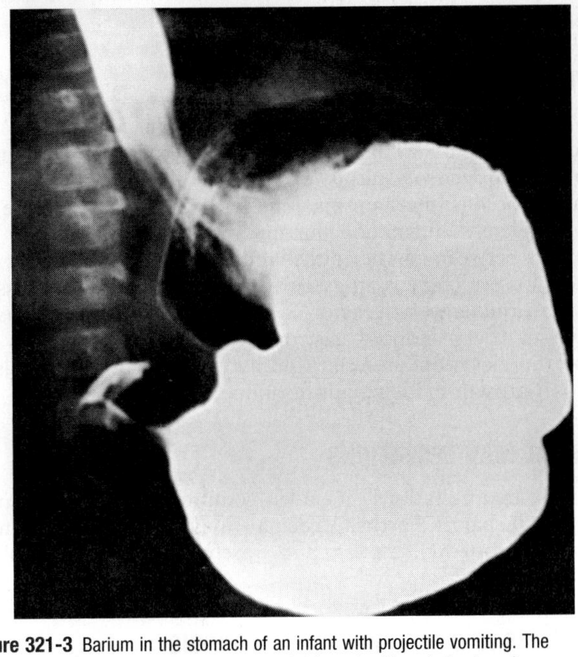

Figure 321-3 Barium in the stomach of an infant with projectile vomiting. The attenuated pyloric canal is typical of congenital hypertrophic pyloric stenosis.

TREATMENT

The preoperative treatment is directed toward correcting the fluid, acid-base, and electrolyte losses. Correction of the alkalosis is essential to prevent postoperative apnea, which may be associated with anesthesia. Most infants can be successfully rehydrated within 24 hr. Vomiting usually stops when the stomach is empty, and only an occasional infant requires nasogastric suction.

The **surgical procedure of choice** is pyloromyotomy. The traditional Ramstedt procedure is performed through a short transverse skin incision. The underlying pyloric mass is cut longitudinally to the layer of the submucosa, and the incision is closed. Laparoscopic technique is equally successful and in one study resulted in a shorter time to full feedings and discharge from the hospital as well as greater parental satisfaction. The success of laparoscopy depends on the skill of the surgeon. Postoperative vomiting occurs in half the infants and is thought to be secondary to edema of the pylorus at the incision site. In most infants, however, feedings can be initiated within 12-24 hr after surgery and advanced to maintenance oral feedings within 36-48 hr after surgery. Persistent vomiting suggests an incomplete pyloromyotomy, gastritis, gastroesophageal reflux disease, or another cause of the obstruction. The surgical treatment of pyloric stenosis is curative, with an operative mortality of 0-0.5%. Endoscopic balloon dilatation has been successful in infants with persistent vomiting secondary to incomplete pyloromyotomy.

Conservative management with nasodudodenal feedings is advisable in patients who are not good surgical candidates. Oral and intravenous atropine sulfate (pyloric muscle relaxant) has also been described when surgical treatment is not available.

BIBLIOGRAPHY

Please visit the Nelson Textbook of Pediatrics *website at* *www.expertconsult.com* *for the complete bibliography.*

321.2 Congenital Gastric Outlet Obstruction

Chris A. Liacouras

Gastric outlet obstruction resulting from pyloric atresia and antral webs is uncommon and accounts for <1% of all the atresias and diaphragms of the alimentary tract. The cause of the defects is unknown. Pyloric atresia has been associated with **epidermolysis bullosa** and usually presents in early infancy. The gender distribution is equal.

CLINICAL MANIFESTATIONS

Infants with pyloric atresia present with nonbilious vomiting, feeding difficulties, and abdominal distention during the 1st day of life. **Polyhydramnios** occurs in the majority of cases, and low birthweight is common. The gastric aspirate at birth is large (>20 mL fluid) and should be removed to prevent aspiration. Rupture of the stomach may occur as early as the 1st 12 hr of life. Infants with antral web may present with less dramatic symptoms, depending on the degree of obstruction. Older children with antral webs present with nausea, vomiting, abdominal pain, and weight loss.

DIAGNOSIS

The diagnosis of congenital gastric outlet obstruction is suggested by the finding of a large, dilated stomach on abdominal plain radiographs or in utero ultrasonography. Upper gastrointestinal (GI) contrast series is usually diagnostic and demonstrates a pyloric dimple. When contrast studies are performed, care must be taken to avoid possible aspiration. An antral web may appear as a thin septum near the pyloric channel. In older children, endoscopy has been helpful in identifying antral webs.

TREATMENT

The treatment of all causes of gastric outlet obstruction in neonates starts with the correction of dehydration and hypochloremic alkalosis. Persistent vomiting should be relieved with nasogastric decompression. Surgical or endoscopic repair should be undertaken when a patient is stable.

321.3 Gastric Duplication

Anna Klaudia Hunter and Chris A. Liacouras

Gastric duplications are uncommon cystic or tubular structures that usually occur within the wall of the stomach. They account for 2-7% of all GI duplications. They are most commonly located on the greater curvature. Most are <12 cm in diameter and do not usually communicate with the stomach lumen; however, they do have common blood supply. Associated anomalies occur in as many as 35% of patients. Several hypotheses for the etiology of the duplication cysts have been developed including the splitting notochord theory, diverticulization, canalization defects, and caudal twinning.

The most common clinical manifestations are associated with partial or complete gastric outlet obstruction. In 33% of patients, the cyst may be palpable. Communicating duplications can cause gastric ulceration and be associated with hematemesis or melena.

Radiographic studies usually show a paragastric mass displacing stomach. Ultrasound can show the inner hyperechoic mucosal and outer hypoechoic muscle layers that are typical of GI duplications. Surgical excision is the treatment for symptomatic gastric duplications.

BIBLIOGRAPHY

Please visit the Nelson Textbook of Pediatrics *website at www.expertconsult.com for the complete bibliography.*

321.4 Gastric Volvulus

Anna Klaudia Hunter and Chris A. Liacouras

The stomach is tethered longitudinally by the gastrohepatic, gastrosplenic, and gastrocolic ligaments. In the transverse axis, it is tethered by the gastrophrenic ligament and the retroperitoneal attachment of the duodenum. A volvulus occurs when 1 of these attachments is absent or elongated, allowing the stomach to rotate around itself. In some children, other associated defects are present, including intestinal malrotation, diaphragmatic defects, hiatal hernia, or adjacent organ abnormalities such as asplenia. Volvulus can occur along the longitudinal axis, producing organoaxial volvulus, or along the transverse axis, producing mesenteroaxial volvulus. Combined volvulus occurs if the stomach rotates around both organoaxial and mesenteroaxial axes.

The clinical presentation of gastric volvulus is nonspecific and suggests high intestinal obstruction. Gastric volvulus in infancy is usually associated with nonbilious vomiting and epigastric distention. It has also been associated with episodes of dyspnea and apnea in this age group. Acute volvulus can advance rapidly to strangulation and perforation. Chronic gastric volvulus is more common in older children; the children present with a history of emesis, abdominal pain and distention, early satiety, and failure to thrive.

The diagnosis is suggested in plain abdominal radiographs by the presence of a dilated stomach. Erect abdominal films demonstrate a double fluid level with a characteristic "beak" near the lower esophageal junction in mesenteroaxial volvulus. The stomach tends to lie in a vertical plane. In organoaxial volvulus, a single air-fluid level is seen without the characteristic beak with stomach lying in a horizontal plane. Upper GI series has also been used to aid the diagnosis.

Treatment of acute gastric volvulus is emergent surgery once a patient is stabilized. Laparoscopic gastropexy is the most common surgical approach. In selected cases of chronic volvulus in older patients, endoscopic correction has been successful.

BIBLIOGRAPHY

Please visit the Nelson Textbook of Pediatrics *website at www.expertconsult.com for the complete bibliography.*

321.5 Hypertrophic Gastropathy

Anna Klaudia Hunter and Chris A. Liacouras

Hypertrophic gastropathy in children is uncommon and, in contrast to that in adults (Ménétrier disease), is usually a transient, benign, and self-limited condition.

PATHOGENESIS

The condition is most often secondary to cytomegalovirus (CMV) infection, but other agents, including herpes simplex virus, *Giardia,* and *Helicobacter pylori* have also been implicated. The pathophysiologic mechanisms underlying the clinical picture are not completely understood but might involve widening of gap junctions between gastric epithelial cells with resultant fluid and protein losses. There is an association with increased expression of transforming growth factor (TGF)-α in gastric mucosal tissue shown in CMV induced gastropathy. *H. pylori* infection can cause the elevation of serum glucagon-like peptide-2 levels, a mucosal growth-inducing gut hormone.

CLINICAL MANIFESTATIONS

Clinical manifestations include vomiting, anorexia, upper abdominal pain, diarrhea, edema (hypoproteinemic protein-losing enteropathy), ascites, and, rarely, hematemesis if ulceration occurs.

DIAGNOSIS AND DIFFERENTIAL DIAGNOSIS

The mean age at diagnosis is 5 yr (range, 2 days-17 yr); the illness usually lasts 2-14 wk, with complete resolution being the rule. Endoscopy with biopsy and tissue CMV polymerase chain reaction (PCR) is diagnostic. The upper GI series might show thickened gastric folds. The differential diagnosis includes eosinophilic gastroenteritis, gastric lymphoma or carcinoma, Crohn disease, and inflammatory pseudotumor.

TREATMENT

Therapy is supportive and should include adequate hydration, H_2 receptor blockade, and albumin replacement if the hypoalbuminemia is symptomatic. When *H. pylori* are detected, appropriate treatment is recommended. Ganciclovir in CMV-positive gastropathy is indicated only in severe cases. Complete recovery is the rule. This is not a chronic condition in children. Disease tends to have much more severe course in adult patients.

BIBLIOGRAPHY

Please visit the Nelson Textbook of Pediatrics *website at www.expertconsult.com for the complete bibliography.*

Chapter 322
Intestinal Atresia, Stenosis, and Malrotation

Christina Bales and Chris A. Liacouras

Approximately 1 in 1,500 children is born with intestinal obstruction. Obstruction may be partial or complete, and it may be characterized as simple or strangulating. Luminal contents fails to progress in an aboral direction in simple obstruction, whereas blood flow to the intestine is also impaired in strangulating obstruction. If strangulating obstruction is not promptly relieved, it can lead to bowel infarction and perforation.

Intestinal obstruction can be further classified as either intrinsic or extrinsic based on underlying etiology. Intrinsic causes include inherent abnormalities of intestinal innervation, mucus production, or tubular anatomy. Among these, congenital disruption of the tubular structure is most common and can manifest as obliteration (atresia) or narrowing (stenosis) of the intestinal lumen. More than 90% of intestinal stenosis and atresia occurs in the duodenum, jejeunum, and ileum. Rare cases occur in the colon, and these may be associated with more proximal atresias.

Extrinsic causes of congenital intestinal obstruction involve compression of the bowel by vessels (e.g., preduodenal portal vein), organs (e.g., annular pancreas), and cysts (e.g. duplication, mesenteric). Abnormalities in intestinal rotation during fetal development also represent a unique extrinsic cause of congenital intestinal obstruction. Malrotation is associated with inadequate mesenteric attachment of the intestine to the posterior abdominal wall, which leaves the bowel vulnerable to auto-obstruction due to intestinal twisting or volvulus. Malrotation is commonly accompanied by congenital adhesions that can compress and obstruct the duodenum as they extend from the cecum to the right upper quadrant.

Obstruction is typically associated with bowel distention, which is caused by an accumulation of ingested food, gas, and intestinal secretions proximal to the point of obstruction. As the bowel dilates, absorption of intestinal fluid is decreased and secretion of fluid and electrolytes is increased. This shift results in isotonic intravascular depletion, which is usually associated with hypokalemia. Bowel distention also results in a decrease in blood flow to the obstructed bowel. As blood flow is shifted away from the intestinal mucosa, there is loss of mucosal integrity. Bacteria proliferate in the stagnant bowel, with a predominance of coliforms and anaerobes. This rapid proliferation of bacteria, coupled with the loss of mucosal integrity, allows bacterial to translocate across the bowel wall and potentially lead to endotoxemia, bacteremia, and sepsis.

The clinical presentation of intestinal obstruction varies with the cause, level of obstruction, and time between the obstructing event and the patient's evaluation. Classic symptoms of obstruction in the neonate include vomiting, abdominal distention, and obstipation. Obstruction high in the intestinal tract results in large-volume, frequent, bilious emesis with little or no abdominal distention. Pain is intermittent and is usually relieved by vomiting. Obstruction in the distal small bowel leads to moderate or marked abdominal distention with emesis that is progressively feculent. Both proximal and distal obstructions are eventually associated with obstipation. However, meconium stools can be passed initially if the obstruction is in the upper part of the intestinal tract or if the obstruction developed late in intrauterine life.

The diagnosis of congenital bowel obstruction relies on a combination of history, physical examination, and radiologic findings. In certain cases, the diagnosis is suggested in the prenatal period. Routine prenatal ultrasound can detect polyhydramnios, which often accompanies high intestinal obstruction. The presence of polyhydramnios should prompt aspiration of the infant's stomach immediately after birth. Aspiration of more than 15-20 mL of fluid, particularly if it is bile stained, is highly indicative of proximal intestinal obstruction.

In the postnatal period, a plain radiograph is the initial diagnostic study and can provide valuable information about potential associated complications. With completely obstructing lesions, plain radiographs reveal bowel distention proximal to the point of obstruction. Upright or cross-table lateral views typically demonstrate a series of air-fluid levels in the distended loops. Caution must be exercised in using plain films to determine the location of intestinal obstruction. Because colonic haustra are not fully developed in the neonate, small and large bowel obstructions may be difficult to distinguish with plain films. In these cases, contrast studies of the bowel or computed tomography images may be indicated. Oral or nasogastric contrast medium may be used to identify obstructing lesions in the proximal bowel, and contrast enemas may be used to diagnose more-distal entities. Indeed, enemas may also play a therapeutic role in relieving distal obstruction due to meconium ileus or meconium plug syndrome.

Initial treatment of infants and children with bowel obstruction must be directed at fluid resuscitation and stabilizing the patient. Nasogastric decompression usually relieves pain and vomiting. After appropriate cultures, broad-spectrum antibiotics are usually started in ill-appearing neonates with bowel obstruction and those with suspected strangulating infarction. Patients with strangulation must have immediate surgical relief before the bowel infarcts, resulting in gangrene and intestinal perforation. Extensive intestinal necrosis results in short bowel syndrome (Chapter 330.7). Nonoperative conservative management is usually limited to children with suspected adhesions or inflammatory strictures that might resolve with nasogastric decompression or anti-inflammatory medications. If clinical signs of improvement are not evident within 12-24 hr, then operative intervention is usually indicated.

BIBLIOGRAPHY

Please visit the Nelson Textbook of Pediatrics *website at www.expertconsult.com for the complete bibliography.*

322.1 Duodenal Obstruction

Christina Bales and Chris A. Liacourus

Congenital duodenal obstruction occurs in 2.5-10/100,000 live births. In most cases, it is caused by atresia, an intrinsic defect of bowel formation. It can also result from extrinsic compression by abnormal neighboring structures (e.g., annular pancreas, preduodenal portal vein), duplication cysts, or congenital bands associated with malrotation. Although intrinsic and extrinsic causes of duodenal obstruction occur independently, they can also coexist. Thus, a high index of suspicion for more than one underlying etiology may be critical to avoiding unnecessary reoperations in these infants.

Duodenal atresia complicates 1/10,000 live births and accounts for 25-40% of all intestinal atresias. In contrast to more-distal atresias, which likely arise from prenatal vascular accidents, duodenal atresia results from failed recanalization of the intestinal lumen during gestation. Throughout the 4th and 5th weeks of normal fetal development, the duodenal mucosa exhibits rapid proliferation of epithelial cells. Persistence of these cells, which should degenerate after the 7th week of gestation, leads to occlusion of the lumen (atresia) in approximately two thirds of cases and narrowing (stenosis) in the remaining one third. Duodenal atresia can take several forms, including a thin membrane that occludes the lumen, a short fibrous cord that connects 2 blind duodenal pouches, or a gap that spans 2 nonconnecting ends of the duodenum. The membranous form is most common, and it almost invariably occurs near the ampulla of Vater. In rare cases, the membrane is distensible and is referred to as a *windsock web*. This unusual form of duodenal atresia causes obstruction several centimeters distal to the origin of the membrane.

Approximately 50% of infants with duodenal atresia are premature. Concomitant congenital anomalies are common and include congenital heart disease (30%), malrotation (20-30%), annular pancreas (30%), renal anomalies (5-15%), esophageal atresia with or without tracheoesophageal fistula (5-10%), skeletal malformations (5%), and anorectal anomalies (5%). Of these anomalies, only complex congenital heart disease has been associated with increased mortality. Annular pancreas has been associated with increased late complications, including gastroesophageal reflux disease, peptic ulcer disease, pancreatitis, gastric outlet and recurrent duodenal obstruction, and gastric cancer. Thus, long-term follow-up of these patients into adulthood is warranted. Nearly half of patients with duodenal atresia have chromosome abnormalities; trisomy 21 is identified in up to one third of patients.

CLINICAL MANIFESTATIONS AND DIAGNOSIS

The hallmark of duodenal obstruction is bilious vomiting without abdominal distention, which is usually noted on the 1st day of life. Peristaltic waves may be visualized early in the disease process. A history of polyhydramnios is present in half the pregnancies and is caused by inadequate absorption of amniotic fluid in the distal intestine. This fluid may be bile stained due to intrauterine vomiting. Jaundice is present in one third of the infants.

The diagnosis is suggested by the presence of a "double-bubble" sign on a plain abdominal radiograph (Fig. 322-1). The appearance is caused by a distended and gas-filled stomach and proximal duodenum, which are invariably connected. Contrast studies are occasionally needed to exclude malrotation and volvulus because intestinal infarction can occur within 6-12 hr if the volvulus is not relieved. Contrast studies are generally not necessary and may be associated with aspiration. Prenatal diagnosis of duodenal atresia is readily made by fetal ultrasonography, which reveals a sonographic double-bubble. Prenatal identification of duodenal atresia is associated with decreased morbidity and fewer hospitalization days.

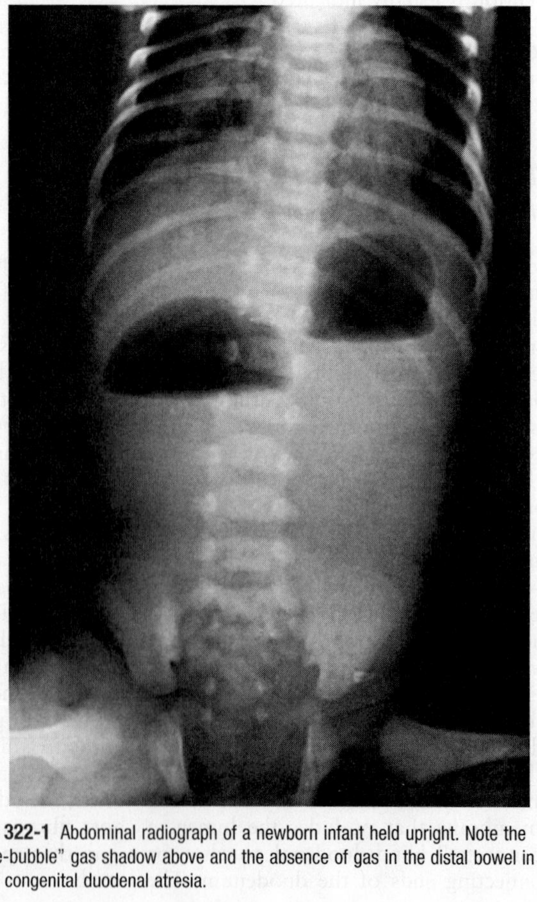

Figure 322-1 Abdominal radiograph of a newborn infant held upright. Note the "double-bubble" gas shadow above and the absence of gas in the distal bowel in this case of congenital duodenal atresia.

TREATMENT

The initial treatment of infants with duodenal atresia includes nasogastric or orogastric decompression and intravenous fluid replacement. Echocardiography, renal ultrasound, and radiology of the chest and spine should be performed to evaluate for associated anomalies. Definitive correction of the atresia is usually postponed until life-threatening anomalies are evaluated and treated.

The typical surgical repair for duodenal atresia is duodenoduodenostomy. This procedure is also preferred in cases of concomitant or isolated annular pancreas. In these instances, the duodenoduodenostomy is performed without dividing the pancreas. The dilated proximal bowel might need to be tapered to improve peristalsis. Postoperatively, a gastrostomy tube can be placed to drain the stomach and protect the airway. Intravenous nutritional support or a transanastomotic jejunal tube is needed until an infant starts to feed orally. Long-term prognosis is excellent, approaching 90% survival in most series.

BIBLIOGRAPHY

Please visit the Nelson Textbook of Pediatrics *website at* *www.expertconsult.com* *for the complete bibliography.*

322.2 Jejunal and Ileal Atresia and Obstruction

Christina Bales and Chris A. Liacouras

The primary etiologies of congenital small bowel obstruction involve intrinsic abnormalities in anatomic development (jejeunoileal stenosis and atresia), mucus secretion (meconium ileus), and bowel wall innervation (long-segment Hirschprung disease).

Jejeunoileal atresias are generally attributed to intrauterine vascular accidents, which result in segmental infarction and resorption of the fetal intestine. Underlying events that potentiate vascular compromise include intestinal volvulus, intussusception, meconium ileus, and strangulating herniation through an abdominal wall defect associated with gastroschisis or omphalocele. Maternal behaviors that promote vasoconstriction, such as cigarette smoking and cocaine use, might also have a role. Only a few cases of familial inheritance have been reported. In these families, multiple intestinal atresias have occurred in an autosomal recessive pattern. Jejunoileal atresias have been linked with multiple births, low birth weight, and prematurity. Unlike atresia in the duodenum, they are not commonly associated with extraintestinal anomalies.

Five types of jejunal and ileal atresias are encountered (Fig. 322-2). In type I, a mucosal web occludes the lumen but continuity is maintained between the proximal and distal bowel. Type II involves a small-diameter solid cord that connects the proximal and distal bowel. Type III is divided into two subtypes. Type IIIa occurs when both ends of the bowel end in blind loops, accompanied by a small mesenteric defect. Type IIIb is similar, but it is associated with an extensive mesenteric defect and a loss of the normal blood supply to the distal bowel. The distal ileum coils around the ileocolic artery, from which it derives its entire blood supply, producing an "apple-peel" appearance. This anomaly is associated with prematurity, an unusually short distal ileum, and significant foreshortening of the bowel. Type IV involves multiple atresias. Types II and IIIa are the most common, each accounting for 30-35% of cases. Type I occurs in approximately 20% of patients. Types IIIb and IV account for the remaining 10-20% of cases, with IIIb being the least common configuration.

Meconium ileus occurs primarily in newborn infants with cystic fibrosis, an exocrine gland defect of chloride transport that results in abnormally viscous secretions. Approximately 80-90% of infants with meconium ileus have cystic fibrosis, but only 10-15% of infants with cystic fibrosis present with meconium ileus. In simple cases, the distal 20-30 cm of ileum is collapsed and filled with pellets of pale stool. The proximal bowel is dilated and filled with thick meconium that resembles sticky syrup or glue. Peristalsis fails to propel this viscid material forward, and it becomes impacted in the ileum. In complicated cases, a volvulus of the dilated proximal bowel can occur, resulting in intestinal ischemia, atresia, and/or perforation. Perforation in utero results in meconium peritonitis, which can lead to potentially obstructing adhesions and calcifications.

Both intestinal atresia and meconium ileus must be distinguished from **long-segment Hirschprung disease.** This condition involves congenital absence of ganglion cells in the myenteric and submucosal plexi of the bowel wall. In a small subset (5%) of patients, the aganglionic segment includes the terminal ileum in addition to the entire length of the colon. Infants with long-segment Hirschprung disease present with a dilated small intestine that is ganglionated but has hypertrophied walls, a funnel-shaped transitional hypoganglionic zone, and a collapsed distal aganglionic bowel.

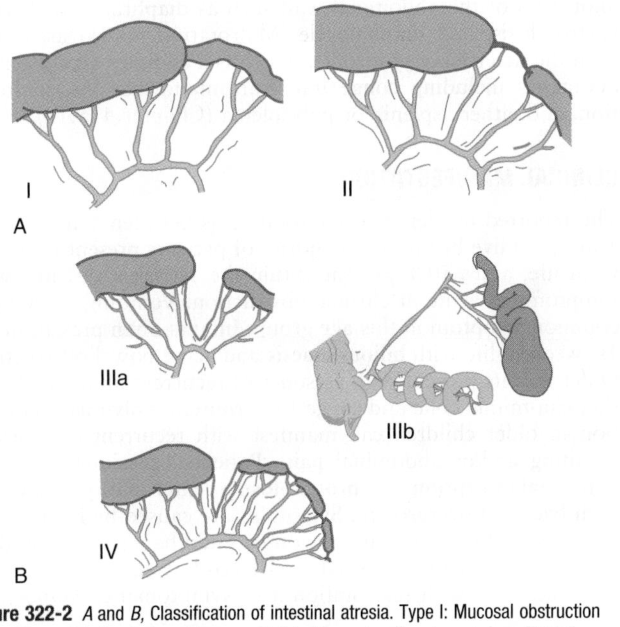

Figure 322-2 *A* and *B*, Classification of intestinal atresia. Type I: Mucosal obstruction caused by an intraluminal membrane with intact bowel wall and mesentery. Type II: Blind ends are separated by a fibrous cord. Type IIIa: Blind ends are separated by a V-shaped mesenteric defect. Type IIIb: "Apple-peel" appearance. Type IV: Multiple atresias. (From Grosfeld J: Jejunoileal atresia and stenosis. In Welch KJ, Randolph JG, Ravitch MM, editors: *Pediatric surgery,* ed 4, Chicago, 1986, Year Book Medical Publishers.)

CLINICAL MANIFESTATION AND DIAGNOSIS

Distal intestinal obstruction is less likely than proximal obstruction to be detected in utero. Polyhydramnios is identified in 20-35% of jejunoileal atresias, and it may be the first sign of intestinal obstruction. Abdominal distention is rarely present at birth, but it develops rapidly after initiation of feeds in the first 12-24 hr. Distention is often accompanied by vomiting, which is often bilious. Up to 80% of infants fail to pass meconium in the first 24 hours of life. Jaundice, associated with unconjugated hyperbilirubinemia, is reported in 20-30% of patients.

In patients with obstruction due to jejunoileal atresia or long-segment Hisrchprung disease, plain radiographs typically demonstrate multiple air-fluid levels proximal to the obstruction in the upright or lateral decubitus positions (Fig. 322-3). These levels may be absent in patients with meconium ileus because the viscosity of the secretions in the proximal bowel prevents layering. Instead, a typical hazy or ground-glass appearance may be appreciated in the right lower quadrant. This haziness is caused by small bubbles of gas that become trapped in inspissated meconium in the terminal ileal region. If there is meconium peritonitis, patchy calcification may also be noted, particularly in the flanks. Plain films can reveal evidence of pneumoperitoneum due to intestinal perforation. Air may be seen in the subphrenic regions on the upright view and over the liver in the left lateral decubitus position.

Because plain radiographs do not reliably distinguish between small and large bowel in neonates, contrast studies are often

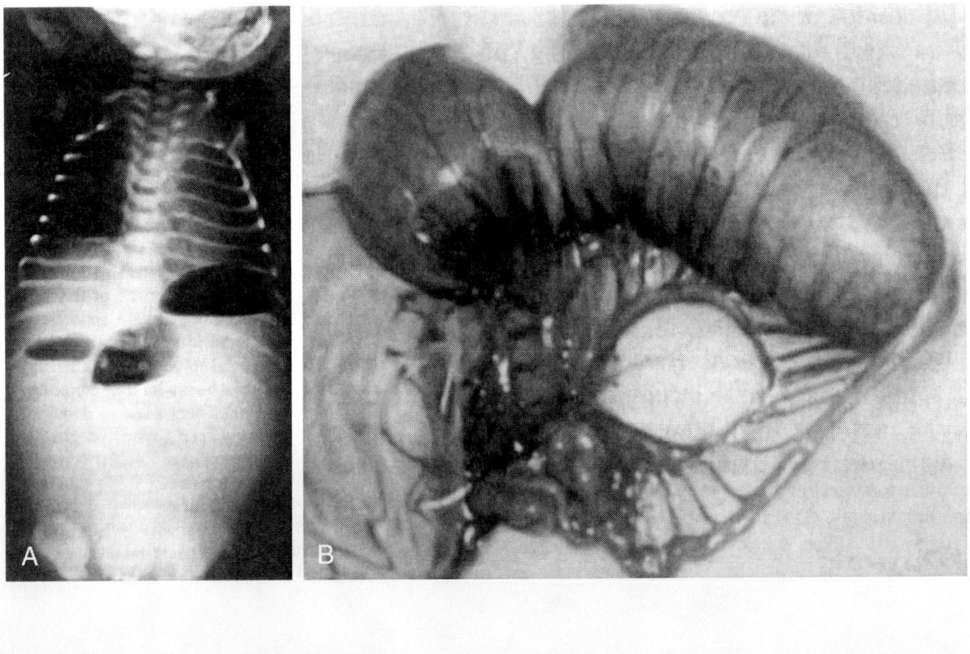

Figure 322-3 *A,* Abdominal radiograph in a neonate with bilious vomiting shows a few loops of dilated intestine with air-fluid levels. *B,* At laparotomy, a type I (mucosal) jejunal atresia was observed. (From O'Neill JA Jr, Grosfeld JL, Fonkalsrud EW, et al, editors: *Principles of pediatric surgery,* ed 2, St Louis, 2003, Mosby, p 493.)

required to localize the obstruction. Water-soluble enemas (Gastrografin, Hypaque) are particularly useful in differentiating atresia from meconium ileus and Hirschprung disease. A small "microcolon" suggests disuse and the presence of obstruction proximal to the ileocecal valve. Abdominal ultrasound may be an important adjunctive study, which can distinguish meconium ileus from ileal atresia and also identify concomitant intestinal malrotation.

TREATMENT

Patients with small bowel obstruction should be stable and in adequate fluid and electrolyte balance before operation or radiographic attempts at disimpaction unless volvulus is suspected. Documented infections should be treated with appropriate antibiotics. Prophylactic antibiotics are usually given before surgery.

Ileal or jejunal atresia requires resection of the dilated proximal portion of the bowel followed by end-to-end anastomosis. If a simple mucosal diaphragm is present, jejunoplasty or ileoplasty with partial excision of the web is an acceptable alternative to resection. In uncomplicated meconium ileus, Gastrografin enemas diagnose the obstruction and wash out the inspissated material. Gastrografin is hypertonic, and care must be taken to avoid dehydration, shock, and bowel perforation. The enema may have to be repeated after 8-12 hr. Resection after reduction is not needed if there have been no ischemic complications.

About 50% of patients with simple meconium ileus do not adequately respond to water-soluble enemas and need laparotomy. Operative management is indicated when the obstruction cannot be relieved by repeated attempts at nonoperative management and for infants with complicated meconium ileus. The extent of surgical intervention depends on the degree of pathology. In simple meconium ileus, the plug can be relieved by manipulation or direct enteral irrigation with *N*-acetylcysteine following an enterotomy. In complicated cases, bowel resection, peritoneal lavage, abdominal drainage, and stoma formation may be necessary. Total parenteral nutrition is generally required.

BIBLIOGRAPHY

Please visit the Nelson Textbook of Pediatrics *website at www.expertconsult.com for the complete bibliography.*

322.3 Malrotation

Melissa Kennedy and Chris A. Liacouras

Malrotation is incomplete rotation of the intestine during fetal development. The gut starts as a straight tube from stomach to rectum. Intestinal rotation and attachment begins in the 5th week of gestation when the mid-bowel (distal duodenum to mid-transverse colon) begins to elongate and progressively protrudes into the umbilical cord until it lies totally outside the confines of the abdominal cavity. As the developing bowel rotates in and out of the abdominal cavity, the superior mesenteric artery, which supplies blood to this section of gut, acts as an axis. The duodenum, on re-entering the abdominal cavity, moves to the region of the ligament of Treitz, and the colon that follows is directed to the left upper quadrant. The cecum subsequently rotates counterclockwise within the abdominal cavity and comes to lie in the right lower quadrant. The duodenum becomes fixed to the posterior abdominal wall before the colon is completely rotated. After rotation, the right and left colon and the mesenteric root become fixed to the posterior abdomen. These attachments provide a broad base of support to the mesentery and the superior mesenteric artery, thus preventing twisting of the mesenteric root and kinking of the vascular supply. Abdominal rotation and attachment are completed by the 12th week of gestation.

Nonrotation occurs when the bowel fails to rotate after it returns to the abdominal cavity. The 1st and 2nd portions of the duodenum are in their normal position, but the remainder of the duodenum, jejunum, and ileum occupy the right side of the abdomen and the colon is located on the left. The most common type of malrotation involves failure of the cecum to move into the right lower quadrant (Fig. 322-4). The usual location of the cecum is in the subhepatic area. Failure of the cecum to rotate properly is associated with failure to form the normal broad-based adherence to the posterior abdominal wall. The mesentery, including the superior mesenteric artery, is tethered by a narrow stalk, which can twist around itself and produce a midgut volvulus. Bands of tissue (**Ladd bands**) can extend from the cecum to the right upper quadrant, crossing and possibly obstructing the duodenum.

Malrotation and nonrotation are often associated with other anomalies of the abdominal wall such as diaphragmatic hernia, gastroschisis, and omphalocele. Malrotation is also associated with the heterotaxy syndrome, which is a complex of congenital anomalies including congenital heart malformations, malrotation, and either asplenia or polysplenia (Chapter 425.11).

CLINICAL MANIFESTATION

The reported incidence of malrotation is between 1 in 500 and 1 in 6,000 live births. The majority of patients present in the 1st yr of life, and >50% present within the 1st month of life, with symptoms of acute or chronic obstruction. Vomiting is the most common symptom in this age group. Infants often present in the 1st week of life with **bilious emesis** and acute bowel obstruction. Older infants present with episodes of recurrent abdominal pain that can mimic colic and suggest intermittent volvulus. Malrotation in older children can manifest with recurrent episodes of vomiting and/or abdominal pain. Patients occasionally present with **malabsorption** or **protein-losing enteropathy** associated with bacterial overgrowth. Symptoms are caused by intermittent volvulus or duodenal compression by Ladd bands or other adhesive bands affecting the small and large bowel. About 25-50% of adolescents with malrotation are asymptomatic. Adolescents

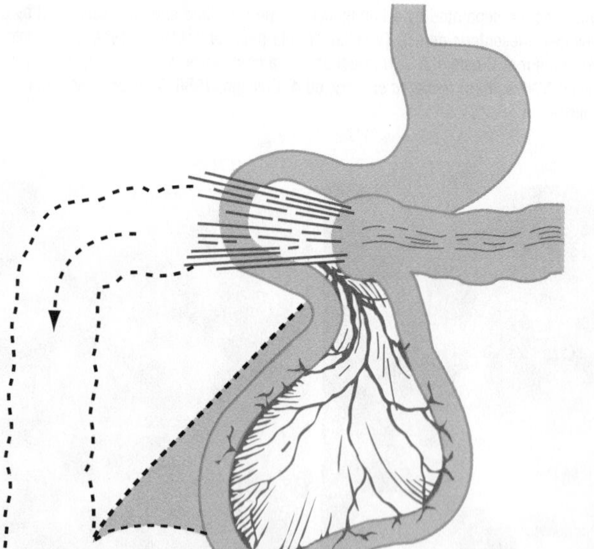

Figure 322-4 The mechanism of intestinal obstruction with incomplete rotation of the midgut (malrotation). The *dotted lines* show the course the cecum should have taken. Failure to rotate has left obstructing bands across the duodenum and a narrow pedicle for the midgut loop, making it susceptible to volvulus. (From Nixon HH, O'Donnell B: *The essentials of pediatric surgery,* Philadelphia, 1961, JB Lippincott.)

who become symptomatic present with acute intestinal obstruction or history of recurrent episodes of abdominal pain with less frequent vomiting and diarrhea. Patients of any age with a rotational anomaly can develop acute bowel-threatening volvulus without pre-existing symptoms.

An acute presentation of small bowel obstruction in a patient without previous bowel surgery is usually a result of **volvulus** associated with malrotation. This is a life-threatening complication of malrotation, which resembles an acute abdomen or sepsis and is the main reason that symptoms suggesting malrotation should always be investigated. Volvulus occurs when the small bowel twists around the superior mesenteric artery leading to vascular compromise of the bowel. The diagnosis may be suggested by ultrasound but is confirmed by contrast radiographic studies. The abdominal plain film is usually nonspecific but might demonstrate a gasless abdomen or evidence of duodenal obstruction with a double-bubble sign. Barium enema usually demonstrates malposition of the cecum but is normal in up to 20% of patients. Upper gastrointestinal series is the imaging test if choice and the gold standard in the evaluation and diagnosis of malrotation and volvulus. It is the best exam to visualize the malposition of the ligament of Treitz and can also reveal a corkscrew appearance of the small bowel or a duodenal obstruction with a "bird's beak" appearance of the duodenum. Ultrasonography demonstrates inversion of the superior mesenteric artery and vein. A superior mesenteric vein located to the left of the superior mesenteric artery suggests malrotation. Malrotation with volvulus is suggested by duodenal obstruction, thickened bowel loops to the right of the spine, and free peritoneal fluid.

Surgical intervention is recommended for any patient with a significant rotational abnormality, regardless of age. If a volvulus is present, surgery is done immediately as an acute emergency, the volvulus is reduced, and the duodenum and upper jejunum are freed of any bands and remain in the right abdominal cavity. The colon is freed of adhesions and placed in the right abdomen with the cecum in the left lower quadrant, usually accompanied by incidental appendectomy. This may be done laparoscopically if gut ischemia is not present, but it is generally done as an open procedure. The purpose of surgical intervention is to minimize the risk of subsequent volvulus rather than to return the bowel to a normal anatomic configuration. Proper surgical management of patients with heterotaxy remains in debate because these patients have a high incidence of malrotation but a low incidence of actual volvulus. It is unclear whether these patients should undergo elective Ladd procedure or whether watchful waiting is appropriate. Extensive intestinal ischemia from volvulus can result in short bowel syndrome (Chapter 330.7). Persistent symptoms after repair of malrotation should suggest a pseudo-obstruction–like motility disorder.

BIBLIOGRAPHY

Please visit the Nelson Textbook of Pediatrics *website at* www.expertconsult.com *for the complete bibliography.*

Chapter 323
Intestinal Duplications, Meckel Diverticulum, and Other Remnants of the Omphalomesenteric Duct

323.1 Intestinal Duplication

Chris A. Liacouras

Duplications of the intestinal tract are rare anomalies that consist of well-formed tubular or spherical structures firmly attached to the intestine with a common blood supply. The lining of the duplications resembles that of the gastrointestinal (GI) tract. Duplications are located on the mesenteric border and can communicate with the intestinal lumen. Duplications can be classified into 3 categories: localized duplications, duplications associated with spinal cord defects and vertebral malformations, and duplications of the colon. Occasionally (10-15% of cases), multiple duplications are found.

Localized duplications can occur in any area of the GI tract but are most common in the ileum and jejunum. They are usually cystic or tubular structures within the wall of the bowel. The cause is unknown, but their development has been attributed to defects in recanalization of the intestinal lumen after the solid stage of embryologic development. Duplication of the intestine occurring in association with **vertebral and spinal cord anomalies** (hemivertebra, anterior spina bifida, band connection between lesion and cervical or thoracic spine) is thought to arise from splitting of the notochord in the developing embryo. **Duplication of the colon** is usually associated with anomalies of the urinary tract and genitals. Duplication of the entire colon, rectum, anus, and terminal ileum can occur. The defects are thought to be secondary to caudal twinning, with duplication of the hindgut, genital, and lower urinary tracts.

CLINICAL MANIFESTATIONS

Symptoms depend on the size, location, and mucosal lining. Duplications can cause bowel obstruction by compressing the adjacent intestinal lumen, or they can act as the lead point of an intussusception or a site for a volvulus. If they are lined by acid-secreting mucosa, they can cause ulceration, perforation, and hemorrhage of or into the adjacent bowel. Patients can present with abdominal pain, vomiting, palpable mass, or acute GI hemorrhage. Intestinal duplications in the thorax (**neuroenteric cysts**) can manifest as respiratory distress. Duplications of the lower bowel can cause constipation or diarrhea or be associated with recurrent prolapse of the rectum.

The diagnosis is suspected on the basis of the history and physical examination. Radiologic studies such as barium studies, ultrasonography, CT, and MRI are helpful but usually nonspecific, demonstrating cystic structures or mass effects. Radioisotope technetium scanning can localize ectopic gastric mucosa. The treatment of duplications is surgical resection and management of associated defects.

323.2 Meckel Diverticulum and Other Remnants of the Omphalomesenteric Duct

Melissa Kennedy and Chris A. Liacouras

A Meckel diverticulum is a remnant of the embryonic yolk sac, which is also referred to as the omphalomesenteric duct or vitelline duct. The omphalomesenteric duct connects the yolk sac to the gut in a developing embryo and provides nutrition until the placenta is established. Between the 5th and 7th wk of gestation, the duct attenuates and separates from the intestine. Just before this involution, the epithelium of the yolk sac develops a lining similar to that of the stomach. Partial or complete failure of involution of the omphalomesenteric duct results in various residual structures. Meckel diverticulum is the most common of these structures and is the most common congenital GI anomaly, occurring in 2-3% of all infants. A typical Meckel diverticulum is a 3-6 cm outpouching of the ileum along the antimesenteric border 50-75 cm from the ileocecal valve (Fig. 323-1). The distance from the ileocecal valve depends on the age of the patient. Other omphalomesenteric duct remnants occur infrequently, including a persistently patent duct, a solid cord, or a cord with a central

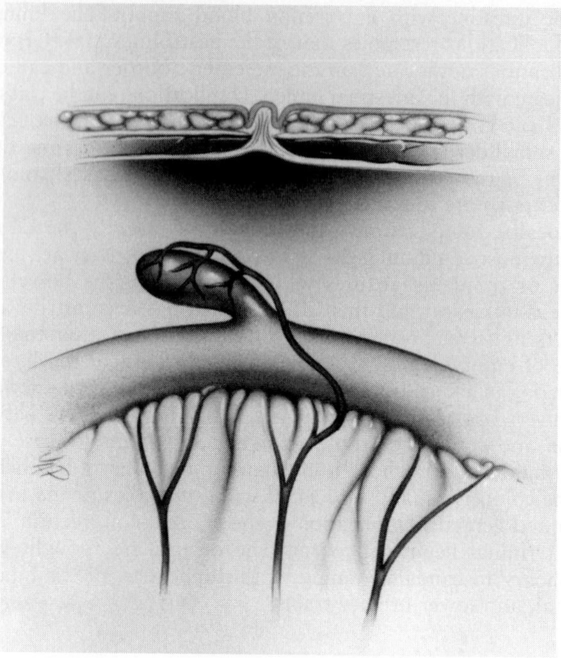

Figure 323-1 Typical Meckel diverticulum located on the antimesenteric border.

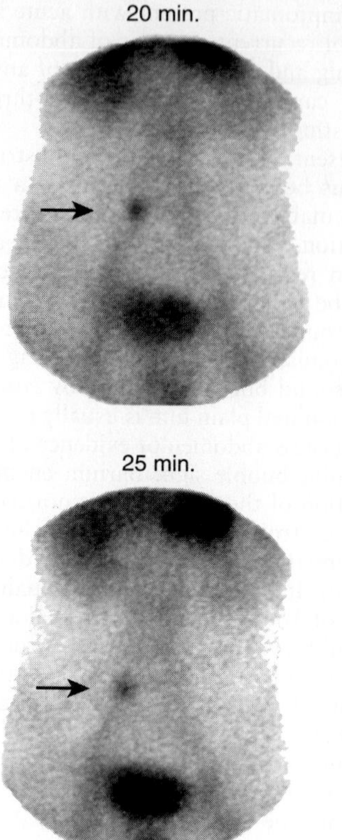

Figure 323-2 Meckel scan demonstrating accumulation of technetium in the stomach superior bladder (inferior) and in the acid-secreting mucosa of a Meckel diverticulum.

cyst or a diverticulum associated with a persistent cord between the diverticulum and the umbilicus.

CLINICAL MANIFESTATIONS

Symptoms of a Meckel diverticulum usually arise in the 1st or 2nd yr of life (average 2.5 yr), but initial symptoms can occur in the 1st decade. The majority of symptomatic Meckel diverticula are lined by an ectopic mucosa, including an acid-secreting mucosa that causes intermittent painless rectal bleeding by ulceration of the adjacent normal ileal mucosa. This ectopic mucosa is most commonly of gastric origin, but it can also be pancreatic, jejunal, or a combination of these tissues. Unlike the upper duodenal mucosa, the acid is not neutralized by pancreatic bicarbonate.

The stool is typically described as brick colored or currant jelly colored. Bleeding can cause significant anemia but is usually self-limited because of contraction of the splanchnic vessels, as patients become hypovolemic. Bleeding from a Meckel diverticulum can also be less dramatic, with melanotic stools.

Less often, a Meckel diverticulum is associated with partial or complete bowel obstruction. The most common mechanism of obstruction occurs when the diverticulum acts as the lead point of an intussusception. The mean age of onset of obstruction is younger than that for patients presenting with bleeding. Obstruction can also result from intraperitoneal bands connecting residual omphalomesenteric duct remnants to the ileum and umbilicus. These bands cause obstruction by internal herniation or volvulus of the small bowel around the band. A Meckel diverticulum occasionally becomes inflamed (**diverticulitis**) and manifests similarly to acute appendicitis. These children are older, with a mean of 8 yr of age. Diverticulitis can lead to perforation and peritonitis.

DIAGNOSIS

The diagnosis of omphalomesenteric duct remnants depends on the clinical presentation. If an infant or child presents with significant painless rectal bleeding, the presence of a Meckel diverticulum should be suspected because Meckel diverticulum accounts for 50% of all lower GI bleeds in children <2 yr of age.

Confirmation of a Meckel diverticulum can be difficult. Plain abdominal radiographs are of no value, and routine barium studies rarely fill the diverticulum. The most sensitive study is a Meckel radionuclide scan, which is performed after intravenous infusion of technetium-99m pertechnetate. The mucus-secreting cells of the ectopic gastric mucosa take up pertechnetate, permitting visualization of the Meckel diverticulum (Fig. 323-2). The uptake can be enhanced with various agents, including cimetidine, ranitidine, glucagon, and pentagastrin. The sensitivity of the enhanced scan is approximately 85%, with a specificity of approximately 95%. A false-negative scan may be seen in anemic patients; although false-positive results are uncommon, they have been reported with intussusception, appendicitis, duplication cysts, arteriovenous malformations, and tumors. Other methods of detection include radio-labeled tagged red blood cell scan (the patient must be actively bleeding), abdominal ultrasound, superior mesenteric angiography, abdominal CT scan, or exploratory laparoscopy. In patients who present with intestinal obstruction or a picture of appendicitis with omphalomesenteric duct remnants, the diagnosis is rarely made before surgery.

The treatment of a symptomatic Meckel diverticulum is surgical excision.

BIBLIOGRAPHY

Please visit the Nelson Textbook of Pediatrics *website at www.expertconsult.com for the complete bibliography.*

Chapter 324 Motility Disorders and Hirschsprung Disease

324.1 Chronic Intestinal Pseudo-Obstruction

Kristin N. Fiorino and Chris A. Liacouras

Chronic intestinal pseudo-obstruction comprises a group of disorders characterized by signs and symptoms of intestinal obstruction in the absence of an anatomic lesion. Pseudo-obstruction can occur as a primary disease or be secondary to a large number of conditions that can transiently or permanently alter bowel motility. Pseudo-obstruction represents a wide spectrum of pathologic disorders from abnormal myoelectric activity to abnormalities of the nerves (**intestinal neuropathy**) or musculature (**intestinal myopathy**) of the gut. The organs involved can include the entire gastrointestinal tract or be limited to certain components, such as the stomach or colon. The distinctive pathologic abnormalities are considered together because of their clinical similarities.

Most congenital forms of pseudo-obstruction occur sporadically. A few clusters of autosomal dominant or recessive patients have been reported as having cases associated with abnormal gut muscle or nerves. Patients with autosomal dominant forms of pseudo-obstruction have variable expressions of the disease. Acquired pseudo-obstruction can follow episodes of acute gastroenteritis, presumably resulting in injury to the myenteric plexus.

In congenital pseudo-obstruction, abnormalities of the muscle or nerves can be demonstrated in most cases. In muscular disease, the outer longitudinal muscle layer is replaced by fibrous material. In neuronal disease, there may be disorganized ganglia, hypoganglionosis, or hyperganglionosis. Abnormalities in the interstitial cells of Cajal (potential gut pacemaker) have been demonstrated in some children and mitochondrial defects have been found in others. Genetic defects have been identified in the transcription factor *SOX10*, the DNA polymerase gamma gene (*POLG*), and a locus on chromosome 8.

CLINICAL MANIFESTATIONS

More than half the children with congenital pseudo-obstruction experience symptoms in the first few months of life. Two thirds of the infants presenting in the first few days of life are born prematurely, and about 40% have malrotation of the intestine. In 75% of all affected children, symptoms occur in the first year of life, and the remainder become symptomatic in the next several years. The **most common symptoms** are abdominal distention and vomiting, which are present in 75% of affected infants. Constipation, growth failure, and abdominal pain occur in about 60% of patients, and diarrhea occurs in 30-40%. The symptoms wax and wane in the majority of the patients; poor nutrition, psychological stress, and intercurrent illness tend to exacerbate symptoms. **Urinary tract and bladder involvement** occurs in 80% of children with myopathic pseudo-obstruction and in 20% of those with neuropathic disease. Symptoms can manifest as recurrent urinary tract infection, megacystis, or obstructive symptoms.

The diagnosis of pseudo-obstruction is based on the presence of compatible symptoms in the absence of anatomic obstruction. Plain abdominal radiographs demonstrate air-fluid levels in the small intestine. Neonates with evidence of obstruction at birth have a microcolon. Contrast studies demonstrate slow passage of barium; water-soluble agents should be considered. Esophageal motility is abnormal in about half the patients. Antroduodenal motility and gastric emptying studies have abnormal results if the upper gut is involved (Table 324-1). Manometric evidence of a normal migrating motor complex and postprandial activity should redirect the diagnostic evaluation. Anorectal motility is normal and differentiates pseudo-obstruction from Hirschsprung disease. Full-thickness intestinal biopsy might show involvement of the muscle layers or abnormalities of the intrinsic intestinal nervous system.

Table 324-1 FINDINGS IN PSEUDO-OBSTRUCTION

GI SEGMENT	FINDINGS*
Esophageal motility	Abnormalities in approximately half of CIPO, although in some series up to 85% demonstrate abnormalities
	Decreased LES pressure
	Failure of LES relaxation
	Esophageal body: low-amplitude waves, poor propagation, tertiary waves, retrograde peristalsis, occasionally aperistalsis
Gastric emptying	May be delayed
ECG	Tachygastria or bradygastria may be seen
ADM	Postprandial antral hypomobility is seen and correlates with delayed gastric emptying
	Myopathic subtype: low-amplitude contractions, <10-20 mm Hg
	Neuropathic subtype: contractions are uncoordinated
	Fed response is absent
	Fasting MMC is absent, or MMC is abnormally propagated
Colonic	No gastric reflex because there is no increased motility in response to a meal
ARM	Normal rectoanal inhibitory reflex (RAIR)

*Findings can vary according to the segment(s) of the gastrointestinal tract that are involved.
ADM, antroduodenal manometry; ARM, anorectal manometry; CIPO, chronic intestinal pseudo-obstruction; EGG, electrogastrography; GI, gastrointestinal; LES, lower esophageal sphincter; MMC, migrating motor complex.
From Wyllie R, Hyams JS, editors: *Pediatric gastrointestinal and liver disease*, ed 3, Philadelphia, 2006, Saunders.

The **differential diagnosis** includes Hirschsprung disease, other causes of mechanical obstruction, psychogenic constipation, neurogenic bladder, and superior mesenteric artery syndrome. Secondary causes of ileus or pseudo-obstruction, such as hypothyroidism, opiates, scleroderma, Chagas disease, hypokalemia, diabetic neuropathy, amyloidosis, porphyria, angioneurotic edema, mitochondrial disorders, and radiation, must be excluded.

TREATMENT

Nutritional support is the mainstay of treatment for pseudo-obstruction. Thirty to 50% require partial or complete parenteral nutrition. Some patients can be treated with intermittent enteral supplementation, whereas others can maintain themselves on selective oral diets. Prokinetic drugs are generally not useful. Isolated gastroparesis can follow episodes of viral gastroenteritis and spontaneously resolves, usually in 6-24 mo. Erythromycin, a motilin receptor agonist, and cisapride, a serotonin 5-HT_4 receptor agonist, can enhance gastric emptying and proximal small bowel motility and may be of use in this selected group of patients. Pain management is difficult and requires a multidisciplinary approach.

Symptomatic small bowel **bacterial overgrowth** is usually treated with oral antibiotics or probiotics. Bacterial overgrowth can be associated with steatorrhea and malabsorption. Although unabsorbable antibiotics remain the treatment of choice, courses of other antibiotics may be introduced and used judiciously to help counteract the possible emergence of drug-resistant bacteria. The long-acting somatostatin analog octreotide has been used in low doses to treat small bowel bacterial overgrowth. Patients with acid peptic symptoms are treated with acid suppressors. Many benefit from a gastrostomy and some benefit from decompressive ileostomies or colostomies. Colectomy with ileorectal anastomosis is beneficial if the large bowel is the primary site of the motility abnormality. Bowel transplantation can benefit selected patients.

BIBLIOGRAPHY

Please visit the Nelson Textbook of Pediatrics *website at www.expertconsult.com for the complete bibliography.*

324.2 Functional Constipation

Kristin N. Fiorino and Chris A. Liacouras

Constipation is defined by a delay or difficulty in defecation present for 2 weeks or longer and significant to cause distress to the patient. Another approach to the definition is noted in Table 324-2. Functional constipation, also known as idiopathic constipation or fecal withholding, can usually be differentiated from constipation secondary to organic causes on the basis of a history and physical examination (Chapter 21.4). Unlike anorectal malformations and Hirschsprung disease, functional constipation typically starts after the neonatal period. Usually, there is an intentional or subconscious withholding of stool. An acute episode usually precedes the chronic course. The acute episode may be a dietary change from human milk to cow's milk, secondary to the change in protein:carbohydrate ratio or an allergy to cow's milk. The stool becomes firm, smaller, and difficult to pass, resulting in anal irritation and often an anal fissure. In toddlers, coercive or inappropriately early toilet training is a factor that can initiate a pattern of stool retention. In older children, retentive constipation can develop after entering a situation that makes stooling inconvenient such as school. Because the passage of bowel movements is painful, voluntary withholding of feces to avoid the painful stimulus develops.

When children have the urge to defecate, typical behaviors include contracting the gluteal muscles by stiffening the legs while lying down, holding onto furniture while standing, or squatting quietly in corners, waiting for the call to stool to pass. The urge to defecate passes as the rectum accommodates to its contents. A vicious cycle of retention develops as increasingly larger volumes of stool need to be expelled. Caregivers might misinterpret these activities as straining, but it is withholding behavior. In functional constipation, daytime encopresis is common, and some children have a history of blood in the stool noted with the passage of a large bowel movement. Findings suggestive of underlying pathology include failure to thrive, weight loss, abdominal pain, vomiting, or persistent anal fissure or fistula.

The physical examination often demonstrates a large volume of stool palpated in the suprapubic area; rectal examination demonstrates a dilated rectal vault filled with guaiac-negative stool. The presence of a hair tuft over the spine or spinal dimple, or failure to elicit a cremasteric reflex or anal wink suggests spinal pathology. A tethered cord is suggested by decreased or absent lower leg reflexes. Spinal cord lesions can occur with overlying skin anomalies. Urinary tract symptoms include recurrent urinary tract infection and enuresis. Children with no evidence of abnormalities on physical examination rarely require radiologic evaluation.

In refractory patients (intractable constipation), specialized testing should be considered to rule out conditions such as hypothyroidism, hypocalcemia, lead toxicity, celiac disease, and allergy testing. Colonic transit studies using radio-opaque markers or scintigraphy techniques may be useful. Selected children can benefit from MRI of the spine to identify an intraspinal process, motility studies to identify underlying myopathic or neuropathic bowel abnormalities, or a barium enema to identify structural abnormalities. Anorectal motility studies can demonstrate a pattern of paradoxical contraction of the external anal sphincter during defecation, which can be treated by behavior modification. Colonic motility can guide therapy in refractory cases, demonstrating segmental problems that might require surgical intervention.

Therapy for functional constipation includes patient education, relief of impaction, and softening of the stool (Chapter 21.4). The parents must understand that soiling associated with overflow incontinence is associated with loss of normal sensation and not a willful act. A regular bowel training program, including sitting on the toilet for 5-10 min after meals and keeping track of the frequency of bowel movements, is often helpful in establishing a regular bowel habit. If an impaction is present on the initial physical examination, an enema is usually required to clear the impaction while bowel softeners are started as maintenance medications. Typical regimens include the use of polyethylene glycol preparations, lactulose, or mineral oil. Prolonged use of stimulants such as senna or bisacodyl should be avoided. Children with behavioral problems that are interfering with successful treatment might benefit from a referral to a mental heath care provider. Maintenance therapy is generally continued until a regular bowel pattern has been established and the association of pain with the passage of stool is abolished. Children with spinal problems can be successfully managed with low volumes of fluid through a cecostomy or sigmoid tube.

Table 324-2 CHRONIC CONSTIPATION: ROME III CRITERIA

INFANTS AND TODDLERS
At least 2 of the following: • ≤2 defecations per week • ≥1 episode of incontinence after the acquisition of toilet training skills • History of excessive stool retention • History of painful or hard bowel movements • Presence of a large fecal mass in the rectum • History of a large-diameter stool that might obstruct the toilet
CHILDREN WITH A DEVELOPMENTAL AGE OF 4-18 YEARS
At least 2 of the following: • ≤2 defecations per week • ≥1 episode of fecal incontinence per week • History of retentive posturing or excessive volitional stool retention • History of painful or hard bowel movements • Presence of a large fecal mass in the rectum • History of a large-diameter stool that might obstruct the toilet

From Carvalho RS, Michail SK, Ashai-Khan F, et al: An update in pediatric gastroenterology and nutrition: a review of some recent advances, *Curr Prob Pediatr Adolesc Health Care* 38:197–234, 2008.

BIBLIOGRAPHY

Please visit the Nelson Textbook of Pediatrics *website at www.expertconsult.com for the complete bibliography.*

324.3 Congenital Aganglionic Megacolon (Hirschsprung Disease)

Kristin Fiorino and Chris A. Liacouras

Hirschsprung disease, or congenital aganglionic megacolon, is a developmental disorder (neurocristopathy) of the enteric nervous system, characterized by the absence of ganglion cells in the submucosal and myenteric plexus. It is the most common cause of lower intestinal obstruction in neonates, with an overall incidence of 1 in 5,000 live births. The male:female ratio for Hirschprung disease is 4 : 1 for short-segment disease and closer to 1 : 1 as the length of the involved segment increase. Prematurity is uncommon.

There is an increased familial incidence in long-segment disease. Hirschsprung disease may be associated with other congenital defects, including Down, Goldberg-Shprintzen, Smith-Lemli-Opitz, Shah-Waardenburg, cartilage-hair hypoplasia, and congenital hypoventilation (Ondine's curse) syndromes and urogenital or cardiovascular abnormalities. Hirschsprung disease has been seen in association with microcephaly, mental retardation, abnormal facies, autism, cleft palate, hydrocephalus, and micrognathia.

PATHOLOGY

Hirschsprung disease is the result of an absence of ganglion cells in the bowel wall, extending proximally and continuously from the anus for a variable distance. The absence of neural innervation is a consequence of an arrest of neuroblast migration from the proximal to distal bowel. Without the myenteric and submucosal plexus, there is inadequate relaxation of the bowel wall and bowel wall hypertonicity, which can lead to intestinal obstruction.

Hirschsprung disease is usually sporadic, although dominant and recessive patterns of inheritance have been demonstrated in family groups. Genetic defects have been identified in multiple genes that encode proteins of the RET signaling pathway (*RET, GDNF,* and *NTN*) and involved in the endothelin (EDN) type B receptor pathway (*EDNRB, EDN3,* and *EVE-1*). Syndromic forms of Hirschsprung disease have been associated with the *L1CAM, SOX10,* and *ZFHX1B* (formerly *SIP1*) genes.

The aganglionic segment is limited to the rectosigmoid in 80% of patients. Approximately 10% to 15% of patients have long-segment disease, defined as disease proximal to the sigmoid colon. Total bowel aganglionosis is rare and accounts for approximately 5% of cases. Observed histologically is an absence of Meissner and Auerbach plexus and hypertrophied nerve bundles with high concentrations of acetylcholinesterase between the muscular layers and in the submucosa.

CLINICAL MANIFESTATIONS

Hirschsprung disease is usually diagnosed in the neonatal period secondary to a distended abdomen, failure to pass meconium, and/or bilious emesis or aspirates with feeding intolerance. In 99% of healthy full-term infants, meconium is passed within 48 hr of birth. Hirschsprung disease should be suspected in any full-term infant (the disease is unusual in preterm infants) with delayed passage of stool. Some neonates pass meconium normally but subsequently present with a history of chronic constipation. Failure to thrive with hypoproteinemia from protein-losing enteropathy is a less common presentation because Hirschsprung disease is usually recognized early in the course of the illness. Breast-fed infants might not suffer disease as severe as formula-fed infants.

Failure to pass stool leads to dilatation of the proximal bowel and abdominal distention. As the bowel dilates, intraluminal pressure increases, resulting in decreased blood flow and deterioration of the mucosal barrier. Stasis allows proliferation of bacteria, which can lead to enterocolitis (*Clostridium difficile, Staphylococcus aureus,* anaerobes, coliforms) with associated diarrhea, abdominal tenderness, sepsis and signs of bowel obstruction. Early recognition of Hirschsprung disease before the onset of enterocolitis is essential in reducing morbidity and mortality.

Hirschsprung disease in older patients must be distinguished from other causes of abdominal distention and chronic constipation (Table 324-3 and Fig. 324-1). The history often reveals constipation starting in infancy that has responded poorly to medical management. Fecal incontinence, fecal urgency, and stool-withholding behaviors are usually not present. The abdomen is tympanitic and distended, with a large fecal mass palpable in the left lower abdomen. Rectal examination demonstrates a normally placed anus that easily allows entry of the finger but feels snug. The rectum is usually empty of feces, and when the finger is removed, there may be an explosive discharge of foul-smelling feces and gas. The stools, when passed, can consist of small pellets, be ribbon-like, or have a fluid consistency, unlike the large stools seen in patients with functional constipation. Intermittent attacks of intestinal obstruction from retained feces may be

Table 324-3 DISTINGUISHING FEATURES OF HIRSCHSPRUNG DISEASE AND FUNCTIONAL CONSTIPATION

VARIABLE	FUNCTIONAL	HIRSCHSPRUNG DISEASE
HISTORY		
Onset of constipation	After 2 yr of age	At birth
Encopresis	Common	Very rare
Failure to thrive	Uncommon	Possible
Enterocolitis	None	Possible
Forced bowel training	Usual	None
EXAMINATION		
Abdominal distention	Uncommon	Common
Poor weight gain	Rare	Common
Rectum	Filled with stool	Empty
Rectal Examination	Stool in rectum	Explosive passage of stool
Malnutrition	None	Possible
INVESTIGATIONS		
Anorectal manometry	Relaxation of internal anal sphincter	Failure of internal anal sphincter relaxation
Rectal biopsy	Normal	No ganglion cells, increased acetylcholinesterase staining
Barium enema	Massive amounts of stool, no transition zone	Transition zone, delayed evacuation (>24 hr)

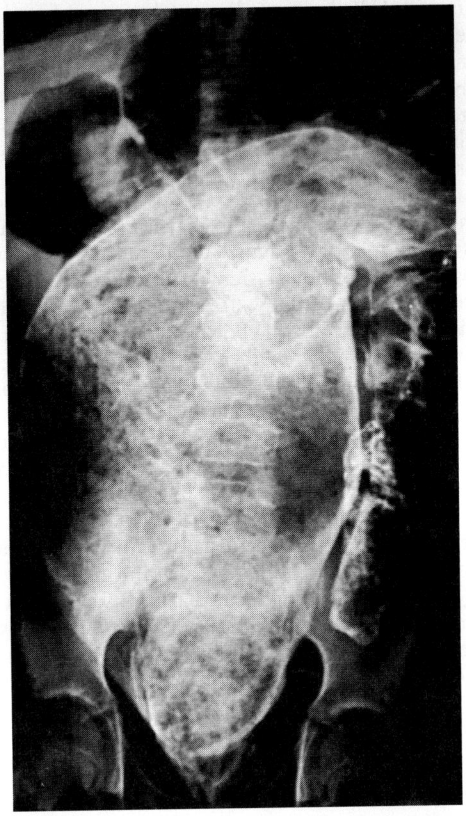

Figure 324-1 Barium enema in a 14 yr old boy with severe constipation. The enormous dilatation of the rectum and distal colon is typical of acquired functional megacolon.

associated with pain and fever. Urinary retention with enlarged balder or hydronephrosis can occur secondary to urinary compression.

In neonates, Hirschsprung disease must be differentiated from meconium plug syndrome, meconium ileus, and intestinal atresia. In older patients, the **Currarino triad** must be considered, which includes **anorectal malformations** (ectopic anus, anal stenosis, imperforate anus), **sacral bone anomalies** (hypoplasia, poor segmentation), and **presacral anomaly** (anterior meningoceles, teratoma, cyst).

DIAGNOSIS

Rectal suction biopsy is the **gold standard** for diagnosing Hirschsprung disease. The biopsy material should contain an adequate amount of submucosa to evaluate for the presence of ganglion cells. To avoid obtaining biopsies in the normal area of hypoganglionosis, which ranges from 3 to 17 mm in length, the suction rectal biopsy should be obtained no closer than 2 cm above the dentate line. The biopsy specimen should be stained for acetylcholinesterase to facilitate interpretation. Patients with aganglionosis demonstrate a large number of hypertrophied nerve bundles that stain positively for acetylcholinesterase with an absence of ganglion cells.

Anorectal manometry measures the pressure of the internal anal sphincter while a balloon is distended in the rectum. In normal patients, rectal distention initiates relaxation of the internal anal sphincter in response to rectal distention with a balloon. In patients with Hirschsprung disease, the internal anal sphincter fails to relax in response to rectal distention. Although the sensitivity and specificity can vary widely, in experienced hands, the test can be quite sensitive. The test, however, can be technically difficult to perform in young infants. A normal response in the course of manometric evaluation precludes a diagnosis of Hirschsprung disease; an equivocal or paradoxical response requires a repeat motility or rectal biopsy.

An unprepared contrast enema is most likely to aid in the diagnosis in children older than 1 mo because the proximal ganglionic segment might not be significantly dilated in the first few weeks of life. Classic findings are based on the presence of an abrupt narrow transition zone between the normal dilated proximal colon and a smaller-caliber obstructed distal aganglionic segment. In the absence of this finding, it is imperative to compare the diameter of the rectum to that of the sigmoid colon, because a rectal diameter that is the same as or smaller than the sigmoid colon suggests Hirschsprung disease. Radiologic evaluation should be performed without preparation to prevent transient dilatation of the aganglionic segment. As many as 10% of newborns with Hirschsprung disease have a normal contrast study. Twenty-four hour delayed films are helpful in showing retained contrast (Fig. 324-2). If significant barium is still present in the colon, it increases the suspicion of Hirschsprung disease even if a transition zone is not identified. Barium enema examination is useful in determining the extent of aganglionosis before surgery and in evaluating other diseases that manifest as lower bowel obstruction in a neonate. Full-thickness rectal biopsies can be performed at the time of surgery to confirm the diagnosis and level of involvement.

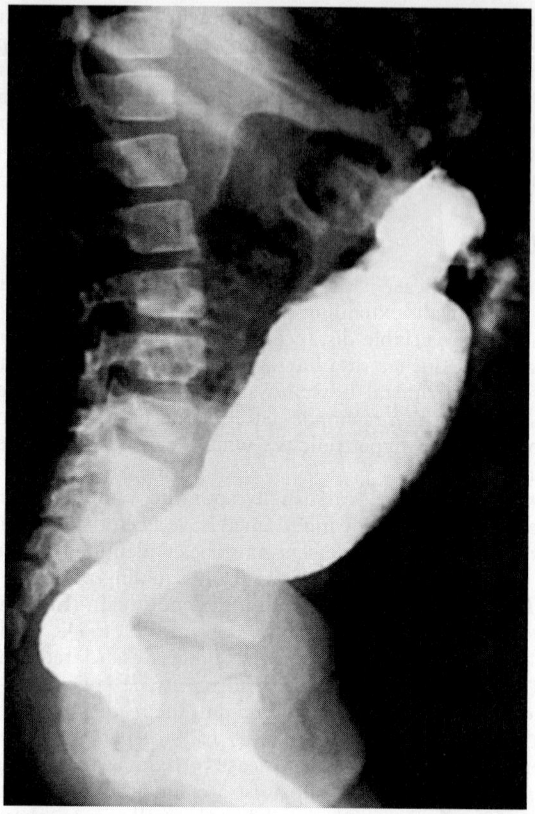

Figure 324-2 Lateral view of a barium enema in a 3 yr old girl with Hirschsprung disease. The aganglionic distal segment is narrow, with distended normal ganglionic bowel above it.

TREATMENT

Once the diagnosis is established, the definitive treatment is operative intervention. Previously, a temporary ostomy was placed and definitive surgery was delayed until the child was older. Currently, many infants undergo a primary pull-through procedure except if there is associated enterocolitis or other complications, when a decompressing ostomy is usually required.

There are 3 basic surgical options. The first successful surgical procedure, described by Swenson, was to excise the aganglionic segment and anastomose the normal proximal bowel to the rectum 1-2 cm above the dentate line. The operation is technically difficult and led to the development of 2 other procedures. Duhamel described a procedure to create a neorectum, bringing down normally innervated bowel behind the aganglionic rectum. The neorectum created in this procedure has an anterior aganglionic half with normal sensation and a posterior ganglionic half with normal propulsion. The endorectal pull-through procedure described by Soave involves stripping the mucosa from the aganglionic rectum and bringing normally innervated colon through the residual muscular cuff, thus bypassing the abnormal bowel from within. *Advances in techniques have led to successful laparoscopic single-stage endorectal pull-through procedures, which are the* ***treatment of choice.***

In **ultrashort-segment** Hirschsprung disease or internal sphincter achalasia, the aganglionic segment is limited to the internal sphincter. The clinical symptoms are similar to those of children with functional constipation. Ganglion cells are present on rectal suction biopsy, but the anorectal manometry is abnormal, with failure of relaxation of the internal anal sphincter in response to rectal distention. Current treatment, although still controversial, includes anal botulism injection to relax the anal sphincter and anorectal myectomy if indicated.

Long-segment Hirschsprung disease involving the entire colon and, at times, part of the small bowel presents a difficult problem. Anorectal manometry and rectal suction biopsy demonstrate findings of Hirschsprung disease, but radiologic studies are difficult to interpret because a colonic transition zone cannot be identified. The extent of aganglionosis can be determined accurately by biopsy at the time of laparotomy. When the entire colon is aganglionic, often together with a length of terminal ileum, ileal-anal anastomosis is the treatment of choice, preserving part of the aganglionic colon to facilitate water absorption, which helps the stools to become firm.

The prognosis of surgically treated Hirschsprung disease is generally satisfactory; the great majority of patients achieve fecal continence. Long-term postoperative problems include constipation, recurrent enterocolitis, stricture, prolapse, perianal abscesses, and fecal soiling. Some children require myectomy or a redo pull-through procedure.

BIBLIOGRAPHY
Please visit the Nelson Textbook of Pediatrics *website at www.expertconsult.com for the complete bibliography.*

324.4 Intestinal Neuronal Dysplasia

Kristin N. Fiorino and Chris A. Liacouras

Intestinal neuronal dysplasia (IND) describes different quantitative (hypo- or hyperganglionosis) and qualitative (immature or heterotropic ganglion cells) abnormalities of the myenteric and/or submucous plexus. The typical histology is that of hyperganglionosis and giant ganglia. **Type A** occurs very rarely and is characterized by congenital aplasia or hypoplasia of the sympathetic innervation. Patients present early in the neonatal period with episodes of intestinal obstruction, diarrhea, and bloody stools. **Type B**, which accounts for >95% of cases, is characterized by malformation of the parasympathetic submucous and myenteric plexus with giant ganglia and thickened nerve fibers, increased acetylcholinesterase staining, and isolated ganglion cells in the lamina propria. IND type B mimics Hirschsprung disease, and patients present with chronic constipation.

For the full continuation of this chapter, please visit the Nelson Textbook of Pediatrics *website at www.expertconsult.com.*

324.5 Superior Mesenteric Artery Syndrome (Wilkie Syndrome, Cast Syndrome, Arteriomesenteric Duodenal Compression Syndrome)

Andrew Chu and Chris A. Liacouras

Superior mesenteric artery syndrome results from compression of the 3rd duodenal segment by the artery against the aorta. Weight loss from malnutrition or catabolic states can cause mesenteric fat depletion, which collapses the duodenum within a narrowed aortomesenteric angle. Other etiologies include extra-abdominal compression (e.g., body cast) and mesenteric tension, as can occur from ileo-anal pouch anastomosis.

For the full continuation of this chapter, please visit the Nelson Textbook of Pediatrics *website at www.expertconsult.com.*

Chapter 325
Ileus, Adhesions, Intussusception, and Closed-Loop Obstructions

325.1 Ileus

Andrew Chu and Chris A. Liacouras

Ileus is the failure of intestinal peristalsis caused by loss of coordinated gut motility without evidence of mechanical obstruction. In children, it is most often associated with abdominal surgery or infection (pneumonia, gastroenteritis, peritonitis). Ileus also accompanies metabolic abnormalities (e.g. uremia, hypokalemia, hypercalcemia, hypermagnesemia, acidosis) or administration of certain drugs, such as opiates, vincristine, and antimotility agents such as loperamide when used during gastroenteritis.

Ileus manifests as increasing abdominal distention, emesis, and pain that worsens with distention. Bowel sounds are minimal or absent, in contrast to early mechanical obstruction, when they are hyperactive. Plain abdominal radiographs demonstrate multiple air-fluid levels throughout the abdomen. Serial radiographs usually do not show progressive distention as they do in mechanical obstruction. Contrast radiographs, if performed, demonstrate slow movement of barium through a patent lumen.

Treatment of ileus involves correcting the underlying abnormality. Nasogastric decompression is used to relieve recurrent vomiting or abdominal distention associated with pain. Ileus after abdominal surgery generally resolves in 24-72 hr. Prokinetic agents such as metoclopramide or erythromycin have been thought to hasten the return of normal bowel motility, but clinical data are inconclusive. The development of selective peripheral opioid antagonists such as methylnaltrexone holds promise in decreasing postoperative ileus, but pediatric data are lacking.

BIBLIOGRAPHY
Please visit the Nelson Textbook of Pediatrics *website at www.expertconsult.com for the complete bibliography.*

325.2 Adhesions

Andrew Chu and Chris A. Liacouras

Adhesions are fibrous tissue bands that result from peritoneal injury. They can constrict hollow organs and are a major cause of postoperative small bowel obstruction. Most remain asymptomatic, but problems can arise anytime after the 2nd postoperative wk to years after surgery, regardless of surgical extent. In 1 study, the 5-year readmission risk due to adhesions varied by operative region (2.1% for colon to 9.2% for ileum) and procedure (0.3% for appendectomy to 25% for ileostomy formation/closure). The overall risk was 5.3% excluding appendectomy and 1.1% when they were included.

The diagnosis is suspected in patients with abdominal pain, constipation, emesis, and a history of intraperitoneal surgery. Nausea and vomiting quickly follow onset of pain. Initially, bowel sounds are hyperactive, and the abdomen is flat. Subsequently, bowel sounds disappear, and bowel dilation can cause abdominal distention. Fever and leukocytosis suggest bowel necrosis and peritonitis. Plain radiographs demonstrate obstructive features, and a CT scan or contrast studies may be needed to define the etiology.

Management includes nasogastric decompression, intravenous fluid resuscitation, and broad-spectrum antibiotics in preparation for surgery. Nonoperative intervention is contraindicated unless a patient is stable with obvious clinical improvement. In children with repeated obstruction, fibrin-glued plication of adjacent small bowel loops can reduce the risk of recurrent problems. Long-term complications include female infertility, failure to thrive, and chronic abdominal and/or pelvic pain.

BIBLIOGRAPHY
Please visit the Nelson Textbook of Pediatrics *website at www.expertconsult.com for the complete bibliography.*

325.3 Intussusception

Melissa Kennedy and Chris A. Liacouras

Intussusception occurs when a portion of the alimentary tract is telescoped into an adjacent segment. It is the most common cause of intestinal obstruction between 3 mo and 6 yr of age and the most common abdominal emergency in children <2 yr. Sixty percent of patients are <1 yr of age, and 80% of the cases occur before age 24 mo; it is rare in neonates. The incidence varies from 1 to 4/1,000 live births. The male:female ratio is 3:1. A few intussusceptions reduce spontaneously, but if left untreated, most lead to intestinal infarction, perforation, peritonitis, and death.

ETIOLOGY AND EPIDEMIOLOGY

Approximately 90% of cases of intussusception in children are idiopathic. The seasonal incidence has peaks in spring and autumn. Correlation with prior or concurrent respiratory adenovirus (type C) infection has been noted, and the condition can complicate otitis media, gastroenteritis, Henoch-Schönlein purpura, or upper respiratory tract infections. The risk of intussusception was increased in infants ≤1 yr of age after receiving a tetravalent rhesus-human reassortant rotavirus vaccine within 2 wk of immunization. The Advisory Committee on Immunization Practices no longer recommends this vaccine, and it is no longer available. Although rotavirus produces an enterotoxin, there is no association between wild-type human rotavirus and intussusception. The currently approved rotavirus vaccines have not been associated with an increased risk of intussusception.

It is postulated that gastrointestinal infection or the introduction of new food proteins results in swollen Peyer patches in the terminal ileum. Lymphoid nodular hyperplasia is another related risk factor. Prominent mounds of lymph tissue lead to mucosal prolapse of the ileum into the colon, thus causing an intussusception. In 2-8% of patients, **recognizable lead points** for the intussusception are found, such as a Meckel diverticulum, intestinal polyp, neurofibroma, intestinal duplication cysts, hemangioma, or malignant conditions such as lymphoma. Lead points are more common in children >2 yr of age; the older the child, the higher the risk of a lead point. Intussusception can complicate mucosal hemorrhage, as in Henoch-Schönlein purpura or hemophilia. Cystic fibrosis is another risk factor. Postoperative intussusception is ileoileal and usually occurs within several days of an abdominal operation. Intrauterine intussusception may be associated with the development of intestinal atresia. Intussusception in premature infants is rare.

PATHOLOGY

Intussusceptions are most often ileocolic, less commonly cecocolic, and rarely exclusively ileal. Very rarely, the appendix forms the apex of an intussusception. The upper portion of bowel, the **intussusceptum,** invaginates into the lower, the **intussuscipiens,** pulling its mesentery along with it into the enveloping loop. Constriction of the mesentery obstructs venous return; engorgement of the intussusceptum follows, with edema, and bleeding from the mucosa leads to a bloody stool, sometimes containing mucus. The apex of the intussusception can extend into the transverse, descending, or sigmoid colon, even to and through the anus in neglected cases. This presentation must be distinguished from rectal prolapse. Most intussusceptions do not strangulate the bowel within the 1st 24 hr but can eventuate in intestinal gangrene and shock.

CLINICAL MANIFESTATIONS

In typical cases, there is sudden onset, in a previously well child, of severe paroxysmal colicky pain that recurs at frequent intervals and is accompanied by straining efforts with legs and knees flexed and loud cries. The infant may initially be comfortable and play normally between the paroxysms of pain; but if the intussusception is not reduced, the infant becomes progressively weaker and lethargic. At times, the **lethargy** is out of proportion to the abdominal signs. Eventually, a shocklike state, with fever, can develop. The pulse becomes weak and thready, the respirations become shallow and grunting, and the pain may be manifested only by moaning sounds. Vomiting occurs in most cases and is usually more frequent in the early phase. In the later phase, the vomitus becomes bile stained. Stools of normal appearance may be evacuated in the 1st few hours of symptoms. After this time, fecal excretions are small or more often do not occur, and little or no flatus is passed. Blood is generally passed in the 1st 12 hr, but at times not for 1-2 days, and infrequently not at all; 60% of infants pass a stool containing red blood and mucus, the currant jelly stool. Some patients have only irritability and alternating or progressive lethargy. The classic triad of pain, a palpable sausage-shaped abdominal mass, and bloody or currant jelly stool is seen in <15% of patients with intussuscpetion.

Palpation of the abdomen usually reveals a slightly tender sausage-shaped mass, sometimes ill defined, which might increase in size and firmness during a paroxysm of pain and is most often in the right upper abdomen, with its long axis cephalocaudal. If it is felt in the epigastrium, the long axis is transverse. About 30% of patients do not have a palpable mass. The presence of bloody mucus on rectal examination supports the diagnosis of intussusception. Abdominal distention and tenderness develop as intestinal obstruction becomes more acute. On rare occasions, the advancing intestine prolapses through the anus. *This prolapse can be distinguished from prolapse of the rectum by the separation between the protruding intestine and the rectal wall, which does not exist in prolapse of the rectum.*

Ileoileal intussusception can have a less-typical clinical picture, the symptoms and signs being chiefly those of small intestinal obstruction. **Recurrent intussusception** is noted in 5-8% and is more common after hydrostatic than surgical reduction. Chronic intussusception, in which the symptoms exist in milder form at recurrent intervals, is more likely to occur with or after acute enteritis and can arise in older children as well as in infants.

DIAGNOSIS

When the clinical history and physical findings suggest intussusception, an ultrasound is typically performed. A plain abdominal radiograph might show a density in the area of the intussusception. Screening ultrasounds for suspected intussusception increases the yield of diagnostic or therapeutic enemas and reduces unnecessary radiation exposure in children with negative ultrasound examinations. The diagnostic findings of intussusception on ultrasound include a tubular mass in longitudinal views and a doughnut or target appearance in transverse images (Fig. 325-1). Ultrasound has a sensitivity of approximately 98-100% and a sensitivity of about 88% in diagnosing intussusception. Air, hydrostatic (saline), and, less often, water-soluble contrast enemas have replaced barium examinations. Contrast enemas demonstrate a filling defect or cupping in the head of the contrast media where its advance is obstructed by the intussusceptum (Fig. 325-2). A central linear column of contrast media may be visible in the compressed lumen of the intussusceptum, and a thin rim of contrast may be seen trapped around the invaginating intestine in the folds of mucosa within the intussuscipiens (coiled-spring sign), especially after evacuation. Retrogression of the intussusceptum under pressure and visualized on x-ray or ultrasound documents successful reduction. Air reduction is associated with fewer complications and lower radiation exposure than traditional contrast hydrostatic techniques.

DIFFERENTIAL DIAGNOSIS

It may be particularly difficult to diagnose intussusception in a child who already has gastroenteritis; a change in the pattern of illness, in the character of pain, or in the nature of vomiting or the onset of rectal bleeding should alert the physician. The bloody stools and abdominal cramps that accompany enterocolitis can

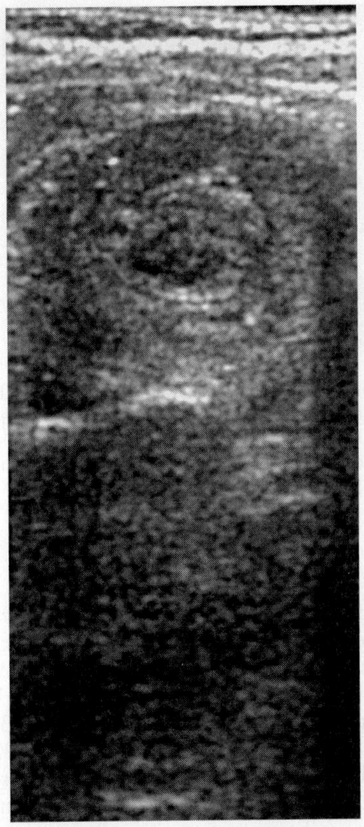

Figure 325-1 Transverse image of an ileocolic intussusception. Note the loops within the loops of bowel.

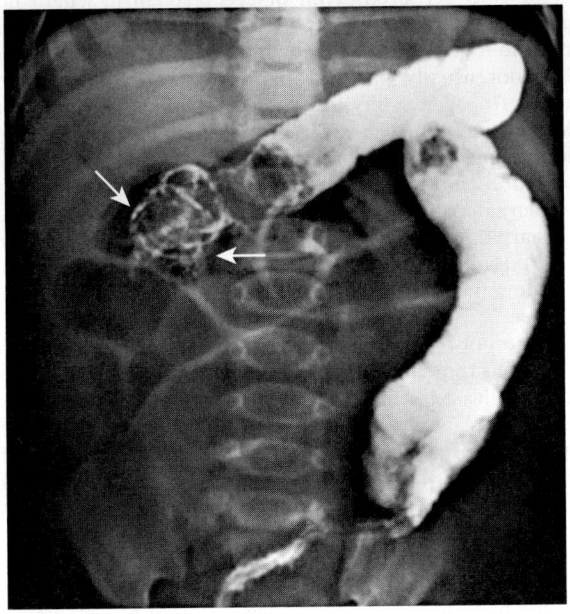

Figure 325-2 Intussusception in an infant. The obstruction is evident in the proximal transverse colon. Contrast material between the intussusceptum and the intussuscipiens is responsible for the coiled-spring appearance.

usually be differentiated from intussusception because in enterocolitis the pain is less severe and less regular, there is diarrhea, and the infant is recognizably ill between pains. Bleeding from a Meckel diverticulum is usually painless. Joint symptoms, purpura, or hematuria usually but not invariably accompany the intestinal hemorrhage of Henoch-Schönlein purpura. Because intussusception can be a complication of this disorder, ultrasonography may be needed to distinguish the conditions.

TREATMENT

Reduction of an acute intussusception is an emergency procedure and should be performed immediately after diagnosis in preparation for possible surgery. In patients with prolonged intussusception and signs of shock, peritoneal irritation, intestinal perforation, or pneumatosis intestinalis, hydrostatic reduction should not be attempted.

The success rate of radiologic hydrostatic reduction under fluoroscopic or ultrasonic guidance is approximately 80-95% in patients with ileocolic intussusception. Spontaneous reduction of intussusception occurs in about 4-10% of patients. Bowel perforations occur in 0.5-2.5% of attempted barium and hydrostatic (saline) reductions. The perforation rate with air reduction is 0.1-0.2%.

An **ileoileal intussusception** is best demonstrated by abdominal ultrasonography. Reduction by instillation of contrast agents, saline, or air might not be possible. Such intussusceptions can develop insidiously after bowel surgery and require reoperation if they do not spontaneously reduce. If manual operative reduction is impossible or the bowel is not viable, resection of the intussusception is necessary, with end-to-end anastomosis.

PROGNOSIS

Untreated intussusception in infants is usually fatal; the chances of recovery are directly related to the duration of intussusception before reduction. Most infants recover if the intussusception is reduced in the 1st 24 hr, but the mortality rate rises rapidly after this time, especially after the 2nd day. Spontaneous reduction during preparation for operation is not uncommon.

The **recurrence rate** after reduction of intussusceptions is about 10%, and after surgical reduction it is 2-5%; none has recurred after surgical resection. Corticosteroids can reduce the frequency of recurrent intussusception. Recurrent intussusception can usually be reduced radiologically. It is unlikely that an intussusception caused by a lesion such as lymphosarcoma, polyp, or Meckel diverticulum will be successfully reduced by radiologic intervention. With adequate surgical management, operative reduction carries a very low mortality rate in early cases.

BIBLIOGRAPHY

Please visit the Nelson Textbook of Pediatrics *website at www.expertconsult.com for the complete bibliography.*

325.4 Closed-Loop Obstructions

Andrew Chu and Chris A. Liacouras

Closed-loop obstructions (i.e., **internal hernia**) are caused by small bowel loops that enter windows created by mesenteric defects or adhesions and become trapped. Vascular engorgement of the strangulated bowel results in intestinal ischemia and necrosis unless promptly relieved. Symptoms include abdominal pain, distention, and bilious emesis. Peritoneal signs suggest ischemic bowel. Plain radiographs demonstrate signs of small bowel obstruction or free air if the bowel has perforated. Supportive management includes intravenous fluids, antibiotics, and nasogastric decompression. Prompt surgical relief of the obstruction is indicated to prevent bowel necrosis. Symptoms occasionally are intermittent if the herniated bowel slides in and out of the defect, spontaneously relieving and regenerating the obstruction.

BIBLIOGRAPHY

Please visit the Nelson Textbook of Pediatrics *website at www.expertconsult.com for the complete bibliography.*

Chapter 326 Foreign Bodies and Bezoars

326.1 Foreign Bodies in the Stomach and Intestine

Judith Kelsen and Chris A. Liacouras

Once in the stomach, 95% of all ingested objects pass without difficulty through the remainder of the gastrointestinal tract. Perforation after ingestion of a foreign body is estimated to be <1% of all objects ingested. Perforation tends to occur in areas of physiologic sphincters (pylorus, ileocecal valve), acute angulation (duodenal sweep), congenital gut malformations (webs, diaphragms, diverticula), or areas of previous bowel surgery.

Most patients who ingest foreign bodies are between the ages of 6 mo and 6 yr. Coins are the most commonly ingested foreign body in children, and meat or food impactions are the most common accidental foreign body in adolescents and adults. Patients with nonfood foreign bodies often describe a history of ingestion. Young children might have a witness to ingestion. Approximately 90% of foreign bodies are opaque. Radiologic examination is routinely performed to determine the type, number, and location of the suspected objects. Contrast radiographs may be necessary to demonstrate some objects, such as plastic parts or toys.

Conservative management is indicated for most foreign bodies that have passed through the esophagus and entered the stomach. Most objects pass though the intestine in 4-6 days, although some take as long as 3-4 wk. While waiting for the object to pass, parents are instructed to continue a regular diet and to observe the stools for the appearance of the ingested object. Cathartics should be avoided. Exceptionally long or sharp objects are usually monitored radiologically. Parents or patients should be instructed to report abdominal pain, vomiting, persistent fever, and hematemesis or melena immediately to their physicians. Failure of the object to progress within 3-4 wk seldom implies an impeding perforation but may be associated with a congenital malformation or acquired bowel abnormality.

Certain objects pose more risk than others. In cases of sharp foreign bodies, such as straight pins, weekly assessments are required. Surgical removal is necessary if the patient develops symptoms or signs of obstruction or perforation or if the foreign body fails to progress for several weeks. Small magnets used to secure earrings have been associated with bowel perforation. When the multiple magnets disperse after ingestion, they may be attracted to each other across bowel wall, leading to pressure necrosis and perforation (Fig. 326-1). Inexpensive toy medallions containing lead can lead to **lead toxicity.** Newer coins can also decompose when subjected to prolonged acid exposure. Unless multiple coins are ingested; however, the metals released are unlikely to pose a clinical risk.

Ingestion of batteries rarely leads to problems, but symptoms can arise from leakage of alkali or heavy metal (mercury) from battery degradation in the gastrointestinal tract. Batteries can also generate electrical current and thereby cause low-voltage electrical burns to the intestine. If patients experience symptoms such as vomiting or abdominal pain, if a large-diameter battery (>20 mm in diameter) remains in the stomach for >48 hr, or if a lithium battery is ingested, the battery should be removed. Batteries >15 mm that do not pass the pylorus within 48 hr are less likely to pass spontaneously and generally require removal. In children <6 yr of age, batteries >15 mm are not likely to pass spontaneously and should be removed endoscopically. If the patient develops peritoneal signs, surgical removal is required. The battery should be identified by size and imprint code or by evaluation of a duplicate measurement of the battery compartment. The National Button Battery Ingestion Hotline can be called for help in identification: 202-625-3333. The Poison Control Center can be called as well: 800-222-1222 for ingestion of batteries and caustic materials. Lithium batteries result in more severe injury than a button alkali battery, with damage occurring in minutes.

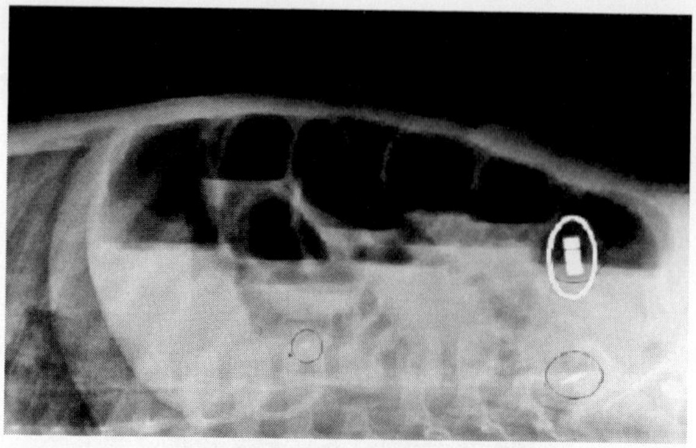

Figure 326-1 Abdominal radiograph of a boy aged 3 yr, noting 3 attached magnets that resulted in volvulus (i.e., twisting of the bowel) and multiple bowel perforations. (Courtesy of the US Consumer Product Safety Commission. From Centers for Disease Control and Prevention: Gastrointestinal injuries from magnet ingestion in children—United States, 2003–2006, *MMWR* 55:1296–1300, 2006.)

In older children and adults, oval objects >5 cm in diameter or 2 cm in thickness tend to lodge in the stomach and should be endoscopically retrieved. Thin objects >10 cm in length fail to negotiate the duodenal sweep and should also be removed. In infants and toddlers, objects >3 cm in length or >20 mm in diameter do not usually pass through the pylorus and should be removed. An open safety pin presents a major problem. Razor blades can be managed with a rigid endoscope by pulling the blade into instrument. The endoscopist can alternatively use a rubber hood on the head of the endoscope to protect the esophagus. Open safety pins should also be endoscopically retrieved, but other sharp objects can be managed conservatively. Drugs (aggregated iron pills, cocaine packing) may need to be surgically removed; initial management can include oral polyethylene glycol lavage.

Ingestion of magnets poses a danger to children. The number of magnets is thought to be critical. If a single magnet is ingested, there is the least likelihood of complications. If ≥2 magnets are ingested, the magnetic poles are attracted to each other and create the risk of obstruction, fistula development, and perforation. Endoscopic retrieval is emergent after films are taken when multiple magnets are ingested. Abdominal pain or peritoneal signs require urgent surgical intervention.

Lead-based foreign bodies can cause symptoms from lead intoxication. Early endoscopic removal is indicated of an object suspected to contain lead. A lead level should be obtained.

Children occasionally place objects in their rectum. Small blunt objects usually pass spontaneously, but large or sharp objects typically need to be retrieved. Adequate sedation is essential to relax the anal sphincter before attempted endoscopic or speculum removal. If the object is proximal to the rectum, observation for 12-24 hr usually allows the object to descend into the rectum.

BIBLIOGRAPHY

Please visit the Nelson Textbook of Pediatrics *website at www.expertconsult.com for the complete bibliography.*

326.2 Bezoars

Judith Kelsen and Chris A. Liacouras

A bezoar is an accumulation of exogenous matter in the stomach or intestine. They are predominantly composed of food or fiber. Most bezoars have been found in females with underlying personality problems or in neurologically impaired persons. Patients who have undergone abdominal surgery are at higher risk for the development of bezoars. The peak age at onset of symptoms is the 2nd decade of life.

Bezoars are classified on the basis of their composition. **Trichobezoars** are composed of the patient's own hair, and **phytobezoars** are composed of a combination of plant and animal material. **Lactobezoars** were previously found most often in premature infants and can be attributed to the high casein or calcium content of some premature formulas. Swallowed chewing gum can occasionally lead to a bezoar.

Trichobezoars can become large and form casts of the stomach; they can enter into the proximal duodenum. They manifest as symptoms of gastric outlet or partial intestinal obstruction including vomiting, anorexia, and weight loss. Patients might complain of abdominal pain, distention, and severe halitosis. Physical examination can demonstrate patchy baldness and a firm mass in the left upper quadrant. Patients occasionally have iron-deficiency anemia, hypoproteinemia, or steatorrhea caused by an associated chronic gastritis. Phytobezoars manifest in a similar manner. Detached segments of the bezoar or trichobezoar can migrate to the small intestine as a ""satellite masses"" and result in small bowel obstruction.

An abdominal plain film can suggest the presence of a bezoar, which can be confirmed on ultrasound or CT examination. On CT a bezoar appears a nonhomogeneous, nonenhancing mass within the lumen of the stomach or intestine. Oral contrast circumscribes the mass.

Bezoars in the stomach can usually be removed endoscopically. If endoscopy is unsuccessful, surgical intervention may be needed. Lactobezoars usually resolve when feedings are withheld for 24-48 hr.

BIBLIOGRAPHY

Please visit the Nelson Textbook of Pediatrics *website at www.expertconsult.com for the complete bibliography.*

Chapter 327
Peptic Ulcer Disease in Children

Samra S. Blanchard and Steven J. Czinn

Peptic ulcer disease, the end result of inflammation due to an imbalance between cytoprotective and cytotoxic factors in the stomach and duodenum, manifests with varying degrees of gastritis or frank ulceration. The pathogenesis of peptic ulcer disease is multifactorial, but the final common pathway for the development of ulcers is the action of acid and pepsin-laden contents of the stomach on the gastric and duodenal mucosa and the inability of mucosal defense mechanisms to allay those effects. Abnormalities in the gastric and duodenal mucosa can be visualized on endoscopy, with or without histologic changes. Deep mucosal lesions that disrupt the muscularis mucosa of the gastric or duodenal wall define **peptic ulcers.** Gastric ulcers are generally located on the lesser curvature of the stomach, and 90% of duodenal ulcers are found in the duodenal bulb. Despite the lack of large population-based pediatric studies, rates of peptic ulcer disease in childhood appear to be low. Large pediatric centers anecdotally report an incidence of 5-7 children with gastric or duodenal ulcers per 2,500 hospital admissions each year.

Table 327-1 ETIOLOGIC CLASSIFICATION OF PEPTIC ULCERS
Positive for *Helicobacter pylori* infection
Drug (NSAID)-induced
H pylori and NSAID positive
H pylori and NSAID negative*
Acid hypersecretory state (Zollinger-Ellison syndrome)
Anastomosis ulcer after subtotal gastric resection
Tumors (cancer, lymphoma)
Rare specific causes
Crohn disease of the stomach or duodenum
Eosinophilic gastroduodenitis
Systemic mastocytosis
Radiation damage
Viral infections (cytomegalovirus or herpes simplex infection, particularly in immunocompromised patients)
Colonization of stomach with *Helicobacter heilmannii*
Severe systemic disease
Cameron ulcer (gastric ulcer where a hiatus hernia passes through the diaphragmatic hiatus)
True idiopathic ulcer

*Requires search for other specific causes.
NSAID, nonsteroidal anti-inflammatory drug.
From Vakil N, Megraud F: Eradication therapy for *Helicobacter pylori*, *Gastroenterology* 133:985–1001, 2007.

Ulcers in children can be classified as **primary** peptic ulcers, which are chronic and more often duodenal, or **secondary,** which are usually more acute in onset and are more often gastric (Table 327-1). Primary ulcers are most often associated with *Helicobacter pylori* infection; idiopathic primary peptic ulcers account for up to 20% of duodenal ulcers in children. Secondary peptic ulcers can result from stress due to sepsis, shock, or an intracranial lesion (Cushing ulcer) or in response to a severe burn injury (Curling ulcer). Secondary ulcers are often the result of using aspirin or nonsteroidal anti-inflammatory drugs (NSAIDs); hypersecretory states like Zollinger-Ellison syndrome (Chapter 327.1), short bowel syndrome, and systemic mastocytosis are rare causes of peptic ulceration.

PATHOGENESIS

Acid Secretion

By 3-4 yr of age, gastric acid secretion approximates adult values. Acid initially secreted by the oxyntic cells of the stomach has a pH of ~0.8, whereas the pH of the stomach contents is 1-2. Excessive acid secretion is associated with a large parietal cell mass, hypersecretion by antral G cells, and increased vagal tone, resulting in increased or sustained acid secretion in response to meals and increased secretion during the night. Control of acid secretion is achieved through multiple different feedback mechanisms involving endocrine, paracrine, and neural pathways. The secretagogues that promote gastric acid production include acetylcholine released by the vagus nerve, histamine secreted by enterochromaffin cells, and gastrin released by the G cells of the antrum. Mediators that decrease gastric acid secretion and enhance protective mucin production include prostaglandins.

Mucosal Defense

A continuous layer of mucous gel that serves as a diffusion barrier to hydrogen ions and other chemicals covers the gastrointestinal (GI) mucosa. Mucus production and secretion are stimulated by prostaglandin E_2. Underlying the mucous coat, the epithelium forms a second-line barrier, the characteristics of which are determined by the biology of the epithelial cells and their tight junctions. Another important function of epithelial cells is to secrete chemokines when threatened by microbial attack. Secretion of bicarbonate into the mucous coat, which is regulated by prostaglandins, is important for neutralization of hydrogen ions. If mucosal injury occurs, active proliferation and migration of mucosal cells occurs rapidly, driven by epithelial growth factor, transforming growth factor-α, insulin-like growth factor, gastrin, and bombesin, and covers the area of epithelial damage.

CLINICAL MANIFESTATIONS

The presenting symptoms of peptic ulcer disease vary with the age of the patient. Hematemesis or melena is reported in up to half of the patients with peptic ulcer disease. School-aged children and adolescents more commonly present with epigastric pain and nausea, presentations generally seen in adults. Dyspepsia, epigastric abdominal pain or fullness, is seen in older children. Infants and younger children usually present with feeding difficulty, vomiting, crying episodes, hematemesis, or melena. In the neonatal period, gastric perforation can be the initial presentation.

The classic symptom of peptic ulceration, epigastric pain alleviated by the ingestion of food, is present only in a minority of children. Many pediatric patients present with poorly localized abdominal pain, which may be periumbilical. The vast majority of patients with periumbilical or epigastric pain or discomfort do not have a peptic ulcer, but rather a functional GI disorder, such as irritable bowel syndrome or nonulcer (functional) dyspepsia. Patients with peptic ulceration rarely present with acute abdominal pain from perforation or symptoms and signs of pancreatitis from a posterior penetrating ulcer. Occasionally, bright red blood per rectum may be seen if the rate of bleeding is brisk and the intestinal transit time is short. Vomiting can be a sign of gastric outlet obstruction.

The pain is often described as dull or aching, rather than sharp or burning, as in adults. It can last from minutes to hours; patients have frequent exacerbations and remissions lasting from weeks to months. Nocturnal pain waking the child is common in older children. A history of typical ulcer pain with prompt relief after taking antacids is found in <33% of children. Rarely, in patients with acute or chronic blood loss, penetration of the ulcer into the abdominal cavity or adjacent organs produces shock, anemia, peritonitis, or pancreatitis. If inflammation and edema are extensive, acute or chronic gastric outlet obstruction can occur.

DIAGNOSIS

Esophagogastroduodenoscopy is the method of choice to establish the diagnosis of peptic ulcer disease. It can be safely performed in all ages by experienced pediatric gastroenterologists. Endoscopy allows the direct visualization of esophagus, stomach, and duodenum, identifying the specific lesions. Biopsy specimens must be obtained from the esophagus, stomach, and duodenum for histologic assessment as well as to screen for the presence of *H. pylori* infection. Endoscopy also provides the opportunity for hemostatic therapy including injection and the use of a heater probe or electrocoagulation if necessary. Fecal enzyme immunoassay tests for *H. pylori* are available and have varying utility in children.

PRIMARY ULCERS

Helicobacter Pylori Gastritis

H. pylori is among the most common bacterial infections in humans. *H. pylori* is a gram-negative, S-shaped rod that produces urease, catalase, and oxidase, which might play a role in the pathogenesis of peptic ulcer disease. The mechanism of acquisition and transmission of *H. pylori* is unclear, although the most likely mode of transmission is fecal-oral or oral-oral. Viable *H. pylori* organisms can be cultured from the stool or vomitus of infected patients. Risk factors such as low socioeconomic status in childhood or affected family members also influence the prevalence. All children infected with *H. pylori* develop histologic chronic active gastritis but are often asymptomatic. In children, *H. pylori* infection can manifest with abdominal pain or vomiting and, less often, refractory iron deficiency anemia or growth retardation. *H. pylori* can be associated, though rarely, with chronic autoimmune thrombocytopenia. Chronic colonization with *H. pylori* can predispose children to a significantly increased risk of developing a duodenal ulcer, gastric cancer such as adenocarcinoma, or MALT (mucosa-associated lymphoid tissue) lymphomas. The relative risk of gastric carcinoma is 2.3-8.7 times greater in infected adults as compared to uninfected subjects. *H. pylori* is classified by the World Health Organization as a group I carcinogen.

Anemia, idiopathic thrombocytopenic purpura, short stature, and sudden infant death syndrome (SIDS) have also been reported as extragastric manifestations of *H. pylori* infection. In one published study, *H. pylori* infection has been correlated with cases of SIDS, but there is no evidence to suggest that *H. pylori* plays a role in the pathogenesis of SIDS.

The **diagnosis** of *H. pylori* infection is made histologically by demonstrating the organism in the biopsy specimens (Fig. 327-1). Although serologic assays using validated immunoglobulin G (IgG) antibody detection may be helpful for screening children for the presence of *H. pylori,* they do not help predict active infection or assess the success of antimicrobial eradication therapy. ^{13}C-urea breath tests and stool antigen tests are also noninvasive methods of detecting *H. pylori* infection. Nonetheless, for children with suspected *H. pylori* infection, an initial upper endoscopy is recommended to evaluate and confirm *H. pylori* disease. The range of endoscopic findings in children with *H. pylori* infection varies from being grossly normal to the presence of nonspecific gastritis with prominent rugal folds, nodularity (Fig. 327-2), or ulcers. Because the antral mucosa appears to be endoscopically normal in a significant number of children with primary *H. pylori* gastritis, gastric biopsies should always be obtained from the body and antrum of the stomach regardless of the endoscopic appearance. If *H. pylori* is identified, even in a child with no symptoms, eradication therapy should be offered (Tables 327-2 and 327-3).

Idiopathic Ulcers

H. pylori–negative duodenal ulcers in children who have no history of taking NSAIDs represent 15-20% of pediatric duodenal ulcers. These patients do not have nodularity in the gastric antrum or histologic evidence of gastritis. In idiopathic

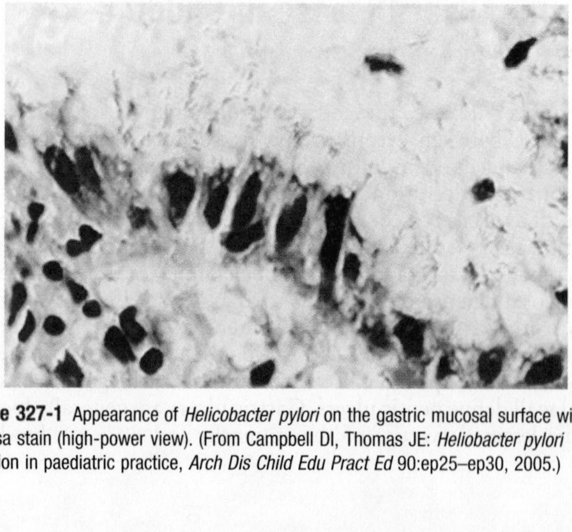

Figure 327-1 Appearance of *Helicobacter pylori* on the gastric mucosal surface with Giemsa stain (high-power view). (From Campbell DI, Thomas JE: *Heliobacter pylori* infection in paediatric practice, *Arch Dis Child Edu Pract Ed* 90:ep25–ep30, 2005.)

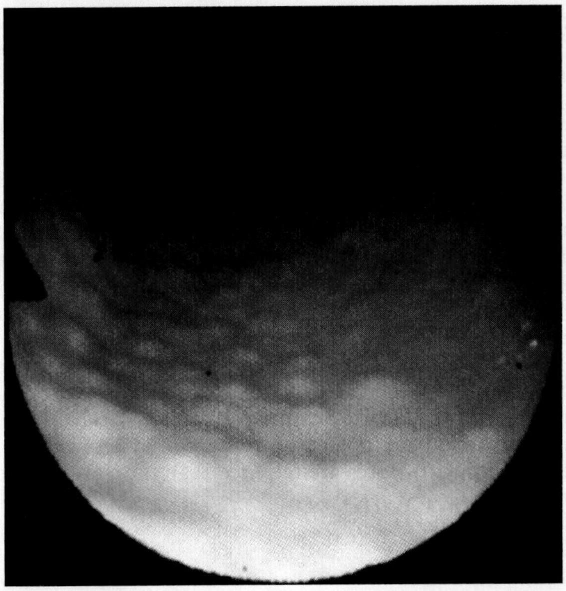

Figure 327-2 Endoscopic view of lymphoid modular hyperplasia of the gastric antrum. (From Campbell DI, Thomas JE: *Heliobacter pylori* infection in paediatric practice, *Arch Dis Child Edu Pract Ed* 90:ep25–ep30, 2005.)

Table 327-2 RECOMMENDED ERADICATION THERAPIES FOR *H. PYLORI*-ASSOCIATED DISEASE IN CHILDREN

MEDICATIONS	DOSE	DURATION OF TREATMENT
Amoxicillin	50 mg/kg/day in 2 divided doses	14 days
Clarithromycin	15 mg/kg/day in 2 divided doses	14 days
Proton pump inhibitor	1 mg/kg/day in 2 divided doses	1 mo
or		
Amoxicillin	50 mg/kg/day in 2 divided doses	14 days
Metronidazole	20 mg/kg/day in 2 divided doses	14 days
Proton pump inhibitor	1 mg/kg/day in 2 divided doses	1 mo
or		
Clarithromycin	15 mg/kg/day in 2 divided doses	14 days
Metronidazole	20 mg/kg/day in 2 divided doses	14 days
Proton pump inhibitor	1 mg/kg/day in 2 divided doses	1 mo

Adapted from Gold BD, Colletti RB, Abbott M, et al: Medical position statement: The North American Society for Pediatric Gastroenterology and Nutrition. *Helicobacter pylori* infection in children: recommendations for diagnosis and treatment, *J Pediatr Gastroenterol Nutr* 31:490–497, 2000.

ulcers, acid suppression alone is the preferred effective treatment. Either proton pump inhibitors (PPIs) or H_2 receptor antagonists may be used. Idiopathic ulcers have a high recurrence rate after discontinuing antisecretory therapy. These children should be followed closely, and if symptoms recur, antisecretory therapy should be restarted. In such cases, if the child is older than 1 yr, PPIs are preferred for maintenance therapy, because they have been shown to be superior to H_2 receptor antagonists in preventing recurrent ulcers.

SECONDARY ULCERS

Aspirin and Other Nonsteroidal Anti-inflammatory Drugs

Nonsteroidal anti-inflammatory drugs (NSAIDs) produce mucosal injury by direct local irritation and by inhibiting cyclooxygenase and prostaglandin formation. Prostaglandins enhance mucosal resistance to injury; therefore, a decrease in prostaglandin production increases the risk of mucosal injury. The severe erosive gastropathy produced by NSAIDs can ultimately result in bleeding ulcers or gastric perforations. The location of these ulcers is more commonly in the stomach than in the duodenum, and usually in the antrum.

Table 327-3 ANTISECRETORY THERAPY WITH PEDIATRIC DOSAGES

MEDICATION	PEDIATRIC DOSE	HOW SUPPLIED
H_2 RECEPTOR ANTAGONISTS		
Cimetidine	20-40 mg/kg/day Divided 2 to 4 × a day	Syrup: 300 mg/mL Tablets: 200, 300, 400, 800 mg
Ranitidine	4-10 mg/kg/day Divided 2 or 3 × a day	Syrup: 75 mg/5 mL Tablets: 75, 150, 300 mg
Famotidine	1-2 mg/kg/day Divided twice a day	Syrup: 40 mg/5 mL Tablets: 20, 40 mg
Nizatidine	10 mg/kg/day Divided twice a day	
PROTON PUMP INHIBITORS		
Omeprazole	1.0-3.3 mg/kg/day<20 kg: 10 mg/day>20 kg: 20 mg/day Approved for use in those >2 yr old	Capsules: 10, 20, 40 mg
Lansoprazole	0.8-4 mg/kg/day<30 kg: 15 mg/day>30 kg: 30 mg/day Approved for use in those >1 yr old	Capsules: 15, 30 mg Powder packet: 15, 30 mg Solu-tab: 15, 30 mg
Rabeprazole	Adult dose: 20 mg/day	Tablet: 20 mg
Pantoprazole	Adult dose: 40 mg/day	Tablet: 40 mg
CYTOPROTECTIVE AGENTS		
Sucralfate	40-80 mg/kg/day	Suspension: 1,000 mg/5 mL Tablet: 1,000 mg

"STRESS" ULCERATION

Stress ulceration usually occurs within 24 hr of onset of a critical illness in which physiologic stress is present. In many cases, the patients bleed from gastric erosions, rather than ulcers. Approximately 25% of the critically ill children in a pediatric intensive care unit (PICU) have macroscopic evidence of gastric bleeding. Preterm and term infants in the neonatal intensive care unit can also develop gastric mucosal lesions and can present with upper GI bleeding or perforated ulcers. Although prophylactic measures to prevent stress ulcers in children are not standardized, drugs that inhibit gastric acid production (see later) are often used in the PICU to reduce the rate of gastric erosions or ulcers.

TREATMENT

The management of acute hemorrhage includes serial monitoring of pulse, blood pressure, and hematocrit to insure hemodynamic stability and avoid significant anemia. Normal saline can be used to resuscitate a patient who has poor intravascular volume status. This can be followed by packed red blood cell transfusions for significant symptomatic anemia. The patient's blood should be typed and cross matched, and a large-bore catheter should be placed for fluid or blood replacement. A nasogastric tube should be placed to determine if the bleeding has stopped. Significant anemia can occur after fluid resuscitation due to equilibration or continued blood loss (which can also cause shock). Fortunately, most acute peptic ulcer bleeding stops spontaneously.

Patients with suspected peptic ulcer hemorrhage should receive high-dose intravenous PPI therapy, which lowers the risk of rebleeding. Some centers also use octreotide, which lowers splanchnic blood flow and gastric acid production.

Once the patient is hemodynamically stable, endoscopy may be indicated to identify the source of bleeding and treat a potential bleeding site. Methods used for vessel hemostasis include pressure, laser, thermal, or electric coagulation; clips; bands; and injections (epinephrine, saline).

Ulcer therapy has two goals: ulcer healing and elimination of the primary cause. Other important considerations are relief of symptoms and prevention of complications. The **first-line drugs** for the treatment of gastritis and peptic ulcer disease in children are H_2 receptor antagonists and PPIs (see Table 327-3). PPIs are more potent in ulcer healing. Cytoprotective agents can also be used as adjunct therapy if mucosal lesions are present. Antibiotics in combination with a PPI must be used for the treatment of *H. pylori*-associated ulcers (see Table 327-2).

H_2 receptor antagonists (cimetidine, ranitidine, famotidine, nizatidine) competitively inhibit the binding of histamine at the H_2 subtype receptor of the gastric parietal cell. PPIs block the gastric parietal cell H^+/K^+ATPase pump in a dose-dependent fashion, reducing basal and stimulated gastric acid secretion. At least 5 PPIs are available in the United States: omeprazole, lansoprazole, pantoprazole, esomeprazole, and rabeprazole. Although not all of them are approved for use in children, they are well tolerated with only minor adverse effects, such as diarrhea (1-4%), headache (1-3%), and nausea (1%). When one considers therapeutic efficacy, the evidence suggests that all PPIs have comparable efficacy in treatment of peptic ulcer disease using standard doses and are superior to H_2-receptor antagonists. PPIs have their greatest effect when given before a meal.

Treatment of *H. Pylori*–Related Peptic Ulcer Disease

In pediatrics, antibiotics and bismuth salts have been used in combination with PPIs to treat *H. pylori* infection (see Table 327-2). Eradication rates in children range from 68% to 92% when the dual or triple therapy is used for 4-6 wk. The ulcer healing rate ranges from 91% to 100%. Triple therapy yields a higher cure rate than dual therapy. The optimal regimen for the eradication of *H. pylori* infection in children has yet to be established, but the use of a PPI in combination with clarithromycin and amoxicillin or metronidazole for 2 wk is a well-tolerated and recommended triple therapy (see Table 327-2). Although children <5 yr of age can become reinfected, the most common reason for treatment failure is poor compliance or antibiotic resistance. *H. pylori* has become more resistant to clarithromycin or metronidazole due to the extensive use of these antibiotics for other infections. In the case of resistant *H. pylori* infection, sequential treatment or rescue therapy with different antibiotics is acceptable options. The sequential treatment regimen is a 10-day treatment consisting of a PPI and amoxicillin (both twice daily) administered for the first 5 days followed by triple therapy consisting of a PPI, clarithromycin, and metronidazole for the remaining 5 days. Levofloxacin, rifabutin, or furazolidone can be used with amoxicillin and bismuth as a rescue therapy depending on the age of the patient. Fidaxomicin has equivalent efficacy to vancomycin in adults. Knowledge of the community's *H. pylori* resistance pattern to clarithromycin or metronidazole might help chose the initial or rescue therapy.

Surgical Therapy

Since the discovery of *H. pylori* and the availability of modern medical management, peptic ulcer disease requiring surgical treatment has become extremely rare. The indications for surgery remain uncontrolled bleeding, perforation, and obstruction. Since the introduction of H_2 receptor antagonists, the recognition and treatment of *H. pylori,* and the use of PPIs, the incidence of surgery for bleeding and perforation has decreased dramatically.

BIBLIOGRAPHY

Please visit the Nelson Textbook of Pediatrics *website at www.expertconsult.com for the complete bibliography.*

327.1 Zollinger-Ellison Syndrome

Samra S. Blanchard and Steven J. Czinn

Zollinger-Ellison syndrome is a rare syndrome characterized by refractory, severe peptic ulcer disease caused by gastric hypersecretion due to the autonomous secretion of gastrin by a neuroendocrine tumor, a gastrinoma. Clinical presentations are similar to those of peptic ulcer disease with the addition of diarrhea. The diagnosis is suspected by the presence of recurrent, multiple, or atypically located ulcers. More than 98% of patients have elevated fasting gastrin levels. Zollinger-Ellison syndrome is common in patients with **multiple endocrine neoplasia** (**MEN1**) and rare with **neurofibromatosis** and **tuberous sclerosis.** Prompt and effective management of increased gastric acid secretion is essential in the management. PPIs are the drug of choice due to their long duration of action and potency. H_2 receptor antagonists are also effective, but higher doses are required than those used in peptic ulcer disease.

BIBLIOGRAPHY

Please visit the Nelson Textbook of Pediatrics *website at www.expertconsult.com for the complete bibliography.*

Chapter 328
Inflammatory Bowel Disease

Andrew B. Grossman and Robert N. Baldassano

The term *inflammatory bowel disease* (IBD) is used to represent 2 distinctive disorders of idiopathic chronic intestinal inflammation: Crohn disease and ulcerative colitis. Their respective etiologies are poorly understood, and both disorders are characterized by unpredictable exacerbations and remissions. The most common time of onset of IBD is during the preadolescent/adolescent era and young adulthood. A bimodal distribution has been shown with an early onset at 10-20 yr of age and a 2nd, smaller peak at 50-80 yr of age. About 25% of patients present before 20 yr of age. IBD may begin as early as the 1st yr of life, and an increased incidence among young children has been observed since the turn of the century. Children with early-onset IBD are more likely to have colonic involvement. In developed countries, these disorders are the major causes of chronic intestinal inflammation in children beyond the 1st few yr of life. A 3rd, less-common category, indeterminate colitis, represents ~10% of pediatric patients.

Genetic and environmental influences are involved in the pathogenesis of IBD. The prevalence of Crohn disease in the United States is much lower for Hispanics and Asians than for whites and blacks. The risk of IBD in family members of an affected person has been reported in the range of 7-30%; a child whose parents both have IBD has a >35% chance of acquiring the disorder. Relatives of a patient with ulcerative colitis have a greater risk of acquiring ulcerative colitis than Crohn disease, whereas relatives of a patient with Crohn disease have a greater risk of acquiring this disorder; the 2 diseases can occur in the same family. The risk of occurrence of IBD among relatives of patients with Crohn disease is somewhat greater than for patients with ulcerative colitis.

The importance of genetic factors in the development of IBD is noted by a higher chance that both twins will be affected if they are monozygotic rather than dizygotic. The concordance rate in twins is higher in Crohn disease (36%) than in ulcerative colitis (16%). Genetic disorders that have been associated with IBD include Turner syndrome, the Hermansky-Pudlak syndrome, glycogen storage disease type Ib, and various immunodeficiency disorders. In 2001 the first IBD gene, *NOD2,* was identified through association mapping. A few months later, the IBD 5 risk haplotype was identified. These early successes were followed by a long period without notable risk factor discovery. Since 2006, the year of the first published genome wide array study on IBD, there has been an exponential growth in the set of validated genetic risk factors for IBD.

A perinuclear antineutrophil antibody (pANCA) is found in ~70% of patients with ulcerative colitis compared with <20% of those with Crohn disease and is believed to represent a marker of genetically controlled immunoregulatory disturbance. About 55% of those with Crohn disease are positive for anti-*Saccharomyces cerevisiae* (ASCA) antibody. Additional markers including antibody to *Escherichia coli* outer membrane porin (anti-OmpC) and anti-flagellin (anti-CBir1) antibodies are associated with Crohn disease.

Environmental factors are also important and presumably explain discordance between twins and changes in risk among the same race in different geographic regions; the precise factors remain unknown. Persons migrating to developed countries often appear to acquire the higher rates of IBD associated with these regions. Cigarette smoking is a risk factor for Crohn disease but paradoxically protects against ulcerative colitis. No specific infectious agent has been reproducibly associated with IBD, although this is an active area of investigation.

An abnormality in intestinal mucosal immunoregulation may be of primary importance in the pathogenesis of IBD. The gut is under constant immunologic stimulation from microbial agents and dietary antigens. In response, the mucosa normally displays "physiologic" inflammation. In IBD, the mechanisms that keep "physiologic" inflammation in check fail and pathologic inflammation ensues. It is not clear if this represents an abnormal response to customary enteric antigens or a normal response to an as-yet-unidentified microbe. Mediators of inflammation (cytokines, arachidonic acid metabolites, reactive oxygen metabolites, growth factors) are involved, leading to tissue destruction and remodeling with fibrosis. Most therapies are aimed at interfering with these mediators.

It is usually possible to distinguish between ulcerative colitis and Crohn disease by the clinical presentation and radiologic, endoscopic, and histopathologic findings (Table 328-1). It is not possible to make a definitive diagnosis in ~10% of patients with chronic colitis; this disorder is called *indeterminate colitis.* Occasionally, a child initially believed to have ulcerative colitis on the basis of clinical findings is subsequently found to have Crohn colitis. This is particularly true for the youngest patients, because Crohn disease in this patient population can more often manifest as exclusively colonic inflammation, mimicking ulcerative colitis. The medical treatments of Crohn disease and ulcerative colitis overlap.

Extraintestinal manifestations occur slightly more commonly with Crohn disease than with ulcerative colitis (Table 328-2). Growth retardation is seen in 15-40% of children with Crohn disease at diagnosis. Of the extraintestinal manifestations that occur with IBD, joint, skin, eye, mouth, and hepatobiliary involvement tend to be associated with colitis, whether ulcerative or Crohn. The presence of some manifestations, such as peripheral arthritis, erythema nodosum, and anemia, correlates with activity of the bowel disease. Activity of pyoderma gangrenosum correlates less well with activity of the bowel disease, whereas sclerosing cholangitis, ankylosing spondylitis, and sacroiliitis do not correlate with intestinal disease. Arthritis occurs in 3 patterns: migratory peripheral arthritis involving primarily large joints, ankylosing spondylitis, and sacroiliitis. The peripheral arthritis of IBD tends to be nondestructive. Ankylosing spondylitis begins in the 3rd decade and occurs most commonly in patients with ulcerative colitis who have the human leukocyte antigen B27 phenotype. Symptoms include low back pain and morning stiffness; back, hips, shoulders, and sacroiliac joints are typically affected. Isolated sacroiliitis is usually asymptomatic but is common when a careful search is performed. Among the skin manifestations, erythema nodosum is most common. Patients with erythema nodosum or pyoderma gangrenosum have a high likelihood of having arthritis as well. Glomerulonephritis, uveitis, and a hypercoagulable state are other rare manifestations that occur in childhood. Cerebral thromboembolic disease has been described in children with IBD.

Table 328-1 COMPARISON OF CROHN DISEASE AND ULCERATIVE COLITIS

FEATURE	CROHN DISEASE	ULCERATIVE COLITIS
Rectal bleeding	Sometimes	Common
Diarrhea, mucus, pus	Variable	Common
Abdominal pain	Common	Variable
Abdominal mass	Common	Not present
Growth failure	Common	Variable
Perianal disease	Common	Rare
Rectal involvement	Occasional	Universal
Pyoderma gangrenosum	Rare	Present
Erythema nodosum	Common	Less common
Mouth ulceration	Common	Rare
Thrombosis	Less common	Present
Colonic disease	50-75%	100%
Ileal disease	Common	None except backwash ileitis
Stomach-esophageal disease	More common	Chronic gastritis can be seen
Strictures	Common	Rare
Fissures	Common	Rare
Fistulas	Common	Rare
Toxic megacolon	None	Present
Sclerosing cholangitis	Less common	Present
Risk for cancer	Increased	Greatly increased
Discontinuous (skip) lesions	Common	Not present
Transmural involvement	Common	Unusual
Crypt abscesses	Less common	Common
Granulomas	Common	None
Linear ulcerations	Uncommon	Common

328.1 Chronic Ulcerative Colitis

Andrew B. Grossman and Robert N. Baldassano

Ulcerative colitis, an idiopathic chronic inflammatory disorder, is localized to the colon and spares the upper gastrointestinal (GI) tract. Disease usually begins in the rectum and extends proximally for a variable distance. When it is localized to the rectum, the disease is ulcerative proctitis, whereas disease involving the entire colon is pancolitis. Approximately 50-80% of pediatric patients have extensive colitis, and adults more commonly have distal disease. Ulcerative proctitis is less likely to be associated with systemic manifestations, although it may be less responsive to treatment than more-diffuse disease. About 30% of children who present with ulcerative proctitis experience proximal spread of the disease. Ulcerative colitis has rarely been noted to present in infancy. Dietary protein intolerance can easily be misdiagnosed as ulcerative colitis in this age group. Dietary protein intolerance (cow's milk protein) is a transient disorder; symptoms are directly associated with the intake of the offending antigen.

The incidence of ulcerative colitis has remained relatively constant, in contrast to an increase in Crohn disease, but varies with country of origin. Incidence rates are highest in northern European countries and the United States (15/100,000) and lowest in Japan and South Africa (1/100,000). The incidence of ulcerative

Table 328-2 EXTRAINTESTINAL COMPLICATIONS OF INFLAMMATORY BOWEL DISEASE

MUSCULOSKELETAL	Peripheral arthritis Granulomatous monoarthritis Granulomatous synovitis Rheumatoid arthritis Sacroiliitis Ankylosing spondylitis Digital clubbing and hypertrophic osteoarthropathy Periosteitis Osteoporosis, osteomalacia Rhabdomyolysis Pelvic osteomyelitis Recurrent multifocal osteomyelitis Relapsing polychondritis
SKIN AND MUCOUS MEMBRANES	Oral lesions Cheilitis Apthous stomatitis, glossitis Granulomatous oral Crohn disease Inflammatory hyperplasia fissures and cobblestone mucosa Peristomatitis vegetans
DERMATOLOGIC	Erythema nodosum Pyoderma gangrenosum Sweet syndrome Metastatic Crohn disease Psoriasis Epidermolysis bullosa acquisita Perianal skin tags Polyarteritis nodosa
OCULAR	Conjunctivitis Uveitis, iritis Episcleritis Scleritis Retrobulbar neuritis Chorioretinitis with retinal detachment Crohn keratopathy Posterior segment abnormalities Retinal vascular disease
BRONCHOPULMONARY	Chronic bronchitis with bronchiectasis Chronic bronchitis with neutrophilic infiltrates Fibrosing alveolitis Pulmonary vasculitis Small airway disease and bronchiolitis obliterans Eosinophilic lung disease Granulomatous lung disease Tracheal obstruction
CARDIAC	Pleuropericarditis Cardiomyopathy Endocarditis Myocarditis
MALNUTRITION	Decreased intake of food • IBD • Dietary restriction Malabsorption • IBD • Bowel resection • Bile salt depletion • Bacterial overgrowth Intestinal losses • Electrolytes • Minerals • Nutrients Increased caloric needs • Inflammation • Fever
HEMATOLOGIC	Anemia: iron deficiency (blood loss) Vitamin B_{12} (ileal disease or resection, bacterial overgrowth, folate deficiency) Anemia of chronic inflammation Anaphylactoid purpura (Crohn disease) Hyposplenism Autoimmune hemolytic anemia Coagulation abnormalities Increased activation of coagulation factors Activated fibrinolysis Anticardiolipin antibody Increased risk of arterial and venous thrombosis with cerebrovascular stroke, myocardial infarction, peripheral arterial, and venous occlusions
RENAL AND GENITOURINARY	Metabolic • Urinary crystal formation (nephrolithiasis, uric acid, oxylate) Hypokalemic nephropathy Inflammation • Retroperitoneal abscess • Fibrosis with ureteral obstruction • Fistula formation Glomerulitis Membranonephritis Renal amyloidosis, nephrotic syndrome
PANCREATITIS	Secondary to medications (sulfasalazine, 6-mercaptopurine, azathioprine, parenteral nutrition) Ampullary Crohn disease Granulomatous pancreatitis Decreased pancreatic exocrine function Sclerosing cholangitis with pancreatitis
HEPATOBILIARY	PSC Small duct PSC (pericholangitis) Carcinoma of the bile ducts Fatty infiltration of the liver Cholelithiasis Autoimmune hepatitis
ENDOCRINE AND METABOLIC	Growth failure, delayed sexual maturation Thyroiditis Osteoporosis, osteomalacia
NEUROLOGIC	Peripheral neuropathy Meningitis Vestibular dysfunction Pseudotumor cerebri

G6PD, glucose-6-phosphate dehydrogenase; IBD, inflammatory bowel disease; PSC, primary sclerosing cholangitis.
Modified from Kugathasan S: Diarrhea. In Kliegman RM, Greenbaum LA, Lye PS, editors: *Practical strategies in pediatric diagnosis and therapy*, ed 2, Philadelphia, 2004, Saunders, p 285.

colitis in Israel varies with the country of origin; those born in Asia or Africa have the lowest risk. The prevalence of ulcerative colitis in northern European countries and the United States varies from 100 to 200/100,000 population. Men are slightly more likely to acquire ulcerative colitis than are women; the reverse is true for Crohn disease.

CLINICAL MANIFESTATIONS

Blood, mucus, and pus in the stool as well as diarrhea are the typical presentation of ulcerative colitis. Constipation may be observed in those with proctitis. Symptoms such as tenesmus, urgency, cramping abdominal pain (especially with bowel movements), and nocturnal bowel movements are common. The mode of onset ranges from insidious with gradual progression of symptoms to acute and fulminant. Fever, severe anemia, hypoalbuminemia, leukocytosis, and more than 5 bloody stools per day for 5 days define **fulminant colitis.** Chronicity is an important part of the diagnosis; it is difficult to know if a patient has a subacute, transient infectious colitis or ulcerative colitis when a child has had 1-2 weeks of symptoms. Symptoms beyond this duration often prove to be secondary to IBD. Anorexia, weight loss, and growth failure may be present, although these complications are more typical of Crohn disease.

Extraintestinal manifestations that tend to occur more commonly with ulcerative colitis than with Crohn disease include pyoderma gangrenosum, sclerosing cholangitis, chronic active hepatitis, and ankylosing spondylitis. Iron deficiency can result from chronic blood loss as well as decreased intake. Folate deficiency is unusual but may be accentuated in children treated with sulfasalazine, which interferes with folate absorption. Chronic inflammation and the elaboration of a variety of inflammatory cytokines can interfere with erythropoiesis and result in the anemia of chronic disease. Secondary amenorrhea is common during periods of active disease.

The clinical course of ulcerative colitis is marked by remission and relapse, often without apparent explanation. After treatment of initial symptoms, ~5% of children with ulcerative colitis have a prolonged remission (>3 yr). About 25% of children presenting with severe ulcerative colitis require colectomy within 5 yr of diagnosis, compared with only 5% of those presenting with mild disease. It is important to consider the possibility of enteric infection with recurrent symptoms; these infections can mimic a flare-up or actually provoke a recurrence. The use of nonsteroidal anti-inflammatory drugs is considered by some to predispose to exacerbation.

It is generally believed that the risk of colon cancer begins to increase after 8-10 yr of disease and can then increase by 0.5-1% per yr. The risk is delayed by ~10 yr in patients with colitis limited to the descending colon. Proctitis alone is associated with virtually no increase in risk over the general population. Because colon cancer is usually preceded by changes of mucosal dysplasia, it is recommended that patients who have had ulcerative colitis for >10 yr be screened with colonoscopy and biopsies every 1-2 yr. Although this is the current standard of practice, it is not clear if morbidity and mortality are changed by this approach. Two competing concerns about this plan of management remain unresolved: The original studies may have overestimated the risk of colon cancer and, therefore, the need for surveillance has been overemphasized; and screening for dysplasia might not be adequate for preventing colon cancer in ulcerative colitis if some cancers are not preceded by dysplasia.

DIFFERENTIAL DIAGNOSIS

The major conditions to exclude are infectious colitis, allergic colitis, and Crohn colitis. Every child with a new diagnosis of ulcerative colitis should have stool cultured for enteric pathogens, stool evaluation for ova and parasites, and perhaps serologic studies for amebae (Table 328-3). In the setting of antibiotic use, pseudomembranous colitis secondary to *Clostridium difficile* should be considered. Cytomegalovirus infection can mimic ulcerative colitis or be associated with an exacerbation of existing disease. The most difficult distinction is from Crohn disease because the colitis of Crohn disease can initially appear identical to that of ulcerative colitis, particularly in younger children. The gross appearance of the colitis or development of small bowel disease eventually leads to the correct diagnosis; this can occur years after the initial presentation.

At the onset, the colitis of hemolytic-uremic syndrome may be identical to that of early ulcerative colitis. Ultimately, signs of microangiopathic hemolysis (the presence of schistocytes on blood smear), thrombocytopenia, and subsequent renal failure should confirm the diagnosis of hemolytic-uremic syndrome. Although Henoch-Schönlein purpura can manifest as abdominal pain and bloody stools, it is not usually associated with colitis. Behçet disease can be distinguished by its typical features (Chapter 155). Other considerations are radiation proctitis, viral colitis in immunocompromised patients, and ischemic colitis (Table 328-4). In infancy, dietary protein intolerance can be confused with ulcerative colitis, although the former is a transient problem that resolves on removal of the offending protein, and ulcerative colitis is extremely rare in this age group. Hirschsprung disease can produce an enterocolitis before or within months after surgical correction; this is unlikely to be confused with ulcerative colitis.

DIAGNOSIS

The diagnosis of ulcerative colitis or ulcerative proctitis requires a typical presentation in the absence of an identifiable specific cause (see Tables 328-3 and 328-4) and typical endoscopic and histologic findings (see Table 328-1). One should be hesitant to make a diagnosis of ulcerative colitis in a child who has experienced symptoms for <2-3 wk until infection has been excluded. When the diagnosis is suspected in a child with subacute symptoms, the physician should make a firm diagnosis only when there is evidence of chronicity on colonic biopsy. Laboratory studies can demonstrate evidence of anemia (either iron deficiency or the anemia of chronic disease) or hypoalbuminemia. Although the sedimentation rate and C-reactive protein are often elevated, they may be normal even with fulminant colitis. An elevated white blood cell count is usually seen only with more-severe colitis. Fecal calprotectin levels are usually elevated. Barium enema is suggestive but not diagnostic of acute (Fig. 328-1) or chronic burned-out disease (Fig. 328-2).

The diagnosis of ulcerative colitis must be confirmed by endoscopic and histologic examination of the colon. Classically, disease starts in the rectum with a gross appearance characterized by erythema, edema, loss of vascular pattern, granularity, and friability. There may be a "cutoff" demarcating the margin between inflammation and normal colon, or the entire colon may be involved. There may be some variability in the intensity of inflammation even in those areas involved. Flexible sigmoidoscopy can confirm the diagnosis; colonoscopy can evaluate the extent of disease and rule out Crohn colitis. A colonoscopy should not be performed when fulminant colitis is suspected because of the risk of provoking *toxic megacolon* or causing a perforation during the procedure. The degree of colitis can be evaluated by the gross appearance of the mucosa. One does not generally see discrete ulcers, which would be more suggestive of Crohn colitis. The endoscopic findings of ulcerative colitis result from microulcers, which give the appearance of a diffuse abnormality. With very severe chronic colitis, pseudopolyps may be seen. Biopsy of involved bowel demonstrates evidence of acute and chronic mucosal inflammation. Typical histologic findings are cryptitis, crypt abscesses, separation of crypts by inflammatory cells, foci of acute inflammatory cells, edema, mucus depletion, and branching of crypts. The last finding is not seen in

Table 328-3 INFECTIOUS AGENTS MIMICKING INFLAMMATORY BOWEL DISEASE

AGENT	MANIFESTATIONS	DIAGNOSIS	COMMENTS
BACTERIAL			
Campylobacter jejuni	Acute diarrhea, fever, fecal blood, and leukocytes	Culture	Common in adolescents, may relapse
Yersinia enterocolitica	Acute → chronic diarrhea, right lower quadrant pain, mesenteric adenitis- pseudoappendicitis, fecal blood, and leukocytes Extraintestinal manifestations, mimics Crohn disease	Culture	Common in adolescents as FUO, weight loss, abdominal pain
Clostridium difficile	Postantibiotic onset, watery → bloody diarrhea, pseudomembrane on sigmoidoscopy	Cytotoxin assay	May be nosocomial Toxic megacolon possible
Escherichia coli 0157:H7	Colitis, fecal blood, abdominal pain	Culture and typing	Hemolytic-uremic syndrome
Salmonella	Watery → bloody diarrhea, food borne, fecal leukocytes, fever, pain, cramps	Culture	Usually acute
Shigella	Watery → bloody diarrhea, fecal leukocytes, fever, pain, cramps	Culture	Dysentery symptoms
Edwardsiella tarda	Bloody diarrhea, cramps	Culture	Ulceration on endoscopy
Aeromonas hydrophila	Cramps, diarrhea, fecal blood	Culture	May be chronic Contaminated drinking water
Plesiomonas	Diarrhea, cramps	Culture	Shellfish source
Tuberculosis	Rarely bovine, now *Mycobacterium tuberculosis* Ileocecal area, fistula formation	Culture, PPD, biopsy	Can mimic Crohn disease
PARASITES			
Entamoeba histolytica	Acute bloody diarrhea and liver abscess, colic	Trophozoite in stool, colonic mucosal flask ulceration, serologic tests	Travel to endemic area
Giardia lamblia	Foul-smelling, watery diarrhea, cramps, flatulence, weight loss; no colonic involvement	"Owl"-like trophozoite and cysts in stool; rarely duodenal intubation	May be chronic
AIDS-ASSOCIATED ENTEROPATHY			
Cryptosporidium	Chronic diarrhea, weight loss	Stool microscopy	Mucosal findings not like IBD
Isospora belli	As in Cryptosporidium		Tropical location
Cytomegalovirus	Colonic ulceration, pain, bloody diarrhea	Culture, biopsy	More common when on immunosuppressive medications

FUO, fever of unknown origin; IBD, inflammatory bowel disease; PPD, purified protein derivative.

Table 328-4 CHRONIC INFLAMMATORY-LIKE INTESTINAL DISORDERS

INFECTION (SEE TABLE 328-3)
Bacterial Parasite
AIDS-ASSOCIATED
TOXIN
IMMUNE-INFLAMMATORY
Congenital immunodeficiency disorders Acquired immunodeficiency diseases Dietary protein enterocolitis Behçet disease Lymphoid nodular hyperplasia Eosinophilic gastroenteritis Graft versus host disease
VASCULAR-ISCHEMIC DISORDERS
Systemic vasculitis (SLE, dermatomyositis) Henoch-Schönlein purpura Hemolytic-uremic syndrome
OTHER
Prestenotic colitis Diversion colitis Radiation colitis Neonatal necrotizing enterocolitis Typhlitis Hirschsprung colitis Intestinal lymphoma Laxative abuse

SLE, systemic lupus erythematosus.

infectious colitis. Granulomas, fissures, or full-thickness involvement of the bowel wall (usually on surgical rather than endoscopic biopsy) suggest Crohn disease.

Perianal disease, with the exception of mild local irritation or anal fissures associated with diarrhea, should make the clinician think of Crohn disease. Plain radiographs of the abdomen might demonstrate loss of haustral markings in an air-filled colon or marked dilation with toxic megacolon. With severe colitis, the colon may become dilated; a diameter of >6 cm, determined radiographically, in an adult suggests toxic megacolon. If it is necessary to examine the colon radiologically in a child with severe colitis (to evaluate the extent of involvement or to try to rule out Crohn disease), it is sometimes helpful to perform an upper GI contrast series with small bowel follow-through and then look at delayed films of the colon. A barium enema is contraindicated in the setting of a potential toxic megacolon.

TREATMENT

Medical

A medical cure for ulcerative colitis is not available; treatment is aimed at controlling symptoms and reducing the risk of recurrence, with a secondary goal of minimizing steroid exposure. The intensity of treatment varies with the severity of the symptoms. About 20-30% of patients with ulcerative colitis have spontaneous improvement in symptoms.

The first drug class to be used with mild colitis is an aminosalicylate. Sulfasalazine is composed of a sulfur moiety linked to the active ingredient 5-aminosalicylate (5-ASA). This linkage prevents the premature absorption of the medication in the upper GI tract, allowing it to reach the colon, where the 2 components are separated by bacterial cleavage. The dose of sulfasalazine is

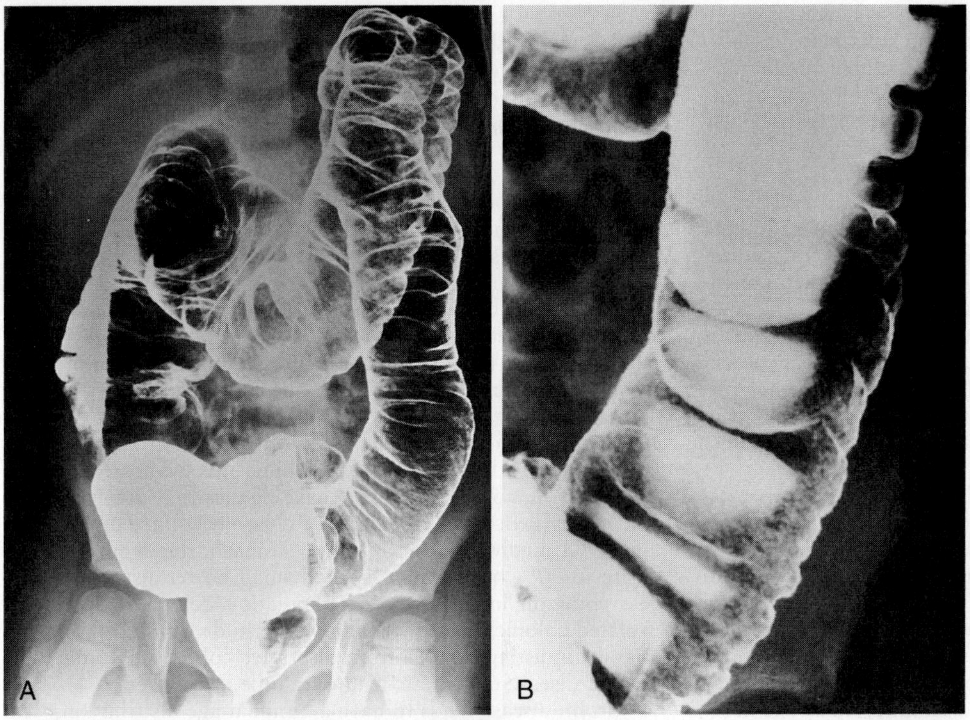

Figure 328-1 Ulcerative colitis. Double-contrast barium enema in a 5 yr old boy who had had intermittent intestinal and extraintestinal symptoms since the age of 3 yr. *A,* Small ulcerations are distributed uniformly about the colonic circumference and continuously from the rectum to the proximal transverse colon. This pattern of involvement is typical of ulcerative colitis. *B,* In this coned view of the sigmoid in the same patient, small ulcerations are represented by fine spiculation of the colonic contour in tangent and by fine stippling of the colon surface en face. (From The child with diarrhea. In Hoffman AD, Hilton SW, Edwards DK, editors: *Practical pediatric radiology,* ed 2, Philadelphia, 1994, WB Saunders, p 260.)

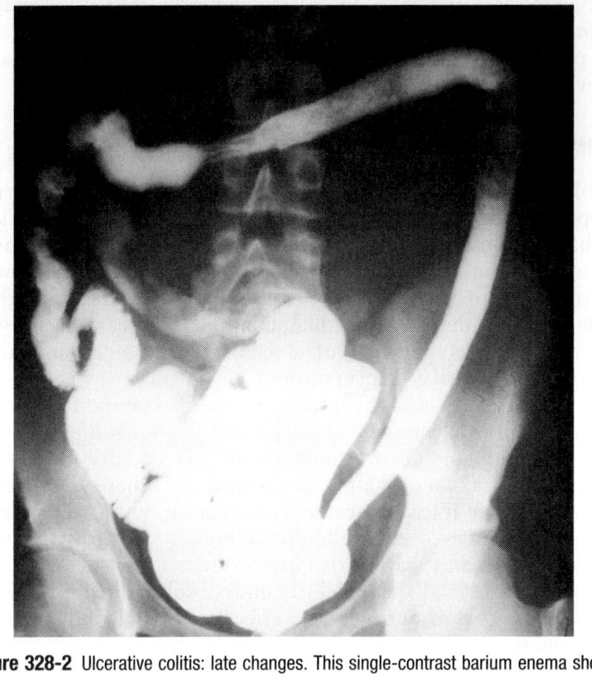

Figure 328-2 Ulcerative colitis: late changes. This single-contrast barium enema shows the late changes of ulcerative colitis in a 15 yr old girl. The colon is featureless, reduced in caliber, and shortened. Dilatation of the terminal ileum (backwash ileitis) is present. (From The child with diarrhea. In Hoffman AD, Hilton SW, Edwards DK, editors: *Practical pediatric radiology,* ed 2, Philadelphia, 1994, WB Saunders, p 262.)

50-75 mg/kg/24 hr (divided into 2-4 doses). Generally, the dose is not more than 2-4 g/24 hr. Hypersensitivity to the sulfa component is the major side effect of sulfasalazine and occurs in 10-20% of patients. Because of poor tolerance, sulfasalazine is used less commonly than other, better tolerated 5-ASA preparations (mesalamine, 50-100 mg/kg/day; balsalazide 110-175 mg/kg/day). Sulfasalazine and the 5-ASA preparations have been shown to effectively treat active ulcerative colitis and to prevent recurrence. It is recommended that the medication be continued even when the disorder is in remission. These medications might also decrease the lifetime risk of colon cancer.

Approximately 5% of patients have an allergic reaction to 5-ASA, manifesting as rash, fever, and bloody diarrhea, which can be difficult to distinguish from symptoms of a flare of ulcerative colitis. 5-ASA can also be given in enema or suppository form and is especially useful for proctitis. Hydrocortisone enemas are used to treat proctitis as well, but they are probably not as effective. Oral and rectal 5-ASA has been shown to be more effective than just oral 5-ASA for distal colitis.

Probiotics have been shown to be effective in adults for maintenance of remission for ulcerative colitis, although they have not been shown to induce remission during an active flare. The most promising role for probiotics has been to prevent pouchitis, a common complication following surgery.

Children with moderate to severe pancolitis or colitis that is unresponsive to 5-ASA therapy should be treated with oral corticosteroids, most commonly, prednisone. The usual starting dose of prednisone is 1-2 mg/kg/24 hr (40-60 mg maximum dose). This medication can be given once daily. With severe colitis, the dose can be divided twice daily and can be given intravenously. Steroids are considered an effective medication for acute flares, but they are not appropriate maintenance medications due to loss of effect and side effects, including growth retardation, adrenal suppression, cataracts, osteopenia, aseptic necrosis of the head of the femur, glucose intolerance, risk of infection, and cosmetic effects. For a hospitalized patient with persistence of symptoms despite intravenous steroid treatment for 5-7 days, escalation of therapy or surgical options should be considered.

With medical management, most children are in remission within 3 mo; however, 5-10% continue to have symptoms unresponsive to treatment beyond 6 mo. Many children with disease requiring frequent corticosteroid therapy are started on immunomodulators such as azathioprine (2.0-2.5 mg/kg/day) or 6-mercaptopurine (1-1.5 mg/kg/day). Uncontrolled data suggest a corticosteroid-sparing effect in many treated patients. Lymphoproliferative disorders are associated with thiopurine use. Cyclosporine, which has been associated with improvement in some children with severe or fulminant colitis, is rarely used owing to high side-effect profile, the inability of this medication to change the natural history of disease, and increasing use of infliximab, a chimeric monoclonal antibody to tumor necrosis factor (TNF)-α, also effective in cases of fulminant colitis. Infliximab has also been shown to be effective for induction and maintenance therapy in adults with moderate to severe disease. TNF blocking agents are associated with an increased risk of infection (particularly tuberculosis) and malignancies (lymphoma, leukemia).

Surgical

Colectomy is performed for intractable disease, complications of therapy, and fulminant disease that is unresponsive to medical management. No clear benefit of the use of total parenteral nutrition or a continuous enteral elemental diet in the treatment of severe ulcerative colitis has been noted. Nevertheless, parenteral nutrition is used if oral intake is insufficient so that the patient will be nutritionally ready for surgery if medical management fails. With any medical treatment for ulcerative colitis, the clinician should always weigh the risk of the medication or therapy against the fact that colitis can be successfully treated surgically.

Surgical treatment for intractable or fulminant colitis is total colectomy. The optimal approach is to combine colectomy with an endorectal pull-through, where a segment of distal rectum is retained and the mucosa is stripped from this region. The distal ileum is pulled down and sutured at the internal anus with a J pouch created from ileum immediately above the rectal cuff. This procedure allows the child to maintain continence. Commonly, a temporary ileostomy is created to protect the delicate anastomosis between the sleeve of the pouch and the rectum. The ileostomy is usually closed within several months, restoring bowel continuity. At that time, stool frequency is often increased but may be improved with loperamide. The major complication of this operation is *pouchitis,* which is a chronic inflammatory reaction in the pouch, leading to bloody diarrhea, abdominal pain, and, occasionally, low-grade fever. The cause of this complication is unknown, although it is more common when the ileal pouch has been constructed for ulcerative colitis than for other indications (e.g., familial polyposis coli). Pouchitis is seen in 30-40% of patients who had ulcerative colitis. It commonly responds to treatment with oral metronidazole or ciprofloxacin. Probiotics have also been shown to decrease the rate of pouchitis as well as the recurrence of pouchitis following antibiotic therapy.

Support

Psychosocial support is an important part of therapy for this disorder. This may include adequate discussion of the disease manifestations and management between patient and physician, psychological counseling for the child when necessary, and family support from a social worker or family counselor. Patient support groups have proved helpful for some families. Children with ulcerative colitis should be encouraged to participate fully in age-appropriate activities; however, activity may need to be reduced during periods of disease exacerbation.

PROGNOSIS

The course of ulcerative colitis is marked by remissions and exacerbations. Most children with this disorder respond initially to medical management. Many children with mild manifestations continue to respond well to medical management and may stay in remission on a prophylactic 5-ASA preparation for long periods. An occasional child with mild onset, however, experiences intractable symptoms at a later time. Beyond the 1st decade of disease, the risk of development of colon cancer begins to increase rapidly. The risk of colon cancer may be diminished with surveillance colonoscopies beginning after 8-10 yr of disease. Detection of significant dysplasia on biopsy would prompt colectomy.

BIBLIOGRAPHY

Please visit the Nelson Textbook of Pediatrics *website at www.expertconsult.com for the complete bibliography.*

328.2 Crohn Disease (Regional Enteritis, Regional Ileitis, Granulomatous Colitis)

Andrew B. Grossman and Robert N. Baldassano

Crohn disease, an idiopathic, chronic inflammatory disorder of the bowel, involves any region of the alimentary tract from the mouth to the anus. Although there are many similarities between ulcerative colitis and Crohn disease, there are also major differences in the clinical course and distribution of the disease in the GI tract (see Table 328-1). The inflammatory process tends to be eccentric and segmental, often with skip areas (normal regions of bowel between inflamed areas). Although inflammation in ulcerative colitis is limited to the mucosa (except in toxic megacolon), GI involvement in Crohn disease is often transmural.

Compared to adult-onset disease, pediatric Crohn disease is more likely to have extensive anatomic involvement. At initial presentation, >50% of patients have disease that involves ileum and colon (ileocolitis), 20% have exclusively colonic disease, and upper GI involvement (esophagus, stomach, duodenum) is seen in up to 30% of children. Isolated small bowel disease is much less common in the pediatric population compared to adults. Isolated colonic disease is common in children <8 yr of age and may be indistinguishable from ulcerative colitis. Anatomic location of disease tends to extend over time in children.

Crohn disease tends to have a bimodal age distribution, with the 1st peak beginning in the teenage years. The incidence of Crohn disease has been increasing, whereas that of ulcerative colitis has been stable. In the United States, the reported incidence of pediatric Crohn disease is 4.56/100,000 and the pediatric prevalence is 43/100,000.

CLINICAL MANIFESTATIONS

Crohn disease can be characterized as inflammatory, stricturing, or penetrating. Patients with small bowel disease are more likely to have an obstructive pattern (most commonly with right lower quadrant pain) characterized by fibrostenosis, and those with colonic disease are more likely to have symptoms resulting from inflammation (diarrhea, bleeding, cramping). Disease phenotypes often change as duration of disease lengthens (inflammatory becomes structuring or penetrating).

Systemic signs and symptoms are more common in Crohn disease than in ulcerative colitis. Fever, malaise, and easy fatigability are common. Growth failure with delayed bone maturation and delayed sexual development can precede other symptoms by 1 or 2 yr and is at least twice as likely to occur with Crohn disease as with ulcerative colitis. Children can present with growth failure as the only manifestation of Crohn disease. Causes of growth failure include inadequate caloric intake, suboptimal absorption or excessive loss of nutrients, the effects of chronic inflammation on bone metabolism and appetite, and the use of corticosteroids during treatment. Primary or secondary amenorrhea and pubertal delay are common. In contrast to ulcerative colitis, perianal disease is common (tags, fistula, abscess). Gastric or duodenal involvement may be associated with recurrent vomiting and epigastric pain. Partial small bowel obstruction, usually secondary to narrowing of the bowel lumen from inflammation or stricture, can cause symptoms of cramping abdominal pain (especially with meals), borborygmus, and intermittent abdominal distention (Fig. 328-3). Stricture should be suspected if the child notes relief of symptoms in association with a sudden sensation of gurgling of intestinal contents through a localized region of the abdomen.

Penetrating disease is demonstrated by fistula formation. Enteroenteric or enterocolonic fistulas (between segments of bowel) are often asymptomatic but can contribute to malabsorption if they have high output or result in bacterial overgrowth (Fig. 328-4). Enterovesical fistulas (between bowel and urinary

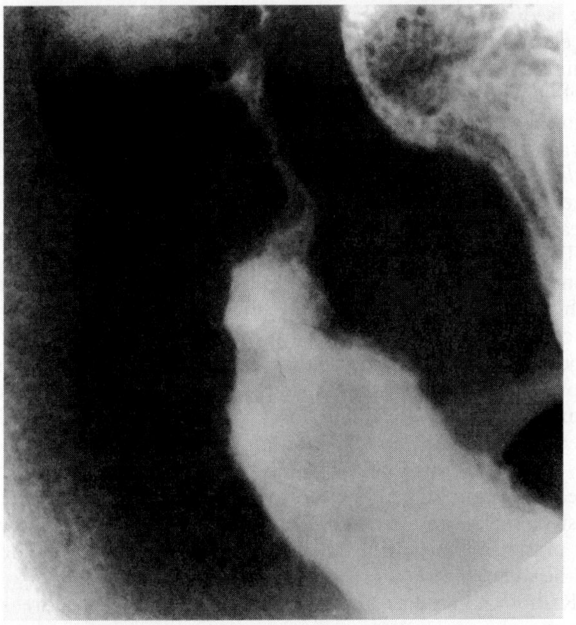

Figure 328-3 Stenotic Crohn disease. Severe stenosis of the terminal ileum is present in this 16 yr old boy. Inflammatory effacement of the mucosal folds and small ulcerations characterize the proximal nonstenotic segment. (From The child with diarrhea. In Hoffman AD, Hilton SW, Edwards DK, editors: *Practical pediatric radiology*, ed 2, Philadelphia, 1994, WB Saunders, p 267.)

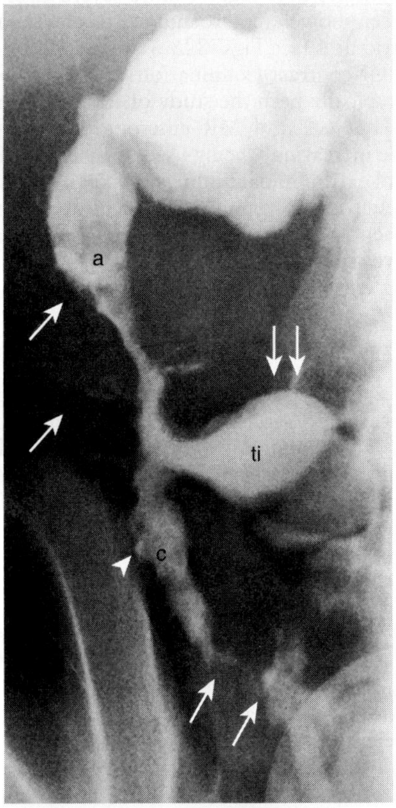

Figure 328-4 Crohn disease: sinuses and fistula. Severe ileocolitis has resulted in an ileocecal fistula *(single arrows, lower)* and sinus formation in the ascending colon (a) *(arrows on platform)*. c, cecum *(arrowhead);* ti, terminal ileum *(paired arrows)*. (From The child with diarrhea. In Hoffman AD, Hilton SW, Edwards DK, editors: *Practical pediatric radiology*, ed 2, Philadelphia, 1994, WB Saunders, p 268.)

bladder) originate from ileum or sigmoid colon and appear as signs of urinary infection, pneumaturia, or fecaluria. Enterovaginal fistulas originate from the rectum, cause feculent vaginal drainage, and are difficult to manage. Enterocutaneous fistulas (between bowel and abdominal skin) often are caused by prior surgical anastomoses with leakage. Intra-abdominal abscess may be associated with fever and pain but might have relatively few symptoms. Hepatic or splenic abscess can occur with or without a local fistula. Anorectal abscesses often originate immediately above the anus at the crypts of Morgagni. The patterns of perianal fistulas are complex because of the different tissue planes. Perianal abscess is usually painful, but perianal fistulas tend to produce fewer symptoms than anticipated. Purulent drainage is commonly associated with perianal fistulas. **Psoas abscess** secondary to intestinal fistula can present as hip pain, decreased hip extension (psoas sign), and fever.

Extraintestinal manifestations occur more commonly with Crohn disease than with ulcerative colitis; those that are especially associated with Crohn disease include oral aphthous ulcers, peripheral arthritis, erythema nodosum, digital clubbing, episcleritis, renal stones (uric acid, oxalate), and gallstones. Any of the extraintestinal disorders described in the section on IBD can occur with Crohn disease (see Table 328-2). The peripheral arthritis is nondeforming. The occurrence of extraintestinal manifestations usually correlates with the presence of colitis.

Extensive involvement of small bowel, especially in association with surgical resection, can lead to short bowel syndrome, which is rare in children. Complications of terminal ileal dysfunction or resection include bile acid malabsorption with secondary diarrhea and vitamin B_{12} malabsorption. Chronic steatorrhea can lead to oxaluria with secondary renal stones. Increasing calcium intake can actually decrease the risk renal stones secondary to ileal inflammation. The risk of cholelithiasis is also increased secondary to bile acid depletion.

A disorder with this diversity of manifestations can have a major impact on an affected child's lifestyle. Fortunately, the majority of children with Crohn disease are able to continue with their normal activities, having to limit activity only during periods of increased symptoms.

DIFFERENTIAL DIAGNOSIS

The most common diagnoses to be distinguished from Crohn disease are the infectious enteropathies (in the case of Crohn disease: acute terminal ileitis, infectious colitis, enteric parasites, and periappendiceal abscess) (see Tables 328-3, 328-4, and 328-5). *Yersinia* can cause many of the radiologic and endoscopic findings in the distal small bowel that are seen in Crohn disease. The symptoms of bacterial dysentery are more likely to be mistaken for ulcerative colitis than for Crohn disease. Celiac disease and *Giardia* infection have been noted to produce a Crohn-like presentation including diarrhea, weight loss, and protein-losing enteropathy. GI tuberculosis is rare but can mimic Crohn disease. Foreign-body perforation of the bowel (toothpick) can mimic a localized region with Crohn disease. Small bowel lymphoma can mimic Crohn disease but tends to be associated with nodular filling defects of the bowel without ulceration or narrowing of the lumen. Bowel lymphoma is much less common in children than is Crohn disease. Recurrent functional abdominal pain can mimic the pain of small bowel Crohn disease. *Lymphoid nodular hyperplasia* of the terminal ileum (a normal finding) may be mistaken for Crohn ileitis. Right lower quadrant pain or mass with fever can be the result of periappendiceal abscess. This entity is occasionally associated with diarrhea as well.

Growth failure may be the only manifestation of Crohn disease; other disorders such as growth hormone deficiency, gluten-sensitive enteropathy (celiac disease), Turner syndrome, or anorexia nervosa must be considered. If arthritis precedes the bowel manifestations, an initial diagnosis of juvenile idiopathic

Table 328-5 DIFFERENTIAL DIAGNOSIS OF PRESENTING SYMPTOMS OF CROHN DISEASE

PRIMARY PRESENTING SYMPTOM	DIAGNOSTIC CONSIDERATIONS
Right lower quadrant abdominal pain, with or without mass	Appendicitis, infection (e.g., *Campylobacter, Yersinia* spp.), lymphoma, intussusception, mesenteric adenitis, Meckel diverticulum, ovarian cyst
Chronic periumbilical or epigastric abdominal pain	Irritable bowel syndrome, constipation, lactose intolerance, peptic disease
Rectal bleeding, no diarrhea	Fissure, polyp, Meckel diverticulum, rectal ulcer syndrome
Bloody diarrhea	Infection, hemolytic-uremic syndrome, Henoch-Schönlein purpura, ischemic bowel, radiation colitis
Watery diarrhea	Irritable bowel syndrome, lactose intolerance, giardiasis, *Cryptosporidium* infection, sorbitol, laxatives
Perirectal disease	Fissure, hemorrhoid (rare), streptococcal infection, condyloma (rare)
Growth delay	Endocrinopathy
Anorexia, weight loss	Anorexia nervosa
Arthritis	Collagen vascular disease, infection
Liver abnormalities	Chronic hepatitis

From Kugathasan S: Diarrhea. In Kliegman RM, Greenbaum LA, Lye PS, editors: *Practical strategies in pediatric diagnosis and therapy*, ed 2, Philadelphia, 2004, Saunders, p 287.

arthritis may be made. Refractory anemia may be the presenting feature and may be mistaken for a primary hematologic disorder. Leukemia can manifest with abdominal pain in association with an abnormal blood cell count and might initially be mistaken for Crohn disease. Chronic granulomatous disease of childhood can cause inflammatory changes in the bowel as well as perianal disease. Antral narrowing in this disorder may be mistaken for a stricture secondary to Crohn disease.

DIAGNOSIS

Crohn disease can manifest as a variety of symptom combinations. At the onset, symptoms may be subtle (growth retardation, abdominal pain alone); this explains why the diagnosis might not be made until 1 or 2 years after the start of symptoms. The diagnosis of Crohn disease depends on finding typical clinical features of the disorder (history, physical examination, laboratory studies, and endoscopic or radiologic findings), ruling out specific entities that mimic Crohn disease, and demonstrating chronicity. The history can include any combination of abdominal pain (especially right lower quadrant), diarrhea, vomiting, anorexia, weight loss, growth retardation, and extraintestinal manifestations. Only 25% initially have the triad of diarrhea, weight loss, and abdominal pain. Most do not have diarrhea, and only 25% have GI bleeding.

Children with Crohn disease often appear chronically ill. They commonly have weight loss and growth failure, and they are often malnourished. The earliest of sign of growth failure is decreased height velocity, which can be present in up to 88% of prepubertal patients with Crohn disease and typically precedes symptoms. Children with Crohn disease often appear pale, with decreased energy level and poor appetite; the latter finding sometimes results from an association between meals and abdominal pain or diarrhea. There may be abdominal tenderness that is either diffuse or localized to the right lower quadrant. A tender mass or fullness may be palpable in the right lower quadrant. Perianal disease, when present, may be characteristic. Large anal skin tags (1-3 cm diameter) or perianal fistulas with purulent drainage suggest Crohn disease. Digital clubbing, findings of arthritis, and skin manifestations may be present.

A complete blood cell count commonly demonstrates anemia, often with a component of iron deficiency. Although the erythrocyte sedimentation rate is often elevated, it may be normal; an elevated platelet count is common. The white blood cell count may be normal or mildly elevated. The serum albumin level may be low, indicating small bowel inflammation or protein-losing enteropathy. Fecal calprotectin or lactoferrin is often elevated. Anti–*Saccharomyces cerevisiae* antibodies, antibody to *Escherichia coli* outer membrane porin (anti-OmpC), and anti-flagellin (anti-CBir1) antibodies are associated with Crohn's disease.

The small and large bowel and the upper GI tract should be examined by both endoscopic and radiologic studies in the child with suspected Crohn disease. Esophagogastroduodenoscopy and ileocolonoscopy should be performed to properly assess the upper GI tract, terminal ileum, and entire colon. Findings on colonoscopy can include patchy, nonspecific inflammatory changes (erythema, friability, loss of vascular pattern), aphthous ulcers, linear ulcers, nodularity, and strictures. Findings on biopsy may be only nonspecific chronic inflammatory changes. Noncaseating granulomas, similar to those of sarcoidosis, are the most characteristic histologic findings, although often they are not present. Transmural inflammation is also characteristic but can be identified only in surgical specimens.

Radiologic studies are necessary to assess the entire small bowel and investigate for evidence of structuring or penetrating disease. A variety of findings may be apparent on radiologic studies. Plain films of the abdomen may be normal or might demonstrate findings of partial small bowel obstruction or thumb-printing of the colon wall. An upper GI contrast study with small bowel follow-through might show aphthous ulceration and thickened, nodular folds as well as narrowing or stricturing of the lumen. Linear ulcers can give a cobblestone appearance to the mucosal surface. Bowel loops are often separated as a result of thickening of bowel wall and mesentery. Other manifestations on radiographic studies that suggest more-severe Crohn disease are fistulas between bowel (enteroenteric or enterocolonic), sinus tracts, and strictures (see Figs. 328-3 and 328-4).

An upper GI contrast examination with small bowel follow-through has typically been the study of choice for imaging of the small bowel, but CT and MR enterography and small bowel ultrasound are increasingly being used to assess for intestinal wall thickening and extraluminal findings such as abscesses or fistulas. MR of the pelvis is also useful for delineating the extent of perianal involvement. Video capsule endoscopy has revealed evidence of small bowel mucosal lesions in some patients with normal radiologic evaluation.

TREATMENT

Crohn disease cannot be cured by medical or surgical therapy. The aim of treatment is to relieve symptoms and prevent complications of chronic inflammation (anemia, growth failure), prevent relapse, minimize corticosteroid exposure, and, if possible, effect mucosal healing.

Medical

The specific therapeutic modalities used depend on geographic localization of disease, severity of inflammation, age of the patient, and the presence of complications (abscess). For mild terminal ileal disease or mild Crohn disease of the colon, an initial trial of mesalamine (50-100 mg/kg/day, maximum 3-4 g) may be attempted. Specific pharmaceutical preparations have been formulated to release the active 5-ASA compound throughout the small bowel, in the ileum and colon, or exclusively in the colon. Rectal preparations are used for distal colonic inflammation. Antibiotics such as metronidazole (10-20 mg/kg/day) are used for infectious complications, are first-line therapy for perianal disease (although perianal disease usually recurs when antibiotic is discontinued), and they may be effective for treatment of mild to moderate Crohn disease.

Corticosteroids continue to be a mainstay of therapy for acute exacerbations of pediatric Crohn disease because they effectively suppress acute inflammation, rapidly relieving symptoms. For more extensive or severe small bowel or colonic disease, most clinicians initiate therapy with corticosteroids (prednisone, 1-2 mg/kg/day, maximum 40-60 mg). The goal is to taper dosing as soon as the disease becomes quiescent. Clinicians vary in their tapering schedules, and the disease can flare during this process. There is no role for continuing corticosteroids as maintenance therapy because, in addition to their side effects, tolerance develops and steroids have not been shown to change disease course or promote healing of mucosa. A special controlled ileal-release formulation of budesonide, a corticosteroid with local anti-inflammatory activity on the bowel mucosa and with high hepatic first-pass metabolism, is also used for mild to moderate ileal or ileocecal disease (adult dose, 9 mg daily). Budesonide appears to be more effective than mesalamine in the treatment of active ileocolonic disease but is less effective than prednisone. Although less effective than traditional corticosteroids, budesonide does cause less steroid-related side effects.

Unfortunately, up to 50% of children with Crohn disease either become refractory to corticosteroid therapy or become dependent on daily dosing and quickly experience flare of the disease when the dose is decreased. Immunomodulators such as azathioprine (2.0-2.5 mg/kg/day) or 6-mercaptopurine (1.0-1.5 mg/kg/day) may be effective in some children who have a poor response to prednisone or who are steroid dependent. Because a beneficial effect of these drugs can be delayed for 3-6 mo after starting therapy, they are not helpful acutely. The early use of these agents can decrease cumulative prednisone dosages over the 1st 1-2 years of therapy. Genetic variations in the enzyme systems responsible for metabolism of these agents (thiopurine *S*-methyltransferase [TPMT]) can affect response rates and potential toxicity. Lymphoproliferative disorders have developed from thiopurine use in patients with IBD. Methotrexate is another immunomodulator that is effective in the treatment of active Crohn's disease and has been shown to improve height velocity in the 1st year of administration. The advantages of this medication include once-weekly dosing by either subcutaneous or oral route (10 mg weekly for 20-29 kg, 15 mg weekly for 30-39 kg, 20 mg weekly for 40-49 kg, 25 mg weekly for >50 kg) and a more-rapid onset of action (6-8 wk) than azathioprine or 6-mercaptopurine. Folic acid is usually administered concomitantly to decrease medication side effects. The immunomodulators are effective for the treatment of perianal fistulas.

Therapy with antibodies directed against mediators of inflammation is used for patients with Crohn disease. Infliximab (5 mg/kg IV), a chimeric monoclonal antibody to TNF-α, has been shown to be effective for the induction and maintenance of remission and mucosal healing in chronically active moderate to severe Crohn disease, healing of perianal fistulas, and steroid sparing. Pediatric data have additionally supported improved growth with the administration of this medication. The onset of action of infliximab is quite rapid and it is initially given as 3 infusions over a 6 wk period (0, 2, and 6 wk). The durability of response to infliximab is variable and can be as short as 4-8 wk, making maintenance therapy necessary. Side effects include infusion reactions, increased incidence of infections (especially reactivation of latent tuberculosis), increased risk of lymphoma, and the development of autoantibodies and autoimmune disorders (leukocytoclastic vasculitis). The development of antibodies to infliximab (ATI) is associated with an increased incidence of infusion reactions and decreased durability of response. Regularly scheduled dosing of infliximab, as opposed to episodic dosing on an as-needed basis, is associated with decreased levels of ATI. A purified protein derivative (PPD) test for tuberculosis should be done before starting infliximab. Active or latent intra-abdominal infection (abscess) is a contraindication to infliximab therapy. Adalimumab, a subcutaneously administered, fully humanized monocloncal antibody against TNF-α, has also been shown to be effective for the treatment of chronically active moderate to severe Crohn's disease in adults, and it has been used extensively in children for this purpose. Antibodies against interleukin 6, 10, 11, 12, 23, and 23/p40 and intracellular adhesion molecules are being tested.

Exclusive enteral nutritional therapy is an effective primary as well as adjunctive treatment. The enteral nutritional approach (elemental or polymeric diets) is as rapid in onset of response and as effective as the other treatments. Pediatric studies have suggested similar efficacy to prednisone for improvement in clinical symptoms, but enteral nutritional therapy is superior to steroids for actual healing of mucosa. Because elemental diets are relatively unpalatable, they are administered via a nasogastric or gastrostomy infusion, usually overnight. Most children are hesitant to use nasogastric infusion, but once it is begun, most find it is not difficult. The advantages are that it is relatively free of side effects, avoids the problems associated with corticosteroid therapy, and simultaneously addresses the nutritional rehabilitation. Children can participate in normal daytime activities. A major disadvantage of this approach is that patients are not able to eat a regular diet because they are receiving all of their calories from formula. In addition, perianal and colon disease does not respond well. For children with growth failure, this approach may be ideal, however.

High-calorie oral supplements, although effective, are often not tolerated because of early satiety or exacerbation of symptoms (abdominal pain, vomiting, or diarrhea). Nonetheless, they should be offered to children whose weight gain is suboptimal even if they are not candidates for exclusive enteral nutritional therapy. The continuous administration of nocturnal nasogastric feedings for chronic malnutrition and growth failure has been effective with a much lower risk of complications than parenteral hyperalimentation. The efficacy of probiotics and omega-3 fatty acids in the treatment of Crohn disease is controversial.

Surgery

Surgical therapy should be reserved for very specific indications. Recurrence rate after bowel resection is high (>50% by 5 yr); the risk of requiring additional surgery increases with each operation. Potential complications of surgery include development of fistula or stricture, anastomotic leak, postoperative partial small bowel obstruction secondary to adhesions, and short bowel syndrome. Surgery is the treatment of choice for localized disease of small bowel or colon that is unresponsive to medical treatment, bowel perforation, fibrosed stricture with symptomatic partial small bowel obstruction, and intractable bleeding. Intra-abdominal or liver abscess sometimes is successfully treated by ultrasonographic or CT-guided catheter drainage and concomitant intravenous antibiotic treatment. Open surgical drainage is necessary if this approach is not successful. Growth retardation was once considered an indication for resection; without other indications, this approach has not been shown to be beneficial, and medical or nutritional therapy, or both, is preferred.

Perianal abscess often requires drainage unless it drains spontaneously. In general, perianal fistulas should be managed by a combined medical and surgical approach. Often, the surgeon places a seton through the fistula to keep the tract open and actively draining while medical therapy is administered, to help prevent the formation of a perianal abscess. A severely symptomatic perianal fistula can require fistulotomy, but this procedure should be considered only if the location allows the sphincter to remain undamaged.

The surgical approach for Crohn disease is to remove as limited a length of bowel as possible. There is no evidence that removing bowel up to margins that are free of histologic disease has a better outcome than removing only grossly involved areas. The latter approach reduces the risk of short bowel syndrome. Laparoscopic approach is increasingly being used, with decreased postoperative recovery time. One approach to symptomatic small bowel stricture has been to perform a strictureplasty rather than resection. The surgeon makes a longitudinal incision across the stricture but then closes the incision with sutures in a transverse fashion. This is ideal for short strictures without active disease. The reoperation rate is no higher with this approach than with resection, whereas bowel length is preserved. Postoperative medical therapy with agents such as mesalamine, metronidazole, azathioprine, and, more recently, infliximab, is often given to decrease the likelihood of postoperative recurrence.

Severe perianal disease can be incapacitating and difficult to treat if unresponsive to medical management. Colon diversion can allow the area to be less active, but on reconnection of the colon, disease activity usually recurs. Therefore, surgical treatment of severe perianal disease can require colectomy. Procedures that create a continent ileostomy or endorectal pull-through are generally discouraged in Crohn disease because of the risk of recurrence of the disease in remaining bowel. With colectomy, a conventional ileostomy is performed.

Support

Psychosocial issues for the child with Crohn disease include a sense of being different, concerns about body image, difficulty in not participating fully in age-appropriate activities, and family conflict brought on by the added stress of this disease. Social support is an important component of the management of Crohn disease. Parents are often interested in learning about other children with similar problems, but children may be hesitant to participate. Social support and individual psychologic counseling are important in the adjustment to a difficult problem at an age that by itself often has difficult adjustment issues. Patients who are socially "connected" fare better. Ongoing education about the disease is an important aspect of management because children generally fare better if they understand and anticipate problems. The Crohn and Colitis Foundation of America has local chapters throughout the United States.

PROGNOSIS

Crohn disease is a chronic disorder that is associated with high morbidity but low mortality. Symptoms tend to recur despite treatment and often without apparent explanation. Weight loss and growth failure can usually be improved with treatment and attention to nutritional needs. Up to 15% of patients with early growth retardation secondary to Crohn disease have a permanent decrease in linear growth. Osteopenia is particularly common in those with chronic poor nutrition and frequent exposure to high doses of corticosteroids. Some of the extraintestinal manifestations can, in themselves, be major causes of morbidity, including sclerosing cholangitis, chronic active hepatitis, pyoderma gangrenosum, and ankylosing spondylitis.

The region of bowel involved often increases with time, although rapid progression typically occurs early and is subsequently slow. Complications of the inflammatory process tend to increase with time and include bowel strictures, fistulas, perianal disease, and intra-abdominal or retroperitoneal abscess. A majority of patients with Crohn disease eventually require surgery for one of its many complications; the rate of reoperation is high. The time between the onset of symptoms and the need for surgery appears to be shorter in children than in adults. Surgery is unlikely to be curative and should be avoided except for the specific indications noted previously. Repeated small bowel resection, which may be unavoidable, can lead to malabsorption secondary to short bowel syndrome (Chapter 330.7). Resection of terminal ileum can result in bile acid malabsorption with diarrhea and vitamin B_{12} malabsorption. The risk of colon cancer in patients with long-standing Crohn colitis approaches that associated with ulcerative colitis, and screening colonoscopy after 10 years of colonic disease is indicated.

Despite these complications, most children with Crohn disease lead active, full lives with intermittent flare-up in symptoms.

BIBLIOGRAPHY

Please visit the Nelson Textbook of Pediatrics *website at www.expertconsult.com for the complete bibliography.*

Chapter 329 Eosinophilic Gastroenteritis

Andrew B. Grossman and Robert N. Baldassano

Eosinophilic gastroenteritis consists of a group of rare and poorly understood disorders that have in common gastric and small intestine infiltration with eosinophils and peripheral eosinophilia. The esophagus and large intestine may also be involved. Tissue eosinophilic infiltration can be seen in mucosa, muscularis, or serosa. Mucosal involvement can produce nausea, vomiting, diarrhea, abdominal pain, gastrointestinal bleeding, protein-losing enteropathy, or malabsorption. Involvement of the muscularis can produce obstruction (especially of the pylorus), whereas serosal activity produces eosinophilic ascites.

This condition clinically overlaps the dietary protein hypersensitivity disorders of the small bowel and colon. The differential diagnosis also includes celiac disease, chronic granulomatous disease, connective tissue disorders and vasculitides, multiple infections (particularly parasites), hypereosinophilic syndrome, early inflammatory bowel disease, and rarely malignancy. Allergies to multiple foods are often seen, and serum IgE is commonly elevated. Peripheral eosinophilia is present in ~75% of patients with this disorder. The mucosal form is most common and is diagnosed by identifying large numbers of eosinophils in biopsy specimens of gastric antrum or small bowel.

The presentation of eosinophilic gastroenteritis is nonspecific. The most common presenting symptoms include weight loss, diarrhea, growth failure, colicky abdominal pain, bloating, dysphagia, and vomiting. Presentation in infants can be similar to pyloric stenosis. Laboratory testing often reveals peripheral eosinophilia, elevated serum IgE levels, hypoalbuminemia, and anemia.

The disease usually runs a chronic, debilitating course with sporadic severe exacerbations. Although almost always effective for the treatment of isolated eosinophilic esophagitis, elemental diets are not always successful for the treatment of eosinophilic gastroenteritis. Orally administered cromolyn sodium and montelukast are sometimes successful. A majority of patients require treatment with systemic corticosteroids.

BIBLIOGRAPHY

Please visit the Nelson Textbook of Pediatrics *website at www.expertconsult.com for the complete bibliography.*

Chapter 330 Disorders of Malabsorption

David Branski

All disorders of malabsorption are associated with diminished intestinal absorption of one or more dietary nutrients. Malabsorption can result from a defect in the nutrient **digestion** in

Table 330-1 MALABSORPTION DISORDERS AND CHRONIC DIARRHEA ASSOCIATED WITH GENERALIZED MUCOSAL DEFECT

Mucosal disorders
Gluten-sensitive enteropathy (celiac disease)
Cow's milk and other protein-sensitive enteropathies
Eosinophilic enteropathy
Protein-losing enteropathy
Lymphangiectasia (congenital and acquired)
Disorders causing bowel mucosal inflammation, Crohn disease
Congenital bowel mucosal defects
Microvillous inclusion disease
Tufting enteropathy
Carbohydrate-deficient glycoprotein syndrome
Enterocyte heparan sulfate deficiency
Enteric anendocrinosis (*NEUROG 3* mutation)
Immunodeficiency disorders
Congenital immunodeficiency disorders
Selective IgA deficiency (can be associated with celiac disease)
Severe combined immunodeficiency
Agammaglobulinemia
X-linked hypogammaglobulinemia
Wiskott-Aldrich syndrome
Common variable immunodeficiency disease
Chronic granulomatous disease
Acquired immune deficiency
HIV infection
Immunosuppressive therapy and post-bone marrow transplantation
Autoimmune enteropathy
IPEX (*i*mmune dysregulation, *p*olyendocrinopathy, *e*nteropathy, *X*-linked inheritance)
Miscellaneous
Immunoproliferative small intestinal disease
Short bowel syndrome
Chronic malnutrition
Radiation enteritis

IgA, immunoglobulin A.

the intestinal lumen or from defective mucosal **absorption.** Malabsorption disorders can be categorized into generalized mucosal abnormalities usually resulting in malabsorption of multiple nutrients (Table 330-1) or malabsorption of specific nutrients (carbohydrate, fat, protein, vitamins, minerals, and trace elements) (Table 330-2). Almost all the malabsorption disorders are accompanied by chronic diarrhea (Chapter 333).

CLINICAL APPROACH

The clinical features depend on the extent and type of the malabsorbed nutrient. The common presenting features, especially in toddlers with malabsorption, are diarrhea, abdominal distention, and failure to gain weight, with a fall in growth chart percentiles. Physical findings include muscle wasting and the disappearance of the subcutaneous fat, with subsequent loose skinfolds (Fig. 330-1). The nutritional consequences of malabsorption are more dramatic in toddlers because of the limited energy reserves and higher proportion of calorie intake being used for weight gain and linear growth. In older children, malnutrition can result in growth retardation, as is commonly seen in children with late diagnosis of celiac disease. If malabsorption is untreated, linear growth slows, and with prolonged malnutrition, death can follow (Chapter 43). This extreme outcome is usually restricted to children living in the developing world, where resources to provide enteral and parenteral nutrition support may be limited. Specific findings on examination can guide toward a specific disorder; edema is usually associated with protein-losing enteropathy, digital clubbing with cystic fibrosis and celiac disease, perianal excoriation and gaseous abdominal distention with carbohydrate malabsorption, perianal and circumoral rash with acrodermatitis enteropathica, abnormal hair with Menkes syndrome, and the typical facial features diagnostic of the Johanson-Blizzard syndrome.

Table 330-2 CLASSIFICATION OF MALABSORPTION DISORDERS AND CHRONIC DIARRHEA BASED ON THE PREDOMINANT NUTRIENT MALABSORBED

CARBOHYDRATE MALABSORPTION
Lactose malabsorption
Congenital lactase deficiency
Hypolactasia (adult type)
Secondary lactase deficiency
Congenital sucrase-isomaltase deficiency
Glucose galactose malabsorption
FAT MALABSORPTION
Abetalipoproteinemia
Lymphangiectasia
Homozygous hypobetalipoproteinemia
Chylomicron retention disease (Anderson disease)
Cystic fibrosis
Shwachman-Diamond syndrome
Blizzard Johanson syndrome
Pearson syndrome
Secondary exocrine pancreatic insufficiency
Isolated enzyme deficiency
Enterokinase deficiency
Trypsinogen deficiency
Lipase/co-lipase deficiency
Chronic pancreatitis
Protein-calorie malnutrition
Decreased pancreozymin/cholecystokinin secretion
Disrupted enterohepatic circulation of bile salts
Cholestatic liver disease
Bile acid synthetic defects
Bile acid malabsorption (terminal ileal disease)
AMINO ACID MALABSORPTION
Lysinuric protein intolerance (defect in dibasic amino acid transport, Chapter 79.13)
Hartnup disease (defect in free neutral amino acids)
Blue diaper syndrome (isolated tryptophan malabsorption)
Oast-house urine disease (defect in methionine absorption)
Lowe syndrome (lysine and arginine malabsorption)
MINERAL AND VITAMIN MALABSORPTION
Congenital chloride diarrhea
Congenital sodium absorption defect
Acrodermatitis enteropathica (zinc malabsorption)
Menkes disease (copper malabsorption)
Vitamin D–dependent rickets
Folate malabsorption
Congenital
Secondary to mucosal damage (celiac disease)
Vitamin B_{12} malabsorption
Autoimmune pernicious anemia
Decreased gastric acid (H_2 blockers or proton pump inhibitors)
Terminal ileal disease (e.g., Crohn disease) or resection
Inborn errors of vitamin B_{12} transport and metabolism
Primary hypomagnesemia
DRUG INDUCED
Sulfasalazine: folic acid malabsorption
Cholestyramine: calcium and fat malabsorption
Anticonvulsant drugs such as phenytoin (causing vitamin D deficiency and calcium malabsorption)

Many children with malabsorption disorders have very good appetites as they try to compensate for the fecal protein and energy losses. In exocrine pancreatic insufficiency, fecal losses of up to 40% of ingested protein and energy do not lead to malnutrition, as long as they are compensated by an increased appetite. In conditions associated with villous atrophy or inflammation (celiac disease, postinfectious enteropathy), fecal protein and energy losses are usually modest, but associated anorexia and reduced food intake results in malnutrition.

The nutritional assessment is an important part of clinical evaluation in children with malabsorptive disorders (Chapter 41).

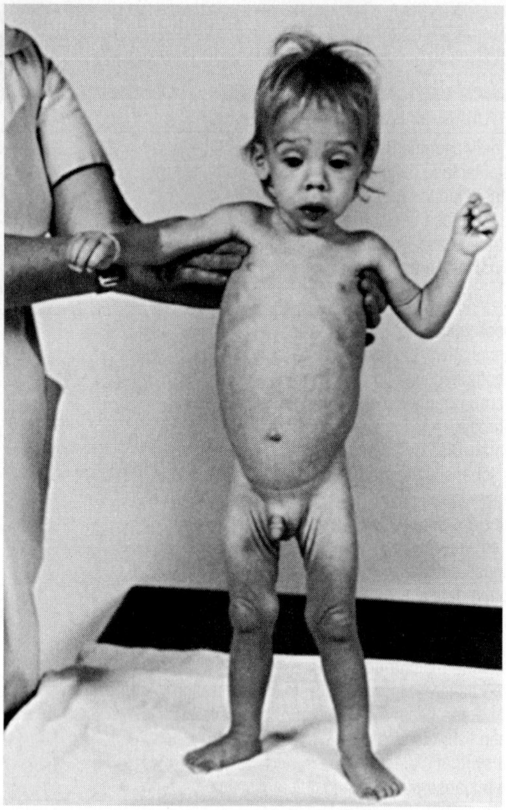

Figure 330-1 An 18 mo old boy with active celiac disease. Note the loose skinfolds, marked proximal muscle wasting, and distended abdomen. The child looks ill.

Long-term calcium and vitamin D malabsorption can lead to reduced bone mineral density and metabolic bone disease, with increased risk of bone fractures. Vitamin K malabsorption, irrespective of the underlying mechanism (fat malabsorption, mucosal atrophy), can result in coagulopathy. Severe protein-losing enteropathy is often associated with malabsorption syndromes (celiac disease, intestinal lymphangiectasia) and causes hypoalbuminemia and edema. Other nutrient deficiencies include iron malabsorption causing microcytic anemia and low reticulocyte count, low serum folate levels in conditions associated with mucosal atrophy, and low serum vitamin A and vitamin E concentrations in fat malabsorption.

Clinical history alone might not be sufficient to make a specific diagnosis, but it can direct the pediatrician toward a more structured and rational investigative approach. Diarrhea is the main clinical expression of malabsorption. Onset of diarrhea in early infancy suggests a congenital defect (Table 330-3). In secretory diarrhea due to disorders such as congenital chloride diarrhea and microvillus inclusion disease, the stool is watery and voluminous and can be mistaken for urine. Onset of symptoms after introduction of a particular food into a child's diet can provide diagnostic clues, such as with sucrose in sucrase-isomaltase deficiency. The nature of the diarrhea may be helpful: explosive watery diarrhea suggests carbohydrate malabsorption; loose, bulky stools are associated with celiac disease; and pasty and yellowish offensive stools suggest an exocrine pancreatic insufficiency. Stool color is usually not helpful; green stool with undigested "peas and carrots" can suggest rapid intestinal transit in toddler's diarrhea, which is a self-limiting condition unassociated with failure to thrive.

Table 330-3 DIARRHEAL DISEASES APPEARING IN THE NEONATAL PERIOD

CONDITION	CLINICAL FEATURES
Microvillus inclusion disease	Secretory watery diarrhea
Tufting enteropathy	Secretory watery diarrhea
Congenital glucose-galactose malabsorption	Acidic diarrhea
Congenital lactase deficiency	Acidic diarrhea
Congenital chloride diarrhea	Hydramnion, secretory watery diarrhea Metabolic alkalosis
Congenital defective jejunal Na^+/H^+ exchange	Hydramnion, secretory watery diarrhea
Congenital bile acid malabsorption	Steatorrhea
Congenital enterokinase deficiency	Failure to thrive, edema
Congenital trypsinogen deficiency	Failure to thrive, edema
Congenital lipase and/or co-lipase deficiency	Failure to thrive, oily stool
Enteric anendocrinosis (*NEUROG 3* mutation)	Hyperchloremic acidosis, failure to thrive

Adapted from Schmitz J: Maldigestion and malabsorption. In Walker WA, Durie PR, Hamilton JR, et al, editors: *Pediatric gastrointestinal disease,* ed 3, Hamilton, Ontario, 2000, BC Decker, p 55.

330.1 Evaluation of Children with Suspected Intestinal Malabsorption

Michael J. Lentze and David Branski

The investigation is guided by the history and physical examination. In a child presenting with chronic or recurrent diarrhea, the initial work-up should include stool cultures and antibody tests for parasites, stool microscopy for ova and parasites such as *Giardia,* and stool occult blood and leukocytes to exclude inflammatory disorders. Stool pH and reducing substances for carbohydrate malabsorption, and quantitative stool fat examination and α_1-antitrypsin to demonstrate fat and protein malabsorption, respectively, should also be determined. Fecal stool elastase-1 can determine exocrine pancreatic insufficiency.

A complete blood count including peripheral smear for microcytic anemia, lymphopenia (lymphangiectasia), neutropenia (Shwachman syndrome), and acanthocytosis (abetalipoproteinemia) is useful. If celiac disease is suspected, serum immunoglobulin A (IgA) and tissue transglutaminase (TG2) antibody levels should be determined. Depending on the initial test results, more-specific investigations can be planned.

INVESTIGATIONS FOR CARBOHYDRATE MALABSORPTION

Measurement of carbohydrate in the stool, using a Clinitest reagent that identifies reducing substances, is a simple screening test. An acidic stool with >2+ reducing substance suggests carbohydrate malabsorption. Sucrose or starch in the stool is not recognized as a reducing sugar until after hydrolysis with hydrochloric acid, which converts them to reducing sugars.

Breath hydrogen test is used to identify the specific carbohydrate that is malabsorbed. After an overnight fast, the suspected sugar (lactose, sucrose, fructose, or glucose) is administered as an oral solution (carbohydrate load 1-2 g/kg, maximum 50 g). In malabsorption, the sugar is not digested or absorbed in the small bowel, passes on to the colon, and is metabolized by the normal bacteria flora. One of the products of this process is hydrogen gas, which is absorbed through the colon mucosa and excreted in the breath. Increased hydrogen concentration in the breath samples suggests carbohydrate malabsorption. A rise in breath hydrogen of 20 ppm above the baseline is considered a positive test. The child should not be on antibiotics at the time of the test, because colonic flora is essential for fermenting the sugar.

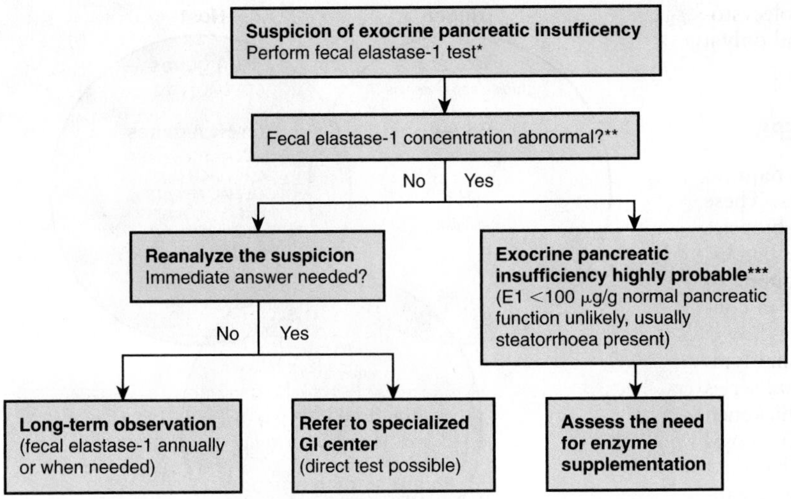

Figure 330-2 Algorithm for assessment of exocrine pancreatic function. *If not available, use other test. Perform appropriate imaging studies of the pancreas. **In case of borderline values, consider repeating the test with three independent samples. ***Consider differential diagnosis (especially consider mucosal villous atrophy and dilution effect of watery stool). GI, gastrointestinal. (Adapted from Walkowiak J, Nousia-Arvanitakis S, Henker J, et al: Indirect pancreatic function tests in children, *J Pediatr Gastroenterol Nutr* 40:107–114, 2005.)

Small bowel mucosal biopsies can measure mucosal disaccharidase (lactase, sucrase, maltase, palatinase) concentrations directly. In primary enzyme deficiencies the mucosal enzyme levels are low and small bowel mucosal morphology is normal. Partial or total villous atrophy due to disorders such as celiac disease, or following rotavirus gastroenteritis can result in secondary disaccharidase deficiency and transient lactose intolerance. The disaccharidase levels revert to normal after mucosal healing.

INVESTIGATIONS FOR FAT MALABSORPTION

The presence of fat globules in the stool suggests fat malabsorption. The ability to assimilate fat varies with age; a premature infant can absorb only 65-75% of dietary fat, a full-term infant absorbs almost 90%, and an older child absorbs >95% of fat while on a regular diet. Quantitative determination of fat malabsorption requires a 3-day stool collection for evaluation of fat excretion and determination of the coefficient of fat absorption:

$$\text{Coefficient of fat absorption (\%)} = (\text{fat intake} - \text{fecal fat losses/fat intake}) \times 100$$

where fat intake and fat losses are in grams. Because fecal fat balance studies are cumbersome, expensive, and unpleasant to perform, simpler tests are often preferred. Among these stool tests, the acid steatocrit test is the most reliable. When bile acid deficiency is suspected of being the cause of fat malabsorption, the evaluation of bile acid levels in duodenal fluid aspirate may be useful.

Fat malabsorption and exocrine pancreatic insufficiency are usually associated with deficiencies of fat-soluble vitamins A, D, E, and K. Serum concentrations of vitamins A, D, and E can be measured. A prolonged prothrombin time is an indirect test to assess vitamin K deficiency.

INVESTIGATIONS FOR PROTEIN LOSING ENTEROPATHY

Dietary and endogenous proteins secreted into the bowel are almost completely absorbed; <1 g of protein from these sources passes into the colon. The majority of the stool nitrogen is derived from gut bacterial proteins. Excessive bowel protein loss usually manifests as **hypoalbuminemia.** However, the most common cause of hypoalbuminemia in children is a renal disorder; therefore, urinary protein excretion must be determined. Other potential causes of hypoalbuminemia include liver disease (reduced production) and inadequate protein intake. Very rarely hypoalbuminemia can result from an extensive skin disorder causing protein loss via the skin. Measurement of stool **α_1-antitrypsin** is a useful screening test for protein-losing enteropathy. This serum protein has a molecular weight similar to albumin's; however, unlike albumin it is resistant to digestion in the gastrointestinal (GI) tract. Excessive α_1-antitrypsin excretion in the stool should prompt further investigations to identify the specific cause of gut or stomach (Menetrier disease) protein loss.

INVESTIGATIONS FOR EXOCRINE PANCREATIC FUNCTION (FIG. 330-2)

Cystic fibrosis is the most common cause of exocrine pancreatic insufficiency in children; therefore, a sweat chloride test must be performed before embarking on invasive tests to investigate possible exocrine pancreatic insufficiency. Many cases of cystic fibrosis are detected by neonatal genetic screening programs; occasional rare mutations are undetected.

Fecal elastase-1 estimation is a sensitive test to assess exocrine pancreatic function in chronic cystic fibrosis and pancreatitis. Elastase-1 is a stable endoprotease unaffected by exogenous pancreatic enzymes. One disadvantage of the fecal elastase-1 test is the lack of full differentiation between primary exocrine pancreatic insufficiency and exocrine pancreatic dysfunction secondary to intestinal villous atrophy. The proximal small bowel is the site for pancreozymin/cholecystokinin production; the latter is the hormone that stimulates enzyme secretion from the exocrine pancreas. Mucosal atrophy can lead to diminished pancreozymin/cholecystokinin secretion and subsequently to exocrine pancreatic insufficiency. Fecal elastase-1 can also give a false-positive result during acute episodes of diarrhea.

Serum trypsinogen concentration can also be used as a screening test for exocrine pancreatic insufficiency. In cystic fibrosis, the levels are greatly elevated early in life, and then they gradually fall, so that by 5-7 yr of age, most patients with cystic fibrosis with pancreatic insufficiency have subnormal levels. Patients with cystic fibrosis and adequate exocrine pancreatic function tend to have normal or elevated levels. In such patients, observing the trend in serial serum trypsinogen estimation may be useful in monitoring exocrine pancreatic function. In Shwachman syndrome, another condition associated with exocrine pancreatic insufficiency, the serum trypsinogen level is low.

Other tests for pancreatic insufficiency (NBT-PABA test and pancreolauryl test) measure urine or breath concentrations of substances released and absorbed across the mucosal surface following pancreatic digestion. These tests lack specificity and are rarely used in clinical practice.

The gold standard test for exocrine pancreatic function is direct analysis of **duodenal aspirate** for volume, bicarbonate, trypsin and lipase upon secretin and pancreozymin/cholecystokinin stimulation. This involves duodenal intubation, and only a few centers perform this test (Chapter 340).

INVESTIGATIONS FOR INTESTINAL MUCOSAL DISORDERS

Establishing a specific diagnosis for malabsorption often requires histologic examination of small bowel mucosal biopsies. These are obtained during endoscopy, which allows multiple biopsies to be performed, because mucosal involvement can be patchy, especially in celiac disease. Periodic acid–Schiff (PAS) staining of mucosal biopsies and electron microscopy are necessary in congenital diarrhea to assess congenital microvillus atrophy. Bowel mucosal lesions can also be segmental in cases of intestinal lymphangiectasia. In these situations radiographic small bowel series or repeated ultrasonographies can identify a region of thickened bowel responsible for protein loss. During endoscopy, mucosal biopsies can be obtained to measure mucosal disaccharidase activities. Duodenal aspirates can be performed to measure pancreatic enzyme concentration as well as quantitative bacterial cultures. Aspirates to demonstrate other infections and infestations such as *Giardia* may be useful.

IMAGING PROCEDURES

Plain radiographs and barium contrast studies might suggest a site and cause of intestinal motility disorders. Although flocculations of barium and dilated bowel with thickened mucosal folds have been attributed to diffuse malabsorptive lesions such as celiac disease, these abnormalities are nonspecific. Diffuse fluid-filled bowel loops during sonography also suggest malabsorption.

330.2 Gluten-Sensitive Enteropathy (Celiac Disease)

David Branski and Riccardo Troncone

ETIOLOGY AND EPIDEMIOLOGY

Celiac disease is an immune-mediated disorder elicited by the ingestion of gluten in genetically susceptible persons and characterized by chronic inflammation of the small intestine. It is considered an autoimmune condition because of the presence of anti–TG2 antibodies and the association with other autoimmune diseases (thyroid, liver, diabetes, adrenal).

Celiac disease is triggered by the ingestion of wheat gluten and related prolamines from rye and barley. In most studies oats proved to be safe; however, a few celiac patients have oats prolamine–reactive mucosal T cells that can cause mucosal inflammation.

Celiac disease is a common disorder (1% prevalence of biopsy-proven disease). It is thought to be rare in Central Africa and East Asia. Environmental factors might affect the risk of developing celiac disease or the timing of its presentation. Prolonged breastfeeding has been associated with a reduced incidence of symptomatic disease. Less clear is the effect of the time of gluten introduction in the infant diet; the ingestion of increased amounts of gluten in the 1st year of life can increase the incidence. Infectious agents have been hypothesized to play a role because frequent rotavirus infections are associated with an increased risk. It is plausible that the contact with gliadin at a time when there is ongoing intestinal inflammation, altered intestinal permeability, and enhanced antigen presentation can increase the risk of developing the disease, at least in a subset of persons (Fig. 330-3).

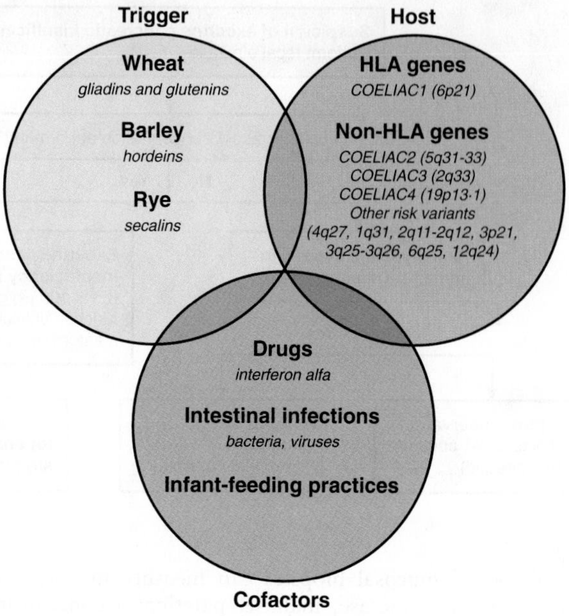

Figure 330-3 Causative factors in celiac disease. HLA, human leukocyte antigen. (From Di Sabatino A, Corazza GR: Coeliac disease, *Lancet* 373:1480-1490, 2009.)

GENETICS AND PATHOGENESIS

A genetic predisposition is suggested by the family aggregation and the concordance in monozygotic twins, which approaches 100%. It is suggested that the primary association of CD is with the DQ $\alpha\beta$ heterodimer encoded by the *DQA1*05* and the *DQB1*02* genes. Such a DQ molecule is present in ≥95% of celiac patients compared with 20-30% of controls. DQ2-negative celiac patients are invariably HLA DQ8 positive *(DQA1*0301/DQB1*0302)*. A gene dosage effect has been suggested, and a molecular hypothesis for such a phenomenon has been proposed, based on the impact of the number and quality of the HLA DQ2 molecules on gluten peptide presentation to T cells. Other non-HLA genes confer susceptibility to celiac disease. Genome-wide association studies have shown risk variants in genes controlling the immune response, some being shared with type 1 diabetes.

Celiac disease is a T cell–mediated chronic inflammatory disorder with an autoimmune component. Altered processing by intraluminal enzymes, changes in intestinal permeability, and activation of innate immunity mechanisms may be involved and precede the activation of the adaptive immune response. Immunodominant epitopes from gliadin are highly resistant to intraluminal and mucosal digestion; incomplete degradation favors the immunostimulatory and toxic effects. Some gliadin peptides (p31-43) can activate innate immunity, and in particular they induce interleukin 15 (IL-15). Others activate lamina propria T cells in the context of HLA-DQ2 or DQ8 molecules. Gliadin-specific T-cell responses are enhanced by the action of TG2; the enzyme converts particular glutamine residues into glutamic acid, which results in higher affinity of these gliadin peptides for HLA-DQ2 or HLA-DQ8. The pattern of cytokines produced following gliadin activation is dominated by interferon-γ (IFN-γ) (Th1 skewed); IFN-α, IL-18, and IL-21 are also upregulated. A complex remodeling of the mucosa then takes place, involving increased levels of metalloproteinases and growth factors, which leads to the classic flat mucosa. Increased density of CD8+ cytotoxic intraepithelial lymphocytes are a hallmark of celiac disease. IL-15 is implicated in the expression of natural killer receptors CD94 and NKG2D, as well as in epithelial expression of stress molecules, thus enhancing cytotoxicity, cell apoptosis, and villous atrophy.

Table 330-4 SOME CLINICAL MANIFESTATIONS OF CELIAC DISEASE IN CHILDREN AND ADOLESCENTS

SYSTEM	MANIFESTATION	(POSSIBLE) CAUSE
Gastrointestinal	Diarrhea Distended abdomen Vomiting Anorexia Weight loss Failure to thrive Aphthous stomatitis	Atrophy of the small bowel mucosa Malabsorption
Hematologic	Anemia	Iron malabsorption
Skeletal	Rickets Osteoporosis Enamel hypoplasia of the teeth	Calcium/vitamin D malabsorption
Muscular	Atrophy	Malnutrition
Neurologic	Peripheral neuropathy Epilepsy Irritability	Thiamine/vitamin B_{12} deficiency
Endocrinologic	Short stature Pubertas tarda Secondary hyperparathyroidism	Malnutrition Calcium/vitamin D malabsorption
Dermatologic	Dermatitis herpetiformis Alopecia areata Erythema nodosum	Autoimmunity
Respiratory	Idiopathic pulmonary hemosiderosis	

Adapted from Mearin ML: Celiac disease among children and adolescents, *Curr Prob Pediatr Adolesc Health Care* 37:81–112, 2007.

The most evident expression of autoimmunity is the presence of serum antibodies to TG2. However, the mechanisms leading to autoimmunity are largely unknown. The finding of IgA deposits on extracellular TG2 in the liver, lymph nodes, and muscles indicates that TG2 is accessible to the gut-derived autoantibodies. Several extraintestinal clinical manifestations of celiac disease (e.g., liver, heart, nervous system) are possibly related to the presence of autoantibodies.

CLINICAL PRESENTATION AND ASSOCIATED DISORDERS

Clinical features of celiac disease vary considerably (Table 330-4). Intestinal symptoms are common in children whose disease is diagnosed within the 1st 2 years of life; failure to thrive, chronic diarrhea, vomiting, abdominal distention, muscle wasting, anorexia, and irritability are present in most cases (see Fig. 330-1). Occasionally there is constipation, rectal prolapse, or intussusception. As the age at presentation of the disease shifts to later in childhood, and with the more liberal use of serologic screening tests, extraintestinal manifestations and associated disorders, without any accompanying digestive symptoms, have increasingly become recognized, affecting almost all organs (Table 330-5).

The most common extraintestinal manifestation of celiac disease is iron-deficiency anemia, unresponsive to iron therapy. Osteoporosis may be present; in contrast to the situation in adults, it can be reversed by a gluten-free diet, with restoration of normal peak bone densitometric values. Other extraintestinal manifestations include short stature, endocrinopathies, arthritis and arthralgia, epilepsy with bilateral occipital calcifications, peripheral neuropathies, cardiomyopathy, chronic lung disease, isolated hypertransaminasemia, dental enamel hypoplasia, aphthous stomatitis, and alopecia. The mechanisms responsible for the severity and the variety of clinical presentations remain obscure. Nutritional deficiencies or abnormal immune responses have been advocated.

Silent celiac disease is being increasingly recognized, mainly in asymptomatic 1st-degree relatives of celiac patients investigated

Table 330-5 RISK GROUPS FOR CELIAC DISEASE CASE-FINDING

1st-degree relatives
Dermatitis herpetiformis
Unexplained iron deficiency anaemia
Autoimmune thyroiditis
Type 1 diabetes
Unexplained infertility
Recurrent abortion
Dental enamel hypoplasia
Cryptic hypertransaminasemia
Autoimmune liver disease
Short stature
Delayed puberty
Down, Williams, and Turner syndromes
Irritable bowel syndrome
Unexplained osteoporosis
Sjögren syndrome
Epilepsy with occipital calcifications
Selective IgA deficiency
Addison disease

IgA, immunoglobulin A.
Modified from Di Sabatino A, Corazza GR: Coeliac disease, *Lancet* 373:1480–1490, 2009.

Table 330-6 CLINICAL SPECTRUM OF CELIAC DISEASE

SYMPTOMATIC
Frank malabsorption symptoms: chronic diarrhea, failure to thrive, weight loss
Extraintestinal manifestations: anemia, fatigue, hypertransaminasemia, neurologic disorders, short stature, dental enamel defects, arthralgia, aphthous stomatitis
SILENT
No apparent symptoms in spite of histologic evidence of villous atrophy
In most cases identified by serologic screening in at-risk groups (see Table 330-1)
LATENT
Subjects who have a normal histology, but at some other time, before or after, have shown a gluten-dependent enteropathy
POTENTIAL
Subjects with positive celiac disease serology but without evidence of altered jejunal histology
It might or might not be symptomatic

during screening studies. However, small bowel biopsy in these people reveals severe mucosal damage consistent with celiac disease. Potential celiac disease is defined when patients are identified by positive screening studies but without documented celiac disease on small bowel biopsy. It is important to follow these patients because they can develop established celiac disease in the future (Table 330-6).

Some diseases, many with an autoimmune pathogenesis, are found with a higher than normal incidence in celiac patients. Among these are type 1 diabetes, autoimmune thyroid disease, Addison disease, Sjögren syndrome, autoimmune cholangitis, autoimmune hepatitis, primary biliary cirrhosis, IgA nephropathy, alopecia, and dilated cardiomyopathy. Such associations have been interpreted as a consequence of the sharing of identical HLA haplotypes. The relation between celiac disease and other autoimmune diseases is poorly defined; once those diseases are established, they are not influenced by a gluten-free diet. Other associated conditions include selective IgA deficiency, Down syndrome, Turner syndrome, and Williams syndrome.

Patients with celiac disease show increased long-term mortality, the risk rising with delayed diagnosis and/or poor dietary compliance. Non-Hodgkin lymphoma is the main cause of death. Adult patients can develop complications such a refractory celiac disease, ulcerative jejunoileitis, or enteropathy-associated T-cell lymphoma.

Table 330-7 OTHER CAUSES OF FLAT MUCOSA
Autoimmune enteropathy
Tropical sprue
Giardiasis
HIV enteropathy
Bacterial overgrowth
Crohn disease
Eosinophilic gastroenteritis
Cow's milk enteropathy
Soy protein enteropathy
Primary immunodeficiency
Graft-versus-host disease
Chemotherapy and radiation
Protein energy malnutrition
Tuberculosis
Lymphoma
Non-gluten food intolerances

Modified from Di Sabatino A, Corazza GR: Coeliac disease, *Lancet* 373:1480–1490, 2009.

DIAGNOSIS

Serologic tests have a crucial role in the diagnosis of celiac disease; sensitivity of the IgA anti-TG2 is 61-100% (mean, 87%), and specificity is 86-100% (mean, 95%). Some 10% of patients whose disease is diagnosed earlier than 2 yr of age show absence of IgA anti-TG2. For them, the measurement of serum antigliadin antibodies is generally advised. Antibodies against gliadin-derived deamidated peptides (D-AGA) have been assessed. Compared with conventional AGA, the peptide antibodies (IgG and IgA) have a greater sensitivity and specificity. A problem with serology is represented by the association of celiac disease with IgA deficiency (10-fold increase compared to the general population). Serum IgA should always be checked, and in the case of IgA deficiency, D-AGA, IgG anti-endomysium, or TG2 should be sought. Negative serology should not preclude a biopsy examination when the clinical suspicion is strong.

Genetic tests have an increasing role in the diagnosis. Less than 2% of celiac patients lack both HLA specificities; at the same time, approximately one third of the "normal" population has one or the other marker; that means that the measurement of HLA DQ2 and/or DQ8 has a strong negative predictive value but a very weak positive predictive value for the diagnosis of celiac disease. With these limitations the test can prove useful to exclude celiac disease when the genetic studies are negative in subjects on a gluten-free diet or in subjects belonging to an at-risk group (e.g., 1st-degree relatives, insulin-dependent diabetics, patients with Down syndrome) to avoid long-term follow-up.

The ultimate diagnosis of celiac disease relies on the demonstration of specific, though not pathognomonic, histopathologic abnormalities in the small bowel mucosa (Table 330-7). According to The European Society for Pediatric Gastroenterology, Hepatology and Nutrition (ESPGHAN) current criteria, the 2 requirements mandatory for the diagnosis of celiac disease are the finding of villous atrophy with hyperplasia of the crypts and abnormal surface epithelium, while the patient is eating adequate amounts of gluten, and a full clinical remission after withdrawal of gluten from the diet. The finding of circulating IgA celiac disease–associated antibodies at the time of diagnosis and their disappearance on a gluten-free diet adds weight to the diagnosis. A control biopsy to verify the consequences of the gluten-free diet on the mucosal architecture is considered mandatory only in patients with an equivocal clinical response to the diet. Gluten challenge is not considered mandatory except in situations where there is doubt about the initial diagnosis, for example, when an initial biopsy was not performed or when the biopsy specimen was inadequate or atypical of celiac disease.

It is now accepted that the spectrum of histologic abnormalities in the celiac small intestine is wider than previously recognized. In some celiac disease patients, only subtle changes of crypt elongation with an increase in intraepithelial lymphocytes may be present. In those cases, it is very important to also evaluate the serology and the HLA typing so as to reach the correct diagnosis. Analysis of multiple biopsies is also very important.

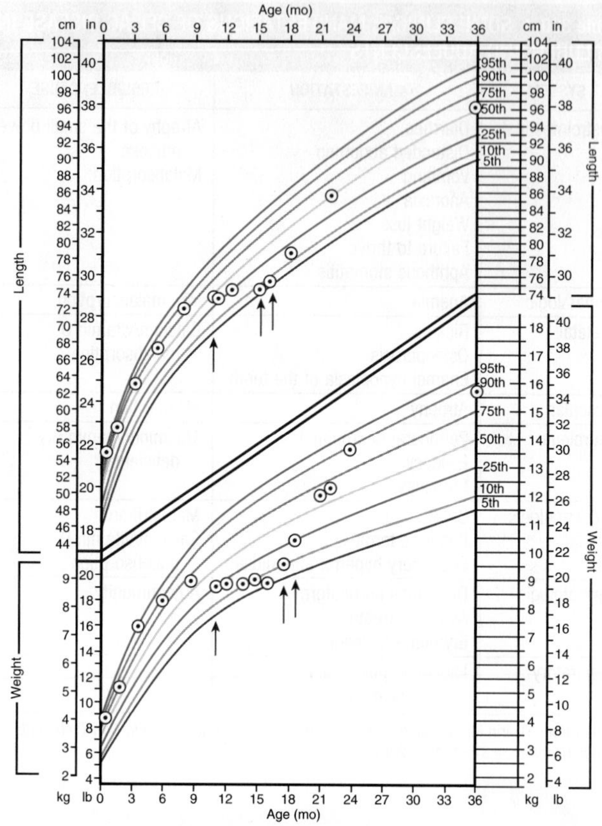

Figure 330-4 Gluten-sensitive enteropathy. Growth curve demonstrates initial normal growth from 0 to 9 mo, followed by onset of poor appetite with intermittent vomiting and diarrhea after initiation of gluten-containing diet *(single arrow).* After biopsy confirmed diagnosis and treatment with gluten-free diet *(double arrow),* growth improves.

Nevertheless, many cases of celiac disease are undiagnosed, and the ratio between patients with diagnosed and with undiagnosed disease may be as high as 1 : 7. Case finding by liberal use of anti-endomysium or anti-TG2 antibodies, followed by confirmatory jejunal biopsy, is more cost effective in primary care than mass screening is. Patients with symptoms or diseases known to be associated with celiac disease should undergo serologic evaluation.

TREATMENT

The only treatment for celiac disease is lifelong strict adherence to a gluten-free diet (Fig. 330-4). This requires a wheat-, barley-, and rye-free diet. Despite evidence that oats are safe for most patients with celiac disease, there is concern regarding the possibility of contamination of oats with gluten during harvesting, milling, and shipping. Nevertheless, it seems wise to add oats to the gluten-free diet only when the latter is well established, so that possible adverse reactions can be readily identified. There is a consensus that all celiac disease patients should be treated with a gluten-free diet regardless of the presence of symptoms. However, whereas it is relatively easy to assess the health improvement after treatment of celiac disease in patients with clinical symptoms of the disease, it proves difficult in persons with asymptomatic celiac disease. The nutritional risks, particularly osteopenia, are those mainly feared for subjects who have silent celiac disease and continue on a gluten-containing diet. Little is known about the health risks in untreated patients with minor enteropathy, which may be clinically silent. There are no guidelines concerning the need for a gluten-free diet in subjects with "potential" celiac disease (patients with positive celiac disease–associated serology but without enteropathy).

The Codex Alimentarius Guidelines define gluten-free as <20 ppm, but, although analytical methods for gluten detection have already reached a satisfactory degree of sensitivity, more information is needed on the daily gluten amount that may be tolerated by celiac disease patients. The data available so far seem to suggest that the threshold should be set to <50 mg/day, although individual variability makes it difficult to set a universal threshold.

It is important that an experienced dietician with specific expertise in celiac disease counseling educates the family and the child about dietary restriction. Compliance with a gluten-free diet can be difficult, especially in adolescents. It is recommended that children with celiac disease be monitored with periodic visits for assessment of symptoms, growth, physical examination, and adherence to the gluten-free diet. Periodic measurements of TG2 antibody levels to document reduction in antibody titers can be helpful as indirect evidence of adherence to a gluten-free diet, although they are inaccurate in detecting slight dietary transgressions.

BIBLIOGRAPHY

Please visit the Nelson Textbook of Pediatrics *website at www.expertconsult.com for the complete bibliography.*

330.3 Other Malabsorptive Syndromes

Philip M. Sherman, David Branski, and Olivier Goulet

CONGENITAL INTESTINAL MUCOSAL DEFECTS

Microvillus Inclusion Disease (Congenital Microvillus Atrophy)

Microvillus inclusion disease is an autosomal recessive disorder, which manifests at birth with **profuse watery secretory diarrhea.** It is the most commonly recognized cause of congenital diarrhea. Light microscopy of the small bowel mucosa demonstrates diffuse thinning of the mucosa, with hypoplastic villus atrophy and no inflammatory infiltrate. Diagnosis may be easily performed with light microscopy using PAS and CD10 staining, which shows a very thin or absent brush border, together with positive PAS and CD10 intracellular inclusions. Electron microscopy shows enterocytes with absent or sparse microvilli. The apical cytoplasm of the enterocytes contains electron-dense secretory granules; the hallmark is presence of microvilli within involutions of the apical membrane. Polyhydramnios is not a classic presentation of MID. Neonates usually present with dehydration and failure to thrive. Despite parenteral nutrition, diarrhea continues and initial fluid management is difficult. The disease is fatal without long-term parenteral nutrition support. Some infants present with rapid onset of liver disease, which is associated with pruritus. Most children die in infancy or early childhood. The long-acting somatostatin analog octreotide has been used as **treatment** and can reduce the volume of stool in some infants (Chapter 331). Intestinal transplantation is the only definitive treatment for this rare disease. Rarely, in milder forms of the disease, the patient can reach young adulthood and enjoy partially oral feeding. The underlying gene defect is a mutation in *MYO5B*, which encodes a protein involved in subcellular protein trafficking. Several types of mutations are involved.

Tufting Enteropathy

Tufting enteropathy (intestinal epithelial dysplasia) manifests in the 1st weeks of life with **persistent watery diarrhea** and accounts for a small fraction of infants with protracted diarrhea of infancy. Symptoms typically do not begin immediately after birth but occur in early infancy. The distinctive feature on small intestinal mucosal biopsy is focal epithelial "tufts" (teardrop-shaped groups of closely packed enterocytes with apical rounding of the plasma membrane) involving 80-90% of the epithelial surface. However, the typical pathology does not appear immediately after birth, and in other known enteropathies tufts are seen on ≤15% of the epithelial surface. Colonic epithelium shows abnormalities that are more difficult to identify. Electron microscopy does not help in the diagnosis.

The pathogenesis of this disorder may be due to a disorder of cell-cell and cell-matrix interactions, because there is an abnormal distribution of $\alpha_2\beta_1$-integrin along the crypt-villus axis, increased expression of desmoglein, and ultrastructural changes of desmosomes. Tufting enteropathy is often associated with punctiform keratitis and conjunctival dysplasia resembling typical pictures of tufts. The genetic basis of tufting enteropathy supports this speculation, because a single amino acid substitution in exon 4 of the *EPCAM* gene encoding an epithelial cell adhesion molecule protein has been described.

No **treatment** has been effective, so management requires permanent parenteral nutrition with possible intestinal transplantation (Chapter 331). Several types of mutations are involved, opening the door to genotype-phenotype analysis.

Enteric Anendocrinosis

Mutations of the *NEUROG3* gene produce generalized mucosal malabsorption, vomiting, diarrhea, failure to thrive, dehydration, and a hyperchloremic metabolic acidosis. Oral alimentation with anything other than water produces diarrhea. Villus-crypt architecture in small bowel biopsies is normal, but staining for neuroendocrine cells (e.g., employing anti-chromogranin antibodies) demonstrates a complete absence of this secretory cell lineage with preservation of goblet cells and Paneth cells. **Treatment** is with total parenteral nutrition and small bowel transplantation.

CARBOHYDRATE-DEFICIENT GLYCOPROTEIN SYNDROME AND ENTEROCYTE HEPARAN SULFATE DEFICIENCY

Congenital disorders of glycosylation (also carbohydrate-deficient glycoprotein, CDG) are genetic disorders of assembly of N-glycans in the cytosol and endoplasmic reticulum, resulting in a variety of manifestations (Chapter 81.6). The subtypes of CDG I are all associated with **protein-losing enteropathy.** Diagnosis can be established by isoelectric focusing of serum transferrin, enzyme analysis, and/or DNA analysis. Oral mannose can provide effective therapy in CDG Ib, so early identification of children presenting with hypoglycemia, hypothyroidism, and/or thyroid binding globulin deficiency is beneficial.

Congenital enterocyte heparan deficiency (CEHD) is a rare cause of intractable diarrhea with protein-losing enteropathy, which may be an unusual presentation of the carbohydrate-deficient glycoprotein syndrome (CDGS) type 1 (also known as Jaeken syndrome) (Chapter 81.6). Heparan sulfate is a glycosaminoglycan with multiple roles in the intestine, including restriction of charged macromolecules, such as albumin, in the vascular lumen.

INTESTINAL LYMPHANGIECTASIA

Obstruction of the lymphatic drainage of the intestine can be due to either congenital defects in lymphatic duct formation or to secondary causes (Table 330-8). The **congenital** form is often associated with lymphatic abnormalities elsewhere in the body, as occur with Turner, Noonan, and Klippel-Trenaunay-Weber syndromes. Causes of **secondary** lymphangiectasia include constrictive pericarditis, heart failure, retroperitoneal fibrosis, abdominal tuberculosis, and retroperitoneal malignancies. Lymph rich in proteins, lipids, and lymphocytes leaks into the bowel lumen, resulting in protein-losing enteropathy, steatorrhea, and

Table 330-8 CAUSES OF PROTEIN-LOSING ENTEROPATHY

Mucosal inflammation
Infection
Cytomegalovirus (CMV)
Bacterial overgrowth
Invasive bacterial infection
Gastric inflammation
Menetrier disease
Eosinophilic gastroenteropathy
Intestinal inflammation
Celiac disease
Crohn disease
Eosinophilic gastroenteropathy
Tropical sprue
Radiation enteritis
Primary intestinal lymphangiectasia
Secondary intestinal lymphangiectasia
Constrictive pericarditis
Congestive heart failure
Post Fontan procedure
Malrotation
Lymphoma
Sarcoidosis
Radiation therapy
Colonic inflammation
Inflammatory bowel diseases
Necrotizing enterocolitis
Congenital disorders of glycosylation

lymphocyte depletion. Hypoalbuminemia, hypogammaglobulinemia, edema, lymphopenia, malabsorption of fat and fat-soluble vitamins, and chylous ascites often occur. Intestinal lymphangiectasia can also manifest with ascites, peripheral edema, and a low serum albumin.

The diagnosis is suggested by the typical findings in association with an elevated fecal α_1-antitrypsin clearance. Radiologic findings of uniform, symmetric thickening of mucosal folds throughout the small intestine are characteristic but nonspecific. Small bowel mucosal biopsy can show dilated lacteals with distortion of villi and no inflammatory infiltrate. A patchy distribution and deeper mucosal involvement on occasion causes false-negative results on small bowel histology. **Treatment** of lymphangiectasia includes restricting the amount of long-chain fat ingested and administering a formula containing protein and medium-chain triglycerides (MCTs). Supplementing a low-fat diet with MCT oil in cooking is used in the management of older children with lymphangiectasia. Rarely, parenteral nutrition is required. If only a portion of the intestine is involved, surgical resection may be considered.

SYNDROMIC DIARRHEA

Syndromic diarrhea (SD), also known as phenotypic diarrhea (PD) or tricho-hepato-enteric (THE) syndrome, is a congenital enteropathy manifesting with early onset of severe diarrhea requiring parenteral nutrition. The estimated prevalence is approximately 1/300,000-400,000 live births in Western Europe. Patients born small for gestational age present with diarrhea starting in the 1st 6 mo of life (<1 mo of age in most cases). They have an abnormal phenotype, including facial dysmorphism with prominent forehead, broad nose, and hypertelorism and a distinct abnormality of hair, **trichorrhexis nodosa**. Hairs are woolly, easily removed, and poorly pigmented. Liver disease affects about half of the patients with extensive fibrosis or cirrhosis. The patients have defective antibody responses despite normal serum immunoglobulin levels and defective antigen-specific skin tests despite positive proliferative responses in vitro. Microscopic analysis shows twisted hair (pili torti), aniso- and poilkilotrichosis, and trichorrhexis nodosa. Histopathologic analysis shows nonspecific villus atrophy with or without mononuclear cell infiltration of the lamina propria, without specific histologic abnormalities involving the epithelium. Recently mutations in the *TTC37* gene were found as the cause of THE syndrome. The common association of the disorder with parental consanguinity and/or affected siblings suggests a genetic origin with an autosomal recessive transmission. Prognosis of this type of intractable diarrhea of infancy is poor because most patients have died between the ages of 2 and 5 yr, some of them with early-onset liver disease.

AUTOIMMUNE ENTEROPATHY

Symptoms of autoimmune enteropathy usually occur after the 1st 6 mo of life with chronic diarrhea, malabsorption, and failure to thrive. Histologic findings in the small bowel include partial or complete villous atrophy, crypt hyperplasia, and an increase in chronic inflammatory cells in the lamina propria. In contrast to gluten-sensitive enteropathy, an increase in intra-epithelial lymphocytes is not a prominent feature of autoimmune enteropathy. Specific serum anti-enterocyte antibodies can be identified in ≥50% of patients by indirect immunofluorescent staining of normal small bowel mucosa and kidney. In some patients anti-goblet cell antibodies can be demonstrated as well. The colon is also often involved, with inflammation and clinical features of colitis.

Extraintestinal autoimmune disorders are usual and include arthritis, membranous glomerulonephritis, insulin-dependent diabetes, thrombocytopenia, autoimmune hepatitis, hypothyroidism, and hemolytic anemia. It is essential to exclude underlying primary immune deficiency, particularly in boys with other autoimmune features (diabetes mellitus), because a proportion have underlying *I*mmune dysregulation, *P*olyendocrinopathy, *E*nteropathy, *X* linked (**IPEX**) **syndrome** (Chapter 120.5). This systemic autoimmune disorder is due to mutations in *FOXP3*, a transcriptional regulator essential for the normal development of regulatory T cells (T_{regs}). Autoimmune enteropathy is reported in cases of Schimke immunoosseous dysplasia.

Treatment for autoimmune enteropathy includes immune suppression drugs including prednisone, azathioprine, cyclophosphamide, cyclosporine, and tacrolimus. Bone marrow transplantation is curative for children with IPEX syndrome.

PROPROTEIN CONVERTASE 1/3 DEFICIENCY

Chronic watery, neonatal onset diarrhea is described in infants with hyperinsulinism, hypoglycemia, hypogonadism, and hypoadrenalism. Small bowel biopsy reveals a nonspecific enteropathy. A clue to the autosomal recessive condition is subsequent onset of marked obesity with hyperphagia in the toddler years in both affected probands and symptomatic siblings.

BILE ACID MALABSORPTION

In primary bile acid malabsorption, mutation of the ileal sodium–bile acid cotransporter gene, *SLC10A2,* results in congenital diarrhea, steatorrhea, interruption of enterohepatic circulation of bile acids, and reduced plasma cholesterol levels. Bile acids are normally synthesized from cholesterol in the liver and secreted into the small intestine, where they facilitate absorption of fat, fat-soluble vitamins, and cholesterol. Bile acids are reabsorbed in the distal ileum, return to the liver via the portal venous circulation, and are resecreted into the bile. Normally, the enterohepatic circulation of bile acids is an extremely efficient process; only 10% of the intestinal bile acids escape reabsorption and are eliminated in feces. Bile acid secretion is largely autoregulated, but there is only a limited capacity to increase bile acid secretion. Reduction in the bile acid pool due to bile acid malabsorption causes steatorrhea, which requires restriction of dietary fat.

Unabsorbed bile acids stimulate chloride excretion in the colon, resulting in diarrhea, which responds to cholestyramine, an anion-binding resin. Secondary bile acid malabsorption can result from ileal disease, such as in Crohn disease, and following an ileal resection.

Chronic neonatal-onset diarrhea has also been described in autosomal recessive **cerebrotendinous xanthomatosis,** which is caused by an inborn error of bile acid synthesis due to 27-hydroxylase deficiency. These children also present with juvenile-onset cataracts and developmental delay. Neonatal cholestasis has also been described as a presenting feature. Tendon xanthomas develop in the second and third decades of life. The diagnosis is important to establish, because **treatment** is effective when employing oral chenodeoxycholic acid.

ABETALIPOPROTEINEMIA

Abetalipoproteinemia is a rare autosomal recessive disorder of lipoprotein metabolism (Bassen Kornsweig syndrome) (Chapter 80). It is associated with severe fat malabsorption from birth. Children fail to thrive during the 1st year of life, with stools that are pale, foul smelling, and bulky. The abdomen is distended and deep tendon reflexes are absent as a result of peripheral neuropathy, which is secondary to vitamin E (fat-soluble vitamin) deficiency. Intellectual development tends to be slow. After 10 yr of age, intestinal symptoms are less severe, ataxia develops, and there is a loss of position and vibration sensation with the onset of intention tremors unless vitamin E levels are maintained in the normal range. These latter symptoms reflect involvement of the posterior columns, cerebellum, and basal ganglia. In adolescence, atypical retinitis pigmentosa develops without adequate supplemental of vitamin E; for instance, using a TPGS formulation of the vitamin.

Diagnosis rests on the presence of acanthocytes in the peripheral blood smear and extremely low plasma levels of cholesterol (<50 mg/dL); triglycerides are also very low (<20 mg/dL). Chylomicrons and very low density lipoproteins are not detectable, and the low-density lipoprotein (LDL) fraction is virtually absent from the circulation. Marked triglyceride accumulation in villus enterocytes occurs in the duodenal mucosa. Steatorrhea occurs in younger patients, but other processes of nutrient assimilation are intact. Rickets may be an unusual initial manifestation of abetalipoproteinemia and hypobetalipoproteinemia. Rickets is caused by steatorrhea-induced calcium losses and vitamin D deficiency. Patients have mutations of the microsomal triglyceride transfer protein (MTP) gene, resulting in absence of MTP function in the small bowel. This protein is required for normal assembly and secretion of very low density lipoproteins and chylomicrons.

Specific **treatment** is not available. Large supplements of the fat-soluble vitamins A, D, E, and K should be given. Vitamin E (100-200 mg/kg/24 hr) appears to arrest neurologic and retinal degeneration. Limiting long-chain fat intake can alleviate intestinal symptoms; medium-chain triglycerides can be used to supplement the fat intake.

HOMOZYGOUS HYPOBETALIPOPROTEINEMIA

Homozygous hypobetalipoproteinemia (Chapter 80) is transmitted as an autosomal dominant trait. The homozygous form is indistinguishable from abetalipoproteinemia. The parents of these patients, as heterozygotes, have reduced plasma LDL and apoprotein-β concentrations, whereas the parents of patients with abetalipoproteinemia have normal levels. On transmission electron microscopy of small bowel biopsies, the size of lipid vacuoles in enterocytes differentiates between abetalipoproteinemia and hypobetalipoproteinemia: Many small vacuoles are present in hypobetalipoproteinemia, and larger vacuoles are seen in abetalipoproteinemia.

CHYLOMICRON RETENTION DISEASE (ANDERSON DISEASE)

In chylomicron retention disease, a rare recessive disorder, there is a defect in chylomicron exocytosis from enterocytes. Sar1-GTP promotes the formation of endoplasmic reticulum to Golgi transport carriers, and *Sar1b* is defective in Anderson disease. These patients have severe intestinal symptoms with steatorrhea, chronic diarrhea, and failure to thrive. Acanthocytosis is rare, and neurologic manifestations are less severe than those observed in abetalipoproteinemia. Plasma cholesterol levels are moderately reduced (<75 mg/dL) and fasting triglycerides are normal, but the fat-soluble vitamins, particularly A and E, are very low. Treatment is early aggressive therapy with fat-soluble vitamins and modification of dietary fat intake, as in the treatment of abetalipoproteinemia.

WOLMAN DISEASE

Wolman disease is a rare, lethal lipid storage disease that leads to lipid accumulation in multiple organs, including the small intestine. In addition to vomiting, severe diarrhea, and hepatosplenomegaly, patients have steatorrhea as a result of lymphatic obstruction. Deficiency of lysosomal acid lipase is the underlying cause of disease (Chapter 80). Successful long-term bone marrow engraftment has resulted in normalization of peripheral blood leukocyte lysosomal enzyme acid lipase activity, with subsequent resolution of diarrhea and the restoration of developmental milestones.

BIBLIOGRAPHY

Please visit the Nelson Textbook of Pediatrics *website at www.expertconsult.com for the complete bibliography.*

330.4 Intestinal Infections and Infestations Associated with Malabsorption

David Branski and Raanan Shamir

Malabsorption is a rare consequence of primary intestinal infection and infestation in immunocompetent children, but it can occur after infection with *Campylobacter, Shigella, Salmonella, Giardia*, cryptosporidium, coccidioidosis, and rotavirus. These infectious causes of malabsorption are more common in immunocompromised children.

POSTINFECTIOUS DIARRHEA

In infants and very young toddlers chronic diarrhea can appear following infectious enteritis, regardless of the nature of the pathogen. The pathogenesis of the diarrhea is not always clear and may be related to secondary lactase deficiency, food protein allergy, antibiotic-associated colitis (including pseudomembranous colitis due to *Clostridium difficile* toxin), or a combination of these.

Treatment is supportive and may include a lactose-free diet in the presence of secondary lactase deficiency; infants might require a semi-elemental diet. The beneficial effect of probiotic should await well-controlled clinical trials.

BACTERIAL OVERGROWTH

Bacteria are normally present in large numbers in the colon (10^{11}-10^{13} colony-forming units [CFU]/gram of feces) and have a symbiotic relationship with the host, providing nutrients and protecting the host from pathogenic organisms. Excessive numbers of bacteria in the small bowel or stomach are harmful.

Bacteria are usually present only in a small number in the stomach and small bowel. Gastric acid pH prevents the ingested organisms from colonizing the small bowel. Small bowel motility and the migrating motor complex cleanse the small bowel between meals and at night; the ileocecal valve prevents colonic bacteria from refluxing into the ileum. Mucosal defenses such as mucin and immunoglobulins prevent bacterial overgrowth in the small bowel. Bacterial overgrowth can result from clinical conditions that alter the gastric pH or small bowel motility, including disorders such as partial bowel obstruction, diverticula, short bowel, intestinal duplications, diabetes mellitus, idiopathic intestinal pseudo-obstruction syndrome, and scleroderma. Prematurity, immunodeficiency, and malnutrition are other factors associated with bacterial overgrowth of the small bowel.

Diagnosis of bacterial overgrowth can be made by culturing small bowel aspirate or by lactulose hydrogen breath test. Lactulose is a synthetic disaccharide, which is not digested by mucosal brush border enzymes but can be fermented by bacteria. High baseline hydrogen and a quick rise in hydrogen in expired breath samples support the diagnosis of bacterial overgrowth, but false-positive tests are common.

Bacterial overgrowth leads to inefficient intraluminal processing of dietary fat and to steatorrhea due to bacterial deconjugation of bile salts, vitamin B_{12} malabsorption, and microvillus brush border damage with malabsorption. Bacterial consumption of vitamin B_{12} and enhanced synthesis of folate result in decreased vitamin B_{12} and increased folate serum levels. Overproduction of D-lactate (the isomer of L-lactate) can cause stupor, neurologic dysfunction, and shock from D-lactic acidosis. Lactic acidosis should be suspected in children at risk of bacterial overgrowth, who show signs of neurologic deterioration and a high anion gap metabolic acidosis not explained by measurable acids such as L-lactate. Measurement of D-lactate is required because standard lactate assay only measures the L-isomer.

Treatment of bacterial overgrowth focuses on correction of underlying causes such as partial obstruction. The oral administration of antibiotics is the mainstay of therapy. Initial treatment with 2-4 wk of metronidazole can provide relief for many months. Cycling of antibiotics including azithromycin, trimethoprim-sulfamethoxazole, ciprofloxacin, and metronidazole is required. Other alternatives are oral nonabsorbable antibiotics such as aminoglycosides. Occasionally, antifungal therapy is required to control fungal overgrowth of the bowel.

TROPICAL SPRUE

Natives and expatriates of certain tropical regions can present with a diffuse lesion of the small intestinal mucosa—tropical sprue, even long after emigration. The endemic regions include South India, the Philippines, and some islands in the Caribbean. It is uncommon in Africa, Jamaica, and Southeast Asia. The etiology of this disorder is unclear; because it follows outbreaks of acute diarrheal disease and improves with antibiotic therapy, an infectious etiology is suspected. The incidence is decreasing worldwide, possibly due to common use of antibiotics for gastroenteritis in developing countries.

Clinical symptoms include fever and malaise followed by watery diarrhea. After about a week the acute features subside, and anorexia, intermittent diarrhea, and chronic malabsorption result in severe malnutrition characterized by glossitis, stomatitis, cheilosis, night blindness, hyperpigmentation, and edema. Muscle wasting is often marked, and the abdomen is often distended. Megaloblastic anemia results from folate and vitamin B_{12} deficiencies.

Diagnosis is made by small bowel biopsy, which shows villous flattening, crypt hyperplasia, and a chronic inflammatory cell infiltrate of the lamina propria with adjacent lipid accumulation in the surface epithelium.

Treatment requires nutritional supplementation, including supplementation of folate and vitamin B_{12}. To prevent recurrence, 6 mo of therapy with oral folic acid (5 mg) and tetracycline or sulfonamides is recommended. Relapses occur in 10-20% of patients who continue to reside in an endemic tropical region; additional courses of antibiotics may be necessary.

WHIPPLE DISEASE

Whipple disease is a chronic multisystem disorder. It is a rare disease, especially in childhood. The disease is caused by an infectious agent, *Tropheryma whipplei,* which can be cultured from a lymph node in the involved tissue. The syndrome encompasses weight loss, diarrhea, abdominal pain, occult bleeding from the bowel mucosa, hepatosplenomegaly, hepatitis, and ascites. Other organs and systems such as the joints, eyes, heart, and kidneys can also be affected and there may be neurologic and psychiatric manifestations as well.

Diagnosis is made upon demonstration of PAS-positive macrophages in the biopsy material and later by positive identification of polymerase chain reaction (PCR) for *T. whipplei.*

Treatment requires antibiotics such as cotrimoxazole for 1-2 yr. Recently a 2-wk course of intravenous ceftriaxone or meropenem, followed by cotrimoxazole for 1 yr, has been recommended.

BIBLIOGRAPHY

Please visit the Nelson Textbook of Pediatrics *website at www.expertconsult.com for the complete bibliography.*

330.5 Immunodeficiency Disorders

Ernest G. Seidman and David Branski

Malabsorption can occur with **congenital immunodeficiency** disorders, and chronic diarrhea with failure to thrive is often the mode of presentation. Defects of humoral and or cellular immunity may be involved, including selective IgA deficiency, agammaglobulinemia, common variable immunodeficiency disease (CVID), severe combined immunodeficiency, Wiskott-Aldrich syndrome, or chronic granulomatous disease. Although most patients with selective IgA deficiency are asymptomatic, malabsorption due to giardiasis or nonspecific enteropathy with bacterial overgrowth can occur. Malabsorption syndrome or chronic noninfectious diarrhea has been reported in 60% of children with CVID, most often in the subgroup with low memory B cell counts. Malabsorption has also been reported in ~10% of patients with late-onset CVID, often secondary to giardiasis. Celiac disease is more common in patients with IgA deficiency and CVID. Paradoxically, it is more difficult to exclude the diagnosis of celiac disease because of the lack of reliability of IgA- and IgG-based serologic tests. Malabsorption due to chronic rotavirus, giardiasis, bacterial overgrowth, and protein-losing enteropathy are well-recognized complications of X-linked agammaglobulinemia. Malabsorption associated with immunodeficiency is exacerbated by villus atrophy and secondary disaccharidase deficiency. In chronic granulomatous disease, phagocytic function is impaired and granulomas develop throughout the GI tract, mimicking Crohn disease. In addition to failure to thrive, it is important to consider that malabsorption associated with immunodeficiency is often complicated by micronutrient deficiencies, including vitamins A, E, and B_{12} and calcium, zinc, and iron.

Overall, immunodeficiencies such as hypogammaglobulinemia in the pediatric age group are more often secondary to other conditions such as cancer and chemotherapy, chronic infections, malabsorption, nephrotic syndrome, or cardiac disease. Malnutrition, diarrhea, and failure to thrive are common in untreated children with **HIV infection.** The risk of GI infection is related to the depression of the CD4 count. Opportunistic infections include *Cryptosporidium parvum,* cytomegalovirus, *Mycobacterium avium-intracellulare, Isospora belli, Enterocytozoon bieneusi, Candida albicans,* astrovirus, calicivirus, adenovirus, and the usual bacterial enteropathogens. In these patients, *Cryptosporidium* can cause a chronic secretory diarrhea.

Cancer chemotherapy can damage the bowel mucosa, leading to secondary malabsorption of disaccharides such as lactose. After bone marrow transplantation, mucosal damage from **graft vs host disease** can cause diarrhea and malabsorption. Small bowel biopsies show nonspecific villus atrophy, mixed inflammatory cell infiltrates, and increased apoptosis. Cancer chemotherapy and bone marrow transplantation have been associated with pancreatic damage leading to exocrine pancreatic insufficiency.

BIBLIOGRAPHY

Please visit the Nelson Textbook of Pediatrics *website at www.expertconsult.com for the complete bibliography.*

330.6 Immunoproliferative Small Intestinal Disease

Ernest G. Seidman and David Branski

Malignant lymphomas of the small intestine are categorized into 3 subtypes: Burkitt lymphoma, non-Hodgkin lymphomas, and Mediterranean lymphoma. Burkitt lymphoma, the most common form in children, characteristically involves the terminal ileum with extensive abdominal involvement. The relatively uncommon "Western" type of non-Hodgkin lymphomas (usually large B-cell type), can involve various parts of the small intestine. **Mediterranean lymphoma** predominantly involves the proximal small intestine. The World Health Organization (WHO) recommended the term *immunoproliferative small intestinal disease* (IPSID) for the syndrome associated with Mediterranean lymphoma, because in its early stages it does not appear to be a truly malignant lymphoma. Many of the patients with "secretory" IPSID syndrome have variable levels of abnormal immunoglobulin in serum or other body fluids, identified as truncated α heavy chain. The WHO classification lists IPSID with heavy chain diseases as a special variant of extranodal marginal zone B-cell small intestinal **mucosa associated lymphoid tissue (MALT) lymphoma.**

IPSID occurs most often in the proximal small intestine in older children and young adults in the Mediterranean basin, Middle East, Asia, and Africa. Poverty and frequent episodes of gastroenteritis during infancy are antecedent risk factors. The initial clinical presentation is intermittent diarrhea and abdominal pain. Later, chronic diarrhea with malabsorption (60-80%), protein-losing enteropathy, weight loss, digital clubbing, and growth failure ensue. Intestinal obstruction, abdominal masses, and ascites are common in advanced stages.

In contrast to primary non-immunoproliferative small intestinal lymphomas, in which the pathology in the intestine is usually focal, involving specific segments of the intestine and leaving the segments between the involved areas free of disease, the pathology in IPSID is diffuse, with a mucosal cellular infiltrate involving large segments of the intestine and sometimes the entire length of the intestine, thus producing malabsorption. Molecular and immunohistochemical studies demonstrated an association with *Campylobacter jejuni* infection. The differential diagnosis includes chronic enteric infections (parasites, tropical sprue), celiac disease, and other lymphomas. Radiologic findings include multiple filling defects, ulcerations, strictures, and enlarged mesenteric lymph nodes on CT scan.

The diagnosis is usually established by endoscopic biopsies and/or laparotomy. Upper endoscopy shows thickening, erythema, and nodularity of the mucosal folds in the duodenum and proximal jejunum. As the disease progresses, tumors usually appear in the proximal small intestine and rarely in the stomach. The diagnosis requires multiple duodenal and jejunal mucosal biopsies showing dense mucosal infiltrates, consisting of centrocyte-like and plasma cells. Progression to higher-grade large-cell lymphoplasmacytic and immunoblastic lymphoma is characterized by increased plasmocytic atypia with formation of aggregates and later sheets of dystrophic plasma cells and immunoblasts invading the submucosa and muscularis propria. A serum marker of IgA, α heavy-chain paraprotein, is present in most cases.

Treatment of early-stage IPSID with antibiotics results in complete remission in 30-70% of cases. However, the majority of untreated IPSID cases progress to lymphoplasmacytic and immunoblastic lymphoma invading the intestinal wall and mesenteric lymph nodes and can metastasize to distant organs, requiring chemotherapy.

BIBLIOGRAPHY

Please visit the Nelson Textbook of Pediatrics *website at www.expertconsult.com for the complete bibliography.*

330.7 Short Bowel Syndrome

Jon A. Vanderhoof and David Branski

Short bowel syndrome results from congenital malformations or resection of the small bowel. Causes of short bowel syndrome are listed in Table 330-9. Loss of >50% of the small bowel, with or without a portion of the large intestine, can result in symptoms of generalized malabsorption disorder or in specific nutrient deficiencies, depending on the region of the bowel resected. At birth, the length of small bowel is 200-250 cm; by adulthood, it grows to 300-800 cm. Bowel resection in an infant has a better prognosis than in an adult because of the potential for intestinal growth. An infant with as little as 15 cm of bowel with an ileocecal valve, or 20 cm without, has the potential to survive and be eventually weaned from total parenteral nutrition (TPN).

In addition to the length of the bowel, the anatomic location of the resection is also important. The jejunum has more circular folds and longer villi. The proximal 100-200 cm of jejunum is the main site for carbohydrate, protein, iron, and water-soluble vitamin absorption, whereas fat absorption occurs over a longer length of the small bowel. Depending on the region of the bowel resected, specific nutrient malabsorption can result. Vitamin B_{12} and bile salts are only absorbed in the distal ileum (Fig. 330-5). Jejunal resections are generally tolerated better than ileal resections because the ileum can adapt to absorb nutrients and fluids. Net sodium and water absorption is relatively much higher in the ileum. Ileal resection has a profound effect on fluid and electrolyte absorption due to malabsorption of sodium and water by the remaining ileum; ileal malabsorption of bile salts stimulates increased colonic secretion of fluid and electrolytes.

Table 330-9 CAUSES OF SHORT BOWEL SYNDROME
CONGENITAL
Congenital short bowel syndrome Multiple atresias Gastroschisis
BOWEL RESECTION
Necrotizing enterocolitis Volvulus with or without malrotation Long segment Hirschsprung disease Meconium peritonitis Crohn disease Trauma

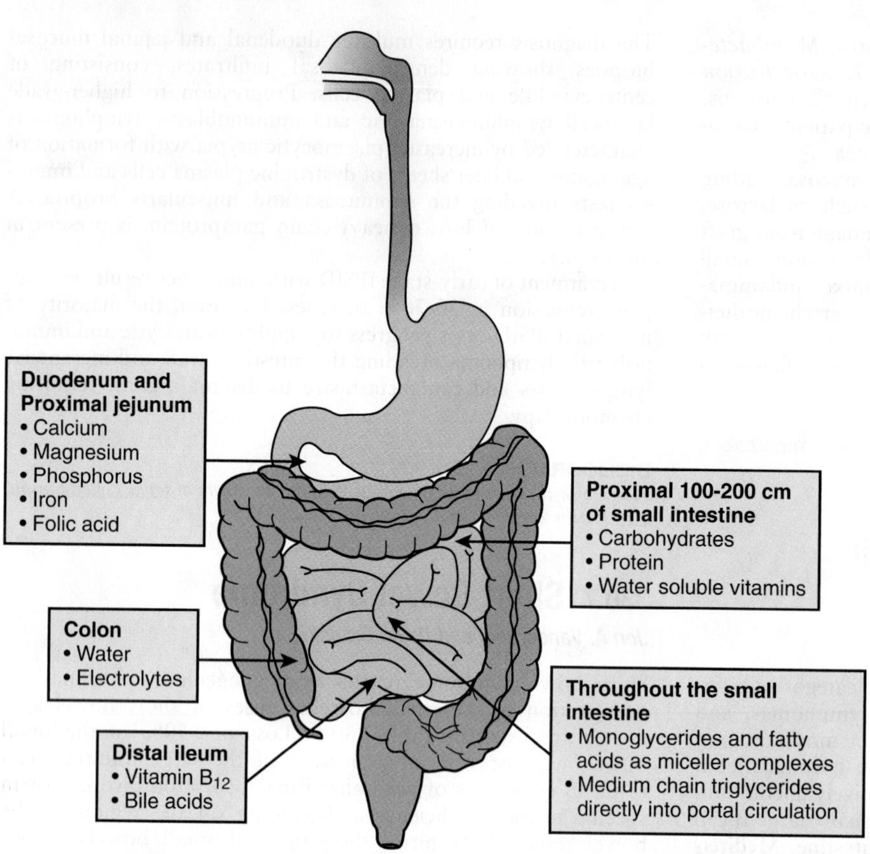

Figure 330-5 Absorption of nutrients in the small bowel varies with the region.

TREATMENT

After bowel resection, treatment of short bowel syndrome is initially focused on repletion of the massive fluid and electrolyte losses while the bowel initially accommodates to absorb these losses. Nutritional support is often provided via parenteral nutrition. A central venous catheter should be inserted to provide parenteral fluid and nutrition support. The ostomy or stool output should be measured and fluid and electrolyte losses adequately replaced. Measurement of urinary Na^+ to assess body Na^+ stores is useful to prevent Na^+ depletion. Maintaining urinary Na^+ higher than K^+ ensures that Na^+ intake is adequate. Use of oral glucose electrolyte solutions improves intestinal sodium absorption, particularly in patients without a colon.

After the initial few weeks following resection, fluid and electrolyte losses stabilize, and the focus of therapy shifts to bowel rehabilitation with the gradual reintroduction of enteral feeds. Continuous small-volume trophic enteral feeding should be initiated with a protein hydrolysate and medium-chain triglyceride–enriched formula to stimulate gut hormones and promote mucosal growth. Enteral feeding also increases pancreatobiliary flow and reduces parenteral nutrition-induced hepatotoxicity. As soon as possible, the infant should be given a small amount of water, and then formula by mouth to maintain an interest in oral feeding and minimize or avoid the development of **oral aversion.** As intestinal adaptation occurs, enteral feeding increases and parenteral supplementation decreases. The bowel mucosa proliferates and bowel lengthens with growth.

After achieving the maximal increase in bowel absorptive capacity, management of specific micronutrient and vitamin deficiencies and treatment of transient problems such as postinfectious mucosal malabsorption are required. GI infections such as rotavirus or small bowel bacterial overgrowth can cause setbacks in the progression to full enteral feeding in patients with marginal absorptive function. A marked increase in stool output or evidence of carbohydrate malabsorption (stool pH <5.5 and positive test for reducing substances) contraindicate further increases in enteral feeds. Slow advancement of continuous enteral feeding rates continues until all nutrients are provided enterally. Then the feeds can be altered to include increased oral or bolus feeding volumes.

In patients with large stool outputs, the addition of soluble fiber and antidiarrheal agents such as loperamide and anticholinergics can be beneficial, although these drugs can increase the risk of bacterial overgrowth. Cholestyramine can be beneficial for patients with distal ileal resection, but its potential depletion of the bile acid pool can increase steatorrhea. Bacterial overgrowth is common in infants with a short bowel and can delay progression of enteral feedings. Empirical treatment with metronidazole or other antibiotics is often useful. Diets high in fat and lower in carbohydrate may be helpful in reducing bacterial overgrowth as well as enhancing adaptation.

COMPLICATIONS

Long-term complications of short bowel syndrome include those of parenteral nutrition: central catheter infection, thrombosis, hepatic cholestasis and cirrhosis, and gallstones. Appropriate care of the central line to prevent infection and catheter-related thrombosis is extremely important. Some patients need long-term parenteral nutritional support, and lack of central line access is potentially life-threatening; inappropriate removal or changes of central lines in the neonatal period should be avoided. Other complications of terminal ileal resection include vitamin B_{12} deficiency, which might not appear until 1-2 yr after parenteral nutrition is withdrawn. Long-term monitoring for deficiencies of vitamin B_{12}, folate, iron, fat-soluble vitamins, and trace minerals such as zinc and copper is important. **Renal stones** can occur as a result of hyperoxaluria secondary to steatorrhea (calcium binds to the excess fat and not to oxalate, so more oxalate is reabsorbed and excreted in the urine). Venous thrombosis and vitamin deficiency have been associated with hyperhomocystinemia in short bowel syndrome. Bloody diarrhea secondary to patchy, mild colitis can develop during the progression of enteral feedings. The pathogenesis of this "feeding colitis" is unknown, but it is usually benign and can improve with a hypoallergenic diet or treatment with sulfasalazine.

In patients who are unable to achieve full enteral feeding after several years of nutritional rehabilitation, surgical bowel lengthening procedures may be considered. In some children with complications of parenteral nutrition, especially impending liver failure, small intestinal and liver transplantation may be considered (Chapter 331).

330.8 Chronic Malnutrition

Raanan Shamir and David Branski

Primary malnutrition (i.e., undernutrition) is very common in developing countries and is directly related to increased disease burden and mortality (Chapter 43). In developed countries, chronic malnutrition occurs mainly as a result of decreased food intake, malabsorption syndromes, and increased nutritional needs in children with chronic diseases, and it affects 11-50% of hospitalized children. Child neglect and improper preparation of formula can result in severe malnutrition. Malnutrition can be identified by evaluating dietary intake, by medical history (anorexia, vomiting, dysphagia, mood and behavioral changes, abdominal pain, diarrhea), by anthropometric measurements (e.g., reduced weight per age and weight per height, BMI <5th percentile) by clinical signs of nutrient deficiencies (atrophic tongue in iron deficiency anemia or alopecia in zinc deficiency).

Malnourished children suffer from impaired immunity, poor wound healing, muscle weakness, and diminished psychologic drive. Malnutrition has short-term consequences (increased disability, morbidity, and mortalitiy) and long-term consequences (final adult size, lower IQ, economic productivity). Undernutrition in hospitalized children is related to increased infectious complications, delayed recovery, increased length of stay and costs, increased readmission rate, and increased mortality.

Nutritional rehabilitation in malnourished children is discussed in Chapter 43.

Chronic malnutrition complicated by diarrheal dehydration is a commonly observed phenomenon. Infectious diarrhea is common in tropical and subtropical countries, in the setting of poor hygiene practices, in immunocompromised hosts (HIV, congenital immunodeficiency), and when impairment of the immune response is due to chronic malnutrition itself. In children with chronic disorders, diarrhea may be related to the underlying disease and should be sought. Examples include noncompliance with a gluten-free diet in celiac disease, noncompliance with pancreatic enzyme treatment in cystic fibrosis, and disease relapse in inflammatory bowel disease (IBD). In the case of IBD, relapse should be diagnosed only after infectious diarrhea and *C. difficile* infection have been ruled out. Malnutrition per se can lead to exocrine pancreatic insufficiency, which, in turn, aggravates malabsorption and diarrhea.

In infants and children with severe malnutrition, many of the signs normally used to assess the state of hydration or shock are unreliable. Severe malnutrition might be accompanied by sepsis; thus, children with septic shock might not have diarrhea, thirst, or sunken eyes, but may be hypothermic, hypoglycemic, or febrile. The electrocardiogram (ECG) often shows tachycardia, low amplitude, and flat or inverted T waves. Cardiac reserve seems lowered, and heart failure is a common complication.

Despite clinical signs of dehydration, urinary osmolality may be low in the chronically malnourished child. Renal acidifying ability is also limited in patients with malnutrition.

Management of the diarrhea in chronically malnourished children is based on 3 principles: oral rehydration to correct dehydration, rapid resumption of regular feeds with avoidance of periods of nothing by mouth, and treating the etiology of the diarrhea.

When treating the dehydration, it must be remembered that in dehydrated and malnourished infants there appears to be overexpansion of the extracellular space accompanied by extracellular and presumably intracellular hypo-osmolality. Thus, reduced or hypotonic osmolarity oral rehydration solutions are indicated in this setting. When oral rehydration is not possible, the route of choice is nasogastric, and intravenous therapy should be avoided if possible.

Initial intravenous therapy in profound dehydration is designed to improve the circulation and expand extracellular volume. For patients with edema, the quality of fluid and the rate of administration might need to be readjusted from recommended levels to avoid overhydration and pulmonary edema. Blood should be given if the patient is in shock or severely anemic. Potassium salts can be given early if urine output is good. Clinical and ECG improvement may be more rapid with magnesium therapy.

Children with chronic malnutrition are at risk for the refeeding syndrome. Therefore, initial calorie provision should not exceed the previous daily intake and is usually begun at 50-75% of estimated resting energy expenditure, with rapid increase to caloric goals once there are no severe abnormalities in sodium, potassium, phosphorus, calcium, or magnesium. Correction of malnutrition and catch-up growth are not part of the primary treatment of these children, but a nutrition rehabilitation plan is necessary.

BIBLIOGRAPHY

Please visit the Nelson Textbook of Pediatrics *website at www.expertconsult.com for the complete bibliography.*

330.9 Enzyme Deficiencies

Michael J. Lentze and David Branski

CARBOHYDRATE MALABSORPTION

Symptoms of carbohydrate malabsorption include loose watery diarrhea, flatulence, abdominal distention, and pain. Some children are asymptomatic unless the malabsorbed carbohydrate is consumed in large amounts. Disaccharidases are present on the brush border membrane of the small bowel. Disaccharidase deficiency can be due to a genetic defect or secondarily due to damage to the small bowel epithelium, as occurs with infection or inflammatory disorders.

Unabsorbed carbohydrates enter the large bowel and are fermented by intestinal bacteria, producing organic acids and gases such as methane and hydrogen. The gases can cause discomfort and the unabsorbed carbohydrate and the organic acids cause osmotic diarrhea characterized by an acidic pH and presence of either reducing or nonreducing sugars in the stool. Hydrogen gas can be detected in the breath as a sign of fermentation of unabsorbed carbohydrates (H_2-breath test).

LACTASE DEFICIENCY

Congenital lactase deficiency is rare and is associated with symptoms occurring on exposure to lactose in milk. Fewer than 50 cases have been reported worldwide. In patients with congenital lactase deficiency, 5 distinct mutations in the coding region of the *LCT* gene were found. In most patients (84%), homozygosity for a nonsense mutation, 4170T-A (Y1390X; OMIM 223000), designated Fin (major), was found.

Primary adult type-hypolactasia is caused by a physiologic decline in lactase actively that occurs following weaning in most mammals. The brush border lactase is expressed at low levels during fetal life; activity increases in late fetal life and peaks from term to 3 yr, after which levels gradually decrease with age. This decline in lactase levels varies between ethnic groups. Lactase deficiency occurs in ~15% of white adults, 40% of Asian adults, and 85% of black adults in the United States. Lactase is encoded by a single gene *(LCT)* of ~50 kb located on chromosome 2q21. C/T (−13910) polymorphisms of the MCM6 gene were found to be related to adult-type hypolactasia in most European populations. In 3 African populations—Tanzanians, Kenyans, and Sudanese—3 SNPs, G/C (−14010), T/G(−13915), and C/G(−13907) were identified with lactase persistence and have derived alleles that significantly enhance transcription from the lactase gene promoter in vitro.

Secondary lactose intolerance follows small bowel mucosal damage (celiac disease, rotavirus infection) and is usually transient, improving with mucosal healing.

Lactase deficiency can be diagnosed by H_2-breath test or by measurement of lactase activity in mucosal tissue retrieved by small bowel biopsy. Diagnostic testing is not mandatory, and often simple dietary changes that reduce or eliminate lactose from the diet relieve symptoms.

Treatment of lactase deficiency consists of a milk-free diet. A lactose-free formula (based on either soy or cow's milk) can be used in infants. In older children, low-lactose milk can be consumed. Addition of lactase to dairy products usually abbreviates the symptoms.

Live-culture yogurt contains bacteria that produce lactase enzymes and is therefore tolerated in most patients with lactase deficiency. Hard cheeses have a small amount of lactose and are generally well tolerated.

FRUCTOSE MALABSORPTION

Children consuming a large quantity of juice rich in fructose, corn syrup, or natural fructose in fruit juices can present with diarrhea, abdominal distention, and slow weight gain. Restricting the amount of juice in the diet resolves the symptoms and helps avoid unnecessary investigations. Fructose H_2 breath test can be helpful in the diagnosis of fructose malabsorption. The reason for fructose malabsorption is the reduced abundance of GLUT-5 transporter on the surface of the intestinal brush border membrane, which occurs in about 5% of the population.

SUCRASE-ISOMALTASE DEFICIENCY

Sucrase-isomaltase deficiency is a rare autosomal recessive disorder with a complete absence of sucrase and reduced maltase digestive activity. The sucrase-isomaltase complex is composed of 1,927 amino acids encoded by a 3,364 bp mRNA. The gene locus on chromosome 3 has 30 exons spanning 106.6 kb. The majority of sucrase-isomaltase mutations result in a lack of enzyme protein synthesis (null mutation). Post-translational processing defects are also identified.

Approximately 2% of Europeans and Americans are mutant heterozygote. Sucrase deficiency is especially common in indigenous Greenlanders (estimated 5%) in whom it is often accompanied by lactase deficiency.

Symptoms of sucrase-isomaltase deficiency usually begin when the infant is exposed to sucrose or a glucose polymer diet. This can occur with ingestion of non–lactose based infant formula or on the introduction of pureed food, especially fruits and sweets. Diarrhea, abdominal pain, and poor growth are observed. Occasional patients present with symptoms in late childhood or even adult life, but careful history often indicates that symptoms appeared earlier. Diagnosis of sucrase-isomaltase malabsorption requires acid hydrolysis of stool for reducing substances because sucrase is a nonreducing sugar. Alternatively, diagnosis can be achieved with hydrogen breath test or direct enzyme assay of small bowel biopsy.

The mainstay of **treatment** is lifelong dietary restriction of sucrose-containing foods. Enzyme replacement with a purified yeast enzyme, sacrosidase (Sucraid), is a highly effective adjunct to dietary restriction.

GLUCOSE-GALACTOSE MALABSORPTION

More than 30 different mutations of the sodium/glucose co-transporter gene *(SGLT1)* are identified. These mutations cause a rare autosomal recessive disorder of intestinal glucose and galactose/Na^+ co-transport system that leads to osmotic diarrhea. Because most dietary sugars are polysaccharides or disaccharides with glucose or galactose moieties, diarrhea follows the ingestion of glucose, breast milk, or conventional lactose-containing formulas. Dehydration and acidosis can be severe, resulting in death.

The stools are acidic and contain sugar. Patients with the defect have normal absorption of fructose, and their small bowel function and structure are normal in all other aspects. Intermittent or permanent glycosuria after fasting or after a glucose load is a common finding due to the transport defect also being present in the kidney. The presence of reducing substances in watery stools and slight glycosuria despite low blood sugar levels is highly suggestive of glucose-galactose malabsorption. Malabsorption of glucose and galactose is easily identified using the breath hydrogen test. It is safe to perform the 1st test with a dose of 0.5 g/kg of glucose; if necessary, a second test can be performed using 2 g/kg. Breath H_2 will rise more than 20 ppm. The small intestinal biopsy is useful to document a normal villous architecture and normal disaccharidase activities. The identification of mutations of *SGLT1* makes it possible to perform prenatal screening in families at risk for the disease.

Treatment consists of rigorous restriction of glucose and galactose. Fructose, the only carbohydrate that can be given safely, should be added to a carbohydrate-free formula at a concentration of 6-8%. Diarrhea immediately ceases when infants are given such a formula. Although the defect is permanent, later in life, limited amounts of glucose, such as starches or sucrose may be tolerated.

EXOCRINE PANCREATIC INSUFFICIENCY

Disorders of exocrine pancreatic insufficiency are discussed in Chapter 341. Cystic fibrosis is the most common congenital disorder associated with exocrine pancreatic insufficiency. Although rare, the next most common cause of pancreatic insufficiency in children is Shwachman-Diamond syndrome. Other rare disorders causing exocrine pancreatic insufficiency are Blizzard-Johanson syndrome (severe steatorrhea, aplasia of alae nasi, deafness, hypothyroidism, scalp defects), Pearson bone marrow syndrome (sideroblastic anemia, variable degree of neutropenia, thrombocytopenia), and isolated pancreatic enzyme deficiency (lipase, colipase and lipase-colipase, trypsinogen, amylase). Deficiency of enterokinase—a key enzyme that is produced in the proximal small bowel and is responsible for the activation of trypsinogen to trypsin—manifests clinically as exocrine pancreatic insufficiency.

Autoimmune polyendocrinopathy syndrome type 1, a rare autosomal recessive disorder, is caused by mutation in the autoimmune regulator gene *(AIRE)*. Chronic mucocutaneous candidiasis is associated with failure of parathyroid gland, adrenal cortex, pancreatic β-cells, gonads, gastric parietal cells, and thyroid gland. Pancreatic insufficiency and steatorrhea have been associated with this condition.

ENTEROKINASE (ENTEROPEPTIDASE) DEFICIENCY

Enterokinase (enteropeptidase) is a brush border enzyme of the small intestine. It is responsible for the activation of trypsinogen into trypsin. Deficiency of this enzyme results in severe diarrhea, malabsorption, failure to thrive, and hypoproteinemic edema after birth.

Enterokinase deficiency is caused by mutation in the serine protease-7 gene *(PRSS7)* on chromosome 21q21. The diagnosis can be established by measuring the enzyme level in intestinal tissue. Treatment of this rare autosomal recessive disorder consists of replacement with pancreatic enzymes and administration of a protein hydrolyzed formula with added MCT oil in infancy.

TRYPSINOGEN DEFICIENCY

Trypsinogen deficiency is a rare syndrome with symptomatology similar to that of enterokinase deficiency. Enterokinase catalyzes the conversion of trypsinogen to trypsin, which, in turn, activates the various pancreatic proenzymes such as chymothrypsin, procaboxypeptidase, and proelastase for their active forms. Deficiency of trypsinogen results in severe diarrhea, malabsorption, failure to thrive and hypoproteinemic edema soon after birth.

The trypsinogen gene is encoded on chromosome 7q35. Treatment is the same as for enterokinase deficiency, with pancreatic enzymes and protein hydrolysate formula with added MCT oil in infancy.

330.10 Liver and Biliary Disorders Causing Malabsorption

Anil Dhawan and David Branski

Absorption of fats and fat-soluble vitamins depends to a great extent on adequate bile flow providing bile acids to the small intestine. Most of the liver and biliary disorders lead to impairment of the bile flow, contributing to malabsorption of long-chain fatty acids and vitamins such as A, D, E, and K. In addition, severe portal hypertension can lead to portal hypertensive enteropathy, resulting in poor absorption of the nutrients. Decompensated liver disease leads to anorexia and increased energy expenditures, further widening the gap between calorie intake and net absorption, leading to severe malnutrition. Adequate management of nutrition is essential to improve the outcome with or without liver transplantation. This is usually achieved by using medium-chain triglyceride-rich milk formula, supplemental vitamins, and continuous or bolus enteral feed where oral intake is poor.

Vitamin D deficiency is commonly observed on biochemical tests, and children rarely present with pathologic fractures. Simultaneous administration of vitamin D with the water-soluble vitamin E preparation (d-α-tocopherol polyethylene glycol 1,000 succinate [TPGS]) enhances absorption of vitamin D. In young infants, oral vitamin D_3 is given at a dose of 1,000 IU/kg/24 hr. After 1 mo, if the serum 25-hydroxyvitamin D level is low, the same dose of oral vitamin D is mixed with TPGS. 25-hydroxyvitamin D is then monitored every 3 mo, with adjustment of doses as necessary.

Vitamin E deficiency in patients with chronic cholestasis is not usually symptomatic, but it can manifest as a progressive neurologic syndrome, which includes peripheral neuropathy (manifesting as loss of deep tendon reflexes and ophthalmoplegia), cerebellar ataxia, and posterior column dysfunction. Early in the course, findings are partially reversible with treatment; late features might not be reversible. It may be difficult to identify vitamin E deficiency because the elevated blood lipid levels in cholestatic liver disease can falsely elevate the serum vitamin E level. Therefore, it is important to measure the ratio of serum vitamin E to total serum lipids; the normal level for patients <12 yr of age is >0.6, and for patients >12 yr it is >0.8. The neurologic disease can be prevented with the use of an oral water-soluble vitamin E preparation (TPGS, Liqui-E) at a dose of 25-50 IU/day in neonates and 1 IU/kg/day in children.

Vitamin K deficiency can occur as a result of cholestasis and poor fat absorption. In children with liver disease it is very important to differentiate between the coagulopathy related to vitamin K deficiency and one secondary to the synthetic failure of the liver. A single dose of vitamin K administered intravenously does not correct the prolonged prothrombin time in liver failure, but the deficiency state responds within a few hours. Easy bruising may be the 1st sign. In neonatal cholestasis, coagulopathy due to vitamin K deficiency can manifest with intracranial bleeds with devastating consequences, and prothrombin time should be routinely measured to monitor for deficiency in children with cholestasis. All children with cholestasis should receive vitamin K supplements.

Vitamin A deficiency is rare and is associated with night blindness, xerophthalmia, and increased mortality if patients contract measles. Serum vitamin A levels should be monitored and adequate supplementation considered.

In practice, children with cholestasis are prescribed twice the recommended daily allowance of the commonly available multivitamin preparations while awaiting blood levels.

330.11 Rare Inborn Defects Causing Malabsorption

Peter Zimmer and David Branski

Some congenital (primary) malabsorption disorders originate from a defect of integral membrane proteins, which fulfill a transport function as receptor or channel across the apical or basolateral membrane of enterocytes for nutritional components. Histologic examination of the small and large bowel is typically normal. Most of these disorders are inherited in an autosomal recessive pattern. Most are rare, and patients present with a broad phenotypic heterogeneity due to modifier genes and nutritional and other secondary factors.

DISORDERS OF CARBOHYDRATE ABSORPTION

Patients with **Fanconi-Bickel syndrome (FBS)** present with tubular nephropathy; rickets; hepatomegaly; glycogen accumulation in liver, kidney, and small bowel; failure to thrive; and fasting hypoglycemia. The disorder is caused by homozygous mutations of GLUT2, the facilitative glucose (and galactose) transporter at the basolateral membrane of enterocytes hepatocytes, renal tubules, pancreatic islet cells, and cerebral neurons. Because severe osmotic diarrhea is not a feature of FBS, a GLUT2-independent basolateral transport for glucose is suggested. GLUT2 seems to modulate insulin secretion, renal reabsorption, and glucose uptake from the apical membrane of enterocytes in response to the (postprandial) sugar environment. Diagnostic signs are elevated galactose levels in the blood (found in the neonatal screening program), neonatal bilateral cataracts, marked glycosuria, generalized aminoaciduria, and excessive renal losses of phosphate and calcium. Liver and kidneys are enlarged. Therapy includes substitution of electrolyte losses and vitamin D and supplying uncooked cornstarch to prevent hypoglycemia. Patients who present in the neonatal period need frequent small meals and galactose-free milk.

DISORDERS OF AMINO ACID AND PEPTIDE ABSORPTION

Owing to their ontogenic origins, enterocytes and renal tubules express amino acid transporter in common. Their highest intestinal transporter activity is found in the jejunum. The transporters causing Hartnup disease, cystinuria, iminoglycinuria, and dicarboxylic aminoaciduria are located in the apical membrane, and those causing lysinuric protein intolerance (LPI) and blue diaper syndrome are anchored in the basolateral membrane of the intestinal epithelium.

Dibasic amino acids, including cystine, ornithine, lysine, and arginine are taken up by the Na-independent SLC3A1/SLC7A9, which is defective in **cystinuria.** The overall prevalence of the disease is 1 in 7,000 newborns. This disorder is not associated with any GI or nutritional consequences because of compensation by alternative transporter. However, hypersecretion of cystine in the urine leads to recurrent cystine stones, which account for up to 1% of all urinary tract stones. Ample hydration, urine alkalinization, and cystine-binding thiol drugs can increase the solubility of cystine. Cystinuria type I is inherited as an autosomal recessive trait, and the transmission of type II is autosomal dominant with incomplete penetrance. Cystinuria type I has been described in association with 2p21 deletion syndrome and hypotonia-cystinuria syndrome.

Hartnup disease is characterized by malabsorption of neutral amino acids, including the essential amino acid tryptophan, with aminoaciduria, photosensitive pellagra-like rash, headaches, cerebellar ataxia, delayed intellectual development, and diarrhea. The clinical spectrum ranges from asymptomatic patients to severely affected patients with progressive neurodegeneration leading to death by adolescence. SLC6A19, which is the major luminal sodium-dependent neutral amino acid transporter of small intestine and renal tubules, has been identified as the defective protein. Its association with collectrin and angiotensin-converting enzyme (ACE) II is likely to be involved in the phenotypic heterogeneity of Hartnup disorder. Tryptophan is a precursor of NAD(P)H biosynthesis; therefore the disorder can be treated by nicotinamide in addition to a diet of 4 g protein/kg. The use of lipid-soluble esters of amino acids and tryptophan ethylester has also been reported.

In the **blue diaper syndrome (indicanuria, Drummond syndrome)** tryptophan is specifically malabsorbed and the defect is expressed only in the intestine and not in the kidney, in contrast to Hartnup disease. Intestinal bacteria convert the unabsorbed tryptophan to indican, which is responsible for the bluish discoloration of the urine after its hydrolysis and oxidation. Symptoms can include digestive disturbances such as vomiting, constipation, poor appetite, failure to thrive, hypercalcemia, nephrocalcinosis, fever, irritability, and ocular abnormalities. The molecular genetic defect of this disorder has not yet been characterized.

The underlying defect of **iminoglycinuria** is the malabsorption of proline, hydroxyproline, and glycine due to the proton amino acid transporter SLC36A2 defect, with a possible participation of modifier genes, one of which (SLC6A20), is present in the intestinal epithelium. This disorder is usually benign, but sporadic cases with encephalopathy, mental retardation, deafness, blindness, kidney stones, hypertension, and gyrate atrophy have been described.

The excitatory amino acid carrier SLC1A1 is affected in **dicarboxylic aminoaciduria.** This carrier is present in the small intestine, kidney, and brain, and transports the anionic acids L-glutamate, L- and D-aspartate, and L-cysteine. There are single case reports indicating that this disorder could be associated with hyperprolinemia and neurologic symptoms such as **POLIP** (polyneuropathy, ophthalmoplegia, leukoencephalopathy, intestinal pseudo-obstruction).

A histidine-specific transport system has also been proposed. A few patients have been reported with an intestinal and renal defect of this carrier. It has not been confirmed that patients with **histidinuria,** who have low plasma histidine levels, in contrast to histidinemia, develop neurologic symptoms (e.g., hearing loss, myoclonic seizures).

A methionine-preferring transporter in the small intestine was suggested to be affected in **Smith-Strang disease (oasthouse urine disease)**, which is characterized by purple, red-brown-colored urine with a cabbage-like odor, containing 2-hydroxybutyric acid, valine, and leucine. The potential symptoms of **methionine malabsorption** include neurologic signs, white hair, and diarrhea. Large amounts of methionine and branched-chain amino acids are present in the feces but not in the urine. A low-methionine diet is recommended to alleviate the symptoms.

Among the diseases (see the earlier discussion of cystinuria) with a membrane transport defect of cationic amino acids (lysine, arginine, ornithine), **lysinuric protein intolerance** (LPI) is the 2nd most common, with a prevalence in Finland of 1 in 60,000. The y^+LAT-1 (SLC7A7) carrier at the basolateral membrane of the intestinal and renal epithelium is affected, with failure to deliver cytosolic dibasic cationic amino acids into the paracellular space in exchange for Na^+ and neutral amino. This defect is not compensated by the SLC3A1/SLC7A9 transporter (at the apical membrane), the latter being affected in cystinuria. The symptoms of LPI, which appear after weaning, include diarrhea, failure to thrive, hepatosplenomegaly, nephritis, respiratory insufficiency, alveolar proteinosis, pulmonary fibrosis, and osteoporosis. Abnormalities of bone marrow have also been described in a subgroup of LPI patients. The disorder is characterized by low plasma concentrations of dibasic amino acids (in contrast to high levels of citrulline, glutamine, and alanine) and massive excretion of lysine (as well as orotic acid, ornithine, and arginine in moderate excess) in the urine. Hyperammonemia and coma usually develop after episodic attacks of vomiting, after fasting, or following administration of large amounts of protein (or alanine load), possibly due to a deficiency of intramitochondrial ornithine. Some patients show moderate retardation. Cutaneous manifestations can include alopecia, perianal dermatitis, and sparse hair. Some patients avoid protein-containing food. Treatment includes orally administered citrulline (200 mg/kg/day), which is well absorbed from the intestine; dietary protein restriction (<1.5 g/kg/day); and carnitine supplementation. One patient with **isolated lysinuria** has been reported with growth failure, seizures, and mental retardation.

DISORDERS OF FAT TRANSPORT

Abetalipoproteinemia, hypobetalipoproteinemia, and chylomicron retention disease are described in Chapter 80. The long-chain fatty acid (FATP4) and cholesterol transporters, the latter being called Niemann-Pick C1-like protein (NPC1L1), have been characterized at the intestinal brush border in knock-out mice models showing a hyperproliferative hyperkeratosis and an impaired fatty acid and cholesterol uptake. NPC1L1 is inhibited by ezetimibe, which is used to restrict the absorption of dietary cholesterol.

Tangier disease is characterized by the absence of high-density lipoprotein cholesterol (HDL-C), which is caused by mutations in the adenosine triphosphate (ATP)-binding cassette transporter A1 (ABCA1) gene. The failure of intracellular phospholipids and cholesterol efflux to lipid-poor apolipoprotein acceptors such as HDL predisposes to premature coronary heart disease and accumulation of cholesterol in liver, spleen, lymph nodes (tonsils), and small intestine.

Features of Tangier disease include orange tonsils, hepatosplenomegaly, relapsing neuropathy, orange-brown spots on the colon and ileum, diarrhea in association with decreased plasma cholesterol levels (apo A-I, apo A-II), and normal or elevated triglyceride levels. Specific therapy for Tangier disease has not yet been established.

In **sitosterolemia** defective efflux of sterol leads to increased absorption of dietary sterols; normally, <5% are retained by the GI tract. Patients carry mutations of the ABCG5 (sterolin-1) and ABCG8 (sterolin-2) transporters. The disorder is associated with tendon xanthomas, increased atherosclerosis, and hemolysis. Plasma levels of phytosterols (mainly sitosterol) are typically >10 mg/dL.

DISORDERS OF VITAMIN ABSORPTION

Transporters and receptors of the intestinal epithelium have been described for water-soluble but not fat-soluble vitamins, the latter being absorbed primarily by enterocytes, by passive diffusion after emulsification of fats by bile salts. Transfer proteins (retinol-binding protein, RBP4 and α-tocopherol transfer protein, TTP1) have been involved in deficiency states of vitamins E (spinocerebellar ataxia) and A (ophthalmologic signs), respectively.

Vitamin B_{12} (cobalamin) is used exclusively by microorganisms and is acquired mostly from meat and milk. Its absorption starts with the removal of cobalamin from dietary protein by gastric acidity and its binding to haptocorrin. In the duodenum, pancreatic proteases hydrolyze the cobalamin-haptocorrin complex, allowing the binding of cobalamin to intrinsic factor (IF), which originates from parietal cells. The receptor of the cobalamin-IF complex is located at the apical membrane of the ileal enterocytes and represents a heterodimer consisting of cubulin and amnionless, with endocytic uptake of this ligand into endosomes, where it binds to megalin and forms a cobalamin–transcobalamin-2 complex (after cleavage of IF) for further transcytosis. As a cofactor for methionine synthase, cobalamin converts homocysteine to methionine. Cobalamin deficiency can be caused by inadequate intake of the vitamin (e.g., breast-feeding by mothers on a vegetarian diet), primary or secondary achlorhydria including autoimmune gastritis, exocrine pancreatic insufficiency, bacterial overgrowth (Chapter 330.4), ileal disease (Crohn disease, Chapter 328), ileal (or gastric) resection, infections (fish tapeworm), and Whipple disease (Chapter 333).

Clinical signs of congenital **cobalamin malabsorption**, which usually appear from a few months to 14 yr of age, are pancytopenia including megaloblastic anemia, fatigue, failure to thrive, and neurologic symptoms including developmental delay. Recurrent infections and bruising may be present. Laboratory evaluation indicates low serum cobalamin, hyperhomocysteinemia, methylmalonicacidemia, and mild proteinuria. The Schilling test is useful to differentiate between lack of IF and malabsorption of cobalamin. Three rare autosomal recessive disorders of congenital cobalamin deficiency affect absorption and transport of cobalamin (in addition to 7 other inherited defects of cobalamin metabolism). These include mutations of the gastric IF (GIF) gene with absence of IF (but normal acid secretion and lack of autoantibodies against IF or parietal cells), mutations of the amnionless *(AMN)* and cubilin *(CUBN)* genes (**Imerslund-Grasbeck syndrome**), and mutations in the transcobalamin 2 cDNA. These disorders require long-term parenteral cobalamin treatment: intramuscular injections of hydroxycobalamin 1 mg daily for 10 days and then once a month. High-dose substitution with oral cyanocobalamin (1 mg biweekly) does not seem to be sufficient for all patients with congenital cobalamin deficiency.

Folate is an essential vitamin required to synthesize methionine from homocysteine. It is found mainly in green leafy vegetables, legumes, and oranges. It is converted to 5-methyltetrahydrofolate (5MTHF) after its uptake by enterocytes. Secondary folate deficiency is caused by insufficient folate intake, villous atrophy (e.g., celiac disease, IBD), treatment with phenytoin, and trimethoprim among others (Chapter 448.1). Several inherited disorders of folate metabolism and transport have been described.

Hereditary **folate malabsorption** is characterized by a defect of the proton-coupled folate transporter (PCFT, formerly reported to be HCP1, a heme carrier) of the brush border, leading to impaired absorption of folate in the upper small intestine as well as impaired transport of folate into the central nervous system. Mutations of the reduced folate carrier (RFC1, SLC19A1) have not been found in this entity. Sulfasalazine and methotrexate are potent inhibitors of PCFT. Symptoms of congenital folate malabsorption are diarrhea, failure to thrive, megaloblastic anemia (in the 1st few months of life), glossitis, infections *(Pneumocystis jirovecii)* with hypoimmunoglobulinemia, and neurologic abnormalities (seizures, mental retardation, and basal ganglia calcifications). Macrocytosis, with or without neutropenia, multilobulated polymorphonuclear cells, increased LDH and bilirubin, increased saturation of transferrin, and decreased cholesterol can be found. Low levels of folate are present in serum and cerebrospinal fluid. Plasma homocysteine concentrations as well as urine excretion of formiminoglutamic acid and orotic acid are elevated. Long-lasting deficiency is best documented using red cell folate. Therapy involves large doses of oral (up to 100 mg/day) or systemic (intrathecal) folate.

The molecular basis of intestinal transport of other water-soluble vitamins such as **vitamin C** (Na^+-dependent vitamin C transporter, SVCT1 and SVCT2), **pyridoxine/vitamin B_6**, and **biotin/vitamin B_5** (Na^+-dependent multivitamin transporter, SMVT) have been described; however congenital defects of these transporter systems have not yet been found in humans. A **thiamine/vitamin B_1**-responsive megaloblastic anemia (TRMA) syndrome, which is associated with early-onset type 1 diabetes mellitus and sensorineural deafness, is caused by mutations of the thiamine transporter protein, THTR-1 (SLC19A2), present in the brush border.

DISORDERS OF ELECTROLYTE AND MINERAL ABSORPTION

Congenital chloride diarrhea belongs to the more common causes of severe congenital diarrhea, with prevalence in Finland of 1: 20,000. It is caused by a defect of the *SLC26A3* gene, which encodes a Na^+-independent Cl^-/HCO_3^- exchanger within the apical membrane of ileal and colonic epithelium. Founder mutations have been described in Finnish, Polish, and Arab patients: V317del, I675-676ins, and G187X, respectively. The Cl^-/HCO_3^- exchanger absorbs chloride originating from gastric acid and the cystic fibrosis transmembrane conductance regulator (CFTR) and secretes bicarbonate into the lumen, neutralizing the acidity of gastric secretion.

Prenatal clinical signs of this disorder are a dilated small bowel that can mislead to a diagnosis of intestinal obstruction. Newborns with congenital chloride diarrhea present with severe life-threatening secretory diarrhea during the 1st weeks of life. Laboratory findings are metabolic alkalosis, hypochloremia, hypokalemia, and hyponatremia (with high plasma renin and aldosterone activities). Fecal chloride concentrations are >90 mmol/L and exceed the sum of fecal sodium and potassium. Early diagnosis and aggressive lifelong enteral substitution of KCl in combination with NaCl (chloride doses of 6-8 mmol/kg/day for infants and 3-4 mmol/kg/day for older patients) prevent mortality and long-term complications (such as urinary infections, hyperuricemia with renal calcifications, renal insufficiency, and hypertension) and allow normal growth and development. Orally administered proton pump inhibitors, cholestyramine, and butyrate can reduce the severity of diarrhea. The diarrheal symptoms usually tend to regress with age. However, febrile diseases are likely to exacerbate symptoms as a consequence of severe dehydration and electrolyte imbalances. (See Chapter 52 for fluid and electrolyte management.)

The classic form of **congenital sodium diarrhea** manifests with polyhydramnios, massive secretory diarrhea, severe metabolic acidosis, alkaline stools (fecal pH >7.5) and hyponatremia as a result of fecal losses of Na^+ (fecal Na^+ >70 mmol/L). Urinary secretion of sodium is low to normal. There is partial villous atrophy. The molecular genetic defect could not be located in the Na^+-H^+ exchangers (NHEs), which were thought to be impaired because they seem to be mainly responsible for Na^+ absorption in the small intestine. In addition, a syndromic form of congenital sodium diarrhea with choanal or anal atresia, hypertelorism, and corneal erosions has been related to mutations of *SPINT2*, encoding a serine-protease inhibitor, whose pathophysiologic action on intestinal Na^+ absorption is unclear. Some patients can be weaned from parenteral nutrition later in childhood but depend on oral sodium citrate supplementation.

The congenital form of **acrodermatitis enteropathica** manifests with severe deficiency of body zinc soon after birth in bottle-fed children or after weaning from breastfeeding. Clinical signs of this disorder are anorexia, diarrhea, failure to thrive, humoral and cell-mediated immunodeficiency (poor wound healing, recurrent infections), male hypogonadism, skin lesions (vesicobullous dermatitis on the extremities and perirectal, perigenital, and perioral regions, and alopecia), and neurologic abnormalities (tremor, apathy, depression, irritability, nystagmus, photophobia, night blindness, and hypogeusia). The genetic defect of acrodermatitis enteropathica is caused by a mutation in the Zrt-Irt-lik protein 4 (ZIP4, SLC39A4), normally expressed on the apical membrane, which enables the uptake of zinc into the cytosol of enterocytes. The zinc-dependent alkaline phosphatase and plasma zinc levels are low. Paneth cells in the crypt of the small intestinal mucosa show inclusion bodies. Acrodermatitis enteropathica requires long-term treatment with elemental zinc 1 mg/kg/day. Maternal zinc deficiency impairs embryonic, fetal, and postnatal development. Acquired forms of zinc deficiency are described in Chapter 51.

Menkes disease and **occipital horn syndrome** are both caused by mutations in the gene encoding Cu^{2+} transporting ATPase, alpha polypeptide (ATP7A), also called Menkes or MNK protein. ATP7A is mainly expressed by enterocytes, placental cells, and CNS and is localized in the trans-Golgi network for copper transfer to enzymes in the secretory pathway or to endosomes to facilitate copper efflux. Copper values in liver and brain are low in contrast to an increase in mucosal cells, including enterocytes and fibroblasts. Plasma copper and ceruloplasmin levels decline postnatally. Clinical features of Menkes disease are progressive cerebral degeneration (convulsions), feeding difficulties, failure to thrive, hypothermia, apnea, infections (urinary tract), peculiar facies, hair abnormalities (kinky hair), hypopigmentation, bone changes, and cutis laxa. Patients with the classic form of Menkes disease usually die before the age of 3 yr. A therapeutic trial with copper-histidinate should start before the age of 6 wk. In contrast to Menkes disease, occipital horn syndrome usually manifests during adolescence with borderline intelligence, craniofacial abnormalities, skeletal dysplasia (short clavicles, pectus excavatum, genu valgum), connective tissue abnormalities, chronic diarrhea, orthostatic hypotension, obstructive uropathy, and osteoporosis. It should be differentiated from Ehlers-Danlos syndrome type V.

Active **calcium** absorption is mediated by the transient receptor potential channel 6 (TRPV6) at the brush border membrane, calbindin, and the CaATPase, or the Na^+-Ca^{++} exchanger for calcium efflux at the basolateral membrane within the proximal small bowel. A congenital defect of these transporters has not yet been described.

Intestinal absorption of dietary magnesium, which occurs via the transient receptor potential channel TRPM6 at the apical membrane, is impaired in familial **hypomagnesemia with secondary hypocalcemia**, which manifests with neonatal seizures and tetany.

Intestinal iron absorption consists of several complex regulated processes starting with the uptake of heme-containing iron by heme carrier protein 1 (HCP1) and Fe^{2+} (after luminal reduction of oxidized Fe^{3+}) by the divalent metal transporter 1 (DMT1) at the apical membrane, followed by the efflux of Fe^{2+} by ferroportin 1 (also called iron-regulated transporter[IREG1]) at the basolateral membrane of duodenal enterocytes. Mutations of the ferroportin 1 gene have been found in the autosomal dominant form of **hemochromatosis type 4**. Mutations of HFE (Cys282 Tyr, His63Asn, Ser65Cys) of classic hemochromatosis reduce the endocytic uptake of diferric transferrin by the transferrin receptor-1 (TfR1) at the basolateral membrane of the intestinal epithelium. Hepcidin antimicrobial peptide (HAMP) encodes hepcidin, a hepatic peptide hormone, which inhibits the efflux of iron through ferroportin and can be induced by IL-6. It is the defective gene of juvenile hemochromatosis (type 2, subtype B).

BIBLIOGRAPHY

Please visit the Nelson Textbook of Pediatrics *website at www.expertconsult.com for the complete bibliography.*

330.12 Malabsorption in Eosinophilic Gastroenteritis

Ernest G. Seidman and David Branski

The diagnosis of eosinophilic gastroenteritis is based on GI symptoms, GI eosinophilic infiltrates, and no demonstrable cause of the eosinophilia such as parasitic infection (most commonly *Enterobius vermicularis* in children) or a specific allergic response. Peripheral eosinophilia is variable and not uniformly considered a criterion for diagnosis. The majority (50-70%) of patients have a history of other allergic disorders, and others might have associated connective tissue diseases. Approximately 10% of patients with this disorder have an immediate family member with this disorder as well, suggesting that eosinophilic GI disorders stem from a genetic predisposition, common environmental factors, or, most likely, a combination. Hypersensitivity to specific food allergens has been postulated as an etiologic factor. Symptoms depend on the severity and location of eosinophilic inflammation. Any region or layer (mucosa, submucosa, and serosa) of the gut may be involved, alone or in combination.

For the full continuation of this chapter, please visit the Nelson Textbook of Pediatrics *website at www.expertconsult.com.*

330.13 Malabsorption in Inflammatory Bowel Disease

Ernest G. Seidman and David Branski

Crohn disease and ulcerative colitis represent the 2 forms of chronic, immune-mediated IBD that commonly affect pediatric patients (Chapter 328). Because the small bowel is involved in the majority of pediatric Crohn disease patients, malabsorption of nutrients is far more of a problem than in ulcerative colitis. At the time of diagnosis, significant weight loss is observed in up to 85% of pediatric patients with Crohn disease and in about 65% with ulcerative colitis, due to inadequate intake of energy and micronutrients as well as diarrhea and malabsorption. Consequently, growth failure due to chronic undernutrition is far more common in Crohn disease than in ulcerative colitis, affecting up to 40% of cases.

For the full continuation of this chapter, please visit the Nelson Textbook of Pediatrics *website at www.expertconsult.com.*

Chapter 331 Intestinal Transplantation in Children with Intestinal Failure

Jorge D. Reyes

The introduction of **tacrolimus** and the development of the abdominal **multiorgan procurement** techniques allowed the tailoring of various types of intestine grafts, which can contain other intra-abdominal organs such as the liver, pancreas, and stomach; this tailoring has been critical to the application of this type of organ transplant, given the wide scope of diseases for which replacement of the intestine may be necessary. Also, the understanding that the liver protects the intestine against rejection had been suggested by previous combinations of liver plus other organs such as the kidney. The first survivors of intestine transplantation would also go on to demonstrate the interaction (host-versus-graft and graft-versus-host) between recipient and donor immunocytes (brought with the allograft), which under the cover of immunosuppression allows varying degrees of graft acceptance and eventual minimization of drug therapy.

For the full continuation of this chapter, please visit the Nelson Textbook of Pediatrics *website at www.expertconsult.com.*

Chapter 332
Acute Gastroenteritis in Children

Zulfiqar Ahmed Bhutta

The term *gastroenteritis* denotes infections of the gastrointestinal (GI) tract caused by bacterial, viral, or parasitic pathogens (Tables 332-1 to 332-3). Many of these infections are foodborne illnesses. The most common manifestations are diarrhea and vomiting, which can also be associated with systemic features such as abdominal pain and fever. The term **gastroenteritis** captures the bulk of infectious cases of diarrhea. The term **diarrheal disorders** is more commonly used to denote infectious diarrhea in public health settings, although several noninfectious causes of GI illness with vomiting and/or diarrhea are well recognized (Table 332-4).

EPIDEMIOLOGY OF CHILDHOOD DIARRHEA

Diarrheal disorders in childhood account for a large proportion (18%) of childhood deaths, with an estimated 1.5 million deaths per year globally, making it the second most common cause of child deaths worldwide. The World Health Organization (WHO) and UNICEF estimate that almost 2.5 billion episodes of diarrhea occur annually in children <5 yr of age in developing countries, with more than 80% of the episodes occurring in Africa and South Asia (46% and 38%, respectively). Global mortality may be declining, but the overall incidence of diarrhea remains unchanged at about 3.6 episodes per child-year (Fig. 332-1), and it is estimated to account for 13% of all childhood disability-adjusted life years (DALYs).

Although the exact etiologic fractions of diarrhea in developing countries are a subject of much research, there are indications that rates of various types of bacterial diarrhea may be decreasing. There are indications that rates of hospitalization and deaths due to *Shigella* infections, especially *Shigella dysenteriae* type 1, the most severe form of shigellosis, may be declining and account for almost 160,000 deaths annually. Enterotoxigenic *Escherichia coli* (ETEC) may be responsible for 300,000-500,000 deaths among children <5 yr annually. Rotavirus infections (the most common identifiable viral cause of gastroenteritis in all children) account for 527,000 deaths annually or 29% of all deaths due to diarrhea among children <5 yr of age. About 23% of deaths due to rotavirus disease occurred in India; 6 countries (India, Nigeria, Congo, Ethiopia, China, and Pakistan) accounted for >50% of deaths due to rotavirus disease.

The decline in diarrheal mortality, despite the lack of significant changes in incidence, is the result of preventive rotavirus vaccination and improved case management of diarrhea, as well as improved nutrition of infants and children. These interventions have included widespread home- and hospital-based oral rehydration therapy and improved nutritional management of children with diarrhea.

Persistently high rates of diarrhea among young children, despite intensive efforts at control, are of particular concern. There is very little information on the long-term consequences of diarrheal diseases, especially persistent or prolonged diarrhea and subsequent malnutrition. Diarrheal illnesses can have a significant impact on psychomotor and cognitive development in young children. Early and repeated episodes of childhood diarrhea during periods of critical development, especially when associated with malnutrition, co-infections, and anemia, can have long-term effects on linear growth, as well as on physical and cognitive functions.

ETIOLOGY OF DIARRHEA

Gastroenteritis is due to infection acquired through the fecal-oral route or by ingestion of contaminated food or water. Gastroenteritis is associated with poverty, poor environmental hygiene, and development indices. Enteropathogens that are infectious in a small inoculum (*Shigella*, enterohemorrhagic *E. coli, Campylobacter jejuni,* noroviruses, rotavirus, *Giardia lamblia, Cryptosporidium parvum, Entamoeba histolytica*) can be transmitted by person-to-person contact, whereas others, such as cholera, are generally a consequence of contamination of food or water supply (see Tables 332-1 to 332-3).

In the United States, rotavirus and the noroviruses (small round viruses such as Norwalk-like virus and caliciviruses) are the most common viral agents, followed by sapovirus, enteric adenoviruses, and astroviruses (see Table 332-2). Food-borne outbreaks of bacterial diarrhea in the United States are most commonly due to *Salmonella, E. coli, Clostridium botulinum, Clostridium perfringens,* and *Staphylococcus aureus* followed much less often by *Campylobacter, Shigella, Cryptosporidium, Yersinia, Listeria, Vibrio,* and *Cyclospora* species, in that order. *Salmonella, Shigella,* and, most notably, the various diarrhea-producing *E. coli* organisms are the most common bacterial pathogens in developing countries (see Table 332-1). *Clostridium difficile* (by toxin production) is linked to antibiotic-associated diarrhea and pseudomembranous colitis, although most cases of antibiotic-associated diarrhea in children are not due to *C. difficile. C. difficile*-negative antibiotic-associated hemorrhagic colitis in adults may be due to cytotoxin-producing *Klebsiella oxytoca.* Waterborne outbreaks are often due to *Cryptosporidium* species (most common), *C. jejuni,* noroviruses, *Shigella* species, *Giardia, E. coli* O157:H7, *Plesiomonas shigelloides,* or *Vibrio* species.

In developed countries, episodes of infectious diarrhea can occur through seasonal exposure to organisms such as rotavirus or exposure to pathogens in settings of close contact (e.g., daycare centers). Children in developing countries become infected with a diverse group of bacterial and parasitic pathogens, whereas all children in developed as well as developing countries acquire rotavirus and, in many cases, other viral enteropathogens as well as *G. lamblia* and *C. parvum* in their 1st 5 yr of life.

PATHOGENESIS OF INFECTIOUS DIARRHEA

Pathogenesis and severity of bacterial disease depend on whether organisms have preformed toxins *(S. aureus, Bacillus cereus)*, produce secretory (cholera, *E. coli, Salmonella, Shigella*) or cytotoxic (*Shigella, S. aureus, Vibrio parahemolyticus, C. difficile, E. coli, C. jejuni*) toxins or are invasive and on whether they replicate in food. Enteropathogens can lead to either an inflammatory or noninflammatory response in the intestinal mucosa (Table 332-5).

Text continued on p. 1330

Table 332-1 FOODBORNE BACTERIAL ILLNESSES

ETIOLOGY	INCUBATION PERIOD	SIGNS AND SYMPTOMS	DURATION OF ILLNESS	ASSOCIATED FOODS	LABORATORY TESTING	TREATMENT
Bacillus anthracis	2 days to weeks	Nausea, vomiting, malaise, bloody diarrhea, acute abdominal pain	Weeks	Insufficiently cooked contaminated meat	Blood	Penicillin is first choice for naturally acquired GI anthrax Ciprofloxacin is 2nd option
Bacillus cereus (preformed enterotoxin)	1-6 hr	Sudden onset of severe nausea and vomiting Diarrhea may be present	24 hr	Improperly refrigerated cooked or fried rice, meats	Normally a clinical diagnosis Clinical laboratories do not routinely identify this organism If indicated, send stool and food specimens to reference laboratory for culture and toxin identification	Supportive care
Bacillus cereus (diarrheal toxin)	10-16 hr	Abdominal cramps, watery diarrhea, nausea	24-48 hr	Meats, stews, gravies, vanilla sauce	Testing not necessary, self-limiting Consider testing food and stool for toxin in outbreaks	Supportive care
Brucella abortus, B. melitensis, and *B. suis*	7-21 days	Fever, chills, sweating, weakness, headache, muscle and joint pain, diarrhea, bloody stools during acute phase	Weeks	Raw milk, goat cheese made from unpasteurized milk, contaminated meats	Blood culture and positive serology	Acute: Rifampin and doxycycline daily for ≥6 wk Infections with complications require combination therapy with rifampin, tetracycline, and an aminoglycoside
Campylobacter jejuni	2-5 days	Diarrhea, cramps, fever, and vomiting; diarrhea may be bloody	2-10 days	Raw and undercooked poultry, unpasteurized milk, contaminated water	Routine stool culture; Campylobacter requires special media and incubation at 42°C to grow	Supportive care For severe cases, antibiotics such as erythromycin and quinolones may be indicated early in the diarrheal disease Guillain-Barré syndrome can be a sequela
Clostridium botulinum: children and adults (preformed toxin)	12-72 hr	Vomiting, diarrhea, blurred vision, diplopia, dysphagia, descending muscle weakness	Variable (days to months) Can be complicated by respiratory failure and death	Home-canned foods with a low acid content, improperly canned commercial foods, home-canned or fermented fish, herb-infused oils, baked potatoes in aluminium foil, cheese sauce, bottled garlic, foods held warm for extended periods (e.g., in a warm oven)	Stool, serum, and food can be tested for toxin Stool and food can also be cultured for the organism These tests can be performed at some state health department laboratories and CDC	Supportive care Botulism antitoxin is helpful if given early in the course of the illness Contact the state health department. The 24-hour number for state health departments to call is (800) 232-4636
Clostridium botulinum: infants	3-30 days	In infants <12 mo, lethargy, weakness, poor feeding, constipation, hypotonia, poor head control, poor gag and sucking reflex	Variable	Honey, home-canned vegetables and fruits, corn syrup	Stool, serum, and food can be tested for toxin Stool and food can also be cultured for the organism These tests can be performed at some state health department laboratories and CDC	Supportive care Botulism immune globulin can be obtained from the Infant Botulism Prevention Program, Health and Human Services, California (510-540-2646) Botulinum antitoxin is generally not recommended for infants
Clostridium perfringens toxin	8-16 hr	Watery diarrhea, nausea, abdominal cramps; fever is rare	24-48 hr	Meats, poultry, gravy, dried or precooked foods, time- and/or temperature-abused food	Stools can be tested for enterotoxin and cultured for organism Because *Clostridium perfringens* can normally be found in stool, quantitative cultures must be done	Supportive care Antibiotics not indicated
Enterohemorrhagic *Escherichia coli* (EHEC) including *E. coli* 0157:H7 and other *Shiga* toxin–producing *E. coli* (STEC)	1-8 days	Severe diarrhea that is often bloody; abdominal pain and vomiting Usually, little or no fever is present More common in children <4 yr old	5-10 days	Undercooked beef especially hamburger, unpasteurized milk and juice, raw fruits and vegetables (e.g., sprouts), salami (rarely), contaminated water	Stool culture; *E. coli* 0157:H7 requires special media to grow. If *E. coli* 0157:H7 is suspected, specific testing must be requested. *Shiga* toxin testing may be done using commercial kits; positive isolates should be forwarded to public health laboratories for confirmation and serotyping.	Supportive care, monitor renal function, hemoglobin, and platelets closely. *E. coli* 0157:H7 infection is also associated with hemolytic uremic syndrome (HUS), which can cause lifelong complications Studies indicate that antibiotics might promote the development of HUS
Enterotoxigenic *E. coli* (ETEC)	1-3 days	Watery diarrhea, abdominal cramps, some vomiting	3 to >7 days	Water or food contaminated with human feces	Stool culture ETEC requires special laboratory techniques for identification Must request specific testing	Supportive care Antibiotics are rarely needed except in severe cases Recommended antibiotics include

	symptoms, 2-6 wk for invasive disease	diarrhea Pregnant women might have mild flulike illness, and infection can lead to premature delivery or stillbirth Elderly or immunocompromised patients can have bacteremia or meningitis		unpasteurized milk, inadequately pasteurized milk, ready-to-eat deli meats, hot dogs	Asymptomatic fecal carriage occurs; therefore, stool culture usually not helpful Antibody to listerolysin O may be helpful to identify outbreak retrospectively	intravenous ampicillin, penicillin, or TMP-SMX are recommended for invasive disease
	At birth and infancy	Infants infected from mother at risk for sepsis or meningitis				
Salmonella spp.	1-3 days	Diarrhea, fever, abdominal cramps, vomiting *S. typhi* and *S. paratyphi* produce typhoid with insidious onset characterized by fever, headache, constipation, malaise, chills, and myalgia; diarrhea is uncommon, and vomiting is not usually severe	4-7 days	Contaminated eggs, poultry, unpasteurized milk or juice, cheese, contaminated raw fruits and vegetables (alfalfa sprouts, melons) *S. typhi* epidemics are often related to fecal contamination of water supplies or street-vended foods	Routine stool cultures	Supportive care Other than for *S. typhi* and *S. paratyphi,* antibiotics are not indicated unless there is extra-intestinal spread, or the risk of extra-intestinal spread, of the infection Consider ampicillin, gentamicin, TMP-SMX, or quinolones if indicated A vaccine exists for *S. typhi*
Shigella spp.	24-48 hr	Abdominal cramps, fever, diarrhea Stools might contain blood and mucus	4-7 days	Food or water contaminated with human fecal material Usually person-to-person spread, fecal-oral transmission Ready-to-eat foods touched by infected food workers, e.g., raw vegetables, salads, sandwiches	Routine stool cultures	Supportive care. TMP-SMX recommended in the USA if organism is susceptible; nalidixic acid or other quinolones may be indicated if organism is resistant, especially in developing countries
Staphylococcus aureus (preformed enterotoxin)	1-6 hr	Sudden onset of severe nausea and vomiting Abdominal cramps Diarrhea and fever may be present	24-48 hr	Unrefrigerated or improperly refrigerated meats, potato and egg salads, cream pastries	Normally a clinical diagnosis Stool, vomitus, and food can be tested for toxin and cultured if indicated	Supportive care
Vibrio cholerae (toxin)	24-72 hr	Profuse watery diarrhea and vomiting, which can lead to severe dehydration and death within hours	3-7 days Causes life-threatening dehydration	Contaminated water, fish, shellfish, street-vended food typically from Latin America or Asia	Stool culture *V. cholerae* requires special media to grow; if *V. cholerae* is suspected, must request specific testing	Supportive care with aggressive oral and intravenous rehydration In cases of confirmed cholera, tetracycline or doxycycline is recommended for adults, and TMP-SMX for children <8 yr
Vibrio parahaemolyticus	2-48 hr	Watery diarrhea, abdominal cramps, nausea, vomiting.	2-5 days	Undercooked or raw seafood, such as fish, shellfish	Stool cultures. *V. parahaemolyticus* requires special media to grow; must request specific testing	Supportive care Antibiotics are recommended in severe cases: tetracycline, doxycycline, gentamicin, and cefotaxime
Vibrio vulnificus	1-7 days	Vomiting, diarrhea, abdominal pain, bactermia, and wound infections More common in the immunocompromised or in patients with chronic liver disease (presenting with bullous skin lesions) Can be fatal in patients with liver disease and the immunocompromised	2-8 days	Undercooked or raw shellfish, especially oysters, other contaminated seafood, and open wounds exposed to seawater	Stool, wound, or blood cultures *V. vulnificus* requires special media to grow; if *V. vulnificus* is suspected, must request specific testing	Supportive care and antibiotics; tetracycline, doxycycline, and ceftazidime are recommended
Yersinia enterocolytica and *Y. pseudotuberculosis*	24-48 hr	Appendicitis-like symptoms (diarrhea and vomiting, fever, abdominal pain) occur primarily in older children and young adults Might have a scarlitiniform rash or erythema nodosum with *Y. pseudotuberculosis*	1-3 wk, usually self-limiting	Undercooked pork, unpasteurized milk, tofu, contaminated water Infection has occurred in infants whose caregivers handled chitterlings	Stool, vomitus, or blood culture *Yersinia* requires special media to grow; must request specific testing Serology is available in research and reference laboratories	Supportive care If septicemia or other invasive disease occurs, antibiotic therapy with gentamicin or cefotaxime (doxycycline and ciprofloxacin also effective)

CDC, Centers for Disease Control and Prevention; GI, gastrointestinal; TMP-SMX, trimethoprim-sulfamethoxazole.
From Centers for Disease Control and Prevention: Diagnosis and management of foodborne illnesses, *MMWR* 53:7–9, 2004.

Table 332-2 FOODBORNE VIRAL ILLNESSES

ETIOLOGY	INCUBATION PERIOD	SIGNS AND SYMPTOMS	DURATION OF ILLNESS	ASSOCIATED FOODS	LABORATORY TESTING	TREATMENT
Hepatitis A	28 days average (15-50 days)	Diarrhea, dark urine, jaundice, and flulike symptoms, i.e., fever, headache, nausea, and abdominal pain	Variable, 2 wk-3 mo	Shellfish harvested from contaminated waters, raw produce, contaminated drinking water, uncooked foods, and cooked foods that are not reheated after contact with infected food handler	Increase in ALT, bilirubin Positive IgM and anti-hepatitis A antibodies	Supportive care Prevention with immunization
Caliciviruses (including norovirses and sapoviruses)	12-48 hr	Nausea, vomiting, abdominal cramping, diarrhea, fever, myalgia, and some headache Diarrhea is more prevalent in adults and vomiting is more prevalent in children Prolonged asymptomatic excretion possible	12-60 hr	Shellfish, fecally contaminated foods, ready-to-eat foods touched by infected food workers (salads, sandwiches, ice, cookies, fruit)	Routine RT-PCR and EM on fresh unpreserved stool samples Clinical diagnosis, negative bacterial cultures Stool is negative for WBCs	Supportive care such as rehydration Good hygiene
Rotavirus (groups A-C)	1-3 days	Vomiting, watery diarrhea, low-grade fever Temporary lactose intolerance can occur Infants and children, elderly, and immunocompromised are especially vulnerable	4-8 days	Fecally contaminated foods Ready-to-eat foods touched by infected food workers (salads, fruits)	Identification of virus in stool via immunoassay	Supportive care Severe diarrhea can require fluid and electrolyte replacement
Other viral agents (astroviruses, adenoviruses, parvoviruses)	10-70 hr	Nausea, vomiting, diarrhea, malaise, abdominal pain, headache, fever	2-9 days	Fecally contaminated foods Ready-to-eat foods touched by infected food workers Some shellfish	Identification of the virus in early acute stool samples Serology Commercial ELISA kits are available for adenoviruses and astroviruses	Supportive care, usually mild, self-limiting Good hygiene

ALT, alanine aminotransferase; ELISA, enzyme linked immunoserbent assay; EM, electron microscopy; IgM, immunoglobulin M; RT-PCR, reverse transcriptase polymerase chain reaction; WBCs, white blood cells.
From Centers for Disease Control and Prevention: Diagnosis and management of foodborne illnesses, *MMWR* 53:9, 2004.

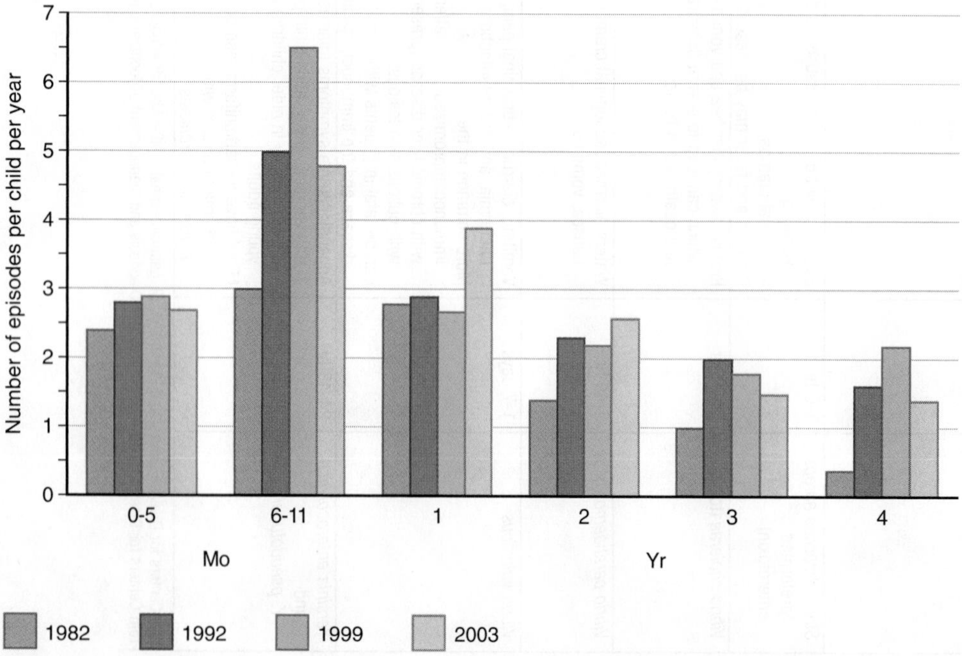

Figure 332-1 Global trends in diarrhea incidence.

Table 332-3 FOODBORNE PARASITIC ILLNESSES

ETIOLOGY	INCUBATION PERIOD	SIGNS AND SYMPTOMS	DURATION OF ILLNESS	ASSOCIATED FOODS	LABORATORY TESTING	TREATMENT
Angiostrongylus cantonensis	1 wk to ≥1 mo	Severe headaches, nausea, vomiting, neck stiffness, paresthesias, hyperesthesias, seizures, and other neurologic abnormalities	Several weeks to several months	Raw or undercooked intermediate hosts (e.g., snails or slugs), infected paratenic (transport) hosts (e.g., crabs, freshwater shrimp), fresh produce contaminated with intermediate or transport hosts	Examination of CSF for elevated pressure, protein, leukocytes, and eosinophils; serologic testing using ELISA to detect antibodies to *Angiostrongylus cantonensis*	Supportive care. Repeat lumbar punctures and use of corticosteroid therapy may be used for more severely ill patients
Cryptosporidium	2-10 days	Diarrhea (usually watery), stomach cramps, upset stomach, slight fever	May be remitting and relapsing over weeks to months	Any uncooked food or food contaminated by an ill food handler after cooking; drinking water	Request specific examination of the stool for *Cryptosporidium* May need to examine water or food	Supportive care, self-limited If severe consider paromomycin for 7 days For children aged 1-11 yr, consider nitazoxanide for 3 days
Cyclospora cayetanensis	1-14 days, usually at ≥1 wk	Diarrhea (usually watery), loss of appetite, substantial loss of weight, stomach cramps, nausea, vomiting, fatigue	May be remitting and relapsing over weeks to months	Various types of fresh produce (imported berries, lettuce)	Request specific examination of the stool for *Cyclospora* May need to examine water or food	TMP-SMX for 7 days
Entamoeba histolytica	2-3 days to 1-4 wk	Diarrhea (often bloody), frequent bowel movements, lower abdominal pain	May be protracted (several weeks to several months)	Any uncooked food or food contaminated by an ill food handler after cooking; drinking water	Examination of stool for cysts and parasites; may need at least 3 samples Serology for long-term infections	Metronidazole and a luminal agent (iodoquinol or paromomycin)
Giardia lamblia	1-2 wk	Diarrhea, stomach cramps, gas, weight loss	Days to weeks	Any uncooked food or food contaminated by an ill food handler after cooking; drinking water	Examination of stool for ova and parasites; may need at least 3 samples	Metronidazole
Toxoplasma gondii	5-23 days	Generally asymptomatic, 20% develop cervical lymphadenopathy and/or a flulike illness In immunocompromised patients: CNS disease, myocarditis, or pneumonitis is often seen	Months	Accidental ingestion of contaminated substances (e.g., soil contaminated with cat feces on fruits and vegetables), raw or partially cooked meat (especially pork, lamb, or venison)	Isolation of parasites from blood or other body fluids; observation of parasites in patient specimens via microscopy or histology Detection of organisms is rare; serology (reference laboratory needed) can be a useful adjunct in diagnosing toxoplasmosis; however, IgM antibodies can persist for 6-18 mo and thus do not necessarily indicate recent infection PCR of bodily fluids	Asymptomatic healthy, but infected, persons do not require treatment Spiramycin or pyrimethamine plus sulfadiazine may be used for pregnant women Pyrimethamine plus sulfadiazine may be used for immunocompromised persons, in specific cases Pyrimethamine plus sulfadiazine (with or without steroids) may be given for ocular disease when indicated Folinic acid is given with pyrimethamine plus sulfadiazine to counteract bone marrow suppression

Continued

Table 332-3 FOODBORNE PARASITIC ILLNESSES—cont'd

ETIOLOGY	INCUBATION PERIOD	SIGNS AND SYMPTOMS	DURATION OF ILLNESS	ASSOCIATED FOODS	LABORATORY TESTING	TREATMENT
Toxoplasma gondii (congenital infection)	In infants at birth	Treatment of the mother can reduce severity and/or incidence of congenital infection Most infected infants have few symptoms at birth; later, they generally develop signs of congenital toxoplasmosis (mental retardation, severely impaired eyesight, cerebral palsy, seizures), unless the infection is treated	Months	Passed from mother (who acquired acute infection during pregnancy) to child	Isolation of *T. gondii* from placenta, umbilical cord, or infant blood; PCR of white blood cells, CSF, or amniotic fluid, or IgM and IgA serology, performed by a reference laboratory	
Trichinella spiralis	1-2 days for initial symptoms; others begin 2-8 wk after infection	Acute: nausea, diarrhea, vomiting, fatigue, fever, abdominal discomfort followed by muscle soreness, weakness, and occasional cardiac and neurologic complications	Months	Raw or undercooked contaminated meat, usually pork or wild game meat (e.g., bear or moose)	Positive serology or demonstration of larvae via muscle biopsy; increase in eosinophils	Supportive care plus mebendazole or albendazole

CNS, central nervous system; CSF, cerebrospinal fluid; ELISA, enzyme linked immunoserbent assay; IgM, immunoglobulin M; PCR, polymerase chain reaction; TMP-SMX, trimethoprim-sulfamethoxazole.
From Centers for Disease Control and Prevention: Diagnosis and management of foodborne illnesses, *MMWR* 53:9–10, 2004.

Table 332-4 FOODBORNE NONINFECTIOUS ILLNESSES

ETIOLOGY	INCUBATION PERIOD	SIGNS AND SYMPTOMS	DURATION OF ILLNESS	ASSOCIATED FOODS	LABORATORY TESTING	TREATMENT
Antimony	5 min–8 hr usually <1 hr	Vomiting, metallic taste	Usually self-limited	Metallic container	Identification of metal in beverage or food	Supportive care
Arsenic	Few hours	Vomiting, colic, diarrhea	Several days	Contaminated food	Urine Can cause eosinophilia	Gastric lavage, BAL (dimercaprol)
Cadmium	5 min–8 hr usually <1 hr	Nausea, vomiting, myalgia, increase in salivation, stomach pain	Usually self-limited	Seafood, oysters, clams, lobster, grains, peanuts	Identification of metal in food	Supportive care
Ciguatera fish poisoning (ciguatera toxin)	2-6 hr	GI: abdominal pain, nausea, vomiting, diarrhea	Days to weeks to months	A variety of large reef fish: grouper, red snapper, amberjack, and barracuda (most common)	Radioassay for toxin in fish or a consistent history	Supportive care, IV mannitol Children more vulnerable
	3 hr	Neurologic: paresthesias, reversal of hot or cold, pain, weakness				
	2-5 days	Cardiovascular: bradycardia, hypotension, increase in T wave abnormalities				
Copper	5 min–8 hr usually <1 hr	Nausea, vomiting, blue or green vomitus	Usually self-limited	Metallic container	Identification of metal in beverage or food	Supportive care
Mercury	1 wk or longer	Numbness, weakness of legs, spastic paralysis, impaired vision, blindness, coma Pregnant women and the developing fetus are especially vulnerable	May be protracted	Fish exposed to organic mercury, grains treated with mercury fungicides	Analysis of blood, hair	Supportive care
Mushroom toxins, short-acting (museinol, muscarine, psilocybin, *Coprius artemetaris*, ibotenic acid)	<2 hr	Vomiting, diarrhea, confusion, visual disturbance, salivation, diaphoresis, hallucinations, disulfiram-like reaction, confusion, visual disturbance	Self-limited	Wild mushrooms (cooking might not destroy these toxins)	Typical syndrome and mushroom identified or demonstration of the toxin	Supportive care

Table 332-4 FOODBORNE NONINFECTIOUS ILLNESSES—cont'd

ETIOLOGY	INCUBATION PERIOD	SIGNS AND SYMPTOMS	DURATION OF ILLNESS	ASSOCIATED FOODS	LABORATORY TESTING	TREATMENT
Mushroom toxins, long-acting (amanitin)	4-8 hr diarrhea; 24-48 hr liver failure	Diarrhea, abdominal cramps, leading to hepatic and renal failure	Often fatal	Mushrooms	Typical syndrome and mushroom identified and/or demonstration of the toxin	Supportive care, life-threatening, may need life support
Nitrite poisoning	1-2 hr	Nausea, vomiting, cyanosis, headache, dizziness, weakness, loss of consciousness, chocolate-brown blood	Usually self-limited	Cured meats, any contaminated foods, spinach exposed to excessive nitrification	Analysis of the food, blood	Supportive care, methylene blue
Pesticides (organophosphates or carbamates)	Few min to few hr	Nausea, vomiting, abdominal cramps, diarrhea, headache, nervousness, blurred vision, twitching, convulsions, salivation, meiosis	Usually self-limited	Any contaminated food	Analysis of the food, blood	Atropine; 2-PAM (Pralidoxime) is used when atropine is not able to control symptoms and is rarely necessary in carbamate poisoning
Puffer fish (tetrodotoxin)	<30 min	Parasthesias, vomiting, diarrhea, abdominal pain, ascending paralysis, respiratory failure	Death usually in 4-6 hr	Puffer fish	Detection of tetrodotoxin in fish	Life-threatening, may need respiratory support
Scombroid (histamine)	1 min-3 hr	Flushing, rash, burning sensation of skin, mouth and throat, dizziness, urticaria, paresthesias	3-6 hr	Fish: bluefin, tuna, skipjack, mackerel, marlin, escolar, and mahi mahi	Demonstration of histamine in food or clinical diagnosis	Supportive care, antihistamines
Shellfish toxins (diarrheic, neurotoxic, amnesic)	Diarrheic shellfish poisoning (DSP): 30 min to 2 hr	Nausea, vomiting, diarrhea, and abdominal pain accompanied by chills, headache, and fever	Hours to 2-3 days	A variety of shellfish, primarily mussels, oysters, scallops, and shellfish from the Florida coast and the Gulf of Mexico	Detection of the toxin in shellfish; high-pressure liquid chromatography	Supportive care, generally self-limiting
	Neurotoxic shellfish poisoning (NSP): few min to hours	Tingling and numbness of lips, tongue, and throat, muscular aches, dizziness, reversal of the sensations of hot and cold, diarrhea, and vomiting				
	Amnesic shellfish poisoning (ASP): 24-48 hr	Vomiting, diarrhea, abdominal pain and neurologic problems such as confusion, memory loss, disorientation, seizure, coma				Elderly are especially sensitive to ASP
Shellfish toxins (paralytic shellfish poisoning)	30 min–3 hr	Diarrhea, nausea, vomiting leading to paresthesias of mouth and lips, weakness, dysphasia, dysphonia, respiratory paralysis	Days	Scallops, mussels, clams, cockles	Detection of toxin in food or water where fish are located; high-pressure liquid chromatography	Life-threatening, may need respiratory support
Sodium fluoride	Few min to 2 hr	Salty or soapy taste, numbness of mouth, vomiting, diarrhea, dilated pupils, spasms, pallor, shock, collapse	Usually self-limited	Dry foods (e.g., dry milk, flour, baking powder, cake mixes) contaminated with NaF-containing insecticides and rodenticides	Testing of vomitus or gastric washings Analysis of the food	Supportive care
Thallium	Few hours	Nausea, vomiting, diarrhea, painful parathesias, motor polyneuropathy, hair loss	Several days	Contaminated food	Urine, hair	Supportive care
Tin	5 min–8 hr usually <1 hr	Nausea, vomiting, diarrhea	Usually self-limited	Metallic container	Analysis of the food	Supportive care
Vomitoxin	Few min to 3 hr	Nausea, headache, abdominal pain, vomiting	Usually self-limited	Grains such as wheat, corn, barley	Analysis of the food	Supportive care
Zinc	Few hours	Stomach cramps, nausea, vomiting, diarrhea, myalgias	Usually self-limited	Metallic container	Analysis of the food, blood and feces, saliva or urine	Supportive care

From Centers for Disease Control and Prevention: Diagnosis and management of foodborne illnesses, *MMWR* 53:11–12, 2004.

Table 332-5 COMPARISON OF THREE TYPES OF ENTERIC INFECTION

PARAMETER	TYPE OF INFECTION I	II	III
Mechanism	Noninflammatory (enterotoxin or adherence/superficial invasion)	Inflammatory (invasion, cytotoxin)	Penetrating
Location	Proximal small bowel	Colon	Distal small bowel
Illness	Watery diarrhea	Dystentery	Enteric fever
Stool examination	No fecal leukocytes Mild or no ↑ lactoferrin	Fecal polymorphonuclear leukocytes ↑↑ Lactoferrin	Fecal mononuclear leukocytes
Examples	*Vibrio cholerae* *Escherichia coli* (ETEC, LT, ST) *Clostridium perfringens* *Bacillus cereus* *Staphylococcus aureus* Also†: *Giardia lamblia* *Rotavirus* Norwalk-like viruses *Cryptosporidium parvum* *E. coli* (EPEC, EAEC) *Microsporidia* *Cyclospora cayetanensis*	*Shigella* *E. coli* (EIEC, EHEC) *Salmonella enteridis* *Vibrio parahaemolyticus* *Clostridium difficile* *Campylobacter jejuni* *Entamoeba histolytica**	*Salmonella typhi* *Yersinia enterocolitica* *?Campylobacter fetus*

*Although amebic dysentery involves tissue inflammation, the leukocytes are characteristically pyknotic or absent, having been destroyed by the virulent amebae.
†Although not typically enterotoxic, these pathogens alter bowel physiology via adherence, superficial cell entry, cytokine induction, or toxins that inhibit cell function.
EAEC, enteroagregative *E. coli*; EHEC, enterohemorrhagic *E. coli*; EIEC, enteroinvasive *E. coli*; EPEC, enteropathogenic *E. coli*; ETEC, enterotoxigenic *E. coli*; LT, heat-labile; ST, heat-stable.
From Mandel GL, Bennett JE, Dolin R, editors: *Principles and practices of infectious diseases*, ed 7, Philadelphia, 2010, Churchill Livingstone.

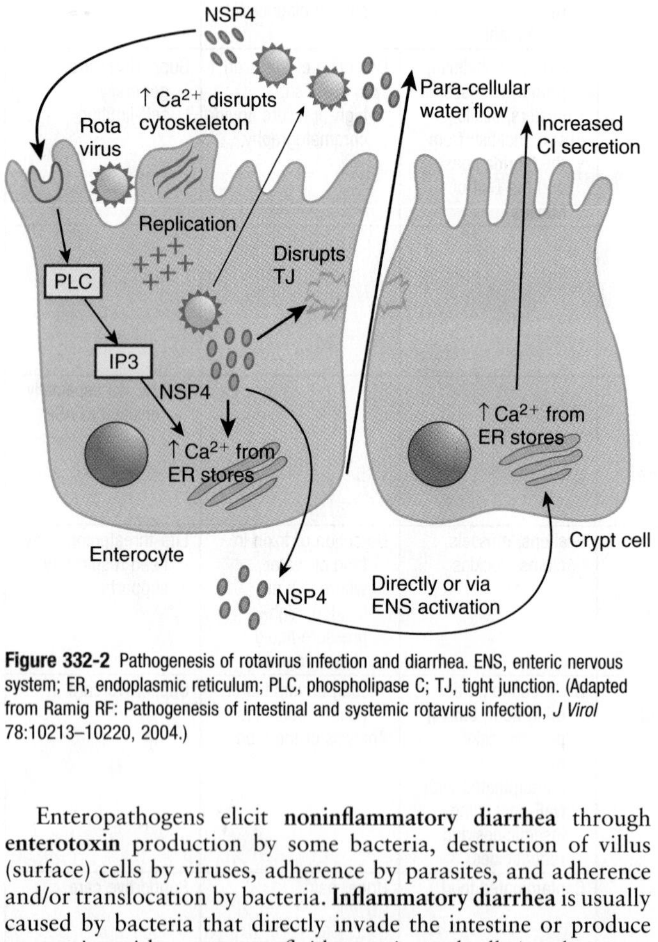

Figure 332-2 Pathogenesis of rotavirus infection and diarrhea. ENS, enteric nervous system; ER, endoplasmic reticulum; PLC, phospholipase C; TJ, tight junction. (Adapted from Ramig RF: Pathogenesis of intestinal and systemic rotavirus infection, *J Virol* 78:10213–10220, 2004.)

Enteropathogens elicit **noninflammatory diarrhea** through **enterotoxin** production by some bacteria, destruction of villus (surface) cells by viruses, adherence by parasites, and adherence and/or translocation by bacteria. **Inflammatory diarrhea** is usually caused by bacteria that directly invade the intestine or produce cytotoxins with consequent fluid, protein, and cells (erythrocytes, leukocytes) that enter the intestinal lumen. Some enteropathogens possess >1 virulence property. Some viruses, such as rotavirus, target the microvillus tips of the enterocytes and can enter the cells by direct invasion or calcium-dependent endocytosis. This can result in villus shortening and loss of enterocyte absorptive surface through cell shortening and loss of microvilli (Fig. 332-2).

Most bacterial pathogens elaborate enterotoxins; the rotavirus protein NSP4 acts as a viral enterotoxin. Bacterial enterotoxins can selectively activate enterocyte intracellular signal transduction and can also affect cytoskeletal rearrangements with subsequent alterations in the water and electrolyte fluxes across enterocytes. In toxigenic diarrhea enterotoxin produced by *Vibrio cholerae*, increased mucosal levels of cAMP inhibit electroneutral NaCl absorption but have no effect on glucose-stimulated Na^+ absorption. In inflammatory diarrhea (e.g., *Shigella* spp. or *Salmonella* spp.) there is extensive histologic damage, resulting in altered cell morphology and reduced glucose-stimulated Na^+ and electroneutral NaCl absorption. The role of 1 or more cytokines in this inflammatory response is critical. In secretory cells from crypts, Cl-secretion is minimal in normal subjects and is activated by cyclic adenosine monophosphate (cAMP) in toxigenic and inflammatory diarrhea (Fig. 332-3).

ETEC colonizes and adheres to enterocytes of the small bowel via its surface fimbriae (pili) and induces hypersecretion of fluids and electrolytes into the small intestine through 1 of 2 toxins: the heat-labile enterotoxin (LT) or the heat-stable enterotoxin. LT is structurally similar to the *V. cholerae* toxin, and activates adenylate cyclase, resulting in an increase in intracellular cyclic guanosine monophosphate (cGMP) (Fig. 332-4). In contrast, *Shigella* spp. cause gastroenteritis via a superficial invasion of colonic mucosa, which they invade through M cells located over Peyer patches. After phagocytosis, a series of events occurs, including apoptosis of macrophages, multiplication and spread of bacteria into adjacent cells, release of inflammatory mediators (interleukin [IL]-1 and IL-8), transmigration of neutrophils into the lumen of the colon, neutrophil necrosis and degranulation, further breach of the epithelial barrier, and mucosal destruction (Fig. 332-5).

RISK FACTORS FOR GASTROENTERITIS

Major risks include environmental contamination and increased exposure to enteropathogens. Additional risks include young age, immunodeficiency, measles, malnutrition, and lack of exclusive or predominant breast-feeding. Malnutrition increases the risk of diarrhea and associated mortality, and moderate to severe stunting increases the odds of diarrhea-associated mortality 1.6- to 4.6-fold. The fraction of such infectious diarrhea deaths that are attributable to nutritional deficiencies

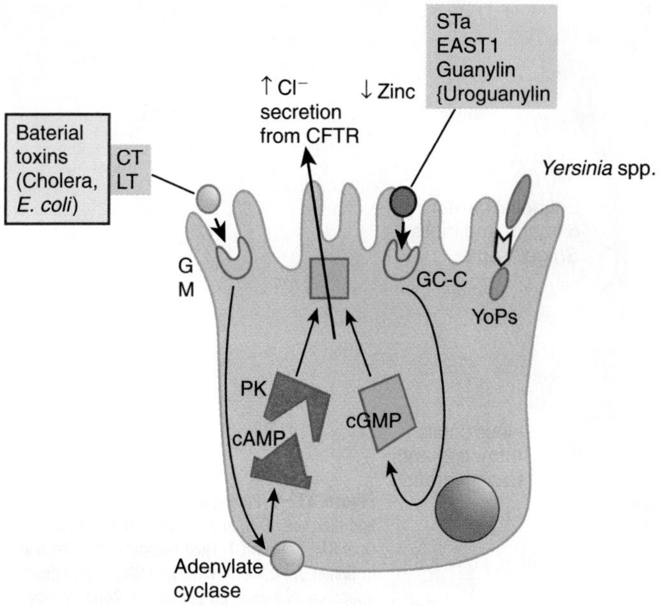

Figure 332-3 Mechanism of cholera toxin. (Adapted from Thapar M, Sanderson IR: Diarrhoea in children: an interface between developing and developed countries, *Lancet* 363:641–653, 2004; and Montes M, DuPont HL: Enteritis, enterocolitis and infectious diarrhea syndromes. In Cohen J, Powderly WG, Opal SM, et al, editors: *Infections diseases,* ed 2, London, 2004, Mosby, pp 31–52.)

varies with the prevalence of deficiencies; the highest attributable fractions are in sub-Saharan Africa, south Asia, and Andean Latin America. The risks are particularly higher with micronutrient malnutrition; in children with **vitamin A deficiency,** the risk of dying from diarrhea, measles, and malaria is increased by 20-24%. **Zinc deficiency** is estimated to increase the risk of mortality from diarrhea, pneumonia, and malaria by 13-21%.

The majority of cases of diarrhea resolve within the 1st wk of the illness. A smaller proportion of diarrheal illnesses fail to resolve and persist for >2 wk. **Persistent diarrhea** is defined as episodes that began acutely but last for ≥14 days. Such episodes account for 3-20% of all diarrheal episodes in children <5 yr of age and up to 50% of all diarrhea-related deaths. Many children (especially infants and toddlers) in developing countries have frequent episodes of acute diarrhea. Although few individual episodes persist beyond 14 days, frequent episodes of acute diarrhea can result in nutritional compromise and can predispose these children to develop persistent diarrhea, protein-calorie malnutrition, and secondary infections. In addition, increasing attention is being focused on prolonged episodes of diarrhea that last 7-13 days and are associated with significant nutritional penalties.

CLINICAL MANIFESTATION OF DIARRHEA

Most of the clinical manifestations and clinical syndromes of diarrhea are related to the infecting pathogen and the dose or

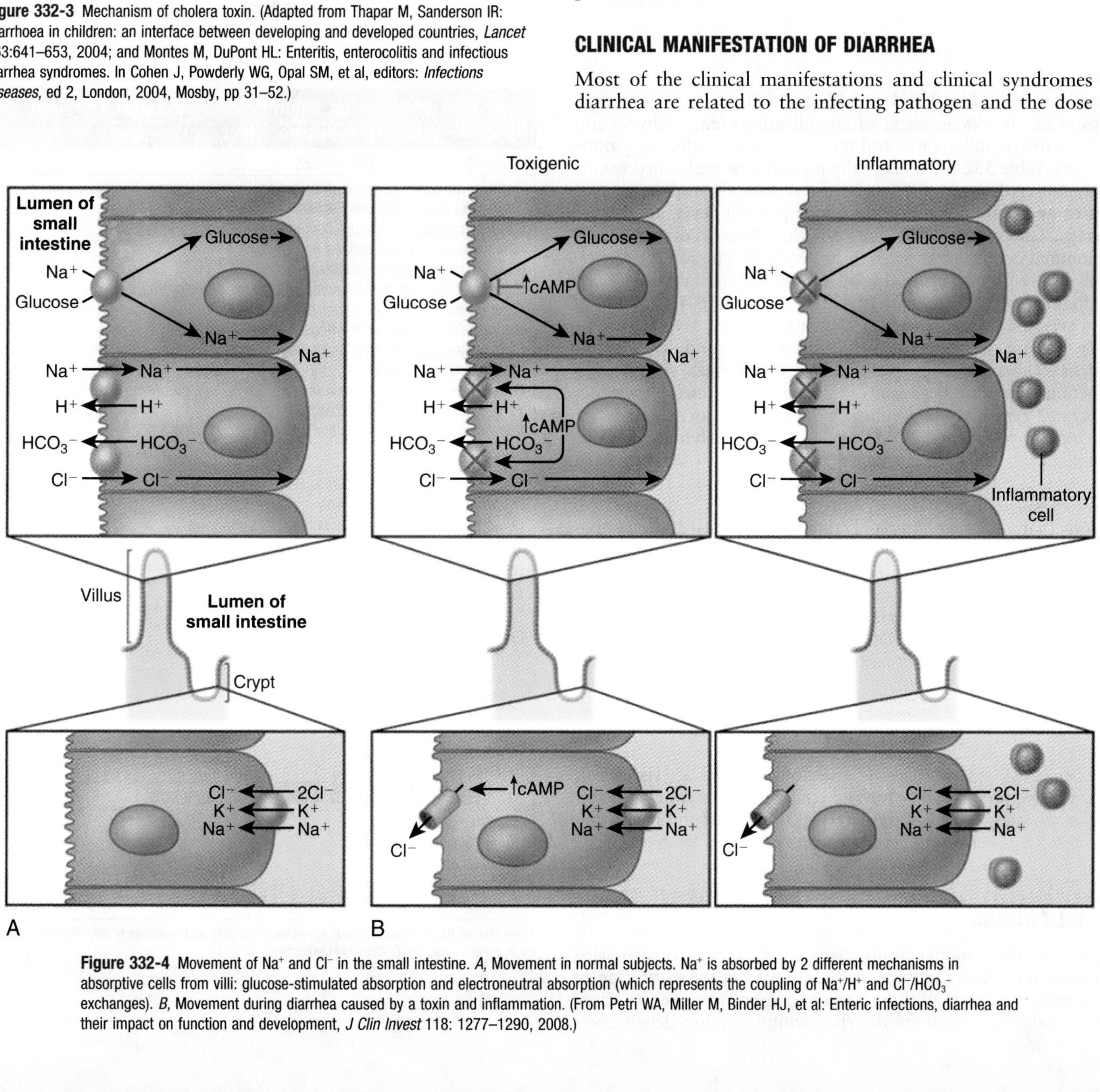

Figure 332-4 Movement of Na^+ and Cl^- in the small intestine. *A,* Movement in normal subjects. Na^+ is absorbed by 2 different mechanisms in absorptive cells from villi: glucose-stimulated absorption and electroneutral absorption (which represents the coupling of Na^+/H^+ and Cl^-/HCO_3^- exchanges). *B,* Movement during diarrhea caused by a toxin and inflammation. (From Petri WA, Miller M, Binder HJ, et al: Enteric infections, diarrhea and their impact on function and development, *J Clin Invest* 118: 1277–1290, 2008.)

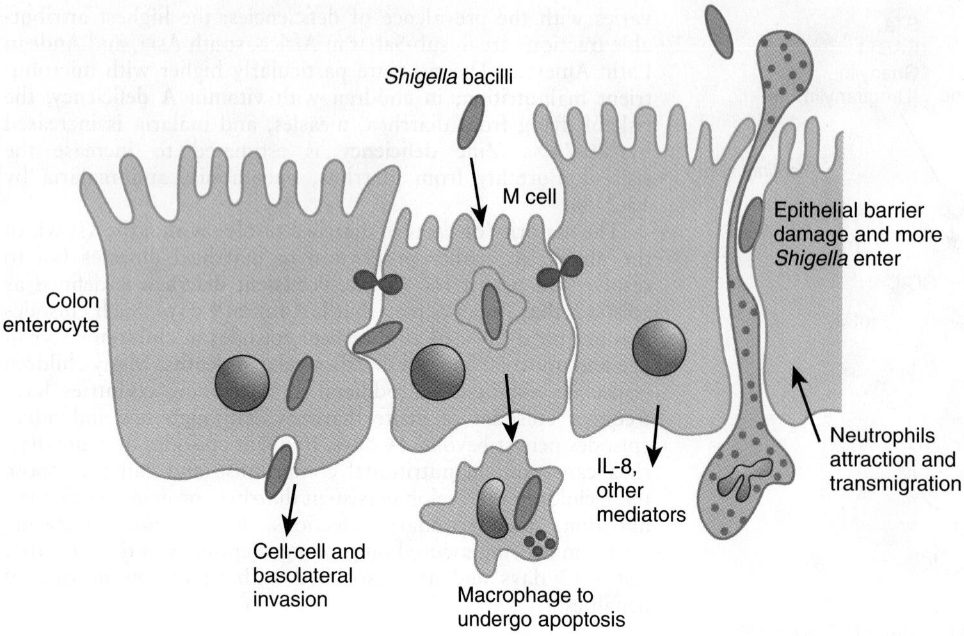

Figure 332-5 Pathogenesis of *Shigella* infection and diarrhea. IL-8, interleukin-8. (Adapted from Opal SM, Keusch GT: Host responses to infection. In Cohen J, Powderly WG, Opal SM, et al, editors: *Infections diseases,* ed 2, London, 2004, Mosby, pp 31–52.)

inoculum (see Tables 332-1 to 332-3). Additional manifestations depend on the development of complications (e.g., dehydration and electrolyte imbalance) and the nature of the infecting pathogen (see Table 332-5). Usually the ingestion of preformed toxins (e.g., those of *S. aureus*) is associated with the rapid onset of nausea and vomiting within 6 hr, with possible fever, abdominal cramps, and diarrhea within 8-72 hr. Watery diarrhea and abdominal cramps after an 8-16 hr incubation period are associated with enterotoxin-producing *C. perfringens* and *B. cereus.* Abdominal cramps and watery diarrhea after a 16-48 hr incubation period can be associated with noroviruses, several enterotoxin-producing bacteria, *Cryptosporidium,* and *Cyclospora* and have also been a notable feature of influenza virus H1N1 infections. Several organisms, including *Salmonella, Shigella, C. jejuni, Yersinia enterocolitica,* enteroinvasive or hemorrhagic (Shigatoxin-producing) *E. coli,* and *V. parahaemolyticus,* produce diarrhea that can contain blood as well as fecal leukocytes in association with abdominal cramps, tenesmus, and fever; these features suggest **bacterial dysentery** and fever (Table 332-6). Bloody diarrhea and abdominal cramps after a 72-120 hr incubation period are associated with infections due to *Shigella* and also Shigatoxin-producing *E. coli,* such as *E. coli* O157:H7. Organisms associated with dysentery or hemorrhagic diarrhea can also cause watery diarrhea alone without fever or that precedes a more complicated course that results in dysentery.

Although many of the manifestations of acute gastroenteritis in children are nonspecific, some clinical features can help identify major categories of diarrhea and allow rapid triage for antibiotic or specific dietary therapy (see Tables 332-1 to 332-3). There is considerable overlap in the symptomatology. The positive predictive values for the features of dysentery are very poor; the negative predictability for bacterial pathogens is much better in the absence of signs of dysentery. If warranted and if facilities and resources permit, the etiology can be verified by appropriate laboratory testing.

COMPLICATIONS

Most of the complications associated with gastroenteritis are related to delays in diagnosis and delays in the institution of appropriate therapy. Without early and appropriate rehydration, many children with acute diarrhea would develop dehydration

Table 332-6 DIFFERENTIAL DIAGNOSIS OF ACUTE DYSENTERY AND INFLAMMATORY ENTEROCOLITIS

SPECIFIC INFECTIOUS PROCESSES
Bacillary dysentery (*Shigella dysenteriae, Shigella flexneri, Shigella sonnei, Shigella boydii;* invasive *Escherichia coli*)
Campylobacteriosis *(Campylobacter jejuni)*
Amebic dysentery *(Entamoeba histolytica)*
Ciliary dysentery *(Balantidium coli)*
Bilharzial dysentery *(Schistosoma japonicum, Schistosoma mansoni)*
Other parasitic infections *(Trichinella spiralis)*
Vibriosis *(Vibrio parahaemolyticus)*
Salmonellosis *(Salmonella typhimurium)*
Thyphoid fever *(Salmonella typhi)*
Enteric fever *(Salmonella choleraesuis, Salmonella paratyhpi)*
Yersiniosis *(Yersinia enterocolitica)*
Spirillar dysentery (*Sprillium* spp.)
PROCTITIS
Gonococcal *(Neisseria gonorrhoeae)*
Herpetic (herpes simplex virus)
Chlamydial *(Chlamydia trachomatis)*
Syphilitic *(Treponema pallidum)*
OTHER SYNDROMES
Necrotizing enterocolitis of the newborn
Enteritis necroticans
Pseudomembranous enterocolitis *(Clostridium difficile)*
Typhlitis
CHRONIC INFLAMMATORY PROCESSES
Enteropathogenic and enteroaggregative *E. coli*
Gastrointestinal tuberculosis
Gastrointestinal mycosis
Parasitic enteritis
SYNDROMES WITHOUT KNOWN INFECTIOUS CAUSE
Idiopathic ulcerative colitis
Crohn disease
Radiation enteritis
Ischemic colitis
Allergic enteritis

From Mandel GL, Bennett JE, Dolin R, editors: *Principles and practices of infectious diseases,* ed 7, Philadelphia, 2010, Churchill Livingstone.

Table 332-7 EXTRAINTESTINAL MANIFESTATIONS OF ENTERIC INFECTIONS

MANIFESTATION	ASSOCIATED ENTERIC PATHOGEN(S)	ONSET AND PROGNOSIS
Focal infections due to systemic spread of bacterial pathogens, including vulvovaginitis, urinary tract infection, endocarditis, osteomyelitis, meningitis, pneumonia, hepatitis, peritonitis, chorioamnionitis, soft tissue infection, and septic thrombophlebitis	All major pathogens can cause such direct extraintestinal infections, including *Salmonella, Shigella, Yersinia, Campylobacter, Clostridium difficile*	Onset usually during the acute infection, but can occur subsequently Prognosis depends on infection site
Reactive arthritis	*Salmonella, Shigella, Yersinia, Campylobacter, Cryptosporidium, Clostridium difficile*	Typically occurs about 1-3 wk after infection Relapses after reinfection can develop in 15-50% of people but most children recover fully within 2-6 mo after the 1st symptoms appear
Guillain-Barré syndrome	*Campylobacter*	Usually occurs a few weeks after the original infection Prognosis is good although 15-20% may have sequelae
Glomerulonephritis	*Shigella, Campylobacter, Yersinia*	Can be of sudden onset in acute, referring to a sudden attack of inflammation, or chronic, which comes on gradually In most cases, the kidneys heal with time
IgA nephropathy	*Campylobacter*	Characterized by recurrent episodes of blood in the urine, this condition results from deposits of the protein immunoglobulin A (IgA) in the glomeruli. IgA nephropathy can progress for years with no noticeable symptoms Men seem more likely to develop this disorder than women
Erythema nodosum	*Yersinia, Campylobacter, Salmonella*	Although painful, is usually benign and more commonly seen in adolescents Resolves with 4-6 wk
Hemolytic uremic syndrome	*Shigella dysenteriae* 1, *Escherichia coli* 0157:H7, others	Sudden onset, short-term renal failure In severe cases, renal failure requires several sessions of dialysis to take over the kidney function, but most children recover without permanent damage to their health
Hemolytic anemia	*Campylobacter, Yersinia*	Relatively rare complication and can have a chronic course

From: Centers for Disease Control and Prevention: Managing acute gastroenteritis among children, *MMWR Recomm Rep* 53:1–33, 2004.

with associated complications (Chapter 54). These can be life-threatening in infants and young children. Inappropriate therapy can lead to prolongation of the diarrheal episodes, with consequent malnutrition and complications such as secondary infections and micronutrient deficiencies (iron, zinc). In developing countries and HIV-infected populations, associated bacteremias are well-recognized complications in malnourished children with diarrhea.

Specific pathogens are associated with extraintestinal manifestations and complications. These are not pathognomonic of the infection, nor do they always occur in close temporal association with the diarrheal episode (Table 332-7).

DIAGNOSIS

The diagnosis of gastroenteritis is based on clinical recognition, an evaluation of its severity by rapid assessment and by confirmation by appropriate laboratory investigations, if indicated.

Clinical Evaluation of Diarrhea

The most common manifestation of GI tract infection in children is diarrhea, abdominal cramps, and vomiting. Systemic manifestations are varied and associated with a variety of causes. The evaluation of a child with acute diarrhea includes:

- Assess the degree of dehydration and acidosis and provide rapid resuscitation and rehydration with oral or intravenous fluids as required (Tables 332-8 and 332-9).
- Obtain appropriate contact, travel, or exposure history. This includes information on exposure to contacts with similar symptoms, intake of contaminated foods or water, child-care center attendance, recent travel of patient or contact with a person who traveled to a diarrhea-endemic area, and use of antimicrobial agents.

Table 332-8 SYMPTOMS ASSOCIATED WITH DEHYDRATION

SYMPTOM	MINIMAL OR NO DEHYDRATION (<3% LOSS OF BODY WEIGHT)	MILD TO MODERATE DEHYDRATION (3-9% LOSS OF BODY WEIGHT)	SEVERE DEHYDRATION (<9% LOSS OF BODY WEIGHT)
Mental status	Well; alert	Normal, fatigued or restless, irritable	Apathetic, lethargic, unconscious
Thirst	Drinks normally; might refuse liquids	Thirsty; eager to drink	Drinks poorly; unable to drink
Heart rate	Normal	Normal to increased	Tachycardia, with bradycardia in most severe cases
Quality of pulses	Normal	Normal to decreased	Weak, thready, or impalpable
Breathing	Normal	Normal; fast	Deep
Eyes	Normal	Slightly sunken	Deeply sunken
Tears	Present	Decreased	Absent
Mouth and tongue	Moist	Dry	Parched
Skinfold	Instant recoil	Recoil in <2 sec	Recoil in >2 sec
Capillary refill	Normal	Prolonged	Prolonged; minimal
Extremities	Warm	Cool	Cold; mottled; cyanotic
Urine output	Normal to decreased	Decreased	Minimal

Adapted from Duggan C, Santosham M, Glass RI: The management of acute diarrhea in children: oral rehydration, maintenance, and nutritional therapy, *MMWR Recomm Rep* 41(RR-16):1–20, 1992; and World Health Organization: *The treatment of diarrhoea: a manual for physicians and other senior health workers,* Geneva, 1995, World Health Organization; Centers for Disease Control and Prevention: Diagnosis and management of foodborne illnesses, *MMWR* 53:5, 2004.

Table 332-9 SUMMARY OF TREATMENT BASED ON DEGREE OF DEHYDRATION

DEGREE OF DEHYDRATION	REHYDRATION THERAPY	REPLACEMENT OF LOSSES	NUTRITION
Minimal or no dehydration	Not applicable	<10 kg body weight: 60-120 mL ORS for each diarrheal stool or vomiting episode>10 kg body weight: 120-240 mL ORS for each diarrheal stool or vomiting episode	Continue breast-feeding, or resume age-appropriate normal diet after initial hydration, including adequate caloric intake for maintenance*
Mild to moderate dehydration	ORS, 50-100 mL/kg body weight over 3-4 hr	Same	Same
Severe dehydration	Lactated Ringer solution or normal saline in 20 mL/kg body weight IV until perfusion and mental status improve; then administer 100 mL/kg body weight ORS over 4 hr or 5% dextrose ½ normal saline IV at twice maintenance fluid rates	Same; if unable to drink, administer through nasogastric tube or administer 5% dextrose in ¼ normal saline with 20 mEq/L potassium chloride IV	Same

*Overly restricted diets should be avoided during acute diarrheal episodes. Breast-fed infants should continue to nurse ad libitum even during acute rehydration. Infants too weak to eat can be given milk or formula through a nasogastric tube. Lactose-containing formulas are usually well tolerated. If lactose malabsorption appears clinically substantial, lactose-free formulas can be used. Complex carbohydrates, fresh fruits, lean meats, yogurt, and vegetables are all recommended. Carbonated drinks or commercial juices with a high concentration of simple carbohydrates should be avoided.
ORS, oral rehydration solution.
From Centers for Disease Control and Prevention: Diagnosis and management of foodborne illnesses, *MMWR* 53:1–33, 2004.

- Clinically determine the etiology of diarrhea for institution of prompt antibiotic therapy, if indicated. Although nausea and vomiting are nonspecific symptoms, they indicate infection in the upper intestine. Fever suggests an inflammatory process but also occurs as a result of dehydration or co-infection (e.g., urinary tract infection, otitis media). Fever is common in patients with inflammatory diarrhea. Severe abdominal pain and tenesmus indicate involvement of the large intestine and rectum. Features such as nausea and vomiting and absent or low-grade fever with mild to moderate periumbilical pain and watery diarrhea indicate small intestine involvement and also reduce the likelihood of a serious bacterial infection.

This clinical approach to the diagnosis and management of diarrhea in young children is a critical component of the **integrated management of childhood illness (IMCI)** package that is being implemented in developing countries with high burden of diarrhea mortality (Fig. 332-6).

Stool Examination
Microscopic examination of the stool and cultures can yield important information on the etiology of diarrhea. Stool specimens should be examined for mucus, blood, and leukocytes. Fecal leukocytes indicate bacterial invasion of colonic mucosa, although some patients with shigellosis have minimal leukocytes at an early stage of infection, as do patients infected with Shigatoxin-producing *E. coli* and *E. histolytica.* In endemic areas, stool microscopy must include examination for parasites causing diarrhea, such as *G. lamblia* and *E. histolytica.*

Stool cultures should be obtained as early in the course of disease as possible from children with **bloody diarrhea** in whom stool microscopy indicates **fecal leukocytes,** in **outbreaks** with suspected **hemolytic-uremic syndrome** (**HUS**), and in **immunosuppressed** children with diarrhea. Stool specimens for culture need to be transported and plated quickly; if the latter is not quickly available, specimens might need to be transported in special media. The yield and diagnosis of bacterial diarrhea is improved by using molecular diagnostic procedures such as PCR. In most previously healthy children with uncomplicated watery diarrhea, no laboratory evaluation is needed except for epidemiologic purposes.

TREATMENT
The broad principles of management of acute gastroenteritis in children include oral rehydration therapy, enteral feeding and diet selection, zinc supplementation, and additional therapies such as probiotics.

Oral Rehydration Therapy
Children, especially infants, are more susceptible than adults to dehydration because of the greater basal fluid and electrolyte requirements per kg and because they are dependent on others to meet these demands. **Dehydration** must be evaluated rapidly and corrected in 4-6 hr according to the degree of dehydration and estimated daily requirements. A small minority of children, especially those in shock or unable to tolerate oral fluids, require initial intravenous rehydration, but oral rehydration is the preferred mode of rehydration and replacement of ongoing losses (see Tables 332-8 and 332-9). Risks associated with severe dehydration that might necessitate intravenous resuscitation include: age <6 mo, prematurity, chronic illness, fever >38°C if <3 mo or >39°C if 3-36 mo, bloody diarrhea, persistent emesis, poor urine output, sunken eyes, and a depressed level of consciousness. The low-osmolality WHO oral rehydration solution (ORS) containing 75 mEq of sodium and 75 mmol of glucose per liter, with total osmolarity of 245 mOsm per liter, is more effective than other formulations in reducing stool output without the risk of hyponatremia, and it is now the global standard of care (Table 332-10).

Cereal-based oral rehydration fluids can also be advantageous in malnourished children and can be prepared at home. Home remedies including decarbonated soda beverages, fruit juices, and tea are not suitable for rehydration or maintenance therapy because they have inappropriately high osmolalities and low sodium concentrations. A clinical evaluation plan and management strategy for children with moderate to severe diarrhea is outlined in Figure 332-6 and Table 332-9. Oral rehydration should be given to infants and children slowly, especially if they have emesis. It can be given initially by a dropper, teaspoon, or syringe, beginning with as little as 5 mL at a time. The volume is increased as tolerated. Replacement for emesis or stool losses is noted in Table 332-9. Oral rehydration can also be given by a nasogastric tube if needed; this is not the usual route.

Limitations to oral rehydration therapy include shock, an ileus, intussusception, carbohydrate intolerance (rare), severe emesis, and high stool output (>10 mL/kg/hr). Ondansetron (oral mucosal absorption preparation) reduces the incidence of emesis, thus permitting more effective oral rehydration.

Enteral Feeding and Diet Selection
Continued enteral feeding in diarrhea aids in recovery from the episode, and a continued age-appropriate diet after rehydration is the norm. Although intestinal brush border surface and luminal enzymes can be affected in children with prolonged diarrhea, there is evidence that satisfactory carbohydrate, protein, and fat absorption can take place on a variety of diets. Once rehydration

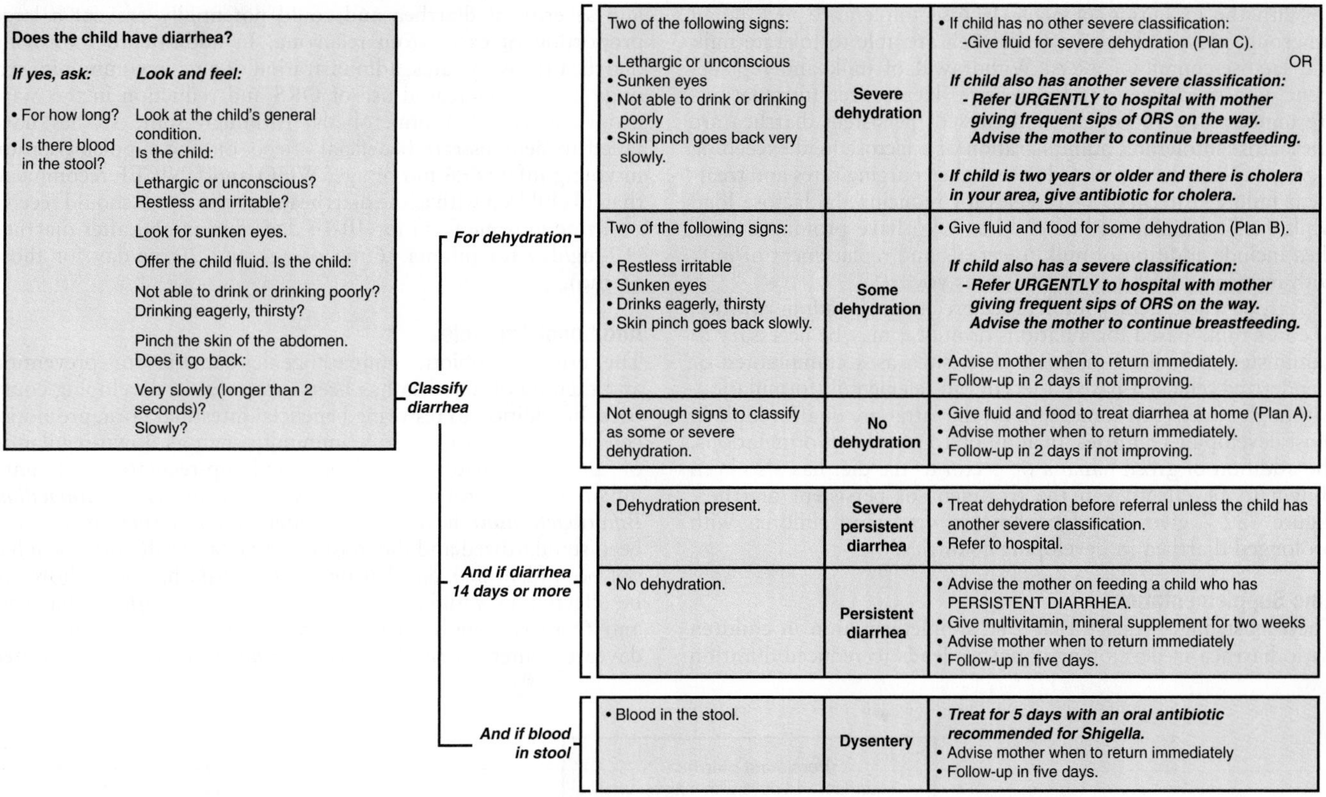

Figure 332-6 Integrated management of childhood illness (IMCI) protocol for the recognition and management of diarrhea in developing countries. ORS, oral rehydration solution.

Table 332-10 COMPOSITION OF COMMERCIAL ORAL REHYDRATION SOLUTIONS AND COMMONLY CONSUMED BEVERAGES

SOLUTION	CARBOHYDRATE (g/L)	SODIUM (mmol/L)	POTASSIUM (mmol/L)	CHLORIDE (mmol/L)	BASE* (mmol/L)	OSMOLARITY (mOsm/L)
ORAL REHYDRATION SOLUTION						
Low osmolality ORS	13.5	75	20	65	10	245
WHO (2005)						
WHO (2002)	13.5	75	20	65	30	245
WHO (1975)	20	90	20	80	10	311
European Society of Paediatric Gastroenterology, Hepatology and Nutrition	16	60	20	60	30	240
Enfalyte†	30	50	25	45	34	200
Pedialyte‡	25	45	20	35	30	250
Rehydralyte§	25	75	20	65	30	305
CeraLyte‖	40	50-90	20	NA	30	220
COMMONLY USED BEVERAGES (NOT APPROPRIATE FOR DIARRHEA TREATMENT)						
Apple juice¶	120	0.4	44	45	NA	730
Coca-Cola** Classic	112	1.6	NA	NA	13.4	650

*Actual or potential bicarbonate (e.g., lactate, citrate, or acetate).
†Mead-Johnson Laboratories, Princeton, New Jersey. Additional information is available at *www.meadjohnson.com/professional/products/enfalyte.html.*
‡Ross Laboratories (Abbott Laboratories), Columbus, Ohio. Data regarding Flavored and Freezer Pop Pedialyte are identical. Additional information is available at *www.pedialyte.com.*
§Ross Laboratories (Abbott Laboratories), Columbus, Ohio. Additional information is available at *www.abbottnutrition.com/products/pedialyte.*
‖Cera Products, LLC, Jessup, Maryland. Additional information is available at *www.ceraproductsinc.com/productline/ceralyte.html.*
¶Meeting U.S. Department of Agriculture minimum requirements.
**Coca-Cola Corporation, Atlanta, Georgia. Figures do not include electrolytes that might be present in local water used for bottling. Base = phosphate.
NA, not applicable; ORS, oral rehydration solution; WHO, World Health Organization.
From Centers for Disease Control and Prevention: Diagnosis and management of foodborne illnesses, *MMWR* 53:1–33, 2004.

is complete, food should be reintroduced while oral rehydration can be continued to replace ongoing losses from emesis or stools and for maintenance. Breast-feeding or nondiluted regular formula should be resumed as soon as possible. Foods with complex carbohydrates (rice, wheat, potatoes, bread, and cereals), lean meats, yogurt, fruits, and vegetables are also tolerated. Fatty foods or foods high in simple sugars (juices, carbonated sodas) should be avoided. The usual energy density of any diet used for the therapy of diarrhea should be around 1 kcal/g, aiming to provide an energy intake of a minimum of 100 kcal/kg/day and a protein intake of 2-3 g/kg/day. In selected circumstances when adequate intake of energy-dense food is problematic, the addition of amylase to the diet through germination techniques can also be helpful.

With the exception of acute lactose intolerance in a small subgroup, most children with diarrhea are able to tolerate milk and lactose-containing diets. Withdrawal of milk and replacement with specialized (and expensive) lactose-free formulations are unnecessary. Although children with persistent diarrhea are not lactose intolerant, administration of a lactose load exceeding 5 g/kg/day may be associated with higher purging rates and treatment failure. Alternative strategies for reducing the lactose load while feeding malnourished children who have prolonged diarrhea include addition of milk to cereals and replacement of milk with fermented milk products such as yogurt.

Rarely, when dietary intolerance precludes the administration of cow's milk–based formulations or milk it may be necessary to administer specialized milk-free diets such as a comminuted or blenderized chicken-based diet or an elemental formulation. Although effective in some settings, the latter are unaffordable in most developing countries. In addition to rice-lentil formulations, the addition of green banana or pectin to the diet has also been shown to be effective in the treatment of persistent diarrhea. Figure 332-7 gives an algorithm for managing children with prolonged diarrhea in developing countries.

Zinc Supplementation

There is strong evidence that zinc supplementation in children with diarrhea in developing countries leads to reduced duration and severity of diarrhea and could potentially prevent a large proportion of cases from recurring. In addition to improving diarrhea recovery rates, administration of zinc in community settings leads to increased use of ORS and reduction in the inappropriate use of antimicrobials. Although some studies have failed to demonstrate beneficial effects of zinc supplementation in young infants <6 mo of age, WHO and UNICEF recommend that all children with acute diarrhea in at-risk areas should receive oral zinc in some form for 10-14 days during and after diarrhea (10 mg/day for infants <6 mo of age and 20 mg/day for those >6 mo).

Additional Therapies

The use of probiotic nonpathogenic bacteria for prevention and therapy of diarrhea has been successful in developing countries. In addition to restoring beneficial intestinal flora, probiotics can enhance host protective immunity such as down-regulation of pro-inflammatory cytokines and up-regulation of anti-inflammatory cytokines. A variety of organisms *(Lactobacillus, Bifidobacterium)* have a good safety record; therapy has not been standardized and the most effective (and safe) organism has not been identified. *Saccharomyces boulardii* has been shown to be effective in antibiotic-associated and in *C. difficile* diarrhea, and there is some evidence that it might prevent diarrhea in daycare centers. *Lactobacillus rhamnosus GG* was associated

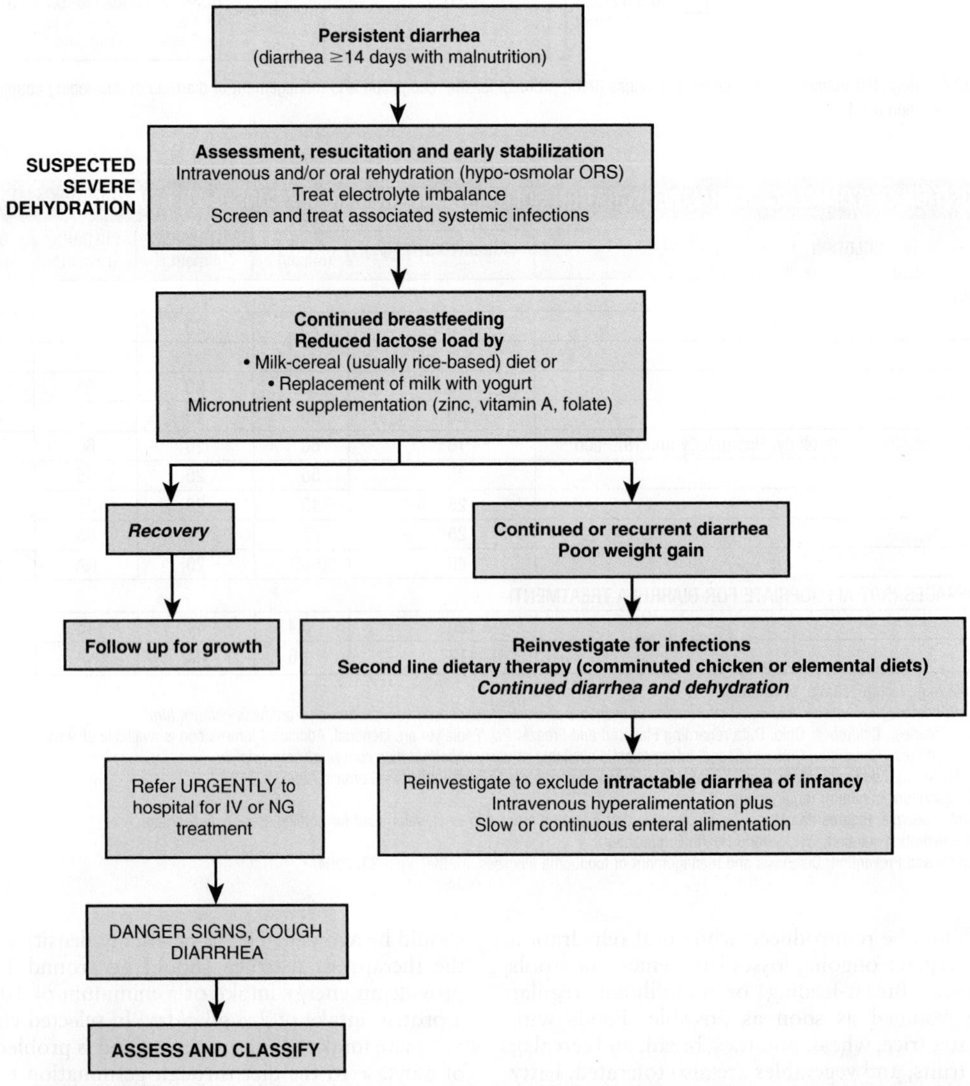

Figure 332-7 Management of persistent diarrhea. IV, intravenous; NG, nasogastric tube; ORS, oral rehydration solution.

with reduced diarrheal duration and severity, more evident in case of childhood rotavirus diarrhea. Similar, although weaker, evidence was obtained with *S. boulardii*. Further work is needed before probiotics can be recommended for routine use in childhood diarrhea and in developing countries.

Antimotility agents (loperamide) are contraindicated in children with dysentery and probably have no role in the management of acute watery diarrhea in otherwise healthy children. Similarly, **antiemetic** agents such as the phenothiazines are of little value and are associated with potentially serious side effects (lethargy, dystonia, malignant hyperpyrexia). Nonetheless, ondansetron is an effective and less-toxic antiemetic agent. Because persistent vomiting can limit oral rehydration therapy, a single sublingual dose of an oral dissolvable tablet of ondansetron (4 mg 4-11 yr and 8 mg for children >11 yr [generally 0.2 mg/kg]) may be given. However, most children do not require specific antiemetic therapy; careful oral rehydration therapy is usually sufficient.

Racecadotril, an enkephalinse inhibitor, has inconsistently been shown to reduce stool output in patients with diarrhea. Experience with this drug in children is limited, and for the average child with acute diarrhea it may be unnecessary.

Antibiotic Therapy

Timely antibiotic therapy in select cases of diarrhea can reduce the duration and severity of diarrhea and prevent complications (Table 332-11). Although these agents are important to use in specific cases, their widespread and indiscriminate use leads to the development of antimicrobial resistance. **Nitazoxanide**, an anti-infective agent, has been effective in the treatment of a wide variety of pathogens including *C. parvum*, *G. lamblia*, *E. histolytica*, *Blastocystis hominis*, *C. difficile*, and rotavirus. Although preliminary data suggest that nitazoxanide may be of use in nonspecific acute secretory diarrhea, these data need replication in further studies.

PREVENTION

In many developed countries, diarrhea due to pathogens such as *C. botulinum*, *E. coli* O157:H7, *Salmonella*, *Shigella*, *V. cholerae*, *Cryptosporidium*, and *Cyclospora* is a notifiable disease and, thus, contact tracing and source identification is important in preventing outbreaks.

Table 332-11 ANTIBIOTIC THERAPY FOR INFECTIOUS DIARRHEA

ORGANISM	DRUG OF CHOICE	DOSAGE AND DURATION OF TREATMENT
Shigella (severe dysentery and EIEC dysentery)	Ciprofloxacin*, ampicillin, ceftriaxone, azit hromycin, or TMP-SMX Most strains are resistant now to several antibiotics	Ceftriaxone 50-100 mg/kg/day IV or IM, qd or bid × 7 days Ciprofloxacin 20-30 mg/kg/day PO bid × 7-10 days Ampicillin PO, IV 50-100 mg/kg/day qid × 7 days
EPEC, ETEC, EIEC	TMP-SMX or ciprofloxacin*	TMP 10 mg/kg/day and SMX 50 mg/kg/day bid × 5 days Ciprofloxacin PO 20-30 mg/kg/day qid for 5-10 days
Salmonella	No antibiotics for uncomplicated gastroenteritis in normal hosts caused by non-typhoidal species **Treatment** indicated in infants <3 mo, and patients with malignancy, chronic GI disease, severe colitis hemoglobinopathies, or HIV infection, and other immunocompromised patients Most strains have become resistant to multiple antibiotics	See treatment of *Shigella*
Aeromonas/Plesiomonas	TMP-SMX Ciprofloxacin*	TMP 10 mg/kg/day and SMX 50 mg/kg/day bid for 5 days Ciprofloxacin PO 20-30 mg/kg/day divided bid × 7-10 days
Yersinia spp.	Antibiotics are not usually required for diarrhea Deferoxamine therapy should be withheld for severe infections or associated bacteremia Treat sepsis as for immunocompromised hosts, using combination therapy with parenteral doxycycline, aminoglycoside, TMP-SMX, or fluoroquinolone	
Campylobacter jejuni	Erythromycin or azithromycin	Erythromycin PO 50 mg/kg/day divided tid × 5 days Azithromycin PO 5-10 mg/kg/day qid × 5 days
Clostridium difficile	Metronidazole (first line)	PO 30 mg/kg/day divided qid × 5 days; max 2 g
	Discontinue initiating antibiotic	
	Vancomycin (2nd line)	PO 40 mg/kg/day qid × 7 days, max 125 mg
Entamoeba histolytica	Metronidazole followed by iodoquinol or paromomycin	Metronidazole PO 30-40 mg/kg/day tid × 7-10 days Iodoquinol PO 30-40 mg/kg/day tid × 20 days Paromomycin PO 25-35 mg/kg/day tid × 7 days
Giardia lamblia	Furazolidone or metronidazole or albendazole or quinacrine	Furazolidone PO 25 mg/kg/day qid × 5-7 days Metronidazole PO 30-40 mg/kg/day tid × 7 days Albendazole PO 200 mg bid × 10 days
Cryptosporidium spp.	Nitazoxanide PO treatment may not be needed in normal hosts In immunocompromised, PO immunoglobulin + aggressively treat HIV, etc.	Children 1-3 yr: 100 mg bid × 3 days Children 4-11 yr: 200 mg bid
Isospora spp.	TMP-SMX	PO TMP 5 mg/kg/day and SMX 25 mg/kg/day, bid × 7-10 days
Cyclospora spp.	TMP/SMX	PO TMP 5 mg/kg/day and SMX 25 mg/kg/day bid × 7 days
Blastocystis hominis	Metronidazole or iodoquinol	Metronidazole PO 30-40 mg/kg/day tid × 7-10 days Iodoquinol PO 40 mg/kg/day tid × 20 days

EIEC, Enteroinvasive *Escherichia coli*; EPEC, enteropathogenic *E. coli*; ETEC, enterotoxigenic *E. coli*; SMX, sulfamethoxazole; TMP, trimethoprim.
*Ciprofloxacin is approved for children ≥16 yr of age.

Many developing countries struggle with huge disease burdens of diarrhea where a wider approach to diarrhea prevention may be required. Preventive strategies may be of relevance to both developed and developing countries.

Promotion of Exclusive Breast-feeding

Exclusive breast-feeding (administration of no other fluids or foods for the 1st 6 mo of life) is not common, especially in many developed countries. Exclusive breast-feeding protects very young infants from diarrheal disease through the promotion of passive immunity and through reduction in the intake of potentially contaminated food and water. Breast milk contains all the nutrients needed in early infancy, and when continued during diarrhea, it also diminishes the adverse impact on nutritional status. Exclusive breast-feeding for the first 6 mo of life is widely regarded as one of the most effective interventions to reduce the risk of premature childhood mortality and the potential to prevent 13% of all deaths of children <5 yr of age.

Improved Complementary Feeding Practices

There is a strong inverse association between appropriate, safe complementary feeding and mortality in children age 6-11 mo; malnutrition is an independent risk for the frequency and severity of diarrheal illness. Complementary foods should be introduced at 6 mo of age, and breast-feeding should continue for up to 1 yr (longer period for developing countries). Complementary foods in developing countries are generally poor in quality and often are heavily contaminated, thus predisposing to diarrhea. Contamination of complementary foods can be potentially reduced through caregivers' education and improving home food storage. Improved vitamin A status has been shown to reduce the frequency of severe diarrhea. Vitamin A supplementation reduces all-cause childhood mortality by 21% and diarrhea-specific mortality by 31% (95% CI, 17-42%).

Rotavirus Immunization

Most infants acquire rotavirus diarrhea early in life; an effective rotavirus vaccine would have a major effect on reducing diarrhea mortality in developing countries. In 1998, a quadrivalent Rhesus rotavirus-derived vaccine was licensed in the United States but subsequently withdrawn due to an increased risk of intussusception. Subsequent development and testing of newer rotavirus vaccines have led to their introduction in most developed countries and approval by the WHO in 2009 for widespread use in developing countries. Emerging evidence indicates that the introduction of these vaccines is associated with a significant reduction in severe diarrhea and associated mortality.

The institution of large-scale rotavirus vaccination programs has led to major reduction in the burden of disease and associated mortality. In an evaluation of large-scale rotavirus vaccine introduction, coverage rate of 74% was achieved in infants <12 mo of age, with 41% reduction (95% CI, 36-47%) in diarrhea-related mortality. In an evaluation of the vaccine in Africa, overall protective efficacy against rotavirus gastroenteritis ranged from 49% to 61%, with 30% protective efficacy against all-cause severe gastroenteritis in infancy. Vaccine (live virus) associated rotavirus infection has been reported in children with severe combined immunodeficiency disease.

Other vaccines that could potentially reduce the burden of severe diarrhea and mortality in young children are vaccines against *Shigella* and ETEC.

Improved Water and Sanitary Facilities and Promotion of Personal and Domestic Hygiene

Much of the reduction in diarrhea prevalence in the developed world is the result of improvement in standards of hygiene, sanitation, and water supply. Strikingly, an estimated 88% of all diarrheal deaths worldwide can be attributed to unsafe water, inadequate sanitation, and poor hygiene. Improved sanitation across a range of studies has been shown to reduce the incidence of diarrhea by 36%. In addition, routine handwashing with plain soap in the home can reduce the incidence of diarrhea in all environments. Behavioral change strategies through promotion of handwashing indicate that handwashing promotion and access to soap reduces the burden of diarrhea in developing countries.

Improved Case Management of Diarrhea

Improved management of diarrhea through prompt identification and appropriate therapy significantly reduces diarrhea duration, its nutritional penalty, and risk of death in childhood. Improved management of acute diarrhea is a key factor in reducing the burden of prolonged episodes and persistent diarrhea. The WHO/UNICEF recommendations to use low-osmolality ORS and zinc supplementation for the management of diarrhea, coupled with selective and appropriate use of antibiotics, have the potential to reduce the number of diarrheal deaths among children. A recent estimate indicated that 22% of all deaths of children <5 yr of age could be prevented by optimal use of ORS, zinc supplements, and antibiotics for dysentery.

BIBLIOGRAPHY

Please visit the Nelson Textbook of Pediatrics *website at* www.expertconsult.com *for the complete bibliography.*

332.1 Traveler's Diarrhea

Zulfiqar Ahmed Bhutta

Traveler's diarrhea is a common complication of visitors to developing countries and is caused by a variety of pathogens, in part depending on the season and the region visited (Table 332-12). Traveler's diarrhea has a high attack rate among travelers from higher-income countries visiting, during the summer, countries in a warmer climate that have a high prevalence of indigenous infectious diarrhea. Traveler's diarrhea can manifest with watery diarrhea or as dysentery.

TREATMENT

Traveler's diarrhea is often self-limiting but requires particular attention to avoid dehydration. For infants and children, rehydra-

Table 332-12 REGIONAL DISTRIBUTION OF THE MOST COMMON PATHOGENS THAT CAUSE TRAVELER'S DIARRHEA

PATHOGEN	ASIA (%)	LATIN AMERICA (%)	AFRICA (%)
BACTERIAL			
Enterotoxigenic *Escherichia coli*	6-37	17-70	8-42
Other *E. coli*	3-4	7-22	2-9
Campylobacter jejuni	9-39	1-5	1-28
Salmonella spp.	1-33	1-16	4-25
Shigella spp.	0-17	2-30	0-9
Plesiomonas shigelloides	3-13	0-6	3-5
Aeromonas spp.	1-57	1-5	0-9
VIRAL			
Rotavirus	1-8	0-6	0-36
PARASITIC			
Entamoeba histolytica	5-11	<1	2-9
Giardia lambia	1-12	1-2	0-1
Cryptosporidium spp.	1-5	<1	2
Cyclospora cayetanensis	1-5?	<1?	<1?
No pathogen identified	10-56	24-62	15-53

From Al-Abri SS, Beeching NJ, Nye FJ: Traveller's diarrhea, *Lancet Infect Dis* 5:349–360, 2005.

tion as discussed in Chapter 332 is appropriate, followed by a standard diet. Adolescents and adults should increase their intake of electrolyte-rich fluids. Kaolin-pectin, anticholinergic agents, *Lactobacillus,* and bismuth salicylate have not been effective therapies. Loperamide, an antimotility and antisecretory agent, reduces the number of stools in older children with watery diarrhea and has been shown to improve outcomes when used in combination with antibiotics in traveler's diarrhea. However, loperamide should be used with great caution or not at all in febrile or toxic patients with dysentery or those with bloody diarrhea.

Antibiotics, with or without loperamide, can also reduce the number of unformed stools. Short-duration (3 days) therapy with fluoroquinolones, trimethoprim-sulfamethoxazole, azithromycin, or rifaximin is effective; the choice of antibiotic depends on the age of the patient, the potential organism, and the organism's local resistance patterns. For up-to-date information on local pathogens and resistant patterns, see *www.cdc.gov/travel.*

PREVENTION

Travelers should drink bottled or canned beverages or boiled water. They should avoid ice, salads, and fruit they did not peel themselves. Food should be eaten hot, if possible. Raw or poorly cooked seafood is a risk, as is eating in a restaurant rather than a private home. Swimming pools and other recreational water sites can also be contaminated.

Chemoprophylaxis is not routinely recommended for previously healthy children or adults. Nonetheless, travelers should bring azithromycin (<16 yr of age) or ciprofloxacin (>16 yr of age) and begin antimicrobial therapy if diarrhea develops.

BIBLIOGRAPHY

Please visit the Nelson Textbook of Pediatrics *website at www.expertconsult.com for the complete bibliography.*

Chapter 333
Chronic Diarrhea

Alfredo Guarino and David Branski

DEFINITION AND EPIDEMIOLOGY

Chronic diarrhea is defined as a diarrheal episode that lasts for ≥14 days. Its epidemiology has 2 distinct patterns. In developing countries, chronic diarrhea is often the result of an intestinal infection that lasts longer than expected. This syndrome is often defined as protracted diarrhea, and there is no clear distinction between protracted and chronic diarrhea. In countries with high socioeconomic conditions, chronic diarrhea is less common and its etiology is more diverse, showing an age-related pattern. The outcome of diarrhea depends on its cause and ranges from benign conditions such as toddler's diarrhea, to severe congenital diseases such as microvillus inclusion disease that can lead to irreversible intestinal failure and ultimately death.

PATHOPHYSIOLOGY

The mechanisms of diarrhea are generally divided into secretory and osmotic, but often diarrhea is the result of both mechanisms. Secretory diarrhea is usually associated with large volumes of watery stools and persists when oral food is withdrawn. Osmotic diarrhea is dependent on oral feeding, and stool volumes are usually not as massive as in secretory diarrhea (Fig. 333-1).

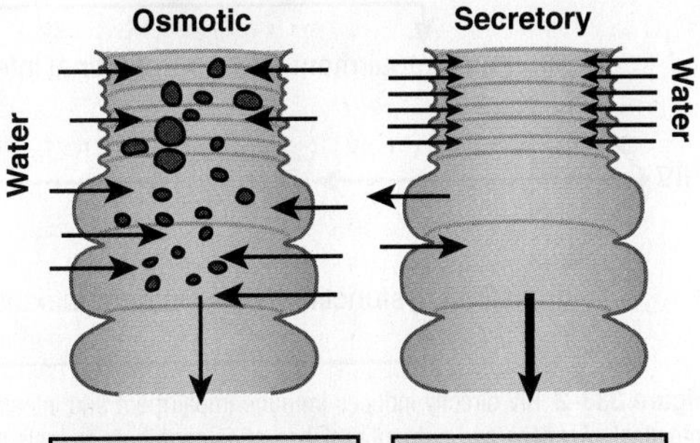

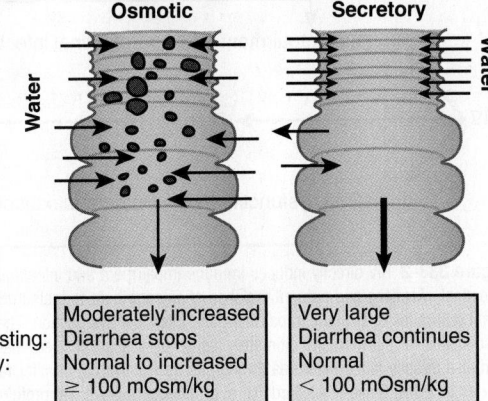

	Osmotic	Secretory
Stool volume:	Moderately increased	Very large
Response to fasting:	Diarrhea stops	Diarrhea continues
Stool osmolality:	Normal to increased	Normal
Ion gap:	≥ 100 mOsm/kg	< 100 mOsm/kg

Figure 333-1 Pathways of osmotic and secretory diarrhea. Osmotic diarrhea is due to functional or structural damage of intestinal epithelium. Nonabsorbed osmotically active solutes drive water into the lumen. Stool osmolality and ion gap are generally increased. Diarrhea stops in children when they are not eating. In secretory diarrhea, ions are actively pumped into the intestine by the action of exogenous and endogenous secretagogues. Usually there is no intestinal damage. Osmolality and ion gap are within normal levels. Large volumes of stools are lost independent of food ingestion.

Secretory diarrhea is characterized by active electrolyte and water fluxes toward the intestinal lumen, resulting from either the inhibition of neutral NaCl absorption in villous enterocytes or an increase in electrogenic chloride secretion in secretory crypt cells due to the opening of the cystic fibrosis transmembrane regulator (CFTR) chloride channel. The other components of the enterocyte ion secretory machinery are the Na-K-2Cl cotransporter for the electroneutral chloride entrance into the enterocyte; the Na-K pump, which decreases the intracellular Na^+ concentration, determining the driving gradient for further Na^+ influx; and the K^+ selective channel, which enables K^+, once it has entered the cell in together with Na^+, to return to the extracellular fluid.

Electrogenic secretion is induced by an increase of intracellular concentration of cyclic adenosine monophosphate (cAMP), cyclic guanosine monophosphate (cGMP), or calcium in response to microbial enterotoxins or to endogenous endocrine or nonendocrine moieties, including inflammatory cytokines. Another mechanism of secretory diarrhea is the inhibition of the electroneutral NaCl-coupled pathway that involves the Na^+/H^+ and the Cl^-/HCO_3^- **exchangers.** Defects in the genes of the Na^+/H^+ and the Cl^-/HCO_3^- **exchangers** are responsible for congenital Na^+ and Cl^- diarrhea, respectively.

Osmotic diarrhea is caused by nonabsorbed nutrients in the intestinal lumen due to one or more of the following mechanisms: intestinal damage (such as in enteric infection), reduced functional absorptive surface (such as in celiac disease), defective digestive enzyme or nutrient carrier (such as in lactase deficiency), decreased intestinal transit time (such as in functional diarrhea), and nutrient overload exceeding the digestive capacity. Osmotic diarrhea occurs whenever digestion or absorption is impaired. Whatever the mechanism, the osmotic force generated by nonabsorbed solutes drives water into the intestinal lumen. An example of osmotic diarrhea is lactose intolerance. Lactose, if not absorbed in the small intestine, reaches the colon, where it is fermented to short-chain organic acids, generating an osmotic overload that overwhelms the absorptive capacity.

In many children, chronic diarrhea is induced by multiple mechanisms, intersecting each other and often producing a vicious cycle. A paradigm of chronic diarrhea generated by multiple mechanisms is provided by HIV infection, in which immune derangement, enteric infections, nutrient malabsorption, and intestinal damage, together with a direct enteropathogenic role of HIV, trigger and maintain chronic diarrhea (Fig. 333-2).

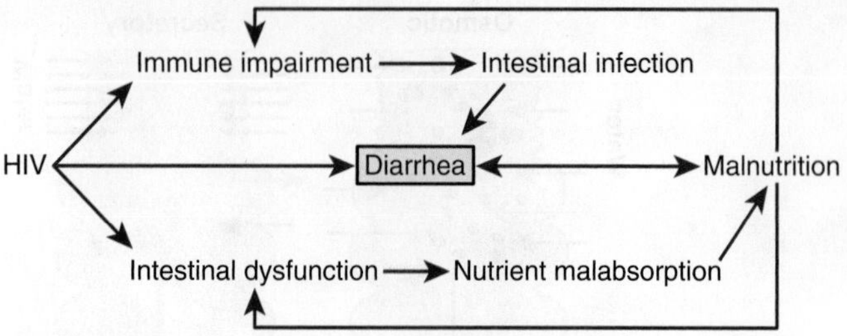

Figure 333-2 HIV directly induces immune impairment and intestinal dysfunction. Intestinal infections and nutrient malabsorption contribute to malnutrition. The latter in turn contributes to immune impairment and intestinal dysfunction. The vicious cycle is responsible for diarrhea and ultimately results in wasting, the terminal stage of AIDS. HIV can also directly induce diarrhea through its transactivating transfer factor Tat. (From Berni Canani R, Cirillo P, Mallardo G, et al: Effects of HIV-1 Tat protein on ion secretion and on cell proliferation in human intestinal epithelial cells, *Gastroenterology* 124:368–376, 2003.)

ETIOLOGY

A list of the main causes of chronic diarrhea is shown in Table 333-1.

Enteric infections are by far the most common cause of chronic diarrhea in developing and industrialized countries, and sequential infections with the same or a different pathogen may be responsible for prolonged symptoms. Entero-adherent *Escherichia coli* and *Cryptosporidium parvum* have been implicated in chronic diarrhea in developing countries. In developed countries chronic infectious diarrhea usually runs a benign course and the etiology is often viral. Rotavirus and Norovirus are often involved, whereas cytomegalovirus and *Clostridium difficile* are emerging agents of severe diarrhea in children.

Opportunistic microorganisms induce diarrhea exclusively, or more severely, or for more-prolonged periods, in specific populations, such as immunocompromised children. Enteric cryptosporidiosis is the most common cause of severe and protracted diarrhea in AIDS, but HIV may be directly responsible for diarrhea and for HIV enteropathy.

In **small intestinal bacterial overgrowth,** diarrhea may be the result of either a direct interaction between the microorganism and the enterocyte or the consequence of the deconjugation and dehydroxylation of bile salts and the hydroxylation of fatty acids due to an abnormal proliferation of bacteria in the proximal intestine (Chapter 330.4).

Postenteritis syndrome is a clinical-pathologic condition in which small intestinal mucosal damage persists after acute gastroenteritis. Sensitization to food antigens, secondary disaccharidase deficiency, or an infection or reinfection with an enteric pathogen is responsible for postenteritis syndrome. A change of the gut microflora due to the infectious agent and/or antibiotic therapy can contribute to postenteritis diarrhea.

A reduction of intestinal absorptive surface is responsible for diarrhea in **celiac disease**, a permanent gluten intolerance that is sustained by a genetic basis affecting as many as 1/100 normal people, depending on geographic origin. Gliadin induces villous atrophy, leading to a reduction of functional absorptive surface area that is reversible upon implementation of a strict gluten-free diet (Chapter 330.2).

Allergy to cow's milk protein and other foods can manifest with chronic diarrhea, especially during infancy. **Eosinophilic gastroenteritis** is characterized by eosinophilic infiltration of the intestinal wall and is strongly associated with atopy.

In older children and adolescents, inflammatory bowel disease including Crohn disease, ulcerative colitis, and indeterminate colitis, are major causes of chronic diarrhea.

Chronic diarrhea may be the manifestation of maldigestion due to exocrine **pancreatic disorders** (Chapter 343). In most

Table 333-1 INFECTIOUS AND NONINFECTIOUS CAUSES OF CHRONIC DIARRHEA

INFECTIOUS ETIOLOGIES
Bacterial
Viral and protozoan agents
Small intestinal bacterial overgrowth
Postenteritis syndrome
Tropical sprue
Whipple disease
DIARRHEA ASSOCIATED WITH EXOGENOUS SUBSTANCES
Excessive intake of carbonated fluid
Dietetic foods containing sorbitol, mannitol, or xylitol
Excessive intake of antacids or laxatives containing lactulose or $Mg(OH)_2$
Excessive intake of drinks containing methylxanthines (cola, tea, coffee)
ABNORMAL DIGESTIVE PROCESSES:
Cystic fibrosis
Shwachman-Diamond syndrome
Isolated pancreatic enzyme deficiency
Chronic pancreatitis
Johanson-Blizzard syndrome
Pearson syndrome
Trypsinogen and enterokinase deficiency
Chronic cholestasis
Use of bile acids sequestrants
Primary bile acid malabsorption
Terminal ileum resection
NUTRIENT MALABSORPTION
Congenital or acquired lactase deficiency
Congenital or acquired sucrase-isomaltase deficiency
Glucose-galactose malabsorption
Fructose malabsorption
Congenital or acquired short bowel
IMMUNE AND INFLAMMATORY
Food allergy (cow's milk or soy proteins, others)
Celiac disease
Eosinophilic gastroenteritis
Inflammatory bowel disease
Autoimmune enteropathy
IPEX syndrome
Primary and secondary immunodeficiencies
STRUCTURAL DEFECTS
Microvillus inclusion disease
Tufting enteropathy
Phenotypic diarrhea
Heparan-sulphate deficiency
$\alpha_2\beta_1$ and $\alpha_6\beta_4$ integrin deficiency
Lymphangiectasia
Enteric anendocrinosis (neorogenin-3 mutation)
DEFECTS OF ELECTROLYTE AND METABOLITE TRANSPORT
Congenital chloride diarrhea
Congenital sodium diarrhea
Acrodermatitis enteropathica
Selective folate deficiency
Abetalipoproteinemia
MOTILITY DISORDERS
Hirschsprung disease
Chronic intestinal pseudo-obstruction (neurogenic and myopathic)
Thyrotoxicosis
NEOPLASTIC DISEASES
Neuroendocrine hormone-secreting tumors (APUDomas such as VIPoma)
Zollinger-Ellison
Mastocytosis
Pheochromocytoma
Lymphoma
CHRONIC NONSPECIFIC DIARRHEA
Functional diarrhea
Toddler's diarrhea
Irritable bowel syndrome

IPEX, immunodysregulation polyendocrinopathy enteropathy X-linked syndrome.

patients with cystic fibrosis, pancreatic insufficiency results in fat and protein malabsorption. In **Shwachman-Diamond syndrome,** exocrine pancreatic hypoplasia may be associated with neutropenia, bone changes, and intestinal protein loss. Specific isolated pancreatic enzyme defects result in fat and/or protein malabsorption. **Familial pancreatitis**, associated with a mutation in the trypsinogen gene, may be associated with pancreatic insufficiency and chronic diarrhea.

Liver disorders can lead to a reduction in the bile salts, resulting in fat malabsorption. Bile acid loss may be associated with terminal ileum diseases, such as Crohn disease or disease following ileal resection. In **primary bile acid malabsorption** neonates and young infants present with chronic diarrhea and fat malabsorption due to mutations of ileal bile transporter.

Carbohydrate malabsorption and lactose intolerance may be due to a molecular deficiency of lactase or sucrase-isomaltase, or to congenital **glucose-galactose malabsorption. Lactose intolerance** is more commonly a consequence of secondary lactase deficiency due to intestinal mucosal damage. A progressive, age-related loss of lactase activity affects about 80% of the non-white population and may be responsible for chronic diarrhea in older children receiving cow's milk.

The most benign etiology is **chronic nonspecific diarrhea** that encompasses **functional diarrhea** (or toddler's diarrhea) in children <4 yr of age and **irritable bowel syndrome** in those ≥5 yr. The disease is the same with a slightly different age presentation, in that abdominal pain is more common and clearly associated with the diarrhea in older children. The hallmark of the syndrome is diarrhea associated with normal weight growth in well-appearing subjects. In younger children diarrhea is often watery, at times containing undigested food particles. It is usually more severe in the morning. If the child's fluid intake is >150 mL/kg/24 hr, fluid intake should be reduced to no more than 90 mL/kg/24 hr. The child is often irritable in the first 2 days after the fluid restriction; however, persistence with this approach for several more days results in a decrease in the stool frequency and volume. If the dietary history suggests that the child is ingesting significant amounts of fruit juices, then the offending juices should be decreased. Sorbitol, which is a nonabsorbable sugar, is found in apple, pear, and prune juices and it can cause diarrhea in toddlers. Apple and pear juices contain higher amounts of fructose than glucose, a feature postulated to cause diarrhea in toddlers. In older children, irritable bowel syndrome is often associated with abdominal pain and may be related to anxiety, depression, and other psychologic disturbances.

The most severe etiology includes a number of heterogeneous conditions leading to the **intractable diarrhea syndrome,** which is often the result of a permanent defect in the structure or function of intestine, leading to progressive, often irreversible intestinal failure, requiring parenteral nutrition for survival. The main etiologies of intractable diarrhea include structural enterocyte defects, disorders of intestinal motility, immune-based disorders, short gut, and multiple food intolerance. The genetic and molecular bases of many etiologies of intractable diarrhea have been recently identified (Table 333-2).

Structural enterocyte defects are due to specific molecular defects responsible for early-onset severe diarrhea. In **microvillus inclusion disease,** microvilli are sequestered in vacuoles as a consequence of autophagocytosis due to a mutation in myosin that impairs apical protein trafficking leading to aberrant brush border development (Fig. 333-3). **Intestinal epithelial dysplasia** (or **tufting enteropathy**) is characterized by disorganization of surface enterocytes with focal crowding and formation of tufts. Abnormal deposition of laminin and heparan sulfate proteoglycan on the basement membrane has been detected in intestinal epithelia. An abnormal intestinal distribution of $\alpha_2\beta_1$ and $\alpha_6\beta_4$ integrins has been implicated in tufting enteropathy. These ubiquitous proteins are involved in cell-cell and cell-matrix interactions, and they play a crucial role in cell development and differentiation.

Electrolyte transport defects are a subgroup of structural enterocyte defects that include **congenital chloride diarrhea,** in which a mutation in the solute carrier family 26 member 3 gene (SLC26A3) leads to severe intestinal Cl^- malabsorption due to a defect or absence of the Cl^-/HCO_3^- exchanger. The consequent defect in bicarbonate secretion leads to metabolic alkalosis and acidification of the intestinal content, with further inhibition of Na^+/H^+ exchanger–dependent Na^+ absorption. Patients with **congenital sodium diarrhea** show similar clinical features because of a defective Na^+/H^+ exchanger in the small and large intestine, leading to massive Na^+ fecal loss and severe acidosis.

Multiple food protein hypersensitivity is regarded as a cause of intractable diarrhea syndrome. However, this is usually a diagnosis of exclusion and is based on a relationship between *any* ingested food and diarrhea. In most cases, multiple food intolerance is not ultimately confirmed by oral challenge, and most children are eventually able to return to a free diet.

Autoimmune processes can target the intestinal epithelium, alone or in association with extraintestinal symptoms. **Autoimmune enteropathy** is characterized by the production of anti-enterocyte and anti-goblet cell antibodies, primarily IgG, directed against components of the enterocyte brush border or cytoplasm and by a cell-mediated autoimmune response with mucosal T-cell activation. An X-linked immune dysregulation, polyendocrinopathy and enteropathy (**IPEX**) **syndrome** is associated with variable phenotypes of chronic diarrhea.

Abnormal immune function, as seen in patients with agammaglobulinemia, isolated immunoglobulin A deficiency, and combined immunodeficiency disorders, can result in persistent infectious diarrhea.

Phenotypic diarrhea, also defined as syndromic diarrhea or tricho-hepato-enteric syndrome, is a rare disease presenting with facial dysmorphism, woolly hair, severe diarrhea, and malabsorption (Fig. 333-4). Half of the patients have liver disease.

Disorders of intestinal motility include derangements of development and function of the enteric nervous system, such as in **Hirschsprung disease and chronic idiopathic intestinal pseudo-obstruction** (which encompass both the neurogenic and the myogenic forms). Other motility disorders may be secondary to extraintestinal disorders, such as in hyperthyroidism and scleroderma. Motility disorders are associated with either constipation or diarrhea or both, with the former usually dominating the clinical picture.

Short bowel syndrome (Chapter 330.7) is the single most common etiology of diarrhea and intestinal failure. Many intestinal abnormalities such as stenosis, segmental atresia, and malrotation can require surgical resection. In these conditions the residual intestine may be insufficient to carry on its digestive-absorptive functions. Alternatively, small bowel bacterial overgrowth can cause diarrhea, such as in the **blind loop syndrome.**

In rare cases of severe chronic diarrhea, the gastrointestinal symptoms may be the initial manifestation of a **mitochondrial disease or another metabolic disorder, namely carbohydrate-deficient glycoproteins.** Finally, when the cause of the diarrhea is undetermined and the clinical course is inconsistent with organic disorders, **factitious disorder by proxy** (formerly Munchausen syndrome by proxy) should be considered.

The natural history of intractable diarrhea is related to the primary intestinal disease. Food intolerances generally resolve in a few weeks or months, as does autoimmune enteropathy when appropriate immune suppression is started. Children with motility disorders have long-lasting stable symptoms that are rarely fatal, whereas those with structural enterocyte defects never recover, undergoing a more-severe course and often becoming candidates for intestinal transplantation.

Table 333-2 Molecular Basis of the Main Forms of Congenital Diarrheal Diseases

DISEASE	GENE	LOCATION	FUNCTION
DEFECTS OF ABSORPTION AND TRANSPORT OF NUTRIENTS AND ELECTROLYTES			
Congenital lactase deficiency	*LCT*	2q21	Lactase-phlorizin hydrolase activity
Disaccharide intolerance	EC 3.2.1.48	3q25-q26	Isomaltase-sucrase
Maltase-glucoamylase deficiency	*MGAM*	7q34	Maltase-glucoamylase activity
Glucose-galactose malabsorption	*SGLT1*	22q13.1	Na^+/glucose cotransporter
Fructose malabsorption	*GLUT5*	1p36	Fructose transporter
Fanconi-Bickel syndrome	*GLUT2*	3q26	Basolateral glucose transporter
Cystic fibrosis	*CFTR*	7q31.2	cAMP-dependent Cl^- channel
Acrodermatitis enteropathica	*SLC39A4*	8q24.3	Zn^{2+} transporter
Congenital chloride diarrhea	*DRA*	7q22-q31.1	Cl^-/base exchanger
Congenital sodium diarrhea	*SPINT2*	Unknown	Na^+/hydrogen exchanger?
Enterokinase deficiency	Serine protease 7	21q21	Serine-protease inhibitor
Trypsinogen deficiency	Trypsinogen	7q35	Proenterokinase: hydrolyzes tripsinogen
Lysinuric protein intolerance	*SLC7A7*	14q11	Hydrolyzes endo- and exopeptidases AA basolateral transport
Pancreatic lipase deficiency	Pancreatic lipase	10q26	Hydrolyzes triglycerides to fatty acids
Abetalipoproteinemia	*MTP*	4q22	Transfer lipids to apolipoprotein B
Hypobetalipoproteinemia	*APOB*	2p24	Apolipoprotein that forms chylomicrons
Chylomicron retention disease	*SARA2*	5q31	Intracellular chylomicron trafficking
Congenital bile acid diarrhea	*ABAT*	13q3	Ileal Na^+/bile salt transporter
DEFECTS OF ENTEROCYTE DIFFERENTIATION AND POLARIZATION			
Microvillous inclusion disease	*EpCAM*	18q21	Myosin Vb. intracellular protein trafficking
Congenital tufting enteropathy	Unknown	2p21	Cell-cell interaction
Syndromic diarrhea	Unknown	Unknown	Unknown
DEFECTS OF ENTEROENDOCRINE CELL DIFFERENTIATION			
Enteric anendocrinosis	*NEUROG3*	10q21.3	Enteroendocrine cell fate determination
Enteric dysendocrinosis	—	—	Enteroendocrine cells function
Proprotein convertase 1 deficiency	Prohormone convertase-1	5q15-q21	Prohormone processing
DEFECTS OF MODULATION OF INTESTINAL IMMUNE RESPONSE			
IPEX	*FOXP3*	Xp11.23-q13.3	Transcription factor
IPEX-like syndrome	Unknown	Unknown	Unknown
Immunodeficiency-associated autoimmune enteropathy	Unknown	Unknown	Unknown
Autoimmune polyglandular syndrome-1 (APS-1)	*AIRE*	21p22.3	Autoimmune regulator protein
Autoimmune enteropathy with colitis-generalized autoimmune gut disorder (GAGD)	Unknown	Unknown	Unknown

cAMP, cyclic adenosine monophosphate; IPEX, immune dysregulation, polyendocrinopathy, enteropathy, X-linked.

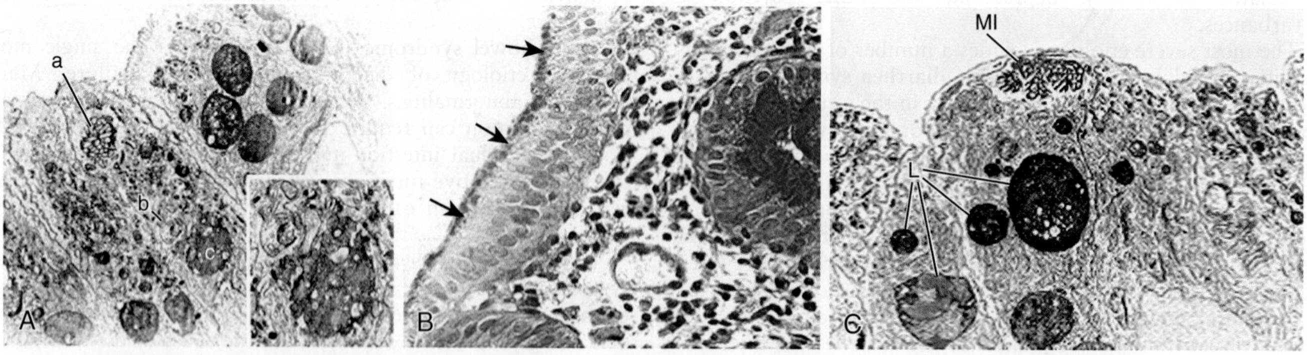

Figure 333-3 Microvillus inclusion disease. *A,* From top to bottom: microvillus inclusion (a), a granule with few microvilli (b), and a lysosome (c) detected in the same enterocyte. *Inset:* higher magnification of b and c ×11,000, inset ×21,500. *B,* PAS staining highlights abundant PAS-positive material *(arrows)* in the apical part of the enterocyte cytoplasm. *C,* The villous enterocyte lack brush-border microvilli, whereas their apical cytoplasm contains a microvillus inclusion *(MI)* and numerous lysosomes *(L)* ×5,500. (*A* From Morroni M, Cangiotti AM, Guarino A, et al: Unusual ultrastructural features in microvillous inclusion disease: a report of two cases, *Virchows Archiv* 448:805–810, 2006.)

EVALUATION OF PATIENTS

Because of the wide spectrum of the etiologies, the medical approach should be based on diagnostic algorithms that begin with the age of the child, evaluate the weight pattern, and then consider clinical and epidemiologic factors, always taking into account the results of microbiologic investigations. The etiology of chronic diarrhea shows an age-related pattern, and an early onset might suggest a congenital and severe condition. In later infancy and up to 2 yr of age, infections and allergies are more

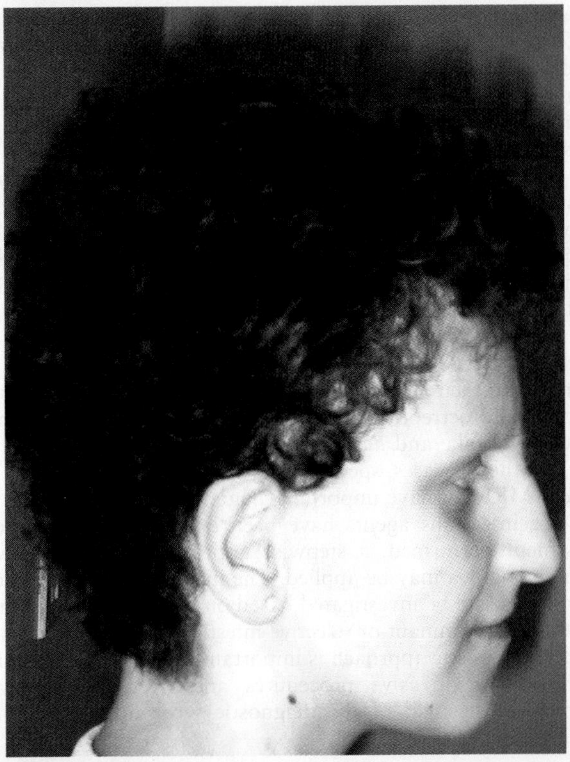

Figure 333-4 A child with phenotypic diarrhea showing facial dysmorphism, hypertelorism, and woolly hair. Etiology is unknown, but the presence of affected siblings suggests an autosomal recessive transmission.

Table 333-3 MAIN CAUSES OF CHRONIC DIARRHEA ACCORDING TO THE AGE OF ONSET*

0-30 DAYS	1-24 MONTHS	2-18 YEARS
Microvillus inclusion disease	Apple juice and pear nectar	Apple juice or pear nectar
	Autoimmune enteropathy	Antibiotic-associated *Clostridium difficile* colitis
	Intestinal infection	Intestinal infection
Congenital short bowel syndrome	Short gut	
Food allergy	Food allergy	Lactose intolerance
	Functional diarrhea†	Irritable bowel syndrome‡
	Celiac disease	Celiac disease
Hirschsprung's disease	Cystic fibrosis	
Malrotation with partial blockage	Post-gastroenteritis diarrhea	Post-gastroenteritis diarrhea
Neonatal lymphangectasia		
	Tufting enteropathy	
Primary bile-salt malabsorption		
Intestinal pseudo-obstruction	Intestinal pseudo-obstruction	

*In addition to all the diseases listed in Table 333-2.
†Age range 0-4 years.
‡Age range 5-18 years.

Table 333-4 DEGREE OF MALNUTRITION AS ESTIMATED BY VISCERAL PROTEIN CONCENTRATIONS IN CHILDREN WITH CHRONIC DIARRHEA

VISCERAL PROTEIN	HALF-LIFE	NORMAL VALUES	MILD MALNUTRITION	MODERATE MALNUTRITION	SEVERE MALNUTRITION
Albumin	20 days	30-45 g/L	3.0-2.9 g/L	2.8-2.5 g/L	<2.5 g/L
Prealbumin	2 days	0.2-04 g/L	0.2-0.18 g/L	0.17-0.1 g/L	<0.1 g/L
Retinol binding protein	12 hr	2.6-7.6 g/L	2.5-2.0 g/L	1.9-1.5 g/L	<1 g/L
Transferrin	8 days	218-411 µg/dL	200-150 µg/dL	149-100 µg/dL	<100 µg/dL
Serum iron	11-19 hr	16-124 µg/dL	15-13 µg/dL	12-10 µg/dL	<10 µg/dL

Consider also the concentrations of the following micronutrients: calcium, zinc, magnesium, iodine, vitamin A, vitamin C, vitamin B_1.

common, whereas inflammatory diseases are more common in older children and adolescents. Celiac disease on the one hand, and chronic nonspecific diarrhea on the other, should always be considered independent of age owing to their relatively high frequency (Table 333-3).

Specific clues in the family and personal history may provide useful indications, suggesting a congenital, allergic or inflammatory etiology. A previous episode of acute gastroenteritis suggests postenteritis syndrome, whereas the association of diarrhea with specific foods can indicate a food allergy. A history of polyhydramnios is consistent with congenital chloride or sodium diarrhea or, conversely, cystic fibrosis. The presence of eczema or asthma is associated with an allergic disorder, whereas specific extraintestinal manifestations (e.g., arthritis, diabetes, thrombocytopenia) might suggest an autoimmune disease. Specific skin lesions can suggest acrodermatitis enteropathica. Typical facial abnormalities and woolly hair are associated with phenotypic diarrhea (see Fig. 333-4).

Anthropometric evaluation is an essential step to evaluate "if, since when, and how much" diarrhea has affected body weight. The combined evaluation of the duration and amount of weight loss provides an estimate of the severity of diarrhea.

Initial clinical examination should include evaluating general and nutritional status. Dehydration, marasmus, or kwashiorkor requires prompt supportive interventions to stabilize the patient. Nutritional evaluation is crucial to establish the need for rapid intervention. It should start with the evaluation of the weight and height curves and of the weight for height index to determine the impact of diarrhea on growth. Weight is generally impaired before height, but with time linear growth also becomes affected, and both parameters may be equally abnormal in the long term. Assessment of nutritional status includes the dietary history and biochemical and nutritional investigations. Caloric intake should be quantitatively determined and the relationship between weight modifications and energy intake should be carefully considered.

Biochemical markers assist in grading malnutrition (Table 333-4). The half -life of serum proteins can differentiate between short-term and long-term malnutrition. Assessment of body composition may be performed by measuring mid-arm circumference and triceps skinfold thickness or, more accurately, by bioelectrical impedance analysis or dual emission x-ray absorptiometry (DEXA) scans.

Diagnosis of functional diarrhea is based on pure clinical grounds using established age-related criteria (see Table 333-3).

Conversely, a child with persistent diarrhea and suspected malabsorption might be inappropriately "treated" with a diluted hypocaloric diet in an effort to reduce the diarrhea, and persistent diarrhea may be an indirect consequence of ongoing malnutrition. One such example of this vicious cycle is exocrine pancreatic insufficiency due to protein calorie malnutrition.

The search for etiology may be based on the pathophysiology of the diarrhea. Fecal electrolyte concentrations discriminate between secretory and osmotic diarrhea, and the results can guide the subsequent diagnostic approach. Microbiologic investigation of stool samples should include a thorough list of bacterial, viral, and protozoan agents. Proximal intestinal bacterial overgrowth may be sought using the hydrogen breath test after an oral glucose load.

Noninvasive assessment of digestive-absorptive functions and of intestinal inflammation plays a key role in the diagnostic work-up (Table 333-5).

Diagnostic work-up of chronic diarrhea usually requires endoscopy and histology. Small intestinal biopsy can detect a primary intestinal etiology in the majority of cases of chronic diarrhea and malabsorption. Colonoscopy should be performed in all cases of chronic diarrhea in which gross blood or leukocytes are detected in the stools or when an increased frequency of mucoid stools and abdominal pain suggest colonic involvement. Abnormalities in the digestive-absorptive function tests suggest small bowel involvement, whereas intestinal inflammation, as demonstrated by increased calprotectin and rectal nitric oxide, supports a distal intestinal localization. Capsule endoscopy allows exploration of the entire intestine looking for morphologic abnormalities, inflammation, and bleeding.

Biopsies should be performed at multiple sites, even in a normal-appearing intestine, because abnormalities can have a patchy distribution. Histology is important to establish the degree of mucosal involvement through grading of intestinal damage and the evaluation of associated abnormalities, such as inflammatory infiltration of the lamina propria. Morphometry provides additional quantitative information of epithelial changes. In selected cases, light microscopy can help to identify specific intracellular agents, such as cytomegalovirus, based on the presence of parasites or of large inclusion bodies in infected cells. Electron microscopy is essential to detect cellular structural abnormalities such as microvillous inclusion disease. Immunohistochemistry allows the study of mucosal immune activation as well as of other cell types (smooth muscle cells and enteric neuronal cells), and the components of the basal membrane.

Imaging has a major role in the diagnostic approach. A preliminary plain abdominal x-ray is useful for detecting gaseous distention that suggests intestinal obstruction. Intramural or portal gas may be seen in necrotizing enterocolitis or intussusception. Structural abnormalities such as diverticula, malrotation, stenosis, blind loop, and inflammatory bowel disease, as well as motility disorders, may be appreciated after a barium meal and an entire bowel follow-through examination. The latter also provides information on transit time. Abdominal ultrasound can help detect liver and pancreatic abnormalities or an increase in intestinal wall thickness that suggests an inflammatory bowel disease.

Specific investigations should be carried out for specific diagnostic dilemmas. Prick and patch test can support a diagnosis of food allergy, although definitive diagnosis requires oral challenge. Bile malabsorption may be explored by the retention of the bile acid analog ^{75}Se–homocholic acid–taurine (^{75}SeHCAT) in the enterohepatic circulation. A scintigraphic examination, with radio-labeled octreotide is indicated in suspected APUD (*a*mine *p*recursor *u*ptake and *d*ecarboxylation) cell neoplastic proliferation. In other diseases, specific imaging techniques such as CT or nuclear MRI can have important diagnostic value.

Once infectious agents have been excluded and nutritional assessment performed, a stepwise approach to the child with chronic diarrhea may be applied. The main etiologies of chronic diarrhea should be investigated based on the features of diarrhea and their predominant or selective intestinal dysfunction. A step-by-step diagnostic approach is important to minimize the unnecessary use of invasive procedures and overall costs, while optimizing the yield of the diagnostic work-up (Table 333-6, Fig. 333-5).

TREATMENT

Chronic diarrhea associated with impaired nutritional status should always be considered a serious disease, and therapy should be started promptly. Treatment includes general supportive measures, nutritional rehabilitation, elimination diet, and drugs. Drug treatment includes therapies for specific etiologies as well as interventions aimed at counteracting fluid secretion and/or promoting restoration of disrupted intestinal epithelium. Because death in most instances is caused by dehydration, replacement of fluid and electrolyte losses is the most important early intervention.

Nutritional rehabilitation is often essential and is based on clinical and biochemical assessment. In moderate to severe malnutrition, caloric intake may be progressively increased to 50% or more above the recommended dietary allowances. The intestinal absorptive capacity should be monitored by digestive function tests. In children with steatorrhea, medium chain triglycerides may be the main source of lipids. A lactose-free diet should be

Table 333-5 NONINVASIVE TESTS FOR INTESTINAL AND PANCREATIC DIGESTIVE-ABSORPTIVE FUNCTIONS AND INTESTINAL INFLAMMATION

TEST	NORMAL VALUES	IMPLICATION	REFERENCE
α1-Antitrypsin concentration	<0.9 mg/g stool	Increased intestinal permeability and protein loss	Catassi C, et al: *J Pediatr* 109:500–502, 1986
Steatocrit	<2.5% (>2 yr old)	Fecal fat loss	Guarino A, et al: *J Pediatr Gastroenterol Nutr* 14:268–274, 1992
Fecal reducing substances	Absent	Carbohydrate malabsorption	Lindquist BL, et al: *Arch Dis Child* 51:319–321, 1976
Elastase concentration	>200 μg/g stool	Exocrine pancreatic dysfunction	Carroccio A, et al: *Gut* 43:558–563, 1998
Chymotrypsin concentration	>7.5 U/g>375 U/24 h	Exocrine pancreatic dysfunction	Carroccio A, et al: *Gastroenterology* 112:1839–1844, 1997
Fecal occult blood	Absent	Fecal blood loss, distal intestinal inflammation	Fine KD: *N Engl J Med* 334:1163–1167, 1996
Calprotectin concentration	100 μg/g stool	Intestinal inflammation	Fagerberg UL, et al: *J Pediatr Gastroenterol Nutr* 37:468–472, 2003
Fecal leukocytes	<5/microscopic field	Colonic inflammation	Harris JC, et al: *Ann Intern Med* 76:697–703, 1972
Nitric oxide in rectal dyalisate	<5 μM of NO_2^-/NO_3^-	Rectal inflammation	Berni Canani R, et al: *Am J Gastroenterol* 97:1574–1576, 2002
Dual sugar (cellobiose/mannitol) absorption test	Urine excretion ratio: 0.010 ±0.018	Increased intestinal permeability	Catassi C, et al: *J Pediatr Gastro Nutr* 46:41–47, 2008

Table 333-6 STEPWISE DIAGNOSTIC WORK-UP FOR CHILDREN WITH CHRONIC DIARRHEA

STEP 1
Intestinal microbiology • Stool cultures • Microscopy for parasites • Viruses • Stool electrolytes • H_2 breath test Screening test for celiac disease (transglutaminase 2 autoantibodies) Noninvasive tests for: • Intestinal function • Pancreatic function and sweat test • Intestinal inflammation Tests for food allergy • Prick/patch tests
STEP 2
Intestinal morphology • Standard jejunal/colonic histology • Morphometry • PAS staining • Electron microscopy
STEP 3
Special investigations • Intestinal immunohistochemistry • Anti-enterocyte antibodies • Serum chromogranin and catecholamines • Autoantibodies • ^{75}SeHCAT measurement • Brush border enzymatic activities • Motility and electrophysiological studies

PAS, periodic acid–Schiff; ^{75}SeHCAT, ^{75}Se–homocholic acid–taurine.

started in all children with chronic diarrhea, as is recommended by the World Health Organization (WHO). Lactose is generally replaced by maltodextrin or a combination of complex carbohydrates. A sucrose-free formula is indicated in sucrase-isomaltase deficiency. Semi-elemental or elemental diets have the double purpose of overcoming food intolerance, which may be the primary cause of chronic diarrhea, and facilitating nutrient absorption. The sequence of elimination should be graded from less to more restricted diets, such as cow's milk protein hydrolysate to amino-acid–based formula, depending on the child's situation. In severely compromised infants it may be convenient to start with amino-acid–based feeding.

Clinical nutrition includes enteral or parenteral nutrition. Enteral nutrition may be delivered via nasogastric or gastrostomy tube and is indicated in a child who cannot be fed through the oral route, either because of primary intestinal diseases or because of extreme weakness. Continuous enteral nutrition is effective in children with a reduced absorptive function, such as short bowel syndrome, because it extends the time of nutrient absorption through the still-functioning surface area. In extreme wasting, enteral nutrition might not be sufficient, and parenteral nutrition is required.

Micronutrient and vitamin supplementation are part of nutritional rehabilitation and prevent further problems, especially in malnourished children from developing countries. Zinc supplementation is an important factor in both prevention and therapy of chronic diarrhea, because it promotes ion absorption, restores epithelial proliferation, and stimulates immune response. Nutritional rehabilitation has a general beneficial effect on the patient's overall condition, intestinal function, and immune response and can break the vicious circle shown in Figure 333-2.

Drug therapy includes anti-infectious drugs, immune suppression, and drugs that can inhibit fluid loss and promote cell growth. If a bacterial agent is detected, specific antibiotics should be prescribed. Empirical antibiotic therapy may be used in

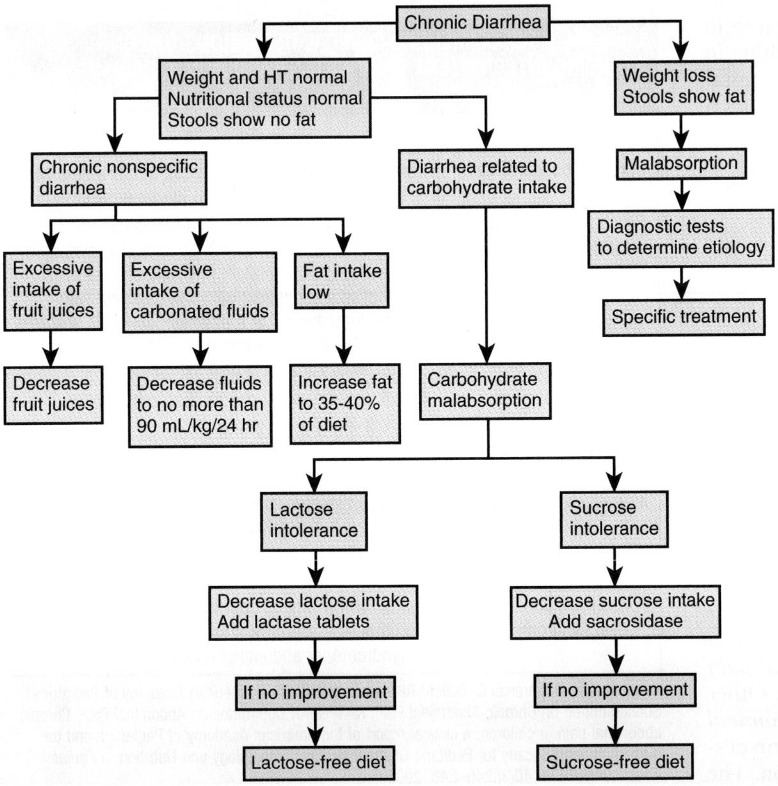

Figure 333-5 General therapeutic approaches to management of chronic diarrhea. HT, height.

children with small bowel bacterial overgrowth or with suspected bacterial diarrhea. Trimethoprim-sulfamethoxazole, metronidazole or albendazole, and nitazoxanide have a broad pattern of targets, including parasites. In Rotavirus-induced severe and protracted diarrhea, oral administration of human immunoglobulins (300 mg/kg) should be considered.

Immune suppression should be considered in selected conditions such as autoimmune enteropathy. In selected cases, biologic immune suppression may be considered.

Treatment may be also directed at modifying specific pathophysiologic processes. Severe ion secretion may be reduced by pro-absorptive agents, such as the enkephalinase inhibitor racecadotril. In diarrhea due to neuroendocrine tumors, microvillus inclusion disease, and enterotoxin-induced severe diarrhea, a trial with the somatostatin analog octreotide may be considered. Zinc or growth hormone promote enterocyte growth and ion absorption and may be effective when intestinal atrophy and ion secretion are associated.

When other attempts have failed, the only option may be parenteral nutrition or intestinal transplantation.

BIBLIOGRAPHY

Please visit the Nelson Textbook of Pediatrics *website at www.expertconsult.com for the complete bibliography.*

333.1 Diarrhea from Neuroendocrine Tumors

Helen Spoudeas and David Branski

Rare tumors of the neuroendocrine cells of the gastroenteropancreatic axis and adrenal and extra-adrenal sites derive from the APUD system. They are characterized by an excessive production of one or several peptides, which when released into the circulation exert their endocrine effects and can be measured by radioimmunologic methods (in the plasma or as their urinary metabolites) and hence act as tumor markers. In clinically functioning tumors, the hypersecretion causes a recognizable syndrome that can include watery diarrhea. Though rare, neuroendocrine tumor (NET) should be considered a potential cause in patients with a particularly severe or chronic course (resulting in electrolyte and fluid depletion), associated flushing or palpitations, or a positive family history of multiple endocrine neoplasia (MEN-1 or MEN-2) syndromes (see Table 333-7 on the *Nelson Textbook of Pediatrics* website at www.expertconsult.com).

For the full continuation of this chapter, please visit the Nelson Textbook of Pediatrics *website at www.expertconsult.com.*

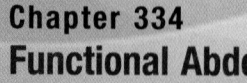

Chapter 334
Functional Abdominal Pain (Nonorganic Chronic Abdominal Pain)

Raman Sreedharan and Chris A. Liacouras

Recurrent abdominal pain (RAP) in children was defined as at least 3 episodes of pain over at least 3 mo that interfered with function. In many situations the term *recurrent abdominal pain* was used synonymously with *functional abdominal pain.* Other terms such as *chronic abdominal pain, nonorganic abdominal pain,* and *psychogenic abdominal pain* that were used for describing abdominal pain in children led to clinical confusion. The American Academy of Pediatrics Subcommittee on Chronic Abdominal Pain and the North American Society for Pediatric Gastroenterology Hepatology and Nutrition Committee on Abdominal Pain suggested that RAP no longer be used. The recommended clinical definitions for long-lasting intermittent or constant abdominal pain by the same committees are outlined in Table 334-1.

Chronic abdominal pain can be organic or nonorganic, depending on whether a specific etiology is identified. Nonorganic abdominal pain or functional abdominal pain refers to pain without evidence of anatomic, inflammatory, metabolic, or neoplastic abnormalities. **Functional gastrointestinal disorders (FGIDs)** are a group of gastrointestinal (GI) disorders that include variable combinations of chronic or recurrent GI symptoms not explained by structural or biochemical abnormalities. The Rome Committee updates and modifies the information on FGIDs for clinical and research purposes. The Rome III process had 2 pediatric subcommittees based on age range: Neonate/Toddler (0-4 yr) and Child/Adolescent (4-18 yr). The Child/Adolescent committee categorized abdominal pain-related FGIDs under Category H2 in Table 334-2. The Rome III criteria for the diagnosis of Childhood Functional Abdominal Pain (category H2d) and Childhood Functional Abdominal Pain Syndrome (category H2d1) is represented in Table 334-3.

The exact incidence and prevalence of chronic abdominal pain is not known. There are reports of chronic abdominal pain affecting 9-15% of children. There are also reports that 13% of middle school and 17% of high school children have weekly complaints of abdominal pain.

PATHOPHYSIOLOGY

The symptoms of FGIDs may be the result of dysfunctions of the intestinal sensory and motor systems. The pathophysiology of functional abdominal pain is complex and not fully understood. Visceral hypersensitivity and motility disturbances are thought to be involved in functional abdominal pain. The traditional concept that motility disorders alone have an important role in functional

Table 334-1 RECOMMENDED CLINICAL DEFINITIONS OF LONG-STANDING INTERMITTENT OR CONSTANT ABDOMINAL PAIN IN CHILDREN

DISORDER	DEFINITION
Chronic abdominal pain	Long-lasting intermittent or constant abdominal pain that is functional or organic (disease based)
Functional abdominal pain	Abdominal pain without demonstrable evidence of pathologic condition, such as anatomic metabolic, infectious, inflammatory or neoplastic disorder. Functional abdominal pain can manifest with symptoms typical of functional dyspepsia, irritable bowel syndrome, abdominal migraine or functional abdominal pain syndrome.
Functional dyspepsia	Functional abdominal pain or discomfort in the upper abdomen
Irritable bowel syndrome	Functional abdominal pain associated with alteration in bowel movements
Abdominal migraine	Functional abdominal pain with features of migraine (paroxysmal abdominal pain associated with anorexia, nausea, vomiting or pallor as well as maternal history of migraine headaches)
Functional abdominal pain syndrome	Functional abdominal pain without the characteristics of dyspepsia, irritable bowel syndrome, or abdominal migraine.

Adapted from Di Lorenzo C, Colletti RB, Lehmann HP, et al; American Academy of Pediatrics Subcommittee on Chronic Abdominal Pain; NASPGHAN Committee on Abdominal Pain: Chronic abdominal pain in children: a clinical report of the American Academy of Pediatrics and the North American Society for Pediatric Gastroenterology, Hepatology and Nutrition, *J Pediatr Gastroenterol Nutr* 40(3):245–248, 2005.

Table 334-2 CHILDHOOD FUNCTIONAL GI DISORDERS: CHILD/ADOLESCENT (CATEGORY H)

H1. Vomiting and aerophagia
- H1a. Adolescent rumination syndrome
- H1b. Cyclic vomiting syndrome
- H1c. Aerophgia

H2. Abdominal pain—related FGIDs
- H2a. Functional dyspepsia
- H2b. Irritable bowel syndrome
- H2c. Abdominal migraine
- H2d. Childhood functional abdominal pain
  - H2d1. Childhood functional abdominal pain syndrome

H3. Constipation and incontinence
- H3a. Functional constipation
- H3b. Nonr-Retentive fecal incontinence

Adapted from Rome Foundation: *Rome III disorders and criteria* (website). www.romecriteria.org/criteria/. Accessed May 7, 2010.

Table 334-3 ROME III CRITERIA FOR CHILDHOOD FUNCTIONAL ABDOMINAL PAIN H2D AND CHILDHOOD FUNCTIONAL ABDOMINAL PAIN SYNDROME H2D1

H2d. CHILDHOOD FUNCTIONAL ABDOMINAL PAIN

Diagnostic criteria* must include **all** of the following:
- Episodic or continuous abdominal pain
- Insufficient criteria for other FGIDs
- No evidence of an inflammatory, anatomic, metabolic or neoplastic process that explains the subject's symptoms

H2d1. CHILDHOOD FUNCTIONAL ABDOMINAL PAIN SYNDROME

Diagnostic criteria* must satisfy criteria for childhood functional abdominal pain and have at least 25% of the time **one or more** of the following:
- Some loss of daily function
- Additional somatic symptoms such as headache, limb pain, or difficulty sleeping.

*Criteria fulfilled at least once per week for ≥2 mo prior to diagnosis
FGID, functional gastrointestinal disorder.
Adapted from Rome Foundation: *Rome III disorders and criteria* (website). www.romecriteria.org/criteria/. Accessed May 7, 2010.

pain has not been confirmed. It is believed that visceral hypersensitivity leading to abnormal bowel sensitivity to stimuli (physiologic, psychologic, noxious) might have a more dominant role in functional abdominal pain. Visceral hypersensitivity could be due to abnormal interpretation of normal signals by the brain or aberrant signals sent to the brain or a combination. Intestinal pain receptors respond to mechanical and/or chemical stimuli. The visceral receptors can respond to both mechanical and chemical stimuli, but the mucosal receptors are primarily stimulated by chemical stimuli.

The viscera are innervated by dual set of nerves (vagal and splanchnic spinal nerves or pelvic and splanchnic spinal nerves). The spinal afferents carry impulses to the spinal cord. The dorsal horn of the spinal cord regulates conduction of impulses from peripheral nociceptive receptors to the spinal cord and brain, and the pain experience is further influenced by cognitive and emotional centers. Chronic peripheral nervous system pain can produce increased neural activity in higher central nervous system centers, leading to perpetuation of pain. Psychosocial stress can affect pain intensity and quality through these mechanisms. The child's response to pain can be influenced by stress, personality type, and the reinforcement of illness behavior within the family. The autonomic and enteric nervous systems can overlie the initiation, perception, and perpetuation of pain.

A normal functioning enteric nervous system (ENS) is important for coordination of intestinal motility, secretion and blood flow. Abnormalities of the enteric nervous system may be an underlying factor for functional abdominal pain. Inflammation of the intestine and its role in the pathogenesis of functional

Table 334-4 ALARM *SYMPTOMS* USUALLY NEEDING FURTHER INVESTIGATIONS

- Pain that wakes up the child from sleep
- Persistent right upper or right lower quadrant pain
- Significant vomiting (bilious vomiting, protracted vomiting, cyclical vomiting or worrisome pattern to the physician)
- Unexplained fever
- Genitourinary tract symptoms
- Dysphagia
- Chronic severe diarrhea or nocturnal diarrhea
- Gastrointestinal blood loss
- Involuntary weight loss
- Deceleration of linear growth
- Delayed puberty
- Family history of inflammatory bowel disease, celiac disease, and peptic ulcer disease

abdominal pain could be due to the effects of the inflammatory mediators and cytokines (released by the various inflammatory cells) on the ENS. The dysregulation in the brain-gut interactions can also lead to functional abdominal pain. The role of certain triggers for pain, such as lactose, sorbitol, fructose, bile acids, or fatty acids, could be due to the altered sensitivity or motor function, because some patients have relief when eliminating these from their diet. Altered intestinal permeability enabling passage of food antigens into the mucosa leading to prolonged stimulation of the intestinal mucosal immune system and the ENS is also a possible cause for functional abdominal pain.

EVALUATION AND DIAGNOSIS

While evaluating a patient with chronic abdominal pain, distinguishing organic pain and functional pain can be challenging. A wide range of potential organic causes of chronic abdominal pain (see Table 298-13) must be considered before establishing a diagnosis of functional pain (nonorganic). Frequently cited causes of chronic abdominal pain include constipation, esophagitis, gastritis, inflammatory bowel disease, and possibly giardiasis. There is little evidence that the frequency, severity, or location of the pain helps to distinguish between organic and nonorganic pain. It is controversial whether nighttime awakening due to pain is concerning for organic disorders or if it can be seen with functional pain syndromes.

Children with chronic abdominal pain might have associated headaches, anorexia, nausea, vomiting, excessive gas, diarrhea or constipation, and joint pain, but this does not help distinguish between functional and organic disorder. Negative lifestyle events and high life stress levels also do not help to distinguish organic and nonorganic pain, despite several reports of higher levels of life stress in children with chronic abdominal pain. Daily stressors may increase the likelihood for pain episodes, but there is no evidence that psychological issues distinguishes between organic and nonorganic abdominal pain. Nonetheless, it is important to investigate and manage the psychologic factors because there is evidence suggesting that children with chronic abdominal pain have more anxiety and depression symptoms. Whether this causes pain or is the result of pain is not known.

Children with functional pain do not have higher levels of conduct disorder or oppositional behavior compared to the controls but they can be more prone to emotional symptoms or psychiatric disorders later in life. Parents of patients with functional abdominal pain have more symptoms of somatization, anxiety, and depression. Both the family and the affected child when an adult have a higher incidence of irritable bowel syndrome (IBS).

A through history and physical examination would identify the alarm symptoms and signs (Tables 334-4 and 334-5). The

Table 334-5 ALARM *SIGNS* USUALLY NEEDING FURTHER INVESTIGATIONS

Localized tenderness in the right upper quadrant
Localized tenderness in the right lower quadrant
Localized fullness or mass
Hepatomegaly
Splenomegaly
Jaundice
Costovertebral angle tenderness
Arthritis
Spinal tenderness
Perianal disease
Abnormal or unexplained physical findings

presence of alarm symptoms and signs warrants further investigation. The absence of alarm symptoms and signs, a normal physical examination, and a normal stool hemoccult test is sufficient for an initial diagnosis of functional abdominal pain. The laboratory, radiologic, or endoscopic approach to children with chronic abdominal pain should be individualized, depending on the findings suggested by a detailed history and physical examination.

Laboratory studies may be unnecessary if the history and physical examination lead to a diagnosis of functional abdominal pain. Nonetheless, medical tests can reassure the patient and family, and at times the physician, if there is significant functional disability and poor quality of life. A complete blood cell count, sedimentation rate, C-reactive protein, basic chemistry panel, celiac panel, stool culture, stool test for ova and parasites, and urinalysis are reasonable screening studies. *The risk of celiac disease may be 4 times higher in these patients compared with the general population.* Elevated stool calprotectin levels usually suggest an inflammatory etiology.

If indicated, an ultrasound examination of the abdomen can give information about kidneys, gallbladder, and pancreas; with lower abdominal pain, a pelvic ultrasonogram may be indicated. An upper GI x-ray series is indicated if one suspects a disorder of the stomach or small intestine.

Helicobacter pylori infection does not seem to be associated with chronic abdominal pain, but in patients with symptoms suggesting gastritis or ulcer, an *H. pylori* test (fecal *H. pylori* antigen) may be performed. Breath hydrogen testing is done for ruling out lactose or sucrose malabsorption. Lactose intolerance is so common that the finding may be coincidental, and the clinician must be cautious in attributing chronic abdominal pain to this condition.

Esophagogastroduodenoscopy is indicated with symptoms suggesting persistent upper GI pathology. In the absence of this suspicion, esophagogastroduodenoscopy is unlikely to identify an abnormality and is usually not necessary.

TREATMENT

Making a positive diagnosis of functional abdominal pain is important and can be done by the primary care pediatrician in most 4-18 yr old children with chronic abdominal pain if there are no alarm symptoms or signs, a normal physical examination, and a negative stool occult blood testing. In practice, on many occasions children do not get a conclusive diagnosis of functional abdominal pain. This can lead to unwarranted referrals and increased anxiety to the patient and the family. Even if a diagnostic evaluation is initiated during the initial office visit, a discussion about functional abdominal pain as the most likely diagnosis during that visit will help the patient and family to understand the diagnosis better. Close following and counseling by one consistent health care provider is essential.

The most important component of the treatment is reassurance and education of the child and family. The child and family need to be reassured that no evidence of a serious underlying disorder is present. The family and the child with functional pain might worry about the inability to identify an organic cause and may be resistant to a diagnosis of nonorganic disease. Explanation in simple language that although the pain is real, there is no underlying serious disorder usually alleviates the anxiety in the patient and family. Children of families that do not accept a functional cause of the symptoms are more likely to have persistent somatic complaints and school absences. The parents should be instructed to avoid reinforcing the symptoms with secondary gain. If children have missed school or have been removed from routine activities because of the pain, it is important that they return to regular activities.

Table 334-6 EFFECTIVENESS OF TREATMENTS FOR ABDOMINAL PAIN IN CHILDREN

THERAPY	DEFINITION OF DISORDER	EFFECTIVENESS
Cognitive behavioral (family) therapy	Recurrent abdominal pain	Beneficial
Famotidine	Recurrent abdominal pain and dyspeptic symptoms	Inconclusive
Added dietary fiber	Recurrent abdominal pain	Unlikely to be beneficial
Lactose-free diet	Recurrent abdominal pain	Unlikely to be beneficial
Peppermint oil	Irritable bowel syndrome	Likely to be beneficial
Amitriptyline	Functional GI disorders, Irritable bowel syndrome	Inconsistent results
Lactobacillus GG	Irritable bowel syndrome using Rome II criteria	Unlikely to be beneficial

The effectiveness of analgesics, antispasmodics, sedatives, and antidepressants is currently unknown.
GI, gastrointestinal.
From Berger MY, Gieteling MJ, Benninga MA: Chronic abdominal pain in children, *BMJ* 334:997–1002, 2007.

Treatment goals should be set for return to function and minimizing pain. Complete disappearance of pain would be an unreasonable goal to set. Cognitive-behavioral therapy is helpful in the short term for managing pain and functional disability (Table 334-6). Biofeedback, guided imagery, and relaxation techniques have been useful in some children with functional pain. Even though studies have not shown consistent benefits from medications, time-limited use of medications is usually part of the multidisciplinary approach. The commonly used medications include acid suppressants for dyspepsia symptoms, antispasmodics, and low-dose amitriptyline. For chronic abdominal pain with IBS symptoms, antidiarrheals and nonstimulating laxatives are used. Peppermint oil for 2 wk improves IBS symptoms in children. There is no evidence that lactose-restricted diet and fiber supplements decrease the frequency of attacks in chronic abdominal pain in children. Proton pump inhibitors or visceral muscle relaxants (anticholinergics) have been used empirically but are often unhelpful in the absence of specific indication.

Irritable Bowel Syndrome

IBS is most often diagnosed in adolescents and young adults and is characterized as a chronic functional bowel disorder associated with abdominal pain or discomfort and altered bowel function. There are multiple diagnostic criteria with varying durations of symptoms ranging from ≥3 mo to >2 yr.

Abdominal pain is episodic, cramping, or aching, usually in the lower abdomen, and often relieved by defecation. There may be abdominal discomfort, bloating, and flatulence. Diarrhea and constipation alone or in an alternating pattern must be present. The diarrhea is often watery and frequent and is associated with pain, the passage of mucus per rectum, and a feeling of incomplete emptying. The constipation is associated with a decreased stooling frequency and the passage of hard stools. Symptoms may be traced back to childhood or following an episode of presumed bacterial or viral gastroenteritis. It is important to rule out organic causes of abdominal pain and altered bowel patterns, especially celiac disease, even in the absence of the classic features of this disease.

Management focuses on the dominant symptoms. Pain has been managed with cognitive-behavioral therapy, pain clinic referrals, peppermint, antispasmodic agents, and tricyclic antidepressant agents (amitriptyline). Diarrhea has been managed with loperamide, oral nonabsorbable antibiotics, and 5-HT_3 antagonists (alosetron). Constipation is managed with fiber (psyllium), increased fluid intake, lactulose, 5-HT_4 agonists (tegaserod), and selective C2 chloride channel–activating agents. In all medication trials, there is often a high response to placebo.

BIBLIOGRAPHY

Please visit the Nelson Textbook of Pediatrics *website at www.expertconsult.com for the complete bibliography.*

Chapter 335
Acute Appendicitis

John J. Aiken and Keith T. Oldham

Acute appendicitis, despite a declining incidence in the United States in the past half century, remains the most common acute surgical condition in children and a major cause of childhood morbidity. Approximately 80,000 children are affected annually in the United States, a rate of 4/1,000 children <14 yr of age. Although since the turn of the century there has been a trend toward shorter hospital stays, appendicitis accounts for >1 million hospital days utilized per year. Mortality is low, but morbidity remains high, mostly in association with perforated appendicitis.

The methods of diagnosis and treatment of appendicitis vary significantly among clinicians and hospitals, and consensus regarding a best practice approach to the child who presents with the chief complaint of abdominal pain and suspected appendicitis has been elusive. Management has changed substantially in the past several decades with improved antibiotics regimens, advances in imaging techniques, percutaneous drainage procedures by interventional radiologists, initial nonoperative management in selected cases, and the use of laparoscopy.

PATHOLOGY

Acute appendicitis is most likely a disease of multiple etiologies, the final common pathway of which involves invasion of the appendiceal wall by bacteria. One pathway to acute appendicitis begins with luminal obstruction; inspissated fecal material, lymphoid hyperplasia, ingested foreign body, parasites, and tumors have been implicated. Obstruction of the appendiceal lumen results in increasing intraluminal pressures from bacterial proliferation and continued secretion of mucus. Elevated intraluminal pressure, in turn, leads to lymphatic and venous congestion and edema followed by impaired arterial perfusion, eventually leading to ischemia of the wall of the appendix, bacterial invasion with inflammatory infiltrate of all layers of the appendiceal wall, and necrosis. This progression correlates with progression from simple appendicitis to gangrenous appendicitis and, thereafter, appendiceal perforation. Submucosal lymphoid follicles, which can obstruct the appendiceal lumen, are few at birth but multiply steadily during childhood, reaching a peak in number during the teen years, when acute appendicitis is most common, and declining after age 30 yr. Fecaliths and appendicitis are more common in developed countries with refined, low-fiber diets than in developing countries with a high-fiber diet; no causal relationship has been established between lack of dietary fiber and appendicitis.

The finding that <50% of specimens from cases of acute appendicitis demonstrate luminal obstruction on pathologic examination has prompted investigations of alternative etiologies. Enteric infection likely plays a role in many cases in association with mucosal ulceration and invasion of the appendiceal wall by bacteria. Bacteria such as *Yersinia*, *Salmonella*, and *Shigella* spp and viruses such as mumps, coxsackievirus B, and adenovirus have been implicated. In addition, case reports demonstrate the occurrence of appendicitis from ingested foreign bodies, in association with carcinoid tumors of the appendix or *Ascaris* and following blunt abdominal trauma. Children with cystic fibrosis have an increased incidence of appendicitis; the cause is believed to be the abnormal thickened mucus. Appendicitis in neonates is rare and warrants evaluation for cystic fibrosis and Hirschsprung disease.

A primary focus in the management of acute appendicitis is avoidance of sepsis and the infectious complications mostly seen in association with perforation. Bacteria can be cultured from the serosal surface of the appendix before microscopic or gross perforation and bacterial invasion of the mesenteric veins can result in portal vein sepsis (pylephlebitis) and liver abscess. Subsequent to perforation, the microbiologic fecal contamination may be localized to the right lower quadrant (RLQ) or pelvis by the omentum and adjacent loops of bowel, resulting in a localized abscess or inflammatory mass (phlegmon), or alternatively, the fecal contamination can spread throughout the peritoneal cavity, causing diffuse peritonitis. Young children typically have a poorly developed omentum and are often unable to control the local infection. Perforation and abscess formation with appendicitis can lead to fistula formation in adjacent organs, scrotal cellulitis and abscess through a patent processus vaginalis (congenital indirect inguinal hernia), or small bowel obstruction.

CLINICAL FEATURES

Appendicitis is most common in older children, with peak incidence between the age of 12 and 18 yr; it is rare in children <5 yr of age (<5% of cases) and extremely rare (<1% of cases) in children <3 yr of age. It affects boys slightly more often than girls and whites more often than blacks in the United States. There is a seasonal peak incidence in autumn and spring. There appears to be a familial predisposition in some cases, particularly in children in whom appendicitis develops before age 6 yr.

Perforation is most common in young children, with rates as high as 82% for children <5 yr and approaching 100% in infants. There is an increased incidence of perforated appendicitis in children of minority race and children with Medicaid health insurance.

Appendicitis in children has an immensely broad spectrum of clinical presentation. The signs and symptoms can be classic or atypical and quite variable depending on the timing of presentation, the patient's age, the position of the appendix, and individual variability in the evolution of the disease process. Children early in the disease process can appear well and have minimal symptoms, subtle findings on physical examination, and normal laboratory studies; those with perforation and advanced peritonitis often demonstrate bowel obstruction, renal failure, and septic shock.

Despite advances in imaging technology and computer-assisted decision-making models and scoring systems, accurate diagnosis can be difficult, and perforation rates have not changed in the past few decades.

Whereas the classic presentation of acute appendicitis is well described, this represents less than half the cases; therefore, most cases of appendicitis have an "atypical" presentation. The illness typically begins insidiously with generalized malaise and anorexia; the child does not appear ill and the family is not likely to seek consultation assuming the child has "stomach flu" or a viral syndrome. Unfortunately, if the diagnosis is appendicitis, the illness escalates rapidly with abdominal pain followed by vomiting; appendiceal perforation is likely to occur within 48 hr of the onset of illness, and the opportunity for diagnosis before perforation is generally brief.

Abdominal pain is consistently the primary and often the first symptom and begins shortly (hours) after the onset of illness. The pain is initially vague, unrelated to activity or position, often colicky, and periumbilical in location as a result of visceral inflammation from a distended appendix. Progression of the inflammatory process in the next 12-24 hr leads to involvement of the adjacent parietal peritoneal surfaces, resulting in somatic pain localized to the RLQ. The pain becomes steady and more severe and is exacerbated by movement. The child often describes marked discomfort with the "bumpy" car ride to the hospital, moves cautiously, and has difficulty getting onto the examining room stretcher. Nausea and vomiting occur in more than half the patients and usually *follow* the onset of abdominal pain by several hours. Anorexia is a classic and consistent finding in acute appendicitis, but occasionally, affected patients are hungry. Diarrhea and urinary symptoms are also common, particularly in cases of perforated appendicitis when there is likely inflammation near the rectum and possible abscess in the pelvis. Because enteric infections can cause appendicitis, diarrhea may be the initial manifestation and gastroenteritis may be the assumed diagnosis. In contrast to gastroenteritis, the abdominal pain in appendicitis is constant (not cramping or relieved by defecation), the emesis may become bile stained and persistent, and the clinical course worsens rather than improves over time. Fever is typically low-grade unless perforation has occurred. Most patients demonstrate at least mild tachycardia.

The temporal progression of symptoms from vague mild pain, malaise, and anorexia to severe localized pain, fever, and vomiting typically occurs rapidly, in 24-48 hr in the majority of cases. If the diagnosis is delayed beyond 36-48 hr, the perforation rate exceeds 65%. A period after perforation of lessened abdominal pain and acute symptoms has been described, presumably with the elimination of pressure within the appendix. If the omentum or adjacent intestine is able to wall off the infectious process, the evolution of illness is less predictable and delay in presentation is likely. If perforation leads to diffuse peritonitis, the child generally has escalating diffuse abdominal pain and rapid development of toxicity evidenced by dehydration and by signs of sepsis including hypotension, oliguria, acidosis, and high-grade fever. When several days have elapsed in the progression of appendicitis, patients often develop signs and symptoms of developing small bowel obstruction. If the appendix is retrocecal, appendicitis predictably evolves more slowly and patients are likely to relate 4-5 days of illness preceding evaluation. The pain is lateral and posterior and can mimic the symptoms associated with septic arthritis of the hip or a psoas muscle abscess.

Atypical clinical features include absence of fever, Rovsing sign, rebound pain, migration of pain, guarding, and anorexia in 30-50% of pediatric patients. Other atypical features include normal to increased bowel sounds and an abrupt onset of pain.

PHYSICAL EXAMINATION

The hallmark of diagnosing acute appendicitis remains a careful and thorough history and physical examination. A primary focus of the initial assessment is attention to the temporal evolution of the illness in relation to specific presenting signs and symptoms. In many children, appendicitis can be confidently diagnosed on clinical examination alone and they can thus be spared the treatment delay, expense, and possible radiation exposure associated with imaging studies.

Physical examination begins with inspection of the child's demeanor as well as the appearance of the abdomen. Because appendicitis most often has an insidious onset, children rarely present <12 hr from the onset of illness, and the children who do present early are likely to have minimal findings. Children with early appendicitis (18-36 hr) typically appear mildly ill and move tentatively, hunched forward and often with a slight limp favoring the right side. Supine, they often lie quietly on their right side with their knees pulled up to relax the abdominal muscles, and when asked to lie flat or sit up, they move cautiously and might use a hand to protect the RLQ.

Early in appendicitis, the abdomen is typically flat; abdominal distention suggests more advanced disease characteristic of perforation or developing small bowel obstruction. Auscultation can reveal normal or hyperactive bowel sounds in early appendicitis, which are replaced by hypoactive bowel sounds as the disease progresses to perforation. *The judicious use of morphine analgesia to relieve abdominal pain does not change diagnostic accuracy or interfere with surgical decision-making, and patients should receive adequate pain control.*

Localized abdominal tenderness is the single most reliable finding in the diagnosis of acute appendicitis. In 1899, McBurney described the classic point of localized tenderness in acute appendicitis, which is the junction of the lateral and middle thirds of the line joining the right anterior-superior iliac spine and the umbilicus, but the tenderness can also localize to any of the aberrant locations of the appendix. Localized tenderness is a later and less-consistent finding when the appendix is retrocecal in position.

A gentle touch on the child's arm at the beginning of the examination with the reassurance that the abdominal examination will be similarly gentle can help to establish trust and increase the chance for a reliable and reproducible examination. The examination is best initiated in the left lower abdomen, so that the immediate part of the exam is not uncomfortable, and conducted in a counterclockwise direction moving to the left upper abdomen, right upper abdomen, and lastly, the right lower abdomen. This should alleviate anxiety, allow relaxation of the abdominal musculature, and enhance trust. The examiner makes several "circles" of the abdomen with sequentially more pressure.

A consistent finding in acute appendicitis is rigidity of the overlying rectus muscle. This rigidity may be voluntary, to protect the area of tenderness from the examiner's hand, or involuntary, secondary to peritonitis causing spasm of the overlying muscle. Physical examination findings must be interpreted relative to the temporal evolution of the illness. Abdominal tenderness may be vague or even absent early in the course of appendicitis and is often diffuse after rupture. Rebound tenderness and referred rebound tenderness (Rovsing sign) are also consistent findings in acute appendicitis but not always present. Rebound tenderness is elicited by deep palpation of the abdomen followed by the sudden release of the examining hand. This is often very painful to the child and has demonstrated poor correlation with peritonitis, so it should be avoided. Gentle finger percussion is a better test for peritoneal irritation. Similarly, digital rectal examination is uncomfortable and unlikely to contribute to the evaluation of appendicitis in most cases. Rectal exam may be helpful in selected cases, including when the diagnosis is in doubt, when a pelvic appendix or abscess is suspected, or in adolescent girls when ovarian pathology is suspected. Psoas and obturator internus signs are pain with passive stretch of these muscles. The psoas sign is elicited with active right thigh flexion or passive extension of the hip and typically positive in cases of a retrocecal appendix. The obturator sign is demonstrated by adductor pain after internal rotation of the flexed thigh and typically positive in cases of a pelvic appendix. Physical examination may demonstrate a mass in the RLQ representing an inflammatory phlegmon around the appendix or a localized abscess.

Table 335-1 PEDIATRIC APPENDICITIS SCORES

FEATURE	SCORE
Fever >38°C	1
Anorexia	1
Nausea/vomiting	1
Cough/percussion/hopping tenderness	2
Right lower quadrant tenderness	2
Migration of pain	1
Leukocytosis >10,000 (10^9/L)	1
Polymorphonuclear-neutrophilia >7,500 (10^9/L)	1
Total	10

From Acheson J, Banerjee J: Management of suspected appendicitis in children, *Arch Dis Child Educ Pract Ed* 95:9–13, 2010.

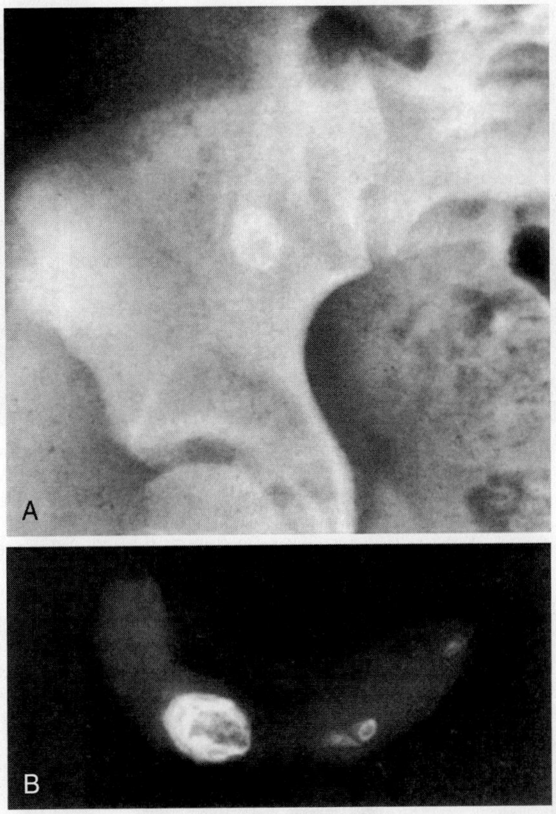

Figure 335-1 Calcified appendicoliths are seen in a coned-down anteroposterior view of the right lower quadrant *(A)* and in the resected appendix of a 10 yr old girl with acute appendicitis *(B)*. (From Kuhn JP, Slovis TL, Haller JO: *Caffrey's pediatric diagnostic imaging,* vol 2, ed 10, Philadelphia, 2004, Mosby, p 1682.)

DIAGNOSTIC STUDIES

Laboratory Findings

A variety of laboratory tests have been used in the evaluation of children with suspected appendicitis. Individually, none are very sensitive or specific for appendicitis, but collectively they can affect the clinician's level of suspicion and decision-making to proceed with pediatric surgery consultation, discharge, or imaging studies. Findings should be interpreted with attention to the temporal evolution of the illness.

A complete blood count with differential and urinalysis are commonly obtained.

The leukocyte count in early appendicitis (<24 hr of illness) may be normal and typically is mildly elevated with a left shift (11,000-16,000/mm^3) as the illness progresses in the 1st 24-48 hr. Whereas a normal white blood cell count (WBC) never completely eliminates appendicitis, a count <8,000/mm^3 in a patient with a history of illness >48 hr should be viewed as highly suspicious for an alternative diagnosis. The leukocyte count may be markedly elevated (>20,000/mm^3) in perforated appendicitis and rarely in nonperforated cases; a markedly elevated WBC, other than in cases of advanced, perforated appendicitis, should raise suspicion of an alternative diagnosis.

Urinalysis often demonstrates a few white or red blood cells, due to proximity of the inflamed appendix to the ureter or bladder, but it should be free of bacteria. The urine is often concentrated and contains ketones from diminished oral intake and vomiting. Gross hematuria is uncommon and suggests primary renal pathology.

Electrolytes and liver chemistries are generally normal unless there has been a delay in diagnosis, leading to severe dehydration and/or sepsis. Amylase and liver enzymes are only helpful to exclude alternative diagnoses such as pancreatitis and cholecystitis and are not obtained if appendicitis is the strongly suspected diagnosis.

C-reactive protein increases in proportion to the degree of appendiceal inflammation but is nonspecific and not widely used. Serum amyloid A protein is consistently elevated in patients with acute appendicitis with a sensitivity and specificity of 86% and 83%, respectively.

The Pediatric Appendicitis score combines history, physical, and laboratory data to assist in the diagnosis (Table 335-1). Scores of ≤2 suggest a very low likelihood of appendicitis, while scores ≥8 are highly associated with appendicitis. Scores between 3 and 7 warrant further diagnostic studies. Nonetheless, no scoring system is perfectly sensitive or specific.

Radiologic Studies

PLAIN FILMS Plain abdominal x-rays can demonstrate several findings in acute appendicitis, including sentinel loops of bowel and localized ileus, scoliosis from psoas muscle spasm, a colonic air-fluid level above the right iliac fossa (colon cutoff sign), or a fecalith (5-10% of cases), but they have a low sensitivity for appendicitis and are not generally recommended (Fig. 335-1). Plain films are most helpful in evaluating complicated cases in which small bowel obstruction or free air is suspected.

ULTRASOUND Ultrasound (US) is often used in the evaluation of acute appendicitis and has demonstrated >90% sensitivity and specificity in pediatric centers experienced with the technique. Graded abdominal compression is used to displace the cecum and ascending colon and identify the appendix, which has a typical target appearance (Fig. 335-2). The ultrasound criteria for appendicitis include wall thickness ≥6 mm, luminal distention, lack of compressibility, a complex mass in the RLQ, or a fecalith. The visualized appendix usually coincides with the site of localized pain and tenderness. Findings that suggest advanced appendicitis on ultrasound include asymmetric wall thickening, abscess formation, associated free intraperitoneal fluid, surrounding tissue edema, and decreased local tenderness to compression.

The main limitation of ultrasound is inability to visualize the appendix, which is reported in up to 20% of cases. **A normal appendix must be visualized to exclude appendicitis by ultrasound.** Certain conditions decrease the sensitivity and reliability of ultrasound for appendicitis, including obesity, bowel distention, and pain.

Major advantages of ultrasound include its low cost and freedom from need for patient preparation and ionizing radiation. Ultrasound can be particularly helpful in adolescent girls, a group with a high negative appendectomy rate (normal appendix found at surgery), because of its ability to evaluate for ovarian pathology without ionizing radiation. A diagnostic or normal ultrasound exam eliminates the need for CT and should be considered the first exam in an experienced center.

CT SCAN CT scan has been the gold standard imaging study for evaluating children with suspected appendicitis. CT examination

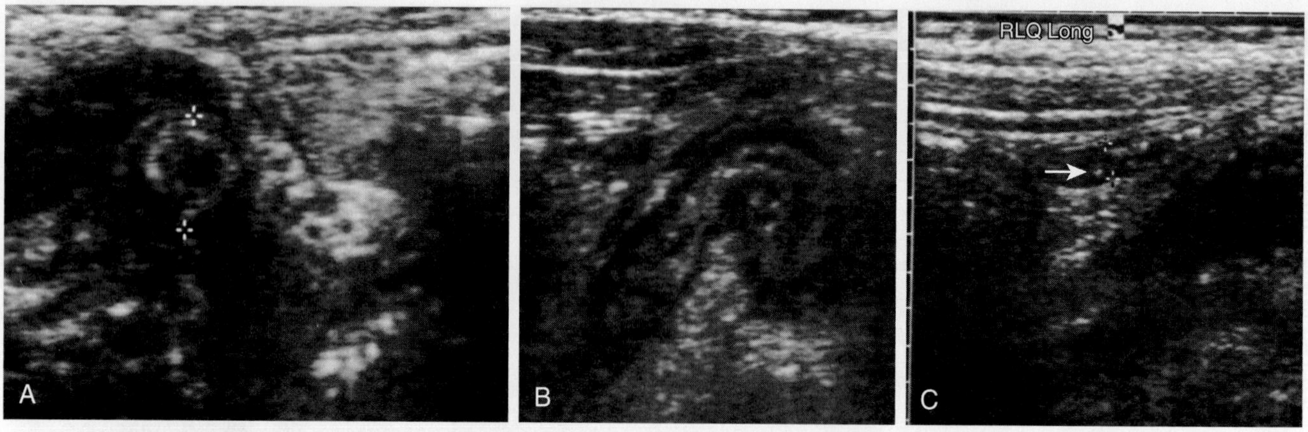

Figure 335-2 Ultrasound examination of patients with appendicitis. *A,* Transverse ultrasound scan of the appendix demonstrates the characteristic "target sign." In this case, the innermost portion is sonolucent, compatible with fluid or pus. *B,* Longitudinal view of another patient demonstrates the alternating hyperechoic and hypoechoic layers with an outermost hypoechoic layer, suggesting periappendiceal fluid. *C,* Longitudinal ultrasound scan of the right lower quadrant (RLQ) demonstrates a dilated, noncompressible appendix. The bright echo within the appendix represents an appendicolith with acoustic shadowing *(arrow).* (From Kuhn JP, Slovis TL, Haller JO: *Caffrey's pediatric diagnostic imaging,* vol 2, ed 10, Philadelphia, 2004, Mosby, p 1684.)

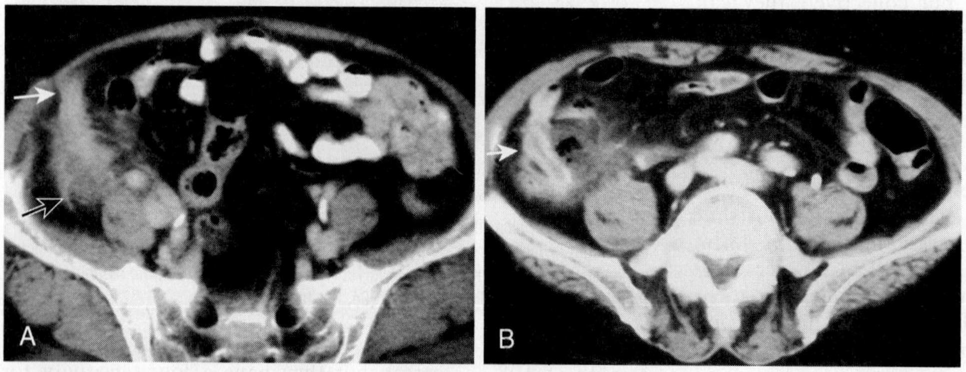

Figure 335-3 *A,* Phlegmon *(open arrow)* is noted around the enlarged appendix *(solid arrow)* in perforated appendicitis. *B,* Extraluminal air is shown adjacent to the wall-enhanced appendix *(arrow)* in perforated appendicitis. (From Yeung KW, Chang MS, Hsiao CP: Evaluation of perforated and nonperforated appendicitis with CT, *J Clin Imag* 28:422–427, 2004.)

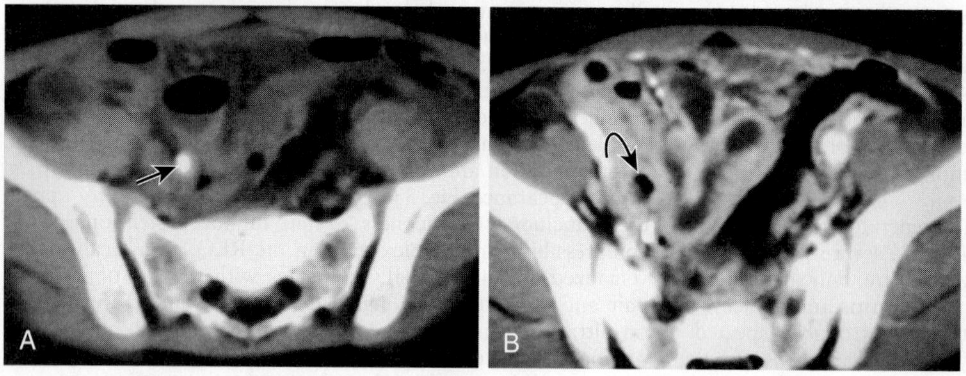

Figure 335-4 *A,* Precontrast-enhanced CT reveals an appendicolith *(arrow)* in perforated appendicitis. *B,* Postcontrast-enhanced CT (1 cm below the level in *A*) reveals intraluminal air in the appendix *(curved arrow)* associated with ileal wall enhancement in perforated appendicitis. (From Yeung KW, Chang MS, Hsiao CP: Evaluation of perforated and nonperforated appendicitis with CT, *J Clin Imag* 28:422–427, 2004.)

can be performed in many ways, including standard CT scan, helical CT scan, with or without oral and intravenous contrast, examination of both the abdomen and pelvis or pelvis alone, focused appendiceal CT scan, and focused appendiceal CT scan with rectal contrast. All of these techniques have demonstrated >95% sensitivity and specificity for acute appendicitis. Findings on CT scan consistent with appendicitis include a distended thick-walled appendix, inflammatory streaking of surrounding mesenteric fat, or a pericecal phlegmon or abscess (Figs. 335-3 and 335-4).

Appendicoliths are more readily demonstrated on CT scan than on plain radiographs. CT scan is also useful in advanced appendicitis to identify and guide percutaneous drainage of fluid collections and identification of an inflammatory mass, which might prompt a plan for initial nonoperative management.

Disadvantages of CT scan include greater cost; radiation exposure; possible need for intravenous, oral, or rectal contrast; and possible need for sedation. Oral contrast is particularly problematic if appendicitis is confirmed, because of the risk for aspiration at induction of anesthesia. Because the finding of fat stranding in surrounding tissues is a key component of CT evaluation for appendicitis, CT is less reliable in thin children with minimal body fat. For this reason, rectal contrast can increase diagnostic accuracy in this group. CT imaging is also helpful in demonstrating nonappendiceal causes of abdominal pain.

MRI/WBC SCAN MRI has been demonstrated to be at least equivalent to CT in diagnostic accuracy for appendicitis and does not involve ionizing radiation. The use of MRI in the evaluation of appendicitis is limited because it is less available, is more costly, most often requires sedation, and does not offer equivalent access for drainage of fluid collections. Radionuclide-labeled WBC scans have also been used in some centers in evaluating atypical cases of possible appendicitis in children and demonstrated a high sensitivity (97%) but only modest specificity (80%).

DIFFERENTIAL DIAGNOSIS

The list of illnesses that can mimic acute appendicitis is extensive because many gastrointestinal, gynecologic, and inflammatory disorders can manifest with similar illness history, signs, and symptoms. Differential diagnosis, even limited to common conditions, includes gastroenteritis, mesenteric adenitis, Meckel diverticulitis, inflammatory bowel disease, diabetes mellitus, sickle cell disease, streptococcal pharyngitis, pneumonia, cholecystitis, pancreatitis, urinary tract infection, infectious enteritis, and, in girls, ovarian torsion, ectopic pregnancy, ruptured ovarian cysts, and pelvic inflammatory disease (including tubo-ovarian abscess). Intestinal tract lymphoma, tumors of the appendix (carcinoid in children), and ovarian tumors are rare but can also masquerade as acute appendicitis.

Children <3 yr of age and adolescent girls have historically proved to be at particularly high risk for an incorrect diagnosis.

Most important is differentiation of the patients with gastroenteritis, which is the most common misdiagnosis in the child with appendicitis, because significant morbidity surrounds this distinction. The time course of illness (hours, days, weeks) leading to presentation is a critical component of the history. The classic patient with acute appendicitis describes abdominal pain as the preeminent symptom. In general, symptoms of systemic illness such as headache, chills, and myalgias indicate that a patient does not have appendicitis. Acute appendicitis most often begins insidiously as generalized malaise or anorexia, but there is early onset of abdominal pain and the illness typically escalates rapidly in the 1st 24-48 hr. Whereas most patients with acute appendicitis have 1 or 2 episodes of vomiting in the 1st 24-48 hr of illness, multiple episodes of vomiting are unusual in early appendicitis. In contrast, when gastroenteritis is the diagnosis, diarrhea and vomiting are more likely to be predominant symptoms early in the illness, and abdominal pains may seem associated with the frequent episodes of diarrhea and vomiting. In patients with an acute presentation (<72 hr of illness), vomiting preceding pain, large-volume diarrhea, large amounts of nonbilious vomiting, and high fever suggest gastroenteritis. In addition, patients with appendicitis typically have normal or hypoactive bowel sounds, whereas gastroenteritis typically produces persistently hyperactive bowel sounds. From the onset of illness, the child with appendicitis typically has a steadily deteriorating clinical course, whereas the child with gastroenteritis may have an undulating course, at times feeling better and other times feeling worse.

In the classic child with acute appendicitis who presents within 48 hr of the onset of illness, the WBC count can be low, normal, or elevated but is only rarely elevated >20,000/mm^3. WBC counts in this range should prompt consideration of alternative diagnoses and further studies.

Children who present with a history of illness >3-4 days are often more challenging. If the diagnosis is appendicitis, perforation has likely occurred and the child's presentation should evidence signs and symptoms of localized abscess/phlegmon in the RLQ or diffuse peritonitis. At this point in the illness, the WBC count should be elevated (>12/000/mm^3) with a left shift; a WBC count <7,000/mm^3 with a lymphocytosis is distinctly unusual and more typical of gastroenteritis.

An abnormal hemogram combined with purpuric skin lesions, arthritis, and nephritis suggests a diagnosis of Henoch-Schönlein purpura or hemolytic-uremic syndrome. Torsion of an undescended testis and epididymitis are common but should be discovered on physical examination. Meckel diverticulitis is an infrequent condition, but the clinical presentation closely mimics appendicitis and the diagnosis is usually made at surgery. Primary spontaneous peritonitis in prepubertal girls is often mistaken for appendicitis.

It should be recognized that "missed" appendicitis is the most common cause of small bowel obstruction in children without history of prior abdominal surgery. Atypical presentations of appendicitis are expected in association with other conditions such as pregnancy, Crohn disease, steroid treatment, or immunosuppressive therapy. Appendicitis in association with Crohn disease often has a protracted presentation with an atypical pattern of recurring but localized abdominal pain.

The diagnosis of appendicitis in adolescent girls is especially challenging, and some series report negative appendectomy rates as high as 30%. Ovarian cysts are often painful as a result of rupture, rapid enlargement, or hemorrhage. Rupture of an ovarian follicle associated with ovulation often causes mid-cycle lateralizing pain (mittelschmerz), but there is no progression of symptoms and systemic illness is absent. Ovarian tumors and torsion can also mimic acute appendicitis, although ovarian torsion is typically characterized by the acute onset of severe pain and is associated with more dramatic nausea and vomiting than is normally seen in early appendicitis. In pelvic inflammatory disease, the pain is typically suprapubic, bilateral, and of longer duration. The need for accurate urgent diagnosis in girls is influenced by concern that perforated appendicitis can predispose the patient to future ectopic pregnancy or tubal infertility, although data have not consistently demonstrated increased incidence of infertility after perforated appendicitis. For these reasons, the majority of adolescent girls warrant further diagnostic studies by ultrasonography, CT, or laparoscopy.

DIAGNOSTIC APPROACH

The diagnosis of appendicitis occasionally humbles even experienced clinicians. A diagnosis of acute appendicitis is made in only 50-70% of children at the time of initial assessment, and delay in diagnosis and treatment leads to substantial increases in morbidity, length of hospitalization, and cost. When patients have perforation due to late presentation, missed diagnosis, or delay in diagnosis, they require longer hospitalizations, often other invasive procedures such as percutaneous drainage of abscesses, and longer courses of antibiotics, and they are at higher risk for the complications of appendicitis including abscess formation, peritonitis, sepsis, wound infection, and small bowel obstruction. The cost of treatment for cases of perforated appendicitis is approximately double the cost for nonperforated cases.

Traditionally, early surgery in equivocal cases was the standard because complications and morbidity rise dramatically in appendicitis after perforation. Negative laparotomy rates of 10-20% were common and were deemed acceptable to keep perforation rates low. Many authors have criticized these high negative laparotomy rates, citing the risks and expense of unnecessary surgery. National databases have become an important resource for benchmarking and standardization of care. The Pediatric Health Information System (PHIS) was created by the Child Health Corporation of America (CHCA) as a national database to support the evaluation and improvement of clinical care in children's hospitals. A review of data collected from this source demonstrated substantial variation in practice patterns and resource utilization in the evaluation and management of appendicitis. Overall rupture rates for appendicitis varied from 20% to 76%, with a median of 36%. The median overall negative laparotomy rate (normal appendix) was 2.6%, significantly lower than traditionally reported rates of 10%-20%. The lack of consensus in management approach is reflected by the fact that the use of diagnostic imaging in cases of suspected appendicitis varied from 18% to 89%.

The diagnostic challenges are many, including the rapid escalation of appendicitis from subtle malaise to perforation (often within 36-48 hr), variable abilities of medical centers and experience among clinicians, and fear of malpractice suits for missed diagnosis. Several reports have described clinical scoring systems and computer-assisted decision-making models incorporating specific elements of the history, physical examination, and laboratory studies designed to improve diagnostic accuracy in acute appendicitis (see Table 335-1). To date, none has demonstrated improved accuracy over experienced clinical judgment.

Some clinicians remain steadfast to the primacy of a careful history and physical examination and rarely order imaging studies. The initial assessment, along with the history and physical examination, may include a complete blood count with differential, urinalysis, and plain films (chest and abdominal series). If the initial assessment leads to a high level of suspicion for appendicitis, pediatric surgical consultation should be the next step, with the likelihood of prompt appendectomy without further studies. If the initial evaluation suggests a nonsurgical diagnosis and a low concern for appendicitis, the child may be discharged with advice to the family to return for repeat evaluation if the child is not improving on liquids and a bland diet in the next 24 hr. This approach has demonstrated high sensitivity and specificity (>90%) at certain institutions, but collective data from many centers have not been able to reproduce this degree of accuracy.

In equivocal cases, some clinicians or centers proceed with a plan of active observation. Many reports substantiate improved diagnostic accuracy by observation and serial examination over a period of 12-24 hr, simplifying the eventual decision to proceed with appendectomy, discharge the patient, or proceed with imaging studies, and report no correlation between surgical morbidity and timing of surgery. The child may be observed with intravenous fluids and planned repeat CBC and physical examination in 6-12 hr. At the end of a period of observation, the clinician should decide to discharge the patient based on improved clinical status, proceed to appendectomy, or proceed to further imaging evaluation. Further imaging in this equivocal group hopefully can minimize the negative laparotomy rate without increasing the perforation rate (missed or delayed diagnosis). Less than 2% of children's appendices perforate while under observation. This approach is cost effective, often avoids radiologic imaging, and is optimized if an observational unit is available that avoids admission costs for the period of observation.

Most centers demonstrate improved diagnostic accuracy for appendicitis in children when using radiologic imaging as an adjunct to history and physical examination, and some have even recommended imaging in all atypical cases to minimize unnecessary surgery (negative appendectomy) and avoid the complications of missed appendicitis, including perforation with abscess formation and peritonitis, sepsis, wound infection, and small bowel obstruction. The consequence of missed appendicitis substantially increases morbidity, length of stay, and cost. With selective imaging, the PHIS review of pediatric centers had an overall negative appendicitis appendectomy rate of 2.6%.

It seems likely that if imaging studies are obtained in all patients with equivocal presentations and a brief duration of illness (<24 hr), the false-negative rate of the imaging studies will increase. Maximum benefit and effectiveness of imaging is obtained when it is used selectively in children for whom the diagnosis is equivocal after careful history and physical examination by an experienced clinician and who are not too early in the temporal evolution of the illness.

A thoughtful approach in equivocal cases of appendicitis is to begin with ultrasound if it is readily available and the hospital has experience with ultrasound for possible appendicitis. Ultrasound in one study decreased the need for CT scan in 22% of patients. CT scan is used if ultrasound is unavailable or inconclusive, or as the first-line test in obese patients, in cases of probable advanced or perforated appendicitis, or when there is gaseous distention of the bowel. This approach has proved highly accurate and cost-effective.

Practice guidelines have decreased both length of stay and cost without increasing complications. One such guideline employing clinical judgment and selective imaging attained a positive and negative predictive value for appendicitis of 94% and 99%, respectively.

TREATMENT

Once the diagnosis of appendicitis is confirmed or highly suspected, the treatment for acute appendicitis is most often prompt appendectomy. Antibiotics and advances in interventional radiology have permitted drainage of fluid collections and initial nonoperative management as an alternative option in late presentations, depending on the patient's general condition and the state of the appendix. Emergency surgery is rarely indicated, and most patients require preoperative supportive measures to stabilize vital signs and to ensure the safety of the procedure and improve outcomes.

Whereas the traditional surgical approach has been to proceed with surgery as soon as the diagnosis is confirmed, appendectomy should rarely be undertaken in the middle of the night. Often, unexpected pathology (appendiceal tumors, intestinal lymphoma, congenital renal anomalies, inflammatory bowel disease) are discovered at operation, and intraoperative consultation and frozen section may be needed. There is no correlation between timing of surgery and perforation rates or postoperative morbidity when the operation proceeds within 24-48 hr of diagnosis. Appendectomy can be a challenging operation, with potential for major complications including injury to adjacent intestine, the iliac vessels, or the right ureter. The operation should proceed semielectively within 12-24 hr of diagnosis. Children with appendicitis are typically at least mildly dehydrated and require preoperative fluid resuscitation to correct hypovolemia and electrolyte abnormalities before anesthesia. Fever, if present, should be treated. Pain management begins even before a definitive diagnosis is made, and consultation of a pain service, if available, is appropriate once a decision is made to proceed to surgery. In the majority of cases, preoperative management can be accomplished during the period of diagnostic evaluation and prompt appendectomy can be performed.

In patients in whom perforated appendicitis is identified at the time of diagnosis, the operation is even less urgent and proper preoperative management is more critical. When the illness is protracted owing to a delay in diagnosis or presentation, patients can demonstrate significant physiologic derangements including severe dehydration, hypotension, acidosis, and renal failure. These patients require a longer period of stabilization with fluid resuscitation and antibiotics, including, in occasional cases, admission to an intensive care unit before proceeding with more definitive management. Based on the patient's status, findings on CT scan, and availability of experienced radiologists, the initial plan may be percutaneous drainage of fluid collections by interventional radiology and continued fluid resuscitation and antibiotics. A phlegmon without an identifiable fluid component might initially respond to nonoperative antibiotic treatment. Placement of one or more drainage catheters under imaging (CT or ultrasound) guidance has been successful in >80% of patients. Most patients still require delayed appendectomy (during the same hospitalization) or interval appendectomy (4-6 weeks after the initial presentation).

If diffuse peritonitis exists, most surgeons proceed promptly with appendectomy after a brief period of intravenous fluids and broad spectrum antibiotics. Others continue nonoperative management provided the patient demonstrates clinical improvement by physiologic criteria including hemodynamic stability, urine output, control of fever, and declining leukocyte count. If the patient demonstrates clinical recovery by resolution of fever, sepsis, and return of bowel function, generally a 2 wk course of oral antibiotics is completed and a decision is made regarding interval appendectomy in 6-8 wk. A child who fails to improve within 24-72 hr needs an urgent appendectomy to control sepsis. Emergency appendectomy should only be performed in the occasional circumstance when physiologic resuscitation requires urgent control of advanced peritoneal sepsis not amenable to interventional drainage or this is not available.

Antibiotics

Antibiotics lower the incidence of postoperative wound infections and intraperitoneal abscesses in perforated appendicitis, but their role is less well defined in simple appendicitis. The antibiotic regimen should be directed against the typical bacterial flora found in the appendix, including anaerobic organisms (*Bacteroides, Clostridia,* and *Peptostreptococcus* spp.) and gram-negative aerobic bacteria (*Escherchia coli, Pseudomonas aeruginosa, Enterobacter,* and *Klebsiella* spp.). Gram-positive organisms are less commonly found in the colon, and the need to provide antibiotic coverage for them (primarily enterococcus) is controversial. Many antibiotic combinations have demonstrated equivalent efficacy in controlled trials in terms of wound infection rate, resolution of fever, length of stay, and incidence of complications.

For simple nonperforated appendicitis, one preoperative dose of a single broad-spectrum agent (cefoxitin) or equivalent is sufficient. In perforated or gangrenous appendicitis, most surgeons prefer either "triple" antibiotics (ampicillin, gentamicin, and clindamycin or metronidazole) or a combination such as ceftriaxone-metronidazole or ticarcillin-clavulanate plus gentamicin, and antibiotic coverage is continued postoperatively for 3-5 days. Oral antibiotics have proved equally effective as intravenous, and therefore the patient can be switched to an oral regimen and discharged once bowel function returns. This transition to oral antibiotics has significantly affected length of stay and cost in the management of perforated appendicitis.

Interval Appendectomy

Appendicitis complicated by a walled-off inflammatory mass or abscess can be treated without immediate appendectomy. This strategy is intended to avoid a predictable higher surgical complication rate and is often useful in children, in whom the overall incidence of perforation approaches 50%. In this group of patients, debate exists over the need for interval appendectomy. The risk of developing recurrent appendicitis if the appendix is not removed is unknown, and published reports vary between 10% and 80% (most are closer to 10%). Most cases of recurrent appendicitis develop within 2 yr of the initial illness. Some authors believe interval appendectomy is unnecessary because of the low risk for recurrent appendicitis. Others support interval appendectomy to avoid recurrent appendicitis and to confirm the original diagnosis, citing an incidence of unexpected pathology in 30% of interval appendectomy specimens. The vast majority of pediatric surgeons perform interval appendectomy routinely (4-6 wk interval) after nonoperative management of perforated appendicitis.

SURGICAL TECHNIQUE Appendectomy is traditionally performed through a RLQ muscle-splitting incision. Laparoscopic appendectomy is also popular among pediatric surgeons for both simple and perforated appendicitis. Studies that have compared the open surgical approach to laparoscopic appendectomy demonstrate differences in administrative factors (cost, resource utilization, length of stay) and clinical outcome measures (wound infection rate, intraabdominal abscess, analgesic requirements, return to full activity) but have failed to establish an evidence-based preference between laparoscopic and open appendectomy in children.

In nonperforated appendicitis, laparoscopic appendectomy appears to have lower narcotic analgesic requirements, decreased wound morbidity, and improved cosmesis, but operative times and costs seem slightly higher when compared to the open procedure. Length of hospitalization is similar for both approaches.

The role of laparoscopy in perforated appendicitis is less well defined. There are no convincing data to recommend one approach in all patients. Most pediatric surgeons use both approaches selectively. The laparoscopic approach is used most often for obese patients, when alternative diagnoses are suspected, and in adolescent girls to better evaluate for ovarian pathology and pelvic inflammatory disease while avoiding the ionizing radiation associated with CT imaging. Injection of bupivacaine into the wound has been shown to reduce postoperative pain significantly in a randomized, controlled trial in children.

Complications

Morbidity rates for appendicitis vary widely in large series from 10% to 45%. The principal determinant of complications is the severity of the appendicitis. In nonperforated appendicitis, an overall complication rate of 5-10% is expected. With perforated appendicitis, the complication rate rises to 15-30%. The most common complications are wound infections (3-10%) and intra-abdominal abscesses; both are more common after perforation. Perforation and abscess formation can also lead to fistula formation in adjacent organs. Perforation rates are consistently >80% in children <5 yr of age. Patients with advanced appendicitis can progress to sepsis and multisystem organ failure, but generally these patients respond promptly to antibiotics, fluids, and other supportive measures. Other potential complications include postoperative ileus, diffuse peritonitis, portal vein pylephlebitis (rare), and adhesive small bowel obstruction.

Mortality with appendicitis is rare (<0.3%) and seen mostly in neonates and immunocompromised patients.

BIBLIOGRAPHY

Please visit the Nelson Textbook of Pediatrics *website at www.expertconsult.com for the complete bibliography.*

Chapter 336
Surgical Conditions of the Anus and Rectum

336.1 Anorectal Malformations

Shawn J. Stafford and Michael D. Klein

In understanding the spectrum of anorectal anomalies, it is necessary to consider the importance of the sphincter complex, a mass of muscle fibers surrounding the anorectum (Fig. 336-1). This complex is the combination of the puborectalis, levator ani, external and internal sphincters, and the superficial external sphincter muscles, all meeting at the rectum. Anorectal malformations are defined by the relationship of the rectum to this complex and include varying degrees of stenosis to complete atresia. The incidence is 1/3,000 live births. Significant long-term concerns focus on bowel control and urinary and sexual functions.

EMBRYOLOGY

The hindgut forms early as the part of the primitive gut tube that extends into the tail fold in the 2nd wk of gestation. At about day 13, it develops a ventral diverticulum, the allantois or primitive bladder. The junction of allantois and hindgut become the cloaca, into which the genital, urinary, and intestinal tubes empty.

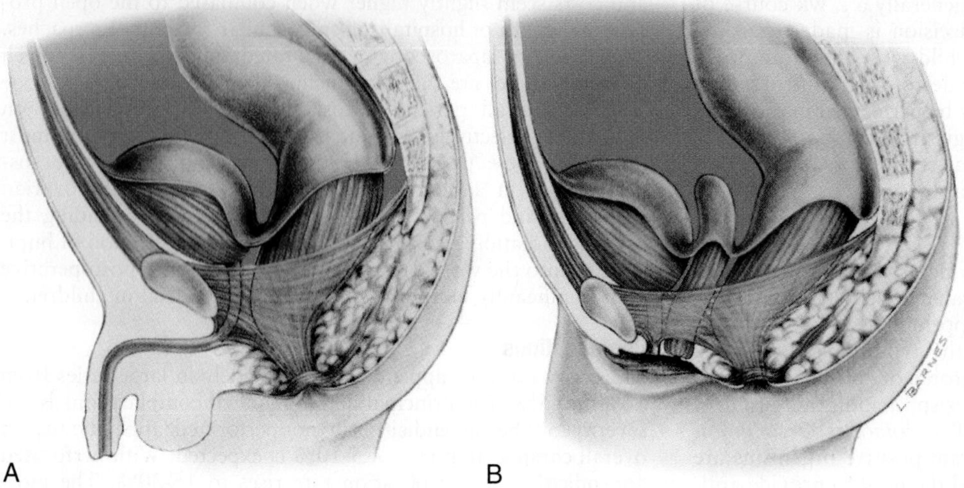

Figure 336-1 Normal anorectal anatomy in relation to pelvic structures. *A*, Male. *B*, Female. (From Peña A: *Atlas of surgical management of anorectal malformations*, New York, 1989, Springer-Verlag, p 3.)

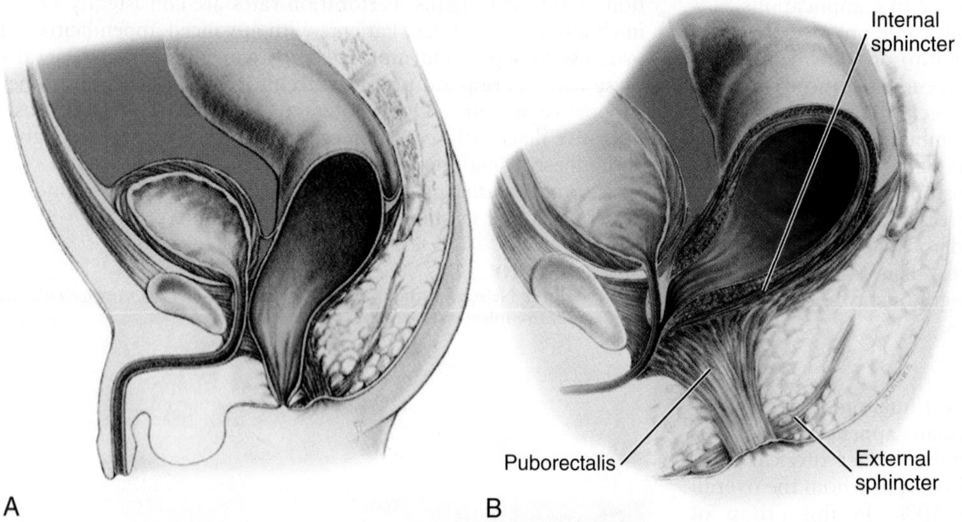

Figure 336-2 Imperforate anus in males. *A*, Low lesions. *B*, High lesions. (From Peña A: *Atlas of surgical management of anorectal malformations*, New York, 1989, Springer-Verlag, pp 7, 26.)

This is covered by a cloacal membrane. The urorectal septum descends to divide this common channel by forming lateral ridges, which grow in and fuse by the middle of the 7th wk. Opening of the posterior portion of the membrane (the anal membrane) occurs in the 8th wk. Failures in any part of these processes can lead to the clinical spectrum of anogenital anomalies.

Imperforate anus can be divided into low lesions, where the rectum has descended through the sphincter complex, and high lesions, where it has not. Most patients with imperforate anus have a fistula. There is a spectrum of malformation in boys and girls. In boys, low lesions usually manifest with meconium staining somewhere on the perineum along the median raphe (Fig. 336-2*A*). Low lesions in girls also manifest as a spectrum from an anus that is only slightly anterior on the perineal body to a fourchette fistula that opens on the moist mucosa of the introitus distal to the hymen (Fig. 336-3*A*). A high imperforate anus in a boy has no apparent cutaneous opening or fistula, but it usually has a fistula to the urinary tract, either the urethra or the bladder (see Fig. 336-2*B*). Although there is occasionally a rectovaginal fistula, in girls, high lesions are usually cloacal anomalies in which the rectum, vagina, and urethra all empty into a common channel or cloacal stem of varying length (see Fig. 336-3*B*). The interesting category of boys with imperforate anus and no fistula occurs mainly in children with trisomy 21.

ASSOCIATED ANOMALIES

There are many anomalies associated with anorectal malformations (Table 336-1). The most common are anomalies of the kidneys and urinary tract in conjunction with abnormalities of the sacrum. This complex is often referred to as the **caudal regression syndrome.** Boys with a rectovesical fistula and patients with a persistent cloaca have a 90% risk of urologic defects. Other common associated anomalies are cardiac anomalies and esophageal atresia with or without tracheoesophageal fistula. These can cluster in any combination in a patient. When combined, they are often accompanied by abnormalities of the radial aspect of the upper extremity and are termed the VATERR (*v*ertebral, *a*nal, *t*racheal, *e*sophageal, *r*adial, *r*enal) or VACTERL (*v*ertebral, *a*nal, *c*ardiac, *t*racheal, *e*sophageal, *r*enal, *l*imb) anomalad.

A good correlation exists between the degree of sacral development and future function. Patients with an absent sacrum usually have permanent fecal and urinary incontinence. Spinal abnormalities and different degrees of dysraphism are often associated with these defects. Tethered cord occurs in ~25% of patients with anorectal malformations. Untethering of the cord can lead to improved urinary and rectal continence in some patients, although it seldom reverses established neurologic defects. The diagnosis of spinal defects can be established in the

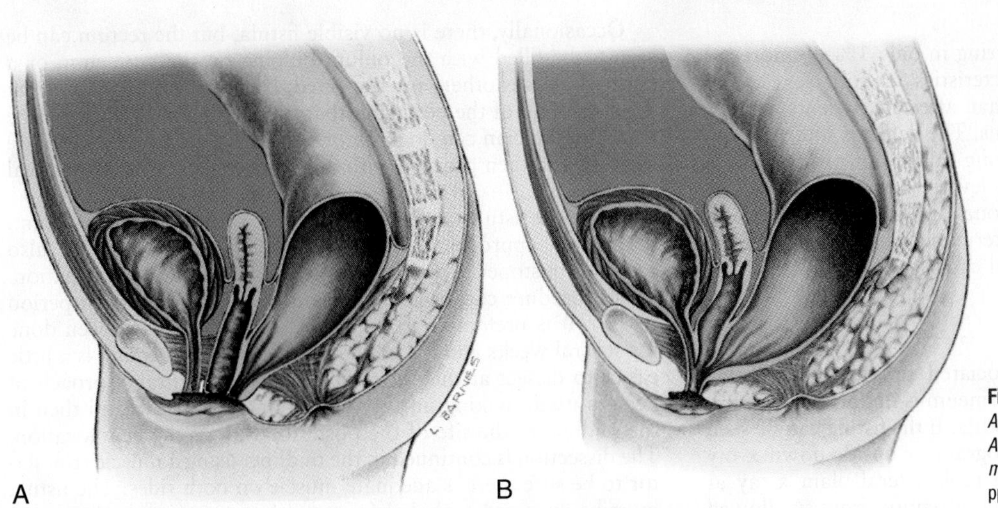

Figure 336-3 Imperforate anus in females. *A*, Vestibular fistula. *B*, Cloaca. (From Peña A: *Atlas of surgical management of anorectal malformations,* New York, 1989, Springer-Verlag, pp 50, 60.)

Table 336-1 ASSOCIATED MALFORMATIONS

GENITOURINARY
Vesicoureteric reflux Renal agenesis Renal dysplasia Ureteral duplication Cryptorchidism Hypospadias Bicornuate uterus Vaginal septums
VERTEBRAL

Spinal dysraphism
  Tethered chord
Presacral masses
  Meningocele
  Lipoma
  Dermoid
  Teratoma

CARDIOVASCULAR
Tetralogy of Fallot Ventricular septal defect Transposition of the great vessels Hypoplastic left heart syndrome
GASTROINTESTINAL
Tracheoesophageal fistula Duodenal atresia Malrotation Hirschsprung's disease
CENTRAL NERVOUS SYSTEM
Spina bifida Tethered cord

1st 3 mo of life by spinal ultrasound. In older patients, MRI is needed.

MANIFESTATIONS AND DIAGNOSIS

Low Lesions

Examination of a newborn includes the inspection of the perineum. The absence of an anal orifice in the correct position leads to further evaluation. Mild forms of imperforate anus are often called *anal stenosis* or *anterior ectopic anus.* These are probably imperforate anus with a perineal fistula. The normal position of the anus on the perineum is approximately halfway (0.5 ratio) between the coccyx and the scrotum or introitus. Although symptoms, primarily constipation, have been attributed to anterior ectopic anus (ratio <0.34 in girls, <0.46 in boys), many patients have no symptoms.

If no anus or fistula is visible, there may be a low lesion or "covered anus." In these cases, there are well-formed buttocks and often a thickened raphe or "bucket handle." After 24 hr, meconium bulging may be seen, creating a blue or black appearance. In these cases, an immediate perineal procedure can often be performed, followed by a dilatation program.

In a boy, the perineal (cutaneous) fistula can track anteriorly along the median raphe across the scrotum and even down the penile shaft. This is usually a thin track, with a normal rectum often just a few millimeters from the skin. Extraintestinal anomalies are seen in <10% of these patients.

In a girl, a low lesion enters the vestibule or fourchette (the moist mucosa outside the hymen but within the introitus). In this case, the rectum has descended through the sphincter complex.

Children with a low lesion can usually be treated initially with perineal manipulation and dilation. Visualizing these low fistulas is so important in the evaluation and treatment that one should avoid passing a nasogastric tube for the 1st 24 hr to allow the abdomen and bowel to distend, pushing meconium down into the distal rectum.

High Lesions

In a boy with a high imperforate anus, the perineum appears flat. There may be air or meconium passed via the penis (urethra) when the fistula is high, entering the bulbar or prostatic urethra, or even the bladder. In **rectobulbarurethral fistulas** (the most common in boys), the sphincter mechanism is satisfactory, the sacrum may be underdeveloped, and an anal dimple is present. In **rectoprostaticurethral fistulas,** the sacrum is poorly developed, the scrotum may be bifid, and the anal dimple is near the scrotum. In **rectovesicular fistulas,** the sphincter mechanism is poorly developed and the sacrum is hypoplastic or absent. In boys with trisomy 21, all the features of a high lesion may be present, but there is no fistula, the sacrum and sphincter mechanisms are usually well developed, and the prognosis is good.

In girls with high imperforate anus, there may be the appearance of a rectovaginal fistula. A true rectovaginal fistula is rare. Most are either the fourchette fistulas described earlier or are forms of a cloacal anomaly.

Persistent Cloaca

In persistent cloaca, the embryologic stage persists in which the rectum, urethra, and vagina communicate in a common orifice, the cloaca. It is important to realize this, because the repair often requires repositioning the urethra and vagina as well as the rectum. Children of both sexes with a high lesion require a colostomy before repair.

Rectal Atresia

Rectal atresia is a rare defect occurring in only 1% of anorectal anomalies. It has the same characteristics in both sexes. The unique feature of this defect is that affected patients have a normal anal canal and a normal anus. The defect is often discovered while rectal temperature is being taken. An obstruction is present about 2 cm above the skin level. These patients need a protective colostomy. The functional prognosis is excellent because they have a normal sphincteric mechanism (and normal sensation), which resides in the anal canal.

APPROACH TO THE PATIENT

Evaluation includes identifying associated anomalies (see Table 336-1). Careful inspection of the perineum is important to determine the presence or absence of a fistula. If the fistula can be seen there, it is a low lesion. The invertogram or upside-down x-ray is of little value, but a prone cross-table lateral plain x-ray at 24 hr of life (to allow time for bowel distention from swallowed air) with a radioopaque marker on the perineum can demonstrate a low lesion by showing the renal gas bubble <1 cm from the perineal skin. A plain x-ray of the entire sacrum, including both iliac wings, is important to identify sacral anomalies and the adequacy of the sacrum. An abdominal-pelvic ultrasound and voiding cystourethrogram (VCUG) must be performed. The clinician should also pass a nasogastric tube to identify esophageal atresia and should obtain an echocardiogram. In boys with a high lesion, the VCUG often identifies the rectourinary fistula. In girls with a high lesion, more invasive evaluation, including vaginogram and endoscopy, is often necessary for careful detailing of the cloacal anomaly.

Good clinical evaluation and a urinalysis provide enough data in 80-90% of **male** patients to determine the need for a colostomy. Voluntary sphincteric muscles surround the most distal part of the bowel in cases of perineal and rectourethral fistulas, and the intralumenal bowel pressure must be sufficiently high to overcome the tone of those muscles before meconium can be seen in the urine or on the perineum. The presence of meconium in the urine and a flat bottom are considered indications for the creation of a colostomy. Clinical findings consistent with the diagnosis of a perineal fistula represent an indication for an anoplasty without a protective colostomy. Ultrasound is valuable not only for the evaluation of the urinary tract, but it can also be used to investigate spinal anomalies in the newborn and to determine how close to the perineum the rectum has descended.

More than 90% of the time, the diagnosis in **girls** can be established on perineal inspection. The presence of a single perineal orifice is a cloaca. A palpable pelvic mass (hydrocolpos) reinforces this diagnosis. A vestibular fistula is diagnosed by careful separation of the labia, exposing the vestibule. The rectal orifice is located immediately behind the hymen within the female genitalia and in the vestibule. A perineal fistula is easy to diagnose. The rectal orifice is located somewhere between the female genitalia and the center of the sphincter and is surrounded by skin. Less than 10% of these patients fail to pass meconium through the genitalia or perineum after 24 hr of observation. Those patients can require a prone cross-table lateral film.

OPERATIVE REPAIR

Sometimes a perineal fistula, if it opens in good position, can be treated by simple dilatation. Hegar dilators are employed, starting with a No. 5 or 6 and letting the baby go home when the mother can use a No. 8. Twice-daily dilatations are done at home, increasing the size every few weeks until a No. 14 is achieved. By 1 yr of age, the stool is usually well formed and further dilation is not necessary. By the time No. 14 is reached, the examiner can usually insert a little finger. If the anal ring is soft and pliable, dilatation can be reduced in frequency or discontinued.

Occasionally, there is no visible fistula, but the rectum can be seen to be filled with meconium bulging on the perineum, or a covered anus is otherwise suspected. If confirmed by plain x-ray or ultrasound of the perineum that the rectum is <1 cm from the skin, the clinician can do a minor perineal procedure to perforate the skin and then proceed with dilatation or do a simple perineal anoplasty.

When the fistula orifice is very close to the introitus or scrotum, it is often appropriate to move it back surgically. This also requires postoperative dilation to prevent stricture formation. This procedure can be done any time from the newborn period to 1 yr. It is preferable to wait until dilatations have been done for several weeks and the child is bigger. The anorectum is a little easier to dissect at this time. The posterior sagittal approach of Peña is used, making an incision around the fistula and then in the midline to the site of the posterior wall of the new location. The dissection is continued in the midline, using a muscle stimulator to be sure there is adequate muscle on both sides. The fistula must be dissected cephalad for several centimeters to allow posterior positioning without tension. If appropriate, some of the distal fistula is resected before the anastomosis to the perineal skin.

In children with a high lesion, a double-barrel colostomy is performed. This effectively separates the fecal stream from the urinary tract. It also allows the performance of an augmented pressure colostogram before repair to identify the exact position of the distal rectum and the fistula. The definitive repair or posterior sagittal anorectoplasty (PSARP) is performed at about 1 yr of age. A midline incision is made, often splitting the coccyx and even the sacrum. Using a muscle stimulator, the surgeon stays strictly in the midline and divides the sphincter complex and identifies the rectum. The rectum is then opened in the midline and the fistula is identified from within the rectum. This allows a division of the fistula without injury to the urinary tract. The rectum is then dissected proximally until enough length is gained to suture it to an appropriate perineal position. The muscles of the sphincter complex are then sutured around (and especially behind) the rectum.

Other operative approaches (such as an anterior approach) are used, but the one that currently rivals the PSARP for popularity is the laparoscopic. This operation allows division of the fistula under direct visualization and identification of the sphincter complex by transillumination of perineum.

A similar procedure can be done for female high anomalies with variations to deal with separating the vagina and rectum from within the cloacal stem. When the stem is longer than 3 cm, this is an especially difficult and complex procedure.

Usually, the colostomy can be closed 6 wks or more after the PSARP. Two weeks after any anal procedure, twice-daily dilatations are performed by the family. By doing frequent dilatations, each one is not so painful and there is less tissue trauma, inflammation, and scarring.

OUTCOME

The ability to achieve rectal continence depends on both motor and sensory elements. There must be adequate muscle in the sphincter complex and proper positioning of the rectum within the complex. There must also be intact innervation of the complex and of sensory elements as well as the presence of these sensory elements in the anorectum. Patients with low lesions are more likely to achieve true continence. They are also, however, more prone to constipation, which leads to overflow incontinence. It is very important that all these patients are followed closely, and that the constipation and anal dilatation are well managed until toilet training is successful. Tables 336-2 and 336-3 outline the results of continence and constipation in relation to the malformation encountered.

Table 336-2 RESULTS OF SURGICAL TREATMENT OF ANORECTAL MALFORMATIONS: TOTAL CONTINENCE*

TYPE	PERCENTAGE
LOW	
Perineal fistula	90
Rectal atresia/stenosis	75
Vestibular fistula	71
HIGH	
Imperforate with no fistula	60
Bulbar urethral fistula	50
Short cloaca	50
Prostatic fistula	31
Long cloaca	29
Bladder neck fistula	12

*Voluntary bowel movements, no soiling.
Modified from Levitt MA, Peña A: Outcomes from the correction of anorectal malformations, *Curr Opin Pediatr* 17:394–401, 2005.

Table 336-3 CONSTIPATION AND TYPE OF ANOGENITAL MALFORMATION

TYPE	PERCENTAGE
Vestibular fistula	61
Bulbar urethral fistula	64
Rectal atresia/stenosis	50
Imperforate with no fistula	55
Perineal fistula	57
Long cloaca	35
Prostatic fistula	45
Short cloaca	40
Bladder neck fistula	16

Modified from Levitt MA, Peña A: Outcomes from the correction of anorectal malformations, *Curr Opin Pediatr* 17:394–401, 2005.

Children with high lesions, especially boys with rectoprostatic urethral fistulas and girls with cloacal anomalies, have a poorer chance of being continent, but they can usually achieve a socially acceptable defecation (without a colostomy) pattern with a bowel management program. Often, the bowel management program consists of a daily enema to keep the colon empty and the patient clean until the next enema. If this is successful, an antegrade continence enema procedure (ACE or Malone procedure) can improve the patient's quality of life. These procedures provide access to the right colon either by bringing the appendix out the umbilicus in a non-refluxing fashion or by putting a plastic button in the right lower quadrant to access the cecum. The patient can then sit on the toilet and administer the enema through the ACE, thus flushing out the entire colon. Antegrade regimens can produce successful 24 hr cleanliness rates of up to 95%. Of special interest is the clinical finding that most patients improve their control with growth. Patients who wore diapers or pull-ups to primary school are often in regular underwear by high school. Some groups have taken advantage of this evidence of psychologic influences to initiate behavior modification early with good results.

BIBLIOGRAPHY

Please visit the Nelson Textbook of Pediatrics *website at www.expertconsult.com for the complete bibliography.*

336.2 Anal Fissure

Shawn J. Stafford and Michael D. Klein

Anal fissure is a laceration of the anal mucocutaneous junction. It is an acquired lesion of unknown yet etiology likely secondary to the forceful passage of a hard stool, yet mainly seen in infants <1 yr of age when the stool is frequently quite soft. Fissures may be the consequence and not the cause of constipation.

CLINICAL MANIFESTATIONS

A history of constipation is often described, with a recent painful bowel movement corresponding to the fissure formation after passing of hard stool. The patient then voluntarily retains stool to avoid another painful bowel movement, exacerbating the constipation, resulting in harder stools. Complaints of pain on defecation and bright red blood on the surface of the stool are often elicited.

The diagnosis is established by inspection of the perineal area. The infant's hips are held in acute flexion, the buttocks are separated to expand the folds of the perianal skin, and the fissure becomes evident as a minor laceration. Often a small skin appendage is noted peripheral to the lesion. This "skin tag" actually represents epithelialized granulomatous tissue, formed in response to chronic inflammation. Findings on rectal examination can include hard stool in the ampulla and rectal spasm.

TREATMENT

The parents must be counseled as to the origin of the laceration and the mechanism of the cycle of constipation. The goal is to ensure that the patient has soft stools to avoid overstretching the anus. The healing process can take several weeks or even several months. A single episode of impaction with passing of hard stool can exacerbate the problem. Treatment requires that the primary cause of the constipation be identified. The use of dietary and behavioral modification and a stool softener is indicated. Parents should titrate the dose of the stool softener based on the patient's response to treatment. Stool softening is best done by increasing water intake or using an oral polyethylene glycolate such as Miralax or Glycolax. Surgical intervention, including stretching of the anus, "internal" anal sphincterotomy, or excision of the fissure, is not indicated or supported by scientific evidence.

Chronic anal fissures in older patients have been associated with constipation, prior rectal surgery, Crohn disease, and chronic diarrhea. They are managed initially like fissures in infants, with stool softeners with the addition of sitz baths. Topical 0.2% glyceryl trinitrate reduces anal spasm and heals fissures, but it is often associated with headaches. In addition, local anesthetics such as 10% lidocaine or EMLA (5% prilocaine, 5% lidocaine) may be effective. Patients who do not respond may be managed with the local injection of botulinum toxin to treat the associated contraction of the sphincter.

BIBLIOGRAPHY

Please visit the Nelson Textbook of Pediatrics *website at www.expertconsult.com for the complete bibliography.*

336.3 Perianal Abscess and Fistula

Shawn J. Stafford and Michael D. Klein

Children account for 0.5-4.3% of all patients presenting with perianal abscesses. These usually manifest in the first year of life and are of unknown etiology. Links to congenitally abnormal crypts of Morgagni have been proposed, suggesting that deeper crypts (3-10 mm rather than the normal 1-2 mm) lead to trapped debris and cryptitis (Fig. 336-4). The most common organisms

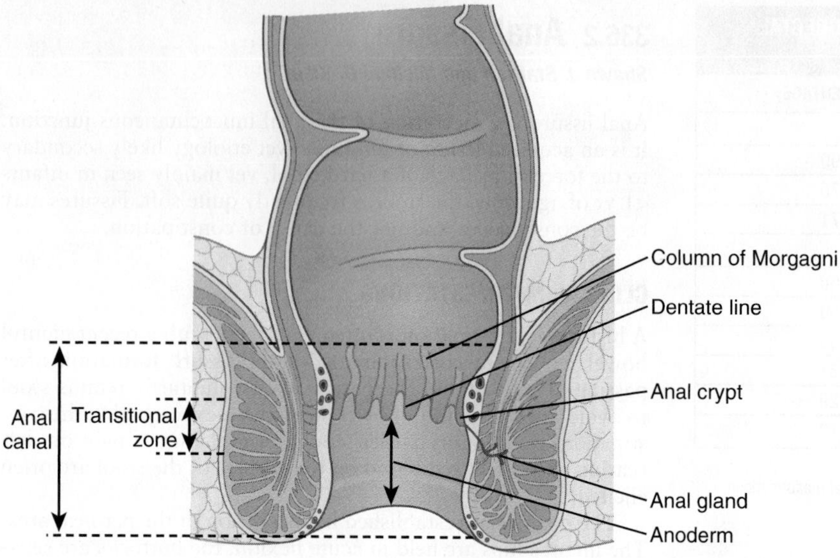

Figure 336-4 Anatomy of the anal canal. (Adapted from Brunicardi FC, Anderson DK, Billar TR, et al: *Schwartz's principles of surgery*, ed 8, New York, 2004, McGraw-Hill.)

isolated from perianal abscesses are mixed aerobic *(Escherichia coli, Klebsiella pneumoniae, Staphylococcus aureus)* and anaerobic (*Bacteroides* spp., *Clostridium, Veillonella*) flora. Ten to 15% yield pure growth of *E. coli, S. aureus,* or *Bacteroides fragilis.* There is a strong male predominance in those affected younger than 2 yr of age. This imbalance corrects in older patients, where the etiology shifts to associated conditions such as inflammatory bowel disease, leukemia, or immunocompromised states.

CLINICAL MANIFESTATIONS

In younger patients, symptoms are usually mild and can consist of low-grade fever, mild rectal pain, and an area of perianal cellulitis. Often these spontaneously drain and resolve without treatment. In older patients with underlying predisposing conditions, the clinical course may be more serious. A compromised immune system can mask fever and allow rapid progression to toxicity and sepsis. Abscesses in these patients may be deeper in the ischiorectal fossa or even supralevator in contrast to those in younger patients, which are usually adjacent to the involved crypt.

Progression to fistula in patients with perianal abscesses occurs in up to 85% of cases and usually manifest with drainage from the perineal skin or multiple recurrences. Similar to abscess formation, fistulas have a strong male predominance. Histologic evaluation of fistula tracts typically reveals an epithelial lining of stratified squamous cells associated with chronic inflammation. It might also reveal an alternative etiology such as the granulomas of Crohn disease or even evidence of tuberculosis.

TREATMENT

Treatment is rarely indicated in infants with no predisposing disease because the condition is often self-limited. Even in cases of fistulization, conservative management (observation) is advocated because the fistula often disappears spontaneously before 2 yr of age. Antibiotics are not useful in these patients. When dictated by extreme patient discomfort, abscesses may be drained under local anesthesia. Fistulas requiring surgical intervention may be treated by fistulotomy (unroofing or opening), fistulectomy (excision of the tract leaving it open to heal secondarily), or placement of a seton (heavy suture threaded through the fistula, brought out the anus and tied tightly to itself).

Older children with predisposing diseases might also do well with minimal intervention. If there is little discomfort and no fever or other sign of systemic illness, local hygiene and antibiotics may be best. The danger of surgical intervention in an immunocompromised patient is the creation of an even larger, nonhealing wound. There certainly are such patients with serious systemic symptoms who require more aggressive intervention along with treatment of the predisposing condition. Broad-spectrum antibiotic coverage must be administered and wide excision and drainage are mandatory in cases involving sepsis and expanding cellulitis.

Fistulas in older patients are mainly associated with Crohn disease, a history of pull-through surgery for the treatment of Hirschsprung disease, or in rare cases, tuberculosis. Those fistulas are often resistant to therapy and require treatment of the predisposing condition.

Complications of treatment include recurrence and, rarely, incontinence.

BIBLIOGRAPHY

Please visit the Nelson Textbook of Pediatrics *website at* www.expertconsult.com *for the complete bibliography.*

336.4 Hemorrhoids

Shawn J. Stafford and Michael D. Klein

Hemorrhoidal disease does occur in children and adolescents, often related to a diet deficient in fiber and poor hydration. In younger children, the presence of hemorrhoids should also raise the suspicion of portal hypertension. A third of patients with hemorrhoids require treatment.

CLINICAL MANIFESTATIONS

Presentation depends on the location of the hemorrhoids. External hemorrhoids occur below the dentate line (Figs. 336-4 and 336-5) and are associated with extreme pain and itching, often due to acute thrombosis. Internal hemorrhoids are located above the dentate line and manifest primarily with bleeding, prolapse, and occasional incarceration.

TREATMENT

In most cases, conservative management with dietary modification, decreased straining, and avoidance of prolonged time spent sitting on the toilet results in resolution of the condition.

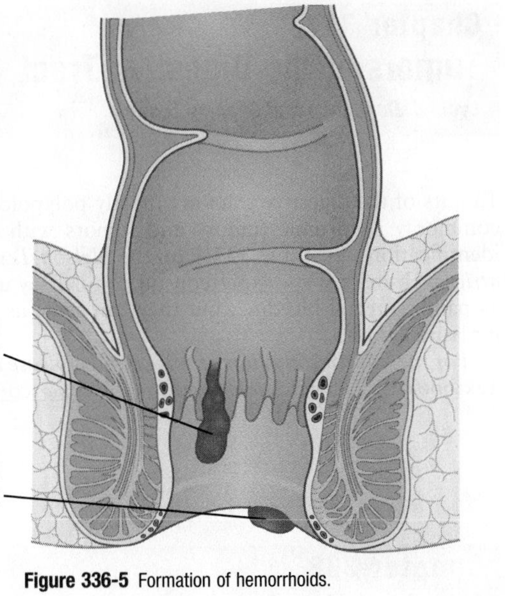

Figure 336-5 Formation of hemorrhoids.

Discomfort may be treated with topical analgesics or anti-inflammatories such as Anusol (pramoxine) and Anusol-HC (hydrocortisone) and sitz baths. The natural course of the disease involves increasing pain, which peaks at 48-72 hr, with gradual remission as the thrombus organizes and involutes over the next 1-2 wk. In cases where the patient with external hemorrhoids presents with excruciating pain soon after the onset of symptoms, thrombectomy may be indicated. This is best accomplished with local infiltration of bupivacaine 0.25% with epinephrine 1:200,000, followed by incision of the vein or skin tag and extraction of the clot. This provides immediate relief; recurrence is rare and further follow-up is unnecessary.

Internal hemorrhoids can become painful when prolapse leads to incarceration and necrosis. Pain usually resolves with reduction of hemorrhoidal tissue. Surgical treatment is reserved for patients failing conservative management. Techniques described include rubber band ligation, open excision, and use of a transanal stapling device.

Complications are rare (<5%) and include recurrence, bleeding, infection, nonhealing wounds, and fistula formation.

BIBLIOGRAPHY

Please visit the Nelson Textbook of Pediatrics *website at www.expertconsult.com for the complete bibliography.*

336.5 Rectal Mucosal Prolapse

Shawn J. Stafford and Michael D. Klein

Rectal mucosal prolapse is the exteriorization of the rectal mucosa through the anus. In the unusual occurrence when all of the layers of the rectal wall are included, it is called **procidentia.** Most cases of rectal tissue protruding through the anus are prolapse and not polyps, intussusception, or other tissue.

Most cases of prolapse are idiopathic. The onset is often between 1 and 5 yr of age. It usually occurs when the child begins standing and then resolves by about 3 to 5 yr of age when the sacrum has taken its more adult shape and the anal lumen is oriented posteriorly. Thus, the entire weight of the abdominal viscera is not pushing down on the rectum as it is earlier in development.

Other predisposing factors include intestinal parasites (particularly in endemic areas), malnutrition, diarrhea, ulcerative colitis, pertussis, Ehlers-Danlos syndrome, meningocele (more often associated with procidentia owing to the lack of perineal muscle support), cystic fibrosis, and chronic constipation. Patients treated surgically for imperforate anus can also have varying degrees of rectal mucosal prolapse. This is particularly common in patients with poor sphincteric development.

CLINICAL MANIFESTATIONS

Rectal mucosal prolapse usually occurs during defecation, especially during toilet training. Reduction of the prolapse may be spontaneous or accomplished manually by the patient or parent. In severe cases, the prolapsed mucosa becomes congested and edematous, making it more difficult to reduce. Rectal prolapse is usually painless or produces mild discomfort. If the rectum remains prolapsed after defecation, it can be traumatized by friction with undergarments, with resultant bleeding, wetness, and potentially, ulceration. The appearance of the prolapse varies from bright red to dark red and resembles a beehive. It can be as long as 10-12 cm. See Chapter 337 for a distinction from a prolapsed polyp.

TREATMENT

Initial evaluation should include tests to rule out any predisposing conditions, especially cystic fibrosis and sacral root lesions. Reduction of protrusion is aided by pressure with warm compresses. An easy method of reduction is to cover the finger with a piece of toilet paper, introduce it into the lumen of the mass, and gently push it into the patient's rectum. The finger is then immediately withdrawn. The toilet paper adheres to the mucous membrane, permitting release of the finger. The paper, when softened, is later expelled.

Conservative treatment consists of careful manual reduction of the prolapse after defecation, attempts to avoid excessive pushing during bowel movements (with patient's feet off the floor), use of laxatives and stool softeners to prevent constipation, avoidance of inflammatory conditions of the rectum, and treatment of intestinal parasitosis when present. If all this fails, surgical treatment may be indicated. Existing surgical options are associated with some morbidity, and therefore medical treatment should always be attempted first.

Sclerosing injections have been associated with complications such as neurogenic bladder. We have found linear cauterization effective and with few complications other than recurrence. In the operating room, the prolapse is recreated by traction on the mucosa. Linear burns are made through nearly the full thickness of the mucosa using electrocautery. One can usually make 8 linear burns on the outside and 4 on the inside of the prolapsed mucosa. In the immediate postoperative period, prolapse can still occur, but in the next several weeks, the burned areas contract and keep the mucosa within the anal canal. The Delorme mucosal sleeve resection addresses mucosal prolapse via a transanal approach by incising, prolapsing, and amputating the redundant mucosa. The resulting mucosal defect is then approximated with absorbable suture.

For patients with procidentia or full-thickness prolapse or intussusception of the rectosigmoid (usually due to myelodysplasia or other sacral root lesions) other, more invasive options exist. Insertion of a Thiersch wire involves placing a subcutaneous wire or stitch in an effort to narrow the anal opening. Complications include obstruction, fecal impaction, and fistula formation. In the Ripstein procedure, a nonabsorbable material is wrapped around the rectum and sutured to the presacral fascia under tension, suspending the redundant bowel within the pelvis. The Frykman-Goldberg procedure consists of a combination of rectosigmoid resection and rectopexy. The redundant sigmoid colon is resected and the descending colon is anastomosed to the rectum. In contrast, the Altemeier perineal rectosigmoidectomy is a transanal, full-thickness resection of redundant bowel with a primary anastomosis to the anus.

BIBLIOGRAPHY
Please visit the Nelson Textbook of Pediatrics *website at www.expertconsult.com for the complete bibliography.*

336.6 Pilonidal Sinus and Abscess

Shawn J. Stafford and Michael D. Klein

The etiology of pilonidal disease remains unknown; 3 hypotheses explaining its origin have been proposed. The first states that trauma, such as can occur with prolonged sitting, impacts hair into the subcutaneous tissue, which serves as a nidus for infection. Another suggests that in some patients, hair follicles exist in the subcutaneous tissues, perhaps due to some embryologic abnormality, and that they serve as a focal point for infection, especially with secretion of hair oils. A third speculates that motion of the buttocks disturbs a particularly deep midline crease and works bacteria and hair beneath the skin. This theory arises from the apparent improved short-term and long-term results of operations that close the wound off the midline, obliterating the deep natal cleft.

Pilonidal disease usually manifests in adolescents or young adults with significant hair over the midline sacral and coccygeal areas. It can occur as an acute abscess with a tender, warm, fluctulent, erythematous swelling or as draining sinus tracts. This disease does not resolve with nonoperative treatment. An acute abscess should be drained and packed open with appropriate anesthesia. Oral broad-spectrum antibiotics covering the usual isolates (*Staphylococcus aureus* and *Bacteroides* species) are prescribed, and the patient's family withdraws the packing over the course of a week. When the packing has been totally removed, the area can be kept clean by a bath or shower. The wound usually heals completely in 6 wk. Once the wound is healed, elective excision should be scheduled to avoid recurrence. Usually, patients who present with sinus tracts may be managed with a single elective excision.

Most surgeons carefully identify the extent of each sinus tract and excise all skin and subcutaneous tissue involved to the fascia covering the sacrum and coccyx. Some close the wound in the midline; others leave it open and packed for healing by secondary intention. Some marsupialize the wound by suturing the skin edges down to the exposed fascia covering the sacrum and coccyx. There appears to be improved success with excision and closure in such a way that the suture line is not in the midline. Studies comparing wide-local excision versus unroofing and marsupialization have submitted that decreased complications and faster healing were observed in the latter group. An additional prospective, randomized trial comparing wide local excision with rhomboid excision and Limberg flap favored the flap procedure. Recurrence or wound-healing problems are relatively common, occurring in 9-27% of cases. Some have treated these with vacuum-assisted closure (VAC) sponge dressings. This is a system that applies continuous suction to a porous dressing. It is usually changed every 3 days and can be done at home with the assistance of a nurse. Recalcitrant cases are treated by a large, full-thickness gluteal flap or skin grafting. Malignant degeneration of pilonidal sinus cyst has been reported only in patients with chronic infections and abscesses.

A simple dimple located in the midline intergluteal cleft, at the level of the coccyx, is seen relatively commonly in normal infants. No evidence indicates that this little sinus provokes any problems for the patient. An open dermal sinus is an asymptomatic, benign condition that does not require operative intervention.

BIBLIOGRAPHY
Please visit the Nelson Textbook of Pediatrics *website at www.expertconsult.com for the complete bibliography.*

Chapter 337
Tumors of the Digestive Tract

Lydia J. Donoghue and Michael D. Klein

Tumors of the digestive tract are mostly polypoid. They are also commonly syndromic tumors and tumors with known genetic identification (see Table 337-1 on the *Nelson Textbook of Pediatrics* website at www.expertconsult.com). They usually manifest as painless rectal bleeding, but they can serve as lead points for intussusception.

For the full continuation of this chapter, please visit the Nelson Textbook of Pediatrics *website at www.expertconsult.com.*

Chapter 338
Inguinal Hernias

John J. Aiken and Keith T. Oldham

Inguinal hernias are one of the most common conditions seen in pediatric practice. The frequency of this condition in concert with its potential morbidity of ischemic injury to the intestine, testis, or ovary makes proper diagnosis and management an important part of daily practice for pediatric practitioners and pediatric surgeons. The overwhelming majority of inguinal hernias in infants and children are congenital indirect hernias (99%) as a consequence of a patent processus vaginalis. The incidence is up to 10 times higher in boys than in girls. Other types of inguinal hernias include direct or acquired (0.5-1.0%) and femoral (<0.5%). Approximately one half of inguinal hernias manifest clinically in the 1st year of life, most in the 1st 6 mo. Premature infants have an incidence of inguinal hernia approaching 30%. The risk of incarceration and possible strangulation of an inguinal hernia is greatest in the 1st year of life (30-40%) and mandates prompt identification and operative repair to minimize morbidity and complications.

EMBRYOLOGY AND PATHOGENESIS

Indirect inguinal hernias in infants and children are congenital and result from an arrest of embryologic development, failure of obliteration of the processus vaginalis, rather than an acquired muscular weakness. The pertinent developmental anatomy of congenital indirect inguinal hernia relates to development of the gonads and descent of the testis through the internal ring and into the scrotum late in gestation. The gonads develop near the kidney as a result of migration of primitive germ cells from the yolk sac to the genital ridge, which is completed by 6 wk of gestation. Differentiation into testis or ovary occurs by 7 or 8 wk of gestation under hormonal influences. The testes descend from the urogenital ridge in the retroperitoneum to the area of the internal ring by about 28 wk of gestation. The final descent of the testes into the scrotum occurs late in gestation between weeks 28 and 36. The testis is preceded in descent to the scrotum by the gubernaculum and the processus vaginalis. The processus vaginalis is present in the developing fetus at 12 wk of gestation as a peritoneal outpouching that extends through the internal inguinal ring and accompanies the testis as it exits the abdomen and descends into the scrotum.

The gubernaculum testis forms from the mesonephros (developing kidney), attaches to the lower pole of the testis, and directs the testis through the internal ring and inguinal canal and into the scrotum. The testis passes through the inguinal canal in a few days but takes about 4 wk to migrate from the external ring to the scrotum. The cordlike structures of the gubernaculum occasionally pass to ectopic locations (perineum or femoral region), resulting in ectopic testes.

In the last few weeks of gestation or shortly after birth, the layers of the processus vaginalis normally fuse together and obliterate the patency from the peritoneal cavity through the inguinal canal to the testis. The processus vaginalis also obliterates just above the testes, and the portion of the processus vaginalis that envelops the testis becomes the tunica vaginalis. In girls, the processus vaginalis obliterates earlier, at about 7 mo of gestation. Failure of the processus vaginalis to close permits fluid or abdominal viscera to escape the peritoneal cavity and accounts for a variety of inguinal-scrotal abnormalities seen in infancy and childhood. The ovaries descend into the pelvis from the urogenital ridge but do not exit from the abdominal cavity. The cranial portion of the gubernaculum in girls differentiates into the ovarian ligament, and the inferior aspect of the gubernaculum becomes the round ligament, which passes through the internal ring and attaches to the labia majora. The processus vaginalis in girls extends into the labia majora through the inguinal canal and is also known as the canal of Nuck.

Androgenic hormones, adequate end-organ receptors, and mechanical factors such as increased intra-abdominal pressure influence complete descent of the testis through the inguinal canal. The testes and spermatic cord structures (spermatic vessels and vas deferens) are located in the retroperitoneum but are affected by increases in intra-abdominal pressure as a consequence of their intimate attachment to the processus vaginalis. The genitofemoral nerve also has an important role: It innervates the cremaster muscle, which develops within the gubernaculum, and experimental division or injury to both nerves in the fetus prevents testicular descent. Failure of regression of smooth muscle (present to provide the force for testicular descent) might have a role in the development of indirect inguinal hernias. Several studies have investigated genes involved in the control of testicular descent for their role in closure of the patent processus vaginalis, for example, hepatocyte growth factor and calcitonin gene-related peptide. Unlike in adult hernias, there does not appear to be any change in collagen synthesis associated with inguinal hernias in children (Fig. 338-1).

GENETICS

The genetics of inguinal hernias in children are not well elucidated. There is some genetic risk incurred for siblings of patients with inguinal hernias; the sisters of affected girls are at the highest risk, with a relative risk of 17.8. In general, the risk of brothers of a sibling is approximately 4-5, as is the risk of a sister of an affected brother. Both a multifactorial threshold model and autosomal dominance with incomplete penetrance and sex influence have been suggested as an explanation for this pattern of inheritance.

PATHOLOGY

Closure of the processus vaginalis is often incomplete at birth; closure continues postnatally, and the rate of patency is inversely proportional to the age of the child. It has been estimated that ~40% close during the first months of life and that ~20% of boys have a persistent patency of the processus vaginalis at 2 yr of age. Patency of the processus vaginalis after birth is a potential hernia, but not all patients with a patent processus vaginalis develop a clinical hernia. An inguinal hernia occurs when intra-abdominal contents escape the abdominal cavity and enter the inguinal region through a patent processus vaginalis. Based on their location in the inguinal canal (lateral to the inferior epigastric vessels), they are indirect inguinal hernias but are rarely associated with a muscular weakness or defect, as is typical of an adult hernia. Depending on the extent of patency of the distal processus, the hernia may be confined to the inguinal region or pass down into the scrotum. Complete failure of obliteration of the processus predisposes to a complete inguinal hernia characterized by a protrusion of abdominal contents into the inguinal canal and possibly extending into the scrotum. Obliteration of the processus vaginalis distally (around the testis) with patency proximally results in the classic indirect inguinal hernia with the protrusion in the inguinal canal.

A **hydrocele** is when only fluid enters the patent processus vaginalis and the swelling may exist only in the scrotum (scrotal hydrocele), only along the spermatic cord in the inguinal region (hydrocele of the spermatic cord), or extend from the scrotum through the inguinal canal and even into the abdomen (abdominal-scrotal hydrocele). A hydrocele is termed a *communicating hydrocele* if it demonstrates fluctuation in size, often increasing in size after activity and, at other times, being smaller when the fluid decompresses into the peritoneal cavity. Occasionally, hydroceles in older children follow trauma, inflammation, or tumors affecting the testis. Although reasons for failure of closure of the processus vaginalis are unknown, it is more common in cases of testicular nondescent and prematurity. In addition, persistent patency of the processus vaginalis is twice as common on the right side, presumably related to later descent of the right testis and interference from the developing inferior vena cava and external iliac vein. Risk factors identified as contributing to the development of congenital inguinal hernia relate to conditions that predispose to failure of obliteration of the processus vaginalis and are listed in Table 338-1. Incidence of inguinal hernia in

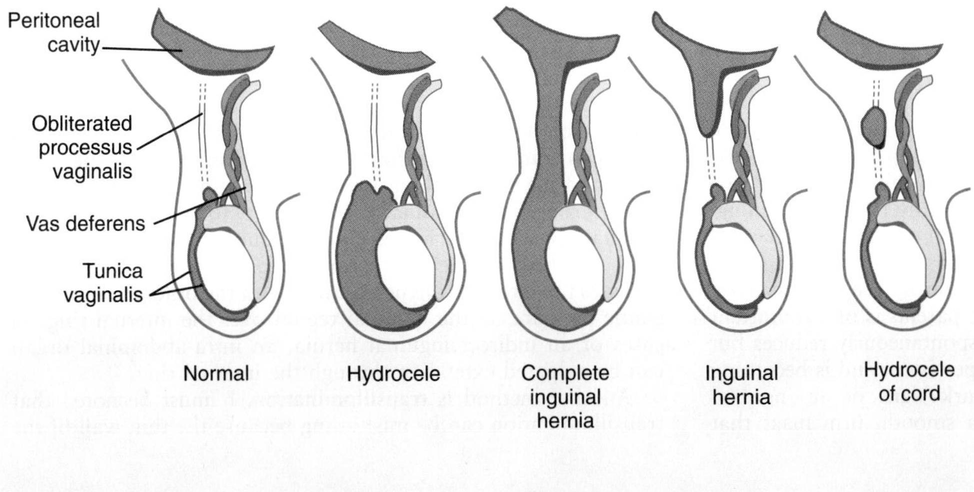

Figure 338-1 Hernia and hydroceles. (Modified from Scherer LR III, Grosfeld JL: Inguinal and umbilical anomalies, *Pediatr Clin North Am* 40: 1121–1131, 1993.)

Table 338-1 PREDISPOSING FACTORS FOR HERNIAS

Prematurity
Urogenital
• Cryptorchidism
• Exstrophy of the bladder or cloaca
• Ambiguous genitalia
• Hypospadius/epispadius
Increased peritoneal fluid
• Ascites
• Ventriculoperitoneal shunt
• Peritoneal dialysis catheter
Increased intra-abdominal pressure
• Repair of abdominal wall defects
• Severe ascites (chylous)
• Meconium peritonitis
Chronic respiratory disease
• Cystic fibrosis
Connective tissue disorders
• Ehlers-Danlos syndrome
• Hunter-Hurler syndrome
• Marfan syndrome
• Mucopolysaccharidosis

patients with cystic fibrosis is ~15%, believed to be related to an altered embryogenesis of the wolffian duct structures, which leads to an absent vas deferens in males with this condition. There is also an increased incidence of inguinal hernia in patients with testicular feminization syndrome and other forms of ambiguous genitalia. The rate of recurrence after repair of an inguinal hernia in patients with a connective tissue disorder approaches 50%, and often the diagnosis of connective tissue disorders in children results from investigation after development of a recurrent inguinal hernia.

INCIDENCE

The incidence of congenital indirect inguinal hernia in full-term newborn infants is estimated at 3.5-5.0%. The incidence of hernia in preterm and low birthweight infants is considerably higher, ranging from 9% to 11%, and approaches 30% in very low birthweight infants (<1,000 g) and preterm infants <28 wk of gestation. Inguinal hernia is much more common in boys than girls, with a male : female ratio of ~6 : 1. About 60% of inguinal hernias occur on the right side, 30% are on the left side, and 10% are bilateral. The incidence of bilateral hernias is higher in girls and appears to be 20-40%. The increased frequency on the right side is presumably related to the later descent of the right testis and interference with obliteration of the processus vaginalis from the developing inferior vena cava. An increased incidence of congenital inguinal hernia has been documented in twins and in family members of patients with inguinal hernia. There is a history of another inguinal hernia in the family in 11.5% of patients.

CLINICAL PRESENTATION

An inguinal hernia typically appears as a bulge in the inguinal region or extending through the inguinal region into the scrotum. In girls, the mass typically occurs in the upper portion of the labia majora. The bulge or mass is most visible at times of irritability or increased intra-abdominal pressure (crying, straining, coughing). It may be present at birth or might not appear until weeks, months, or years later. The bulge is most often 1st noted by the parents or on routine examination by the primary care physician. The classic history from the parents is of intermittent groin, labial, or scrotal swelling that spontaneously reduces but that is gradually enlarging or is more persistent and is becoming more difficult to reduce. The **hallmark signs** of an inguinal hernia on physical examination are a smooth, firm mass that emerges through the external inguinal ring lateral to the pubic tubercle and enlarges with increased intra-abdominal pressure. When the child relaxes, the hernia typically reduces spontaneously or can be reduced by gentle pressure, 1st posteriorly to free it from the external ring and then upward toward the peritoneal cavity.

Methods used to demonstrate the hernia on examination vary depending on the age of the child. A quiet infant can be made to strain the abdominal muscles by stretching him or her out supine on the bed with legs extended and arms held straight above the head. Most infants struggle to get free, thus increasing the intra-abdominal pressure and pushing out the hernia. Older patients can be asked to perform the Valsalva maneuver by blowing up a balloon or coughing. The older child should be examined while standing, and examination after voiding can also be helpful. With increased intra-abdominal pressure, the protruding mass is obvious on inspection of the inguinal region or can be palpated by an examining finger invaginating the scrotum to palpate at the external ring. In the female infant, the ovary and fallopian tube can be contained within the hernia sac, presenting as a firm, discrete, nontender mass in the labia. Another test is the **"silk glove sign,"** which describes the feeling of the layers of the hernia sac (processus vaginalis) as they slide over the spermatic cord structures, with rolling of the spermatic cord beneath the index finger at the pubic tubercle; this physical finding has a sensitivity of 91% and a specificity of 97.3%. If the bulge is located below the inguinal canal on the medial aspect of the thigh, a femoral hernia should be suspected. In the absence of a bulge, the finding of increased thickness of the inguinal canal structures on palpation also suggests the diagnosis of an inguinal hernia. It is important on examination to note the position of the testes because retractile testes are common in infants and young children and can mimic an inguinal hernia with a bulge in the region of the external ring. Because in the female patient ~20-25% of inguinal hernias are sliding hernias (the contents of the hernia sac are adherent within the sac and therefore not reducible), a fallopian tube or ovary can be palpated in the inguinal canal.

EVALUATION OF ACUTE INGUINAL-SCROTAL SWELLING

Occasionally, an inguinal-scrotal mass appears suddenly in an infant or child and is associated with discomfort. The **differential diagnosis** includes incarcerated inguinal hernia, acute hydrocele, torsion of an undescended testis, and suppurative inguinal lymphadenitis. Differentiating between the incarcerated inguinal hernia and the acute hydrocele is probably the most difficult. The infant or child with an incarcerated inguinal hernia is likely to have associated findings suggesting intestinal obstruction, such as colicky abdominal pain, abdominal distention, vomiting, and cessation of stool, and might appear ill. The infant with an acute hydrocele might have discomfort but is consolable and tolerates feedings without signs or symptoms suggesting intestinal obstruction. When the diagnosis is incarcerated inguinal hernia, plain radiographs typically demonstrate multiple air-fluid levels.

On examination of the child with the acute hydrocele, the clinician may note that the mass is somewhat mobile. In addition, in the area between the suspected hydrocele mass and the internal ring, the cord structures can appear only slightly thickened. With the incarcerated hernia, there is a lack of mobility of the groin mass and marked swelling or mass extending from the scrotal mass through the inguinal area and up to and including the internal ring. An experienced clinician can use a bimanual examination to help differentiate groin abnormalities. The examiner palpates the internal ring per rectum, with the other hand placing gentle pressure on the inguinal region over the internal ring. In cases of an indirect inguinal hernia, an intra-abdominal organ can be palpated extending through the internal ring.

Another method is **transillumination.** It must be noted that transillumination can be misleading because the thin wall of the infant's intestine can approximate that of the hydrocele wall and both might transilluminate. This is also the reason aspiration to determine the contents of a groin mass is discouraged. **Ultrasonography** can help distinguish between a hernia and a hydrocele. An expeditious diagnosis is important to avoid the potential complications of an incarcerated hernia, which can develop rapidly. Diagnostic laparoscopy has emerged as an effective and reliable tool in this setting but requires general anesthesia.

The occurrence of suppurative adenopathy in the inguinal region can be confused with an incarcerated inguinal hernia. Examination of the watershed area of the inguinal lymph node might reveal a superficial infected or crusted lesion. In addition, the swelling associated with inguinal lymphadenopathy is typically located more inferior and lateral than the mass of an inguinal hernia, and there may be other associated nodes in the area. Torsion of an undescended testis can manifest as a painful erythematous mass in the groin. The absence of a gonad in the scrotum in the ipsilateral side should clinch this diagnosis.

Incarcerated Hernia

With incarcerated hernia, the contents of the hernia sac cannot be reduced into the abdominal cavity. Contained structures can include small bowel, appendix, omentum, colon, or, rarely, Meckel diverticulum. In girls, the ovary, fallopian tube, or both are commonly incarcerated. Rarely, the uterus in infants can also be pulled into the hernia sac. A **strangulated hernia** is one that is tightly constricted in its passage through the inguinal canal and, as a result, the hernia contents have become ischemic or gangrenous.

Although incarceration may be tolerated in adults for years, most nonreducible inguinal hernias in children, unless treated, rapidly progress to strangulation with potential infarction of the hernia contents. Initially, pressure on the herniated viscera as they pass through the internal ring, inguinal canal, and external ring leads to impaired lymphatic and venous drainage. This leads, in turn, to swelling of the herniated viscera, which further increases the compression in the inguinal canal, ultimately resulting in total occlusion of the arterial supply to the trapped viscera. Progressive ischemic changes take place, culminating in gangrene and/or perforation of the herniated viscera. The testis is also at risk of ischemia because of compression of the spermatic cord structures by the strangulated hernia. In girls, herniation of the ovary places it at risk of strangulation and torsion. The incidence of incarceration of an inguinal hernia is between 12% and 17%. Two thirds of incarcerated hernias occur in the 1st year of life. The greatest risk is in infancy, with reported incidences of between 25% and 30% for infants <6 mo of age. The incidence of incarceration is slightly less in premature infants, although the reasons are unclear.

The symptoms of an incarcerated hernia are irritability, pain in the groin and abdomen, abdominal distention, and vomiting. A somewhat tense, nonfluctuant mass is present in the inguinal region and can extend down into the scrotum or labia majora. The mass is well defined, may be tender, and does not reduce. With the onset of ischemic changes, the pain intensifies, and the vomiting becomes bilious or feculent. Blood may be noted in the stools. The mass is typically tender, and there is often edema and erythema of the overlying skin, with fever and signs of intestinal obstruction. The testes may be normal or may be swollen and hard on the affected side because of venous congestion resulting from compression of the spermatic veins and lymphatic channels at the inguinal ring by the tightly strangulated hernia mass. Abdominal radiographs demonstrate features of partial or complete intestinal obstruction, and gas within the incarcerated bowel segments may be seen below the inguinal ligament or within the scrotum.

Ambiguous Genitalia

Infants with disorders of sexual development commonly present with inguinal hernias, often containing a gonad, and require special consideration. In female infants with inguinal hernias, particularly if the presentation is bilateral inguinal masses, **testicular feminization syndrome** should be suspected because >50% of patients with testicular feminization have an inguinal hernia (Chapter 577). Conversely, the true incidence of testicular feminization in all female infants with inguinal hernias is difficult to determine but is ~1%. In phenotypic females, if the diagnosis of testicular feminization is suspected preoperatively, the child should be screened with a buccal smear for Barr bodies and appropriate genetic evaluation before proceeding with the hernia repair. The diagnosis of testicular feminization is occasionally made at the time of operation by identifying an abnormal gonad (testis) within the hernia sac or absence of the uterus on rectal examination. In the normal female infant, the uterus is easily palpated as a distinct midline structure beneath the symphysis pubis on rectal examination. Preoperative diagnosis of testicular feminization syndrome or other disorders of sexual development such as mixed gonadal dysgenesis and selected pseudohermaphrodites enables the family to receive counseling, and gonadectomy can be accomplished at the time of the hernia repair.

MANAGEMENT

The presence of an inguinal hernia in the pediatric age group constitutes the indication for operative repair. An inguinal hernia does not resolve spontaneously, and early repair eliminates the risk of incarceration and the associated potential complications, particularly in the 1st 6-12 mo of life. The timing of operative repair depends on several factors including age, general condition of the patient, and comorbid conditions. In infants <1 yr of age with an inguinal hernia, repair should proceed promptly because as many as 70% of incarcerated inguinal hernias requiring emergency operation for reduction and repair occur in the 1st year of life. In addition, the incidence of testicular atrophy after incarceration in infants <3 mo of age has been reported as high as 30%. In children >1 yr, the risk of incarceration is less and the repair can be scheduled with less urgency. For the routine reducible hernia, the operation should be carried out electively shortly after diagnosis. Elective inguinal hernia repair can be safely performed in an outpatient setting with an expectation for full recovery within 48 hr. The operation should be performed at a facility with the ability to admit the patient to an inpatient unit as needed. Certain conditions can dictate postponement of repair, such as marked prematurity, intercurrent pneumonia (especially respiratory syncytial virus [RSV]), other infections, or severe congenital heart disease. In cases of marked prematurity (1,800-2,000 g), repair is typically performed before discharge from the neonatal intensive care unit.

The operation is most often performed under general anesthesia, but it can be performed under spinal or caudal anesthesia if avoidance of intubation is preferable due to chronic lung disease or bronchopulmonary dysplasia. Prophylactic antibiotics are not routinely used except for associated conditions such as congenital heart disease or the presence of a venticuloperitoneal shunt. Preterm infants mandate special consideration because of their higher risk for apnea and bradycardia after general anesthesia (Chapter 70). Infants <44 wk postconceptional age and full-term infants <3 mo of age and with comorbid conditions should be observed overnight with appropriate apnea and cardiorespiratory monitors.

An incarcerated, irreducible hernia without evidence of strangulation in a clinically stable patient should initially be managed nonoperatively. Unless there is clear peritonitis or bowel compromise, incarcerated hernias can usually be reduced manually using a technique called *taxis*. Manual reduction is performed first with traction caudad and posteriorly to free the mass from the external inguinal ring, and then upward to reduce the contents back into the peritoneal cavity. The attempt should not be continued if the infant is crying and resisting the pressure on the hernia. The use of sedation or analgesia before attempting reduction can be helpful; this reduces intra-abdominal pressure and relieves the pressure on the neck of the hernia sac at the inguinal ring. Care must be taken to avoid respiratory depression, especially in the premature infant. Other techniques advocated to assist in the nonoperative reduction of an incarcerated inguinal hernia include elevation of the lower torso and legs and brief exposure to an ice pack. Many practitioners do not favor the use of an ice pack in infants because of the risk of hypothermia. If reduction is successful but difficult, the patient should be observed to ensure that feedings are tolerated and there is no concern that necrotic intestine was reduced. Because of the high risk for early recurrent incarceration, surgical repair is performed 24-48 hr later, by which time there is less edema, handling of the sac is easier, and the risk of complications is reduced.

A common presentation in female patients is an irreducible ovary in the inguinal hernia in an otherwise asymptomatic patient. The inguinal mass is soft and nontender to gentle exam, and there is no swelling or edema; thus, there are no findings suggesting strangulation. This represents a "sliding" hernia with the fallopian tube and ovary fused to the posterior-medial wall of the hernia sac. Overzealous attempts to reduce the hernia are unwarranted and potentially harmful to the tube and ovary. The risk that incarceration of the ovary in this setting will lead to strangulation is not known. Most pediatric surgeons recommend elective repair of the hernia within 24-48 hr. For any patient who presents with a prolonged history of incarceration, signs of peritoneal irritation, or small bowel obstruction, surgery and operative reduction and repair of the hernia should be performed.

Operative Management

When the hernia cannot be reduced or is strangulated, immediate operation is indicated to prevent further damage to the contents of the hernia sac or testis. If there are signs of intestinal obstruction or strangulation, initial management includes nasogastric intubation, intravenous fluids, and administration of broad-spectrum antibiotics. When fluid and electrolyte imbalance has been corrected and the child's condition is satisfactory, exploration is undertaken. The operation consists of reduction of the contents of the hernia sac, separation of the hernia sac from the spermatic cord vessels and vas deferens in the inguinal canal, and high ligation of the hernia sac at the internal ring. Resection of nonviable structures within the hernia sac or of an infarcted testis may be indicated based on the experience and judgment of the surgeon. Although the testis might appear ischemic, most patients recover after the incarceration is relieved and do not require removal.

The elective operative repair of a congenital indirect inguinal hernia is straightforward and consists of high ligation of the hernia sac (patent processus vaginalis) at the level of the internal ring, thus preventing protrusion of abdominal contents into the inguinal canal. In boys, this requires careful separation of the sac from the spermatic cord structures and avoidance of injury to these vital structures. An associated hydrocele, present ~20% of the time, is released anteriorly to avoid injury to the spermatic cord structures located posteriorly. In girls, surgical repair is simpler because the hernia sac and round ligament can be ligated without concern for injury to the ovary and its blood supply, which generally remain within the abdomen. The fallopian tube is routinely visualized to rule out testicular feminization syndrome. If the ovary and fallopian tube are within the sac and not reducible, most often the sac is ligated distal to these structures and the internal ring is closed after reducing the sac and its contents to the abdominal cavity.

LAPAROSCOPIC INGUINAL HERNIA REPAIR Although the classic open inguinal hernia repair is most commonly performed, laparoscopic repair is increasingly used by pediatric surgeons experienced in the technique. Like the open technique, the laparoscopic technique is fundamentally a high ligation of the indirect inguinal hernia sac (processus vaginalis). Proponents of the laparoscopic approach cite ease of examining the contralateral internal ring, decreased manipulation of the vas deferens and spermatic vessels, decreased operative time, and an ability to identify unsuspected direct or femoral hernias. In a prospective, randomized study of 97 patients, the laparoscopic approach was associated with decreased pain, parental perception of faster recovery, and parental perception of better wound cosmesis; however, to date complication and recurrence rates have been slightly higher for the laparoscopic approach.

Contralateral Inguinal Exploration

Controversy exists regarding when to proceed with contralateral groin exploration in infants and children with a unilateral indirect inguinal hernia. The only purpose of contralateral exploration is to avoid the occurrence of a hernia on that side at a later date (metachronous hernia). The incidence of a contralateral patent processus vaginalis is ~60% at 2 mo of age and decreases to ~20% at 2 yr of age. A patent processus represents only a potential hernia, and many risk factors influence the likelihood of development of an actual inguinal hernia.

The advantages of contralateral exploration include avoidance of parental anxiety and possibly a second anesthesia, the cost of additional surgery, and the risk of contralateral incarceration. The disadvantages include potential injury to the spermatic cord vessels, vas deferens, and testis; increased operative time; and the fact that, in many infants, it is an unnecessary procedure. The relevant issues in the debate revolve around the frequency of occurrence of contralateral hernias after one-sided hernia repair and the relation of this to age, gender, and side of the clinically apparent hernia. Historically, most large series noted a chance of developing a contralateral hernia as 30-40% in children <2 yr of age, leading most pediatric surgeons to recommend routine contralateral exploration in this age group. The risk of injury to the spermatic cord or vas deferens with inguinal exploration has been estimated in some studies to be as low as 1% and by others as high as 30%. When boys were studied 8 to 20 yr after inguinal hernia repair, 5.8% of them had decreased testicular size on the side of the repair and 1% had testicular atrophy. Most pediatric surgeons believe that routine open contralateral exploration is indicated selectively in high-risk patients for contralateral hernia. In girls, because of the higher incidence of bilateral inguinal hernias and elimination of concern for injury to the spermatic cord or testis, routine contralateral exploration has been recommended up to age 5 or 6 yr. Infants and children with risk factors for development of an inguinal hernia or with medical conditions that increase the risk of general anesthesia should be approached with a low threshold for routine contralateral exploration.

Laparoscopy enables assessment of the contralateral side without risk of injury to the spermatic cord structures or testis. This procedure can be performed through an umbilical incision or by passing a 30-degree or 70-degree oblique scope through the open hernia sac just before ligation of the hernia sac on the involved side. If patency of the contralateral side is demonstrated, the surgeon can proceed with bilateral hernia repair, and if the contralateral side is properly obliterated, exploration and potential complications are avoided. The downside of this approach is that laparoscopy cannot differentiate between a patent processus vaginalis and a true hernia (Figs. 338-2 and 338-3).

DIRECT INGUINAL HERNIA

Direct inguinal hernias are rare in children. Direct hernias appear as groin masses that extend toward the femoral vessels with exertion or straining. The etiology is from a muscular defect or weakness in the floor of the inguinal canal medial to the epigastric vessels. Thus, direct inguinal hernias in children are generally considered an acquired defect. In one third of cases, the patient has a history of a prior indirect hernia repair on the side of the

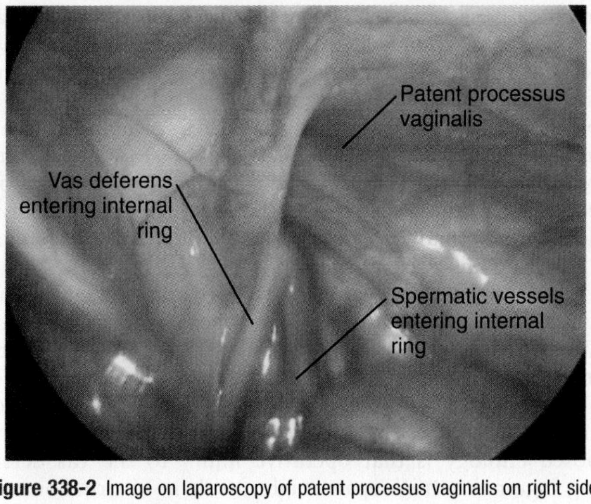

Figure 338-2 Image on laparoscopy of patent processus vaginalis on right side.

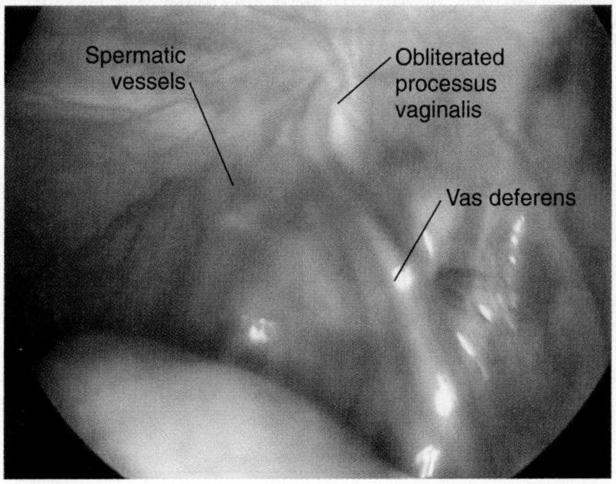

Figure 338-3 Image on diagnostic laparoscopy of obliterated processus vaginalis on left side.

direct hernia, which suggests a possible injury to the floor muscles of the inguinal canal at the time of the first herniorrhaphy. Patients with **connective tissue disorders** such as Ehlers-Danlos syndrome or Marfan syndrome and mucopolysaccharidosis such as Hunter-Hurler syndrome are at increased risk for the development of direct inguinal hernias either independently or after indirect inguinal hernia repair.

Operative repair of a direct inguinal hernia involves strengthening of the floor of the inguinal canal, and many standard techniques have been described, similar to repair techniques used in adults. The repair can be performed through a single limited incision and, therefore, laparoscopic repair does not offer any significant advantage. Recurrence after repair, in contrast to that in adults, is extraordinarily rare. Because typically the area of muscular weakness is small and pediatric tissues have greater elasticity, primary repair is usually possible. Prosthetic material for direct hernia repair or other approaches, such as preperitoneal repair, are rarely required in the pediatric age group. The older child with a direct inguinal hernia and a connective tissue disorder may be the exception, and a laparoscopic approach and prosthetic material in such a case can be useful for repair.

FEMORAL HERNIA

Femoral hernias are also rare in children (<1% of groin hernias in children). They are more common in girls than boys, with a ratio of 2:1. They are extremely rare in infancy and occur typically in older children. Femoral hernias represent a protrusion through the femoral canal. The bulge of a femoral hernia is located below the inguinal ligament and typically projects toward the medial aspect of the thigh. Femoral hernias are more often missed clinically than direct hernias on physical examination or at the time of indirect hernia repair. Repair of a femoral hernia involves closure of the defect at the femoral canal, generally suturing the inguinal ligament to the pectineal ligament and pectineal fascia.

COMPLICATIONS

Complications after elective inguinal hernia repair are uncommon (1.5%) but significantly higher in association with incarceration (10%). Some complications are related to technical factors (recurrence, iatrogenic cryptorchidism), whereas others are related to the underlying process, such as bowel ischemia, gonadal infarction, and testicular atrophy related to an incarcerated hernia. The majority of complications are related to episodes of incarceration or occur after emergency operative reduction and hernia repair.

Wound Infection

Wound infection occurs in <1% of elective inguinal hernia repairs in infants and children, but the incidence increases to 5-7% in association with incarceration and emergent repair. The patient typically develops fever and irritability 3-5 days after the surgery, and the wound demonstrates warmth, erythema, and fluctuance. Management consists of opening and draining the wound, a short course of antibiotics, and a daily wound dressing. Most common organisms are gram-positive (*Staphylococcus* and *Streptococcus* spp.), and consideration should be given to coverage of methicillin-resistant *Staphlococcus aureus.* The wound generally heals in 1-2 wk with low morbidity and a good cosmetic result.

Recurrent Hernia

The recurrence rate of inguinal hernias after elective inguinal hernia repairs is generally reported as 0.5-1.0%, with rates as high as 2% for premature infants. The rate of recurrence after emergency repair of an incarcerated hernia is significantly higher, reported as 3-6% in most large series. The true incidence of recurrence is most certainly even higher, given the problem of accurate long-term follow-up. In the group of patients who develop recurrent inguinal hernia, the recurrence occurs in 50% within 1 yr of the initial repair and in 75% by 2 yr.

Recurrence of an indirect hernia is most likely due to a technical problem in the original procedure, such as failure to identify the sac properly, failure to perform high ligation of the sac at the level of the internal ring, or a tear in the sac that leaves a strip of peritoneum along the cord structures. Recurrence as a direct hernia can result from injury to the inguinal floor (transversalis fascia) during the original procedure or failure to identify a direct hernia during the original exploration. Patients with connective tissue disorders (collagen deficiency) or conditions that cause increased intra-abdominal pressure (ventriculoperitoneal shunts, ascites, peritoneal catheter for dialysis) are at increased risk for recurrence.

Iatrogenic Cryptorchidism

Iatrogenic cryptorchidism describes malposition of the testis after inguinal hernia repair. This complication is usually related to disruption of the testicular attachment or failure to recognize an undescended testis during the original procedure, allowing the testis to retract, typically to the region of the external ring. At the completion of inguinal hernia repair, the testis should be placed in a dependent intrascrotal position. If the testis will not remain in this position, an orchiopexy should be performed at the time of the hernia repair.

Incarceration

Incarceration of an inguinal hernia can result in injury to the intestines, the fallopian tube and ovary, or the ipsilateral testis. The incidence of incarceration of a congenital indirect inguinal hernia is reported as 6-18% and as high as 30% for infants <3 mo of age. Intestinal injury requiring bowel resection is uncommon, occurring in 1-2% of incarcerated hernias. In cases of incarceration in which the hernia is reduced nonoperatively, the likelihood of intestinal injury is low, but these patients should be observed closely for persistent signs and symptoms of intestinal obstruction, such as fever, vomiting, abdominal distention, or bloody stools.

The reported incidence of testicular infarction and subsequent testicular atrophy with incarceration is 4-12%, with higher rates among the irreducible cases. The testicular insult can be caused by compression of the gonadal vessels by the incarcerated hernia mass or as a result of damage incurred during operative repair. Young infants are at higher risk, with testicular infarction rates reported as high as 30% in infants <2-3 mo of age. These problems underscore the need for prompt reduction of incarcerated hernias and early repair once the diagnosis is known to avoid repeat episodes of incarceration.

Injury to the Vas Deferens and Male Fertility

Similar to the gonadal vessels, the vas deferens can be injured as a consequence of compression from an incarcerated hernia or during operative repair. This injury is almost certainly underreported because it is unlikely to be recognized until adulthood and, even then, possibly only if the injury is bilateral. Although the vulnerability of the vas deferens has been documented in many studies, no good data exist as to the actual incidence of this problem. One review reported an incidence of injury to the vas deferens of 1.6% based on pathology demonstrating segments of the vas deferens in the hernia sac specimen; this may be overstated, because others have shown that small glandular inclusions found in the hernia sac can represent müllerian duct remnants and are of no clinical importance.

The relationship between male fertility and previous inguinal hernia repair is also unknown. There appears to be an association between infertile males with testicular atrophy and abnormal sperm count and a previous hernia repair. A relationship has also been reported between infertile males with spermatic autoagglutinating antibodies and previous inguinal hernia repair. The proposed etiology is that operative injury to the vas deferens during inguinal hernia repair might result in obstruction of the vas with diversion of spermatozoa to the testicular lymphatics, and this breach of the blood-testis barrier produces an antigenic challenge, resulting in formation of spermatic autoagglutinating antibodies.

BIBLIOGRAPHY

Please visit the Nelson Textbook of Pediatrics *website at www.expertconsult.com for the complete bibliography.*

Section 5 EXOCRINE PANCREAS

Chapter 339 Embryology, Anatomy, and Physiology

Steven L. Werlin

The human pancreas develops from the ventral and dorsal domains of the primitive duodenal endoderm beginning at about the 5th wk of gestation (see Fig. 339-1 on the *Nelson Textbook of Pediatrics* website at www.expertconsult.com). The larger dorsal anlage, which develops into the tail, body, and part of the head of the pancreas, grows directly from the duodenum. The smaller ventral anlage develops as 1 or 2 buds from the primitive liver and eventually forms the major portion of the head of the pancreas. At about the 17th wk of gestation, the dorsal and ventral anlagen fuse as the buds develop and the gut rotates. The ventral duct forms the proximal portion of the major pancreatic duct of Wirsung, which opens into the ampulla of Vater. The dorsal duct forms the distal portion of the duct of Wirsung and the accessory duct of Santorini, which empties independently in ~5% of people. Variations in fusion might account for pancreatic developmental anomalies. Pancreatic agenesis has been associated with a base pair deletion in the *ipf1* HOX gene, *PDX1*, and possibly in the *PTF1A* and *FS123TER* genes. Other recessive genes involved in pancreatic organogenesis include the *IHH*, *SHH* or sonic hedgehog gene, *SMAD2*, and transforming growth factor (TGF)-1β genes.

For the full continuation of this chapter, please visit the Nelson Textbook of Pediatrics *website at www.expertconsult.com.*

339.1 Anatomic Abnormalities

Steven L. Werlin

Complete or partial **pancreatic agenesis** is a rare condition. Complete agenesis is associated with severe neonatal diabetes and usually death at an early age (Chapter 583).

For the full continuation of this chapter, please visit the Nelson Textbook of Pediatrics *website at www.expertconsult.com.*

339.2 Physiology

Steven L. Werlin

The acinus is the functional unit of the exocrine pancreas. Acinar cells are arrayed in a semicircle around a lumen. Ducts that drain the acini are lined by centroacinar and ductular cells. This arrangement allows the secretions of the various cell types to mix.

For the full continuation of this chapter, please visit the Nelson Textbook of Pediatrics *website at www.expertconsult.com.*

Chapter 340
Pancreatic Function Tests
Steven L. Werlin

Pancreatic function can be measured by direct and indirect methods. An indirect test, the measurement of *fecal elastase*, which has become the standard screening test for pancreatic insufficiency, has a sensitivity and specificity >90%. Falsely abnormal results can occur in many enteropathies. The activity of other pancreatic enzymes in stool is now rarely measured.

For the full continuation of this chapter, please visit the Nelson Textbook of Pediatrics *website at www.expertconsult.com.*

Chapter 341
Disorders of the Exocrine Pancreas
Steven L. Werlin

DISORDERS ASSOCIATED WITH PANCREATIC INSUFFICIENCY

Other than cystic fibrosis, conditions that cause pancreatic insufficiency are rare in children. They include Shwachman-Diamond syndrome, isolated enzyme deficiencies, enterokinase deficiency (Chapter 330), chronic pancreatitis, and protein-calorie malnutrition (Chapters 43 and 330).

Cystic Fibrosis (Chapter 395)

Cystic fibrosis is the most common lethal genetic disease and the most common cause of malabsorption among white American or European children. By the end of the 1st yr of life, 85-90% of children with cystic fibrosis (CF) have pancreatic insufficiency, which, if untreated, can lead to malnutrition. Treatment of the associated pancreatic insufficiency leads to improvement in absorption, better growth, and normalized stools. Pancreatic function can be monitored in children with CF with serial measurements of fecal elastase. Certain mutations in the cystic fibrosis gene have been associated with idiopathic chronic pancreatitis. CF is part of the newborn screen in every state in the United States.

Shwachman-Diamond Syndrome (Chapter 125)

Shwachman-Diamond syndrome (SDS) is an autosomal recessive syndrome (1/20,000 births) due in 90-95% of patients to a mutation of the Shwachman-Bodian-Diamond *(SBDS)* gene on chromosome 7 causing ribosomal dysfunction. Signs and symptoms of SDS include pancreatic insufficiency; neutropenia, which may be cyclic; neutrophil chemotaxis defects; metaphyseal dysostosis; failure to thrive; and short stature. Some patients with SDS have liver or kidney involvement, dental disease, or learning difficulty. SDS is one of the most common causes of congenital neutropenia.

Patients typically present in infancy with poor growth and greasy, foul-smelling stools that are characteristic of malabsorption. These children can be readily differentiated from those with cystic fibrosis by their normal sweat chloride levels, lack of the cystic fibrosis gene, characteristic metaphyseal lesions, and fatty pancreas characterized by a hypodense appearance on CT and MRI scans.

Despite adequate pancreatic replacement therapy and correction of malabsorption, poor growth commonly continues. Pancreatic insufficiency is often transient, and steatorrhea might spontaneously improve with age. Recurrent pyogenic infections (otitis media, pneumonia, osteomyelitis, dermatitis, sepsis) are common and are a common cause of death. Thrombocytopenia is found in 70% of patients and anemia in 50%. Development of a *myelodysplastic syndrome* can occur, and transformation to *acute myeloid leukemia* has been reported in ~3% and 24% of patients, respectively. Pathologically, the pancreatic acini are replaced by fat with little fibrosis. Islet cells and ducts are normal.

Pearson Syndrome

Pearson syndrome is caused by a mitochondrial DNA mutation affecting oxidative phosphorylation that manifests in infants with severe macrocytic anemia and variable thrombocytopenia. The bone marrow demonstrates vacuoles in erythroid and myeloid precursors as well as ringed sideroblasts. In addition to its role in severe bone marrow failure, pancreatic insufficiency contributes to growth failure. Mitochondrial DNA mutations are transmitted through maternal inheritance to both sexes or are sporadic.

Isolated Enzyme Deficiencies

Isolated deficiencies of trypsinogen, enterokinase, lipase, and colipase have been reported. Although enterokinase is a brush border enzyme, deficiency causes pancreatic insufficiency because pancreatic proteases remain inactive. Deficiencies of trypsinogen or enterokinase manifest with failure to thrive, hypoproteinemia, and edema. Isolated amylase deficiency is typically developmental and resolves by age 2-3 yr.

SYNDROMES ASSOCIATED WITH PANCREATIC INSUFFICIENCY

Pancreatic agenesis, the Johanson-Blizzard syndrome (pancreatic insufficiency, deafness, low birthweight, microcephaly, midline ectodermal scalp defects, psychomotor retardation, hypothyroidism, dwarfism, absent permanent teeth, and aplasia of the alae nasae), congenital pancreatic hypoplasia, and congenital rubella are rare causes of pancreatic insufficiency. Some children with both syndromic (Alagille) and nonsyndromic paucity of intrahepatic bile ducts also have pancreatic insufficiency associated with their liver disease. Pancreatic insufficiency has also been reported in duodenal atresia and stenosis and may also be seen in an infant with familial or nonfamilial hyperinsulinemic hypoglycemia, who requires 95-100% pancreatectomy to control hypoglycemia.

BIBLIOGRAPHY

Please visit the Nelson Textbook of Pediatrics *website at www.expertconsult.com for the complete bibliography.*

Chapter 342
Treatment of Pancreatic Insufficiency
Steven L. Werlin

Treatment of exocrine pancreatic insufficiency by oral enzyme replacement usually corrects creatorrhea, but steatorrhea is difficult to correct completely. This may be due to inadequate dosage, incorrect timing of doses in relation to food consumption or gastric emptying, lipase inactivation by gastric acid, and the observation that *chymotrypsin* in the enzyme preparation digests and thus inactivates *lipase*. In 2010 the FDA removed all pre-existing enzyme preparations from the U.S. market. The previous practice of overfilling capsules was banned. To date, 3 new preparations have been approved. All have been tested and shown to reduce malabsorption in cystic fibrosis patients. Modern enzyme products are enteric-coated to resist gastric acid inactivation.

The dosage of pancreatic replacement for children depends on the amount of food eaten and is established by trial and error. Because these products contain excess protease compared with lipase, the dosage is estimated from the lipase requirement of 500-2,500 IU/kg/meal, with a maximum of 10,000 IU/kg/day. An adequate dose is one that is followed by the return of the stools to normal fat content, which can be verified by a 72-hour fecal fat collection, and normalization of stool consistency color, and odor. Enzyme replacement should be given at the beginning of and with the meal. In children unable to swallow enzyme capsules, the granules can be mixed with a small quantity of food, typically applesauce. Enzymes should not be chewed, crushed or dissolved in food, which would allow gastric acid to penetrate the enteric coating and destroy the enzymes. Enzymes must also be given with snacks. Increasing enzyme supplements beyond the recommended dose does not improve absorption, might retard growth, and can cause fibrosing colonopathy.

When adequate fat absorption is not achieved, gastric acid neutralization with an H_2-receptor antagonist or, more commonly, a proton pump inhibitor decreases enzyme inactivation by gastric acid and improves delivery of lipase into the intestine. Enteric coating also protects lipase from acid inactivation.

Untoward effects secondary to pancreatic enzyme replacement therapy include allergic reactions, increased uric acid levels, and kidney stones. Fibrosing colonopathy, consisting of colonic fibrosis and strictures, can occur 7-12 mo after high-dose pancreatic supplement therapy (6,500-58,000 IU lipase/kg/meal).

BIBLIOGRAPHY

Please visit the Nelson Textbook of Pediatrics *website at www.expertconsult.com for the complete bibliography.*

Chapter 343 Pancreatitis

343.1 Acute Pancreatitis

Steven L. Werlin

Acute pancreatitis, the most common pancreatic disorder in children, is increasing in incidence. At least 30-50 cases are now seen in major pediatric centers per year. In children, blunt abdominal injuries, multisystem disease, biliary stones or microlithiasis (sludging), and drug toxicity are the most common etiologies. Although many drugs and toxins can induce acute pancreatitis in susceptible persons, in children, valproic acid, L-asparaginase, 6-mercaptopurine, and azathioprine are the most common causes of drug-induced pancreatitis. Other cases follow organ transplantation or are due to infections, metabolic disorders, and mutations in susceptibility genes (Chapter 343.2). Less than 5% of cases are idiopathic (Table 343-1).

After an initial insult, such as ductal disruption or obstruction, there is premature activation of trypsinogen to trypsin within the acinar cell. Trypsin then activates other pancreatic proenzymes, leading to autodigestion, further enzyme activation, and release of active proteases. Lysosomal hydrolases co-localize with pancreatic proenzymes within the acinar cell. Pancreastasis (similar in concept to cholestasis) with continued synthesis of enzymes occurs. Lecithin is activated by phospholipase A2 into the toxic lysolecithin. Prophospholipase is unstable and can be activated by minute quantities of trypsin. After the insult, cytokines and other proinflammatory mediators are released.

The healthy pancreas is protected from autodigestion by pancreatic proteases that are synthesized as inactive proenzymes;

Table 343-1 ETIOLOGY OF ACUTE PANCREATITIS IN CHILDREN

DRUGS AND TOXINS
Acetaminophen overdose
Alcohol
L-Asparaginase
Azathioprine
Carbamazipine
Cimetidine
Corticosteroids
Enalapril
Erythromycin
Estrogen
Furosemide
Isoniazid
Lisinopril
6-Mercaptopurine
Methyldopa
Metronidazole
Octreotide
Organophosphate poisoning
Pentamidine
Retrovirals: DDC, DDI, tenofovir
Sulfonamides: Mesalamine, 5-aminosalicytates, sulfasalazine, trimethoprim/sulfmethoxazole
Sulindac
Tetracycline
Thiazides
Valproic acid
Venom (spider, scorpion, Gila monster lizard)
Vincristine
GENETIC
Cationic trypsinogen gene (*PRSS1*)
Chymotrypsin C gene (*CTRC*)
Cystic fibrosis gene (*CFTR*)
Trypsin inhibitor gene (*SPINK1*)
INFECTIOUS
Ascariasis
Coxsackie B virus
Epstein-Barr virus
Hepatitis A, B
Influenza A, B
Leptospirosis
Malaria
Measles
Mumps
Mycoplasma
Rubella
Rubeola
Reye syndrome: varicella, influenza B
Septic shock
OBSTRUCTIVE
Ampullary disease
Ascariasis
Biliary tract malformations
Choledochal cyst
Choledochocele
Cholelithiasis, microlithiasis, and choledocholithiasis (stones or sludge)
Duplication cyst
Endoscopic retrograde cholangiopancreatography (ERCP) complication
Pancreas divisum
Pancreatic ductal abnormalities
Postoperative
Sphincter of Oddi dysfunction
Tumor

Table 343-1 ETIOLOGY OF ACUTE PANCREATITIS IN CHILDREN—cont'd

SYSTEMIC DISEASE
Autoimmune pancreatitis Brain tumor Collagen vascular diseases Crohn disease Diabetes mellitus Head trauma Hemochromatosis Hemolytic uremic syndrome Hyperlipidemia: type I, IV, V Hyperparathyroidism/Hypercalcemia Kawasaki disease Malnutrition Organic academia Peptic ulcer Periarteritis nodosa Renal failure Systemic lupus erythematosus Transplantation: bone marrow, heart, liver, kidney, pancreas Vasculitis
TRAUMATIC
Blunt injury Burns Child abuse Hypothermia Surgical trauma Total body cast

Table 343-2 DIFFERENTIAL DIAGNOSIS OF HYPERAMYLASEMIA

PANCREATIC PATHOLOGY
Acute or chronic pancreatitis Complications of pancreatitis (pseudocyst, ascites, abscess) Factitious pancreatitis
SALIVARY GLAND PATHOLOGY
Parotitis (mumps, *Staphylococcus aureus,* cytomegalovirus, HIV, Epstein-Barr virus) Sialadenitis (calculus, radiation) Eating disorders (anorexia nervosa, bulimia)
INTRA-ABDOMINAL PATHOLOGY
Biliary tract disease (cholelithiasis) Peptic ulcer perforation Peritonitis Intestinal obstruction Appendicitis
SYSTEMIC DISEASES
Metabolic acidosis (diabetes mellitus, shock) Renal insufficiency, transplantation Burns Pregnancy Drugs (morphine) Head injury Cardiopulmonary bypass

digestive enzymes that are segregated into secretory granules at pH 6.2 by low calcium concentration, which minimizes trypsin activity; the presence of protease inhibitors both in the cytoplasm and zymogen granules; and enzymes that are secreted directly into the ducts.

Histopathologically, interstitial edema appears early. Later, as the episode of pancreatitis progresses, localized and confluent necrosis, blood vessel disruption leading to hemorrhage, and an inflammatory response in the peritoneum can develop.

CLINICAL MANIFESTATIONS

Mild Acute Pancreatitis

The patient with acute pancreatitis has severe abdominal pain, persistent vomiting, and possibly fever. The pain is epigastric or in either upper quadrant and steady, often resulting in the child's assuming an antalgic position with hips and knees flexed, sitting upright, or lying on the side. The child is very uncomfortable and irritable and appears acutely ill. The abdomen may be distended and tender and a mass may be palpable. The pain can increase in intensity for 24-48 hr, during which time vomiting may increase and the patient can require hospitalization for dehydration and might need fluid and electrolyte therapy. The prognosis for complete recovery in the acute uncomplicated case is excellent. The incidence of acute pancreatitis is increasing.

Severe Acute Pancreatitis

Severe acute pancreatitis is rare in children. In this life-threatening condition, the patient is acutely ill with severe nausea, vomiting, and abdominal pain. Shock, high fever, jaundice, ascites, hypocalcemia, and pleural effusions can occur. A bluish discoloration may be seen around the umbilicus (***Cullen*** sign) or in the flanks (***Grey Turner*** sign). The pancreas is necrotic and can be transformed into an inflammatory hemorrhagic mass. The mortality rate, which is ~20%, is related to the systemic inflammatory response syndrome with multiple organ dysfunction, shock, renal failure, acute respiratory distress syndrome, disseminated intravascular coagulation, massive gastrointestinal bleeding, and systemic or intra-abdominal infection. The percentage of necrosis seen on CT scan and failure of pancreatic tissue to enhance on CT scan (suggesting necrosis) predicts the severity of the disease.

DIAGNOSIS

Acute pancreatitis is usually diagnosed by measurement of serum lipase and amylase activities. Serum lipase is now considered the test of choice for acute pancreatitis as it is more specific than amylase for acute inflammatory pancreatic disease and should be determined when pancreatitis is suspected. The serum lipase rises by 4-8 hr, peaks at 24-48 hr, and remains elevated 8-14 days longer than serum amylase. Serum lipase can be elevated in nonpancreatic diseases. The serum amylase level is typically elevated for up to 4 days. A variety of other conditions can also cause hyperamylasemia without pancreatitis (Table 343-2). Elevation of salivary amylase can mislead the clinician to diagnose pancreatitis in a child with abdominal pain. The laboratory can separate amylase isoenzymes into pancreatic and salivary fractions. Initially, serum amylase levels are normal in 10-15% of patients.

Other laboratory abnormalities that may be present in acute pancreatitis include hemoconcentration, coagulopathy, leukocytosis, hyperglycemia, glucosuria, hypocalcemia, elevated γ-glutamyl transpeptidase, and hyperbilirubinemia.

X-ray of the chest and abdomen might demonstrate nonspecific findings. The chest x-ray might demonstrate platelike atelectasis, basilar infiltrates, elevation of the hemidiaphragm, left- (rarely right-) sided pleural effusions, pericardial effusion, and pulmonary edema. Abdominal x-rays might demonstrate a sentinel loop, dilation of the transverse colon (cutoff sign), ileus, pancreatic calcification (if recurrent), blurring of the left psoas margin, a pseudocyst, diffuse abdominal haziness (ascites), and peripancreatic extraluminal gas bubbles.

CT scanning has a major role in the diagnosis and follow-up of children with pancreatitis. Findings can include pancreatic enlargement, a hypoechoic, sonolucent edematous pancreas, pancreatic masses, fluid collections, and abscesses (Fig. 343-1); ≥20% of children with acute pancreatitis initially have normal imaging studies. In adults, CT findings are the basis of a widely accepted prognostic system. Ultrasonography is more sensitive than CT scanning for the diagnosis of biliary stones. Magnetic

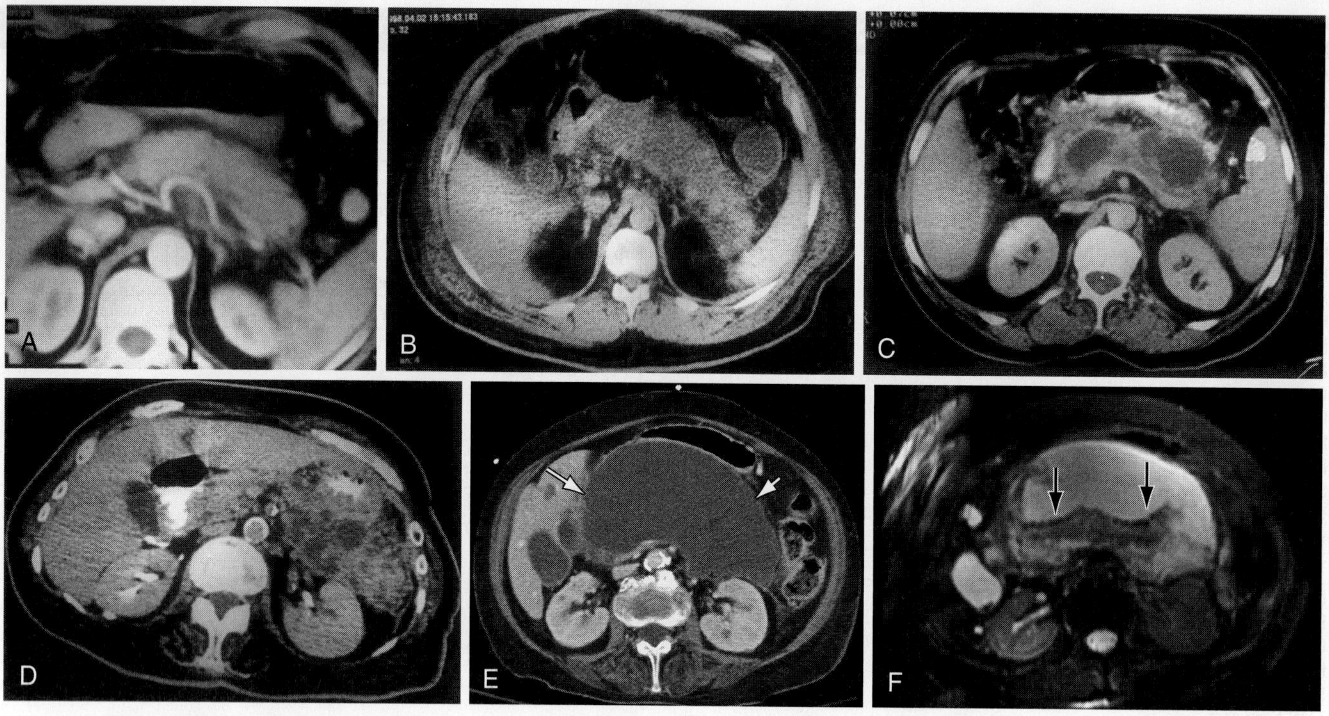

Figure 343-1 Computed tomography (CT) and magnetic resonance imaging (MRI) appearance of pancreatitis. *A,* Mild acute pancreatitis. Arterial phase spiral CT. Diffuse enlargement of pancreas without fluid accumulation. *B,* Severe acute pancreatitis. Lack of enhancement of the pancreatic parenchyma due to the necrosis of the entire pancreatic gland. *C,* Pancreatic pseudocyst. A round fluid collection with thin capsule is seen within the lesser sac. *D,* Acute severe pancreatitis and peripancreatic abscess formation. Peripancreatic abscess formation is observed within the peripancreatic and the left anterior pararenal space. *E,* Pancreatic necrosis. A well-defined fluid attenuation collection in the pancreatic bed (*white arrows*) seen on CECT imaging. *F,* The same collection is more complex appearing on the corresponding T2-weighted MR image. The internal debris and necrotic tissue are better appreciated because of the superior soft tissue contrast of MR imaging (*black arrows*). (*A-D,* From Elmas N: The role of diagnostic radiology in pancreatitis, *Eur J Radiol* 38[2]:120–132, 2001, Figs 1, 3b, 4a, and 5. *E-F,* From Soakar A, Rabinowitz CB, Sahani DV: Cross-sectional imaging in acute pancreatitis, *Radiol Clin North Am* 45[3]:447–460, 2007, Fig 14.)

resonance cholangiopancreatography (MRCP) and endoscopic retrograde cholangiopancreatography (ERCP) are essential in the investgation of recurrent pancreatitis, nonresolving pancreatitis, and disease associated with gallbladder pathology. Endoscopic ultrasonography also helps visualize the pancreaticobiliary system.

TREATMENT

The aims of medical management are to relieve pain and restore metabolic homeostasis. Analgesia should be given in adequate doses. Fluid, electrolyte, and mineral balance should be restored and maintained. Nasogastric suction is useful in patients who are vomiting. While vomiting, the patient should be maintained with nothing by mouth. Recovery is usually complete within 4-5 days. Refeeding can commence when vomiting has resolved. Early refeeding decreases the complication rate and length of stay.

In severe pancreatitis, prophylactic antibiotics are used to prevent infected pancreatic necrosis or to treat infected necrosis. Gastric acid is suppressed. Endoscopic therapy can be of benefit when pancreatitis is caused by anatomic abnormalities, such as strictures or stones. Enteral alimentation by mouth, nasogastric tube, or nasojejunal tube (in severe cases or for those intolerant of oral or nasogastric feedings), within 2-3 days of onset, reduces the length of hospitalization. In children, surgical therapy of nontraumatic, acute pancreatitis is rarely required but may include drainage of necrotic material or abscesses.

PROGNOSIS

Children with uncomplicated acute pancreatitis do well and recover within 4-5 days. When pancreatitis is associated with trauma or systemic disease, the prognosis is typically related to the associated medical conditions.

BIBLIOGRAPHY

Please visit the Nelson Textbook of Pediatrics *website at www.expertconsult.com for the complete bibliography.*

343.2 Chronic Pancreatitis

Steven L. Werlin

Chronic pancreatitis in children is often due to genetic mutations or due to congenital anomalies of the pancreatic or biliary ductal system. Mutations in the *PRSS1* gene (cationic trypsinogen) located on the long arm of chromosome 7, *SPINK 1* gene (pancreatic trypsin inhibitor) located on chromosome 5, in the cystic fibrosis gene (*CFTR*), and chymotrypsin C all lead to chronic pancreatitis (see Table 343-1).

Cationic trypsinogen has a trypsin-sensitive cleavage site. Loss of this cleavage site in the abnormal protein permits uncontrolled activation of trypsinogen to trypsin, which leads to autodigestion of the pancreas. Mutations in *PRSS1* act in an autosomal dominant fashion with incomplete penetrance and variable expressivity. Symptoms often begin in the 1st decade but are usually mild at the onset. Although spontaneous recovery from each attack

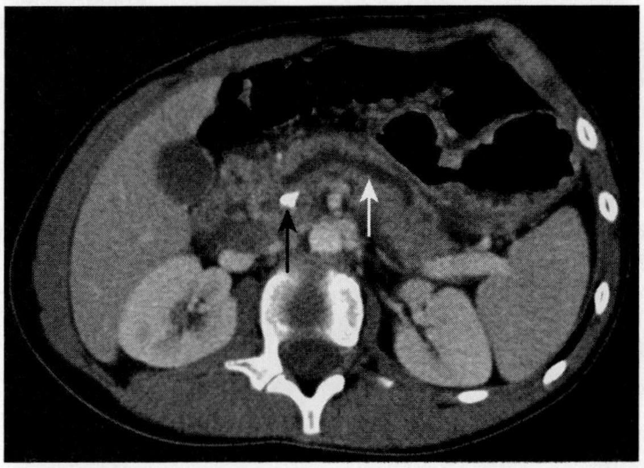

Figure 343-2 Chronic pancreatitis. Computed tomogram showing calcification in the head of the pancreas *(black arrow)* and dilated pancreatic duct *(white arrow)* in a 12 yr old patient. (Courtesy of Dr. Janet Reid.) (From Wyllie R, Hyams JS, editors: *Pediatric gastrointestinal and liver disease,* ed 3, Philadelphia, 2006, Saunders.)

occurs in 4-7 days, episodes become progressively severe. Clinically, hereditary pancreatitis may be diagnosed by the presence of the disease in successive generations of a family. An evaluation during symptom-free intervals may be unrewarding until calcifications, pseudocysts, or pancreatic exocrine and endocrine insufficiency develops (Fig. 343-2). Chronic pancreatitis is a risk factor for future development of pancreatic cancer. Multiple mutations of the *PRSS1* gene associated with hereditary pancreatitis have been described.

Trypsin inhibitor acts as a fail-safe mechanism to prevent uncontrolled autoactivation of trypsin. Mutations in the *SPINK1* gene have been associated with recurrent or chronic pancreatitis. In *SPINK1* mutations, this fail-safe mechanism is lost; this gene may be a modifier gene and not the direct etiologic factor.

Mutations of the cystic fibrosis gene *(CFTR),* which cause cystic fibrosis with pancreatic sufficiency or which do not typically produce pulmonary disease, can cause chronic pancreatitis, possibly due to ductal obstruction. A mutation in the *Chymotrypsin C* gene, causing a gain of function, is a newly described genetic etiology of recurrent pancreatitis. Indications for genetic testing include recurrent episodes of acute pancreatitis, chronic pancreatitis, a family history of pancreatitis, or unexplained pancreatitis in children.

Other conditions associated with chronic, relapsing pancreatitis are hyperlipidemia (types I, IV, and V), hyperparathyroidism, and ascariasis. Previously, most cases of recurrent pancreatitis in childhood were considered idiopathic; with the discovery of at least 4 gene families associated with recurrent pancreatitis, this has changed. Congenital anomalies of the ductal systems, such as pancreas divisum are more common than previously recognized.

Autoimmune pancreatitis typically manifests with jaundice, abdominal pain, and weight loss. The pancreas is typically enlarged and the pancreas is hypodense on CT. The pathogenesis is unknown. Treatment is with steroids. There have been only a few case reports of this condition in children.

Juvenile tropical pancreatitis is the most common form of chronic pancreatitis in developing equatorial countries. The highest prevalence is in the Indian state of Kerala. Tropical pancreatitis occurs during late childhood or early adulthood, manifesting with abdominal pain and irreversible pancreatic insufficiency followed by diabetes mellitus within 10 years. The pancreatic ducts are obstructed with inspissated secretions, which later calcify. This condition is associated with mutations in the *SPINK* gene in 50% of cases.

A thorough diagnostic evaluation of every child with >1 episode of pancreatitis is indicated. Serum lipid, calcium, and phosphorus levels are determined. Stools are evaluated for ascaris, and a sweat test is performed. Plain abdominal films are evaluated for the presence of pancreatic calcifications. Abdominal ultrasound or CT scanning is performed to detect the presence of a pseudocyst. The biliary tract is evaluated for the presence of stones. After genetic counseling, evaluation of *PRSS1*, *SPINK1*, *CFTR*, and *CRTC* genotypes can be measured.

MRCP and ERCP are techniques that can be used to define the anatomy of the gland and are mandatory if surgery is considered. MRCP is the test of choice when endotherapy is not being considered and should be performed as part of the evaluation of any child with idiopathic, nonresolving, or recurrent pancreatitis and in patients with a pseudocyst before drainage. In these cases a previously undiagnosed anatomic defect that may be amenable to endoscopic or surgical therapy may be detected. Endoscopic treatments include sphincterotomy, stone extraction, drainage on pseudocysts, and insertion of pancreatic or biliary endoprosthetic stents. These treatments allow successful nonsurgical management of conditions previously requiring surgical intervention.

BIBLIOGRAPHY

Please visit the Nelson Textbook of Pediatrics *website at* www.expertconsult.com *for the complete bibliography.*

Chapter 344
Pseudocyst of the Pancreas

Steven L. Werlin

Pancreatic pseudocyst formation is an uncommon sequela to acute or chronic pancreatitis. Pseudocysts are sacs delineated by a fibrous wall in the lesser peritoneal sac. They can enlarge or extend in almost any direction, thus producing a wide variety of symptoms (see Fig. 343-1C).

A pancreatic pseudocyst is suggested when an episode of pancreatitis fails to resolve or when a mass develops after an episode of pancreatitis. Clinical features usually include pain, nausea, and vomiting, but many patients are asymptomatic. The most common signs are a palpable mass in 50% of patients and jaundice in 10%. Other findings include ascites and pleural effusions (usually left-sided).

Pancreatic pseudocysts can be detected by transabdominal ultrasonography, CT scanning, magnetic resonance cholangiopancreatography (MRCP), endoscopic retrograde cholangiopancreatography (ERCP), and endoscopic ultrasound (EUS). Because of its ease, availability, and reliability, ultrasonography is the 1st choice. Sequential ultrasonography studies have demonstrated that most small pseudocysts (<6 cm) resolve spontaneously. It is recommended that the patient with acute pancreatitis undergo an ultrasonographic evaluation 2-4 wk after resolution of the acute episode for an evaluation of possible pseudocyst formation.

Percutaneous or endoscopic drainage of pseudocysts has replaced open surgical drainage, except for complicated or recurrent pseudocysts. Whereas a pseudocyst must be allowed to mature for 4-6 wk before surgical drainage is attempted, percutaneous or endoscopic drainage can be attempted earlier. In some cases, endoscopic creation of a cyst-gastrostomy is performed. MRCP or ERCP should precede surgical treatment to help the surgeon plan the approach and define anatomic abnormalities. EUS is helpful when an endoscopic approach is chosen.

BIBLIOGRAPHY

Please visit the Nelson Textbook of Pediatrics *website at* www.expertconsult.com *for the complete bibliography.*

Chapter 345
Pancreatic Tumors
Steven L. Werlin

Pancreatic tumors can be of either endocrine or nonendocrine origin. Tumors of endocrine origin include insulinomas and gastrinomas. These and other functioning tumors occur in the autosomal dominantly inherited multiple endocrine neoplasia type 1 (MEN-1). Hypoglycemia accompanied by higher than expected insulin levels or refractory gastric ulcers (Zollinger-Ellison syndrome) indicate the possibility of a pancreatic tumor (Chapter 337). Most gastrinomas arise outside of the pancreas. The treatment of choice is surgical removal. If the primary tumor cannot be found or if it has metastasized, cure might not be possible. Treatment with high dose of a proton pump inhibitor to inhibit gastric acid secretion is then indicated.

For the full continuation of this chapter, please visit the Nelson Textbook of Pediatrics *website at www.expertconsult.com.*

Section 6 THE LIVER AND BILIARY SYSTEM

Chapter 346
Morphogenesis of the Liver and Biliary System
Alexander G. Miethke and William F. Balistreri

Morphogenesis of the liver and biliary system is a complex process. It follows that altered development has significant consequences, including cholestatic disorders such as Alagille syndrome and biliary atresia.

For the full continuation of this chapter, please visit the Nelson Textbook of Pediatrics *website at www.expertconsult.com.*

Chapter 347
Manifestations of Liver Disease
Lynelle M. Boamah and William F. Balistreri

PATHOLOGIC MANIFESTATIONS

Alterations in hepatic structure and function can be acute or chronic, with varying patterns of reaction of the liver to cell injury. Hepatocyte injury can result in inflammatory cell infiltration or cell death (necrosis), which may be followed by a healing process of scar formation (fibrosis) and, potentially, nodule formation (regeneration). Cirrhosis is the end result of any progressive liver disease.

Injury to individual hepatocytes can result from viral infection, drugs or toxins, hypoxia, immunologic disorders, or inborn errors of metabolism. The evolving process leads to repair, continuing injury with chronic changes, or, in rare cases, to massive hepatic damage.

Cholestasis is an alternative or concomitant response to injury caused by extrahepatic or intrahepatic obstruction to bile flow. Substances that are normally excreted in bile, such as conjugated bilirubin, cholesterol, bile acids, and trace elements, accumulate in serum. Bile pigment accumulation in liver parenchyma can be seen in liver biopsy. In extrahepatic obstruction, bile pigment may be visible in the intralobular bile ducts or throughout the parenchyma as bile lakes or infarcts. In intrahepatic cholestasis, an injury to hepatocytes or an alteration in hepatic physiology leads to a reduction in the rate of secretion of solute and water. Likely causes include alterations in enzymatic or canalicular transporter activity, permeability of the bile canalicular apparatus, organelles responsible for bile secretion, or ultrastructure of the cytoskeleton of the hepatocyte. The end result can be clinically indistinguishable from obstructive cholestasis.

Cirrhosis, defined histologically by the presence of bands of fibrous tissue that link central and portal areas and form parenchymal nodules, is a potential end stage of any acute or chronic liver disease. Cirrhosis can be *posthepatitic* (after acute or chronic hepatitis) or *postnecrotic* (after toxic injury), or it can follow chronic biliary obstruction *(biliary cirrhosis)*. Cirrhosis can be macronodular, with nodules of various sizes (up to 5 cm) separated by broad septa, or micronodular, with nodules of uniform size (<1 cm) separated by fine septa; mixed forms occur. The progressive scarring of cirrhosis results in altered hepatic blood flow, with further impairment of liver cell function. Increased intrahepatic resistance to portal blood flow leads to portal hypertension.

The liver can be secondarily involved in neoplastic (metastatic) and non-neoplastic (storage diseases, fat infiltration) processes as well as a number of systemic conditions and infectious processes. The liver can also be affected by chronic passive congestion or acute hypoxia, with hepatocellular damage.

CLINICAL MANIFESTATIONS

Hepatomegaly

Enlargement of the liver can be due to several mechanisms (Table 347-1). Normal liver size estimations are based on age-related clinical indices, such as the degree of extension of the liver edge below the costal margin, the span of dullness to percussion, or the length of the vertical axis of the liver, as estimated from imaging techniques. In children, the normal liver edge can be felt up to 2 cm below the right costal margin. In a newborn infant, extension of the liver edge >3.5 cm below the costal margin in the right midclavicular line suggests hepatic enlargement. Measurement of liver span is carried out by percussing the upper margin of dullness and by palpating the lower edge in the right midclavicular line. This may be more reliable than an extension of the liver edge alone. The 2 measurements can correlate poorly.

The liver span increases linearly with body weight and age in both sexes, ranging from ~4.5-5.0 cm at 1 wk of age to ~7-8 cm in boys and 6.0-6.5 cm in girls by 12 yr of age. The lower edge of the right lobe of the liver extends downward (Riedel lobe) and

Table 347-1 MECHANISMS OF HEPATOMEGALY

INCREASE IN THE NUMBER OR SIZE OF THE CELLS INTRINSIC TO THE LIVER
Storage
Fat: malnutrition, obesity, metabolic liver disease (diseases of fatty acid oxidation and Reye syndrome–like illnesses), lipid infusion (total parenteral nutrition), cystic fibrosis, diabetes mellitus, medication related, pregnancy Specific lipid storage diseases: Gaucher, Niemann-Pick, Wolman disease Glycogen: glycogen storage diseases (multiple enzyme defects); total parenteral nutrition; infant of diabetic mother, Beckwith syndrome Miscellaneous: α_1-antitrypsin deficiency, Wilson disease, hypervitaminosis A, neonatal iron storage disease
Inflammation
Hepatocyte enlargement (hepatitis) • Viral: acute and chronic • Bacterial: sepsis, abscess, cholangitis • Toxic: drugs • Autoimmune Kupffer cell enlargement • Sarcoidosis • Systemic lupus erythematosus • Macrophage activating syndrome
INFILTRATION OF CELLS
Primary Liver Tumors: Benign
Hepatocellular • Focal nodular hyperplasia • Nodular regenerative hyperplasia • Hepatocellular adenoma Mesodermal • Infantile hemangioendothelioma • Mesenchymal hamartoma Cystic masses • Choledochal cyst • Hepatic cyst • Hematoma • Parasitic cyst • Pyogenic or amebic abscess
Primary Liver Tumors: Malignant
Hepatocellular • Hepatoblastoma • Hepatocellular carcinoma Mesodermal • Angiosarcoma • Undifferentiated embryonal sarcoma Secondary or metastatic processes • Lymphoma • Leukemia • Histiocytosis • Neuroblastoma • Wilms tumor
INCREASED SIZE OF VASCULAR SPACE
Intrahepatic obstruction to hepatic vein outflow • Veno-occlusive disease • Hepatic vein thrombosis (Budd-Chiari syndrome) • Hepatic vein web Suprahepatic • Congestive heart failure • Pericardial disease • Tamponade Constrictive pericarditis Hematopoietic: sickle cell anemia, thalassemia
INCREASED SIZE OF BILIARY SPACE
Congenital hepatic fibrosis Caroli disease Extrahepatic obstruction
IDIOPATHIC
Various • Riedel lobe • Normal variant • Downward displacement of diaphragm

can be palpated as a broad mass normally in some people. An enlarged left lobe of the liver is palpable in the epigastrium of some patients with cirrhosis. Downward displacement of the liver by the diaphragm (hyperinflation) or thoracic organs can create an erroneous impression of hepatomegaly.

Examination of the liver should note the consistency, contour, tenderness, and presence of any masses or bruits, as well as assessment of spleen size. Documentation of the presence of ascites and any stigmata of chronic liver disease is important.

Ultrasonography (US) is useful in assessment of liver size and consistency, as well as gallbladder size. Hyperechogenic hepatic parenchyma can be seen with metabolic disease (glycogen storage disease) or fatty liver (obesity, malnutrition, hyperalimentation, corticosteroids).

Gallbladder length normally varies from 1.5-5.5 cm (average, 3.0 cm) in infants to 4-8 cm in adolescents; width ranges from 0.5 to 2.5 cm for all ages. Gallbladder distention may be seen in infants with sepsis. The gallbladder is often absent in infants with biliary atresia.

Jaundice (Icterus)

Yellow discoloration of the sclera, skin, and mucous membranes is a sign of hyperbilirubinemia (Chapter 96.3). Clinically apparent jaundice in children and adults occurs when the serum concentration of bilirubin reaches 2-3 mg/dL (34-51 μmol/L); the neonate might not appear icteric until the bilirubin level is >5 mg/dL (>85 μmol/L). Jaundice may be the earliest and only sign of hepatic dysfunction. Liver disease must be suspected in the infant who appears only mildly jaundiced but has dark urine or acholic (light-colored) stools. Immediate evaluation to establish the cause is required.

Measurement of the total serum bilirubin concentration allows quantitation of jaundice. Bilirubin occurs in plasma in 4 forms: *unconjugated* bilirubin tightly bound to albumin; *free or unbound bilirubin* (the form responsible for kernicterus, because it can cross cell membranes); *conjugated bilirubin* (the only fraction to appear in urine); and *δ fraction* (bilirubin covalently bound to albumin), which appears in serum when hepatic excretion of conjugated bilirubin is impaired in patients with hepatobiliary disease. The δ fraction permits conjugated bilirubin to persist in the circulation and delays resolution of jaundice. Although the terms *direct* and *indirect* bilirubin are used equivalently with *conjugated* and *unconjugated* bilirubin, this is not quantitatively correct, because the direct fraction includes both conjugated bilirubin and δ bilirubin. An elevation of the serum bile acid level is often seen in the presence of any form of cholestasis.

Investigation of jaundice in an infant or older child must include determination of the accumulation of both unconjugated and conjugated bilirubin. Unconjugated hyperbilirubinemia might indicate increased production, hemolysis, reduced hepatic removal, or altered metabolism of bilirubin (Table 347-2). Conjugated hyperbilirubinemia reflects decreased excretion by damaged hepatic parenchymal cells or disease of the biliary tract, which may be due to obstruction, sepsis, toxins, inflammation, and genetic or metabolic disease (Table 347-3).

Pruritus

Intense generalized itching, often with skin excoriation, can occur in patients with cholestasis (conjugated hyperbilirubinemia). Pruritus is unrelated to the degree of hyperbilirubinemia; deeply jaundiced patients can be asymptomatic. Although retained components of bile are likely important, the cause is probably multifactorial, as evidenced by the symptomatic relief of pruritus after administration of various therapeutic agents including bile acid-binding agents (cholestyramine), choleretic agents (ursodeoxycholic acid), opiate antagonists, antihistamines, and antibiotics (rifampin). Surgical diversion of bile (partial external biliary diversion) can also provide relief for medically refractory pruritus.

Table 347-2 DIFFERENTIAL DIAGNOSIS OF UNCONJUGATED HYPERBILIRUBINEMIA

INCREASED PRODUCTION OF UNCONJUGATED BILIRUBIN FROM HEME
Hemolytic Disease (Hereditary or Acquired)
Isoimmune hemolysis (neonatal; acute or delayed transfusion reaction; autoimmune)
• Rh incompatibility
• ABO incompatibility
• Other blood group incompatibilities
Congenital spherocytosis
Hereditary elliptocytosis
Infantile pyknocytosis
Erythrocyte enzyme defects
Hemoglobinopathy
• Sickle cell anemia
• Thalassemia
• Others
Sepsis
Microangiopathy
• Hemolytic-uremic syndrome
• Hemangioma
• Mechanical trauma (heart valve)
Ineffective erythropoiesis
Drugs
Infection
Enclosed hematoma
Polycythemia
• Diabetic mother
• Fetal transfusion (recipient)
• Delayed cord clamping
DECREASED DELIVERY OF UNCONJUGATED BILIRUBIN (IN PLASMA) TO HEPATOCYTE
Right-sided congestive heart failure
Portacaval shunt
DECREASED BILIRUBIN UPTAKE ACROSS HEPATOCYTE MEMBRANE
Presumed enzyme transporter deficiency
Competitive inhibition
• Breast milk jaundice
• Lucey-Driscoll syndrome
• Drug inhibition (radiocontrast material)
Miscellaneous
• Hypothyroidism
• Hypoxia
• Acidosis
DECREASED STORAGE OF UNCONJUGATED BILIRUBIN IN CYTOSOL (DECREASED Y AND Z PROTEINS)
Competitive inhibition
Fever
DECREASED BIOTRANSFORMATION (CONJUGATION)
Neonatal jaundice (physiologic)
Inhibition (drugs)
Hereditary (Crigler-Najjar)
• Type I (complete enzyme deficiency)
• Type II (partial deficiency)
Gilbert disease
Hepatocellular dysfunction
ENTEROHEPATIC RECIRCULATION
Breast milk jaundice
Intestinal obstruction
• Ileal atresia
• Hirschsprung disease
• Cystic fibrosis
• Pyloric stenosis
Antibiotic administration

Spider Angiomas
Vascular spiders (telangiectasias), characterized by central pulsating arterioles from which small, wiry venules radiate, may be seen in patients with chronic liver disease; these are usually most prominent on the face and chest. They presumably reflect altered estrogen metabolism in the presence of hepatic dysfunction.

Palmar Erythema
Blotchy erythema, most noticeable over the thenar and hypothenar eminences and on the tips of the fingers, is also noted in patients with chronic liver disease. This may be due to vasodilation and increased blood flow.

Xanthomas
The marked elevation of serum cholesterol levels (to >500 mg/dL) associated with some forms of chronic cholestasis can cause the deposition of lipid in the dermis and subcutaneous tissue. Brown nodules can develop, 1st over the extensor surfaces of the extremities; rarely, xanthelasma of the eyelids develops.

Portal Hypertension
The portal vein drains the splanchnic area (abdominal portion of the gastrointestinal tract, pancreas, and spleen) into the hepatic sinusoids. Normal portal pressure gradient, the pressure difference between the portal vein and the systemic veins (hepatic veins or inferior vena cava), is 3-6 mm Hg. Clinically significant portal hypertension exists when pressure exceeds a threshold of 10 mm Hg. Portal hypertension is the main complication of cirrhosis, directly responsible for 2 of its most common and potentially lethal complications: ascites and variceal hemorrhage.

Ascites
The onset of ascites in the child with chronic liver disease means that the 2 prerequisite conditions for ascites are present: portal hypertension and hepatic insufficiency. Ascites can also be associated with nephrotic syndrome and other urinary tract abnormalities, metabolic diseases (such as lysosomal storage diseases), congenital or acquired heart disease, and hydrops fetalis. Factors favoring the intra-abdominal accumulation of fluid include decreased plasma colloid osmotic pressure, increased capillary hydrostatic pressure, increased ascitic colloid osmotic fluid pressure, and decreased ascitic fluid hydrostatic pressure. Abnormal renal sodium retention must be considered (Chapter 362).

Variceal Hemorrhage
Gastroesophageal varices are the more clinically significant portosystemic collaterals because of their propensity to rupture and cause life-threatening hemorrhage. Variceal hemorrhage results from increased pressure within the varix, which leads to changes in the diameter of the varix and increased wall tension. When the variceal wall strength is exceeded, physical rupture of the varix results. Given the high blood flow and pressure in the portosystemic collateral system, coupled with the lack of a natural mechanism to tamponade variceal bleeding, the rate of hemorrhage can be striking.

Encephalopathy
Hepatic encephalopathy can involve any neurologic function, and it can be prominent or present in subtle forms such as deterioration of school performance, depression, or emotional outbursts. It can be recurrent and precipitated by intercurrent illness, drugs, bleeding, or electrolyte and acid-base disturbances. The appearance of hepatic encephalopathy depends on the presence of portosystemic shunting, alterations in the blood-brain barrier, and the interactions of toxic metabolites with the central nervous system. Postulated causes include altered ammonia metabolism, synergistic neurotoxins, or false neurotransmitters with plasma amino acid imbalance.

Endocrine Abnormalities
Endocrine abnormalities are more common in adults with hepatic disease than in children. They reflect alterations in hepatic synthetic, storage, and metabolic functions, including those concerned with hormonal metabolism in the liver. Proteins that bind hormones in plasma are synthesized in the liver, and steroid hormones are conjugated in the liver and excreted in the urine;

Table 347-3 DIFFERENTIAL DIAGNOSIS OF NEONATAL AND INFANTILE CHOLESTASIS

INFECTIOUS Generalized bacterial sepsis Viral hepatitis • Hepatitis A, B, C, D • Cytomegalovirus • Rubella virus • Herpesvirus: herpes simplex, human herpesvirus 6 and 7 • Varicella virus • Coxsackievirus • Echovirus • Reovirus type 3 • Parvovirus B19 • HIV • Adenovirus Others • Toxoplasmosis • Syphilis • Tuberculosis • Listeriosis • Urinary tract infection	**GENETIC OR CHROMOSOMAL** Trisomy 17, 18, 21 Donahue syndrome **INTRAHEPATIC CHOLESTASIS SYNDROMES** "Idiopathic" neonatal hepatitis Alagille syndrome (arteriohepatic dysplasia) Nonsyndromic bile duct paucity syndrome Intrahepatic cholestasis (PFIC) • FIC-1 deficiency • BSEP deficiency • MDR3 deficiency Familial benign recurrent cholestasis associated with lymphedema (Aagenaes) Congenital hepatic fibrosis Caroli disease (cystic dilatation of intrahepatic ducts) **EXTRAHEPATIC DISEASES** Biliary atresia Sclerosing cholangitis Bile duct stricture/stenosis Choledochal-pancreaticoductal junction anomaly Spontaneous perforation of the bile duct Choledochal cyst Mass (neoplasia, stone) Bile/mucous plug ("inspissated bile")
TOXIC Sepsis Parenteral nutrition related Drug related **METABOLIC** Disorders of amino acid metabolism • Tyrosinemia Disorders of lipid metabolism • Wolman disease • Niemann-Pick disease (type C) • Gaucher disease Cholesterol ester storage disease Disorders of carbohydrate metabolism • Galactosemia • Fructosemia • Glycogenosis IV Disorders of bile acid biosynthesis Other metabolic defects • α1-Antitrypsin deficiency • Cystic fibrosis • Hypopituitarism • Hypothyroidism • Zellweger (cerebrohepatorenal) syndrome • Neonatal iron storage disease • Indian childhood cirrhosis/infantile copper overload • Congenital disorders of glycosylation • Mitochondrial hepatopathies • Citrin deficiency	**MISCELLANEOUS** Shock and hypoperfusion Associated with enteritis Associated with intestinal obstruction Neonatal lupus erythematosus Myeloproliferative disease (trisomy 21) Hemophagocytic lymphohistiocytosis (HLH) Arthrogryposis cholestatic pigmentary (ARC) syndrome

failure of such functions can have clinical consequences. Endocrine abnormalities can also result from malnutrition or specific deficiencies.

Renal Dysfunction

Systemic disease or toxins can affect the liver and kidneys simultaneously, or parenchymal liver disease can produce secondary impairment of renal function. In hepatobiliary disorders, there may be renal alterations in sodium and water economy, impaired renal concentrating ability, and alterations in potassium metabolism. Ascites in patients with cirrhosis may be related to inappropriate retention of sodium by the kidneys and expansion of plasma volume, or it may be related to sodium retention mediated by diminished effective plasma volume. **Hepatorenal syndrome** (HRS) is defined as functional renal failure in patients with end-stage liver disease. The pathophysiology of HRS is poorly defined, but the hallmark is intense renal vasoconstriction (mediated by hemodynamic, humoral, or neurogenic mechanisms) with coexistent systemic vasodilation. The diagnosis is supported by the findings of oliguria (<1 mL/kg/day), a characteristic pattern of urine electrolyte abnormalities (urine sodium <10 mEq/L, fractional excretion of sodium of <1%, urine : plasma creatinine ratio <10, and normal urinary sediment), absence of hypovolemia, and exclusion of other kidney pathology. The best treatment of HRS is timely liver transplantation, because complete renal recovery can be expected.

Pulmonary Involvement

Hepatopulmonary syndrome is characterized by the typical triad of hypoxemia, intrapulmonary vascular dilations, and liver disease. There is intrapulmonic right-to-left shunting of blood, which results in systemic desaturation. It should be suspected and investigated in the child with chronic liver disease with history of shortness of breath or exercise intolerance and clinical examination findings of cyanosis (particularly of the lips and fingers), digital clubbing, and oxygen saturations <96%, particularly in the upright position. Treatment is timely liver transplantation; successful pulmonary resolution follows.

Recurrent Cholangitis

Ascending infection of the biliary system is often seen in pediatric cholestatic disorders, due most commonly to gram-negative enteric organisms, such as *Escherichia coli, Klebsiella, Pseudomonas,* and *Enterococcus.* Liver transplantation is the definitive treatment for recurrent cholangitis, especially when medical therapy is not effective.

Miscellaneous Manifestations of Liver Dysfunction

Nonspecific signs of acute and chronic liver disease include anorexia, which often affects patients with anicteric hepatitis and with cirrhosis associated with chronic cholestasis; abdominal pain or distention resulting from ascites, spontaneous peritonitis, or visceromegaly; malnutrition and growth failure; and bleeding, which may be due to altered synthesis of coagulation factors (biliary obstruction with vitamin K deficiency or excessive hepatic damage) or to portal hypertension with hypersplenism. In the presence of hypersplenism, there can be decreased synthesis of specific clotting factors, production of qualitatively abnormal proteins, or alterations in platelet number and function. Altered drug metabolism can prolong the biologic half-life of commonly administered medications.

BIBLIOGRAPHY

Please visit the Nelson Textbook of Pediatrics *website at www.expertconsult.com for the complete bibliography.*

347.1 Evaluation of Patients with Possible Liver Dysfunction

Lynelle M. Boamah and William F. Balistreri

Adequate evaluation of an infant, child, or adolescent with suspected liver disease involves an appropriate and accurate history, a carefully performed physical examination, and skillful interpretation of signs and symptoms. Further evaluation is aided by judicious selection of diagnostic tests, followed by the use of imaging modalities or a liver biopsy. Most of the so-called liver function tests do not measure specific hepatic functions: a rise in serum aminotransferase levels reflects liver cell injury, an increase in immunoglobulin levels reflects an immunologic response to injury, or an elevation in serum bilirubin levels can reflect any of several disturbances of bilirubin metabolism (see Tables 347-2 and 347-3). Any single biochemical assay provides limited information, which must be placed in the context of the entire clinical picture. The most cost-efficient approach is to become familiar with the rationale, implications, and limitations of a selected group of tests so that specific questions can be answered. Young infants with cholestatic jaundice should be evaluated promptly to identify patients needing surgical intervention.

For a patient with suspected liver disease, evaluation addresses the following issues in sequence: Is liver disease present? If so, what is its nature? What is its severity? Is specific treatment available? How can we monitor the response to treatment? What is the prognosis?

BIOCHEMICAL TESTS

Laboratory tests commonly used to screen for or to confirm a suspicion of liver disease include measurements of serum aminotransferase, bilirubin (total and fractionated), and alkaline phosphatase (AP) levels, as well as determinations of prothrombin time (PT) or international normalized ratio (INR) and albumin level. These tests are complementary, provide an estimation of synthetic and excretory functions, and might suggest the nature of the disturbance (inflammation or cholestasis).

The severity of the liver disease may be reflected in clinical signs or biochemical alterations. Clinical signs include encephalopathy, variceal hemorrhage, worsening jaundice, apparent shrinkage of liver mass owing to massive necrosis, or onset of ascites. Biochemical alterations include hypoglycemia, acidosis, hyperammonemia, electrolyte imbalance, continued hyperbilirubinemia, marked hypoalbuminemia, or a prolonged PT or INR that is unresponsive to parenteral administration of vitamin K.

Acute liver cell injury (parenchymal disease) due to viral hepatitis, drug- or toxin-induced liver disease, shock, hypoxemia, or metabolic disease is best reflected by a marked increase in serum aminotransferase levels. Cholestasis (obstructive disease) involves regurgitation of bile components into serum; the serum levels of total and conjugated bilirubin and serum bile acids are elevated. Elevations in serum AP, 5′ nucleotidase (5′NT), and γ-glutamyl transpeptidase (GGT) levels are also sensitive indicators of obstruction or inflammation of the biliary tract. Fractionation of the total serum bilirubin level into conjugated and unconjugated bilirubin fractions helps to distinguish between elevations caused by processes such as hemolysis and those caused by hepatic dysfunction. A predominant elevation in the conjugated bilirubin level provides a relatively sensitive index of hepatocellular disease or hepatic excretory dysfunction.

Alanine aminotransferase (ALT, serum glutamate pyruvate transaminase) is liver specific, whereas aspartate aminotransferase (AST, serum glutamic-oxaloacetic transaminase) is derived from other organs in addition to the liver. The most marked rises of AST and ALT levels can occur with acute hepatocellular injury; a several thousand–fold elevation can result from acute viral hepatitis, toxic injury, hypoxia, or hypoperfusion. After blunt abdominal trauma, parallel elevations in aminotransferase levels can provide an early clue to hepatic injury. A differential rise or fall in AST and ALT levels sometimes provides useful information. In acute hepatitis, the rise in ALT may be greater than the rise in AST. In alcohol-induced liver injury, fulminant echovirus infection, and various metabolic diseases, more predominant rises in the AST level are reported. In chronic liver disease or in intrahepatic and extrahepatic biliary obstruction, AST and ALT elevations may be less marked. Elevated serum aminotransferase levels are seen in nonalcoholic fatty liver disease (NAFLD) and nonalcoholic steatohepatitis (NASH), chronic liver disorders seen in obese children; the notable characteristic is histology similar to alcoholic-induced liver injury in the absence of alcohol abuse.

Hepatic synthetic function is reflected in serum albumin and protein levels and in the PT or INR. Examination of serum globulin concentration and of the relative amounts of the globulin fractions may be helpful. Patients with autoimmune hepatitis often have high gamma-globulin levels and increased titers of anti–smooth muscle, antinuclear, and anti–liver-kidney-microsome antibodies. Antimitochondrial antibodies may also be found in patients with autoimmune hepatitis. A resurgence in α-fetoprotein levels can suggest hepatoma, hepatoblastoma, or hereditary tyrosinemia. Hypoalbuminemia caused by depressed synthesis can complicate severe liver disease and serve as a prognostic factor. Deficiencies of factor V and of the vitamin K–dependent factors (II, VII, IX, and X) can occur in patients with severe liver disease or fulminant hepatic failure. If the PT or INR is prolonged as a result of intestinal malabsorption of vitamin K (resulting from cholestasis) or decreased nutritional intake of vitamin K, parenteral administration of vitamin K should correct the coagulopathy, leading to normalization within 12-24 hr. Unresponsiveness to vitamin K suggests severe hepatic disease. Persistently low levels of factor VII are evidence of a poor prognosis in fulminant liver disease.

Interpretation of results of biochemical tests of hepatic structure and function must be made in the context of age-related changes. The activity of AP varies considerably with age. Normal growing children have significant elevations of serum AP activity originating from influx into serum of the isoenzyme that originates in bone, particularly in rapidly growing adolescents. An isolated increase in AP does not indicate hepatic or biliary disease if other liver function test results are normal. Other enzymes such as 5′NT and GGT are increased in cholestatic conditions, and may be more specific for hepatobiliary disease. 5′NT is not found in bone. GGT exhibits high enzyme activity in early life that declines rapidly with age. Cholesterol concentrations increase throughout life. Cholesterol levels may be markedly elevated in patients with intra- or extrahepatic cholestasis and decreased in severe acute liver disease such as hepatitis.

Interpretation of serum ammonia values must be carried out with caution because of variability in their physiologic determinants and the inherent difficulty in laboratory measurement.

LIVER BIOPSY

Liver biopsy combined with clinical data can suggest a cause for hepatocellular injury or cholestatic disease in most cases. Specimens of liver tissue can be used to determine a precise histologic diagnosis in patients with neonatal cholestasis, chronic hepatitis, NAFLD or NASH, metabolic liver disease, intrahepatic cholestasis, congenital hepatic fibrosis, or undefined portal hypertension; for enzyme analysis to detect inborn errors of metabolism; and for analysis of stored material such as iron, copper, or specific metabolites. Liver biopsies can monitor responses to therapy or detect complications of treatment with potentially hepatotoxic agents, such as aspirin, anti-infectives (erythromycin, minocycline, ketoconazole, isoniazid), antimetabolites, antineoplastics, or anticonvulsant agents.

In infants and children, needle biopsy of the liver is easily accomplished percutaneously. The amount of tissue obtained, even in small infants, is usually sufficient for histologic interpretation and for biochemical analyses, if the latter are deemed necessary. Percutaneous liver biopsy can be performed safely in infants as young as 1 wk of age. Patients usually require only conscious sedation and local anesthesia. Contraindications to the percutaneous approach include prolonged PT or INR; thrombocytopenia; suspicion of a vascular, cystic, or infectious lesion in the path of the needle; and severe ascites. If administration of fresh frozen plasma or of platelet transfusions fails to correct a prolonged PT, INR, or thrombocytopenia, a tissue specimen can be obtained via alternative techniques. Considerations include either the open laparotomy (wedge) approach by a general surgeon or the transjugular approach under US and fluoroscopic guidance by an experienced pediatric interventional radiologist in an appropriately equipped fluoroscopy suite. The risk of development of a complication such as hemorrhage, hematoma, creation of an arteriovenous fistula, pneumothorax, or bile peritonitis is small.

HEPATIC IMAGING PROCEDURES

Various techniques help define the size, shape, and architecture of the liver and the anatomy of the intrahepatic and extrahepatic biliary trees. Although imaging might not provide a precise histologic and biochemical diagnosis, specific questions can be answered, such as whether hepatomegaly is related to accumulation of fat or glycogen or is due to a tumor or cyst. These studies can direct further evaluation such as percutaneous biopsy and make possible prompt referral of patients with biliary obstruction to a surgeon. Choice of imaging procedure should be part of a carefully formulated diagnostic approach, with avoidance of redundant demonstrations by several techniques.

A plain x-ray study can suggest hepatomegaly, but a carefully performed physical examination gives a more reliable assessment of liver size. The liver might appear less dense than normal in patients with fatty infiltration or more dense with deposition of heavy metals such as iron. A hepatic or biliary tract mass can displace an air-filled loop of bowel. Calcifications may be evident in the liver (parasitic or neoplastic disease), in the vasculature (portal vein thrombosis), or in the gallbladder or biliary tree (gallstones). Collections of gas may be seen within the liver (abscess), biliary tract, or portal circulation (necrotizing enterocolitis).

US provides information about the size, composition, and blood flow of the liver. Increased echogenicity is observed with fatty infiltration; mass lesions as small as 1-2 cm may be shown. US has replaced cholangiography in detecting stones in the gallbladder or biliary tree. Even in neonates, US can assess gallbladder size, detect dilatation of the biliary tract, and define a choledochal cyst. In infants with biliary atresia, US findings might include small or absent gallbladder; nonvisualization of the common duct; and presence of the triangular cord sign, a triangular or tubular-shaped echogenic density in the bifurcation of the portal vein, representing fibrous remnants at the porta hepatis. In patients with portal hypertension, Doppler US can evaluate patency of the portal vein, demonstrate collateral circulation, and assess size of spleen and amount of ascites. Relatively small amounts of ascitic fluid can also be detected. The use of Doppler US has been helpful in determining vascular patency after liver transplantation.

CT scanning provides information similar to that obtained by US but is less suitable for use in patients <2 yr of age because of the small size of structures, the paucity of intra-abdominal fat for contrast, and the need for heavy sedation or general anesthesia. MRI is a useful alternative. Magnetic resonance cholangiography can be of value in differentiating biliary tract lesions. CT scan or MRI may be more accurate than US in detecting focal lesions such as tumors, cysts, and abscesses. When enhanced by contrast medium, CT scanning can reveal a neoplastic mass density only slightly different from that of a normal liver. When a hepatic tumor is suspected, CT scanning is the best method to define anatomic extent, solid or cystic nature, and vascularity. CT scanning can also reveal subtle differences in density of liver parenchyma, the average liver attenuation coefficient being reduced with fatty infiltration. Increases in density can occur with diffuse iron deposition or with glycogen storage. In differentiating obstructive from nonobstructive cholestasis, CT scanning or MRI identifies the precise level of obstruction more often than US. Either CT scanning or US may be used to guide percutaneously placed fine needles for biopsies, aspiration of specific lesions, or cholangiography.

Radionuclide scanning relies on selective uptake of a radiopharmaceutical agent. Commonly used agents include technetium 99m-labeled sulfur colloid, which undergoes phagocytosis by Kupffer cells; ^{99m}Tc-iminodiacetic acid agents, which are taken up by hepatocytes and excreted into bile in a fashion similar to bilirubin; and gallium-67, which is concentrated in inflammatory and neoplastic cells. The anatomic resolution possible with hepatic scintiscans is generally less than that obtained with CT scanning, MRI, or US.

The ^{99m}Tc-sulfur colloid scan can detect focal lesions (tumors, cysts, abscesses) >2-3 cm in diameter. This modality can help to evaluate patients with possible cirrhosis and with patchy hepatic uptake and a shift of colloid uptake from liver to bone marrow.

The ^{99m}Tc-substituted iminodiacetic acid dyes can differentiate intrahepatic cholestasis from extrahepatic obstruction in neonates. Imaging results are best when scanning is preceded by a 5-7 day period of treatment with phenobarbital to stimulate bile flow. After intravenous injection, the isotope is normally detected in the bowel within 1-2 hr. In the presence of extrahepatic obstruction, excretion of the isotope is delayed; accordingly, serial scans should be made for up to 24 hr after injection. Early in the course of biliary atresia, hepatocyte function is usually good; uptake (clearance) occurs rapidly, but excretion into the intestine is absent. In contrast, uptake is poor in parenchymal liver disease, such as neonatal hepatitis, but excretion into the bile and intestine eventually ensues.

Cholangiography, direct visualization of the intrahepatic and extrahepatic biliary tree after injection of opaque material, may be required in some patients to evaluate the cause, location, or extent of biliary obstruction. Percutaneous transhepatic cholangiography with a fine needle is the technique of choice in infants and young children. The likelihood of opacifying the biliary tract is excellent in patients in whom CT scanning, MRI,

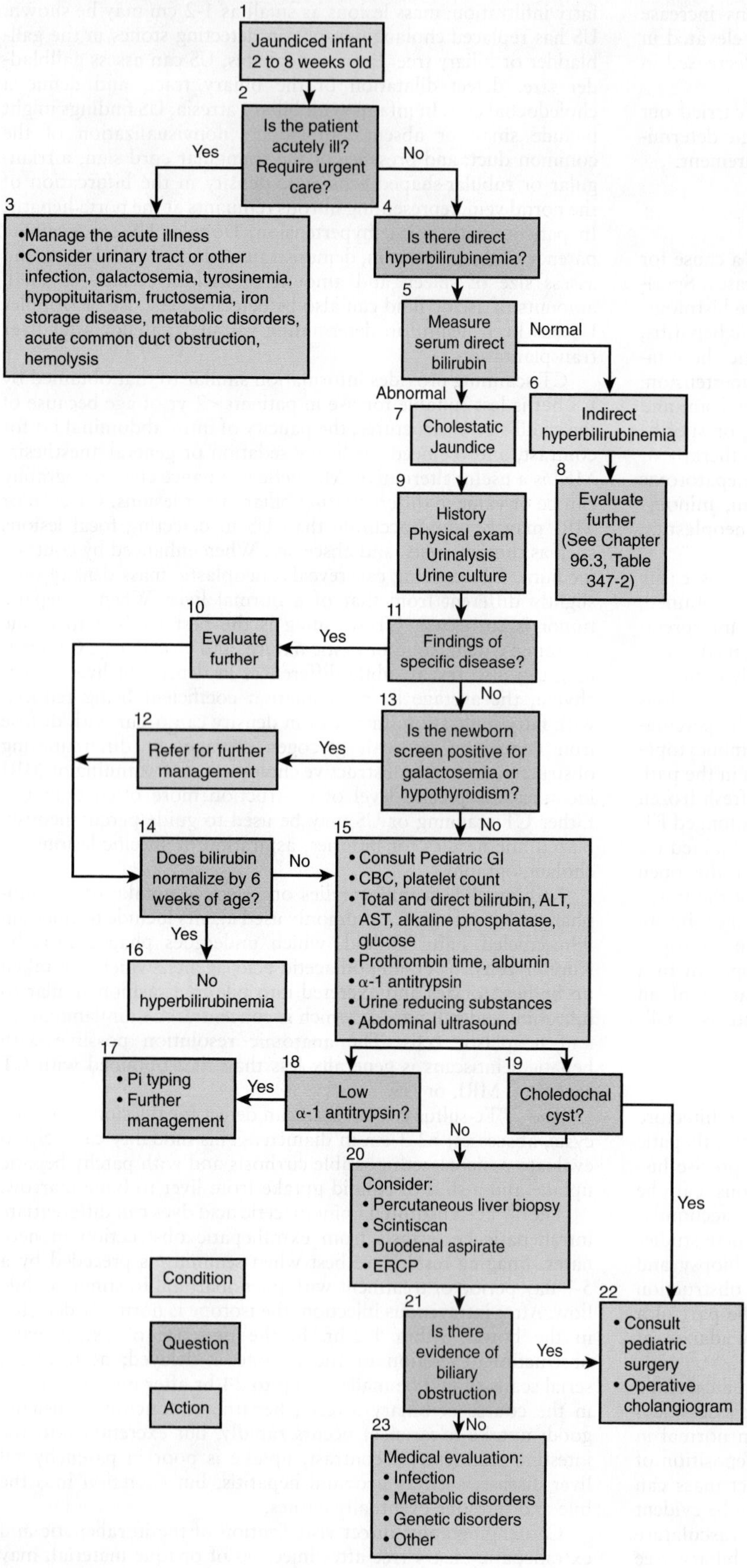
1
Jaundiced infant 2 to 8 weeks old
2
Is the patient acutely ill? Require urgent care?
Yes
No
3
•Manage the acute illness
•Consider urinary tract or other infection, galactosemia, tyrosinemia, hypopituitarism, fructosemia, iron storage disease, metabolic disorders, acute common duct obstruction, hemolysis
4
Is there direct hyperbilirubinemia?
5
Measure serum direct bilirubin
Normal
Abnormal
6
Indirect hyperbilirubinemia
7
Cholestatic Jaundice
8
Evaluate further (See Chapter 96.3, Table 347-2)
9
History
Physical exam
Urinalysis
Urine culture
10
Evaluate further
Yes
11
Findings of specific disease?
No
12
Refer for further management
Yes
13
Is the newborn screen positive for galactosemia or hypothyroidism?
No
14
Does bilirubin normalize by 6 weeks of age?
No
Yes
15
• Consult Pediatric GI
• CBC, platelet count
• Total and direct bilirubin, ALT, AST, alkaline phosphatase, glucose
• Prothrombin time, albumin
• α-1 antitrypsin
• Urine reducing substances
• Abdominal ultrasound
16
No hyperbilirubinemia
17
• Pi typing
• Further management
18
Yes
Low α-1 antitrypsin?
No
19
Choledochal cyst?
Yes
20
Consider:
• Percutaneous liver biopsy
• Scintiscan
• Duodenal aspirate
• ERCP
Condition
Question
Action
21
Is there evidence of biliary obstruction?
Yes
22
• Consult pediatric surgery
• Operative cholangiogram
No
23
Medical evaluation:
• Infection
• Metabolic disorders
• Genetic disorders
• Other

Figure 347-1 Cholestasis clinical practice guideline. Algorithm for a 2-8 wk old. ALT, alanine aminotransferase; AST, aspartate aminotransferase; ERCP, endoscopic retrograde cholangiopancreatography. (Moyer V, Freese DK, Whitington PF, et al; North American Society for Pediatric Gastroenterology, Hepatology and Nutrition: Guideline for the evaluation of cholestatic jaundice in infants: recommendations of the North American Society for Pediatric Gastroenterology, Hepatology and Nutrition, *J Pediatr Gastroenterol Nutr* 39:115–128, 2004.)

or ultrasonography demonstrates dilated ducts. Percutaneous transhepatic cholangiography has been used to outline the biliary ductal system.

Endoscopic retrograde cholangiopancreatography (ERCP) is an alternative method of examining the bile ducts in older children. The papilla of Vater is cannulated under direct vision through a fiberoptic endoscope, and contrast material is injected into the biliary and pancreatic ducts to outline the anatomy.

Selective angiography of the celiac, superior mesenteric, or hepatic artery can be used to visualize the hepatic or portal circulation. Both arterial and venous circulatory systems of the liver can be examined. Angiography is often required to define the blood supply of tumors before surgery and is useful in the study of patients with known or presumed portal hypertension. The patency of the portal system, the extent of collateral circulation, and the caliber of vessels under consideration for a shunting procedure can be evaluated. MRI can provide similar information.

DIAGNOSTIC APPROACH TO INFANTS WITH JAUNDICE

The North American Society for Pediatric Gastroenterology, Hepatology and Nutrition has published an algorithm for the evaluation of cholestatic jaundice in neonates and young infants. Well-appearing infants can have cholestatic jaundice. Biliary atresia and neonatal hepatitis are the most common causes of cholestasis in early infancy. Biliary atresia portends a poor prognosis unless it is identified early. The best outcome for this disorder is with early surgical reconstruction (45-60 days of age). History, physical examination, and the detection of a conjugated hyperbilirubinemia via examination of total and direct bilirubin are the 1st steps in evaluating the jaundiced infant (Fig. 347-1). Consultation with a pediatric gastroenterologist should be sought early in the course of the evaluation.

BIBLIOGRAPHY

Please visit the Nelson Textbook of Pediatrics *website at www.expertconsult.com for the complete bibliography.*

Chapter 348
Cholestasis

348.1 Neonatal Cholestasis

H. Hesham A-kader and William F. Balistreri

Neonatal cholestasis is defined biochemically as prolonged elevation of the serum levels of conjugated bilirubin beyond the 1st 14 days of life. Jaundice that appears after 2 wk of age, progresses after this time, or does not resolve at this time should be evaluated and a conjugated bilirubin level determined. Cholestasis in a newborn can be due to infectious, genetic, metabolic, or undefined abnormalities giving rise to *mechanical* obstruction of bile flow or to *functional* impairment of hepatic excretory function and bile secretion (see Table 347-3). Mechanical lesions include stricture or obstruction of the common bile duct; biliary atresia is the prototypic obstructive abnormality. Functional impairment of bile secretion can result from congenital defects or damage to liver cells or to the biliary secretory apparatus.

Neonatal cholestasis can be divided into extrahepatic and intrahepatic disease (Fig. 348-1). The clinical features of any form of cholestasis are similar. In an affected neonate, the diagnosis of certain entities, such as galactosemia, sepsis, or hypothyroidism, is relatively simple and a part of most neonatal screening programs. In most cases, the cause of cholestasis is more obscure. Differentiation among biliary atresia, idiopathic neonatal hepatitis, and intrahepatic cholestasis is particularly difficult.

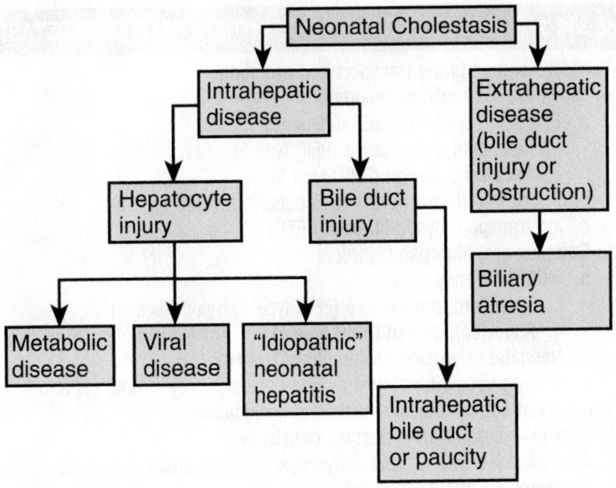

Figure 348-1 Neonatal cholestasis. Conceptual approach to the group of diseases presenting as cholestasis in the neonate. There are areas of overlap: patients with biliary atresia might have some degree of intrahepatic injury. Patients with "idiopathic" neonatal hepatitis might, in the future, be determined to have a primary metabolic or viral disease.

MECHANISMS

Metabolic liver disease caused by inborn errors of bile acid metabolism or transport is associated with accumulation of atypical toxic primitive bile acids and failure to produce normal choleretic and trophic bile acids. The clinical and histologic manifestations are nonspecific and are similar to those in other forms of neonatal hepatobiliary injury. Autoimmune mechanisms may also be responsible for some of the enigmatic forms of neonatal liver injury.

Some of the histologic manifestations of hepatic injury in early life are not seen in older patients. Giant cell transformation of hepatocytes occurs commonly in infants with cholestasis and can occur in any form of neonatal liver injury. It is more common and more severe in intrahepatic forms of cholestasis. The clinical and histologic findings that exist in patients with neonatal hepatitis and in those with biliary atresia are quite disparate; the basic process is an undefined initiating insult causing inflammation of the liver cells or of the cells within the biliary tract. If bile duct epithelium is the predominant site of disease, cholangitis can result and lead to progressive sclerosis and narrowing of the biliary tree, the ultimate state being complete obliteration (biliary atresia). Injury to liver cells can present the clinical and histologic picture of "neonatal hepatitis." This concept does not account for the precise mechanism, but it offers an explanation for well-documented cases of unexpected postnatal evolution of these disease processes; infants initially regarded as having neonatal hepatitis, with a patent biliary system shown on cholangiography, can later develop biliary atresia.

Functional abnormalities in the generation of bile flow can also have a role in neonatal cholestasis. Bile flow is directly dependent on effective hepatic bile acid excretion by the hepatocytes. During the phase of relatively inefficient liver cell transport and metabolism of bile acids in early life, minor degrees of hepatic injury can further decrease bile flow and lead to production of atypical and potentially toxic bile acids. Selective impairment of a single step in the series of events involved in hepatic excretion produces the full expression of a cholestatic syndrome. Specific defects in bile acid synthesis are found in infants with various forms of intrahepatic cholestasis (Table 348-1). Severe forms of familial cholestasis have been associated with neonatal hemochromatosis and an aberration in the contractile proteins that compose the cytoskeleton of the hepatocyte. Neonatal hemo-

Table 348-1 PROPOSED SUBTYPES OF INTRAHEPATIC CHOLESTASIS

A. Disorders of membrane transport and secretion
  1. Disorders of canalicular secretion
    a. Bile acid transport: BSEP deficiency
      i. Persistent, progressive (PFIC type 2)
      ii. Recurrent, benign (BRIC type 2)
    b. Phospholipid transport: MDR3 deficiency (PFIC type 3)
    c. Ion transport: cystic fibrosis (CFTR)
  2. Complex or multiorgan disorders
    a. FIC1 deficiency
      i. Persistent, progressive (PFIC type 1, Byler disease)
      ii. Recurrent, benign (BRIC type 1)
    b. Neonatal sclerosing cholangitis *(CLDN1)*
    c. Arthrogryposis-renal dysfunction-cholestasis syndrome (*VPS33B*)
B. Disorders of bile acid biosynthesis and conjugation
  1. 3-oxoΔ-4-steroid 5β-reductase deficiency
  2. 3β-hydroxy-5-C27-steroid dehydrogenase/isomerase deficiency
  3. Oxysterol 7α-hydroxylase deficiency
  4. Bile acid-CoA Ligase deficiency
  5. BAAT deficiency (familial hypercholanemia)
C. Disorders of embryogenesis
  1. Alagille syndrome (Jagged1 defect, syndromic bile duct paucity)
  2. Ductal plate malformation (ARPKD, ADPLD, Caroli disease)
D. Unclassified (idiopathic "neonatal hepatitis"): mechanism unknown

Note: FIC1 deficiency, BSEP deficiency, and some of the disorders of bile acid biosynthesis are characterized clinically by low levels of serum GGT despite the presence of cholestasis. In all other disorders listed, the serum GGT level is elevated.
ADPLD, autosomal dominant polycystic liver disease (cysts in liver only); ARPKD, autosomal recessive polycystic kidney disease (cysts in liver and kidney); BAAT, bile acid transporter; BRIC, benign recurrent intrahepatic cholestasis; BSEP, bile salt export pump in; GGT, γ-glutamyl transpeptidase; PFIC, progressive familial intrahepatic cholestasis.
From Balistreri WF, Bezerra JA, Jansen P, et al: Intrahepatic cholestasis: summary of an American Association for the Study of Liver Diseases single-topic conference, *Hepatology* 42:222–235, 2005.

Table 348-2 VALUE OF SPECIFIC TESTS IN THE EVALUATION OF PATIENTS WITH SUSPECTED NEONATAL CHOLESTASIS

TEST	RATIONALE
Serum bilirubin fractionation (i.e., assessment of the serum level of conjugated bilirubin)	Indicates cholestasis
Assessment of stool color (does the baby have pigmented or acholic stools?)	Indicates bile flow into intestine
Urine and serum bile acids measurement	Confirms cholestasis; might indicate inborn error of bile acid biosynthesis
Hepatic synthetic function (albumin, coagulation profile)	Indicates severity of hepatic dysfunction
α1-Antitrypsin phenotype	Suggests (or excludes) PiZZ
Thyroxine and TSH	Suggests (or excludes) endocrinopathy
Sweat chloride and mutation analysis	Suggests (or excludes) cystic fibrosis
Urine and serum amino acids and urine reducing substances	Suggests (or excludes) metabolic liver disease
Ultrasonography	Suggests (or excludes) choledochal cyst; might detect the triangular cord (TC) sign, suggesting biliary atresia
Hepatobiliary scintigraphy	Documents bile duct patency or obstruction
Liver biopsy	Distinguishes biliary atresia; suggests alternative diagnosis

PiZZ, protease inhibitor ZZ phenotype; TSH, thyroid-stimulating hormone.

chromatosis can also be an alloimmune-mediated gestational (maternal antibodies against fetal hepatocytes) disease responsive to maternal intravenous immunoglobulin (IVIG). Sepsis is known to cause cholestasis, presumably mediated by an endotoxin produced by *Escherichia coli.*

EVALUATION

The evaluation of the infant with jaundice should follow a logical, cost-effective sequence in a multistep process (Table 348-2). Although cholestasis in the neonate may be the initial manifestation of numerous and potentially serious disorders, the clinical manifestations are usually similar and provide very few clues about etiology. Affected infants have icterus, dark urine, light or acholic stools, and hepatomegaly, all resulting from decreased bile flow due to either hepatocyte injury or bile duct obstruction. Hepatic synthetic dysfunction can lead to hypoprothrombinemia and bleeding. Administration of vitamin K should be included in the initial treatment of cholestatic infants to prevent hemorrhage.

In contrast to unconjugated hyperbilirubinemia, which can be physiologic, cholestasis (conjugated bilirubin elevation of any degree) in the neonate is **always pathologic** and prompt differentiation is imperative. Thus the initial step is to identify the infant who has cholestasis. The next step is to recognize conditions that cause cholestasis and for which specific therapy is available to prevent further damage and avoid long-term complications such as sepsis, an endocrinopathy (hypothyroidism, panhypopituitarism), nutritional hepatotoxicity caused by a specific metabolic illness (galactosemia), or other metabolic diseases (tyrosinemia).

Hepatobiliary disease can be the initial manifestation of homozygous α_1-antitrypsin deficiency or of cystic fibrosis. Neonatal liver disease can also be associated with congenital syphilis and specific viral infections, notably echovirus and herpesviruses including cytomegalovirus (CMV). These account for a small percentage of cases of neonatal hepatitis syndrome The hepatitis viruses (A, B, C) rarely cause neonatal cholestasis.

The final and critical step in evaluating neonates with cholestasis is to differentiate extrahepatic biliary atresia from neonatal hepatitis.

INTRAHEPATIC CHOLESTASIS

Neonatal Hepatitis

The term *neonatal hepatitis* implies intrahepatic cholestasis (see Fig. 348-1), which has various forms (Tables 348-1 and 348-3).

Idiopathic neonatal hepatitis, which can occur in either a sporadic or a familial form, is a disease of unknown cause. Patients with the sporadic form presumably have a specific yet undefined metabolic or viral disease. Familial forms, on the other hand, presumably reflect a genetic or metabolic aberration; in the past, patients with α_1-antitrypsin deficiency were included in this category.

Aagenaes syndrome is a form of idiopathic familial intrahepatic cholestasis associated with lymphedema of the lower extremities. The relationship between liver disease and lymphedema is not understood and may be attributable to decreased hepatic lymph flow or hepatic lymphatic hypoplasia. Affected patients usually present with episodic cholestasis with elevation of serum aminotransferases, alkaline phosphatase, and bile acids. Between episodes, the patients are usually asymptomatic and biochemical indices improve. Compared to other types of hereditary neonatal cholestasis, patients with Aagenaes syndrome have a relatively good prognosis because >50% can expect a normal life span. The locus for Aagenaes syndrome is mapped to a 6.6cM interval on chromosome 15q.

Zellweger (cerebrohepatorenal) syndrome is a rare autosomal recessive genetic disorder marked by progressive degeneration of the liver and kidneys (Chapter 80.2). The incidence is estimated to be 1/100,000 births; the disease is usually fatal in 6-12 mo. Affected infants have severe, generalized hypotonia and markedly

Table 348-3 MOLECULAR DEFECTS CAUSING LIVER DISEASE

GENE	PROTEIN	FUNCTION, SUBSTRATE	DISORDER
ATP8b1	FIC1	P-type ATPase; aminophospholipid translocase that flips phosphatidylserine and phosphatidylethanolamine from the outer to the inner layer of the canalicular membrane	PFIC 1 (Byler disease), BRIC 1, GFC
ABCB11	BSEP	Canalicular protein with ATP-binding cassette (ABC family of proteins); works as a pump transporting bile acids through the canalicular domain	PFIC 2, BRIC 2
ABCB4	MDR3	Canalicular protein with ATP-binding cassette (ABC family of proteins); works as a phospholipid flippase in canalicular membrane	PFIC 3, ICP, cholelithiasis
AKR1D1	5β-reductase	3-oxoΔ-4-steroid 5β-reductase gene; regulates bile acid synthesis	BAS: neonatal cholestasis with giant cell hepatitis
HSD3B7	C27-3β-HSD	3β-hydroxy-5-C27-steroid oxido-reductase (C27-3β-HSD) gene; regulates bile acid synthesis	BAS: chronic intrahepatic cholestasis
CYP7BI	CYP7BI	Oxysterol 7α-hydroxylase; regulates the acidic pathway of bile acid synthesis	BAS: neonatal cholestasis with giant cell hepatitis
JAG1	JAG1	Transmembrane, cell-surface proteins that interact with Notch receptors to regulate cell fate during embryogenesis	Alagille syndrome
TJP2	Tight junction protein	Belongs to the family of membrane-associated guanylate kinase homologs that are involved in the organization of epithelial and endothelial intercellular junction; regulates paracellular permeability	FHC
BAAT	BAAT	Enzyme that transfers the bile acid moiety from the acyl coenzyme A thioester to either glycine or taurine	FHC
EPHX1	Epoxide hydrolase	Microsomal epoxide hydrolase regulates the activation and detoxification of exogenous chemicals	FHC
ABCC2	MRP2	Canalicular protein with ATP-binding cassette (ABC family of proteins); regulates canalicular transport of GSH conjugates and arsenic	Dubin-Johnson syndrome
ATP7B	ATP7B	P-type ATPase; function as copper export pump	Wilson disease
CLDN1	Claudin 1	Tight junction protein	NSC
CIRH1A	Cirhin	Cell signaling?	NAICC
CFTR	CFTR	Chloride channel with ATP-binding cassette (ABC family of proteins); regulates chloride transport	Cystic fibrosis
PKHD1	Fibrocystin	Protein involved in ciliary function and tubulogenesis	ARPKD
PRKCSH	Hepatocystin	Assembles with glucosidase II α subunit in endoplasmic reticulum	ADPLD
VPS33B	Vascular Protein sorting 33	Regulates fusion of proteins to cellular membrane	ARC

ADPLD, autosomal dominant polycystic liver disease; ARC, arthrogryposis–renal dysfunction–cholestasis syndrome*; ARPKD, autosomal recessive polycystic kidney disease; ATP, adenosine triphosphate; BAAT, bile acid transporter; BAS, bile acid synthetic defect; BRIC, benign recurrent intrahepatic cholestasis; BSEP, bile salt export pump; CFTR, cystic fibrosis transmembrane conductance regulator; FHC, familial hypercholanemia; GFC, Greenland familial cholestasis; GSH, glutathione; ICP, intrahepatic cholestasis of pregnancy; NAICC, North American Indian childhood cirrhosis; NSC, neonatal sclerosing cholangitis with ichthyosis, leukocyte vacuoles, and alopecia; PFIC, progressive familial intrahepatic cholestasis.*

*Low GGT (PFIC types 1 and 2, BRIC types 1 and 2, ARC).

From Balistreri WF, Bezerra JA, Jansen P, et al: Intrahepatic cholestasis: summary of an American Association for the Study of Liver Diseases single-topic conference, *Hepatology* 42:222–235, 2005.

impaired neurologic function with psychomotor retardation. Patients have an abnormal head shape and unusual facies, hepatomegaly, renal cortical cysts, stippled calcifications of the patellas and greater trochanter, and ocular abnormalities. Hepatic cells on ultrastructural examination show an absence of peroxisomes. MRI performed in the 3rd trimester can allow analysis of cerebral gyration and myelination, facilitating the prenatal diagnosis of Zellweger syndrome.

Neonatal iron storage disease (NISD; neonatal hemochromatosis) is a rapidly progressive disease characterized by increased iron deposition in the liver, heart, and endocrine organs without increased iron stores in the reticuloendothelial system. Patients have multiorgan failure and shortened survival. Familial cases are reported, and repeated affected neonates in the same family are common. This is an alloimmune disorder with maternal antibodies directed against the fetal liver. Laboratory findings include hypoglycemia, hyperbilirubinemia, hypoalbuminemia, and profound hypoprothrombinemia. Serum aminotransferase levels may be high initially but normalize with the progression of the disease. The diagnosis is usually confirmed by buccal mucosal biopsy or MRI demonstrating extrahepatic siderosis. The prognosis is poor; liver transplantation can be curative. Despite initially encouraging reports, the use of a combination of antioxidants and prostaglandin infusion with chelation might not uniformly improve outcome in patients with NISD. Although recovery from NISD either spontaneously or with medical therapy is unusual, the potential for histologic recovery with regression of fibrosis has been reported.

Neonatal hemochromatosis seems to be a gestational alloimmune disease, and reoccurrence of severe neonatal hemochromatosis in at-risk pregnancies may be reduced by maternal treatment with weekly (beginning gestational age 18 wk) high-dose IVIG (1 g/kg) during gestation. After birth, affected neonates are treated with exchange transfusions and IVIG (1 g/kg), which improves survival and reduces the need for liver transplantation.

Disorders of Transport, Secretion, Conjugation, and Biosynthesis of Bile Acids

Progressive familial intrahepatic cholestasis type 1 (PFIC 1) or FIC1 disease (formerly known as **Byler disease**) is a severe form of intrahepatic cholestasis. The disease was initially described in the Amish kindred of Jacob Byler. Affected patients present with steatorrhea, pruritus, vitamin D–deficient rickets, gradually developing cirrhosis, and **low** γ-glutamyl transpeptidase (GGT) levels. The absence of bile duct paucity and extrahepatic features differentiate this disorder from Alagille syndrome.

PFIC 1 (FIC-1 deficiency) has been mapped to chromosome 18q12 and results from defect in the gene for F1C1 (*ATP8B1*; Tables 348-3 and 348-4). F1C1 is a P-type adenosine triphosphatase (ATPase) that functions as aminophospholipid flippase, facilitating the transfer of phosphatidyl serine and phosphatidyl

Table 348-4 PROGRESSIVE FAMILIAL INTRAHEPATIC CHOLESTASIS

	PFIC1	PFIC2	PFIC3
Transmission	Autosomal recessive	Autosomal recessive	Autosomal recessive
Chromosome	18q21-22	2q24	7q21
Gene	*ATP8B1/F1C1*	*ABCB11/BSEP*	*ABCB4/MDR3*
Protein	FIC1	BSEP	MDR3
Location	Hepatocyte, colon, intestine, pancreas; on apical membranes	Hepatocyte canalicular membrane	Hepatocyte canalicular membrane
Function	ATP-dependent aminophospholipid flippase; unknown effects on intracellular signaling	ATP-dependent bile acid transport	ATP-dependent phosphatidylcholine translocation
Phenotype	Progressive cholestasis, diarrhea, steatorrhea, growth failure, severe pruritus	Rapidly progressive cholestatic giant cell hepatitis, growth failure, pruritus	Later-onset cholestasis, portal hypertension, minimal pruritus, intraductal and gallbladder lithiasis
Histology	Initial bland cholestatic; coarse, granular canalicular bile on EM	Neonatal giant cell hepatitis, amorphous canalicular bile on EM	Proliferation of bile ductules, periportal fibrosis, eventually biliary cirrhosis
Biochemical features	Normal serum γGT; high serum, low biliary bile acid concentrations	Normal serum γGT; high serum, low biliary bile acid concentrations	Elevated serum γGT; low to absent biliary PC; absent serum LPX; normal biliary bile acid concentrations
Treatment	Biliary diversion, ileal exclusion, liver transplantation, but post-OLT diarrhea, steatorrhea, fatty liver	Biliary diversion, liver transplantation	UDCA if residual PC secretion; liver transplantation

ATP, adenosine triphosphate; BCEP, B-cell epitope peptide; EM, electron microscopy; γGT, γ-glutamyl transpeptidase; LPX, lipoprotein X; OLT, orthotopic liver transplantation; PC, phosphatidylcholine; PFIC, progressive familial intrahepatic cholestasis; UDCA, ursodeoxycholic acid.
From Suchy FJ, Sokol RJ, Balistreri WF, editors: *Liver disease in children*, ed 3, New York, 2007, Cambridge University Press.

ethanolamine from the outer to inner hemileaflet of the cellular membrane. F1C1 might also play a role in intestinal bile acid absorption, as suggested by the high level of expression in the intestine. Defective F1C1 might also result in another form of intrahepatic cholestasis: **benign recurrent intrahepatic cholestasis (BRIC) type I.** The disease is characterized by recurrent bouts of cholestasis, jaundice, and severe pruritus lasting from a 2 wk to 6 mo period; it can last up to 5 yr. The episodes vary from few episodes per year to 1 episode per decade and can profoundly affect the quality of life. Nonsense, frame shift, and deletional mutations cause PFIC type I; missense and split type mutations result in BRIC type I. Typically, patients with BRIC type I have normal cholesterol and GGT levels.

PFIC type 2 (BSEP deficiency) is mapped to chromosome 2q24 and is similar to PFIC 1 but is present in non-Amish families (Middle Eastern and European). The disease results from defects in the canalicular ATP-dependent bile acid transporter BSEP (*ABCB11*). The progressive liver disease results from accumulation of bile acids secondary to reduction in canalicular bile acid secretion. Mutation in *ABC11* is also described in another disorder, BRIC type 2, characterized by recurrent bouts of cholestasis.

In contrast to PFIC 1 and 2, patients with **PFIC type 3** (MDR3 disease) have **high** levels of GGT. The disease results from defects in a canalicular phospholipids flippase, MDR3 (*ABCB4*), which results in deficient translocation of phosphatidylcholine across the canalicular membrane. Mothers who are heterozygous for this gene can develop intrahepatic cholestasis during pregnancy.

Familial hypercholanemia (FHC) is characterized by elevated serum bile acid concentration, pruritus, failure to thrive, and coagulopathy. FHC is a complex genetic trait associated with mutation of bile acid coenzyme A (CoA): amino acid *N*-acyltransferase (encoded by *BAAT*) as well as mutations in tight junction protein 2 (encoded by *TJP 2*, also known as *ZO-2*). Mutation of BAAT, which is a bile acid–conjugating enzyme, abrogates the enzyme activity. Patients who are homozygous for this mutation have only unconjugated bile acids in their bile. Mutation of both BAAT and TJP 2 can disrupt bile acid transport and circulation. Patients with FHC usually respond to the administration of ursodeoxycholic acid.

Defective bile acid biosynthesis has been postulated to be an initiating or perpetuating factor in neonatal cholestatic disorders; the hypothesis is that inborn errors in bile acid biosynthesis lead to absence of normal trophic or choleretic primary bile acids and accumulation of atypical (hepatotoxic) metabolites. Inborn errors of bile acid biosynthesis cause acute and chronic liver disease; early recognition allows institution of targeted bile acid replacement, which reverses the hepatic injury. Several specific defects have been described, as follows.

Deficiency of Δ^4-3-oxosteroid-5β reductase, the 4th step in the pathway of cholesterol degradation to the primary bile acids, manifests with significant cholestasis and liver failure developing shortly after birth, with coagulopathy and metabolic liver injury resembling tyrosinemia. Hepatic histology is characterized by lobular disarray with giant cells, pseudoacinar transformation, and canalicular bile stasis. Mass spectrometry is required to document increased urinary bile acid excretion and the predominance of oxo-hydroxy and oxo-dihydroxy cholenoic acids. **Treatment** with cholic acid and ursodeoxycholic acid is associated with normalization of biochemical, histologic, and clinical features.

Deficiency of 3β-hydroxy C_{27}-steroid dehydrogenase (3β-HSD) isomerase, the 2nd step in bile acid biosynthesis, causes progressive familial intrahepatic cholestasis. Affected patients usually have jaundice with increased aminotransferase levels and hepatomegaly; GGT levels and serum cholylglycine levels are **normal.** The histology is variable, ranging from giant cell hepatitis to chronic hepatitis. The diagnosis, suggested by mass spectrometry detection of C^{24} bile acids in urine, which retain the 3β-hydroxy-Δ^5 structure, can be confirmed by determination of 3β-HSD activity in cultured fibroblasts using 7α-hydroxy-Δ^5 cholesterol as a substrate. Primary bile acid therapy, administered orally to downregulate cholesterol 7α-hydroxylase activity, to limit the production of 3β-hydroxy-Δ^5 bile acids, and to facilitate hepatic clearance, has been effective in reversing hepatic injury.

Deficiency of oxysterol 7α-hydroxylase deficiency has been reported in a 10 wk old boy of parents who were first cousins. The patient presented with severe progressive cholestasis, hepatosplenomegaly, cirrhosis, and liver failure during early infancy. Although serum ALT and AST were markedly elevated, serum GGT was normal. Liver biopsy showed cholestasis with impressive giant cell transformation, bridging fibrosis, and proliferating bile ductules. Administration of cholic acid was therapeutically ineffective and UDCA resulted in deterioration in liver function tests. The patient received orthotopic liver transplant at 4½ months of age but subsequently died from disseminated Epstein-Barr virus–related lymphoproliferative disease.

BILE ACID CoA LIGASE DEFICIENCY

Conjugation with the amino acids glycine and taurine is the final step in bile acid synthesis. Two enzymes catalyze the amidation of bile acids. In the first reaction, a CoA thioester is formed by the rate-limiting bile acid-CoA ligase. The other reaction involves the coupling of glycine or taurine and is catalyzed by a cytosolic bile acid-CoA:amino acid *N*-acyltransferase. Several patients with bile acid-CoA ligase deficiency have been reported. The patients present with conjugated hyperbilirubinemia, growth failure, or fat-soluble vitamin deficiency and have been identified with mutation of bile acid-CoA ligase gene. Administration of conjugates of the primary bile acid, glycocholic acid may be beneficial and can correct the fat-soluble vitamin malabsorption and improve growth.

DISORDERS OF EMBRYOGENESIS

Alagille syndrome (arteriohepatic dysplasia) is the most common syndrome with intrahepatic bile duct paucity. Bile duct "paucity" (often erroneously called *intrahepatic biliary atresia*) designates an absence or marked reduction in the number of interlobular bile ducts in the portal triads, with normal-sized branches of portal vein and hepatic arteriole. Biopsy in early life often reveals an inflammatory process involving the bile ducts; subsequent biopsy specimens then show subsidence of the inflammation, with residual reduction in the number and diameter of bile ducts, analogous to the "disappearing bile duct syndrome" noted in adults with immune-mediated disorders. Serial assessment of hepatic histology often suggests progressive destruction of bile ducts.

Clinical manifestations of Alagille syndrome are expressed in various degrees and can be nonspecific; they include unusual facial characteristics (broad forehead; deep-set, widely spaced eyes; long, straight nose; and an underdeveloped mandible). There may also be ocular abnormalities (posterior embryotoxon, microcornea, optic disk drusen, shallow anterior chamber), cardiovascular abnormalities (usually peripheral pulmonic stenosis, sometimes tetralogy of Fallot, pulmonary atresia, VSD, ASD, aortic coarctation), vertebral defects (butterfly vertebrae, fused vertebrae, spina bifida occulta, rib anomalies), and tubulointerstitial nephropathy. Other findings such as short stature, pancreatic insufficiency, and defective spermatogenesis can reflect or produce nutritional deficiency. The prognosis for prolonged survival is good, but patients are likely to have pruritus, xanthomas with markedly elevated serum cholesterol levels, and neurologic complications of vitamin E deficiency if untreated. Mutations in human Jagged1 gene (*JAG1*), which encodes a ligand for the notch receptor, are linked to Alagille syndrome.

BILIARY ATRESIA

The term *biliary atresia* is imprecise because the anatomy of abnormal bile ducts in affected patients varies markedly. A more appropriate terminology would reflect the pathophysiology, namely, progressive obliterative cholangiopathy. Patients can have distal segmental bile duct obliteration with patent extrahepatic ducts up to the porta hepatis. This is a surgically correctable lesion, but it is uncommon. The most common form of biliary atresia, accounting for ~85% of the cases, is obliteration of the entire extrahepatic biliary tree at or above the porta hepatis. This presents a much more difficult problem in surgical management. Most patients with biliary atresia (85-90%) are normal at birth and have a postnatal progressive obliteration of bile ducts; the embryonic or fetal-onset form manifests at birth and is associated with other congenital anomalies (situs inversus, polysplenia, intestinal malrotation, complex congenital heart disease) within the polysplenia spectrum (biliary atresia splenic malformation [BASM]) (Fig. 348-2) (Chapter 425.11). The postnatal onset may be an immune- or infection-mediated process.

Biliary atresia has been detected in 1/10,000-15,000 live births.

Differentiation of Idiopathic Neonatal Hepatitis from Biliary Atresia

It may be difficult to clearly differentiate infants with biliary atresia, who require surgical correction, from those with intrahepatic disease (neonatal hepatitis) and patent bile ducts. No single biochemical test or imaging procedure is entirely satisfactory. Diagnostic schemas incorporate clinical, historical, biochemical, and radiologic features.

Idiopathic neonatal hepatitis has a familial incidence of ~20%, whereas biliary atresia is unlikely to recur within the same family. A few infants with fetal onset of biliary atresia have an increased incidence of other abnormalities, such as the polysplenia syndrome with abdominal heterotaxia, malrotation, levocardia, and intra-abdominal vascular anomalies. Neonatal hepatitis appears to be more common in infants who are premature or small for gestational age. Persistently acholic stools suggest biliary obstruction (biliary atresia), but patients with severe idiopathic neonatal hepatitis can have a transient severe impairment of bile excretion. Consistently pigmented stools rule against biliary atresia. The finding of bile-stained fluid on duodenal intubation also excludes biliary atresia. Palpation of the liver might find an abnormal size or consistency in patients with biliary atresia; this is less common with idiopathic neonatal hepatitis.

Abdominal ultrasound is a helpful diagnostic tool in evaluating neonatal cholestasis because it identifies choledocholithiasis, perforation of the bile duct, or other structural abnormalities of the biliary tree such as a choledochal cyst. In patients with biliary atresia, ultrasound can detect associated anomalies such as abdominal polysplenia and vascular malformations. The gallbladder either is not visualized or is a microgallbladder in patients with biliary atresia. Children with intrahepatic cholestasis caused by idiopathic neonatal hepatitis, cystic fibrosis, or total parenteral nutrition can have similar ultrasonographic findings. Ultrasonographic triangular cord (TC) sign, which represents a cone-shaped fibrotic mass cranial to the bifurcation of the portal vein, may be seen in patients with biliary atresia (Figs. 348-3 and 348-4). The echogenic density, which represents the fibrous remnants at the porta hepatis of biliary atresia cases at surgery, may be a helpful diagnostic tool in evaluating patients with neonatal cholestasis.

Hepatobiliary scintigraphy with technetium-labeled iminodiacetic acid derivatives is used to differentiate biliary atresia from nonobstructive causes of cholestasis. The hepatic uptake of the agent is normal in patients with biliary atresia, but excretion into the intestine is absent. Although the uptake may be impaired in neonatal hepatitis, excretion into the bowel eventually occurs. Obtaining a follow-up scan after 24 hr is of value to determine the patency of the biliary tree. The administration of phenobarbital (5 mg/kg/day) for 5 days before the scan is recommended because it can enhance biliary excretion of the isotope. Hepatobiliary scintigraphy is a sensitive but not specific test for biliary atresia. It fails to identify other structural abnormalities of the biliary tree or vascular anomalies. The lack of the specificity of the test and the need to wait for 5 days makes this procedure less practical and of limited usefulness in the evaluation of children with suspected biliary atresia.

Percutaneous liver biopsy is the most valuable procedure in the evaluation of neonatal hepatobiliary diseases and provides the most reliable discriminatory evidence. Biliary atresia is characterized by bile ductular proliferation, the presence of bile plugs, and portal or perilobular edema and fibrosis, with the basic hepatic lobular architecture intact. In neonatal hepatitis, there is severe, diffuse hepatocellular disease, with distortion of lobular architecture, marked infiltration with inflammatory cells, and

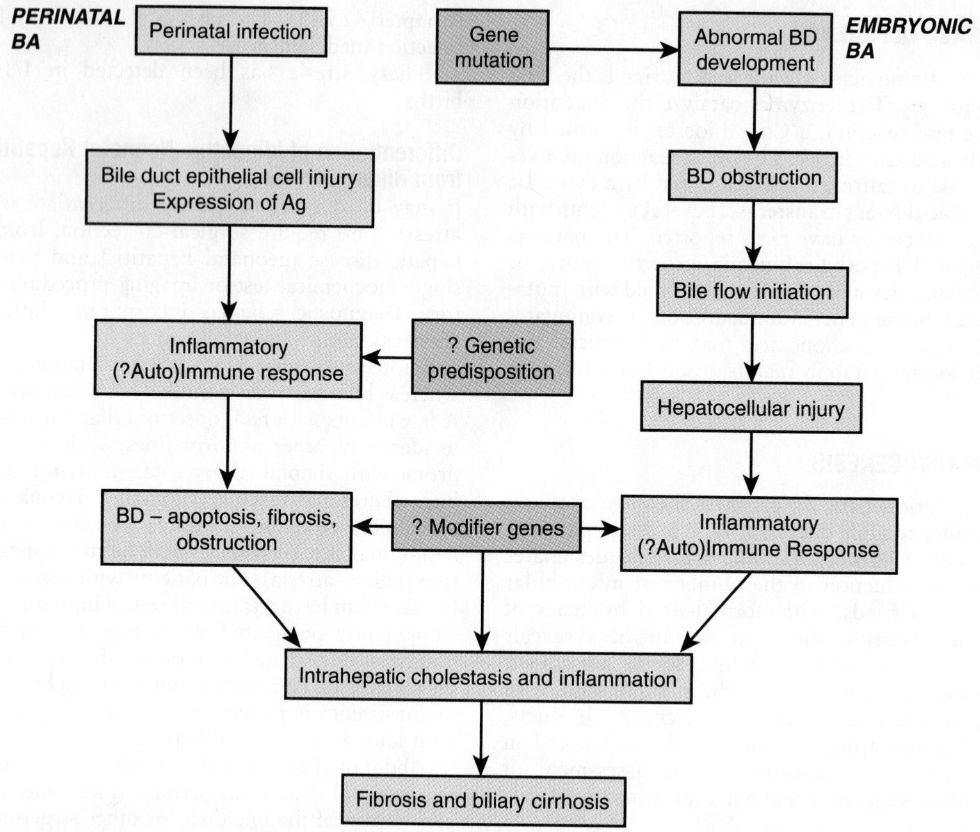

Figure 348-2 Proposed pathways for pathogenesis of 2 forms of biliary atresia (BA). *Perinatal* BA can develop when a perinatal insult, such as a cholangiotropic viral infection, triggers bile duct (BD) epithelial cell injury and exposure of self-antigens or neoantigens that elicit a subsequent immune response. The resulting inflammation induces apoptosis and necrosis of extrahepatic BD epithelium, resulting in fibro-obliteration of the lumen and obstruction of the BD. Intrahepatic bile ducts can also be targets in the ongoing TH1 immune (autoimmune?) attack and the cholestatic injury, resulting in progressive portal fibrosis and culminating in biliary cirrhosis. *Embryonic* BA may be the result of mutations in genes controlling normal bile duct formation or differentiation, which secondarily induces an inflammatory/immune response within the common bile duct and liver after the initiation of bile flow at ~11-13 wk of gestation. Secondary hepatocyte and intrahepatic bile duct injury ensue either as a result of cholestatic injury or as targets for the immune (autoimmune?) response that develops. The end result is intrahepatic cholestasis and portal tract fibrosis, culminating in biliary cirrhosis. Other major factors may be the role played by genetic predisposition to autoimmunity and modifier genes that determine the extent and type of cellular and immune response and the generation of fibrosis. (From Mack CL, Sokol RJ: Unraveling the pathogenesis and etiology of biliary atresia, *Pediatr Res* 57:87R–94R, 2005.)

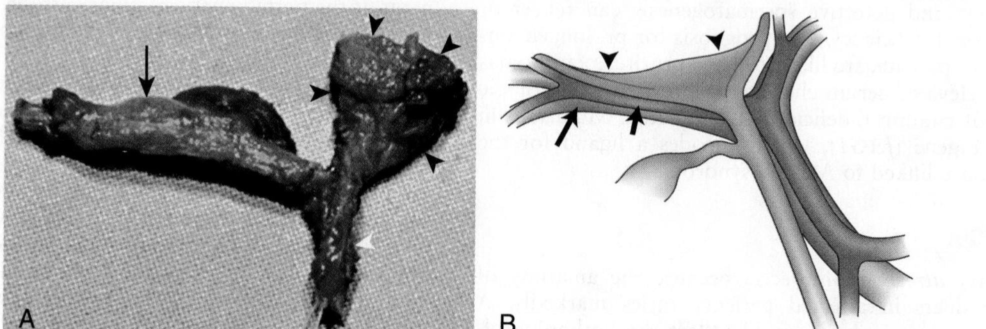

Figure 348-3 Surgical findings of biliary atresia. *A,* Photograph of surgical specimen of obliterated extrahepatic bile ducts shows the fibrous ductal remnant *(black arrowheads)* in the porta hepatis, atretic gallbladder *(arrow),* and fibrous common bile duct *(white arrowhead).* The fibrous ductal remnant is a triangular cone-shaped mass. *B,* Schematic drawing represents the anatomic relationship between the fibrous ductal remnant and blood vessels around the porta hepatis. The triangular, cone-shaped, fibrous ductal remnant *(black arrowheads, green)* is positioned anterior and slightly superior to the portal vein *(long arrow, blue)* and the hepatic artery *(short arrow, red).* (*A,* From Park WH, Choi SO, Lee HJ, et al: A new diagnostic approach to biliary atresia with emphasis on the ultrasonographic triangular cord sign: comparison of ultrasonography, hepatobiliary scintigraphy, and liver needle biopsy in the evaluation of infantile cholestasis, *J Pediatr Surg* 32:1555–1559, 1997.)

focal hepatocellular necrosis; the bile ductules show little alteration. Giant cell transformation is found in infants with either condition and has no diagnostic specificity.

The histologic changes seen in patients with idiopathic neonatal hepatitis can occur in other diseases, including α_1-antitrypsin deficiency, galactosemia, and various forms of intrahepatic cholestasis. Although paucity of intrahepatic bile ductules may be detected on liver biopsy even in the 1st few weeks of life, later biopsies in such patients reveal a more characteristic pattern.

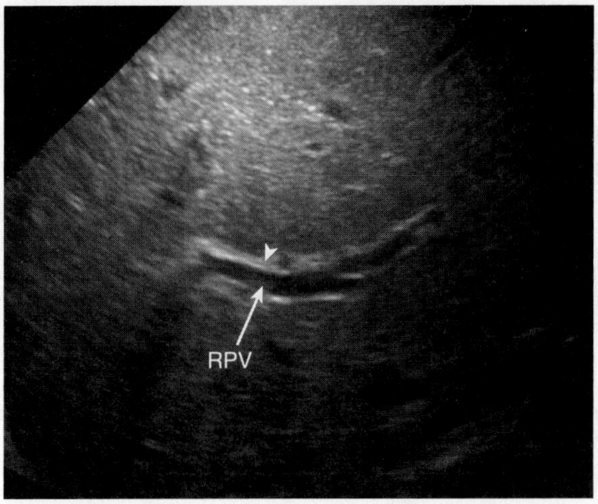

Figure 348-4 Biliary atresia in an 8 wk old male with elevated direct bilirubin. Transverse sonogram shows the triangular cord sign seen as a linear cord of echogenicity *(arrowhead)* along the right portal vein (RPV). (From Lowe LH: Imaging hepatobiliary disease in children, *Semin Roentgenol* 43:39–49, 2008, Fig 1B.)

Management of Patients with Suspected Biliary Atresia

All patients with suspected biliary atresia should undergo exploratory laparotomy and direct cholangiography to determine the presence and site of obstruction. Direct drainage can be accomplished in the few patients with a correctable lesion. When no correctable lesion is found, an examination of frozen sections obtained from the transected porta hepatis can detect the presence of biliary epithelium and determine the size and patency of the residual bile ducts. In some cases, the cholangiogram indicates that the biliary tree is patent but of diminished caliber, suggesting that the cholestasis is not due to biliary tract obliteration but to bile duct paucity or markedly diminished flow in the presence of intrahepatic disease. In these cases, transection of or further dissection into the porta hepatis should be avoided.

For patients in whom no correctable lesion is found, the **hepatoportoenterostomy (Kasai) procedure** should be performed. The rationale for this operation is that minute bile duct remnants, representing residual channels, may be present in the fibrous tissue of the porta hepatis; such channels may be in direct continuity with the intrahepatic ductule system. In such cases, transection of the porta hepatis with anastomosis of bowel to the proximal surface of the transection might allow bile drainage. If flow is not rapidly established in the 1st months of life, progressive obliteration and cirrhosis ensue. If microscopic channels of patency >150 μm in diameter are found, postoperative establishment of bile flow is likely. The success rate for establishing good bile flow after the Kasai operation is much higher (90%) if performed before 8 wk of life. Therefore, early referral and prompt evaluation of infants with suspected biliary atresia is important.

Some patients with biliary atresia, even of the "noncorrectable" type, derive long-term benefits from interventions such as the Kasai procedure. In most, a degree of hepatic dysfunction persists. Patients with biliary atresia usually have persistent inflammation of the intrahepatic biliary tree, which suggests that biliary atresia reflects a dynamic process involving the entire hepatobiliary system. This might account for the ultimate development of complications such as portal hypertension. The short-term benefit of hepatoportoenterostomy is decompression and drainage sufficient to forestall the onset of cirrhosis and sustain growth until a successful liver transplantation can be done (Chapter 360).

MANAGEMENT OF CHRONIC CHOLESTASIS

With any form of neonatal cholestasis, whether the primary disease is idiopathic neonatal hepatitis, intrahepatic cholestasis, or biliary atresia, affected patients are at increased risk for progression and complications of chronic cholestasis. These reflect various degrees of residual hepatic functional capacity and are due directly or indirectly to diminished bile flow. Any substance normally excreted into bile is retained in the liver, with subsequent accumulation in tissue and in serum. Involved substances include bile acids, bilirubin, cholesterol, and trace elements. Decreased delivery of bile acids to the proximal intestine leads to inadequate digestion and absorption of dietary long-chain triglycerides and fat-soluble vitamins. Impairment of hepatic metabolic function can alter hormonal balance and utilization of nutrients. Progressive liver damage can lead to biliary cirrhosis, portal hypertension, and liver failure.

Table 348-5 SUGGESTED MEDICAL MANAGEMENT OF PERSISTENT CHOLESTASIS

CLINICAL IMPAIRMENT	MANAGEMENT
Malnutrition resulting from malabsorption of dietary long-chain triglycerides	Replace with dietary formula or supplements containing medium-chain triglycerides
Fat-soluble vitamin malabsorption:	
Vitamin A deficiency (night blindness, thick skin)	Replace with 10,000-15,000 IU/day as Aquasol A
Vitamin E deficiency (neuromuscular degeneration)	Replace with 50-400 IU/day as oral α-tocopherol or TPGS
Vitamin D deficiency (metabolic bone disease)	Replace with 5,000-8,000 IU/day of D_2 or 3-5 μg/kg/day of 25-hydroxycholecalciferol
Vitamin K deficiency (hypoprothrombinemia)	Replace with 2.5-5.0 mg every other day as water-soluble derivative of menadione
Micronutrient deficiency	Calcium, phosphate, or zinc supplementation
Deficiency of water-soluble vitamins	Supplement with twice the recommended daily allowance
Retention of biliary constituents such as cholesterol (itch or xanthomas)	Administer choleretic bile acids (ursodeoxycholic acid, 15-30 mg/kg/day)
Progressive liver disease; portal hypertension (variceal bleeding, ascites, hypersplenism)	Interim management (control bleeding; salt restriction; spironolactone)
End-stage liver disease (liver failure)	Transplantation

TPGS, D-tocopherol polyethylene glycol 1000 succinate.

Treatment of such patients is empirical, and is guided by careful monitoring (Table 348-5). No therapy is known to be effective in halting the progression of cholestasis or in preventing further hepatocellular damage and cirrhosis.

Growth failure is a major concern and is related in part to malabsorption and malnutrition resulting from ineffective digestion and absorption of dietary fat. Use of a medium-chain triglyceride-containing formula can improve caloric balance.

With chronic cholestasis and prolonged survival, children with hepatobiliary disease can experience deficiencies of the fat-soluble vitamins (A, D, E, K). Inadequate absorption of fat and fat-soluble vitamins may be exacerbated by administration of the bile acid binder cholestyramine. Metabolic bone disease is common.

Serum vitamin A concentration can usually be maintained at normal levels in patients who have chronic cholestasis and who receive oral supplementation of vitamin A esters. It is essential to monitor the vitamin A status in such patients.

A degenerative neuromuscular syndrome is found with chronic cholestasis, caused by malabsorption and vitamin E deficiency; affected children experience progressive areflexia, cerebellar ataxia, ophthalmoplegia, and decreased vibratory sensation. Specific morphologic lesions have been found in the central nervous system, peripheral nerves, and muscles. These lesions are potentially reversible in children <3-4 yr of age. Affected children have low serum vitamin E concentrations, increased hydrogen peroxide hemolysis, and low ratios of serum vitamin E to total serum lipids (<0.6 mg/g for children <12 yr and <0.8 mg/g for older patients). Vitamin E deficiency may be prevented by oral administration of large doses (up to 1,000 IU/day); patients unable to absorb sufficient quantities may require administration of D-α-tocopheryl polyethylene glycol 1000 succinate orally. Serum levels may be monitored as a guide to efficacy.

Pruritus is a particularly troublesome complication of chronic cholestasis, often with the appearance of xanthomas. Both features seem to be related to the accumulation of cholesterol and bile acids in serum and in tissues. Elimination of these retained compounds is difficult when bile ducts are obstructed, but if there is any degree of bile duct patency, administration of ursodeoxycholic acid can increase bile flow or interrupt the enterohepatic circulation of bile acids and thus decrease the xanthomas and ameliorate the pruritus (see Table 348-5). Ursodeoxycholic acid therapy can also lower serum cholesterol levels. The recommended initial dose is 15 mg/kg/24 hr.

Partial external biliary diversion is efficacious in managing pruritus refractory to medical therapy and provides a favorable outcome in a select group of patients with chronic cholestasis who have not yet developed cirrhosis. The surgical technique involves resecting a segment of intestine to be used as a biliary conduit. One end of the conduit is attached to the gallbladder and the other end is brought out to the skin, forming a stoma. The main drawback of the procedure is the need to use an ostomy bag.

Progressive fibrosis and cirrhosis lead to the development of portal hypertension and consequently to ascites and variceal hemorrhage. The presence of ascites is a risk factor for the development of spontaneous bacterial peritonitis (SBP). The first step in the management of patients with ascites is to rule out SBP and restrict sodium intake to 0.5 g (~1-2 mEq/kg/24 hr). There is no need for fluid restriction in patients with adequate renal output. Should this be ineffective, diuretics may be helpful. The diuretic of choice is spironolactone (3-5 mg/kg/24 hr in 4 doses). If spironolactone alone does not control ascites, the addition of another diuretic such as thiazide or furosemide may be beneficial. Patients with ascites but without peripheral edema are at risk for reduced plasma volume and decreased urine output during diuretic therapy. Tense ascites alters renal blood flow and systemic hemodynamics. Paracentesis and intravenous albumin infusion can improve hemodynamics, renal perfusion, and symptoms. Follow-up includes dietary counseling and monitoring of serum and urinary electrolyte concentrations (Chapters 356 and 359).

In patients with portal hypertension, variceal hemorrhage and the development of hypersplenism are common. It is important to ascertain the cause of bleeding because episodes of gastrointestinal hemorrhage in patients who have chronic liver disease may be due to gastritis or peptic ulcer disease. Because the management of these various complications differs, differentiation, perhaps via endoscopy, is necessary before treatment is initiated (Chapter 359). If the patient is volume depleted, blood transfusion should be carefully administered, avoiding overtransfusion, which can precipitate further bleeding. Balloon tamponade is not recommended in children because it can be associated with significant complications. Sclerotherapy or endoscopic variceal ligation may be useful palliative measures in the management of bleeding varices and may be superior to surgical alternatives.

For patients with advanced liver disease, hepatic transplantation has a success rate >85% (Chapter 360). If the operation is technically feasible, it will prolong life and might correct the metabolic error in diseases such as α_1-antitrypsin deficiency, tyrosinemia, and Wilson disease. Success depends on adequate intraoperative, preoperative, and postoperative care and on cautious use of immunosuppressive agents. Scarcity of donors of small livers severely limits the application of liver transplantation for infants and children. The use of reduced-size transplants and living donors increases the ability to treat small children successfully.

PROGNOSIS

For patients with idiopathic neonatal hepatitis, the variable prognosis might reflect the heterogeneity of the disease. In sporadic cases, 60-70% recover with no evidence of hepatic structural or functional impairment. Approximately 5-10% have persistent fibrosis or inflammation, and a smaller percentage have more severe liver disease, such as cirrhosis. Infants usually die early in the course of the illness, owing to hemorrhage or sepsis. Of infants with idiopathic neonatal hepatitis of the familial variety, only 20-30% recover; 10-15% acquire chronic liver disease with cirrhosis. Liver transplantation may be required.

348.2 Cholestasis in the Older Child

Robert M. Kliegman

Cholestasis with onset after the neonatal period is most often caused by acute viral hepatitis or exposure to hepatotoxic drugs. However, many of the conditions causing neonatal cholestasis can also cause chronic cholestasis in older patients. Therefore, older children and adolescents with conjugated hyperbilirubinemia should be evaluated for acute and chronic viral hepatitis, α_1-antitrypsin deficiency, Wilson disease, liver disease associated with inflammatory bowel disease, autoimmune hepatitis, and the syndromes of intrahepatic cholestasis. Other causes include obstruction caused by cholelithiasis, abdominal tumors, enlarged lymph nodes, or hepatic inflammation resulting from drug ingestion. Management of cholestasis in the older child is similar to that proposed for neonatal cholestasis (see Table 348-5).

BIBLIOGRAPHY

Please visit the Nelson Textbook of Pediatrics *website at www.expertconsult.com for the complete bibliography.*

Chapter 349
Metabolic Diseases of the Liver

William F. Balistreri and Rebecca G. Carey

Because the liver has a central role in synthetic, degradative, and regulatory pathways involving carbohydrate, protein, lipid, trace element, and vitamin metabolism, many metabolic abnormalities or specific enzyme deficiencies affect the liver primarily or secondarily (Table 349-1). Much has been learned in the past few years about the biochemical basis, molecular biology, and molecular genetics of metabolic liver diseases. This information has led to more precise diagnostic strategies and novel therapeutic approaches. Liver disease can arise when absence of an enzyme produces a block in a metabolic pathway, when unmetabolized substrate accumulates proximal to a block, when deficiency of an essential substance produced distal to an aberrant chemical reaction develops, or when synthesis of an abnormal metabolite occurs. The spectrum of pathologic changes includes: **hepatocyte injury,** with subsequent failure of other metabolic functions, often eventuating in cirrhosis, liver tumors, or both; **storage** of lipid, glycogen, or other products manifested as hepatomegaly, often with complications specific to deranged metabolism (hypoglycemia with glycogen storage disease); and absence of structural

Table 349-1 INBORN ERRORS OF METABOLISM THAT AFFECT THE LIVER

DISORDERS OF CARBOHYDRATE METABOLISM
Disorders of galactose metabolism
Galactosemia (galactose-1-phosphate uridylyltransferase deficiency)
Disorders of fructose metabolism
Hereditary fructose intolerance (aldolase deficiency)
Fructose-1,6 diphosphatase deficiency
Glycogen storage diseases
Type I
Von Gierke Ia (glucose-6-phosphatase deficiency)
Type Ib (glucose-6-phosphatase transport defect)
Type III Cori/Forbes (glycogen debrancher deficiency)
Type IV Andersen (glycogen branching enzyme deficiency)
Type VI Hers (liver phosphorylase deficiency)
Congenital disorders of glycosylation (multiple subtypes)
DISORDERS OF AMINO ACID AND PROTEIN METABOLISM
Disorders of tyrosine metabolism
Hereditary tyrosinemia type I (fumarylacetoacetate deficiency)
Tyrosinemia, type II (tyrosine aminotransferase deficiency)
Inherited urea cycle enzyme defects
CPS deficiency (carbamoyl phosphate synthetase I deficiency)
OTC deficiency (ornithine transcarbamoylase deficiency)
Citrullinemia type I (argininosuccinate synthetase deficiency)
Argininosuccinic aciduria (argininosuccinate deficiency)
Argininemia (arginase deficiency)
N-AGS deficiency (N-acetylglutamate synthetase deficiency)
Maple serum urine disease (multiple possible defects*)
DISORDERS OF LIPID METABOLISM
Wolman disease (lysosomal acid lipase deficiency)
Cholesteryl ester storage disease (lysosomal acid lipase deficiency)
Homozygous familial hypercholesterolemia (low density lipoprotein receptor deficiency)
Gaucher disease type I (beta-glucocerebrosidase deficiency)
Niemann-Pick type C (NPC 1 and 2 mutations)
DISORDERS OF BILE ACID METABOLISM
Isomerase deficiency
Reductase deficiency
Zellweger syndrome-cerebrohepatorenal (multiple mutations in peroxisome biogenesis genes)
DISORDERS OF METAL METABOLISM
Wilson disease (ATP7B mutations)
Hepatic copper overload
Indian childhood cirrhosis
Neonatal iron storage disease
DISORDERS OF BILIRUBIN METABOLISM
Crigler-Najjar (bilirubin-uridinediphosphoglucuronate glucuronosyltransferase mutations)
Type I
Type II
Gilbert disease (bilirubin-uridinediphosphoglucuronate glucuronosyltransferase polymorphism)
Dubin-Johnson syndrome (multiple drug-resistant protein 2 mutation)
Rotor syndrome
MISCELLANEOUS
α_1-Antitrypsin deficiency
Citrullinemia type II (citrin deficiency)
Cystic fibrosis (cystic fibrosis transmembrane conductance regulator mutations)
Erythropoietic protoporphyria (ferrochelatase deficiency)
Polycystic kidney disease

*Maple syrup urine disease can be caused by mutations in branched-chain alpha keto dehydrogenase, keto acid decarboxylase, lioamide dehydrogenase, or dihydrolipoamide dehydrogenase.

Table 349-2 CLINICAL MANIFESTATIONS THAT SUGGEST THE POSSIBILITY OF METABOLIC DISEASE

Recurrent vomiting, failure to thrive, short stature, dysmorphic features, edema/anasarca
Jaundice, hepatomegaly (± splenomegaly), fulminant hepatic failure
Hypoglycemia, organic acidemia, lactic acidemia, hyperammonemia, bleeding (coagulopathy)
Developmental delay/psychomotor retardation, hypotonia, progressive neuromuscular deterioration, seizures
Cardiac dysfunction/failure, unusual odors, rickets, cataracts

change despite profound **metabolic effects,** as with urea cycle defects. Clinical manifestations of metabolic diseases of the liver mimic infections, intoxications, and hematologic and immunologic diseases (Table 349-2). Many metabolic diseases are detected in expanded newborn metabolic screening programs (Chapter 78). Clues are provided by family history of a similar illness or by the observation that the onset of symptoms is closely associated with a change in dietary habits; for example, in patients with hereditary fructose intolerance, symptoms follow ingestion of fructose. Clinical and laboratory evidence often guides the evaluation. Liver biopsy offers morphologic study and permits enzyme assays, as well as quantitative and qualitative assays of various other constituents. Genetic/molecular diagnostic approaches are also available. Such studies require cooperation of experienced laboratories and careful attention to collection and handling of specimens. Treatment depends on the specific type of metabolic defect, and although individually rare when taken together, metabolic diseases of the liver account for up to 10% of the indications for liver transplantation in children.

349.1 Inherited Deficient Conjugation of Bilirubin (Familial Nonhemolytic Unconjugated Hyperbilirubinemia)

Rebecca G. Carey and William F. Balistreri

Bilirubin is the metabolic end product of heme. Before excretion into bile, it is first glucuronidated by the enzyme bilirubin-uridinediphosphoglucuronate glucuronosyltransferase (UDPGT). UDPGT activity is deficient or altered in 3 genetically and functionally distinct disorders (Crigler-Najjar [CN] syndromes type I and II and Gilbert syndrome), producing congenital nonobstructive, nonhemolytic, **unconjugated** hyperbilirubinemia. UGT1A1 is the primary UDPGT isoform needed for bilirubin glucuronidation, and complete absence of UGT1A1 activity causes CN type I. CN type II is due to decreased UGT1A1 activity. **Gilbert syndrome** is caused by a common polymorphism, a TA insertion in the promoter region of UGT1A1 that leads to decreased binding of the TATA binding protein and decreases normal gene activity but only to ~30%. Unlike the Crigler-Najjar syndromes, Gilbert syndrome usually occurs after puberty; it is not associated with chronic liver disease and no treatment is required. However, it is more common, affecting up to 5-10% of the white population with total serum bilirubin concentrations that fluctuate from 1 to 6 mg/dL. Because UGT1A1 is involved in glucuronidation of multiple substrates other than bilirubin (e.g., pharmaceutical drugs, endogenous hormones, environmental toxins, and aromatic hydrocarbons) and glucuronidation leads to inactivation of these substrates, mutations in the UGT1A1 gene have been implicated in cancer risk and the disposition to drug toxicity.

CRIGLER-NAJJAR SYNDROME TYPE I (GLUCURONYL TRANSFERASE DEFICIENCY)

CN type I is inherited as an autosomal recessive trait and is usually secondary to mutations that cause a premature stop codon or frameshift mutation and thereby abolish UGT1A1 activity. More than 35 mutations have been identified to date. Parents of affected children have partial defects in conjugation as determined by hepatic specific enzyme assay or by measurement of glucuronide formation; their serum unconjugated bilirubin concentrations are normal.

Clinical Manifestations

Severe unconjugated hyperbilirubinemia develops in homozygous affected infants in the 1st 3 days of life, and without treatment, serum unconjugated bilirubin concentrations of 25-35 mg/dL are reached in the 1st month. Kernicterus, an almost universal complication of this disorder, is usually 1st noted in the early neonatal period; some treated infants have survived childhood without clinical sequelae. Stools are pale yellow. Persistence of unconjugated hyperbilirubinemia at levels >20 mg/dL after the 1st wk of life in the absence of hemolysis should suggest the syndrome.

Diagnosis

The diagnosis of CN type I is based on the early age of onset and the extreme level of bilirubin elevation in the absence of hemolysis. In the bile, bilirubin concentration is <10 mg/dL compared with normal concentrations of 50-100 mg/dL; there is no bilirubin glucuronide. Definitive diagnosis is established by measuring hepatic glucuronyl transferase activity in a liver specimen obtained by a closed biopsy; open biopsy should be avoided because surgery and anesthesia can precipitate kernicterus. DNA diagnosis is also available and may be preferable. Identification of the heterozygous state in parents also strongly suggests the diagnosis. The differential diagnosis of unconjugated hyperbilirubinemia is discussed in Chapter 96.3.

Treatment

The serum unconjugated bilirubin concentration should be kept to <20 mg/dL for at least the 1st 2-4 wk of life; in low birth-weight infants, the levels should be kept lower. This usually requires repeated exchange transfusions and phototherapy. Phenobarbital therapy should be considered to determine responsiveness and differentiation between type I and II (see later).

The risk of kernicterus persists into adult life, although the serum bilirubin levels required to produce brain injury beyond the neonatal period are considerably higher (usually >35 mg/dL). Therefore, phototherapy is generally continued through the early years of life. In older infants and children, phototherapy is used mainly during sleep so as not to interfere with normal activities. Despite the administration of increasing intensities of light for longer periods, the serum bilirubin response to phototherapy decreases with age. Adjuvant therapy using agents that bind photobilirubin products such as calcium phosphate, cholestyramine, or agar can be used to interfere with the enterohepatic recirculation of bilirubin.

Prompt treatment of intercurrent infections, febrile episodes, and other types of illness might help prevent the later development of kernicterus, which can occur at bilirubin levels of 45-55 mg/dL. All patients with CN type I have eventually experienced severe kernicterus by young adulthood.

Orthotopic liver transplantation cures the disease and has been successful in a small number of patients; isolated hepatocyte transplantation has been reported in fewer than 10 patients, but all patients eventually required orthotopic transplantation. Other therapeutic modalities have included plasmapheresis and limitation of bilirubin production. The latter option, inhibiting bilirubin generation, is possible via inhibition of heme oxygenase using metalloporphyrin therapy.

CRIGLER-NAJJAR SYNDROME TYPE II (PARTIAL GLUCURONYL TRANSFERASE DEFICIENCY)

Like CN type I, CN type II is an autosomal recessive disease; it is caused by homozygous missense mutations in UGT1A1, resulting in reduced (partial) enzymatic activity. More than 18 mutations have been identified to date. Type II disease can be distinguished from type I by the marked decline in serum bilirubin level that occurs in type II disease after treatment with phenobarbital secondary to an inducible phenobarbital response element on the UGT1A1 promoter.

Clinical Manifestations

When this disorder appears in the neonatal period, unconjugated hyperbilirubinemia usually occurs in the 1st 3 days of life; serum bilirubin concentrations can be in a range compatible with physiologic jaundice or can be at pathologic levels. The concentrations characteristically remain elevated into and after the 3rd wk of life, persisting in a range of 1.5-22 mg/dL; concentrations in the lower part of this range can create uncertainty about whether chronic hyperbilirubinemia is present. Development of kernicterus is unusual. Stool color is normal, and the infants are without clinical signs or symptoms of disease. There is no evidence of hemolysis.

Diagnosis

Concentration of bilirubin in bile is nearly normal in CN type II. Jaundiced infants and young children with type II syndrome respond readily to 5 mg/kg/24 hr of oral phenobarbital, with a decrease in serum bilirubin concentration to 2-3 mg/dL in 7-10 days.

Treatment

Long-term reduction in serum bilirubin levels can be achieved with continued administration of phenobarbital at 5 mg/kg/24 hr. The cosmetic and psychosocial benefit should be weighed against the risks of an effective dose of the drug because there is a small long-term risk of kernicterus even in the absence of hemolytic disease. Orlistat, an irreversible inhibitor of intestinal lipase, induces a mild decrease in plasma bilirubin levels (~10%) in patients with CN I and II.

INHERITED CONJUGATED HYPERBILIRUBINEMIA

Conjugated hyperbilirubinemia can be due to a small number of rare autosomal recessive conditions characterized by mild jaundice. The transfer of bilirubin and other organic anions from the liver cell to bile is defective. Chronic mild conjugated hyperbilirubinemia is usually detected during adolescence or early adulthood but can occur as early as the second year of life. The results of routine liver function tests are normal. Jaundice can be exacerbated by infection, pregnancy, oral contraceptives, alcohol consumption, and surgery. There is usually no morbidity and life expectancy is normal, but these disorders can initially present difficult problems in the differential diagnosis of more serious diseases.

Dubin-Johnson Syndrome

Dubin-Johnson syndrome is an autosomal recessive inherited defect with variable penetrance in hepatocyte secretion of bilirubin glucuronide. The defect in hepatic excretory function is not limited to conjugated bilirubin excretion but also involves several organic anions normally excreted from the liver cell into bile. Absent function of multiple drug-resistant protein 2 (MRP2), an adenosine triphosphate (ATP)-dependent canalicular transporter, is the responsible defect. More than 10 different mutations have been identified and either affect localization of MRP2 with resultant increased degradation or impair MRP2 transport activity in the canalicular membrane. Bile acid excretion and serum bile acid levels are normal. Total urinary coproporphyrin excretion is normal in quantity but coproporphrin I excretion increases to ~80% with a concomitant decrease in coproporphyrin III excretion. Normally, coproporphyrin III is >75% of the total. Cholangiography fails to visualize the biliary tract and x-ray of the gallbladder is also abnormal. Liver histology demonstrates normal architecture, but hepatocytes contain black pigment similar to melanin.

Rotor Syndrome

Patients with Rotor syndrome have an additional deficiency in organic anion uptake; however, the genetic defect has not yet been elucidated. Unlike Dubin-Johnson syndrome, total urinary coproporphyrin excretion is elevated, with a relative increase in the amount of the coproporphyrin I isomer. The gallbladder is normal by roentgenography, and liver cells contain no black pigment. In Dubin-Johnson and Rotor syndromes, sulfobromophthalein excretion is often abnormal.

BIBLIOGRAPHY
Please visit the Nelson Textbook of Pediatrics *website at* www.expertconsult.com *for the complete bibliography.*

349.2 Wilson Disease

William F. Balistreri and Rebecca G. Carey

Wilson disease (hepatolenticular degeneration) is an autosomal recessive disorder that can be associated with degenerative changes in the brain, liver disease, and Kayser-Fleischer rings in the cornea. The incidence is 1/50,00 to 1/100,000 births. It is progressive and potentially fatal if untreated; specific effective treatment is available. Rapid diagnostic investigation of the possibility of Wilson disease in a patient presenting with any form of liver disease, particularly if >5 yr of age, not only facilitates early institution of management of Wilson disease and related genetic counseling but also allows appropriate treatment of non-Wilsonian liver disease once copper toxicosis is ruled out.

PATHOGENESIS

The abnormal gene for Wilson disease is localized to the long arm of chromosome 13 (13q14.3). The Wilson disease gene encodes a copper transporting P-type ATPase, ATP7B, which is mainly but not exclusively expressed in hepatocytes and is critical for biliary copper excretion and for copper incorporation into ceruloplasmin. Absence or malfunction of ATP7B results in decreased biliary copper excretion and diffuse accumulation of copper in the cytosol of hepatocytes. With time, liver cells become overloaded and copper is redistributed to other tissues, including the brain and kidneys, causing toxicity, primarily as a potent inhibitor of enzymatic processes. Ionic copper inhibits pyruvate oxidase in brain and ATPase in membranes, leading to decreased ATP-phosphocreatine and potassium content of tissue.

More than 250 mutations in the gene have been identified, making diagnosis by DNA mutational analysis a difficult task unless a proband mutation is known. Most patients are compound heterozygotes. Mutations that completely knock out gene function are associated with an onset of disease symptoms as early as 2-3 yr of age, when Wilson disease might not typically be considered in the differential diagnosis. Milder mutations can be associated with neurologic symptoms or liver disease as late as 70 yr of age. Cloning of the gene for Wilson disease raises the prospect of precise presymptomatic detection of Wilson disease, timely initiation of therapy, and, ultimately, gene therapy.

CLINICAL MANIFESTATIONS

Forms of Wilsonian hepatic disease include asymptomatic hepatomegaly (with or without splenomegaly), subacute or chronic hepatitis, and acute hepatic failure (with or without hemolytic anemia). Cryptogenic cirrhosis, portal hypertension, ascites, edema, variceal bleeding, or other effects of hepatic dysfunction (delayed puberty, amenorrhea, coagulation defect) can be manifestations of Wilson disease.

Disease presentations are variable, with a tendency to familial patterns. The younger the patient, the more likely hepatic involvement will be the predominant manifestation. Girls are 3 times more likely than boys to present with acute hepatic failure. After 20 yr of age, neurologic symptoms predominate.

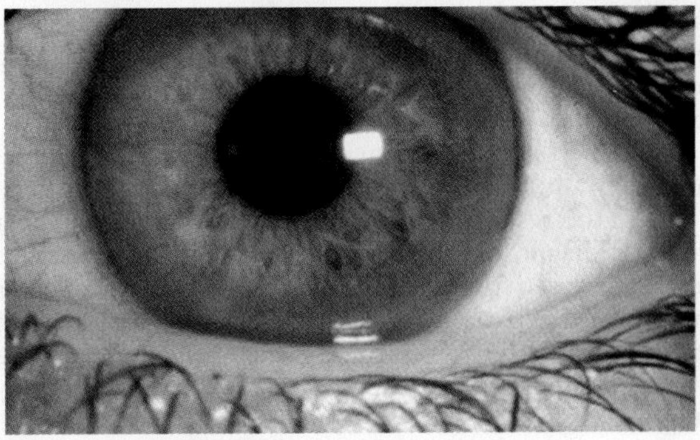

Figure 349-1 Kayser-Fleischer (K-F) ring. There is a brown discoloration at the outer margin of the cornea because of the deposition of copper in Descemet's membrane. Here it is clearly seen against the light green iris. Slit lamp examination is required for secure detection. (From Ala A, Walker AP, Ashkan K, et al: Wilson's disease, *Lancet* 369:397–408, 2007.)

Neurologic disorders can develop insidiously or precipitously, with intention tremor, dysarthria, rigid dystonia, parkinsonism, choreiform movements, lack of motor coordination, deterioration in school performance, or behavioral changes. Kayser-Fleischer rings may be absent in young patients with liver disease but are always present in patients with neurologic symptoms (Fig. 349-1). **Psychiatric manifestations** include depression, personality changes, anxiety, or psychosis.

Coombs-negative hemolytic anemia may be an initial manifestation, possibly related to the release of large amounts of copper from damaged hepatocytes; this form of Wilson disease is usually fatal without transplantation. During hemolytic episodes, urinary copper excretion and serum copper levels (not ceruloplasmin bound) are markedly elevated. Manifestations of renal Fanconi syndrome and progressive renal failure with alterations in tubular transport of amino acids, glucose, and uric acid may be present. Unusual manifestations include arthritis, infertility or recurrent miscarriages, cardiomyopathy, and endocrinopathies (hypoparathyroidism).

PATHOLOGY

All grades of hepatic injury occur with steatosis, heptocellular ballooning and degeneration, glycogen granules, minimal inflammation, and enlarged Kupffer cells. The lesion may be indistinguishable from that of autoimmune hepatitis. With progressive parenchymal damage, fibrosis and cirrhosis develop. Ultrastructural changes primarily involve the mitochondria and include increased density of the matrix material, inclusions of lipid and granular material, and increased intracristal space with dilatation of the tips of the cristae.

DIAGNOSIS

Wilson disease should be considered in children and teenagers with unexplained acute or chronic liver disease, neurologic symptoms of unknown cause, acute hemolysis, psychiatric illnesses, behavioral changes, Fanconi syndrome, or unexplained bone (osteoporosis, fractures) or muscle disease (myopathy, arthralgia). The clinical suspicion is confirmed by study of indices of copper metabolism.

Most patients with Wilson disease have decreased ceruloplasmin levels (<20 mg/dL). The failure of copper to be incorporated into ceruloplasmin leads to a plasma protein with a shorter half-life and, therefore, a reduced steady-state concentration of ceruloplasmin in the circulation. Caution should be used in interpreting serum ceruloplasmin levels, because they may be elevated in acute inflammation and in states of elevated estrogen such as pregnancy, estrogen supplementation, or oral contraceptive use. The serum copper level may be elevated in early Wilson disease, and urinary copper excretion (usually <40 µg/day) is increased to >100 µg/day and often up to 1,000 µg or more per day. In equivocal cases, the response of urinary copper output to chelation may be of diagnostic help. During the 24 hr urine collection patients are given two 500 mg oral doses of D-penicillamine 12 hr apart; affected patients excrete >1,600 µg/24 hr. Demonstration of Kayser-Fleischer rings, which might not be present in younger children, requires a slit-lamp examination by an ophthalmologist.

Liver biopsy is of value for determining the extent and severity of liver disease and for measuring the hepatic copper content (normally <10 µg/g dry weight). In Wilson disease, hepatic copper content exceeds 250 µg/g dry weight. In healthy heterozygotes, levels may be intermediate. In later stages of Wilson disease hepatic copper content can be unreliable because cirrhosis leads to variable hepatic copper distribution and sampling error.

Family members of patients with proven cases require screening for presymptomatic Wilson disease. Such screening should include determination of the serum ceruloplasmin level and urinary copper excretion. If these results are abnormal or equivocal, liver biopsy should be carried out to determine morphology and hepatic copper content. Genetic screening by either linkage analysis or direct DNA mutation analysis is possible, especially if the mutation for the proband case is known or the patient is from an area where a specific mutation is known (in central and eastern Europe, the *H1069Q* mutation is present in 50-80% of patients).

TREATMENT

A major attempt should be made to restrict dietary copper intake to <1 mg/day. Foods such as liver, shellfish, nuts, and chocolate should be avoided. If the copper content of the drinking water exceeds 0.1 mg/L, it may be necessary to demineralize the water.

The initial treatment in symptomatic patients is the administration of copper-chelating agents, which leads to rapid excretion of excess deposited copper. Chelation therapy is managed with oral administration of D-penicillamine (β,β-dimethylcysteine) in a dose of 1 g/day in 2 doses before meals for adults and 20 mg/kg/day for pediatric patients or triethylene tetramine dihydrochloride (Trien, TETA, trientine) at a dose of 0.5-2.0 g/day for adults and 20 mg/kg/day for children. In response to chelation, urinary copper excretion markedly increases, and with continued administration, urinary copper levels can become normal, with marked improvement in hepatic and neurologic function and the disappearance of Kayser-Fleischer rings.

Approximately 10-50% of patients initially treated with penicillamine for neurologic symptoms have a worsening of their condition. Toxic effects of penicillamine occur in 10-20% and consist of hypersensitivity reactions (Goodpasture syndrome, systemic lupus erythematosus, polymyositis), interaction with collagen and elastin, deficiency of other elements such as zinc, and aplastic anemia and nephrosis. Because penicillamine is an antimetabolite of vitamin B_6, additional amounts of this vitamin are necessary. For these reasons, triethylene tetramine dihydrochloride is a preferred alternative, and is considered 1st-line therapy for some patients.

Trientine has few known side effects. Ammonium tetrathiomolybdate is another alternative chelating agent under investigation for patients with neurologic disease; initial results suggest that significantly fewer patients experience neurologic deterioration with this drug compared to penicillamine. The initial dose is 120 mg/day (20 mg between meals tid and 20 mg with meals tid). Side effects include anemia, leukopenia, thrombocytopenia, and mild elevations of transaminases.

Zinc has also been used as adjuvant therapy, maintenance therapy, or primary therapy in presymptomatic patients, owing to its unique ability to impair the gastrointestinal absorption of copper. Zinc acetate is given in adults at a dose of 25-50 mg of elemental zinc 3 times a day, and 25 mg 3 times a day in children >5 yr of age. Side effects are mostly limited to gastric upset.

PROGNOSIS

Untreated patients with Wilson disease can die of hepatic, neurologic, renal, or hematologic complications. The prognosis for patients receiving prompt and continuous penicillamine is variable and depends on the time of initiation of and the individual response to chelation. Liver transplantation should be considered for patients with fulminant liver disease, decompensated cirrhosis, or progressive neurologic disease; the last indication remains controversial. Liver transplantation is curative, with a survival rate of ~85-90%. In asymptomatic siblings of affected patients, early institution of chelation or zinc therapy can prevent expression of the disease.

BIBLIOGRAPHY

Please visit the Nelson Textbook of Pediatrics *website at* *www.expertconsult.com* *for the complete bibliography.*

349.3 Indian Childhood Cirrhosis

William F. Balistreri and Rebecca G. Carey

Indian childhood cirrhosis (ICC) is a chronic liver disease of young children unique to the Indian subcontinent. ICC manifests with jaundice, pruritus, lethargy, and hepatosplenomegaly. Untreated ICC has a mortality of 40-50% within 4 wk. Histologically, it is characterized by hepatocyte necrosis, Mallory bodies, intralobular fibrosis, and inflammation.

The etiology has remained elusive; it was once believed that excess copper ingestion in the setting of a genetic susceptibility to copper toxicosis was the most likely cause. Epidemiological data demonstrated that the copper toxicity theory is unlikely. The increased hepatic copper content, usually >700 µg/g dry weight, seen in ICC is only seen in the late stages of disease and is accompanied by even higher levels of zinc, a nonhepatotoxic metal. The copper-contaminated utensils used to feed babies and implicated in excess copper ingestion are found in only 10-15% of all cases. The current hypothesis implicates the postnatal use of local hepatotoxic therapeutic remedies, although the exact causative agent is unknown.

Over the last few decades, as the awareness of the disease has increased, the incidence of ICC has decreased and has even been virtually eliminated in some areas of India. Variants of this syndrome have been named according to the population where it has been described, such as Tyrolean childhood cirrhosis. It has also been reported in the Middle East, West Africa, and North and Central America.

BIBLIOGRAPHY

Please visit the Nelson Textbook of Pediatrics *website at* *www.expertconsult.com* *for the complete bibliography.*

349.4 Neonatal Iron Storage Disease

Rebecca G. Carey and William F. Balistreri

Neonatal iron storage disease (NISD), also known as **neonatal hemochromatosis**, is a rare form of fulminant liver disease that manifests in the 1st few days of life. It is unrelated to the familial forms of hereditary hemochromatosis that occur later in life. NISD has a high rate of recurrence in families, with ~80% probability that subsequent infants will be affected. NISD is postulated to be a gestational alloimmune disease and has also been classified as **congenital alloimmune hepatitis.** Alloimmunity develops in the pregnant mother of the affected infant when she is exposed to an unknown fetal hepatocyte cell surface antigen that she does not recognize as *self*. Maternal IgG to this fetal antigen then crosses the placenta and induces hepatic injury via immune system activation. Additional evidence of a gestational insult is given by the fact that affected infants may be born prematurely or with intrauterine growth restriction. Several infants with NISD also have renal dysgenesis.

NISD is a rapidly fatal, progressive illness characterized by hepatomegaly, hypoglycemia, hypoprothrombinemia, hypoalbuminemia, hyperferritinemia, and hyperbilirubinemia. The coagulopathy is refractory to therapy with vitamin K. Liver pathology demonstrates severe liver injury with acute and chronic inflammation, fibrosis, and cirrhosis. The diagnosis can be confirmed in the neonate with severe liver injury and extrahepatic siderosis (biopsy material of buccal mucosal glands is laden with iron) or MRI determination of iron storage in organs such as the pancreas.

The prognosis for affected infants is generally poor, but some patients with NISD have been successfully treated with iron-chelating agents (deferoxamine) combined with aggressive antioxidant therapy. Combining this therapy with double volume exchange transfusion followed by administration of intravenous immunoglobulin (IVIG) has also been shown to remove the injury-causing maternal IgG. Liver transplantation should also be an early consideration. Recurrences of NISD may be modified with IVIG administered to the mother once a week from the 18th week of gestation until delivery. The largest experience reports 48 women with previous infants with NISD who successfully delivered 52 babies after IVIG treatment. The majority of infants had biochemical evidence of liver disease with elevated serum α-fetoprotein and ferritin. All infants survived with medical therapy or no therapy.

BIBLIOGRAPHY

Please visit the Nelson Textbook of Pediatrics *website at* *www.expertconsult.com* *for the complete bibliography.*

349.5 Miscellaneous Metabolic Diseases of the Liver

William F. Balistreri and Rebecca G. Carey

α_1-ANTITRYPSIN DEFICIENCY

A small percentage of patients homozygous for deficiency of the major serum protease inhibitor α_1-antitrypsin manifest neonatal cholestasis or later-onset childhood cirrhosis. α_1-Antitrypsin, a protease inhibitor synthesized by the liver, protects lung alveolar tissues from destruction by neutrophil elastase (Chapter 385). α_1-Antitrypsin is present in >20 different co-dominant alleles, only a few of which are associated with defective protease inhibitors. The most common allele of the protease inhibitor (Pi) system is M, and the normal phenotype is PiMM. The Z allele predisposes to clinical deficiency; patients with liver disease are usually PiZZ homozygotes and have serum α_1-antitrypsin levels <2 mg/mL (~10-20% of normal). The incidence of the PiZZ genotype in the white population is estimated at 1/2,000-4,000. Compound heterozygotes PiZ-, PiSZ, PiZI are not a cause of liver disease alone but can act as modifier genes, increasing the risk of progression in other liver disease such as nonalcoholic fatty liver disease and hepatitis C. The null phenotype due to stop codons in the coding exon of the α_1-antitrypsin gene or complete deletion of α_1-antitrypsin coding exons leads to the complete absence of any protein and causes only lung disease.

Newly formed α_1-antitrypsin peptide normally enters the endoplasmic reticulum (ER), where it undergoes enzymatic modification and folding before transport to the plasma membrane, where it is excreted as a 55 kDa glycoprotein. In affected patients with PiZZ, the rate at which the α_1-antitrypsin peptide folds is decreased, and this delay allows the formation of polymers that are retained in the ER. How the polymers cause liver damage has not been completely elucidated, but research indicates that accumulation of abnormally folded protein leads to activation of stress and proinflammatory pathways in the ER and hepatocyte programmed cell death. In liver biopsies from patients, polymerized α_1-antitrypsin peptides can be seen by electron microscopy and histochemically as periodic acid–Schiff (PAS)-positive diastase-resistant globules primarily in periportal hepatocytes but also in Kupffer cells and biliary epithelial cells. The pattern of neonatal liver injury can be highly variable, and liver biopsies might demonstrate heptocellular necrosis, inflammatory cell infiltration, bile duct proliferation, periportal fibrosis, or cirrhosis.

In affected patients, the course of liver disease is also highly variable. Prospective studies in Sweden have shown that only 10% of patients develop clinically significant liver disease by their 4th decade. Genetic traits or environmental factors must influence the development of disease in α_1-antitrypsin–deficient patients. Infants with liver disease are indistinguishable from other infants with "idiopathic" neonatal hepatitis, of whom they constitute ~5-10%. Jaundice, acholic stools, and hepatomegaly are present in the 1st wk of life, but the jaundice usually clears in the 2nd-4th mo. Complete resolution, persistent liver disease, or the development of cirrhosis can follow. Older children can present with asymptomatic hepatomegaly or manifestations of chronic liver disease or cirrhosis, with evidence of portal hypertension. Long-term patients are at risk for hepatocellular carcinoma.

Therapy is supportive; liver transplantation has been curative.

BIBLIOGRAPHY

Please visit the Nelson Textbook of Pediatrics *website at* *www.expertconsult.com* *for the complete bibliography.*

Chapter 350
Viral Hepatitis

Nada Yazigi and William F. Balistreri

Viral hepatitis continues to be is a major health problem in both developing and developed countries. This disorder is caused by at least 5 pathogenic hepatotropic viruses recognized to date: hepatitis A, B, C, D, and E viruses (Table 350-1). Many other viruses (and diseases) can cause hepatitis, usually as 1 component of a multisystem disease. These include herpes simplex virus

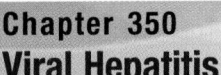

Table 350-1 FEATURES OF THE HEPATOTROPIC VIRUSES

VIROLOGY	HAV RNA	HBV DNA	HCV RNA	HDV RNA	HEV RNA
Incubation (days)	15-19	60-180	14-160	21-42	21-63
Transmission					
• Parenteral	Rare	Yes	Yes	Yes	No
• Fecal-oral	Yes	No	No	No	Yes
• Sexual	No	Yes	Yes	Yes	No
• Perinatal	No	Yes	Rare	Yes	No
Chronic infection	No	Yes	Yes	Yes	No
Fulminant disease	Rare	Yes	Rare	Yes	Yes

(HSV), cytomegalovirus (CMV), Epstein-Barr virus (EBV), varicella-zoster virus, HIV, rubella, adenoviruses, enteroviruses, parvovirus B19, and arboviruses (Table 350-2).

The hepatotropic viruses are a heterogeneous group of infectious agents that cause similar acute clinical illness. In most pediatric patients, the acute phase causes no or mild clinical disease. Morbidity is related to rare cases of **acute liver failure (ALF)** triggered in susceptible patients and to the chronic disease state and attendant complications that three of these viruses (hepatides B, C, and D) can cause.

Table 350-2 CAUSES AND DIFFERENTIAL DIAGNOSIS OF HEPATITIS IN CHILDREN

INFECTIOUS
Hepatotropic viruses • HAV • HBV • HCV • HDV • HEV • Hepatitis non-A-E viruses Systemic infection that can include hepatitis • Adenovirus • Arbovirus • Coxsackievirus • Cytomegalovirus • Enterovirus • Epstein-Barr virus • "Exotic" viruses (e.g., yellow fever) • Herpes simplex virus • Human immunodeficiency virus • Paramyxovirus • Rubella • Varicella zoster Other
NON-VIRAL LIVER INFECTIONS
Abscess Amebiasis Bacterial sepsis Brucellosis Fitz-Hugh-Curtis syndrome Histoplasmosis Leptospirosis Tuberculosis Other
AUTOIMMUNE
Autoimmune hepatitis Sclerosing cholangitis Other (e.g., systemic lupus erythematosus, juvenile rheumatoid arthritis)
METABOLIC
α1-Antitrypsin deficiency Tyrosinemia Wilson disease Other
TOXIC
Iatrogenic or drug induced (e.g., acetaminophen) Environmental (e.g., pesticides)
ANATOMIC
Choledochal cyst Biliary atresia Other
HEMODYNAMIC
Shock Congestive heart failure Budd-Chiari syndrome Other
NON-ALCOHOLIC FATTY LIVER DISEASE
Idiopathic Reye syndrome Other

From Wyllie R, Hyams JS, editors: *Pediatric gastrointestinal and liver disease,* ed 3, Philadelphia, 2006, Saunders.

ISSUES COMMON TO ALL FORMS OF VIRAL HEPATITIS

Differential Diagnosis

Often what brings the patient with hepatitis to medical attention is clinical icterus, which is a mixed or conjugated (direct) reacting hyperbilirubinemia.

Symptomatic infection results in icteric skin and mucous membranes. The liver is usually enlarged and tender to palpation and percussion. Splenomegaly and lymphadenopathy can be present. Extrahepatic symptoms are more readily seen in HBV and HCV infections (rashes, arthritis). Clinical signs of altered sensorium and hyperreflexivity should be carefully sought, because they mark the onset of encephalopathy and ALF.

The differential diagnosis varies with age of presentation.

In the **newborn period,** infection is a common cause of conjugated hyperbilirubinemia; the infectious cause is either a bacterial agent *(Escherichia coli, Listeria, Syphilis)* or one of the nonhepatotropic viruses (HSV, enteroviruses, CMV). Metabolic and anatomic causes (tyrosinemia, biliary atresia, genetic forms of intrahepatic cholestasis, and choledochal cysts) should always be excluded.

In later **childhood,** extrahepatic obstruction (gallstones, primary sclerosing cholangitis, pancreatic pathology), inflammatory conditions (autoimmune hepatitis, juvenile rheumatoid arthritis, Kawasaki disease, immune dysregulation), infiltrative disorders (malignancies), toxins and medications, metabolic disorders (Wilson disease, cystic fibrosis), and infection (EBV, varicella, malaria, leptospirosis, syphilis) should be ruled out.

Pathogenesis

The acute response of the liver to hepatotropic viruses involves a direct cytopathic and an immune-mediated injury. The entire liver is involved. Necrosis is usually most marked in the centrilobular areas. An acute mixed inflammatory infiltrate predominates in the portal areas but also affects the lobules. The lobular architecture remains intact, although balloon degeneration and necrosis of single or groups of parenchymal cells occurs commonly. Fatty change is rare except with HCV infection. Bile duct proliferation but not bile duct damage is common. Diffuse Kupffer cell hyperplasia is noticeable in the sinusoids. Neonates often respond to hepatic injury by forming **giant cells.**

In **fulminant hepatitis,** parenchymal collapse occurs on the just-described background.

With recovery, the liver morphology returns to normal within 3 mo of the acute infection. If chronic hepatitis develops, the inflammatory infiltrate settles in the periportal areas and often leads to progressive scarring. Both of these hallmarks of chronic hepatitis are seen in cases of HBV and HCV.

Common Biochemical Profiles in the Acute Infectious Phase

Acute liver injury caused by the hepatotropic viruses manifests in 3 main functional liver biochemical profiles. These serve as an important guide to supportive care and monitoring in the acute phase of the infection for all viruses.

As a reflection of *cytopathic injury* to the hepatocytes, there is a rise in serum levels of alanine aminotransferase (ALT) and aspartate aminotransferase (AST). The magnitude of enzyme elevation does not correlate with the extent of hepatocellular necrosis and has little prognostic value. There is usually slow improvement over several weeks, but AST and ALT levels lag behind the serum bilirubin level, which tends to normalize first. Rapidly falling aminotransferase levels can predict a poor outcome, particularly if their decline occurs in conjunction with a rising bilirubin level and a prolonged prothrombin time; this combination of findings usually indicates that massive hepatic injury has occurred.

Cholestasis, defined by elevated serum conjugated bilirubin levels, results from abnormal bile flow at the canalicular and cellular level due to hepatocyte damage and inflammatory mediators. Elevation of serum alkaline phosphatase (ALP), 5′-nucleotidase, γ-glutamyl transpeptidase (GGT), and urobilinogen all mark cholestasis. Improvement tends to parallel the acute hepatitis phase. Absence of cholestatic markers does not rule out progression to chronicity in HCV or HBV infections.

The most important marker of liver injury is altered *synthetic function*. Monitoring of synthetic function should be the main focus in clinical follow-up to define the severity of the disease. In the acute phase, the degree of liver synthetic dysfunction guides treatment and helps to establish intervention criteria. Abnormal liver synthetic function is a marker of liver failure and is an indication for prompt referral to a transplant center. Serial assessment is necessary because liver dysfunction does not progress linearly. Synthetic dysfunction is reflected by a combination of abnormal protein synthesis (prolonged prothrombin time, high international normalized ratio [INR], low serum albumin levels), metabolic disturbances (hypoglycemia, lactic acidosis, hyperammonemia), poor clearance of medications dependent on liver function, and altered sensorium with increased deep tendon reflexes (hepatic encephalopathy; Chapter 356).

HEPATITIS A

Hepatitis A virus (HAV) infection is the most prevalent of the 5. This virus is also responsible for most forms of acute and benign hepatitis; although fulminant hepatic failure can occur, it is rare and occurs more often in adults than in children.

Etiology

HAV is an RNA virus, a member of the picornavirus family. It is heat stable and has limited host range—namely, the human and other primates.

Epidemiology

HAV infection occurs throughout the world but is most prevalent in developing countries. In the United States, 30-40% of the adult population has evidence of previous HAV infection. Hepatitis A is thought to account for ~50% of all clinically apparent acute viral hepatitis in the United States. As a result of aggressive implementation of a childhood vaccination strategy, the prevalence of symptomatic HAV cases in the United States has declined significantly. However, outbreaks in daycare centers (where the spread from young, nonicteric, infected children can occur easily) as well as multiple foodborne and waterborne outbreaks have justified the implementation of a universal vaccination program.

HAV is highly contagious. Transmission is almost always by person-to-person contact through the fecal-oral route. Perinatal transmission occurs rarely. No other form of transmission is recognized. HAV infection during pregnancy or at the time of delivery does not appear to result in increased complications of pregnancy or clinical disease in the newborn. In the USA, increased risk of infection is found in contacts with infected persons, child-care centers, and household contacts. Infection has also been associated with contact with contaminated food or water and after travel to endemic areas. Common source foodborne and waterborne outbreaks have occurred, including several due to contaminated shellfish, frozen berries, and raw vegetables; no known source is found in about half of the cases. The mean incubation period for HAV is ~3 wk. Fecal excretion of the virus starts late in the incubation period, reaches its peak just before the onset of symptoms, and resolves by 2 wk after the onset of jaundice in older subjects. The duration of viral excretion is prolonged in infants. The patient is therefore contagious before clinical symptoms are apparent and remains so until viral shedding ceases.

Clinical Manifestations

HAV is responsible for acute hepatitis only. Often, this is an anicteric illness, with clinical symptoms indistinguishable from other forms of viral gastroenteritis, particularly in young children.

The illness is much more likely to be symptomatic in older adolescents or adults, in patients with underlying liver disorders, and in those who are immunocompromised. It is characteristically an acute febrile illness with an abrupt onset of anorexia, nausea, malaise, vomiting, and jaundice. The typical duration of illness is 7-14 days (Fig. 350-1).

Other organ systems can be affected during acute HAV infection. Regional lymph nodes and the spleen may be enlarged. The bone marrow may be moderately hypoplastic, and aplastic anemia has been reported. Tissue in the small intestine might show changes in villous structure, and ulceration of the gastrointestinal tract can occur, especially in fatal cases. Acute pancreatitis and myocarditis have been reported, though rarely, and nephritis, arthritis, vasculitis, and cryoglobulinemia can result from circulating immune complexes.

Diagnosis

Acute HAV infection is diagnosed by detecting antibodies to HAV, specifically, anti-HAV (IgM) by radioimmunoassay or, rarely, by identifying viral particles in stool. A viral polymerase chain reaction (PCR) assay is available for research use (Table 350-3). Anti-HAV is detectable when the symptoms are clinically apparent, and it remains positive for 4-6 mo after the acute infection. A neutralizing anti-HAV (IgG) is usually detected within 8 wk of symptom onset and is measured as part of a total anti-HAV in the serum. Anti-HAV (IgG) confers long-term protection.

Rises in serum levels of ALT, AST, bilirubin, ALP, 5′-nucleotidase, and GGT are almost universally found and do not help to differentiate the cause of hepatitis.

Complications

Although most patients achieve full recovery, two distinct complications can occur.

ALF from HAV infection is a rare but not infrequent complication of HAV. Those at risk for this complication are adolescents and adults, but also patients with underlying liver disorders or those who are immunocompromised. The height of HAV viremia may be linked to the severity of hepatitis. Whereas in the United States, HAV represents <0.5% of pediatric-aged ALF, it

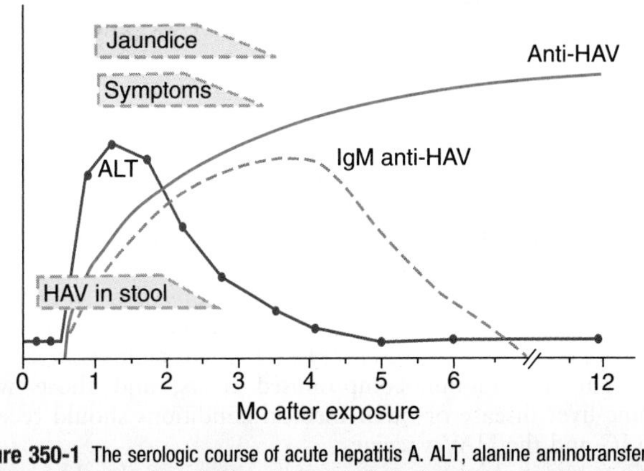

Figure 350-1 The serologic course of acute hepatitis A. ALT, alanine aminotransferase; HAV, hepatitis A virus. (From Goldman L, Ausiello D: *Cecil textbook of medicine*, ed 22, Philadelphia, 2004, Saunders, p 913.)

Table 350-3 DIAGNOSTIC BLOOD TESTS: SEROLOGY AND VIRAL PCR

HAV	HBV	HCV	HDV	HEV
ACUTE INFECTION				
Anti-HAV IgM+	Anti-HBc IgM+	Anti-HCV+	Anti-HDV IgM+	Anti-HEV IgM+
Blood PCR positive*	HBsAg+ Anti-HBs HBV DNA+ (PCR)	HCV RNA+ (PCR)	Blood PCR positive HBsAg+ Anti-HBs−	Blood PCR positive
PAST INFECTION (RECOVERED)				
Anti-HAV IgG+	Anti-HBs+ Anti-HBc IgG+	Anti-HCV− Blood PCR negative	Anti-HDV IgG+ Blood PCR negative	Anti-HEV IgG+ Blood PCR negative
CHRONIC INFECTION				
N/A	Anti-HBc IgG+ HBsAg+ Anti-HBs PCR positive or negative	Anti-HCV+ Blood PCR positive	Anti-HDV IgG+ Blood PCR negative HBsAg+	N/A
VACCINE RESPONSE				
Anti-HAV IgG+	Anti-HBs+ Anti-HBc−	N/A	N/A	N/A

*Research tool.
HAV, hepatitis A virus; HBs, hepatitis B surface; HBsAg, hepatitis B surface antigen; Ig, immunoglobulin; PCR, polymerase chain reaction.

Table 350-4 HEPATITIS A VIRUS PROPHYLAXIS

PRE-EXPOSURE PROPHYLAXIS (TRAVELERS TO ENDEMIC REGIONS)		
Age	**Exposure**	**Dose**
<1 yr of age	Expected <3 mo	Ig 0.02 mL/kg
	Expected 3-5 mo	Ig 0.06 mL/kg
	Expected long term	Ig 0.06 mL/kg at departure and every 5 mo thereafter
≥1 yr of age	Healthy host	HAV vaccine
	Immunocompromised host, or one with chronic liver disease or chronic health problems	HAV vaccine and Ig 0.02 mL/kg

POSTEXPOSURE PROPHYLAXIS*	
Exposure	**Recommendations**
≤2 wk since exposure	< 1 y of age: IG 0.02 mL/kg Immunocompromised host, or host with chronic liver disease or chronic health problems: IG 0.02 mL/kg and HAV vaccine >1 yr and healthy host: HAV vaccine, IG remains optional Sporadic non-household or close contact exposure: prophylaxis not indicated*
>2 wk since exposure	None

*Decision for prophylaxis in non-household contacts should be tailored to individual exposure and risk.
Ig, immunoglobulin.

is responsible for up to 3% mortality in the adult population with ALF. In endemic areas of the world, HAV constitutes up to 40% of all cases of pediatric ALF.

HAV can progress to a prolonged cholestatic syndrome that waxes and wanes over several months. Pruritus and fat malabsorption are problematic and require symptomatic support with antipruritic medications and fat-soluble vitamins. This syndrome occurs in the absence of any liver synthetic dysfunction and resolves with no sequelae.

Treatment

There is no specific treatment for hepatitis A. Supportive treatment consists of intravenous hydration as needed and antipruritic agents and fat-soluble vitamins for the prolonged cholestatic form of disease. Serial monitoring for signs of ALF and, if ALF is diagnosed, a prompt referral to a transplantation center can be lifesaving.

Prevention

Patients infected with HAV are contagious for 2 wk before and ~7 days after the onset of jaundice and should be excluded from school, child care, or work during this period. Careful handwashing is necessary, particularly after changing diapers and before preparing or serving food. In hospital settings, contact and standard precautions are recommended for 1 wk after onset of symptoms.

IMMUNOGLOBULIN Indications for intramuscular administration of immunoglobulin (IG) (0.02 mL/kg) include pre-exposure and postexposure prophylaxis (Table 350-4).

IG is recommended for pre-exposure prophylaxis for susceptible travelers to countries where HAV is endemic, and it provides effective protection for up to 3 mo. *HAV vaccine given any time before travel is preferred for pre-exposure prophylaxis in healthy persons, but IG ensures an appropriate prophylaxis in children <1 yr of age, patients allergic to a vaccine component, or those who elect not to receive the vaccine.* If travel is planned in <2 wk, older patients, immunocompromised hosts, and those with chronic liver disease or other medical conditions should receive both IG and the HAV vaccine.

IG as prophylaxis in postexposure situations should be used as soon as possible (not effective >2 wk after exposure). It is exclusively used for children <12 mo of age, immunocompromised hosts, those with chronic liver disease or in whom vaccine is contraindicated; IG is preferably used in patients > 40 yr of age. IG is optional in healthy persons 12 mo-40 yr, in whom HAV vaccine is preferred. *An alternative approach is to immunize previously unvaccinated patients who are ≥12 mo at the age-appropriate vaccine dosage as soon as possible.* IG is not routinely recommended for sporadic nonhousehold exposure (e.g., protection of hospital personnel or schoolmates).

VACCINE The availability of two inactivated, highly immunogenic, and safe HAV vaccines has had a major impact on the prevention of HAV infection. Both vaccines are approved for children >1 yr of age. They are administered intramuscularly in a 2-dose schedule, with the 2nd dose given 6-12 mo after the 1st dose. Seroconversion rates in children exceed 90% after an initial dose and approach 100% after the 2nd dose; protective antibody titer persists at least for 10 yr. The immune response in immunocompromised persons, older patients, and those with chronic illnesses may be suboptimal; in those patients, combining the vaccine with IG for pre- and postexposure prophylaxis is indicated. HAV vaccine may be administered simultaneously with other vaccines. A combination HAV and HBV vaccine is currently undergoing trials in adults. For healthy persons >1 yr of age, vaccine is preferable to immunoglobulin for pre-exposure and postexposure prophylaxis (see Table 350-3).

In the USA and some other countries, universal vaccination is now recommended for all children >1 yr of age. Prior to implementing universal HAV vaccination, mass immunization of school children has been used when epidemics have been school centered. The vaccine is effective in curbing outbreaks of hepatitis A due to rapid seroconversion and the long incubation period of the disease.

Prognosis

The prognosis for the patient with hepatitis A is excellent, with no long-term sequelae. The only feared complication is ALF. HAV infection remains a cause of major morbidity, however, and has a high socioeconomic impact during epidemics and in endemic areas.

HEPATITIS B

Etiology

HBV is a member of the Hepadnaviridae family. HBV has a circular, partially double-stranded DNA genome composed of ~3,200 nucleotides. Four genes have been identified: the S (surface), C (core), X, and P (polymer) genes. The surface of the virus includes particles designated *hepatitis B surface antigen (HBsAg),* which is a 22 nm diameter spherical particle and a 22 nm wide tubular particle with a variable length of up to 200 nm. The inner portion of the virion contains hepatitis B core antigen (HBcAg), the nucleocapsid that encodes the viral DNA, and a nonstructural antigen called hepatitis B e antigen (HBeAg), a nonparticulate soluble antigen derived from HBcAg by proteolytic self-cleavage. HBeAg serves as a marker of active viral replication and usually correlates with HBV DNA levels. Replication of HBV occurs predominantly in the liver but also occurs in the lymphocytes, spleen, kidney, and pancreas.

Epidemiology

HBV has been detected worldwide, with an estimated 400 million persons chronically infected. The areas of highest prevalence of HBV infection are sub-Saharan Africa, China, parts of the Middle East, the Amazon basin, and the Pacific Islands. In the United States, the native population in Alaska had the highest prevalence rate before the implementation of universal vaccination programs. An estimated 1.25 million persons in the United States are chronic HBV carriers, with ~300,000 new cases of HBV occurring each year, the highest incidence being among adults 20-39 yr of age. One in 4 chronic HBV carriers will develop serious sequelae in their lifetime. The number of new cases in children reported each year is thought to be low but is difficult to estimate because many infections in children are asymptomatic. In the United States, since 1982 when the first vaccine for HBV was introduced, the overall incidence of HBV infection has been reduced by more than half. Since the implementation of universal vaccination programs in Taiwan and the United States, substantial progress has been made toward eliminating HBV infection in children in these countries.

HBV is present in high concentrations in blood, serum, and serous exudates and in moderate concentrations in saliva, vaginal fluid, and semen. Efficient transmission occurs through blood exposure and sexual contact. Risk factors for HBV infection in children and adolescents include acquisition by intravenous drugs or blood products and by acupuncture or tattoos, sexual contact, institutional care, and intimate contact with carriers. No risk factors are identified in ~40% of cases. HBV is not thought to be transmitted via indirect exposure such as sharing toys.

In children, the most important risk factor for acquisition of HBV remains perinatal exposure to an HBsAg-positive mother. The risk of transmission is greatest if the mother is also HBeAg positive; up to 90% of these infants become chronically infected if untreated. Intrauterine infection occurs in 2.5% of these infants. In most cases, serologic markers of infection and antigenemia appear 1-3 mo after birth, suggesting that transmission occurred at the time of delivery. Virus contained in amniotic fluid or in maternal feces or blood may be the source. Immunoprophylaxis of those infants is very effective in preventing infection and protects >95% of neonates. Of the 22,000 infants born each year to HBsAg-positive mothers in the United States, >98% receive immunoprophylaxis and are thus protected.

HBsAg is inconsistently recovered in human milk of infected mothers. Breast-feeding of nonimmunized infants by infected mothers does not confer a greater risk of hepatitis than does formula feeding.

The risk of developing **chronic HBV** infection, defined as being positive for HBsAg for >6 mo, is inversely related to age of acquisition. In the United States, although <10% of infections occurs in children, these infections account for 20-30% of all chronic cases. This risk of chronic infection is 90% in children <1 yr; the risk is 30% for those 1-5 yr and 2% for adults. Chronic infection is associated with the development of chronic liver disease and hepatocellular carcinoma. The carcinoma risk is independent of the presence of cirrhosis and was the most prevalent cancer-related death in young adults in Asia where HBV was endemic.

HBV has 8 genotypes (A-H). A is pandemic, B and C are prevalent in Asia, D is seen in Southern Europe, E in Africa, F in the United States, G in the United States and France, and H in Central America. Genetic variants have become resistant to antiviral agents. After infection, the incubation period ranges from 45 to 160 days, with a mean of ~120 days.

Pathogenesis

The acute response of the liver to HBV is the same as for all hepatotropic viruses. Persistence of histologic changes in patients with hepatitis B indicates development of chronic liver disease. HBV, unlike the other hepatotropic viruses, is a predominantly non-cytopathogenic virus that causes injury mostly by immune-mediated processes. The severity of hepatocyte injury reflects the degree of the immune response, with the most complete immune response being associated with the greatest likelihood of viral clearance but also the most severe injury to hepatocytes. The first step in the process of **acute hepatitis** is infection of hepatocytes by HBV, resulting in expression of viral antigens on the cell surface. The most important of these viral antigens may be the nucleocapsid antigens HBcAg and HBeAg. These antigens, in combination with class I major histocompatibility (MHC) proteins, make the cell a target for cytotoxic T-cell lysis.

The mechanism for development of **chronic hepatitis** is less well understood. To permit hepatocytes to continue to be infected, the core protein or MHC class I protein might not be recognized, the cytotoxic lymphocytes might not be activated, or some other, yet unknown mechanism might interfere with destruction of hepatocytes. This **tolerance** phenomenon predominates in the cases acquired perinatally, resulting in a high incidence of persistent infection in children with no or little inflammation in the liver. Although end-stage liver disease rarely develops in those patients, the inherent hepatocellular carcinoma risk is very high, possibly related, in part, to uncontrolled viral replication cycles.

ALF has been seen in infants of chronic carrier mothers who have anti-HBe or are infected with a precore-mutant strain. This fact led to the postulate that HBeAg exposure in utero in infants of chronic carriers likely induces tolerance to the virus once infection occurs postnatally. In the absence of this tolerance, the liver is massively attacked by T cells and the patient presents with ALF.

Immune-mediated mechanisms are also involved in the **extrahepatic conditions** that can be associated with HBV infections. **Circulating immune complexes** containing HBsAg can occur in patients who develop associated polyarteritis nodosa, membranous or membranoproliferative glomerulonephritis, polymyalgia rheumatica, leukocytoclastic vasculitis, and Guillain-Barré syndrome.

Clinical Manifestations

Many acute cases of HBV infection in children are asymptomatic, as evidenced by the high carriage rate of serum markers in persons who have no history of acute hepatitis. The usual acute symptomatic episode is similar to that of HAV and HCV infections but may be more severe and is more likely to include involvement of skin and joints (Fig. 350-2). The first biochemical evidence of HBV infection is elevation of serum ALT levels, which begin to rise just before development of fatigue, anorexia, and malaise, which occurs about 6-7 wk after exposure. The illness is preceded

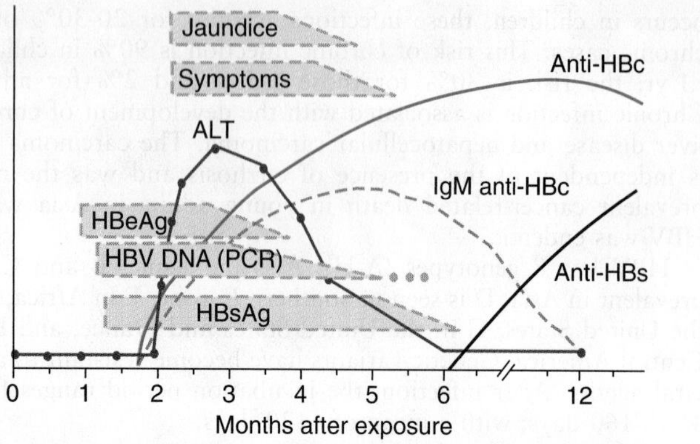

Figure 350-2 The serologic course of acute hepatitis B. HBc, hepatitis B core; HBeAg, hepatitis B e antigen; HBs, hepatitis B surface; HBsAg, hepatitis B surface antigen; HBV, hepatitis B virus; PCR, polymerase chain reaction. (From Goldman L, Ausiello D: *Cecil textbook of medicine,* ed 22, Philadelphia, 2004, Saunders, p 914.)

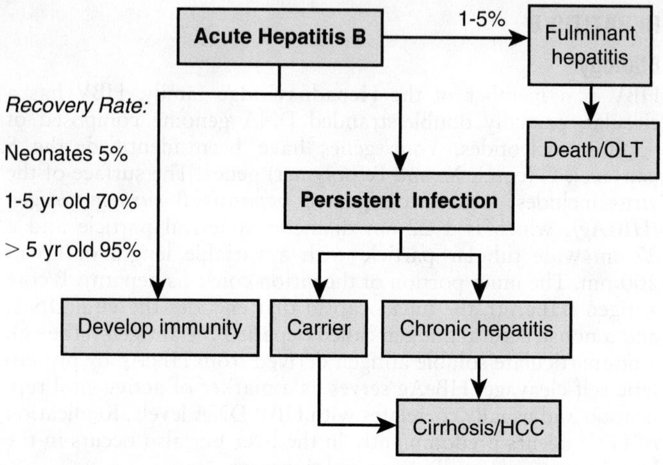

Figure 350-3 Natural history of hepatitis B virus infection. HCC, hepatocellular carcinoma; OLT, orthotopic liver transplant.

in a few children by a serum sickness–like prodrome marked by arthralgia or skin lesions, including urticarial, purpuric, macular, or maculopapular rashes. Papular acrodermatitis, the Gianotti-Crosti syndrome, can also occur. Other extrahepatic conditions associated with HBV infections in children include polyarteritis, glomerulonephritis, and aplastic anemia. Jaundice, which is present in ~25% of acutely infected patients, usually begins ~8 wk after exposure and lasts for ~4 wk.

In the usual course of resolving HBV infection, symptoms are present for 6-8 wk. The percentage of children in whom clinical evidence of hepatitis develops is higher for HBV than for HAV, and the rate of ALF is also greater. Most patients do recover, but the "chronic carrier state" complicates up to 10% of cases acquired in adulthood. The rate of acquisition of chronic infection depends largely on the mode and age of acquisition and is up to 90% in the perinatal cases. Chronic hepatitis, cirrhosis, and hepatocellular carcinoma are only seen with chronic infection. Chronic HBV infection has 3 identified phases: immune tolerant, immune active, and inactive. Most children fall in the immune-tolerant phase, against which no effective therapy is yet developed, but most treatments target the immune active phase of the disease, characterized by active inflammation, elevated ALT/AST levels, and progressive fibrosis. Spontaneous HBeAg seroconversion occurs in the immune-tolerant phase, albeit at low rates of 4-5% per year. It is more common in childhood-acquired HBV rather than in vertically transmitted infections. Seroconversion can last many years, during which significant damage to the liver can happen. There are no large studies that help accurately assess the lifelong risks and morbidities of children with chronic HBV infection, making the timing of still less-than-ideal treatments ever so hard to decide. Reactivation of chronic infection has been reported in immunosuppressed children (treated with chemotherapy, biologic immunomodulators, T-cell depleting agents), leading to an increased risk of ALF or to rapidly progressing fibrotic liver disease.

Diagnosis

The serologic profile of HBV infection is more complex than for HAV infection and differs depending on whether the disease is acute or chronic (Fig. 350-3). Several antigens and antibodies are used to confirm the diagnosis of acute HBV infection (see Table 350-3). Routine screening for HBV infection requires assay of ≥3 serologic markers (HBsAg, anti-HBc, anti-HBs). HBsAg is the first serologic marker of infection to appear and is found in almost all infected persons; its rise closely coincides with the onset of symptoms. Persistence of HBsAg beyond 6 mo defines the chronic infection state. During recovery from acute infection, because HBsAg levels fall before symptoms wane, IgM antibody to HBcAg (anti-HBc IgM) might be the only marker of acute infection. Anti-HBc IgM rises early after the infection and remains positive for many months before being replaced by anti-HBc IgG, which then persists for years. Anti-HBc is therefore a valuable serologic marker of acute HBV infection. Anti-HBs marks serologic recovery and protection. Only anti-HBs is present in persons immunized with hepatitis B vaccine, whereas both anti-HBs and anti-HBc are detected in persons with resolved infection. HBeAg is present in active acute or chronic infection and is a marker of infectivity. The development of anti-HBe marks improvement and is a goal of therapy in chronically infected patients. HBV DNA can be detected in the serum of acutely infected patients and chronic carriers. High DNA titers are seen in patients with HBeAg, and they typically fall once anti-HBe develops.

Complications

ALF with coagulopathy, encephalopathy, and cerebral edema occurs more commonly with HBV than with the other hepatotropic viruses. The risk of ALF is further increased when there is co-infection or super-infection with HDV and in an immunosuppressed host. Mortality due to ALF is >30%, and liver transplantation is the only effective intervention. Supportive care aimed at sustaining patients and early referral to a liver transplantation center can be lifesaving. As mentioned, HBV infection can also result in **chronic hepatitis,** which can lead to cirrhosis, end-stage liver disease complications, and primary **hepatocellular carcinoma. Membranous glomerulonephritis** with deposition of complement and HBeAg in glomerular capillaries is a rare complication of HBV infection.

Treatment

Treatment of *acute* HBV infection is largely supportive. Close monitoring for liver failure and extrahepatic morbidities is key.

Treatment of *chronic* HBV infection is in evolution; no one drug currently achieves reliably complete eradication of the virus. The natural history of HBV chronic infection in children is complex, and there is a lack of reliable long-term outcome data on which to base treatment recommendation. Treatment of chronic HBV infection in children should be individualized and done under the care of a pediatric gastroenterologist experienced in treating liver disease.

The goal of treatment is to reduce viral replication as defined by undetectable HBV DNA in the serum and development of anti-HBe. This seroconversion transforms the disease into an inactive form, therefore decreasing active liver injury and inflammation, fibrosis progression, and infectivity as well as the risk of hepatocellular carcinoma.

Currently, treatment is only indicated for patients in the immune-active form of the disease, with evidence of ongoing inflammation and fibrosis putting the child at higher risk for cirrhosis during childhood.

TREATMENT STRATEGIES *Interferon-α-2b (IFN-α2b)* has immunomodulatory and antiviral effects. It has been used in children, with long-term viral response rates similar to the 25% rate reported in adults. IFN use is limited by its subcutaneous administration, duration of treatment for 24 weeks, and possible side effects (marrow suppression, depression, retinal changes, autoimmune disorders). IFN is further contraindicated in decompensated cirrhosis.

Lamivudine is an oral synthetic nucleoside analog that inhibits the viral enzyme reverse transcriptase. In children >2 yr, its use for 52 wk resulted in HBeAg clearance in 34% of patients with an ALT >2 times normal; 88% remained in remission at 1 yr. It has a good safety profile. Lamivudine has to be used for ≥6 mo after viral clearance, and the emergence of a mutant viral strain (YMDD) poses a barrier to its long-term use. Combination therapy in children using IFN and lamivudine did not seem to improve the rates of response in most series.

Adefovir (a purine analog that inhibits viral replication) is approved for use in children >12 yr of age, in whom a prospective 1-yr study showed 23% seroconversion. No viral resistance was noted in that study but has been reported in adults.

Peginterferon-α2 and several new nucleotide/nucleoside analogs (Telbivudine, Tenofevir, and Entecavir) are approved for use in adults. They seem to have an improved efficacy and less viral resistance than IFN-α2b or Lamivudine in the adult population. No data are yet available on their use in children <16 yr of age.

Patients most likely to respond to currently available drugs have low serum HBV DNA titers, are HBeAg positive, have active hepatic inflammation (ALT greater than twice the upper limit of normal), and recently acquired disease.

Immunotolerant patients are currently not considered for treatment, although the emergence of new treatment paradigms are promising for this large, yet hard to treat, subgroup of patients.

Prevention

Hepatitis B vaccine and hepatitis B immunoglobulin (HBIG) are available for prevention of HBV infection. Two recombinant DNA vaccines are available in the United States; both are highly immunogenic in children. The safety profile of HBV vaccine is excellent. The most reported side effects are pain at the injection site (up to 29% of cases) and fever (up to 6% of cases).

Household, sexual, and needle-sharing contacts should be identified and vaccinated if they are susceptible to HBV infection. Patients should be advised about the perinatal and intimate contact risk of transmission of HBV. HBV is not spread by breast-feeding, kissing, hugging, or sharing water or utensils. Children with HBV should not be excluded from school, play, child care, or work, unless they are prone to biting. A support group might help children to cope better with their disease. All patients positive for HBsAg should be reported to the state or local health department, and chronicity is diagnosed if they remain positive past 6 mo.

HEPATITIS B IMMUNOGLOBULIN HBIG is indicated only for specific postexposure circumstances and provides only temporary protection (3-6 mo) (Table 350-5). It plays a pivotal role in preventing perinatal transmission when administered within 12 h of birth.

UNIVERSAL VACCINATION In 2005, the Centers for Disease Control and Prevention (CDC) Advisory Committee on Immunization Practices revised its recommendations regarding HBV vaccination. These recommendations have been incorporated into the American Academy of Pediatrics Revised Vaccine schedule.

Table 350-5 INDICATIONS AND DOSING SCHEDULE FOR HEPATITIS B VACCINE AND HEPATITIS B IMMUNOGLOBULIN

	VACCINE DOSE		
	Recombivax HB (μg)	Engerix-B (μg)	SCHEDULE
UNIVERSAL PROPHYLAXIS			
Infants of HBsAg⁻ women	5	10	Birth, 1-2, 6-18 mo
Children and adolescents (11-19 yr)	5	10	0, 1, and 6 mo
POSTEXPOSURE PROPHYLAXIS IN SUSCEPTIBLE INDIVIDUALS			
Contact with HBsAg-Positive Source			
Infants of HBsAg⁺ women	5	10	Birth* (+HBIG†), 1 and 6 mo
Intimate or Identifiable Blood Exposure			
0-19 yr old	5	10	Exposure (+HBIG†), 1 and 6 mo
>19 yr old	10	20	Exposure (+HBIG†), 1 and 6 mo
Household			
0-19 yr old	5	10	Exposure, 1 and 6 mo
>19 yr old	10	20	Exposure, 1 and 6 mo
Casual	None	None	None
Immunocompromised‡	40	40	Exposure (+HBIG†), 1 and 6 mo
Contact with Unknown HBsAg Status; Intimate or Identifiable Blood Exposure			
>19 yr old	10	20	Exposure, 1 and 6 mo
Immunocompromised‡	40	40	Exposure (+HBIG†), 1 and 6 mo

*Both HBIG and vaccine should be administered within 12 hr of the infant's birth and within 24 hr of identifiable blood exposure. HBIG can be given up to 14 days after sexual exposure.
†HBIG dose: 0.5 μL for newborns of HBsAg-positive mothers, and 0.0 6 μL/kg for all others when recommended.
‡Seroconversion status of immunocompromised patients should be checked 1-2 mo after the last dose of vaccine, and yearly thereafter. Booster doses of vaccine should be administered if the anti-HBs titer is <10 mIU/mL. Nonresponsive patients should be considered at high risk for HBV acquisition and counseled about preventive measures.
HBs, hepatitis B surface; HBsAg, hepatitis B surface antigen; HBV, hepatitis B virus.

A main focus is **universal infant vaccination,** beginning at birth, to provide a safety net for preventing perinatal infection, prevent early childhood infection, facilitate implementation of universal vaccine recommendations, and prevent infection in adolescents and adults. The ultimate goal is to eliminate HBV transmission in the United States and to integrate HBV vaccination in a harmonized childhood vaccination.

Two single antigen vaccines (Recombivax HB and Engerix-B) are approved for children and are the only preparations approved for infants <6 mo old. Three combination vaccines can be used for subsequent immunization dosing and enable integration of the HBV vaccine into the regular immunization schedule. Seropositivity is >95% with all vaccines, achieved after the 2nd dose in most patients. The 3rd dose serves as a booster and may have an effect on maintaining long-term immunity. In immunosuppressed patients and infants <2,000 g birthweight, a 4th dose is recommended, as is checking for seroconversion. Despite declines in the anti-HBs titer in time, most healthy vaccinated persons remain protected against HBV infection.

Current HBV vaccination recommendations are as follows (see Table 350-5):

- For all medically stable infants weighing >2,000 g at birth and born to HBsAg-*negative* mothers, the first dose of HBV vaccine should be administered before hospital discharge. Single-dose antigen HBV vaccine should be used for the birth dose. Subsequent doses to complete the series are given at 1-4 mo and at 6-18 mo of age. Routine post-vaccination testing of immunized infants born to HBsAg-negative women or with anti-HBs is not recommended.

- In rare circumstances (on a case-by-case basis), the 1st dose may be delayed (up to 2 mo) until after hospital discharge. When a decision to delay is made, however, a physician's order to withhold the birth dose, along with a copy of the original laboratory report indicating that the mother was HBsAg *negative,* should be placed on the medical record.
- Preterm infants weighing <2,000 g at birth and born to HBsAg-*negative* mothers should have their initial dose delayed until 1 mo of age or before hospital discharge.
- To increase coverage of children and adolescents not previously vaccinated, many states have made immunization a requirement for entry into junior high school (middle school).
- To prevent perinatal transmission through improved maternal screening and immunoprophylaxis of infants born to HbsAg-positive mothers, infants born to HBsAg-positive women should receive vaccine at birth, 1-2 mo, and 6 mo of age (see Table 350-4). The first dose should be accompanied by administration of 0.5 mL of HBIG as soon after delivery as possible (within 12 hr) because the effectiveness decreases rapidly with increased time after birth. Post-vaccination testing for HBsAg and anti-HBs should be done at 9-18 mo. If the result is positive for anti-HBs, the child is immune to HBV. If the result is positive for HBsAg only, the parent should be counseled and the child evaluated by a pediatric gastroenterologist. If the result is negative for both HBsAg and anti-HBs, a 2nd complete hepatitis B vaccine series should be administered, followed by testing for anti-HBs to determine if subsequent doses are needed.

Administration of 4 doses of vaccine is permissible when combination vaccines are used after the birth dose; this does not increase vaccine response.

Postexposure Prophylaxis

Recommendations for postexposure prophylaxis for prevention of hepatitis B infection depend on the conditions under which the person is exposed to HBV (see Table 350-5). Vaccination should never be postponed if written records of the exposed person's immunization history are not available, but every effort should still be made to obtain those records.

Prognosis

In general, the outcome after acute HBV infection is favorable, despite a risk of ALF. The risk of developing chronic infection brings the risks of liver cirrhosis and hepatocellular carcinoma to the forefront. Perinatal transmission leading to chronicity is responsible for the high incidence of hepatocellular carcinoma in young adults in the endemic areas. Importantly, HBV infection and its complications are effectively controlled and prevented with vaccination.

HEPATITIS C

Etiology

HCV is a single-stranded RNA virus, classified as a separate genus within the Flaviviridae family, with marked genetic heterogeneity. It has 6 major genotypes and numerous subtypes and quasi-species, which permit the virus to escape host immune surveillance. Genotype variation might partially explain the differences in clinical course and response to treatment. Genotype 1b is the most common genotype in the United States and is the least responsive to the currently available medications.

Epidemiology

In the United States, HCV infection is the most common cause of chronic liver disease in adults and causes 8,000-10,000 deaths per year. About 4 million people in the United States and 170 million people worldwide are estimated to be infected with HCV. Approximately 85% of infected adults remain chronically infected. In children, seroprevalence of HCV is 0.2% in children <11 yr of age and 0.4% in children ≥11 yr of age.

Risk factors for HCV transmission in the United States previously included blood transfusion as the most common route of infection, but, with the current screening practices, the risk of HCV transmission is now about 0.001% per unit transfused. Illegal drug use with exposure to blood or blood products from HCV-infected persons accounts for more than half of adult cases in the United States. Sexual transmission, especially through multiple sexual partners, is the second most common cause of infection. Other risk factors include occupational exposure; ~10% of new infections has no known transmission source. In children, perinatal transmission is the most prevalent mode of transmission (see Table 350-1). Perinatal transmission occurs in up to 5% of infants born to viremic mothers. HIV co-infection and high viremia titers (HCV RNA positive) in the mother can increase the transmission rate to 20%. The incubation period is 7-9 wk (range, 2-24 wk).

Pathogenesis

The pattern of acute hepatic injury is indistinguishable from that of other hepatotropic viruses. In chronic cases, lymphoid aggregates or follicles in portal tracts are found, either alone or as part of a general inflammatory infiltration of the tracts. Steatosis is also often seen in these liver specimens. HCV appears to cause injury primarily by cytopathic mechanisms, but immune-mediated injury can also occur. The cytopathic component appears to be mild, because the acute illness is typically the least severe of all hepatotropic virus infections.

Clinical Manifestations

Acute HCV infection tends to be mild and insidious in onset (Fig. 350-4; see also Table 350-1). ALF rarely occurs. HCV is the most likely hepatotropic virus to cause chronic infection (Fig. 350-5). Of affected adults, <15% clear the virus; the rest develop chronic hepatitis. In pediatric studies, 6-19% of children achieved spontaneous sustained clearance of the virus during a 6 yr follow-up.

Chronic HCV infection is also clinically silent until a complication develops. Serum aminotransferase levels fluctuate and are sometimes normal, but histologic inflammation is universal. Progression of liver fibrosis is slow over several years, unless comorbid factors are present, which can accelerate fibrosis progression. About 25% of infected patients ultimately progress to cirrhosis, liver failure, and, occasionally, primary hepatocellular carcinoma

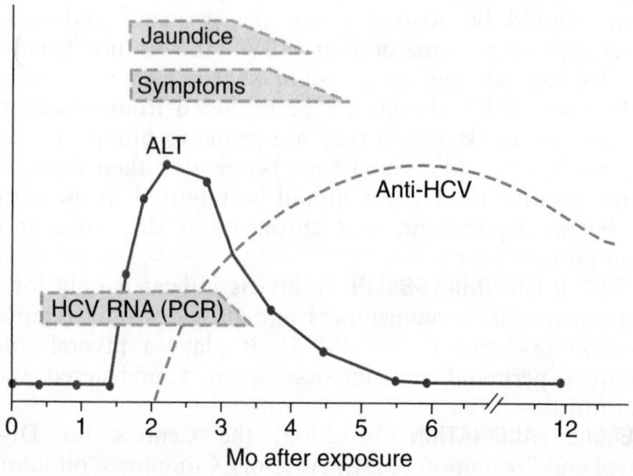

Figure 350-4 The serologic course of acute hepatitis C. ALT, alanine aminotransferase; HCV, hepatitis C virus; PCR, polymerase chain reaction. (From Goldman L, Ausiello D: *Cecil textbook of medicine,* ed 22, Philadelphia, 2004, Saunders, p 915.)

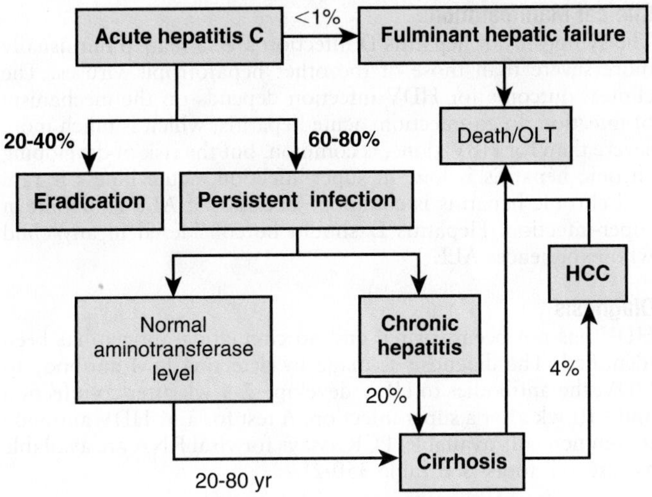

Figure 350-5 Natural history of hepatitis C virus infection. HCC, hepatocellular carcinoma; OLT, orthotopic liver transplant. (From Hochman JA, Balistreri WF: Chronic viral hepatitis: always be current! *Pediatr Rev* 24:399–410, 2003.)

(HCC) within 20-30 yr of the acute infection. Although progression is rare within the pediatric age range, cirrhosis and HCC from HCV have been reported in children. The long-term morbidities constitute the rationale for diagnosis and treatment in children with HCV.

Chronic HCV infection can be associated with **small vessel vasculitis** and is a common cause of essential mixed cryoglobulinemia. Other extrahepatic manifestations predominantly seen in adults include cutaneous vasculitis, peripheral neuropathy, cerebritis, membranoproliferative glomerulonephritis, and nephrotic syndrome. Antibodies to smooth muscle, antinuclear antibodies, and low thyroid hormone levels may also be present.

Diagnosis

Clinically available assays for detection of HCV infection are based on detection of antibodies to HCV antigens or detection of viral RNA (see Table 350-3); neither can predict the severity of liver disease.

The most widely used **serologic test** is the third-generation enzyme immunoassay (EIA) to detect anti-HCV. The predictive value of this assay is greatest in high-risk populations, but the false-positive rate can be as high as 50-60% in low-risk populations. False-negative results also occur because antibodies remain negative for as long as 1-3 mo after clinical onset of illness. Anti-HCV is not a protective antibody and does not confer immunity; it is usually present simultaneously with the virus.

The most commonly used **virologic assay** for HCV is a PCR assay, which permits detection of small amounts of **HCV RNA** in serum and tissue samples within days of infection. The qualitative PCR detection is especially useful in patients with recent or perinatal infection, hypogammaglobulinemia, or immunosuppression and is very sensitive. The quantitative PCR aids in identifying patients who are likely to respond to therapy and in monitoring response to therapy.

Screening for HCV should include all patients with the following risk factors: history of illegal drug use (even if only once), receiving clotting factors made before 1987 (when inactivation procedures were introduced) or blood products before 1992, hemodialysis, idiopathic liver disease, and children born to HCV-infected women (qualitative PCR in infancy and anti-HCV after 12 mo of age). Routine screening of all *pregnant women* is not recommended.

Determining HCV **genotype** is also important, particularly when therapy is considered, because the response to the current therapeutic agents varies greatly. Genotype 1 is poorly responsive; genotypes 2 and 3 are more reliably responsive to therapy (as discussed later).

Aminotransferase levels typically fluctuate during HCV infection and do not correlate with the degree of liver fibrosis.

A liver biopsy is the only means to assess the presence and extent of hepatic fibrosis, outside of overt signs of chronic liver disease. A liver biopsy is indicated only before starting any treatment and to rule out other causes of overt liver disease.

Complications

The risk of ALF due to HCV is low, but the risk of **chronic hepatitis** is the highest of all the hepatotropic viruses. In adults, risk factors for progression to hepatic fibrosis include older age, obesity, male sex, and even moderate alcohol ingestion (two 1 oz drinks per day). Progression to cirrhosis or HCC is a major cause of morbidity and the most common indication for liver transplantation in adults in the United States.

Treatment

In adults, peginterferon (subcutaneous, weekly) combined with oral daily ribavirin is the most effective therapy. Studies incorporate, in addition, nucleoside analogs. Patients most likely to respond have mild hepatitis, shorter duration of infection, and low viral titers. Genotypes 2 and 3 are the most sensitive to treatment; patients with genotype 1 virus respond poorly. The goal of treatment is to achieve a sustained viral response (SVR), as defined by the absence of viremia 6 mo after stopping the medications; SVR is associated with improved histology and decreased risk of morbidities.

The natural history of HCV infection in children is still being defined. It is believed that children have a higher rate of spontaneous clearance than in adults (up to 45% by age 19 yr). A multicenter study followed 359 children infected with HCV over 10 yr. Only 7.5% had cleared the virus, and 1.8% progressed to decompensated cirrhosis. Treatment in adults with acute HCV in a pilot study showed an 88% sustained viral response (SVR) in genotype 1 subjects (treated with IFN and ribavarin for 24 wk). Such data, if confirmed, could actually raise the question whether children, with shorter duration of infection and fewer comorbid conditions than their adult counterparts, could be "ideal" candidates for treatment. Given the adverse effects of currently available therapy, this strategy is not recommended outside of clinical trials.

Peginterferon (Schering), IFN-α2b, and ribavirin are approved by the Food and Drug Administration (FDA) for use in children >3 yr of age with HCV hepatitis. Studies of IFN monotherapy in children have shown a higher SVR than in adults, with better compliance and fewer side effects. An SVR up to 49% for genotype 1 was achieved in multiple studies. Factors associated with a higher likelihood of response are age <12 yr, genotypes 2 and 3, and, in patients with genotype 1b, an RNA titer <2 million copies/mL of blood, and viral response (PCR at weeks 4 and 12 of treatment). Side effects of medications lead to discontinuation of treatment in a high proportion of patients; these include anemia, neutropenia, and influenza-like symptoms.

Treatment should be considered for all children infected with genotypes 2 and 3, because they have a high response rate to therapy. If the child has genotype type 1b virus, the treatment choice remains more controversial. Treatment should be considered for patients with evidence of advanced fibrosis or injury on liver biopsy. A consensus recommendation paper suggested considering treatment in all patients with evidence of active inflammation on a liver biopsy along with biochemical anomalies.

Treatment consists of 48 wk of IFN and ribavarin (therapy should be stopped if still detectable on viral PCR at 24 wk of therapy). A liver biopsy was recommended before treatment. Close monitoring for treatment side effects was encouraged. Treatment of children with normal biochemical profile and mild histologic inflammation should be reserved to a clinical study context.

NEWER TREATMENTS Peginterferon and an antiviral telaprevir (NS3 viral protease inhibitor) have shown a much improved SVR success in adults. Studies are pending in pediatrics. Combination therapy schemes and staggered therapy is also being explored in adults.

Prevention

No vaccine is available to prevent HCV. Current immunoglobulin preparations are not beneficial, likely because immunoglobulin preparations produced in the United States do not contain antibodies to HCV because blood and plasma donors are screened for anti-HCV and excluded from the donor pool. Broad neutralizing antibodies to HCV were found to be protective and might pave the road for vaccine development.

Once HCV infection is identified, patients should be screened yearly with a liver ultrasound and serum α-fetoprotein for HCC, as well as for any clinical evidence of liver disease. Vaccinating the affected patient against HAV and HBV will prevent super-infection with these viruses and the increased risk of developing severe liver failure.

Prognosis

Viral titers should be checked yearly to document spontaneous remission. Most patients develop chronic hepatitis. Progressive liver damage is higher in those with additional comorbid factors such as alcohol consumption, viral genotypic variations, obesity, and underlying genetic predispositions. Referral to a pediatric gastroenterologist is strongly advised to take advantage of up-to-date monitoring regimens and to optimize their enrollment in treatment protocols when available.

HEPATITIS D

Etiology

HDV, the smallest known animal virus, is considered defective because it cannot produce infection without concurrent HBV infection. The 36 nm diameter virus is incapable of making its own coat protein; its outer coat is composed of excess HBsAg from HBV. The inner core of the virus is single-stranded circular RNA that expresses the HDV antigen.

Epidemiology

HDV can cause an infection at the same time as the initial HBV infection (**co-infection**), or HDV can infect a person who is already infected with HBV (**super-infection**). Transmission usually occurs by intrafamilial or intimate contact in areas of high prevalence, which are primarily developing countries (see Table 350-1). In areas of low prevalence, such as the United States, the parenteral route is far more common. HDV infections are uncommon in children in the United States but must be considered when ALF occurs. The incubation period for HDV super-infection is about 2-8 wk; with co-infection, the incubation period is similar to that of HBV infection.

Pathogenesis

Liver pathology in HDV hepatitis has no distinguishing features except that damage is usually quite severe. In contrast to HBV, HDV causes injury directly by cytopathic mechanisms. Many of the most severe cases of HBV infection appear to be a result of co-infection of HBV and HDV.

Clinical Manifestations

The symptoms of hepatitis D infection are similar to but usually more severe than those of the other hepatotropic viruses. The clinical outcome for HDV infection depends on the mechanism of infection. In co-infection, acute hepatitis, which is much more severe than for HBV alone, is common, but the risk of developing chronic hepatitis is low. In super-infection, acute illness is rare and chronic hepatitis is common. The risk of ALF is highest in super-infection. Hepatitis D should be considered in any child who experiences ALF.

Diagnosis

HDV has not been isolated and no circulating antigen has been identified. The diagnosis is made by detecting IgM antibody to HDV; the antibodies to HDV develop ~2-4 wk after co-infection and ~10 wk after a super-infection. A test for anti-HDV antibody is commercially available. PCR assays for viral RNA are available as research tools (see Table 350-2).

Complications

HDV must be considered in all cases of ALF. Co-infection with HBV can also result in a more severe chronic disease.

Treatment

The treatment is based on supportive measures once an infection is identified. There are no specific HDV-targeted treatments to date. The treatment is mostly based on controlling and treating HBV infection, without which HDV cannot induce hepatitis.

Prevention

There is no vaccine for hepatitis D. Because HDV replication cannot occur without hepatitis B co-infection, immunization against HBV also prevents HDV infection. Hepatitis B vaccines and HBIG are used for the same indications as for hepatitis B alone.

HEPATITIS E

Etiology

HEV has not been isolated but has been cloned using molecular techniques. This RNA virus has a nonenveloped sphere shape with spikes and is similar in structure to the caliciviruses.

Epidemiology

Hepatitis E is the epidemic form of what was formerly called non-A, non-B hepatitis. Transmission is fecal-oral (often water-borne) and is associated with shedding of 27-34 nm particles in the stool (see Table 350-1). The highest prevalence of HEV infection has been reported in the Indian subcontinent, the Middle East, Southeast Asia, and Mexico, especially in areas with poor sanitation. The mean incubation period is ~40 days (range, 15-60 days).

Pathogenesis

HEV appears to act as a cytopathic virus. The pathologic findings are similar to those of the other hepatitis viruses.

Clinical Manifestations

The clinical illness associated with HEV infection is similar to that of HAV but is often more severe. As with HAV, chronic illness does not occur. In addition to often causing a more severe episode than HAV, HEV tends to affect older patients, with a peak age between 15 and 34 yr. HEV is a major pathogen in pregnant women, in whom it causes ALF with a high fatality incidence. HEV could also lead to decompensation of pre-existing chronic liver disease.

Complications

HEV is associated with a high risk of death in pregnant women. No other complications are recognized in association with this virus.

Diagnosis

Recombinant DNA technology has resulted in development of antibodies to HEV particles, and IgM and IgG assays are available to distinguish between acute and resolved infections (see Table 350-3). IgM antibody to viral antigen becomes positive after ~1 wk of illness. Viral RNA can be detected in stool and serum by PCR.

Prevention

A recombinant hepatitis E vaccine is highly effective in adults. No evidence suggests that immunoglobulin is effective in preventing HEV infections. Immunoglobulin pooled from patients in endemic areas might prove to be effective.

APPROACH TO ACUTE OR CHRONIC HEPATITIS

Although new treatment modalities for chronic viral hepatitis are continuously being developed, and treatment outcomes have improved, the major medical breakthrough in regard to the pediatric population is prevention, with the availability of effective and safe vaccines for the HAV and HBV infections. The availability of more sensitive and reliable diagnostic tools may lead to improved care for affected patients. The primary care physician is at the forefront of the care and control of patients exposed to these viruses. Aggressive perinatal, childhood, and adolescent immunization strategies have already had a major impact in endemic HAV and HBV areas.

Identifying deterioration of the patient with acute hepatitis and the development of ALF is a major contribution of the primary pediatrician (Fig. 350-6). If ALF is identified, the clinician should immediately refer the patient to a transplant center; this can be lifesaving.

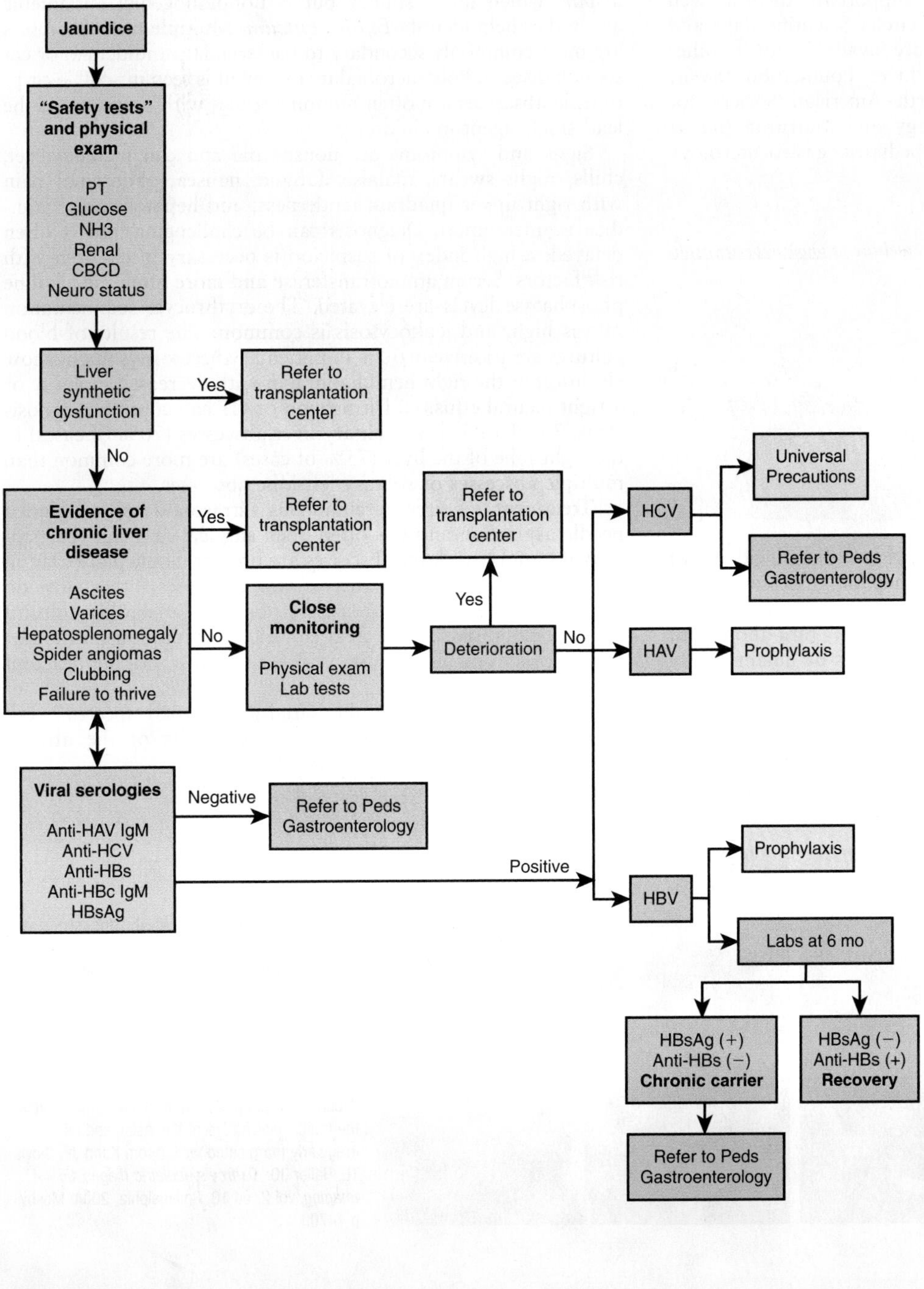

Figure 350-6 Clinical approach to viral hepatitis. CBCD, complete blood count with differential; HAV, hepatitis A virus; HBs, hepatitis B surface; HBsAg, hepatitis B surface antigen; HBV, hepatitis B virus; HCV, hepatitis C virus; IgM, immunoglobulin M; NH_3, ammonia; PT, prothrombin time.

Once chronic infection is identified, close follow-up and referral to a pediatric gastroenterologist is recommended to enroll the patient in appropriate treatment trials. Treatment of chronic HBV and HCV in children should preferably be delivered within controlled trials, because indications, timing, regimen, and outcomes remain to be defined and cannot simply be extrapolated from adult data. All patients with chronic viral hepatitis should avoid, as much as possible, further insult to the liver: HAV vaccine is recommended; patients must avoid alcohol consumption and obesity, and they should exercise care when taking new medications, including over-the-counter drugs and herbal medications.

International adoption and ease of travel continue to change the epidemiology of hepatitis viruses. In the United States, chronic HBV and HCV have a high prevalence among international adoptee patients; vigilance is required to establish early diagnosis in order to offer appropriate treatment as well as prophylactic measures to limit viral spread.

Chronic hepatitis can be a stigmatizing disease for children and their families. The pediatrician should offer, with proactive advocacy, appropriate support for them as well as needed education for their social circle. Scientific data and information about support groups are available for families on the websites for the American Liver Foundation (*www.liverfoundation-ne.org*) and the North American Society for Pediatric Gastroenterology, Hepatology and Nutrition (*www.naspghan.org*), as well as through pediatric gastroenterology centers.

BIBLIOGRAPHY

Please visit the Nelson Textbook of Pediatrics *website at www.expertconsult.com for the complete bibliography.*

Chapter 351
Liver Abscess

Robert M. Kliegman

Pyogenic liver abscesses are rare in children, with an incidence of 10/100,000 hospitalizations. Pyogenic hepatic abscesses can be caused by bacteria entering the liver via the portal circulation in cases of omphalitis, portal vein pylephlebitis, intra-abdominal infection, or abscess secondary to appendicitis or inflammatory bowel disease; a primary bacteremia (sepsis, endocarditis); ascending cholangitis associated with biliary tract obstruction caused by gallstones or sclerosing cholangitis, after a Kasai procedure, or secondary to choledochal cysts; contiguous infection or penetrating trauma; and cryptogenic biliary tract infections. Very rarely, liver abscesses occur after percutaneous liver biopsy. Hepatic abscesses can also occur in neonates in association with sepsis, umbilical vein infection, or cannulation; 50% are seen in children < 6 yr old. In adults with pyogenic liver abscesses, liver transplantation is a significant risk factor; it is not known if pediatric liver transplant patients are also at increased risk. Children with chronic granulomatous disease, Job syndrome or cancer are also at increased risk for a hepatic abscess.

In children with pyogenic liver abscesses, the most common pathogenic organisms include *Staphylococcus aureus, Streptococcus* spp; *Escherichia coli, Klebsiella pneumoniae, Salmonella,* and anaerobic organisms; *Entamoeba histolytica* or *Toxocara canis*–associated liver abscesses have also been reported in developing countries or in highly endemic areas.

Amebic disease is rare in the USA and is associated with immigrants from or travel to highly endemic areas. Recovery of *E. histolytica* from the stool is pathogenic and highly suggestive of an amebic abscess, but this must be distinguished from *E. dispar*, which looks similar but is nonpathogenic; antiamebic antibodies help identify *E. histolyticum*. Multiple microabscesses are most commonly secondary to bacteremia, candidemia, or cat scratch disease. Polymicrobial involvement is seen in ~50%; cryptogenic abscesses are often monomicrobial with *S. aureus* as the lead single agent in children.

Signs and symptoms are nonspecific and can include fever, chills, night sweats, malaise, fatigue, nausea, abdominal pain with right upper quadrant tenderness, and hepatomegaly; jaundice is uncommon. Diagnosis can be challenging and is often delayed; a high index of suspicion is necessary in children with risk factors. Serum aminotransferase and more often the alkaline phosphatase levels are elevated. The erythrocyte sedimentation rate is high, and leukocytosis is common. The results of blood cultures are positive in 50% of patients. Chest x-rays might show elevation of the right hemidiaphragm with decreased mobility or a right pleural effusion. Ultrasound or CT can confirm diagnosis (Figs. 351-1 to 351-3). Solitary liver abscesses (70% of cases) in the right lobe of the liver (75% of cases) are more common than multiple abscesses or solitary left lobe abscesses.

Treatment requires percutaneous ultrasound- or CT-guided needle aspiration and less often open surgical drainage, particularly if multiple or large abscesses are present. Some place a drain and leave it in until the abscess wall collapses, others just do single or repeated aspirations. Aerobic and anaerobic cultures should be obtained. Some treat empirically without aspiration or drainage. If amebic disease is present, most do not attempt aspiration.

Antibiotic therapy should initially be broad spectrum but then narrowed, based on the culture results of the abscess

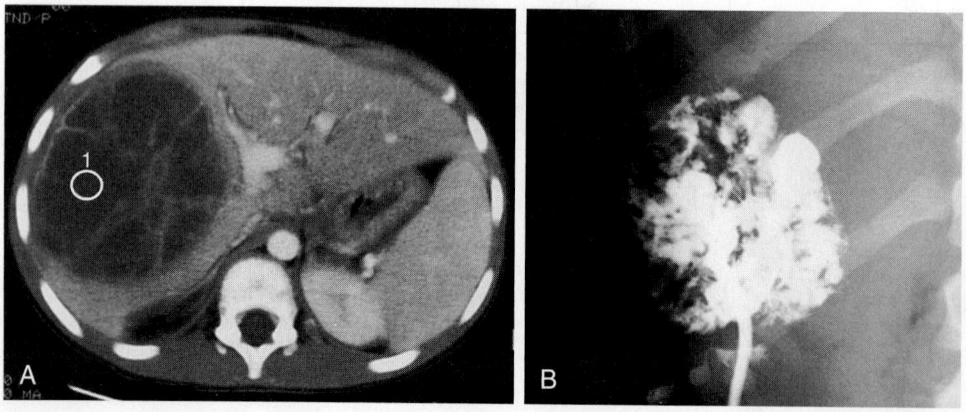

Figure 351-1 Liver abscess. *A,* Contrast-enhanced CT scan demonstrates a multioculated septated mass of decreased attenuation in the right lobe of the liver. There is increased attenuation of the septa. There is also faintly visible edema between the abscess and the enhanced normal liver. *B,* Injection of contrast material after percutaneous drainage of this documented streptococcal abscess demonstrates the multiocular nature of the lesion and its irregularly marginated wall. (From Kuhn JP, Slovis TL, Haller JO: *Caffrey's pediatric diagnostic imaging,* vol 2, ed 10, Philadelphia, 2004, Mosby, p 1470.)

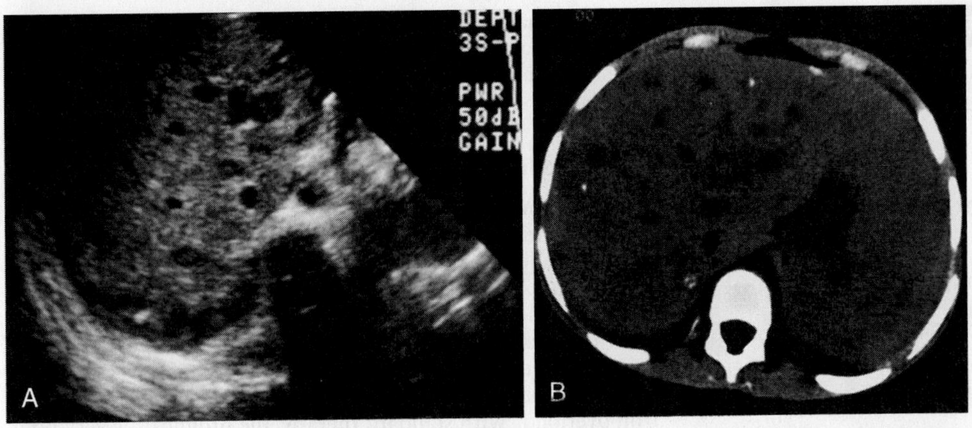

Figure 351-2 Hepatic candidiasis. Transverse sonogram *(A)* and CT scan *(B)* of the upper abdomen demonstrate "bull's-eye" lesions in the right lobe of the liver in an immunocompromised patient. The calcifications seen on the CT scan are presumed to represent sequelae of prior infection. Liver biopsy demonstrated candidiasis. (From Kuhn JP, Slovis TL, Haller JO: *Caffrey's pediatric diagnostic imaging,* vol 2, ed 10, Philadelphia, 2004, Mosby, p 1472.)

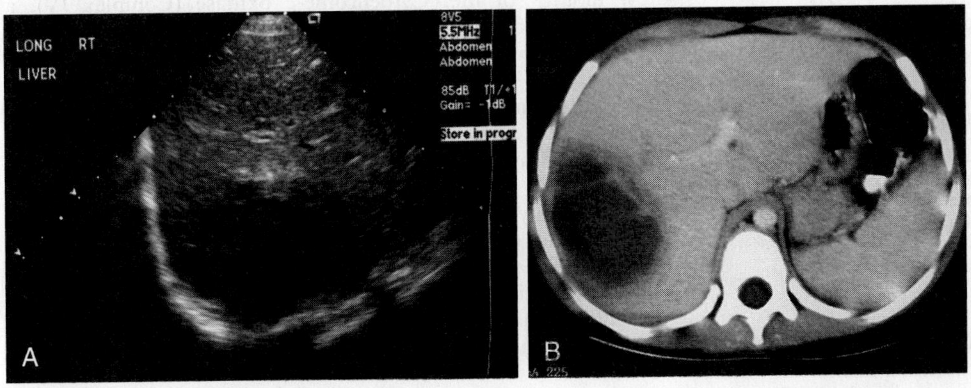

Figure 351-3 Amebic abscess. *A,* Sonogram demonstrates a hypoechogenic mass in the right lobe of the liver with a more hypoechoic surrounding rim. *B,* CT scan demonstrates a low-attenuation mass in the right lobe of the liver with a prominent halo. (From Kuhn JP, Slovis TL, Haller JO: *Caffrey's pediatric diagnostic imaging,* vol 2, ed 10, Philadelphia, 2004, Mosby, p 1473.)

fluid. Empirical initial antibiotic regimens include ampicillin/sulbactam, ticarcillin/clavulanic acid, or piperacillin/tazobactam. Others recommend a combination of a third-generation cephalosporin plus metronidazole. Amebic abscesses are treated with metronidazole or tinidazole plus paromomycin (oral nonabsorbable to treat the associated intestinal amebic infection). Antibiotic therapy for pyogenic abscess is intravenous for 2-3 wk followed by oral therapy to complete a 4-6 wk course. Mortality has decreased significantly since the 1980s with early diagnosis and initiation of appropriate therapy.

BIBLIOGRAPHY

Please visit the Nelson Textbook of Pediatrics *website at* *www.expertconsult.com* *for the complete bibliography.*

Chapter 352
Liver Disease Associated with Systemic Disorders

Kathryn D. Moyer and William F. Balistreri

Liver disease is found in a wide variety of systemic illnesses, both as a result of the primary pathologic process and as a secondary complication of the disease or associated therapy.

For the full continuation of this chapter, please visit the Nelson Textbook of Pediatrics *website at* *www.expertconsult.com*.

Chapter 353
Mitochondrial Hepatopathies

Rebecca G. Carey and William F. Balistreri

Hepatocytes are rich in mitochondria due to the energy required for the process of metabolism and are a target organ for disorders in mitochondrial function. Defects in mitochondrial function can lead to impaired oxidative phosphorylation (OXPHOS), increased generation of reactive oxygen species, impairment of other metabolic pathways, and activation of mechanisms of cellular death. Mitochondrial disorders can be divided into primary, in which the mitochondrial defect is the primary cause of the disorder, and secondary, in which mitochondrial function is affected by exogenous injury or a genetic mutation in a nonmitochondrial gene (Chapter 81.4). Primary mitochondrial disorders can be caused by mutations affecting mitochondrial DNA (mtDNA) or by nuclear genes that encode mitochondrial proteins or cofactors (Table 353-1). Secondary mitochondrial disorders include diseases with an uncertain etiology such as Reye syndrome; disorders caused by endogenous or exogenous toxins, drugs, or metals; and other conditions in which mitochondrial oxidative injury may be involved in the pathogenesis of liver injury.

EPIDEMIOLOGY

More than 200 gene mutations that involve mtDNA and nuclear DNA that encodes mitochondrial proteins are identified. Mitochondrial genetics are unique because mitochondria are able to replicate, transcribe, and translate their mitochondrial derived DNA independently. The mitochondrial genome encodes 2 ribosomal RNAs, 22 transfer RNAs, and 13 proteins of complex I, III, IV, and V of the respiratory chain. OXPHOS (the process

Table 353-1 PRIMARY MITOCHONDRIAL HEPATOPATHIES

Electron transport (respiratory chain) defects
Neonatal liver failure
Complex I deficiency (NADH: ubiquinone oxidoreductase), complex IV deficiency (cytochrome-*c* oxidase)
Complex III deficiency (ubiquinol: cytochrome c oxidoreductase)
Multiple complex deficiencies
Mitochondrial DNA depletion syndrome (DGUOK, MPV17 and POLG)
Alpers disease (complex I deficiency, POLG)
Pearson marrow-pancreas syndrome (mtDNA deletion)
Mitochondrial neurogastrointestinal encephalomyopathy (thymidine phosphorylase, tryptophan tRNA)
Chronic diarrhea (villous atrophy) with hepatic involvement (complex III deficiency)
Navajo neurohepatopathy (mt DNA depletion, MPV17)
Mitochondrial translation defects (elongation factor G1)
Fatty acid oxidation and transport defects
Carnitine palmitoyltransferase I and II deficiencies
Carnitine-acylcarnitine translocase deficiency
Long-chain hydroxyacyl CoA dehydrogenase deficiency
Acute fatty liver of pregnancy (AFLP)
Urea cycle enzyme deficiencies
Electron-transfer flavoprotein (EFT) and EFT-dehydrogenase deficiencies
Phosphoenolpyruvate carboxykinase (PEPCK) deficiency (mitochondrial)
Nonketotic hyperglycinemia (glycine cleavage enzyme deficiency)

DGUOK, deoxyguanosine kinase; MPV17; POLG, polymerase γ; CoA, coenzyme A; mtDNA, mitochondrial DNA; NADH, nicotinamide adenine dinucleotide.
Adapted from Lee WS, Sokol RJ: Mitochondrial hepatopathies: advances in genetics and pathogenesis, *Hepatology* 45:1555–1565, 2007.

of adenosine triphosphate [ATP] production) occurs in the respiratory chain located in the inner mitochondrial membrane and is divided into 5 multienzyme complexes: reduced nicotinamide adenine dinucleotide (NADH) coenzyme Q (CoQ) reductase (complex I), succinate-CoQ reductase (complex II), reduced CoQ-cytochrome c reductase (complex III), cytochrome-*c* oxidase (complex IV), and ATP synthase (complex V). The polypeptides that form these complexes are transcribed from both mitochondrial and nuclear DNA; mutations in either genome can result in disorders of OXPHOS.

Expression of mitochondrial disorders is complex and epidemiologic studies are hampered by technical difficulties collecting and processing tissue specimens needed to make accurate diagnoses, the variability in clinical presentation, and the fact that most disorders display maternal inheritance with variable penetrance (Chapter 75). mtDNA mutates 10 times more frequently than nuclear DNA secondary to a lack of introns, protective histones, and an effective repair system in mitochondria. Mitochondrial genetics also display a threshold effect in that the type and severity of mutation required for clinical expression varies among people and organ systems. Despite this, it has been estimated that mitochondrial diseases have a prevalence of 11.5 cases per 100,000 populations. Treatments for mitochondrial hepatopathies are supportive. The role of liver transplantation is controversial given the multisystemic involvement.

CLINICAL MANIFESTATIONS

Defects in OXPHOS can affect any tissue to a variable degree, with the most energy-dependent organs being the most vulnerable. One should consider the diagnosis of a mitochondrial disorder in a patient of any age who presents with progressive, multisystem involvement that cannot be explained by a specific diagnosis. Gastrointestinal (GI) complaints include vomiting, diarrhea, constipation, failure to thrive (FTT), and abdominal pain; certain mitochondrial disorders have characteristic GI presentations. Pearson marrow-pancreas syndrome manifests with sideroblastic anemia and exocrine pancreatic insufficiency, whereas mitochondrial neurogastrointestinal encephalomyopathy (MNGIE) manifests with chronic intestinal pseudo-obstruction and cachexia. Hepatic presentations range from chronic cholestasis, hepatomegaly, or steatosis to fulminant hepatic failure and death.

PRIMARY MITOCHONDRIAL HEPATOPATHIES

A common presentation of respiratory chain defects is severe liver failure in the 1st few months of life, characterized by lactic acidosis, jaundice, hypoglycemia, renal dysfunction, and hyperammonemia. Symptoms are nonspecific and include lethargy and vomiting. Most patients additionally have neurologic involvement manifested as a weak suck, recurrent apnea, or myoclonic epilepsy. Liver biopsy shows predominantly microvesicular steatosis, cholestasis, bile duct proliferation, glycogen depletion, and iron overload. With standard therapy, the prognosis is very poor, and most patients die from liver failure or infection in the 1st few months of life. **Cytochrome-*c* oxidase** (Complex IV), a nuclear encoded gene, is the most common deficiency in these infants although complex I and III have also been implicated (see Table 353-1).

Alpers syndrome (Alpers-Huttenlocher syndrome or Alpers hepatopathic poliodystrophy) also manifest from infancy up to 8 yr of age with seizures, hypotonia, feeding difficulties, psychomotor regression, and ataxia. Patients typically develop hepatomegaly and jaundice and have a slower progression to liver failure than those with cytochrome-*c* oxidase deficiency. The disease is inherited in an autosomal recessive fashion; mutations in the catalytic subunit of the nuclear gene mtDNA polymerase-γA (POLG) have been identified in multiple families with Alpers syndrome, leading to the advent of molecular diagnosis for Alpers syndrome.

Mitochondrial DNA Depletion Syndrome

Mitochondrial DNA depletion syndrome (MDS) is characterized by a tissue-specific reduction in mtDNA copy number, leading to deficiencies in complexes I, III, IV, and V. MDS manifests with phenotypic heterogeneity, and multisystem and localized disease forms include myopathic, hepatocerebral, and liver-restricted presentations.

Infants with the hepatocerebral form present in the neonatal period with progressive liver failure, neurologic abnormalities, hypoglycemia, and lactic acidosis. Death usually occurs by 1 yr of age. Spontaneous recovery has been reported in 1 patient with liver-restricted disease. Inheritance is autosomal recessive and mutations in the **deoxyguanosine kinase *(dGK)*** gene have been identified in many patients with hepatocerebral MDS. *dGK* is a nuclear gene whose protein product phosphorylates deoxyguanosine to deoxyguanosine monophosphate, confirming the importance of nucleotide pool homeostasis in mtDNA stability and maintenance. **Thymidine kinase 2 (TK2)** is also involved in deoxynucleotide phosphorylation and has been implicated in the myopathic form; no known genetic defect has been identified in liver-restricted MDS. Multiple other genes including ***DGUOK, POLG,*** and ***MPV17*** have been implicated in hepatocerebral MDS.

Liver biopsies of patients with MDS show microvesicular steatosis, cholestasis, focal cytoplasmic biliary necrosis, and cytosiderosis in hepatocytes and sinusoidal cells. Ultrastructural changes are characteristic with oncocytic transformation of mitochondria, which is characterized by mitochondria with sparse cristae, granular matrix, and dense or vesicular inclusions. **Diagnosis** is established by demonstration of a low ratio of mtDNA (<10%) to nuclear DNA in affected tissues and/or genetic testing. Importantly, the sequence of the mitochondrial genome is normal.

Navajo Neurohepatopathy

Navajo neurohepatopathy (NNH) is an autosomal recessive sensorimotor neuropathy with progressive liver disease found only in Navajo Indians of the southwestern United States. The incidence is 1/1,600 live births. Diagnostic criteria have been defined and include sensory neuropathy; motor neuropathy; corneal anesthesia; liver disease; metabolic or infectious complications including FTT, short stature, delayed puberty, or systemic infection; and evidence of central nervous system (CNS) demyelination on radiographic imaging. A definite case requires 4 of these criteria or 3 with a sibling previously diagnosed with NNH. A founder effect is possible with the identification of a homozygous R50Q mutation in the *MPV17* gene in 6 patients with NNH from 5 different families. Interestingly, this is the same gene implicated in MDS (see earlier), demonstrating that NNH may be a specific type of MDS found only in Navajo Indians.

NNH has been divided into 3 phenotypic variations based on age of presentation and clinical findings. Different presentations have been noted within single families. First, **classic NNH** appears in infancy with severe progressive neurologic deterioration manifesting clinically as weakness, hypotonia, loss of sensation with accompanying acral mutilation and corneal ulcerations, and poor growth. Liver disease, present in the majority of patients, is secondary and variable and includes asymptomatic elevations of liver function tests, Reye syndrome–like episodes, hepatocellular carcinoma, or cirrhosis. γ-Glutamyl transpeptidase (GGT) levels tend to be higher than in other forms of NNH. Liver biopsy might show chronic portal tract inflammation and cirrhosis, but it shows less cholestasis, hepatocyte ballooning, and giant cell transformation than other forms of NNH.

Infantile NNH manifests between the ages of 1 and 6 mo with jaundice and failure to thrive and progresses to liver failure and death by 2 yr of age. Patients have hepatomegaly with moderate elevations in aspartate aminotransferase (AST or SGOT), alanine aminotransferase (ALT or SGPT), and GGT. Liver biopsy demonstrates pseudo-acinar formation, multinucleate giant cells, portal and lobular inflammation, canalicular cholestasis, and microvesicular steatosis. Progressive neurologic symptoms are not usually noticed at presentation but do develop later.

Childhood NNH manifests from age 1-5 yr with the acute onset of fulminant hepatic failure that leads to death within months. Most patients also have evidence of neuropathy at presentation. Liver biopsies are similar to those in infantile NNH, except significant hepatocyte ballooning and necrosis, bile duct proliferation, and cirrhosis are also seen.

Nerve biopsy in all types might show reduction of large- and small-caliber myelinated nerve fibers and degeneration and regeneration of unmyelinated nerve fibers. There is no effective treatment for any of the forms of NNH, and neurologic symptoms often preclude liver transplantation. The identical ***MPV17*** mutation is seen in patients with both the infantile and classic form of NNH highlighting the clinical heterogeneity of NNH.

SECONDARY MITOCHONDRIAL HEPATOPATHIES

Secondary mitochondrial hepatopathies are caused by a hepatotoxic metal, drug, toxin, or endogenous metabolite. In the past, the most common secondary mitochondrial hepatopathy was **Reye syndrome,** the prevalence of which peaked in the 1970s and had a mortality rate of >40%. Even though mortality has not changed, the prevalence has decreased from >500 cases in 1980 to ~35 cases per yr since. It is precipitated in a genetically susceptible person by the interaction of a viral infection (influenza, varicella) and salicylate use. Clinically, it is characterized by a preceding viral illness that appears to be resolving and the acute onset of vomiting and encephalopathy (Table 353-2). Neurologic symptoms can rapidly progress to seizures, coma, and death. Liver dysfunction is invariably present when vomiting develops, with coagulopathy and elevated serum levels of AST, ALT, and ammonia. Importantly, patients remain anicteric and serum bilirubin levels are normal. Liver biopsies show microvesicular steatosis without evidence of liver inflammation or necrosis. Death is usually secondary to increased intracranial pressures and herniation. Patients who survive have full recovery of liver function but should be carefully screened for fatty-acid oxidation and fatty-acid transport defects (Table 353-3).

Table 353-2 CLINICAL STAGING OF REYE SYNDROME AND REYE-LIKE DISEASES

Symptoms at the time of admission:

I. Usually quiet, **lethargic** and sleepy, vomiting, laboratory evidence of liver dysfunction
II. Deep lethargy, **confusion,** delirium, combativeness, hyperventilation, hyperreflexia
III. Obtunded, **light coma** ± seizures, decorticate rigidity, intact pupillary light reaction
IV. Seizures, deepening coma, **decerebrate rigidity,** loss of oculocephalic reflexes, fixed pupils
V. Coma, loss of deep tendon reflexes, respiratory arrest, fixed dilated pupils, **flaccidity/decerebration** (intermittent); isoelectric electroencephalogram

Table 353-3 DISEASES THAT PRESENT A CLINICAL OR PATHOLOGIC PICTURE RESEMBLING REYE SYNDROME

Metabolic disease
- Organic aciduria
- Disorders of oxidative phosphorylation
- Urea cycle defects (carbamoyl phosphate synthetase, ornithine transcarbamylase)
- Defects in fatty acid oxidation metabolism
- Acyl-CoA dehydrogenase deficiencies
- Systemic carnitine deficiency
- Hepatic carnitine palmitoyltransferase deficiency
- 3-OH, 3-methylglutaryl-CoA lyase deficiency
- Fructosemia

Central nervous system infections or intoxications (meningitis), encephalitis, toxic encephalopathy

Hemorrhagic shock with encephalopathy

Drug or toxin ingestion (salicylate, valproate)

CoA, coenzyme A.

Acquired abnormalities of mitochondrial function can be caused by several drugs and toxins, including valproic acid, cyanide, amiodarone, chloramphenicol, iron, antimycin A, the emetic toxin of *Bacillus cereus,* and nucleoside analogs. Valproic acid is a branched fatty acid that can be metabolized into the mitochondrial toxin 4-envalproic acid. Children with underlying respiratory chain defects appear more sensitive to the toxic effects of this drug and valproic acid has been reported to precipitate liver failure in patients with **Alpers syndrome** and **cytochrome-*c* oxidase deficiency.** Nucleoside analogs directly inhibit mitochondrial respiratory chain complexes. Fialuridine, used to treat hepatitis B infection, can produce fatal lactic acidosis and liver failure. The mechanism of mitochondrial injury involves the direct incorporation of fialuridine into mtDNA, replacing thymidine and thereby directly inhibiting DNA transcription, which leads to acquired mtDNA depletion syndrome. The reverse transcriptase inhibitors zidovudine, didanosine, stavudine, and zalcitabine used to treat HIV-infected patients inhibit DNA polymerase-γ of mitochondria and can block elongation of mtDNA, leading to mtDNA depletion. Other conditions that can lead to mitochondrial oxidative stress include cholestasis, nonalcoholic steatohepatitis, α_1-antitrypsin deficiency, and Wilson disease.

There is no effective therapy for most patients with mitochondrial hepatopathies; neurologic involvement often precludes orthotopic liver transplantation. Several drug mixtures that include antioxidants, vitamins, cofactors, and electron acceptors have been proposed, but no randomized, controlled trials have been completed to evaluate these drug combinations. Therefore, current treatment strategies are supportive.

BIBLIOGRAPHY

Please visit the Nelson Textbook of Pediatrics *website at www.expertconsult.com for the complete bibliography.*

Chapter 354
Autoimmune Hepatitis

Benjamin L. Shneider and Frederick J. Suchy

Autoimmune hepatitis is a chronic hepatic inflammatory process manifested by elevated serum aminotransaminase concentrations, liver-associated serum autoantibodies, and/or hypergammaglobulinemia. The target of the inflammatory process can include hepatocytes and to a lesser extent bile duct epithelium. Chronicity is determined either by duration of liver disease (typically >3-6 mo) or by evidence of chronic hepatic decompensation (hypoalbuminemia, thrombocytopenia) or physical stigmata of chronic liver disease (clubbing, spider telangiectasia, hepatosplenomegaly). The severity is variable; the affected child might have only biochemical evidence of liver dysfunction, might have stigmata of chronic liver disease, or can present in hepatic failure.

Chronic hepatitis can also be caused by persistent viral infection (Chapter 350), drugs (Chapter 355), metabolic diseases (Chapter 353), or unknown and autoimmune disorders (Table 354-1). Approximately 15-20% of chronic cases are associated with hepatitis B infection; unusually severe disease may be caused by superimposed infection with hepatitis D (a defective RNA virus that is dependent on replicating hepatitis B virus [HBV]). More than 90% of hepatitis B infections in the 1st yr of life become chronic, compared with 5-10% among older children and adults. Chronic hepatitis develops in >50% of acute hepatitis C virus infections. Patients receiving blood products or who have had massive transfusions are at increased risk. Hepatitis A or E viruses do not cause chronic hepatitis. **Drugs** that are commonly used in children and can cause chronic liver injury include isoniazid, methyldopa, pemoline, nitrofurantoin, dantrolene, minocycline, pemoline, and the sulfonamides. **Metabolic diseases** can lead to chronic hepatitis including α_1-antitrypsin deficiency, inborn errors of bile acid biosynthesis, and Wilson disease. **Nonalcoholic steatohepatitis,** usually associated with obesity and insulin resistance, is another common cause of chronic hepatitis; it is relatively benign and responds to weight reduction and/or vitamin E therapy. Progression to cirrhosis has been described in adults and some children. In most cases, the cause of chronic hepatitis is unknown; in many, an autoimmune mechanism is suggested by the finding of serum antinuclear and anti–smooth muscle antibodies and by multisystem involvement (arthropathy, thyroiditis, rashes, Coombs-positive hemolytic anemia).

Histologic features help characterize chronic hepatitis. Subdivision of chronic hepatitis into a persistent vs active form on the basis of histologic findings is not as useful as once thought. The finding of inflammation contained within the limiting plate of the portal tract (chronic persistent hepatitis) and the absence of fibrosis or cirrhosis suggest a more benign course. The finding of activity on biopsy can predict response to antiviral therapy if hepatitis B infection is present and is a criterion used in the diagnosis of autoimmune hepatitis. Histologic features help identify the etiology; characteristic periodic acid–Schiff (PAS)-positive, diastase-resistant granules are seen in α_1-antitrypsin deficiency, and macrovesicular and microvesicular neutral fat accumulation within hepatocytes is a feature of steatohepatitis. Bile duct injury can suggest an autoimmune cholangiopathy. Ultrastructural analysis might suggest distinct types of storage disorders.

Autoimmune hepatitis is a clinical constellation that suggests an immune-mediated process; it is responsive to immunosuppressive therapy (Table 354-2). Autoimmune hepatitis typically refers

Table 354-1 DISORDERS PRODUCING CHRONIC HEPATITIS

Chronic viral hepatitis
- Hepatitis B
- Hepatitis C
- Hepatitis D

Autoimmune hepatitis
- Antiactin antibody positive
- Anti-liver-kidney microsomal antibody positive
- Antisoluble liver antigen antibody positive
- Others (includes antibodies to liver-specific lipoproteins or asialoglycoprotein)
- Overlap syndrome with sclerosing cholangitis and autoantibodies
- Systemic lupus erythematosus
- Celiac disease

Drug-induced hepatitis

Metabolic disorders associated with chronic liver disease
- Wilson disease
- α_1-Antitrypsin deficiency
- Tyrosinemia
- Niemann-pick disease type 2
- Glycogen storage disease type iv
- Cystic fibrosis
- Galactosemia

Bile acid biosynthetic abnormalities

Table 354-2 CLASSIFICATION OF AUTOIMMUNE HEPATITIS

VARIABLE	TYPE 1 AUTOIMMUNE HEPATITIS	TYPE 2 AUTOIMMUNE HEPATITIS
Characteristic autoantibodies	Antinuclear antibody*	Antibody against liver-kidney microsome 1*
	Smooth-muscle antibody*	
	Antiactin antibody†	Antibody against liver cytosol 1*
	Autoantibodies against soluble liver antigen and liver-pancreas antigen‡	
	Atypical perinuclear antineutrophil cytoplasmic antibody	
Geographic variation	Worldwide	Worldwide; rare in North America
Age at presentation	Any age	Predominantly childhood and young adulthood
Sex of patients	Female in ~75% of cases	Female in ~95% of cases
Association with other autoimmune diseases	Common	Common§
Clinical severity	Broad range	Generally severe
Histopathologic features at presentation	Broad range	Generally advanced
Treatment failure	Infrequent	Frequent
Relapse after drug withdrawal	Variable	Common
Need for long-term maintenance	Variable	~100%

*The conventional method of detection is immunofluorescence.
†Tests for this antibody are rarely available in commercial laboratories.
‡This antibody is detected by enzyme-linked immunosorbent assay.
§Autoimmune polyendocrinopathy-candidiasis-ectodermal dystrophy is seen only in patients with type 2 disease.
From Krawitt EL: Autoimmune hepatitis, *N Engl J Med* 354:54–66, 2006.

to a primarily hepatocyte-specific process, whereas autoimmune cholangiopathy and sclerosing cholangitis are predominated by intra- and extrahepatic bile duct injury. Overlap of the process involving both hepatocyte and bile duct directed injury may be common in children. De novo hepatitis is seen in a subset of liver transplant recipients whose initial disease was not autoimmune.

ETIOLOGY

In **autoimmune hepatitis (AIH)** a dense portal mononuclear cell infiltrate invades the surrounding parenchyma and comprises T and B lymphocytes, macrophages, and plasma cells. The immunopathogenic mechanisms underlying autoimmune hepatitis are unsettled. Triggering factors can include infections, drugs, and the environment (toxins) in a genetically susceptible host. Several HLA class II molecules, particularly DR3 isoforms, confer susceptibility to autoimmune hepatitis and present antigens from outside of the cell to T-lymphocytes. Cytochrome P450 (CYP) 2D6 is the main autoantigen in type 2 autoimmune hepatitis. $CD4^+$ T lymphocytes recognizing a self-antigenic liver peptide orchestrate liver injury. Cell-mediated injury by cytokines released by CD8+ cytotoxic T cells and/or antibody-mediated cytotoxicity can be operative. Antibody-coated hepatocytes may be lysed by complement or Fc-bearing natural killer (NK) lymphocytes. Heterozygous mutations in the **autoimmune regulator gene (*AIRE*)**, which encodes a transcription factor controlling the negative selection of autoreactive thymocytes, can be found in some children with autoimmune hepatitis types 1 and 2. *AIRE* mutations also cause autoimmune polyendocrinopathy-candidiasis-ectodermal dystrophy in which autoimmune hepatitis occurs in about 20% of patients.

PATHOLOGY

The histologic features common to untreated cases include inflammatory infiltrates, consisting of lymphocytes and plasma cells that expand portal areas and often penetrate the lobule; moderate to severe piecemeal necrosis of hepatocytes extending outward from the limiting plate; variable necrosis, fibrosis, and zones of parenchymal collapse spanning neighboring portal triads or between a portal triad and central vein (bridging necrosis); and variable degrees of bile duct epithelial injury. Distortion of hepatic architecture can be severe; cirrhosis may be present in children at the time of diagnosis. Histologic features in acute liver failure may be obscured by massive necrosis.

CLINICAL MANIFESTATIONS

The clinical features and course of autoimmune hepatitis are extremely variable. Signs and symptoms at the time of presentation comprise a wide spectrum of disease including a substantial number of asymptomatic patients and some who have an acute, even fulminant, onset. In 25-30% of patients with autoimmune hepatitis, particularly children, the illness mimics acute viral hepatitis. In most, the onset is insidious. Patients can be asymptomatic or have fatigue, malaise, behavioral changes, anorexia, and amenorrhea, sometimes for many months before jaundice or stigmata of chronic liver disease are recognized. Extrahepatic manifestations can include arthritis, vasculitis, nephritis, thyroiditis, Coombs-positive anemia, and rash. Some patients' initial clinical features reflect cirrhosis (ascites, bleeding esophageal varices, or hepatic encephalopathy).

There is usually mild to moderate jaundice. Spider telangiectasias and palmar erythema may be present. The liver is often tender and slightly enlarged but might not be felt in patients with cirrhosis. The spleen is commonly enlarged. Edema and ascites may be present in advanced cases. Evidence of involvement of other organ systems may be found.

LABORATORY FINDINGS

The findings are related to the severity of presentation. In many asymptomatic cases, serum aminotransferase ranges between 100 and 300 IU/L, whereas levels in excess of 1,000 IU/L can be seen in symptomatic young patients. Serum bilirubin concentrations (predominantly the direct-reacting fraction) are commonly 2-10 mg/dL. Serum alkaline phosphatase (ALP) and γ-glutamyl transpeptidase (GGT) activities are normal to slightly increased but may be more significantly elevated in autoimmune cholangiopathy. Serum gamma-globulin levels can show marked polyclonal elevations. Hypoalbuminemia is common. The prothrombin time is prolonged, most often as a result of vitamin K deficiency but also as a reflection of impaired hepatocellular function. A normochromic normocytic anemia, leukopenia, and thrombocytopenia are present and become more severe with the development of portal hypertension and hypersplenism.

Most patients with autoimmune hepatitis have hypergammaglobulinemia. Serum immunoglobulin (Ig) G levels usually exceed 16 g/L. Characteristic patterns of serum **autoantibodies** define several subgroups of autoimmune hepatitis (see Table 354-2). The most common pattern is the formation of non–organ-specific antibodies, such as antiactin (smooth muscle) and antinuclear antibodies. Approximately 50% of these patients are 10-20 yr of age. High titers of a liver-kidney microsomal (LKM) antibody are detected in another form that usually affects children 2-14 yr of age. A subgroup of primarily young women might demonstrate autoantibodies against a soluble liver antigen but not against nuclear or microsomal proteins. Antineutrophil cytoplasmic antibodies may be seen more commonly in autoimmune cholangiopathy. Autoantibodies are rare in healthy children so that titers as low as 1:40 may be significant, although nonspecific elevation in autoantibodies can be observed in a variety of liver diseases. Up to 20% of patients with apparent autoimmune hepatitis might not have autoantibodies at presentation. Antibodies to a cytochrome P450 component of LKM are commonly found in adult patients with chronic hepatitis C infection. Homologies in antigenic peptide epitopes between the hepatitis C virus and cytochrome P450 might explain this. Other, less-common autoantibodies include rheumatoid factor, anti-parietal cell antibodies, and antithyroid antibodies. A Coombs-positive hemolytic anemia may be present.

DIAGNOSIS

Autoimmune hepatitis is a clinical diagnosis based on certain diagnostic criteria; no single test will make this diagnosis. Diagnostic criteria with scoring systems have been developed for adults and modified slightly for children, although these scoring systems were developed as research and not diagnostic tools. Important positive features include female gender, primary elevation in transaminases and not ALP, elevated gamma-globulin levels, the presence of autoantibodies (most commonly antinuclear, smooth muscle, or liver-kidney microsome), and characteristic histologic findings (Fig. 354-1). Important negative features include the absence of viral markers (hepatitis B, C, D) of infection, absence of a history of drug or blood product exposure, and negligible alcohol consumption.

All other conditions that might lead to chronic hepatitis should be excluded (see Table 354-1). The differential diagnosis includes α_1-antitrypsin deficiency (Chapter 349) and Wilson disease (Chapter 349.2). The former disorder must be excluded by performing α_1-antitrypsin phenotyping and the latter by measuring serum ceruloplasmin and 24 hr urinary copper excretion and/or hepatic copper levels. Chronic hepatitis may occur in patients with inflammatory bowel disease, but liver dysfunction in such patients is more commonly due to pericholangitis or sclerosing cholangitis. Celiac disease (Chapter 330.2) is associated with liver disease that is akin to autoimmune hepatitis, and

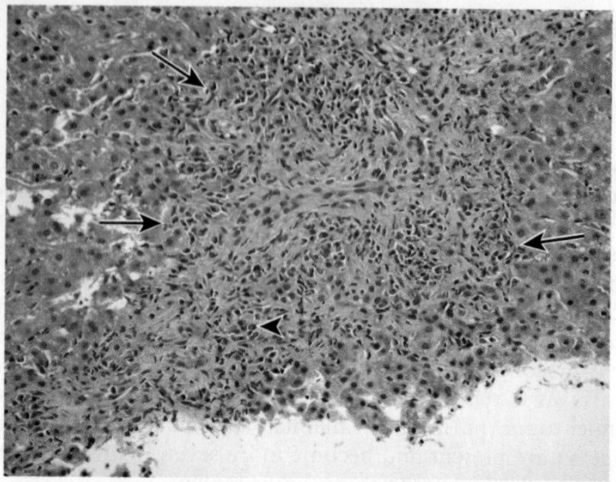

Figure 354-1 Autoimmune hepatitis. Liver biopsy showing fibrous expansion of the portal tracts with moderate portal lymphocytic infiltrates rich in plasma cells *(arrowhead)*. There is extensive interface hepatitis *(arrows)*. Original magnification ×20. (Courtesy of Margret Magid, Mount Sinai School of Medicine.)

appropriate serologic testing should be performed, including assays for tissue transglutaminase. An ultrasonogram should be done to identify a choledochal cyst or other structural disorders of the biliary system. MR cholangiography may be very useful for screening for evidence of sclerosing cholangitis. Dilated or obliterated veins on ultrasonography suggest the possibility of the Budd-Chiari syndrome.

TREATMENT

Prednisone, with or without azathioprine or 6-mercaptopurine, improves the clinical, biochemical, and histologic features in most patients with autoimmune hepatitis and prolongs survival in most patients with severe disease. The choleretic agent ursodeoxycholic acid may be particularly useful in patients with biliary features of their disease.

The goal is to suppress or eliminate hepatic inflammation with minimal side effects. Prednisone at an initial dose of 1-2 mg/kg/24 hr is continued until aminotransferase values return to less than twice the upper limit of normal. The dose should then be lowered in 5 mg decrements over 2-4 mo until a maintenance dose of 0.1-0.3 mg/kg/24 hr is achieved. In patients who respond poorly, who experience severe side effects, or who cannot be maintained on low-dose steroids, azathioprine (1.5-2.0 mg/kg/24 hr, up to 100 mg/24 hr) can be added, with frequent monitoring for bone marrow suppression. Monitoring of metabolites of azathioprine may be useful in tailoring therapy for an individual patient. Single-agent therapy with alternate-day corticosteroids should be used with great caution, although addition of azathioprine to alternate-day steroids can be an effective approach that minimizes corticosteroid-related toxicity. In patients with a mild and relatively asymptomatic presentation, some favor a lower starting dose of prednisone (10-20 mg) coupled with the simultaneous early administration of either 6-mercaptopurine (1.0-1.5 mg/kg/24 hr) or azathioprine (1.5-2.0 mg/kg/24 hr). Anecdotal reports have shown a potential for budesonide, cyclosporine, tacrolimus, mycophenylate mofetil, and sirolimus in the management of cases refractory to standard therapy. Use of these agents should be reserved for practitioners with extensive experience in their administration, because the agents have a more restricted therapeutic to toxic ratio.

Histologic progress does not necessarily need to be assessed by sequential liver biopsies, although biochemical remission does not ensure histologic resolution. Follow-up liver biopsy is therefore especially important in patients for whom consideration is given to discontinuing corticosteroid therapy. In patients with disappearance of symptoms and biochemical abnormalities and resolution of the necroinflammatory process on biopsy, an attempt at gradual discontinuation of medication is justified. There is a high rate of relapse after discontinuation of therapy. Relapse can require reinstitution of high levels of immunosuppression to control disease.

PROGNOSIS

The initial response to therapy in autoimmune hepatitis is generally prompt, with a >75% rate of remission. Transaminases and bilirubin fall to near-normal levels, often in the 1st 1-3 mo. When present, abnormalities in serum albumin and prothrombin time respond over a longer period (3-9 mo). In patients meeting the criteria for tapering and then withdrawal of treatment (25-40% of children), 50% are weaned from all medication; in the other 50%, relapse occurs after a variable period. Relapse usually responds to retreatment. Many children will not meet the criteria for an attempt at discontinuation of immunosuppression and should be maintained on the smallest dose of prednisone that minimizes biochemical activity of the disease. A careful balance of the risks of continued immunosuppression and ongoing hepatitis must be continually evaluated. This requires continual screening for complications of medical therapy (ophthalmologic examination, bone density measurement, blood pressure monitoring). Intermittent flares of hepatitis can occur and can necessitate recycling of prednisone therapy.

Some children have a relatively steroid-resistant form of hepatitis. More extensive evaluations of the etiology of their hepatitis should be undertaken, directed particularly at reassessing for the presence of either sclerosing cholangitis or Wilson disease. Progression to cirrhosis can occur in autoimmune hepatitis despite a good response to drug therapy and prolongation of life. Corticosteroid therapy in fulminant autoimmune disease may be useful, although it should be administered with caution, given the predisposition of these patients to systemic bacterial and fungal infections.

Orthotopic liver transplantation has been successful in patients with end-stage liver disease associated with autoimmune hepatitis (Chapter 360). Disease can recur after transplantation. Indication for transplantation should include evidence of hepatic decompensation.

BIBLIOGRAPHY

Please visit the Nelson Textbook of Pediatrics *website at www.expertconsult.com for the complete bibliography.*

Chapter 355
Drug- and Toxin-Induced Liver Injury

Frederick J. Suchy

The liver is the main site of drug metabolism and is particularly susceptible to structural and functional injury after ingestion, parenteral administration, or inhalation of chemical agents, drugs, plant derivatives (home remedies), or environmental toxins. The possibility of drug use or toxin exposure at home or in the parents' workplace should be explored for every child with liver dysfunction. The clinical spectrum of illness can vary from asymptomatic biochemical abnormalities of liver function to fulminant failure. Liver injury may be the only clinical feature of an adverse drug reaction or may be accompanied by systemic manifestations and damage to other organs. In hospitalized patients, clinical and laboratory findings may be confused with the underlying illness.

Hepatic metabolism of drugs and toxins is mediated by a sequence of enzymatic reactions that in large part transform hydrophobic, less-soluble molecules into more nontoxic, hydrophilic compounds that can be readily excreted in urine or bile (Chapter 56). Relative liver size, liver blood flow, and extent of protein binding also influence drug metabolism. Phase 1 of the process involves enzymatic activation of the substrate to reactive intermediates containing a carboxyl, phenol, epoxide, or hydroxyl group. Mixed-function mono-oxygenase, cytochrome-*c* reductase, various hydrolases, and the cytochrome P450 (CYP) system are involved in this process. Nonspecific induction of these enzymatic pathways, which can occur during intercurrent viral infection, with starvation, and with administration of certain drugs such as anticonvulsants, can alter drug metabolism and increase the potential for hepatotoxicity. A single agent can be metabolized by >1 biochemical reaction. The reactive intermediates that are potentially damaging to the cell are enzymatically conjugated in phase 2 reactions with glucuronic acid, sulfate, acetate, glycine, or glutathione. Some drugs may be directly metabolized by these conjugating reactions without 1st undergoing phase 1 activation. Phase 3 is the energy-dependent excretion of drug metabolites and their conjugates by an array of membrane transporters such as the multiple drug resistant protein 1 (MDR-1).

Pathways for biotransformation are expressed early in the fetus and infant, but many phase 1 and 2 enzymes are immature, particularly in the 1st yr of life. CYP3A4 is the primary hepatic CYP expressed postnatally and metabolizes >75 commonly used therapeutic drugs and several environmental pollutants and procarcinogens. Hepatic CYP3A4 activity is poorly expressed in the fetus but increases after birth to reach 30% of adult values by 1 mo and 50% of adult values between 6 and 12 mo of age. CYP3A4 can be induced by a number of drugs, including phenytoin, phenobarbital, and rifampin. Enhanced production of toxic metabolites can overwhelm the capacity of phase 2 reactions. Conversely, numerous inhibitors of CYP3A4 from several different drug classes, such as erythromycin and cimetidine, can lead to toxic accumulations of CYP3A4 substrates. By contrast, although CYP2D6 is also developmentally regulated (maturation by 10 yr of age), its activity depends more on genetic polymorphisms than on sensitivity to inducers and inhibitors because >70 allelic variants of CYP2D6 significantly influence the metabolism of many drugs. UDP-glucuronosyltransferase 1A6, a phase 2 enzyme that glucuronidates acetaminophen, is also absent in the human fetus, increases slightly in the neonate, but does not reach adult levels until sometime after 10 yr of age. Mechanisms for the uptake and excretion of organic ions can also be deficient early in life. Impaired drug metabolism via phrase 1 and 2 reactions present in the 1st few months of life is followed by a period of enhanced metabolism of many drugs in children through 10 yr of age compared with adults.

Genetic polymorphisms in genes encoding enzymes and transporters mediating phase 1, 2, and 3 reactions can also be associated with impaired drug metabolism and an increased risk of hepatotoxicity. Some cases of idiosyncratic hepatotoxicity can occur as a result of aberrations (polymorphisms) in phase 1 drug metabolism, producing intermediates of unusual hepatotoxic potential combined with developmental, acquired, or relative inefficiency of phase 2 conjugating reactions. Children may be more or less susceptible than adults to hepatotoxic reactions; liver injury after the use of the anesthetic halothane is rare in children, and acetaminophen toxicity is less common in infants than in adolescents, whereas most cases of fatal hepatotoxicity associated with sodium valproate use have been reported in children. Excessive or prolonged therapeutic administration of acetaminophen combined with reductions in caloric or protein intake can produce hepatotoxicity in children. In this setting, acetaminophen metabolism may be impaired by reduced synthesis of sulfated and glucuronated metabolites and reduced stores of glutathione. Immaturity of hepatic drug metabolic pathways can prevent degradation of a toxic agent; under other circumstances, the same immaturity might limit the formation of toxic metabolites.

Chemical hepatotoxicity can be predictable or idiosyncratic. Predictable hepatotoxicity implies a high incidence of hepatic injury in exposed persons, with dose dependence. It is understandable that only a few drugs in clinical use fall into this category. These agents might damage the hepatocyte directly through alteration of membrane lipids (peroxidation) or through denaturation of proteins; such agents include carbon tetrachloride and trichloroethylene. Indirect injury can occur through interference with metabolic pathways essential for cell integrity or through distortion of cellular constituents by covalent binding of a reactive metabolite; examples include the liver injury produced by acetaminophen or by antimetabolites such as methotrexate or 6-mercaptopurine.

Idiosyncratic hepatotoxicity is uncommon and unpredictable but accounts for the majority of adverse reactions. The likelihood of injury is not dose dependent and can occur at any time during exposure to the agent. Idiosyncratic drug reactions in certain patients can reflect aberrant pathways for drug metabolism, possibly related to genetic polymorphisms, with production of toxic intermediates (isoniazid and sodium valproate can cause liver damage through this mechanism). Duration of drug use before liver injury varies (weeks to ≥1 yr) and the response to re-exposure may be delayed.

An idiosyncratic reaction can also be immunologically mediated as a result of prior sensitization (hypersensitivity); extrahepatic manifestations of hypersensitivity can include fever, rash, arthralgia, and eosinophilia. Duration of exposure before reaction is generally 1-4 wk, with prompt recurrence of injury on re-exposure. Studies indicate that arene oxides, generated through oxidative (cytochrome P450) metabolism of aromatic anticonvulsants (phenytoin, phenobarbital, carbamazepine), can initiate the pathogenesis of some hypersensitivity reactions. Arene oxides, formed in vivo, can bind to cellular macromolecules, thus perturbing cell function and possibly initiating immunologic mechanisms of liver injury.

Although the generation of chemically reactive metabolites has received great attention in the pathogenesis of hepatoxicity, increasing evidence now exists for the multifactorial nature of the process, in particular the role played by the host immune system. Activation of liver nonparenchymal Kupffer cells and infiltration by neutrophils perpetuate toxic injury by many drugs by release of reactive oxygen and nitrogen species as well as cytokines. Stellate cells can also be activated, potentially leading to hepatic fibrosis and cirrhosis.

The pathologic spectrum of drug-induced liver disease is extremely wide, is rarely specific, and can mimic other liver diseases (Table 355-1). Predictable hepatotoxins such as acetaminophen produce centrilobular necrosis of hepatocytes. Steatosis is an important feature of tetracycline (microvesicular) and ethanol (macrovesicular) toxicities. A cholestatic hepatitis can be observed, with injury caused by erythromycin estolate and chlorpromazine. Cholestasis without inflammation may be a toxic effect of estrogens and anabolic steroids. Use of oral contraceptives and androgens has also been associated with benign and malignant liver tumors. Some idiosyncratic drug reactions can produce mixed patterns of injury, with diffuse cholestasis and cell necrosis. Some herbal supplements have been associated with hepatic failure (Table 355-2). Chronic hepatitis has been associated with the use of methyldopa and nitrofurantoin.

Clinical manifestations can be mild and nonspecific, such as fever and malaise. Fever, rash, and arthralgia may be prominent in cases of hypersensitivity. In ill hospitalized patients, the signs and symptoms of hepatic drug toxicity may be difficult to separate from the underlying illness. The differential diagnosis should include acute and chronic viral hepatitis, biliary tract disease,

Table 355-1 PATTERNS OF HEPATIC DRUG INJURY

DISEASE	DRUG
Centrilobular necrosis	Acetaminophen Halothane
Microvesicular steatosis	Valproic acid
Acute hepatitis	Isoniazid
General hypersensitivity	Sulfonamides Phenytoin
Fibrosis	Methotrexate
Cholestasis	Chlorpromazine Erythromycin Estrogens
Veno-occlusive disease	Irradiation plus busulfan Cyclophosphamide
Portal and hepatic vein thrombosis	Estrogens Androgens
Biliary sludge	Ceftriaxone
Hepatic adenoma or hepatocellular carcinoma	Oral contraceptives Anabolic steroids

Table 355-2 POTENTIALLY HEPATOTOXIC HERBAL OR DIETARY SUPPLEMENTS

Kava (*Kava kava*, awa, kew)
Chaparral (creosote bush, greasewood, *Larrea tridentata*)
Ma huang *(Ephedra)*
Comfrey leaves (pyrrolizidine alkaloids)
Germander extracts *(Trucrium chamaedrys)*
Valerian with skullcap
Mushroom *(Amanita phalloides, Galerina)*
LipoKinetix (phenylpropanolamine, sodium usinate, diiodothyronine, yohimbine, caffeine)

septicemia, ischemic and hypoxic liver injury, malignant infiltration, and inherited metabolic liver disease.

The laboratory features of drug- or toxin-related liver disease are extremely variable. Hepatocyte damage can lead to elevations of serum aminotransferase activities and serum bilirubin levels and to impaired synthetic function as evidenced by decreased serum coagulation factors and albumin. Hyperammonemia can occur with liver failure or with selective inhibition of the urea cycle (sodium valproate). Toxicologic screening of blood and urine specimens can aid in the detecting drug or toxin exposure. Percutaneous liver biopsy may be necessary to distinguish drug injury from complications of an underlying disorder or from intercurrent infection.

Slight elevation of serum aminotransferase activities (generally <2-3 times normal) can occur during therapy with drugs, particularly anticonvulsants, capable of inducing microsomal pathways for drug metabolism. Liver biopsy reveals proliferation of smooth endoplasmic reticulum but no significant liver injury. Liver test abnormalities often resolve with continued drug therapy.

TREATMENT

Treatment of drug- or toxin-related liver injury is mainly supportive. Contact with the offending agent should be avoided. Corticosteroids might have a role in immune-mediated disease. *N*-Acetylcysteine therapy, by stimulating glutathione synthesis, is effective in preventing hepatotoxicity when administered within 16 hr after an acute overdose of acetaminophen and appears to improve survival in patients with severe liver injury even up to 36 hr after ingestion (Chapter 58). Intravenous L-carnitine may be of value in treating valproic acid–induced hepatotoxicity. Orthotopic liver transplantation may be required for treatment of drug- or toxin-induced hepatic failure.

PROGNOSIS

The prognosis of drug- or toxin-induced liver injury depends on its type and severity. Injury is usually completely reversible when the hepatotoxic factor is withdrawn. The mortality of submassive hepatic necrosis with fulminant liver failure can, however, exceed 50%. With continued use of certain drugs, such as methotrexate, effects of hepatoxicity can proceed insidiously to cirrhosis. Neoplasia can follow long-term androgen therapy. Rechallenge with a drug suspected of having caused previous liver injury is rarely justified and can result in fatal hepatic necrosis.

PREVENTION

The prevention of drug-induced liver injury remains a challenge. Monitoring of liver biochemical tests may be useful in some cases, but it can prove difficult to sustain for agents used for many years. Such testing may be particularly important in patients with pre-existing liver disease. For drugs with particular hepatotoxic potential, even if episodes are infrequent in children, such as with the use of isoniazid, patients should be advised to immediately stop the medication with onset of nausea, vomiting, abdominal pain, and fatigue until liver damage is excluded. Obvious symptoms of liver disease such as jaundice and dark urine can lag behind severe hepatocellular injury. Monitoring for toxic metabolites and genotyping can be effective in preventing severe toxicity with the use of azathioprine. Advances in pharmacogenomics, such as the use of gene chips to detect variants in some of the cytochrome P450 enzymes, hold promise of a personalized approach to prevent hepatotoxicity.

BIBLIOGRAPHY

Please visit the Nelson Textbook of Pediatrics *website at* *www.expertconsult.com* *for the complete bibliography.*

Chapter 356
Fulminant Hepatic Failure

Frederick J. Suchy

Fulminant hepatic failure (acute liver failure) is a clinical syndrome resulting from massive necrosis of hepatocytes or from severe functional impairment of hepatocytes. Synthetic, excretory, and detoxifying functions of the liver are all severely impaired. In adults, hepatic encephalopathy has been an essential diagnostic feature. This narrow definition may be problematic because early hepatic encephalopathy can be difficult to detect in infants and children. The currently accepted definition in children includes biochemical evidence of acute liver injury (usually <8 wk duration); no evidence of chronic liver disease; and hepatic-based coagulopathy defined as a prothrombin time (PT) >15 sec or international normalized ratio (INR) >1.5 not corrected by vitamin K in the presence of clinical hepatic encephalopathy, or a PT >20 sec or INR >2 regardless of the presence of clinical hepatic encephalopathy. Liver failure in the perinatal period can be associated with prenatal liver injury and even cirrhosis. Examples include neonatal iron storage (hemochromatosis) disease, tyrosinemia, and some cases of congenital viral infection. Liver disease may be noticed at birth or after several days of apparent well-being. Fulminant Wilson disease also occurs in older children who were previously asymptomatic but, by definition, have pre-existing liver disease. In some cases of liver failure, particularly in the idiopathic form of acute hepatic failure, the onset of encephalopathy occurs later, from 8 to 28 wk after the onset of jaundice.

ETIOLOGY

Fulminant hepatic failure can be a complication of viral hepatitis (A, B, D, E). An unusually high risk of fulminant hepatic failure occurs in young people who have combined infections with the hepatitis B virus (HBV) and hepatitis D. Mutations in the precore and/or promoter region of HBV DNA have been associated with fulminant and severe hepatitis. HBV is also responsible for some cases of fulminant liver failure in the absence of serologic markers of HBV infection but with HBV DNA found in the liver. Hepatitis C and E viruses are uncommon causes of fulminant hepatic failure in the United States. Patients with chronic HCV are at risk if they have superinfection with HAV. Epstein-Barr virus, herpes simplex virus (HSV), adenovirus, enteroviruses, cytomegalovirus, parvovirus B19, human herpesvirus-6, and varicella-zoster infections can also produce fulminant hepatitis in children.

Fulminant hepatic failure can also be caused by autoimmune hepatitis in ~5% of cases. Patients have a positive autoimmune marker (e.g., antinuclear antibody, anti–smooth muscle antibody, liver-kidney microsomal antibody, or soluble liver antigen) and possibly an elevated serum IgG level. Liver histology, if a biopsy can be safely done, might support the diagnosis.

Acute liver failure is a common feature of hemophagocytic lymphohistocytosis (HLH) caused by several gene defects, infections by mostly viruses of the herpes group, and a variety of other conditions including organ transplantation and malignancies. Impaired function of natural killer (NK) cells and cytotoxic T-cells (CTL) with uncontrolled hemophagocytosis and cytokine overproduction is characteristic for genetic and acquired forms of HLH. Biochemical markers include elevated ferritin and triglycerides and low fibrinogen.

An idiopathic form of fulminant hepatic failure accounts for 40-50% of cases in children. The disease occurs sporadically and usually without the risk factors for common causes of viral hepatitis. It is likely that the etiology of these cases is heterogeneous, including unidentified or variant viruses and undiagnosed metabolic disorders.

Various hepatotoxic drugs and chemicals can also cause fulminant hepatic failure. Predictable liver injury can occur after exposure to carbon tetrachloride or *Amanita phalloides* mushroom or after acetaminophen overdose. Acetaminophen is the most common etiology of acute hepatic failure in children and adolescents in the United States and England. In addition to the acute intentional ingestion of a massive dose, a therapeutic misadventure leading to severe liver injury can also occur in ill children given doses of acetaminophen exceeding weight-based recommendations for many days. Such patients can have reduced stores of glutathione after a prolonged illness and a period of poor nutrition. Idiosyncratic damage can follow the use of drugs such as halothane, isoniazid, or sodium valproate. Herbal supplements are additional causes of hepatic failure (see Table 355-2).

Ischemia and hypoxia resulting from hepatic vascular occlusion, severe heart failure, cyanotic congenital heart disease, or circulatory shock can produce liver failure. Metabolic disorders associated with hepatic failure include Wilson disease, acute fatty liver of pregnancy, galactosemia, hereditary tyrosinemia, hereditary fructose intolerance, neonatal iron storage disease, defects in β-oxidation of fatty acids, and deficiencies of mitochondrial electron transport.

PATHOLOGY

Liver biopsy usually reveals patchy or confluent massive necrosis of hepatocytes. Multilobular or bridging necrosis can be associated with collapse of the reticulin framework of the liver. There may be little or no regeneration of hepatocytes. A zonal pattern of necrosis may be observed with certain insults. (Centrilobular damage is associated with acetaminophen hepatotoxicity or with circulatory shock.) Evidence of severe hepatocyte dysfunction rather than cell necrosis is occasionally the predominant histologic finding (microvesicular fatty infiltrate of hepatocytes is observed in Reye syndrome, β-oxidation defects, and tetracycline toxicity).

PATHOGENESIS

The mechanisms that lead to fulminant hepatic failure are poorly understood. It is unknown why only about 1-2% of patients with viral hepatitis experience liver failure. Massive destruction of hepatocytes might represent both a direct cytotoxic effect of the virus and an immune response to the viral antigens. One third to one half of patients with HBV-induced liver failure become negative for serum hepatitis B surface antigen within a few days of presentation and often have no detectable HBV antigen or HBV DNA in serum. These findings suggest a hyperimmune response to the virus that underlies the massive liver necrosis. Formation of hepatotoxic metabolites that bind covalently to macromolecular cell constituents is involved in the liver injury produced by drugs such as acetaminophen and isoniazid; fulminant hepatic failure can follow depletion of intracellular substrates involved in detoxification, particularly glutathione. Whatever the initial cause of hepatocyte injury, various factors can contribute to the pathogenesis of liver failure, including impaired hepatocyte regeneration, altered parenchymal perfusion, endotoxemia, and decreased hepatic reticuloendothelial function.

The pathogenesis of hepatic encephalopathy can relate to increased serum levels of ammonia, false neurotransmitters, amines, increased γ-aminobutyric acid (GABA) receptor activity, or increased circulating levels of endogenous benzodiazepine-like compounds. Decreased hepatic clearance of these substances can produce marked central nervous system dysfunction.

CLINICAL MANIFESTATIONS

Fulminant hepatic failure can be the presenting feature of liver disease or it can complicate previously known liver disease. A history of developmental delay and/or neuromuscular dysfunction can indicate an underlying mitochondrial or β-oxidation defect. A child with fulminant hepatic failure has usually been previously healthy and most often has no risk factors for liver disease such as exposure to toxins or blood products. Progressive jaundice, fetor hepaticus, fever, anorexia, vomiting, and abdominal pain are common. A rapid decrease in liver size without clinical improvement is an ominous sign. A hemorrhagic diathesis and ascites can develop.

Patients should be closely observed for hepatic encephalopathy, which is initially characterized by minor disturbances of consciousness or motor function. Irritability, poor feeding, and a change in sleep rhythm may be the only findings in infants; asterixis may be demonstrable in older children. Patients are often somnolent, confused, or combative on arousal and can eventually become responsive only to painful stimuli. Patients can rapidly progress to deeper stages of coma in which extensor responses and decerebrate and decorticate posturing appear. Respirations are usually increased early, but respiratory failure can occur in stage IV coma (Table 356-1).

LABORATORY FINDINGS

Serum direct and indirect bilirubin levels and serum aminotransferase activities may be markedly elevated. Serum aminotransferase activities do not correlate well with the severity of the illness and can actually decrease as a patient deteriorates. The blood ammonia concentration is usually increased, but hepatic coma can occur in patients with a normal blood ammonia level. PT and

Table 356-1 STAGES OF HEPATIC ENCEPHALOPATHY

	STAGES I	II	III	IV
Symptoms	Periods of lethargy, euphoria; reversal of day-night sleeping; may be alert	Drowsiness, inappropriate behavior, agitation, wide mood swings, disorientation	Stupor but arousable, confused, incoherent speech	Coma IVa responds to noxious stimuli IVb no response
Signs	Trouble drawing figures, performing mental tasks	Asterixis, fetor hepaticus, incontinence	Asterixis, hyperreflexia, extensor reflexes, rigidity	Areflexia, no asterixis, flaccidity
Electroencephalogram	Normal	Generalized slowing, q waves	Markedly abnormal, triphasic waves	Markedly abnormal bilateral slowing, d waves, electric-cortical silence

the INR are prolonged and often do not improve after parenteral administration of vitamin K. Hypoglycemia can occur, particularly in infants. Hypokalemia, hyponatremia, metabolic acidosis, or respiratory alkalosis can develop.

TREATMENT

Specific therapies for identifiable causes of acute liver failure include *N*-acetylcysteine (acetaminophen), acyclovir (HSV), penicillin (*Amanita* mushrooms), lamivudine (HBV), prednisone (autoimmune hepatitis), and pleconaril (enteroviruses). Management of other types of fulminant hepatic failure is supportive. No therapy is known to reverse hepatocyte injury or to promote hepatic regeneration.

An infant or child with acute hepatic failure should be cared for in an institution able to perform a liver transplantation if necessary and managed in an intensive care unit with continuous monitoring of vital functions. Endotracheal intubation may be required to prevent aspiration, to reduce cerebral edema by hyperventilation, and to facilitate pulmonary toilet. Mechanical ventilation and supplemental oxygen are often necessary in advanced coma. Sedatives should be avoided unless needed in the intubated patient because these agents can aggravate or precipitate encephalopathy. Opiates may be better tolerated than benzodiazepines. Prophylactic use of proton pump inhibitors should be considered because of the high risk of gastrointestinal bleeding.

Hypovolemia should be avoided and treated with cautious infusions of isotonic fluids and blood products. Renal dysfunction can result from dehydration, acute tubular necrosis, or functional renal failure (hepatorenal syndrome). Electrolyte and glucose solutions should be administered intravenously to maintain urine output, to correct or prevent hypoglycemia, and to maintain normal serum potassium concentrations. Hyponatremia is common and should be avoided, but it is usually dilutional and not a result of sodium depletion. Parenteral supplementation with calcium, phosphorus, and magnesium may be required. Hypophosphatemia, probably a reflection of liver regeneration, and early phosphorus administration are associated with a better prognosis in acute liver failure, whereas hyperphosphatemia predicts a failure of spontaneous recovery.

Coagulopathy should be treated with parenteral administration of vitamin K and can require infusion of fresh frozen plasma, cryoprecipitate, and platelets to treat clinically significant bleeding; disseminated intravascular coagulation can also occur. Plasmapheresis can permit temporary correction of the bleeding diathesis without resulting in volume overload. Recombinant factor VIIa has been used for transient correction of coagulopathy refractory to fresh frozen plasma infusions and can facilitate the performance of invasive procedures such as placement of a central line or an intracranial pressure monitor. Continuous hemofiltration is useful for managing fluid overload and acute renal failure.

Patients should be monitored closely for infection, including sepsis, pneumonia, peritonitis, and urinary tract infections. At least 50% of patients experience serious infection. Gram-positive organisms *(Staphylococcus aureus, S. epidermidis)* are the most common pathogens, but gram-negative and fungal infections are also observed.

Gastrointestinal hemorrhage, infection, constipation, sedatives, electrolyte imbalance, and hypovolemia can precipitate encephalopathy and should be identified and corrected. Protein intake should be initially restricted or eliminated, depending on the degree of encephalopathy. The gut should be purged with several enemas. Lactulose should be given every 2-4 hr orally or by nasogastric tube in doses (10-50 mL) sufficient to cause diarrhea. The dose is then adjusted to produce several acidic, loose bowel movements daily. Lactulose syrup diluted with 1-3 volumes of water can also be given as a retention enema every 6 hr. Lactulose, a nonabsorbable disaccharide, is metabolized to organic acids by colonic bacteria; it probably lowers blood ammonia levels through decreasing microbial ammonia production and through trapping of ammonia in acidic intestinal contents. Oral or rectal administration of a nonabsorbable antibiotic such as rifaximin or neomycin can reduce enteric bacteria responsible for ammonia production. Oral antibiotics may be more effective than lactulose in lowering serum ammonia levels. Flumazenil, a benzodiazepine antagonist, can temporally reverse early hepatic encephalopathy. *N*-Acetylcysteine has also been effective in improving the outcome of patients with acute liver failure not associated with acetaminophen.

Cerebral edema is an extremely serious complication of hepatic encephalopathy that responds poorly to measures such as corticosteroid administration and osmotic diuresis. Monitoring intracranial pressure can be useful in preventing severe cerebral edema, in maintaining cerebral perfusion pressure, and in establishing the suitability of a patient for liver transplantation. Controlled trials have shown a worsened outcome of fulminant hepatic failure in patients treated with corticosteroids.

Temporary liver support continues to be evaluated as a bridge for the patient with liver failure to liver transplantation or regeneration. Nonbiologic systems, essentially a form of liver dialysis with an albumin-containing dialysate, and biologic liver support devices that involve perfusion of the patient's blood through a cartridge containing liver cell lines or porcine hepatocytes can remove some toxins, improve serum biochemical abnormalities, and, in some cases, improve neurologic function, but there has been little evidence of improved survival, and few children have been treated.

Orthotopic liver transplantation (OLT) can be lifesaving in patients who reach advanced stages (III, IV) of hepatic coma. Reduced-size allografts and living donor transplantation have been important advances in the treatment of infants with hepatic failure. Partial auxiliary orthotopic or heterotopic liver transplantation is successful in a small number of children, and in some cases it has allowed regeneration of the native liver and eventual withdrawal of immunosuppression. OLT should not be done in patients with liver failure and neuromuscular dysfunction secondary to a mitochondrial disorder because progressive neurologic deterioration is likely to continue after transplant.

PROGNOSIS

Children with hepatic failure might fare somewhat better than adults, but overall mortality with supportive care alone exceeds 70%. The prognosis varies considerably with the cause of liver failure and stage of hepatic encephalopathy. With intensive medical support, survival rates of 50-60% occur with hepatic failure, complicating acetaminophen overdose (may be as high as 90%) and with fulminant HAV or HBV infection. By contrast, spontaneous recovery can be expected in only 10-20% of patients with liver failure caused by the idiopathic form of acute liver failure or an acute onset of Wilson disease. In patients who progress to stage IV coma (see Table 356-1), the prognosis is extremely poor. Brainstem herniation is the most common cause of death. Major complications such as sepsis, severe hemorrhage, or renal failure increase the mortality. The prognosis is particularly poor in patients with liver necrosis and multiorgan failure. Age <1 yr, stage 4 encephalopathy, an INR >4, and the need for dialysis before transplantation have been associated with increased mortality. Pretransplant serum bilirubin concentration or the height of hepatic enzymes is not predictive of post-transplant survival. Children with acute hepatic failure are more likely to die while on the waiting list compared to children with other diagnoses. Owing to the severity of their illness, the 6 mo post–liver transplantation survival of ~75% is significantly lower than the 90% achieved in children with chronic liver disease. Patients who recover from fulminant hepatic failure with only supportive care do not usually develop cirrhosis or chronic liver disease. Aplastic anemia occurs in ~10% of children with the idiopathic form of fulminant hepatic failure and is often fatal.

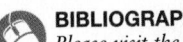

BIBLIOGRAPHY

Please visit the Nelson Textbook of Pediatrics *website at www.expertconsult.com for the complete bibliography.*

Chapter 357
Cystic Diseases of the Biliary Tract and Liver
Frederick J. Suchy

Cystic lesions of liver may be initially recognized during infancy and childhood (see Table 357-1 on the *Nelson Textbook of Pediatrics* website at www.expertconsult.com). Hepatic fibrosis can also occur as part of an underlying developmental defect (see Table 357-2 on the *Nelson Textbook of Pediatrics* website at www.expertconsult.com). Cystic renal disease is usually associated and often determines the clinical presentation and prognosis. Virtually all proteins encoded by genes mutated in combined cystic diseases of the liver and kidney are at least partially localized to primary cilia in renal tubular cells and cholangiocytes.

For the full continuation of this chapter, please visit the Nelson Textbook of Pediatrics *website at www.expertconsult.com.*

Chapter 358
Diseases of the Gallbladder
Frederick J. Suchy

ANOMALIES

The gallbladder is congenitally absent in about 0.1% of the population. Hypoplasia or absence of the gallbladder can be associated with extrahepatic biliary atresia or cystic fibrosis. Duplication of the gallbladder occurs rarely. Gallbladder ectopia can occur with a transverse, intrahepatic, left-sided, or retroplaced location. Multiseptate gallbladder, characterized by the presence of multiple septa dividing the gallbladder lumen, is another rare congenital anomaly of the gallbladder.

For the full continuation of this chapter, please visit the Nelson Textbook of Pediatrics *website at www.expertconsult.com.*

Chapter 359
Portal Hypertension and Varices
Frederick J. Suchy

Portal hypertension, defined as an elevation of portal pressure >10-12 mm Hg, is a major cause of morbidity and mortality in children with liver disease. The normal portal venous pressure is ~7 mm Hg. The clinical features of the various forms of portal hypertension may be similar, but the associated complications, management, and prognosis can vary significantly and depend on whether the process is complicated by hepatic insufficiency.

For the full continuation of this chapter, please visit the Nelson Textbook of Pediatrics *website at www.expertconsult.com.*

Chapter 360
Liver Transplantation
Jorge D. Reyes

Development of liver transplantation requires continuous refinements in the management of end organ disease, surgical technique, and perioperative care. The development of better immunosuppressive management (cyclosporine in 1978 and tacrolimus in 1989) and enhancements in our understanding of the relationship between recipient and host immune systems have resulted in better long-term survival. Paralleling this, advancements in the abdominal organ procurement techniques and organ preservation solutions have made possible the procurement and transportation of organs over long distances, with the creation of a national system for matching these donor organs with waiting recipients (the Organ Procurement and Transplantation Network [OPTN] and the United Network for Organ Sharing[UNOS]).

For the full continuation of this chapter, please visit the Nelson Textbook of Pediatrics *website at www.expertconsult.com.*

Section 7 PERITONEUM

Chapter 361
Malformations

Melissa Kennedy and Chris A. Liacouras

Congenital peritoneal bands may be responsible for intestinal obstruction; numerous other anomalies can occur in the course of the development of the peritoneum but are rarely of clinical importance. Intra-abdominal herniations infrequently occur through ring-like formations produced by anomalous peritoneal bands. Absence of the omentum or its duplication occurs rarely. Omental cysts arise in obstructed lymphatic channels within the omentum. They may be congenital or can result from trauma and are usually asymptomatic. Abdominal pain or partial small bowel obstruction can result from compression or torsion of the small bowel from traction on the omentum.

Chapter 362
Ascites

Melissa Kennedy and Chris A. Liacouras

Ascites is an accumulation of serous fluid within the peritoneal cavity. Multiple causes of ascites have been described (see Table 362-1 on the *Nelson Textbook of Pediatric* website at www.expertconsult.com). In children, hepatic, renal, and cardiac disease are the most common causes.

For the full continuation of this chapter, please visit the Nelson Textbook of Pediatrics *website at www.expertconsult.com.*

362.1 Chylous Ascites

Jessica Wen and Chris A. Liacouras

Chylous ascites can result from an anomaly, injury, or obstruction of the intra-abdominal portion of the thoracic duct. Although uncommon, it can occur at any age. Causes include congenital malformations, peritoneal bands, generalized lymphangiomatosis, chronic inflammatory processes of the bowel, tumors, enlarged lymph nodes, previous abdominal surgery, and trauma. Congenital anomalies of the lymphatic system are associated with Turner, Noonan, yellow nail, and Klippel-Trenaunay-Weber syndromes.

For the full continuation of this chapter, please visit the Nelson Textbook of Pediatrics *website at www.expertconsult.com.*

Chapter 363
Peritonitis

Jessica Wen and Chris A. Liacouras

Inflammation of the peritoneal lining of the abdominal cavity can result from infectious, autoimmune, neoplastic, and chemical processes. Infectious peritonitis is usually defined as primary (spontaneous) or secondary. In primary peritonitis, the source of infection originates outside the abdomen and seeds the peritoneal cavity via hematogenous, lymphatic, or transmural spread. Secondary peritonitis arises from the abdominal cavity itself through extension from or rupture of an intra-abdominal viscus or an abscess within an organ. Tertiary peritonitis refers to recurrent diffuse or localized disease and is associated with poorer outcomes than secondary peritonitis.

Clinically, patients have abdominal pain, abdominal tenderness, and rigidity on exam. Peritonitis can result from rupture of a hollow viscus, such as the appendix or a Meckel diverticulum; disruption of the peritoneum from trauma or peritoneal dialysis catheter; chemical peritonitis from other bodily fluid, including bile and urine; and infection. Meconium peritonitis is described in Chapters 96.1 and 322. Peritonitis is considered a surgical emergency and requires exploration and lavage of the abdomen except in spontaneous bacterial peritonitis.

BIBLIOGRAPHY

Please visit the Nelson Textbook of Pediatrics *website at www.expertconsult.com for the complete bibliography.*

363.1 Acute Primary Peritonitis

Jessica Wen and Chris A. Liacouras

ETIOLOGY AND EPIDEMIOLOGY

Primary peritonitis usually refers to bacterial infection of the peritoneal cavity without a demonstrable intra-abdominal source. Most cases occur in children with ascites resulting from nephrotic syndrome or cirrhosis. Infection can result from translocation of gut bacteria as well as immune dysfunction. Rarely, primary peritonitis occurs in previously healthy children. Pneumococci (most common), group A streptococci, enterococci, staphylococci, and gram-negative enteric bacteria, especially *Escherichia coli* and *Klebsiella pneumoniae,* are also commonly found. The sexes are affected equally; most cases occur before 6 yr of age. *Mycobacterium tuberculosis* and *M. bovis* are rare causes.

CLINICAL MANIFESTATIONS

Onset may be insidious or rapid and is characterized by fever, abdominal pain, vomiting, diarrhea, and a toxic appearance. Hypotension and tachycardia are common along with shallow, rapid respirations because of discomfort associated with breathing. Abdominal palpation might demonstrate rebound tenderness and rigidity. Bowel sounds are hypoactive or absent. The prior use of corticosteroids can diminish the clinical expression of peritonitis and delay diagnosis.

DIAGNOSIS AND TREATMENT

Peripheral leukocytosis with a marked predominance of polymorphonuclear cells is common, although the white blood cell (WBC) count can be affected by pre-existing hypersplenism in patients with cirrhosis. Subjects with nephrotic syndrome generally have proteinuria, and low serum albumin in these patients is associated with increased risk of peritonitis. X-ray examination of the abdomen reveals dilatation of the large and small intestines, with increased separation of loops secondary to bowel wall thickening. Distinguishing primary peritonitis from appendicitis may be impossible in patients without a history of nephrotic syndrome or cirrhosis; accordingly, the diagnosis of primary peritonitis is made by CT scan, laparoscopy, or laparotomy. In a child with known renal or hepatic disease and ascites, the presence of peritoneal signs should prompt diagnostic paracentesis. Infected fluid usually reveals a white blood cell (WBC) count of ≥250 cells/mm^3, with >50% polymorphonuclear cells.

Other peritoneal fluid findings suggestive of primary peritonitis include a pH <7.35, arterial:ascitic fluid pH gradient >0.1, and elevated lactate. Gram stain of the ascitic fluid characteristically reveals a single species of gram-positive or, less often, gram-negative bacteria. The presence of mixed bacterial flora on ascitic fluid examination or free air on abdominal roentgenogram in children with presumed primary peritonitis mandates laparotomy to localize a perforation as a likely intra-abdominal source of the infection. Inoculation of ascitic fluid obtained at paracentesis directly into blood culture bottles increases the yield of positive cultures. Parenteral antibiotic therapy with cefotaxime and an aminoglycoside should be started promptly, with subsequent changes dependent on sensitivity testing (vancomycin for resistant pneumococci). Therapy should be continued for 10-14 days.

Culture-negative neutrocytic ascites is a variant of primary peritonitis with a WBC count of 500 cells/mm^3, a negative culture, no intra-abdominal source of infection, and no prior treatment with antibiotics. It should be treated in a similar manner as primary peritonitis.

BIBLIOGRAPHY

Please visit the Nelson Textbook of Pediatrics *website at* *www.expertconsult.com* *for the complete bibliography.*

363.2 Acute Secondary Peritonitis

Jessica Wen and Chris A. Liacouras

Acute secondary peritonitis most often results from entry of enteric bacteria into the peritoneal cavity through a necrotic defect in the wall of the intestines or other viscus as a result of obstruction or infarction or after rupture of an intra-abdominal visceral abscess. It most commonly follows perforation of the appendix. Other gastrointestinal (GI) causes include incarcerated hernias, rupture of a Meckel diverticulum, midgut volvulus, intussusception, hemolytic uremic syndrome, peptic ulceration, inflammatory bowel disease, necrotizing cholecystitis, necrotizing enterocolitis, typhlitis, and traumatic perforation. Peritonitis in the neonatal period most often occurs as a complication of necrotizing enterocolitis but may be associated with meconium ileus or spontaneous (or indomethacin-induced) rupture of the stomach or intestines. In postpubertal girls, bacteria from the genital tract *(Neisseria gonorrhoeae, Chlamydia trachomatis)* can gain access to the peritoneal cavity via the fallopian tubes, causing secondary peritonitis. The presence of a foreign body, such as a ventriculoperitoneal catheter or peritoneal dialysis catheter, can predispose to peritonitis, with skin microorganisms, such as *Staphylococcus epidermidis, S. aureus,* and *Candida albicans,* contaminating the shunt. Secondary peritonitis results from direct toxic effects of bacteria as well as local and systemic release of inflammatory mediators in response to organisms and their products (lipopolysaccharide endotoxin). The development of sepsis depends on various host and disease factors, as well as promptness of antimicrobial and surgical intervention.

CLINICAL MANIFESTATIONS

Similar to primary peritonitis, characteristic symptoms include fever (≥39.5°C), diffuse abdominal pain, nausea, and vomiting. Physical findings of peritoneal inflammation include rebound tenderness, abdominal wall rigidity, a paucity of body motion (lying still), and decreased or absent bowel sounds from a paralytic ileus. Massive exudation of fluid into the peritoneal cavity, along with the systemic release of vasodilative substances, can lead to the rapid development of shock. A toxic appearance, irritability, and restlessness are common. Basilar atelectasis as well as intrapulmonary shunting can develop, with progression to acute respiratory distress syndrome.

Laboratory studies reveal a peripheral WBC count >12,000 cells/mm^3, with a marked predominance of polymorphonuclear forms. X-rays of the abdomen can reveal free air in the peritoneal cavity, evidence of ileus or obstruction, peritoneal fluid, and obliteration of the psoas shadow.

TREATMENT

Aggressive fluid resuscitation and support of cardiovascular function should begin immediately. Stabilization of the patient before surgical intervention is mandatory. Antibiotic therapy must provide coverage for organisms that predominate at the site of presumed origin of the infection. For perforation of the lower GI tract, a regimen of ampicillin, gentamicin, and clindamycin will adequately address infection by *E. coli, Klebsiella,* and *Bacteroides* spp. and enterococci. Alternative therapy could include ticarcillin-clavulanic acid and an aminoglycoside. Surgery to repair a perforated viscus should proceed after the patient is stabilized and antibiotic therapy is initiated. Intraoperative peritoneal fluid cultures will indicate whether a change in the antibiotic regimen is warranted. Empirical treatment for peritoneal dialysis (PD) catheter-related peritonitis may include cefazolin plus ceftazidime, imipenem/cilastin, or vancomycin/ciprofloxacin. Serious infection from PD catheters can generally be prevented with good catheter hygiene and prompt removal and replacement with signs of progressive infection.

BIBLIOGRAPHY

Please visit the Nelson Textbook of Pediatrics *website at* *www.expertconsult.com* *for the complete bibliography.*

363.3 Acute Secondary Localized Peritonitis (Peritoneal Abscess)

Jessica Wen and Chris A. Liacouras

ETIOLOGY

Intra-abdominal abscesses occur less commonly in children and infants than in adults but can develop in visceral intra-abdominal organs (hepatic, splenic, renal, pancreatic, tubo-ovarian abscesses) or in the interintestinal, periappendiceal, subdiaphragmatic, subhepatic, pelvic, or retroperitoneal spaces. Most commonly, periappendiceal and pelvic abscesses arise from a perforation of the appendix. Transmural inflammation with fistula formation can result in intra-abdominal abscess formation in children with Crohn disease.

CLINICAL MANIFESTATIONS

Prolonged fever, anorexia, vomiting, and lassitude suggest the development of an intra-abdominal abscess. The peripheral WBC count is elevated, as is the erythrocyte sedimentation rate. With an appendiceal abscess, there is localized tenderness and a palpable mass in the right lower quadrant.

A pelvic abscess is suggested by abdominal distention, rectal tenesmus with or without the passage of small-volume mucous stools, and bladder irritability. Rectal examination might reveal a tender mass anteriorly. Subphrenic gas collection, basal atelectasis, elevated hemidiaphragm, and pleural effusion may be present with a subdiaphragmatic abscess. Psoas abscess can develop from extension of infection from a retroperitoneal appendicitis, Crohn disease, or perirenal or intrarenal abscess. Abdominal findings may be minimal, and presentation can include a limp, hip pain, and fever. Ultrasound examination, CT scanning, and MRI may be used to localize intra-abdominal abscesses; MRI gives the best resolution of disease involvement.

TREATMENT

An abscess should be drained and appropriate antibiotic therapy provided. Drainage can be performed under radiologic control (ultrasonogram or CT guidance) and an indwelling drainage catheter left in place. Initial broad-spectrum antibiotic coverage such as a combination of ampicillin, gentamicin, and clindamycin should be started and can be modified depending on the results of sensitivity testing. The treatment of appendiceal rupture complicated by abscess formation may be problematic because intestinal phlegmon formation can make surgical resection more difficult. Intensive antibiotic therapy for 4-6 wk followed by an interval appendectomy is often the treatment course followed.

BIBLIOGRAPHY

Please visit the Nelson Textbook of Pediatrics *website at www.expertconsult.com for the complete bibliography.*

Chapter 364
Epigastric Hernia

John J. Aiken and Keith T. Oldham

Epigastric hernias are ventral hernias in the midline of the abdominal wall between the xyphoid and the umbilicus. Epigastric hernias result from defects in the decussating fibers of the linea alba and are more likely congenital than acquired. Most epigastric hernias are small and asymptomatic; therefore, the true incidence is unknown, but the reported incidence in childhood varies from <1% to as high as 5%. Epigastric hernias may be single or multiple and are 2-3 times more common in males than females. The defect typically contains only preperitoneal fat without a peritoneal sac or abdominal viscera. Epigastric (incisional) hernias can occur in a previous incision site or be associated with ventricular-peritoneal shunts.

For the full continuation of this chapter, please visit the Nelson Textbook of Pediatrics *website at www.expertconsult.com.*

364.1 Incisional Hernia

John J. Aiken and Keith T. Oldham

Hernia formation at the site of a previous laparotomy is uncommon in childhood. Factors associated with an increased risk of incisional hernia include increased intra-abdominal pressure, wound infection, and midline incision. Transverse abdominal incisions are favored because of their increased strength and blood supply, which reduce the likelihood of wound infection and incisional hernia. Although most incisional hernias require repair, operation should be deferred until the child is in optimal medical condition. Some incisional hernias resolve, especially those occurring in infants. Some recommend elastic bandaging to discourage enlargement of the hernia and to promote spontaneous healing. Newborns with abdominal wall defects represent the largest group of children with incisional hernias. Initial management should be conservative, with repair deferred until about 1 yr of age. Incarceration is very uncommon but is an indication for prompt repair.

BIBLIOGRAPHY

Please visit the Nelson Textbook of Pediatrics *website at www.expertconsult.com for the complete bibliography.*

PART XIX Respiratory System

Section 1 DEVELOPMENT AND FUNCTION

Chapter 365
Respiratory Pathophysiology and Regulation

Ashok P. Sarnaik and Sabrina M. Heidemann

The main function of the respiratory system is to supply sufficient oxygen to meet metabolic demands and remove carbon dioxide. A variety of processes including ventilation, perfusion, and diffusion are involved in tissue oxygenation and carbon dioxide removal. Abnormalities in any one of these mechanisms can lead to respiratory failure. The pathophysiologic manifestations of respiratory disease processes are profoundly influenced by age- and growth-dependent changes in the physiology and anatomy of the respiratory control mechanisms, airway dynamics, and lung parenchymal characteristics. Smaller airways, a more compliant chest wall, and poor hypoxic drive render a younger infant more vulnerable compared to an older child with similar severity of disease.

For the full continuation of this chapter, please visit the Nelson Textbook of Pediatrics *website at www.expertconsult.com.*

365.1 Lung Volumes and Capacities in Health and Disease

Ashok P. Sarnaik and Sabrina M. Heidemann

Traditionally, lung volumes are measured with a spirogram (Fig. 365-1). **Tidal volume** (V_T) is the amount of air moved in and out of the lungs during each breath; at rest, tidal volume is normally 6-7 mL/kg body weight. **Inspiratory capacity (IC)** is the amount of air inspired by maximum inspiratory effort after tidal expiration. **Expiratory reserve volume (ERV)** is the amount of air exhaled by maximum expiratory effort after tidal expiration. The volume of gas remaining in the lungs after maximum expiration is **residual volume (RV)**. **Vital capacity (VC)** is defined as the amount of air moved in and out of the lungs with maximum inspiration and expiration. VC, IC, and ERV are decreased in lung pathology but are also effort dependent. **Total lung capacity** (TLC) is the volume of gas occupying the lungs after maximum inhalation.

For the full continuation of this chapter, please visit the Nelson Textbook of Pediatrics *website at www.expertconsult.com.*

365.2 Chest Wall

Ashok P. Sarnaik and Sabrina M. Heidemann

The chest wall and diaphragm of an infant are mechanically disadvantaged compared to that of an adult when required to increase thoracic (and therefore the lung) volume. The infant's ribs are oriented much more horizontally and the diaphragm is flatter and less domed. The infant is therefore unable to duplicate the efficiency of upward and outward movement of obliquely oriented ribs and downward displacement of the domed diaphragm in an adult to expand the thoracic capacity. Additionally, the infant's rib cage is softer and thus more compliant compared to an adult's. Although a soft, highly compliant chest wall is beneficial to a baby in its passage through the birth canal and allows future lung growth, it places the young infant in a vulnerable situation under certain pathologic conditions. Chest wall compliance is a major determinant of FRC. Because the chest wall and the lungs recoil in opposite directions at rest, FRC is reached at the point where the outward elastic recoil of the thoracic cage counterbalances the inward lung recoil. This balance is attained at a lower lung volume in a young infant because of the extremely high thoracic compliance compared to older children (see Fig. 365-7 on the *Nelson Textbook of Pediatrics* website at www.expertconsult.com). The measured FRC in infants is higher than expected because respiratory muscles of infants maintain the thoracic cage in an inspiratory position at all times. Additionally, some amount of air trapping during expiration occurs in young infants.

For the full continuation of this chapter, please visit the Nelson Textbook of Pediatrics *website at www.expertconsult.com.*

365.3 Pulmonary Mechanics and Work of Breathing in Health and Disease

Ashok P. Sarnaik and Sabrina M. Heidemann

The movement of air in and out of the lungs requires a sufficient pressure gradient between alveoli and atmosphere during inspiration and expiration. Part of the pressure gradient is required to overcome the lung and chest wall elastance; another part is needed to overcome airway resistance. **Elastance** refers to the property of a substance to oppose deformation or stretching. It is calculated as a change in pressure (ΔP) ÷ change in volume (ΔV). Elastic recoil is a property of a substance that enables it to return to its original state after it is no longer subjected to pressure. **Compliance** ($\Delta V \div \Delta P$) is the reciprocal of elastance. In the context of the pulmonary parenchyma, airways, and the chest wall, the compliance refers to their distensibilty. **Resistance** is calculated as the amount of pressure required to generate flow of gas across the airways. Resistance to laminar flow is governed by *Poiseuille's law* stated as:

$$R = 8l\eta \div \Pi r^4$$

where R is resistance, l is length, η is viscosity, and r is the radius. The practical implication of pressure-flow relationship is that airway resistance is inversely proportional to its radius raised to the 4th power. If the airway lumen is decreased in half, the resistance increases 16-fold. Newborns and young infants with their inherently smaller airways are especially prone to marked increase in airway resistance from inflamed tissues and secretions. In diseases in which airway resistance is increased, flow often becomes turbulent. **Turbulence** depends to a great extent on the *Reynolds number* (Re), a dimensionless entity, which is calculated as

$$Re = 2rvd \div \eta$$

where r is radius, v is velocity, d is density, and η is viscosity. Turbulence in gas flow is most likely to occur when Re exceeds 2000. Resistance to turbulent flow is greatly influenced by density. A low-density gas such as helium-oxygen mixture decreases turbulence in obstructive airway diseases such as viral laryngotracheobronchitis and asthma. Neonates and young infants are predominantly nose breathers and therefore even a minimal amount of nasal obstruction is poorly tolerated.

For the full continuation of this chapter, please visit the Nelson Textbook of Pediatrics *website at www.expertconsult.com.*

365.4 Airway Dynamics in Health and Disease

Ashok P. Sarnaik and Sabrina M. Heidemann

Because the trachea and airways of an infant are much more compliant than those of older children and adults, changes in intrapleural pressure result in much greater changes in airway diameter. The airway can be divided into 3 anatomic parts: the **extrathoracic airway** extends from the nose to the thoracic inlet, the **intrathoracic-extrapulmonary airway** extends from the thoracic inlet to the main stem bronchi, and the **intrapulmonary airway** is within the lung parenchyma. During normal respirations, intrathoracic airways expand in inspiration as intrapleural pressure becomes more negative and narrow in expiration as they return to their baseline at FRC. The changes in diameter are of little significance in normal respiration. In diseases characterized by airway obstruction, much greater changes in intrapleural pressure are required to generate adequate airflow, resulting in greater changes in airway lumen. The changes in the size of airway during respiration are accentuated in young infants with their softer, more compliant airways.

For the full continuation of this chapter, please visit the Nelson Textbook of Pediatrics *website at www.expertconsult.com.*

365.5 Interpretation of Clinical Signs to Localize the Site of Pathology

Ashok P. Sarnaik and Sabrina M. Heidemann

The 1st step in establishing the diagnosis of respiratory disease is appropriate interpretation of clinical findings. Respiratory distress can occur without respiratory disease, and severe respiratory failure can be present without significant respiratory distress. Diseases characterized by CNS excitation, such as encephalitis, and neureoexcitatory drugs are associated with central neurogenic hyperventilation. Similarly, diseases that produce metabolic acidosis, such as diabetic ketoacidosis, salicylism, and shock, result in hyperventilation as a compensatory response. Patients in either group could be considered clinically to have respiratory distress; they are distinguished from patients with respiratory disease by their increased tidal volume as well as the respiratory rate. Their blood gas values reflect a low $PaCO_2$ and a normal PaO_2. Patients with neuromuscular diseases, such as Guillain-Barré syndrome or myasthenia gravis, and those with an abnormal respiratory drive can develop severe respiratory failure but are not able to mount sufficient effort to appear in respiratory distress. In these patients, respirations are ineffective or can even appear normal in the presence of respiratory acidosis and hypoxemia.

For the full continuation of this chapter, please visit the Nelson Textbook of Pediatrics *website at www.expertconsult.com.*

365.6 Ventilation-Perfusion Relationship in Health and Disease

Ashok P. Sarnaik and Sabrina M. Heidemann

Alveoli and airways in the nondependent parts (the upper lobes in upright position) of the lung are subjected to greater negative intrapleural pressure during tidal respiration and are therefore kept relatively more inflated compared to the dependent alveoli and airways (the lower lobes in upright position). Gravitational force pulls the lung away from the nondependent part of the parietal pleura. The nondependent alveoli are less compliant because they are already more inflated. During tidal inspiration, ventilation therefore occurs preferentially in the dependent portions of the lung that are more amenable to expansion. Although perfusion is also greater in the dependent portions of the lung because of greater pulmonary arterial hydrostatic pressure due to gravity, the increase in perfusion is greater than the increase in ventilation in the dependent portions of the lung. Thus, the $\dot{V}/\dot{Q}$ ratios favor ventilation in the nondependent portions and perfusion in the dependent portions. Because the airways in the dependent portion of the lung are narrower, they close earlier during expiration. The lung volume at which the dependent airways start to close is referred to as the **closing capacity.** In normal children, the FRC is greater than the closing capacity. During tidal respiration, airways remain patent both in the dependent and the nondependent portions of the lung. In newborns, the closing capacity is greater than the FRC, resulting in perfusion of poorly ventilated alveoli during tidal respiration; therefore, normal neonates have a lower PaO_2 compared to older children.

For the full continuation of this chapter, please visit the Nelson Textbook of Pediatrics *website at www.expertconsult.com.*

365.7 Gas Exchange in Health and Disease

Ashok P. Sarnaik and Sabrina M. Heidemann

The main function of the respiratory system is to remove carbon dioxide from and add oxygen to the systemic venous blood brought to the lung. The composition of the inspired gas, ventilation, perfusion, diffusion, and tissue metabolism have a significant influence on the arterial blood gases.

For the full continuation of this chapter, please visit the Nelson Textbook of Pediatrics *website at www.expertconsult.com.*

365.8 Interpretation of Blood Gases

Ashok P. Sarnaik and Sabrina M. Heidemann

Clinical observations and interpretation of blood gas values are critical in localizing the site of the lesion and estimating its severity (see Table 365-2 on the *Nelson Textbook of Pediatrics* website at www.expertconsult.com). In airway obstruction above the carina (subglottic stenosis, vascular ring), blood gases reflect overall alveolar hypoventilation. This is manifested by an elevated $PACO_2$ and a proportionate decrease in PAO_2 as determined by the alveolar air equation. A rise in $PACO_2$ of 20 torr decreases PAO_2 by 20 × 1.25 or 25 torr. In the absence of significant parenchymal disease and intrapulmonary shunting, such lesions respond very well to supplemental oxygen in reversing hypoxemia. Similar blood gas values, demonstrating alveolar hypoventilation and response to supplemental oxygen, are observed in patients with a depressed respiratory center and ineffective neuromuscular function, resulting in respiratory insufficiency. Such patients can be easily distinguished from those with airway obstruction by their poor respiratory effort.

For the full continuation of this chapter, please visit the Nelson Textbook of Pediatrics *website at www.expertconsult.com.*

365.9 Pulmonary Vasculature in Health and Disease

Ashok P. Sarnaik and Sabrina M. Heidemann

The tunica media of the pulmonary arteries of the fetus become more muscular in the last trimester of pregnancy (Chapter 95.1). Up to 90% of the systemic venous return is shunted away from the pulmonary arterial circulation to the systemic arterial circulation through the foramen ovale and the ductus arteriosus. After birth, with functional closure of the foramen ovale and the ductus arteriosus, and dilatation of the pulmonary arterial circulation with consequent decrease in **pulmonary vascular resistance (PVR)**, all of the right ventricular output passes through the lung. The PVR is ~50% of the systemic arterial resistance 3 days after birth. In the next several wk after birth as pulmonary arterial musculature in the tunica media involutes, there is a further decline in PVR and therefore in pulmonary artery pressure. Two to 3 mo after birth, the PVR and the pulmonary artery pressure are ~15% of the systemic values, a relationship that exists through childhood and adolescence. Pulmonary vasculature constricts in response to hypoxemia, acidosis, and hypercarbia and dilates with increased alveolar and arterial PO_2, alkalosis, and hypocarbia. Younger infants, with their relatively muscular pulmonary arteries, are especially susceptible to pulmonary vasoconstrictive stimuli.

For the full continuation of this chapter, please visit the Nelson Textbook of Pediatrics *website at www.expertconsult.com.*

365.10 Immune Response of the Lung to Injury

Ashok P. Sarnaik and Sabrina M. Heidemann

Local and systemic diseases can potentially induce an inflammatory response in the lung. Local diseases of the lung capable of inducing the inflammatory response include infectious processes, aspiration, asphyxia, pulmonary contusion, and inhalation of chemical irritants; systemic diseases include sepsis, shock, trauma, and cardiopulmonary bypass. This inflammatory response is mediated through the release of cytokines and other mediators. In the lung, alveolar macrophages are the chief architects of the early cytokine response, producing **tumor necrosis factor-α** (TNF-α) and **interleukin-1β** (IL-1β). These cytokines are involved in initiating the inflammatory cascade, resulting in the production of other cytokines, prostaglandins, reactive oxygen species, and upregulating cell adhesion molecules, which, in turn, leads to white cell migration into the lung tissue. The pathophysiologic consequences of the inflammatory response include injury to pulmonary capillary endothelium and the alveolar epithelial cells. Various cytokines and eicosanoids produce pulmonary vasoconstriction, resulting in pulmonary hypertension and increased right ventricular afterload. Injury to the capillary endothelium results in increased permeability and exudation of protein-rich fluid into the pulmonary interstitium and alveoli. Cellular debris and fibrin form the characteristic eosinophilic hyaline membranes along the walls of the alveolar duct. There is sloughing of type 1 pneumocytes. Interstitial and alveolar edema results in decreased FRC, diffusion barrier, intrapulmonary right-to-left shunting across poorly ventilating alveoli, and increase in the alveolar-arterial ($A\text{-}aO_2$) gradient. Clinically, $A\text{-}aO_2$ gradient >200 is characterized as *acute lung injury* and a gradient >300 is termed **acute respiratory distress syndrome (ARDS)** (Chapter 65).

For the full continuation of this chapter, please visit the Nelson Textbook of Pediatrics *website at www.expertconsult.com.*

365.11 Regulation of Respiration

Ashok P. Sarnaik and Sabrina M. Heidemann

The main function of respiration is to maintain normal blood gas homeostasis to match the metabolic needs of the body with the least amount of energy expenditure. Respiratory rate and tidal volume are regulated by a complex interaction of **controllers, sensors,** and **effectors.** The central respiratory controller consists of a group of neurons in the CNS that receives and integrates the afferent information from sensors and sends motor impulses to effectors to initiate and maintain respiration. Sensors are a variety of receptors located throughout the body. They gather chemical and physical information that is sent to the controller either to stimulate or to inhibit its activity. Effectors are the various muscles of respiration that, under the influence of the controller, move air in and out of the lung at a given tidal volume and rate. The respiratory regulatory mechanism itself undergoes a significant maturation process from the neonatal period throughout infancy and early childhood. **Sleep states** have the potential for profound influences on the control of respiration.

For the full continuation of this chapter, please visit the Nelson Textbook of Pediatrics *website at www.expertconsult.com.*

Chapter 366 Diagnostic Approach to Respiratory Disease

Gabriel G. Haddad and Thomas P. Green

A careful history and physical examination are the critical components in determining a diagnosis in a child presenting with respiratory signs and symptoms. In some patients, additional diagnostic tests and modalities are required.

For the full continuation of this chapter, please visit the Nelson Textbook of Pediatrics *website at www.expertconsult.com.*

Chapter 367 Sudden Infant Death Syndrome

Carl E. Hunt and Fern R. Hauck

The sudden, unexpected death of an infant that is unexplained by a thorough postmortem examination, which includes a complete autopsy, investigation of the scene of death, and review of the medical history, constitutes sudden infant death syndrome (SIDS). An autopsy is essential to identify possible natural explanations for sudden, unexpected death such as congenital anomalies or infection and to diagnose traumatic child abuse (Tables 367-1, 367-2, 367-3). The autopsy typically cannot distinguish between SIDS and intentional suffocation, but the scene investigation and medical history may be of help if inconsistencies are evident.

Table 367-1 DIFFERENTIAL DIAGNOSIS OF SUDDEN UNEXPECTED DEATH IN INFANCY

CAUSE OF DEATH	PRIMARY DIAGNOSTIC CRITERIA	CONFOUNDING FACTOR(S)	FREQUENCY DISTRIBUTION (%)
EXPLAINED AT AUTOPSY			
Natural			18-20*
Infections	History, autopsy, and cultures	If minimal findings: SIDS	35-46†
Congenital anomaly	History and autopsy	If minimal findings: SIDS or intentional suffocation	14-24†
Unintentional injury	History, scene investigation, autopsy	Traumatic child abuse	15*
Traumatic child abuse	Autopsy and scene investigation	Unintentional injury	13-24*
Other natural causes	History and autopsy	If minimal findings: SIDS or intentional suffocation	12-17*
UNEXPLAINED AT AUTOPSY			
SIDS	History, scene investigation, absence of explainable cause at autopsy	Intentional suffocation	80-82%
Intentional suffocation (filicide)	Perpetrator confession, absence of explainable cause at autopsy	SIDS	Unknown

*As a percentage of all sudden unexpected infant deaths explained at autopsy.
†As a percentage of all natural causes of sudden unexpected infant deaths explained at autopsy.
SIDS, sudden infant death syndrome.
Adapted from Hunt CE: Sudden infant death syndrome and other causes of infant mortality: diagnosis, mechanisms and risk for recurrence in siblings, *Am J Respir Crit Care Med* 164:346–357, 2001.

EPIDEMIOLOGY

SIDS is the 3rd leading cause of infant mortality in the USA, accounting for 8% of all infant deaths. It is the most common cause of postneonatal infant mortality, accounting for 40-50% of all deaths between 1 mo and 1 yr of age. The annual rate of SIDS in the USA was stable at 1.3-1.4/1,000 live births (about 7,000 infants/yr) before 1992, when the American Academy of Pediatrics (AAP) recommended that infants sleep nonprone as a way to reduce risk for SIDS. Since then, particularly after initiation of the national Back to Sleep campaign in 1994, the rate of SIDS progressively declined and then leveled off in 2001 at 0.55/1,000 live births (2,234 infants). The rates have remained stagnant since that time; in 2006 it was 0.55/1,000 live births (2,323 infants). The decline in the number of SIDS deaths in the USA and other countries has been attributed to the increasing use of the supine position for sleep. In 1992, 82% of sampled infants in the USA were placed prone for sleep. Several other countries have decreased prone sleeping prevalence to ≤2%, but in the USA in 2008, 15% of infants were still being placed prone for sleeping.

PATHOLOGY

There are no autopsy findings pathognomonic for SIDS and no findings required for the diagnosis, although there are some common findings. Petechial hemorrhages are found in 68-95% of cases and are more extensive than in explained causes of infant mortality. Pulmonary edema is often present and may be substantial. The reasons for these findings are unknown.

SIDS victims have several identifiable changes in the lungs and other organs and in brainstem structure and function. Nearly 65% of SIDS victims have structural evidence of pre-existing, chronic low-grade asphyxia, and other studies have identified biochemical markers of asphyxia. SIDS victims have higher levels of vascular endothelial growth factor (VEGF) in the cerebrospinal fluid (CSF). These increases may be related to VEGF polymorphisms (see Genetic Risk Factors) or might indicate recent hypoxemic events, because VEGF is upregulated by hypoxia. Brainstem findings include a persistent increase of dendritic spines and delayed maturation of synapses in the medullary respiratory centers, and decreased tyrosine hydroxylase immunoreactivity and catecholaminergic neurons. Decreases in serotonin 1A (5-HT_{1A}) and 5-HT_{2A} receptor immunoreactivity have been observed in the dorsal nucleus of the vagus, solitary nucleus, and ventrolateral medulla, whereas increases are present in periaqueductal gray matter of the midbrain. The decreased immunoreactivity of receptors is accompanied by brainstem gliosis, and it is therefore unclear whether the decreases are secondary to hypoxia or ischemia or whether they reflect primary alterations in 5-HT metabolism or transport (see Genetic Risk Factors) (Table 367-4).

The ventral medulla has been a particular focus for studies in SIDS victims. It is an integrative area for vital autonomic functions including breathing, arousal, and chemosensory function. Quantitative 3-dimensional (3D) anatomic studies indicate that some SIDS infants have hypoplasia of the arcuate nucleus and up to 60% have histopathologic evidence of less extensive bilateral or unilateral hypoplasia. Considering the apparent overlap between putative mechanisms for SIDS and unexpected late fetal deaths, ~30% of late unexpected and unexplained stillbirths also have hypoplasia of the arcuate nucleus.

Neurotransmitter studies of the arcuate nucleus have also identified receptor abnormalities in some SIDS infants that involve several receptor types relevant to state-dependent autonomic control overall and to ventilatory and arousal responsiveness in particular. These deficits include significant decreases in binding to kainate, muscarinic cholinergic, and 5-HT receptors. Studies of the ventral medulla have identified morphologic and biochemical deficits in 5-HT neurons. Immunohistochemical analyses have revealed an increased number of 5-HT neurons and an increase in the fraction of 5-HT neurons showing an immature morphology, suggesting a failure or delay in the maturation of these neurons. It is not known whether such deficits in ventral medullary 5-HT neurons are sufficient to result in fatal autonomic dysfunction. High neuronal levels of interleukin 1β (IL-1β) are present in the arcuate and dorsal vagal nuclei in SIDS victims compared to controls, perhaps contributing to molecular interactions affecting cardiorespiratory and arousal responses.

The neuropathologic data provide compelling evidence for altered 5-HT homeostasis, creating an underlying vulnerability contributing to SIDS. 5-HT is an important neurotransmitter and the 5-HT neurons in the medulla project extensively to neurons in the brainstem and spinal cord that influence respiratory drive and arousal, cardiovascular control including blood pressure, circadian regulation and non-REM sleep, thermoregulation, and upper airway reflexes. Medullary 5-HT neurons may be respiratory chemosensors and may be involved with respiratory responses to intermittent hypoxia and respiratory rhythm generation. Decreases in 5-HT_{1A} and 5-HT_{2A} receptor immunoreactivity have been observed in the dorsal nucleus of the vagus, solitary nucleus, and ventrolateral medulla. There are extensive serotoninergic brainstem abnormalities in SIDS infants, including increased

Table 367-2 CONDITIONS THAT CAN CAUSE APPARENT LIFE-THREATENING EVENTS OR SUDDEN DEATH

CENTRAL NERVOUS SYSTEM
Arteriovenous malformation Subdural hematoma Seizures Congenital central hypoventilation Neuromuscular disorders (Werdnig-Hoffmann disease) Arnold-Chiari crisis Leigh syndrome
CARDIAC
Subendocardial fibroelastosis Aortic stenosis Anomalous coronary artery Myocarditis Cardiomyopathy Arrhythmias (prolonged Q-T syndrome, Wolff-Parkinson-White syndrome, congenital heart block)
PULMONARY
Pulmonary hypertension Vocal cord paralysis Aspiration Laryngotracheal disease
GASTROINTESTINAL
Pancreatitis Diarrhea and/or dehydration Gastroesophageal reflux Volvulus
ENDOCRINE-METABOLIC
Congenital adrenal hyperplasia Malignant hyperpyrexia Long- or medium-chain acyl coenzyme A deficiency Hyperammonemias (urea cycle enzyme deficiencies) Glutaricaciduria Carnitine deficiency (systemic or secondary) Glycogen storage disease type I Maple syrup urine disease Congenital lactic acidosis Biotinidase deficiency
INFECTION
Sepsis Meningitis Encephalitis Brain abscess Hepatitis Pyelonephritis Bronchiolitis (respiratory syncytial virus) Infant botulism Pertussis
TRAUMA
Child abuse Suffocation Physical trauma Factitious syndrome (formerly Munchausen syndrome) by proxy
POISONING
Boric acid Carbon monoxide Salicylates Barbiturates Ipecac Cocaine Insulin Others Intentional or unintentional

From Kliegman RM, Greenbaum LA, Lye PS: *Practical strategies in pediatric diagnosis and therapy*, ed 2, Philadelphia, 2004, Elsevier Saunders, p 98.

Table 367-3 DIFFERENTIAL DIAGNOSIS OF RECURRENT SUDDEN INFANT DEATH IN A SIBSHIP

IDIOPATHIC
Recurrent true sudden infant death syndrome
CENTRAL NERVOUS SYSTEM
Congenital central hypoventilation Neuromuscular disorders Leigh syndrome
CARDIAC
Endocardial fibroelastosis Wolff-Parkinson-White syndrome Prolonged Q-T syndrome Congenital heart block
PULMONARY
Pulmonary hypertension
ENDOCRINE-METABOLIC
See Table 367-2
INFECTION
Disorders of immune host defense
CHILD ABUSE
Filicide Infanticide Factitious syndrome (formerly Munchausen syndrome) by proxy

From Kliegman RM, Greenbaum LA, Lye PS: *Practical strategies in pediatric diagnosis and therapy*, ed 2, Philadelphia, 2004, Elsevier Saunders, p 101.

Table 367-4 IDENTIFIED GENES FOR WHICH THE DISTRIBUTION OF POLYMORPHISMS DIFFERS IN SUDDEN INFANT DEATH SYNDROME INFANTS COMPARED TO CONTROL INFANTS

CARDIA CHANNELOPATHIES (7)
Sodium ion channel gene *(SCN5A)* (long QT syndrome 3, Brugada syndrome) Potassium ion channel genes *(KCNE2, KCNH2, KCNQ1)* *CAV3* (long QT syndrome 9) *GPD1-L* (Brugada syndrome) *RyR2* (catecholaminergic polymorphic ventricular tachycardia)
SEROTONIN (5-HT) (3)
5-HT transporter protein *(5-HTT)* Intron 2 of *SLC6A4* (variable numer tandem repeat [VNTR] polymorphism) 5-HT FEV gene
GENES PERTINENT TO DEVELOPMENT OF AUTONOMIC NERVOUS SYSTEM (8)
Paired-like homeobox 2a *(PHOX2A)* *PHOX2B* Rearranged during transfection factor *(RET)* Endothelin converting enzyme-1 *(ECE1)* T-cell leukemia homeobox *(TLX3)* Engrailed-1 *(EN1)* Tyrosine hydroxylase *(THO1)* Monamine oxidase A *(MAOA)*
INFECTION AND INFLAMMATION (6)
Complement C4A Complement C4B Interleukin-10 (IL-10) Interleukin-6 (IL-6) (pro-inflammatory) Vascular endothelial growth factor (VEGF) (pro-inflammatory) Tumor necrosis factor (TNF)-α (pro-inflammatory)
ENERGY PRODUCTION (1)
Mitochondrial DNA (mtDNA) polymorphisms

Adapted from Hunt CE, Hauck FR: Sudden infant death syndrome: gene-environment interactions. In Brugada R, Brugada J, Brugada P, editors: *Clinical care in inherited cardiac syndromes*, Guildford, UK, 2009, Springer-Verlag London.

5-HT neuronal count, a lower density of 5-HT_{1A} receptor-binding sites in regions of the medulla involved in homeostatic function, and a lower ratio of 5-HT transporter (5-HTT) binding density to 5-HT neuronal count in the medulla. Male SIDS infants have lower receptor-binding density than female SIDS infants. These findings suggest that the synthesis and availability of 5-HT is altered within 5-HT pathways and hence alters neuronal firing. These neuropathologic data could be explained by an increased number of 5-HT neurons, leading to an excess of extracellular 5-HT and secondary down-regulation of 5-HT_{1A} receptors. It is also possible that 5-HT synthesis and/or release may be deficient, leading to a deficiency of extracellular 5-HT despite a compensatory overabundance of 5-HT neurons. Although the neuropathologic data thus do not clarify whether medullary 5-HT levels are increased or decreased in SIDS infants, the 5-HTT polymorphism data are consistent with decreased extracellular or synaptic 5-HT concentrations.

ENVIRONMENTAL RISK FACTORS

Declines of 50% or more in rates of SIDS in the USA and around the world have occurred in the past decade, at least in part as a result of national education campaigns directed at reducing risk factors associated with SIDS. The reductions in risk appear to be related primarily to decreases in placing infants prone for sleep and increases in placing them supine. A number of other risk factors also have significant associations with SIDS (Table 367-5); although many are nonmodifiable and most of the modifiable factors have not changed appreciably, self-reported maternal smoking prevalence during pregnancy has decreased by 25% in the past decade.

NONMODIFIABLE RISK FACTORS

Although SIDS affects infants from all social strata, lower socioeconomic status is consistently associated with higher risk. In the USA, African-American, Native American, and Alaskan Native infants are 2 to 3 times more likely than white infants to die of SIDS, whereas Asian, Pacific Islander, and Hispanic infants have the lowest incidence. Some of this disparity may be related to the higher concentration of poverty and other adverse environmental factors found within the communities with higher incidence.

Infants are at greatest risk of SIDS at 2-4 months of age, with most deaths having occurred by 6 months. This characteristic age has decreased in some countries as the SIDS incidence has declined, with deaths occurring at earlier ages and with a flattening of the peak incidence. Similarly, the commonly found winter seasonal predominance of SIDS has declined or disappeared in some countries as prone prevalence has decreased, supporting prior findings of an interaction between sleep position and factors more common in colder months (overheating, infection). Male infants are 30-50% more likely to be affected than female infants.

Table 367-5 ENVIRONMENTAL FACTORS ASSOCIATED WITH INCREASED RISK FOR SUDDEN INFANT DEATH SYNDROME

MATERNAL AND ANTENATAL RISK FACTORS
Elevated 2nd trimester serum α-fetoprotein
Smoking
Alcohol use
Drug use (cocaine, heroin)
Nutritional deficiency
Inadequate prenatal care
Low socioeconomic status
Younger age
Lower education
Single marital status
Shorter interpregnancy interval
Intrauterine hypoxia
Fetal growth restriction
INFANT RISK FACTORS:
Age (peak 2-4 mo, but may be decreasing)
Male gender
Race and ethnicity (African-American and Native American)
Growth failure
No breast-feeding
No pacifier (dummy)
Prematurity
Prone and side sleep position
Recent febrile illness (mild infections)
Inadequate immunizations
Smoking exposure (prenatal and postnatal)
Soft sleeping surface, soft bedding
Bed sharing with parent(s) or other children
Thermal stress, overheating
Colder season, no central heating

MODIFIABLE RISK FACTORS

Pregnancy-Related Factors

An increased SIDS risk is associated with numerous obstetric factors, suggesting that the in utero environment of future SIDS victims is suboptimal. SIDS infants are more commonly of higher birth order, independent of maternal age, and of gestations after shorter interpregnancy intervals. Mothers of SIDS infants generally receive less prenatal care and initiate care later in pregnancy. Additionally, low birthweight, preterm birth, and slower intrauterine and postnatal growth rates are risk factors.

Cigarette Smoking

There is a major association between intrauterine exposure to cigarette smoking and risk for SIDS. The incidence of SIDS is about 3 times greater among infants of mothers who smoke in studies conducted before SIDS risk-reduction campaigns and 5 times higher in studies after implementation of risk-reduction campaigns. The risk of death is progressively greater as daily cigarette use increases. The effects of smoking by the father and other household members are more difficult to interpret because they are highly correlated with maternal smoking. There appears to be a small independent effect of paternal smoking, but data on other household members have been inconsistent.

It is very difficult to assess the independent effect of infant exposure to environmental tobacco smoke (ETS) because parental smoking behavior during and after pregnancy are also highly correlated. An increased risk of SIDS is also found for infants exposed to only postnatal maternal ETS. There is a dose response for the number of household smokers, number of people smoking in the same room as the infant, and the number of cigarettes smoked. These data suggest that keeping the infant free of ETS can further reduce an infant's risk of SIDS.

Drug and Alcohol Use

Most studies link maternal prenatal drug use, especially opiates, with an increased risk of SIDS, ranging from 2-15-fold increased risk. Most studies have not found an association between maternal alcohol use prenatally or postnatally and SIDS. However, in one study of Northern Plains Indians, periconceptional alcohol use and binge drinking in the 1st trimester were associated with a 6-fold and an 8-fold increased risk of SIDS, respectively. A Danish cohort study found that mothers admitted to the hospital at any time before or after the birth of their infants for an alcohol- or drug-related disorder had a 3-times higher risk of their infant dying from SIDS, and a Dutch study reported that maternal alcohol consumption in the 24 hr before the infant died carried a 2-8-fold increased risk of SIDS. Siblings of infants with fetal alcohol syndrome have a 10-fold increased risk of SIDS compared to controls.

Infant Sleep Environment

Sleeping prone has consistently been shown to increase the risk of SIDS. As rates of prone positioning have decreased in the general population, the odds ratios for SIDS in infants still sleeping prone have increased. The highest risk of SIDS might occur in infants who are usually placed nonprone but placed prone for last sleep ("unaccustomed prone") or found prone ("secondary prone"). The "unaccustomed prone" position is more likely to occur in daycare or other settings outside the home and highlights the need for all infant caretakers to be educated about appropriate sleep positioning.

The initial SIDS risk-reduction campaign recommendations considered side sleeping to be nearly equivalent to the supine position in reducing the risk of SIDS. Subsequent studies have indicated that although it is safer than the prone position, side-sleeping infants are twice as likely to die of SIDS as infants sleeping supine. This increased risk might relate to the relative instability of the position, with some infants placed on the side rolling to the prone position. The **current recommendations** call for **supine position for sleeping for all infants except those few with specific medical conditions** for which recommending a different position may be justified.

Many parents and health care providers were initially concerned that supine sleeping would be associated with an increase in adverse consequences, such as difficulty sleeping, vomiting, or aspiration. Evidence suggests that the risk of regurgitation and choking is highest for prone-sleeping infants. Some newborn nursery staff still tend to favor side positioning, which models inappropriate infant care practice to parents. Infants sleeping on their backs do not have more episodes of cyanosis or apnea; reports of apparent life-threatening events decreased in Scandinavia after increased use of the supine position. Among infants in the USA who maintained the same sleep position at 1, 3, and 6 mo of age, no clinical symptoms or reasons for outpatient visits (including fever, cough, wheezing, trouble breathing or sleeping, vomiting, diarrhea, or respiratory illness) are more common in infants sleeping supine or on their sides compared with infants sleeping prone. Three symptoms are actually less common in infants sleeping supine or on their sides: fever at 1 month, stuffy nose at 6 months, and trouble sleeping at 6 months. Outpatient visits for ear infection are less common at 3 and 6 months for infants sleeping supine and also less common at 3 months for infants sleeping on their sides. These results provide reassurance for parents and health care providers and should contribute to universal acceptance of supine as the safest and optimal sleep position for infants.

Soft sleep surfaces or bedding, such as comforters, pillows, sheepskins, polystyrene bean pillows, and older or softer mattresses are associated with increased risk of SIDS. Head and face covering by loose bedding, particularly heavy comforters, is also associated with increased risk. Overheating has been associated with increased risk for SIDS based on indicators such as higher room temperature, high body temperature, sweating, and excessive clothing or bedding. Some studies have identified an interaction between overheating and prone sleeping, with overheating increasing the risk of SIDS only when infants are sleeping prone. Higher external environmental temperatures have not been associated with increased SIDS incidence in the USA.

Several studies have implicated **bed sharing** as a risk factor for SIDS. Bed sharing is particularly hazardous when other children are in the same bed, when the parent is sleeping with an infant on a couch or other soft or confining sleeping surface, and when the mother smokes. Infants <4 mo of age are at increased risk even when mothers are nonsmokers. Risk is also increased with longer duration of bed sharing during the night; returning the infant to his or her own crib is not associated with increased risk. Room sharing without bed sharing is associated with lower SIDS rates; the safest place for an infant to sleep may be in his or her own crib in the parents' room.

One study found that having a fan on in the room during sleep was associated with a reduced risk of SIDS. This effect was more pronounced in adverse sleep environments. Other studies will need to confirm this finding before recommendations can be made about this factor.

Infant-Feeding Care Practices and Exposures

A number of studies have demonstrated a protective effect of breast-feeding, but others have found that this protective effect is not present after adjusting for potentially confounding factors. A large study from Germany found a reduced risk of SIDS among breast-fed infants, even after adjusting for socioeconomic and other confounding factors. *This study and several others now provide strong evidence of benefit from breast-feeding.*

Pacifier (dummy) use lowers the risk of SIDS in the majority of studies when used for last or reference sleep. Although it is not known if this is a direct effect of the pacifier itself or from associated infant or parental behavior, there is increasing evidence that pacifier use and dislodgment can increase the arousability of infants during sleep. Concerns have been expressed about recommending pacifiers as a means of reducing the risk of SIDS for fear of adverse consequences, particularly interference with breast-feeding. Well-designed studies have found no association between pacifiers and breast-feeding duration. A small increased incidence of otitis media and of respiratory and gastrointestinal illness has been reported for pacifier users compared with nonusers. The Netherlands (for bottle-fed babies) and Germany have recommended pacifier use as a potential way to reduce the risk of SIDS. *The most recent AAP guidelines recommend pacifier use for all infants, delaying introduction for nursing infants until after breast-feeding has been well established.*

Upper respiratory tract infections have generally not been found to be an independent risk factor for SIDS. These and other minor infections might play a role in the pathogenesis of SIDS. Risk for SIDS has been found to be increased after illness among prone sleepers, those who were heavily wrapped, and those whose heads were covered during sleep.

No adverse association between immunizations and SIDS has been found. SIDS infants are less likely to be immunized than control infants; in immunized infants, no temporal relationship between vaccine administration and death has been identified. In a meta-analysis of case-control studies that adjusted for potentially confounding factors, the risk of SIDS for infants immunized with diphtheria, tetanus, and pertussis was half that for nonimmunized infants.

SIDS rates remain higher among Native Americans, Alaskan Natives, and African-Americans. This may be due, in part, to group differences in adopting supine sleeping or other risk-reduction practices. Greater efforts are needed to address this persistent disparity and to ensure that SIDS risk-reduction education reaches all parents and all other care providers, including other family members and personnel at daycare centers.

GENETIC RISK FACTORS

As shown in Table 367-4, there are numerous genetic differences identified among healthy infants, infants dying from other causes, and SIDS infants. Polymorphisms occurring at higher incidence in SIDS compared to controls have been identified for 7 cardiac ion channelopathy genes that are proarrhythmic, 3 5-HT genes, 8 autonomic nervous system (ANS) development genes, 6 genes related to infection and inflammation that are pro-inflammatory, and 1 gene related to energy production.

Long Q-T syndrome (LQTS) is a known cause of sudden unexpected death in adults and children, due to a prolonged cardiac action potential by either increasing depolarization or decreasing repolarization current. The first evidence supporting a causal role for LQTS in SIDS was a large Italian study in which having a corrected QT interval >440 ms on an electrocardiogram performed on day 3-4 of life was associated with a 41.3 odds ratio for SIDS. Several case reports have provided proof-of-concept that cardiac channelopathy polymorphisms are associated with SIDS. LQTS has been associated with polymorphisms related to mainly gain-of-function mutations in the sodium channel gene *(SCN5A)* that encode critical channel pore-forming alpha subunits or essential channel interacting proteins. LQTS has also been associated with mainly loss-of-function polymorphisms in 3 potassium channel genes (*KCNE2, KCNH2, KCNQ1*). The mechanism by which potassium channel variants can contribute to SIDS is thought to be mediated at least in part through increased sympathetic activity during sleep, including REM sleep, and associated sleep-related hypoxemia and chemoreceptive reflexes. Short QTS (SQTS) is more recently recognized as another cause of life-threatening arrhythmia or sudden death, often during rest or sleep. Gain-of-function mutations in genes including *KCNH2* and *KCNQ1* have been causally linked to SQTS, and some of these deaths have occurred in infants, suggesting that SQTS may also be causally linked to SIDS.

Both LQTS and SQTS are pro-arrhythmic and associated with cardiac arrest and sudden death. However, some of these polymorphisms are associated with concealed phenotypes in which perturbation by a stressor such as acidosis, hypoxemia, or adrenergic stress is required to elicit electrocardiographic evidence of the pro-arrhythmic dysfunction. The other cardiac ion-related channelopathy polymorphisms are also pro-arrhythmic, including Brugada syndrome (*BrS1, BrS2*), and catecholaminergic paroxysmal ventricular tachycardia (*CPVT1*). Collectively, these mutations in cardiac ion channels provide a lethal arrhythmogenic substrate in some infants at risk for SIDS (Fig. 367-1) and might account for as many as 10% of SIDS.

Many genes are involved in the control of 5-HT synthesis, storage, membrane uptake, and metabolism. Polymorphisms have been identified in the promotor region of the 5-HT transporter (5-HTT) protein gene located on chromosome 17 that occur in greater frequency in SIDS than control infants. The long "L" allele increases effectiveness of the promotor and reduces extracellular 5-HT concentrations at nerve endings compared to the short "S" allele. White, African-American, and Japanese SIDS infants are more likely than controls to have the "L" (long) allele. There is also a negative association between SIDS and the S/S genotype. The L/L genotype is associated with increased serotonin transporters on neuroimaging and postmortem binding studies.

An association has also been observed between SIDS and a 5-HTT intron 2 polymorphism, which differentially regulates *5-HTT* expression. There are positive associations between SIDS and the intron 2 genotype distributions in African-American infants compared to African-American controls. The human fifth Ewing variant (FEV) gene is specifically expressed in central 5-HT neurons in the brain, with a predicted role in specification and maintenance of the serotoninergic neuronal phenotype. An insertion mutation has been identified in intron 2 of the FEV gene, and the distribution of this mutation differs significantly in SIDS compared to control infants.

Molecular genetic studies in SIDS victims have also identified mutations pertinent to early embryologic development of the autonomic nervous system (ANS). The relevant genes include mammalian achaete-scute homolog-1 *(MASH1)*, bone morphogenic protein-2 *(BMP2)*, paired-like homeobox 2a *(PHOX2a)*, *PHOX 2b*, rearranged during transfection factor *(RET)*, endothelin converting enzyme-1 *(ECE 1)*, T-cell leukemia homeobox *(TLX3)*, engrailed-1 *(EN1)*, tyrosine hydroxylase *(THO1)*, and monamine oxidase A *(MAOA)*. Eleven protein-changing rare mutations have been identified in 14/92 SIDS cases among the *PHOX 2a, RET, ECE1, TLX3,* and *EN1* genes. Only one of these mutations *(TLX3)* was found in 2/92 controls. African-American infants accounted for 10/11 mutations in SIDS infants and in both affected controls with protein-changing mutations. Eight polymorphisms in the *PHOX2B* gene occurred significantly more frequently in SIDS compared to control infants.

Genetic differences in SIDS infants compared to control infants have been reported for 2 complement *C4* genes. Among SIDS infants, infant deaths attributed to infection, and healthy infant controls, SIDS infants with mild upper respiratory infection prior to death are more likely to have deletion of either the *C4A* or the *C4B* gene compared to SIDS victims without infection or to living controls. Among living infants, there are no differences in the *C4* gene in those with versus without an upper

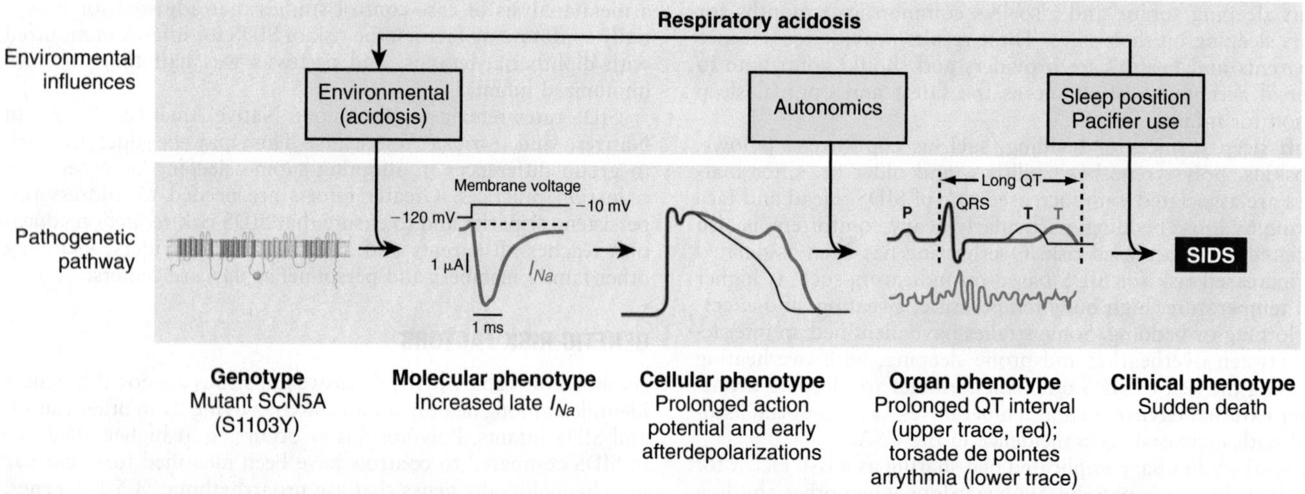

Figure 367-1 An arrhythmogenic pathogenetic pathway for sudden infant death syndrome (SIDS) from patient genotype to clinical phenotype, with environmental influences noted. The genetic abnormality—in this instance, a polymorphism in the cardiac Na^+ channel SCN5A—causes a molecular phenotype of increased late Na^+ current (I_{Na}) under the influence of environmental factors such as acidosis. Interacting with other ion currents that may themselves be altered by genetic and environmental factors, the late Na^+ current causes a cellular phenotype of prolonged action potential duration as well as early after-depolarizations. Prolonged action potential in the cells of the ventricular myocardium and further interaction with environmental factors such as autonomic innervation, which, in turn, may be affected by genetic factors, produce a tissue-organ phenotype of a prolonged Q-T interval on the electrocardiogram (ECG) and torsades de pointes arrhythmia in the whole heart. If this is sustained or degenerates to ventricular fibrillation, the clinical phenotype of SIDS results. Environmental and multiple genetic factors can interact at many different levels to produce the characteristic phenotypes at the molecular, cellular, tissue, organ, and clinical levels. (From Makielski JC: SIDS: genetic and environmental influences may cause arrhythmia in this silent killer, *J Clin Invest* 116:297–299, 2006.)

respiratory infection. These data suggest that partial deletions of *C4* in combination with a mild upper respiratory infection place these relatively hypoimmune infants at increased risk for sudden unexpected death. Some SIDS infants have loss-of-function polymorphisms in the gene promoter region for interleukin-10 (IL-10), another anti-inflammatory cytokine. Among SIDS infants compared to living controls, sudden infant death is strongly associated with the IL-10 polymorphism. These IL-10 polymorphisms are associated with decreased IL-10 levels and hence could contribute to SIDS by delaying initiation of protective antibody production or reducing capacity to inhibit inflammatory cytokine production. A larger study did not find differences in IL-10 genes in SIDS compared to control infants, but it did identify an association with the ATA haplotype in sudden and unexpected infant deaths classified as resulting from infection.

Significant associations with SIDS have been reported for polymorphisms in vascular endothelial growth factor (VEGF), IL-6, and tumor necrosis factor-α (TNF-α). These 3 cytokines are pro-inflammatory, and these gain-of-function polymorphisms would result in increased inflammatory response to infectious or inflammatory stimuli and hence contribute to an imbalance between pro-inflammatory and anti-inflammatory cytokines. As apparent proof of principle, elevated levels of IL-6 and VEGF have been reported from cerebrospinal fluid in SIDS infants. There were no group differences in the IL6-174G/C polymorphism in a Norwegian SIDS study, but the aggregate evidence nevertheless suggests an activated immune system in SIDS and thus implicates genes involved in the immune system.

Several studies of mtDNA in SIDS infants have demonstrated significant differences in mutations compared to control infants, including a high substitution rate in the HVR-1 region of the D-loop and an association between a high number of these substitutions and mutations in coding areas of mtDNA. Another study of mitochondrial tRNA genes and flanking regions did not demonstrate an association between a specific mitochondrial tRNA gene mutation and SIDS, or a higher mtDNA mutation frequency in SIDS versus control infants. Cardiac arrhythmias, including prolonged QT intervals, have been observed in families with mitochondrial disease. Although the mtDNA polymorphism T3394C that is associated with cardiac arrhythmia has not been observed to occur with greater frequency in SIDS compared to control infants, it is nevertheless possible that mtDNA mutations such as T3394C may be genetic variants that when combined with environmental risk factors not present in healthy infants could predispose to sudden death.

GENE-AND-ENVIRONMENT INTERACTIONS

Interactions between genetic and environmental risk factors determine the actual risk for SIDS in individual infants (Fig. 367-2). There appears to be an interaction between prone sleep position and impaired ventilatory and arousal responsiveness. Facedown or nearly facedown sleeping does occasionally occur in prone-sleeping infants and can result in episodes of airway obstruction and asphyxia in healthy full-term infants. Healthy infants arouse before such episodes become life-threatening, but infants with insufficient arousal responsiveness to asphyxia may be at risk for sudden death. There may also be links between modifiable risk factors such as soft bedding, prone sleep position and thermal stress, and links between genetic risk factors such as ventilatory and arousal abnormalities and temperature or metabolic regulation deficits. Cardiorespiratory control deficits could be related to 5-HTT polymorphisms, for example, or to polymorphisms in genes pertinent to ANS development. Affected infants could be at increased risk for sleep-related hypoxemia and hence more susceptible to adverse effects associated with unsafe sleep position or bedding. Infants at increased risk for sleep-related hypoxemia could also be at greater risk for fatal arrhythmias in the presence of a cardiac ion channelopathy polymorphism.

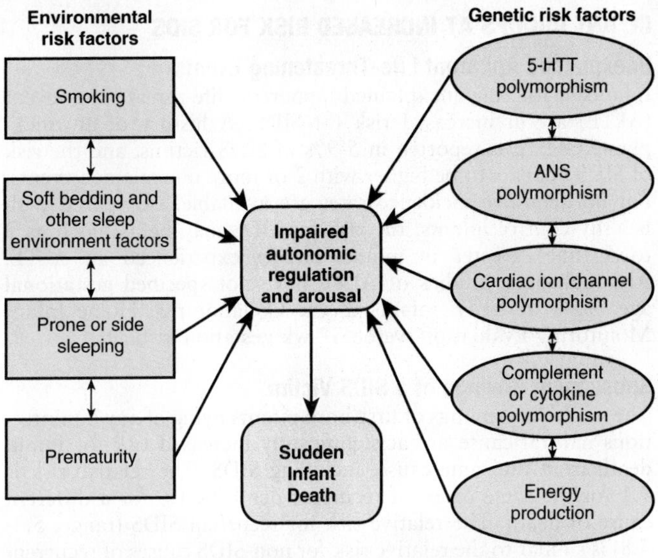

Figure 367-2 Schematic illustration of potential interactions between representative environmental and genetic risk factors for sudden unexpected death in infancy (SUDI) and sudden infant death syndrome (SIDS). ANS, autonomic nervous system; 5-HTT, serotonin (5-HT) transporter. (Adapted from Hunt CE, Hauck FR: Sudden infant death syndrome: gene-environment interactions. In Brugada R, Brugada J, Brugada P, editors: *Clinical care in inherited cardiac syndromes,* Guildford, UK, 2009, Springer-Verlag London.)

In >50% of SIDS victims, recent febrile illnesses, often related to upper respiratory infection, have been documented (see Table 367-5). Otherwise benign infections might increase risk for SIDS if interacting with genetically determined impaired immune responses including those due to partial deletions in the complement C4 gene or to interleukin polymorphisms (see Table 367-4). Deficient inflammatory responsiveness can also occur due to mast cell degranulation, which has been reported in SIDS infants; this is consistent with an anaphylactic reaction to a bacterial toxin, and some family members of SIDS infants also have mast cell hyper-releasability and degranulation, suggesting that increased susceptibility to an anaphylactic reaction is another genetic factor influencing fatal outcomes to otherwise minor infections in infants. Interactions between upper respiratory infections or other minor illnesses and other factors such as prone sleeping might also play a role in the pathogenesis of SIDS.

The increased risk for SIDS associated with fetal and postnatal exposure to cigarette smoke may be related at least in part to genetic or epigenetic factors, including those affecting brainstem autonomic control. Although no genetic studies have yet identified any polymorphism affecting nicotine or tobacco metabolism, both animal and human infant studies document decreased ventilatory and arousal responsiveness to hypoxia following fetal nicotine exposure, and impaired autoresuscitation after apnea has been associated with postnatal nicotine exposure. Decreased brain stem immunoreactivity to selected protein kinase C and neuronal nitric oxide synthase isoforms occurs in rats exposed to cigarette smoke prenatally, another potential cause of impaired hypoxic responsiveness. Smoking exposure also increases susceptibility to viral and bacterial infections and increases bacterial binding after passive coating of mucosal surfaces with smoke components, implicating interactions between smoking, cardiorespiratory control, and immune status.

In infants with a cardiac ion channelopathy, risk for a fatal arrhythmia during sleep may be substantially enhanced by predisposing perturbations that increase electrical instability. These perturbations could include REM sleep with bursts of vagal and sympathetic activation, minor respiratory infections, or any other cause of sleep-related hypoxemia or hypercarbia, especially those resulting in acidosis. The prone sleeping position is associated with increased sympathetic activity.

INFANT GROUPS AT INCREASED RISK FOR SIDS

Unexplained Apparent Life-Threatening Events

Infants with an unexplained apparent life-threatening event (ALTE) are at increased risk for SIDS. A history of an unexplained ALTE is reported in 5-9% of SIDS victims, and the risk of SIDS appears to be higher with 2 or more unexplained events, but no definitive incidence rates are available. Compared with healthy control infants, the risk for SIDS may be as much as 3 to 5 times greater in infants having experienced an ALTE. Although most studies of ALTE have not specified gestational age, 30% of ALTE infants in the Collaborative Home Infant Monitoring Evaluation were ≤37 wk gestation at birth.

Subsequent Siblings of a SIDS Victim

The next-born siblings of first-born infants dying of any noninfectious natural cause are at significantly increased risk for infant death from the same cause, including SIDS. The relative risk is 9.1 for the same cause of recurrent death vs 1.6 for a different cause of death. The relative risk for recurrent SIDS (range, 5.4-5.8) is similar to the relative risk for non-SIDS causes of recurrent death (range, 4.6-12.5). The risk for recurrent infant mortality from the same cause as in the index sibling thus appears to be increased to a similar degree in subsequent siblings for both explained causes and for SIDS. This increased risk in SIDS families is consistent with genetic risk factors interacting with environmental risk factors (Table 367-5 and Fig. 367-2).

Controversy as to the extent to which risk for SIDS may be increased in subsequent siblings prevails as a result of uncertainty about the frequency with which intentional suffocation is misclassified as SIDS and continued limits of understanding of the role of genetic risk factors. Clarification of the role of intentional suffocation has been impaired by the lack of objective criteria for diagnosis. Although some health professionals have in the past stated that all subsequent cases of sudden unexpected infant deaths in a family should be investigated for possible homicide, there are substantial data in support of genetic and environmental factors leading to increased natural risk for recurrent SIDS in some families. In addition to genetic evidence consistent with increased risk for SIDS in subsequent siblings, epidemiologic data from the United Kingdom confirm that 2nd infant deaths in families are not rare and that at least 80-90% are natural. The proportion of recurrent infant death from SIDS in subsequent siblings was 5.9 times greater than the proportion of probable homicides.

Prematurity

There is an inverse relationship between risk for SIDS and gestational age. The environmental risk factors associated with SIDS in preterm infants are not substantially different from those observed in full-term infants, including prone and side sleeping. The postnatal age of preterm infants dying of SIDS is 5-7 wk older than that of full-term infants, and the postconceptional age is 4-6 wk younger than that of full-term infants. Compared with infants with birthweight >2,500 g, infants with birthweight of 1,000-1,499 g and 1,500-2,499 g are approximately 4 and 3 times more likely to die of SIDS, respectively.

Physiologic Studies

Physiologic studies have been performed on healthy infants in early infancy, a few of whom later died of SIDS. Physiologic studies have also been performed on infant groups at increased risk for SIDS, especially those with ALTE and subsequent siblings of SIDS. In the aggregate, these studies indicate brainstem abnormalities in neuroregulation of cardiorespiratory control or other autonomic functions and are consistent with the autopsy findings and genetic studies in SIDS victims (see the "Pathology" and "Genetic Risk Factors" sections).

Brainstem muscarinic cholinergic pathways develop from the neural crest and are important in ventilatory responsiveness to CO_2. The muscarinic system develops from the neural crest, and the *RET* gene is important for this development. *RET* knockout mice have a depressed ventilatory response to hypercarbia. In addition to chemoreceptor sensitivity, these observed physiologic abnormalities also affect respiratory patterns, control of heart and respiratory rate or variability, and asphyxic arousal responsiveness. A deficit in arousal responsiveness may be a necessary prerequisite for SIDS to occur but may be insufficient to cause SIDS in the absence of other genetic or environmental risk factors. **Autoresuscitation (gasping)** is a critical component of the asphyxic arousal response, and a failure of autoresuscitation in SIDS infants may be the final and most devastating physiologic failure. Most full-term infants <9 wk of age arouse in response to mild hypoxia, but only 10-15% of normal infants >9 wk of age arouse. These data thus suggest that as infants mature, their ability to arouse to mild to moderate hypoxic stimuli diminishes as they reach the age range of greatest risk for SIDS.

The ability to shorten the QT interval as heart rate increases appears to be impaired in some SIDS victims, suggesting that such infants may be predisposed to ventricular arrhythmia. This is consistent with the observations of cardiac ion channel gene polymorphisms in other SIDS victims (Table 367-4), but there are no antemortem QT interval data in the SIDS infants having postmortem channelopathy polymorphisms. Infants studied physiologically and dying of SIDS a few weeks later have higher heart rates in all sleep-wake states, diminished heart rate variability during wakefulness, and significantly lower heart rate variability at the respiratory frequency across all sleep-wake cycles. Also, these SIDS infants have longer QT intervals than control infants in both REM and non-REM sleep, especially in the late hours of the night when most SIDS likely occurs. In only 1 of these SIDS infants, however, did the QT interval exceed 440 ms.

Part of the decreased heart rate variability and increased heart rate observed in infants who later die of SIDS may be related to decreased vagal tone. This decreased tone appears, at least in part, to be related to vagal neuropathy or to brainstem damage in areas responsible for parasympathetic cardiac control. In a comparison of heart rate power spectra before and after obstructive apneas in infants, future SIDS infants do not have the decreases in low-frequency to high-frequency power ratios observed in control infants. Some future SIDS victims thus have different autonomic responsiveness to obstructive apnea, perhaps indicating impaired ANS control associated with higher vulnerability to external or endogenous stress factors and hence to reduced electrical stability of the heart.

Sweating during sleep has been observed in some infants with an unexplained ALTE or SIDS. Although overheating may be the cause of this sweating, it might also be caused by hypoventilation and secondary asphyxia or by autonomic dysfunction as part of a more generalized deficiency in brainstem function.

Home cardiorespiratory monitors with memory capability have recorded the terminal events in some SIDS victims. These recordings have not included pulse oximetry and do not permit identification of obstructed breaths due to reliance on transthoracic impedance for breath detection. In most instances, there has been sudden and rapid progression of severe bradycardia that is either unassociated with central apnea or appears to occur too soon to be explained by the central apnea. These observations are consistent with an abnormality in autonomic control of heart rate variability, or with obstructed breaths and associated bradycardia or hypoxemia.

CLINICAL STRATEGIES

Home Monitoring

SIDS cannot be prevented in individual infants because it is not possible to identify prospective SIDS infants, and no effective intervention has been established even if SIDS infants could be prospectively identified. Studies of cardiorespiratory pattern or other autonomic abnormalities do not have sufficient sensitivity and specificity to be clinically useful as screening tests. Home electronic surveillance using existing technology does not reduce the risk of SIDS. Although a prolonged QT interval in an infant may be treated if diagnosed, neither the role of routine postnatal electrocardiographic (ECG) screening nor the cost-effectiveness of diagnosis and treatment and safety of treatment has been established (Chapter 429.5). Parental ECG screening is not helpful because spontaneous mutations are common.

Reducing the Risk of SIDS

Reducing risk behaviors and increasing protective behaviors among infant caregivers to achieve further reductions and eventual elimination of SIDS is a critical goal. Recent increases in placing infants prone for sleep in the USA are cause for concern and require renewed educational efforts. The AAP guidelines to reduce the risk of SIDS in individual infants are appropriate for most infants, but physicians and other health care providers might, on occasion, need to consider alternative approaches. The major components are as follows:

- Full-term and premature infants should be placed for sleep in the supine position. There are no adverse health outcomes from supine sleeping. Side sleeping is not recommended.
- It is recommended that infants sleep in the same room as their parents but in their own crib or bassinette that conforms to the safety standards of the Consumer Product Safety Commission. Placing the crib or bassinette near the mother's bed facilitates nursing and contact.
- Infants should be put to sleep on a firm mattress. Waterbeds, sofas, soft mattresses, or other soft surfaces should not be used.
- Soft materials in the infant's sleep environment—over, under, or near the infant—should be avoided. These include pillows, comforters, quilts, sheepskins, cushion-like bumper pads, and stuffed toys. Because loose bedding may be hazardous, blankets, if used, should be tucked in around the crib mattress. Sleeping clothing, such as a sleep sack, can be used in place of blankets.
- Avoid overheating and overbundling. The infant should be lightly clothed for sleep and the thermostat set at a comfortable temperature.
- Infants should have some time in the prone position (tummy time) while awake and observed. Alternating the placement of the infant's head as well as his or her orientation in the crib can also minimize the risk of head flattening from supine sleeping (positional plagiocephaly).
- Devices advertised to maintain sleep position, "protect" a bed-sharing infant, or reduce the risk of rebreathing are not recommended.
- Home respiratory, cardiac, and O_2 saturation monitoring may be of value for selected infants who have extreme instability, but there is no evidence that monitoring decreases the incidence of SIDS and it is therefore not recommended for this purpose.
- Consider offering a pacifier at bedtime and naptime. The pacifier should be used when placing the infant down for sleep and not be reinserted once it falls out. For breast-fed infants, delay introduction of the pacifier until breast-feeding is well established.
- Mothers should not smoke during pregnancy and infants should not be exposed to secondhand smoke.
- The national Back to Sleep campaign should continue and be expanded to emphasize the multiple characteristics of a safe sleeping environment and to focus on the groups who continue to have higher rates of SIDS. Educational strategies must be tailored to each racial or ethnic group to ensure acceptance within that cultural context. Secondary care providers need to be targeted to receive these educational messages, including daycare providers, grandparents, foster parents, and babysitters. Health care professionals in intensive care and normal newborn nurseries should implement these recommendations well before anticipated discharge.

BIBLIOGRAPHY

Please visit the Nelson Textbook of Pediatrics *website at www.expertconsult.com for the complete bibliography.*

Section 2 DISORDERS OF THE RESPIRATORY TRACT

Chapter 368 Congenital Disorders of the Nose

Joseph Haddad, Jr.

NORMAL NEWBORN NOSE

Children and adults preferentially breathe through their nose unless nasal obstruction interferes. Most newborn infants are obligate nasal breathers and significant nasal obstruction presenting at birth, such as choanal atresia, may be a life-threatening situation for the infant unless an alternative to the nasal airway is established. Nasal congestion with obstruction is common in the 1st year of life and can affect the quality of breathing during sleep; it may be associated with a narrow nasal airway, viral or bacterial infection, enlarged adenoids, or maternal estrogenic stimuli similar to rhinitis of pregnancy. The internal nasal airway doubles in size in the 1st 6 mo of life, leading to resolution of symptoms in many infants. Supportive care with a bulb syringe and saline nose drops, topical nasal decongestants, and antibiotics, when indicated, improve symptoms in affected infants.

PHYSIOLOGY

The nose is responsible for olfaction and initial warming and humidification of inspired air. In the anterior nasal cavity, turbulent airflow and coarse hairs enhance the deposition of large particulate matter; the remaining nasal airways filter out particles as small as 6 µm in diameter. In the turbinate region, the airflow becomes laminar and the airstream is narrowed and directed superiorly, enhancing particle deposition, warming, and humidification. Nasal passages contribute as much as 50% of the total resistance of normal breathing. Nasal flaring, a sign of respiratory distress, reduces the resistance to inspiratory airflow through the nose and can improve ventilation (Chapter 365).

Although the nasal mucosa is more vascular, especially in the turbinate region than in the lower airways, the surface epithelium is similar, with ciliated cells, goblet cells, submucosal glands, and a covering blanket of mucus. The nasal secretions contain lysozyme and secretory immunoglobulin A (IgA), both of which have antimicrobial activity, and IgG, IgE, albumin, histamine, bacteria, lactoferrin, and cellular debris, as well as mucous glycoproteins, which provide viscoelastic properties. Aided by the ciliated cells, mucus flows toward the nasopharynx, where the airstream widens, the epithelium becomes squamous, and secretions are

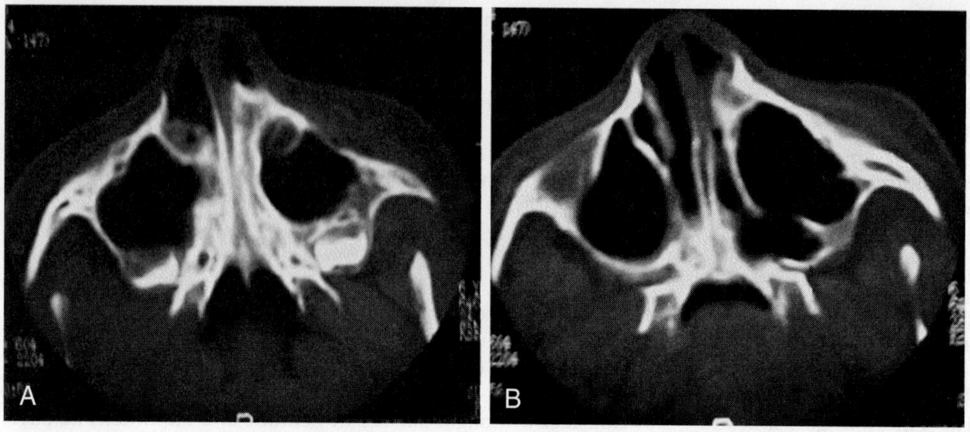

Figure 368-1 CT scan showing *(A)* hypoplastic nasal cavities, and *(B)* bony and mucosal choanal atresia. (From Altuntas A, Yilmaz MD, Kahveci OK, et al: Coexistence of choanal atresia and Tessier's facial cleft number 2, *Int J Pediatr Otorhinolaryngol* 68:1081–1085, 2004.)

wiped away by swallowing. Replacement of the mucous layers occurs about every 10-20 min. Estimates of daily mucus production vary from 0.1-0.3 mg/kg/24 hr, with most of the mucus being produced by the submucosal glands.

CONGENITAL DISORDERS

Congenital *structural nasal malformations* are uncommon compared with acquired abnormalities. The nasal bones can be congenitally absent so that the bridge of the nose fails to develop, resulting in *nasal hypoplasia.* Congenital absence of the nose *(arhinia),* complete or partial duplication, or a single centrally placed nostril can occur in isolation but is usually part of a malformation syndrome. Rarely, *supernumerary teeth* are found in the nose, or teeth grow into it from the maxilla.

Nasal bones can be sufficiently malformed to produce severe narrowing of the nasal passages. Often, such narrowing is associated with a high and narrow hard palate. Children with these defects can have significant obstruction to airflow during infections of the upper airways and are more susceptible to the development of chronic or recurrent hypoventilation (Chapter 17). Rarely, the alae nasi are sufficiently thin and poorly supported to result in inspiratory obstruction, or there may be congenital nasolacrimal duct obstruction with cystic extension into the nasopharynx, causing respiratory distress.

CHOANAL ATRESIA

This is the most common congenital anomaly of the nose and has a frequency of ~1/7,000 live births. It consists of a unilateral or bilateral bony (90%) or membranous (10%) septum between the nose and the pharynx; most cases are a combination of bony and membranous atresia. About 50-70% of affected infants have other congenital anomalies, with the anomalies occurring more often in bilateral cases. The **CHARGE syndrome** (*c*oloboma, *h*eart disease, *a*tresia choanae, *r*etarded growth and development or CNS anomalies or both, *g*enital anomalies or hypogonadism or both, and *e*ar anomalies or deafness or both) is one of the more common anomalies associated with choanal atresia. Most patients with CHARGE syndrome have mutations in the *CHD7* gene, which is involved in chromatin organization. Approximately 10-20% of patients with choanal atresia have the CHARGE syndrome.

Clinical Manifestations

Newborn infants have a variable ability to breathe through their mouths, so nasal obstruction does not produce the same symptoms in every infant. When the obstruction is unilateral, the infant may be asymptomatic for a prolonged period, often until the 1st respiratory infection, when unilateral nasal discharge or persistent nasal obstruction can suggest the diagnosis. Infants with bilateral choanal atresia who have difficulty with mouth breathing make vigorous attempts to inspire, often suck in their lips, and develop cyanosis. Distressed children then cry (which relieves the cyanosis) and become calmer, with normal skin color, only to repeat the cycle after closing their mouths. Those who are able to breathe through their mouths at once experience difficulty when sucking and swallowing, becoming cyanotic when they attempt to feed.

Diagnosis

Diagnosis is established by the inability to pass a firm catheter through each nostril 3-4 cm into the nasopharynx. The atretic plate may be seen directly with fiberoptic rhinoscopy. The anatomy is best evaluated by using high-resolution CT (Fig. 368-1).

Treatment

Initial treatment consists of prompt placement of an oral airway, maintaining the mouth in an open position, or intubation. A standard oral airway (such as that used in anesthesia) can be used, or a feeding nipple can be fashioned with large holes at the tip to facilitate air passage. Once an oral airway is established, the infant can be fed by gavage until breathing and eating without the assisted airway is possible. In bilateral cases, intubation or, less often, tracheotomy may be indicated. If the child is free of other serious medical problems, operative intervention is considered in the neonate; transnasal repair is the treatment of choice, with the introduction of small magnifying endoscopes and smaller surgical instruments and drills. Stents are usually left in place for weeks after the repair to prevent closure or stenosis. Tracheotomy should be considered in cases of bilateral atresia in which the child has other potentially life-threatening problems and in whom early surgical repair of the choanal atresia may not be appropriate or feasible. Operative correction of unilateral obstruction may be deferred for several years. In both unilateral and bilateral cases, restenosis necessitating dilation or reoperation, or both, is common. Mitomycin C has been used to help prevent the development of granulation tissue and stenosis.

CONGENITAL DEFECTS OF THE NASAL SEPTUM

Perforation of the septum is most commonly acquired after birth secondary to infection, such as syphilis, tuberculosis, or trauma; rarely, it is developmental. Continuous positive airway pressure cannulas are a cause of iatrogenic perforation. Trauma from delivery is the most common cause of septal deviation noted at birth. When recognized early, it can be corrected with immediate realignment using blunt probes, cotton applicators, and topical anesthesia. Formal surgical correction, when required, is usually postponed to avoid disturbance of midface growth.

Mild septal deviations are common and usually asymptomatic; abnormal formation of the septum is uncommon unless other malformations are present, such as cleft lip or palate.

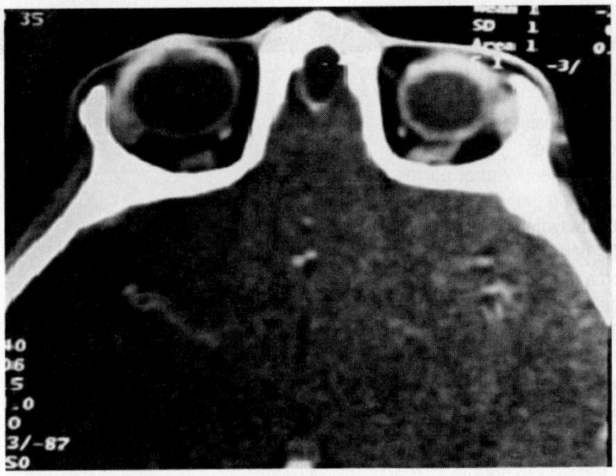

Figure 368-2 CT axial view showing nasal dermoid extension into the anterior cranial fossa through a defect in the cribriform plate. (From Meher R, Singh I, Aggarwal S: Nasal dermoid with intracranial extension, *J Postgrad Med* 51:39–40, 2005.)

PYRIFORM APERTURE STENOSIS

Infants with this bony abnormality of the anterior nasal aperture present with severe nasal obstruction at birth or shortly thereafter. Diagnosis is made by CT of the nose; surgical repair by means of an anterior, sublabial approach may be needed if the child cannot feed or breathe without difficulty. A drill is used to enlarge the stenotic anterior bone apertures.

CONGENITAL MIDLINE NASAL MASSES

Dermoids, gliomas, and *encephaloceles* (in descending order of frequency) occur intranasally or extranasally and can have intracranial connections. Nasal dermoids often have a dimple or pit on the nasal dorsum, sometimes with hair being present, and can predispose to intracranial infections if an intracranial fistula or sinus is present. Recurrent infection of the dermoid itself is more common. Gliomas or heterotopic brain tissue are firm, whereas encephaloceles are soft and enlarge with crying or the Valsalva maneuver. Diagnosis is based on physical examination findings and results from imaging studies. CT provides the best bony detail, but MRI allows sagittal views, which may be needed to further define intracranial extension (Fig. 368-2). Surgical excision of these masses is generally required, with the extent and surgical approach based on the type and size of the mass.

Other nasal masses include *hemangiomas, congenital nasolacrimal duct obstruction* (which can occur as an intranasal mass), nasal polyps, and tumors such as rhabdomyosarcoma (Chapter 494). Nasal polyps are rarely present at birth, but the other masses often present at birth or in early infancy (Chapter 370).

Poor development of the paranasal sinuses and a narrow nasal airway are associated with recurrent or chronic upper airway infection in Down syndrome (Chapter 76).

DIAGNOSIS AND TREATMENT

In children with congenital nasal disorders, supportive care of the airway is given until the diagnosis is established. Diagnosis is made through a combination of flexible scoping and imaging studies, primarily CT scan. In the case of surgically correctable congenital problems such as choanal atresia, surgery is performed once the child is deemed healthy and free of life-threatening problems such as congenital heart disease.

BIBLIOGRAPHY

Please visit the Nelson Textbook of Pediatrics *website at* *www.expertconsult.com* *for the complete bibliography.*

Chapter 369
Acquired Disorders of the Nose

Joseph Haddad, Jr.

Tumors, septal perforations, and other acquired abnormalities of the nose and paranasal sinuses can manifest with epistaxis. Midface trauma with a nasal or facial fracture may be accompanied by epistaxis. Trauma to the nose can cause a *septal hematoma;* if treatment is delayed, this can lead to necrosis of septal cartilage and a resultant *saddle-nose deformity.* Other abnormalities that can cause a change in the shape of the nose and paranasal bones, with obstruction but few other symptoms, include *fibro-osseus lesions* (ossifying fibroma, fibrous dysplasia, cementifying fibroma) and *mucoceles of the paranasal sinuses.* These conditions may be suspected on physical examination and confirmed by CT scan and biopsy. Although these are considered benign lesions, they can all greatly change the anatomy of surrounding bony structures and often require surgical intervention for management.

369.1 Foreign Body

Joseph Haddad, Jr.

ETIOLOGY

Foreign bodies (food, beads, crayons, small toys, erasers, paper wads, buttons, batteries, beans, stones, pieces of sponge, and other small objects) are often placed in the nose by small children and developmentally delayed children and constitute ≤1% of pediatric emergency department visits. Initial symptoms are unilateral obstruction, sneezing, relatively mild discomfort, and rarely pain. Presenting clinical symptoms include history of insertion of foreign bodies (86%), mucopurulent nasal discharge (24%), foul nasal odor (9%), epistaxis (6%), nasal obstruction (3%), and mouth breathing (2%). Irritation results in mucosal swelling because some foreign bodies are hygroscopic and increase in size as water is absorbed; signs of local obstruction and discomfort can increase with time. The patient might also present with a generalized body odor known as *bromhidrosis.*

DIAGNOSIS

Unilateral nasal discharge and obstruction should suggest the presence of a foreign body, which can often be seen on examination with a nasal speculum or wide otoscope placed in the nose. Purulent secretions may need to be cleared so that the foreign object can actually be seen; a headlight, suction, and topical decongestants are often needed. The object is usually situated anteriorly, but unskilled attempts at removal can force the object deeper into the nose. A long-standing foreign body can become embedded in granulation tissue or mucosa and appear as a nasal mass. A lateral skull radiograph assists in diagnosis if the foreign body is metallic or radiopaque.

TREATMENT

A quick examination of the nose is made to determine if a foreign body is present, and whether it needs to be removed emergently. Planning is then made for office or operating room extrication of the foreign body. Prompt removal minimizes the danger of aspiration and local tissue necrosis. This can usually be performed with topical anesthesia, using either forceps or nasal suction. If there is marked swelling, bleeding, or tissue overgrowth, general anesthesia may be needed to remove the object. Infection usually clears promptly after the removal of the object and, generally, no further therapy is necessary.

COMPLICATIONS

Infection often follows and gives rise to a purulent, malodorous, or bloody discharge. Local tissue damage from long-standing foreign body, or alkaline injury from a disk battery, can lead to local tissue loss and cartilage destruction. A synechia or scar band can then form, causing nasal obstruction. Loss of septal mucosa and cartilage can cause a septal perforation. Disk batteries are dangerous when placed in the nose; they leach base, which causes pain and local tissue destruction in a matter of hours.

Tetanus is a rare complication of long-standing nasal foreign bodies in nonimmunized children (Chapter 203). Toxic shock syndrome is also rare, and most commonly occurs from nasal surgical packing (Chapter 174.2); oral antibiotics should be administered when nasal surgical packing is placed.

PREVENTION

Tempting objects such as round, shiny beads should only be used under adult supervision. Disk batteries should be stored away from the reach of small children.

BIBLIOGRAPHY

Please visit the Nelson Textbook of Pediatrics *website at* *www.expertconsult.com* *for the complete bibliography.*

369.2 Epistaxis

Joseph Haddad, Jr.

Nosebleeds are rare in infancy and common in childhood. Their incidence decreases after puberty and rises again after age 50 yr. Diagnosis and treatment depend on the location and cause of the bleeding.

ANATOMY

The most common site of bleeding is the Kiesselbach plexus, an area in the anterior septum where vessels from both the internal carotid (anterior and posterior ethmoid arteries) and external carotid (sphenopalatine and terminal branches of the internal maxillary arteries) converge. The thin mucosa in this area, as well as the anterior location, makes it prone to exposure to dry air and trauma.

ETIOLOGY

Common causes of nosebleeds from the anterior septum include digital trauma, foreign bodies, dry air, and inflammation, including upper respiratory tract infections, sinusitis, and allergic rhinitis (Table 369-1). There is often a family history of childhood epistaxis. Nasal steroid sprays are commonly used in children, and their chronic use may be associated with bleeding. Young infants with significant gastroesophageal reflux into the nose rarely present with epistaxis secondary to mucosal inflammation. Susceptibility is increased during respiratory infections and in the winter when dry air irritates the nasal mucosa, resulting in formation of fissures and crusting. Severe bleeding may be encountered with congenital vascular abnormalities, such as *hereditary hemorrhagic telangiectasia* (Chapter 426.3), varicosities, hemangiomas, and, in children with thrombocytopenia, deficiency of clotting factors, particularly von Willebrand disease, hypertension, renal failure, or venous congestion. Nasal polyps or other intranasal growths may be associated with epistaxis. Recurrent, and often severe, nosebleeds may be the initial presenting symptom in **juvenile nasal angiofibromas,** which occur in adolescent boys.

Table 369-1 COMMON CAUSES OF EPISTAXIS
Epistaxis digitorum (nose picking)
Rhinitis
Chronic sinusitis
Foreign bodies
Intranasal neoplasm or polyps
Irritants (e.g., cigarette smoke)
Septal deviation
Septal perforation
Trauma including child abuse
Vascular malformation or telangiectasia
Hemophilia
Platelet dysfunction
Thrombocytopenia
Hypertension
Leukemia
Liver disease (e.g., cirrhosis)
Medications (e.g., aspirin, anticoagulants, nonsteroidal anti-inflammatory drugs, topical corticosteroids)
Cocaine abuse

From Kucik CJ, Clenney T: Management of epistaxis, *Am Fam Physician* 71(2):305–311, 2005.

CLINICAL MANIFESTATIONS

Epistaxis usually occurs without warning, with blood flowing slowly but freely from one nostril or occasionally from both. In children with nasal lesions, bleeding might follow physical exercise. When bleeding occurs at night, the blood may be swallowed and become apparent only when the child vomits or passes blood in the stools. Posterior epistaxis can manifest as anterior nasal bleeding or, if bleeding is copious, the patient might vomit blood as the initial symptom.

TREATMENT

Most nosebleeds stop spontaneously in a few minutes. The nares should be compressed and the child kept as quiet as possible, in an upright position with the head tilted forward to avoid blood trickling back into the throat. Cold compresses applied to the nose can also help. If these measures do not stop the bleeding, local application of a solution of oxymetazoline (Afrin or Neo-Synephrine) (0.25-1%) may be useful. If bleeding persists, an anterior nasal pack might need to be inserted; if bleeding originates in the posterior nasal cavity, combined anterior and posterior packing is necessary. After bleeding has been controlled, and if a bleeding site is identified, its obliteration by cautery with silver nitrate may prevent further difficulties. Because the septal cartilage derives its nutrition from the overlying mucoperichondrium, only 1 side of the septum should be cauterized at a time to reduce the chance of a septal perforation. During the winter, or in a dry environment, a room humidifier, saline drops, and petrolatum (Vaseline) applied to the septum can help to prevent epistaxis.

In patients with severe or repeated epistaxis, blood transfusions may be necessary. Otolaryngologic evaluation is indicated for these children and for those with bilateral bleeding or with hemorrhage that does not arise from the Kiesselbach plexus. Hematologic evaluation (for coagulopathy and anemia), along with nasal endoscopy and diagnostic imaging, may be needed to make a definitive diagnosis in cases of severe recurrent epistaxis. Replacement of deficient clotting factors may be required for patients who have an underlying hematologic disorder (Chapter 470). Profuse unilateral epistaxis associated with a nasal mass in an adolescent boy near puberty might signal a **juvenile nasopharyngeal angiofibroma.** This unusual tumor has also been reported in a 2 yr old and in 30-40 yr olds, but the incidence peaks in adolescent and preadolescent boys. CT with contrast medium enhancement and MRI are part of the initial evaluation; arteriography, embolization, and extensive surgery may be needed.

Surgical intervention may also be needed for bleeding from the internal maxillary artery or other vessels that can cause bleeding in the posterior nasal cavity.

PREVENTION

The discouragement of nose picking, and attention to proper humidification of the bedroom during dry winter months helps to prevent many nosebleeds. Prompt attention to nasal infections and allergies is beneficial to nasal hygiene. Prompt cessation of nasal steroid sprays prevents ongoing bleeding.

BIBLIOGRAPHY
Please visit the Nelson Textbook of Pediatrics *website at www.expertconsult.com for the complete bibliography.*

Chapter 370
Nasal Polyps

Joseph Haddad, Jr.

ETIOLOGY

Nasal polyps are benign pedunculated tumors formed from edematous, usually chronically inflamed nasal mucosa. They commonly arise from the ethmoidal sinus and occur in the middle meatus. Occasionally, they appear within the maxillary antrum and can extend to the nasopharynx (antrochoanal polyp).

It is estimated that between 0.2% and 1% of the population will develop nasal polyps at some time; the incidence of nasal polyps increases with age. Antrochoanal polyps represent only 4-6% of all nasal polyps in the general population but account for approximately one third of polyps in the pediatric population. Large or multiple polyps can completely obstruct the nasal passage. The polyps originating from the ethmoidal sinus are usually smaller and multiple, as compared with the large and usually single antrochoanal polyp.

Cystic fibrosis is the most common childhood cause of nasal polyposis and should be suspected in any child <12 yr old with nasal polyps, even in the absence of typical respiratory and digestive symptoms; as many as 30% of children with cystic fibrosis acquire nasal polyps (Chapter 395). Nasal polyposis is also associated with chronic sinusitis and allergic rhinitis. In the uncommon Samter triad, nasal polyps are associated with aspirin sensitivity and asthma.

CLINICAL MANIFESTATIONS

Obstruction of nasal passages is prominent, with associated hyponasal speech and mouth breathing. Profuse unilateral mucoid or mucopurulent rhinorrhea may also be present. An examination of the nasal passages shows glistening, gray, grapelike masses squeezed between the nasal turbinates and the septum.

DIAGNOSIS AND DIFFERENTIAL DIAGNOSIS

Examination of the external nose and rhinoscopy is performed. Ethmoidal polyps can be readily distinguished from the well-vascularized turbinate tissue, which is pink or red; antrochoanal polyps may have a more fleshy appearance (Fig. 370-1). Antrochoanal polyps may prolapse into the nasopharynx; flexible nasopharyngoscopy can assist in making this diagnosis. Prolonged presence of ethmoidal polyps in a child can widen the bridge of the nose and erode adjacent osseous structures. Tumors of the nose cause more local destruction and distortion of the anatomy. CT scan of the midface is key to diagnosis and planning for surgical treatment (Fig. 370-2).

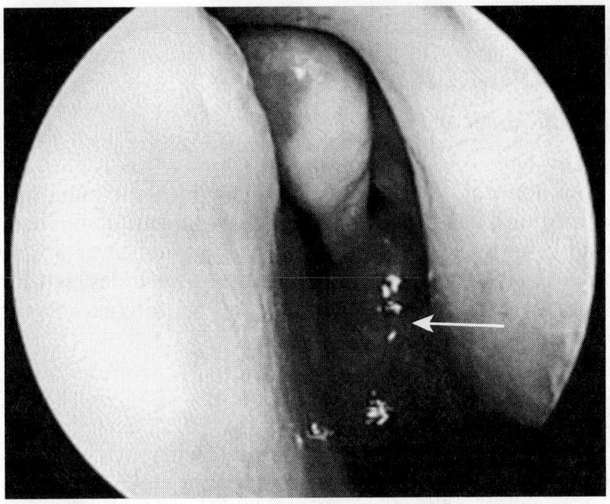

Figure 370-1 Antrochoanal polyp viewed endoscopically *(arrow).* (From Basak S, Karaman CZ, Akdilli A, et al: Surgical approaches to antro-choanal polyps in children, *Int J Pediatr Otorhinolaryngol* 46:197–205, 1998.)

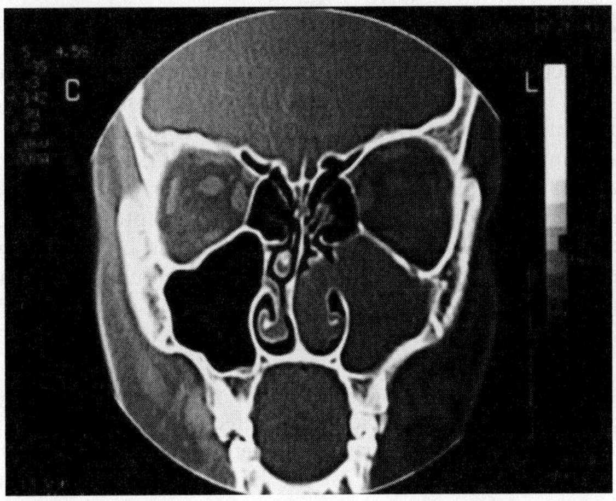

Figure 370-2 A typical CT image of an isolated antrochoanal polyp on the left side. (From Basak S, Karaman CZ, Akdilli A, et al: Surgical approaches to antrochoanal polyps in children, *Int J Pediatr Otorhinolaryngol* 46:197–205, 1998.)

TREATMENT

Local or systemic decongestants are not usually effective in shrinking the polyps, although they may provide symptomatic relief from the associated mucosal edema. Intranasal steroid sprays, and sometimes systemic steroids, can provide some shrinkage of nasal polyps with symptomatic relief and have proved useful in children with cystic fibrosis and adults with nasal polyps. Polyps should be removed surgically if complete obstruction, uncontrolled rhinorrhea, or deformity of the nose appears. If the underlying pathogenic mechanism cannot be eliminated (cystic fibrosis), the polyps may soon return. Functional endoscopic sinus surgery provides more complete polyp removal and treatment of other associated nasal disease; in some cases, this has reduced the need for frequent surgeries. Nasal steroid sprays should also be started preventively, once postsurgical healing occurs.

Antrochoanal polyps do not respond to medical measures and must be removed surgically. Because these types of polyps are not associated with any underlying disease process, the recurrence rate is much less than for other types of polyps.

BIBLIOGRAPHY
Please visit the Nelson Textbook of Pediatrics *website at www.expertconsult.com for the complete bibliography.*

Chapter 371
The Common Cold
Ronald B. Turner and Gregory F. Hayden

The common cold is a viral illness in which the symptoms of rhinorrhea and nasal obstruction are prominent; systemic symptoms and signs such as headache, myalgia, and fever are absent or mild. It is often termed *rhinitis* but includes self-limited involvement of the sinus mucosa and is more correctly termed *rhinosinusitis*.

ETIOLOGY

The most common pathogens associated with the common cold are the rhinoviruses (Chapter 255), but the syndrome can be caused by many different viruses (Table 371-1). The role of bocavirus as a cause of colds is uncertain because the virus is often isolated from patients who are co-infected with other recognized pathogens.

EPIDEMIOLOGY

Colds occur year-round, but the incidence is greatest from the early fall until the late spring, reflecting the seasonal prevalence of the viral pathogens associated with cold symptoms. The highest incidence of rhinovirus infection occurs in the early fall (August-October) and in the late spring (April-May). The seasonal incidence for parainfluenza viruses (Chapter 251) usually peaks in the late fall and late spring and is highest between December and April for respiratory syncytial virus (RSV; Chapter 252) and influenza viruses (Chapter 250).

Young children have an average of 6-8 colds per year, but 10-15% of children have at least 12 infections per year. The incidence of illness decreases with age, with 2 to 3 illnesses per year by adulthood. The incidence of infection is primarily a function of exposure to the virus. Children in out-of-home daycare centers during the 1st year of life have 50% more colds than children cared for only at home. The difference in the incidence of illness between these groups of children decreases as the length of time spent in daycare increases, although the incidence of illness remains higher in the daycare group through at least the 1st 3 yr of life. Mannose-binding lectin deficiency with impaired innate immunity may be associated with an increased incidence of colds in children.

PATHOGENESIS

Viruses that cause the common cold are spread by small-particle aerosols, large-particle aerosols, and direct contact. Although the different common cold pathogens can presumably be spread by any of these mechanisms, some routes of transmission appear to be more efficient than others for particular viruses. Studies of rhinoviruses and RSV suggest that direct contact is an efficient mechanism of transmission of these viruses, although transmission by large-particle aerosols can also occur. In contrast to rhinoviruses and RSV, influenza viruses appear to be most efficiently spread by small-particle aerosols.

Table 371-1 PATHOGENS ASSOCIATED WITH THE COMMON COLD

ASSOCIATION	PATHOGEN	RELATIVE FREQUENCY*
Agents primarily associated with colds	Rhinoviruses	Frequent
	Coronaviruses	Occasional
Agents primarily associated with other clinical syndromes that also cause common cold symptoms	Respiratory syncytial viruses	Occasional
	Human metapneumovirus	Occasional
	Influenza viruses	Uncommon
	Parainfluenza viruses	Uncommon
	Adenoviruses	Uncommon
	Enteroviruses	Uncommon
	Bocavirus	Uncommon

*Relative frequency of colds caused by the agent.

The respiratory viruses have evolved different mechanisms to avoid host defenses. Infections with rhinoviruses and adenoviruses result in the development of serotype-specific protective immunity. Repeated infections with these pathogens occur because there are a large number of distinct serotypes of each virus. Influenza viruses have the ability to change the antigens presented on the surface of the virus and thus behave as though there were multiple viral serotypes. The interaction of coronaviruses (Chapter 256) with host immunity is not well defined, but it appears that multiple distinct strains of coronaviruses are capable of inducing at least short-term protective immunity. The parainfluenza viruses and RSV each have a small number of distinct serotypes. Reinfection with these viruses occurs because protective immunity to these pathogens does not develop after an infection. Although reinfection is not prevented by the adaptive host response to these viruses, the severity of subsequent illness is moderated by pre-existing immunity.

Viral infection of the nasal epithelium can be associated with destruction of the epithelial lining, as with influenza viruses and adenoviruses, or there can be no apparent histologic damage, as with rhinoviruses and RSV. Regardless of the histopathologic findings, infection of the nasal epithelium is associated with an acute inflammatory response characterized by release of a variety of inflammatory cytokines and infiltration of the mucosa by inflammatory cells. This acute inflammatory response appears to be responsible, at least in part, for many of the symptoms associated with the common cold. Inflammation can obstruct the sinus ostium or eustachian tube and predispose to bacterial sinusitis or otitis media.

CLINICAL MANIFESTATIONS

The onset of common cold symptoms typically occurs 1-3 days after viral infection. The 1st symptom noted is often sore or scratchy throat, followed closely by nasal obstruction and rhinorrhea. The sore throat usually resolves quickly and, by the 2nd and 3rd day of illness, nasal symptoms predominate. Cough is associated with ~30% of colds and usually begins after the onset of nasal symptoms. Influenza viruses, RSV, and adenoviruses are more likely than rhinoviruses or coronaviruses to be associated with fever and other constitutional symptoms. The usual cold persists for about 1 wk, although 10% last for 2 wk.

The physical findings of the common cold are limited to the upper respiratory tract. Increased nasal secretion is usually obvious; a change in the color or consistency of the secretions is common during the course of the illness and does not indicate sinusitis or bacterial superinfection. Examination of the nasal cavity might reveal swollen, erythematous nasal turbinates, although this finding is nonspecific and of limited diagnostic value.

DIAGNOSIS

The most important task of the physician caring for a patient with a cold is to exclude other conditions that are potentially more serious or treatable. The differential diagnosis of the common cold includes noninfectious disorders as well as other upper respiratory tract infections (Table 371-2).

Table 371-2 CONDITIONS THAT CAN MIMIC THE COMMON COLD

CONDITION	DIFFERENTIATING FEATURES
Allergic rhinitis	Prominent itching and sneezing Nasal eosinophils
Foreign body	Unilateral, foul-smelling secretions Bloody nasal secretions
Sinusitis	Presence of fever, headache or facial pain, or periorbital edema or persistence of rhinorrhea or cough for >14 days
Streptococcosis	Mucopurulent nasal discharge that excoriates the nares
Pertussis	Onset of persistent or severe cough
Congenital syphilis	Persistent rhinorrhea with onset in the 1st 3 mo of life

LABORATORY FINDINGS

Routine laboratory studies are not helpful for the diagnosis and management of the common cold. A nasal smear for eosinophils may be useful if allergic rhinitis is suspected (Chapter 137). A predominance of polymorphonuclear leukocytes in the nasal secretions is characteristic of uncomplicated colds and does not indicate bacterial superinfection.

The viral pathogens associated with the common cold can be detected by polymerase chain reaction (PCR), culture, antigen detection, or serologic methods. These studies are generally not indicated in patients with colds because a specific etiologic diagnosis is useful only when treatment with an antiviral agent is contemplated. Bacterial cultures or antigen detection are useful only when group A streptococcus (Chapter 176), *Bordetella pertussis* (Chapter 189), or nasal diphtheria (Chapter 180) is suspected. The isolation of other bacterial pathogens is not an indication of bacterial nasal infection and is not a specific predictor of the etiologic agent in sinusitis.

TREATMENT

The management of the common cold consists primarily of symptomatic treatment.

Antiviral Treatment

Specific antiviral therapy is not available for rhinovirus infections. Ribavirin, which is approved for treatment of RSV infections, has no role in the treatment of the common cold. The neuraminidase inhibitors oseltamivir and zanamivir have a modest effect on the duration of symptoms associated with influenza viral infections in children. Oseltamivir also reduces the frequency of influenza-associated otitis media. The difficulty of distinguishing influenza from other common cold pathogens and the necessity that therapy be started early in the illness (within 48 hr of onset of symptoms) to be beneficial are practical limitations to the use of these agents for mild upper respiratory tract infections. Antibacterial therapy is of no benefit in the treatment of the common cold.

Symptomatic Treatment

The use of symptomatic therapies in children is controversial; although some of these medications are effective in adults, no studies have demonstrated a significant effect in children. Young children cannot assist in the assessment of symptom severity, so studies of these treatments in children have generally been based on observations by parents or other observers, a method that is likely to be insensitive for detection of treatment effects. The use of symptomatic oral over-the-counter (OTC) therapies (often containing antihistamines, antitussives, and decongestants) in children can only be based on an assumption that the effects of symptomatic treatments may be similar in adults and children. As a result of the lack of direct evidence for effectiveness and the potential for unwanted side effects, the FDA recommends that OTC cough and cold products not be used for infants and children <2 yr of age. Further studies have shown that OTC cough and cold products are ineffective in treating symptoms of children <6 yr of age. A decision whether to use these medications in older children must balance the likelihood of clinical benefit against the potential adverse effects of these drugs. The prominent or most bothersome symptoms of colds vary in the course of the illness and, therefore, if symptomatic treatments are used, it is reasonable to target therapy to specific bothersome symptoms. If symptomatic treatments are recommended, care should be taken to ensure that caregivers understand the intended effect and can determine the proper dosage of the medications.

FEVER Fever is not usually associated with an uncomplicated common cold, and antipyretic treatment is generally not indicated.

NASAL OBSTRUCTION Either topical or oral adrenergic agents can be used as nasal decongestants. Effective topical adrenergic agents such as xylometazoline, oxymetazoline, or phenylephrine are available as either intranasal drops or nasal sprays. Reduced-strength formulations of these medications are available for use in younger children, although they are not approved for use in children <2 yr old. Systemic absorption of the imidazolines (oxymetazoline, xylometazoline) has very rarely been associated with bradycardia, hypotension, and coma. Prolonged use of the topical adrenergic agents should be avoided to prevent the development of **rhinitis medicamentosa,** an apparent rebound effect that causes the sensation of nasal obstruction when the drug is discontinued. The oral adrenergic agents are less effective than the topical preparations and are occasionally associated with systemic effects such as central nervous system stimulation, hypertension, and palpitations. Saline nose drops (wash, irrigation) can improve nasal symptoms.

RHINORRHEA The first-generation antihistamines reduce rhinorrhea by 25-30%. The effect of the antihistamines on rhinorrhea appears to be related to the anticholinergic rather than the antihistaminic properties of these drugs, and therefore the second-generation or "nonsedating" antihistamines have no effect on common cold symptoms. The major adverse effect associated with the use of the antihistamines is sedation, although there is some evidence that this adverse effect is less bothersome in children than in adults. Rhinorrhea may also be treated with ipratropium bromide, a topical anticholinergic agent. This drug produces an effect comparable to the antihistamines but is not associated with sedation. The most common side effects of ipratropium are nasal irritation and bleeding.

SORE THROAT The sore throat associated with colds is generally not severe, but treatment with mild analgesics is occasionally indicated, particularly if there is associated myalgia or headache. The use of acetaminophen during rhinovirus infection has been associated with suppression of neutralizing antibody responses, but this observation has no apparent clinical significance. Aspirin should not be given to children with respiratory infections because of the risk of Reye syndrome in children with influenza (Chapter 591).

COUGH Cough suppression is generally not necessary in patients with colds. Cough in some patients appears to be due to upper respiratory tract irritation associated with postnasal drip. Cough in these patients is most prominent during the time of greatest nasal symptoms, and treatment with a first-generation antihistamine may be helpful. Sugar-containing cough drops or honey as a demulcent may be temporarily effective. In other patients, cough may be a result of virus-induced reactive airways disease. These patients can have cough that persists for days to weeks after the acute illness and might benefit from bronchodilator therapy. Codeine or dextromethorphan hydrobromide has no effect on cough from colds. Expectorants such as guaifenesin are not effective antitussive agents. The combination of camphor, menthol, and eucalyptus oils may relieve nocturnal cough.

Ineffective Treatments

Vitamin C, guaifenesin, and inhalation of warm, humidified air are no more effective than placebo for the treatment of cold symptoms.

Zinc, given as oral lozenges, has been evaluated in several studies as a treatment for common cold symptoms. The function of the rhinovirus 3C protease, an essential enzyme for rhinovirus replication, is inhibited by zinc, but there has been no evidence of an antiviral effect of zinc in vivo. The effect of zinc on symptoms has been inconsistent, with some studies reporting dramatic treatment effects (in adults), whereas other studies find no benefit. A synthesis of these disparate results is difficult, but it appears unlikely that zinc has a clinically significant impact on common cold symptoms in children.

Echinacea is a popular herbal treatment for the common cold. Although echinacea extracts have been shown to have biologic effects, echinacea is not effective as a common cold treatment. The lack of standardization of commercial products containing echinacea also presents a formidable obstacle to the rational evaluation or use of this therapy.

COMPLICATIONS

The most common complication of a cold is **otitis media** (Chapter 632), which is reported in 5-30% of children who have a cold, with the higher incidence occurring in children cared for in a group daycare setting. Symptomatic treatment has no effect on the development of acute otitis media, but treatment with oseltamivir might reduce the incidence of otitis media in patients with influenza.

Sinusitis is another complication of the common cold (Chapter 372). Self-limited sinus inflammation is a part of the pathophysiology of the common cold, but 0.5-2% of viral upper respiratory tract infections in adults, and 5-13% in children, are complicated by acute bacterial sinusitis. The differentiation of common cold symptoms from bacterial sinusitis may be difficult. The diagnosis of bacterial sinusitis should be considered if rhinorrhea or daytime cough persists without improvement for at least 10-14 days or if signs of more-severe sinus involvement such as fever, facial pain, or facial swelling develop. There is no evidence that symptomatic treatment of the common cold alters the frequency of development of bacterial sinusitis.

Exacerbation of **asthma** is a relatively uncommon but potentially serious complication of colds. The majority of asthma exacerbations in children are associated with the common cold. There is no evidence that treatment of common cold symptoms prevents this complication.

Although not a complication, another important consequence of the common cold is the inappropriate use of antibiotics for these illnesses and the associated contribution to the problem of increasing antibiotic resistance of pathogenic respiratory bacteria. In 1998 in the USA, there were an estimated 25 million primary care office visits for the common cold, with 30% of these visits resulting in an inappropriate prescription for antibiotics.

PREVENTION

Chemoprophylaxis or immunoprophylaxis is generally not available for the common cold. Immunization or chemoprophylaxis against influenza can prevent colds caused by this pathogen; influenza is responsible for only a small proportion of all colds. Vitamin C and echinacea do not prevent the common cold.

Hand-to-hand transmission of rhinoviruses followed by self-inoculation can theoretically be blocked by virucidal agents. In the experimental setting, virucidal tissues prevent the contamination of hands with virus during nose-blowing, and hand sanitizers can remove infectious virus from the hands. Under natural conditions, however, neither of these interventions prevents common colds. Handwashing is commonly recommended for prevention of colds, but convincing data for effectiveness are not available.

BIBLIOGRAPHY

Please visit the Nelson Textbook of Pediatrics *website at www.expertconsult.com for the complete bibliography.*

Chapter 372
Sinusitis

Diane E. Pappas and J. Owen Hendley

Sinusitis is a common illness of childhood and adolescence with significant acute and chronic morbidity as well as the potential for serious complications. There are 2 types of acute sinusitis: viral and bacterial. The common cold produces a viral, self-limited rhinosinusitis (Chapter 371). Approximately 0.5-2% of viral upper respiratory tract infections in children and adolescents are complicated by acute bacterial sinusitis. Some children with underlying predisposing conditions have chronic sinus disease that does not appear to be infectious. The means for appropriate diagnosis and optimal treatment of sinusitis remain controversial.

Both the **ethmoidal** and **maxillary** sinuses are present at birth, but only the ethmoidal sinuses are pneumatized (Fig. 372-1). The maxillary sinuses are not pneumatized until 4 yr of age. The **sphenoidal** sinuses are present by 5 yr of age, whereas the **frontal sinuses** begin development at age 7-8 yr and are not completely developed until adolescence. The ostia draining the sinuses are narrow (1-3 mm) and drain into the ostiomeatal complex in the middle meatus. The **paranasal sinuses** are normally sterile, maintained by the mucociliary clearance system.

ETIOLOGY

The bacterial pathogens causing acute bacterial sinusitis in children and adolescents include *Streptococcus pneumoniae* (~30%; Chapter 176), nontypable *Haemophilus influenzae* (~20%; Chapter 186), and *Moraxella catarrhalis* (~20%; Chapter 188). Approximately 50% of *H. influenzae* and 100% of *M. catarrhalis* are β-lactamase positive. About 25% of *S. pneumoniae* may be penicillin resistant. *Staphylococcus aureus*, other streptococci, and anaerobes are uncommon causes of acute bacterial sinusitis in children. Although *Staphylococcus aureus* is an uncommon

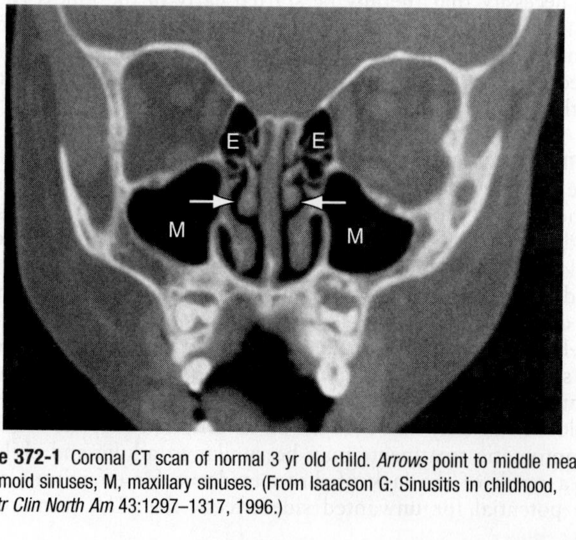

Figure 372-1 Coronal CT scan of normal 3 yr old child. *Arrows* point to middle meatus. E, ethmoid sinuses; M, maxillary sinuses. (From Isaacson G: Sinusitis in childhood, *Pediatr Clin North Am* 43:1297–1317, 1996.)

pathogen for acute sinusitis in children, the increasing prevalence of methicillin-resistant *Staphylococcus aureus* (MRSA) is a significant concern. *H. influenzae,* α- and β-hemolytic streptococci, *M. catarrhalis, S. pneumoniae,* and coagulase-negative staphylococci are commonly recovered from children with **chronic sinus disease.**

EPIDEMIOLOGY

Acute bacterial sinusitis can occur at any age. Predisposing conditions include viral upper respiratory tract infections (associated with out-of-home daycare or a school-aged sibling), allergic rhinitis, and cigarette smoke exposure. Children with immune deficiencies particularly of antibody production (immunoglobulin G [IgG], IgG subclasses, IgA) (Chapter 118), cystic fibrosis (Chapter 395), ciliary dysfunction (Chapter 396), abnormalities of phagocyte function, gastroesophageal reflux, anatomic defects (cleft palate), nasal polyps, cocaine abuse, and nasal foreign bodies (including nasogastric tubes) can develop chronic sinus disease. Immunosuppression for bone marrow transplantation or malignancy with profound neutropenia and lymphopenia predisposes to severe fungal (aspergillus, mucor) sinusitis, often with intracranial extension. Patients with nasotracheal intubation or nasogastric tubes may have obstruction of the sinus ostia and develop sinusitis with the multiple-drug resistant organisms of the intensive care unit (ICU).

PATHOGENESIS

Acute bacterial sinusitis typically follows a viral upper respiratory tract infection. Initially, the viral infection produces a viral rhinosinusitis; MRI evaluation of the paranasal sinuses demonstrates major abnormalities (mucosal thickening, edema, inflammation) of the paranasal sinuses in 68% of healthy children in the normal course of the common cold. Nose blowing has been demonstrated to generate sufficient force to propel nasal secretions into the sinus cavities. Bacteria from the nasopharynx that enter the sinuses are normally cleared readily, but during viral rhinosinusitis, inflammation and edema can block sinus drainage and impair mucociliary clearance of bacteria. The growth conditions are favorable, and high titers of bacteria are produced.

CLINICAL MANIFESTATIONS

Children and adolescents with sinusitis can present with nonspecific complaints, including nasal congestion, purulent nasal discharge (unilateral or bilateral), fever, and cough. Less-common symptoms include bad breath (halitosis), a decreased sense of smell (hyposmia), and periorbital edema. Complaints of headache and facial pain are rare in children. Additional symptoms include maxillary tooth discomfort and pain or pressure exacerbated by bending forward. Physical examination might reveal erythema and swelling of the nasal mucosa with purulent nasal discharge. Sinus tenderness may be detectable in adolescents and adults. Transillumination reveals an opaque sinus that transmits light poorly.

DIAGNOSIS

The clinical diagnosis of acute bacterial sinusitis is based on history. Persistent symptoms of upper respiratory tract infection, including nasal discharge and cough, for >10-14 days without improvement, or severe respiratory symptoms, including temperature of at least 102°F (39°C) and purulent nasal discharge for 3-4 consecutive days, suggest a complicating acute bacterial sinusitis. Bacteria are recovered from maxillary sinus aspirates in 70% of children with such persistent or severe symptoms studied. Children with chronic sinusitis have a history of persistent respiratory symptoms, including cough, nasal discharge, or nasal congestion, lasting >90 days.

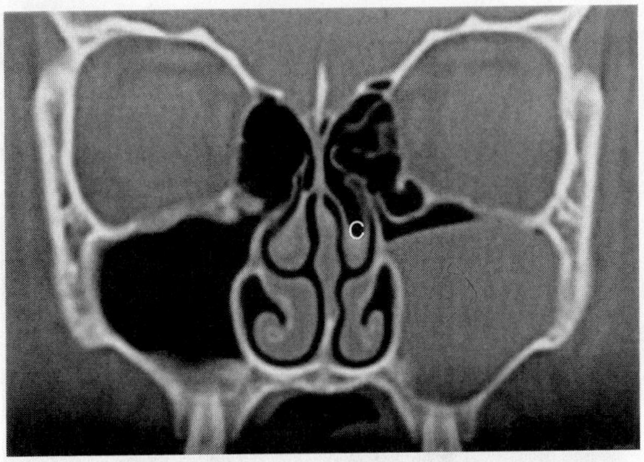

Figure 372-2 Acute left maxillary sinusitis with an air-fluid level. Note concha bullosa *(C).* (From Isaacson G: Sinusitis in childhood, *Pediatr Clin North Am* 43:1297–1317, 1996.)

Sinus aspirate culture is the only accurate method of diagnosis but is not practical for routine use for immunocompetent patients. It may be a necessary procedure for immunosuppressed patients with suspected fungal sinusitis. In adults, *rigid nasal endoscopy* is a less-invasive method for obtaining culture material from the sinus but detects a great excess of positive cultures compared to aspirates. *Transillumination* of the sinus cavities can demonstrate the presence of fluid but cannot reveal whether it is viral or bacterial in origin. In children, transillumination is difficult to perform and is unreliable. Findings on radiographic studies (sinus plain films, CT scans) including opacification, mucosal thickening, or presence of an air-fluid level are not totally diagnostic (Fig. 372-2). Such findings can confirm the presence of sinus inflammation but cannot be used to differentiate among viral, bacterial, or allergic causes of inflammation.

Given the nonspecific clinical picture, differential diagnostic considerations include viral upper respiratory tract infection, allergic rhinitis, nonallergic rhinitis, and nasal foreign body. Viral upper respiratory tract infections are characterized by clear and usually nonpurulent nasal discharge, cough, and initial fever; symptoms do not usually persist beyond 10-14 days, although a few children (10%) have persistent symptoms even at 14 days. Allergic rhinitis can be seasonal; evaluation of nasal secretions should reveal significant eosinophilia.

TREATMENT

It is unclear whether antimicrobial treatment of clinically diagnosed acute bacterial sinusitis offers any substantial benefit. A randomized, placebo-controlled trial comparing 14-day treatment of children with clinically diagnosed sinusitis with amoxicillin, amoxicillin-clavulanate, or placebo found that antimicrobial therapy did not affect resolution of symptoms, duration of symptoms, or days missed from school. Guidelines from the American Academy of Pediatrics recommend antimicrobial treatment for acute bacterial sinusitis to promote resolution of symptoms and prevent suppurative complications, although 50-60% of children with acute bacterial sinusitis recover without antimicrobial therapy.

Initial therapy with amoxicillin (45 mg/kg/day) is adequate for the majority of children with uncomplicated acute bacterial sinusitis. Alternative treatments for the penicillin-allergic patient include trimethoprim-sulfamethoxazole, cefuroxime axetil, cefpodoxime, clarithromycin, or azithromycin. For children with risk factors (antibiotic treatment in the preceding 1-3 mo, daycare attendance, or age <2 yr) for the presence of resistant bacterial species, and for children who fail to respond to initial therapy with amoxicillin within 72 hr, treatment with high-dose amoxicillin-clavulanate (80-90 mg/kg/day of amoxicillin) should

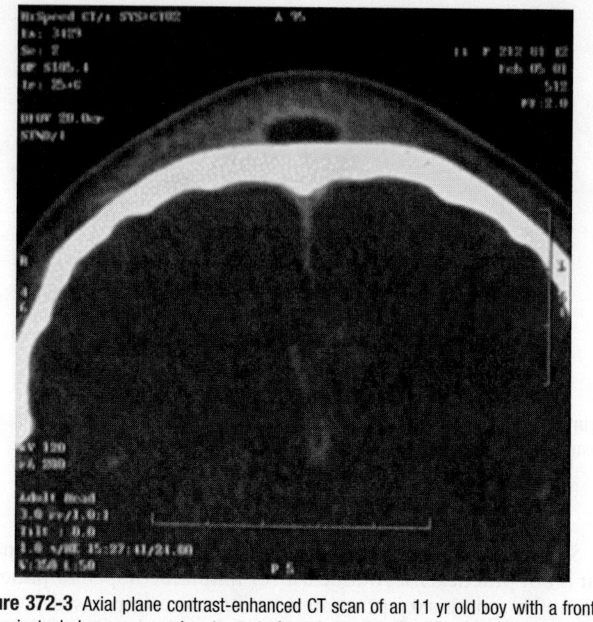

Figure 372-3 Axial plane contrast-enhanced CT scan of an 11 yr old boy with a frontal subperiosteal abscess secondary to acute frontal sinusitis. The CT scan demonstrates a ring-enhancing midline fluid density over the frontal bone. (From Parikh SR, Brown SM: Image-guided frontal sinus surgery in children, *Operative Tech Otolaryngol Head Neck Surg* 15:37–41, 2004.)

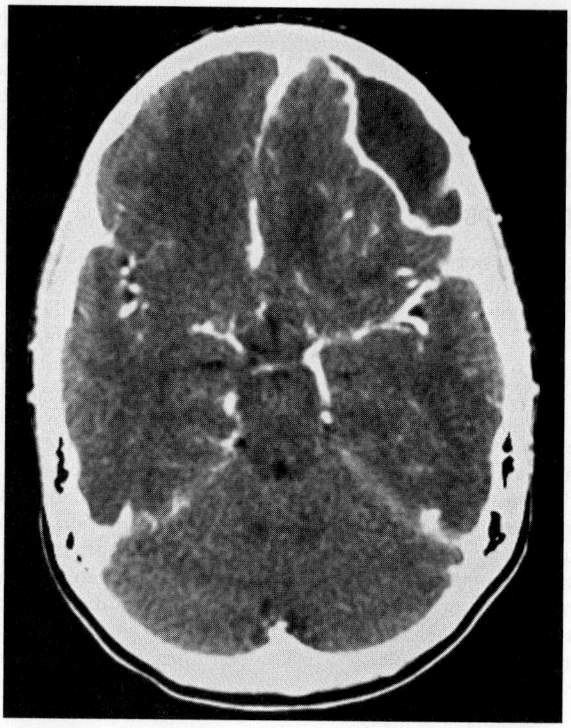

Figure 372-4 Axial plane contrast-enhanced CT scan of an 11 yr old obtunded girl with a subfrontal lobe abscess secondary to frontal sinusitis. The CT scan demonstrates an eliptiform ring-enhancing fluid-filled cavity adjacent to the frontal lobe with contralateral shift of the midline. (From Parikh SR, Brown SM: Image-guided frontal sinus surgery in children, *Operative Tech Otolaryngol Head Neck Surg* 15:37–41, 2004.)

be initiated. Azithromycin (or in older children, levofloxacin) is an alternative antibiotic. Failure to respond to this regimen necessitates referral to an otolaryngologist for further evaluation because maxillary sinus aspiration for culture and susceptibility testing may be necessary. The appropriate duration of therapy for sinusitis has yet to be determined; individualization of therapy is a reasonable approach, with treatment recommended for 7 days after resolution of symptoms.

Frontal sinusitis can rapidly progress to serious intracranial complications and necessitates initiation of parenteral ceftriaxone until substantial clinical improvement is achieved (Figs. 372-3 and 372-4). Treatment is then completed with oral antibiotic therapy.

The use of decongestants, antihistamines, mucolytics, and intranasal corticosteroids has not been adequately studied in children and is not recommended for the treatment of acute uncomplicated bacterial sinusitis. Likewise, saline nasal washes or nasal sprays can help to liquefy secretions and act as a mild vasoconstrictor, but the effects have not been systematically evaluated in children.

COMPLICATIONS

Because of the close proximity of the paranasal sinuses to the brain and eyes, serious orbital and/or intracranial complications can result from acute bacterial sinusitis and progress rapidly. Orbital complications, including *periorbital cellulitis* and *orbital cellulitis* (Chapter 626) are most often secondary to acute bacterial ethmoiditis. Infection can spread directly through the lamina papyracea, the thin bone that forms the lateral wall of the ethmoidal sinus. Periorbital cellulitis produces erythema and swelling of the tissues surrounding the globe, whereas orbital cellulitis involves the intraorbital structures and produces proptosis, chemosis, decreased visual acuity, double vision and impaired extraocular movements, and eye pain. Evaluation should include CT scan of the orbits and sinuses with ophthalmology and otolaryngology consultations. Treatment with intravenous antibiotics should be initiated. Orbital cellulitis can require surgical drainage of the ethmoidal sinuses.

Intracranial complications can include epidural abscess, meningitis, cavernous sinus thrombosis, subdural empyema, and brain abscess (Chapter 595). Children with altered mental status, nuchal rigidity, or signs of increased intracranial pressure (headache, vomiting) require immediate CT scan of the brain, orbits, and sinuses to evaluate for the presence of intracranial complications of acute bacterial sinusitis. Treatment with broad-spectrum intravenous antibiotics (usually cefotaxime or ceftriaxone combined with vancomycin) should be initiated immediately, pending culture and susceptibility results. In 50% the abscess is a polymicrobial infection. Abscesses can require surgical drainage. Other complications include osteomyelitis of the frontal bone (**Pott puffy tumor**), which is characterized by edema and swelling of the forehead (see Fig. 372-3), and **mucoceles,** which are chronic inflammatory lesions commonly located in the frontal sinuses that can expand, causing displacement of the eye with resultant diplopia. Surgical drainage is usually required.

PREVENTION

Prevention is best accomplished by frequent handwashing and avoiding persons with colds. Because acute bacterial sinusitis can complicate influenza infection, prevention of influenza infection by yearly influenza vaccine will prevent some cases of complicating sinusitis. Immunization or chemoprophylaxis against influenza with oseltamivir or zanamivir may be useful for prevention of colds caused by this pathogen and the associated complications; influenza is responsible for only a small proportion of all colds.

BIBLIOGRAPHY

Please visit the Nelson Textbook of Pediatrics *website at* *www.expertconsult.com* *for the complete bibliography.*

Chapter 373
Acute Pharyngitis

Gregory F. Hayden and Ronald B. Turner

Upper respiratory tract infections account for a substantial portion of visits to pediatricians. Approximately 30% of such illnesses feature a sore throat as the primary symptom.

ETIOLOGY

The most important agents causing pharyngitis are viruses, (adenoviruses, coronaviruses, enteroviruses, rhinoviruses, respiratory syncytial virus [RSV], Epstein-Barr virus [EBV], herpes simplex virus [HSV], metapneumovirus) and group A β-hemolytic streptococcus (GABHS; Chapter 176). Other organisms sometimes associated with pharyngitis include group C streptococcus (especially *Streptococcus equisimilis*), *Arcanobacterium haemolyticum, Francisella tularensis, Mycoplasma pneumoniae, Neisseria gonorrhoeae, Fusobacterium necrophorum*, and *Corynebacterium diphtheriae.* Other bacteria, such as *Haemophilus influenzae* and *Streptococcus pneumoniae,* may be cultured from the throats of children with pharyngitis, but their role in causing pharyngitis has not been established. Primary infection with HIV can also manifest with pharyngitis and a mononucleosis-like syndrome.

EPIDEMIOLOGY

Viral upper respiratory tract infections are spread by close contact and occur most commonly in fall, winter, and spring. Streptococcal pharyngitis is relatively uncommon before 2-3 yr of age, has a peak incidence in the early school years, and declines in late adolescence and adulthood. Illness occurs most often in winter and spring and spreads among siblings and classmates. Pharyngitis from group C streptococcus and *Arcanobacterium haemolyticum* occurs most commonly among adolescents and adults.

PATHOGENESIS

Colonization of the pharynx by GABHS can result in either asymptomatic carriage or acute infection. The M protein is the major virulence factor of GABHS and facilitates resistance to phagocytosis by polymorphonuclear neutrophils. Type-specific immunity develops following most infections and provides protective immunity to subsequent infection with that particular M serotype.

Scarlet fever is caused by GABHS that produces 1 of 3 streptococcal erythrogenic exotoxins (A, B, and C) that can induce a fine papular rash (Chapter 176). Exotoxin A appears to be most strongly associated with scarlet fever. Exposure to each exotoxin confers specific immunity only to that toxin and, therefore, scarlet fever can occur up to 3 times.

Clinical Manifestations

The onset of streptococcal pharyngitis is often rapid, with prominent sore throat and fever in the absence of cough. Headache and gastrointestinal symptoms (abdominal pain, vomiting) are common. The pharynx is red, and the tonsils are enlarged and classically covered with a yellow, blood-tinged exudate. There may be petechiae or "doughnut" lesions on the soft palate and posterior pharynx, and the uvula may be red, stippled, and swollen. The anterior cervical lymph nodes are enlarged and tender. The incubation period is 2-5 days. Some patients demonstrate the additional stigmata of scarlet fever: circumoral pallor, strawberry tongue, and a red, finely papular rash that feels like sandpaper and resembles sunburn with goose pimples (Chapter 176).

The onset of viral pharyngitis may be more gradual, and symptoms more often include rhinorrhea, cough, and diarrhea. A viral etiology is suggested by the presence of conjunctivitis, coryza, hoarseness, and cough. Adenovirus pharyngitis can feature concurrent conjunctivitis and fever (pharyngoconjunctival fever; Chapter 254). Coxsackievirus pharyngitis can produce small (1-2 mm) grayish vesicles and punched-out ulcers in the posterior pharynx (herpangina), or small (3-6 mm) yellowish-white nodules in the posterior pharynx (acute lymphonodular pharyngitis; Chapter 242). In EBV pharyngitis, there may be prominent tonsillar enlargement with exudate, cervical lymphadenitis, hepatosplenomegaly, rash, and generalized fatigue as part of the infectious mononucleosis syndrome (Chapter 246). Primary HSV infections in young children often manifest as high fever and gingivostomatitis, but pharyngitis may be present (Chapter 244).

The illnesses attributed to group C streptococcus and *A. haemolyticum* are generally similar to those caused by GABHS. Infections with *A. haemolyticum* are sometimes accompanied by a blanching, erythematous, maculopapular rash. Gonococcal pharyngeal infections are usually asymptomatic but can cause acute pharyngitis with fever and cervical lymphadenitis. **Lemierre syndrome** is a serious complication of *F. necrophorum* pharyngitis and is characterized by septic thrombophlebitis of the internal jugular veins with septic pulmonary emboli, producing hypoxia and pulmonary infiltrates (Chapters 374, 375).

DIAGNOSIS

The clinical presentations of streptococcal and viral pharyngitis show considerable overlap. Physicians relying solely on clinical judgment often overestimate the likelihood of a streptococcal etiology, so laboratory testing is useful in identifying children who are most likely to benefit from antibiotic therapy. Throat culture remains an imperfect gold standard for diagnosing streptococcal pharyngitis. False-positive cultures can occur if other organisms are misidentified as GABHS, and children who are streptococcal carriers can also have positive cultures. False-negative cultures are attributed to a variety of causes, including inadequate throat swab specimens and patients' surreptitious use of antibiotics. The specificity of rapid tests to detect group A streptococcal antigen is high, so if a rapid test is positive, throat culture is unnecessary and appropriate treatment is indicated. Because rapid tests are generally less sensitive than culture, confirming a negative rapid test with a throat culture has been recommended, especially if the clinical suspicion of GABHS is high. Special culture media and a prolonged incubation are required to detect *A. haemolyticum.* Viral cultures are often unavailable and are generally too expensive and slow to be clinically useful. Viral polymerase chain reaction (PCR) is more rapid and may be useful but is not always necessary. A complete blood cell (CBC) count showing many atypical lymphocytes and a positive slide agglutination (or "spot") test can help to confirm a clinical diagnosis of EBV infectious mononucleosis.

TREATMENT

Most untreated episodes of streptococcal pharyngitis resolve uneventfully in a few days, but early antibiotic therapy hastens clinical recovery by 12-24 hr. The primary benefit of treatment is the prevention of acute rheumatic fever, which is almost completely successful if antibiotic treatment is instituted within 9 days of illness. Antibiotic therapy should be started immediately without culture for children with symptomatic pharyngitis and a positive rapid streptococcal antigen test, a clinical diagnosis of scarlet fever, a household contact with documented streptococcal pharyngitis, a past history of acute rheumatic fever, or a recent history of acute rheumatic fever in a family member.

A variety of antimicrobial agents are effective. GABHS remains universally susceptible to penicillin, which has a narrow spectrum and few adverse effects. Penicillin V is inexpensive and is given bid or tid for 10 days: 250 mg/dose for children <27 kg (60 lb) and 500 mg/dose for larger children and adults. Oral amoxicillin is often preferred for children because of taste, availability as chewable tablets, and convenience of once-daily dosing (750 mg fixed dose or 50 mg/kg, maximum 1 g) given orally for 10 days. A single intramuscular dose of benzathine penicillin (600,000U for children <27 kg [60 lb]; 1.2 million U for larger children and adults) or a benzathine-procaine penicillin G combination is painful but ensures compliance and provides adequate blood levels for more than 10 days. For patients allergic to penicillin, treatment options include

- Erythromycin: erythromycin ethyl succinate 40 mg/kg/day divided bid, tid, or qid orally for 10 days; or erythromycin estolate 20-40 mg/kg/day divided bid, tid, or qid orally for 10 days; maximum dose for either drug 1 g/24 hr
- Azithromycin: 12 mg/kg once daily for 5 days, maximum daily dose 500 mg
- Clarithromycin: 15 mg/kg/day divided bid for 10 days, maximum dose 250 mg bid
- Clindamycin: 20 mg/kg/day divided in 3 doses for 10 days, maximum daily dose 1.8 g

The increased use of macrolide antibiotics has been correlated with increased rates of resistance to erythromycin among group A streptococci. A narrow-spectrum cephalosporin (cephalexin or cefadroxil) is another treatment option so long as a patient's previous reaction to penicillin was not an immediate, type I hypersensitivity reaction. Based on the proportion of cultures that remain positive for GABHS after therapy, cephalosporins appear to be as good as, or better than, penicillin, perhaps because these drugs are more effective in eradicating streptococcal carriage. Current evidence is not sufficient to recommend shorter courses of cephalosporins for routine therapy.

Follow-up cultures are unnecessary unless symptoms recur. Some treated patients continue to harbor GABHS in their pharynx and become streptococcal carriers. Carriage generally poses little risk to patients and their contacts, but it can confound the test results used to determine the etiology of subsequent episodes of sore throat. The treatment regimen most effective for eradicating streptococcal carriage is clindamycin, 20 mg/kg/day divided in 3 doses (adult dose: 150-450 mg tid or qid; maximum dose 1.8 g/day) orally for 10 days.

Specific therapy is unavailable for most viral pharyngitis. On the basis of in vitro susceptibility data, oral penicillin is often suggested for patients with group C streptococcal isolates and oral erythromycin is recommended for patients with *A. haemolyticum,* but the clinical benefit of such treatment is uncertain.

Nonspecific, symptomatic therapy can be an important part of the overall treatment plan. An oral antipyretic/analgesic agent (acetaminophen or ibuprofen) can relieve fever and sore throat pain. Gargling with warm salt water is often comforting, and anesthetic sprays and lozenges (often containing benzocaine, phenol, or menthol) can provide local relief.

RECURRENT PHARYNGITIS

Recurrent streptococcal pharyngitis can represent relapse with an identical strain if type-specific antibody has not yet developed. If compliance with antibiotic treatment has been poor, intramuscular benzathine penicillin is suggested. The possibility of resistance should be considered if a nonpenicillin treatment such as erythromycin was given. Recurrences can also be caused by a different strain resulting from new exposures or can represent pharyngitis of another cause accompanied by streptococcal carriage. This last possibility is likely if the illnesses are mild and otherwise atypical for streptococcal pharyngitis. If GABHS is detected by repeat culture a few days after completing treatment, therapy to eliminate carriage is recommended. Prolonged pharyngitis (>1-2 wk) suggests another disorder such as neutropenia or recurrent fever syndromes.

Tonsillectomy lowers the incidence of pharyngitis for 1-2 yr among children with recurrent, culture-positive GABHS pharyngitis that has been severe and frequent (>7 episodes in the previous year, or >5 in each of the preceding 2 yr). Most children spontaneously have fewer episodes over time, however, so the anticipated clinical benefit must be balanced against the risks of anesthesia and surgery. Undocumented histories of recurrent pharyngitis are an inadequate basis for recommending tonsillectomy.

COMPLICATIONS AND PROGNOSIS

Viral respiratory tract infections can predispose to bacterial middle ear infections. The complications of streptococcal pharyngitis include local suppurative complications, such as parapharyngeal abscess, and later nonsuppurative illnesses, such as acute rheumatic fever (Chapter 176.1) and acute postinfectious glomerulonephritis (Chapter 505.1).

PREVENTION

Multivalent streptococcal vaccines based on M protein peptides are under development. Antimicrobial prophylaxis with daily oral penicillin prevents recurrent GABHS infections but is recommended only to prevent recurrences of acute rheumatic fever (Chapter 176.1).

BIBLIOGRAPHY

Please visit the Nelson Textbook of Pediatrics *website at* *www.expertconsult.com* *for the complete bibliography.*

Chapter 374
Retropharyngeal Abscess, Lateral Pharyngeal (Parapharyngeal) Abscess, and Peritonsillar Cellulitis/Abscess

Diane E. Pappas and J. Owen Hendley

The neck contains deeply located lymph nodes including *retropharyngeal nodes* and *lateral pharyngeal nodes* that drain the mucosal surfaces of the upper airway and digestive tracts. These nodes lie within the *retropharyngeal space* (located between the pharynx and the cervical vertebrae and extending down into the superior mediastinum) and the *lateral pharyngeal space* (bounded by the pharynx medially, the carotid sheath posteriorly, and the muscles of the styloid process laterally), which are interconnected. The lymph nodes in these deep neck spaces communicate with each other, allowing bacteria from either cellulitis or node abscess to spread to other nodes. Infection of the nodes usually occurs as a result of extension from a localized infection of the oropharynx. Retropharyngeal abscess can also result from penetrating trauma to the oropharynx, dental infection, and vertebral osteomyelitis. Once infected, the nodes may progress through three stages: *cellulitis, phlegmon,* and *abscess.* Infection in the retropharyngeal and lateral pharyngeal spaces can result in airway compromise or posterior mediastinitis, making timely diagnosis important.

RETROPHARYNGEAL AND LATERAL PHARYNGEAL ABSCESS

Retropharyngeal abscess occurs most commonly in children <3-4 yr of age, with boys affected more often than girls. Up to

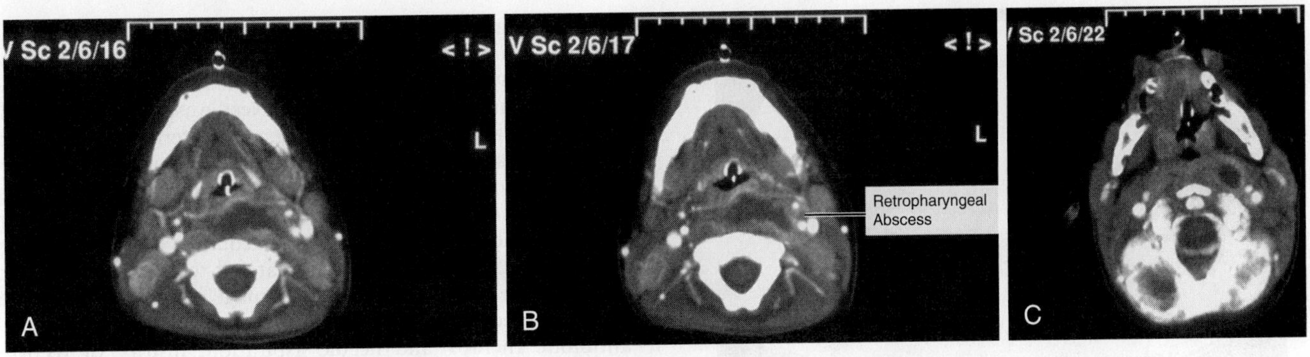

Figure 374-1 CT of retropharyngeal abscess. *A,* CT image at level of epiglottis. *B,* Sequential CT slice exhibiting ring-enhancing lesion. *C,* Further sequential CT slice demonstrating inferior extent of lesion. (From Philpott CM, Selvadurai D, Banerjee AR: Paediatric retropharyngeal abscess, *J Laryngol Otol* 118:925, 2004.)

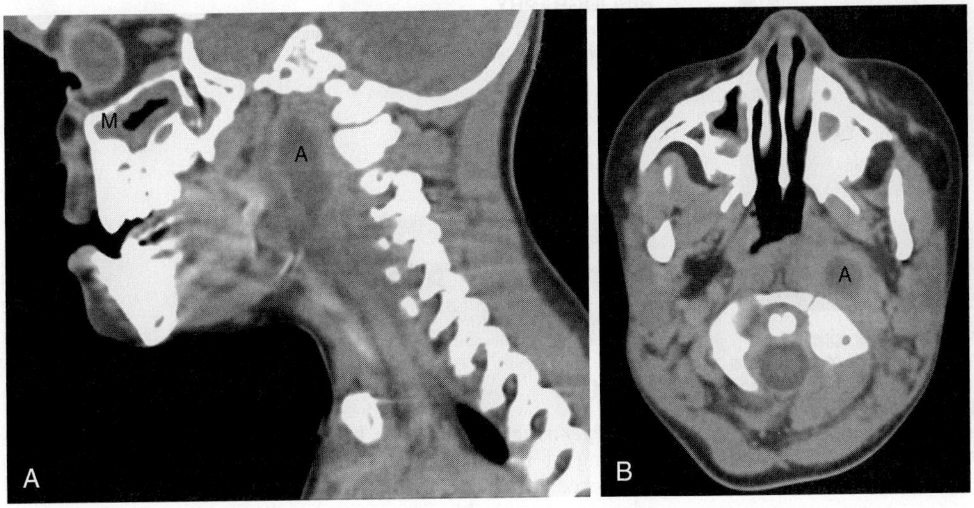

Figure 374-2 CT of parapharyngeal abscess in a 3 yr old child. *A,* Sagittal section demonstrating parapharyngeal abscess (A) and mucosal swelling (M) in the maxillary sinus. *B,* Coronal section of parapharyngeal abscess (A).

67% of patients have a history of recent ear, nose, or throat infection. The retropharyngeal nodes involute after 5 yr of age and, therefore, infection in older children and adults is much less common.

Clinical manifestations of retropharyngeal abscess are nonspecific and include fever, irritability, decreased oral intake, and drooling. Neck stiffness, torticollis, and refusal to move the neck may also be present. The verbal child might complain of sore throat and neck pain. Other signs can include muffled voice, stridor, respiratory distress, or even obstructive sleep apnea. Physical examination can reveal bulging of the posterior pharyngeal wall, although this is present in <50% of infants with retropharyngeal abscess. Cervical lymphadenopathy may also be present. Lateral pharyngeal abscess commonly presents as fever, dysphagia, and a prominent bulge of the lateral pharyngeal wall, sometimes with medial displacement of the tonsil.

The differential diagnosis includes acute epiglottitis and foreign body aspiration. In the young child with limited neck mobility, meningitis must also be considered. Other possibilities include lymphoma, hematoma, and vertebral osteomyelitis.

Incision for drainage and culture of an abscessed node provides the definitive diagnosis, but CT can be useful in identifying the presence of a retropharyngeal, lateral pharyngeal, or parapharyngeal abscess (Figs. 374-1 and 374-2). With CT scans, deep neck infections can be accurately identified and localized, but CT accurately identifies abscess formation in only 63% of patients. Soft tissue neck films taken during inspiration with the neck extended might show increased width or an air-fluid level in the retropharyngeal space. CT with contrast medium enhancement can reveal central lucency, ring enhancement, or scalloping of the walls of a lymph node. Scalloping of the abscess wall is thought to be a late finding and predicts abscess formation.

Retropharyngeal and lateral pharyngeal infections are most often polymicrobial; the usual pathogens include group A streptococcus (Chapter 176), oropharyngeal anaerobic bacteria (Chapter 205), and *Staphylococcus aureus* (Chapter 174.1). Studies have documented an increased incidence of group A streptococcus recovered from such abscesses. Other pathogens can include *Haemophilus influenzae, Klebsiella,* and *Mycobacterium avium-intracellulare.*

Treatment options include intravenous antibiotics with or without surgical drainage. A 3rd-generation cephalosporin combined with ampicillin-sulbactam or clindamycin to provide anaerobic coverage is effective. The increasing prevalence of methicillin-resistant *Staphylococcus aureus* can influence empiric antibiotic therapy. Studies have shown that >50% of children with retropharyngeal or lateral pharyngeal abscess as identified by CT can be successfully treated without surgical drainage. Drainage is necessary in the patient with respiratory distress or failure to improve with intravenous antibiotic treatment. The optimal duration of treatment is unknown, but therapy for several days with intravenous antibiotics until the patient has begun to improve followed by a course of oral antibiotic is typically used.

Complications of retropharyngeal or lateral pharyngeal abscess include significant upper airway obstruction, rupture leading to aspiration pneumonia, and extension to the mediastinum. Thrombophlebitis of the internal jugular vein and erosion of the carotid artery sheath can also occur.

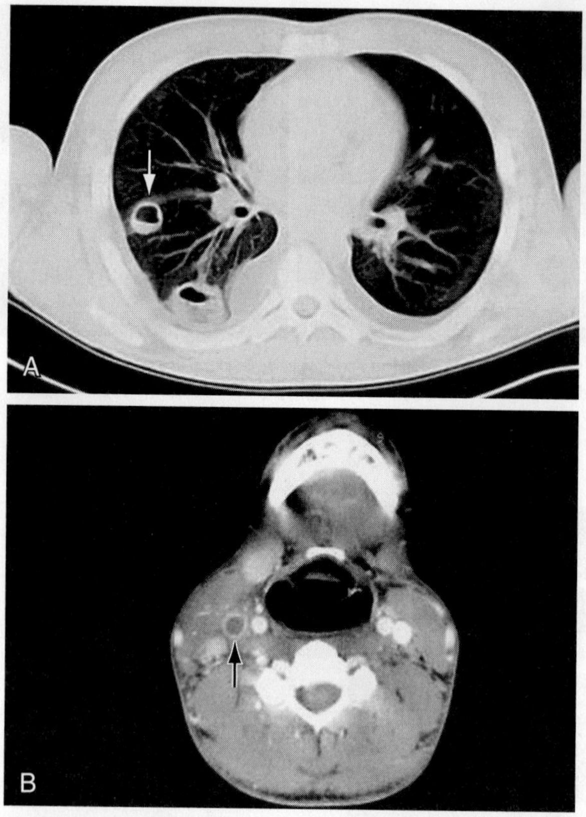

Figure 374-3 CT of Lemierre disease. *A,* CT demonstrating nodular appearance of pulmonary infiltrates *(arrow). B,* CT of neck demonstrating thrombosis of right internal jugular vein *(arrow).* (From Plymyer MR, Zoccola DC, Tallarita G: An 18 year old man presenting with sepsis following a recent pharyngeal infection, *Arch Pathol Lab Med* 128:813, 2004. Reprinted with permission from Archives of Pathology & Laboratory Medicine. Copyright 2004. College of American Pathologists.)

An uncommon but characteristic infection of the parapharyngeal space is **Lemierre disease,** in which infection from the oropharynx extends to cause septic thrombophlebitis of the internal jugular vein and embolic abscesses in the lungs (Fig. 374-3). The causative pathogen is *Fusobacterium necrophorum,* an anaerobic bacterial constituent of the oropharyngeal flora. The typical presentation is that of a previously healthy adolescent or young adult with a history of recent pharyngitis who becomes acutely ill with fever, hypoxia, tachypnea, and respiratory distress. Chest radiography demonstrates multiple cavitary nodules, often bilateral and often accompanied by pleural effusion. Blood culture may be positive. Treatment involves prolonged intravenous antibiotic therapy with penicillin or cefoxitin; surgical drainage of extrapulmonary metastatic abscesses may be necessary (Chapters 373, 375).

PERITONSILLAR CELLULITIS AND/OR ABSCESS

Peritonsillar cellulitis and/or abscess, which is relatively common compared to the deep neck infections, is caused by bacterial invasion through the capsule of the tonsil, leading to cellulitis and/or abscess formation in the surrounding tissues. The typical patient with a peritonsillar abscess is an adolescent with a recent history of acute pharyngotonsillitis. Clinical manifestations include sore throat, fever, trismus, and dysphagia. Physical examination reveals an asymmetric tonsillar bulge with displacement of the uvula. An asymmetric tonsillar bulge is diagnostic, but it may be poorly visualized because of trismus. CT is helpful for revealing the abscess. Group A streptococci and mixed oropharyngeal anaerobes are the most common pathogens, with more than 4 bacterial isolates per abscess typically recovered by needle aspiration.

Treatment includes surgical drainage and antibiotic therapy effective against group A streptococci and anaerobes. Surgical drainage may be accomplished through needle aspiration, incision and drainage, or tonsillectomy. Needle aspiration can involve aspiration of the superior, middle, and inferior aspects of the tonsil to locate the abscess. General anesthesia may be required for the uncooperative patient. Approximately 95% of peritonsillar abscesses resolve after needle aspiration and antibiotic therapy. A small percentage of these patients require a repeat needle aspiration. The 5% with infections that fail to resolve after needle aspiration require incision and drainage. Tonsillectomy should be considered if there is failure to improve within 24 hours of antibiotic therapy and needle aspiration, history of recurrent peritonsillar abscess or recurrent tonsillitis, or complications from peritonsillar abscess. The feared, albeit rare, complication is rupture of the abscess, with resultant aspiration pneumonitis. There is a 10% recurrence risk for peritonsillar abscess.

BIBLIOGRAPHY

Please visit the Nelson Textbook of Pediatrics *website at www.expertconsult.com for the complete bibliography.*

Chapter 375
Tonsils and Adenoids

Ralph F. Wetmore

ANATOMY

Waldeyer ring refers to the lymphoid tissue that surrounds the opening of the oral and nasal cavities into the pharynx. It is composed of the palatine tonsils, the pharyngeal tonsil or adenoid, lymphoid tissue surrounding the eustachian tube orifice in the lateral walls of the nasopharynx, the lingual tonsil at the base of the tongue, and scattered lymphoid tissue throughout the remainder of the pharynx, particularly behind the posterior pharyngeal pillars and along the posterior pharyngeal wall. Lymphoid tissue located between the palatoglossal fold (anterior tonsillar pillar) and the palatopharyngeal fold (posterior tonsillar pillar) forms the *palatine tonsil.* This lymphoid tissue is separated from the surrounding pharyngeal musculature by a thick fibrous capsule. The *adenoid* is a single aggregation of lymphoid tissue that occupies the space between the nasal septum and the posterior pharyngeal wall. A thin fibrous capsule separates it from the underlying structures; the adenoid does not contain the complex crypts that are found in the palatine tonsils but rather more simple crypts. Lymphoid tissue at the base of the tongue forms the *lingual tonsil* that also contains simple tonsillar crypts.

NORMAL FUNCTION

Situated at the opening of the pharynx to the external environment, the tonsils and adenoid are in a position to provide primary defense against foreign matter. The immunologic role of the tonsils and adenoids is to induce secretory immunity and to regulate the production of the secretory immunoglobulins. Deep crevices within tonsillar tissue form tonsillar crypts that are lined with squamous epithelium but have a concentration of lymphocytes at their bases. Lymphoid tissue of Waldeyer ring is most immunologically active between 4 and 10 yr of age, with a decrease after puberty. No major immunologic deficiency has been demonstrated after removal of either or both of the tonsils and adenoid.

PATHOLOGY

Acute Infection

Most episodes of acute pharyngotonsillitis are caused by viruses (Chapter 373). Group A β-hemolytic streptococcus (GABHS) is the most common cause of bacterial infection in the pharynx (Chapter 176).

Chronic Infection

The tonsils and adenoids can be chronically infected by multiple microbes, which can include a high incidence of β-lactamase–producing organisms. Both aerobic species, such as streptococci and *Haemophilus influenzae,* and anaerobic species, such as *Peptostreptococcus, Prevotella,* and *Fusobacterium,* predominate. The tonsillar crypts can accumulate desquamated epithelial cells, lymphocytes, bacteria, and other debris, causing cryptic tonsillitis. With time, these cryptic plugs can calcify into tonsillar concretions or tonsillolith. There is growing evidence that biofilms might also play a role in chronic inflammation of the tonsils.

Airway Obstruction

Both the tonsils and adenoids are a major cause of upper airway obstruction in children. Airway obstruction in children is typically manifested in sleep-disordered breathing, including obstructive sleep apnea, obstructive sleep hypopnea, and upper airway resistance syndrome (Chapter 17). Sleep-disordered breathing secondary to adenotonsillar breathing is a cause of growth failure (Chapter 38).

Tonsillar Neoplasm

Rapid enlargement of one tonsil is highly suggestive of a tonsillar malignancy, typically lymphoma in children.

CLINICAL MANIFESTATIONS

Acute Infection

Symptoms of GABHS infection include odynophagia, dry throat, malaise, fever and chills, dysphagia, referred otalgia, headache, muscular aches, and enlarged cervical nodes. Signs include dry tongue, erythematous enlarged tonsils, tonsillar or pharyngeal exudate, palatine petechiae, and enlargement and tenderness of the jugulodigastric lymph nodes (Fig. 375–1; Chapters 176 and 373).

Chronic Infection

Children with chronic or cryptic tonsillitis often present with halitosis, chronic sore throats, foreign body sensation, or a history of expelling foul-tasting and foul-smelling cheesy lumps. Examination can reveal tonsils of almost any size and often they contain copious debris within the crypts. Because the offending organism is not usually GABHS, streptococcal culture is usually negative.

Airway Obstruction

In many children, the diagnosis of airway obstruction (Chapters 17 and 365) can be made by history and physical examination. Daytime symptoms of airway obstruction, secondary to adenotonsillar hypertrophy, include chronic mouth breathing, nasal obstruction, hyponasal speech, hyposmia, decreased appetite, poor school performance, and, rarely, symptoms of right-sided heart failure. Nighttime symptoms consist of loud snoring, choking, gasping, frank apneas, restless sleep, abnormal sleep positions, somnambulism, night terrors, diaphoresis, enuresis, and sleep talking. Large tonsils are typically seen on examination, although the absolute size might not indicate the degree of obstruction. The size of the adenoid tissue can be demonstrated on a lateral neck radiograph or with flexible endoscopy. Other signs that can contribute to airway obstruction include the presence of a craniofacial syndrome or hypotonia.

Tonsillar Neoplasm

The rapid unilateral enlargement of a tonsil, especially if accompanied by systemic signs of night sweats, fever, weight loss, and lymphadenopathy, is highly suggestive of a tonsillar malignancy. The diagnosis of a tonsillar malignancy should also be entertained if the tonsil appears grossly abnormal. Among 54,901 patients undergoing tonsillectomy, 54 malignancies were identified (0.087% prevalence); all but 6 malignancies had been suspected based on suspicious anatomic features preoperatively.

TREATMENT

Medical Management

The treatment of acute pharyngotonsillitis is discussed in Chapter 373 and antibiotic treatment of GABHS in Chapter 176. Because co-pathogens such as staphylococci or anaerobes can produce β-lactamase that can inactivate penicillin, the use of cephalosporins or clindamycin may be more efficacious in the treatment of chronic throat infections. Tonsillolith or debris may be expressed manually with either a cotton-tipped applicator or a water jet. Chronically infected tonsillar crypts can be cauterized using silver nitrate.

Tonsillectomy

Tonsillectomy alone is usually performed for recurrent or chronic pharyngotonsillitis. Indications for surgery remain uncertain;

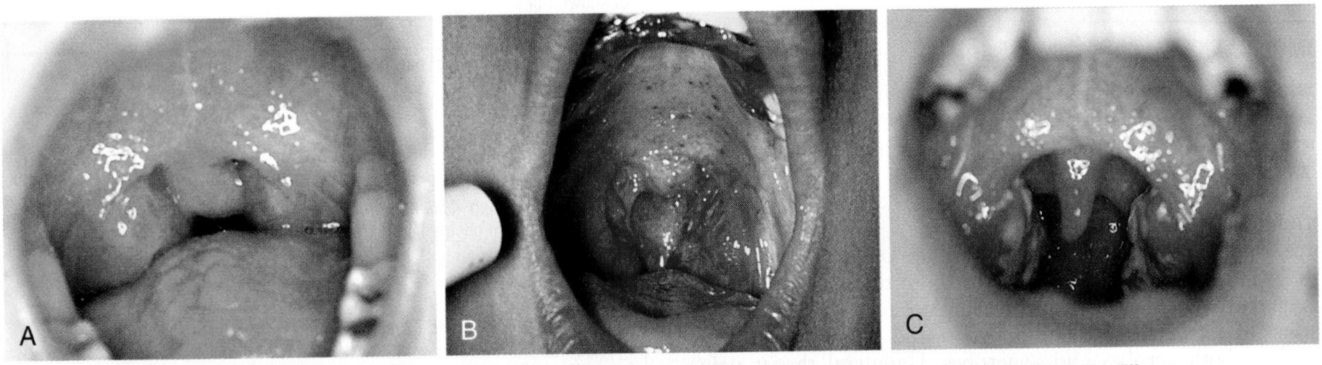

Figure 375–1 Pharyngotonsillitis. This common syndrome has a number of causative pathogens and a wide spectrum of severity. *A,* The diffuse tonsillar and pharyngeal erythema seen here is a nonspecific finding that can be produced by a variety of pathogens. *B,* This intense erythema, seen in association with acute tonsillar enlargement and palatal petechiae, is highly suggestive of group A β-streptococcal infection, though other pathogens can produce these findings. *C,* This picture of exudative tonsillitis is most commonly seen with either group A streptococcal or Epstein-Barr virus infection. (*B,* Courtesy of Michael Sherlock, MD, Lutherville, MD.) (From Yellon RF, McBride TP, Davis HW: Otolaryngology. In Zitelli BJ, Davis HW, editors: *Atlas of pediatric physical diagnosis,* ed 4, Philadelphia, 2002, Mosby, p 852.)

there are large variations in surgical rates among children across countries: 144/10,000 in Italy; 115/10,000 in the Netherlands; 65/10,000 in England; and 50/10,000 in the United States. Rates are generally higher in boys. Potential but nonevidenced based indications include 7 or more throat infections treated with antibiotics in the preceding yr, 5 or more throat infections treated in each of the preceding 2 yr, or 3 or more throat infections treated with antibiotics in each of the preceding 3 yr. The American Academy of Otolaryngology—Head and Neck Surgery offers guidelines of 3 or more infections of tonsils and/or adenoids per yr despite adequate medical therapy; the Scottish Intercollegiate Tonsillectomy Guidelines Network recommends 5 or more episodes per yr of tonsillitis with disabling symptoms and lasting for longer than 1 yr. Tonsillectomy has been shown to be effective in reducing the number of infections and the symptoms of chronic tonsillitis such as halitosis, persistent or recurrent sore throats, and recurrent cervical adenitis. In resistant cases of cryptic tonsillitis, tonsillectomy may be curative. Rarely in children, tonsillectomy is indicated for biopsy of a unilaterally enlarged tonsil to exclude a neoplasm or to treat recurrent hemorrhage from superficial tonsillar blood vessels. Tonsillectomy has not been shown to offer clinical benefit over conservative treatment in children with mild symptoms.

Adenoidectomy

Adenoidectomy alone may be indicated for the treatment of chronic nasal infection (chronic adenoiditis), chronic sinus infections that have failed medical management, and recurrent bouts of acute otitis media, including those in children with tympanostomy tubes who suffer from recurrent otorrhea. Adenoidectomy may be helpful in children with chronic or recurrent otitis media with effusion. Adenoidectomy alone may be curative in the management of patients with nasal obstruction, chronic mouth breathing, and loud snoring suggesting sleep-disordered breathing. Adenoidectomy may also be indicated for children in whom upper airway obstruction is suspected of causing craniofacial or occlusive developmental abnormalities.

Tonsillectomy and Adenoidectomy

The criteria for both tonsillectomy and adenoidectomy for recurrent infection are the same as those for tonsillectomy alone. The other major indication for performing both procedures together is upper airway obstruction secondary to adenotonsillar hypertrophy that results in sleep-disordered breathing, failure to thrive, craniofacial or occlusive developmental abnormalities, speech abnormalities, or, rarely, cor pulmonale. A high proportion of children with failure to thrive in the context of adenotonsillar hypertrophy resulting in sleep disorder experience significant growth acceleration after adenotonsillectomy.

COMPLICATIONS

Acute Pharyngotonsillitis

The 2 major complications of untreated GABHS infection are post-streptococcal glomerulonephritis and acute rheumatic fever (Chapters 176 and 505.1).

Peritonsillar Infection

Peritonsillar infection can occur as either cellulitis or a frank abscess in the region superior and lateral to the tonsillar capsule (Chapter 374). These infections usually occur in children with a history of recurrent tonsillar infection and are polymicrobial, including both aerobes and anaerobes. Unilateral throat pain, referred otalgia, drooling, and trismus are presenting symptoms. The affected tonsil is displaced down and medial by swelling of the anterior tonsillar pillar and palate. The diagnosis of an abscess can be confirmed by CT or by needle aspiration, the contents of which should be sent for culture.

Retropharyngeal Space Infection

Infections in the retropharyngeal space develop in the lymph nodes that drain the oropharynx, nose, and nasopharynx. (See Chapter 374).

Parapharyngeal Space Infection

Tonsillar infection can extend into the parapharyngeal space, causing symptoms of fever, neck pain and stiffness, and signs of swelling of the lateral pharyngeal wall and neck on the affected side. The diagnosis is confirmed by contrast medium–enhanced CT, and treatment includes intravenous antibiotics and external incision and drainage if an abscess is demonstrated on CT (Chapter 374). Septic thrombophlebitis of the jugular vein, **Lemierre syndrome,** manifests with fever, toxicity, neck pain and stiffness, and respiratory distress due to multiple septic pulmonary emboli and is a complication of a parapharyngeal space or odontogenic infection from *Fusobacterium necrophorum.* Concurrent Epstein-Barr virus mononucleosis can be a predisposing event before the sudden onset of fever, chills, and respiratory distress in an adolescent patient. Treatment includes high-dose intravenous antibiotics (ampicillin-sulbactam, clindamycin, penicillin, or ciprofloxacin) and heparinization.

Recurrent or Chronic Pharyngotonsillitis

See Chapter 373.

Table 375-1 RISKS AND POTENTIAL BENEFITS OF TONSILLECTOMY OR ADENOIDECTOMY OR BOTH

RISKS
Cost*
Risk of anesthetic accidents
Malignant hyperthermia
Cardiac arrhythmia
Vocal cord trauma
Aspiration with resulting bronchopulmonary obstruction or infection
Risk of miscellaneous surgical or postoperative complications
Hemorrhage
Airway obstruction due to edema of tongue, palate, or nasopharynx, or retropharyngeal hematoma
Central apnea
Prolonged muscular paralysis
Dehydration
Palatopharyngeal insufficiency
Otitis media
Nasopharyngeal stenosis
Refractory torticollis
Facial edema
Emotional upset
Unknown risks
POTENTIAL BENEFITS
Reduction in frequency of ear, nose, throat illness and thus in
Discomfort
Inconvenience
School absence
Parental anxiety
Work missed by parents
Costs of physician visits and drugs
Reduction in nasal obstruction with improved
Respiratory function
Comfort
Sleep
Craniofacial growth and development
Appearance
Reduction in hearing impairment
Improved growth and overall well-being
Reduction in long-term parental anxiety

*Cost for tonsillectomy alone and adenoidectomy alone are somewhat lower.
Modified from Bluestone CD, editor: *Pediatric otolaryngology,* ed 4, Philadelphia, 2003 Saunders, p. 1213.

CHRONIC AIRWAY OBSTRUCTION

Although rare, children with chronic airway obstruction from enlarged tonsils and adenoids can present with cor pulmonale.

The effects of chronic airway obstruction (Chapter 17) and mouth breathing on facial growth remain a subject of controversy. Studies of chronic mouth breathing, both in humans and animals, have shown changes in facial development, including prolongation of the total anterior facial height and a tendency toward a retrognathic mandible, the so-called adenoid facies. Adenotonsillectomy can reverse some of these abnormalities. Other studies have disputed these findings.

Tonsillectomy and Adenoidectomy

The risks and potential benefits of surgery must be considered (Table 375–1). Bleeding can occur in the immediate postoperative period or be delayed after separation of the eschar. Bleeding is more common after high dose dexamethasone (0.5 mg/kg), although postoperative nausea and emesis is reduced. The risk of bleeding is lower with lower-dose dexamethasone (0.15 mg/kg), which also has a lowered risk of postoperative nausea and emesis. Swelling of the tongue and soft palate can lead to acute airway obstruction in the 1st few hours after surgery. Children with underlying hypotonia or craniofacial anomalies are at greater risk for suffering this complication. Dehydration from odynophagia is not uncommon in the 1st postoperative week. Rare complications include velopharyngeal insufficiency, nasopharyngeal or oropharyngeal stenosis, and psychologic problems.

BIBLIOGRAPHY

Please visit the Nelson Textbook of Pediatrics *website at* *www.expertconsult.com* *for the complete bibliography.*

Chapter 376
Chronic or Recurrent Respiratory Symptoms

Thomas F. Boat and Thomas P. Green

Cough, wheeze, stridor, and other respiratory tract symptoms occur frequently or persist for long periods in a substantial number of children; others have persistent or recurring lung infiltrates with or without symptoms. Determining the cause of these chronic findings can be difficult because symptoms can be caused by a close succession of unrelated acute respiratory tract infections or by a single pathophysiologic process. Specific and easily performed diagnostic tests do not exist for many acute and chronic respiratory conditions. Pressure from the affected child's family for a quick remedy because of concern over symptoms related to breathing may complicate diagnostic and therapeutic efforts.

For the full continuation of this chapter, please visit the Nelson Textbook of Pediatrics *website at* *www.expertconsult.com*.

Chapter 377
Acute Inflammatory Upper Airway Obstruction (Croup, Epiglottitis, Laryngitis, and Bacterial Tracheitis)

Genie E. Roosevelt

The lumen of an infant's or child's airway is narrow; because airway resistance is inversely proportional to the 4th power of the radius (Chapter 365), minor reductions in cross-sectional area due to mucosal edema or other inflammatory processes cause an exponential increase in airway resistance and a significant increase in the work of breathing. The larynx is composed of 4 major cartilages (**epiglottic**, **arytenoid**, **thyroid**, and **cricoid cartilages**, ordered from superior to inferior) and the soft tissues that surround them. The cricoid cartilage encircles the airway just below the vocal cords and defines the narrowest portion of the upper airway in children <10 yr of age.

Inflammation involving the vocal cords and structures inferior to the cords is called **laryngitis, laryngotracheitis**, or **laryngotracheobronchitis**, and inflammation of the structures superior to the cords (i.e., arytenoids, aryepiglottic folds ["false cords"], epiglottis) is called **supraglottitis**. The term **croup** refers to a heterogeneous group of mainly acute and infectious processes that are characterized by a bark-like or brassy cough and may be associated with hoarseness, inspiratory stridor, and respiratory distress. **Stridor** is a harsh, high-pitched respiratory sound, which is usually inspiratory but can be biphasic and is produced by turbulent airflow; it is not a diagnosis but a sign of upper airway obstruction (Chapter 366). Croup typically affects the larynx, trachea, and bronchi. When the involvement of the larynx is sufficient to produce symptoms, they dominate the clinical picture over the tracheal and bronchial signs. Traditionally, a distinction has been made between spasmodic or recurrent croup and laryngotracheobronchitis. Some clinicians believe that spasmodic croup might have an allergic component and improves rapidly without treatment, whereas laryngotracheobronchitis is always associated with a viral infection of the respiratory tract. Others believe that the signs and symptoms are similar enough to consider them within the spectrum of a single disease, in part because studies have documented viral etiologies in both acute and recurrent croup.

377.1 Infectious Upper Airway Obstruction

Genie E. Roosevelt

ETIOLOGY AND EPIDEMIOLOGY

With the exceptions of diphtheria, bacterial tracheitis, and epiglottitis, most acute infections of the upper airway are caused by viruses. The parainfluenza viruses (types 1, 2, and 3; Chapter 251) account for ~75% of cases; other viruses associated with croup include influenza A and B, adenovirus, respiratory syncytial virus (RSV), and measles. Influenza A has been associated with severe laryngotracheobronchitis. *Mycoplasma pneumoniae* has rarely been isolated from children with croup and causes mild disease (Chapter 215). Most patients with croup are between the ages of 3 mo and 5 yr, with the peak in the 2nd yr of life. The incidence of croup is higher in boys; it occurs most commonly in the late fall and winter but can occur throughout the year. Recurrences are frequent from 3-6 yr of age and decrease with growth of the airway. Approximately 15% of patients have a strong family history of croup.

In the past, *Haemophilus influenzae* type b was the most commonly identified etiology of acute epiglottitis. Since the widespread use of the HiB vaccine, invasive disease due to *H. influenzae* type b in pediatric patients has been reduced by 80-90% (Chapter 186). Therefore, other agents, such as *Streptococcus pyogenes*, *Streptococcus pneumoniae*, and *Staphylococcus aureus*, now represent a larger portion of pediatric cases of epiglottitis in vaccinated children. In the prevaccine era, the typical patient with epiglottitis due to *H. influenza* type b was 2-4 yr of age, although cases were seen in the 1st year of life and in patients as old as 7 yr of age. The typical patient with epiglottitis is an adult with a sore throat, although cases still do occur in underimmunized children; vaccine failures have been reported.

CLINICAL MANIFESTATIONS

Croup (Laryngotracheobronchitis)

Viruses most commonly cause croup, the most common form of acute upper respiratory obstruction. The term **laryngotracheobronchitis** refers to viral infection of the glottic and subglottic regions. Some clinicians use the term **laryngotracheitis** for the most common and most typical form of croup and reserve the term **laryngotracheobronchitis** for the more severe form that is considered an extension of laryngotracheitis associated with bacterial superinfection that occurs 5-7 days into the clinical course.

Most patients have an upper respiratory tract infection with some combination of rhinorrhea, pharyngitis, mild cough, and low-grade fever for 1-3 days before the signs and symptoms of upper airway obstruction become apparent. The child then develops the characteristic "barking" cough, hoarseness, and inspiratory stridor. The low-grade fever can persist, although temperatures can reach 39-40°C (102.2-104°F); some children are afebrile. Symptoms are characteristically worse at night and often recur with decreasing intensity for several days and resolve completely within a week. Agitation and crying greatly aggravate the symptoms and signs. The child may prefer to sit up in bed or be held upright. Older children usually are not seriously ill. Other family members might have mild respiratory illnesses with laryngitis. Most young patients with croup progress only as far as stridor and slight dyspnea before they start to recover.

Physical examination can reveal a hoarse voice, coryza, normal to moderately inflamed pharynx, and a slightly increased respiratory rate. Patients vary substantially in their degrees of respiratory distress. Rarely, the upper airway obstruction progresses and is accompanied by an increasing respiratory rate; nasal flaring; suprasternal, infrasternal, and intercostal retractions; and continuous stridor. Croup is a disease of the upper airway, and alveolar gas exchange is usually normal. Hypoxia and low oxygen saturation are seen only when complete airway obstruction is imminent. The child who is hypoxic, cyanotic, pale, or obtunded needs immediate airway management. Occasionally, the pattern of severe laryngotracheobronchitis is difficult to differentiate from epiglottitis, despite the usually more acute onset and rapid course of the latter.

Croup is a clinical diagnosis and does not require a radiograph of the neck. Radiographs of the neck can show the typical subglottic narrowing, or steeple sign, of croup on the posteroanterior view (Fig. 377-1). However, the steeple sign may be absent in patients with croup, may be present in patients without croup as a normal variant, and may rarely be present in patients with epiglottitis. The radiographs do not correlate well with disease severity. Radiographs should be considered only after airway stabilization in children who have an atypical presentation or clinical course. Radiographs may be helpful in distinguishing between severe laryngotracheobronchitis and epiglottitis, but airway management should always take priority.

Acute Epiglottitis (Supraglottitis)

This dramatic, potentially lethal condition is characterized by an acute rapidly progressive and potentially fulminating course of high fever, sore throat, dyspnea, and rapidly progressing respiratory obstruction. The degree of respiratory distress at presentation is variable. The initial lack of respiratory distress can deceive the unwary clinician; respiratory distress can also be the 1st manifestation. Often, the otherwise healthy child suddenly develops a sore throat and fever. Within a matter of hours, the patient appears toxic, swallowing is difficult, and breathing is labored. Drooling is usually present and the neck is hyperextended in an attempt to maintain the airway. The child may assume the tripod position, sitting upright and leaning forward with the chin up and mouth open while bracing on the arms. A brief period of air hunger with restlessness may be followed by rapidly increasing cyanosis and coma. Stridor is a late finding and suggests near-complete airway obstruction. Complete obstruction of the airway and death can ensue unless adequate treatment is provided. The barking cough typical of croup is rare. Usually, no other family members are ill with acute respiratory symptoms.

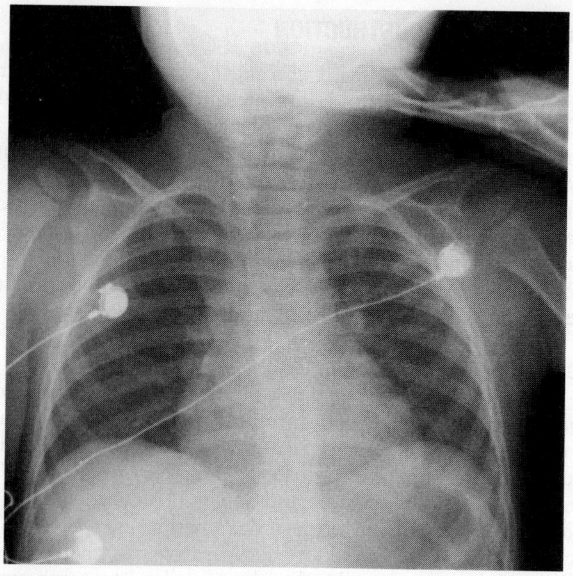

Figure 377-1 Radiograph of an airway of a patient with croup, showing typical subglottic narrowing (steeple sign).

The diagnosis requires visualization of a large, cherry red, swollen epiglottis by laryngoscopy. Occasionally, the other supraglottic structures, especially the aryepiglottic folds, are more involved than the epiglottis itself. In a patient in whom the diagnosis is certain or probable based on clinical grounds, laryngoscopy should be performed expeditiously in a controlled environment such as an operating room or intensive care unit. Anxiety-provoking interventions such as phlebotomy, intravenous line placement, placing the child supine, or direct inspection of the oral cavity should be avoided until the airway is secure. If epiglottitis is thought to be possible but not certain in a patient with acute upper airway obstruction, the patient can undergo lateral radiographs of the upper airway first. Classic radiographs of a child who has epiglottitis show the thumb sign (Fig. 377-2). Proper positioning of the patient for the lateral neck radiograph is crucial in order to avoid some of the pitfalls associated with interpretation of the film. Adequate hyperextension of the head and neck is necessary. In addition, the epiglottis can appear to be round if the lateral neck is taken at an oblique angle. If the concern for epiglottitis still exists after the radiographs, direct visualization should be performed. A physician skilled in airway management and use of intubation equipment should accompany patients with suspected epiglottitis at all times. An older cooperative child might voluntarily open the mouth wide enough for a direct view of the inflamed epiglottis.

Establishing an airway by nasotracheal intubation or, less often, by tracheostomy is indicated in patients with epiglottitis, regardless of the degree of apparent respiratory distress, because as many as 6% of children with epiglottitis without an artificial airway die, compared with <1% of those with an artificial airway. No clinical features have been recognized that predict mortality. Pulmonary edema can be associated with acute airway obstruction. The duration of intubation depends on the clinical course of the patient and the duration of epiglottic swelling, as determined by frequent examination using direct laryngoscopy or flexible fiberoptic laryngoscopy. In general, children with acute epiglottitis are intubated for 2-3 days, because the response

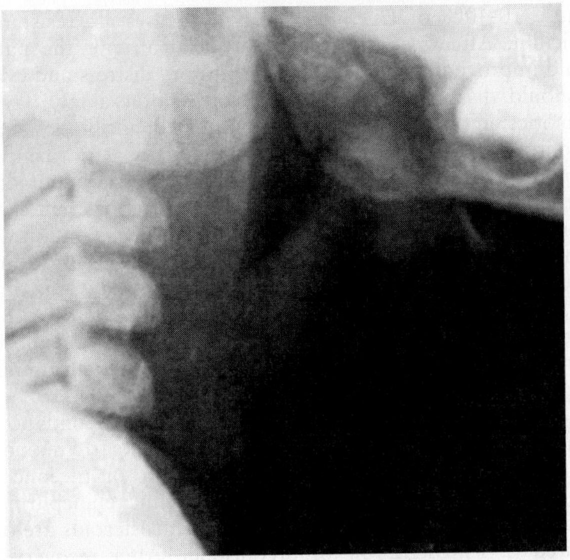

Figure 377-2 Lateral roentgenogram of the upper airway reveals the swollen epiglottis (thumb sign).

to antibiotics is usually rapid (see later). Most patients have concomitant bacteremia; occasionally, other infections are present, such as pneumonia, cervical adenopathy, or otitis media. Meningitis, arthritis, and other invasive infections with *H. influenzae* type b are rarely found in conjunction with epiglottitis.

Acute Infectious Laryngitis

Laryngitis is a common illness. Viruses cause most cases; diphtheria is an exception but is extremely rare in developed countries (Chapter 180). The onset is usually characterized by an upper respiratory tract infection during which sore throat, cough, and hoarseness appear. The illness is generally mild; respiratory distress is unusual except in the young infant. Hoarseness and loss of voice may be out of proportion to systemic signs and symptoms. The physical examination is usually not remarkable except for evidence of pharyngeal inflammation. Inflammatory edema of the vocal cords and subglottic tissue may be demonstrated laryngoscopically. The principal site of obstruction is usually the subglottic area.

Spasmodic Croup

Spasmodic croup occurs most often in children 1-3 yr of age and is clinically similar to acute laryngotracheobronchitis, except that the history of a viral prodrome and fever in the patient and family are often absent. The cause is viral in some cases, but allergic and psychologic factors may be important in others.

Occurring most commonly in the evening or nighttime, spasmodic croup begins with a sudden onset that may be preceded by mild to moderate coryza and hoarseness. The child awakens with a characteristic barking, metallic cough, noisy inspiration, and respiratory distress and appears anxious and frightened. The patient is usually afebrile. Usually, the severity of the symptoms diminishes within several hr, and the following day, the patient often appears well except for slight hoarseness and cough. Similar, but usually less severe, attacks without extreme respiratory distress can occur for another night or 2. Such episodes often recur several times. Spasmodic croup might represent more of an allergic reaction to viral antigens than direct infection, although the pathogenesis is unknown.

DIFFERENTIAL DIAGNOSIS

These 4 syndromes must be differentiated from one another and from a variety of other entities that can present as upper airway obstruction. **Bacterial tracheitis** is the most important differential diagnostic consideration and has a high risk of airway obstruction. Diphtheritic croup is extremely rare in North America, although a major epidemic of diphtheria occurred in countries of the former Soviet Union beginning in 1990 from the lack of routine immunization. Early symptoms of diphtheria include malaise, sore throat, anorexia, and low-grade fever. Within 2-3 days, pharyngeal examination reveals the typical gray-white membrane, which can vary in size from covering a small patch on the tonsils to covering most of the soft palate. The membrane is adherent to the tissue, and forcible attempts to remove it cause bleeding. The course is usually insidious, but respiratory obstruction can occur suddenly. Measles croup almost always coincides with the full manifestations of systemic disease and the course may be fulminant (Chapter 238).

Sudden onset of respiratory obstruction can be caused by aspiration of a **foreign body** (Chapter 379). The child is usually 6 mo-3 yr of age. Choking and coughing occur suddenly, usually without prodromal signs of infection, although children with a viral infection can also aspirate a foreign body. A **retropharyngeal** or **peritonsillar abscess** can mimic respiratory obstruction (Chapter 374). CT scans of the upper airway are helpful in evaluating the possibility of a retropharyngeal abscess. A peritonsillar abscess is often a clinical diagnosis. Other possible causes of upper airway obstruction include extrinsic compression of the airway (laryngeal web, vascular ring) and intraluminal obstruction from masses (laryngeal papilloma, subglottic hemangioma); these tend to have chronic or recurrent symptoms.

Upper airway obstruction is occasionally associated with **angioedema** of the subglottic areas as part of anaphylaxis and generalized allergic reactions, edema after endotracheal intubation for general anesthesia or respiratory failure, hypocalcemic tetany, infectious mononucleosis, trauma, and tumors or malformations of the larynx. A croupy cough may be an early sign of asthma. Vocal cord dysfunction can also occur. Epiglottitis, with the characteristic manifestations of drooling or dysphagia and stridor, can also result from the accidental ingestion of very hot liquid.

COMPLICATIONS

Complications occur in ~15% of patients with viral croup. The most common is extension of the infectious process to involve other regions of the respiratory tract, such as the middle ear, the terminal bronchioles, or the pulmonary parenchyma. Bacterial tracheitis may be a complication of viral croup rather than a distinct disease. If associated with *S. aureus,* toxic shock syndrome can develop. Bacterial tracheitis can produce a two-phased illness, with the second phase associated with high fever, toxicity, and airway obstruction. Alternatively, the onset of tracheitis occurs without a second phase and appears as continued but higher fever and worsening respiratory distress rather than the usual recovery after 2-3 days of viral croup. Pneumonia, cervical lymphadenitis, otitis media, or, rarely, meningitis or septic arthritis can occur in the course of epiglottitis. Mediastinal emphysema and pneumothorax are the most common complications of tracheotomy.

TREATMENT

The mainstay of treatment for children with **croup** is airway management and treatment of hypoxia. Treatment of the respiratory distress should take priority over any testing. Most children with either acute spasmodic croup or infectious croup can be managed safely at home. Despite the observation that cold night air is beneficial, a Cochrane review has found no evidence supporting the use of cool mist in the emergency department for the treatment of croup. Children with both wheezing and croup can experience worsening of their bronchospasm with cool mist.

Nebulized racemic epinephrine is an accepted treatment for moderate or severe croup. The mechanism of action is believed to be constriction of the precapillary arterioles through the β-adrenergic receptors, causing fluid resorption from the interstitial space and a decrease in the laryngeal mucosal edema. Traditionally, racemic epinephrine, a 1:1 mixture of the D- and L-isomers of epinephrine, has been administered. A dose of 0.25-0.5 mL of 2.25% racemic epinephrine in 3 mL of normal saline can be used as often as every 20 min. Racemic epinephrine was initially chosen over the more active and more readily available L-epinephrine to minimize anticipated cardiovascular side effects such as tachycardia and hypertension. There is evidence that L-epinephrine (5 mL of 1:1,000 solution) is equally effective as racemic epinephrine and does not carry the risk of additional adverse effects. This information is both practical and important, because racemic epinephrine is not available outside the USA.

The indications for the administration of nebulized epinephrine include moderate to severe **stridor at rest,** the possible need for intubation, respiratory distress, and hypoxia. The duration of activity of racemic epinephrine is <2 hr. Therefore, observation is mandated. The symptoms of croup might reappear, but racemic epinephrine does not cause rebound worsening of the obstruction. Patients can be safely discharged home after a 2-3 hr period of observation provided they have no stridor at rest; have normal air entry, normal pulse oximetry, and normal level of consciousness; and have received steroids (see later). Nebulized epinephrine should still be used cautiously in patients with tachycardia, heart conditions such as tetralogy of Fallot, or ventricular outlet obstruction because of possible side effects.

The effectiveness of oral corticosteroids in viral croup is well established. Corticosteroids decrease the edema in the laryngeal mucosa through their anti-inflammatory action. Oral steroids are beneficial, even in mild croup, as measured by reduced hospitalization, shorter duration of hospitalization, and reduced need for subsequent interventions such as epinephrine administration. Most studies that demonstrated the efficacy of oral dexamethasone used a *single dose of 0.6 mg/kg*; a dose as low as 0.15 mg/kg may be just as effective. Intramuscular dexamethasone and nebulized budesonide have an equivalent clinical effect; oral dosing of dexamethasone is as effective as intramuscular administration. A single dose of oral prednisolone is less effective. There are no controlled studies examining the effectiveness of multiple doses of corticosteroids. The only adverse effect in the treatment of croup with corticosteroids is the development of *Candida albicans* laryngotracheitis in a patient who received dexamethasone, 1 mg/kg/24 hr, for 8 days. Corticosteroids should not be administered to children with varicella or tuberculosis (unless the patient is receiving appropriate antituberculosis therapy) because they worsen the clinical course.

Antibiotics are not indicated in croup. Over-the-counter cough and cold medications should not be used in children <4 yr of age. A helium-oxygen mixture (Heliox) may be effective in children with severe croup for whom intubation is being considered. Children with croup should be hospitalized for any of the following: progressive stridor, severe stridor at rest, respiratory distress, hypoxia, cyanosis, depressed mental status, poor oral intake, or the need for reliable observation.

Epiglottitis is a medical emergency and warrants immediate treatment with an **artificial airway** placed under controlled conditions, either in an operating room or intensive care unit. All patients should receive oxygen en route unless the mask causes excessive agitation. Racemic epinephrine and corticosteroids are ineffective. Cultures of blood, epiglottic surface, and, in selected cases, cerebrospinal fluid should be collected after the airway is stabilized. *Ceftriaxone, cefotaxime,* or *meropenum* should be given parenterally, pending culture and susceptibility reports, because 10-40% of *H. influenzae* type b cases are resistant to ampicillin. After insertion of the artificial airway, the patient should improve immediately, and respiratory distress and cyanosis should disappear. Epiglottitis resolves after a few days of antibiotics, and the patient may be extubated; antibiotics should be continued for 7-10 days. Chemoprophylaxis is not routinely recommended for household, child-care, or nursery contacts of patients with invasive *H. influenzae* type b infections, but careful observation is mandatory, with prompt medical evaluation when exposed children develop a febrile illness. **Indications for rifampin prophylaxis** (20 mg/kg orally once a day for 4 days; maximum dose, 600 mg) for all household members are any contact <48 mo of age who is incompletely immunized, any contact <12 mo who has not received the primary vaccination series, or an immunocompromised child in the household.

Acute laryngeal swelling on an allergic basis responds to epinephrine (1:1,000 dilution in dosage of 0.01 mL/kg to a maximum of 0.5 mL/dose) administered intramuscularly or racemic epinephrine (dose of 0.5 mL of 2.25% racemic epinephrine in 3 mL of normal saline) (Chapter 143). Corticosteroids are often required (2-4 mg/kg/24 hr of prednisone). After recovery, the patient and parents should be discharged with a preloaded syringe of epinephrine to be used in emergencies. Reactive mucosal swelling, severe stridor, and respiratory distress unresponsive to mist therapy may follow endotracheal intubation for general anesthesia in children. Racemic epinephrine and corticosteroids are helpful.

Tracheotomy and Endotracheal Intubation

With the introduction of routine nasotracheal intubation or, less often, tracheotomy for epiglottitis, the mortality rate for epiglottis has dropped to almost zero. Both procedures should always be performed in an operating room or intensive care unit if time permits; prior intubation and general anesthesia greatly facilitate performing a tracheotomy without complications. The use of a nasotracheal tube that is 0.5-1.0 mm smaller than estimated by age is recommended to facilitate intubation and reduce long-term sequelae. The choice of procedure should be based on the local expertise and experience with the procedure and the postoperative care involved with each.

Endotracheal intubation or tracheotomy is required for most patients with bacterial tracheitis and all young patients with epiglottitis. It is rarely required for patients with laryngotracheobronchitis, spasmodic croup, or laryngitis. Severe forms of laryngotracheobronchitis that require intubation in a high proportion of patients have been reported during severe measles and influenza A virus epidemics. Assessing the need for these procedures requires experience and judgment because they should not be delayed until cyanosis and extreme restlessness have developed (Chapter 65).

The endotracheal tube or tracheostomy must remain in place until edema and spasm have subsided and the patient is able to handle secretions satisfactorily. It should be removed as soon as possible, usually within a few days. Adequate resolution of epiglottic inflammation that has been accurately confirmed by fiberoptic laryngoscopy, permitting much more rapid extubation, often occurs within 24 hr. Racemic epinephrine and dexamethasone (0.5 mg/kg/dose every 6 hr as needed) may be useful in the treatment of croup associated with extubation.

PROGNOSIS

In general, the length of hospitalization and the mortality rate for cases of acute infectious upper airway obstruction increase as the infection extends to involve a greater portion of the respiratory tract, except in epiglottitis, in which the localized infection itself can prove to be fatal. Most deaths from croup are caused by a laryngeal obstruction or by the complications of tracheotomy. Rarely, fatal out-of-hospital arrests due to viral laryngotracheobronchitis have been reported, particularly in infants and in patients whose course has been complicated by bacterial tracheitis. Untreated epiglottitis has a mortality rate of 6% in some series, but if the diagnosis is made and appropriate treatment is initiated before the patient is moribund, the prognosis is excellent. The outcome of acute laryngotracheobronchitis, laryngitis, and spasmodic croup is also excellent. As a group, children who need to be hospitalized for croup have somewhat increased bronchial reactivity compared with normal children when tested several yr later, but the significance is uncertain.

BIBLIOGRAPHY

Please visit the Nelson Textbook of Pediatrics *website at www.expertconsult.com for the complete bibliography.*

377.2 Bacterial Tracheitis

Genie E. Roosevelt

Bacterial tracheitis is an acute bacterial infection of the upper airway that is potentially life threatening. *Staphylococcus aureus* is the most commonly isolated pathogen. *Moraxella catarrhalis,* nontypable *H. influenzae,* and anaerobic organisms have also been implicated. The mean age is between 5 and 7 yr. Incidence and severity do not differ by sex. Bacterial tracheitis often follows a viral respiratory infection (especially laryngotracheitis), so it may be considered a bacterial complication of a viral disease, rather than a primary bacterial illness. This life-threatening entity is more common than epiglottitis in vaccinated populations.

CLINICAL MANIFESTATIONS

Typically, the child has a brassy cough, apparently as part of a viral laryngotracheobronchitis. High fever and "toxicity" with respiratory distress can occur immediately or after a few days of apparent improvement. The patient can lie flat, does not drool, and does not have the dysphagia associated with epiglottitis. The usual treatment for croup (racemic epinephrine) is ineffective. Intubation or tracheostomy may be necessary, but only 50-60% of patients require intubation for management; younger patients are more likely to need intubation. The major pathologic feature appears to be mucosal swelling at the level of the cricoid cartilage, complicated by copious, thick, purulent secretions, sometimes causing pseudomembranes. Suctioning these secretions, although occasionally affording temporary relief, usually does not sufficiently obviate the need for an artificial airway.

DIAGNOSIS

The diagnosis is based on evidence of bacterial upper airway disease, which includes high fever, purulent airway secretions, and an absence of the classic findings of epiglottitis. X-rays are not needed but can show the classic findings (Fig. 377-3); purulent material is noted below the cords during endotracheal intubation (Fig. 377-4).

TREATMENT

Appropriate antimicrobial therapy, which usually includes antistaphylococcal agents, should be instituted in any patient whose

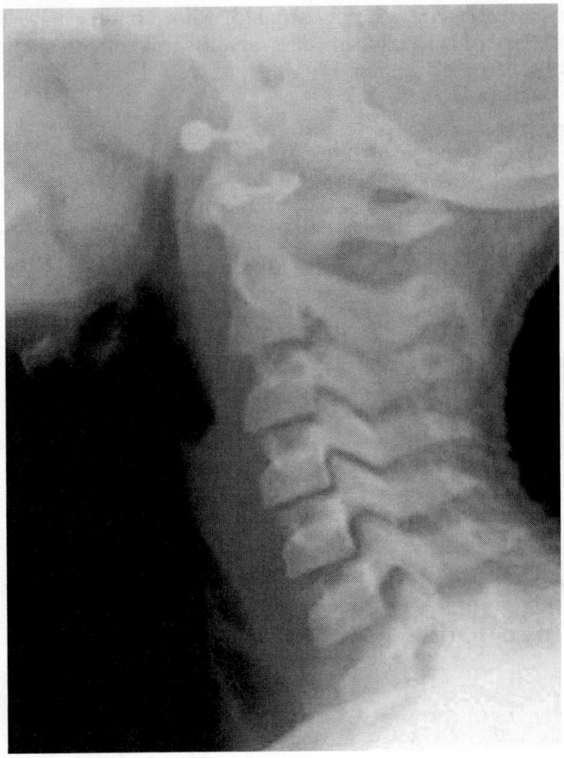

Figure 377-3 Lateral radiograph of the neck of a patient with bacterial tracheitis, showing pseudomembrane detachment in the trachea. (From Stroud RH, Friedman NR: An update on inflammatory disorders of the pediatric airway: epiglottitis, croup, and tracheitis, *Am J Otolaryngol* 22:268–275, 2001. Photo courtesy of the Department of Radiology, University of Texas Medical Branch at Galveston.)

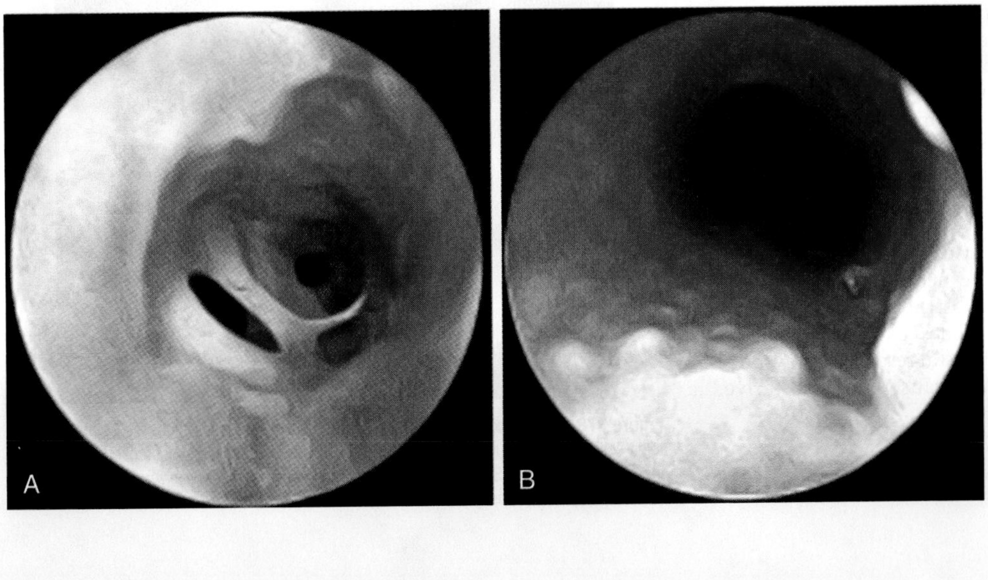

Figure 377-4 Thick tracheal membranes seen on rigid bronchoscopy. The supraglottis was normal. *A,* Thick adherent membranous secretions. *B,* The distal tracheobronchial tree is unremarkable. In contrast to croup, tenacious secretions are seen throughout the trachea, and in contrast to bronchitis, the bronchi are not affected. (From Salamone FN, Bobbitt DB, Myer CM, et al: Bacterial tracheitis reexamined: is there a less severe manifestation? *Otolaryngol Head Neck Surg* 131:871–876, 2004. © 2004 American Academy of Otolaryngology—Head and Neck Surgery Foundation, Inc.)

course suggests bacterial tracheitis. Current empiric therapy recommendations for life-threatening infections such as bacterial tracheitis include vancomycin and a β-lactamase–resistant β-lactam antimicrobial agent (e.g., naficillin or oxacillin). When bacterial tracheitis is diagnosed by direct laryngoscopy or is strongly suspected on clinical grounds, an artificial airway should be strongly considered. Supplemental oxygen is usually necessary.

COMPLICATIONS

Chest radiographs often show patchy infiltrates and can show focal densities. Subglottic narrowing and a rough and ragged tracheal air column can often be demonstrated radiographically. If airway management is not optimal, cardiorespiratory arrest can occur. Toxic shock syndrome has been associated with staphylococcal tracheitis (Chapter 174.2).

PROGNOSIS

The prognosis for most patients is excellent. Patients usually become afebrile within 2-3 days of the institution of appropriate antimicrobial therapy, but prolonged hospitalization may be necessary. In recent years, there appears to be a trend toward a less-morbid condition. With a decrease in mucosal edema and purulent secretions, extubation can be accomplished safely, and the patient should be observed carefully while antibiotics and oxygen therapy are continued.

BIBLIOGRAPHY

Please visit the Nelson Textbook of Pediatrics *website at www.expertconsult.com for the complete bibliography.*

Chapter 378
Congenital Anomalies of the Larynx, Trachea, and Bronchi

Lauren D. Holinger

Because the larynx functions as a breathing passage, a valve to protect the lungs, and the primary organ of communication, symptoms of laryngeal anomalies are those of airway obstruction, difficulty feeding, and abnormalities of phonation (Chapter 365). Obstruction of the pharyngeal airway (due to enlarged tonsils, adenoids, tongue, or syndromes with midface hypoplasia) typically produces worse obstruction during sleep than during waking. Obstruction that is worse when awake is typically laryngeal, tracheal, or bronchial and is exacerbated by exertion. Congenital anomalies of the trachea and bronchi can create serious respiratory difficulties from the first minutes of life. Intrathoracic lesions typically cause **expiratory** wheezing and stridor, often masquerading as asthma. The expiratory wheezing contrasts to the **inspiratory** stridor caused by the extrathoracic lesions of congenital laryngeal anomalies, specifically laryngomalacia and bilateral vocal cord paralysis.

With airway obstruction, the severity of the obstructing lesion, the work of breathing, determines the necessity for diagnostic procedures and surgical intervention. Obstructive symptoms vary from mild to severe stridor with episodes of apnea, cyanosis, suprasternal (tracheal tugging) and subcostal retractions, dyspnea, and tachypnea. Chronic obstruction can cause failure to thrive.

BIBLIOGRAPHY

Please visit the Nelson Textbook of Pediatrics *website at www.expertconsult.com for the complete bibliography.*

378.1 Laryngomalacia

Lauren D. Holinger

CLINICAL MANIFESTATIONS

Laryngomalacia is the most common congenital laryngeal anomaly and the most common cause of stridor in infants and children. Sixty percent of congenital laryngeal anomalies in children with stridor are due to laryngomalacia. Stridor is inspiratory, low-pitched, and exacerbated by any exertion: crying, agitation, or feeding. Stridor results from the collapse of supraglottic structures inwards during inspiration. Symptoms usually appear within the first 2 wk of life and increase in severity for up to 6 mo, although gradual improvement can begin at any time. Laryngopharyngeal reflux is commonly associated with laryngomalacia.

DIAGNOSIS

The diagnosis is confirmed by outpatient flexible laryngoscopy (Fig. 378-1). When the work of breathing is moderate to severe, airway films and chest radiographs are indicated. With associated dysphagia, a contrast swallow study and esophagram may be considered. Because 15-60% of infants with laryngomalacia have synchronous airway anomalies, complete bronchoscopy is undertaken for patients with moderate to severe obstruction.

TREATMENT

Expectant observation is suitable for most infants because most symptoms resolve spontaneously as the child and airway grow. Laryngopharyngeal reflux is managed aggressively. For the few patients who have such severe obstruction that surgical intervention is unavoidable (patients with apparent life-threatening events, cor pulmonale, cyanosis, failure to thrive) endoscopic supraglottoplasty can be used to avoid tracheotomy.

BIBLIOGRAPHY

Please visit the Nelson Textbook of Pediatrics *website at www.expertconsult.com for the complete bibliography.*

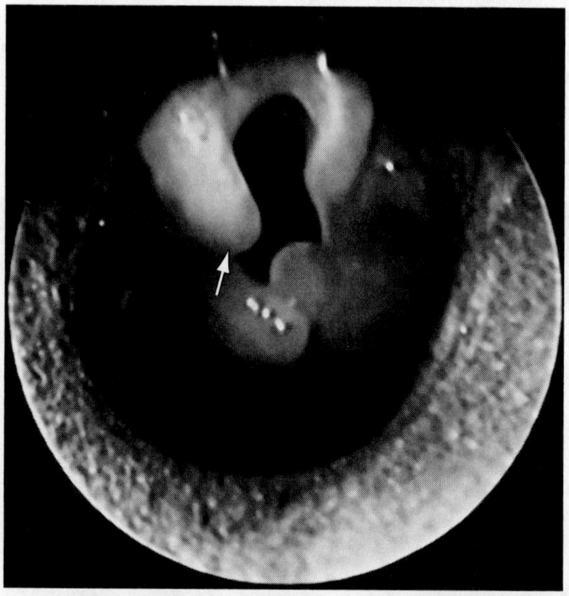

Figure 378-1 Endoscopic example of laryngomalacia. On inspiration, the epiglottic folds collapse into the airway. The lateral tips of the epiglottis are also collapsing inward *(arrow)*. (From Slovis TL, editor: *Caffey's pediatric diagnostic imaging,* ed 11, Philadelphia, 2008, Mosby.)

378.2 Congenital Subglottic Stenosis

Lauren D. Holinger

CLINICAL MANIFESTATIONS

Congenital subglottic stenosis is the 2nd most common cause of stridor. Stridor is biphasic or primarily inspiratory. Recurrent or persistent croup is typical. First symptoms often occur with a respiratory tract infection as the edema and thickened secretions of a common cold narrow an already compromised airway.

DIAGNOSIS

The diagnosis made by airway radiographs is confirmed by direct laryngoscopy. As with all cases of upper airway obstruction, tracheostomy is avoided when possible. Dilation and endoscopic laser surgery are rarely effective because most congenital stenoses are cartilaginous. Anterior laryngotracheal decompression (cricoid split) or laryngotracheal reconstruction with cartilage grafting is usually effective in avoiding tracheostomy. The differential diagnosis includes other anatomic anomalies as well as a hemangioma or papillomatosis.

BIBLIOGRAPHY

Please visit the Nelson Textbook of Pediatrics *website at www.expertconsult.com for the complete bibliography.*

378.3 Vocal Cord Paralysis

Lauren D. Holinger

CLINICAL MANIFESTATIONS

Vocal cord paralysis is the 3rd most common congenital laryngeal anomaly that produces stridor in infants and children. Congenital central nervous system lesions such as myelomeningocele, Arnold-Chiari malformation, and hydrocephalus may be associated with bilateral paralysis.

Unilateral paralysis may be a result of recurrent laryngeal nerve injury following surgical management of congenital cardiac anomalies or tracheoesophageal fistula.

Bilateral vocal cord paralysis produces airway obstruction manifested by high-pitched inspiratory stridor: a phonatory sound or inspiratory cry. Unilateral paralysis causes aspiration, coughing, and choking; the cry is weak and breathy, but stridor and other symptoms of airway obstruction are less common.

DIAGNOSIS

The diagnosis of vocal cord paralysis is made by awake flexible laryngoscopy. A thorough investigation for the underlying primary cause is indicated. Because of the association with other congenital lesions, evaluation includes neurology and cardiology consultations as well as diagnostic endoscopy of the larynx, trachea, and bronchi.

TREATMENT

Vocal cord paralysis in infants usually resolves spontaneously within 6-12 mo. Bilateral paralysis can require temporary tracheotomy. For unilateral vocal cord paralysis with aspiration, injection laterally to the paralyzed vocal cord moves it medially to reduce aspiration and related complications.

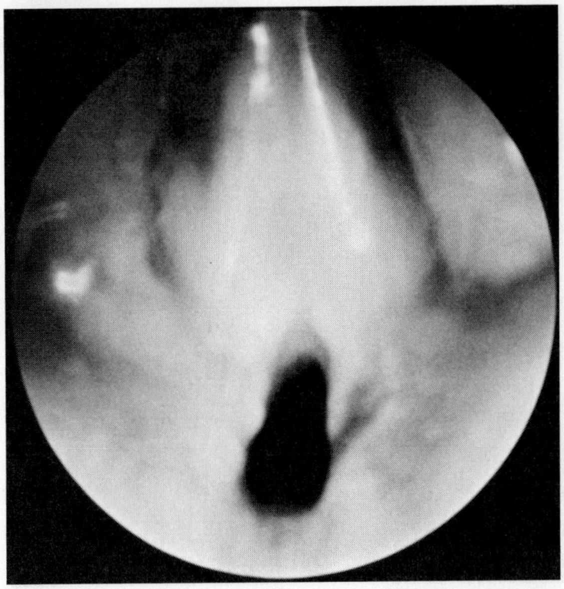

Figure 378-2 Anterior glottic web. Most of the membranous true vocal cords are involved. (From Milczuk HA, Smith JD, Evans EC: Congenital laryngeal webs: surgical management and clinical embryology, *Int J Pediatr Otorhionlaryngol* 52(1):1–9, 2000.)

378.4 Congenital Laryngeal Webs and Atresia

Lauren D. Holinger

Most congenital laryngeal webs are glottic with subglottic extension and associated subglottic stenosis. Airway obstruction is not always present and may be related to the subglottic stenosis. Thick webs may be suspected in lateral radiographs of the airway. Diagnosis is made by direct laryngoscopy (Fig. 378-2). Treatment might require only incision or dilation. Webs with associated subglottic stenosis are likely to require cartilage augmentation of the cricoid cartilage (laryngotracheal reconstruction). Laryngeal atresia occurs as a complete glottic web and commonly is associated with tracheal agenesis and tracheoesophageal fistula.

378.5 Congenital Subglottic Hemangioma

Lauren D. Holinger

Symptoms of airway obstruction typically occur within the 1st 2 mo. of life. Stridor is biphasic but usually more prominent during inspiration. A barking cough, hoarseness, and symptoms of recurrent or persistent croup are typical. A facial hemangioma is not always present, but when it is evident, it is in the beard distribution. Chest and neck radiographs can show the characteristic asymmetric narrowing of the subglottic larynx. Treatment is discussed in Chapter 382.3.

BIBLIOGRAPHY

Please visit the Nelson Textbook of Pediatrics *website at www.expertconsult.com for the complete bibliography.*

378.6 Laryngoceles and Saccular Cysts

Lauren D. Holinger

A laryngocele is an abnormal air-filled dilation of the laryngeal saccule. It communicates with the laryngeal lumen and, when intermittently filled with air, causes hoarseness and dyspnea. A saccular cyst (congenital cyst of the larynx) is distinguished from the laryngocele in that its lumen is isolated from the interior of

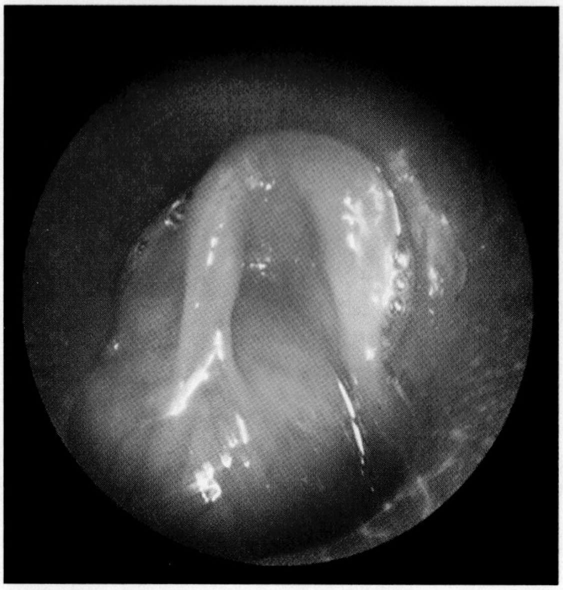

Figure 378-3 Endoscopic photograph of a saccular cyst. (From Ahmad SM, Soliman AMS: Congenital anomalies of the larynx, *Otolaryngol Clin North Am* 40:177–191, 2007, Fig 3.)

the larynx and it contains mucus, not air. A saccular cyst may be visible on radiography, but the diagnosis is made by laryngoscopy (Fig. 378-3). Needle aspiration of the cyst confirms the diagnosis but rarely provides a cure. Approaches include endoscopic CO_2 laser excision, endoscopic extended ventriculotomy, or, traditionally, external excision.

BIBLIOGRAPHY

Please visit the Nelson Textbook of Pediatrics *website at* *www.expertconsult.com* *for the complete bibliography.*

378.7 Posterior Laryngeal Cleft and Laryngotracheoesophageal Cleft

Lauren D. Holinger

The posterior laryngeal cleft (PLC) is characterized by aspiration and is due to a deficiency in the midline of the posterior larynx. In severe cases the cleft extends inferiorly into the cervical or thoracic trachea so there is no separation between the trachea and esophagus, creating a laryngotracheoesophageal cleft (LTEC). Laryngeal clefts can occur in families and are likely to be associated with tracheal agenesis, tracheoesophageal fistula, and multiple congenital anomalies, as with G syndrome, Opitz-Frias syndrome, and Pallister-Hall syndrome.

Initial symptoms are those of aspiration and respiratory difficulties. Esophagogram is undertaken with extreme caution. Confirmation of the diagnosis is made by direct laryngoscopy and bronchoscopy. Stabilization of the airway is the 1st priority. Gastroesophageal reflux must be controlled and a careful assessment for other congenital anomalies is undertaken before repair.

BIBLIOGRAPHY

Please visit the Nelson Textbook of Pediatrics *website at* *www.expertconsult.com* *for the complete bibliography.*

378.8 Vascular and Cardiac Anomalies

Lauren D. Holinger

The aberrant innominate artery is the most common cause of secondary tracheomalacia (Chapter 426). Expiratory wheezing and cough occur and, rarely, reflex apnea or "dying spells." Surgical intervention is rarely necessary. Infants are treated expectantly because the problem is self-limited.

The term *vascular ring* is used to describe vascular anomalies that result from abnormal development of the aortic arch complex. The double aortic arch is the most common complete vascular ring, encircling both the trachea and esophagus, compressing both. With few exceptions, these patients are symptomatic by 3 mo of age. Respiratory symptoms predominate, but dysphagia may be present. The diagnosis is established by barium esophagram that shows a posterior indentation of the esophagus by the vascular ring (Fig. 426-2). CT scan with contrast or MRI with angiography provides the surgeon the information needed (Chapter 426).

Other vascular anomalies include the pulmonary artery sling, which also requires surgical correction. The most common open (incomplete) vascular ring is the aberrant right subclavian artery. Although common, it is usually asymptomatic and of academic interest only.

Congenital cardiac defects are likely to compress the left main bronchus or lower trachea. Any condition that produces significant pulmonary hypertension increases the size of the pulmonary arteries, which in turn cause compression of the left main bronchus. Surgical correction of the underlying pathology to relieve pulmonary hypertension relieves the airway compression.

BIBLIOGRAPHY

Please visit the Nelson Textbook of Pediatrics *website at* *www.expertconsult.com* *for the complete bibliography.*

378.9 Tracheal Stenoses, Webs, and Atresia

Lauren D. Holinger

Long-segment congenital tracheal stenosis with complete tracheal rings typically occurs within the 1st yr of life, usually after a crisis has been precipitated by an acute respiratory illness. The diagnosis may be suggested by plain radiographs. CT with contrast delineates associated intrathoracic anomalies such as the pulmonary artery sling, which occurs in one third of patients; one fourth have associated cardiac anomalies. Bronchoscopy is the best method to define the degree and extent of the stenosis and the associated abnormal bronchial branching pattern. Treatment of clinically significant stenosis involves tracheal resection of short segment stenosis, slide tracheoplasty for long segment stenosis. Congenital soft tissue stenoses and thin webs are rare. Dilation may be all that is required.

378.10 Foregut Cysts

Lauren D. Holinger

The bronchogenic cyst, intramural esophageal cyst (esophageal duplication), and enteric cyst can all produce symptoms of respiratory obstruction and dysphagia. The diagnosis is suspected when chest radiographs or CT scan delineate the mass, and, in the case of enteric cyst, the associated vertebral anomaly. The treatment of all foregut cysts is surgical excision.

378.11 Tracheomalacia and Bronchomalacia

(See Chapter 381).

Chapter 379
Foreign Bodies of the Airway
Lauren D. Holinger

EPIDEMIOLOGY AND ETIOLOGY

Infants and toddlers use their mouths to explore their surroundings. Most victims of foreign body aspiration are older infants and toddlers (Fig. 379-1). Children <3 yr of age account for 73% of cases. Preambulatory toddlers can aspirate objects given to them by older siblings. One third of aspirated objects are nuts, particularly peanuts. Fragments of raw carrot, apple, dried beans, popcorn, and sunflower or watermelon seeds are also aspirated, as are small toys or toy parts.

The most serious complication of foreign body aspiration is complete obstruction of the airway. Globular or round food objects such as hotdogs, grapes, nuts, and candies are the most frequent offenders. Hot dogs are rarely seen as airway foreign bodies because toddlers who choke on hot dogs asphyxiate at the scene unless treated immediately. Complete airway obstruction is recognized in the conscious child as sudden respiratory distress followed by inability to speak or cough.

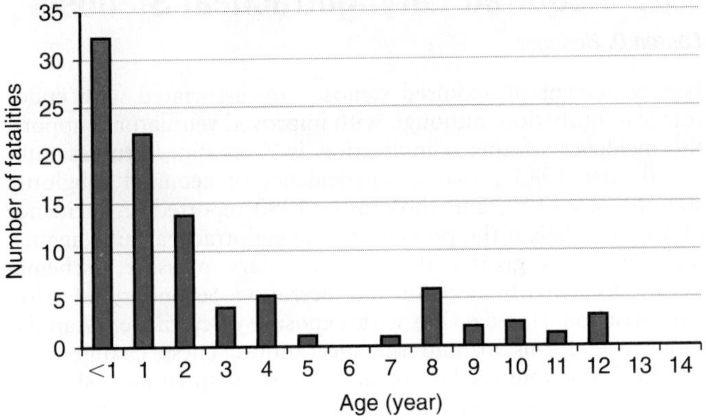

Figure 379-1 Number of fatalities vs victim age, all fatalities. (From Milkovich SM, Altkorn R, Chen X, et al: Development of the small parts cylinder: lessons learned, *Laryngoscope* 118[11]:2082–2086, 2008.)

CLINICAL MANIFESTATIONS

Three stages of symptoms may result from aspiration of an object into the airway:

1. Initial event: Violent paroxysms of coughing, choking, gagging, and possibly airway obstruction occur immediately when the foreign body is aspirated.
2. Asymptomatic interval: The foreign body becomes lodged, reflexes fatigue, and the immediate irritating symptoms subside. This stage is most treacherous and accounts for a large percentage of delayed diagnoses and overlooked foreign bodies. It is during this 2nd stage, when the child is first seen, that the possibility of a foreign body aspiration is minimized, the physician being reassured by the absence of symptoms that no foreign body is present.
3. Complications: Obstruction, erosion, or infection develops to direct attention again to the presence of a foreign body. In this 3rd stage, complications include fever, cough, hemoptysis, pneumonia, and atelectasis.

DIAGNOSIS

A positive history must never be ignored. A negative history may be misleading. Choking or coughing episodes accompanied by wheezing are highly suggestive of an airway foreign body. Because nuts are the most common bronchial foreign body, the physician specifically questions the toddler's parents about nuts. If there is any history of eating nuts, bronchoscopy is carried out promptly.

Most airway foreign bodies lodge in a bronchus (right bronchus ~58% of cases); the location is the larynx or trachea in ~10% of cases. An esophageal foreign body can compress the trachea and be mistaken for an airway foreign body. The patient is asymptomatic and the radiograph is normal in 15-30% of cases. Opaque foreign bodies occur in only 10-25% of cases. CT can help define radiolucent foreign bodies such as fish bones. If there is a high index of suspicion, bronchoscopy should be performed despite negative imaging studies. History is the most important factor in determining the need for bronchoscopy.

TREATMENT

The treatment of choice for airway foreign bodies is prompt endoscopic removal with rigid instruments. Bronchoscopy is deferred only until preoperative studies have been obtained and the patient has been prepared by adequate hydration and

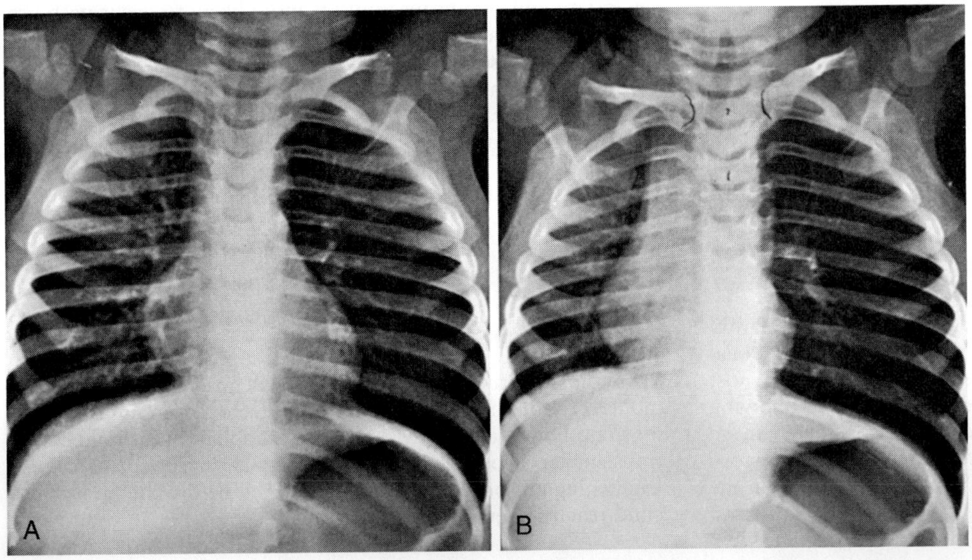

Figure 379-2 *A,* Normal inspiratory chest radiograph in a toddler with a peanut fragment in the left main bronchus. *B,* Expiratory radiograph of the same child showing the classic obstructive emphysema (air trapping) on the involved (left) side. Air leaves the normal right side allowing the lung to deflate. The medium shifts toward the unobstructed side.

emptying of the stomach. Airway foreign bodies are usually removed the same day the diagnosis is first considered.

379.1 Laryngeal Foreign Bodies

Lauren D. Holinger

Complete obstruction asphyxiates the child unless it is promptly relieved with the Heimlich maneuver (Chapter 62 and Figs. 62-6 and 62-7). Objects that are partially obstructive are usually flat and thin. They lodge between the vocal cords in the sagittal plane, causing symptoms of croup, hoarseness, cough, stridor, and dyspnea.

379.2 Tracheal Foreign Bodies

Lauren D. Holinger

Choking and aspiration occurs in 90% of patients with tracheal foreign bodies, stridor in 60%, and wheezing in 50%. Posteroanterior and lateral soft tissue neck radiographs (airway films) are abnormal in 92% of children, whereas chest radiographs are abnormal in only 58%.

379.3 Bronchial Foreign Bodies

Lauren D. Holinger

Radiologic evaluation—posteroanterior and lateral chest radiographs—are standard in the assessment of infants and children suspected of having aspirated a foreign object. The abdomen is included. A good expiratory posteroanterior chest film is most helpful. During expiration the bronchial foreign body obstructs the exit of air from the obstructed lung, producing obstructive emphysema, air trapping, with persistent inflation of the obstructed lung and shift of the mediastinum toward the opposite side (Fig. 379-2). Air trapping is an immediate complication, in contrast to atelectasis, which is a late finding. Lateral decubitus chest films or fluoroscopy can provide the same information but are unnecessary. History and physical examination, not radiographs, determine the indication for bronchoscopy.

BIBLIOGRAPHY

Please visit the Nelson Textbook of Pediatrics *website at www.expertconsult.com for the complete bibliography.*

Chapter 380 Laryngotracheal Stenosis and Subglottic Stenosis

Lauren D. Holinger

Laryngotracheal stenosis is the most common cause of airway obstruction requiring tracheostomy in infants. The glottis (vocal cords) and the upper trachea are also compromised in most laryngeal stenoses, particularly those that develop following endotracheal intubation. Subglottic stenosis is considered to be congenital when there is no other apparent cause such as a history of laryngeal trauma; approximately 90% of cases manifest in the 1st yr of life.

380.1 Congenital Subglottic Stenosis

Lauren D. Holinger

CLINICAL MANIFESTATIONS

Biphasic or primarily inspiratory stridor is the typical presenting symptom for congenital subglottic stenosis. Recurrent or persistent croup usually occurs in these children at 6 mo of age or younger. The edema associated with an upper respiratory tract infection or laryngopharyngeal reflux events compromises the underlying narrowed airway.

TREATMENT

Treatment is dictated by the severity of the obstruction and is the same as acquired subglottic stenosis. Because most cases of congenital stenosis are cartilaginous, dilatation or laser surgery are not uniformly effective. Anterior laryngotracheal decompression (cricoid split) or laryngotracheal reconstruction with cartilage grafting usually avoids tracheostomy.

BIBLIOGRAPHY

Please visit the Nelson Textbook of Pediatrics *website at www.expertconsult.com for the complete bibliography.*

380.2 Acquired Laryngotracheal Stenosis

Lauren D. Holinger

Ninety percent of acquired stenoses are associated with endotracheal intubation, although with improved ventilatory support, the incidence of this complication is decreasing. Studies published after 1983 reported an incidence of neonatal subglottic stenosis of <4.0%, and those after 1990 reported an incidence of <0.63%. When the pressure of the endotracheal tube against the mucosa is greater than the capillary pressure, ischemia occurs, followed by necrosis and ulceration. Secondary infection and perichondritis develop with exposure of cartilage. Granulation tissue forms around the ulcerations. These changes and edema throughout the larynx usually resolve spontaneously after extubation. Chronic edema and fibrous stenosis develop in only a small percentage of cases. A number of factors predispose to the development of laryngeal stenosis. Laryngopharyngeal reflux of acid and pepsin from the stomach exacerbates endotracheal tube trauma. More damage is caused in areas left unprotected, owing to loss of mucosa. Congenital subglottic stenosis narrows the larynx and significant injury is more likely to occur with use of an endotracheal tube of age-appropriate size. Other patient factors include sepsis and infection, dehydration, malnutrition, chronic inflammatory disorders, and immunosuppression. An oversized endotracheal tube is the most common factor contributing to laryngeal injury. A tube that allows a small air leak at the end of the inspiratory cycle minimizes potential trauma. Other extrinsic factors—traumatic intubation, multiple reintubations, movement of the endotracheal tube, and duration of intubation—can contribute to varying degrees in individual patients.

CLINICAL MANIFESTATIONS

Symptoms of acquired and congenital stenosis are similar. Spasmodic croup, the sudden onset of severe croup in the early morning hours, is usually due to laryngopharyngeal reflux with transient laryngospasm and subsequent laryngeal edema. These frightening episodes resolve rapidly, often before the family and child reach the emergency department.

DIAGNOSIS

The diagnosis is confirmed by direct laryngoscopy and bronchoscopy. High-resolution CT imaging is of limited value.

TREATMENT

The severity, location, and type (cartilaginous or soft tissue) of the stenosis determine the treatment. Mild cases can be managed without operative intervention because the airway will improve as the child grows. Moderate soft tissue stenosis is treated by endoscopy using gentle dilations or CO_2 laser. Severe laryngotracheal stenosis is likely to require laryngotracheal expansion surgery or resection of the narrowed portion of the laryngeal and tracheal airway (partial cricotracheal resection). Every effort is made to avoid tracheotomy using endoscopic techniques or open surgical procedures.

BIBLIOGRAPHY

Please visit the Nelson Textbook of Pediatrics *website at www.expertconsult.com for the complete bibliography.*

Chapter 381
Bronchomalacia and Tracheomalacia

Jonathan D. Finder

Chondromalacias of the trachea or of a main bronchus occur when there is insufficient cartilage to maintain airway patency throughout the respiratory cycle and are common causes of persistent wheezing in infancy. Tracheomalacia and bronchomalacia can be either primary or secondary (see Table 381-1 on the *Nelson Textbook of Pediatrics* website at www.expertconsult.com). Although primary tracheomalacia and bronchomalacia are often seen in premature infants, most affected patients are born at term. Secondary tracheomalacia and bronchomalacia refers to the situation in which the central airway is compressed by adjacent structure (e.g., vascular ring, Chapter 426) or deficient in cartilage due to tracheoesophageal fistula. Laryngomalacia can accompany primary bronchomalacia or tracheomalacia. Involvement of the entire central airway (laryngotracheobronchomalacia) is also seen.

For the full continuation of this chapter, please visit the Nelson Textbook of Pediatrics *website at www.expertconsult.com.*

Chapter 382
Neoplasms of the Larynx, Trachea, and Bronchi

382.1 Vocal Nodules

Lauren D. Holinger

Vocal nodules are the most common cause of chronic hoarseness in children. They are not true neoplasms. Chronic vocal abuse or misuse produces nodules at the junction of the anterior and middle thirds of the phonating edge of the vocal cords. These symmetric, bilateral swellings interfere with voice production and cause children to strain the voice. Vocal nodules can occur in infants and are exacerbated by laryngopharyngeal reflux.

For the full continuation of this chapter, please visit the Nelson Textbook of Pediatrics *website at www.expertconsult.com.*

382.2 Recurrent Respiratory Papillomatosis

Lauren D. Holinger

Papillomas are the most common respiratory tract neoplasms in children, occurring in 4.3/100,000. They are simply warts—benign tumors—caused by the human papillomavirus (HPV) (Chapter 258); the same pathology is found in condylomata acuminata (vaginal warts). HPV types 6 and 11 are most commonly associated with laryngeal disease. Fifty percent of recurrent respiratory papillomatosis (RRP) cases occur in children <5 yr, but the diagnosis may be made at any age; 67% of children with RRP are born to mothers who had condylomata during pregnancy or parturition. The risk for transmission is ~1/500 vaginal births in mothers with active condylomata. Neonates have been reported to have RRP, suggesting intrauterine transmission of HPV.

For the full continuation of this chapter, please visit the Nelson Textbook of Pediatrics *website at www.expertconsult.com.*

382.3 Congenital Subglottic Hemangioma

Lauren D. Holinger

CLINICAL MANIFESTATIONS

Typically, congenital subglottic hemangiomas are symptomatic within the 1st 2 mo of life, almost all occurring before 6 mo of age. Stridor is biphasic but usually more prominent during inspiration. The infant may be hoarse, have a barking cough, and present with croup. Fifty percent of congenital subglottic hemangiomas are associated with facial lesions. Radiographs classically delineate an asymmetric subglottic narrowing. The diagnosis is made by direct laryngoscopy.

For the full continuation of this chapter, please visit the Nelson Textbook of Pediatrics *website at www.expertconsult.com.*

382.4 Vascular Anomalies

Lauren D. Holinger

Vascular malformations are not true neoplastic lesions. They have a normal rate of endothelial turnover and various channel abnormalities. They are categorized by their predominant type (capillary, venous, arterial, lymphatic, or a combination thereof). Slow-flow malformations have capillary, lymphatic, or venous components. These incorrectly were called capillary hemangiomas, cystic hygromas or lymphangiomas, and cavernous hemangiomas, respectively.

For the full continuation of this chapter, please visit the Nelson Textbook of Pediatrics *website at www.expertconsult.com.*

382.5 Other Laryngeal Neoplasms

Lauren D. Holinger

Neurofibromatosis rarely involves the larynx. When children are affected, limited local resection is undertaken to maintain an airway and optimize the voice. Complete surgical extirpation is virtually impossible without debilitating resection of vital laryngeal structures. Most surgeons select the option of less-aggressive symptomatic surgery because of the poorly circumscribed and infiltrative nature of these fibromas. **Rhabdomyosarcoma** and other malignant tumors of the larynx are rare. Symptoms of hoarseness and progressive airway obstruction prompt initial evaluation by flexible laryngoscopy in the office.

382.6 Tracheal Neoplasms

Lauren D. Holinger

Tracheal tumors include malignant and benign neoplasms. The two most common benign tumors are inflammatory pseudotumor and hamartoma. The **inflammatory pseudotumor** is probably a reaction to a previous bronchial infection or traumatic insult. Growth is slow and the tumor may be locally invasive. Hamartomas are tumors of primary tissue elements that are abnormal in proportion and arrangement.

For the full continuation of this chapter, please visit the Nelson Textbook of Pediatrics *website at www.expertconsult.com.*

382.7 Bronchial Tumors

Lauren D. Holinger

Bronchial tumors are rare. Two thirds are malignant. Bronchial "adenomas" are the most common, representing 30% of all lung tumors. Bronchogenic carcinoma is the second most common and occurs in approximately 20% of cases. Bronchial carcinoid also occurs. The diagnosis is confirmed at bronchoscopy and biopsy; treatment depends on the histopathology.

Chapter 383 Wheezing, Bronchiolitis, and Bronchitis

383.1 Wheezing in Infants: Bronchiolitis

Kimberly Danieli Watts and Denise M. Goodman

DEFINITIONS AND GENERAL PATHOPHYSIOLOGY (SEE ALSO CHAPTER 365)

A **wheeze** is a musical and continuous sound that originates from oscillations in narrowed airways. Wheezing is heard mostly on expiration as a result of critical airway obstruction. Wheezing is **polyphonic** when there is widespread narrowing of the airways, causing various pitches or levels of obstruction to airflow as seen in asthma. **Monophonic** wheezing refers to a single-pitch sound that is produced in the larger airways during expiration, as in distal tracheomalacia or bronchomalacia. When obstruction occurs in the extrathoracic airways during inspiration, the noise is referred to as **stridor.**

Infants are prone to wheeze, owing to a differing set of lung mechanics in comparison to older children and adults. The obstruction to flow is affected by the airway caliber and compliance of the infant lung. Resistance to airflow through a tube is inversely related to the radius of the tube to the 4th power. In children <5 yr old, small-caliber peripheral airways can contribute up to 50% of the total airway resistance. Marginal additional narrowing can cause further flow limitation and a subsequent wheeze.

With the very compliant newborn chest wall, the inward pressure produced in expiration subjects the intrathoracic airways to collapse. Flow limitation is further affected in infants by the differences in tracheal cartilage composition and airway smooth muscle tone, causing further increase in airway compliance in comparison to older children. All of these mechanisms combine to make the infant more susceptible to airway collapse, increased resistance, and subsequent wheezing. Many of these conditions are outgrown in the 1st yr of life.

Immunologic and molecular influences can contribute to the infant's propensity to wheeze. In comparison to older children and adults, infants tend to have higher levels of lymphocytes and neutrophils, rather than mast cells and eosinophils, in bronchoalveolar lavage fluid. The childhood wheezing phenotype has been linked to many early exposures including fetal nutrition, maternal smoking, prenatal and birth maternal complications, prenatal and neonatal exposure to antibiotics, exposure to high levels of environmental allergens, and high infant adiposity. Infections during infancy have been cited as risk factors for later wheezing, including respiratory syncytial virus (RSV), rhinovirus, cytomegalovirus, human metapneumovirus, bocavirus, adenovirus, and *Chlamydia pneumoniae.*

A variety of inflammatory mediators have also been implicated in the wheezing infant such as histamine, cytokines, leukotrienes, and interleukins. Taken together, these fetal and/or early postnatal exposures can cause a "programming" of the lung that ultimately affects structure and function.

ETIOLOGY

Most wheezing in infants is caused by inflammation (generally bronchiolitis), but many other entities can manifest with wheezing (Table 383-1).

Acute Bronchiolitis and Inflammation of the Airway

Infection can cause obstruction to flow by internal narrowing of the airways.

Acute bronchiolitis is predominantly a viral disease. RSV is responsible for >50% of cases (Chapter 252). Other agents include parainfluenza (Chapter 251), adenovirus, and *Mycoplasma.* Emerging pathogens include human metapneumovirus (Chapter 253) and human bocavirus, which may be a primary cause of viral respiratory infection or occur as a co-infection with RSV. There is no evidence of a bacterial cause for bronchiolitis, although bacterial pneumonia is sometimes confused clinically with bronchiolitis, but bronchiolitis is rarely followed by bacterial superinfection. Concurrent infection with viral bronchiolitis and pertussis has been described.

Approximately 75,000-125,000 children <1 yr old are hospitalized annually in the United States due to RSV infection. Increasing rates of hospitalization might reflect increased attendance of infants in daycare centers, changes in criteria for hospital admission, and/or improved survival of premature infants and others at risk for severe RSV-associated disease.

Bronchiolitis is more common in boys, in those who have not been breast-fed, and in those who live in crowded conditions. Risk is higher for infants with young mothers or mothers who smoked during pregnancy. Older family members are a common source of infection; they might only experience minor upper respiratory symptoms (colds). The clinical manifestations of lower respiratory tract illness (LRTI) seen in young infants may be minimal in older patients, in whom bronchiolar edema is better tolerated.

Not all infected infants develop LRTI. Host anatomic and immunologic factors play a significant role in the severity of the clinical syndrome, as does the nature of the viral pathogen. Infants with pre-existent smaller airways and diminished lung function have a more-severe course. In addition, RSV infection incites a complex immune response. Eosinophils degranulate and

Table 383-1 DIFFERENTIAL DIAGNOSIS OF WHEEZING IN INFANCY

INFECTION
Viral
Respiratory syncytial virus (RSV) Human metapneumovirus Parainfluenza Adenovirus Influenza Rhinovirus Bocavirus
Other
Chlamydia trachomatis Tuberculosis Histoplasmosis Papillomatosis
ASTHMA
Transient wheezer • Initial risk factor is primarily diminished lung size Persistent wheezers • Initial risk factors include passive smoke exposure, maternal asthma history, and an elevated immunoglobulin E (IgE) level in the 1st year of life • At increased risk of developing clinical asthma Late-onset wheezer
ANATOMIC ABNORMALITIES
Central Airway Abnormalities
Malacia of the larynx, trachea, and/or bronchi Tracheoesophageal fistula (specifically H-type fistula) Laryngeal cleft (resulting in aspiration)
Extrinsic Airway Anomalies Resulting in Airway Compression
Vascular ring or sling Mediastinal lymphadenopathy from infection or tumor Mediastinal mass or tumor Esophageal foreign body
Intrinsic Airway Anomalies
Airway hemangioma, other tumor Cystic adenomatoid malformation Bronchial or lung cyst Congenital lobar emphysema Aberrant tracheal bronchus Sequestration Congenital heart disease with left-to-right shunt (increased pulmonary edema) Foreign body
Immunodeficiency States
Immunoglobulin A deficiency B-cell deficiencies Primary ciliary dyskinesia AIDS Bronchiectasis
MUCOCILIARY CLEARANCE DISORDERS
Cystic fibrosis Primary ciliary dyskinesias Bronchiectasis
ASPIRATION SYNDROMES
Gastroesophageal reflux disease Pharyngeal/swallow dysfunction
OTHER
Bronchopulmonary dysplasia Interstitial lung disease, including bronchiolitis obliterans Heart failure Anaphylaxis Inhalation injury—burns

release eosinophil cationic protein, which is cytotoxic to airway epithelium. Innate immunity plays a significant role and can depend on polymorphisms in toll-like receptor (TLR), interferon (IF), interleukins (IL), and nuclear factor κB (NFκB). Chemokines and cytokines such as tumor necrosis factor α (TNF-α) may be differentially expressed depending on the inciting virus. Co-infection with >1 virus can also alter the clinical manifestations and/or severity of presentation.

Acute bronchiolitis is characterized by bronchiolar obstruction with edema, mucus, and cellular debris. Even minor bronchiolar wall thickening significantly affects airflow because resistance is inversely proportional to the 4th power of the radius of the bronchiolar passage. Resistance in the small air passages is increased during both inspiration and exhalation, but because the radius of an airway is smaller during expiration, the resultant respiratory obstruction leads to early air trapping and overinflation. If obstruction becomes complete, trapped distal air will be resorbed and the child will develop atelectasis.

Hypoxemia is a consequence of ventilation-perfusion mismatch early in the course. With severe obstructive disease and tiring of respiratory effort, hypercapnia can develop.

Chronic infectious causes of wheezing should be considered in infants who seem to fall out of the range of a normal clinical course. Cystic fibrosis is one such entity; suspicion increases in a patient with persistent respiratory symptoms, digital clubbing, malabsorption, failure to thrive, electrolyte abnormalities, or a resistance to bronchodilator treatment (Chapter 395).

Allergy and asthma are important causes of wheezing and probably generate the most questions by the parents of a wheezing infant. Asthma is characterized by airway inflammation, bronchial hyperreactivity, and reversibility of obstruction (Chapter 138). Three identified patterns of infant wheezing are the transient early wheezer, the persistent wheezer, and the late-onset wheezer. Transient early wheezers constituted 19.9% of the general population, and they had wheezing at least once with a lower respiratory infection before the age of 3 yr but never wheezed again. The persistent wheezer constituted 13.7% of the general population, had wheezing episodes before age 3 yr, and were still wheezing at 6 yr of age. The late-onset wheezer constituted 15% of the general population, had no wheezing by 3 yr, but was wheezing by 6 yr. The other ½ of the children had never wheezed by 6 yr. Of all the infants who wheezed before 3 yr old, almost 60% stopped wheezing by 6 yr.

Multiple studies have tried to predict which early wheezers will go on to have asthma in later life. Risk factors for persistent wheezing include parental history of asthma and allergies, maternal smoking, persistent rhinitis (apart from acute upper respiratory tract infections), eczema at <1 yr of age, and frequent episodes of wheezing during infancy.

Other Causes

Congenital malformations of the respiratory tract cause wheezing in early infancy. These findings can be diffuse or focal and can be from an external compression or an intrinsic abnormality. *External vascular compression* includes a vascular ring, in which the trachea and esophagus are surrounded completely by vascular structures, or a vascular sling, in which the trachea and esophagus are not completely encircled (Chapter 426). *Cardiovascular causes* of wheezing include dilated chambers of the heart including massive cardiomegaly, left atrial enlargement, and dilated pulmonary arteries. Pulmonary edema caused by heart failure can also cause wheezing by lymphatic and bronchial vessel engorgement that leads to obstruction and edema of the bronchioles and further obstruction (Chapter 436).

Foreign body aspiration (Chapter 379) can cause acute or chronic wheezing. It is estimated that 78% of those who die from foreign body aspiration are between 2 mo and 4 yr old. Even in young infants, a foreign body can be ingested if given to the infant by another person such as an older sibling. Infants who have atypical histories or misleading clinical and radiologic findings can receive a misdiagnosis of asthma or another obstructive disorder as inflammation and granulation develop around the foreign body. Esophageal foreign body can transmit pressure to the membranous trachea, causing compromise of the airway lumen.

Gastroesophageal reflux (Chapter 315.1) can cause wheezing with or without direct aspiration into the tracheobronchial tree. Without aspiration, the reflux is thought to trigger a vagal or neural reflex, causing increased airway resistance and airway reactivity. Aspiration from gastroesophageal reflux or from the direct aspiration from oral liquids can also cause wheezing.

Trauma and tumors are much rarer causes of wheezing in infants. Trauma of any type to the tracheobronchial tree can cause an obstruction to airflow. Accidental or nonaccidental aspirations, burns, or scalds of the tracheobronchial tree can cause inflammation of the airways and subsequent wheezing. Any space-occupying lesion either in the lung itself or extrinsic to the lung can cause tracheobronchial compression and obstruction to airflow.

CLINICAL MANIFESTATIONS

History and Physical Examination

Initial history of a wheezing infant should include accounts of the recent event including onset, duration, and associated factors (Table 383-2). *Birth history* includes weeks of gestation, neonatal intensive care unit admission, history of intubation or oxygen requirement, maternal complications including infection with herpes simplex virus (HSV) or HIV, and prenatal smoke exposure. Past medical history includes any comorbid conditions including syndromes or associations. *Family history* of cystic fibrosis, immunodeficiencies, asthma in a 1st-degree relative, or any other recurrent respiratory conditions in children should be obtained. *Social history* should include an environmental history including any smokers at home, inside or out, daycare exposure, number of siblings, occupation of inhabitants of the home, pets, tuberculosis exposure, and concerns regarding home environment (e.g., dust mites, construction dust, heating and cooling techniques, mold, cockroaches).

On **physical examination,** evaluation of the patient's vital signs with special attention to the respiratory rate and the pulse oximetry reading for oxygen saturation is an important initial step. There should also be a thorough review of the patient's growth chart for signs of failure to thrive. Wheezing produces an expiratory whistling sound that can be polyphonic or monophonic. Expiratory time may be prolonged. Biphasic wheezing can occur if there is a central, large airway obstruction. *The lack of audible wheezing is not reassuring if the infant shows other signs of respiratory distress because complete obstruction to airflow can eliminate the turbulence that causes the sound to resonate.* Aeration should be noted and a trial of a bronchodilator may be warranted to evaluate for any change in wheezing after treatment. Listening to breath sounds over the neck helps differentiate upper airway from lower airway sounds. The absence or presence of stridor should be noted and appreciated on inspiration. Signs of respiratory distress include tachypnea, increased respiratory effort, nasal flaring, tracheal tugging, subcostal and intercostal retractions, and excessive use of accessory muscles. In the upper airway, signs of atopy, including boggy turbinates and posterior oropharynx cobblestoning, can be evaluated in older infants. It is also useful to evaluate the skin of the patient for eczema and any significant hemangiomas; midline lesions may be associated with an intrathoracic lesion. Digital clubbing should be noted (Chapter 366).

Table 383-2 PERTINENT MEDICAL HISTORY IN THE WHEEZING INFANT
Did the onset of symptoms begin at birth or thereafter?
Is the infant a noisy breather and when is it most prominent?
Is there a history of cough apart from wheezing?
Was there an earlier lower respiratory tract infection?
Have there been any emergency department visits, hospitalizations, or intensive care unit admissions for respiratory distress?
Is there a history of eczema?
Does the infant cough after crying or cough at night?
How is the infant growing and developing?
Is there associated failure to thrive?
Is there failure to thrive without feeding difficulties?
Is there a history of electrolyte abnormalities?
Are there signs of intestinal malabsorption including frequent, greasy, or oily stools?
Is there a maternal history of genital herpes simplex virus (HSV) infection?
What was the gestational age at delivery?
Was the patient intubated as a neonate?
Does the infant bottle-feed in the bed or the crib, especially in a propped position?
Are there any feeding difficulties including choking, gagging, arching, or vomiting with feeds?
Is there any new food exposure?
Is there a toddler in the home or lapse in supervision in which foreign body aspiration could have occurred?
Change in caregivers or chance of nonaccidental trauma?

Acute bronchiolitis is usually preceded by exposure to an older contact with a minor respiratory syndrome within the previous week. The infant 1st develops a mild upper respiratory tract infection with sneezing and clear rhinorrhea. This may be accompanied by diminished appetite and fever of 38.5-39°C (101-102°F), although the temperature can range from subnormal to markedly elevated. Gradually, respiratory distress ensues, with paroxysmal wheezy cough, dyspnea, and irritability. The infant is often tachypneic, which can interfere with feeding. The child does not usually have other systemic complaints, such as diarrhea or vomiting. Apnea may be more prominent than wheezing early in the course of the disease, particularly with very young infants (<2 mo old) or former premature infants.

The **physical examination** is often dominated by wheezing. The degree of tachypnea does not always correlate with the degree of hypoxemia or hypercarbia, so pulse oximetry and noninvasive determination of carbon dioxide is essential. Work of breathing may be markedly increased, with nasal flaring and retractions. Auscultation might reveal fine crackles or overt wheezes, with prolongation of the expiratory phase of breathing. Barely audible breath sounds suggest very severe disease with nearly complete bronchiolar obstruction. Hyperinflation of the lungs can permit palpation of the liver and spleen.

Diagnostic Evaluation

Initial evaluation depends on likely etiology; a baseline chest radiograph, including posteroanterior and lateral films, is warranted in many cases and for any infant in acute respiratory distress. Infiltrates are most often found in wheezing infants who have a pulse oximetry reading <93%, grunting, decreased breath sounds, prolonged inspiratory to expiratory ratio, and crackles. The chest radiograph may also be useful for evaluating hyperinflation (common in bronchiolitis and viral pneumonia), signs of chronic disease such as bronchiectasis, or a space-occupying lesion causing airway compression. A trial of bronchodilator may be diagnostic as well as therapeutic because these medications can reverse conditions such as bronchiolitis (occasionally) and asthma but will not affect a fixed obstruction. Bronchodilators potentially can worsen a case of wheezing caused by tracheal or bronchial malacia. A sweat test to evaluate for cystic fibrosis and evaluation of baseline immune status are reasonable in infants with recurrent wheezing or complicated courses. Further evaluation such as upper gastrointestinal (GI) contrast x-rays, chest CT, bronchoscopy, infant pulmonary function testing, video swallow study, and pH probe can be considered second-tier diagnostic procedures in complicated patients.

The diagnosis of **acute bronchiolitis** is clinical, particularly in a previously healthy infant presenting with a first-time wheezing episode during a community outbreak. Chest radiography can reveal hyperinflated lungs with patchy atelectasis. The white blood cell and differential counts are usually normal. Viral testing (polymerase chain reaction, rapid immunofluorescence, or viral culture) is helpful if the diagnosis is uncertain or for epidemiologic purposes. Because concurrent bacterial infection (sepsis, pneumonia, meningitis) is highly unlikely, confirmation of viral bronchiolitis can obviate the need for a sepsis evaluation in a febrile infant and assist with respiratory precautions and isolation if the patient requires hospitalization.

TREATMENT

Treatment of an infant with wheezing depends on the underlying etiology. Response to bronchodilators is unpredictable, regardless of cause, but suggests a component of bronchial hyperreactivity. It is appropriate to administer albuterol aerosol and objectively observe the response. For children <3 yr of age, it is acceptable to continue to administer inhaled medications through a metered-dose inhaler (MDI) with mask and spacer if a therapeutic benefit is demonstrated. Therapy should be continued in all patients with asthma exacerbations from a viral illness.

The use of ipratropium bromide in this population is controversial, but it appears to be somewhat effective as an adjunct therapy. It is also useful in infants with significant tracheal and bronchial malacia who may be made worse by β_2 agonists such as albuterol because of the subsequent decrease in smooth muscle tone.

A trial of inhaled steroids may be warranted in a patient who has responded to multiple courses of oral steroids and who has moderate to severe wheezing or a significant history of atopy including food allergy or eczema. Inhaled corticosteroids are appropriate for maintenance therapy in patients with known reactive airways but are controversial when used for episodic or acute illnesses. Intermittent, high-dose inhaled corticosteroids are not recommended for intermittent wheezing. Early use of inhaled corticosteroids has not been shown to prevent the progression of childhood wheezing or affect the natural history of asthma in children.

Oral steroids are generally reserved for atopic wheezing infants thought to have asthma that is refractory to other medications. Their use in first-time wheezing infants or in infants who do not warrant hospitalization is controversial.

Infants with **acute bronchiolitis** who are experiencing respiratory distress (hypoxia, inability to take oral feedings, extreme tachypnea) should be hospitalized; risk factors for severe disease include age <12 wk, preterm birth, or underlying comorbidity such as cardiovascular, pulmonary, or immunologic disease. The mainstay of treatment is supportive. Hypoxemic children should receive cool humidified oxygen. Sedatives are to be avoided because they can depress respiratory drive. The infant is sometimes more comfortable if sitting with head and chest elevated at a 30-degree angle with neck extended. The risk of aspiration of oral feedings may be high in infants with bronchiolitis, owing to tachypnea and the increased work of breathing. The infant may be fed through a nasogastric tube. If there is any risk for further respiratory decompensation potentially necessitating tracheal intubation, the infant should not be fed orally but be maintained with parenteral fluids. Frequent suctioning of nasal and oral secretions often provides relief of distress or cyanosis. Suctioning of secretions is an essential part of the treatment of bronchiolitis. Oxygen is definitely indicated in all infants with hypoxia. High-flow nasal cannula therapy can reduce the need for intubation in patients with impending respiratory failure.

A number of agents have been proposed as adjunctive therapies for bronchiolitis. Bronchodilators can produce modest short-term improvement in clinical features. This must be placed in context of potential adverse effects and the lack of any evidence indicating improvement in overall course of the disease. A trial dose of inhaled bronchodilator may be reasonable, with further therapy predicated on response in the individual patient. Corticosteroids, whether parenteral, oral, or inhaled, have been used for bronchiolitis despite conflicting and often negative studies. Corticosteroids are not recommended in previously healthy infants with RSV. Ribavirin, an antiviral agent administered by aerosol, has been used for infants with congenital heart disease or chronic lung disease. There is no convincing evidence of a positive impact on clinically important outcomes such as mortality and duration of hospitalization. Antibiotics have no value unless there is coexisting bacterial infection. Likewise, there is no support for RSV immunoglobulin administration during acute episodes of RSV bronchiolitis in previously healthy children. Combined therapy with nebulized epinephrine and dexamethasone has been used but is not currently recommended. Nebulized hypertonic saline has also been reported to have some benefit.

PROGNOSIS

Infants with **acute bronchiolitis** are at highest risk for further respiratory compromise in the 1st 48-72 hr after onset of cough and dyspnea; the child may be desperately ill with air hunger, apnea, and respiratory acidosis. The case fatality rate is <1%, with death attributable to apnea, respiratory arrest, or severe dehydration. After this critical period, symptoms can persist. The median duration of symptoms in ambulatory patients is ~12 days. There is a higher incidence of wheezing and asthma in children with a history of bronchiolitis unexplained by family history or other atopic syndromes. It is unclear whether bronchiolitis incites an immune response that manifests as asthma later or whether those infants have an inherent predilection for asthma that is merely unmasked by their episode of RSV. Approximately 60% of infants who wheeze will stop wheezing.

PREVENTION

Reduction in the severity and incidence of **acute bronchiolitis** due to RSV is possible through the administration of pooled hyperimmune RSV intravenous immunoglobulin and palivizumab, an intramuscular monoclonal antibody to the RSV F protein, before and during RSV season. Palivizumab should be considered for infants <2 yr of age with chronic lung disease, a history of prematurity, and some forms of congenital heart disease. Meticulous hand hygiene is the best measure to prevent nosocomial transmission.

BIBLIOGRAPHY

Please visit the Nelson Textbook of Pediatrics *website at* *www.expertconsult.com* *for the complete bibliography.*

383.2 Bronchitis

Denise M. Goodman

Nonspecific bronchial inflammation is termed **bronchitis** and occurs in multiple childhood conditions. **Acute bronchitis** is a syndrome, usually viral in origin, with cough as a prominent feature.

Acute tracheobronchitis is a term used when the trachea is prominently involved. Nasopharyngitis may also be present, and a variety of viral and bacterial agents, such as those causing influenza, pertussis, and diphtheria, may be responsible. Isolation of common bacteria such as pneumococcus, *Staphylococcus aureus,* and *Streptococcus pneumoniae* from the sputum might not imply a bacterial cause that requires antibiotic therapy.

ACUTE BRONCHITIS

Clinical Manifestations

Acute bronchitis often follows a viral upper respiratory tract infection. It is more common in the winter when respiratory viral syndromes predominate. The tracheobronchial epithelium is invaded by the infectious agent, leading to activation of inflammatory cells and release of cytokines. Constitutional symptoms including fever and malaise follow. The tracheobronchial epithelium can become significantly damaged or hypersensitized, leading to a protracted cough lasting 1-3 wk.

The child 1st presents with nonspecific upper respiratory infectious symptoms, such as rhinitis. Three to 4 days later, a frequent, dry, hacking cough develops, which may or may not be productive. After several days, the sputum can become purulent, indicating leukocyte migration but not necessarily bacterial infection. Many children swallow their sputum, and this can produce emesis. Chest pain may be a prominent complaint in older children and is exacerbated by coughing. The mucus gradually thins, usually within 5-10 days, and then the cough gradually abates. The entire episode usually lasts about 2 wk and seldom >3 wk.

Findings on physical examination vary with the age of the patient and stage of the disease. Early findings are absent or are low-grade fever and upper respiratory signs such as nasopharyngitis, conjunctivitis, and rhinitis. Auscultation of the chest may be unremarkable at this early phase. As the syndrome progresses and cough worsens, breath sounds become coarse, with coarse and fine crackles and scattered high-pitched wheezing. Chest radiographs are normal or can have increased bronchial markings.

The principal objective of the clinician is to exclude pneumonia, which is more likely caused by bacterial agents requiring antibiotic therapy. In adults, absence of abnormality of vital signs (tachycardia, tachypnea, fever) and a normal physical examination of the chest reduce the likelihood of pneumonia.

Differential Diagnosis

Persistent or recurrent symptoms should lead the clinician to consider entities other than acute bronchitis. Many entities manifest with cough as a prominent symptom (Table 383-3).

Treatment

There is no specific therapy for acute bronchitis. The disease is self-limited, and antibiotics, although often prescribed, do not hasten improvement. Frequent shifts in position can facilitate pulmonary drainage in infants. Older children are sometimes more comfortable with humidity, but this does not shorten the disease course. Cough suppressants can relieve symptoms but can also increase the risk of suppuration and inspissated secretions and, therefore, should be used judiciously. Antihistamines dry secretions and are not helpful; expectorants are likewise not indicated.

Table 383-3 DISORDERS WITH COUGH AS A PROMINENT FINDING

CATEGORY	DIAGNOSES
Inflammatory	Asthma
Chronic pulmonary processes	Bronchopulmonary dysplasia Postinfectious bronchiectasis Cystic fibrosis Tracheomalacia or bronchomalacia Ciliary abnormalities Other chronic lung diseases
Other chronic disease or congenital disorders	Laryngeal cleft Swallowing disorders Gastroesophageal reflux Airway compression (such as a vascular ring or hemangioma) Congenital heart disease
Infectious or immune disorders	Immunodeficiency Tuberculosis Allergy Sinusitis Tonsillitis or adenoiditis *Chlamydia, Ureaplasma* (infants) *Bordetella pertussis* *Mycoplasma pneumoniae*
Acquired	Foreign body aspiration, tracheal or esophageal

CHRONIC BRONCHITIS

Chronic bronchitis is well recognized in adults, formally defined as ≥3 mo of productive cough each year for ≥2 yr. The disease can develop insidiously, with episodes of acute obstruction alternating with quiescent periods. A number of predisposing conditions can lead to progression of airflow obstruction or chronic obstructive pulmonary disease (COPD), with smoking as the major factor (up to 80% of patients have a smoking history). Other conditions include air pollution, occupational exposures, and repeated infections. In children, cystic fibrosis, bronchopulmonary dysplasia, and bronchiectasis must be ruled out.

The applicability of this definition to children is unclear. The existence of chronic bronchitis as a distinct entity in children is controversial. Like adults, however, children with chronic inflammatory diseases or those with toxic exposures can develop damaged pulmonary epithelium. Thus, chronic or recurring cough in children should lead the clinician to search for underlying pulmonary or systemic disorders (see Table 383-3). One proposed entity is persistent or protracted bacterial bronchitis, which may be mistaken for asthma and shares some characteristics with other forms of suppurative lung disease.

CIGARETTE SMOKING AND AIR POLLUTION

Exposure to environmental irritants, such as tobacco smoke and air pollution, can incite or aggravate cough. There is a well-established association between tobacco exposure and pulmonary disease, including bronchitis and wheezing. This can occur through cigarette smoking or by exposure to passive smoke. Marijuana smoke is another irritant sometimes overlooked when eliciting a history. There is some evidence that women may be particularly susceptible to long-term pulmonary disease as a consequence of childhood smoking.

A number of pollutants compromise lung development and likely precipitate lung disease, including particulate matter, ozone, acid vapor, and nitrogen dioxide. Because these substances coexist in the atmosphere, the relative contribution of any 1 to pulmonary symptoms is difficult to discern. Proximity to motor vehicle traffic is an important source of these pollutants.

BIBLIOGRAPHY

Please visit the Nelson Textbook of Pediatrics *website at www.expertconsult.com for the complete bibliography.*

Chapter 384
Emphysema and Overinflation

Steven R. Boas and Glenna B. Winnie

Pulmonary emphysema is distention of air spaces with irreversible disruption of the alveolar septa. It can be generalized or localized, involving part or all of a lung. **Overinflation** is distention with or without alveolar rupture and is often reversible. **Compensatory overinflation** can be acute or chronic and occurs in normally functioning pulmonary tissue when, for any reason, a sizable portion of the lung is removed or becomes partially or completely airless, which can occur with pneumonia, atelectasis, empyema, and pneumothorax. **Obstructive overinflation** results from partial obstruction of a bronchus or bronchiole, when it becomes more difficult for air to leave the alveoli than to enter; there is a gradual accumulation of air distal to the obstruction, the so-called bypass, ball valve, or check valve type of obstruction.

LOCALIZED OBSTRUCTIVE OVERINFLATION

When a ball-valve type of obstruction partially occludes the main stem bronchus, the entire lung becomes overinflated; individual lobes are affected when the obstruction is in lobar bronchi. Segments or subsegments are affected when their individual bronchi are blocked. Localized obstructions that can be responsible for overinflation include foreign bodies and the inflammatory reaction to them, abnormally thick mucus (cystic fibrosis, Chapter 395), endobronchial tuberculosis or tuberculosis of the tracheobronchial lymph nodes (Chapter 207), and endobronchial or mediastinal tumors. When most or all of a lobe is involved, the percussion note is hyperresonant over the area, and the breath sounds are decreased in intensity. The distended lung can extend across the mediastinum into the opposite hemithorax. Under fluoroscopic scrutiny during exhalation, the overinflated area does not decrease, and the heart and the mediastinum shift to the opposite side because the unobstructed lung empties normally.

Unilateral Hyperlucent Lung

Unilateral hyperlucent lung can be associated with a variety of cardiac and pulmonary diseases of children, but in some patients, it occurs without demonstrable underlying active disease. More than half the cases follow one or more episodes of pneumonia; a rising titer to adenovirus (Chapter 254) has been documented in several children. This condition can follow bronchiolitis obliterans and can include obliterative vasculitis as well, accounting for the greatly diminished perfusion and vascular marking on the affected side.

Patients with unilateral hyperlucent lung can present with **clinical manifestations** of pneumonia, but in some patients the condition is discovered only when a chest radiograph is obtained for an unrelated reason. A few patients have hemoptysis. Physical findings can include hyperresonance and a small lung with the mediastinum shifted toward the more abnormal lung. This condition has been labeled **Swyer-James** or **Macleod syndrome.** The condition is thought to result from an insult to the lower respiratory tract. Some patients show a mediastinal shift away from the lesion with exhalation. CT scanning or bronchography can demonstrate bronchiectasis. In some patients, previous chest radiographs have been normal or have shown only an acute pneumonia, suggesting that a hyperlucent lung is an acquired lesion. No specific treatment is known; it may become less symptomatic with time. Indications as to which children would benefit from surgery remain controversial.

Congenital Lobar Emphysema

Congenital lobar emphysema (CLE) can result in severe respiratory distress in early infancy and can be caused by localized obstruction. Familial occurrence has been reported. In 50% of cases, a cause of CLE can be identified. Congenital deficiency of the bronchial cartilage, external compression by aberrant vessels, bronchial stenosis, redundant bronchial mucosal flaps, and kinking of the bronchus caused by herniation into the mediastinum have been described as leading to bronchial obstruction and subsequent CLE and commonly affects the left upper lobe.

Clinical manifestations usually become apparent in the neonatal period but are delayed for as long as 5-6 mo in 5% of patients. Many cases are diagnosed by antenatal ultrasonography. Babies with prenatally diagnosed cases are not always symptomatic at birth. In some patients, CLE remains undiagnosed until school age or beyond. Signs range from mild tachypnea and wheeze to severe dyspnea with cyanosis. CLE can affect one or more lobes; it affects the upper and middle lobes, and the left upper lobe is the most common site. The affected lobe is essentially nonfunctional because of the overdistention, and atelectasis of the ipsilateral normal lung can ensue. With further distention, the mediastinum is shifted to the contralateral side, with impaired function seen as well (Fig. 384-1). A radiolucent lobe and a mediastinal shift are often revealed by radiographic examination. A CT scan can demonstrate the aberrant anatomy of the lesion, and MRI or MR angiography can demonstrate any vascular lesions, which might be causing extraluminal compression. Nuclear imaging studies are useful to demonstrate perfusion defects in the affected lobe. Figure 384-2 outlines evaluation of an infant presenting with suspected CLE. The differential diagnosis includes pneumonia with or without an effusion, pneumothorax, and cystic adenomatoid malformation.

Treatment by immediate surgery and excision of the lobe may be lifesaving when cyanosis and severe respiratory distress are present, but some patients respond to medical treatment. Selective intubation of the unaffected lung may be of value. Some children with apparent congenital lobar emphysema have reversible overinflation, without the classic alveolar septal rupture implied in the term *emphysema*. Bronchoscopy can reveal an endobronchial lesion.

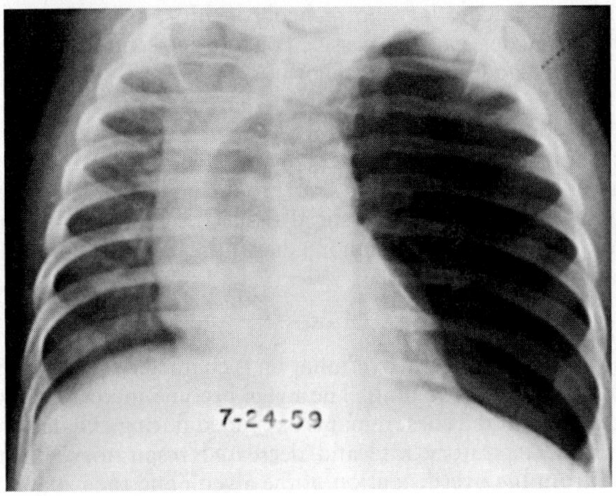

Figure 384-1 Congenital left upper lobe emphysema. Note the extension of the emphysematous lobe into the left lower lobe and its displacement of the mediastinum toward the right.

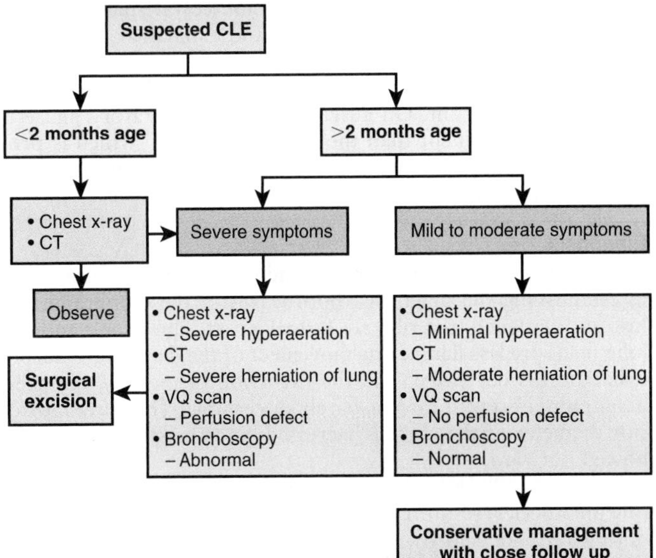

Figure 384-2 Algorithm for evaluation and treatment of congenital lobar emphysema (CLE). (Adapted from Senocak ME, Ciftci AO, et al: Congenital lobar emphysema: diagnostic and therapeutic considerations, *J Pediatr Surg* 34:1347–1351, 1999. Cited in Chao MC, Karamzadeh AM, Ahuja G: Congenital lobar emphysema: an otolaryngologic perspective, *Int J Pediatr Otorhinolaryngol* 69:553, 2005.)

Overinflation of All Three Lobes of the Right Lung

Overinflation of all three lobes of the right lung has been produced by anomalous location of the left pulmonary artery, which impinges on the right main stem bronchus. Hyperinflation also occurs in patients with the absent pulmonary valve type of tetralogy of Fallot (Chapter 424.1) and secondary aneurysmal dilatation of the pulmonary artery, which partially compresses the main stem bronchi. A number of neonates have lobar overinflation while being treated for hyaline membrane disease with assisted ventilation, suggesting an acquired cause. Medical management with selective intubation of the unaffected bronchus or high-frequency ventilation has occasionally been successful and lobectomy avoided.

GENERALIZED OBSTRUCTIVE OVERINFLATION

Acute generalized overinflation of the lung results from widespread involvement of the bronchioles and is usually reversible. It occurs more commonly in infants than in children and may be secondary to a number of clinical conditions, including asthma, cystic fibrosis, acute bronchiolitis, interstitial pneumonitis, atypical forms of acute laryngotracheobronchitis, aspiration of zinc stearate powder, chronic passive congestion secondary to a congenital cardiac lesion, and miliary tuberculosis.

Pathology

In chronic overinflation, many of the alveoli are ruptured and communicate with one another, producing distended saccules. Air can also enter the interstitial tissue (i.e., interstitial emphysema), resulting in pneumomediastinum and pneumothorax (Chapters 405 and 406).

Clinical Manifestations

Generalized obstructive overinflation is characterized by dyspnea, with difficulty in exhaling. The lungs become increasingly overdistended, and the chest remains expanded during exhalation. An increased respiratory rate and decreased respiratory excursion result from the overdistention of the alveoli and their inability to be emptied normally through the narrowed bronchioles. Air hunger is responsible for forced respiratory movements. Overaction of the accessory muscles of respiration results in retractions at the suprasternal notch, the supraclavicular spaces, the lower margin of the thorax, and the intercostal spaces. Unlike the flattened chest during inspiration and exhalation in cases of laryngeal obstruction, minimal reduction in the size of the overdistended chest during exhalation is observed. The percussion note is hyperresonant. On auscultation, the inspiratory phase is usually less prominent than the expiratory phase, which is prolonged and roughened. Fine or medium crackles may be heard. Cyanosis is more common in the severe cases.

Diagnosis

Radiographic and fluoroscopic examinations of the chest assist in establishing the diagnosis. Both leaves of the diaphragm are low and flattened, the ribs are farther apart than usual, and the lung fields are less dense. The movement of the diaphragm during exhalation is decreased, and the excursion of the low, flattened diaphragm in severe cases is barely discernible. The anteroposterior diameter of the chest is increased, and the sternum may be bowed outward.

BULLOUS EMPHYSEMA Bullous emphysematous blebs or cysts (pneumatoceles) result from overdistention and rupture of alveoli during birth or shortly thereafter, or they may be sequelae of pneumonia and other infections. They have been observed in tuberculosis lesions during specific antibacterial therapy. These emphysematous areas presumably result from rupture of distended alveoli, forming a single or multiloculated cavity. The cysts can become large and might contain some fluid; an air-fluid level may be demonstrated on the radiograph (Fig. 384-3). The cysts should be differentiated from pulmonary abscesses. In most cases, the cysts disappear spontaneously within a few mo, although they can persist for a yr or more. Aspiration or surgery is not indicated except in cases of severe respiratory and cardiac compromise.

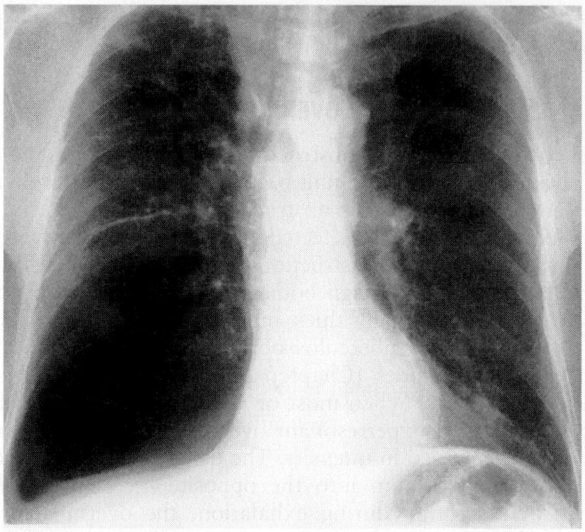

Figure 384-3 Increased transradiancy in the right lower zone. A large emphysematous bulla occupies the lower half of the right lung, and the apical changes are in keeping with previous tuberculosis. (From Padley SPG, Hansell DM: Imaging techniques. In Albert RK, Spiro SG, Jett JR, editors: *Clinical respiratory medicine,* ed 3, Philadelphia, 2008, Mosby, Fig 1-48.)

SUBCUTANEOUS EMPHYSEMA Subcutaneous emphysema results from any process that allows free air to enter into the subcutaneous tissue. The most common causes include pneumomediastinum or pneumothorax. Additionally, it can be a complication of fracture of the orbit, which permits free air to escape from the nasal sinuses. In the neck and thorax, subcutaneous emphysema can follow tracheotomy, deep ulceration in the pharyngeal region, esophageal wounds, or any perforating lesion of the larynx or trachea. It is occasionally a complication of thoracentesis, asthma, or abdominal surgery. Rarely, air is formed in the subcutaneous tissues by gas-producing bacteria.

Tenderness over the site of emphysema and a crepitant quality on palpation of the skin are classic manifestations. Subcutaneous emphysema is usually a self-limited process and requires no specific treatment. Minimization of activities that can increase airway pressure (cough, performance of high-pressure pulmonary function testing maneuvers) is recommended. Resolution occurs by resorption of subcutaneous air after elimination of its source. Rarely, dangerous compression of the trachea by air in the surrounding soft tissue requires surgical intervention.

BIBLIOGRAPHY

Please visit the Nelson Textbook of Pediatrics *website at* www.expertconsult.com *for the complete bibliography.*

Chapter 385
α_1-Antitrypsin Deficiency and Emphysema

Glenna B. Winnie and Steven R. Boas

Although it rarely causes lung disease in children, homozygous deficiency of α_1-antitrypsin (α-AT) is an important cause of early-onset severe panacinar pulmonary emphysema in adults in the

3rd and 4th decades of life and an important cause of liver disease in children (Chapter 349.5). It has been associated with panniculitis and vasculitis in adults.

For the full continuation of this chapter, please visit the Nelson Textbook of Pediatrics *website at www.expertconsult.com.*

Chapter 386 Other Distal Airway Diseases

386.1 Bronchiolitis Obliterans

Steven R. Boas

EPIDEMIOLOGY

Bronchiolitis obliterans (BO) is a rare chronic obstructive lung disease of the bronchioles and smaller airways. An insult to the lower respiratory tract occurs, resulting in fibrosis of the small airways. In the nontransplant patient, BO most commonly occurs in the pediatric population after respiratory infections, particularly adenovirus, but also *Mycoplasma,* measles, legionella, influenza, and pertussis; other causes include inflammatory diseases (juvenile rheumatoid arthritis, systemic lupus erythematosus [Chapter 152], scleroderma [Chapter 154], Stevens-Johnson syndrome [Chapter 146]), and inhalation of toxin fumes (NO_2, NH_3) (see Table 386-1 on the *Nelson Textbook of Pediatrics* website at www.expertconsult.com). Bronchiolitis obliterans syndrome (BOS), a clinical entity that relates to graft deterioration after transplantation due to progressive airway, is increasingly recognized as a long-term complication of lung and bone marrow transplantation; more than one third of survivors of lung transplant can develop this disorder. BO occurs in all age groups, and the prevalence in 1 pediatric autopsy series was 2/1,000. BOS appears to be more common among older children and adolescents than infants and toddlers. There is some evidence that postinfectious obliterans may be more common in the southern hemisphere and among persons of Asian descent.

For the full continuation of this chapter, please visit the Nelson Textbook of Pediatrics *website at www.expertconsult.com.*

386.2 Follicular Bronchitis

Steven R. Boas

Follicular bronchitis (FB) is a lymphoproliferative lung disorder characterized by the presence of lymphoid follicles coursing alongside the airways (bronchi or bronchioles) and infiltration of the walls of bronchi and bronchioles. Although the cause is unknown, an infectious etiology (viral) has been proposed. It can occur in adults and children; in children, onset of symptoms generally occurs by 6 wk of age and peaks between 6 and 18 mo. Cough, moderate respiratory distress, fever, and fine crackles are common clinical findings. Fine crackles generally persist over time, and recurrence of symptoms is common. Chest radiographs may be relatively benign initially (air trapping, peribronchial thickening) but evolve into the typical interstitial pattern. Chest CT can show a fine reticular pattern. Definitive diagnosis is made by open lung biopsy. Some patients with FB respond to therapy with corticosteroids. Prognosis is variable, with some patients having significant progression of pulmonary disease and others developing only mild obstructive airway disease. In children it is generally associated with immunodeficiency; the differential diagnosis includes the pulmonary complications of HIV infection.

BIBLIOGRAPHY

Please visit the Nelson Textbook of Pediatrics *website at www.expertconsult.com for the complete bibliography.*

386.3 Pulmonary Alveolar Microlithiasis

Steven R. Boas

Approximately 400 cases of pulmonary alveolar microlithiasis (PAM), an unusual disorder, have been reported. Although the underlying cause of PAM is unknown, the disease is characterized by the formation of lamellar concretions of calcium phosphate or "microliths" within the alveoli, creating a classic pattern on the radiograph (see Fig. 386-2 on the *Nelson Textbook of Pediatrics* website at www.expertconsult.com).

For the full continuation of this chapter, please visit the Nelson Textbook of Pediatrics *website at www.expertconsult.com.*

Chapter 387 Congenital Disorders of the Lung

387.1 Pulmonary Agenesis and Aplasia

Jonathan D. Finder

ETIOLOGY AND PATHOLOGY

Pulmonary agenesis differs from hypoplasia in that agenesis entails the complete absence of a lung. Agenesis differs from aplasia by the absence of a bronchial stump or carina that is seen in aplasia. Bilateral pulmonary agenesis is incompatible with life, manifesting as severe respiratory distress and failure. Based on reports of patients with parental consanguinity, pulmonary agenesis is thought to be an autosomal recessive trait. The incidence is estimated to be 1 in 10,000-15,000 births.

CLINICAL MANIFESTATIONS AND PROGNOSIS

Unilateral agenesis or hypoplasia can have few symptoms and nonspecific findings, resulting in only 33% of the cases being diagnosed while the patient is living. Symptoms tend to be related to associated central airway complications of compression, stenosis, and/or tracheobronchomalacia. In patients in whom the right lung is absent, the aorta can compress the trachea and lead to symptoms of central airway compression. Right lung agenesis has a higher morbidity and mortality than left lung agenesis. Pulmonary agenesis is often seen in association with other congenital anomalies such as the VACTERL sequence (*v*ertebral anomalies, *a*nal atresia, *c*ongenital heart disease, *t*racheoesophageal fistula, *r*enal anomalies, and *l*imb anomalies), ipsilateral facial and skeletal malformations, and central nervous system and cardiac malformations. Compensatory growth of the remaining lung allows improved gas exchange, but the mediastinal shift can lead to scoliosis and airway compression. Scoliosis can result from unequal thoracic growth.

DIAGNOSIS AND TREATMENT

Chest radiographic findings of unilateral lung or lobar collapse with a shift of mediastinal structures toward the affected side can prompt referral for suspected foreign body aspiration, mucous plug occlusion, or other bronchial mass lesions. The diagnosis requires a high index of suspicion to avoid the unnecessary risks of bronchoscopy, including potential perforation of the rudimentary bronchus. CT of the chest is diagnostic, although the diagnosis may be suggested by chronic changes in the contralateral aspect of the chest wall and lung expansion on chest radiographs. Conservative treatment is usually recommended, although surgery has offered benefit in selected cases.

BIBLIOGRAPHY

Please visit the Nelson Textbook of Pediatrics *website at www.expertconsult.com for the complete bibliography.*

387.2 Pulmonary Hypoplasia

Jonathan D. Finder

ETIOLOGY AND PATHOLOGY

Pulmonary hypoplasia involves a decrease in both the number of alveoli and the number of airway generations. The hypoplasia may be bilateral in the setting of bilateral lung constraint, as in oligohydramnios or thoracic dystrophy. Pulmonary hypoplasia is usually secondary to other intrauterine disorders that produce an impairment of normal lung development (Chapter 95). Conditions such as deformities of the thoracic spine and rib cage (thoracic dystrophy), pleural effusions with fetal hydrops, cystic adenomatoid malformation, and congenital diaphragmatic hernia physically constrain the developing lung. Any condition that produces oligohydramnios (fetal renal insufficiency or prolonged premature rupture of membranes) can also lead to diminished lung growth. In these conditions, airway and arterial branching are inhibited, thereby limiting the capillary surface area. Large unilateral lesions, such as congenital diaphragmatic hernia and cystic adenomatoid malformation, can displace the mediastinum and thereby produce a contralateral hypoplasia, although usually not as severe as that seen on the ipsilateral side.

CLINICAL MANIFESTATIONS

Pulmonary hypoplasia is usually recognized in the newborn period, owing to either the respiratory insufficiency or the presentation of persistent pulmonary hypertension. Later presentation (tachypnea) with stress or respiratory viral infection can be seen in infants with mild pulmonary hypoplasia.

TREATMENT

Mechanical ventilation and oxygen may be required to support gas exchange. Specific therapy to control associated pulmonary hypertension, such as inhaled nitric oxide, may be useful. In cases of severe hypoplasia, the limited capacity of the lung for gas exchange may be inadequate to sustain life. Extracorporeal membrane oxygenation can provide gas exchange for a critical period of time and permit survival. Rib-expanding devices (vertically expansible prosthetic titanium ribs) can improve the survival of patients with thoracic dystrophies (Chapter 671).

387.3 Cystic Adenomatoid Malformation

Jonathan D. Finder

PATHOLOGY

Congenital cystic adenomatoid malformation (CCAM) consists of hamartomatous or dysplastic lung tissue mixed with more normal lung, generally confined to one lobe. This congenital pulmonary disorder occurs in ~1-4/100,000 births. Three histologic patterns have been described. **Type 1** (50%) is macrocystic and consists of a single or several large (>2 cm in diameter) cysts lined with ciliated pseudostratified epithelium. The wall of the cyst contains smooth muscle cells and elastic tissue. One third of cases have mucus-secreting cells. Cartilage is rarely seen in the wall of the cyst. This type has a good prognosis for survival. **Type 2** (40%) is microcystic and consists of multiple small cysts with histology similar to that of the type 1 lesion. Type 2 is associated with other congenital anomalies and carries a poor prognosis. In **type 3** (<10%), the lesion is solid with bronchiole-like structures lined with cuboidal ciliated epithelium and separated by areas of nonciliated cuboidal epithelium. This lesion carries the poorest prognosis and can be fatal. Prenatal ultrasonographic findings are classified as macrocystic (single or multiple cysts >5 mm) or microcystic (echogenic cysts <5 mm).

ETIOLOGY

The lesion probably results from an embryologic insult before the 35th day of gestation, with maldevelopment of terminal bronchiolar structures. Histologic examination reveals little normal lung and many glandular elements. Cysts are very common; cartilage is rare. The presence of cartilage might indicate a somewhat later embryologic insult, perhaps extending into the 10th-24th wk. Although growth factor interactions and signaling mechanisms have been implicated in altered lung-branching morphogenesis, the exact roles in the maldevelopment seen here remain obscure.

DIAGNOSIS

Cystic adenomatoid malformations can be diagnosed in utero by ultrasonography (Fig. 387-1). Fetal cystic lung abnormalities can include cystic adenomatoid malformations (40%), pulmonary sequestration (14%) (Chapter 387.4), or both (26%); the median age at diagnosis is usually 21 wk gestation. In 1 series, only 7% had severe signs of fetal distress including hydrops, pleural effusion, polyhydramnios, ascites, or severe facial edema; 96% of the fetuses were born alive, 2 of whom died in the neonatal period. Lesions causing fetal hydrops have a poor prognosis. Large lesions, by compressing adjacent lung, can produce pulmonary hypoplasia in nonaffected lobes (Chapter 387.2). Even lesions that appear large in early gestation can regress considerably or decrease in relative size and be associated with good pulmonary function in childhood. CT allows accurate diagnosis and sizing of the lesion.

CLINICAL MANIFESTATIONS

Patients can present in the newborn period or early infancy with respiratory distress, recurrent respiratory infection, and pneumothorax. The lesion may be confused with a diaphragmatic hernia (Chapter 95.8). Patients with smaller lesions are usually asymptomatic until mid-childhood, when episodes of recurrent or persistent pulmonary infection or chest pain occur. Breath sounds may be diminished, with mediastinal shift away from the lesion on physical examination. Chest radiographs reveal a cystic mass, sometimes with mediastinal shift (Fig. 387-2). Occasionally, an air-fluid level suggests a lung abscess.

TREATMENT

Antenatal intervention in severely affected infants is controversial but can include excision of the affected lobe for microcystic lesions, aspiration of macrocystic lesions, and, rarely, open fetal surgery. In the postnatal period, surgery is indicated for symptomatic patients. Although surgery may be delayed for

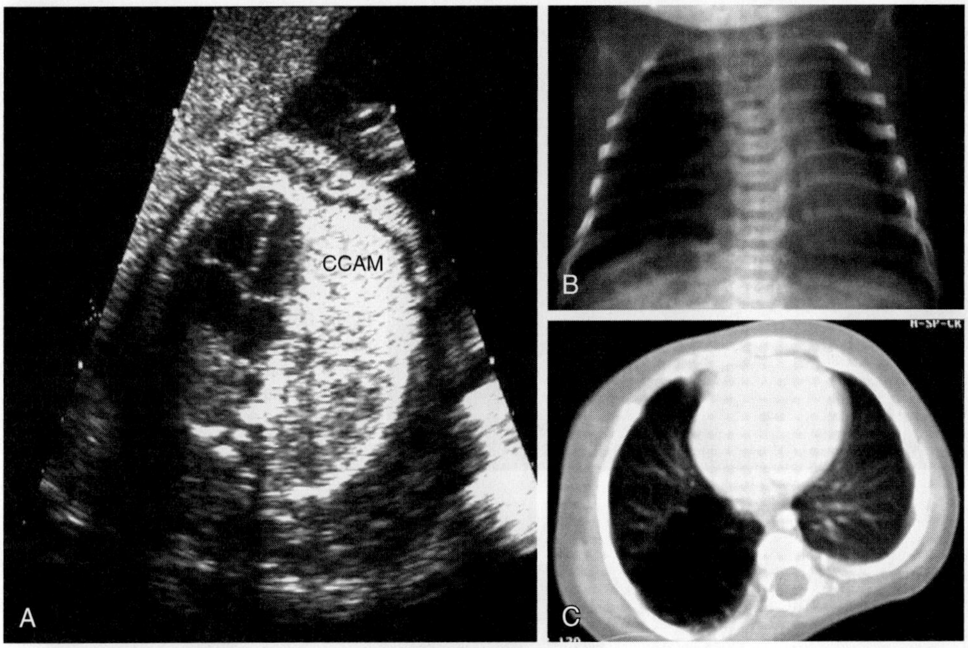

Figure 387-1 Imaging of congenital cystic adenomatous malformation of the lung (CCAM) on the same patient with prenatal ultrasound scan *(A)*, chest radiograph *(B)*, and CT scan *(C)*. Note that the lesion is not visible on the chest radiograph. (From Lakhoo K: Management of congenital cystic adenomatous malformations of the lung, *Arch Dis Child Fetal Neonatal Ed* 94:F73–F76, 2009.)

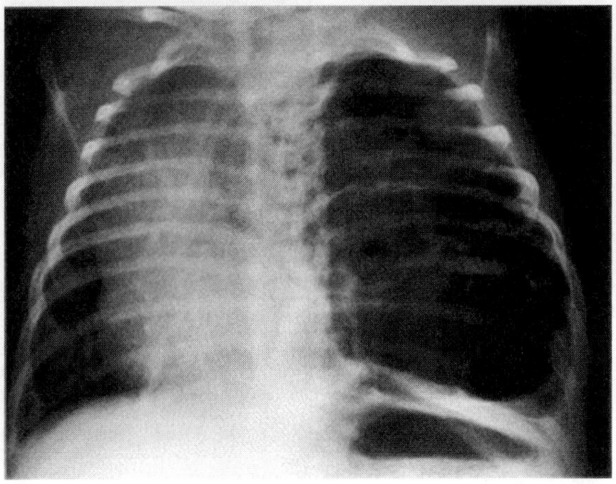

Figure 387-2 Neonatal chest x-ray showing large multicystic mass in the left hemithorax with mediastinal shift due to congenital cystic adenomatoid malformation (CCAM). (From Williams HJ, Johnson KJ: Imaging of congenital cystic lung lesions, *Paediatr Resp Rev* 3:120–127, 2002.)

asymptomatic infants because postnatal resolution has been reported, true resolution appears to be very rare in that abnormalities usually remain detectable on CT or MRI. Sarcomatous and carcinomatous differentiation has been described in patients with CCAM, so surgical resection by 1 yr of age is recommended to limit malignant potential. The mortality rate is <10%. Another indication for surgery is to rule out pleuropulmonary blastoma, a malignancy that can appear radiologically similar to type I CCAM.

BIBLIOGRAPHY

Please visit the Nelson Textbook of Pediatrics *website at* *www.expertconsult.com* *for the complete bibliography.*

387.4 Pulmonary Sequestration

Jonathan D. Finder

Pulmonary sequestration is a congenital anomaly of lung development that can be intrapulmonary or extrapulmonary, according to the location within the visceral pleura. The majority of sequestrations are intrapulmonary.

PATHOPHYSIOLOGY

The lung tissue in a sequestration does not connect to a bronchus and receives its arterial supply from the systemic arteries (commonly off the aorta) and returns its venous blood to the right side of the heart through the inferior vena cava (extralobar) or pulmonary veins (intralobar). The sequestration functions as a space-occupying lesion within the chest; it does not participate in gas exchange and does not lead to a left-to-right shunt or alveolar dead space. Communication with the airway can occur as the result of rupture of infected material into an adjacent airway. Collateral ventilation within intrapulmonary lesions via pores of Kohn can occur. Pulmonary sequestrations can arise through the same pathoembryologic mechanism as a remnant of a diverticular outgrowth of the esophagus. Some propose that intrapulmonary sequestration is an acquired lesion primarily caused by infection and inflammation; inflammation leads to cystic changes and hypertrophy of a feeding systemic artery. This is consistent with the rarity of this lesion in autopsy series of newborns. Gastric or pancreatic tissue may be found within the sequestration. Cysts also may be present. Other associated congenital anomalies, including CCAM (Chapter 387.3), diaphragmatic hernia (Chapter 95.8), and esophageal cysts, are not uncommon. Some believe that intrapulmonary sequestration is often a manifestation of cystic adenomatoid malformation and have questioned the existence of intrapulmonary sequestration as a separate entity.

CLINICAL MANIFESTATIONS AND DIAGNOSIS

Physical findings in patients with sequestration include an area of dullness to percussion and decreased breath sounds over the lesion. During infection, crackles may also be present. A continuous or purely systolic murmur may be heard over the back. If findings on routine chest radiographs are consistent with the diagnosis, further delineation is indicated before surgical intervention (Fig. 387-3). CT with contrast can demonstrate both the extent of the lesion and its vascular supply. Magnetic resonance angiography (MRA) is also useful. Ultrasonography can help rule out a diaphragmatic hernia and demonstrate the systemic artery.

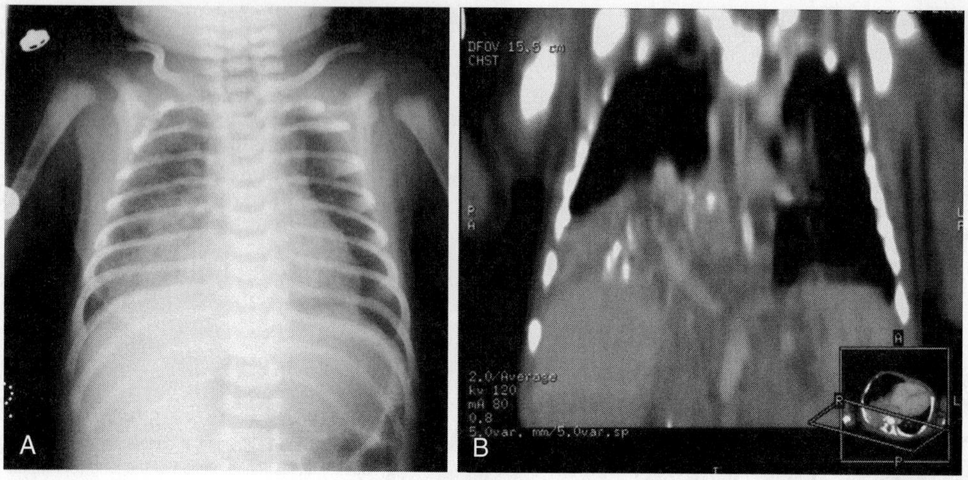

Figure 387-3 *A,* Plain chest x-ray showing changes in the region of the right lower/middle lobe of the lung. *B,* CT showing parenchymal changes in the right lower lobe of the lung in keeping with a sequestration. (From Corbett HJ, Humphrey GME: Pulmonary sequestration, *Paediatr Resp Rev* 5:59–68, 2004.)

Surgical removal is recommended. Identifying the blood supply before surgery avoids inadvertently severing its systemic artery.

Intrapulmonary sequestration is generally found in a lower lobe and does not have its own pleura. Patients usually present with infection. In older patients, hemoptysis is common. A chest radiograph during a period when there is no active infection reveals a mass lesion; an air-fluid level may be present. During infection, the margins of the lesion may be blurred. There is no difference in the incidence of this lesion in each lung.

Extrapulmonary sequestration is much more common in boys and almost always involves the left lung. This lesion is enveloped by a pleural covering and is associated with diaphragmatic hernia and other abnormalities such as colonic duplication, vertebral abnormalities, and pulmonary hypoplasia. Many of these patients are asymptomatic when the mass is discovered by routine chest radiography. Other patients present with respiratory symptoms or heart failure. Subdiaphragmatic extrapulmonary sequestration can manifest as an abdominal mass on prenatal ultrasonography. The advent of prenatal ultrasonography has also enabled evidence that fetal pulmonary sequestrations can spontaneously regress.

TREATMENT

Treatment of intrapulmonary sequestration is surgical removal of the lesion, a procedure that usually requires excision of the entire involved lobe. Segmental resection occasionally suffices. Surgical resection of the involved area is recommended for extrapulmonary sequestration.

BIBLIOGRAPHY

Please visit the Nelson Textbook of Pediatrics *website at* *www.expertconsult.com* *for the complete bibliography.*

387.5 Bronchogenic Cysts

Jonathan D. Finder

ETIOLOGY AND PATHOLOGY

Bronchogenic cysts arise from abnormal budding of the tracheal diverticulum of the foregut before the 16th wk of gestation and are originally lined with ciliated epithelium. They are more commonly found on the right and near a midline structure (trachea, esophagus, carina), but peripheral lower lobe and perihilar intrapulmonary cysts are not infrequent. Diagnosis may be precipitated by enlargement of the cyst, which causes symptoms by

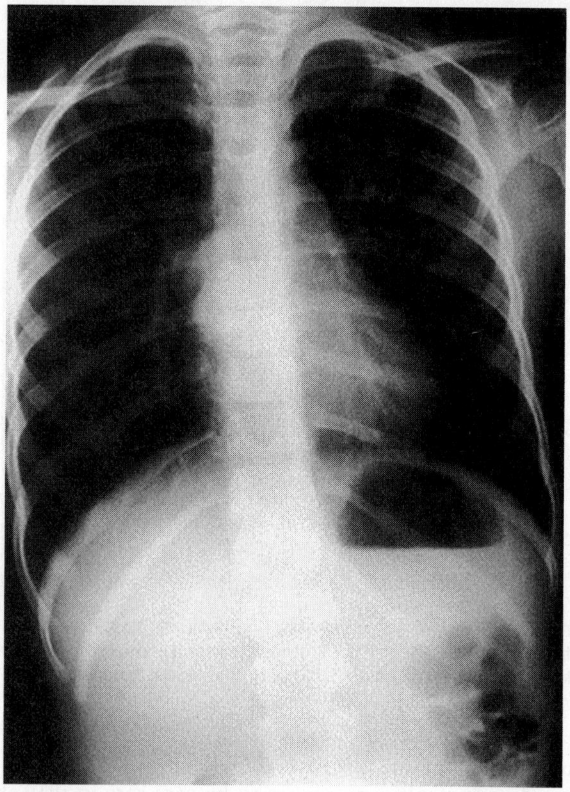

Figure 387-4 Chest x-ray showing an ovoid, well-defined, soft-tissue density causing splaying of the carina due to bronchogenic cyst. (From Williams HJ, Johnson KJ: Imaging of congenital cystic lung lesions, *Paediatr Resp Rev* 3:120–127, 2002.)

pressure on an adjacent airway. When the diagnosis is delayed until an infection occurs, the ciliated epithelium may be lost, and accurate pathologic diagnosis is then impossible. Cysts are rarely demonstrable at birth. Later, some cysts become symptomatic by becoming infected or by enlarging and compromising the function of an adjacent airway.

CLINICAL MANIFESTATIONS AND TREATMENT

Fever, chest pain, and productive cough are the most common presenting symptoms. Dysphagia may be present; some bronchogenic cysts are asymptomatic. A chest radiograph reveals the cyst, which can contain an air-fluid level (Fig. 387-4). CT scan or MRI is obtained in most cases to better demonstrate anatomy and extent of lesion before surgical resection. Treatment of symptomatic cysts is surgical excision after appropriate antibiotic management. Asymptomatic cysts are generally excised in view of the high rate of infection.

BIBLIOGRAPHY
Please visit the Nelson Textbook of Pediatrics *website at www.expertconsult.com for the complete bibliography.*

387.6 Congenital Pulmonary Lymphangiectasia

Jonathan D. Finder

ETIOLOGY AND PATHOLOGY

Congenital pulmonary lymphangiectasia is characterized by greatly dilated lymphatic ducts throughout the lung. It can occur in 3 pathologic circumstances: pulmonary venous obstruction that produces an elevated transvascular pressure and engorges the pulmonary lymphatics; generalized lymphangiectasia, as a generalized disease of several organ systems, including lungs and the intestines (can be associated with Noonan syndrome); and primary lymphangiectasia limited to the lung as a manifestation of an abnormality in lymphatic development.

CLINICAL MANIFESTATIONS AND TREATMENT

Children with pulmonary venous obstruction or severe pulmonary lymphangiectasia present with dyspnea and cyanosis in the newborn period. Hydrops fetalis may be diagnosed antenatally. Chest radiographs reveal diffuse, dense, reticular densities with prominence of Kerley B lines. Pleural effusions are common; thoracentesis will reveal chylothorax in this setting. If the lung is not completely involved, the spared areas appear hyperlucent. Respiration is compromised because of impaired diffusion and decreased pulmonary compliance. The diagnosis can be suggested by CT scan and/or cardiac catheterization; definitive diagnosis requires lung biopsy (either thoracoscopic or open).

Treatment is supportive and includes administration of oxygen, mechanical ventilation, nutritional support (including gastrostomy placement and use of feedings containing medium-chain triglycerides), and careful fluid management with diuretics. Primary pulmonary lymphangiectasia can produce severe pulmonary dysfunction that can require long-term mechanical ventilation; long-term survival and resolution of respiratory insufficiency is possible even in severe cases. Occasionally, the pulmonary venous obstruction is secondary to left-sided cardiac lesions; relief of the latter can produce improvement in pulmonary dysfunction. Generalized lymphangiectasia generally produces milder pulmonary dysfunction, and survival to mid-childhood and beyond is not unusual.

BIBLIOGRAPHY
Please visit the Nelson Textbook of Pediatrics *website at www.expertconsult.com for the complete bibliography.*

387.7 Lung Hernia

Jonathan D. Finder

ETIOLOGY AND PATHOLOGY

A lung hernia is a protrusion of the lung beyond its normal thoracic boundaries. About 20% are congenital, with the remainder being noted after chest trauma or thoracic surgery or in patients with pulmonary diseases such as cystic fibrosis (Chapter 395) or asthma (Chapter 138), which cause frequent cough and generate high intrathoracic pressure. A congenital weakness of the suprapleural membrane (Sibson's fascia) or musculature of the neck can play a role in the appearance of a lung hernia. More than half of congenital lung hernias and almost all acquired hernias are **cervical.** Congenital cervical hernias usually occur anteriorly through a gap between the scalenus anterior and sternocleidomastoid muscles. Cervical herniation is usually prevented by the trapezius muscle (posteriorly, at the thoracic inlet) and by the three scalene muscles (laterally).

CLINICAL MANIFESTATIONS AND TREATMENT

The presenting sign of a cervical hernia (Sibson hernia) is usually a neck mass noticed while straining or coughing. Some lesions are asymptomatic and detected only when a chest film is taken for another reason. Findings on physical examination are normal except during Valsalva maneuver, when a soft bulge may be noticed in the neck. In most cases, no treatment is necessary, although these hernias can cause problems during attempts to place a central venous catheter through the jugular or subclavian veins. They can resolve spontaneously.

Paravertebral or parasternal hernias are usually associated with rib anomalies. Intercostal hernias usually occur parasternally, where the external intercostal muscle is absent. Posteriorly, despite the seemingly inadequate internal intercostal muscle, the paraspinal muscles usually prevent herniation. Straining, coughing, or playing a musical instrument can have a role in causing intercostal hernias, but in most cases, there is probably a preexisting defect in the thoracic wall.

Surgical treatment for lung hernia is occasionally justified for cosmetic reasons. In patients with severe chronic pulmonary disease and chronic cough and for whom cough suppression is contraindicated, permanent correction might not be achieved.

BIBLIOGRAPHY
Please visit the Nelson Textbook of Pediatrics *website at www.expertconsult.com for the complete bibliography.*

387.8 Other Congenital Malformations of the Lung

Jonathan D. Finder

CONGENITAL LOBAR EMPHYSEMA AND PULMONARY CYSTS

See Chapter 384.

PULMONARY ARTERIOVENOUS MALFORMATION

See Chapters 426 and 438.

BRONCHOBILIARY FISTULA

A bronchobiliary fistula consists of a fistulous connection between the right middle lobe bronchus and the left hepatic ductal system. Although diagnosis can be delayed until adulthood, this rare anomaly typically manifests with life-threatening bronchopulmonary infections in early infancy. Girls are more commonly affected. *Definitive diagnosis* requires endoscopy and bronchography or exploratory surgery. *Treatment* includes surgical excision of the entire intrathoracic portion of the fistula. If the hepatic portion of the fistula does not communicate with the biliary system or duodenum, the involved segment might also have to be resected. Bronchobiliary communications also occur as acquired lesions resulting from hepatic disease complicated by infection.

Chapter 388
Pulmonary Edema

Robert Mazor and Thomas P. Green

Pulmonary edema is an excessive accumulation of fluid in the interstitium and air spaces of the lung resulting in oxygen desaturation, decreased lung compliance, and respiratory distress. It is a common problem in the acutely ill child and a sequela of several different pathologic processes.

PATHOPHYSIOLOGY

Although pulmonary edema is traditionally separated into two categories according to cause (*cardiogenic* and *noncardiogenic*), the end result of both processes is a net fluid accumulation within the interstitial and alveolar spaces. Noncardiogenic pulmonary edema, in its most severe state, is also known as **acute respiratory distress syndrome** (**ARDS**) (Chapters 65 and 365).

The hydrostatic pressure and colloid osmotic (oncotic) pressure on either side of a pulmonary vascular wall, along with vascular permeability, are the forces and physical factors that determine fluid movement through the vessel wall. Baseline conditions lead to a net filtration of fluid from the intravascular space into the interstitium. This "extra" interstitial fluid is usually rapidly reabsorbed by pulmonary lymphatics. Conditions that lead to altered vascular permeability, increased pulmonary vascular pressure, and decreased intravascular oncotic pressure increase the net flow of fluid out of the vessel (Table 388-1). Once the capacity of the lymphatics for fluid removal is exceeded, water accumulates in the lung.

Table 388-1 ETIOLOGY OF PULMONARY EDEMA

INCREASED PULMONARY CAPILLARY PRESSURE
Cardiogenic, such as left ventricular failure Noncardiogenic, as in pulmonary venoocclusive disease, pulmonary venous fibrosis, mediastinal tumors
INCREASED CAPILLARY PERMEABILITY
Bacterial and viral pneumonia Acute respiratory distress syndrome (ARDS) Inhaled toxic agents Circulating toxins Vasoactive substances such as histamine, leukotrienes, thromboxanes Diffuse capillary leak syndrome, as in sepsis Immunologic reactions, such as transfusion reactions Smoke inhalation Aspiration pneumonia/pneumonitis Drowning and near drowning Radiation pneumonia Uremia
LYMPHATIC INSUFFICIENCY
Congenital and acquired
DECREASED ONCOTIC PRESSURE
Hypoalbuminemia, as in renal and hepatic diseases, protein-losing states, and malnutrition
INCREASED NEGATIVE INTERSTITIAL PRESSURE
Upper airway obstructive lesions, such as croup and epiglottitis Reexpansion pulmonary edema
MIXED OR UNKNOWN CAUSES
Neurogenic pulmonary edema High-altitude pulmonary edema Eclampsia Pancreatitis Pulmonary embolism Heroin (narcotic) pulmonary edema

Modified from Robin E, Carroll C, Zelis R: Pulmonary edema, *N Engl J Med* 288:239, 292, 1973; and Desphande J, Wetzel R, Rogers M: In Rogers M, editor: *Textbook of pediatric intensive care*, ed 3, Baltimore, 1996, Williams & Wilkins, pp 432–442.

To understand the sequence of lung water accumulation, it is helpful to consider its distribution among 4 distinct compartments, as follows:

Vascular compartment: This compartment consists of all blood vessels that participate in fluid exchange with the interstitium. The vascular compartment is separated from the interstitium by capillary endothelial cells. Several endogenous inflammatory mediators, as well as exogenous toxins, are implicated in the pathogenesis of pulmonary capillary endothelial damage, leading to the "leakiness" seen in several systemic processes.

Interstitial compartment: The importance of this space lies in its interposition between the alveolar and vascular compartments. As fluid leaves the vascular compartment, it collects in the interstitium before overflowing into the air spaces of the alveolar compartment.

Alveolar compartment: This compartment is lined with type 1 and type 2 epithelial cells. These epithelial cells have a role in active fluid transport from the alveolar space, and they act as a barrier to exclude fluid from the alveolar space. The potential fluid volume of the alveolar compartment is many times greater than that of the interstitial space, perhaps providing another reason that alveolar edema clears more slowly than interstitial edema.

Pulmonary lymphatic compartment: There is an extensive network of pulmonary lymphatics. Excess fluid present in the alveolar and interstitial compartments is drained via the lymphatic system. When the capacity for drainage of the lymphatics is surpassed, fluid accumulation occurs.

ETIOLOGY

The specific clinical findings vary according to the underlying mechanism (see Table 388-1).

Increases in pulmonary vascular pressure *(capillary hydrostatic pressure)* lead to increases in transudation of fluid. *Cardiac processes* that lead to myocardial dysfunction and decreased left-sided output and those that lead to mitral valve regurgitation cause increased "back-pressure" in the pulmonary vasculature. In addition, abnormalities of the pulmonary veins often obstruct venous drainage and also result in an *increase in pulmonary capillary pressure.*

Increased capillary permeability is usually secondary to endothelial damage. Such damage can occur secondary to direct injury to the alveolar epithelium or indirectly through systemic processes that deliver circulating inflammatory mediators or toxins to the lung. Inflammatory mediators (tumor necrosis factor, leukotrienes, thromboxanes) and vasoactive agents (nitric oxide, histamine) formed during pulmonary and systemic processes potentiate the altered capillary permeability that occurs in many disease processes, with sepsis being a common cause.

Fluid homeostasis in the lung largely depends on drainage via the lymphatics. Experimentally, pulmonary edema occurs with obstruction of the lymphatic system. Increased lymph flow and dilation of lymphatic vessels occur in chronic edematous states.

A decrease in intravascular oncotic pressure leads to pulmonary edema by altering the forces promoting fluid reentry into the vascular space. This occurs in dilutional disorders such as fluid overload with hypotonic solutions and in protein-losing states such as nephrotic syndrome and malnutrition.

The excessive negative interstitial pressure seen in upper airway diseases, such as croup and laryngospasm, may promote pulmonary edema. Aside from the physical forces present in these diseases, other mechanisms may also be involved. Theories implicate an increase in CO_2 tension, decreased O_2 tension, and extreme increases in cardiac afterload, leading to transient cardiac insufficiency.

The mechanism causing neurogenic pulmonary edema is not clear. A massive sympathetic discharge secondary to a cerebral injury may produce increased pulmonary and systemic vasoconstriction, resulting in a shift of blood to the pulmonary vasculature, an increase in capillary pressure, and edema formation.

The mechanism responsible for high-altitude pulmonary edema is unclear, but it may also be related to sympathetic outflow, increased pulmonary vascular pressures, and hypoxia-induced increases in capillary permeability.

Active ion transport followed by passive, osmotic water movement is important in clearing the alveolar space of fluid. Interindividual genetic differences in the rates of these transport processes may be important in determining which individuals are susceptible to altitude-related pulmonary edema. Although the existence of these mechanisms suggests that therapeutic interventions may be developed to promote resolution of pulmonary edema, no such therapies currently exist.

CLINICAL MANIFESTATIONS

The clinical features depend on the mechanism of edema formation. In general, interstitial edema and alveolar edema prevent the inflation of alveoli, leading to atelectasis and decreased surfactant production. This results in diminished pulmonary compliance and tidal volume. The patient must increase respiratory effort and/or the respiratory rate in order to maintain minute ventilation. The earliest clinical signs of pulmonary edema include increased work of breathing, tachypnea, and dyspnea. As fluid accumulates in the alveolar space, auscultation reveals fine crackles and wheezing, especially in dependent lung fields. In cardiogenic pulmonary edema, a gallop may be present as well as peripheral edema and jugular venous distention.

Chest radiographs can provide useful ancillary data, although findings of initial radiographs may be normal. Early radiographic signs that represent accumulation of interstitial edema include peribronchial and perivascular cuffing. Diffuse streakiness reflects interlobular edema and distended pulmonary lymphatics. Diffuse, patchy densities, the so-called butterfly pattern, represent bilateral interstitial or alveolar infiltrates and are a late sign. Cardiomegaly is often seen with causes that involve left ventricular dysfunction. Heart size is usually normal in noncardiogenic pulmonary edema (Table 388-2). Chest tomography demonstrates edema accumulation in the dependent areas of the lung. As a result, changing the patient's position can alter regional differences in lung compliance and alveolar ventilation.

Measurement of brain natriuretic peptide (BNP), often elevated in heart disease, can help differentiate cardiac from pulmonary causes of pulmonary edema. A BNP level >500 pg/mL suggests heart disease; a level <100 pg/mL suggests lung disease.

Table 388-2 RADIOGRAPHIC FEATURES THAT MAY HELP DIFFERENTIATE CARDIOGENIC FROM NONCARDIOGENIC PULMONARY EDEMA

RADIOGRAPHIC FEATURE	CARDIOGENIC EDEMA	NONCARDIOGENIC EDEMA
Heart size	Normal or greater than normal	Usually normal
Width of the vascular pedicle*	Normal or greater than normal	Usually normal or less than normal
Vascular distribution	Balanced or inverted	Normal or balanced
Distribution of edema	Even or central	Patchy or peripheral
Pleural effusions	Present	Not usually present
Peribronchial cuffing	Present	Not usually present
Septal lines	Present	Not usually present
Air bronchograms	Not usually present	Usually present

*The width of the vascular pedicle in adults is determined by dropping a perpendicular line from the point at which the left subclavian artery exits the aortic arch and measuring across to the point at which the superior vena cava crosses the right mainstem bronchus. A vascular-pedicle width >70 mm on a portable digital anteroposterior radiograph of the chest obtained when the patient is supine is optimal for differentiating high from normal-to-low intravascular volume.

From Ware LB, Matthay MA: Acute pulmonary edema, *N Engl J Med* 353:2788–2796, 2005.

TREATMENT

The treatment of a patient with noncardiogenic pulmonary edema is largely supportive, with the primary goal to ensure adequate ventilation and oxygenation. Additional therapy is directed toward the underlying cause. Patients should receive supplemental oxygen to increase alveolar oxygen tension and pulmonary vasodilation. Patients with pulmonary edema of cardiogenic causes should be managed with inotropic agents and systemic vasodilators to reduce left ventricular afterload (Chapter 436). Diuretics are valuable in the treatment of pulmonary edema associated with total body fluid overload (sepsis, renal insufficiency). Morphine is often helpful as a vasodilator and a mild sedative.

Positive airway pressure improves gas exchange in patients with pulmonary edema. In tracheally intubated patients, **positive end-expiratory pressure (PEEP)** can be used to optimize pulmonary mechanics. Noninvasive forms of ventilation, such as mask or nasal prong continuous positive airway pressure (CPAP), are also effective. The mechanism by which positive airway pressure improves pulmonary edema is not entirely clear but is not associated with decreasing lung water. Rather, CPAP prevents complete closure of alveoli at the low lung volumes present at the end of expiration. It may also recruit already collapsed alveolar units. This leads to increased functional residual capacity (FRC) and improved pulmonary compliance, improved surfactant function, and decreased pulmonary vascular resistance. The net effect is to decrease the work of breathing, improve oxygenation, and decrease cardiac afterload (Chapter 365).

When mechanical ventilation becomes necessary, especially in noncardiogenic pulmonary edema, care must be taken to minimize the risk of development of complications from barotrauma, including pneumothorax, pneumomediastinum, and primary alveolar damage (Chapter 65.1). Lung protective strategies include setting low tidal volumes, relatively high PEEPs, and allowing for permissive hypercapnia.

High-altitude pulmonary edema (HAPE) should be managed with altitude descent and supplemental oxygen. Portable CPAP or a portable hyperbaric chamber is also helpful. Nifedipine (10 mg initially, and then 20-30 mg by slow release every 12-24 hr) in adults is also helpful. If there is a history of HAPE, nifedipine and β-adrenergic agonists (inhaled) may prevent recurrence.

BIBLIOGRAPHY

Please visit the Nelson Textbook of Pediatrics *website at* *www.expertconsult.com* *for the complete bibliography.*

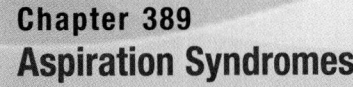

Chapter 389 Aspiration Syndromes

John L. Colombo

Aspiration includes a wide clinical spectrum from an asymptomatic condition to acute life-threatening events, such as occur with massive aspiration of gastric contents or hydrocarbon products. Other chapters discuss mechanical obstruction of large or intermediate-sized airways (as occurs with foreign bodies; Chapter 379) and infectious complications of aspiration and recurrent microaspiration (Chapter 390), such as may occur with gastroesophageal reflux (Chapter 315.1) or dysphagia (Chapter 298). Occult aspiration of nasopharyngeal secretions into the lower respiratory tract is a normal event in healthy people, usually without apparent clinical significance.

GASTRIC CONTENTS

Large-volume aspiration of gastric contents usually occurs in the context of vomiting. It is an infrequent complication of general anesthesia, gastroenteritis, and altered level of consciousness. Among 63,180 pediatric patients undergoing general anesthesia, 24 cases of aspiration occurred, but symptoms developed in only 9. Pathophysiologic consequences can vary, depending primarily on the pH and volume of the aspirate and the amount of particulate material. Increased clinical severity is noted with volumes greater than approximately 0.8 mL/kg and/or pH <2.5. Hypoxemia, hemorrhagic pneumonitis, atelectasis, intravascular fluid shifts, and pulmonary edema all occur rapidly after massive aspiration. These occur earlier, become more severe, and last longer with acid aspiration. Most clinical changes are present within minutes to 1-2 hr after the aspiration event. In the next 24-48 hr, there is a marked increase in lung parenchymal neutrophil infiltrations, mucosal sloughing, and alveolar consolidation that often correlates with increasing infiltrates on chest radiographs. These changes tend to occur significantly later and are more prolonged after aspiration of particulate material. Infection usually does not have a role in initial lung injury after aspiration of gastric contents; aspiration may impair pulmonary defenses, predisposing the patient to secondary bacterial pneumonia. In the patient who has shown clinical improvement but then demonstrates clinical worsening, especially with fever and leukocytosis, secondary bacterial pneumonia should be suspected.

Treatment

If large-volume or highly toxic substance aspiration occurs in a patient who already has an artificial airway in place, it is important to perform immediate suctioning of the airway. If immediate suctioning cannot be performed, later suctioning or bronchoscopy is usually of limited therapeutic value. An exception to this policy is suspicion of significant particulate aspiration. Attempts at acid neutralization are not warranted because acid is rapidly neutralized by the respiratory epithelium. Patients in whom large-volume or toxic aspiration is suspected should be observed, should undergo oxygenation measurement by oximetry or blood gas analysis, and should undergo a chest radiograph, even if they are asymptomatic. If the chest radiograph findings and oxygen saturation are normal, and the patient remains asymptomatic, home observation, after a period of observation in the hospital or office, is adequate. No treatment is indicated at that time, but the caregivers should be instructed to bring the child back in for medical attention should respiratory symptoms or fever develop. For patients who present with abnormal findings or in whom such findings develop during observation, oxygen therapy is given to correct hypoxemia. Endotracheal intubation and mechanical ventilation are often necessary for more severe cases. Bronchodilators may be tried, although they are usually of limited benefit. Animal studies indicate that treatment with corticosteroids does not appear to have any benefit, unless given nearly simultaneously with the aspiration event; use of these agents may increase the risk of secondary infection. Prophylactic antibiotics are not indicated, although in the patient with very limited reserve, early antibiotic coverage may be appropriate. If used, antibiotics should be selected that cover for anaerobic microbes. If the aspiration event occurs in a hospitalized or chronically ill patient, coverage of *Pseudomonas* and enteric gram-negative organisms should also be considered. A mortality rate of ≤5% is seen if 3 or fewer lobes are involved. Unless complications develop, such as infection or barotrauma, most patients recover in 2-3 wk, although prolonged lung damage may persist, with scarring, bronchiolitis obliterans, and bronchiectasis.

Prevention

Prevention of aspiration should always be the goal when airway manipulation is necessary for intubation or other invasive procedures. Feeding with enteral tubes passed beyond the pylorus, elevating the head of the bed 30-45 degrees in mechanically ventilated patients, and oral decontamination, have been shown to reduce the incidence of aspiration complications in the intensive care unit. Minimizing use of sedation, monitoring for gastric residuals, and gastric acid suppression may all help prevent aspiration. Any patient with altered consciousness, especially one who is receiving tube feedings, should be considered at high risk for aspiration.

HYDROCARBON ASPIRATION

The most dangerous consequence of acute hydrocarbon ingestion is usually aspiration and resulting pneumonitis (Chapter 58). Although significant pneumonitis occurs in <2% of all hydrocarbon ingestions, an estimated 20 deaths occur annually from hydrocarbon aspiration in both children and adults. Some of these deaths represent suicides. Hydrocarbons with lower surface tensions (gasoline, turpentine, naphthalene) have more potential for aspiration toxicity than heavier mineral or fuel oils. Ingestion of >30 mL (approximate volume of an adult swallow) of hydrocarbon is associated with an increased risk of severe pneumonitis. Clinical findings such as chest retractions, grunting, cough, and fever may occur as soon as 30 min after aspiration or may be delayed for several hours. Lung radiographic changes usually occur within 2-8 hr, peaking in 48-72 hr (Fig. 389-1). Pneumatoceles and pleural effusions may occur. Patients presenting with cough, shortness of breath, or hypoxemia are at high risk for pneumonitis. Persistent pulmonary function abnormalities can be present many years after hydrocarbon aspiration. Other organ

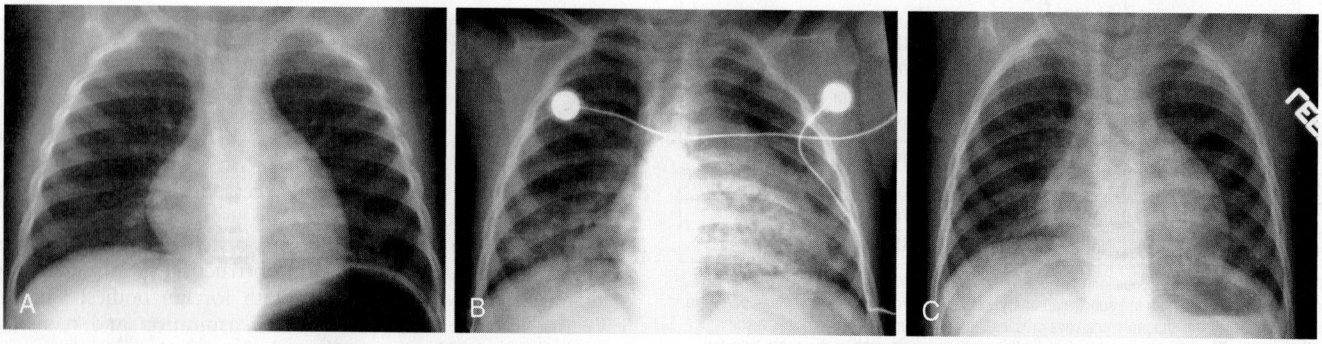

Figure 389-1 Chest radiographs of a 17 mo old who ingested furniture polish. *A,* Three hours after ingestion, the lungs are clear. *B,* At 24 hours, there are bibasilar coalescing nodular opacities. *C,* Three days later, there is much clearing. (From Slovis TL, editor: *Caffey's pediatric diagnostic imaging,* ed 11, Philadelphia, 2008, Mosby/Elsevier, p 1287.)

systems, especially the liver, central nervous system, and heart, may suffer serious injury. Cardiac dysrhythmias may occur and may be exacerbated by hypoxia and acid-base or electrolyte disturbances.

Treatment

Gastric emptying is nearly always contraindicated because the risk of aspiration is greater than any systemic toxicity. Treatment is generally supportive, consisting of oxygen, fluids, and ventilatory support as necessary. The child who has no symptoms and normal chest radiograph findings should be observed for 6-8 hr to ensure safe discharge. Certain hydrocarbons have more inherent systemic toxicity. The pneumonic **CHAMP** refers collectively to the following hydrocarbons: camphor, **h**alogenated carbons, aromatic hydrocarbons, and those associated with **m**etals and pesticides. Patients who ingest these compounds in volumes >30 mL, such as might occur with intentional overdose, may benefit from gastric emptying. This is still a high-risk procedure that can result in further aspiration. If a cuffed endotracheal tube can be placed without inducing vomiting, this procedure should be considered, especially in the presence of altered mental status. Treatment of each case should be considered individually, with guidance from a poison control center.

Other substances that are particularly toxic and cause significant lung injury when aspirated or inhaled include baby powder, chlorine, shellac, beryllium, and mercury vapors. Repeated exposure to low concentrations of these agents can lead to chronic lung disease, such as interstitial pneumonitis and granuloma formation. Corticosteroids may help reduce fibrosis development and improve pulmonary function, although the evidence for this benefit is limited.

BIBLIOGRAPHY
Please visit the Nelson Textbook of Pediatrics *website at* www.expertconsult.com *for the complete bibliography.*

Chapter 390
Chronic Recurrent Aspiration

John L. Colombo

ETIOLOGY

The recurrent aspiration of small quantities of gastric, nasal, or oral contents can lead to several clinical presentations, including recurrent bronchitis or bronchiolitis; recurrent pneumonia; atelectasis; wheezing; cough; apnea; and/or laryngospasm. Pathologic outcomes include granulomatis inflammation, interstitial inflammation, fibrosis, lipoid pneumonia, and bronchiolitis obliterans. Most cases, although associated with significant morbidity, do not come to pathologic inspection, but clinically manifest as airway inflammation. Underlying disorders that are frequently associated with recurrent aspiration are listed in Table 390-1. Oropharyngeal incoordination is reportedly the most common underlying problem associated with recurrent pneumonias in hospitalized children. In one series of 238 children hospitalized with recurrent pneumonia, 48% were found to have dysphagia as the underlying problem. Lipoid pneumonia may occur after the use of home/folk remedies involving oral or nasal administration of animal or vegetable oils to treat various childhood illnesses. Lipoid pneumonia has been reported as a complication of these practices in the Middle East, Asia, India, Brazil, and Mexico. The initial underlying disease, language barriers, and a belief that these are not "medications" may delay the diagnosis.

Gastroesophageal reflux disease (GERD) is also a common underlying finding that may predispose to recurrent respiratory

Table 390-1 CONDITIONS PREDISPOSING TO ASPIRATION LUNG INJURY IN CHILDREN

ANATOMICAL AND MECHANICAL
Tracheoesophageal fistula
Laryngeal cleft
Vascular ring
Cleft palate
Micrognathia
Macroglossia
Achalasia
Esophageal foreign body
Tracheostomy
Endotracheal tube
Nasoenteric tube
Collagen vascular disease (scleroderma, dermatomyositises)
Gastroesophageal reflux disease
Obesity
NEUROMUSCULAR
Altered consciousness
Immaturity of swallowing/Prematurity
Dysautonomia
Increased intracranial pressure
Hydrocephalus
Vocal cord paralysis
Cerebral palsy
Muscular dystrophy
Myasthenia gravis
Guillain-Barré syndrome
Werdnig-Hoffmann disease
Ataxia-telangiectasia
Cerebral vascular accident
MISCELLANEOUS
Poor oral hygiene
Gingivitis
Prolonged hospitalization
Gastric outlet or intestinal obstruction
Poor feeding techniques (bottle propping, overfeeding, inappropriate foods for toddlers)
Bronchopulmonary dysplasia
Viral infection

disease, but it is less frequently associated with recurrent pneumonia than dysphagia. GERD is discussed in Chapter 315.1. Aspiration has also been observed in infants with respiratory symptoms but no other apparent abnormalities. Recurrent microaspiration has been reported in otherwise apparently normal newborns, especially premature infants. Aspiration is also a risk in patients suffering from acute respiratory illness from other causes, especially respiratory syncytial virus infection. These patients, when studied with modified barium swallow and videofluoroscopy, have been seen to have silent aspiration. This finding emphasizes the need for a high degree of clinical suspicion for ongoing aspiration in a child with an acute respiratory illness, being fed enterally, who deteriorates unexpectedly.

DIAGNOSIS

Some underlying predisposing factors (see Table 390-1) are frequently clinically apparent but may require specific further evaluation. Initial assessment begins with a detailed history and physical examination. The caregiver should be asked about spitting, vomiting, arching, or epigastric discomfort in an older child, the timing of symptoms in relation to feedings, positional changes, and nocturnal symptoms such as coughing and wheezing. It is important to remember that coughing or gagging may be minimal or absent in a child with a depressed cough or gag reflex. Observation of a feeding is an essential part of the exam when a diagnosis of recurrent aspiration is being considered. Particular attention should be given to nasopharyngeal reflux, difficulty with sucking or swallowing, and associated coughing and choking. The oral cavity should be inspected for gross abnormalities and stimulated to assess the gag reflex. Drooling or excessive accumulation of secretions in the mouth suggests dysphagia. Lung auscultation may reveal transient crackles or wheezes after feeding, particularly in the dependent lung segments.

The diagnosis of recurrent microaspiration is challenging because of the lack of highly specific and sensitive tests (Table 390-2). A plain chest radiograph is the usual initial study for a child in whom recurrent aspiration is suspected.The classic findings of segmental or lobar infiltrates localized to dependent areas may be found (Fig. 390-1), but there are a wide variety of radiographic findings. These findings include diffuse infiltrates, lobar infiltrates, bronchial wall thickening, hyperinflation, and even no detectable abnormalities. CT scans, though generally not indicated to establish a diagnosis of aspiration, may show infiltrates with decreased attenuation suggestive of lipoid pneumonia (Fig. 390-2). A carefully performed barium esophagram is useful in looking for anatomic abnormalities such as vascular ring, stricture, hiatal hernia, and tracheoesophageal fistula. It also yields qualitative information about esophageal motility and, when extended, of gastric emptying. However, primarily because of the very short viewing time, the esophagram is quite insensitive and nonspecific for aspiration or GERD. A modified barium swallow study with video fluoroscopy (video fluoroscopic swallowing study) is generally considered the gold standard for evaluating the swallowing mechanism. This study is preferably done with the assistance of a pediatric feeding specialist and a caregiver in the attempt to simulate the usual feeding technique of the child. The child is seated in normal eating position, and various consistencies of barium or barium impregnated foods are offered. This

Table 390-2 SUMMARY OF DIAGNOSTIC TESTS OF ASPIRATION

EVALUATION	BENEFITS	LIMITATIONS
Chest radiograph	Inexpensive and widely available Assesses accumulation of injury over time	Insensitive to early subtle changes of lung injury
HRCT	Sensitive in detecting lung injury, such as bronchiectasis, tree-in-bud opacities, and bronchial thickening Less radiation than conventional CT Assesses accumulation of injury over time	More radiation exposure than plain radiograph Expensive
VSS	Evaluates all phases of swallowing Evaluates multiple consistencies Feeding recommendations made at time of study	Information limited if child consumes only small quantities Difficult to perform in child who has not been feeding by mouth Radiation exposure proportional to study duration Cannot be performed at bedside Limited evaluation of anatomy Evaluates one moment in time Expensive
FEES/with sensory testing	Ability to thoroughly evaluate functional anatomy Evaluates multiple consistencies Can assess risk of aspiration in nonorally feeding child; airway protective reflexes can be assessed Feeding recommendations made at time of study Visual feedback for caregivers Can be performed at bedside No radiation exposure	Blind to oesophageal phase and actual swallow Invasive and may not represent physiological swallowing conditions Evaluates one moment in time Not widely available Expensive
BAL	Evaluates anatomy of entire upper and lower airways Samples the endorgan of damage Sample available for multiple cytological and microbiological tests Becoming more widely available	Uncertainty regarding interpretation of lipid-laden macrophage index Index cumbersome to calculate Requires sedation or anaesthesia Invasive Expensive
Esophageal pH monitoring	Current gold standard for diagnosis of GOR Established normative data in children	Blind to majority of reflux events Difficult to establish causal relationship between GOR and aspiration Somewhat invasive Evaluates one moment in time
Esophageal impedance monitoring	Likely future gold standard for diagnosis of GERD with supra-esophageal manifestations Able to detect acid and nonacid reflux events Detects proximal reflux events Able to evaluate for GERD without stopping medications	Lack of normative data for children Somewhat invasive Expensive and cumbersome to interpret Not widely available Evaluates one moment in time
Gastroesophageal scintigraphy	Performed under physiological conditions Low radiation exposure	Poor sensitivity May not differentiate between aspiration from dysphagia or GERD
Radionuclide salivagram	Child does not have to be challenged with food bolus Low radiation exposure	Unknown sensitivity Unknown relationship to disease outcomes Evaluates one moment in time
Dye studies	Can be constructed as screening test or confirmatory test Can evaluate aspiration of secretions or feeds Repeating over time allows for broader evaluation	Uncertainty in interpretation owing to variability of technique Can only be performed in children with tracheostomies

HRCT: high-resolution computed tomography; VSS: videofluoroscopic swallow study; FEES: fibreoptic-endoscopic evaluation of swallowing; BAL: bronchoalveolar lavage; CT: computed tomography; GERD, gastroesophageal reflux disease.
From Boesch RP, Daines C, Willging JP, et al: Advances in the diagnosis and management of chronic pulmonary aspiration in children, *Eur Respir J* 28:847–861, 2006.

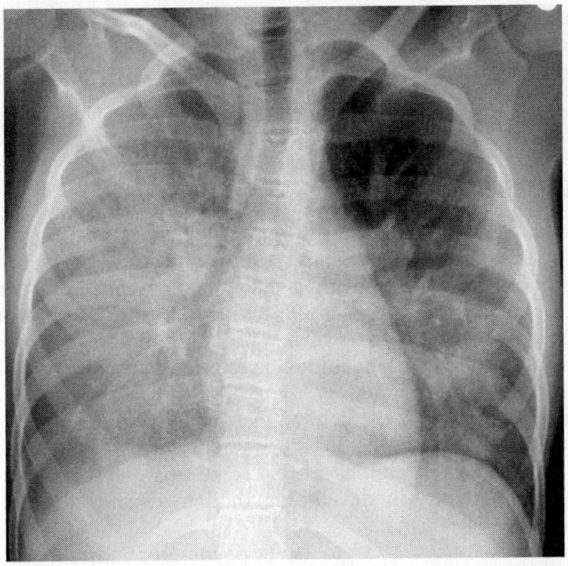

Figure 390-1 Chest radiograph of a developmentally delayed 15 yr old with chronic aspiration of oral formula. Note posterior (dependent areas) distribution with sparing of heart borders.

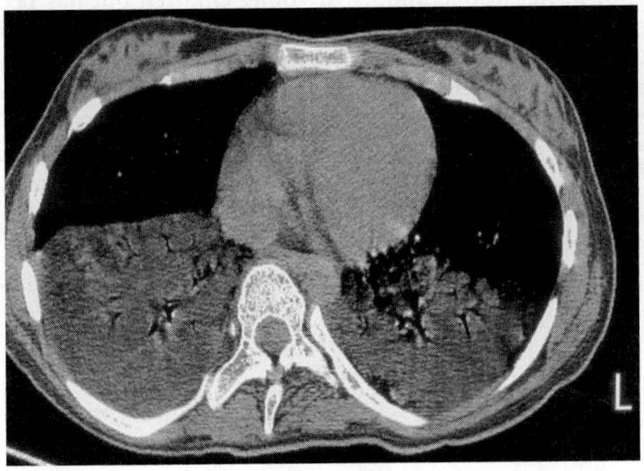

Figure 390-2 Chest CT scan of same patient as in Figure 390-1. Note lung consolidation in dependent region is of similar density to subcutaneous fat.

study is more sensitive for demonstrating aspiration than bedside assessment or a traditional barium swallow study. The sensitivity of the modified barium swallow study is such that it occasionally detects aspiration in patients without apparent respiratory abnormalities.

A gastroesophageal "milk" scintiscan offers theoretical advantages over a barium swallow in being more physiologic and giving a longer window of viewing than the barium esophagram for detecting aspiration and GERD. However, this form of study provides relatively little anatomic detail. Another radionuclide scan termed the "salivagram" may also be useful to assess aspiration of esophageal contents. When this scan is performed by experienced personnel, its sensitivity appears to be comparable to that of the modified barium swallow study. The use of fiberoptic endoscopic evaluation of swallowing (FEES) is useful in pediatric patients to observe swallowing directly without radiation exposure. The child's reaction to placement of the endoscope may alter the assessment of function, depending on level of comfort and cooperation.

Tracheobronchial aspirates can be examined for numerous entities to evaluate for aspiration. For patients with artificial airways, the use of an oral dye and visual examination of tracheal secretions is useful. However, this test should not be done on a chronic basis, such as in tube feedings, due to possible dye toxicity. In using this test acutely, the best method is to place a few drops of dye on the patient's tongue and perform subsequent suctioning of the airway over the next several minutes. Quantitation of lipid-laden alveolar macrophages from bronchial aspirates has been shown to be a sensitive test for aspiration in children, but false positive tests occur, especially with endobronchial obstruction, use of intravenous lipids, sepsis, and pulmonary bleeding. Bronchial washings may also be examined for various food substances, including lactose, glucose, food fibers, and milk antigens. Specificity and sensitivity of these tests have not been well studied.

TREATMENT

If chronic aspiration is associated with another underlying medical condition, treatment should be directed toward that problem. The level of morbidity from respiratory problems should determine the level of intervention. Often milder dysphagia can be treated with alteration of feeding position, limiting texture of foods to those best tolerated on modified barium esophagram (usually thicker foods), or limiting quantity per feeding. Nasogastric tube feedings can be utilized temporarily during periods of transient vocal cord dysfunction or other dysphagia. Post-pyloric feedings may also be helpful, especially if gastroesophageal reflux is present. There are several surgical procedures that may be considered. Tracheostomy, although sometimes predisposing to aspiration, may provide overall benefit from improved bronchial hygiene and the ability to suction aspirated material. Fundoplication with gastrostomy or jejunostomy feeding tube will reduce the probability of gastroesophageal reflux-induced aspiration, but recurrent pneumonias often persist because of dysphagia and presumed aspiration of upper airway secretions. Medical treatment with anticholinergics, such as glycopyrrolate or scopolamine, may significantly reduce morbidity from salivary aspiration but often has side effects. Aggressive surgical intervention with salivary gland excision, ductal ligation, laryngotracheal separation, or esophagogastric disconnection can be considered in severe, unresponsive cases. Although usually reserved for the most severe cases, surgical therapy may significantly improve quality of life and ease of care for some patients.

BIBLIOGRAPHY

Please visit the Nelson Textbook of Pediatrics *website at www.expertconsult.com for the complete bibliography.*

Chapter 391
Parenchymal Disease with Prominent Hypersensitivity, Eosinophilic Infiltration, or Toxin-Mediated Injury

391.1 Hypersensitivity to Inhaled Materials

Oren Lakser

Extrinsic allergic alveolitis or hypersensitivity pneumonitis (HP) is an immunologically mediated diffuse inflammatory disease of the pulmonary interstitium caused by inhalation of a variety (>200) of different organic antigens. Antigens are typically of animal or vegetable origin and ~1-5 µm in size and therefore deposit in the alveoli. Reactive antigens, such as a variety of drugs, can occasionally cause HP.

For the full continuation of this chapter, please visit the Nelson Textbook of Pediatrics *website at www.expertconsult.com.*

391.2 Silo Filler Disease

Oren Lakser

Silo filler disease (also referred as **silage gas poisoning** or **silo filler pneumoconiosis**) is typically caused by nitrogen dioxide toxicity. Nitrogen dioxide is produced in silos (particularly corn silos) within a few hr of filling and reaches a maximum concentration within about 2 days. Dangerous concentrations of gas can remain in a closed silo for as long as 2 wk. After entering a silo within this time frame without proper protection, a person may experience various degrees of silo filler disease.

For the full continuation of this chapter, please visit the Nelson Textbook of Pediatrics *website at www.expertconsult.com.*

391.3 Paraquat Lung

Oren Lakser

Paraquat is the most toxic dipyridilium herbicide. Concentrated solutions (12-20%) tend to be more dangerous than dilute solutions. Its toxic effects result from the production of superoxides and other highly reactive free radicals that cause the peroxidation of cell membranes and selective mitochondrial damage, resulting in cell death. Paraquat selectively concentrates in the lungs because of an amine uptake process that exists in alveolar epithelial cells. Additionally, paraquat-induced injury is significantly increased in the presence of high concentrations of oxygen. Although its use is banned or restricted in some countries, paraquat is still used extensively, particularly in many developing and transitional countries including tourist destinations. Most cases of paraquat intoxication are self-inflicted (suicide attempts). There have been case reports of fetal poisoning after maternal ingestion of paraquat (readily crosses placenta) with poor prognosis for the fetus.

For the full continuation of this chapter, please visit the Nelson Textbook of Pediatrics *website at www.expertconsult.com.*

391.4 Eosinophilic Lung Disease

Oren Lakser

The findings of pulmonary infiltrates and circulating or tissue eosinophilia describe the heterogenous group of disorders referred to as **eosinophilic lung diseases** or **pulmonary infiltrates with eosinophilia** (PIE) (see Table 391-2 the *Nelson Textbook of Pediatrics* website at www.expertconsult.com). There are numerous classification schemes for these types of lung disease. PIE syndromes can be divided into primary (idiopathic) and secondary eosinophilic lung diseases. Primary eosinophilic lung diseases include simple pulmonary eosinophilia (Löffler syndrome), acute eosinophilic pneumonia, chronic eosinophilic pneumonia, and idiopathic hypereosinophilic syndrome. Secondary eosinophilic lung diseases include tropical pulmonary eosinophilia, pulmonary eosinophilia with asthma, polyarteritis nodosa, Churg-Strauss syndrome, allergic bronchopulmonary aspergillosis (ABPA), and drug-induced eosinophilic lung disease. Additional lung diseases such as idiopathic pulmonary fibrosis, Langerhans cell granuloma, and other interstitial lung diseases may have associated eosinophilia but are better classified elsewhere.

For the full continuation of this chapter, please visit the Nelson Textbook of Pediatrics *website at www.expertconsult.com.*

Chapter 392 Community-Acquired Pneumonia

Thomas J. Sandora and Theodore C. Sectish

EPIDEMIOLOGY

Pneumonia—inflammation of the parenchyma of the lungs—is a substantial cause of morbidity and mortality in childhood throughout the world, rivaling diarrhea as a cause of death in developing countries (Fig. 392-1). With ≈158 million episodes of pneumonia per year, of which ≈154 million are occurring in developing countries, pneumonia is estimated to cause ≈3 million deaths, or an estimated 29% of all deaths, among children younger than 5 yr worldwide. The incidence of pneumonia is more than 10-fold higher (0.29 episodes versus 0.03 episodes), and the number of childhood-related deaths due to pneumonia ≈2000-fold higher, in developing than in developed countries (Table 392-1).

In the USA from 1939 to 1996, pneumonia mortality in children declined by 97%. It is hypothesized that this decline is attributable to the introduction of antibiotics, vaccines, and the expansion of medical insurance coverage for children. *Haemophilus influenzae* type b (Hib) (Chapter 186) was an important cause of bacterial pneumonia in young children but has become uncommon with the routine use of effective vaccines. The introduction of heptavalent pneumococcal conjugate vaccine and its impact on pneumococcal disease (Chapter 175) has reduced the overall incidence of pneumonia in infants and children in the USA by ≈30% in the 1st yr of life, ≈20% in the 2nd yr of life, and ≈10% in children >2 yr of age. In developing countries, the introduction of measles vaccine has greatly reduced the incidence of measles-related pneumonia deaths.

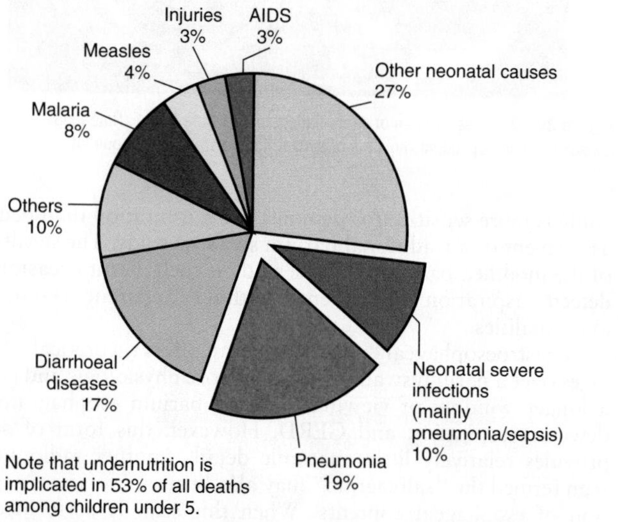

Figure 392-1 Pneumonia is the leading killer of children worldwide, as shown by this illustration of global distribution of cause-specific mortality among children <5 yr in 2004. Pneumonia causes 19% of all under-5 deaths. This illustration, however, does not include deaths due to pneumonia during the neonatal period. It is estimated that 26% of neonatal deaths, or 10% of under-5 deaths, are caused by severe infections. Large proportions of these infections are caused by pneumonia/sepsis. If these deaths were added to the overall estimate, pneumonia would account for up to 3 million, or as many as one third (29%), of under-5 deaths worldwide. (Sources of data: Cause-specific mortality estimates from WHO. World Health Report 2005: Make Every Mother and Child Count. Geneva: World Health Organization, 2005; under-five mortality estimates from UNICEF. The state of the world's children 2006. New York: United Nations Children's Fund, 2005. From Wardlaw T, Salama P, Johansson EW: Pneumonia: the leading killer of children, *Lancet* 368:1048–1050, 2006.)

Table 392-1 INCIDENCE OF PNEUMONIA CASES AND PNEUMONIA DEATHS AMONG CHILDREN UNDER FIVE, BY UNICEF REGION*

UNICEF REGIONS	NUMBER OF CHILDREN UNDER FIVE YEARS OF AGE (IN THOUSANDS)	NUMBER OF CHILDHOOD PNEUMONIA DEATHS (IN THOUSANDS)	INCIDENCE OF PNEUMONIA CASES (EPISODES PER CHILD PER YEAR)	TOTAL NUMBER OF PNEUMONIA EPISODES (IN THOUSANDS)
South Asia	169,300	702	0.36	61,300
Sub-Saharan Africa	117,300	1,022	0.30	35,200
Middle East and North Africa	43,400	82	0.26	11,300
East Asia and Pacific	146,400	158	0.24	34,500
Latin America and Caribbean	56,500	50	0.22	12,200
Central and Eastern Europe and the Commonwealth of Independent States	26,400	29	0.09	2,400
Developing countries	533,000	2,039	0.29	154,500
Industrialized countries	54,200	1	0.03	1,600
World	**613,600**	**2,044**	**0.26**	**158,500**

*Regional estimates in Columns 2, 3, and 5 do not add up to the world total because of rounding.

Table 392-2 CAUSES OF INFECTIOUS PNEUMONIA

BACTERIAL	
Common	
Streptococcus pneumoniae	Consolidation, empyema
Group B streptococci	Neonates
Group A streptococci	Empyema
*Mycoplasma pneumoniae**	Adolescents; summer-fall epidemics
*Chlamydophila pneumoniae**	Adolescents
Chlamydia trachomatis	Infants
Mixed anaerobes	Aspiration pneumonia
Gram-negative enterics	Nosocomial pneumonia
Uncommon	
Haemophilus influenzae type b	Unimmunized
Staphylococcus aureus	Pneumatoceles, empyema; infants
Moraxella catarrhalis	
Neisseria meningitidis	
Francisella tularensis	Animal, tick, fly contact; bioterrorism
Nocardia species	Immunosuppressed persons
*Chlamydophila psittaci**	Bird contact (especially parakeets)
Yersinia pestis	Plague; rat contact; bioterrorism
Legionella species*	Exposure to contaminated water; nosocomial
*Coxiella burnetii**	Q fever; animal (goat, sheep, cattle) exposure
VIRAL	
Common	
Respiratory synctial virus	Bronchiolitis
Parainfluenza types 1-3	Croup
Influenza A, B	High fever; winter months
Adenovirus	Can be severe; often occurs between January and April
Human metapneumovirus	Similar to respiratory syncytial virus
Uncommon	
Rhinovirus	Rhinorrhea
Enterovirus	Neonates
Herpes simplex	Neonates
Cytomegalovirus	Infants, immunosuppressed persons
Measles	Rash, coryza, conjunctivitis
Varicella	Adolescents or unimmunized
Hantavirus	Southwestern USA, rodents
Coronavirus (severe acute respiratory syndrome)	Asia
FUNGAL	
Histoplasma capsulatum	Ohio/Mississippi River valley; bird, bat contact
Blastomyces dermatitidis	Ohio/Mississippi River valley
Coccidioides immitis	Southwest USA
Cryptococcus neoformans	Bird contact
Aspergillus species	Immunosuppressed persons; nodular lung infection
Mucormycosis	Immunosuppressed persons
Pneumocystis jiroveci	Immunosuppressed, steroids
RICKETTSIAL	
Rickettsia rickettsiae	Tick bite
MYCOBACTERIAL	
Mycobacterium tuberculosis	Travel to endemic region; exposure to high-risk persons
Mycobacterium avium complex	Immunosuppressed persons
PARASITIC	
Various parasites (e.g., Ascaris, *Strongyloides* species)	Eosinophilic pneumonia

*Atypical pneumonia syndrome; may have extrapulmonary manifestations, low-grade fever, patchy diffuse infiltrates, poor response to beta-lactam antibiotics, and negative sputum Gram stain.
From Kliegman RM, Greenbaum LA, Lye PS: *Practical strategies in pediatric diagnosis & therapy*, ed 2, 2004, Philadelphia, Elsevier, p 29.

ETIOLOGY

Although most cases of pneumonia are caused by microorganisms, noninfectious causes include aspiration of food or gastric acid, foreign bodies, hydrocarbons, and lipoid substances, hypersensitivity reactions, and drug- or radiation-induced pneumonitis. The cause of pneumonia in an individual patient is often difficult to determine because direct culture of lung tissue is invasive and rarely performed. Cultures performed on specimens obtained from the upper respiratory tract or "sputum" often do not accurately reflect the cause of lower respiratory tract infection. With the use of state-of-the-art diagnostic testing, a bacterial or viral cause of pneumonia can be identified in 40-80% of children with community-acquired pneumonia. *Streptococcus pneumoniae* (pneumococcus) is the most common bacterial pathogen in children 3 wk to 4 yr of age, whereas *Mycoplasma pneumoniae* and *Chlamydophila pneumoniae* are the most frequent pathogens in children 5 yr and older. In addition to pneumococcus, other bacterial causes of pneumonia in previously healthy children in the USA include group A streptococcus (*Streptococcus pyogenes*) and *Staphylococcus aureus* (Chapter 174.1) (Table 392-2).

S. pneumoniae, H. influenzae, and *S. aureus* are the major causes of hospitalization and death from bacterial pneumonia

Table 392-3 ETIOLOGIC AGENTS GROUPED BY AGE OF THE PATIENT

AGE GROUP	FREQUENT PATHOGENS (IN ORDER OF FREQUENCY)
Neonates (<3 wk)	Group B streptococcus, *Escherichia coli*, other gram-negative bacilli, *Streptococcus pneumoniae*, *Haemophilus influenzae* (type b,* nontypable)
3 wk-3 mo	Respiratory syncytial virus, other respiratory viruses (parainfluenza viruses, influenza viruses, adenovirus), *S. pneumoniae*, *H. influenzae* (type b,* nontypable); if patient is afebrile, consider *Chlamydia trachomatis*
4 mo-4 yr	Respiratory syncytial virus, other respiratory viruses (parainfluenza viruses, influenza viruses, adenovirus), *S. pneumoniae*, *H. influenzae* (type b,* nontypable), *Mycoplasma pneumoniae*, group A streptococcus
≥5 yr	*M. pneumoniae*, *S. pneumoniae*, *Chlamydophila pneumoniae*, *H. influenzae* (type b,* nontypable), influenza viruses, adenovirus, other respiratory viruses, *Legionella pneumophila*

**H. influenzae* type b is uncommon with routine *H. influenzae* type b immunization.
From Kliegman RM, Marcdante KJ, Jenson HJ, et al: *Nelson essentials of pediatrics*, ed 5, Philadelphia, 2006, Elsevier, p 504.

among children in developing countries, although in children with HIV infection, *Mycobacterium tuberculosis* (Chapter 207), atypical mycobacteria, *Salmonella* (Chapter 190), *Escherichia coli* (Chapter 192), and *Pneumocystis jiroveci* (Chapter 236) must be considered. The incidence of *H. influenzae* has been significantly reduced in areas where routine Hib immunization has been implemented.

Viral pathogens are a prominent cause of lower respiratory tract infections in infants and children <5 yr of age. Viruses are responsible for 45% of the episodes of pneumonia identified in hospitalized children in Dallas. Unlike bronchiolitis, for which the peak incidence is in the 1st yr of life, the highest frequency of viral pneumonia occurs between the ages of 2 and 3 yr, decreasing slowly thereafter. Of the respiratory viruses, influenza virus (Chapter 250), and respiratory syncytial virus (RSV) (Chapter 252) are the major pathogens, especially in children <3 yr of age. Other common viruses causing pneumonia include parainfluenza viruses, adenoviruses, rhinoviruses, and human metapneumovirus. The age of the patient may help identify possible pathogens (Table 392-3).

Lower respiratory tract viral infections in the USA are much more common in the fall and winter, in relation to the seasonal epidemics of respiratory viral infection that occur each year. The typical pattern of these epidemics usually begins in the fall, when parainfluenza infections appear and most often manifest as croup. Later in winter, RSV, human metapneumovirus, and influenza viruses cause widespread infection, including upper respiratory tract infections, bronchiolitis, and pneumonia. RSV attacks infants and young children, whereas influenza virus causes disease and excess hospitalization for acute respiratory illness in all age groups. Knowledge of the prevailing viral epidemic may lead to a presumptive initial diagnosis.

Immunization status is relevant because children fully immunized against *H. influenzae* type b and *S. pneumoniae* are less likely to be infected with these pathogens. Children who are immunosuppressed or who have an underlying illness may be at risk for specific pathogens, such as *Pseudomonas* spp. in patients with cystic fibrosis.

PATHOGENESIS

The lower respiratory tract is normally kept sterile by physiologic defense mechanisms, including mucociliary clearance, the properties of normal secretions such as secretory immunoglobulin A (IgA), and clearing of the airway by coughing. Immunologic defense mechanisms of the lung that limit invasion by pathogenic organisms include macrophages that are present in alveoli and bronchioles, secretory IgA, and other immunoglobulins. Additional factors that promote pulmonary infection include trauma, anesthesia, and aspiration.

Viral pneumonia usually results from spread of infection along the airways, accompanied by direct injury of the respiratory epithelium, which results in airway obstruction from swelling, abnormal secretions, and cellular debris. The small caliber of airways in young infants makes such patients particularly susceptible to severe infection. Atelectasis, interstitial edema, and ventilation-perfusion mismatch causing significant hypoxemia often accompany airway obstruction. Viral infection of the respiratory tract can also predispose to secondary bacterial infection by disturbing normal host defense mechanisms, altering secretions, and modifying the bacterial flora.

Bacterial pneumonia most often occurs when respiratory tract organisms colonize the trachea and subsequently gain access to the lungs, but pneumonia may also result from direct seeding of lung tissue after bacteremia. When bacterial infection is established in the lung parenchyma, the pathologic process varies according to the invading organism. *M. pneumoniae* attaches to the respiratory epithelium, inhibits ciliary action, and leads to cellular destruction and an inflammatory response in the submucosa. As the infection progresses, sloughed cellular debris, inflammatory cells, and mucus cause airway obstruction, with spread of infection occurring along the bronchial tree, as it does in viral pneumonia.

S. pneumoniae produces local edema that aids in the proliferation of organisms and their spread into adjacent portions of lung, often resulting in the characteristic focal lobar involvement.

Group A streptococcus infection of the lower respiratory tract results in more diffuse infection with interstitial pneumonia. The pathology includes necrosis of tracheobronchial mucosa; formation of large amounts of exudate, edema, and local hemorrhage, with extension into the interalveolar septa; and involvement of lymphatic vessels and the increased likelihood of pleural involvement.

S. aureus pneumonia manifests in confluent bronchopneumonia, which is often unilateral and characterized by the presence of extensive areas of hemorrhagic necrosis and irregular areas of cavitation of the lung parenchyma, resulting in pneumatoceles, empyema, or, at times, bronchopulmonary fistulas.

Recurrent pneumonia is defined **as 2 or more** episodes in a single year **or 3 or more** episodes ever, with radiographic clearing between occurrences. An underlying disorder should be considered if a child experiences recurrent pneumonia (Table 392-4).

CLINICAL MANIFESTATIONS

Viral and bacterial pneumonias are often preceded by several days of symptoms of an upper respiratory tract infection, typically rhinitis and cough. In viral pneumonia, fever is usually present; temperatures are generally lower than in bacterial pneumonia. Tachypnea is the most consistent clinical manifestation of pneumonia. Increased work of breathing accompanied by intercostal, subcostal, and suprasternal retractions, nasal flaring, and use of accessory muscles is common. Severe infection may be accompanied by cyanosis and respiratory fatigue, especially in infants. Auscultation of the chest may reveal crackles and wheezing, but it is often difficult to localize the source of these adventitious sounds in very young children with hyperresonant chests. It is often not possible to distinguish viral pneumonia clinically from disease caused by *Mycoplasma* and other bacterial pathogens.

Bacterial pneumonia in adults and older children typically begins suddenly with a shaking chill followed by a high fever, cough, and chest pain. Other symptoms that may be seen include drowsiness with intermittent periods of restlessness; rapid respirations; anxiety; and, occasionally, delirium. Circumoral cyanosis

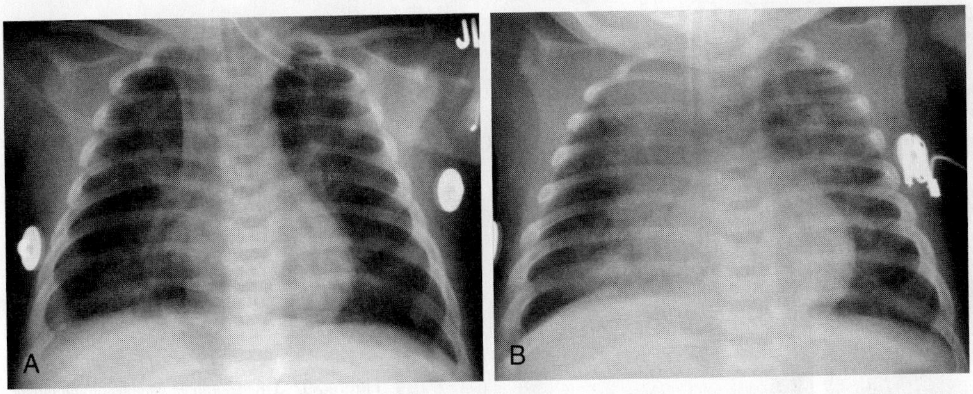

Figure 392-2 *A,* Radiographic findings characteristic of respiratory syncytial virus pneumonia in a 6 mo old infant with rapid respirations and fever. Anteroposterior radiograph of the chest shows hyperexpansion of the lungs with bilateral fine air space disease and streaks of density, indicating the presence of both pneumonia and atelectasis. An endotracheal tube is in place. *B,* One day later, the AP radiograph of the chest shows increased bilateral pneumonia.

Table 392-4 DIFFERENTIAL DIAGNOSIS OF RECURRENT PNEUMONIA

HEREDITARY DISORDERS
Cystic fibrosis Sickle cell disease
DISORDERS OF IMMUNITY
HIV/AIDS Bruton's agammaglobulinemia Selective immunoglobulin G subclass deficiencies Common variable immunodeficiency syndrome Severe combined immunodeficiency syndrome Chronic granulomatous disease Hyperimmunoglobulin E syndrome (Job syndrome) Leukocyte adhesion defect
DISORDERS OF CILIA
Immotile cilia syndrome Kartagener syndrome
ANATOMIC DISORDERS
Pulmonary sequestration Lobar emphysema Gastroesophageal reflux Foreign body Tracheoesophageal fistula (H type) Bronchiectasis Aspiration (oropharyngeal incoordination)

From Kliegman RM, Marcdante KJ, Jenson HJ, et al: *Nelson essentials of pediatrics,* ed 5, Philadelphia, 2006, Elsevier, p 507.

may be observed. In many children, splinting on the affected side to minimize pleuritic pain and improve ventilation is noted; such children may lie on one side with the knees drawn up to the chest.

Physical findings depend on the stage of pneumonia. Early in the course of illness, diminished breath sounds, scattered crackles, and rhonchi are commonly heard over the affected lung field. With the development of increasing consolidation or complications of pneumonia such as effusion, empyema, and pyopneumothorax, dullness on percussion is noted and breath sounds may be diminished. A lag in respiratory excursion often occurs on the affected side. Abdominal distention may be prominent because of gastric dilation from swallowed air or ileus. Abdominal pain is common in lower lobe pneumonia. The liver may seem enlarged because of downward displacement of the diaphragm secondary to hyperinflation of the lungs or superimposed congestive heart failure.

Symptoms described in adults with pneumococcal pneumonia may be noted in older children but are rarely observed in infants and young children, in whom the clinical pattern is considerably more variable. In infants, there may be a prodrome of upper respiratory tract infection and diminished appetite, leading to the abrupt onset of fever, restlessness, apprehension, and respiratory distress. These infants appear ill, with respiratory distress manifested as grunting; nasal flaring; retractions of the supraclavicular, intercostal, and subcostal areas; tachypnea; tachycardia; air hunger; and often cyanosis. Results of physical examination may be misleading, particularly in young infants, with meager findings disproportionate to the degree of tachypnea. Some infants with bacterial pneumonia may have associated gastrointestinal disturbances characterized by vomiting, anorexia, diarrhea, and abdominal distention secondary to a paralytic ileus. Rapid progression of symptoms is characteristic in the most severe cases of bacterial pneumonia.

DIAGNOSIS

An infiltrate on chest radiograph supports the diagnosis of pneumonia; the film may also indicate a complication such as a pleural effusion or empyema. Viral pneumonia is usually characterized by hyperinflation with bilateral interstitial infiltrates and peribronchial cuffing (Fig. 392-2). Confluent lobar consolidation is typically seen with pneumococcal pneumonia (Fig. 392-3). The radiographic appearance alone is not diagnostic, and other clinical features must be considered. Repeat chest radiographs are not required for proof of cure for patients with uncomplicated pneumonia.

The peripheral white blood cell (WBC) count can be useful in differentiating viral from bacterial pneumonia. In viral pneumonia, the WBC count can be normal or elevated but is usually not higher than 20,000/mm^3, with a lymphocyte predominance. Bacterial pneumonia is often associated with an elevated WBC count, in the range of 15,000-40,000/mm^3, and a predominance of granulocytes. A large pleural effusion, lobar consolidation, and a high fever at the onset of the illness are also suggestive of a bacterial etiology. **Atypical pneumonia** due to *C. pneumoniae* or *M. pneumoniae* is difficult to distinguish from pneumococcal pneumonia on the basis of radiographic and laboratory findings, and although pneumococcal pneumonia is associated with a higher WBC count, erythrocyte sedimentation rate (ESR), and C-reactive protein (CRP) level, there is considerable overlap.

The definitive diagnosis of a viral infection rests on the isolation of a virus or detection of the viral genome or antigen in respiratory tract secretions. Growth of respiratory viruses in conventional viral culture usually requires 5-10 days, although shell vial cultures can reduce this "turnaround time" to 2-3 days. Reliable DNA or RNA tests for the rapid detection of RSV, parainfluenza, influenza, and adenoviruses are available and accurate. Serologic techniques can also be used to diagnose a recent respiratory viral infection but generally require testing of acute and convalescent serum samples for a rise in antibodies to a specific viral agent. This diagnostic technique is laborious, slow, and not generally clinically useful because the infection usually resolves by the time it is confirmed serologically. Serologic testing may be valuable as an epidemiologic tool to define

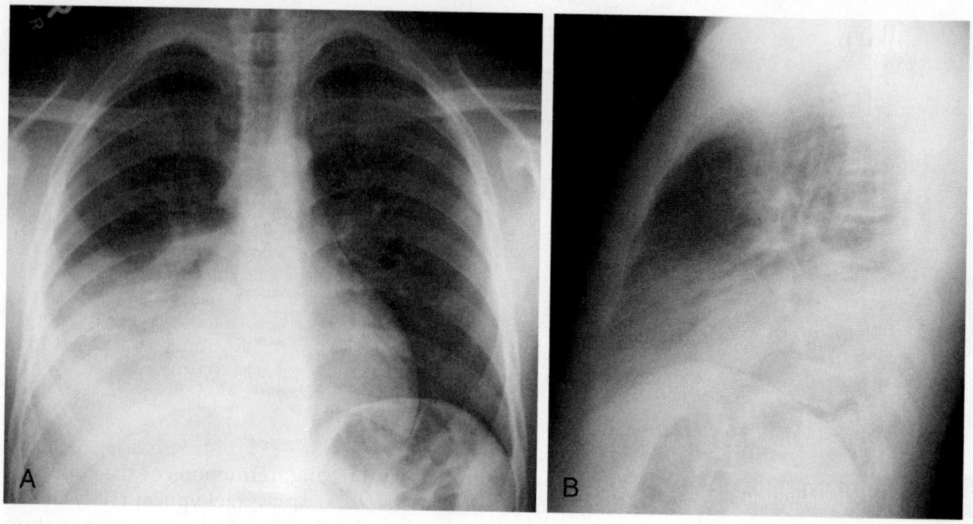

Figure 392-3 Radiographic findings characteristic of pneumococcal pneumonia in a 14 yr old boy with cough and fever. Posteroanterior *(A)* and lateral *(B)* chest radiographs reveal consolidation in the right lower lobe, strongly suggesting bacterial pneumonia.

the incidence and prevalence of the various respiratory viral pathogens.

The definitive diagnosis of a bacterial infection requires isolation of an organism from the blood, pleural fluid, or lung. Culture of sputum is of little value in the diagnosis of pneumonia in young children. Blood culture results are positive in only 10% of children with pneumococcal pneumonia. Cold agglutinins at titers >1:64 are found in the blood in ≈50% of patients with *M. pneumoniae* infections. Cold agglutinin findings are nonspecific because other pathogens such as influenza viruses may also cause increases. Acute infection caused by *M. pneumoniae* can be diagnosed on the basis of a positive polymerase chain reaction (PCR) test result or seroconversion in an IgG assay. Serologic evidence, such as the antistreptolysin O (ASO) titer, may be useful in the diagnosis of group A streptococcal pneumonia.

Table 392-5 FACTORS SUGGESTING NEED FOR HOSPITALIZATION OF CHILDREN WITH PNEUMONIA

Age <6 mo
Sickle cell anemia with acute chest syndrome
Multiple lobe involvement
Immunocompromised state
Toxic appearance
Moderate to severe respiratory distress
Requirement for supplemental oxygen
Dehydration
Vomiting or inability to tolerate oral fluids or medications
No response to appropriate oral antibiotic therapy
Social factors (e.g., inability of caregivers to administer medications at home or follow up appropriately)

Adapted from Baltimore RS: Pneumonia. In Jenson HB, Baltimore RS, editors: *Pediatric infectious diseases: principles and practice,* Philadelphia, 2002, WB Saunders, p 801.

TREATMENT

Treatment of suspected bacterial pneumonia is based on the presumptive cause and the age and clinical appearance of the child. For mildly ill children who do not require hospitalization, amoxicillin is recommended. In communities with a high percentage of penicillin-resistant pneumococci, high doses of amoxicillin (80-90 mg/kg/24 hr) should be prescribed. Therapeutic alternatives include cefuroxime axetil and amoxicillin/clavulanate. For school-aged children and in children in whom infection with *M. pneumoniae* or *C. pneumoniae* is suggested, a macrolide antibiotic such as azithromycin is an appropriate choice. In adolescents, a respiratory fluoroquinolone (levofloxacin, moxifloxacin, gemifloxacin) may be considered as an alternative. In developing countries only ≈54% of children with pneumonia (≈41% in sub-Saharan Africa) are taken to an appropriate caregiver. In response, the World Health Organization and other international groups have developed systems to train mothers and local health care providers in the recognition and treatment of pneumonia.

The empiric treatment of suspected bacterial pneumonia in a hospitalized child requires an approach based on the clinical manifestations at the time of presentation. Parenteral cefotaxime or ceftriaxone is the mainstay of therapy when bacterial pneumonia is suggested. If clinical features suggest staphylococcal pneumonia (pneumatoceles, empyema), initial antimicrobial therapy should also include vancomycin or clindamycin.

If viral pneumonia is suspected, it is reasonable to withhold antibiotic therapy, especially for those patients who are mildly ill, have clinical evidence suggesting viral infection, and are in no respiratory distress. Up to 30% of patients with known viral infection may have coexisting bacterial pathogens. Therefore, if the decision is made to withhold antibiotic therapy on the basis of presumptive diagnosis of a viral infection, deterioration in clinical status should signal the possibility of superimposed bacterial infection, and antibiotic therapy should be initiated.

Indications for admission to a hospital are noted in Table 392-5. In developing countries, oral zinc (20 mg/day) helps accelerate recovery from severe pneumonia. The optimal duration of antibiotic treatment for pneumonia has not been well-established in controlled studies. For pneumococcal pneumonia, antibiotics should probably be continued until the patient has been afebrile for 72 hours, and the total duration should not be less than 10 to 14 days (or 5 days if azithromycin is used). Available data do not support prolonged courses of treatment for uncomplicated pneumonia.

PROGNOSIS

Typically, patients with uncomplicated community-acquired bacterial pneumonia show response to therapy, with improvement in clinical symptoms (fever, cough, tachypnea, chest pain), within 48-96 hr of initiation of antibiotics. Radiographic evidence of improvement lags substantially behind clinical improvement. A number of factors must be considered when a patient does not improve with appropriate antibiotic therapy: (1) complications, such as empyema; (2) bacterial resistance; (3) nonbacterial etiologies such as viruses and aspiration of foreign bodies or food; (4) bronchial obstruction from endobronchial lesions, foreign body, or mucous plugs; (5) pre-existing diseases such as immunodeficiencies, ciliary dyskinesia, cystic fibrosis, pulmonary sequestration, or cystic adenomatoid malformation; and (6) other noninfectious causes (including bronchiolitis obliterans, hypersensitivity

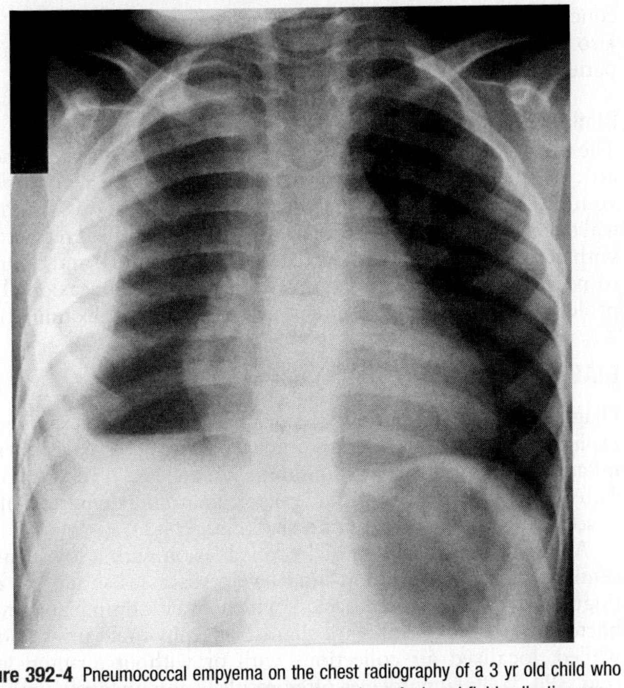

Figure 392-4 Pneumococcal empyema on the chest radiography of a 3 yr old child who has had upper respiratory symptoms and fever for 3 days. A pleural fluid collection can be seen on the right side. The patient had a positive pleural tap and blood culture result for pneumococci. The child recovered completely within 3 wk. (From Kuhn JP, Slovis TL, Haller JO: *Caffrey's pediatric diagnostic imaging,* vol 1, ed 10, Philadelphia, 2004, Mosby/Elsevier, p 1002.)

pneumonitis, eosinophilic pneumonia, aspiration, and Wegener's granulomatosis). A repeat chest radiograph is the 1st step in determining the reason for delay in response to treatment.

Mortality from community-acquired pneumonia in developed nations is rare, and most children with pneumonia do not experience long-term pulmonary sequelae. Some data suggest that up to 45% of children have symptoms of asthma 5 yr after hospitalization for pneumonia; this finding may reflect either undiagnosed asthma at the time of presentation or a propensity for development of asthma after pneumonia.

COMPLICATIONS

Complications of pneumonia are usually the result of direct spread of bacterial infection within the thoracic cavity (pleural effusion, empyema, pericarditis) or bacteremia and hematologic spread (Fig. 392-4). Meningitis, suppurative arthritis, and osteomyelitis are rare complications of hematologic spread of pneumococcal or *H. influenzae* type b infection.

S. aureus, S. pneumoniae, and *S. pyogenes* are the most common causes of parapneumonic effusions and of empyema (Table 392-6). The treatment of empyema is based on the stage (exudative, fibrinopurulent, organizing). Imaging studies including ultrasonography and CT are helpful in determining the stage of empyema. The mainstays of therapy include antibiotic therapy and drainage with tube thoracostomy. Additional approaches include the use of intrapleural fibrinolytic therapy (urokinase, streptokinase, tissue plasminogen activator) and selected video-assisted thoracoscopy (VATS) to debride or lyse adhesions, and drain loculated areas of pus. Early diagnosis and intervention, particularly with fibrinolysis or VATS, may obviate the need for thoracotomy and open debridement. Fibrinolysis may be more cost effective than VATS.

PREVENTION

Some evidence exists to suggest that vaccination has reduced the incidence of pneumonia hospitalizations. The annual rate of all-cause pneumonia hospitalization among children <2 yr of age in the USA during the period 1997-1999 was 12.5 per 1000 children. In February 2000 the 7-valent pneumococcal conjugate vaccine (PCV7) was licensed and recommended. In 2006 the pneumonia hospitalization rate in this age group was 8.1 per 1,000 children, a 35% decrease from the pre-vaccine rate. Although these data do not establish that PCV7 directly reduced pneumonia hospitalization rates, they do suggest that vaccination has resulted in a sustained benefit in preventing hospitalization for young children with pneumonia.

Currently, the 13-valent pneumococcal conjugate vaccine (PCV13) is licensed; it may prevent even more cases of pneumococcal disease not covered by the PCV7 vaccine.

The expansion of influenza vaccine recommendations to include all children >6 mo of age might be expected to affect pneumonia hospitalization rates in a similar fashion, and ongoing surveillance is warranted.

Table 392-6 DIFFERENTIATION OF PLEURAL FLUID

	TRANSUDATE	EMPYEMA
Appearance	Clear	Cloudy or purulent
Cell count (per mm^3)	<1000	Often >50,000 (cell count has limited predictive value)
Cell type	Lymphocytes, monocytes	Polymorphonuclear leukocytes (neutrophils)
Lactate dehydrogenase	<200 U/L	>1000 U/L
Pleural fluid/serum LDH ratio	<0.6	>0.6
Protein >3g	Unusual	Common
Pleural fluid/serum protein ratio	<0.5	>0.5
Glucose*	Normal	Low (<40 mg/dL)
pH*	Normal (7.40-7.60)	<7.10
Gram stain	Negative	Occasionally positive (less than one-third of cases)

*Low glucose or pH may be seen in malignant effusion, tuberculosis, esophageal rupture, pancreatitis (positive pleural amylase), and rheumatologic diseases (e.g., systemic lupus erythematosus).
From Kliegman RM, Greenbaum LA, Lye PS: *Practical strategies in pediatric diagnosis & therapy,* ed 2, Philadelphia, 2004, Elsevier, p 30.

BIBLIOGRAPHY

Please visit the Nelson Textbook of Pediatrics *website at* www.expertconsult.com *for the complete bibliography.*

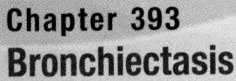

Chapter 393
Bronchiectasis

Oren Lakser

Bronchiectasis, a disease characterized by irreversible abnormal dilatation and anatomic distortion of the bronchial tree, likely represents a common end stage of a number of nonspecific and unrelated antecedent events. Its incidence has been decreasing overall in developed countries, but it persists as a problem in developing countries and among some ethnic groups in industrialized nations. In at least 1 series of children with bronchiectasis (not due to cystic fibrosis), the male : female ratio was 2 : 1.

For the full continuation of this chapter, please visit the Nelson Textbook of Pediatrics *website at* www.expertconsult.com.

Chapter 394
Pulmonary Abscess

Oren Lakser

Pulmonary abscesses are localized areas composed of thick-walled purulent material formed as a result of lung infection that lead to destruction of lung parenchyma, cavitation, and central necrosis. Lung abscesses are much less common in children than in adults. A **primary lung abscess** occurs in a previously healthy patient with no underlying medical disorders. A **secondary lung abscess** occurs in a patient with underlying or predisposing conditions.

PATHOLOGY AND PATHOGENESIS

A number of conditions predispose children to the development of pulmonary abscesses, including aspiration, pneumonia, cystic fibrosis (Chapter 395), gastroesophageal reflux (Chapter 315.1), tracheoesophageal fistula (Chapter 311), immunodeficiencies, postoperative complications of tonsillectomy and adenoidectomy, seizures, and a variety of neurologic diseases. In children, aspiration of infected materials or a foreign body is the predominant source of the organisms causing abscesses. Initially, pneumonitis impairs drainage of fluid or the aspirated material. Inflammatory vascular obstruction occurs, leading to tissue necrosis, liquefaction, and abscess formation. Abscess can also occur as a result of pneumonia and hematogenous seeding from another site.

If the aspiration event occurred while the child was recumbent, the right and left upper lobes and apical segment of the right lower lobes are the dependent areas most likely to be affected. In a child who was upright, the posterior segments of the upper lobes were dependent and therefore are most likely to be affected. Primary abscesses are found most often on the right side, whereas secondary lung abscesses, particularly in immunocompromised patients, have a predilection for the left side.

Both anaerobic and aerobic organisms can cause lung abscesses. Common anaerobic bacteria that can cause a pulmonary abscess include *Bacteroides* spp, *Fusobacterium* spp, and *Peptostreptococcus* spp. Abscesses can be caused by aerobic organisms such as *Streptococcus* spp, *Staphylococcus aureus, Escherichia coli, Klebsiella pneumoniae,* and *Pseudomonas aeruginosa.* Aerobic and anaerobic cultures should be part of the work-up for all patients with lung abscess. Occasionally, concomitant viral-bacterial infection can be detected. Fungi can also cause lung abscesses, particularly in immunocompromised patients.

Clinical Manifestations

The most common symptoms of pulmonary abscess in the pediatric population are cough, fever, tachypnea, dyspnea, chest pain, vomiting, sputum production, weight loss, and hemoptysis. Physical examination typically reveals tachypnea, dyspnea, retractions with accessory muscle use, decreased breath sounds, and dullness to percussion in the affected area. Crackles and, occasionally, a prolonged expiratory phase may be heard on lung examination.

DIAGNOSIS

Diagnosis is most commonly made on the basis of chest radiography. Classically, the chest radiograph shows a parenchymal inflammation with a cavity containing an air-fluid level (Fig. 394-1). A chest CT scan can provide better anatomic definition of an abscess, including location and size (Fig. 394-2).

An abscess is usually a thick-walled lesion with a low-density center progressing to an air-fluid level. Abscesses should be distinguished from pneumatoceles, which often complicate severe bacterial pneumonias and are characterized by thin- and smooth-walled, localized air collections with or without air-fluid level (Fig. 394-3). Pneumatoceles often resolve spontaneously with the treatment of the specific cause of the pneumonia.

The determination of the etiologic bacteria in a lung abscess can be very helpful in guiding antibiotic choice. Although Gram stain of sputum can provide an early clue as to the class of bacteria involved, sputum cultures typically yield mixed bacteria and are therefore not always reliable. Attempts to avoid contamination from oral flora include direct lung puncture, percutaneous (aided by CT guidance) or transtracheal aspiration, and bronchoalveolar lavage specimens obtained bronchoscopically. Bronchoscopic aspiration should be avoided as it can be complicated by massive intrabronchial aspiration, and great care should therefore be taken during the procedure. To avoid invasive procedures in previously normal hosts, empiric therapy can be initiated in the absence of culturable material.

TREATMENT

Conservative management is recommended for pulmonary abscess. Most experts advocate a 2- to 3-wk course of parenteral

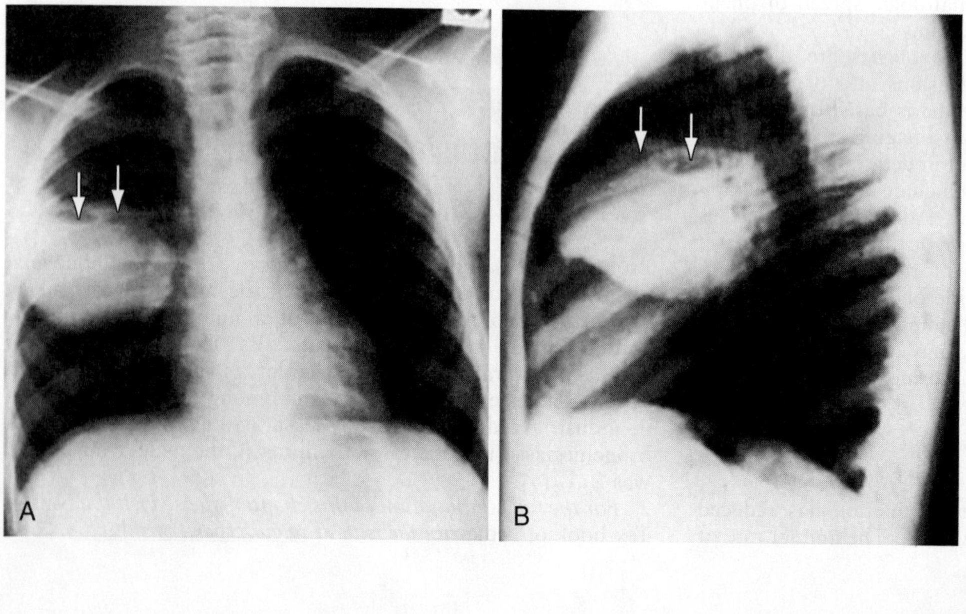

Figure 394-1 *A* and *B,* Multiloculated lung abscess *(arrows).* (From Brook I: Lung abscess and pulmonary infections due to anaerobic bacteria. In Chernick V, Boat TF, Wilmott RW, et al, editors: *Kendig's disorders of the respiratory tract in children,* ed 7, Philadelphia, 2006, Saunders, p 482.)

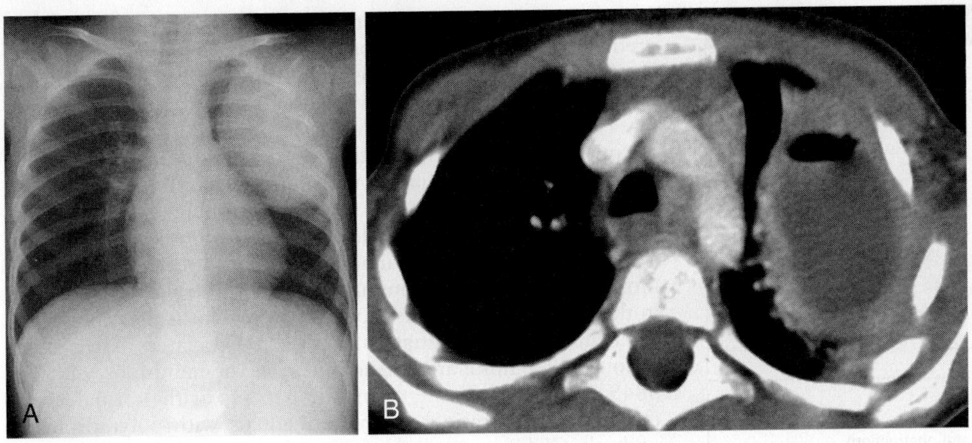

Figure 394-2 Pulmonary abscess in a 2 yr old boy with persistent cough. *A,* Chest radiograph shows large oval mass in the left upper lobe. *B,* CT scan demonstrates an abscess with a thick enhancing wall that contains both air and fluid. (From Slovis TL, editor: *Caffey's pediatric diagnostic imaging,* ed 11, Philadelphia, 2008, Mosby, p 1297.)

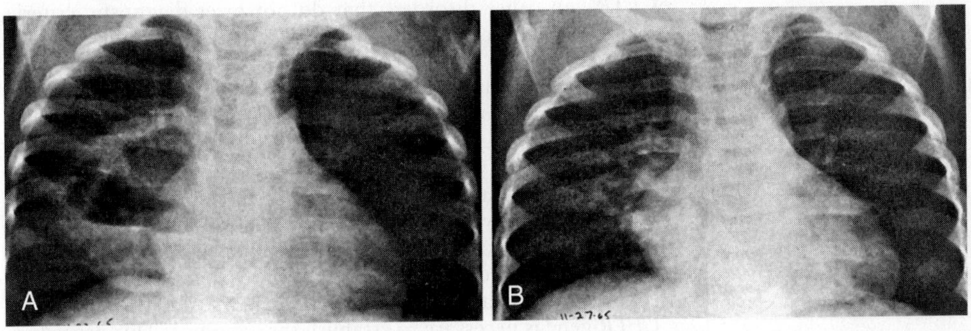

Figure 394-3 Appearance over a period of 5 days of a large multiloculated pneumonocele in a segment of alveolar consolidation. *A,* There is a large cavity with two air-fluid levels in a segment of alveolar pneumonia in the right upper lobe. *B,* Five days later, the cavity and most of the pneumonic consolidation have disappeared. (From Silverman FN, Kuhn JP: *Essentials of Caffrey's pediatric x-ray diagnosis,* Chicago, 1990, Year Book, p 303.)

antibiotics for uncomplicated cases, followed by a course of oral antibiotics to complete a total of 4-6 wk. Antibiotic choice should be guided by results of Gram stain and culture but initially should include agents with aerobic and anaerobic coverage. Treatment regimens should include a penicillinase-resistant agent active against *S. aureus* and anaerobic coverage, typically with clindamycin or ticarcillin/clavulanic acid. If gram-negative bacteria are suspected or isolated, an aminoglycoside should be added. Early CT-guided percutaneous drainage has been advocated as it can hasten the recovery and shorten the course of parenteral antibiotic therapy needed.

For severely ill patients or those whose status fails to improve after 7-10 days of appropriate antimicrobial therapy, surgical intervention should be considered. Minimally invasive percutaneous aspiration techniques, often with CT guidance, are the initial and, often, only intervention required. In rare complicated cases, thoracotomy with surgical drainage or lobectomy and/or decortication may be necessary.

PROGNOSIS

Overall, prognosis for children with primary pulmonary abscesses is excellent. The presence of aerobic organisms may be a negative prognostic indicator, particularly in those with secondary lung abscesses. Most children become asymptomatic within 7-10 days, although the fever can persist for as long as 3 wk. Radiologic abnormalities usually resolve in 1-3 mo but can persist for years.

BIBLIOGRAPHY

Please visit the Nelson Textbook of Pediatrics *website at* *www.expertconsult.com* *for the complete bibliography.*

Chapter 395
Cystic Fibrosis

Marie Egan

Characterized by obstruction and infection of airways and by maldigestion and its consequences, cystic fibrosis (CF) is an inherited multisystem disorder of children and adults; it is the most common life-limiting recessive genetic trait among white persons. Dysfunction of the *cystic fibrosis transmembrane conductance regulator protein* (CFTR), the primary defect, leads to a wide and variable array of presenting manifestations and complications.

CF is responsible for most cases of exocrine pancreatic insufficiency in early life and is the major cause of severe chronic lung disease in children. It is also responsible for many cases of salt depletion, nasal polyposis, pansinusitis, rectal prolapse, pancreatitis, cholelithiasis, and insulin-dependent hyperglycemia. CF may manifest as failure to thrive and, occasionally, as cirrhosis or other forms of hepatic dysfunction. Therefore, this disorder enters into the differential diagnosis of many pediatric conditions (Table 395-1).

GENETICS

CF occurs most frequently in white populations of northern Europe, North America, and Australia/New Zealand. The prevalence in these populations varies but approximates 1/3,500 live births (1/9,200 individuals of Hispanic descent and 1/15,000 in African Americans). Although less frequent in African, Hispanic,

Table 395-1 COMPLICATIONS OF CYSTIC FIBROSIS

RESPIRATORY
Bronchiectasis, bronchitis, bronchiolitis, pneumonia
Atelectasis
Hemoptysis
Pneumothorax
Nasal polyps
Sinusitis
Reactive airway disease
Cor pulmonale
Respiratory failure
Mucoid impaction of the bronchi
Allergic bronchopulmonary aspergillosis
GASTROINTESTINAL
Meconium ileus, meconium plug (neonate)
Meconium peritonitis (neonate)
Distal intestinal obstruction syndrome (non-neonatal obstruction)
Rectal prolapse
Intussusception
Volvulus
Fibrosing colonopathy (strictures)
Appendicitis
Intestinal atresia
Pancreatitis
Biliary cirrhosis (portal hypertension: esophageal varices, hypersplenism)
Neonatal obstructive jaundice
Hepatic steatosis
Gastroesophageal reflux
Cholelithiasis
Inguinal hernia
Growth failure (malabsorption)
Vitamin deficiency states (vitamins A, K, E, D)
Insulin deficiency, symptomatic hyperglycemia, diabetes
Malignancy (rare)
OTHER
Infertility
Delayed puberty
Edema-hypoproteinemia
Dehydration–heat exhaustion
Hypertrophic osteoarthropathy-arthritis
Clubbing
Amyloidosis
Diabetes mellitus
Aquagenic palmoplantar keratoderma (skin wrinkling)

Adapted from Silverman FN, Kuhn JP: *Essentials of Caffrey's pediatric x-ray diagnosis,* 1990, Chicago, Year Book, p 649.

Middle Eastern, South Asian, and eastern Asian populations, the disorder does exist in these populations as well (Fig. 395-1).

CF is inherited as an autosomal recessive trait. The CF gene codes for the CFTR protein, which is 1,480 amino acids. CFTR is expressed largely in epithelial cells of airways, the gastrointestinal tract (including the pancreas and biliary system), the sweat glands, and the genitourinary system. CFTR is a member of the adenosine triphosphate (ATP)–binding cassette superfamily of proteins. It functions as a chloride channel and has other regulatory functions that are perturbed variably by the different mutations. More than 1,500 *CFTR* polymorphisms grouped into 5 main classes of mutations that affect protein function are associated with the CF syndrome (Table 395-2). The most prevalent mutation of *CFTR* is the deletion of a single phenylalanine residue at amino acid 508 (ΔF508). This mutation is responsible for the high incidence of CF in northern European populations and is considerably less frequent in other populations, such as those of southern Europe and Israel. Approximately 50% of individuals with CF who are of northern European ancestry are homozygous for ΔF508, and >80% carry at least one ΔF508 gene. The remainder of patients has an extensive array of mutations, none of which has a prevalence of more than several percentage points, except in circumscribed populations; the W1282X mutation occurs in 60% of Ashkenazi Jews with CF. The relationship between CFTR genotype and clinical phenotype is highly complex and is not predictable for individual patients. Mutations categorized as "severe" are associated almost uniformly with pancreatic insufficiency but only in general with more rapid progression of lung disease. Modifier gene polymorphisms appear to be responsible for much of the variation in the progression of lung disease. The most compelling association with more severe disease is with a single nucleotide change in the transforming growth factor-β1(TGF-β1) gene. Variant alleles of the mannose-binding lectin, a key factor in systemic innate immunity, are associated with more serious lung infections and reduced survival. Polymorphism in the $IRFD_1$ gene, a transcriptional co-regulator that is essential for neutrophil differentiation, has been associated with a more serious CF pulmonary phenotype. Several mutations, such as 3849 + 10kbC→T, are found in patients with normal sweat chloride concentrations. Some individuals with polymorphisms of both *CFTR* genes have few or no CF manifestations until adolescence or adulthood, when they present with pancreatitis, sinusitis, diffuse bronchiectasis, or male infertility. Whereas *CFTR* mutations are a sine qua non for CF, two mutations of *CFTR* can cause disorders that do not meet diagnostic criteria for CF and, occasionally, do not cause discernible clinical problems.

Occurrence of liver disease cannot be predicted by CFTR genotype. This finding suggests a major environmental (acquired) component of organ system dysfunction and the presence of other genes that modify the CF phenotype.

Through the use of probes for 40 of the most common mutations, the genotype of 80-90% of Americans with CF can be ascertained. Genotyping using a discreet panel of mutation probes is quick and less costly than more comprehensive sequencing and is commercially available. In special cases, sequencing the entire *CFTR* gene is necessary to establish the genotype. This procedure is also available commercially although relatively expensive and can identify polymorphisms and unique mutations of unknown clinical importance.

The high frequency of *CFTR* mutations has been ascribed to resistance to the morbidity and mortality associated with infectious dysenteries through the ages. In support of this hypothesis, cultured CF intestinal epithelial cells homozygous for the ΔF508 mutation are unresponsive to the secretory effects of cholera toxin. The heterozygote (for CFTR) mice experience less mortality when treated with cholera toxin than their unaffected wild type littermates.

PATHOGENESIS

A number of long-standing observations of CF are of fundamental pathophysiologic importance; they include failure to clear mucous secretions, a paucity of water in mucous secretions, an elevated salt content of sweat and other serous secretions, and chronic infection limited to the respiratory tract. Additionally, there is a greater negative potential difference across the respiratory epithelia of patients with CF than across the respiratory epithelia of control subjects. Aberrant electrical properties are also demonstrated for CF sweat gland duct and rectal epithelia. The membranes of CF epithelial cells are unable to secrete chloride ions in response to cyclic adenosine monophosphate (cAMP)–mediated signals, and at least in the respiratory tract, excessive amounts of sodium are absorbed through these membranes (Fig. 395-2). These defects can be traced to a dysfunction of CFTR (Figs. 395-3 and 395-4).

Cyclic AMP–stimulated protein kinase A (PKA) regulation of chloride conductance is the primary function of CFTR; this function is absent in epithelial cells with many different mutations of the *CFTR* gene. *CFTR* mutations fall into 6 classes in another classification system, albeit with some overlap (see Fig. 395-4). Individuals with class I, II, and III mutations, on average, have shorter survival than those with "mild" genotypes (class IV or

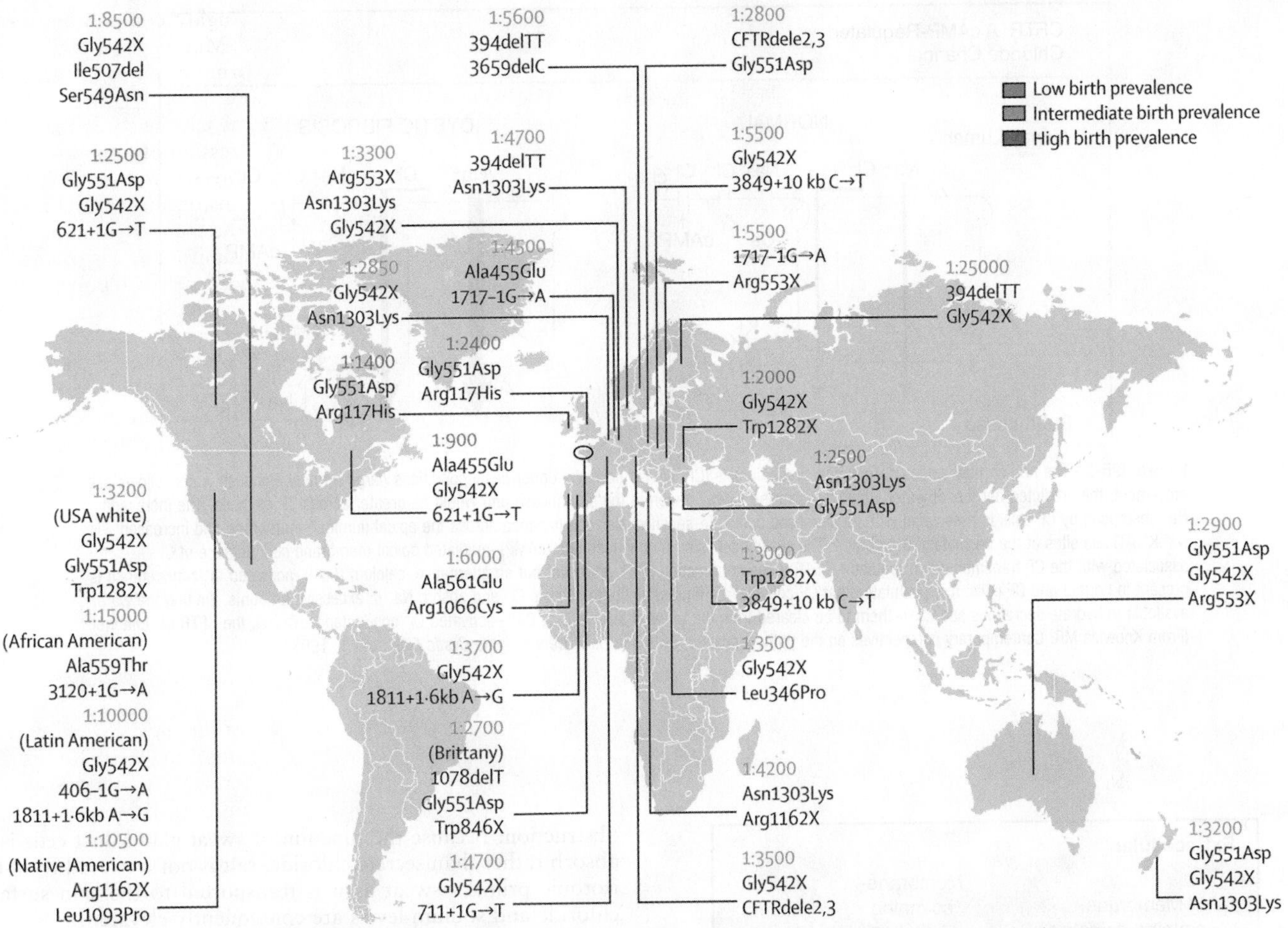

Figure 395-1 Approximate cystic fibrosis birth prevalence and common mutations for selected countries. Birth prevalence is reported as number of live births per case of cystic fibrosis. Common/important mutations in each region are listed below the prevalence figures. The birth prevalence can vary greatly among ethnic groups in a country. (From O'Sullivan BP, Freedman SD: Cystic fibrosis, *Lancet* 373:1891–1902, 2009.)

Table 395-2 ONE PROPOSED CLASSIFICATION OF CYSTIC FIBROSIS TRANSMEMBRANE CONDUCTANCE REGULATOR (CFTR) MUTATIONS

CLASS	EFFECT ON CFTR	FUNCTIONAL CFTR PRESENT?	SAMPLE MUTATIONS
I	Lack of protein production	No	Stop codons (designation in X; e.g., Trp1282X, Gly542X); splicing defects with no protein production (e.g., 711=1G→T, 1717-1G→A)
II	Defect in protein trafficking with ubiquitination and degradation in endoplasmic reticulum/Golgi body	No/substantially reduced	Phe508del, Asn1303Lys, Gly85Gly, leu1065Pro, Asp507, Ser549Arg
III	Defective regulation; CFTR not activated by adenosine triphosphate or cyclic adenosine monophosphate	No (nonfunction CFTR present in apical membrane)	Gly551Asp, Ser49Phe, Val520Phe, Arg553Gly, Arg560Thr, Arg 560Ser
IV	Reduced chloride transport through CFTR at the apical membrane	Yes	Ala455Glu, Arg117Cyst, asp1152His, Leu227Arg, Arg334Trp, Arg117His*
V	Splicing defect with reduced production of	Yes	3849+10kbC→T, 1811+1-6kbA→G, IVS8-5T, 2789+5G→A

*Function of Arg117His depends on the length of the polythymidine track on the same chromosome in intron 8 (IVS8): 5T, 7T, or 9T. There is more normal CFTR function with a longer poly-T tract.
From O'Sullivan BP, Freedman SD: Cystic fibrosis, *Lancet* 373:1891–1902, 2009.

V). The clinical importance of these functional categories is limited because they do not uniformly correlate with specific clinical features or their severity. Rather, clinical features correlate with the residual CFTR activity.

Many hypotheses have been postulated to explain how CFTR dysfunction results in the clinical phenotype. It is likely that no one hypothesis explains the full spectrum of disease. Most believe that the epithelial pathophysiology in airways involves an inability to secrete salt and secondarily to secrete water in the presence of excessive reabsorption of salt and water. The proposed outcome is insufficient water on the airway surface to hydrate secretions. Desiccated secretions become more viscous and elastic (rubbery) and are harder to clear by mucociliary and other mechanisms. In addition it has been suggested that CFTR dysfunction results in an altered microenvironment with low HCO_3^- and a more acidic pH, thus altering mucus rheology and aggravating poor mucociliary clearance. The result is that these secretions are retained and obstruct airways, starting with those of the smallest caliber, the bronchioles. Airflow obstruction at the level of small airways is the earliest observable physiologic abnormality of the respiratory system.

It is plausible that similar pathophysiologic events take place in the pancreatic and biliary ducts (and in the vas deferens), leading to desiccation of proteinaceous secretions and

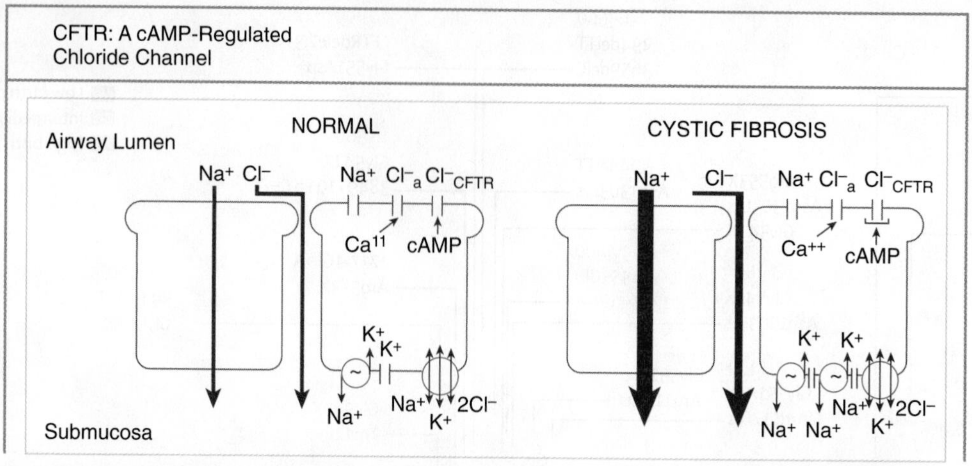

Figure 395-2 The net ion flow across normal and cystic fibrosis (CF) airway epithelia under basal conditions *(large arrows).* Because water follows salt movement, the predicted net flux of water would be from the airway lumen to the submucosa and would be greater across CF epithelia. The increased Na^+ absorption by CF cells is associated with an increased amiloride-sensitive Na^+ conductance across the apical (luminal) membrane and increased Na^+,K^+-ATPase sites at the basolateral membrane. The cyclic adenosine monophosphate (cAMP)–mediated apical membrane conductance of Cl^- associated with the CF transmembrane regulator (CFTR) does not function in CF epithelia, but an alternative, calcium (Ca^{++})–activated Cl^- conductance is present in normal and CF cells. It is postulated that CF cells have a limited ability to secrete Cl^- and absorb Na^+ in excessive amounts, limiting the water available to hydrate secretions and allow them to be cleared from the airways lumen. Cl^-_a, Ca^{++}–activated Cl^- conductance: Cl^-_{CTFR}, the CFTR Cl^- channel. (From Knowles MR: Contemporary perspectives on the pathogenesis of cystic fibrosis, *New Insights Cystic Fibrosis* 1:1, 1993.)

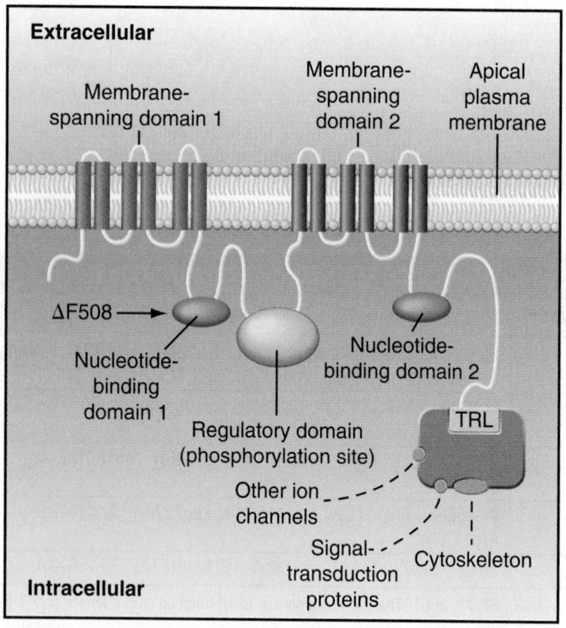

Figure 395-3 Hypothesized structure of cystic fibrosis transmembrane regulator (CFTR). The protein contains 1,480 amino acids and a number of discrete globular and transmembrane domains. Activation of CFTR relies on phosphorylation, particularly through protein kinase A but probably involving other kinases as well. Channel activity is governed by the 2 nucleotide-binding domains, which regulate channel gating. The carboxyl terminal (consisting of threonine, arginine, and leucine [TRL]) of CFTR is anchored through a PDZ-type binding interaction with the cytoskeleton and is kept in close approximation *(dashed lines)* to a number of important proteins. These associated proteins influence CFTR functions, including conductance, regulation of other channels, signal transduction, and localization at the apical plasma membrane. Each membrane-spanning domain contains 6 membrane-spanning α helixes, portions of which form a chloride-conductance pore. The regulatory domain is a site of protein kinase A phosphorylation. The common ΔF508 mutation occurs on the surface of nucleotide-binding domain 1. (From Rowe SM, Miller S, Sorscher EJ: Cystic fibrosis, *N Engl J Med* 352:1992–2001, 2005.)

obstruction. Because the function of sweat gland duct cells is to absorb rather than secrete chloride, salt is not retrieved from the isotonic primary sweat as it is transported to the skin surface; chloride and sodium levels are consequently elevated.

Chronic infection in CF is limited to the airways. A likely explanation for infection is a sequence of events starting with failure to clear inhaled bacteria promptly and then proceeding to persistent colonization and an inflammatory response in airway walls. In addition, it has been proposed that abnormal CFTR creates a proinflammatory state or amplifies the inflammatory response to initial infections (viral or bacterial). Some investigators have identified primary differences in CF-affected immune cells and have suggested that these alterations contribute to this proinflammatory state. It appears that inflammatory events occur first in small airways, perhaps because clearance of altered secretions and microorganisms from these regions is more difficult. Chronic bronchiolitis and bronchitis are the initial lung manifestations (Chapter 383), but after months to years, structural changes in airway walls produce bronchiolectasis and bronchiectasis.

The agents of airway injury include neutrophil products, such as oxidative radicals and proteases, and immune reaction products. With advanced lung disease, infection may extend to peribronchial lung parenchyma.

A finding that is not readily explained by CFTR dysfunction is the high prevalence in patients with CF of airway colonization with *Staphylococcus aureus* (Chapter 174.1), *Pseudomonas aeruginosa* (Chapter 197.1), and *Burkholderia cepacia* (Chapter 197.2), organisms that rarely infect the lungs of other individuals. It has been postulated that the CF airway epithelial cells or surface liquids may provide a favorable environment for harboring these organisms. CF airway epithelium may be compromised in its innate defenses against these organisms, through either acquired or genetic alterations. Antimicrobial activity is diminished in CF secretions; this diminution may be related to hyperacidified surface liquids or other effects on innate immunity. Another puzzle is the propensity for *P. aeruginosa* to undergo mucoid transformation in the CF airways. The complex

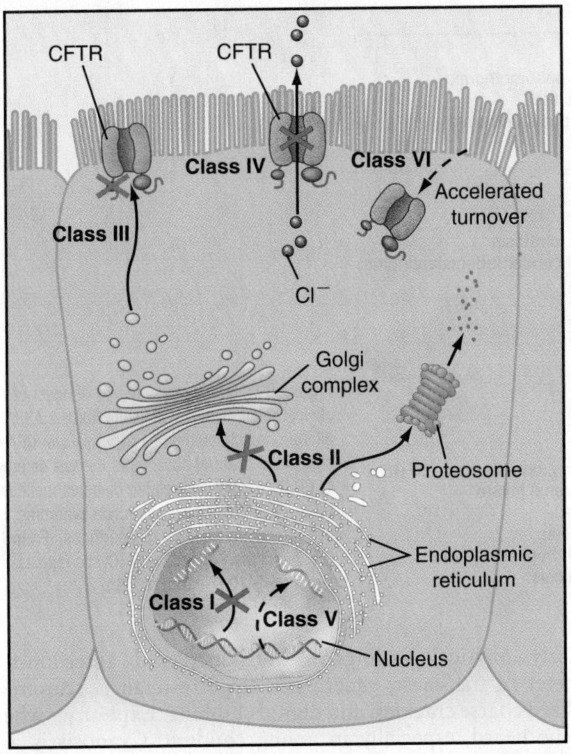

Figure 395-4 Categories of *CFTR* (cystic fibrosis transmembrane regulator) mutations. Classes of defects in the *CFTR* gene include the absence of synthesis (class I); defective protein maturation and premature degradation (class II); disordered regulation, such as diminished adenosine triphosphate (ATP) binding and hydrolysis (class III); defective chloride conductance or channel gating (class IV); a reduced number of CFTR transcripts due to a promoter or splicing abnormality (class V); and accelerated turnover from the cell surface (class VI). (From Rowe SM, Miller S, Sorscher EJ: Cystic fibrosis, *N Engl J Med* 352:1992–2001, 2005.)

polysaccharide produced by these organisms generates a biofilm that provides a hypoxic environment and thereby protects *Pseudomonas* against antimicrobial agents.

Nutritional deficits, including fatty acid deficiency, have been implicated as predisposing factors for respiratory tract infection. More specifically, concentrations of lipoxins—molecules that suppress neutrophilic inflammation—are suppressed in CF airways. In support of this idea it the observation that the 10-15% of individuals with CF who retain substantial exocrine pancreatic function have delayed onset of colonization with *P. aeruginosa* and slower deterioration of lung function. It appears that nutritional factors are only contributory because preservation of pancreatic function does not preclude development of typical lung disease.

PATHOLOGY

The earliest pathologic lesion in the lung is that of **bronchiolitis** (mucous plugging and an inflammatory response in the walls of the small airways); with time, mucus accumulation and inflammation extend to the larger airways (**bronchitis**) (Chapter 383). Goblet cell hyperplasia and submucosal gland hypertrophy become prominent pathologic findings, which is most likely a response to chronic airway infection. Organisms appear to be confined to the endobronchial space; invasive bacterial infection is not characteristic. With long-standing disease, evidence of airway destruction such as **bronchiolar obliteration, bronchiolectasis,** and **bronchiectasis** (Chapter 393) becomes prominent. Imaging modalities demonstrate both increased airway wall thickness and luminal cross-sectional area relatively early in lung disease evaluation. Bronchiectatic cysts and emphysematous bullae or subpleural blebs are frequent with advanced lung disease, the upper lobes being most commonly involved. These enlarged air spaces may rupture and cause pneumothorax. Interstitial disease is not a prominent feature, although areas of fibrosis appear eventually. Bronchial arteries are enlarged and tortuous, contributing to a propensity for **hemoptysis** in bronchiectatic airways. Small pulmonary arteries eventually display medial hypertrophy, which would be expected in secondary pulmonary hypertension.

The **paranasal sinuses** are uniformly filled with secretions containing inflammatory products, and the epithelial lining displays hyperplastic and hypertrophied secretory elements (Chapter 372). Polypoid lesions within the sinuses and erosion of bone have been reported. The nasal mucosa may form large or multiple polyps, usually from a base surrounding the ostia of the maxillary and ethmoidal sinuses.

The **pancreas** is usually small, occasionally cystic, and often difficult to find at postmortem examination. The extent of involvement varies at birth. In infants, the acini and ducts are often distended and filled with eosinophilic material. In 85-90% of patients, the lesion progresses to complete or almost complete disruption of acini and replacement with fibrous tissue and fat. Infrequently, foci of calcification may be seen on radiographs of the abdomen. The islets of Langerhans contain normal appearing β cells, although they may begin to show architectural disruption by fibrous tissue in the 2nd decade of life.

The **intestinal tract** shows only minimal changes. Esophageal and duodenal glands are often distended with mucous secretions. Concretions may form in the appendiceal lumen or cecum. Crypts of the appendix and rectum may be dilated and filled with secretions.

Focal biliary cirrhosis secondary to blockage of intrahepatic bile ducts is uncommon in early life, although it is responsible for occasional cases of prolonged neonatal jaundice. This lesion becomes much more prevalent and extensive with age and is found in 70% of patients at postmortem examination. This process can proceed to symptomatic multilobular biliary cirrhosis that has a distinctive pattern of large irregular parenchymal nodules and interspersed bands of fibrous tissue. Approximately 30-70% of patients have fatty infiltration of the liver, in some cases despite apparently adequate nutrition. At autopsy, hepatic congestion secondary to cor pulmonale is frequently observed. The gallbladder may be hypoplastic and filled with mucoid material and often contains stones. The epithelial lining often displays extensive mucous metaplasia. Atresia of the cystic duct and stenosis of the distal common bile duct have been observed.

Mucus-secreting salivary glands are usually enlarged and display focal plugging and dilatation of ducts.

Glands of the **uterine cervix** are distended with mucus, copious amounts of which collect in the cervical canal. Endocervicitis may be prevalent in teenagers and young women. In >95% of males, the body and tail of the epididymis, the vas deferens, and the seminal vesicles are obliterated or atretic.

CLINICAL MANIFESTATIONS

Mutational heterogeneity and environmental factors appear responsible for highly variable involvement of the lungs, pancreas, and other organs. A list of presenting manifestations is lengthy, although pulmonary and gastrointestinal presentations predominate (Fig. 395-5). With inclusion of CF newborn screening panels, an increasing proportion of children are diagnosed before symptoms appear (Table 395-3).

Respiratory Tract

Cough is the most constant symptom of pulmonary involvement. At first, the cough may be dry and hacking, but eventually it becomes loose and productive. In older patients, the cough is most prominent upon arising in the morning or after activity.

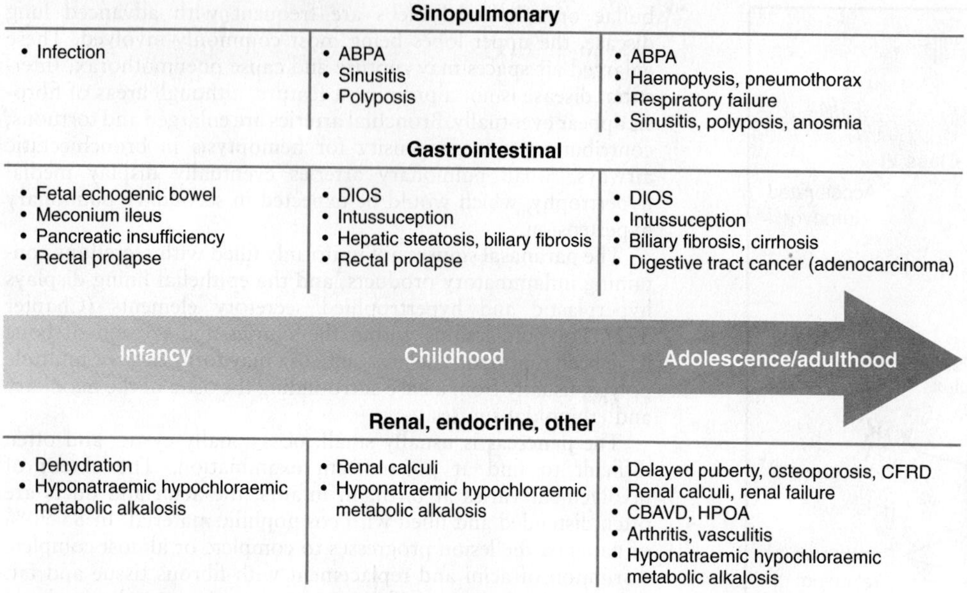
Sinopulmonary
• Infection
• ABPA
• Sinusitis
• Polyposis
• ABPA
• Haemoptysis, pneumothorax
• Respiratory failure
• Sinusitis, polyposis, anosmia
Gastrointestinal
• Fetal echogenic bowel
• Meconium ileus
• Pancreatic insufficiency
• Rectal prolapse
• DIOS
• Intussuception
• Hepatic steatosis, biliary fibrosis
• Rectal prolapse
• DIOS
• Intussuception
• Biliary fibrosis, cirrhosis
• Digestive tract cancer (adenocarcinoma)
Infancy
Childhood
Adolescence/adulthood
Renal, endocrine, other
• Dehydration
• Hyponatraemic hypochloraemic metabolic alkalosis
• Renal calculi
• Hyponatraemic hypochloraemic metabolic alkalosis
• Delayed puberty, osteoporosis, CFRD
• Renal calculi, renal failure
• CBAVD, HPOA
• Arthritis, vasculitis
• Hyponatraemic hypochloraemic metabolic alkalosis

Figure 395-5 Approximate age of onset of clinical manifestations of cystic fibrosis ABPA, allergic bronchopulmonary aspergillosis; CBAVD, congenital bilateral absence of the vas deferens; CFRD, cystic fibrosis-related diabetes mellitus; DIOS, distal intestinal obstruction syndrome; HPOA, hypertrophic pulmonary osteoarthritis. (From O'Sullivan BP, Freedman SD: Cystic fibrosis, *Lancet* 373:1891–1902, 2009.)

Table 395-3 PRESENTING FEATURES OF MORE THAN 25,000 PATIENTS WITH CYSTIC FIBROSIS IN THE USA

FEATURE	%	% of Patients Presenting in 2007
Acute or persistent respiratory symptoms	45.6	31.2
Failure to thrive, malnutrition	37.5	18.7
Abnormal stools	28.8	13.8
Meconium ileus, intestinal obstruction	19.9	14
Family history	16.0	12
Newborn Screening	6.4	30.7
Electrolyte, acid-base abnormality	4.2	1.1
Rectal prolapse	3.3	3.3
Nasal polyps, sinus disease	3.3	4.6
Hepatobiliary disease	1.2	1.4
Other*	3-4	6.7

*Includes pseudotumor cerebri, azoospermia, acrodermatitis-like rash, vitamin deficiency states, hypoproteinemic edema, hypoprothrombinemia with bleeding, and meconium plug syndrome.
Data from the Patient Registry, Cystic Fibrosis Foundation, Bethesda, MD.

Expectorated mucus is usually purulent. Some patients remain asymptomatic for long periods or seem to have prolonged but intermittent acute respiratory infections. Others acquire a chronic cough in the first weeks of life, or they have pneumonia repeatedly. Extensive bronchiolitis accompanied by wheezing is a frequent symptom during the first years of life. As lung disease slowly progresses, exercise intolerance, shortness of breath, and failure to gain weight or grow are noted. Exacerbations of lung symptoms, presumably owing to more active airways infection, often require repeated hospitalizations for effective treatment. Cor pulmonale, respiratory failure, and death eventually supervene unless lung transplantation is accomplished. Colonization with *B. cepacia* and other multidrug-resistant organisms may be associated with particularly rapid pulmonary deterioration and death.

The rate of progression of lung disease is the chief determinant of morbidity and mortality. The course of lung disease is largely independent of genotype. Severe mutations tend to be associated with more rapid progression. A few mutations may substantially or even fully spare the lungs. Male gender and exocrine pancreatic sufficiency are also associated with a slower rate of pulmonary function decline.

Early **physical findings** include increased anteroposterior diameter of the chest, generalized hyperresonance, scattered or localized coarse crackles, and digital clubbing. Expiratory wheezes may be heard, especially in young children. Cyanosis is a late sign. Common pulmonary complications include atelectasis, hemoptysis, pneumothorax, and cor pulmonale; these usually appear beyond the 1st decade of life.

Even though the paranasal sinuses are virtually always opacified radiographically, acute sinusitis is infrequent. Nasal obstruction and rhinorrhea are common, caused by inflamed, swollen mucous membranes or, in some cases, nasal polyposis. **Nasal polyps** are most troublesome between 5 and 20 yr of age.

Intestinal Tract

In 15-20% of newborn infants with CF, the ileum is completely obstructed by meconium (**meconium ileus**). The frequency is greater (≈30%) among siblings born subsequent to a child with meconium ileus and is particularly striking in monozygotic twins, reflecting a genetic contribution from one or more modifying genes. Abdominal distention, emesis, and failure to pass meconium appear in the 1st 24-48 hr of life (Chapters 96.1 and 322.2). Abdominal radiographs (Fig. 395-6) show dilated loops of bowel with air-fluid levels and, frequently, a collection of granular, "ground-glass" material in the lower central abdomen. Rarely, **meconium peritonitis** results from intrauterine rupture of the bowel wall and can be detected radiographically as the presence of peritoneal or scrotal calcifications. **Meconium plug syndrome** occurs with increased frequency in infants with CF but is less specific than meconium ileus. Ileal obstruction with fecal material (distal intestinal obstruction syndrome [DIOS]) occurs in older patients, causing cramping abdominal pain and abdominal distention.

More than 85% of affected children show evidence of maldigestion from exocrine pancreatic insufficiency. Symptoms include frequent, bulky, greasy stools and failure to gain weight even when food intake appears to be large. Characteristically, stools contain readily visible droplets of fat. A protuberant abdomen, decreased muscle mass, poor growth, and delayed maturation are typical physical signs. Excessive flatus may be a problem. A number of mutations are associated with preservation of some exocrine pancreatic function, including R117H and 3849 + 10kbC→T. Virtually all individuals homozygous for ΔF508 have pancreatic insufficiency.

Less common gastrointestinal manifestations include intussusception, fecal impaction of the cecum with an asymptomatic

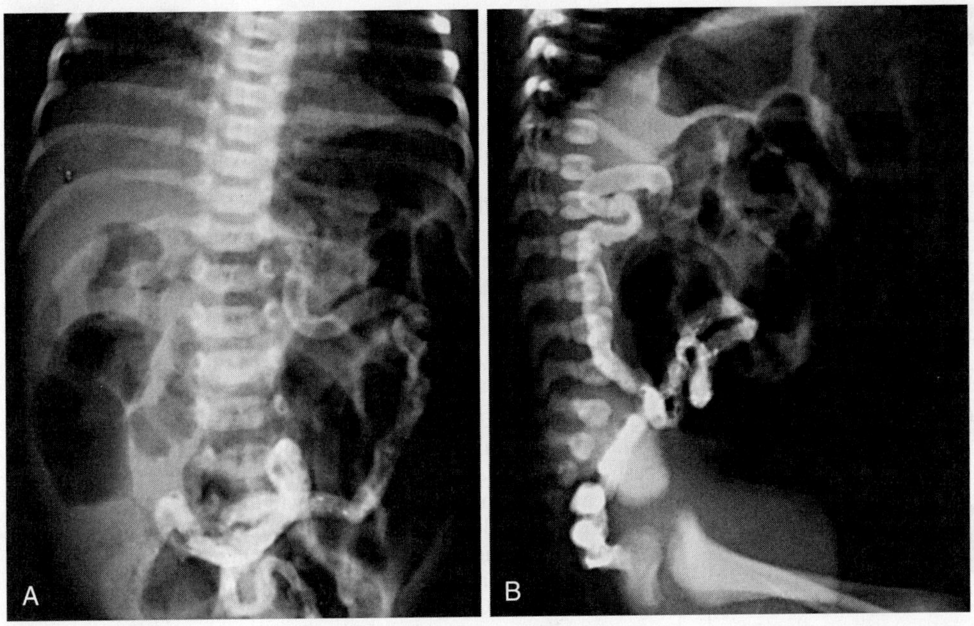

Figure 395-6 *A* and *B*, Contrast enema study in a newborn infant with abdominal distention and failure to pass meconium. Notice the small diameter of the sigmoid and ascending colon and dilated, air-filled loops of small intestine. Several air-fluid levels in the small bowel are visible on the upright lateral view.

right lower quadrant mass, and epigastric pain owing to duodenal inflammation. Acid or bile reflux with esophagitis symptoms is common in older children and adults. Subacute appendicitis and periappendiceal abscess have been encountered. Historically a relatively common event, rectal prolapse now occurs much less frequently as the result of earlier diagnosis and initiation of pancreatic enzyme replacement therapy. Occasionally, hypoproteinemia with anasarca appears in malnourished infants, especially if children are fed soy-based preparations. Neurologic dysfunction (dementia, peripheral neuropathy) and hemolytic anemia may occur because of **vitamin E deficiency.** Deficiency of other fat-soluble vitamins is occasionally symptomatic. **Hypoprothrombinemia** due to vitamin K deficiency may result in a bleeding diathesis. Clinical manifestations of other fat-soluble vitamin deficiencies, such as decreased bone density and night blindness, have been noted. Rickets is rare.

Biliary Tract
Evidence for liver dysfunction is most often detected in the 1st 15 yr of life and can be found in up to 30% of individuals. Biliary cirrhosis becomes symptomatic in only 5-7% of patients. Manifestations can include icterus, ascites, hematemesis from esophageal varices, and evidence of hypersplenism. A neonatal hepatitis–like picture and massive hepatomegaly owing to steatosis have been reported. Biliary colic secondary to cholelithiasis may occur in the 2nd decade or later. Liver disease occurs independent of genotype but is associated with meconium ileus and pancreatic insufficiency.

Pancreas
In addition to exocrine pancreatic insufficiency, evidence for hyperglycemia and glycosuria, including polyuria and weight loss, may appear, especially in the 2nd decade of life. Eight percent of 11-17 yr old patients and 30% of patients >25 yr of age have CF-related diabetes. Ketoacidosis usually does not occur, but eye, kidney, and other vascular complications have been noted in patients living ≥10 yr after the onset of hyperglycemia. Recurrent, acute pancreatitis occurs occasionally in individuals who have residual exocrine pancreatic function and may be the sole manifestation of two *CFTR* mutations.

Genitourinary Tract
Sexual development is often delayed but only by an average of 2 yr. More than 95% of males are azoospermic because of failure of development of wolffian duct structures, but sexual function is generally unimpaired. The incidence of inguinal hernia, hydrocele, and undescended testis is higher than expected. Adolescent females may experience secondary amenorrhea, especially with exacerbations of pulmonary disease. Cervicitis and accumulation of tenacious mucus in the cervical canal have been noted. The female fertility rate is diminished. Pregnancy is generally tolerated well by women with good pulmonary function but may accelerate pulmonary progression in those with moderate or advanced lung problems.

Sweat Glands
Excessive loss of salt in the sweat predisposes young children to salt depletion episodes, especially during episodes of gastroenteritis and during warm weather. These children present with **hypochloremic alkalosis.** Frequently, parents notice salt "frosting" of the skin or a salty taste when they kiss the child. A few genotypes are associated with normal sweat chloride values.

DIAGNOSIS AND ASSESSMENT

The diagnosis of CF has been based on a positive quantitative sweat test ($Cl^- \geq 60$ mEq/L) in conjunction with 1 or more of the following features: typical chronic obstructive pulmonary disease, documented exocrine pancreatic insufficiency, and a positive family history. With newborn screening, diagnosis is often made prior to obvious clinical manifestations such as failure to thrive and chronic cough (Table 395-3). Diagnostic criteria have been recommended to include additional testing procedures (Table 395-4).

Sweat Testing
The sweat test, which involves using pilocarpine iontophoresis to collect sweat and performing chemical analysis of its chloride content, is the standard approach to diagnosis of CF. The procedure requires care and accuracy. An electric current is used to carry pilocarpine into the skin of the forearm and locally stimulate the sweat glands. If an adequate amount of sweat is collected, the specimens are analyzed for chloride concentration. Testing may be difficult in the 1st 2 wk of life because of low sweat rates but is recommended any time after the 1st 48 hr of life. Positive results should be confirmed; for a negative result, the test should be repeated if suspicion of the diagnosis remains.

Table 395-4 DIAGNOSTIC CRITERIA FOR CYSTIC FIBROSIS (CF)

Presence of typical clinical features (respiratory, gastrointestinal, or genitourinary)
OR
A history of CF in a sibling
OR
A positive newborn screening test
PLUS
Laboratory evidence for CFTR (CF transmembrane regulator) dysfunction:
Two elevated sweat chloride concentrations obtained on separate days
OR
Identification of two CF mutations
OR
An abnormal nasal potential difference measurement

Table 395-5 CONDITIONS ASSOCIATED WITHFALSE-POSITIVE AND FALSE-NEGATIVE SWEAT TEST RESULTS

WITH FALSE-POSITIVE RESULTS
Eczema (atopic dermatitis)
Ectodermal dysplasia
Malnutrition/failure to thrive/deprivation
Anorexia nervosa
Congenital adrenal hyperplasia
Adrenal insufficiency
Glucose-6-phosphatase deficiency
Mauriac syndrome
Fucosidosis
Familial hypoparathyroidism
Hypothyroidism
Nephrogenic diabetes insipidus
Pseudohypoaldosteronism
Klinefelter syndrome
Familial cholestasis syndrome
Autonomic dysfunction
Prostaglandin E infusions
Munchausen syndrome by proxy
WITH FALSE-NEGATIVE RESULTS
Dilution
Malnutrition
Edema
Insufficient sweat quantity
Hyponatremia
Cystic fibrosis transmembrane conductance regulator (CFTR) mutations with preserved sweat duct function

More than 60 mEq/L of chloride in sweat is diagnostic of CF when 1 or more other criteria are present. Threshold levels of 30-40 mEq/L for infants have been suggested. Borderline (or intermediate) values of 40 to 60 mEq/L have been reported in patients of all ages who have CF with atypical involvement and require further testing. Chloride concentrations in sweat are somewhat lower in individuals who retain exocrine pancreatic function but usually remain within the diagnostic range. Conditions associated with false-negative and false-positive results are noted in Table 395-5.

DNA Testing

Several commercial laboratories test for 30-96 of the most common *CFTR* mutations. This testing identifies ≥90% of individuals who carry 2 CF mutations. Some children with typical CF manifestations are found to have 1 or no detectable mutations by this methodology. Some laboratories perform comprehensive mutation analysis screening for all of the >1,500 identified mutations.

Other Diagnostic Tests

The finding of increased potential differences across nasal epithelium, the loss of this difference with topical amiloride application, and the absence of a voltage response to a β-adrenergic agonist have been used to confirm the diagnosis of CF in patients with equivocal or frankly normal sweat chloride values.

Pancreatic Function

Exocrine pancreatic dysfunction is clinically apparent in many patients. Documentation is desirable if there are questions about the functional status of the pancreas. Measurement of fat balances with a 3-day stool collection or direct documentation of enzyme secretion after duodenal intubation and pancreozymin-secretin stimulation provides a reliable measure, but the fat collection is cumbersome and duodenal intubation is very invasive and rarely performed. A simpler test that can be used to screen pancreatic function, the quantification of elastase-1 activity in a fresh stool sample, is used routinely. Other indirect measures of pancreatic enzyme secretion are available but have limited or unproven clinical value. Endocrine pancreatic dysfunction may be more prevalent than previously recognized. Many authorities advocate yearly monitoring with a modified 2-hr oral glucose tolerance test (OGTT) after 10 yr of age. This approach is more sensitive than spot checks of blood and urine glucose levels and glycosylated hemoglobin levels.

Radiology

Pulmonary radiologic findings suggest the diagnosis but are not specific. Hyperinflation of lungs occurs early and may be overlooked in the absence of infiltrates or streaky densities. Bronchial thickening and plugging and ring shadows suggesting bronchiectasis usually appear first in the upper lobes. Nodular densities, patchy atelectasis, and confluent infiltrate follow. Hilar lymph nodes may be prominent. With advanced disease, impressive hyperinflation with markedly depressed diaphragms, anterior bowing of the sternum, and a narrow cardiac shadow are noted. Cyst formation, extensive bronchiectasis, dilated pulmonary artery segments, and segmental or lobar atelectasis are often apparent with advanced disease. Typical progression of lung disease is seen in Figure 395-7. Most CF centers obtain chest radiographs (posteroanterior [PA] and lateral) at least annually. Standardized scoring of roentgenographic changes has been used to follow progression of lung disease. CT of the chest can detect and localize thickening of bronchial airway walls, mucous plugging, focal hyperinflation, and early bronchiectasis (Fig. 395-8); it is generally not used for routine evaluation of chest disease. Many children with normal lung function have bronchiectasis on CT, indicating that this imaging modality is sensitive to early lung changes.

Radiographs of paranasal sinuses reveal panopacification and, often, failure of frontal sinus development. CT provides better resolution of sinus changes if this information is required clinically. Fetal ultrasonography may suggest ileal obstruction with meconium early in the 2nd trimester, but this finding is not predictive of meconium ileus at birth.

Pulmonary Function

Standard pulmonary function studies are not obtained until patients are 4-6 yr of age, by which time many patients show the typical pattern of obstructive pulmonary involvement (Chapter 376). Decrease in the midmaximal flow rate is an early functional change, reflecting small airway obstruction. This lesion also affects the distribution of ventilation and increases the alveolar-arterial oxygen difference. The findings of obstructive airway disease and modest responses to a bronchodilator are consistent with the diagnosis of CF at all ages. Residual volume and functional residual capacity are increased early in the course of lung disease. Restrictive changes, characterized by declining total lung capacity and vital capacity, correlate with extensive lung injury

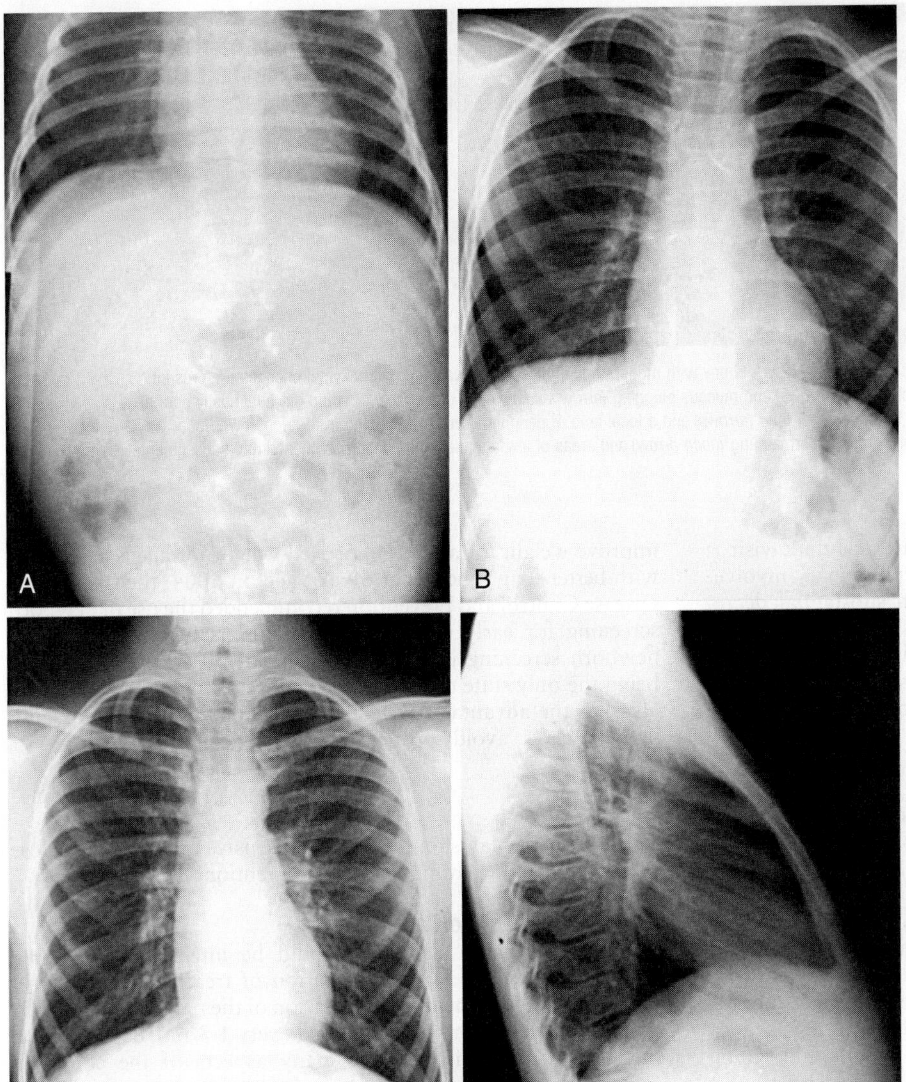

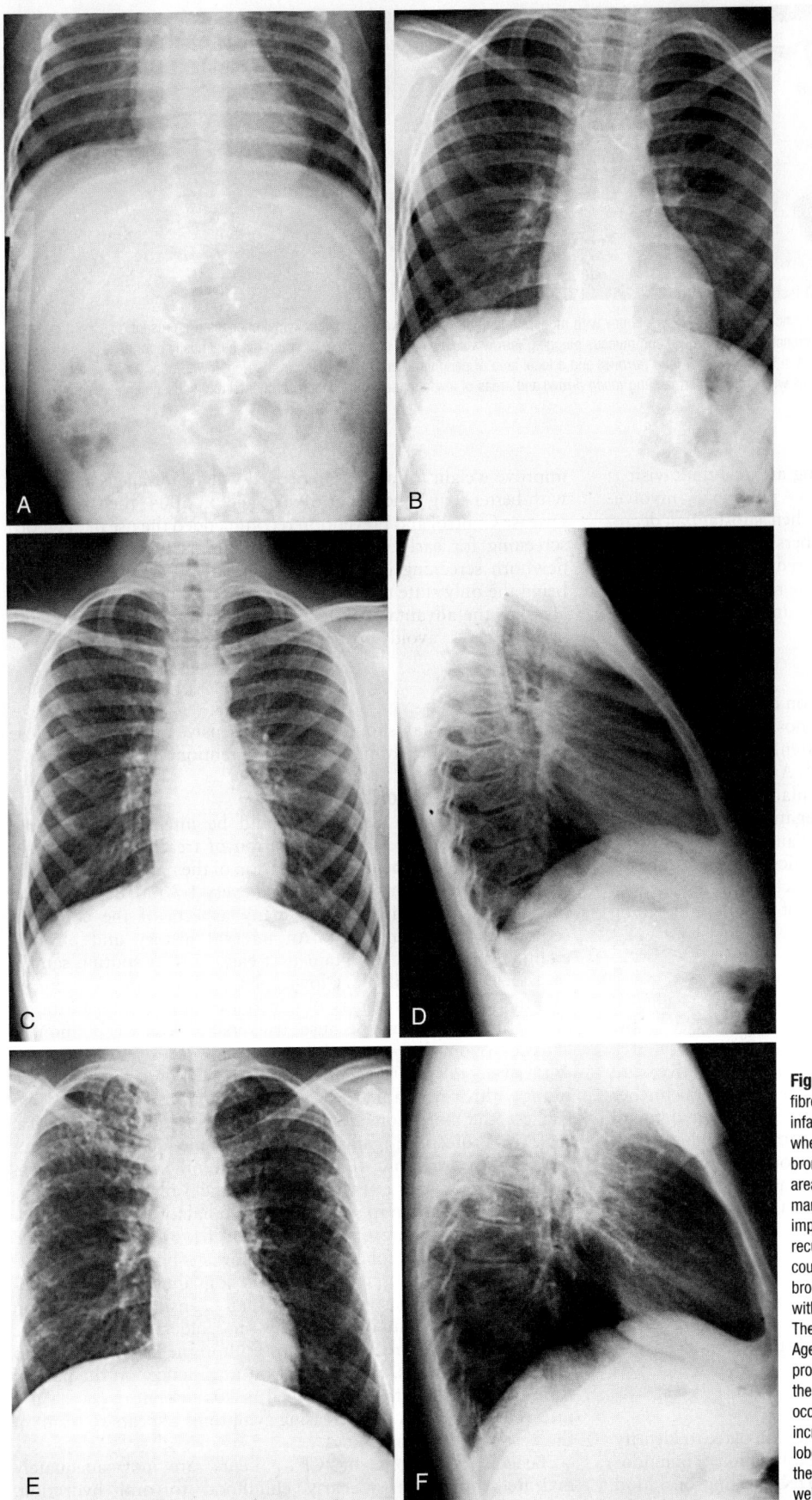

Figure 395-7 Roentgenographic progression of cystic fibrosis lung disease in one patient, from the diagnosis in infancy to 18 yr of age. *A,* Patient admitted with cough and wheezing at 2 mo of age. Notice the mild increase in bronchovascular markings, especially in the upper lobe areas. *B,* At age 4 yr, cough was minimal. Bronchovascular markings were mildly increased, and there was some improvement in the upper lobes. The wheeze never recurred. *C* and *D,* At age 13 yr, the patient had minimal cough and occasional sputum production. The bronchovascular markings were generally further increased, with early bronchiectatic changes in the right upper lobe. The lateral view does not suggest overinflation. *E* and *F,* Age 18 yr. During adolescence, cough and sputum production increased even though outpatient antibiotic therapy was intensified. Small-volume hemoptysis, occasional paroxysms of cough, and weight loss as well as increased nodular infiltrates (especially in the right upper lobe) and hyperinflation (as seen on the lateral view) led to the patient's 1st hospitalization since infancy. Height and weight were maintained in the 25th-50th percentile range.

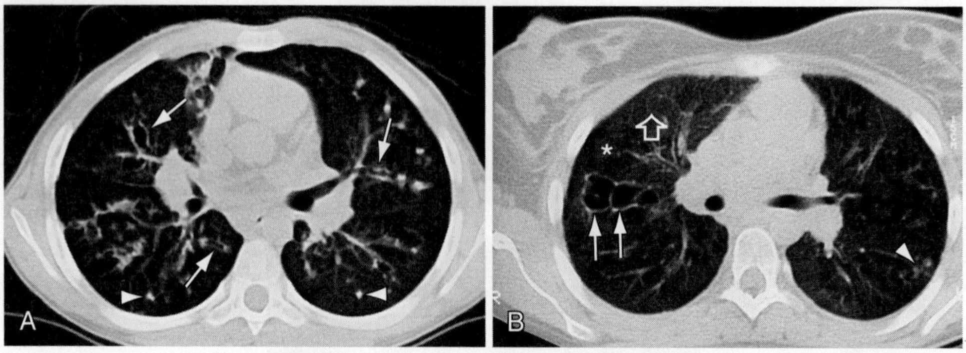

Figure 395-8 CT scans of the chest in cystic fibrosis. *A,* A 12 yr old boy with moderate lung disease. Airway and parenchymal changes are present throughout both lungs. Multiple areas of bronchiectasis *(arrows)* and mucous plugging *(arrowheads)* can be seen. *B,* A 19 yr old girl has mostly normal lung with 1 area of saccular bronchiectasis in the right upper lobe *(arrows)* and a focal area of peripheral mucous plugging in the right lower lobe *(arrowhead).* Lung density is heterogeneous with areas of normal lung *(open arrow)* and areas of low attenuation reflecting segmental and subsegmental air trapping *(asterisk).*

and fibrosis and are a late finding. Testing at each clinic visit is recommended to evaluate the course of the pulmonary involvement and allow for early intervention when substantial decrements are documented. Increasing numbers of CF centers are equipped to measure airflow patterns of sedated infants (infant pulmonary function tests). Some patients reach adolescent or adult life with normal pulmonary function and without evidence of overinflation.

Microbiologic Studies

The finding of *S. aureus* or *P. aeruginosa* on culture of the lower airways (sputum) strongly suggests a diagnosis of CF. In particular, mucoid forms of *P. aeruginosa* are often recovered from CF lungs. *B. cepacia* recovery also suggests CF. A wide range of other organisms are frequently recovered, particularly in advanced lung disease; they include a variety of gram-negative rods, fungi, and nontuberculous mycobacterial species. Failure of respiratory symptom flares to respond to usual antibiotics triggers testing for *Mycoplasma* and viruses. Fiberoptic bronchoscopy is used to gather lower respiratory tract secretions of infants and young children who do not expectorate.

Heterozygote Detection and Prenatal Diagnosis

Mutation analysis should be fully informative for testing of potential carriers or a fetus, provided that mutations within the family have been previously identified. Testing a spouse of a carrier with a standard panel of probes is ≈90% sensitive, and full CFTR sequence analysis is commercially available if further testing is warranted. Prenatal testing should be offered to all couples planning to have children in addition to individuals with a family history of CF and partners of CF women. The American College of Medical Genetics and the American College of Obstetricians and Gynecologists recommend that CF carrier screening be offered to individuals of Ashkenazi Jewish or white descent and be made available to individuals of other ethnic and racial groups; in one large series, 14% of carrier screening referrals were from Hispanic and African-American individuals, and 12% from individuals with ethnicities other than white or Ashkenazi Jewish. Screening of the siblings of an affected child is also suggested.

Newborn Screening

A variety of newborn screening algorithms are in place to identify infants with CF. Most algorithms utilize a combination of immunoreactive trypsinogen results and limited DNA testing on blood spots, which are then coupled with confirmatory sweat analysis. This screening test is ≈95% sensitive. Newborn diagnoses can prevent early nutritional deficiencies and improve long-term growth and may improve cognitive function. Early diagnosis may improve weight for age; an improved weight for age is associated with better lung function at 6 yr of age. In 2004, the Centers for Disease Control and Prevention recommended the use of newborn screening for early identification of infants with CF. In 2009, newborn screening is mandated in 49 of 50 states, with Texas being the only state that does not require testing. Early diagnosis also has the advantage of genetic counseling for the family and, in some cases, avoids protracted diagnostic efforts.

TREATMENT

The treatment plan should be comprehensive and linked to close monitoring and early, aggressive intervention.

General Approach to Care

Initial efforts after diagnosis should be intensive and should include baseline assessment, initiation of treatment, clearing of pulmonary involvement, and education of the patient and parents. Follow-up evaluations are scheduled every 1-3 mo, depending on the age at diagnosis, because many aspects of the condition require careful monitoring. An interval history and physical examination should be obtained at each visit. A sputum sample or, if that is not available, a lower pharyngeal swab taken during or after a forced cough is obtained for culture and antibiotic susceptibility studies. Because irreversible loss of pulmonary function from low-grade infection can occur gradually and without acute symptoms, emphasis is placed on a thorough pulmonary history. Table 395-6 lists symptoms and signs that suggest the need for more intensive antibiotic and physical therapy. Protection against exposure to methicillin-resistant *S. aureus, P. aeruginosa, B. cepacia,* and other resistant gram-negative organisms is essential, including isolation procedures and careful attention to sterilization of inhalation therapy equipment. A nurse, respiratory therapist, social worker, dietitian, and psychologist, as members of the multidisciplinary care team, should evaluate children regularly and contribute to the development of a comprehensive daily care plan. Considerable education and programs to empower families and older children to take responsibility for care are likely to result in the best adherence to daily care programs. Standardization of practice, on the part of both caregivers and families, as well as close monitoring and early intervention for new or increasing symptoms appears to result in the best long-term outcomes.

Because secretions of CF patients are not adequately hydrated, attention in early childhood to oral hydration, especially during warm weather or with acute gastroenteritis, may minimize complications associated with impaired mucus clearance. Intravenous therapy for dehydration should be initiated early.

Table 395-6 SYMPTOMS AND SIGNS ASSOCIATED WITH EXACERBATION OF PULMONARY INFECTION IN PATIENTS WITH CYSTIC FIBROSIS

SYMPTOMS
Increased frequency and duration of cough
Increased sputum production
Change in appearance of sputum
Increased shortness of breath
Decreased exercise tolerance
Decreased appetite
Feeling of increased congestion in the chest
SIGNS
Increased respiratory rate
Use of accessory muscles for breathing
Intercostal retractions
Change in results of auscultatory examination of chest
Decline in measures of pulmonary function consistent with the presence of obstructive airway disease
Fever and leukocytosis
Weight loss
New infiltrate on chest radiograph

From Ramsey B: Management of pulmonary disease in patients with cystic fibrosis, *N Engl J Med* 335:179, 1996.

Table 395-7 COMPLICATIONS OF THERAPY FOR CYSTIC FIBROSIS*

COMPLICATION	AGENT
Gastrointestinal bleeding	Ibuprofen
Hyperglycemia	Corticosteroids (systemic)
Growth retardation	Corticosteroids (systemic, inhaled)
Renal dysfunction:	
Tubular	Aminoglycosides
Interstitial nephritis	Semisynthetic penicillins, nonsteroidal anti-inflammatory drugs
Hearing loss, vestibular dysfunction	Aminoglycosides
Peripheral neuropathy or optic atrophy	Chloramphenicol (prolonged course)
Hypomagnesemia	Aminoglycosides
Hyperuricemia, colonic stricture	Pancreatic extracts (very large doses)
Goiter	Iodine-containing expectorants
Gynecomastia	Spironolactone
Enamel hypoplasia or staining	Tetracyclines (used in 1st 8 yr of life)

**Note:* Common hypersensitivity reactions to drugs are not included.

The goal of therapy is to maintain a stable condition for prolonged periods. This can be accomplished for most patients by interval evaluation and adjustments of the home treatment program. Some children have episodic acute or low-grade chronic lung infection that progresses. For these patients, intensive inhalation and airway clearance and intravenous antibiotics are indicated. Improvement is most reliably accomplished in a hospital setting; selected patients have demonstrated successful outcomes while completing these treatments at home. Intravenous antibiotics may be required infrequently or as often as every 2-3 mo. The goal of treatment is to return patients to their previous pulmonary and functional status.

The basic daily care program varies according to the age of the child, the degree of pulmonary involvement, other system involvement, and the time available for therapy. The major components of this care are pulmonary and nutritional therapies. Because therapy is medication-intensive, iatrogenic problems frequently arise. Monitoring for these complications is also an important part of management (Table 395-7).

Pulmonary Therapy

The object of pulmonary therapy is to clear secretions from airways and to control infection. When a child is not doing well, every potentially useful aspect of therapy should be reconsidered.

INHALATION THERAPY Aerosol therapy is used to deliver medications and hydrate the lower respiratory tract. Metered-dose inhalers can deliver some agents, such as bronchodilators and corticosteroids, with a spacer for younger children. Alternately, these medications can be delivered with a compressor that drives a handheld nebulizer. In some patients β-agonists may decrease Pa_{O_2} acutely by increasing ventilation-perfusion mismatch, a concern if the Pa_{O_2} is marginal.

Human recombinant DNase (2.5 mg), given as a single daily aerosol dose, improves pulmonary function, decreases the number of pulmonary exacerbations, and promotes a sense of well-being in patients who have moderate disease and purulent secretions. Benefit for those with normal forced expiratory volume in 1 sec (FEV_1) values or advanced lung disease has also been documented. Improvement is sustained for ≥12 mo with continuous therapy. Another mucolytic agent, *N*-acetylcysteine, is toxic to ciliated epithelium, and its repeated administration should be avoided.

Nebulized hypertonic saline, acting as a hyperosmolar agent, is believed to draw water into the airway and rehydrate mucus and the peri ciliary fluid layer, resulting in improved mucociliary clearance. A number of studies have reported 7% hypertonic saline nebulized 2-4 times daily results in increased mucus clearance and improved pulmonary function.

Aerosolized antibiotics are often used when the airways are colonized with *Pseudomonas* as part of daily therapy. Aerosolized tobramycin, TOBI, used as a suppressive therapy (on 1 month, off 1 month) may reduce symptoms, improve pulmonary function, and alleviate the need for hospitalization (see Aerosolized Antibiotic Therapy).

AIRWAY CLEARANCE THERAPY Airway clearance treatment usually consists of chest percussion combined with postural drainage and derives its rationale from the idea that cough clears mucus from large airways but chest vibrations are required to move secretions from small airways, where expiratory flow rates are low. **Chest physical therapy (PT)** can be particularly useful for patients with CF because they accumulate secretions in small airways first, even before the onset of symptoms. Although immediate improvement of pulmonary function generally cannot be demonstrated after PT, cessation of chest PT in children with mild to moderate airflow limitation results in deterioration of lung function within 3 wk, and prompt improvement of function occurs when therapy is resumed. Chest PT is recommended 1-4 times a day, depending on the severity of lung dysfunction. Cough, huffing, or forced expirations are encouraged after each lung segment is "drained." Vest-type mechanical percussors are also useful. Voluntary coughing, repeated forced expiratory maneuvers with and without positive expiratory pressure, patterned breathing, and use of an array of handheld oscillatory devices are additional aids to clearance of mucus. Routine aerobic exercise appears to slow the rate of decline of pulmonary function, and benefit has also been documented with weight training. No one airway clearance technique (ACT) is superior to any other, so all modes should be considered in the development of an airway clearance prescription. Adherence to daily therapy is essential therefore ACT plans are individualized for each patient.

ANTIBIOTIC THERAPY Antibiotics are the mainstay of therapy designed to control progression of lung infection. The goal is to reduce the intensity of endobronchial infection and to delay progressive lung damage. The usual guidelines for acute chest infections, such as fever, tachypnea, or chest pain, are often absent. Consequently, all aspects of the patient's history and examination, including anorexia, weight loss, and diminished activity, must be used to guide the frequency and duration of therapy. Antibiotic treatment varies from intermittent short courses of 1 antibiotic to nearly continuous treatment with 1 or more antibiotics. Dosages for some antibiotics are often 2 to 3 times the amount recommended for minor infections because patients with CF have proportionately more lean body mass and higher clearance rates for many antibiotics than other individuals. In addition, it is difficult to achieve effective drug levels of many antimicrobials in respiratory tract secretions.

ORAL ANTIBIOTIC THERAPY Indications for oral antibiotic therapy in a patient with CF include the presence of respiratory tract symptoms and identification of pathogenic organisms in respiratory tract cultures. Whenever possible, the choice of antibiotics should be guided by in vitro sensitivity testing. Common organisms, include *S. aureus,* nontypable *Haemophilus influenzae, P. aeruginosa; B. cepacia* and other gram-negative rods, are encountered with increasing frequency. The first 2 can be eradicated from the respiratory tract in CF with use of oral antibiotics, but *Pseudomonas* is more difficult to treat. The usual course of therapy is ≥2 wk, and maximal doses are recommended. Useful oral antibiotics are listed in Table 395-8. The quinolones are the only broadly effective oral antibiotics for *Pseudomonas* infection, but resistance against these agents emerges rapidly. Infection with mycoplasmal or chlamydial organisms has been documented, providing a rationale for the use of macrolides on an empirical basis for flare of symptoms. Macrolides may reduce the virulence properties of *P. aeruginosa,* such as biofilm production, and contribute anti-inflammatory effects. Long-term therapy with azithromycin times a week has been shown to improve lung function in patients with chronic *P. aeruginosa* infection.

AEROSOLIZED ANTIBIOTIC THERAPY *P. aeruginosa* and other gram-negative organisms are frequently resistant to all oral antibiotics. Aerosol delivery of antibiotics has been used as an option for home delivery of additional agents, such as tobramycin, colistin, and gentamicin. Although these therapies are used, the evidence to support aerosolized antibiotics for an acute pulmonary exacerbation is limited. However, there is good evidence to support the use of inhaled tobramycin as a long-term suppressive therapy in a patient colonized with *P. aeruginosa.* When tobramycin is given at a dose of 300 mg twice daily on alternate months for 6 mo, *Pseudomonas* density in sputum decreases, fewer hospitalizations are required, and pulmonary function can improve by ≥10%. Toxicity is negligible. On the basis of available evidence, this therapy is recommended in patients with chronic colonization with *P. aeruginosa,* to lessen symptoms and/or to improve long-term function in patients with moderate to severe disease. Other antimicrobials, such as colistin (75-150 mg), have been given in aerosolized 2 to 4 times a day; however, their efficacy has not been established. Sensitization and resistance to inhaled antibiotics can occur, but both developments are surprisingly infrequent. Bronchospasm may complicate aerosolized colistin therapy. Another indication for aerosolized antibiotic therapy is the acquisition of *P. aeruginosa* in the airways. Early infection may be eliminated for months to several years by oral ciprofloxacin with aerosolized colistin or tobramycin. Established infection is rarely eradicated.

INTRAVENOUS ANTIBIOTIC THERAPY For the patient who has progressive or unrelenting symptoms and signs despite intensive home measures, intravenous antibiotic therapy is indicated. This therapy is usually initiated in the hospital but may be completed on an ambulatory basis. Although many patients show improvement within 7 days, it is usually advisable to extend the period of treatment to at least 14 days. Permanent intravenous access can be provided for long-term or frequent courses of therapy in the hospital or at home. Thrombophilia screening should be

Table 395-8 ANTIMICROBIAL AGENTS FOR CYSTIC FIBROSIS LUNG INFECTION

ROUTE	ORGANISMS	AGENTS	DOSAGE (mg/kg/24 hr)	NO. DOSES/24 hr
Oral	*Staphylococcus aureus*	Dicloxacillin	25-50	4
		Linezolid	20	2
		Cephalexin	50	4
		Clindamycin	10-30	3-4
		Amoxicillin-clavulanate	25-45	2-3
	Haemophilus influenzae	Amoxicillin	50-100	2-3
	Pseudomonas aeruginosa	Ciprofloxacin	20-30	2-3
	Burkholderia cepacia	Trimethoprim-sulfamethoxazole	8-10*	2-4
	Empirical	Azithromycin	10, day 1; 5, days 2-5	1
		Erythromycin	30-50	3-4
Intravenous	*S. aureus*	Nafcillin	100-200	4-6
		Vancomycin	40	3-4
	P. aeruginosa	Tobramycin	8-12	1-3
		Amikacin	15-30	2-3
		Ticarcillin	400	4
		Piperacillin	300-400	4
		Ticarcillin-clavulanate	400†	4
		Piperacillin-Tazobactam	240-400‡	3
		Meropenem	60-120	3
		Imipenem-cilastatin	45-100	3-4
		Ceftazidime	150	3
		Aztreonam	150-200	4
	B. cepacia	Chloramphenicol	50-100	4
		Meropenem	60-120	3
Aerosol		Tobramycin (inhaled)	300§	2

*Quantity of trimethoprim.
†Quantity of ticarcillin.
‡Quantity of piperacillin.
§In mg per dose.

considered before the use of totally implantable intravenous devices or for recurring problems with venous catheters.

Commonly used intravenous antibiotics are listed in Table 395-8. In general, treatment of *Pseudomonas* infection requires 2-drug therapy. A 3rd agent may be required for optimal coverage of *S. aureus* or other organisms. The aminoglycosides have a relatively short half-life in many patients with CF. The initial parenteral dose, noted in Table 395-8, is generally given every 8 hr. After blood levels have been determined, the total daily dose should be adjusted. Peak levels of 10-15 mg/L are desirable, and trough levels should be kept at <2 mg/L to minimize the risk of ototoxicity and nephrotoxicity. Once- or twice-daily aminoglycoside dosing may have advantages over dosing every 8 hr. Changes in therapy should be guided by lack of improvement and by culture results. If patients do not show improvement, complications such as heart failure and reactive airways or infection with viruses, *Aspergillus fumigatus* (Chapter 229), nontuberculous mycobacteria (Chapter 209), or other unusual organisms should be considered. *B. cepacia* is the most frequent of a growing list of gram-negative rods that may be particularly refractory to antimicrobial therapy.

Bronchodilator Therapy

Reversible airway obstruction occurs in many children with CF, sometimes in conjunction with frank asthma or acute bronchopulmonary aspergillosis. Reversible obstruction is defined as improvement of ≥15% in flow rates after inhalation of a bronchodilator. In many patients with CF, flow rates may improve by only 5-10%, however. Nevertheless, subjective benefit is claimed by many following use of a β-adrenergic agonist aerosol. Cromolyn sodium and ipratropium hydrochlorides are alternative agents, but there is no evidence to support their use.

Anti-Inflammatory Agents

Corticosteroids are useful for the treatment of allergic bronchopulmonary aspergillosis and severe reactive airway disease occasionally encountered in children with CF. Prolonged treatment of standard CF lung disease using an alternate-day regimen initially appeared to improve pulmonary function and diminish hospitalization rates. However, a 4-yr double-blind, multicenter study of this regimen for patients with mild to moderate lung disease found only modest efficacy and prohibitive side effects, including growth retardation, cataracts, and abnormalities of glucose tolerance at a dose of 2 mg/kg and growth retardation at 1 mg/kg. Inhaled corticosteroids have theoretical appeal, but there are few data documenting their efficacy and safety; it appears that discontinuing inhaled corticosteroids in patients with CF had no effect on lung function, antibiotic use, or bronchodilator use. Ibuprofen, given long term (dose adjusted to achieve a peak serum concentration of 50-100 µg/mL) for 4 yr, is associated with a slowing of disease progression, particularly in younger patients with mild lung disease. Side effects of nonsteroidal anti-inflammatory drugs have been encountered (see Table 395-7); therefore, this therapy has not gained broad acceptance even though ibuprofen is the only anti-inflammatory agent with documented efficacy in the patient population.

Endoscopy and Lavage

Treatment of obstructed airways sometimes includes tracheobronchial suctioning or lavage, especially if atelectasis or mucoid impaction is present. Bronchopulmonary lavage can be performed by the instillation of saline or a mucolytic agent through a fiberoptic bronchoscope. Antibiotics (usually gentamicin or tobramycin) can also be instilled directly at lavage in order to transiently achieve a much higher endobronchial concentration than can be obtained by using intravenous therapy. There is no evidence for sustained benefit from repeated endoscopic or lavage procedures.

Other Therapies

Expectorants such as iodides and guaifenesin do not effectively assist with the removal of secretions from the respiratory tract. Inspiratory muscle training can enhance maximum oxygen consumption during exercise as well as FEV_1.

EMERGING THERAPIES A number of potential therapies are under development, including promising mutation-specific therapies in clinical trials. For class 1 mutations (nonsense or premature stop-codon mutations) that result in a premature termination of the mRNA that leads to no protein production, PTC124 has been shown to suppress the termination codon, allowing for read through and partial correction of the defect in approximately 30% of subjects with CF. Additional studies are under way to further evaluate PTC124's efficacy. Several molecules have been identified that allow for proper processing of class 2 mutations; clinical trials are planned to evaluate a number of these substances. Significant progress has been made on a group of small molecules referred to as "potentiators," including VX-770 (Vertex Pharmaceuticals, Cambridge, MA), that activate CFTR mutants (G551D-CFTR) that traffic to the plasma membrane but do not appropriately activate. Therapies including denufosol and Moli1901 (lancovutide, Lantibio/AOP Orphan Pharmaceuticals AG, Vienna) are directed at bypassing the primary CFTR defect by regulating alternative ion channels and normalizing the ion transport properties of affected tissue, thus correcting the mucociliary abnormality observed in the respiratory tract of the patient with CF.

TREATMENT OF PULMONARY COMPLICATIONS

Atelectasis

Lobar atelectasis occurs relatively infrequently; it may be asymptomatic and noted only at the time of a routine chest radiograph. Aggressive intravenous therapy with antibiotics and increased chest PT directed at the affected lobe may be effective. If there is no improvement in 5-7 days, bronchoscopic examination of the airways may be indicated. If the atelectasis does not resolve, continued intensive home therapy is indicated, because atelectasis may resolve during a period of weeks or months. Persistent atelectasis may be asymptomatic. Lobectomy should be considered only if expansion is not achieved and the patient has progressive difficulty from fever, anorexia, and unrelenting cough (Chapter 402).

Hemoptysis

Endobronchial bleeding usually reflects airway wall erosion secondary to infection. With increasing numbers of older patients, hemoptysis has become a relatively frequent complication. Blood streaking of sputum is particularly common. Small-volume hemoptysis (<20 mL) should not trigger panic and is usually viewed as a need for intensified antimicrobial therapy and chest PT. When the hemoptysis is persistent or increases in severity, hospital admission is indicated. **Massive hemoptysis,** defined as total blood loss of ≥250 mL in a 24-hr period, is rare in the 1st decade and occurs in <1% of adolescents, but it requires close monitoring and the capability to replace blood losses rapidly. Chest PT is often discontinued until 12-24 hr after the last brisk bleeding episode and is then gradually re-instituted. Patients should receive vitamin K for an abnormal prothrombin time. During brisk hemoptysis, the child and parents require a great deal of reassurance that the bleeding will stop. Blood transfusion is not indicated unless there is hypotension or the hematocrit is significantly reduced. Ticarcillin, salicylates, and nonsteroidal anti-inflammatory drugs interfere with platelet function and may aggravate hemoptysis. Bronchoscopy rarely reveals the site of bleeding. Lobectomy is to be avoided, if possible, because functioning lung should be preserved. Bronchial artery embolization can be useful to control persistent, significant hemoptysis.

Pneumothorax

Pneumothorax (Chapter 405) is encountered in <1% of children and teenagers with CF, although it is more frequently encountered in older patients and may be life-threatening. The episode may be asymptomatic but is often attended by chest and shoulder pain, shortness of breath, or hemoptysis. A small air collection that does not grow can be observed closely. Chest tube placement with or without pleurodesis is often the initial therapy. Intravenous antibiotics are also begun on admission. An open thoracotomy or video-assisted thoracoscopy (VATS) with plication of blebs, apical pleural stripping, and basal pleural abrasion should be considered if the air leak persists. Surgical intervention is usually well tolerated even in cases of advanced lung disease. The thoracotomy tube is removed as soon as possible, usually on the 2nd or 3rd postoperative day. The patient can then be mobilized, and full postural drainage therapy resumed. Previous pneumothorax with or without pleurodesis is not a contraindication to subsequent lung transplantation.

Allergic Aspergillosis

Allergic aspergillosis occurs in 5-10% of patients with CF and may manifest as wheezing, increased cough, shortness of breath, and marked hyperinflation (Chapters 229 and 391). In some patients, a chest radiograph shows new, focal infiltrates. The presence of rust-colored sputum, the recovery of *Aspergillus* organisms from the sputum, the demonstration of serum precipitating and specific immunoglobulin E (IgE) and IgG antibodies against *A. fumigatus*, or the presence of eosinophils in a fresh sputum sample supports the diagnosis. The serum IgE level is usually high. Treatment is directed at controlling the inflammatory reaction with oral corticosteroids and preventing central bronchiectasis. For refractory cases, oral antifungals may be required.

Nontuberculous Mycobacteria Infection (Chapter 209)

Injured airways with poor clearance may be colonized by *Mycobacterium avium-complex* but also *Mycobacterium abscessus* and *Mycobacterium kansasii*. Distinguishing endobronchial colonization (frequent) from invasive infection (infrequent) is challenging. Persistent fevers and new infiltrates or cystic lesions coupled with the finding of acid-fast organisms on sputum smear suggest infection. Treatment is prolonged and requires multiple antimicrobial agents. Symptoms may improve, but the nontuberculous mycobacteria (NTM) are not usually cleared from the lungs.

Bone and Joint Complications

Hypertrophic osteoarthropathy causes elevation of the periosteum over the distal portions of long bones and bone pain, overlying edema, and joint effusions. Acetaminophen or ibuprofen may provide relief. Control of lung infection usually reduces symptoms. Intermittent arthropathy unrelated to other rheumatologic disorders occurs occasionally, has no recognized pathogenesis, and usually responds to nonsteroidal anti-inflammatory agents. Back pain or rib fractures from vigorous coughing may require pain management to permit adequate airway clearance. These and other fractures may stem from diminished bone mineralization, the result of reduced vitamin D absorption, corticosteroid therapy, diminished weight-bearing exercises, and, perhaps, other factors. There may be a bone phenotype in CF that is unrelated to therapies or nutritional status and may be due to CFTR dysfunction.

Sleep-Disordered Breathing

Particularly with advanced pulmonary disease and during chest exacerbations, individuals with CF may experience more sleep arousals, less time in rapid eye movement (REM) sleep, nocturnal hypoxemia, hypercapnia, and associated neurobehavioral impairment. Nocturnal hypoxemia may hasten the onset of pulmonary hypertension and right-sided heart failure. Efficacy of specific interventions for this complication of CF has not been systematically assessed. Prompt treatment of airway symptoms and nocturnal oxygen supplementation or bilevel positive airway pressure (BiPAP) support should be considered in selected cases.

Acute Respiratory Failure

Acute respiratory failure (Chapter 65) rarely occurs in patients with mild to moderate lung disease and is usually the result of a severe viral or other infectious illness. Because patients with this complication can regain their previous status, intensive therapy is indicated. In addition to aerosol, postural drainage, and intravenous antibiotic treatment, oxygen is required to raise the arterial Pa_{O_2}. An increasing Pc_{O_2} may require ventilatory assistance. Endotracheal or bronchoscopic suction may be necessary to clear airway inspissated secretions and can be repeated daily. Right-sided heart failure should be treated vigorously. Recovery is often slow. Intensive intravenous antibiotic therapy and postural drainage should be continued for 1-2 wk after the patient has regained baseline status.

Chronic Respiratory Failure

Patients with CF acquire chronic respiratory failure after prolonged deterioration of lung function. Although this complication can occur at any age, it is now seen most frequently in adult patients. Because a long-standing Pa_{O_2} <50 mm Hg promotes the development of right-sided heart failure, patients usually benefit from low-flow oxygen to raise arterial P_{O_2} to ≥55 mm Hg. Increasing hypercapnia may prevent the use of optimal F_{IO_2}. Most patients improve somewhat with intensive antibiotic and pulmonary therapy measures and can be discharged from the hospital. Low-flow oxygen therapy is needed at home, especially with sleep. Noninvasive ventilatory support can improve gas exchange and has been documented to enhance quality of life. Ventilatory support may be particularly useful for patients awaiting lung transplantation. These patients usually display cor pulmonale and should reduce their salt intake and be given diuretics. Caution should be exercised to avoid ventilation-suppressing metabolic alkalosis that results from CF-related chloride depletion and, in many cases, from diuretic-induced bicarbonate retention. Chronic pain (headache, chest pain, abdominal pain, and limb pain) is frequent at the end of life and responds to judicious use of analgesics, including opioids. Dyspnea has been ameliorated with nebulized fentanyl.

Lung transplantation is an option for end-stage lung disease (Chapter 437) but a topic of vigorous debate. Criteria for referral continue to be a subject of investigation and ideally include estimates of longevity with and without transplant based on lung function and exercise tolerance data. Because of bronchiolitis obliterans (Chapter 386.1) and other complications, transplanted lungs cannot be expected to function for the lifetime of a recipient, and repeat transplantation is increasingly common. The demand for donor lungs exceeds the supply, and waiting lists as well as duration of waits continue to grow. The protocol for matching donor organs with lung transplant recipients has been revised to account for the severity of the patients' lung disease. In a review of lung transplantation in children with CF between 1992 and 2002, pre-transplantation colonization with *B. cepacia*, diabetes, and older age decreased post-transplantation survival. The review suggests that transplantation is often associated with many complications and may not prolong life nor significantly improve its quality.

Heart Failure

Some patients experience reversible right-sided heart failure (Chapter 436) as the result of an acute event such as a viral infection or pneumothorax. Individuals with long-standing, advanced pulmonary disease, especially those with severe hypoxemia (Pa_{O_2} <50 mm Hg), often acquire chronic right-sided heart failure. The mechanisms include hypoxemic pulmonary arterial constriction and loss of the pulmonary vascular bed. Pulmonary arterial wall changes contribute to increased vascular resistance with time. Evidence for concomitant left ventricular dysfunction is often found. Cyanosis, increased shortness of breath, increased liver size with a tender margin, ankle edema, jugular venous distention, an unusual weight gain, increased heart size seen on chest radiograph, or evidence for right-sided heart enlargement on electrocardiogram or echocardiogram helps to confirm the diagnosis. Diuresis induced by furosemide (1 mg/kg administered intravenously) confirms the suspicion of fluid retention. Repeated doses are often required at 24- to 48-hr intervals to reduce fluid accumulation and accompanying symptoms. Concomitant use of spironolactone may protect against potassium depletion and facilitate long-term diuresis. Hypochloremic alkalosis complicates the long-term use of loop diuretics. Digitalis is not effective in pure right-sided failure but may be useful when there is an associated left-sided dysfunction. The arterial P_{O_2} should be maintained at >50 mm Hg if possible. Intensive pulmonary therapy, including intravenous antibiotics, is most important. Initially, the salt intake should be limited. Volume overload and antibiotics with high sodium content should be avoided. No clear-cut long-term benefit from pulmonary vasodilators has been demonstrated. The prognosis for heart failure is poor, but a number of patients survive for ≥5 yr after the appearance of heart failure. Heart-lung transplantation may be an option (see preceding section).

NUTRITIONAL THERAPY Up to 90% of patients with CF have loss of exocrine pancreatic function as well as inadequate digestion and absorption of fats and proteins. They require dietary adjustment, pancreatic enzyme replacement, and supplementary vitamins. In general, children with CF need to exceed the usual required daily caloric intake to grow. The target has been set at 130 kcal per kg of body weight. Daily supplements of the fat-soluble vitamins are required.

Diet

Historically, at the time of diagnosis many infants presented with nutritional deficits; this situation is changing because of newborn screening. Sometimes young infants with a history of wheezy breathing were often started on soy-protein formulas prior to their evaluation; they did not use this protein well and often acquired hypoproteinemia with anasarca. Although in the past a low-fat, high-protein, high-calorie diet was generally recommended for older children, it resulted in deficiencies of essential fatty acids and poor growth. With the advent of improved pancreatic enzyme products, increased amounts of fat in the diet are well tolerated and preferred.

Most individuals with CF have a higher than normal caloric need because of increased work of breathing and perhaps because of increased metabolic activity related to the basic defect. When anorexia of chronic infection supervenes, weight loss occurs. Encouragement to eat high-calorie foods is important, but weight gain is not generally realized unless lung infection is controlled. Weight stabilization or gain sometimes requires nocturnal feeding via nasogastric tube or percutaneous enterostomy or with short-term intravenous hyperalimentation. Not infrequently, parent-child interactions at feeding time are maladaptive, and behavioral interventions can improve caloric intake. Long-term benefits of these interventions include improved quality of life and psychologic well-being. In addition there is good correlation between improved BMI and maintenance of FEV_1.

Recombinant growth hormone therapy (3 times per week) has improved nutritional outcomes, including positive effects on nitrogen balance and improved height and weight velocities.

Pancreatic Enzyme Replacement

Extracts of animal pancreas given with ingested food reduce but do not fully correct stool fat and nitrogen losses. Enzyme dosage and product should be individualized for each patient. Enteric-coated, pH-sensitive enzyme microspheres are most often prescribed. Several strengths up to 20,000 IU of lipase/capsule are available. Administration of excessive doses has been linked to **colonic strictures** requiring surgery. Consequently, enzyme replacement should not exceed 2,500 lipase units/kg/meal in most circumstances. In general, infants need 2,000-4,000 lipase units per feeding, which is most easily given mixed with applesauce. Snacks should also be covered. The dose of enzymes required usually increases with age, but some patients have lower requirements as teenagers and young adults.

Vitamin and Mineral Supplements

Because pancreatic insufficiency results in malabsorption of fat-soluble vitamins (A, D, E, K), vitamin supplementation is recommended. Several vitamin preparations containing all 4 vitamins for patients with CF are available. They should be taken daily. Replacement doses may be required when low serum levels are documented or the patient is symptomatic. Infants with zinc deficiency and an acrodermatitis enteropathica–like rash have been described. In addition, attention should be paid to iron status; in one study, almost 30% of children with CF had low serum ferritin concentrations.

TREATMENT OF INTESTINAL COMPLICATIONS

Meconium Ileus

When meconium ileus (Chapter 96.1) is suspected, a nasogastric tube is placed for suction and the newborn is hydrated. In many cases, diatrizoate (Gastrografin) enemas with reflux of contrast material into the ileum not only confirm the diagnosis but have also resulted in the passage of a meconium plug and clearing of the obstruction. Use of this hypertonic solution requires careful correction of water losses into the bowel. Children in whom this procedure fails require operative intervention. Children who are successfully treated generally have a prognosis similar to that of other patients with severe CF mutations. Infants with meconium ileus should be treated as if they have CF until adequate diagnostic testing can be carried out.

Distal Intestinal Obstruction Syndrome (Meconium Ileus Equivalent) and Other Causes of Abdominal Symptoms

Despite appropriate pancreatic enzyme replacement, 2-5% of patients accumulate fecal material in the terminal portion of the ileum and in the cecum, which may result in partial or complete obstruction. For intermittent symptoms, pancreatic enzyme replacement should be continued or even increased, and stool softeners (polyethylene glycol [MiraLAX] or docusate sodium [Colace]) given. Increased fluid intake is also recommended. Failure to relieve symptoms signals the need for large-volume bowel lavage with a balanced salt solution containing polyethylene glycol taken by mouth or by nasogastric tube. When there is complete obstruction, a diatrizoate enema, accompanied by large amounts of intravenous fluids, can be therapeutic. Intussusception (Chapter 325.3) and volvulus (Chapter 321.4) must also be considered in the differential diagnosis. Intussusception, usually ileocolic, occurs at any age and often follows a 1- to 2-day history of "constipation." It can often be diagnosed and reduced via a diatrizoate enema. If a nonreducible intussusception or a volvulus is present, laparotomy is required. Repeated episodes of intussusception may be an indication for cecectomy.

Chronic appendicitis with or without periappendiceal abscess may manifest as recurrent or persistent abdominal pain, raising the question of need for a laparotomy. A lack of acid buffering in the duodenum appears to promote duodenitis and ulcer formation in some children. Other reasons for surgical procedures include carcinoma of the colon or biliary tract and sclerosing colonopathy.

Gastroesophageal Reflux (Chapter 315)

Because several factors raise intra-abdominal pressure, including cough and obstructed airways, pathologic gastroesophageal reflux is not uncommon and may exacerbate lung disease secondary to reflex wheezing and repeated aspiration. Dietary, positional, and medication therapies should be considered. Cholinergic agonists are contraindicated because they trigger mucus secretion and progressive respiratory difficulty. Reduction of stomach acid secretion can help, with proton pump inhibitors being the most effective agents. Fundoplication is a procedure of last resort.

Rectal Prolapse (Chapter 336.5)

Though uncommon, rectal prolapse occurs most often in infants with CF and less frequently in older children with the disease. It is usually related to steatorrhea, malnutrition, and repetitive cough. The prolapsed rectum can usually be replaced manually by continuous gentle pressure with the patient in the knee-chest position. Sedation may be helpful. To prevent an immediate recurrence, the buttocks can be taped closed. Adequate pancreatic enzyme replacement, decreased fat and roughage in the diet, stool softener, and control of pulmonary infection result in improvement. Occasionally, a patient may continue to have rectal prolapse and may require sclerotherapy or surgery.

Hepatobiliary Disease

Liver function abnormalities associated with biliary cirrhosis can be improved by treatment with ursodeoxycholic acid. The ability of bile acids to prevent progression of cirrhosis has not been clearly documented. Portal hypertension with esophageal varices, hypersplenism, or ascites occurs in ≤8% of children with CF (Chapter 359). The acute management of bleeding esophageal varices includes nasogastric suction and cold saline lavage. Sclerotherapy is recommended after an initial hemorrhage. In the past, significant bleeding has also been treated successfully with portosystemic shunting. Splenorenal anastomosis has been the most effective treatment. Pronounced hypersplenism may require splenectomy. Cholelithiasis should prompt surgical consultation. The management of ascites is discussed in Chapter 362.

Obstructive jaundice in newborns with CF needs no specific therapy. Hepatomegaly with steatosis requires careful attention to nutrition and may respond to carnitine repletion. Rarely, biliary cirrhosis proceeds to hepatocellular failure, which should be treated as in patients without CF (Chapters 356 and 359). End-stage liver disease is an indication for liver transplantation in children with CF, especially if pulmonary function is good (Chapter 360).

Pancreatitis

Pancreatitis can be precipitated by fatty meals, alcohol ingestion, or tetracycline therapy. Serum amylase and lipase values may remain elevated for long periods. Treatment of this disorder is discussed in Chapter 343.

Hyperglycemia

Onset of hyperglycemia occurs most frequently after the 1st decade. Approximately 20% of young adults are treated for hyperglycemia, although the incidence of CF-related diabetes (CFRD) may be higher. Prevalence is greater in females and in ΔF508 homozygotes. Ketoacidosis is rarely encountered. The pathogenesis includes both impaired insulin secretion and insulin resistance. Routine screening consists of an annual modified 2-hr oral glucose tolerance test after the child reaches age 8-10 yr. Glucose intolerance without urine glucose losses is usually not treated; glycosylated hemoglobin levels should be followed at least annually. With persistent glycosuria and symptoms, insulin treatment should be instituted. Oral hypoglycemic agents, with or without drugs that reduce insulin resistance, may also be effective. Exocrine pancreatic insufficiency and malabsorption make strict dietary control of hyperglycemia difficult. Corticosteroid therapy should be avoided. The development of significant hyperglycemia favors acquisition of *P. aeruginosa* and *B. cepacia* in the airways and may adversely affect pulmonary function. Thus, careful control of blood glucose level is an important goal. Long-term vascular complications of diabetes can occur, providing an additional rationale for good control of blood glucose levels.

OTHER THERAPY

Nasal Polyps

Nasal polyps (Chapter 370) occur in 15-20% of patients with CF and are most prevalent in the 2nd decade of life. Local corticosteroids and nasal decongestants occasionally provide some relief. When the polyps completely obstruct the nasal airway, rhinorrhea becomes constant, or widening of the nasal bridge is noticed, surgical removal of the polyps is indicated; polyps may recur promptly or after a symptom-free interval of months to years. Polyps inexplicably stop developing in many adults.

Rhinosinusitis

Opacification of paranasal sinuses is not an indication for intervention. Acute or chronic sinus-related symptoms are treated initially with antimicrobials, with or without maxillary sinus aspiration for culture. Functional endoscopic sinus surgery has anecdotally provided benefit.

Salt Depletion

Sweat salt losses in patients with CF can be high, especially in warm arid climates. Children should have free access to salt, and precautions against overdressing infants should be observed. Salt supplements are often prescribed to newborns identified through newborn screening and to children who live in hot weather climates. Hypochloremic alkalosis should be suspected in any infant who has had symptoms of gastroenteritis, and prompt fluid and electrolyte therapy should be instituted as needed.

Growth and Maturation

Delayed growth should be vigorously addressed by enhancing nutrition, treating lung disease more vigorously, and, in selected instances, endocrine evaluation and, possibly, growth hormone therapy. The risk : benefit ratio for anabolic steroid therapy does not support its use for undersized children with CF. Delayed sexual maturation, often associated with short stature, occurs fairly frequently in children with CF. Although many patients have severe pulmonary infection or poor nutrition, delayed puberty also occurs in those with otherwise mild disease and is not well explained. Adolescents with CF should receive specific counseling throughout their developing years concerning sexual maturation and reproductive potential.

Surgery

Minor surgical procedures, including dental work, should be performed with the use of local anesthesia if possible in children with CF. Patients with good or excellent pulmonary status can tolerate general anesthesia without any intensive pulmonary measures before the procedure. Those with moderate or severe pulmonary infection usually do better with a 1- to 2-wk course of intensive antibiotic treatment and increased airway clearance before surgery. If this approach is impossible, prompt intravenous antibiotic therapy is indicated once it is recognized that major surgery is required. The total time of anesthesia should be kept to a minimum. After induction, tracheal suctioning is useful and should be repeated. Patients with severe disease require monitoring of blood gas values and may need ventilatory assistance in the immediate postoperative period.

After major surgery, cough should be encouraged and airway clearance treatments should be re-instituted as soon as possible, usually within 24 hr. Adequate analgesia is important if early effective therapy is to be achieved. For those with significant pulmonary involvement, intravenous antibiotics are continued for 7-14 days postoperatively. Early ambulation and intermittent deep breathing are important; an incentive spirometer can also be helpful. After open thoracotomy for treatment of pneumothorax or lobectomy, the chest tube is the greatest single obstacle to effective pulmonary therapy and should be removed as soon as possible so that full postural drainage therapy can resume.

PROGNOSIS

CF remains a life-limiting disorder, although survival has improved dramatically in the past 30-40 yr. Infants with severe lung disease occasionally succumb, but most children survive this difficult period and are relatively healthy into adolescence or adulthood. The slow progression of lung disease eventually reaches disabling proportions, however. Life table data now indicate a median cumulative survival exceeding 35 yr. Male survival is somewhat better than female survival for reasons that are not readily apparent. Children in socioeconomically disadvantaged families have, on average, a poorer prognosis.

Children with CF usually have good school attendance records and should not be restricted in their activities. A high percentage eventually attend and graduate from college. Most adults with CF find satisfactory employment, and an increasing number marry. Transitioning care from pediatric to adult care centers by 21 yr of age is an important objective and requires a thoughtful, supportive approach involving both the pediatric and internal medicine specialists.

With increasing life span for patients with CF, a new set of psychosocial considerations has emerged, including dependence-independence issues, self-care, peer relationships, sexuality, reproduction, substance abuse, educational and vocational planning, medical care costs and other financial burdens, and anxiety concerning health and prognosis. Many of these issues are best addressed in an anticipatory fashion, before the onset of psychosocial dysfunction. With appropriate medical and psychosocial support, children and adolescents with CF generally cope well. Achievement of an independent and productive adulthood is a realistic goal for many.

BIBLIOGRAPHY

Please visit the Nelson Textbook of Pediatrics *website at* *www.expertconsult.com* *for the complete bibliography.*

Chapter 396
Primary Ciliary Dyskinesia (Immotile Cilia Syndrome)

Thomas Ferkol

Primary ciliary dyskinesia (PCD) is an inherited disorder characterized by impaired ciliary function leading to diverse clinical manifestations, including chronic sinopulmonary disease, persistent middle ear effusions, laterality defects, and infertility. Although PCD is thought to be a rare lung disease, its prevalence in children with repeated respiratory infections is estimated to be as high as 5%. Ultrastructural defects of cilia are linked to the clinical presentation of PCD.

For the full continuation of this chapter, please visit the Nelson Textbook of Pediatrics *website at* *www.expertconsult.com*.

Chapter 397
Interstitial Lung Diseases

Young-Jee Kim and Michelle S. Howenstine

Pediatric interstitial lung diseases (ILDs) are a group of uncommon, heterogeneous, familial, or sporadic diseases that cause disruption of alveolar interstitium and sometimes involve airway pathology. Knowledge regarding pediatric ILDs is limited because of their rare occurrence, the varied spectrum of disease, and the lack of controlled clinical trials investigating the disease process and treatment measures. The pathophysiology is believed to be more complex than that of adult disease because the injury occurs during the process of lung growth and differentiation. In ILD, the initial injury causes damage to the alveolar epithelium and capillary endothelium. Abnormal healing of injured tissue may be more prominent than inflammation in the initial steps of the development of chronic ILD. Some familial cases, especially surfactant dysfunction disorders, involve a specific gene.

For the full continuation of this chapter, please visit the Nelson Textbook of Pediatrics *website at* *www.expertconsult.com*.

Chapter 398
Pulmonary Alveolar Proteinosis

Aaron Hamvas, Lawrence M. Nogee, and F. Sessions Cole

Pulmonary alveolar proteinosis (PAP) is a rare cause of interstitial lung disease characterized by the intra-alveolar accumulation of pulmonary surfactant. Histopathologic examination shows distal air spaces to be filled with a granular, eosinophilic material that stains positively with periodic acid–Schiff reagent and is diastase resistant. Two clinically distinct forms of PAP have been described in children: a fulminant, usually fatal form manifesting shortly after birth (termed congenital PAP) and a gradually progressive type manifesting in older infants and children that is similar to the PAP observed in adults. PAP in older individuals has historically been classified as either primary or secondary to a number of recognized conditions, although this terminology is evolving as specific etiologies for PAP are identified. In the congenital form, alveolar proteinosis is a histologic feature that is found along with alveolar type II cell hyperplasia, interstitial thickening and inflammation, and alveolar macrophage accumulation in what are now being classified as disorders of surfactant metabolism or surfactant dysfunction (Chapter 399).

For the full continuation of this chapter, please visit the Nelson Textbook of Pediatrics *website at* *www.expertconsult.com*.

Chapter 399
Inherited Disorders of Surfactant Metabolism

Aaron Hamvas, Lawrence M. Nogee, and F. Sessions Cole

Pulmonary surfactant is a mixture of phospholipids and proteins synthesized, packaged, and secreted by type II pneumocytes that line the distal air spaces. This mixture forms a monolayer at the air-liquid interface that lowers surface tension at end-expiration of the respiratory cycle and thereby prevents atelectasis and ventilation-perfusion mismatch. Four surfactant-associated proteins have been described: surfactant proteins A and D (SP-A, SP-D) participate in host defense in the lung, whereas surfactant proteins B and C (SP-B, SP-C) contribute to the surface tension–lowering activity of the pulmonary surfactant. The ATP (adenosine triphosphate) binding cassette protein member A3, ABCA3, is a transporter located on the limiting membrane of lamellar bodies, the storage organelle for surfactant within alveolar type II cells, and has an essential role in surfactant phospholipids metabolism. Two genes for SP-A [*SFTPA1*, *SFTPA2*] and one gene for SP-D [*SFTPD*] are located on human chromosome 10, whereas single genes encode SP-B [*SFTPB*] and SP-C [*SFTPC*] and ABCA3 [*ABCA3*], which are located on human chromosomes 2, 8, and 16, respectively. Genetically engineered mice deficient in SP-A or SP-D are susceptible to viral and bacterial infections, and lineages deficient in SP-D accumulate lipids and foamy macrophages in their lungs and demonstrate emphysema as they age. Although inherited deficiencies of SP-D have not been identified in humans, mutations in the gene encoding SP-A2 may result in pulmonary fibrosis and lung cancer, although the disease did not manifest until adulthood in these cases. Inherited disorders of SP-B, SP-C, and ABCA3 have been identified in humans (see Table 399-1 on the *Nelson Textbook of Pediatrics* website at www.expertconsult.com).

For the full continuation of this chapter, please visit the Nelson Textbook of Pediatrics *website at www.expertconsult.com.*

Chapter 400
Pulmonary Hemosiderosis

Mary A. Nevin

The diagnosis of pulmonary hemosiderosis refers to the chronic and diffuse alveolar process diffuse **alveolar hemorrhage (DAH)**, rather than focal or self-limited pulmonary hemorrhage. Pulmonary hemosiderosis has classically been characterized by the triad consisting of iron-deficiency anemia, hemoptysis, and multiple alveolar infiltrates on chest radiographs. A high level of clinical suspicion may be required for the diagnosis, because any or all of these features of the disease can be absent at any point in the course of the disease. Pulmonary hemosiderosis can exist in isolation, but more commonly, it occurs in association with an underlying condition. A precise etiology for hemorrhage is not always found. A diagnosis of **idiopathic pulmonary hemosiderosis (IPH)** is made when alveolar hemorrhage occurs in isolation and an exhaustive evaluation for underlying disease is found to be negative.

ETIOLOGY

Most cases of DAH are associated with an underlying immunologic, rheumatologic, or vasculitic disorder but other diagnoses may manifest as recurrent or chronic pulmonary bleeding (Table 400-1).

Pulmonary hemosiderosis has historically been classified as primary or secondary. **Primary pulmonary hemosiderosis (PPH)** is described as encompassing the diagnoses of IPH, **Goodpasture syndrome** (Chapter 511), and **Heiner syndrome** (cow's milk hyperreactivity); Goodpasture syndrome (or anti–basement membrane antibody disease) appears to be the most common among these entities as a cause of pulmonary hemorrhage.

Secondary pulmonary hemosiderosis refers to the remaining, diverse group of potential etiologies. Among these are cardiac causes of pulmonary hemosiderosis, such as congestive heart failure, pulmonary hypertension, and mitral valve stenosis. Vasculitic and collagen vascular diseases such as systemic lupus erythematosus (SLE; Chapter 152), rheumatoid arthritis (Chapter 148), Wegener granulomatosis (Chapter 161.4), and Henoch-Schönlein purpura (HSP; Chapter 161.1) are another important group to consider in the differential diagnosis. Coagulopathies are encountered and may be either inherited or acquired. Prematurity is also a recognized risk factor for hemorrhage. Pulmonary hemosiderosis has been well described in association with celiac disease. Postinfectious processes such as hemolytic-uremic syndrome (Chapter 478.4) and immunodeficiency syndromes, including chronic granulomatous disease (CGD; Chapter 124) have also been implicated. Numerous medications, environmental exposures, chemicals, and food allergens have been reported as potential causes.

Trends in disease classification are based on the finding of pulmonary capillaritis. The pathologic appearance of pulmonary capillaritis includes inflammation and cellular disruption of the pulmonary interstitial capillary network. This finding is nonspecific with regard to underlying diagnosis, but pulmonary capillaritis, when present, appears to be an important negative prognostic factor in DAH. Newer classification protocols divide the variable causes of DAH into 3 categories. Disorders with pulmonary capillaritis (including SLE, HSP, drug-induced capillaritis, Wegener granulomatosis, and Goodpasture syndrome) are distinguished from those without pulmonary capillaritis. Those disorders in which the pathologic finding of capillary network disruption is absent are further divided into cardiac (pulmonary hypertension, mitral stenosis) and noncardiac (immunodeficiency, Heiner syndrome, coagulopathy, IPH) etiologies.

Table 400-1 CLASSIFICATION OF DIFFUSE ALVEOLAR HEMORRHAGE SYNDROMES

CLASSIFICATION	SYNDROME
Disorders with pulmonary capillaritis	Idiopathic pulmonary capillaritis Wegener granulomatosis Microscopic polyangiitis Systemic lupus erythematosus Goodpasture syndrome Antiphospholipid antibody syndrome Henoch-Schönlein purpura Immunoglobulin A nephropathy Polyarteritis nodosa Behçet syndrome Cryoglobulinemia Drug-induced capillaritis Idiopathic pulmonary-renal syndrome
Disorders without pulmonary capillaritis:	
Noncardiovascular causes	Idiopathic pulmonary hemosiderosis Heiner syndrome Acute idiopathic pulmonary hemorrhage of infancy Bone marrow transplantation Immunodeficiency Coagulation disorders Celiac disease Infanticide (child abuse)
Cardiovascular causes	Mitral stenosis Pulmonary veno-occlusive disease Arteriovenous malformations Pulmonary lymphangioleiomyomatosis Pulmonary hypertension Pulmonary capillary hemangiomatosis Chronic heart failure Vascular thrombosis with infarction

From Susarla SC, Fan LL: Diffuse alveolar hemorrhage syndromes in children, *Curr Opin Pediatr* 19:314–320, 2007.

EPIDEMIOLOGY

Because of the variety of disorders that can manifest with alveolar hemorrhage as a component, the frequency with which DAH occurs is difficult to quantify. Similarly, the prevalence of IPH is largely unknown. In fact, in many children and young adults who were diagnosed with IPH in the past, the etiology of the hemorrhage might have been discovered if they had been studied with the newer and more advanced diagnostics available today. Estimates of prevalence obtained from Swedish and Japanese retrospective case analyses vary from 0.24 to 1.23 cases per million. In general, the manifestations of IPH are seen before age 10 yr. Nearly 80% of cases occur in this age group. The remaining 20% of cases, which occur in adult patients, are typically diagnosed before age 30 yr. The ratio of affected males to females is 1 : 1 in the childhood diagnosis group, and men are only slightly more affected in the group diagnosed as adults.

PATHOLOGY

With repeated episodes of pulmonary hemorrhage, lung tissue appears brown secondary to the presence of **hemosiderin.** The finding of blood in the airways or alveoli is representative of a recent hemorrhage. Hemosiderin-laden macrophages (HLMs) are seen with recovering, recurrent, or chronic pulmonary hemorrhage. It takes 48-72 hr for the alveolar macrophages to convert iron from erythrocytes into hemosiderin. HLMs may be detectable for weeks after a hemorrhagic event. Other nonspecific pathologic findings include thickening of alveolar septa and hypertrophy of type II pneumocytes. Fibrosis may be seen with chronic disease (Chapter 408).

PATHOPHYSIOLOGY

In Goodpasture syndrome, anti–basement membrane antibody (ABMA) binds to the basement membrane of both the alveolus and the glomerulus. At the alveolar level, immunoglobulin G (IgG), IgM, and complement are deposited at alveolar septa. Electron microscopy shows disruption of basement membranes and vascular integrity, which allows blood to escape into alveolar spaces.

Pulmonary hemosiderosis in association with **cow's milk hypersensitivity** was first reported by Heiner in 1962. This condition is characterized by variable symptoms of milk intolerance. Symptoms can include grossly bloody or heme-positive stools, vomiting, failure to thrive, symptoms of gastroesophageal reflux, and/or upper airway congestion. Pathologic findings have included elevations of IgE and peripheral eosinophilia as well as alveolar deposits of IgG, IgA, and C3. High titers to cow's milk protein are also typically found in cow's milk hypersensitivity.

Alveolar hemorrhage, seen rarely in association with **SLE,** is often severe and potentially life-threatening. Pathologic vasculitic features may be absent. Some immunofluorescent studies have revealed IgG and C3 deposits at the alveolar septa. A clear link between immune complex formation and alveolar hemorrhage has not been established, however.

In **HSP,** pulmonary hemorrhage is a rare but recognized complication. Pathologic findings have included transmural neutrophilic infiltration of small vessels, alveolar septal inflammation, and intra-alveolar hemorrhage. Vasculitis is the proposed mechanism for hemorrhage.

Wegener granulomatosis is a rare etiology for hemorrhage in children. Pulmonary granuloma formation (with or without cavitation) and a necrotizing vasculitis may be appreciated. In children, presentations attributable to the upper airway, including subglottic stenosis, may suggest the diagnosis. Results of testing for antineutrophil cytoplasmic antibody (ANCA) are generally positive.

A premature infant's neonatal course can frequently be complicated by pulmonary hemorrhage. The alveolar and vascular networks are immature and particularly prone to inflammation and damage by ventilator mechanics, oxidative stress, and infection. Pulmonary hemorrhage may be unrecognized if the volume of blood is insufficient to reach the proximal airways. The chest radiographic findings in pulmonary hemorrhage may be appreciated instead as a worsening picture of respiratory distress syndrome, edema, or infection.

A number of additional associated conditions and exposures exist, as outlined previously. These occur infrequently in the pediatric population, and suggested mechanisms for hemorrhage are variable. The diagnosis of IPH is made when there is evidence of chronic or recurrent diffuse alveolar hemorrhage and when exhaustive evaluations for primary or secondary etiologies have negative results. A biopsy specimen should not reveal any evidence of granulomatous disease, vasculitis, infection, infarction, immune complex deposition, malignancy, or any other features of associated primary or secondary conditions.

CLINICAL MANIFESTATIONS

The clinical presentation of pulmonary hemosiderosis is highly variable. Symptoms may be reflective of an underlying and associated disease process rather than specifically related to pulmonary hemorrhage. Presentations can vary widely from a relative lack of symptoms to shock or sudden death. Hemorrhage may be significant without remarkable symptomatology. Hemoptysis may not occur. Bleeding may occasionally be recognized from the presence of alveolar infiltrates on a chest radiograph. It should be noted that the absence of an infiltrate does not rule out an ongoing hemorrhagic process.

Because the presence of blood in the lung is typically a source of significant irritation and inflammation, the patient may present after an episode of hemorrhage with wheezing, cough, dyspnea, and alterations in gas exchange, reflecting bronchospasm, edema, mucus plugging, and inflammation. On physical examination, the patient may be pale with tachycardia and tachypnea. During an acute exacerbation, children are frequently febrile. Examination of the chest may reveal retractions and differential or decreased aeration, with crackles or wheezes. The patient may present in shock with respiratory failure from massive hemoptysis. Children in particular may present with symptoms of chronic anemia, such as failure to thrive.

LABORATORY FINDINGS AND DIAGNOSIS

Pulmonary hemorrhage is associated with a decrease in hemoglobin and hematocrit. The classic finding is a microcytic, hypochromic anemia. The reticulocyte count is elevated. The anemia of IPH can mimic a hemolytic anemia. Elevations of plasma bilirubin are caused by absorption and breakdown of hemoglobin in the alveoli. The serum iron level is reduced. Iron-binding capacity is generally elevated. Any or all hematologic manifestations may be absent in the presence of recent hemorrhage.

White blood cell count and differential should be evaluated for evidence of infection and eosinophilia. A stool specimen can be heme-positive secondary to swallowed blood. Renal and liver functions should be reviewed. A urinalysis should be obtained to assess for evidence of nephritis. A coagulation profile, quantitative immunoglobulins (including IgE), and complement studies are recommended.

Testing for ANCA, antinuclear antibody (ANA), anti–double stranded DNA, rheumatoid factor, antiphospholipid antibody, and anti–glomerular basement membrane antibody (antiGBM) evaluates for a number of primary and secondary etiologies of DAH. An elevated erythrocyte sedimentation rate (ESR) is a nonspecific finding.

Sputum or pulmonary secretions should be analyzed for significant evidence of blood or HLMs. Gastric secretions may also reveal HLMs. Flexible bronchoscopy provides visualization of any areas of active bleeding. With bronchoalveolar lavage, pulmonary secretions may be sent for pathologic review and culture analysis. The ability to perform flexible bronchoscopy will be limited if there are large amounts of blood or clots in the airway. A patient with respiratory failure can be ventilated more effectively through a rigid bronchoscope.

Lung biopsy is warranted when DAH occurs without discernible etiology, extrapulmonary disease, or circulating ABMAs. Pulmonary tissue when obtained should be evaluated for evidence of vasculitis, immune complex deposition, and granulomatous disease.

A chest radiograph may reveal evidence of acute or chronic disease. Hyperaeration is frequently seen, especially during an acute hemorrhage. Infiltrates are typically symmetric and may spare the apices of the lung. Atelectasis may also be appreciated. With chronic disease, fibrosis, lymphadenopathy and nodularity may be seen. CT findings may demonstrate a subclinical and contributory disease process.

Pulmonary function testing will likely reveal primarily obstructive disease in the acute period. With more chronic disease, fibrosis and restrictive disease tend to predominate. Oxygen saturation levels may be decreased. Lung volumes may reveal air trapping acutely and decreases in total lung capacity chronically. The diffusing capacity of carbon monoxide (DLCO) may be low or normal in the chronic phase but is likely to be elevated in the setting of an acute hemorrhage, because carbon monoxide binds to the hemoglobin in extravasated red blood cells.

TREATMENT

Supportive therapy, including volume resuscitation, ventilatory support, supplemental oxygen, and transfusion of blood products, may be warranted in the patient with pulmonary hemosiderosis. Surgical or medical therapy should be directed at any treatable underlying condition. In IPH, early treatment with systemic corticosteroids is the treatment of choice. Therapy is generally initiated at 2-5 mg/kg/day and decreased to 1 mg/kg every other day after resolution of acute symptoms. Early treatment with corticosteroids appears to decrease episodes of hemorrhage. This therapy may also modulate the neutrophil influx and inflammation associated with hemorrhage, thereby decreasing progression toward fibrotic disease.

The goal of gradually tapering the systemic steroid dose may not be tolerated. In addition, a subgroup of patients may not respond optimally to corticosteroid therapy alone. In these cases, immunosuppressive agents such as cyclophosphamide, azathioprine, and chloroquine have been utilized. The indications for and effectiveness of long-term immunosuppressive therapies is unclear. The numerous potential long-term side effects of corticosteroids and other immunosuppressive agents may limit therapy.

In chronic disease, progression to debilitating pulmonary fibrosis has been described. Lung transplantation has been performed in patients with IPH refractory to immunosuppressive therapy. In one reported case study, IPH recurred in the transplanted lung.

PROGNOSIS

The outcome of patients suffering from DAH is highly dependent on the underlying disease process. Some conditions, such as cow's milk hypersensitivity, respond well to removal of the offending agent. Other syndromes, especially those with an immunologic mechanism, tend to carry a poor prognosis. In IPH, mortality is often related to massive hemorrhage or, alternatively, to progressive fibrosis, respiratory insufficiency, and right-sided heart failure.

Long-term prognosis in patients with IPH varies among studies. Initial case study reviews suggested an average survival after symptom onset of only 2.5 yr. In this early review, a minority of patients were treated with steroids. A later review reported a 5-yr survival rate of 86%. Whether this improvement in survival is related to primarily overall advances in care or long-term immunosuppressive therapy is not established at this time. Spontaneous remissions have been documented.

BIBLIOGRAPHY

Please visit the Nelson Textbook of Pediatrics *website at www.expertconsult.com for the complete bibliography.*

Chapter 401
Pulmonary Embolism, Infarction, and Hemorrhage

401.1 Pulmonary Embolus and Infarction

Mary A. Nevin

Venous thromboembolic disease (VTE) is well described in children and adolescents with or without risk factors (Table 401-1). Improvements in therapeutics for childhood illnesses and increased survival with chronic illness may contribute to the larger number of children presenting with thromboembolic events, which can be a significant source of morbidity and mortality.

ETIOLOGY

Commonly appreciated risk factors for thromboembolic disease in adults include immobility, malignancy, pregnancy, infection, and hypercoagulability; up to 20% of adults with this disorder may have no identifiable risk factor (see Table 401-1). Children with deep venous thrombosis (DVT) and pulmonary embolism (PE) are much more likely to have 1 or more identifiable conditions or circumstances placing them at risk. In a large Canadian registry, 96% of pediatric patients were found to have 1 risk factor and 90% had 2 or more risk factors.

Embolic disease has variable etiologies in children. An embolus can contain thrombus, air, amniotic fluid, septic material, or metastatic neoplastic tissue; thromboemboli are most commonly encountered. A commonly encountered risk factor for DVT and PE in the pediatric population is the presence of a central venous catheter. The presence of a catheter in a vessel lumen as well as instilled medications can induce endothelial damage and favor thrombus formation.

Children with malignancies are also at considerable risk. The risk of PE is more significant in children with solid rather than hematologic malignancies. PE has been described in children with Wilms tumor (tumor embolism) as well as leukemia. A child with malignancy may have numerous risk factors related to the primary disease process and the therapeutic interventions. Infection from chronic immunosuppression may interact with hypercoagulability of malignancy and chemotherapeutic effects on the endothelium.

In the neonatal period, thromboembolic disease and PE are often related to indwelling catheters used for parenteral nutrition and medication delivery. Emboli in neonates may occasionally reflect maternal risk factors, such as diabetes and toxemia of pregnancy. Infants with congenitally acquired homozygous deficiencies of antithrombin, protein C, and protein S are also

Table 401-1 RISK FACTORS FOR PULMONARY EMBOLISM

ENVIRONMENTAL
Long-haul air travel Obesity Cigarette smoking Hypertension Immobility
WOMEN'S HEALTH
Oral contraceptives, including progesterone-only and, especially, third-generation pills Pregnancy Hormone replacement therapy Septic abortion
MEDICAL ILLNESS
Previous pulmonary embolism or deep venous thrombosis Cancer Congestive heart failure Chronic obstructive pulmonary disease Diabetes mellitus Inflammatory bowel disease Antipsychotic drug use Long-term indwelling central venous catheter Permanent pacemaker Internal cardiac defibrillator Stroke with limb paresis Spinal cord injury Nursing home confinement or current or repeated hospital admission
SURGICAL
Trauma Orthopedic surgery General surgery Neurosurgery, especially craniotomy for brain tumor
THROMBOPHILIA
Factor V Leiden mutation Prothrombin gene mutation Hyperhomocysteinanemia (including mutation in methylenetetrahydrofolate reductase) Antiphospholipid antibody syndrome Deficiency of antithrombin III, protein C, or protein S High concentrations of factor VIII or XI Increased lipoprotein (a)
NONTHROMBOTIC
Air Foreign particles (e.g., hair, talc, as a consequence of intravenous drug misuse) Amniotic fluid Bone fragments, bone marrow Fat Tumors (Wilms tumor)

Modified from Goldhaber SZ: Pulmonary embolism, *Lancet* 363:1295–1305, 2004.

Table 401-2 THROMBOEMBOLIC DISEASE IN CHILDREN: 1979-2001

DISEASE	AGE GROUP (YR)	RATE OF DIAGNOSIS/100,000 CHILDREN/YR		
		All	Boys	Girls
Pulmonary embolism	0-1	2.2*	—‡	—
	2-14	0.4	—	—
	15-17	2.0*	—	—
	All	0.9	—	—
Deep venous thrombosis	0-1	8.7†	9.3	8.0
	2-14	2.1	2.0	2.2
	15-17	9.9†	6.5	13.5
	All	4.2	3.6	4.8
Venous thrombolic disease	0-1	10.5†	11.3	9.7
	2-14	2.4	2.3	2.6
	15-17	11.4†	8.1	14.9
	All	4.9	4.3	5.5

*$P < .05$ age 0-1 vs age 2-14, and age 15-17 vs age 2-14.
†$P < .001$ age 0-1 vs age 2-14, and age 15-17 vs age 2-14.
‡Insufficient data for interpretation according to age and sex.
From Stein P, Kayali F, Olson R: Incidence of venous thromboembolism in infants and children: data from the National Hospital Discharge Survey, *J Pediatr* 145:563–565, 2004.

likely to present with thromboembolic disease in the neonatal period.

Prothrombotic disease can also manifest in older infants and children. Disease can be congenital or acquired; DVT/PE may be the initial presentation. *Factor V Leiden mutation* (Chapter 472), *hyperhomocysteinemia* (Chapter 79.3), *prothrombin 20210A mutation* (Chapter 472), *anticardiolipin antibody,* and elevated values of *lipoprotein A* have all been linked to thromboembolic disease. Children with sickle cell disease are also at high risk for pulmonary embolus and infarction. Acquired prothrombotic disease is represented by *nephrotic syndrome* (Chapter 521) and *antiphospholipid antibody syndrome.* From one quarter to one half of children with *systemic lupus erythematosus* (Chapter 152) have thromboembolic disease.

Other risk factors include infection, cardiac disease, recent surgery, and trauma. Surgical risk is thought to be more significant when immobility will be a prominent feature of the recovery. Use of oral contraceptives confers additional risk, although the level of risk in patients taking these medications appears to be decreasing, perhaps as a result of the lower amounts of estrogen in current formulations.

Septic emboli are rare in children but may be caused by osteomyelitis, cellulitis, urinary tract infection, jugular vein or umbilical thrombophlebitis, and right-sided endocarditis.

EPIDEMIOLOGY

Younger age appears to be somewhat protective in thromboembolic disease. The DVT incidence in 1 study of hospitalized children was 5.3/10,000 admissions. A study that analyzed data from 1979 through 2001 found 0.9 cases of PE per 100,000 children per yr, 4.2 cases of DVT per 100,000 children per yr, and 4.9 cases of VTE per 100,000 children per yr (Table 401-2).

Pediatric autopsy reviews have estimated the incidence of thromboembolic disease in children as between 1% and 4%. Not all of these embolic findings were clinically significant. Thromboembolic pulmonary disease is often unrecognized, and antemortem studies may underestimate the true incidence. Pediatric deaths from isolated pulmonary emboli are rare. Most thromboemboli are related to central venous catheters. The source of the emboli may be lower or upper extremity veins as well as the pelvis and right heart. The most common location for an embolus unassociated with the presence of an indwelling venous catheter is the lower extremity.

PATHOPHYSIOLOGY

Favorable conditions for thrombus formation include injury to the vessel endothelium, hemostasis, and hypercoagulability. Once an embolus develops and travels to the pulmonary circulation, symptoms of presentation are largely attributable to unequal ventilation and perfusion. The occlusion of the involved vessel prevents perfusion of distal alveolar units, thereby creating an increase in dead space and hypoxia with an elevated alveolar-arterial oxygen tension difference, or a-Ao_2 (PAo_2 - Pao_2). Most patients are hypocarbic secondary to hyperventilation, which often persists even when oxygenation is optimized. Abnormalities of oxygenation and ventilation are likely to be less significant in the pediatric population, possibly owing to less underlying cardiopulmonary disease and greater reserve. The vascular supply to lung tissue is abundant, and pulmonary infarction is unusual with pulmonary embolus but may result from distal arterial occlusion and alveolar hemorrhage. In rare instances of death from massive pulmonary embolus, marked increases in pulmonary vascular resistance and heart failure are usually present. Most of these severe outcomes are expectedly found in those with pre-existing cardiopulmonary disease.

CLINICAL MANIFESTATIONS

Presentation is variable, and many pulmonary emboli are silent. Rarely, a massive PE may manifest as cardiopulmonary failure. Children are more likely to have underlying disease processes or risk factors but might still present asymptomatically with small emboli. Common symptoms and signs of PE include hypoxia (cyanosis), tachypnea, dyspnea, cough, diaphoresis, and chest pain. Localized crackles may occasionally be appreciated on examination. These are nonspecific complaints and may be attributed to an underlying disease process or an unrelated/incorrect diagnosis in many cases. A high level of clinical suspicion is required because the diagnosis of pulmonary embolus is infrequently considered in children. A large number of diagnoses can cause similar symptoms. Therefore, confirmatory testing should follow a clinical diagnosis of PE. In addition, clinical risk scoring systems may help raise the likelihood of a PE. High-risk findings include surgery or lower extremity fractures, malignancy, hemoptysis, lower extremity signs of a DVT (pain, swelling), tachycardia, and hypoxia.

LABORATORY FINDINGS AND DIAGNOSIS

Radiographic images of the chest are often normal in a child with PE. Any abnormalities found on chest radiographs are likely to be nonspecific. Patients with septic emboli may have multiple areas of nodularity and cavitation, which are typically located peripherally in both lung fields. Many patients with PE have hypoxemia. The a-Ao_2 gradient is more sensitive in detecting gas exchange derangements. A review of results of a complete blood count (CBC), urinalysis, and coagulation profile is warranted. Prothrombotic diseases should be highly suspected on the basis of past medical or family history; therefore, additional laboratory evaluations include fibrinogen assays, protein C, protein S, and antithrombin III studies, and analysis for factor V Leiden mutation as well as evaluation for lupus anticoagulant and anticardiolipin antibodies.

Electrocardiographs may reveal ST segment changes or evidence of pulmonary hypertension with right ventricular failure (cor pulmonale). These changes are nonspecific and nondiagnostic. Echocardiograms may be warranted to assess ventricular size and function. A transAmerican Thoracic Society/European Respiratory Society International Multidisciplinary Consensus echocardiogram is required if there is any suspicion of intracardiac thrombi or endocarditis.

Noninvasive venous ultrasound testing with Doppler flow can be used to confirm DVT in the lower extremities; ultrasonography may not detect thrombi in the upper extremities or pelvis. In patients with significant venous thrombosis, D dimers are usually elevated. When a high level of suspicion exists, confirmatory testing with venography should be pursued. DVT can be recurrent and multifocal and may lead to repeated episodes of pulmonary embolism.

Although a ventilation-perfusion ($\dot{V}$-$\dot{Q}$) radionuclide scan is a noninvasive and potentially sensitive method of pulmonary embolus detection, the interpretation of $\dot{V}$-$\dot{Q}$ scans can be problematic. Helical or spiral CT with an intravenous contrast agent is valuable and the diagnostic test of choice to detect a PE. Specificity exceeds 90%. CT studies detect emboli in lobar and segmental vessels with acceptable sensitivities. Poorer sensitivities may be encountered in the evaluation of the subsegmental pulmonary vasculature. Pulmonary angiography is the gold standard for diagnosis of PE, but with current availability of multidetector spiral CT angiography, it is not necessary except in unusual cases.

TREATMENT

Initial treatment should always be directed toward stabilization of the patient. Careful approaches to ventilation, fluid resuscitation, and inotropic support are always indicated, because improvement in one area of decompensation can often exacerbate coexisting pathology.

After the patient with a PE has been stabilized, the next therapeutic step is anticoagulation. Evaluations for prothrombotic disease must precede anticoagulation. Treatment is generally initiated with heparin. Anticoagulation is usually achieved when the activated partial thromboplastin time (PTT) is 1.5-2 times the control. Long-term therapy with heparin should be avoided whenever possible. Complications of heparin include bleeding and acquired thrombocytopenia.

Heparin therapy continues for several days before oral therapy with warfarin is begun. Anticoagulation may be required for 3-6 mo in the setting of acute thromboembolic disease. Longer treatment is indicated in patients with ongoing thrombotic disease. Coagulation profiles are obtained regularly to guide warfarin and heparin therapies.

In adults, therapy with low molecular weight (LMW) heparin is considered equivalent to that with heparin. The longer half-life of LMW heparin allows discontinuous dosing, and effectiveness appears comparable. Minimal monitoring is involved with drug administration. Other advantages may include decreased risks of both osteoporosis and thrombocytopenia. At this time, LMW heparin is being used in many pediatric patients. Studies of LMW heparin use in children and neonates have suggested similarities to its use in adults in terms of success of thrombolysis, rate of recurrence, and complications.

Thrombolytic agents can be combined with anticoagulants in the early stages of treatment. Thrombolytic agents include urokinase, streptokinase, and, most often, recombinant tissue plasminogen activator. Combined therapy may reduce the incidences of progressive thromboembolism, pulmonary embolus, and postphlebitic syndrome. Mortality rate appears to be unaffected by additional therapies; nonetheless, the additional theoretic risk of hemorrhage limits the use of combination therapy in all but the most compromised patients. The use of thrombolytic agents in patients with active bleeding, recent cerebrovascular accidents, or trauma is contraindicated.

Surgical embolectomy is invasive and is associated with significant mortality. Its application should be limited to those with persistent hemodynamic compromise refractory to standard therapy.

PROGNOSIS

Mortality in pediatric patients with PE is likely to be attributable to an underlying disease process rather than to the embolus itself. Conditions associated with a poorer prognosis include malignancy, infection, and cardiac disease. The mortality rate in children from PE is 2.2%. Recurrent thromboembolic disease may complicate recovery. The practitioner must conduct an extensive evaluation for underlying pathology so as to prevent progressive disease. Postphlebitic syndrome is another recognized complication of pediatric thrombotic disease. Venous valvular damage can be initiated by the presence of DVT, leading to persistent venous hypertension with ambulation and valvular reflux. Symptoms include edema, pain, increases in pigmentation, and ulcerations. Affected pediatric patients may suffer lifelong disability.

BIBLIOGRAPHY

Please visit the Nelson Textbook of Pediatrics *website at www.expertconsult.com for the complete bibliography.*

401.2 Pulmonary Hemorrhage and Hemoptysis

Mary A. Nevin

Pulmonary hemorrhage is relatively uncommon but potentially fatal in children. Diffuse, slow bleeding in the lower airways may become severe and manifest as anemia, fatigue, or respiratory compromise without the patient ever experiencing episodes of hemoptysis. Hemoptysis must always be separated from episodes of hematemesis or epistaxis, all of which have similar presentations in the young patient.

ETIOLOGY

Conditions that can manifest as pulmonary hemorrhage or hemoptysis in children are found in Table 401-3. The chronic (opposed to an acute) presence of a foreign body can lead to inflammation and/or infection, thereby inducing hemorrhage. Hemorrhage most commonly reflects chronic inflammation and infection such as that seen in cystic fibrosis with bronchiectasis or in tuberculosis with cavitary disease, although it may also reflect an acute condition such as bronchitis and bronchopneumonia. Other relatively common etiologies are congenital heart disease and trauma. Traumatic irritation or damage of the airway is often accidental in nature. Bleeding can also be related to instrumentation of the airway as is commonly seen in a child with a tracheostomy. It is important to note, however, that children who have been victims of nonaccidental trauma or deliberate suffocation can also be found to have blood in the mouth or airway. Less commonly, syndromes associated with vasculitic, autoimmune, and idiopathic disorders can be associated with diffuse alveolar hemorrhage (DAH). The mechanisms of DAH are multiple and are discussed further in Chapter 400.

Table 401-3 ETIOLOGY OF PULMONARY HEMORRHAGE (HEMOPTYSIS)

FOCAL HEMORRHAGE
Bronchitis and bronchiectasis (especially cystic fibrosis–related)
Infection (acute or chronic), pneumonia, abscess
Tuberculosis
Trauma
Pulmonary arteriovenous malformation
Foreign body (chronic)
Neoplasm including hemangioma
Pulmonary embolus with or without infarction
Bronchogenic cysts
DIFFUSE HEMORRHAGE
Idiopathic of infancy
Congenital heart disease (including pulmonary hypertension, veno-occlusive disease, congestive heart failure)
Prematurity
Cow's milk hyperreactivity (Heiner syndrome)
Goodpasture syndrome
Collagen vascular diseases (systemic lupus erythematosus, rheumatoid arthritis)
Henoch-Schönlein purpura and vasculitic disorders
Granulomatous disease (Wegener granulomatosis)
Celiac disease
Coagulopathy (congenital or acquired)
Malignancy
Immunodeficiency
Exogenous toxins
Hyperammonemia
Pulmonary hypertension
Pulmonary alveolar proteinosis
Idiopathic pulmonary hemosiderosis
Tuberous sclerosis
Lymphangiomyomatosis or lymphangioleiomyomatosis
Physical injury or abuse

Acute idiopathic pulmonary hemorrhage (AIPH) occurs in young infants as a distinct entity, but the disorders in Table 401-3 must also be considered.

EPIDEMIOLOGY

The frequency with which pulmonary hemorrhage occurs in the pediatric population is difficult to define. This difficulty is largely related to the variability in disease presentation. Chronic bronchiectasis as seen in cystic fibrosis or ciliary dyskinesia can cause hemoptysis but usually in children >10 yr of age. The incidence of pulmonary hemorrhage may be significantly underestimated because many children and young adults swallow rather than expectorate mucus, a behavior that may prevent recognition of hemoptysis, the primary presenting symptom of the disorder.

AIPH is defined as evidence of blood in the airway in a child age ≤1 yr, with no medical conditions predisposing to pulmonary hemorrhage and severe respiratory distress leading to respiratory failure. This entity may be more common than previously thought. Most cases are idiopathic, but some have been associated with von Willebrand disease. There is no association between the disorder and house contamination with molds.

PATHOPHYSIOLOGY

Pulmonary hemorrhage can be localized or diffuse. Focal hemorrhage from an isolated bronchial lesion is often secondary to infection or chronic inflammation. Erosion through a chronically inflamed airway into the adjacent bronchial artery is a mechanism for potentially massive hemorrhage. Bleeding from such a lesion is more likely to be bright red, brisk, and secondary to enlarged bronchial arteries and systemic arterial pressures. The severity of more diffuse hemorrhage can be difficult to ascertain. The rate of blood loss may be insufficient to reach the proximal airways. Therefore, the patient may present without hemoptysis. The diagnosis of pulmonary hemorrhage is generally achieved by finding evidence of blood or hemosiderin in the lung. Within 48-72 hr of an episode of bleeding, alveolar macrophages convert the iron from erythrocytes into hemosiderin. It may take weeks to clear these hemosiderin-laden macrophages completely from the alveolar spaces. This fact may allow differentiation between acute and chronic hemorrhage. Hemorrhage is often followed by the influx of neutrophils and other proinflammatory mediators. With repeated or chronic hemorrhage, pulmonary fibrosis can become a prominent pathologic finding.

CLINICAL MANIFESTATIONS

The severity of presentation in patients with hemoptysis and pulmonary hemorrhage is highly variable. Older children and young adults with a focal hemorrhage may complain of warmth or a "bubbling" sensation in the chest wall. This can occasionally aid the clinician in locating the area involved. Rapid and large-volume blood loss manifests as symptoms of cyanosis, respiratory distress, and shock. Chronic, subclinical blood loss may manifest as anemia, fatigue, dyspnea, or altered activity tolerance. Less commonly, patients present with persistent infiltrates on chest radiograph or symptoms of chronic illness such as failure to thrive.

LABORATORY FINDINGS AND DIAGNOSIS

Every patient with suspected hemorrhage should have a laboratory evaluation with CBC and coagulation studies. The CBC result may demonstrate a microcytic, hypochromic anemia. Other laboratory findings are highly dependent on the underlying diagnosis. A urinalysis may show evidence of nephritis in patients with concomitant pulmonary and renal diseases. The classic finding, which defines pulmonary hemorrhage, is that of hemosiderin-laden macrophages in pulmonary secretions. These can be detected by sputum analysis with Prussian blue staining. Chest radiographs may demonstrate fluffy bilateral densities, as seen in AIPH of infancy (Fig. 401-1) or the patchy consolidation seen in idiopathic pulmonary hemosiderosis (Fig. 401-2). Alveolar infiltrates seen on chest radiograph may be regarded as a representation of recent bleeding, but their absence does not rule out a hemorrhage. Infiltrates, when present, are often symmetric and diffuse. CT may be indicated to assess for underlying disease processes.

Flexible bronchoscopy with bronchoalveolar lavage is frequently utilized to obtain pulmonary secretions in a child or young adult who is not able to expectorate secretions. Lung biopsy is rarely necessary unless bleeding is chronic or an etiology cannot be determined with other methods. Pulmonary function testing, including a determination of gas exchange, is important to assess the severity of the ventilatory defect. In older children, spirometry may demonstrate evidence of predominantly obstructive disease in the acute period. Restrictive disease secondary to fibrosis is typically seen with more chronic disease. DLCO measurements are typically elevated in the setting of pulmonary hemorrhage because of the strong affinity of hemoglobin for carbon monoxide.

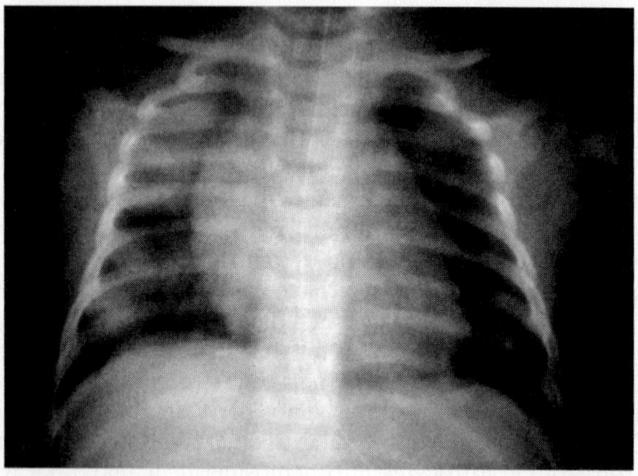

Figure 401-1 Radiographic appearance of acute idiopathic pulmonary hemorrhage in infancy. (From Brown CM, Redd SC, Damon SA; Centers for Disease Control and Prevention [CDC]: Acute idiopathic pulmonary hemorrhage among infants: recommendations from the Working Group for Investigation and Surveillance, *MMWR Recomm Rep* 53:1–12, 2004.)

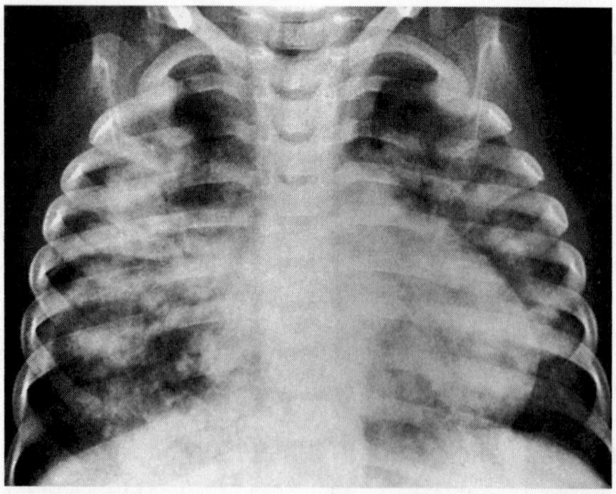

Figure 401-2 Diffuse pulmonary hemorrhage that was thought to be the result of idiopathic pulmonary hemosiderosis in a 3 yr old boy. Frontal radiograph reveals bilateral airspace consolidation that is patchy. Tracheal washing contained large numbers of macrophages filled with hemosiderin. Ten days later, most of the consolidative changes in the lungs had cleared. The patient's anemia was successfully treated with blood transfusion. (From Slovis T, editor: *Caffey's pediatric diagnostic imaging,* ed 11, Philadelphia, 2008, Mosby/Elsevier; courtesy of Bertram Girdany, MD, Pittsburgh, PA.)

TREATMENT

In the setting of massive blood loss, volume resuscitation and transfusion of blood products are necessary. Maintenance of adequate ventilation and circulatory function is crucial. Rigid bronchoscopy may be utilized for removal of debris or the application of topical vasoconstrictive agents. Ideally, treatment is directed at the specific pathologic process responsible for the hemorrhage. When bronchiectasis is a known entity and a damaged artery can be localized, bronchial artery embolization is often the therapy of choice. If embolization fails, total or partial lobectomy may be required. In circumstances of diffuse hemorrhage, corticosteroids and other immunosuppressive agents have been shown to be of benefit. Prognosis depends largely on the underlying disease process.

BIBLIOGRAPHY

Please visit the Nelson Textbook of Pediatrics *website at www.expertconsult.com for the complete bibliography.*

Chapter 402
Atelectasis
Ranna A. Rozenfeld

Atelectasis, the incomplete expansion or complete collapse of air-bearing tissue, results from obstruction of air intake into the alveolar sacs. Segmental, lobar, or whole lung collapse is associated with the absorption of air contained in the alveoli, which are no longer ventilated.

For the full continuation of this chapter, please visit the Nelson Textbook of Pediatrics *website at www.expertconsult.com.*

Chapter 403
Pulmonary Tumors
Susanna A. McColley

ETIOLOGY

Primary tumors of the lung are rare in children and adolescents. An accurate estimate of frequency is difficult because the literature is limited primarily to case reports and case series. A high incidence of "inflammatory pseudotumors" further clouds the statistics. **Bronchial adenomas (including bronchial carcinoid, adenoid cystic carcinoma** and **mucoepidermoid carcinomas**) are the most common primary tumors; bronchial carcinoid tumors represent ≈ 80%. Carcinoids are low-grade malignancies; carcinoid syndrome is rare in children. Metastatic lesions are the most common forms of pulmonary malignancy in children; primary processes include Wilms tumor, osteogenic sarcoma, and hepatoblastoma (Part XXII). Adenocarcinoma and undifferentiated histology are the most common pathologic findings in primary lung cancer; pulmonary blastoma is rarer and frequently occurs in the setting of cystic lung disease. Mediastinal involvement with lymphoma is more common than primary pulmonary malignancies.

For the full continuation of this chapter, please visit the Nelson Textbook of Pediatrics *website at www.expertconsult.com.*

Chapter 404
Pleurisy, Pleural Effusions, and Empyema

Glenna B. Winnie and Steven V. Lossef

Pleurisy or inflammation of the pleura is often accompanied by an effusion. The most common cause of pleural effusion in children is bacterial pneumonia (Chapter 392); heart failure (Chapter 436), rheumatologic causes, and metastatic intrathoracic malignancy are the next most common causes. A variety of other diseases account for the remaining cases, including tuberculosis (Chapter 207), lupus erythematosus (Chapter 152), aspiration pneumonitis (Chapter 389), uremia, pancreatitis, subdiaphragmatic abscess, and rheumatoid arthritis. Males and females are affected equally.

Inflammatory processes in the pleura are usually divided into 3 types: dry or plastic, serofibrinous or serosanguineous, and purulent pleurisy or empyema.

404.1 Dry or Plastic Pleurisy (Pleural Effusion)

Glenna B. Winnie and Steven V. Lossef

ETIOLOGY

Plastic pleurisy may be associated with acute bacterial or viral pulmonary infections or may develop during the course of an acute upper respiratory tract illness. The condition is also associated with tuberculosis and connective tissue diseases such as rheumatic fever.

PATHOLOGY AND PATHOGENESIS

The process is usually limited to the visceral pleura, with small amounts of yellow serous fluid and adhesions between the pleural surfaces. In tuberculosis, the adhesions develop rapidly and the pleura are often thickened. Occasionally, fibrin deposition and adhesions are severe enough to produce a fibrothorax that markedly inhibits the excursions of the lung.

CLINICAL MANIFESTATIONS

The primary disease often overshadows signs and symptoms. Pain, the principal symptom, is exaggerated by deep breathing, coughing, and straining. Occasionally, pleural pain is described as a dull ache, which is less likely to vary with breathing. The pain is often localized over the chest wall and is referred to the shoulder or the back. Pain with breathing is responsible for grunting and guarding of respirations, and the child often lies on the affected side in an attempt to decrease respiratory excursions. Early in the illness, a leathery, rough, inspiratory and expiratory friction rub may be audible, but it usually disappears rapidly. If the layer of exudate is thick, increased dullness to percussion and decreased breath sounds may be heard. Pleurisy may be asymptomatic. Chronic pleurisy is occasionally encountered with conditions such as atelectasis, pulmonary abscess, connective tissue diseases, and tuberculosis.

LABORATORY FINDINGS

Plastic pleurisy may be detected on radiographs as a diffuse haziness at the pleural surface or a dense, sharply demarcated shadow (Figs. 404-1 and 404-2). The latter finding may be indistinguishable from small amounts of pleural exudate. Chest radiographic findings may be normal, but ultrasonography or CT findings will be positive.

DIFFERENTIAL DIAGNOSIS

Plastic pleurisy must be distinguished from other diseases, such as epidemic pleurodynia, trauma to the rib cage (rib fracture), lesions of the dorsal root ganglia, tumors of the spinal cord, herpes zoster, gallbladder disease, and trichinosis. Even if evidence of pleural fluid is not found on physical or radiographic examination, a CT- or ultrasound-guided pleural tap in suspected cases often results in the recovery of a small amount of exudate, which when cultured may reveal the underlying bacterial cause in patients with an acute pneumonia. Patients with pleurisy and pneumonia should always be screened for tuberculosis.

TREATMENT

Therapy should be aimed at the underlying disease. When pneumonia is present, neither immobilization of the chest with adhesive plaster nor therapy with drugs capable of suppressing the cough reflex is indicated. If pneumonia is not present or is under good therapeutic control, strapping of the chest to restrict expansion may afford relief from pain. Analgesia with nonsteroidal anti-inflammatory agents may be helpful.

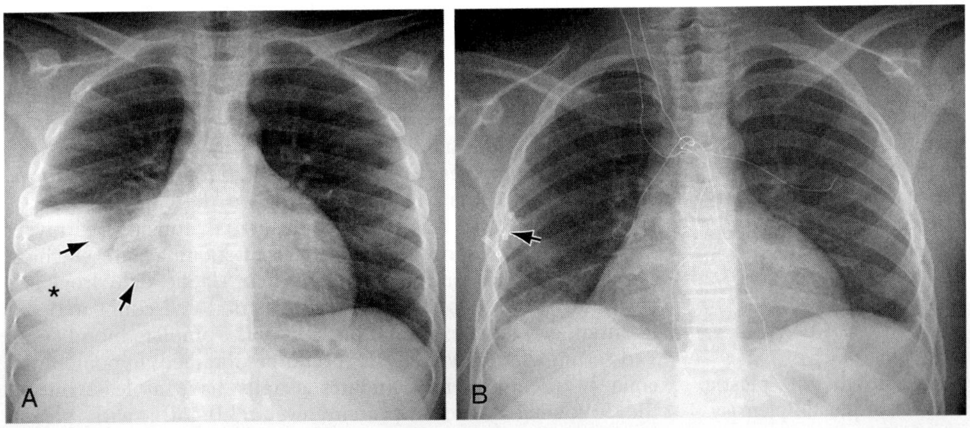

Figure 404-1 *A,* Right pleural effusion (*asterisk*) due to lupus erythematosus in a 12 yr old child. Note compressed middle and lower lobes of the right lung (*arrows*). *B,* The effusion was evacuated and the right lung was completely reexpanded after insertion of the pigtail chest tube (*arrow*).

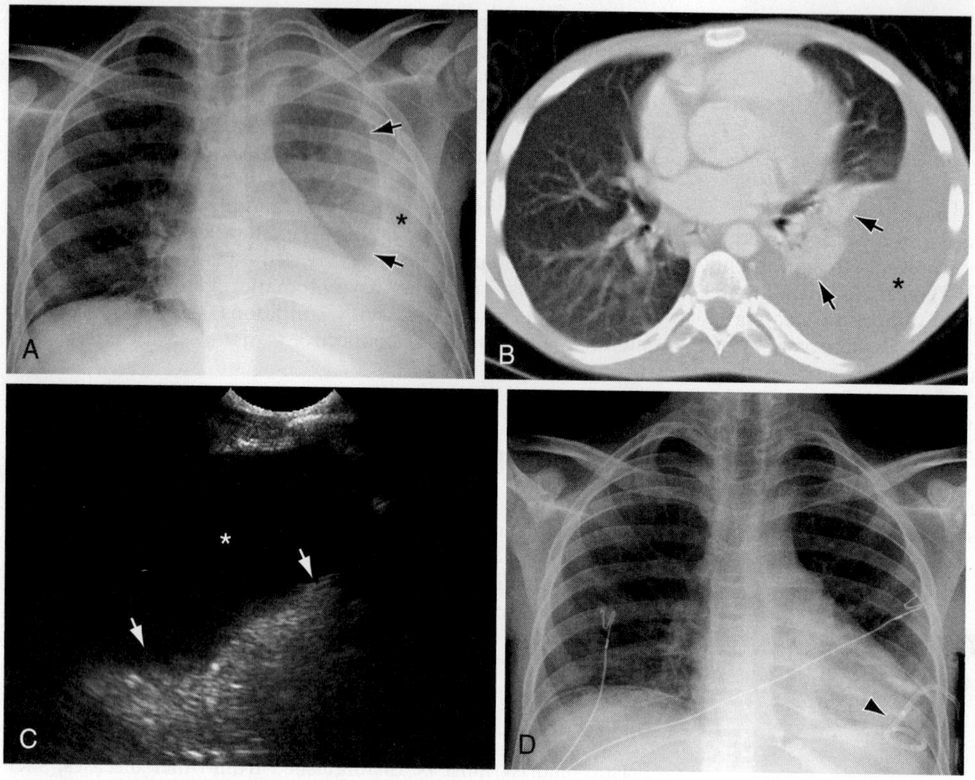

Figure 404-2 Left pleural effusion in a teenager with AIDS and mycoplasma avium intracellulare infection. The pleural effusion (*asterisk*) is clearly seen on the chest radiograph (*A*), CT scan (*B*), and ultrasonogram (*C*) of the left chest. *Arrows* point to the compressed and atelectatic left lung. *D*, A pigtail chest tube (*arrowhead*) was inserted, resulting in reexpansion of the left lung.

404.2 Serofibrinous or Serosanguineous Pleurisy (Pleural Effusion)

Glenna B. Winnie and Steven V. Lossef

ETIOLOGY

Serofibrinous pleurisy is defined by a fibrinous exudate on the pleural surface and an exudative effusion of serous fluid into the pleural cavity. Typically it is associated with infections of the lung or with inflammatory conditions of the abdomen or mediastinum. Occasionally, it is found with connective tissue diseases such as lupus erythematosus, periarteritis, and rheumatoid, arthritis and it may be seen with primary or metastatic neoplasms of the lung, pleura, or mediastinum; tumors are commonly associated with a hemorrhagic pleurisy.

PATHOGENESIS

Pleural fluid originates from the capillaries of the parietal pleura and is absorbed from the pleural space via pleural stomas and the lymphatics of the parietal pleura. The rate of fluid formation is dictated by the Starling law, by which fluid movement is determined by the balance of hydrostatic and osmotic pressures in the pleural space and pulmonary capillary bed, and the permeability of the pleural membrane. Normally, only 4-12 mL of fluid is present in the pleural space, but if formation exceeds clearance, fluid accumulates. Pleural inflammation increases the permeability of the plural surface, with increased proteinaceous fluid formation; there may also be some obstruction to lymphatic absorption.

CLINICAL MANIFESTATIONS

Because serofibrinous pleurisy is often preceded by the plastic type, early signs and symptoms may be those of plastic pleurisy. As fluid accumulates, pleuritic pain may disappear. The patient may become asymptomatic if the effusion remains small, or there may be only signs and symptoms of the underlying disease. Large fluid collections can produce cough, dyspnea, retractions, tachypnea, orthopnea, or cyanosis.

Physical findings depend on the amount of effusion. Dullness to flatness may be found on percussion. Breath sounds are decreased or absent, and there are a diminution in tactile fremitus, a shift of the mediastinum away from the affected side, and, occasionally, fullness of the intercostal spaces. If the fluid is not loculated, these signs may shift with changes in position. If extensive pneumonia is present, crackles and rhonchi may also be audible. Friction rubs are usually detected only during the early or late plastic stage. In infants, physical signs are less definite, and bronchial breathing may be heard instead of decreased breath sounds.

LABORATORY FINDINGS

Radiographic examination shows a generally homogeneous density obliterating the normal markings of the underlying lung. Small effusions may cause obliteration of only the costophrenic or cardiophrenic angles or a widening of the interlobar septa. Examinations should be performed with the patient both supine and upright, to demonstrate a shift of the effusion with a change in position; the decubitus position may be helpful. Ultrasonographic examinations are useful and may guide thoracentesis if the effusion is loculated. Examination of the fluid is essential to differentiate exudates from transudates and to determine the type of exudate (Chapter 392). Depending on the clinical scenario, pleural fluid is sent for culture for bacterial, fungal, and mycobacterial cultures; antigen testing; Gram staining; and chemical evaluation of content, including protein, lactic dehydrogenase and glucose, amylase, specific gravity, total cell count and differential, cytologic examination, and pH. Complete blood count and serum chemistry analysis should be obtained; hypoalbuminemia is often present. **Exudates** usually have at least one of the following features: protein level >3.0 g/dL, with pleural fluid:serum protein ratio >0.5; pleural fluid lactic dehydrogenase values >200 IU/L; or fluid:serum lactic dehydrogenase ratio >0.6. Although systemic acidosis reduces the usefulness of pleural fluid pH measurements, pH <7.20 suggests an exudate. Glucose is usually <60 mg/dL in malignancy, rheumatoid disease, and tuberculosis; the finding of many small lymphocytes and a pH <7.20 suggest tuberculosis. The fluid of serofibrinous pleurisy is clear or slightly cloudy and contains relatively few leukocytes and, occasionally, some erythrocytes. Gram staining may occasionally show bacteria; however, acid-fast staining rarely demonstrates tubercle bacilli.

DIAGNOSIS AND DIFFERENTIAL DIAGNOSIS

Thoracentesis should be performed when pleural fluid is present or is suggested, unless the effusion is small and the patient has a classic-appearing lobar pneumococcal pneumonia. Thoracentesis can differentiate serofibrinous pleurisy, empyema, hydrothorax, hemothorax, and chylothorax. Exudates are usually associated with an infectious process. In hydrothorax, the fluid has a specific gravity <1.015, and evaluation reveals only a few mesothelial cells rather than leukocytes. Chylothorax and hemothorax usually have fluid with a distinctive appearance, but differentiating serofibrinous from purulent pleurisy is impossible without microscopic examination of the fluid. Cytologic examination may reveal malignant cells. Serofibrinous fluid may rapidly become purulent.

COMPLICATIONS

Unless the fluid becomes purulent, it usually disappears relatively rapidly, particularly with appropriate treatment of bacterial pneumonia. It persists somewhat longer if due to tuberculosis or a connective tissue disease and may recur or remain for a long time if due to a neoplasm. As the effusion is absorbed, adhesions often develop between the 2 layers of the pleura, but usually little or no functional impairment results. Pleural thickening may develop and is occasionally mistaken for small quantities of fluid or for persistent pulmonary infiltrates. Pleural thickening may persist for months, but the process usually disappears, leaving no residua.

TREATMENT

Therapy should address the underlying disease. With a large effusion, draining the fluid makes the patient more comfortable. When a diagnostic thoracentesis is performed, as much fluid as possible should be removed for therapeutic purposes. Rapid removal of ≥1 L of pleural fluid may be associated with the development of reexpansion pulmonary edema (Chapter 388). If the underlying disease is adequately treated, further drainage is usually unnecessary, but if sufficient fluid reaccumulates to cause respiratory embarrassment, chest tube drainage should be performed. In older children with suspected parapneumonic effusion, tube thoracostomy is considered necessary if the pleural fluid pH is <7.20 or the pleural fluid glucose level is <50 mg/dL. If the fluid is clearly purulent, tube drainage with thrombolytic therapy or video-assisted thoracoscopic surgery (VATS) is indicated. Patients with pleural effusions may need analgesia, particularly after thoracentesis or insertion of a chest tube. Those with acute pneumonia may need supplemental oxygen in addition to specific antibiotic treatment.

BIBLIOGRAPHY

Please visit the Nelson Textbook of Pediatrics *website at www.expertconsult.com for the complete bibliography.*

404.3 Purulent Pleurisy or Empyema

Glenna B. Winnie and Steven V. Lossef

ETIOLOGY

Empyema is an accumulation of pus in the pleural space. It is most often associated with pneumonia (Chapter 392) due to *Streptococcus pneumoniae,* although *Staphylococcus aureus* is most common in developing nations and Asia as well as in post-traumatic empyema. The relative incidence of *Haemophilus influenzae* empyema has decreased since the introduction of the Hib vaccination. Group A streptococcus, gram-negative organisms, tuberculosis, fungi, and malignancy are less common causes. The disease can also be produced by rupture of a lung abscess into the pleural space, by contamination introduced from trauma or thoracic surgery, or, rarely, by mediastinitis or the extension of intra-abdominal abscesses.

EPIDEMIOLOGY

Empyema is most frequently encountered in infants and preschool children. It is increasing in frequency. It occurs in 5-10% of children with bacterial pneumonia and in up to 86% of children with necrotizing pneumonia.

PATHOLOGY

Empyema has 3 stages: exudative, fibrinopurulent, and organizational. During the **exudative stage,** fibrinous exudate forms on the pleural surfaces. In the **fibrinopurulent stage,** fibrinous septa form, causing loculation of the fluid and thickening of the parietal pleura. If the pus is not drained, it may dissect through the pleura into lung parenchyma, producing bronchopleural fistulas and pyopneumothorax, or into the abdominal cavity. Rarely, the pus dissects through the chest wall (i.e., empyema necessitatis). During the **organizational stage,** there is fibroblast proliferation; pockets of loculated pus may develop into thick-walled abscess cavities or the lung may collapse and become surrounded by a thick, inelastic envelope (peel).

CLINICAL MANIFESTATIONS

The initial signs and symptoms are primarily those of bacterial pneumonia. Children treated with antibiotic agents may have an interval of a few days between the clinical pneumonia phase and the evidence of empyema. Most patients are febrile, develop increased work of breathing or respiratory distress, and often appear more ill. Physical findings are identical to those described for serofibrinous pleurisy, and the 2 conditions are differentiated only by thoracentesis, which should always be performed when empyema is suspected.

LABORATORY FINDINGS

Radiographically, all pleural effusions appear similar, but the absence of a shift of the fluid with a change of position indicates a loculated empyema (Figs. 404-3 to 404-5). Septa may be confirmed by ultrasonography or CT. The maximal amount of fluid obtainable should be withdrawn by thoracentesis and studied as described in Chapter 404.2. The effusion is empyema if bacteria are present on Gram staining, the pH is <7.20, and there are >100,000 neutrophils/μL. The appearance of pus produced by different organisms is not distinctive; cultures of the fluid must always be performed. In pneumococcal empyema, the culture is positive in 58% of cases. In patients with negative culture results for pneumococcus, the pneumococcal polymerase chain reaction (PCR) analysis is most helpful to making a diagnosis. Blood

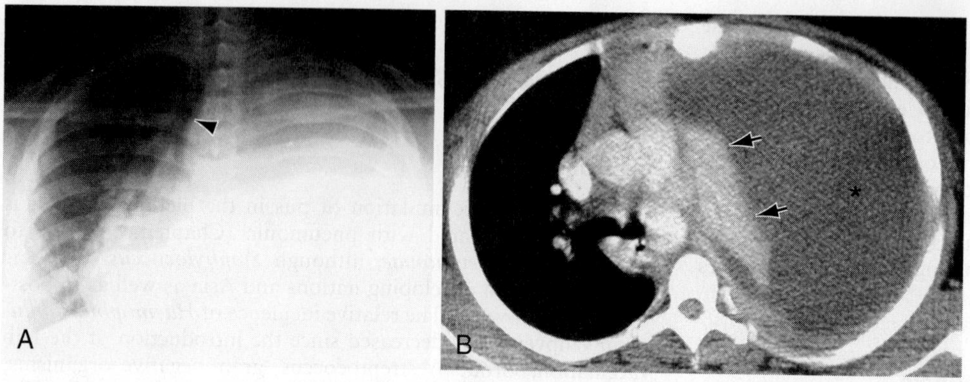

Figure 404-3 Empyema and pneumonia in a teenager. *A,* Chest radiograph shows opacification of the left thorax. Note shift of mediastinum and trachea (*arrowhead*) to right. *B,* Thoracic CT scan shows massive left pleural effusion (*asterisk*). Note the compression and atelectasis of the left lung (*arrows*) and shift of the mediastinum to the right.

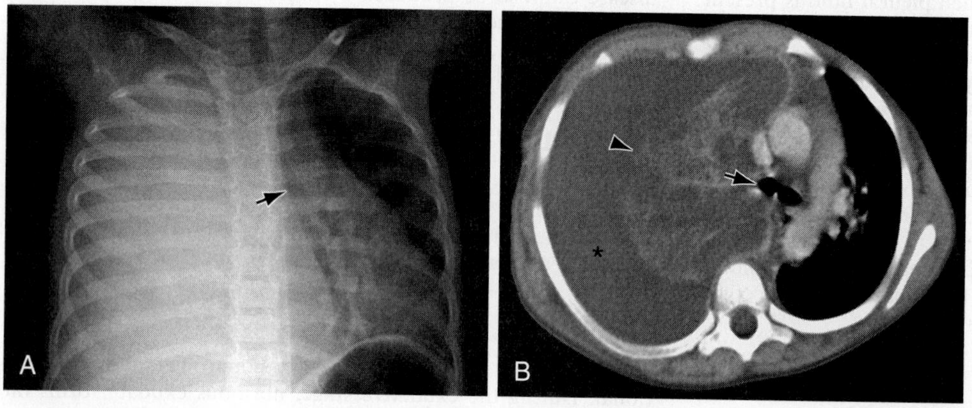

Figure 404-4 Pneumonia and parapneumonic effusion in a 4 yr old child. *A,* Chest radiograph shows complete opacification of the right thorax due to a large pleural effusion. Note the shift of the mediastinum and trachea (*arrow*) to the left. *B,* Thoracic CT scan shows a large right pleural effusion (*asterisk*) surrounding and compressing the consolidated right lung (*arrowhead*). Note the shift of the mediastinum and tracheal carina (*arrow*) to the left.

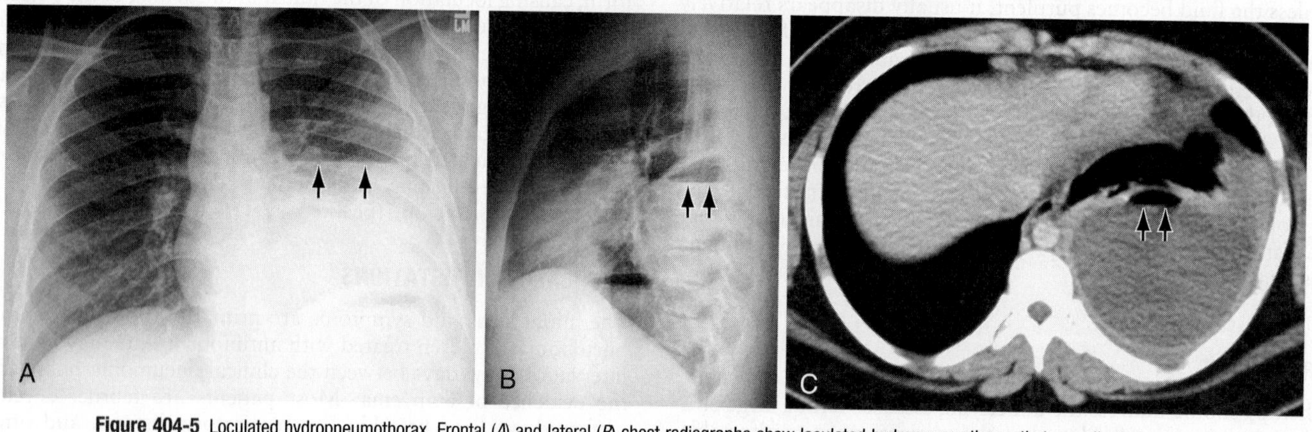

Figure 404-5 Loculated hydropneumothorax. Frontal (*A*) and lateral (*B*) chest radiographs show loculated hydropneumothorax that complicated pneumonia in a 14 yr old child. *Arrows* point to the horizontal air-fluid level at the interface between the intrapleural effusion and air. *C,* Thoracic CT scan helps to localize the loculated hydropneumothorax, with its air-fluid level (*arrows*).

cultures have a high yield, possibly higher than cultures of the pleural fluid. Leukocytosis and an elevated sedimentation rate may be found.

COMPLICATIONS

With staphylococcal infections, bronchopleural fistulas and pyopneumothorax commonly develop. Other local complications include purulent pericarditis, pulmonary abscesses, peritonitis from extension through the diaphragm, and osteomyelitis of the ribs. Septic complications such as meningitis, arthritis, and osteomyelitis may also occur. Septicemia is often encountered in *H. influenzae* and pneumococcal infections. The effusion may organize into a thick "peel," which may restrict lung expansion and may be associated with persistent fever and temporary scoliosis.

TREATMENT

Treatment includes systemic antibiotics and thoracentesis and possibly chest tube drainage with or without a fibrinolytic agent, video-assisted thoracoscopic surgery (VATS), or open decortication (Chapter 392); controlled studies are needed. If empyema is diagnosed early, antibiotic treatment plus thoracentesis achieves a complete cure. The selection of antibiotic should be based on the in vitro sensitivities of the responsible organism. See Chapters 174, 175, and 186 for treatment of infections by *Staphylococcus, S. pneumoniae,* and *H. influenzae,* respectively. Clinical response in empyema is slow; even with optimal treatment, there may be little improvement for as long as 2 wk. With staphylococcal infections, resolution is very slow, and systemic antibiotic therapy is required for 3-4 wk. Instillation of antibiotics into the pleural cavity does not improve results.

When pus is obtained by thoracentesis, it is unclear whether optimal management is closed-chest tube drainage or VATS followed by chest tube drainage. Multiple aspirations of the pleural cavity should not be attempted. If pleural fluid septa are detected on ultrasound, immediate VATS can be associated with a shortened hospital course. Closed-chest tube drainage is controlled by an underwater seal or continuous suction; sometimes more than 1 tube is required to drain loculated areas. Closed drainage is usually continued for about 1 wk. Chest tubes that are no longer draining are removed.

Instillation of fibrinolytic agents into the pleural cavity via the chest tube may promote drainage, decrease fever, lessen need for surgical intervention, and shorten hospitalization; it does not shorten the course of disease when used after VATS, however. The optimal drug and dosage have not been determined. Streptokinase 15,000 U/kg in 50 mL of 0.9% saline daily for 3-5 days and urokinase 40,000 U in 40 mL saline every 12 hr for 6 doses have been evaluated in randomized trials in children. There is a risk of anaphylaxis with streptokinase, and both drugs can be associated with hemorrhage and other complications.

Extensive fibrinous changes may take place over the surface of the lungs owing to empyema, but they eventually resolve. In the child who remains febrile and dyspneic >72 hr after initiation of therapy with intravenous antibiotics and thoracostomy tube drainage, surgical decortication via VATS or, less often, open thoracotomy may speed recovery. If pneumatoceles form, no attempt should be made to treat them surgically or by aspiration, unless they reach sufficient size to cause respiratory embarrassment or become secondarily infected. Pneumatoceles usually resolve spontaneously with time. The long-term clinical prognosis for adequately treated empyema is excellent, and follow-up pulmonary function studies suggest that residual restrictive disease is uncommon, with or without surgical intervention.

BIBLIOGRAPHY

Please visit the Nelson Textbook of Pediatrics *website at www.expertconsult.com for the complete bibliography.*

Table 405-1 CAUSES OF PNEUMOTHORAX IN CHILDREN

SPONTANEOUS
Primary idiopathic—usually resulting from ruptured subpleural blebs
Secondary blebs
Congenital lung disease:
Congenital cystic adenomatoid malformation
Bronchogenic cysts
Pulmonary hypoplasia*
Conditions associated with increased intrathoracic pressure:
Asthma
Bronchiolitis
Air-block syndrome in neonates
Cystic fibrosis
Airway foreign body
Infection:
Pneumatocele
Lung abscess
Bronchopleural fistula
Diffuse lung disease:
Langerhans cell histiocytosis
Tuberous sclerosis
Marfan syndrome
Ehlers-Danlos syndrome
Metastatic neoplasm—usually osteosarcoma (rare)
TRAUMATIC
Noniatrogenic
Penetrating trauma
Blunt trauma
Loud music (air pressure)
Iatrogenic
Thoracotomy
Thoracoscopy, thoracentesis
Tracheostomy
Tube or needle puncture
Mechanical ventilation

*Associated with renal agenesis, diaphragmatic hernia, amniotic fluid leaks.
From Kuhn JP, Slovis TL, Haller JO: *Caffey's pediatric diagnostic imaging,* vol 1, ed 10, Philadelphia, 2004, Mosby.

Chapter 405
Pneumothorax

Glenna B. Winnie and Steven V. Lossef

Pneumothorax is the accumulation of extrapulmonary air within the chest, most commonly from leakage of air from within the lung. Air leaks can be primary or secondary and can be spontaneous, traumatic, iatrogenic, or catamenial (Table 405-1). Pneumothorax in the neonatal period is also discussed in Chapter 95.12.

ETIOLOGY AND EPIDEMIOLOGY

A **primary spontaneous pneumothorax** occurs without trauma or underlying lung disease. Spontaneous pneumothorax with or without exertion occurs occasionally in teenagers and young adults, most frequently in males who are tall, thin, and thought to have subpleural blebs. Familial cases of spontaneous pneumothorax occur and have been associated with mutations in the folliculin gene. Patients with collagen synthesis defects, such as Ehlers-Danlos disease (Chapter 651) and Marfan syndrome (Chapter 693) are unusually prone to the development of pneumothorax.

A pneumothorax arising as a complication of an underlying lung disorder but without trauma is a **secondary spontaneous pneumothorax.** Pneumothorax can occur in pneumonia, usually with empyema; it can also be secondary to pulmonary abscess, gangrene, infarct, rupture of a cyst or an emphysematous bleb (in asthma), or foreign bodies in the lung. In infants with staphylococcal pneumonia, the incidence of pneumothorax is relatively high. It is found in ≈5% of hospitalized asthmatic children and usually resolves without treatment. Pneumothorax is a serious complication in cystic fibrosis (CF; Chapter 395). Pneumothorax also occurs in patients with lymphoma or other malignancies, and in graft versus host disease with bronchiolitis obliterans.

External chest or abdominal blunt or penetrating trauma can tear a bronchus or abdominal viscus, with leakage of air into the pleural space. Ecstasy (methylenedioxymethamphetamine) abuse has been associated with pneumothorax.

Iatrogenic pneumothorax can complicate transthoracic needle aspiration, tracheotomy, subclavian line placement, thoracentesis, or transbronchial biopsy. It may occur during mechanical or noninvasive ventilation, acupuncture, and other diagnostic or therapeutic procedures.

Catamenial pneumothorax, an unusual condition that is related to menses, is associated with diaphragmatic defects and pleural blebs.

Pneumothorax can be associated with a serous effusion (hydropneumothorax), a purulent effusion (pyopneumothorax), or blood (hemopneumothorax). Bilateral pneumothorax is rare after the neonatal period but has been reported after lung transplantation and with *Mycoplasma pneumoniae* infection and tuberculosis.

PATHOGENESIS

The tendency of the lung to collapse, or elastic recoil, is balanced in the normal resting state by the inherent tendency of the chest

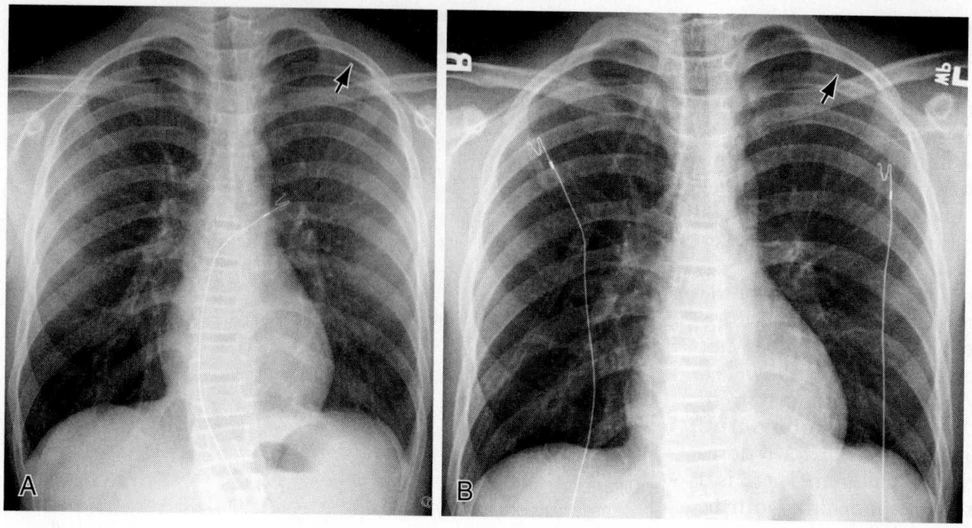

Figure 405-1 Utility of an expiratory film in detection of a small pneumothorax. *A,* Teenage boy with stab wound and subtle radiolucency in the left apical region (*arrow*) on inspiratory chest radiograph. The margin of the visceral pleura is very faintly visible. *B,* On an expiratory film, the pneumothorax (*arrow*) is more obvious as the right lung has deflated and become more opaque, providing better contrast with the air in the pleural space.

wall to expand outward, creating negative pressure in the intrapleural space. When air enters the pleural space, the lung collapses. Hypoxemia occurs because of alveolar hypoventilation, ventilation-perfusion mismatch, and intrapulmonary shunt. In simple pneumothorax, intrapleural pressure is atmospheric, and the lung collapses up to 30%. In complicated, or tension, pneumothorax, continuing leak causes increasing positive pressure in the pleural space, with further compression of the lung, shift of mediastinal structures toward the contralateral side, and decreases in venous return and cardiac output.

CLINICAL MANIFESTATIONS

The onset of pneumothorax is usually abrupt, and the severity of symptoms depends on the extent of the lung collapse and on the amount of pre-existing lung disease. Pneumothorax may cause dyspnea, pain, and cyanosis. When it occurs in infancy, symptoms and physical signs may be difficult to recognize. Moderate pneumothorax may cause little displacement of the intrathoracic organs and few or no symptoms. The severity of pain usually does not directly reflect the extent of the collapse.

Usually, there is respiratory distress, with retractions, markedly decreased breath sounds, and a tympanitic percussion note over the involved hemithorax. The larynx, trachea, and heart may be shifted toward the unaffected side. When fluid is present, there is usually a sharply limited area of tympany above a level of flatness to percussion. The presence of amphoric breathing or, when fluid is present in the pleural cavity, of gurgling sounds synchronous with respirations suggests an open fistula connecting with air-containing tissues.

DIAGNOSIS AND DIFFERENTIAL DIAGNOSIS

The diagnosis of pneumothorax is usually established by radiographic examination (Figs. 405-1 to 405-6). The amount of air outside the lung varies with time. A radiograph that is taken early shows less lung collapse than one taken later if the leak continues. Expiratory views accentuate the contrast between lung markings and the clear area of the pneumothorax (see Fig. 405-1). When the possibility of diaphragmatic hernia is being considered, a small amount of barium may be necessary to demonstrate that it is not free air but is a portion of the gastrointestinal tract that is in the thoracic cavity. Ultrasound can also be used to establish the diagnosis.

It may be difficult to determine whether a pneumothorax is under tension. **Evidence of tension** includes shift of mediastinal structures away from the side of the air leak. A shift may be

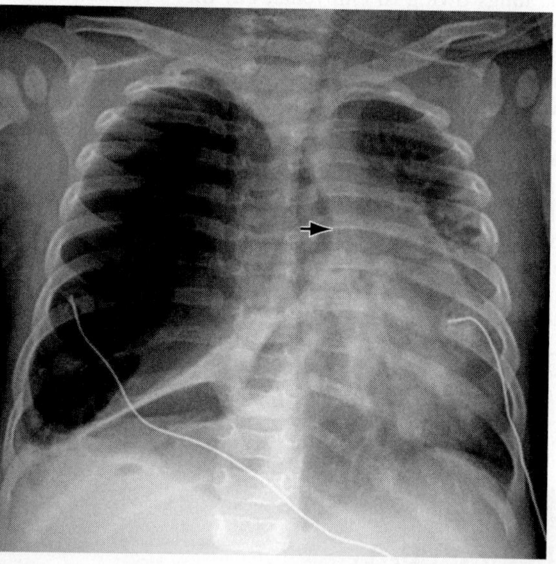

Figure 405-2 Right pneumothorax, with lung collapse of a compliant lung. Shift of the mediastinum to the left (*arrow*) indicates that this is a tension pneumothorax.

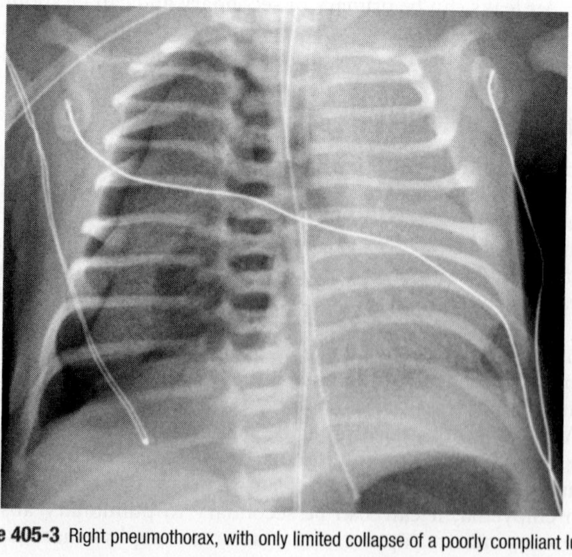

Figure 405-3 Right pneumothorax, with only limited collapse of a poorly compliant lung.

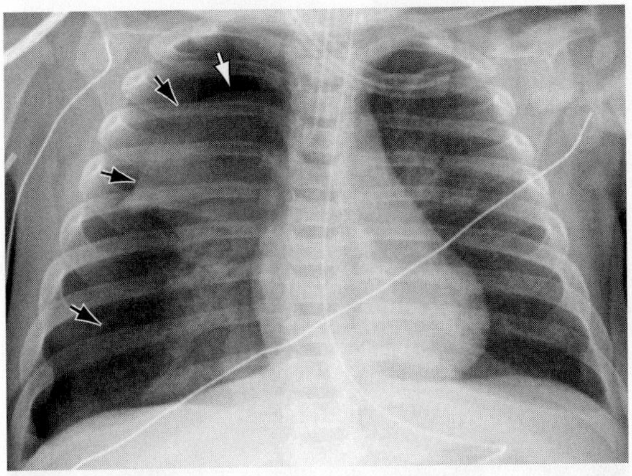

Figure 405-4 Pneumothorax, with collapse of right lung (*arrows*) caused by barotrauma in a 7 month old child who was intubated for respiratory failure.

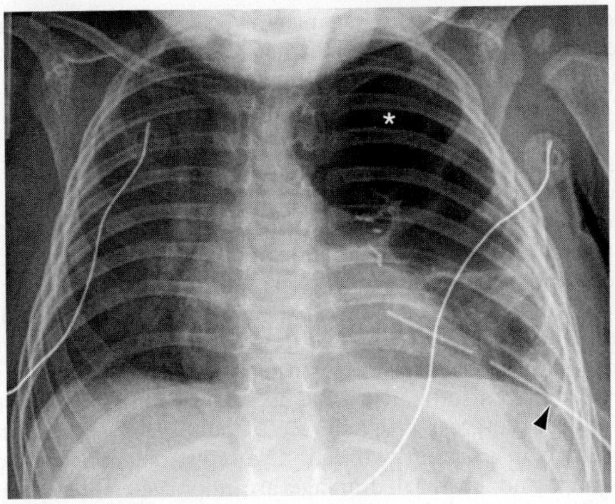

Figure 405-6 Bronchopleural fistula following surgical resection of the left upper lobe due to congenital lobar emphysema. Chest radiograph shows localized pneumothorax (*asterisk*) that persisted despite prior insertion of a large-bore chest tube (*arrowhead*).

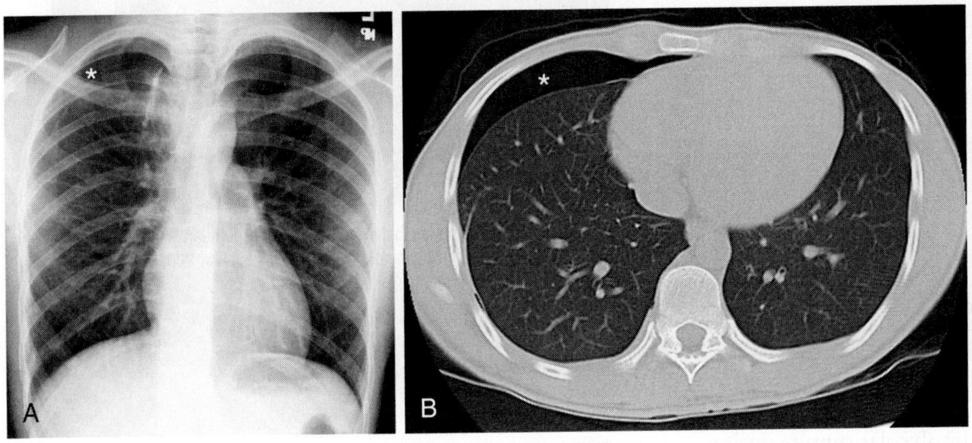

Figure 405-5 Teenager in whom a spontaneous right pneumothorax developed because of a bleb. He had a persistent air leak despite recent surgical resection of the causative apical bleb. Chest radiograph (*A*) and CT scan (*B*) clearly show the persistent pneumothorax (*asterisk*).

absent in situations in which the other hemithorax resists the shift, such as in the case of bilateral pneumothorax. When the lungs are both stiff, such as in CF or respiratory distress syndrome, the unaffected lung may not collapse easily and shift may not occur (see Fig. 405-3). On occasion, the diagnosis of tension pneumothorax is made only on the basis of evidence of circulatory compromise or on hearing a "hiss" of rapid exit of air under tension with the insertion of the thoracostomy tube.

Pneumothorax must be differentiated from localized or generalized emphysema, an extensive emphysematous bleb, large pulmonary cavities or other cystic formations, diaphragmatic hernia, compensatory overexpansion with contralateral atelectasis, and gaseous distention of the stomach. In most cases, chest radiography or CT differentiates among these possibilities.

TREATMENT

Therapy varies with the extent of the collapse and the nature and severity of the underlying disease. A small (<5%) or even moderate-sized pneumothorax in an otherwise normal child may resolve without specific treatment, usually within about 1 wk. A small pneumothorax complicating asthma may also resolve spontaneously. Administering 100% oxygen may hasten resolution, but patients with chronic hypoxemia should be monitored closely during administration of supplemental oxygen. Pleural pain deserves analgesic treatment. Needle aspiration may be required on an emergency basis for tension pneumothorax and is as effective as tube thoracostomy in the emergency room management of primary spontaneous pneumothorax. If the pneumothorax is recurrent, secondary, or under tension, or there is >5% collapse, chest tube drainage is necessary. Pneumothorax complicating CF frequently recurs, and definitive treatment may be justified with the 1st episode. Similarly, if pneumothorax complicating malignancy does not improve rapidly with observation, chemical pleurodesis or surgical thoracotomy is often necessary.

Closed thoracotomy (simple insertion of a chest tube) and drainage of the trapped air through a catheter, the external opening of which is kept in a dependent position under water, is adequate to reexpand the lung in most patients; pigtail catheters are frequently used. When there have been previous pneumothoraces, it may be indicated to induce the formation of strong adhesions between the lung and chest wall by a sclerosing procedure to prevent recurrence. This can be carried out by the introduction of talc, doxycycline, or iodopovidone into the pleural space (**chemical pleurodesis**). Open thoracotomy through a limited incision, with plication of blebs, closure of fistula, stripping of the pleura (usually in the apical lung, where the surgeon has direct vision), and basilar pleural abrasion is also an effective treatment for recurring pneumothorax. Stripping and abrading the pleura leaves raw, inflamed surfaces that heal with sealing adhesions. Postoperative pain is comparable to that with chemical pleurodesis, but the chest tube can usually be removed in 24-48 hr, compared with the usual 72-hr minimum for closed thoracotomy and pleurodesis. VATS is a preferred therapy for blebectomy, pleural stripping, pleural brushing, and instillation of sclerosing agents, with somewhat less morbidity than occurs with traditional open thoracotomy.

Pleural adhesions help prevent recurrent pneumothorax, but they also make subsequent thoracic surgery difficult. When lung transplantation may be a future consideration (e.g., in CF), a stepwise approach to treatment of pneumothorax has been proposed. This approach begins with observation and progresses through chest tube drainage and thoracoscopic and then open surgery, and finally to chemical or mechanical pleurodesis. At any step during this approach, the patient and family are given the option of the definitive procedure if they understand that its performance may make lung transplantation difficult or impossible. It should also be kept in mind that the longer a chest tube is in place, the greater the chance of pulmonary deterioration, particularly in a patient with CF, in whom strong coughing, deep breathing, and postural drainage are important. These are all difficult to accomplish with a chest tube in place.

Treatment of the underlying pulmonary disease should begin on admission and should be continued throughout the course of treatment directed at the air leak.

BIBLIOGRAPHY

Please visit the Nelson Textbook of Pediatrics *website at www.expertconsult.com for the complete bibliography.*

Chapter 406
Pneumomediastinum

Glenna B. Winnie

Pneumomediastinum is the presence or air or gas in the mediastinum.

ETIOLOGY

Pneumomediastinum is usually caused by alveolar rupture during acute or chronic pulmonary disease. A diverse group of nonrespiratory entities can also cause it, and the lung is not always the source of the air. Pneumomediastinum has been reported after dental extractions, adenotonsillectomy, normal menses, obstetric delivery, diabetes mellitus with ketoacidosis, acupuncture, anorexia nervosa, and acute gastroenteritis. It can also result from esophageal perforation, penetrating chest trauma, or inhaled foreign body. Occasionally, no underlying cause is found. Acute asthma is the most common cause of pneumomediastinum in older children and teenagers. Simultaneous pneumothorax is unusual in these patients.

PATHOGENESIS

After intrapulmonary alveolar rupture, air dissects through the perivascular sheaths and other soft tissue, planes toward the hilum, and enters the mediastinum.

CLINICAL MANIFESTATIONS

Transient stabbing chest pain that may radiate to the neck is the principal feature of pneumomediastinum. Isolated abdominal pain and sore throat also occur. The patient may have dyspnea and cough. Pneumomediastinum is difficult to detect by physical examination alone. Subcutaneous emphysema, if present, is diagnostic. Cardiac dullness to percussion may be decreased, but the chests of many patients with pneumomediastinum are chronically overinflated, and it is unlikely that the clinician can be sure of this finding. A mediastinal "crunch" (Hamman sign) is occasionally heard but is easily confused with a friction rub.

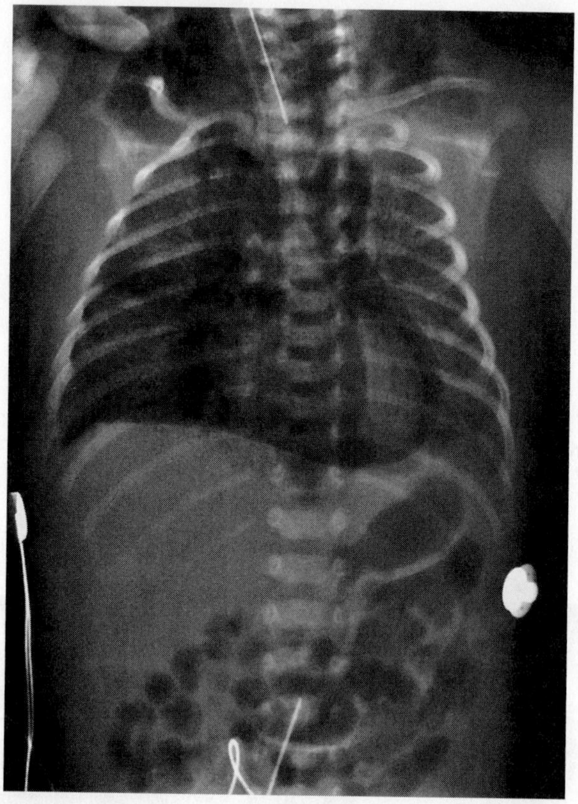

Figure 406-1 Large pneumomediastinum surrounding the heart and dissecting into the neck. (From Clark DA: *Atlas of neonatology,* ed 7, Philadelphia, 2000, WB Saunders.)

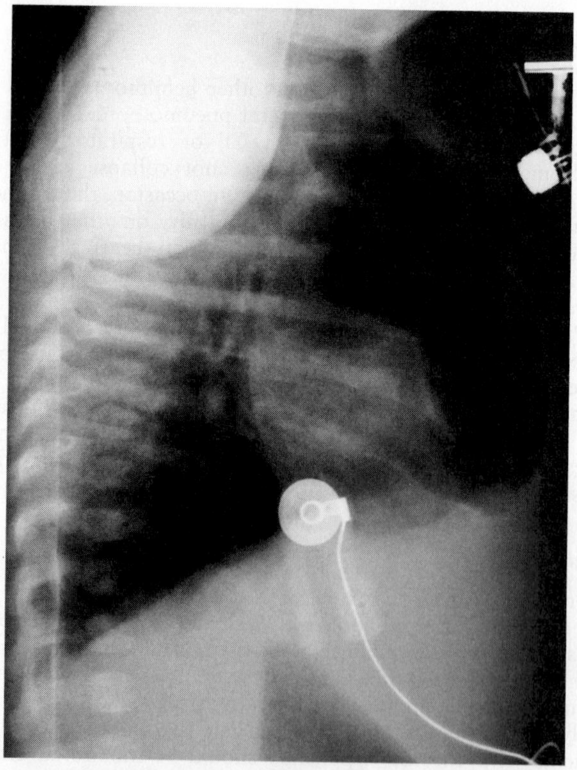

Figure 406-2 Lateral radiograph: upper mediastinal air. (From Clark DA: *Atlas of neonatology,* ed 7, Philadelphia, 2000, WB Saunders, p 94.)

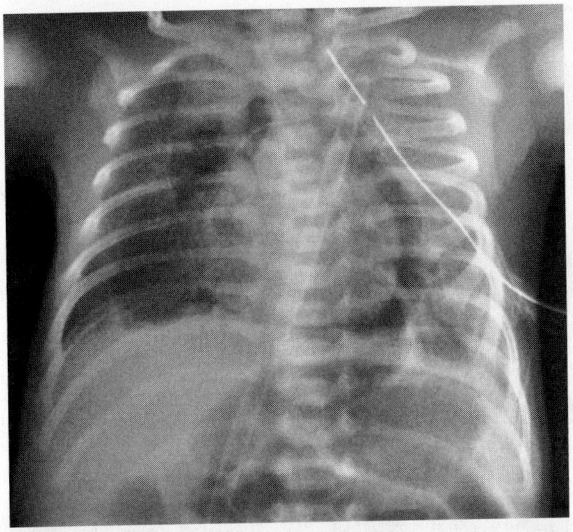

Figure 406-3 Sail sign—thymic elevation. (From Clark DA: *Atlas of neonatology,* ed 7, Philadelphia, 2000, WB Saunders, p 94.)

LABORATORY FINDINGS

Chest radiography reveals mediastinal air, with a more distinct cardiac border than normal (Figs. 406-1 to 406-3). On the lateral projection, the posterior mediastinal structures are clearly defined, there may be a lucent ring around the right pulmonary artery, and retrosternal air can usually be seen (see Fig. 406-2). Vertical streaks of air in the mediastinum and subcutaneous air are often observed (see Fig. 406-1).

COMPLICATIONS

Pneumomediastinum is rarely a major problem in older children because the mediastinum can be depressurized by escape of air into the neck or abdomen. In the newborn, however, the rate at which air can leave the mediastinum is limited, and pneumomediastinum can lead to dangerous cardiovascular compromise or pneumothorax (Chapters 95.12 and 405).

TREATMENT

Treatment is directed primarily at the underlying obstructive pulmonary disease or other precipitating condition. Analgesics are occasionally needed for chest pain. Rarely, subcutaneous emphysema can cause sufficient tracheal compression to justify tracheotomy; the tracheotomy also decompresses the mediastinum. Collar mediastinotomy and percutaneous drainage catheter placement are other treatment modalities.

BIBLIOGRAPHY
Please visit the Nelson Textbook of Pediatrics *website at* *www.expertconsult.com* *for the complete bibliography.*

Chapter 407
Hydrothorax

Glenna B. Winnie and Steven V. Lossef

Hydrothorax is a transudative pleural effusion usually caused by abnormal pressure gradients in the lung.

ETIOLOGY

Hydrothorax is most often associated with cardiac, renal, or hepatic disease. It can also be a manifestation of severe nutritional edema and hypoalbuminemia. Rarely, it results from vascular obstruction by neoplasms, enlarged lymph nodes, pulmonary embolism, or adhesions. It may occur from a ventriculoperitoneal shunt or peritoneal dialysis and has been reported in congenital parvovirus B19 infection.

CLINICAL MANIFESTATIONS

Hydrothorax is usually bilateral, but in cardiac disease it can be limited to the right side or greater on the right than on the left side. The physical signs are the same as those described for serofibrinous pleurisy (Chapter 404.2), but in hydrothorax, there is more rapid shifting of the level of dullness with changes of position. It is usually associated with an accumulation of fluid in other parts of the body.

LABORATORY FINDINGS

The fluid is noninflammatory, has few cells, and has a lower specific gravity (<1.015) than that of a serofibrinous exudate. The ratio of pleural fluid to serum total protein is <0.5, the ratio of pleural fluid to serum lactic dehydrogenase is <0.6, and the pleural fluid lactic dehydrogenase value is less than 66% of the upper limit of the normal serum lactic dehydrogenase range.

TREATMENT

Therapy is directed at the underlying disorder; aspiration may be necessary when pressure symptoms are notable.

BIBLIOGRAPHY
Please visit the Nelson Textbook of Pediatrics *website at* *www.expertconsult.com* *for the complete bibliography.*

Chapter 408
Hemothorax

Glenna B. Winnie and Steven V. Lossef

Hemothorax is an accumulation of blood in the pleural cavity. It is rare in children.

ETIOLOGY

Bleeding into the chest cavity most commonly occurs after chest trauma, either blunt or penetrating. It can be the result of iatrogenic trauma, including surgical procedures and venous line insertion. Hemothorax can also result from erosion of a blood vessel in association with inflammatory processes such as tuberculosis and empyema. It may complicate a variety of congenital anomalies, including sequestration, patent ductus arteriosus, and pulmonary arteriovenous malformation. It is also an occasional manifestation of intrathoracic neoplasms, costal exostoses, blood dyscrasias, bleeding diatheses, or thrombolytic therapy. Rupture of an aneurysm is unlikely during childhood. Hemothorax may occur spontaneously in neonates and older children. A pleural hemorrhage associated with a pneumothorax is a *hemopneumothorax*; it is usually due to a ruptured bulla with lung volume loss causing a torn pleural adhesion.

CLINICAL MANIFESTATIONS

In addition to the symptoms and signs of pleural effusion (Chapter 404.2), hemothorax is associated with hemodynamic compromise related to the amount and rapidity of bleeding.

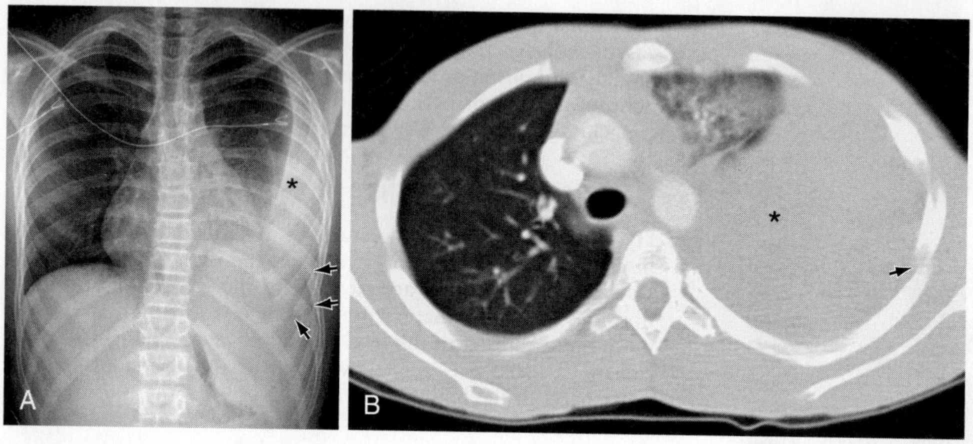

Figure 408-1 Hemothorax (*asterisk*) and associated rib fractures (*arrows*) in a teenager involved in a motor vehicle accident. *A,* Chest radiograph. *B,* CT scan.

DIAGNOSIS

The diagnosis of a hemothorax is initially suspected from radiographs or CT scans but can be made only with thoracentesis (Fig. 408-1). In every case, an effort must be made to determine and treat the cause.

TREATMENT

Initial therapy is tube thoracostomy. Surgical intervention may be required to control active bleeding, and transfusion may be indicated. Inadequate removal of blood in extensive hemothorax may lead to substantial restrictive disease secondary to organization of fibrin; fibrinolytic therapy or a decortication procedure may then be necessary.

BIBLIOGRAPHY

Please visit the Nelson Textbook of Pediatrics *website at* *www.expertconsult.com* *for the complete bibliography.*

Chapter 409
Chylothorax

Glenna B. Winnie and Steven V. Lossef

Chylothorax is a pleural collection of fluid formed by the escape of chyle from the thoracic duct or lymphatics into the thoracic cavity.

ETIOLOGY

Chylothorax in children occurs most frequently because of thoracic duct injury as a complication of cardiothoracic surgery (Fig. 409-1). Other cases are associated with chest injury (Fig. 409-2) or with primary or metastatic intrathoracic malignancy (Fig. 409-3), particularly lymphoma. In newborns, rapidly increased venous pressure during delivery may lead to thoracic duct rupture. Less common causes include lymphangiomatosis; restrictive pulmonary diseases; thrombosis of the duct, superior vena cava, or subclavian vein; tuberculosis or histoplasmosis; and congenital anomalies of the lymphatic system (Fig. 409-4). Refractory chylothorax in the fetus has been associated with a missense mutation in integrin $a\alpha_9$. Chylothorax can occur in trauma and child abuse (Chapter 37). It is important to establish the etiology, because treatment varies with the cause. In some patients, no specific cause is identified.

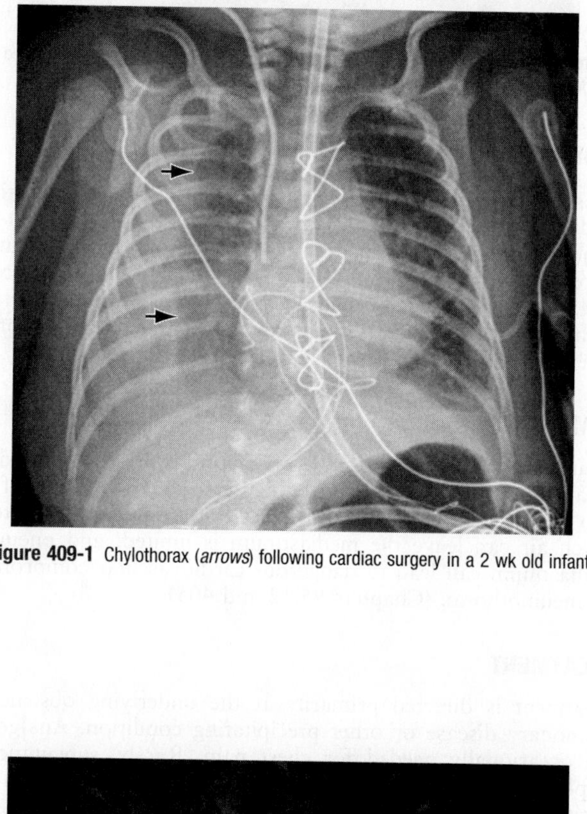

Figure 409-1 Chylothorax (*arrows*) following cardiac surgery in a 2 wk old infant.

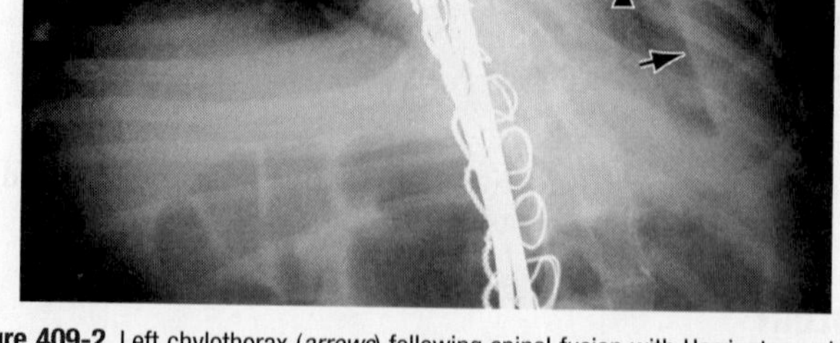

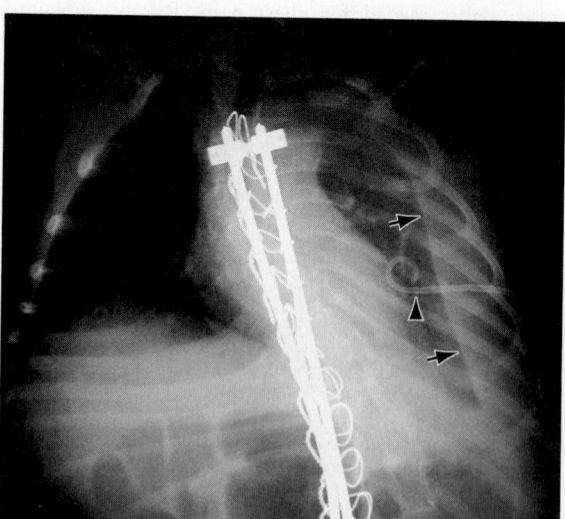

Figure 409-2 Left chylothorax (*arrows*) following spinal fusion with Harrington rods. It is postulated that the thoracic duct was injured during spine surgery. The pigtail chest tube (*arrowhead*) needed to be retracted to better drain the effusion.

CLINICAL MANIFESTATIONS

The signs and symptoms of chylothorax are the same as those due to pleural effusion of similar size. Chyle is not irritating, so pleuritic pain is uncommon. Onset is often gradual. However, after trauma to the thoracic duct chyle may accumulate in the posterior mediastinum for days and then rupture into the pleural space with sudden onset of dyspnea, hypotension, and hypoxemia. About 50% of newborns with chylothorax present with respiratory distress in the 1st day of life. Chylothorax is rarely bilateral and usually occurs on the right side.

LABORATORY FINDINGS

Thoracentesis demonstrates a chylous effusion, a milky fluid containing fat, protein, lymphocytes, and other constituents of chyle; fluid may be yellow or bloody. In newborn infants or those who are not ingesting food, the fluid may be clear. A pseudochylous milky fluid may be present in chronic serous effusion, in which fatty material arises from degenerative changes in the fluid and not from lymph. In chylothorax, the fluid triglyceride level is >110 mg/dL, the pleural fluid:serum triglyceride ratio is >1.0, and pleural fluid:serum cholesterol ratio is <1.0; lipoprotein analysis reveals chylomicrons. The cells are primarily T lymphocytes. Chest radiographs show an effusion; CT scans show normal pleural thickness and may reveal a lymphoma as the etiology of the chylothorax. A lymphangiogram can localize the site of the leak, and lymphoscintigraphy may demonstrate abnormalities of the lymphatic trunks and peripheral lymphatics.

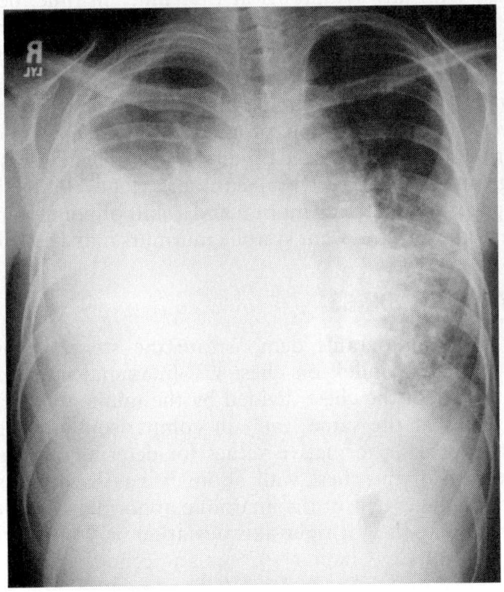

Figure 409-3 Large right chylous effusion opacifying much of the right thorax in a teenager with pulmonary lymphangiomatosis and hemangiomatosis. Note the associated interstitial lung disease.

COMPLICATIONS

Repeated aspirations may be required to relieve the symptoms of pressure. Chyle reaccumulates quickly, and repeated thoracentesis may cause malnutrition with significant loss of calories, protein, and electrolytes. Immunodeficiencies, including hypogammaglobulinemia and abnormal cell-mediated immune responses, have been associated with repeated and chronic thoracenteses for chylothorax. The loss of T lymphocytes is associated with increased risk of infection in neonates; otherwise, infection is uncommon, but patients should not receive live virus vaccines. Lack of resolution of chylothorax can lead to inanition, infection, and death.

TREATMENT

Spontaneous recovery occurs in >50% of cases of neonatal chylothorax. Initial therapy includes enteral feedings with a low-fat or medium-chain triglyceride, high-protein diet or parenteral nutrition. Thoracentesis is repeated as needed to relieve pressure symptoms; tube thoracostomy is often performed. If there is no resolution in 1-2 wk, total parenteral nutrition is instituted; if this measure is unsuccessful, a pleuroperitoneal shunt, thoracic duct ligation, or application of fibrin glue is considered. Surgery should be considered earlier in neonates with massive chylothorax and chyle output of >50 mL/kg/day despite maximum medical therapy for 3 days. Parenteral octreotide at a dose of 80 to 100 μg/kg/day intravenously has been used to manage chylothorax, but further study is needed. Other therapeutic approaches include pressure control ventilation with positive end-expiratory pressure, talc or iodopovidone pleurodesis, and inhalation of nitric oxide. Treatment is similar for traumatic chylothorax. Chemical pleurodesis or irradiation is used in malignant chylothorax. OK432 (picibanil) has been used to treat fetal and newborn chylothorax.

BIBLIOGRAPHY

Please visit the Nelson Textbook of Pediatrics *website at www.expertconsult.com for the complete bibliography.*

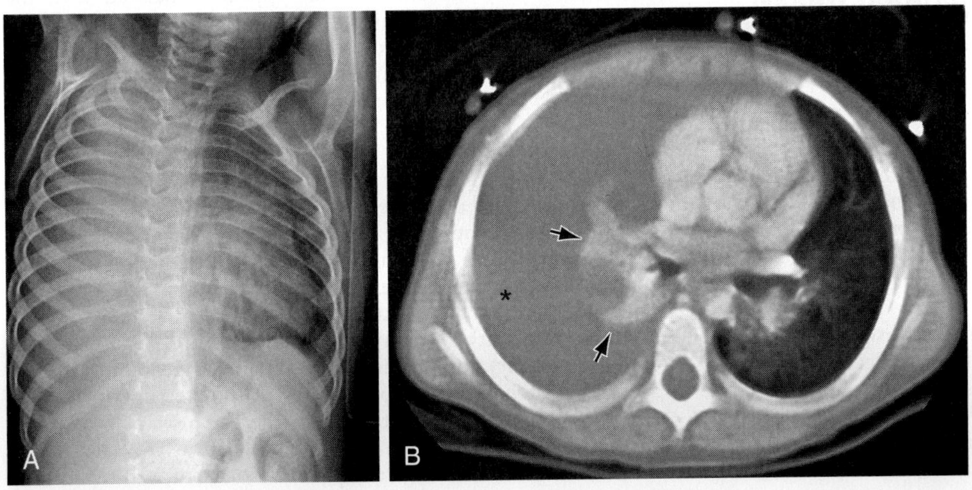

Figure 409-4 Spontaneous chylothorax in a 4 yr old with a duplication of chromosome 6. *A,* Chest radiograph shows opacification of the right thorax. *B,* CT scan shows the chylous pleural effusion (*asterisk*) compressing the atelectatic right lung (*arrows*).

Chapter 410
Bronchopulmonary Dysplasia
Steven Lestrud

Bronchopulmonary dysplasia (BPD) is a syndrome characterized by signs and symptoms of chronic lung disease that originates in the neonatal period (Chapter 95). The pathogenesis of the lung disease was originally thought to arise from mechanical and oxidant injury to the airways and interstitium leading to edema, inflammation, and fibrosis with characteristic radiographic and pathologic stages. The pathogenesis of lung disease in the population of neonates <1000 g also includes the contribution of immature development of airway and vascular structures of the lung. This fact has led to a change in recognized radiographic, pathologic, and clinical findings in BPD and an evolution in its definition. An accepted definition includes an oxygen requirement for 28 days postnatally, and the disorder is graded as mild, moderate or severe on the basis of supplemental oxygen requirement and gestational age (see Table 410-1 on the *Nelson Textbook of Pediatrics* website at www.expertconsult.com).

For the full continuation of this chapter, please visit the Nelson Textbook of Pediatrics *website at www.expertconsult.com.*

Chapter 411
Skeletal Diseases Influencing Pulmonary Function
Steven R. Boas

Pulmonary function is influenced by the structure of the chest wall (Chapter 365). Chest wall abnormalities can lead to restrictive or obstructive pulmonary disease, impaired respiratory muscle strength, and decreased ventilatory performance in response to physical stress. The congenital chest wall deformities include pectus excavatum, pectus carinatum, sternal clefts, Poland syndrome, and skeletal and cartilage dysplasias. Vertebral anomalies such as kyphoscoliosis can alter pulmonary function in children and adolescents.

411.1 Pectus Excavatum (Funnel Chest)
Steven R. Boas

EPIDEMIOLOGY

Pectus excavatum occurs in 1:400 births with a 9:1 male preponderance and accounts for >90% of congenital chest wall anomalies. There is a positive family history in one third of cases.

ETIOLOGY

Midline narrowing of the thoracic cavity is usually an isolated skeletal abnormality. The cause is unknown. Pectus excavatum can occur in isolation or it may be associated with a connective tissue disorder (Marfan [Chapter 693] or Ehlers-Danlos syndrome [Chapter 651]). It may be acquired secondarily to chronic lung disease, neuromuscular disease, or trauma.

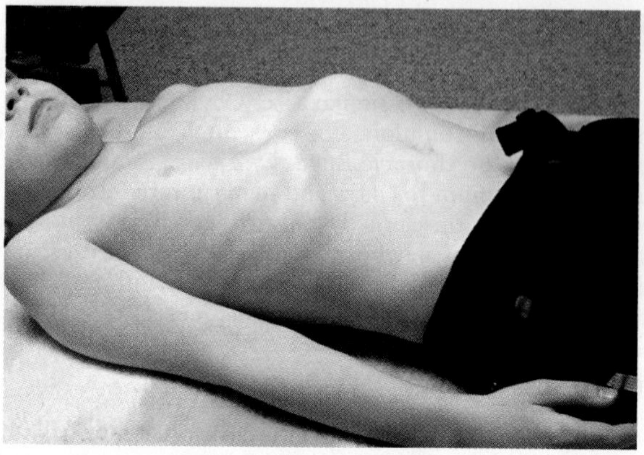

Figure 411-1 Pectus excavatum.

CLINICAL MANIFESTATIONS

The deformity is present at or shortly after birth but is usually not associated with any symptoms at that time. In time, decreased exercise tolerance, fatigue, chest pain, palpitations, recurrent respiratory infections, wheezing, stridor, and cough may be present. Because of the cosmetic nature of this deformity, children may experience significant psychologic stress. Physical examination may reveal sternal depression, protracted shoulders, kyphoscoliosis, inferior rib flares, rib cage rigidity, forward head tilt, scapular winging, and loss of vertebral contours (Fig. 411-1). Patients exhibit paroxysmal sternal motion and a shift of point of maximal impulse to the left. Innocent systolic murmurs may be heard.

LABORATORY FINDINGS

Lateral chest radiograms demonstrate the sternal depression. Use of the Haller index on chest CT (maximal internal transverse diameter of the chest divided by the minimal anteroposterior diameter at the same level) in comparison with age- and gender-appropriate normative values for determining the extent of depression of the chest wall anomaly has become useful in determining the extent of the anatomic abnormality. An electrocardiogram may show a right-axis deviation or Wolff-Parkinson-White syndrome (Chapter 429); an echocardiogram may demonstrate mitral valve prolapse (Chapter 422.3) and ventricular compression. Results of static pulmonary function tests may be normal but commonly show an obstructive defect in the lower airways and, less commonly, a restrictive defect due to abnormal chest wall mechanics. Exercise testing may demonstrate either normal tolerance or limitations from underlying cardiopulmonary dysfunction that appear associated with the severity of the defect. Ventilatory limitations are commonly seen in younger children and adolescents, whereas cardiac limitations secondary to stroke volume impairments are more commonly seen in older adolescents and young adults.

TREATMENT

Treatment is based on the severity of the deformity and the extent of physiologic compromise. Therapeutic options include careful observation, use of physical therapy to address musculoskeletal compromise, and corrective surgery. For patients with significant physiologic compromise, surgical correction may improve the cosmetic deformity and may help minimize or even improve the cardiopulmonary compromise. The 2 main surgical interventions are the Ravitch and Nuss procedures. Although superiority of 1 approach has not been established, there is now >20 years of successful experience with the minimally invasive Nuss procedure. For teenagers with exercise limitations, surgical repair may result in improved exercise tolerance. Normalization of lung perfusion scans and maximal voluntary ventilation have also been observed after surgery. Ongoing treatment to address the secondary musculoskeletal findings is commonly employed before and after the operation.

BIBLIOGRAPHY
Please visit the Nelson Textbook of Pediatrics *website at www.expertconsult.com for the complete bibliography.*

411.2 Pectus Carinatum and Sternal Clefts

Steven R. Boas

PECTUS CARINATUM

Etiology/Epidemiology

Pectus carinatum is a sternal deformity accounting for 5-15% of congenital chest wall anomalies. Anterior displacements of the mid and lower sternum and adjacent costal cartilages are the most common types. They are most commonly associated with protrusion of the upper sternum; depression of the lower sternum occurs in only 15% of patients. Asymmetry of the sternum is common, and localized depression of the lower anterolateral chest is also often observed. Males are affected 4 times more often than females. There is a high familial occurrence and a common association of mild to moderate scoliosis. Mitral valve disease and coarctation of the aorta are associated with this anomaly. Three types of anatomic deformity occur (upper, lower, and lateral pectus carinatum), with corresponding physiologic changes and treatment algorithms.

Clinical Manifestations

In early childhood, symptoms appear minimal. School-aged children and adolescents, however, commonly complain of dyspnea with mild exertion, decreased endurance with exercise, and exercise-induced wheezing. The incidence of increased respiratory infections and use of asthma medication is higher than in nonaffected subjects. On physical examination, a marked increase in the anteroposterior chest diameter is seen, with resultant reduction in chest excursion and expansion. The increased residual volume results in tachypnea and diaphragmatic respirations. Chest radiographs show an increased anteroposterior diameter of the chest wall, emphysematous-appearing lungs, and a narrow cardiac shadow. The pectus severity score (width of chest divided by distance between sternum and spine; analogous to the Haller index) is reduced.

Treatment

For symptomatic patients with pectus carinatum, newer, less invasive surgical correction procedures result in improvement of the clinical symptoms. Surgery is often performed for cosmetic and psychologic reasons.

STERNAL CLEFTS

Sternal clefts are rare congenital malformations that result from the failure of the fusion of the sternum. Partial sternal clefts are more common and may involve the superior sternum in association with other lesions, such as vascular dysplasias and supraumbilical raphe, or the inferior sternal clefts, which are often associated with other midline defects (pentalogy of Cantrell). Complete sternal clefts with complete failure of sternal fusion are rare. These disorders may also occur in isolation. The paradoxic movement of thoracic organs with respiration may alter pulmonary mechanics. Rarely, respiratory infections and even significant compromise result. Surgery is required early in life, before fixation and immobility occur.

BIBLIOGRAPHY
Please visit the Nelson Textbook of Pediatrics *website at www.expertconsult.com for the complete bibliography.*

411.3 Asphyxiating Thoracic Dystrophy (Thoracic-Pelvic-Phalangeal Dystrophy)

Steven R. Boas

PATHOGENESIS

A multisystem autosomal recessive disorder, asphyxiating thoracic dystrophy results in a constricted and narrow rib cage. Also known as Jeune syndrome, the disorder is associated with a characteristic skeletal abnormalities as well as variable involvement of other systems, including renal, hepatic, neurologic, pancreatic, and retinal abnormalities. Several genetic loci have been identified in affected individuals.

CLINICAL MANIFESTATIONS

Most patients with this disorder die shortly after birth from respiratory failure, although less aggressive forms have been reported in older children. For those who survive the neonatal period, progressive respiratory failure often ensues, owing to impaired lung growth, recurrent pneumonia, and atelectasis originating from the rigid chest wall.

DIAGNOSIS

Physical examination reveals a narrowed thorax that, at birth, is much smaller than the head circumference. The ribs are horizontal, and the child has short extremities. Chest radiographs demonstrate a bell-shaped chest cage with short, horizontal, flaring ribs and high clavicles.

TREATMENT

No specific treatment exists, although thoracoplasty to enlarge the chest wall and long-term mechanical ventilation have been tried. Rib-expanding procedures have resulted in improved survival.

PROGNOSIS

For some children with asphyxiating thoracic dystrophy, improvement in the bony abnormalities occurs with age. However, children <1 yr old often succumb to respiratory infection and failure. Progressive renal disease often occurs with older children. Use of vaccines for influenza and other respiratory pathogens is warranted, as is aggressive use of antibiotics for respiratory infections.

BIBLIOGRAPHY
Please visit the Nelson Textbook of Pediatrics *website at www.expertconsult.com for the complete bibliography.*

411.4 Achondroplasia

Steven R. Boas

Achondroplasia is the most common condition characterized by disproportionate short stature. This condition is inherited as an autosomal dominant disorder that results in disordered growth (Chapter 687). Much has been learned about this disorder, including its genetic origins and how to minimize its serious complications.

CLINICAL MANIFESTATIONS

Restrictive pulmonary disease, affecting <5% of children with achondroplasia who are younger than 3 yr, is more likely at high elevation. Recurrent infections, cor pulmonale, and dyspnea are commonly associated. There is an increased risk of obstructive sleep apnea, although most patients are not affected. Hypoxemia during sleep is a common feature. Onset of restrictive lung disease can begin at a very young age. On examination, the breathing pattern is rapid and shallow, with associated abdominal breathing. The anteroposterior diameter of the thorax is reduced. Special growth curves for chest circumference of patients with achondroplasia from birth to 7 yr are available. **Three distinct phenotypes** exist: phenotypic group 1 patients possess relative adenotonsillar hypertrophy, group 2 patients have muscular upper airway obstruction and progressive hydrocephalus, and group 3 patients have upper airway obstruction without hydrocephalus. Kyphoscoliosis may develop during infancy.

DIAGNOSIS

Pulmonary function tests reveal a reduced vital capacity that is more pronounced in males. The lungs are small but functionally normal. Chest radiographs demonstrate the decreased anteroposterior diameter along with anterior cupping of the ribs. The degree of foramen magnum involvement correlates with the extent of respiratory dysfunction.

TREATMENT

Treatment of sleep apnea, if present, is supportive (Chapter 17). Physiotherapy and bracing may minimize the complications of both kyphosis and severe lordosis. Aggressive treatment of respiratory infections and scoliosis is warranted.

PROGNOSIS

The life span is normal for most children with this condition, except for the phenotypic groups with hydrocephalus or with severe cervical or lumbar spinal compression.

BIBLIOGRAPHY

Please visit the Nelson Textbook of Pediatrics *website at www.expertconsult.com for the complete bibliography.*

411.5 Kyphoscoliosis: Adolescent Idiopathic Scoliosis and Congenital Scoliosis

Steven R. Boas

PATHOGENESIS

Adolescent idiopathic scoliosis (AIS) is characterized by lateral bending of the spine (Chapter 671). It commonly affects children during their teen years as well as during periods of rapid growth. The cause is unknown. Congenital scoliosis is uncommon, affecting girls more than boys, and is apparent in the 1st year of life (Chapter 671.2).

CLINICAL MANIFESTATIONS

The pulmonary manifestations of scoliosis may include chest wall restriction, leading to a reduction in total lung capacity. The angle of scoliosis deformity has been correlated with the degree of lung impairment only for patients with thoracic curves. Vital capacity, forced expiratory volume in 1 sec (FEV_1), work capacity, diffusion capacity, chest wall compliance, and Pao_2 decrease as the severity of thoracic curve increases. These findings can be seen in even mild to moderate AIS (Cobb angle <30 degrees) but do not occur in other, nonthoracic curves. Reduction in peripheral muscle function has been associated with AIS through either intrinsic mechanisms or deconditioning. Severe impairment can lead to cor pulmonale or respiratory failure and can occur before age 20 yr. Children with severe scoliosis, especially boys, may have abnormalities of breathing during sleep, and the resultant periods of hypoxemia may contribute to the eventual development of pulmonary hypertension.

DIAGNOSIS

Physical examination and an upright, posteroanterior radiograph with subsequent measurement of the angle of curvature (Cobb technique) remain the gold standard for assessment. Curves >10 degrees define the presence of scoliosis.

TREATMENT

Depending on the extent of the curve and the degree of skeletal maturation, treatment options include reassurance, observation, bracing, and surgery (spinal fusion). Influenza vaccine should be administered, given the extent of pulmonary compromise that may coexist. Because vital capacity is a strong predictor for the development of respiratory failure in untreated AIS, surgical goals are to diminish the scoliotic curve, maintain the correction, and prevent deterioration in pulmonary function. Abnormalities of vital capacity and total lung capacity, exercise intolerance, and the rate of change of these variables over time should be taken into consideration for the timing of surgical correction. Preoperative assessment of lung function may assist in predicting postsurgical pulmonary difficulties. Many patients undergoing surgical correction may be managed postoperatively without mechanical ventilation. Even patients with mild scoliosis may have pulmonary compromise immediately after spinal fusion, secondary to pain and a body cast that may restrict breathing and interfere with coughing. Children with a preoperative FEV_1 <40% predicted are at risk for requiring prolonged postoperative mechanical ventilation. Rib-expanding procedures have been successful in severe cases of congenital scoliosis.

BIBLIOGRAPHY

Please visit the Nelson Textbook of Pediatrics *website at www.expertconsult.com for the complete bibliography.*

411.6 Congenital Rib Anomalies

Steven R. Boas

CLINICAL MANIFESTATIONS

Isolated defects of the highest and lowest ribs have minimal clinical pulmonary consequences. Missing midthoracic ribs are associated with the absence of the pectoralis muscle, and lung function can become compromised. Associated kyphoscoliosis and hemivertebrae may accompany this defect. If the rib defect is small, no significant sequelae ensue. When the 2nd to 5th ribs are absent anteriorly, lung herniation and significant abnormal respiration ensue. The lung is soft and nontender and may be easily reducible on examination. Complicating sequelae include severe lung restriction (secondary to scoliosis), cor pulmonale, and congestive heart failure. Symptoms are often minimal but can cause dyspnea. Respiratory distress is rare in infancy.

DIAGNOSIS

Chest radiographs demonstrate the deformation and absence of ribs with secondary scoliosis. Most rib abnormalities are discovered as incidental findings on a chest film.

TREATMENT

If symptoms are severe enough to cause clinical compromise or significant lung herniation, then homologous rib grafting can be performed. Rib-expanding procedures are also of great value. Adolescent girls with congenital rib anomalies may require cosmetic breast surgery.

BIBLIOGRAPHY

Please visit the Nelson Textbook of Pediatrics *website at www.expertconsult.com for the complete bibliography.*

Chapter 412 Chronic Severe Respiratory Insufficiency

Zehava Noah and Cynthia Etzler Budek

Improvements in the treatment of acute respiratory failure and advancements in invasive and noninvasive ventilation have led to an increase in the number of pediatric patients receiving long-term mechanical ventilation. Infants, children, and adolescents with disorders of central control of breathing, disease of the airways, residual lung disease after severe respiratory illness, and neuromuscular disorders may experience hypercarbic and/or hypoxemic chronic respiratory failure. Although it is generally possible to identify a primary cause for the respiratory failure, many children have multiple causative factors. **Chronic respiratory failure** is pulmonary insufficiency for a protracted period, usually 28 days or longer. Patients are maintained on long-term ventilation until they recover from the initial pulmonary insult. Patients with conditions such as central hypoventilation, progressive neuromuscular disease, and high quadriplegia may need ventilatory support indefinitely. The preferred site for a patient's care after initial discharge with a ventilator is within the family home. When social circumstances do not allow this placement, patients may be placed in a highly skilled nursing facility.

Less than 1% of patients admitted to pediatric intensive care units require long-term noninvasive or invasive ventilatory assistance. A survey from Massachusetts by Graham, Fleegler, and Robinson (2007) identified 197 children undergoing long-term ventilatory support, a threefold increase over a 15-year period. The majority of the primary diagnoses (54%) were congenital or perinatal-acquired neurologic or neuromuscular disorders. Chronic lung disease of prematurity represented only 7% of the sample, a significant shift downward, presumably a result of improvement in neonatal care over the same period. Seventy percent of the patients were cared for at home.

412.1 Neuromuscular Diseases

Zehava Noah and Cynthia Etzler Budek

Neuromuscular diseases (NMDs) of childhood include muscular dystrophies, metabolic and congenital myopathies, anterior horn cell disorders, peripheral neuropathies, and diseases that affect the neuromuscular junction. Decreases in muscle strength and endurance resulting from neuromuscular disorders can affect any skeletal muscle, including muscles involved in respiratory function. Of particular concern are those muscles mediating upper airway patency, generation of cough, and lung inflation. Acute respiratory insufficiency is often the most prominent clinical manifestation of several acute neuromuscular disorders, such as high-level spinal cord injury, poliomyelitis, Guillain-Barré syndrome (Chapter 608), and botulism (Chapter 202). Although much more insidious in its clinical course, respiratory dysfunction constitutes the leading cause of morbidity and mortality in progressive neuromuscular disorders (e.g., Duchenne muscular dystrophy [Chapter 601], spinal muscular atrophy, congenital myotonic dystrophy, myasthenia gravis [Chapter 604], and Charcot-Marie-Tooth disease [Chapter 605]).

Two of the most common and best understood NMDs of childhood are **Duchenne muscular dystrophy** (DMD) and **spinal muscular atrophy** (SMA). Principles utilized to evaluate and treat respiratory insufficiency in these disorders are often based on medical consensus rather than research. Despite this limitation, these principles are useful in the management of DMD and SMA as well as other less common NMDs.

PATHOGENESIS

Early onset of NMD can lead to chest wall deformity and lung disease due to developmental factors. In infancy the chest wall is very compliant with relatively stiff lungs and small airways. With progressive weakness of the intercostal muscles, the chest wall becomes even more compliant. Small airways have a tendency to become obstructed, leading to micro-atelectasis and decreased functional residual capacity. The compliant chest wall with initial sparing of diaphragm function leads to development of a small bell-shaped chest with depressed sternum, protruding abdomen, and paradoxical breathing, typically seen in SMA type 1. As the disease progresses, chest wall muscles shorten and lose elasticity, costosternal and costovertebral joints contract, and lung volumes decrease as a result of severe hypotonia. Inspiratory and expiratory pressures decrease, expiratory pressures more so than inspiratory, causing ineffective cough and poor airway clearance. As the child with NMD ages, kyphoscoliosis commonly develops, increasing the severity of restrictive lung disease. Although central control of breathing remains normal, response to central chemoreceptors may decrease because of chronic hypercapnia.

TREATMENT

Even though gene-targeted therapies are being developed for some NMDs, current interventions are primarily supportive rather than curative. Close surveillance through periodic review of the history and physical examination is critical. The development of personality changes, such as irritability, decreased attention span, fatigue, and somnolence, may point to the presence of sleep-associated gas exchange abnormalities and sleep fragmentation. Changes in speech and voice characteristics, nasal flaring, and the use of other accessory muscles during quiet breathing at rest may provide sensitive indicators of progressive muscle dysfunction and respiratory compromise. Although the frequency of periodic re-evaluation needs to be tailored to the individual patient, tentative guidelines were developed for patients with DMD; an abbreviated summary of such recommendations, applicable to all children with NMDs, is provided in Table 412-1.

Guidelines for evaluation and management of patients with SMA were developed on the basis of expert consensus. Four classifications of SMA, based on age of onset and level of function, are recognized (Table 412-2). Treatment of SMA is focused on level of function (non-sitter, sitter, or walker) rather than SMA type. Unlike patients with DMD, patients with SMA do not demonstrate correlation between pulmonary function and need for mechanical ventilatory support. Rather, longitudinal

Table 412-1 PROPOSED GUIDELINES FOR INITIAL EVALUATION AND FOLLOW-UP OF PATIENTS WITH NEUROMUSCULAR DISEASE

INITIAL EVALUATION	BASIC INTERVENTION/TRAINING
History/physical/anthropometrics	Nutritional consultation and guidance
Lung function and maximal respiratory pressures (PFTs)	Regular chest physiotherapy
Arterial blood gases	Use of percussive devices
Polysomnography*	Respiratory muscle training
Exercise testing (in selected cases)	Annual influenza vaccine
If vital capacity >60% predicted or maximal respiratory pressures >60 cm H_2O	Evaluate PFTs every 6 mo
	CXR and polysomnography every year
If vital capacity <60% predicted or maximal respiratory pressures <60 cm H_2O	Evaluate PFTs every 3-4 mo
	CXR, MIP/MEP every 6 mo
	Polysomnography every 6 mo to every year

CXR, chest x-ray; MEP, maximal expiratory pressure; MIP, maximal inspiratory pressure; PFT, pulmonary function test.
*Please note that if polysomnography is not readily available, multichannel recordings including oronasal airflow, nocturnal oximetry, and end-tidal carbon dioxide levels may provide an adequate alternative.

Table 412-2 CLINICAL CLASSIFICATION OF SPINAL MUSCULAR ATROPHY (SMA)

SMA TYPE	AGE OF ONSET	HIGHEST FUNCTION	NATURAL AGE OF DEATH
Type 1 (severe)	0-6 mo	Never sits	<2 yr
Type 2 (intermediate)	7-18 mo	Never stands	<2 yr
Type 3 (mild)	>18 mo	Stands and walks	Adult
Type 4 (adult)	Second or third decade	Walks during adult years	Adult

From Wang CH, Finkel RS, Bertini ES, et al: Consensus statement for standard of care in spinal muscular atrophy, *J Child Neurol* 22:1027–1049, 2007.

monitoring for signs and symptoms of sleep-disordered breathing and ineffective airway clearance should be utilized to direct patient care.

BIBLIOGRAPHY

Please visit the Nelson Textbook of Pediatrics *website at www.expertconsult.com for the complete bibliography.*

412.2 Congenital Central Hypoventilation Syndrome

Zehava Noah, Cynthia Etzler Budek, Pallavi P. Patwari, and Debra E. Weese-Mayer

Congenital central hypoventilation syndrome (CCHS) is a clinically complex disorder of respiratory and autonomic regulation. In the classic case of CCHS, symptoms of alveolar hypoventilation are manifest during sleep only, but in more severe cases, the symptoms are manifest during sleep and wakefulness. The classic syndrome is further characterized by ventilatory failure to respond to hypercarbia and hypoxemia during wakefulness and sleep as well as physiologic and/or anatomic autonomic nervous system (ANS) dysregulation (ANSD). The physiologic ANSD may include all organ systems affected by the ANS, specifically the respiratory, cardiac, sudomotor, ophthalmologic, neurologic, enteric systems, and more. The anatomic or structural ANSD in CCHS includes Hirschsprung disease and tumors of neural crest origin (neuroblastoma, ganglioneuroma, or ganglioneuroblastoma). Most patients with CCHS present in the neonatal period, although later-onset CCHS (LO-CCHS) may manifest in infancy, childhood, and even adulthood. The initial symptoms include diminished tidal volume and a typically monotonous respiratory rate with cyanosis and hypercarbia. Diagnosis and management of children with CCHS have improved considerably, owing to greater knowledge in genetic testing, comprehensive care, and availability of technology for the home.

GENETICS

In 2003, the paired-like homeobox 2B (*PHOX2B*) gene was identified as the disease-defining gene for CCHS. This gene, which is essential to the embryologic development of the ANS from the neural crest, is expressed in key regions that explain much of the CCHS phenotype. Individuals with CCHS are heterozygous for either a polyalanine repeat expansion mutation (PARM) in exon 3 of the *PHOX2B* gene (normal number of alanines is 20 with normal genotype 20/20), such that individuals with CCHS have 24-33 alanines on the affected allele (genotype range is 20/24-20/33), or a non–polyalanine repeat expansion mutation (NPARM) resulting from a missense, nonsense, or frameshift mutation. Roughly 90% of the cases of CCHS have PARMs and the remaining ≈10% of cases have NPARMs. The specific type of *PHOX2B* mutation is clinically significant as it can help with anticipatory guidance in patient management.

The majority of CCHS cases occur because of a *de novo PHOX2B* mutation, but 5-10% of children with CCHS inherit the mutation from an asymptomatic parent who is mosaic for the *PHOX2B* mutation. CCHS is inherited in an autosomal dominant manner. Therefore, an individual with CCHS has a 50% chance of transmitting the mutation, and resulting disease phenotype, to each child. Mosaic parents have up to a 50% chance of transmitting the *PHOX2B* mutation to each offspring. Genetic counseling is essential for family planning and for preparedness in the delivery room for an anticipated CCHS birth. *PHOX2B* testing is advised for both parents of a child with CCHS to anticipate risk of recurrence in subsequent pregnancies. Further, prenatal testing for *PHOX2B* mutation is clinically available (*www.genetests.org*) for families with a known *PHOX2B* mutation.

Ventilator Dependence

A correlation between the *PHOX2B* genotype and ventilator dependence has been reported. The greater the number of extra alanines, the more likely the need for continuous ventilatory support. Thus patients with the 20/25 genotype seldom require awake ventilatory support, although they do require support during sleep. Patients with the 20/26 genotype have variable awake support needs, and patients with 20/27-20/33 genotypes and those with NPARMs are likely to need continuous ventilatory support.

Hirschsprung Disease (Chapter 324.3)

Overall, 20% of children with CCHS also have Hirschsprung disease, and any infant or child with CCHS who presents with constipation should undergo rectal biopsy to screen for absence of ganglion cells. The type of *PHOX2B* mutation can help the primary physician anticipate which children are at higher risk. The frequency of Hirschsprung disease seems to increase with the longer polyalanine tracts (genotypes 20/27-20/33) and in those with NPARMs. Thus far no children with the 20/25 genotype have been reported to have Hirschsprung disease.

Tumors of Neural Crest Origin

Tumors of neural crest origin are more frequent in patients with NPARMs (50%) than in those with PARMs (1%). These extracranial tumors are more often neuroblastomas in individuals with NPARMs, rather than ganglioneuromas and ganglioneuroblastomas, which have been reported in patients with longer PARMs (20/29 and 20/33 genotype only).

Cardiac Asystole

Transient, abrupt, and prolonged sinus pauses have been identified in patients with CCHS, necessitating implantation of cardiac pacemakers when the pauses are ≥3 seconds. Among patients with the *PHOX2B* genotypes, 19% of those with the 20/26 genotype and 83% of those with the 20/27 genotype have pauses in the heartbeat of 3 sec or longer. Children with the 20/25 genotype have not been noted to have prolonged asystole, though one adult diagnosed with LO-CCHS has demonstrated a prolonged asystole.

Autonomic Nervous System Dysregulation

A higher number of polyalanine repeats among the PARMs is associated with an increased number of physiologic symptoms of ANSD. A higher frequency of anatomic ANSD findings is seen in individuals with CCHS who have NPARMs than in those who have PARMs. In addition, there is a spectrum of physiologic ANSD symptoms, including decreased heart rate variability, esophageal/gastric/colonic dysmotility, decreased pupillary response to light, reduced basal body temperature, altered distribution and amount of diaphoresis, lack of perception of shortness of breath, and altered perception of anxiety.

Facial Phenotype

Children with CCHS and PARMs have a characteristic faciès that is boxy in appearance, flattened on profile, and short relative to its width. The following five variables correctly predict 86% of CCHS cases: upper lip height, binocular width, upper facial height, nasal tip protrusion, and inferior inflection of the upper lip vermillion border (lip trait).

Neuropathology

Anatomic findings in the brains of individuals with CCHS from early MRI studies were unremarkable, and those from autopsies were inconsistent. In a small cohort of adolescents with suspected CCHS, though without *PHOX2B* mutation confirmation, neuropathologic brainstem changes were identified by diffusion tensor imaging (DTI) in structures known to mediate central chemosensitivity and to link a network of cardiovascular, respiratory, and affective responses. The neuroanatomic defects in CCHS are likely the result of focal *PHOX2B* (mis)expression coupled with, in the suboptimally managed patient, sequelae of recurrent hypoxemia/hypercarbia. On the basis of rodent studies and functional MRI (fMRI) in humans, the following regions pertinent to respiratory control show *PHOX2B* expression in the pons and medulla of the brainstem: locus coeruleus, dorsal respiratory group, nucleus ambiguus, parafacial respiratory group, among other areas. Physiologic evidence suggests that the respiratory failure in these children is mostly based on defects in central mechanisms, but peripheral mechanisms (mainly carotid bodies) are also important.

Patients with CCHS have deficient carbon dioxide sensitivity during wakefulness and sleep; they do not respond with increased ventilation or arousal to hypercarbia during sleep. During wakefulness, a subset of patients may respond sufficiently to avoid hypercarbia, but most individuals with CCHS have hypoventilation that is severe enough that hypercarbia is apparent in the resting awake state. Children with CCHS also have altered sensitivity to hypoxia while awake and asleep. A key feature of CCHS is the lack of respiratory distress or sense of asphyxia with physiologic compromise. This lack of responsiveness to hypercarbia and/or hypoxemia with subsequent respiratory failure does not improve with advancing age. A subset of older children with CCHS may show an increase in ventilation (specifically increase in respiratory rate rather than increase in tidal volume) when they are exercised at various work rates, a response that is possibly secondary to neural reflexes from rhythmic limb movements—although the increase in minute ventilation is often insufficient to avoid physiologic compromise.

CLINICAL MANIFESTATIONS

Patients with CCHS usually present in the first few hours after birth. Most children are the products of uneventful pregnancies and are term infants with appropriate weight for gestational age; Apgar scores have been variable. They do not show signs of respiratory distress, but their shallow respirations and respiratory pauses (apnea) evolve to respiratory failure with apparent cyanosis in the first day of life. In neonates with CCHS, the $Pa{CO_2}$ accumulates during sleep to very high levels, sometimes >90 mm Hg, and may decline to normal levels after the infants awaken. This problem becomes most apparent with failure of multiple attempts at extubation in an intubated neonate (who appears well with ventilatory support but in whom respiratory failure develops after removal of the support). However, the more severely affected infants hypoventilate awake and asleep; thus the previously described difference in $Pa{CO_2}$ between states is not apparent. Often, the respiratory rate is higher in rapid eye movement (REM) sleep than in non-REM sleep in individuals with CCHS.

LO-CCHS should be suspected in infants, children, and adults who have unexplained hypoventilation, especially subsequent to the use of anesthetic agents, sedation, acute respiratory illness, and potentially treated obstructive sleep apnea. These individuals may have other evidence of chronic hypoventilation, including pulmonary hypertension, polycythemia, and elevated bicarbonate concentration.

Besides treatment for these respiratory symptoms, children with CCHS require comprehensive evaluation and coordinated care to optimally manage associated abnormalities such as Hirschsprung disease, tumors of neural crest origin, symptoms of physiologic ANSD, and cardiac asystole, among other findings.

DIFFERENTIAL DIAGNOSIS

Studies should be performed to rule out primary neuromuscular, lung, and cardiac disease as well as an identifiable brainstem lesion that could account for the constellation of symptoms characteristic of CCHS. Introduction of clinically available *PHOX2B* genetic testing allows for early and definitive diagnosis of CCHS. Because CCHS mimics many treatable and/or genetic diseases, the following disorders should be considered: X-linked myotubular myopathy, multiminicore disease, congenital myasthenic syndrome, altered airway or intrathoracic anatomy (diagnosis made with bronchoscopy and chest CT), diaphragm dysfunction (diagnosis made with diaphragm fluoroscopy), congenital cardiac disease, a structural hindbrain or brainstem abnormality (diagnosis made with MRI of the brain and brainstem), Möbius syndrome (diagnosis made with MRI of the brain and brainstem and neurologic examination), and specific metabolic diseases, such as Leigh syndrome, pyruvate dehydrogenase deficiency, and discrete carnitine deficiency.

Rapid-Onset Obesity with Hypothalamic Dysfunction, Hypoventilation, and Autonomic Dysregulation

Previously referred to as late-onset central hypoventilation syndrome with hypothalamic dysfunction (LO-CHS/HD), rapid-onset obesity with hypothalamic dysfunction, hypoventilation, and autonomic dysregulation (ROHHAD) is a very rare disorder that was renamed in 2007 to clarify that it is distinct from LO-CCHS. The acronym is intended to describe the general sequence of presenting symptoms, which can evolve over years. Most dramatic is that these children are seemingly normal, and then demonstrate rapid weight gain (often >20 lb), which occurs within 6-12 mo. The diagnosis is based on clinical criteria that include onset of obesity and alveolar hypoventilation after the age of 1.5 yr (typically between 1.5 and 7 yr) and evidence of hypothalamic dysfunction as defined by ≥1 of the following findings: rapid-onset obesity, hyperprolactinemia, central hypothyroidism, disordered water balance, failure of response to growth hormone stimulation, corticotropin deficiency, and delayed/precocious puberty. Though it may not be apparent early in the course, all children with ROHHAD have hypoventilation. Considering the high prevalence of cardiorespiratory arrest and multisystem involvement, children with this disorder require coordinated comprehensive care with attention to development of hypoventilation (such as with repeated sleep studies and initiation of supported ventilation), bradycardia (via Holter monitor), treatment of hypothalamic dysfunction (with involvement of an endocrinologist), tumors of neural crest origin (often ganglioneuromas or ganglioneuroblastomas), and behavioral/intellectual decline (with annual neurocognitive testing).

Although children with ROHHAD can present with obstructive sleep apnea after development of obesity, it is distinct from obstructive sleep apnea hypoventilation syndrome (OSAHS) and obesity hypoventilation syndrome (OHS). In children, the existence of OHS is controversial and is often referred to as OSAHS because it describes chronic obstructive sleep apnea with resulting overnight hypercarbia, hypoxemia, and frequent arousals that lead to an altered set point of the central control of breathing (insensitivity to hypercarbia). Therefore, children with OSAHS experience awake hypoventilation and daytime sleepiness. The management is simply relief of the obstruction, such as tonsillectomy and/or initiation of noninvasive ventilation. If these interventions are unsuccessful, tracheostomy must be considered. In children with OSAHS, treatment of the upper airway obstruction would be expected to result in complete resolution of hypoventilation and daytime sleepiness. In contrast, in children with ROHHAD, relief of the upper airway obstruction unveils the central alveolar hypoventilation that requires lifelong ventilatory support. Both are distinguished from LO-CCHS by the absence of *PHOX2B* mutation and the presence of (often morbid) obesity.

MANAGEMENT

Supported Ventilation—Diaphragm Pacing

Depending on the severity of respiratory control deficit, the child with CCHS can have various means of ventilatory support: noninvasive positive pressure ventilation or mechanical ventilation via tracheostomy (see later section on long-term mechanical ventilation). Diaphragm pacing offers another mode of supported ventilation; it involves bilateral surgical implantation of electrodes beneath the phrenic nerves, with connecting wires to subcutaneously implanted receivers. The external transmitter, which is much smaller and lighter than a ventilator, sends a signal to donut-shaped antennae that are placed on the skin, over the subcutaneously implanted receivers. A signal can now travel from the external transmitter, ultimately, to the phrenic nerve to stimulate contraction of the diaphragm. A tracheostomy is typically required, at least initially, because the pacers induce a negative pressure on inspiration as a result of the contraction of the diaphragm being unopposed by pharyngeal dilatation. Individuals with CCHS who are ventilator dependent 24 hr/day are ideal candidates for diaphragm pacing, which provides increased ambulatory freedom (without the "ventilator tether") while they are awake and mechanical ventilator support while they are asleep. This balance between awake pacing and asleep mechanical ventilation allows for a rest from phrenic nerve stimulation at night.

Monitoring in the Home

Home monitoring for children with CCHS is distinctly different from and more conservative than that for other children requiring long-term ventilation because children with CCHS lack innate ventilatory and arousal responses to hypoxemia and hypercarbia. In the event of physiologic compromise, other children likely are able to show clinical signs of respiratory distress. By contrast, for children with CCHS, the only means of determining adequate ventilation and oxygenation is with objective measures from a pulse oximeter, end-tidal carbon dioxide monitor, and close supervision of these values by a trained registered nurse (RN). At a minimum, it is essential that individuals with CCHS have continuous monitoring with pulse oximetry and end-tidal carbon dioxide with RN supervision during all sleep time, but ideally 24 hr per day. While awake, they are not able to sense or adequately respond to a respiratory challenge as may occur with ensuing respiratory illness, increased activity, or even the simple activity of eating.

BIBLIOGRAPHY

Please visit the Nelson Textbook of Pediatrics *website at www.expertconsult.com for the complete bibliography.*

412.3 Other Conditions

Zehava Noah and Cynthia Etzler Budek

MYELOMENINGOCELE WITH ARNOLD-CHIARI TYPE II MALFORMATION

Arnold-Chiari type II malformation (Chapter 585.11) is associated with myelomeningocele, hydrocephalus, and herniation of the cerebellar tonsils, caudal brainstem, and the fourth ventricle through the foramen magnum.

Sleep-disordered breathing, including obstructive sleep apnea and hypoventilation, has been reported. Direct pressure on the respiratory centers or brainstem nuclei, or increased intracranial pressure because of the hydrocephalus may be responsible. Vocal cord paralysis, apnea, hypoventilation, and bradyarrhythmias have also been reported.

Patients with Arnold-Chiari type II malformation have blunted responses to hypercapnia, and to a lesser degree, hypoxia.

Management

An acute change in the ventilatory state of a patient with this malformation requires immediate evaluation. Consideration must be given to posterior fossa decompression and/or treatment of the hydrocephalus. If this treatment is unsuccessful in resolving central hypoventilation or apnea, tracheostomy and long-term mechanical ventilation should be considered.

RAPID-ONSET OBESITY, HYPOTHALAMIC DYSFUNCTION, AND AUTONOMIC DYSREGULATION (CHAPTER 412.2)

Obesity Hypoventilation Syndrome

As its name implies, obesity hypoventilation syndrome is a syndrome of central hypoventilation during wakefulness in obese patients with sleep-disordered breathing. Although it was initially described mainly in adult obese patients, obese children have also demonstrated the syndrome. Sleep-disordered breathing is a combination of obstructive sleep apnea, hypopnea, and/or sleep hypoventilation syndrome. Patients are hypercapnic with cognitive impairment, morning headache, and hypersomnolence during the day. Chronic hypoxemia may lead to pulmonary hypertension and cor pulmonale.

Obesity is associated with reduced respiratory system compliance, increased airway resistance, reduced functional residual capacity, and increased work of breathing. Affected patients are unable to increase their respiratory drive in response to hypercapnia. Leptin may have a role in this syndrome. The sleep-disordered breathing leads to compensatory metabolic alkalosis. Because of the long half-life of bicarbonate, its elevation causes compensatory respiratory acidosis during wakefulness with elevated Pa_{CO_2}.

MANAGEMENT The use of continuous positive airway pressure (CPAP) during sleep may be sufficient for many patients. Patients with hypoxemia may require bilevel positive airway pressure (BiPAP) and supplemental oxygen. Tracheostomy may be considered for patients who do not tolerate mask ventilation.

ACQUIRED ALVEOLAR HYPOVENTILATION

Traumatic, ischemic, and inflammatory injuries to the brainstem, brainstem infarction, brain tumors, bulbar polio, and viral paraneoplastic encephalitis may also result in central hypoventilation.

OBSTRUCTIVE SLEEP APNEA

Epidemiology

Habitual snoring during sleep is extremely common during childhood, and up to 27% of children are affected. The current obesity epidemic has affected the epidemiology of this condition. Peak prevalence is at 2-8 yr. The ratio between habitual snoring and obstructive sleep apnea (OSA) is 4:1 to 6:1.

Pathophysiology

OSA occurs when the luminal cross-sectional area of the upper airway is significantly reduced during inspiration. With increased airway resistance and reduced activation of pharyngeal dilators, negative pressure leads to upper airway collapse. The site of upper airway closure in children with OSA is at the level of tonsils and adenoids. The size of tonsils and adenoids increases throughout childhood up to 12 yr of age. Environmental irritants such as cigarette smoke or allergic rhinitis may accelerate the process. Reports now suggest that early viral infections may affect adenotonsillar proliferation.

Clinical Presentation

Snoring during sleep, behavioral disturbances, learning difficulties, excessive daytime sleepiness, metabolic issues, and cardiovascular morbidity may alert the parent or physician to the presence of OSA.

Diagnosis is made with the help of a polysomnogram and airway radiograms.

Treatment

When adenotonsillar hypertrophy is suspected, a consultation with an ear, nose, and throat specialist for adenoid tonsillectomy may be indicated. For patients who are not candidates for this treatment or who persist with OSA, CPAP or BiPAP during sleep may alleviate the obstruction (Chapter 17).

SPINAL CORD INJURY (SCI)

Epidemiology

Spinal cord injury (SCI) occurs at a rate of 30-40 per million population per year, resulting in 10,000 new cases each year. Spinal cord injury is relatively rare in pediatric patients, with an incidence of 1-13% of all SCI patients. The incidence in infancy and early childhood is similar for boys and girls. There is male preponderance in children >13 yr of age. Motor vehicle accidents, falls, sports injuries, and assaults are the main causes. SCI usually leads to lifelong disability.

Pathophysiology

In children with SCI there is disproportionately higher involvement of the upper cervical spine, a high frequency of spinal cord injury without radiographic abnormality, delayed onset of neurologic deficits, and a higher proportion of complete injury. Sixty percent of pediatric SCI cases involve C1-C3 and 30-40% involve C4-C7. Thus, there is a high likelihood in a child with SCI of quadriplegia with intercostal muscle and/or diaphragmatic paralysis leading to respiratory failure.

Management

Immobilization and stabilization of the spine must be accomplished simultaneously with resuscitation and stabilization. Patients with high SCI in many instances require lifelong ventilation. Depending on the patient's age and general condition, tracheostomy with mechanical ventilation or diaphragmatic pacing may be indicated. Often patients with diaphragmatic pacing need tracheostomy placement if there is no coordination between pacing and glottis opening. Muscle spasms occur frequently in these patients and are treated with muscle relaxants. Occasionally the muscle spasms involve the chest and present a serious impediment to ventilation. Continuous intrathecal infusion of muscle relaxant may be indicated (Chapter 598.5).

METABOLIC DISEASE

Mucopolysaccharidoses (Chapter 82)

Mucopolysaccharidoses (MPSs) are a group of progressive hereditary disorders that lack the lysosomal enzymes that degrade glycosaminoglycans. Incompletely catabolized mucopolysaccharides accumulate in connective tissue throughout the body. The incidence is 1:30,000 to 1:150,000 live births. The inheritance is autosomal recessive except for Hunt syndrome, which is X-linked. The diagnosis is suggested by a pattern of glycosaminuria and is confirmed by a lysosomal enzyme assay.

I-cell disease mucolipidosis type II is an inherited lysosomal disorder with accumulation of mucolipids. Phenotypically, it is similar to MPS but the age of onset is earlier and there is no mucopolysacchariduria.

Mucopolysaccharide deposits are frequently found in the head and neck and cause airway obstruction. Typically, the affected patient has a coarse face and large tongue. Significant deposits are found in the adenoids, tonsils, and cartilage. A polysomnogram and airway radiograms may help define the severity of the upper airway obstruction.

Treatment has been attempted with enzyme replacement therapy and stem cell transplantation, with limited success. Adenoidotonsillectomy may be indicated but seldom solves the problem. Noninvasive positive end expiratory pressure or ventilation may be helpful. Tracheostomy may be indicated with CPAP or ventilatory support.

Dysplasias

Camptomelic dysplasia and thanatophoric dysplasia affect rib cage size, shape, and compliance, leading to respiratory failure. Most patients with these disorders do not survive beyond early infancy. Tracheostomy and ventilation may prolong life.

Lung Disease

Common metabolic lung conditions include bronchopulmonary dysplasia (BPD) and recuperation from acute respiratory distress syndrome (ARDS). Former premature infants recuperating from respiratory distress syndrome may experience BPD (Chapters 95.3 and 410). Volutrauma, barotrauma, and air leak syndromes incurred during mechanical ventilation contribute to lung injury. When extreme, BPD may progress to respiratory failure. Increased pulmonary vascular resistance, pulmonary hypertension, cor pulmonale, and lower airway obstruction are known complications.

Treatment of patients with these conditions may include mechanical ventilation, diuretics, bronchodilators, inhaled steroids, intermittent systemic steroids, and pulmonary vasodilators.

Glycogenosis Type II (Chapter 81.1)

Glycogenosis type II is an autosomal recessive disorder. Clinical manifestations include cardiomyopathy and muscle weakness.

Cardiac issues may include heart failure and arrhythmias. Muscle weakness leads to respiratory insufficiency and sleep-disordered breathing. Treatment includes emerging therapies such as enzyme replacement therapy, chaperone molecules, and gene therapy. Supportive therapy may consist of either noninvasive ventilation, or tracheostomy and mechanical ventilation. Cardiac medications, protein-rich nutrition, and judicious physical therapy are additional measures that can be utilized.

Severe Tracheomalacia and/or Bronchomalacia (Airway Malacia)

Conditions associated with airway malacia include tracheoesophageal fistula, innominate artery compression, and pulmonary artery sling after surgical repair (Chapter 381). Patients with tracheobronchomalacia present with cough, lower airway obstruction, and wheezing. Diagnosis is made via bronchoscopy, preferably with the patient breathing spontaneously. Positive end-expiratory pressure (PEEP) titration during the bronchoscopy helps identify the airway pressure required to maintain airway patency and prevent tracheobronchial collapse.

Neuromyopathy of Severe Illness

Children recuperating from severe illness in the intensive care unit often have neuromuscular weakness from suboptimal nutrition. This neuromuscular weakness can be devastating when coupled with the catabolic effects of severe illness and the residual effects of sedatives, analgesics, and muscle relaxants, particularly if corticosteroids were administered. Children with neuromuscular disease have limited ability to increase ventilation and usually do so by increasing respiratory rate. Because of weakness, sternal retractions may not be observed. In severe illness, some of these children respond to increased respiratory load by becoming apneic. A look of panic, a change in vital signs such as significant tachycardia or bradycardia, and cyanosis may be the only signs of respiratory failure.

BIBLIOGRAPHY

Please visit the Nelson Textbook of Pediatrics *website at www.expertconsult.com for the complete bibliography.*

412.4 Long-Term Mechanical Ventilation

Zehava Noah and Cynthia Etzler Budek

Some children with chronic severe respiratory insufficiency benefit from long-term ventilatory support. The goals of such support are to maintain normal oxygenation and ventilation and to minimize the work of breathing. Long-term ventilation in the home is a complex, physically demanding, emotionally taxing, and expensive process for the family and for society. It changes the family's way of life, priorities, and relationships. It may adversely affect intrafamilial and extrafamilial relationships.

The prognosis of the disease is a critical factor in the decision to initiate long-term ventilation. The discharge process for a child undergoing ventilatory support should start as soon as the child is medically stable and supported by equipment that can be maintained in the home. Children with degenerative neuromuscular disease, such as type I SMA, suffer from respiratory failure very early in life, often triggered by the first respiratory illness. Although some parents decide to provide only palliative end-of-life care (Chapter 40) for the child with SMA, others choose long-term invasive or noninvasive ventilatory support. Young children with chronic lung disease and airway malacia have the potential to improve their pulmonary function and to wean successfully off ventilator support if provided with adequate ventilation, good nutrition, and measures to promote development and prevent further lung injury.

Successful home discharge of a patient receiving mechanical ventilation depends on whether there are adequate resources in the community to support the family. Some hospital programs that transition children home on ventilators utilize professional nurses in the home to assist with round-the-clock care. This measure depends on funding as well as availability of nursing agencies in the community. Housing can be a significant barrier to home discharge because there must be adequate space for the child and caretakers, equipment, and supplies, environmental safety, including compliance with building and electrical codes, and home modifications for mobility, including ramping and lifts.

Funding for home care is usually a difficult issue for this population of children. Even if they have private insurance, coverage for home care benefits is frequently limited. In the USA, for children eligible for public aid, most states have funds available to meet the special needs of children who are ventilator dependent, although the extent of coverage varies considerably among geographic areas.

RESPIRATORY EQUIPMENT FOR HOME CARE

Modes of mechanical ventilation support are discussed in Chapter 65.1.

Noninvasive Equipment

Supplemental oxygen and positive pressure can be administered by nasal cannula. This system delivers heated, supersaturated, high-flow gases. A number of devices are available for the delivery of CPAP and biPAP. These machines attach to nasal and full-face masks or to nasal pillows and are best suited for the treatment of obstructive sleep apnea. Long-term use of these devices in small children may result in midface dysplasia or pressure wounds. This type of ventilation has also been used in less severely affected patients with recurrent atelectasis and/or nocturnal hypoventilation, as well as for palliation in more severely affected patients.

Rocker Bed

A rocker bed moves in a longitudinal seesaw motion at a set rate. The child is secured to the bed with a strap. Movement of the bed promotes diaphragm movement. The bed may be an option for children with mild neuromuscular weakness, for instance, during recuperation from Guillain-Barré syndrome. This device should not be placed in a home with toddlers or young children, who may get trapped in its mechanism.

Cuirasse

The cuirasse is a negative-pressure device that resembles a turtle shell. It is designed to fit over the anterior chest and provide a tight seal. Cycled negative pressure is applied to the child's chest through a hole in the cuirasse. The device is suitable only for infants and children with mild neuromuscular weakness. A plastic bag–like device that fits snugly around the chest applies the same principle.

Iron Lung

The iron lung is a device that applies negative pressure to the child's body. The child is placed in the iron lung cylinder with the head extending outside the device. A cuff is placed around the neck to minimize air leaks. Negative pressure is cycled within the iron lung, facilitating chest wall movement. Ventilation is disrupted when the device is opened to deliver care. This device is suitable for children with muscular weakness who require ventilation for part of the day. Its main advantage is that it does not require a tracheostomy; however, upper airway obstruction may occur, and this risk requires ongoing evaluation. A smaller, lightweight version of this device is available for travel.

Diaphragmatic Pacing

Detailed in the management section of Ch. 412.2, diaphragm pacers may also be considered in children with spinal cord injury involving a level above C3, though the immediate advantages are less apparent than in CCHS.

Positive Pressure Ventilation

Ideally, a ventilator intended for home use is lightweight and small, is able to entrain room air, preferably has continuous flow, and has a wide range of settings (pressure, volume, pressure support, and rate) that would allow ventilation from infancy to adulthood. Battery support for the ventilator, both internal and external, should be sufficient to permit unrestricted portability in the home and community. The equipment must also be impervious to electromagnetic interference and must be relatively easy to understand and troubleshoot. A variety of ventilators that can be used in the home are available, and familiarity with these devices is necessary to choose the best option for the child.

AIRWAY CLEARANCE

Thick, copious secretions may contribute to increased airway resistance and may provide substrate for bacterial and fungal growth. Respiratory infections in turn lead to an increase in the amount of secretions and may increase viscosity, contributing to problems in airway clearance. Patients with neuromuscular weakness often have discoordination or absence of swallow, putting them at risk for aspiration of oral secretions or food. Reflux resulting in aspiration is also common. Additionally, many patients have poor or nonexistent cough; some of them may have ciliary dysfunction.

Modalities that help with clearance of secretions include postural drainage, manual or mechanical percussion or vibration, and vest or wrap percussion therapy. Cough effort may be enhanced with a cough assist device and/or abdominal binder. In addition, oropharyngeal or tracheal suctioning to remove secretions may promote airway clearance.

Control of oral secretions can be achieved pharmacologically with anticholinergic drugs or by localized injection of botulinum toxin (Botox) or surgical ligation of selected salivary ducts. In extreme cases, surgical tracheolaryngeal separation may be indicated. If thick, tenacious secretions are problematic, patient hydration and dosing of anticholinergic medication should be reviewed. Administration of DNAase or *N*-acetylcysteine may be considered to thin secretions. In selected cases, bronchoscopy may be indicated for the removal of inspissated secretions and/or re-expansion of atelectatic pulmonary lobe or segment.

PHYSICAL THERAPY, OCCUPATIONAL THERAPY, AND SPEECH THERAPY

Therapies are very important in chronic respiratory failure. Potential goals for physical therapy are mobilization of the patient and strengthening of muscles, particularly truncal and abdominal muscles essential to pulmonary rehabilitation. Occupational therapy goals revolve around achieving or maintaining developmental milestones. Child life/developmental therapy focuses on provision of developmentally appropriate environmental stimulation and age-appropriate play. Speech therapy goals deal with oromotor skills for feeding and communication. Evaluation of swallow is a key component of therapy for children with chronic respiratory failure. Sign language is frequently utilized for communication, because of delayed speech or hearing loss. Audiology specialists should be involved in the assessment of hearing, as there is a higher incidence of hearing loss in the patients undergoing long-term ventilation.

INFECTIONS

Infections—tracheitis (Chapter 377.2), bronchitis (Chapter 383.2), pneumonia (Chapter 392)—are common in patients with chronic respiratory failure. They may be due to community-acquired viruses (adenovirus, influenza, respiratory syncytial virus, parainfluenza) or community- or hospital-acquired bacteria. Many of the latter organisms are gram-negative, highly antimicrobial-resistant pathogens that cause further deterioration in pulmonary function. Bacterial infection is most likely in the presence of fever, deteriorating lung function (hypoxia, hypercarbia, tachypnea, retractions), leukocytosis, and mucopurulent sputum. The presence of leukocytes and organisms on Gram stain of tracheal aspirate, as well as the visualization of new infiltrates on radiographs, may be consistent with bacterial infection. Infection must be distinguished from tracheal colonization, which is asymptomatic and associated with normal amounts of clear tracheal secretions. If infection is suspected, it must be treated with antibiotics, based on the culture and sensitivities of organisms recovered from the tracheal aspirate. Inhaled tobramycin, started early, may avert more serious infection. Infections should be prevented by appropriate immunizations (influenza, pneumococcus, *Haemophilus influenzae* type b), passive immunity (respiratory syncytial virus), and good tracheostomy care. Antibiotics should be used judiciously to prevent further colonization with drug-resistant organisms. However, some patients who have recurrent infections may benefit from prophylaxis with inhaled antibiotics.

MONITORING IN THE HOME

A patient who is ventilated in the home must be monitored at all times. The patient must be under direct observation of the caregivers. Continuous monitoring of O_2 saturation and heart rate is recommended during sleep, and either continuous or intermittent monitoring during the daytime, depending on patient stability. Patients with CCHS or pulmonary hypertension are particularly vulnerable to episodes of hypoxemia and/or hypercarbia. Patients with pulmonary hypertension may experience a rapid drop in O_2 saturation.

Patients followed up in pulmonary clinics should be monitored at each clinic visit for heart rate, O_2 saturation, and transcutaneous and/or end-tidal CO_2. Pulmonary function tests should be considered for those patients who are old enough and able to cooperate, usually after 5 yr of age.

Enhanced monitoring and surveillance are recommended for patients whose pulmonary status has improved and are in the process of being weaned completely off ventilator support. A polysomnogram may be useful when total liberation from mechanical ventilation is being contemplated. In addition to physiologic parameters, patients must be monitored for signs of stress, agitation, and fatigue. Often these signs appear one or more days after the ventilator parameter changes.

DISCHARGE PROCESS

The initial discharge process for a child going home on a ventilator is complex. A multidisciplinary, coordinated team approach is needed to develop a comprehensive plan that addresses medical, psychosocial, developmental, educational, and safety issues. The ventilated child must demonstrate medical stability that can be safely managed at home; interventions to maintain stability should be minimal before discharge. The child should be transitioned to a ventilator suitable for home use that allows portability as well as adequate ventilation. Medical management should also focus on transitioning oxygen and ventilator parameters to settings appropriate for home care. Depending on the type of ventilation employed, a tracheostomy may be placed to promote comfort and a stable airway as soon as the decision for long-term ventilation is made.

Nutrition should be optimized to promote growth yet minimize excessive weight gain and carbon dioxide production. The nutritional requirements of a ventilated child are frequently decreased due to the supported work of breathing. The ventilated child often has problems with swallowing from discoordination and oral aversion secondary to intubation. Speech therapy should be introduced early to begin oromotor therapy and return of swallow. Many children require gastrostomy tube placement to replace or supplement oral intake. Evaluation and management of reflux and the risk of aspiration should also be considered. Some children with severe reflux may require jejunal feeding. Communication devices to augment speech and introduction of sign language for speech and hearing impaired should be part of the planning.

Training of caregivers should be initiated early in the discharge process and should be provided by nurses, respiratory care practitioners, and physical, occupational, and speech therapists. Caregivers must be trained in all aspects of the child's care, including tracheostomy care, ventilator management, and cardiopulmonary resuscitation. Their independence in delivery of care at the bedside and while transporting the child should be emphasized. Special focus should be placed on safety and the appropriate response in the event of an emergency. An emergency bag containing critical supplies should accompany the patient at all times. Caregivers must demonstrate their proficiency before the child is discharged.

Community agencies should be identified for provision of home support services. They may include a nursing agency to provide private duty nursing services. It is ideal to train home care nurses about the ventilator and the child's care before home discharge. An equipment vendor who can provide the ventilator equipment, supplies, and service should be selected. A care conference involving the hospital team, funding agency, home nursing agency, equipment vendor, and family caregivers should take place before discharge. The conference is important for coordination of last-minute details and facilitation of a smooth transition to home.

Providing continued support to the child and family after discharge is essential. The pediatrician in the community has a central role in providing coordination of care, well child care, and all other medical services, with the possible exception of ventilatory management. Equally important is the establishment of lines of communication to the medical center and the provision of timely access for advice and troubleshooting during the intervals between multidisciplinary clinic visits.

BIBLIOGRAPHY

Please visit the Nelson Textbook of Pediatrics *website at www.expertconsult.com for the complete bibliography.*

Chapter 413
Extrapulmonary Diseases with Pulmonary Manifestations

Susanna A. McColley

Respiratory symptoms commonly originate from extrapulmonary processes. The respiratory system adapts to metabolic demands and is exquisitely responsive to cortical input; therefore, **tachypnea** is common in the presence of metabolic stress such as fever, whereas dyspnea may be related to anxiety. **Cough** most commonly arises from upper or lower respiratory tract disorders, but it can originate from the central nervous system, as with cough tic or psychogenic cough, and it can be a prominent symptom in children with gastroesophageal reflux disease. **Chest pain** does not commonly arise from pulmonary processes in otherwise healthy children but more often has a neuromuscular or inflammatory etiology. **Cyanosis** can be caused by cardiac or hematologic disorders, and **dyspnea** and **exercise intolerance** can have a number of extrapulmonary causes. These disorders may be suspected on the basis of the history and physical examination, or they may be considered in children in whom diagnostic studies have atypical findings or who show poor response to usual therapy. More common causes of such symptoms are listed in Table 413-1 on the *Nelson Textbook of Pediatrics* website at www.expertconsult.com.

For the full continuation of this chapter, please visit the Nelson Textbook of Pediatrics *website at www.expertconsult.com.*

PART XX The Cardiovascular System

Section 1 DEVELOPMENTAL BIOLOGY OF THE CARDIOVASCULAR SYSTEM

Chapter 414 Cardiac Development

Daniel Bernstein

Knowledge of the cellular and molecular mechanisms of cardiac development is necessary in understanding congenital heart defects and will be even more important in developing strategies for prevention, whether cell or molecular therapies or fetal cardiac interventional procedures. Cardiac defects have traditionally been grouped by common morphologic patterns: for example, abnormalities of the outflow tracts (conotruncal lesions such as tetralogy of Fallot and truncus arteriosus) and abnormalities of atrioventricular septation (primum atrial septal defect, complete atrioventricular canal defect). These morphologic categories may be revised or eventually supplanted by new categories as our understanding of the genetic basis of congenital heart disease progresses.

414.1 Early Cardiac Morphogenesis

Daniel Bernstein

In the early presomite embryo, the 1st identifiable cardiac progenitor cell clusters are arranged in the anterior lateral plate mesoderm on both sides of the embryo's central axis; these clusters form paired cardiac tubes by 18 days of gestation. The paired tubes fuse in the midline on the ventral surface of the embryo to form the primitive heart tube by 22 days. This straight heart tube is composed of an outer myocardial layer, an inner endocardium, and a middle layer of extracellular matrix known as the cardiac jelly. There are 2 distinct cell lineages: the primary heart field provides precursor cells for the left ventricle, whereas the secondary heart field provides precursors for the atria and right ventricle. Premyocardial cells, including epicardial cells and cells derived from the neural crest, continue their migration into the region of the heart tube. Regulation of this early phase of cardiac morphogenesis is controlled in part by the interaction of specific signaling molecules or ligands, usually expressed by 1 cell type, with specific receptors, usually expressed by another cell type. Positional information is conveyed to the developing cardiac mesoderm by factors such as retinoids (isoforms of vitamin A), which bind to specific nuclear receptors and regulate gene transcription. Migration of epithelial cells into the developing heart tube is directed by extracellular matrix proteins (such as fibronectin) interacting with cell surface receptors (the integrins). Other important regulatory molecules include bone morphogenetic protein 2 (BMP2); fibroblast growth factor 4 (FGF4), the transcription factors Nkx2.5, GATA4, Mesp1, and Mesp2; and members of the Wnt/β-catenin signaling pathway. The clinical importance of these ligands is revealed by the spectrum of **cardiac teratogenic** effects caused by the retinoid-like drug isotretinoin.

For the full continuation of this chapter, please visit the Nelson Textbook of Pediatrics *website at www.expertconsult.com.*

414.2 Cardiac Looping

Daniel Bernstein

At ≈22-24 days, the heart tube begins to bend ventrally and toward the right (see Web Fig. 414-1). The heart is the 1st organ to escape from the bilateral symmetry of the early embryo. Looping brings the future left ventricle leftward and in continuity with the sinus venosus (future left and right atria), whereas the future right ventricle is shifted rightward and in continuity with the truncus arteriosus (future aorta and pulmonary artery). This pattern of development explains the relatively common occurrence of the cardiac anomalies double-outlet right ventricle and double-inlet left ventricle and the extreme rarity of double-outlet left ventricle and double-inlet right ventricle (Chapter 424.5). When cardiac looping is abnormal (situs inversus, heterotaxia), the incidence of serious cardiac malformations is high and there are usually associated abnormalities in the L-R patterning of the lungs and abdominal viscera.

For the full continuation of this chapter, please visit the Nelson Textbook of Pediatrics *website at www.expertconsult.com.*

414.3 Cardiac Septation

Daniel Bernstein

When looping is complete, the external appearance of the heart is similar to that of a mature heart; internally, the structure resembles a single tube, although it now has several bulges resulting in the appearance of primitive chambers. The common atrium (comprising both the right and left atria) is connected to the primitive ventricle (future left ventricle) via the atrioventricular canal. The primitive ventricle is connected to the bulbus cordis (future right ventricle) via the bulboventricular foramen. The distal portion of the bulbus cordis is connected to the truncus arteriosus via an outlet segment (the conus).

For the full continuation of this chapter, please visit the Nelson Textbook of Pediatrics *website at www.expertconsult.com.*

414.4 Aortic Arch Development

Daniel Bernstein

The aortic arch, head and neck vessels, proximal pulmonary arteries, and ductus arteriosus develop from the aortic sac, arterial arches, and dorsal aortae. When the straight heart tube develops, the distal outflow portion bifurcates into the right and left 1st aortic arches, which join the paired dorsal aortae (Fig. 414-1). The dorsal aortae will fuse to form the descending aorta. The proximal aorta from the aortic valve to the left carotid artery arises from the aortic sac. The 1st and 2nd arches largely regress by about 22 days, with the 1st aortic arch giving rise to the maxillary artery and the 2nd to the stapedial and hyoid arteries. The 3rd arches participate in the formation of the innominate

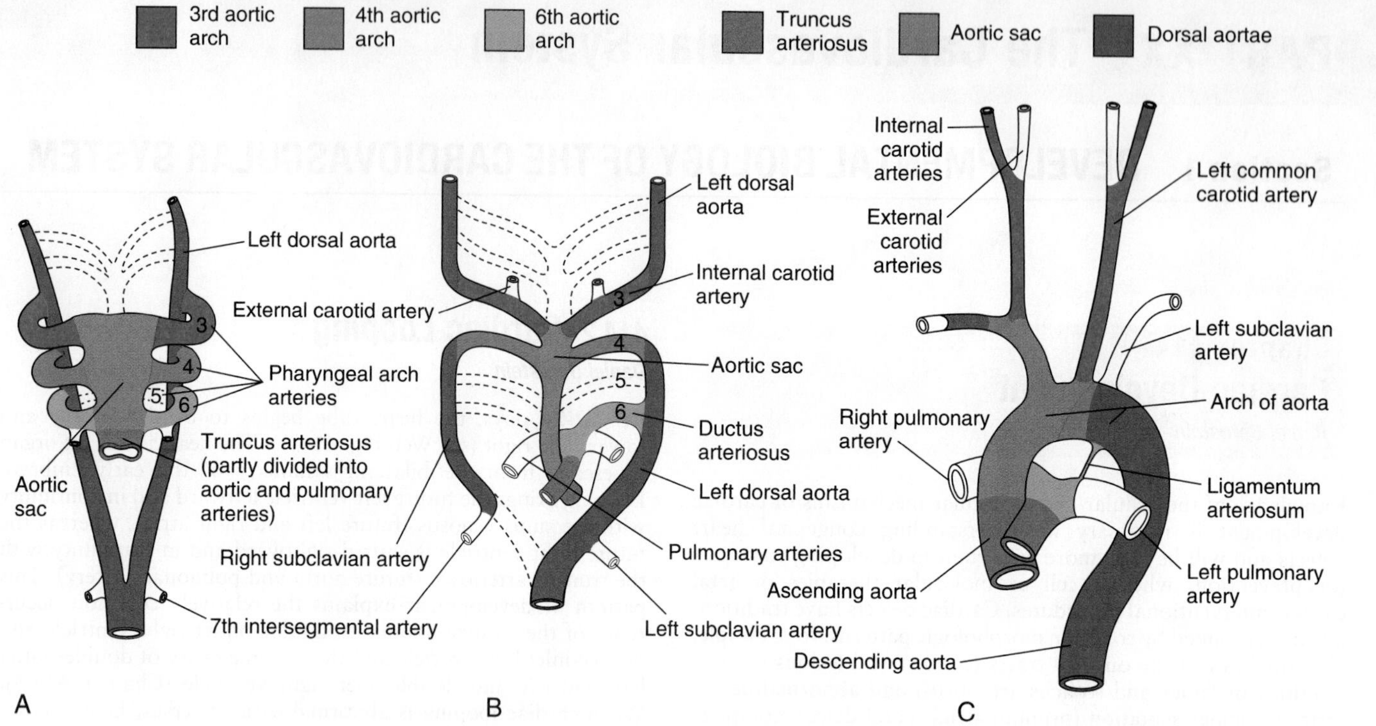

Figure 414-1 Schematic drawings illustrating the changes that result during transformation of the truncus arteriosus, aortic sac, aortic arches, and dorsal aortae into the adult arterial pattern. The vessels that are not shaded or colored are not derived from these structures. *A,* Aortic arches at 6 wk; by this stage the 1st 2 pairs of aortic arches have largely disappeared. *B,* Aortic arches at 7 wk; the parts of the dorsal aortae and aortic arches that normally disappear are indicated by *broken lines. C,* Arterial vessels of a 6 mo old infant. (From Moore KL, Persaud TVN, Torchia M: *The developing human,* Philadelphia, 2007, Elsevier.)

artery and the common and internal carotid arteries. The right 4th arch gives rise to the innominate and right subclavian arteries, and the left 4th arch participates in formation of the segment of the aortic arch between the left carotid artery and the ductus arteriosus. The 5th arch does not persist as a major structure in the mature circulation. The 6th arches join the more distal pulmonary arteries, with the right 6th arch giving rise to a portion of the proximal right pulmonary artery and the left 6th arch giving rise to the ductus arteriosus. The aortic arch between the ductus arteriosus and the left subclavian artery is derived from the left-sided dorsal aorta, whereas the aortic arch distal to the left subclavian artery is derived from the fused right and left dorsal aortae. Abnormalities in development of the paired aortic arches are responsible for **right aortic arch, double aortic arch,** and **vascular rings** (Chapter 426.1).

414.5 Cardiac Differentiation

Daniel Bernstein

The process by which the totipotential cells of the early embryo become committed to specific cell lineages is differentiation. Precardiac mesodermal cells differentiate into mature cardiac muscle cells with an appropriate complement of cardiac-specific contractile elements, regulatory proteins, receptors, and ion channels. Expression of the contractile protein myosin occurs at an early stage of cardiac development, even before fusion of the bilateral heart primordia. Differentiation in these early mesodermal cells is regulated by signals from the anterior endoderm, a process known as *induction.* Several putative early signaling molecules include fibroblast growth factor, activin, and insulin. Signaling molecules interact with receptors on the cell surface; these receptors activate 2nd messengers, which, in turn, activate specific nuclear transcription factors (GATA-4, MEF2, Nkx, bHLH, and the retinoic acid receptor family) that induce the expression of specific gene products to regulate cardiac differentiation. Some of the primary disorders of cardiac muscle, the **cardiomyopathies,** may be related to defects in some of these signaling molecules (Chapter 433).

For the full continuation of this chapter, please visit the Nelson Textbook of Pediatrics *website at www.expertconsult.com.*

414.6 Developmental Changes in Cardiac Function

Daniel Bernstein

During development, the composition of the myocardium undergoes profound changes that result in an increase in the number and size of myocytes. During prenatal life, this process involves myocyte division (hyperplasia), whereas after the 1st few postnatal weeks, subsequent cardiac growth occurs by an increase in myocyte size (hypertrophy). The myocytes themselves change shape from round to cylindrical, the proportion of myofibrils (which contain the contractile apparatus) increases, and the myofibrils become more regular in their orientation.

For the full continuation of this chapter, please visit the Nelson Textbook of Pediatrics *website at www.expertconsult.com.*

BIBLIOGRAPHY

Please visit the Nelson Textbook of Pediatrics *website at www.expertconsult.com for the complete bibliography.*

Chapter 415
The Fetal to Neonatal Circulatory Transition

415.1 The Fetal Circulation

Daniel Bernstein

The human fetal circulation and its adjustments after birth are similar to those of other large mammals, although rates of maturation differ. In the fetal circulation, the right and left ventricles exist in a parallel circuit, as opposed to the series circuit of a newborn or adult (see Fig. 415-1*A* on the *Nelson Textbook of Pediatrics* website at www.expertconsult.com). In the fetus, the placenta provides for gas and metabolite exchange. Since the lungs do not provide gas exchange, the pulmonary vessels are vasoconstricted, diverting blood away from the pulmonary circulation. Three cardiovascular structures unique to the fetus are important for maintaining this parallel circulation: the ductus venosus, foramen ovale, and ductus arteriosus.

For the full continuation of this chapter, please visit the Nelson Textbook of Pediatrics *website at www.expertconsult.com.*

415.2 The Transitional Circulation

Daniel Bernstein

At birth, mechanical expansion of the lungs and an increase in arterial Po_2 result in a rapid decrease in pulmonary vascular resistance. Concomitantly, removal of the low-resistance placental circulation leads to an increase in systemic vascular resistance. The output from the right ventricle now flows entirely into the pulmonary circulation, and because pulmonary vascular resistance becomes lower than systemic vascular resistance, the shunt through the ductus arteriosus reverses and becomes left to right. In the course of several days, the high arterial Po_2 constricts and eventually closes the ductus arteriosus, which eventually becomes the ligamentum arteriosum. The increased volume of pulmonary blood flow returning to the left atrium from the lungs increases left atrial volume and pressure sufficiently to close the flap of the foramen ovale functionally, although the foramen may remain probe patent for several years.

For the full continuation of this chapter, please visit the Nelson Textbook of Pediatrics *website at www.expertconsult.com.*

415.3 The Neonatal Circulation

Daniel Bernstein

At birth, the fetal circulation must immediately adapt to extrauterine life as gas exchange is transferred from the placenta to the lungs (Chapter 95.1). Some of these changes are virtually instantaneous with the 1st breath, whereas others develop over a period of hours or weeks. With the onset of ventilation, pulmonary vascular resistance is markedly decreased as a consequence of both active (Po_2-related) and passive (mechanical related) pulmonary vasodilation. In a normal neonate, closure of the ductus arteriosus and the fall in pulmonary vascular resistance decreases pulmonary arterial and right ventricular pressures. The largest decline in pulmonary resistance from the high fetal levels to the low "adult" levels in the human infant at sea level usually occurs within the 1st 2-3 days but may be prolonged for 7 days or more. Over the next several weeks of life, pulmonary vascular resistance decreases even further, secondary to a remodeling of the pulmonary vasculature, including thinning of the vascular smooth muscle and recruitment of new vessels. This decrease in pulmonary vascular resistance significantly influences the timing of the clinical appearance of many congenital heart lesions that are dependent on the relative levels of systemic and pulmonary vascular resistances. The left-to-right shunt through an large ventricular septal defect may be minimal in the 1st wk after birth when pulmonary vascular resistance is still high. As pulmonary resistance decreases in the next week or two, the volume of the left-to-right shunt through the ventricular septal defect increases and eventually leads to symptoms of heart failure within the 1st month or two of life.

For the full continuation of this chapter, please visit the Nelson Textbook of Pediatrics *website at www.expertconsult.com.*

415.4 Persistent Pulmonary Hypertension of the Neonate (Persistence of Fetal Circulatory Pathways)

See Chapter 95.7.

BIBLIOGRAPHY

Please visit the Nelson Textbook of Pediatrics *website at www.expertconsult.com for the complete bibliography.*

Section 2 EVALUATION OF THE CARDIOVASCULAR SYSTEM

Chapter 416
History and Physical Examination

Daniel Bernstein

The importance of the history and physical examination cannot be overemphasized in the evaluation of infants and children with suspected cardiovascular disorders. Patients may require further laboratory evaluation and eventual treatment, or the family may be reassured that no significant problem exists. Although the ready availability of echocardiography may entice the clinician to skip these preliminary steps, an initial evaluation by a skilled cardiologist is preferred for several reasons: (1) a cardiac examination allows the cardiologist to guide the echocardiographic evaluation toward confirming or eliminating specific diagnoses, thereby increasing its accuracy; (2) because most childhood murmurs are innocent, evaluation by a pediatric cardiologist can eliminate unnecessary and expensive laboratory tests; and (3) the cardiologist's knowledge and experience are important in reassuring the patient's family and preventing unnecessary restrictions on healthy physical activity. An experienced pediatric cardiologist can differentiate an innocent murmur from serious congenital heart disease by history and physical alone with a high sensitivity and specificity.

HISTORY

A comprehensive cardiac history starts with details of the perinatal period including the presence of cyanosis, respiratory distress, or prematurity. Maternal complications such as gestational diabetes, teratogenic medications, systemic lupus erythematosus, or substance abuse can be associated with cardiac problems. If cardiac symptoms began during infancy, the timing of the initial symptoms should be noted to provide important clues about the specific cardiac condition.

Many of the symptoms of **heart failure** in infants and children are age specific. In infants, feeding difficulties are common. Inquiry should be made about the frequency of feeding and either the volume of each feeding or the time spent on each breast. An infant with heart failure often takes less volume per feeding and becomes dyspneic or diaphoretic while sucking. After falling asleep exhausted, the baby, inadequately fed, will awaken for the next feeding after a brief time. This cycle continues around the clock and must be carefully differentiated from colic or other feeding disorders. Additional symptoms and signs include those of respiratory distress: rapid breathing, nasal flaring, cyanosis, and chest retractions. In older children, heart failure may be manifested as exercise intolerance, difficulty keeping up with peers during sports or need for a nap after coming home from school, poor growth, or chronic abdominal complaints. Eliciting a history of fatigue in an older child requires questions about age-specific activities, including stair climbing, walking, bicycle riding, physical education class, and competitive sports; information should be obtained regarding more severe manifestations such as orthopnea and nocturnal dyspnea.

Cyanosis at rest is often overlooked by parents; it may be mistaken for a normal individual variation in color. Cyanosis during crying or exercise, however, is more often noted as abnormal by observant parents. Many infants and toddlers turn "blue around the lips" when crying vigorously or during breath-holding spells; this condition must be carefully differentiated from cyanotic heart disease by inquiring about inciting factors, the length of episodes, and whether the tongue and mucous membranes also appear cyanotic. Newborns often have cyanosis of their extremities (acrocyanosis) when undressed and cold; this response to cold must be carefully differentiated from true cyanosis, where the mucous membranes are also blue.

Chest pain is an unusual manifestation of cardiac disease in pediatric patients, although it is a frequent cause for referral to a pediatric cardiologist, especially in adolescents. Nonetheless, a careful history, physical examination, and, if indicated, laboratory or imaging tests will assist in identifying the cause of chest pain (Table 416-1). For patients with some forms of repaired congenital heart disease or those with a history of Kawasaki disease (Chapter 438.1); however, chest pain should be evaluated carefully for a coronary etiology.

Cardiac disease may be a manifestation of a known congenital malformation syndrome with typical physical findings (Table 416-2) or a manifestation of a generalized disorder affecting the heart and other organ systems (Table 416-3). Extracardiac malformations may be noted in 20-45% of infants with congenital heart disease. Between 5 and 10% of patients have a known chromosomal abnormality; the importance of genetic evaluation will increase as our knowledge of specific gene defects linked to congenital heart disease increases.

A careful family history may also reveal early (at age less than 50 yr) coronary artery disease or stroke (suggestive of familial hypercholesterolemia or thrombophilia), sudden death (suggestive of cardiomyopathy or familial arrhythmic disorder), generalized muscle disease (suggestive of one of the muscular dystrophies, dermatomyositis, or familial or metabolic cardiomyopathy), or first-degree relatives with congenital heart disease.

Table 416-1 DIFFERENTIAL DIAGNOSIS OF CHEST PAIN IN PEDIATRIC PATIENTS

MUSCULOSKELETAL (COMMON)
Trauma (accidental, abuse)
Exercise, overuse injury (strain, bursitis)
Costochondritis (Tietze syndrome)
Herpes zoster (cutaneous)
Pleurodynia
Fibrositis
Slipping rib
Precordial catch
Sickle cell anemia vasoocclusive crisis
Osteomyelitis (rare)
Primary or metastatic tumor (rare)
PULMONARY (COMMON)
Pneumonia
Pleurisy
Asthma
Chronic cough
Pneumothorax
Infarction (sickle cell anemia)
Foreign body
Embolism (rare)
Pulmonary hypertension (rare)
Tumor (rare)
Bronchiectasis
GASTROINTESTINAL (LESS COMMON)
Esophagitis (gastroesophageal reflux, infectious, pill)
Esophageal foreign body
Esophageal spasm
Cholecystitis
Subdiaphragmatic abscess
Perihepatitis (Fitz-Hugh-Curtis syndrome)
Peptic ulcer disease
Pancreatitis
CARDIAC (LESS COMMON)
Pericarditis
Postpericardiotomy syndrome
Endocarditis
Cardiomyopathy
Mitral valve prolapse
Aortic or subaortic stenosis
Arrhythmias
Marfan syndrome (dissecting aortic aneurysm)
Kawasaki disease
Cocaine, sympathomimetic ingestion
Angina (familial hypercholesterolemia, anomalous coronary artery)
IDIOPATHIC (COMMON)
Anxiety, hyperventilation
Panic disorder
OTHER (LESS COMMON)
Spinal cord or nerve root compression
Breast-related pathologic condition (mastalgia)
Castleman disease (lymph node neoplasm)

GENERAL PHYSICAL EXAMINATION

A general assessment of the patient is always the first part of the examination, with specific attention directed toward the presence of cyanosis, abnormalities in growth, chest wall abnormalities, and any evidence of respiratory distress. Although the murmur may be the most prominent part of the overall examination, any murmur must be placed in context of other physical findings. Frequently, associated findings, such as the quality of the pulses, the presence of a ventricular heave or thrill, or the splitting of the second heart sound, provide important clues to a specific cardiac diagnosis.

Accurate measurement of height and weight and plotting on a standard growth chart are important because both cardiac failure and chronic cyanosis can result in **failure to thrive.** Growth failure is manifested predominantly by poor weight gain; if length

Table 416-2 CONGENITAL MALFORMATION SYNDROMES ASSOCIATED WITH CONGENITAL HEART DISEASE

SYNDROME	FEATURES	SYNDROME	FEATURES
CHROMOSOMAL DISORDERS		Polysplenia syndrome	Acyanotic lesions with increased pulmonary blood flow, azygos continuation of inferior vena cava, partial anomalous pulmonary venous return, dextrocardia, single ventricle, common atrioventricular valve
Trisomy 21 (Down syndrome)	Endocardial cushion defect, VSD, ASD	PHACE syndrome (*p*osterior brain fossa anomalies, facial *h*emangiomas, *a*rterial anomalies, *c*ardiac anomalies and aortic coarctation, *e*ye anomalies)	VSD, PDA, coarctation of aorta, arterial aneurysms
Trisomy 21p (cat eye syndrome)	Miscellaneous, total anomalous pulmonary venous return	**TERATOGENIC AGENTS**	
Trisomy 18	VSD, ASD, PDA, coarctation of aorta, bicuspid aortic or pulmonary valve	Congenital rubella	PDA, peripheral pulmonic stenosis
Trisomy 13	VSD, ASD, PDA, coarctation of aorta, bicuspid aortic or pulmonary valve	Fetal hydantoin syndrome	VSD, ASD, coarctation of aorta, PDA
Trisomy 9	Miscellaneous	Fetal alcohol syndrome	ASD, VSD
XXXXY	PDA, ASD	Fetal valproate effects	Coarctation of aorta, hypoplastic left side of heart, aortic stenosis, pulmonary atresia, VSD
Penta X	PDA, VSD	Maternal phenylketonuria	VSD, ASD, PDA, coarctation of aorta
Triploidy	VSD, ASD, PDA	Retinoic acid embryopathy	Conotruncal anomalies
XO (Turner syndrome)	Bicuspid aortic valve, coarctation of aorta	**OTHERS**	
Fragile X	Mitral valve prolapse, aortic root dilatation	Apert syndrome	VSD
Duplication 3q2	Miscellaneous	Autosomal dominant polycystic kidney disease	Mitral valve prolapse
Deletion 4p	VSD, PDA, aortic stenosis	Carpenter syndrome	PDA
Deletion 9p	Miscellaneous	Conradi syndrome	VSD, PDA
Deletion 5p (cri du chat syndrome)	VSD, PDA, ASD	Crouzon disease	PDA, coarctation of aorta
Deletion 10q	VSD, TOF, conotruncal lesions*	Cutis laxa	Pulmonary hypertension, pulmonic stenosis
Deletion 13q	VSD	de Lange syndrome	VSD
Deletion 18q	VSD	Ellis–van Creveld syndrome	Single atrium, VSD
SYNDROME COMPLEXES		Holt-Oram syndrome	ASD, VSD, 1st-degree heart block
CHARGE association (*c*oloboma, *h*eart, *a*tresia choanae, *r*etardation, *g*enital, and *e*ar anomalies)	VSD, ASD, PDA, TOF, endocardial cushion defect	Infant of diabetic mother	Hypertrophic cardiomyopathy, VSD, conotruncal anomalies
DiGeorge sequence, CATCH 22 (*c*ardiac defects, *a*bnormal facies, *t*hymic aplasia, *c*left palate, and *h*ypocalcemia)	Aortic arch anomalies, conotruncal anomalies	Kartagener syndrome	Dextrocardia
Alagille syndrome (arteriohepatic dysplasia)	Peripheral pulmonic stenosis, PS, TOF	Meckel-Gruber syndrome	ASD, VSD
VATER association (*v*ertebral, *a*nal, *t*racheo *e*sophageal, *r*adial, and *r*enal anomalies)	VSD, TOF, ASD, PDA	Noonan syndrome	Pulmonic stenosis, ASD, cardiomyopathy
FAVS (*f*acio-*a*uriculo-*v*ertebral *s*pectrum)	TOF, VSD	Pallister-Hall syndrome	Endocardial cushion defect
CHILD (*c*ongenital *h*emidysplasia with *i*chthyosiform *e*rythroderma, *l*imb *d*efects)	Miscellaneous	Rubinstein-Taybi syndrome	VSD
Mulibrey nanism (*mu*scle, *li*ver, *br*ain, *ey*e)	Pericardial thickening, constrictive pericarditis	Scimitar syndrome	Hypoplasia of right lung, anomalous pulmonary venous return to inferior vena cava
Asplenia syndrome	Complex cyanotic heart lesions with decreased pulmonary blood flow, transposition of great arteries, anomalous pulmonary venous return, dextrocardia, single ventricle, single atrioventricular valve	Smith-Lemli-Opitz syndrome	VSD, PDA
		TAR syndrome (*t*hrombocytopenia and *a*bsent *r*adius)	ASD, TOF
		Treacher Collins syndrome	VSD, ASD, PDA
		Williams syndrome	Supravalvular aortic stenosis, peripheral pulmonic stenosis

ASD, atrial septal defect; AV, aortic valve; PDA, patent ductus arteriosus; PS, pulmonary stenosis; TOF, tetralogy of Fallot; VSD, ventricular septal defect.
*Conotruncal includes TOF, pulmonary atresia, truncus arteriosus, and transposition of great arteries.

or head circumference is also affected, additional congenital malformations or metabolic disorders should be suspected.

Mild cyanosis may be too subtle for early detection, and clubbing of the fingers and toes is not usually manifested until late in the 1st yr of life, even in the presence of severe arterial oxygen desaturation. **Cyanosis** is best observed over the nail beds, lips, tongue, and mucous membranes. Differential cyanosis, manifested as blue lower extremities and pink upper extremities (usually the right arm), is seen with right-to-left shunting across a ductus arteriosus in the presence of coarctation or an interrupted aortic arch. Circumoral cyanosis or blueness around the forehead may be the result of prominent venous plexuses in these areas, rather than decreased arterial oxygen saturation. The extremities of infants often turn blue when the infant is unwrapped and cold (acrocyanosis), and this condition can be distinguished from central cyanosis by examination of the tongue and mucous membranes.

Heart failure in infants and children usually results in some degree of hepatomegaly and occasionally splenomegaly. The sites of **peripheral** edema are age dependent. In infants, edema is usually seen around the eyes and over the flanks, especially on initially waking. Older children and teenagers manifest both periorbital edema and pedal edema. A not uncommon initial complaint in these older patients is that their clothes no longer fit.

The heart rate of newborn infants is rapid and subject to wide fluctuations (Table 416-4). The average rate ranges from 120 to

Table 416-3 CARDIAC MANIFESTATIONS OF SYSTEMIC DISEASES

SYSTEMIC DISEASE	CARDIAC COMPLICATIONS
INFLAMMATORY DISORDERS	
Sepsis	Hypotension, myocardial dysfunction, pericardial effusion, pulmonary hypertension
Juvenile rheumatoid arthritis	Pericarditis, rarely myocarditis
Systemic lupus erythematosus	Pericarditis, Libman-Sacks endocarditis, coronary arteritis, coronary atherosclerosis (with steroids), congenital heart block
Scleroderma	Pulmonary hypertension, myocardial fibrosis, cardiomyopathy
Dermatomyositis	Cardiomyopathy, arrhythmias, heart block
Kawasaki disease	Coronary artery aneurysm and thrombosis, myocardial infarction, myocarditis, valvular insufficiency
Sarcoidosis	Granuloma, fibrosis, amyloidosis, biventricular hypertrophy, arrhythmias
Lyme disease	Arrhythmias, myocarditis
Löffler hypereosinophilic syndrome	Endomyocardial disease
INBORN ERRORS OF METABOLISM	
Refsum disease	Arrhythmia, sudden death
Hunter or Hurler syndrome	Valvular insufficiency, heart failure, hypertension
Fabry disease	Mitral insufficiency, coronary artery disease with myocardial infarction
Glycogen storage disease IIa (Pompe disease)	Short P-R interval, cardiomegaly, heart failure, arrhythmias
Carnitine deficiency	Heart failure, cardiomyopathy
Gaucher disease	Pericarditis
Homocystinuria	Coronary thrombosis
Alkaptonuria	Atherosclerosis, valvular disease
Morquio-Ullrich syndrome	Aortic incompetence
Scheie syndrome	Aortic incompetence
CONNECTIVE TISSUE DISORDERS	
Arterial calcification of infancy	Calcinosis of coronary arteries, aorta
Marfan syndrome	Aortic and mitral insufficiency, dissecting aortic aneurysm, mitral valve prolapse
Congenital contractural arachnodactyly	Mitral insufficiency or prolapse
Ehlers-Danlos syndrome	Mitral valve prolapse, dilatated aortic root
Osteogenesis imperfecta	Aortic incompetence
Pseudoxanthoma elasticum	Peripheral arterial disease
NEUROMUSCULAR DISORDERS	
Friedreich ataxia	Cardiomyopathy
Duchenne dystrophy	Cardiomyopathy, heart failure
Tuberous sclerosis	Cardiac rhabdomyoma
Familial deafness	Occasionally arrhythmia, sudden death
Neurofibromatosis	Pulmonic stenosis, pheochromocytoma, coarctation of aorta
Riley-Day syndrome	Episodic hypertension, postural hypotension
Von Hippel–Lindau disease	Hemangiomas, pheochromocytomas
ENDOCRINE-METABOLIC DISORDERS	
Graves disease	Tachycardia, arrhythmias, heart failure
Hypothyroidism	Bradycardia, pericardial effusion, cardiomyopathy, low-voltage electrocardiogram
Pheochromocytoma	Hypertension, myocardial ischemia, myocardial fibrosis, cardiomyopathy
Carcinoid	Right-sided endocardial fibrosis
HEMATOLOGIC DISORDERS	
Sickle cell anemia	High-output heart failure, cardiomyopathy, pulmonary hypertension
Thalassemia major	High-output heart failure, hemochromatosis
Hemochromatosis (1° or 2°)	Cardiomyopathy
OTHERS	
Appetite suppressants (fenfluramine and dexfenfluramine)	Cardiac valvulopathy, pulmonary hypertension
Cockayne syndrome	Atherosclerosis
Familial dwarfism and nevi	Cardiomyopathy
Jervell and Lange-Nielsen syndrome	Prolonged QT interval, sudden death
Kearns-Sayre syndrome	Heart block
LEOPARD syndrome (lentiginosis)	Pulmonic stenosis, prolonged Q-T interval
Progeria	Accelerated atherosclerosis
Osler-Weber-Rendu disease	Arteriovenous fistula (lung, liver, mucous membrane)
Romano-Ward syndrome	Prolonged Q-T interval, sudden death
Weill-Marchesani syndrome	Patent ductus arteriosus
Werner syndrome	Vascular sclerosis, cardiomyopathy

LEOPARD, *multiple* lentigines, *electrocardiographic conduction abnormalities,* ocular *hypertelorism,* pulmonary *stenosis,* abnormal *genitals,* retardation *of growth,* sensorineural *deafness.*

Table 416-4 PULSE RATES AT REST

AGE	LOWER LIMITS OF NORMAL		AVERAGE		UPPER LIMITS OF NORMAL	
Newborn	70/min		125/min		190/min	
1–11 mo	80		120		160	
2 yr	80		110		130	
4 yr	80		100		120	
6 yr	75		100		115	
8 yr	70		90		110	
10 yr	70		90		110	
	GIRLS	BOYS	GIRLS	BOYS	GIRLS	BOYS
12 yr	70	65	90	85	110	105
14 yr	65	60	85	80	105	100
16 yr	60	55	80	75	100	95
18 yr	55	50	75	70	95	90

140 beats/min and may increase to 170+ beats/min during crying and activity or drop to 70-90 beats/min during sleep. As the child grows older, the average pulse rate decreases and may be as low as 40 beats/min at rest in athletic adolescents. Persistent tachycardia (>200 beats/min in neonates, 150 beats/min in infants, or 120 beats/min in older children), bradycardia, or an irregular heartbeat other than sinus arrhythmia requires investigation to exclude pathologic arrhythmias (Chapter 429). Sinus arrhythmia can usually be distinguished by the rhythmic nature of the heart rate variations, occurring in concert with the respiratory cycle, and with a P wave before every QRS complex.

Careful evaluation of the character of the **pulses** is an important early step in the physical diagnosis of congenital heart disease. A wide pulse pressure with bounding pulses may suggest an aortic runoff lesion such as patent ductus arteriosus, aortic insufficiency, an arterial-venous communication, or increased cardiac output secondary to anemia, anxiety, or conditions associated with increased catecholamine or thyroid hormone secretion. The presence of diminished pulses in all extremities is associated with pericardial tamponade, left ventricular outflow obstruction, or cardiomyopathy. The radial and femoral pulses should always be palpated simultaneously. Normally, the femoral pulse should be appreciated immediately before the radial pulse. In infants with coarctation of the aorta, the femoral pulses may be decreased. However, in older children with coarctation of the aorta, blood flow to the descending aorta may channel through collateral vessels and results in the femoral pulse being palpable but delayed until after the radial pulse (**radial-femoral delay**).

Blood pressure should be measured in the legs as well as in the arms to be certain that coarctation of the aorta is not overlooked. Palpation of the femoral or dorsalis pedis pulse, or both, is not reliable alone to exclude coarctation. In older children, a mercury sphygmomanometer with a cuff that covers approximately two thirds of the upper part of the arm or leg may be used for blood pressure measurement. A cuff that is too small results in falsely high readings, whereas a cuff that is too large records slightly decreased pressure. Pediatric clinical facilities should be equipped with 3, 5, 7, 12, and 18 cm cuffs to accommodate the large spectrum of pediatric patient sizes. The 1st Korotkoff sounds indicate systolic pressure. As cuff pressure is slowly decreased, the sounds usually become muffled before they disappear. Diastolic pressure may be recorded when the sounds become muffled (preferred) or when they disappear altogether; the former is usually slightly higher and the latter slightly lower than true diastolic pressure. For lower extremity blood pressure determination, the stethoscope is placed over the popliteal artery. Ordinarily, the pressure recorded in the legs with the cuff technique is about 10 mm Hg higher than that in the arms.

In infants, blood pressure can be determined by auscultation, palpation, or an oscillometric (Dinamap) device that, when properly used, provides accurate measurements in infants as well as older children.

Blood pressure varies with the age of the child and is closely related to height and weight. Significant increases occur during adolescence, and many temporary variations take place before the more stable levels of adult life are attained. Exercise, excitement, coughing, crying, and struggling may raise the systolic pressure of infants and children as much as 40-50 mm Hg greater than their usual levels. Variability in blood pressure in children of approximately the same age and body build should be expected, and serial measurements should always be obtained when evaluating a patient with hypertension (Figs. 416-1 and 416-2).

Though of little use in infants, in cooperative older children, inspection of the **jugular venous pulse** wave provides information about central venous and right atrial pressure. The neck veins should be inspected with the patient sitting at a 90-degree angle. The external jugular vein should not be visible above the clavicles unless central venous pressure is elevated. Increased venous pressure transmitted to the internal jugular vein may appear as venous pulsations without visible distention; such pulsation is not seen in normal children reclining at an angle of 45 degrees. Because the great veins are in direct communication with the right atrium, changes in pressure and the volume of this chamber are also transmitted to the veins. The one exception occurs in superior vena cava obstruction, in which venous pulsatility is lost.

CARDIAC EXAMINATION

The heart should be examined in a systematic manner, starting with inspection and palpation. A **precordial bulge** to the left of the sternum with increased precordial activity suggests cardiac enlargement; such bulges can often best be appreciated by having the child lay supine with the examiner looking up from the child's feet. A **substernal thrust** indicates the presence of right ventricular enlargement, whereas an apical heave is noted with left ventricular enlargement. A hyperdynamic precordium suggests a volume load such as that found with a large left-to-right shunt, although it may be normal in a thin patient. A overly silent precordium with a barely detectable apical impulse suggests pericardial effusion or severe cardiomyopathy, but may be normal in an obese patient.

The relationship of the **apical impulse** to the midclavicular line is also helpful in the estimation of cardiac size: the apical impulse moves laterally and inferiorly with enlargement of the left ventricle. Right-sided apical impulses signify dextrocardia, tension pneumothorax, or left-sided thoracic space-occupying lesions (e.g., diaphragmatic hernia).

Thrills are the palpable equivalent of murmurs and correlate with the area of maximal auscultatory intensity of the murmur. It is important to palpate the suprasternal notch and neck for aortic bruits, which may indicate the presence of aortic stenosis or, when faint, pulmonary stenosis. Right lower sternal border and apical systolic thrills are characteristic of ventricular septal defect and mitral insufficiency, respectively. Diastolic thrills are occasionally palpable in the presence of atrioventricular valve stenosis. The timing and localization of thrills should be carefully noted.

Auscultation is an art that improves with practice. The diaphragm of the stethoscope is placed firmly on the chest for high-pitched sounds; a lightly placed bell is optimal for low-pitched sounds. The physician should initially concentrate on the characteristics of the individual heart sounds and their variation with respirations and later concentrate on murmurs. The patient should be supine, lying quietly, and breathing normally. The **1st heart sound** is best heard at the apex, whereas the **2nd heart sound** should be evaluated at the upper left and right sternal borders. The 1st heart sound is caused by closure of the atrioventricular valves (mitral and tricuspid); the 2nd sound is caused by closure of the semilunar valves (aortic and pulmonary) (Fig. 416-3). During inspiration, the decrease in intrathoracic pressure results in increased filling of the right side of the heart, which leads to an increased right ventricular ejection time and thus delayed closure of the pulmonary valve; consequently, **splitting of the 2nd heart** sound increases during inspiration and decreases during expiration.

Often, the 2nd heart sound seems to be single during expiration. The presence of a normally split 2nd sound is strong evidence against the diagnosis of atrial septal defect, defects associated with pulmonary arterial hypertension, severe pulmonary valve stenosis, aortic and pulmonary atresia, and truncus arteriosus. Wide splitting is noted in atrial septal defect, pulmonary stenosis, Ebstein anomaly, total anomalous pulmonary venous return, and right bundle branch block. An accentuated pulmonic component of the 2nd sound with narrow splitting is a sign of pulmonary hypertension. A single 2nd sound occurs in pulmonary or aortic atresia or severe stenosis, truncus arteriosus, and, often, transposition of the great arteries.

A **3rd heart sound** is best heard with the bell at the apex in mid-diastole. A **4th sound** occurring in conjunction with atrial contraction may be heard just before the 1st heart sound in late diastole. The 3rd sound may be normal in an adolescent with a relatively slow heart rate, but in a patient with the clinical signs of heart failure and tachycardia, it may be heard as a gallop rhythm and may merge with a 4th heart sound, a finding known as a summation gallop. A gallop rhythm is attributed to poor compliance of the ventricle, and exaggeration of the normal 3rd sound is associated with ventricular filling.

Ejection clicks, which are heard in early systole, are usually due to a mildly to moderately stenotic aortic or pulmonary valve or to a dilated ascending aorta or pulmonary artery. They are heard so close to the 1st heart sound that they may be mistaken for a split 1st sound. Aortic ejection clicks are best heard at the left middle to right upper sternal border and are constant in intensity. They occur in conditions in which the aortic valve is stenotic or the aorta is dilated (tetralogy of Fallot, truncus

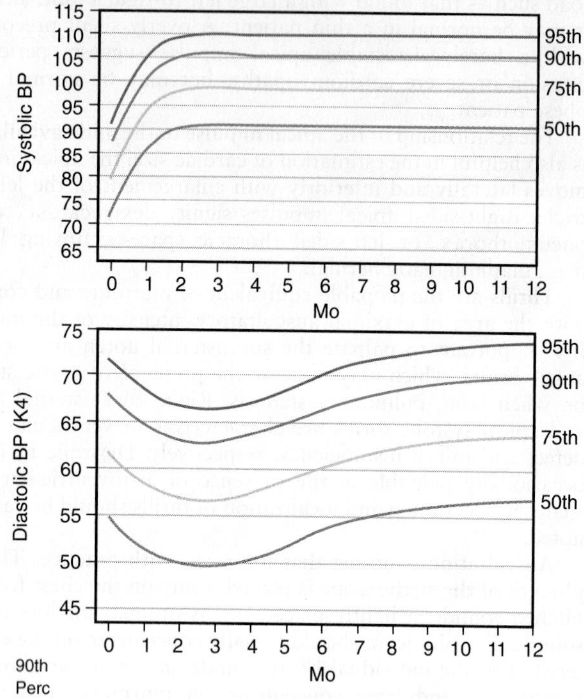

90th Perc													
Sys BP	87	101	106	106	106	105	105	105	105	105	105	105	105
Dias BP	68	65	63	63	63	65	66	67	68	68	69	69	69
Ht cm	51	59	63	66	68	70	72	73	74	76	77	78	80
Wt kg	4	4	5	5	6	7	8	9	9	10	10	11	11

A

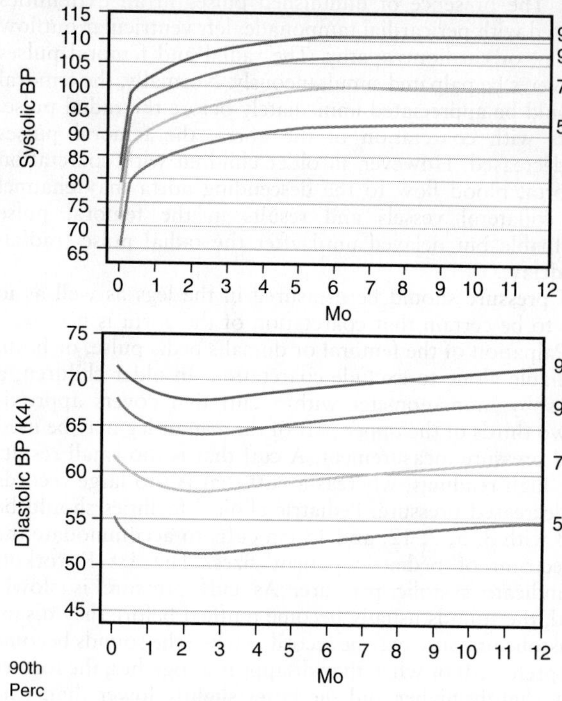

90th Perc													
Sys BP	76	98	101	104	105	106	106	106	106	106	106	105	105
Dias BP	68	65	64	64	65	65	66	66	66	67	67	67	67
Ht cm	54	55	56	58	61	63	66	68	70	72	74	75	77
Wt kg	4	4	4	5	5	6	7	8	9	9	10	10	11

B

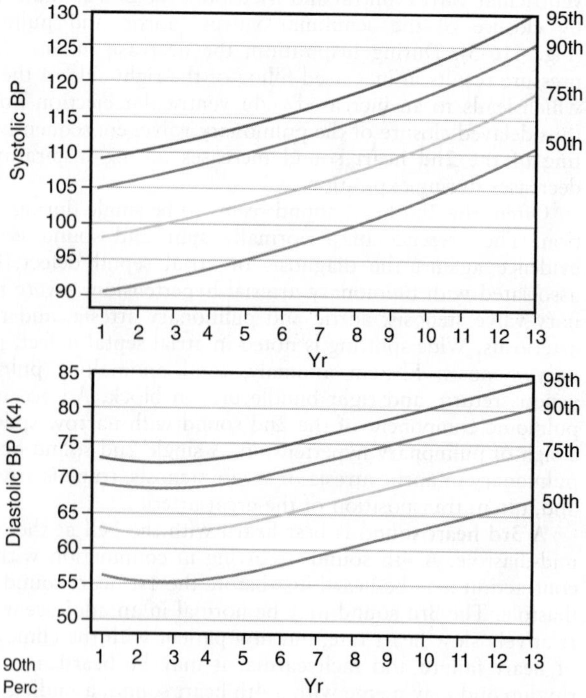

90th Perc													
Sys BP	105	106	107	108	109	111	112	114	115	117	119	121	124
Dias BP	69	68	68	69	69	70	71	73	74	75	76	77	79
Ht cm	80	91	100	108	115	122	129	135	141	147	153	159	165
Wt kg	11	14	16	18	22	25	29	34	39	44	50	55	62

C

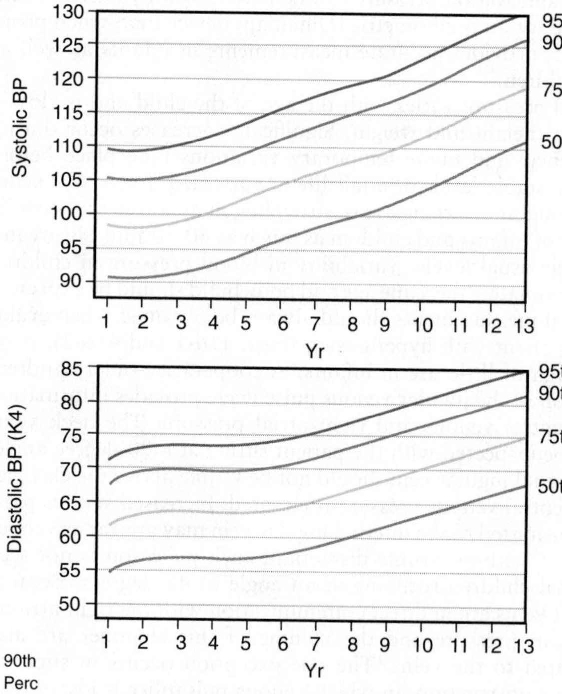

90th Perc													
Sys BP	105	105	106	107	109	111	112	114	115	117	119	122	124
Dias BP	67	69	69	69	69	70	71	72	74	75	77	78	80
Ht cm	77	89	98	107	115	122	129	135	142	148	154	160	165
Wt kg	11	13	15	18	22	25	30	35	40	45	51	58	63

D

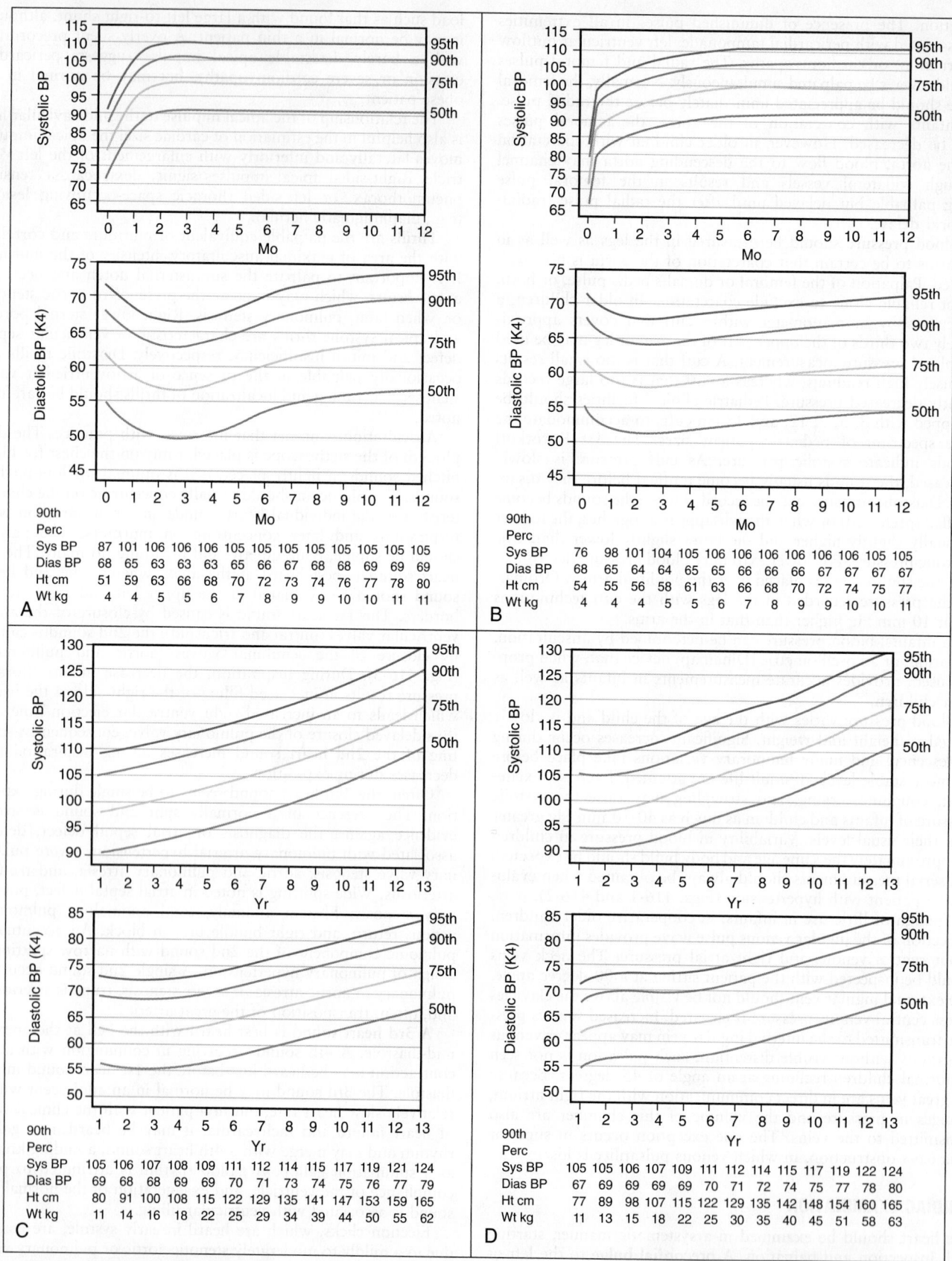

Figure 416-1 *A,* Age-specific percentiles of blood pressure (BP) measurements in boys from birth to 12 mo of age. *B,* Age-specific percentiles of BP measurements in girls from birth to 12 mo of age. *C,* Age-specific percentiles of BP measurements in boys 1-13 yr of age. *D,* Age-specific percentiles of BP measurements in girls 1-13 yr of age; Korotkoff phase IV (K4) used for diastolic BP. Dias, diastolic; Ht, height; Perc, percentile; Sys, systolic; Wt, weight. (From [no authors listed]: Report of the Second Task Force on Blood Pressure Control in Children—1987. National Heart, Lung, and Blood Institute, Bethesda, MD, *Pediatrics* 79:1–25, 1987.Copyright 1987 by the American Academy of Pediatrics.)

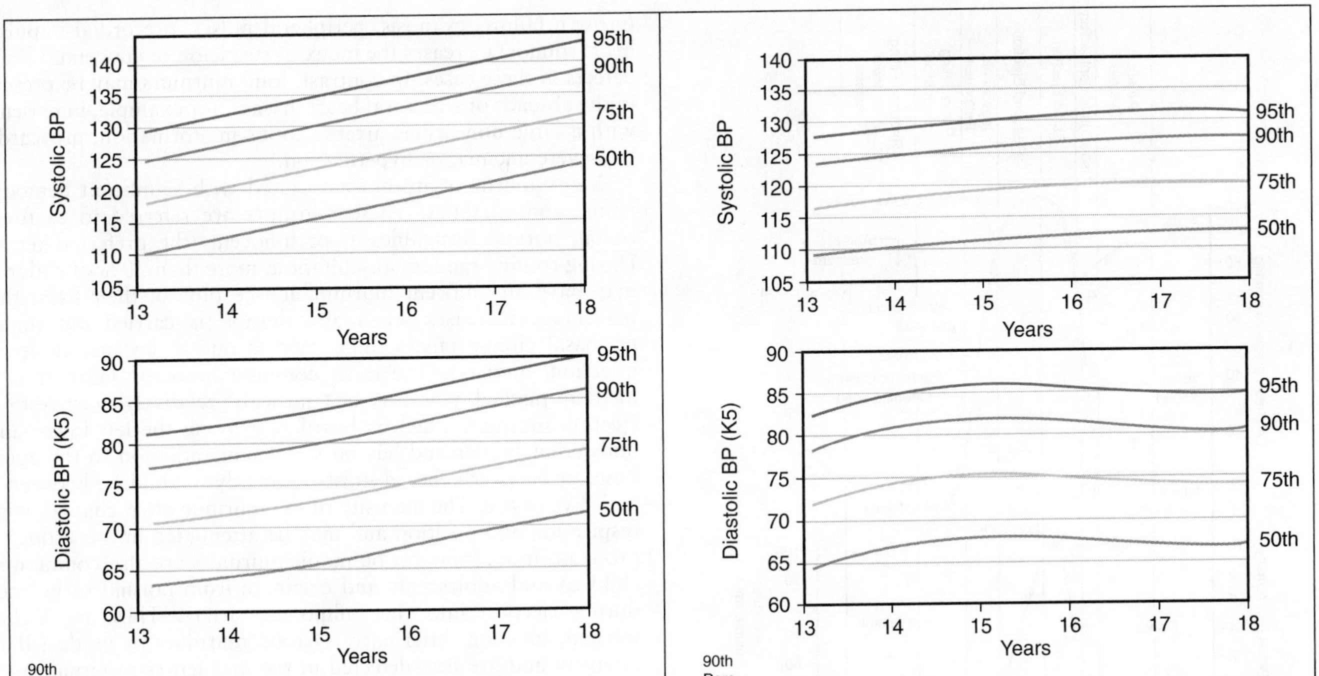

A

90th Perc	13	14	15	16	17	18
Sys BP	124	126	129	131	134	136
Dias BP	77	78	79	81	83	84
Ht cm	165	172	178	182	184	184
Wt kg	62	68	74	80	84	86

B

90th Perc	13	14	15	16	17	18
Sys BP	124	126	126	127	127	127
Dias BP	78	81	82	81	80	80
Ht cm	165	168	169	170	170	170
Wt kg	63	67	70	72	73	74

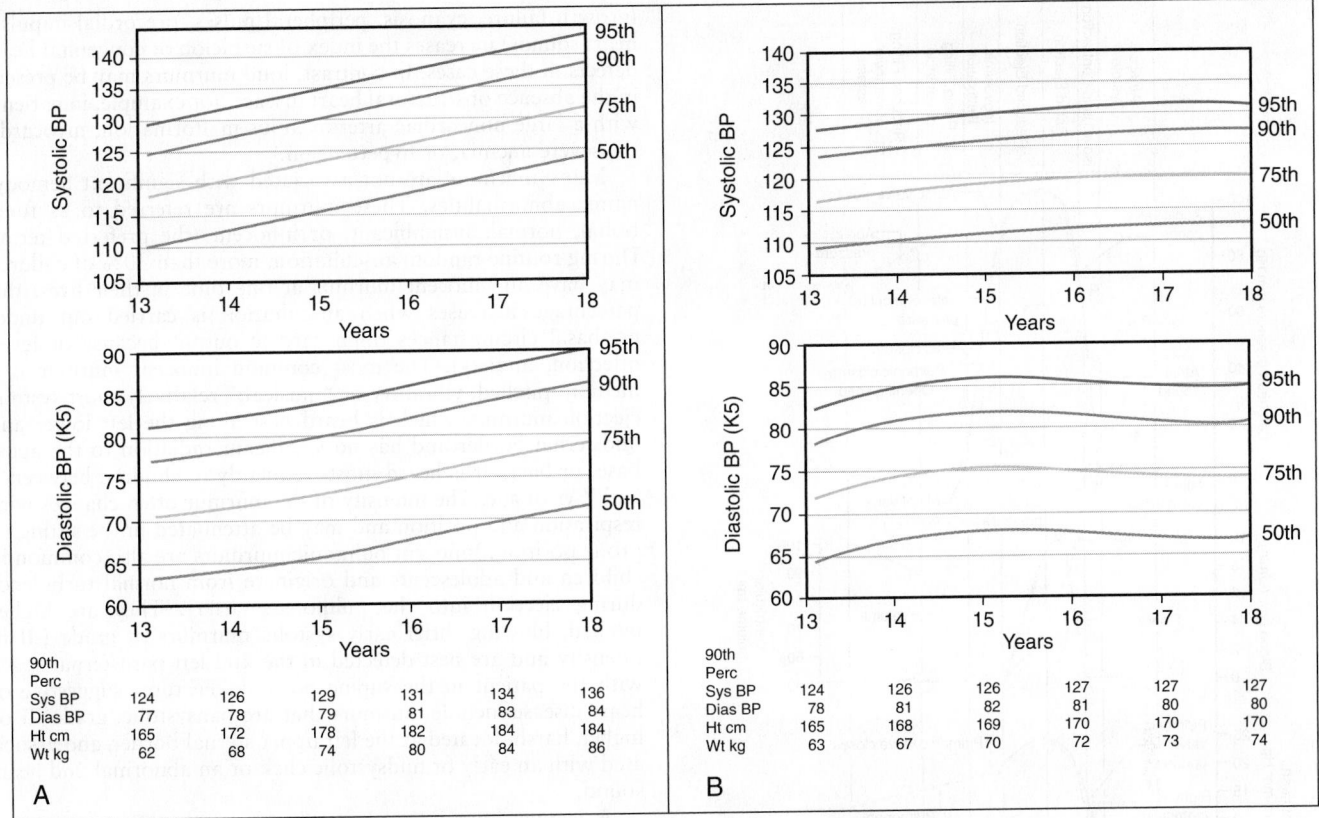

Figure 416-2 *A,* Age-specific percentiles of blood pressure (BP) measurements in boys 13-18 yr of age. *B,* Age-specific percentiles of BP measurements in girls 13-18 yr of age; Korotkoff phase V (K5) used for diastolic BP. Dias, diastolic; Ht, height; Perc, percentile; Sys, systolic; Wt, weight. (From [no authors listed]: Report of the Second Task Force on Blood Pressure Control in Children—1987. National Heart, Lung, and Blood Institute, Bethesda, MD, *Pediatrics* 79:1–25, 1987. Copyright 1987 by the American Academy of Pediatrics.)

arteriosus). Pulmonary ejection clicks, which are associated with mild to moderate pulmonary stenosis, are best heard at the left middle to upper sternal border and vary with respirations, often disappearing with inspiration. Split 1st heart sounds are usually heard best at the lower left sternal border. A midsystolic click heard at the apex, often preceding a late systolic murmur, suggests mitral valve prolapse.

Murmurs should be described according to their intensity, pitch, timing (systolic or diastolic), variation in intensity, time to peak intensity, area of maximal intensity, and radiation to other areas. Auscultation for murmurs should be carried out across the upper precordium, down the left or right sternal border, and out to the apex and left axilla. Auscultation should also always be performed in the right axilla and over both sides of the back. Systolic murmurs are classified as ejection, pansystolic, or late systolic according to the timing of the murmur in relation to the 1st and 2nd heart sounds. The intensity of systolic murmurs is graded from I to VI: I, barely audible; II, medium intensity; III, loud but no thrill; IV, loud with a thrill; V, very loud but still requiring positioning of the stethoscope at least partly on the chest; and VI, so loud that the murmur can be heard with the stethoscope off the chest. In patients who have undergone prior heart surgery, a murmur of grade IV or greater may be heard in the absence of a thrill.

Systolic ejection murmurs start a short time after a well-heard 1st heart sound, increase in intensity, peak, and then decrease in intensity; they usually end before the 2nd sound. In patients with severe pulmonary stenosis, however, the murmur may extend beyond the 1st component of the 2nd sound, thus obscuring it. **Pansystolic or holosystolic murmurs** begin almost simultaneously with the 1st heart sound and continue throughout systole, on occasion becoming gradually decrescendo. It is helpful to remember that after closure of the atrioventricular valves (the 1st heart sound), a brief period occurs during which ventricular pressure increases but the semilunar valves remain closed (isovolumic contraction; see Fig. 416-3). Thus, pansystolic murmurs (heard during both isovolumic contraction and the ejection phases of systole) cannot be caused by flow across the semilunar valves because these valves are closed during isovolumic contraction. Pansystolic murmurs must therefore be related to blood exiting the contracting ventricle via either an abnormal opening (a ventricular septal defect) or atrioventricular (mitral or tricuspid) valve insufficiency. Systolic ejection murmurs usually imply increased flow or stenosis across one of the ventricular outflow tracts (aortic or pulmonic). In infants with rapid heart rates, it is often difficult to distinguish between ejection and pansystolic murmurs. If a clear and distinct 1st heart sound can be appreciated, the murmur is most likely ejection in nature.

A **continuous murmur** is a systolic murmur that continues or "spills" into diastole and indicates continuous flow, such as in the presence of a patent ductus arteriosus or other aortopulmonary communication. This murmur should be differentiated from a to-and-fro murmur, where the systolic component of the murmur ends at or before the 2nd sound and the diastolic murmur begins after semilunar valve closure (aortic or pulmonary stenosis combined with insufficiency). A late systolic murmur begins well beyond the 1st heart sound and continues until the end of systole. Such murmurs may be heard after a midsystolic click in patients with mitral valve prolapse and insufficiency.

Several types of **diastolic murmurs** (graded I-IV) can be identified. A decrescendo diastolic murmur is a blowing murmur along the left sternal border that begins with S_2 and diminishes toward mid-diastole. When high-pitched, this murmur is associated with aortic valve insufficiency or pulmonary insufficiency related to pulmonary hypertension. When low-pitched, this murmur is associated with pulmonary valve insufficiency in the absence of

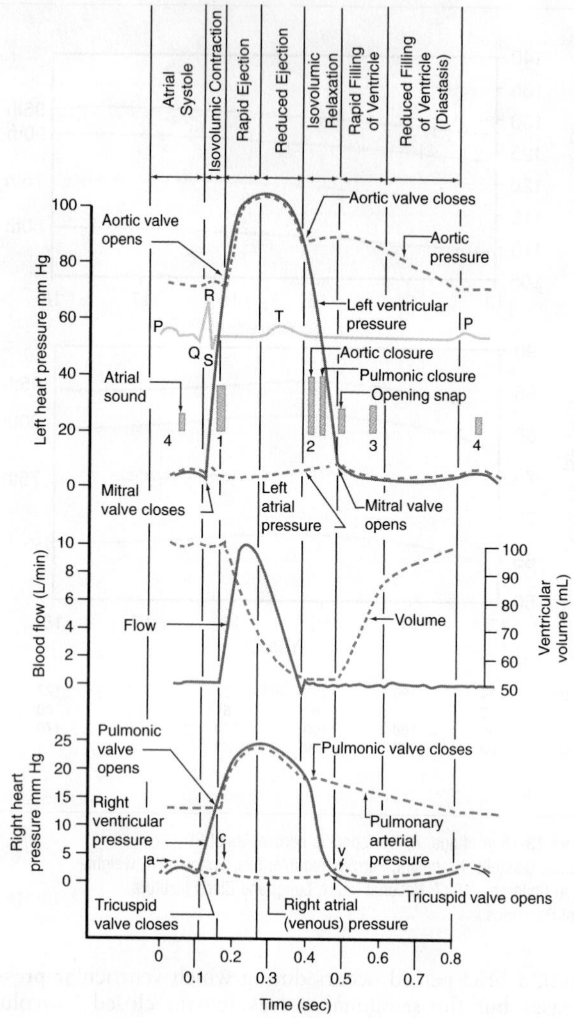

Figure 416-3 Idealized diagram of the temporal events of a cardiac cycle.

pulmonary hypertension. A low-pitched decrescendo diastolic murmur is typically noted after surgical repair of the pulmonary outflow tract in defects such as tetralogy of Fallot or in patients with absent pulmonary valves. A rumbling mid-diastolic murmur at the left middle and lower sternal border may be due to increased blood flow across the tricuspid valve, such as occurs with an atrial septal defect or, less often, because of actual stenosis of this valve. When this murmur is heard at the apex, it is caused by increased flow across the mitral valve, such as occurs with large left-to-right shunts at the ventricular level (ventricular septal defects), at the great vessel level (patent ductus arteriosus, aorto-pulmonary shunts), or with increased flow because of mitral insufficiency. When an apical diastolic rumbling murmur is longer and is accentuated at the end of diastole (presystolic), it usually indicates anatomic mitral valve stenosis.

The absence of a precordial murmur does not rule out significant congenital or acquired heart disease. Congenital heart defects, some of which are ductal dependent, may not demonstrate a murmur if the ductus arteriosus closes. These lesions include pulmonary or tricuspid valve atresia and transposition of the great arteries. Murmurs may seem insignificant in patients with severe aortic stenosis, atrial septal defects, anomalous pulmonary venous return, atrioventricular septal defects, coarctation of the aorta, or anomalous insertion of a coronary artery. Careful attention to other components of the physical examination (growth failure, cyanosis, peripheral pulses, precordial impulse, heart sounds) increases the index of suspicion of congenital heart defects in these cases. In contrast, loud murmurs may be present in the absence of structural heart disease, for example, in patients with a large noncardiac arteriovenous malformation, myocarditis, severe anemia, or hypertension.

Many murmurs are not associated with significant hemodynamic abnormalities. These murmurs are referred to as functional, normal, insignificant, or innocent (the preferred term). During routine random auscultation, more than 30% of children may have an innocent murmur at one time in their lives; this percentage increases when auscultation is carried out under nonbasal circumstances (high cardiac output because of fever, infection, anxiety). The most **common innocent murmur** is a medium-pitched, vibratory or "musical," relatively short systolic ejection murmur, which is heard best along the left lower and midsternal border and has no significant radiation to the apex, base, or back. It is heard most frequently in children between 3 and 7 yr of age. The intensity of the murmur often changes with respiration and position and may be attenuated in the sitting or prone position. Innocent pulmonic murmurs are also common in children and adolescents and originate from normal turbulence during ejection into the pulmonary artery. They are higher pitched, blowing, brief early systolic murmurs of grade I-II in intensity and are best detected in the 2nd left parasternal space with the patient in the supine position. Features suggestive of heart disease include murmurs that are pansystolic, grade III or higher, harsh, located at the left upper sternal border, and associated with an early or midsystolic click or an abnormal 2nd heart sound.

A **venous hum** is another example of a common innocent murmur heard during childhood. Such hums are produced by turbulence of blood in the jugular venous system; they have no pathologic significance and may be heard in the neck or anterior portion of the upper part of the chest. A venous hum consists of a soft humming sound heard in both systole and diastole; it can be exaggerated or made to disappear by varying the position of the head, or it can be decreased by lightly compressing the jugular venous system in the neck. These simple maneuvers are sufficient to differentiate a venous hum from the murmurs produced by organic cardiovascular disease, particularly a patent ductus arteriosus.

The lack of significance of an innocent murmur should be discussed with the child's parents. It is important to offer complete reassurance because lingering doubts about the importance of a cardiac murmur may have profound effects on child-rearing practices, most often in the form of overprotectiveness. An underlying fear that a cardiac abnormality is present may negatively affect a child's self-image and subtly influence personality development. The physician should explain that an innocent murmur is simply a "noise" and does not indicate the presence of a significant cardiac defect. When asked, "Will it go away?" the best response is to state that because the murmur has no clinical significance, it therefore does not matter whether it "goes away." Parents should be warned that the intensity of the murmur might increase during febrile illnesses, a time when, typically, another physician examines the child. With growth, however, innocent murmurs are less well heard and often disappear completely. At times, additional studies may be indicated to rule out a congenital heart defect, but "routine" electrocardiographic, chest roentgenographic, and echocardiographic examinations should be avoided in well children with innocent murmurs.

BIBLIOGRAPHY

Please visit the Nelson Textbook of Pediatrics *website at www.expertconsult.com for the complete bibliography.*

Chapter 417
Laboratory Evaluation

417.1 Radiologic Assessment

Daniel Bernstein

The chest x-ray may provide information about cardiac size and shape, pulmonary blood flow (vascularity), pulmonary edema, and associated lung and thoracic anomalies that may be associated with congenital syndromes (skeletal dysplasias, extra or deficient number of ribs, abnormal vertebrae, previous cardiac surgery). Variations are due to differences in body build, the phase of respiration or the cardiac cycle, abnormalities of the thoracic cage, position of the diaphragm, or pulmonary disease.

The most frequently used measurement of cardiac size is the maximal width of the cardiac shadow in a posteroanterior chest film taken mid-inspiration. A vertical line is drawn down the middle of the sternal shadow, and perpendicular lines are drawn from the sternal line to the extreme right and left borders of the heart; the sum of the lengths of these lines is the maximal cardiac width. The maximal chest width is obtained by drawing a horizontal line between the right and left inner borders of the rib cage at the level of the top of the right diaphragm. When the maximal cardiac width is more than half the maximal chest width (cardiothoracic ratio >50%), the heart is usually enlarged. Cardiac size should be evaluated only when the film is taken during inspiration with the patient in an upright position. A diagnosis of "cardiac enlargement" on expiratory or prone films is a common cause of unnecessary referrals and laboratory studies.

The cardiothoracic ratio is a less useful index of cardiac enlargement in infants than in older children because the horizontal position of the heart may increase the ratio to >50% in the absence of true enlargement. Furthermore, the thymus may overlap not only the base of the heart but also virtually the entire mediastinum, thus obscuring the true cardiac silhouette.

A lateral chest roentgenogram may be helpful in infants as well as in older children with pectus excavatum or other conditions that result in a narrow anteroposterior chest dimension. In these situations, the heart may appear small in the lateral view and suggest that the apparent enlargement in the posteroanterior projection was due to either the thymic image (anterior mediastinum only) or flattening of the cardiac chambers as a result of a structural chest abnormality.

In the posteroanterior view, the left border of the cardiac shadow consists of three convex shadows produced, from above downward, by the aortic knob, the main and left pulmonary arteries, and the left ventricle (Fig. 417-1). In cases of moderate to marked left atrial enlargement, the atrium may project between the pulmonary artery and the left ventricle. The outflow tract of the right ventricle does not contribute to the shadows formed by the left border of the heart. The aortic knob is not as easily seen in infants and children as in adults. The side of the aortic arch (left or right) can often be inferred as being opposite the side of the midline from which the air-filled trachea is visualized. This observation is important because a right-sided aortic arch is often present in cyanotic congenital heart disease, particularly in tetralogy of Fallot. Three structures contribute to the right border of the cardiac silhouette. In the view from above, they are the superior vena cava, the ascending aorta, and the right atrium.

Enlargement of cardiac chambers or major arteries and veins results in prominence of the areas in which these structures are normally outlined on the chest x-ray. In contrast, the electrocardiogram (ECG) is a more sensitive and accurate index of **ventricular hypertrophy.**

The chest roentgenogram is also an important tool for assessing the degree of pulmonary vascularity. Angiocardiographic studies have shown that the hilar shadows seen on the plain chest roentgenogram are mainly vascular. Pulmonary overcirculation is usually associated with left-to-right shunt lesions, whereas pulmonary undercirculation is associated with obstruction of the outflow tract of the right ventricle.

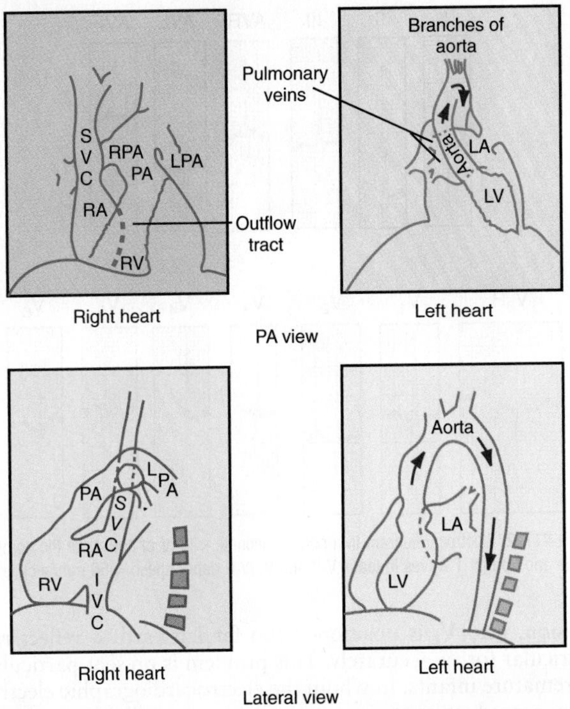

Figure 417-1 Idealized diagrams showing normal position of the cardiac chambers and great blood vessels. IVC, inferior vena cava; LA, left atrium; LPA, left pulmonary artery; LV, left ventricle; PA, pulmonary artery; RA, right atrium; RPA, right pulmonary artery; RV, right ventricle; SVC, superior vena cava. (Adapted and redrawn from Dotter CT, Steinberg I: Angiocardiographic interpretation, *Radiology* 153:513, 1949.)

The esophagus is closely related to the great vessels, and a barium esophagogram can help delineate these structures in the initial evaluation of suspected vascular rings, although this has largely been supplanted by CT. Echocardiographic examination best defines the morphologic features of intracardiac chambers, cardiac valves, and intracardiac shunts. CT is used as an adjunct to echo to evaluate extracardiac vascular morphology. MRI is used to quantitate ventricular volumes, cardiac function, and shunt and regurgitant fractions.

417.2 Electrocardiography

Daniel Bernstein

DEVELOPMENTAL CHANGES

The marked changes that occur in cardiac physiology and chamber dominance during the perinatal transition (Chapter 415) are reflected in the evolution of the ECG during the neonatal period. Because vascular resistance in the pulmonary and systemic circulations is nearly equal in a term fetus, the intrauterine work of the heart results in an equal mass of both the right and left ventricles. After birth, systemic vascular resistance rises when the placental circulation is eliminated, and pulmonary vascular resistance falls when the lungs expand. These changes are reflected in the ECG as the right ventricular wall begins to thin.

The ECG demonstrates these anatomic and hemodynamic features principally by changes in QRS and T-wave morphologic features. It is recommended that a 13-lead ECG be performed in pediatric patients, including either lead V_3R or V_4R, which are important in the evaluation of right ventricular hypertrophy. On

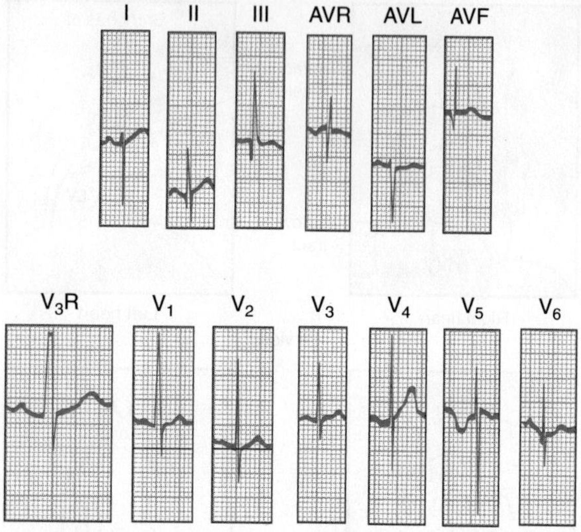

Figure 417-2 Electrocardiogram in a normal neonate <24 hr of age. Note the dominant R wave and upright T waves in leads V_3R and V_1 (V_3R paper speed = 50 mm/sec).

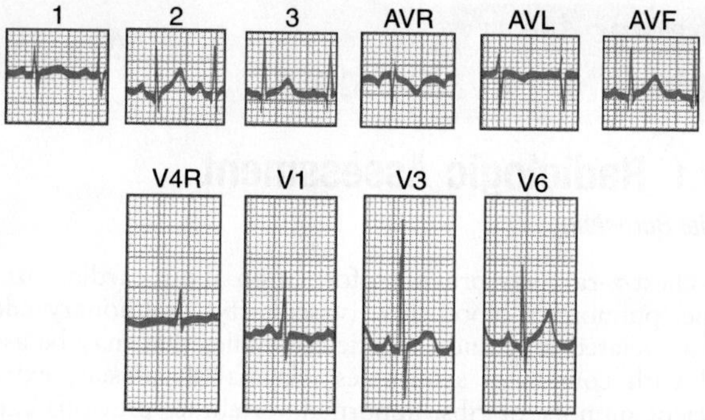

Figure 417-3 Electrocardiogram of a normal infant. Note the tall R and small S waves in V_4R and V_1 and the inverted T wave in these leads. A dominant R wave is also present in V_6.

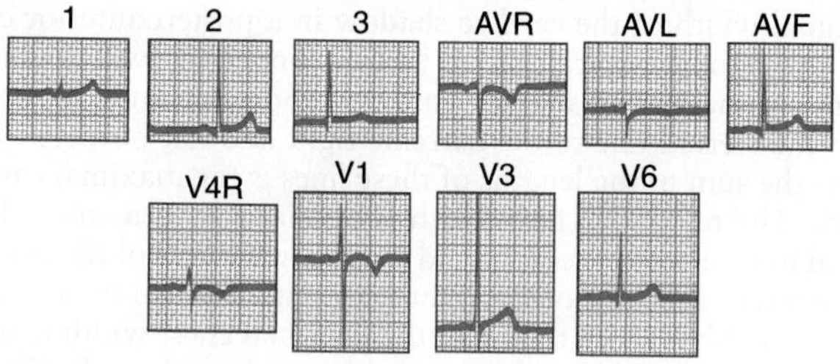

Figure 417-4 Electrocardiogram of a normal child. Note the relatively tall R waves and inversion of the T waves in V_4R and V_1.

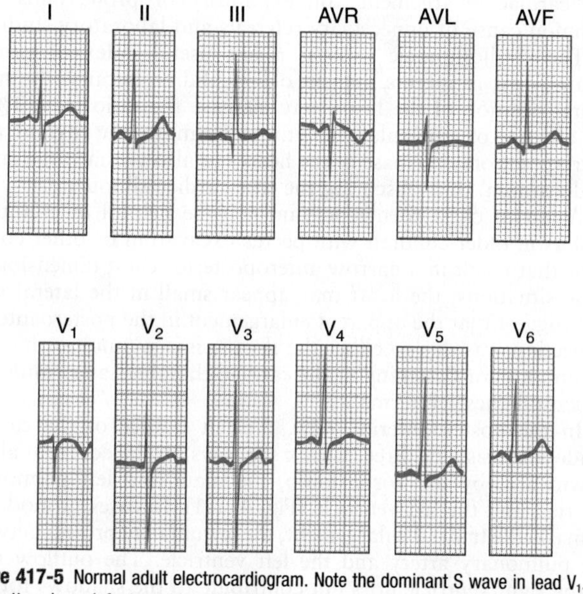

Figure 417-5 Normal adult electrocardiogram. Note the dominant S wave in lead V_1. This pattern in an infant would indicate the presence of left ventricular hypertrophy.

occasion, lead V_1 is positioned too far leftward to reflect right ventricular forces accurately. This problem is present particularly in premature infants, in whom the electrocardiographic electrode gel may produce contact among all the precordial leads.

During the 1st days of life, right axis deviation, large R waves, and upright T waves in the right precordial leads (V_3R or V_4R and V_1) are the norm (Fig. 417-2). As pulmonary vascular resistance decreases in the 1st few days after birth, the right precordial T waves become negative. In the great majority of instances, this change occurs within the 1st 48 hr of life. Upright T waves that persist in leads V_3R, V_4R, or V_1 beyond 1 wk of life are an abnormal finding indicating right ventricular hypertrophy or strain, even in the absence of QRS voltage criteria. The T wave in V_1 should never be positive before 6 yr of age and may remain negative into adolescence. This finding represents one of the most important, yet subtle differences between pediatric and adult ECGs and is a common source of error when adult cardiologists interpret pediatric ECGs.

In a newborn, the mean **QRS frontal-plane axis** normally lies in the range of +110 to +180 degrees. The right-sided chest leads reveal a larger positive (R) than negative (S) wave and may do so for months because the right ventricle remains relatively thick throughout infancy. Left-sided leads (V_5 and V_6) also reflect right-sided dominance in the early neonatal period, when the R : S ratio in these leads may be <1. A dominant R wave in V_5 and V_6 reflecting left ventricular forces quickly becomes evident within the 1st few days of life (Fig. 417-3). Over the years, the QRS axis gradually shifts leftward, and the right ventricular forces slowly regress. Leads V_1, V_3R, and V_4R display a prominent R wave until 6 mo to 8 yr of age. Most children have an R : S ratio >1 in lead V_4R until they are 4 yr of age. The T waves are inverted in leads V_4R, V_1, V_2, and V_3 during infancy and may remain so into the middle of the 2nd decade of life and beyond. The processes of right ventricular thinning and left ventricular growth are best reflected in the QRS-T pattern over the right precordial leads. The diagnosis of right or left ventricular hypertrophy in a pediatric patient can be made only with an understanding of the normal developmental physiology of these chambers at various ages until adulthood is reached. As the left ventricle becomes dominant, the ECG evolves to the characteristic pattern of older children (Fig. 417-4) and adults (Fig. 417-5).

Ventricular hypertrophy may result in increased voltage in the R and S waves in the chest leads. The height of these deflections is governed by the proximity of the specific electrode to the surface of the heart; by the sequence of electrical activation through the ventricles, which can result in variable degrees of cancellation of forces; and by hypertrophy of the myocardium. Because the chest wall in infants and children, as well as in adolescents, may be relatively thin, the diagnosis of ventricular hypertrophy should not be based on voltage changes alone.

The diagnosis of pathologic right ventricular hypertrophy is difficult in the 1st wk of life because physiologic right ventricular hypertrophy is a normal finding. Serial tracings are often necessary to determine whether marked right axis deviation and potentially abnormal right precordial forces or T waves, or both, will persist beyond the neonatal period (Fig. 417-6). In contrast, an adult electrocardiographic pattern (see Fig. 417-5) seen in a neonate suggests left ventricular hypertrophy. The exception is a premature infant, who may display a more "mature" ECG than a full-term infant (Fig. 417-7) as a result of lower pulmonary vascular resistance secondary to underdevelopment of the medial

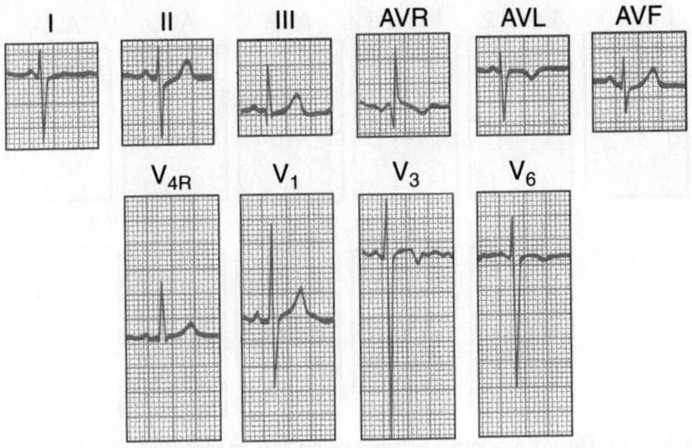

Figure 417-6 Electrocardiogram of an infant with right ventricular hypertrophy (tetralogy of Fallot). Note the tall R waves in the right precordium and deep S waves in V_6. The positive T waves in V_4R and V_1 are also characteristic of right ventricular hypertrophy.

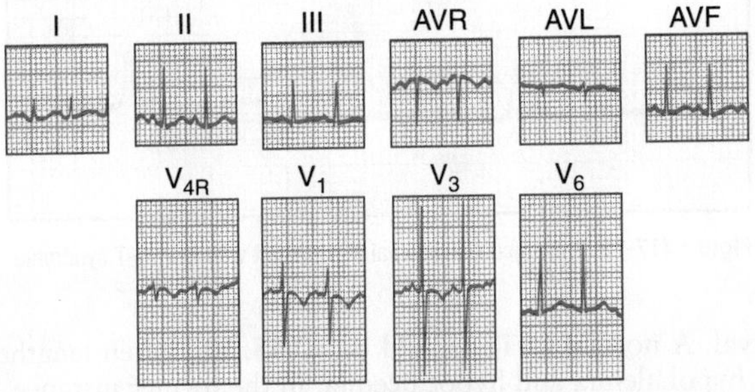

Figure 417-7 Electrocardiogram of a premature infant (weight 2 kg and age 5 wk at the time of the tracing). The cardiovascular system was clinically normal. Left ventricular dominance is manifested by R-wave progression across the chest, similar to tracings obtained from older children. Compare with the tracing from a normal full-term infant (see Fig. 417-3).

muscular layer of the pulmonary arterioles. Some premature infants display a pattern of generalized low voltage across the precordium.

The ECG should always be evaluated systematically to avoid the possibility of overlooking a minor, but important abnormality. One approach is to begin with an assessment of rate and rhythm, followed by a calculation of the mean frontal-plane QRS axis, measurements of segment intervals, assessment of voltages, and, finally, assessment of ST and T-wave abnormalities.

RATE AND RHYTHM

A brief rhythm strip should be examined to assess whether a P wave always precedes each QRS complex. The P-wave axis should then be estimated as an indication of whether the rhythm is originating from the sinus node. If the atria are situated normally in the chest, the P wave should be upright in leads I and aVF and inverted in lead aVR. With atrial inversion (situs inversus), the P wave may be inverted in lead I. Inverted P waves in leads II and aVF are seen in low atrial, nodal, or junctional rhythms. The absence of P waves indicates a rhythm originating more distally in the conduction system. In this case, the morphologic features of the QRS complexes are important in differentiating a junctional (usually a narrow QRS complex) from a ventricular (usually a wide QRS complex) rhythm.

P WAVES

Tall (>2.5 mm), narrow, and spiked P waves are indicative of **right atrial enlargement** and are seen in congenital pulmonary stenosis, Ebstein anomaly of the tricuspid valve, tricuspid atresia, and sometimes cor pulmonale. These abnormal waves are most obvious in leads II, V_3R, and V_1 (Fig. 417-8*A*). Similar waves are

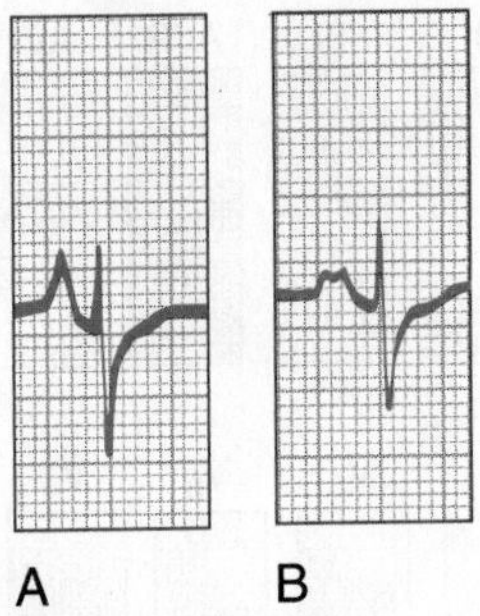

Figure 417-8 Atrial enlargement. *A,* Peaked narrow P waves characteristic of right atrial enlargement. *B,* Wide bifid M-shaped P waves typical of left atrial enlargement.

sometimes seen in thyrotoxicosis. **Broad P waves,** commonly **bifid** and sometimes **biphasic,** are indicative of left atrial enlargement (Fig. 417-8*B*). They are seen in some patients with large left-to-right shunts (ventricular septal defect [VSD], patent ductus arteriosus [PDA]) and with severe mitral stenosis or regurgitation. Flat P waves may be encountered in hyperkalemia.

QRS COMPLEX

Right Ventricular Hypertrophy

For the most accurate assessment of ventricular hypertrophy, pediatric ECGs should include the right precordial lead V_3R or V_4R, or both. The diagnosis of right ventricular hypertrophy depends on demonstration of the following changes (see Fig. 417-6): (1) a qR pattern in the right ventricular surface leads; (2) a positive T wave in leads V_3R-V_4R and V_1-V_3 between the ages of 6 days and 6 yr; (3) a monophasic R wave in V_3R, V_4R, or V_1; (4) an rsR′ pattern in the right precordial leads with the 2nd R wave taller than the initial one; (5) age-corrected increased voltage of the R wave in leads V_3R-V_4R or the S wave in leads V_6-V_7, or both; (6) marked right axis deviation (>120 degrees in patients beyond the newborn period); and (7) complete reversal of the normal adult precordial RS pattern. At least 2 of these changes should be present to support a diagnosis of right ventricular hypertrophy.

Abnormal ventricular loading can be characterized as either systolic (as a result of obstruction of the right ventricular outflow tract, as in pulmonic stenosis) or diastolic (as a result of increased volume load, as in atrial septal defects [ASDs]). These two types of abnormal loads result in distinct electrocardiographic patterns. The **systolic overload pattern** is characterized by tall, pure R waves in the right precordial leads. In older children, the T waves in these leads are initially upright and later become inverted. In infants and children <6 yr, the T waves in V_3R-V_4R and V_1 are abnormally upright. The **diastolic overload pattern** (typically seen in patients with ASDs) is characterized by an rsR′ pattern (Fig. 417-9) and a slightly increased QRS duration (minor right ventricular conduction delay). Patients with mild to moderate pulmonary stenosis may also exhibit an rsR′ pattern in the right precordial leads.

Left Ventricular Hypertrophy

The following features indicate the presence of left ventricular hypertrophy (Fig. 417-10): (1) depression of the ST segments and inversion of the T waves in the left precordial leads (V_5, V_6, and V_7), known as a *left ventricular strain* pattern—these findings suggest the presence of a severe lesion; (2) a deep Q wave in the left precordial leads; and (3) increased voltage of the S wave in V_3R and V_1 or the R wave in V_6-V_7, or both. It is important to emphasize that evaluation of left ventricular hypertrophy should not be based on voltage criteria alone. The concepts of systolic and diastolic overload, though not always consistent, are also useful in evaluating left ventricular enlargement. Severe systolic overload of the left ventricle is suggested by straightening of the

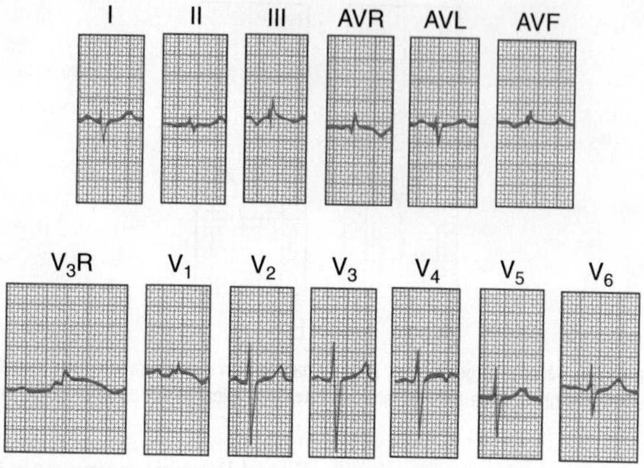

Figure 417-9 Electrocardiogram showing right ventricular conduction delay characterized by an rsR′ pattern in V_1 and a deep S wave in V_6 (V_3R paper speed = 50 mm/sec).

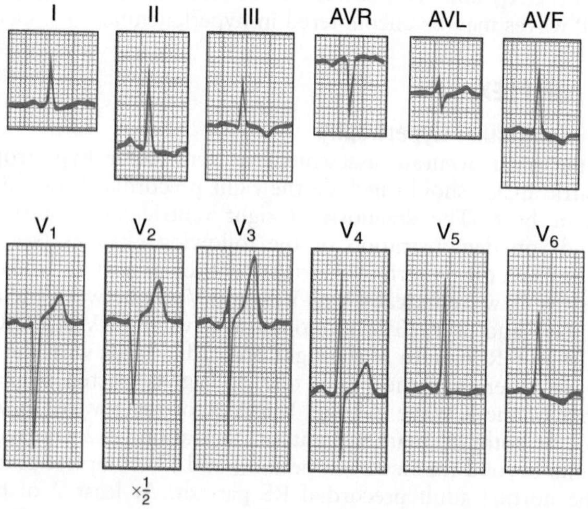

Figure 417-10 Electrocardiogram showing left ventricular hypertrophy in a 12 yr old child with aortic stenosis. Note the deep S wave in V_1-V_3 and tall R in V_5. In addition, T-wave inversion is present in leads II, III, aVF, and V_6.

ST segments and inverted T waves over the left precordial leads; diastolic overload may result in tall R waves, a large Q wave, and normal T waves over the left precordium. Finally, an infant with an ECG that would be considered "normal" for an older child may, in fact, have left ventricular hypertrophy.

Bundle Branch Block

A complete right bundle branch block may be congenital or may be acquired after surgery for congenital heart disease, especially when a right ventriculotomy has been performed, as in repair of the tetralogy of Fallot. Congenital left bundle branch block is rare; this pattern is occasionally seen with cardiomyopathy. A bundle branch block pattern may be indicative of a bypass tract associated with one of the pre-excitation syndromes (Chapter 429).

P-R AND Q-T INTERVALS

The duration of the P-R interval shortens with increasing heart rate; thus, assessment of this interval should be based on age- and rate-corrected nomograms. A long P-R interval is diagnostic of a **1st-degree heart block,** the cause of which may be congenital, postoperative, inflammatory (myocarditis, pericarditis, rheumatic fever), or pharmacologic (digitalis).

The duration of the Q-T interval varies with the cardiac rate; a corrected Q-T interval (Q-Tc) can be calculated by dividing the measured Q-T interval by the square root of the preceding R-R

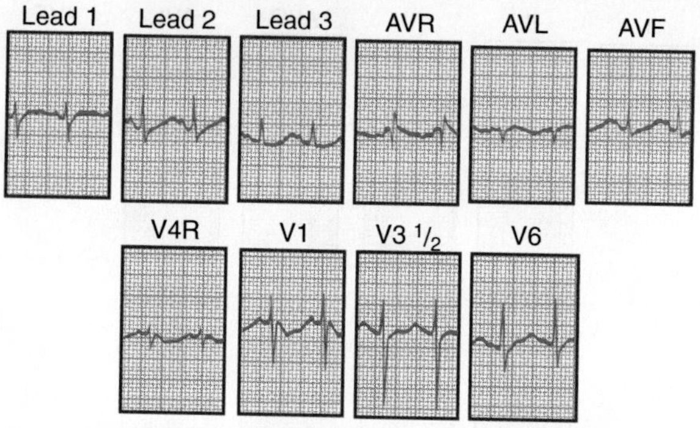

Figure 417-11 Electrocardiogram in hypokalemia (serum potassium, 2.7 mEq/L; serum calcium, 4.8 mEq/L at the time of the tracing). Note the prolongation of electrical systole as evidenced by a widened TU wave, as well as depression of the ST segment in V_4R, V_1, and V_6.

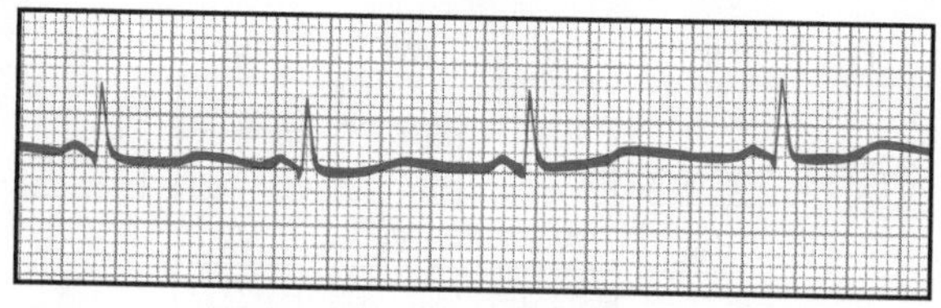

Figure 417-12 Prolonged Q-T interval in a patient with long Q-T syndrome.

interval. A normal Q-Tc should be <0.45. It is often lengthened with hypokalemia and hypocalcemia; in the former instance, a U wave may be noted at the end of the T wave (Fig. 417-11). There are a number of medications that can also lengthen the Q-T interval. A congenitally prolonged Q-T interval (Fig. 417-12) may also be seen in children with one of the long Q-T syndromes. These patients are at high risk for ventricular arrhythmias, including a form of ventricular tachycardia known as torsades de pointes, and sudden death (Chapter 429.5).

ST SEGMENT AND T-WAVE ABNORMALITIES

A slight elevation of the ST segment may occur in normal teenagers and is attributed to early repolarization of the heart. In pericarditis, irritation of the epicardium may cause elevation of the ST segment followed by abnormal T-wave inversion as healing progresses. Administration of digitalis is sometimes associated with sagging of the ST segment and abnormal inversion of the T wave.

Depression of the ST segment may also occur in any condition that produces myocardial damage or ischemia, including severe anemia, carbon monoxide poisoning, aberrant origin of the left coronary artery from the pulmonary artery, glycogen storage disease of the heart, myocardial tumors, and mucopolysaccharidoses. An aberrant origin of the left coronary artery from the pulmonary artery may lead to changes indistinguishable from those of acute myocardial infarction in adults. Similar changes may occur in patients with other rare abnormalities of the coronary arteries and in those with cardiomyopathy, even in the presence of normal coronary arteries. These patterns are often misread in young infants because of the unfamiliarity of pediatricians with this "infarct" pattern, and thus a high index of suspicion must be maintained in infants with dilated cardiomyopathy or with symptoms compatible with coronary ischemia (e.g., inconsolable crying).

T-wave inversion may occur in myocarditis and pericarditis, or it may be a sign of either right or left ventricular hypertrophy and strain. Hypothyroidism may produce flat or inverted T waves in association with generalized low voltage. In hyperkalemia, the T waves are commonly of high voltage and are tent-shaped (Fig. 417-13).

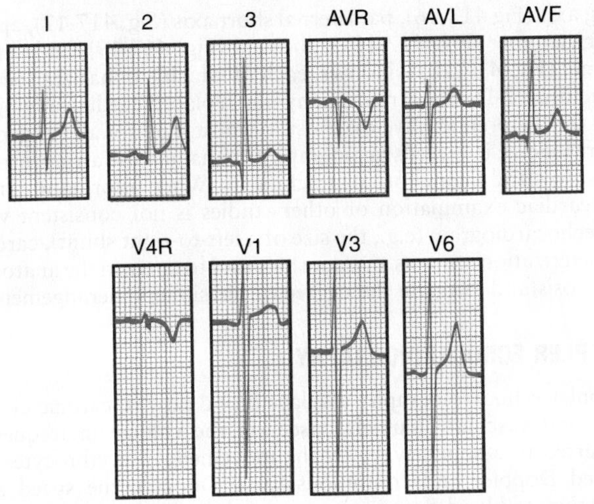

Figure 417-13 Electrocardiogram in hyperkalemia (serum potassium, 6.5 mEq/L; serum calcium, 5.1 mEq/L). Note the tall, tent-shaped T waves, especially in leads I, II, and V_6.

BIBLIOGRAPHY

Please visit the Nelson Textbook of Pediatrics *website at www.expertconsult.com for the complete bibliography.*

417.3 Hematologic Data

Daniel Bernstein

In acyanotic infants with large left-to-right shunts, the onset of heart failure often coincides with the nadir of the normal physiologic anemia of infancy. Increasing the hematocrit in these patients to >40% may decrease shunt volume and result in an improvement in symptoms; this form of treatment is reserved for infants who are not otherwise surgical candidates (extremely premature infants or those with exceedingly complex congenital heart disease for whom only palliative surgery is possible). In these select infants, regular evaluation of the hematocrit and booster transfusions when appropriate may be helpful in improving growth. In some patients, particularly those who are anemic but stable hemodynamically, erythropoietin (Epogen) can be used to more gradually increase hemoglobin and thus oxygen-carrying capacity.

Polycythemia is frequently noted in cyanotic patients with right-to-left shunts. Patients with severe polycythemia are in a delicate balance between the risks of intravascular thrombosis and a bleeding diathesis. The most frequent abnormalities include accelerated fibrinolysis, thrombocytopenia, abnormal clot retraction, hypofibrinogenemia, prolonged prothrombin time, and prolonged partial thromboplastin time. The preparation of cyanotic, polycythemic patients for elective noncardiac surgery, such as dental extraction, includes evaluation and treatment of abnormal coagulation.

Because of the high viscosity of polycythemic blood (hematocrit >65%), patients with cyanotic congenital heart disease are at risk for the development of vascular thromboses, especially of cerebral veins. Dehydration increases the risk of thrombosis, and thus adequate fluid intake must be maintained during hot weather or intercurrent gastrointestinal illnesses. Diuretics should be used with caution in these patients and may need to be decreased if fluid intake is a concern. Polycythemic infants with concomitant **iron deficiency** are at even greater risk for cerebrovascular accidents, probably because of the decreased deformability of microcytic red blood cells. Iron therapy may reduce this risk somewhat, but surgical treatment of the cardiac anomaly is the best therapy.

Severely cyanotic patients should have periodic determinations of hemoglobin and hematocrit. Increasing polycythemia, often associated with headache, fatigue, dyspnea, or a combination of these conditions, is one indication for palliative or corrective surgical intervention. In cyanotic patients with inoperable conditions, partial exchange transfusion may be required to treat symptomatic individuals whose hematocrit has risen to the 65-70% level. This procedure is not without risk, especially in patients with an extreme elevation in pulmonary vascular resistance. Because these patients do not tolerate wide fluctuations in circulating blood volume, blood should be replaced with fresh frozen plasma or albumin.

417.4 Echocardiography

Daniel Bernstein

Transthoracic echocardiography has replaced invasive studies such as cardiac catheterization for the *initial diagnosis* of most forms of congenital heart disease. The echocardiographic examination can be used to evaluate cardiac structure in congenital heart lesions, estimate intracardiac pressures and gradients across stenotic valves and vessels, quantitate cardiac contractile function (both systolic and diastolic), determine the direction of flow across a defect, examine the integrity of the coronary arteries, and detect the presence of vegetations from endocarditis, as well as the presence of pericardial fluid, cardiac tumors, and chamber thrombi. Echocardiography may also be used to assist in the performance of interventional procedures, including pericardiocentesis, balloon atrial septostomy (Chapter 425.2), atrial or ventricular septal defect closure and endocardial biopsy, and in the placement of flow-directed pulmonary artery (Swan-Ganz) monitoring catheters. **Transesophageal echocardiography** is used routinely to monitor ventricular function in patients during difficult surgical procedures and can provide an immediate assessment of the results of surgical repair of congenital heart lesions. A complete transthoracic echocardiographic examination usually entails a combination of M-mode and two-dimensional (2-D) imaging, as well as pulsed, continuous, and color Doppler flow studies. Doppler tissue imaging and other new technologies provide more quantitative assessments of ventricular function. Three-dimensional (3-D) echocardiography provides valuable information regarding cardiac morphology.

M-MODE ECHOCARDIOGRAPHY

M-mode echocardiography displays a one-dimensional slice of cardiac structure varying over time (Fig. 417-14). It is used mostly for the measurement of cardiac dimensions (wall thickness and chamber size) and cardiac function (fractional shortening, wall thickening). M-mode echocardiography is also useful for assessing the motion of intracardiac structures (opening and closing of valves, movement of free walls and septa) and the anatomy of valves (Fig. 417-15). The most frequently used index of cardiac function in children is percent fractional shortening (%FS), which is calculated as (LVED − LVES)/LVED, where LVED is left ventricular (LV) dimension at end-diastole and LVES is LV dimension at end-systole. Normal fractional shortening is approximately 28-40%. Other M-mode indices of cardiac function include the mean velocity of fiber shortening (mean V_{CF}), systolic time intervals (LVPEP = LV pre-ejection period, LVET = LV ejection time), and isovolemic contraction time. More sophisticated indices of cardiac function can be derived noninvasively with the assistance of echocardiography (pressure-volume relationship, end-systolic wall stress-strain relationship).

TWO-DIMENSIONAL ECHOCARDIOGRAPHY

2-D echocardiography provides a real-time image of cardiac structures. With 2-D echocardiography, the contracting heart is imaged in real time using several standard views, including parasternal

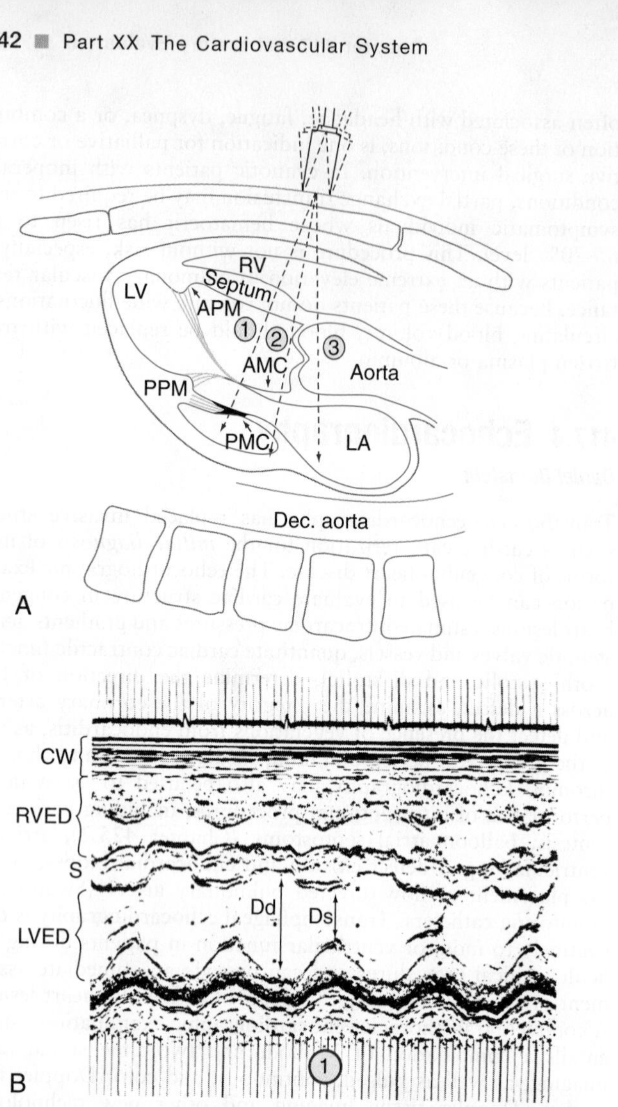

Figure 417-14 M-mode echocardiogram. *A,* Diagram of a sagittal section of a heart showing the structures traversed by the echo beam as it is moved superiorly to positions (*1*), (*2*), and (*3*). AMC, anterior mitral cusp; APM, anterior papillary muscle; Dec. aorta, descending aorta; LA, left atrium; LV, left ventricle; PMC, posterior mitral cusp; PPM, posterior papillary muscle; RV, right ventricle. *B,* Echocardiogram from transducer position (*1*); this view is the best one for measuring cardiac dimensions and fractional shortening. Fractional shortening is calculated as (LVED–LVES)/LVED. CW, chest wall; Ds, LV dimension in systole; LVED, LV dimension at end-diastole (Dd); RVED, RV dimension at end-diastole.

long axis (Fig 417-16), parasternal short axis (Fig. 417-17), apical four chamber (Fig. 417-18), subcostal (Fig. 417-19), and suprasternal (Fig. 417-20) windows, each of which emphasizes specific structures. 2-D echocardiography has replaced cardiac angiography for the preoperative diagnosis of most, but not all congenital heart lesions; it exceeds angiography in imaging the atrioventricular valves and their chordal attachments. When information from the cardiac examination or other studies is not consistent with the echocardiogram (e.g., the size of a left-to-right shunt), cardiac catheterization remains an important tool to confirm the anatomic diagnosis and evaluate the degree of physiologic derangement.

DOPPLER ECHOCARDIOGRAPHY

Doppler echocardiography displays blood flow in cardiac chambers and vascular channels based on the change in frequency imparted to a sound wave by the movement of erythrocytes. In pulsed Doppler and continuous wave Doppler, the speed and direction of blood flow in the line of the echo beam change the transducer's reference frequency. This frequency change can be translated into volumetric flow (L/min) data for estimating systemic or pulmonary blood flow and into pressure (mm Hg) data for estimating gradients across the semilunar or atrioventricular valves or across septal defects or vascular communications such

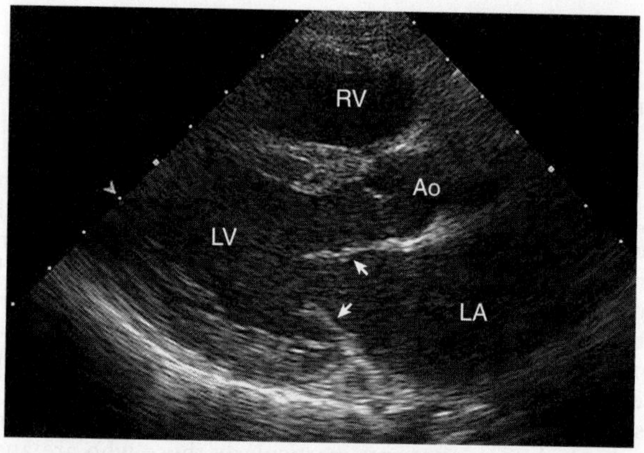

Figure 417-16 Normal parasternal long axis echocardiographic window. The transducer is angulated slightly posteriorly, imaging the left-sided cardiac structures. If the transducer were to be angulated more anteriorly, the right ventricular structures would be imaged. The mitral valve leaflets can be seen in partially open position in early diastole *(arrowheads).* The closed aortic valve leaflets can be seen just below the label *Ao.* Ao, aorta; LA, left atrium; LV, left ventricle; RV, right ventricle.

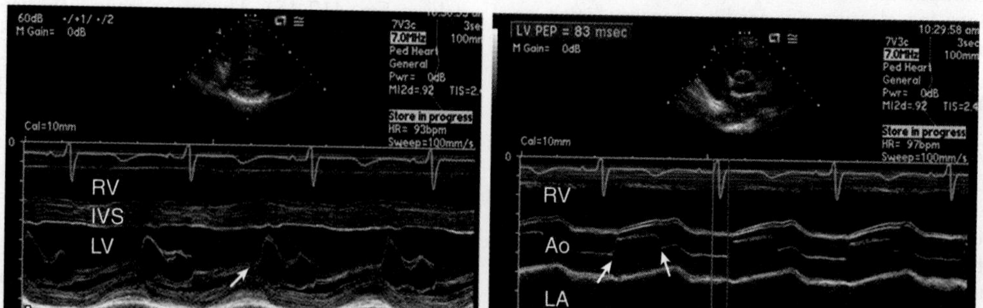

Figure 417-15 M-mode echocardiograms. The small figure at the top of each panel shows the 2-D parasternal short axis echo image from which the M-modes are derived. The cursor can be seen midway through the image, indicating the one-dimensional line through which the M-mode is being sampled. *A,* M-mode echocardiogram of a normal mitral valve. *Arrow* shows the opening of the anterior leaflet in early diastole (see ECG tracing above for reference). *B,* M-mode echocardiogram of a normal aortic valve. The opening and closing of the aortic leaflets in systole are outlined by the two *arrows.* Ao, aorta; IVS, interventricular septum; LV, left ventricle; RV, right ventricle.

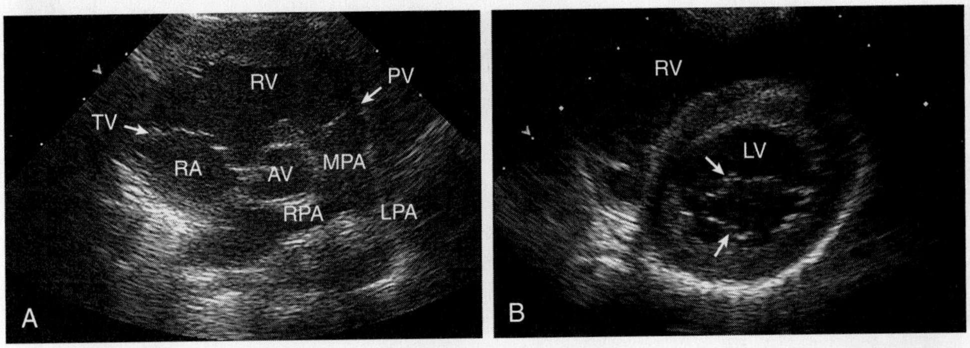

Figure 417-17 Normal parasternal short axis echocardiographic windows. *A,* With the transducer angled superiorly and rightwards, the aortic valve *(AV)* is imaged, surrounded by both inflow and outflow portions of the right ventricle *(RV).* LPA, left pulmonary artery; MPA, main pulmonary artery; PV, pulmonary valve; RA, right atrium; RPA, right pulmonary artery; TV, tricuspid valve. *B,* With the transducer angled inferiorly and leftwards, the left ventricular chamber is imaged along with cross-sectional view of the mitral valve *(arrows).* LV, left ventricle; RV, right ventricle.

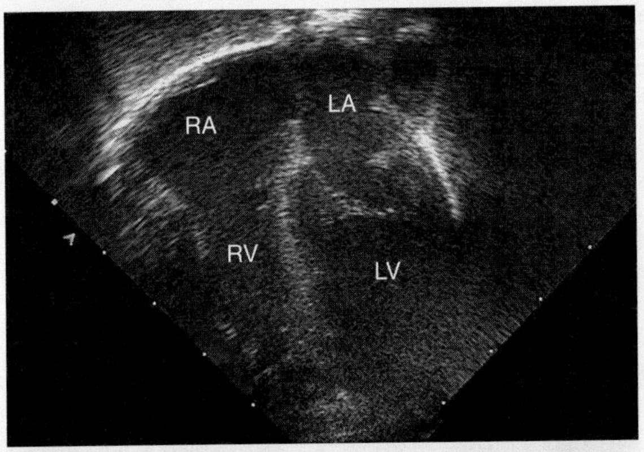

Figure 417-18 Normal apical four chamber echocardiographic window showing all four cardiac chambers and both atrioventricular valves opened in diastole. LA, left atrium; LV, left ventricle; RA, right atrium; RV, right ventricle.

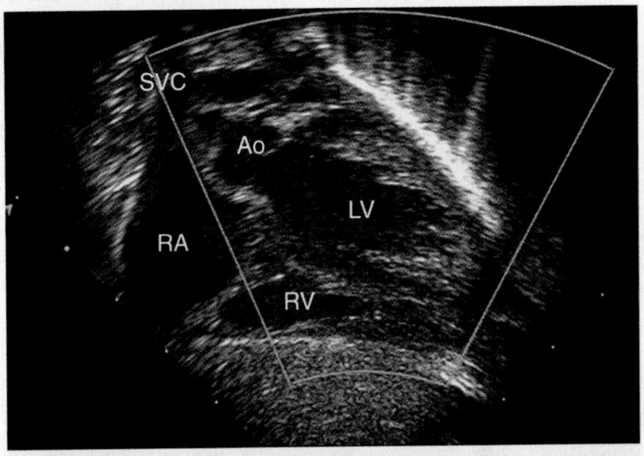

Figure 417-19 Normal subcostal echocardiographic window showing the left ventricular outflow tract. The right-sided structures are not fully imaged in this view. Ao, ascending aorta; LV, left ventricle; RA, right atrium; RV, right ventricle; SVC, superior vena cava.

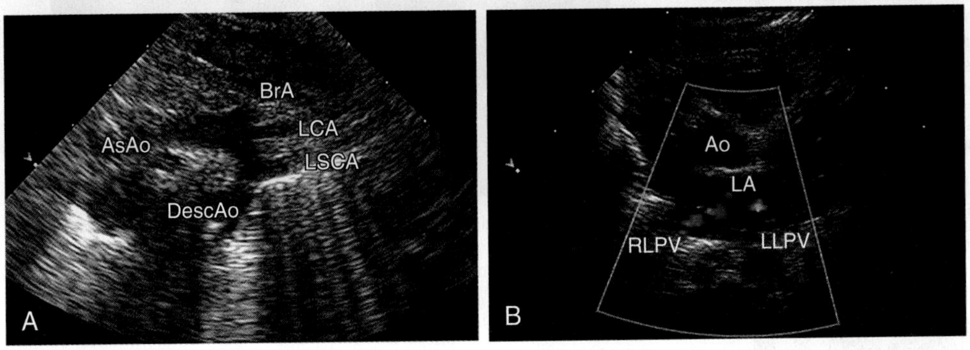

Figure 417-20 *A,* Normal suprasternal echocardiographic window showing the aortic arch and its major branches. AsAo, ascending aorta; BrA, brachiocephalic artery; DescAo, descending aorta; LCA, left carotid artery; LSCA, left subclavian artery. *B,* Normal high parasternal window showing color Doppler imaging of normal pulmonary venous return to the left atrium (LA) of both right (RLPV) and left (LLPV) lower pulmonary veins.

as shunts. Color Doppler permits highly accurate assessment of the presence and direction of intracardiac shunts and allows identification of small or multiple left-to-right or right-to-left shunts (Fig. 417-21). The severity of valvular insufficiency can be evaluated with both pulsed and color Doppler (Fig. 417-22). Alterations in venous Doppler flow patterns can be used to detect abnormalities of systemic and pulmonary veins and alterations of atrioventricular valve Doppler flow patterns can be used to assess ventricular diastolic functional abnormalities.

Sophisticated M-mode, 2-D, and Doppler echocardiographic methods of assessing left ventricular systolic and diastolic function (e.g., end-systolic wall stress, dobutamine stress echocardiography, and Doppler tissue imaging) have proved useful in the serial assessment of patients at risk for the development of both systolic and diastolic ventricular dysfunction and ventricular dyssynchrony (where the coordination of left and right ventricular contraction is abnormal). Such patients include those with cardiomyopathies, those receiving anthracycline drugs for cancer chemotherapy, those at risk for iron overload, and those being monitored for rejection or coronary artery disease after heart transplantation.

THREE-DIMENSIONAL ECHOCARDIOGRAPHY

Real-time 3-D echocardiographic reconstruction is valuable for the assessment of cardiac morphology (Fig. 417-23). Details of valve structure, the size and location of septal defects, abnormalities of the ventricular myocardium, and details of the great vessels, which may not be as readily apparent using 2-D imaging, can often be appreciated on 3-D echo. Reconstruction of the view that the surgeon will encounter in the operating room makes this technique a valuable adjunct for preoperative imaging.

TRANSESOPHAGEAL ECHOCARDIOGRAPHY

Transesophageal echocardiography is an extremely sensitive imaging technique that produces a clearer view of smaller lesions such as vegetations in endocarditis, especially in larger patients.

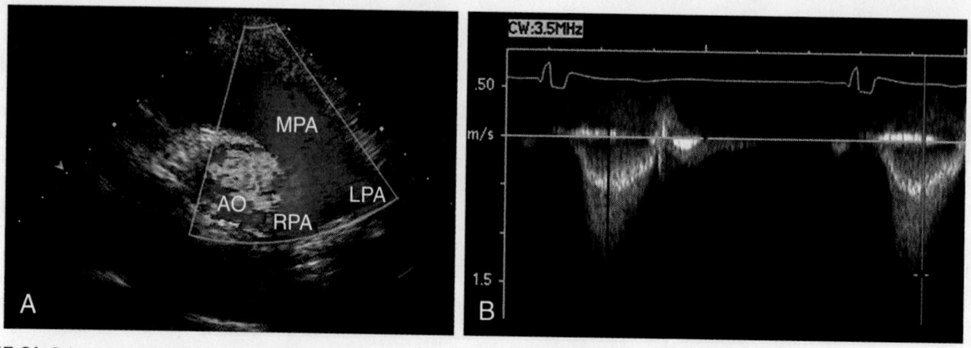

Figure 417-21 Color and pulsed Doppler evaluation of pulmonary arterial flow. *A*, Color Doppler evaluation of a parasternal short axis view showing normal flow through the pulmonary valve to the main and branch pulmonary arteries. The color of the Doppler flow is blue, indicating that the flow is moving away from the transducer (which is located at the top of the figure, at the apex of the triangular ultrasound window). Note that the color assigned to the Doppler signal does not indicate the oxygen saturation of the blood. Ao, aorta; LPA, left pulmonary artery; MPA, main pulmonary artery; RPA, right pulmonary artery. *B*, Pulsed wave Doppler flow pattern through the pulmonary valve showing a low velocity of flow (<1.5 m/sec), indicating the absence of a pressure gradient across the valve. The envelope of the flow signal is below the line, indicating that the flow is moving away from the transducer.

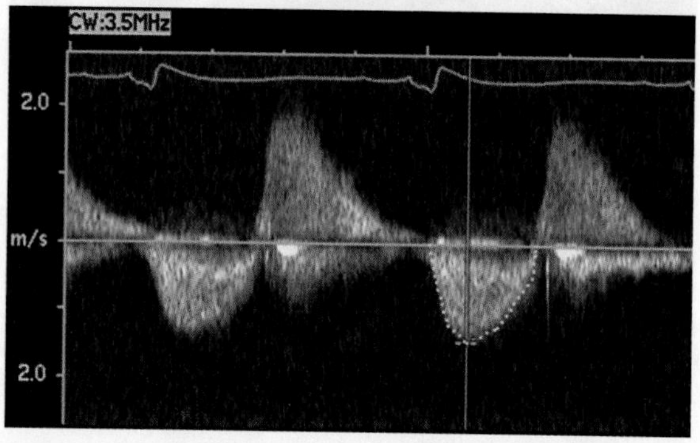

Figure 417-22 Doppler evaluation of a patient who had previously undergone repair of tetralogy of Fallot and who has mild pulmonary stenosis and moderate pulmonary regurgitation. The tracing shows the to-and-fro flow across the pulmonary valve with the signal below the line representing forward flow in systole (see ECG tracing for reference) and the signal above the line representing regurgitation during diastole.

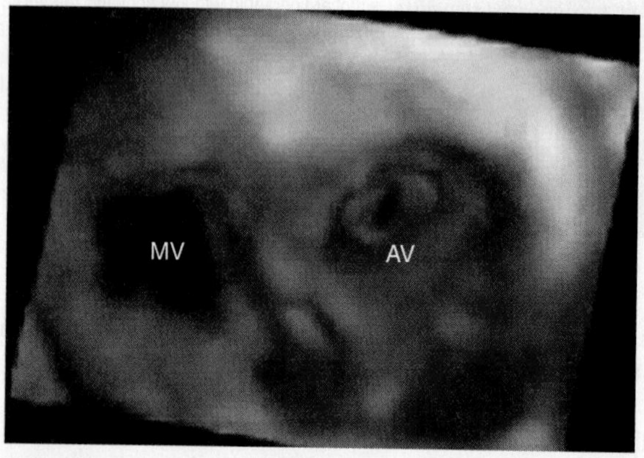

Figure 417-23 3-D echocardiogram showing a short axis view of the left ventricle. AV, aortic valve; MV, mitral valve. (Courtesy of Dr. Norman Silverman, Stanford University, Stanford, CA.)

It is useful in visualizing posteriorly located structures such as the atria, aortic root, and atrioventricular valves. Transesophageal echocardiography is extremely useful as an intraoperative technique for monitoring cardiac function during both cardiac and noncardiac surgery and for screening for residual cardiac defects after the patient in initially weaned from cardiopulmonary bypass. This technique has been especially helpful in evaluating the degree of residual regurgitation after valve repairs and in searching for small muscular VSDs that may have been missed during the closure of larger defects.

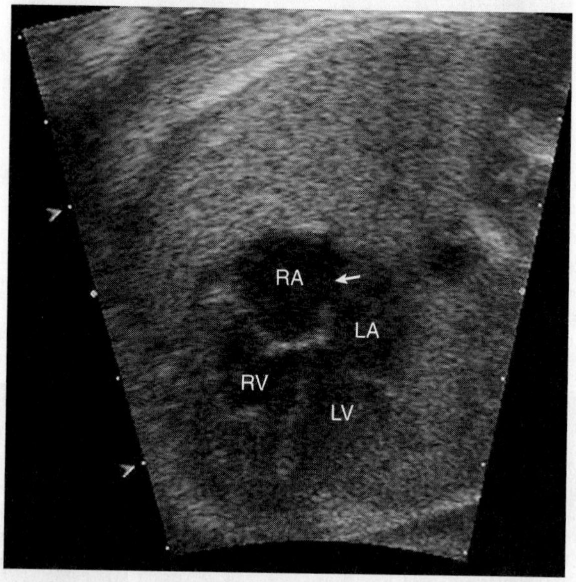

Figure 417-24 Normal four chamber view echocardiogram on a fetus at 20 wk of gestation. The foramen ovale *(arrow)* can be seen between the right and left atria. LA, left atrium; LV, left ventricle; RA, right atrium; RV, right ventricle.

FETAL ECHOCARDIOGRAPHY

Fetal echocardiography can be used to evaluate cardiac structures or disturbances in cardiac rhythm (Fig. 417-24). Perinatologists often detect gross abnormalities in cardiac structure on routine obstetric ultrasonography or may refer the patient because of unexplained hydrops fetalis, a family history of congenital heart disease, or a maternal condition associated with fetal cardiac pathology such as gestational diabetes. Fetal echocardiography is capable of diagnosing most significant congenital heart lesions as early as 17-19 wk of gestation; however, accuracy at this early stage is still limited and families should understand that these studies cannot totally eliminate the possibility of congenital heart disease. Serial fetal echocardiograms have also demonstrated the importance of flow disturbance in the pathogenesis of congenital heart disease; such studies can show the intrauterine progression of a moderate lesion, such as aortic stenosis, into a more severe lesion, such as hypoplastic left heart syndrome. M-mode echocardiography can diagnose rhythm disturbances in the fetus and can determine the success of antiarrhythmic therapy administered to the mother. A screening fetal echocardiogram is recommended for women with a previous child or 1st-degree relative with congenital heart disease, for those who are at higher risk of having a child with cardiac disease (insulin-dependent diabetics, patients with exposure to teratogenic drugs during early pregnancy), and in any fetus in which a chromosomal abnormality is suspected or confirmed.

Early detection provides the opportunity to counsel and educate the parents about the severity of the cardiac lesion and potential therapeutic or palliative care options. Referral to a high risk perinatal service is then performed, for further ultrasound screening for associated anomalies of other organs and potential amniocentesis for karyotyping. For those fetuses with ductal dependent lesions, delivery can be planned at a tertiary care center, avoiding the requirement for postnatal transport of an unstable infant.

BIBLIOGRAPHY

Please visit the Nelson Textbook of Pediatrics *website at www.expertconsult.com for the complete bibliography.*

417.5 Exercise Testing

Daniel Bernstein

The normal cardiorespiratory system adapts to the extensive demands of exercise with a several-fold increase in oxygen consumption and cardiac output. Because of the large reserve capacity for exercise, significant abnormalities in cardiovascular performance may be present without symptoms at rest or during ordinary activities. When patients are evaluated in a resting state, significant abnormalities in cardiac function may not be appreciated, or if detected, their implications for quality of life may not be recognized. Permission for children with cardiovascular disease to participate in various forms of physical activity is frequently based on totally subjective criteria. As the importance of aerobic exercise is increasingly recognized, even for children with complex congenital heart lesions, exercise testing can provide a quantitative evaluation of the child's ability to safely participate in both competitive and noncompetitive sports. Exercise testing can also play an important role in evaluating symptoms and quantitating the severity of cardiac abnormalities.

In older children, exercise studies are generally performed on a graded treadmill apparatus with timed intervals of increasing grade and speed. In younger children, exercise studies are often performed on a bicycle ergometer. Many laboratories have the capacity to measure both cardiac and pulmonary function noninvasively during exercise. This allows measurement of both resting and maximal oxygen consumption (Vo_2max) and the point at which anaerobic threshold (AT) is reached, important indicators of cardiovascular fitness.

As a child grows, the capacity for work is enhanced with increased body size and skeletal muscle mass. All indices of cardiopulmonary function do not increase in a uniform manner. A major response to exercise is an increase in cardiac output, principally achieved through an increase in heart rate, but stroke volume, systemic venous return, and pulse pressure is also increased. Systemic vascular resistance is greatly decreased as the blood vessels in working muscle dilate in response to increasing metabolic demands. As the child becomes older and larger, the response of the heart rate to exercise remains prominent, but cardiac output increases because of growing cardiac volume capacity and, hence, stroke volume. Responses to dynamic exercise are not dependent solely on age. For any given body surface area, boys have a larger stroke volume than size-matched girls. This increase is also mediated by posture. Augmentation of stroke volume with upright, dynamic exercise is facilitated by the pumping action of working muscles, which overcomes the static effect of gravity and increases systemic venous return.

Dynamic exercise testing defines not only endurance and exercise capacity but also the effect of such exercise on myocardial blood flow and cardiac rhythm. Significant ST segment depression reflects abnormalities in myocardial perfusion, for example, the subendocardial ischemia that commonly occurs during exercise in children with hypertrophied left ventricles. The **exercise ECG** is considered abnormal if the ST segment depression is >2 mm and extends for at least 0.06 sec after the J point (onset of the ST segment) in conjunction with a horizontal-, upward-, or downward-sloping ST segment. Provocation of rhythm disturbances during an exercise study is an important method of evaluating selected patients with known or suspected rhythm disorders. The effect of pharmacologic management can also be tested in this manner.

BIBLIOGRAPHY

Please visit the Nelson Textbook of Pediatrics *website at www.expertconsult.com for the complete bibliography.*

417.6 MRI, MRA, CT, and Radionuclide Studies

Daniel Bernstein

Magnetic resonance imaging (MRI) and **magnetic resonance angiography (MRA)** are extremely helpful in the diagnosis and management of patients with congenital heart disease. These techniques produce tomographic images of the heart in any projection (Fig. 417-25), with excellent contrast resolution of fat, myocardium, and lung, as well as moving blood from blood vessel walls. MRI has been useful in evaluating areas that are less well visualized by echocardiography, such as distal branch pulmonary artery anatomy and anomalies in systemic and pulmonary venous return.

MRA allows the acquisition of images in several tomographic planes. Within each plane, images are obtained at different phases of the cardiac cycle. Thus, when displayed in a dynamic

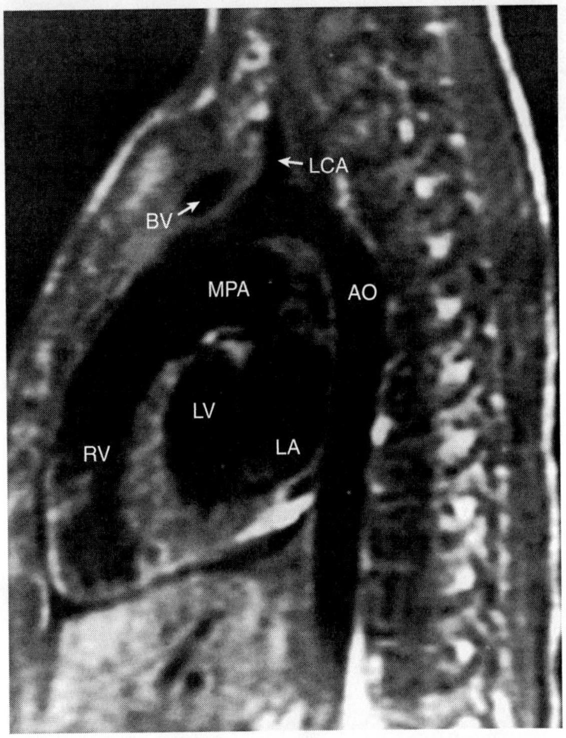

Figure 417-25 Sagittal normal MRI. Ao, aorta; BV, brachiocephalic vein; LA, left atrium; LCA, left coronary artery; LV, left ventricle; MPA, main pulmonary artery; RV, right ventricle. (From Bisset GS III: Cardiac and great vessel anatomy. In El-Khoury GY, Bergman RA, Montgomery WJ, editors: *Sectional anatomy by MRI/CT,* New York, 1990, Churchill Livingstone.)

"cine" format, changes in wall thickening, chamber volume, and valve function can be displayed and analyzed. Blood flow velocity and blood flow volume can be calculated. MRA is an excellent technique for following patients serially after repair of complex congenital heart disease, such as tetralogy of Fallot. In these patients, MRA can be used to assess right ventricular volume and mass as well as quantify the amount of regurgitation through either the pulmonary or tricuspid valve. Other MRI techniques, such as myocardial delayed enhancement, can be used to quantify areas of myocardial scar in patients with cardiomyopathy or in patients after congenital heart disease repair, especially tetralogy of Fallot. **Magnetic resonance spectroscopy (MRS)**, predominantly a research tool at present, provides a means of demonstrating relative concentrations of high-energy metabolites (adenosine triphosphate, adenosine diphosphate, inorganic phosphate, and phosphocreatine) within regions of the working myocardium.

Computer processing of MRA images allows the noninvasive visualization of the cardiovascular system from inside of the heart or vessels, a technique known as fly-through imaging. These images allow the cardiologist to image the interiors of various cardiovascular structures (Fig. 417-26). These imaging techniques are especially helpful in imaging complex peripheral arterial stenoses, especially after balloon angioplasty.

CT scanning can now be used to perform rapid, respiration-gated cardiac imaging in children with resolutions down to 0.5 mm. 3-D reconstruction of CT images (Fig. 417-27) are especially useful in evaluating branch pulmonary arteries, anomalies in systemic and pulmonary venous return, and great vessel anomalies such as coarctation of the aorta.

Radionuclide angiography may be used to detect and quantify shunts and to analyze the distribution of blood flow to each lung. This technique is particularly useful in quantifying the volume of blood flow distribution between the two lungs in patients with abnormalities of the pulmonary vascular tree or after a shunt operation (Blalock-Taussig or Glenn), or to quantify the success of balloon angioplasty and intravascular stenting procedures. Gated blood pool scanning can be used to calculate hemodynamic measurements, quantify valvular regurgitation, and detect regional wall motion abnormalities. Thallium imaging can be performed to evaluate cardiac muscle perfusion. These methods can be used at the bedside of seriously ill children and can be performed serially, with minimal discomfort and low radiation exposure.

BIBLIOGRAPHY

Please visit the Nelson Textbook of Pediatrics *website at www.expertconsult.com for the complete bibliography.*

417.7 Diagnostic and Interventional Cardiac Catheterization

Daniel Bernstein

As echocardiography, MRI, and CT have become the standards for the diagnosis of most forms of congenital heart disease, the catheterization laboratory has become the site of high-technology interventional procedures, allowing for the nonsurgical repair or palliation of heart defects that once required open heart surgery.

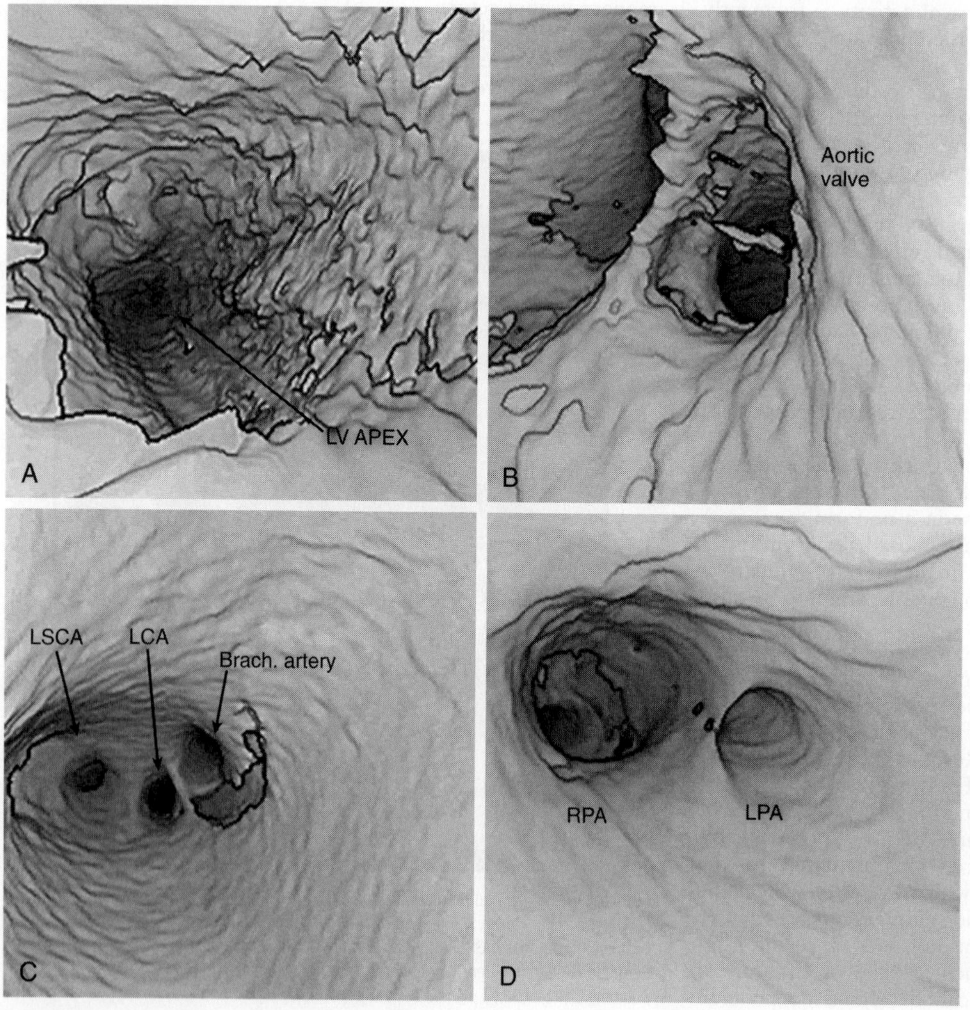

Figure 417-26 Fly-through imaging in a patient with an aortopulmonary window. This series of still frames shows the progression from the left ventricular (LV) chamber *(A)*, through the aortic valve *(B)*, out to the ascending aorta *(C)*, and then through the defect to the branch pulmonary arteries *(D)*. Brach., brachiocephalic artery; LCA, left carotid artery; LPA, left pulmonary artery; LSCA, left subclavian artery; RPA, right pulmonary artery.

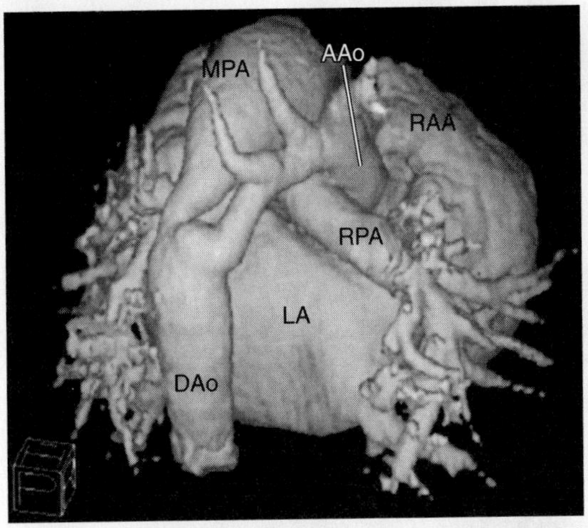

Figure 417-27 3-D reconstruction of electron beam CT images from a neonate with severe coarctation of the aorta. The patent ductus arteriosus can be seen toward the left leading from the main pulmonary artery to the descending aorta. The tortuous and narrow coarctated segment is just to the right of the ductus. The transverse aorta is hypoplastic as well. AAo, ascending aorta; DAo, descending aorta; LA, left atrium; MPA, main pulmonary artery; RAA, right atrial appendage; RPA, right pulmonary artery. (Image courtesy of Dr. Paul Pitlick, Stanford University, Stanford, CA.)

Some centers have developed hybrid catheterization laboratories, combining standard fluoroscopic imaging with an operating suite, allowing combined approaches to treat complex congenital heart lesions.

DIAGNOSTIC CARDIAC CATHETERIZATION

Diagnostic catheterization is still performed: (1) to assist in the initial diagnosis of some complex congenital heart lesions (e.g., tetralogy of Fallot with pulmonary atresia and major aortopulmonary collateral arteries [MAPCAs], pulmonary atresia with intact ventricular septum and coronary sinusoids, hypoplastic left heart syndrome with mitral stenosis); (2) in cases in which other imaging studies are equivocal; (3) in patients for whom hemodynamic assessment is critical (to determine the size of a left-to-right shunt in borderline cases, or to determine the presence or absence of pulmonary vascular disease in an older patient with a left-to-right shunt); (4) between stages of repair of complex congenital heart disease (e.g., hypoplastic left or right heart syndromes); (5) for myocardial biopsy in the diagnosis of cardiomyopathy or in screening for cardiac rejection after cardiac transplantation; and (6) for electrophysiologic study in the evaluation of cardiac arrhythmias (Chapter 429).

Cardiac catheterization should be performed with the patient in as close to a basal state as possible. Conscious sedation is routine; if a deeper level of general anesthesia is required, careful choice of an anesthetic agent is warranted to avoid depression of cardiovascular function and subsequent distortion of the calculations of cardiac output, pulmonary and systemic vascular resistance, and shunt ratios.

Cardiac catheterization in critically ill infants with congenital heart disease should be performed in a center where a pediatric cardiovascular surgical team is available in the event that an operation is required immediately afterward. The complication rate of cardiac catheterization and angiography is greatest in critically ill infants; they must be studied in a thermally neutral environment and treated quickly for hypothermia, hypoglycemia, acidosis, or excessive blood loss.

Catheterization may be limited to the right-sided cardiac structures, the left-sided structures, or both the right and left sides of the heart. The catheter is passed into the heart under fluoroscopic guidance through a percutaneous entry point in a femoral or jugular vein. In infants and in a number of older children, the left side of the heart can be accessed by passing the catheter across a patent foramen ovale to the left atrium and left ventricle. If the foramen is closed, the left side of the heart can be catheterized by passing the catheter retrograde via a percutaneous entry site in the femoral artery, or if necessary, via a trans-atrial septal puncture. The catheter can be manipulated through abnormal intracardiac defects (ASDs, VSDs). Blood samples are obtained for measuring oxygen saturation and calculating shunt volumes, pressures are measured for calculating gradients and valve areas, and radiopaque contrast is injected to delineate cardiac and vascular structures. A catheter with a thermosensor tip can be utilized for measurement of cardiac output by thermodilution. Specialized catheters can be utilized to measure more sophisticated indices of cardiac function: Those with pressure-transducer tips can be utilized to measure the first derivative of left ventricular pressure (dP/dt); and conductance catheters can be used to generate pressure-volume loops, from which indices of both contractility (end-systolic elastance) and relaxation can be derived. Complete hemodynamics can be calculated, including cardiac output, intracardiac left-to-right and right-to-left shunts, and systemic and pulmonary vascular resistances. Normal circulatory dynamics are depicted in Figure 417-28.

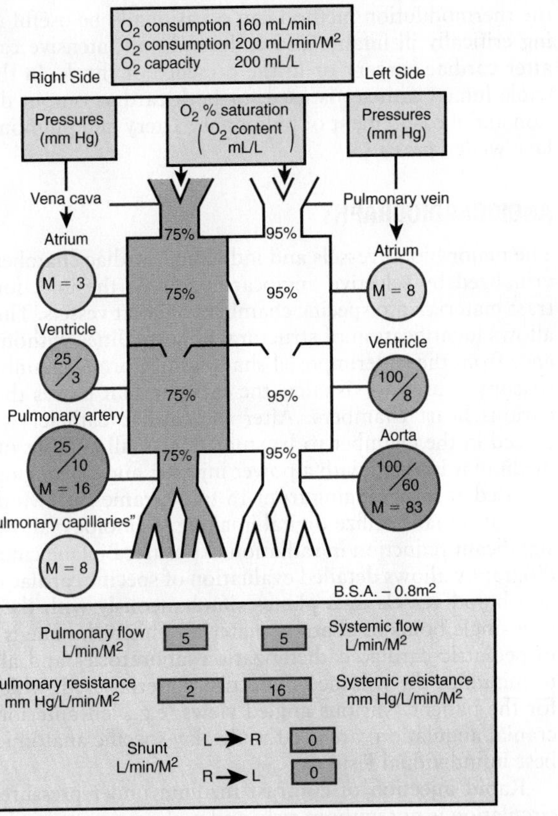

Figure 417-28 Diagram of normal circulatory dynamics with pressure readings, oxygen content, and percent saturation. B.S.A., body surface area. (Modified from Nadas AS, Fyler DC: *Pediatric cardiology,* ed 3, Philadelphia, 1972, WB Saunders.)

THERMODILUTION MEASUREMENT OF CARDIAC OUTPUT

The thermodilution method for measuring cardiac output is performed with a flow-directed, thermistor-tipped, pulmonary artery (Swan-Ganz) catheter. A known change in the heat content of the blood is induced at one point in the circulation (usually the right atrium or inferior vena cava) by injecting room temperature saline, and the resultant change in temperature is detected at a point downstream (usually the pulmonary artery). This method is used to measure cardiac output in the catheterization laboratory in patients without shunts. Monitoring cardiac output by the thermodilution method can occasionally be useful in managing critically ill infants and children in an intensive care setting after cardiac surgery or in the presence of shock. In this case, a triple-lumen catheter is used for both cardiac output determination and measurement of pulmonary artery and pulmonary capillary wedge pressure.

ANGIOCARDIOGRAPHY

The major blood vessels and individual cardiac chambers may be visualized by selective angiocardiography, the injection of contrast material into specific chambers or great vessels. This method allows identification of structural abnormalities without interference from the superimposed shadows of normal chambers. Fluoroscopy is used to visualize the catheter as it passes through the various heart chambers. After the cardiac catheter is properly placed in the chamber to be studied, a small amount of contrast medium is injected with a power injector, and cineangiograms are exposed at rates ranging from 15 to 60 frames/sec. Modern catheterization labs utilize digital imaging technology, allowing for a significant reduction in radiation exposure. Biplane cineangiocardiography allows detailed evaluation of specific cardiac chambers and blood vessels in 2 planes simultaneously with the injection of a single bolus of contrast material. This technique is standard in pediatric cardiac catheterization laboratories and allows one to minimize the volume of contrast material used, which is safer for the patient. Various angled views (e.g., left anterior oblique, cranial angulation) are used to display specific anatomic features best in individual lesions.

Rapid injection of contrast medium under pressure into the circulation is not without risk, and each injection should be carefully planned. Contrast agents consist of hypertonic solutions, with some containing organic iodides, which can cause complications, including nausea, a generalized burning sensation, central nervous system symptoms, renal insufficiency, and allergic reactions. Intramyocardial injection is generally avoided by careful placement of the catheter before injection. Hypertonicity of the contrast medium may result in transient myocardial depression and a drop in blood pressure, followed soon afterward by tachycardia, an increase in cardiac output, and a shift of interstitial fluid into the circulation. This shift can transiently increase the symptoms of heart failure in critically ill patients.

INTERVENTIONAL CARDIAC CATHETERIZATION

The miniaturization of catheter delivery systems has allowed for the safe application of many of these interventional catheterization techniques, even in neonates and premature infants. Catheter treatment is now the standard of practice for most cases of isolated pulmonary or aortic valve stenosis (see Fig. 421-4) as well as for re-coarctation of the aorta. A special catheter with a sausage-shaped balloon at the distal end is passed through the obstructed valve. Rapid filling of the balloon with a mixture of contrast material and saline solution results in tearing of the stenotic valve tissue, usually at the site of inappropriately fused raphe. Valvular pulmonary stenosis can be treated successfully by balloon angioplasty; in most patients, angioplasty has replaced surgical repair as the initial procedure of choice. The clinical results of this procedure are similar to those obtained by open heart surgery, but without the need for sternotomy or prolonged hospitalization. Balloon valvuloplasty for aortic stenosis has also yielded excellent results, although, as with surgery, aortic stenosis often recurs as the child grows and multiple procedures may thus be required. One complication of both valvuloplasty and surgery is the creation of valvular insufficiency. This complication has more serious implications when it occurs on the aortic vs the pulmonary side of the circulation because regurgitation is less well tolerated at systemic arterial pressures. Balloon angioplasty is the procedure of choice for patients with re-stenosis of

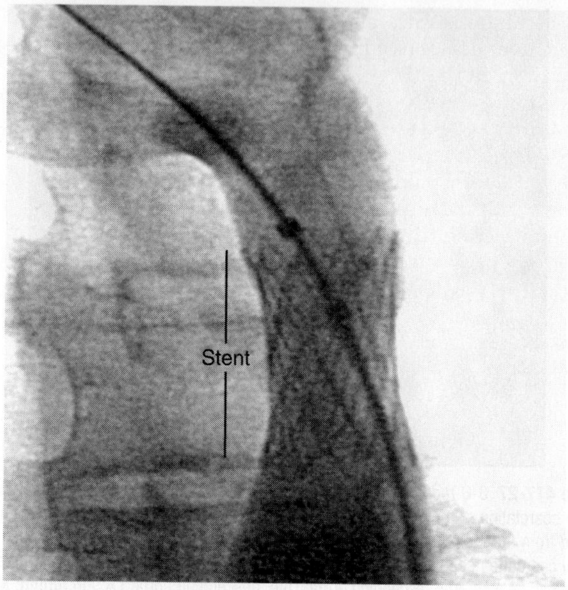

Figure 417-29 Intravascular stent placed in the descending aorta for treatment of recurrent coarctation of the aorta.

coarctation of the aorta after earlier surgery. It is controversial whether angioplasty is the best procedure for native (unoperated) coarctation of the aorta because of reports of later aneurysm formation and most centers still refer primary coarctation in infants and young children for surgical repair. However, in older patients with previously undiagnosed coarctation, especially those with decreased left ventricular function, primary angioplasty with possible stent placement, may be considered. Other applications of the balloon angioplasty technique include amelioration of mitral stenosis, dilatation of surgical conduits (Mustard or Senning atrial baffles), relief of branch pulmonary artery narrowing, dilatation of systemic or pulmonary venous obstructions, and the long-used balloon atrial septostomy (Rashkind procedure) for transposition of the great arteries (Chapter 425.2).

Interventional catheterization techniques are being adapted for use in the **fetus** with lesions such as aortic stenosis in an attempt to prevent their progression to more complex lesions such as hypoplastic left heart syndrome. In these procedures, after administration of appropriate anesthesia, a needle is passed through the maternal abdominal wall, the uterine wall, and the fetal chest wall and directly into the fetal left ventricle (see Fig. 425-13). A coronary angioplasty balloon catheter is passed through the needle and across the stenotic aortic valve, which is then dilated. With the restoration of normal left ventricular blood flow, it is to be hoped that normal left ventricular growth potential is restored. Mid-term results with this technique in a growing number of patients show mixed results with good ventricular growth leading to a two-ventricle circulation in approximately 25% of patients.

In patients with branch pulmonary artery stenoses, the previously mixed results with balloon angioplasty alone have been enhanced with the use of **intravascular stents** (Fig. 417-29) delivered over a balloon catheter and expanded within the vessel lumen. Once placed, they can often be dilated to successively greater sizes as the patient grows, although their use in younger infants and children is limited by the extent to which they can be further expanded. Research into biodissolvable stents may solve this problem in the future. Stents are also being utilized in adolescents and young adults with coarctation of the aorta.

Closure of a small PDA is now routinely achieved with catheter-delivered coils (see Fig. 420-11), whereas a larger PDA can be closed with a variety of sandwich-type devices. Closure of anomalous vascular connections (coronary fistulas, veno-venous collaterals in cyanotic heart lesions) can also be achieved using coils. Secundum ASDs are now routinely closed with a double disc occluder device (see Fig. 420-3). Versions of these devices are currently in clinical trials for closure of surgically hard-to-reach muscular VSDs and even for the more common perimembranous VSD. Catheter-delivered devices may also be used as an adjunct to complex surgical repairs (dilation or stenting of branch pulmonary artery or pulmonary vein stenosis or closure of a difficult to reach muscular VSD). High-risk patients undergoing the Fontan operation (Chapter 430.4) often have a small fenestration created between the right and left sides of the circulation to serve as a "popoff valve" for high right-sided pressure in the early surgical period. Patients with these "fenestrated Fontans" are usually candidates for subsequent closure of the fenestration with a catheter-delivered device.

BIBLIOGRAPHY

Please visit the Nelson Textbook of Pediatrics *website at www.expertconsult.com for the complete bibliography.*

Section 3 CONGENITAL HEART DISEASE

Chapter 418
Epidemiology and Genetic Basis of Congenital Heart Disease

Daniel Bernstein

PREVALENCE

Congenital heart disease occurs in approximately 0.8% of live births. The incidence is higher in stillborns (3-4%), spontaneous abortuses (10-25%), and premature infants (about 2% excluding patent ductus arteriosus [PDA]). This overall incidence does not include mitral valve prolapse, PDA of preterm infants, and bicuspid aortic valves (present in 1-2% of adults). Congenital cardiac defects have a wide spectrum of severity in infants: about 2-3 in 1,000 newborn infants will be symptomatic with heart disease in the 1st yr of life. The diagnosis is established by 1 wk of age in 40-50% of patients with congenital heart disease and by 1 mo of age in 50-60% of patients. With advances in both palliative and corrective surgery, the number of children with congenital heart disease surviving to adulthood has increased dramatically. Despite these advances, congenital heart disease remains the leading cause of death in children with congenital malformations. Table 418-1 summarizes the relative frequency of the most common congenital cardiac lesions.

Table 418-1 RELATIVE FREQUENCY OF MAJOR CONGENITAL HEART LESIONS*

LESION	% OF ALL LESIONS
Ventricular septal defect	35-30
Atrial septal defect (secundum)	6-8
Patent ductus arteriosus	6-8
Coarctation of aorta	5-7
Tetralogy of Fallot	5-7
Pulmonary valve stenosis	5-7
Aortic valve stenosis	4-7
d-Transposition of great arteries	3-5
Hypoplastic left ventricle	1-3
Hypoplastic right ventricle	1-3
Truncus arteriosus	1-2
Total anomalous pulmonary venous return	1-2
Tricuspid atresia	1-2
Single ventricle	1-2
Double-outlet right ventricle	1-2
Others	5-10

*Excluding patent ductus arteriosus in preterm neonates, bicuspid aortic valve, physiologic peripheral pulmonic stenosis, and mitral valve prolapse.

For the full continuation of this chapter, please visit the Nelson Textbook of Pediatrics *website at www.expertconsult.com.*

Chapter 419
Evaluation of the Infant or Child with Congenital Heart Disease

Daniel Bernstein

The initial evaluation for suspected congenital heart disease involves a systematic approach with three major components. First, congenital cardiac defects can be divided into 2 major groups based on the presence or absence of cyanosis, which can be determined by physical examination aided by pulse oximetry. Second, these 2 groups can be further subdivided according to whether the chest radiograph shows evidence of increased, normal, or decreased pulmonary vascular markings. Finally, the electrocardiogram can be used to determine whether right, left, or biventricular hypertrophy exists. The character of the heart sounds and the presence and character of any murmurs further narrow the differential diagnosis. The final diagnosis is then confirmed by echocardiography, CT or MRI, or cardiac catheterization.

ACYANOTIC CONGENITAL HEART LESIONS

Acyanotic congenital heart lesions can be classified according to the predominant physiologic load that they place on the heart. Although many congenital heart lesions induce more than one physiologic disturbance, it is helpful to focus on the primary load abnormality for purposes of classification. The most common lesions are those that produce a volume load, and the most common of these are left-to-right shunt lesions. Atrioventricular (AV) valve regurgitation and some of the cardiomyopathies are other causes of increased volume load. The second major class of lesions causes an increase in pressure load, most commonly secondary to ventricular outflow obstruction (pulmonic or aortic valve stenosis) or narrowing of one of the great vessels (coarctation of the aorta). The chest radiograph and electrocardiogram are useful tools for differentiating between these major classes of volume and pressure overload lesions.

Lesions Resulting in Increased Volume Load

The most common lesions in this group are those that cause left-to-right shunting (see Chapter 420): atrial septal defect, ventricular septal defect (VSD), AV septal defects (AV canal), and patent ductus arteriosus. The pathophysiologic common denominator in this group is communication between the systemic and pulmonary sides of the circulation, which results in shunting of fully oxygenated blood back into the lungs. This shunt can be quantitated by calculating the ratio of pulmonary to systemic blood flow, or Qp:Qs. Thus, a 2:1 shunt implies twice the normal pulmonary blood flow.

The direction and magnitude of the shunt across such a communication depend on the size of the defect, the relative pulmonary and systemic pressure and vascular resistances, and the compliances of the 2 chambers connected by the defect. These factors are dynamic and may change dramatically with age: Intracardiac defects may grow smaller with time; pulmonary vascular resistance, which is high in the immediate newborn period, decreases to normal adult levels by several weeks of life; and chronic exposure of the pulmonary circulation to high pressure and blood flow results in a gradual increase in pulmonary vascular resistance (Eisenmenger physiology, Chapter 427.2). Thus, a lesion such as a large VSD may be associated with little shunting and few symptoms during the initial weeks of life. When pulmonary vascular resistance declines in the next several weeks, the volume of the left-to-right shunt increases, and symptoms begin to appear.

The increased volume of blood in the lungs decreases pulmonary compliance and increases the work of breathing. Fluid leaks into the interstitial space and alveoli and causes pulmonary edema. The infant acquires the symptoms we refer to as **heart failure,** such as tachypnea, chest retractions, nasal flaring, and wheezing. The term *heart failure* is a misnomer, however; total left ventricular output is actually several times greater than normal, although much of this output is ineffective because it returns directly to the lungs. To maintain this high level of left ventricular output, heart rate and stroke volume are increased, mediated by an increase in sympathetic nervous system activity. The increase in circulating catecholamines, combined with the increased work of breathing, results in an elevation in total body oxygen consumption, often beyond the oxygen transport ability of the circulation. Sympathetic activation leads to the additional symptoms of sweating and irritability and the imbalance between oxygen supply and demand lead to failure to thrive. Remodeling of the heart occurs, with predominantly dilatation and a lesser degree of hypertrophy. If left untreated, pulmonary vascular resistance eventually begins to rise and, by several years of age, the shunt volume will decrease and eventually reverse to right to left (Eisenmenger physiology, Chapter 427.2).

Additional lesions that impose a volume load on the heart include regurgitant lesions (Chapter 422) and the cardiomyopathies (Chapter 433). Regurgitation through the AV valves is most commonly encountered in patients with partial or complete AV septal defects (AV canal, endocardial cushion defects). In these lesions, the combination of a left-to-right shunt with AV valve regurgitation increases the volume load on the heart and often leads to more severe symptoms. Isolated regurgitation through the tricuspid valve is seen in mild to moderate forms of Ebstein anomaly (Chapter 424.7). Regurgitation involving one of the semilunar valves is usually also associated with some degree of stenosis; however, aortic regurgitation may be encountered in patients with a VSD directly under the aortic valve (supracristal VSD) and in patients with membranous subaortic stenosis.

In contrast to left-to-right shunts, in which intrinsic cardiac muscle function is generally either normal or increased, heart muscle function is decreased in the cardiomyopathies. **Cardiomyopathies** may affect systolic contractility or diastolic relaxation, or both. Decreased cardiac function results in increased atrial and ventricular filling pressure, and pulmonary edema occurs secondary to increased capillary pressure. Poor cardiac output leads to decreased organ blood flow, sympathetic activation, and the symptoms of poor perfusion and decreased urine output. The major causes of cardiomyopathy in infants and children include viral myocarditis, metabolic disorders, and genetic defects (Chapter 433).

Lesions Resulting in Increased Pressure Load

The pathophysiologic common denominator of these lesions is an obstruction to normal blood flow. The most frequent are obstructions to ventricular outflow: valvular pulmonic stenosis, valvular aortic stenosis, and coarctation of the aorta (Chapter 421). Less common are obstruction to ventricular inflow: tricuspid or mitral stenosis, cor triatriatum and obstruction of the pulmonary veins. Ventricular outflow obstruction can occur at the valve, below the valve (double-chambered right ventricle, subaortic membrane), or above it (branch pulmonary stenosis or supravalvular aortic stenosis). Unless the obstruction is severe, cardiac output will be maintained and the clinical symptoms of heart failure will be either subtle or absent. This compensation predominantly involves an increase in cardiac wall thickness (hypertrophy), but in later stages it also involves dilatation and can progress to ventricular dilation and failure.

The clinical picture is different when obstruction to outflow is severe, which is usually encountered in the immediate newborn period. The infant may become critically ill within several hours of birth. Severe pulmonic stenosis in the newborn period (critical pulmonic stenosis) results in signs of right-sided heart failure (hepatomegaly, peripheral edema), as well as cyanosis from right-to-left shunting across the foramen ovale. Severe aortic stenosis in the newborn period (critical aortic stenosis) is characterized by signs of left-sided heart failure (pulmonary edema, poor perfusion) and right-sided failure (hepatomegaly, peripheral edema), and it may progress rapidly to total circulatory collapse. In older children, severe pulmonic stenosis leads to symptoms of right-sided heart failure, but not to cyanosis unless a pathway persists for right-to-left shunting (e.g., patency of the foramen ovale).

Coarctation of the aorta in older children and adolescents is usually manifested as upper body hypertension and diminished pulses in the lower extremities. In the immediate newborn period, however, the clinical presentation of coarctation may be delayed because of the presence of a patent ductus arteriosus. In these patients, the open aortic end of the ductus may serve as a conduit for blood flow to partially bypass the obstruction. These infants then become symptomatic, often dramatically, when the ductus finally closes, usually within the 1st 2 mo of life.

CYANOTIC CONGENITAL HEART LESIONS

This group of congenital heart lesions can also be further divided according to pathophysiology: whether pulmonary blood flow is decreased (tetralogy of Fallot, pulmonary atresia with an intact septum, tricuspid atresia, total anomalous pulmonary venous return with obstruction) or increased (transposition of the great vessels, single ventricle, truncus arteriosus, total anomalous pulmonary venous return without obstruction). The chest radiograph is a valuable tool for initial differentiation between these two categories.

Cyanotic Lesions with Decreased Pulmonary Blood Flow

These lesions must include both an obstruction to pulmonary blood flow (at the tricuspid valve or right ventricular or pulmonary valve level) and a pathway by which systemic venous blood can shunt from right to left and enter the systemic circulation (via a patent foramen ovale, atrial septal defect, or VSD). Common lesions in this group include tricuspid atresia, tetralogy of Fallot, and various forms of single ventricle with pulmonary stenosis (Chapter 424). In these lesions, the degree of cyanosis depends on the degree of obstruction to pulmonary blood flow. If the obstruction is mild, cyanosis may be absent at rest. These patients may have hypercyanotic ("tet") spells during conditions of stress. In contrast, if the obstruction is severe, pulmonary blood flow may be totally dependent on patency of the ductus arteriosus. When the ductus closes in the 1st few days of life, the neonate experiences profound hypoxemia and shock.

Cyanotic Lesions with Increased Pulmonary Blood Flow

This group of lesions is not associated with obstruction to pulmonary blood flow. Cyanosis is caused by either abnormal ventricular-arterial connections or total mixing of systemic venous and pulmonary venous blood within the heart (Chapter 425). Transposition of the great vessels is the most common of the former group of lesions. In this condition, the aorta arises from the right ventricle and the pulmonary artery arises from the left ventricle. Systemic venous blood returning to the right atrium is pumped directly back to the body, and oxygenated blood returning from the lungs to the left atrium is pumped back into the lungs. The persistence of fetal pathways (foramen ovale and ductus arteriosus) allows for a small degree of mixing in the immediate newborn period; when the ductus begins to close, these infants become extremely cyanotic.

Total mixing lesions include cardiac defects with a common atrium or ventricle, total anomalous pulmonary venous return, and truncus arteriosus (Chapter 425). In this group, deoxygenated systemic venous blood and oxygenated pulmonary venous blood mix completely in the heart and, as a result, oxygen saturation is equal in the pulmonary artery and aorta. If pulmonary blood flow is not obstructed, these infants have a combination of cyanosis and heart failure. In contrast, if pulmonary stenosis is present, these infants may have cyanosis alone, similar to patients with tetralogy of Fallot.

BIBLIOGRAPHY

Please visit the Nelson Textbook of Pediatrics *website at www.expertconsult.com for the complete bibliography.*

Chapter 420
Acyanotic Congenital Heart Disease: The Left-to-Right Shunt Lesions

420.1 Atrial Septal Defect

Daniel Bernstein

Atrial septal defects (ASDs) can occur in any portion of the atrial septum (secundum, primum, or sinus venosus), depending on which embryonic septal structure has failed to develop normally (Chapter 414). Less commonly, the atrial septum may be nearly absent, with the creation of a functional single atrium. Isolated secundum ASDs account for ≈7% of congenital heart defects. The majority of cases of ASD are sporadic; autosomal dominant inheritance does occur as part of the Holt-Oram syndrome (hypoplastic or absent radii, 1st-degree heart block, ASD) or in families with secundum ASD and heart block.

An isolated valve-incompetent patent foramen ovale (PFO) is a common echocardiographic finding during infancy. It is usually of no hemodynamic significance and is not considered an ASD; a PFO may play an important role if other structural heart defects are present. If another cardiac anomaly is causing increased right atrial pressure (pulmonary stenosis or atresia, tricuspid valve abnormalities, right ventricular dysfunction), venous blood may shunt across the PFO into the left atrium with resultant cyanosis. Because of the anatomic structure of the PFO, left-to-right shunting is unusual outside the immediate newborn period. In the presence of a large volume load or a hypertensive left atrium (secondary to mitral stenosis), the foramen ovale may be sufficiently dilated to result in a significant atrial left-to-right shunt. A valve-competent but probe-patent foramen ovale may be present in 15-30% of adults. An isolated PFO does not require surgical treatment, although it may be a risk for paradoxical (right to left) systemic embolization. Device closure of these defects has been considered in young adults with a history of thromboembolic stroke.

BIBLIOGRAPHY

Please visit the Nelson Textbook of Pediatrics *website at www.expertconsult.com for the complete bibliography.*

420.2 Ostium Secundum Defect

Daniel Bernstein

An ostium secundum defect in the region of the fossa ovalis is the most common form of ASD and is associated with structurally normal atrioventricular (AV) valves. Mitral valve prolapse has been described in association with this defect but is rarely an important clinical consideration. Secundum ASDs may be single or multiple (fenestrated atrial septum), and openings ≥2 cm in diameter are common in symptomatic older children. Large defects may extend inferiorly toward the inferior vena cava and ostium of the coronary sinus, superiorly toward the superior vena cava, or posteriorly. Females outnumber males 3:1 in incidence. Partial anomalous pulmonary venous return, most commonly of the right upper pulmonary vein, may be an associated lesion.

PATHOPHYSIOLOGY

The degree of left-to-right shunting is dependent on the size of the defect, the relative compliance of the right and left ventricles, and the relative vascular resistance in the pulmonary and systemic circulations. In large defects, a considerable shunt of oxygenated blood flows from the left to the right atrium (Fig. 420-1). This blood is added to the usual venous return to the right atrium and is pumped by the right ventricle to the lungs. With large defects, the ratio of pulmonary to systemic blood flow (Qp:Qs) is usually between 2:1 and 4:1. The paucity of symptoms in infants with ASDs is related to the structure of the right ventricle in early life when its muscular wall is thick and less compliant, thus limiting the left-to-right shunt. As the infant becomes older and pulmonary vascular resistance drops, the right ventricular wall becomes thinner and the left-to-right shunt across the ASD increases. The increased blood flow through the right side of the heart results

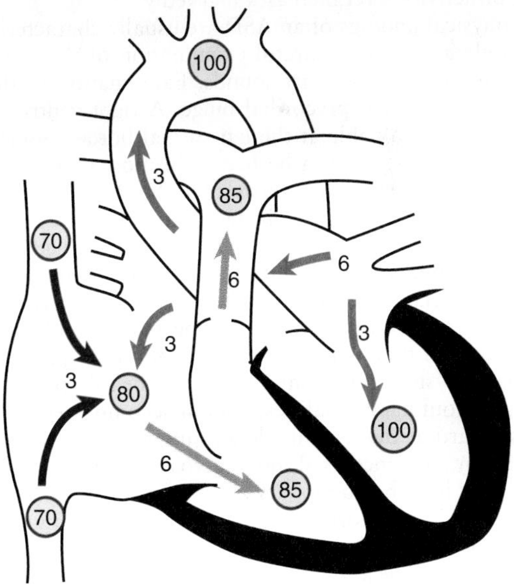

Figure 420-1 Physiology of atrial septal defect (ASD). *Circled numbers* represent oxygen saturation values. The *numbers next to the arrows* represent volumes of blood flow (in L/min/m²). This illustration shows a hypothetical patient with a pulmonary-to-systemic blood flow ratio (Qp:Qs) of 2:1. Desaturated blood enters the right atrium from the vena cavae at a volume of 3 L/min/m² and mixes with an additional 3 L of fully saturated blood shunting left to right across the ASD; the result is an increase in oxygen saturation in the right atrium. Six liters of blood flows through the tricuspid valve and causes a mid-diastolic flow rumble. Oxygen saturation may be slightly higher in the right ventricle because of incomplete mixing at the atrial level. The full 6 L flows across the right ventricular outflow tract and causes a systolic ejection flow murmur. Six liters returns to the left atrium, with 3 L shunting left to right across the defect and 3 L crossing the mitral valve to be ejected by the left ventricle into the ascending aorta (normal cardiac output).

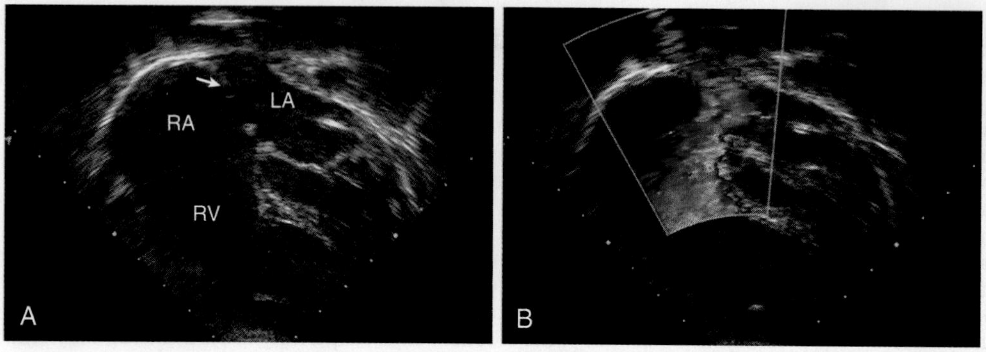

Figure 420-2 Echocardiographic findings in a secundum atrial septal defect (ASD). *A,* 2-D echocardiogram (apical four-chamber view) shows a moderate-sized secundum ASD *(arrow). B,* Color flow Doppler imaging shows left-to-right shunting (the red color represents blood moving toward the ultrasound transducer and does not indicate the level of oxygenation of the blood). LA, left atrium; RA, right atrium; RV, right ventricle.

in enlargement of the right atrium and ventricle and dilatation of the pulmonary artery. The left atrium may also be enlarged, but the left ventricle and aorta are normal in size. Despite the large pulmonary blood flow, pulmonary arterial pressure is usually normal because of the absence of a high-pressure communication between the pulmonary and systemic circulations. Pulmonary vascular resistance remains low throughout childhood, although it may begin to increase in adulthood and may eventually result in reversal of the shunt and clinical cyanosis.

CLINICAL MANIFESTATIONS

A child with an ostium secundum ASD is most often asymptomatic; the lesion is often discovered inadvertently during physical examination. Even an extremely large secundum ASD rarely produces clinically evident heart failure in childhood. However, on closer evaluation, in younger children, subtle failure to thrive may be present; in older children, varying degrees of exercise intolerance may be noted. Often, the degree of limitation may go unnoticed by the family until after surgical repair, when the child's growth or activity level increases markedly.

The physical findings of an ASD are usually characteristic but fairly subtle and require careful examination of the heart, with special attention to the heart sounds. Examination of the chest may reveal a mild left precordial bulge. A right ventricular systolic lift may be palpable at the left sternal border. Sometimes a pulmonic ejection click can be heard. In most patients with an ASD, the characteristic finding is that the 2nd heart sound is **widely split and fixed in its splitting** during all phases of respiration. Normally, the duration of right ventricular ejection varies with respiration, with inspiration increasing right ventricular volume and delaying closure of the pulmonary valve. With an ASD, right ventricular diastolic volume is constantly increased and the ejection time is prolonged throughout all phases of respiration. A systolic ejection murmur is heard; it is medium pitched, without harsh qualities, seldom accompanied by a thrill, and best heard at the left middle and upper sternal border. It is produced by the increased flow across the right ventricular outflow tract into the pulmonary artery, not by low-pressure flow across the ASD. A short, rumbling mid-diastolic murmur produced by the increased volume of blood flow across the tricuspid valve is often audible at the lower left sternal border. This finding, which may be subtle and is heard best with the bell of the stethoscope, usually indicates a Qp:Qs ratio of at least 2:1.

DIAGNOSIS

The chest roentgenogram shows varying degrees of enlargement of the right ventricle and atrium, depending on the size of the shunt. The pulmonary artery is enlarged, and pulmonary vascularity is increased. These signs vary and may not be conspicuous in mild cases. Cardiac enlargement is often best appreciated on the lateral view because the right ventricle protrudes anteriorly as its volume increases. The electrocardiogram shows volume overload of the right ventricle; the QRS axis may be normal or exhibit right axis deviation, and a minor right ventricular conduction delay (rsR′ pattern in the right precordial leads) may be present.

The echocardiogram shows findings characteristic of right ventricular volume overload, including an increased right ventricular end-diastolic dimension and flattening and abnormal motion of the ventricular septum (Fig. 420-2). A normal septum moves posteriorly during systole and anteriorly during diastole. With right ventricular overload and normal pulmonary vascular resistance, septal motion is either flattened or reversed—that is, anterior movement in systole. The location and size of the atrial defect are readily appreciated by two-dimensional scanning, with a characteristic brightening of the echo image seen at the edge of the defect (T-artifact). The shunt is confirmed by pulsed and color flow Doppler. The normal entry of all pulmonary veins into the left atrium should be confirmed.

Patients with the classic features of a hemodynamically significant ASD on physical examination and chest radiography, in whom echocardiographic identification of an isolated secundum ASD is made, need undergo diagnostic catheterization before repair, with the exception of an older patient, in whom pulmonary vascular resistance may be a concern. If pulmonary vascular disease is suspected, cardiac catheterization confirms the presence of the defect and allows measurement of the shunt ratio and pulmonary pressure and resistance.

If catheterization is performed, the oxygen content of blood from the right atrium will be much higher than that from the superior vena cava. This feature is not specifically diagnostic because it may occur with partial anomalous pulmonary venous return to the right atrium, with a ventricular septal defect (VSD) in the presence of tricuspid insufficiency, with AV septal defects associated with left ventricular to right atrial shunts, and with aorta to right atrial communications (ruptured sinus of Valsalva aneurysm). Pressure in the right side of the heart is usually normal, but small to moderate pressure gradients (<25 mm Hg) may be measured across the right ventricular outflow tract because of functional stenosis related to excessive blood flow. In children and adolescents, the pulmonary vascular resistance is almost always normal. The shunt is variable and depends on the size of the defect, but it may be of considerable volume (as high as 20 L/min/m^2). Cineangiography, performed with the catheter through the defect and in the right upper pulmonary vein, demonstrates the defect and the location of the right upper pulmonary venous drainage. Alternatively, pulmonary angiography demonstrates the defect on the levophase (return of contrast to the left side of the heart after passing through the lungs).

COMPLICATIONS

Secundum ASDs are usually isolated, although they may be associated with partial anomalous pulmonary venous return, pulmonary valvular stenosis, VSD, pulmonary artery branch stenosis, and persistent left superior vena cava, as well as mitral valve

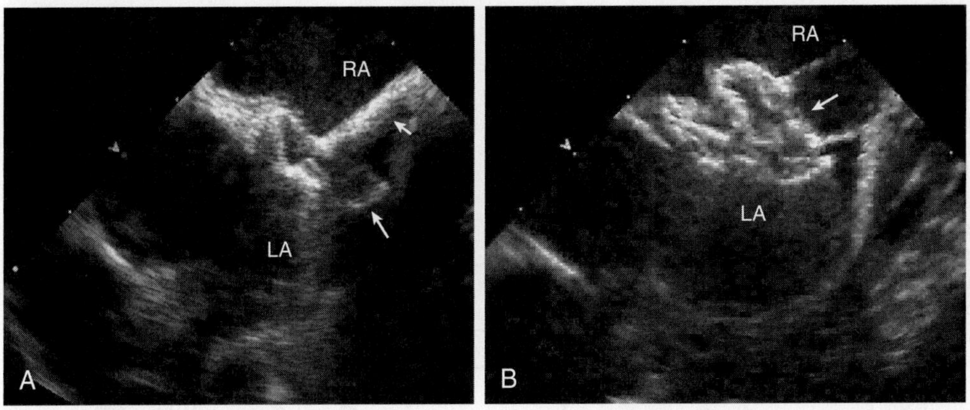

Figure 420-3 Intravascular ultrasound imaging of transcatheter occlusion of an atrial septal defect. *A,* A catheter *(small arrow)* has been advanced across the atrial defect, and the left-sided disk of the device *(large arrow)* has been extruded from the sheath into the left atrium (LA). *B,* The right atrial disk *(arrow)* has now been extruded into the right atrium (RA). The two halves of the device are then locked together and the catheter detached from the occluder device and removed.

prolapse and insufficiency. Secundum ASDs are associated with the autosomal dominant Holt-Oram syndrome. The gene responsible for this syndrome, situated in the region 12q21-q22 of chromosome 12, is *TBX5,* a member of the T-box transcriptional family. A familial form of secundum ASD associated with AV conduction delay has been linked to mutations in another transcription factor, Nkx2.5. Patients with familial ASD without heart block may carry a mutation in the transcription factor GATA4, located on chromosome 8p22-23.

TREATMENT

Surgical or transcatheter device closure is advised for all symptomatic patients and also for asymptomatic patients with a Qp:Qs ratio of at least 2:1 or those with right ventricular enlargement. The timing for elective closure is usually after the 1st yr and before entry into school. Closure carried out at open heart surgery is associated with a mortality rate of <1%. Repair is preferred during early childhood because surgical mortality and morbidity are significantly greater in adulthood; the long-term risk of arrhythmia is also greater after ASD repair in adults. For most patients, the procedure of choice is percutaneous catheter device closure using an atrial septal occlusion device, implanted transvenously in the cardiac catheterization laboratory (Fig. 420-3). The results are excellent and patients are discharged the following day. With the latest generation of devices, the incidence of serious complications such as device erosion is 0.1% and can be decreased by identifying high-risk patients such as those with a deficient rim of septum around the device. Echocardiography can usually determine whether a patient is a good candidate for device closure. In patients with small secundum ASDs and minimal left-to-right shunts without right ventricular enlargement, the consensus is that closure is not required. It is unclear at present whether the persistence of a small ASD into adulthood increases the risk for stroke enough to warrant prophylactic closure of all these defects.

PROGNOSIS

Small- to moderate-sized ASDs detected in term infants may close spontaneously. Secundum ASDs are well tolerated during childhood, and symptoms do not usually appear until the 3rd decade or later. Pulmonary hypertension, atrial dysrhythmias, tricuspid or mitral insufficiency, and heart failure are late manifestations; these symptoms may initially appear during the increased volume load of pregnancy. Infective endocarditis is extremely rare, and antibiotic prophylaxis for isolated secundum ASDs is not recommended.

The results after surgical or device closure in children with moderate to large shunts are excellent. Symptoms disappear rapidly, and growth is frequently enhanced. Heart size decreases to normal, and the electrocardiogram shows decreased right ventricular forces. Late right heart failure and arrhythmias are less frequent in patients who have had early surgical repair, becoming more common in patients who undergo surgery after 20 yr of age. Although early and midterm results with device closure are excellent, the long-term effects are not yet known. Reports of resolution of migraine headaches in patients after device closure of ASD or PFO are intriguing, suggesting a possible thromboembolic etiology; there are also paradoxical reports of patients whose migraines began or worsened after placement of one of these devices.

420.3 Sinus Venosus Atrial Septal Defect

Daniel Bernstein

A sinus venosus ASD is situated in the upper part of the atrial septum in close relation to the entry of the superior vena cava. Often, one or more pulmonary veins (usually from the right lung) drain anomalously into the superior vena cava. The superior vena cava sometimes straddles the defect; in this case, some systemic venous blood enters the left atrium, but only rarely does it cause clinically evident cyanosis. The hemodynamic disturbance, clinical picture, electrocardiogram, and roentgenogram are similar to those seen in secundum ASD. The diagnosis can usually be made by two-dimensional echocardiography. If there are questions regarding pulmonary venous drainage, cardiac CT or MRI is usually diagnostic. Cardiac catheterization is rarely required, with the exception being in adult patients where assessment of pulmonary vascular resistance may be important. Anatomic correction generally requires the insertion of a patch to close the defect while incorporating the entry of anomalous veins into the left atrium. If the anomalous vein drains high in the superior vena cava, the vein can be left intact and the ASD closed to incorporate the mouth of the superior vena cava into the left atrium. The superior vena cava proximal to the venous entrance is then detached and anastomosed directly to the right atrium. This procedure avoids direct suturing of the pulmonary vein with less chance of future stenosis. Surgical results are generally excellent. Rarely, sinus venosus defects involve the inferior vena cava.

420.4 Partial Anomalous Pulmonary Venous Return

Daniel Bernstein

One or several pulmonary veins may return anomalously to the superior or inferior vena cava, the right atrium, or the coronary sinus and produce a left-to-right shunt of oxygenated blood. Partial anomalous pulmonary venous return usually involves some or all of the veins from only one lung, more often the right one. When an associated ASD is present, it is generally of the sinus venosus type, although can be of the secundum type

(Chapter 420.3). When an ASD is detected by echocardiography, one must always search for associated partial anomalous pulmonary venous return. The history, physical signs, and electrocardiographic and roentgenographic findings are indistinguishable from those of an isolated ostium secundum ASD. Occasionally, an anomalous vein draining into the inferior vena cava is visible on chest radiography as a crescentic shadow of vascular density along the right border of the cardiac silhouette (**scimitar syndrome**); in these cases, an ASD is not usually present, but **pulmonary sequestration** and anomalous arterial supply to that lobe are common findings. Total anomalous pulmonary venous return is a cyanotic lesion and is discussed in Chapter 425.7. Echocardiography generally confirms the diagnosis. MRI and CT are also useful if there is a question regarding pulmonary venous drainage or in cases of scimitar syndrome. If cardiac catheterization is performed, the presence of anomalous pulmonary veins is demonstrated by selective pulmonary arteriography and anomalous pulmonary arterial supply to the right lung is demonstrated by descending aortography.

The prognosis is excellent, similar to that for ostium secundum ASDs. When a large left-to-right shunt is present, surgical repair is performed. The associated ASD should be closed in such a way that pulmonary venous return is directed to the left atrium. A single anomalous pulmonary vein without an atrial communication may be difficult to redirect to the left atrium; if the shunt is small, it may be left unoperated.

420.5 Atrioventricular Septal Defects (Ostium Primum and Atrioventricular Canal or Endocardial Cushion Defects)

Daniel Bernstein

The abnormalities encompassed by AV septal defects are grouped together because they represent a spectrum of a basic embryologic abnormality, a deficiency of the AV septum. An **ostium primum** defect is situated in the lower portion of the atrial septum and overlies the mitral and tricuspid valves. In most instances, a **cleft** in the **anterior leaflet** of the **mitral valve** is also noted. The tricuspid valve is usually functionally normal, although some anatomic abnormality of the septal leaflet is generally present. The ventricular septum is intact.

An **AV septal defect,** also known as an **AV canal defect** or an **endocardial cushion defect**, consists of contiguous atrial and ventricular septal defects with markedly abnormal AV valves. The severity of the valve abnormalities varies considerably; in the complete form of AV septal defect, a single AV valve is common to both ventricles and consists of an anterior and a posterior bridging leaflet related to the ventricular septum, with a lateral leaflet in each ventricle. The lesion is common in children with **Down syndrome**.

Transitional varieties of these defects also occur and include ostium primum defects with clefts in the anterior mitral and septal tricuspid valve leaflets and small ventricular septal defects, and, less commonly, ostium primum defects with normal AV valves. In some patients, the atrial septum is intact, but an inlet VSD is similar to that found in the full AV septal defect. Sometimes AV septal defects are associated with varying degrees of hypoplasia of one of the ventricles, known as either *left-* or *right-dominant AVSD*. If the affected ventricular chamber is too small to establish a two ventricle circulation, then surgical palliation, aiming for an eventual Fontan procedure, is performed (Chapters 424.4 and 425.10).

PATHOPHYSIOLOGY

The basic abnormality in patients with ostium primum defects is the combination of a left-to-right shunt across the atrial defect and mitral (or occasionally tricuspid) insufficiency. The shunt is usually moderate to large, the degree of mitral insufficiency is generally mild to moderate, and pulmonary arterial pressure is typically normal or only mildly increased. The physiology of this lesion is therefore similar to that of an ostium secundum ASD.

In complete AV septal defects, the left-to-right shunt occurs at both the atrial and ventricular levels (Fig. 420-4). Additional shunting may occur directly from the left ventricle to the right atrium because of absence of the AV septum. Pulmonary hypertension and an early tendency to increase pulmonary vascular resistance are common. AV valvular insufficiency increases the volume load on one or both ventricles. If the defect is large enough, some right-to-left shunting may also occur at both the atrial and ventricular levels and lead to mild arterial desaturation. With time, progressive pulmonary vascular disease increases the right-to-left shunt so that clinical cyanosis develops (Eisenmenger physiology, Chapter 427.2).

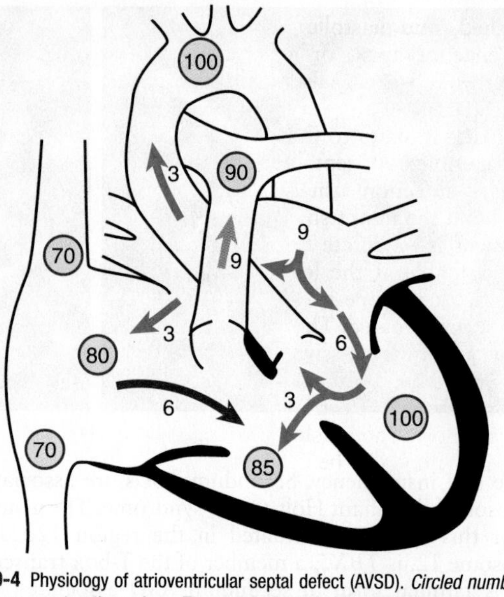

Figure 420-4 Physiology of atrioventricular septal defect (AVSD). *Circled numbers* represent oxygen saturation values. The *numbers next to the arrows* represent volumes of blood flow (in L/min/m^2). This illustration shows a hypothetical patient with a pulmonary-to-systemic blood flow ratio (Qp : Qs) of 3 : 1. Desaturated blood enters the right atrium from the vena cavae at a volume of 3 L/min/m^2 and mixes with 3 L of fully saturated blood shunting left to right across the atrial septal defect; the result is an increase in oxygen saturation in the right atrium. Six liters of blood flows through the right side of the common AV valve, joined by an additional 3 L of saturated blood shunting left to right at the ventricular level, further increasing oxygen saturation in the right ventricle. The full 9 L flows across the right ventricular outflow tract into the lungs. Nine liters returns to the left atrium, with 3 L shunting left to right across the defect and 6 L crossing the left side of the common AV valve and causing a mid-diastolic flow rumble. Three liters of this volume shunts left to right across the VSD, and 3 L is ejected into the ascending aorta (normal cardiac output).

CLINICAL MANIFESTATIONS

Many children with ostium primum defects are asymptomatic, and the anomaly is discovered during a general physical examination. In patients with moderate shunts and mild mitral insufficiency, the physical signs are similar to those of the secundum ASD, but with an additional apical holosystolic murmur caused by mitral insufficiency.

A history of exercise intolerance, easy fatigability, and recurrent pneumonia may be obtained, especially in infants with large left-to-right shunts and severe mitral insufficiency. In these patients, cardiac enlargement is moderate or marked, and the precordium is hyperdynamic. Auscultatory signs produced by the left-to-right shunt include a normal or accentuated 1st heart sound; wide, fixed splitting of the 2nd sound; a pulmonary systolic ejection murmur sometimes preceded by a click; and a low-pitched, mid-diastolic rumbling murmur at the lower left sternal edge or apex, or both, as a result of increased flow through the AV valves. Mitral insufficiency may be manifested by a harsh (occasionally very high pitched) apical holosystolic murmur that radiates to the left axilla.

With complete AV septal defects, heart failure and intercurrent pulmonary infection usually appear in infancy. The liver is enlarged and the infant shows signs of failure to thrive. Cardiac enlargement is moderate to marked, and a systolic thrill is frequently palpable at the lower left sternal border. A precordial bulge and lift may be present as well. The 1st heart sound is normal or accentuated. The 2nd heart sound is widely split if the pulmonary flow is massive. A low-pitched, mid-diastolic rumbling murmur is audible at the lower left sternal border, and a pulmonary systolic ejection murmur is produced by the large pulmonary flow. The harsh apical holosystolic murmur of mitral insufficiency may also be present.

DIAGNOSIS

Chest radiographs of children with complete AV septal defects often show moderate to severe cardiac enlargement caused by the prominence of both ventricles and atria. The pulmonary artery is large, and pulmonary vascularity is increased.

The electrocardiogram in patients with a complete AV septal defect is distinctive. The principal abnormalities are (1) superior orientation of the mean frontal QRS axis with left axis deviation to the left upper or right upper quadrant, (2) counterclockwise inscription of the superiorly oriented QRS vector loop (often manifest by a Q wave in leads I and aVL), (3) signs of biventricular hypertrophy or isolated right ventricular hypertrophy, (4) right ventricular conduction delay (rSR′ pattern in leads V_3R and V_1), (5) normal or tall P waves, and (6) occasional prolongation of the P-R interval (Fig. 420-5).

The echocardiogram (Fig. 420-6) is characteristic and shows signs of right ventricular enlargement with encroachment of the mitral valve echo on the left ventricular outflow tract; the abnormally low position of the AV valves results in a "gooseneck" deformity of the left ventricular outflow tract. In normal hearts, the tricuspid valve inserts slightly more toward the apex than the mitral valve does. In AV septal defects, both valves insert at the same level because of absence of the AV septum. In complete AV septal defects, the ventricular septum is also deficient and the common AV valve is readily appreciated. Pulsed and color flow Doppler echocardiography will demonstrate left-to-right shunting at the atrial, ventricular, or left ventricular to right atrial levels and semiquantitate the degree of AV valve insufficiency. Echocardiography is useful for determining the insertion points of the chordae of the common AV valve and for evaluating the presence of associated lesions such as patent ductus arteriosus (PDA) or coarctation of the aorta.

Cardiac catheterization and angiocardiography is rarely required in the modern era to confirm the diagnosis unless pulmonary vascular disease is suspected, such as in a patient in whom diagnosis has been delayed beyond early infancy, especially in those with Down syndrome in whom the development of pulmonary vascular disease may be more rapid. Catheterization demonstrates the magnitude of the left-to-right shunt, the degree of elevation of pulmonary vascular resistance, and the severity of insufficiency of the common AV valve. By oximetry, the shunt is usually demonstrable at both the atrial and ventricular levels. Arterial oxygen saturation is normal or only mildly reduced unless severe pulmonary vascular disease is present. Children with ostium primum defects generally have normal or only moderately elevated pulmonary arterial pressure. Conversely, complete AV septal defects are associated with right ventricular and pulmonary hypertension and, in older patients, with increased pulmonary vascular resistance (Chapter 427.2).

Selective left ventriculography will demonstrate deformity of the mitral or common AV valve and the distortion of the left ventricular outflow tract caused by this valve (gooseneck deformity). The abnormal anterior leaflet of the mitral valve is serrated, and mitral insufficiency is noted, usually with regurgitation of blood into both the left and right atria. Direct shunting of blood from the left ventricle to the right atrium may also be demonstrated.

TREATMENT

Ostium primum defects are approached surgically from an incision in the right atrium. The cleft in the mitral valve is located through the atrial defect and is repaired by direct suture. The defect in the atrial septum is usually closed by insertion of a patch prosthesis. The surgical mortality rate for ostium primum defects is very low. Surgical treatment of complete AV septal defects is more difficult, especially in infants with cardiac failure and pulmonary hypertension. Because of the risk of **pulmonary vascular**

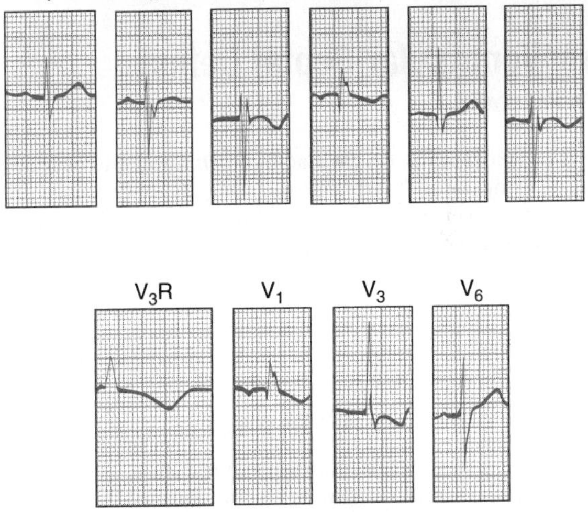

Figure 420-5 Electrocardiogram from a child with an atrioventricular septal defect. Note the QRS axis of −60 degrees and the right ventricular conduction delay with an RSR′ pattern in V_1 and V_3R (V_3R paper speed = 50 mm/sec).

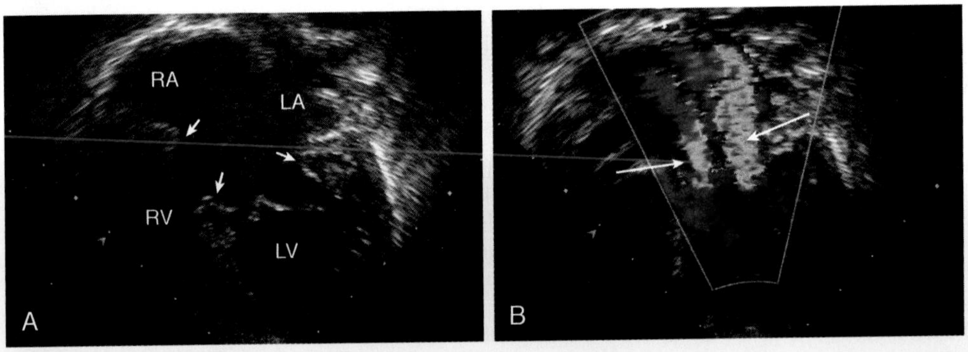

Figure 420-6 Echocardiogram of an atrioventricular septal defect. *A,* Subcostal four-chamber view demonstrating the common atrioventricular valve *(arrows)* spanning the atrial and ventricular septal defects. *B,* Doppler imaging shows 2 jets of regurgitation through the left side of the common atrioventricular valve *(arrows).* LA, left atrium; LV, left ventricle; RA, right atrium; RV, right ventricle.

disease developing as early as 6-12 mo of age, surgical intervention must be performed during infancy. With modern surgical techniques, full correction of these defects can be readily accomplished in infancy; palliation with pulmonary arterial banding is reserved for the subset of patients who have other associated lesions that make early corrective surgery too risky. The atrial and ventricular defects are patched and the AV valves reconstructed. Complications include surgically induced heart block requiring placement of a permanent pacemaker, excessive narrowing of the left ventricular outflow tract requiring surgical revision, and eventual worsening of mitral regurgitation requiring replacement with a prosthetic valve.

PROGNOSIS

The prognosis for unrepaired complete AV septal defects depends on the magnitude of the left-to-right shunt, the degree of elevation of pulmonary vascular resistance, and the severity of AV valve insufficiency. Death from cardiac failure during infancy used to be frequent before the advent of early corrective surgery. In patients who survived without surgery, pulmonary vascular obstructive disease usually developed. Most patients with ostium primum defects and minimal AV valve involvement are asymptomatic or have only minor, nonprogressive symptoms until they reach the 3rd-4th decade of life, similar to the course of patients with secundum ASDs. Late postoperative complications include atrial arrhythmias and heart block, progressive narrowing of the left ventricular outflow tract requiring surgical revision, and eventual worsening of atrioventricular valve regurgitation (usually on the left side) requiring replacement with a prosthetic valve.

BIBLIOGRAPHY

Please visit the Nelson Textbook of Pediatrics *website at www.expertconsult.com for the complete bibliography.*

420.6 Ventricular Septal Defect

Daniel Bernstein

VSD is the most common cardiac malformation and accounts for 25% of congenital heart disease. Defects may occur in any portion of the ventricular septum, but most are of the membranous type. These defects are in a posteroinferior position, anterior to the septal leaflet of the tricuspid valve. VSDs between the crista supraventricularis and the papillary muscle of the conus may be associated with pulmonary stenosis and other manifestations of tetralogy of Fallot (Chapter 424.1). VSDs superior to the crista supraventricularis (supracristal) are less common; they are found just beneath the pulmonary valve and may impinge on an aortic sinus and cause aortic insufficiency. VSDs in the midportion or apical region of the ventricular septum are muscular in type and may be single or multiple (Swiss cheese septum).

PATHOPHYSIOLOGY

The physical size of the VSD is a major, but not the only determinant of the size of the left-to-right shunt. The level of pulmonary vascular resistance in relation to systemic vascular resistance also determines the shunt's magnitude. When a small communication is present (usually <5 mm), the VSD is pressure **restrictive**, meaning that right ventricular pressure is normal. The higher pressure in the left ventricle drives the shunt left to right and the size of the defect limits the magnitude of the shunt. In large **nonrestrictive VSDs** (usually >10 mm), right and left ventricular pressures are equalized. In these defects, the direction of shunting and the shunt magnitude are determined by the ratio of pulmonary to systemic vascular resistance (Fig. 420-7).

After birth in patients with a large VSD, pulmonary vascular resistance may remain elevated, delaying the normal postnatal

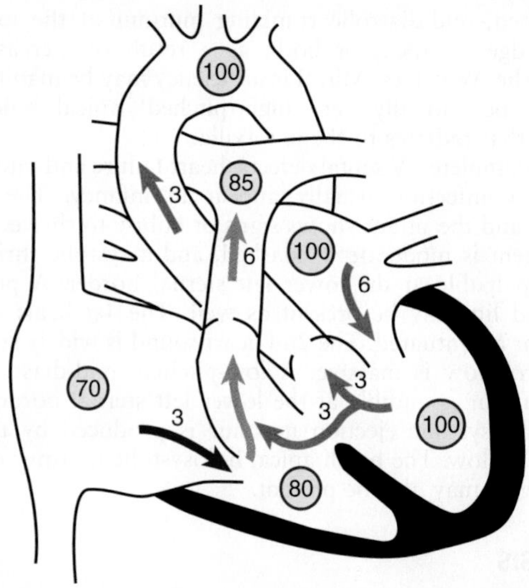

Figure 420-7 Physiology of a large ventricular septal defect (VSD). *Circled numbers* represent oxygen saturation values. The *numbers next to the arrows* represent volumes of blood flow (in L/min/m^2). This illustration shows a hypothetical patient with a pulmonary-to-systemic blood flow ratio (Qp : Qs) of 2 : 1. Desaturated blood enters the right atrium from the vena cava at a volume of 3 L/min/m^2 and flows across the tricuspid valve. An additional 3 L of blood shunts left to right across the VSD, the result being an increase in oxygen saturation in the right ventricle. Six liters of blood is ejected into the lungs. Pulmonary arterial saturation may be further increased because of incomplete mixing at right ventricular level. Six liters returns to the left atrium, crosses the mitral valve, and causes a mid-diastolic flow rumble. Three liters of this volume shunts left to right across the VSD, and 3 L is ejected into the ascending aorta (normal cardiac output).

decrease, and thus the size of the left-to-right shunt may initially be limited. Because of normal involution of the media of small pulmonary arterioles, pulmonary vascular resistance begins to fall in the 1st few weeks after birth and the size of the left-to-right shunt increases. Eventually, a large left-to-right shunt develops, and clinical symptoms become apparent. In most cases during early infancy, pulmonary vascular resistance is only slightly elevated, and the major contribution to pulmonary hypertension is the large communication allowing exposure of the pulmonary circulation to systemic pressure and the large pulmonary blood flow. With continued exposure of the pulmonary vascular bed to high systolic pressure and high flow, pulmonary vascular obstructive disease eventually develops. When the ratio of pulmonary to systemic resistance approaches 1 : 1, the shunt becomes bidirectional, signs of heart failure abate, and the patient begins to show signs of cyanosis (Eisenmenger physiology, Chapter 427.2). In rare infants with a large VSD, usually those with Down syndrome, pulmonary vascular resistance never decreases, and symptoms may remain minimal until Eisenmenger physiology becomes evident.

The magnitude of intracardiac shunts is usually described by the Qp : Qs ratio. If the left-to-right shunt is small (Qp : Qs <1.5 : 1), the cardiac chambers are not appreciably enlarged and the pulmonary vascular bed is probably normal. If the shunt is large (Qp : Qs >2 : 1), left atrial and ventricular volume overload occurs, as does right ventricular and pulmonary arterial hypertension. The main pulmonary artery, left atrium, and left ventricle are enlarged.

CLINICAL MANIFESTATIONS

The clinical findings of patients with a VSD vary according to the size of the defect and pulmonary blood flow and pressure. Small VSDs with trivial left-to-right shunts and normal pulmonary arterial pressure are the most common. These patients are asymptomatic, and the cardiac lesion is usually found during routine physical examination. Characteristically, a loud, harsh, or blowing holosystolic murmur is present and heard best over the lower left sternal border, and it is frequently accompanied by a thrill. In a few instances, the murmur ends before the 2nd sound, presumably because of closure of the defect during late systole. A short, harsh systolic murmur localized to the apex in a neonate is often a sign of a tiny VSD in the apical muscular septum. In premature infants, the murmur may be heard early because pulmonary vascular resistance decreases more rapidly.

Large VSDs with excessive pulmonary blood flow and pulmonary hypertension are responsible for dyspnea, feeding difficulties, poor growth, profuse perspiration, recurrent pulmonary infections, and cardiac failure in early infancy. Cyanosis is usually absent, but duskiness is sometimes noted during infections or crying. Prominence of the left precordium is common, as are a palpable parasternal lift, a laterally displaced apical impulse and apical thrust, and a systolic thrill. The holosystolic murmur of a large VSD is generally less harsh than that of a small VSD and more blowing in nature because of the absence of a significant pressure gradient across the defect. It is even less likely to be prominent in the newborn period. The pulmonic component of the 2nd heart sound may be increased as a result of pulmonary hypertension. The presence of a mid-diastolic, low-pitched rumble at the apex is caused by increased blood flow across the mitral valve and indicates a Qp:Qs ratio of ≥2:1. This murmur is best appreciated with the bell of the stethoscope.

DIAGNOSIS

In patients with small VSDs, the chest x-ray is usually normal, although minimal cardiomegaly and a borderline increase in pulmonary vasculature may be observed. The electrocardiogram is generally normal but may suggest left ventricular hypertrophy. The presence of right ventricular hypertrophy is a warning that the defect is not small and that the patient has pulmonary hypertension or an associated lesion such as pulmonic stenosis. In large VSDs, the chest x-ray shows gross cardiomegaly with prominence of both ventricles, the left atrium, and the pulmonary artery (Fig. 420-8). Pulmonary vascular markings are increased, and frank pulmonary edema, including pleural effusions, may be present. The electrocardiogram shows biventricular hypertrophy; P waves may be notched or peaked.

The two-dimensional echocardiogram (Fig. 420-9) shows the position and size of the VSD. In small defects, especially those of the muscular septum, the defect itself may be difficult to image and is visualized only by color Doppler examination. In defects of the **membranous septum,** a thin membrane (called a **ventricular septal aneurysm** but consisting of tricuspid valve tissue) can partially cover the defect and limit the volume of the left-to-right shunt. Echocardiography is also useful for estimating shunt size by examining the degree of volume overload of the left atrium and left ventricle; in the absence of associated lesions, the extent of their increased dimensions is a good reflection of the size of the left-to-right shunt. Pulsed Doppler examination shows whether the VSD is pressure restrictive by calculating the pressure gradient across the defect. Such calculation allows an estimation of right ventricular pressure and helps determine whether the patient is at risk for the development of early pulmonary vascular disease. The echocardiogram can also be useful to determine the presence of aortic valve insufficiency or aortic leaflet prolapse in the case of supracristal VSDs.

The hemodynamics of a VSD can also be demonstrated by cardiac catheterization, although catheterization is today performed only when laboratory data do not fit well with the clinical findings or when pulmonary vascular disease is suspected. Oximetry demonstrates increased oxygen content in the right ventricle; because some defects eject blood almost directly into the pulmonary artery (streaming), the full magnitude of the oxygen saturation increase is occasionally apparent only when pulmonary arterial blood is sampled. Small, restrictive VSDs are associated with normal right heart pressures and pulmonary vascular resistance. Large, nonrestrictive VSDs are associated with equal or

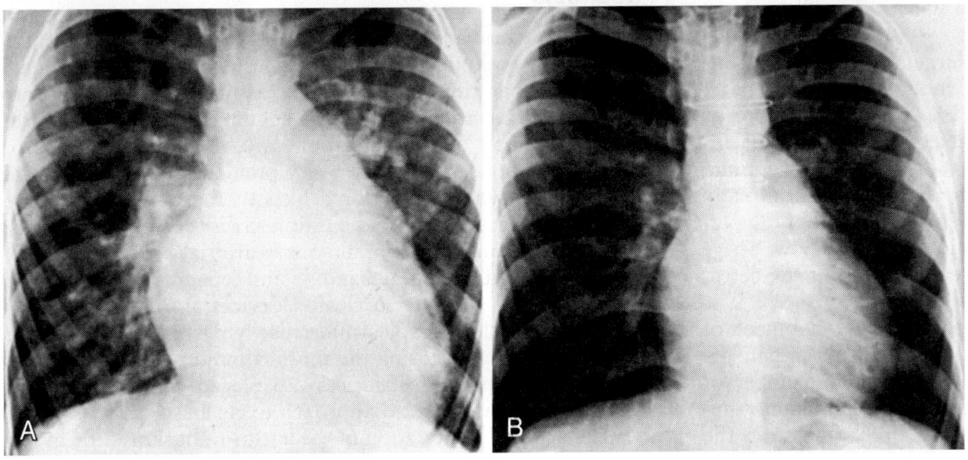

Figure 420-8 *A,* Preoperative roentgenogram in a patient with a ventricular septal defect with a large left-to-right shunt and pulmonary hypertension. Significant cardiomegaly, prominence of the pulmonary arterial trunk, and pulmonary overcirculation are evident. *B,* Three years after surgical closure of the defect, heart size is markedly decreased, and the pulmonary vasculature is normal.

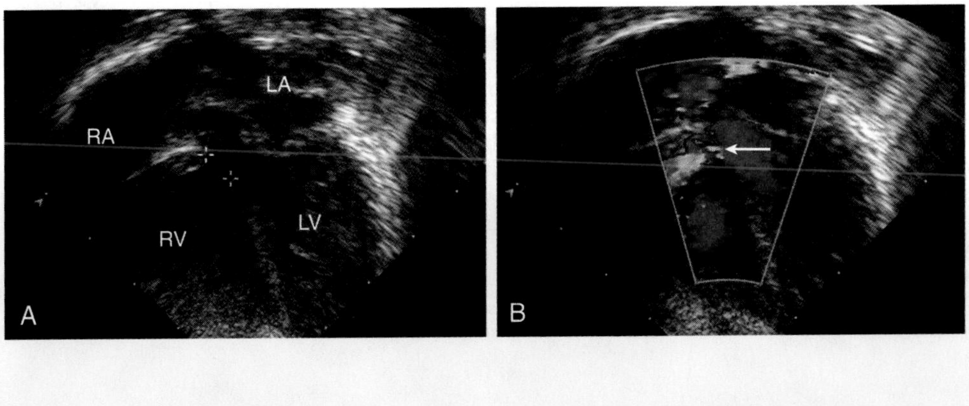

Figure 420-9 Echocardiogram in a patient with a perimembranous ventricular septal defect (VSD). *A,* Apical four-chamber view showing the location of the defect (outlined between two *crosshatches*) beneath the aortic valve. *B,* Color Doppler imaging shows the left-to-right shunt *(arrow)* through the defect (the red color represents blood moving toward the ultrasound transducer and does not indicate the level of oxygenation of the blood). LA, left atrium; LV, left ventricle; RA, right atrium; RV, right ventricle.

nearly equal pulmonary and systemic systolic pressure and variable elevations in pulmonary vascular resistance. Pulmonary blood flow may be 2 to 4 times systemic blood flow. In patients with such "**hyperdynamic pulmonary hypertension,**" pulmonary vascular resistance is only minimally elevated because resistance is equal to pressure divided by flow. However, if left untreated until Eisenmenger syndrome is present, pulmonary artery systolic and diastolic pressure will be elevated but the degree of left-to-right shunting minimal. In these cases, desaturation of blood in the left ventricle is usually encountered. The size, location, and number of ventricular defects can be demonstrated by left ventriculography. Contrast medium passes across the defect or defects to opacify the right ventricle and pulmonary artery. Administration of 100% oxygen with and without nitric oxide can be used to determine whether the pulmonary vascular resistance, if elevated, is still reactive and therefore more likely to drop after surgical repair.

TREATMENT

The natural course of a VSD depends to a large degree on the size of the defect. A significant number (30-50%) of small defects close spontaneously, most frequently during the 1st 2 yr of life. Small muscular VSDs are more likely to close (up to 80%) than membranous VSDs (up to 35%). The vast majority of defects that close do so before the age of 4 yr, although spontaneous closure has been reported in adults. VSDs that close often have ventricular septal aneurysm (accessory tricuspid valve) tissue that limits the magnitude of the shunt. Most children with small defects remain asymptomatic, without evidence of an increase in heart size, pulmonary arterial pressure, or resistance. A long-term risk is infective endocarditis. Some long-term studies of adults with unoperated small VSDs show an increased incidence of arrhythmia, subaortic stenosis, and exercise intolerance. The Council on Cardiovascular Disease in the Young of the American Heart Association states that an isolated, small, hemodynamically insignificant VSD is not an indication for surgery. The declining risk of open heart surgery has led others to suggest that all VSDs be closed electively by mid-childhood.

It is less common for moderate or large VSDs to close spontaneously, although even defects large enough to result in heart failure may become smaller and up to 8% may close completely. More commonly, infants with large defects have repeated episodes of respiratory infection and heart failure despite optimal medical management. Heart failure may be manifested in many of these infants primarily as failure to thrive. Pulmonary hypertension occurs as a result of high pulmonary blood flow. These patients are at risk for pulmonary vascular disease if the defect is not repaired during early infancy.

Patients with VSD are also at risk for the development of aortic valve regurgitation, the greatest risk occurring in patients with a supracristal VSD (Chapter 420.7). A small number of patients with VSD develop **acquired infundibular pulmonary stenosis,** which then protects the pulmonary circulation from the short-term effects of pulmonary overcirculation and the long-term effects of pulmonary vascular disease. In these patients, the clinical picture changes from that of a VSD with a large left-to-right shunt to a VSD with pulmonary stenosis. The shunt may diminish in size, become balanced, or even become a net right-to-left shunt. These patients must be carefully distinguished from those in whom an Eisenmenger physiology develops (Chapter 427.2).

In patients with small VSDs, parents should be reassured of the relatively benign nature of the lesion, and the child should be encouraged to live a normal life, with no restrictions on physical activity. Surgical repair is currently not recommended. As protection against infective endocarditis, the integrity of primary and permanent teeth should be carefully maintained; with the latest revision of the American Heart Association guidelines, antibiotic prophylaxis is no longer recommended for dental visits or surgical procedures (Chapter 431). These patients can be monitored by a combination of clinical examination and noninvasive laboratory tests until the VSD has closed spontaneously. Echocardiography is used to estimate pulmonary artery pressure, screen for the development of left ventricular outflow tract pathology (subaortic membrane or aortic regurgitation), and to confirm spontaneous closure.

In infants with a large VSD, management has 2 aims: to get the symptoms of heart failure under control (Chapter 436) and prevent the development of pulmonary vascular disease. If early treatment is successful, sometimes the shunt may diminish in size with spontaneous improvement, especially during the 1st yr of life. The clinician must be alert not to confuse clinical improvement caused by a decrease in defect size with clinical changes caused by the development of Eisenmenger physiology. Because surgical closure can be carried out at low risk in most infants, medical management should not be pursued in symptomatic infants after an initial unsuccessful trial. Since pulmonary vascular disease can usually be prevented when surgery is performed within the 1st yr of life, even infants with well controlled heart failure should not have surgery delayed inordinately unless there is evidence that the defect is becoming pressure restrictive.

Indications for surgical closure of a VSD include patients at any age with large defects in whom clinical symptoms and failure to thrive cannot be controlled medically; infants between 6 and 12 mo of age with large defects associated with pulmonary hypertension, even if the symptoms are controlled by medication; and patients older than 24 mo with a Qp:Qs ratio greater than 2:1. Patients with a supracristal VSD of any size are usually referred for surgery because of the high risk for aortic valve regurgitation (Chapter 420.7). Severe pulmonary vascular disease nonresponsive to pulmonary vasodilators is a contraindication to closure of a VSD.

PROGNOSIS

The results of primary surgical repair are excellent, and complications leading to long-term problems (residual ventricular shunts requiring reoperation or heart block requiring a pacemaker) are rare. Pulmonary arterial palliative banding with repair in later childhood, once the standard of care, is now reserved for extremely complicated cases or very premature infants. Surgical risks are somewhat higher for defects in the muscular septum, particularly apical defects and multiple (Swiss cheese–type) VSDs. These patients may require pulmonary arterial banding if symptomatic, with subsequent debanding and repair of multiple VSDs at an older age. **Catheter occlusion devices** are in clinical trials as a means of closing apical muscular VSDs and other devices are being tested for closing the more common perimembranous defects. Sometimes these devices are placed during surgery in what is known as a hybrid approach to repair.

After surgical obliteration of the left-to-right shunt, the hyperdynamic heart becomes quiet, cardiac size decreases toward normal (see Fig. 420-8), thrills and murmurs are abolished, and pulmonary artery hypertension regresses. The patient's clinical status improves markedly. Most infants begin to thrive, and cardiac medications are no longer required. Catch-up growth occurs in most patients within the next 1-2 yr. In some instances after successful surgery, systolic ejection murmurs of low intensity persist for months. The long-term prognosis after surgery is excellent. Patients with a small VSD and those who have undergone surgical closure without residua are considered to be at standard risk for health and life insurance.

BIBLIOGRAPHY

Please visit the Nelson Textbook of Pediatrics *website at* *www.expertconsult.com* *for the complete bibliography.*

420.7 Supracristal Ventricular Septal Defect with Aortic Insufficiency

Daniel Bernstein

A supracristal VSD is complicated by prolapse of the aortic valve into the defect and aortic insufficiency, which may eventually occur in 50-90% of patients. Although supracristal VSD accounts for ≈5% of all patients with VSD, the incidence is higher in Asian children. The VSD, which may be small or moderate in size, is located anterior to and directly below the pulmonary valve in the outlet septum, superior to the muscular ridge known as the *crista supraventriculari,* which separates the trabecular body of the right ventricle from the smooth outflow portion. The right or, less often, the noncoronary aortic cusp prolapses into the defect and may partially or even completely occlude it. Such occlusion may limit the amount of left-to-right shunting and give the false impression that the defect is not large. Aortic insufficiency is most often not recognized until late in the 1st decade of life or beyond. Of note, aortic insufficiency is occasionally associated with VSDs located in the membranous septum.

Early heart failure secondary to a large left-to-right shunt rarely occurs, but without surgery, severe aortic insufficiency and left ventricular failure may ensue. The murmur of a supracristal VSD is usually heard at the mid to upper left sternal border, as opposed to the lower left sternal border, and it is sometimes confused with that of pulmonic stenosis. A decrescendo diastolic murmur will be appreciated at the upper right or mid left sternal borders if there is aortic insufficiency. More advanced degrees of aortic insufficiency will be associated with a wide pulse pressure. These clinical findings must be distinguished from PDA or other defects associated with aortic runoff.

The clinical manifestations vary widely from trivial aortic regurgitation and small left-to-right shunts in asymptomatic children to florid aortic insufficiency and massive cardiomegaly in symptomatic adolescents. Closure of all supracristal ventricular VSDs at the time of diagnosis is commonly recommended to prevent the development of aortic regurgitation, even in an asymptomatic child. Patients who already have significant aortic insufficiency require surgical intervention to prevent irreversible left ventricular dysfunction. Surgical options depend on the degree of damage to the valve. If the insufficiency is mild, they may include simple closure of the defect to bolster the valve apparatus without touching the valve itself, valvuloplasty for more significant degrees of involvement, and replacement with a prosthesis or homograft or aortopulmonary translocation for severe involvement.

420.8 Patent Ductus Arteriosus

Daniel Bernstein

During fetal life, most of the pulmonary arterial blood is shunted right-to-left through the ductus arteriosus into the aorta (Chapter 415). Functional closure of the ductus normally occurs soon after birth, but if the ductus remains patent when pulmonary vascular resistance falls, aortic blood then is shunted left-to-right into the pulmonary artery. The aortic end of the ductus is just distal to the origin of the left subclavian artery, and the ductus enters the pulmonary artery at its bifurcation. Female patients with patent ductus arteriosus (PDA) outnumber males 2 : 1. PDA is also associated with maternal rubella infection during early pregnancy, a now uncommon occurrence. However, PDA is a common problem in premature infants, as the smooth muscle in the wall of the preterm ductus is less responsive to high Po_2 and therefore less likely to constrict after birth. In these infants, it can cause severe hemodynamic derangements and several major sequelae (Chapter 95.3).

When a term infant is found to have a PDA, the wall of the ductus is deficient in both the mucoid endothelial layer and the muscular media, whereas in the premature infant, the PDA usually has a normal structure. Thus, a PDA persisting beyond the 1st few weeks of life in a term infant rarely closes spontaneously or with pharmacologic intervention, whereas if early pharmacologic or surgical intervention is not required in a premature infant, spontaneous closure occurs in most instances. A PDA is seen in 10% of patients with other congenital heart lesions and often plays a critical role in providing a source of pulmonary blood flow when the right ventricular outflow tract is stenotic or atretic (Chapter 421.6) or in providing systemic blood flow in the presence of aortic coarctation or interruption (Chapter 421.8).

PATHOPHYSIOLOGY

As a result of the higher aortic pressure postnatally, blood shunts left to right through the ductus, from the aorta to the pulmonary artery. The extent of the shunt depends on the size of the ductus and on the ratio of pulmonary to systemic vascular resistance. If the PDA is small, pressures within the pulmonary artery, the right ventricle, and the right atrium are normal. If the PDA is large, pulmonary artery pressure may be elevated to systemic levels during both systole and diastole. Thus, patients with a large PDA are at high risk for the development of pulmonary vascular disease if left unoperated.

CLINICAL MANIFESTATIONS

A small PDA is usually asymptomatic. A large PDA will result in heart failure similar to that encountered in infants with a large VSD. Retardation of physical growth may be a major manifestation in infants with large shunts. A small PDA is associated with normal peripheral pulses, and a large PDA results in bounding peripheral arterial pulses and a wide pulse pressure, due to runoff of blood into the pulmonary artery during diastole. The heart is normal in size when the ductus is small, but moderately or grossly enlarged in cases with a large communication. In these cases, the apical impulse is prominent and, with cardiac enlargement, is heaving. A thrill, maximal in the 2nd left interspace, is often present and may radiate toward the left clavicle, down the left sternal border, or toward the apex. It is usually systolic but may also be palpated throughout the cardiac cycle. The classic continuous murmur is described as being like machinery in quality. It begins soon after onset of the 1st sound, reaches maximal intensity at the end of systole, and wanes in late diastole. It may be localized to the 2nd left intercostal space or radiate down the left sternal border or to the left clavicle. When pulmonary vascular resistance is increased, the diastolic component of the murmur may be less prominent or absent. In patients with a large left-to-right shunt, a low-pitched mitral mid-diastolic murmur may be audible at the apex as a result of the increased volume of blood flow across the mitral valve.

DIAGNOSIS

If the left-to-right shunt is small, the electrocardiogram is normal; if the ductus is large, left ventricular or biventricular hypertrophy is present. The diagnosis of an isolated, uncomplicated PDA is untenable when right ventricular hypertrophy is present.

Radiographic studies in patients with a large PDA show a prominent pulmonary artery with increased pulmonary vascular markings. Cardiac size depends on the degree of left-to-right shunting; it may be normal or moderately to markedly enlarged. The chambers involved are the left atrium and left ventricle. The aortic knob may be normal or prominent.

The echocardiographic view of the cardiac chambers is normal if the ductus is small. With large shunts, left atrial and left ventricular dimensions are increased. The ductus can easily be visualized directly and its size estimated. Color and pulsed Doppler examinations demonstrate systolic or diastolic (or both)

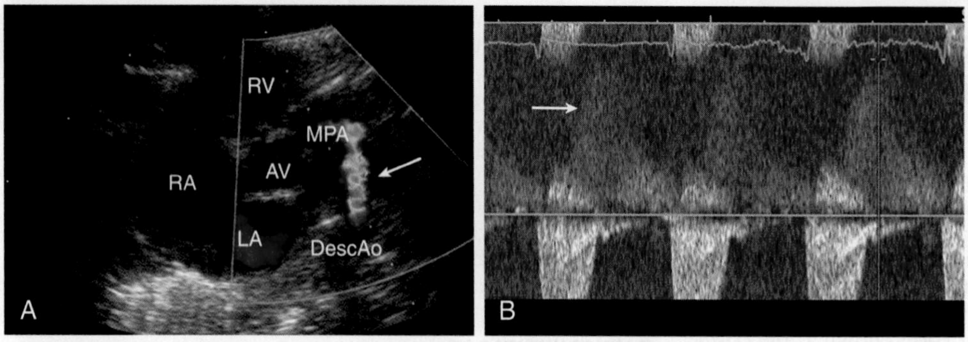

Figure 420-10 Echocardiogram in a newborn with a small- to moderate-sized patent ductus arteriosus (PDA). *A,* Color Doppler performed in a parasternal short axis view shows flow *(arrow)* from the aorta into the main pulmonary artery. *B,* Doppler evaluation demonstrates retrograde diastolic flow into the pulmonary artery. AV, aortic valve; DescAo, descending aorta; LA, left atrium; MPA, main pulmonary artery; RA, right atrium; RV, right ventricle.

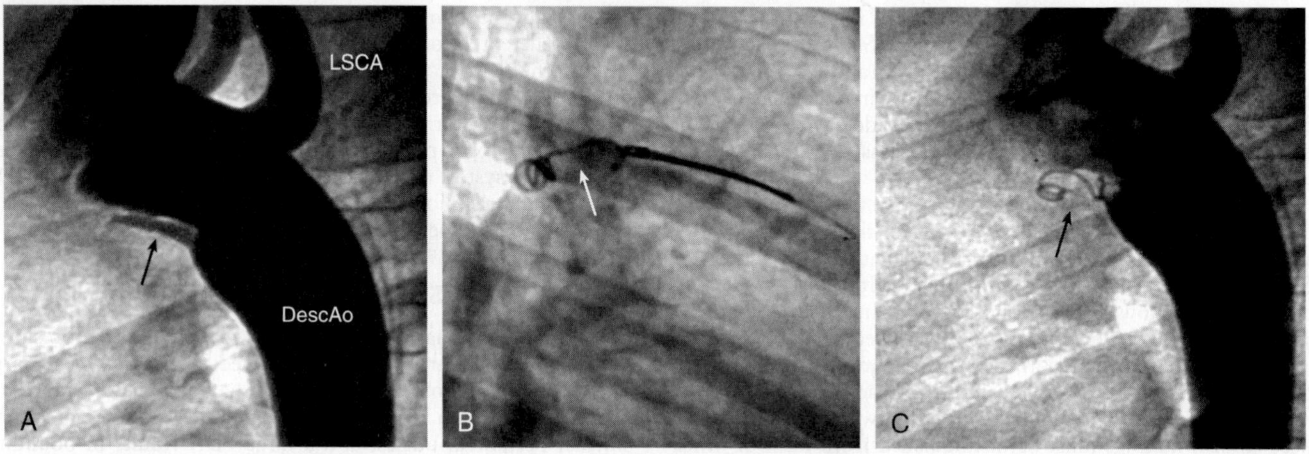

Figure 420-11 Transcatheter closure of a small patent ductus arteriosus (PDA) using a coil. *A,* Angiogram of transverse and descending aorta shows small PDA *(arrow). B,* Coil *(arrow)* has been extruded from sheath and is being positioned in ductal lumen. *C,* Angiogram demonstrating total occlusion of PDA by coil *(arrow).* DescAo, descending aorta; LSCA, left subclavian artery.

retrograde turbulent flow in the pulmonary artery, and aortic retrograde flow in diastole (Fig. 420-10) in the presence of a large shunt.

The clinical pattern is sufficiently distinctive to allow an accurate diagnosis by noninvasive methods in most patients. In patients with atypical findings, cardiac catheterization may be indicated. Cardiac catheterization will demonstrate either normal or increased pressure in the right ventricle and pulmonary artery, depending on the size of the ductus. The presence of oxygenated blood shunting into the pulmonary artery confirms the left-to-right shunt. The catheter may pass from the pulmonary artery through the ductus into the descending aorta. Injection of contrast medium into the ascending aorta shows opacification of the pulmonary artery from the aorta and identifies the ductus.

Other conditions can produce systolic and diastolic murmurs in the pulmonic area in an acyanotic patient and are described in Chapter 416. An **aorticopulmonary window** defect may rarely be clinically indistinguishable from a patent ductus, although, in most cases, the murmur is only systolic and is loudest at the right rather than the left upper sternal border. A sinus of Valsalva aneurysm that has ruptured into the right side of the heart or pulmonary artery, coronary arteriovenous fistulas, and an aberrant left coronary artery with massive collaterals from the right coronary display dynamics similar to that of a PDA with a continuous murmur and a wide pulse pressure. Truncus arteriosus with torrential pulmonary flow also has an "aortic runoff" physiology. A peripheral arteriovenous fistula also results in a wide pulse pressure, but the distinctive precordial murmur of a PDA is not present. VSD with aortic insufficiency, repaired tetralogy of Fallot, and combined aortic and mitral insufficiency (usually due to rheumatic fever) may be confused with a PDA, but the murmurs should be differentiated by their to-and-fro rather than continuous nature. The combination of a large VSD and a PDA results in findings more like those of an isolated VSD. Echocardiography should be able to eliminate these other diagnostic possibilities.

PROGNOSIS AND COMPLICATIONS

Spontaneous closure of the ductus after infancy is extremely rare. Patients with a small PDA may live a normal span with few or no cardiac symptoms, but late manifestations may occur. In patients with a large PDA, cardiac failure most often occurs in early infancy but may occur later in life, even with a moderate-sized communication.

Infective endarteritis may be seen at any age. Pulmonary or systemic emboli may occur. Rare complications include aneurysmal dilatation of the pulmonary artery or the ductus, calcification of the ductus, noninfective thrombosis of the ductus with embolization, and paradoxical emboli. Pulmonary hypertension (Eisenmenger syndrome) usually develops in patients with a large PDA who do not undergo ductal closure (Chapter 427.2).

TREATMENT

Irrespective of age, patients with PDA require surgical or catheter closure. In patients with a small PDA, the rationale for closure is prevention of bacterial endarteritis or other late complications. In patients with a moderate to large PDA, closure is accomplished to treat heart failure or prevent the development of pulmonary vascular disease, or both. Once the diagnosis of a moderate to large PDA is made, treatment should not be unduly postponed after adequate medical therapy for cardiac failure has been instituted.

Transcatheter PDA closure is routinely performed in the cardiac catheterization laboratory (Fig. 420-11). Small PDAs are generally closed with intravascular coils. Moderate to large PDAs may be closed with an umbrella-like device or with a catheter-introduced sac into which several coils are released. Surgical closure of PDA can be accomplished by a standard left thoracotomy or using thoracoscopic minimally invasive techniques. Because the case fatality rate with interventional or surgical treatment is considerably less than 1% and the risk without it is greater, closure of the ductus is indicated in asymptomatic patients, preferably before 1 yr of age. Pulmonary hypertension is not a contraindication to surgery at any age if it can be demonstrated at cardiac catheterization that the shunt flow is still predominantly left to right and that severe pulmonary vascular disease is not present. After closure, symptoms of cardiac failure rapidly disappear. Infants who had failed to thrive usually have immediate improvement in physical development. The pulse and blood pressure return to normal, and the machinery-like murmur disappears. A functional systolic murmur over the pulmonary area may persist; it may represent turbulence in a persistently dilated pulmonary artery. The radiographic signs of cardiac enlargement and pulmonary overcirculation disappear over a period of several months, and the electrocardiogram becomes normal.

PATENT DUCTUS ARTERIOSUS IN LOW BIRTHWEIGHT INFANTS

See Chapter 95.

BIBLIOGRAPHY

Please visit the Nelson Textbook of Pediatrics *website at www.expertconsult.com for the complete bibliography.*

420.9 Aorticopulmonary Window Defect

Daniel Bernstein

An aorticopulmonary (AP) window defect consists of a communication between the ascending aorta and the main pulmonary artery. The presence of pulmonary and aortic valves and an intact ventricular septum distinguishes this anomaly from truncus arteriosus (Chapter 425.8). Symptoms of heart failure appear during early infancy; occasionally, minimal cyanosis is present. The defect is usually large, and the cardiac murmur is usually systolic with an apical mid-diastolic rumble as a result of the increased blood flow across the mitral valve. In the rare instance when the communication is smaller and pulmonary hypertension is absent, the findings on examination can mimic those of a PDA (wide pulse pressure and a continuous murmur at the upper sternal borders). The electrocardiogram shows either left ventricular or biventricular hypertrophy. Radiographic studies demonstrate cardiac enlargement and prominence of the pulmonary artery and intrapulmonary vasculature. The echocardiogram shows enlarged left-sided heart chambers; the window defect can best be delineated with color flow Doppler. CT or MRI angiography can also be utilized to visualize the defect (see Fig. 417-20).

Cardiac catheterization, usually performed in older children to evaluate pulmonary vascular resistance, reveals a left-to-right shunt at the level of the pulmonary artery, as well as hyperkinetic pulmonary hypertension, because the defect is almost always large. Selective aortography with injection of contrast medium into the ascending aorta demonstrates the lesion, and manipulation of the catheter from the main pulmonary artery directly to the ascending aorta is also diagnostic.

An aorticopulmonary window defect is surgically corrected during infancy. If surgery is not carried out in infancy, survivors carry the risk of progressive pulmonary vascular obstructive disease, similar to that of other patients who have large intracardiac or great vessel communications.

420.10 Coronary-Cameral Fistula

Daniel Bernstein

A congenital fistula may exist between a coronary artery and an atrium, ventricle (especially the right), or pulmonary artery. Sometimes, multiple fistulas exist. Regardless of the recipient chamber, the clinical signs are similar to those of PDA, although the machinery-like murmur may be more diffuse. If the flow is substantial, the involved coronary artery may be dilated or aneurysmal. The anatomic abnormality is usually demonstrable by color flow Doppler echocardiography and, during catheterization, by injection of contrast medium into the ascending aorta. Small fistulas may be hemodynamically insignificant and may even close spontaneously. If the shunt is large, treatment consists of either transcatheter coil embolization or, for lesions not amenable to catheter intervention, surgical closure of the fistula.

BIBLIOGRAPHY

Please visit the Nelson Textbook of Pediatrics *website at www.expertconsult.com for the complete bibliography.*

420.11 Ruptured Sinus of Valsalva Aneurysm

Daniel Bernstein

When one of the sinuses of Valsalva of the aorta is weakened by congenital or acquired disease, an aneurysm may form and eventually rupture, usually into the right atrium or ventricle. This condition is extremely rare in childhood. The onset is usually sudden. The diagnosis should be suspected in a patient in whom symptoms of acute heart failure develop in association with a new loud to-and-fro murmur. Color Doppler echocardiography and cardiac catheterization demonstrate the left-to-right shunt at the atrial or ventricular level. Urgent surgical repair is generally required. This condition is often associated with infective endocarditis of the aortic valve.

Chapter 421 Acyanotic Congenital Heart Disease: The Obstructive Lesions

421.1 Pulmonary Valve Stenosis with Intact Ventricular Septum

Daniel Bernstein

Of the various forms of right ventricular outflow obstruction with an intact ventricular septum, the most common is isolated valvular pulmonary stenosis, which accounts for 7-10% of all congenital heart defects. The valve cusps are deformed to various degrees and, as a result, the valve opens incompletely during systole. The valve may be bicuspid or tricuspid and the leaflets partially fused together with an eccentric outlet. This fusion may be so severe that only a pinhole central opening remains. If the valve is not severely thickened, it produces a dome-like obstruction to right ventricular outflow during systole. Isolated infundibular or subvalvular stenosis, supravalvular pulmonary stenosis, and branch pulmonary artery stenosis are also encountered. In cases where pulmonary valve stenosis is associated with a ventricular septal defect (VSD) but without anterior deviation of the infundibular septum and overriding aorta, this condition is better classified as pulmonary stenosis with VSD rather than as tetralogy of Fallot

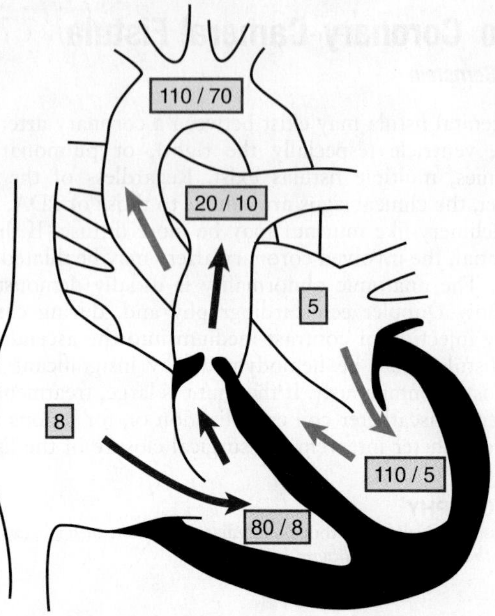

Figure 421-1 Physiology of valvular pulmonary stenosis. Boxed numbers represent pressure in mm Hg. Because of the absence of right-to-left or left-to-right shunting, blood flow through all cardiac chambers is normal at 3 L/min/m^2. The pulmonary-to-systemic blood flow ratio (Qp : Qs) is 1 : 1. Right atrial pressure is increased slightly as a result of decreased right ventricular compliance. The right ventricle is hypertrophied, and systolic and diastolic pressure is increased. The pressure gradient across the thickened pulmonary valve is 60 mm Hg. The main pulmonary artery pressure is slightly low, and poststenotic dilatation is present. Left heart pressure is normal. Unless right-to-left shunting is occurring through a foramen ovale, the patient's systemic oxygen saturation will be normal.

(Chapter 424.1). Pulmonary stenosis and an atrial septal defect (ASD) are also occasionally seen as associated defects. The clinical and laboratory findings reflect the dominant lesion, but it is important to rule out any associated anomalies. Pulmonary stenosis as a result of valve dysplasia is the most common cardiac abnormality in **Noonan syndrome** (Chapter 76), and is associated in about 50% of cases with a mutation in the gene *PTPN11,* encoding the protein tyrosine phosphotase SHP-2 on chromosome 12. The mechanism for pulmonic stenosis is unknown, although maldevelopment of the distal portion of the bulbus cordis and the sequelae of fetal endocarditis have been suggested as etiologies. Pulmonary stenosis, either of the valve or the branch pulmonary arteries, is a common finding in patients with arteriohepatic dysplasia, also known as **Alagille syndrome** (Chapter 348). In this syndrome and in some patients with isolated pulmonic stenosis, a mutation is present in the *Jagged1* gene.

PATHOPHYSIOLOGY

The obstruction to outflow from the right ventricle to the pulmonary artery results in increased right ventricular systolic pressure and wall stress, which leads to hypertrophy of the right ventricle (Fig. 421-1). The severity of these abnormalities depends on the size of the restricted valve opening. In severe cases, right ventricular pressure may be higher than systemic arterial systolic pressure, whereas with milder obstruction, right ventricular pressure is only mildly or moderately elevated. Pulmonary artery pressure (distal to the obstruction) is normal or decreased. Arterial oxygen saturation will be normal even in cases of severe stenosis, unless an intracardiac communication such as a VSD or ASD is allowing blood to shunt from right to left. When severe pulmonic stenosis occurs in a neonate, decreased right ventricular compliance often leads to cyanosis due to right-to-left shunting through a patent foramen ovale, a condition termed **critical pulmonic stenosis.**

CLINICAL MANIFESTATIONS AND LABORATORY FINDINGS

Patients with mild or moderate stenosis usually do not have any symptoms. Growth and development are most often normal. If the stenosis is severe, signs of right ventricular failure such as hepatomegaly, peripheral edema, and exercise intolerance may be present. In a neonate or young infant with critical pulmonic stenosis, signs of right ventricular failure may be more prominent, and cyanosis is often present because of right-to-left shunting at the foramen ovale.

With **mild pulmonary stenosis,** venous pressure and pulse are normal. The heart is not enlarged, the apical impulse is normal, and the right ventricular impulse is not palpable. A sharp pulmonic ejection click immediately after the 1st heart sound is heard at the left upper sternal border during expiration. The 2nd heart sound is split, with a pulmonary component of normal intensity that may be slightly delayed. A relatively short, low- or medium-pitched systolic ejection murmur is maximally audible over the pulmonic area and radiates minimally to the lung fields bilaterally. The electrocardiogram is normal or characteristic of mild right ventricular hypertrophy; inversion of the T waves in the right precordial leads may be seen. (Remember that the T wave in lead V_1 should normally be inverted until at least 6-8 yr of age. Therefore, a positive T wave in V_1 in a young child is a sign of right ventricular hypertrophy.) The only abnormality demonstrable radiographically is usually poststenotic dilatation of the pulmonary artery. Two-dimensional echocardiography shows right ventricular hypertrophy and a slightly thickened pulmonic valve, which domes in systole; Doppler studies demonstrate a right ventricle to pulmonary artery gradient of ≤30 mm Hg.

In **moderate pulmonic stenosis,** venous pressure may be slightly elevated; in older children, a prominent *a* wave may be noted in the jugular pulse. A right ventricular lift may be palpable at the lower left sternal border. The 2nd heart sound is split, with a delayed and soft pulmonary component. As valve motion becomes more limited with more severe degrees of stenosis, both the pulmonic ejection click and the pulmonic 2nd sound may become inaudible. With increasing degrees of stenosis, the peak of the systolic ejection murmur is prolonged later into systole, and its quality becomes louder and harsher (higher frequency). The murmur radiates more prominently to both lung fields.

The electrocardiogram reveals right ventricular hypertrophy, sometimes with a prominent spiked P wave. Radiographically, the heart can vary from normal size to mildly enlarged with uptilting of the apex due to prominence of the right ventricle; pulmonary vascularity may be normal or slightly decreased. The echocardiogram shows a thickened pulmonic valve with restricted systolic motion. Doppler examination demonstrates a right ventricle to pulmonary artery pressure gradient in the 30-60 mm Hg range. Mild tricuspid regurgitation may be present and allows Doppler confirmation of right ventricular systolic pressure.

In **severe stenosis,** mild to moderate cyanosis may be noted in patients with an interatrial communication (atrial septal defect or patent foramen ovale). If hepatic enlargement and peripheral edema are present, they are an indication of right ventricular failure. Elevation of venous pressure is common and is caused by a large presystolic jugular *a* wave. The heart is moderately or greatly enlarged, and a conspicuous parasternal right ventricular lift is present and frequently extends to the left midclavicular line. The pulmonary component of the 2nd sound is usually inaudible. A loud, long, and harsh systolic ejection murmur, usually accompanied by a thrill, is maximally audible in the pulmonic area and may radiate over the entire precordium, to both lung fields, into the neck, and to the back. The peak of the murmur occurs later in systole as valve opening becomes more restricted. The murmur frequently encompasses the aortic component of the 2nd sound but is not preceded by an ejection click.

The electrocardiogram shows gross right ventricular hypertrophy, frequently accompanied by a tall, spiked P wave.

Radiographic studies confirm the presence of cardiac enlargement with prominence of the right ventricle and right atrium. Prominence of the main pulmonary artery segment may be seen due to poststenotic dilatation (Fig. 421-2). Intrapulmonary vascularity is decreased. The two-dimensional echocardiogram shows severe deformity of the pulmonary valve and right ventricular hypertrophy (Fig. 421-3). In the late stages of the disease, systolic dysfunction of the right ventricle may be seen, and in these cases the ventricle may become dilated, with prominent tricuspid regurgitation. Doppler studies demonstrate a high gradient (>60 mm Hg) across the pulmonary valve. The classic findings of severe pulmonary stenosis in older children are rarely seen because of early intervention. Signs of critical pulmonic stenosis, with all of the features of severe pulmonic stenosis plus cyanosis, are usually encountered in the neonatal period.

Cardiac catheterization is not generally required for diagnostic purposes but is undertaken as part of a **balloon valvuloplasty** procedure. Catheterization demonstrates an abrupt pressure gradient across the pulmonary valve. Pulmonary artery pressure is either normal or low. The severity of the stenosis is graded based on the ratio of right ventricular systolic pressure to systemic systolic pressure or the right ventricle to pulmonary artery pressure gradient: a gradient of 10-30 mm Hg in mild cases, 30-60 mm Hg in moderate cases, and >60 mm Hg or with right ventricular pressure greater than systemic pressure in severe cases. If cardiac output is low or a significant right-to-left shunt exists across the atrial septum, the pressure gradient may underestimate the degree of valve stenosis. Selective right ventriculography demonstrates the thickened, poorly mobile valve. In mild to moderate stenosis, doming of the valve in systole is readily seen. Flow of contrast medium through the stenotic valve in ventricular systole produces a narrow jet of dye that fills the dilated main pulmonary artery. Subvalvular hypertrophy that may intensify the obstruction may be present.

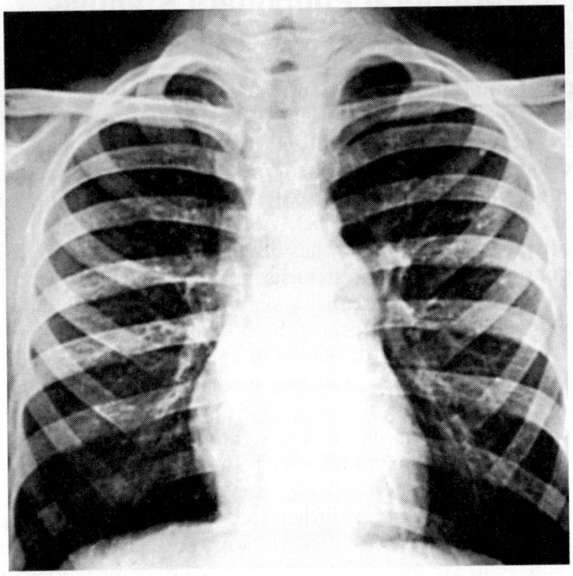

Figure 421-2 Roentgenogram in a patient with valvular pulmonary stenosis and a normal aortic root. The heart size is within normal limits, but poststenotic dilatation of the pulmonary artery is present.

TREATMENT

Patients with moderate or severe isolated pulmonary stenosis require relief of the obstruction. Balloon valvuloplasty is the initial treatment of choice for the majority of patients (Fig. 421-4). Patients with severely thickened pulmonic valves, especially common in those with Noonan syndrome, may require surgical intervention. In a neonate with critical pulmonic stenosis, urgent treatment by either balloon valvuloplasty or surgical valvotomy is warranted.

Excellent results are obtained in most instances. The gradient across the pulmonary valve is markedly reduced or abolished. In the early period after balloon valvuloplasty, a small to moderate residual gradient may remain because of muscular infundibular narrowing; it usually resolves with time. A short, early decrescendo diastolic murmur may be heard at the mid to upper left sternal border as a result of pulmonary valvular insufficiency. The degree of insufficiency is not usually clinically significant. No difference in patient status after valvuloplasty or surgery is noted at late follow-up; recurrence is unusual after successful treatment except in those patients with extremely dysplastic valves.

PROGNOSIS AND COMPLICATIONS

Heart failure occurs only in severe cases and most often during the 1st mo of life. The development of cyanosis from a right-to-left shunt across a foramen ovale is almost exclusively seen in the neonatal period when the stenosis is severe. Infective endocarditis is a risk but is not common in childhood.

Children with mild stenosis can lead a normal life, but their progress should be evaluated at regular intervals. Patients who have small gradients rarely show progression and do not need intervention, but a significant gradient is more likely to develop in children with moderate stenosis as they grow older. Worsening of obstruction may also be due to the development of secondary subvalvular muscular and fibrous tissue hypertrophy. In untreated severe stenosis, the course may abruptly worsen with the development of right ventricular dysfunction and cardiac failure. Infants with critical pulmonic stenosis require urgent catheter balloon valvuloplasty or surgical valvotomy. Development of right ventricular failure many years after pulmonary balloon valvuloplasty is uncommon. Nonetheless, patients should be followed serially for worsening pulmonary insufficiency and right ventricular dilation.

BIBLIOGRAPHY

Please visit the Nelson Textbook of Pediatrics *website at* *www.expertconsult.com* *for the complete bibliography.*

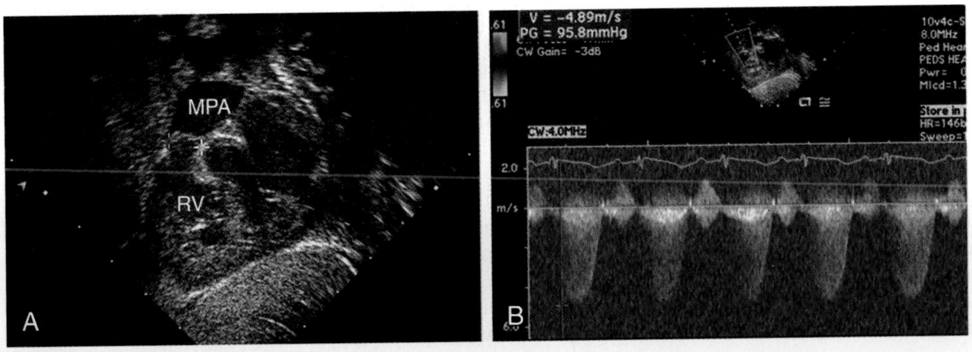

Figure 421-3 Echocardiogram demonstrating valvar pulmonic stenosis. *A*, Subcostal view showing thickened pulmonary valve leaflets (between *crosshatches*). *B*, Doppler study indicating a 95 mm Hg peak pressure gradient across the stenotic valve. MPA, main pulmonary artery; RV, right ventricle.

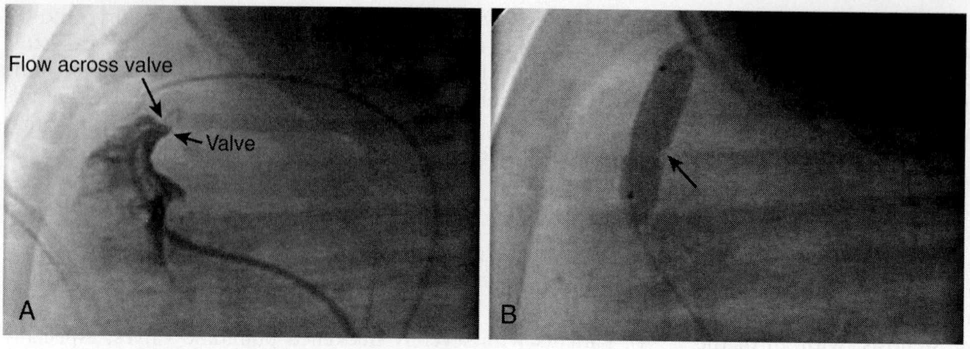

Figure 421-4 Valvar pulmonary stenosis and balloon valvuloplasty. *A,* Right ventricular angiogram showing severely stenotic pulmonary valve with narrow jet of blood flowing across. *B,* Inflation of the balloon catheter showing the indentation *(arrow)* made on the balloon from the stenotic valve. (Photos courtesy of Dr. Jeffrey Feinstein, Stanford University, Stanford, CA.)

421.2 Infundibular Pulmonary Stenosis and Double-Chamber Right Ventricle

Daniel Bernstein

Infundibular pulmonary stenosis is caused by muscular or fibrous obstruction in the outflow tract of the right ventricle. The site of obstruction may be close to the pulmonary valve or well below it; an infundibular chamber may be present between the right ventricular cavity and the pulmonary valve. In many cases, a VSD may have been present initially and later closed spontaneously. When the pulmonary valve is also stenotic, the combined defect is primarily classified as valvular stenosis with secondary infundibular hypertrophy. The hemodynamics and clinical manifestations of patients with isolated infundibular pulmonary stenosis are similar, for the most part, to those described in the discussion of isolated valvular pulmonary stenosis (Chapter 421.1).

A common variation in right ventricular outflow obstruction below the pulmonary valve is that of a double-chambered right ventricle. In this condition, a muscular band is present in the mid-right ventricular region; the band divides the chamber into two parts and creates obstruction between the inlet and outlet portions. An associated VSD that may close spontaneously is often noted. Obstruction is not usually seen early in life but may progress rapidly in a similar manner to the progressive infundibular obstruction observed with tetralogy of Fallot (Chapter 424.1).

The diagnosis of isolated right ventricular infundibular stenosis or double-chambered right ventricle is usually made by echocardiography. The ventricular septum must be evaluated carefully to determine whether an associated VSD is present. The prognosis for untreated cases of severe right ventricular outflow obstruction is similar to that for valvular pulmonary stenosis. When the obstruction is moderate to severe, surgery is indicated. After surgery, the pressure gradient is abolished or markedly reduced and the long-term outlook is excellent.

421.3 Pulmonary Stenosis in Combination with an Intracardiac Shunt

Daniel Bernstein

Valvular or infundibular pulmonary stenosis, or both, may be associated with either an ASD or a VSD. In these patients, the clinical features depend on the degree of pulmonary stenosis, which determines whether the net shunt is from left to right or from right to left.

The presence of a large left-to-right shunt at the atrial or ventricular level is evidence that the pulmonary stenosis is mild. These patients have symptoms similar to those of patients with an isolated ASD or VSD. With increasing age, worsening of the obstruction may limit the shunt and result in a gradual improvement in symptoms. Eventually, particularly in patients with pulmonary stenosis and VSD, a further increase in obstruction may lead to right-to-left shunting and cyanosis. When a patient with a VSD has evidence of decreasing heart failure and increased right ventricular forces on the electrocardiogram, one must differentiate between the development of increasing pulmonary stenosis versus the onset of pulmonary vascular disease (Eisenmenger syndrome, Chapter 427.2).

These anomalies are readily repaired surgically. Defects in the atrial or ventricular septum are closed, and the pulmonary stenosis is relieved by resection of infundibular muscle or pulmonary valvotomy, or both, as indicated. Patients with a predominant right-to-left shunt have symptoms similar to those of patients with **tetralogy of Fallot** (Chapter 424.1).

421.4 Peripheral Pulmonary Stenosis

Daniel Bernstein

Single or multiple constrictions may occur anywhere along the major branches of the pulmonary arteries and may range from mild to severe and from localized to extensive. Frequently, these defects are associated with other types of congenital heart disease, including valvular pulmonic stenosis, tetralogy of Fallot, patent ductus arteriosus (PDA), VSD, ASD, and supravalvular aortic stenosis. A familial tendency has been recognized in some patients with peripheral pulmonic stenosis. A high incidence is found in infants with congenital rubella syndrome. The combination of supravalvular aortic stenosis with pulmonary arterial branch stenosis, idiopathic hypercalcemia of infancy, elfin facies, and mental retardation is known as **Williams syndrome,** a condition associated with deletion of the elastin gene in region 7q11.23 on chromosome 7. Peripheral pulmonary stenosis is also associated with the **Alagille syndrome,** which may be associated with a mutation in the *Jagged1* gene.

A mild constriction has little effect on the pulmonary circulation. With multiple severe constrictions, pressure is increased in the right ventricle and in the pulmonary artery proximal to the site of obstruction. When the anomaly is isolated, the diagnosis is suspected by the presence of murmurs in widespread locations over the chest, either anteriorly or posteriorly. These murmurs are usually systolic ejection in quality but may be continuous. Most often, the physical signs are dominated by the associated anomaly, such as tetralogy of Fallot (Chapter 424.1).

In the immediate newborn period, a mild and transient form of peripheral pulmonic stenosis may be present. Physical findings are generally limited to a soft systolic ejection murmur, which can be heard over either or both lung fields. It is the absence of other physical findings of valvular pulmonic stenosis (right ventricular lift, soft pulmonic 2nd sound, systolic ejection click, murmur loudest at the upper left sternal border) that supports this diagnosis. This murmur usually disappears by 1-2 mo.

If the stenosis is severe, the electrocardiogram shows evidence of right ventricular and right atrial hypertrophy, and the chest radiograph shows cardiomegaly and prominence of the main pulmonary artery. The pulmonary vasculature is usually normal; in some cases, however, small intrapulmonary vascular shadows are seen that represent areas of poststenotic dilatation. Echocardiography is limited in its ability to visualize the distal branch pulmonary arteries. Doppler examination demonstrates the acceleration of blood flow through the stenoses and, if tricuspid regurgitation is present, allows an estimation of right ventricular systolic pressure. MRI and CT are extremely helpful in delineating distal obstructions; if moderate to severe disease is suspected, the diagnosis is usually confirmed by cardiac catheterization.

Severe obstruction of the main pulmonary artery and its primary branches can be relieved during corrective surgery for associated lesions such as the tetralogy of Fallot or valvular pulmonary stenosis. If peripheral pulmonic stenosis is isolated, it may be treated by catheter balloon dilatation, sometimes with placement of an intravascular stent (Fig. 417-29).

421.5 Aortic Stenosis

Daniel Bernstein

PATHOPHYSIOLOGY

Congenital aortic stenosis accounts for ≈5% of cardiac malformations recognized in childhood; a bicuspid aortic valve, one of the most common congenital heart lesions overall, is identified in up to 1.5% of adults and may be asymptomatic in childhood. Aortic stenosis is more frequent in males (3:1). In the most common form, valvular aortic stenosis, the leaflets are thickened and the commissures are fused to varying degrees. Left ventricular systolic pressure is increased as a result of the obstruction to outflow. The left ventricular wall hypertrophies in compensation; as its compliance decreases, end-diastolic pressure increases as well.

Subvalvular (subaortic) stenosis with a discrete fibromuscular shelf below the aortic valve is also an important form of left ventricular outflow tract obstruction. This lesion is frequently associated with other forms of congenital heart disease such as mitral stenosis and coarctation of the aorta (**Shone syndrome**) and may progress rapidly in severity. It is less commonly diagnosed during early infancy and may develop despite previous documentation of no left ventricular outflow tract obstruction. Subvalvular aortic stenosis may become apparent after successful surgery for other congenital heart defects (coarctation of the aorta, PDA, VSD), may develop in association with mild lesions that have not been surgically repaired, or may occur as an isolated abnormality. Subvalvular aortic stenosis may also be due to a markedly hypertrophied ventricular septum in association with hypertrophic cardiomyopathy (Chapter 433.2).

Supravalvular aortic stenosis, the least common type, may be sporadic, familial, or associated with **Williams syndrome,** which includes mental retardation (IQ range 41-80), elfin facies (full face, broad forehead, flattened bridge of the nose, long upper lip, and rounded cheeks) (Fig. 421-5), and idiopathic hypercalcemia of infancy. Additional features include loquacious personality, hypersensitivity to sound, spasticity, hypoplastic nails, dental anomalies (partial anodontia, microdontia enamel hypoplasia), joint hypermobility, nephrocalcinosis, hypothyroidism, and poor weight gain. Narrowing of the coronary artery ostia can occur in patients with supravalvar aortic stenosis and should be carefully evaluated. Stenosis of other arteries, in particular, the branch pulmonary arteries, may also be present. Williams syndrome has been shown to be due to a deletion involving the elastin gene on chromosome 7q11.23.

CLINICAL MANIFESTATIONS

Symptoms in patients with aortic stenosis depend on the severity of the obstruction. Severe aortic stenosis that occurs in early infancy is termed **critical aortic stenosis** and is associated with left ventricular failure and signs of low cardiac output. Heart failure, cardiomegaly, and pulmonary edema are severe, the pulses are weak in all extremities, and the skin may be pale or grayish. Urine output may be diminished. If cardiac output is significantly decreased, the intensity of the murmur at the right upper sternal border may be minimal. Most children with less severe forms of aortic stenosis remain asymptomatic and display normal growth and development. The murmur is usually discovered during routine physical examination. Rarely, fatigue, angina, dizziness, or syncope may develop in an older child with previously undiagnosed severe obstruction to left ventricular outflow. Sudden death has been reported with aortic stenosis but usually occurs in patients with severe left ventricular outflow obstruction in whom surgical relief has been delayed.

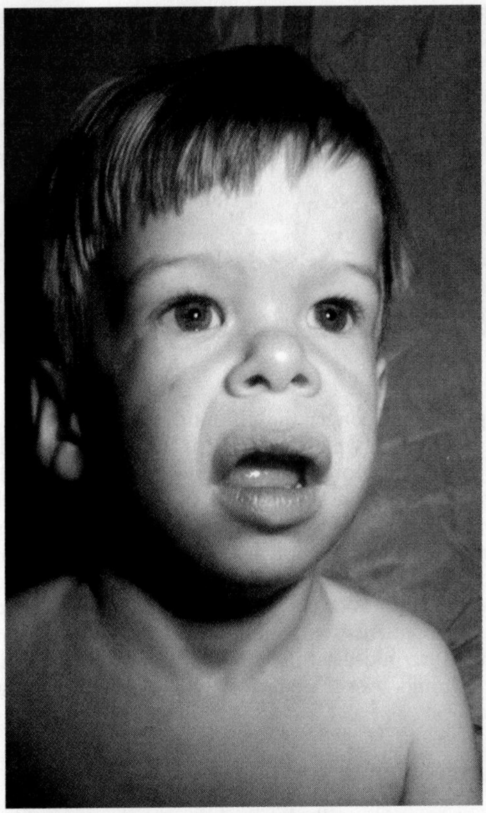

Figure 421-5 Williams syndrome. (From Jones KL, Smith DW: The Williams elfin facies syndrome: a new perspective, *J Pediatr* 86:718, 1975.)

The physical findings are dependent on the degree of obstruction to left ventricular outflow. In mild stenosis, the pulses, heart size, and apical impulse are all normal. With increasing degrees of severity, the pulses become diminished in intensity and the heart may be enlarged, with a left ventricular apical thrust. Mild to moderate valvular aortic stenosis is usually associated with an early systolic ejection click, best heard at the apex and left sternal edge. Unlike the click in pulmonic stenosis, its intensity does not vary with respiration. Clicks are unusual in more severe aortic stenosis or in discrete subaortic stenosis. If the stenosis is severe, the 1st heart sound may be diminished because of decreased compliance of the thickened left ventricle. Normal splitting of the 2nd heart sound is present in mild to moderate obstruction. In patients with severe obstruction, the intensity of aortic valve closure is diminished, and, rarely in children, the 2nd sound may be split paradoxically (becoming wider in expiration). A 4th heart sound may be audible when the obstruction is severe due to decreased left ventricular compliance.

The intensity, pitch, and duration of the systolic ejection murmur are other indications of severity. The louder, harsher

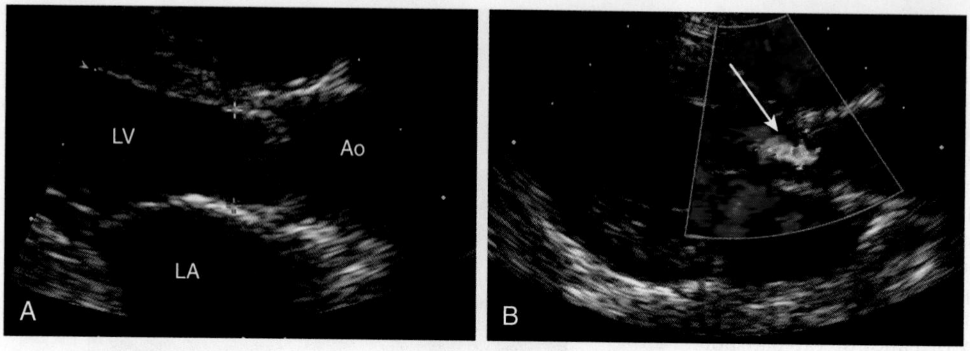

Figure 421-6 Echocardiogram showing valvar aortic stenosis with regurgitation. *A,* In this parasternal long axis view, the stenotic aortic valve can be seen doming in systole. The *crosshatch* marks delineate the aortic annulus. *B,* Doppler study shows the presence of aortic regurgitation *(arrow).* Ao, aorta; LA, left atrium; LV, left ventricle.

(higher pitch), and longer the murmur, the greater the degree of obstruction is. The typical murmur is audible maximally at the right upper sternal border and radiates to the neck and the left midsternal border. It is usually accompanied by a thrill in the suprasternal notch. In patients with subvalvular aortic stenosis, the murmur may be maximal along the left sternal border or even at the apex. A soft decrescendo diastolic murmur indicative of aortic insufficiency is often present when the obstruction is subvalvular or in patients with a bicuspid aortic valve. Occasionally, an apical short mid-diastolic rumbling murmur is audible; this murmur should raise suspicion of associated mitral valve stenosis.

LABORATORY FINDINGS AND DIAGNOSIS

The diagnosis can usually be made on the basis of the physical examination and the severity of obstruction confirmed by laboratory tests. If the pressure gradient across the aortic valve is mild, the electrocardiogram is likely to be normal. The electrocardiogram may occasionally be normal even with more severe obstruction, but evidence of left ventricular hypertrophy and strain (inverted T waves in the left precordial leads) is generally present if severe stenosis is long-standing. The chest radiograph frequently shows a prominent ascending aorta, but the aortic knob is normal. Heart size is typically normal. Valvular calcification has been noted only in older children and adults. Echocardiography identifies both the site and the severity of the obstruction. Two-dimensional imaging shows left ventricular hypertrophy and the thickened and domed aortic valve (Fig. 421-6). The echo will also demonstrate the number of valve leaflets and their morphology, and the presence of a subaortic membrane or supravalvar stenosis. Associated anomalies of the mitral valve or aortic arch or a VSD or PDA are present in up to 20% of cases. In the absence of left ventricular failure, the shortening fraction of the left ventricle may be increased because the ventricle is hypercontractile. In infants with critical aortic stenosis, the left ventricular shortening fraction is usually decreased and may be quite poor. The endocardium may appear bright, indicative of the development of endocardial fibrous scarring, known as **endocardial fibroelastosis.** Doppler studies show the specific site of obstruction and determine the peak and mean systolic left ventricular outflow tract gradients. When severe aortic obstruction is associated with left ventricular dysfunction, the Doppler-derived valve gradient may markedly underestimate the severity of the obstruction because of the low cardiac output across the valve.

Left heart catheterization, usually performed in conjunction with aortic balloon valvuloplasty, demonstrates the magnitude of the pressure gradient from the left ventricle to the aorta. The aortic pressure curve is abnormal if the obstruction is severe. In patients with severe obstruction and decreased left ventricular compliance, left atrial pressure is increased and pulmonary hypertension may be present. When a critically ill infant with left ventricular outflow tract obstruction undergoes cardiac catheterization, left ventricular function is often markedly decreased. As with the echocardiogram, the gradient measured across the stenotic aortic valve may underestimate the degree of obstruction because of low cardiac output. Actual measurement of cardiac output by thermodilution and calculation of the aortic valve area may be helpful.

TREATMENT

Balloon valvuloplasty is indicated for children with moderate to severe valvular aortic stenosis to prevent progressive left ventricular dysfunction and the risk of syncope and sudden death. It is generally agreed that valvuloplasty should be advised when the peak-to-peak systolic gradient between the left ventricle and aorta exceeds 60-70 mm Hg at rest, assuming normal cardiac output, or for lesser gradients when symptoms or electrocardiographic changes are present. For more rapidly progressive subaortic obstructive lesions, a gradient of 40-50 mm Hg or the presence of aortic insufficiency is considered an indication for surgery. With the development of low-profile balloons and smaller catheters that cause less injury to peripheral arteries, balloon valvuloplasty has become the procedure of choice even in the neonatal period. Surgical treatment is usually reserved for extremely dysplastic aortic valves that are not amenable to balloon therapy or in patients who also have subvalvar or valvar (also known as *supravalvar*) stenosis.

Discrete subaortic stenosis can be resected without damage to the aortic valve, the anterior leaflet of the mitral valve, or the conduction system. This type of obstruction is not usually amenable to catheter treatment. Relief of supravalvular stenosis is also achieved surgically, and the results are excellent if the area of obstruction is discrete and not associated with a hypoplastic aorta. In association with supravalvular aortic stenosis, one or both coronary arteries may be stenotic at their origins because of a thick supra-aortic fibrous ridge. For patients who have aortic stenosis in association with severe tunnel-like subaortic obstruction, the left ventricular outflow tract can be enlarged by "borrowing" space anteriorly from the right ventricular outflow tract (the Konno procedure).

Regardless of whether surgical or catheter treatment has been carried out, aortic insufficiency or calcification with re-stenosis is likely to occur years or even decades later and eventually require reoperation and often aortic valve replacement. When recurrence develops, it may not be associated with early symptoms. Signs of recurrent stenosis include electrocardiographic signs of left ventricular hypertrophy, an increase in the Doppler echocardiographic gradient, deterioration in echocardiographic indices of left ventricular function, and recurrence of signs or symptoms during graded treadmill exercise. Evidence of significant aortic regurgitation includes symptoms of heart failure, cardiac enlargement on roentgenogram, and left ventricular dilatation on echocardiogram. The choice of reparative procedure depends on the relative degree of stenosis and regurgitation.

When **aortic valve replacement** is necessary, the choice of procedure often depends on the age of the patient. Homograft valves tend to calcify more rapidly in younger children, but they do not require chronic anticoagulation. Mechanical prosthetic valves are much longer lasting, yet they require anticoagulation, which can be difficult to manage in young children. In adolescent girls who are nearing childbearing age, consideration of the teratogenic effects of warfarin may warrant the use of a homograft valve. None of these options are perfect for a younger child who requires valve replacement because neither homograft nor mechanical valves grow with the patient. An alternative operation is **aortopulmonary translocation (Ross procedure)**; it involves removing the patient's own pulmonary valve and using it to replace the abnormal aortic valve. A homograft is then placed in the pulmonary position. The potential advantage of this procedure is the possibility for growth of the translocated living "neoaortic" valve and the increased longevity of the homograft valve when placed in the lower pressure pulmonary circulation. The long-term success of this operation, especially in young children, is still being investigated. Stent valves, which are tissue valves sewn into the inside of an expandable metal stent, are currently in clinical trials in adults. These can be implanted in the cardiac catheterization laboratory using a percutaneous approach. Tissue-engineered replacement valves grown in the laboratory from the patient's own arterial endothelial cells are the best hope for long-term palliation and are currently under development in animal models.

PROGNOSIS

Neonates with critical aortic stenosis may have severe heart failure and deteriorate rapidly to a low-output shock state. Emergency surgery or balloon valvuloplasty is lifesaving, but the mortality risk is not trivial. Neonates who die of critical aortic stenosis frequently have significant left ventricular endocardial fibroelastosis. Those who survive may develop signs of left ventricular diastolic muscle dysfunction (restrictive cardiomyopathy) and require cardiac transplantation (Chapter 433.3).

In older infants and children with mild to moderate aortic stenosis, the prognosis is reasonably good, although disease progression over a period of 5-10 yr is common. Patients with aortic valve gradients <40-50 mm Hg are considered to have mild disease; those with gradients of 40-70 mm Hg have moderate disease. These patients usually respond well to treatment (either surgery or valvuloplasty), although reoperations on the aortic valve are often required later in childhood or in adult life, and many patients eventually require valve replacement. In unoperated patients with severe obstruction, sudden death is a significant risk and often occurs during or immediately after exercise. Aortic stenosis is one of the causes of sudden cardiac death in the pediatric age group.

Patients with moderate to severe degrees of aortic stenosis should not participate in active competitive sports. In those with milder disease, sports participation is less severely restricted. The status of each patient should be reviewed at least annually and intervention advised if progression of signs or symptoms occurs. Prophylaxis against infective endocarditis is no longer recommended unless a prosthetic valve has been inserted.

Older children and adults with isolated bicuspid aortic valve are at increased risk for developing dilation of their ascending aorta, even in the absence of significant stenosis. This risk increases with age, and the rate of increase is greatest in those with the largest aortic roots. In children, this dilation is usually mild and remains stable over many years of observation, but in older patients the aorta can dilate substantially and progressively. Whether these patients have some undiagnosed form of connective tissue disorder remains to be determined (since this form of dilation is similar to that seen in Marfan syndrome). Patients with Turner syndrome and bicuspid aortic valve do have an increased risk of aortic dilation. Although dissection and rupture are described complications of severe aortic root dilation in adults, there is not yet sufficient data to determine these risks in children. Only isolated cases have been reported.

BIBLIOGRAPHY

Please visit the Nelson Textbook of Pediatrics *website at* *www.expertconsult.com* *for the complete bibliography.*

421.6 Coarctation of the Aorta

Daniel Bernstein

Constrictions of the aorta of varying degrees may occur at any point from the transverse arch to the iliac bifurcation, but 98% occur just below the origin of the left subclavian artery at the origin of the ductus arteriosus (juxtaductal coarctation). The anomaly occurs twice as often in males as in females. Coarctation of the aorta may be a feature of **Turner syndrome** (Chapters 76 and 580.1) and is associated with a bicuspid aortic valve in more than 70% of patients. Mitral valve abnormalities (a supravalvular mitral ring or parachute mitral valve) and subaortic stenosis are potential associated lesions. When this group of left-sided obstructive lesions occurs together, they are referred to as the **Shone complex.**

PATHOPHYSIOLOGY

Coarctation of the aorta can occur as a discrete juxtaductal obstruction or as tubular hypoplasia of the transverse aorta starting at one of the head or neck vessels and extending to the ductal area (previously referred to as *preductal* or *infantile-type coarctation;* Fig. 421-7). Often, both components are present. It is postulated that coarctation may be initiated in fetal life by the presence of a cardiac abnormality that results in decreased blood flow anterograde through the aortic valve (e.g., bicuspid aortic

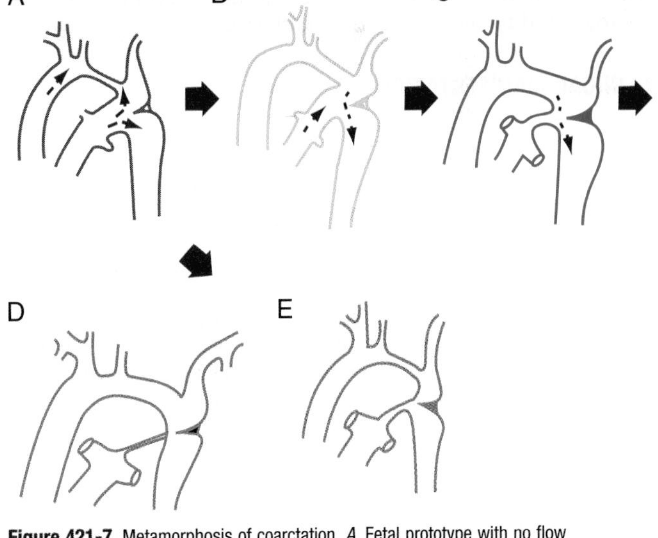

Figure 421-7 Metamorphosis of coarctation. *A,* Fetal prototype with no flow obstruction. *B,* Late gestation. The aortic ventricle increases its output and dilates the hypoplastic segment. Antegrade aortic flow bypasses the shelf via the ductal orifice. *C,* Neonate. Ductal constriction initiates the obstruction by removing the bypass and increasing antegrade arch flow. *D,* Mature juxtaductal stenosis. The bypass is completely obliterated, and intimal hypoplasia on the edge of the shelf is aggravating the stenosis. Collaterals develop. *E,* Persistence of the infantile-type fetal prototype. An intracardiac left-sided heart obstruction precludes an increase in antegrade aortic flow before or after birth. Both isthmus hypoplasia and a contraductal shelf are present. Lower body flow often depends on patency of the ductus. (From Gersony WM: Coarctation of the aorta. In Adams FH, Emmanouilides GC, Riemenshneider T, editors: *Moss heart disease in infants, children, and adolescents,* ed 4, Baltimore, 1989, Williams & Wilkins.)

valve, VSD). Alternatively, coarctation may be due to abnormal extension of contractile ductal tissue into the aortic wall.

In patients with discrete juxtaductal coarctation, ascending aortic blood flows through the narrowed segment to reach the descending aorta, although left ventricular hypertension and hypertrophy result. In the 1st few days of life, the PDA may serve to widen the juxtaductal area of the aorta and provide temporary relief from the obstruction. Net left-to-right ductal shunting occurs in these acyanotic infants. With more severe juxtaductal coarctation or in the presence of transverse arch hypoplasia, right ventricular blood is ejected through the ductus to supply the descending aorta. Perfusion of the lower part of the body is then dependent on right ventricular output (see Fig. 421-7). In this situation, the femoral pulses are palpable, and differential blood pressures may not be helpful in making the diagnosis. The ductal right-to-left shunting is manifested as differential cyanosis, with the upper extremities being pink and the lower extremities blue.

Such infants may have severe pulmonary hypertension and high pulmonary vascular resistance. Signs of heart failure are prominent. Occasionally, severely hypoplastic segments of the aortic isthmus may become completely atretic and result in an interrupted aortic arch, with the left subclavian artery arising either proximal or distal to the interruption. Coarctation associated with arch hypoplasia was once referred to as infantile type because its severity usually led to recognition of the condition in early infancy. Adult type referred to isolated juxtaductal coarctation, which, if mild, was not usually recognized until later childhood. These terms have been replaced with the more accurate anatomic terms describing the location and severity of the defect.

Blood pressure is elevated in the vessels that arise proximal to the coarctation; blood pressure as well as pulse pressure is lower below the constriction. The hypertension is not due to the mechanical obstruction alone but also involves neurohumoral mechanisms. Unless operated on in infancy, coarctation of the aorta usually results in the development of an extensive collateral circulation, chiefly from branches of the subclavian, superior intercostal, and internal mammary arteries, to create channels for arterial blood to bypass the area of coarctation. The vessels contributing to the collateral circulation may become markedly enlarged and tortuous by early adulthood.

CLINICAL MANIFESTATIONS

Coarctation of the aorta recognized after infancy is not usually associated with significant symptoms. Some children or adolescents complain about weakness or pain (or both) in the legs after exercise, but in many instances, even patients with severe coarctation are asymptomatic. Older children are frequently brought to the cardiologist's attention when they are found to be hypertensive on routine physical examination.

The classic sign of coarctation of the aorta is a disparity in pulsation and blood pressure in the arms and legs. The femoral, popliteal, posterior tibial, and dorsalis pedis pulses are weak (or absent in up to 40% of patients), in contrast to the bounding pulses of the arms and carotid vessels. The radial and femoral pulses should always be palpated simultaneously for the presence of a radial-femoral delay. Normally, the femoral pulse occurs slightly before the radial pulse. A radial-femoral delay occurs when blood flow to the descending aorta is dependent on collaterals, in which case the femoral pulse is felt after the radial pulse. In normal persons (except neonates), systolic blood pressure in the legs obtained by the cuff method is 10-20 mm Hg higher than that in the arms. In coarctation of the aorta, blood pressure in the legs is lower than that in the arms; frequently, it is difficult to obtain. This differential in blood pressures is common in patients with coarctation who are older than 1 yr, about 90% of whom have systolic hypertension in an upper extremity greater than the 95th percentile for age. It is important to determine the blood pressure in each arm; a pressure higher in the right than the left arm suggests involvement of the left subclavian artery in the area of coarctation. Occasionally, the right subclavian may arise anomalously from below the area of coarctation and result in a left arm pressure that is higher than the right. With exercise, a more prominent rise in systemic blood pressure occurs, and the upper-to-lower extremity pressure gradient will increase.

The precordial impulse and heart sounds are usually normal; the presence of a systolic ejection click or thrill in the suprasternal notch suggests a bicuspid aortic valve (present in 70% of cases). A short systolic murmur is often heard along the left sternal border at the 3rd and 4th intercostal spaces. The murmur is well transmitted to the left infrascapular area and occasionally to the neck. Often, the typical murmur of mild aortic stenosis can be heard in the 3rd right intercostal space. Occasionally, more significant degrees of obstruction are noted across the aortic valve. The presence of a low-pitched mid-diastolic murmur at the apex suggests mitral valve stenosis. In older patients with well-developed collateral blood flow, systolic or continuous murmurs may be heard over the left and right sides of the chest laterally and posteriorly. In these patients, a palpable thrill can occasionally be appreciated in the intercostal spaces on the back.

Neonates or infants with more severe coarctation, usually including some degree of transverse arch hypoplasia, initially have signs of lower body hypoperfusion, acidosis, and severe heart failure. These signs may be delayed days or weeks until after closure of the ductus arteriosus. If detected before ductal closure, patients may exhibit differential cyanosis, best demonstrated by simultaneous oximetry of the upper and lower extremities. On physical examination, the heart is large, and a systolic murmur is heard along the left sternal border with a loud 2nd heart sound.

DIAGNOSIS

Findings on roentgenographic examination depend on the age of the patient and on the effects of hypertension and the collateral circulation. Cardiac enlargement and pulmonary congestion are noted in infants with severe coarctation. During childhood, the findings are not striking until after the 1st decade, when the heart tends to be mildly or moderately enlarged because of left ventricular prominence. The enlarged left subclavian artery commonly produces a prominent shadow in the left superior mediastinum. **Notching** of the **inferior border of the ribs** from pressure erosion by enlarged collateral vessels is common by late childhood. In most instances, the descending aorta has an area of poststenotic dilatation.

The electrocardiogram is usually normal in young children but reveals evidence of left ventricular hypertrophy in older patients. Neonates and young infants display right or biventricular hypertrophy. The segment of coarctation can generally be visualized by two-dimensional echocardiography (Fig. 421-8); associated anomalies of the mitral and aortic valve can also be demonstrated. The descending aorta is hypopulsatile. Color Doppler is useful for demonstrating the specific site of the obstruction. Pulsed and continuous wave Doppler studies determine the pressure gradient directly at the area of coarctation; in the presence of a PDA, however, the severity of the narrowing may be underestimated. CT and MRI are valuable noninvasive tools for evaluation of coarctation when the echocardiogram is equivocal. Cardiac catheterization with selective left ventriculography and aortography is useful in occasional patients with additional anomalies and as a means of visualizing collateral blood flow. In cases that are well defined by echocardiography, CT, or MRI, diagnostic catheterization is not usually required before surgery.

TREATMENT

In neonates with severe coarctation of the aorta, closure of the ductus often results in hypoperfusion, acidosis, and rapid

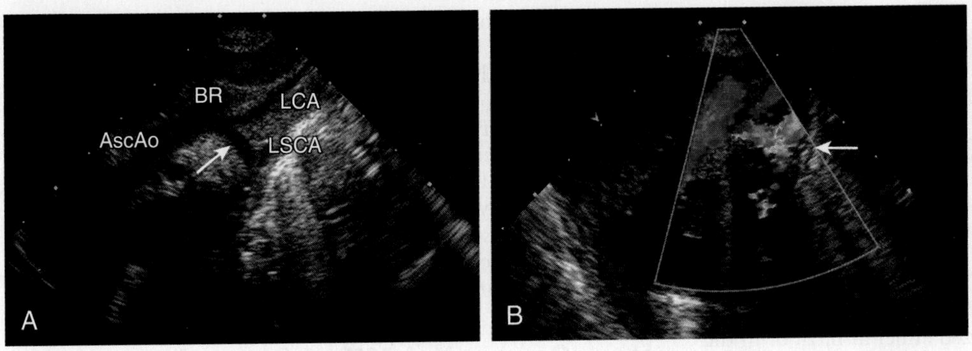

Figure 421-8 Echocardiogram demonstrating coarctation of the aorta with hypoplastic transverse arch. *A,* Suprasternal notch two-dimensional echocardiogram showing marked narrowing beginning just distal to the brachiocephalic artery. *B,* Color Doppler demonstrates turbulent flow in the juxtductal area *(arrow).* AscAo, ascending aorta; BR, brachiocephalic artery; LCA, left carotid artery; LSCA, left subclavian artery.

deterioration. These patients should be given an infusion of **prostaglandin E_1** to reopen the ductus and re-establish adequate lower extremity blood flow. Once a diagnosis has been confirmed and the patient stabilized, surgical repair should be performed. Older infants with heart failure but good perfusion should be managed with anticongestive measures to improve their clinical status before surgical intervention. There is usually no reason to delay surgical repair waiting for patient growth; successful repairs have been performed in small premature infants.

Older children with significant coarctation of the aorta should be treated relatively soon after diagnosis. Delay is unwarranted, especially after the 2nd decade of life, when the operation may be less successful because of decreased left ventricular function and degenerative changes in the aortic wall. Nevertheless, if cardiac reserve is sufficient, satisfactory repair is possible well into mid-adult life.

The procedure of choice for isolated juxtaductal coarctation of the aorta is controversial. Surgery remains the treatment of choice at most centers, and several surgical techniques are used. The area of coarctation can be excised and a primary re-anastomosis performed. Often, the transverse aorta is splayed open and an "extended end-to-end" anastomosis performed to increase the effective cross-sectional area of the repair. The subclavian flap procedure, which involves division of the left subclavian artery and incorporation of it into the wall of the repaired coarctation, is used by some, although has grown out of favor due to a higher degree of residual stenosis. Others favor a patch aortoplasty, in which the area of coarctation is enlarged with a roof of prosthetic material. The use of primary angioplasty for native coarctation remains controversial, although is useful in conditions where surgical intervention may be associated with increased risk in patients with severe left ventricular dysfunction.

After surgery, a striking increase in the amplitude of pulsations in the lower extremities is noted. In the immediate postoperative course, **"rebound" hypertension** is common and requires medical management. This exaggerated acute hypertension gradually subsides and, in most patients, antihypertensive medications can be discontinued. Residual murmurs are common and may be due to associated cardiac anomalies, to a residual flow disturbance across the repaired area, or to collateral blood flow. Rare operative problems include spinal cord injury from aortic cross-clamping if the collaterals are poorly developed, chylothorax, diaphragm injury, and laryngeal nerve injury. If a left subclavian flap is used, the radial pulse and blood pressure in the left arm are diminished or absent.

POSTCOARCTECTOMY SYNDROME

Postoperative **mesenteric arteritis** may be associated with acute hypertension and abdominal pain in the immediate postoperative period. The pain varies in severity and may occur in conjunction with anorexia, nausea, vomiting, leukocytosis, intestinal hemorrhage, bowel necrosis, and small bowel obstruction. Relief is usually obtained with antihypertensive drugs (nitroprusside, esmolol, captopril) and intestinal decompression; surgical exploration is rarely required for bowel obstruction or infarction.

PROGNOSIS

Although re-stenosis in older patients after coarctectomy is rare, a significant number of infants operated on before 1 yr of age require revision later in childhood. All patients should be monitored carefully for the development of recoarctation and an aortic anastomotic aneurysm. Should recoarctation occur, **balloon angioplasty** is the procedure of choice. In these patients, scar tissue from previous surgery may make reoperation more difficult yet makes balloon angioplasty safer because of the lower incidence of aneurysm formation. Relief of obstruction with this technique is usually excellent. **Intravascular stents** are commonly used, especially in adolescents and young adults, with generally excellent results.

Repair of coarctation in the 2nd decade of life or beyond may be associated with a higher incidence of premature cardiovascular disease, even in the absence of residual cardiac abnormalities. Early onset of adult chronic hypertension may occur, even in patients with adequately resected coarctation.

Abnormalities of the aortic valve are present in most patients. Bicuspid aortic valves are common but do not generally produce clinical signs unless the stenosis is significant. The association of a PDA and coarctation of the aorta is also common. VSDs and ASDs may be suspected by signs of a left-to-right shunt; they are exacerbated by the increased resistance to flow through the left side of the heart. Mitral valve abnormalities are also occasionally seen, as is subvalvular aortic stenosis.

Severe neurologic damage or even death may rarely occur from associated cerebrovascular disease. Subarachnoid or intracerebral hemorrhage may result from rupture of congenital aneurysms in the circle of Willis, rupture of other vessels with defective elastic and medial tissue, or rupture of normal vessels; these accidents are secondary to hypertension. Children with **PHACE syndrome** (posterior brain fossa anomalies, facial hemangiomas, arterial anomalies, cardiac anomalies and aortic coarctation, eye anomalies) may have strokes (Table 416-2). Abnormalities of the subclavian arteries may include involvement of the left subclavian artery in the area of coarctation, stenosis of the orifice of the left subclavian artery, and anomalous origin of the right subclavian artery.

Untreated, the great majority of older patients with coarctation of the aorta would succumb between the ages of 20 and 40 yr; some live well into middle life without serious disability. The common serious complications are related to systemic hypertension, which may result in premature coronary artery disease, heart failure, hypertensive encephalopathy, or intracranial hemorrhage. Heart failure may be worsened by associated anomalies. Infective endocarditis or endarteritis is a significant complication in adults. Aneurysms of the descending aorta or the enlarged collateral vessels may develop.

BIBLIOGRAPHY
Please visit the Nelson Textbook of Pediatrics *website at www.expertconsult.com for the complete bibliography.*

421.7 Coarctation with Ventricular Septal Defect

Daniel Bernstein

Coarctation in the presence of a VSD results in both increased preload and afterload on the left ventricle, and patients with this combination of defects will be recognized either at birth or in the 1st mo of life and often have intractable cardiac failure. The magnitude of the left-to-right shunt through a VSD is dependent on the ratio of pulmonary to systemic vascular resistance. In the presence of coarctation, resistance to systemic outflow is enhanced by the obstruction, and the volume of the shunt is markedly increased. The clinical picture is that of a seriously ill infant with tachypnea, failure to thrive, and typical findings of heart failure. Often, the difference in blood pressure between the upper and lower extremities is not very marked because cardiac output may be low. Medical management should be used to stabilize the patient initially; however, it should not be used to delay corrective surgery inordinately.

In most cases, coarctation is the major anomaly causing the severe symptoms, and resection of the coarcted segment results in striking improvement. Many centers routinely repair both the VSD and coarctation at the same operation through a midline sternotomy using cardiopulmonary bypass. Some centers repair the coarctation through a left lateral thoracotomy and, at the same time, place a pulmonary artery band to decrease the ventricular-level shunt. This may be performed when a complicated VSD is present (multiple VSDs, apical muscular VSD), to avoid open heart surgery during infancy for these complex ventricular septal abnormalities.

421.8 Coarctation with Other Cardiac Anomalies and Interrupted Aortic Arch

Daniel Bernstein

Coarctation often occurs in infancy in association with other major cardiovascular anomalies, including hypoplastic left heart, severe mitral or aortic valve disease, transposition of the great arteries, and variations of double-outlet or single ventricle. The clinical manifestations depend on the effects of the associated malformations, as well as on the coarctation itself.

Coarctation of the aorta associated with severe mitral and aortic valve disease may have to be treated within the context of the hypoplastic left heart syndrome (Chapter 425.10), even if the left ventricular chamber is not severely hypoplastic. Such patients usually have a long segment of narrow transverse aortic arch in addition to an isolated coarctation at the site of the ductus arteriosus. Coarctation of the aorta with transposition of the great arteries or single ventricle may be repaired alone or in combination with other corrective or palliative measures.

Complete interruption of the aortic arch is the most severe form of coarctation and is usually associated with other intracardiac pathology. Interruption may occur at any level, although it is most commonly seen between the left subclavian artery and the insertion of the ductus arteriosus (type A), followed in frequency by those between the left subclavian and left carotid arteries (type B), or between the left carotid and brachiocephalic arteries (type C). In newborns with an interrupted aortic arch, the ductus arteriosus provides the sole source of blood flow to the descending aorta, and differential oxygen saturations between the right arm (normal saturation) and the legs (decreased saturation) is noted. When the ductus begins to close, severe congestive heart failure, lower extremity hypoperfusion, anuria, and shock usually develops. Patients with an interrupted aortic arch can be supported with prostaglandin E_1 to keep the ductus patent before surgical repair. As one of the conotruncal malformations, an interrupted aortic arch, especially type B, can be associated with DiGeorge syndrome (cardiac defects, abnormal facies, thymic hypoplasia, cleft palate, hypocalcemia). Cytogenetic analysis using fluorescence in situ hybridization demonstrates deletion of a segment of chromosome 22q11 known as the DiGeorge critical region.

421.9 Congenital Mitral Stenosis

Daniel Bernstein

Congenital mitral stenosis is a rare anomaly that can be isolated or associated with other defects, the most common being subvalvar and valvar aortic stenosis and coarctation of the aorta (**Shone complex**). The mitral valve may be funnel-shaped, with thickened leaflets and chordae tendineae that are shortened and deformed. Other mitral valve anomalies associated with stenosis include parachute mitral valve, caused by a single papillary muscle, and double-orifice mitral valve.

For the full continuation of this chapter, please visit the Nelson Textbook of Pediatrics *website at www.expertconsult.com.*

421.10 Pulmonary Venous Hypertension

Daniel Bernstein

A variety of lesions may give rise to chronic pulmonary venous hypertension, which when extreme may result in pulmonary arterial hypertension and right-sided heart failure. These lesions include congenital mitral stenosis, mitral insufficiency, total anomalous pulmonary venous return with obstruction, left atrial myxomas, cor triatriatum (stenosis of a common pulmonary vein), individual pulmonary vein stenosis, and supravalvular mitral rings. Early symptoms can be confused with chronic pulmonary disease such as asthma because of a lack of specific cardiac findings on physical examination. Subtle signs of pulmonary hypertension may be present. The electrocardiogram shows right ventricular hypertrophy with spiked P waves. Roentgenographic studies reveal cardiac enlargement and prominence of the pulmonary veins in the hilar region, the right ventricle and atrium, and the main pulmonary artery; the left atrium is normal in size or only slightly enlarged.

The echocardiogram may demonstrate left atrial myxoma, cor triatriatum, stenosis of one or more pulmonary veins, or a mitral valve abnormality, especially supravalvar mitral ring. Cardiac catheterization excludes the presence of a shunt and demonstrates pulmonary hypertension with elevated pulmonary arterial wedge pressure. Left atrial pressure is normal if the lesion is at the level of the pulmonary veins, but it is elevated if the lesion is at the level of the mitral valve. Selective pulmonary arteriography usually delineates the anatomic lesion. Cor triatriatum, left atrial myxoma, and supravalvular mitral rings can all be successfully managed surgically.

The **differential diagnosis** includes pulmonary veno-occlusive disease, an idiopathic process that produces obstructive lesions in 1 or more pulmonary veins. The cause is uncertain and disease that begins in 1 vein can spread to others. Although it is usually encountered in patients after repair of obstructed total anomalous pulmonary venous return (Chapter 425.7), it can occur in the absence of congenital heart disease. The patient initially presents with left-sided heart failure on the basis of congested lungs with apparent pulmonary edema. Dyspnea, fatigue, and pleural effusions are common. Left atrial pressure is normal, but pulmonary arterial wedge pressure is usually elevated. A normal wedge pressure may be encountered if collaterals have formed or the wedge recording is performed in an uninvolved segment. Angiographically, the pulmonary veins return normally to the left atrium, but one or more pulmonary veins are narrowed, either focally or diffusely.

Studies using lung biopsy have demonstrated pulmonary venous and, occasionally, arterial involvement. Pulmonary veins and venules demonstrate fibrous narrowing or occlusion, and pulmonary artery thrombi may be present. Attempts at surgical repair, balloon dilatation, and transcatheter stenting have not significantly improved the generally poor prognosis of these patients. Clinical trials of antiproliferative chemotherapy are currently in progress. Combined heart-lung transplantation (Chapter 437.2) is often the only alternative therapeutic option.

Chapter 422 Acyanotic Congenital Heart Disease: Regurgitant Lesions

422.1 Pulmonary Valvular Insufficiency and Congenital Absence of the Pulmonary Valve

Daniel Bernstein

Pulmonary valvular insufficiency most often accompanies other cardiovascular diseases or may be secondary to severe pulmonary hypertension. Incompetence of the valve is an expected result after surgery for right ventricular outflow tract obstruction, for example, pulmonary valvotomy in patients with valvular pulmonic stenosis or valvotomy with infundibular resection in patients with tetralogy of Fallot. Isolated congenital insufficiency of the pulmonary valve is rare. These patients are usually asymptomatic because the insufficiency is generally mild.

The prominent physical sign is a decrescendo diastolic murmur at the upper and midleft sternal border, which has a lower pitch than the murmur of aortic insufficiency because of the lower pressure involved. Roentgenograms of the chest show prominence of the main pulmonary artery and, if the insufficiency is severe, right ventricular enlargement. The electrocardiogram is normal or shows minimal right ventricular hypertrophy. Pulsed and color Doppler studies demonstrate retrograde flow from the pulmonary artery to the right ventricle during diastole. Cardiac magnetic resonance angiography (MRA) is useful for quantifying both right ventricular volume and the regurgitant fraction. Isolated pulmonary valvular insufficiency is generally well tolerated and does not require surgical treatment. When pulmonary insufficiency is severe, especially if significant tricuspid insufficiency has begun to develop, replacement with a homograft valve may become necessary to preserve right ventricular function.

Congenital absence of the pulmonary valve is usually associated with a ventricular septal defect, often in the context of tetralogy of Fallot (Chapter 424.1). In many of these neonates, the pulmonary arteries become widely dilated and compress the bronchi, with subsequent recurrent episodes of wheezing, pulmonary collapse, and pneumonitis. The presence and degree of cyanosis are variable. Florid pulmonary valvular incompetence may not be well tolerated, and death may occur from a combination of bronchial compression, hypoxemia, and heart failure. Correction involves plication of the massively dilated pulmonary arteries, closure of the ventricular septal defect, and placement of a homograft across the right ventricular outflow tract.

BIBLIOGRAPHY

Please visit the Nelson Textbook of Pediatrics *website at www.expertconsult.com for the complete bibliography.*

422.2 Congenital Mitral Insufficiency

Daniel Bernstein

Congenital mitral insufficiency is rare as an isolated lesion and is more often associated with other anomalies. It is most commonly encountered in combination with an atrioventricular septal defect, either an ostium primum defect, or a complete AV septal defect (Chapter 420.5). Mitral insufficiency is also seen in patients with dilated cardiomyopathy (Chapter 433.1) as their left ventricular function deteriorates, secondary to dilatation of the valve ring. Mitral insufficiency may also be encountered in conjunction with coarctation of the aorta, ventricular septal defect, corrected transposition of the great vessels, anomalous origin of the left coronary artery from the pulmonary artery, or Marfan syndrome. In the absence of other congenital heart disease, endocarditis or rheumatic fever should be suspected in a patient with isolated severe mitral insufficiency (Table 422-1).

In isolated mitral insufficiency, the mitral valve annulus is usually dilated, the chordae tendineae are short and may insert anomalously, and the valve leaflets are deformed. When mitral insufficiency is severe enough to cause clinical symptoms, the left atrium enlarges as a result of the regurgitant flow, and the left ventricle becomes hypertrophied and dilated. Pulmonary venous pressure is increased, and the increased pressure ultimately results in pulmonary hypertension and right ventricular hypertrophy and dilatation. Mild lesions produce no symptoms; the only abnormal sign is the apical holosystolic murmur of mitral regurgitation. Severe regurgitation results in symptoms that can appear at any age, including poor physical development, frequent respiratory infections, fatigue on exertion, and episodes of pulmonary edema or congestive heart failure. Often, a diagnosis of reactive airway disease will have been made because of the similarity in pulmonary symptoms, including wheezing, which may be a dominant finding in infants and young children.

The typical murmur of mitral insufficiency is a high-pitched, apical holosystolic murmur. If the insufficiency is moderate to severe, it is usually associated with a low-pitched, apical

Table 422-1 CAUSES AND MECHANISMS OF MITRAL REGURGITATION

	ORGANIC			FUNCTIONAL
	Type I*	Type II†	Type IIIa‡	Type I*/Type IIIb‡
Non-ischemic	Endocarditis (perforation); degenerative (annular calcification); congenital (cleft leaflet)	Degenerative (billowing/flail leaflets); endocarditis (ruptured chordae); traumatic (ruptured chord/PM); rheumatic (acute RF)	Rheumatic (chronic RF); iatrogenic (radiation/drug); inflammatory (lupus/anticardiolipin), eosinophilic endocardial disease, endomyocardial fibrosis)	Cardiomyopathy; myocarditis; left-ventricular dysfunction (any cause)

*Mechanism involves normal leaflet movement.
†Mechanism involves excessive valve movement.
‡Restricted valve movement, IIIa in diastole, IIIb in systole.
MR, mitral regurgitation; PM, papillary muscle; RF, rheumatic fever;
Modified from Sarano ME, Akins CW, Vahanian A: Mitral regurgitation, *Lancet* 373:1382–1394, 2009, p 1383, Table 1.

mid-diastolic rumbling murmur indicative of increased diastolic flow across the mitral valve. The pulmonary component of the 2nd heart sound will be accentuated in the presence of pulmonary hypertension. The electrocardiogram usually shows bifid P waves consistent with left atrial enlargement, signs of left ventricular hypertrophy, and sometimes signs of right ventricular hypertrophy. Roentgenographic examination shows enlargement of the left atrium, which at times is massive. The left ventricle is prominent, and pulmonary vascularity is normal or prominent. The echocardiogram demonstrates the enlarged left atrium and ventricle. Color Doppler demonstrates the extent of the insufficiency, and pulsed Doppler of the pulmonary veins detects retrograde flow when mitral insufficiency is severe. Cardiac catheterization shows elevated left atrial pressure. Pulmonary artery hypertension of varying severity may be present. Selective left ventriculography reveals the severity of mitral regurgitation.

Mitral valvuloplasty can result in striking improvement in symptoms and heart size, but in some patients, installation of a prosthetic mechanical mitral valve may be necessary. Before surgery, associated anomalies must be identified.

422.3 Mitral Valve Prolapse

Daniel Bernstein

Mitral valve prolapse results from an abnormal mitral valve mechanism that causes billowing of one or both mitral leaflets, especially the posterior cusp, into the left atrium toward the end of systole. The abnormality is predominantly congenital but may not be recognized until adolescence or adulthood. Mitral valve prolapse is usually sporadic, is more common in girls, and may be inherited as an autosomal dominant trait with variable expression. It is common in patients with Marfan syndrome, straight back syndrome, pectus excavatum, scoliosis, Ehlers-Danlos syndrome, osteogenesis imperfecta, and pseudoxanthoma elasticum. The dominant abnormal signs are auscultatory, although occasional patients may have chest pain or palpitations. The apical murmur is late systolic and may be preceded by a click, but these signs may vary in the same patient and, at times, only the click is audible. In the standing or sitting position, the click may occur earlier in systole, and the murmur may be more prominent in late systole. Arrhythmias may occur and are primarily unifocal or multifocal premature ventricular contractions.

The electrocardiogram is usually normal but may show biphasic T waves, especially in leads II, III, aVF, and V_6; the T-wave abnormalities may vary at different times in the same patient. The chest roentgenogram is normal. The echocardiogram shows a characteristic posterior movement of the posterior mitral leaflet during mid- or late systole or demonstrates pansystolic prolapse of both the anterior and posterior mitral leaflets. These echocardiographic findings must be interpreted cautiously because the appearance of minimal mitral prolapse may be a normal variant. Prolapse is more precisely defined by single or bileaflet prolapse of >2 mm beyond the long axis annular plane with or without leaflet thickening. Prolapse with valve thickening >5 mm is "classic," a lesser degree is "non-classic." Two-dimensional real-time echocardiography shows that both the free edge and the body of the mitral leaflets move posteriorly in systole toward the left atrium. Doppler can assess the presence and severity of mitral regurgitation.

This lesion is not progressive in childhood, and specific therapy is not indicated. Antibiotic prophylaxis is no longer recommended during surgery and dental procedures (Chapter 431).

Adults (men more often than women) with mitral valve prolapse are at increased risk for cardiovascular complications (sudden death, arrhythmia, cerebrovascular accidents, progressive valve dilatation, heart failure, and endocarditis) in the presence of **thickened** (>5 mm) and **redundant** mitral valve leaflets. Risk factors for morbidity also include poor left ventricular function, moderate to severe mitral regurgitation, and left atrial enlargement.

Often, confusion exists concerning the diagnosis of mitral valve prolapse. The high frequency of mild prolapse on the echocardiogram in the absence of clinical findings suggests that, in these cases, true mitral valve prolapse syndrome is not present. These patients and their parents should be reassured of this fact, and no special recommendations should be made regarding management or frequent laboratory studies.

BIBLIOGRAPHY

Please visit the Nelson Textbook of Pediatrics *website at www.expertconsult.com for the complete bibliography.*

422.4 Tricuspid Regurgitation

Daniel Bernstein

Isolated tricuspid regurgitation is generally associated with Ebstein anomaly of the tricuspid valve. Ebstein anomaly may occur either without cyanosis or with varying degrees of cyanosis, depending on the severity of the tricuspid regurgitation and the presence of an atrial-level communication (patent foramen ovale or atrial septal defect). Older children tend to have the acyanotic form, whereas if detected in the newborn period, Ebstein anomaly is usually associated with severe cyanosis (Chapter 424.7).

Tricuspid regurgitation often accompanies right ventricular dysfunction. When the right ventricle becomes dilated because of volume overload or intrinsic myocardial disease, or both, the tricuspid annulus also enlarges, with resultant valve insufficiency. This form of regurgitation may improve if the cause of the right ventricular dilatation is corrected, or it may require surgical plication of the valve annulus. Tricuspid regurgitation is also encountered in newborns with perinatal asphyxia. The cause may be related to an increased susceptibility of the papillary muscles to ischemic damage and subsequent transient papillary muscle dysfunction. Finally, tricuspid regurgitation is seen in up to 30% of children after heart transplantation, which can be a risk factor for graft dysfunction but is also seen as a consequence of valve injury due to endomyocardial biopsy.

BIBLIOGRAPHY

Please visit the Nelson Textbook of Pediatrics *website at www.expertconsult.com for the complete bibliography.*

Chapter 423
Cyanotic Congenital Heart Disease: Evaluation of the Critically Ill Neonate with Cyanosis and Respiratory Distress

Daniel Bernstein

See also Chapter 95.

A severely ill neonate with cardiorespiratory distress and cyanosis is a diagnostic challenge. The clinician must perform a rapid evaluation to determine whether congenital heart disease is a cause so that potentially lifesaving measures can be instituted. The differential diagnosis of neonatal cyanosis is presented in Table 95-1.

CARDIAC DISEASE

Congenital heart disease produces cyanosis when obstruction to right ventricular outflow causes intracardiac right-to-left shunting or when complex anatomic defects, many unassociated with pulmonary stenosis, cause an admixture of pulmonary and systemic venous return in the heart. Cyanosis from pulmonary edema may also develop in patients with heart failure caused by left-to-right shunts, although the degree is usually less severe. Cyanosis may be caused by persistence of fetal pathways, for example, right-to-left shunting across the foramen ovale and ductus arteriosus in the presence of pulmonary outflow tract obstruction or persistent pulmonary hypertension of the newborn (PPHN) (Chapter 95.8).

DIFFERENTIAL DIAGNOSIS

The **hyperoxia test** is one method of distinguishing cyanotic congenital heart disease from pulmonary disease. Neonates with cyanotic congenital heart disease are usually not able to significantly raise their arterial Pa_{O_2} during administration of 100% oxygen. If the Pa_{O_2} rises above 150 mm Hg during 100% oxygen administration, an intracardiac right-to-left shunt can usually be excluded, although this is not 100% confirmative, as some patients with cyanotic congenital heart lesions may be able to increase their Pa_{O_2} to >150 mm Hg because of favorable intracardiac streaming patterns. In patients with pulmonary disease, Pa_{O_2} generally increases significantly with 100% oxygen as ventilation-perfusion inequalities are overcome. In infants with cyanosis due to a CNS disorder, the Pa_{O_2} usually normalizes completely during artificial ventilation. Hypoxia in many heart lesions is profound and constant, whereas in respiratory disorders and in persistent pulmonary hypertension of the neonate (PPHN), arterial oxygen tension often varies with time or changes in ventilator management. Hyperventilation may improve the hypoxia in neonates with PPHN and only occasionally in those with cyanotic congenital heart disease.

Although a significant heart murmur usually suggests a cardiac basis for the cyanosis, several of the more severe cardiac defects (transposition of the great vessels) may not initially be associated with a murmur. The chest roentgenogram may be helpful in the differentiation of pulmonary and cardiac disease; in the latter, it indicates whether pulmonary blood flow is increased, normal, or decreased.

Two-dimensional echocardiography is the definitive noninvasive test to determine the presence of congenital heart disease. Cardiac catheterization is less often used for diagnostic purposes, and is usually performed to examine structures that are sometime less well visualized by echocardiography, such as distal branch pulmonary arteries or aortopulmonary collateral arteries in patients with tetralogy of Fallot with pulmonary atresia (Chapter 424.2), coronary arteries and right ventricular sinusoids in patients with pulmonary atresia and intact ventricular septum (Chapter 424.3). If echocardiography is not immediately available, the clinician caring for a newborn with possible cyanotic heart disease should not hesitate to start a prostaglandin infusion (for a possible ductal-dependent lesion). Because of the risk of hypoventilation associated with prostaglandins, a practitioner skilled in neonatal endotracheal intubation must be available.

Chapter 424
Cyanotic Congenital Heart Lesions: Lesions Associated with Decreased Pulmonary Blood Flow

424.1 Tetralogy of Fallot

Daniel Bernstein

Tetralogy of Fallot is one of the conotruncal family of heart lesions in which the primary defect is an anterior deviation of the infundibular septum (the muscular septum that separates the aortic and pulmonary outflows). The consequences of this deviation are the 4 components: (1) obstruction to right ventricular outflow (pulmonary stenosis), (2) a malalignment type of ventricular septal defect (VSD), (3) dextroposition of the aorta so that it overrides the ventricular septum, and (4) right ventricular hypertrophy (Fig. 424-1). Obstruction to pulmonary arterial blood flow is usually at both the right ventricular infundibulum (subpulmonic area) and the pulmonary valve. The main pulmonary artery may be small, and various degrees of branch pulmonary artery stenosis may be present. Complete obstruction of right ventricular outflow (pulmonary atresia with VSD) is classified as an extreme form of tetralogy of Fallot (Chapter 424.2). The degree of pulmonary outflow obstruction determines the degree of the patient's cyanosis and the age of first presentation.

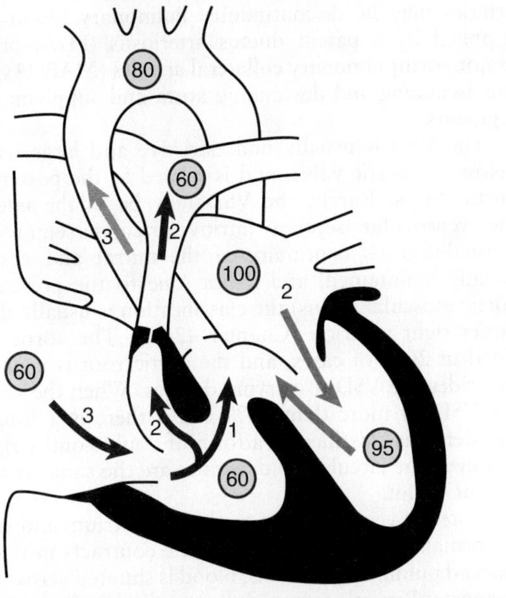

Figure 424-1 Physiology of the tetralogy of Fallot. Circled numbers represent oxygen saturation values. The numbers next to the *arrows* represent volumes of blood flow (in L/min/m²). Atrial (mixed venous) oxygen saturation is decreased because of the systemic hypoxemia. A volume of 3 L/min/m² of desaturated blood enters the right atrium and traverses the tricuspid valve. Two liters flows through the right ventricular outflow tract into the lungs, whereas 1 L shunts right to left through the ventricular septal defect (VSD) into the ascending aorta. Thus, pulmonary blood flow is two thirds normal (Qp:Qs [pulmonary-to-systemic blood flow ratio] of 0.7 : 1). Blood returning to the left atrium is fully saturated. Only 2 L of blood flows across the mitral valve. Oxygen saturation in the left ventricle may be slightly decreased because of right-to-left shunting across the VSD. Two liters of saturated left ventricular blood mixing with 1 L of desaturated right ventricular blood is ejected into the ascending aorta. Aortic saturation is decreased, and cardiac output is normal.

PATHOPHYSIOLOGY

The pulmonary valve annulus may range from being nearly normal in size to being severely hypoplastic. The valve itself is often bicuspid or unicuspid and, occasionally, is the only site of stenosis. More commonly, the subpulmonic or infundibular muscle, known as the *crista supraventricularis,* is hypertrophic, which contributes to the subvalvar stenosis and results in an infundibular chamber of variable size and contour. When the right ventricular outflow tract is completely obstructed (**pulmonary atresia**), the anatomy of the branch pulmonary arteries is extremely variable. A main pulmonary artery segment may be in continuity with right ventricular outflow, separated by a fibrous but imperforate pulmonary valve; the main pulmonary artery may be moderately or severely hypoplastic but still supply part or all of the pulmonary bed; or the entire main pulmonary artery segment may be absent. Occasionally, the branch pulmonary arteries may be discontinuous. Pulmonary blood flow may be supplied by a patent ductus arteriosus (PDA) or by multiple **major aortopulmonary collateral arteries (MAPCAs)** arising from the ascending and descending aorta and supplying various lung segments.

The VSD is usually nonrestrictive and large, is located just below the aortic valve, and is related to the posterior and right aortic cusps. Rarely, the VSD may be in the inlet portion of the ventricular septum (atrioventricular septal defect). The normal fibrous continuity of the mitral and aortic valves is usually maintained, and if not (due to the presence of a subaortic muscular conus) the classification is usually that of double outlet right ventricle (Chapter 424.5). The aortic arch is right sided in 20% of cases, and the aortic root is usually large and overrides the VSD to varying degrees. When the aorta overrides the VSD by more than 50% and if there is a subaortic conus, this defect is classified as a form of double-outlet right ventricle; however, the circulatory dynamics are the same as that of tetralogy of Fallot.

Systemic venous return to the right atrium and right ventricle is normal. When the right ventricle contracts in the presence of marked pulmonary stenosis, blood is shunted across the VSD into the aorta. Persistent arterial desaturation and cyanosis result, the degree dependent on the severity of the pulmonary obstruction. Pulmonary blood flow, when severely restricted by the obstruction to right ventricular outflow, may be supplemented by a PDA. Peak systolic and diastolic pressures in each ventricle are similar and at systemic level. A large pressure gradient occurs across the obstructed right ventricular outflow tract, and pulmonary arterial pressure is either normal or lower than normal. The degree of right ventricular outflow obstruction determines the timing of the onset of symptoms, the severity of cyanosis, and the degree of right ventricular hypertrophy. When obstruction to right ventricular outflow is mild to moderate and a balanced shunt is present across the VSD, the patient may not be visibly cyanotic (**acyanotic** or **"pink"** tetralogy of Fallot). When obstruction is severe, cyanosis will be present from birth and worsen when the ductus begins to close.

CLINICAL MANIFESTATIONS

Infants with mild degrees of right ventricular outflow obstruction may initially be seen with heart failure caused by a ventricular-level left-to-right shunt. Often, cyanosis is not present at birth; but with increasing hypertrophy of the right ventricular infundibulum as the patient grows, cyanosis occurs later in the 1st yr of life. In infants with severe degrees of right ventricular outflow obstruction, neonatal cyanosis is noted immediately. In these infants, pulmonary blood flow may be partially or nearly totally dependent on flow through the ductus arteriosus. When the ductus begins to close in the 1st few hours or days of life, severe cyanosis and circulatory collapse may occur. Older children with long-standing cyanosis who have not undergone surgery may have dusky blue skin, gray sclerae with engorged blood vessels, and marked clubbing of the fingers and toes. Extracardiac manifestations of long-standing cyanotic congenital heart disease are described in Chapter 428.

In older children with unrepaired tetralogy, dyspnea occurs on exertion. They may play actively for a short time and then sit or lie down. Older children may be able to walk a block or so before stopping to rest. Characteristically, children assume a squatting position for the relief of dyspnea caused by physical effort; the child is usually able to resume physical activity after a few minutes of squatting. These findings occur most often in patients with significant cyanosis at rest.

Paroxysmal hypercyanotic attacks (hypoxic, **"blue,"** or **"tet" spells**) are a particular problem during the 1st 2 yr of life. The infant becomes hyperpneic and restless, cyanosis increases, gasping respirations ensue, and syncope may follow. The spells occur most frequently in the morning on initially awakening or after episodes of vigorous crying. Temporary disappearance or a decrease in intensity of the systolic murmur is usual as flow across the right ventricular outflow tract diminishes. The spells may last from a few minutes to a few hours. Short episodes are followed by generalized weakness and sleep. Severe spells may progress to unconsciousness and, occasionally, to convulsions or hemiparesis. The onset is usually spontaneous and unpredictable. Spells are associated with reduction of an already compromised pulmonary blood flow, which, when prolonged, results in severe systemic hypoxia and metabolic acidosis. Infants who are only mildly cyanotic at rest are often more prone to the development of hypoxic spells because they have not acquired the homeostatic mechanisms to tolerate rapid lowering of arterial oxygen saturation, such as polycythemia.

Depending on the frequency and severity of hypercyanotic attacks, one or more of the following procedures should be instituted in sequence: (1) placement of the infant on the abdomen in the knee-chest position while making certain that the infant's clothing is not constrictive, (2) administration of oxygen (although increasing inspired oxygen will not reverse cyanosis caused by intracardiac shunting), and (3) injection of morphine subcutaneously in a dose not in excess of 0.2 mg/kg. Calming and holding the infant in a knee-chest position may abort progression of an early spell. Premature attempts to obtain blood samples may cause further agitation and be counterproductive.

Because metabolic acidosis develops when arterial Po_2 is <40 mm Hg, rapid correction (within several minutes) with intravenous administration of sodium bicarbonate is necessary if the spell is unusually severe and the child shows a lack of response to the foregoing therapy. Recovery from the spell is usually rapid once the pH has returned to normal. Repeated blood pH measurements may be necessary because rapid recurrence of acidosis may ensue. For spells that are resistant to this therapy, intubation and sedation are often sufficient to break the spell. Drugs that increase systemic vascular resistance, such as intravenous phenylephrine, can improve right ventricular outflow, decrease the right-to-left shunt, and improve the symptoms. β-Adrenergic blockade by the intravenous administration of propranolol (0.1 mg/kg given slowly to a maximum of 0.2 mg/kg) has also been used. Growth and development may be delayed in patients with severe untreated tetralogy of Fallot, particularly when their oxygen saturation is chronically <70%. Puberty may also be delayed in patients who have not undergone surgery.

The pulse is usually normal, as are venous and arterial pressures. In older infants and children, the left anterior hemithorax may bulge anteriorly because of long-standing right ventricular hypertrophy. A substernal right ventricular impulse can usually be detected. A systolic thrill may be felt along the left sternal border in the 3rd and 4th parasternal spaces. The systolic murmur is usually loud and harsh; it may be transmitted widely, especially to the lungs, but is most intense at the left sternal border. The murmur is generally ejection in quality at the upper sternal border, but it may sound more holosystolic toward the lower sternal border. It may be preceded by a click. The murmur is caused by turbulence through the right ventricular outflow tract. It tends to become louder, longer, and harsher as the severity of pulmonary stenosis increases from mild to moderate; however, it can actually become less prominent with severe obstruction, especially during a hypercyanotic spell due to shunting of blood away from the right ventricular outflow through the aortic valve. Either the 2nd heart sound is single, or the pulmonic component is soft. Infrequently, a continuous murmur may be audible, especially if prominent collaterals are present.

DIAGNOSIS

Roentgenographically, the typical configuration as seen in the anteroposterior view consists of a narrow base, concavity of the

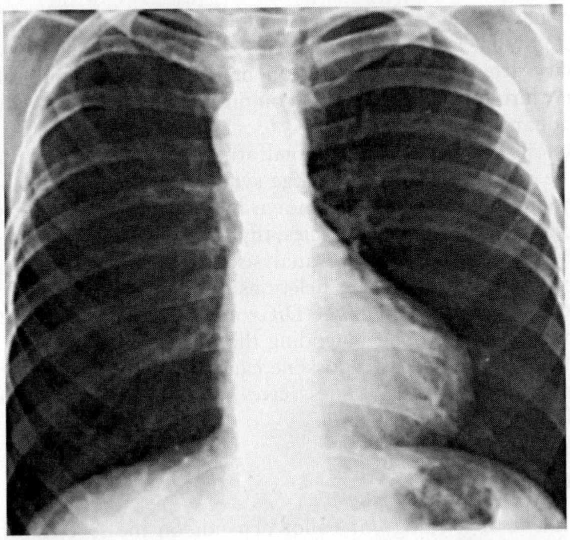

Figure 424-2 Chest x-ray of an 8 yr old boy with the tetralogy of Fallot. Note the normal heart size, some elevation of the cardiac apex, concavity in the region of the main pulmonary artery, right-sided aortic arch, and diminished pulmonary vascularity.

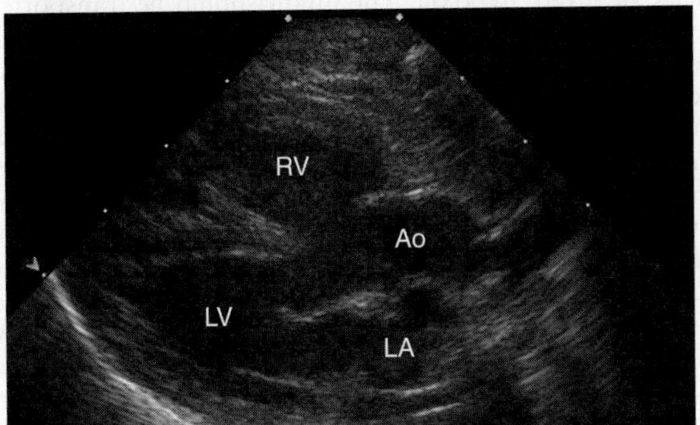

Figure 424-3 Echocardiogram in a patient with the tetralogy of Fallot. This parasternal long-axis two-dimensional view demonstrates anterior displacement of the outflow ventricular septum that resulted in stenosis of the subpulmonic right ventricular outflow tract, overriding of the aorta, and an associated ventricular septal defect. Ao, overriding aorta; LA, left atrium; LV, left ventricle; RV, right ventricle.

left heart border in the area usually occupied by the pulmonary artery, and normal overall heart size. The hypertrophied right ventricle causes the rounded apical shadow to be uptilted so that it is situated higher above the diaphragm than normal and pointing horizontally to the left chest wall. The cardiac silhouette has been likened to that of a boot or wooden shoe ("coeur en sabot") (Fig. 424-2). The hilar areas and lung fields are relatively clear because of diminished pulmonary blood flow or the small size of the pulmonary arteries, or both. The aorta is usually large, and in about 20% of patients it arches to the right, which results in an indentation of the leftward-positioned air-filled tracheobronchial shadow in the anteroposterior view.

The electrocardiogram demonstrates right axis deviation and evidence of right ventricular hypertrophy. A dominant R wave appears in the right precordial chest leads (Rs, R, qR, qRs) or an RSR′ pattern. In some cases, the only sign of right ventricular hypertrophy may initially be a positive T wave in leads V_3R and V_1. The P wave is tall and peaked suggesting right atrial enlargement (see Fig. 417-6).

Two-dimensional echocardiography establishes the diagnosis (Fig. 424-3) and provides information about the extent of aortic override of the septum, the location and degree of the right ventricular outflow tract obstruction, the size of the pulmonary valve

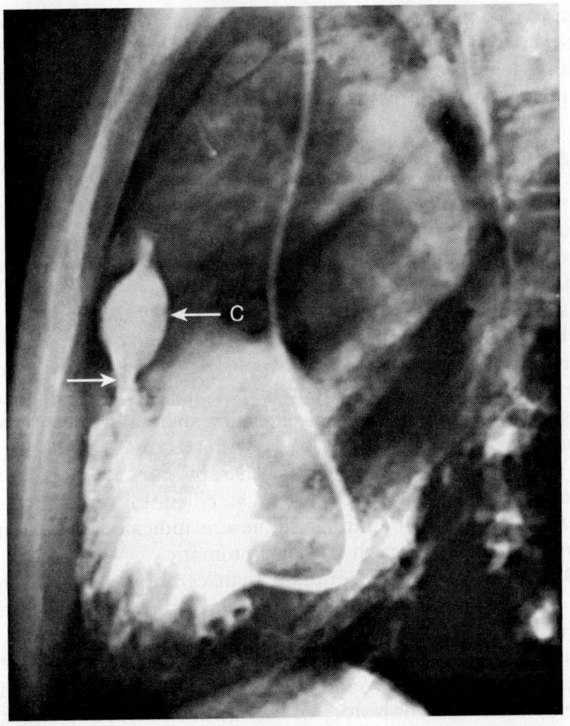

Figure 424-4 Lateral view of a selective right ventriculogram in a patient with the tetralogy of Fallot. The *arrow* points to an infundibular stenosis that is below the infundibular chamber *(C)*. The narrowed pulmonary valve orifice is seen at the distal end of the infundibular chamber.

annulus and main and proximal branch pulmonary arteries, and the side of the aortic arch. The echocardiogram is also useful in determining whether a PDA is supplying a portion of the pulmonary blood flow. In a patient without pulmonary atresia, echocardiography usually obviates the need for catheterization before surgical repair.

Cardiac catheterization demonstrates a systolic pressure in the right ventricle equal to the systemic pressure, since the right ventricle is connected directly to the overriding aorta. If the pulmonary artery is entered, the pressure is markedly decreased, although crossing the right ventricular outflow tract, especially in severe cases, may precipitate a tet spell. Pulmonary arterial pressure is usually lower than normal, in the range of 5-10 mm Hg. The level of arterial oxygen saturation depends on the magnitude of the right-to-left shunt; in "pink tets," the systemic oxygen saturation may be normal, whereas in a moderately cyanotic patient at rest, it is usually 75-85%.

Selective right ventriculography will demonstrate all of the anatomical features. Contrast medium outlines the heavily trabeculated right ventricle. The infundibular stenosis varies in length, width, contour, and distensibility (Fig. 424-4). The pulmonary valve is usually thickened, and the annulus may be small. In patients with pulmonary atresia and VSD, echocardiography alone is not adequate to assess the anatomy of the pulmonary arteries and MAPCAs. Cardiac CT is extremely helpful, and cardiac catheterization with injection into each arterial collateral is indicated. Complete and accurate information regarding the size and peripheral distribution of the main pulmonary arteries and any collateral vessels (MAPCAs) is important when evaluating these children as surgical candidates.

Aortography or coronary arteriography outlines the course of the coronary arteries. In 5-10% of patients with the tetralogy of Fallot, coronary artery abnormalities may be present, most commonly an aberrant coronary artery crossing over the right ventricular outflow tract; this artery must not be cut during surgical repair. Verification of normal coronary arteries is important when considering surgery in young infants who may need a patch across the pulmonary valve annulus. Echocardiography can usually delineate the coronary artery anatomy; angiography is reserved for cases in which questions remain.

COMPLICATIONS

Before the age of corrective surgery, patients with tetralogy of Fallot were susceptible to several serious complications. For this reason, most children undergo complete repair (or in some cases palliation) in infancy, and therefore these days these complications are rare. **Cerebral thromboses,** usually occurring in the cerebral veins or dural sinuses and occasionally in the cerebral arteries, are a sequelae of extreme polycythemia and dehydration. Thromboses occur most often in patients younger than 2 yr. These patients may have iron-deficiency anemia, frequently with hemoglobin and hematocrit levels in the normal range (but too low for cyanotic heart disease). Therapy consists of adequate hydration and supportive measures. Phlebotomy and volume replacement with albumin or saline are indicated in extremely **polycythemic** patients who are symptomatic.

Brain abscess is less common than cerebral vascular events and extremely rare today. Patients with a brain abscess are usually older than 2 yr. The onset of the illness is often insidious and consists of low-grade fever or a gradual change in behavior, or both. Some patients have an acute onset of symptoms that may develop after a recent history of headache, nausea, and vomiting. Seizures may occur; localized neurologic signs depend on the site and size of the abscess and the presence of increased intracranial pressure. CT or MRI confirms the diagnosis. Antibiotic therapy may help keep the infection localized, but surgical drainage of the abscess is usually necessary (Chapter 596).

Bacterial endocarditis may occur in the right ventricular infundibulum or on the pulmonic, aortic, or, rarely, tricuspid valves. Endocarditis may complicate palliative shunts or, in patients with corrective surgery, any residual pulmonic stenosis or VSD. Heart failure is not a usual feature in patients with tetralogy of Fallot, with the exception of some young infants with "pink" or acyanotic tetralogy of Fallot. As the degree of pulmonary obstruction worsens with age, the symptoms of heart failure resolve and eventually the patient experiences cyanosis, often by 6-12 mo of age. These patients are at increased risk for hypercyanotic spells at this time.

ASSOCIATED ANOMALIES

A PDA may be present, and defects in the atrial septum are occasionally seen. A right aortic arch occurs in ≈20% of patients, and other anomalies of the pulmonary arteries and aortic arch may also be seen. Persistence of a left superior vena cava draining into the coronary sinus is common but not a concern. Multiple VSDs are occasionally present and must be diagnosed before corrective surgery. Coronary artery anomalies are present in 5-10% and can complicate surgical repair. Tetralogy of Fallot may also occur with an atrioventricular septal defect, often associated with Down syndrome.

Congenital absence of the pulmonary valve produces a distinct syndrome that is usually marked by signs of upper airway obstruction (Chapter 422.1). Cyanosis may be absent, mild, or moderate; the heart is large and hyperdynamic; and a loud to-and-fro murmur is present. Marked aneurysmal dilatation of the main and branch pulmonary arteries results in compression of the bronchi and produces stridulous or wheezing respirations and recurrent pneumonia. If the airway obstruction is severe, reconstruction of the trachea at the time of corrective cardiac surgery may be required to alleviate the symptoms.

Absence of a branch pulmonary artery, most often the left, should be suspected if the roentgenographic appearance of the pulmonary vasculature differs on the two sides; absence of a pulmonary artery is often associated with hypoplasia of the affected lung. It is important to recognize the absence of a pulmonary artery because occlusion of the remaining pulmonary artery during surgery seriously compromises the already reduced pulmonary blood flow.

As one of the conotruncal malformations, tetralogy of Fallot can be associated with **DiGeorge syndrome** or **Shprintzen velocardiofacial syndrome**, also known by the acronym CATCH 22 (cardiac defects, abnormal facies, thymic hypoplasia, cleft palate, hypocalcemia). Cytogenetic analysis using fluorescence in situ hybridization demonstrates deletions of a large segment of chromosome 22q11 known as the *DiGeorge critical region.* Deletion or mutation of the gene encoding the transcription factor *Tbx1* has been implicated as a possible cause of DiGeorge syndrome, although several other genes have been identified as possible candidates or modifier genes.

TREATMENT

Treatment of tetralogy of Fallot depends on the severity of the right ventricular outflow tract obstruction. Infants with severe tetralogy require urgent medical treatment and surgical intervention in the neonatal period. Therapy is aimed at providing an immediate increase in pulmonary blood flow to prevent the sequelae of severe hypoxia. The infant should be transported to a medical center adequately equipped to evaluate and treat neonates with congenital heart disease under optimal conditions. Prolonged, severe hypoxia may lead to shock, respiratory failure, and intractable acidosis and will significantly reduce the chance of survival, even when surgically amenable lesions are present. It is critical that normal body temperature be maintained during the transfer since cold increases oxygen consumption, which places additional stress on a cyanotic infant, whose oxygen delivery is already limited. Blood glucose levels should be monitored because hypoglycemia is more likely to develop in infants with cyanotic heart disease.

Neonates with marked right ventricular outflow tract obstruction may deteriorate rapidly because, as the ductus arteriosus begins to close, pulmonary blood flow is further compromised. The intravenous administration of prostaglandin E_1 (0.01-0.20 μg/kg/min), a potent and specific relaxant of ductal smooth muscle, causes dilatation of the ductus arteriosus and usually provides adequate pulmonary blood flow until a surgical procedure can be performed. This agent should be administered intravenously as soon as cyanotic congenital heart disease is clinically suspected and continued through the preoperative period and during cardiac catheterization. Because prostaglandin can cause apnea, an individual skilled in neonatal intubation should be readily available.

Infants with less severe right ventricular outflow tract obstruction who are stable and awaiting surgical intervention require careful observation. Acyanotic patients can fairly quickly progress to having cyanotic episodes. Prevention or prompt treatment of dehydration is important to avoid hemoconcentration and possible thrombotic episodes. Oral propranolol (0.5-1 mg/kg every 6 hr) had been used in the past to decrease the frequency and severity of hypercyanotic spells, but with the excellent surgical results available today, surgical treatment is now indicated as soon as spells begin.

Infants with symptoms and severe cyanosis in the 1st mo of life usually have marked obstruction of the right ventricular outflow tract. Two options are available in these infants. The first is corrective open heart surgery performed in early infancy and even in the newborn period in critically ill infants. This approach has widespread acceptance today with excellent short- and long-term results and has supplanted palliative shunts (see later) for most cases. Early total repair carries the theoretical advantage that early physiologic correction allows for improved growth of the branch pulmonary arteries. In infants with less severe

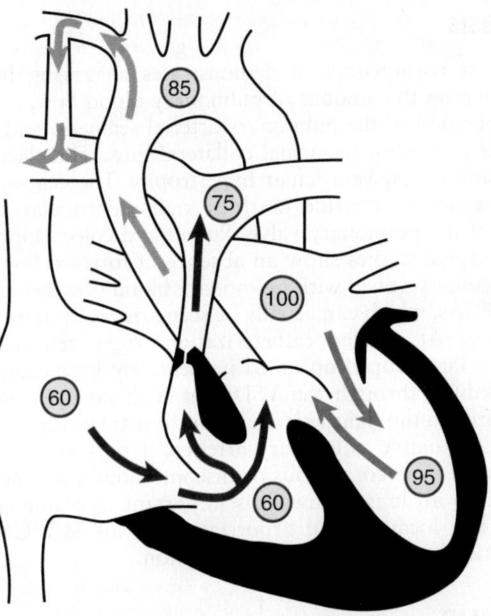

Figure 424-5 Physiology of a Blalock-Taussig shunt in a patient with the tetralogy of Fallot. *Circled numbers* represent oxygen saturation values. The intracardiac shunting pattern is as described for Figure 424-1. Blood shunting left to right across the shunt from the right subclavian artery to the right pulmonary artery increases total pulmonary blood flow and results in a higher oxygen saturation than would exist without the shunt (see Fig. 424-1).

cyanosis who can be maintained with good growth and absence of hypercyanotic spells, primary repair is performed electively at between 4 and 6 mo of age.

Corrective surgical therapy consists of relief of the right ventricular outflow tract obstruction by resecting obstructive muscle bundles and by patch closure of the VSD. If the pulmonary valve is stenotic, as it usually is, a valvotomy is performed. If the pulmonary valve annulus is too small or the valve is extremely thickened, a valvectomy may be performed, the pulmonary valve annulus split open, and a transannular patch placed across the pulmonary valve ring. The surgical risk of total correction in major centers is <5%. A right ventriculotomy was once the standard approach; a transatrial-transpulmonary approach is routinely performed to reduce the long-term risks of a large right ventriculotomy. In patients in whom repair has been delayed to childhood, increased bleeding in the immediate postoperative period may be a complicating factor due to their extreme polycythemia.

The second option, more common in previous years, is a palliative systemic-to-pulmonary artery shunt (**Blalock-Taussig shunt**) performed to augment pulmonary artery blood flow. The rationale for this surgery, previously the only option for these patients, is to augment pulmonary blood flow to decrease the amount of hypoxia and improve linear growth, as well as augment growth of the branch pulmonary arteries. The modified Blalock-Taussig shunt is currently the most common aortopulmonary shunt procedure and consists of a Gore-Tex conduit anastomosed side to side from the subclavian artery to the homolateral branch of the pulmonary artery (Fig. 424-5). Sometimes the shunt is brought directly from the ascending aorta to the main pulmonary artery and in this case is called a central shunt. The Blalock-Taussig operation can be successfully performed in the newborn period with shunts 3-4 mm in diameter and has also been used successfully in premature infants.

Postoperative complications after a Blalock-Taussig shunt include chylothorax, diaphragmatic paralysis, and Horner syndrome. Postoperative pulmonary overcirculation leading to symptoms of cardiac failure may be caused by too large a shunt; its treatment is described in Chapter 436. Vascular problems other than a diminished radial pulse and occasional long-term arm length discrepancy are rarely seen in the upper extremity supplied by the subclavian artery used for the anastomosis.

After a successful shunt procedure, cyanosis diminishes. The development of a continuous murmur over the lung fields after the operation indicates a functioning anastomosis. A good continuous shunt murmur may not be heard until several days after surgery. The duration of symptomatic relief is variable. As the child grows, more pulmonary blood flow is needed and the shunt eventually becomes inadequate. When increasing cyanosis develops rapidly, thrombosis of the shunt should be suspected, often requiring emergent surgery.

PROGNOSIS

After successful total correction, patients are generally asymptomatic and are able to lead unrestricted lives. Uncommon immediate postoperative problems include right ventricular failure, transient heart block, residual VSD with left-to-right shunting, and myocardial infarction from interruption of an aberrant coronary artery. Postoperative heart failure (particularly in patients with a large transannular outflow patch) may require anticongestive therapy. The long-term effects of isolated, surgically induced pulmonary valvular insufficiency are still being defined as more patients with repaired tetralogy of Fallot reach middle age, but insufficiency is generally well tolerated through adolescence. Many patients after tetralogy repair and all of those with transannular patch repairs have a to-and-fro murmur at the left sternal border, usually indicative of mild outflow obstruction and mild to moderate pulmonary insufficiency. Patients with more marked pulmonary valve insufficiency also have moderate to marked heart enlargement and may develop tricuspid regurgitation as the tricuspid valve annulus dilates. These patients will develop a holosystolic murmur at the lower left sternal border. Patients with a severe residual gradient across the right ventricular outflow tract may require reoperation, but mild to moderate obstruction is usually present and does not require reintervention.

Follow-up of patients 5-20 yr after surgery indicates that the marked improvement in symptoms is generally maintained. Asymptomatic patients nonetheless have lower than normal exercise capacity, maximal heart rate, and cardiac output. These abnormal findings are more common in patients who underwent placement of a transannular outflow tract patch and may be less frequent when surgery is performed at an early age. As these children move into adolescence and adulthood, some (more commonly those with transannular patches) will develop right ventricular dilation due to severe pulmonary regurgitation. After reaching adulthood, careful lifelong follow-up by a specialist in adult congenital heart disease is important. Serial echocardiography and magnetic resonance angiography (MRA) are valuable tools for assessing the degree of right ventricular dilation, the presence of right ventricular dysfunction, and for quantifying the regurgitant fraction. Valve replacement is indicated for those patients with increasing right ventricular dilation and tricuspid regurgitation.

Conduction disturbances can occur after surgery. The atrioventricular node and the bundle of His and its divisions are in close proximity to the VSD and may be injured during surgery; however, permanent complete heart block after tetralogy repair is rare. When present, it should be treated by placement of a permanently implanted pacemaker. Even transient complete heart block in the immediate postoperative period is rare; it may be associated with an increased incidence of late-onset complete heart block and sudden death. In contrast, right bundle branch block is quite common on the postoperative electrocardiogram. The duration of the QRS interval has been shown to predict both the presence of residual hemodynamic derangement and the long-term risk of arrhythmia and sudden death. Research is ongoing to determine the effectiveness of biventricular pacing (in which a pacemaker is used to resynchronize the activation of the right and left ventricles) in improving hemodynamics in those patients with long ventricular conduction delays.

A number of children have premature ventricular beats after repair of the tetralogy of Fallot. These beats are of concern in patients with residual hemodynamic abnormalities; 24-hr electrocardiographic (Holter) monitoring studies should be performed to be certain that occult short episodes of ventricular tachycardia are not occurring. Exercise studies may be useful in provoking cardiac arrhythmias that are not apparent at rest. In the presence of complex ventricular arrhythmias or severe residual hemodynamic abnormalities, prophylactic antiarrhythmic therapy, catheter ablation, or implantation of an implantable defibrillator is warranted. Re-repair is indicated if significant residual right ventricular outflow obstruction or severe pulmonary insufficiency is present, because arrhythmias may improve after hemodynamics are restored to a more normal level.

BIBLIOGRAPHY

Please visit the Nelson Textbook of Pediatrics *website at www.expertconsult.com for the complete bibliography.*

424.2 Tetralogy of Fallot with Pulmonary Atresia

Daniel Bernstein

PATHOPHYSIOLOGY

Tetralogy of a Fallot with pulmonary atresia is the most extreme form of the tetralogy of Fallot. The pulmonary valve is atretic (absent), and the pulmonary trunk may be hypoplastic or atretic as well. The entire right ventricular output is ejected into the aorta. Pulmonary blood flow is then dependent on collateral vessels or major aortopulmonary collateral arteries (MAPCAs) or, less commonly, on a PDA. The ultimate prognosis depends on the degree of development of the branch pulmonary arteries, which needs to be assessed by cardiac catheterization. If the pulmonary arteries are severely hypoplastic and fail to grow after palliative shunt procedures, heart-lung transplantation may be the only therapy (Chapter 437.2). Pulmonary atresia with VSD is also associated with the CATCH 22 deletion and DiGeorge syndrome. The association of severe **tracheomalacia** or **bronchomalacia** with these severe forms of tetralogy/pulmonary atresia may complicate postoperative recovery.

CLINICAL MANIFESTATIONS

Patients with pulmonary atresia and VSD have findings similar to those in patients with severe tetralogy of Fallot. Cyanosis usually appears within the 1st few hr or days after birth; however, the prominent systolic murmur associated with the tetralogy is usually absent. The 1st heart sound may be followed by an ejection click caused by the enlarged aortic root, the 2nd heart sound is single and loud, and continuous murmurs of a PDA or bronchial collateral flow may be heard over the entire precordium, both anteriorly and posteriorly. Most patients are moderately cyanotic and are initially stabilized with a prostaglandin E_1 infusion pending cardiac catheterization or CT scan to further delineate the anatomy. Patients with several large MAPCAs may be less cyanotic and, once the diagnosis is confirmed, can be taken off prostaglandin while awaiting palliative surgical intervention. Some patients may even develop symptoms of heart failure caused by increased pulmonary blood flow via these collateral vessels.

DIAGNOSIS

The chest roentgenogram demonstrates a varying heart size, depending on the amount of pulmonary blood flow, a concavity at the position of the pulmonary arterial segment, and often the reticular pattern of bronchial collateral flow. The electrocardiogram shows right ventricular hypertrophy. The echocardiogram identifies aortic override, a thick right ventricular wall, and atresia of the pulmonary valve. Pulsed and color Doppler echocardiographic studies show an absence of forward flow through the pulmonary valve, with pulmonary blood flow being supplied by MAPCAs, which can usually be seen arising from the descending aorta. At cardiac catheterization, right ventriculography reveals a large aorta, opacified immediately by passage of contrast medium through the VSD, but with no dye entering the lungs through the right ventricular outflow tract. Careful delineation of the native pulmonary arteries, if present, to determine whether they are continuous or discontinuous and whether they arborize to all lung segments is important in planning surgical repair. The location and arborization of all MAPCAs is also determined by selective contrast injection.

TREATMENT

The surgical procedure of choice depends on whether the main pulmonary artery segment is present and, if so, on the size and branching pattern of the branch pulmonary arteries. If these arteries are well developed, a one-stage surgical repair with a homograft conduit between the right ventricle and pulmonary arteries and closure of the VSD is feasible. If the pulmonary arteries are hypoplastic, extensive reconstruction may be required. This usually involves several staged surgical procedures. If the native pulmonary artery is small, a connection made between the aorta and the hypoplastic native pulmonary artery (aortopulmonary window) in the newborn period induces growth. At 3-4 mo of age, the multiple MAPCAs are gathered together (unifocalization procedure) and eventually incorporated into the final repair along with the native pulmonary arteries. This may be accomplished through successive lateral thoracotomies, or through a single midline sternotomy if the anatomy is more favorable.

To be a candidate for full repair, the pulmonary arteries must be of adequate size to accept the full volume of right ventricular output. Complete repair includes closure of the VSD and placement of a homograft conduit from the right ventricle to the pulmonary artery. At the time of reparative surgery, previous shunts are taken down. Because of patient growth as well as homograft narrowing due to proliferation of intimal tissue and calcification, replacement of the homograft conduit replacement is usually required in later life, and multiple replacements may be needed. Patients with obstruction of the very distal branches of the pulmonary arteries may undergo transcatheter balloon dilatation of the multiple branch pulmonary arterial stenoses, as these distal branches may be difficult to reach surgically.

424.3 Pulmonary Atresia with Intact Ventricular Septum

Daniel Bernstein

PATHOPHYSIOLOGY

In pulmonary atresia with an intact ventricular septum, the pulmonary valve leaflets are completely fused to form a membrane and the right ventricular outflow tract is atretic. Because no VSD is present, no egress of blood from the right ventricle can occur. Any blood that enters the right ventricle will regurgitate back across the tricuspid valve into the right atrium. Right atrial

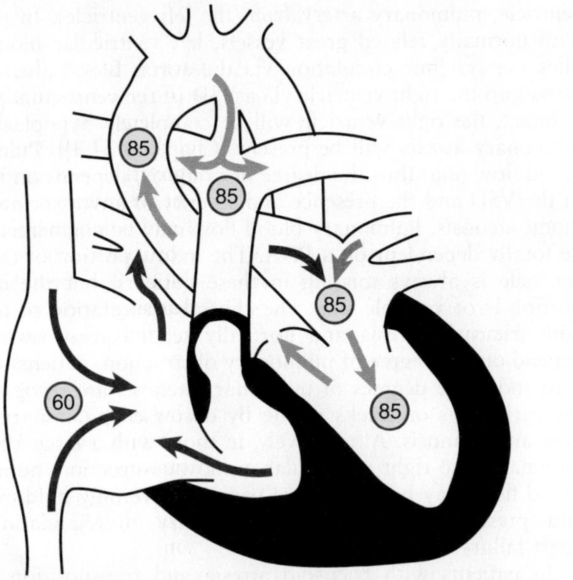

Figure 424-6 Physiology of pulmonary atresia with an intact ventricular septum. *Circled numbers* represent oxygen saturation values. Right atrial (mixed venous) oxygen saturation is decreased secondary to systemic hypoxemia. A small amount of the blood entering the right atrium may cross the tricuspid valve, which is often stenotic as well. The right ventricular cavity is hypertrophied and may be hypoplastic. No outlet from the right ventricle exists because of the atretic pulmonary valve; thus, any blood entering the right ventricle returns to the right atrium via tricuspid regurgitation. Most of the desaturated blood shunts right to left via the foramen ovale into the left atrium, where it mixes with fully saturated blood returning from the lungs. The only source of pulmonary blood flow is via the patent ductus arteriosus. Aortic and pulmonary arterial oxygen saturation will be identical (definition of a total mixing lesion).

pressure increases, and blood shunts via the foramen ovale into the left atrium, where it mixes with pulmonary venous blood and enters the left ventricle (Fig. 424-6). The combined left and right ventricular output is pumped solely by the left ventricle into the aorta. In a newborn with pulmonary atresia, the only source of pulmonary blood flow occurs via a **PDA.** The right ventricle and tricuspid valve are usually hypoplastic, although the degree of hypoplasia varies considerably. Patients who have a small right ventricular cavity also tend to be those with the smallest tricuspid valve annulus, which limits right ventricular inflow. Patients with pulmonary atresia and intact ventricular septum may have **coronary sinusoidal channels** within the right ventricular wall that communicate directly with the coronary arterial circulation. The high right ventricular pressure results in desaturated blood flowing retrograde via these channels into the coronary arteries. Sometimes there are also stenoses of the coronary arteries proximal to where the sinusoids enter, so that distal coronary artery flow is dependent on flow from the right ventricle (known as *RV dependent coronary circulation*). The prognosis in patients with these sinusoids and proximal stenosis of the coronary arteries is more guarded than in those patients without sinusoids or with sinusoids but no coronary stenoses. Rarely, the proximal coronary artery may be totally absent.

CLINICAL MANIFESTATIONS

As the ductus arteriosus closes in the 1st hours/days of life, infants with pulmonary atresia and an intact ventricular septum become markedly cyanotic since their only source of pulmonary blood flow is removed. Untreated, most patients die within the 1st wk of life. Physical examination reveals severe cyanosis and respiratory distress. The 2nd heart sound, representing only aortic closure, is single and loud. Often, no murmurs are audible; sometimes a systolic or continuous murmur can be heard secondary to ductal blood flow. A harsh holosytolic murmur may be heard at the lower left sternal border if there is significant tricuspid regurgitation.

DIAGNOSIS

The electrocardiogram shows a frontal QRS axis between 0 and +90 degrees, the amount of leftward shift reflecting the degree of hypoplasia of the right ventricle. Tall, spiked P waves indicate right atrial enlargement. QRS voltages are consistent with left ventricular dominance or hypertrophy; right ventricular forces are decreased in proportion to the decreased size of the right ventricular cavity. Most patients with small right ventricles have decreased right ventricular forces, but, occasionally, patients with larger, thickened right ventricular cavities may have evidence of right ventricular hypertrophy. The chest roentgenogram shows decreased pulmonary vascularity, the degree depending on the size of the branch pulmonary arteries and the patency of the ductus. Unlike in patients with pulmonary atresia and tetralogy of Fallot, the presence of major collateral vessels (MAPCAs) is rare.

The two-dimensional echocardiogram is useful in estimating right ventricular dimensions and the size of the tricuspid valve annulus, which have been shown to be of prognostic value. Echocardiography can often suggest the presence of sinusoidal channels but cannot be used to evaluate coronary stenoses. Thus, cardiac catheterization is necessary for complete evaluation. Pressure measurements reveal right atrial and right ventricular hypertension. Ventriculography demonstrates the size of the right ventricular cavity, the atretic right ventricular outflow tract, the degree of tricuspid regurgitation, and the presence or absence of intramyocardial sinusoids filling the coronary vessels. Aortography shows filling of the pulmonary arteries via the PDA and is helpful in determining the size and branching patterns of the pulmonary arterial bed. An aortogram, or if necessary, selective coronary angiography is performed to evaluate for the presence of proximal coronary artery stenosis (right ventricular dependent coronary circulation).

TREATMENT

Infusion of prostaglandin E_1 (0.01-0.20 μg/kg/min) is usually effective in keeping the ductus arteriosus open before intervention, thus reducing hypoxemia and acidemia before surgery. The choice of surgical procedure depends on whether there is an RV dependent coronary circulation and on the size of the right ventricular cavity. In patients with only mild to moderate right ventricular hypoplasia without sinusoids, or in patients with sinusoids but no evidence of coronary stenoses, a surgical pulmonary valvotomy is carried out to relieve outflow obstruction. Often, the right ventricular outflow tract is widened with a patch. To preserve adequate pulmonary blood flow, an aortopulmonary shunt may also be performed during the same procedure. An alternative approach utilizes interventional catheterization, in which the imperforate pulmonary valve is first punctured either with a wire or a radiofrequency ablation catheter, followed by a balloon valvuloplasty. If this course is taken, it may take days to weeks before the right ventricular muscle regresses enough for the patient to be weaned from prostaglandin, and many of these patients will still require surgical intervention. The aim of surgery or interventional catheterization is to encourage growth of the right ventricular chamber by allowing some forward flow through the pulmonary valve while using the shunt to ensure adequate pulmonary blood flow. Later, if the tricuspid valve annulus and right ventricular chamber grow to adequate size, the shunt is taken down and any remaining atrial level shunt can be closed. If the right ventricular chamber remains too small for use as a pulmonary ventricle, then the patient is treated as a single ventricle circulation, with a **Glenn procedure** followed by a modified **Fontan procedure** (Chapter 424.4) allowing blood to bypass the hypoplastic right ventricle by flowing to the pulmonary arteries directly from the venae cavae. When coronary artery stenoses are present and retrograde coronary perfusion occurs from the right ventricle via myocardial sinusoids, the prognosis is more guarded because of a higher risk of arrhythmias, coronary ischemia, and sudden death. It is important for these patients not to try to open the right ventricular outflow tract, as dropping the right ventricular pressure will reduce coronary perfusion, leading to ischemia. These patients are usually treated with an aortopulmonary shunt, followed by the Glenn and Fontan procedure. Although at higher risk than those without coronary stenoses, recent reports suggest that these palliative procedures can still be successful. Some of these infants, especially those with total atresia of a proximal coronary artery, are referred instead for heart transplantation.

BIBLIOGRAPHY

Please visit the Nelson Textbook of Pediatrics *website at www.expertconsult.com for the complete bibliography.*

424.4 Tricuspid Atresia

Daniel Bernstein

PATHOPHYSIOLOGY

In tricuspid atresia, no outlet from the right atrium to the right ventricle is present; the entire systemic venous return leaves the right atrium and enters the left side of the heart by means of the foramen ovale or, most often, through an atrial septal defect (Fig. 424-7). The physiology of the circulation and the clinical presentation will depend on the presence of other congenital heart defects, most notably on whether the great vessels are normally related or are transposed (aorta arising from the right ventricle, pulmonary artery from the left ventricle). In patients with normally related great vessels, left ventricular blood supplies the systemic circulation via the aorta. Blood also usually flows into the right ventricle via a VSD (if the ventricular septum is intact, the right ventricle will be completely hypoplastic and pulmonary atresia will be present [Chapter 424.3]). Pulmonary blood flow (and thus the degree of cyanosis) depends on the size of the VSD and the presence and severity of any associated pulmonic stenosis. Pulmonary blood flow may be augmented by or be totally dependent on a PDA. The inflow portion of the right ventricle is always missing in these patients, but the outflow portion is of variable size. The clinical presentation of patients with tricuspid atresia and normally related great vessels will depend on the degree of pulmonary obstruction. Patients with at least moderate degrees of pulmonary stenosis are recognized in the early days or weeks of life by decreased pulmonary blood flow and cyanosis. Alternatively, in those with a large VSD and minimal or no right ventricular outflow obstruction, pulmonary blood flow may be high; these patients have only mild cyanosis and present with signs of pulmonary overcirculation and heart failure.

In patients with tricuspid atresia and transposition of the great arteries, left ventricular blood flows directly into the pulmonary artery, whereas systemic blood must traverse the VSD and right ventricle to reach the aorta. In these patients, pulmonary blood flow is usually massively increased and heart failure develops early. If the VSD is restrictive, aortic blood flow may be compromised. Coarctation of the aorta is not uncommon in this setting.

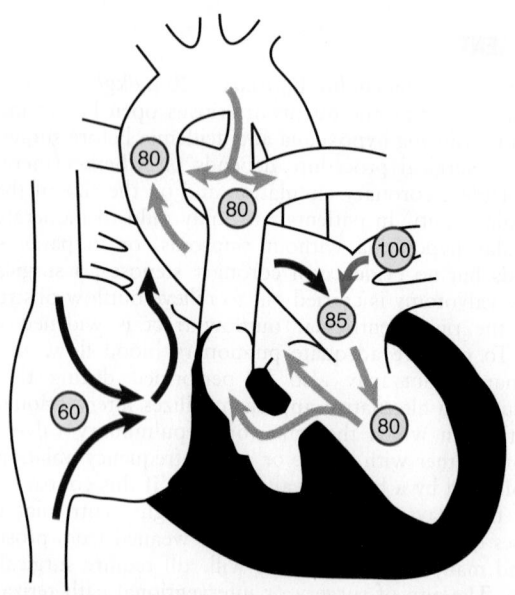

Figure 424-7 Physiology of tricuspid atresia with normally related great vessels. *Circled numbers* represent oxygen saturation values. Right atrial (mixed venous) oxygen saturation is decreased secondary to systemic hypoxemia. The tricuspid valve is nonpatent, and the right ventricle may manifest varying degrees of hypoplasia. The only outlet from the right atrium involves shunting right to left across an atrial septal defect or patent foramen ovale to the left atrium. There, desaturated blood mixes with saturated pulmonary venous return. Blood enters the left ventricle and is ejected either through the aorta or via a ventricular septal defect (VSD) into the right ventricle. In this example, some pulmonary blood flow is derived from the right ventricle, the rest from a patent ductus arteriosus (PDA). In patients with tricuspid atresia, the PDA may close or the VSD may grow smaller and result in a marked decrease in systemic oxygen saturation.

CLINICAL MANIFESTATIONS

Some degree of cyanosis is usually evident at birth, with the extent depending on the degree of limitation to pulmonary blood flow (as noted above). An increased left ventricular impulse may be noted, in contrast to most other causes of cyanotic heart disease, in which an increased right ventricular impulse is usually present. The majority of patients have holosystolic murmurs audible along the left sternal border; the 2nd heart sound is usually single. Pulses in the lower extremities may be weak or absent in the presence of transposition with coarctation of the aorta. Patients with tricuspid atresia are at risk for spontaneous narrowing or even closure of the VSD, which can occasionally occur rapidly and lead to a marked increase in cyanosis.

DIAGNOSIS

Roentgenographic studies show either pulmonary under circulation (usually in patients with normally related great vessels) or over circulation (usually in patients with transposed great vessels). Left axis deviation and left ventricular hypertrophy are generally noted on the electrocardiogram (except in those patients with transposition of the great arteries), and these features distinguish tricuspid atresia from most other cyanotic heart lesions. Thus the combination of cyanosis and left axis deviation on the electrocardiogram is highly suggestive of tricuspid atresia. In the right precordial leads, the normally prominent R wave is replaced by an rS complex. The left precordial leads show a qR complex, followed by a normal, flat, biphasic, or inverted T wave. RV_6 is normal or tall, and SV_1 is generally deep. The P waves are usually biphasic, with the initial component tall and spiked in lead II. Two-dimensional echocardiography reveals the presence of a fibromuscular membrane in place of a tricuspid valve, a variably small right ventricle, VSD, and the large left ventricle (Fig. 424-8). The relationship of the great vessels (normal or transposed) can be determined. The degree of obstruction at the level of the VSD or at the right ventricular outflow tract can be determined by Doppler examination. Blood flow through a patent ductus can be evaluated by color flow and pulsed Doppler.

Cardiac catheterization, indicated usually only if questions remain after echocardiography, shows normal or slightly elevated right atrial pressure with a prominent *a* wave. If the right ventricle is entered through the VSD, the pressure may be lower than on the left if the VSD is restrictive in size. Right atrial angiography shows immediate opacification of the left atrium from the right atrium followed by left ventricular filling and visualization of the aorta. Absence of direct flow to the right ventricle results in an angiographic filling defect between the right atrium and the left ventricle.

TREATMENT

Management of patients with tricuspid atresia depends on the adequacy of pulmonary blood flow. Severely cyanotic neonates should be maintained on an intravenous infusion of prostaglandin E_1 (0.01-0.20 µg/kg/min) until a surgical aortopulmonary shunt procedure can be performed to increase pulmonary blood flow. The Blalock-Taussig procedure (Chapter 424.1) or a variation is the preferred anastomosis. Rare patients with restrictive atrial-level communications also benefit from a Rashkind balloon atrial septostomy (Chapter 425.2) or surgical septectomy.

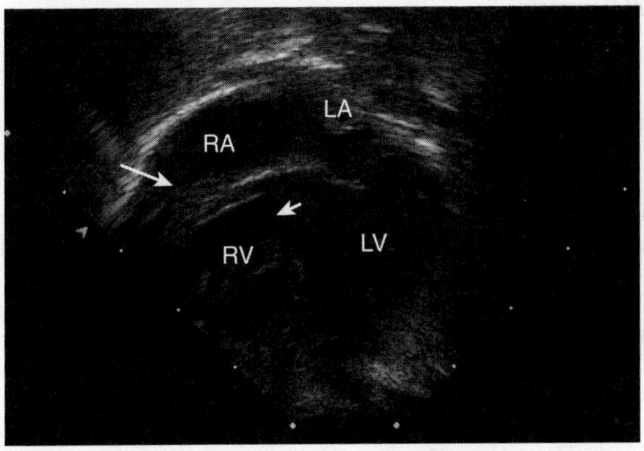

Figure 424-8 Echocardiogram demonstrating tricuspid atresia. The floor of the right atrium consists of a fibromuscular membrane *(large arrow)* instead of the normal tricuspid valve apparatus. The large secundum atrial septal defect can be seen between the right and left atria. The *small arrow* shows the ventricular septal defect. LA, left atrium; LV, left ventricle; RA, right atrium; RV, right ventricle.

Infants with increased pulmonary blood flow because of an unobstructed pulmonary outflow tract (more often patients with aortopulmonary transposition) may require pulmonary arterial banding to decrease the symptoms of heart failure and protect the pulmonary bed from the development of pulmonary vascular disease. Infants with just adequate pulmonary blood flow who are well balanced between cyanosis and pulmonary overcirculation can be watched closely for the development of increasing cyanosis, which may occur as the VSD begins to get smaller or the pulmonary outflow becomes narrower and is an indication for surgery.

The next stage of palliation for patients with tricuspid atresia involves the creation of an anastomosis between the superior vena cava and the pulmonary arteries (**bidirectional Glenn shunt;** Fig. 424-9*A*). This procedure is performed at usually between 3 and 6 mo of age. The benefit of the Glenn shunt is that it reduces the volume load on the left ventricle and may lessen the chance of left ventricular dysfunction developing later in life.

The **modified Fontan operation** is the preferred approach to later surgical management. It is usually performed between 1.5 and 3 yr of age, usually after the patient is ambulatory. Initially, this procedure was performed by anastomosing the right atrium or atrial appendage directly to the pulmonary artery. A modification of the Fontan procedure, known as a *cavopulmonary isolation procedure,* involves anastomosing the inferior vena cava to the pulmonary arteries, either via a baffle that runs along the lateral wall of the right atrium (lateral tunnel Fontan; see Fig. 424-9*B*) or via a homograft or Gore-Tex tube running outside the heart (external conduit Fontan). The advantage of these later approaches is that blood flows by a more direct route into the pulmonary arteries, thereby decreasing the possibility of right atrial dilatation and markedly reducing the incidence of postoperative pleural effusions, which were common with the earlier method. In a completed Fontan repair, desaturated blood flows from both venae cavae directly into the pulmonary arteries. Oxygenated blood returns to the left atrium, enters the left ventricle, and is ejected into the systemic circulation. The volume load is completely removed from the left ventricle, and the right-to-left shunt is abolished. Because of the reliance on passive filling of the pulmonary circulation, the Fontan procedure is contraindicated in patients with elevated pulmonary vascular resistance, in those with pulmonary artery hypoplasia, and in patients with left ventricular dysfunction. The patient must also not have significant mitral insufficiency. Patients who are not in

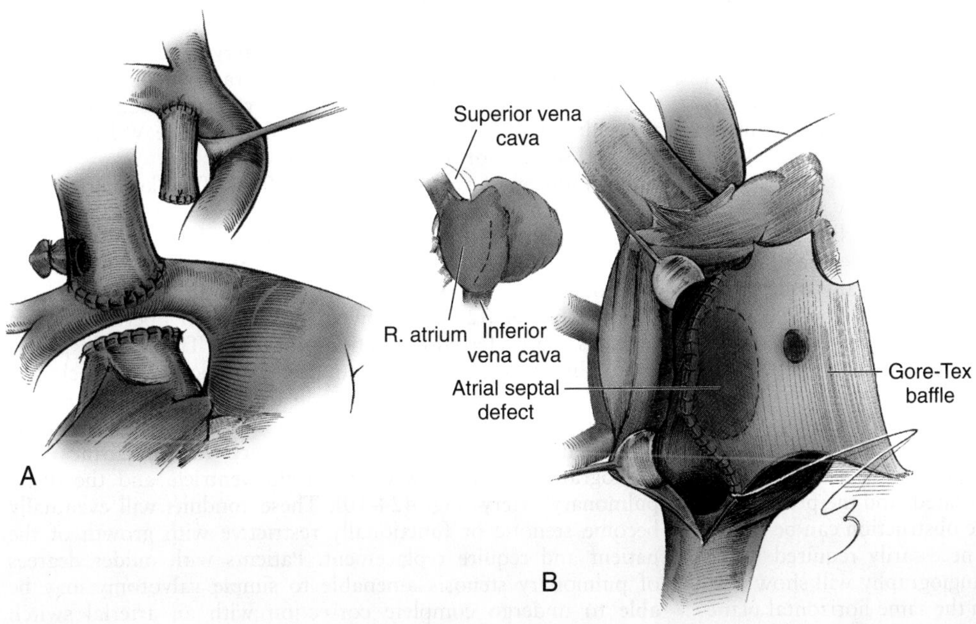

Figure 424-9 *A,* Bidirectional Glenn shunt showing the superior vena cava–right pulmonary anastomosis. *B,* A modified Fontan procedure (cavopulmonary isolation) is completed with placement of a baffle to convey inferior vena cava blood along the lateral wall of the right atrium to the superior vena cava orifice. A 4 mm fenestration is sometimes made on the medial aspect of the polytetrafluoroethylene baffle. (From Castañeda AR, Jonas RA, Mayer JE Jr, et al: Single-ventricle tricuspid atresia. In *Cardiac surgery of the neonate and infant,* Philadelphia, 1994, WB Saunders.)

normal sinus rhythm are at increased risk and if a pacemaker is required in these patients, dual chamber pacing is the preferred approach.

Postoperative problems after the Fontan procedure include marked elevation of systemic venous pressure, fluid retention, and pleural or pericardial effusions. In the past, pleural effusions were a problem in 30-40% of patients using the standard Fontan procedure, but the cavopulmonary isolation procedure now in use reduces this risk to about 5%. Some centers use a fenestration at the time of the Fontan, consisting of a small communication between the inferior vena cava and the pulmonary artery conduit and the left atrium. This serves as a "pop-off" during early postoperative recovery and may hasten hospital discharge. The fenestration will result in some amount of right-to-left shunting, and is therefore usually closed with a catheter closure device after the immediate postoperative period.

Late complications of the Fontan procedure include baffle obstruction causing superior or inferior vena cava syndrome, vena cava or pulmonary artery thromboembolism, protein-losing enteropathy, supraventricular arrhythmias (atrial flutter, paroxysmal atrial tachycardia), and hepatic cirrhosis due to persistently elevated central venous pressures. Left ventricular dysfunction may be a late occurrence, usually not until adolescence or young adulthood. Heart transplantation is a successful treatment option for pediatric patients with "failed" Fontan circuits but is a somewhat riskier procedure in adults.

BIBLIOGRAPHY

Please visit the Nelson Textbook of Pediatrics *website at* *www.expertconsult.com* *for the complete bibliography.*

424.5 Double-Outlet Right Ventricle

Daniel Bernstein

Double-outlet right ventricle (DORV) is characterized when both the aorta and pulmonary artery arise from the right ventricle. The outlet from the left ventricle is through VSD into the right ventricle. Normally, the aortic and mitral valves are in fibrous continuity; however, in DORV, the aortic and mitral valves are separated by a smooth muscular conus, similar to that seen under the normal pulmonary valve. In DORV, the great arteries may be normally related, with the aorta closer to the VSD, or malposed, with the pulmonary artery closer to the VSD. The great artery closest to the VSD may override the defect by a variable amount but is at least 50% committed to the right ventricle. When the VSD is subaortic, the defect may be viewed as part of a continuum with the tetralogy of Fallot, and the physiology as well as the history, physical examination, electrocardiogram, and roentgenograms are depending on the degree of pulmonary stenosis, similar to the situation in tetralogy of Fallot (Chapter 424.1). If the VSD is subpulmonic, there may be subvalvar, valvar, or supravalvar aortic stenosis, and coarctation is a possibility as well. This is known as the **Taussig-Bing malformation.** The clinical presentation of these patients will be dependent on the degree of aortic obstruction, but since the pulmonary artery is usually wide open, will usually include some degree of pulmonary overcirculation and heart failure. If the aortic obstruction is severe or there is a coarctation, poor pulses, hypoperfusion, and cardiovascular collapse are possible presenting signs.

The two-dimensional echocardiogram demonstrates both great vessels arising from the right ventricle and mitral-aortic valve discontinuity. The relationships between the aorta and pulmonary artery to the VSD can be delineated, and the presence of either pulmonary obstruction or aortic obstruction can be evaluated. Cardiac catheterization is not necessarily required if the echocardiogram is straightforward. Angiography will show that the aortic and pulmonary valves lie in the same horizontal plane and that both arise predominantly or exclusively from the right ventricle.

Surgical correction depends on the relationship of the great vessels to the VSD. If the VSD is subaortic, the repair may be similar to that used for tetralogy of Fallot, or consist of creating an intraventricular tunnel so that the left ventricle ejects blood through the VSD, into the tunnel, and into the aorta. The pulmonary obstruction is relieved either with an outflow patch or with a right ventricular to pulmonary artery homograft conduit (**Rastelli operation**). If the VSD is subpulmonic, the great vessels can be switched (Chapter 424.6) and the Rastelli operation performed. However, if there is substantial aortic obstruction, or if one of the ventricles is hypoplastic, then a Norwood-style single ventricle repair may be necessary (Chapter 425.10). In small infants, palliation with an aortopulmonary shunt provides symptomatic improvement and allows for adequate growth before corrective surgery is performed.

424.6 Transposition of the Great Arteries with Ventricular Septal Defect and Pulmonary Stenosis

Daniel Bernstein

This combination of anomalies may mimic tetralogy of Fallot in its clinical features (Chapter 424.1). However, because of the transposed great vessels, the site of obstruction is in the left as opposed to the right ventricle. The obstruction can be either valvular or subvalvular; the latter type may be dynamic, related to the interventricular septum or atrioventricular valve tissue, or acquired, as in patients with transposition and VSD after pulmonary arterial banding.

The age at which clinical manifestations initially appear varies from soon after birth to later infancy, depending on the degree of pulmonic stenosis. Clinical findings include cyanosis, decreased exercise tolerance, and poor physical development, similar to those described for tetralogy of Fallot; the heart is usually more enlarged. The pulmonary vasculature as seen on the roentgenogram is dependent on the degree of pulmonary obstruction. The electrocardiogram usually shows right axis deviation, right and left ventricular hypertrophy, and sometimes tall, spiked P waves. Echocardiography confirms the diagnosis and is useful in sequential evaluation of the degree and progression of the left ventricular outflow tract obstruction. Cardiac catheterization, if necessary, shows that pulmonary arterial pressure is low and that oxygen saturation in the pulmonary artery exceeds that in the aorta. Selective right and left ventriculography demonstrates the origin of the aorta from the right ventricle, the origin of the pulmonary artery from the left ventricle, the VSD, and the site and severity of the pulmonary stenosis.

An infusion of prostaglandin E_1 (0.01-0.20 μg/kg/min) should be started in neonates who present with cyanosis. When necessary, balloon atrial septostomy is performed to improve atrial-level mixing and to decompress the left atrium (Chapter 425.2). Cyanotic infants may be palliated with an aortopulmonary shunt (Chapter 424.1) followed by a Rastelli operation when older as the preferred corrective procedure. The Rastelli procedure achieves physiologic and anatomic correction by (1) closure of the VSD using an interventricular tunnel so that left ventricular blood flow is directed to the aorta, and (2) connection of the right ventricle to the pulmonary artery via an extracardiac homograft conduit between the right ventricle and the distal pulmonary artery (Fig. 424-10). These conduits will eventually become stenotic or functionally restrictive with growth of the patient and require replacement. Patients with milder degrees of pulmonary stenosis amenable to simple valvotomy may be able to undergo complete correction with an arterial switch

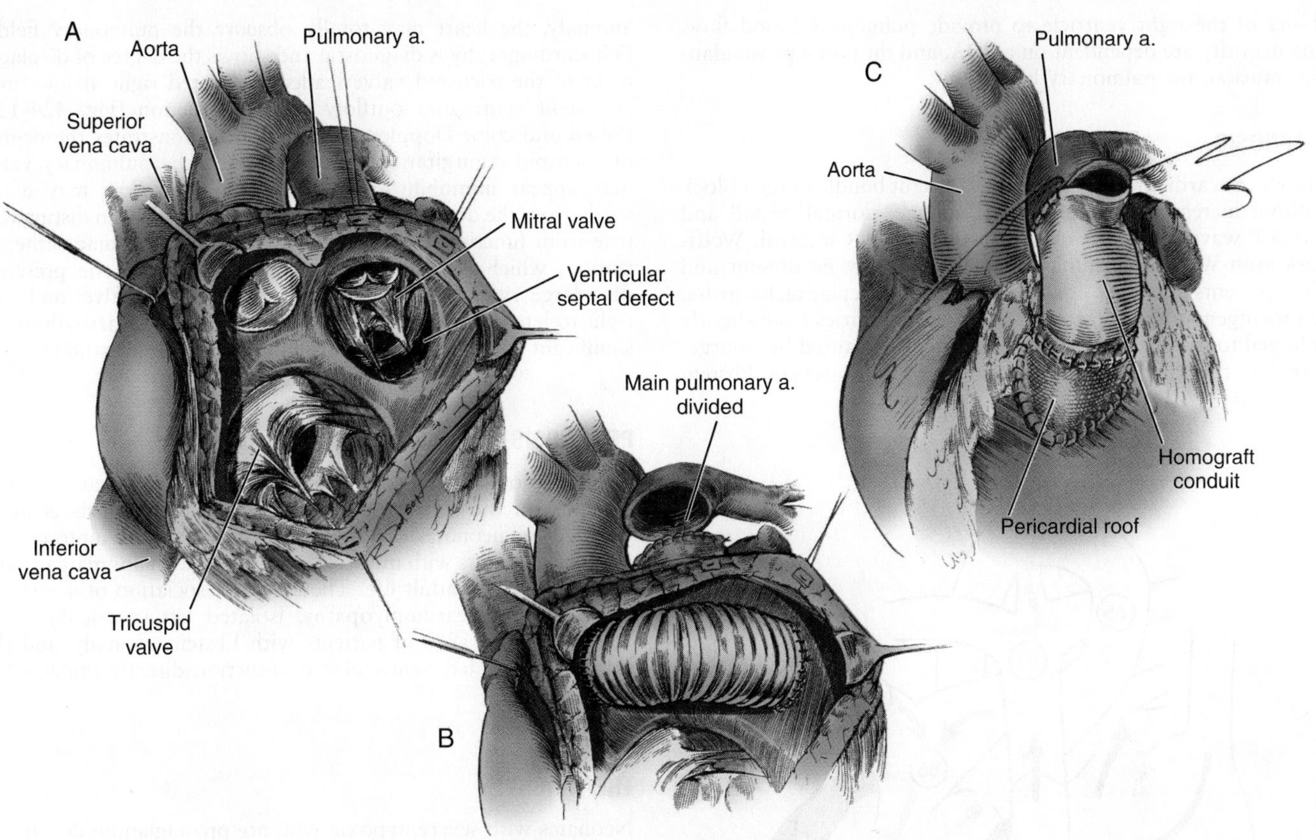

Figure 424-10 *A,* Taussig-Bing type of double-outlet right ventricle with subpulmonary stenosis necessitating repair by the Rastelli technique. *B,* The main pulmonary artery is divided and oversewn proximally. The pulmonary valve lies within the baffle pathway. *C,* Completion of the Rastelli repair with a right ventricle-pulmonary artery allograft conduit. (From Castañeda AR, Jonas RA, Mayer JE Jr, et al: Single-ventricle tricuspid atresia. In *Cardiac surgery of the neonate and infant,* Philadelphia, 1994, WB Saunders.)

procedure (Chapter 425.2) and closure of the VSD. Surgical correction by the Mustard operation (Chapter 425.2) with simultaneous closure of the VSD and relief of left ventricular outflow obstruction may be an alternative when the position of the VSD is not suitable for a Rastelli operation; however, this procedure leaves the right ventricle as the systemic pumping chamber and has fallen out of favor.

424.7 Ebstein Anomaly of the Tricuspid Valve

Daniel Bernstein

PATHOPHYSIOLOGY

Ebstein anomaly consists of downward displacement of an abnormal tricuspid valve into the right ventricle. The defect arises from failure of the normal process by which the tricuspid valve is separated from the right ventricular myocardium (Chapter 414). The anterior cusp of the valve retains some attachment to the valve ring, but the other leaflets are adherent to the wall of the right ventricle. The right ventricle is thus divided into 2 parts by the abnormal tricuspid valve: the 1st, a thin-walled "atrialized" portion, is continuous with the cavity of the right atrium; the 2nd, often smaller portion consists of normal ventricular myocardium. The right atrium is enlarged as a result of tricuspid valve regurgitation, although the degree is extremely variable. In more severe forms of Ebstein anomaly, the effective output from the right side of the heart is decreased due to a combination of the poorly functioning small right ventricle, tricuspid valve regurgitation, and obstruction of the right ventricular outflow tract produced by the large, sail-like, anterior tricuspid valve leaflet. In newborns, right ventricular function may be so compromised that it is unable to generate enough force to open the pulmonary valve in systole, thus producing "functional" pulmonary atresia. Some infants have true anatomic pulmonary atresia. The increased volume of right atrial blood shunts through the foramen ovale (or through an associated atrial septal defect) to the left atrium and produces cyanosis (Fig. 424-11).

CLINICAL MANIFESTATIONS

The severity of symptoms and the degree of cyanosis are highly variable and depend on the extent of displacement of the tricuspid valve and the severity of right ventricular outflow tract obstruction. In many patients, symptoms are mild and may be delayed until the teenage years or young adult life; the patient may initially have fatigue or palpitations as a result of cardiac dysrhythmias. The atrial right-to-left shunt is responsible for cyanosis and polycythemia. Jugular venous pulsations, a index of central venous pressure, may be normal or increased in those with tricuspid insufficiency. On palpation, the precordium is quiet. A holosystolic murmur caused by tricuspid regurgitation is audible over most of the anterior left side of the chest. A gallop rhythm is common and often associated with multiple clicks at the lower left sternal border. A scratchy diastolic murmur may also be heard at the left sternal border. This murmur may mimic a pericardial friction rub.

Newborns with severe forms of Ebstein anomaly have marked cyanosis, massive cardiomegaly, and long holosystolic murmurs. Death may result from cardiac failure, hypoxemia, and pulmonary hypoplasia. Spontaneous improvement may occur in some neonates as pulmonary vascular resistance falls and improves the ability of the right ventricle to provide pulmonary blood flow. The majority are dependent on a PDA, and thus on a prostaglandin infusion, for pulmonary blood flow.

DIAGNOSIS

The electrocardiogram usually shows a right bundle branch block without increased right precordial voltage, normal or tall and broad P waves, and a normal or prolonged P-R interval. **Wolff-Parkinson-White syndrome** (Chapter 429) may be present and these patients may have episodes of supraventricular tachycardia. On roentgenographic examination, heart size varies from slightly enlarged to massive box-shaped cardiomegaly caused by enlargement of the right atrium. In newborns with severe Ebstein anomaly, the heart may totally obscure the pulmonary fields. Echocardiography is diagnostic and shows the degree of displacement of the tricuspid valve leaflets, a dilated right atrium, and any right ventricular outflow tract obstruction (Fig. 424-12). Pulsed and color Doppler examination demonstrates the degree of tricuspid regurgitation. In severe cases, the pulmonary valve may appear immobile and pulmonary blood flow may come solely from the ductus arteriosus. It may be difficult to distinguish true from functional pulmonary valve atresia. Cardiac catheterization, which is not usually necessary, confirms the presence of a large right atrium, an abnormal tricuspid valve, and any right-to-left shunt at the atrial level. The risk of arrhythmia is significant during catheterization and angiographic studies.

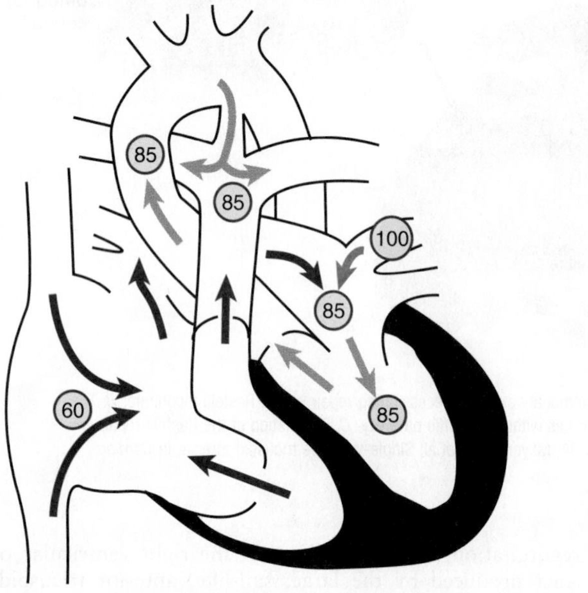

Figure 424-11 Physiology of Ebstein anomaly of the tricuspid valve. *Circled numbers* represent oxygen saturation values. Inferior displacement of the tricuspid valve leaflets into the right ventricle has resulted in a thin-walled, low-pressure "atrialized" segment of right ventricle. The tricuspid valve is grossly insufficient *(clear arrow).* Right atrial blood flow is shunted right to left across an atrial septal defect or patent foramen ovale into the left atrium. Some blood may cross the right ventricular outflow tract and enter the pulmonary artery; however, in severe cases, the right ventricle may generate insufficient force to open the pulmonary valve, and "functional pulmonary atresia" results. In the left atrium, desaturated blood mixes with saturated pulmonary venous return. Blood enters the left ventricle and is ejected via the aorta. In this example, some pulmonary blood flow is derived from the right ventricle, the rest from a patent ductus arteriosus (PDA). Severe cyanosis will develop in neonates with a severe Ebstein anomaly when the PDA closes.

PROGNOSIS AND COMPLICATIONS

The prognosis in Ebstein anomaly is extremely variable and depends on the severity of the defect. The prognosis is more guarded for neonates or infants with intractable symptoms and cyanosis. Patients with milder degrees of Ebstein anomaly usually survive well into adult life. There is an association of a form of left ventricular cardiomyopathy, isolated left ventricular noncompaction, in 18% of patients with Ebstein anomaly, and the severity of the left ventricular dysfunction directly impacts the prognosis.

TREATMENT

Neonates with severe hypoxia who are prostaglandin dependent have been treated with an aortopulmonary shunt alone, by repair of the tricuspid valve, or by surgical patch closure of the tricuspid valve, atrial septectomy, and placement of an aortopulmonary shunt (with eventual single ventricle repair using the Fontan procedure [Chapter 424.4]). Many infants with Ebstein anomaly who have undergone valve repair will still have enough regurgitation that a Glenn shunt is performed to reduce the volume load on the right ventricle (Chapter 424.4). In older children with mild or moderate disease, control of supraventricular dysrhythmias is of primary importance; surgical treatment may not be necessary until adolescence or young adulthood. In patients with severe tricuspid regurgitation, repair or replacement of the abnormal tricuspid valve along with closure of the atrial septal defect is carried out. In some older patients, a bidirectional Glenn shunt is also performed, with the superior vena cava anastomosed to the pulmonary arteries. This procedure reduces the volume of blood that the dysfunctional right side of the heart has to pump, thus creating a "one-and-one-half ventricle repair."

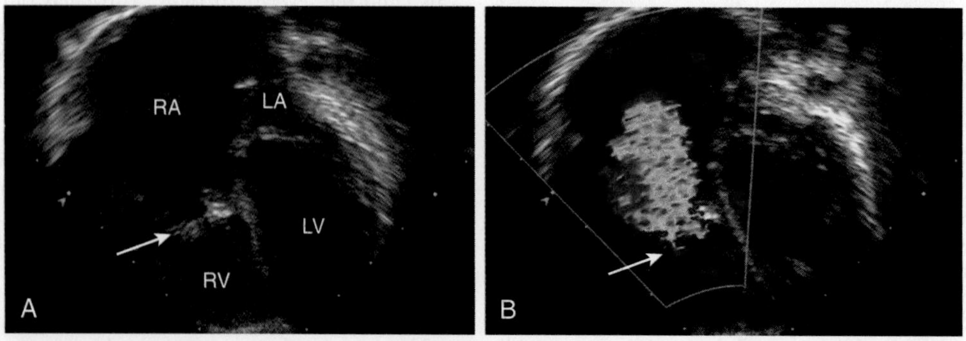

Figure 424-12 Echocardiographic demonstration of Ebstein anomaly of the tricuspid valve. *A,* Subcostal, four-chamber, two-dimensional view showing severe displacement of the tricuspid valve leaflets *(large arrow)* inferiorly into the right ventricle. The location of the tricuspid valve annulus is outlined by the two *arrowheads.* The portion of the right ventricle between the valve annulus and the valve leaflets is the "atrialized" component. *B,* Color Doppler examination showing severe regurgitation of the dysplastic tricuspid valve. Note that the regurgitant turbulent flow *(arrow)* begins halfway into the right ventricular chamber, at the location of the displaced valve leaflets. LA, left atrium; LV, left ventricle; RA, right atrium; RV, right ventricle.

BIBLIOGRAPHY
Please visit the Nelson Textbook of Pediatrics *website at www.expertconsult.com for the complete bibliography.*

Chapter 425
Cyanotic Congenital Heart Disease: Lesions Associated with Increased Pulmonary Blood Flow

425.1 D-Transposition of the Great Arteries

Daniel Bernstein

Transposition of the great vessels, a common cyanotic congenital anomaly, accounts for ≈5% of all congenital heart disease. In this anomaly, the systemic veins return normally to the right atrium and the pulmonary veins return to the left atrium. The connections between the atria and ventricles are also normal (atrioventricular concordance). The aorta arises from the right ventricle and the pulmonary artery from the left ventricle (Fig. 425-1). In normally related great vessels, the aorta is posterior and to the right of the pulmonary artery; in d-transposition of the great arteries (d-TGA), the aorta is anterior and to the right of the pulmonary artery (the *d* indicates a dextropositioned aorta, transposition indicates that it arises from the anterior right ventricle). Desaturated blood returning from the body to the right side of the heart goes inappropriately out the aorta and back to the body again, whereas oxygenated pulmonary venous blood returning to the left side of the heart is returned directly to the lungs. Thus, the systemic and pulmonary circulations exist as two parallel circuits. Survival in the immediate newborn period is provided by the foramen ovale and the ductus arteriosus, which permit some mixture of oxygenated and deoxygenated blood. About 50% of patients with d-TGA also have a ventricular septal defect (VSD), which usually provides for better mixing. The clinical findings and hemodynamics vary in relation to the presence or absence of associated defects (e.g. VSD or pulmonary stenosis). d-TGA is more common in infants of diabetic mothers and in males (3 : 1). d-TGA, especially when accompanied by other cardiac defects such as pulmonic stenosis or right aortic arch, can be associated with deletion of chromosome 22q11 (DiGeorge syndrome [Chapter 418]). Before the modern era of corrective or palliative surgery, mortality was >90% in the 1st yr of life.

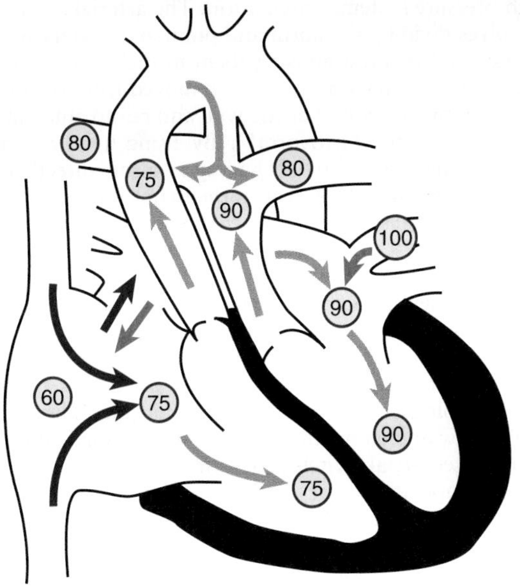

Figure 425-1 Physiology of d-transposition of the great arteries (d-TGA). *Circled numbers* represent oxygen saturation values. Right atrial (mixed venous) oxygen saturation is decreased secondary to systemic hypoxemia. Desaturated blood enters the right atrium, flows through the tricuspid valve into the right ventricle, and is ejected into the transposed aorta with resultant severe aortic desaturation. Fully saturated pulmonary venous blood flows into the left atrium, across the mitral valve into the left ventricle, and across the transposed pulmonary artery into the lungs. Pulmonary arterial oxygen saturation is thus increased. This lesion would not be compatible with life were it not for the ability of blood to shunt via two fetal pathways: the patent foramen ovale (PFO) and patent ductus arteriosus (PDA). Blood may shunt left to right or bidirectionally at the PFO. Because systemic vascular resistance tends to be higher than pulmonary vascular resistance, blood tends to shunt across the PDA mostly from the aorta to the pulmonary artery. As pulmonary resistance drops in the 1st few weeks of life, pulmonary blood flow will gradually increase in patients with d-TGA.

425.2 D-Transposition of the Great Arteries with Intact Ventricular Septum

Daniel Bernstein

D-TGA with an intact ventricular septum is also referred to as simple TGA or isolated TGA. Before birth, oxygenation of the fetus is only slightly abnormal, but after birth, once the ductus arteriosus begins to close, the minimal mixing of systemic and pulmonary blood via the patent foramen ovale is usually insufficient and severe hypoxemia ensues, generally within the 1st few days of life.

CLINICAL MANIFESTATIONS

Cyanosis and tachypnea are most often recognized within the 1st hrs or days of life. Untreated, the vast majority of these infants would not survive the neonatal period. Hypoxemia is usually moderate to severe, depending on the degree of atrial level shunting and whether the ductus is partially open or totally closed. This condition is a medical emergency, and only early diagnosis and appropriate intervention can avert the development of prolonged severe hypoxemia and acidosis, which lead to death. Physical findings, other than cyanosis, may be remarkably nonspecific. The precordial impulse may be normal, or a parasternal heave may be present. The 2nd heart sound is usually single and loud, although it may be split. Murmurs may be absent, or a soft systolic ejection murmur may be noted at the midleft sternal border.

DIAGNOSIS

The electrocardiogram is usually normal, showing the expected neonatal right-sided dominant pattern. Roentgenograms of the chest may show mild cardiomegaly, a narrow mediastinum (the classic "egg-shaped heart"), and normal to increased pulmonary blood flow. In the early newborn period, the chest roentgenogram is generally normal. As pulmonary vascular resistance drops during the 1st several weeks of life, evidence of increased pulmonary blood flow becomes apparent. Arterial Po_2 is low and does not rise appreciably after the patient breathes 100% oxygen (hyperoxia test), although this test may not be totally reliable. Echocardiography is diagnostic and confirms the transposed ventricular-arterial connections (Fig. 425-2). The size of the interatrial communication and the ductus arteriosus can be visualized and the degree of mixing assessed by pulsed and color Doppler examination. The presence of any associated lesion, such as left ventricular outflow tract obstruction or a VSD, can also be assessed. The origins of the coronary arteries can be imaged, although echocardiography is generally not as accurate as catheterization for this purpose. Cardiac catheterization may be performed in patients for whom noninvasive imaging is

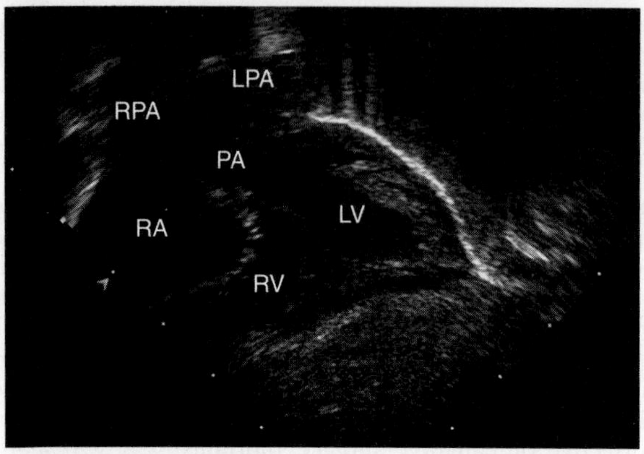

Figure 425-2 Subcostal four-chamber two-dimensional echocardiographic demonstration of d-transposition of the great arteries. The pulmonary artery (PA) can be seen arising directly from the left ventricle (LV). The immediate bifurcation of this great vessel into the branch pulmonary arteries differentiates it from the aorta, which branches more distally from the heart. LPA, left pulmonary artery; RA, right atrium; RPA, right pulmonary artery; RV, right ventricle.

diagnostically inconclusive, where an unusual coronary artery anomaly is suspected, or in patients who require emergency balloon atrial septostomy. Catheterization will show right ventricular pressure to be systemic because this ventricle is supporting the systemic circulation. The blood in the left ventricle and pulmonary artery has a higher oxygen saturation than that in the aorta. Depending on the age at catheterization, left ventricular and pulmonary arterial pressure can vary from systemic level to <50% of systemic-level pressure. Right ventriculography demonstrates the anterior and rightward aorta originating from the right ventricle, as well as the intact ventricular septum. Left ventriculography shows that the pulmonary artery arises exclusively from the left ventricle.

Anomalous coronary arteries are noted in 10-15% of patients and defined by an aortic root injection or by selective coronary arteriography.

TREATMENT

When transposition is suspected, an infusion of prostaglandin E_1 should be initiated immediately to maintain patency of the ductus arteriosus and improve oxygenation (dosage, 0.01-0.20 µg/kg/min). Because of the risk of apnea associated with prostaglandin infusion, an individual skilled in neonatal endotracheal intubation should be available. Hypothermia intensifies the metabolic acidosis resulting from hypoxemia, and thus the patient should be kept warm. Prompt correction of acidosis and hypoglycemia is essential.

Infants who remain severely hypoxic or acidotic despite prostaglandin infusion should undergo **Rashkind balloon atrial septostomy** (Fig. 425-3). A Rashkind atrial septostomy is also usually performed in all patients in whom any significant delay in surgery is necessary. If surgery is planned during the 1st 2 wk of life, and the patient is stable, catheterization and atrial septostomy may be avoided.

A successful Rashkind atrial septostomy should result in a rise in $Pa{O_2}$ to 35-50 mm Hg and elimination of any pressure gradient across the atrial septum. Some patients with TGA and VSD (Chapter 425.3) may require balloon atrial septostomy because of poor mixing, even though the VSD is large. Others may benefit from decompression of the left atrium to alleviate the symptoms of increased pulmonary blood flow and left-sided heart failure.

The **arterial switch (Jatene) procedure** is the surgical **treatment of choice** for neonates with d-TGA and an intact ventricular septum and is usually performed within the 1st 2 wk of life. The reason for this time frame is that as pulmonary vascular resistance declines after birth, pressure in the left ventricle (connected to the

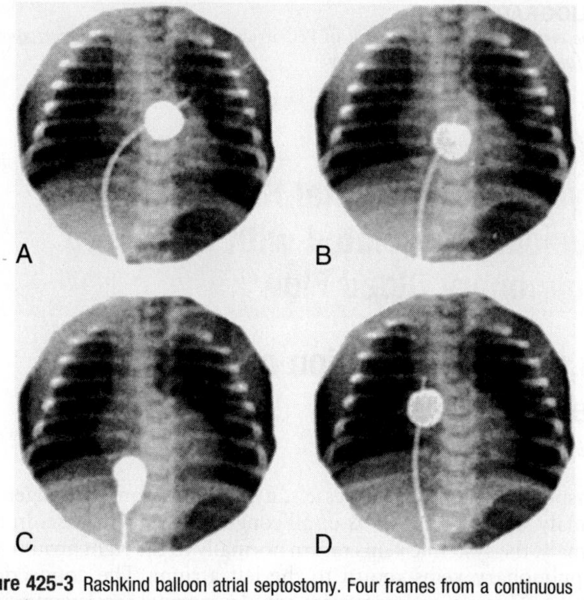

Figure 425-3 Rashkind balloon atrial septostomy. Four frames from a continuous cineangiogram show the creation of an atrial septal defect in a hypoxemic newborn infant with transposition of the great arteries and an intact ventricular septum. *A*, Balloon inflated in the left atrium. *B*, The catheter is jerked suddenly so that the balloon ruptures the foramen ovale. *C*, Balloon in the inferior vena cava. *D*, Catheter advanced to the right atrium to deflate the balloon. The time from A to C is <1 sec.

pulmonary vascular bed) also declines. This drop in pressure results in a decrease in left ventricular mass over the 1st few weeks of life. If the arterial switch operation is attempted after left ventricular pressure (and mass) has declined too far, the left ventricle will be unable to generate adequate pressure to pump blood to the high pressure systemic circulation. The arterial switch operation involves dividing the aorta and pulmonary artery just above the sinuses and re-anastomosing them in their correct anatomic positions. The coronary arteries are removed from the old aortic root along with a button of aortic wall and reimplanted in the old pulmonary root (the "neoaorta"). By using a button of great vessel tissue, the surgeon avoids having to suture directly onto the coronary artery (Fig. 425-4); this is the major innovation that has allowed the arterial switch to replace previous atrial switch operations for d-TGA. Rarely, a two-stage arterial switch procedure, with initial placement of a pulmonary artery band, may be used in patients presenting late who already have had a reduction in left ventricular muscle mass and pressure.

In experienced centers, the arterial switch procedure has a survival rate of 95% for uncomplicated d-TGA. It restores the normal physiologic relationships of systemic and pulmonary arterial blood flow and eliminates the long-term complications of the previously used atrial switch procedure.

Previous operations for d-TGA consisted of some form of **atrial switch procedure** (**Mustard** or **Senning** operation). These procedures produced excellent early survival (≈85-90%), but had significant long-term morbidities. Atrial switch procedures reverse blood flow at the atrial level by the creation of an inter-atrial baffle that directs systemic venous blood returning from the vena cavae to the left atrium, where it will enter the left ventricle and then, via the pulmonary artery, the lungs. The same baffle also permits oxygenated pulmonary venous blood to cross over to the right atrium, right ventricle, and aorta. Atrial switch procedures involve significant atrial surgery and have been associated with the late development of atrial conduction disturbances, sick sinus syndrome with bradyarrhythmia and tachyarrhythmia, atrial flutter, sudden death, superior or inferior vena cava syndrome, edema, ascites, and protein-losing enteropathy. The atrial switch procedure also leaves the right ventricle as the systemic pumping chamber and these "systemic" right ventricles often begin to fail

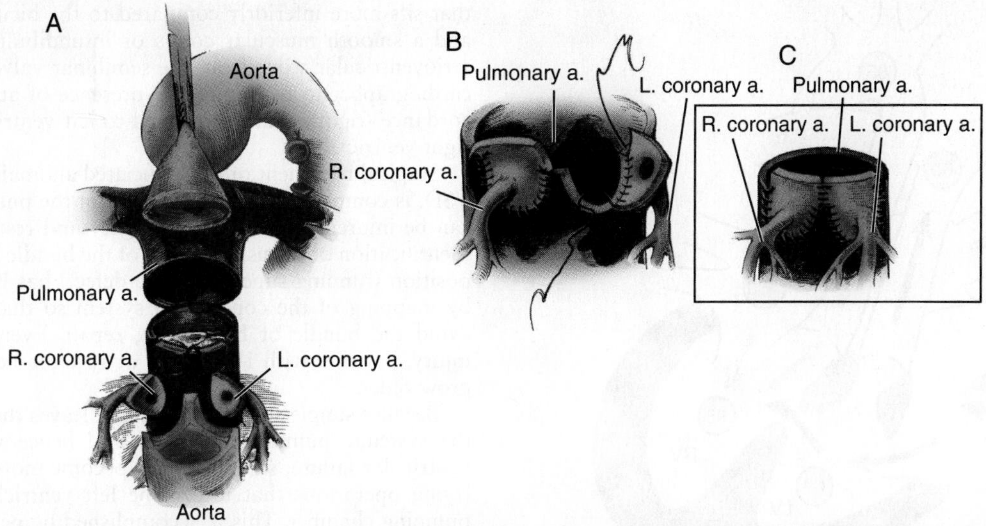

Figure 425-4 Method for translocating the coronary arteries in the arterial switch (Jantene) procedure. *A,* The aorta (anterior) and the pulmonary artery (posterior) have been transected to allow visualization of the left and right coronary arteries. The coronaries have been excised from their respective sinuses, including a large flap (button) of arterial wall. Equivalent segments of the wall of the pulmonary artery (which will become the neoaorta) are also removed. *B,* The aortocoronary buttons are sutured into the proximal portion of the neoaorta. With this technique all sutures are placed in the button of aortic wall rather than directly on the coronary arteries. *C,* Completed anastomosis of the left and right coronary arteries to the neoaorta. (Adapted from Castañeda AR, Jonas RA, Mayer JE Jr, et al: *Cardiac surgery of the neonate and infant,* Philadelphia, 1994, WB Saunders.)

in young adulthood. Atrial switch operations are currently reserved for patients whose anatomy is such that they are not candidates for the arterial switch procedure.

425.3 Transposition of the Great Arteries with Ventricular Septal Defect

Daniel Bernstein

If the VSD associated with d-TGA is small, the clinical manifestations, laboratory findings, and treatment are similar to those described previously for transposition with an intact ventricular septum. A harsh systolic murmur is audible at the lower left sternal border, resulting from flow through the defect. Many of these small defects eventually close spontaneously and may not be addressed at the time of surgery.

When the VSD is large and not restrictive to ventricular ejection, significant mixing of oxygenated and deoxygenated blood usually occurs and clinical manifestations of cardiac failure are seen. The degree of cyanosis may be subtle and sometimes may not be recognized until an oxygen saturation measurement is performed. The murmur is holosystolic and generally indistinguishable from that produced by a large VSD in patients with normally related great arteries. The heart is usually significantly enlarged.

Cardiomegaly, a narrow mediastinal waist, and increased pulmonary vascularity are demonstrated on the chest roentgenogram. The electrocardiogram shows prominent P waves and isolated right ventricular hypertrophy or biventricular hypertrophy. Occasionally, dominance of the left ventricle is present. Usually, the QRS axis is to the right, but it can be normal or even to the left. The diagnosis is confirmed by echocardiography, and the extent of pulmonary blood flow can also be assessed by the degree of enlargement of the left atrium and ventricle. In equivocal cases, the diagnosis can be confirmed by cardiac catheterization. Right and left ventriculography indicate the presence of arterial transposition and demonstrate the site and size of the VSD. Systolic pressure is equal in the 2 ventricles, the aorta, and the pulmonary artery. Left atrial pressure may be much higher than right atrial pressure, a finding indicative of a restrictive communication at the atrial level. At the time of cardiac catheterization, Rashkind balloon atrial septostomy may be performed to decompress the left atrium, even when adequate mixing is occurring at the ventricular level.

Surgical treatment is advised soon after diagnosis, because heart failure and failure to thrive are difficult to manage and pulmonary vascular disease can develop unusually rapidly in these patients. Preoperative management with diuretics lessens the symptoms of heart failure and stabilizes the patient prior to surgery.

Patients with d-TGA and a VSD without pulmonic stenosis can be treated with an arterial switch procedure combined with VSD closure. In these patients, the arterial switch operation can be safely performed after the 1st 2 wk of life because the VSD results in equal pressure in both ventricles and prevents regression of left ventricular muscle mass. At major centers, however, there is no reason to delay repair, as results are excellent whether the surgery is performed in the neonatal period or later.

425.4 L-Transposition of the Great Arteries (Corrected Transposition)

Daniel Bernstein

In l-transposition (l-TGA), the atrioventricular relationships are discordant: the right atrium is connected to the left ventricle and the left atrium to the right ventricle (also known as *ventricular inversion*). The great arteries are also transposed, with the aorta arising from the right ventricle and the pulmonary artery from the left. In contrast to d-TGA, the aorta arises to the left of the pulmonary artery (hence the designation *l* for levo-transposition). The aorta may be anterior to the pulmonary artery, although often they are nearly side by side.

The physiology of l-TGA is quite different from that of d-TGA. Desaturated systemic venous blood returns via the vena cavae to a normal right atrium, from which it passes through a bicuspid atrioventricular (mitral) valve into a right-sided ventricle that has the architecture and smooth wall morphologic features of the normal left ventricle (Fig. 425-5). Because transposition is also present, however, the desaturated blood ejected from this left ventricle enters the transposed pulmonary artery and flows into the lungs, as it would in the normal circulation. Oxygenated

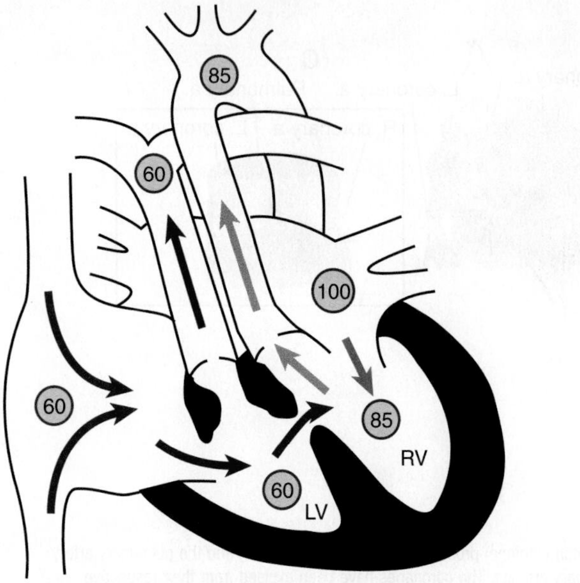

Figure 425-5 Physiology of l- or corrected transposition of the great arteries (l-TGA) with a ventricular septal defect and pulmonic stenosis (VSD + PS). *Circled numbers* represent oxygen saturation values. Right atrial (mixed venous) oxygen saturation is decreased secondary to systemic hypoxemia. Blood from the right atrium flows through the mitral valve into the "inverted" left ventricle. The left ventricle is, however, attached to the transposed pulmonary artery. Therefore, despite the anomalies, desaturated blood still winds up in the pulmonary circulation. Saturated blood returns to the left atrium, traverses the tricuspid valve into the "inverted" right ventricle, and is pumped into the transposed aorta. This circulation would be totally "corrected" were it not for the frequent association of other congenital anomalies, in this case, VSD + PS. Because of the stenotic pulmonary valve, some left ventricular blood flow crosses the VSD and into the right ventricle and the ascending aorta, and systemic desaturation results.

pulmonary venous blood returns to a normal left atrium, passes through a tricuspid atrioventricular valve into a left-sided ventricle, which has the trabeculated morphologic features of a normal right ventricle, and is then ejected into the transposed aorta. The double inversion of the atrioventricular and ventriculoarterial relationships result in desaturated right atrial blood appropriately flowing to the lungs and oxygenated pulmonary venous blood appropriately flowing to the aorta. The circulation is thus physiologically **"corrected."** Without other defects, the hemodynamics would be nearly normal. In most patients, however, associated anomalies coexist: VSD, Ebstein-like abnormalities of the left-sided atrioventricular (tricuspid) valve, pulmonary valvular or subvalvular stenosis (or both), and atrioventricular conduction disturbances (complete heart block, accessory pathways such as Wolff-Parkinson-White syndrome).

CLINICAL MANIFESTATIONS

Symptoms and signs are widely variable and are determined by the associated lesions. If pulmonary outflow is unobstructed, the clinical signs are similar to those of an isolated VSD. If l-TGA is associated with pulmonary stenosis and a VSD, the clinical signs are more similar to those of tetralogy of Fallot.

DIAGNOSIS

The chest roentgenogram may suggest the abnormal position of the great arteries; the ascending aorta occupies the upper left border of the cardiac silhouette and has a straight profile. The electrocardiogram, in addition to any atrioventricular conduction disturbances, may show abnormal P waves; absent Q waves in V_6; abnormal Q waves in leads III, aVR, aVF, and V_1; and upright T waves across the precordium. The echocardiogram is diagnostic. The characteristic echocardiographic features of the right ventricle (moderator band, coarser trabeculations, tricuspid valve that sits more inferiorly compared to the bicuspid mitral valve, and a smooth muscular conus or infundibulum separating the atrioventricular valve from the semilunar valve) allow the echocardiographer to determine the presence of atrioventricular discordance (right atrium connected to left ventricle; left atrium to right ventricle).

Surgical treatment of the associated anomalies, most often the VSD, is complicated by the position of the bundle of His, which can be injured at the time of surgery and result in heart block. Identification of the usual course of the bundle in corrected transposition (running superior to the defect) has been accomplished by mapping of the conduction system so that the surgeon can avoid the bundle of His during repair. Even without surgical injury, patients with l-TGA are at risk for heart block as they grow older.

Because simple surgical correction leaves the right ventricle as the systemic pumping chamber, and hence vulnerable to late ventricular failure, surgeons have become more aggressive about trying operations that utilize the left ventricle as the systemic pumping chamber. This is accomplished by performing an atrial switch operation, to reroute the systemic and pulmonary venous returns, in combination with an arterial switch operation to reroute the ventricular outflows (**double switch procedure**). The long-term benefit of this approach in preserving systemic ventricular function is still under investigation.

BIBLIOGRAPHY

Please visit the Nelson Textbook of Pediatrics *website at* *www.expertconsult.com* *for the complete bibliography.*

425.5 Double-Outlet Right Ventricle without Pulmonary Stenosis

Daniel Bernstein

In double-outlet right ventricle without pulmonary stenosis, both the aorta and the pulmonary artery arise from the right ventricle (Chapter 424.5). The only outlet from the left ventricle is through a VSD. In the absence of obstruction to pulmonary blood flow, clinical manifestations are similar to those of an uncomplicated VSD with a large left-to-right shunt, although mild systemic desaturation may be present because of mixing of oxygenated and deoxygenated blood in the right ventricle. The electrocardiogram usually shows biventricular hypertrophy. Echocardiography is diagnostic and shows the right ventricular origin of both great arteries, their anteroposterior relationship, as well as the relationship of the VSD to each of the great arteries. Surgical correction is dependent on these relationships. If the VSD is subaortic, it is accomplished by creation of an intracardiac tunnel. Blood is then ejected from the left ventricle via the VSD into the aorta. If the VSD is subpulmonic, an arterial switch may be performed in combination with an intracardiac tunnel. If pulmonary blood flow is excessive enough to cause congestive heart failure, pulmonary arterial banding may be required in infancy, followed by surgical correction when the child is bigger. When associated pulmonary stenosis is present, cyanosis is more marked, pulmonary blood flow is decreased, and clinical presentation may be similar to that of tetralogy of Fallot (Chapter 425.5).

425.6 Double-Outlet Right Ventricle with Malposition of the Great Arteries (Taussig-Bing Anomaly)

Daniel Bernstein

In double-outlet right ventricle with malposed great arteries, the VSD is usually directly subpulmonary and the aorta distant from

the left ventricle. Sometimes both the pulmonary and aortic valves may be located close to the VSD (doubly committed VSD) and sometimes neither is (doubly uncommitted VSD). The term malposition is used instead of transposition since both great arteries arise from the right ventricle. Aortic obstructive lesions are common, including valvular and subvalvular aortic stenosis, coarctation of the aorta, and interruption of the aortic arch. Because pulmonary blood flow is unobstructed, patients experience cardiac failure early in infancy and are at risk for the development of pulmonary vascular disease and cyanosis. If aortic obstructive lesions are a component, patients can present with poor systemic output and cardiovascular collapse, particularly after the ductus begins to close. Cardiomegaly is usual, and a parasternal systolic ejection murmur is audible, sometimes preceded by an ejection click and loud closure of the pulmonary valve. The electrocardiogram shows right axis deviation and right, left, or biventricular hypertrophy. The roentgenogram shows cardiomegaly and prominence of the pulmonary vasculature. The anatomic features of the anomaly and associated abnormalities are usually demonstrated by echocardiography, augmented if necessary by either cardiac catheterization, MRI, or CT. Palliation may be achieved by pulmonary arterial banding in infancy and surgical correction at a later age, which may be accomplished by an arterial switch procedure (Chapter 425.2) combined with an intracardiac baffle, or some modification of the Rastelli procedure (Chapter 425.8).

425.7 Total Anomalous Pulmonary Venous Return

Daniel Bernstein

PATHOPHYSIOLOGY

Abnormal development of the pulmonary veins may result in either partial or complete anomalous drainage into the systemic venous circulation. Partial anomalous pulmonary venous return is usually an acyanotic lesion (Chapter 420.4). Total anomalous pulmonary venous return (TAPVR) is associated with total mixing of systemic venous and pulmonary venous blood flow within the heart and thus produces cyanosis.

In TAPVR, the heart has no direct pulmonary venous connection into the left atrium. The pulmonary veins may drain above the diaphragm into the right atrium directly, into the coronary sinus, or into the superior vena cava via a "vertical vein," or they may drain below the diaphragm and join into a "descending vein" that enters into the inferior vena cava or one of its major tributaries, often via the ductus venosus. This latter form of anomalous venous drainage is most commonly associated with obstruction to venous flow, usually as the ductus venosus closes soon after birth, although supracardiac anomalous veins may also become obstructed. Occasionally, the drainage may be mixed, with some veins draining above and others below the diaphragm.

All forms of TAPVR involve mixing of oxygenated and deoxygenated blood before or at the level of the right atrium (total mixing lesion). This mixed right atrial blood either passes into the right ventricle and pulmonary artery or passes through an atrial septal defect (ASD) or patent foramen ovale into the left atrium, which will be the only source of systemic blood flow. The right atrium and ventricle and the pulmonary artery are generally enlarged, whereas the left atrium and ventricle may be normal or small. The clinical manifestations of TAPVR depend on the presence or absence of obstruction of the venous channels (Table 425-1). If pulmonary venous return is obstructed, severe pulmonary congestion and pulmonary hypertension develop; rapid deterioration occurs without surgical intervention. Obstructed TAPVR is a pediatric cardiac surgical emergency because prostaglandin therapy is usually not effective.

Table 425-1 TOTAL ANOMALOUS PULMONARY VENOUS RETURN

SITE OF CONNECTION (% OF CASES)	% WITH SIGNIFICANT OBSTRUCTION
Supracardiac (50)	
Left superior vena cava (40)	40
Right superior vena cava (10)	75
Cardiac (25)	
Coronary sinus (20)	10
Right atrium (5)	5
Infracardiac (20)	95-100
Mixed (5)	

CLINICAL MANIFESTATIONS

Two major clinical patterns of TAPVR are seen, depending on the presence or absence of obstruction. Those neonates with severe obstruction to pulmonary venous return, most prevalent in the infracardiac group (see Table 425-1), present with severe cyanosis and respiratory distress. Murmurs may not be present. These infants are severely ill and fail to respond to mechanical ventilation. Rapid diagnosis and surgical correction are necessary for survival. In contrast, those with mild or no obstruction to pulmonary venous return are usually characterized by the development of heart failure as the pulmonary vascular resistance falls, with mild to moderate degrees of desaturation. Systolic murmurs may be audible along the left sternal border, and a gallop rhythm may be present. Some infants may have mild obstruction in the neonatal period and develop worsening obstruction as time passes.

DIAGNOSIS

The electrocardiogram demonstrates right ventricular hypertrophy (usually a qR pattern in V_3R and V_1, and the P waves are frequently tall and spiked). In neonates with marked pulmonary venous obstruction, the chest roentgenogram demonstrates a very dramatic perihilar pattern of pulmonary edema and a small heart. This appearance can sometimes be confused with primary pulmonary disease and the differential diagnosis includes persistent pulmonary hypertension of the newborn, respiratory distress syndrome, pneumonia (bacterial, meconium aspiration), pulmonary lymphangiectasia, and other heart defects (hypoplastic left heart syndrome). In older children, if the anomalous pulmonary veins enter the innominate vein and persistent left superior vena cava (Fig. 425-6), a large supracardiac shadow can be seen, which together with the normal cardiac shadow forms a **"snowman"** appearance. In most cases without obstruction, the heart is enlarged, the pulmonary artery and right ventricle are prominent, and pulmonary vascularity is increased.

The echocardiogram demonstrates a large right ventricle and usually identifies the pattern of abnormal pulmonary venous connections (Fig. 425-7). The demonstration of any vein with Doppler flow away from the heart is pathognomonic of TAPVR since normal venous flow is usually towards the heart. Shunting occurs from right to left at the atrial level. The size of the left atrium and left ventricle can be measured and the presence of any associated cardiac defects determined.

Echocardiography should be adequate to demonstrate TAPVR in most cases, however, if there is question about the drainage of one or more pulmonary veins, cardiac catheterization, MRI, or CT is performed. Catheterization shows that the oxygen saturation of blood in both atria, both ventricles, and the aorta is similar, indicative of a total mixing lesion. An increase in systemic venous saturation occurs at the site of entry of the abnormal

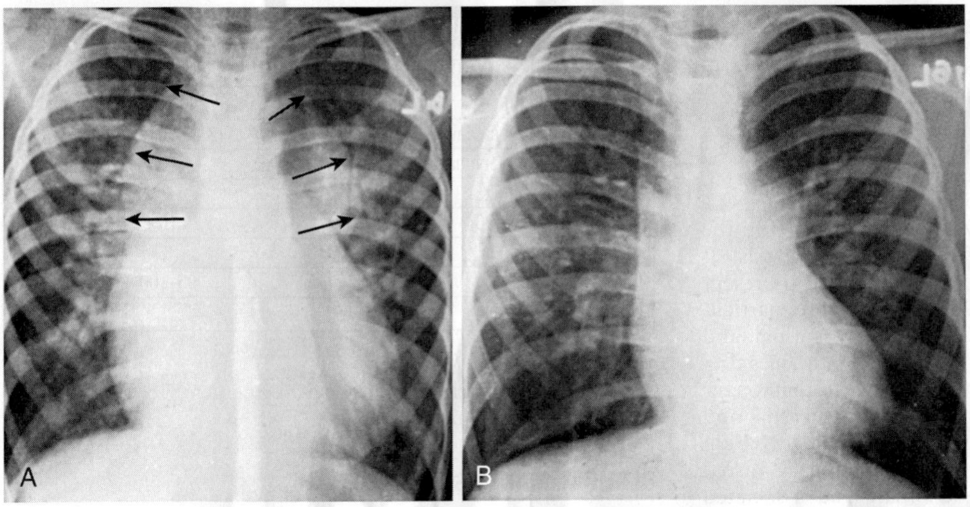

Figure 425-6 Chest x-ray of total anomalous pulmonary venous return to the left superior vena cava. *A,* Preoperative image. *Arrows* point to the supracardiac shadow, which produces the snowman or figure 8 configuration. Cardiomegaly and increased pulmonary vascularity are evident. *B,* Postoperative image showing a decrease in the size of the heart and the supracardiac shadow.

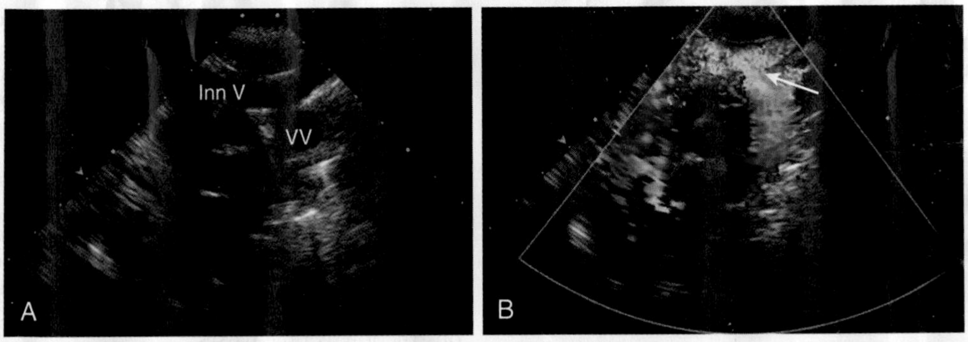

Figure 425-7 Suprasternal two-dimensional echocardiographic views demonstrating supracardiac total anomalous pulmonary venous return (type I). *A,* The large vertical ascending vein can be seen entering the innominate vein. There is a moderate narrowing where the anomalous vein enters the upper body venous system. *B,* Color Doppler examination shows a venous flow signal (*red color*) indicating that blood is moving away toward the transducer and thus from the heart (all venous flow should normally return toward the heart), diagnostic of anomalous pulmonary venous return. The turbulent acceleration of flow can be seen (*arrow*) where the vertical vein enters the innominate. Inn V, innominate vein; VV, vertical vein.

pulmonary venous channel, either above or below the diaphragm. In older patients, pulmonary arterial and right ventricular pressure may be only moderately elevated, but in infants with pulmonary venous obstruction, pulmonary hypertension is usual. Selective pulmonary arteriography shows the anatomy of the pulmonary veins and their point of entry into the systemic venous circulation.

TREATMENT

Surgical correction of TAPVR is indicated during infancy, with emergent repair performed for those patients with venous obstruction. If surgery cannot be performed urgently, extracorporeal membrane oxygenation (ECMO) may be required to maintain oxygenation. Surgically, the pulmonary venous confluence is anastomosed directly to the left atrium, the ASD is closed, and any connection to the systemic venous circuit is interrupted. Early results are generally good, even for critically ill neonates. The postoperative period may be complicated by pulmonary vascular hypertensive crises. In some patients, especially those in whom the diagnosis was delayed or the obstruction was severe, recurrent stenosis and development of pulmonary veno-occlusive disease may occur. Attempts have been made to treat recurrent stenosis with surgery, balloon angioplasty, stents, and antiproliferative chemotherapy. To date, the long-term prognosis in these patients is very guarded and in those with veno-occlusive disease **heart-lung transplantation** may be the only option (Chapter 437.2).

BIBLIOGRAPHY

Please visit the Nelson Textbook of Pediatrics *website at* *www.expertconsult.com* *for the complete bibliography.*

425.8 Truncus Arteriosus

Daniel Bernstein

PATHOPHYSIOLOGY

In truncus arteriosus, a single arterial trunk (truncus arteriosus) arises from the heart and supplies the systemic, pulmonary, and coronary circulations. A VSD is always present, with the truncus overriding the defect and receiving blood from both the right and left ventricles (Fig. 425-8). The number of truncal valve cusps varies from 2 to as many as 6 and the valve may be stenotic, regurgitant, or both. The pulmonary arteries can arise together from the posterior left side of the persistent truncus arteriosus and then divide into left and right pulmonary arteries (**type I**). In **types II** and **III** truncus arteriosus, no main pulmonary artery is present, and the right and left pulmonary arteries arise from separate orifices on the posterior (**type II**) or lateral (**type III**) aspects of the truncus arteriosus. **Type IV** truncus is a term no longer used, since in this case there is no identifiable connection between the heart and pulmonary arteries, and pulmonary blood flow is derived from major aortopulmonary collateral arteries (MAPCAs) arising from the transverse or

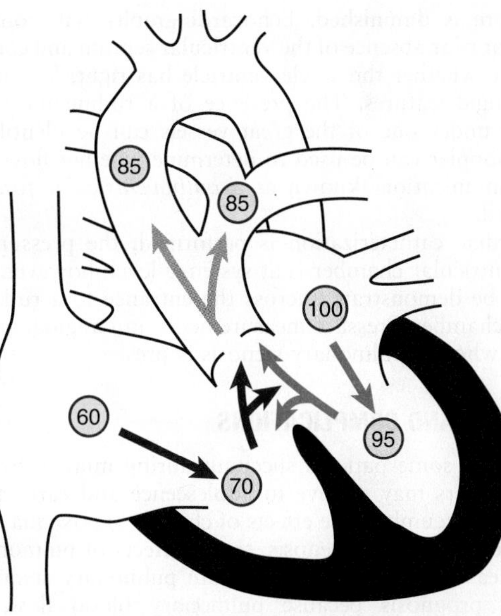

Figure 425-8 Physiology of truncus arteriosus. *Circled numbers* represent oxygen saturation values. Right atrial (mixed venous) oxygen saturation is decreased secondary to systemic hypoxemia. Desaturated blood enters the right atrium, flows through the tricuspid valve into the right ventricle, and is ejected into the truncus. Saturated blood returning from the left atrium enters the left ventricle and is also ejected into the truncus. The common aortopulmonary trunk gives rise to the ascending aorta and to the main or branch pulmonary arteries. Oxygen saturation in the aorta and pulmonary arteries is usually the same (definition of a total mixing lesion). As pulmonary vascular resistance decreases in the 1st few weeks of life, pulmonary blood flow increases dramatically and mild cyanosis and congestive heart failure result.

descending aorta; this is essentially a form of pulmonary atresia (Chapter 424.2).

Both ventricles are at systemic pressure and both eject blood into the truncus. When pulmonary vascular resistance is relatively high immediately after birth, pulmonary blood flow may be normal; as pulmonary resistance drops in the 1st mo of life, blood flow to the lungs is greatly increased and heart failure ensues. Truncus arteriosus is a total mixing lesion with complete admixture of pulmonary and systemic venous return. Because of the large volume of pulmonary blood flow, clinical cyanosis is usually mild. If the lesion is left untreated, pulmonary resistance eventually increases, pulmonary blood flow decreases, and cyanosis becomes more prominent (Eisenmenger physiology; Chapter 427.2).

CLINICAL MANIFESTATIONS

The clinical signs of truncus arteriosus vary with age and depend on the level of pulmonary vascular resistance. In the immediate newborn period, signs of heart failure are usually absent; a murmur and minimal cyanosis may be the only initial findings. Over the next 1-2 mo of life, pulmonary blood flow begins to become torrential and the clinical picture is dominated by heart failure, with still mild cyanosis. Runoff of blood from the truncus to the pulmonary circulation may result in a wide pulse pressure and bounding pulses. These findings will be further exaggerated if truncal valve insufficiency is present. The heart is usually enlarged, and the precordium is hyperdynamic. The 2nd heart sound is loud and single. A systolic ejection murmur, sometimes accompanied by a thrill, is generally audible along the left sternal border. The murmur is frequently preceded by an early systolic ejection click due to the abnormal truncal valve. In the presence of truncal valve insufficiency, a high-pitched early diastolic decrescendo murmur is heard at the mid-left sternal border. An apical mid-diastolic rumbling murmur caused by increased flow through the mitral valve is often audible with the bell of the stethoscope,

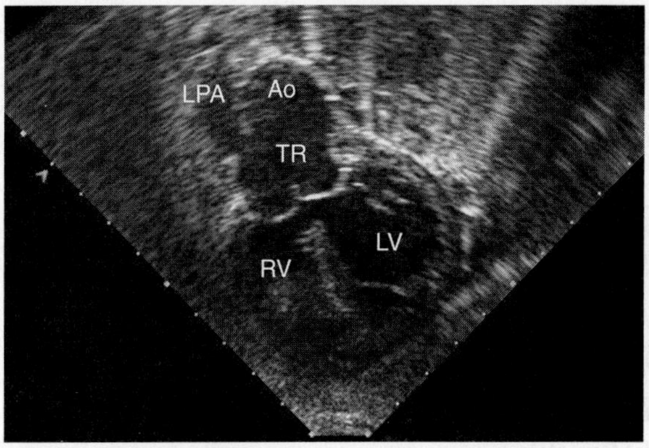

Figure 425-9 Subcostal two-dimensional echocardiographic demonstration of truncus arteriosus. The large truncal valve can be seen overriding the ventricular septal defect. In this case, only the left pulmonary artery (*LPA*) arises from the truncus (*TR*). The pulmonary arteries are discontinuous and the right pulmonary artery arises from the descending aorta via the ductus arteriosus (not shown). Ao, aorta; LV, left ventricle; RV, right ventricle.

especially as heart failure develops. Truncus arteriosus is a conotruncal malformation and may be associated with **DiGeorge syndrome,** linked to a deletion of a large region of chromosome 22q11 (Chapter 418).

DIAGNOSIS

The electrocardiogram shows right, left, or combined ventricular hypertrophy. The chest roentgenogram also shows considerable variation. Cardiac enlargement will develop over the 1st several weeks of life, and is due to prominence of both ventricles. The truncus may produce a prominent shadow that follows the normal course of the ascending aorta and aortic knob; the aortic arch is right-sided in 50% of patients. Sometimes a high bulge left of the aortic knob is produced by the main or left pulmonary artery. Pulmonary vascularity is increased after the 1st few weeks of life. Echocardiography is diagnostic and demonstrates the large truncal artery overriding the VSD and the pattern of origin of the branch pulmonary arteries (Fig. 425-9). Associated anomalies such as an interrupted aortic arch may be noted. Pulsed and color Doppler studies are used to evaluate truncal valve regurgitation. If required, cardiac catheterization shows a left-to-right shunt at the ventricular level, with right-to-left shunting into the truncus. Systolic pressure in both ventricles and the truncus is similar. Angiography reveals the large truncus arteriosus and more defines the origin of the pulmonary arteries.

PROGNOSIS AND COMPLICATIONS

Surgical results have been excellent, and many patients with repaired truncus are now entering adulthood. The need to replace the right ventricular to pulmonary artery conduit as the child grows means that these patients will need to undergo multiple operations by the time they reach adulthood. When truncus arteriosus is associated with DiGeorge syndrome, the associated endocrine, immunologic, craniofacial, and airway abnormalities may complicate recovery.

TREATMENT

In the 1st few weeks of life, many of these infants can be managed with anticongestive medications; as pulmonary vascular resistance falls, heart failure symptoms worsen and surgery is indicated, usually within the 1st few months. Delay of surgery much beyond this time period may increase the likelihood of pulmonary vascular disease; many centers now perform routine neonatal repair at the time of diagnosis. At surgery, the VSD is closed, the pulmonary arteries are separated from the truncus, and continuity is established between the right ventricle and the pulmonary arteries with a homograft conduit. Immediate surgical results are excellent, but these conduits will develop either regurgitation or stenosis over time, and must be replaced, often several times, as the child grows.

BIBLIOGRAPHY

Please visit the Nelson Textbook of Pediatrics *website at www.expertconsult.com for the complete bibliography.*

425.9 Single Ventricle (Double-Inlet Ventricle, Univentricular Heart)

Daniel Bernstein

PATHOPHYSIOLOGY

With a single ventricle, both atria empty through a common atrioventricular valve or via 2 separate valves into a single ventricular chamber, with total mixing of systemic and pulmonary venous return. This chamber may have left, right, or indeterminate ventricular anatomic characteristics. The aorta and pulmonary artery both arise from this single chamber, although 1 of the great vessels may originate from a rudimentary outflow chamber. The aorta may be posterior, anterior (malposition), or side by side with the pulmonary artery and either to the right or to the left. Pulmonary stenosis or atresia is common.

CLINICAL MANIFESTATIONS

The clinical picture is variable and depends on the associated intracardiac anomalies. If pulmonary outflow is obstructed, the findings are usually similar to those of tetralogy of Fallot: marked cyanosis without heart failure. If pulmonary outflow is unobstructed, the findings are similar to those of transposition with VSD: minimal cyanosis with increasing heart failure.

In patients with pulmonary stenosis, cyanosis is present in early infancy. Cardiomegaly is mild or moderate, a left parasternal lift is palpable, and a systolic thrill is common. The systolic ejection murmur is usually loud; an ejection click may be audible, and the 2nd heart sound is single and loud. In patients with unobstructed pulmonary flow, as pulmonary vascular resistance drops, torrential pulmonary blood flow develops, and these patients present with tachypnea, dyspnea, failure to thrive, and recurrent pulmonary infections. Cyanosis is only mild or moderate. Cardiomegaly is generally marked, and a left parasternal lift is palpable. A systolic ejection murmur is present but is not usually loud or harsh, and the 2nd heart sound is loud and closely split. A 3rd heart sound is common and may be followed by a short mid-diastolic rumbling murmur caused by increased flow through the atrioventricular valves. The eventual development of pulmonary vascular disease reduces pulmonary blood flow so that the cyanosis increases and signs of cardiac failure appear to improve (Eisenmenger physiology; Chapter 427.2).

DIAGNOSIS

Findings on the electrocardiogram are nonspecific. P waves are normal, spiked, or bifid. The precordial lead pattern suggests right ventricular hypertrophy, combined ventricular hypertrophy, or sometimes left ventricular dominance. The initial QRS forces are usually to the left and anterior. Roentgenographic examination confirms the degree of cardiomegaly. If present, a rudimentary outflow chamber may produce a bulge on the upper left border of the cardiac silhouette in the posteroanterior projection. In the absence of pulmonary stenosis, pulmonary vasculature is increased, whereas in the presence of pulmonary stenosis, pulmonary vasculature is diminished. Echocardiography will confirm the absence or near absence of the ventricular septum and can usually determine whether the single ventricle has right, left, or mixed morphologic features. The presence of a rudimentary outflow chamber under one of the great vessels can be identified, and pulsed Doppler can be used to determine whether flow through this communication (known as a *bulboventricular foramen*) is obstructed.

If cardiac catheterization is performed, the pressure in the single ventricular chamber is at systemic level; however, a gradient may be demonstrated across the entrance to a rudimentary outflow chamber. Pressure measurements and angiography demonstrate whether pulmonary stenosis is present.

PROGNOSIS AND COMPLICATIONS

Unoperated, some patients succumb during infancy from heart failure. Others may survive to adolescence and early adult life but finally succumb to the effects of chronic hypoxemia or, in the absence of pulmonary stenosis, to the effects of pulmonary vascular disease. Patients with moderate pulmonary stenosis have the best prognosis because pulmonary blood flow, though restricted, is still adequate. Surgical palliation, eventually leading to Fontan-type circulatory physiology (Chapter 424.4), has very good short- and intermediate-term results.

TREATMENT

If pulmonary stenosis is severe, a **Blalock-Taussig aortopulmonary shunt** is performed to provide a reliable source of pulmonary blood flow (Chapter 424.1). If pulmonary blood flow is unrestricted, pulmonary arterial banding is used to control heart failure and prevent progressive pulmonary vascular disease. The **bidirectional Glenn shunt** is usually performed at between 2 and 6 mo of age, followed by a **modified Fontan operation** (cavopulmonary isolation procedure, Chapter 424.4) at 2-3 yr of age. If subaortic stenosis is present because of a restrictive connection to a rudimentary outflow chamber, (restrictive bulboventricular foramen) surgical relief can be provided by anastomosing the proximal pulmonary artery to the side of the ascending aorta (**Damus-Stansyl-Kaye operation**).

425.10 Hypoplastic Left Heart Syndrome

Daniel Bernstein

PATHOPHYSIOLOGY

The term hypoplastic left heart is used to describe a related group of anomalies that include underdevelopment of the left side of the heart (atresia of the aortic or mitral orifice) and hypoplasia of the ascending aorta. The left ventricle may be moderately hypoplastic, very small and nonfunctional, or totally atretic; in the immediate neonatal period the right ventricle maintains both the pulmonary circulation and the systemic circulation via the ductus arteriosus (Fig. 425-10). Pulmonary venous blood passes through an atrial septal defect or dilated foramen ovale from the left to the right side of the heart, where it mixes with systemic venous blood (**total mixing lesion**). When the ventricular septum is intact, which is usually the case, all the right ventricular blood is ejected into the main pulmonary artery; the descending aorta is supplied via the ductus arteriosus, and flow from the ductus also fills the ascending aorta and coronary arteries in a retrograde fashion. The major hemodynamic abnormalities are inadequate maintenance of the systemic circulation and, depending on the size of the atrial-level communication, either pulmonary venous hypertension (restrictive foramen ovale) or pulmonary overcirculation (moderate or large ASD).

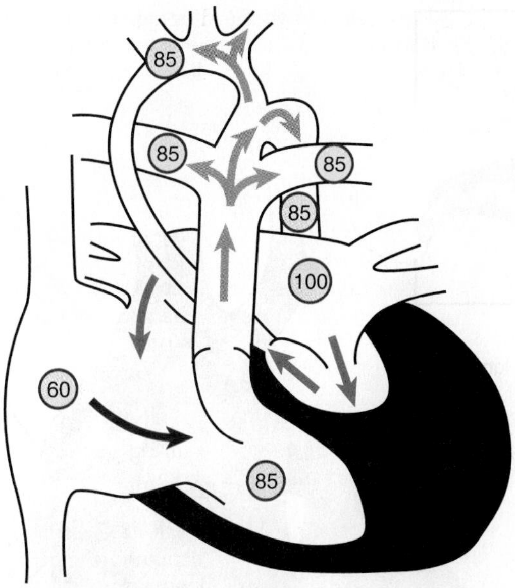

Figure 425-10 Physiology of hypoplastic left heart syndrome (HLHS). *Circled numbers* represent oxygen saturation values. HLHS is not a single lesion but a constellation of different degrees of hypoplasia of the left-sided heart structures. This drawing shows a patent mitral valve, a small left ventricular cavity, and a diminutive ascending aorta. Right atrial (mixed venous) oxygen saturation is decreased secondary to systemic hypoxemia. Desaturated blood enters the right atrium, flows through the tricuspid valve into the right ventricle, and is ejected into the pulmonary artery. Because of the markedly decreased left ventricular compliance, most of the pulmonary venous blood returning to the left atrium shunts left to right at the atrial level. A small amount of left atrial blood will cross the mitral valve and be ejected into the tiny ascending aorta. The right ventricular oxygen saturation represents a mixing of desaturated systemic venous blood and saturated pulmonary venous blood. Pulmonary artery blood flows into the pulmonary arteries as well as right to left across the patent ductus arteriosus (PDA) into the aorta. Ductal blood flows prograde to the descending aorta as well as retrograde to the ascending aorta, where it supplies the head and neck vessels in addition to the coronary arteries (which arise off the small ascending aorta). Closure of the PDA results in profound hypoxia and circulatory collapse.

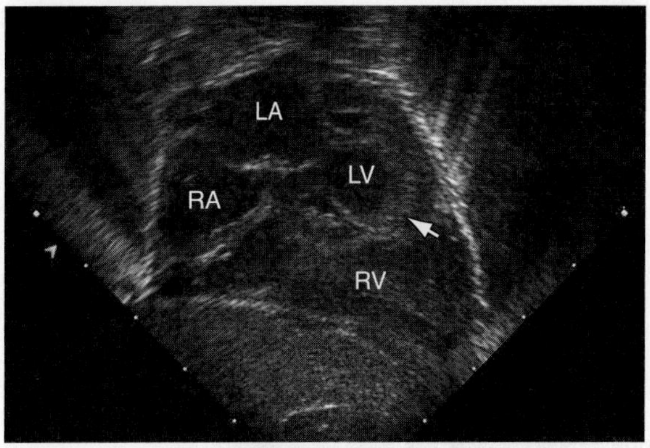

Figure 425-11 Subcostal two-dimensional echocardiographic diagnosis of hypoplastic left heart syndrome. The small left ventricular chamber can be seen, the apex of which *(arrowhead)* does not form the apex of the heart. The atrial septum can be seen bowing from the left to the right, indicating that the communication between the two atria is pressure restrictive. LA, left atrium; LV, left ventricle; RA, right atrium; RV, right ventricle.

CLINICAL MANIFESTATIONS

Although cyanosis may not always be obvious in the 1st 48 hr of life, a grayish-blue color of the skin is soon apparent and denotes a mix of cyanosis and poor perfusion. The condition is diagnosed in most infants in the 1st few hours or days of life. Once the ductus arteriosus begins to closes, signs of poor systemic perfusion and shock predominate. All of the peripheral pulses may be weak or absent. A palpable right ventricular parasternal lift may be present along with a nondescript systolic murmur.

This lesion may be isolated or associated in 5-15% of patients with known genetic syndromes, such as Turner syndrome, trisomy 13 or 18, Jacobsen syndrome (11q deletion), Holt-Oram syndrome, and Rubinstein-Taybi syndrome. In these circumstances, noncardiac manifestations of the syndrome may be evident and influence the clinical outcomes.

DIAGNOSIS

On the chest roentgenogram, the heart is variable in size in the 1st days of life, but cardiomegaly develops rapidly and is associated with increased pulmonary vascularity. The initial electrocardiogram may show only the normal neonatal pattern of right ventricular dominance, but later, P waves become prominent and right ventricular hypertrophy is usual with reduced left ventricular forces. The echocardiogram is diagnostic and demonstrates absence or hypoplasia of the mitral valve and aortic root, a variably small left atrium and left ventricle, and a large right atrium and right ventricle (Fig. 425-11). The size of the atrial communication, by which pulmonary venous blood leaves the left atrium, can be assessed directly and by pulsed and color flow Doppler studies. The small ascending aorta and transverse aortic arch are identified and a discrete coarctation of the aorta in the juxtaductal area may be present, although in the presence of a large ductus, it may be difficult to identify. Doppler echocardiography demonstrates the absence of anterograde flow in the ascending aorta, which is supplied by retrograde flow via the ductus arteriosus. The diagnosis of hypoplastic left heart syndrome can usually be made without need for cardiac catheterization. If catheterization is necessary, the hypoplastic ascending aorta is demonstrated by angiography.

PROGNOSIS AND COMPLICATIONS

Untreated patients most often succumb during the 1st months of life, usually during the 1st or 2nd wk. Occasionally, unoperated patients may live for months or rarely years. Up to 30% of infants with hypoplastic left heart syndrome have evidence of either a major or minor central nervous system abnormality. Other dysmorphic features may be found in up to 40% of patients. Thus, careful preoperative evaluation (genetic, neurologic, ophthalmologic) should be performed in patients being considered for surgical therapy.

Long-term follow up after the Norwood procedure demonstrates reduced neurodevelopmental outcomes and poor exercise tolerance. Whether the poor neurodevelopmental outcome is due to prenatal associated central nervous system injury or malformation, the alterations of cerebral hemodynamics during bypass surgery, or poor postoperative perfusion is unknown.

TREATMENT

Surgical therapy for hypoplastic left heart syndrome has been associated with improving survival rates, reported as high as 95% for the 1st-stage palliation in experienced centers. The 1st-stage repair is designed to construct a reliable source of systemic blood flow arising from the single right ventricle using a combination of aortic and pulmonary arterial tissue, and to limit pulmonary blood flow to avoid heart failure and prevent the development of pulmonary vascular disease. The 2 surgical procedures most commonly utilized are the **Norwood procedure** (Fig. 425-12) or the **Sano procedure.** Primary heart transplantation, previously advocated by a few centers, is much less common due to the substantially improved survival rates with standard surgery and the limited supply of donor organs in this age group.

If a Norwood or Sano procedure is to be performed, preoperative medical management includes correction of acidosis and

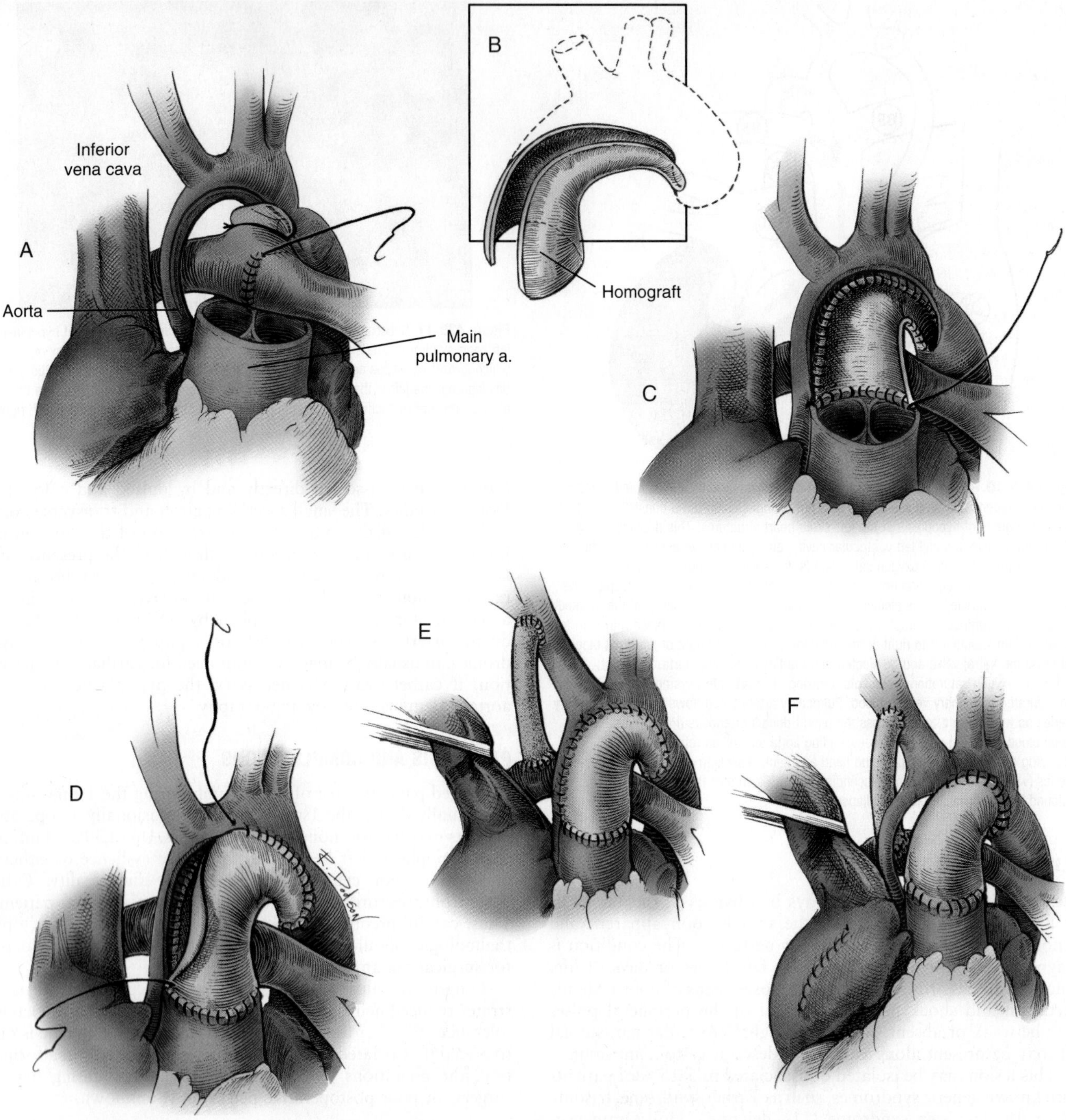

Figure 425-12 The Norwood procedure, one of the two current techniques for 1st-stage palliation of hypoplastic left heart syndrome. *A,* Incisions used for the procedure incorporate a cuff of arterial wall allograft. The distal divided main pulmonary artery may be closed by direct suture or with a patch. *B,* Dimensions of the cuff of the arterial wall allograft. *C,* The arterial wall allograft is used to supplement the anastomosis between the proximal divided main pulmonary artery and the ascending aorta, aortic arch, and proximal descending aorta. *D* and *E,* The procedure is completed by an atrial septectomy and a 3.5-mm modified right Blalock shunt. *F,* When the ascending aorta is particularly small, an alternative procedure involves placement of a complete tube of arterial allograft. The tiny ascending aorta may be left in situ, as indicated, or implanted into the side of the neoaorta. (From Castañeda AR, Jonas RA, Mayer JE Jr, et al: Single-ventricle tricuspid atresia. In *Cardiac surgery of the neonate and infant,* Philadelphia, 1994, WB Saunders.)

hypoglycemia, maintenance of ductus arteriosus patency with prostaglandin E_1 (0.01-0.20 μg/kg/min) to support systemic blood flow, and prevention of hypothermia. Preoperative management should avoid excessive pulmonary blood flow; either through management of ventilator settings, increasing the concentration of inspired CO_2, or decreasing the concentration of inspired O_2. Balloon dilatation of the atrial septum may be indicated.

The Norwood procedure is usually performed in 3 stages. **Stage I** (see Fig. 425-12) includes an atrial septectomy and transection and ligation of the distal main pulmonary artery; the proximal pulmonary artery is then connected to the transversely opened hypoplastic aortic arch to form a neoaorta, extending through the coarcted segment of the juxtaductal aortic arch. A synthetic aortopulmonary (Blalock-Taussig) shunt connects the

aorta to the main pulmonary artery to provide controlled pulmonary blood flow. In the Sano modification, a right ventricle to pulmonary artery conduit is used instead of an aortopulmonary shunt to provide pulmonary blood flow, temporarily creating a double-outlet right ventricle. The operative risk for these 1st-stage procedures has improved dramatically in the past 2 decades and the best reported results demonstrate a 90-95% survival rate.

Stage II consists of a Glenn anastomosis to connect the superior vena cava to the pulmonary arteries (Chapter 425.4), at between 2 and 6 mo of age. **Stage III**, usually performed at 2-3 yr of age, consists of a modified Fontan procedure (cavopulmonary isolation) to connect the inferior vena cava to the pulmonary arteries via either an intra-atrial or external baffle. After **stage III**, all systemic venous return enters the pulmonary circulation directly. Pulmonary venous flow enters the left atrium and is directed across the atrial septum to the tricuspid valve and subsequently to the right (now the systemic) ventricle. Blood leaves the right ventricle via the neoaorta, which supplies the systemic circulation. The old aortic root now attached to the neoaorta provides coronary blood flow. The risks associated with stages II and III are even less than those of stage I; interstage mortality (usually between stages I and II) has been reduced with the use of home monitoring programs. The short- and long-term benefits of using the Norwood vs the Sano procedure remain to be demonstrated.

An alternative therapy is **cardiac transplantation**, either in the immediate neonatal period, thereby obviating stage I of the Norwood procedure, or after a successful stage I Norwood procedure is performed as a bridge to transplantation. After transplantation, patients usually have normal cardiac function and no symptoms of heart failure; however, these patients have the chronic risk of organ rejection and lifelong immunosuppressive therapy (Chapter 437.1). The combination of donor shortage and improved results with standard surgical procedures has caused most centers to stop recommending transplantation except when associated lesions make the Norwood operation an exceptionally high-risk procedure, or for patients who develop poor ventricular function at some time after the standard surgical approach.

PREVENTION

Serial fetal echocardiographic studies demonstrate that in some fetuses, hypoplastic left heart syndrome may be a progressive lesion, beginning with simple valvar aortic stenosis in midgestation. The decreased flow through the stenotic aortic valve reduces flow through the left ventricle during development, resulting in gradual ventricular chamber hypoplasia. The potential for preventing this hypoplasia has been demonstrated by performing in utero aortic balloon valvuloplasty in midgestation fetuses (Fig. 425-13). Early results are encouraging, although even if the aortic valve is successfully opened, adequate ventricular growth occurs in only about 30% of patients. At present, this procedure is regarded as experimental.

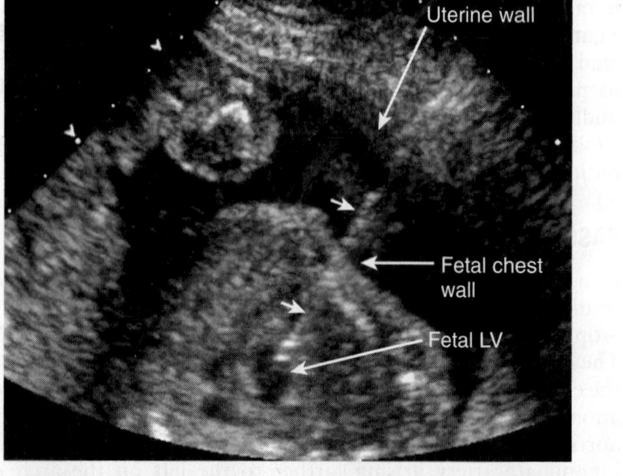

Figure 425-13 Fetal treatment of critical aortic stenosis to prevent development of hypoplastic left heart syndrome. Fetal ultrasound showing insertion of a needle *(arrowheads)* via the maternal abdominal wall, through the uterus and the fetal chest wall, and into the fetal left ventricle (LV). A balloon catheter is next inserted via the needle into the left ventricular chamber and across the stenotic aortic valve. The balloon is inflated to dilate the valve, the catheter and needle are removed. (Courtesy of Dr. Stanton Perry, Stanford University, Stanford, CA.)

BIBLIOGRAPHY

Please visit the Nelson Textbook of Pediatrics *website at www.expertconsult.com for the complete bibliography.*

425.11 Abnormal Positions of the Heart and the Heterotaxy Syndromes (Asplenia, Polysplenia)

Daniel Bernstein

Classification and diagnosis of abnormal cardiac position are best performed via a segmental approach, with the position of the viscera and atria defined first, and then the ventricles, followed by the great vessels. Determination of **visceroatrial situs** can be made by roentgenographic demonstration of the position of the abdominal organs and the tracheal bifurcation for recognition of the right and left bronchi and by echocardiography. The atrial situs is usually similar to the situs of the viscera and lungs. In **situs solitus**, the viscera are in their normal positions (stomach and spleen on the left, liver on the right), the 3-lobed right lung is on the right, and the 2-lobed left lung on the left; the right atrium is on the right, and the left atrium is on the left. When the abdominal organs and lung lobation are reversed, an arrangement known as **situs inversus** occurs, the left atrium is on the right and the right atrium on the left. If the visceroatrial situs cannot be readily determined, a condition known as situs indeterminus or **heterotaxia** exists. The 2 major variations are (1) **asplenia syndrome** (right isomerism or bilateral right-sidedness), which is associated with a centrally located liver, absent spleen, and 2 morphologic right lungs; and (2) **polysplenia syndrome** (left isomerism or bilateral left-sidedness), which is associated with multiple small spleens, absence of the intrahepatic portion of the inferior vena cava, and 2 morphologic left lungs. The heterotaxia syndromes are usually associated with severe congenital heart lesions: ASD, VSD, atrioventricular septal defect, hypoplasia of 1 of the ventricles, pulmonary stenosis or atresia, and anomalous systemic venous or pulmonary venous return (Table 425-2).

The next segment is localization of the ventricles, which depends on the direction of development of the embryonic cardiac loop. Initial protrusion of the loop to the right (d-loop) carries the future right ventricle anteriorly and to the right, whereas the left ventricle remains posterior and on the left. With situs solitus, a d-loop yields normal atrioventricular connections (right atrium connecting to the right ventricle, left atrium to the left ventricle). Protrusion of the loop to the left (l-loop) carries the future right ventricle to the left and the left ventricle to the right. In this case, in the presence of situs solitus, the right atrium connects with the left ventricle and the left atrium with the right ventricle (**ventricular inversion**).

The final segment is that of the great vessels. With each type of cardiac loop, the ventricular-arterial relationships may be regarded as either normal (right ventricle to the pulmonary artery, left ventricle to the aorta) or transposed (right ventricle to the aorta, left ventricle to the pulmonary artery). A further classification can be based on the position of the aorta (normally to the right and posterior) relative to the pulmonary artery. In trans-

Table 425-2 COMPARISON OF CARDIOSPLENIC HETEROTAXY SYNDROMES

FEATURE	ASPLENIA (RIGHT ISOMERISM)	POLYSPLENIA (LEFT ISOMERISM)
Spleen	Absent	Multiple
Sidedness (isomerism)	Bilateral right	Bilateral left
Lungs	Bilateral trilobar with eparterial bronchi	Bilateral bilobar with hyparterial bronchi
Sex	Male (65%)	Female ≥ male
Right-sided stomach	Yes	Less common
Symmetric liver	Yes	Yes
Partial intestinal rotation	Yes	Yes
Dextrocardia (%)	30-40	30-40
Pulmonary blood flow	Decreased (usually)	Increased (usually)
Severe cyanosis	Yes	No
Transposition of great arteries (%)	60-75	15
Total anomalous pulmonary venous return (%)	70-80	Rare
Common atrioventricular valve (%)	80-90	20-40
Single ventricle (%)	40-50	10-15
Absent inferior vena cava with azygos continuation	No	Characteristic
Bilateral superior vena cava	Yes	Yes
Other common defects	PA, PS	Partial anomalous pulmonary venous return, ventricular septal defect, double-outlet right ventricle
Risk of sepsis	Yes	No
Howell-Jolly and Heinz bodies, pitted erythrocytes	Yes	No
Absent gallbladder; biliary atresia	No	Yes

PA, pulmonary atresia; PS, pulmonary stenosis.

position, the aorta is usually anterior and either to the right of the pulmonary artery (**d-transposition**) or to the left (**l-transposition**). These segmental relationships can usually be determined by echocardiographic studies demonstrating both atrioventricular and ventriculoarterial relationships. The clinical manifestations of these syndromes of abnormal cardiac position are determined primarily by their associated cardiovascular anomalies.

Dextrocardia occurs when the heart is in the right side of the chest; **levocardia** (the normal situation) is present when the heart is in the left side of the chest. Dextrocardia without associated situs inversus and levocardia in the presence of situs inversus are most often complicated by other severe cardiac malformations. Surveys of older children and adults indicate that dextrocardia with situs inversus and normally related great arteries ("mirror-image" dextrocardia) is often associated with a functionally normal heart, although congenital heart disease of a less severe nature is common.

Anatomic or functional abnormalities of the lungs, diaphragm, and thoracic cage may result in displacement of the heart to the right (**dextroposition**). In this case, however, the cardiac apex is pointed normally to the left. This anatomic position is less often associated with congenital heart lesions, although hypoplasia of a lung may be accompanied by anomalous pulmonary venous return from that lung (**scimitar syndrome** [Chapter 420.4]).

The electrocardiogram is difficult to interpret in the presence of lesions with discordant atrial, ventricular, and great vessel anatomy. Diagnosis usually requires detailed echocardiographic and sometimes MRI, CT, or cardiac catheterization studies. The prognosis and treatment of patients with one of the cardiac positional anomalies are determined by the underlying defects and are covered in their respective chapters. Asplenia increases the risk of serious infections such as bacterial sepsis and thus requires daily antibiotic prophylaxis. Patients with polysplenia frequently have poor splenic function and may also require prophylaxis against pneumococcal sepsis.

BIBLIOGRAPHY

Please visit the Nelson Textbook of Pediatrics *website at www.expertconsult.com for the complete bibliography.*

Chapter 426
Other Congenital Heart and Vascular Malformations

426.1 Anomalies of the Aortic Arch

Daniel Bernstein

RIGHT AORTIC ARCH

In this abnormality, the aorta curves to the right and, if it descends on the right side of the vertebral column, is usually associated with other cardiac malformations. It is found in 20% of cases of tetralogy of Fallot and is also common in truncus arteriosus. A right aortic arch without other cardiac anomalies is not associated with symptoms. It can often be visualized on the chest roentgenogram. The trachea is deviated slightly to the left of the midline rather than to the right, as in the presence of a normal left arch. On a barium esophagogram, the esophagus is indented on its right border at the level of the aortic arch.

VASCULAR RINGS

Congenital abnormalities of the aortic arch and its major branches result in the formation of vascular rings around the trachea and esophagus with varying degrees of compression (Table 426-1). The origin of these lesions can best be appreciated by reviewing the embryology of the aortic arch (Fig. 414-1). The most common anomalies include (1) double aortic arch (Fig. 426-1A), (2) right aortic arch with a left ligamentum arteriosum, (3) anomalous innominate artery arising farther to the left on the arch than usual, (4) anomalous left carotid artery arising farther to the right than usual and passing anterior to the trachea, and (5) anomalous left pulmonary artery (vascular sling). In the latter anomaly, the abnormal vessel arises from an elongated main pulmonary artery or from the right pulmonary artery. It courses between and compresses the trachea and the esophagus. Associated congenital

Table 426-1 VASCULAR RINGS

LESION	SYMPTOMS	PLAIN FILM	BARIUM SWALLOW	BRONCHOSCOPY	MRI ECHOCARDIOGRAPHY	TREATMENT
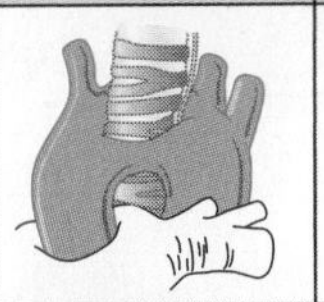 DOUBLE ARCH	Stridor Respiratory distress Swallowing dysfunction Reflex apnea	AP-wider base of heart Lat.-narrowed trachea displaced forward at C3-C4	Bilateral indentation of esophagus	Bilateral tracheal compression-both pulsatile	Diagnostic	Ligate and divide smaller arch (usually left)
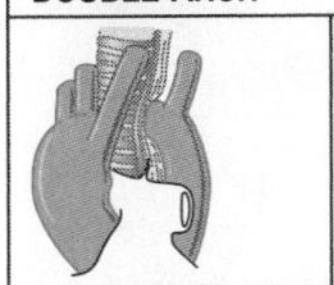 RIGHT ARCH AND LIGAMENTUM/DUCTUE	Respiratory distress Swallowing dysfunction	AP-tracheal deviation to left (right arch)	Bilateral indentation of esophagus R > L	Bilateral tracheal compression-r. pulsatile	Diagnostic	Ligate ligamentum or ductus
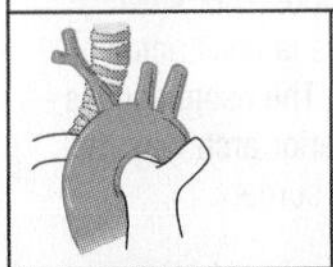 ANOMALOUS INNOMINATE	Cough Stridor Reflex apnea	AP-normal Lat.-anterior tracheal compression	Normal	Pulsatile anterior tracheal compression	Unnecessary	Conservative apnea, then suspend
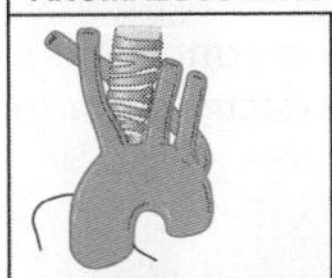 ABERRANT RIGHT SUBCLAVIAN	Occasional swallowing dysfunction	Normal	AP-oblique defect upward to right Lat.-small defect on right posterior wall	Usually normal	Diagnostic	Ligate artery
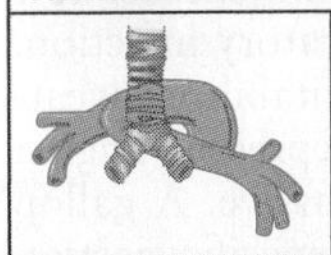 PULMONARY SLING	Expiratory stridor Rrespiratory distress	AP-low l. hilum, r. emphysema/atelectasis Lat.-anterior bowing of right bronchus and trachea	±Anterior indentation above carina between esophagus and trachea	Tracheal displacement to left Compression of right main bronchus	Diagnostic	Detach and reanastornose to main pulmonary artery in front of trachea

AP, anteroposterior; L and l., Left; Lat. Lateral; MRI, magnetic resonance imaging; R and r., right.
From Kliegman RM, Greenbaum LA, Lye PS: *Practical strategies in pediatric diagnosis and therapy*, ed 2, Philadelphia, 2004, Elsevier, p 88.

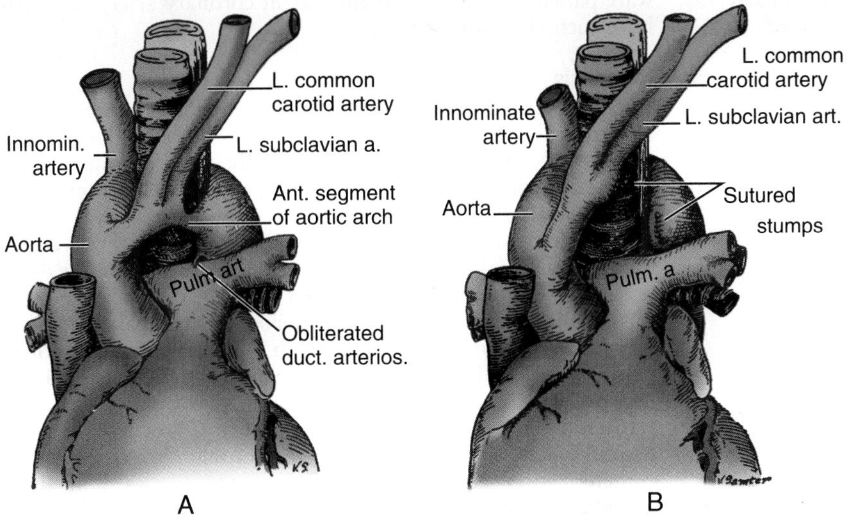

Figure 426-1 Double aortic arch. *A,* Small anterior segment of the double aortic arch (most common type). *B,* Operative procedure for release of the vascular ring.

heart disease may be present in 5-50% of patients, depending on the vascular anomaly.

Clinical Manifestations

If the vascular ring produces compression of the trachea and esophagus, symptoms are frequently present during infancy. Chronic wheezing is exacerbated by crying, feeding, and flexion of the neck. Extension of the neck tends to relieve the noisy respiration. Vomiting may also be a component. Affected infants may have a brassy cough, pneumonia, or rarely, sudden death from aspiration.

Diagnosis

Standard roentgenographic examination is not usually helpful, however, in the past, performing a barium esophagogram was the standard method of diagnosis (Fig. 426-2). Echocardiography in combination with either MRI or CT will usually define the lesion.

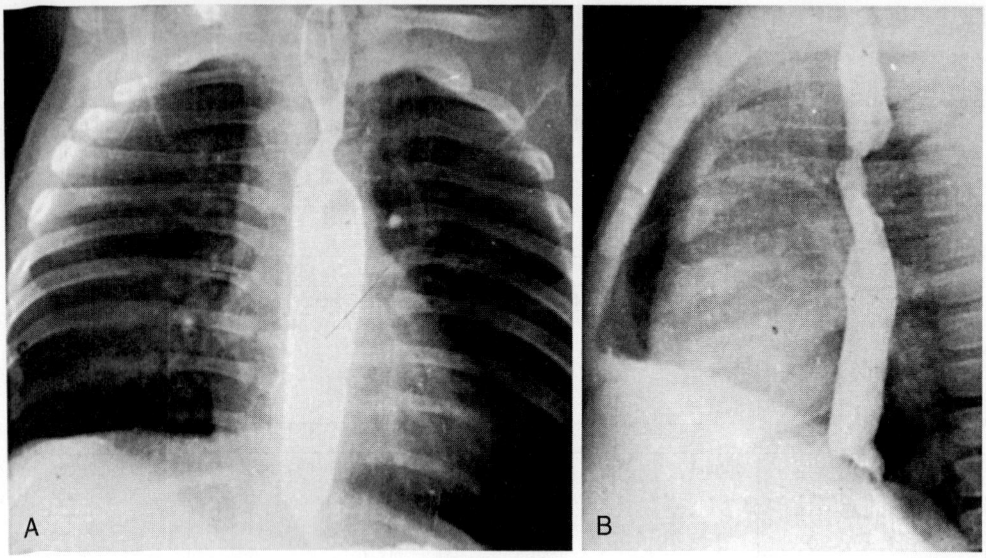

Figure 426-2 Double aortic arch in an infant aged 5 mo. *A,* Anteroposterior view. The barium-filled esophagus is constricted on both sides. *B,* Lateral view. The esophagus is displaced forward. The anterior arch was the smaller and was divided at surgery.

Cardiac catheterization is reserved for cases with associated anomalies or in rare cases where these other modalities are not diagnostic. Bronchoscopy may be helpful in more severe cases to determine the extent of airway narrowing.

Treatment

Surgery is advised for symptomatic patients who have evidence of tracheal compression. The anterior vessel is usually divided in patients with a double aortic arch (see Fig. 426-1B). Compression produced by a right aortic arch and left ligamentum arteriosum is relieved by division of the latter. Anomalous innominate or carotid arteries cannot be divided; attaching the adventitia of these vessels to the sternum usually relieves the tracheal compression. An anomalous left pulmonary artery is corrected by division at its origin and re-anastomosis to the main pulmonary artery after it has been brought in front of the trachea. Severe tracheomalacia, if present, may require reconstruction of the trachea as well.

BIBLIOGRAPHY

Please visit the Nelson Textbook of Pediatrics *website at www.expertconsult.com for the complete bibliography.*

426.2 Anomalous Origin of the Coronary Arteries

Daniel Bernstein

ANOMALOUS ORIGIN OF THE LEFT CORONARY ARTERY FROM THE PULMONARY ARTERY (ALCAPA)

In anomalous origin of the left coronary artery from the pulmonary artery, the blood supply to the left ventricular myocardium is severely compromised. Soon after birth, as pulmonary arterial pressure falls, perfusion pressure to the left coronary artery becomes inadequate; myocardial ischemia, infarction, and fibrosis result. In some cases, interarterial collateral anastomoses develop between the right and left coronary arteries. Blood flow in the left coronary artery is then reversed, and it empties into the pulmonary artery, a condition known as the "myocardial steal" syndrome. The left ventricle becomes dilated, and its performance is decreased. Mitral insufficiency is a frequent complication secondary to a dilated valve ring or infarction of a papillary muscle. Localized aneurysms may also develop in the left ventricular free wall. Occasional patients have adequate myocardial blood flow during childhood and, later in life, a continuous murmur and a small left-to-right shunt via the dilated coronary system (aorta to right coronary to left coronary to pulmonary artery).

Clinical Manifestations

Evidence of heart failure becomes apparent within the 1st few months of life, and may be exacerbated by respiratory infection. Recurrent attacks of discomfort, restlessness, irritability, sweating, dyspnea, and pallor occur and probably represent angina pectoris. Cardiac enlargement is moderate to massive. A gallop rhythm is common. Murmurs may be of the nonspecific ejection type or may be holosystolic due to mitral insufficiency. Older patients with abundant intercoronary anastomoses may have continuous murmurs and minimal left ventricular dysfunction. During adolescence, they may experience angina during exercise. Rare patients with an anomalous right coronary artery may also have such clinical findings.

Diagnosis

Roentgenographic examination confirms the cardiomegaly. The electrocardiogram resembles the pattern described in lateral wall myocardial infarction in adults. A QR pattern followed by inverted T waves is seen in leads I and aVL. The left ventricular surface leads (V_5 and V_6) may also show deep Q waves and exhibit elevated ST segments and inverted T waves (Fig. 426-3). Two-dimensional echocardiography can usually suggest the diagnosis; however, echocardiography is not always reliable in diagnosing this condition. On two-dimensional imaging alone, the left coronary artery may appear as though it is arising from the aorta. Color Doppler ultrasound examination has improved the accuracy of diagnosis of this lesion, demonstrating the presence of retrograde flow in the left coronary artery. CT or MRI may be helpful in confirming the origin of the coronary arteries. Cardiac catheterization is diagnostic; aortography shows immediate opacification of the right coronary artery only. This vessel is large and tortuous. After filling of the intercoronary anastomoses, the left coronary artery is opacified, and contrast can be seen to enter the pulmonary artery. Pulmonary arteriography may also opacify the origin of the anomalous left coronary artery. Selective left ventriculography usually demonstrates a dilated left ventricle that empties poorly and mitral regurgitation.

Treatment and Prognosis

Untreated, death often occurs from heart failure within the 1st 6 mo of life. Those who survive generally have abundant intercoronary collateral anastomoses. Medical management

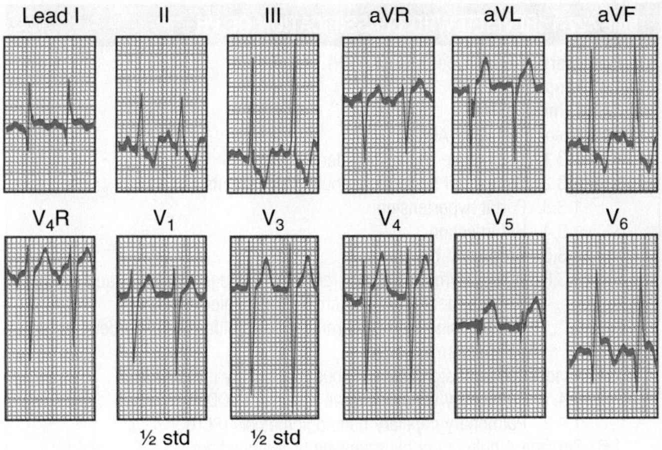

Figure 426-3 Electrocardiogram of a 3 mo old child with anomalous origin of the left coronary artery from the pulmonary artery. Lateral myocardial infarction is present as evidenced by abnormally large and wide Q waves in leads I, V_5, and V_6; an elevated ST segment in V_5 and V_6; and inversion of TV_6.

includes standard therapy for heart failure (diuretics, angiotensin-converting enzyme inhibitors) and for controlling ischemia (nitrates, β-blocking agents).

Surgical treatment consists of detaching the anomalous coronary artery from the pulmonary artery and anastomosing it to the aorta to establish normal myocardial perfusion. A seriously ill infant with a tiny left coronary artery may present a difficult technical problem. In patients who have already sustained a significant myocardial infarction, cardiac transplantation may be the best option (Chapter 437.1).

ANOMALOUS ORIGIN OF THE RIGHT CORONARY ARTERY FROM THE PULMONARY ARTERY

Anomalous origin of the right coronary artery from the pulmonary artery is rarely manifested in infancy or early childhood. The left coronary artery is enlarged, whereas the right is thin-walled and mildly enlarged. In early infancy, perfusion of the right coronary artery is from the pulmonary artery, whereas later, perfusion is from collaterals of the left coronary vessels. Angina and sudden death can occur in adolescence or adulthood. When recognized, this anomaly should be repaired by re-anastomosis of the right coronary artery to the aorta.

ECTOPIC ORIGIN OF THE CORONARY ARTERY FROM THE AORTA WITH ABERRANT PROXIMAL COURSE

In ectopic origin of the coronary artery from the aorta with an aberrant proximal course, the aberrant artery may be a left, right, or major branch coronary artery. The site of origin may be the wrong sinus of Valsalva or a proximal coronary artery. The ostium may be hypoplastic, slitlike, or of normal caliber. The aberrant vessel may pass anteriorly, posteriorly, or between the aorta and right ventricular outflow tract; it may tunnel in the conal or interventricular septal tissue. Obstruction resulting from hypoplasia of the ostia, tunneling between the aorta and right ventricular outflow tract or interventricular septum, and acute angulation produces myocardial infarction. Unobstructed vessels produce no symptoms. Patients with this extremely rare abnormality are often initially seen with severe myocardial infarction, ventricular arrhythmias, angina pectoris, or syncope; sudden death may occur, especially in young athletes.

Diagnostic modalities include an electrocardiogram, stress testing, two-dimensional echocardiography, CT or MRI, radionuclide perfusion scan, and cardiac catheterization with selective coronary angiography.

Treatment is indicated for obstructed vessels and consists of aortoplasty with re-anastomosis of the aberrant vessel or, occasionally, coronary artery bypass grafting. The management of asymptomatic infants with these forms of ectopic coronary origin remains controversial.

BIBLIOGRAPHY

Please visit the Nelson Textbook of Pediatrics *website at www.expertconsult.com for the complete bibliography.*

426.3 Pulmonary Arteriovenous Fistula

Daniel Bernstein

Fistulous vascular communications in the lungs may be large and localized or multiple, scattered, and small. The most common form of this unusual condition is the **Osler-Weber-Rendu syndrome** (hereditary hemorrhagic telangiectasia type I), which is also associated with angiomas of the nasal and buccal mucous membranes, gastrointestinal tract, or liver. Mutations in the endoglin gene, a cell surface component of the transforming growth factor-β receptor complex causes this syndrome. The usual communication is between the pulmonary artery and pulmonary vein; direct communication between the pulmonary artery and left atrium is extremely rare. Desaturated blood in the pulmonary artery is shunted through the fistula into the pulmonary vein, thus bypassing the lungs, and then enters the left side of the heart resulting in systemic arterial desaturation and, sometimes, clinically detectable cyanosis. The shunt across the fistula is at low pressure and resistance, so pulmonary arterial pressure is normal; cardiomegaly and heart failure are not present.

For the full continuation of this chapter, please visit the Nelson Textbook of Pediatrics *website at www.expertconsult.com.*

426.4 Ectopia Cordis

Daniel Bernstein

In the most common thoracic form of ectopia cordis, the sternum is split and the heart protrudes outside the chest. In other forms, the heart protrudes through the diaphragm into the abdominal cavity or may be situated in the neck. Associated intracardiac anomalies are common. **Pentalogy of Cantrell** consists of ectopia cordis, midline supraumbilical abdominal defect, deficiency of the anterior diaphragm, defect of the lower sternum, and an intracardiac defect (either a ventricular septal defect, tetralogy of Fallot or diverticulum of the left ventricle). Death may occur early in life, usually from infection, cardiac failure, or hypoxemia. Surgical therapy for neonates without overwhelmingly severe cardiac anomalies consists of covering the heart with skin without compromising venous return or ventricular ejection. Repair or palliation of associated defects is also necessary.

426.5 Diverticulum of the Left Ventricle

Daniel Bernstein

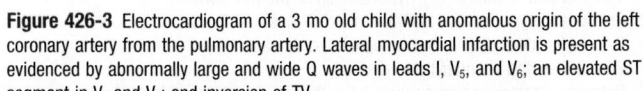

Left ventricular diverticulum is a rare anomaly, where the diverticulum protrudes into the epigastrium. The lesion may be isolated or associated with complex cardiovascular anomalies. A pulsating mass is usually visible and palpable in the epigastrium. Systolic or systolic-diastolic murmurs produced by blood flow into and out of the diverticulum may be audible over the lower part of the sternum and the mass. The electrocardiogram shows a pattern of complete or incomplete left bundle branch block. Roentgenograms of the chest may or may not show the mass. Associated abnormalities include defects of the sternum, abdominal wall, diaphragm, and pericardium (see earlier). Surgical treatment of the diverticulum and associated cardiac defects can be performed in selected cases. Occasionally, a diverticulum may be small and not associated with clinical signs or symptoms. These small diverticula are diagnosed at the time of echocardiographic examination for other indications.

Chapter 427 Pulmonary Hypertension

427.1 Primary Pulmonary Hypertension

Daniel Bernstein

PATHOPHYSIOLOGY

Primary pulmonary hypertension is characterized by pulmonary vascular obstructive disease and right-sided heart failure. It occurs at any age, although in pediatric patients the diagnosis is usually made in adolescence. In older patients, females outnumber males 1.7:1; in younger patients, both genders are represented equally. Some patients have evidence of either an immunologic disorder or a hypercoagulable state. Mutations in the gene for bone morphogenetic protein receptor-2 (BMPR-2, a member of the transforming growth factor-β receptor family) on chromosome 2q33 have been identified in patients with autosomal dominant familial primary pulmonary hypertension (known as *PPH1*). This genetic variant demonstrates a female preponderance and is found in 60% of patients with a family history and up to 25% of patients with sporadic disease. Other potential disease causing genes have been identified, including chromosome 2q31 (PPH2) and 12q13 (ALK1). Viral infection, such as with the vasculotropic human herpesvirus 8 (HHV8), has been suggested as a trigger factor in many patients. Diet pills, particularly fenfluramine, have also been implicated. Pulmonary hypertension is a common complication of sickle cell anemia and other hemolytic anemias. Pulmonary hypertension is associated with precapillary obstruction of the pulmonary vascular bed as a result of hyperplasia of the muscular and elastic tissues and a thickened intima of the small pulmonary arteries and arterioles. Atherosclerotic changes may be found in the larger pulmonary arteries as well. In children, pulmonary veno-occlusive disease may account for some cases of primary pulmonary hypertension. Before a diagnosis of primary pulmonary hypertension can be made, other causes of elevated pulmonary arterial pressure must be eliminated (chronic pulmonary parenchymal disease, persistent obstruction of the upper airway, congenital cardiac malformations, recurrent pulmonary emboli, alveolar capillary dysplasia, liver disease, autoimmune disease, and moyamoya disease). A classification system is noted in Table 427-1. Pulmonary hypertension places an afterload burden on the right ventricle, which results in right ventricular hypertrophy. Dilatation of the pulmonary artery is present, and pulmonary valve insufficiency may occur. In the later stages of the disease, the right ventricle dilates, tricuspid insufficiency develops, and cardiac output is decreased. Arrhythmias, syncope, and sudden death are common.

Table 427-1 REVISED WHO CLASSIFICATION OF PH

1. Pulmonary arterial hypertension (PAH)
   - 1.1. Idiopathic (IPAH)
   - 1.2. Familial (FPAH)
   - 1.3. Associated with (APAH):
     - 1.3.1. Connective tissue disorder
     - 1.3.2. Congenital systemic-to-pulmonary shunts
     - 1.3.3. Portal hypertension
     - 1.3.4. HIV infection
     - 1.3.5. Drugs and toxins
     - 1.3.6. Other (thyroid disorders, glycogen storage disease, Gaucher disease, hereditary hemorrhagic telangiectasia, hemoglobinopathies, chronic myeloproliferative disorders, splenectomy)
   - 1.4. Associated with significant venous or capillary involvement
     - 1.4.1. Pulmonary veno-occlusive disease (PVOD)
     - 1.4.2. Pulmonary capillary hemangiomatosis (PCH)
   - 1.5. Persistent pulmonary hypertension of the newborn
2. Pulmonary hypertension with left heart disease
   - 2.1. Left-sided atrial or ventricular heart disease
   - 2.2. Left-sided valvular heart disease
3. Pulmonary hypertension associated with lung diseases and/or hypoxemia
   - 3.1. Chronic obstructive pulmonary disease
   - 3.2. Interstitial lung disease
   - 3.3. Sleep disordered breathing
   - 3.4. Alveolar hypoventilation disorders
   - 3.5. Chronic exposure to high altitude
   - 3.6. Developmental abnormalities
4. Pulmonary hypertension due to chronic thrombotic and/or embolic disease (CTEPH)
   - 4.1. Thromboembolic obstruction of proximal pulmonary arteries
   - 4.2. Thromboembolic obstruction of distal pulmonary arteries
   - 4.3. Nonthrombotic pulmonary embolism (tumor, parasites, foreign material)
5. Miscellaneous: sarcoidosis, histiocytosis X, lymphangiomatosis, compression of pulmonary vessels (adenopathy, tumor, fibrosing mediastinitis)

From ACCF/AHA: 2009 Expert consensus document on pulmonary hypertension: a report of the American College of Cardiology Foundation Task Force on Expert Consensus Documents and the American Heart Association developed in collaboration with the American College of Chest Physicians; American Thoracic Society, Inc.; and the Pulmonary Hypertension Association, *J Am Coll Cardiol* 53:1573–1619, 2009.

CLINICAL MANIFESTATIONS

The predominant symptoms include exercise intolerance and fatigability; occasionally, precordial chest pain, dizziness, syncope, or headaches are noted. Peripheral cyanosis may be present, especially in patients with a patent foramen ovale through which blood can shunt from right to left; in the late stages of disease, patients may have cold extremities and a gray appearance associated with low cardiac output. Arterial oxygen saturation is usually normal unless there is an associated intracardiac shunt. If right-sided heart failure has supervened, jugular venous pressure is elevated, and hepatomegaly and edema are present. Jugular venous *a* waves are present, and in those with functional tricuspid insufficiency, a conspicuous jugular *cv* wave and systolic hepatic pulsations are manifested. The heart is moderately enlarged, and a right ventricular heave can be noted. The 1st heart sound is often followed by an ejection click emanating from the dilated pulmonary artery. The 2nd heart sound is narrowly split, loud, and sometimes booming in quality; it is frequently palpable at the upper left sternal border. A presystolic gallop rhythm may be audible at the lower left sternal border. The systolic murmur is soft and short and is sometimes followed by a blowing decrescendo diastolic murmur caused by pulmonary insufficiency. In later stages, a holosystolic murmur of tricuspid insufficiency is appreciated at the lower left sternal border.

DIAGNOSIS

Chest roentgenograms reveal a prominent pulmonary artery and right ventricle (Fig. 427-1). The pulmonary vascularity in the hilar areas may be prominent, in contrast to the peripheral lung fields in which pulmonary markings are decreased. The electrocardiogram shows right ventricular hypertrophy, often with spiked P waves. Echocardiography is used to screen for any congenital cardiac malformations. Doppler evaluation of the tricuspid valve, if insufficiency is present, will allow estimation of the right ventricular (and hence pulmonary arterial) systolic pressure.

At cardiac catheterization, the presence of left-sided obstructive lesions (pulmonary venous stenosis, mitral stenosis,

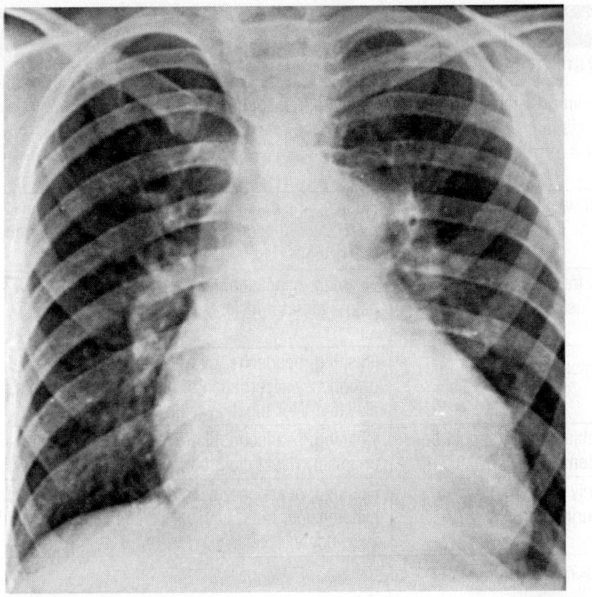

Figure 427-1 Roentgenogram in primary pulmonary hypertension. Note the moderate cardiac enlargement, dilatation of the pulmonary artery, and relative pulmonary undervascularity in the outer two thirds of the lung fields.

restrictive cardiomyopathy) that result in pulmonary venous hypertension can be evaluated (Chapters 421.9, 425.7, and 433.3). The presence of pulmonary arterial hypertension with a normal pulmonary capillary wedge pressure is diagnostic of primary pulmonary hypertension. If the wedge pressure is elevated and left ventricular end-diastolic pressure is normal, obstruction at the level of the pulmonary veins, left atrium, or mitral valve should be suspected. If left ventricular end-diastolic pressure is also elevated, the diagnosis of restrictive cardiomyopathy should be entertained. The risks associated with cardiac catheterization are increased in severely ill patients with primary pulmonary hypertension.

PROGNOSIS AND TREATMENT

Primary pulmonary hypertension is progressive, and no cure is currently available. Some success has been reported with oral calcium channel blocking agents such as nifedipine in children who demonstrate pulmonary vasoreactivity when these agents are administered during catheterization. Continuous intravenous infusion of the arachidonic acid metabolite, prostacyclin (epoprostenol), provides relief as long as the infusion is continued. Despite the success of prostacyclin in reducing symptoms and improving quality of life, it slows but does not stop the progression of the disease. Treprostinil, a prostacyclin analogue with a longer half-life has also been shown to be effective. Continuous administration of nitric oxide via nasal cannula, nebulized forms of prostacyclin (iloprost), and orally administered pulmonary vasodilators (bosentan, an antagonist of endothelin receptors; or sildenafil, a phosphodiesterase type 5 inhibitor) have been used with success in adults, although clinical studies in children are of small numbers (Table 427-2). Anticoagulation may be of value in patients with previous pulmonary thromboemboli, and some of these patients will respond to balloon angioplasty of narrowed pulmonary artery segments. Despite many advances, definitive therapy is still heart-lung or lung transplantation (Chapter 437.2). In patients with severe pulmonary hypertension and low cardiac output, the terminal event is often sudden and related to a lethal arrhythmia. Patients with primary pulmonary hypertension diagnosed in infancy often have rapid progression and high mortality.

427.2 Pulmonary Vascular Disease (Eisenmenger Syndrome)

Daniel Bernstein

PATHOPHYSIOLOGY

The term **Eisenmenger syndrome** refers to patients with a ventricular septal defect in which blood is shunted partially or totally from right to left as a result of the development of pulmonary vascular disease. This physiologic abnormality can also occur with atrioventricular septal defect, ventricular septal defect, patent ductus arteriosus or any other communication between the aorta and pulmonary artery, and in many forms of complex congenital heart disease with unrestricted pulmonary blood flow. Pulmonary vascular disease with an isolated atrial septal defect can occur, but is less common and does not occur until late in adulthood.

In Eisenmenger syndrome, pulmonary vascular resistance after birth either remains high or, after having decreased during early infancy, rises thereafter because of increased shear stress on pulmonary arterioles. Factors playing a role in the rapidity of development of pulmonary vascular disease include increased pulmonary arterial pressure, increased pulmonary blood flow, and the presence of hypoxia or hypercapnia. Early in the course of disease, pulmonary hypertension (elevated pressure in the pulmonary arteries) is the result of markedly increased pulmonary blood flow (hyperkinetic pulmonary hypertension). This form of pulmonary hypertension decreases with the administration of pulmonary vasodilators such as nitric oxide, or oxygen, or both. With the development of Eisenmenger syndrome, pulmonary hypertension is the result of pulmonary vascular disease (obstructive pathologic changes in the pulmonary vessels). This form of pulmonary hypertension is usually only minimally responsive to pulmonary vasodilators or oxygen or not at all.

PATHOLOGY AND PATHOPHYSIOLOGY

The pathologic changes of Eisenmenger syndrome occur in the small pulmonary arterioles and muscular arteries (<300 μm) and are graded on the basis of histologic characteristics (Heath-Edwards classification): **Grade I** changes involve medial hypertrophy alone, **grade II** consists of medial hypertrophy and intimal hyperplasia, **grade III** involves near obliteration of the vessel lumen, **grade IV** includes arterial dilatation, and **grades V and VI** include plexiform lesions, angiomatoid formation, and fibrinoid necrosis. Grades IV-VI indicate irreversible pulmonary vascular obstructive disease. Eisenmenger physiology is usually defined by an absolute elevation in pulmonary arterial resistance to greater than 12 Wood units (resistance units indexed to body surface area) or by a ratio of pulmonary to systemic vascular resistance of ≥1.0.

Pulmonary vascular disease occurs more rapidly in patients with trisomy 21 who have left-to-right shunts. It also complicates the natural history of patients with elevated pulmonary venous pressure secondary to mitral stenosis or left ventricular dysfunction, especially in those patients with restrictive cardiomyopathy (Chapter 439.3). Pulmonary vascular disease can also occur in any patient with transmission of systemic pressure to the pulmonary circulation via a shunt at the interventricular or great vessel level, and in patients chronically exposed to low Po_2 (because of high altitude). Patients with cyanotic congenital heart lesions associated with unrestricted pulmonary blood flow are at particularly high risk.

CLINICAL MANIFESTATIONS

Symptoms do not usually develop until the 2nd or 3rd decade of life, although a more fulminant course may occur. Intracardiac

Table 427-2 SUMMARY OF DRUGS USED TO TREAT PULMONARY HYPERTENSION*

DRUG AND MECHANISM OF ACTION	DOSES USED IN PEDIATRIC STUDIES	COMMON SIDE EFFECTS
Epoprostenol (prostacyclin PGI_2, a potent vasodilator; also inhibits platelet aggregation)	1 ng/kg/min initially. Increase based on clinical course and tolerance to 5-50 ng/kg/min. Some patients may require even higher doses. Must be given by continuous infusion that is not interrupted.	Flushing, headache, nausea, diarrhea, hypotension, chest pain, jaw pain.
Iloprost (synthetic analogue of prostacyclin PGI_2)	2.5-5.0 µg 6-9 times daily (not more frequently than every 2 hr) via inhalation.	Flushing, headache, diarrhea, hypotension, jaw pain, exacerbation of pulmonary symptoms (cough, wheezing).
Treprostinil (synthetic analogue of prostacyclin)	1 ng/kg/min initially. Target dose ranges from 20-80 ng/kg/min. Given either i.v. or s.c. via continuous infusion. Longer half-life than epoprostenol.	Flushing, headache, diarrhea, hypotension, jaw pain. Pain at infusion site when given s.c.
Bosentan (endothelin receptor ET_A and ET_B antagonist)	2 mg/kg/dose BID. Use ½ dose for 1st month and check for LFT abnormalities prior to up-titrating.	Flushing, headache, diarrhea, hypotension, fluid retention, exacerbation of heart failure, anemia, elevated liver function tests, palpitations.
Sildenafil (inhibitor of cGMP specific phosphodiesterase PDE5)	1.0 mg/kg/dose given 3-4 times daily. Initial dosing should be ½ final target dose to evaluate for hypotension.	Flushing, headache, diarrhea, myalgia, hypotension, priapism, visual disturbance (blue coloration).
Calcium channel blockers (e.g., diltiazem, nifedipine)	Previously widely used. Now indicated only for patients who show a strong response to nitric oxide during cardiac catheterization.	Flushing, headache, edema, arrhythmia, headache, hypotension, rash, nausea, constipation, elevated liver function tests.

*These medications should only be administered under the direction of a specialist in pulmonary hypertension.

or extracardiac communications that would normally shunt from left to right are converted to right-to-left shunting as pulmonary vascular resistance exceeds systemic vascular resistance. Cyanosis becomes apparent, and dyspnea, fatigue, and a tendency toward dysrhythmias begin to occur. In the late stages of the disease, heart failure, chest pain, headaches, syncope, and hemoptysis may be seen. Physical examination reveals a right ventricular heave and a narrowly split 2nd heart sound with a loud pulmonic component. Palpable pulmonary artery pulsation may be present at the left upper sternal border. A holosystolic murmur of tricuspid regurgitation may be audible along the left sternal border. An early decrescendo diastolic murmur of pulmonary insufficiency may also be heard along the left sternal border. The degree of cyanosis depends on the stage of the disease.

DIAGNOSIS

Roentgenographically, the heart varies in size from normal to greatly enlarged; the latter usually occurs late in the course of the disease. The main pulmonary artery is generally prominent, similar to primary pulmonary hypertension (see Fig. 427-1). The pulmonary vessels are enlarged in the hilar areas and taper rapidly in caliber in the peripheral branches. The right ventricle and atrium are prominent. The electrocardiogram shows marked right ventricular hypertrophy. The P wave may be tall and spiked. Cyanotic patients have various degrees of polycythemia that depend on the severity and duration of hypoxemia.

The echocardiogram shows a thick-walled right ventricle and demonstrates the underlying congenital heart lesion. Two-dimensional echocardiography assists in eliminating from consideration lesions such as obstructed pulmonary veins, supramitral membrane, mitral stenosis, and restrictive cardiomyopathy. Doppler studies demonstrate the direction of the intracardiac shunt and the presence of a typical hypertension waveform in the main pulmonary artery. Tricuspid and pulmonary regurgitation can be used in the Doppler examination to estimate pulmonary arterial systolic and diastolic pressures.

Cardiac catheterization usually shows a bidirectional shunt at the site of the defect. Systolic pressure is generally equal in the systemic and pulmonary circulations. Pulmonary capillary wedge pressure is normal unless a left-sided heart obstructive lesion or left ventricular failure is the cause of the pulmonary arterial hypertension. Arterial oxygen saturation is decreased depending on the magnitude of the right-to-left shunt. The response to vasodilator therapy (oxygen, prostacyclin, nitric oxide) may identify patients with hyperdynamic pulmonary hypertension. Selective pulmonary artery injections may be necessary if pulmonary venous obstruction is suspected because of high wedge pressure and low left ventricular end-diastolic pressure.

TREATMENT

The best management for patients who are at risk for the development of late pulmonary vascular disease is prevention by early surgical elimination of large intracardiac or great vessel communications during infancy. Some patients may be missed because they have not shown early clinical manifestations. Rarely, pulmonary vascular resistance never decreases at birth in these infants, and therefore they never acquire enough left-to-right shunting to become clinically apparent. Such delayed recognition is a particular risk in patients with congenital heart disease who live at high altitude. It is also a risk in infants with trisomy 21, who have a propensity for earlier development of pulmonary vascular disease. Because of the high incidence of congenital heart disease associated with trisomy 21, routine echocardiography is recommended at the time of initial diagnosis, even in the absence of other clinical findings.

Medical treatment of Eisenmenger syndrome is primarily symptomatic. Many patients benefit substantially from either oral (calcium channel blocker, endothelin antagonist, phosphodiesterase inhibitors) or chronic intravenous (prostacyclin) therapy. Combined heart-lung or bilateral lung transplantation is the only surgical option for many of these patients (Chapter 437.2).

BIBLIOGRAPHY

Please visit the Nelson Textbook of Pediatrics *website at* *www.expertconsult.com* *for the complete bibliography.*

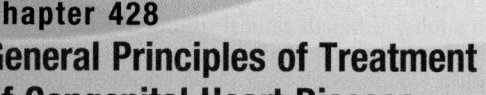

Chapter 428
General Principles of Treatment of Congenital Heart Disease

Daniel Bernstein

Most patients who have mild congenital heart disease require no treatment. The parents and child should be made aware that a normal life is expected and that no restriction of the child's activities is necessary. Overprotective parents may use the presence of a mild congenital heart lesion or even a functional heart murmur as a means to exert excessive control over their child's activities. Although fears may not be expressed overtly, the child may become anxious regarding early death or debilitation, especially when an adult member of the family acquires unrelated symptomatic heart disease. The family may have an unexpressed fear of sudden death, and the rarity of this manifestation should be emphasized in discussions directed at improving their understanding of the child's congenital heart defect. The difference between congenital heart disease and degenerative coronary disease in adults should be emphasized. General health maintenance, including a well-balanced, "heart-healthy" diet; aerobic exercise; and avoidance of smoking, should be encouraged.

Even patients with moderate to severe heart disease need not be markedly restricted in physical activity. **Physical education** should be modified appropriately to the child's capacity to participate. The extent of such modification can generally be determined best by formal exercise testing. Competitive sports for many of these patients is discouraged, but decisions are usually made on an individual basis. Patients with severe heart disease and decreased exercise tolerance usually tend to limit their own activities. Dyspnea, headache, and fatigability in cyanotic patients may be a sign of increasing hypoxemia and may require limitation of activity in those for whom specific medical or surgical treatment is not available. **Routine immunizations** should be given, with the inclusion of influenza vaccine during the appropriate season; patients who might be considered candidates for heart or heart-lung transplantation should not receive live-virus vaccinations just before transplantation.

Bacterial infections should be treated vigorously, but the presence of congenital heart disease is not an appropriate reason to use antibiotics indiscriminately. Prophylaxis against infective endocarditis should be carried out during dental procedures for appropriate patients. The American Heart Association has recently significantly revised these recommendations, with most patients no longer requiring routine prophylaxis (Chapter 431).

Cyanotic patients need to be monitored for a multitude of noncardiac manifestations of oxygen deficiency (Table 428-1). Treatment of iron deficiency anemia is important in cyanotic patients, who will show improved exercise tolerance and general well-being with adequate hemoglobin levels. These patients should also be carefully observed for excessive polycythemia. Cyanotic patients should avoid situations in which dehydration may occur, which leads to increased viscosity and increases the risk of stroke. Diuretics may need to be decreased or temporarily discontinued during episodes of acute gastroenteritis. High altitudes and sudden changes in the thermal environment should also be avoided. Phlebotomy with partial exchange transfusion is carried out only in symptomatic patients with severe **polycythemia** (usually those hematocrit >65%). Patients with moderate to severe forms of congenital heart disease or a history of rhythm disturbance should be carefully monitored during anesthesia for even routine surgical procedures. Consultation with an anesthesiologist experienced in the care of children with congenital heart disease is encouraged. Women with nonrepaired severe congenital heart disease should be counseled on the risks associated with childbearing and on the use of contraceptives and tubal ligation. Pregnancy may be dangerous for patients with chronic cyanosis or pulmonary arterial hypertension. Women with mild to moderate heart disease and many of those who have had corrective surgery can have normal pregnancies, although those with residual hemodynamic derangements or with systemic right ventricles should optimally be followed by a high-risk perinatologist and a cardiologist with expertise in caring for adults with congenital heart disease.

Table 428-1 EXTRACARDIAC COMPLICATIONS OF CYANOTIC CONGENITAL HEART DISEASE AND EISENMENGER PHYSIOLOGY

PROBLEM	ETIOLOGY	THERAPY
Polycythemia	Persistent hypoxia	Phlebotomy
Relative anemia	Nutritional deficiency	Iron replacement
CNS abscess	Right-to-left shunting	Antibiotics, drainage
CNS thromboembolic stroke	Right-to-left shunting or polycythemia	Phlebotomy
Low-grade DIC, thrombocytopenia	Polycythemia	None for DIC unless bleeding, then phlebotomy
Hemoptysis	Pulmonary infarct, thrombosis, or rupture of pulmonary artery plexiform lesion	Embolization
Gum disease	Polycythemia, gingivitis, bleeding	Dental hygiene
Gout	Polycythemia, diuretic agent	Allopurinol
Arthritis, clubbing	Hypoxic arthropathy	None
Pregnancy complications: abortion, fetal growth retardation, prematurity increase, maternal illness	Poor placental perfusion, poor ability to increase cardiac output	Bed rest, pregnancy prevention counseling
Infections	Associated asplenia, DiGeorge syndrome, endocarditis	Antibiotics
	Fatal RSV pneumonia with pulmonary hypertension	Ribavirin; RSV immunoglobulin (prevention)
Failure to thrive	Increased oxygen consumption, decreased nutrient intake	Treat heart failure; correct defect early; increase caloric intake
Psychosocial adjustment	Limited activity, cyanotic appearance, chronic disease, multiple hospitalizations	Counseling

CNS, central nervous system; DIC, disseminated intravascular coagulation; RSV, respiratory syncytial virus.

POSTOPERATIVE MANAGEMENT

After successful open heart surgery, the severity of the congenital heart defect, the age and condition (nutritional status) of the patient before surgery, the events in the operating room, and the quality of the postoperative care influence the patient's course. Intraoperative factors that influence survival and that should be noted when a patient returns from the operating room include the duration of cardiopulmonary bypass, the duration of aortic cross-clamping (the time during which the heart is not being perfused), and the duration of profound hypothermia (used in some newborns: the period during which the entire body is not being perfused).

Immediate postoperative care should be provided in an intensive care unit staffed by a team of physicians, nurses, and technicians experienced with the unique problems encountered after open heart surgery in childhood. In most major centers, this occurs in a dedicated pediatric cardiovascular intensive care unit. Preparation for postoperative monitoring begins in the operating room, where the anesthesiologist or surgeon places an arterial catheter to allow direct arterial pressure measurements and arterial sampling for blood gas determination. A central venous catheter is also placed for measuring central venous pressure and for infusions of cardioactive medications. In more complex cases, right or left atrial or pulmonary artery catheters may be inserted directly into these cardiac structures and used for pressure monitoring purposes. Flow-directed thermodilution monitoring (Swan-Ganz) catheters are sometimes used for monitoring pulmonary capillary wedge pressure and the cardiac index, although this modality is not commonly used in children. Temporary pacing wires are placed on the atrium or ventricle, or both, in case temporary postoperative heart block occurs. Transcutaneous oximetry provides for continuous monitoring of arterial oxygen saturation.

Functional failure of one organ system may cause profound physiologic and biochemical changes in another. Respiratory insufficiency, for example, leads to hypoxia, hypercapnia and acidosis, which, in turn, compromise cardiac, vascular, and renal function. The latter problems cannot be managed successfully until adequate ventilation is re-established. Thus, it is essential that the primary source of each postoperative problem be identified and treated.

Respiratory failure is a serious postoperative complication encountered after open heart surgery. Cardiopulmonary bypass carried out in the presence of pulmonary congestion results in decreased lung compliance, copious tracheal and bronchial secretions, atelectasis, and increased breathing effort. Because fatigue and, subsequently, hypoventilation and acidosis may rapidly ensue, mechanical positive pressure endotracheal ventilation may be continued after open heart surgery for a minimum of several hours in relatively stable patients and for up to 2-3 days or longer in severely ill patients, especially infants. Patients with certain congenital heart lesions, particularly those with DiGeorge syndrome, may also have airway abnormalities (micrognathia, tracheomalacia, bronchomalacia) that can make extubation more difficult.

The electrocardiogram should be monitored continuously during the postoperative period. A change in heart rate, even without arrhythmia, may be the first indication of a serious complication such as hemorrhage, hypothermia, hypoventilation, or heart failure. **Cardiac rhythm disorders** must be diagnosed quickly because a prolonged untreated arrhythmia may add a severe hemodynamic burden to the heart in the critical early postoperative period (Chapter 429). Injury to the heart's conduction system during surgery can result in postoperative complete heart block. This complication is usually temporary and is treated with surgically placed pacing wires that can later be removed. Occasionally, complete heart block is permanent. If heart block persists beyond 10-14 days postoperatively, insertion of a permanent pacemaker is required. Tachyarrhythmias are a common problem in postoperative patients. Junctional ectopic tachycardia (JET) can be a particularly troublesome rhythm to manage (Chapter 429), although it usually responds to intravenous amiodarone.

Heart failure with poor cardiac output after cardiac surgery may be secondary to respiratory failure, serious arrhythmias, myocardial injury, blood loss, hypovolemia, a significant residual hemodynamic abnormality, or any combination of these factors. Treatment specific to the cause should be instituted. Catecholamines, phosphodiesterase inhibitors, nitroprusside and other afterload-reducing agents, and diuretics are the cardioactive agents most often used in patients with myocardial dysfunction in the early postoperative period (Chapter 436). Postoperative pulmonary hypertension can be managed with hyperventilation and inhaled nitric oxide. In patients who are unresponsive to standard pharmacologic treatment, various ventricular assist devices are available, depending on the patient's size. If pulmonary function is adequate, a left ventricular assist device (LVAD) may be used. If pulmonary function is inadequate, extracorporeal membrane oxygenation (ECMO) may be used. These extraordinary measures are helpful in maintaining the circulation until cardiac function improves, usually within 2-3 days. They have also been used with moderate success as a bridge to transplantation in patients with severe nonremitting postoperative cardiac failure.

Acidosis secondary to low cardiac output, renal failure, or hypovolemia must be prevented or if present, promptly corrected. Serial monitoring of arterial blood gases and lactate concentrations is performed. An arterial pH <7.3 may result in a decrease in cardiac output with an increase in lactic acid production and may be the forerunner of arrhythmias or cardiac arrest.

Renal function may be compromised by congestive heart failure and further impaired by prolonged cardiopulmonary bypass. Blood and fluid replacement, cardiac inotropic agents, and vasodilators will usually re-establish normal urine flow in patients with hypovolemia or cardiac failure. Renal failure secondary to tubular injury may require temporary peritoneal or hemodialysis or hemofiltration.

Neurologic abnormalities can develop after cardiopulmonary bypass, especially in the neonatal period. Seizures may occur when the patient awakens from sedation and can usually be controlled with anticonvulsant medications. In the absence of other neurologic signs, self-limited isolated seizures in the immediate postoperative period usually carry a good long-term prognosis. Thromboembolism and stroke are rarer but serious complications of open heart surgery. In the long term, both subtle and more substantial learning disabilities may develop. Patients who have undergone surgery entailing the use of cardiopulmonary bypass, especially in the newborn period, should be watched carefully during their early school years for signs of mild to moderate learning disabilities, which are often amenable to early remedial intervention. The risk is higher in patients who have undergone repair using hypothermic total circulatory arrest than in those where systemic blood flow is maintained using cardiopulmonary bypass.

The **postpericardiotomy syndrome** may occur toward the end of the 1st postoperative week or may sometimes be delayed until weeks or months after surgery. This febrile illness is characterized by fever, decreased appetite, listlessness, nausea, and vomiting. Chest pain is not always present, so a high index of suspicion should be maintained in any recently postoperative patient. Echocardiography is diagnostic. In most instances, the postpericardiotomy syndrome is self-limited; however, when pericardial fluid accumulates rapidly, the potential danger of cardiac tamponade should be recognized (Chapter 434). Rarely, arrhythmias may also occur. Symptomatic patients usually respond to salicylates or indomethacin and bed rest. Occasionally, steroid therapy or pericardiocentesis is required. Late recurrences can occur but are less usual.

Hemolysis of mechanical origin is seen, although rarely, after repair of certain cardiac defects, for example, atrioventricular septal defects (AVSDs), or after the insertion of a mechanical prosthetic valve. It is due to unusual turbulence of blood at increased pressure. Reoperation may be necessary in rare patients with severe and progressive hemolysis who require frequent blood transfusions, but in most instances the problem slowly regresses.

Infection is another potentially serious postoperative problem. Patients usually receive a broad-spectrum antibiotic for the initial postoperative period. Potential sites of infection include the lungs (generally related to postoperative atelectasis), the subcutaneous tissues at the incision site, the sternum, and the urinary tract (especially after an indwelling catheter has been in place). Sepsis with infective endocarditis is an infrequent complication, and can be difficult to manage, especially if prosthetic material was placed at the time of surgery (Chapter 431).

LONG-TERM MANAGEMENT

Patients who have undergone surgery for congenital heart disease can be divided into several major categories: (1) lesions for which total repair has been achieved; (2) lesions for which both anatomic and physiologic correction has been achieved; and (3) lesions for which only palliation, albeit potentially long-term, has been achieved. There is some disagreement among cardiologists as to exactly which categories a particular congenital heart lesion might fall, and to some degree every case should be considered individually. Many argue that only for isolated patent ductus arteriosus is total repair really achieved, with no requirement for long-term follow-up. Patients who are able to undergo anatomic and physiologic correction include many of the left-to-right shunt lesions (atrial and ventricular septal defects) and milder forms of obstructive lesions (e.g., valvar pulmonic stenosis, some forms of valvar aortic stenosis, and coarctation of the aorta), and some forms of

cyanotic heart disease, for example, uncomplicated tetralogy of Fallot and simple transposition of the great arteries. These patients usually have achieved total or near-total physiologic correction of their lesion; however, they are still at some risk of long-term sequelae, including late heart failure or arrhythmia, or recurrence of a significant physiologic abnormality (e.g., recoarctation of the aorta, worsening mitral regurgitation in patients with AVSDs, or long-standing pulmonary regurgitation in patients with tetralogy of Fallot repaired with a transannular patch). These patients require regular follow-up with a pediatric cardiologist (and when old enough, with an adult congenital heart disease specialist [Chapter 428.1]), however, their long-term prognosis is generally very good. Patients with more complex lesions, such as those with single ventricle physiology, are at much higher risk of long-term sequelae and require even closer follow-up. These patients, particularly those who have undergone the Fontan procedure, are at risk long-term for arrhythmia, thrombosis, protein losing enteropathy, end-organ (especially hepatic) dysfunction, and heart failure. Some may eventually require cardiac transplantation.

Physical limitations are variable, ranging from minimal to none in patients with physiologic correction, to mild to moderate in patients with palliative procedures. The extent to which a patient should be allowed to participate in athletics, both recreational and competitive, can best be determined by the cardiologist, often with the assistance of the data that can be derived from cardiopulmonary exercise testing (Chapter 417.5).

Long-term morbidities affecting neurologic function and behavior are influenced by many factors, including the effects of any genetic alterations on the developing central nervous system. Data suggest a greater role for prenatal central nervous system abnormalities (anatomic or secondary to alterations in cerebral blood flow or oxygenation) than previously suspected; these include microcephaly, cerebral atrophy, altered cerebral biochemistry (lactate, choline, *N*-acetylaspartate) average diffusivity, and fractional anisotropy of white matter tracts. Chronic hypoxemia and failure to thrive also may influence the developing brain, and there is evidence that the type of intervention required (cardiopulmonary bypass, hypothermic total circulatory arrest, catheter-based therapy) plays a substantial role. In general, in the absence of a significant genetic syndrome or major perioperative complication, most children function at a fairly high level after repair of congenital heart defects and are able to attend regular school. Group mean scores on standard cognitive tests are not different from the general population; however, some areas appear to be more at risk than others, including certain aspects of motor function, speech, visual-motor tracking, and phonological awareness. Awareness of these potential issues is critical to obtaining prompt remedial assistance if a child is found to be struggling in school.

BIBLIOGRAPHY

Please visit the Nelson Textbook of Pediatrics *website at www.expertconsult.com for the complete bibliography.*

428.1 Congenital Heart Disease in Adults

Michael G. Earing

The advent of cardiac surgical procedures such as ligation of patent ductus arteriosus, resection of coarctation of aorta, and the Blalock-Taussig shunt, as well as advances in diagnostic, interventional, and critical care skills have resulted in survival of approximately 90% of children with congenital heart disease to adulthood. More adults than children are living with congenital heart disease in the USA, with a 5% increase every year.

LONG-TERM MEDICAL CONSIDERATIONS

About 25% of adults with congenital heart disease have a mild form that has allowed them to survive into adulthood without surgical or interventional cardiac catheterization. The most common lesions in this category include mild aortic valve stenosis (usually in setting of bicuspid aortic valve), small restrictive ventricular septal defects, mild pulmonary valve stenosis, and mitral valve prolapse (Table 428-2). These patients need less frequent follow-up to assess for progression of disease and to identify associated complications. The majority of adults with congenital heart disease living in the USA are patients who have had previous intervention (Table 428-3). Although the majority of children who undergo surgical intervention will survive to adulthood, with few exceptions, "total correction" is not the rule. The few exceptions include patent ductus arteriosus, ventricular septal defects, and atrial septal defects; this is true only if they are closed early before the development of irreversible pulmonary vascular changes and no residual lesions exist. Because adult patients with congenital heart disease are surviving longer than ever, it is becoming increasingly apparent that even the simplest lesions can be associated with long-term complications. These long-term complications include both cardiac and noncardiac problems (Tables 428-4 and 428-5, Fig. 428-1). Cardiac complications include arrhythmias and conduction defects, ventricular dysfunction, residual shunts, valvular lesions (regurgitation and stenosis), hypertension, and aneurysms. Noncardiac sequelae include developmental abnormalities such as developmental delay, somatic abnormalities such as facial dysmorphism (cleft palate/lip), central nervous abnormalities such as seizure disorders from previous thromboembolic events or cerebrovascular accidents, disturbances of the senses such as hearing loss or vision loss, and pulmonary sequelae such as both restrictive and obstructive lung disease. Psychosocial problems involving employment, life and health insurance, participation in sports, sexual activity, and contraception are common. As result of these long-term complications, the majority of adults with congenital heart disease need lifelong follow-up.

Table 428-2 CONGENITAL HEART DEFECTS ASSOCIATED WITH SURVIVAL INTO ADULTHOOD WITHOUT SURGERY OR INTERVENTIONAL CARDIAC CATHETERIZATION

Mild pulmonary valve stenosis
Bicuspid aortic valve
Small to moderate size atrial septal defect
Small ventricular septal defect
Small patent ductus arteriosus
Mitral valve prolapse
Partial atrioventricular canal (ostium primum atrial septal defect and cleft mitral valve)
Marfan syndrome
Ebstein anomaly
Congenitally corrected transposition (atrioventricular & ventriculoarterial discordance)

Table 428-3 MOST COMMON CONGENITAL HEART DEFECTS SURVIVING TO ADULTHOOD AFTER SURGERY OR INTERVENTIONAL CATHETERIZATION

Aortic valve disease following balloon valvuloplasty or surgical valvotomy
Pulmonary valve stenosis following balloon valvuloplasty or surgical valvotomy
Tetralogy of Fallot
Ventricular septal defect
Completer atrioventricular canal
Transposition of the great arteries
Coarctation of the aorta
Complex single ventricles after the modified Fontan procedure

SPECIFIC LESIONS

Left-to-Right Shunts

If the shunt is large and nonrestrictive (allowing transmission of near systemic pressure to the pulmonary arteries), irreversible

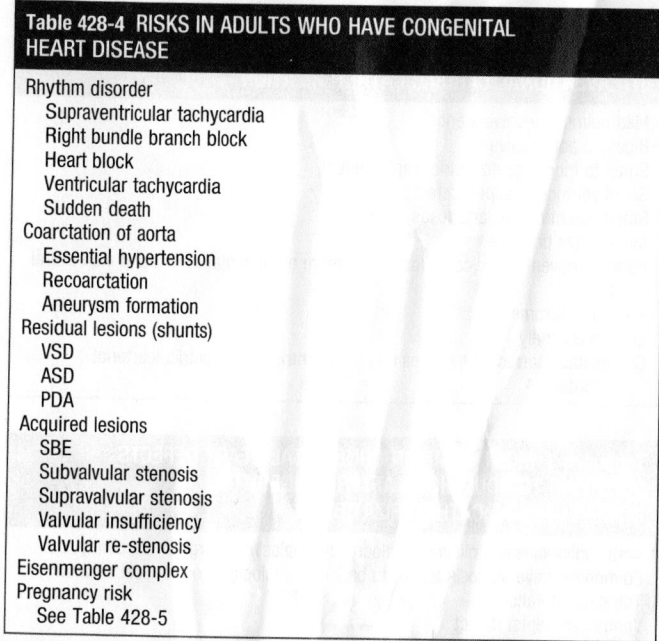

Table 428-4 RISKS IN ADULTS WHO HAVE CONGENITAL HEART DISEASE

- Rhythm disorder
  - Supraventricular tachycardia
  - Right bundle branch block
  - Heart block
  - Ventricular tachycardia
  - Sudden death
- Coarctation of aorta
  - Essential hypertension
  - Recoarctation
  - Aneurysm formation
- Residual lesions (shunts)
  - VSD
  - ASD
  - PDA
- Acquired lesions
  - SBE
  - Subvalvular stenosis
  - Supravalvular stenosis
  - Valvular insufficiency
  - Valvular re-stenosis
- Eisenmenger complex
- Pregnancy risk
  - See Table 428-5

ASD, atrial septal defect; PDA, patent ductus arteriosus; SBE, subacute bacterial endocarditis; VSD, ventricular septal defect.

Table 428-5 LESION SPECIFIC RISKS OF MATERNAL AND NEONATAL COMPLICATIONS OF PREGNANCY

No additional risk	Small septal defects
	Surgically closed ASD, VSD, PDA
	Mild to moderate aortic regurgitation
	Mild to moderate pulmonary stenosis
Slightly increased risk	Postoperative repair of tetralogy of Fallot
	Transposition of the great arteries, s/p arterial switch procedure
Moderate risk	Transposition of the great arteries, s/p atrial switch procedure
	Congenitally corrected transposition of the great arteries
	Single ventricle physiology, s/p Fontan procedure
Severe risk	Cyanotic congenital heart disease, unoperated or palliated
	Marfan syndrome
	Prosthetic valves
	Obstructive lesions including coarctation
Pregnancy contraindicated	Severe pulmonary hypertension
	Severe obstructive lesions
	Marfan syndrome, aortic root >40 mm

ASD, atrial septal defect; PDA, patent ductus arteriosus; s/p, status post (after); VSD, ventricular septal defect.

pulmonary vascular changes can occur, resulting in pulmonary hypertension at systemic levels with reversed or bidirectional shunting at the level of the defect (Eisenmenger syndrome) (Chapter 427.2).

Atrial Septal Defects (ASDs) (Chapter 420.1)

Although, most individuals with an ASD are diagnosed during childhood after a murmur is noted, a minority of patients present with symptoms for the first time as adults. Most patients are asymptomatic during the 1st and 2nd decades of life. In the 3rd decade, an increasing number of patients then develop exercise intolerance, palpitations due to atrial arrhythmias, and cardiac enlargement on chest x-ray. While survival into adulthood is the rule, life expectancy is not normal and there is significant

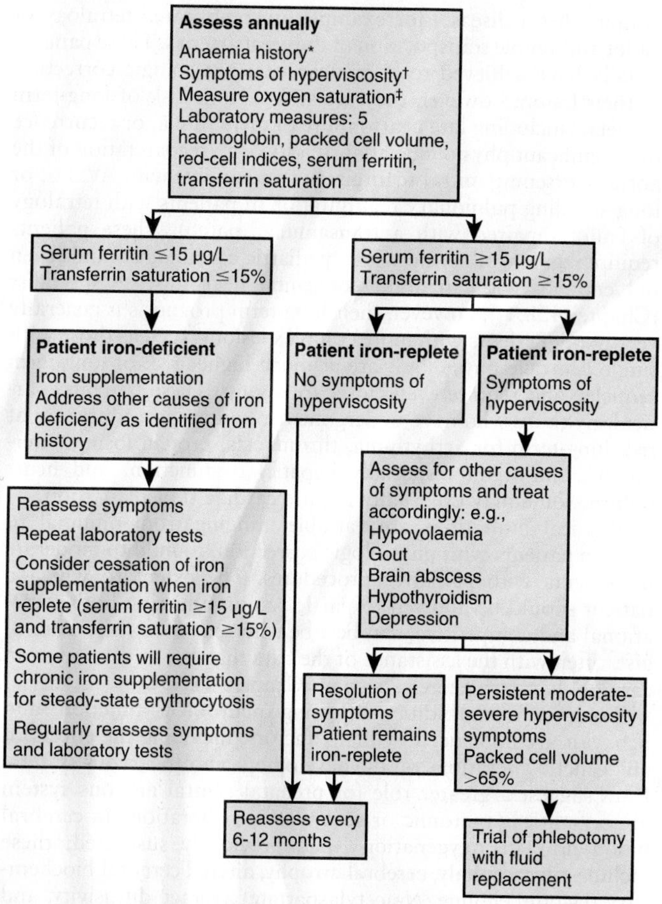

Figure 428-1 Important issues that are crucial to address at time of transition. (From Spence MS, Balaratnam MS, Gatzoulis MA: Clinical update: cyanotic adult congenital heart disease, *Lancet* 370:1530–1532, 2007, p 1531.)

long-term morbidity. After the age of 40 yr, the mortality rate increases by 6% per year, and more than 20% of patients will have developed atrial fibrillation. By age 60 yr, the number of patients with atrial fibrillation will have increased to more than 60%.

LATE OUTCOME FOLLOWING CLOSURE OF ASD Most patients who have undergone early closure of a defect will have excellent long-term survival with low morbidity if repair is undertaken before age 25 yr. Older age of repair is associated with decreased late survival with an associated increased risk for the development of atrial arrhythmias, thromboembolic event, and pulmonary hypertension.

Long-term late complications and survival following transcatheter device closure remain unknown.

Ventricular Septal Defects (VSDs) (Chapter 420.6)

Although isolated VSDs are one of the most common forms of congenital heart disease, the diagnosis of a VSD in an adult is rare. The primary reason for this is that most patients with a hemodynamically significant VSD will have undergone repair in childhood or will have died earlier in life. As result, the spectrum of isolated VSD in adults is limited to (1) those with small restrictive defects, (2) those with Eisenmenger syndrome, and (3) those who had their defects closed in childhood.

For patients with small restrictive VSD, the long-term survival is excellent with estimated 25-yr survival of 96%. In addition, the long-term morbidity for patients with a restrictive VSD also appears to be low. Their clinical course is not completely benign. Reported long-term complications include endocarditis, progressive aortic regurgitation secondary to prolapse of aortic valve into the defect (highest risk is with supracristal type, but also can

occur in setting of perimembranous defect), and the development of both right and left outflow tract obstruction from a double chamber right ventricle or a subaortic membrane.

For those patients who develop Eisenmenger syndrome, survival into the 3rd decade is common. With increasing age, the long-term complications of right heart failure, paradoxical emboli, and erythrocytosis usually result in progressive decline in survival, with an average age of death of 37 yr.

Adults with previous VSD closure, without pulmonary hypertension or residual defects, live a normal life expectancy.

Because patients with small VSDs are asymptomatic, these patients should be managed conservatively. Given the long-term risks, they do need intermittent follow-up for life to monitor for the development of late complications. The exception to this rule is patients with small supracristal or perimembranous VSD with associated prolapse of the aortic cusp into the defect resulting in progressive aortic regurgitation. These patients should be considered for surgical repair at the time of diagnosis to prevent progressive aortic valve damage.

Complete Atrioventricular Canal (Chapter 420.5)

The natural history for patients with complete AVSD is characterized by the early development of pulmonary vascular disease, leading to irreversible damage often by age 1 yr (especially in children with Down syndrome). Surgery needs to be undertaken early if it is to be successful. Thus, patients who present in adulthood can be categorized into two groups (1) those with Eisenmenger syndrome or (2) those who had their defects closed in childhood.

Overall, for those patients who underwent early repair before the development of pulmonary vascular disease, the long-term prognosis is good. The most common long-term complication is left AV valve regurgitation, with approximately 5-10% of patients requiring surgical revision for left AV valve repair or replacement during follow-up. The second most common long-term complication for this patient group is subaortic stenosis, occurring in up to 5% of patients after repair. Other long-term complications include residual atrial or ventricular level shunts, complete heart block, atrial and ventricular arrhythmias, and endocarditis.

For those patients who have developed Eisenmenger syndrome, all are symptomatic with exertional dyspnea, fatigue, palpitations, edema, and syncope. Survival is similar to other forms of Eisenmenger syndrome, with a mean age of death of 37 yr. Strong predictors for death in retrospective studies include syncope, age at presentation of symptoms, poor functional class, low oxygen saturation (<85%), serum creatinine, serum uric acid concentration, and Down syndrome.

Patients who underwent previous repair with significant left AV valve regurgitation causing symptoms, atrial arrhythmias, or deterioration in ventricular function should undergo elective repair or replacement. Those previously repaired patients who develop significant subaortic stenosis (defined as a peak cardiac catheterization or echo gradient of >50 mm Hg) should undergo surgical repair.

Patent Ductus Arteriosus (PDA) (Chapter 420.8)

A PDA is usually an isolated lesion in the adult patient. Like with VSDs, the size of the defect is the primary determinant of clinical course in the adult patient. These clinical courses can be grouped into 5 main categories: (1) silent PDAs, (2) small hemodynamically insignificant PDAs, (3) moderate size PDAs, (4) large PDAs, and (5) previously repaired PDAs.

A silent PDA is a tiny defect that cannot be heard by auscultation and is only detected by other nonclinical means such as echocardiography. Life expectancy is always normal in this population and the risk for endocarditis is extremely low.

Patients with a small PDA have an audible long-ejection or continuous murmur heard best at the left upper sternal border that radiates to the back. In addition, they have normal peripheral pulses. Because there is negligible left to right shunting these patients have normal left aorta (LA) and left ventricle (LV) size and normal pulmonary artery pressure by echocardiography and chest x-ray. These patients like those with silent PDAs are aysmptomatic and live a normal life expectancy. They have a higher risk for endocarditis.

Patients with moderate size PDAs may present during adulthood. These patients often will have wide, bouncy peripheral pulses and an audible continuous murmur. These patients all have significant volume overload and develop some degree of LA and LV enlargement and some degree of pulmonary hypertension. These patients are symptomatic with dyspnea, palpitations, and heart failure.

Patients with large PDAs typically present with signs of severe pulmonary hypertension and Eisenmenger syndrome. By adulthood, the continuous murmur is typically absent and there is differential cyanosis (lower extremity saturations lower than the right arm saturation). These patients have a similar prognosis as other patients with Eisenmenger syndrome.

Patients who underwent repair of a PDA prior to the development of pulmonary hypertension, have a normal life expectancy without restrictions.

All patients with clinical evidence of a PDA are at increased risk for endocarditis. As result, all PDAs except for small silent PDAs and those patients with severe irreversible pulmonary hypertension should be considered for closure. Catheter device closure is the preferred method in most centers today. Surgical closure is reserved for patients with PDAs too large for device closure or when the anatomy is distorted, such as in the setting of a large ductal aneurysm.

Cyanotic Heart Disease (Chapters 423, 424, 425)

Unlike the acyanotic forms of congenital heart disease, the majority of patients with cyanotic congenital heart disease will have had at least 1 and often several previous interventions prior to adulthood. The most frequent defects seen in the outpatient adult congenital setting is tetralogy of Fallot, complete transposition of the great arteries (TGA, also known as d-transposition), pulmonary valve stenosis, and various forms of single ventricles. Other defects include total anomalous pulmonary venous return, truncus arteriosus, and double outlet right ventricle.

Tetralogy of Fallot (TOF) (Chapter 424.1)

In the developed world, the unoperated adult patient with tetralogy of Fallot has become a rarity because the majority of patients will have undergone palliation or, more often, repair in childhood. Survival in the unoperated patient to the 7th decade has been described but is rare. In general, only 11% of patients are alive by age 20 yr and only 3% by age 40 yr.

Late survival following repair of TOF is excellent. Repair is typically performed at 3-12 mo of age and consists of patch closure of the VSD and relief of the pulmonary outflow tract obstruction by patch augmentation of the right ventricular outflow tract, pulmonary valve annulus, or both. Survival rates at 32 and 35 yr have been reported to be 86% and 85% respectively, compared to 95% in age- and sex-matched controls. Most patients lived an unrestricted life. Many patients do develop late symptoms that include exertional dyspnea, palpitations, syncope, and sudden cardiac death. Late complications include endocarditis, aortic regurgitation with or without aortic root dilation (typically due to damage of the aortic valve during VSD closure or secondary to an intrinsic aortic root abnormality), LV dysfunction (secondary to inadequate myocardial protection during previous repair or chronic left ventricular volume overload due to long-standing palliative arterial shunts), residual pulmonary obstruction, residual pulmonary valve regurgitation, right ventricular (RV) dysfunction (due to pulmonary regurgitation or pulmonary stenosis), atrial arrhythmias (typically atrial flutter), ventricular arrhythmias, and heart block.

Reintervention is necessary in approximately 10% of patients following reparative surgery at 20-year follow-up. With longer follow-up, the incidence of reintervention continues to increase. The most common indication for reintervention is pulmonary valve replacement for severe pulmonary valve regurgitation.

Transposition of the Great Arteries (TGA) (Chapter 425.1)

The natural history of patients with unrepaired TGA is so poor that very few patients survive past childhood without intervention. The first definitive operations for TGA were described by Dr. Senning in 1959 and Dr. Mustard in 1964 (atrial switch procedures). With these procedures, the systemic and pulmonary venous returns are rerouted in the atrium by constructing baffles. The systemic venous return from the superior and inferior vena cavae is directed through the mitral valve and into the left ventricle (connected to the pulmonary artery). The pulmonary venous return is then directed through the tricuspid valve into the RV (connected to the aorta). These procedures can be performed with low mortality but leave the left ventricle as the pulmonary ventricle and the right ventricle as the systemic ventricle. Long-term follow-up studies after the atrial switch procedure show a small but ongoing attrition rate with numerous other intermediate and long-term complications. Two specific problems after the atrial switch procedure are most concerning. These include the loss of sinus rhythm with the development of atrial arrhythmias, occurring at an incidence of 50% by age 25 yr, and the development of systemic ventricular dysfunction, occurring at an incidence of 50% by age 35 yr. Other long-term complications include endocarditis, baffle leaks, baffle obstruction, tricuspid valve regurgitation, and sinus node dysfunction requiring pacemaker placement.

As result of these long-term complications, the arterial switch operation has become the procedure of choice to treat these patients since 1985. During the arterial switch procedure, the great arteries are transected and re-anastomosed to the correct ventricle (LV to the aorta and the RV to the pulmonary artery) with coronary artery transfer. Operative survival after the arterial switch procedure in the current surgical era is very good, with a surgical mortality rate of 2-5%. Long-term data on survival and complications does not exist but intermediate results are promising. Reported intermediate complications include endocarditis, pulmonary outflow tract obstruction (at the supravalvular level or at the takeoff of the peripheral pulmonary arteries), aortic valve regurgitation, and coronary artery compromise (ranging from minor stenosis to complete occlusion).

Because of the high incidence of observed and potential medical problems, all patients who have had both atrial and arterial repair of transposition of the great arteries should have lifelong follow-up by a cardiologist at a center specializing in adult congenital heart disease.

Pulmonary Valve Stenosis (Chapter 421.1)

Most patients with pulmonary valve stenosis are asymptomatic and present with a cardiac murmur. Survival into adult life and the need for intervention however is directly correlated to the degree of obstruction. Patients with trivial stenosis (defined as a peak gradient <25 mm Hg) followed for 25 yr remain asymptomatic and had no significant progression of obstruction over time. For those patients with moderate pulmonary valve stenosis (defined as a peak gradient of 25-49 mm Hg), there is an approximately 20% chance of requiring intervention by age 25 yr. For those patients with severe stenosis (defined as a peak gradient of >50 mm Hg), the majority ultimately require an intervention, either surgery or balloon valvuloplasty by age 25 yr.

Following surgical valvotomy for isolated pulmonary stenosis, long-term survival is excellent. With longer follow-up the incidence of late complications and the need for reintervention do increase. The most common indication for reintervention is pulmonary valve replacement for severe pulmonary regurgitation. Other long-term complications include recurrent atrial arrhythmias, endocarditis, and residual right ventricular outflow tract obstruction.

Patients with moderate to severe pulmonary stenosis (defined as a peak gradient of >50 mm Hg) should be considered for intervention even in the absence of symptoms. Since 1985, percutaneous balloon valvuloplasty has been the accepted treatment for patients of all ages. Prior to 1985, surgical valvotomy had been the gold standard. Surgical valvotomy is reserved for those patients that are unlikely to have successful results from balloon valvuloplasty, such as those with an extremely dysplastic or calcified valve.

Left-Sided Obstructive Lesions

COARCTATION OF THE AORTA (CHAPTER 421.6) The clinical presentation of coarctation of the aorta depends on the severity of obstruction and the associated anomalies. Unrepaired coarctation of the aorta typically presents with symptoms prior to adulthood. These symptoms include headaches related to hypertension, leg fatigue or cramps, exercise intolerance, and systemic hypertension. Those untreated patients surviving to adulthood thus typically have only mild coarctation of the aorta. In the era prior to surgery, without treatment the mean age of death was 32 yr. Causes of death included left ventricular failure, intracranial hemorrhage, endocarditis, aortic rupture/dissection, and premature coronary artery disease.

Following surgical repair, long-term survival is good but is directly correlated with the age at repair, with those repaired after age 14 yr having a lower 20 yr survival than those repaired earlier, 91% compared to 79%. Like almost all forms of repaired congenital heart disease, with longer follow-up the incidence of long-term complications continues to rise. The most common long-term complication is persistent or new systemic hypertension at rest or during exercise. Other long-term complications include aneurysms of the ascending or descending aorta, recoarctation at the site of previous repair, coronary artery disease, aortic stenosis or regurgitation (in setting of bicuspid aortic valve), rupture of an intracranial aneurysm, and endocarditis.

Patients with significant native or residual coarctation of the aorta (symptomatic patients with a peak gradient across the coarctation of >30 mm Hg) should be considered for intervention, either surgery or catheter intervention with balloon angioplasty with or without stent placement. Surgical repair in the adult patient is technically difficult and is associated with high morbidity. Catheter based intervention has become the preferred method in most experienced adult congenital heart disease centers.

Aortic Valve Stenosis (Chapter 421.5)

The natural history of aortic valve stenosis in adults is quite variable but is characterized by progressive stenosis over time. By age 45 yr, approximately 50% of bicuspid aortic valves will have some degree of stenosis.

Most patients with aortic valve stenosis are asymptomatic and are diagnosed after a murmur is detected. The severity of obstruction at the time of diagnosis correlates with the pattern of progression. Symptoms are rare until patients have severe aortic valve stenosis (mean gradient by echocardiography of >50 mm Hg). Symptoms include chest pain, exertional dyspnea, near syncope, and syncope. When any of these symptoms are present, the risk of sudden cardiac death is very high and as result, surgical intervention is mandated.

For patients requiring surgical valvotomy to relieve the stenosis prior to adulthood, the majority of patients do well. However, at 25 yr follow-up, up to 40% of patients will have required a 2nd operation for residual stenosis or regurgitation.

Patients with symptoms and severe aortic valve stenosis should be considered for intervention. Treatment involves manipulating the valve to reduce stenosis. This can be accomplished by transvenous balloon dilation of the valve, open surgical valvotomy, or valve replacement. In absence of significant aortic regurgitation, most centers favor balloon dilation or surgical valvotomy for children and young adults who have pliable valves with fusion of commissures. In older adults, aortic valve replacement is the treatment of choice.

Endocarditis Prophylaxis (Chapter 431)

The American Heart Association found that very few cases of endocarditis are prevented with antibiotic prophylaxis. Only patients with cardiac conditions associated with the highest risk for adverse outcomes should continue follow antibiotic prophylaxis before surgery: patients with previous endocarditis, unrepaired cyanotic congenital heart disease (CHD), including palliative shunts and conduits; completely repaired congenital heart defects with prosthetic material or device, whether placed by surgery or by catheter intervention, during the first 6 months after the procedure; and repaired CHD with residual defects at the site or adjacent to the site of a prosthetic patch or prosthetic device (which inhibit endothelialization). Except for the conditions just listed, antibiotic prophylaxis is no longer recommended for other forms of CHD.

PREGNANCY AND CONGENITAL HEART DISEASE

CHD is the most common form of heart disease encountered during pregnancy in developed countries. Heart disease does not preclude a successful pregnancy but increases the risk to both the mother and the baby. During pregnancy there are substantial hemodynamic changes that occur. The hemodynamic changes in pregnancy result in a steady increase in cardiac output during pregnancy until the 32nd week of gestation, at which time, the cardiac output reaches a plateau at 30-50% above the prepregnancy level. At time of delivery, with uterine contractions an additional 300-500 ml of blood enters the circulation. This in conjunction with increased blood pressure and heart rate during labor increases the cardiac output at delivery to 80% the prepregnancy level.

Despite these hemodynamic changes, the outcome of pregnancy is favorable in most women with CHD provided that functional class and systemic ventricular function are good (see Table 428-5). Pulmonary artery hypertension presents a serious risk during pregnancy, particularly when the pulmonary pressure exceeds 70% of systemic pressure, regardless of functional class. Other contraindications to pregnancy include severe obstructive left-sided lesions (coarctation of the aorta, aortic valve stenosis, mitral valve stenosis, hypertrophic cardiomyopathy), Marfan syndrome with coexisting dilated ascending aorta (defined as >4.0 cm), persistent cyanosis, and systemic ventricular dysfunction (ejection fraction of ≤40%). The need for full anticoagulation during pregnancy, although not a contraindication, poses an increased risk to both mother and fetus. The relative risks and benefits of the different anticoagulant approaches need to be discussed fully with the prospective mother.

Pregnancy counseling should begin early in adolescence and should be part of the routine cardiac follow-up visit. During counseling, a discussion about the risk of CHD in the offspring should take place. In the general population, the incidence of CHD is 1%. In the offspring of a mother with CHD, the risk increases to 5-6%. Often the cardiac lesion in the offspring is not the same as that in the mother, except for in the case of a syndrome with autosomal dominant inheritance (Marfan syndrome, hypertrophic cardiomyopathy). Risk stratification should include the specific CHD lesion but also needs to take in account the maternal functional class. While the specific CHD lesion is important, multiple studies have demonstrated that the maternal functional class prior to pregnancy is highly predictive of both maternal and fetal outcomes, with those having the best functional class having the best outcomes.

CONTRACEPTION

A critical part of caring for adults with congenital heart disease is to provide or make available advice on contraception. Unfortunately, there are limited data on the safety of various contraceptive techniques in ACHD patients. The estrogen-containing oral contraceptive pill can be used in many ACHD patients but is not recommended in ACHD patients at risk of thromboembolism, such as those with cyanosis, prior Fontan procedure, atrial fibrillation, or pulmonary artery hypertension. In addition, this form of contraceptive therapy may upset anticoagulation control. While slightly less effective than combined estrogen/progesterone containing contraceptive pills, medroxyprogesterone, the progesterone-only pills, and levonorgestrel are good options for most ACHD patients. They however can cause fluid retention and as result, need to be used with caution in patients with heart failure. These medications have also been associated with depression and often breakthrough bleeding. Tubal ligation, although the most secure method of contraception, can be a high-risk procedure in patients with complex CHD or those with pulmonary hypertension. Hysteroscopic sterilization (Essure) may be reasonable for high-risk patients. In the past intrauterine devices were seldom used in cardiac patients because of the associated risk of bacteremia, pelvic inflammatory disease, and endocarditis. Newer intrauterine devices such as the Mirena, however appear to be safe and effective, and are rapidly becoming one of the most commonly used form of contraception in the ACHD population.

ADOLESCENT TRANSITION

It is well recognized that, as part of the process of obtaining independence, adolescents or young adults must develop a forward-looking, independent approach to their medical care. For children with heart disease, the transition process must begin during early adolescence and should be encouraged by both the primary care provider and the pediatric cardiologist, who must identify an appropriate adult congenital heart program to which transition and transfer will be made at an appropriate time (Table 428-6).

A successful transition program includes the following elements:

- Development of a written transition plan that should begin by the age of 14 yr.
- Because adolescents and young adults are frequently unaware of the details of their cardiac diagnosis and history, a complete, concise, portable medical record, including all pertinent aspects of cardiac care, should be shared with adolescents and their families and prepared for transmittal to the eventual adult care destination.
- The primary care provider and cardiologist must address unique adolescent medical issues as they impact the cardiovascular system. In addition to medical problems, education, vocational planning, psychosocial issues, and access to medical care

Table 428-6 ISSUES THAT REQUIRE COORDINATION OF CARE BETWEEN THE CARDIOLOGIST AND THE PRIMARY CARE PHYSICIAN
Antibiotic prophylaxis for endocarditis
Medications and drug interactions
Anticoagulation with prosthetic valves
Exercise and sports participation
Educational and vocational planning
Contraception and pregnancy
Drug, alcohol, and tobacco use
Noncardiac surgical planning
Anesthetic issues
New symptoms or acute illnesses
Coexistent medical conditions
Travel

are all topics that should be discussed with adolescents and their families.

- There is a tendency for young adults to avoid medical care because of lack of education, denial, or difficulty with access to the medical care system. Thus, a critical goal of the adolescent transition process is to identify an appropriate site for ongoing medical care and ensure maintenance of the medical record and continuity of care for the young adult. The site of care for a young adult with congenital heart disease may be a pediatric program or facility, or may be a specialized center or program for the adult with congenital heart disease. The critical issues are the continuity of care, the preparation of the patient, and the patient's participation in the process.

BIBLIOGRAPHY

Please visit the Nelson Textbook of Pediatrics *website at www.expertconsult.com for the complete bibliography.*

Section 4 CARDIAC ARRHYTHMIAS

Chapter 429 Disturbances of Rate and Rhythm of the Heart

George F. Van Hare

The term "arrhythmia" refers to a disturbance in heart rate or rhythm. Such disturbances can lead to heart rates that are abnormally fast, slow, or irregular. They may be transient or incessant, in-born or acquired, or caused by a toxin or by drugs. They may be a complication of surgical correction of congenital heart disease, a result of congenital metabolic disorders of mitochondria, or fetal inflammation as in maternal systemic lupus erythematosus (SLE). The principal risk of any arrhythmia, either slow or fast, is decreased cardiac output, or degeneration into a more critical arrhythmia such as ventricular fibrillation. Such arrhythmias may lead to syncope or to sudden death. When a patient has an arrhythmia, it is important to determine whether the particular rhythm is likely to lead to severe symptoms or to deteriorate into a life-threatening condition. Rhythm abnormalities, such as single premature atrial and ventricular beats, are common in children without heart disease and in the great majority of instances do not pose a risk to the patient.

A number of effective pharmacologic agents are available for treating arrhythmias in adults; many have not been studied extensively in children. Insufficient data are available regarding pharmacokinetics, pharmacodynamics, and efficacy in the pediatric population, and therefore the selection of an appropriate agent is often necessarily empirical. Fortunately, the majority of rhythm disturbances in children can be reliably controlled with a single agent (Table 429-1). Transcatheter ablation is acceptable therapy not only for life-threatening or drug-resistant tachyarrhythmias but also for the elective definitive treatment of arrhythmias. For patients with bradycardia, implantable pacemakers are small enough for use in premature infants. Implantable cardioverter-defibrillators (ICDs) are available for use in high-risk patients with malignant ventricular arrhythmias and an increased risk of sudden death.

429.1 Principles of Antiarrhythmic Therapy

George F. Van Hare

When considering drug therapy in the pediatric population, it is important to recognize that there are marked differences in pharmacokinetics by age and in comparison with adults. Infants may have slower absorption, slow gastric emptying, and differing sizes of drug tissue compartments affecting the volume of distribution. Hepatic metabolism and renal excretion may vary within the pediatric age group as well as in comparison to adults. When considering antiarrhythmic therapy, it is important to recognize that the likely arrhythmia mechanism may be different for the pediatric vs. adult population.

There are many antiarrhythmic agents available for rhythm control. The majority have not been approved by the U.S. Food and Drug Administration (FDA) for use in children; their use is usually considered "off-label," Pediatric cardiologists have experience with these drugs, and there are well-recognized standards regarding dosing.

With the availability of potentially curative ablation procedures, medical therapy has become less important. Clinicians and patients accept fewer drug side effects. Intolerable side effects, as well as the potential for a proarrhythmia induced by an antiarrhythmic drug, can seriously limit medical therapy and will lead the physician and family toward a potentially curative ablation procedure.

Antiarrhythmic drugs are commonly categorized using the Vaughan Williams classification system. This system comprises 4 classes: Class I includes agents that primarily block the sodium channel, class II includes the β-blockers, class III includes those agents that prolong repolarization, and class IV are the calcium channel blockers. Class I is further divided by the strength of the sodium channel blockade (see Table 429-1).

429.2 Sinus Arrhythmias and Extrasystoles

George F. Van Hare

Phasic sinus arrhythmia represents a normal physiologic variation in impulse discharges from the sinus node related to respirations. The heart rate slows during expiration and accelerates during inspiration. Occasionally, if the sinus rate becomes slow enough, an escape beat arises from the atrioventricular (AV) junction region (Fig. 429-1). Normal phasic sinus arrhythmia can be quite prominent in children and may mimic frequent premature contractions, but the relationship to the phases of respiration can be appreciated with careful auscultation. Drugs that increase vagal tone, such as digoxin, may exaggerate sinus arrhythmia; it is usually abolished by exercise. Other irregularities in sinus rhythm, especially bradycardia associated with periodic apnea are commonly seen in premature infants.

Sinus bradycardia is due to slow discharge of impulses from the sinus node, the heart's natural pacemaker. A sinus rate <90 beats/min in neonates and <60 beats/min in older children is considered to be sinus bradycardia. It is commonly seen in

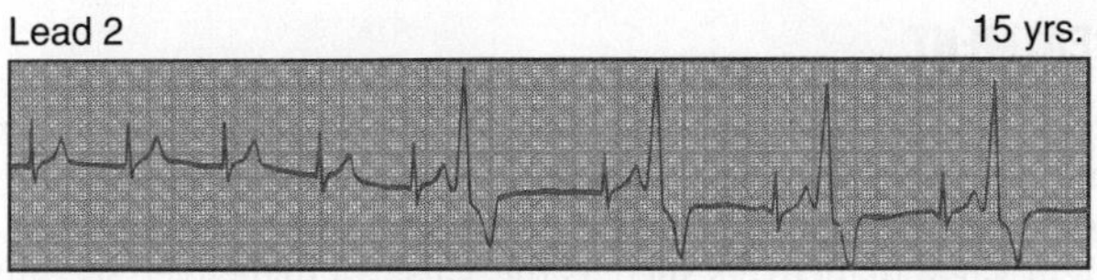

Figure 429-4 Premature ventricular contractions (PVCs) in a bigeminal rhythm, in a patient who is hyperventilating. Note that the premature beat is wide and has a completely different morphology from that of the sinus beat. The premature beat is not preceded by a discernable premature P wave or any appreciable deformation of the preceding T wave.

uniform, suggesting origin from a common site. When PVCs vary in contour, they are designated as multiform, suggesting origin from more than 1 ventricular site. Ventricular extrasystoles are often, but not always, followed by a full compensatory pause. The presence of fusion beats, that is, complexes with morphologic features that are intermediate between those of normal sinus beats and those of PVCs, proves the ventricular origin of the premature beat. Extrasystoles produce a smaller stroke and pulse volume than normal and, if quite premature, may not be audible with a stethoscope or palpable at the radial pulse. When frequent, extrasystoles may assume a definite rhythm, for example, alternating with normal beats (**bigeminy**) or occurring after 2 normal beats (**trigeminy**). Most patients are unaware of single premature ventricular contractions, although some may be aware of a "skipped beat" over the precordium. This sensation is due to the increased stroke volume of the normal beat after a compensatory pause. Anxiety, a febrile illness, or ingestion of various drugs or stimulants may exacerbate PVCs.

It is important to distinguish PVCs that are benign from those that are likely to lead to more severe arrhythmias. The former usually disappear during the tachycardia of exercise. If they persist or become more frequent during exercise, the arrhythmia may have greater significance. The following criteria are indications for further investigation of PVCs that could require **suppressive therapy:** (1) 2 or more ventricular premature beats in a row, (2) multiform PVCs, (3) increased ventricular ectopic activity with exercise, (4) R on T phenomenon (premature ventricular depolarization occurs on the T wave of the preceding beat), and (5) most importantly, the presence of underlying heart disease, a history of heart surgery, or both. The best therapy for benign PVCs is reassurance that the arrhythmia is not life threatening, although very symptomatic individuals may benefit from suppressive therapy. Malignant PVCs are usually secondary to another medical problem (electrolyte imbalance, hypoxia, drug toxicity, cardiac injury, or an intraventricular catheter). Successful treatment includes correction of the underlying abnormality. An intravenous lidocaine bolus and drip is the 1st line of therapy, with more effective drugs such as amiodarone reserved for refractory cases or for patients underlying ventricular dysfunction or hemodynamic compromise.

429.3 Supraventricular Tachycardia

George F. Van Hare

Supraventricular tachycardia (SVT) is a general term that includes essentially all forms of paroxysmal or incessant tachycardia except ventricular tachycardia. The category of SVT can be divided into 3 major subcategories: re-entrant tachycardias using an accessory pathway, re-entrant tachycardias without an accessory pathway, and ectopic or automatic tachycardias. Atrioventricular reciprocating tachycardia (AVRT) involves an accessory pathway and is the most common mechanism of SVT in infants. Atrioventricular node re-entry tachycardia (AVNRT) is rare in infancy but there is an increasing incidence of AVNRT in childhood and into adolescence. Atrial flutter is rarely seen in children with normal hearts, whereas intra-atrial re-entry tachycardia (IART) is common in patients following cardiac surgery. Atrial and junctional ectopic tachycardias are more commonly associated with abnormal hearts (cardiomyopathy) and in the immediate postoperative period following surgery for congenital heart disease.

CLINICAL MANIFESTATIONS

Re-entrant SVT is characterized by an abrupt onset and cessation; it usually occurs when the patient is at rest, although in infants it may be precipitated by an acute infection. Attacks may last only a few seconds or may persist for hours. The heart rate usually exceeds 180 beats/min and may occasionally be as rapid as 300 beats/min. The only complaint may be awareness of the rapid heart rate. Many children tolerate these episodes extremely well, and it is unlikely that short paroxysms are a danger to life. If the rate is exceptionally rapid or if the attack is prolonged, precordial discomfort and heart failure may occur. In children, SVT may be exacerbated by exposure to over-the-counter decongestants or by bronchodilators.

In young infants, the diagnosis may be more obscure because of the inability to communicate their symptoms. The heart rate at this age is normally higher than in older children and it increases greatly with crying. Infants with SVT on occasion initially present with heart failure, because the tachycardia may go unrecognized for a long time. The heart rate during episodes is frequently in the range of 240-300 beats/min. If the attack lasts 6-24 hr or more, heart failure may be recognized, and the infant will have an ashen color, and be restless and irritable, with tachypnea and hepatomegaly. When tachycardia occurs in the fetus, it can cause hydrops fetalis, which is the in utero manifestation of heart failure.

In neonates, SVT is usually manifested as a narrow QRS complex (<0.08 sec). The P wave is visible on a standard electrocardiogram in only 50-60% of neonates with SVT, but it is detectable with a transesophageal lead in most patients. **Differentiation from sinus tachycardia** may be difficult, but is important, as sinus tachycardia requires treatment of the underlying problem (e.g., sepsis, hypovolemia) rather than antiarrhythmic medication. If the rate is >230 beats/min with an abnormal P-wave axis (a normal P wave is positive in leads I and aVF), sinus tachycardia is not likely. The heart rate in SVT also tends to be *unvarying*, whereas in sinus tachycardia the heart rate *varies* with changes in vagal and sympathetic tone. AV reciprocating tachycardia uses a bypass tract that may either be able to conduct bidirectionally (**Wolff-Parkinson-White [WPW] syndrome**) or retrograde only (**concealed accessory pathway**). Patients with WPW syndrome have a small, but real risk of sudden death. If the accessory pathway rapidly conducts in antegrade fashion, the patient is at risk for atrial fibrillation begetting ventricular fibrillation. Risk stratification, including 24 hr Holter monitoring and exercise study, may help differentiate patients at higher risk for sudden death from WPW. Syncope is an ominous symptom in WPW and any patient with syncope and WPW syndrome should have an electrophysiology study and likely catheter ablation.

The typical electrocardiographic features of the Wolff-Parkinson-White syndrome are seen when the patient is not having tachycardia. These features include a short P-R interval and slow upstroke of the QRS (delta wave) (Fig. 429-5). Though most often present in patients with a normal heart, this syndrome may also be associated with Ebstein anomaly of the tricuspid valve, or hypertrophic cardiomyopathy. The critical anatomic structure is an accessory pathway consisting of a muscular bridge connecting atrium to ventricle on either the right or the left side of the AV ring (Fig. 429-6). During sinus rhythm, the impulse is carried over both the AV node and the accessory pathway; it produces some degree of fusion of the 2 depolarization fronts that results in an abnormal QRS. During AVRT, an

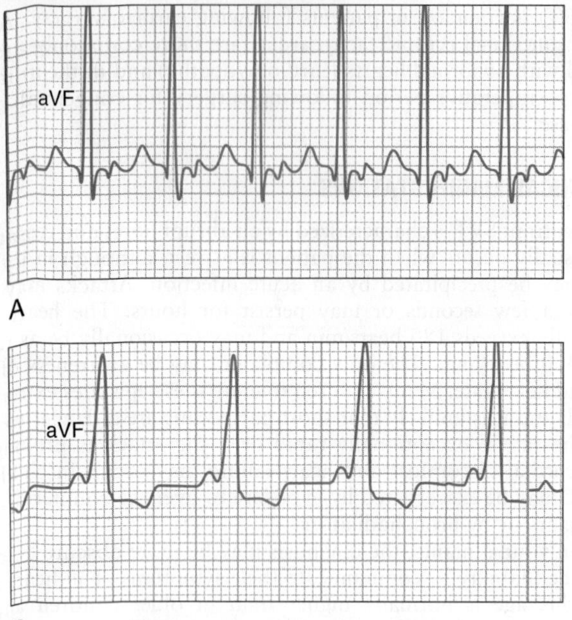

Figure 429-5 *A,* Supraventricular tachycardia in a child with Wolff-Parkinson-White (WPW) syndrome. Note the normal QRS complexes during the tachycardia, as well as clear retrograde P waves seen on the upstroke of the T waves. *B,* Later, the typical features of WPW syndrome are apparent (short P-R interval, delta wave, and wide QRS).

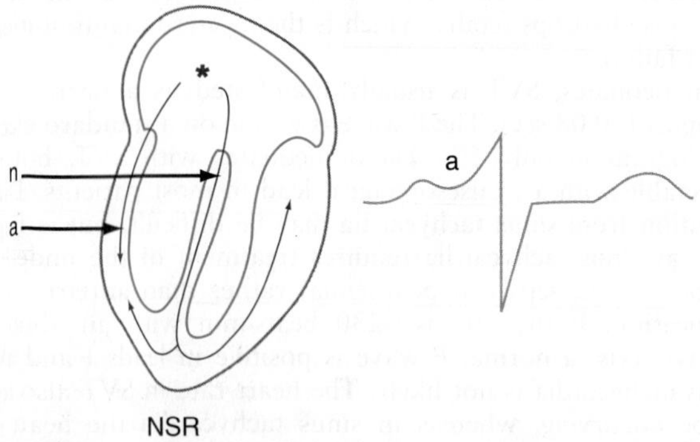

Figure 429-6 Schematic representation of the heart with a right-sided accessory pathway (Wolff-Parkinson-White syndrome). The *asterisk* indicates initiation of the sinus beat. The *arrows* indicate the direction and spread of excitation. The electrocardiographic complex shown represents a fusion beat that combines activation over the normal *(n)* and accessory *(a)* pathways. The latter inscribes the delta wave. NSR, normal sinus rhythm.

impulse is carried in antegrade fashion through the AV node (**orthodromic conduction**), which results in a normal QRS complex, and in retrograde fashion through the accessory pathway to the atrium, thereby perpetuating the tachycardia. In these cases, only after cessation of the tachycardia are the typical ECG features of WPW syndrome recognized (see Fig. 429-5). When rapid antegrade conduction occurs through the pre-excitation pathway during tachycardia and the retrograde re-entry pathway to the atrium is via the AV node (**antidromic conduction**), the QRS complexes are wide and the potential for more serious arrhythmias (ventricular fibrillation) is greater, especially if atrial fibrillation occurs.

AV nodal re-entrant tachycardia (AVNRT) involves the use of 2 pathways within the AV node. This arrhythmia is more commonly seen in adolescence. It is one of the few SVTs that is occasionally associated with syncope. This arrhythmia is usually amenable to antiarrhythmic therapy, such as β-blockers, or to catheter ablation therapy.

TREATMENT

Vagal stimulation by placing of the face in ice water (in older children) or by placing an ice bag over the face (in infants) may abort the attack. To terminate the attack, older children may be taught vagal maneuvers such as the Valsalva maneuver, straining, breath holding, or standing on their head. Ocular pressure must never be performed, and carotid sinus massage is very rarely effective. When these measures fail, several pharmacologic alternatives are available (see Table 429-1). In stable patients, adenosine by rapid intravenous push is the **treatment of choice** because of its rapid onset of action and minimal effects on cardiac contractility. The dose may need to be increased if no effect on the tachycardia is seen. Because of the potential for adenosine to initiate atrial fibrillation, it should not be administered without a means for DC cardioversion near at hand. Calcium channel blockers such as verapamil have also been used in the initial treatment of SVT in older children. Verapamil may reduce cardiac output and produce hypotension and cardiac arrest in infants younger than 1 yr; it is therefore contraindicated in this age group. In urgent situations when symptoms of severe heart failure have already occurred, synchronized DC cardioversion (0.5-2 J/kg) is recommended as the initial management (Chapter 62).

Once the patient has been converted to sinus rhythm, a longer acting agent may is selected for maintenance therapy. In patients without an antegrade accessory pathway (non-WPW), the β-blockers are the mainstay of therapy. Digoxin is also popular, and is effective in infants, but less so in older children. In children with WPW, digoxin or calcium channel blockers may increase the rate of antegrade conduction of impulses through the bypass tract, with the possibility of ventricular fibrillation, and are therefore contraindicated. These patients are usually managed in the long term with β-blockers. In patients with resistant tachycardias, procainamide, quinidine, flecainide, propafenone, sotalol, and amiodarone have all been used. Most antiarrhythmic agents have the potential of causing new dangerous arrhythmias (**proarrhythmia**) and decreasing heart function. Flecainide and propafenone in particular should be limited to use in patients with otherwise normal hearts.

If cardiac failure occurs because of prolonged tachycardia in an infant with a normal heart, cardiac function usually returns to normal after sinus rhythm is reinstituted, although it may take days to weeks. Infants with SVT diagnosed within the 1st 3-4 mo of life have a lower incidence of recurrence than do those in whom it is initially diagnosed at a later age. These patients have an 80% chance of resolution by the 1st yr of life, although about 30% will have recurrences later in childhood; if medical therapy is required; it can be tapered within a year and the patient watched for signs of recurrence. Parents should be taught to measure the heart rate in their infants, so that prolonged unapparent episodes of SVT may be detected before heart failure occurs.

Twenty-four hour electrocardiographic (Holter) recordings are useful in monitoring the course of therapy and in detecting brief runs of asymptomatic tachycardia, particularly in younger children and infants. Some centers use **transesophageal pacing** to evaluate the effects of therapy in infants. More detailed electrophysiologic studies performed in the cardiac catheterization laboratory are often indicated in patients with refractory SVTs who are candidates for **catheter ablation**. During an electrophysiologic study, multiple electrode catheters are placed transvenously in different locations in the heart. Pacing is performed to evaluate the conduction characteristics of the accessory pathway and to initiate the tachyarrhythmia, and mapping is performed to locate the accessory pathway. **Catheter ablation** of an accessory pathway is often used electively in children and teenagers, as well as in patients who require multiple agents or find drug side effects intolerable or for whom arrhythmia control is poor. Ablation may be performed either by radiofrequency ablation, which creates tissue heating, or cryoablation, in which tissue is frozen.

The overall initial success rate for catheter ablation ranges from approximately 80% to 95%, depending on the location of the accessory pathway. Surgical ablation of bypass tracts may also be successful in selected patients.

The management of SVT due to **atrioventricular node re-entry tachycardia (AVNRT)** is nearly identical to that for AVRT. Children with AVNRT are not at increased risk of sudden death, as they do not have a manifest accessory pathway. In practice, their episodes are more likely to be brought on by exercise or other forms of stress, and the heart rates can be quite fast, leading to chest pain, dizziness, and occasionally syncope. The choice of chronic antiarrhythmic medications is with β-blockers being the drugs of choice; AVNRT does respond to adenosine. Less is known about the natural history, but patients with AVNRT are seen quite commonly in adulthood, so spontaneous resolution seems unlikely. Patients are quite amenable to catheter ablation, either using radiofrequency energy or cryoablation, with high success rates and low complication rates.

Atrial ectopic tachycardia is an uncommon tachycardia in childhood. It is characterized by a variable rate (seldom >200 beats/min), identifiable P waves with an abnormal axis, and either a sustained or incessant nonsustained tachycardia. This form of atrial tachycardia has a single automatic focus. Identification of this mechanism is aided by monitoring the electrocardiogram while initiating vagal or pharmacologic therapy. Re-entry tachycardias "break" suddenly, whereas automatic tachycardias gradually slow down and then gradually speed up again. Atrial ectopic tachycardias are usually more difficult to control pharmacologically than are the more common re-entrant tachycardias. If pharmacologic therapy with a single agent is unsuccessful, catheter ablation is suggested and has a success rate >90%.

Chaotic or multifocal atrial tachycardia is defined as atrial tachycardia with ≥3 ectopic P waves, frequent blocked P waves, and varying P-R intervals of conducted beats. This arrhythmia occurs most often in infants younger than 1 yr, usually without cardiac disease, although some evidence suggests an association with viral myocarditis or pulmonary disease. The goal of drug treatment is slowing of the ventricular rate, as conversion to sinus may not be possible, and multiple agents are often required. When this arrhythmia occurs in infancy, it usually terminates spontaneously by 3 yr of age.

Accelerated junctional ectopic tachycardia (JET) is an automatic (non–re-entry) arrhythmia in which the junctional rate exceeds that of the sinus node and AV dissociation results. This arrhythmia is most often recognized in the early postoperative period after cardiac surgery and may be extremely difficult to control. Reduction of the infusion rate of catecholamines and control of fever are important adjuncts to management. Congenital JET may be seen in the absence of surgery. It is incessant, and can lead to dilated cardiomyopathy. Intravenous amiodarone is effective in the treatment of postoperative JET. Patients who require chronic therapy may respond to amiodarone or sotalol. Congenital JET can be cured by catheter ablation, but long-term AV block requiring a pacemaker is a prominent complication.

Atrial flutter, also known as *intra-atrial re-entrant tachycardia,* is an atrial tachycardia characterized by atrial activity at a rate of 250-300 beats/min in children and adolescents, and 400-600 in neonates. The mechanism of common atrial flutter consists of a re-entrant or rhythm originating in the right atrium circling the tricuspid valve annulus. Because the AV node cannot transmit such rapid impulses, some degree of **AV block** is virtually always present, and the ventricles respond to every 2nd-4th atrial beat (Fig. 429-7). Occasionally, the response is variable and the rhythm appears irregular.

In older children, atrial flutter usually occurs in the setting of congenital heart disease; neonates with atrial flutter frequently have normal hearts. Atrial flutter may occur during acute infectious illnesses but is most often seen in patients with large stretched atria, such as those associated with long-standing mitral

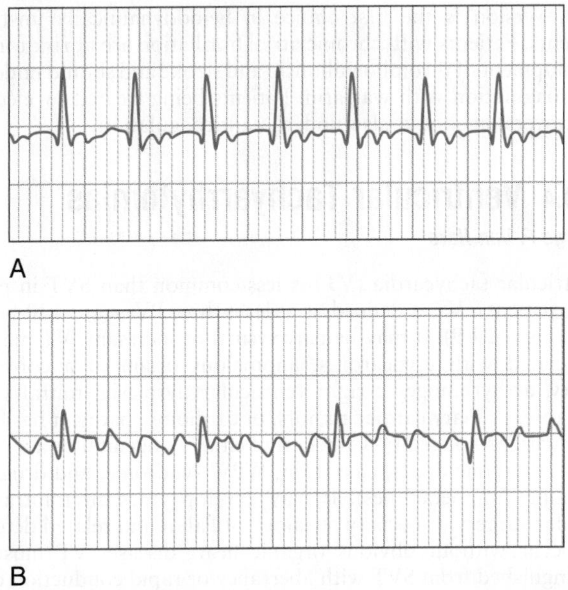

Figure 429-7 Neonatal atrial flutter. Note that the flutter waves are not obvious in the first tracing *(A)* but once a dose of adenosine is given, flutter waves at a rate of about 450 beats/min emerge *(B).*

or tricuspid insufficiency, tricuspid atresia, Ebstein anomaly, or rheumatic mitral stenosis. Atrial flutter can also occur after palliative or corrective intra-atrial surgery. Uncontrolled atrial flutter may precipitate heart failure. Vagal maneuvers (such as carotid sinus pressure or iced saline submersion) or adenosine generally produce a temporary slowing of the heart rate due to increased AV block. The **diagnosis** is confirmed by electrocardiography, which demonstrates the rapid and regular atrial saw-toothed flutter waves. Atrial flutter usually converts immediately to sinus rhythm by **synchronized DC cardioversion,** which is most often the **treatment of choice.** Patients with chronic atrial flutter in the setting of congenital heart disease may be at increased risk for **thromboembolism** and stroke and should thus undergo anticoagulation before elective cardioversion. Digoxin, β-blockers, or calcium channel blockers may be used to slow the ventricular response in atrial flutter by prolonging the AV node refractory period. Other agents may be used to maintain sinus rhythm, and choices include type I agents such as procainamide or propafenone, type III agents such as amiodarone and sotalol. Other modalities, including catheter and surgical ablation, have been used in older patients with congenital heart disease with moderate success. Following cardioversion, neonates with normal hearts may be treated with digoxin for 6-12 mo, after which the medication can usually be discontinued, as neonatal atrial flutter generally does not recur.

Atrial fibrillation is uncommon in children and is rare in infants. The atrial excitation is chaotic and more rapid (400-700 beats/min) and produces an irregularly irregular ventricular response and pulse (Fig. 429-8). This rhythm disorder is often associated with atrial enlargement or disease. Atrial fibrillation may be seen in older children with rheumatic mitral valve stenosis. It is also seen rarely as a complication of atrial surgery, in patients with left atrial enlargement secondary to left AV valve insufficiency, and in patients with WPW syndrome. Thyrotoxicosis, pulmonary embolism, pericarditis, or cardiomyopathy may be suspected in a previously normal older child or adolescent with atrial fibrillation. Very rarely, atrial fibrillation may be familial. The best initial treatment is **rate control,** most effectively with calcium channel blockers, to limit the ventricular rate during atrial fibrillation. Digoxin is not given if WPW syndrome is present. Normal sinus rhythm may be restored with intravenous procainamide or amiodarone, or by DC cardioversion, and DC cardioversion is the first choice in hemodynamically unstable patients. Patients with chronic atrial fibrillation are at risk for the development of thromboembolism and stroke and should undergo anticoagulation with warfarin. Patients being treated by elective cardioversion should also undergo anticoagulation.

429.4 Ventricular Tachyarrhythmias

George F. Van Hare

Ventricular tachycardia (VT) is less common than SVT in pediatric patients. VT is defined as at least three PVCs at >120 beats/min (Fig. 429-9). It may be paroxysmal or incessant. VT may be associated with myocarditis, anomalous origin of a coronary artery, arrhythmogenic right ventricular dysplasia, mitral valve prolapse, primary cardiac tumors, or cardiomyopathy. It has been seen with prolonged Q-T interval of either congenital or acquired (proarrhythmic drugs) causation, WPW syndrome, and drug use (cocaine, amphetamines). It may develop years after intraventricular surgery (especially tetralogy of Fallot and related defects) or occur without obvious organic heart disease. VT must be distinguished from SVT with aberrancy or rapid conduction over an accessory pathway (Table 429-2). The presence of clear capture and fusion beats confirms the diagnosis of VT. Although some children tolerate rapid ventricular rates for many hours, this arrhythmia should be promptly treated because hypotension and degeneration into ventricular fibrillation may result. For patients who are hemodynamically stable, intravenous amiodarone, lidocaine, or procainamide are the initial drugs of choice. If treatment is to be successful, it is critical to search for and correct any underlying abnormalities such as electrolyte imbalance, hypoxia, or drug toxicity. Amiodarone is the **treatment of choice** during cardiac arrest (Chapter 62). Hemodynamically unstable patients with VT should be immediately treated with DC cardioversion. Overdrive ventricular pacing, through temporary pacing wires or a permanent pacemaker, may also be effective, although it may cause the arrhythmia to deteriorate into ventricular fibrillation. In the neonatal period, ventricular tachycardia may be associated with an anomalous left coronary artery (Chapter 426.2) or a myocardial tumor.

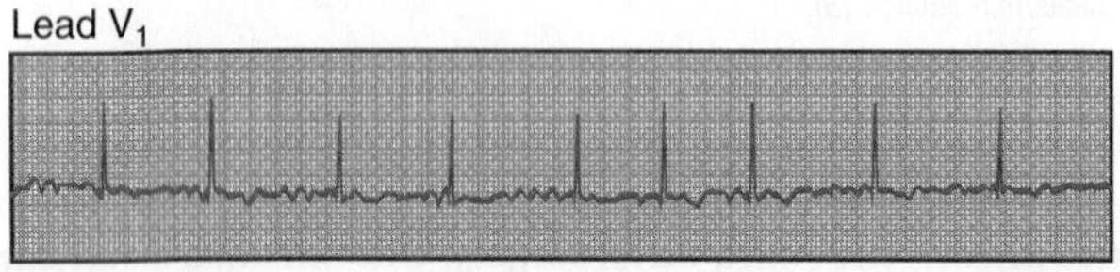

Figure 429-8 Atrial fibrillation, characterized by the absence of clear P waves and an irregularly irregular ventricular response. One can appreciate the irregular, rapid undulations (F waves). Fibrillatory waves may not be visible in all leads and should be carefully sought in every tracing with irregular R-R intervals. Note that no two R-R intervals are the same.

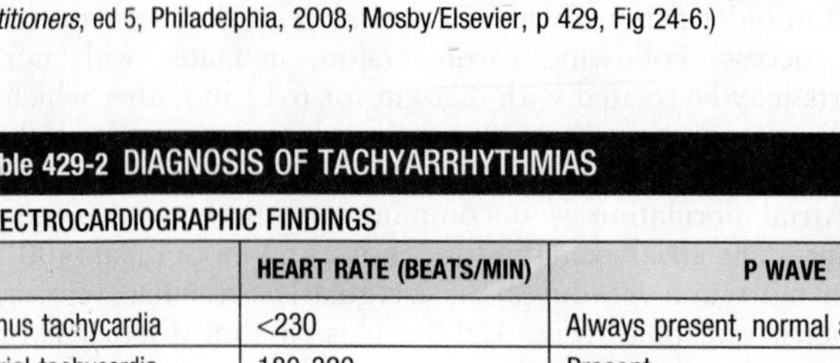

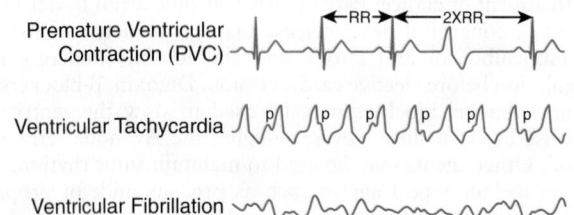

Figure 429-9 Ventricular arrhythmias. (From Park MY: *Pediatric cardiology for practitioners*, ed 5, Philadelphia, 2008, Mosby/Elsevier, p 429, Fig 24-6.)

Unless a clearly reversible cause is identified, electrophysiologic study is usually indicated for patients in whom VT has developed, and depending on the findings, catheter ablation and/or ICD implantation may be indicated.

A related arrhythmia, **ventricular accelerated rhythm**, is occasionally seen in infants. It is defined the same way as VT, but the rate is only slightly faster than the coexisting sinus rate (within 10%). It is generally benign.

Ventricular fibrillation is a chaotic rhythm that results in death unless an effective ventricular beat is rapidly re-established (see Fig. 429-9). A thump on the chest may occasionally restore sinus rhythm. Usually, cardiopulmonary resuscitation and DC defibrillation is necessary. If defibrillation is ineffective or fibrillation recurs, amiodarone or lidocaine may be given intravenously and defibrillation repeated (Chapter 62). After recovery from ventricular fibrillation, a search should be made for the underlying cause. **Electrophysiologic study** is indicated for patients who have survived ventricular fibrillation unless a clearly reversible cause is identified. If WPW syndrome is noted, catheter ablation should be performed. For patients in whom no correctable abnormality can be found, an ICD is nearly always indicated, because of the high risk of sudden death.

429.5 Long Q-T Syndromes

George F. Van Hare

Long Q-T syndromes (LQTS) are genetic abnormalities of ventricular repolarization, with an estimated incidence of about 1 per 10,000 births (Table 429-3). They present as a long Q-T

Table 429-2 DIAGNOSIS OF TACHYARRHYTHMIAS

ELECTROCARDIOGRAPHIC FINDINGS

	HEART RATE (BEATS/MIN)	P WAVE	QRS DURATION	REGULARITY
Sinus tachycardia	<230	Always present, normal axis	Normal	Rate varies with respiration
Atrial tachycardia	180-320	Present Abnormal P wave morphology and axis	Normal or prolonged (with aberration)	Usually regular but ventricular response may be variable due to Wenckebach conduction
Atrial fibrillation	120-180	Fibrillatory waves	Normal or prolonged (with aberration)	Irregularly irregular (no two R-R intervals alike)
Atrial flutter	Atrial: 250-400 Ventricular response variable: 100-320	Saw-toothed flutter waves	Normal or prolonged (with aberration)	Regular ventricular response (e.g., 2:1, 3:1, 3:2, and so on)
Junctional tachycardia	120-280	Atrioventricular dissociation with no fusion, and normal QRS capture beats	Normal or prolonged (with aberration)	Regular (except with capture beats)
Ventricular tachycardia	120-300	Atrioventricular dissociation with capture beats and fusion beats	Prolonged for age	Regular (except with capture beats)

Table 429-3 INHERITED CHANNEL MUTATIONS IN LONG AND SHORT Q-T SYNDROMES

	CHROMOSOME	GENE	PROTEIN	ION CURRENT AFFECTED	TRIGGER	SPECIAL FEATURES/OCCURRENCE
LQTS TYPE						
1	11p15.5	*KCNQ1*	KvLQT1 (Kv7.1)	I_{Ks}	Exercise (swimming), emotion	42-54%
2	7q35-36	*KCNH2*	HERG, (Kv11.1)	I_{Kr}	Rest, emotion, exercise (acoustic, post partum)	35-45%
3	3p24-21	*SCN5A*	Nav1.5	I_{Na}	Rest, sleep, emotion	1.7-8%; High lethality
4	4q24-27	*ANK2*	Ankyrin-B	$I_{Na\text{-}K}$, $I_{Na\text{-}Ca}$, I_{Na}	Exercise	<1%
5	21q22	*KCNE1*	MinK	I_{Ks}	Exercise, emotion	<1%
6	21q22	*KCNE2*	MiRP1	I_{Kr}	Rest, exercise	<1%
7	17q23	*KCNJ2*	Kir2.1	I_{K1}	Rest, exercise	Periodic paralysis, dysmorphic feature
8	12p13.3	*CACNA1C*	Cav1.2	I_{Ca}	Exercise, emotion	Rare, syndactyly
9	3p25.3	*CAV3*	Caveolin-3	I_{Na}	Nonexertional, sleep	Rare
10	11q23.3	*SCN4B*	NaVβ4	I_{Na}	Exercise, postpartum	<0.1%
SHORT Q-T SYNDROME TYPE						
1	7q35-36	*KCNH2*	HERG (Kv11.1)	I_{Kr}	Exercise, rest (acoustic)	—
2	11p15.5	*KCNQ1*	KvLQT1 (Kv7.1)	I_{Ks}	—	—
3	17q23	*KCNJ2*	Kir2.1	I_{K1}	Sleep	—
4	12p13.3	*CACNA1C*	Cav1.2	I_{Ca}	—	—
5	10p12.33	*CACNB2b*	CaVβ2b	I_{Ca}	—	—
JERVELL AND LANGE-NIELSEN SYNDROME TYPE						
1	11p15.5	*KCNQ1*	KvLQT1 (Kv7.1)	I_{Ks}	Exercise (swimming), emotion	1-7%; deafness
2	21q22	*KCNE1*	MinK	I_{Ks}	Exercise (swimming), emotion	<1%; deafness

From Morita H, Wu J, Zipes DP: The QT syndromes: long and short, *Lancet* 372:750–762, 2008, p 751, Table 1.

interval on the surface ECG and are associated with malignant ventricular arrhythmias (torsades de pointes and ventricular fibrillation). They are a cause of syncope and sudden death and may be associated with sudden infant death syndrome or drowning. At least 50% of cases are familial, but due to variable penetrance, this may be an underestimate. The old distinction between dominant and recessive forms of the disease (Romano-Ward syndrome [RWS] vs Jervell and Lange-Nielsen syndrome [JLNS]) is no longer commonly made, as the latter "recessive" condition is known to be due to the homozygous state. JLNS is associated with congenital sensorineural deafness. Asymptomatic patients carrying the gene mutation may not all have a prolonged Q-T duration. Q-T interval prolongation may become apparent with exercise or during catecholamine infusions.

Genetic studies have identified mutations in cardiac potassium and sodium channels (see Table 429-3). Additional forms of LQTS have been described, but these are much more uncommon. JLNS has been seen in patients who have homozygous mutations of KVLQT1 and minK, whereas the heterozygous state is manifested as RWS. Genotype may predict clinical manifestations; for example, **LQT1 events are usually stress induced,** whereas events in **LQT3 often occur during sleep.** LQT2 events have an intermediate pattern. LQT3 has the highest probability for sudden death, followed by LQT2 and then LQT1. Drugs may prolong the Q-T interval directly but more often do so when drugs such as erythromycin or ketoconazole inhibit their metabolism (Table 429-4).

The **clinical manifestation** of LQTS in children is most often a syncopal episode brought on by exercise, fright, or a sudden startle; some events occur during sleep (LQT3). Patients can initially be seen with seizures, presyncope, or palpitations; about 10% are initially in cardiac arrest. The diagnosis is based on electrocardiographic and clinical criteria. Not all patients with long Q-T intervals have LQTS, and patients with normal Q-T intervals on a resting electrocardiogram may have LQTS. A heart rate–corrected Q-T interval of >0.47 sec is highly indicative, whereas a Q-T interval of >0.44 sec is suggestive. Other features include notched T waves, T wave alternans, a low heart rate for age, a history of syncope (especially with stress), and a familial

Table 429-4 ACQUIRED CAUSES OF Q-T PROLONGATION*

DRUGS
Antibiotics—erythromycin, clarithromycin, telithromycin, azithromycin, trimethoprim/sulfamethoxazole
Antifungal agents—fluconazole, itraconazole, ketoconazole
Antiprotozoal agents—pentamidine isethionate
Antihistamines—astemizole, terfenadine (Seldane) (Seldane has been removed from the market for this reason)
Antidepressants—tricyclics such as imipramine (Tofranil), amitriptyline (Elavil), desipramine (Norpramin), and doxepin (Sinequan)
Antipsychotics—haloperidol, risperidone, phenothiazines such as thioridazine (Mellaril) and chlorpromazine (Thorazine)
Antiarrhythmic agents
Class 1A (sodium channel blockers)—quinidine, procainamide, disopyramide
Class III (prolong depolarization)—amiodarone (rare), bretylium, dofetilide, *N*-acetyl-procainamide, sotalol
Lipid-lowering agents—probucol
Antianginals—bepridil
Diuretics (through K^+ loss)—furosemide (Lasix), ethacrynic acid (bumetanide [Bumex])
Oral hypoglycemic agents—glibenclamide, glyburide
Organophosphate insecticides
Promotility agents—cisapride
Vasodilators—prenylamine
ELECTROLYTE DISTURBANCES
Hypokalemia—diuretics, hyperventilation
Hypocalcemia
Hypomagnesemia
UNDERLYING MEDICAL CONDITIONS
Bradycardia—complete atrioventricular block, severe bradycardia, sick sinus syndrome
Myocardial dysfunction—anthracycline cardiotoxicity, congestive heart failure, myocarditis, cardiac tumors
Endocrinopathy—hyperparathyroidism, hypothyroidism, pheochromocytoma
Neurologic—encephalitis, head trauma, stroke, subarachnoid hemorrhage
Nutritional—alcoholism, anorexia nervosa, starvation

*A more exhaustive updated list of medications that can prolong the QTc interval is available at the University of Arizona Center for Education and Research of Therapeutics website (*www.azcert.org*).

From Park MY: *Pediatric cardiology for practitioners*, ed 5, Philadelphia, 2008, Mosby/Elsevier, p 433, Box 24-1.

history of either LQTS or unexplained sudden death. Twenty-four hour Holter monitoring and exercise testing are adjuncts to the diagnosis. Genotyping is available and can identify the mutation is about 75% of patients known to have LQTS by clinical criteria. Genotyping is not useful in ruling out the diagnosis in individuals suspected of having the disease, but when positive is very useful in identifying asymptomatic affected relatives of the index case.

Short Q-T syndromes (see Table 429-3) manifest with atrial or ventricular fibrillation and are associated with syncope and sudden death.

Treatment of LQTS includes the use of **β-blocking agents** at doses that blunt the heart rate response to exercise. Some patients require a **pacemaker** because of drug-induced profound bradycardia. In patients with continued syncope despite treatment, an implantable cardiac defibrillator is indicated for those who do not respond to β-blocking drugs and those who have experienced cardiac arrest. Genotype-phenotype correlative studies have suggested that β-blocking agents are not effective in patients with LQT3, and in those individuals, an ICD is usually indicated.

429.6 Sinus Node Dysfunction

George F. Van Hare

Sinus arrest and **sinoatrial block** may cause a sudden pause in the heartbeat. The former is presumably caused by failure of impulse formation within the sinus node and the latter by a block between the sinus pacemaker complex and the surrounding atrium. These arrhythmias are rare in childhood except as manifestations of digoxin toxicity or in patients who have had extensive atrial surgery.

Sick sinus syndrome is the result of abnormalities in the sinus node or atrial conduction pathways, or both. This syndrome may occur in the absence of congenital heart disease and has been reported in siblings, but it is most commonly seen after surgical correction of congenital heart defects, especially the Fontan procedure and the atrial switch (Mustard or Senning) operation for transposition of the great arteries. Clinical manifestations depend on the heart rate. Most patients remain asymptomatic without treatment, but dizziness and syncope can occur during periods of marked sinus slowing with failure of junctional escape (Fig. 429-10). Pacemaker therapy is indicated in patients who experience symptoms such as exercise intolerance or syncope.

Patients with sinus node dysfunction may also have episodes of SVT (**"tachy-brady syndrome"**) with symptoms of palpitations, exercise intolerance, or dizziness. Treatment must be individualized. Drug therapy to control tachyarrhythmias (propranolol, sotalol, amiodarone) may suppress sinus and AV node function to such a degree that further symptomatic bradycardia may be produced. Therefore, insertion of a pacemaker in conjunction with drug therapy is usually necessary for such patients, even in the absence of symptoms ascribable to low heart rate.

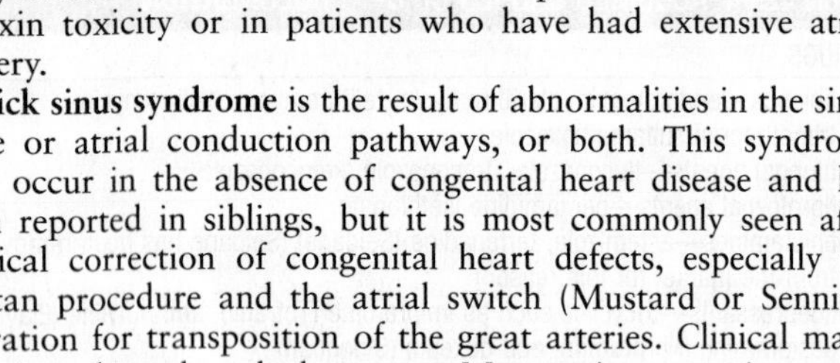

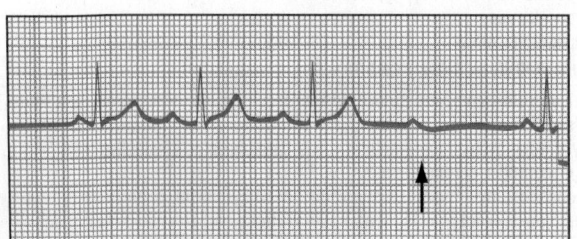

Figure 429-10 The "tachy-brady" syndrome with sinus node dysfunction. Note the bursts of supraventricular tachycardia, probably multifocal atrial in origin, followed by long periods of sinus arrest and by sinus bradycardia. Often, symptoms are due to the long sinus pauses following termination of tachycardia, rather than to the tachycardia itself.

429.7 AV Block

George F. Van Hare

AV block may be divided into 3 forms. In **1st-degree AV block,** the PR interval is prolonged, but all the atrial impulses are conducted to the ventricle (Fig. 429-11). In **2nd-degree AV block,** not every atrial impulse is conducted to the ventricle. In 1 variant of 2nd-degree block known as the **Wenckebach type** (also called **Mobitz type I**), classically the PR interval increases progressively until a P wave is not conducted. In the cycle following the dropped beat, the PR interval normalizes (see Fig. 429-11). In **Mobitz type II,** there is no progressive conduction delay and subsequent shortening of the PR interval after a blocked beat. This conduction defect is less common but has more potential to cause syncope and may be progressive. A related condition is **high-grade 2nd-degree AV block,** in which more than 1 P wave in a row fails to conduct. This is even more worrisome. In **3rd-degree AV block (complete heart block),** no impulses from the atria reach the ventricles (see Fig. 429-11). Generally, an independent escape rhythm is present, but may not be reliable, leading to symptoms such as syncope.

Congenital complete AV block in children is presumed to be caused by autoimmune injury of the fetal conduction system by maternally derived IgG antibodies (anti-SSA/Ro, anti-SSB/La) in a mother with overt or, more often, asymptomatic SLE or Sjögren syndrome. Autoimmune disease accounts for 60-70% of all cases of congenital complete heart block and ≈80% of cases in which the heart is structurally normal (Fig. 429-12). A homeobox gene

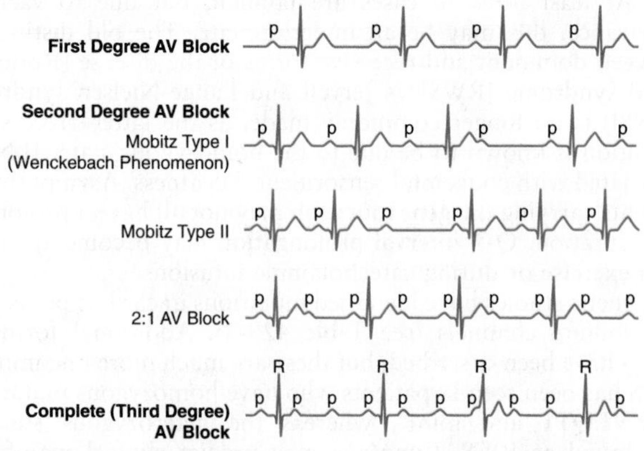

Figure 429-11 Atrioventricular (AV) block. (From Park MY: *Pediatric cardiology for practitioners*, ed 5, Philadelphia, 2008, Mosby/Elsevier, p 446, Fig. 25-1.)

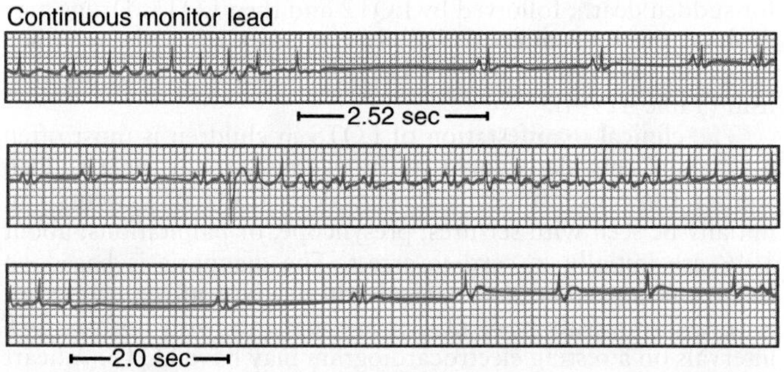

Figure 429-12 Congenital complete atrioventricular (AV) block. The ventricular rate is regular at 53 beats/min. The atrial rate is somewhat variable, from 65 to 95 beats/min, and completely dissociated from the ventricle. The QRS morphology is normal, which is common in congenital complete AV block.

mutation, NKX2-5, is described in which congenital AV block is seen most commonly in association with atrial septal defects. Complete AV block is also seen in patients with complex congenital heart disease and abnormal embryonic development of the conduction system. It has been associated with myocardial tumors and myocarditis. It is a known complication of myocardial abscess secondary to endocarditis. It is also seen in genetic abnormalities including LQTS and Kearn-Sayre syndrome. It is also a complication of congenital heart disease repair and, in particular, repairs involving VSD closure.

The incidence of congenital complete heart block is 1/20,000-25,000 live births; a high fetal loss rate may cause an underestimation of its true incidence. In some infants of mothers with SLE, complete heart block is not present at birth but develops within the 1st 3-6 mo after birth. The arrhythmia is often diagnosed in the fetus (secondary to the dissociation between atrial and ventricular contractions seen on fetal echocardiography) and may produce hydrops fetalis. Infants with associated congenital heart disease and heart failure have a high mortality rate.

In older children with otherwise normal hearts, the condition is commonly asymptomatic, although syncope and sudden death may occur. Infants and toddlers may have night terrors, tiredness with frequent naps, and irritability. The peripheral pulse is prominent as a result of the compensatory large ventricular stroke volume and peripheral vasodilatation; systolic blood pressure is elevated. Jugular venous pulsations occur irregularly and may be large when the atrium contracts against a closed tricuspid valve (cannon wave). Exercise and atropine may produce an acceleration of ≥10-20 beats/min. Systolic murmurs are frequently audible along the left sternal border, and apical mid-diastolic murmurs are not unusual. The first heart sound is variable, due to variable ventricular filing with AV dissociation. AV block results in enlargement of the heart on the basis of increased diastolic ventricular filling.

The **diagnosis** is confirmed by electrocardiography; the P waves and QRS complexes have no constant relationship (see Fig. 429-12). The QRS duration may be prolonged, or it may be normal if the heartbeat is initiated high in the AV node or bundle of His.

The **prognosis** for congenital complete heart block is usually favorable; patients who have been observed to the age of 30-40 yr have lived normal, active lives. Some patients have episodes of exercise intolerance, dizziness, and syncope (Stokes-Adams attacks); this symptom requires the implantation of a permanent cardiac pacemaker. Pacemaker implantation should be considered for patients who develop symptoms such as progressive cardiac enlargement, prolonged pauses, or daytime average heart rates of ≤50 beats/min. In addition, prophylactic pacemaker implantation in adolescents is reasonable considering the low risk of the implant procedure and the difficulty in predicting who will develop sudden severe symptoms.

Cardiac pacing is recommended in neonates with low ventricular rates (≤50 beats/min), evidence of heart failure, wide complex rhythms, or congenital heart disease. Isoproterenol, atropine, or epinephrine may be used to try to increase the heart rate temporarily until pacemaker placement can be arranged. Transthoracic epicardial pacemaker implants have traditionally been used in infants; transvenous placement of pacemaker leads is available for young children.

Postsurgical complete AV block can occur after any open heart procedure requiring suturing near the AV valves or crest of the ventricular septum. Postoperative heart block is initially managed with temporary pacing wires. The likelihood of a return to sinus rhythm after 10-14 days is low; a permanent pacemaker is recommended after that time.

BIBLIOGRAPHY

Please visit the Nelson Textbook of Pediatrics *website at* *www.expertconsult.com* *for the complete bibliography.*

Chapter 430 Sudden Death

George F. Van Hare

Sudden death other than sudden infant death syndrome (SIDS; Chapter 367) is rare in children younger than 18 yr. Sudden death can be divided into either traumatic or nontraumatic origin. Traumatic causes of sudden death are the most common in children; these include motor vehicle crashes, violent deaths, recreational deaths, and occupational deaths. Nontraumatic sudden deaths are often due to specific cardiac causes. The incidence of sudden death varies from 0.8 to 6.2 per 100,000 per year in children and adolescents as opposed to the higher incidence of sudden cardiac death in adults of 1 per 1,000. Approximately 65% of sudden deaths are due to heart-related problems in patients with either normal or congenitally (corrected, palliated, or unoperated) abnormal hearts. Competitive high-school sports (basketball, football) are high-risk environmental factors. The most common cause of death in competitive athletes is hypertrophic cardiomyopathy, with or without obstruction to left ventricular outflow. Other potential causes are listed in Table 430-1. These can be classified as structural abnormalities, including aortic stenosis and coronary artery abnormalities; myocardial disease, such as myocarditis; conduction system disease, including long Q-T syndrome (LQTS); and miscellaneous causes, including pulmonary hypertension and commotio cordis. Symptoms may be absent before the event but, if present, include syncope, chest pain, dyspnea, and palpitations. Patients may have a family history of heart disease (dilated or hypertrophic cardiomyopathy, long Q-T interval, arrhythmogenic right ventricular dysplasia, Marfan syndrome) or sudden death. Death often follows exertion or exercise.

MECHANISM OF SUDDEN DEATH

There are 3 mechanisms of sudden death: arrhythmic, nonarrhythmic cardiac (circulatory and vascular causes), and noncardiac. Ventricular fibrillation (VF), while the most common final cause of sudden death in adults, is only the final cause in 10-20% of children with sudden cardiac death. More commonly, bradycardia leads either to VF or asystole (Chapter 429).

CONGENITAL HEART DISEASE

Valvar aortic stenosis is the congenital defect most commonly associated with sudden death in children. Historically, approximately 5% of children with this disease die. A history of syncope, chest pain, and evidence of severe obstruction and left ventricular hypertrophy are risk factors (Chapter 421.5).

Coronary artery anomalies are also commonly associated with sudden death in children and adolescents. The most common abnormality associated with sudden death is the origin of the left main coronary artery from the right sinus of Valsalva. The coronary artery therefore courses between the aorta and pulmonary artery, and may also be intramural in course. Exercise results in a rise in pulmonary and aortic pressure, which compresses the left main coronary artery and results in ischemia due to compression or kinking.

CARDIOMYOPATHY

All 3 major types of cardiomyopathy (hypertrophic, dilated, and restrictive) are associated with sudden death in the pediatric population; sudden death may be the initial manifestation of the cardiomyopathy (Chapter 433).

Hypertrophic cardiomyopathy (HCM) is the most common cause of sudden death in the athletic adolescent. The annual risk

Table 430-1 POTENTIAL CAUSES OF SUDDEN DEATH IN INFANTS, CHILDREN, AND ADOLESCENTS

SIDS AND SIDS "MIMICS"
SIDS Long Q-T syndromes* Inborn errors of metabolism Child abuse Myocarditis Duct-dependent congenital heart disease
CORRECTED OR UNOPERATED CONGENITAL HEART DISEASE
Aortic stenosis Tetralogy of Fallot Transposition of great vessels (postoperative atrial switch) Mitral valve prolapse Hypoplastic left heart syndrome Eisenmenger syndrome
CORONARY ARTERIAL DISEASE
Anomalous origin* Anomalous tract (tunneled) Kawasaki disease Periarteritis Arterial dissection Marfan syndrome (rupture of aorta) Myocardial infarction
MYOCARDIAL DISEASE
Myocarditis Hypertrophic cardiomyopathy* Dilated cardiomyopathy Arrhythmogenic right ventricular dysplasia
CONDUCTION SYSTEM ABNORMALITY/ARRHYTHMIA
Long Q-T syndromes* Brugada syndrome Proarrhythmic drugs Preexcitation syndromes Heart block Commotio cordis Idiopathic ventricular fibrillation Arrhythmogenic right ventricular dysplasia Heart tumor
MISCELLANEOUS
Pulmonary hypertension Pulmonary embolism Heat stroke Cocaine and other stimulant drugs or medications Anorexia nervosa Electrolyte disturbances

*Common.
SIDS, sudden infant death syndrome.

of sudden death in young patients with HCM is 2% per year. Risk factors for sudden death include a family history of sudden death, symptoms, ventricular arrhythmias, and presentation at an early age. Many patients with HCM have obstruction to the left ventricular outflow tract. The mechanism of sudden death is arrhythmic and may be secondary to development of dynamic obstruction with exercise and resultant loss of cardiac output, or may be related to cardiac ischemia.

The **dilated cardiomyopathies** are also associated with sudden cardiac death. Arrhythmogenic right ventricular dysplasia (ARVD) is a specific form of cardiomyopathy associated with exercise-induced ventricular arrhythmias and sudden death. The diagnosis can be difficult; MRI, electrophysiology study, or endomyocardial biopsy is used with limited reliability. Pathology includes transmural fatty replacement of right ventricular myocardium, with patchy areas of fibrosis.

Myocarditis has been found commonly on pathology of patients with sudden death of unknown etiology. Symptoms prior to sudden death may be absent, or may include overt heart failure or subtle findings such as a high heart rate. Pediatric patients may

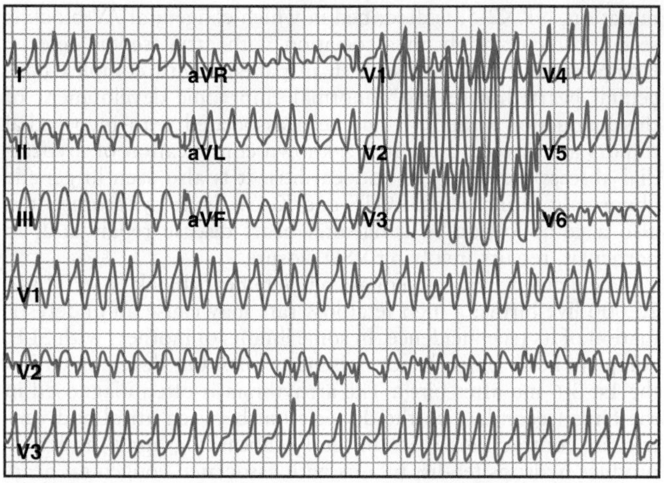

Figure 430-1 Atrial fibrillation in a patient with Wolff-Parkinson-White (WPW) syndrome and rapid conduction to the ventricle. Note the wide QRS complexes, due to full preexcitation, and the irregularly irregular ventricular response, due to the atrial fibrillation.

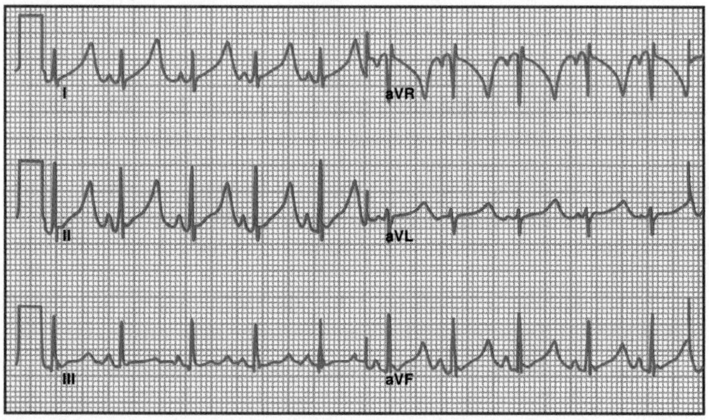

Figure 430-2 Long Q-T syndrome in a neonate. QTc is markedly prolonged. T waves are also peaked and abnormal in appearance.

have complete heart block or ventricular arrhythmias with this disease.

CARDIAC ARRHYTHMIA

A primary conduction system abnormality may result in sudden death. Causes include Wolff-Parkinson-White (WPW) syndrome and long Q-T syndrome. Besides causing supraventricular tachycardia (SVT), WPW syndrome can result in atrial fibrillation with rapid conduction across the accessory pathway leading to ventricular fibrillation and sudden death (Fig. 430-1) (Chapter 429). This is unusual in pediatric patients but has an increasing incidence in adolescence. In adults, there is an incidence of sudden death in asymptomatic patients of 1 per 1,000 patient-years, but this rate may well be higher in children, who by definition have not survived to adulthood. As digoxin and verapamil can augment conduction down accessory pathways, these drugs are contraindicated in WPW syndrome.

Long Q-T syndrome (Chapter 429), a group of channelopathies that affect ventricular repolarization, is also associated with sudden death (Fig. 430-2). The mechanism of sudden death is polymorphic VT (torsades de pointes) (Fig. 430-3). An initial presentation of sudden cardiac death is found in 9% of patients. Thus, treatment of asymptomatic patients with a long Q-T interval on electrocardiogram (ECG) and positive family history is advised.

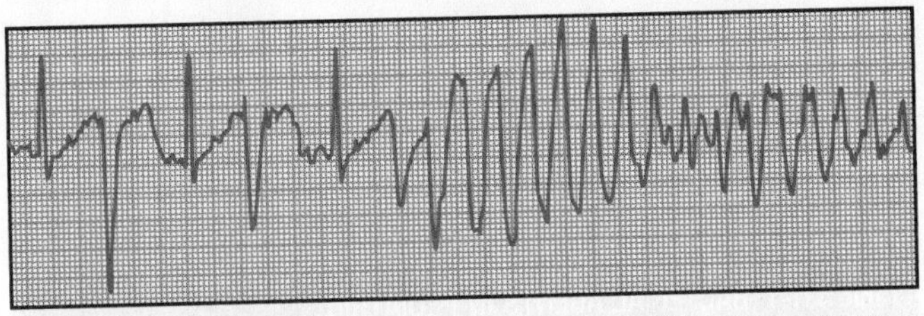

Figure 430-3 Episode of torsades de pointes in a patient with long Q-T syndrome.

Acquired long Q-T intervals may be seen in patients with marked electrolyte abnormalities, CNS injury, or starvation (including bulimia and anorexia nervosa). Medications can also result in prolongation of the Q-T interval (Table 429-4). These patients are also at risk of malignant ventricular arrhythmias, and correction of the underlying problem may be necessary to reduce the risk of sudden death.

MISCELLANEOUS CAUSES

Commotio cordis is a nearly universally fatal condition that follows blunt nonpenetrating trauma to the chest (e.g., from a baseball or hockey puck). Occasionally, innocent-appearing chest blows incurred at home or at a playground may be fatal. Patients experience immediate ventricular fibrillation in the absence of identifiable cardiac trauma (contusion, hematoma, lacerated coronary artery). Historically death results from ventricular fibrillation that is unresponsive to resuscitative efforts in 85-90% of children. Immediate DC defibrillation should be effective, if available.

EVALUATION AND THERAPY FOR RESUSCITATED PATIENTS

It is important to focus therapy on potentially reversible causes of sudden death. These include correction of major hemodynamic defects, pacing therapy for a patient with bradycardia, or supportive therapy for myocarditis. Unfortunately, reversible causes are not always found in young cardiac arrest survivors. Added to this dilemma is the fact that there is a limited ability to predict antiarrhythmic drug response or risk of recurrence. Thus, the implantable cardioverter defibrillator (ICD) has become the **therapy of choice** for survivors of arrhythmic sudden death.

MEDICATION FOR ATTENTION-DEFICIT DISORDER (ADD)

There has been some concern about the possibility that stimulant medications prescribed for the treatment of children with attention-deficit disorder could potentially increase the risk of sudden death. The concern arises from a limited number of reports to the U.S. Food and Drug Administration of sudden death of unknown etiology in individuals taking stimulant medications, most of whom are adults. In a few cases, left ventricular hypertrophy due to hypertension, coarctation of the aorta or hypertrophic cardiomyopathy has been identified at postmortem examination. There are no prospective studies to support the notion that these medications increase the risk, and little or no evidence that electrocardiographic screening will reliably identify a subgroup at risk. Some have suggested ECG screening of children prior to starting these medications, but there is no consensus that such an approach will be effective.

Table 430-2 CARDIAC SCREENING QUESTIONS INCLUDED IN THE *PREPARTICIPATION PHYSICAL EVALUATION*

Have you ever passed out or nearly passed out during exercise?
Have you ever passed out or nearly passed out after exercise?
Have you ever had discomfort, pain, or pressure in your chest during exercise?
Does your heart race or skip beats during exercise?
Has a doctor ever told you that you have high blood pressure, high cholesterol, a heart murmur, or a heart infection?
Has a doctor ever ordered a test for your heart?
Has anyone in your family ever died for no apparent reason?
Does anyone in your family have a heart problem?
Has any family member or relative died of heart problems or sudden death before age 50?
Does anyone in your family have Marfan syndrome?

Reprinted with permission from "Preparticipation Physical Evaluation." Copyright © American Academy of Family Physicians. All Rights Reserved.

PREVENTION OF SUDDEN DEATH

The probability of survival to hospital discharge for a young patient who experiences an out-of-hospital cardiac arrest is <20%. The presence of immediate automatic external defibrillators (AEDs), when combined with standard cardiopulmonary resuscitation at the site of exercise (gym, track, basketball, or football arena), may improve survival substantially. Thus, identifying patients at risk is extremely important.

Many of the more common causes of sudden death in children and adolescents can be identified from the patient's history (prodromal symptoms), the family history, and physical examination (Table 430-2). Of paramount importance is the careful evaluation of any child who experiences syncope in association with exercise, as this may be the last opportunity to diagnose a life-threatening condition in such a patient.

Patient avoidance of high-risk behavior (cocaine use, anorexia nervosa) and acquisition of knowledge of drug side effects (tricyclic antidepressants) or drug interactions (terfenadine [Seldane] and erythromycin) is critical. Chest-protecting equipment may not prevent commotio cordis. Prompt cardiopulmonary resuscitation and rapid defibrillation by an AED or by an emergency medical services rescue team should improve survival. Family survivors of victims of sudden death should be evaluated for genetic causes such as LQTS and hypertrophic cardiomyopathy.

There is evidence that a sports preparticipation ECG, in addition to a cardiac specific history and physical, may add to the detection of those athletes at risk for sudden death. Because many athletes either have no pre-event symptoms or are unwilling to volunteer cardiac manifestations for fear of not being able to play, the ECG may identify a small but at-risk group with hypertrophic cardiomyopathy or the prolonged QT, Brugada, or Wolff-Parkinson-White syndromes. Various authoritative groups consider preparticipation ECG cost-effective with the potential of saving lives following more definitive evaluation with echocardiography for those with a positive ECG. ECG testing is routine in many European countries but not in the USA.

BIBLIOGRAPHY

Please visit the Nelson Textbook of Pediatrics *website at www.expertconsult.com for the complete bibliography.*

Section 5 ACQUIRED HEART DISEASE

Chapter 431
Infective Endocarditis

Daniel Bernstein

Infective endocarditis includes acute and subacute bacterial endocarditis, as well as nonbacterial endocarditis caused by viruses, fungi, and other microbiologic agents. It is a significant cause of morbidity and mortality in children and adolescents despite advances in the management and prophylaxis of the disease with antimicrobial agents. The inability to eradicate infective endocarditis by prevention or early treatment stems from several factors. The disease represents a complex interplay between a pathogen and host factors such as endothelial disruption and immune function that is still not completely understood; the nature of the infecting organism has changed over time; diagnosis may be difficult during early stages and is thus often delayed until a more serious infection has set in; and special risk groups have emerged, including intravenous drug users; survivors of cardiac surgery, especially those with mechanical prosthesis; patients taking immunosuppressant medications; and patients who require chronic intravascular catheters. Some patients get endocarditis on what was thought to be a previously healthy native valve, although on surgical inspection is found to have mild structural abnormalities.

ETIOLOGY

Viridans-type streptococci (α-hemolytic streptococci) and *Staphylococcus aureus* remain the leading causative agents for endocarditis in pediatric patients. Other organisms cause endocarditis less frequently and, in ≈6% of cases, blood cultures are negative for any organisms (Table 431-1). No relationship exists between the infecting organism and the type of congenital defect, the duration of illness, or the age of the child. Staphylococcal endocarditis is more common in patients with no underlying heart disease; viridans group streptococcal infection is more common after dental procedures; group D enterococci are seen more often after lower bowel or genitourinary manipulation; *Pseudomonas aeruginosa* or *Serratia marcescens* is seen more frequently in intravenous drug users; and fungal organisms are encountered after open heart surgery. Coagulase-negative staphylococci are common in the presence of an indwelling central venous catheter.

Table 431-1 BACTERIAL AGENTS IN PEDIATRIC INFECTIVE ENDOCARDITIS

COMMON: NATIVE VALVE OR OTHER CARDIAC LESIONS
Viridans group streptococci *(Streptococcus mutans, Streptococcus sanguinis, Streptococcus mitis)*
Staphylococcus aureus
Group D streptococcus (enterococcus) *(Streptococcus bovis, Streptococcus faecalis)*
UNCOMMON: NATIVE VALVE OR OTHER CARDIAC LESIONS
Streptococcus pneumoniae
Haemophilus influenzae
Coagulase-negative staphylococci
*Coxiella burnetii (Q fever)**
Neisseria gonorrhoeae
*Brucella**
*Chlamydia psittaci**
*Chlamydia trachomatis**
*Chlamydia pneumoniae**
*Legionella**
*Bartonella**
HACEK group†
*Streptobacillus moniliformis**
*Pasteurella multocida**
Campylobacter fetus
Culture negative (6% of cases)
PROSTHETIC VALVE
Staphylococcus epidermidis
Staphylococcus aureus
Viridans group streptococcus
Pseudomonas aeruginosa
Serratia marcescens
Diphtheroids
Legionella species*
HACEK group†
Fungi‡

*These fastidious bacteria plus some fungi may produce culture-negative endocarditis. Detection may require special media, incubation for more than 7 days, or serologic tests.
†The HACEK group includes *Haemophilus* species *(H. paraphrophilus, H. parainfluenzae, H. aphrophilus), Actinobacillus actinomycetemcomitans, Cardiobacterium hominis, Eikenella corrodens,* and *Kingella* species.
‡*Candida* species, *Aspergillus* species, *Pseudallescheria boydii, Histoplasma capsulatum.*

EPIDEMIOLOGY

Infective endocarditis is often a complication of congenital or rheumatic heart disease but can also occur in children without any abnormal valves or cardiac malformations. In developed countries, congenital heart disease is the overwhelming predisposing factor. Endocarditis is rare in infancy; in this age group, it usually follows open heart surgery or is associated with a central venous line.

Patients with congenital heart lesions where there is turbulent blood flow due to a hole or stenotic orifice, especially if there is a high pressure gradient across the defect, are most susceptible to endocarditis. This turbulent flow traumatizes the vascular endothelium, creating a substrate for deposition of fibrin and platelets, leading to the formation of a nonbacterial thrombotic embolus (NBTE) that is thought to be the initiating lesion for infective endocarditis. Biofilms form on the surface of implanted mechanical devices such as valves, catheters, or pacemaker wires that also serve as the adhesive substrate for infection. The development of transient bacteremia then colonizes this NBTE or biofilm, leading to proliferation of bacteria within the lesion. Bacterial surface proteins, such as the FimA antigen in viridans streptococci, act as adhesion factors to the NBTE or biofilm, after which bacteria can rapidly proliferate within the vegetation. Given the heavy colonization of mucosal surfaces (the oropharynx, or gastrointestinal, vaginal, or urinary tracts) by potentially pathogenic bacteria, these surfaces are thought to be the origin of this transient bacteremia. There is controversy over the extent to which daily activities (such as brushing or flossing the teeth) vs invasive procedures (such as dental cleanings or surgery) contribute to this bacteremia. Transient bacteremia has been reported to occur in 20-68% of patients after tooth brushing and flossing, and even in 7-51% of patients after chewing food. The magnitude of this bacteremia is also similar to that resulting from dental procedures. Maintenance of good oral hygiene may be a more important factor in decreasing the frequency and magnitude of bacteremia.

Children at **highest risk** of adverse outcome after infective endocarditis include those with: prosthetic cardiac valves or other prosthetic material used for cardiac valve repair, unrepaired cyanotic congenital heart disease (including those palliated with shunts and conduits), completely repaired defects with prosthetic material or device during the 1st 6 mo after repair, repaired congenital heart disease with residual defects at or adjacent to the site of a prosthetic patch or device, valve stenosis or insufficiency occurring after heart transplantation, and previous infective endocarditis. Patients with high velocity blood flow lesions such as ventricular septal defects and aortic stenosis are also at high risk. In older patients, congenital bicuspid aortic valves and mitral valve prolapse with regurgitation pose additional risks for endocarditis. Surgical correction of congenital heart disease may reduce but does not eliminate the risk of endocarditis, with the exception of repair of a simple atrial septal defect or patent ductus arteriosus without prosthetic material.

In ≈30% of patients with infective endocarditis, a predisposing factor is presumably recognized. Although a preceding dental procedure may be identified in 10-20% of patients, the time of the procedure may range from 1 to 6 mo prior to the onset of symptoms, hence the continued controversy over the absolute risk of infective endocarditis after dental procedures. Primary bacteremia with *Staphylococcus aureus* is thought to be another risk for endocarditis. The occurrence of endocarditis directly after most routine heart surgery is relatively low, but it can be an antecedent event, especially if prosthetic material is utilized.

CLINICAL MANIFESTATIONS (TABLE 431-2)

Early manifestations are usually mild, especially when viridans group streptococci are the infecting organisms. Prolonged fever without other manifestations (except, occasionally, weight loss) that persists for as long as several months may be the only symptom. Alternatively, the onset may be acute and severe, with high, intermittent fever and prostration. Usually, the onset and course vary between these two extremes. The symptoms are often nonspecific and consist of low-grade fever with afternoon elevations, fatigue, myalgia, arthralgia, headache, and, at times, chills, nausea, and vomiting. **New or changing heart murmurs** are common, particularly with associated heart failure. Splenomegaly and petechiae are relatively common. Serious neurologic complications such as embolic strokes, cerebral abscesses, mycotic aneurysms, and hemorrhage are most often associated with staphylococcal disease and may be late manifestations. Meningismus, increased intracranial pressure, altered sensorium, and focal neurologic signs are manifestations of these complications. Myocardial abscesses may occur with staphylococcal disease and may damage the cardiac conducting system, causing heart block, or may rupture into the pericardium and produce purulent pericarditis. Pulmonary and other systemic emboli are infrequent, except with fungal disease. Many of the classic skin findings develop late in the course of the disease; they are seldom seen in appropriately treated patients. Such manifestations include **Osler nodes** (tender, pea-sized intradermal nodules in the pads of the fingers and toes), **Janeway lesions** (painless small erythematous or hemorrhagic lesions on the palms and soles), and **splinter hemorrhages** (linear lesions beneath the nails). These lesions may represent vasculitis produced by circulating antigen-antibody complexes.

Identification of infective endocarditis is most often based on a high index of suspicion during evaluation of an infection in a child with an underlying risk factor.

DIAGNOSIS

The critical information for appropriate treatment of infective endocarditis is obtained from blood cultures. All other laboratory data are secondary in importance (see Table 431-2). Blood specimens for culture should be obtained as promptly as possible, even if the child feels well and has no other physical findings. Three to five separate blood collections should be obtained after careful preparation of the phlebotomy site. Contamination presents a special problem inasmuch as bacteria found on the skin may themselves cause infective endocarditis. The timing of collections is not important because bacteremia can be expected to be relatively constant. In 90% of cases of endocarditis, the causative agent is recovered from the 1st 2 blood cultures. The laboratory should be notified that endocarditis is suspected so that, if necessary, the blood can be cultured on enriched media for longer than usual (>7 days) to detect nutritionally deficient and fastidious bacteria or fungi. Antimicrobial pretreatment of the patient reduces the yield of blood cultures to 50-60%. The microbiology laboratory should be notified if the patient has received antibiotics so that more sophisticated methods can be used to recover the offending agent. Other specimens that may be cultured include scrapings from cutaneous lesions, urine, synovial fluid, abscesses, and, in the presence of manifestations of meningitis, cerebrospinal fluid.

Table 431-2 MANIFESTATIONS OF INFECTIVE ENDOCARDITIS

HISTORY
Prior congenital or rheumatic heart disease
Preceding dental, urinary tract, or intestinal procedure
Intravenous drug use
Central venous catheter
Prosthetic heart valve
SYMPTOMS
Fever
Chills
Chest and abdominal pain
Arthralgia, myalgia
Dyspnea
Malaise, weakness
Night sweats
Weight loss
CNS manifestations (stroke, seizures, headache)
SIGNS
Elevated temperature
Tachycardia
Embolic phenomena (Roth spots, petechiae, splinter nail bed hemorrhages, Osler nodes, CNS or ocular lesions)
Janeway lesions
New or changing murmur
Splenomegaly
Arthritis
Heart failure
Arrhythmias
Metastatic infection (arthritis, meningitis, mycotic arterial aneurysm, pericarditis, abscesses, septic pulmonary emboli)
Clubbing
LABORATORY
Positive blood culture
Elevated erythrocyte sedimentation rate; may be low with heart or renal failure
Elevated C-reactive protein
Anemia
Leukocytosis
Immune complexes
Hypergammaglobulinemia
Hypocomplementemia
Cryoglobulinemia
Rheumatoid factor
Hematuria
Renal failure: azotemia, high creatinine (glomerulonephritis)
Chest radiograph: bilateral infiltrates, nodules, pleural effusions
Echocardiographic evidence of valve vegetations, prosthetic valve dysfunction or leak, myocardial abscess, new-onset valve insufficiency

CNS, central nervous system.

Table 431-3 DIAGNOSTIC APPROACH TO UNCOMMON PATHOGENS CAUSING ENDOCARDITIS

PATHOGEN	DIAGNOSTIC PROCEDURE
Brucella spp.	Blood cultures; serology; culture, immunohistology, and PCR of surgical material
Coxiella burnetti	Serology (IgG phase I >1 in 800); tissue culture, immunohistology, and PCR of surgical material
Bartonella spp.	Blood cultures; serology; culture, immunohistology, and PCR of surgical material
Chlamydia spp.	Serology; culture, immunohistology, and PCR of surgical material
Mycoplasma spp.	Serology; culture, immunohistology, and PCR of surgical material
Legionella spp.	Blood cultures; serology; culture, immunohistology, and PCR of surgical material
Tropheryma whipplei	Histology and PCR of surgical material

PCR, polymerase chain reaction.
From Moreillon P, Que YA: Infective endocarditis, *Lancet* 363:139–148, 2004.

Serologic diagnosis or PCR of resected valve tissues is necessary in patients with unusual or fastidious microorganisms (Table 431-3).

The index of suspicion should be high when evaluating infection in a child with an underlying contributing factor. The combination of transthoracic and transesophageal echocardiography enhances the ability to diagnose endocarditis. Two-dimensional echocardiography can identify the size, shape, location, and mobility of the lesion; when combined with Doppler studies, the presence of valve dysfunction (regurgitation, obstruction) can be determined and its effect on left ventricular performance quantified. Echocardiography may also be helpful in predicting embolic complications, given that lesions >1 cm and fungating masses are at greatest risk for embolization. The absence of vegetations does not exclude endocarditis, and vegetations are often not visualized in the early phases of the disease or in patients with complex congenital heart lesions.

The **Duke criteria** help in the diagnosis of endocarditis. **Major criteria** include (1) positive blood cultures (2 separate cultures for a usual pathogen, 2 or more for less typical pathogens), and (2) evidence of endocarditis on echocardiography (intracardiac mass on a valve or other site, regurgitant flow near a prosthesis, abscess, partial dehiscence of prosthetic valves, or new valve regurgitant flow). **Minor criteria** include predisposing conditions, fever, embolic-vascular signs, immune complex phenomena (glomerulonephritis, arthritis, rheumatoid factor, Osler nodes, Roth spots), a single positive blood culture or serologic evidence of infection, and echocardiographic signs not meeting the major criteria. Two major criteria, one major and three minor, or five minor criteria suggest definite endocarditis. A modification of the Duke criteria may increase sensitivity while maintaining specificity. The following minor criteria are added to those already listed: the presence of newly diagnosed clubbing, splenomegaly, splinter hemorrhages, and petechiae; a high erythrocyte sedimentation rate; a high C-reactive protein level; and the presence of central nonfeeding lines, peripheral lines, and microscopic hematuria.

PROGNOSIS AND COMPLICATIONS

Despite the use of antibiotic agents, mortality is at 20-25%. Serious morbidity occurs in 50-60% of children with documented infective endocarditis; the most common is heart failure caused by vegetations involving the aortic or mitral valve. Myocardial abscesses and toxic myocarditis may also lead to heart failure without characteristic changes in auscultatory findings and, occasionally, to life-threatening arrhythmias. Systemic emboli, often with central nervous system manifestations, are a major threat. Pulmonary emboli may occur in children with ventricular septal defect or the tetralogy of Fallot, although massive life-threatening pulmonary embolization is rare. Other complications include mycotic aneurysms, rupture of a sinus of Valsalva, obstruction of a valve secondary to large vegetations, acquired ventricular septal defect, and heart block as a result of involvement (abscess) of the conduction system. Additional complications include meningitis, osteomyelitis, arthritis, renal abscess, purulent pericarditis, and immune complex-mediated glomerulonephritis.

TREATMENT

Antibiotic therapy should be instituted immediately once a definitive diagnosis is made. When virulent organisms are responsible, small delays may result in progressive endocardial damage and are associated with a greater likelihood of severe complications. The choice of antibiotics, method of administration, and length of treatment should be coordinated with consultants from both cardiology and infectious diseases (Tables 431-4 and 431-5). Empirical therapy before the identifiable agent is recovered may be initiated with vancomycin plus gentamicin in patients without a prosthetic valve and when there is a high risk of *S. aureus* enterococcus or viridans streptococci (the 3 most common organisms). High serum bactericidal levels must be maintained long enough to eradicate organisms that are growing in relatively inaccessible avascular vegetations. Between 5 and 20 times the minimal in vitro inhibiting concentration must be produced at the site of infection to destroy bacteria growing at the core of these lesions. Several weeks are required for a vegetation to organize completely; therapy must be continued through this period so that recrudescence can be avoided. A total of 4-6 wk of treatment is usually recommended. Depending on the clinical and laboratory responses, antibiotic therapy may require modification and, in some instances, more prolonged treatment is required. With highly sensitive viridans group streptococcal infections, shortened regimens that include oral penicillin for some portion have been recommended. In nonstaphylococcal disease, bacteremia usually resolves in 24-48 hr, whereas fever resolves in 5-6 days with appropriate antibiotic therapy. Resolution with staphylococcal disease takes longer.

If the infection occurs on a valve and induces or increases symptoms and signs of heart failure, appropriate therapy should be instituted, including diuretics, afterload reducing agents, and in some cases, digitalis. Surgical intervention for infective endocarditis is indicated for severe aortic or mitral valve involvement with intractable heart failure. Rarely, a mycotic aneurysm, rupture of an aortic sinus, intraseptal abscess causing complete heart block, or dehiscence of an intracardiac patch requires an emergency operation. Other surgical indications include failure to sterilize the blood despite adequate antibiotic levels, myocardial abscess, recurrent emboli, and increasing size of vegetations while receiving therapy. Although antibiotic therapy should be administered for as long as possible before surgical intervention, active infection is not a contraindication if the patient is critically ill as a result of severe hemodynamic deterioration from infective endocarditis. Removal of vegetations and, in some instances, valve replacement may be lifesaving, and sustained antibiotic administration will most often prevent reinfection. Replacement of infected prosthetic valves carries a higher risk.

Fungal endocarditis is difficult to manage and has a poorer prognosis. It has been encountered after cardiac surgery, in severely debilitated or immunosuppressed patients, and in patients on prolonged courses of antibiotics. The drugs of choice are amphotericin B (liposomal or standard preparation) and 5-fluorocytosine. Surgery to excise infected tissue is occasionally attempted, though often with limited success. Recombinant tissue

Table 431-4 THERAPY OF NATIVE VALVE ENDOCARDITIS CAUSED BY HIGHLY PENICILLIN-SUSCEPTIBLE VIRIDANS GROUP STREPTOCOCCI AND *STREPTOCOCCUS BOVIS*

REGIMEN	DOSAGE* AND ROUTE	DURATION, WK	COMMENTS
Aqueous crystalline penicillin G sodium	12-18 million U/24 hr IV either continuously or in 4 or 6 equally divided doses	4	Preferred in patients with impairment of 8th cranial nerve function or renal function
or			
Ceftriaxone sodium	2 g/24 hr IV/IM in 1 dose	4	
	***Pediatric dose*†**: penicillin 200,000 U/kg per 24 hr IV in 4-6 equally divided doses; ceftriaxone 100 mg/kg per 24 hr IV/IM in 1 dose		
Aqueous crystalline penicillin G sodium	12-18 million U/24 hr IV either continuously or in 6 equally divided doses	2	2 wk regimen not intended for patients with known cardiac or extracardiac abscess or for those with creatinine clearance of <20 ml/min, impaired 8th cranial nerve function, or *Abiotrophia, Granulicatella,* or *Gemella* spp infection; gentamicin dosage should be adjusted to achieve peak serum concentration of 3-4 μg/ml and trough serum concentration of <1 μg/ml when 3 divided doses are used; nomogram used for single daily dosing
or			
Ceftriaxone sodium	2 g/24 hr IV/IM in 1 dose	2	
plus			
Gentamicin sulfate‡	3 mg/kg per 24 hr IV/IM in 1 dose, or 3 equally divided doses ***Pediatric dose:*** penicillin 200,000 U/kg per 24 hr IV in 4-6 equally divided doses; ceftriaxone 100 mg/kg per 24 hr IV/IM in 1 dose; gentamicin 3 mg/kg per 24 hr IV/IM in 1 dose or 3 equally divided doses§	2	
Vancomycin hydrochloride¶	30 mg/kg per 24 hr IV in 2 equally divided doses not to exceed 2 g/24 hr unless concentrations in serum are inappropriately low ***Pediatric dose:*** 40 mg/kg per 24 hr IV in 2-3 equally divided doses	4	Vancomycin therapy recommended only for patients unable to tolerate penicillin or ceftriaxone; vancomycin dosage should be adjusted to obtain peak (1 hr after infusion completed) serum concentration of 30-45 μg/ml and a trough concentration range of 10-15 μg/ml

*Dosages recommended are for patients with normal renal function.
†Pediatric dose should not exceed that of a normal adult.
‡Other potentially nephrotoxic drugs (e.g., nonsteroidal antiinflammatory drugs) should be used with caution in patients receiving gentamicin therapy.
§Data for once-daily dosing of aminoglycosides for children exist, but no data for treatment of infective endocarditis exist.
¶Vancomycin dosages should be infused during course of at least 1 hr to reduce risk of histamine-release "red man" syndrome.
Minimum inhibitory concentration ≤0.12 μg/ml.
From Baddour LM, Wilson WR, Bayer AS, et al: Infective endocarditis: diagnosis, antimicrobial therapy, and management of complications, *Circulation* 111:e394–e433, 2005; correction: *Circulation* 112:2373, 2005.

Table 431-5 THERAPY FOR ENDOCARDITIS CAUSED BY STAPHYLOCOCCI IN THE ABSENCE OF PROSTHETIC MATERIALS

REGIMEN	DOSAGE* AND ROUTE	DURATION	COMMENTS
OXACILLIN-SUSCEPTIBLE STRAINS			
Nafcillin or oxacillin†	12 g/24 hr IV in 4-6 equally divided doses	6 wk	For complicated right-sided IE and for left-sided IE; for uncomplicated right-sided IE, 2 wk
with			
Optional addition of gentamicin sulfate‡	3 mg/kg per 24 hr IV/IM in 2 or 3 equally divided doses	3-5 day	
	***Pediatric dose*§**: Nafcillin or oxacillin 200 mg/kg per 24 hr IV in 4-6 equally divided doses; gentamicin 3 mg/kg per 24 hr IV/IM in 3 equally divided doses		Clinical benefit of aminoglycosides has not been established
For penicillin-allergic (nonanaphylactoid type) patients:			Consider skin testing for oxacillin-susceptible staphylococci and questionable history of immediate-type hypersensitivity to penicillin
Cefazolin	6 g/24 hr IV in 3 equally divided doses	6 wk	Cephalosporins should be avoided in patients with anaphylactoid-type hypersensitivity to β-lactams; vancomycin should be used in these cases§
with			
Optional addition of gentamicin sulfate	3 mg/kg per 24 hr IV/IM in 2 or 3 equally divided doses	3-5 day	Clinical benefit of aminoglycosides has not been established
	Pediatric dose: cefazolin 100 mg/kg per 24 hr IV in 3 equally divided doses; gentamicin 3 mg/kg per 24 hr IV/IM in 3 equally divided doses		
OXACILLIN-RESISTANT STRAINS			
Vancomycin¶	30 mg/kg per 24 hr IV in 2 equally divided doses ***Pediatric dose:*** 40 mg/kg per 24 hr IV in 2 or 3 equally divided doses	6 wk	Adjust vancomycin dosage to achieve 1 hr serum concentration of 30-45 μg/ml and trough concentration of 10-15 μg/ml

*Dosages recommended are for patients with normal renal function.
†Penicillin G 24 million U/24 hr IV in 4 to 6 equally divided doses may be used in place of nafcillin or oxacillin if strain is penicillin susceptible (minimum inhibitory concentration ≤0.1 μg/ml) and does not produce β-lactamase.
‡Gentamicin should be administered in close temporal proximity to vancomycin, nafcillin, or oxacillin dosing.
§Pediatric dose should not exceed that of a normal adult.
¶For specific dosing adjustment and issues concerning vancomycin, see Table 431-4 footnotes.
IE, infective endocarditis.
From Baddour LM, Wilson WR, Bayer AS, et al: Infective endocarditis: diagnosis, antimicrobial therapy, and management of complications, *Circulation* 111:e394–e433, 2005; corrections *Circulation* 112:2373, 2005.

plasminogen activation may help lyse intracardiac vegetations and avoid surgery in some high-risk patients.

PREVENTION

Recommendations by the American Heart Association for antimicrobial prophylaxis before dental and other surgical procedures received a major revision in 2007. A substantial reduction in the number of patients who require prophylactic treatment and the procedures requiring coverage was recommended. The primary reasons for these revised recommendations were that (1) infective endocarditis is much more likely to result from exposure to the more frequent random bacteremias associated with daily activities than from a dental or surgical procedure; (2) routine prophylaxis may prevent "an exceedingly small" number of cases; and (3) the risk of antibiotic-related adverse events exceeds the benefits of prophylactic therapy. Improving general dental hygiene was felt to be a more important factor in reducing the risk of infective endocarditis resulting from routine daily bacteremias. The current recommendations limit the use of prophylaxis to those patients with cardiac conditions associated with the greatest risk of an adverse outcome from infective endocarditis (Table 431-6). Prophylaxis for these patients is recommended for "all dental procedures that involve manipulation of gingival tissue or the periapical region of teeth or perforation of the oral mucosa." Furthermore, "placement of removable prosthodontic or endodontic appliances, adjustment of orthodontic appliances, placement of orthodontic brackets, shedding of deciduous teeth and bleeding from trauma to the lips or oral mucosa" are not indications for prophylaxis. Given that many invasive respiratory tract procedures do cause bacteremia, prophylaxis for many of these procedures in considered reasonable. In contrast to prior recommendations, prophylaxis for gastrointestinal or genitourinary procedures is no longer recommended in the majority of cases. Prophylaxis for patients undergoing cardiac surgery with placement of prosthetic material is still recommended. Given the highly individual nature of these recommendations and the continued concern amongst some cardiologists over their adoption, direct consultation with the child's cardiologist is still the best method for determining a specific patient's ongoing need for prophylaxis (Table 431-7).

Continuing education regarding both oral hygiene and, in appropriate cases, the need for prophylaxis is important, especially in teenagers and young adults. Vigorous treatment of sepsis and local infections and careful asepsis during heart surgery and catheterization reduce the incidence of infective endocarditis.

Table 431-6 2007 STATEMENT OF THE AMERICAN HEART ASSOCIATION (AHA): CARDIAC CONDITIONS ASSOCIATED WITH THE HIGHEST RISK OF AN ADVERSE OUTCOME FROM INFECTIVE ENDOCARDITIS FOR WHICH PROPHYLAXIS WITH DENTAL PROCEDURES IS REASONABLE

Prosthetic cardiac valve or prosthetic material used for cardiac valve repair Previous infective endocarditis
CONGENITAL HEART DISEASE (CHD)* Unrepaired cyanotic CHD, including palliative shunts and conduits Completely repaired CHD with prosthetic material or device, whether placed by surgery **or** catheter intervention, during the first 6 mo after the procedure† Repaired CHD with residual defects at the site or adjacent to the site of a prosthetic patch, **or** prosthetic device (which inhibit endothelization)
Cardiac transplantation recipients who develop cardiac valulopathy

*Except for the conditions listed here, antibiotic prophylaxis is no longer recommended by the AHA for any other form of CHD.
†Prophylaxis is reasonable because endothelization of prosthetic material occurs within 6 mo after the procedure.
From Wilson W, Taubert KA, Gewitz M, et al: Prevention of infective endocarditis. Guidelines from the American Heart Association, *Circulation* 116:1736–1754, 2007.

BIBLIOGRAPHY

Please visit the Nelson Textbook of Pediatrics *website at* www.expertconsult.com *for the complete bibliography.*

Chapter 432
Rheumatic Heart Disease
Daniel Bernstein

Rheumatic involvement of the valves and endocardium is the most important manifestation of rheumatic fever (Chapter 176). The valvular lesions begin as small verrucae composed of fibrin and blood cells along the borders of one or more of the heart valves. The mitral valve is affected most often, followed in frequency by the aortic valve; right-sided heart manifestations are rare. As the inflammation subsides, the verrucae tend to disappear and leave scar tissue. With repeated attacks of rheumatic fever, new verrucae form near the previous ones, and the mural endocardium and chordae tendineae become involved.

Table 431-7 2007 STATEMENT OF THE AMERICAN HEART ASSOCIATION (AHA): PROPHYLACTIC ANTIBIOTIC REGIMENS FOR A DENTAL PROCEDURE

SITUATION	AGENT	ADULTS	CHILDREN
Oral	Amoxicillin	2 g	50 mg/kg
Unable to take oral medication	Ampicillin OR cefazolin or ceftriaxone	2 g IM or IV 1 g IM or IV	50 mg/kg IM or IV 50 mg/kg IM or IV
Allergic to penicillins or ampicillin—oral	Cephalexin*† OR Clindamycin OR Azithromycin or clarithromycin	2 g 600 mg 500 mg	50 mg/kg 20 mg/kg 15 mg/kg
Allergic to penicillins or ampicillin and unable to take oral medication	Cefazolin or ceftriaxone† OR clindamycin	1 g IM or IV 600 mg IM or IV	50 mg/kg IM or IV 20 mg/kg IM or IV

*Or other first- or second-generation oral cephalosporin in equivalent adult or pediatric dosage.
†Cephalosporins should not be used in an individual with a history of anaphylaxis, angioedema, urticaria with penicillins or ampicillin.
IM, intramuscular; IV, intravenous.
From Wilson W, Taubert KA, Gewitz M, et al: Prevention of infective endocarditis. Guidelines from the American Heart Association, *Circulation* 116:1736–1754, 2007.

PATTERNS OF VALVULAR DISEASE

Mitral Insufficiency

PATHOPHYSIOLOGY Mitral insufficiency is the result of structural changes that usually include some loss of valvular substance and shortening and thickening of the chordae tendineae. During acute rheumatic fever with severe cardiac involvement, heart failure is caused by a combination of mitral insufficiency coupled with inflammatory disease of the pericardium, myocardium, endocardium, and epicardium. Because of the high volume load and inflammatory process, the left ventricle becomes enlarged. The left atrium dilates as blood regurgitates into this chamber. Increased left atrial pressure results in pulmonary congestion and symptoms of left-sided heart failure. Spontaneous improvement usually occurs with time, even in patients in whom mitral insufficiency is severe at the onset. The resultant chronic lesion is most often mild or moderate in severity, and the patient is asymptomatic. More than half of patients with acute mitral insufficiency no longer have the mitral murmur 1 yr later. In patients with severe chronic mitral insufficiency, pulmonary arterial pressure becomes elevated, the right ventricle and atrium become enlarged, and right-sided heart failure subsequently develops.

CLINICAL MANIFESTATIONS The physical signs of mitral insufficiency depend on its severity. With mild disease, signs of heart failure are not present, the precordium is quiet, and auscultation reveals a high-pitched holosystolic murmur at the apex that radiates to the axilla. With severe mitral insufficiency, signs of chronic heart failure may be noted. The heart is enlarged, with a heaving apical left ventricular impulse and often an apical systolic thrill. The 2nd heart sound may be accentuated if pulmonary hypertension is present. A 3rd heart sound is generally prominent. A holosystolic murmur is heard at the apex with radiation to the axilla. A short mid-diastolic rumbling murmur is caused by increased blood flow across the mitral valve as a result of the insufficiency. Auscultation of a diastolic murmur does not necessarily mean that mitral stenosis is present. The latter lesion takes many years to develop and is characterized by a diastolic murmur of greater length, usually with presystolic accentuation.

The electrocardiogram and roentgenograms are normal if the lesion is mild. With more severe insufficiency, the electrocardiogram shows prominent bifid P waves, signs of left ventricular hypertrophy, and associated right ventricular hypertrophy if pulmonary hypertension is present. Roentgenographically, prominence of the left atrium and ventricle can be seen. Congestion of perihilar vessels, a sign of pulmonary venous hypertension, may also be evident. Calcification of the mitral valve is rare in children. Echocardiography shows enlargement of the left atrium and ventricle, an abnormally thickened mitral valve, and Doppler studies demonstrate the severity of the mitral regurgitation. Heart catheterization and left ventriculography are considered only if diagnostic questions are not totally resolved by noninvasive assessment.

COMPLICATIONS Severe mitral insufficiency may result in cardiac failure that may be precipitated by progression of the rheumatic process, the onset of atrial fibrillation, or infective endocarditis. The effects of chronic mitral insufficiency may become manifest after many years and include right ventricular failure and atrial and ventricular arrhythmias.

TREATMENT In patients with mild mitral insufficiency, prophylaxis against recurrences of rheumatic fever is all that is required. Treatment of complicating heart failure (Chapter 436), arrhythmias (Chapter 429), and infective endocarditis (Chapter 431) is described elsewhere. Afterload-reducing agents (ACE inhibitors or angiotensin receptor blockers) may reduce the regurgitant volume and preserve left ventricular function. Surgical treatment is indicated for patients who despite adequate medical therapy have persistent heart failure, dyspnea with moderate activity, and progressive cardiomegaly, often with pulmonary hypertension. Although annuloplasty provides good results in some children and adolescents, valve replacement may be required. In patients with a prosthetic mitral valve replacement, prophylaxis against bacterial endocarditis is warranted for dental procedures, as the routine antibiotics taken by these patients for rheumatic fever prophylaxis are insufficient to prevent endocarditis.

Mitral Stenosis

PATHOPHYSIOLOGY Mitral stenosis of rheumatic origin results from fibrosis of the mitral ring, commissural adhesions, and contracture of the valve leaflets, chordae, and papillary muscles over time. It usually takes 10 yr or more for the lesion to become fully established, although the process may occasionally be accelerated. Rheumatic mitral stenosis is seldom encountered before adolescence and is not usually recognized until adult life. Significant mitral stenosis results in increased pressure and enlargement and hypertrophy of the left atrium, pulmonary venous hypertension, increased pulmonary vascular resistance, and pulmonary hypertension. Right ventricular hypertrophy and right atrial dilatation ensue and are followed by right ventricular dilation, tricuspid regurgitation, and clinical signs of right-sided heart failure.

CLINICAL MANIFESTATIONS Generally, the correlation between symptoms and the severity of obstruction is good. Patients with mild lesions are asymptomatic. More severe degrees of obstruction are associated with exercise intolerance and dyspnea. Critical lesions can result in orthopnea, paroxysmal nocturnal dyspnea, and overt pulmonary edema, as well as atrial arrhythmias. When pulmonary hypertension has developed, right ventricular dilatation may result in functional tricuspid insufficiency, hepatomegaly, ascites, and edema. Hemoptysis caused by rupture of bronchial or pleurohilar veins and, occasionally, by pulmonary infarction may occur.

Jugular venous pressure is increased in severe disease with heart failure, tricuspid valve disease, or severe pulmonary hypertension. In mild disease, heart size is normal; however, moderate cardiomegaly is usual with severe mitral stenosis. Cardiac enlargement can be massive when atrial fibrillation and heart failure supervene. A parasternal right ventricular lift is palpable when pulmonary pressure is high. The principal auscultatory findings are a loud 1st heart sound, an opening snap of the mitral valve, and a long, low-pitched, rumbling mitral diastolic murmur with presystolic accentuation at the apex. The mitral diastolic murmur may be virtually absent in patients who are in significant heart failure. A holosystolic murmur secondary to tricuspid insufficiency may be audible. In the presence of pulmonary hypertension, the pulmonic component of the 2nd heart sound is accentuated. An early diastolic murmur may be caused by associated rheumatic aortic insufficiency or pulmonary valvular insufficiency secondary to pulmonary hypertension.

Electrocardiograms and roentgenograms are normal if the lesion is mild; as the severity increases, prominent and notched P waves and varying degrees of right ventricular hypertrophy become evident. Atrial fibrillation is a common late manifestation. Moderate or severe lesions are associated with roentgenographic signs of left atrial enlargement and prominence of the pulmonary artery and right-sided heart chambers; calcifications may be noted in the region of the mitral valve. Severe obstruction is associated with a redistribution of pulmonary blood flow so that the apices of the lung have greater perfusion (the reverse of normal). Echocardiography shows thickening of the mitral valve, distinct narrowing of the mitral orifice during diastole and left atrial enlargement. Doppler can estimate the transmitral pressure gradient. Cardiac catheterization quantitates the diastolic gradient across the mitral valve, allows for the calculation of valve area, and assesses the degree of elevation of pulmonary arterial pressure.

TREATMENT Intervention is indicated in patients with clinical signs and hemodynamic evidence of severe obstruction but before

the severe manifestations outlined earlier. Surgical valvotomy or balloon catheter mitral valvuloplasty generally yields good results; valve replacement is avoided unless absolutely necessary. Balloon valvuloplasty is indicated for symptomatic, stenotic, pliable, noncalcified valves of patients without atrial arrhythmias or thrombi.

Aortic Insufficiency

In chronic rheumatic aortic insufficiency, sclerosis of the aortic valve results in distortion and retraction of the cusps. Regurgitation of blood leads to volume overload with dilatation and hypertrophy of the left ventricle. Combined mitral and aortic insufficiency is more common than aortic involvement alone.

CLINICAL MANIFESTATIONS Symptoms are unusual except in severe aortic insufficiency. The large stroke volume and forceful left ventricular contractions may result in palpitations. Sweating and heat intolerance are related to excessive vasodilation. Dyspnea on exertion can progress to orthopnea and pulmonary edema; angina may be precipitated by heavy exercise. Nocturnal attacks with sweating, tachycardia, chest pain, and hypertension may occur.

The pulse pressure is wide with bounding peripheral pulses. Systolic blood pressure is elevated, and diastolic pressure is lowered. In severe aortic insufficiency, the heart is enlarged, with a left ventricular apical heave. A diastolic thrill may be present. The typical murmur begins immediately with the 2nd heart sound and continues until late in diastole. The murmur is heard over the upper and midleft sternal border with radiation to the apex and upper right sternal border. Characteristically, it has a high-pitched blowing quality and is easily audible in full expiration with the diaphragm of the stethoscope placed firmly on the chest and the patient leaning forward. An aortic systolic ejection murmur is frequent because of the increased stroke volume. An apical presystolic murmur (**Austin Flint murmur**) resembling that of mitral stenosis is sometimes heard and is a result of the large regurgitant aortic flow in diastole preventing the mitral valve from opening fully.

Roentgenograms show enlargement of the left ventricle and aorta. The electrocardiogram may be normal, but in advanced cases it reveals signs of left ventricular hypertrophy and strain with prominent P waves. The echocardiogram shows a large left ventricle and diastolic mitral valve flutter or oscillation caused by regurgitant flow hitting the valve leaflets. Doppler studies demonstrate the degree of aortic runoff into the left ventricle. Magnetic resonance angiography (MRA) can be useful in quantitating regurgitant volume. Cardiac catheterization is necessary only when the echocardiographic data are equivocal.

PROGNOSIS AND TREATMENT Mild and moderate lesions are well tolerated. Unlike mitral insufficiency, aortic insufficiency does not regress. Patients with combined lesions during the episode of acute rheumatic fever may have only aortic involvement 1-2 yr later. Treatment consists of afterload reducers (ACE inhibitors or angiotensin receptor blockers) and prophylaxis against recurrence of acute rheumatic fever. Surgical intervention (valve replacement) should be carried out well in advance of the onset of heart failure, pulmonary edema, or angina, when signs of decreasing myocardial performance become evident as manifested by increasing left ventricular dimensions on the echocardiogram. Surgery is considered when early symptoms are present, ST-T wave changes are seen on the electrocardiogram, or evidence of decreasing left ventricular ejection fraction is noted.

Tricuspid Valve Disease

Primary tricuspid involvement is rare after rheumatic fever. Tricuspid insufficiency is more common secondary to right ventricular dilatation resulting from unrepaired left-sided lesions. The signs produced by tricuspid insufficiency include prominent pulsations of the jugular veins, systolic pulsations of the liver, and a blowing holosystolic murmur at the lower left sternal border that increases in intensity during inspiration. Concomitant signs of mitral or aortic valve disease, with or without atrial fibrillation, are frequent. In these cases, signs of tricuspid insufficiency decrease or disappear when heart failure produced by the left-sided lesions is successfully treated. Tricuspid valvuloplasty may be required in rare cases.

Pulmonary Valve Disease

Pulmonary insufficiency usually occurs on a functional basis secondary to pulmonary hypertension and is a late finding with severe mitral stenosis. The murmur (**Graham Steell murmur**) is similar to that of aortic insufficiency, but peripheral arterial signs (bounding pulses) are absent. The correct diagnosis is confirmed by two-dimensional echocardiography and Doppler studies.

BIBLIOGRAPHY

Please visit the Nelson Textbook of Pediatrics *website at www.expertconsult.com for the complete bibliography.*

Section 6 DISEASES OF THE MYOCARDIUM AND PERICARDIUM

Chapter 433 Diseases of the Myocardium

Robert Spicer and Stephanie Ware

The extremely heterogeneous groups of heart muscle diseases that are associated with structural and/or functional cardiac dysfunction (cardiomyopathy) are important causes of morbidity and mortality in the pediatric population. Certain anatomic and physiologic conditions such as congenital heart disease, hypertension, and coronary artery disease may result in heart muscle dysfunction, but are distinct from the conditions presented in this chapter. Several classification schemes have been formulated in an effort to provide logical, useful, and scientifically based etiologies for the cardiomyopathies. Insight into the molecular genetic basis of cardiomyopathies has increased exponentially and it is likely that etiologic classification schemes will continue to evolve.

Table 433-1 classifies the cardiomyopathies based on their anatomic (ventricular morphology) and functional pathophysiology. Dilated cardiomyopathy, the most common form of cardiomyopathy, is characterized predominantly by left ventricular dilation and decreased left ventricular systolic function (Fig. 433-1). Hypertrophic cardiomyopathy demonstrates increased ventricular myocardial wall thickness, normal or increased systolic function, and often, diastolic (relaxation) abnormalities (Table 433-2). Restrictive cardiomyopathy is characterized by nearly normal ventricular chamber size and wall thickness with preserved systolic function, but dramatically impaired diastolic function leading to elevated filling pressures and atrial enlargement (see Fig. 433-3). Arrhythmogenic right ventricular cardiomyopathy and left ventricular

Table 433-1 ETIOLOGY OF PEDIATRIC MYOCARDIAL DISEASE

CARDIOMYOPATHY	
Dilated Cardiomyopathy (DCM)	
Neuromuscular diseases	Muscular dystrophies (Duchenne, Becker, limb girdle, Emery- Dreifuss, congenital muscular dystrophy, etc.), myotonic dystrophy, myofibrillar myopathy
Inborn errors of metabolism	Fatty acid oxidation disorders (trifunctional protein, VLCAD), carnitine abnormalities (carnitine transport, CPTI, CPTII), mitochondrial disorders (including Kearns-Sayre syndrome), organic acidemias (propionic acidemia)
Genetic mutations in cardiomyocyte structural apparatus	Familial or sporadic DCM
Genetic syndromes	Alstrom syndrome, Barth syndrome (phospholipid disorders)
Ischemic	Most common in adults
Chronic tachyarrhythmias	
Hypertrophic Cardiomyopathy (HCM)	
Inborn errors of metabolism	Mitochondrial disorders (including Friedreich ataxia, mutations in nuclear or mitochondrial genome), storage disorders (glycogen storage disorders, especially Pompe; mucopolysaccharidoses; Fabry disease; sphingolipidoses; hemochromatosis; Danon disease)
Genetic mutations in cardiomyocyte structural apparatus	Familial or sporadic HCM
Genetic syndromes	Noonan, Costello, cardio-faciocutaneous, Beckwith-Wiedemann syndrome
Infant of a diabetic mother	Transient hypertrophy
Restrictive Cardiomyopathy (RCM)	
Neuromuscular disease	Myofibrillar myopathies
Metabolic	Storage disorders
Genetic mutations in cardiomyocyte structural apparatus	Familial or sporadic RCM
Arrhythmogenic Right Ventricular Cardiomyopathy (ARVC)	
Genetic mutations in cardiomyocyte structural apparatus	Familial or sporadic ARVC
Left Ventricular Noncompaction (LVNC)	X-linked (Barth syndrome), autosomal dominant, autosomal recessive, mitochondrial inheritance, or sporadic LVNC Sporadic LVNC
SECONDARY OR ACQUIRED MYOCARDIAL DISEASE	
Myocarditis	**Viral:** parvovirus B19, adenovirus, coxsackievirus A and B, echovirus, rubella, varicella, influenza, mumps, Epstein-Barr virus, cytomegalovirus, measles, poliomyelitis, smallpox vaccine, hepatitis C virus, HIV virus, or opportunistic infections **Rickettsial:** psittacosis, *Coxiella*, Rocky Mountain spotted fever, typhus **Bacterial:** diphtheria, mycoplasma, meningococcus, leptospirosis, Lyme disease, typhoid fever, tuberculosis, streptococcus, listeriosis **Parasitic:** Chagas disease, toxoplasmosis, *Loa loa, Toxocara canis,* schistosomiasis, cysticercosis, echinococcus, trichinosis **Fungal:** histoplasmosis, coccidioidomycosis, actinomycosis
Systemic Inflammatory Disease	Systemic lupus erythematosus (SLE), infant of mother with SLE, scleroderma, Churg-Strauss vasculitis, rheumatoid arthritis, rheumatic fever, sarcoidosis, dermatomyositis, periarteritis nodosa, hypereosinophilic syndrome (Löffler syndrome), acute eosinophilic necrotizing myocarditis, giant cell myocarditis
Nutritional Deficiency	Beriberi (thiamine deficiency), kwashiorkor, Keshan disease (selenium deficiency)
Drugs, Toxins	Doxorubicin (Adriamycin), cyclophosphamide, chloroquine, ipecac (emetine), sulfonamides, mesalazine, chloramphenicol, alcohol, hypersensitivity reaction, envenomations, irradiation, herbal remedy (blue cohosh)
Coronary Artery Disease	Kawasaki disease, medial necrosis, anomalous left coronary artery from the pulmonary artery (ALCAPA), other congenital coronary anomalies (anomalous right coronary, coronary ostial stenosis), familial hypercholesterolemia
Hematology-Oncology	Anemia, sickle cell disease, leukemia
Endocrine-Neuroendocrine	Hyperthyroidism, carcinoid tumor, pheochromocytoma

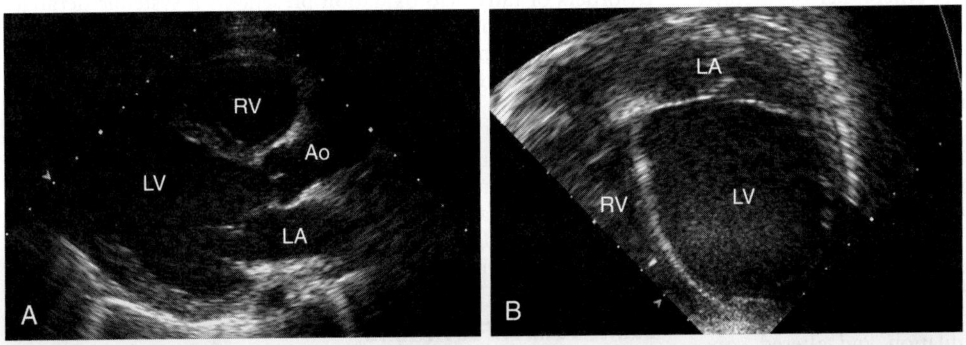

Figure 433-1 Echocardiogram of a patient with dilated cardiomyopathy. *A,* Parasternal long-axis view showing the enlarged left ventricle. *B,* Apical four-chamber view showing the large left ventricle compressing the right ventricle. Ao, ascending aorta; LA, left atrium; LV, left ventricle; RV, right ventricle.

Table 433-2 CARDIOMYOPATHIES

	DCM	HCM	RCM	LVNC	ARVC
Prevalence	50/100,000	1/500	Unknown	Unknown	1/2000
Familial	30–50% AD, AR, X-L, Mt	50% AD, Mt	AD, % unknown	AD, X-L, Mt, % unknown	30-50% AD, rare AR (Naxos disease; Carvajal syndrome)
Genes*	Sarcomere: MYH7, MYBPC3, TNNI3, TNNT2, TNNC1, MYH6, TPM1, ACTC1 Cytoskeleton or Z-disc: DMD, TTN, CSRP3, TCAP, VCL, ACTN2, DES, LDB3, SGCD, MYPN Nuclear envelope: LMNA, EMD, TMPO Cardiolipin metabolism: TAZ Mitochondrial function: mt DNA depletion; Mt genome mutations/deletions Other: CRYAB, SCN5A, EYA4, ABCC9, PLN, PSEN1, PSEN2, FCMD, ALMS1	Sarcomere: MYH7, MYBPC3, MYL2, MYL3, TNNT2, TNNI3, TNNC1, MYH6, TPM1, ACTC1 Cytoskeleton or Z-disc: TTN, CSRP3, LDB3, TCAP, VCL, ACTN2, MYOZ2, Storage: PRKAG2, LAMP2, GLA, GAA, AGL Mitochondrial function: FRDA, SCO2, SURF1, COX genes, ANT1, Mt genome mutations/deletions Cell signaling: PTPN11, RAF1, SOS1, KRAS, HRAS, BRAF, MEK1, MEK2 Other: PLN, JPH2	Sarcomere: MYH7, TNNT2, TNNI3, ACTC1 Cytoskeleton or Z-disc: DES	Cytoskeletal or Z-disc: DTNA, LDB3 Cardiolipin metabolism: TAZ Sarcomere: MYH7, ACTC1 Mitochondrial function: see HCM and DCM	Desmosome: DSP2, PKP2, DSG2, DSC2, JUP Other: TMEM43, TGFB3, RYR2
Sudden death	Yes	Yes	Yes	Yes	Yes
Arrhythmias	Atrial, ventricular, and conduction disturbances	Atrial and ventricular	Atrial fibrillation		Ventricular and conduction disturbances
Ventricular function	Systolic and diastolic dysfunction	Diastolic dysfunction Dynamic systolic outflow obstruction	Diastolic dysfunction Normal systolic function	Systolic or diastolic dysfunction	Normal-reduced systolic and diastolic function

*Genes are listed using the human gene symbol.
ACE, angiotensin-converting enzyme; AD, autosomal dominant inheritance; AR, autosomal recessive inheritance; ICD, implantable cardioverter-defibrillator; Mt, mitochondrial inheritance; X-L, X-linked inheritance.

non-compaction are characterized by specific morphologic abnormalities and heterogeneous functional disturbances.

BIBLIOGRAPHY

Please visit the Nelson Textbook of Pediatrics *website at www.expertconsult.com for the complete bibliography.*

433.1 Dilated Cardiomyopathy

Robert Spicer and Stephanie Ware

ETIOLOGY AND EPIDEMIOLOGY

Dilated cardiomyopathy (DCM), the most common form of cardiomyopathy in children, is the cause of significant morbidity and mortality as well as a common indication for cardiac transplantation. The etiologies are diverse. Unlike adult patients with dilated cardiomyopathy, ischemic etiologies are rare in children, although these include anomalous origin of the left coronary artery from the pulmonary artery, premature coronary atherosclerosis (homozygous type II hypercholesterolemia), and coronary inflammatory diseases, such as Kawasaki disease. It is estimated that up to 50% of cases are genetic, including some with metabolic causes (see Table 433-1). Although the most common etiology of dilated cardiomyopathy remains idiopathic, it is likely that undiagnosed familial/genetic conditions and myocarditis predominate. The annual incidence of DCM in children younger than 18 yr is 0.57 cases per 100,000 per year. Incidence is higher in males, African Americans, and in infants less than 1 yr old.

PATHOGENESIS

The pathogenesis of the ventricular dilation and altered contractility seen in dilated cardiomyopathy varies depending on the underlying etiology. Genetic abnormalities of several components of the cardiac muscle including sarcomere protein, the cytoskeleton, and the proteins that bridge the contractile apparatus to the cytoskeleton, have been identified in autosomal dominant and X-linked inherited disorders. Dilated cardiomyopathy can occur following viral myocarditis and, although the primary pathogenesis varies from direct myocardial injury to viral-induced inflammatory injury, the resulting myocardial damage, ventricular enlargement, and poor function likely occur by a final common pathway similar to that which occurs in genetic disorders.

In 20-50% of cases, the DCM is familial with autosomal dominant inheritance most common (see Table 433-2). **Duchenne and Becker muscular dystrophies** (Chapter 601.1) are X-linked cardiomyopathies that account for 5-10% of familial dilated cardiomyopathy cases. These dystrophinopathies result in an abnormal sarcomere-cytoskeleton connection, causing impaired myocardial force generation, myocyte damage/scarring, chamber enlargement, and altered function.

Mitochondrial myopathies, like the muscular dystrophies, may present clinically with a predominance of extra cardiac findings and are inherited in a recessive or mitochondrial pattern. Disorders of **fatty acid oxidation** present with systemic derangements of metabolism (hypoketotic hypoglycemia, acidosis, liver dysfunction), some with peripheral myopathy and neuropathy, and others with sudden death or life-threatening cardiac arrhythmias

Anthracycline cardiotoxicity (doxorubicin [Adriamycin]) on rare occasion causes acute inflammatory myocardial injury, but more classically results in dilated cardiomyopathy and occurs in up to 30% of patients given a cumulative dose of doxorubicin exceeding 550 mg/m^2. The risk of toxicity appears to be exacerbated by concomitant radiation therapy.

CLINICAL MANIFESTATIONS

Although more prevalent in patients less than 1 yr of age, all age groups may be affected. Clinical manifestations of dilated cardiomyopathy are most commonly those of congestive heart failure, but can also include palpitations, syncope, and sudden death. Irritability or lethargy can be accompanied by additional nonspecific complaints of failure to thrive, nausea, vomiting, or abdominal pain. Respiratory symptoms (tachypnea, wheezing, cough, or dyspnea on exertion) are often present. Uncommonly, patients may present acutely with pallor, altered mentation, hypotension, and shock. Patients can be tachycardic with narrow pulse pressure and have hepatic enlargement, and rales or wheezing. The precordial cardiac impulse is increased and the heart may be enlarged to palpation or percussion. Auscultation may reveal a gallop rhythm in addition to tachycardia and occasionally murmurs of mitral or, less commonly, tricuspid insufficiency may be present. The presence of hypoglycemia, acidosis, hypotonia, or signs of liver failure suggests an inborn error of metabolism. Neurologic or skeletal muscle deficits are associated with mitochondrial disorders or muscular dystrophies.

LABORATORY FINDINGS

Electrocardiographic screening reveals atrial or ventricular hypertrophy, nonspecific T-wave abnormalities, and occasionally atrial or ventricular arrhythmias. The chest x-ray demonstrates cardiomegaly and may reveal pulmonary vascular prominence or pleural effusions. The echocardiogram is often diagnostic, demonstrating the characteristic findings of left ventricular enlargement, decreased ventricular contractility, and occasionally a globular (remodeled) left ventricular contour (see Fig. 433-1). Right ventricular enlargement and depressed function are occasionally noted. Echo Doppler studies can reveal evidence of pulmonary hypertension, mitral regurgitation, or other structural cardiac or coronary abnormalities.

Additional testing should include CBC, renal and liver function tests, CPK, cardiac troponin I, lactate, plasma amino acids, urine organic acids, and an acylcarnitine profile. Additional genetic and enzymatic testing may be useful (see Table 433-2). Cardiac catheterization and endomyocardial biopsy are not routine but may be useful in patients with acute dilated cardiomyopathy. Biopsy samples can also be assessed for the presence of mononuclear cell infiltrates, myocardial damage, storage abnormalities, and viral infection or genomes. It is important to consider screening of 1st-degree family members utilizing echocardiography and ECG.

PROGNOSIS AND MANAGEMENT

The 1- and 5-yr rates of death or need for transplantation in patients diagnosed with DCM is 31% and 46%, respectively. Independent risk factors at DCM diagnosis for subsequent death or transplantation include older age, congestive heart failure, lower left ventricular fractional shortening *z* score, and underlying etiology. Dilated cardiomyopathy is the most common cause for cardiac transplantation in pediatric and adult studies.

The therapeutic approach to patients with dilated cardiomyopathy includes a careful assessment to uncover possible treatable etiologies, screening of family members, and rigorous pharmacologic therapy. Decongestive therapy may improve symptoms of heart failure, prolong survival, and occasionally results in complete resolution of dysfunction. Patients are often treated with diuretics and angiotensin-converting enzyme (ACE) inhibitors. The use of digitalis and angiotensin receptor blockers may be of additional benefit. β-Adrenergic blockade with carvedilol or metoprolol is often utilized in patients with chronic congestive heart failure although pediatric specific outcome data have failed to show effectiveness. In patients presenting with extreme degrees of heart failure or circulatory collapse, intensive care measures are often required, including intravenous inotropes and diuretics, mechanic ventilatory support, and on occasion, mechanical circulatory support, which may include ECMO, ventricular assist devices, and ultimately cardiac transplantation. In patients with dilated cardiomyopathy and atrial or ventricular arrhythmias, specific antiarrhythmic therapy should be instituted.

BIBLIOGRAPHY

Please visit the Nelson Textbook of Pediatrics *website at www.expertconsult.com for the complete bibliography.*

433.2 Hypertrophic Cardiomyopathy

Robert Spicer and Stephanie Ware

ETIOLOGY AND EPIDEMIOLOGY

Hypertrophic cardiomyopathy (HCM) is a heterogeneous, relatively common, and potentially severe form of cardiomyopathy. The causes of hypertrophic cardiomyopathy are heterogeneous and include inborn errors of metabolism, neuromuscular disorders, syndromic conditions, and genetic abnormalities of the structural components of the cardiomyocyte (see Table 433-1). Both the age of onset and associated features are helpful in identifying the underlying etiology.

HCM is a genetic disorder and frequently occurs as a result of mutations in sarcomere or cytoskeletal components of the cardiomyocyte. Mutations of the genes encoding cardiac β-myosin heavy-chain *(MYH7)* and myosin-binding protein C *(MYBPC3)* are the most common (see Table 433-2). Mutations are inherited in an autosomal dominant pattern with widely variable penetrance; many cases represent de novo mutations. Some patients have mutations in more than 1 gene; this may result in early onset and more severe symptoms. Additional genetic causes for HCM include nonsarcomeric protein mutations, such as the γ-2-regulatory subunit of AMP-activated protein kinase *(PRKAG2)* and the lysosome-associated membrane protein 2α-galactosidase (Danon disease, a form of glycogen storage disease). Syndromic conditions, such as Noonan syndrome, may manifest with hypertrophic cardiomyopathy at birth and recognition of extracardiac manifestations is important in making the diagnosis.

Glycogen storage disorders such as Pompe disease often present in infancy with a heart murmur, abnormal ECG, systemic signs and symptoms, and occasionally heart failure. The characteristic electrocardiogram in Pompe disease demonstrates prominent P waves, a short P-R interval, and massive QRS voltages; the echocardiogram confirms severe, often concentric, left ventricular hypertrophy.

PATHOGENESIS

Hypertrophic cardiomyopathy is characterized by the presence of an increased left ventricular wall thickness in the absence of structural heart disease or hypertension. Often the interventricular septum is disproportionately involved, leading to the previous designation of idiopathic hypertrophic subaortic stenosis (IHSS) or the current term of asymmetric septal hypertrophy. In the presence of a resting or provocable outflow tract gradient, the term hypertrophic obstructive cardiomyopathy (HOCM) is used. Although the left ventricle is predominantly affected, the right ventricle may be involved, particularly in infancy. The mitral valve can demonstrate systolic anterior motion of the mitral valve and mitral insufficiency. Left ventricular outflow tract obstruction occurs in 25% of patients, is dynamic in nature, and may in part be secondary to the abnormal position of the mitral valve as well as the obstructing subaortic hypertrophic cardiac muscle. The cardiac myofibrils and myofilaments demonstrate disarray and myocardial fibrosis.

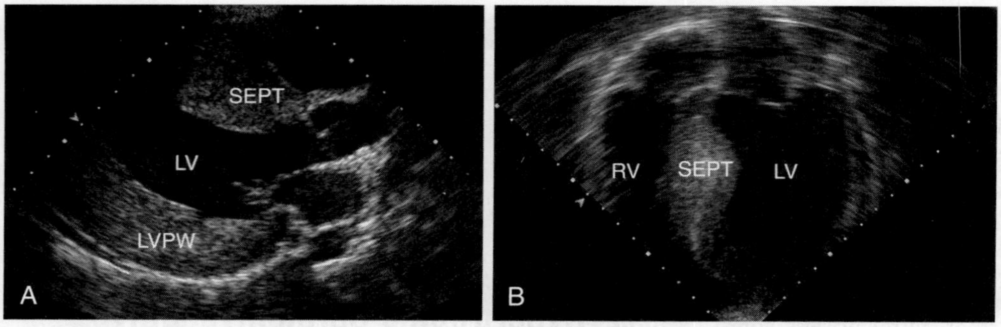

Figure 433-2 Echocardiograms demonstrating hypertrophic cardiomyopathy. *A,* Parasternal long-axis view of a patient with severe concentric left ventricular hypertrophy. *B,* Four-chamber view of a patient with asymmetric septal hypertrophy. LV, left ventricle; LVPW, left ventricular posterior wall; RV, right ventricle; SEPT, septum.

Typically, systolic pump function is preserved or even hyperdynamic, though systolic dysfunction may occur late. Outflow tract obstruction with or without mitral insufficiency may be provoked by physiologic manipulations such as the Valsalva maneuver, positional changes, and physical activity. Frequently, the hypertrophic and fibrosed cardiac muscle demonstrates relaxation abnormalities (diminished compliance) and left ventricular filling may be impaired (diastolic dysfunction).

CLINICAL MANIFESTATIONS

Many patients are asymptomatic, and 50% of cases present with a heart murmur or during screening when another family member has been diagnosed with HCM. Symptoms of HCM may include palpitations, chest pain, easy fatigability, dyspnea, dizziness, and syncope. Sudden death is a well-recognized but uncommon manifestation that often occurs during physical exertion.

Characteristic physical examination findings include an overactive precordial impulse with a lift or heave, abnormal peripheral pulses (hyperdynamic or diminished), a systolic ejection murmur in the aortic region *not* associated with an ejection click, and an apical blowing murmur of mitral insufficiency.

DIAGNOSIS

The electrocardiogram typically demonstrates left ventricular hypertrophy with ST segment and T-wave abnormalities. Intraventricular conduction delays and signs of ventricular preexcitation (Wolff-Parkinson-White syndrome) may be present and should raise the possibility of Danon disease or Pompe disease. Chest radiography demonstrates normal or mildly increased heart size with a prominence of the left ventricle. Echocardiography is diagnostic in identifying, localizing, and quantifying the degree of myocardial hypertrophy (Fig. 433-2). Doppler interrogation defines, localizes, and quantifies the degree of ventricular outflow tract obstruction and also demonstrates and quantifies the degree of mitral insufficiency. Diastolic dysfunction can be confirmed by M-mode, flow, and tissue Doppler techniques.

Cardiac catheterization may be indicated in some cases of hypertrophic cardiomyopathy to define the left ventricular outflow gradient with and without pharmacologic provocation, to perform electrophysiologic investigation for assessment of arrhythmia risk, or in rare cases, endomyocardial biopsy.

Additional diagnostic studies include metabolic testing, genetic testing for specific syndromic conditions, or genetic testing for mutations in genes known to cause isolated HCM (see Table 433-2). The clinical availability of these tests is expanding. In adults, where isolated HCM is a common genetic diagnosis, it has been possible to identify a subset of mutations that confer an increased risk for arrhythmia or sudden death. As identification of the molecular basis of disease in children increases, similar correlations are expected to emerge. In addition, genetic diagnosis is useful to identify at risk family members that require ongoing surveillance.

PROGNOSIS AND MANAGEMENT

Children under 1 yr of age or with inborn errors of metabolism or malformation syndromes have a significantly poorer prognosis. The risk of sudden death in older patients is greater in those with a history of cardiac arrest, ventricular tachycardia, exercise hypotension, syncope, excessive (>3 cm) ventricular wall thickness, and a ventricular obstruction gradient over 30 mm Hg. Although intrafamilial variability in symptoms occurs, a family history of sudden death is a highly significant predictor of risk.

Competitive sports and strenuous physical activity should be prohibited as most sudden deaths in patients with HCM occur during or immediately after vigorous physical exertion. β-Adrenergic blocking agents (propranolol, atenolol) or calcium channel blocking agents (verapamil) may be useful in diminishing ventricular outflow tract obstruction, modifying ventricular hypertrophy, and improving ventricular filling. Although significant symptomatic improvement occurs in some patients, the risk for development of heart failure or sudden death has not been lessened. In patients with atrial or ventricular arrhythmias, specific antiarrhythmic therapy should be utilized. Patients with documented ventricular arrhythmias, strong family histories of arrhythmias or sudden death, or patients with syncope should be treated with an implantable cardioverter defibrillator (ICD).

Innovative interventional procedures to anatomically or physiologically reduce the degree of LV outflow tract obstruction have been utilized. Dual chamber pacing, alcohol septal ablation, surgical septal myomectomy, and mitral valve replacement have all met with limited success.

First-degree relatives of patients identified as having HCM should be screened with electrocardiography and echocardiography. Genetic testing is available clinically. It is important to first test the affected individual in the family rather than "at risk" individuals since 20-40% of cases of HCM will not demonstrate mutations in currently available panels of genes. If a causative mutation is identified, "at risk" members of the family can be effectively tested. In families with HCM without demonstrable gene mutations, repeat noninvasive cardiac screening with ECG and echo should be undertaken in at risk individuals every 3-5 yr for patients under 12 yr of age and yearly throughout the teenage years and young adulthood. The clinical course of other affected family members and the results of genetic testing may be of some use in stratifying risk in an affected child.

BIBLIOGRAPHY

Please visit the Nelson Textbook of Pediatrics *website at www.expertconsult.com for the complete bibliography.*

433.3 Restrictive Cardiomyopathy

Robert Spicer and Stephanie Ware

ETIOLOGY AND EPIDEMIOLOGY

RCM accounts for <5% of cardiomyopathy cases. Incidence increases with age, and it is more common in females. In equatorial Africa, RCM accounts for a large number of deaths. Infiltrative myocardial causes and storage disorders frequently result in associated LV hypertrophy and may represent HCM with restrictive physiology. Noninfiltrative causes include mutations in genes encoding sarcomeric or cytoskeletal proteins. The majority of RCM cases are considered idiopathic.

PATHOGENESIS

Restrictive cardiomyopathy is characterized by normal ventricular chamber dimensions, normal myocardial wall thickness, and preserved systolic function. The abnormal myocardium demonstrates impaired ventricular compliance and filling. Filling pressures in the ventricle are typically elevated and are transmitted to the atria which become dilated. Autosomal dominant inheritance has been demonstrated for families with mutations in sarcomeric and cytoskeletal genes.

CLINICAL MANIFESTATIONS

Abnormal ventricular filling, sometimes referred to as *diastolic heart failure,* is manifest in the systemic venous circulation with edema, hepatomegaly, or ascites. Elevation of left-sided filling pressures result in cough, dyspnea, or pulmonary edema. With activity, patients may experience chest pain, shortness of breath, syncope/near syncope, or even sudden death. Pulmonary hypertension and pulmonary vascular disease develop and may progress rapidly. Heart murmurs are typically absent, but a gallop rhythm may be prominent. In the presence of pulmonary hypertension, an overactive right ventricular impulse and pronounced pulmonary component of the second heart sound are present.

DIAGNOSIS

The characteristic electrocardiographic finding of prominent P waves is usually associated with normal QRS voltages and nonspecific ST and T-wave changes. Right ventricular hypertrophy occurs in patients with pulmonary hypertension. The chest x-ray may be normal or demonstrate a prominent atrial shadow and pulmonary vascular redistribution. The echocardiogram is often diagnostic, demonstrating normal-sized ventricles with preserved systolic function and dramatic enlargement of the atria (Fig. 433-3). Flow and tissue Doppler interrogation reveal abnormal filling parameters. Differential diagnosis from constrictive pericarditis is critical, as the latter can be treated surgically. Magnetic resonance imaging may be necessary to demonstrate the thickened or calcified pericardium often present in constrictive pericardial disease.

PROGNOSIS AND MANAGEMENT

Pharmacologic treatment modalities are of limited use and the prognosis of patients with restrictive cardiomyopathy is generally poor with rapid clinical deterioration. Sudden death is common, with a 2-yr survival of 50%. When signs of heart failure exist, judicious use of diuretics can result in clinical improvement. As a result of the dramatic atrial enlargement, these patients are predisposed to the development of atrial tachyarrhythmias and thromboemboli. As a result, antiarrhythmic agents may be necessary and anticoagulation with platelet inhibitors or coumadin is indicated.

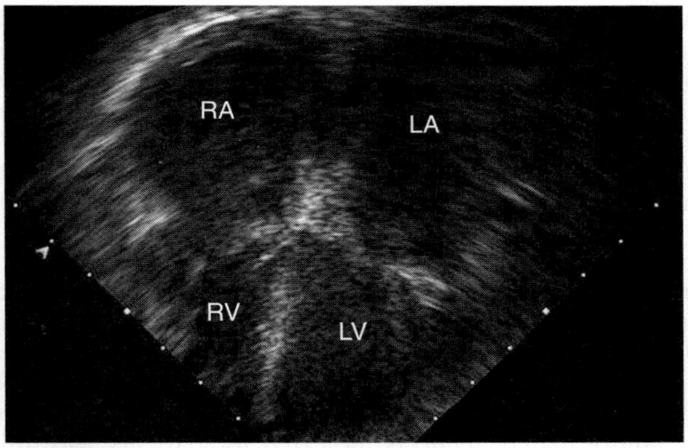

Figure 433-3 Echocardiogram of a patient with restrictive cardiomyopathy. The apical four-chamber view shows the markedly enlarged right and left atria, compared to the normal sized left and right ventricular chambers. LA, left atrium; LV, left ventricle; RA, right atrium; RV, right ventricle.

Cardiac transplantation is the treatment of choice in many centers for patients with restrictive cardiomyopathy, and the results are excellent in patients without pulmonary hypertension, pulmonary vascular disease, or severe congestive heart failure.

BIBLIOGRAPHY

Please visit the Nelson Textbook of Pediatrics *website at www.expertconsult.com for the complete bibliography.*

433.4 Left Ventricular Noncompaction, Arrhythmogenic Right Ventricular Cardiomyopathy, and Endocardial Fibroelastosis

Robert Spicer and Stephanie Ware

Left ventricular noncompaction (LVNC) was initially believed to be a rare disorder found only in children, but is now known to affect individuals of all ages. LVNC is characterized by a distinctive trabeculated or spongy appearing left ventricle (Fig. 433-4) commonly associated with left ventricular hypertrophy and/or dilation, and at times, systolic or diastolic dysfunction. LVNC may be isolated or associated with structural congenital cardiac defects. Patients may present with signs of heart failure, arrhythmias, syncope, sudden death, or as an asymptomatic finding during screening of family members.

Imaging studies utilizing ultrasound or magnetic resonance can demonstrate the characteristic pattern of deeply trabeculated LV myocardium, most characteristically within the apex of the left ventricle. ECG findings are nonspecific and include chamber hypertrophy, ST and T wave changes, or arrhythmias. In some patients, preexcitation is notable and giant voltages occur in approximately 30% of younger children. Metabolic screening should be considered, especially in young children. Elevated serum lactate and urine 3-methylglutaconic acid may be seen in Barth syndrome, an X-linked disorder of phospholipid metabolism caused by a mutation in the tafazzin (*TAZ*) gene. Clinical testing for *TAZ* mutations is available and should be considered, especially in males. Patients with mitochondrial disorders frequently demonstrate signs of LVNC. These children are at risk for atrial or ventricular arrhythmias and thromboembolic complications. Treatment includes anticoagulation, antiarrhythmic therapy if needed, and treatment of heart failure if present. In patients refractory to medical therapy, cardiac transplantation has been used successfully.

Arrhythmogenic right ventricular cardiomyopathy (ARVC) has been thought to be uncommon in North America but is among the most common forms of cardiomyopathy in Europe, especially Italy. Autosomal dominant inheritance is common. In addition, recessive forms associated with severe ARVC and skin manifestations are known. Comprehensive genetic screening has been reported to identify a cause in up to 50% of cases. ARVC is typically characterized by a dilated right ventricle (RV) with fibrofatty infiltration of the RV wall; increasingly, LV involvement is being recognized. Global and regional right and left ventricular dysfunction and ventricular tachyarrhythmias are the major clinical findings. Syncope or aborted sudden death can occur and should be treated with antiarrhythmic medications and placement of a defibrillator. In patients with ventricular dysfunction, heart failure management as indicated for patients with dilated cardiomyopathy may be of use.

Endocardial fibroelastosis (EFE), at one time an important cause of heart failure in children, has become uncommon. The decline in primary EFE is likely related to the abolition of mumps virus infections by immunization practices. Rare familial cases exist, but the causative genes are unknown. In secondary EFE, severe congenital heart disease of the left-sided obstructive type (aortic stenosis or atresia, forms of hypoplastic left heart syndrome, or severe coarctation of the aorta) is present. EFE is characterized by an opaque, white, fibroelastic thickening on the endocardial surface of the ventricle, which leads to systolic or diastolic dysfunction. Standard heart failure management or cardiac transplantation has been utilized in the management of EFE.

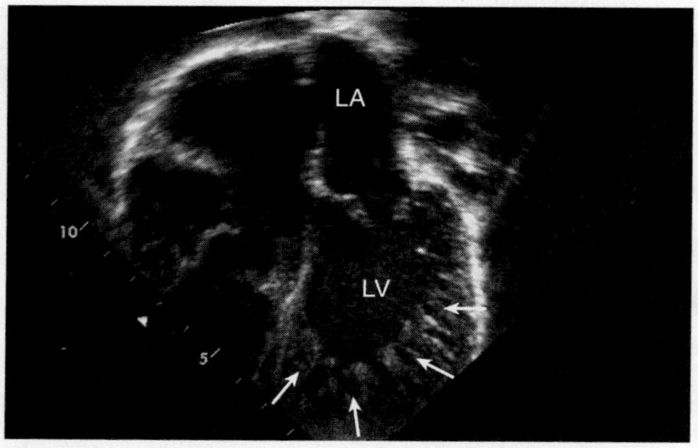

Figure 433-4 Echocardiogram of a patient with left ventricular noncompaction cardiomyopathy. Apical view showing the abnormal trabeculations of the left ventricle at the apex *(arrows)*. For comparison, see the smooth walled LV in Fig. 433-1. LA, left atrium; LV, left ventricle.

BIBLIOGRAPHY

Please visit the Nelson Textbook of Pediatrics *website at www.expertconsult.com for the complete bibliography.*

433.5 Myocarditis

Robert Spicer and Stephanie Ware

Acute or chronic inflammation of the myocardium is characterized by inflammatory cell infiltrates, myocyte necrosis, or myocyte degeneration and may be caused by infectious, connective tissue, granulomatous, toxic, or idiopathic processes. There may be associated systemic manifestations of the disease and on occasion the endocardium or pericardium is involved, though coronary pathology is uniformly absent. Patients may be asymptomatic, have nonspecific prodromal symptoms, or present with overt congestive heart failure, compromising arrhythmias, or sudden death. It is thought that viral infections are the most common etiology though myocardial toxins, drug exposures, hypersensitivity reactions, and immune disorders may also lead to myocarditis (Table 433-3).

ETIOLOGY AND EPIDEMIOLOGY

Viral Infections

Coxsackievirus and other enteroviruses, adenovirus, parvovirus, Epstein-Barr virus, and cytomegalovirus are the most common causative agents in children, though most known viral agents have been reported. In Asia, hepatitis C virus appears to be significant as well. The true incidence of viral myocarditis is unknown as mild cases likely very often go undetected. The disease is typically sporadic but may be epidemic. Manifestations are, to some degree, age dependent: in infants, viral myocarditis can be fulminant; in children, it often will occur as an acute, myopericarditis with congestive heart failure; and in older children and adolescents, it may present with signs and symptoms of acute or chronic congestive heart failure.

Bacterial Infections

Bacterial myocarditis has become far less common with the advent of advanced public health measures, which have minimized infectious causes such as diphtheria. Diphtheritic

Table 433-3 COMMON CAUSES OF MYOCARDITIS

INFECTIOUS		IMMUNE-MEDIATED		TOXIC
Viral	Adenovirus Parvovirus Coxsackievirus Hepatitis C virus Human immunodeficiency virus	Autoantigens	Churg-Strauss syndrome Inflammatory bowel disease Giant cell myocarditis Diabetes mellitus Sarcoidosis Systemic lupus erythematosus Thyrotoxicosis Takayasu arteritis	Anthracyclines Cocaine Interleukin-2 Ethanol Heavy metals
Bacterial	*Mycobacteria* *Streptococcus* spp. *Mycoplasma pneumoniae* *Treponema pallidum*			
Fungal	*Aspergillus* *Candida* *Coccidioides* *Cryptococcus* *Histoplasma*	Hypersensitivity	Wegener granulomatosis Sulfonamides Cephalosporins Diuretics Tricyclic antidepressants Dobutamine	
Protozoal	*Trypanosoma cruzi*			
Parasitic	Schistosomiasis Larva migrans			

Data from Feldman AM, McNamara D: Myocarditis, *N Engl J Med* 343:1388–1398, 2000; Magnani JW, Dec GW: Myocarditis: current trends in diagnosis and treatment, *Circulation* 113:876–990, 2006.

myocarditis (Chapter 180) is unique as bacterial toxin may produce circulatory collapse and toxic myocarditis characterized by atrioventricular block, bundle branch block, or ventricular ectopy. Any overwhelming systemic bacterial infection can manifest with circulatory collapse and shock with evidence of myocardial dysfunction characterized by tachycardia, gallop rhythm, and low cardiac output. Additional nonviral infectious causes of myocarditis include rickettsia, protozoa, parasitic infections, and fungal disease.

PATHOPHYSIOLOGY

Myocarditis is characterized by myocardial inflammation, injury or necrosis, and ultimately fibrosis. Cardiac enlargement and diminished systolic function occur as a direct result of the myocardial damage. Typical signs of congestive heart failure occur and may progress rapidly to shock, atrial or ventricular arrhythmias, and sudden death. Viral myocarditis may also become a chronic process with persistence of viral nucleic acid in the myocardium, and the perpetuation of chronic inflammation secondary to altered host immune response including activated T lymphocytes (cytotoxic and natural killer cells) and antibody-dependent cell mediated damage. Additionally, persistent viral infection may alter the expression of major histocompatibility complex antigens with resultant exposure of neoantigens to the immune system. Some viral proteins share antigenic epitopes with host cells, resulting in autoimmune damage to the antigenically related myocyte. Cytokines such as tumor necrosis factor-α and interleukin-1 are inhibitors of myocyte response to adrenergic stimuli and result in diminished cardiac function. The final result of viral-associated inflammation can be dilated cardiomyopathy.

CLINICAL MANIFESTATIONS

Manifestations of myocarditis range from asymptomatic or nonspecific generalized illness to acute cardiogenic shock and sudden death. Infants and young children more often have a fulminant presentation with fever, respiratory distress, tachycardia, hypotension, gallop rhythm, and cardiac murmur. Associated findings may include a rash or evidence of end organ involvement such as hepatitis or aseptic meningitis.

Patients with acute or chronic myocarditis may present with chest discomfort, fever, palpitations, easy fatigability, or syncope/near syncope. Cardiac findings include overactive precordial impulse, gallop rhythm, and an apical systolic murmur of mitral insufficiency. In patients with associated pericardial disease, a rub may be noted. Hepatic enlargement, peripheral edema, and pulmonary findings such as wheezes or rales may be present in patients with decompensated congestive heart failure.

DIAGNOSIS

Electrocardiographic changes are nonspecific and may include sinus tachycardia, atrial or ventricular arrhythmias, heart block, diminished QRS voltages, and nonspecific ST and T-wave changes, often suggestive of acute ischemia. Chest roentgenograms in severe, symptomatic cases reveal cardiomegaly, pulmonary vascular prominence, overt pulmonary edema, or pleural effusions. Echocardiography often shows diminished ventricular systolic function, cardiac chamber enlargement, mitral insufficiency, and occasionally, evidence of pericardial infusion.

Endomyocardial biopsy may be useful in identifying inflammatory cell infiltrates or myocyte damage and performing molecular viral analysis using polymerase chain reaction (PCR) techniques. Catheterization and biopsy, although not without risk (perforation and arrhythmias), should be performed by experienced personnel in patients suspected to have myocarditis or if there is strong suspicion for unusual forms of cardiomyopathy such as storage diseases or mitochondrial defects. Supportive but nonspecific tests include sedimentation rate, CPK isoenzymes, cardiac troponin I, and brain natriuretic peptide (BNP) levels.

DIFFERENTIAL DIAGNOSIS

The predominant diseases mimicking acute myocarditis include carnitine deficiency, other metabolic disorders of energy generation, hereditary mitochondrial defects, idiopathic dilated cardiomyopathy, pericarditis, EFE, and anomalies of the coronary arteries (see Table 433-1).

TREATMENT

Primary therapy for acute myocarditis is supportive (Chapter 436). Acutely, the use of inotropic agents, preferably milrinone, should be entertained but used with caution because of their proarrhythmic potential. Diuretics are often required as well. If in extremis, mechanical ventilatory support and mechanical circulatory support with ventricular assist device implantation or ECMO may be needed to stabilize the patient's hemodynamic status and act as a bridge to recovery or cardiac transplantation. Diuretics, angiotensin-converting enzyme inhibitors, and angiotensin receptor blockers are of use in patients with compensated congestive heart failure in the outpatient setting, but may be contraindicated in those presenting with fulminant heart failure and cardiovascular collapse. In patients manifesting with significant atrial or ventricular arrhythmias, specific antiarrhythmic agents (for example, amiodarone) should be administered and ICD placement considered.

Immunomodulation of patients with myocarditis is controversial. Intravenous immune globulin may have a role in the treatment of acute or fulminant myocarditis and corticosteroids have been reported to improve cardiac function, but the data are not convincing in children. Relapse has been noted in patients receiving immunosuppression who have been weaned from support. There are no studies to recommend specific antiviral therapies for myocarditis.

PROGNOSIS

The prognosis of symptomatic acute myocarditis in newborns is poor, and 75% mortality has been reported. The prognosis is better for children and adolescents, although patients who have persistent evidence of dilated cardiomyopathy often progress to need for cardiac transplantation. Recovery of ventricular function has been reported in 10-50% of patients, however.

BIBLIOGRAPHY

Please visit the Nelson Textbook of Pediatrics *website at www.expertconsult.com for the complete bibliography.*

Chapter 434
Diseases of the Pericardium

Robert Spicer and Stephanie Ware

The heart is enveloped in a bilayer membrane, the pericardium, which normally contains a small amount of serous fluid. The pericardium is not vital to normal function of the heart, and primary diseases of the pericardium are uncommon. However, the pericardium may be affected by a variety of conditions (Table 434-1), often as a manifestation of a systemic illness and can result in serious, even life-threatening, cardiac compromise.

Table 434-1 ETIOLOGY OF PERICARDIAL DISEASE

CONGENITAL
Absence (partial, complete) Cysts Mulibrey nanism (*TRIM 37* gene mutation) Camptodactyly-arthropathy-coxa vara-pericarditis syndrome (*PRG4* gene mutation)
INFECTIOUS
Viral (coxsackievirus B, Epstein-Barr virus, influenza, adenovirus, parvovirus) Bacterial (*Haemophilus influenzae*, streptococcus, pneumococcus, staphylococcus, meningococcus, mycoplasma, tularemia, listeria, leptospirosis) Immune complex (meningococcus, *H. influenzae*) Tuberculosis Fungal Parasitic
NONINFECTIOUS
Systemic inflammatory diseases (acute rheumatic fever, juvenile rheumatoid arthritis, systemic lupus erythematosus, mixed connective tissue disorders, systemic sclerosis, Wegener granulomatosis) Metabolic (uremia, hypothyroidism, Gaucher disease, very long chain acyl CoA dehydrogenase deficiency) Traumatic (surgical, catheter, nonmedical) Lymphomas, leukemia, radiation therapy Primary pericardial tumors

434.1 Acute Pericarditis

Robert Spicer and Stephanie Ware

PATHOGENESIS

Inflammation of the pericardium may have only minor pathophysiologic consequences in the absence of significant fluid accumulation in the pericardial space. When the amount of fluid in the nondistensible pericardial space becomes excessive, pressure within the pericardium increases and is transmitted to the heart resulting in impaired filling. Although small to moderate amounts of pericardial effusion can be well tolerated and clinically silent, once the noncompliant pericardium has been distended maximally, any further fluid accumulation causes abrupt impairment of cardiac filling and is termed cardiac tamponade. When untreated, tamponade can lead to shock and death. Pericardial effusions may be serous/transudative, exudative/purulent, fibrinous, or hemorrhagic.

CLINICAL MANIFESTATIONS

The most common symptom of acute pericarditis is chest pain, typically described as sharp/stabbing, positional, radiating, worse with inspiration, and relieved by sitting upright or prone. Cough, fever, dyspnea, abdominal pain, and vomiting are nonspecific symptoms associated with pericarditis. Additionally, signs and symptoms of organ system involvement may occur in the presence of generalized systemic disease.

Muffled or distant heart sounds, tachycardia, narrow pulse pressure, jugular venous distension, and a pericardial friction rub provide clues to the diagnosis of acute pericarditis. Cardiac tamponade is recognized by the excessive fall of systolic blood pressure (>10 mm Hg) with inspiration. This pulsus paradoxus can be assessed by careful auscultatory blood pressure determination (automated blood pressure cuffs are inadequate), arterial pressure line wave form, or pulse oximeter tracing inspection. Conditions other than cardiac tamponade, which may result in pulsus paradoxus include severe dyspnea, obesity, and positive pressure ventilator support.

DIAGNOSIS

The electrocardiogram is often abnormal in acute pericarditis although the findings are nonspecific. Low voltage QRS amplitude may be seen as a result of pericardial fluid accumulation. Tachycardia and abnormalities of the ST segments, PR segments, and T waves may be present as well.

Although the chest x-ray findings in a patient with pericarditis without effusion are usually normal, in the presence of a significant effusion, cardiac enlargement will be seen and cardiac contour may be unusual (Erlenmeyer flask). Echocardiography is the most sensitive technique for identifying the size and location of a pericardial effusion. Compression and collapse of the right atrium and/or right ventricle are present with cardiac tamponade (Fig. 434-1). Abnormal diastolic filling parameters have also been described in cases of tamponade.

DIFFERENTIAL DIAGNOSIS

Chest pain similar to that present in pericarditis can occur with lung diseases, especially pleuritis, and with gastroesophageal reflux. Pain related to myocardial ischemia is usually more severe, more prolonged, and occurs with exercise, allowing distinction from pericarditis-induced pain. The presence of a pericardial effusion by echocardiography is virtually diagnostic of pericarditis.

Infectious Pericarditis

A number of viral agents are known to cause pericarditis, and the clinical course of the majority of these infections is mild and spontaneously resolving. The term acute benign pericarditis is synonymous for viral pericarditis. Agents identified as causing pericarditis include the enteroviruses, influenza, adenovirus, respiratory syncytial virus, and parvovirus. As the course of this illness is usually benign, symptomatic treatment with nonsteroidal antiinflammatory agents is often sufficient. Patients with large effusions and tamponade may require pericardiocentesis. If the condition becomes chronic or relapsing, surgical pericardiectomy or creation of a pericardial window may be necessary.

Echocardiography is useful in differentiating pericarditis from myocarditis, the latter of which will show evidence of diminished myocardial contractility or valvular dysfunction. Pericarditis and myocarditis may occur together in some cases of viral infection.

Purulent pericarditis, often caused by bacterial infections, has become much less common with the advent of new immunizations for haemophilus and pneumococcal disease. Historically, purulent pericarditis was seen in association with severe pneumonias, epiglottitis, meningitis, or osteomyelitis. Patients with purulent pericarditis are acutely ill. Unless the infection is recognized and treated expeditiously, the course can be fulminant, leading to tamponade and death. Tuberculous pericarditis is rare in developed countries, but can be seen as a relatively common complication of HIV infection in regions where tuberculosis is endemic and access to anti-retroviral therapy is limited. Immune-complex mediated pericarditis is a rare complication that may result in a nonpurulent (sterile) effusion following systemic bacterial infections such as meningococcus or haemophilus.

Noninfectious Pericarditis

Systemic inflammatory diseases including autoimmune, rheumatologic, and connective tissue disorders may involve the pericardium and result in serous pericardial effusions. Pericardial inflammation may be a component of the type II hypersensitivity reaction seen in patients with acute rheumatic fever. It is often associated with rheumatic valvulitis and responds quickly to antiinflammatory agents including steroids. Tamponade is very uncommon (Chapters 176.1 and 432).

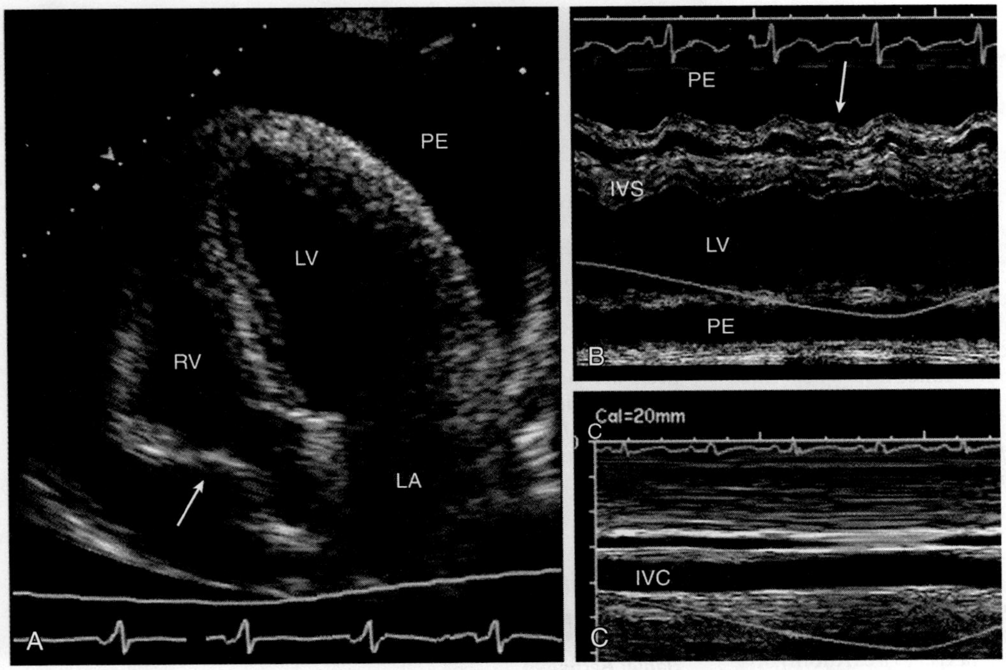

Figure 434-1 Echocardiographic images of large pericardial effusion with features of tamponade. *A,* Apical four-chamber view of LV, LA, and RV that shows large PE with diastolic right-atrial collapse *(arrow). B,* M-mode image with cursor placed through RV, IVS, and LV in parasternal long axis. The view shows circumferential PE with diastolic collapse of RV free wall *(arrow)* during expiration. *C,* M-mode image from subcostal window in same patient that shows IVC plethora without inspiratory collapse. IVC, inferior vena cava; IVS, interventricular septum; LA, left atrium; LV, left ventricle; PE, pericardial effusion; RV, right ventricle. (From Troughton RW, Asher CR, Klein AL: Pericarditis, *Lancet* 363:717–727, 2004.)

Juvenile rheumatoid arthritis, usually systemic onset disease, can manifest with pericarditis. Differentiating rheumatoid pericardial inflammation from that seen with systemic lupus erythematosus is difficult and requires careful rheumatologic evaluation. Aspirin and/or corticosteroids can result in rapid resolution of a pericardial effusion but may be needed on a chronic basis to prevent relapse.

Patients with chronic renal failure or hypothyroidism may have pericardial effusions and should be carefully screened with physical exam, and, if indicated, imaging studies, during the course of their illness should clinical suspicion arise.

Especially common in referral centers with hematology/oncology units is the presence of pericardial effusion related to neoplastic disease. Conditions resulting in effusion include Hodgkin disease, lymphomas, and leukemia. Radiation therapy directed to the mediastinum of patients with malignancy can result in pericarditis and later constrictive pericardial disease.

The postpericardiotomy syndrome occurs in patients having undergone cardiac surgery and is characterized by fever, lethargy, anorexia, irritability, and chest/abdominal discomfort beginning 7-14 days postoperatively. There can be associated pleural effusions and serologic evidence of elevated antiheart antibodies. Postpericardiotomy syndrome is effectively treated with aspirin, nonsteroidal inflammatory agents, and in severe cases, corticosteroids. Pericardial drainage is necessary in those patients with cardiac tamponade.

434.2 Constrictive Pericarditis

Robert Spicer and Stephanie Ware

Rarely, chronic pericardial inflammation can result in fibrosis, calcification, and thickening of the pericardium. Pericardial scarring may lead to impaired cardiac distensibility and filling and is termed constrictive pericarditis. Constrictive pericarditis can occur following recurrent or chronic pericarditis, cardiac surgery, or radiation to the mediastinum as a treatment for malignancies, most commonly Hodgkin disease or lymphoma.

Clinical manifestations of systemic venous hypertension predominate in cases of restrictive pericarditis. Jugular venous distension, peripheral edema, hepatomegaly, and ascites may precede signs of more significant cardiac compromise such as tachycardia, hypotension, and pulsus paradoxus. A pericardial knock, rub, and distant heart sounds might be present on auscultation. Abnormalities of liver function tests, hypoalbuminemia, hypoproteinemia, and lymphopenia may be present. On occasion, x-rays of the chest demonstrate calcifications of the pericardium.

Constrictive pericarditis may be difficult to distinguish clinically from restrictive cardiomyopathy as both conditions result in impaired myocardial filling (Chapter 433.3). Echocardiography may be helpful in distinguishing constrictive pericardial disease from restrictive cardiomyopathy, but magnetic resonance imaging and computed tomographic imaging are more sensitive in detecting abnormalities of the pericardium. In rare instances, exploratory thoracotomy with direct examination of the pericardium may be required to confirm the diagnosis.

Although acute pericardial constriction is reported to respond to antiinflammatory agents, the more typical chronic constrictive pericarditis will respond only to surgical pericardiectomy with extensive resection of the pericardium.

BIBLIOGRAPHY

Please visit the Nelson Textbook of Pediatrics *website at* *www.expertconsult.com* *for the complete bibliography.*

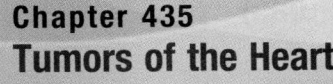

Chapter 435
Tumors of the Heart

Robert Spicer and Stephanie Ware

Although cardiac tumors occur rarely in pediatric patients, they may result in serious hemodynamic or electrophysiologic abnormalities depending on tumor type and location.

For the full continuation of this chapter, please visit the Nelson Textbook of Pediatrics *website at* *www.expertconsult.com.*

Section 7 CARDIAC THERAPEUTICS

Chapter 436
Heart Failure
Daniel Bernstein

Heart failure occurs when the heart cannot deliver adequate cardiac output to meet the metabolic needs of the body. In the early stages of heart failure, various compensatory mechanisms are evoked to maintain normal metabolic function. When these mechanisms become ineffective, increasingly severe clinical manifestations result (Chapter 64).

For the full continuation of this chapter, please visit the Nelson Textbook of Pediatrics *website at www.expertconsult.com.*

436.1 Cardiogenic Shock
Daniel Bernstein

Cardiogenic shock (Chapter 64) may occur as a complication of (1) severe cardiac dysfunction before or after cardiac surgery, (2) septicemia, (3) severe burns, (4) anaphylaxis, (5) cardiomyopathy, (6) myocarditis, (7) myocardial infarction or stunning, and (8) acute central nervous system disorders. It is characterized by low cardiac output and hypotension and therefore results in inadequate tissue perfusion.

For the full continuation of this chapter, please visit the Nelson Textbook of Pediatrics *website at www.expertconsult.com.*

Chapter 437
Pediatric Heart and Heart-Lung Transplantation

437.1 Pediatric Heart Transplantation
Daniel Bernstein

Pediatric heart transplantation is standard therapy for children with end-stage cardiomyopathy and other lesions not amenable to surgical repair. As of 2005, >6,900 heart transplants had been performed on children in the USA, with ≈375 transplants annually. Survival rates among children compare favorably with those of adults. For children transplanted in the 1980s and early 1990s, 1 yr survival has been 75-80%, whereas for those transplanted after 2000, 1 yr survival is now in the range of 90%; during the same time periods, 5 yr survival has improved from 60-65% to 75% (see Fig. 437-1 on the *Nelson Textbook of Pediatrics* website at www.expertconsult.com). A growing number of children are now reaching their 15, 20, and 30 yr post-transplant anniversaries.

For the full continuation of this chapter, please visit the Nelson Textbook of Pediatrics *website at www.expertconsult.com.*

437.2 Heart-Lung and Lung Transplantation
Daniel Bernstein

More than 700 heart-lung and lung (single or double) transplants have been performed in children in the USA, with ≈60 procedures performed annually. Primary indications for heart-lung transplantation include cystic fibrosis, primary pulmonary hypertension, complex congenital heart disease with pulmonary hypoplasia or Eisenmenger syndrome, congenital lung abnormalities, and end-stage parenchymal lung disease (bronchopulmonary dysplasia, chronic lung disease, and interstitial fibrosis). Many of these patients with normal hearts may also be candidates for single- or double-lung transplantation if right ventricular function is preserved. In some patients with Eisenmenger physiology, double-lung transplantation can be performed in combination with repair of intracardiac defects. Patients with cystic fibrosis are not candidates for single-lung grafts because of the risk of infection from the diseased contralateral lung. Patients are selected according to many of the same criteria as for heart transplant recipients (Chapter 437.1).

For the full continuation of this chapter, please visit the Nelson Textbook of Pediatrics *website at www.expertconsult.com.*

Section 8 DISEASES OF THE PERIPHERAL VASCULAR SYSTEM

Chapter 438
Diseases of the Blood Vessels (Aneurysms and Fistulas)

438.1 Kawasaki Disease
Daniel Bernstein

(See also Chapter 160.)

Aneurysms of the coronary or systemic arteries may complicate Kawasaki disease and are the leading cause of morbidity in this disease (Figs. 438-1 and 438-2 on the *Nelson Textbook of Pediatrics* website at www.expertconsult.com). Other than in Kawasaki disease, aneurysms are not common in children and occur most frequently in the aorta in association with coarctation of the aorta, patent ductus arteriosus, and Marfan syndrome and in intracranial vessels (Chapter 594). They may also occur secondary to an infected embolus; infection contiguous to a blood vessel; trauma; congenital abnormalities of vessel structure, especially the medial wall; and arteritis, for example, polyarteritis nodosa, Behçet syndrome, and Takayasu arteritis (Chapter 161.2).

438.2 Arteriovenous Fistulas
Daniel Bernstein

Arteriovenous fistulas may be limited to small cavernous hemangiomas or may be extensive (Chapters 499 and 642). The most common sites in infants and children are within the cranium, in the liver, in the lung, in the extremities, and in vessels in or near the thoracic wall. These fistulas, though usually congenital, may follow trauma or be a manifestation of hereditary hemorrhagic telangiectasia (Osler-Weber-Rendu disease). Femoral arteriovenous fistulas are a rare complication of percutaneous femoral catheterization.

For the full continuation of this chapter, please visit the Nelson Textbook of Pediatrics *website at www.expertconsult.com.*

Chapter 439
Systemic Hypertension

Marc B. Lande

Primary (essential) hypertension occurs commonly in adults and, if untreated, is a major risk factor for myocardial infarction, stroke, and renal failure. In adults with hypertension, a 5 mm Hg increase in diastolic blood pressure (BP) increased the risk of coronary artery disease by 20% and the risk of stroke by 35%. Furthermore, hypertension is implicated in the etiology of nearly 50% of adults with end-stage renal disease. The prevalence of adult hypertension increases with age, ranging from 15% in young adults to 60% in individuals older than 65 yr.

While such late hypertension-related cardiovascular events from essential hypertension do not usually occur in childhood, hypertensive children, although usually asymptomatic, already manifest evidence of target organ damage. Up to 40% of hypertensive children have left ventricular hypertrophy and hypertensive children have increased carotid intima-media thickness, a marker of early atherosclerosis. Primary hypertension during childhood often tracks into adulthood. Children with BP >90th percentile have a 2.4-fold greater risk of having hypertension as adults. Similarly, nearly half of hypertensive adults had a BP >90th percentile as children. There is also an association between childhood hypertension and early atherosclerosis in young adulthood. The phenomenon of BP tracking into adulthood and the demonstration of the beginnings of hypertensive target organ damage during childhood, together with the increased prevalence of childhood essential hypertension, have raised concern of an impending epidemic of cardiovascular morbidity and mortality.

PREVALENCE OF HYPERTENSION IN CHILDREN

In infants and young children, systemic hypertension is uncommon, with a prevalence of <1%, but when present, it is often indicative of an underlying disease process (**secondary hypertension**). *Severe and symptomatic hypertension in children is usually due to secondary hypertension.* In contrast, the prevalence of primary essential hypertension, mostly in older school age children and adolescents, has increased in prevalence in parallel with the obesity epidemic. Approximately 10% of U.S. youth overall have prehypertension and 4% have hypertension. The influence of obesity on elevated BP is evident in children as young as 2-5 yr old. Approximately 20% of American youth are obese, and up to 10% of obese youth have hypertension.

DEFINITION OF HYPERTENSION

The definition of hypertension in adults is BP ≥140/90 mm Hg, regardless of body size, sex, or age. This is a functional definition relating level of BP elevation with the likelihood of subsequent cardiovascular events. Since hypertension-associated cardiovascular events such as myocardial infarction or stroke usually do not occur in childhood, the definition of hypertension in children is statistical rather than functional. The National High Blood Pressure Education Program Working Group on High Blood Pressure in Children and Adolescents published the Fourth Report on the Diagnosis, Evaluation, and Treatment of High Blood Pressure in Children and Adolescents (Fourth Report) in 2004. This report established normal values based on the normative distribution of BP in healthy children and included tables with systolic and diastolic values for the 50th, 90th, 95th, and 99th percentile by age, sex, and height percentile. These normative tables can be obtained free online at *www.nhlbi.nih.gov/guidelines/hypertension/child_tbl.htm*. The Fourth Report defined hypertension as average systolic blood pressure (SBP) and/or diastolic blood pressure (DBP) that is ≥95th percentile for age, sex, and height on ≥3 occasions. **Prehypertension** was defined as average SBP or DBP that are ≥90th percentile but <95th percentile. In adolescents beginning at age 12 yr, prehypertension is defined as BP between 120/80 mm Hg and the 95th percentile. A child with BP levels ≥95th percentile in a medical setting but normal BP outside of the office has **white coat hypertension.**

The Fourth Report further recommended that if BP is ≥95th percentile, then the hypertension should be staged. Children with BP between the 95th and 99th percentile plus 5 mm Hg are categorized as **stage 1 hypertension,** and children with BP above the 99th percentile plus 5 mm Hg have **stage 2 hypertension**. Stage 1 hypertension, if asymptomatic and without target organ damage, allows time for evaluation before starting treatment; whereas stage 2 hypertension calls for more prompt evaluation and pharmacologic therapy (Fig. 439-1).

MEASUREMENT OF BP IN CHILDREN

The Fourth Report recommended that children 3 yr or older should have their BP checked during every health care episode. Selected children <3 yr old should also have their BP checked, including those with a history of prematurity, congenital heart disease, renal disease, solid organ transplant, cancer, treatment with drugs known to raise BP, other illnesses associated with hypertension, or evidence of increased intracranial pressure. The preferred method is by auscultation and a BP cuff appropriate for the size of the child's arm should be used. Elevated readings should be confirmed on repeat visits before determining that a child is hypertensive. The BP should be measured with the child in the sitting position after a period of quiet for at least 5 min. Careful attention to cuff size is necessary to avoid overdiagnosis, as a cuff that is too short or narrow artificially increases BP readings. A wide variety of bladder sizes should be available in any medical office where children are routinely seen. An appropriate sized cuff has an inflatable bladder that is at least 40% of the arm circumference at a point midway along the upper arm. The inflatable bladder should cover at least two thirds of the upper arm length and 80-100% of its circumference.

Systolic pressure is indicated by appearance of the 1st Korotkoff sound. Diastolic pressure has been defined by consensus as the 5th Korotkoff sound. Palpation is useful for rapid assessment of SBP, although the palpated pressure is generally about 10 mm Hg less than that obtained via auscultation. Oscillometric techniques are used frequently in infants and young children, but they are susceptible to artifacts and are best for measuring mean BP.

Ambulatory blood pressure monitoring (ABPM) is a procedure where the child wears a device that records BP frequently, usually every 20-30 min, throughout a 24 hr period while the child goes about usual daily activities, including sleep. This allows calculation of the mean daytime BP, sleep BP, and mean BP over 24 hr. The physician can also determine the proportion of BP measurements that are in the hypertensive range (BP load) and whether there is an appropriate decrease in BP during sleep (nocturnal dip). ABPM is particularly useful in the evaluation for white coat hypertension and may also be useful for determining

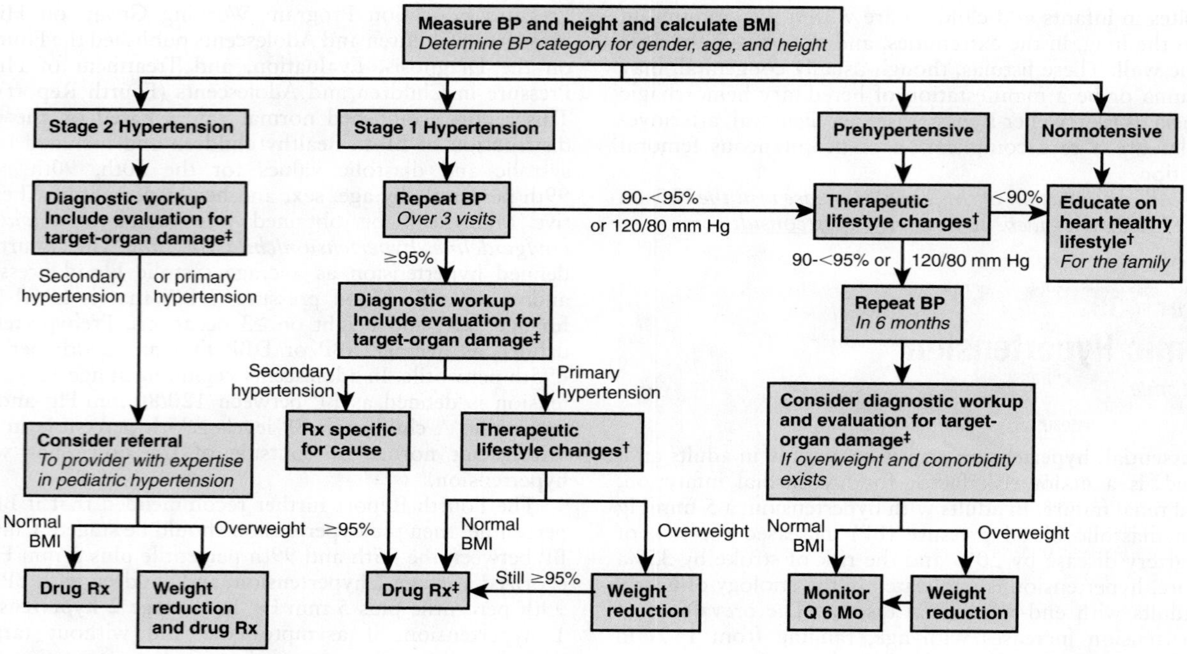

Figure 439-1 Management algorithm. BMI, body mass index; BP, blood pressure; Q, every; Rx, prescription; † diet modification and physical activity; ‡ especially if younger, very high BP, little or no family history, diabetic, or other risk factors. (From National High Blood Pressure Education Program Working Group on High Blood Pressure in Children and Adolescents. The fourth report on the diagnosis, evaluation, and treatment of high blood pressure in children and adolescents, *Pediatrics* 114[2 Suppl 4th Report]:571, 2004.)

risk of hypertensive target organ damage, evaluating resistance to pharmacologic therapy, and evaluating patients with hypotensive episodes on antihypertensive medication. ABPM is also useful for certain special populations, such as children with chronic kidney disease, where it may provide important information on cardiovascular risk that cannot be determined as well by office measurements.

ETIOLOGY AND PATHOPHYSIOLOGY

BP is the product of cardiac output and peripheral vascular resistance. An increase in either cardiac output or peripheral resistance results in an increase in BP; if one of these factors increases while the other decreases, BP may not increase. When hypertension is the result of another disease process, it is referred to as secondary hypertension. When no identifiable cause can be found, it is referred to as primary (essential) hypertension. Many factors, including heredity, diet, stress, and obesity, may play a role in the development of primary hypertension. Secondary hypertension is most common in infants and younger children. In general, the younger the child, the higher the BP and the presence of symptoms related to hypertension, the more likely there will be an underlying secondary cause of hypertension. Many childhood diseases can be responsible for chronic hypertension (Table 439-1) or acute/intermittent hypertension (Table 439-2). The most likely cause varies with age. Hypertension in the premature infant is most often associated with umbilical artery catheterization and renal artery thrombosis. Hypertension during early childhood may be due to renal disease, coarctation of the aorta, endocrine disorders, or medications. In older school-aged children and adolescents, primary hypertension becomes increasingly common.

Secondary hypertension in children is most commonly due to renal abnormalities; cardiovascular disease or endocrinopathies are additional etiologies. Renal (chronic glomerulonephritis, reflux or obstructive nephropathy, hemolytic uremic syndrome, polycystic or dysplastic renal diseases), or renovascular hypertension account for approximately 90% of children with secondary hypertension. Renal parenchymal disease and renal artery stenosis lead to water and sodium retention thought to be, in part, secondary to increased renin secretion. Coarctation of the aorta should always be considered. Several endocrinopathies are associated with hypertension, usually those involving the thyroid, parathyroid, and adrenal glands. Systolic hypertension and tachycardia are common in hyperthyroidism; diastolic pressure is not usually elevated. Hypercalcemia, whether secondary to hyperparathyroidism or other causes, often results in mild elevation in BP because of an increase in vascular tone. Adrenocortical disorders (aldosterone-secreting tumors, sodium retaining congenital adrenal hyperplasia, Cushing syndrome) may produce hypertension in patients with increased mineralocorticoid secretion. Pheochromocytomas are catecholamine-secreting tumors that give rise to hypertension because of the cardiac and peripheral vascular effects of epinephrine and norepinephrine. Children with pheochromocytoma usually have sustained rather than intermittent or exercise-induced hypertension. Pheochromocytoma develops in approximately 5% of patients with neurofibromatosis. Rarely, secondary hypertension can be due to pseudohyperaldosteronism, which leads to elevated BP in the face of a suppressed renin level. Such disorders include Liddle syndrome, apparent mineralocorticoid excess, and dexamethasone suppressible aldosteronism. Altered sympathetic tone can be responsible for acute or intermittent elevation of BP in children with Guillain-Barré syndrome, poliomyelitis, burns, and Stevens-Johnson syndrome. Sympathetic outflow from the central nervous system is also affected by intracranial lesions.

A number of drugs of abuse, therapeutic agents, and toxins may cause hypertension. Cocaine may provoke a rapid increase in BP and can result in seizures or intracranial hemorrhage. Phencyclidine causes transient hypertension that may become persistent in chronic abusers. Tobacco use may also increase BP. Sympathomimetic agents used as nasal decongestants, appetite suppressants, and stimulants for attention deficit disorder produce peripheral vasoconstriction and varying degrees of cardiac stimulation. Individuals vary in their susceptibility to these effects. Oral contraceptives should be suspected as a cause of hypertension in

Table 439-1 CONDITIONS ASSOCIATED WITH CHRONIC HYPERTENSION IN CHILDREN

RENAL
Chronic pyelonephritis
Chronic glomerulonephritis
Hydronephrosis
Congenital dysplastic kidney
Multicystic kidney
Solitary renal cyst
Vesicoureteral reflux nephropathy
Segmental hypoplasia (Ask-Upmark kidney)
Ureteral obstruction
Renal tumors
Renal trauma
Rejection damage following transplantation
Postirradiation damage
Systemic lupus erythematosus (other connective tissue diseases)
VASCULAR
Coarctation of thoracic or abdominal aorta
Renal artery lesions (stenosis, fibromuscular dysplasia, thrombosis, aneurysm)
Umbilical artery catheterization with thrombus formation
Neurofibromatosis (intrinsic or extrinsic narrowing for vascular lumen)
Renal vein thrombosis
Vasculitis
Arteriovenous shunt
Williams-Beuren syndrome
Moyamoya disease
Takayasu arteritis
ENDOCRINE
Hyperthyroidism
Hyperparathyroidism
Congenital adrenal hyperplasia (11β-hydroxylase and 17-hydroxylase defect)
Cushing syndrome
Primary aldosteronism
Dexamethasone-suppressible hyperaldosteronism
Pheochromocytoma
Other neural crest tumors (neuroblastoma, ganglioneuroblastoma, ganglioneuroma)
Liddle syndrome
CENTRAL NERVOUS SYSTEM
Intracranial mass
Hemorrhage
Residual following brain injury
Quadriplegia

Table 439-2 CONDITIONS ASSOCIATED WITH TRANSIENT OR INTERMITTENT HYPERTENSION IN CHILDREN

RENAL
Acute postinfectious glomerulonephritis
Anaphylactoid (Henoch-Schönlein) purpura with nephritis
Hemolytic-uremic syndrome
Acute tubular necrosis
After renal transplantation (immediately and during episodes of rejection)
After blood transfusion in patients with azotemia
Hypervolemia
After surgical procedures on the genitourinary tract
Pyelonephritis
Renal trauma
Leukemic infiltration of the kidney
Obstructive uropathy associated with Crohn disease
DRUGS AND POISONS
Cocaine
Oral contraceptives
Sympathomimetic agents
Amphetamines
Phencyclidine
Corticosteroids and adrenocorticotropic hormone
Cyclosporine or sirolimus treatment post-transplantation
Licorice (glycyrrhizic acid)
Lead, mercury, cadmium, thallium
Antihypertensive withdrawal (clonidine, methyldopa, propranolol)
Vitamin D intoxication
CENTRAL AND AUTONOMIC NERVOUS SYSTEM
Increased intracranial pressure
Guillain-Barré syndrome
Burns
Familial dysautonomia
Stevens-Johnson syndrome
Posterior fossa lesions
Porphyria
Poliomyelitis
Encephalitis
MISCELLANEOUS
Preeclampsia
Fractures of long bones
Hypercalcemia
After coarctation repair
White cell transfusion
Extracorporeal membrane oxygenation
Chronic upper airway obstruction

adolescent girls, although the incidence is lower with the use of low-estrogen preparations. Immunosuppressant agents such as cyclosporine and tacrolimus cause hypertension in organ transplant recipients, and the effect is exacerbated by the co-administration of steroids. BP may be elevated in patients with poisoning by a heavy metal.

Children and adolescents with primary (essential) hypertension are commonly overweight, often have a strong family history of hypertension, and usually have BP values at or only slightly above the 95th percentile for age. Primary hypertension is the most common form of hypertension in adults, and it is recognized more often in adolescents than in young children. The cause of primary hypertension is likely to be multifactorial; obesity, genetic alterations in calcium and sodium transport, vascular smooth muscle reactivity, the renin-angiotensin system, sympathetic nervous system overactivity, and insulin resistance have been implicated in this disorder. Elevated uric acid levels may play a role in the pathophysiology of primary hypertension. Some children and adolescents demonstrate salt-sensitive hypertension, a factor that is ameliorated with weight loss and sodium restriction.

Normotensive children of hypertensive parents may show abnormal physiologic responses that are similar to those of their parents. When subjected to stress or competitive tasks, the offspring of hypertensive adults, as a group, respond with greater increases in heart rate and BP than do children of normotensive parents. Similarly, some children of hypertensive parents may excrete higher levels of urinary catecholamine metabolites or may respond to sodium loading with greater weight gain and increases in BP than do those without a family history of hypertension. The abnormal responses in children with affected parents tend to be greater in the black population than among white individuals.

Tracking of BP is the process by which individuals maintain their relative ranking of BP over time with respect to their peers. Children and young adolescents with BP greater than the 90th percentile for age have a nearly threefold greater likelihood of becoming adults with hypertension than do children with BP at the 50th percentile. Adolescents with primary hypertension may progress from high cardiac output and normal systemic vascular resistance to the adult pattern of normal cardiac output with elevated systemic vascular resistance.

CLINICAL MANIFESTATIONS

Children and adolescents with primary hypertension are usually asymptomatic; the BP elevation is usually mild and is detected during a routine examination or evaluation before athletic participation. These children may also be obese. Children with secondary hypertension can have BP elevations ranging from mild to severe. Unless the pressure has been sustained or is rising rapidly, hypertension does not usually produce symptoms. Therefore, clinical manifestations may instead reflect the underlying disease process, such as growth failure in children with chronic kidney disease. With substantial hypertension, headache, dizziness, epistaxis, anorexia, visual changes, and seizures may occur. Hypertensive encephalopathy (generalized or posterior reversible encephalopathy syndrome [PRES]) is suggested by the presence of vomiting, temperature elevation, ataxia, stupor, CT abnormalities, and seizures. Cardiac failure, pulmonary edema, and renal dysfunction (malignant hypertension) may occur in the face of marked hypertension. Bell palsy may be seen in asymptomatic or symptomatic patients; the etiology is unknown. Hypertensive crisis may manifest with decreased vision (retinal hemorrhages of hypertensive retinopathy) and papilledema, encephalopathy (headache, seizures, depressed level of consciousness), heart failure, or accelerated deterioration of renal function.

Subclinical hypertensive target-organ injury is a common clinical manifestation in children with essential hypertension. With the use of echocardiography utilizing pediatric normative data, left ventricular hypertrophy is detected in up to 40% of hypertensive children. Other markers of target organ damage that have been demonstrated in hypertensive children include increased carotid intima-media thickness, hypertensive retinopathy, and microalbuminuria.

DIAGNOSIS

The evaluation of the child with chronic hypertension should be directed toward uncovering potential underlying causes of the hypertension, evaluating for co-morbidities, and screening for evidence of target organ damage. The extent of the evaluation for underlying causes of hypertension depends on the type of hypertension that is suspected. When secondary hypertension is a strong consideration, as in younger children with severe and symptomatic hypertension, an extensive evaluation may be necessary (Fig. 439-2). Alternatively, overweight adolescents with a family history of hypertension who have mild elevations of BP may need only a limited number of tests.

In all cases, a careful history and physical examination are warranted. A family history for early cardiovascular events should be obtained. Growth parameters should be determined to detect evidence of chronic disease. BP should be obtained in all 4 extremities to detect coarctation (thoracic or abdominal) of the aorta. Other features of the physical examination that may provide evidence of an underlying cause of hypertension are noted in Table 439-3. Unless the history and physical examination suggest another cause, children with confirmed hypertension should have an evaluation to detect renal disease, including urinalysis, electrolytes, BUN, creatinine, complete blood count, urine culture, and renal ultrasound. A more complete list of tests to consider in the clinical evaluation of a child with confirmed hypertension is given in Table 439-4.

Renovascular hypertension is often associated with other diseases (Table 439-5) but may be isolated. Doppler ultrasonography as well as captopril renography and MR or spiral CT angiography are helpful screening tests, but invasive angiography is often needed especially to detect intrarenal arterial stenosis (Fig. 439-3).

Primary hypertension often clusters with other risk factors. All hypertensive children should be screened for co-morbidities that may increase cardiovascular risk, including hyperlipidemia and glucose intolerance. A fasting lipid panel and fasting glucose level should be obtained. In addition, a sleep history should be obtained in children with confirmed hypertension to screen for disordered sleep breathing, an entity that is associated with high BP, particularly in overweight children.

Left ventricular hypertrophy (LVH) is the most common manifestation of target organ damage in hypertensive children. All children with confirmed hypertension should have

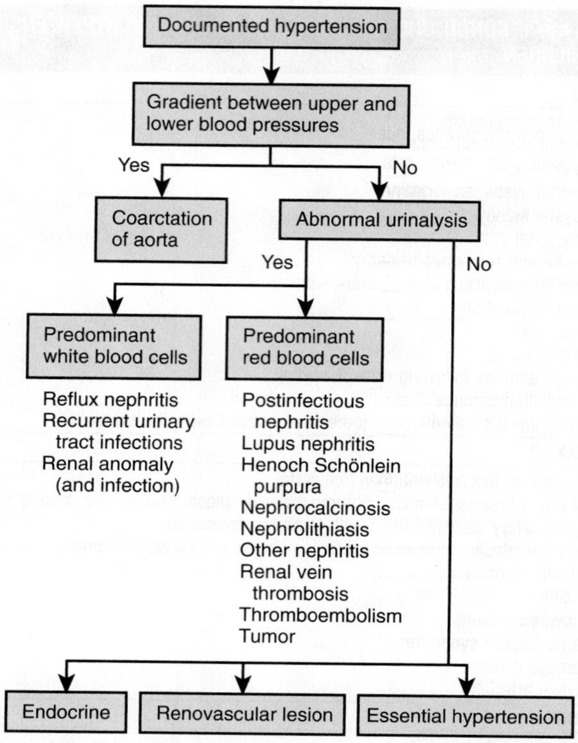

Figure 439-2 Initial diagnostic algorithm in the evaluation of hypertension. (From Kliegman RM, Greenbaum LA, Lye PS: *Practical strategies in pediatric diagnosis and therapy,* ed 2, Philadelphia, 2004, Elsevier, p 222.)

echocardiography to evaluate for the presence of LVH. Left ventricular mass measurements should be indexed to height ($m^{2.7}$) to account for the effect of body size. The presence of LVH is an indication to treat the hypertension with pharmacologic therapy.

PREVENTION

Prevention of high BP may be viewed as part of the prevention of cardiovascular disease and stroke, the leading cause of death in adults in the USA. Other risk factors for cardiovascular disease include obesity, elevated serum cholesterol levels, high dietary sodium intake, a sedentary lifestyle, as well as alcohol and tobacco use. The increase in arterial wall rigidity and blood viscosity that is associated with exposure to the components of tobacco may exacerbate hypertension. Population approaches to prevention of primary hypertension include a reduction in obesity, reduced sodium intake, and an increase in physical activity through school and community-based programs.

TREATMENT

The Fourth Report recommended a management algorithm for children with confirmed hypertension according to whether the child has prehypertension, stage 1 hypertension, or stage 2 hypertension (Figs. 439-1 and 439-4). The mainstay of therapy for children with asymptomatic mild hypertension without evidence of target organ damage is therapeutic lifestyle modification with dietary changes and regular exercise. Weight loss is the primary therapy in obesity-related hypertension. It is recommended that all hypertensive children have a diet increased in fresh fruits, fresh vegetables, fiber, and nonfat dairy and reduced in sodium. In addition, regular aerobic physical activity for at least 30-60 min on most days along with a reduction of sedentary activities to less than 2 hr per day is recommended. Indications for pharmacologic therapy include symptomatic hypertension, secondary

Table 439-3 FINDINGS TO LOOK FOR ON PHYSICAL EXAMINATION

PHYSICAL FINDINGS	POTENTIAL RELEVANCE
GENERAL	
Pale mucous membranes, edema, growth retardation	Chronic renal disease
Elfin facies, poor growth, retardation	Williams syndrome
Webbing of neck, low hairline, widespread nipples, wide carrying angle	Turner syndrome
Moon face, buffalo hump, hirsutism, truncal obesity, striae	Cushing syndrome
HABITUS	
Thinness	Pheochromocytoma, renal disease, hyperthyroidism
Virilization	Congenital adrenal hyperplasia
Rickets	Chronic renal disease
SKIN	
Café-au-lait spots, neurofibromas	Neurofibromatosis, pheochromocytoma
Tubers, "ash-leaf" spots	Tuberous sclerosis
Rashes	SLE, vasculitis (HSP), impetigo with acute nephritis
Pallor, evanescent flushing, sweating	Pheochromocytoma
Needle tracks	Illicit drug use
Bruises, striae	Cushing syndrome
EYES	
Extraocular muscle palsy	Nonspecific, chronic, severe
Fundal changes	Nonspecific, chronic, severe
Proptosis	Hyperthyroidism
HEAD AND NECK	
Goiter	Thyroid disease
CARDIOVASCULAR SIGNS	
Absent of diminished femoral pulses, low leg pressure relative to arm pressure	Aortic coarctation
Heart size, rate, rhythm; murmurs; respiratory difficulty, hepatomegaly	Aortic coarctation, congestive heart failure
Bruits over great vessels	Arteritis or arteriopathy
Rub	Pericardial effusion secondary to chronic renal disease
PULMONARY SIGNS	
Pulmonary edema	Congestive heart failure, acute nephritis
Picture of bronchopulmonary dysplasia (BPD)	BPD-associated hypertension
ABDOMEN	
Epigastric bruit	Primary renovascular disease or in association with Williams syndrome, neurofibromatosis, fibromuscular dysplasia, or arteritis
Abdominal masses	Wilms tumor, neuroblastoma, pheochromocytoma, polycystic kidneys, hydronephrosis
NEUROLOGIC SIGNS	
Neurologic deficits	Chronic or severe acute hypertension with stroke
GENITALIA	
Ambiguous, virilized	Congenital adrenal hyperplasia

HSP, Henoch-Schönlein purpura; SLE, systemic lupus erythematosus.
From Kliegman RM, Greenbaum LA, Lye PS: *Practical strategies in pediatric diagnosis and therapy,* ed 2, Philadelphia, 2004, Elsevier, p 200.

Table 439-4 CLINICAL EVALUATION OF CONFIRMED HYPERTENSION

STUDY OR PROCEDURE	PURPOSE	TARGET POPULATION
EVALUATION FOR IDENTIFIABLE CAUSES		
History, including sleep history, family history, risk factors, diet, and habits such as smoking and drinking alcohol; physical examination	History and physical examination help focus subsequent evaluation	All children with persistent BP ≥95th percentile
BUN, creatinine, electrolytes, urinalysis, and urine culture	R/O renal disease and chronic pyelonephritis	All children with persistent BP ≥95th percentile
CBC	R/O anemia, consistent with chronic renal disease	All children with persistent BP ≥95th percentile
Renal U/S	R/O renal scar, congenital anomaly, or disparate renal size	All children with persistent BP ≥95th percentile
EVALUATION FOR CO-MORBIDITY		
Fasting lipid panel, fasting glucose	Identify hyperlipidemia, identify metabolic abnormalities	Overweight patients with BP at 90th-94th percentile; all patients with BP ≥95th percentile; family history of hypertension or CVD; child with chronic renal disease
Drug screen	Identify substances that might cause hypertension	History suggestive of possible contribution by substances or drugs.
Polysomnography	Identify sleep disorder in association with hypertension	History of loud, frequent snoring

Continued

Table 439-4 CLINICAL EVALUATION OF CONFIRMED HYPERTENSION—cont'd

STUDY OR PROCEDURE	PURPOSE	TARGET POPULATION
EVALUATION FOR TARGET-ORGAN DAMAGE		
Echocardiogram	Identify LVH and other indications of cardiac involvement	Patients with co-morbid risk factors* and BP 90th-94th percentile; all patients with BP ≥95th percentile
Retinal exam	Identify retinal vascular changes	Patients with co-morbid risk factors and BP 90th-94th percentile; all patients with BP ≥95th percentile
ADDITIONAL EVALUATION AS INDICATED		
ABPM	Identify white coat hypertension, abnormal diurnal BP pattern, BP load	Patients in whom white coat hypertension is suspected, and when other information on BP pattern is needed
Plasma renin determination	Identify low renin, suggesting mineralocorticoid-related disease	Young children with stage 1 hypertension and any child or adolescent with stage 2 hypertension
		Positive family history of severe hypertension
Renovascular imaging Isotopic scintigraphy (renal scan) MRA Duplex Doppler flow studies 3-Dimensional CT	Identify renovascular disease	Young children with stage 1 hypertension and any child or adolescent with stage 2 hypertension
Arteriography: DSA or classic		
Plasma and urine steroid levels	Identify steroid-mediated hypertension	Young children with stage 1 hypertension and any child or adolescent with stage 2 hypertension
Plasma and urine catecholamines	Identify catecholamine-mediated hypertension	Young children with stage 1 hypertension and any child or adolescent with stage 2 hypertension

*Co-morbid risk factors also include diabetes mellitus and kidney disease.
BUN, blood urea nitrogen; CBC, complete blood count; R/O, rule out; U/S, ultrasound.
From National High Blood Pressure Education Program Working Group on High Blood Pressure in Children and Adolescents. The fourth report on the diagnosis, evaluation, and treatment of high blood pressure in children and adolescents, *Pediatrics* 114(2 Suppl 4th Report):562, 2004.

Table 439-5 CAUSES OF RENOVASCULAR HYPERTENSION IN CHILDREN

Fibromuscular dysplasia
Syndromic
- Neurofibromatosis type 1
- Tuberous sclerosis
- Williams syndrome
- Marfan syndrome
- Other syndromes

Vasculitis
- Takayasu disease
- Polyarteritis nodosa
- Kawasaki disease
- Other systemic vasculitides

Extrinsic compression
- Neuroblastoma
- Wilms tumor
- Other tumors

Other causes
- Radiation
- Umbilical artery catheterization
- Trauma
- Congenital rubella syndrome
- Transplant renal artery stenosis

From Tullus K, Brennan E, Hamilton G, et al: Renovascular hypertension in children, *Lancet* 371:1453–1463, 2008; p 1454, Panel 1.

hypertension, hypertensive target organ damage, diabetes (types 1 and 2), and persistent hypertension despite nonpharmacologic measures (Table 439-6). When indicated, antihypertensive medication should be initiated as a single agent at low dose (see Fig. 439-4). The dose can then be increased until the goal BP is achieved. Once the highest recommended dose is reached or if the child develops side effects, then a second drug from a different class can be added. Acceptable drug classes for use in children include ACE inhibitors, angiotensin receptor blockers, β-blockers, calcium channel blockers, and diuretics. Details on recommended doses of different classes of antihypertensive medications for children can be found in the Fourth Report available free online at *www.nhlbi.nih.gov/health/prof/heart/hbp/hbp_ped.pdf*.

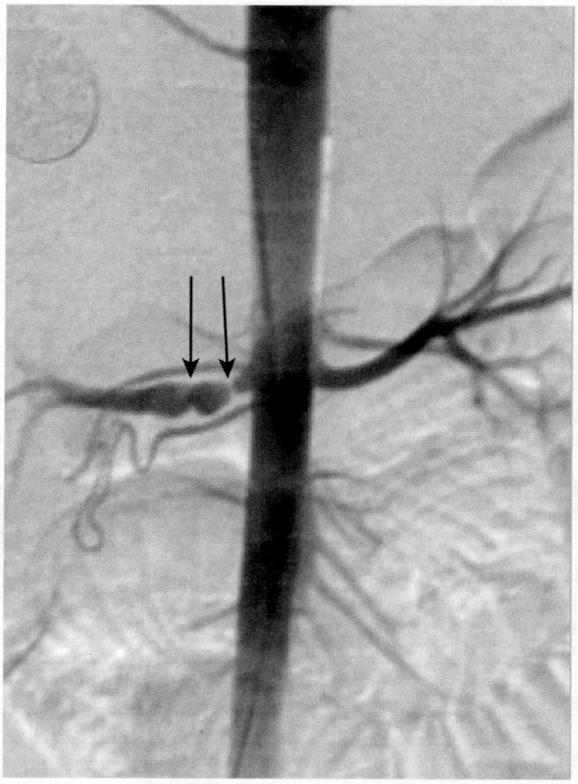

Figure 439-3 Renal angiogram in 7 yr old boy with hypertension. Right renal artery is visible with a string-of-beads appearance characteristic of fibromuscular dysplasia *(arrows)*. The aorta and left renal artery appear normal. (From Tullus K, Brennan E, Hamilton G, et al: Renovascular hypertension in children, *Lancet* 371:1453–1463, 2008; p 1454, Fig 1.)

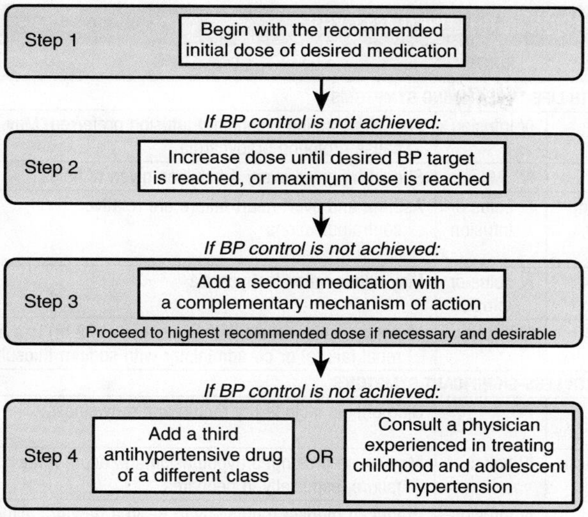
Step 1
Begin with the recommended initial dose of desired medication
If BP control is not achieved:
Step 2
Increase dose until desired BP target is reached, or maximum dose is reached
If BP control is not achieved:
Step 3
Add a second medication with a complementary mechanism of action
Proceed to highest recommended dose if necessary and desirable
If BP control is not achieved:
Step 4
Add a third antihypertensive drug of a different class
OR
Consult a physician experienced in treating childhood and adolescent hypertension

Figure 439-4 Stepped-care approach to antihypertensive therapy in children and adolescents. BP, blood pressure. (From Flynn JT, Daniels SR: Pharmacologic treatment of hypertension in children and adolescents, *J Pediatr* 149:746–754, 2006; p 751, Fig 2.)

The goal of therapy for hypertension should be to reduce BP below the 95th percentile, except in the presence of chronic kidney disease, diabetes, or target organ damage, when the goal should be to reduce BP to less than the 90th percentile. ACE inhibitors or angiotensin receptor blockers should be used for children with diabetes and microalbuminuria or proteinuric renal disease. β-Blockers or calcium channel blockers should be considered for hypertensive children with migraine headaches.

Severe, symptomatic hypertension is a hypertensive emergency that is often accompanied by cardiac failure, retinopathy, renal failure, encephalopathy, and seizures. Intravenous administration is often preferred so that the fall in BP can be carefully titrated (Table 439-7). Drug choices include labetalol, nicardipine, and sodium nitroprusside. Because too rapid a reduction in BP may interfere with adequate organ perfusion, a stepwise reduction in pressure should be planned. In general, the pressure should be reduced by 10% in the 1st hour, and 15% more in the next 3-12 hr, but not to normal during the acute phase of treatment. Hypertensive urgencies, usually accompanied by few serious symptoms such as severe headache or vomiting, can be treated either orally or intravenously. The Fourth Report also includes detailed information on antihypertensive drugs used for the management of severe hypertension in children.

Table 439-6 RECOMMENDED DOSES FOR SELECTED ANTIHYPERTENSIVE AGENTS FOR USE IN HYPERTENSIVE CHILDREN AND ADOLESCENTS

CLASS	DRUG	STARTING DOSE	INTERVAL	MAXIMUM DOSE*
Angiotensin-converting enzyme inhibitors	Benazepril†	0.2 mg/kg/day up to 10 mg/day	QD	0.6 mg/kg/day up to 40 mg/day
	Captopril†	0.3-0.5 mg/kg/dose	BID-TID	6 mg/kg/day up to 450 mg/day
	Enalapril†	0.08 mg/kg/day	QD	0.6 mg/kg/day up to 40 mg/day
	Fosinopril	0.1 mg/kg/day up to 10 mg/day	QD	0.6 mg/kg/day up to 40 mg/day
	Lisinopril†	0.07 mg/kg/day up to 5 mg/day	QD	0.6 mg/kg/day up to 40 mg/day
	Quinapril	5-10 mg/day	QD	80 mg/day
	Ramipril	2.5 mg/day	QD	20 mg/day
Angiotensin-receptor blockers	Candesartan	4 mg/day	QD	32 mg/day
	Irbesartan	75-150 mg/day	QD	300 mg/day
	Losartan†	0.75 mg/kg/day up to 50 mg/day	QD	1.4 mg/kg/day up to 100 mg/day
α- and β-Adrenergic antagonists	Labetalol†	2-3 mg/kg/day	BID	10-12 mg/kg/day up to 1.2 g/day
	Carvedilol	0.1 mg/kg/dose up to 12.5 mg BID	BID	0.5 mg/kg/dose up to 25 mg BID
β-Adrenergic antagonists	Atenolol†	0.5-1 mg/kg/day	QD-BID	2 mg/kg/day up to 100 mg/day
	Bisoprolol/HCTZ	0.04 mg/kg/day up to 2.5/6.25 mg/day	QD	10/6.25 mg/day
	Metoprolol	1-2 mg/kg/day	BID	6 mg/kg/day up to 200 mg/day
	Propranolol	1 mg/kg/day	BID-TID	16 mg/kg/day up to 640 mg/day
Calcium channel blockers	Amlodipine†	0.06 mg/kg/day up to 5 mg/day	QD	0.6 mg/kg/day up to 10 mg/day
	Felodipine	2.5 mg/day	QD	10 mg/day
	Isradipine†	0.05-0.15 mg/kg/dose	TID-QID	0.8 mg/kg/day up to 20 mg/day
	Extended-release nifedipine	0.25-0.50 mg/kg/day	QD-BID	3 mg/kg/day up to 120 mg/day
Central α-agonists	Clonidine†	5-10 µg/kg/day	BID-TID	25 µg/kg/day up to 0.9 mg/day
	Methyldopa†	5 mg/kg/day	BID-QID	40 mg/kg/day up to 3 g/day
Diuretics	Amiloride	5-10 mg/day	QD	20 mg/day
	Chlorothiazide	10 mg/kg/day	BID	20 mg/kg/day up to 1.0 gram/day
	Chlorthalidone	0.3 mg/kg/day	QD	2 mg/kg/day up to 50 mg/day
	Furosemide	0.5-2.0 mg/kg/dose	QD-BID	6 mg/kg/day
	HCTZ	0.5-1 mg/kg/day	QD	3 mg/kg/day up to 50 mg/day
	Sprionolactone†	1 mg/kg/day	QD-BID	3.3 mg/kg/day up to 100 mg/day
	Triamterene	1-2 mg/kg/day	BID	3-4 mg/kg/day up to 300 mg/day
Peripheral α-antagonists	Doxazosin	1 mg/day	QD	4 mg/day
	Prazosin	0.05-0.1 mg/kg/day	TID	0.5 mg/kg/day
	Terazosin	1 mg/day	QD	20 mg/day
Vasodilators	Hydralazine	0.25 mg/kg/dose	TID-QID	7.5 mg/kg/day up to 200 mg/day
	Minoxidil	0.1-0.2 mg/kg/day	BID-TID	1 mg/kg/day up to 50 mg/day

*The maximum recommended adult dose should never be exceeded.
†Information on preparation of a stable extemporaneous suspension is available for these agents.
BID, twice daily; HCTZ, hydrochlorothiazide; QD, once daily; QID, 4 times daily; TID, 3 times daily.
From Flynn JT, Daniels SR: Pharmacologic treatment of hypertension in children and adolescents, *J Pediatr* 149:746–754, 2006; p752, Table 2.

Table 439-7 ANTIHYPERTENSIVE DRUGS FOR MANAGEMENT OF SEVERE HYPERTENSION IN CHILDREN 1-17 YRS

DRUG	CLASS	DOSE	ROUTE	COMMENTS
USEFUL FOR SEVERELY HYPERTENSIVE PATIENTS WITH LIFE-THREATENING SYMPTOMS				
Esmolol	β-adrenergic blocker	100-500 μg/kg per min	IV infusion	Very short-acting—constant infusion preferred. May cause profound bradycardia
Hydralazine	Direct vasodilator	0.2-0.6 mg/kg per dose	IV, IM	Should be given every 4 hr when given IV bolus
Labetalol	α- and β-adrenergic blocker	Bolus: 0.20-1.0 mg/kg per dose, up to 40 mg per dose Infusion: 0.25-3.0 mg/kg/hr	IV bolus or infusion	Asthma and overt heart failure are relative contraindications
Nicardipine	Calcium channel blocker	Bolus: 30 μg/kg up to 2 mg/dose Infusion: 0.5-4 μg/kg per min	IV bolus or infusion	May cause reflex tachycardia
Sodium nitroprusside	Direct vasodilator	0.5-10 μg/kg per min	IV infusion	Monitor cyanide levels with prolonged (>72 hr) use or in renal failure, or co-administer with sodium thiosulfate
USEFUL FOR SEVERELY HYPERTENSIVE PATIENTS WITH LESS-SIGNIFICANT SYMPTOMS				
Clonidine	Central α-agonist	0.05-0.1 mg/dose, may be repeated up to 0.8 mg total dose	PO	Side effects include dry mouth and drowsiness
Enalaprilat	ACE inhibitor	0.05-0.10 mg/kg per dose up to 1.25 mg/dose	IV bolus	May cause prolonged hypotension and acute renal failure, especially in neonates
Fenoldopam	Dopamine receptor agonist	0.2-0.8 μg/kg per min	IV infusion	Produced modest reductions in BP in a pediatric clinical trial in patients up to 12 yr
Hydralazine	Direct vasodilator	0.25 mg/kg per dose up to 25 mg/dose	PO	Extemporaneous suspension stable for only 1 wk
Isradipine	Calcium channel blocker	0.05-0.1 mg/kg per dose up to 5 mg/dose	PO	Stable suspension can be compounded
Minoxidil	Direct vasodilator	0.1-0.2 mg/kg per dose up to 10 mg/dose	PO	Most potent oral vasodilator; long-acting

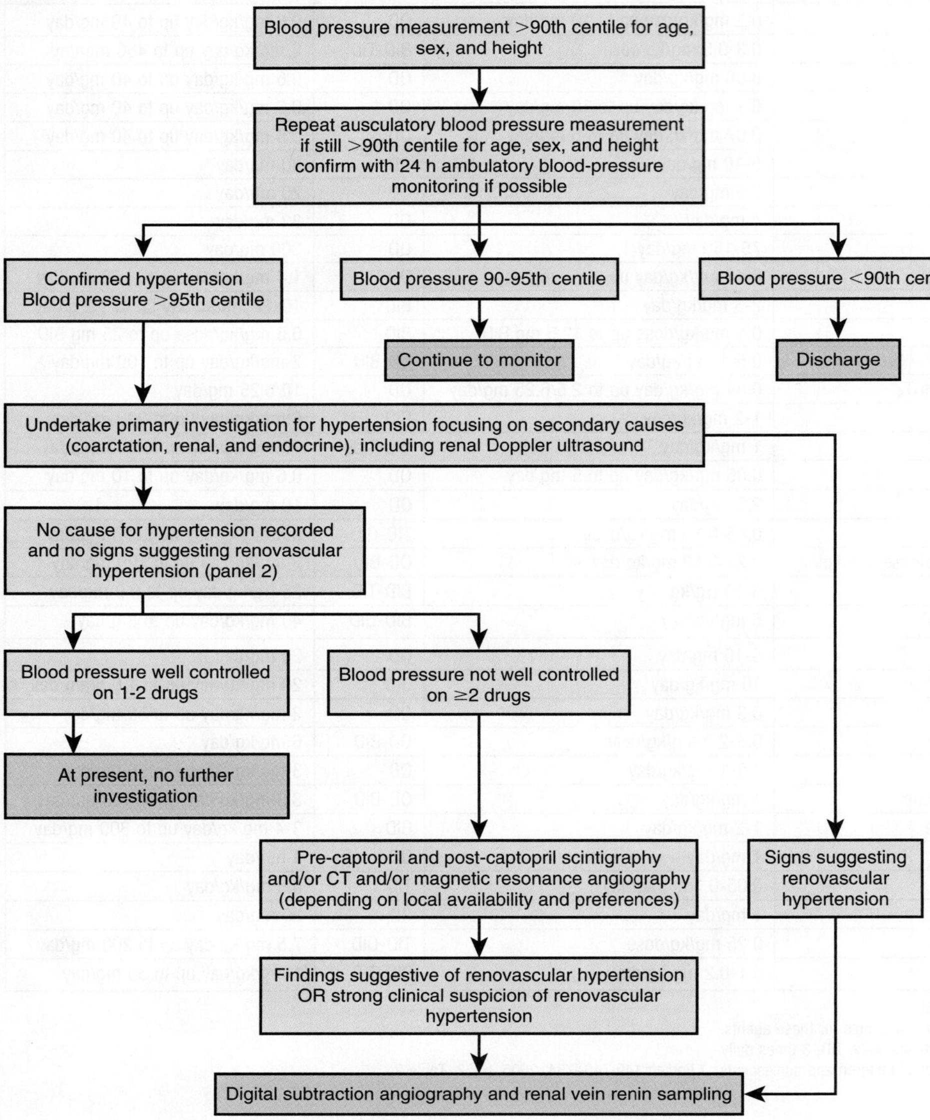

Figure 439-5 Treatment pathway for renovascular hypertension. (From Tullus K, Brennan E, Hamilton G, et al: Renovascular hypertension in children, *Lancet* 371:1453–1463, 2008; p 1458, Fig 6.)

Treatment of secondary hypertension must also focus on the underlying disease such as chronic renal disease, hyperthyroidism, adrenal-genital syndrome, pheochromocytoma, coarctation of the aorta, or renovascular hypertension. The treatment of renovascular stenosis includes antihypertensive medications, angioplasty, or surgery (Fig. 439-5). If bilateral renovascular hypertension or renovascular disease in a solitary kidney is suspected, drugs acting on the renin-angiotensin axis are usually contraindicated because they may reduce glomerular filtration rates and produce renal failure. Balloon angioplasty or surgical revascularization should then be attempted.

BIBLIOGRAPHY

Please visit the Nelson Textbook of Pediatrics *website at www.expertconsult.com for the complete bibliography.*

PART XXI Diseases of the Blood

Section 1 THE HEMATOPOIETIC SYSTEM

Chapter 440
Development of the Hematopoietic System

Robert D. Christensen and Robin K. Ohls

HEMATOPOIESIS IN THE HUMAN EMBRYO AND FETUS

Hematopoiesis is the process by which the cellular elements of blood are formed. In the developing human embryo and fetus, hematopoiesis is conceptually divided into 3 anatomic stages: mesoblastic, hepatic, and myeloid. Mesoblastic hematopoiesis occurs in extraembryonic structures, principally in the yolk sac, and begins between the 10th and 14th days of gestation. By 6-8 wk of gestation the liver replaces the yolk sac as the primary site of blood cell production, and during this time the placenta also contributes as a hematopoietic site. By 10-12 wk extraembryonic hematopoiesis has essentially ceased. Hepatic hematopoiesis occurs through the remainder of gestation, although hepatic production diminishes during the 2nd trimester while bone marrow (myeloid) hematopoiesis increases. The liver remains the predominant erythropoietic organ (few if any neutrophils are produced in the human fetal liver) through 20-24 wk of gestation.

For the full continuation of this chapter, please visit the Nelson Textbook of Pediatrics *website at* *www.expertconsult.com*.

Chapter 441
The Anemias

Norma B. Lerner

Anemia is defined as a reduction of the hemoglobin concentration or red blood cell (RBC) volume below the range of values occurring in healthy persons. "Normal" hemoglobin and hematocrit (packed red cell volume) vary substantially with age and sex (Table 441-1). There are also racial differences, with significantly lower hemoglobin levels in African-American children than in white non-Hispanic children of comparable age (Table 441-2).

Physiologic adjustments to anemia include increased cardiac output, augmented oxygen extraction (increased arteriovenous oxygen difference), and a shunting of blood flow toward vital organs and tissues. In addition, the concentration of 2,3-diphosphoglycerate (2,3-DPG) increases within the RBC. The resultant "shift to the right" of the oxygen dissociation curve reduces the affinity of hemoglobin for oxygen and results in more complete transfer of oxygen to the tissues. (The same shift in the oxygen dissociation curve can also occur at high altitude.) Higher levels of erythropoietin (EPO) and consequent increased red cell production by the bone marrow further assist the body to adapt.

Table 441-1 NORMAL MEAN AND LOWER LIMITS OF NORMAL FOR HEMOGLOBIN, HEMATOCRIT, AND MEAN CORPUSCULAR VOLUME

AGE (YR)	HEMOGLOBIN (G/DL)		HEMATOCRIT (%)		MEAN CORPUSCULAR VOLUME (μM³)	
	Mean	Lower Limit	Mean	Lower Limit	Mean	Lower Limit
0.5-1.9	12.5	11.0	37	33	77	70
2-4	12.5	11.0	38	34	79	73
5-7	13.0	11.5	39	35	81	75
8-11	13.5	12.0	40	36	83	76
12-14 female	13.5	12.0	41	36	85	78
12-14 male	14.0	12.5	43	37	84	77
15-17 female	14.0	12.0	41	36	87	79
15-17 male	15.0	13.0	46	38	86	78
18-49 female	14.0	12.0	42	37	90	80
18-49 male	16.0	14.0	47	40	90	80

From Brugnara C, Oski FJ, Nathan DG: *Nathan and Oski's hematology of infancy and childhood*, ed 7, Philadelphia, 2009, WB Saunders, p 456.

Table 441-2 NHANES III HEMOGLOBIN VALUES FOR NON-HISPANIC WHITES AND AFRICAN AMERICANS AGED 2-18 YEARS

AGE (YR)	WHITE NON-HISPANIC		AFRICAN AMERICAN	
	Mean	−2 SD	Mean	−2 SD
2-5	12.21	10.8	11.95	10.37
6-10	12.87	11.31	12.40	10.74
11-15 male	13.76	11.76	13.06	10.88
11-15 female	13.32	11.5	12.61	10.85
16-18 male	15.00	13.24	14.18	12.42
16-18 female	13.39	11.61	12.37	10.37

Sample size is 5,142 (white, 2,264; African American, 2,878).
Modified from Robbins EB, Blum S: Hematologic reference values for African American children and adolescents, *Am J Hematol* 82:611–614, 2007.

HISTORY AND PHYSICAL EXAMINATION

As with any medical condition, a detailed history and thorough physical exam are essential when evaluating an anemic child. Important historical facts should include age, sex, race and ethnicity, diet, medications, chronic diseases, infections, travel, and exposures. A family history of anemia and/or associated difficulties such as splenomegaly, jaundice, or early-age onset of gallstones is also of consequence. There often are few physical symptoms or signs that result solely from a low hemoglobin, particularly when the anemia develops slowly. Clinical findings generally do not become apparent until the hemoglobin level falls to <7-8 g/dL. Clinical features can include pallor, sleepiness, irritability, and decreased exercise tolerance. Pallor can involve the tongue, nail beds, palms, or palmar creases. A flow murmur is often present. Ultimately, weakness, tachypnea, shortness of breath on exertion, tachycardia, cardiac dilatation, and high-output heart failure will result from increasingly severe anemia, regardless of its cause. Unusual physical findings linked to

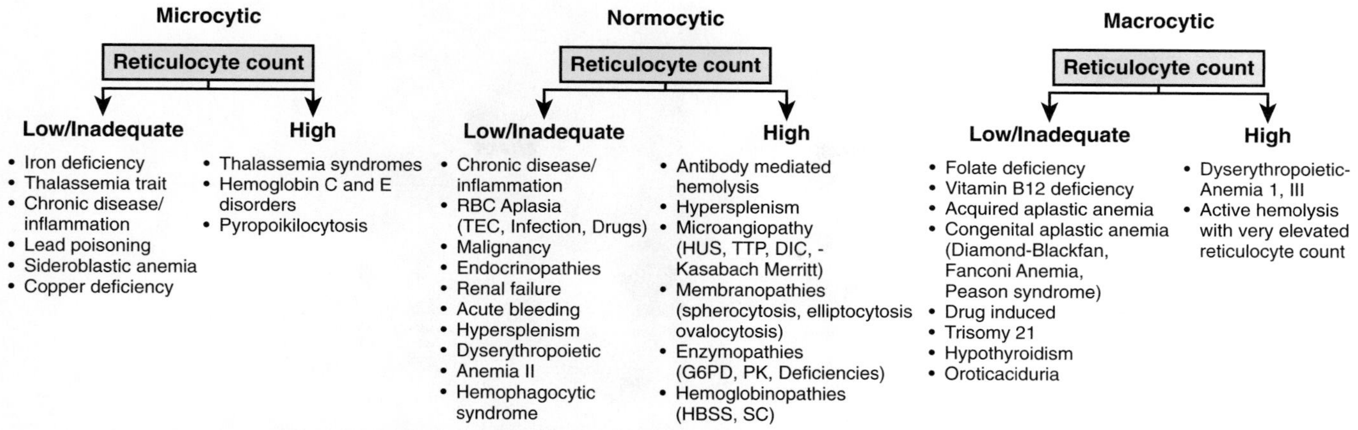

Figure 441-1 Use of the mean corpuscular volume (MCV) and reticulocyte count in the diagnosis of anemia. (Adapted from From Brunetti M, Cohen J: *The Harriet Lane handbook*, ed 17, Philadelphia, 2005, Elsevier Mosby, p 338.)

particular underlying disease etiologies are discussed in detail in sections describing the associated disorders.

LABORATORY STUDIES

Initial laboratory testing should include hemoglobin, hematocrit, and red cell indices as well as a white blood cell count and differential, platelet count, reticulocyte count, and examination of the peripheral blood smear. The need for additional laboratory studies is dictated by the history, the physical, and the results of this initial testing.

DIFFERENTIAL DIAGNOSIS

Anemia is not a specific entity but rather can result from any of number of underlying pathologic processes. In order to narrow the diagnostic possibilities, anemias may be classified on the basis of their morphology and/or physiology (Fig. 441-1).

Anemias may be morphologically categorized on the basis of RBC size (mean corpuscular volume [MCV]), and microscopic appearance. They can be classified as microcytic, normocytic, or macrocytic based on whether the MCV is low, normal, or high, respectively. RBC size also changes with age, and normal developmental changes in MCV should be recognized before a designation is made (see Table 441-1). Examination of a peripheral blood smear often reveals changes in RBC appearance that will help to further narrow the diagnostic categories (Fig. 441-2). Details regarding morphologic changes associated with particular disorders are described in subsequent sections.

Anemias may also be further divided on the basis of underlying physiology. The two major categories are decreased production and increased destruction or loss. The two groups are not always mutually exclusive. Decreased RBC production may be a consequence of ineffective erythropoiesis or a complete or relative failure of erythropoiesis. Increased destruction or loss may be secondary to hemolysis, sequestration, or bleeding. The peripheral blood reticulocyte percentage or absolute number will help to make a distinction between the two physiologic categories. The normal reticulocyte percentage of total RBCs during most of childhood is about 1.0%, with an absolute reticulocyte count of 25,000-75,000/mm^3. In the presence of anemia, EPO production and the absolute number of reticulocytes should rise. Low or normal numbers of reticulocytes generally represent an inadequate response to anemia that is associated with relative bone marrow failure or ineffective erythropoiesis. Increased numbers of reticulocytes represent a normal bone marrow response to ongoing RBC destruction (hemolysis), sequestration, or loss (bleeding).

Figure 441-1 presents a useful approach to assessing the common causes of anemia in the pediatric age group. Children with microcytic anemia and low or normal reticulocyte counts most often have defects in erythroid maturation or ineffective erythropoiesis. *Iron deficiency* (Chapter 449) is the most common cause. *Thalassemia trait* (Chapter 456) constitutes the primary differential diagnosis when iron deficiency is suspected. Distinctions between these entities are presented in Table 449-1 (Chapter 449). *Chronic disease or inflammation (more often normocytic), lead poisoning, and sideroblastic anemias* should also be considered and are discussed in other chapters. Microcytosis and elevated reticulocyte counts are associated with thalassemia syndromes and hemoglobin C and E (Chapter 456). Notably, thalassemias and hemoglobinopathies are most commonly seen in patients of Mediterranean, Middle Eastern, African, or Asian background.

Normocytic anemia and low reticulocyte count characterize a large number of anemias. The *anemia of chronic disease/inflammation* (Chapter 445) is usually normocytic. The anemia associated with renal failure, caused by reduced erythropoietin production, will invariably be associated with clinical and laboratory evidence of significant kidney disease. Decreased or absent red cell production secondary to transient erythroblastopenia of childhood (TEC), infection, drugs, or endocrinopathy usually results in a normocytic anemia, as does bone marrow infiltration by malignancy. In the case of invading leukemia or malignancy, abnormal leukocytes or tumor cells in association with thrombocytopenia or reduced or elevated white cell counts may be seen. Acute bleeding, hypersplenism, and congenital dyserythropoietic anemia (CDA) type II (Chapter 446) are also normocytic.

In children with normocytic anemia and an appropriate (high) reticulocyte response, the anemia is usually a consequence of bleeding, hypersplenism, or ongoing hemolysis. In hemolytic conditions, reticulocytosis, indirect hyperbilirubinemia, and increased serum lactate dehydrogenase are indicators of accelerated erythrocyte destruction. There are many causes of hemolysis, resulting from conditions that are extrinsic (usually acquired) or intrinsic (usually congenital) to the red cell. Abnormal RBC morphology (e.g., spherocytes, sickle forms, microangiopathy) identified on the peripheral smear is often helpful in ascertaining the cause.

The anemia seen in children with macrocytic blood cells is sometimes megaloblastic (Chapter 448), resulting from impaired DNA synthesis and nuclear development. The peripheral blood smear in megaloblastic anemias contains large macrovalocytes, and the neutrophils often show nuclear hypersegmentation. The major causes of megaloblastic anemia include folate deficiency, vitamin B_{12} deficiency, and rare inborn errors of metabolism.

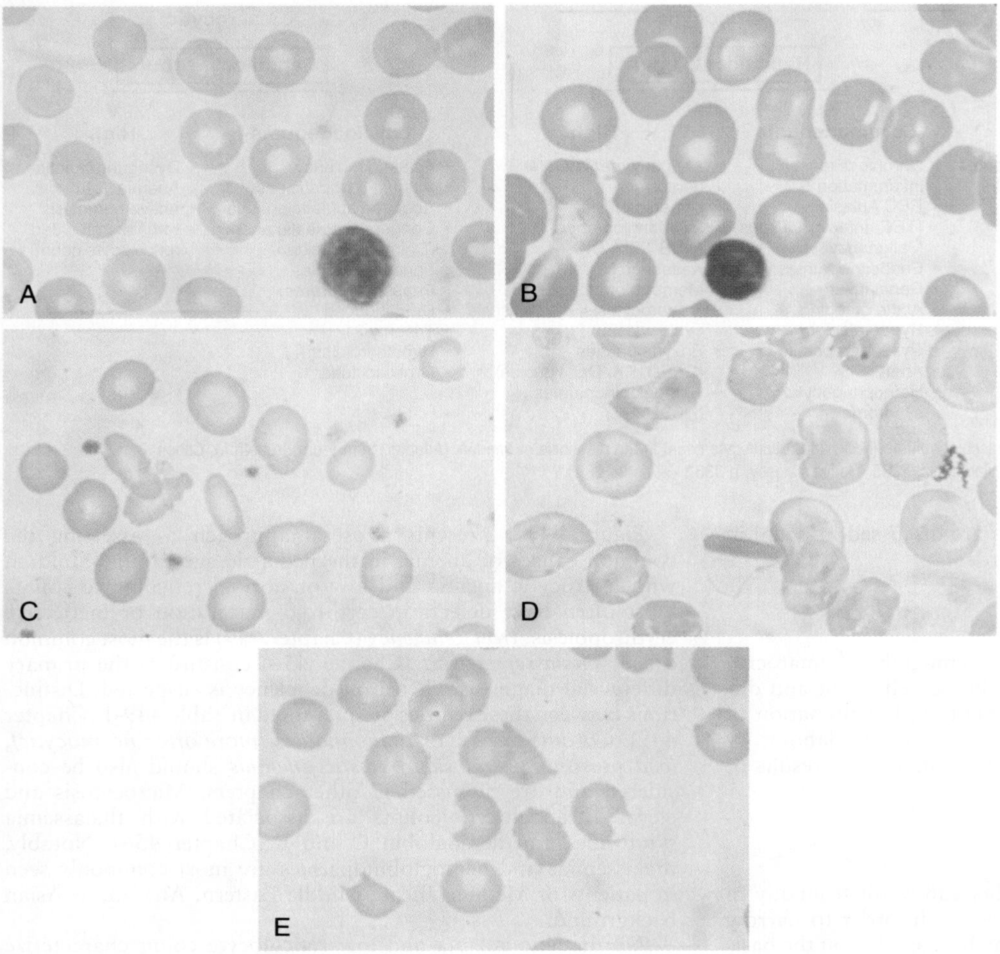

Figure 441-2 Morphologic abnormalities of the red blood cell. *A,* Normal. *B,* Macrocytes (folic acid or vitamin B_{12} deficiency). *C,* Hypochromic microcytes (iron deficiency). *D,* Target cells (HbCC disease). *E,* Schizocytes (hemolytic-uremic syndrome). (Courtesy of Dr. E. Schwartz.)

Other macrocytic anemias with low or normal reticulocyte counts include acquired and congenital (Diamond-Blackfan and Fanconi) aplastic anemias and hypothyroidism. Patients with trisomy 21 have macrocytic cells, although an accompanying anemia is generally not present. High MCV and reticulocytosis is seen in CDA I and III and in situations wherein hemolysis results in such a large outpouring of young red cells that the mean MCV is abnormally high.

BIBLIOGRAPHY

Please visit the Nelson Textbook of Pediatrics *website at* www.expertconsult.com *for the complete bibliography.*

Section 2 ANEMIAS OF INADEQUATE PRODUCTION

Chapter 442 Congenital Hypoplastic Anemia (Diamond-Blackfan Anemia)

Norma B. Lerner

Congenital hypoplastic anemia (Diamond-Blackfan anemia, DBA) is a rare condition that usually becomes symptomatic in early infancy, often presenting with pallor in the neonatal period. More than 90% of cases are recognized in the 1st year of life. Occasionally the disorder is first diagnosed later in childhood. The most characteristic hematologic features are anemia, usually macrocytic, reticulocytopenia, and a deficiency or absence of red blood cell (RBC) precursors in an otherwise normally cellular bone marrow.

ETIOLOGY

The primary defect in DBA is intrinsic to the erythroid progenitor cell and results in increased apoptosis (programmed cell death). High levels of erythropoietin (EPO) are present in serum and urine, although mutations in the EPO receptor gene have not been identified. In about 25% of cases, mutations are seen in the gene *RPS19,* which codes for a ribosomal protein mapped to chromosome 19q13.2. De novo mutations have also been found in the genes *RPS24* and *RPS17,* located at chromosome 10q22-q23 and 15q25.2, respectively, and also coding for ribosomal proteins. Mutations have also been found in large ribosomal subunit proteins.

EPIDEMIOLOGY

Approximately 40-45% of cases of DBA are familial, with an autosomal dominant pattern of inheritance. The others are either sporadic or familial, with varying inheritance patterns.

CLINICAL MANIFESTATIONS

Although hematopoiesis is usually adequate in fetal life, some affected infants appear pale at birth or in the first days after birth; rarely, hydrops fetalis occurs. Profound anemia usually becomes evident by 2-6 mo of age, occasionally somewhat later. Growth retardation (short stature) is recognized in about 30% of children, and congenital malformations are noted in about 35-45%. Craniofacial abnormalities are the most common anomalies and include hypertelorism and snub nose. Thumb abnormalities, including flattening of the thenar eminence and triphalangeal thumb, may be bilateral or unilateral. The radial pulse may be absent. Ophthalmologic, urogenital, cardiac, musculoskeletal, and neuromotor anomalies have also been identified. Overall, the abnormalities are diverse, with no specific pattern emerging among most of those affected.

LABORATORY FINDINGS

The RBCs are usually macrocytic for age, but no hypersegmented neutrophils or other characteristics of megaloblastic anemia are appreciated on the peripheral blood smear. Chemical evaluation of the RBCs reveals an enzyme pattern similar to that of a "fetal" RBC population with increased expression of "i" antigen and elevated fetal hemoglobin (HbF). Erythrocyte adenosine deaminase (ADA) activity is increased in most patients with this disorder, a finding that helps distinguish congenital RBC aplasia from acquired *transient erythroblastopenia of childhood* (Chapter 444). Because elevated ADA activity is not a fetal RBC feature, measurement of this enzyme may be particularly helpful when diagnosing DBA in very young infants. Thrombocytosis or rarely thrombocytopenia and occasionally neutropenia also may be present. Reticulocyte percentages are characteristically very low despite severe anemia. RBC precursors in the marrow are markedly reduced in most patients; other marrow elements are usually normal. Serum iron levels are elevated. Bone marrow chromosome studies are normal and, unlike in Fanconi anemia, there is no increase in chromosomal breaks when lymphocytes are exposed to alkylating agents.

DIFFERENTIAL DIAGNOSIS

DBA must be differentiated from other anemias with low reticulocyte counts. The syndrome of transient erythroblastopenia of childhood (TEC) is often the primary alternative diagnosis. Table 444-1 in Chapter 444 shows a useful comparison of findings in these two disorders. TEC often is differentiated from DBA by its relatively late onset, although it occasionally develops in infants <6 mo of age (Chapter 444). Macrocytosis, congenital anomalies, fetal red cell characteristics, and elevated erythrocyte ADA are generally associated with DBA and not with TEC.

Hemolytic disease of the newborn can have a protracted course, and the associated anemia is occasionally coupled with markedly reduced erythropoiesis; the anemia usually resolves spontaneously at 5-8 wk of age. Aplastic anemic crisis characterized by reticulocytopenia and by decreased numbers of RBC precursors, often caused by parvovirus B19 infection, can complicate various types of chronic hemolytic disease but usually occurs after the first several months of life (Chapter 444). Infection with parvovirus B19 (Chapter 243) in utero can also cause pure RBC aplasia in infancy, even with hydrops fetalis at birth. The absence of parvovirus B19 detected by polymerase chain reaction (PCR) is an essential feature in establishing the diagnosis of DBA in young infants. Other inherited macrocytic bone marrow failure syndromes should be considered, particularly Fanconi anemia and Schwachman-Diamond syndrome. Other infections, including HIV, as well as drugs, immune processes, and Pearson syndrome (Chapter 443) should also be ruled out.

TREATMENT

Corticosteroids are the mainstay of therapy, and about 80% of patients respond initially. The mechanism of the effect remains unknown. Owing to concerns regarding possible detrimental properties and the lack of evidence that a delay of corticosteroids is associated with poor response, this therapy is generally not recommended for children <6 mo of age. Many hematologists recommend not beginning corticosteroids before age 1 yr. Prednisone or prednisolone in doses totaling 2 mg/kg/24 hr is used as an initial trial. An increase in RBC precursors is usually seen in the bone marrow 1-3 wk after therapy is begun and is followed by peripheral reticulocytosis. The hemoglobin can reach normal levels in 4-6 wk, although the rate of response is quite variable. Once it is established that the hemoglobin concentration is increasing, the dose of corticosteroid may be reduced gradually by tapering and then by eliminating all except a single, lowest effective daily dose. This dose may then be doubled, used on alternate days, and tapered still further while maintaining the hemoglobin level at ≥9 g/dL. In some patients, very small amounts of prednisone, as low as 2.5 mg twice a week, may be sufficient to sustain adequate erythropoiesis. Many children with DBA who are initially started on corticosteroids stop taking the drug, usually because of unacceptable side effects or the evolution of corticosteroid refractoriness at acceptable doses. In as many as 20% of cases, there is spontaneous remission of anemia with independence from steroid or red cell transfusion therapy.

In patients who do not respond to corticosteroid therapy, transfusions at intervals of 4-8 wk are necessary to sustain normal growth and activities. Chelation therapy needs to be instituted as excess iron accumulates. Other therapies, including androgens, cyclosporine, cyclophosphamide, antithymocyte globulin (ATG), high-dose intravenous immunoglobulin, high-dose methylprednisolone, EPO, and interleukin-3 have not had consistent beneficial effects and can have a high incidence of side effects.

Hematopoietic stem cell transplantation can be curative but remains a controversial treatment option for DBA. Transfusion dependence is the most common indication, although some practitioners would consider this alternative for any young child with DBA who has an HLA-matched related donor. When allogeneic sibling and alternative donor transplants are compared, survival is 72% vs. 17% at ≥5 yr from transplant. Survival for patients <10 yr of age who received transplants from HLA matched siblings is 92%.

PROGNOSIS

Among patients with DBA approximately 40% are transfusion dependent, 40% are steroid dependent, and 20% require neither therapy to maintain an acceptable hemoglobin level. Most remissions occur in the first decade. The Diamond-Blackfan Anemia Registry (DBAR) is accumulating data to ascertain responses to therapy and survival (*www.dbar.org/*). An analysis of North American DBAR data revealed an overall actuarial survival at >40 years to be 75.1%. About 70% of deaths were treatment related (opportunistic infection secondary to corticosteroid therapy, iron overload, transplant complications, etc.) and about 30% were disease related (aplastic anemia and malignancy). DBA may be a premalignant syndrome, with acute leukemia (usually myeloid) and myelodysplasia occurring in a small proportion (~5%) of patients. Solid tumor malignancies are also reported, especially osteosarcoma.

BIBLIOGRAPHY

Please visit the Nelson Textbook of Pediatrics *website at* *www.expertconsult.com* *for the complete bibliography.*

Chapter 443
Pearson's Syndrome
Norma B. Lerner

Pearson's syndrome is a form of congenital hypoplastic anemia that may be confused initially with Diamond-Blackfan syndrome or transient erythroblastopenia of childhood. It also involves the pancreas, kidney, and liver. The marrow failure usually appears in the neonatal period and is characterized by a macrocytic anemia and, occasionally, neutropenia and thrombocytopenia. The hemoglobin F level is elevated, and there are vacuolated erythroblasts and myeloblasts in the marrow. This very rare disorder is considered a unique variant of congenital sideroblastic anemia because the marrow also contains ringed sideroblasts. Associated clinical features include failure to thrive, pancreatic fibrosis with insulin-dependent diabetes and exocrine pancreatic deficiency, muscle and neurologic impairment, villous atrophy with chronic diarrhea, and often early death.

This multiorgan disorder is due to sporadic, mitochondrial DNA deletions. There is heterogeneity in different tissues and between patients, accounting for the variable clinical picture. The proportion of deleted mtDNA in the bone marrow correlates with the severity of the hematologic picture, and a change in the percentage of tissue mtDNA types over time may be associated with spontaneous improvement of red blood cell hypoproliferation. Therapy includes transfusions of red blood cells as needed. Granulocyte colony-stimulating factor can reverse episodes of severe neutropenia.

BIBLIOGRAPHY

Please visit the Nelson Textbook of Pediatrics *website at www.expertconsult.com for the complete bibliography.*

Chapter 444
Acquired Pure Red Blood Cell Anemia
Norma B. Lerner

TRANSIENT ERYTHROBLASTOPENIA OF CHILDHOOD

Transient erythroblastopenia of childhood (TEC) is the most common *acquired red cell aplasia* occurring in children. It is more prevalent than congenital hypoplastic (Diamond-Blackfan) anemia. This syndrome of severe, transient hypoplastic anemia occurs mainly in previously healthy children between 6 mo and 3 yr of age, and most of the children are older than 12 mo at onset. Only 10% of affected patients are >3 yr of age. The annual incidence is estimated to be up to 4.3 cases per 100,000 children, although it is likely higher, because many cases might go undiagnosed and resolve spontaneously. The suppression of erythropoiesis has been linked to immunoglobulin (Ig)G, IgM, and cell-mediated mechanisms. Familial cases have been reported, suggesting a hereditary component. TEC often follows a viral illness, although no specific virus has been implicated consistently. A study of acute cases found no proof that human herpesvirus (HHV)-6, parvovirus B19, Epstein-Barr virus (EBV), or cytomegalovirus (CMV) is a causative agent.

The temporary suppression of erythropoiesis results in reticulocytopenia and moderate to severe normocytic anemia. Some degree of neutropenia occurs in up to 20% of cases. Platelet numbers are normal or elevated. Similar to the situation observed in iron-deficiency anemia and other red blood cell (RBC) hypoplasias, thrombocytosis is presumably caused by increased erythropoietin, which has some homology with thrombopoietin. Mean corpuscular volume (MCV) is characteristically normal for age, and fetal hemoglobin (HbF) levels are normal before the recovery phase. RBC adenosine deaminase (ADA) levels are normal in this disorder, thus contrasting with the elevation noted in most cases of congenital hypoplastic anemia (Table 444-1). Differentiation from the latter disease is sometimes difficult, but differences in age at onset and in age-related MCV, HbF, and ADA are usually helpful. The peak occurrence of TEC coincides with that of iron-deficiency anemia in infants receiving milk as their main caloric source; differences in MCV should help to distinguish between these 2 disorders.

Table 444-1 COMPARISON OF DIAMOND-BLACKFAN ANEMIA AND TRANSIENT ERYTHROBLASTOPENIA OF CHILDHOOD

FEATURE	DBA	TEC
Male : female	1.1	1.3
Age at diagnosis, male (mo)		
Mean	10	26
Median	2	23
Range	0-408	1-120
Age at diagnosis, female (mo)		
Mean	14	26
Median	3	23
Range	0-768	1-192
Boys >1 yr	9%	82%
Girls >1 yr	12%	80%
Etiology	Genetic	Acquired
Antecedent history	None	Viral illness
Physical examination abnormal	25%	0%
Laboratory		
Hemoglobin (g/dL)	1.2-14.8	2.2-12.5
WBCs <5,000/µL	15%	20%
Platelets >400,000/µL	20%	45%
Adenosine deaminase	Increased	Normal
MCV increased at diagnosis	80%	5%
MCV increased during recovery	100%	90%
MCV increased in remission	100%	0%
HbF increased at diagnosis	100%	20%
HbF increased during recovery	100%	100%
HbF increased in remission	85%	0%
i Antigen increased	100%	20%
i Antigen increased during recovery	100%	60%
i Antigen increased in remission	90%	0%

DBA, Diamond-Blackfan anemia; HbF, fetal hemoglobin; MCV, mean cell volume; TEC, transient erythroblastopenia of childhood; WBC, white blood cell.
From Nathan DG, Orkin SH, Ginsburg D, et al, editors: *Nathan and Oski's hematology of infancy and childhood*, ed 6, vol 1, Philadelphia, 2003, WB Saunders, p 329. Adapted from Alter BP: The bone marrow failure syndromes. In Nathan DG, Oski FA, editors: *Hematology of infancy and childhood*, ed 3, Philadelphia, 1987, WB Saunders, p 159; and Link MP, Alter BP: Fetal erythropoiesis during recovery from transient erythroblastopenia of childhood (TEC), *Pediatr Res* 15:1036–1039, 1981.

Virtually all children recover within 1-2 mo. RBC transfusions may be necessary for severe anemia in the absence of signs of early recovery. The anemia develops slowly, and significant symptoms usually develop only with severe anemia. Corticosteroid therapy is of no value in this disorder. Any child with presumed TEC who requires >1 transfusion should be re-evaluated for another possible diagnosis. In rare instances, a prolonged case of apparent TEC may be caused by parvovirus-induced RBC aplasia, occurring in children with *congenital* or *acquired immunodeficiencies*.

RED CELL APLASIA ASSOCIATED WITH PARVOVIRUS B19 INFECTION

Parvovirus B19 is a common infectious agent that causes erythema infectiosum (fifth disease) (Chapter 243). It is also the best-documented viral cause of RBC aplasia in patients with chronic hemolysis, patients who are immunocompromised, and fetuses in utero. The virus is particularly infective and cytotoxic in marrow erythroid progenitor cells, interacting specifically with the RBC P antigen. In addition to decreased or absent erythroid precursors, characteristic nuclear inclusions in erythroblasts and giant pronormoblasts may be seen under the light microscope in bone marrow specimens.

CHRONIC HEMOLYSIS

Because parvovirus infection is usually transient, with recovery occurring in <2 wk, anemia is either not present or not appreciated in otherwise normal children whose peripheral RBC life span is 100-120 days. The RBC life span is much shorter in patients with hemolysis secondary to conditions such as hereditary spherocytosis or sickle cell disease. In these children, a brief cessation of erythropoiesis can cause severe anemia, a condition known as an **aplastic crisis.** When a definitive diagnosis is required, the work-up should include serum parvovirus IgM and IgG titers and, if needed, viral detection using polymerase chain reaction (PCR) techniques. Recovery from moderate to severe anemia is usually spontaneous, heralded by a wave of nucleated RBCs and subsequent reticulocytosis in the peripheral blood. A RBC transfusion may be necessary if the anemia is associated with significant symptoms. Notably, parvovirus-induced aplastic crisis usually occurs only once in children with chronic hemolysis. In families with >1 child affected with a hemolytic disorder, parents should be warned that a similar aplastic episode can occur in the other children if they have not been previously infected.

IMMUNODEFICIENCY

Persistent parvovirus infection rarely occurs in children with congenital immunodeficiency diseases, those being treated with immunosuppressive agents, and those with HIV/AIDS, because these children may be unable to mount an adequate antibody response. The resultant pure RBC aplasia may be severe, and affected children often are thought to have TEC. This type of RBC aplasia differs from TEC in that there is no spontaneous recovery and >1 transfusion is often needed. The diagnosis of parvovirus infection is made by PCR of peripheral blood or bone marrow DNA because the usual serologic responses, reflected by parvovirus serum Ig M or Ig G titers, are impaired in immunodeficient children. In chronically infected patients, the disease may be treated with high doses of intravenous immunoglobulin (IVIG), which contains neutralizing antibody to parvovirus.

MISCARRIAGE AND HYDROPS FETALIS

Parvovirus infection and destruction of erythroid precursors can also occur in utero. Such events are associated with increased fetal wastage in the first and second trimesters. Infants may be born with hydrops fetalis (Chapter 97) and viremia. The presence of persistent congenital parvovirus infection is detected by PCR of peripheral blood and/or bone marrow DNA, because immunologic tolerance to the virus can prevent the usual development of specific antibodies.

OTHER RED CELL APLASIAS IN CHILDREN

Acquired red cell aplasia in adults is usually mediated by a chronic antibody and often associated with disorders such as chronic lymphocytic leukemia, lymphoma, thymoma, lymphoproliferative disorders, and systemic lupus erythematosus. This chronic antibody-mediated type of RBC aplasia is extremely rare in childhood. Alemtuzumab (humanized anti-CD52 antibody) has been used to treat adult-onset pure red cell aplasia when treatment with corticosteroids and other immunosuppressive agents was unsuccessful.

Certain drugs, such as chloramphenicol, also can inhibit erythropoiesis in a dose-dependent manner. Reticulocytopenia, erythroid hypoplasia, and vacuolated pronormoblasts in the bone marrow are reversible effects of this drug. These effects are distinct from the idiosyncratic and rare development of severe aplastic anemia in chloramphenicol recipients. Acquired antibody-mediated pure red cell aplasia is also a rare complication in patients who are chronically treated with recombinant human erythropoietin (EPO), usually for chronic renal failure. In addition to discontinuing EPO, treatment may include immunosuppression and renal transplantation.

BIBLIOGRAPHY

Please visit the Nelson Textbook of Pediatrics *website at www.expertconsult.com for the complete bibliography.*

Chapter 445
Anemia of Chronic Disease and Renal Disease

445.1 Anemia of Chronic Disease

Norma B. Lerner

The anemia of chronic disease (ACD), also referred to as "anemia of inflammation," is found in conditions where there is chronic immune activation. This anemia thus complicates a number of systemic diseases associated with infection (e.g., HIV, bronchiectasis, osteomyelitis) or autoimmunity (e.g., rheumatoid arthritis, systemic lupus erythematosus, inflammatory bowel disease) as well as some hematologic and solid malignancies. Despite diverse underlying causes, the erythroid abnormalities are similar, although incompletely understood. Erythrocytes have a mildly decreased life span, felt to be, at least in part, secondary to erythrophagocytosis by activated macrophages. However, it is the relative failure of the bone marrow to respond adequately to the increased destruction that perpetuates the anemia. Erythropoietin (EPO) levels are modestly increased but are often inadequate. More importantly, inflammation induces a blunted response and relative resistance to EPO.

For the full continuation of this chapter, please visit the Nelson Textbook of Pediatrics *website at www.expertconsult.com.*

445.2 Anemia of Renal Disease

Norma B. Lerner

Anemia is common in children with chronic renal disease. The anemia is usually normocytic, and the absolute reticulocyte count is normal or low. Although the anemia seen in chronic renal disease shares some features with the anemia of chronic disease, its major cause is decreased EPO production by diseased kidneys. The second important cause of the anemia is absolute and/or functional iron deficiency due to chronic blood loss (from blood sampling, surgeries, and dialysis) as well as disturbances in the iron metabolic pathway. In adults, lower glomerular filtration rate (GFR) has been associated with lower hemoglobin concentration, and hemoglobin has been reported to decline below a GFR threshold of 40-60 mL/min/1.73 m^2. In children with chronic kidney disease hemoglobin levels decline as the GFR decreases below 43 mL/min/1.73 m^2.

For the full continuation of this chapter, please visit the Nelson Textbook of Pediatrics *website at www.expertconsult.com.*

Chapter 446
Congenital Dyserythropoietic Anemias
Norma B. Lerner

The congenital dyserythropoietic anemias (CDA) are a heterogeneous class of genetic disorders characterized by unique morphologic abnormalities in marrow erythroblasts: multinuclearity, abnormal nuclear fragments, and intrachromatin bridges between cells, associated with ineffective erythropoiesis. Three major types of CDA (types I, II, and III) are defined (see Table 446-1 on the *Nelson Textbook of Pediatrics* website at www.expertconsult.com), although additional subgroups and variants have also been identified. These rare disorders are characterized by variable degrees of anemia, increased marrow erythroid activity (ineffective erythropoiesis), and secondary hemochromatosis.

For the full continuation of this chapter, please visit the Nelson Textbook of Pediatrics *website at www.expertconsult.com.*

Chapter 447
Physiologic Anemia of Infancy
Norma B. Lerner

At birth, normal full-term infants have higher hemoglobin and hematocrit levels and larger red blood cells (RBCs) than do older children and adults. However, within the 1st wk of life, a progressive decline in hemoglobin level begins and then persists for 6-8 wk. The resulting anemia is known as the **physiologic anemia of infancy.** Several factors appear to be involved.

With the onset of respiration at birth, considerably more oxygen becomes available for binding to hemoglobin, and, as a consequence, the hemoglobin-oxygen saturation increases from 50% to 95% or more. There is also a gradual, normal developmental switch from fetal to adult hemoglobin synthesis after birth that results in the replacement of high-oxygen-affinity fetal hemoglobin with lower-affinity adult hemoglobin, capable of delivering more oxygen to tissues. The increase in blood oxygen content and delivery results in the downregulation of erythropoietin (EPO) production, leading to suppression of erythropoiesis. Because there is no erythropoiesis, aged RBCs that are removed from the circulation are not replaced and the hemoglobin level decreases. The hemoglobin concentration continues to decline until tissue oxygen needs become greater than oxygen delivery. Normally, this point is reached between 8 and 12 wk of age, when the hemoglobin concentration is about 11 g/dL. At this juncture, EPO production increases and erythropoiesis resumes. The supply of stored reticuloendothelial iron, derived from previously degraded RBCs, remains sufficient for this renewed hemoglobin synthesis, even in the absence of dietary iron intake, until approximately 20 wk of age. In all, this "anemia" should be viewed as a physiologic adaptation to extrauterine life, reflecting the excess oxygen delivery relative to tissue oxygen requirements. There is no hematologic problem, and no therapy is required.

Premature infants also develop a physiologic anemia, known as *physiologic anemia of prematurity*. The hemoglobin decline is both more extreme and more rapid. Minimal hemoglobin levels of 7-9 g/dL commonly are reached by 3-6 wk of age, and levels may be even lower in very small premature infants (Chapter 97). The same physiologic factors at play in term infants are operative in preterm infants but are exaggerated. In premature infants, the physiologic hemoglobin decline may be intensified by blood loss from repeated phlebotomies obtained to monitor ill neonates. Demands on erythropoiesis are further heightened by the premature infant's shortened RBC lifespan (40-60 days) and the accelerated expansion of RBC mass that accompanies the premature baby's rapid rate of growth. Nonetheless, plasma EPO levels are lower than would be expected for the degree of anemia, resulting in a suboptimal erythropoietic response. The reason for diminished EPO levels is not fully understood. During fetal life, EPO synthesis is handled primarily by the liver, whose oxygen sensor is relatively insensitive to hypoxia when compared to the oxygen sensor of the kidney. The developmental switch from liver to kidney EPO production is not accelerated by early birth, and thus the preterm infant must rely on the liver as the primary site for synthesis, leading to diminished responsiveness to anemia. An additional mechanism thought to contribute to diminished EPO levels may be accelerated EPO metabolism.

Physiologic anemia of infancy may be exacerbated by other ongoing processes. A late hyporegenerative anemia, with absence of reticulocytes, can occur in infants with mild hemolytic disease of the newborn. The persistence of maternally derived anti-RBC antibodies in the infant's circulation can lead to an ongoing low-grade hemolytic anemia that can exaggerate the physiologic anemia. Lower-than-expected hemoglobin at the "physiologic" nadir has also been seen in infants after intrauterine or neonatal RBC transfusions. When infants are transfused with adult blood containing HbA, the associated shift of the oxygen dissociation curve facilitates oxygen delivery to the tissues. Accordingly, the definition of anemia and the need for transfusion should be based not only on the infant's hemoglobin level but also oxygen requirements and the ability of circulating RBCs to release oxygen to the tissues.

Some dietary factors, such as folic acid deficiency, can aggravate physiologic anemia. Unless there has been significant blood loss, iron stores should be sufficient to maintain erythropoiesis early on. Notably, despite past suggestions to the contrary, vitamin E deficiency does not appear to play a role in anemia of prematurity. A controlled and blinded study of oral administration of vitamin E to infants weighing <1,500 g showed no difference in hemoglobin levels, reticulocytes, RBC morphology, or platelet counts. Breast milk and modern infant formulas appear to provide adequate vitamin E.

TREATMENT
In the full-term infant, physiologic anemia requires no therapy beyond ensuring that the infant's diet contains essential nutrients for normal hematopoiesis. In premature infants an optimal hematocrit has not been established and is usually dictated by the infant's overall clinical condition. Transfusions may be needed to maintain the hematocrit at what is considered safe for that child. Premature infants who are feeding well and growing normally rarely need transfusion unless iatrogenic blood loss has been significant. Although factors such as poor weight gain, respiratory difficulties, and abnormal heart rate have prompted transfusion, the beneficial effect has not been documented. Laboratory tests such as blood lactate, erythropoietin, and mixed venous oxygen saturation have poor predictive value. Liberal and restrictive transfusion strategies have been compared in this population. Although a restrictive strategy did not result in increased morbidity or mortality, it might have resulted in poorer neuroprotection than that provided by a liberal approach. For now, most consensus-based transfusion guidelines advise the liberal approach. When transfusions are necessary, an RBC volume of 10-15 mL/kg is recommended. It is good practice to split units derived from a single donor so that sequential transfusions can be given as required and donor exposure can be minimized. In early preterm infants (<1,250 g), the half-life of transfused RBCs is about 30 days.

Because premature infants are known to have low plasma erythropoietin levels, recombinant human erythropoietin (rEPO) has been studied as an alternative to transfusion for the treatment of symptomatic preterm infants with anemia of prematurity. Infants have been shown to require higher dosages per kilogram than adults and supplementation with adequate protein, vitamin E, and iron to achieve the full benefit of the medication. Although rEPO has been associated with reduced numbers of red cell transfusions, it is unclear whether it reliably reduces donor exposures. Reports of adverse effects such as a possible increase in retinopathy of prematurity have further limited a willingness to use this expensive treatment. Its routine use in this population might have to await further clinical trials.

BIBLIOGRAPHY

Please visit the Nelson Textbook of Pediatrics *website at www.expertconsult.com for the complete bibliography.*

Chapter 448 Megaloblastic Anemias

Norma B. Lerner

Megaloblastic anemia is a macrocytic anemia characterized by ineffective erythropoiesis, a kinetic term that describes active erythropoiesis associated with premature cell death and decreased red blood cell (RBC) output from the bone marrow. The RBCs are larger than normal at every developmental stage, and maturational asynchrony between the nucleus and cytoplasm of erythrocytes is present. The delayed nuclear development becomes increasingly evident as cell divisions proceed. Myeloid and platelet precursors are also affected, and giant metamyelocytes and neutrophil bands are often present in the bone marrow. *There is usually an associated thrombocytopenia and leukopenia.* The peripheral blood smear is notable for large, often oval, RBCs, with increased mean corpuscular volume (MCV). Neutrophils are characteristically hypersegmented, with many having >5 lobes. Almost all cases of childhood megaloblastic anemia result from folic acid or vitamin B_{12} deficiency; rarely, they may be caused by inborn errors of metabolism. Because folate and vitamin B_{12} are both required for the manufacture of nucleoproteins, deficiencies result in defective DNA and, to a lesser extent, RNA and protein synthesis. Megaloblastic anemias resulting from malnutrition are relatively uncommon in the USA but are important worldwide (Chapters 1 and 43).

448.1 Folic Acid Deficiency

Norma B. Lerner

Folic acid, or pteroylglutamic acid, consists of pteroic acid conjugated to glutamic acid. Biologically active folates are derived from folic acid and serve as one-carbon donors and acceptors in many biosynthetic pathways. As such, they are essential for DNA replication and cellular proliferation. Like other mammals, humans cannot synthesize folate and depend on dietary sources, including green vegetables, fruits, and animal organs (e.g., liver, kidney). Folates are heat labile and water soluble, and consequently boiling or heating folate sources leads to decreased amounts of vitamin. Naturally occurring folates are in a polyglutamated form that is less-efficiently absorbed than the monoglutamate species (i.e., folic acid). Dietary folate polyglutamates are hydrolyzed to simple folates that are absorbed primarily in the proximal small intestine by a specific carrier-mediated system. There is an active enterohepatic circulation. Folic acid is not biologically active and is reduced by dihydrofolate reductase to tetrahydrofolate, which is transported into tissue cells and polyglutamated. Because body stores of folate are limited, megaloblastic anemia will occur after 2-3 mo on a folate-free diet.

For the full continuation of this chapter, please visit the Nelson Textbook of Pediatrics *website at www.expertconsult.com.*

448.2 Vitamin B_{12} (Cobalamin) Deficiency

Norma B. Lerner

Because cobalamin is synthesized exclusively by certain microorganisms, animals must rely on dietary sources for their needs. Animal protein is the major source of vitamin B_{12} in nonvegetarians. Vitamin B_{12} serves as a cofactor in 2 essential metabolic reactions, namely methylation of homocysteine to methionine and conversion of methylmalonyl coenzyme A (CoA) to succinyl CoA. It is necessary for the production of tetrahydrofolate, which is important in DNA synthesis. In contrast to the situation with folate stores, older children and adults have sufficient vitamin B_{12} stores to last 3-5 yr. However, in young infants born to mothers with low vitamin B_{12} stores, clinical signs of cobalamin deficiency can become apparent in the first 6-18 mo of life.

For the full continuation of this chapter, please visit the Nelson Textbook of Pediatrics *website at www.expertconsult.com.*

448.3 Other Rare Megaloblastic Anemias

Norma B. Lerner

Orotica ciduria is a rare autosomal recessive disorder that usually appears in the 1st year of life and is characterized by growth failure, developmental retardation, megaloblastic anemia, and increased urinary excretion of orotic acid (Chapter 83). This defect is the most common metabolic error in the de novo synthesis of pyrimidines and therefore affects nucleic acid synthesis. The usual form of hereditary orotic aciduria is caused by a deficiency (in all body tissues) of orotic phosphoribosyl transferase (OPT) and orotidine-5-phosphate decarboxylase (ODC), two sequential enzymatic steps in pyrimidine nucleotide synthesis. The diagnosis is suggested by the presence of severe megaloblastic anemia with normal serum B_{12} and folate levels and no evidence of TC-II deficiency. A presumptive diagnosis is made by finding increased urinary orotic acid. However, confirmation of the diagnosis requires assay of the transferase and decarboxylase enzymes in the patient's erythrocytes. Physical and mental retardation often accompany this condition. The anemia is refractory to vitamin B_{12} or folic acid but responds promptly to administration of uridine.

For the full continuation of this chapter, please visit the Nelson Textbook of Pediatrics *website at www.expertconsult.com.*

Chapter 449 Iron-Deficiency Anemia

Norma B. Lerner and Richard Sills

Iron deficiency is the most widespread and common nutritional disorder in the world. It is estimated that 30% of the global population suffers from iron-deficiency anemia, and most of them live in developing countries. In the USA, 9% of children ages 12-36 mo are iron deficient, and 30% of this group have progressed to iron-deficiency anemia.

The incidence of iron-deficiency relates to basic aspects of iron metabolism and nutrition. The body of a full-term newborn infant contains about 0.5 g of iron, compared to 5 g of iron in adults. This change in quantity of iron from birth to adulthood means that an average of 0.8 mg of iron must be absorbed each day during the first 15 years of life. A small additional amount is necessary to balance normal losses of iron by shedding of cells. It is therefore necessary to absorb approximately 1 mg daily to maintain positive iron balance in childhood. Because <10% of dietary iron usually is absorbed, a dietary intake of 8-10 mg of iron daily is necessary to maintain iron levels. During infancy, when growth is most rapid, the approximately 1 mg/L of iron in bovine and breast milk makes it difficult to maintain body iron. Breast-fed infants have an advantage because they absorb iron 2-3 times more efficiently than infants fed bovine milk.

ETIOLOGY

Most iron in neonates is in circulating hemoglobin. As the relatively high hemoglobin concentration of the newborn infant falls during the first 2-3 mo of life, considerable iron is reclaimed and stored. These reclaimed stores usually are sufficient for blood formation in the first 6-9 mo of life in term infants. Stores are depleted sooner in low-birthweight infants or infants with perinatal blood loss because their iron stores are smaller. Delayed clamping of the umbilical cord can improve iron status and reduce the risk of iron deficiency. Dietary sources of iron are especially important in these infants. In term infants, anemia caused solely by inadequate dietary iron usually occurs at 9-24 mo of age and is relatively uncommon thereafter. The usual dietary pattern observed in infants and toddlers with nutritional iron-deficiency anemia in developed countries is excessive consumption of bovine milk (low iron content, blood loss from milk protein colitis) in a child who is often overweight. Worldwide, undernutrition is usually responsible for iron deficiency.

Blood loss must be considered as a possible cause in every case of iron-deficiency anemia, particularly in older children. Chronic iron-deficiency anemia from occult bleeding may be caused by a lesion of the gastrointestinal (GI) tract, such as peptic ulcer, Meckel diverticulum, polyp, hemangioma, or inflammatory bowel disease. Infants can have chronic intestinal blood loss induced by exposure to a heat-labile protein in whole bovine milk. This GI reaction is not related to enzymatic abnormalities in the mucosa, such as lactase deficiency, or to a typical milk allergy. Involved infants characteristically develop anemia that is more severe and occurs earlier than would be expected simply from an inadequate intake of iron. The ongoing loss of blood in the stools can be prevented either by breast-feeding or by delaying the introduction of whole bovine milk in the 1st year of life and then limiting the quantity of whole bovine milk to <24 oz/24 hr. Unrecognized blood loss also can be associated with chronic diarrhea and rarely with pulmonary hemosiderosis. In developing countries, infections with hookworm, *Trichuris trichiura, Plasmodium,* and *Helicobacter pylori* often contribute to iron deficiency.

About 2% of adolescent girls have iron-deficiency anemia, due in large part to their adolescent growth spurt and menstrual blood loss. The highest risk of iron deficiency is among teenagers who are or have been pregnant; >30% of these girls have iron-deficiency anemia.

CLINICAL MANIFESTATIONS

Most children with iron deficiency are asymptomatic and are identified by recommended laboratory screening at 12 months of age or sooner if at high risk. Pallor is the most important clinical sign of iron deficiency but is not usually visible until the hemoglobin falls to 7-8 g/dL. It is most readily noted as pallor of the palms, palmar creases, nail beds, or conjunctivae. Parents often fail to note the pallor because of the typical slow drop over time. Often a visiting friend or relative is the first to notice. In mild to moderate iron deficiency (i.e., hemoglobin levels of 6-10 g/dL), compensatory mechanisms, including increased levels of 2,3-diphosphoglycerate (2,3-DPG) and a shift of the oxygen dissociation curve, may be so effective that few symptoms of anemia aside from mild irritability are noted. When the hemoglobin level falls to <5 g/dL, irritability, anorexia, and lethargy develop, and systolic flow murmurs are often heard. As the hemoglobin continues to fall, tachycardia and high output cardiac failure can occur.

Table 449-1 LABORATORY STUDIES DIFFERENTIATING THE MOST COMMON MICROCYTIC ANEMIAS

STUDY	IRON DEFICIENCY ANEMIA	α OR β THALASSEMIA	ANEMIA OF CHRONIC DISEASE
Hemoglobin	Decreased	Decreased	Decreased
MCV	Decreased	Decreased	Normal-decreased
RDW	Increased	Normal	Normal-increased
RBC	Decreased	Normal-increased	Normal-decreased
Serum ferritin	Decreased	Normal	Increased
Total Fe binding capacity	Increased	Normal	Decreased
Transferrin saturation	Decreased	Normal	Decreased
FEP	Increased	Normal	Increased
Transferrin receptor	Increased	Normal	Increased
Reticulocyte hemoglobin concentration	Decreased	Normal	Normal-decreased

FEP, free erythrocyte protoporphyrin; MCV, mean corpuscular volume; RBC, red blood cell; RDW, red cell distribution width.

Iron deficiency has nonhematologic systemic effects. The most concerning effects in infants and adolescents are impaired intellectual and motor functions that can occur early in iron deficiency before anemia develops. There is evidence that these changes might not be completely reversible after treatment with iron, increasing the importance of prevention. Pica, the desire to ingest non-nutritive substances, and **pagophagia,** the desire to ingest ice, are other systemic symptoms of iron deficiency. The pica can result in the ingestion of lead-containing substances and result in concomitant **plumbism** (Chapter 702).

LABORATORY FINDINGS

In progressive iron deficiency, a sequence of biochemical and hematologic events occurs (Tables 449-1 and 449-2). Clinically, iron deficiency anemia is not difficult to diagnose. First, tissue iron stores are depleted. This depletion is reflected by reduced serum ferritin, an iron-storage protein, which provides an estimate of body iron stores in the absence of inflammatory disease. Next, serum iron levels decrease, the iron-binding capacity of the serum (serum transferrin) increases, and the transferrin saturation falls below normal. As iron stores decrease, iron becomes unavailable to complex with protoporphyrin to form heme. Free erythrocyte protoporphyrins (FEPs) accumulate, and hemoglobin synthesis is impaired. At this point, iron deficiency progresses to iron-deficiency anemia. With less available hemoglobin in each cell, the red cells become smaller. This morphologic characteristic is best quantified by the decrease in mean corpuscular volume (MCV) and mean corpuscular hemoglobin (MCH). Developmental changes in MCV require the use of age-related standards for diagnosis of microcytosis (see Table 441-1). Increased variation in cell size occurs as normocytic red cells are replaced by microcytic ones; this variation is quantified by an elevated RBC distribution width (RDW). The red cell count (RBC) also decreases. The reticulocyte percentage may be normal or moderately elevated, but absolute reticulocyte counts indicate an insufficient response to the degree of anemia. The blood smear reveals hypochromic, microcytic red cells with substantial variation in cell size. Elliptocytic or cigar-shaped red cells are often seen (Fig. 449-1). Detection of increased transferrin receptor and decreased reticulocyte hemoglobin concentration provides supporting diagnostic information when these studies are available.

White blood cell count (WBC) is normal, and thrombocytosis is often present. Thrombocytopenia is occasionally seen with very severe iron deficiency, potentially confusing the diagnosis with

Table 449-2 INDICATORS OF IRON-DEFICIENCY ANEMIA

INDICATOR	SELECTED CUTOFF VALUES TO DEFINE IRON DEFICIENCY	COMMENTS
Hemoglobin (g/L)	6 mo-5 yr <110 6-11 yr <115 Nonpregnant women <120 Pregnant women <110	When used alone, it has low specificity and sensitivity
Mean corpuscular volume (MCV) (µm³)	Children older than 11 yr and adults <82	A reliable, but late indicator of iron deficiency Low values can also be due to thalassemia
Reticulocyte hemoglobin content (CHr) (pg)	In infants and young children <27.5 In adults ≤28.0	A sensitive indicator that falls within days of onset of iron-deficient erythropoiesis False normal values can occur when MCV is increased and in thalassemia Wider use is limited because it can only be measured on a few analyzer models
Erythrocyte zinc protoporphyrin (ZPP) (µmol/mol heme)	≤5 yr >70 Children >5 yr >80 Children >5 yr on washed red cells >40	It can be measured directly on a drop of blood with a portable hematofluorometer A useful screening test in field surveys, particularly in children, in whom uncomplicated iron deficiency is the primary cause of anemia Red cells should be washed before measurement because circulating factors, including serum bilirubin, can spuriously increase values Lead poisoning can increase values, particularly in urban and industrial settings
Transferrin saturation	<16%	It is inexpensive, but its use is limited by diurnal variation in serum iron and by many clinical disorders that affect transferrin concentrations
Serum ferritin (SF) (µg/L)	≤5 yr <12 Children >5 yr <15 In all age groups in the presence of infection <30	It is probably the most useful laboratory measure of iron status; a low value of SF is diagnostic of iron-deficiency anemia in a patient with anemia In healthy persons, SF is directly proportional to iron stores: 1 µg/L SF corresponds to 8-10 mg body iron or 120 µg storage iron per kg body weight As an acute-phase protein, SF increases independent of iron status by acute or chronic inflammation; it is also unreliable in patients with malignancy, hyperthyroidism, liver disease, or heavy alcohol intake
Serum transferrin receptor (sTfR)	Cutoff varies with assay and with patient's age and ethnic origin	Main determinants are the erythroid mass in the bone marrow and iron status; thus, sTfR is increased by enhanced erythropoiesis and iron deficiency sTfR is not substantially affected by the acute-phase response, but it might be affected by malaria, age, and ethnicity Its application is limited by high cost of commercial assays and lack of an international standard
sTfR : SF ratio		This ratio is a quantitative estimate of total body iron; the logarithm of this ratio is directly proportional to the amount of stored iron in iron-replete patients and the tissue iron deficit in iron deficiency In elderly people, this ratio might be more sensitive than other laboratory tests for iron deficiency This ratio cannot be used in patients with inflammation because SF might be high independent of iron stores This ratio is assay specific Although it is only validated for adults, this ratio has been used in children

From Zimmermann MB, Hurrell RF: Nutritional iron deficiency, *Lancet* 370:511–520, 2007.

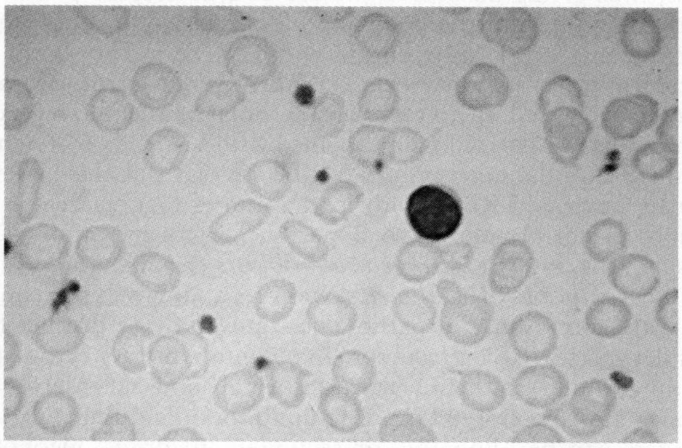

Figure 449-1 This is the peripheral blood smear from a patient with severe iron-deficiency anemia. The hypochromia is marked. A normal lymphocyte that is comparable in size to a normocytic red cell serves to document many microcytic erythrocytes. The elliptocytic ("cigar-forms") red cells are typical of iron deficiency. Note the variation in red cell size. (Courtesy of the University of Washington/American Society of Hematology Slide Bank.)

bone marrow failure disorders. Stool for occult blood should be checked to exclude blood loss as the cause of iron deficiency.

In most instances, a complete blood count demonstrating a microcytic anemia with a high RDW, reduced RBC, normal WBC, and normal or elevated platelet count is sufficient for a presumptive diagnosis. Other laboratory studies, such as reduced ferritin, reduced serum iron, and increased total iron-binding capacity, are not usually necessary unless severe anemia requires a more rapid diagnosis, other complicating clinical factors are present, or the anemia does not respond to iron therapy.

DIFFERENTIAL DIAGNOSIS

The most common alternative causes of microcytic anemia are α or β thalassemia and hemoglobinopathies, including hemoglobin E and C (Chapter 456). The thalassemia traits are most common and are associated with an elevated as opposed to decreased red blood cell count and a normal as opposed to elevated RDW. The anemia of chronic disease is usually normocytic but can be microcytic in a minority of cases (Chapter 445). Lead poisoning can cause microcytic anemia, but more often iron deficiency anemia causes pica, which then results in lead intoxication (Chapter 702). Table 449-1 compares the use of laboratory studies in the diagnosis of the most common microcytic anemias. Other etiologies of microcytic anemia are found in Table 449-3.

PREVENTION

Iron deficiency is best prevented to avoid both its systemic manifestations and the anemia. Breast-feeding should be encouraged, with the addition of iron-fortified cereals after 4-6 mo of age. Infants who are not breast-fed should only receive iron-fortified formula (12 mg of iron per liter) for the first year, and thereafter bovine milk should be limited to <20-24 oz daily. This approach

Table 449-3 DIFFERENTIAL DIAGNOSIS OF MICROCYTIC ANEMIA THAT FAILS TO RESPOND TO ORAL IRON

Poor compliance (true intolerance of Fe is uncommon)
Incorrect dose or medication
Malabsorption of administered iron
Ongoing blood loss including gastrointestinal, menstrual, and pulmonary
Concurrent infection or inflammatory disorder inhibiting the response to iron
Concurrent vitamin B_{12} or folate deficiency
Diagnosis other than iron deficiency
- Thalassemias
- Hemoglobin C and E disorders
- Anemia of chronic disease
- Lead poisoning
- Sickle thalassemias, hemoglobin SC disease
- Rare microcytic anemias (Chapter 450)

Table 449-4 RESPONSES TO IRON THERAPY IN IRON-DEFICIENCY ANEMIA

TIME AFTER IRON ADMINISTRATION	RESPONSE
12-24 hr	Replacement of intracellular iron enzymes; subjective improvement; decreased irritability; increased appetite
36-48 hr	Initial bone marrow response; erythroid hyperplasia
48-72 hr	Reticulocytosis, peaking at 5-7 days
4-30 days	Increase in hemoglobin level
1-3 mo	Repletion of stores

encourages the ingestion of foods richer in iron and prevents blood loss due to bovine milk–induced enteropathy.

When these preventive measures fail, routine screening helps prevent the development of severe anemia. Routine screening using hemoglobin or hematocrit is done at 12 mo of age, or earlier if at 4 mo of age the child is assessed to be at high risk for iron deficiency.

TREATMENT

The regular response of iron-deficiency anemia to adequate amounts of iron is a critical diagnostic and therapeutic feature (Table 449-4). Oral administration of simple ferrous salts (most often ferrous sulfate) provides inexpensive and effective therapy. There is no evidence that the addition of any trace metal, vitamin, or other hematinic substance significantly increases the response to simple ferrous salts. Aside from the unpleasant taste of iron, intolerance to oral iron is uncommon in young children. In contrast, older children and adolescents sometimes have GI complaints.

The therapeutic dose should be calculated in terms of elemental iron. A daily total dose of 3-6 mg/kg of elemental iron in 3 divided doses is adequate, with the higher dose used in more severe cases. Ferrous sulfate is 20% elemental iron by weight and is ideally given between meals with juice, although this issue is usually not critical with a therapeutic dose. Parenteral iron preparations are only used when malabsorption is present or when compliance is poor, because oral therapy is otherwise as fast, as effective, and much less expensive and less toxic. When necessary, parenteral iron sucrose and ferric gluconate complex have a lower risk of serious reactions than iron dextran.

In addition to iron therapy, dietary counseling is usually necessary. Excessive intake of milk, particularly bovine milk, should be limited. Iron deficiency in adolescent girls secondary to abnormal uterine blood flow loss is treated with iron and hormone therapy (Chapter 110.2).

If the anemia is mild, the only additional study is to repeat the blood count approximately 4 wk after initiating therapy. At this point the hemoglobin has usually risen by at least 1-2 g/dL and has often normalized. If the anemia is more severe, earlier confirmation of the diagnosis can be made by the appearance of a reticulocytosis usually within 48-96 hr of instituting treatment. The hemoglobin will then begin to increase 0.1-0.4 g/dL per day depending on the severity of the anemia. Iron medication should be continued for 8 wk after blood values normalize to re-establish iron stores. Good follow-up is essential to ensure a response to therapy. When the anemia responds poorly or not at all to iron therapy, there are multiple considerations, including diagnoses other than iron deficiency (see Table 449-3).

Because a rapid hematologic response can be confidently predicted in typical iron deficiency, blood transfusion is rarely necessary. It should only be used when congestive heart failure is eminent or if the anemia is severe with evidence of substantial ongoing blood loss.

BIBLIOGRAPHY

Please visit the Nelson Textbook of Pediatrics *website at* *www.expertconsult.com* *for the complete bibliography.*

Chapter 450
Other Microcytic Anemias

Richard Sills

Sideroblastic anemias result from acquired and hereditary disorders of heme synthesis. The anemias are characterized by hypochromic microcytic red blood cells (RBCs) mixed with normal RBCs, thus giving an overall picture of a dimorphic population of erythrocytes, and the complete blood cell count indicates an extremely high RBC distribution width (RDW). The serum iron concentration usually is elevated, and the transferrin saturation of iron is increased. In all cases of sideroblastic anemia, regardless of the specific cause, impaired heme synthesis leads to retention of iron within the mitochondria. Morphologically, this is seen in marrow nucleated RBCs with iron granules (aggregates of iron in mitochondria) that have a perinuclear distribution. These unusual cells, known as *ringed sideroblasts* (see Fig. 450-1 on the *Nelson Textbook of Pediatrics* website at www.expertconsult.com), are found only in pathologic states and are distinct from the sideroblasts (RBC precursors that contain diffuse cytoplasmic ferritin granules) in the marrow of normal subjects. Sideroblastic anemias most commonly occur in adulthood, and these acquired disorders can be idiopathic or secondary to drugs, alcohol, or myelodysplastic disorders. A few sideroblastic anemias are seen in children.

For the full continuation of this chapter, please visit the Nelson Textbook of Pediatrics *website at* *www.expertconsult.com*.

Section 3 HEMOLYTIC ANEMIAS

Chapter 451 Definitions and Classification of Hemolytic Anemias

George B. Segel

Hemolysis is defined as the premature destruction of red blood cells (RBCs). Anemia results when the rate of destruction exceeds the capacity of the marrow to produce RBCs. Normal RBC survival time is 110-120 days (half-life, 55-60 days), and approximately 0.85% of the most senescent RBCs are removed and replaced each day. During hemolysis, RBC survival is shortened, the RBC count falls, erythropoietin is increased, and the stimulation of marrow activity results in heightened RBC production, reflected in an increased percentage of reticulocytes in the blood. Thus, hemolysis should be suspected as a cause of anemia if an elevated reticulocyte count is present. The reticulocyte count also may be elevated as a response to acute blood loss or for a short period after replacement therapy for iron, vitamin B_{12}, or folate deficiency. The marrow can increase its output 2- to 3-fold acutely, with a maximum of 6- to 8-fold in long-standing hemolysis. The reticulocyte percentage can be corrected to measure the magnitude of marrow production in response to hemolysis as follows:

$$\text{Reticulocyte index} = \text{reticulocyte\%} \times \frac{\text{Observed hematocrit}}{\text{Normal hematocrit}} \times \frac{1}{\mu}$$

where μ is a maturation factor of 1-3 related to the severity of the anemia (see Fig. 451-1 on the *Nelson Textbook of Pediatrics* website at www.expertconsult.com). The normal reticulocyte index is 1.0; therefore, the index measures the fold increase in erythropoiesis (e.g., 2-fold, 3-fold).

For the full continuation of this chapter, please visit the Nelson Textbook of Pediatrics *website at www.expertconsult.com.*

Chapter 452 Hereditary Spherocytosis

George B. Segel

Hereditary spherocytosis is a common cause of hemolysis and hemolytic anemia, with a wide spectrum of severity and with a prevalence of approximately 1/5,000 in people of Northern European descent. It is the most common inherited abnormality of the red blood cell (RBC) membrane. Affected patients may be asymptomatic, without anemia and with minimal hemolysis, or they may have severe hemolytic anemia. Hereditary spherocytosis has been described in most ethnic groups but is most common among persons of Northern European origin.

ETIOLOGY

Hereditary spherocytosis usually is transmitted as an autosomal dominant or, less commonly, as an autosomal recessive disorder. As many as 25% of patients have no previous family history. Of these patients, most represent new mutations, and a few cases result from recessive inheritance or represent nonpaternity. The most common molecular defects are abnormalities of spectrin or ankyrin, which are major components of the cytoskeleton responsible for RBC shape. A recessive defect has been described in α-spectrin. Dominant defects have been described in β-spectrin and protein 3. Dominant and recessive defects have been described in ankyrin (Table 452-1). A deficiency in spectrin, protein 3, or ankyrin results in uncoupling in the "vertical" interactions of the lipid bilayer skeleton and the loss of membrane microvesicles (Figs. 452-1 and 452-2). The loss of membrane surface area without a proportional loss of cell volume causes sphering of the RBCs and an associated increase in cation permeability, cation transport, adenosine triphosphate (ATP) use, and glycolysis. The decreased deformability of the spherocytic RBCs impairs cell passage from the splenic cords to the splenic sinuses, and the spherocytic RBCs are destroyed prematurely in the spleen. Splenectomy markedly improves RBC life span and cures the anemia.

Table 452-1 COMMON GENE MUTATIONS IN HEREDITARY SPHEROCYTOSIS

PROTEIN	SEVERITY	GENE	PATIENTS WITH HEREDITARY SPHEROCYTOSIS (%)	INHERITANCE
Ankyrin-1	Mild to moderate	*ANK1*	50-67	Dominant and recessive
Band 3	Mild to moderate	*AE1 (SLC4A1)*	15-20	Mostly dominant
β Spectrin	Mild to moderate	*SPTB*	15-20	Dominant
α Spectrin	Severe	*SPTA1*	<5	Recessive
Protein 4.2	Mild to moderate	*EPB42*	<5	Recessive

Mild: normal hemoglobin, reticulocytes <6%; moderate: hemoglobin >8 g/dL, reticulocytes >6%; severe: hemoglobin <6 g/dL, reticulocytes >10%.

CLINICAL MANIFESTATIONS

Hereditary spherocytosis may be a cause of hemolytic disease in the newborn and can manifest as anemia and hyperbilirubinemia sufficiently severe to require phototherapy or exchange transfusions. Hemolysis may be more prominent in the newborn because hemoglobin F binds 2,3-diphosphoglycerate poorly, and the increased level of free 2,3-diphosphoglycerate destabilizes interactions among spectrin, actin, and protein 4.1 in the RBC membrane (see Fig. 452-1).

The severity of symptoms in infants and children is variable. Some patients remain asymptomatic into adulthood, but others have severe anemia with pallor, jaundice, fatigue, and exercise intolerance. Severe cases may be marked by expansion of the diploë of the skull and the medullary region of other bones, but to a lesser extent than in thalassemia major. After infancy, the spleen is usually enlarged, and pigmentary (bilirubin) gallstones can form as early as age 4-5 years. At least 50% of unsplenectomized patients ultimately form gallstones, although they may be asymptomatic.

Because of the high RBC turnover and heightened erythroid marrow activity, children with hereditary spherocytosis are susceptible to aplastic crisis, primarily as a result of parvovirus B19 infection, and to hypoplastic crises associated with various other infections (Fig. 452-3). The erythroid marrow failure can rapidly result in profound anemia (hematocrit <10%), high-output heart failure, hypoxia, cardiovascular collapse, and death. White blood cell and platelet counts can also fall (see Fig. 452-3).

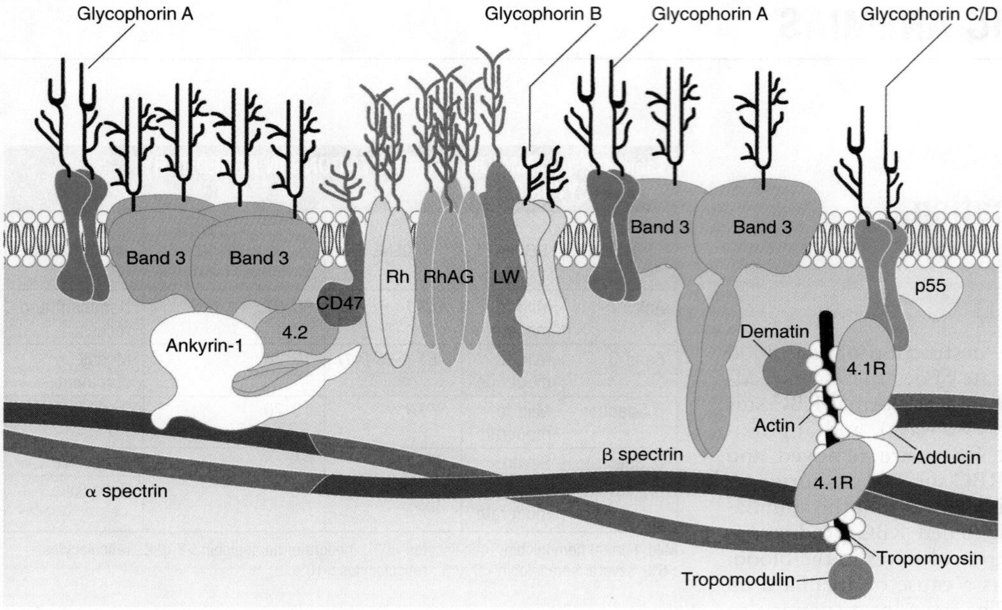

Figure 452-1 A simplified cross-section of the red blood cell (erythrocyte) membrane. The lipid bilayer forms the equator of the cross-section with its polar heads *(small circles)* turned outward. 4.1 R, protein; 4.2, protein 4.2; LW, Landsteiner-Wiener glycoprotein; Rh, Rhesus polypeptide; RhAG, Rh-associated glycoprotein. (From Perrotta S, Gallagher PG, Mohandas N: Hereditary spherocytosis, *Lancet* 372:1411–1426, 2008.)

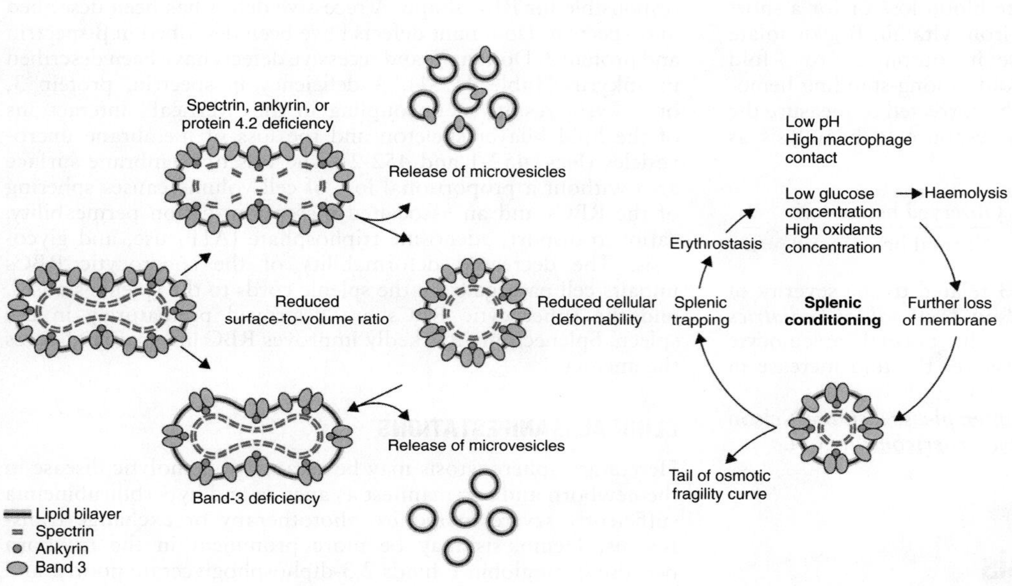

Figure 452-2 Pathophysiologic effects of hereditary spherocytosis. (From Perrotta S, Gallagher PG, Mohandas N: Hereditary spherocytosis, *Lancet* 372:1411–1426, 2008.)

Long-term complications include gout, myopathy, and spinocerebellar degenerations.

LABORATORY FINDINGS

Evidence of hemolysis includes reticulocytosis and indirect hyperbilirubinemia. The hemoglobin level usually is 6-10 g/dL, but it can be in the normal range. The reticulocyte percentage often is increased to 6-20%, with a mean of approximately 10%. The mean corpuscular volume (MCV) is normal, although the mean corpuscular hemoglobin concentration often is increased (36-38 g/dL RBCs). The RBCs on the blood film vary in size and include polychromatophilic reticulocytes and spherocytes (Fig. 452-4). The spherocytes are smaller in diameter and appear hyperchromic on the blood film as a result of the high hemoglobin concentration. The central pallor is less conspicuous than in normal cells. Spherocytes may be the predominant cells or may be relatively sparse, depending on the severity of the disease, but they usually account for >15-20% of the cells when hemolytic anemia is present. Erythroid hyperplasia is evident in the marrow aspirate or biopsy. Marrow expansion may be evident on routine roentgenographic examination. Other evidence of hemolysis can include decreased haptoglobin and the presence of gallstones on ultrasonography.

The diagnosis of hereditary spherocytosis usually is established clinically from the blood film, which shows many spherocytes and reticulocytes, from the family history, and from splenomegaly. The presence of spherocytes in the blood can be confirmed with an osmotic fragility test (Fig. 452-5). The RBCs are incubated in progressive dilutions of an iso-osmotic buffered salt solution. Exposure to hypotonic saline causes the RBCs to swell, and the spherocytes lyse more readily than biconcave cells in hypotonic solutions. This feature is accentuated by depriving the cells of glucose overnight at 37°C, known as the *incubated osmotic fragility test*. Unfortunately, this test is not specific for hereditary spherocytosis, and results may be abnormal in immune and other hemolytic anemias. A normal test result also may be found in 10-20% of patients. Other tests, such as the cryohemolysis test, osmotic gradient ektacytometry, and the eocin-5-maleimide test, may be more sensitive but are not readily available.

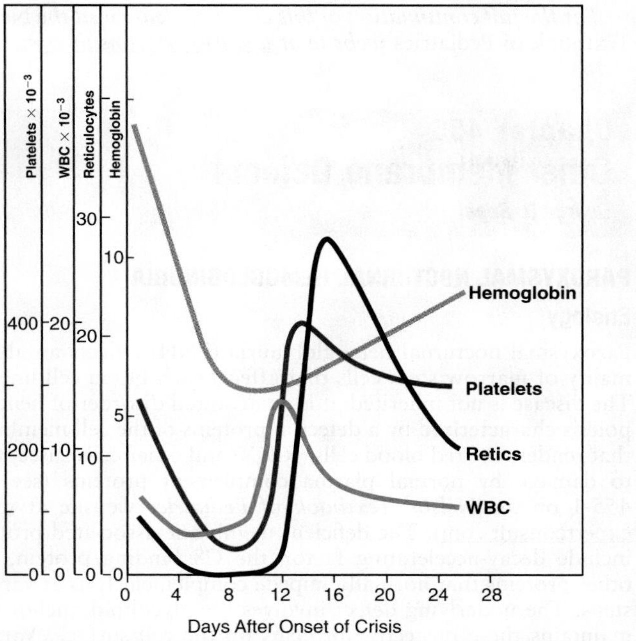

Figure 452-3 Parvovirus-induced aplastic crisis. Progression of the changes in blood count is shown for a patient with hereditary spherocytosis and infection with parvovirus. Note that the fall in baseline reticulocytosis is associated with a rapid fall in hemoglobin. White blood cells (WBC) and platelets are also affected. (Modified from Nathan DG, Orkin SH, Ginsburg D, et al, editors: *Hematology of infancy and childhood,* ed 6, Philadelphia, 2003, WB Saunders.)

Detection of a population of hyperdense RBCs using a laser-based instrument or a Coulter counter may prove more convenient as an approach to diagnosis.

As a research tool, the specific protein abnormality can be established in 80% of these patients by RBC membrane protein analysis using gel electrophoresis and densitometric quantitation. The protein abnormalities are more evident in patients who have had a splenectomy. Studies to define the underlying defects in the cytoskeleton might require assessment of protein synthesis, stability, assembly, and binding to the other membrane proteins. Molecular diagnosis also is possible. Most patients have family-specific private mutations that can be detected by DNA analysis. De novo mutations in the β-spectrin and ankyrin genes have been described in 50% of patients with unaffected parents.

DIFFERENTIAL DIAGNOSIS

The major alternative considerations when large numbers of spherocytes are seen on the blood film are isoimmune and autoimmune hemolysis. Isoimmune hemolytic disease of the newborn, particularly due to ABO incompatibility, mimics hereditary spherocytosis. The detection of antibody on an infant's RBCs using a direct antiglobulin (Coombs) test should establish the diagnosis of immune hemolysis. Autoimmune hemolytic anemias also are characterized by spherocytes, and there may be evidence of previously normal values for hemoglobin, hematocrit, and reticulocyte count. Rare causes of spherocytosis include thermal injury, clostridial septicemia with exotoxemia, and Wilson disease, each of which can manifest as transient hemolytic anemia (see Table 451-1).

TREATMENT

Because the spherocytes in hereditary spherocytosis are destroyed almost exclusively in the spleen, splenectomy eliminates most of the hemolysis associated with this disorder. After splenectomy, osmotic fragility often improves because of diminished splenic conditioning and less RBC membrane loss; the anemia, reticulocytosis, and hyperbilirubinemia then resolve. Whether all patients with hereditary spherocytosis should undergo splenectomy is controversial. Some do not recommend splenectomy for patients whose hemoglobin values exceed 10 g/dL and whose reticulocyte percentage is <10%. Folic acid, 1 mg daily, should be administered to prevent deficiency and the resultant decrease in erythropoiesis. For patients with more severe anemia and reticulocytosis or those with hypoplastic or aplastic crises, poor growth, or cardiomegaly, splenectomy is recommended after age 5-6 yr to avoid the heightened risk of postsplenectomy sepsis in younger children. Laparoscopic splenectomy decreases the length of hospital stay and has replaced open splenectomy for many patients.

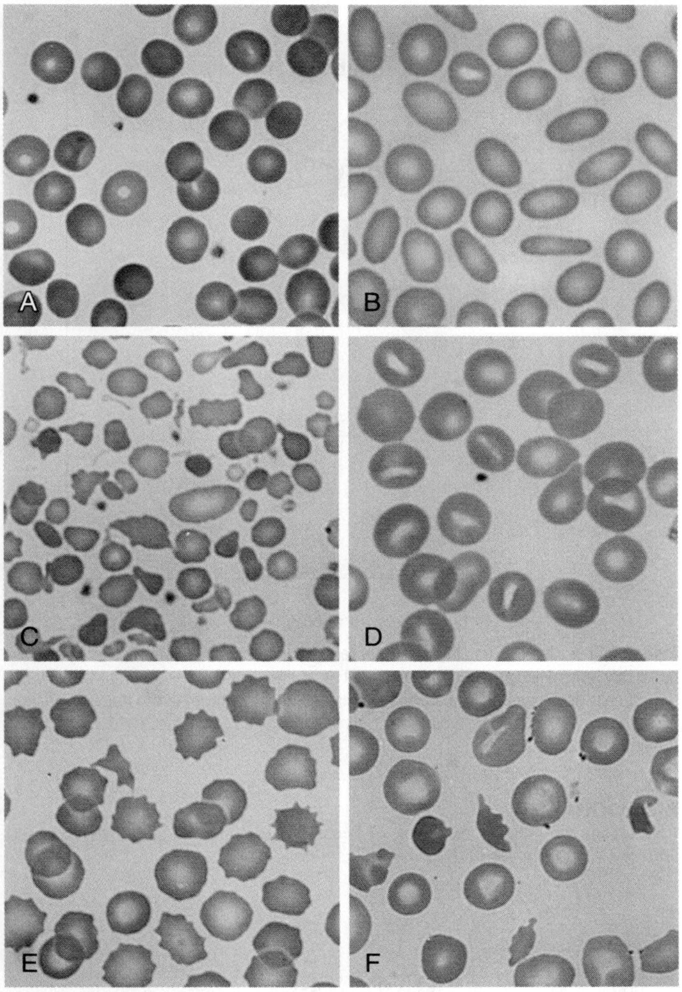

Figure 452-4 Morphology of abnormal red cells. *A,* Hereditary spherocytosis. *B,* Hereditary elliptocytosis. *C,* Hereditary pyropoikilocytosis. *D,* Hereditary stomatocytosis. *E,* Acanthocytosis. *F,* Fragmentation hemolysis.

Vaccines (conjugated and/or capsular) for encapsulated organisms, such as pneumococcus, meningococcus, and *Haemophilus influenzae* type b, should be administered before splenectomy, and prophylactic oral penicillin V (age <5 yr, 125 mg twice daily; age 5 yr through adulthood, 250 mg twice daily) should be administered thereafter. Postsplenectomy thrombocytosis is commonly observed, but it needs no treatment and usually resolves spontaneously. Partial (near total) splenectomy also may be useful in children younger than age 5 yr and can provide some increase in hemoglobin and reduction in the reticulocyte count, with potential maintenance of splenic phagocytic and immune function.

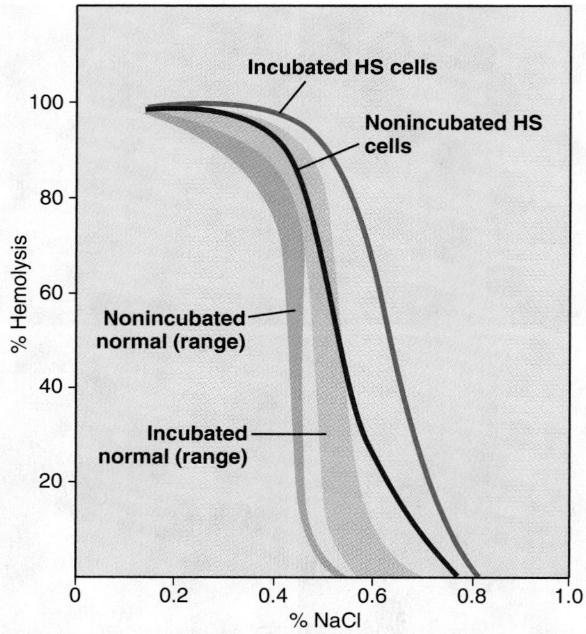

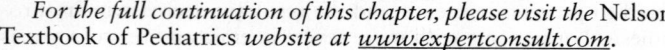

Figure 452-5 Osmotic fragility of normal red cells and red cells from a patient with hereditary spherocytosis (HS). The accentuation of the osmotic sensitivity, particularly of the HS cells, is shown after incubation overnight without glucose. (From Reich PR, editor: *Hematology: pathophysiologic basis for clinical practice,* ed 2, Boston, 1984, Little, Brown, with permission.)

BIBLIOGRAPHY

Please visit the Nelson Textbook of Pediatrics *website at* *www.expertconsult.com* *for the complete bibliography.*

Chapter 453
Hereditary Elliptocytosis

George B. Segel

Hereditary elliptocytosis is a less common disorder than spherocytosis and also varies markedly in severity. Mild hereditary elliptocytosis produces no symptoms; more severe varieties can result in neonatal poikilocytosis (shape variation) and hemolysis, chronic or sporadic hemolytic anemia, or hereditary pyropoikilocytosis (HPP), which is a severe disorder with microspherocytosis and poikilocytosis. Hereditary elliptocytosis is rare in Western populations and is more common among West Africans.

For the full continuation of this chapter, please visit the Nelson Textbook of Pediatrics *website at* *www.expertconsult.com*.

Chapter 454
Hereditary Stomatocytosis

George B. Segel and Lisa R. Hackney

Hereditary stomatocytosis includes a rare group of dominantly inherited hemolytic anemias in which there are characteristic morphologic changes in the RBCs and increased red cell cation permeability. The RBCs are cup shaped, creating a mouth-shaped area (stoma) of central pallor instead of the usual circular area of central pallor. Hereditary stomatocytosis is classified by the RBC hydration status. The two major varieties are either overhydrated (hydrocytosis) or dehydrated (xerocytosis).

For the full continuation of this chapter, please visit the Nelson Textbook of Pediatrics *website at* *www.expertconsult.com*.

Chapter 455
Other Membrane Defects

George B. Segel

PAROXYSMAL NOCTURNAL HEMOGLOBINURIA

Etiology

Paroxysmal nocturnal hemoglobinuria (PNH) reflects an abnormality of marrow stem cells that affects each blood cell lineage. The disease is not inherited; it is an acquired disorder of hematopoiesis characterized by a defect in proteins of the cell membrane that renders the red blood cells (RBCs) and other cells susceptible to damage by normal plasma complement proteins (see Fig. 455-1 on the *Nelson Textbook of Pediatrics* website at www.expertconsult.com). The deficient membrane-associated proteins include decay-accelerating factor, the C8 binding protein, and other proteins that normally impede complement lysis at various steps. The underlying defect involves the glycolipid anchor that maintains these protective proteins on the cell surface. Various mutations in the *PIGA* gene that are involved in glycosylphosphatidylinositol biosynthesis have been identified in patients with PNH. More than one *PIGA* gene mutation often occurs in an individual patient, suggesting multiclonality. Glycosylphosphatidylinositol-deficient cells are found at low frequency in normal persons, suggesting that injury to the normal marrow stem cells provides a selective advantage to the progeny of PNH clones in the genesis of this disease.

For the full continuation of this chapter, please visit the Nelson Textbook of Pediatrics *website at* *www.expertconsult.com*.

Chapter 456
Hemoglobinopathies

Michael R. DeBaun, Melissa Frei-Jones, and Elliott Vichinsky

HEMOGLOBIN DISORDERS

Hemoglobin is a tetramer consisting of 2 pairs of globin chains. Abnormalities in these proteins are referred to as *hemoglobinopathies*.

There are ~800 variant hemoglobins. The most common and useful clinical classification of hemoglobinopathies is based on nomenclature associated with alteration of the involved globin chain. Two hemoglobin gene clusters are involved in the production of hemoglobin and are located at the end of the short arms of chromosomes 16 and 11. Their control is complex, including an upstream locus control region on each respective chromosome and an X-linked control site. On chromosome 16, there are 3 genes within the α gene cluster, namely zeta (ζ), alpha 1 (α1), and alpha 2 (α2). On chromosome 11, there are 5 genes within the beta gene cluster, namely epsilon (ε), 2 gamma genes (γ), a delta gene (δ), and a beta gene (β).

The order of the gene expression within each cluster roughly follows the order of expression during the embryonic period, fetal period, and eventually childhood. After 8 wk of fetal life the embryonic hemoglobins, Gower-1 ($\zeta_2\varepsilon_2$), Gower-2 ($\alpha_2\varepsilon_2$), and Portland ($\zeta_2\gamma_2$), are formed. At 9 wk of fetal life, the major hemoglobin is Hb F ($\alpha_2\gamma_2$). Hb A ($\alpha_2\beta_2$) appears at ~1 mo of fetal life but does not become the dominant hemoglobin until after birth, when Hb F levels start to decline. Hb A_2 ($\alpha_2\delta_2$) is a minor hemoglobin that appears shortly before birth and remains at a low level after birth. The final hemoglobin distribution pattern that occurs in childhood is not achieved until at least 6 mo of age and sometimes later. The normal hemoglobin pattern is ≥95% Hb A, ≤3.5 Hb A_2, and <2.5% Hb F.

456.1 Sickle Cell Disease

Michael R. DeBaun, Melissa Frei-Jones, and Elliott Vichinsky

Hemoglobin S (Hb S) is the result of a single base-pair change, thymine for adenine, at the sixth codon of the β globin gene. This change encodes valine instead of glutamine in the sixth position in the β globin molecule. Sickle cell anemia, homozygous Hb S, occurs when both β globin genes have the sickle cell mutation. Sickle cell disease refers to not only patients with sickle cell anemia but also to compound heterozygotes where one β globin gene mutation includes the sickle cell mutation and the second β globin allele includes a gene mutation other than the sickle cell mutation, such as mutations associated with Hb C, Hb S β-thalassemia, Hb D, and Hb O Arab. In sickle cell anemia, Hb S is commonly as high as 90% of the total hemoglobin. In sickle cell disease, Hb S is >50% of all hemoglobin.

In the United States, sickle cell disease is the most common genetic disease identified through the state-mandated newborn screening program, occurring in 1:2,647 births and exceeding the incidence of primary congenital hypothyroidism (1:3,000), cystic fibrosis (1:3,900), and clinically significant hyperphenylalaninemia (1:14,000). In regard to race in the United States, sickle cell disease occurs in African Americans at a rate of 1:396 births and in Hispanics at a rate of 1:36,000 births.

Children with sickle cell disease should be followed by experts in the management of this disease, most often by pediatric hematologists. Comprehensive medical care with evidence-based strategies delivered by experts in sickle cell disease and anticipatory guidance of the parents about the most common complications has dramatically decreased sickle cell disease–related mortality and morbidity since the 1990s. Medical care provided by a pediatric hematologist is also associated with a decreased frequency of emergency department visits and length of hospitalization when compared to patients who were not seen by a hematologist within the last year.

CLINICAL MANIFESTATIONS AND TREATMENT OF SICKLE CELL ANEMIA

Infants with sickle cell anemia have abnormal immune function and, as early as 6 mo of age, may have functional asplenia. Bacterial sepsis is one of the greatest causes for morbidity and mortality in this patient population. By 5 yr of age, most children with sickle cell anemia have functional asplenia. Children with sickle cell anemia have an additional risk factor, the deficiency of alternative complement pathway serum opsonins against pneumococci. Regardless of age, all patients with sickle cell anemia are at increased risk of infection and death from bacterial infection, particularly encapsulated organisms such as *Streptococcus pneumoniae* and *Haemophilus influenzae* type b. Children with sickle cell anemia should receive prophylactic oral penicillin VK until at least 5 yr of age (125 mg twice a day up to age 3 yr, and then 250 mg twice a day). No established guidelines exist for penicillin prophylaxis beyond 5 yr of age, and some clinicians continue penicillin prophylaxis, whereas others recommend discontinuation. Continuation of penicillin prophylaxis should be considered for children beyond 5 yr of age with previous diagnosis of pneumococcal infection, due to the increased risk of a recurrent infection. An alternative for children who are allergic to penicillin is erythromycin ethyl succinate 10 mg/kg twice a day. In addition to penicillin prophylaxis, routine childhood immunizations as well as the annual administration of influenza vaccine are highly recommended.

Table 456-1 CLINICAL FACTORS ASSOCIATED WITH INCREASED RISK OF BACTEREMIA REQUIRING ADMISSION IN FEBRILE CHILDREN WITH SICKLE CELL DISEASE

Seriously ill appearance
Hypotension: systolic BP <70 mm Hg at 1 year of age or <70 mm Hg + 2 × the age in yr for older children
Poor perfusion: capillary-refill time >4 sec
Temperature >40.0°C
A corrected white-cell count >30,000/mm³ or <500/mm³
Platelet count <100,000/mm³
History of pneumococcal sepsis
Severe pain
Dehydration: poor skin turgor, dry mucous membranes, history of poor fluid intake, or decreased output of urine
Infiltration of a segment or a larger portion of the lung
Hemoglobin level <5.0 g/dL

BP, blood pressure.

From Williams JA, Flynn PM, Harris S et al: A randomized study of outpatient treatment with ceftriaxone for selected febrile children with sickle cell disease, *N Engl J Med* 329:472–476, 1993.

Human parvovirus B19 poses a unique threat for patients with sickle cell anemia because such infections limit the production of reticulocytes. Any child with reticulocytopenia should be considered to have parvovirus B19 until proved otherwise. Acute infection with parvovirus B19 is associated with red cell aplasia (aplastic crisis), fever, pain, splenic sequestration, acute chest syndrome (ACS), **glomerulonephritis,** and strokes.

Fever and Bacteremia

Fever in a child with sickle cell anemia is a medical emergency, requiring prompt medical evaluation and delivery of antibiotics due to the increased risk of bacterial infection and concomitant high fatality rate with infection. Several clinical management strategies have been developed for children with fever, ranging from admitting all patients with a fever for IV antimicrobial therapy to administering a 3rd-generation cephalosporin in an outpatient setting to patients without any of the previously established risk factors for occult bacteremia (Table 456-1). Given the observation that the average time for a positive blood culture with a bacterial pathogen is <20 hr in children with sickle cell anemia, admission for 24 hr is probably the most prudent strategy for children and families without a telephone or transportation, or with a history of inadequate follow-up. Outpatient management should be considered only for those with the lowest risk for bacteremia, and treatment choice should be considered carefully.

Children who have sickle cell disease and who are treated with ceftriaxone can develop severe, rapid, and life-threatening immune hemolysis; the established risks of outpatient management must be balanced against the perceived benefits. Regardless of the clinical management strategy, all patients with any type of sickle cell disease and fever should be evaluated and treated immediately for occult bacteremia with either IV or IM antibiotics. Those with poor adherence, limited financial resources, or established risk factors for bacteremia should be admitted for at least 24 hr. For patients with positive blood cultures, pathogen-specific therapy should be considered. In the event that *Salmonella* spp. or *Staphylococcus aureus* bacteremia occurs, strong consideration should be given to evaluation of osteomyelitis with a bone scan, given the increased risk of osteomyelitis in children with sickle cell anemia when compared to the general population.

Dactylitis

Dactylitis, often referred to as **hand-foot syndrome,** is often the first manifestation of pain in children with sickle cell anemia,

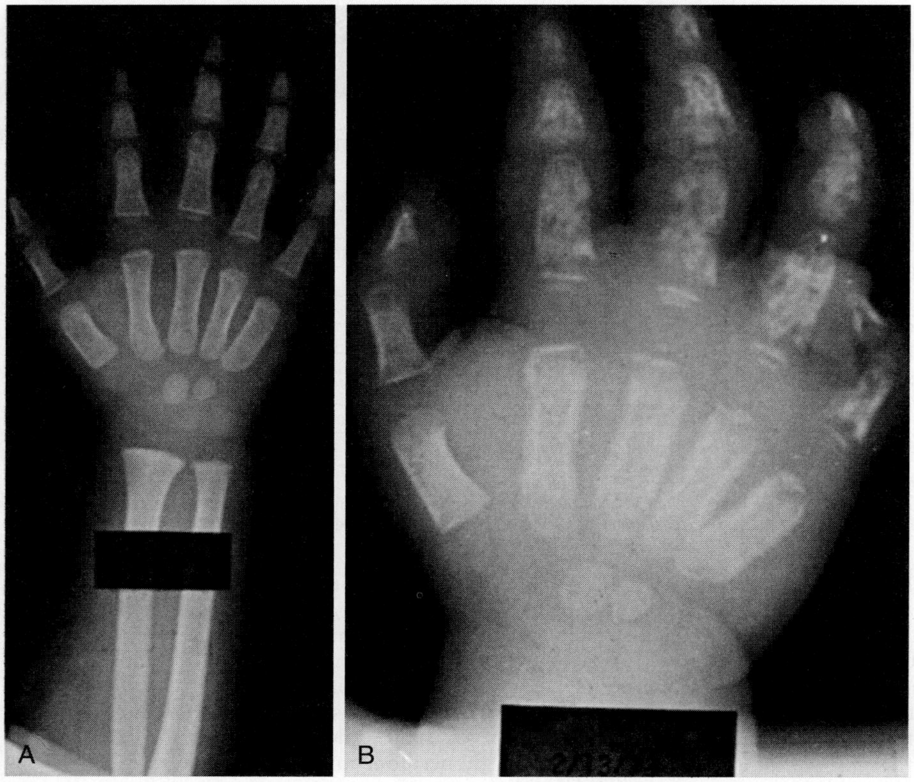

Figure 456-1 Roentgenograms of an infant with sickle cell anemia and acute dactylitis. *A,* The bones appear normal at the onset of the episode. *B,* Destructive changes and periosteal reaction are evident 2 wk later.

occurring in 50% of children by their 2nd year (Fig. 456-1). Dactylitis often manifests with symmetric or unilateral swelling of the hands and/or feet. Unilateral dactylitis can be confused with osteomyelitis, and careful evaluation to distinguish between the two is important, because treatment differs significantly. Dactylitis requires palliation with pain medications, such as acetaminophen with codeine, whereas osteomyelitis requires at least 4-6 wk of IV antibiotics.

Splenic Sequestration

Acute splenic sequestration is a life-threatening complication occurring primarily in infants and can occur as early as 5 wk of age. Approximately 30% of children with sickle cell anemia have a severe splenic sequestration episode, and a significant percentage of these episodes are fatal.

Appropriate anticipatory guidance should include teaching parents and primary caregivers how to palpate the spleen to determine if the spleen is enlarging. The etiology of splenic sequestration is unknown. Clinically, splenic sequestration is associated with engorgement of the spleen, subsequent increase in spleen size, evidence of hypovolemia, and decline in hemoglobin of ≥2 g/dL from the patient's baseline hemoglobin; reticulocytosis and a decrease in the platelet count may be present. These events can be accompanied by upper respiratory tract infections, bacteremia, or viral infection. Treatment includes early intervention and maintenance of hemodynamic stability using isotonic fluid or blood transfusions. If blood is required, typically 5 mL/kg of packed red blood cells (RBCs) is given. Repeated episodes of splenic sequestration are common, occurring in ~50% of patients. Most recurrent episodes develop within 6 mo of the previous episode. Prophylactic splenectomy performed after an acute episode has resolved is the only effective strategy for preventing future life-threatening episodes. Although blood transfusion therapy has been used to prevent subsequent episodes, evidence strongly suggests this strategy does not reduce the risk of recurrent splenic sequestration when compared to no transfusion therapy.

Pain

The cardinal clinical feature of sickle cell anemia is **pain.** No written definition can describe the visual picture of a child with sickle cell anemia in pain. The pain is characterized as unremitting discomfort that can occur in any part of the body but most often occurs in the chest, abdomen, or extremities. These painful episodes are often abrupt and can cause disruption of daily life activities and anguish for children and their families. The only measure for pain is the patient. Health care providers working with children with sickle cell anemia should develop a consistent, validated pain scale, such as the Wong-Baker FACES Scale for determining the magnitude of the pain. Although pain scales have proved useful for some children, others require prenegotiated activities to determine when opioid therapy should be initiated and decreased. For instance, sleeping through the night might be an indication for decreasing pain medication by 20% the following morning. The majority of painful episodes in patients with sickle cell anemia are managed at home with comfort measures, such as heating blanket, relaxation techniques, massage, and pain medication. A patient with sickle cell anemia has ~1 painful episode per year that requires medical attention.

The exact etiology of pain is unknown, but the pathogenesis is initiated when blood flow is disrupted in the microvasculature by sickle cells, resulting in tissue ischemia. Precipitating causes of painful episodes can include physical stress, infection, dehydration, hypoxia, local or systemic acidosis, exposure to cold, and swimming for prolonged periods. Successful treatment of painful episodes requires education of both the parents and the patients regarding the recognition of symptoms and the optimal management strategy. Given the absence of any reliable objective laboratory or clinical parameter associated with pain, trust between the patient and the treating physician is paramount to a successful clinical management strategy. Specific therapy for pain varies greatly but generally includes the use of acetaminophen or a nonsteroidal agent early in the course of pain, followed by escalation to acetaminophen with codeine or a short- or long-acting oral opioid.

Table 456-2 SUMMARY OF THE CHRONOLOGY OF PAIN IN CHILDREN WITH SICKLE CELL DISEASE

PHASE	PAIN CHARACTERISTICS	SUGGESTED COMFORT MEASURES USED
1 (Baseline)	No vaso-occlusive pain; pain of complications may be present, such as that connected with avascular necrosis of the hip	No comfort measures used
2 (Pre-pain)	No vaso-occlusive pain; pain of complications may be present; prodromal signs of impending vaso-occlusive episode may appear, e.g., "yellow eyes" and/or fatigue	No comfort measures used; caregivers may encourage child to increase fluids to prevent pain event from occurring
3 (Pain start point)	First signs of vaso-occlusive pain appear, usually in mild form	Mild oral analgesic often given; fluids increased; child usually maintains normal activities
4 (Pain acceleration)	Intensive of pain increases from mild to moderate Some children skip this level or move quickly from phase 3 to phase 5	Stronger oral analgesic are given; rubbing, heat, or other activities are often used; child usually stays in school until the pain becomes more severe, then stays home and limits activities; is usually in bed; family searches for ways to control the pain
5 (Peak pain experience)	Pain accelerates to high moderate or severe levels and plateaus; pain can remain elevated for extended period Child's appearance, behavior, and mood are significantly different from normal	Oral analgesics are given around the clock at home; combination of comfort measures is used; family might avoid going to the hospital; if pain is very distressing to the child, parent takes the child to the emergency department After child enters the hospital, families often turn over comforting activities to health care providers and wait to see if the analgesics work Family caregivers are often exhausted from caring for the child for several days with little or no rest
6 (Pain decrease start point)	Pain finally begins to decrease in intensity from the peak pain level	Family caregivers again become active in comforting the child but not as intensely as during phases 4 and 5
7 (Steady pain decline)	Pain decreases more rapidly, become more tolerable for the child Child and family are more relaxed	Health care providers begin to wean the child from the IV analgesic; oral opioids given; discharge planning is started Children may be discharged before they are pain free
8 (Pain resolution)	Pain intensity is at a tolerable level, and discharge is imminent Child looks and acts like "normal" self Mood improves	May receive oral analgesics

Adapted from Beyer JE, Simmons LE, Woods GM, et al: A chronology of pain and comfort in children with sickle cell disease, *Arch Pediatr Adolesc Med* 153:913–920, 1999.

Some patients require hospitalization for administration of IV morphine or derivatives of morphine. The incremental increase and decrease in the use of the medication to relieve pain roughly parallels the 8 phases associated with a chronology of pain and comfort (Table 456-2). The average hospital length of stay for children admitted in pain is 4.4 days. The American Pain Society has published clinical guidelines for treating acute and chronic pain in patients with sickle cell disease of any type. These recommendations are comprehensive and represent a starting point for treating pain (*www.ampainsoc.org/pub/sc.htm*).

Several myths have been propagated regarding the treatment of pain in sickle cell anemia. The concept that painful episodes in children should be managed without opioids is without foundation and results in unwarranted suffering on the part of the patient. There is no evidence that blood transfusion therapy during an existing painful episode decreases the intensity or duration of the painful episode. Blood transfusion should be reserved for patients with a decrease in hemoglobin resulting in hemodynamic compromise, respiratory distress, or a falling hemoglobin concentration, with no expectation that a safe nadir will be reached, such as when the child has both a falling hemoglobin level and reticulocyte count with a parvovirus B19 infection. IV hydration does not relieve or prevent pain and is appropriate when the patient is unable to drink as a result of the severe pain or is dehydrated. Opioid dependency in children with sickle cell anemia is rare and should never be used as a reason to withhold pain medication. However, patients with multiple painful episodes requiring hospitalization within a year or with pain episodes that require hospital stays >7 days should be evaluated for comorbidities and psychosocial stressors that might contribute to the frequency or duration of pain.

Hydroxyurea, a myelosuppressive agent, is the only effective drug proved to reduce the frequency of painful episodes. A clinical trial in adults with sickle cell anemia and ≥3 painful episodes per year demonstrated the efficacy of hydroxyurea. Hydroxyurea was found to decrease the rate of painful episodes by 50% and the rate of ACS episodes and blood transfusions by ~50%. In children with sickle cell anemia, only a safety feasibility trial of hydroxyurea has been conducted. This study demonstrated that hydroxyurea was safe and well tolerated in children >5 yr of age. No clinical adverse events were identified in this study; the primary toxicities were limited to myelosuppression that reversed upon cessation of the drug.

Given the short-term safety profile in children and the established efficacy in adults, hydroxyurea is commonly used in children with multiple painful episodes. The long-term toxicity associated with hydroxyurea in children has not been established, but all evidence to date suggests that the benefits far outweigh the risks. For these reasons and others, children >5 yr of age receiving hydroxyurea require well-informed parents and medical care by pediatric hematologists or at least comanagement by a physician with expertise in managing chemotherapy. The typical starting dose of hydroxyurea is 15-20 mg/kg given daily, with an incremental dosage increase every 8 wk of 2.5-5.0 mg/kg, if no toxicities occur, up to a maximum of 35 mg/kg per dose. Achievement of the therapeutic effect of hydroxyurea can require several months. Monitoring children on hydroxyurea is labor intensive, with initial visits every 2 wk to monitor for hematologic toxicity with dose escalations and then monthly after a therapeutic dose has been identified. Close monitoring of the patient requires a commitment by the parents and patient as well as diligence by a physician to monitor for toxicity.

Priapism

Priapism is defined as an involuntary penile erection lasting for longer than 30 minutes and is a common problem in sickle cell anemia. The persistence of a painful erection beyond several hr suggests priapism. On examination, the penis is erect. The ventral portion and the glans of the penis are typically not involved, and their involvement necessitates urologic consultation based on the

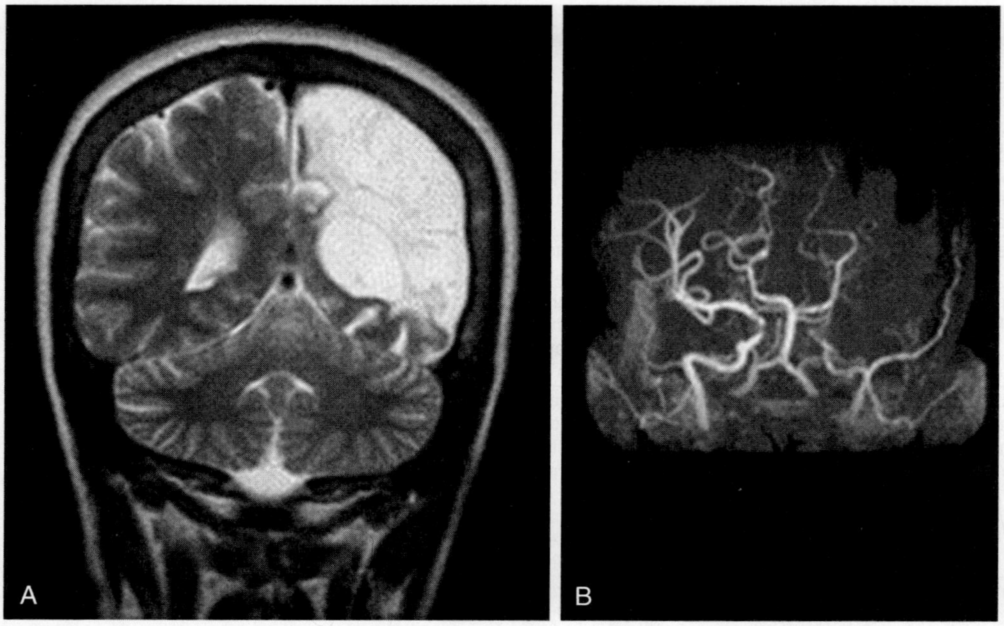

Figure 456-2 T2-weighted MRI and magnetic resonance angiography (MRA) of the brain. *A,* T2-weighted MRI shows remote infarction of the territories of the left anterior cerebral artery and middle cerebral artery. *B,* MRA shows occlusion of the left internal carotid artery siphon distal to the takeoff of the ophthalmic artery.

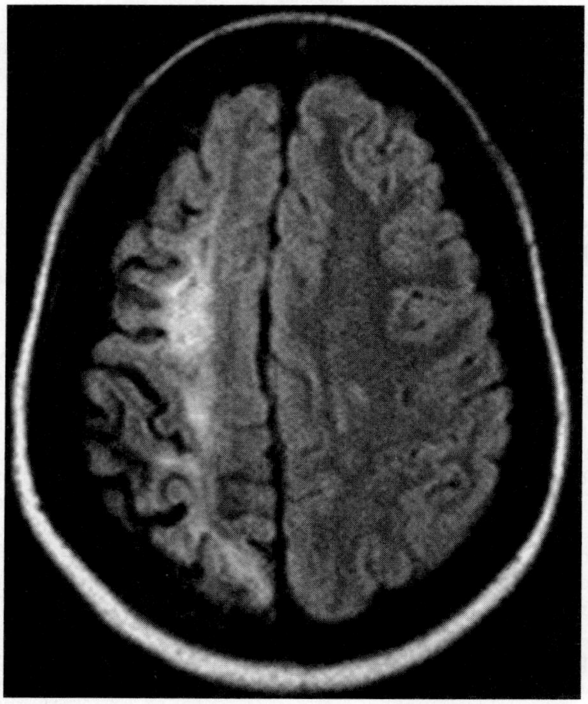

Figure 456-3 Fast fluid-attenuated inversion-recovery-sequence (FLAIR) MRI of the brain showing a right hemisphere border-zone cerebral infarction in a child with sickle cell anemia. (From Switzer JA, Hess DC, Nichols F, et al: Pathophysiology and treatment of stoke in sickle-cell disease: present and future, *Lancet Neurol* 5:501–512, 2006.)

poor prognosis for spontaneous resolution. Priapism occurs in 2 patterns, stuttering and refractory, with both types occurring in patients from early childhood to adulthood. No formal definitions have been established for these terms, but generally stuttering priapism is defined as self-limited, intermittent bouts of priapism with several episodes over a defined period. Refractory priapism is defined as prolonged priapism beyond several hours.

Approximately 20% of patients between 5 and 20 yr of age report having at least 1 episode of priapism. Most episodes occur between 3 AM and 9 AM. The mean age at first episode is 12 yr, and the mean number of episodes per patient is ~16, with a mean duration of ~2 hr. The actuarial probability of a patient's experiencing priapism is ~90% by 20 yr of age.

The optimal treatment for priapism is unknown, but treatment strategies can be divided into acute treatment and preventive therapy. For acute treatment, supported therapy, such as sitz bath or pain medication, is commonly employed. Priapism lasting >4 hr should be treated by aspiration of blood from the corpora cavernosa followed by irrigation with dilute epinephrine to produce immediate and sustained detumescence. Urology consultation is required to initiate this procedure, with appropriate input from a hematologist. Either simple blood transfusion therapy or exchange transfusion has been proposed for the acute treatment of priapism. However, evidence suggests that exchange transfusion therapy is not effective in enhancing detumescence.

For the prevention of recurrent priapism, hydroxyurea appears to have promise; the use of etilefrine, a sympathomimetic amine with both α_1 and β_1 adrenergic effects, appears safe and promising in the secondary prevention of priapism. The long-term effects of recurrent or prolonged priapism episodes in prepubertal children are not known. In adults, infertility and impotence are potential consequences.

Neurologic Complications

Neurologic complications associated with sickle cell anemia are varied and complex. Approximately 11% and 20% of children with sickle cell anemia will have overt and silent strokes, respectively, before their 18th birthday (Figs. 456-2 and 456-3). An overt stroke is defined as a focal neurologic deficit lasting >24 hr. However, this definition is outdated because many patients with sickle cell anemia will be treated with blood therapy that can hasten their recovery to baseline. A more functional definition is the presence of a focal neurologic deficit that lasts for >24 hr and/or increased signal intensity with a T2-weighted MRI of the brain indicating a cerebral infarct, corresponding to the focal neurologic deficit. The definition of silent cerebral infarct is the absence of a focal neurologic deficit lasting >24 hr in the presence of a lesion on T2-weighted MRI indicating a cerebral infarct. Evidence of a stroke can be found as early as 1 yr of age. Other neurologic complications include headaches that may or may not be related to sickle cell anemia, seizures, cerebral venous thrombosis, and reversible posterior leukoencephalopathy syndrome (RPLS). Children with other types of sickle cell disease such as

Hb SC or Hb Sβ-thalassemia plus might have overt or silent cerebral infarcts as well.

For patients presenting with an acute focal neurologic deficit, a prompt pediatric neurologic evaluation is recommended. In addition, oxygen administration to keep oxygen saturations >96% and simple blood transfusion within 1 hr of presentation with a goal of increasing the hemoglobin to a maximum of 10 g/dL is warranted. To exceed this hemoglobin threshold might limit oxygen delivery to the brain because hyperviscosity of the blood can decrease oxygen delivery. Subsequently, prompt treatment with an exchange transfusion should be considered, either manually or with erythrocytapheresis, to reduce the Hb S percentage to at least <50% and ideally <30%. CT to exclude cerebral hemorrhage should be performed as soon as possible, and if available, MRI of the brain with diffusion-weighted imaging should be performed to distinguish between ischemic infarcts and RPLS. MR venography is also useful to evaluate the possibility of cerebral venous thrombosis.

The clinical presentation of RPLS or central venous thrombosis can mimic a stroke. The diagnosis of either RPLS or cerebral venous thrombosis requires a different course of treatment than a stroke. For both RPLS and cerebral venous thrombosis, the optimal management has not been defined in patients with sickle cell disease, resulting in the need for consultation with both a pediatric neurologist and a pediatric hematologist.

Primary prevention of stroke can be accomplished by transcranial Doppler (TCD) assessment of the blood velocity in the terminal portion of the internal carotid and the proximal portion of the middle cerebral artery. Children with sickle cell anemia with a time-averaged mean maximum (TAMM) blood-flow velocity ≥200 cm/sec are at increased risk for a cerebrovascular event. This value defines the transfusion threshold, and chronic blood transfusion therapy is instituted to maintain Hb S levels <30%. This strategy results in an 85% reduction in the rate of overt strokes. Once transfusion therapy is initiated, patients are expected to continue it indefinitely. The optimal age to start and end TCD measurement in children with sickle cell anemia has not been established; many hematologists initiate TCD screening at 2 yr of age when most patients no longer require sedation. A TAMM measurement of <200 cm/sec but ≥180 cm/sec represents a conditional threshold. A repeat measurement is suggested within several months because of the high rate of conversion to a TCD velocity >200 cm/sec in this group of patients. The optimal interval for TCD measurements is not known, but most experts advise measurements every 12-18 mo from 2 yr of age up to 16 yr of age. TCD measurement for patients >16 yr of age has not been proved to have any benefit. Given that blood transfusion therapy and acute illness can alter the TCD measurements, patients are commonly screened when their hemoglobin is near their baseline and when they are not acutely ill.

Two distinct methods of measuring TCD velocity exist, a nonimaging and an imaging technique. The nonimaging technique was the method used in the TCD trial sponsored by the National Institutes of Health; however, the imaging technique is more commonly used by pediatric radiologists in practice. When compared to each other, the imaging technique has values that are 10-15% below that of the nonimaging technique. The imaging technique uses the time-averaged mean of the maximum velocity (TAMX), and this measure is believed to be equivalent to the nonimaging calculation of TAMM. A downward adjustment for the transfusion threshold is appropriate for centers that conduct the imaging method to assess TCD velocity. The magnitude of the downward adjustment is unclear, but for the imaging technique, a transfusion threshold of a TAMX of 185 cm/sec and a conditional threshold of TAMX of 165 cm/sec seems reasonable.

The primary approach for secondary prevention of strokes is blood transfusion therapy aimed at keeping the maximum Hb S concentration <30% in the first 2 yr following any new stroke and <50% thereafter. Despite regular blood transfusion therapy, ~20% of patients will have a second stroke and 30% of this group will have a third stroke. The primary toxic effect of blood transfusion therapy relates to excessive iron stores, which can result in organ damage and premature death. A unit of blood contains ~200 mg of iron. In the United States, 2 chelating agents are commercially available and approved for use in transfusional iron overload. Deferoxamine is administered subcutaneously 5 of 7 nights per week for 10 hr a night, and deferasirox is an effervescent tablet that is dissolved in liquid and taken by mouth daily. Deferasirox, the newest and only orally administered chelator, was approved by the FDA in 2005 for use in patients age ≥2 yr.

Excessive Iron Stores

The assessment of **excessive iron stores** in children receiving regular blood transfusions is difficult. The gold standard involves biopsy of the liver, which is an invasive procedure exposing children to the risk of general anesthesia, bleeding, and pain. Liver biopsy alone does not accurately estimate total body iron because the amount of iron deposited in the liver is not homogenous and the degree of iron deposition varies among the affected organs; for example, the amount of iron in the liver is not the same as the amount of iron in cardiac tissues. The most commonly used and least-invasive method of estimating total body iron involves serum ferritin levels; however, ferritin measurements have significant limitations, because ferritin levels rise during acute inflammation and correlate poorly with excessive iron in specific organs after 2 yr of regular blood transfusion therapy. MRI of the liver is a reasonable alternative to biopsy and more accurate than serum ferritin in measuring iron content in heart and liver, the two most commonly affected organs associated with increased total body iron stores. MRI T2* and MRI R2 and R2* sequences are used to estimate iron levels in the heart and liver.

Three methods of blood transfusion therapy are available: erythrocytapheresis, manual exchange transfusions (phlebotomy of a set amount of the patient's blood followed by rapid administration of donated packed RBCs), and simple transfusion. Erythrocytapheresis is the preferred method because there is a minimum net iron balance after the procedure. Simple transfusion therapy is the least preferable method because this strategy results in the highest net positive iron balance after the procedure. Despite being the preferred method, erythrocytapheresis is less commonly performed because of the requirement for technical expertise, access to a large vein, and an available pheresis machine.

For patients who either will not or cannot continue blood transfusion therapy to prevent subsequent strokes, hydroxyurea therapy may be a reasonable alternative. The efficacy and toxicity of hydroxyurea as an option for preventing secondary stroke is being addressed in a clinical trial setting. Alternatively, human leukocyte antigen (HLA) matched hematopoietic stem cell transplantation from a sibling donor is a reasonable approach for patients with strokes, although only a few children have suitable donors. Hematopoietic stem cell transplantation using unrelated donors is the subject of an open clinical trial that is too premature to comment on.

Lung Disease

Lung disease in children with sickle cell anemia is the second most common reason for admission to the hospital and a common cause of death. ACS refers to a constellation of findings that include a new radiodensity on chest radiograph, fever, respiratory distress, and pain that occurs often in the chest, but it can also include the back and/or abdomen only (Fig. 456-4). Even in the absence of respiratory symptoms, all patients with fever should receive a chest radiograph to identify ACS because clinical examination alone is insufficient to identify patients with a new radiographic density, and early detection of acute syndrome will alter clinical management. The radiographic findings in ACS are variable but can include involvement of a single lobe (predominantly

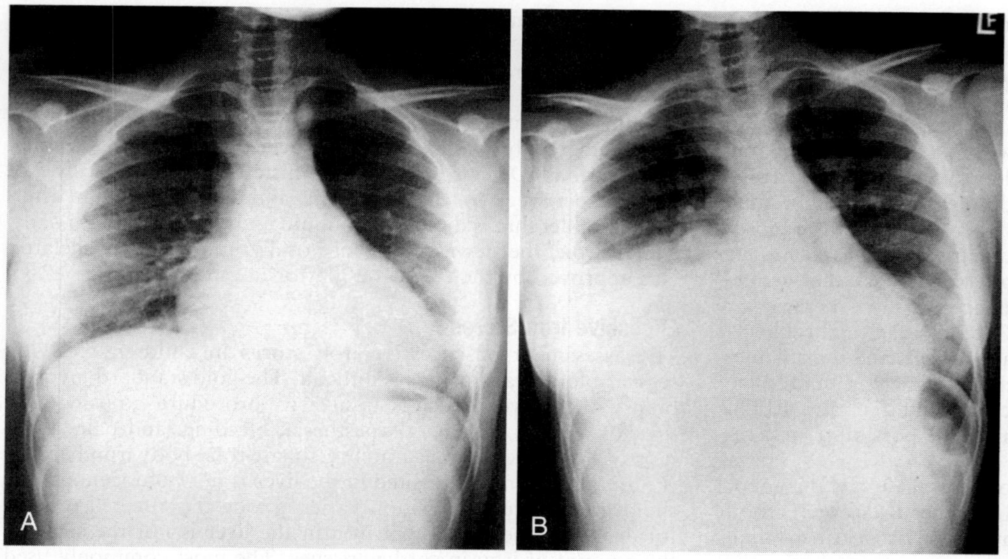

Figure 456-4 Probable pulmonary infarction in a 15 yr old patient with sickle cell anemia. *A,* Frontal radiograph shows consolidation and a small pleural effusion posteriorly in the right lower lobe. *B,* Radiograph obtained <24 hr later shows massive right middle and lower lobe consolidation and effusion. No organisms could be cultured. The diagnosis of probable pulmonary infarction was established clinically. (Courtesy of Dr. Thomas L. Slovis, Children's Hospital of Michigan, Detroit, MI. From Kuhn JP, Slovis TL, Haller JO: *Caffey's pediatric diagnostic imaging,* vol 1, ed 10, Philadelphia, 2004, Mosby, p 1087.)

Table 456-3 OVERALL STRATEGIES FOR THE MANAGEMENT OF ACUTE CHEST SYNDROME

PREVENTION
Incentive spirometry and periodic ambulation in patients admitted for vaso-occlusive crises, surgery, or febrile episodes
Watchful waiting in any hospitalized child or adult with sickle cell disease (pulse oximetry monitoring and frequent respiratory assessments)
Avoidance of overhydration
Intense education and optimum care of patients who have sickle cell anemia and asthma
DIAGNOSTIC TESTING AND LABORATORY MONITORING
Blood cultures
Nasopharyngeal samples for viral culture (respiratory syncytial virus, influenza)
Blood counts every day and appropriate chemistries
Continuous pulse oximetry
Chest radiographs
TREATMENT
Blood transfusion (simple or exchange)
Supplemental O_2 for drop in pulse oximetry by 4% over baseline, or values <90%
Empirical antibiotics (cephalosporin and macrolide)
Continued respiratory therapy (incentive spirometry and chest physiotherapy as necessary)
Bronchodilators and steroids for patients with asthma
Optimum pain control and fluid management

the left lower lobe) or multiple lobes (most often both lower lobes) and pleural effusions (either unilateral or bilateral).

Given the clinical overlap between ACS and common pulmonary complications such as bronchiolitis, asthma, and pneumonia, a wide range of therapeutic strategies have been used (Table 456-3). Oxygen administration and blood transfusion therapy, either simple or exchange (manual or automated), are the most common interventions used to treat ACS. Supplemental oxygen should be administered when the room air oxygen saturation is >90%. The decision about when to give blood and whether the transfusion should be a simple or exchange transfusion is less clearly defined. Commonly, blood transfusions are given when at least one of the following clinical features is present: decreasing oxygen saturation, increase work of breathing, rapid change in respiratory effort either with or without a worsening chest radiograph, or previous history of severe ACS requiring admission to the intensive care unit.

The majority of patients with ACS do not have an identifiable cause. Infection is the best-known etiology, but only ~30% of ACS episodes are associated with positive sputum or bonchoalveolar culture. The most common illness preceding ACS is a painful episode requiring opioids. The risk of ACS is influenced by the type of opioid (morphine conveys a greater risk than nalbuphine hydrochloride) and the route of administration of the opioid (oral carries a greater risk than IV opioid). Under no circumstance should opioid administration be limited in order to prevent ACS. In patients with chest pain, regular use of an incentive spirometer at 10-12 breaths every 2 hr can significantly reduce the frequency of subsequent acute chest pain episodes. Fat emboli have also been implicated as a cause of ACS, are believed to arise from infarcted bone marrow, and can be life threatening if large amounts are released to the lungs. As a result of the clinical overlap between pneumonia and ACS, *all episodes should be treated promptly with antimicrobial therapy*, including at least a macrolide and a third-generation cephalosporin to treat the most common pathogens associated with ACS, namely *Streptococcus pneumoniae*, *Mycoplasma pneumoniae*, and *Chlamydia* spp. A previous diagnosis of asthma should prompt treatment with steroids and bronchodilators even when the patient does not have evidence of wheezing. Lower respiratory symptoms alone are sufficient to initiate such therapy in a patient with only asthma. The presence of ACS does not negate the recommended management of a patient with asthma who has findings suggestive of an asthma exacerbation.

The diagnosis of pulmonary hypertension has been identified as a major risk factor for death in adults with sickle cell anemia. The natural history of pulmonary hypertension in children with sickle cell anemia is unknown, and therefore the optimal diagnostic and therapeutic strategy for pulmonary hypertension has not been identified.

Kidney Disease

Renal disease among patients with sickle cell anemia is a major comorbid condition that can lead to premature death. Seven sickle cell anemia associated nephropathies have been identified: gross hematuria, papillary necrosis, nephrotic syndrome, renal infarction, hyposthenuria, pyelonephritis, and renal medullary carcinoma. The presentation of these entities is varied but can include hematuria, proteinuria, renal insufficiency, concentrating defects, or hypertension. The treatment of asymptomatic proteinuria with angiotensin-converting enzyme (ACE) inhibitors can decrease renal insufficiency. Suspicion of renal medullary carcinoma, an aggressive malignant epithelial neoplasm, is important because most patients present with late-stage disseminated disease that responds poorly to chemotherapy and radiation therapy. The youngest reported patient with medullary carcinoma was a 6 yr old African-American with *sickle cell trait*, presenting with gross hematuria.

Cognitive and Psychological Complications

As with any child with a chronic illness, good health maintenance must include psychological and social assessment. Ongoing evaluation of the family unit and identification of the resources available to cope with a chronic illness are critical for optimal management. Further, children with sickle cell anemia are at great risk for academic failure and have a poor high school graduation rate, ~20%. One of the reasons behind the low high school graduation rate is that ~30% of children with sickle cell anemia have had a cerebral infarct, either a silent cerebral infarct or an overt stroke. Children with cerebral infarcts require ongoing cognitive and school performance assessment so that education resources can be focused to optimize educational attainment. Relevant support groups and attendance in group activities such as camps for children with sickle cell anemia may be of direct benefit by improving self-esteem and establishing peer relationships.

Other Complications

In addition to organ dysfunctions, patients with sickle cell anemia can have other significant complications. Examples of these complications include sickle cell retinopathy, delayed onset of puberty, avascular necrosis of the femoral and humeral heads, and leg ulcers. Optimal treatment for each of these entities has not been determined, and individual management requires consultation with the disease-specific specialist, a hematologist, and the primary care physician. Preparation for surgery for children with sickle cell disease requires a coordinated effort between the hematologist, surgeon, and primary care provider. ACS and pain are the two most common postoperative complications, and ACS is a significant risk factor for postoperative death.

Blood transfusion before surgery for children with sickle cell anemia designed to raise the hemoglobin level preoperatively to 10 g/dL is desirable; however, achieving a level of at least 10 g/dL is not necessary to provide benefit from simple transfusion. When preparing a child with sickle cell anemia for surgery with a simple blood transfusion, caution must be used to avoid elevating the hemoglobin beyond 10.5 g/dL because of the risk of hyperviscosity syndrome. For children with sickle cell anemia, exchange transfusion before surgery is of no greater benefit than simple blood transfusion and carries significantly higher risk of RBC alloimmunization. For children with Hb SC disease or other sickle syndromes with hemoglobins >10.0 g/dL, a decision must be made on a case-by-case basis as to whether an exchange transfusion is warranted because a simple transfusion can raise the hemoglobin to an unacceptable level.

DIAGNOSIS

Every state in the United States has instituted a mandatory newborn screening program for sickle cell disease. Such programs identify newborns with the disease, provide prompt diagnosis and anticipatory guidance for parents, and are responsible for initiating penicillin before 4 mo of age.

The most commonly used procedures for newborn diagnosis include thin layer/isoelectric focusing and high-performance liquid chromatography (HPLC). A 2-step system is recommended, with all patients who have initially abnormal screens being retested during the first clinical visit and after 6 mo of age to determine the final hemoglobin phenotype. In addition, a complete blood cell count (CBC) and hemoglobin analysis are recommended on both parents to confirm the diagnosis and to provide an opportunity for genetic counseling. Table 456-4 correlates the initial hemoglobin phenotype at birth with the type of hemoglobinopathy, baseline hemoglobin range, and requirement for a hematologist.

Table 456-4 VARIOUS NEWBORN SICKLE CELL DISEASE SCREENING RESULTS WITH BASELINE HEMOGLOBIN

NEWBORN SCREENING RESULTS: SICKLE CELL DISEASE*	POSSIBLE HEMOGLOBIN PHENOTYPE†	BASELINE HEMOGLOBIN RANGE	EXPERTISE IN HEMATOLOGY CARE REQUIRED
FS	SCD-SS	6-11 g/dL	Yes
	SCD-S β^0 thal	6-10 g/dL	Yes
	SCD-S β^+ thal	9-12 g/dL	Yes
	SCD-S $\delta\beta^-$ thal	10-12 g/dL	Yes
FSC	S HPFH	12-14 g/dL	Yes
FSA	SCD-SC	10-15 g/dL	Yes
FS other	SCD-S β^0 thal	6-10 g/dL	Yes
	SCD-SD, SO^{Arab}, SC^{Harlem}, S Lepare		Yes
AFS	SCD-SS	6-10 g/dL	Yes
	SCD-S β+ thal	6-9 g/dL	Yes
	SCD-S β^0 thal‡	7-13 g/dL variable	Yes

*Hemoglobins are reported in order of quantity.
†Requires confirmatory hemoglobin analysis after at least 6 mo of age and, if possible, hemoglobin analysis from both parents for accurate diagnosis of hemoglobin phenotype.
‡Impossible to determine the diagnosis because the infant received a blood transfusion before testing.
A, normal hemoglobin; C, hemoglobin C; F, fetal hemoglobin; HPFH, hereditary persistence of fetal hemoglobin; O, hemoglobin O; S, sickle hemoglobin; SC, heterozygous sickle cell disease; SCD, sickle cell disease; SS, homozygous sickle cell disease.

In newborn screening programs, the hemoglobin with the greatest quantity is reported first followed by the other hemoglobins in decreasing quantity. In newborns with a hemoglobin analysis result of FS, the pattern supports Hb SS, hereditary persistent fetal hemoglobin, or Hb S β-thalassemia zero. In a newborn with a hemoglobin analysis of FSA, the pattern is supportive of diagnosis Hb S β-thalassemia+. The diagnosis of Hb S β-thalassemia+ is confirmed if at least 50% of the hemoglobin is Hb S, HbA is present, and the amount of Hb A_2 is elevated (typically >3.5%), although Hb A_2 is not elevated in the newborn period. In newborns with a hemoglobin analysis of FSC, the pattern supports a diagnosis of Hb SC. In newborns with a hemoglobin analysis of FAS, the pattern supports a diagnosis of Hb AS (sickle cell trait).

A newborn with a hemoglobin analysis of AFS has been transfused with red blood cells before obtaining the laboratory test because the amount of Hb A is greater than the amount of Hb F or there has been an error. The patient may have either sickle cell disease or sickle cell trait, and should be started on penicillin prophylaxis until the final diagnosis can be determined. Given the implications of a diagnosis of either sickle cell disease or sickle cell trait in a newborn, repeating the hemoglobin analysis in the patient and obtaining a hemoglobin analysis and CBC to evaluate the smear and RBC parameters in the parents for genetic counseling cannot be overemphasized. Unintended mistakes do occur in state newborn screening programs. Newborns who have the initial phenotype of Hb FS but whose final true phenotype included Hb S β-thalassemia+ have been described as one of the more common errors identified in newborn screening hemoglobinopathy programs.

OTHER SICKLE CELL SYNDROMES

The most commonly occurring sickle cell syndromes besides Hb SS are Hb SC, Hb S/β-thalassemia zero, and Hb S/β-thalassemia+. The other syndromes—Hb SD, Hb SO Arab, hereditary persistence of fetal hemoglobin (HPFH), and other variants—are much less common. Patients with Hb S/β-thalassemia zero have a clinical course like the course in patients with Hb SS. Hb SC does not polymerize like Hb SS, but crystals of Hb C interact with the membrane ion transport, dehydrating red cells and inducing sickling. Children who have Hb SC disease can experience the same symptoms and complications as those with severe Hb SS disease, but the frequency is less. Children with Hb SC also have increased incidence of retinopathy, chronic hypersplenism, splenic sequestration, and renal medullary carcinoma. The natural history of the other sickle cell syndromes is variable and difficult to predict due to the lack of systematic evaluation.

There is no validated model that can predict the clinical course of an individual with sickle cell disease. A patient with Hb SC can have a more-severe clinical course than a patient with Hb SS. Management of end-organ dysfunction in children with sickle cell syndromes requires the same general principles as managing patients with sickle cell anemia; however, each situation should be managed on a case-by-case basis and requires consultation with a pediatric hematologist.

BIBLIOGRAPHY

Please visit the Nelson Textbook of Pediatrics *website at* *www.expertconsult.com* *for the complete bibliography.*

456.2 Sickle Cell Trait (Hemoglobin AS)

Michael R. DeBaun, Melissa Frei-Jones, and Elliott Vichinsky

The prevalence of sickle cell trait varies throughout the world; in the United States the incidence is 7-10% of African-Americans. Because screening for sickle cell disease is performed by all state newborn programs, sickle cell trait status is first identified on newborn screening, allowing early communication to parents and health care providers. Tracking of the sickle cell trait status from infancy to young adulthood for the patient, family, and health care providers has been inconsistent.

The amount of Hb S is influenced by the number of α-thalassemia genes present, and the amount in most persons with sickle cell trait (Hb AS) is <50%. The life span of people with sickle cell trait is normal, and serious complications are very rare. The CBC is within the normal range. Hemoglobin analysis is diagnostic, revealing a predominance of Hb A, typically >50%, and Hb S <50%. Complications of sickle cell trait include sudden death during rigorous exercise, splenic infarcts at high altitude, hematuria, hyposthenuria, bacteriuria, and susceptibility to eye injury with formation of a hyphema (Table 456-5). Renal medullary carcinoma is also associated with sickle cell trait and occurs predominantly in young adults and children.

In general, children with sickle cell trait should not have any restrictions on activities. Sudden death in persons with sickle cell trait while exercising under extreme conditions has been reported. It is unclear whether this association is causal. All patients with sickle cell trait who participate in rigorous athletic activities should receive maximum hydration and appropriate rest during exertion. The presence of sickle cell trait should never be a reason to exclude a person from athletic participation but rather should serve as an indication that prudent surveillance is necessary to ensure appropriate hydration and prevention of exhaustion from heat or other strenuous exercise. These requirements are applicable to all athletes during rigorous training and should not be limited to athletes with sickle cell trait.

The National Association of Athletic Trainers (NATA) has made specific recommendations for the training of athletes with sickle cell trait, including the rapid recognition and treatment of exertional sickling or sickling collapse, which occurs when sickled RBCs occlude vessels and lead to ischemic rhabdomyolysis (Table 456-6). An important component of the screening of athletes is that adequate knowledge about sickle cell trait status identified at birth is later communicated to the adolescent before transitioning to adulthood.

Table 456-5 COMPLICATIONS ASSOCIATED WITH SICKLE CELL TRAIT

DEFINITE ASSOCIATIONS
Renal medullary cancer
Hematuria
Renal papillary necrosis
Hyposthenuria
Splenic infarction
Exertional rhabdomyolysis
Exercise-related sudden death
Protection against severe falciparum malaria
PROBABLE ASSOCIATIONS
Complicated hyphema
Venous thromboembolic events
Fetal loss/demise
Low birthweight
POSSIBLE ASSOCIATIONS
Acute chest syndrome
Asymptomatic bacteriuria in pregnancy
Proliferative retinopathy
UNLIKELY OR UNPROVEN ASSOCIATIONS
Stroke
Cholelithiasis
Priapism
Leg ulcers
Avascular necrosis of the femoral head

From Tsaras G, Owusu-Ansah A, Boateng O, et al: Complications associated with sickle cell trait: a brief narrative review, *Am J Med* 122:507–512, 2009.

456.3 Other Hemoglobinopathies

Michael R. DeBaun, Melissa Frei-Jones, and Elliott Vichinsky

HEMOGLOBIN C

The mutation for Hb C is at the same site as Hb S, with lysine instead of valine substituted for glutamine. In the USA, Hb AC occurs in 1 : 50 and Hb CC occurs in 1 : 5,000 African-Americans. Hb AC is asymptomatic. Hb CC can result in a mild anemia, splenomegaly, and cholelithiasis; rare cases of spontaneous splenic rupture have been reported. Sickling does not occur. This condition is usually diagnosed through newborn screening programs. Hb C crystallizes, disrupting the red cell membrane.

HEMOGLOBIN Eβ

Hb Eβ is the second most common globin mutation worldwide. In California, Hb Eβ-thalassemia is found almost exclusively in Southeast Asians, with a prevalence of 1 : 2,600 births.

HEMOGLOBIN D

At least 16 variants of Hb D exist. Hb D-Punjab (Los Angeles) is a rare hemoglobin that is seen in 1-3% of Western Indians and in some Europeans with Asian Indian ancestry and produces symptoms of sickle cell disease when present in combination with Hb S. Heterozygous Hb D is clinically silent. Homozygous Hb DD produces a mild to moderate anemia with splenomegaly.

456.4 Unstable Hemoglobin Disorders

Michael R. DeBaun, Melissa Frei-Jones, and Elliott Vichinsky

At least 200 rare unstable hemoglobins have been identified; the most common is Hb Köln. Most patients seem to have de novo mutations rather than inherited hemoglobin disorders. Unstable hemoglobins whose mutation causes unstable heme

Table 456-6 NATIONAL ATHLETIC TRAINER'S ASSOCIATION GUIDELINES FOR ATHLETES WITH SICKLE CELL TRAIT

GENERAL RECOMMENDATIONS FOR ATHLETES WITH SICKLE CELL TRAIT
There is no contraindication to participation in sport for the athlete with sickle cell trait.
Red blood cells can sickle during intense exertion, blocking blood vessels and posing a grave risk for athletes with sickle cell trait.
Screening and simple precautions may prevent deaths and help athletes with sickle cell trait thrive in their sport.
Efforts to document newborn screening results should be made during the pre-sports physical exam (PPE).
In the absence of newborn screening results, institutions should carefully weigh the decision to screen based on the potential to provide key clinical information and targeted education that may save lives.
Irrespective of screening, institutions should educate staff, coaches, and athletes on the potentially lethal nature of this condition.
Education and precautions work best when targeted at those athletes who need it most; therefore, institutions should carefully weigh this factor in deciding whether to screen. All told, the case for screening is strong.

SYMPTOMS OF SICKLING COLLAPSE* VERSUS HEAT CRAMPING	
Sickling Collapse	**Heat Cramping**
No prodrome	Prodrome of muscle twinges
Pain is less excruciating	Pain is more excruciating
Sickling players slump to the ground with weak muscles	Athletes stop due to "locked-up" muscles
Athletes with sickling lie fairly still, not yelling in pain, with muscles that look and feel normal	Athletes writhe and yell in pain, with muscles visibly contracted and rock-hard
If caught early, sickling players recover faster	Even with treatment heat cramping has delayed resolution

PREVENTION OF SICKLING COLLAPSE*
Build up slowly in training with paced progressions, allowing longer periods of rest and recovery between repetitions.
Encourage participation in preseason strength and conditioning programs to enhance the preparedness of athletes for performance testing, which should be sports-specific. Athletes with sickle cell trait should be excluded from participation in performance tests such as mile runs, serial sprints, etc., as several deaths have occurred from participation in this setting.
Cessation of activity with onset of symptoms: muscle "cramping," pain, swelling, weakness, tenderness, inability to "catch breath," or fatigue
If sickle-trait athletes can set their own pace, they seem to do fine.
All athletes should participate in a year-round, periodized strength and conditioning program that is consistent with individual needs, goals, abilities, and sport-specific demands. Athletes with sickle cell trait who perform repetitive high speed sprints and/or interval training that induces high levels of lactic acid should be allowed extended recovery between repetitions since this type of conditioning poses special risk to these athletes.
Ambient heat stress, dehydration, asthma, illness, and altitude predispose the athlete with sickle trait to an onset of crisis in physical exertion.
• Adjust work/rest cycles for environmental heat stress • Emphasize hydration • Control asthma • No workout if an athlete with sickle trait is ill • Watch closely the athlete with sickle cell trait who is new to altitude. Modify training and have supplemental oxygen available for competitions.
Educate to create an environment that encourages athletes with sickle cell trait to report any symptoms immediately; any signs or symptoms such as fatigue, difficulty breathing, leg or low back pain, or leg or low back cramping in an athlete with sickle cell trait should be assumed to be sickling.

TREATMENT OF SICKLING COLLAPSE*
Check vital signs.
Administer high-flow oxygen, 15 L/min (if available), with a non-rebreather face mask.
Cool the athlete, if necessary.
If the athlete is obtunded or as vital signs decline, call 911, attach an automated external defibrillator, start an IV, and get the athlete to the hospital fast.
Tell the doctors to expect explosive rhabdomyolysis and grave metabolic complications.
Proactively prepare by having an emergency action plan and appropriate emergency equipment for all practices and competitions.

*Sickling collapse or exertional sickling occurs when sickled red blood cells accumulate in the blood stream during intense exercise and cause ischemic rhabdomyolysis, precipitating severe metabolic consequences.

binding eventually leading to the denaturation of the hemoglobin molecule are the best studied. The denatured hemoglobin can be visualized during severe hemolysis or after splenectomy as Heinz bodies. Unlike the Heinz bodies seen after toxic exposure, in unstable hemoglobins, Heinz bodies are present in reticulocytes and older red cells (Fig. 456-5). Heterozygotes are asymptomatic.

Children with homozygous gene mutations can present in early childhood with anemia and splenomegaly or with unexplained hemolytic anemia. Hemolysis is increased with febrile illness and with the ingestion of oxidant medications (similar to glucose-6-phosphate dehydrogenase [G6PD] deficiency) with some unstable hemoglobins. If the spleen is functional, the blood smear can appear almost normal or have only hypochromasia and basophilic stippling. A diagnosis may be made by demonstrating Heinz bodies, hemoglobin instability, or an abnormal electrophoresis (although some unstable hemoglobins have normal mobility and are not detected on an electrophoresis).

Treatment is supportive. Transfusion may be required during hemolytic episodes in severe cases. Oxidative drugs should be avoided, and folate supplementation should be provided. Splenectomy has been performed, but the complications of splenectomy, including bacterial sepsis and the possibility of developing pulmonary hypertension, should be considered before this therapy.

456.5 Abnormal Hemoglobins with Increased Oxygen Affinity

Michael R. DeBaun, Melissa Frei-Jones, and Elliott Vichinsky

More than 110 high-affinity hemoglobins have been characterized. These mutations affect the state of hemoglobin configuration during oxygenation and deoxygenation. Hemoglobin changes structure when in the oxygenated versus the deoxygenated state. The deoxygenated state is termed the T (tense) state and is stabilized by 2,3-diphosphoglycerate (2,3-DPG). When fully oxygenated, hemoglobin assumes the R (relaxed) state. The exact molecular interactions between these 2 states are not known. High-affinity hemoglobins contain mutations that either stabilize the R form or destabilize the T form. The interactions between these 2 forms are complex, and the mechanisms of the mutations are not known. In most cases, the high-affinity hemoglobins can be identified by hemoglobin analysis; about 20% must be characterized under controlled conditions of measurements of the P_{50}, which are 9-21 mm Hg (normal: 23-29 mm Hg). The decrease in P_{50} causes most of these hemoglobins to produce an erythrocytosis with hemoglobin levels of 17-20 g/dL. Levels of erythropoietin and 2,3-DPG are normal. Patients are usually asymptomatic and do not need phlebotomy. If phlebotomy is performed, oxygen delivery could be problematic owing to a lowered hemoglobin.

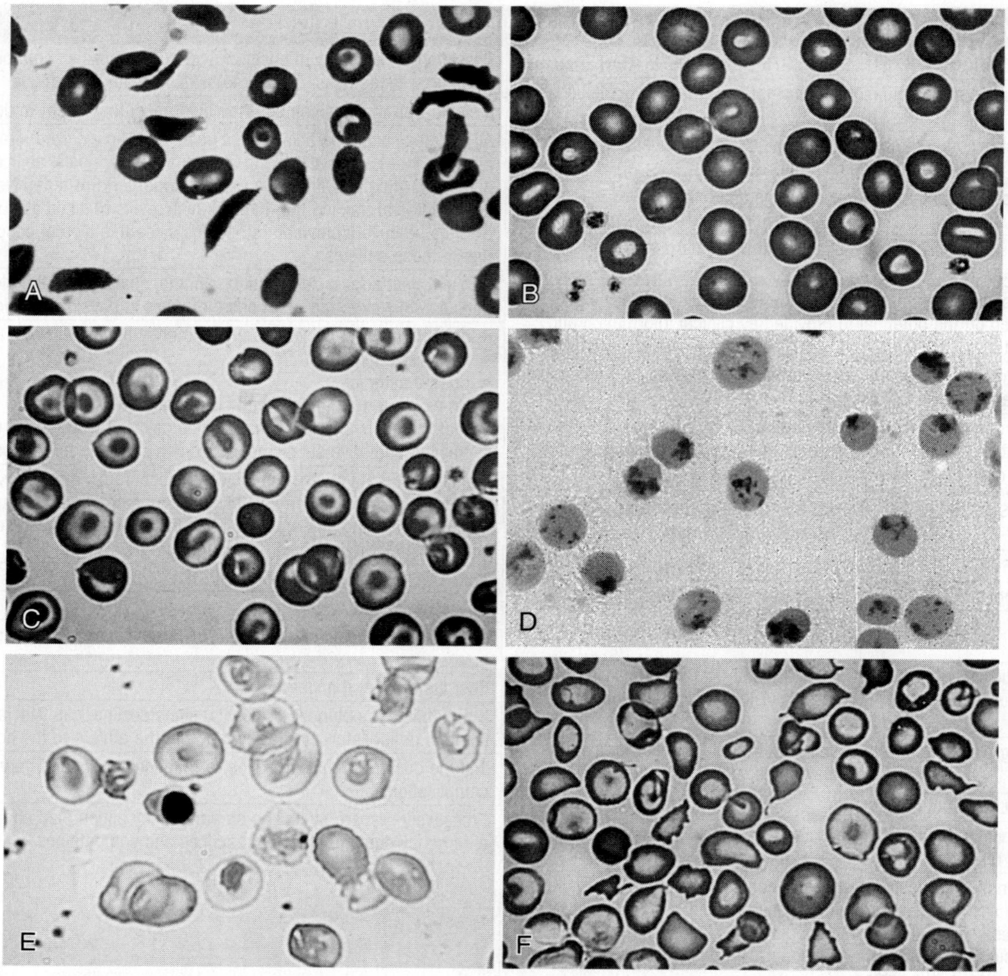

Figure 456-5 Red blood cell (RBC) morphology associated with hemoglobin disorders. *A,* Sickle cell anemia (Hb SS): target cells and fixed (irreversibly sickled) cells. *B,* Sickle cell trait (Hb AS): normal RBC morphology. *C,* Hemoglobin CC: target cells and occasional spherocytes. *D,* Congenital Heinz body anemia (unstable hemoglobin): RBCs stained with supravital stain (brilliant cresyl blue) reveal intracellular inclusions. *E,* Homozygous β^0-thalassemia: severe hypochromia with deformed RBCs and normoblasts. *F,* Hemoglobin H disease (α-thalassemia): anisopoikilocytosis with target cells. (Courtesy of Dr. John Bolles, The ASH Collection, University of Washington, Seattle.)

456.6 Abnormal Hemoglobins Causing Cyanosis

Michael R. DeBaun, Melissa Frei-Jones, and Elliott Vichinsky

Abnormal hemoglobins causing cyanosis are rare. The major group is the M hemoglobins, of which there are seven. Hb M variants have mutations in either the α or the β chain, confined to the heme pocket of the hemoglobin molecule. Six of the seven have a tyrosine residue that covalently binds to the heme iron, stabilizing it in the oxidized form. These unstable hemoglobins lead to a hemolytic anemia, most pronounced in the β forms. Clinically, these children are cyanotic from birth without other signs or symptoms of disease if the tyrosine is on the α chain (Hb M Boston, Hb M Iwate). Infants with β-chain mutations become cyanotic later in infancy owing to the fetal hemoglobin switch (Hb M Saskatoon, Hb M Hyde Park, Hb M Milwaukee). The abnormal hemoglobins are autosomal dominant and are diagnosed by hemoglobin analysis using special techniques and HPLC. There is no specific treatment. Children with the β form should avoid oxidant drugs.

Low-affinity hemoglobins have less cyanosis than the M hemoglobins. The amino acid substitutions destabilize the oxyhemoglobin and lead to decreased oxygen saturation. The best characterized are Hb Kansas and Hb Beth Israel.

456.7 Hereditary Methemoglobinemia

Michael R. DeBaun, Melissa Frei-Jones, and Elliott Vichinsky

The iron molecule in hemoglobin is normally in the ferrous state (Fe^{2+}), which is essential for its oxygen-transporting function. Under physiologic conditions there is a slow, constant loss of electrons to released oxygen, and the ferric (Fe^{3+}) form combines with water, producing methemoglobin (MetHb). The predominant intracellular mechanism for the reduction of MetHb is cytochrome 5b. This mechanism is >100-fold more efficient than the production of MetHb, and only 1% of hemoglobin is in the ferric state normally.

MetHb may be increased in the red cell owing to exposure to toxic substances or to absence of reductive pathways, such as NADH-cytochrome b5 reductase deficiency. Toxic methemoglobinemia is much more common than hereditary methemoglobinemia (Table 456-7). Infants are particularly vulnerable to hemoglobin oxidation because their RBCs have half the amount of cytochrome b5 reductase seen in adults; fetal hemoglobin is more susceptible to oxidation than hemoglobin A; and the more alkaline infant gastrointestinal tract promotes the growth of nitrite-producing gram-negative bacteria. When MetHb levels are >1.5 g/24 hr, cyanosis is visible (15% MetHb); a level of 70% MetHb is lethal. The level is usually reported as a percentage of normal hemoglobin, and the toxic level is lower at a lower

Table 456-7 KNOWN ETIOLOGIES OF ACQUIRED METHEMOGLOBINEMIA

MEDICATIONS
Benzocaine Chloroquine Dapsone EMLA (eutectic mixture of local anesthetics) topical anesthetic (lidocaine 2.5% and prilocaine 2.5%) Flutamide Lidocaine Metoclopramide Nitrates Nitric oxide Nitroglycerin Nitroprusside Nitrous oxide Phenazopyridine Prilocaine Primaquine Riluzole Silver nitrate Sodium nitrate Sulfonamides
MEDICAL CONDITIONS
Pediatric gastrointestinal infection, sepsis Recreational drug overdose with amyl nitrate ("poppers") Sickle cell disease-related painful episode
MISCELLANEOUS
Aniline dyes Fume inhalation (automobile exhaust, burning of wood and plastics) Herbicides Industrial chemicals: nitrobenzene, nitroethane (found in nail polish, resins, rubber adhesives) Pesticides Gasoline octane booster

From Ash-Bernal R, Wise R, Wright SM: Acquired methemoglobinemia, *Medicine* 83:265–273, 2004.

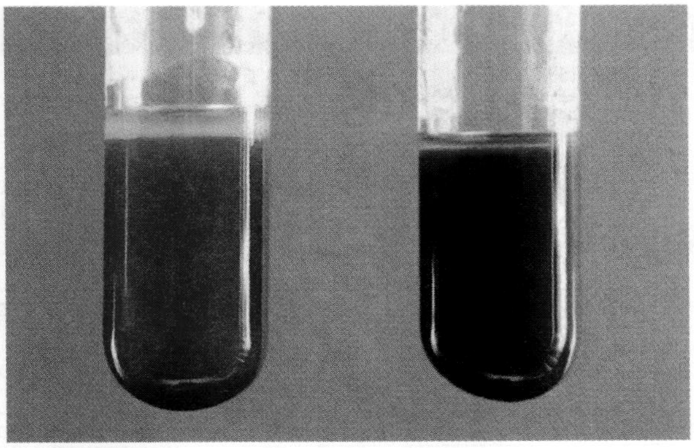

Figure 456-6 Normal arterial blood vs methemoglobulinemia. Arterial whole blood with 1% methemoglobin *(left)* vs arterial whole blood with 72% methemoglobin *(right)*. Note the characteristic chocolate-brown color of the sample with an elevated methemoglobin level. Both samples were briefly exposed to 100% oxygen and shaken. This quick analysis is a good bedside test for methemoglobulinemia. The sample on the *left* turned bright red, whereas the sample on the *right* remained chocolate-brown. Methods: Whole blood samples were drawn at the same time from the same person. The measured hemoglobin concentration was 11.7 g/dL. Calculated concentration of methemoglobin: $11.7\ g/dL \times 0.01 = 0.117\ g/dL$ *(left)* and $11.7\ g/dL \times 0.72 = 8.42\ g/dL$ *(right)*. An elevated methemoglobin level was made in vitro by adding 0.1 mL of a 0.144 molar solution of sodium nitrate *(right)*, and 0.1 mL of normal saline was added as a control *(left)*. Co-oximetry measurements were taken on both samples shortly after the blood was drawn and 20 min after the addition of sodium nitrate solution. Both blood samples were exposed to 100% oxygen before the 2nd measurement. (Protocol based on personal communication with Dr. Ali Mansouri, December 2002.)

hemoglobin level. Methemoglobinemia has been described in infants who ingested foods and water high in nitrates, who were exposed to aniline teething gels or other chemicals, and in some infants with severe gastroenteritis and acidosis. Methemoglobin can color the blood brown (Fig. 456-6).

HEREDITARY METHEMOGLOBINEMIA WITH DEFICIENCY OF NADH CYTOCHROME B5 REDUCTASE

Hereditary methemoglobinemia with deficiency of NADH cytochrome b5 reductase is a group of rare disorders classified into 4 types. In type I, the most common form, the deficiency of NADH cytochrome b5 activity is found only in RBCs. In type II, the enzyme deficiency is present in all tissues and therefore has more significant symptoms beginning in infancy with encephalopathy, mental retardation, spasticity, microcephaly, and growth retardation. In type III, the deficiency occurs in leukocytes, platelets, and RBCs. In type IV, deficiency is localized to only RBC cytochrome b5.

Clinically, cyanosis varies in intensity with season and diet. Methemoglobin can color the blood brown (see Fig. 456-6). The time at onset of cyanosis also varies; in some patients it appears at birth, in others as late as adolescence. Although as much as 50% of the total circulating hemoglobin may be in the form of nonfunctional methemoglobin, little or no cardiorespiratory distress occurs in these patients, except on exertion.

Daily oral treatment with ascorbic acid (200-500 mg/day in divided doses) gradually reduces the methemoglobin to about 10% of the total pigment and alleviates the cyanosis as long as therapy is continued. Chronic high doses of ascorbic acid have been associated with hyperoxaluria and renal stone formation. Ascorbic acid should not be used to treat toxic methemoglobinemia. When immediately available, poison control should be contacted to verify the most up-to-date therapeutic strategies. Methylene blue given IV (1-2 mg/kg initially) is used to treat toxic methemoglobinemia. An oral dose can be administered (100-300 mg PO per day) as maintenance therapy.

Methylene blue should not be used in patients with G6PD deficiency. This treatment is ineffective and can cause severe oxidative hemolysis. In the event that methylene blue is given to a patient that has G6PD deficiency, there will be no change in the clinical status of the patient. Given the observation that G6PD deficiency status is rarely available at the time of treatment, a careful history should be elicited. When the history is negative for symptoms of G6PD deficiency, treatment should be initiated judiciously, and the patient should be evaluated for improvement shortly afterward.

BIBLIOGRAPHY

Please visit the Nelson Textbook of Pediatrics *website at* *www.expertconsult.com* *for the complete bibliography.*

456.8 Syndromes of Hereditary Persistence of Fetal Hemoglobin

Michael R. DeBaun, Melissa Frei-Jones, and Elliott Vichinsky

HPFH syndromes are a form of thalassemia; mutations are associated with a decrease in the production of either or both β- and δ-globins. There is an imbalance in the α:non-α synthetic ratio (Chapter 456.9) characteristic of thalassemia. More than 20 variants of HPFH have been described. They are deletional, $\delta\beta^0$ (Black, Ghanaian, Italian), nondeletional (Tunisian, Japanese, Australian), linked to the β-globin-gene cluster (British, Italian-Chinese, Black), or unlinked to the β-globin-gene cluster (Atlanta, Czech, Seattle). The $\delta\beta^0$ forms have deletions of the entire δ- and β-gene sequences, and the most common form in the United States is the Black (HPFH 1) variant. As a result of the δ and β gene deletions, there is production only of γ-globin and formation

Table 456-8 THE THALASSEMIAS

THALASSEMIA	GLOBIN GENOTYPE	FEATURES	EXPRESSION	HEMOGLOBIN ANALYSIS
α-THALASSEMIA				
1 gene deletion	-,α/α,α	Normal	Normal	Newborn: Bart's 1-2%
2 gene deletion trait	-,α/-,α -, -/α,α	Microcytosis, mild hypochromasia	Normal, mild anemia	Newborn: Bart's: 5-10%
3 gene deletion hemoglobin H	-,-/-,α	Microcytosis, hypochromic	Mild anemia, transfusions not required	Newborn: Bart's: 20-30%
2 gene deletion + Constant Spring	$-,-/\alpha,\alpha^{\text{Constant Spring}}$	Microcytosis, hypochromic	Moderate to severe anemia, transfusion, splenectomy.	2-3% Constant Spring, 10-15% hemoglobin H
4 gene deletion	-,-/-,-	Anisocytosis, poikilocytosis	Hydrops fetalis	Newborn: 89-90% Bart's with Gower 1 and 2 and Portland
Nondeletional	$\alpha,\alpha/\alpha,\alpha^{\text{variant}}$	Microcytosis, mild anemia	Normal	1-2% variant hemoglobin
β-THALASSEMIA				
β^0 or β^+ heterozygote: trait	$\beta^0/A,\beta^+/A$	Variable microcytosis	Normal	Elevated A_2, variable elevation of F
β^0-Thalassemia	β^0/β^0, β^+/β^0, E/β^0	Microcytosis, nucleated RCB	Transfusion dependent	F 98% and A_2 2% E 30-40%
β^+-Thalassemia severe	β^+/β^+	Microcytosis nucleated RBC	Transfusion dependent/ thalassemia intermedia	F 70-95%, A_2 2%, trace A
Silent	β^+/A	Microcytosis	Normal with only microcytosis	A_2 3.3-3.5%
β^+/β^+	Hypochromic, microcytosis	Mild to moderate anemia	A_2 2-5%, F 10-30%	
Dominant (rare)	B^0/A	Microcytosis, abnormal RBCs	Moderately severe anemia, splenomegaly	Elevated F and A_2
δ-Thalassemia	A/A	Normal	Normal	A_2 absent
$(\delta\beta)^0$-Thalassemia	$(\delta\beta)^0/A$	Hypochromic	Mild anemia	F 5-20%
$(\delta\beta)^+$-Thalassemia Lepore	β^{Lepore}/A	Microcytosis	Mild anemia	Lepore 8-20%
Lepore	$\beta^{\text{Lepore}}/\beta^{\text{Lepore}}$	Microcytic, hypochromic	Thalassemia intermedia	F 80%, Lepore 20%
γδβ-Thalassemia	$(\gamma^A\delta\beta)^{0/}A$	Microcytosis,microcytic, hypochromic	Moderate anemia, Splenomegaly, Homozygote: thalassemia intermedia	Decreased F and A2 compared with δβ-thalassemia
γ-Thalassemia	$(\gamma^A\gamma^G)^0/A$	Microcytosis	Insignificant unless homozygote	Decreased F
HEREDITARY PERSISTENCE OF FETAL HEMOGLOBIN				
Deletional	A/A	Microcytic	Mild anemia	F 100% homozygotes
Nondeletional	A/A	Normal	Normal	F 20-40%

of Hb F. In the homozygous form, no manifestations of thalassemia are present. There is only Hb F with very mild anemia and slight microcytosis. When inherited with other variant hemoglobins, Hb F is elevated into the 20-30% range; when inherited with Hb S, there is an amelioration of sickle cell disease with fewer complications.

456.9 Thalassemia Syndromes

Michael R. DeBaun, Melissa Frei-Jones, and Elliott Vichinsky

Thalassemia refers to genetic disorders in globin chain production. In individuals with beta thalassemia, there is either a complete absence of β globin production (β-thalassemia major) or a partial reduction in β globin production (β thalassemia minor). In alpha thalassemia, there is an absence of or partial reduction in α globin production. The primary pathology in thalassemia stems from the quantity of globin production, whereas the primary pathology in sickle cell disease is related to the quality of globin produced.

EPIDEMIOLOGY

There are >200 mutations for β-thalassemia, although most are rare. About 20 common alleles constitute 80% of the known thalassemias worldwide; 3% of the world's population carry genes for β-thalassemia, and in Southeast Asia 5-10% of the population carry genes for α-thalassemia. In a particular region, there are fewer common alleles. In the United States, an estimated 2,000 persons have β-thalassemia.

PATHOPHYSIOLOGY

Two related features contribute to the sequelae of β-thalassemia: inadequate β-globin gene production leading to decreased levels of normal hemoglobin (Hb A) and unbalanced α- and β-globin chain production. Selected features of thalassemia can be seen in Table 456-8. In the bone marrow, thalassemia mutations disrupt the maturation of erythrocytes, resulting in ineffective erythropoiesis; the marrow is hyperactive, but there are relatively few reticulocytes and severe anemia exists. In β-thalassemia, there is an excess of α-globin chains relative to β- and γ-globin chains, and α-globin tetramers (α_4) are formed. These inclusions interact with the red cell membrane and shorten red cell survival, leading to anemia and increased erythroid production. The γ-globin chains are produced in increased amounts, leading to an elevated Hb F ($\alpha_2\gamma_2$). The δ-globin chains are also produced in increased amounts, leading to an elevated Hb A_2 ($\alpha_2\delta_2$) in β-thalassemia.

In α-thalassemia there are relatively fewer α-globin chains and an excess of β- and γ-globin chains. These excess chains form Bart's hemoglobin (γ_4) in fetal life and Hb H (β_4) after birth. These abnormal tetramers are not lethal but lead to extravascular hemolysis. Prenatally a fetus with α-thalassemia can become symptomatic because Hb F requires sufficient of α-globin gene production, whereas postnatally infants with β-thalassemia become symptomatic because Hb A requires sufficient production of β-globin genes.

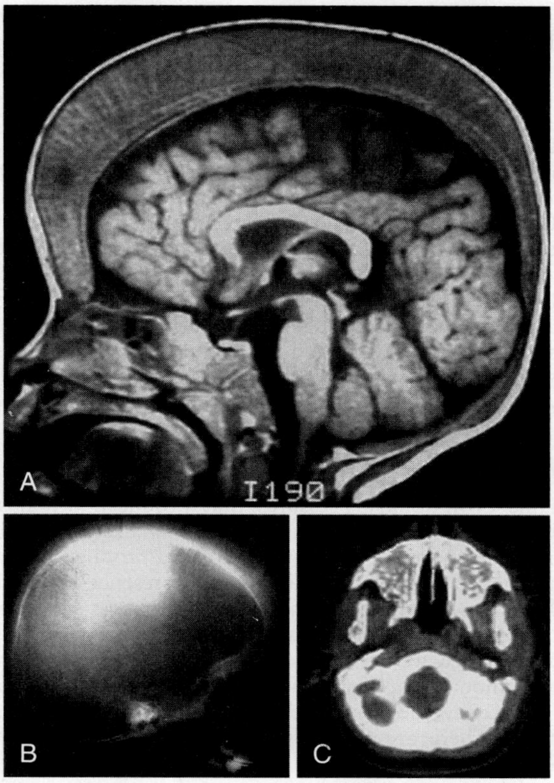

Figure 456-7 Ineffective erythropoiesis in a 3 yr old patient who has thalassemia major and has not received a transfusion. *A,* Massive widening of the diploic spaces of the skull as seen on MRI. *B,* Radiographic appearance of the trabeculae as seen on plain radiograph. *C,* Obliteration of the maxillary sinuses with hematopoietic tissue as seen on CT scan.

HOMOZYGOUS β-THALASSEMIA (THALASSEMIA MAJOR, COOLEY ANEMIA)

Clinical Manifestations

If not treated, children with β-thalassemia usually become symptomatic from progressive hemolytic anemia, with profound weakness and cardiac decompensation during the 2nd 6 mo of life. Depending on the mutation and degree of fetal hemoglobin production, transfusions in β-thalassemia major are necessary beginning in the 2nd mo to 2nd yr of life, but rarely later. The decision to transfuse depends on the child's ability to compensate for the degree of anemia.

Most infants and children have cardiac decompensation at hemoglobins of 4 g/dL or less. Generally, fatigue, poor appetite, and lethargy are late findings of severe anemia in an infant or child and were more common before transfusions were standard therapy. The classic presentation of children with severe disease includes thalassemic facies (maxilla hyperplasia, flat nasal bridge, frontal bossing), pathologic bone fractures, marked hepatosplenomegaly, and cachexia and is now primarily seen in developing countries. The spleen can become so enlarged that it causes mechanical discomfort and secondary hypersplenism. The features of ineffective erythropoiesis include expanded medullary spaces (with massive expansion of the marrow of the face and skull producing the characteristic thalassemic facies), extramedullary hematopoiesis, and higher metabolic needs (Fig. 456-7). The hepatosplenomegaly can interfere with nutritional support. Pallor, hemosiderosis, and jaundice can combine to produce a greenish brown complexion.

The chronic anemia produces an increase in iron absorption from the gastrointestinal tract, with toxicity leading to further complications. Many of these features become less severe and infrequent with transfusion therapy, but excessive iron stores associated with transfusional iron overload is a major concern in patients with β-thalassemia. Many of the complications of thalassemia seen in developed countries today are the result of increased iron deposition. Most of these complications can be avoided by the consistent use of an iron chelator. However, chelation therapy also has associated complications, including hearing loss, peripheral neuropathy, and poor growth.

Endocrine and cardiac pathology are often associated with excessive iron stores in patients with β-thalassemia major who are chronically transfused. Endocrine dysfunction can include hypothyroidism, hypogonadotrophic gonadism, growth hormone deficiency, hypoparathyroidism, and diabetes mellitus. Congestive heart failure and cardiac arrhythmias are potentially lethal complications of excessive iron stores in children with thalassemia.

Laboratory Findings

The infant is born only with Hb F or, in some cases, Hb F and Hb E (heterozygosity for β-thalassemia zero). Eventually, there is severe anemia, reticulocytopenia, numerous nucleated erythrocytes, and microcytosis with almost no normal-appearing erythrocytes on the peripheral smear (see Fig. 456-5E). The hemoglobin level falls progressively to <5 g/dL unless transfusions are given. The reticulocyte count is commonly <8% and is inappropriately low when compared to the degree of anemia due to ineffective erythropoiesis. The unconjugated serum bilirubin level is usually elevated, but other chemistries may be normal at an early stage. Even if the child does not receive transfusions, eventually there is iron accumulation with elevated serum ferritin and transferrin saturation. Bone marrow hyperplasia can be seen on radiographs (see Fig. 456-7).

Treatment

Before initiating chronic transfusions, the diagnosis of β-thalassemia major should be confirmed and the parents counseled concerning this life-long therapy. Beginning transfusion and chelation therapy are difficult challenges for parents to face early in their child's life. Before beginning transfusion therapy, a red-cell phenotype is obtained; blood products that are leukoreduced and phenotypically matched for the Rh and Kell antigens are required for transfusion. If a bone marrow transplant is a possibility, the blood for transfusion should be negative for cytomegalovirus unless the child has had a previous cytomegalovirus infection. Transfusion therapy promotes general health and well-being and avoids the consequences of ineffective erythropoiesis. A transfusion program generally requires monthly transfusions, with the pretransfusion hemoglobin level between 9.5 and 10.5 g/dL. In patients with cardiac disease, higher pretransfusion hemoglobin levels may be beneficial. Some blood centers have donor programs, pairing donors and recipients, which decreases the exposure to multiple red cell antigens.

Excessive iron stores from transfusion cause many of the complications of β-thalassemia major. Accurate assessment of excessive iron stores is essential to optimal therapy. The serum ferritin is useful in assessing iron balance trends but does not accurately predict quantitative iron stores. Undertreatment or overtreatment of presumed excessive iron stores can occur in managing a patient based on serum ferritin alone. Quantitative iron by liver biopsy is the standard method for accurately determining iron store for patients. T2* MRI software is now being used to estimate iron stores in the liver and heart among patients with β-thalassemia major. One reason for the preference of T2* MRI over liver biopsy is that liver iron stores might not accurately reflect cumulative changes in cardiac iron. Patients can have cardiac iron overload at the time of a safe liver iron measurement. Many thalassemia centers now monitor cardiac iron with T2* MRI imaging.

Excessive iron stores can be prevented by the use of deferoxamine (Desferal) or deferasirox (Exjade). Deferoxamine chelates iron and some other divalent cations, allowing their excretion in the urine and the stool. Deferoxamine is given subcutaneously over 10-12 hr, 5-6 days a week. The side effects include ototoxicity with high-frequency hearing loss, retinal changes, and bone dysplasia with truncal shortening. The number of hours that deferoxamine is used daily is more important than the daily dosage. High dose, short-term infusions increase toxicity with little efficacy. Plasma non–transferrin bound iron (NTBI) is most likely responsible for serious iron injury. When deferoxamine is infusing, it binds NTBI. When deferoxamine is stopped, there are rebound increases in NTBI levels and risk for injury. In patients with excessive iron stores in the heart resulting in symptomatic congestive heart failure, 24-hr deferoxamine has been shown to reverse cardiomyopathy.

The oral iron chelator deferasirox (Exjade) is commercially available in the United States. For many patients and families, deferasirox has replaced deferoxamine because the latter must be given subcutaneously for 10 hr a night, typically 5 of 7 nights a week. Although the optimal dose of deferasirox is well defined, some patients have a less-than-expected response to the maximum approved doses (30 mg/kg/day). The optimal dose beyond 30 mg/kg/day is not known, but it should be evaluated carefully if evidence of a positive iron balance continues to occur while the patient is adherent to the medication.

Hematopoietic stem cell transplantation has cured >1,000 patients who have β-thalassemia major. Most success has been in children younger than 15 yr of age without excessive iron stores and hepatomegaly who undergo sibling HLA-matched allogeneic transplantation. All children who have an HLA-matched sibling should be offered the option of bone marrow transplantation.

OTHER β-THALASSEMIA SYNDROMES

The β-thalassemia syndromes are broken into six groups: β-thalassemia, δβ-thalassemias, γ-thalassemias, δ-thalassemias, εγδβ-thalassemias, and the HPFH syndrome. Most of these thalassemias are relatively rare, some being found only in family groups. The β-thalassemias can also be classified clinically as thalassemia trait, minima, minor, intermedia, and major, reflecting the degree of anemia. The genetic classification does not necessarily define the phenotype, and the degree of anemia does not always predict the genetic classification.

Thalassemia intermedia can be any combination of β-thalassemia mutations (β^0/β^+, $\beta^0/\beta^{variant}$, E/β^0), which will lead to a phenotype of microcytic anemia with hemoglobin of about 7 g/dL. There is controversy about whether these children should receive transfusions. They will certainly develop a degree of medullary hyperplasia, nutritional hemosiderosis perhaps requiring chelation, splenomegaly, and other complications of β-thalassemia associated with excessive iron stores. Extramedullary hematopoiesis can occur in the vertebral canal, compressing the spinal cord and causing neurologic symptoms; the latter is a medical emergency requiring immediate local radiation therapy to halt erythropoiesis. Transfusion alleviates the thalassemic manifestations; the decision to transfuse must be balanced against the future need for chelation therapy.

Splenectomy may be indicated for patients with thalassemia intermedia who have a falling steady-state hemoglobin and for transfused patients with rising transfusion requirements. However, splenectomy can have serious consequences, including infection, pulmonary hypertension, and thrombosis. All patients should be fully immunized against encapsulated bacteria before splenectomy and subsequently should be on long-term penicillin prophylaxis with appropriate instructions regarding fever management.

The thalassemias classified as minima and minor are usually heterozygotes (β^0/β, β^+/β^+), having a phenotype more severe than trait but not as severe as intermedia. These children should be investigated for their genotype and monitored for iron accumulation. The β-thalassemias are influenced by the presence of α-thalassemia: α-thalassemia trait leading to less severe anemia and duplicated α genes (ααα/αα) leading to a more severe thalassemia. Often, patients who are in these groups require transfusions in adolescence or adulthood; some may be candidates for chemotherapy such as hydroxyurea.

Thalassemia trait is often misdiagnosed as iron deficiency in children because the 2 produce similar hematologic abnormalities on CBC, and iron deficiency is much more prevalent. A short course of iron and re-evaluation is all that is required to identify children who will need further evaluation. Children who have β-thalassemia trait have a persistently normal red cell distribution width and low mean corpuscular volume (MCV). On hemoglobin analysis, they have an elevated Hb F and diagnostically elevated Hb A_2. There are "silent" forms of β-thalassemia trait, and if the family history is suggestive, further studies may be indicated.

α-THALASSEMIA

The same evolutionary pressures that produced β-thalassemia and sickle cell disease produced α-thalassemia. Infants are identified in the newborn period by the increased production of Bart's hemoglobin (γ_4) during fetal life and its presence at birth. The α-thalassemias occur most commonly in Southeast Asia. Deletion mutations are common in α-thalassemia. In addition to deletional mutations, there are nondeletional α-globin gene mutations, the most common being Constant Spring ($\alpha^{CS}\alpha$); these mutations cause a more severe anemia and clinical course than the deletional mutations. There are four α-globin genes and four deletional α-thalassemia phenotypes.

The deletion of one α-globin gene (silent trait) is not identifiable hematologically. Specifically, no alterations are noted in the mean corpuscular volume (MCV) and mean corpuscular hemoglobin (MCH). Persons with this deletion are usually diagnosed after the birth of a child with a 2-gene deletion or Hb H (β_4). During the newborn period, <3% Hb Bart's is observed. The deletion of one α-globin gene is common in African-Americans.

The deletion of 2 α-globin genes results in α-thalassemia trait. The α-globin genes can be lost in a *trans*-(−α/−α) or *cis*- ($\alpha,\alpha/^{-SEA}$) configuration. The *trans* or *cis* mutations can combine with other mutations and lead to Hb H or α-thalassemia major. In persons from Africa or of African descent the most common α-globin gene deletion is in the *trans* configuration, whereas in persons from Asia or the Mediterranean region the *cis* deletion is most common.

The α-thalassemia traits manifest as a microcytic anemia that can be mistaken for iron-deficiency anemia (see Fig. 456-5F). The hemoglobin analysis is normal, except during the newborn period, when Hb Bart's is commonly <8% but >3%. Children with a deletion of 2 α-globin genes are commonly thought to have iron deficiency, given the presence of both low MCV and MCH. The simplest approach to distinguish between iron deficiency and α-thalassemia trait is with a good dietary history. Children with iron-deficiency anemia often have a diet that is low in iron. Alternatively, a brief course of iron supplementation along with monitoring of erythrocyte parameters might confirm the diagnosis of iron deficiency, or α-globin gene deletion analysis may be necessary.

The deletion of three α-globin genes leads to the diagnosis of Hb H disease. In California, where a large population of Asians resides, ~1 : 15,000 newborns have Hb H disease. The simplest manner of diagnosing Hb H disease is during the newborn period, when excess in γ-tetramers are present and Hb Bart's is commonly >25%. Obtaining supporting evidence from the parents is also necessary. Later in childhood, there is an excess in β-globin chain tetramers that results in Hb H. A definitive diagnosis of Hb H disease requires DNA analysis with supporting evidence. Brilliant cresyl blue can stain Hb H, but it is rarely used for diagnosis. Patients with Hb H disease have a marked microcytosis, anemia, mild splenomegaly, and, occasionally, scleral icterus or cholelithiasis. Transfusion is not commonly used for therapy because the range of hemoglobin is 7-11 g/dL, with MCV 51-73 fl.

The deletion of all four α-globin genes causes profound anemia during fetal life, resulting in hydrops fetalis; the ζ-globin gene must be present for fetal survival. There are no normal hemoglobins present at birth (primarily Hb Bart's, with Hb Gower 1, Gower 2, and Portland). If the fetus survives, immediate exchange transfusion is indicated. These infants with α-thalassemia major are transfusion dependent, and hematopoietic stem cell transplant is the only cure.

The presence of a nondeletional α-globin mutation with a 2-gene deletion results in a more severe anemia, increased hepatosplenomegaly, increased jaundice, and a much more severe clinical course than Hb H disease. Hb H Constant Spring is the most common form ($-\alpha/\alpha,\alpha^{CS}$).

Treatment of the α-thalassemia deletion syndromes consists of folate supplementation, possible splenectomy (with the attendant risks), intermittent transfusion during severe anemia for the nondeletional Hb H diseases, and chronic transfusion therapy or bone marrow transplant for survivors of hydrops fetalis. These children also should not be exposed to oxidative medications.

BIBLIOGRAPHY

Please visit the Nelson Textbook of Pediatrics *website at www.expertconsult.com for the complete bibliography.*

Chapter 457 Enzymatic Defects

457.1 Pyruvate Kinase Deficiency

George B. Segel

Congenital hemolytic anemia occurs in persons homozygous or compound heterozygous for autosomal recessive genes that cause either a marked reduction in red blood cell (RBC) pyruvate kinase (PK) or production of an abnormal enzyme with decreased activity. Generation of adenosine triphosphate (ATP) within RBCs is impaired, and low levels of ATP, pyruvate, and the oxidized form of nicotinamide adenine dinucleotide (NAD^+) are found (Fig. 457-1). The concentration of 2,3-diphosphoglycerate is increased; this isomer is beneficial in facilitating oxygen release from hemoglobin but detrimental in inhibiting hexokinase and enzymes of the hexose monophosphate shunt. In addition, an unexplained decrease occurs in the sum of the adenine (ATP, adenosine diphosphate, and adenosine monophosphate) and pyridine (NAD^+ and the reduced form of NAD) nucleotides, further impairing glycolysis. As a consequence of decreased ATP, RBCs cannot maintain their potassium and water content; the cells become rigid, and their life span is considerably reduced.

ETIOLOGY

There are 2 mammalian PK genes, but only the *PKLR* gene is expressed in red cells. The human *PKLR* gene is located on chromosome 1q21. More than 180 mutations are reported in this structural gene, which codes for a 574–amino acid protein that forms a functional tetramer. These mutations include missense, splice site, and insertion-deletion alterations. Most affected patients are compound heterozygotes for 2 different PK gene defects. The many possible combinations likely account for the variability in clinical severity. The mutations 1456 C to T and 1529 G to A are the most common mutations in the white population.

CLINICAL MANIFESTATIONS AND LABORATORY FINDINGS

The clinical manifestations of PK deficiency vary from severe neonatal hemolytic anemia to mild, well-compensated hemolysis first noted in adulthood. Severe jaundice and anemia may occur in the neonatal period, and kernicterus has been reported. The hemolysis in older children and adults varies in severity, with hemoglobin values ranging from 8 to 12 g/dL associated with some pallor, jaundice, and splenomegaly. Patients with these findings usually do not require transfusion. A severe form of the disease has a relatively high incidence among the Amish of the Midwestern United States. PK deficiency may provide protection against falciparum malaria; there is no demographic support for this observation, however.

Polychromatophilia and mild macrocytosis reflect the elevated reticulocyte count. Spherocytes are uncommon, but a few spiculated pyknocytes may be found. The non-incubated osmotic fragility is normal. Diagnosis relies on demonstration of a marked reduction of RBC PK activity or an increase in the Michaelis-Menten dissociation constant (K_m) for its substrate, phosphoenolpyruvate (high K_m variant). Other RBC enzyme activity is normal or elevated, reflecting the reticulocytosis. No abnormalities of hemoglobin are noted. The white cells have normal PK activity and must be rigorously excluded from the red cell hemolysates used to measure PK activity. Heterozygous carriers usually have moderately reduced levels of PK activity.

TREATMENT

Phototherapy and exchange transfusions may be indicated for hyperbilirubinemia in newborns. Transfusions of packed RBCs are necessary for severe anemia or for aplastic crises. If the anemia is consistently severe or if frequent transfusions are required, splenectomy should be performed after the child is 5-6 yr of age. Although it is not curative, splenectomy may be followed by higher hemoglobin levels and by strikingly high (30-60%) reticulocyte counts. Death resulting from overwhelming pneumococcal sepsis has followed splenectomy; thus, immunization with vaccines for encapsulated organisms should be given before splenectomy, and prophylactic penicillin should be administered after the procedure.

457.2 Other Glycolytic Enzyme Deficiencies

George B. Segel

Chronic nonspherocytic hemolytic anemias of varying severity have been associated with deficiencies of other enzymes in the glycolytic pathway, including hexokinase, glucose phosphate isomerase, and aldolase, which are inherited as autosomal recessive disorders. **Phosphofructokinase deficiency,** which occurs primarily in Ashkenazi Jews in the USA, results in hemolysis associated with a myopathy classified as glycogen storage disease type VII (Chapter 81.1). Clinically, hemolytic anemia is complicated by muscle weakness, exercise intolerance, cramps, and possibly myoglobinuria. Enzyme assays for phosphofructokinase yield low values for RBCs and muscle.

Triose phosphate isomerase (TPI) deficiency is an autosomal recessive disorder affecting many systems. Affected patients have hemolytic anemia, cardiac abnormalities, and lower motor neuron and pyramidal tract impairment, with or without evidence of cerebral impairment. They usually die in early childhood. The gene for TPI has been cloned and sequenced and is located on chromosome 12.

Phosphoglycerate kinase (PGK) is the first ATP-generating step in glycolysis. At least 23 kindreds with PGK deficiency have been

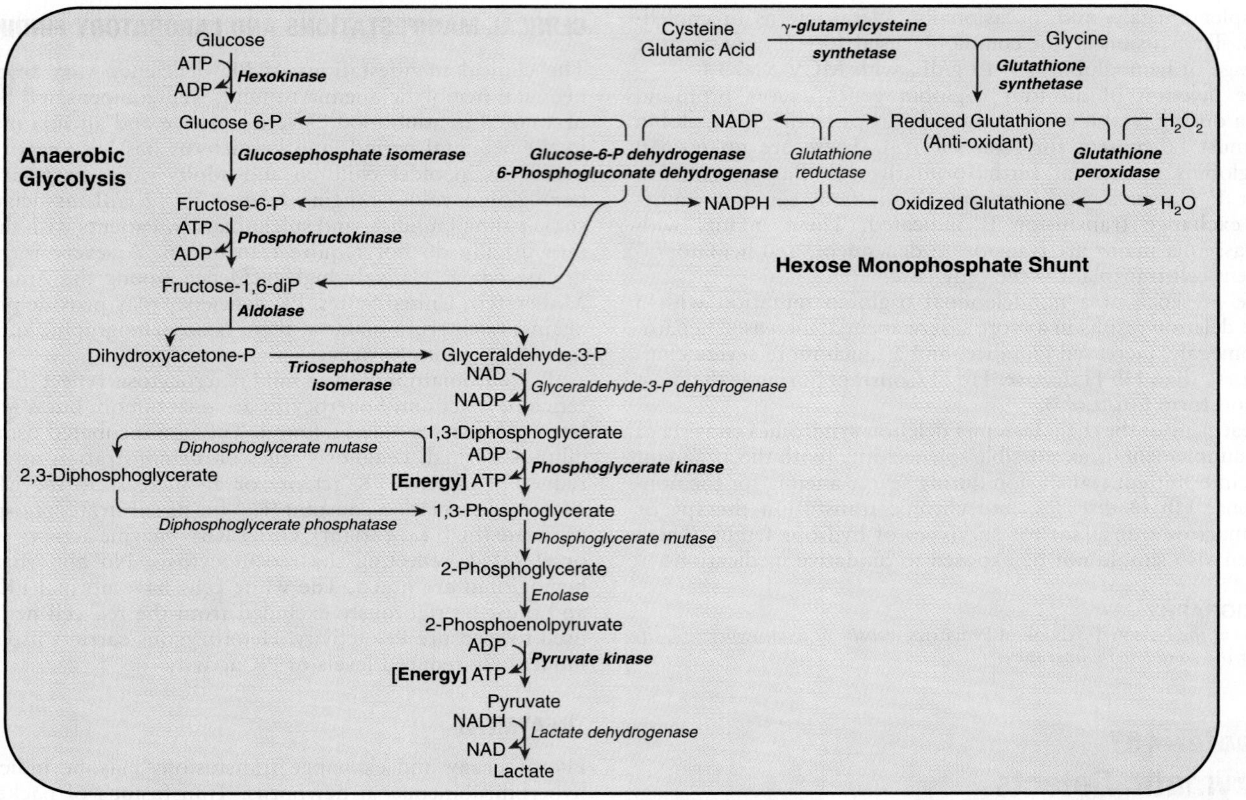

Figure 457-1 Red blood cell metabolism. Glycolysis and the hexose monophosphate pathway. The enzyme deficiencies clearly associated with hemolysis are shown in bold type. ATP, adenosine triphosphate; ADP, adenosine diphosphate; NADP, nicotinamide-adenine dinucleotide phosphate; NADPH, reduced form of NADP.

described. PGK is the only glycolytic enzyme inherited on the X chromosome. Affected males may have progressive extrapyramidal disease, myopathy, seizures, and variable mental retardation in conjunction with hemolytic anemia. Nine Japanese patients had neural or myopathic symptoms with hemolysis; 6 had hemolysis alone; 7 had neural or myopathic symptoms alone; and 1 had no symptoms. The gene for PGK is particularly large, spanning 23 kb, and various genetic abnormalities, including nucleotide substitutions, gene deletions, missense, and splicing mutations, result in PGK deficiency.

DEFICIENCIES OF ENZYMES OF THE HEXOSE MONOPHOSPHATE PATHWAY

The most important function of the hexose monophosphate pathway is to maintain glutathione in its reduced state (GSH) as protection against the oxidation of RBCs (see Fig. 457-1). Approximately 10% of the glucose taken up by RBCs passes through this pathway to provide the reduced form of nicotinamide adenine dinucleotide phosphate (NADPH) necessary for the conversion of oxidized glutathione to GSH. Maintenance of GSH is essential for the physiologic inactivation of oxidant compounds, such as hydrogen peroxide, that are generated within RBCs. If glutathione, or any compound or enzyme necessary for maintaining it in the reduced state, is decreased, the SH groups of the RBC membrane are oxidized and the hemoglobin becomes denatured and may precipitate into RBC inclusions called Heinz bodies. Once Heinz bodies have formed, an acute hemolytic process results from damage to the RBC membrane by the precipitated hemoglobin, the oxidant agent, and the action of the spleen. The damaged RBCs then are rapidly removed from the circulation.

457.3 Glucose-6-Phosphate Dehydrogenase Deficiency and Related Deficiencies

George B. Segel and Lisa R. Hackney

Glucose-6-phosphate dehydrogenase (G6PD) deficiency, the most frequent disease involving enzymes of the hexose monophosphate pathway, is responsible for 2 clinical syndromes, episodic hemolytic anemia, and chronic nonspherocytic hemolytic anemia. The most common manifestations of this disorder are neonatal jaundice and episodic acute hemolytic anemia, which is induced by infections, certain drugs, and, rarely, fava beans. This X-linked deficiency affects more than 400 million people worldwide, representing an overall 4.9% global prevalence. The global distribution of this disorder parallels that of malaria, representing an example of "balanced polymorphism," in which there is an evolutionary advantage of resistance to falciparum malaria in heterozygous females that outweighs the small negative effect of affected hemizygous males.

The deficiency is caused by inheritance of any of a large number of abnormal alleles of the gene responsible for the synthesis of the G6PD protein. About 140 mutations have been described in the gene responsible for the synthesis of the G6PD protein. Many of these mutations are single base changes leading to amino acid substitutions and destabilization of the G6PD enzyme. The gene for G6PD has been cloned and sequenced. A web-accessible database catalogs G6PD mutations (*www.bioinf.org.uk/g6pd*). Some of the mutations that cause episodic vs chronic hemolysis are shown in Figure 457-2. Milder disease is associated with mutations near the amino terminus of the G6PD molecule, and chronic nonspherocytic hemolytic anemia is

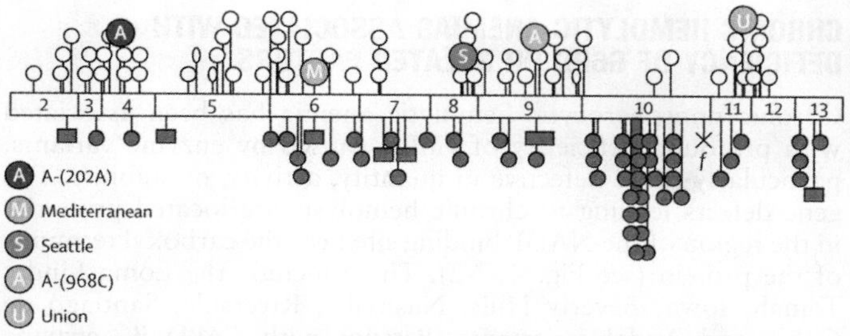

Figure 457-2 Most common mutations along coding sequence of *G6PD* gene. Exons are shown as *open numbered boxes. Open circles* are mutations causing classes II and III variants. *Filled circles* represent sporadic mutations giving rise to severe variants (class I). *Open ellipses* are mutations causing class IV variants. *Cross,* a nonsense mutation; *f,* a splice site mutation; *filled square,* small deletion. 202A and 968C are the two sites of base substitution in G6PD-A. (From Cappellini MD, Fiorelli G: Glucose-6-phosphate dehydrogenase deficiency, *Lancet* 371:64–74, 2008.)

associated with mutations clustered near the carboxyl terminus. The normal enzyme found in most populations is designated G6PD B+. A normal variant, designated G6PD A+, is common in Americans of African descent.

EPISODIC OR INDUCED HEMOLYTIC ANEMIA

Etiology

G6PD catalyzes the conversion of glucose 6-phosphate to 6-phosphogluconic acid. This reaction produces NADPH, which maintains glutathione in the reduced, functional state (see Fig. 457-1). Reduced glutathione provides protection against oxidant threats from certain drugs and infections that would otherwise cause precipitation of hemoglobin (Heinz bodies) or damage the RBC membrane.

Synthesis of RBC G6PD is determined by a gene on the X chromosome. Thus, heterozygous females have intermediate enzymatic activity and have 2 populations of RBCs: one is normal, and the other is deficient in G6PD activity. Because they have fewer susceptible cells, most heterozygous females do not have evident clinical hemolysis after exposure to oxidant drugs. Rarely, the majority of RBCs is G6PD deficient in heterozygous females because the inactivation of the normal X chromosome is random and sometimes exaggerated (Lyon-Beutler hypothesis).

Disease involving this enzyme therefore occurs more frequently in males than in females. Approximately 13% of male Americans of African descent have a mutant enzyme (**G6PD A–**) that results in a deficiency of RBC G6PD activity (5-15% of normal). Italians, Greeks, and other Mediterranean, Middle Eastern, African, and Asian ethnic groups also have a high incidence, ranging from 5% to 40%, of a variant designated **G6PD B–** (**G6PD Mediterranean**). In these variants, the G6PD activity of homozygous females or hemizygous males is <5% of normal. Therefore, the defect in Americans of African descent is less severe than that in Americans of European descent. A third mutant enzyme with markedly reduced activity (**G6PD Canton**) occurs in approximately 5% of the Chinese population.

Clinical Manifestations

Most individuals with G6PD deficiency are asymptomatic, with no clinical manifestations of illness unless triggered by infection, drugs, or ingestion of fava beans. Typically, hemolysis ensues in about 24-48 hr after a patient has ingested a substance with oxidant properties. In severe cases, hemoglobinuria and jaundice result, and the hemoglobin concentration may fall precipitously. Drugs that elicit hemolysis in these individuals include aspirin, sulfonamides, rasburicase, and antimalarials, such as primaquine (Table 457-1). The degree of hemolysis varies with the inciting agent, amount ingested, and severity of the enzyme deficiency. In some individuals, ingestion of fava beans also produces an acute,

Table 457-1 AGENTS PRECIPITATING HEMOLYSIS IN GLUCOSE-6-PHOSPHATE DEHYDROGENASE DEFICIENCY

MEDICATIONS
Antibacterials
Sulfonamides
Dapsone
Trimethoprim-sulfamethoxazole
Nalidixic acid
Chloramphenicol
Nitrofurantoin
Antimalarials
Primaquine
Pamaquine
Chloroquine
Quinacrine
Others
Acetanilide
Vitamin K analogs
Methylene blue
Probenecid
Acetylsalicylic acid
Phenazopyridine
CHEMICALS
Phenylhydrazine
Benzene
Naphthalene
2,4,6-Trinitrotoluene
ILLNESS
Diabetic acidosis
Hepatitis
Sepsis

From Asselin BL, Segel GB: In Rakel R, editor: *Conn's current therapy,* Philadelphia, 1994, WB Saunders, p 341.

severe hemolytic syndrome, known as *favism.* Fava beans contain divicine, isouramil, and convicine, which ultimately lead to production of hydrogen peroxide and other reactive oxygen products. Favism is thought to be more frequently associated with the G6PD B– variant.

In the G6PD A– variant, the stability of the folded protein dimer is impaired, and this defect is accentuated as the RBCs age. Thus, hemolysis decreases as older red cells are destroyed, even if administration of the drug is continued. This recovery results from the age-labile enzyme, which is abundant and more stable in younger RBCs. The associated reticulocytosis produces a compensated hemolytic process in which the blood hemoglobin may be only slightly decreased, despite continued exposure to the offending agent.

G6PD deficiency can produce hemolysis in the neonatal period. In G6PD A–, spontaneous hemolysis and hyperbilirubinemia have been observed in preterm infants. In newborns with the G6PDB– and G6PD Canton varieties, hyperbilirubinemia and even kernicterus may occur. Neonates with coinheritance of G6PD deficiency and a mutation of the promoter of uridine-diphosphate-glucuronyl transferase (UGT1A1), seen in Gilbert syndrome, have more severe neonatal jaundice. When a pregnant woman ingests oxidant drugs, they may be transmitted to her G6PD-deficient fetus, and hemolytic anemia and jaundice may be apparent at birth.

Laboratory Findings

The onset of acute hemolysis usually results in a precipitous fall in hemoglobin and hematocrit. If the episode is severe, the hemoglobin binding proteins, such as haptoglobin, are saturated, and free hemoglobin may appear in the plasma and subsequently in the urine. Unstained or supravital preparations of RBCs reveal precipitated hemoglobin, known as Heinz bodies. The RBC inclusions are not visible on the Wright-stained blood

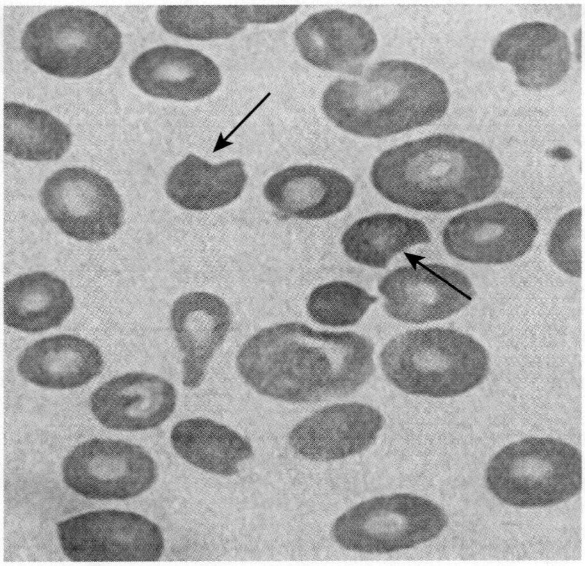

Figure 457-3 Morphologic erythrocyte changes (anisopoikilocytosis, bite cells) during acute hemolysis in a G6PD-deficient patient. *Arrows* show bite cells. Anisopoikilocytosis is abnormality in the shape or size of erythrocytes. (From Cappellini MD, Fiorelli G: Glucose-6-phosphate dehydrogenase deficiency, *Lancet* 371:64–74, 2008.)

film. Cells that contain these inclusions are seen only within the first 3-4 days of illness because they are rapidly cleared from the blood. Also, the blood film may contain red cells with what appears to be a bite taken from their periphery and polychromasia (evidence of bluish, larger RBCs), representing reticulocytosis (Fig. 457-3).

Diagnosis

The diagnosis depends on direct or indirect demonstration of reduced G6PD activity in RBCs. By direct measurement, enzyme activity in affected persons is ≤10% of normal, and the reduction of enzyme activity is more extreme in Americans of European descent and in Asians than in Americans of African descent. Satisfactory screening tests are based on decoloration of methylene blue, reduction of methemoglobin, or fluorescence of NADPH. Immediately after a hemolytic episode, reticulocytes and young RBCs predominate. These young cells have significantly higher enzyme activity than do older cells in the A– variety. Testing may therefore have to be deferred for a few weeks before a diagnostically low level of enzyme can be shown. The diagnosis can be suspected when G6PD activity is within the low-normal range in the presence of a high reticulocyte count. G6PD variants also can be detected by electrophoretic and molecular analysis.

Prevention and Treatment

Prevention of hemolysis constitutes the most important therapeutic measure. When possible, males belonging to ethnic groups with a significant incidence of G6PD deficiency (e.g., Greeks, southern Italians, Sephardic Jews, Filipinos, southern Chinese, Americans of African descent, and Thais) should be tested for the defect before known oxidant drugs are given. The usual doses of aspirin and trimethoprim-sulfamethoxazole do not cause clinically relevant hemolysis in the A– variety. Aspirin administered in doses used for acute rheumatic fever (60-100 mg/kg/24 hr) may produce a severe hemolytic episode. Infants with severe neonatal jaundice who belong to these ethnic groups also require testing for G6PD deficiency because of their heightened risk for this defect. If severe hemolysis has occurred, supportive therapy may require blood transfusions, although recovery is the rule when the oxidant agent is discontinued.

CHRONIC HEMOLYTIC ANEMIAS ASSOCIATED WITH DEFICIENCY OF G6PD OR RELATED FACTORS

Chronic nonspherocytic hemolytic anemia has been associated with profound deficiency of G6PD caused by enzyme variants, particularly those defective in quantity, activity, or stability. The gene defects leading to chronic hemolysis are located primarily in the region of the NADP binding site near the carboxyl terminus of the protein (see Fig. 457-2). These include the Loma Linda, Tomah, Iowa, Beverly Hills, Nashville, Riverside, Santiago de Cuba, and Andalus variants. Persons with G6PD B– enzyme deficiency occasionally have chronic hemolysis, and the hemolytic process may worsen after ingestion of oxidant drugs. Splenectomy is of little value in these types of chronic hemolysis.

Other enzyme defects may impair the regeneration of GSH as an oxidant "sump" (see Fig. 457-1). Mild, chronic nonspherocytic anemia has been reported in association with decreased RBC GSH, resulting from γ-glutamylcysteine or glutathione synthetase deficiencies. Deficiency of 6-phosphogluconate dehydrogenase (6PDG) has been associated primarily with drug-induced hemolysis, and hemolysis with hyperbilirubinemia has been related to a deficiency of glutathione peroxidase in newborn infants.

BIBLIOGRAPHY

Please visit the Nelson Textbook of Pediatrics *website at www.expertconsult.com for the complete bibliography.*

Chapter 458
Hemolytic Anemias Resulting from Extracellular Factors—Immune Hemolytic Anemias

George B. Segel and Charles H. Packman

AUTOIMMUNE HEMOLYTIC ANEMIAS

A number of extrinsic agents and disorders may lead to premature destruction of red blood cells (RBCs) (Table 458-1). Among the most clearly defined are antibodies associated with immune hemolytic anemias. The hallmark of this group of diseases is the positive result of the direct antiglobulin (Coombs) test, which detects a coating of immunoglobulin or components of complement on the RBC surface. The most important immune hemolytic disorder in pediatric practice is hemolytic disease of the newborn (erythroblastosis fetalis), caused by transplacental transfer of maternal antibody active against the RBCs of the fetus, that is, isoimmune hemolytic anemia (Chapter 97.2). Various other immune hemolytic anemias are autoimmune (see Table 458-1) and may be idiopathic or related to various infections (Epstein-Barr virus, rarely HIV, cytomegalovirus, and mycoplasma), immunologic diseases (systemic lupus erythematosus [SLE], rheumatoid arthritis), immunodeficiency diseases (agammaglobulinemia, autoimmune lymphoproliferative disorder, dysgammaglobulinemias), neoplasms (lymphoma, leukemia, and Hodgkin disease), or drugs (methyldopa, L-dopa). Other drugs (penicillins, cephalosporins) cause hemolysis by means of "drug-dependent antibodies—that is antibodies directed toward the drug and in some cases toward an RBC membrane antigen as well.

AUTOIMMUNE HEMOLYTIC ANEMIAS ASSOCIATED WITH "WARM" ANTIBODIES

Etiology

In the autoimmune hemolytic anemias, abnormal antibodies are directed against RBC membrane antigens, but the pathogenesis of antibody induction is uncertain. The autoantibody may be produced as an inappropriate immune response to an RBC antigen or to another antigenic epitope similar to an RBC antigen, known as *molecular mimicry.* Alternatively, an infectious agent may alter the RBC membrane so that it becomes "foreign" or antigenic to the host. The antibodies usually react to epitopes (antigens) that are "public" or common to all human RBCs, such as Rh proteins.

In most instances of warm antibody hemolysis, no underlying cause can be found; this is the primary or idiopathic type (see Table 458-1). If the autoimmune hemolysis is associated with an underlying disease, such as a lymphoproliferative disorder, SLE, or immunodeficiency, it is secondary. In as many as 20% of cases of immune hemolysis, drugs may be implicated (Table 458-2).

Drugs (penicillin or sometimes cephalosporins) that cause hemolysis via the "hapten" mechanism (immune but not autoimmune) bind tightly to the RBC membrane (see Table 458-1). Antibodies to the drug, either newly or previously formed, bind to the drug molecules on RBCs, mediating their destruction in the spleen. In other cases, certain drugs, such as quinine and quinidine, do not bind to RBCs but, rather, form part of a "ternary complex," consisting of the drug, an RBC membrane antigen, and an antibody that recognizes both (see Table 458-1). Methyldopa and sometimes cephalosporins may, by unknown mechanisms, incite true autoantibodies to RBC membrane antigens, so that the presence of the drug is not required to cause hemolysis.

Table 458-1 DISEASES CHARACTERIZED BY IMMUNE-MEDIATED RED BLOOD CELL DESTRUCTION

AUTOIMMUNE HEMOLYTIC ANEMIA DUE TO WARM REACTIVE AUTOANTIBODIES
Primary (idiopathic) Secondary Lymphoproliferative disorders Connective tissue disorders (especially systemic lupus erythematosus) Nonlymphoid neoplasms (e.g., ovarian tumors) Chronic inflammatory diseases (e.g., ulcerative colitis) Immunodeficiency disorders
AUTOIMMUNE HEMOLYTIC ANEMIA DUE TO COLD REACTIVE AUTOANTIBODIES (CRYOPATHIC HEMOLYTIC SYNDROMES)
Primary (idiopathic) cold agglutinin disease Secondary cold agglutinin disease Lymphoproliferative disorders Infections (*Mycoplasma pneumoniae*, Epstein-Barr virus) Paroxysmal cold hemoglobinuria Primary (idiopathic) Viral syndromes (most common) Congenital or tertiary syphilis
DRUG-INDUCED IMMUNE HEMOLYTIC ANEMIA (see Table 458-2)
Hapten/drug adsorption (e.g., penicillin) Ternary (immune) complex (e.g., quinine or quinidine) True autoantibody induction (e.g., methyldopa)

Modified from Packman CH: Autoimmune hemolytic anemias. In Rakel R, editor: *Conn's current therapy*, Philadelphia, 1995, WB Saunders, p 305.

Clinical Manifestations

Autoimmune hemolytic anemias may occur in either of 2 general clinical patterns. The first, an acute transient type lasting 3-6 mo and occurring predominantly in children ages 2-12 yr, accounts for 70-80% of patients. It is frequently preceded by an infection, usually respiratory. Onset may be acute, with prostration, pallor, jaundice, fever, and hemoglobinuria, or more gradual, with primarily fatigue and pallor. The spleen is usually enlarged and is the primary site of destruction of immunoglobulin G (IgG)–coated RBCs. Underlying systemic disorders are unusual. A consistent response to glucocorticoid therapy, a low mortality rate, and full recovery are characteristic of the acute form. The other clinical pattern involves a prolonged and chronic course, which is more frequent in infants and in children >12 yr old. Hemolysis may continue for many months or years. Abnormalities involving other blood elements are common, and the response to glucocorticoids is variable and inconsistent. The mortality rate is approximately 10%, and death is often attributable to an underlying systemic disease.

Table 458-2 SELECTED DRUGS THAT CAUSE IMMUNE-MEDIATED HEMOLYSIS

MECHANISM	DRUG ADSORPTION (HAPTEN)	TERNARY (IMMUNE) COMPLEX	AUTOANTIBODY INDUCTION
Direct antiglobulin test	Positive (anti-IgG)	Positive (anti-C3)	Positive (anti-IgG)
Site of hemolysis	Extravascular	Intravascular	Extravascular
Medications	Penicillin	Quinidine	α-Methyldopa
	Ampicillin	Phenacetin	Mefenamic acid
	Methicillin	Hydrochlorothiazide	(Ponstel)
	Carbenicillin	Rifampin (Rifadin)	L-Dopa
	Cephalothin (Keflin)*	Sulfonamides	Procainamide
	Cephaloridine (Loridine)	Isoniazid	Ibuprofen
		Quinine	Diclofenac (Voltaren)
		Insulin	Interferon alfa
		Tetracycline	
		Melphalan (Alkeran)	
		Acetaminophen	
		Hydralazine (Apresoline)	
		Probenecid	
		Chlorpromazine (Thorazine)	
		Streptomycin	
		Fluorouracil (Adrucil)	
		Sulindac (Clinoril)	

*Not available in the USA.

Ig, immunoglobulin.

Adapted from Schwartz RS, Berkman EM, Silberstein LE: Autoimmune hemolytic anemias. In Hoffman R, Benz EJ Jr, Schattil SJ, et al, editors: *Hematology: basic principles and practice*, ed 3, Philadelphia, 2000, Churchill Livingstone, p 624. Reproduced from Dhaliwal G, Cornett PA, Tierney LM: Hemolytic anemia, *Am Family Physician* 69:2599–2606, 2004.

Laboratory Findings

In many cases, anemia is profound, with hemoglobin levels <6 g/dL. Considerable spherocytosis and polychromasia (reflecting the reticulocyte response) are present. More than 50% of the circulating RBCs may be reticulocytes, and nucleated RBCs usually are present. In some cases, a low reticulocyte count may be found, particularly early in the episode. Leukocytosis is common. The platelet count is usually normal, but concomitant immune thrombocytopenic purpura sometimes occurs (**Evans syndrome**). The prognosis for patients with Evans syndrome is guarded, because many have or eventually have a chronic disease, including SLE, an immunodeficiency syndrome, or an autoimmune lymphoproliferative disorder.

Results of the direct antiglobulin test are strongly positive, and free antibody can sometimes be demonstrated in the serum (indirect Coombs test). These antibodies are active at 35-40°C ("warm" antibodies) and most often belong to the IgG class. They do not require complement for activity and are usually *incomplete* antibodies that do not produce agglutination in vitro. Antibodies from the serum and those eluted from the RBCs react with the RBCs of many persons in addition to those of the patient. They often have been regarded as nonspecific panagglutinins, but careful studies have revealed specificity for RBC antigens of the Rh system in 70% of patients (≈50% of adult patients). Complement, particularly fragments of C3b, may be detected on the RBCs in conjunction with IgG. The Coombs test result is *rarely* negative *because of* the limited sensitivity of the Coombs reaction. A minimum of 260-400 molecules of IgG per cell is necessary on the RBC membrane to produce a positive reaction. Special tests are required to detect the antibody in cases of "Coombs-negative" autoimmune hemolytic anemia. In warm antibody hemolytic anemia, the direct Coombs test may detect IgG alone, both IgG– and complement fragments, or solely complement fragments if the level of RBC-bound IgG is below the detection limit of the anti-IgG Coombs reagent.

Treatment

Transfusions may provide only transient benefit but may be lifesaving in cases of severe anemia by providing delivery of oxygen until the effect of other treatment is observed. In general, all tested units for transfusion are serologically incompatible. It is important to identify the patient's ABO blood group in order to avoid a hemolytic transfusion reaction mediated by anti-A or anti-B. The blood bank should also test for the presence of an underlying allo-antibody, which could cause rapid hemolysis of transfused red cells. Patients who have neither been previously transfused nor pregnant are unlikely to harbor an alloantibody. Early consultation between the clinician and the blood bank physician is essential. Failure to transfuse a profoundly anemic infant or child may lead to serious morbidity and even death.

Patients with mild disease and compensated hemolysis may not require any treatment. If the hemolysis is severe and results in significant anemia or symptoms, treatment with glucocorticoids is initiated. Glucocorticoids decrease the rate of hemolysis by blocking macrophage function by down regulating Fcγ receptor expression, decreasing the production of the autoantibody, and perhaps enhancing the elution of antibody from the RBCs. Prednisone or its equivalent is administered at a dose of 2 mg/kg/24 hr. In some patients with severe hemolysis, doses of prednisone of up to 6 mg/kg/24 hr may be required to reduce the rate of hemolysis. Treatment should be continued until the rate of hemolysis decreases, and then the dose gradually reduced. If relapse occurs, resumption of the full dosage may be necessary. The disease tends to remit spontaneously within a few weeks or months. The Coombs test result may remain positive even after the hemoglobin level returns to normal. In general, it is safe to discontinue prednisone once the direct Coombs test result becomes negative. When hemolytic anemia remains severe despite glucocorticoid therapy, or if very large doses are necessary to maintain a reasonable hemoglobin level, IV immunoglobulin may be tried. Rituximab, a monoclonal antibody that targets B lymphocytes, the source of antibody production, has been useful in chronic cases refractory to conventional therapy. Plasmapheresis has been used in refractory cases but generally is not helpful. Splenectomy may be beneficial but is complicated by a heightened risk of infection with encapsulated organisms, particularly in patients <6 yr. Prophylaxis is indicated with appropriate vaccines (pneumococcal, meningococcal, and *Haemophilus influenzae* type b) before splenectomy and with oral penicillin after splenectomy.

Course and Prognosis

Acute idiopathic autoimmune hemolytic disease in childhood varies in severity but is self-limited; death from untreatable anemia is rare. Approximately 30% of patients have chronic hemolysis, often associated with an underlying disease, such as SLE, lymphoma, or leukemia. The presence of antiphospholipid antibodies in adult patients with immune hemolysis predisposes to thrombosis. Mortality in chronic cases depends on the primary disorder.

AUTOIMMUNE HEMOLYTIC ANEMIAS ASSOCIATED WITH "COLD" ANTIBODIES

"Cold" antibodies agglutinate RBCs at temperatures <37°C. They are primarily of the IgM class and require complement for hemolytic activity. The highest temperature at which RBC agglutination occurs is called the *thermal amplitude*. A higher thermal amplitude antibody—that is—one that can bind to RBCs at temperatures achievable in the body, results in hemolysis with exposure to a cold environment. High antibody titers are associated with a high thermal amplitude.

Cold Agglutinin Disease

Cold antibodies usually have specificity for the oligosaccharide antigens of the I/i system. They may occur in primary or idiopathic cold agglutinin disease, secondary to infections such as those from *Mycoplasma pneumoniae* and Epstein-Barr virus, or secondary to lymphoproliferative disorders. After *M. pneumoniae* infection, the anti-I levels may increase considerably, and occasionally, enormous increases may occur to titers ≥1/30,000. The antibody has specificity for the I antigen and thus reacts poorly with human cord RBCs, which possess the i antigen but exhibit low levels of I. Patients with infectious mononucleosis occasionally have cold agglutinin disease, and the antibodies in these patients often have anti-i specificity. This antibody causes less hemolysis in adults than in children because adults have fewer i molecules on their RBCs. Spontaneous RBC agglutination is observed in the cold and in vitro, and RBC aggregates are seen on the blood film. Mean corpuscular volume may be spuriously elevated because of RBC agglutination. The severity of the hemolysis is related to the thermal amplitude of the antibody, which itself partly depends on the IgM antibody titer.

When very high titers of cold antibodies are present and active near body temperature, severe intravascular hemolysis with hemoglobinemia and hemoglobinuria may occur and may be heightened on a patient's exposure to cold (external temperature or ingested foods). Each IgM molecule has the potential to activate a C1 molecule so that large amounts of complement are found on the RBCs in cold agglutinin disease. These sensitized RBCs may undergo intravascular complement-mediated lysis or may be destroyed in the liver and spleen.

Cold agglutinin disease is less common in children than in adults and more frequently results in an acute, self-limited episode of hemolysis. Glucocorticoids are much less effective in cold agglutinin disease than in disease with warm antibodies. Patients should avoid exposure to cold and should be treated for underlying disease. In the uncommon patients with severe hemolytic disease, treatment includes immunosuppression and plasmapheresis. Successful treatment of cold agglutinin disease has been reported with the monoclonal antibody rituximab, which effectively depletes B lymphocytes. Splenectomy is not useful in cold agglutinin disease.

Paroxysmal Cold Hemoglobinuria

Paroxysmal cold hemoglobinuria is mediated by the Donath-Landsteiner hemolysin, which is an IgG cold-reactive autoantibody with anti-P specificity. This antibody fixes large amounts of complement in the cold, and the RBCs are lysed as the temperature is increased. Most reported cases are self-limited and are usually associated with nonspecific viral infections. They are now rarely found in association with congenital or acquired syphilis. This disorder may account for 30% of immune hemolytic episodes among children. Treatment includes transfusion for severe anemia and avoidance of cold ambient temperatures.

BIBLIOGRAPHY

Please visit the Nelson Textbook of Pediatrics *website at www.expertconsult.com for the complete bibliography.*

Chapter 459 Hemolytic Anemias Secondary to Other Extracellular Factors

George B. Segel

FRAGMENTATION HEMOLYSIS (SEE TABLE 451-1)

Red blood cell (RBC) destruction may occur in hemolytic anemias because of mechanical injury as the cells traverse a damaged vascular bed. Damage may be microvascular when RBCs are sheared by fibrin in the capillaries during intravascular coagulation or when renovascular disease accompanies the hemolytic-uremic syndrome (Chapter 512) or thrombotic thrombocytopenic purpura (Chapter 478.5). Larger vessels may be involved in Kasabach-Merritt syndrome (giant hemangioma and thrombocytopenia; Chapter 499) or when a replacement heart valve is poorly epithelialized. The blood film shows many "schistocytes," or fragmented cells, as well as polychromatophilia, reflecting the reticulocytosis (see Fig. 452-4*F*). Secondary iron deficiency may complicate the intravascular hemolysis because of urinary hemoglobin and hemosiderin iron loss (see Fig. 451-2). Treatment should be directed toward the underlying condition, and the prognosis depends on the effectiveness of this treatment. The benefit of transfusion is transient because the transfused cells are destroyed as quickly as those produced by the patient.

For the full continuation of this chapter, please visit the Nelson Textbook of Pediatrics *website at www.expertconsult.com.*

Section 4 POLYCYTHEMIA (ERYTHROCYTOSIS)

Chapter 460 Polycythemia

Amanda M. Brandow and Bruce M. Camitta

Polycythemia exists when the red blood cell (RBC) count, hemoglobin level, and total RBC volume all exceed the upper limits of normal. In postpubertal individuals, an RBC mass > 25% above the mean normal value (based on body surface area), or a hematocrit level > 60 (in males) or > 56 (in females) indicate absolute erythrocytosis. A decrease in plasma volume, such as occurs in acute dehydration and burns, may result in a high hemoglobin value. These situations are more accurately designated as *hemoconcentration* or *relative polycythemia* because the RBC mass is not increased and normalization of the plasma volume restores hemoglobin to normal levels. Once the diagnosis of true polycythemia is made, sequential studies should be done to determine the underlying etiology (see Fig. 460-1 on the *Nelson Textbook of Pediatrics* website at www.expertconsult.com).

For the full continuation of this chapter, please visit the Nelson Textbook of Pediatrics *website at www.expertconsult.com.*

Chapter 461 Secondary Polycythemia

Amanda M. Brandow and Bruce M. Camitta

PATHOGENESIS

Secondary polycythemia is diagnosed when true polycythemia is caused by a physiologic process that is not clonal in nature (see Table 461-1 on the *Nelson Textbook of Pediatrics* website at www.expertconsult.com). Secondary polycythemia can be congenital or acquired.

For the full continuation of this chapter, please visit the Nelson Textbook of Pediatrics *website at www.expertconsult.com.*

Section 5 THE PANCYTOPENIAS

Chapter 462
The Inherited Pancytopenias

Melvin H. Freedman

Pancytopenia refers to a reduction below normal values of all 3 peripheral blood lineages: leukocytes, platelets, and erythrocytes. Pancytopenia requires microscopic examination of a bone marrow biopsy specimen and a marrow aspirate to assess overall cellularity and morphology. There are 3 general categories of pancytopenia depending on the marrow findings.

Hypocellular marrow on biopsy is seen with inherited ("constitutional") marrow failure syndromes, acquired aplastic anemia of varied etiologies (Chapter 463), the hypoplastic variant of myelodysplastic syndrome (MDS; Chapter 124), and some cases of paroxysmal nocturnal hemoglobinuria with pancytopenia.

Cellular marrow is seen (1) with primary bone marrow disease, such as acute leukemia (Chapter 489), and MDS, and (2) secondary to systemic disease, such as autoimmune disorders (systemic lupus erythematosus; Chapter 152), vitamin B_{12} or folate deficiency (Chapters 46 and 448), storage disease (Gaucher and Niemann-Pick diseases; Chapter 80), overwhelming infection, sarcoidosis, and hypersplenism.

Bone marrow infiltration can cause pancytopenia in myelofibrosis, osteopetrosis (Chapter 698), hemophagocytic lymphohistiocytosis (Chapter 501), and metastatic solid tumors.

Inherited ("constitutional") pancytopenia is defined as a decrease in marrow production of the 3 major hematopoietic lineages that occurs on an inherited basis, resulting in anemia, neutropenia, and thrombocytopenia. Any of these conditions (Table 462-1) can be transmitted as a simple mendelian disorder by mutant genes with inherited patterns of autosomal dominant, autosomal recessive, or X-linked types. Modifying genes and acquired factors may also be operative. Inherited pancytopenias account for approximately 30% of cases of pediatric marrow failure. Fanconi anemia is the most common of these disorders.

FANCONI ANEMIA

Etiology and Epidemiology

Fanconi anemia (FA) is primarily inherited in an autosomal recessive manner (one uncommon form is X-linked recessive). It occurs in all racial and ethnic groups. At presentation, patients with FA may have: (1) typical physical anomalies but normal hematologic findings; (2) normal physical features but abnormal hematologic findings; or (3) physical anomalies and abnormal hematologic findings, which constitute the classic phenotype (39% of cases). There can be sibling discordance in clinical and hematologic findings, even in affected monozygotic twins. Approximately 75% of patients are 3-14 yr of age at the time of diagnosis.

Table 462-1 INHERITED PANCYTOPENIA SYNDROMES

Fanconi anemia
Shwachman-Diamond syndrome
Dyskeratosis congenita
Congenital amegakaryocytic thrombocytopenia
Unclassified inherited bone marrow failure syndromes
Other genetic syndromes
Down syndrome
Dubowitz syndrome
Seckel syndrome
Reticular dysgenesis
Schimke immunoosseous dysplasia
Familial aplastic anemia (non-Fanconi)
Cartilage-hair hypoplasia
Noonan syndrome

Pathology

Patients have abnormal chromosome fragility, which is seen in metaphase preparations of peripheral blood lymphocytes cultured with phytohemagglutinin and enhanced by adding clastogenic agents such as diepoxybutane (DEB) and mitomycin C. Cell fusion of FA cells with normal cells or with cells from some unrelated patients with FA produces a corrective effect on chromosomal fragility, a process called *complementation.* This phenomenon allows subtyping of cases of FA into discrete complementation groups. Fourteen separate complementation groups have been identified, and 14 mutant FA (*FANC*) genes have been cloned so far (A, B, C, D1/BRCA2, D2, E, F, G, I, J, L, M, N, and O) all prefixed with *FANC*, e.g. *FANCA*, *FANCB* and so on); *FANCD1* is identical to the breast cancer susceptibility protein BRCA2. The protein products of wild-type *FANC* genes are involved in the DNA damage recognition and repair biochemical pathways. Therefore, mutant gene proteins lead to genomic instability, chromosome fragility, and FA. An inability of FA cells to remove oxygen-free radicals, resulting in oxidative damage, is a contributing factor in the pathogenesis. Additional factors are also operative. Leukocyte telomere length is significantly shortened but telomerase activity is increased, suggesting a high proliferative rate of marrow progenitors that ultimately leads to their premature senescence. Increased marrow cell apoptosis occurs and is mediated by Fas, a membrane glycoprotein receptor containing an integral death domain. A consistent finding is diminished cellular interleukin-6 production along with markedly heightened tumor necrosis factor-α generation.

Clinical Manifestations

The most common anomaly in FA is hyperpigmentation of the trunk, neck, and intertriginous areas, as well as café-au-lait spots and vitiligo, alone or in combination (Fig. 462-1 and Table 462-2). Half the patients have short stature. Growth failure may be associated with abnormal growth hormone secretion or with hypothyroidism. Absence of radii and thumbs that are hypoplastic, supernumerary, bifid, or absent are common. Anomalies of the feet, congenital hip dislocation, and leg abnormalities are seen. A male patient with FA may have an underdeveloped penis; undescended, atrophic, or absence of the testes; and hypospadias or phimosis. Females can have malformations of the vagina, uterus, and ovary. Many patients have a FA "facies," including microcephaly, small eyes, epicanthal folds, and abnormal shape, size, or positioning of the ears (see Fig. 462-1). Ectopic, pelvic, or horseshoe kidneys are detected by imaging and may show other organs as duplicated, hypoplastic, dysplastic, or absent kidneys. Cardiovascular and gastrointestinal malformations also occur. Approximately 10% of patients with FA are cognitively delayed.

Laboratory Findings

Marrow failure usually ensues in the 1st decade of life. Thrombocytopenia often appears initially, with subsequent onset of granulocytopenia and then macrocytic anemia. Severe aplasia develops in most cases, but its full expression is variable and evolves over a period of months to years. The marrow becomes progressively

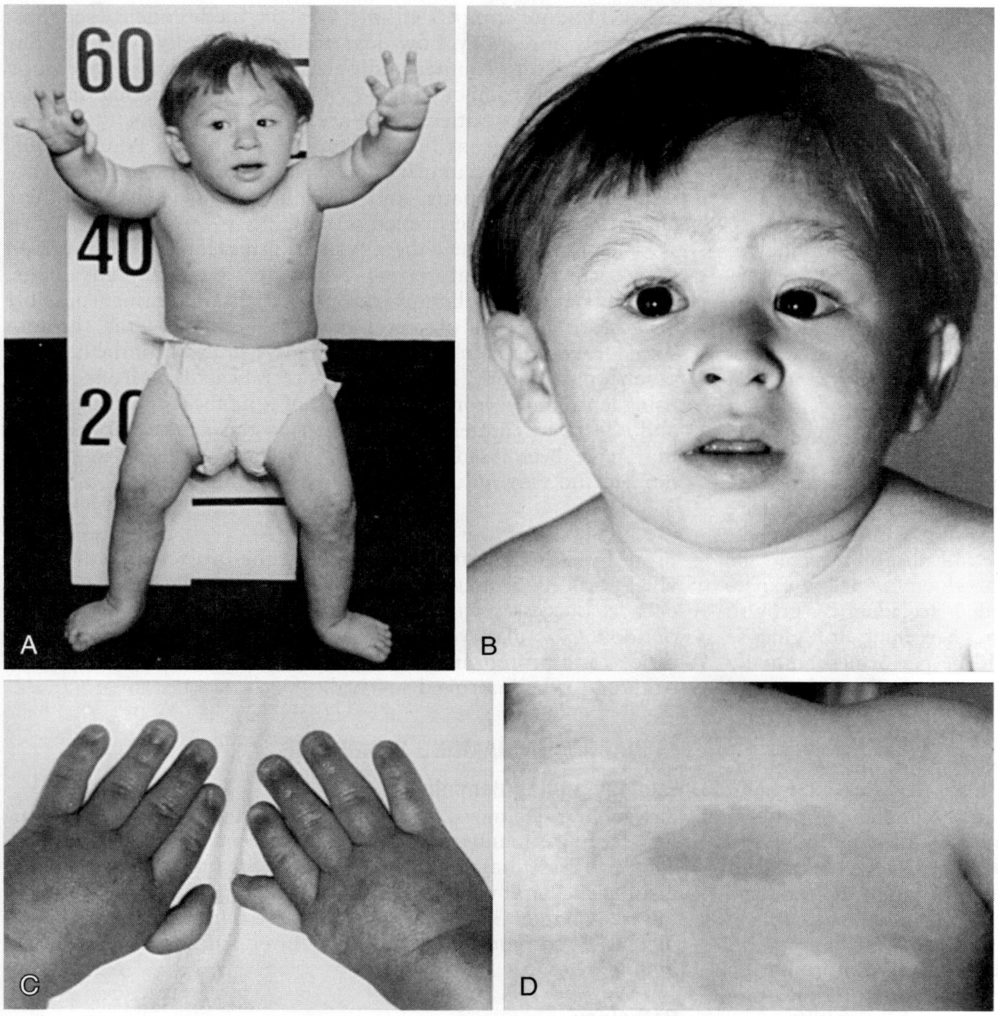

Figure 462-1 A 3 yr old boy with Fanconi anemia who exhibits several classic phenotype features. *A,* Front view. *B,* Face. *C,* Hands. *D,* Back right shoulder. The features to be noted include short stature, dislocated hips, microcephaly, a broad nasal base, epicanthal folds, micrognathia, thumbs attached by a thread, and café-au-lait spots with hypopigmented areas beneath. (From Nathan DC, Orkin SH, Ginsburg D, et al, editors: *Nathan and Oski's hematology of infancy and childhood,* ed 6, vol I, Philadelphia, 2003, WB Saunders, p 285.)

Table 462-2 CHARACTERISTIC PHYSICAL ANOMALIES IN FANCONI ANEMIA

ANOMALY	APPROXIMATE FREQUENCY (% OF PATIENTS)
Skin pigment changes ± café-au-lait spots	55
Short stature	51
Upper limb abnormalities (thumbs, hands, radii, ulnas)	43
Hypogonadal and genital changes (mostly male)	35
Other skeletal findings (head/face, neck, spine)	30
Eye/lid/epicanthal fold anomalies	23
Renal malformations	21
Gastrointestinal/cardiopulmonary malformations	11
Hip, leg, foot, toe abnormalities	10
Ear anomalies (external and internal), deafness	9

hypocellular and fatty, like that in severe acquired aplastic anemia. Chromosome fragility is indicated by spontaneously occurring chromatid breaks, rearrangements, gaps, endoreduplications, and chromatid exchanges in blood lymphocytes cultured with phytohemagglutinin as well as in cultured skin fibroblasts, underscoring the constitutional nature of the disorder. With addition of DEB, fragility is strikingly enhanced in lymphocyte cultures of patients with FA in comparison with those of controls. For prenatal diagnosis, abnormal chromosome breakage can be tested for in amniotic fluid cells or in tissue from a chorionic villus biopsy.

Complications

A major feature of the phenotype of FA is the propensity for cancer. The most frequent solid tumors are squamous cell carcinomas of the head, neck, and upper esophagus, followed by carcinomas of the vulva and/or anus, cervix, and lower esophagus. Human papilloma virus is suspected in the pathogenesis. Some patients experience oral cancer after bone marrow transplantation. Benign and malignant liver tumors occur (adenomas, hepatomas) and are usually associated with androgen therapy for aplastic anemia. Androgens are also implicated in the etiology of peliosis hepatis (blood-filled hepatic sinusoids). Peliosis hepatis is reversible when androgen therapy is discontinued, and tumors may regress. Approximately 15% of patients with FA are at risk for acute leukemia or MDS.

Diagnosis

FA should be considered in all children and young adults with unexplained cytopenias. Abnormal hematologic findings and characteristic physical anomalies suggest the diagnosis, which is confirmed with a lymphocyte chromosomal breakage study using DEB. No other inherited pancytopenia is associated with an abnormal DEB chromosomal breakage study result. Ten percent to 15% of patients with suspected FA have "somatic mosaicism" and do not show abnormal lymphocyte chromosomal fragility because of mixed populations of somatic cells, some with 2 abnormal alleles and some with 1. Testing on skin fibroblast cultures instead of lymphocytes confirms the diagnosis.

Most patients have stable elevations of serum α-fetoprotein expressed constitutively, independent of liver complications or androgen therapy. The laboratory measurement of serum α-fetoprotein can be used as a rapid screening diagnostic test.

Specialized laboratories can perform an accurate diagnostic and mutant gene subtyping assay, whereby patient lymphocytes or fibroblasts are studied after exposure to mitomycin C or radiation by immunoblotting for *FANCD2*. Alternatively, wild-type *FANC* genes can be transvected into patient T cells by means of retroviral vectors, and if a specific wild-type *FANC* gene corrects the abnormal T-cell chromosome fragility, the specific mutant gene is deduced.

Treatment

A hematologist and a multidisciplinary team should supervise patients with FA. If the hematologic findings are stable and there are no transfusion requirements, observation is indicated. Subspecialty consultations for anomalies and disabilities can be arranged during this interval. If growth velocity is below expectations, endocrine evaluation is needed to identify growth hormone deficiency or hypothyroidism. Screening for glucose intolerance and hyperinsulinemia should be performed annually or biannually, depending on the degree of hyperglycemia found on initial testing. Blood counts should be performed every 1-3 mo; bone marrow aspiration and biopsy are indicated annually for leukemia and MDS surveillance by means of morphology and cytogenetics. Patients should be assessed for solid tumors at least annually. Beginning at menarche, female patients should be screened annually for gynecologic cancer. Administration of human papilloma virus quadrivalent vaccine to prevent squamous cell carcinoma will likely become a standard intervention.

Hematopoietic stem cell transplantation (HSCT; Chapter 129) is the only curative therapy for the hematologic abnormalities. Patients with FA <10 yr old who undergo transplantation using an HLA–identical sibling donor have a survival rate >80%. Survival rates are lower for patients undergoing the procedure when >10 yr. Preparative regimens are continuously evaluated, refined, and improved worldwide. For patients who do not have a matched sibling donor, a search for a matched unrelated donor (including a search of umbilical cord blood banks) might be initiated. Because of the heightened graft vs host response in patients with FA, the survival and cure rates have not been as good as those for matched sibling donor HSCT (≈ 30% survival). Molecular technology has led to preimplantation genetic diagnosis on parent-derived blastomeres to find an HLA-matched sibling donor without FA.

The potential for recombinant growth factor (cytokine) therapy for FA has not been defined. Granulocyte colony-stimulating factor (G-CSF) can usually induce an increase in the absolute neutrophil count and occasionally may boost platelet counts and hemoglobin levels. However, there may be a heightened risk of marrow cell cytogenetic clonal expansion with monosomy 7. Combination therapy consisting of G-CSF given subcutaneously daily or every 2 days along with erythropoietin given subcutaneously or IV 3 times/wk results in improved neutrophil counts in almost all patients and a sustained rise in platelets and hemoglobin levels in approximately one third of patients, although most patients lose the response after 1 yr owing to progression of marrow failure.

Androgens produce a response in 50% of patients, heralded by reticulocytosis and a rise in hemoglobin within 1-2 mo. White blood cell counts may increase next, followed by platelet counts, but it may take many months to achieve the maximum response. When the response plateaus, androgen dosage can be slowly tapered but not stopped entirely. Oral oxymetholone is used most frequently once a day. Low-dose prednisone orally every 2nd day may be added to counter androgen-induced growth acceleration and prevent thrombocytopenic bleeding by promoting vascular stability. In many patients who are taking androgens, the disease becomes refractory as marrow failure progresses. Potential side effects include masculinization, elevated hepatic enzymes, cholestasis, peliosis hepatis, and liver tumors. Screening for these changes should be performed serially.

The premise for gene therapy in FA is based on the assumption that corrected hematopoietic cells offer a growth advantage. Attempts at gene therapy have been disappointing, possibly because of the type of vector but also because of the chromosomal fragility and impaired proliferative function of the hematopoietic progenitors. Encouraging preclinical data from studies using lentiviral vectors offer hope that gene therapy will be a safe and effective treatment for FA. Transposons are nonviral vectors that have been used successfully for gene delivery in murine models and may hold promise for use in humans.

Prognosis

From FA cases reported in the 1990s, the projected median survival was >30 yr of age, an improvement over that in the previous decade. Successes with HSCT have dramatically improved the outlook. Careful surveillance for known complications, especially cancer, and prompt intervention on their detection has also contributed to the improved survival.

SHWACHMAN-DIAMOND SYNDROME

Etiology and Epidemiology

Shwachman-Diamond syndrome (SDS) is inherited in an autosomal recessive manner; it occurs in all racial and ethnic groups. The two essential diagnostic criteria are exocrine pancreatic insufficiency and variable hematologic cytopenias due to marrow failure (Chapter 341). Chromosomes are normal, and there is no increased chromosomal breakage after DEB testing of SDS lymphocytes.

Pathology

The mutant gene *SBDS* maps to chromosome 7q11 and in 90% of cases is responsible for the multisystem, pleiotropic phenotype. The wild-type gene protein product is involved in ribosomal biogenesis or function. Pancreatic insufficiency is due to failure of pancreatic acinar development. Fatty replacement of pancreatic tissue is prominent. Bone marrow failure is characterized by dysfunctional marrow stem cells and a defective marrow microenvironment that does not support and maintain normal hematopoiesis.

Clinical Manifestations

Most patients with SDS have symptoms of fat malabsorption from birth that are caused by pancreatic insufficiency, but steatorrhea is not always obvious. Approximately 50% of patients appear to exhibit a modest improvement in pancreatic enzyme secretion as they age. The clinical picture can be dominated by complications from anemia, neutropenia, or thrombocytopenia. Bacterial and fungal infections secondary to neutropenia, neutrophil dysfunction, and immune deficiency can occur. Short stature is a consistent feature of the syndrome; most patients show normal growth velocity yet remain consistently below the 3rd percentile for height and weight. The occasional SDS adult achieves the 25th percentile for height. Although skeletal abnormalities are variable, classic findings are delayed bone maturation, metaphyseal dysplasia, short or flared ribs, thoracic dystrophy, and bifid thumb. Some patients have unexplained hepatomegaly and elevations of liver enzymes. Most patients have dental abnormalities and poor oral health. Many have neurocognitive problems and poor social skills.

Laboratory Findings

Fatty replacement of pancreatic tissue can be visualized by CT scan or ultrasound. Fat malabsorption is proven by assay on a 72-hour stool collection. Pancreatic function tests show markedly impaired enzyme secretion, but with preservation of ductal function. Serum trypsinogen and isoamylase levels are reduced. Neutropenia is present in 100% of patients with SDS on at least 1 occasion. It can be chronic, cyclic, or intermittent. It has been identified in some neonates during an episode of sepsis. Neutrophils may have a defect in mobility, migration, and chemotaxis owing to alterations in neutrophil cytoskeletal or microtubular function. Anemia, thrombocytopenia, and pancytopenia are seen in 66%, 60%, and up to 44% of cases, respectively. Pancytopenia can be severe as a result of full-blown aplastic anemia. Bone marrow biopsy specimens and aspirates usually show varying degrees of marrow hypoplasia and fat infiltration. Patients may also have B-cell defects with 1 or more of the following: low immunoglobulin (Ig) G or IgG subclasses, low percentage of circulating B lymphocytes, decreased in vitro B-cell proliferation, and lack of specific antibody production. Patients may have a low percentage of circulating T cells, subsets, or natural killer cells, and decreased in vitro T-cell proliferation.

Diagnosis

Mutational analysis for *SBDS* is definitive in 90% of cases. Pearson syndrome (Chapter 443), consisting of refractory sideroblastic anemia, cytoplasmic vacuolization of bone marrow precursors, metabolic acidosis, exocrine pancreatic insufficiency, and a diagnostic mitochondrial DNA mutation is similar to SDS, but the clinical course, morphologic features of the bone marrow, and gene mutation are different. Also, severe anemia requiring transfusion, rather than neutropenia, is present from birth to 1 yr of age. SDS shares some manifestations with Fanconi anemia, such as marrow dysfunction and growth failure, but patients with SDS are readily distinguished because of pancreatic insufficiency with fat malabsorption, fatty changes within the pancreatic body that can be visualized by imaging, characteristic skeletal abnormalities not seen in Fanconi anemia, and a normal chromosomal breakage study with DEB.

Complications

Patients with SDS are predisposed to MDS and leukemic transformation. The crude rate of MDS or acute leukemia in patients with SDS is 8-33%. Marrow cell clonal cytogenetic abnormalities are an isolated finding, occurring in up to 41% of patients. Isochromosome 7 [i(7q)] is particularly common, suggesting that it is a fairly specific clonal marker of SDS and probably related to the presence of mutant *SBDS* on 7q11. Other clonal chromosome abnormalities include monosomy 7, i(7q) combined with monosomy 7, deletions or translocations involving part of 7q, and deletions of 20q [Del(20q)]. Although i(7q) and Del(20q) are rarely related to leukemic transformation or MDS, the prognostic significance of all marrow clonal changes requires prospective monitoring.

Treatment

Fat malabsorption responds to oral pancreatic enzyme replacement and supplemental fat-soluble vitamins, administered according to guidelines similar to those for cystic fibrosis (Chapter 395). A long-term plan should be initiated to monitor changes in peripheral blood counts that require corrective action and to look for early evidence of malignant myeloid transformation. The latter requires serial bone marrow aspirations for smears and cytogenetics and marrow biopsy. One recommendation is to perform marrow testing annually.

Daily subcutaneous G-CSF for profound neutropenia is effective in inducing a sustained increase in neutrophils. Some patients require transfusion support for management of severe anemia or thrombocytopenia. Experience with erythropoietin is limited. Small numbers of patients have been treated with corticosteroids, and hematologic improvement has been seen in approximately 50%. In some patients who received androgens plus steroids, blood counts have improved. The only curative option for severe marrow failure in SDS is allogeneic HSCT, although experience has been limited. About 50% of patients with SDS who underwent transplantation have died of complications related to the preparative therapy. The risk of cardiotoxicity has been noted. Fludarabine-based protocols using reduced-intensity conditioning appear to be safer and effective for SDS HSCT.

Prognosis

Published literature cites a median survival for patients with SDS as 35 years, but the number of undiagnosed patients with mild or asymptomatic disease is unknown. Hence, overall prognosis may be better than previously thought. Approximately 50% of patients experience spontaneous conversion from pancreatic insufficiency to pancreatic sufficiency as a result of improvement in pancreatic enzyme secretion. Enzyme replacement therapy is then no longer needed. Although all patients have some degree of hematologic cytopenia, the changes in most patients are mild to moderate and do not require therapeutic intervention. Severe neutropenia responds well to G-CSF, but there is concern that the predisposition to MDS and acute leukemia can be heightened by the agent's powerful growth stimulus on marrow cells. HSCT for severe marrow failure has produced a 50% survival rate, but safer protocols are being introduced. Malignant marrow transformation remains ominous.

DYSKERATOSIS CONGENITA

Etiology and Epidemiology

Dyskeratosis congenita (DC) is an inherited multisystem disorder characterized by mucocutaneous abnormalities, bone marrow failure, and a predisposition to cancer and MDS. The diagnostic mucocutaneous (ectodermal) triad is reticulate skin pigmentation of the upper body, mucosal leukoplakia, and nail dystrophy (Fig. 462-2). Skin and nail findings usually become apparent in the 1st 10 yr of life, whereas oral leukoplakia is seen later. These manifestations tend to progress as patients get older. Aplastic anemia occurs in approximately 50% of cases, usually in the 2nd decade of life. About 73% of patients with DC are male, a finding compatible with X-linked recessive inheritance. The remainder has either an autosomal dominant or autosomal recessive mode of inheritance.

Pathology

DC is genetically heterogeneous, and patients have mutations in genes that encode components of the telomerase complex (*DKC1*, *TERC*, *TERT*, *NOP*10, and *NHP*2), and the telomere shelterin complex (*TINF2*), all components critical for telomere maintenance. The **X-linked recessive form** of DC maps to Xq28, and many mutations have been identified in the *DKC1* gene, which codes for the nuclear protein dyskerin. The **autosomal dominant form** is due to mutations in *TINF2,* or in *TERC* or *TERT*, the RNA and enzymatic components of telomerase, respectively. **Autosomal recessive** DC is linked to mutations in *NOP10* or *NHP2*. Because of impaired telomere maintenance in all 3 inherited forms of DC, short telomeres are demonstrated in the peripheral blood cells of all patients and are a cardinal marker for DC and for marrow failure. The failure is likely due to progressive attrition and depletion of hematopoietic stem cells because of premature senescence, which manifests as pancytopenia.

Clinical Manifestations

Skin pigmentation and nail changes typically appear first, mucosal leukoplakia and excessive ocular tearing appear later, and by the

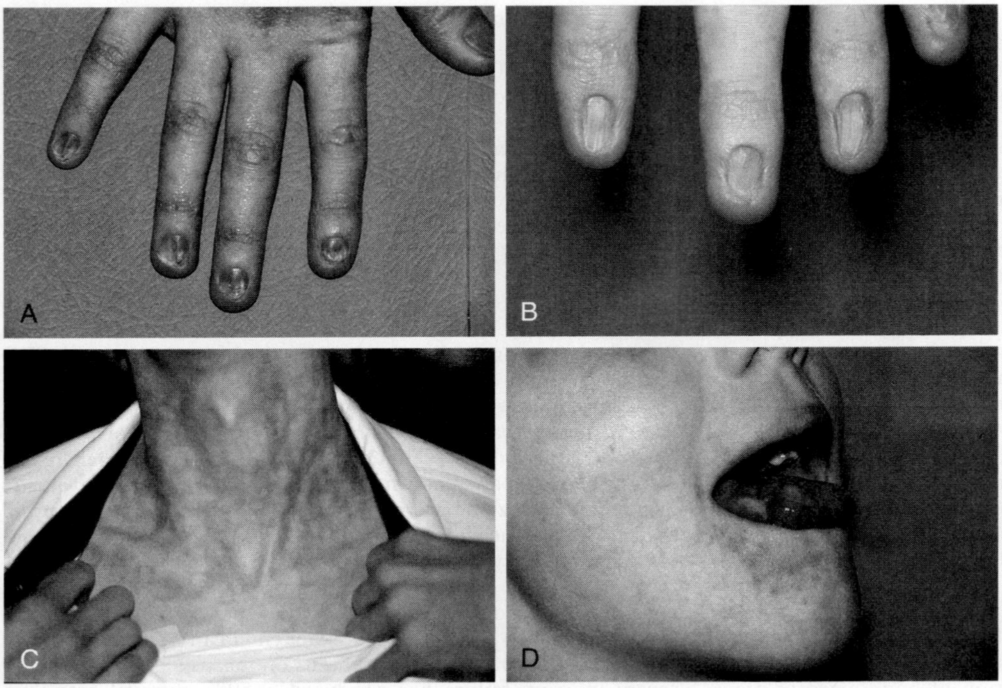

Figure 462-2 Physical findings in patients with dyskeratosis congenita. *A* and *B*, Dystrophic fingernails in 2 different patients. *C*, Lacy reticular pigmentation. *D*, Leukoplakia on the tongue. (From Nathan DG, Orkin SH, Ginsburg D, et al, editors: *Nathan and Oski's hematology of infancy and childhood*, ed 6, vol I, Philadelphia, 2003, WB Saunders, p 300.)

mid-teens, patients with DC have bone marrow failure and malignancy. Many female patients have the same features as male patients. In males, cutaneous findings are the most consistent feature. Lacy reticulated skin pigmentation affecting the face, neck, chest, and arms is a common finding (89%). The degree of pigmentation increases with age and can involve the entire skin surface. There may also be a telangiectatic erythematous component. Nail dystrophy of both hands and feet is the next most common finding (88%). It usually starts with longitudinal ridging, splitting, or pterygium formation and may progress to complete nail loss. Leukoplakia usually involves the oral mucosa (78%), especially the tongue, but may also be seen in the conjunctiva and the anal, urethral, or genital mucosa. Hyperhidrosis of the palms and soles is common, and hair loss is sometimes seen. Eye abnormalities are observed in approximately 50% of cases. Excessive tearing (epiphora) secondary to nasolacrimal duct obstruction is common. Other ophthalmologic manifestations include conjunctivitis, blepharitis, loss of eyelashes, strabismus, cataracts, and optic atrophy. An increased rate of dental decay and early loss of teeth are common. Skeletal abnormalities, such as osteoporosis, avascular necrosis, abnormal bone trabeculation, scoliosis, and mandibular hypoplasia, are seen in approximately 20% of cases. Genitourinary abnormalities include hypoplastic testes, hypospadias, phimosis, urethral stenosis, and horseshoe kidney. Gastrointestinal findings, such as esophageal strictures, hepatomegaly, and cirrhosis, are seen in 10% of cases. A subset of patients has pulmonary complications, with reduced diffusion capacity and/or a restrictive defect. In fatal cases, lung tissue shows pulmonary fibrosis and abnormalities of the pulmonary vasculature.

Laboratory Findings

The initial hematologic change in DC is usually thrombocytopenia, anemia, or both, followed by full-blown pancytopenia and aplastic anemia. The red cells are often macrocytic, and the fetal hemoglobin value can be elevated initially. Initial bone marrow specimens may be hypercellular, but with time, a symmetric depletion of all hematopoietic lineages ensues. Some patients have immunologic abnormalities, including reduced or elevated immunoglobulin values, decreased B- and/or T-lymphocyte count, and reduction of or absence of lymphocyte proliferative responses to phytohemagglutinin. Unlike patients with FA, patients with DC show no abnormal chromosomal breakage in phytohemagglutinin-stimulated lymphocytes upon exposure to DEB. However, primary skin fibroblasts in culture have abnormal morphologic features and doubling rate and show numerous unbalanced chromosome rearrangements, such as dicentrics, tricentrics, and translocations, in the absence of DEB. These findings provide evidence of a defect that predisposes patient cells to chromosomal rearrangements and possibly to DNA damage.

Diagnosis

The following abnormalities are seen in patients with DC but not in those with FA: nail dystrophy, leukoplakia, and tooth abnormalities, hyperhidrosis of the palms and soles, and hair loss. There are overlap syndromes that share some of the features of DC. Hoyeraal-Hreidarsson syndrome is a multisystem disorder comprising aplastic anemia, immunodeficiency, microcephaly, growth retardation, and cerebellar hypoplasia. The syndrome is genetically heterogeneous; some cases are X-linked recessive and caused by mutations in *DKC1*, and others are autosomal recessive owing to homozygous *TERT* mutations. Revesz syndrome consists of dystrophic nails, leukoplakia, aplastic anemia, cerebellar hypoplasia, growth retardation, microcephaly, and bilateral exudative retinopathy. *TINF2* is mutated in Revesz syndrome, which hence is an autosomal dominant variant of DC.

Complications

Cancer develops in approximately 10-15% of patients with DC, usually in the 3rd and 4th decades of life. Patients with DC are predisposed to MDS as well as to solid tumors. Forty percent of the cancers in such patients are squamous cell carcinomas of the head and neck (tongue, mouth, pharynx). Cancer of the skin and gastrointestinal tract (esophagus, stomach, colon, and especially the anorectal site) is also common.

Treatment

Androgens, usually combined with low-dose prednisone, can induce improvement of marrow function in approximately 50% of patients. When the response is maximal, the androgen dose can be slowly tapered but not stopped. DC can become refractory to androgens as the aplastic anemia progresses. There is no published information on the use of immunosuppressive therapy for this disorder. Although reports are scanty, cytokine therapy with granulocyte-macrophage colony stimulating factor (GM-CSF) or with G-CSF alone or combined with erythropoietin appears to offer potential benefit, at least in the short term, especially for improving neutrophil numbers.

Allogeneic HSCT has been used to correct marrow failure in patients with DC, but with only a 50% survival rate. Inherent telomere shortening in DC may underlie many of the complications. Vascular lesions and fibrosis involving various organs occur early and late after transplantation and carry a high mortality rate. Patients with DC may be more susceptible to endothelial damage that occurs after HSCT as a result of various factors, including the conditioning regimen, infectious disease, and graft versus host disease. Up to 40% of patients with DC experience fatal pulmonary complications after transplantation.

Although the mutated genes for most cases of DC are known, prospects for gene therapy are not imminent.

Prognosis
Considerable heterogeneity exists in DC. Patients with autosomal dominant disease have milder clinical manifestations. Patients with autosomal recessive disease appear to have more physical anomalies and a higher incidence of aplastic anemia and cancer. The mean age of death for patients with DC is approximately 30 yr. The main causes of death are bone marrow failure, complications of HSCT, cancer, and fatal pulmonary problems.

AMEGAKARYOCYTIC THROMBOCYTOPENIA

Etiology and Epidemiology
Congenital amegakaryocytic thrombocytopenia (CAMT) is the rarest of the 4 major inherited pancytopenias. It is transmitted in an autosomal recessive manner. CAMT manifests in infancy as isolated thrombocytopenia due to reduction or absence of marrow megakaryocytes with initial preservation of granulopoietic and erythroid lineages. Pancytopenia due to aplastic anemia often ensues in the first few years of life. The defect in CAMT is directly related to mutations in *MPL,* the gene for the receptor of thrombopoietin, the growth factor that stimulates megakaryocyte proliferation and maturation. Carriers of the mutant gene have normal hematology; affected individuals have mutations in both alleles. Genotype-phenotype correlations predict disease course and prognosis. **Nonsense mutations** produce a complete loss of function of the thrombopoietin receptor, causing persistently low platelet counts due to absence of megakaryocytes and a fast progression to pancytopenia and aplastic anemia. Because thrombopoietin also has an anti-apoptotic and cell survival effect on stem cells, impaired stem cell survival with *MPL* nonsense mutations explains the evolution of CAMT into aplastic anemia. **Missense mutations** of *MPL* are associated with a milder course, a transient increase in platelets during the first years of life, and delayed onset, if any, of pancytopenia, indicating residual receptor function. Biologically active plasma thrombopoietin is consistently elevated in all patients with CAMT.

Clinical Manifestations
Patients with CAMT have petechial rash, bruising, or bleeding at birth or in the 1st year of life. Patients with proven *MPL* mutations appear thus far to have normal physical and imaging features. About 40% of published phenotypic CAMT cases involved physical anomalies, but *MPL* mutation analyses were not available in these earlier cases, and CAMT was not confirmed genotypically. The most common anomalies in the published cases are neurologic and cardiac. Findings related to cerebellar and cerebral atrophy are frequent, and developmental delay is a prominent feature. Congenital heart disease includes atrial septal defects, ventricular septal defects, patent ductus arteriosus, tetralogy of Fallot, and coarctation of the aorta. Some of these occur in combinations. Other anomalies include abnormal hips or feet, kidney malformations, eye anomalies, and cleft or high-arched palate. Some patients have microcephaly and an abnormal facies.

Laboratory Findings
Thrombocytopenia is the major laboratory finding in CAMT, with normal hemoglobin levels and white blood cell counts initially. Peripheral blood platelets are reduced or totally absent. As in other inherited bone marrow failure syndromes, red blood cells may be macrocytic. Hemoglobin F may be elevated, and there may be increased expression of i antigen. Bone marrow aspirates and biopsy specimens show normal cellularity with marked reduction or absence of megakaryocytes. In patients in whom aplastic anemia develops, marrow cellularity is decreased, with fatty replacement; erythropoietic and granulopoietic lineages are also symmetrically reduced.

Diagnosis
If CAMT manifests beyond the neonatal period, marrow aspirate and biopsy will demonstrate deficient megakaryocytes and suggest the diagnosis; mutational analysis will confirm it. If CAMT occurs at birth or shortly after, it must be distinguished from other causes of inherited and acquired neonatal thrombocytopenia (Chapter 478). Thrombocytopenia with absent radii (TAR syndrome) is distinguished from CAMT because in TAR the radii are absent. CAMT blood lymphocytes do not show increased chromosomal breakage when exposed to DEB, distinguishing the disease it from FA.

Complications
In some patients, clonal marrow cell cytogenetic abnormalities appear such as monosomy 7 and trisomy 8 but without evidence of leukemia. CAMT can evolve into MDS and also acute leukemia, but the true risk cannot be defined because of the rarity of the disease and the paucity of published data.

Therapy and Prognosis
The mortality rate in patients with *MPL* **nonsense** mutations from thrombocytopenic bleeding, complications of aplastic anemia, or leukemic transformation has been very close to 100%. Patients with **missense** mutations have a milder course but may still have serious complications. HSCT is the only curative option. The majority of patients with CAMT who undergo HSCT are cured, especially if the procedure is performed with HLA-matched sibling donors. Before transplantation, platelet transfusion should be used discretely. Platelet count should not always be the sole indication; clinical bleeding is an appropriate trigger. Single-donor filtered platelets are preferred to minimize sensitization, and in a patient for whom HSCT is a possibility, all blood products should be free of cytomegalovirus. Corticosteroids do not appear to be effective for treatment of the thrombocytopenia. For aplastic anemia, androgens in combination with corticosteroids may induce a temporary partial improvement. Interleukin-3 may be an important adjunct to the medical management of CAMT, but it was not adopted broadly and is no longer available. Thrombopoietin has not been tried for the treatment of CAMT and would likely fail, because endogenous thrombopoietin levels are markedly increased and thrombopoietin receptors are either nonfunctional or functioning poorly.

OTHER GENETIC SYNDROMES

Pancytopenia and bone marrow failure can occur in the context of several nonhematologic syndromes and familial settings that do not exactly correspond to the entities already described.

Down Syndrome
Down syndrome (trisomy 21; Chapter 76) has a unique association with aberrant hematologic findings. In addition to the propensity for acute lymphoblastic and myeloblastic leukemias,

especially acute megakaryoblastic leukemia, a few patients with Down syndrome have been reported as having pancytopenia due to aplastic anemia.

Dubowitz Syndrome

Dubowitz syndrome is an autosomal recessive disorder characterized by a peculiar facies, infantile eczema, small stature, and mild microcephaly. The face is small, with a shallow supraorbital ridge, a nasal bridge at the same level as the forehead, short palpebral fissures, variable ptosis, and micrognathia. There is a predilection to cancer as well as to bone marrow dysfunction in these patients. Approximately 10% of patients have hematopoietic disorders, including hypoplastic anemia, moderate pancytopenia, and full-blown aplastic anemia.

Seckel Syndrome

Seckel syndrome, sometimes called "bird-headed dwarfism," is an autosomal recessive developmental disorder characterized by marked growth failure and mental deficiency, microcephaly, a hypoplastic face with a prominent nose, and low-set and/or malformed ears. Approximately 25% of patients have aplastic anemia or malignancies. One form of Seckel syndrome is caused by a mutant *ATR* gene, and another is caused by a mutant *PCNT2* gene. Different loci for 2 additional forms have also been identified, demonstrating genetic heterogeneity.

Reticular Dysgenesis

Reticular dysgenesis (Chapter 120) is an immunologic deficiency syndrome coupled with congenital agranulocytosis. The mode of inheritance is probably autosomal recessive, but an X-linked mode is also possible in some cases. The disorder is a variant of severe combined immune deficiency in which cellular and humoral immunity are absent and severe lymphopenia and neutropenia are also seen. Anemia and thrombocytopenia may also be present. Bone marrow specimens are hypocellular, with markedly reduced myeloid and lymphoid elements. The only curative therapy is HSCT.

Schimke Immunoosseous Dysplasia

Schimke immunoosseous dysplasia is an autosomal recessive disorder caused by mutations in the chromatin remodeling protein *SMARCAL1*. Patients have spondyloepiphyseal dysplasia with exaggerated lumbar lordosis and a protruding abdomen. There are pigmentary skin changes and abnormally discolored and configured teeth. Renal dysfunction can be problematic, with proteinuria and nephrotic syndrome. Approximately 50% of patients have hypothyroidism, 50% have cerebral ischemia, and 10% have bone marrow failure with neutropenia, thrombocytopenia, and anemia. Lymphopenia and altered cellular immunity are present in almost all patients. In 1 published case, a patient underwent successful bone marrow transplantation.

Noonan Syndrome

Noonan syndrome is a developmental disorder characterized by the "Noonan facies" (hypertelorism, ptosis, short neck, low-set ears), short stature, congenital heart disease, and multiple skeletal and hematologic abnormalities. It is an autosomal dominant disorder composed of at least 5 genetic types. Heterozygous mutations in *PTPN11* cause about 50% of cases of the syndrome; others are caused by a mutant *NF1* gene, by a germline *KRAS* mutation, by mutant *SOS1*, or by mutant *RAF1*. In addition to an association with juvenile myelomonocytic leukemia, amegakaryocytic thrombocytopenia, as well as pancytopenia and a hypocellular marrow can develop in patients with Noonan syndrome.

Cartilage-Hair Hypoplasia

Cartilage-hair hypoplasia, an autosomal recessive syndrome seen mostly in Finnish or Amish populations, is characterized by metaphyseal dysostosis, short-limbed dwarfism, and fine, sparse hair. Additional skeletal findings are scoliosis, lordosis, chest deformity, and varus lower limbs. Gastrointestinal abnormalities also occur. Mutations in the *RMRP* gene cause CHH. Macrocytic anemia is seen in most patients and is sometimes severe and persistent. Neutropenia, lymphopenia, and a predisposition to lymphoma and other cancers are also features.

Table 462-3 CANADIAN INHERITED MARROW FAILURE REGISTRY CRITERIA FOR UNCLASSIFIED INHERITED BONE MARROW FAILURE SYNDROMES

FULFILLS CRITERIA 1 AND 2:
1. Does not fulfill criteria for any categorized inherited bone marrow failure syndrome* 2. Fulfills both of the following
FULFILLS AT LEAST 2 OF THE FOLLOWING:
a. Chronic cytopenia(s) detected on at least 2 occasions over at least 3 mo[†] b. Reduced marrow progenitors or reduced clonogenic potential of hematopoietic progenitor cells or evidence of ineffective hematopoiesis[‡] c. High fetal hemoglobin for age[‡] d. Red blood cell macrocytosis (not caused by hemolysis or a nutritional deficiency)
FULFILLS AT LEAST 1 OF THE FOLLOWING:
a. Family history of bone marrow failure b. Presentation at age <1 yr c. Anomalies involving multiple systems to suggest an inherited syndrome

*The Canadian Inherited Marrow Failure Registry diagnostic guidelines for selected syndromes were adapted from the literature and are available at *www.sickkids.ca/cimfr*.

†Cytopenia was defined as follows: neutropenia, neutrophil count of $<1.5 \times 10^9$/L; thrombocytopenia, platelet count of $<150 \times 10^9$/L; anemia, hemoglobin concentration of <2 standard deviations below mean, adjusted for age.

‡Hemoglobinopathies with ineffective erythropoiesis and high hemoglobin F should be excluded by clinical or laboratory testing.

Modified from Teo JT, Klaassen R, Fernandez CV, et al: Clinical and genetic analysis of unclassifiable inherited bone marrow failure syndromes. *Pediatrics* 22:e139–e148, 2008.

Familial Aplastic Anemia

Bone marrow failure can cluster in families, but many of these cases cannot be readily classified into discrete diagnostic entities such as FA. The phenotype of these conditions can be complex, with varying combinations of hematologic abnormalities, immunologic deficiency, physical malformations, and predisposition to leukemia. Both autosomal dominant and autosomal recessive inheritances have been observed; both patterns occur with or without associated physical anomalies. An X-linked type is described with physical anomalies; additionally, the X-linked lymphoproliferative syndrome associated with Epstein-Barr virus is associated with pancytopenia.

UNCLASSIFIED INHERITED BONE MARROW FAILURE SYNDROMES

Unclassified inherited bone marrow failure syndromes are heterogeneous disorders that may be either atypical presentations of identifiable diseases or new syndromes. Characterized by various cytopenias, with or without physical manifestations, they do not fit into a classic genetic bone marrow failure disease because all features may not be evident at the time of presentation. Compared with classic disorders (presentation ≈ 1 mo of age), infants with unclassified disorders present later (≈ 9 mo) and manifest single or multilineage cytopenia, aplastic anemia, myelodysplasia, or malignancy with variable expression of malformations. Criteria for the diagnosis are seen in Table 462-3. With follow-up, some may demonstrate typical physical features of known syndromes, such as Shwachman-Diamond syndrome, although without obvious mutations in the *SBDS* gene.

BIBLIOGRAPHY

Please visit the Nelson Textbook of Pediatrics *website at* www.expertconsult.com *for the complete bibliography.*

Chapter 463
The Acquired Pancytopenias

Jeffrey D. Hord

ETIOLOGY AND EPIDEMIOLOGY

Drugs, chemicals, toxins, infectious agents, radiation, and immune disorders can result in pancytopenia by direct destruction of hematopoietic progenitors, disruption of the marrow microenvironment, or immune-mediated suppression of marrow elements (Table 463-1). A careful history of exposure to known risk factors should be obtained for every child presenting with pancytopenia. Even in the absence of the classic associated physical findings, the possibility of a genetic predisposition to bone marrow failure should always be considered (Chapter 462). The majority of cases of acquired marrow failure in childhood are "idiopathic," in that no causative agent is identified. These are probably immune-mediated through activated T lymphocytes and cytokine destruction of marrow progenitor cells. The overall incidence of acquired aplastic anemia is relatively low, with an approximate incidence in both children and adults in the USA and Europe of 2-6 cases/million/yr. The incidence is higher in Asia, with as many as 14 cases/million/yr in Japan.

Severe bone marrow suppression can develop after exposure to many different drugs and chemicals, including certain chemotherapeutic agents, insecticides, antibiotics, anticonvulsants, nonsteroidal anti-inflammatory agents, and recreational drugs. Some of the most notable agents are benzene, chloramphenicol, gold, and, most recently, 3,4,-methylenedioxymethamphetamine (Ecstasy).

A number of viruses can either directly or indirectly result in bone marrow failure. Parvovirus B19 is classically associated with isolated red blood cell (RBC) aplasia, but in patients with sickle cell disease or immunodeficiency, it can result in transient pancytopenia (Chapters 243 and 462). Prolonged pancytopenia can occur after infection with many of the hepatitis viruses, herpes viruses, Epstein-Barr virus (Chapter 246), cytomegalovirus (Chapter 247), and HIV (Chapter 268).

Patients with evidence of bone marrow failure should also be evaluated for paroxysmal nocturnal hemoglobinuria (PNH; Chapter 458) and collagen vascular diseases, although these are uncommon causes of pancytopenia in childhood. Pancytopenia without peripheral blasts may be caused by bone marrow replacement by leukemic blasts or neuroblastoma cells.

Table 463-1 ETIOLOGY OF ACQUIRED APLASTIC ANEMIA

Radiation drugs and chemicals:
- Predictable: chemotherapy, benzene
- Idiosyncratic: chloramphenicol, antiepileptics, gold; 3,4-methylenedioxymethamphetamine

Viruses:
- Cytomegalovirus
- Epstein-barr
- Hepatitis b
- Hepatitis c
- Hepatitis non-A, non-B, non-C (seronegative hepatitis)
- HIV

Immune diseases:
- Eosinophilic fasciitis
- Hypoimmunoglobulinemia
- Thymoma

Pregnancy

Paroxysmal nocturnal hemoglobinuria

Marrow replacement:
- Leukemia
- Myelodysplasia
- Myelofibrosis

Autoimmune

Other:
- Cryptic dyskeratosis congenita (no physical stigmata)
- Telomerase reverse transcriptase haploinsufficiency

PATHOLOGY AND PATHOGENESIS

The hallmark of aplastic anemia is peripheral pancytopenia, coupled with hypoplastic or aplastic bone marrow. The severity of the clinical course is related to the degree of myelosuppression. **Severe aplastic anemia** is defined as a condition in which 2 or more cell components have become seriously compromised (absolute neutrophil count [ANC] <500/mm^3, platelet count <20,000/mm^3, reticulocyte count <1% after correction for hematocrit) in a patient whose bone marrow biopsy material is moderately or severely hypocellular. Approximately 65% of patients who first present with **moderate aplastic anemia** (ANC 500-1,500/mm^3, platelet count 20,000-100,000/mm^3, reticulocyte count <1%) eventually progress to meet the criteria for severe disease if they are simply observed. Bone marrow failure may be a consequence of a direct cytotoxic effect on hematopoietic stem cells from a drug or chemical or may result from either cell-mediated or antibody-dependent cytotoxicity. There is strong evidence that many cases of idiopathic aplastic anemia are caused by an immune-mediated process, with increased circulating activated T lymphocytes producing cytokines (interferon-γ) that suppress hematopoiesis. Abnormal telomere length and telomerase activity in granulocytic precursors and increased expression of cell surface Flt3 ligand (a member of the class III receptor tyrosine kinase family) in the lymphocytes of patients with aplastic anemia suggest that early apoptosis of hematopoietic progenitors may play a role in the pathogenesis of this disease.

CLINICAL MANIFESTATIONS, LABORATORY FINDINGS, AND DIFFERENTIAL DIAGNOSIS

Pancytopenia results in increased risks of cardiac failure, infection, bleeding, and fatigue. Acquired pancytopenia is typically characterized by anemia, leukopenia, and thrombocytopenia in the setting of elevated serum cytokine values. Other treatable disorders, such as cancer, collagen vascular disorders, PNH, and infections that may respond to specific therapies (IV immune globulin for parvovirus), should be considered in the differential diagnosis. Careful examination of the peripheral blood smear for RBC, leukocyte, and platelet morphologic features is important. A reticulocyte count should be performed to assess erythropoietic activity. In children, the possibility of congenital pancytopenia must always be considered, and chromosomal breakage analysis should be performed to evaluate for Fanconi anemia (Chapter 462). The presence of fetal hemoglobin suggests congenital pancytopenia but is not diagnostic. To assess for the possibility of PNH, flow cytometric analysis of erythrocytes for CD55 and CD59 is the most sensitive test. Bone marrow examination should include both aspiration and a biopsy, and the marrow should be carefully evaluated for morphologic features, cellularity, and cytogenetic findings.

TREATMENT

The treatment of children with acquired pancytopenia requires comprehensive supportive care coupled with an attempt to treat the underlying marrow failure. For patients with an HLA-identical sibling marrow donor, allogeneic bone marrow transplantation (BMT) offers a 90% chance of long-term survival. The risks associated with this approach include the immediate complications of transplantation, graft failure, and graft versus host disease. Late adverse effects associated with transplantation may include secondary cancers, cataracts, short stature, hypothyroidism, and gonadal dysfunction (Chapters 131-133). Only 1 in 5 patients has an HLA-matched sibling donor, so matched-related BMT is not an option for the majority of patients.

For patients without a sibling donor, the major form of therapy is immunosuppression with antithymocyte globulin (ATG) and cyclosporine, with a response rate of 60-80%. The median time to response is 6 mo. As many as 25-30% of "responders" experience relapse after discontinuation of immunosuppression, and some patients must continue cyclosporine for several years to maintain a hematologic response. Among those who have relapse after immunosuppression, about 50% show response to a second course of ATG and cyclosporine. There is an increased risk of clonal bone marrow disease, such as leukemia, myelodysplasia (MDS), or PNH after immunosuppression. The exact risk of clonal disease after immunosuppression is probably <10%, and the abnormal karyotypes most frequently involve chromosomes 6, 7, and 8. To accelerate neutrophil recovery, a hematopoietic colony-stimulating factor (e.g., granulocyte colony-stimulating factor, granulocyte-macrophage colony-stimulating factor) is sometimes added to ATG and cyclosporine for treatment of patients with very severe neutropenia (absolute neutrophil count <200/mm^3), but there is no clear evidence that this treatment influences response rate or survival. In a few cases, tacrolimus has been given successfully with ATG for treatment of aplastic anemia in a patient unable to tolerate cyclosporine.

For patients who show no response to immunosuppression or who experience relapse after immunosuppression, matched unrelated donor marrow/stem cell transplant is a treatment option, with a response rate approaching 80% in later studies. Cord blood transplants have rarely lead to successful outcomes because of problems with non-engraftment. High-dose cyclophosphamide has been used successfully in the treatment of patients with newly diagnosed aplastic anemia and in patients without adequate response to immunosuppression. This therapy leads to prolonged severe pancytopenia, increasing the risk of life-threatening infection, especially fungal. Other therapies that have been used in the past with inconsistent results include androgens, corticosteroids, and plasmapheresis.

COMPLICATIONS

The major complications of severe pancytopenia are predominantly related to the risk of life-threatening bleeding from prolonged thrombocytopenia or to infection secondary to protracted neutropenia. Patients with protracted neutropenia due to bone marrow failure are at risk not only for serious bacterial infections but also for invasive mycoses. The general principles of supportive care that have evolved from the use of chemotherapy-related myelosuppression to treat patients with cancer should be fully extended to the care of patients with acquired pancytopenia (Chapter 171).

PROGNOSIS

Spontaneous recovery from pancytopenia rarely occurs. If left untreated, severe pancytopenia has an overall mortality rate of approximately 50% within 6 mo of diagnosis and of >75% overall, with infection and hemorrhage being the major causes of morbidity and mortality. The majority of children with acquired severe aplastic anemia show response to allogeneic marrow transplantation or immunosuppression, leaving them with normal or near-normal blood cell counts.

PANCYTOPENIA CAUSED BY MARROW REPLACEMENT

Processes that either infiltrate or replace the bone marrow can manifest as acquired pancytopenia. Infiltration can be caused by malignancy (classically, neuroblastoma or leukemia) or occur as a consequence of myelofibrosis, MDS, or osteoporosis. Although uncommon, evidence of hypoplastic anemia can precede the onset of acute leukemia, generally by a few months. This relationship is important to appreciate in evaluating and monitoring children who present with what appears to be acquired aplastic anemia. Morphologic examination of the peripheral blood and bone marrow and marrow cytogenetic studies are critically important in making the diagnoses of leukemia, myelofibrosis, and MDS.

MDS is very rare in children, but when it occurs, its clinical course is more aggressive than the same category of MDS in adults. A number of inherited conditions are associated with an increased risk for development of MDS, including Down syndrome, Kostmann syndrome, Noonan syndrome, Fanconi anemia, trisomy 8 mosaicism, neurofibromatosis, and Schwachman syndrome. Significant clonal abnormalities are found within the marrow of approximately 50% of patients with MDS, with monosomy 7 and trisomy 8 being most common. The transition time from pediatric MDS to acute leukemia is relatively short, at 14-26 mo, so aggressive treatment, such as BMT, must be considered shortly after diagnosis. With allogeneic BMT, the survival rate is approximately 50%. One exception to such an aggressive therapeutic approach is MDS and acute myelocytic leukemia in children with Down syndrome, because this disease in this specific population is very responsive to conventional chemotherapy, with long-term survival rates >80%.

The decision on how to treat a child with MDS who lacks a suitable marrow donor should be made with the specific clonal abnormality found within the child's marrow taken into consideration. Lenalidomide produces the best responses among patients who have the chromosomal abnormality, 5q–. Immunosuppressive therapy with ATG and cyclosporine is most effective in patients with trisomy 8, especially in the presence of a PNH clone. Imatinib mesylate targets mutations in the tyrosine kinase receptor family of genes found in patients with t(5;12) and del(4q12). The DNA hypomethylating agents azacitidine and decitabine have also been used in treating MDS without a known molecular target and have some effect.

BIBLIOGRAPHY

Please visit the Nelson Textbook of Pediatrics *website at www.expertconsult.com for the complete bibliography.*

Section 6 BLOOD COMPONENT TRANSFUSIONS

Chapter 464
Red Blood Cell Transfusions and Erythropoietin Therapy

Ronald G. Strauss

Red blood cells (RBCs) are transfused to increase the oxygen-carrying capacity of the blood and, in turn, to maintain satisfactory tissue oxygenation. Guidelines for RBC transfusions in children and adolescents are similar to those for adults (see Table 464-1 on the *Nelson Textbook of Pediatrics* website at www.expertconsult.com). However, transfusions may be given more stringently to children, because normal hemoglobin levels are lower in healthy children than in adults and, often, children do not have the underlying multiorgan, cardiorespiratory, and vascular diseases that develop with aging in adults. Thus, children often compensate better for RBC loss and, as is true for patients of all ages, there is increasing enthusiasm for conservative practices (i.e., low pre-transfusion hematocrit values).

For the full continuation of this chapter, please visit the Nelson Textbook of Pediatrics *website at www.expertconsult.com.*

Chapter 465
Platelet Transfusions
Ronald G. Strauss

Guidelines for platelet (PLT) support of children and adolescents with quantitative and qualitative PLT disorders are similar to those for adults (see Table 465-1 on the *Nelson Textbook of Pediatrics* website at www.expertconsult.com), in whom the risk of life-threatening bleeding after injury or occurring spontaneously can be related to the severity of thrombocytopenia. PLT transfusions should be given to patients with PLT counts $< 50 \times 10^9/L$ when they are bleeding or are scheduled for an invasive procedure, and the PLT count should be maintained $> 50 \times 10^9/L$ until bleeding ceases or the patient is stable after the procedure.

For the full continuation of this chapter, please visit the Nelson Textbook of Pediatrics *website at www.expertconsult.com.*

Chapter 466
Neutrophil (Granulocyte) Transfusions
Ronald G. Strauss

Guidelines for granulocyte transfusion (GTX) are listed in Table 466-1 on the *Nelson Textbook of Pediatrics* website at www.expertconsult.com. Although GTX has been used sparingly in the past, the ability to collect markedly higher numbers of neutrophils from donors stimulated with recombinant granulocyte colony-stimulating factor (G-CSF) plus dexamethasone has led to renewed interest, particularly for recipients of hematopoietic progenitor cell transplantation. GTX should be reconsidered at institutions where neutropenic patients continue to die of progressive bacterial and fungal infections or to suffer substantial morbidity despite the optimal use of antimicrobial agents (i.e., "antibiotics") and recombinant myeloid growth factors.

For the full continuation of this chapter, please visit the Nelson Textbook of Pediatrics *website at www.expertconsult.com.*

Chapter 467
Plasma Transfusions
Ronald G. Strauss

Guidelines for plasma transfusion in children (see Table 467-1 on the *Nelson Textbook of Pediatrics* website at www.expertconsult.com) are similar to those for adults. Plasma is transfused to replace clinically significant deficiencies of plasma proteins (nearly always clotting proteins) for which more highly purified concentrates are not available. Two interchangeable plasma products are available for transfusion, plasma frozen within 8 hr of collection (fresh frozen plasma) and plasma frozen within 24 hr of collection. Although levels of factors V and VIII are lower in the latter plasma product, they are equally efficacious for literally all indications for plasma transfusions (see Table 467-1). Requirements for plasma vary with the specific protein being replaced, but a starting dose of 15 mL/kg is usually satisfactory.

For the full continuation of this chapter, please visit the Nelson Textbook of Pediatrics *website at www.expertconsult.com.*

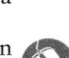

Chapter 468
Risks of Blood Transfusions
Ronald G. Strauss

The greatest risk of a blood transfusion is receiving a transfusion intended for another patient. This risk is particularly high for infants, because identification bands may not be attached to their bodies, difficulties in drawing pretransfusion compatibility testing blood sample may lead to deviations in usual policies, and infants cannot speak to identify themselves. Thus, particular care must be taken to ensure accurate patient and blood sample identification.

For the full continuation of this chapter, please visit the Nelson Textbook of Pediatrics *website at www.expertconsult.com.*

Section 7 HEMORRHAGIC AND THROMBOTIC DISEASES

Chapter 469
Hemostasis
J. Paul Scott, Leslie J. Raffini, and Robert R. Montgomery

Hemostasis is the active process that clots blood in areas of blood vessel injury yet simultaneously limits the clot size only to the areas of injury. Over time, the clot is lysed by the fibrinolytic system, and normal blood flow is restored. If clotting is impaired, hemorrhage occurs. If clotting is excessive, thrombotic complications ensue. The hemostatic response needs to be rapid and regulated such that trauma does not trigger a systemic reaction but must initiate a rapid, localized response. Key to the speed and coordination of response is that when a platelet adheres to a site of vascular injury, the platelet surface provides a reaction surface where clotting factors bind. The active enzyme is brought together with its substrate and a catalytic cofactor on a reaction surface, accelerating reaction rates and providing activated products for reaction with clotting factors further down the coagulation cascade. Active clotting is controlled by negative feedback loops that inhibit the clotting process when the procoagulant process comes in contact with intact endothelium. The main components of the hemostatic process are the **vessel wall, platelets, coagulation proteins, anticoagulant proteins,** and **fibrinolytic system.** Most components of hemostasis are multifunctional; fibrinogen serves as the ligand between platelets during platelet aggregation and also serves as the substrate for thrombin that forms the fibrin clot. Platelets provide the reaction surface on which clotting reactions occur, form the plug at the site of vessel injury, and contract to constrict and limit clot size.

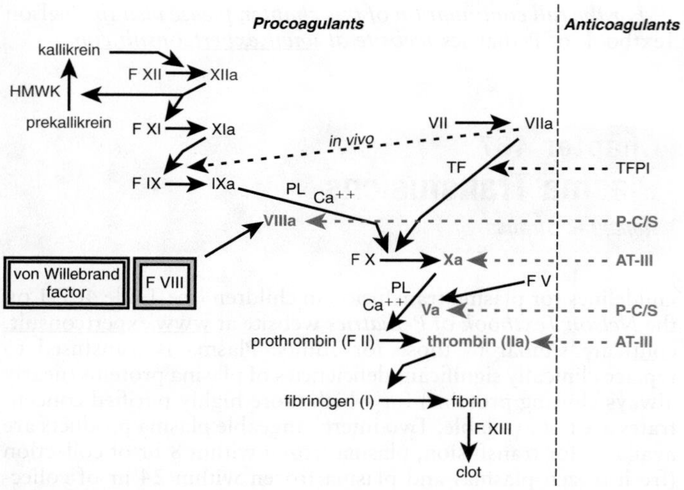

Figure 469-1 The clotting cascade, with sequential activation and amplification of clot formation. Many of the factors (F) are activated by the clotting factors shown above them in the cascade. The activated factors are designated by the addition of an *a.* On the *right side,* the major anticoagulants and the sites that they regulate are shown: Tissue factor pathway inhibitor (TFPI) regulates tissue factor (TF]); factor VIIa, protein C, and protein S (P-C/S) regulate factors VIII and V; and antithrombin III (AT-III) regulates factor Xa and thrombin (factor IIa). The *dotted line* shows that, in vivo, TF and factor VIIa activate both factors IX and X but that, in vitro, only the activation of factor X is measured. Unactivated factor VIII, when bound to its carrier protein, von Willebrand factor, is protected from protein C inactivation. When thrombin, or factor Xa activates factor VIII, it becomes unbound from von Willebrand factor, whereupon it can participate with factor IXa in the activation of factor X in the presence of phospholipid (PL) and Ca^{2+} (the "tenase" complex). Factor XIIIa cross links the fibrin clot and thereby makes it more stable. Prekallikrein, high molecular weight kininogen (HMWK), and factor XII are shown in *blue* because they do not have a physiologic role in coagulation, although they contribute to the clotting time in partial thromboplastin time (PTT).

THE PROCESS

The intact vascular endothelium is the primary barrier against hemorrhage. The endothelial cells that line the vessel wall normally inhibit coagulation and provide a smooth surface that permits rapid blood flow.

After vascular injury, vasoconstriction occurs and flowing blood comes in contact with the subendothelial matrix (Fig. 469-1). In flowing blood, when exposed to subendothelial matrix proteins, von Willebrand factor (VWF) changes conformation and provides the glue to which the platelet VWF receptor, the glycoprotein Ib complex, binds, tethering platelets to sites of injury. When the VWF receptor binds its ligand, complex signaling occurs from the outside membrane receptor to intracellular pathways, activating the platelets and triggering secretion of storage granules containing adenosine diphosphate (ADP), serotonin, and stored plasma and platelet membrane proteins. Upon activation, the platelet receptor for fibrinogen, $\alpha 2b\beta 3$, is switched on ("inside out" signaling) to bind fibrinogen and triggers the aggregation and recruitment of other platelets to form the platelet plug. Multiple physiologic agonists can trigger platelet activation and aggregation, including ADP, collagen, thrombin, and arachidonic acid. Aggregation involves the interaction of specific receptors on the platelet surface with plasma hemostatic proteins, primarily fibrinogen.

One of the subendothelial matrix proteins that are exposed after vascular injury is tissue factor. Just as exposed subendothelial matrix proteins bind VWF, exposed tissue factor binds to factor VII and activates the clotting cascade, as shown in Figure 469-2. The activated clotting factor then initiates the activation of the next sequential clotting factor in a systematic manner. Our understanding of the sequence of steps in the cascade followed assignment of the numerals for the clotting factors for the participant proteins, and thus the sequence seems "out of numerical order." During the process of platelet activation, internalized platelet phospholipids (primarily phosphatidylserine) become externalized and interact at 2 specific, rate-limiting steps in the clotting process—those involving the cofactors factor VIII (X-ase complex) and factor V (prothrombinase complex). Both of these reactions are localized to the platelet surface and bring together the active enzyme, an activated cofactor, and the zymogen that will form the next active enzyme in the cascade. This sequence results in amplification of the process, which supplies a burst of clotting where it is physiologically needed. In vivo, autocatalysis of factor VII generates small amounts of VIIa continuously, so the system is always poised to act. Near the bottom of the cascade, the multipotent enzyme thrombin is formed. Thrombin converts fibrinogen into fibrin, activates factors V, VIII, and XI, and aggregates platelets. Activation of factor XI by thrombin amplifies further thrombin generation and contributes to inhibition of fibrinolysis. Thrombin also activates factor XIII. The stable fibrin-platelet plug is ultimately formed through clot retraction and cross linking of the fibrin clot by factor XIIIa.

Virtually all procoagulant proteins are balanced by an anticoagulant protein that regulates or inhibits procoagulant function. Four clinically important, naturally occurring anticoagulants regulate the extension of the clotting process. They are antithrombin III (AT-III), protein C, protein S, and tissue factor pathway inhibitor (TFPI). AT-III is a serine protease inhibitor that regulates factor Xa and thrombin primarily and factors IXa, XIa, and XIIa to a lesser extent. When thrombin in flowing blood encounters intact endothelium, thrombin binds to thrombomodulin, its endothelial receptor. The thrombin-thrombomodulin complex then converts protein C into activated protein C. In the presence of the cofactor protein S, activated protein C proteolyses and inactivates factor Va and factor VIIIa. Inactivated factor Va is, in fact, a functional anticoagulant that inhibits clotting. TFPI limits activation of factor X by factor VIIa and tissue factor and shifts the activation site of tissue factor and factor VIIa to that of factor IX (see Figs. 469-1 and 469-2).

Once a stable fibrin-platelet plug is formed, the fibrinolytic system limits its extension and also lyses the clot (fibrinolysis) to reestablish vascular integrity. Plasmin, generated from plasminogen by either urokinase-like or tissue-type plasminogen activator, degrades the fibrin clot. In the process of dissolving the fibrin clot, fibrin degradation products (FDPs) are produced. The fibrinolytic pathway is regulated by plasminogen activator inhibitors and α_2-antiplasmin as well as by the thrombin-activatable fibrinolysis inhibitor (TAFI). Finally, the flow of blood in and around the clot is crucial, because flowing blood returns to the liver, where activated clotting factor complexes are removed and new procoagulant and anticoagulant proteins are synthesized to maintain homeostasis of the hemostatic system.

PATHOLOGY

Congenital deficiency of an individual procoagulant protein leads to a bleeding disorder, whereas deficiency of an anticoagulant (clotting factor inhibitor) predisposes the patient to excessive thrombosis. In acquired hemostatic disorders, there are frequently multiple problems with homeostasis that perturb and dysregulate hemostasis. A primary illness (sepsis) and its secondary effects (shock and acidosis) activate coagulation and fibrinolysis and impair the host's ability to restore normal hemostatic function. When sepsis triggers **disseminated intravascular coagulation (DIC)**, platelets, procoagulant clotting factors, and anticoagulant proteins are consumed, leaving the hemostatic system unbalanced and prone to bleeding or clotting. Similarly, newborn infants and patients with severe liver disease have synthetic deficiencies of both procoagulant and anticoagulant proteins. Such dysregulation causes the patient to be predisposed to both hemorrhage and thrombosis with mild or moderate triggers that result in major alterations in the hemostatic process.

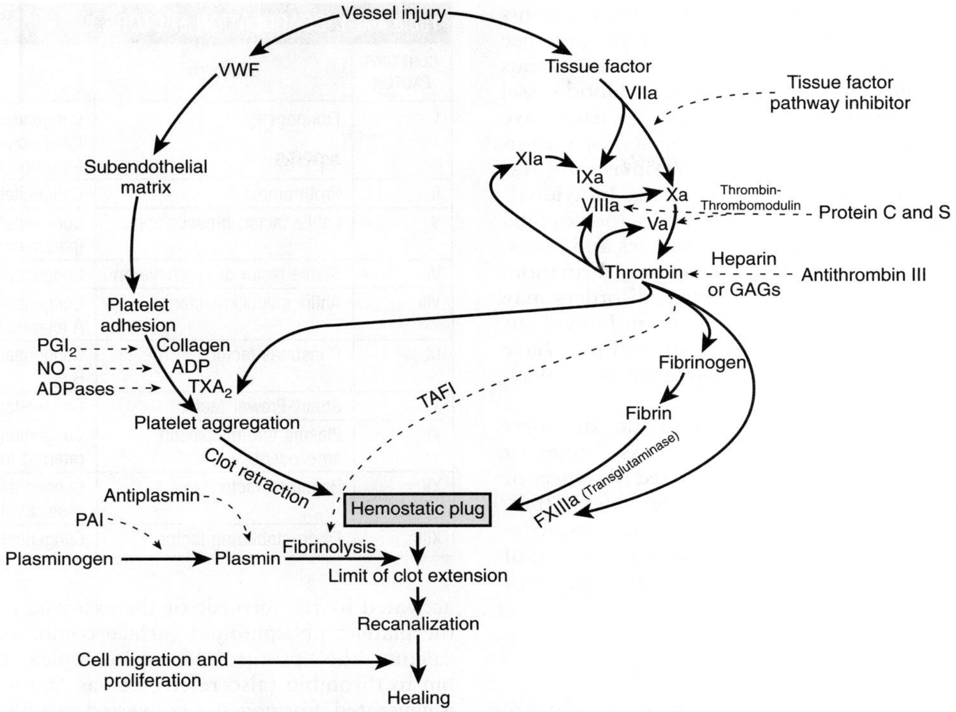

Figure 469-2 The hemostatic mechanism. ADP, adenosine diphosphate; GAGs, glycosaminoglycans; NO, nitric oxide; PGI_2, prostacyclin; PAI, plasminogen activator inhibitor; TAFI, thrombin-activated fibrinolytic inhibitor; TXA_2, thromboxane A_2; VWF, von Willebrand factor.

In the laboratory evaluation of hemostasis, parameters are manipulated to allow assessment of isolated aspects of hemostasis and limit the multifunctionality of some of its components. The coagulation process is studied in plasma anticoagulated with citrate to bind calcium, with added phospholipid to mimic the reaction surface normally provided by the platelet membrane and with a stimulus to trigger clotting. Calcium is added to restart the clotting process. This results in anomalies such that the in vivo physiologic pathway of clotting in which factor VIIa activates factor IX is bypassed; instead, in prothrombin time (PT), factor VIIa activates factor X. If this were truly the physiologic situation, then there would be an in vivo bypass mechanism that would ameliorate severe factor VIII and factor IX deficiencies, the 2 most common severe bleeding disorders.

BIBLIOGRAPHY

Please visit the Nelson Textbook of Pediatrics *website at* www.expertconsult.com *for the complete bibliography.*

469.1 Clinical and Laboratory Evaluation of Hemostasis

J. Paul Scott, Leslie J. Raffini, and Robert R. Montgomery

HISTORY

For most hemostatic disorders, the clinical history provides the most useful information. To evaluate for a bleeding disorder, the history should determine the site or sites of bleeding, the severity and duration of hemorrhage, and the age at onset. Was the bleeding spontaneous, or did it occur after trauma? Was there a previous personal or family history of similar problems? Did the symptoms correlate with the degree of injury or trauma? Does bruising occur spontaneously? Are there lumps with bruises for which there is minimal trauma? If the patient had previous surgery or significant dental procedures, was there any increased bleeding? If a child or adolescent has had surgery that affects the mucosal surfaces, such as a tonsillectomy or major dental extractions, the absence of bleeding usually rules out a hereditary bleeding disorder. Delayed or slow healing of superficial injuries may suggest a hereditary bleeding disorder. In postpubertal females, it is important to take a careful menstrual history. Because some common bleeding disorders, such as von Willebrand disease (VWD), have a fairly high prevalence, mothers and family members may have the same mild bleeding disorder and may not be cognizant that the child's menstrual history is abnormal. Women with mild VWD who have a moderate history of bruising frequently have a reduction of that bruising during pregnancy or after administration of oral contraceptives. Some medications, such as aspirin and other nonsteroidal anti-inflammatory drugs, inhibit platelet function and increase bleeding symptoms in patients with a low platelet count or abnormal hemostasis. Standardized bleeding scores have been developed and are undergoing investigation for their sensitivity and specificity in children.

Outside the neonatal period, thrombotic disorders are relatively rare until adulthood. In the neonate, physiologic deficiencies of procoagulants and anticoagulants cause the hemostatic mechanism to be dysregulated, and clinical events can lead to either hemorrhage or thrombosis. If a child or teenager presents with deep venous thrombosis or pulmonary emboli, a detailed family history must be obtained to evaluate for deep venous thrombosis, pulmonary emboli, myocardial infarction, or stroke in other family members. Even in the absence of a family history, the presence of thrombosis in the child or teenager should trigger consideration whether the individual should be evaluated for a hereditary or acquired predisposition to thrombosis.

PHYSICAL EXAMINATION

The physical examination should focus on whether bleeding symptoms are associated primarily with the mucous membranes or skin (mucocutaneous bleeding) or with the muscles and joints (deep bleeding). The examination should determine the presence of petechiae, ecchymoses, hematomas, hemarthroses, or mucous membrane bleeding. Patients with defects in platelet-blood vessel wall interaction (VWD or platelet function defects) usually have mucocutaneous bleeding, which may include epistaxis, menorrhagia, petechiae, ecchymoses, occasional hematomas, and less commonly, hematuria and gastrointestinal bleeding. Individuals with a clotting factor deficiency of factor VIII or IX (hemophilia A or B) have symptoms of deep bleeding into muscles and joints, with much more extensive ecchymoses and hematoma formation. Patients with mild VWD or other mild bleeding disorders may have no abnormal findings on physical examination. Individuals with disorders of the collagen matrix and vessel wall may have loose joints and lax skin associated with easy bruising (Ehlers-Danlos syndrome).

Patients undergoing evaluation for thrombotic disorders should be asked about swollen, warm, tender extremities or internal organs (venous thrombosis), unexplained dyspnea or persistent "pneumonia," especially in the absence of fever (pulmonary emboli), and varicosities and postphlebitic changes. Arterial thrombi usually cause an acute, dramatic impairment of organ function, such as stroke, myocardial infarction, or a painful, white, cold extremity.

Table 469-1 COAGULATION FACTORS

CLOTTING FACTOR	SYNONYM	DISORDER
I	Fibrinogen	Congenital deficiency (afibrinogenemia) or dysfunction (dysfibrinogenemia)
II	Prothrombin	Congenital deficiency or dysfunction
V	Labile factor, proaccelerin	Congenital deficiency (parahemophilia)
VII	Stable factor or proconvertin	Congenital deficiency
VIII	Antihemophilic factor	Congenital deficiency is hemophilia A (classic hemophilia)
IX	Christmas factor	Congenital deficiency is hemophilia B
X	Stuart-Prower factor	Congenital deficiency
XI	Plasma thromboplastin antecedent	Congenital deficiency, sometimes referred to as hemophilia C
XII	Hageman factor	Congenital deficiency is not associated with clinical symptoms
XIII	Fibrin-stabilizing factor	Congenital deficiency

LABORATORY TESTS

In patients who have a positive bleeding history or who are actively hemorrhaging, a platelet count, PT, and partial thromboplastin time (PTT) should be performed. If the results are normal, a thrombin time to evaluate fibrinogen function and VWF testing should be considered. In individuals with abnormal screening test results, further specific factor work-up should be undertaken. In a patient with an abnormal bleeding history and a positive family history, normal screening tests should not preclude further laboratory evaluation.

There are no useful routine screening tests for hereditary thrombotic disorders. If the family history is positive or clinical thrombosis is unexplained, specific anticoagulant assays should be undertaken. Thrombosis is rare in children, and when it is present, the possibility of a hereditary predisposition should be considered.

Platelet Count

Platelet count is essential in the evaluation of the child with a positive bleeding history because thrombocytopenia is the most common acquired cause of a bleeding diathesis in children. Patients with a platelet count of > 50,000/mm^3 rarely have significant clinical bleeding. Thrombocytosis in children is usually reactive and is not associated with bleeding or thrombotic complications. Persistent, severe thrombocytosis in the absence of an underlying illness may require evaluation for the very rare pediatric presentation of essential thrombocythemia or polycythemia vera.

Prothrombin Time and Activated Partial Thromboplastin Time

Because clotting factors were named in the order of discovery, they do not necessarily reflect the sequential order of activation (Table 469-1). In fact, factors III, IV, and VI were not subsequently found to be independent proteins; thus, these terms are no longer used. The dual mechanisms of activating clotting have been termed the **intrinsic** (surface activation) and **extrinsic** (tissue factor–mediated) pathways. Study of the hemostatic mechanism is further complicated in that the interactions in vivo may use different pathways from those studied in clinical laboratory testing. PT measures the activation of clotting by tissue factor (thromboplastin) in the presence of calcium. Addition of tissue factor causes a burst of factor VIIa generation. The tissue factor–factor VIIa complex activates factor X. Whether factor X is activated by the intrinsic or the extrinsic pathway, factor Xa on the platelet phospholipid surface complexes with factor V and calcium (the "prothrombinase" complex) to activate prothrombin to thrombin (also referred to as *factor IIa*). Once thrombin is generated, fibrinogen is converted to a fibrin clot, the end-point of the reaction (see Fig. 469-2). PT is not prolonged with deficiencies of factors VIII, IX, XI, and XII. In most laboratories, the normal PT value is 10-13 sec. PT has been standardized using the **International Normalized Ratio (INR)** so that values can be compared from 1 laboratory or instrument to another. This ratio is used to determine similar degrees of anticoagulation with warfarin (Coumadin)–like medications.

Partial Thromboplastin Time

The intrinsic pathway involves the initial activation of factor XII, which is accelerated by 2 other plasma proteins, prekallikrein and high molecular weight kininogen. In the clinical laboratory, factor XII is activated using a surface (silica or glass) or a contact activator, such as ellagic acid. Factor XIIa, in turn, activates factor XI to factor XIa, which then catalyzes factor IX to factor IXa. On the platelet phospholipid surface, factor IXa complexes with factor VIII and calcium to activate factor X ("tenase" complex).

This process is accelerated by interaction with phospholipid and calcium at the steps involving factors V and VIII. An isolated deficiency of a single clotting factor may result in isolated prolongation of PT, PTT, or both, depending on the location of the factor in the clotting cascade. This approach is useful in determining hereditary clotting factor deficiencies; however, in acquired hemostatic disorders encountered in clinical practice, > 1 clotting factor is frequently deficient, so the relative prolongation of PT and PTT must be assessed.

Measurement of PTT as performed in the clinical laboratory is actually "activated" PTT; however, most refer to it as *PTT.* This test measures the initiation of clotting at the level of factor XII through sequential steps to the final clot end-point. It does not measure factor VII, factor XIII, or anticoagulants. PTT uses a contact activator (silica, kaolin, or ellagic acid) in the presence of calcium and phospholipid. Because of differences in reagents and laboratory instruments, the normal range for PTT varies among hospital laboratories. Normal ranges for PTT are much more variable from laboratory to laboratory than those for PT.

Thus, the mechanisms studied by PT and PTT allow the evaluation of clotting factor deficiencies, even though these pathways may not be the same as those occurring physiologically In vivo, factor VIIa activates factors IX and X, but as routinely studied in the clinical laboratory, the pathway through which factor VIIa activates factor IX is not evaluated. If the tissue factor–factor VIIa complex activated only factor X, it would be difficult to explain why the most severe bleeding disorders are deficiencies of factor VIII (hemophilia A) and factor IX (hemophilia B). In vivo, thrombin is generated and feeds back to activate factor XI and accelerate the clotting process. Clotting in PTT can be prolonged by deficiencies of factor XII, prekallikrein, and high molecular weight kininogen, yet these deficiencies are asymptomatic conditions.

Thrombin Time

Thrombin time measures the final step in the clotting cascade, in which fibrinogen is converted to fibrin. The normal thrombin time varies between laboratories but is usually 11-15 sec. Prolongation of thrombin time occurs with reduced fibrinogen levels (*hypofibrinogenemia* or *afibrinogenemia*), with dysfunctional fibrinogen (*dysfibrinogenemia*), or in the presence of substances that interfere with fibrin polymerization, such as heparin and fibrin split products. If heparin contamination is a potential cause of prolonged thrombin time, a reptilase time is usually ordered.

Reptilase Time

Reptilase time uses snake venom to clot fibrinogen. Unlike thrombin time, reptilase time is not sensitive to heparin and is prolonged only by reduced or dysfunctional fibrinogen and fibrin split products. Therefore, if thrombin time is prolonged but reptilase time is normal, the prolonged thrombin time is due to heparin and does not indicate the presence of fibrin split products or reduced concentration or function of fibrinogen.

Mixing Studies

If there is unexplained prolongation of PT, PTT, or thrombin time, a mixing study is usually performed. Normal plasma is added to the patient's plasma, and the PT or PTT is repeated. Correction of PT or PTT by 1:1 mixing with normal plasma suggests deficiency of a clotting factor, because a 50% level of individual clotting proteins is sufficient to produce normal PT or PTT. If the clotting time is not corrected or only partially corrected, an inhibitor is usually present. An inhibitor of clotting may be either a chemical similar to heparin that delays coagulation or an antibody directed against a specific clotting factor or the phospholipid used in clotting tests. In the inpatient setting, the most common cause of this finding is heparin contamination of the sample. The presence of heparin in the sample can be ruled in or out with the use of thrombin time and reptilase time, as noted earlier. If the mixing study is not corrected or if its result becomes more prolonged and the patient has clinical bleeding, an inhibitor of a specific clotting factor (antibody directed against the factor), most commonly factor VIII, factor IX, or factor XI, may be present. If the patient has no bleeding symptoms and both PTT and the mixing study are prolonged, a lupus-like anticoagulant (Chapter 476) is often present. Patients with these findings usually have a long PTT, do not bleed, and may have a clinical predisposition to excessive clotting.

Bleeding Time

Bleeding time assesses the function of platelets and their interaction with the vascular wall. Disposable standardized devices have been developed that control the length and depth of the skin incision. A blood pressure cuff is applied to the upper arm and inflated to 40 mm Hg for children and adults. In term newborns and younger children, a modified device has been developed that is used with a lower blood pressure cuff pressure. Bleeding time is a difficult laboratory test to standardize, and there is much interlaboratory and interindividual variation. Although platelet counts of < 100,000/mm^3 are associated with prolonged bleeding time, disproportionate prolongation of bleeding time may suggest a qualitative platelet defect or VWD. After an incision is made with the bleeding time device, blood is blotted from the margin of the incision at 30-sec intervals until bleeding ceases. Although each laboratory must establish its own normal range, bleeding usually stops within 4-8 min. Accurate evaluation of bleeding time requires the cooperation of the patient (often a challenge in the young child) and a skilled technician. Use of the bleeding time is declining in many centers.

Platelet Function Analyzer

In an attempt to evaluate the early stages of hemostasis (platelet function and VWF interaction under high shear), several in vitro platelet analyzers have been developed. The greatest experience has been with the platelet function analyzer (PFA-100, Siemens Healthcare Diagnostics, Inc., Deerfield, IL). The PFA-100 measures platelet adhesion-aggregation in whole blood at high shear when exposed to either collagen-epinephrine or collagen-ADP. Results are reported as the closure time measured in sec. The PFA-100 appears to be sensitive to severe forms of VWD and platelet dysfunction. The PFA-100 has variable sensitivity, particularly in the detection of mild VWD and some platelet function defects. Its use as a preoperative screening tool has been disappointing in some studies.

D-Dimer

D-dimer is formed by plasmin degradation of cross-linked fibrin, produced when fibrinogen is clotted by thrombin and cross-linked by factor XIIIa, and is more specific for fibrinolysis than FDPs. D-dimer is elevated in patients with DIC or acute deep vein thrombosis but is relatively nonspecific, in that other ill hospitalized patients often have elevated levels of D-dimer. Adult studies show that the D-dimer can be useful to help exclude venous thrombosis and pulmonary embolus because of its high negative predictive value; for example, a patient with a normal D-dimer value is unlikely to have an acute thrombosis.

Clotting Factor Assays

Each of the clotting factors can be measured in the clinical laboratory using individual factor–deficient plasmas. For most clotting factors, activity is measured against pooled normal plasma or against a standard, by which 100% activity is expressed as 100 IU/dL. By definition, 1 international unit (IU) of each factor is defined as that amount in 1 mL of normal plasma referenced against a standard established by the World Health Organization (WHO). For most clotting factors, the normal range is 50-150 IU/dL (50-150%) (Table 469-2).

In patients with hemophilia A or hemophilia B, inhibitors of factor VIII or factor IX may develop after exposure to replacement therapy. To quantitate the amount of inhibitor present, the standardized clinical assay of these clotting inhibitors is the Bethesda assay. One Bethesda unit is defined as the amount that will inhibit 50% of the clotting factor in normal plasma.

Platelet Aggregation

When a qualitative platelet function defect is suspected, platelet aggregation testing is usually ordered. Platelet-rich plasma from the patient is activated with 1 of a series of agonists (ADP, epinephrine, collagen, thrombin or thrombin-receptor peptide, and ristocetin). Some platelet aggregometers measure specific ATP release from the platelets, as reflected in generating luminescence (lumiaggregometer), and are more sensitive in detecting abnormalities of the platelet release reaction from storage granules. Repeat testing or testing of other symptomatic family members can help to determine the hereditary nature of the defect. Many medications, especially aspirin, other nonsteroidal anti-inflammatory drugs, and valproic acid, alter platelet function testing.

Testing for Thrombotic Predisposition

Hereditary predisposition to thrombosis is associated with a reduction of anticoagulant function (protein C, protein S, AT-III);

Table 469-2 REFERENCE VALUES FOR COAGULATION TESTS IN HEALTHY CHILDREN*

TEST	28-31 WK GESTATION	30-36 WK GESTATION	FULL TERM	1-5 YR	6-10 YR	11-18 YR	ADULT
SCREENING TESTS							
Prothrombin time (PT) (sec)	15.4 (14.6-16.9)	13.0 (10.6-16.2)	13.0 (10.1-15.9)	11 (10.6-11.4)	11.1 (10.1-12.0)	11.2 (10.2-12.0)	12 (11.0-14.0)
Activated partial thromboplastin time (APTT) (sec)	108 (80-168)	53.6 (27.5-79.4)[‡§]	42.9 (31.3-54.3)[‡]	30 (24-36)	31 (26-36)	32 (26-37)	33 (27-40)
Bleeding time (BT) (min)				6 (2.5-10)[‡]	7 (2.5-13)[‡]	5 (3-8)[‡]	4 (1-7)
PROCOAGULANTS							
Fibrinogen	256 (160-550)	243 (150-373)[‡§]	283 (167-399)	276 (170-405)	279 (157-400)	300 (154-448)	278 (156-40)
Factor II	31 (19-54)	45 (20-77)[‡]	48 (26-70)[‡]	94 (71-116)[‡]	88 (67-107)[‡]	83 (61-104)[‡]	108 (70-146)
Factor V	65 (43-80)	88 (41-144)[§]	72 (34-108)[‡]	103 (79-127)	90 (63-116)[‡]	77 (55-99)[‡]	106 (62-150)
Factor VII	37 (24-76)	67 (21-113)[‡]	66 (28-104)[‡]	82 (55-116)[‡]	86 (52-120)[‡]	83 (58-115)[‡]	105 (67-143)
Factor VIII procoagulant	79 (37-126)	111 (5-213)	100 (50-178)	90 (59-142)	95 (58-132)	92 (53-131)	99 (50-149)
von Willebrand factor (VWF)	141 (83-223)	136 (78-210)	153 (50-287)	82 (60-120)	95 (44-144)	100 (46-153)	92 (50-158)
Factor IX	18 (17-20)	35 (19-65)[‡§]	53 (15-91)[†‡]	73 (47-104)[‡]	75 (63-89)[‡]	82 (59-122)[‡]	109 (55-163)
Factor X	36 (25-64)	41 (11-71)[‡]	40 (12-68)[‡]	88 (58-116)[‡]	75 (55-101)[‡]	79 (50-117)	106 (70-152)
Factor XI	23 (11-33)	30 (8-52)[‡§]	38 (40-66)[‡]	30 (8-52)[‡]	38 (10-66)	74 (50-97)[‡]	97 (56-150)
Factor XII	25 (5-35)	38 (10-66)[‡§]	53 (13-93)[‡]	93 (64-129)	92 (60-140)	81 (34-137)[‡]	108 (52-164)
Prekallikrein (PK)	26 (15-32)	33 (9-89)[‡]	37 (18-69)[‡]	95 (65-130)	99 (66-131)	99 (53-145)	112 (62-162)
High molecular weight kininogen (HMWK)	32 (19-52)	49 (9-89)[‡]	54 (6-102)[‡]	98 (64-132)	93 (60-130)	91 (63-119)	92 (50-136)
Factor XIIIa[ǀ]		70 (32-108)[‡]	79 (27-131)[‡]	108 (72-143)	109 (65-151)	99 (57-140)	105 (55-155)
Factor XIIIb[ǀ]		81 (35-127)[‡]	76 (30-122)[‡]	113 (69-156)[‡]	116 (77-154)[‡]	102 (60-143)	98 (57-137)
ANTICOAGULANTS							
Antithrombin-III (AT-III)	28 (20-38)	38 (14-62)[‡§]	63 (39-87)[‡]	111 (82-139)	111 (90-131)	106 (77-132)	100 (74-126)
Protein C		28 (12-44)[‡§]	35 (17-53)[‡]	66 (40-92)[‡]	69 (45-93)[‡]	83 (55-111)[‡]	96 (64-128)
Protein S:							
Total (U/mL)		26 (14-38)[‡§]	36 (12-60)[‡]	86 (54-118)	78 (41-114)	72 (52-92)	81 (61-113)
Free (U/mL)				45 (21-69)	42 (22-62)	38 (26-55)	45 (27-61)
Plasminogen (U/mL)		170 (112-248)	195 (125-265)	98 (78-118)	92 (75-108)	86 (68-103)	99 (77-122)
Tissue type plasminogen activator (TPA) (ng/mL)		8.48 (3.00-16.70)	9.6 (5.0-18.9)	2.15 (1.0-4.5)[‡]	2.42 (1.0-5.0)[‡]	2.16 (1.0-4.0)[‡]	1.02 (0.68-1.36)
Antiplasmin (α_2AP) (U/mL)		78 (40-116)	85 (55-115)	105 (93-117)	99 (89-110)	98 (78-118)	102 (68-136)
Plasminogen activator inhibitor-I (PAI-1)		5.4 (0.0-12.2)[‡]	6.4 (2.0-15.1)	5.42 (1.0-10.0)	6.79 (2.0-12.0)[‡]	6.07 (2.0-10.0)[‡]	3.60 (0.0-11.0)

*All factors except fibrinogen are expressed as units/mL (fibrinogen in mg/mL), in which pooled normal plasma contains 1 U/mL. All data are expressed as the mean, followed by the upper and lower boundaries encompassing 95% of the normal population (shown in parentheses).

[†]Levels for 19-27 wk and 28-31 wk gestation are from multiple sources and cannot be analyzed statistically.

[‡]Values are significantly different from those of adults.

[§]Values are significantly different from those of full-term infants.

[ǀ]Value given as CTA (Committee on Thrombolytic Agents) units/mL.

Data from Andrew M, Paes B, Johnston M: Development of the hemostatic system in the neonate and young infant, *Am J Pediatr Hematol Oncol* 12:95, 1990; and Andrew M, Vegh P, Johnston M, et al: Maturation of the hemostatic system during childhood, *Blood* 80:1998, 1992.

the presence of a factor V molecule that is resistant to inactivation by protein C (factor V Leiden); elevated levels of procoagulants (a mutation of the prothrombin gene); or a deficiency of fibrinolysis (plasminogen deficiency). When patients are being screened for prothrombotic tendencies, specific tests of the natural anticoagulants are warranted. Although both immunologic and functional tests are usually available, functional assays of protein C, protein S, and AT-III are clinically more useful.

Factor V Leiden is a common mutation in factor V that is associated with an increased risk of thrombosis. A point mutation in the factor V molecule prevents the inactivation of factor Va by activated protein C and, thereby, the persistence of factor Va. This defect, also known as *activated protein C resistance,* is easily diagnosed with DNA testing.

The **prothrombin gene mutation (G20210A)** is a mutation in the noncoding portion of the prothrombin gene, with a glycine (G) at position 20210 being replaced by an alanine (A). This mutation increases the amount of prothrombin messenger RNA, is associated with elevations of prothrombin, and causes a predisposition to thrombosis. This abnormality is easily identified with molecular diagnostic (DNA) testing.

Elevated Homocysteine

Levels of homocysteine may be increased as a result of genetic mutations, causing homocystinuria. Patients with homocysteine elevation are predisposed to arterial and venous thrombosis as well as to an increase in arteriosclerosis.

Tests of the Fibrinolytic System

Euglobulin clot lysis time is a screening test used in some laboratories to assess fibrinolysis. More specific tests are available in most laboratories to determine the levels of plasminogen, plasminogen activator, and inhibitors of fibrinolysis. An increase in fibrinolysis may be associated with hemorrhagic symptoms, and a delay in fibrinolysis is associated with thrombosis.

DEVELOPMENTAL HEMOSTASIS

The normal newborn infant has reduced levels of most procoagulants and anticoagulants (see Table 469-1). In general, there is a more marked abnormality in the preterm infant. Although major differences exist in the normal ranges for newborn and preterm infants, these ranges vary greatly among laboratories. During gestation, there is progressive maturation and increase of the clotting factors synthesized by the liver. The extremely premature infant has prolonged PT and PTT values as well as a marked reduction in anticoagulant protein levels (protein C, protein S, and AT-III). Levels of fibrinogen, factors V and VIII, VWF, and platelets are near-normal throughout the later stages of gestation (Chapter 97.4). Because protein C and protein S are physiologically reduced, the normal factors V and VIII are not balanced with their regulatory proteins. In contrast, the physiologic deficiency of vitamin K–dependent procoagulant proteins (factors II, VII, IX, and X) is partially balanced by the physiologic reduction of AT-III. The net effect is that newborns (especially premature infants) are at increased risk for complications of bleeding, clotting, or both.

BIBLIOGRAPHY

Please visit the Nelson Textbook of Pediatrics *website at www.expertconsult.com for the complete bibliography.*

Chapter 470
Hereditary Clotting Factor Deficiencies (Bleeding Disorders)

J. Paul Scott and Robert R. Montgomery

Hemophilia A (factor VIII deficiency) and **hemophilia B** (factor IX deficiency) are the most common and serious congenital coagulation factor deficiencies. The clinical findings in hemophilia A and hemophilia B are virtually identical. **Hemophilia C** is the bleeding disorder associated with reduced levels of factor XI (Chapter 470.2). Reduced levels of the *contact factors* (factor XII, high molecular weight kininogen, and prekallikrein) are associated with significant prolongation of activated partial thromboplastin time (APTT; also referred to as *PTT*), but are not associated with hemorrhage, as discussed in Chapter 470.3. Other coagulation factor deficiencies that are less common are briefly discussed in subsequent subchapters.

470.1 Factor VIII or Factor IX Deficiency (Hemophilia A or B)

J. Paul Scott and Robert R. Montgomery

Deficiencies of factors VIII and IX are the most common severe inherited bleeding disorders. Recombinant factor VIII and factor IX concentrates are available to treat patients with hemophilia and thereby avoid the infectious risk of plasma-derived transfusion-transmitted diseases.

PATHOPHYSIOLOGY

Factors VIII and IX participate in a complex required for the activation of factor X. Together with phospholipid and calcium, they form the "tenase," or factor X–activating, complex. Figure 469-1 shows the clotting process as it occurs in the test tube, with factor X being activated by either the complex of factors VIII and IX or the complex of tissue factor and factor VII. In vivo, the complex of factor VIIa and tissue factor activates factor IX to initiate clotting. In the laboratory, prothrombin time (PT) measures the activation of factor X by factor VII and is therefore normal in patients with factor VIII or factor IX deficiency.

After injury, the initial hemostatic event is formation of the platelet plug, together with the generation of the fibrin clot that prevents further hemorrhage. In hemophilia A or B, clot formation is delayed and is not robust. Inadequate thrombin generation leads to failure to form a tightly cross-linked fibrin clot to support the platelet plug. Patients with hemophilia slowly form a soft, friable clot. When untreated bleeding occurs in a closed space, such as a joint, cessation of bleeding may be the result of tamponade. With open wounds, in which tamponade cannot occur, profuse bleeding may result in significant blood loss. The clot that is formed may be friable, and rebleeding occurs during the physiologic lysis of clots or with minimal new trauma.

CLINICAL MANIFESTATIONS

Neither factor VIII nor factor IX crosses the placenta; bleeding symptoms may be present from birth or may occur in the fetus. Only 2% of neonates with hemophilia sustain intracranial hemorrhages, and 30% of male infants with hemophilia bleed with circumcision. Thus, in the absence of a positive family history (hemophilia has a high rate of spontaneous mutation), hemophilia may go undiagnosed in the newborn. Obvious symptoms such as easy bruising, intramuscular hematomas, and hemarthroses begin when the child begins to cruise. Bleeding from minor traumatic lacerations of the mouth (a torn frenulum) may persist for hours or days and may cause the parents to seek medical evaluation. Even in patients with severe hemophilia, only 90% have evidence of increased bleeding by 1 yr of age. Although bleeding may occur in any area of the body, the hallmark of hemophilic bleeding is **hemarthrosis.** Bleeding into the joints may be induced by minor trauma; many hemarthroses are spontaneous. The earliest joint hemorrhages appear most commonly in the ankle. In the older child and adolescent, hemarthroses of the knees and elbows are also common. Whereas the child's early joint hemorrhages are recognized only after major swelling and fluid accumulation in the joint space, older children are frequently able to recognize bleeding before the physician does. They complain of a warm, tingling sensation in the joint as the first sign of an early joint hemorrhage. Repeated bleeding episodes into the same joint in a patient with severe hemophilia may become a "target" joint. Recurrent bleeding may then become spontaneous because of the underlying pathologic changes in the joint.

Although most muscular hemorrhages are clinically evident owing to localized pain or swelling, bleeding into the iliopsoas muscle requires specific mention. A patient may lose large volumes of blood into the **iliopsoas muscle,** verging on hypovolemic shock, with only a vague area of referred pain in the groin. The hip is held in a flexed, internally rotated position owing to irritation of the iliopsoas. The diagnosis is made clinically from the inability to extend the hip but must be confirmed with ultrasonography or CT (Fig. 470-1). Life-threatening bleeding in the patient with hemophilia is caused by bleeding into vital structures (central nervous system, upper airway) or by exsanguination (external trauma, gastrointestinal or iliopsoas hemorrhage). Prompt treatment with clotting factor concentrate for these life-threatening hemorrhages is imperative. If head trauma is of sufficient concern

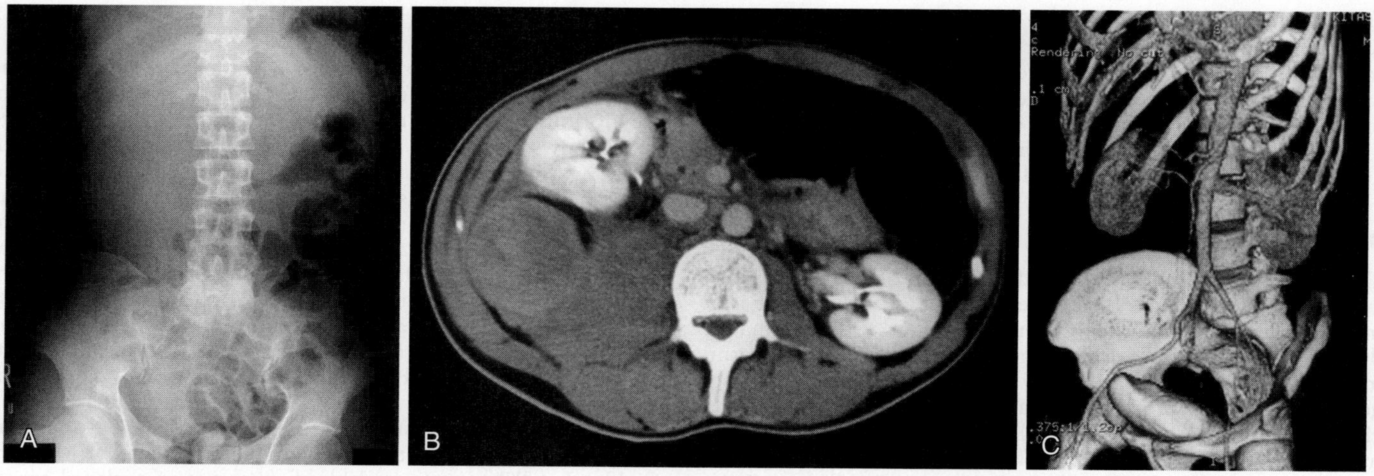

Figure 470-1 Massive hematoma into the iliopsoas muscle in a patient with hemophilia B. A 38-yr-old man with severe deficiency of factor IX (hemophilia B) was admitted for right lower abdominal pain of progressively increasing severity and tenderness. He had had a common cold with severe cough and loss of appetite for approximately 1 wk. *A,* Abdominal radiograph shows presence of the psoas sign on the right side and left-shifted colon gas. *B,* CT scan shows massive hematoma in the right iliopsoas muscle, resulting in anterior translocation of the right kidney. *C,* Reconstructed 3-dimensional image shows more clearly the kidney translocation and the extended, but intact large vessels. These are useful findings for the diagnostic procedures, because progressive right lower abdominal pain may closely simulate acute appendicitis. The hemorrhage was successfully managed by replacement of factor IX for 1 wk without any recurrence. The patient did not have any inhibitors to factor IX. (From Miyazaki K, Higashihara M: Massive hemorrhage into the iliopsoas muscle, *Intern Med* 44:158, 2005.)

to suggest radiologic evaluation, factor replacement should precede radiologic evaluation. Simply put: "Treat first, image second!" Life-threatening hemorrhages require replacement therapy to achieve a level equal to that of normal plasma (100 IU/dL, or 100%).

Patients with mild hemophilia who have factor VIII or factor IX levels > 5 IU/dL usually do not have spontaneous hemorrhages. These individuals may experience prolonged bleeding after dental work, surgery, or injuries from moderate trauma.

LABORATORY FINDINGS AND DIAGNOSIS

The laboratory screening test that is affected by a reduced level of factor VIII or factor IX is PTT. In severe hemophilia, the PTT value is usually 2-3 times the upper limit of normal. Results of the other screening tests of the hemostatic mechanism (platelet count, bleeding time, prothrombin time, and thrombin time) are normal. Unless the patient has an inhibitor to factor VIII or IX, the mixing of normal plasma with patient plasma results in correction of PTT value. The specific assay for factors VIII and IX will confirm the diagnosis of hemophilia. If correction does not occur on mixing, an inhibitor may be present. In 25-35% of patients with hemophilia who receive infusions of factor VIII or factor IX, a factor-specific antibody may develop. These antibodies are directed against the active clotting site and are termed *inhibitors*. In such patients, the quantitative Bethesda assay for inhibitors should be performed to measure the antibody titer.

DIFFERENTIAL DIAGNOSIS

In young infants with severe bleeding manifestations, the differential diagnosis includes severe thrombocytopenia; severe platelet function disorders, such as Bernard-Soulier syndrome and Glanzmann Thrombasthenia; type 3 (severe) von Willebrand disease; and vitamin K deficiency. Hemostatic screening tests should differentiate these entities from hemophilia.

GENETICS AND CLASSIFICATION

Hemophilia occurs in approximately 1:5,000 males, with 85% having factor VIII deficiency and 10-15% having factor IX deficiency. Hemophilia shows no apparent racial predilection, appearing in all ethnic groups. The severity of hemophilia is classified on the basis of the patient's baseline level of factor VIII or factor IX, because factor levels usually correlate with the severity of bleeding symptoms. By definition, 1 IU of each factor is defined as that amount in 1 mL of normal plasma referenced against a standard established by the World Health Organization (WHO); thus, 100 mL of normal plasma has 100 IU/dL (100% activity) of each factor. For ease of discussion, henceforth in this chapter, we use the term *% activity* to refer to the percentage found in normal plasma (100% activity). Factor concentrates are also referenced against an international WHO standard, so treatment doses are usually referred to in IU. **Severe hemophilia** is characterized as having <1% activity of the specific clotting factor, and bleeding is often spontaneous. Patients with **moderate hemophilia** have factor levels of 1-5% and usually require mild trauma to induce bleeding. Individuals with **mild hemophilia** have levels >5%, may go many years before the condition is diagnosed, and frequently require significant trauma to cause bleeding. The hemostatic level for factor VIII is >30-40%, and for factor IX, it is >25-30%. The lower limit of levels for factors VIII and IX in normal individuals is approximately 50%.

The genes for factors VIII and IX are carried near the terminus of the long arm of the X chromosome and are therefore X-linked traits. The majority of patients with hemophilia have reduced clotting factor protein; 5-10% of those with hemophilia A and 40-50% of those with hemophilia B make a dysfunctional protein. Approximately 45-50% of patients with severe hemophilia A have the same mutation, in which there is an internal inversion within the factor VIII gene that results in production of no protein. This mutation can be detected in the blood of patients or carriers and in the amniotic fluid by molecular techniques. African Americans often have a different FVIII haplotype, and this difference may be the reason that African Americans have higher inhibitor formation (see later). Because of the multiple genetic causes of either factor VIII or factor IX deficiency, most cases of hemophilia are classified according to the amount of factor VIII or factor IX clotting activity. In the newborn, factor VIII values may be artificially elevated because of the acute-phase response elicited by the birth process. This artificial elevation may cause a mildly affected patient to have normal or near-normal

Table 470-1 TREATMENT OF HEMOPHILIA

TYPE OF HEMORRHAGE	HEMOPHILIA A	HEMOPHILIA B
Hemarthrosis*	50 IU/kg factor VIII concentrate† on day 1; then 20IU/kg on days 2, 3, 5 until joint function is normal or back to baseline. Consider additional treatment every other day for 7-10 days. Consider prophylaxis.	80-100 IU/kg on day 1; then 40 IU/kg on days 2, 4. Consider additional treatment every other day for 7-10 days. Consider prophylaxis.
Muscle or significant subcutaneous hematoma	50 IU/kg factor VIII concentrate; 20 IU/kg every-other-day treatment may be needed until resolved.	80 IU/kg factor IX concentrate‡; treatment every 2-3 days may be needed until resolved.
Mouth, deciduous tooth, or tooth extraction	20 IU/kg factor VIII concentrate; antifibrinolytic therapy; remove loose deciduous tooth.	40 IU/kg factor IX concentrate‡; antifibrinolytic therapy§; remove loose deciduous tooth.
Epistaxis	Apply pressure for 15-20 min; pack with petrolatum gauze; give antifibrinolytic therapy; 20 IU/kg factor VIII concentrate if this treatment fails.ǀ	Apply pressure for 15-20 min; pack with petrolatum gauze; antifibrinolytic therapy; 30 IU/kg factor IX concentrate‡ if this treatment fails.
Major surgery, life-threatening hemorrhage	50-75 IU/kg factor VIII concentrate, then initiate continuous infusion of 2-4 IU/kg/hr to maintain factor VIII >100 IU/dL for 24 hr‘ then give 2-3 IU/kg/hr continuously for 5-7 days to maintain the level at >50 IU/dL and an additional 5-7 days to maintain the level at >30 IU/dL.¶	120 IU/kg factor IX concentrate‡, then 50-60 IU/kg every 12-24 hr to maintain factor IX at >40 IU/dL for 5-7 days, and then at >30 IU/dL for 7 days.
Iliopsoas hemorrhage	50 IU/kg factor VIII concentrate, then 25 IU/kg every 12 hr until asymptomatic, then 20 IU/kg every other day for a total of 10-14 days.**	120 IU/kg factor IX concentrate‡; then 50-60 IU/kg every 12-24 hr to maintain factor IX at >40 IU/dL until patient is asymptomatic; then 40-50 IU every other day for a total of 10-14 days.**††
Hematuria	Bed rest; 1½ × maintenance fluids; if not controlled in 1-2 days, 20 IU/kg factor VIII concentrate; if not controlled, give prednisone (unless patient is HIV-infected).	Bed rest; 1½ × maintenance fluids; if not controlled in 1-2 days, 40 IU/kg factor IX concentrate‡; if not controlled, give prednisone (unless patient is HIV-infected).
Prophylaxis	20-40 IU/kg factor VIII concentrate every other day to achieve a trough level ≥1%.	30-50 IU/kg factor IX concentrate‡ every 2-3 days to achieve a trough level ≥1%.

*For hip hemarthrosis, orthopedic evaluation for possible aspiration is advisable to prevent avascular necrosis of the femoral head.
†For mild or moderate hemophilia, desmopressin, 0.3 μg/kg, should be used instead of factor VIII concentrate, if the patient is known to respond with a hemostatic level of factor VIII; if repeated doses are given, monitor factor VIII levels for tachyphylaxis.
‡Stated doses apply for recombinant factor IX concentrate; for plasma-derived factor IX concentrate, use 70% of the stated dose.
§Do not give antifibrinolytic therapy until 4-6 hr after a dose of prothrombin complex concentrate.
ǀOver-the-counter coagulation-promoting products may be helpful.
¶Alternatively, give 25 IU/kg every 12 hr to maintain a trough level >50% for 5-7 days followed by 25-30 IU/kg for an additional 5-7 days to maintain trough >25%.
**Repeat radiologic assessment should be performed before discontinuation of therapy.
††If repeated doses of factor IX concentrate are required, use highly purified, specific factor IX concentrate.
Adapted from Montgomery RR, Gill JC, Scott JP: Hemophilia and von Willebrand disease. In Nathan DG, Orkin SH, editors: *Nathan and Oski's hematology of infancy and childhood*, ed 5, Philadelphia, 1998, WB Saunders.

levels of factor VIII. Patients with severe hemophilia do not have detectable levels of factor VIII. In contrast, factor IX levels are physiologically low in the newborn. If severe hemophilia is present in the family, an undetectable level of factor IX is diagnostic of severe hemophilia B. In some patients with mild factor IX deficiency, the presence of hemophilia can be confirmed only after several weeks of life.

Through lyonization of the X chromosome, some **female carriers** of hemophilia A or B have sufficient reduction of factor VIII or factor IX to produce mild bleeding disorders. Levels of these factors should be determined in all known or potential carriers to assess the need for treatment in the event of surgery or clinical bleeding.

Because factor VIII is carried in plasma by von Willebrand factor, the ratio of factor VIII to von Willebrand factor is sometimes used to diagnose carriers of hemophilia. When possible, specific genetic mutations should be identified in the propositus and used to test other family members who are at risk of either having hemophilia or being carriers.

TREATMENT

Early, appropriate therapy is the hallmark of excellent hemophilia care. When mild to moderate bleeding occurs, values of factor VIII or factor IX must be raised to hemostatic levels, in the 35-50% range. For life-threatening or major hemorrhages, the dose should aim to achieve levels of 100% activity.

Calculation of the dose of recombinant factor VIII (FVIII) or recombinant factor IX (FIX) is as follows:

$$\text{Dose of FVII (IU)} = \%\text{ desired (rise in FVII)} \times \text{Body weight (kg)} \times 0.5$$

$$\text{Dose of FIX (IU)} = \%\text{ desired (rise in plasma FIX)} \times \text{Body weight (kg)} \times 1.4$$

For factor VIII, the correction factor is based on the volume of distribution of factor VIII. For factor IX, the correction factor is based on the volume of distribution and the observed rise in plasma level after infusion of recombinant factor IX.

Table 470-1 summarizes the treatment of some common types of hemorrhage in a patient with hemophilia.

With the availability of recombinant replacement products, **prophylaxis is the standard of care** for most children with severe hemophilia, to prevent spontaneous bleeding and early joint deformities. A study comparing prophylaxis with aggressive episodic treatment provides evidence for the superiority of prophylaxis in preventing debilitating joint disease. If target joints develop, "secondary" prophylaxis is often initiated.

With mild factor VIII hemophilia, the patient's endogenously produced factor VIII can be released by the administration of desmopressin acetate (DDAVP). In patients with moderate or severe factor VIII deficiency, the stored levels of factor VIII in the body are inadequate, and desmopressin treatment is ineffective. The risk of exposing the patient with mild hemophilia to transfusion-transmitted diseases and the cost of recombinant products warrant the use of desmopressin, if it is effective. A concentrated intranasal form of **desmopressin acetate**, not the enuresis or pituitary replacement dose, can also be used to treat patients with mild hemophilia A. The dose is 150 μg (1 puff) for children weighing <50 kg and 300 μg (2 puffs) for children and young adults weighing >50 kg. Most centers administer a trial of desmopressin to determine the level of factor VIII achieved after its infusion. Desmopressin is not effective in the treatment of factor IX–deficient hemophilia.

PROPHYLAXIS

Many patients are now given lifelong prophylaxis to prevent spontaneous joint bleeding. The National Hemophilia Foundation recommends that prophylaxis be considered optimal therapy for children with severe hemophilia. Usually, such programs are initiated with the first joint hemorrhage. Young children often require the insertion of a central catheter to ensure venous access. Such programs are expensive but are highly effective in preventing or greatly limiting the degree of joint pathology. Treatment is usually provided every 2-3 days to maintain a measurable plasma level of clotting factor (1-2%) when assayed just before the next infusion (trough level). Whether prophylaxis should be continued into adulthood has not yet been adequately studied. If moderate arthropathy develops, prevention of future bleeding will require higher plasma levels of clotting factors. In the older child who is not given primary prophylaxis, secondary prophylaxis is frequently initiated if a target joint develops.

SUPPORTIVE CARE

Although it is easy to tell parents that their child should avoid trauma, this advice is practically useless. Toddlers are active, are curious about everything, and injure themselves easily. Effective measures include anticipatory guidance, including the use of car seats, seatbelts, and bike helmets, and the importance of avoiding high-risk behaviors. Older boys should be counseled to avoid violent contact sports, but this issue is a challenge. Boys with severe hemophilia often sustain hemorrhages in the absence of known trauma. Early psychosocial intervention helps the family achieve a balance between overprotection and permissiveness. Patients with hemophilia should avoid aspirin and other nonsteroidal anti-inflammatory drugs that affect platelet function. The child with a bleeding disorder should receive the appropriate vaccinations against hepatitis B, even though recombinant products may avoid exposure to transfusion-transmitted diseases. Patients exposed to plasma-derived products should be screened periodically for hepatitis B and C, HIV, and abnormalities in liver function.

CHRONIC COMPLICATIONS

Long-term complications of hemophilia A and B include chronic arthropathy, the development of an inhibitor to either factor VIII or factor IX, and the risk of transfusion-transmitted infectious diseases. Although an aggressive, or prophylactic, approach to treatment has reduced the problems of chronic arthropathy, these problems have not been eliminated.

Historically, chronic arthropathy has been the major long-term disability associated with hemophilia. The natural history of untreated hemophilia is one of cyclic recurrent hemorrhages into specific joints, including hemorrhages into the same (target) joint. In young children, the joint distends easily and a large volume of blood may fill the joint until tamponade ensues or therapy intervenes. After joint hemorrhage, proteolytic enzymes are released by white blood cells into the joint space, and heme iron induces macrophage proliferation, leading to inflammation of the synovium. The synovium thickens and develops frondlike projections into the joint that are susceptible to being pinched and may induce further hemorrhage. The cartilaginous surface becomes eroded and ultimately may even expose raw bone, leaving the joint susceptible to articular fusion. In the older patient with advanced arthropathy, bleeding into the target joint, with its thickened synovium, causes severe pain, because the joint may have little space to accommodate blood. Once a target joint is seen to be developing, the patient is usually given short-or long-term prophylaxis to prevent progression of the arthropathy and reduce inflammation.

Inhibitor Formation

Infusion of the deficient clotting factor may initiate an immune response in patients with either factor VIII or factor IX deficiency. Inhibitors are antibodies directed against factor VIII or factor IX that block the clotting activity. Failure of a bleeding episode to respond to appropriate replacement therapy is usually the first sign of an inhibitor. Less often, inhibitors are identified during routine follow-up testing. Inhibitors develop in approximately 25-35% of patients with hemophilia A; the percentage is somewhat lower in patients with hemophilia B, many of whom make an inactive dysfunctional protein that renders them less susceptible to an immune response. Highly purified factor IX or recombinant factor IX seems to increase the frequency of inhibitor development, and some anti–factor IX inhibitors induce anaphylaxis. Many patients who have an inhibitor lose it with continued regular infusions. Others have a higher titer of antibody with subsequent infusions and may need to go through **desensitization** programs, in which high doses of factor VIII for hemophilia A or factor IX for hemophilia B are infused in an attempt to saturate the antibody and permit the body to develop tolerance. Factor IX immune tolerance programs have resulted in nephrotic syndrome in some patients. Rituximab has been used, off label (i.e., in a use not approved by the U.S. Food and Drug Administration [FDA]), as an alternate therapy for patients with high inhibitor titers in whom immune tolerance programs have failed. If desensitization fails, bleeding episodes are treated with either recombinant factor VIIa or activated prothrombin complex concentrates. The use of these products bypasses the inhibitor in many instances but may increase the risk of thrombosis. Patients with inhibitors require referral to a center that cares for many such patients and has a comprehensive hemophilia program.

In the past, plasma-derived treatment products transmitted hepatitis B and C as well as HIV to large numbers of patients with hemophilia. In the era of recombinant products, the risk of acquiring such infections should be minimal, but patients should receive appropriate immunizations against hepatitis B. Those who are exposed to blood products should be monitored for transfusion-related infections. Reports have also identified the transmission of variant Creutzfeldt-Jakob disease to patients receiving therapeutic plasma and may warrant study of patients with hemophilia for prion transmission from plasma-derived factor concentrates.

COMPREHENSIVE CARE

Today, patients with hemophilia are best managed through comprehensive hemophilia care centers. Such centers are dedicated to patient and family education as well as to the prevention and/or treatment of the complications of hemophilia, including chronic joint disease and inhibitor development as well as infection, such as hepatitis B and C or HIV. Such centers involve a team of physicians, nurses, orthopedists, physical therapists, and psychosocial workers, among others. Education remains crucial in hemophilia care, because patients who are receiving prophylaxis may be less "experienced" in recognizing bleeding episodes than affected children from previous eras.

BIBLIOGRAPHY

Please visit the Nelson Textbook of Pediatrics *website at www.expertconsult.com for the complete bibliography.*

470.2 Factor XI Deficiency (Hemophilia C)

J. Paul Scott and Robert R. Montgomery

Factor XI deficiency is an autosomal deficiency associated with mild to moderate bleeding symptoms. It is frequently encountered in Ashkenazi Jews but has been found in many other ethnic groups. In Israel, 1-3/1,000 individuals are homozygous for this deficiency.

The bleeding tendency is not as severe as in factor VIII or factor IX deficiency. The bleeding associated with factor XI deficiency is not correlated with the amount of factor XI. Some patients with severe deficiency may have minimal or no symptoms at the time of major surgery. Because factor XI augments thrombin generation and leads to activation of the fibrinolytic inhibitor thrombin-activatable fibrinolysis inhibitor (TAFI), surgical bleeding is more prominent in sites of high fibrinolytic activity like the oral cavity. Unless the patient previously had surgery without bleeding, replacement therapy should be considered and given preoperatively, depending on the nature of the surgical procedure. No approved concentrate of factor XI is available in the USA; therefore, the physician must use fresh frozen plasma (FFP).

Bleeding during minor surgery can be controlled with local pressure. Patients undergoing dental extractions can be monitored closely and may benefit from treatment with fibrinolytic inhibitors like aminocaproic acid, with plasma replacement therapy used only if hemorrhage occurs. In a patient with homozygous deficiency of factor XI, PTT is often longer than it is in patients with either severe factor VIII or factor IX deficiency. The paradox of fewer clinical symptoms in combination with longer PTT is surprising, but it occurs because factor VIIa can activate factor IX in vivo. The deficiency of factor XI can be confirmed by specific factor XI assays. Plasma infusions of 1 IU/kg usually increase the plasma concentration by 2%. Thus, infusion of plasma at 10-15 mL/kg will result in a plasma level of 20-30%, which is usually sufficient to control moderate hemorrhage. Frequent infusions of plasma would be necessary to achieve higher levels of factor XI. Because the half-life of factor XI is usually ≥48 hr, maintaining adequate levels of factor XI commonly is not difficult.

Chronic joint bleeding is rarely a problem in factor XI deficiency, and for most patients, the deficiency is a concern only at the time of major surgery unless there is a second underlying hemostatic defect (e.g., von Willebrand disease).

BIBLIOGRAPHY

Please visit the Nelson Textbook of Pediatrics *website at* *www.expertconsult.com* *for the complete bibliography.*

470.3 Deficiencies of the Contact Factors (Nonbleeding Disorders)

J. Paul Scott and Robert R. Montgomery

Deficiency of the "contact factors" (factor XII, prekallikrein, and high molecular weight kininogen) causes prolonged PTT but no bleeding symptoms. Because these contact factors function at the step of initiation of the intrinsic clotting system by the reagent used to determine PTT, the PTT is markedly prolonged when these factors are absent. Thus, there is the paradoxical situation in which PTT is extremely prolonged with no evidence of clinical bleeding. It is important that individuals with these findings be well informed about the meaning of their clotting factor deficiency because they do not need treatment, even for major surgery.

470.4 Factor VII Deficiency

J. Paul Scott and Robert R. Montgomery

Factor VII deficiency is a rare autosomal bleeding disorder usually detected only in the homozygous state. Severity of bleeding varies from mild to severe with hemarthroses, spontaneous intracranial hemorrhage, and mucocutaneous bleeding, especially nosebleeds and menorrhagia. Patients with this deficiency have markedly prolonged PT but normal PTT. Factor VII assays show a marked reduction in factor VII. Because the plasma half-life of factor VII is 2-4 hr, therapy with FFP is difficult and is often complicated by fluid overload. A commercial concentrate of recombinant factor VIIa has been shown in case reports to be effective in treating some patients with factor VII deficiency, but this concentrate has not been approved by the FDA for this indication.

470.5 Factor X Deficiency

J. Paul Scott and Robert R. Montgomery

Factor X deficiency is a rare (estimated 1/1,000,000) autosomal disorder with variable severity. Mild deficiency results in mucocutaneous and post-traumatic bleeding, whereas severe deficiency results in spontaneous hemarthroses and intracranial hemorrhages. Factor X deficiency is the result of either a quantitative deficiency or a dysfunctional molecule. A reduced factor X level is associated with prolongation of both PT and PTT. In patients with hereditary factor X deficiency, factor X levels can be increased with use of either FFP or prothrombin complex concentrate. The half-life of factor X is approximately 30 hr, and its volume of distribution is similar to that of factor IX. Thus, 1 U/kg will increase the plasma level of factor X by 1%.

Although it is rarely a problem in pediatric patients, systemic amyloidosis may be associated with factor X deficiency, owing to the adsorption of factor X on the amyloid protein. In the setting of amyloidosis, transfusion therapy often is not successful because of the rapid clearance of factor X.

470.6 Prothrombin (Factor II) Deficiency

J. Paul Scott and Robert R. Montgomery

Prothrombin deficiency is caused either by a markedly reduced prothrombin level (hypoprothrombinemia) or by functionally abnormal prothrombin (dysprothrombinemia). Laboratory testing in homozygous patients shows prolonged PT and PTT. Factor II, or prothrombin, assays show a markedly reduced prothrombin level. Mucocutaneous bleeding in infancy and post-traumatic bleeding later are common. Patients are treated with either FFP or, rarely, prothrombin complex concentrates. In prothrombin deficiency, FFP is useful, because the half-life of prothrombin is 3.5 days. Administration of 1 IU/kg of prothrombin will increase the plasma activity by 1%.

BIBLIOGRAPHY

Please visit the Nelson Textbook of Pediatrics *website at* *www.expertconsult.com* *for the complete bibliography.*

470.7 Factor V Deficiency

J. Paul Scott and Robert R. Montgomery

Deficiency of factor V is an autosomal recessive, mild to moderate bleeding disorder that has also been termed **parahemophilia.** Hemarthroses occur rarely; mucocutaneous bleeding and hematomas are the most common symptoms. Severe menorrhagia is a frequent symptom in women. Laboratory evaluation shows prolonged PTT and PT. Specific assays for factor V show a reduction in factor V levels. FFP is the only currently available therapeutic product that contains factor V. Factor V is lost rapidly from stored FFP. Patients with severe factor V deficiency are treated with infusions of FFP at 10 mL/kg every 12 hr. Rarely, a patient with a negative family history of bleeding has an acquired antibody to factor V. Often, such a patient does not bleed because the factor V in platelets prevents excessive bleeding.

BIBLIOGRAPHY
Please visit the Nelson Textbook of Pediatrics *website at www.expertconsult.com for the complete bibliography.*

470.8 Combined Deficiency of Factors V and VIII

J. Paul Scott and Robert R. Montgomery

Combined deficiency of factors V and VIII occurs secondary to the absence of an intracellular transport protein that is responsible for transporting factors V and VIII from the endoplasmic reticulum to the Golgi compartments. This explains the paradoxical deficiency of 2 factors, one encoded on chromosome 1 and the other on the X chromosome. Bleeding symptoms are often milder than for hemophilia A and are treated with FFP to replace both factors V and VIII.

470.9 Fibrinogen (Factor I) Deficiency

J. Paul Scott and Robert R. Montgomery

Congenital afibrinogenemia is a rare autosomal recessive disorder in which there is an absence of fibrinogen. Patients with this disorder do not bleed as frequently as patients with hemophilia and rarely have hemarthroses. Affected patients may present in the neonatal period with gastrointestinal hemorrhage or hematomas after vaginal delivery. In addition to marked prolongation of PT and PTT, thrombin time is prolonged. In the absence of consumptive coagulopathy, an unmeasurable fibrinogen level is diagnostic. In addition to the quantitative deficiency of fibrinogen, a number of dysfunctional fibrinogens have been reported (**dysfibrinogenemia**). Rarely patients with dysfibrinogenemia present with thrombosis. Currently, no fibrinogen concentrates are commercially available. Because the plasma half-life of fibrinogen is 2-4 days, treatment with either FFP or cryoprecipitate is effective. The hemostatic level of fibrinogen is >60 mg/dL. Each bag of cryoprecipitate contains 100-150 mg of fibrinogen. Some clinical assays for fibrinogen are inhibited by high doses of heparin. Thus, a markedly prolonged thrombin time associated with a low fibrinogen level should be evaluated with determination of reptilase time. Prolonged reptilase time confirms that functional levels of fibrinogen are low and that heparin is not present.

470.10 Factor XIII Deficiency (Fibrin-Stabilizing Factor or Transglutaminase Deficiency)

J. Paul Scott and Robert R. Montgomery

Because factor XIII is responsible for the cross linking of fibrin to stabilize the fibrin clot, symptoms of delayed hemorrhage are secondary to instability of the clot. Typically, patients have trauma 1 day and then have a bruise or hematoma the next day. Clinical symptoms include mild bruising, delayed separation of the umbilical stump beyond 4 wk in neonates, poor wound healing, and recurrent spontaneous abortions in women. Rare kindreds with XIII deficiency with hemarthroses and intracranial hemorrhage have been described. Results of the usual screening tests for hemostasis are normal in patients with factor XIII deficiency. Screening tests for factor XIII deficiency are based on the observation that there is increased solubility of the clot because of the failure of cross linking. The normal clot remains insoluble in the presence of 5M urea, whereas in a patient with XIII deficiency, the clot dissolves. More specific assays for factor XIII are immunologic. Because the half-life of factor XIII is 5-7 days and the hemostatic level is 2-3% activity, infusion of FFP or cryoprecipitate will correct the deficiency in patients with factor XIII deficiency. Plasma contains 1 IU/dL, and cryoprecipitate contains 75 IU/bag. In patients with significant bleeding symptoms, prophylaxis can be achieved with infusion of cryoprecipitate every 3-4 wk.

BIBLIOGRAPHY
Please visit the Nelson Textbook of Pediatrics *website at www.expertconsult.com for the complete bibliography.*

470.11 Antiplasmin or Plasminogen Activator Inhibitor Deficiency

J. Paul Scott and Robert R. Montgomery

Deficiency of either antiplasmin or plasminogen activator inhibitor, both of which are antifibrinolytic proteins, results in increased plasmin generation and premature lysis of fibrin clots. Affected patients have a mild bleeding disorder characterized by mucocutaneous bleeding but rarely have joint hemorrhages. Because results of the usual hemostatic tests are normal, further work-up of a patient with a positive bleeding history should include euglobulin clot lysis time (if available), which measures fibrinolytic activity and yields a shortened result in the presence of these deficiencies. Specific assays for α_2-antiplasmin and plasminogen activator inhibitor are available. Bleeding episodes are treated with FFP; bleeding in the oral cavity may respond to aminocaproic acid.

BIBLIOGRAPHY
Please visit the Nelson Textbook of Pediatrics *website at www.expertconsult.com for the complete bibliography.*

Chapter 471 von Willebrand Disease

Robert R. Montgomery and J. Paul Scott

The most common hereditary bleeding disorder is von Willebrand disease (VWD), and some reports suggest that it is present in 1-2% of the general population. VWD is inherited autosomally, but most centers report more affected women than men. Because menorrhagia is a major symptom, women may be more likely to seek treatment and thus to be diagnosed. VWD is classified on the basis of whether the protein is quantitatively reduced, but not absent (type 1); qualitatively abnormal (type 2); or absent (type 3) (Fig. 471-1). Mutations in different loci that code for different functional domains of the von Willebrand factor (VWF) protein cause the different variants of VWD.

PATHOPHYSIOLOGY

A large multimeric glycoprotein that is synthesized in megakaryocytes and endothelial cells, VWF is stored in platelet α-granules and endothelial cell Weibel-Palade bodies. The highest molecular weight multimers of VWF are responsible for the normal interaction of VWF with the subendothelial matrix and platelets. During normal hemostasis, VWF adheres to the subendothelial matrix after vascular damage. When VWF binds to the subendothelial matrix, the conformation of VWF is altered by shear so that it causes platelets to adhere to VWF through their glycoprotein IB (GPIb) receptor. These platelets are then activated, causing the recruitment of additional platelets and exposing platelet membrane phosphatidylserine, which is an important regulatory step for factor V– and factor VIII–dependent steps in the clotting

	Normal	Type 1	Type 3	Type 2A	Type 2B	Type 2N	Type 2M	PT-VWD	BSS
VWF:Ag	N	↓	absent	↓	↓	N or ↓	↓ or N	↓	N
VWF:RCo	N	↓	absent	↓↓↓	↓	N or ↓	↓↓↓	↓	N
FVIII	N	↓ or N	1-3%	N or ↓	N or ↓	↓↓	N	N	N
RIPA	N	often normal	absent	↓	often normal	N	↓	N	absent
LD-RIPA	absent	absent	absent	absent	↑↑↑	absent	absent	↑↑↑	absent
PFA	N	↑	↑↑↑	↑	↑	N	↑	↑	↑↑↑
BT	N	N or ↑	↑↑↑	↑	↑	N	↑	↑	↑↑↑
Platelet count	N	N	N	N	↓	N	N	↓	↓
Usual Tx		DDAVP VWF conc	VWF conc	VWF conc (DDAVP)	VWF conc (DDAVP)	VWF conc (DDAVP)	VWF conc (DDAVP)	platelets	platelets
Response to DDAVP		good	none	variable	decreases platelets	variable	variable	decreases platelets	none or modest
Response to VWF Conc		good	good	good	good	good	good	decreases platelets	no response
Frequency in general population		? (reported 1-2%)	very rare 1:250,000	rare	rare	rare	rare	rare	rare
VWF multimers	N	N but ↓	absent	abnormal	abnormal	N but ↓	N but ↓	abnormal	normal

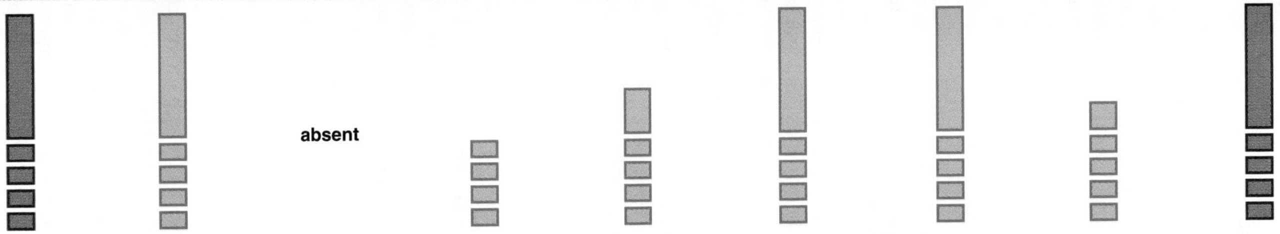

Figure 471-1 Common variants of von Willebrand disease (VWD) and other related disorders. Laboratory testing is listed on the *left*, and the results most commonly identified in patients with these conditions are shown. A graphic representation of von Willebrand factor (VWF) multimers is shown at the *bottom* of each column. A *lighter shade* illustrates a reduction in staining intensity, and *figure length* represents the relative size of the multimers. BSS, Bernard-Soulier syndrome; BT, bleeding time; DDAVP, desmopressin; FVIII, factor VIII; N, normal; PFA, platelet function analyzer; LD-RIPA, ristocetin induced platelet aggregation to low dose ristocetin; PT-VWD, platelet-type pseudo-VWD; RIPA, ristocetin reduced platelet aggregation to standard dose ristocetin; Tx, treatment; VWF:Ag, von Willebrand antigen; VWF:RCo, ristocetin cofactor activity; VWF conc, VWF concentrate; ↑, degree of increase; ↓, degree of decrease.

cascade. VWF also serves as the carrier protein for plasma factor VIII. A severe deficiency of VWF causes a secondary deficiency in factor VIII, even though the gene for factor VIII is normal, explaining autosomal deficiency of factor VIII, now known to be a molecular abnormality of VWF and known as *type 2N VWD*.

CLINICAL MANIFESTATIONS

Patients with VWD usually have symptoms of **mucocutaneous hemorrhage,** including excessive bruising, epistaxis, menorrhagia, and postoperative hemorrhage, particularly after mucosal surgery, such as tonsillectomy or wisdom tooth extraction. Because a teenager's menstrual history is usually put in the context of other family members, excessive menstrual bleeding is not always recognized as being abnormal, because others in the family may be affected with the same disorder. If a menstruating female has iron deficiency, a detailed history of bruising and other bleeding symptoms should be elicited and further hemostatic evaluation undertaken.

Because VWF is an acute-phase protein, stress will increase its level. Thus, patients may not bleed with procedures that incur major stress, such as appendectomy and childbirth, but may bleed excessively at the time of cosmetic or mucosal surgery. Bruising symptoms may diminish during pregnancy, because VWF levels may physiologically double or triple as an acute phase response. Rarely, patients with VWD may have gastrointestinal telangiectasia. This combination results in major bleeding and accounts for numerous hospital admissions for patients with severe disease. In patients with type 3, or homozygous, VWD, bleeding symptoms are much more profound. These patients are usually diagnosed early in life and may have severe epistaxis or menorrhagia that results in major blood loss and possibly shock. Patients with severe type 3 VWD may have joint hemorrhages or spontaneous central nervous system hemorrhages.

LABORATORY FINDINGS

Although patients with VWD were described historically as having a long bleeding time and a long partial thromboplastin time, these findings are frequently normal in patients with type 1 VWD. Normal results on screening tests do not preclude the diagnosis of VWD. Because there is no single assay that has demonstrated the ability to rule out VWD, if the history is suggestive of a mucocutaneous bleeding disorder, VWD testing should be undertaken, including a quantitative assay for VWF antigen, testing for VWF activity (ristocetin cofactor activity), testing for plasma factor VIII activity, determination of VWF structure (VWF multimers), and a platelet count. Although the platelet count is usually normal in most patients, those with type 2B disease or platelet-type disease (pseudo-VWD) may have lifelong thrombocytopenia. Figure 471-1 lists the variants of VWD and summarizes their laboratory findings. Levels of VWF vary with blood type (type O < A < B < AB), which can confound the clinical diagnosis of hereditary VWD, but most clinicians feel bleeding is related to the plasma level of VWF. In addition, there is controversy regarding the clinical definition of "true" VWD. Molecular genetics may clarify the diagnosis of type 1 VWD, but other genetic modifiers may exist outside the gene for VWF and significantly influence the diagnosis. The milder the patient's phenotype, the greater the difficulty in diagnosis.

GENETICS

Chromosome 12 contains the gene for VWF. In each of the type 2 variants listed in Figure 471-1, specific areas of the molecule are affected. The phenotype can guide the genetic diagnosis of the specific mutation. Investigations are underway to clarify whether all cases of type 1 VWD are related to mutations in the VWF gene on chromosome 12 or if there are genetic modifiers, such as blood type, that cause phenotypic VWD. Clinical genetic testing for VWD variants is only available in a few referral laboratories.

VON WILLEBRAND DISEASE VARIANTS

Type 1 VWD is the most common form and accounts for 85% of cases. NHLBI VWD guidelines restrict the diagnosis of VWD to those with VWF levels of <30 IU/dL. Those with levels >30 IU/dL but below the normal range are referred to as having "possible VWD" or as having "low VWF." Bleeding symptoms include epistaxis, bruising, and menorrhagia. If bleeding is excessive, desmopressin (DDAVP) administration at a dose of 0.3 µg/kg IV will increase the level of VWF and factor VIII by 3- to 5-fold. Intranasal DDAVP (Stimate) is particularly helpful for the outpatient treatment of bleeding episodes. The dose is 150 µg (1 puff) for children weighing <50 kg and 300 µg (2 puffs) for those weighing >50 kg. A new subtype of type 1 VWD has been referred to as type 1C because the plasma VWF is low from accelerated clearance, hence the 1C designation. Such patients can be diagnosed by doing VWF:Ag levels 1 and 4 hours after desmopressin infusion to demonstrate the shortened half-life of VWF (2-4 hr) in this variant. Alternatively, determining VWF propeptide level, VWFpp, at baseline demonstrates an elevated VWFpp/VWF:Ag ratio of >2 that is caused by the accelerated clearance of VWF (and not VWFpp). In these patients, desmopressin releases adequate VWF, but levels are not maintained for the normal half-life and may require VWF concentrate infusion, with this VWF $T_{1/2}$ being normal.

Type 2A VWD is caused either by the abnormal proteolysis of VWF by ADAMTS13 or by abnormal synthesis and reduced secretion. In either, only the smallest VWF multimers are present, resulting in a reduction in VWF antigen with a much greater reduction in VWF activity. Although desmopressin is safe in these patients, it is not always effective, because normal multimers are not maintained in plasma. Significant bleeding should be treated with VWF replacement therapy.

Type 2B VWD may be caused by 1 of several mutations resulting in "hyperactive" VWF. The abnormal VWF binds spontaneously to platelets, with resulting rapid clearance of VWF and platelets. The higher molecular weight multimers of VWF are preferentially cleared from the circulation, and moderate to severe thrombocytopenia is common. The laboratory diagnosis is based on the finding that the hyperactive 2B VWF binds to platelets and agglutinates them at low concentrations of ristocetin, a concentration that would not agglutinate normal platelets. If desmopressin is given to these patients, the abnormal hyperactive 2B VWF will be released and more profound thrombocytopenia might occur. Patients with 2B VWD usually respond to the infusion of VWF.

Type 2M VWD is caused by mutations that result in reduction of the platelet-binding function of VWF. Thus, levels of VWF activity are significantly lower than the levels of VWF antigen. Binding of this protein to factor VIII is normal; thus, factor VIII levels are similar to those of VWF antigen. Desmopressin will increase VWF and factor VIII levels, but the released type 2M VWF may not have sufficient activity to cause cessation of bleeding. Thus, VWF replacement therapy may need to be used if desmopressin is not clinically effective.

Type 2N VWD is caused by the reduction of factor VIII binding by VWF. This disorder has also been termed **autosomal hemophilia.** With this variant, platelet interaction with VWF is normal, but type 2N VWF binds weakly (or not at all) to factor VIII, resulting in rapid clearance of factor VIII. Thus, the factor VIII level is reduced much more than VWF levels. Commonly, patients who have symptomatic bleeding are compound heterozygotes who have inherited a gene for type 1 VWD from 1 parent and a gene for type 2N VWD from the other. Rarely, type 2N mutations are inherited from both parents and VWF levels are normal. In the patient who is compound heterozygous for types 1 and 2N, 1 allele makes no protein and the other allele makes a functionally abnormal protein, and as a result, all of the VWF is dysfunctional. Although desmopressin will release type 2N VWF, sustained factor VIII levels occasionally may be inadequate for normal hemostasis. A trial of desmopressin is indicated to assess the response and half-life of VWF and factor VIII after infusion. VWF replacement therapy is usually effective and because that VWF is normal, endogenous factor VIII can bind to the normal VWF with a longer maintenance of plasma factor VIII levels. Recombinant VWF is currently undergoing clinical trials.

Platelet-type (pseudo-) VWD is actually an abnormality of the GPIb receptor on platelets. This form can be considered the converse abnormality of type 2B, in that the GPIb receptor on platelets is hyperfunctional and binds plasma VWF spontaneously, resulting in **thrombocytopenia** and a loss of high molecular weight VWF multimers, which are indistinguishable from those seen in type 2B VWD. However, specific testing shows that this is a platelet abnormality rather than a plasma abnormality. Treatment is with transfusion of normal platelets, but if VWF level and function is particularly low, infusion with normal VWF may also be required initially for major hemorrhage.

Type 3 VWD is the homozygous or compound heterozygous inheritance of VWF deficiency. Patients exhibit undetectable plasma levels of VWF and low, but measurable, levels of factor VIII. These patients will have major hemorrhage but only rarely have joint hemorrhages. This severe, very rare form occurs in approximately 1:500,000 individuals. Intracranial hemorrhage, major epistaxis, and menorrhagia in women are the major features. Bleeding episodes require treatment with VWF-containing concentrates. VWF is both a plasma and a platelet protein. Because treatment with VWF-containing concentrate only corrects the plasma VWF level, patients with severe bleeding may need to be transfused with platelet concentrates to correct the deficiency of platelet VWF. Desmopressin is not effective in type 3 VWD.

Diagnosis and Differential Diagnosis

The diagnosis of VWD is dependent on the finding of a low level of at least 1 of the laboratory measures of VWF noted in Figure 471-1. The differential diagnosis of mucocutaneous bleeding includes abnormalities of platelet number, platelet function, or the vessel wall (Chapter 478). In caring for children, it is important to remember that the most common cause of such findings is trauma, especially nonaccidental trauma—child abuse.

Complications

Complications of bleeding due to VWD are rare. In adolescent females, blood loss due to menorrhagia can lead to severe anemia, either acutely, with signs and symptoms of hypovolemia, or chronically from iron deficiency. Individuals with type 3 VWD can manifest joint or muscle bleeding similar to individuals with hemophilia.

Treatment

Treatment of VWD is directed toward increasing the plasma level of VWF and factor VIII. Because the gene for factor VIII is normal in patients with VWD, elevating the plasma concentration of VWF permits normal recovery and survival of endogenously produced factor VIII. The most common form of VWD is type 1. In these patients, the synthetic drug desmopressin induces the release of VWF from the patient's endothelial cells. In some patients with type 2 or 1C variants, desmopressin may be similarly effective, but in other circumstances, the released VWF is dysfunctional. Patients with VWD may not respond adequately to desmopressin because they release an abnormal VWF molecule (most type 2 variants); because they have type 3 disease, in which there is no VWF to be released; or because they have accelerated clearance of released VWF (type 1C VWD). A small subset of children and adults, especially infants, do not release VWF in response to desmopressin. In these cases, replacement therapy must be used. Current replacement therapy uses plasma-derived VWF containing concentrates that also contain factor VIII. VWF distributes only to the intravascular space, because it is so large. During plasma fractionation, VWF multimers are altered to a variable extent. Therefore, 1 U/kg will increase the plasma level by 1.5%. The plasma half-life of both factor VIII and VWF is 12 hr, but the alteration of VWF during fractionation results in half-lives of 8-10 hr when concentrates are infused. Purified or recombinant VWF concentrates (containing no factor VIII) may become available in the near future. These will be useful in prophylaxis or in presurgical management. However, when used for acute bleeding, these VWF concentrates may need to be supplemented by an infusion of recombinant factor VIII for the 1st infusion, as they contain little or no factor VIII. Both VWF and factor VIII are required for normal hemostasis. If only VWF is replaced, endogenous correction of the factor VIII level takes 12-24 hr. Dental extractions and sometimes nosebleeds can be managed with both desmopressin and an antifibrinolytic agent, such as ε-aminocaproic acid (Amicar).

BIBLIOGRAPHY

Please visit the Nelson Textbook of Pediatrics *website at www.expertconsult.com for the complete bibliography.*

Chapter 472 Hereditary Predisposition to Thrombosis

Leslie J. Raffini and J. Paul Scott

Pediatricians are frequently asked to evaluate children for inherited risk factors for thrombosis with symptomatic thrombosis or asymptomatic children who have relatives affected with either thrombosis or thrombophilia. The clinical utility of thrombophilia testing is debated, both in adults and children.

Thrombophilia testing rarely influences the acute management of a child with a thrombotic event. The association between inherited thrombophilia and pediatric thrombosis varies based on the clinical scenario: children with unprovoked thrombotic events have a high prevalence of inherited defects, while the role of thrombophilic defects in children with catheter-related thrombotic events is questionable. Although some thrombophilic defects are associated with a higher risk of recurrent venous thromboembolism in children, how to use these results to guide the duration of therapy has not been determined. Prospective longitudinal analyses of such patients to determine outcome and response to treatment as well as the impact of known thrombophilic states on these outcomes are clearly needed.

The decision to perform thrombophilia testing in an otherwise healthy child with a family history of thrombosis or thrombophilia should be carefully considered, weighing the potential advantages and limitations of such an approach. Given that the absolute risk of thrombosis in children is extremely low (0.07/100,000), it is unlikely that an inherited thrombophilia will have any impact on clinical decision-making for a young child. The risk of thrombosis increases with age, so that identification of a thrombophilic defect in an adolescent may guide thromboprophylaxis in high-risk situations (lower extremity casting or prolonged immobility), inform the discussion about estrogen-based contraceptives, and may promote lifestyle modification to avoid behavioral prothrombotic risk factors (sedentary lifestyle, dehydration, obesity, and smoking). Limitations of such testing

Table 472-1 INHERITED THROMBOTIC DISORDERS

CLASSIFICATION AND DISORDERS	INHERITANCE	CLINICAL FEATURES
DEFICIENCY OR QUALITATIVE ABNORMALITIES OF INHIBITORS OF ACTIVATED COAGULATION FACTORS		
AT deficiency	AD	Venous thromboembolism (usual and unusual sites), heparin resistance
TM deficiency	AD	Venous thromboembolism
Protein C deficiency	AD	Venous thromboembolism
Protein S deficiency	AD	Venous and arterial thromboembolism
APC resistance	AD	Venous and arterial thromboembolism
IMPAIRED CLOT LYSIS		
Dysfibrinogenemia	AD	More venous thrombosis than arterial thrombosis
Plasminogen deficiency	AD, AR	Venous thromboembolism
TPA deficiency	AD	Venous thromboembolism
Excess PAI-1 activity	AD	Venous thromboembolism and arterial thrombosis
METABOLIC DEFECT		
Hyperhomocysteinemia	Not known	Venous thromboembolism and premature atherosclerotic vascular disease
ABNORMALITY OF COAGULATION ZYMOGEN OR COFACTOR		
Prothrombin mutation	AD	Venous thromboembolism
Elevated factor VIII levels	Not known	Venous thromboembolism
Elevated factor IX levels	Not known	Venous thromboembolism
Elevated factor X levels	Not known	Venous thromboembolism
Elevated factor XI levels	Not known	Venous thromboembolism

AD, autosomal dominant; APC, activated protein C; AR, autosomal recessive; AT, antithrombin; PAI-1, plasminogen activator inhibitor-1; TM, thrombomodulin; TPA, tissue plasminogen activator.

From Robetorye RS, Rodgers GM: Update on selected inherited venous thrombic disorders, *Am J Hematol* 68:256–268, 2001.

Modified with permission from Rodgers GM, Chandler WL: Laboratory and clinical aspects of inherited thrombotic disorders, *Am J Hematol* 41:113–122, 1992. Reprinted with permission of Wiley-Liss, Inc., a subsidiary of John Wiley & Sons, Inc.

include the cost as well as the potential for causing unnecessary anxiety or false reassurance.

The most common inherited thrombophilias are listed in Table 472-1. The inherited defects in which the pathogenic link is best understood include the factor V Leiden mutation, the prothrombin gene mutation, and deficiencies of protein C, protein S, and antithrombin (AT). Elevated levels of factor VIII, lipoprotein (a), and homocysteine are associated with thrombosis, though these are less well characterized and not necessarily genetically determined. Although there are additional alterations in coagulation that have been associated with thrombotic risk, including elevated concentrations of factors IX and XI, heparin cofactor II deficiency, and dysfibrinogenemia, none has gained widespread acceptance in routine testing of children for inherited thrombophilia.

The **factor V Leiden mutation** is the result of a single nucleotide change at nucleotide 1765 within the factor V gene. This mutation causes factor Va to become resistant to inactivation by activated protein C and is the most common inherited risk factor for thrombosis. Approximately 5% of the U.S. white population is heterozygous for this mutation, and it is less prevalent in other ethnic groups. Individuals who are heterozygous have a 5- to 7-fold increase in risk of venous thrombosis, while homozygotes have a relative risk of 80-100. The baseline annual risk of thrombosis for young women of reproductive age is 1 per 12,500 and increases to 1 per 3,500 for those on oral contraceptives. For young women who are heterozygous for the factor V Leiden mutation and are taking oral contraceptives, this baseline annual risk is increased 20- to 30-fold (relative risk) to approximately to 1 per 500 women.

The **prothrombin 20210 gene mutation** is a G to A transition in the 3′ untranslated region of the gene that results in elevated levels of prothrombin. This variant is present in approximately 2% of U.S. whites. It is a weaker risk factor for venous thrombosis than factor V Leiden, with a relative risk of 2-3.

Deficiencies of protein C, protein S, and AT, the natural anticoagulant proteins, are more rare than the common genetic mutations described previously but are associated with a stronger risk of thrombosis. Although heterozygous deficiencies do not often present during childhood, homozygous defects may result in significant symptoms in infancy. Neonates with homozygous deficiencies of AT, protein C, or protein S may present with purpura fulminans. This condition is characterized by rapidly spreading purpuric skin lesions resulting from thromboses of the small dermal vessels followed by bleeding into the skin. In addition, these infants may also develop cerebral thrombosis, ophthalmic thrombosis, disseminated intravascular coagulation (DIC), and large vessel thrombosis. An infant with purpuric skin lesions of unknown cause should receive initial replacement with fresh frozen plasma. Definitive diagnosis can be difficult in the sick premature neonate who may have undetectable levels of these factors but not have a true genetic deficiency. Protein C and AT concentrates are also available and have been demonstrated to be effective.

Neonates have decreased concentrations of protein C, protein S, and AT that increase rapidly over the first 6 mo of life; protein C concentrations remain below adult levels throughout much of childhood. Multiple acquired conditions may affect plasma concentrations of these anticoagulants. Patients with single ventricle congenital heart disease and hepatic dysfunction may have decreased concentrations of all 3 anticoagulants; vitamin K deficiency and warfarin result in a reduction of the vitamin K–dependent factors, including protein C and protein S; nephrotic syndrome, severe burns, and asparaginase all disproportionately decrease AT; and protein S may be decreased during pregnancy and in the presence of antiphospholipid antibodies.

Both venous and arterial thromboses are common in young patients with **homocystinuria,** an inborn error of metabolism due to deficiency of cystathione β-synthase. In this very rare condition, plasma levels of homocysteine exceed 100 μmol/L. Much more common are mild to moderate elevations of homocysteine, which may be acquired or associated with a polymorphism in the methylenetetrahydrofolate reductase (MTHFR) gene. Although moderate elevations of homocysteine have been associated with both venous and arterial thrombotic events, testing for polymorphisms in the MTHFR gene are not indicated, because these polymorphisms are not associated with venous thromboembolism. The pathogenic mechanisms for thrombosis in homocystinemia are not well understood.

Increased plasma concentrations of **factor VIII** (>150 IU/dL) appear to be regulated by both genetic and environmental factors and are associated with an increased risk of thrombosis. While there is a strong component of heritability contributing to factor VIII levels, the molecular mechanisms responsible for elevated factor VIII are not well understood. Factor VIII is also considered to be an acute phase reactant, and may increase transiently during periods of inflammation.

Lipoprotein (a) [Lp(a)] is a low-density lipoprotein particle that has been linked to atherothrombosis in adults, with elevated levels associated with premature myocardial infarction and stroke. Levels of Lp(a) >30 mg/dL have been demonstrated to be an independent risk factor for stroke and venous thrombosis in children in small studies. Lp(a) has a structure that is similar to plasminogen and it is postulated that elevated levels may inhibit fibrinolysis, though this has not been proven.

BIBLIOGRAPHY

Please visit the Nelson Textbook of Pediatrics *website at www.expertconsult.com for the complete bibliography.*

Chapter 473
Thrombotic Disorders in Children

Leslie J. Raffini and J. Paul Scott

Compared to adults, children are generally protected from venous and arterial thromboses. Advancements in the treatment and supportive care of critically ill children, coupled with a heightened awareness of genetic risk factors for thrombosis, have led to an increase in the diagnosis of thromboembolic events (TEs) in children. As a result, TEs are not infrequent in pediatric tertiary care centers and may result in significant acute and chronic morbidity. Despite the fact that TEs in children are increasing in relative terms, they are still rare. This rarity has been the major impediment to prospective clinical trials, resulting in a deficit of evidence-based medicine. Diagnosis and treatment is often extrapolated from adult data.

EPIDEMIOLOGY

Studies have confirmed a significant increase in the diagnosis of venous thromboembolism (VTE) in pediatric tertiary hospitals across the United States. Although the overall incidence of thrombosis in the general pediatric population is quite low (0.07/100,000), the rate of VTE in hospitalized children is 60/10,000 admissions. Infants less than 1 yr old account for the largest proportion of pediatric VTEs, with a 2nd peak during adolescence.

The majority of children who develop a TE have multiple risk factors that may be acquired, inherited, and/or anatomic (Table 473-1). The presence of a central venous catheter (CVC) is the single most important risk factor for venous thromboembolism (VTE) in pediatric patients, associated with approximately 90% of neonatal VTE and 60% of childhood VTE. These catheters are often necessary for the care of premature neonates and children with acute and chronic diseases and are used for intravenous hyperalimentation, chemotherapy, dialysis, antibiotics, or supportive therapy. CVCs may damage the endothelial lining and/or cause blood flow disruption, increasing the risk of thrombosis. There are multiple other acquired risk factors that are associated with thrombosis, including trauma, infection, chronic medical illnesses, and medications. Cancer, congenital heart disease, and prematurity are the most common medical conditions associated with TEs.

Antiphospholipid antibody syndrome (APS) is a well-described syndrome in adults characterized by recurrent fetal loss and/or thrombosis. Antiphospholipid antibodies (APA) are associated with both venous and arterial thrombosis. The mechanism by which these antibodies cause thrombosis is not well understood. A diagnosis of APS requires the presence of both clinical and laboratory abnormalities (see under Laboratory Testing). The laboratory abnormalities must be persistent for 12 wk. Because of the high risk of recurrence, patients with APS often require long-term anticoagulation. It is important to note that healthy children may have a transient lupus anticoagulant, often diagnosed because of a prolonged PTT on routine preoperative testing. These antibodies may be associated with a recent viral infection and are not a risk factor for thrombosis.

Anatomic abnormalities that impede blood flow also predispose patients to thrombosis at an earlier age. Atresia of the inferior vena cava has been described in association with acute and chronic lower extremity deep venous thrombosis (DVT). May-Thurner syndrome (compression of the left iliac vein by the overlying right iliac artery) should be considered in patients who present spontaneously with left iliofemoral thrombosis, and thoracic outlet obstruction (Paget-Schroetter syndrome) frequently presents with effort-related axillary-subclavian vein thrombosis.

Table 473-1 POTENTIAL PROTHROMBOTIC STATES

CONGENITAL
Deficiency of anticoagulants
AT-III, protein C or protein S, plasminogen
Resistance to cofactor proteolysis
Factor V Leiden
High levels of procoagulants
Prothrombin 20210 mutation
Elevated factor VIII levels
Damage to endothelium
Homocystinemia
ACQUIRED
Obstruction to flow
Indwelling lines
Pregnancy
Polycythemia/dehydration
Immobilization
Injury
Trauma, surgery, exercise
Inflammation
IBD, vasculitis, infection, Behçet syndrome
Hypercoagulability
Pregnancy
Malignancy
Antiphospholipid syndrome
Nephrotic syndrome
Oral contraceptives
L-Asparaginase
Elevated factor VIII levels
RARE OTHER ENTITIES
Congenital
Dysfibrinogenemia
Acquired
Paroxysmal nocturnal hemoglobinuria
Thrombocythemia
Vascular grafts

AT-III, antithrombin III; IBD, inflammatory bowel disease.

CLINICAL MANIFESTATIONS

Extremity deep vein thrombosis (DVT): Children with acute DVT often present with extremity pain, swelling, and discoloration. A history of a current or recent CVC in that extremity should be very suggestive. Many times, symptoms of CVC-associated thrombosis are more subtle and chronic, including repeated CVC occlusion or sepsis, or prominent venous collaterals on the chest, face, and neck.

Pulmonary embolism (PE): Symptoms of PE include shortness of breath, pleuritic chest pain, cough, hemoptysis, fever, and, in the case of massive PE, hypotension and right heart failure. Based on autopsy studies, PEs are often not diagnosed, perhaps because young children are unable to accurately describe their symptoms and their respiratory deterioration may be masked by other conditions (Chapter 401.1).

Cerebral sinovenous thrombosis (CSVT): Symptoms may be subtle and may develop over many hours or days. Neonates often present with seizures, whereas older children often complain of headache, vomiting, seizures, and focal signs. They may also have papilledema and abducens palsy. Some patients may have a concurrent sinusitis or mastoiditis that has contributed to the thrombosis.

Renal vein thrombosis: Renal vein thrombosis is the most common spontaneous TE in neonates. Affected infants may present with hematuria, an abdominal mass, and/or thrombocytopenia. Infants of diabetic mothers are at increased risk, although the mechanism for this increased risk is unknown. Approximately 25% of cases are bilateral.

Peripheral arterial thrombosis: With the exception of stroke, the majority of arterial TEs in children are secondary to catheters, often in neonates related to umbilical artery lines or in patients with cardiac defects undergoing cardiac catheterization. Patients with an arterial thrombosis affecting blood flow to an extremity will present with a cold, pale, blue extremity with poor or absent pulses.

Stroke: Ischemic stroke commonly presents with hemiparesis, loss of consciousness, or seizures. This condition may occur secondary to pathology that affects the intracranial arteries (i.e., sickle cell disease, vasculopathy, or traumatic arterial dissection) or may be due to venous thrombi that embolize to the arterial circulation (placental thrombi, children with congenital heart disease or patent foramen ovale).

DIAGNOSIS

Ultrasound with Doppler flow is the most commonly employed imaging study due for the diagnosis of upper or more often lower extremity VTE. Spiral CT is used most frequently for the diagnosis of PE (Fig. 473-1). Other diagnostic imaging options include CT and MR venography, which are noninvasive, although the sensitivity and specificity of these studies is not known. They may be particularly helpful in evaluating proximal thrombosis. For the diagnosis of cerebral sinovenous thrombosis and acute ischemic stroke, the most sensitive imaging study is brain magnetic resonance imaging with venography (MRV) or diffusion weighted imaging.

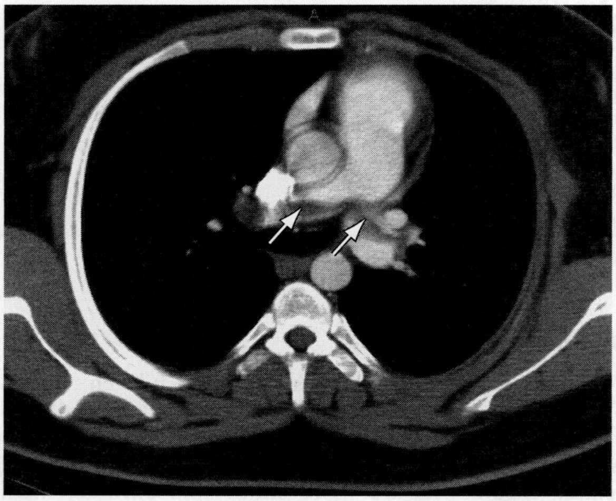

Figure 473-1 Chest CT from a 15 yr old male with a large pulmonary embolism. There are large filling defects in both the right and left main pulmonary arteries.

LABORATORY TESTING

All children with a TE should have a complete blood count and a baseline PT and aPTT to assess their coagulation status. In adults suspected to have a DVT, the D-dimer level has a high negative predictive value. The D-dimer is a fragment produced when fibrin is degraded by plasmin and is a measure of fibrinolysis. Based on the clinical scenario, other laboratory studies such as renal and hepatic function may be indicated. Testing for APS includes evaluation for the lupus anticoagulant as well as anticardiolipin and antiβ2-glycoprotein antibodies.

There is some debate regarding which patients should have testing for inherited risk factors. Thrombophilia testing rarely influences the acute management of a child with a thrombotic event. Identification of an inherited thrombophilia may influence the duration of treatment, particularly for those with combined defects, and may aid in counseling the patient about their risk of recurrence.

The evaluation of coagulation studies in pediatric patients is often complicated due to the differences in normal ranges that have been established for infants and for older children/adults. In addition, there is often significant variation in the laboratory assays used to test anticoagulant levels. It is critical to refer to the age-related normal ranges when interpreting pediatric coagulation studies. One limitation of these normal ranges is that they were performed many years ago, using assays that may not be equivalent to those used today. Molecular assays are not age dependent.

TREATMENT

Therapeutic options for children with thrombosis include anticoagulation, thrombolysis, surgery, and observation. The goal of **anticoagulation** is to reduce the risk of embolism, halt clot extension, and prevent recurrence. In premature neonates and critically ill children who may have an increased risk of bleeding, the potential benefits must be weighed against the risks. Options for acute anticoagulation include unfractionated heparin (uFH) or low molecular weight heparin (LMWH), though LMWH is more frequently used because of the ease of dosing and need for less monitoring (Table 473-2). Both drugs act by catalyzing the action of antithrombin. Thrombolytic therapy, using a plasminogen activator, will hasten thrombus resolution but at the risk of increased bleeding. Surgery may be necessary for life- or limb-threatening

Table 473-2 COMPARISON OF ANTITHROMBOTIC AGENTS

	THROMBOLYTIC THERAPY	UNFRACTIONATED HEPARIN*	WARFARIN	LMW HEPARIN (ENOXAPARIN)
Indication	Recent onset of life- or limb-threatening thrombus	Thrombus of indeterminate age	Long-term oral anticoagulation	Thrombus of indeterminate age
Dose	rTPA 0.1-0.2 mg/kg/hr IV	75 U/kg/bolus, 20-28* U/kg/hr by continuous infusion IV	0.1-0.2 mg/kg/day PO	1.0-1.5* mg/kg q12hr SC
Adjustment	Increase dose for lack of clinical effect	↑ dose by 5-10% q6hr until adequate level or PTT is achieved	↑ dose q 2 days by 20-30% until appropriate, stable INR	↑ or ↓ by 10-20%
Course	6-12 hr	5-14 days	Weeks to months	5 days-6 mo
Monitors/goal	"Lytic state": FDP or D-dimer (TPA)	PTT $2\frac{1}{2}$ times control; thrombin time infinity; heparin level 0.3-0.7 U/mL	INR 2.0-3.0	LMW heparin level 4 hr after 4th dose = 0.5-1.0 U/mL
Mechanism	Activation of plasminogen to plasmin	Accelerates AT-III–dependent inactivation of thrombin, FXa	Impairs vitamin K–dependent carboxylation of FII, FVII, FIX, FX, proteins C and S	Accelerates AT-III–dependent inactivation of FXa and thrombin
Risk of bleeding	Medium to high	Low	Low	Low

*Higher dose is required in newborns.

AT-III, antithrombin III; F, factor; FDP, fibrin degradation product; INR, international normalized ratio; LMW, low molecular weight; PTT, partial thromboplastin time; rTPA, recombinant tissue-type plasminogen activator; U, unit.

Aspirin is the only commonly used antiplatelet agent, and the usual dose is 80 mg/day (1 baby aspirin daily). There is no need to monitor aspirin therapy.

thrombosis when there is a contraindication to thrombolysis. The optimal treatment for a child with acute ischemic stroke depends on the likely etiology and the size of the infarct. Children with sickle cell disease who develop stroke are treated with chronic red blood cell transfusions to reduce recurrence.

COMPLICATIONS

Complications of VTE include recurrent thrombosis (either local or distant), and development of post-thrombotic syndrome (PTS). A thrombosed blood vessel may partially or fully recanalize or may remain occluded. Over time, an occluded deep vein may cause venous hypertension, resulting in blood flow being directed from the deep system into the superficial veins and potentially producing pain, swelling, edema, discoloration, and ulceration. This clinical picture is known as *post-thrombotic syndrome* (PTS) and may be chronically disabling. Several prospective studies in adults have shown PTS to be present in 17-50% of patients with a history of thrombosis. The likelihood of developing PTS is highest in the 1st 2 yr but continues to increase over time. Graduated compression stockings reduce the risk of PTS in adults and can be used in children.

473.1 Anticoagulant and Thrombolytic Therapy

Leslie J. Raffini and J. Paul Scott

Table 473-2 provides an outline of commonly used anticoagulant agents.

Unfractionated (Standard) Heparin

Heparin enhances the rate by which antithrombin III neutralizes the activity of several activated clotting proteins, especially factor Xa and thrombin. The average half-life of heparin administered IV is approximately 60 min in adults and can be as short as 30 min in the newborn. Heparin does not cross the placenta. The half-life of heparin is dose-dependent; the higher the dose, the longer the circulating half-life. In thrombotic disease, the half-life may be shorter than normal in patients with significant thromboembolism (pulmonary embolism) and longer than normal in patients with cirrhosis and uremia.

Anticoagulation with heparin is **contraindicated** in the following circumstances: a recent central nervous system hemorrhage; bleeding from inaccessible sites; malignant hypertension; bacterial endocarditis; recent surgery of the eye, brain, or spinal cord; and current administration of regional or lumbar block anesthesia. A pre-existing coagulation defect or bleeding abnormality is a relative contraindication. Despite these precautions, the frequency of bleeding in patients given heparin anticoagulation is 0.2-1.0%.

Guidelines for therapy using unfractionated heparin are shown in Table 473-1. In newborns with low levels of clotting factors, in patients with a lupus inhibitor, or in patients with elevated levels of factor VIII (as a result of stress or surgery), PTT may not reflect the correct degree of anticoagulation, and specific heparin levels should be obtained so that the heparin level is 0.35-0.70 U/mL by anti–factor Xa assay or 0.2-0.4 U/mL by protamine sulfate assay.

Heparin can be neutralized immediately by using protamine sulfate. Because of the rapid clearance rate of heparin, however, stopping the infusion is adequate treatment for most patients. One milligram of protamine sulfate neutralizes 90-110 U of heparin. Because heparin has rapid in vivo metabolic decay, only one half of the total dose of protamine should be administered. A clotting test is performed to determine whether adequate neutralization has occurred; if not, the additional protamine can be given. Protamine itself is an anticoagulant; thus, if too much is given, clotting time may be prolonged. Although excess protamine has an anticoagulant effect, it rarely (if ever) is a cause of clinical bleeding. Once heparin is neutralized, the patient is returned to the original "prothrombotic" state.

Low Molecular Weight Heparin

LMWH is an effective, convenient alternative to standard heparin therapy, and its use is described in Table 473-1. Several heparins and heparinoids are undergoing clinical trials. Most pediatric experience is with enoxaparin. Adult patients receiving LMW heparin rarely need to have their heparin levels monitored, but in pediatric patients, there is more diversity of response. Monitoring is critical to ensure that a therapeutic level is achieved. PTT cannot be used to monitor LMW heparin; a specific assay should be used. Once a therapeutic range is achieved, routine monitoring is not required or is required only infrequently. When LMW heparin is used for prophylaxis against thrombosis, the dose is 0.5 mg/kg q12hr subcutaneously, with the goal of achieving a level of 0.3 U/mL 4 hr after injection.

Warfarin

Coumarin derivatives are oral anticoagulant drugs that act by decreasing the functional levels of the vitamin K–dependent coagulation factors: II, VII, IX, and X, as well as protein C and protein S (vitamin K–dependent anticoagulants). These drugs inhibit vitamin K–dependent carboxylation of the precursor coagulation proteins. Warfarin probably acts by competitively inhibiting vitamin K metabolism. After the administration of warfarin, levels of factors II, VII, IX, and X decrease gradually, according to each factor's plasma half-life. Because factor VII has the shortest half-life, its level is the 1st to decrease, followed by factors IX and X, and finally, factor II. It generally takes 4-5 days to reduce the levels of all 4 coagulation factors consistent with effective anticoagulation.

Prothrombin time (PT) is the clotting test used to assess warfarin anticoagulation. Current recommendations are based on the International Normalized Ratio (INR), which permits comparison of PT using a wide variety of reagents or instruments. The INR for standard treatment of thrombosis is 2.0-3.0. Table 473-1 provides guidelines for the administration of warfarin to children. For patients with mechanical heart valves and those with homozygous protein C deficiency, the INR should be 3.0-4.0.

The most serious side effect of warfarin is hemorrhage. This is often related to changes in the dose or metabolism of the drug. The addition or removal of certain drugs in the patient's therapeutic regimen can have significant effects on oral anticoagulation. The effect of warfarin can be enhanced by the administration of antibiotics, salicylates, anabolic steroids, chloral hydrate, laxatives, allopurinol, vitamin E, and methylphenidate hydrochloride; its effect can be diminished by barbiturates, vitamin K, oral contraceptives, phenytoin, and other agents. Warfarin-induced bleeding is treated by discontinuation of the drug and oral administration of vitamin K. Generally, the amount of vitamin K given is equal to the amount of the daily warfarin dose. Vitamin K can be administered orally, subcutaneously, or IV (not IM), but the parenteral forms have a much longer half-life and may overshoot the correction. Correction of coagulopathy begins within 6-8 hr and should be complete in 24-48 hr. If the patient is having a significant or life-threatening hemorrhage, fresh frozen plasma (15 mL/kg) should be given when the vitamin K is administered.

Contraindications to coumarin anticoagulants are essentially the same as those for heparin therapy. The oral anticoagulants are teratogenic, cross the placenta, and should not be given during pregnancy, particularly during the 1st trimester. Although breast milk contains warfarin, the quantity is insignificant and the drug can be used to treat the lactating mother without a significant effect on the infant.

Thrombolytic Therapy

Thrombolytic agents, such as recombinant tissue-type plasminogen activator (rTPA), activate plasminogen to lyse blood clots by enzymatic digestion; rTPA is most often used in pediatrics for thrombolytic therapy, as described in Table 473-1. For this therapy to be effective, the patient should have a relatively fresh clot (<3-5 days old), the clot must be accessible to the lytic agent, and there must be an adequate amount of plasminogen. Once plasmin has been formed, it lyses fibrin. Relatively more fibrin-specific than the older thrombolytic agents urokinase and streptokinase, rTPA activates plasminogen within or on a fibrin clot. Clinical trials with rTPA suggest that it rarely produces a systemic hyperfibrinolytic state. The initial dose of rTPA is 0.1 mg/kg/hr. It may be useful to monitor for a therapeutic effect by looking for an increase in the concentration of D-dimers or fibrin degradation products. Higher doses or more prolonged courses of thrombolytic therapy are likely to be associated with an increased risk of bleeding complications. Low doses of rTPA have been efficacious in restoring patency in occluded vascular access catheters.

PREVENTION

There have been no formal trials of prevention of venous thromboembolic disease in children. Children with known prothrombotic conditions who are going to be immobilized for a protracted time probably should receive prophylactic treatment with enoxaparin 0.5 mg/kg q12hr while immobile. More controversial is the use of such therapy for children who are immobilized for a prolonged period due to a severe medical illness, especially if it is associated with inflammation or trauma.

BIBLIOGRAPHY

Please visit the Nelson Textbook of Pediatrics *website at* *www.expertconsult.com* *for the complete bibliography.*

Chapter 474
Postneonatal Vitamin K Deficiency

J. Paul Scott and Robert R. Montgomery

Although "late" hemorrhagic disease has been reported in breast-fed children, vitamin K deficiency occurring after the neonatal period is usually secondary to a lack of oral intake of vitamin K, alterations in the gut flora due to the long-term use of broad-spectrum antibiotics, liver disease, or malabsorption of vitamin K. Intestinal malabsorption of fats may accompany cystic fibrosis or biliary atresia and result in a deficiency of fat-soluble dietary vitamins, with reduced synthesis of vitamin K–dependent clotting factors (factors II, VII, IX, and X, and protein C and protein S). Prophylactic administration of water-soluble vitamin K orally is indicated in these cases (2-3 mg/24 hr for children and 5-10 mg/24 hr for adolescents and adults), or vitamin K may be administered at 1-2 mg IV. In patients with advanced cirrhosis, synthesis of many of the clotting factors may be reduced because of hepatocellular damage. In these patients, vitamin K may be ineffective. The anticoagulant properties of warfarin (Coumadin) and related anticoagulants depend on interference with vitamin K, with a concomitant reduction of factors II, VII, IX, and X. Rat poison (superwarfarin) produces a similar deficiency; vitamin K is a specific antidote.

BIBLIOGRAPHY

Please visit the Nelson Textbook of Pediatrics *website at* *www.expertconsult.com* *for the complete bibliography.*

Chapter 475
Liver Disease

J. Paul Scott and Robert R. Montgomery

Because all of the clotting factors except factor VIII are produced exclusively in the liver, coagulation abnormalities are very common in patients with severe liver disease. Only 15% of such patients have significant clinical bleeding states. The severity of the coagulation abnormality appears to be directly proportional to the extent of hepatocellular damage. The most common mechanism causing the defect is decreased synthesis of coagulation factors. Patients with severe liver disease characteristically have normal to increased (not reduced) levels of factor VIII activity in plasma. In some instances, disseminated intravascular coagulation (Chapter 477) or hyperfibrinolysis may complicate liver disease, making laboratory differentiation of severe liver disease from disseminated intravascular coagulation difficult.

For the full continuation of this chapter, please visit the Nelson Textbook of Pediatrics *website at* *www.expertconsult.com*.

Chapter 476
Acquired Inhibitors of Coagulation

J. Paul Scott and Robert R. Montgomery

Acquired circulating anticoagulants (inhibitors) are antibodies that react or cross react with clotting factors or components used in coagulation screening tests (phospholipids), thereby prolonging screening tests, such as prothrombin time and partial thromboplastin time. Some of these anticoagulants are autoantibodies that react with phospholipid and thereby interfere with clotting in vitro but not in vivo. The most common form of these antiphospholipid antibodies has been referred to as the *lupus anticoagulant* (Chapter 473). This anticoagulant is found in patients with systemic lupus erythematosus (Chapter 152), in those with other collagen-vascular diseases, and in association with HIV. In otherwise healthy children, spontaneous lupus-like inhibitors have developed transiently after incidental viral infection. These transient inhibitors are usually not associated with either bleeding or thrombosis.

Although the classic lupus anticoagulant is more often associated with a predisposition to thrombosis than with bleeding symptoms, bleeding symptoms in a patient with the lupus anticoagulant may be caused by thrombocytopenia, as a manifestation of the antiphospholipid syndrome or of lupus itself, or rarely, by a coexistent specific autoantibody against prothrombin (factor II). This antiprothrombin antibody does not inactivate prothrombin, but causes accelerated clearance of the protein, resulting in low levels of prothrombin.

Rarely, antibodies may arise spontaneously against a specific clotting factor, such as factor VIII or von Willebrand factor, similar to those seen more frequently in elderly patients. These patients are prone to excessive hemorrhage and may require specific treatment. In patients with a hereditary deficiency of a clotting factor (factor VIII or factor IX), antibodies may develop after exposure to transfused factor concentrates. These hemophilic inhibitory antibodies are discussed in Chapter 470.1.

LABORATORY FINDINGS

Inhibitors against specific coagulation factors usually affect factors VIII, IX, and XI, or rarely, prothrombin. Depending on the target of the antibody, prothrombin time, partial thromboplastin time, or both may be prolonged. The mechanism by which the inhibitory antibody functions determines whether mixing patient plasma with normal plasma will normalize (correct) the clotting time. Patient plasma containing antibodies directed against the active site of the clotting factor (factor VIII or factor IX) will not correct on 1 : 1 mixing with normal plasma, whereas antibodies that lead to increased clearance of the factor (prothrombin) will correct on 1 : 1 mixing. Specific factor assays are used to determine which factor is involved.

TREATMENT

Management of the patient with an inhibitor against factor VIII or IX is the same as for the patient with hemophilia who has an alloantibody against factor VIII or factor IX. Infusions of recombinant factor VIIa or activated prothrombin complex concentrate may be needed to control significant bleeding. Acute bleeding due to an antiprothrombin antibody can often be treated with a plasma infusion and may benefit from a short course of corticosteroid therapy.

Asymptomatic spontaneous inhibitors that arise after a viral infection tend to disappear within a few wk to mo. Inhibitors seen with an underlying disease, such as systemic lupus erythematosus, often disappear when the primary disease is effectively treated.

BIBLIOGRAPHY

Please visit the Nelson Textbook of Pediatrics *website at www.expertconsult.com for the complete bibliography.*

Chapter 477 Disseminated Intravascular Coagulation

J. Paul Scott, Leslie J. Raffini, and Robert R. Montgomery

Thrombotic microangiopathy refers to a heterogeneous group of conditions, including disseminated intravascular coagulation (DIC), that result in consumption of clotting factors, platelets, and anticoagulant proteins. Consequences of this process include widespread intravascular deposition of fibrin, leading to tissue ischemia and necrosis, a generalized hemorrhagic state, and hemolytic anemia.

ETIOLOGY

Any life-threatening severe systemic disease associated with hypoxia, acidosis, tissue necrosis, shock, and/or endothelial damage may trigger DIC. A large number of conditions have been reported to be associated with DIC (Table 477-1). Although the clinical symptoms are more often hemorrhagic, the initiating event is usually excessive activation of clotting that consumes both the physiologic anticoagulants (protein C, protein S, and antithrombin III) and procoagulants, resulting in a deficiency of factor V, factor VIII, prothrombin, fibrinogen, and platelets. Commonly, the clinical result of this sequence of events is hemorrhage. The hemostatic dysregulation may also result in thromboses in the skin, kidneys, and other organs. Better understanding of the pathophysiology of hemostasis has lead to an appreciation of the critical interaction of the coagulation pathways with the innate immune system and inflammatory response that likely contributes to the widespread dysregulation present in DIC.

Table 477-1 CAUSES OF DISSEMINATED INTRAVASCULAR COAGULATION

INFECTIOUS
Meningococcemia (purpura fulminans)
Bacterial sepsis (staphylococcal, streptococcal, *Escherichia coli*, *Salmonella*)
Rickettsia (Rocky Mountain spotted fever)
Virus (cytomegalovirus, herpes simplex, hemorrhagic fevers)
Malaria
Fungus
TISSUE INJURY
Central nervous system trauma (massive head injury)
Multiple fractures with fat emboli
Crush injury
Profound shock or asphyxia
Hypothermia or hyperthermia
Massive burns
MALIGNANCY
Acute promyelocytic leukemia
Acute monoblastic or promyelocytic leukemia
Widespread malignancies (neuroblastoma)
VENOM OR TOXIN
Snake bites
Insect bites
MICROANGIOPATHIC DISORDERS
"Severe" thrombotic thrombocytopenic purpura or hemolytic-uremic syndrome
Giant hemangioma (Kasabach-Merritt syndrome)
GASTROINTESTINAL DISORDERS
Fulminant hepatitis
Severe inflammatory bowel disease
Pancreatitis
HEREDITARY THROMBOTIC DISORDERS
Antithrombin III deficiency
Homozygous protein C deficiency
NEWBORN
Maternal toxemia
Bacterial or viral sepsis (group B streptococcus, herpes simplex)
Abruptio placentae
Severe respiratory distress syndrome
Necrotizing enterocolitis
Erythroblastosis fetalis
Fetal demise of a twin
MISCELLLANEOUS
Severe acute graft rejection
Acute hemolytic transfusion reaction
Severe collagen-vascular disease
Kawasaki disease
Heparin-induced thrombosis
Infusion of "activated" prothrombin complex concentrates
Hyperpyrexia/encephalopathy, hemorrhagic shock syndrome
Placental abruption

Modified from Montgomery RR, Scott IP: Hemostasis: diseases of the fluid phase. In Nathan DG, Oski FA, editors: *Hematology of infancy and childhood*, vol 2, ed 4, Philadelphia, 1993, WB Saunders.

CLINICAL MANIFESTATIONS

DIC accompanies a severe systemic disease process, usually with shock. Bleeding frequently first occurs from sites of venipuncture or surgical incision. The skin may show petechiae and ecchymoses. Tissue necrosis may involve many organs and can be most spectacularly seen as infarction of large areas of skin, subcutaneous tissue, or kidneys. Anemia caused by hemolysis may develop rapidly, owing to microangiopathic hemolytic anemia.

LABORATORY FINDINGS

There is no well-defined sequence of events. Certain coagulation factors (factors II, V, and VIII, and fibrinogen) and platelets may be consumed by the ongoing intravascular clotting process, with resultant prolongation of the prothrombin, partial thromboplastin, and thrombin times. Platelet counts may be profoundly depressed. The blood smear may contain fragmented and burr- and helmet-shaped red blood cells (schistocytes). In addition, because the fibrinolytic mechanism is activated, fibrinogen degradation products (FDPs, D-dimers) appear in the blood. The D-dimer is formed by fibrinolysis of a cross-linked fibrin clot. The D-dimer assay is as sensitive as the FDP test and more specific for activation of coagulation and fibrinolysis.

TREATMENT

The 1st 2 steps in the treatment of DIC are the most critical: (1) treat the trigger that caused DIC and (2) restore normal homeostasis by correcting the shock, acidosis, and hypoxia that usually complicate DIC. If the underlying problem can be controlled and the patient stabilized, bleeding quickly ceases, and there is improvement of the abnormal laboratory findings. Blood components are used for replacement therapy in patients with hemorrhage and may consist of platelet infusions (for thrombocytopenia), cryoprecipitate (for hypofibrinogenemia), and/or fresh frozen plasma (for replacement of other coagulation factors and natural inhibitors).

In DIC associated with sepsis, a controlled trial of drotrecogin alpha (activated protein C concentrate [APC]) in adults with sepsis showed a statistically significant survival advantage in those treated with APC. Clinical trials using protein C concentrate in purpura fulminans and APC in children with sepsis syndrome have not shown a statistically significant improvement.

The role of heparin in DIC is limited to patients who have vascular thrombosis in association with DIC or who require prophylaxis because they are at high risk for venous thromboembolism. Such individuals should be treated as outlined in Chapter 473.1, with careful attention to replacement therapy to maintain an adequate platelet count and thus limit bleeding complications.

The prognosis of patients with DIC is primarily dependent on the outcome of the treatment of the primary disease and prevention of end-organ damage.

BIBLIOGRAPHY

Please visit the Nelson Textbook of Pediatrics *website at* www.expertconsult.com *for the complete bibliography.*

Chapter 478
Platelet and Blood Vessel Disorders

J. Paul Scott and Robert R. Montgomery

MEGAKARYOPOIESIS

Platelets are non-nucleated cellular fragments produced by megakaryocytes within the bone marrow and other tissues. Megakaryocytes are large polyploid cells. When the megakaryocyte approaches maturity, budding of the cytoplasm occurs and large numbers of platelets are liberated. Platelets circulate with a life span of 10-14 days. **Thrombopoietin** (TPO) is the primary growth factor that controls platelet production (Fig. 478-1). Levels of TPO appear to correlate inversely with platelet number and megakaryocyte mass. Levels of TPO are highest in the thrombocytopenic states associated with decreased marrow megakaryopoiesis and may be variable in states of increased platelet production.

The platelet plays multiple hemostatic roles. The platelet surface possesses a number of important receptors for adhesive proteins, including von Willebrand factor (VWF) and fibrinogen, as well as receptors for agonists that trigger platelet aggregation, such as thrombin, collagen, and adenosine diphosphate (ADP). After injury to the blood vessel wall, subendothelial collagen binds VWF. VWF undergoes a conformational change that induces binding of the platelet glycoprotein Ib (GPIb) complex (the VWF receptor). This process is called *platelet adhesion.* Platelets then undergo activation. During the process of activation, the platelets generate thromboxane A_2 from arachidonic acid via the enzyme cyclo-oxygenase. After activation, platelets release agonists, such as ADP, adenosine triphosphate (ATP), Ca^{2+}, serotonin, and coagulation factors, into the surrounding milieu. Binding of VWF to the GPIb complex triggers a complex signaling cascade that results in activation of the fibrinogen receptor, the major platelet integrin glycoprotein α_{IIb}-β_3 (GPIIb-IIIa). Circulating fibrinogen binds to its receptor on the activated platelets, complex linking platelets together in a process called *aggregation.* This series of events forms a hemostatic plug at the site of vascular injury. The serotonin and histamine that are liberated during activation increase local vasoconstriction. In addition to acting in concert with the vessel wall to form the platelet plug, the platelet provides the catalytic surface on which coagulation factors assemble and eventually generate thrombin through a sequential series of enzymatic cleavages. Last, the platelet contractile proteins and cytoskeleton mediate clot retraction.

THROMBOCYTOPENIA

The normal platelet count is 150-450 × 10^9/L. *Thrombocytopenia* refers to a reduction in platelet count to <150 × 10^9/L. Causes of thrombocytopenia include: (1) decreased production on either a congenital or an acquired basis; (2) sequestration of the platelets within an enlarged spleen or other organ; and (3) increased destruction of normally synthesized platelets on either an immune or a nonimmune basis (Chapter 469; Tables 478-1 and 478-2 and Fig. 478-2).

BIBLIOGRAPHY

Please visit the Nelson Textbook of Pediatrics *website at* www.expertconsult.com *for the complete bibliography.*

478.1 Idiopathic (Autoimmune) Thrombocytopenic Purpura

J. Paul Scott and Robert R. Montgomery

The most common cause of acute onset of thrombocytopenia in an otherwise well child is (autoimmune) idiopathic thrombocytopenic purpura (ITP).

Epidemiology

In a small number of children, estimated about 1 in 20,000, 1-4 wk after exposure to a common viral infection, an autoantibody directed against the platelet surface develops with resultant sudden onset of thrombocytopenia. A recent history of viral illness is described in 50-65% of cases of childhood ITP. The peak age is 1-4 yr, although the age ranges from early in infancy to the elderly. In childhood, males and females are equally affected. ITP seems to occur more often in late winter and spring after the peak season of viral respiratory illness.

Pathogenesis

Why some children develop the acute presentation of an autoimmune disease is unknown. The exact antigenic target for most such antibodies in most cases of childhood acute ITP remains undetermined. although in chronic ITP most patients demonstrate antibodies against the platelet glycoprotein complexes, α11b-B3 and GPIb. After binding of the antibody to the platelet surface, circulating antibody-coated platelets are recognized by the Fc receptor on splenic macrophages, ingested, and destroyed. Most common viruses have been described in association with

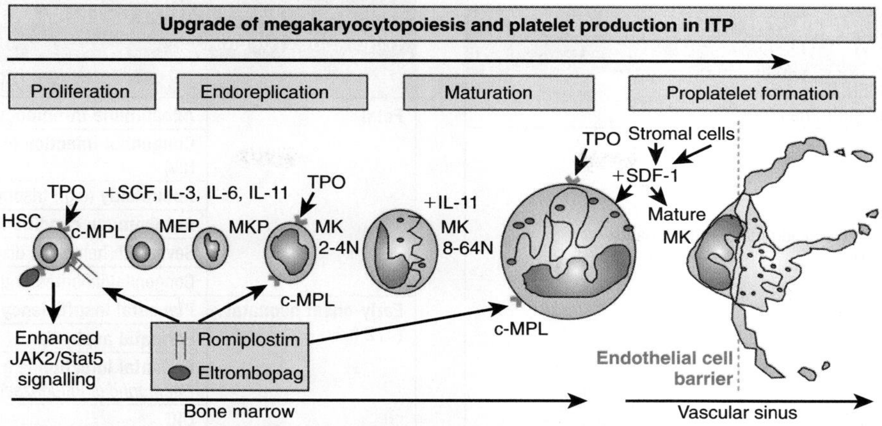

Figure 478-1 Scheme of megakaryocytopoiesis and platelet production in idiopathic thrombocytopenic purpura (ITP). Hematopoietic stem cells (HSC) are mobilized and megakaryocyte (MK) and erythroid progenitors (MEP) accumulate with MK-committed progenitors (MKP) giving rise to mature MKs under control of thrombopoietin (TPO) working with chemokines, cytokines, and growth factors, including stem cell factor (SCF) and interleukin (IL)-3, IL-6, and IL-11. Endoreplication results in ploidy changes in MKs and increased chromosome number (up to 64N). Mature MKs migrate to the endothelial cell barrier delimiting the vascular sinus and, under the influence of stromal-derived factor-1 (SDF-1), give rise to proplatelets that protrude into the circulation and produce large numbers of platelets under hemodynamic determinants. Therapeutically given romiplostim and eltrombopag enter the marrow and join with TPO to stimulate megakaryocytopoiesis and platelet production. (From Nurden AT, Viallard JF, Nurden P: New-generation drugs that stimulate platelet production in chronic immune thrombocytopenic purpura, *Lancet* 373:1562–1568, 2009, p 1563.)

ITP, including Epstein-Barr virus (Chapter 246) and HIV (Chapter 268). Epstein-Barr virus-related ITP is usually of short duration and follows the course of infectious mononucleosis. HIV-associated ITP is usually chronic. In some patients ITP appears to arise in children infected with *Helicobacter pylori* or rarely following the measles, mumps, rubella vaccine.

Clinical Manifestations

The classic presentation of ITP is a previously healthy 1-4 yr old child who has sudden onset of generalized petechiae and purpura. The parents often state that the child was fine yesterday and now is covered with bruises and purple dots. Often there is bleeding from the gums and mucous membranes, particularly with profound thrombocytopenia (platelet count <10 × 10^9/L). There is a history of a preceding viral infection 1-4 wk before the onset of thrombocytopenia. Findings on physical examination are normal, other than the finding of petechiae and purpura. Splenomegaly, lymphadenopathy, bone pain, and pallor are rare. An easy to use classification system has been proposed from the U.K. to characterize the severity of bleeding in ITP on the basis of symptoms and signs, but not platelet count:

1. No symptoms
2. Mild symptoms: bruising and petechiae, occasional minor epistaxis, very little interference with daily living
3. Moderate: more severe skin and mucosal lesions, more troublesome epistaxis and menorrhagia
4. Severe: bleeding episodes—menorrhagia, epistaxis, melena—requiring transfusion or hospitalization, symptoms interfering seriously with the quality of life

The presence of abnormal findings such as hepatosplenomegaly, bone or joint pain, or remarkable lymphadenopathy suggests other diagnoses (leukemia). When the onset is insidious, especially in an adolescent, chronic ITP or the possibility of a systemic illness, such as systemic lupus erythematosus (SLE), is more likely.

Outcome

Severe bleeding is rare (<3% of cases in 1 large international study). In 70-80% of children who present with acute ITP, spontaneous resolution occurs within 6 mo. Therapy does not appear to affect the natural history of the illness. Fewer than 1% of patients develop an intracranial hemorrhage. Those who favor interventional therapy argue that the objective of early therapy is to raise the platelet count to >20 × 10^9/L and prevent the rare development of intracranial hemorrhage. There is no evidence that therapy prevents serious bleeding. Approximately 20% of children who present with acute ITP go on to have chronic ITP. The outcome/prognosis may be related more to age, as ITP in younger children is more likely to resolve whereas the development of chronic ITP in adolescents approaches 50%.

Laboratory Findings

Severe thrombocytopenia (platelet count <20 × 10^9/L) is common, and platelet size is normal or increased, reflective of increased platelet turnover (Fig. 478-3). In acute ITP, the hemoglobin value, white blood cell (WBC) count, and differential count should be normal. Hemoglobin may be decreased if there have been profuse nosebleeds or menorrhagia. Bone marrow examination shows normal granulocytic and erythrocytic series, with characteristically normal or increased numbers of megakaryocytes. Some of the megakaryocytes may appear to be immature and are reflective of increased platelet turnover. **Indications for bone marrow** aspiration/biopsy include an abnormal WBC count or differential or unexplained anemia as well as findings on history and physical examination suggestive of a bone marrow failure syndrome or malignancy. Other laboratory tests should be performed as indicated by the history and physical examination. In adolescents with new-onset ITP, an antinuclear antibody test should be done to evaluate for SLE. HIV studies should be done in at-risk populations, especially sexually active teens. Platelet antibody testing is seldom useful in acute ITP. A direct antiglobulin test (Coombs) should be done if there is unexplained anemia to rule out Evans syndrome (autoimmune hemolytic anemia and thrombocytopenia) (Chapter 458) or before instituting therapy with IV anti-D.

Diagnosis/Differential Diagnosis

The well-appearing child with moderate to severe thrombocytopenia, an otherwise normal complete blood cell count (CBC), and normal findings on physical examination has a limited differential diagnosis that includes exposure to medication that induces drug-dependent antibodies, splenic sequestration due to previously unappreciated portal hypertension, and rarely, early aplastic processes, such as Fanconi anemia (Chapter 462). Other than congenital thrombocytopenia syndromes (Chapter 478.8), such as thrombocytopenia-absent radius (TAR) syndrome and

Table 478-1 DIFFERENTIAL DIAGNOSIS OF THROMBOCYTOPENIA IN CHILDREN AND ADOLESCENTS

DESTRUCTIVE THROMBOCYTOPENIAS
Primary Platelet Consumption Syndromes
Immune thrombocytopenias
Acute and chronic ITP
Autoimmune diseases with chronic ITP as a manifestation
Cyclic thrombocytopenia
Autoimmune lymphoproliferative syndrome and its variants
Systemic lupus erythematosus
Evans syndrome
Antiphospholipid antibody syndrome
Neoplasia-associated immune thrombocytopenia
Thrombocytopenia associated with HIV
Neonatal immune thrombocytopenia
Alloimmune
Autoimmune (e.g., maternal ITP)
Drug-induced immune thrombocytopenia (including heparin-induced thrombocytopenia)
Post-transfusion purpura
Allergy and anaphylaxis
Post-transplant thrombocytopenia
Nonimmune thrombocytopenias
Thrombocytopenia of infection
Bacteremia or fungemia
Viral infection
Protozoan
Thrombotic microangiopathic disorders
Hemolytic-uremic syndrome
Eclampsia, HELLP syndrome
Thrombotic thrombocytopenic purpura
Bone marrow transplantation-associated microangiopathy
Drug-induced
Platelets in contact with foreign material
Congenital heart disease
Drug-induced via direct platelet effects (ristocetin, protamine)
Type 2B VWD or platelet-type VWD
Combined Platelet and Fibrinogen Consumption Syndromes
Disseminated intravascular coagulation
Kasabach-Merritt syndrome
Virus-associated hemophagocytic syndrome
IMPAIRED PLATELET PRODUCTION
Hereditary disorders
Acquired disorders
Aplastic anemia
Myelodysplastic syndrome
Marrow infiltrative process—neoplasia
Osteopetrosis
Nutritional deficiency states (iron, folate, vitamin B_{12}, anorexia nervosa)
Drug- or radiation-induced thrombocytopenia
Neonatal hypoxia or placental insufficiency
SEQUESTRATION
Hypersplenism
Hypothermia
Burns

HIV, human immunodeficiency virus; ITP, immune thrombocytopenic purpura; VWD, von Willebrand disease.
From Wilson DB: Acquired platelet defects. In Orkin SH, Nathan DG, Ginsburg D, et al, editors: *Nathan and Oski's hematology of infancy and childhood*, ed 7, Philadelphia, 2009, WB Saunders, p 1555, Box 33-1.

Table 478-2 CLASSIFICATION OF FETAL AND NEONATAL THROMBOCYTOPENIAS*

	CONDITION
Fetal	**Alloimmune thrombocytopenia**
	Congenital infection (e.g., CMV, toxoplasma, rubella, HIV)
	Aneuploidy (e.g., trisomy 18, 13, or 21, or triploidy)
	Autoimmune condition (e.g., ITP, SLE)
	Severe Rh hemolytic disease
	Congenital/inherited (e.g., Wiskott-Aldrich syndrome)
Early-onset neonatal (<72 hr)	**Placental insufficiency** (e.g., PET, IUGR, diabetes)
	Perinatal asphyxia
	Perinatal infection (e.g., *Escherichia coli*, GBS, *Haemophilus influenzae*)
	DIC
	Alloimmune thrombocytopenia
	Autoimmune condition (e.g., ITP, SLE)
	Congenital infection (e.g., CMV, toxoplasma, rubella, HIV)
	Thrombosis (e.g., aortic, renal vein)
	Bone marrow replacement (e.g., congenital leukemia)
	Kasabach-Merritt syndrome
	Metabolic disease (e.g., proprionic and methylmalonic acidemia)
	Congenital/inherited (e.g., TAR, CAMT)
Late-onset neonatal (>72 hr)	**Late-onset sepsis**
	NEC
	Congenital infection (e.g., CMV, toxoplasma, rubella, HIV)
	Autoimmune
	Kasabach-Merritt syndrome
	Metabolic disease (e.g., proprionic and methylmalonic acidemia)
	Congenital/inherited (e.g., TAR, CAMT)

*The most common conditions are shown in bold.
CAMT, congenital amegakaryocytic thrombocytopenia; CMV, cytomegalovirus; DIC, disseminated intravascular coagulation; GBS, group B streptococcus; ITP, idiopathic thrombocytopenic purpura; IUGR, intrauterine growth restriction; NEC, necrotizing enterocolitis; PET, preeclampsia; SLE, systemic lupus erythematosus; TAR, thrombocytopenia with absent radii.
From Roberts I, Murray NA: Neonatal thrombocytopenia: causes and management, *Arch Dis Child Fetal Neonatal Ed* 88:F359–F364, 2003.

MYH9-related thrombocytopenia, most marrow processes that interfere with platelet production eventually cause abnormal synthesis of red blood cells (RBCs) and WBCs and therefore manifest diverse abnormalities on the CBC. Disorders that cause increased platelet destruction on a nonimmune basis are usually serious systemic illnesses with obvious clinical findings (e.g., hemolytic-uremic syndrome [HUS], disseminated intravascular coagulation [DIC]) [see Table 477-1 and Fig. 478-2]. Isolated enlargement of the spleen suggests the potential for hypersplenism owing to either liver disease or portal vein thrombosis. Autoimmune thrombocytopenia may be an initial manifestation of SLE, HIV infection, common variable immunodeficiency, or rarely lymphoma. Wiskott-Aldrich syndrome (WAS; Chapter 120.2) must be considered in young males found to have thrombocytopenia with small platelets, particularly if there is a history of eczema and recurrent infection.

Treatment

There are no data showing that treatment affects either short- or long-term clinical outcome of ITP. Many patients with new-onset ITP have mild symptoms, with findings limited to petechiae and purpura on the skin, despite severe thrombocytopenia. Compared with untreated control subjects, treatment appears to be capable of inducing a more rapid rise in platelet count to the theoretically safe level of $>20 \times 10^9$/L, although there are no data indicating that early therapy prevents intracranial hemorrhage. Antiplatelet antibodies bind to transfused platelets as well as they do to autologous platelets. Thus, platelet transfusion in ITP is usually contraindicated unless life-threatening bleeding is present. Initial approaches to the management of ITP include the following:

1. No therapy other than education and counseling of the family and patient for patients with minimal, mild, and moderate symptoms, as defined earlier. This approach emphasizes the usually benign nature of ITP and avoids the therapeutic roller

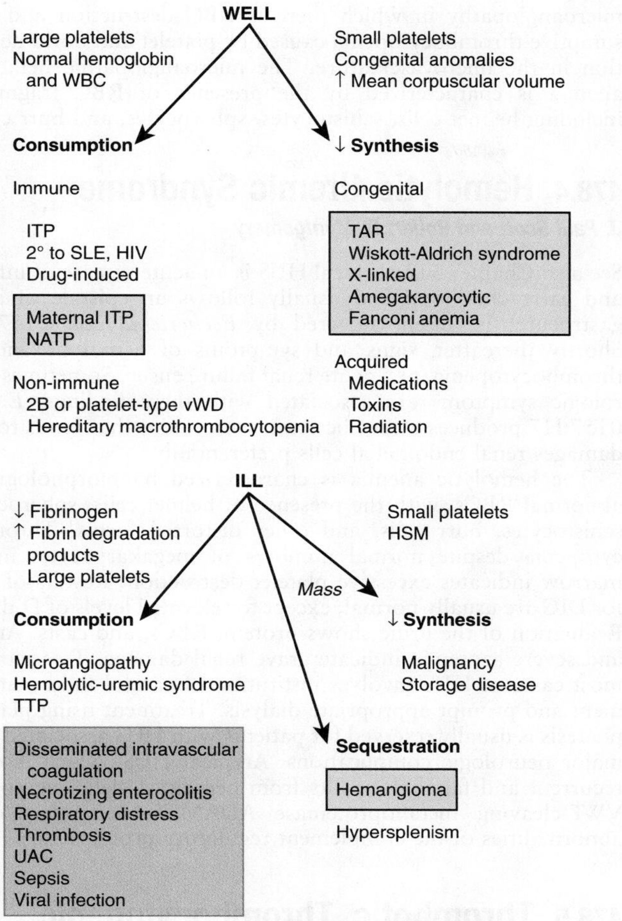

Figure 478-2 Differential diagnosis of childhood thrombocytopenic syndromes. The syndromes initially are separated by their clinical appearance. Clues leading to the diagnosis are shown in *italics.* The mechanisms and common disorders leading to these findings are shown in the *lower part* of the figure. Disorders that commonly affect neonates are listed in the *shaded boxes.* HSM, hepatosplenomegaly; ITP, idiopathic immune thrombocytopenic purpura; NATP, neonatal alloimmune thrombocytopenic purpura; SLE, systemic lupus erythematosus; TAR, thrombocytopenia-absent radius; TTP, thrombotic thrombocytopenic purpura; UAC, umbilical artery catheter; VWD, von Willebrand disease; WBC, white blood cell. (From Scott JP: Bleeding and thrombosis. In Kliegman RM, editor: *Practical strategies in pediatric diagnosis and therapy,* Philadelphia, 1996, WB Saunders, p 849; Kliegman RM, Marcdante KJ, Jenson HB, et al, editors: *Nelson essentials of pediatrics,* ed 5, Philadelphia, 2006, Elsevier/Saunders, p 716.)

coaster that ensues once interventional therapy is begun. This approach is far less costly, and side effects are minimal.

2. Intravenous immunoglobulin (IVIG). IVIG at a dose of 0.8-1.0 g/kg/day for 1-2 days induces a rapid rise in platelet count (usually >20 × 10^9/L) in 95% of patients within 48 hr. IVIG appears to induce a response by downregulating Fc-mediated phagocytosis of antibody-coated platelets. IVIG therapy is both expensive and time-consuming to administer. Additionally, after infusion, there is a high frequency of headaches and vomiting, suggestive of IVIG-induced aseptic meningitis.
3. Intravenous anti-D therapy. For Rh positive patients, IV anti-D at a dose of 50-75 µg/kg causes a rise in platelet count to >20 × 10^9/L in 80-90% of patients within 48-72 hr. When given to Rh positive individuals, IV anti-D induces mild hemolytic anemia. RBC-antibody complexes bind to macrophage Fc receptors and interfere with platelet destruction, thereby causing a rise in platelet count. IV anti-D is ineffective in Rh negative patients. Rare life-threatening episodes of intravascular hemolysis have occurred in children and adults following infusion of IV anti-D.
4. Prednisone. Corticosteroid therapy has been used for many years to treat acute and chronic ITP in adults and children. Doses of prednisone of 1-4 mg/kg/24 hr appear to induce a more rapid rise in platelet count than in untreated patients with ITP. Whether bone marrow examination should be performed to rule out other causes of thrombocytopenia, especially acute lymphoblastic leukemia, before institution of prednisone therapy in acute ITP is controversial. Corticosteroid therapy is usually continued for 2-3 wk or until a rise in platelet count to >20 × 10^9/L has been achieved, with a rapid taper to avoid the long-term side effects of corticosteroid therapy, especially growth failure, diabetes mellitus, and osteoporosis.

Each of these medications may be used to treat ITP exacerbations, which commonly occur several weeks after an initial course of therapy. In the special case of intracranial hemorrhage, multiple modalities should be used, including platelet transfusion, IVIG, high-dose corticosteroids, and prompt consultation by neurosurgery and surgery.

There is no consensus regarding the management of acute childhood ITP, except that patients who are bleeding significantly should be treated, representing less than 5% of children with ITP. Intracranial hemorrhage remains rare, and there are no data showing that treatment actually reduces its incidence.

The role of splenectomy in ITP should be reserved for 1 of 2 circumstances. The older child (≥4 yr) with severe ITP that

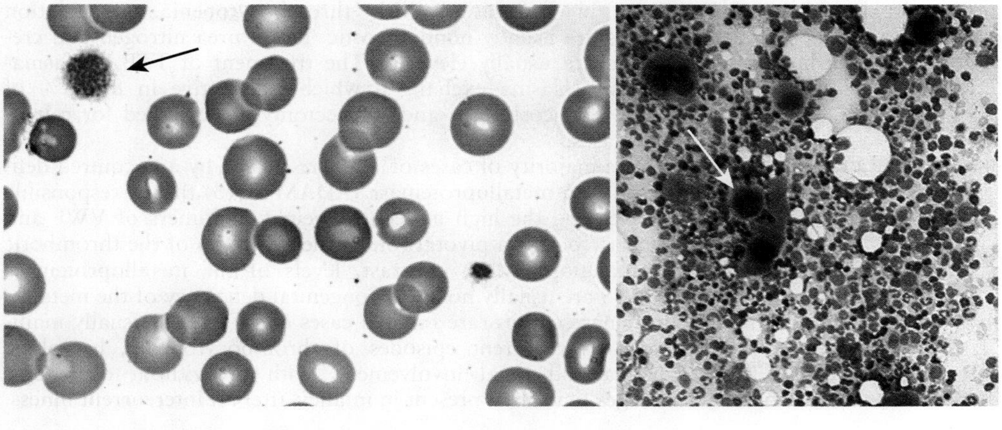

Figure 478-3 Blood smear and bone marrow aspirate from a child who had ITP showing large platelets (blood smear [*left*]) and increased numbers of megakaryocytes, many of which appear immature (bone marrow aspirate [*right*]). (From Blanchette V, Bolton-Maggs P: Childhood immune thrombocytopenic purpura: diagnosis and management, *Pediatr Clin North Am* 55:393–420, 2008, p 400, Fig 4.)

has lasted >1 yr (chronic ITP) and whose symptoms are not easily controlled with therapy is a candidate for splenectomy. Splenectomy must also be considered when life-threatening hemorrhage (intracranial hemorrhage) complicates acute ITP, if the platelet count cannot be corrected rapidly with transfusion of platelets and administration of IVIG and corticosteroids. Splenectomy is associated with a lifelong risk of overwhelming postsplenectomy infection caused by encapsulated organisms and the potential development of pulmonary hypertension in adulthood.

Chronic Idiopathic Thrombocytopenic Purpura

Approximately 20% of patients who present with acute ITP have persistent thrombocytopenia for **>12 mo** and are said to have chronic ITP. At that time, a careful re-evaluation for associated disorders should be performed, especially for autoimmune disease, such as SLE; chronic infectious disorders, such as HIV; and nonimmune causes of chronic thrombocytopenia, such as type 2B and platelet-type von Willebrand disease, X-linked thrombocytopenia, autoimmune lymphoproliferative syndrome, common variable immunodeficiency syndrome, autosomal macrothrombocytopenia, and WAS (also X-linked). The presence of co-existing *H. pylori* infection should be explored and, if found, treated. Therapy should be aimed at controlling symptoms and preventing serious bleeding. In ITP, the spleen is the primary site of both antiplatelet antibody synthesis and platelet destruction. Splenectomy is successful in inducing complete remission in 64-88% of children with chronic ITP. This effect must be balanced against the lifelong risk of overwhelming postsplenectomy infection. This decision is often affected by lifestyle issues as well as the ease with which the child can be managed using medical therapy, such as IVIG, corticosteroids, IV anti-D. Rituximab, a chimeric monoclonal anti–B cell antibody, effectively induces a remission in 30-50% of children with chronic ITP. Two new effective agents that act to stimulate thrombopoiesis, romiplastin and eltrombopag (see Fig. 478-1), have been approved by the Federal Drug Administration to treat adults with chronic ITP. There are no data regarding either drug's safety or efficacy in children.

BIBLIOGRAPHY

Please visit the Nelson Textbook of Pediatrics *website at www.expertconsult.com for the complete bibliography.*

478.2 Drug-Induced Thrombocytopenia

J. Paul Scott and Robert R. Montgomery

A number of drugs are associated with immune thrombocytopenia as the result of either an immune process or megakaryocyte injury. Some common drugs used in pediatrics that cause thrombocytopenia include valproic acid, phenytoin, carbamazepine, sulfonamides, vancomycin, and trimethoprim-sulfamethoxazole. Heparin-induced thrombocytopenia (and rarely, thrombosis) is seldom seen in pediatrics, but it occurs when, after exposure to heparin, the patient has an antibody directed against the heparin–platelet factor 4 complex.

BIBLIOGRAPHY

Please visit the Nelson Textbook of Pediatrics *website at www.expertconsult.com for the complete bibliography.*

478.3 Nonimmune Platelet Destruction

J. Paul Scott and Robert R. Montgomery

The syndromes of DIC (Chapter 477), HUS (Chapters 478.4 and 512), and thrombotic thrombocytopenic purpura (TTP) (Chapter 478.5) share the hematologic picture of a thrombotic microangiopathy in which there is RBC destruction and consumptive thrombocytopenia caused by platelet and fibrin deposition in the microvasculature. The microangiopathic hemolytic anemia is characterized by the presence of RBC fragments, including helmet cells, schistocytes, spherocytes, and burr cells.

478.4 Hemolytic-Uremic Syndrome

J. Paul Scott and Robert R. Montgomery

See also Chapter 512. Typical HUS is an acute disease of infancy and early childhood and usually follows an episode of acute gastroenteritis, often triggered by *Escherichia coli* 0157:H7. Shortly thereafter, signs and symptoms of hemolytic anemia, thrombocytopenia, and acute renal failure ensue. Sometimes neurologic symptoms are associated with these findings. *E. coli* 0157:H7 produces a specific toxin (verotoxin) that binds to and damages renal endothelial cells preferentially.

The hemolytic anemia is characterized by morphologically abnormal RBCs, with the presence of helmet cells, spherocytes, schistocytes, burr cells, and other distorted forms. Thrombocytopenia despite normal numbers of megakaryocytes in the marrow indicates excessive platelet destruction. Results of tests for DIC are usually normal, except for elevated levels of D-dimer. Evaluation of the urine shows protein, RBCs, and casts. Anuria and severe azotemia indicate grave renal damage. Treatment of most cases of HUS involves institution of careful fluid management and prompt appropriate dialysis. Treatment using plasmapheresis is usually reserved for patients with HUS associated with major neurologic complications. Atypical HUS, which is often recurrent and familial, results from hereditary deficiency of the VWF-cleaving metalloproteinase ADAMTS-13 or less often abnormalities of the complement regulatory proteins.

478.5 Thrombotic Thrombocytopenic Purpura

J. Paul Scott and Robert R. Montgomery

Thrombotic thrombocytopenic purpura (TTP) is a rare pentad of **fever, microangiopathic hemolytic anemia, thrombocytopenia, abnormal renal function,** and **central nervous system changes** that is clinically similar to HUS, although TTP usually presents in adults and occasionally in adolescents. Microvascular thrombi within the central nervous system cause subtle, shifting neurologic signs that vary from changes in affect and orientation to aphasia, blindness, and seizures. Initial manifestations are often nonspecific (weakness, pain, emesis); prompt recognition of this disorder is critical. Laboratory findings provide important clues to the diagnosis and show microangiopathic hemolytic anemia characterized by morphologically abnormal RBCs, with schistocytes, spherocytes, helmet cells, and an elevated reticulocyte count in association with thrombocytopenia. Coagulation studies are usually nondiagnostic. Blood urea nitrogen and creatinine are usually elevated. The treatment of TTP is plasmapheresis (plasma exchange), which is effective in 80-95% of cases. Corticosteroids and splenectomy are reserved for refractory cases.

The majority of cases of TTP are caused by an acquired deficiency of a metalloproteinase (ADAMTS-13) that is responsible for cleaving the high molecular weight multimers of VWF and appears to play a pivotal role in the evolution of the thrombotic microangiopathy. In contrast, levels of the metalloproteinase in HUS are usually normal. Congenital deficiency of the metalloproteinase causes rare familial cases of TTP/HUS, usually manifested as recurrent episodes of thrombocytopenia, hemolytic anemia and renal involvement, with or without neurologic changes that often present in infancy after an intercurrent illness.

Abnormalities of the complement system have now also been implicated in rare cases of familial TTP. ADAMTS-13 deficiency can be treated by repeated infusions of fresh frozen plasma.

BIBLIOGRAPHY

Please visit the Nelson Textbook of Pediatrics *website at* *www.expertconsult.com* *for the complete bibliography.*

478.6 Kasabach-Merritt Syndrome

J. Paul Scott and Robert R. Montgomery

See also Chapter 642. The association of a giant hemangioma with localized intravascular coagulation causing thrombocytopenia and hypofibrinogenemia is called *Kasabach-Merritt syndrome.* In most patients, the site of the hemangioma is obvious, but retroperitoneal and intra-abdominal hemangiomas may require body imaging for detection. Inside the hemangioma there is platelet trapping and activation of coagulation, with fibrinogen consumption and generation of fibrin(ogen) degradation products. Arteriovenous malformation within the lesions can cause heart failure. Pathologically Kasabach-Merritt syndrome appears to develop more often as a result of a kaposiform hemangioendothelioma or tufted hemangioma rather than a simple hemangioma. The peripheral blood smear shows microangiopathic changes. Multiple modalities have been used to treat Kasabach-Merritt syndrome, including surgical excision (if possible), laser photocoagulation, high-dose corticosteroids, local radiation therapy, antiangiogenic agents, such as interferon-α_2, and vincristine. Over time, most patients who present in infancy have regression of the hemangioma. Treatment of the associated coagulopathy may benefit from a trial of antifibrinolytic therapy with ε-aminocaproic acid (Amicar).

478.7 Sequestration

J. Paul Scott and Robert R. Montgomery

Thrombocytopenia develops in individuals with massive splenomegaly because the spleen acts as a sponge for platelets and sequesters large numbers. Most such patients also have mild leukopenia and anemia on CBC. Individuals who have thrombocytopenia caused by splenic sequestration should undergo a work-up to diagnose the etiology of splenomegaly, including infectious, inflammatory, infiltrative, neoplastic, obstructive, and hemolytic causes.

478.8 Congenital Thrombocytopenic Syndromes

J. Paul Scott and Robert R. Montgomery

See Table 478-2. **Congenital amegakaryocytic thrombocytopenia** (CAMT) usually manifests within the 1st few days to wk of life, when the child presents with petechiae and purpura caused by profound thrombocytopenia. CAMT is caused by a rare defect in hematopoiesis due to a mutation in the stem cell TPO receptor (MPL). Other than skin and mucous membrane abnormalities, findings on physical examination are normal. Examination of the bone marrow shows an absence of megakaryocytes. These patients often progress to marrow failure (aplasia) over time. Hematopoietic stem cell transplantation is curative.

Thrombocytopenia-absent radius (TAR) syndrome consists of thrombocytopenia (absence or hypoplasia of megakaryocytes) that presents in early infancy with bilateral radial anomalies of variable severity, ranging from mild changes to marked limb shortening (Fig. 478-4). Many such individuals also have other skeletal abnormalities of the ulna, radius, and lower extremities.

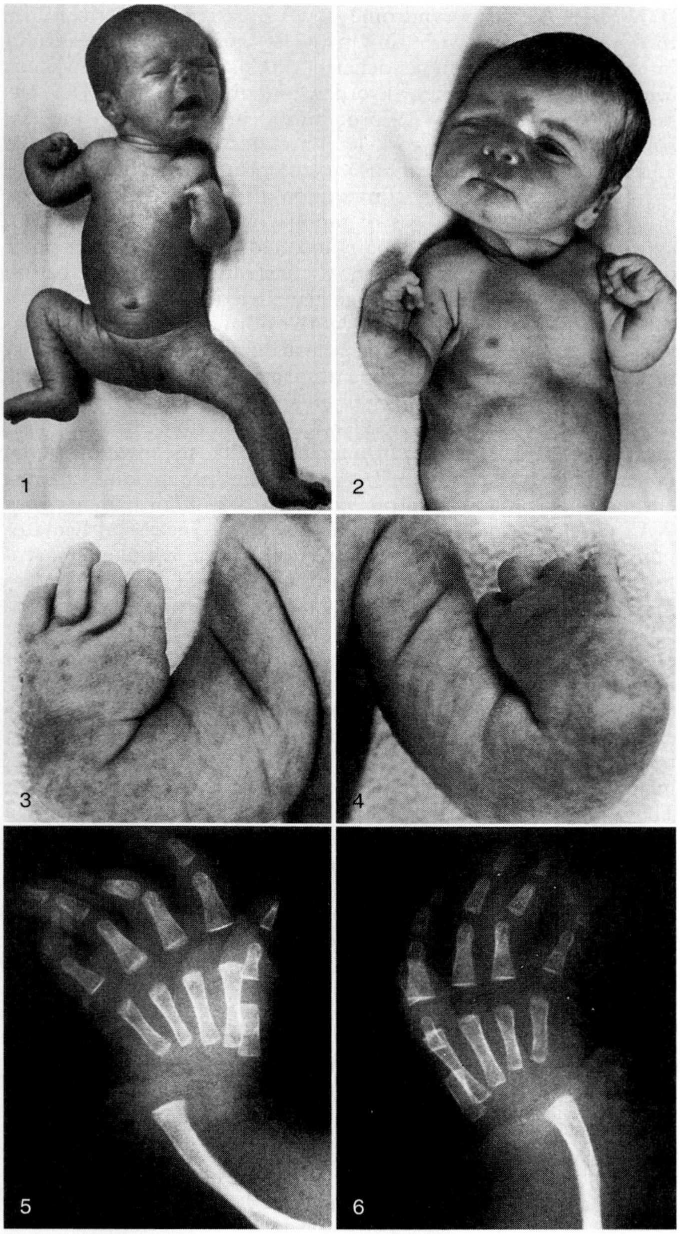

Figure 478-4 A newborn, the 1st child of young, healthy parents, with fully expressed thrombocytopenia-absent radius syndrome, including thrombocytopenia, hypereosinophilia, and anemia. Hypoplasia of the distal humeri and the shoulder girdles, bilateral hip dysplasia, mild talipes calcaneus, and clinodactyly of both little fingers are seen. This patient had a pronounced allergy to cow's milk, with exposure followed by diarrhea, vomiting, and decreased weight and platelet count, making a cow's milk–free diet mandatory. A persistent depressed nasal bridge and development of pronounced bowed legs are seen. (From Wiedemann H-R, Kunze J, Grosse F-R, editors: *Clinical syndromes,* ed 3, [English translation], London, 1997, Mosby-Wolfe, p 430.)

Thumbs are present. Intolerance to cow's milk formula (present in 50%) may complicate management by triggering gastrointestinal bleeding, increased thrombocytopenia, eosinophilia, and a leukemoid reaction. The thrombocytopenia of TAR syndrome frequently remits over the 1st few yr of life. The molecular basis of TAR syndrome remains to be defined. A few patients have been reported to have a syndrome of **amegakaryocytic thrombocytopenia with radioulnar synostosis** due to a mutation in the *HOXA11* gene. Different from TAR syndrome, this mutation causes marrow aplasia.

Wiskott-Aldrich syndrome (WAS) is characterized by thrombocytopenia, with tiny platelets, eczema, and recurrent infection due to immune deficiency (Chapter 120.2). WAS is inherited as an X-linked disorder, and the gene for WAS has been sequenced. The WAS protein appears to play an integral role in regulating the cytoskeletal architecture of both platelets and T lymphocytes in response to receptor-mediated cell signaling. The WAS protein is common to all cells of hematopoietic lineage. Molecular analysis of families with X-linked thrombocytopenia has shown that many affected members have a point mutation within the WAS gene, whereas individuals with the full manifestation of WAS have large gene deletions. Examination of the bone marrow in WAS shows the normal number of megakaryocytes, although they may have bizarre morphologic features. Transfused platelets have a normal life span. Splenectomy often corrects the thrombocytopenia, suggesting that the platelets formed in WAS have accelerated destruction. After splenectomy, these patients are at increased risk for overwhelming infection and require lifelong antibiotic prophylaxis against encapsulated organisms. Approximately 5-15% of patients with WAS develop lymphoreticular malignancies. Successful hematopoietic stem cell transplantation cures WAS. **X-linked macrothrombocytopenia and dyserythropoiesis** have been linked to mutations in the *GATA-1* gene, an erythroid and megakaryocytic transcription factor.

MYH9-related thrombocytopenia: A diverse number of hereditary thrombocytopenia syndromes, given names such as Sebastian, Epstein, May-Hegglin, and Fechtner syndromes, are characterized by autosomal dominant macrothrombocytopenia, neutrophil inclusion bodies, and a variety of physical anomalies, including sensorineural deafness, renal disease, and/or eye disease. These have all been shown to be due to different mutations in the *MYH9* gene (nonmuscle myosin-IIa heavy chain). The thrombocytopenia is usually mild and not progressive. Some other individuals with recessively inherited macrothrombocytopenia have abnormalities in chromosome 22q11. Mutations in the gene for glycoprotein Ibβ, an essential component of the platelet von Willebrand factor receptor, can result in Bernard-Soulier syndrome (Chapter 478.13).

BIBLIOGRAPHY

Please visit the Nelson Textbook of Pediatrics *website at* www.expertconsult.com *for the complete bibliography.*

478.9 Neonatal Thrombocytopenia

J. Paul Scott and Robert R. Montgomery

See also Chapter 97.4.

Thrombocytopenia in the newborn rarely is indicative of a primary disorder of megakaryopoiesis but more often is the result of either systemic illness or transfer of maternal antibodies directed against fetal platelets (see Table 478-2). Neonatal thrombocytopenia often occurs in association with congenital viral infection, especially rubella; cytomegalovirus; protozoal infection, such as toxoplasmosis; syphilis; and perinatal bacterial infection, especially those caused by gram-negative bacilli. Thrombocytopenia associated with DIC may be responsible for severe spontaneous bleeding. The constellation of marked thrombocytopenia and abnormal abdominal findings is common in necrotizing enterocolitis and other causes of necrotic bowel. Thrombocytopenia in an ill child requires a prompt search for viral and bacterial pathogens.

Antibody-mediated thrombocytopenia in the newborn occurs because of transplacental transfer of maternal antibodies directed against fetal platelets. Neonatal alloimmune thrombocytopenic purpura (NATP) is caused by the development of maternal antibodies against antigens present on fetal platelets that are shared with the father and recognized as foreign by the maternal immune system. This is the platelet equivalent of Rh disease of the newborn. The incidence of NATP is 1/4,000-5,000 live births. The clinical manifestations of NATP are those of an apparently well child who, within the 1st few days after delivery, has generalized petechiae and purpura. Laboratory studies show a normal maternal platelet count, yet moderate to severe thrombocytopenia in the newborn. Detailed review of the history should show no evidence of maternal thrombocytopenia. Up to 30% of infants with severe NATP may have intracranial hemorrhage, either prenatally or in the perinatal period. Unlike Rh disease, 1st pregnancies may be severely affected. Subsequent pregnancies may be even more severely affected than the 1st.

The **diagnosis** of NATP is made by checking for the presence of maternal alloantibodies directed against the father's platelets. Specific studies can be done to identify the target alloantigen. The most common cause is incompatibility for the platelet alloantigen HPA-1a. Specific DNA sequence polymorphisms have been identified that permit informative prenatal testing to identify at-risk pregnancies. The differential diagnosis of NATP includes transplacental transfer of maternal antiplatelet autoantibodies (maternal ITP), and more commonly, viral or bacterial infection.

Treatment of NATP requires the administration of IVIG prenatally to the mother. Therapy usually begins in the 2nd trimester and is continued throughout the pregnancy. Fetal platelet count can be monitored by percutaneous umbilical blood sampling. Delivery should be performed by cesarean section. After delivery, if severe thrombocytopenia persists, transfusion of 1 unit of platelets that share the maternal alloantigens (e.g., washed maternal platelets) will cause a rise in platelet counts to provide effective hemostasis. After there has been 1 affected child, genetic counseling is critical to inform the parents of the high risk of thrombocytopenia in subsequent pregnancies.

Children born to mothers with ITP (**maternal ITP**) appear to have a lower risk of serious hemorrhage than infants born with NATP, although severe thrombocytopenia may occur. The mother's pre-existing platelet count may have some predictive value in that severe maternal thrombocytopenia before delivery appears to predict a higher risk of fetal thrombocytopenia. In mothers who have had splenectomy for ITP, the maternal platelet count may be normal and is not predictive of fetal thrombocytopenia.

Treatment includes prenatal administration of corticosteroids to the mother and administration of IVIG and sometimes corticosteroids to the infant after delivery. Thrombocytopenia in an infant, whether due to NATP or maternal ITP, usually resolves within 2-4 mo after delivery. The period of highest risk is the immediate perinatal period.

Two syndromes of congenital failure of platelet production often present in the newborn period. In congenital **amegakaryocytic thrombocytopenia (CAMT)**, the newborn manifests petechiae and purpura shortly after birth. Findings on physical examination are otherwise normal. Megakaryocytes are absent from the bone marrow. This syndrome is caused by a mutation in the megakaryocyte TPO receptor that is essential for development of all hematopoietic cell lines. Pancytopenia eventually develops, and hematopoietic stem cell transplantation is curative. **TAR syndrome** consists of thrombocytopenia that presents in early infancy, with bilateral radial anomalies of variable severity, ranging from mild changes to marked limb shortening. Thumbs are present. In many such individuals, there are also other skeletal abnormalities of the lower extremities. Intolerance to cow's milk formula is present in 50% of patients. TAR syndrome frequently remits over the 1st few yr of life (Chapter 478.8) (see Fig. 478-4).

BIBLIOGRAPHY

Please visit the Nelson Textbook of Pediatrics *website at* www.expertconsult.com *for the complete bibliography.*

478.10 Thrombocytopenia Due to Acquired Disorders Causing Decreased Production

J. Paul Scott and Robert R. Montgomery

Disorders of the bone marrow that inhibit megakaryopoiesis usually affect RBC and WBC production. Infiltrative disorders, including malignancies, such as acute lymphocytic leukemia, histiocytosis, lymphomas, and storage disease, usually cause either abnormalities on physical examination (lymphadenopathy, hepatosplenomegaly, or masses) or abnormalities of the WBC count, or anemia. Aplastic processes may present as isolated thrombocytopenia, although there are usually clues on the CBC (leukopenia, neutropenia, anemia, or macrocytosis). Children with constitutional aplastic anemia (Fanconi anemia) often have abnormalities on examination, including radial anomalies, other skeletal anomalies, short stature, microcephaly, and hyperpigmentation. Bone marrow examination should be performed when thrombocytopenia is associated with abnormalities found on physical examination or on examination of the other blood cell lines.

478.11 Platelet Function Disorders

J. Paul Scott and Robert R. Montgomery

Bleeding time and the platelet function analyzer (PFA-100) are the only commonly available tests to screen for abnormal platelet function. Bleeding time measures the interaction of platelets with the blood vessel wall and thus is affected by both platelet count and platelet function. The predictive value of bleeding time is problematic because bleeding time is dependent on a number of other factors, including the skill of the technician and the cooperation of the patient, often a challenge in the infant or young child. A normal bleeding time does not rule out a mild platelet function defect in a clinically symptomatic individual. The PFA-100 measures platelet adhesion and aggregation in whole blood at high shear when the blood is exposed to either collagen-epinephrine or collagen-ADP. Results are reported as the closure time measured in sec. Many clinical laboratories have replaced bleeding time with the use of the PFA-100. Both the PFA-100 and bleeding time are sensitive to moderate/severe VWD and platelet dysfunction. Both are variably insensitive to mild platelet function abnormalities and mild VWD. The use of the PFA-100 as a screening test remains controversial and, like the bleeding time, lacks specificity. Bleeding time is the only commonly available test to assess platelet-vessel wall interaction. For patient with a positive history of bleeding suggestive of von Willebrand disease or platelet dysfunction, specific von Willebrand factor testing and platelet function studies should be done irrespective of the results of the bleeding time or PFA-100.

Platelet function in the clinical laboratory is currently measured using platelet aggregometry. In the aggregometer, agonists, such as collagen, ADP, ristocetin, epinephrine, arachidonic acid, and thrombin (or the thrombin receptor peptide), are added to platelet-rich plasma, and the clumping of platelets over time is measured by an automated machine. At the same time, other instruments measure the release of granular contents, such as ATP, from the platelets after activation. The ability of platelets to aggregate and their metabolic activity can be assessed simultaneously. When a patient is being evaluated for possible platelet dysfunction, it is critically important to exclude the presence of other exogenous agents and to study the patient, if possible, off all medications for 2 wk.

478.12 Acquired Disorders of Platelet Function

J. Paul Scott and Robert R. Montgomery

A number of systemic illnesses are associated with platelet dysfunction, most commonly, liver disease, kidney disease (uremia), and disorders that trigger increased amounts of fibrin degradation products. These disorders frequently cause prolonged bleeding time and are often associated with other abnormalities of the coagulation mechanism. The most important element of management is to treat the primary illness. If treatment of the primary process is not feasible, infusions of desmopressin have been helpful in augmenting hemostasis and correcting bleeding time. In some patients, transfusions of platelets and/or cryoprecipitate have also been helpful in improving hemostasis.

Many drugs alter platelet function. The most commonly used drug in adults that alters platelet function is acetylsalicylic acid (aspirin). Aspirin irreversibly acetylates the enzyme cyclooxygenase, which is critical in the formation of thromboxane A_2. Aspirin usually causes moderate platelet dysfunction that becomes more prominent if there is another abnormality of the hemostatic mechanism. In children, commonly used drugs that affect platelet function include other nonsteroidal anti-inflammatory drugs, valproic acid, and high-dose penicillin. Specific agents to inhibit platelet function therapeutically include those that block the platelet ADP receptor (clopidogrel), α11b-β3 receptor antagonists as well as aspirin.

478.13 Congenital Abnormalities of Platelet Function

J. Paul Scott and Robert R. Montgomery

Severe platelet function defects usually present with petechiae and purpura shortly after birth, especially after vaginal delivery. Defects in the platelet GPIb complex (the VWF receptor) or the αIIb-β3 complex (the fibrinogen receptor) cause severe congenital platelet dysfunction.

Bernard-Soulier syndrome, a severe congenital platelet function disorder, is caused by absence or severe deficiency of the VWF receptor (GPIb complex) on the platelet membrane. This syndrome is characterized by thrombocytopenia, with giant platelets and markedly prolonged bleeding time (>20 min) or PFA-100 closure time. Platelet aggregation tests show absent ristocetin-induced platelet aggregation, but normal aggregation to all other agonists. Ristocetin induces the binding of VWF to platelets and agglutinates platelets. Results of studies of VWF are normal. The GPIb complex interacts with the platelet cytoskeleton; a defect in this interaction is believed to be the cause of the large platelet size. Bernard-Soulier syndrome is inherited as an autosomal recessive disorder. Genetic mutations causing Bernard-Soulier syndrome are usually identified in the genes forming the GPIb complex of glycoproteins Ibα, Ibβ, V, and IX.

Glanzmann thrombasthenia is a congenital disorder associated with severe platelet dysfunction that yields prolonged bleeding time and a normal platelet count. Platelets have normal size and morphologic features on the peripheral blood smear, and closure times for PFA-100 or bleeding time are markedly abnormal. Aggregation studies show abnormal or absent aggregation with all agonists used except ristocetin, because ristocetin agglutinates platelets and does not require a metabolically active platelet. This disorder is caused by deficiency of the platelet fibrinogen receptor αIIb-β3, the major integrin complex on the platelet surface that undergoes conformational changes by inside out signaling when platelets are activated. Fibrinogen binds to this complex when the platelet is activated and causes platelets to aggregate. Caused by identifiable mutations in the genes for αIIb or β3, this disorder is inherited in an autosomal recessive manner. For both Bernard-Soulier syndrome and Glanzmann thrombasthenia, the diagnosis is confirmed by flow cytometric analysis of the patient's platelet glycoproteins.

Hereditary deficiency of platelet storage granules occurs in 2 well-characterized but rare syndromes that involve deficiency of intracytoplasmic granules. **Dense body deficiency** is characterized by absence of the granules that contain ADP, ATP, Ca^{2+}, and serotonin. This disorder is diagnosed by the finding that ATP is not released on platelet aggregation studies and ideally is characterized by electron microscopic studies. **Gray platelet syndrome** is caused by the absence of platelet α granules, resulting in platelets that appear gray on Wright stain of peripheral blood. In this rare syndrome, aggregation and release are absent with most agonists other than thrombin and ristocetin. Electron microscopic studies are diagnostic.

OTHER HEREDITARY DISORDERS OF PLATELET FUNCTION

Abnormalities in the pathways of platelet activation and release of granular contents cause a heterogeneous group of platelet function defects that are usually manifested as increased bruising, epistaxis, and/or menorrhagia. Symptoms may be subtle and are often made more obvious by high-risk surgery, such as tonsillectomy or adenoidectomy, or by administration of nonsteroidal anti-inflammatory drugs. In the laboratory, bleeding time is variable and closure time as measured by the PFA-100 is frequently, but not always, prolonged. Platelet aggregation studies show deficient aggregation with 1 or 2 agonists and/or abnormal release of granular contents.

The formation of thromboxane from arachidonic acid after the activation of phospholipase is critical to normal platelet function. Deficiency or dysfunction of enzymes, such as cyclo-oxygenase and thromboxane synthase, which metabolize arachidonic acid, causes abnormal platelet function. In the aggregometer, platelets from such patients do not aggregate in response to arachidonic acid.

The most common platelet function defects are those characterized by variable bleeding time/PFA closure times and abnormal aggregation with 1 or 2 agonists, usually ADP and/or collagen. These patients have normal aggregation with thrombin receptor peptide. Some of these individuals have only decreased release of ATP from intracytoplasmic granules; the significance of this finding is debated.

TREATMENT OF PATIENTS WITH PLATELET DYSFUNCTION

Successful treatment depends on the severity of both the diagnosis and the hemorrhagic event. In all but severe platelet function defects, desmopressin 0.3 μg/kg IV may be used for mild to moderate bleeding episodes. In addition to its effect on stimulating levels of VWF and factor VIII, desmopressin corrects bleeding time and augments hemostasis in many individuals with mild to moderate platelet function defects. For individuals with Bernard-Soulier syndrome or Glanzmann thrombasthenia, platelet transfusions of 1 U/5-10 kg corrects the defect in hemostasis and may be lifesaving. Rarely, antibodies develop to the deficient platelet protein, rendering the patient refractory to the transfused platelets. In such patients, the off-label use of recombinant factor VIIa has been effective, and this treatment is undergoing clinical trials. In both conditions, hematopoietic stem cell transplantation has been curative.

BIBLIOGRAPHY

Please visit the Nelson Textbook of Pediatrics *website at www.expertconsult.com for the complete bibliography.*

478.14 Disorders of the Blood Vessels

J. Paul Scott and Robert R. Montgomery

Disorders of the vessel walls or supporting structures mimic the findings of a bleeding disorder although coagulation studies are usually normal. The findings of petechiae and purpuric lesions in such patients are often due to an underlying vasculitis/vasculopathy. Skin biopsy can be particularly helpful in elucidating the type of vascular pathology.

HENOCH-SCHÖNLEIN PURPURA

Henoch-Schönlein purpura (HSP) is characterized by the sudden development of a purpuric rash, arthritis, abdominal pain, and renal involvement (Chapter 509). The characteristic rash, consisting of petechiae and often palpable purpura, usually involves the lower extremities and buttocks. Results of coagulation studies are normal. The pathologic lesions in the skin, intestines, and synovium are leukocytoclastic angiitis, inflammatory damage to the endothelium of the capillary and postcapillary venules mediated by WBCs and macrophages. The trigger for HSP is unknown. In the kidney, the lesion is focal glomerulonephritis with deposition of immunoglobulin A. Results of coagulation studies as well as platelet count are normal in HSP.

EHLERS-DANLOS SYNDROME

Ehlers-Danlos syndrome is a common disorder of collagen structure that causes easy bruising and poor wound healing (Chapter 651). Suggestive findings on physical examination include soft, velvety skin that is hyperelastic; lax joints that are easily subluxed; and unusual scarring. More than 10 variants of Ehlers-Danlos syndrome have been described. The most serious forms have been associated with sudden rupture of visceral organs. Results of coagulation screening tests are usually normal, although bleeding time may be mildly prolonged. Results of platelet aggregation studies are either normal or mildly abnormal, with deficient aggregation to collagen.

OTHER ACQUIRED DISORDERS

Scurvy, chronic corticosteroid therapy, and severe malnutrition are associated with "weakening" of the collagen matrix that supports the blood vessels. Therefore, these factors are associated with easy bruising, and particularly in the case of scurvy, bleeding gums and loosening of the teeth. Lesions of the skin that initially appear to be petechiae and purpura may be seen in vasculitic syndromes, such as SLE.

BIBLIOGRAPHY

Please visit the Nelson Textbook of Pediatrics *website at www.expertconsult.com for the complete bibliography.*

Section 8 THE SPLEEN

Chapter 479
Anatomy and Function of the Spleen
Amanda M. Brandow and Bruce M. Camitta

ANATOMY

The splenic precursor is recognizable by 5 wk of gestation. At birth, the spleen weighs approximately 11 g. Thereafter, it enlarges until puberty, reaching an average weight of 135 g, and then diminishes in size during adulthood. Approximately 15% of patients will have an accessory spleen. The major splenic components are a lymphoid compartment *(white pulp)* and a filtering system *(red pulp)*. The white pulp consists of periarterial lymphatic sheaths of T lymphocytes with embedded germinal centers containing B lymphocytes. The red pulp has a skeleton of fixed reticular cells, mobile macrophages, partially collapsed endothelial passages (cords of Billroth), and splenic sinuses. A *marginal zone* rich in dendritic (antigen-presenting) cells separates the red pulp from the white pulp. The splenic capsule contains smooth muscle and contracts in response to epinephrine. Approximately 10% of the blood delivered to the spleen flows rapidly through a closed vascular network. The other 90% flows more slowly through an open system (the *splenic cords*), where it is filtered through 1-5 μm slits before entering the splenic sinuses.

For the full continuation of this chapter, please visit the Nelson Textbook of Pediatrics *website at www.expertconsult.com.*

Chapter 480
Splenomegaly
Amanda M. Brandow and Bruce M. Camitta

CLINICAL MANIFESTATIONS

A soft, thin spleen is palpable in 15% of neonates, 10% of normal children, and 5% of adolescents. In most individuals, the spleen must be 2-3 times its normal size before it is palpable. The spleen is best examined when standing on the right side of a supine patient by palpating across the abdomen as the patient inspires deeply. A splenic edge felt more than 2 cm below the left costal margin is abnormal. An enlarged spleen might descend into the pelvis; when splenomegaly is suspected, the abdominal examination should begin at a lower starting point. Superficial abdominal venous distention may be present when splenomegaly is a result of portal hypertension. Radiologic detection or confirmation of splenic enlargement is done with ultrasonography, CT, or technetium-99 sulfur colloid scan. The latter also assesses splenic function.

For the full continuation of this chapter, please visit the Nelson Textbook of Pediatrics *website at www.expertconsult.com.*

Chapter 481
Hyposplenism, Splenic Trauma, and Splenectomy
Amanda M. Brandow and Bruce C. Camitta

HYPOSPLENISM

Congenital absence of the spleen is associated with complex cyanotic heart defects, dextrocardia, bilateral trilobed lungs, and heterotopic abdominal organs (Ivemark syndrome; Chapter 425.11). Splenic function is usually normal in children with **congenital polysplenia. Functional hyposplenism** may occur in normal neonates, especially premature infants. Children with sickle cell hemoglobinopathies (Chapter 456.1) may have splenic hypofunction as early as 6 mo of age. Initially, this is caused by vascular obstruction, which can be reversed with red blood cell (RBC) transfusion or hydroxyurea. The spleen eventually autoinfarcts and becomes fibrotic and permanently nonfunctioning. Functional hyposplenism may also occur in malaria (Chapter 280), after irradiation to the left upper quadrant, and when the reticuloendothelial function of the spleen is overwhelmed (as in severe hemolytic anemia or metabolic storage disease). Splenic hypofunction has been reported occasionally in patients with vasculitis, nephritis, inflammatory bowel disease, celiac disease, Pearson syndrome, Fanconi anemia, and graft vs host disease.

For the full continuation of this chapter, please visit the Nelson Textbook of Pediatrics *website at www.expertconsult.com.*

Section 9 THE LYMPHATIC SYSTEM

Chapter 482
Anatomy and Function of the Lymphatic System
Richard L. Tower II and Bruce M. Camitta

The lymphatic system participates in many biologic processes, including fluid homeostasis, absorption of dietary fat, and initiation of specific immune responses. This system includes circulating lymphocytes, lymphatic vessels, lymph nodes, spleen, tonsils, adenoids, Peyer patches, and thymus. Lymph is an ultrafiltrate of blood and is collected by lymphatic capillaries that are present in all organs except the brain, bone marrow, retina, cartilage, epidermis, hair, and nails. These capillaries join to form progressively larger vessels that drain regions of the body. During their course, the lymphatic vessels carry lymph to the lymph nodes. In the nodes, lymph is filtered through sinuses, where particulate matter and infectious organisms are phagocytosed, processed, and presented as antigens to surrounding lymphocytes. These actions stimulate antibody production, T-cell responses, and cytokine secretion (Chapter 117). Lymph is ultimately returned to the intravascular circulation.

For the full continuation of this chapter, please visit the Nelson Textbook of Pediatrics *website at www.expertconsult.com.*

Chapter 483
Abnormalities of Lymphatic Vessels
Richard L. Tower II and Bruce M. Camitta

Abnormalities of the lymph vessels may be congenital or acquired. Signs and symptoms result from increased lymphatic tissue mass or from leakage of lymph. **Lymphangiectasia** is dilation of the lymphatics. Pulmonary lymphangiectasia causes respiratory distress (Chapter 387.6). Involvement of the intestinal lymphatics causes hypoproteinemia and lymphocytopenia secondary to loss of lymph into the intestines (Chapter 330). Therapy includes minimizing the hydrostatic pressure in the lymphatic system, leading to decreased protein loss. Reducing dietary intake of long chain fatty acids and substituting medium chain triglycerides via formula accomplishes this goal. **Lymphangioma** is a congenital lymphatic malformation, usually detected by the age of 2 yr. **Lymphangioma circumscriptum** is defined as the presence of many small, superficial lymphangiomas. Deeper lymphangiomas are classified as either **cavernous lymphangiomas** or **cystic hygromas. Lymphangiomatosis** is the presence of multiple or disseminated malformations. Some of these lesions also have a hemangiomatous component (Chapter 499). Emergent surgical treatment is infrequently necessary due to mass effects. Most lesions may be observed for 18-24 mo to assess for involution. Surgery is effective for superficial lesions, but is complicated by a high incidence of recurrence when used for deeper lesions. Intralesional sclerosing with a streptococcal derivative called OK-432 has been used successfully in selected patients. Other sclerotherapy agents include pure ethanol and bleomycin. Macrocystic lesions appear to respond better than microcystic lymphangiomas to sclerotherapy. Radiofrequency ablation has been used for lymphatic lesions of the tongue. **Lymphatic dysplasia** may cause multisystem problems, including lymphedema, chylous ascites, chylothorax, and lymphangiomas of the bone, lung, or other sites.

For the full continuation of this chapter, please visit the Nelson Textbook of Pediatrics *website at www.expertconsult.com.*

Chapter 484
Lymphadenopathy
Richard L. Tower II and Bruce M. Camitta

Palpable lymph nodes are common in pediatrics. Lymph node enlargement is caused by proliferation of normal lymphoid elements or by infiltration with malignant or phagocytic cells. In most patients, a careful history and a complete physical examination suggest the proper diagnosis. A few key questions significantly aid in determining a diagnosis.

For the full continuation of this chapter, please visit the Nelson Textbook of Pediatrics *website at www.expertconsult.com.*

484.1 Kikuchi-Fujimoto Disease (Histiocytic Necrotizing Lymphadenitis)
Richard L. Tower II and Bruce M. Camitta

Kikuchi-Fujimoto disease is a rare, usually self-limiting disease that was originally reported in patients of Asian heritage. Cases are now described in all ethnic groups. Familial cases have been reported. Presentation is varied and may include fever of unknown origin, but more often, it occurs in children 8-16 yr of age as unilateral posterior cervical adenitis, fever, malaise, elevated erythrocyte sedimentation rate, and leukopenia. Nodes range in size from 0.5-6.0 cm, are painful or tender in 50% of cases, may be multiple, and must be differentiated from lymphoma.

For the full continuation of this chapter, please visit the Nelson Textbook of Pediatrics *website at www.expertconsult.com.*

484.2 Sinus Histiocytosis with Massive Lymphadenopathy (Rosai-Dorfman Disease)
Richard L. Tower II and Bruce M. Camitta

This uncommon, benign, and usually self-limited disease has a worldwide distribution but is more common in Africa and the Caribbean. The etiology is unknown, but immune dysfunction is suspected. Patients present with massive symmetric, painless, cervical adenopathy, along with fever, leukocytosis, high erythrocyte sedimentation rate, and polyclonal elevation of immunoglobulin G. Night sweats and weight loss are frequently present. It rarely occurs at birth or in siblings, and males are affected more often than females.

For the full continuation of this chapter, please visit the Nelson Textbook of Pediatrics *website at www.expertconsult.com.*

484.3 Castleman Disease
Richard L. Tower II and Bruce M. Camitta

Castleman disease is an uncommon lymphoproliferative disease and is also called *angiofollicular lymph node hyperplasia.* The underlying etiology is unknown, although an association with human herpesvirus 8 has been identified. Human herpesvirus 8 may stimulate excessive production of interleukin 6 (IL-6). The disease usually presents in adolescents or young adults. Enlargement of a single node, most often in the mediastinum or abdomen, is the most common localized presentation. Some patients may have fever, night sweats, weight loss, and fatigue. Management includes surgery and/or radiation therapy.

For the full continuation of this chapter, please visit the Nelson Textbook of Pediatrics *website at www.expertconsult.com.*

PART XXII Cancer and Benign Tumors

Chapter 485
Epidemiology of Childhood and Adolescent Cancer

Barbara L. Asselin

Cancer in patients <19 yr of age is uncommon, with an age-adjusted annual incidence rate of 16.6/100,000, representing only about 1% of all new cancer cases in a year in the USA or 18,000 new cases/yr in 2006. Although relative 5-yr survival rates have improved from 61% in 1977 to 81.6% in 2005 in all age groups (Fig 485-1), malignant neoplasms remain the leading cause of disease-related (noninjury) mortality (12.8%) among persons 1-14 yr of age. There are 1500-1600 cancer-related deaths annually in the USA among children <15 yr of age. The relative contribution of cancer to the overall mortality in 15-19 yr olds is lower. Multi-institutional cooperative clinical trials investigating novel therapies and investigating ways to improve survival rates even further and to decrease treatment-related long-term complications are ongoing. Because increasingly more patients survive their disease, clinical investigation also is focusing on the quality of life among survivors and the late outcomes of therapy experienced by pediatric and adult survivors of childhood cancer. The National Cancer Institute estimates that in 1977 there were 269,700 persons alive (in all age groups) who had survived childhood cancer, corresponding to 1/810 of persons <20 yr of age and 1/1,000 of persons 20-39 yr of age in the US population.

Pediatric cancers differ markedly from adult malignancies in both prognosis and distribution by histology and tumor site. Lymphohematopoietic cancers (i.e., acute lymphoblastic leukemia, lymphomas) account for ~40%, nervous system cancers for ~30%, and embryonal tumors and sarcomas for ~10% each among the broad categories of childhood cancers (Table 485-1). In contrast, epithelial tumors of organs such as lung, colon, breast, and prostate, which are commonly seen among adults, are rare malignancies in children. Unlike incidence patterns in adults, where cancer rates tend to increase rapidly with increasing age, a relatively wide age range exists in the pediatric age group, with 2 peaks: the 1st in early childhood and the 2nd in adolescence (Fig 485-2). During the 1st year of life, embryonal tumors such as neuroblastoma, nephroblastoma, retinoblastoma, rhabdomyosarcoma, hepatoblastoma, and medulloblastoma are most common (Figs 485-3 and 485-4). These tumors are much less common in older children and adults after cell differentiation processes have slowed considerably. Embryonal tumors, acute leukemias, non-Hodgkin lymphomas, and gliomas peak in incidence from 2-5 yr of age. As children age, bone malignancies, Hodgkin disease, gonadal germ cell malignancies (testicular and ovarian carcinomas), and other carcinomas increase in incidence. Adolescence is a transitional period between the common early childhood malignancies and characteristic carcinomas of adulthood (see Fig 485-4).

Childhood neoplasms include a diverse array of malignant tumors, termed "cancers," and nonmalignant tumors arising from disorders of genetic processes involved in control of cellular growth and development. Although many genetic conditions are associated with increased risks for childhood cancer, such conditions are believed to account for <5% of all occurrences (Chapter 486). The most notable genetic conditions that impart susceptibility to childhood cancer are neurofibromatosis types 1 and 2, Down syndrome, Beckwith-Wiedemann syndrome, tuberous sclerosis, von Hippel-Lindau disease, xeroderma pigmentosum, ataxia-telangiectasia, nevus basal cell carcinoma syndrome, and Li-Fraumeni (p53) syndrome. The varying incidence patterns of individual childhood cancers around the world imply additional genetic and epidemiologic risk factors that remain uncharacterized.

Compared with adult epithelial tumors, an extremely small fraction of pediatric cancers appear to be explained by known environmental exposures (Table 485-2). Ionizing radiation exposure and several chemotherapeutic agents explain only a small number of pediatric cases (Chapter 699). The association between fetal exposures and pediatric cancer is largely not established, with the exception of maternal diethylstilbestrol intake during pregnancy and subsequent vaginal adenocarcinoma in adolescent daughters. Environmental exposures that have been studied without convincing evidence for a causal role include non-ionizing power frequency electromagnetic fields, pesticides, parental occupational chemical exposures, dietary factors, and environmental cigarette smoke. Viruses have been associated with certain pediatric cancers, such as polyomaviruses (BK, JC, SV40) associated with brain cancer and Epstein-Barr virus with non-Hodgkin lymphoma, but the etiologic importance remains unclear. Because the etiology of cancer in children still is poorly understood, for the most part, epidemiology studies have recognized that the likely mechanism is multifactorial, possibly resulting from potential interactions between genetic susceptibility traits and environmental exposures. Ongoing studies are investigating the role of polymorphisms of genes encoding enzymes, which function in the activation or metabolism of xenobiotics, protection of cells against oxidative stress, DNA repair, and/or immune modulation.

Curative therapy with chemotherapy, radiation, and/or surgery can adversely affect a child's development and result in serious long-term medical and psychosocial effects in childhood and adulthood. Potential adverse late effects include subsequent second malignancy, early mortality, infertility, reduced stature, cardiomyopathy, pulmonary fibrosis, osteoporosis, neurocognitive impairment, affective mood disorders, and altered social functioning. Much has been learned about the incidence of late effects from large multisite cohort studies such as the Childhood Cancer Survivor Study, an ongoing study of medical and psychosocial outcomes in survivors (*www.cancer.umn.edu/ltfu*).

Given the relative rarity of specific types of childhood cancer and the sophisticated technology and expertise required for diagnosis, treatment, and monitoring of late effects, all children with cancer should be treated on standardized clinical protocols in pediatric clinical research settings whenever possible. Promoting such treatment, the Children's Oncology Group is a multi-institutional research consortium that facilitates cooperative clinical, biologic, and epidemiologic research in more than 200 affiliated institutions in the United States, Canada, and other countries (*www.curesearch.org/*). Coordinated participation in such research trials has been a major factor in the increased survival for many children with cancer. Such ongoing efforts are critical to better understand the etiology of childhood cancers, improve survival for malignancies with a poor prognosis, and maximize the quality of life for survivors.

INFLUENCING THE INCIDENCE OF CANCER

Pediatricians have a unique opportunity to educate children and adolescents, and their parents, regarding means of

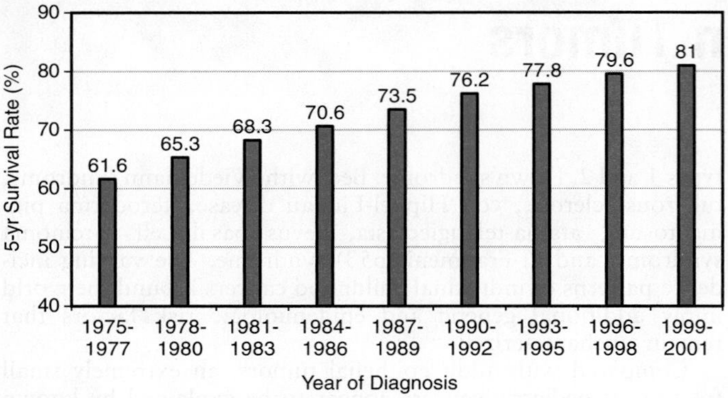

Figure 485-1 Five-year relative survival rates (%) by year of diagnosis of all cancers in children <19 yr of age. Rates based on follow-up of patients from 1999-2005. (From Horner MJ, Ries LAG, Krapcho M, et al, editors: *SEER cancer statistics review*, 1975-2006, Bethesda, MD, 2008, National Cancer Institute.)

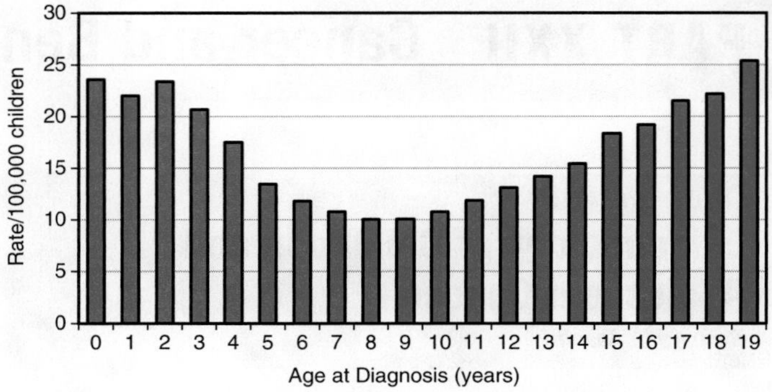

Figure 485-2 Age-specific cancer incidence rates per 100,000 children between 2002-2006 within the USA. (From Horner MJ, Ries LAG, Krapcho M, et al, editors: *SEER cancer statistics review*, 1975-2006, Bethesda, MD, 2008, National Cancer Institute.)

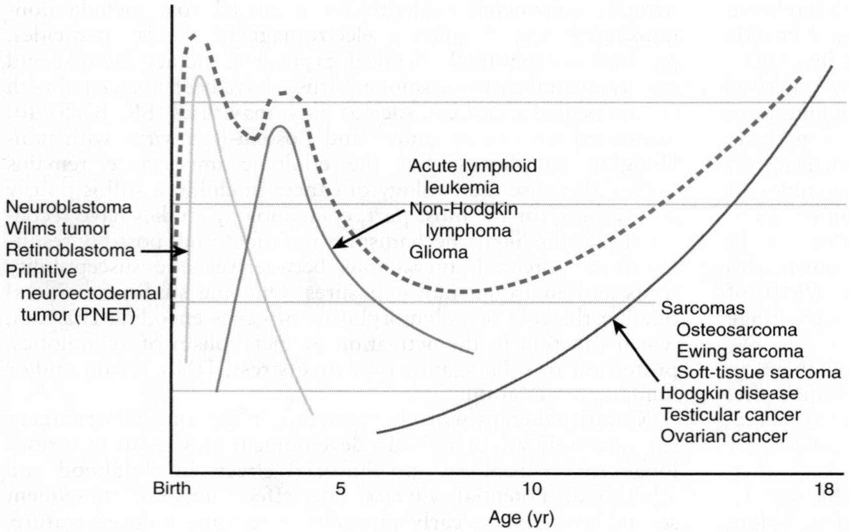

Figure 485-3 Generalized incidence of the most common types of cancer in children by age. The cumulative incidence of all cancers is shown as a *dashed line.* (Courtesy of Archie Bleyer, MD.)

Table 485-1 AGE-ADJUSTED INCIDENCE AND SURVIVAL RATES OF MALIGNANT NEOPLASMS BY TUMOR TYPE AMONG US CHILDREN

	ANNUAL INCIDENCE RATES PER MILLION CHILDREN, 2002-2006					5-YR SURVIVAL (%) ≤19 YR AT DIAGNOSIS, 1999-2005
	<1 Yr	1-4 Yr	5-9 Yr	10-14 Yr	15-19 Yr	
All malignancies combined	241	210	112	131	213	79.4
Leukemia (ALL/AML)	53 (20/20.5)	93 (78/11)	41 (33/4)	32 (21/8)	33 (18/10)	78 (84/57)
Lymphoma (Hodgkin)	8	9 (—)	13 (4.5)	24 (12)	48 (29)	88 (94.5)
CNS tumors	40	47	39	36	42	71
Neuroblastoma	52	19	3	2	0.8	73
Nephroblastoma and Wilms	15	18	4	1	—	87.9
Bone	—	1.5	6	13	15	68
Soft tissue sarcomas	19	11	7	12	16	70
Retinoblastoma	26	9	—	—	—	97
Hepatoblastoma	12	4.5	0.6	—	—	69
Germ cell tumors	21	3	2	8	29	89.5
Malignant epithelial cancer	—	1.9	3.5	13	46	91 (99*/94†)

*Thyroid carcinoma.
†Malignant melanoma.
ALL, acute lymphoid leukemia; AML, acute myeloid leukemia; CNS, central nervous system.
Based on the International Classification of Childhood Cancer (ICCC). Rates are per 1,000,000 children and are age-adjusted to the 2000 US standard population. —indicates that the rate could not be calculated with <6 cases for the age interval. (Data compiled From Horner MJ, Ries LAG, Krapcho M, et al, editors: *SEER Cancer Statistics Review, 1975-2006* (website). http://seer.cancer.gov/csr/1975_2006/. Accessed July 10, 2010.)

Table 485-2 KNOWN RISK FACTORS FOR SELECTED CHILDHOOD CANCERS

CANCER TYPE	RISK FACTOR	COMMENTS
Acute lymphoid leukemia	Ionizing radiation	Although primarily of historical significance, prenatal diagnostic x-ray exposure increases risk. Therapeutic irradiation for cancer treatment also increases risk.
	Race	White children have a 2-fold higher rate than black children in the USA.
	Genetic factors*	Down syndrome is associated with an estimated 10- to 20-fold increased risk. NF1, Bloom syndrome, ataxia-telangiectasia, and Langerhans cell histiocytosis, among others, are associated with an elevated risk.
Acute myeloid leukemias	Chemotherapeutic agents	Alkylating agents and epipodophyllotoxins increase risk.
	Genetic factors*	Down syndrome and NF1 are strongly associated. Familial monosomy 7 and several other genetic syndromes are also associated with increased risk.
Brain cancers	Therapeutic ionizing radiation to the head	With the exception of cancer radiation therapy, higher risk from radiation treatment is essentially of historical importance.
	Genetic factors*	NF1 is strongly associated with optic gliomas, and, to a lesser extent, with other central nervous system tumors. Tuberous sclerosis and several other genetic syndromes are associated with increased risk.
Hodgkin disease	Family history	Monozygotic twins and siblings are at increased risk.
	Infections	EBV is associated with increased risk.
Non-Hodgkin lymphoma	Immunodeficiency	Acquired and congenital immunodeficiency disorders and immunosuppressive therapy increase risk.
	Infections	EBV is associated with Burkitt lymphoma in Africa.
Osteosarcoma	Ionizing radiation	Cancer radiation therapy and high radium exposure increase risk.
	Chemotherapy	Alkylating agents increase risk.
	Genetic factors*	Increased risk is apparent with Li-Fraumeni syndrome and hereditary retinoblastoma.
Ewing sarcoma	Race	White children have about a 9-fold higher incidence rate than black children in the USA.
Neuroblastoma		No established risk factors.
Retinoblastoma	Genetic factors*	No established other risk factors.
Wilms tumor	Congenital anomalies	Aniridia, Beckwith-Wiedemann syndrome, and other congenital and genetic conditions are associated with increased risk.
	Race	Asian children reportedly have about half the rates of white and black children.
Renal medullary carcinoma	Sickle cell trait	Etiology unknown.
Rhabdomyosarcoma	Congenital anomalies and genetic conditions	Li-Fraumeni syndrome and NF1 are believed to be associated with increased risk. There is some concordance with major birth defects.
Hepatoblastoma	Genetic factors*	Beckwith-Wiedemann syndrome, hemihypertrophy, Gardner syndrome, and family history of adenomatous polyposis are associated with increased risk.
Leiomyosarcoma	Immunosuppression and EBV infection	EBV is associated with leiomyosarcoma for all forms of congenital and acquired immunosuppression but not leiomyosarcoma among immunocompetent persons.
Malignant germ cell tumors	Cryptorchidism	Cryptorchidism is a risk factor for testicular germ cell tumors.

EBV, Epstein-Barr virus; NF1, neurofibromatosis type 1.
From Gurney JG, Bondy ML: Epidemiology of childhood cancer. In Pizzo PA, Poplack DG, editors: *Principles and practice of pediatric oncology,* ed 5, Philadelphia, 2006, Lippincott Williams & Wilkins, p 11.
*See Chapter 486, Table 486-2.

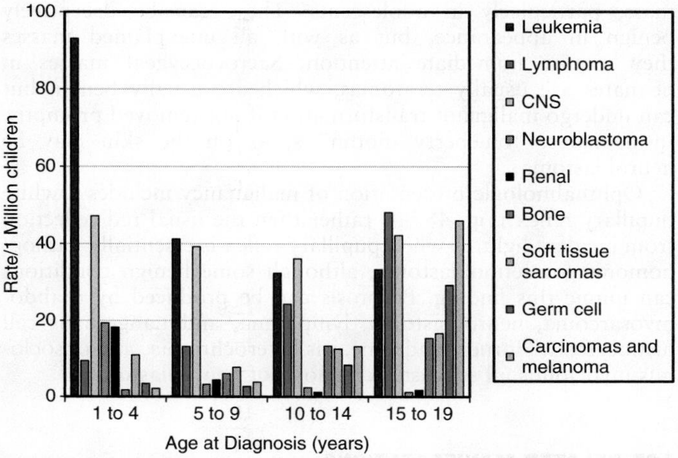

Figure 485-4 Surveillance Epidemiology and End Results (SEER) incidence rates by International Classification of Childhood Cancer (ICCC) and age group <20 years. CNS, central nervous system. (From Horner MJ, Ries LAG, Krapcho M, et al, editors: *SEER Cancer Statistics Review, 1975-2006* (website). http://seer.cancer.gov/csr/1975_2006/. Accessed July 10, 2010.)

preventing cancer. There are only a few recognized environmental causes of childhood cancer that can be avoided. One example is immunization against hepatitis B, which does decrease the risk of hepatocellular carcinoma in adolescence and adulthood; another is HPV vaccination against cervical cancer. An objective of pediatric medicine is to teach children how to adopt healthy lifestyles to reduce their risk of cancer during adulthood, such as avoiding tobacco, alcohol, high-fat diets, and obesity. The earlier these habits are instilled, the greater the lifelong benefit and the more likely it is to be present and sustained during adulthood.

ACKNOWLEDGMENT
The author would like to acknowledge the work of Nina S. Kadin-Lottick on Chapter 491, "Epidemiology of Childhood and Adolescent Cancer," in the previous editions of this work.

BIBLIOGRAPHY
Please visit the Nelson Textbook of Pediatrics *website at www.expertconsult.com for the complete bibliography.*

Chapter 486
Molecular and Cellular Biology of Cancer
Laura L. Worth

Cancer is a complex of diseases arising from alterations that can occur in a wide variety of genes. Alterations in normal cellular processes such as signal transduction, cell cycle control, DNA repair, cellular growth and differentiation, translational regulation, senescence, and apoptosis (programmed cell death) can result in a malignant phenotype.

For the full continuation of this chapter, please visit the Nelson Textbook of Pediatrics *website at www.expertconsult.com.*

Chapter 487
Principles of Diagnosis
A. Kim Ritchey

Childhood cancer is uncommon and can manifest with symptoms seen with benign illnesses. The challenge for the pediatrician is to be alert to the clues suggesting a diagnosis of cancer. In addition to the classic manifestations, any persistent, unexplained symptom or sign should be evaluated as potentially emanating from a cancerous or precancerous condition. As part of the diagnostic evaluation, the pediatrician and pediatric oncologist must convey the possible diagnosis to the patient and family in a sensitive and informative manner.

SIGNS AND SYMPTOMS

The symptoms and signs of cancer are variable and nonspecific in pediatric patients. The types of cancer that occur during the first 20 yr of life vary dramatically as a function of age—more so than at any other comparable age range (Chapter 485). Unlike cancers in adults, childhood cancers usually originate from the deeper, visceral structures and from the parenchyma of organs rather than from the epithelial layers that line the ducts and glands of organs and compose the skin. In children, dissemination of disease at diagnosis is common, and presenting symptoms or signs are often caused by systemic involvement. Pain was one of the initial presenting symptoms in more than 50% of children with cancer in one study. Infants and young children cannot express or localize their symptoms well. Another factor is the variability in the physiology and biology of the host related to growth and development during infancy, childhood, and adolescence.

The signs of cancer in children often are often attributed to other causes before the malignancy is recognized. Delays in diagnosis are particularly problematic during late adolescence and are due to a variety of factors prominent in this age group, including loss of health insurance coverage.

Although there is no clearly established set of warning signs of cancer in young people, the most common cancers in children suggest some guidelines that may be helpful in early recognition of signs and symptoms of cancer (Tables 487-1, 487-2, 487-3). Most of the symptoms and signs are not specific and might represent other possibilities in a differential diagnosis. Nonetheless, these hints encompass the common cancers of childhood and have been very useful in early detection.

PHYSICAL EXAMINATION

Physical examination findings in a child with malignancy are dependent on whether the cancer is systemic (see Table 487-2) or localized. The cancers most common in children involve the lymphohematopoietic system. When the bone marrow is compromised by malignancy (e.g., leukemia, disseminated neuroblastoma), typical findings include pallor from anemia, bleeding, petechiae, or purpura from thrombocytopenia or coagulopathy; cellulitis or other localized infection from leukopenia; skin nodules (especially in infants) and hepatosplenomegaly from malignant leukocytosis. Abnormalities found in lymphatic malignancies include peripheral adenopathy (Fig. 487-1) and signs of superior vena cava syndrome from an anterior mediastinal mass (Fig. 487-2) including respiratory distress, and facial and neck plethora and edema. Enlargement of cervical lymph nodes is common in children, but when persistent, progressive, and painless it often suggests lymphoma. In particular, supraclavicular adenopathy suggests underlying malignancy.

Table 487-1 THE MOST COMMON SIGNS AND SYMPTOMS OF CANCER IN CHILDREN

Pallor, bruising, persistent fever or infection; pancytopenia
Pain: persistent and unexplained; metastasis, bone marrow malignancy, primary bone tumor
Headache with neurologic deficit
Morning headache and vomiting; increased intracranial pressure
Lymphadenopathy: persistent and unexplained
Abdominal mass
Mass or persistent swelling
Eye changes: proptosis, white papillary reflex

Abnormalities of the central nervous system that can indicate cancer include decreased level of consciousness, cranial nerve palsies, ataxia, afebrile seizures, ptosis, decreased visual activity, neuroendocrine deficits, and increased intracranial pressure, which may be diagnosed by the presence of papilledema (Fig. 487-3). Any focal neurologic deficit in the motor or sensory system, especially a decrease in cranial nerve function, should prompt further investigation for malignancy.

Abdominal masses can be divided into upper, mid, and lower locations. Malignancies in the upper abdomen include Wilms tumor, neuroblastoma, hepatoblastoma, germ cell tumors, and sarcomas. Enlargement of the liver or spleen from leukemia can be mistaken for an upper abdominal mass. Mid-abdominal masses include non-Hodgkin lymphoma, neuroblastoma, germ cell tumors, and sarcomas. Lower abdominal masses include ovarian tumors, germ cell tumors, and sarcomas.

Rhabdomyosarcoma commonly appears as an extremity mass, particularly in adolescents. These can be deceptively benign in appearance, but as with all unexplained masses they require immediate attention. Sacrococcygeal masses in neonates are usually teratomas, which are usually benign but can undergo malignant transformation if not removed promptly. In neonates, "blueberry muffin" spots on the skin may be neuroblastoma.

Ophthalmologic presentation of malignancy includes a white pupillary reflex (Fig. 487-4) rather than the usual red reflection from incident light. A white pupillary reflex is essentially pathognomonic for retinoblastoma, although some benign conditions can mimic this finding. Proptosis can be produced by rhabdomyosarcoma, neuroblastoma, lymphoma, and Langerhans cell histiocytosis. Horner syndrome, iris heterochromia, and opsoclonus-myoclonus all suggest a diagnosis of neuroblastoma.

AGE-RELATED MANIFESTATIONS

Because various types of cancer in children occur at specific ages, the physician should tailor the history and physical examination based on the age of the child. The embryonal tumors, including neuroblastoma, Wilms tumor, retinoblastoma,

Table 487-2 COMMON MANIFESTATIONS OF CHILDHOOD MALIGNANCIES

SIGNS AND SYMPTOMS	SIGNIFICANCE	EXAMPLE
HEMATOLOGIC		
Pallor, anemia	Bone marrow infiltration	Leukemia, neuroblastoma
Petechiae, thrombocytopenia	Bone marrow infiltration	Leukemia, neuroblastoma
Fever, persistent or recurrent infection, neutropenia	Bone marrow infiltration	Leukemia, neuroblastoma
SYSTEMIC		
Bone pain, limp, arthralgia	Primary bone tumor, metastasis to bone	Osteosarcoma, Ewing sarcoma, leukemia, neuroblastoma
Fever of unknown origin, weight loss, night sweats	Lymphoma	Hodgkin and non-Hodgkin lymphoma
Painless lymphadenopathy	Lymphoma, metastatic solid tumor	Leukemia, Hodgkin lymphoma, non-Hodgkin lymphoma, Burkitt lymphoma, thyroid carcinoma
Abdominal mass	Adrenal, renal, or lymphoid tumor	Neuroblastoma, Wilms tumor, lymphoma
Hypertension	Renal or adrenal tumor	Neuroblastoma, pheochromocytoma, Wilms tumor
Diarrhea	Vasoactive intestinal polypeptide	Neuroblastoma, ganglioneuroma
Soft tissue mass	Local or metastatic tumor	Ewing sarcoma, osteosarcoma, neuroblastoma, thyroid carcinoma, rhabdomyosarcoma, Langerhans cell histiocytosis
Diabetes insipidus, galactorrhea, poor growth	Neuroendocrine involvement of hypothalamus or pituitary gland	Adenoma, craniopharyngioma, prolactinoma, Langerhans' cell histiocytosis
Emesis, visual disturbances, ataxia, headache, papilledema, cranial nerve palsies	Increased intracranial pressure	Primary brain tumor; metastasis
OPHTHALMOLOGIC SIGNS		
Leukokoria (white pupil)	Retinal mass	Retinoblastoma
Periorbital ecchymosis	Metastasis	Neuroblastoma
Miosis, ptosis, heterochromia	Horner syndrome: compression of cervical sympathetic nerves	Neuroblastoma
Opsomyoclonus, ataxia	Neurotransmitters? Autoimmunity?	Neuroblastoma
Exophthalmos, proptosis	Orbital tumor	Rhabdomyosarcoma, lymphoma, Langerhans cell histiocytosis
THORACIC MASS		
Cough, stridor, pneumonia, tracheal-bronchial compression; superior vena cava syndrome	Anterior mediastinal	Germ cell tumor, non-Hodgkin lymphoma, Hodgkin lymphoma
Vertebral or nerve root compression; dysphagia	Posterior mediastinal	Neuroblastoma, neuroenteric cyst

Modified from Kliegman RM, Marcdante KJ, Jenson HB, et al, editors: *Nelson essentials of pediatrics*, ed 5, Philadelphia, 2006, WB Saunders, p 729.

Table 487-3 UNCOMMON SIGNS AND SYMPTOMS OF CANCER IN CHILDREN

RELATED DIRECTLY TO TUMOR
Superior vena cava syndrome
Subcutaneous nodules
Leukemoid reaction
Myasthenia gravis
Heterochromia
NOT RELATED DIRECTLY TO TUMOR GROWTH
Chronic diarrhea
Polymyoclonus-opsoclonus
Failure to thrive
Cushing syndrome
Pseudomuscular dystrophy

Modified from Vietti TJ, Steuber CP: Clinical assessment and differential diagnosis of the child with suspected cancer. In Pizzo PA, Poplack DG, editors: *Principles and practice of pediatric oncology*, ed 4, Philadelphia, 2002, Lippincott Williams & Wilkins, pp 149–160.

hepatoblastoma, and rhabdomyosarcoma, usually occur during the first 2 yr of life (see Fig. 485-4). From 1-4 yr of age, acute lymphoblastic leukemia peaks in incidence. Brain tumors have a peak incidence in the first decade of life. Non-Hodgkin lymphomas are uncommon earlier than 5 years of age and steadily increase thereafter. During adolescence, bone tumors, Hodgkin disease, and the gonadal and soft tissue sarcomas predominate. Hence, for infants and toddlers, special attention should be paid to the possibility of embryonal and intra-abdominal tumors. Preschool-aged and early school-aged children showing compatible signs and symptoms should be specifically evaluated for leukemia. School-aged children might present with lymphoma or with brain tumors. Adolescents require assessment for bone and soft tissue sarcomas and gonadal malignancies, as well as for Hodgkin lymphoma.

EARLY DETECTION

The prognosis of malignancy in children depends primarily on tumor type, extent of disease at diagnosis, and rapidity of response to treatment. Early diagnosis helps to ensure that appropriate therapy is given in a timely fashion and hence optimizes the chances of cure. Because most physicians in general practice rarely encounter children with undiagnosed cancer, they should remember to investigate the possibility of malignancy, especially when they encounter an atypical course of a common childhood condition, unusual manifestations that do not fit common conditions, and any persistent symptom that defies diagnosis.

Delays in diagnosis are particularly likely in certain clinical situations. The cardinal symptom of both osteosarcoma and Ewing sarcoma is localized and usually persistent pain. Because these tumors occur during the second decade of life, a time of increased physical activity, patients often assume the pain results from trauma. Prompt radiologic evaluation can help confirm the diagnosis. Lymphoma, especially during adolescence, often manifests as an anterior mediastinal mass. Symptoms such as chronic cough, unexplained shortness of breath, or "new-onset asthma" are typical with this presentation and are often overlooked. Tumors of the nasopharynx or middle ear can mimic infection. Prolonged, unexplained ear pain, nasal discharge,

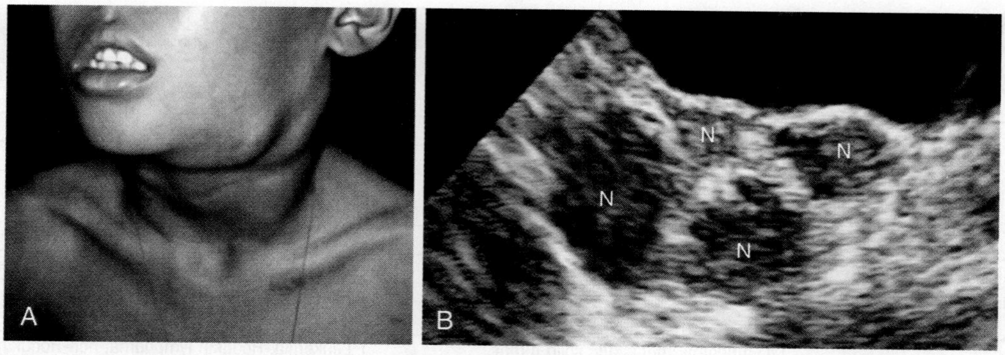

Figure 487-1 Cervical lymphadenopathy. Manifestations on physical examination (*A*) and on ultrasound examination (*B*). N, abnormally enlarged lymph nodes. (From Sinniah D, D'Angio GJ, Chatten J, et al: *Atlas of pediatric oncology,* London, 1996, Arnold.)

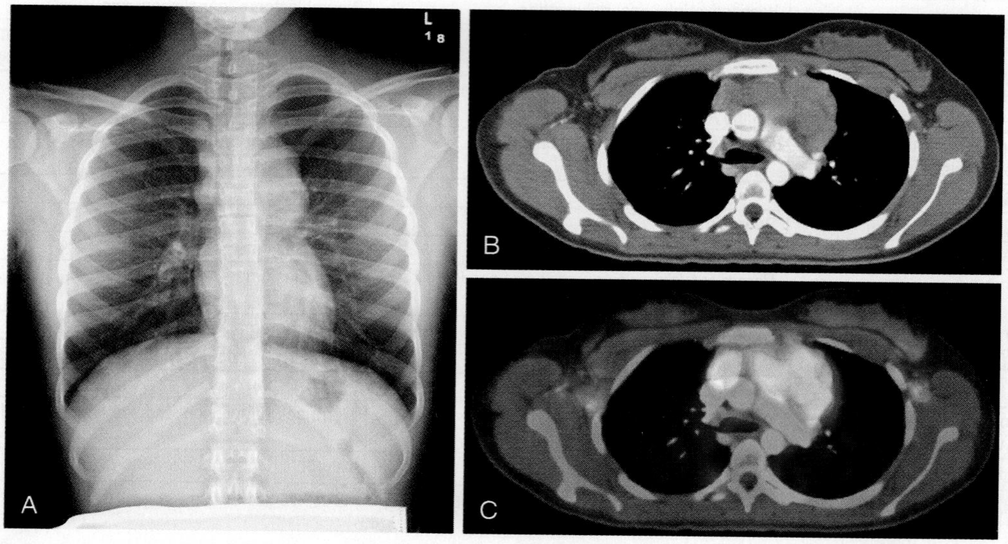

Figure 487-2 Anterior upper mediastinal mass from non-Hodgkin lymphoma. *A,* Plain chest X-ray. *B,* CT scan. *C,* positron-emission tomography (PET) scan.

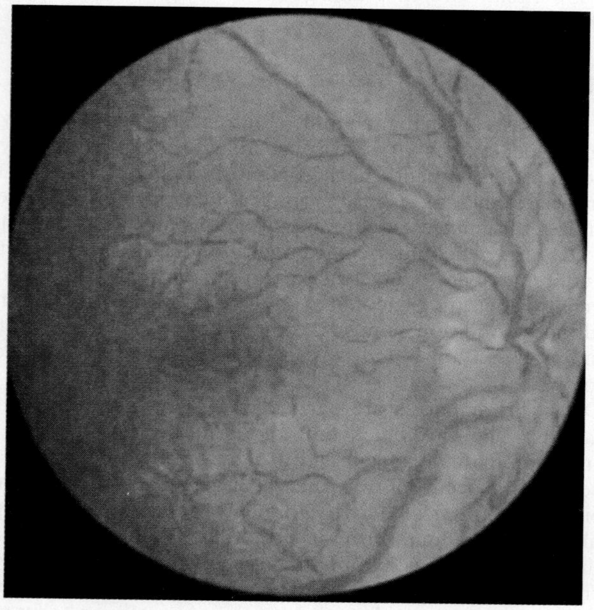

Figure 487-3 Papilledema on funduscopic examination. (From Sinniah D, D'Angio GJ, Chatten J, et al: *Atlas of pediatric oncology,* London, 1996, Arnold.)

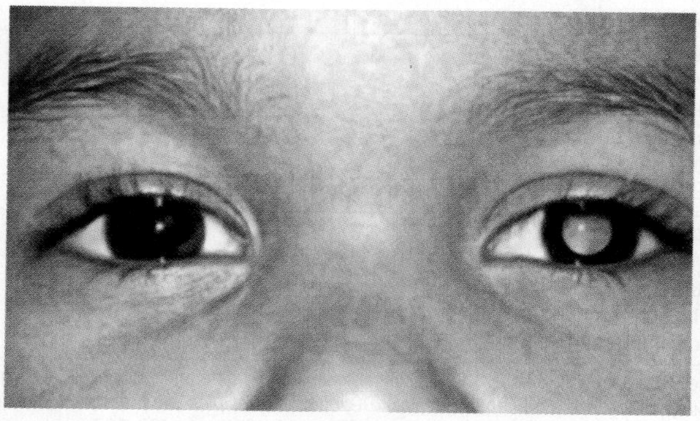

Figure 487-4 White pupillary reflex in the left eye. (From Sinniah D, D'Angio GJ, Chatten J, et al: *Atlas of pediatric oncology,* London, 1996, Arnold.)

retropharyngeal swelling, and trismus should be investigated as possible signs of malignancy.

Early symptoms of leukemia may be limited to prolonged or unexplained low-grade fever or bone and joint pain. Blood counts with two or more cell lines abnormal might indicate the need for bone marrow examination, even when leukemic blast cells are not seen in the blood smear (see Tables 487-1 and 487-2).

Mass screening for children with malignancy is not feasible. A screening program to detect early-stage neuroblastoma was

Table 487-4 WORK-UP OF COMMON PEDIATRIC MALIGNANCIES TO ASSESS PRIMARY TUMOR AND POTENTIAL METASTASES

MALIGNANCY	BONE MARROW ASPIRATE OR BIOPSY	CHEST X-RAY	CT SCAN	MRI	PET SCAN	BONE SCAN	CSF ANALYSIS	SPECIFIC MARKERS	OTHER TESTS
Leukemia	Yes (includes flow cytometry, cytogenetics, molecular studies)	Yes	—	—	—	—	Yes	—	—
Non-Hodgkin lymphoma	Yes (includes flow cytometry, cytogenetics, molecular studies)	Yes	Yes	—	Yes	Yes (selected cases)	Yes	—	—
Hodgkin lymphoma	Yes (in advanced stage)	Yes	Yes	—	Yes	Yes (selected cases)	—	—	—
CNS tumors	—	—	—	Yes	—	—	Yes (selected tumors)	—	—
Neuroblastoma	Yes (includes cytogenetics, molecular studies)	—	Yes	—	—	Yes	—	VMA, HVA	MIBG scan; bone x-rays
Wilms tumor	—	Yes	Yes	—	—	—	—	—	—
Rhabdomyosarcoma	Yes	Yes	Yes	Yes (selected sites)	—	Yes	Yes (for parameningeal tumors only)	—	—
Osteosarcoma	—	Yes	Yes (of chest)	Yes (for primary tumors)	—	Yes	—	—	—
Ewing sarcoma	Yes	Yes	Yes (of chest)	Yes (for primary tumors)	—	Yes	—	—	—
Germ cell tumors	—	Yes	Yes	Consider MRI of brain	—	—	—	AFP, HCG	—
Liver tumors	—	Yes	Yes	—	—	—	—	AFP	—
Retinoblastoma	Selected cases	—	Yes	Yes (includes brain)	—	Selected cases	Selected cases	—	—

Modified from Kliegman RM, Marcdante KJ, Jenson HB, et al, editors: *Nelson essentials of pediatrics,* ed 5, Philadelphia, 2006, WB Saunders, p 730.
AFP, alpha-fetoprotein; CNS, central nervous system; CSF, cerebrospinal fluid; HCG, human chorionic gonadotropin; HVA, homovanillic acid; MIBG, metaiodobenzylguanidine; VMA, vanillylmandelic acid.

successful in documenting more cases of the disease, but it had no impact on overall outcome. However, certain children are at increased risk for cancer and require an individualized plan to ensure early detection of malignancy. Selected examples include children with certain chromosome abnormalities, such as Down syndrome, Klinefelter syndrome, WAGR syndrome (Wilms tumor, aniridia, genital abnormalities, and mental retardation); children with overgrowth syndromes, such as Beckwith-Wiedemann syndrome, and hemihypertrophy; children with certain inherited single-gene disorders, including retinoblastoma, *p53* mutations (Li-Fraumeni syndrome), familial adenomatous polyposis, and neurofibromatosis. (See Table 486-2 for complete list.)

ENSURING THE DIAGNOSIS

When a malignant neoplasm is suspected, the immediate goal is to confirm the diagnosis. A tentative diagnosis can often be established on the basis of the patient's age, symptoms, and location of masses. Selected imaging techniques and tumor markers can facilitate the diagnostic approach (Table 487-4). Especially when a solid tumor is present, the pediatric oncologist, surgeon, and pathologist should work as a team to determine the site of biopsy, amount of tissue required, and whether fine-needle aspiration, percutaneous image-guided biopsy, incisional biopsy, or excisional biopsy and tumor resection are indicated. For selected situations, at the time of the initial diagnostic procedure, plans for bone marrow aspiration and biopsy and placement of central venous access may be appropriate.

Modern pathologic evaluation of pediatric malignancies requires appropriate handling of tissue so that multiple different techniques can be used. It is important that fresh tissue not be placed in formalin. Besides routine light microscopy, pathologic evaluation may include immunochemistry, flow cytometry, cytogenetics, and molecular genetic studies (fluorescence in situ hybridization [FISH], referse-transcriptase polymerase chain reaction [RT-PCR]). An emerging technology is DNA microarray analysis, which can identify specific gene expression patterns of tumors. In time, this technology might ensure more accurate classification and treatment.

STAGING

Once a specific diagnosis is confirmed, studies to define the extent of the malignancy are necessary to determine prognosis and treatment. Table 487-4 outlines minimum evaluation for common pediatric malignancies. In addition, for many tumors (e.g., Wilms tumor, neuroblastoma, rhabdomyosarcoma) a surgical staging system is used. Surgical stage can be determined at the time of the initial diagnostic procedure or subsequently. For example, a patient who has abdominal surgery for possible Wilms tumor or neuroblastoma should have careful evaluation and biopsy of all adjacent lymph nodes. A child with rhabdomyosarcoma can require a subsequent biopsy of sentinel lymph nodes as determined by scintigraphy or dye injection adjacent to the primary tumor. The pathologist facilitates staging by examining margins of the specimen to determine residual tumor.

BIBLIOGRAPHY
Please visit the Nelson Textbook of Pediatrics *website at* www.expertconsult.com *for the complete bibliography.*

Chapter 488
Principles of Treatment

Archie Bleyer and A. Kim Ritchey

Treatment of children with cancer is one of the most complex endeavors in pediatrics. It begins with an absolute requirement for the correct diagnosis (including subtype), proceeds through accurate and thorough staging of the extent of disease and determination of prognostic subgroup, provides appropriate multidisciplinary and usually multimodal therapy, and requires assiduous evaluation of the possibilities of recurrent disease and of adverse late effects of the disease and the therapies rendered. Throughout treatment, every child with cancer should have the benefit of the expertise of specialized teams of providers of pediatric cancer care, including pediatric oncologists, pathologists, radiologists, surgeons, radiotherapists, nurses, and support staff, including nutritionists, social workers, psychologists, pharmacists, other medical specialists, and teachers trained to work with seriously ill children.

For the full continuation of this chapter, please visit the Nelson Textbook of Pediatrics *website at www.expertconsult.com.*

Chapter 489
The Leukemias

David G. Tubergen, Archie Bleyer, and A. Kim Ritchey

The leukemias are the most common malignant neoplasms in childhood, accounting for about 31% of all malignancies that occur in children <15 yr of age. Each year leukemia is diagnosed in approximately 3,250 children <15 yr of age in the USA, an annual incidence of 4.5 cases per 100,000 children. Acute lymphoblastic leukemia (ALL) accounts for about 77% of cases of childhood leukemia, acute myelogenous leukemia (AML) for about 11%, chronic myelogenous leukemia (CML) for 2-3%, and juvenile myelomonocytic leukemia (JMML) for 1-2%. The remaining cases consist of a variety of acute and chronic leukemias that do not fit classic definitions for ALL, AML, CML, or JMML.

The leukemias may be defined as a group of malignant diseases in which genetic abnormalities in a hematopoietic cell give rise to an unregulated clonal proliferation of cells. The progeny of these cells have a growth advantage over normal cellular elements, because of their increased rate of proliferation and a decreased rate of spontaneous apoptosis. The result is a disruption of normal marrow function and, ultimately, marrow failure. The clinical features, laboratory findings, and responses to therapy vary depending on the type of leukemia.

BIBLIOGRAPHY

Please visit the Nelson Textbook of Pediatrics *website at www.expertconsult.com for the complete bibliography.*

489.1 Acute Lymphoblastic Leukemia

David G. Tubergen, Archie Bleyer, and A. Kim Ritchey

Childhood ALL was the first disseminated cancer shown to be curable and consequently has represented the model malignancy for the principles of cancer diagnosis, prognosis, and treatment. It actually is a heterogeneous group of malignancies with a number of distinctive genetic abnormalities that result in varying clinical behaviors and responses to therapy.

EPIDEMIOLOGY

ALL is diagnosed in approximately 2,400 children <15 yr of age in the USA each year. ALL has a striking peak incidence at 2-3 yr of age and occurs more in boys than in girls at all ages. This peak age incidence was apparent decades ago in white populations in advanced socioeconomic countries, but it has since been confirmed in the black population of the USA as well. The disease is more common in children with certain chromosomal abnormalities, such as Down syndrome, Bloom syndrome, ataxia-telangiectasia, and Fanconi anemia. Among identical twins, the risk to the second twin if one develops leukemia is greater than that in the general population. The risk is >70% if ALL is diagnosed in the first twin during the first year of life and the twins shared the same (monochorionic) placenta. If the first twin develops ALL by 5-7 yr of age, the risk to the second twin is at least twice that in the general population, regardless of zygosity.

Table 489-1 FACTORS PREDISPOSING TO CHILDHOOD LEUKEMIA

GENETIC CONDITIONS
Down syndrome
Fanconi anemia
Bloom syndrome
Diamond-Blackfan anemia
Schwachman-Diamond syndrome
Kostmann syndrome
Neurofibromatosis type 1
Ataxia-telangiectasia
Severe combined immune deficiency
Paroxysmal nocturnal hemoglobinuria
Li-Fraumeni syndrome
ENVIRONMENTAL FACTORS
Ionizing radiation
Drugs
Alkylating agents
Nitrosourea
Epipodophyllotoxin
Benzene exposure
Advanced maternal age (?)

ETIOLOGY

In virtually all cases, the etiology of ALL is unknown, although several genetic and environmental factors are associated with childhood leukemia (Table 489-1). Exposure to medical diagnostic radiation both in utero and in childhood has been associated with an increased incidence of ALL. In addition, published descriptions and investigations of geographic clusters of cases have raised concern that environmental factors can increase the incidence of ALL. Thus far, no such factors other than radiation have been identified in the USA. In certain developing countries, there has been an association between B-cell ALL and Epstein-Barr viral infections.

CELLULAR CLASSIFICATION

The classification of ALL depends on characterizing the malignant cells in the bone marrow to determine the morphology, phenotypic characteristics as measured by cell membrane markers, and cytogenetic and molecular genetic features. **Morphology** alone usually is adequate to establish a diagnosis, but the other studies are essential for disease classification, which can have a major influence on the prognosis and the choice of appropriate therapy. The most important distinguishing morphologic feature is the French-American-British (FAB) L3 subtype, which is evidence of a mature B-cell leukemia. The L3 type, also known as Burkitt leukemia, is one of the most rapidly growing cancers in humans and requires a different therapeutic approach than other subtypes of ALL. Phenotypically, surface markers show that about 85% of cases of ALL are derived from progenitors of B cells, about 15% are derived from T cells, and about 1% are derived from B cells. A small percentage of children with leukemia have a disease characterized by surface markers of both lymphoid and myeloid derivation. Immunophenotypes often correlate to disease manifestations (Table 489-2).

Chromosomal and genetic abnormalities are found in most patients with ALL (Table 489-3, Fig. 489-1). The abnormalities,

Table 489-2 CORRELATION OF IMMUNOPHENOTYPE WITH CLINICAL CHARACTERISTICS

	PRO-B, CD10⁻	PRECURSOR-B, CD10⁺	PRE-B	MATURE B (BURKITT)	T-CELL
No. of patients	52	635	156	39	124
Sex (% male)	39	53	50	85	75
Age (yr)					
<1 (%)	33	1	6	3	1
1-<10 (%)	50	82	80	64	62
≥10 (%)	17	17	14	33	37
Leukocyte count < 100×10^9/L					
Median	38	33	42	77	87
≤20 (%)	38	75	53	69	23
>50 (%)	44	11	21	5	57
Platelet count <100×10^9/L (%)	77	75	81	56	56
Hemoglobin ≤8 g/dL (%)	58	40	60	21	15
Splenomegaly (%)*	50	34	46	28	57
Hepatomegaly (%)*	56	46	48	36	61
Mediastinal mass (%)	0	0	1	0	72
Lymphadenopathy	35	36	41	54	78
CNS disease	10	1	1	0	11

*>4 cm below the costal margin.
CNS, central nervous system.
From Nathan DG, Orkin SH, Ginsburg D, et al, editors: *Nathan and Oski's hematology of infancy and childhood,* ed 6, Philadelphia, 2003, WB Saunders, p 1139. Data from Reiter A, Schrappe M, Ludwig WD, et al: Chemotherapy in 998 unselected childhood acute lymphoblastic leukemia patients. Results and conclusions of the multicenter trial ALL-BFM 86. *Blood* 84:3122–3123, 1994.

Table 489-3 COMMON CHROMOSOMAL ABNORMALITIES IN THE ACUTE LEUKEMIAS OF CHILDHOOD

SUBTYPE	CHROMOSOMAL ABNORMALITY	INFLUENCE ON PROGNOSIS	INCIDENCE
ACUTE LYMPHOBLASTIC LEUKEMIA			
Precursor-B	Trisomy 4,10, and 17	Favorable	25%
Precursor-B	t(12;21)	Favorable	20-25%
Precursor-B	t(1;19)	None	5-6%
Precursor-B	t(4;11)	Unfavorable	2%
Precursor-B	t(9;22)	Unfavorable	3%
Mature B-cell (Burkitt)	t(8;14)	None	1-2%
Precursor-B	Hyperdiploidy	Favorable	20-25%
Precursor-B	Hypodiploidy	Unfavorable	1%
ACUTE MYELOGENOUS LEUKEMIA			
M1*	t(8;21)	Favorable	5-15%
M4*	inv(16)	Favorable	2-11%
M3*	t(5;17)	Favorable	6-15%
General	del(7)	Unfavorable	2-7%
Infant	11q23	Unfavorable	2-10%

*Per the French-American-British classification of acute myelogenous leukemia (see Table 489-4).

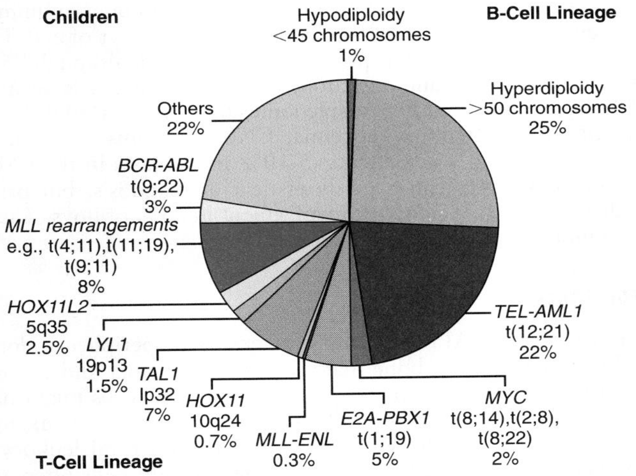

Figure 489-1 Estimated frequency of specific genotypes of acute lymphoblastic leukemia (ALL) in children. The genetic lesions that are exclusively seen in cases of T-cell-lineage leukemias are indicated in *purple.* All other genetic subtypes are either exclusively or primarily seen in cases of B-cell-lineage ALL. (From Pui CH, Relling MV, Downing JR: Acute lymphoblastic leukemia, *N Engl J Med* 350:1535–1548, 2004.)

which may be related to chromosomal number, translocations, or deletions, provide important prognostic information. The identification of the leukemia-specific fusion-gene sequences in archived neonatal blood spots of some children who develop ALL at a later date indicates the importance of in utero events in the initiation of the malignant process, but the long lag period before the onset of the disease in some children, reported to be as long as 14 yr, supports the concept that additional genetic modifications also are required for disease expression. The polymerase chain reaction and fluorescence in situ hybridization techniques offer the ability to pinpoint molecular genetic abnormalities and to detect small numbers of malignant cells during follow-up and are of proven clinical utility. The development of DNA microanalysis makes it possible to analyze the expression of thousands of genes in the leukemic cell. This technique promises to further enhance the understanding of the fundamental biology and to provide clues to the therapeutic approach of ALL. Some effectors of critical signal transduction pathways have already been implicated in the pathogenesis of ALL using this technique.

CLINICAL MANIFESTATIONS

The initial presentation of ALL usually is nonspecific and relatively brief. Anorexia, fatigue, malaise, and irritability often are present, as is an intermittent, low-grade fever. Bone or, less often, joint pain, particularly in the lower extremities, may be present. Patients often have a history of an upper respiratory tract infection in the preceding 1-2 mo. Less commonly, symptoms may be of several months' duration, may be localized predominantly to the bones or joints, and can include joint swelling. Bone pain is severe and can wake the patient at night. As the disease progresses, signs and symptoms of bone marrow failure become more obvious with the occurrence of pallor, fatigue, exercise intolerance, bruising, or epistaxis, as well as fever, which may be caused by infection or the disease. Organ infiltration can cause lymphadenopathy, hepatosplenomegaly, testicular enlargement, or central nervous system (CNS) involvement (cranial neuropathies headache, seizures). Respiratory distress may be due to severe anemia or mediastinal node comparison of the airways.

On **physical examination,** findings of pallor, listlessness, purpuric and petechial skin lesions, or mucous membrane hemorrhage can reflect bone marrow failure (Chapter 487). The proliferative nature of the disease may be manifested as lymphadenopathy, splenomegaly, or, less commonly, hepatomegaly. In patients with bone or joint pain, there may be exquisite tenderness over the bone or objective evidence of joint swelling and effusion. Nonetheless, with marrow involvement, deep bone pain may be present but tenderness will not be elicited. Rarely, patients show signs of increased intracranial pressure that indicate leukemic involvement of the CNS. These include papilledema (see Fig. 487-3), retinal hemorrhages, and cranial nerve palsies. Respiratory distress usually is related to anemia but can occur in patients with an obstructive airway problem (wheezing) due to a large anterior mediastinal mass (e.g., in the thymus or nodes). This problem is most typically seen in adolescent boys with T-cell ALL. T-cell ALL also has a higher leukocyte count.

Precursor B-cell ALL ($CD10^+$ or common acute lymphoblastic leukemia antigen [CALLA] positive) is the most common immunophenotype (see Table 489-2), with onset at 1-10 yr of age. The median leukocyte count at presentation is 33,000, although 75% of patients have counts <20,000; thrombocytopenia is seen in 75% of patients, and hepatosplenomegaly is seen in 30-40% of patients. In all types of leukemia, CNS symptoms are seen at presentation in 5% of patients (5-10% have blasts in the CSF). Testicular involvement is rarely evident at diagnosis, but prior studies have indicated occult involvement in 25% of boys. There is no indication for testicular biopsy.

DIAGNOSIS

The diagnosis of ALL is strongly suggested by peripheral blood findings that indicate bone marrow failure. Anemia and thrombocytopenia are seen in most patients. Leukemic cells might not be reported in the peripheral blood in routine laboratory examinations. Many patients with ALL present with total leukocyte counts of <10,000/μL. In such cases, the leukemic cells often are reported initially to be atypical lymphocytes, and it is only on further evaluation that the cells are found to be part of a malignant clone. When the results of an analysis of peripheral blood suggest the possibility of leukemia, the bone marrow should be examined promptly to establish the diagnosis. It is important that all studies necessary to confirm a diagnosis and adequately classify the type of leukemia be performed, including bone marrow aspiration and biopsy, flow cytometry, cytogenetics, and molecular studies.

ALL is diagnosed by a bone marrow evaluation that demonstrates >25% of the bone marrow cells as a homogeneous population of lymphoblasts. Staging of ALL is based partly on a cerebrospinal fluid (CSF) examination. If lymphoblasts are found and the CSF leukocyte count is elevated, overt CNS or meningeal leukemia is present. This finding reflects a worse stage and indicates the need for additional CNS and systemic therapies. The staging lumbar puncture may be performed in conjunction with the first dose of intrathecal chemotherapy, if the diagnosis of leukemia has been previously established from bone marrow evaluation. The initial lumbar puncture should be performed by an experienced proceduralist, because a traumatic lumbar puncture is associated with an increased risk of CNS relapse.

DIFFERENTIAL DIAGNOSIS

The diagnosis of leukemia is readily made in the patient with typical signs and symptoms, anemia, thrombocytopenia, and elevated white blood count with blasts present on smear. Elevation of the lactate dehydrogenase (LDH) is often a clue to the diagnosis of ALL. When only pancytopenia is present, aplastic anemia (congenital or acquired) and myelofibrosis should be considered. Failure of a single cell line, as seen in transient erythroblastopenia of childhood, immune thrombocytopenia, and congenital or acquired neutropenia, sometimes produces a clinical picture that is difficult to distinguish from ALL and that can require bone marrow examination. A high index of suspicion is required to differentiate ALL from infectious mononucleosis in patients with acute onset of fever and lymphadenopathy and from rheumatoid arthritis in patients with fever, bone pain but often no tenderness, and joint swelling. These presentations also can require bone marrow examination.

ALL must be differentiated from acute myelogenous leukemia (AML) and other malignant diseases that invade the bone marrow and can have clinical and laboratory findings similar to ALL, including neuroblastoma, rhabdomyosarcoma, Ewing sarcoma, and retinoblastoma.

TREATMENT

The single most important prognostic factor in ALL is the treatment: Without effective therapy, the disease is fatal. The survival rates of children with ALL since the 1970s have improved as the results of clinical trials have improved the therapies and outcomes (Fig. 489-2). Survival is also related to age (Fig. 489-3) and subtype (Fig. 489-4).

The choice of treatment of ALL is based on the estimated clinical risk of relapse in the patient, which varies widely among the subtypes of ALL. Three of the most important predictive factors are the age of the patient at the time of diagnosis, the initial leukocyte count, and the speed of response to treatment (i.e., how rapidly the leukemic cells can be cleared from the marrow or peripheral blood). Different study groups use various factors to define risk, but age between 1 and 10 yr and a leukocyte count of <50,000/μL are widely used to define average risk. Children who are >10 yr of age or who have an initial leukocyte count of >50,000/μL are considered to be at higher risk. The outcome for patients at higher risk can be improved by administration of more-intensive therapy despite the greater toxicity of such therapy. Infants with ALL, along with patients who present with specific chromosomal abnormalities, such as t(9;22) or t(4;11), have an even higher risk of relapse despite intensive therapy. Clinical trials have demonstrated that the prognosis for patients with a slower response to initial therapy may be improved by therapy that is more intensive than the therapy considered necessary for patients who respond more rapidly.

Most children with ALL are treated in clinical trials conducted by national or international cooperative groups. In general, the initial therapy is designed to eradicate the leukemic cells from the bone marrow; this is known as **remission induction.** During this phase, therapy usually is given for 4 wk and consists of vincristine weekly, a corticosteroid such as dexamethasone or prednisone, and either repeated doses of native L-asparaginase or a single dose of a long-acting, pegylated asparaginase preparation. Intrathecal cytarabine and/or methotrexate also may be given. Patients at higher risk also receive daunomycin at weekly intervals. With this approach, 98% of patients are in **remission,** as defined by <5% blasts in the marrow and a return of neutrophil and platelet counts to near-normal levels after 4-5 wk of treatment. Intrathecal chemotherapy is usually given at the start of treatment and once more during induction.

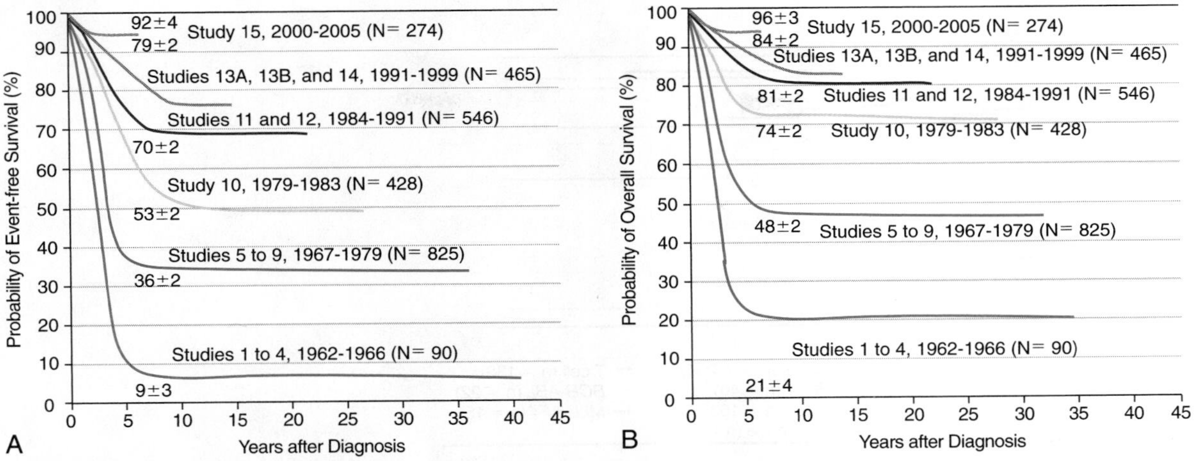

Figure 489-2 Kaplan-Meier analyses of event-free survival (*A*) and overall survival (*B*) in 2628 children with newly diagnosed ALL. The patients participated in 15 consecutive studies conducted at St. Jude Children's Research Hospital from 1962-2005. The 5-year event-free and overall survival estimates (±SE) are shown, except for Study 15, for which preliminary results at 4 years are provided. The results demonstrate steady improvement in clinical outcome over the past 4 decades. The difference in event-free and overall survival rates has narrowed in the more recent periods, suggesting that relapses or second cancers that occur after contemporary therapy are more refractory to treatment. (From Pui CH, Evans WE: Treatment of acute lymphoblastic leukemia, *N Engl J Med* 354:166–178, 2006.)

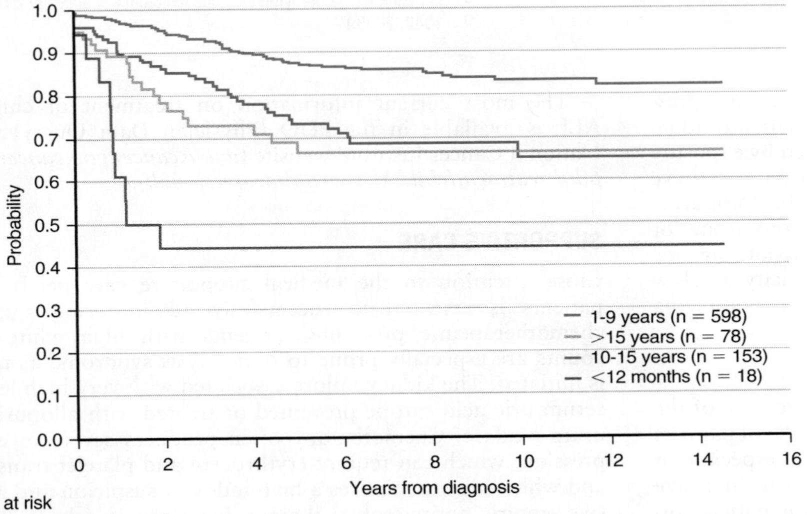

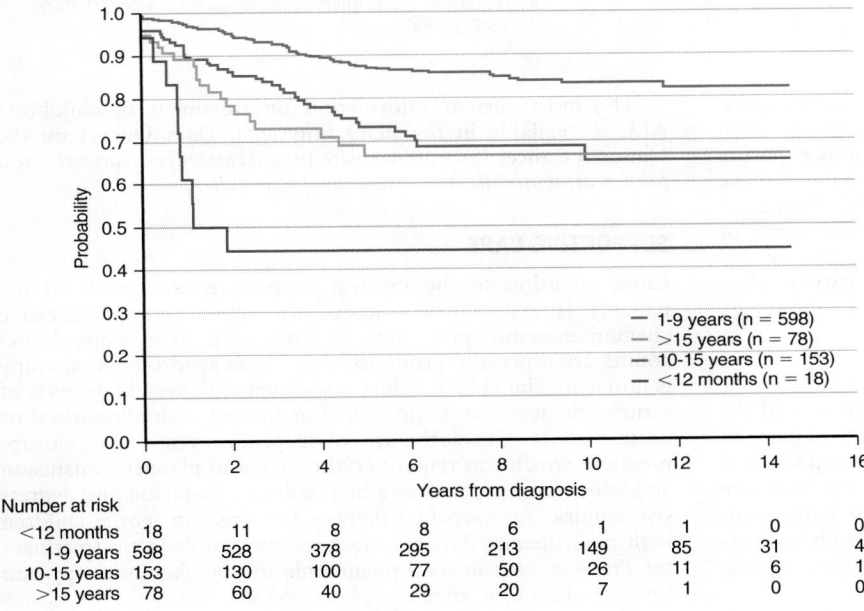

Number at risk									
<12 months	18	11	8	8	6	1	1	0	0
1-9 years	598	528	378	295	213	149	85	31	4
10-15 years	153	130	100	77	50	26	11	6	1
>15 years	78	60	40	29	20	7	1	0	0

Figure 489-3 Kaplan-Meier estimates of event-free survival according to age at diagnosis of acute lymphoblastic leukemia. (From Pui CH, Robinson LL, Look AT: Acute lymphoblastic leukaemia, *Lancet* 371:1030–1042, 2008.)

The second phase of treatment focuses on **CNS therapy** in an effort to prevent later CNS relapses. Intrathecal chemotherapy is given repeatedly by lumbar puncture in conjunction with intensive systemic chemotherapy. The likelihood of later CNS relapse is thereby reduced to <5%. A small percentage of patients with features that predict a high risk of CNS relapse may receive irradiation to the brain. This includes patients who, at the time of diagnosis, have lymphoblasts in the CSF and either an elevated CSF leukocyte count or physical signs of CNS leukemia, such as cranial nerve palsy.

After remission has been induced, in conjunction with CNS therapy, many regimens provide 14-28 wk of multiagent therapy, with the drugs and schedules used varying depending on the risk group of the patient. This period of treatment is termed **consolidation** and **intensification.** Many patients benefit from administration of a delayed intensive phase of treatment (**delayed intensification**), approximately 5-7 mo after the beginning of therapy, and after a relatively nontoxic phase of treatment (interim maintenance) to allow recovery from the prior intensive therapy. Finally, patients are given daily mercaptopurine and weekly methotrexate, usually with intermittent doses of vincristine and a corticosteroid. This period, known as the **maintenance phase** of therapy, lasts for 2-3 yr, depending on the protocol used.

A small number of patients with particularly poor prognostic features, such as those with the t(9;22) translocation known as the Philadelphia chromosome or extreme hypodiploidy, may undergo bone marrow transplantation during the first remission.

Adolescents and young adults with ALL usually have adverse prognostic factors at the time of diagnosis and require more-intensive therapy. A number of studies have proved that patients in this age group have a superior outcome when treated on pediatric as opposed to adult treatment protocols. Although the explanation for these findings may be multifactoral, it is important that these patients be treated on pediatric treatment protocols, ideally in a pediatric cancer center.

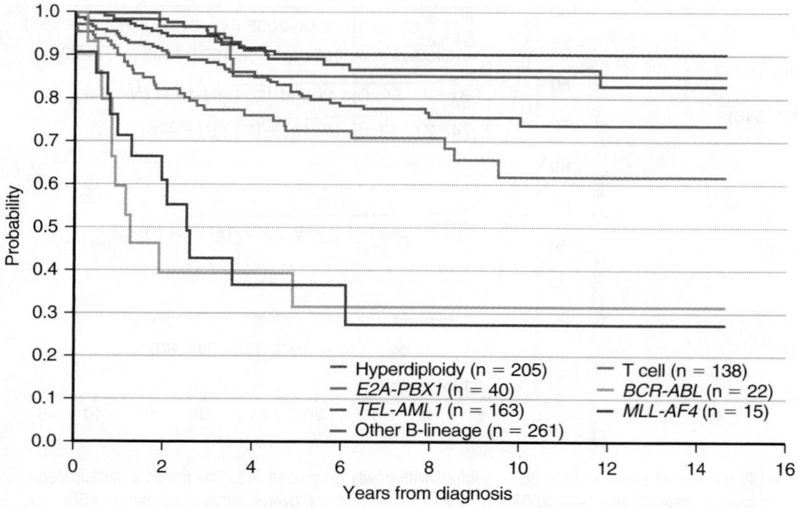

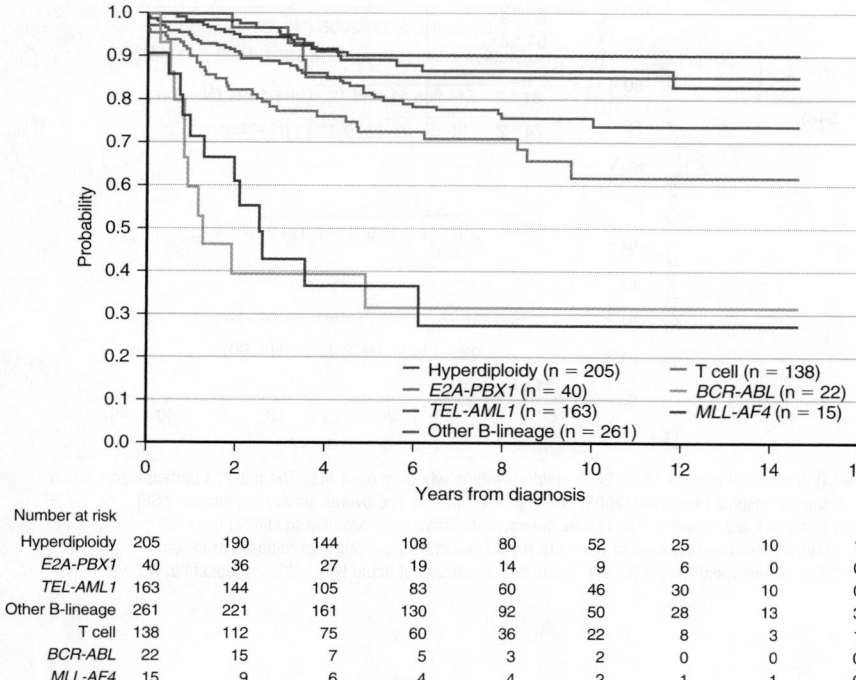

Number at risk									
Hyperdiploidy	205	190	144	108	80	52	25	10	1
E2A-PBX1	40	36	27	19	14	9	6	0	0
TEL-AML1	163	144	105	83	60	46	30	10	0
Other B-lineage	261	221	161	130	92	50	28	13	3
T cell	138	112	75	60	36	22	8	3	1
BCR-ABL	22	15	7	5	3	2	0	0	0
MLL-AF4	15	9	6	4	4	2	1	1	0

Figure 489-4 Kaplan-Meier analysis of event-free survival according to biological subtype of leukemia. (From Pui CH, Robinson LL, Look AT: Acute lymphoblastic leukaemia, *Lancet* 371:1030–1042, 2008.)

In the future, treatment also may be stratified by gene expression profiles of leukemic cells or the presence of minimal residual disease. In particular, gene expression arrays induced by exposure to the chemotherapeutic agent can predict which patients have drug-resistant ALL. **Pharmacogenetic testing** of the thiopurine *S*-methyltransferase gene, which converts mercaptopurine or thioguanine (both prodrugs) into active chemotherapeutic agents, can identify rapid metabolizers (associated with toxicity) or slow metabolizers (associated with treatment failure), thus optimizing drug dosing (Chapter 56).

Treatment of Relapse

The major impediment to a successful outcome is relapse of the disease. Relapse occurs in the bone marrow in 15-20% of patients with ALL and carries the most serious implications, especially if it occurs during or shortly after completion of therapy. Intensive chemotherapy with agents not previously used in the patient followed by allogeneic stem cell transplantation can result in long-term survival for some patients with bone marrow relapse (Chapter 129).

The incidence of CNS relapse has decreased to <10% since introduction of preventive CNS therapy. CNS relapse may be discovered at the time of a routine lumbar puncture in the asymptomatic patient. Symptomatic patients with relapse in the CNS usually present with signs and symptoms of increased intracranial pressure and can present with isolated cranial nerve palsies. The diagnosis is confirmed by demonstrating the presence of leukemic cells in the CSF. The treatment includes intrathecal medication and cranial or craniospinal irradiation. Systemic chemotherapy also must be used, because these patients are at high risk for subsequent bone marrow relapse. Most patients with leukemic relapse confined to the CNS do well, especially those in whom the CNS relapse occurs longer than 18 mo after initiation of chemotherapy.

Testicular relapse occurs in about 2% of boys with ALL, usually after completion of therapy. Such relapse occurs as painless swelling of one or both testes. The diagnosis is confirmed by biopsy of the affected testis. Treatment includes systemic chemotherapy and possibly local irradiation. A high proportion of boys with a testicular relapse can be successfully re-treated, and the survival rate of these patients is good.

The most current information on treatment of childhood ALL is available in the PDQ (Physician Data Query) on the National Cancer Institute website (*www.cancer.gov/cancertopics/pdq/treatment/childALL/healthprofessional/*).

SUPPORTIVE CARE

Close attention to the medical supportive care needs of the patients is essential in successfully administering aggressive chemotherapeutic programs. Patients with high white blood counts are especially prone to tumor lysis syndrome as therapy is initiated. The kidney failure associated with very high levels of serum uric acid can be prevented or treated with allopurinol or urate oxidase. Chemotherapy often produces severe myelosuppression, which can require erythrocyte and platelet transfusion and which always requires a high index of suspicion and aggressive empiric antimicrobial therapy for sepsis in febrile children with neutropenia. Patients must receive prophylactic treatment for *Pneumocystis jiroveci* pneumonia during chemotherapy and for several months after completing treatment.

The successful therapy of ALL is a direct result of intensive and often toxic treatment. However, such intensive therapy can incur substantial academic, developmental, and psychosocial costs for children with ALL and considerable financial costs and stress for their families. Both long-term and acute toxicity effects can occur. An array of cancer care professionals with training and experience in addressing the myriad of problems that can arise is essential to minimize the complications and achieve an optimal outcome.

PROGNOSIS

Most children with ALL can now be expected to have long-term survival, with the survival rate >80% at 5 yr from diagnosis (see Fig. 489-2). The most important prognostic factor is the choice of appropriate risk-directed therapy, with the type of treatment chosen according to the subtype of ALL, the initial white blood count, the age of the patient, and the rate of response to initial therapy. Characteristics generally believed to adversely affect outcome include age <1 yr or >10 yr at diagnosis, a leukocyte count of >50,000/μL at diagnosis, T-cell immunophenotype, or a slow response to initial therapy. Chromosomal abnormalities, including hypodiploidy, the Philadelphia chromosome, and MLL gene rearrangements, and certain mutations, including deletion of the *IKZF1* gene, portend a poorer outcome. More-favorable characteristics include a rapid response to therapy, hyperdiploidy, trisomy of specific chromosomes, and rearrangements of the *TEL/AML1* genes.

Patients in clinical remission can have **minimal residual disease (MRD)** that can only be detected with specific molecular probes to translocations and other DNA markers contained in leukemic cells or specialized flow cytometry. MRD can be quantitative and can provide an estimate of the burden of leukemic cells present in the marrow. Higher levels of MRD present at the end of induction suggest a poorer prognosis and higher risk of subsequent relapse. MRD of 0.01-0.1% on the marrow on day 29 of induction is a significant risk factor for shorter event-free survival for all risk categories, when compared with patients with no MRD.

BIBLIOGRAPHY

Please visit the Nelson Textbook of Pediatrics *website at* *www.expertconsult.com* *for the complete bibliography.*

489.2 Acute Myelogenous Leukemia

David G. Tubergen, Archie Bleyer, and A. Kim Ritchey

EPIDEMIOLOGY

AML accounts for 11% of the cases of childhood leukemia in the USA; it is diagnosed in approximately 370 children annually. The relative frequency of AML increases in adolescence, representing 36% of cases of leukemia in 15-19 yr olds. One subtype, acute promyelocytic leukemia (APL), is more common in certain other regions of the world, but incidence of the other types is generally uniform. Several chromosomal abnormalities associated with AML have been identified, but no predisposing genetic or environmental factors can be identified in most patients (see Table 489-1). Nonetheless, a number of risk factors have been identified, including ionizing radiation, chemotherapeutic agents (e.g., alkylating agents, epipodophyllotoxin), organic solvents, paroxysmal nocturnal hemoglobinuria, and certain syndromes: Down syndrome, Fanconi anemia, Bloom syndrome, Kostmann syndrome, Shwachman-Diamond syndrome, Diamond-Blackfan syndrome, Li-Fraumeni syndrome, and neurofibromatosis type 1.

CELLULAR CLASSIFICATION

The characteristic feature of AML is that >20% of bone marrow cells on bone marrow aspiration or biopsy touch preparations constitute a fairly homogeneous population of blast cells, with features similar to those that characterize early differentiation states of the myeloid-monocyte-megakaryocyte series of blood cells. The most common classification of the subtypes of AML is the FAB system (Table 489-4). Although this system is based on morphologic criteria alone, current practice also requires the use of flow cytometry to identify cell surface antigens and use of chromosomal and molecular genetic techniques for additional diagnostic precision and also to aid the choice of therapy. The World Health Organization (WHO) has proposed a new classification system that incorporates morphology, chromosome abnormalities, and specific gene mutations. This system provides significant biologic and prognostic information.

CLINICAL MANIFESTATIONS

The production of symptoms and signs of AML, as in ALL, is due to replacement of bone marrow by malignant cells and due to secondary bone marrow failure. Thus, patients with AML can present with any or all of the findings associated with **marrow failure** in ALL. In addition, patients with AML present with signs and symptoms that are uncommon in ALL, including **subcutaneous nodules** or "blueberry muffin" lesions (especially in infants), infiltration of the gingiva (especially in M4 and M5 subtypes), signs and laboratory findings of **disseminated intravascular coagulation** (especially indicative of acute promyelocytic leukemia), and discrete masses, known as **chloromas** or **granulocytic sarcomas.** These masses can occur in the absence of apparent bone marrow involvement and typically are associated with the M2 subcategory of AML with a t(8;21) translocation. Chloromas also may be seen in the orbit and epidural space.

Table 489-4 FRENCH-AMERICAN-BRITISH (FAB) CLASSIFICATION OF ACUTE MYELOGENOUS LEUKEMIA

SUBTYPE	COMMON NAME
M0	Acute myeloblastic leukemia without differentiation
M1	Acute myeloblastic leukemia without maturation
M2	Acute myeloblastic leukemia with maturation
M3	Acute promyeloblastic leukemia
M4	Acute myelomonocytic leukemia
M5	Acute monocytic leukemia
M6	Erythroleukemia
M7	Acute megakaryocytic leukemia

DIAGNOSIS

Analysis of bone marrow aspiration and biopsy specimens of patients with AML typically reveals the features of a hypercellular marrow consisting of a monotonous pattern of cells with features that permit FAB subclassification of disease. Flow cytometry and special stains assist in identifying myeloperoxidase-containing cells, thus confirming both the myelogenous origin of the leukemia and the diagnosis. Some chromosomal abnormalities and molecular genetic markers are characteristic of specific subtypes of disease (see Tables 489-3 and 489-5).

TREATMENT

Aggressive multiagent chemotherapy is successful in inducing remission in about 85-90% of patients. Targeting therapy to genetic markers may be beneficial (see Table 489-5). Up to 5% of patients die of either infection or bleeding before a remission can be achieved. Matched-sibling bone marrow or stem cell transplantation after remission has been shown to achieve long-term disease-free survival in 60-70% of patients. Continued chemotherapy for patients who do not have a matched sibling donor is generally less effective than marrow transplantation but nevertheless is curative in about 45-50% of patients. However, for selected patients with favorable prognostic features [t(8;21); t(15;17); inv(16); FAB M3] and improved outcome with chemotherapy, matched sibling stem cell transplantation is recommended only after a relapse. Matched unrelated donor (MUD) stem cell transplants may be effective therapy, but they carry the risk of significant graft versus host disease as well as the complications associated with intensive myeloablative therapy. MUD transplants are usually reserved for patients who have a relapse. However, patients with unfavorable prognostic features (e.g., monosomy 7 and 5, 5q-, and 11q23 abnormalities) who have inferior outcome with chemotherapy might benefit from MUD stem cell transplant in first remission.

Acute promyelocytic leukemia (FAB-M3), characterized by a gene rearrangement involving the retinoic acid receptor [t(15;17); PML-RARA], is very responsive to **all-*trans*-retinoic acid (tretinoin)** combined with anthracyclines and cytarabine. The success

Table 489-5 THERAPEUTIC IMPLICATIONS OF COMMON CHROMOSOMAL ABNORMALITIES IN PEDIATRIC ACUTE MYELOGENOUS LEUKEMIA AND MYELODYSPLASTIC SYNDROMES

CHROMOSOMAL ABNORMALITY	ALTERED GENES	USUAL MORPHOLOGY	PROGNOSIS	RECOMMENDED TREATMENT
t(8;21)	*AML1-ETO*	FAB AML-M2	Favorable	Intensive chemotherapy, including high-dose cytarabine
inv(16), t(16;16)	*CBFB-MYHII*	FAB AML-M4Eo	Favorable	Intensive chemotherapy, including high-dose cytarabine
t(15;17)	*PML-RARA*	FAB AML-M3	Favorable	Intensive chemotherapy, including tretinoin, cytarabine, and anthracyclines
t(11;17)	*PLZF-RARA*	FAB AML-M3	Unfavorable	Intensive chemotherapy, including tretinoin (?), cytarabine, and anthracyclines
11q23 abnormalities	*MLL* rearrangements	FAB AML-M4 or AML-M5	Unfavorable	Intensive chemotherapy, with high-dose cytarabine and MRD HSCT
t(3;v)	*EVI1*	MDS/AML	Unfavorable	Intensive chemotherapy with or without HSCT
t(3;5)	*NPM-MLF*	MDS/AMS	Unfavorable (?)	Intensive chemotherapy with or without HSCT
del(7q), -7	Unknown	MDS/FAB AML-M0	Unfavorable	Intensive chemotherapy with or without HSCT
del(5q), -5	Unknown	MDS/FAB AML-M0	Unfavorable	Intensive chemotherapy with or without HSCT

Modified from Nathan DG, Orkin SH, Ginsburg D, et al, editors: *Nathan and Oski's hematology of infancy and childhood,* ed 6, Philadelphia, 2003, WB Saunders, p 1177.
AML, acute myelogenous leukemia; FAB, French-American-British; HSCT, hematopoietic stem cells transplantation; MDS, myelodysplastic syndromes; MRD, matched related donor.

of this therapy makes marrow transplantation in first remission unnecessary for patients with this disease.

The supportive care needs of patients with AML are basically the same as those for patients with ALL. However, the very intensive therapy required in AML produces prolonged bone marrow suppression with a very high incidence of serious infections, especially streptococcal viridans sepsis and fungal infection.

The most current information on treatment of AML is available in the PDQ (Physician Data Query) on the National Cancer Institute website (*www.cancer.gov/cancertopics/pdq/treatment/childAML/healthprofessional/*).

BIBLIOGRAPHY

Please visit the Nelson Textbook of Pediatrics *website at* *www.expertconsult.com* *for the complete bibliography.*

489.3 Down Syndrome and Acute Leukemia and Transient Myeloproliferative Disorder

David G. Tubergen, Archie Bleyer, and A. Kim Ritchey

Acute leukemia occurs about 15-20 times more frequently in children with Down syndrome than in the general population (Chapter 76). The ratio of ALL to AML in patients with Down syndrome is the same as that in the general population. The exception is during the first 3 yr of life, when AML is more common. In children with Down syndrome who have ALL, the expected outcome of treatment is slightly inferior to that for other children. Patients with Down syndrome demonstrate a remarkable sensitivity to methotrexate and other antimetabolites, which can result in substantial toxicity if standard doses are administered. In AML, however, patients with Down syndrome have much better outcomes than non–Down syndrome children, with a >80% long-term survival rate. After induction therapy, these patients receive therapy that is less intensive to achieve better results.

Approximately 10% of neonates with Down syndrome develop a transient leukemia or **myeloproliferative disorder** characterized by high leukocyte counts, blast cells in the peripheral blood, and associated anemia, thrombocytopenia, and hepatosplenomegaly. These features usually resolve within the first 3 mo of life. Although these neonates can require temporary transfusion support, they do not require chemotherapy unless there is evidence of life-threatening complications. However, patients who have Down syndrome and who develop

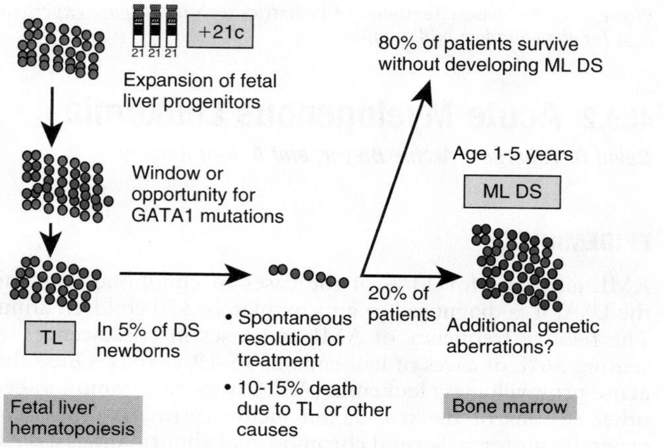

Figure 489-5 Stepwise development of myeloid leukemia in Down syndrome (ML DS) following transient leukemia (TL). TL arises from expanded fetal liver progenitors as a result of constitutional trisomy 21, providing a window of opportunity for the occurrence of acquired mutations in the hematopoietic transcription factor GATA1. In most cases TL spontaneously disappears, but some children need treatment because of severe TL-related symptoms. Approximately 20% of children with TL subsequently develop ML DS, which requires additional hits. (From Zwaan MC, Reinhardt D, Hitzler J, Vyas P: Acute leukemias in children with Down syndrome, *Pediatr Clin North Am* 55:53–70, 2008.)

this transient leukemia or myeloproliferative disorder require close follow-up, because 20-30% will develop typical leukemia (often acute megakaryocytic leukemia) by 3 yr of life (mean onset, 16 mo). *GATA1* mutations (a transcription factor that controls megakaryopoiesis) are present in blasts from patients with Down syndrome who have transient myeloproliferative disease and also in those with leukemia (Fig. 489-5 and see Table 489-5). Transient myeloproliferative disease also can occur in patients who do not have phenotypic features of Down syndrome. Blasts from these patients might have trisomy 21, suggesting a mosaic state.

BIBLIOGRAPHY

Please visit the Nelson Textbook of Pediatrics *website at* *www.expertconsult.com* *for the complete bibliography.*

489.4 Chronic Myelogenous Leukemia

David G. Tubergen, Archie Bleyer, and A. Kim Ritchey

CML is a clonal disorder of the hematopoietic tissue that accounts for 2-3% of all cases of childhood leukemia. About 99% of the cases are characterized by a specific translocation, t(9;22)(q34;q11), known as the **Philadelphia chromosome,** resulting in a *BCR-ABL* fusion protein. The disease is characterized clinically by an initial chronic phase in which the malignant clone produces an elevated leukocyte count with a predominance of mature forms but with increased numbers of immature granulocytes. The **spleen** is often greatly enlarged, resulting in pain in the left upper quadrant of the abdomen. In addition to leukocytosis, blood counts can reveal mild anemia and thrombocytosis.

Typically, the chronic phase terminates 3-4 yr after onset, when the CML moves into the accelerated or "blast crisis" phase. At this point, the blood counts rise dramatically and the clinical picture is indistinguishable from acute leukemia. Additional manifestations can occur, including hyperuricemia and neurologic symptoms from hyperleukocytosis, which causes increased blood viscosity with decreased CNS perfusion.

The presenting symptoms of CML are nonspecific and can include fever, fatigue, weight loss, and anorexia. Splenomegaly also may be present. The diagnosis is suggested by a high white blood count with myeloid cells at all stages of differentiation in the peripheral blood and bone marrow and is confirmed by cytogenetic and molecular studies that demonstrate the presence of the characteristic Philadelphia chromosome and the *BCR-ABL* gene rearrangement. This translocation, although characteristic of CML, is also found in a small percentage of patients with ALL.

Imatinib mesylate (Gleevec), an agent designed specifically to inhibit the *BCR-ABL* tyrosine kinase, has been used in adults and has shown an ability to produce major cytogenetics responses in >70% of patients (see Table 488-1). Experience in children suggests it can be used safely with results comparable to those seen in adults. While waiting for a response with imatinib, disabling or threatening signs and symptoms of CML can be controlled during the chronic phase with hydroxyurea, which gradually returns the leukocyte count to normal. Prolonged morphologic and cytogenetic responses are expected, but the opportunity for cure is enhanced by HLA-matched family donor allogeneic stem cell transplant, with up to 80% of children achieving a cure.

BIBLIOGRAPHY

Please visit the Nelson Textbook of Pediatrics *website at www.expertconsult.com for the complete bibliography.*

489.5 Juvenile Myelomonocytic Leukemia

David G. Tubergen, Archie Bleyer, and A. Kim Ritchey

Juvenile myelomonocytic leukemia (JMML), formerly termed **juvenile chronic myelogenous leukemia,** is a clonal proliferation of hematopoietic stem cells that typically affects children <2 yr of age. Patients with this disease do not have the Philadelphia chromosome that is characteristic of CML. Patients with JMML present with rashes, lymphadenopathy, splenomegaly, and hemorrhagic manifestations. Analysis of the peripheral blood often shows an elevated leukocyte count with increased monocytes, thrombocytopenia, and anemia with the presence of erythroblasts. The bone marrow shows a myelodysplastic pattern, with blasts accounting for <30% of cells. No distinctive cytogenetic abnormalities are seen. JMML is rare, constituting <1% of all cases of childhood leukemia. Patients with neurofibromatosis type 1 and Noonan syndrome have a predilection for this type of leukemia. Therapeutic reports are largely anecdotal. Stem cell transplantation offers the best opportunity for cure but much less so than for classic CML.

BIBLIOGRAPHY

Please visit the Nelson Textbook of Pediatrics *website at www.expertconsult.com for the complete bibliography.*

489.6 Infant Leukemia

David G. Tubergen, Archie Bleyer, and A. Kim Ritchey

About 2% of cases of leukemia during childhood occur before the age of 1 yr. In contrast to older children, the ratio of ALL to AML is 2:1. Some cases may be due to maternal exposure to naturally occurring DNA topoisomerase II inhibitors. Leukemic clones have been noted in cord blood at birth before symptoms apear, and in one case the same clone was noted in maternal cells (maternal to fetal transmission). Chromosome translocations can also occur in utero during fetal hematopoiesis, thus leading to malignant clone formation.

Several unique biologic features and a particularly poor prognosis are characteristic of ALL during infancy. More than 80% of the cases demonstrate rearrangements of the *MLL* gene, found at the site of the 11q23 band translocation, the majority of which are the t(4;11). This subset of patients largely accounts for the very high relapse rate. These patients often present with hyperleukocytosis and extensive tissue infiltration producing organomegaly, including CNS disease. Subcutaneous nodules, known as **leukemia cutis,** and tachypnea due to diffuse pulmonary infiltration by leukemic cells are observed more often in infants than in older children. The leukemic cell morphology is usually that of large irregular lymphoblasts (FAB L2), with a phenotype negative for the CD10 (cALLa) marker (pro-B).

Very intensive chemotherapy programs including stem cell transplantation are being explored in infants with MLL gene rearrangements, but none has yet proved satisfactory. Infants with leukemia who lack the 11q23 rearrangements have a prognosis similar to that of older children with ALL.

Infants with AML often present with CNS or skin involvement and have the FAB M4 subtype, which is commonly known as **acute myelomonocytic leukemia.** The treatment may be the same as that for older children with AML, with similar outcome. Meticulous supportive care is necessary because of the young age and aggressive therapy needed in these patients.

BIBLIOGRAPHY

Please visit the Nelson Textbook of Pediatrics *website at www.expertconsult.com for the complete bibliography.*

Chapter 490*
Lymphoma

Ian M. Waxman, Jessica Hochberg, and Mitchell S. Cairo

Lymphoma is the third most common cancer among U.S. children (age ≤14 yr), with an annual incidence of 15 cases per million children. It is the most common cancer in adolescents, accounting for >25% of newly diagnosed cancers in persons 15 to 19 yr old. The two broad categories of lymphoma, Hodgkin lymphoma (HL) and non-Hodgkin lymphoma (NHL), have different clinical manifestations and treatments.

490.1 Hodgkin Lymphoma

Ian M. Waxman, Jessica Hochberg, and Mitchell S. Cairo

HL is a malignant process of the lymphoreticular system that accounts for 6% of childhood cancers. In the USA, HL accounts for about 5% of cancers in persons ≤14 yr of age and for about

*The views expressed are the result of independent work and do not necessarily represent the views or findings of the U.S. Food and Drug Administration or the United States.

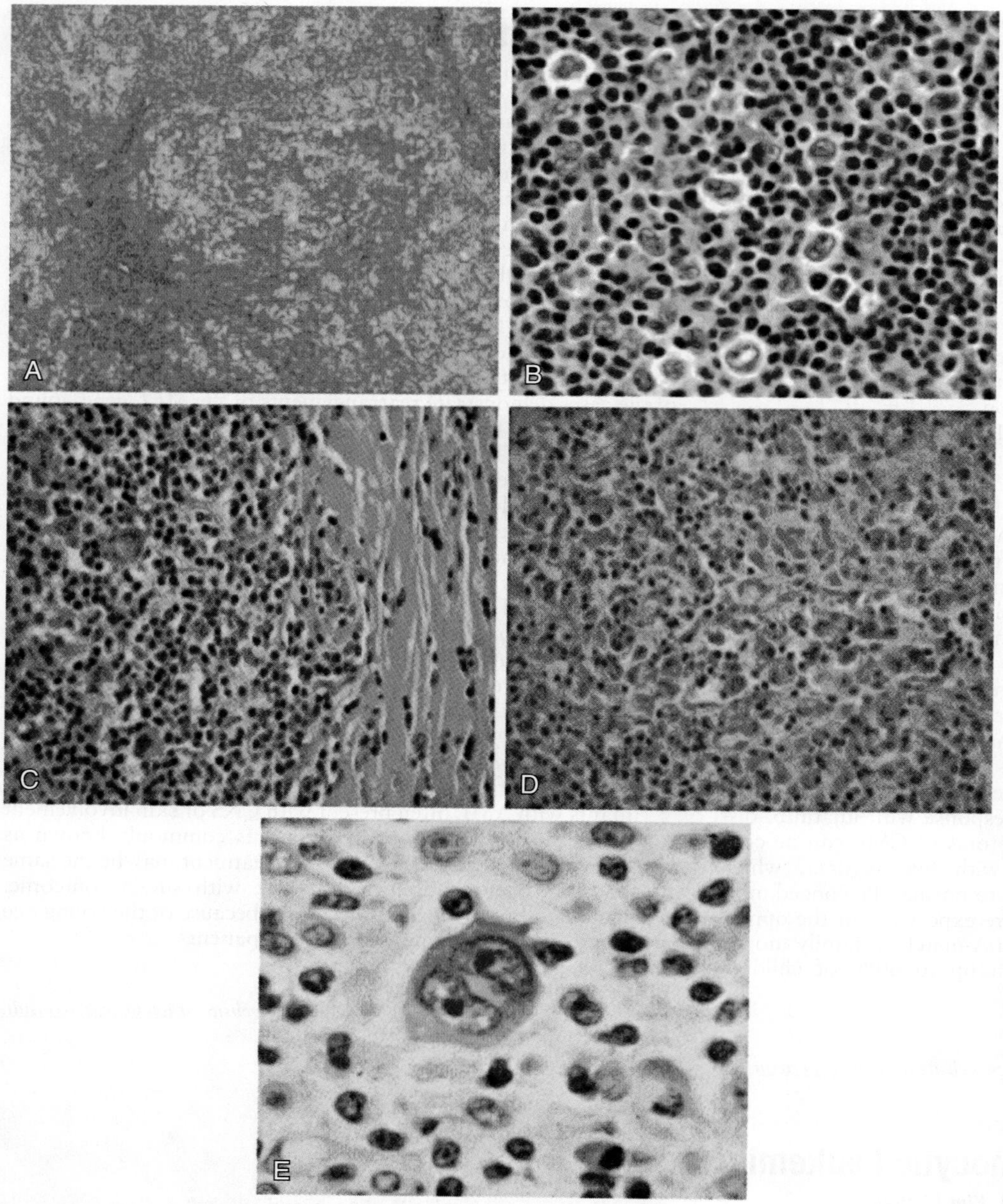

Figure 490-1 Histologic subtypes of Hodgkin lymphoma. *A,* Hematoxylin & eosin stains of nodular lymphocyte-predominant Hodgkin lymphoma (NLPHL) demonstrating a nodular proliferation with a moth-eaten appearance. *B,* High-power view demonstrating the neoplastic L and H cells found in NLPHL. *C,* Classic Hodgkin lymphoma, nodular sclerosis subtype. Large mononuclear and binucleate Reed-Sternberg cells are seen admixed in the inflammatory cell background. *D,* Classic Hodgkin lymphoma, mixed cellularity subtype, demonstrating increased numbers of Reed-Sternberg cells in a mixed inflammatory background without sclerotic changes. *E,* High-power view of a classic Reed-Sternberg cell showing binucleate cells with prominent eosinophilic nucleoli and relatively abundant cytoplasm.

15% of cancers in adolescents, making HL the most common malignancy in this age group (15-19 yr). It is rare in children <10 yr of age.

EPIDEMIOLOGY

The worldwide incidence of HL is approximately 2-4 new cases/100,000 population/year; there is a bimodal age distribution, with peaks at 15-35 yr of age and again after 50 yr. In developing countries, the early peak tends to occur prior to adolescence. A male:female predominance is found among young children but lessens with age. Several studies suggest that infectious agents may be involved, such as human herpes virus 6, cytomegalovirus, and **Epstein-Barr virus (EBV)**. The role of EBV is supported by prospective serologic studies and confers a fourfold higher risk of developing HL and may precede the diagnosis by years. EBV antigens have been demonstrated in HL tissues, although EBV status is not prognostic of outcome.

PATHOGENESIS

The **Reed-Sternberg (RS) cell,** a pathognomonic feature of HL, is a large cell (15-45 µm in diameter) with multiple or multilobulated nuclei. This cell type is considered the hallmark of HL, although similar cells are seen in infectious mononucleosis, NHL, and other conditions. The Reed-Sternberg cell is clonal in origin and arises from the germinal center B cells. HL is characterized by a variable number of RS cells surrounded by an inflammatory infiltrate of lymphocytes, plasma cells, and eosinophils in different proportions, depending on the HL histologic subtype. Other features that distinguish the histologic subtypes include various degrees of fibrosis and the presence of collagen bands, necrosis, or malignant reticular cells (Fig. 490-1). The distribution of subtypes varies with age (Fig. 490-2).

The **Revised World Health Organization (WHO) Classification of Lymphoid Neoplasms** (Table 490-1) includes two modifications of the older Rye system. HL appears to arise in lymphoid

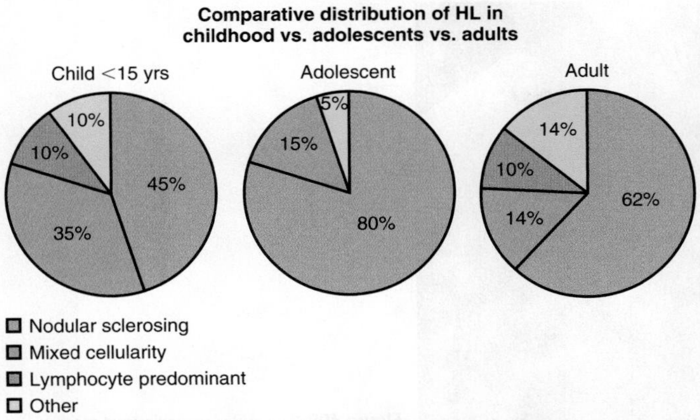

Figure 490-2 Comparative distribution of Hodgkin lymphoma in children, adolescents, and adults. (Adapted from Hochberg J, Waxman IM, Kelly KM, et al: Adolescent non-Hodgkin lymphoma and Hodgkin lymphoma: state of the science, *Br J Haematol* 144:24–40, 2008.)

Table 490-1 NEW WORLD HEALTH ORGANIZATION/REVISED EUROPEAN-AMERICAN CLASSIFICATION OF LYMPHOID NEOPLASMS CLASSIFICATION SYSTEM FOR HODGKIN LYMPHOMA

Nodular lymphocyte predominance
Classical Hodgkin lymphoma
Lymphocyte rich
Mixed cellularity
Nodular sclerosis
Lymphocyte depletion

From Harris NL, Jaffe ES, Diebold J, et al: The World Health Organization classification of neoplastic diseases of the haematopoietic and lymphoid tissues: report of the Clinical Advisory Committee Meeting, Airlie House, Virginia, November 1997, *Histopathology* 36:69–87, 2000.

tissue and spreads to adjacent lymph node areas in a relatively orderly fashion. Hematogenous spread also occurs, leading to involvement of the liver, spleen, bone, bone marrow, or brain, and is usually associated with systemic symptoms.

CLINICAL MANIFESTATIONS

Patients commonly present with painless, nontender, firm, rubbery, cervical or supraclavicular lymphadenopathy and usually some degree of mediastinal involvement. Clinically detectable hepatosplenomegaly is rarely encountered. Depending on the extent and location of nodal and extranodal disease, patients may present with symptoms and signs of airway obstruction (dyspnea, hypoxia, cough), pleural or pericardial effusion, hepatocellular dysfunction, or bone marrow infiltration (anemia, neutropenia, or thrombocytopenia). Disease manifesting below the diaphragm is rare and occurs in approximately 3% of all cases. Systemic symptoms, classified as **B symptoms** that are considered important in staging, are unexplained fever >39°C, weight loss >10% total body weight over 3 mo, and drenching night sweats. Less common and not considered of prognostic significance are symptoms of pruritus, lethargy, anorexia, or pain that worsens after ingestion of alcohol. Patients also exhibit immune system abnormalities that often persist during and after therapy.

DIAGNOSIS

Any patient with persistent, unexplained lymphadenopathy unassociated with an obvious underlying inflammatory or infectious process should undergo chest radiography to identify the presence of a large mediastinal mass before undergoing lymph node biopsy. Formal excisional biopsy is preferred over needle biopsy to ensure that adequate tissue is obtained, both for light microscopy and for appropriate immunohistochemical and molecular

Table 490-2 ANN ARBOR STAGING CLASSIFICATION FOR HODGKIN LYMPHOMA*

STAGE	DEFINITION
I	Involvement of a single lymph node (I) or of a single extralymphatic organ or site (I_E)
II	Involvement of two or more lymph node regions on the same side of the diaphragm (II) or localized involvement of an extralymphatic organ or site and one or more lymph node regions on the same side of the diaphragm (II_E)
III	Involvement of lymph node regions on both sides of the diaphragm (III), which may be accompanied by involvement of the spleen (III_S) or by localized involvement of an extralymphatic organ or site (III_E) or both (III_{SE})
IV	Diffuse or disseminated involvement of one or more extralymphatic organs or tissues with or without associated lymph node involvement

*The absence or presence of fever >38°C for 3 consecutive days, drenching night sweats, or unexplained loss of ≥10% of body weight in the 6 months preceding admission are to be denoted in all cases by the suffix letter A or B, respectively.
From Lister TA, Crowther D, Sutcliffe SB, et al: Report of a committee convened to discuss the evaluation and staging of patients with Hodgkin's disease: Cotswolds meeting, *J Clin Oncol* 7:1630–1636, 1989.

studies. Once the diagnosis of HL is established, extent of disease (stage) should be determined to allow selection of appropriate therapy (Table 490-2). Evaluation includes history, physical examination, and imaging studies, including chest radiograph; CT scans of the chest, abdomen, and pelvis; and either gallium scan or positron emission tomography (PET) scan. Laboratory studies should include a complete blood cell count (CBC) to identify abnormalities that might suggest marrow involvement; erythrocyte sedimentation rate (ESR); and measurement of serum ferritin, which is of some prognostic significance and, if abnormal at diagnosis, serves as a baseline to evaluate the effects of treatment. A chest radiograph is particularly important for measuring the size of the mediastinal mass in relation to the maximal diameter of the thorax (Fig. 490-3). This determines "bulk" disease and becomes prognostically significant. Chest CT more clearly defines the extent of a mediastinal mass if present and identifies hilar nodes and pulmonary parenchymal involvement, which may not be evident on chest radiographs (Fig. 490-4). Bone marrow aspiration and biopsy should be performed to rule out advanced disease. Bone scans are performed in patients with bone pain and/or elevation of alkaline phosphatase. Gallium scan can be particularly helpful in identifying areas of increased uptake, which can then be re-evaluated at the end of treatment. Fluorodeoxyglucose (FDG)–PET imaging has advantages over gallium scanning, as it is a 1-day procedure with higher resolution, better dosimetry, less intestinal activity, and the potential to quantify disease. PET scans are being evaluated as a prognostic tool in HL enabling therapy to be reduced in those predicted to have a good outcome.

The staging classification currently used for HL was adopted at the **Ann Arbor Conference** in 1971 and was revised in 1989 (see Table 490-2). HL can be subclassified into A or B categories: *A* is used to identify asymptomatic patients and *B* is for patients who exhibit any B symptoms. Extralymphatic disease resulting from direct extension of an involved lymph node region is designated by category E. A complete response in HL is defined as the complete resolution of disease on clinical examination and imaging studies or at least 70-80% reduction of disease and a change from initial positivity to negativity on either gallium or PET scanning because residual fibrosis is common.

TREATMENT

Multiple agents allow different mechanisms of action to have non-overlapping toxicities so that full doses can be given to each patient. Chemotherapy and radiation therapy are both effective

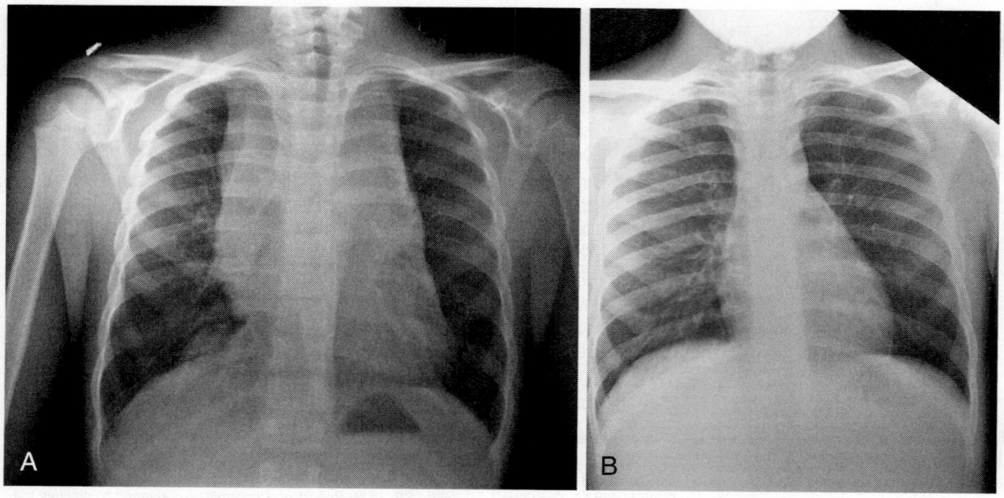

Figure 490-3 *A,* Anterior mediastinal mass in a patient with Hodgkin disease before therapy. *B,* After 2 mo of chemotherapy, the mediastinal mass has disappeared.

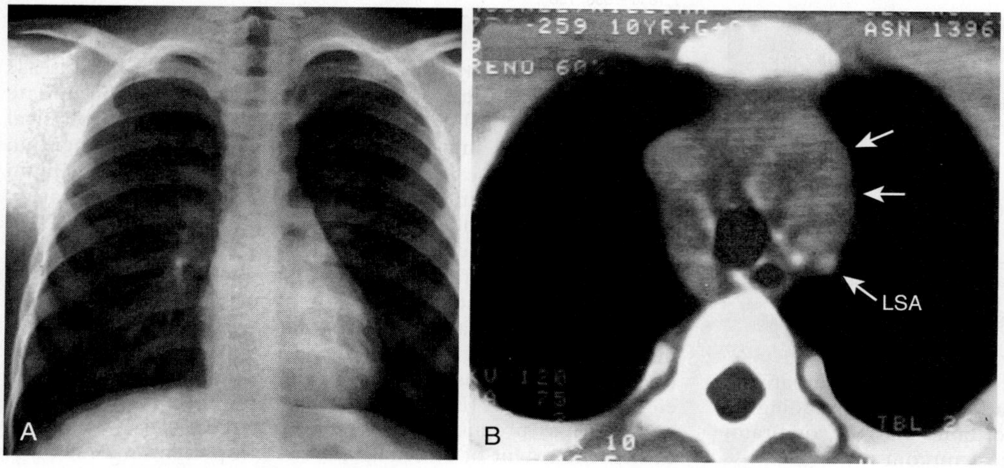

Figure 490-4 CT for the diagnosis of mediastinal disease in Hodgkin lymphoma. *A,* Chest radiograph, findings of which were interpreted as normal. *B,* Contrast-enhanced CT scan reveals marked widening of the mediastinum by an irregular enhancing mass (*arrows*) that is displacing the great vessels posteriorly. Right-sided paratracheal adenopathy is also present posterior to the superior vena cava. LSA, left subclavian artery. (From Slovis TL, editor: *Caffey's pediatric diagnostic imaging,* ed 11, vol 1, Philadelphia, 2008, Mosby/Elsevier.)

in the treatment of HL. Current treatment of HL in pediatric patients is risk adapted and involves the use of combined chemotherapy with or without low-dose involved-field radiation therapy based on response. Treatment is determined largely by disease stage, presence or absence of B symptoms, and the presence of bulky nodal disease. Radiation therapy alone, once given at higher doses, initially resulted in prolonged remission and cure rates in patients with low-stage HL. However, this treatment approach also caused significant long-term morbidity in pediatric patients, including growth retardation, thyroid dysfunction, and cardiac and pulmonary toxicity. The development of effective multiagent combination chemotherapy was a major milestone in the treatment of HL resulting in a complete response rate of 70-80% and cure rate of 40-50% in patients with advanced stage disease. However, as with radiation therapy, this regimen also led to significant acute and long-term toxicity. The desire to reduce side effects and morbidity has stimulated attempts to reduce the intensity of chemotherapy as well as radiation dose and volume. Newer combinations of chemotherapy have reduced the risk of secondary cancers. Also, current radiation therapy utilizes lower amounts of overall radiation in addition to narrowing the radiation treatment field to either involved-field or even involved-node irradiation. The current Children's Oncology Group trials are investigating whether radiation therapy can be eliminated altogether in patients who have a very good rapid early response to pre-radiation induction chemotherapy.

Chemotherapy agents commonly used to treat children and adolescents with HL include cyclophosphamide, procarbazine, vincristine or vinblastine, prednisone or dexamethasone, doxorubicin, bleomycin, dacarbazine, etoposide, methotrexate, and cytosine arabinoside. The combination chemotherapy regimens in current use are based on **COPP** (cyclophosphamide, vincristine [Oncovin], procarbazine, and prednisone) or **ABVD** (doxorubicin [Adriamycin], bleomycin, vinblastine, and dacarbazine), with the addition of prednisone, cyclophosphamide and etoposide (**ABVE-PC** and **BEACOPP**) in various combinations for intermediate- and high-risk groups (Table 490-3). "Risk-adapted" protocols are based on staging criteria as well as rapidity of response to initial chemotherapy. The aim is to reduce total drug doses and treatment duration and to eliminate radiation therapy if possible.

Newer agents such as those that disrupt the nuclear factor-κB (NF-κB) pathway or monoclonal antibodies that target RS tumor cells as well as the benign reactive cells that surround them are currently being investigated. Ongoing clinical trials report encouraging results with the use of anti-CD20 antibody (rituximab). In addition, anti-CD30 agents are being used that are targeted to the RS cells themselves, where CD30 is abundantly expressed. EBV-specific cytotoxic lymphocytes (CTLs) can be generated from patients with advanced HL. In clinical trials, these show promising results, with enhanced antiviral activity and stabilization of disease even though all patients have continued to have persistent disease. Still, this approach represents an exciting direction in adoptive cellular tumor immunology, and success may come with CTLs that have improved cytotoxicity that can overcome inhibitory signals.

Table 490-3 CHEMOTHERAPY REGIMENS COMMONLY USED FOR CHILDREN, ADOLESCENTS, AND YOUNG ADULTS WITH HODGKIN LYMPHOMA

CHEMOTHERAPY REGIMEN	CORRESPONDING AGENTS
ABVD	Doxorubicin (Adriamycin), bleomycin, vinblastine, dacarbazine
ABVE (DBVE)	Doxorubicin (Adriamycin), bleomycin, vincristine, etoposide
VAMP	Vincristine, doxorubicin (Adriamycin), methotrexate, prednisone
OPPA ± COPP (females)	Vincristine (Oncovin), prednisone, procarbazine, doxorubicin (Adriamycin), cyclophosphamide, vincristine (Oncovin), prednisone, procarbazine
OEPA ± COPP (males)	Vincristine (Oncovin), etoposide, prednisone, doxorubicin (Adriamycin), cyclophosphamide, vincristine (Oncovin), prednisone, procarbazine
COPP/ABV	Cyclophosphamide, vincristine (Oncovin), prednisone, procarbazine, doxorubicin (Adriamycin), bleomycin, vinblastine
BEACOPP (advanced stage)	Bleomycin, etoposide, doxorubicin (Adriamycin), cyclophosphamide, vincristine (Oncovin), prednisone, procarbazine
COPP	Cyclophosphamide, vincristine (Oncovin), prednisone, procarbazine
CHOP	Cyclophosphamide, doxorubicin (Adriamycin), vincristine (Oncovin), prednisone
ABVE-PC (DBVE-PC)	Doxorubicin (Adriamycin), bleomycin, vincristine, etoposide, prednisone, cyclophosphamide

RELAPSE

Most relapses occur within the first 3 yr after diagnosis, but relapses as late as 10 yr have been reported. Relapse cannot be predicted accurately with this disease. Poor prognostic features include tumor bulk, stage at diagnosis, and presence of B symptoms. Patients who never achieve remission or suffer relapse <12 mo after initiation of therapy are candidates for myeloablative chemotherapy and autologous stem cell transplantation with or without the addition of radiation therapy. This treatment is most successful in patients with chemoresponsive disease. Myeloablative allogeneic stem cell transplantation reduces the relapse rate in patients with high-risk relapsed or refractory HL. There was no improvement in overall survival in the studies reported, owing to a high transplant-related mortality. These results do suggest a graft versus HL effect. The use of nonmyeloablative, nontoxic regimens to reduce regimen-related morbidity and mortality associated with myeloablative allogeneic stem cell transplantation but still achieve a graft versus HL effect is under investigation.

PROGNOSIS

With the use of current therapeutic regimens, patients with favorable prognostic factors and early-stage disease have an event-free survival (EFS) of 85-90% and an overall survival (OS) at 5 yr >95%. Patients with advanced stage disease have slightly lower EFS (80-85%) and OS o (90%), respectively, although OS has approached 100% with dose-intense chemotherapy (Table 490-4). Prognosis after relapse depends on the time from completion of treatment to recurrence, site of relapse (nodal vs. extranodal), and presence of B symptoms at relapse. Patients whose disease relapses >12 mo after chemotherapy alone or combined-modality therapy have the best prognosis, and their relapses usually respond to additional standard therapy, resulting in a long-term survival of 60-70%. A myeloablative autologous stem cell transplantation in patients with refractory disease or relapse within 12 mo of therapy results in a long-term survival rate of 40-50%.

BIBLIOGRAPHY

Please visit the Nelson Textbook of Pediatrics *website at www.expertconsult.com for the complete bibliography.*

490.2 Non-Hodgkin Lymphoma

Ian M. Waxman, Jessica Hochberg, and Mitchell S. Cairo

NHL accounts for approximately 60% of all lymphomas in children and adolescents. It represents 8-10% of all malignancies in children between 5 and 19 yr of age, with an annual incidence in the USA of 750-800 cases/yr in children ≤19 yr of age. Although >70% of patients present with advanced disease at diagnosis, the prognosis has improved dramatically, with survival rates of 90-95% for localized disease and 60-90% with advanced disease.

EPIDEMIOLOGY

Although most children and adolescents with NHL present with de novo disease, a small number of patients have NHL secondary to specific etiologies, including inherited or acquired immune deficiencies (e.g., severe combined immunodeficiency syndrome, Wiskott-Aldrich syndrome), viruses (e.g., HIV, EBV), and as part of genetic syndromes (e.g., ataxia-telangiectasia, Bloom syndrome). Most children in whom NHL develops have no obvious genetic or environmental etiology.

PATHOGENESIS

The four major pathologic subtypes of childhood and adolescent NHL are **Burkitt lymphoma (BL), lymphoblastic lymphoma (LL), diffuse large B-cell lymphoma (DLBCL),** and **anaplastic large cell lymphoma** (ALCL; Figs. 490-5 and 490-6). DLBCL is further divided into several subtypes: the germinal center B-cell like (GCB), which carries a favorable prognosis and accounts for the vast majority of pediatric cases of DLBCL, and the subtypes with poorer prognosis, activated B cell–like (ABC) and primary mediastinal B-cell (PMB) subtypes. Pediatric NHL is usually high grade and very aggressive, whereas adult NHL is generally less aggressive or indolent. Almost all forms of BL and DLBCL are of B-cell origin; 80% cases of LL are of T-cell origin, and 20% of B-cell origin; and 70% of cases of ALCL are of T-cell origin, 20% of null-cell origin, and 10% of B-cell origin. Some pathologic subtypes have specific cytogenetic aberrations. Children with BL commonly have a t(8;14) translocation (90%) or, less commonly, a t(2;8) or t(8;22) translocation (10%), whereas those with DLBCL may have a t(8;14) translocation (30%) and often have a complex (80%) and aneuploid (80%) karyotype. Patients with ALCL commonly have a t(2;5) translocation (90%), which results in the formation of a fusion gene encoding the constitutively active NPM-ALK tyrosine kinase. Variant ALK translocations, all with a breakpoint at 2p23, have also been reported. T-cell LBL harbors many of the same cytogenetic abnormalities as T-cell acute lymphoblastic leukemia (ALL), including rearrangements with breakpoints at 14q11.2 involving the T-cell receptor, and t(5;14) translocation (20%), which does not involve the 14q11.2 breakpoint.

CLINICAL MANIFESTATIONS

The clinical manifestations of childhood and adolescent NHL depend primarily on pathologic subtype and primary and secondary sites of involvement. Tumors grow rapidly and can cause symptoms based on size and location. Approximately 70% of patients with NHL present with advanced disease, at stage III or IV (Table 490-5), including extranodal disease with gastrointestinal, bone marrow, and central nervous system (CNS)

Table 490-4 Treatment Regimens and Outcome by Disease Staging

		LOCALIZED/LOW STAGE	INTERMEDIATE	ADVANCED
Hodgkin lymphoma	Treatment	*POG study 9426/ GPOH-HD 95:* ABVD type therapy ± IFRT (risk adapted based on early response to chemotherapy)	*Stanford/DAL-HD-90:* COPP-based or dose intense multiagent chemotherapy + low-dose RT *POG 9426/CCG 5942:* ABVD type therapy ± IFRT (risk adapted)	*POG 8725/ DAL-HD-90:* Dose intense multiagent chemotherapy + low-dose RT *HD9/HD12/CCG 59704:* Dose intense BEACOPP ± IFRT
	Prognosis	5-yr EFS: 85-90% 5-yr OS: 95%	*Stanford/DAL-HD-90:* 5-yr EFS: 89-92% *POG 9426/CCG 5942:* 5-yr EFS: 84% 5-yr OS: 91%	*POG 8725:* 5-yr EFS: 72-89% (age based) *DAL-HD-90:* 5-yr EFS: 86% 5-yr OS: 85-90% *HD9/HD12/ CCG 59704:* 5-yr EFS/OS: 88-93/~100%
Burkitt lymphoma & diffuse large B-cell lymphoma	Treatment	*FAB/LMB 96 Group A therapy:* Complete surgical resection followed by 2 cycles of chemotherapy	*FAB/LMB 96 Group B* therapy with reduced cyclophosphamide and no maintenance therapy	*FAB/LMB 96:* standard-intensity Group C therapy: Reduction, induction, intensification, and maintenance therapy
	Prognosis	4-yr EFS: 98% (CI_{95} 94-99.5%) 4-yr OS: 99% (CI_{95} 96-99.9%)	4-yr EFS: 92% (CI_{95} 90-94%) 4-yr OS: 95% (CI_{95} 93-96%) *PMB DLBCL has worse prognosis (OS: 70%)	4-yr EFS: BM+/CNS−: 91% ± 3% BM−/CNS+: 85% ± 6% BM+/CNS+: 66% ± 7%
Lymphoblastic lymphoma	Treatment	*NHL-BFM86/90/95:* *COG A5971:* ALL-type therapy × 2 yr without prophylactic cranial RT	No intermediate group; disease classified as localized (stage I/II) or advanced (stage III/IV)	*NHL-BFM86/90/95, St. Jude NHL 13:* ALL-type therapy × 2 yr ± px CRT *CCG 5941:* Intensive chemotherapy × 1 yr + cranial RT if CNS + at diagnosis
	Prognosis	*COG A5971:* 5-yr EFS: 85 ± 7.5% 5-yr OS: 94 ± 4%	No intermediate group; see above	*NHL-BFM95:* 5-yr EFS: 90% ± 3% (III), 95 ± 5% (IV) *St. Jude NHL 13:* 5-yr EFS/OS: 83% ± 6%/90% ± 5% *CCG 5941:* 5-yr EFS/OS: 78% ± 5%/85% ± 4%
Anaplastic large cell lymphoma	Treatment	*EICHNL ALCL 99:* Short intensive chemotherapy + HD MTX *Completely resected stage I disease may be treated with surgery alone	No intermediate group; disease classified as standard-risk (no skin, visceral or mediastinal involvement) or high-risk (presence of skin, mediastinal, or visceral involvement)	*EICHNL ALCL 99, CCG 5941:* Short intensive chemo + HD MTX
	Prognosis	*EICHNL database:* 5-yr PFS: 89% (CI_{95} 82-96%) 5-yr OS: 94% (CI_{95} 89-99%)	No intermediate group; see above	*EICHNL database:* 5-yr PFS: 61%(CI_{95} 53-59%) 5-yr OS: 73% (CI_{95} 90-94%)

ABVD, doxorubicin (Adriamycin), bleomycin, vinblastine, dacarbazine; ALCL, anaplastic large cell lymphoma; BEACOPP, bleomycin, etoposide, doxorubicin (Adriamycin), cyclophosphamide, vincristine (Oncovin), prednisone, procarbazine; BM, bone marrow (involvement); CI_{95}, 95% confidence interval; CNS, central nervous system (involvement); COPP, cyclophosphamide, vincristine (Oncovin), prednisone, procarbazine; CRT, chemoradiotherapy; EFS, event-free survival; EICHNL, European Intergroup for Childhood Non-Hodgkin Lymphoma; HD MTX, high-dose methotrexate; IFRT, involved field radiation therapy; MTX, methotrexate; NHL-BFM, non-Hodgkin lymphoma Berlin-Frankfurt-Munster; OS, overall survival; PFS, progression-free survival; px, prophylactic; RT, radiation therapy; PMB DLBCL, primary mediastinal B-cell diffuse large B-cell lymphoma.

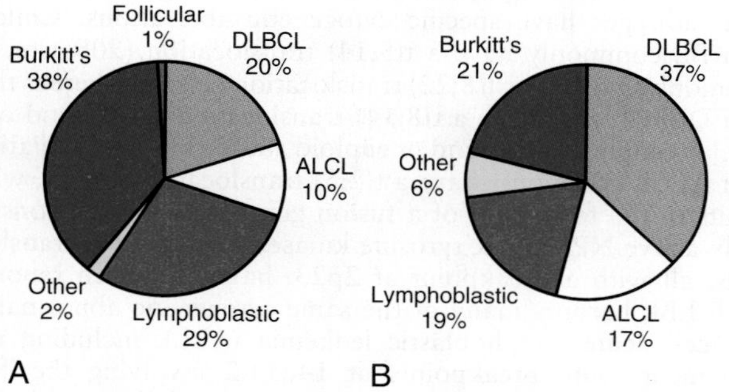

Figure 490-5 Incidence of non-Hodgkin lymphoma subtypes in *(A)* 0-14 yr age group and *(B)* 15-19 yr age group. ALCL, anaplastic large cell lymphoma; DLBCL, diffuse large B-cell lymphoma. (Adapted from Hochberg J, Waxman IM, Kelly KM, et al: Adolescent non-Hodgkin lymphoma and Hodgkin lymphoma: state of the science, *Br J Haematol* 144:24–40, 2008.)

involvement. BL commonly manifests as abdominal (sporadic type) or head and neck (endemic type) disease with involvement of the bone marrow or CNS. LL commonly manifests as an intrathoracic or mediastinal supradiaphragmatic mass and also has a predilection for spreading to the bone marrow and CNS. DLBCL commonly manifests as either an abdominal or mediastinal (PMB subtype) primary and, rarely, dissemination to the bone marrow or CNS. ALCL manifests either as a primary cutaneous manifestation (10%) or as systemic disease (fever, weight loss) with dissemination to liver, spleen, lung, mediastinum, or skin; spread to the bone marrow or CNS is rare. Patients have also been staged according to risk classification in pediatric international cooperative group trials Table 490-6.

Site-specific manifestations include painless, rapid lymph node enlargement; cough, superior mediastinal syndrome (SMS), dyspnea with thoracic involvement; abdominal (massive and rapidly enlarging) mass, intestinal obstruction, intussusception-like symptoms, ascites with abdominal involvement; nasal stuffiness, earache, hearing loss, tonsil enlargement with Waldeyer ring involvement; and localized bone pain (primary or metastatic).

Three **clinical manifestations that require special alternative treatment strategies** are SMS symptoms secondary to a large mediastinal mass obstructing blood flow or respiratory airways; acute paraplegias secondary to spinal cord or CNS compression from neighboring tumor; and tumor lysis syndrome (TLS) secondary to severe metabolic abnormalities, including hyperuricemia, hyperphosphatemia, hyperkalemia, and hypocalcemia from massive tumor cell lysis.

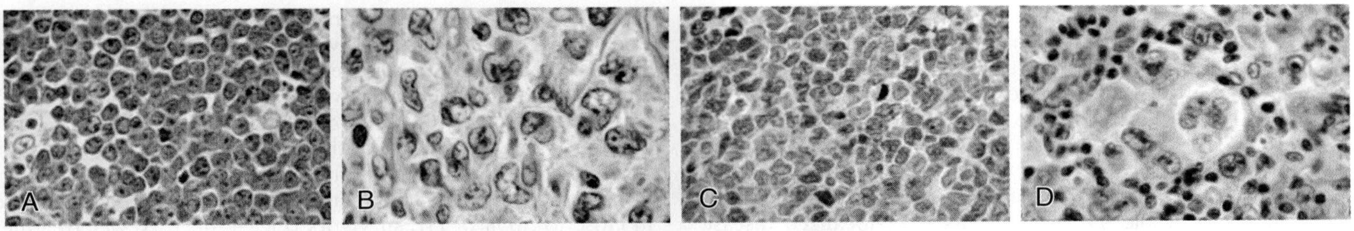

Figure 490-6 Distribution of childhood and adolescent non-Hodgkin lymphoma. Hematoxylin & eosin stains showing morphology of Burkitt lymphoma (*A,* high power), diffuse large B-cell lymphoma (*B,* high power), precursor T-lymphoblastic lymphoma (*C,* high power), and anaplastic large cell lymphoma (*D,* high power). (From Cairo MS, Raetz E, Lim MS, et al: Childhood and adolescent non-Hodgkin lymphoma: new insights in biology and critical challenges for the future, *Pediatr Blood Cancer* 45:753–769, 2005.)

Table 490-5 ST. JUDE STAGING SYSTEM FOR CHILDHOOD NON-HODGKIN LYMPHOMA

STAGE	DESCRIPTION
I	A single tumor (extranodal) or single anatomic area (nodal), with the exclusion of mediastinum or abdomen
II	A single tumor (extranodal) with regional node involvement
	Two or more nodal areas on the same side of the diaphragm
	Two single (extranodal) tumors with or without regional node involvement on the same side of the diaphragm
	A primary gastrointestinal tract tumor, usually in the ileocecal area, with or without involvement of associated mesenteric nodes only, which must be grossly (>90%) resected
III	Two single tumors (extranodal) on opposite sides of the diaphragm
	Two or more nodal areas above and below the diaphragm
	Any primary intrathoracic tumor (mediastinal, pleural, or thymic)
	Any extensive primary intra-abdominal disease
IV	Any of the above, with initial involvement of central nervous system or bone marrow at time of diagnosis

From Murphy SB: Classification, staging and end results of treatment of childhood non-Hodgkin's lymphomas: dissimilarities from lymphomas in adults, *Semin Oncol* 7:332–339, 1980.

Table 490-6 RISK STRATIFICATION GROUPS FOR PEDIATRIC B-CELL NHL

	Berlin-Frankfurt-Munster (BFM)	French-American-British (FAB)
Low Risk	**R1** Stage I or II, completely resected	**Group A** Resected stage I and abdominal completely resected stage II
↓	**R2** Stage I or II, not resected; Stage III with LDH <500 U/L	
	R3 Stage III with LDH ≥500 to <1000 U/L or Stage IV with LDH <1000 U/L and CNS-negative	**Group B** All patients not in Group A or C
High Risk	**R4** Stage III or IV with LDH ≥1000 U/L and/or CNS-positive	**Group C** Bone marrow disease (≥25% L3 blasts) and/or CNS-positive

CNS, central nervous system; LDH, lactate dehydrogenase.

LABORATORY FINDINGS

Recommended laboratory and radiologic testing includes: CBC; measurements of electrolytes, uric acid, calcium, phosphorus, blood urea nitrogen, creatinine, bilirubin, alanine aminotransferase, and aspartate aminotransferase; bone marrow aspiration and biopsy; lumbar puncture with cerebrospinal fluid (CSF) cytology, cell count and protein; chest radiographs; and neck, chest, abdominal, and pelvic CT scans (head CT for suspicion of CNS disease), and PET scan. Tumor tissue (i.e., biopsy, bone marrow, CSF, or pleurocentesis/paracentesis fluid) should be tested by flow cytometry for immunophenotypic origin (T, B, or null) and cytogenetics (karyotype). Additional tests might include fluorescent in situ hybridization (FISH) or quantitative reverse transcription polymerase chain reaction (RT-PCR) for specific genetic translocations, T- and B-cell gene rearrangement studies, and molecular profiling by oligonucleotide microarray.

TREATMENT

The primary modality of treatment for childhood and adolescent NHL is **multiagent systemic chemotherapy with intrathecal chemotherapy**. Surgery is used mainly for diagnosis and staging. Radiation therapy is used only in special circumstances, such as when there is CNS involvement in LL or, occasionally, BL and in the presence of acute SMS and acute paraplegias. Newly diagnosed patients and those otherwise at risk for TLS (usually advanced/bulky BL or LL) require vigorous hydration and either a xanthine oxidase inhibitor (allopurinol, 10 mg/kg/day PO divided tid) or, more often, recombinant urate oxidase (rasburicase, 0.2 mg/kg/day IV once daily up to 5 days).

Specific treatment for localized and advanced disease is similar for BL and DLBCL (see Table 490-4). Localized BL or DLBCL requires 6 wk to 6 mo of multiagent chemotherapy. Complete surgical resection followed by 2 cycles of COPAD (cyclophosphamide, vincristine, prednisone, and doxorubicin) led to a 4-yr overall survival (OS) in the international FAB/LMB 96 (French-American-British Lymphoma, mature B cell) trial. Advanced disease is usually treated with a 4- to 6-mo regimen of multiagent chemotherapy, such as FAB/LMB 96 protocol therapy or NHL-BFM (Berlin-Frankfurt-Munich) 95 protocol therapy.

Localized or advanced LL usually requires almost 24 mo of therapy. The best results in advanced LL have been obtained using the NHL-BFM90 protocol, which uses therapeutic approaches similar to those for childhood acute leukemia, including induction, consolidation, interim maintenance, and re-induction (advanced disease only) phases as well as a year-long maintenance phase with 6-mercaptopurine and methotrexate.

Localized ALCL may require only cutaneous excision or more aggressive therapy similar to that for advanced ALCL. Advanced ALCL is commonly treated with NHL-BFM90 protocol–type therapy.

Intrathecal chemotherapy is administered in the presence of moderate to advanced disease in all subtypes of childhood and adolescent NHL and may include methotrexate, hydrocortisone, or Ara-C.

Patients with NHL in whom progressive or relapsed disease develops require re-induction chemotherapy and either allogeneic or autologous stem cell transplantation. The specific re-induction regimen or transplant type depends on the pathologic subtype, previous therapy, site or reoccurrence, and stem cell donor availability.

COMPLICATIONS

Patients receiving multiagent chemotherapy for advanced disease are at acute risk for serious mucositis, infections, cytopenias that require red blood cell and platelet blood product transfusions, electrolyte imbalances, and poor nutrition. Long-term complications may include growth retardation, cardiac toxicity, gonadal toxicity with infertility, and secondary malignancies.

PROGNOSIS

The prognosis is excellent for most forms of childhood and adolescent NHL (see Table 490-4). Patients with localized disease have a 90-100% chance of survival, and those with advanced disease have a 60-95% chance of survival. The variation in survival depends on pathologic subtype, tumor burden at diagnosis as reflected in serum lactate dehydrogenase (LDH) level, presence or absence of CNS disease, and specific sites of metastatic spread. Specific cytogenetic and molecular genetic subtyping may also be important in predicting outcome and influencing specific therapeutic strategies.

BIBLIOGRAPHY

Please visit the Nelson Textbook of Pediatrics *website at www.expertconsult.com for the complete bibliography.*

490.3 Late Effects in Children and Adolescents with Lymphoma

Ian M. Waxman, Jessica Hochberg, and Mitchell S. Cairo

The majority of patients with newly diagnosed HL and NHL have overall survival rates well above 90%. However, this survival has often been achieved at the expense of an increased relative risk of long-term complications, including solid tumors, leukemia, cardiac disease, pulmonary complications, thyroid disease, and infertility. An analysis of >1,000 long-term childhood NHL survivors found increased rates of death >20 yr after treatment. A review of Surveillance, Epidemiology and End Results (SEER) data over a 25-yr follow-up period has demonstrated that the relative survival curves do not plateau after 10 yr following diagnosis of HL but, rather, accelerate. This finding highlights the importance of late morbidity and mortality among survivors of lymphoma. The first Childhood Cancer Survivor Study, a retrospective cohort study of 10,397 cancer survivors, showed that 62.3% of survivors report at least one chronic condition; with 27.5% reporting severe or life-threatening conditions. The survivor's adjusted relative risk of a severe or life-threatening chronic condition, compared with that of a sibling, was 8.2 (95% confidence interval [CI], 6.9- 9.7). When disease-specific health outcomes were looked at, both HL and NHL were found to be associated with a cumulative incidence of chronic health conditions approaching 70-80%, with severe conditions being reported in close to 50% of HL survivors (Fig. 490-7). Newer treatment strategies continue to be investigated to address the morbidity and consequences survivors of childhood lymphoma must face when undergoing treatment.

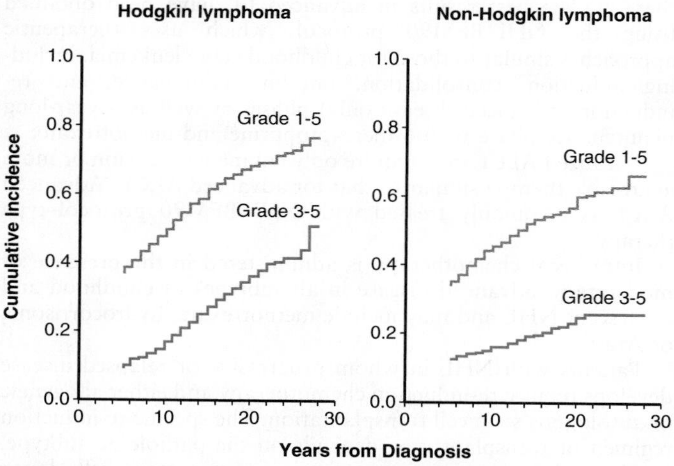

Figure 490-7 Incidence of chronic health conditions in adult survivors of pediatric cancer. Among the survivors of Hodgkin lymphoma and non-Hodgkin lymphoma, the severity of subsequent health conditions was scored according to the National Cancer Institute's Common Terminology Criteria for Adverse Events (version 3) as either mild (grade 1), moderate (grade 2), severe (grade 3), life-threatening or disabling (grade 4), or fatal (grade 5). (Adapted from Oeffinger KC, Mertens AC, Sklar CA, et al: Chronic health conditions in adult survivors of childhood cancer, *N Engl J Med* 355:1572–1582, 2006.)

Chapter 491 Brain Tumors in Childhood

John F. Kuttesch, Jr., Sarah Zieber Rush, and Joann L. Ater

Primary central nervous system (CNS) tumors are a heterogeneous group of diseases that are, collectively, the second most common malignancy in childhood and adolescence. The overall mortality among this group approaches 4.5%. Patients with CNS tumors have the highest morbidity—primarily neurologic—of all children with malignancies. Outcomes have improved over time with innovations in neurosurgery and radiation therapy as well as introduction of chemotherapy as a therapeutic modality. The treatment approach for these tumors is multimodal. Surgery with complete resection, if feasible, is the foundation, with radiation therapy and chemotherapy utilized according to the diagnosis, patient age, and other factors.

ETIOLOGY

The etiology of pediatric brain tumors is not well defined. A male predominance is noted in the incidence of medulloblastoma and ependymoma. Familial and hereditary syndromes associated with increased incidence of brain tumors account for approximately 5% of cases (Table 491-1). Cranial exposure to ionizing radiation also is associated with a higher incidence of brain tumors. There are sporadic reports of brain tumors within families without evidence of a heritable syndrome. The molecular events associated with tumorigenesis of pediatric brain tumors are not known.

EPIDEMIOLOGY

Approximately 3700 primary brain tumors are diagnosed each year in children and adolescents, with an overall annual incidence of approximately 45 cases/million children <20 yr of age. The incidence of CNS tumors is highest in infants and children ≤5 yr of age (approximately 52 cases/million children).

PATHOGENESIS

More than 100 histologic categories and subtypes of primary brain tumors are described in the World Health Organization (WHO) classification of tumors of the CNS. In children 0-14 yr, the most common tumors are pilocytic astrocytomas (PAs) and medulloblastoma/primitive neuroectodermal tumors (PNETs). In adolescents (15-19 yr), the most common tumors are pituitary tumors and PAs (Fig. 491-1).

The Childhood Brain Tumor Consortium reported a slight predominance of infratentorial tumor location (43.2%), followed by the supratentorial location (40.9%), spinal cord (4.9%), and multiple sites (11%) (Fig. 491-2, Table 491-2). There are age-related differences in primary location of tumor. During the first year of life, supratentorial tumors predominate and include, most commonly, choroid plexus complex tumors and teratomas. In children 1-10 yr of age, infratentorial tumors predominate, owing to the high incidence of juvenile pilocytic astrocytoma and medulloblastoma. After 10 yr of age, supratentorial tumors again predominate, with diffuse astrocytomas most common. Tumors of the optic pathway and hypothalamus region, the brainstem, and the pineal-midbrain region are more common in children and adolescents than in adults.

CLINICAL MANIFESTATIONS

The clinical presentation of the patient with a brain tumor depends on the tumor location, the tumor type, and the age of the child. Signs and symptoms are related to obstruction of cerebrospinal fluid (CSF) drainage paths by the tumor, leading to **increased intracranial pressure** (**ICP**) or causing focal brain dysfunction. Subtle changes in personality, mentation, and speech may precede these classic signs and symptoms; such changes often occur with supratentorial (cortical) lesions. In young children, the diagnosis of a brain tumor may be delayed because the symptoms are similar to those of more common illnesses, such as gastrointestinal disorders. Infants with open cranial sutures may present with signs of increased ICP, such as vomiting, lethargy, and irritability, as well as the later finding of macrocephaly. The **classic triad** headache, nausea, and vomiting as well as papilledema are associated with midline or infratentorial tumors. Disorders of equilibrium, gait, and coordination occur with infratentorial tumors. **Torticollis** may result in cerebellar tonsil herniation. Blurred vision, diplopia, and nystagmus also are associated with infratentorial tumors. Tumors of the brainstem region may be associated with gaze palsy, multiple cranial nerve palsies, and upper motor neuron deficits (e.g., hemiparesis, hyperreflexia, clonus). **Supratentorial tumors** are more commonly associated with focal disorders such as motor weaknesses, sensory changes, speech disorders, seizures, and reflex abnormalities. Infants with supratentorial tumors may present with hand preference. Optic pathway tumors manifest as visual disturbances, such as decreased visual acuity, Marcus Gunn pupil (afferent pupillary defect), nystagmus, and/or visual field defects. Suprasellar region tumors and third ventricular region tumors may manifest initially as **neuroendocrine deficits,** such as diabetes insipidus, galactorrhea, precocious puberty, delayed puberty, and hypothyroidism. The **diencephalic syndrome,** which manifests as failure to thrive, emaciation, increased appetite, and euphoric affect, occurs in infants and young children with tumors in these regions. **Parinaud syndrome** is seen with pineal region tumors and is manifested by paresis of upward gaze, pupillary dilation reactive to accommodation but not to light, nystagmus to convergence or retraction, and eyelid retraction. Spinal cord tumors and spinal cord dissemination of brain tumors may manifest as long nerve tract motor and/or sensory deficits, bowel and bladder deficits, and back or radicular pain. The signs and symptoms of meningeal metastatic disease from brain tumors or leukemia are similar to those of infratentorial tumors.

Table 491-1 FAMILIAL SYNDROMES ASSOCIATED WITH PEDIATRIC BRAIN TUMORS

SYNDROME	CENTRAL NERVOUS SYSTEM MANIFESTATIONS	CHROMOSOME	GENE
Neurofibromatosis type 1 (autosomal dominant)	Optic pathway gliomas, astrocytoma, malignant peripheral nerve sheath tumors, neurofibromas	17q11	*NF1*
Neurofibromatosis type 2 (autosomal dominant)	Vestibular schwannomas, meningiomas, spinal cord ependymoma, spinal cord astrocytoma, hamartomas	22q12	*NF2*
von Hippel–Lindau (autosomal dominant)	Hemangioblastoma	3p25-26	*VHL*
Tuberous sclerosis (autosomal dominant)	Subependymal giant cell astrocytoma, cortical tubers	9q34	*TSC1*
		16q13	*TSC2*
Li-Fraumeni (autosomal dominant)	Astrocytoma, primitive neuroectodermal tumor	17q13	*TP53*
Cowden (autosomal dominant)	Dysplastic gangliocytoma of the cerebellum (Lhermitte-Duclos disease)	10q23	*PTEN*
Turcot (autosomal dominant)	Medulloblastoma	5q21	*APC*
	Glioblastoma	3p21	*hMLH1*
		7p22	*hPSM2*
Nevoid basal cell carcinoma (autosomal dominant)	Medulloblastoma	9q31	*PTCH*

Modified from Kleihues P, Cavenee WK: *World Health Organization classification of tumors: pathology and genetics of tumors of the nervous system,* Lyon, 2000, IARC Press.

DIAGNOSIS

The evaluation of a patient in whom a brain tumor is suspected is an emergency. Initial evaluation should include a complete

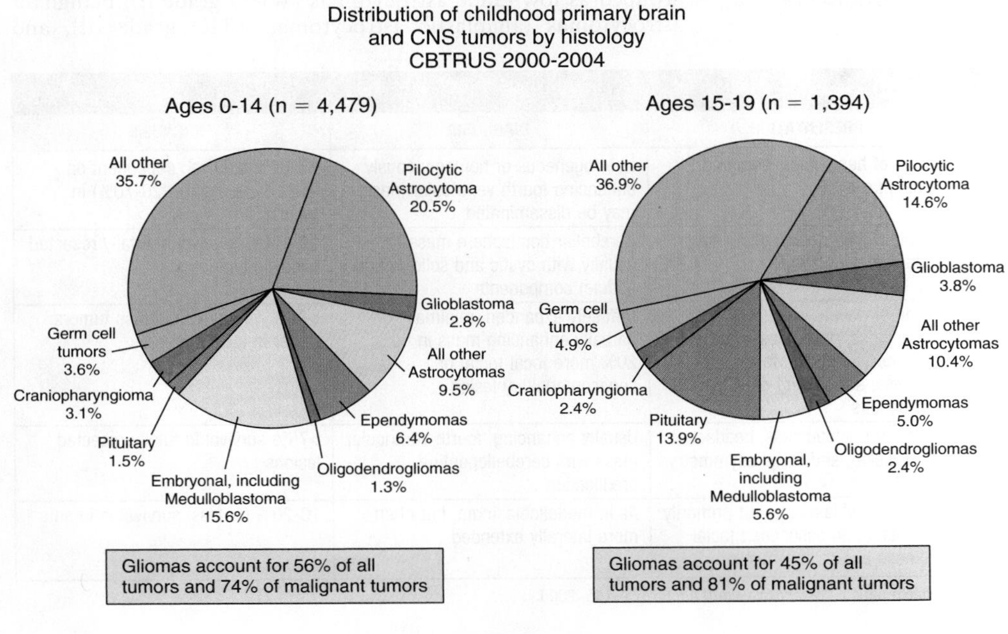

Figure 491-1 Distribution of childhood primary brain and CNS tumors by histology. (From Central Brain Tumor Registry of the United States [CBTRUS]: *CBTRUS statistical report: primary brain and central nervous system tumors diagnosed in the United States in 2004-2006: February 2010* (PDF file). www.cbtrus.org/2010-NPCR-SEER/CBTRUS-WEBREPORT-Final-3-2-10.pdf. Accessed March 19, 2011.)

history, physical (including ophthalmic) examination, and neurologic assessment with neuroimaging. For primary brain tumors, **MRI** is the neuroimaging standard. Tumors in the pituitary/suprasellar region, optic path, and infratentorium are better delineated with MRI than with CT. Patients with tumors of the midline and the pituitary/suprasellar/optic chiasmal region should undergo evaluation for **neuroendocrine dysfunction.** Formal ophthalmologic examination is beneficial in patients with optic path region tumors to document the impact of the disease on oculomotor function, visual acuity, and fields of vision. The suprasellar region and pineal region are preferential sites for germ cell tumors. Both serum and CSF measurements of **β-human chorionic gonadotropin** and **α-fetoprotein** can assist in the diagnosis of germ cell tumors. In tumors with a propensity for spreading to the leptomeninges, such as medulloblastoma/PNET, ependymoma, and germ cell tumors, lumbar puncture with cytologic analysis of the CSF is indicated; lumbar puncture is contraindicated in individuals with newly diagnosed hydrocephalus secondary to CSF flow obstruction, in tumors that cause supratentorial midline shift, and in individuals with infratentorial tumors. Lumbar puncture in these individuals may lead to brain herniation, resulting in neurologic compromise and death. Therefore,

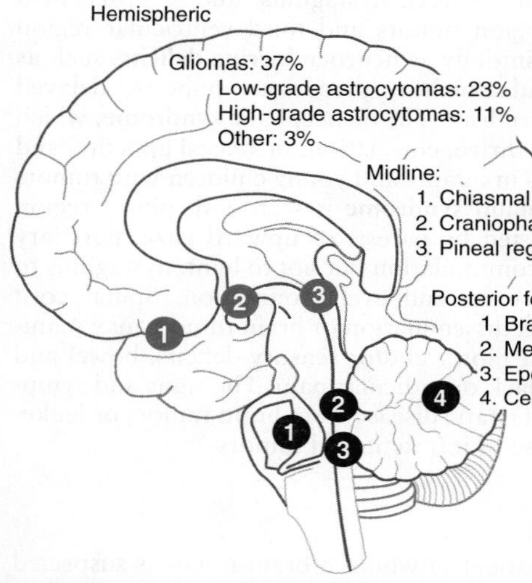

Figure 491-2 Childhood brain tumors occur at any location within the central nervous system. The relative frequency of brain tumor histologic types and the anatomic distribution are shown. (Redrawn from Albright AL: Pediatric brain tumors, *CA Cancer J Clin* 43:272–288, 1993.)

in children with newly diagnosed intracranial tumors and signs of increased ICP, the lumbar puncture usually is delayed until surgery or shunt placement.

SPECIFIC TUMORS

Astrocytomas

Astrocytomas are a heterogeneous group of pediatric CNS tumors that account for approximately 40% of cases. These tumors occur throughout the CNS.

Low-grade astrocytomas (LGAs), the predominant group of astrocytomas in childhood, are characterized by an indolent clinical course. **PA** is the most common astrocytoma in children, accounting for about 20% of all brain tumors (Fig. 491-3). On the basis of clinicopathologic features using the WHO Classification System, PA is classified as a WHO grade I tumor. Although PA can occur anywhere in the CNS, the classic site is the **cerebellum.** Other common sites include the hypothalamic/third ventricular region and the optic nerve and chiasmal region. The classic but not exclusive neuroradiologic finding in PA is the presence of a contrast medium–enhancing nodule within the wall of a cystic mass (see Fig. 491-3). The microscopic findings include the biphasic appearance of bundles of compact fibrillary tissue interspersed with loose microcystic, spongy areas. The presence of **Rosenthal fibers,** which are condensed masses of glial filaments occurring in the compact areas, helps establish the diagnosis. PA has a low metastatic potential and is rarely invasive. A small proportion of these tumors can progress and develop leptomeningeal spread, particularly when they occur in the optic path region. A PA very rarely undergoes malignant transformation to a more aggressive tumor. A PA of the optic nerve and chiasmal region is a relatively common finding in patients with neurofibromatosis type 1 (15% incidence). Unlike in diffuse fibrillary astrocytomas, there are no characteristic cytogenetic abnormalities in PA nor are there any known molecular abnormalities. Other tumors occurring in the pediatric age group with clinicopathologic characteristics similar to those of PA include pleomorphic xanthoastrocytoma, desmoplastic cerebral astrocytoma of infancy, and subependymal giant cell astrocytoma.

The second most common astrocytoma is **fibrillary infiltrating astrocytoma,** which consists of a group of tumors characterized by a pattern of diffuse infiltration of tumor cells among normal neural tissue and potential for anaplastic progression. On the basis of their clinicopathologic characteristics, they are grouped as low-grade astrocytomas (WHO grade II), malignant astrocytomas (anaplastic astrocytoma; WHO grade III), and

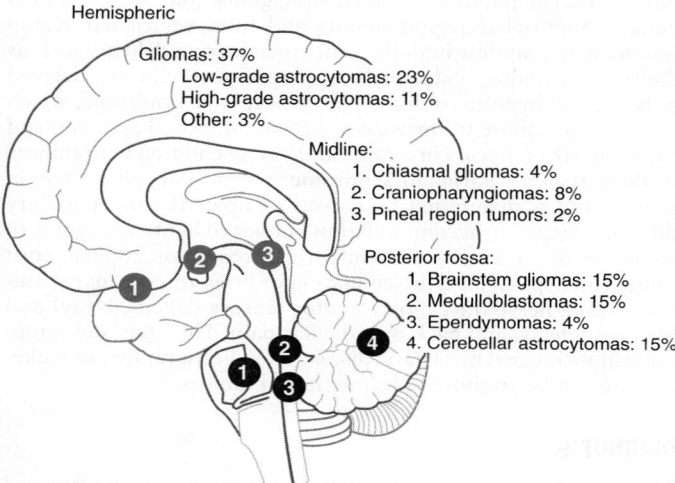

Table 491-2 POSTERIOR FOSSA TUMORS OF CHILDHOOD

TUMOR	RELATIVE INCIDENCE (%)	PRESENTATION	DIAGNOSIS	PROGNOSIS
Medulloblastoma	35-40	2-3 mo of headaches, vomiting, truncal ataxia	Heterogeneous or homogeneously enhancing fourth ventricular mass; may be disseminated	65-85% survival; dependent on stage/type; poorer (20-70%) in infants
Cerebellar astrocytoma	35-40	3-6 mo of limb ataxia; secondary headaches, vomiting	Cerebellar hemisphere mass, usually with cystic and solid (mural nodule) components	90-100% survival in totally resected pilocytic type
Brain stem glioma	10-15	1-4 mo of double vision, unsteadiness, weakness, and other cranial nerve deficits, facial weakness, swallowing deficits, and other deficits	Diffusely expanded, minimally or partially enhancing mass in 80%; 20% more focal tectal or cervicomedullary lesion	>90% mortality in diffuse tumors; better in localized
Ependymoma	10-15	2-5 mo of unsteadiness, headaches, double vision, and facial asymmetry	Usually enhancing, fourth ventricular mass with cerebellopontine predilection	>75% survival in totally resected lesions
Atypical teratoid/rhabdoid	>5 (10-15% of infantile malignant tumors)	As in medulloblastoma, but primarily in infants; often associated facial weakness and strabismus	As in medulloblastoma, but often more laterally extended	10-20% (or less) survival in infants

Modified from Packer RJ, MacDonald T, Vezina G: Central nervous system tumors, *Pediatr Clin North Am* 55:121–145, 2008.

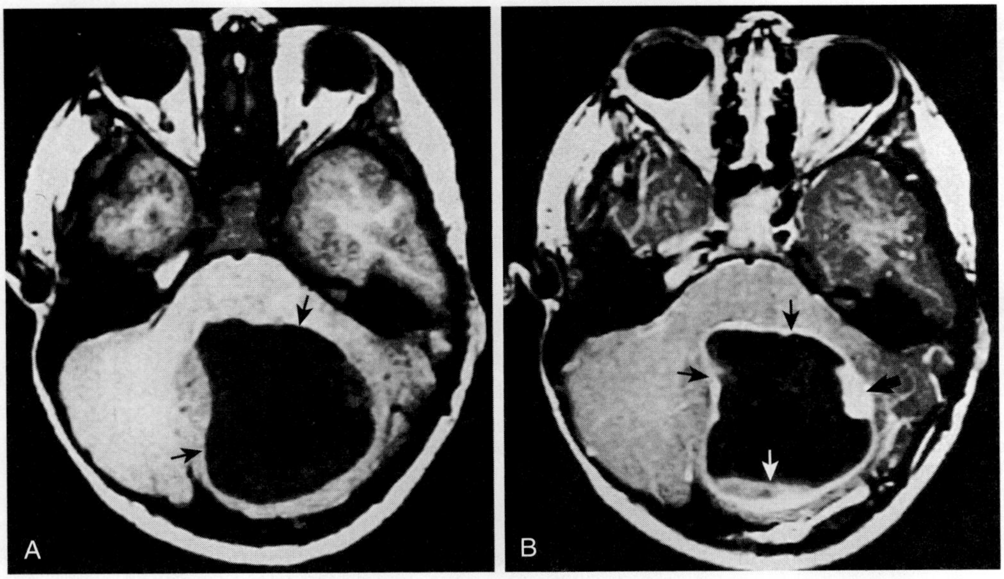

Figure 491-3 *A,* Axial T1-weighted MR image of a patient with cerebellar pilocytic astrocytoma, demonstrating predominantly cystic (hypointense) component *(arrows)* involving the left cerebellar hemisphere and vermis. *B,* Gadolinium-enhanced axial T1-weighted MR image in the same child demonstrates enhancement of the solid component *(large arrow),* enhancement of the capsule *(small black arrows),* and layering of contrast material *(white arrow)* at the bottom of the cyst. (From Kuhn JP, Slovis TL, Haller JO: *Caffey's pediatric diagnostic imaging,* ed 10, Philadelphia, 2004, Mosby, p 576.)

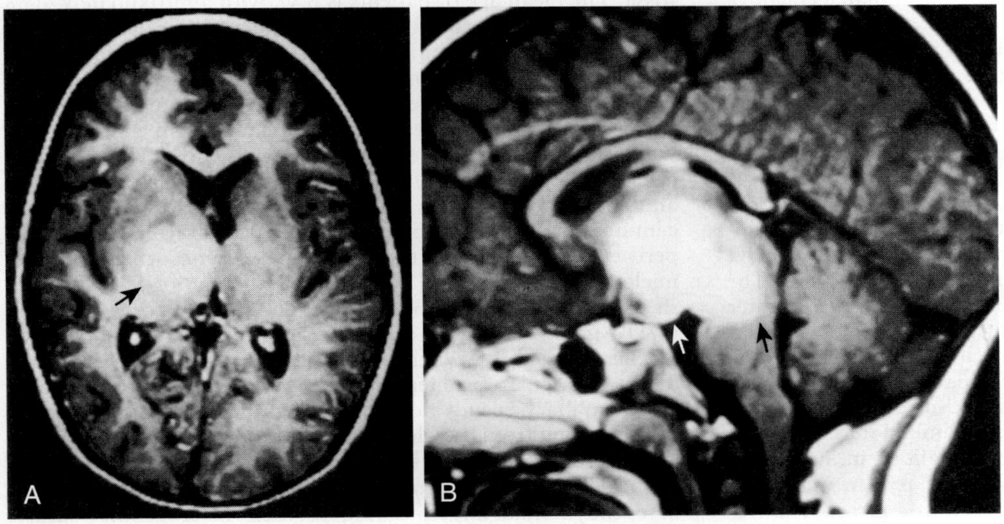

Figure 491-4 *A,* Gadolinium-enhanced axial T1-weighted MR image of grade III astrocytoma of the right thalamus demonstrating diffuse enhancement *(arrow). B,* Gadolinium-enhanced sagittal T1-weighted MR image showing enhancement of grade III astrocytoma of the thalamus with extension into the midbrain *(black arrow)* and hypothalamus *(white arrow).* (From Kuhn JP, Slovis TL, Haller JO: *Caffey's pediatric diagnostic imaging,* ed 10, Philadelphia, 2004, Mosby, p 595.)

glioblastoma multiforme (GBM; WHO grade IV). Of this group, the fibrillary LGA is the second most common astrocytoma in children, accounting for 15% of brain tumors. Histologically, these low-grade tumors demonstrate greater cellularity than normal brain parenchyma, with few mitotic figures, nuclear pleomorphism, and microcysts. The characteristic MRI finding is a lack of enhancement after contrast agent infusion (Fig. 491-4). Molecular genetic abnormalities found among low-grade diffuse infiltrating astrocytomas include mutations of p53 and overexpression of platelet-derived growth factor α-chain and platelet-derived growth factor receptor-α. **Fibrillary infiltrating astrocytoma** has the potential to evolve into malignant astrocytoma, a development that is associated with cumulative acquisition of multiple molecular abnormalities.

Pilomyxoid astrocytoma occurs most commonly in the hypothalamic/optic chiasmic region and carries a high risk of local as well as cerebrospinal spread. This astrocytoma affects young children and infants. It is classified as a WHO grade II tumor.

The **clinical management** of LGAs focuses on a multimodal approach incorporating surgery as the primary treatment as well as radiation therapy and chemotherapy. The outcome of PA is better than with fibrillary LGAs. With complete surgical resection the overall survival approaches 80-100%. In patients with partial resection (<80% resection), overall survival varies from 50% to 95%, depending on the anatomic location of the tumor. In the patient who has undergone partial tumor resection and has stable neurologic status, the current approach is to follow the patient closely by examination and imaging. With evidence of progression, and second surgical resection should be considered. In patients in whom a second procedure was less than complete or is not feasible, radiation therapy is beneficial. Radiation therapy is delivered to the tumor bed at a total cumulative dose ranging from 50 to 55 Gy given on a daily schedule over 6 wk. Historically, patients with deep midline tumors were treated empirically, with radiation therapy and without surgery or biopsy, with variable survival rates from 33% to 75%. Modern surgical techniques and innovative radiation therapy methodology may have a positive impact on the survival and clinical outcome of these patients. The role of chemotherapy in the management of LGAs is evolving. Because of concerns regarding morbidity from radiation therapy in young children, several chemotherapy approaches have been evaluated, especially in children <5 yr of age. Complete response to chemotherapy is uncommon; however, these approaches have yielded durable control of disease in 70-100% of patients. Patients with midline tumors in the hypothalamic/optic chiasmatic region have tended to do less well. Taken together, the chemotherapy approaches have permitted delay and, potentially, avoidance of radiation therapy. Chemotherapy agents

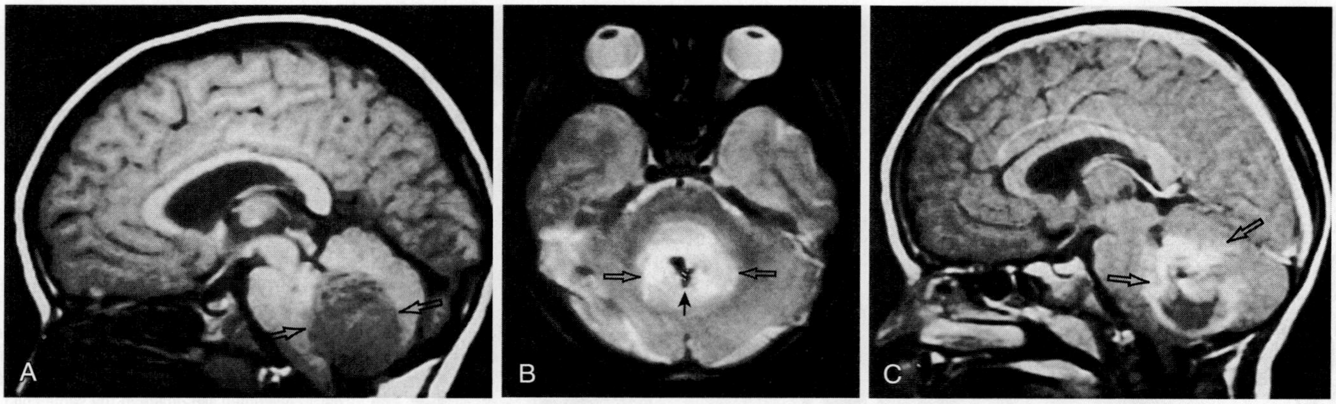

Figure 491-5 *A,* Sagittal T1-weighted MR image of a patient with ependymoma, demonstrating a hypointense mass *(arrows)* within the fourth ventricle. *B,* Axial T2-weighted image of an ependymoma showing a hyperintense mass *(open arrows)* and a hypointense central area of calcification *(closed arrow)* within the fourth ventricle. *C,* Gadolinium-enhanced sagittal T1-weighted image demonstrating an ependymoma *(arrows).* (From Kuhn JP, Slovis TL, Haller JO: *Caffey's pediatric diagnostic imaging,* ed 10, Philadelphia, 2004, Mosby, p 579.)

given singly or in combination in LGA include carboplatin, vincristine, temozolomide, vinblastine, lomustine, and procarbazine. Observation is the primary approach in clinical management of selected patients with LGAs that are biologically indolent. One such group includes patients with neurofibromatosis type 1, in whom an LGA of the optic chiasm/optic pathway or brainstem may develop; it is found incidentally. Another group includes patients with midbrain astrocytomas who have resolution of clinical symptoms after ventricular shunting and do not require further intervention.

Malignant astrocytomas are much less common in children and adolescents than in adults, accounting for 7-10% of all childhood tumors. Among this group, **anaplastic astrocytoma** (WHO grade III) is more common than **GBM** (WHO grade IV). The histopathology of anaplastic astrocytomas demonstrates greater cellularity than that of low-grade diffuse astrocytomas, cellular and nuclear atypia, presence of mitoses, and, variably, microvascular proliferation. Characteristic histopathologic findings in GBM include dense cellularity, high mitotic index, microvascular proliferation, and foci of tumor necrosis. Limited information is available regarding the molecular abnormalities in malignant astrocytomas in children. Overexpression of p53 in malignant astrocytoma in a child is an adverse prognostic factor. The frequency of mutations in p53 as well as loss of heterozygosity at 19q and 22q in childhood malignant astrocytomas is similar to that noted in adults, although the frequency of such mutations in malignant astrocytomas of children <3 yr of age is lower. This finding suggests differing mechanisms of oncogenesis in younger and older children. Optimal therapeutic approaches for malignant astrocytomas have yet to be defined. Standard therapy continues to be surgical resection followed by involved-field radiation therapy. A study of adult glioblastoma showed significantly better survival with temozolomide during and after irradiation than with irradiation alone. Current therapeutic approaches incorporate novel therapeutic agents with radiation therapy.

Oligodendrogliomas are uncommon tumors of childhood. These infiltrating tumors occur predominantly in the cerebral cortex and originate in the white matter. Histologically, oligodendrogliomas consist of rounded cells with little cytoplasm and microcalcifications. Observation of a **calcified cortical mass** on CT in a patient presenting with a seizure is suggestive of oligodendroglioma. Treatment approaches are similar to those for infiltrating astrocytomas.

Ependymal Tumors

Ependymal tumors are derived from the ependymal lining of the ventricular system. Ependymoma (WHO grade II) is the most common of these neoplasms, occurring predominantly in childhood and accounting for 10% of childhood tumors. Approximately 70% of ependymomas in childhood occur in the posterior fossa. The mean age of patients is 6 yr, with approximately 40% of cases occurring in children <4 yr of age. The incidence of leptomeningeal spread approaches 10% overall. Clinical presentation can be insidious and often depends on the anatomic location of the tumor. MRI demonstrates a well-circumscribed tumor with variable and complex patterns of gadolinium enhancement, with or without cystic structures (Fig. 491-5). These tumors usually are noninvasive, extending into the ventricular lumen and/or displacing normal structures, sometimes leading to significant obstructive hydrocephalus. Histologic characteristics include perivascular pseudorosettes, ependymal rosettes, monomorphic nuclear morphology, and occasional nonpalisading foci of necrosis. Other histologic subtypes include anaplastic ependymoma (WHO grade III), which is much less common in childhood and is characterized by a high mitotic index and histologic features of microvascular proliferation and pseudopalisading necrosis. Myxopapillary ependymoma (WHO grade I) is a slow-growing tumor arising from the filum terminale and conus medullaris and appears to be a biologically different subtype. There are no well-defined characteristic cytogenetic or molecular genetic alterations in ependymoma, largely owing to their heterogenous nature, although various pathways have been implicated. Preliminary studies suggest that there are genetically distinct subtypes, exemplified by an association between alterations in the *NF2* gene and spinal ependymoma. Surgery is the primary treatment modality, with extent of surgical resection a major prognostic factor. Two other major prognostic factors are age, with younger children having poorer outcomes, and tumor location, with localization in the posterior fossa, which often is seen in young children, associated with poorer outcomes. Surgery alone is rarely curative. Multimodal therapy incorporating irradiation with surgery has resulted in long-term survival in approximately 40% of patients with ependymoma undergoing gross total resection. Recurrence is predominantly local. Ependymoma is sensitive to a spectrum of chemotherapeutic agents; the role of chemotherapy in multimodal therapy of ependymoma is still unclear. Current investigations are directed toward identification of optimal radiation dose, surgical questions addressing the use of second-look procedures after chemotherapy, and further evaluation of classic as well as novel chemotherapeutic agents.

Choroid Plexus Tumors

Choroid plexus tumors account for 2-4% of childhood CNS tumors. They are the most common CNS tumor in children <1 yr of age and account for 10-20% of CNS tumors in infants. These tumors are intraventricular epithelial neoplasms arising from the

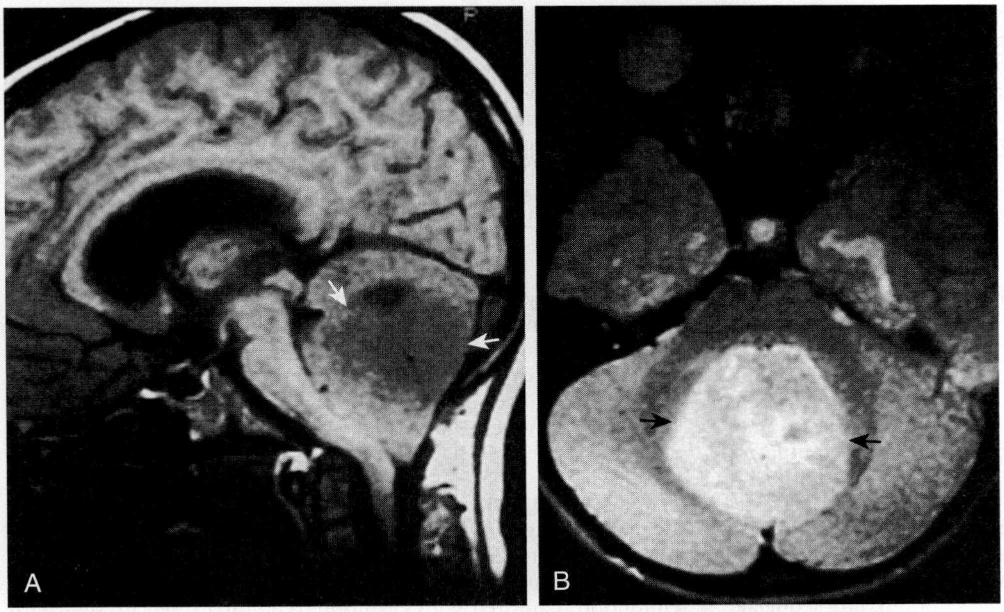

Figure 491-6 MRI of medulloblastoma. *A,* Sagittal T1-weighted image shows hypointense mass involving the vermis *(arrows). B,* Axial T2-weighted image shows hyperintense mass *(arrows)* with areas of hypointensity representing acute hemorrhagic infarction within the medulloblastoma involving the vermis. (From Kuhn JP, Slovis TL, Haller JO: *Caffey's pediatric diagnostic imaging,* ed 10, Philadelphia, 2004, Mosby, p 574.)

choroid plexus. Children present with signs and symptoms of increased ICP. Infants may present with macrocephaly and focal neurologic deficits. In children, these tumors predominantly occur supratentorially in the lateral ventricles. **Choroid plexus papilloma** (WHO grade I), the most common of this group, is a well-circumscribed lesion on neuroimaging and closely resembles normal choroid plexus histologically. **Choroid plexus carcinoma** (WHO grade III) is a malignant tumor with metastatic potential to seed into the CSF pathways. This malignancy has the following histologic characteristics: nuclear pleomorphism, high mitotic index, and increased cell density. Immunopositivity for transthyretin (prealbumin) is useful in confirming the diagnosis of choroid plexus tumors. The tumors are associated with the **Li-Fraumeni syndrome. Simian virus 40 (SV40)** may play an etiologic role in choroid plexus tumors. After complete surgical resection, the frequency of cure for choroid plexus papilloma approaches 100%, whereas the frequency of cure for choroid plexus carcinoma approaches 20-40%. Reports suggest that radiation therapy and/or chemotherapy may lead to better disease control for choroid plexus carcinoma.

Embryonal Tumors

Embryonal tumors or **primitive neuroectodermal tumors (PNETs)** are the most common group of malignant CNS tumors of childhood, accounting for ≈20 % of pediatric CNS tumors. They have the potential to metastasize to the neuraxis and beyond. The group includes medulloblastoma, supratentorial PNET, ependymoblastoma, medulloepithelioblastoma, and atypical teratoid/rhabdoid tumor (ATRT), all of which are histologically classified as WHO grade IV tumors.

Medulloblastoma, which accounts for 90% of embryonal tumors, is a cerebellar tumor occurring predominantly in males and at a median age of 5-7 yr. Most of these tumors occur in the midline cerebellar vermis; however, older patients may present with tumors in the cerebellar hemisphere. CT and MRI demonstrate a solid, homogeneous, contrast medium–enhancing mass in the posterior fossa causing 4th ventricular obstruction and hydrocephalus. Up to 30% of patients with medulloblastoma present with neuroimaging evidence of leptomeningeal spread. Among a variety of diverse histologic patterns of this tumor, the most common is a monomorphic sheet of undifferentiated cells classically noted as small, blue, round cells. Neuronal differentiation is more common among these tumors and is characterized histologically by the presence of Homer Wright rosettes and by immunopositivity for synaptophysin. An anaplastic variant is often more aggressive and may be associated with worse prognosis. Patients present with signs and symptoms of increased ICP (i.e., headache, nausea, vomiting, mental status changes, and hypertension) and cerebellar dysfunction (i.e., ataxia, poor balance, dysmetria). Standard clinical staging evaluation includes MRI of the brain and spine, both preoperatively and postoperatively, as well as lumbar puncture after the increased ICP has resolved (Fig. 491-6). The Chang staging system, originally based on surgical information, has been modified to incorporate information from neuroimaging to identify risk categories. Clinical features that have consistently demonstrated prognostic significance include age at diagnosis, extent of disease, and extent of surgical resection. Patients <4 yr of age have a poor outcome, partly as the result of a higher incidence of disseminated disease on presentation and past therapeutic approaches that have used less intense therapies. Patients with disseminated disease at diagnosis (M >0), including positive CSF cytologic result alone (M1), have a markedly worse outcome than those patients with no dissemination (M0). Similarly, patients with gross residual disease after surgery have worse outcomes than those in whom surgery achieved gross total resection of disease.

Cytogenetic and molecular genetic studies have demonstrated multiple abnormalities in medulloblastoma. The most common abnormality involves chromosome 17p deletions, which occur in 30-40% of all cases. These deletions are not associated with p53 mutations. Several signaling pathways have been shown to be active in medulloblastomas, including Sonic Hedgehog pathway, predominately associated with the desmoplastic variants, and the WNT pathway, which can occur in up to 15% of cases and has been associated with improved survival. Amplification of the *MYCC* oncogene as well as increased expression of the tyrosine kinase receptor ERBB2 have been associated with poorer outcomes, whereas improved survival is demonstrated in patients with overexpression of the neurotrophin-3 receptor (TRKC). Two risk stratification systems for medulloblastoma combining molecular markers with clinical factors have been proposed. One system is based on retrospective analysis of information about histologic variants (classic, nodular desmoplastic, anaplastic large cell); TRKC, *MYCC,* and ERBB2 expression; and clinical characteristics in children with medulloblastoma. One study found that the combination of clinical characteristics and ERBB2 expression provided a highly accurate means of discriminating disease risk. Another study found that gene expression profiling predicted medulloblastoma outcome independent of clinical variables. Both approaches still must be validated in larger prospective studies. With the evolution of gene array technology, preliminary studies have identified clusters of genes/gene expression that appear to be associated with metastatic medulloblastoma and outcome.

A multimodal treatment approach is pursued in medulloblastoma, with surgery the starting point of treatment. Medulloblastoma is sensitive to both chemotherapy and radiation therapy. Historically, surgery alone was ineffective. In the 1940s radiation therapy was found to be effective, improving overall outcome to a 30% survival rate. With technologic advances in neurosurgery, neuroradiology, and radiation therapy, as well as identification of chemotherapy as an effective modality, overall outcome among all patients approaches 60-70%. Standard radiation treatment in medulloblastoma incorporates craniospinal radiation at a total cumulative dose of 24 Gy, with a cumulative dose of 50-55 Gy to the tumor bed. Craniospinal radiation at this dose in children <3 yr of age results in severe late neurologic sequelae, including microcephaly, learning disabilities, mental retardation, neuroendocrine dysfunction (growth failure, hypothyroidism, hypogonadism, and absence/delay of puberty), and/or second malignancies. Similarly, in older children, late sequelae, such as learning disabilities, neuroendocrine dysfunction, and/or second malignancies, can occur. These observations have resulted in stratification of treatment approaches into the following three strata: (1) patients <3 yr of age; (2) standard-risk patients >3 yr of age with surgical total resection and no disease dissemination (M0); and (3) high-risk patients >3 yr of age with disease dissemination (M >0) and/or bulky residual disease after surgery. With the risk-based approach to treatment, children with high-risk medulloblastoma receive high-dose cranial-spinal radiation (36 Gy) with chemotherapy during and after radiation therapy, and those with standard-risk (nonmetastatic) disease receive lower dose craniospinal radiation (24 Gy) with chemotherapy during and after radiation therapy. Approaches in young children (<4 yr of age) incorporate high-dose chemotherapy with peripheral stem cell re-infusion and exclude radiation therapy. Overall survival in children with nonmetastatic medulloblastoma and gross total tumor resection approaches 85%. The presence of bulky residual tumor (56% survival) or metastases (38%) confers a poor prognosis.

Supratentorial primitive neuroectodermal tumors (SPNETs) account for 2-3% of childhood brain tumors, primarily in children within the first decade of life. These tumors are similar histologically to medulloblastoma and are composed of undifferentiated or poorly differentiated neuroepithelial cells. Historically, patients with SPNETs have had poorer outcomes than those with medulloblastoma after combined-modality therapy. In current clinical trials, children with SPNETs are considered among the high-risk group and receive dose-intense chemotherapy with craniospinal radiation therapy.

Atypical teratoid/rhabdoid tumor is a very aggressive embryonal malignancy that occurs predominantly in children <5 yr of age and can occur at any location in the neuraxis. The histology demonstrates a heterogeneous pattern of cells, including rhabdoid cells that express epithelial membrane antigen and neurofilament antigen. The characteristic cytogenetic pattern is partial or complete deletion of chromosome 22q11.2 that has been associated with mutation in the *INI1* gene. The relation between this mutation and tumorigenesis is unclear. Outcome after combined-modality therapy with intensive chemotherapy is very poor, but long-term survival has been reported in some children.

Pineal Parenchymal Tumors

The pineal parenchymal tumors are the most common malignancies after germ cell tumors that occur in the pineal region. These include pineoblastoma, occurring predominantly in childhood, pineocytoma, and the mixed pineal parenchymal tumors. The therapeutic approach in this group of diseases is multimodal. There was significant concern regarding the location of these masses and the potential complications of surgical intervention. With developments in neurosurgical technique and surgical technology, the morbidity and mortality associated with these approaches have markedly decreased. Stereotactic biopsy of these tumors may be adequate to establish diagnosis; however, consideration should be pursued for total resection of the lesion before institution of additional therapy. Pineoblastoma, the more malignant variant, is considered a subgroup of childhood PNETs. Chemotherapy regimens incorporate cisplatin, cyclophosphamide (Cytoxan), etoposide (VP-16), and vincristine and/or lomustine. Data have shown that survival outcome of combined modality therapy of chemotherapy and radiation in pineal region PNETs approaches 70% at 5 yr, similar to that noted for medulloblastoma. Pineocytoma usually is approached with surgical resection.

Craniopharyngioma

Craniopharyngioma (WHO grade I) is a common tumor of childhood, accounting for 7-10% of all childhood tumors. The adamantinomatous variant of craniopharyngioma predominates in childhood. Children with craniopharyngioma often present with endocrinologic abnormalities such as growth failure and delayed sexual maturation. Visual changes can occur and may include decrease acuity or visual field deficits. These tumors are often quite large and heterogenous, displaying both solid and cystic components, and occur within the suprasellar region. They are minimally invasive, adhere to adjacent brain parenchyma, and engulf normal brain structures. MRI demonstrates the solid tumor with cystic structures containing fluid of intermediate density. CT may show calcifications associated with the solid and cystic wall components. Surgery is the primary treatment modality, with gross total resection curative in small lesions. Controversy exists regarding the relative roles of surgery and radiation therapy in large, complex tumors. Significant morbidity (panhypopituitarism, growth failure, visual loss) is associated with these tumors and their therapy, owing to the anatomic location. There is no role for chemotherapy in craniopharyngioma.

Germ Cell Tumors

Germ cell tumors of the CNS are a heterogeneous group of tumors that are primarily tumors of childhood, arising predominantly in midline structures of the pineal and suprasellar regions. They account for 3-5% of pediatric brain tumors. The peak incidence of these tumors is in children 10-12 yr of age. Overall, there is a male preponderance, although there is a female preponderance for suprasellar tumors. Germ cell tumors occur multifocally in 5-10% of cases. This group of tumors is much more prevalent in Asian populations than European populations. Delays in diagnosis can occur because these tumors have a particularly insidious course; the initial presenting symptoms may be subtle, including poor school performance and behavior problems. As in peripheral germ cell tumors, the analysis of protein markers, **α-fetoprotein,** and **β-human chorionic gonadotropin** may be useful in establishing the diagnosis and monitoring treatment response. Surgical biopsy is recommended to establish the diagnosis; however, nongerminomatous germ cell tumors may be diagnosed on the basis of protein marker elevations. Therapeutic approaches to germinomas and mixed germ cell tumors are different. The survival proportion among patients with pure germinoma exceeds 90%. The postsurgical treatment of pure germinomas is somewhat controversial in defining the relative roles of chemotherapy and radiation therapy. Clinical trials have investigated the use of chemotherapy and reduced-dose radiation after surgery in pure germinomas. The therapeutic approach to nongerminomatous germ cell tumors is more aggressive, combining more intense chemotherapy regimens with craniospinal radiation therapy.

Survival rates among patients with these tumors are markedly less than those noted in patients with germinoma, ranging from 40% to 70% at 5 yr. Trials have shown benefit of the use of high doses of chemotherapy with blood stem cell rescue.

Tumors of the Brainstem

Tumors of the brainstem are a heterogeneous group of tumors that account for 10-15% of childhood primary CNS tumors. Outcome depends on tumor location, imaging characteristics, and the patient's clinical status. Patients with these tumors may present with motor weakness, cranial nerve deficits, cerebellar deficits, and/or signs of increased ICP. On the basis of MRI evaluation and clinical findings, tumors of the brainstem can be classified into four types: focal (5-10% of patients); dorsally exophytic (5-10%); cervicomedullary (5-10%); and diffuse intrinsic (70-85%) (Fig. 491-7). Surgical resection is the primary treatment approach for focal and dorsally exophytic tumors and leads to a favorable outcome. Histologically, these two groups usually are low-grade gliomas. Cervicomedullary tumors, owing to their location, may not be amenable to surgical resection but are sensitive to radiation therapy. Diffuse intrinsic tumors, characterized by the diffuse infiltrating pontine glioma, are associated with very poor outcome independent of histologic diagnosis. These tumors are not amenable to surgical resection. Biopsy in children in whom MRI shows a diffuse intrinsic tumor is controversial and is not recommended unless there is suspicion of another diagnosis, such as infection, demyelination, vascular malformation, multiple sclerosis, or metastatic tumor. These diagnoses are much more common in adults. The standard approach for treatment of diffuse infiltrating pontine gliomas has been radiation therapy, and median survival with this treatment is 12 mo, at best. Use of chemotherapy, including high-dose chemotherapy with blood stem cell rescue, has not yet been of survival benefit in this group of patients. Current approaches include evaluation of investigational agents alone or in combination with radiation therapy, similar to approaches being pursued in patients with malignant gliomas.

Metastatic Tumors

Metastatic spread of other childhood malignancies to the brain is uncommon. Childhood acute lymphoblastic leukemia and non-Hodgkin lymphoma can spread to the leptomeninges, causing symptoms of communicating hydrocephalus. **Chloromas,** which are collections of myeloid leukemia cells, can occur throughout the neuraxis. Rarely, brain parenchymal metastases occur from lymphoma, neuroblastoma, rhabdomyosarcoma, Ewing sarcoma, osteosarcoma, and clear cell sarcoma of the kidney. Therapeutic approaches are based on the specific histologic diagnosis and may incorporate radiation therapy, intrathecal administration of chemotherapy, and/or systemic administration of chemotherapy. Medulloblastoma is the childhood brain tumor that most commonly metastasizes extraneuronally. Less commonly, extraneuronal metastases from malignant glioma, PNET, and ependymoma can occur. Ventriculoperitoneal shunts have been known to allow extraneural metastases, primarily within the peritoneal cavity but also systemically.

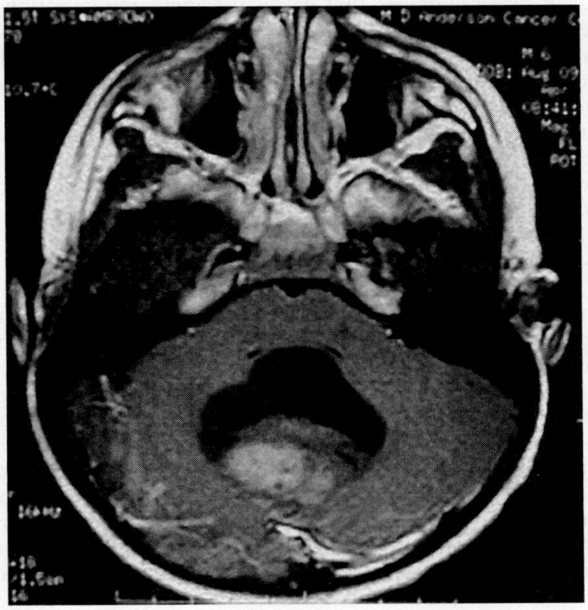

Figure 491-7 T1-weighted sequence post-gadolinium sagittal MR image of a pontine diffuse infiltrating glioma in a 10 yr old girl presenting with headache, cranial nerve palsies, and left-sided weakness.

COMPLICATIONS AND LONG-TERM MANAGEMENT

Data from the National Cancer Institute Surveillance, Epidemiology and End Results (SEER) Program indicate that >70% of patients with childhood brain tumors will be long-term survivors. At least 50% of these survivors will experience chronic problems as a direct result of their tumors and treatment. These problems include chronic neurologic deficits such as focal motor and sensory abnormalities, seizure disorders, neurocognitive deficits (e.g., developmental delays, learning disabilities), and neuroendocrine deficiencies (e.g., hypothyroidism, growth failure, delay or absence of puberty). These patients are also at significant risk for secondary malignancies. Supportive multidisciplinary interventions for children with brain tumors both during and after therapy may help improve their ultimate outcome. Optimal seizure management, physical therapy, endocrine management with timely growth hormone and thyroid replacement therapy, tailored educational programs, and vocational interventions may enhance the childhood brain tumor survivor's quality of life.

BIBLIOGRAPHY

Please visit the Nelson Textbook of Pediatrics *website at www.expertconsult.com for the complete bibliography.*

Chapter 492
Neuroblastoma

Peter E. Zage and Joann L. Ater

Neuroblastomas are embryonal cancers of the peripheral sympathetic nervous system with heterogeneous clinical presentation and course, ranging from tumors that undergo spontaneous regression to very aggressive tumors unresponsive to very intensive multimodal therapy. The causes of most cases remain unknown, and although significant advances have been made in the treatment of children with the tumor, the outcomes for aggressive forms of neuroblastoma remain poor.

EPIDEMIOLOGY

Neuroblastoma is the most common extracranial solid tumor in children and the most commonly diagnosed malignancy in infants. Approximately 600 new cases are diagnosed each year in the USA, accounting for 8-10% of childhood malignancies and one third of cancers in infants. Neuroblastoma accounts for >15% of the mortality from cancer in children. The median age of children at diagnosis of neuroblastoma is 22 months, and 90% of cases are diagnosed by 5 years of age. The incidence is slightly higher in boys and in whites.

Table 492-1 SYNDROMES ASSOCIATED WITH NEUROBLASTOMA

EPONYM	FEATURES
Pepper syndrome	Massive involvement of the liver with metastatic disease with or without respiratory distress.
Horner syndrome	Unilateral ptosis, myosis, and anhidrosis associated with a thoracic or cervical primary tumor. Symptoms do not resolve with tumor resection.
Hutchinson syndrome	Limping and irritability in young child associated with bone and bone marrow metastases.
Opsoclonus-myoclonus-ataxia syndrome	Myoclonic jerking and random eye movement with or without cerebellar ataxia. Often associated with a biologically favorable and differentiated tumor. The condition is likely immune mediated, may not resolve with tumor removal, and often exhibits progressive neuropsychological sequelae.
Kerner-Morrison syndrome	Intractable secretory diarrhea due to tumor secretion of vasointestinal peptides. Tumors are generally biologically favorable.
Neurocristopathy syndrome	Neuroblastoma associated with other neural crest disorders, including congenital hypoventilation syndrome or Hirschsprung disease. Germline mutations in the paired homeobox gene *PHOX2B* have been identified in a subset of patients with this disease.

From Park JR, Eggert A, Caron H: Neuroblastoma: biology, prognosis, and treatment, *Pediatr Clin North Am* 55:97-120, 2008.

PATHOLOGY

Neuroblastoma, which is derived from primordial neural crest cells, consists of a spectrum of tumors with variable degrees of neural differentiation, ranging from tumors with primarily undifferentiated small round cells (neuroblastoma) to tumors containing mature and maturing schwannian stroma with ganglion cells (ganglioneuroblastoma or ganglioneuroma). The tumors may resemble other **small round blue cell tumors,** such as rhabdomyosarcoma, Ewing sarcoma, and non-Hodgkin lymphoma. The prognosis of children with neuroblastoma varies with the histologic features of the tumor, and prognostic factors include the presence and amount of schwannian stroma, the degree of tumor cell differentiation, and the mitosis-karyorrhexis index.

PATHOGENESIS

The etiology of neuroblastoma in most cases remains unknown. Familial neuroblastoma accounts for 1-2% of all cases, is associated with a younger age at diagnosis, and has been linked to mutations in the *Phox2B* and *ALK* genes. Neuroblastoma is associated with other neural crest disorders, including Hirschsprung disease, central hypoventilation syndrome, and neurofibromatosis type I, and potentially congenital cardiovascular malformations (Table 492-1). Children with Beckwith-Wiedemann syndrome and hemihypertrophy also have a higher incidence of neuroblastoma. Increased incidence of neuroblastoma is associated with some maternal and paternal occupational chemical exposures, farming, and work related to electronics, although no single environmental exposure has been shown to cause neuroblastomas.

Genetic characteristics of neuroblastoma tumor tissue that are of prognostic importance include amplification of the *MYCN* (*N-myc*) proto-oncogene and tumor cell DNA content, or ploidy (Tables 492-2 to 492-4). Amplification of *MYCN* is strongly associated with advanced tumor stage and poor outcomes. Hyperdiploidy confers better prognosis if the child is <1 yr of age at diagnosis. Other chromosomal abnormalities, including loss of heterozygosity (LOH) of 1p, 11q, and 14q, and gain of 17q, are commonly found in neuroblastoma tumors and are associated with worse outcomes. In addition, many other biologic factors have been shown to be associated with neuroblastoma outcomes, including tumor histology and vascularity and the expression levels of nerve growth factor receptor (TrkA, TrkB), ferritin, lactate dehydrogenase, ganglioside GD2, neuropeptide Y, chromogranin A, CD44, multidrug resistance–associated protein, and telomerase. These factors and many others are under investigation in clinical trials to determine whether they can be used to reduce therapy for children predicted to fare well with minimal therapy and to intensify therapy for those predicted to be at high risk for relapse.

CLINICAL MANIFESTATIONS

Neuroblastoma may develop at any site of sympathetic nervous system tissue. Approximately half of neuroblastoma tumors arise in the adrenal glands, and most of the remainder originate in the paraspinal sympathetic ganglia. Metastatic spread, which is more common in children >1 yr of age at diagnosis, occurs via local invasion or distant hematogenous or lymphatic routes. The most common sites of metastasis are the regional or distant lymph nodes, long bones and skull, bone marrow, liver, and skin. Lung and brain metastases are rare, occurring in less than 3% of cases.

Neuroblastoma can mimic many other disorders and may be difficult to diagnose. The signs and symptoms of neuroblastoma reflect the tumor site and extent of disease. Metastatic disease can cause a variety of signs and symptoms, including fever, irritability, failure to thrive, bone pain, cytopenias, bluish subcutaneous nodules, orbital proptosis, and periorbital ecchymoses (Fig. 492-1). Localized disease can manifest as an asymptomatic mass or as mass-related symptoms, including spinal cord compression, bowel obstruction, and superior vena cava syndrome.

Children with neuroblastoma can also present with neurologic signs and symptoms. Neuroblastoma originating in the superior cervical ganglion can result in **Horner syndrome.** Paraspinal neuroblastoma can invade the neural foramina, causing spinal cord and nerve root compression. Neuroblastoma can also be associated with a paraneoplastic syndrome of autoimmune origin, termed opsoclonus-myoclonus-ataxia syndrome. Some tumors produce catecholamines that can cause increased sweating and hypertension, and some release vasoactive intestinal peptide, causing a profound secretory diarrhea. Children with extensive tumors can also experience tumor lysis syndrome and disseminated intravascular coagulation. Infants <1 yr of age also can present in unique fashion, termed stage 4S, with widespread subcutaneous tumor nodules, massive liver involvement, limited bone marrow disease, and a small primary tumor without bone involvement or other metastases.

DIAGNOSIS

Neuroblastoma is usually discovered as a mass or multiple masses on plain radiography, CT, or MRI (Fig. 492-2). On plain radiography or CT, the mass often contains calcification and hemorrhage. Prenatal diagnosis of neuroblastoma on maternal ultrasound scans is sometimes possible. Tumor markers, including catecholamine metabolites homovanillic acid (HVA) and vanillylmandelic acid (VMA) in urine, are elevated in 95% of cases and help to confirm the diagnosis. A pathologic diagnosis is established from tumor tissue obtained by biopsy. Neuroblastoma can be diagnosed without a primary tumor biopsy if small round blue tumor cells are observed in bone marrow samples (Fig. 492-3) and an elevation of VMA or HVA is found in the urine.

Evaluations for metastatic disease should include CT or MRI of the chest and abdomen, bone scans to detect cortical bone

Table 492-2 CHILDREN'S ONCOLOGY GROUP NEUROBLASTOMA RISK STRATIFICATION

RISK GROUP	STAGE	AGE	MYCN AMPLIFICATION STATUS	PLOIDY	SHIMADA
Low risk	1	Any	Any	Any	Any
Low risk	2A/2B	Any	Not amplified	Any	Any
High risk	2A/2B	Any	Amplified	Any	Any
Intermediate risk	3	<547 d	Not amplified	Any	any
Intermediate risk	3	≥547 d	Not amplified	Any	FH
High risk	3	Any	Amplified	Any	Any
High risk	3	≥547 d	Not amplified	Any	UH
High risk	4	<365 d	Amplified	Any	Any
Intermediate risk	4	<365 d	Not amplified	Any	Any
High risk	4	365 to <547 d	Amplified	Any	Any
High Risk	4	365 to <547 d	Any	DNA index = 1	Any
High risk	4	365 to <547 d	Any	Any	UH
Intermediate risk	4	365 to <547 d	Not amplified	DNA index > 1	FH
High risk	4	≥547 d	Any	Any	Any
Low risk	4S	<365 d	Not amplified	DNA index > 1	FH
Intermediate risk	4S	<365 d	Not amplified	DNA index = 1	Any
Intermediate risk	4S	<365 d	Not amplified	Any	UH
High risk	4S	<365 d	Amplified	Any	Any

FH, favorable histology; UH, unfavorable histology.
Courtesy of Children's Oncology Group; from Park JR, Eggert A, Caron H: Neuroblastoma: biology, prognosis, and treatment, *Pediatr Clin North Am* 55:97–120, 2008.

Table 492-3 INTERNATIONAL NEUROBLASTOMA STAGING SYSTEM

STAGE	DEFINITION	INCIDENCE (%)	SURVIVAL AT 5 YR* (%)
1	Localized tumor with complete gross excision, with or without microscopic residual disease; representative ipsilateral lymph nodes negative for tumor microscopically (nodes attached to and removed with the primary tumor may be positive)	5	≥90
2A	Localized tumor with incomplete gross excision; representative ipsilateral nonadherent lymph nodes negative for tumor microscopically	10	70-80
2B	Localized tumor with or without complete gross excision, with ipsilateral nonadherent lymph nodes positive for tumor; enlarged contralateral lymph nodes must be negative microscopically	10	70-80
3	Unresectable unilateral tumor infiltrating across the midline,† with or without regional lymph node involvement; *or* localized unilateral tumor with contralateral regional lymph node involvement; *or* midline tumor with bilateral extension by infiltration (resectable) or by lymph node involvement	25	40-70
4	Any primary tumor with dissemination to distant lymph nodes; bone, bone marrow, liver, skin, and other organs (except as defined for stage 4S)	60	85-90 if age at diagnosis is <18 mo 30-40 if age at diagnosis is >18 mo
4S	Localized primary tumor (as defined for stage 1, 2A, or 2B), with dissemination limited to skin, liver, and bone marrow‡ (limited to infants <1 yr of age)	5	>80

*Survival is influenced by other characteristics, such as *MYCN* amplification. Percentages are approximate.
†The *midline* is defined as the vertebral column. Tumors originating on one side and crossing the midline must infiltrate to or beyond the other side of the vertebral column.
‡Marrow involvement in stage 4S should be minimal (i.e., <10% of total nucleated cells identified as malignant on bone marrow biopsy or on marrow aspirate). More extensive marrow involvement would be considered stage 4. Results of the meta-iodobenzylguanidine (MIBG) scan (if performed) should be negative in the marrow.
Modified from Kliegman RM, Marcdante KJ, Jenson HB, et al, editors: *Nelson essentials of pediatrics*, ed 5, Philadelphia, 2006, WB Saunders, p 746; and Brodeur GM, Pritchard J, Berthold F, et al: Revisions of the international criteria for neuroblastoma diagnosis, staging, and response to treatment, *J Clin Oncol* 11:1466–1477, 1993.

Table 492-4 PHENOTYPIC AND GENETIC FEATURES OF NEUROBLASTOMA, TREATMENT, AND SURVIVAL ACCORDING TO PROGNOSTIC CATEGORY

VARIABLE	PROGNOSTIC CATEGORY*			
	Low Risk	Intermediate Risk	High Risk	Tumor Stage 4S
Pattern of disease	Localized tumor	Localized tumor with locoregional lymph-node extension; metastases to bone marrow and bone in infants	Metastases to bone marrow and bone (except in infants)	Metastases to liver and skin (with minimal bone marrow involvement) in infants
Tumor genomics	Whole-chromosome gains	Whole-chromosome gains	Segmental chromosomal aberrations	Whole-chromosome gains
Treatment	Surgery†	Moderate-intensity chemotherapy; surgery†	Dose-intensive chemotherapy, surgery, and external-beam radiotherapy to primary tumor and resistant metastatic sites; myeloablative chemotherapy with autologous hematopoietic stem cell rescue; isotretinoin with anti–ganglioside GD2 immunotherapy	Supportive care‡
Survival rate	>98%	90-95%	40-50%	>90%

*Patients are assigned to prognostic groups according to risk, as described by the Children's Oncology Group, with the level of risk defining the likelihood of death from disease. Stage 4S disease is considered separately here because of the unique phenotype of favorable biologic features and relentless early progression but ultimately full and complete regression of the disease.
†The goal of surgery is to safely debulk the tumor mass and avoid damage to surrounding normal structures while also obtaining sufficient material for molecular diagnostic studies. Some localized tumors may spontaneously regress without surgery.
‡Low-dose chemotherapy, radiation therapy, or both are used in patients with life-threatening hepatic involvement, especially in infants >2 mo of age, who are at much higher risk for life-threatening complications from massive hepatomegaly.
From Maris JM: Recent advances in neuroblastoma, *N Engl J Med* 326:2202–2210, 2010.

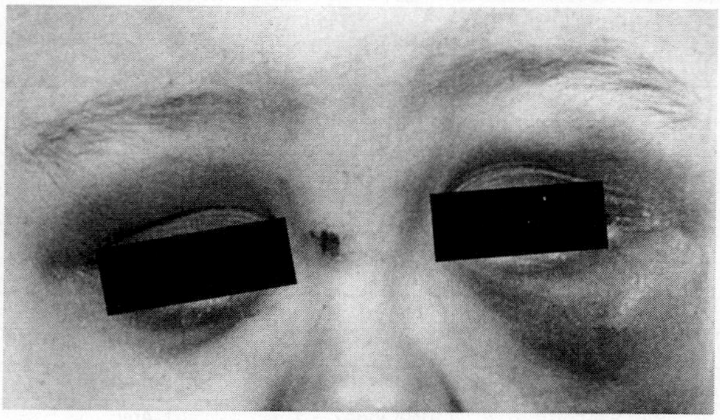

Figure 492-1 Periorbital metastases of neuroblastoma with proptosis and ecchymoses.

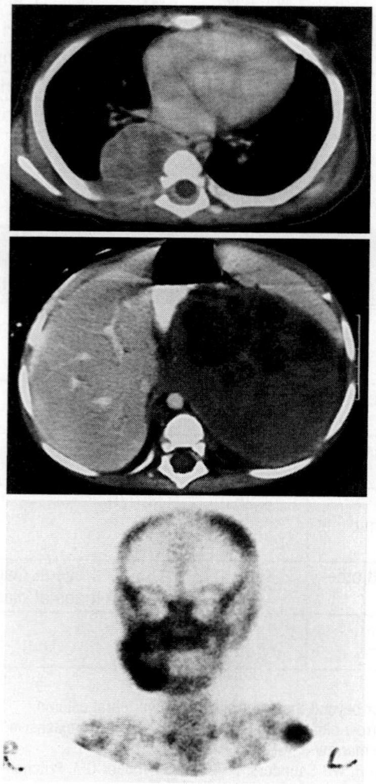

Figure 492-2 *Top,* CT scan of a thoracic neuroblastoma with intraspinal extension at diagnosis. *Middle,* CT scan of an adrenal primary with extensive lymph node involvement. *Bottom,* Bone scintigraphy scan with technetium diphosphonate demonstrating diffuse skeletal involvement.

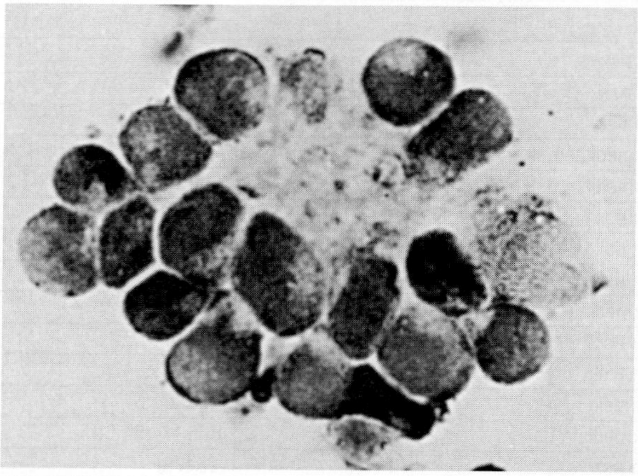

Figure 492-3 Neuroblastoma cells aspirated from the bone marrow. Clumps of cells often contain ≥3 cells with or without evidence of rosette formation. Rosettes of cells surrounding an inner mass of fibrillary material are characteristic of neuroblastoma.

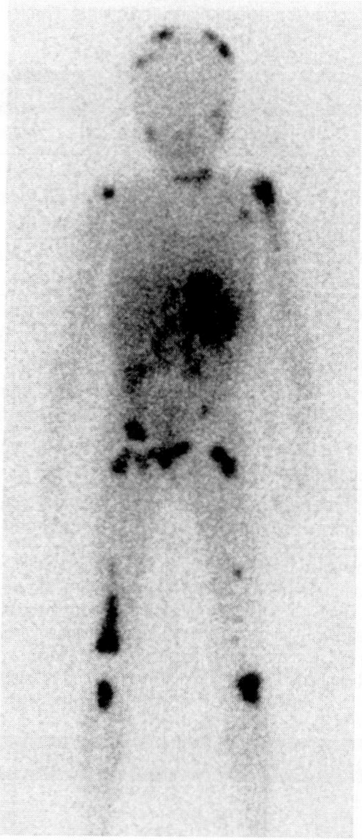

Figure 492-4 Metaiodobenzylguanidine (MIBG)–avid neuroblastoma. Increased uptake of radiolabeled tracer can be detected in multiple sites of disease, including bone and soft tissue. (Figure provided by K Matthay, University of California, San Francisco; from Maris JM, Hogarty MD, Bagatell R, et al: Neuroblastoma, *Lancet* 369:2106–2120, 2007.)

involvement, and at least two independent bone marrow aspirations and biopsies to evaluate for marrow disease. **Iodine-123 meta-iodobenzylguanidine** (123I-MIBG) studies may also be used to better define the extent of disease (Fig. 492-4). MRI of the spine should be performed in cases with suspected or potential spinal cord compression, but imaging of the brain with either CT or MRI is not routinely performed unless dictated by the clinical presentation.

The **International Neuroblastoma Staging System** (INSS) now is currently used to stage patients with neuroblastoma after initial surgical resection (see Table 492-3). INSS stage 1 tumors are confined to the organ or structure of origin and are completely resected. INSS stage 2 tumors extend beyond the structure of origin but not across the midline, either with (stage 2B) or without (stage 2A) ipsilateral lymph node involvement. INSS stage 3 tumors extend beyond the midline, with or without bilateral lymph node involvement, whereas INSS stage 4 tumors are disseminated, with metastases to bones, bone marrow, liver, distant lymph nodes, and other organs. INSS stage 4S refers to neuroblastoma in children less <1 yr of age with dissemination to liver, skin, and/or bone marrow without bone involvement and with a primary tumor that would otherwise be staged as INSS stage 1 or 2. A new International Neuroblastoma Risk Group Staging System (INRGSS) is currently being developed to allow for more effective comparisons of treatments and outcomes worldwide.

TREATMENT

Treatment strategies for neuroblastoma have changed dramatically over the past 20 years, with significant reduction in treatment intensity for children who have localized, low-risk tumors and continued increased treatment intensity and addition of new agents for treatment of children who have high-risk neuroblastoma. Currently the patient's age and tumor stage are combined with cytogenetic and molecular features of the tumor to determine the treatment risk group and estimated prognosis for each patient (see Tables 492-2 to 492-4). The usual treatment for low-risk neuroblastoma is surgery for stages 1 and 2 and observation for stage 4S with cure rates generally >90% without further therapy. Treatment with chemotherapy or radiation for the rare child with local recurrence can still be curative. Children with spinal cord compression at diagnosis also may require urgent treatment with chemotherapy, surgery, or irradiation to avoid neurologic damage. Stage 4S neuroblastomas have a very favorable prognosis, because many regress spontaneously. Chemotherapy or resection of the primary tumor does not improve survival rates, but for infants with massive liver involvement and respiratory compromise, small doses of cyclophosphamide or low-dose hepatic irradiation may alleviate symptoms. For children with stage 4S neuroblastoma who require treatment for symptoms, the survival rate is 81%.

Treatment of intermediate-risk neuroblastoma includes surgery, chemotherapy, and, in some cases, radiation therapy. The chemotherapy usually includes moderate doses of cisplatin or carboplatin, cyclophosphamide, etoposide, and doxorubicin given for several months. Radiation therapy is used for tumors with incomplete response to chemotherapy. Children with intermediate-risk neuroblastoma, including children with stage 3 disease and infants with stage 4 disease and favorable characteristics, have an excellent prognosis and >90% survival with this moderate treatment. In this intermediate-risk group, obtaining adequate diagnostic material for determination of the underlying biologic features of the tumor, such as the Shimada pathologic classification and *MYCN* gene amplification, is critical, so that children with unfavorable characteristics can receive more aggressive treatment and those with favorable features can be spared excessive toxic therapy.

Children with high-risk neuroblastoma have long-term survival rates between 25% and 35% with current treatment that consists of intensive chemotherapy, autologous stem cell transplantation (ASCT), surgery, irradiation, and 13-*cis*-retinoic acid (isotretinoin, Accutane). Current induction chemotherapy for children with high-risk neuroblastoma includes combinations of cyclophosphamide, topotecan, doxorubicin, vincristine, cisplatin, and etoposide. After completion of induction chemotherapy, resection of the residual primary tumor is followed by focal irradiation to areas with residual tumor. Induction chemotherapy is then followed by high-dose chemotherapy with ASCT. A national cooperative group trial demonstrated significantly better survival with ASCT and chemotherapy than with chemotherapy alone. The further addition of 13-cis-retinoic acid after ASCT resulted in further improvements in survival rates.

Cases of high-risk neuroblastoma are associated with frequent relapses, and children with recurrent neuroblastoma have a <50% response rate to alternative chemotherapy regimens. New treatment strategies and agents are needed for children with both high-risk and recurrent neuroblastoma. Therapies currently under investigation include new chemotherapeutic agents, radiolabeled targeted agents (such as ^{131}I-MIBG), monoclonal antibodies (anti–tumor-associated GD2) combined with growth factors (GM-CSF), and antitumor vaccines. It also is hoped that biologic studies of neuroblastoma will eventually lead to the identification of new molecular and genetic targets for therapy.

BIBLIOGRAPHY
Please visit the Nelson Textbook of Pediatrics *website at* www.expertconsult.com *for the complete bibliography.*

Chapter 493
Neoplasms of the Kidney

493.1 Wilms Tumor

Peter M. Anderson, Chetan Anil Dhamne, and Vicki Huff

Wilms tumor, also known as nephroblastoma, is the most common primary malignant renal tumor of childhood; other tumors are very rare. Use of multimodality treatment and multi-institutional cooperative group trials has dramatically improved the Wilms tumor cure rate from <30% to ≈90% (Table 493-1).

ETIOLOGY: GENETICS AND MOLECULAR BIOLOGY

Wilms tumor is an embryonal malignancy of the kidney. Most cases are sporadic, although 1-2% of patients have a familial predisposition to Wilms tumor. Familial cases of Wilms tumor are inherited in an autosomal dominant manner with variable penetrance; they are associated with an earlier age at diagnosis and increased frequency of bilateral disease. Models of Wilms tumor development propose that a genetic mutation predisposes to nephrogenic rests. These are benign foci of embryonal kidney cells that persist abnormally into postnatal life in approximately 1% of newborn kidneys and usually regress or differentiate by early childhood. The nephrogenic rests that persist may sustain additional mutations and transform into Wilms tumor. Nephrogenic rests may be intralobar, as in Wilms tumor aniridia genitourinary abnormalities and mental retardation (WAGR) and Denys-Drash syndrome, or perilobar and often multiple, as in Beckwith-Wiedemann syndrome (BWS).

Wilms tumor is genetically heterogeneous (Table 493-2). Familial Wilms tumors have been linked to *FWT1* gene at

Table 493-1 TEN-YEAR WILMS TUMOR OUTCOMES

HISTOLOGY	STAGE	RECURRENCE-FREE SURVIVAL (%)	OVERALL SURVIVAL(%)
Favorable	I	91	96
Favorable	II	85	93
Favorable	III	84	89
Favorable	IV	75	81
Favorable	V	65	78
Anaplastic	II-III	43	49
Anaplastic	IV	18	18

From Children's Oncology Group Data: National Wilms Tumor Study IV.

Table 493-2 SYNDROMES ASSOCIATED WITH WILMS TUMOR

SYNDROME	CLINICAL CHARACTERISTICS	GENETIC ANOMALIES
Wilms tumor, aniridia, genitourinary abnormalities, and mental retardation (WAGR syndrome)	Aniridia, genitourinary abnormalities, mental retardation	Del 11p13 (*WT1* and *PAX6*)
Denys-Drash syndrome	Early-onset renal failure with renal mesangial sclerosis, male pseudohermaphrodism	*WT1* missense mutation
Beckwith-Wiedemann syndrome (BWS)	Organomegaly (liver, kidney, adrenal, pancreas) macroglossia, omphalocele, hemihypertrophy	Unilateral paternal disomy, duplication of 11p15.5 loss of imprinting, mutation of *p57KIP57* Del 11p15.5 *IGF2* and *H19* imprinting control region

chromosome 17q and *FWT2* gene at chromosome 19q13. However, some families carry neither of these mutations, suggesting that additional Wilms tumor loci exist.

So far the best characterized Wilms tumor gene is *WT1*, located at 11p13. The *WT1* gene encodes a zinc finger transcription factor that is critical to normal development of the kidneys and gonads. WAGR is caused by deletion at chromosome 11p13 that includes both *PAX6* and *WT1* loci. Aniridia arises from the deletion of *PAX6* gene that lies telomeric to the *WT1* gene. Individuals with WAGR are diagnosed with Wilms tumor at an earlier age and generally have a favorable histology; their tumors respond well to treatment but are associated with increased risk of end-stage renal disease (ESRD) as they approach adulthood. Individuals with intragenic *WT1* germline mutation display the same Wilms tumor predisposition and range of genitourinary anomalies as patients with WAGR. Individuals with specific *WT1* missense mutations additionally have early-onset renal failure (Denys-Drash syndrome). *WT1* is homozygously inactivated in 10-20% of Wilms tumors, by either somatic alterations or a combination of germline and somatic *WT1* alterations.

WT2 is a localized to a cluster of imprinted genes at 11p15. Altered expression of one or more of these genes due to duplication or loss of imprinting is observed in BWS. Loss of heterozygosity (LOH) or loss of imprinting (LOI) at 11p15 is observed in approximately 70% of Wilms tumors. Candidate genes in this region include *IGF2*, *H19*, *CDKN1*/p57kip, and *KCNQ1OT1/LIT1*. Uniparental isodisomy of 11p15 and hypermethylation of *H19* are associated with development of Wilms tumor only, whereas alterations in *KCNQ1OT1* are associated with other tumors, macrosomia, and abdominal wall defects in addition to Wilms tumor. Identification of inherited microdeletions within the *H19/IGF2* imprinting control region (ICR) in BWS and BWS/Wilms tumor further strengthen the association between aberrant expressions of *IGF2* and Wilms tumor development. *WTX* at X11.1 has now been reported to be somatically mutated in 20-30% of Wilms tumors. *CTNNB1*, located at 3p22.1, encodes β-catenin and is also somatically mutated in about 15% of Wilms tumors. The WNT signaling pathway seems to be commonly involved in Wilms tumorigenesis. In addition to these genes, loci at 1p, 7p, 16q, and 17p (p53 tumor suppressor gene) are also believed to harbor genes involved in the biology of Wilms tumor.

EPIDEMIOLOGY

The incidence of Wilms tumor is approximately 8 cases/million children <15 yr of age with about 500 new cases in North America per year. It accounts for nearly 6% of pediatric malignancies and is the second most common malignant abdominal tumor in childhood. Although peak incidence is between 2 and 5 yr of age, Wilms tumor has also been encountered in neonates, adolescents, and adults. It can arise in one or both kidneys. The incidence of bilateral Wilms tumors is 7%, and individuals with horseshoe kidney are at twice the risk for development of Wilms tumor as the general population. Wilms tumor may be associated with hemihypertrophy, aniridia, genitourinary anomalies, and a variety of rare syndromes (see Table 493-2), including **BWS** and **Denys Drash syndrome**.

CLINICAL PRESENTATION

The most common initial clinical presentation for Wilms tumor is the incidental discovery of an asymptomatic **abdominal mass** by parents while bathing or clothing an affected child or by a physician during the course of a routine physical examination (Table 493-3). At presentation the mass can be quite large because retroperitoneal masses can grow unhampered by strict anatomic boundaries. Functional defects in paired organs like the kidney, with good functional reserve, are also unlikely to be detected early. **Hypertension** is detected in about 25% of tumors at presentation. Renin production by the tumor itself has been suggested as the cause. Elevated renin values are also attributed to renal ischemia caused by either pressure from the tumor directly on the renal artery or indirectly as a result of tumor compression within the renal capsule or by intrarenal arteriovenous fistula formation. But the etiology remains unknown in majority of the cases. Some patients present with **abdominal pain**. About 15- 25% of cases have **hematuria,** usually asymptomatic. Occasionally rapid **abdominal enlargement and anemia** occur as a result of bleeding into the renal parenchyma or pelvis. Wilms tumor thrombus extends into the inferior vena cava in 4-10% of patients, and rarely into the right atrium. Patients might also have microcytic anemia from iron deficiency or anemia of chronic disease, polycythemia, elevated platelet count, and acquired deficiency of von Willebrand factor or factor VII deficiency.

Table 493-3 DIFFERENTIAL DIAGNOSIS OF ABDOMINAL AND PELVIC TUMORS IN CHILDREN

TUMOR	PATIENT AGE	CLINICAL SIGNS	LABORATORY FINDINGS
Wilms	Preschool	Unilateral flank mass, aniridia, hemihypertrophy	Hematuria, polycythemia, thrombocytosis, elevated partial thromboplastin time value
Neuroblastoma	Preschool	Gastrointestinal/genitourinary obstruction, raccoon eyes, myoclonus opsoclonus diarrhea, skin nodules	Increased urinary vanillylmandelic acid, or homovanillic acid, or ferritin, stippled calcification in the mass
Non-Hodgkin lymphoma	>1 yr	Intussusception in >2 yr old	Increased lactic dehydrogenase, bone marrow positive
Rhabdomyosarcoma	All	Gastrointestinal/genitourinary obstruction, sarcoma botryoides, vaginal bleeding, paratesticular mass	
Germ cell tumor/teratoma	Preschool, teenage	Girls: Abdominal pain, vaginal bleeding Boys: testicular mass, new-onset hydrocele, sacrococcygeal mass/dimple	Increased human chorionic gonadotropin and increased α-fetoprotein
Hepatoblastoma	Birth-3 yr	Large firm liver	Increased α-fetoprotein
Hepatoma	School age, teenage	Large firm nodule, hepatitis B, cirrhosis	Increased α-fetoprotein

DIAGNOSIS AND DIFFERENTIAL DIAGNOSIS

An abdominal mass in a child should be considered malignant until diagnostic imaging, laboratory finding, and/or pathology can define its true nature (see Table 493-3). Imaging studies include abdominal flat plate radiography, abdominal ultrasonography (US), CT, and/or MRI of the abdomen to define the intrarenal origin of the mass and differentiate it from adrenal masses (e.g., neuroblastoma) and other masses in the abdomen. Abdominal US helps differentiate solid from cystic masses. Wilms tumor might show focal areas of necrosis or hemorrhage and hydronephrosis due to obstruction of the renal pelvis by the tumor. US

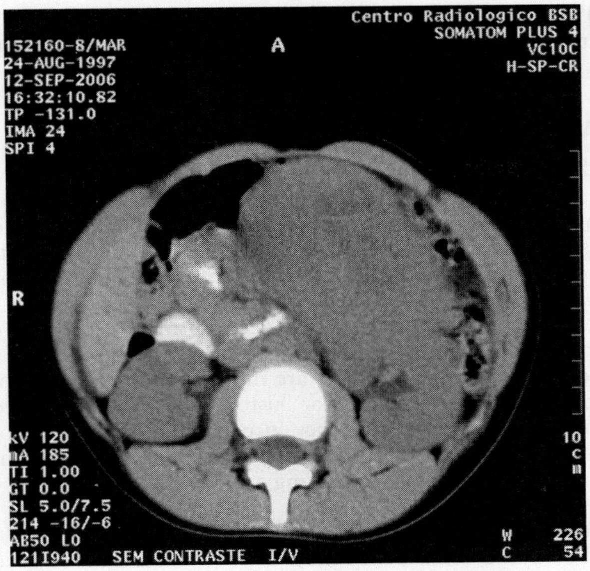

Figure 493-1 Abdominal CT scan with Wilms tumor arising from left kidney. Because of their retroperitoneal location, such tumors can become very large (e.g., >10 cm) before clinical symptoms occur.

with Doppler imaging of renal veins and the inferior vena cava is a useful first study that can not only look for Wilms tumor but also evaluate the collecting system and demonstrate tumor thrombi in the renal veins and/or inferior vena cava.

CT (Fig. 493-1) and/or MRI is useful to define the extent of the disease, integrity of the contralateral kidney, and metastasis. In bilateral cases, MRI may be a better guide to nephron-sparing surgery. If histologic diagnosis confirms clear cell sarcoma of the kidney, a bone scan is indicated. A brain MRI is indicated in case of rhabdoid tumor of the kidney, to look for metastasis. Chest CT is more sensitive than chest radiography to screen for and characterize pulmonary metastasis in Wilms tumor and other solid tumors.

Wilms tumor lesions are metabolically active and concentrate fluorodeoxyglucose (FDG). Regional spread and metastatic lesions are often visualized on positron emission tomography (PET)/CT scanning, which is a useful modality to monitor response to therapy in or patients with relapsed Wilms tumor, in patients with regional lymph node involvement, pelvic soft tissue involvement, and liver metastasis, and in patients with recurrent disease.

TREATMENT

There are two major schools of thought in the management of Wilms tumor. The Children's Oncology Group (COG), formerly National Wilms Tumor Study Group, advocates upfront surgery prior to initiating treatment. On the other hand, the International Society of Pediatric Oncology (SIOP) recommends preoperative chemotherapy. Each approach has advantages and limitations but they have similar outcomes. Early surgery has 100% accurate diagnosis and can facilitate risk-adapted therapy. Preoperative chemotherapy can make surgery easier and reduces the frequency of intraoperative tumor rupture and spillage.

Prognostic factors for risk-adapted therapy include age, stage, tumor weight, and loss of heterozygosity at chromosomes 1p and 16q (Table 493-4). Histology plays a major role in risk stratification of Wilms tumor. Absence of anaplasia is considered a favorable histologic finding. Presence of anaplasia is further classified as focal or diffuse, both of which are unfavorable histologic findings.

The COG has very specific drug dose and schedule recommendations for risk-adapted treatment of Wilms tumor. Therapy is generally performed in the outpatient clinic. Patients <2 yr of age and with a tumor weight <550 g are classified as having very low risk and are treated with nephrectomy only followed by close observation. Patients with stage I and II disease receive two drugs, vincristine and actinomycin D, a regimen (EE-4A) that takes 18 weeks. Actinomycin D (also called dactinomycin) is given every 3 weeks. Vincristine is given weekly for 10 weeks, and then every 3 weeks until week 18. Vincristine doses are adapted for age and weight in order to avoid neurotoxicity; children rarely have alopecia from the vincristine and dactinomycin regimen.

Table 493-4 STAGING OF WILMS TUMOR

Stage I	Tumor *confined to the kidney* and completely resected. Renal capsule or sinus vessels not involved. Regional lymph nodes dissected and negative.
Stage II	Tumor extends *beyond the kidney* but is completely resected with negative margins and lymph nodes. At least one of the following has occurred: (a) penetration of renal capsule, (b) invasion of renal sinus vessels.
Stage III	*Residual tumor* present following surgery confined to the abdomen, including inoperable tumor; positive surgical margins; spillage of tumor preoperatively or intraoperatively; biopsy prior to nephrectomy, regional lymph node metastases; extension of tumor thrombus into the inferior vena cava including thoracic vena cava and heart.
Stage IV	*Metastases* outside the abdomen, for example, lung.
Stage V	*Bilateral* renal tumor.

Source: Children's Oncology Group Protocol AREN 0532.

Doxorubicin is used in higher-risk patients and results in alopecia. Currently in North America, doxorubicin is alternated every 3 weeks with dactinomycin for a total of 24 weeks (regimen DD4A) if LOH is present at both 1p and 16q in patients with stage I and II disease. Patients with stage III disease receive intensive chemotherapy with three drugs and radiation therapy. Patients with presence of LOH at 1p and 16q are treated as being at high risk along with patients with stage IV and favorable histology; these two groups receive two cycles of three drug regimen followed by nephrectomy and then irradiation. Wilms tumors with focal and anaplastic histology have been treated with multiple regimens that included irinotecan, carboplatin and ifosfamide in addition to the standard agents, vincristine, doxorubicin, and actinomycin D.

RECURRENT DISEASE

Patients with recurrent Wilms tumor who previously received only actinomycin D and vincristine had a 4 year recurrence-free survival (RFS) of about 70%, whereas those who previously received the 3-drug regimen of vincristine, actinomycin D, and doxorubicin had an RFS of only 40%. Patients with metachronous relapse (i.e., new disease in the other kidney) are treated with kidney-sparing surgery and chemotherapy in order to try to avoid chronic renal failure. Other agents used to treat recurrent Wilms tumor have included doxorubicin, carboplatin, ifosfamide, topotecan, irinotecan, docetaxel, and etoposide.

PROGNOSIS

Despite some adverse risk factors that decrease prognosis (metastases, unfavorable histology, recurrent disease, and loss of heterozygosity of both 1p and 16q), most children with Wilms tumor have a very favorable prognosis. Overall the survival of children with Wilms tumor approaches 90%, with some risk factors (low stage, favorable histology, young age, low tumor weight) conferring even better outcomes. Thus, Wilms tumor is at the top of the list for best outcome of the common pediatric solid tumors.

LATE EFFECTS

Current strategies are successful with relatively few long-term effects of therapy. Rare late effects in survivors have included secondary malignant neoplasms, cardiac toxicity, pulmonary disease, and renal failure.

493.2 Other Pediatric Renal Tumors

Peter M. Anderson, Chetan Anil Dhamne, and Vicki Huff

MESOBLASTIC NEPHROMA

The most likely diagnosis of a solid renal tumor in a neonate is congenital mesoblastic nephroma. Many cases are diagnosed with prenatal ultrasound and can manifest as polyhydramnios, hydrops, and premature delivery. Most of the patients are diagnosed before 3 mo of age. Wilms tumor is rarely diagnosed before 6 mo of age. Ninety-five percent of mesoblastic nephromas are benign. Radical nephrectomy is the treatment of choice and may be sufficient by itself. Although rare, malignant variants do occur, marked by metastases to the lung, liver, heart, and brain.

CLEAR CELL SARCOMA OF THE KIDNEY

Clear cell sarcoma of the kidney (CCSK) is a rare pediatric tumor with around 20 cases per year diagnosed in North America. Peak incidence is between 1 and 4 years of age, usually presenting as an abdominal mass. CCSK has a high metastatic potential with predilection to involve the bone. Therefore, it is important to get a bone scan in CCSK patients. Early stage disease has excellent prognosis, especially with the addition of doxorubicin.

RHABDOID TUMOR OF THE KIDNEY

Malignant rhabdoid tumor of the kidney (RTK) has rhabdomyoblast-like morphology. It is a rare but aggressive cancer. Hematuria is a common presenting feature. Both rhabdoid tumor of the kidney and CNS atypical teratoid rhabdoid tumors (ATRT) have deletions and mutations of the *hSNF5/INI1* gene and are considered to be related. Prognosis is poor with current therapeutic protocols.

RENAL CELL CARCINOMA

Renal call carcinoma (RCC) is rare in children, accounting for <5% of all renal tumors of childhood. Patients may present with frank hematuria, flank pain, and/or a palpable mass, although RCC can be asymptomatic and detected incidentally. It has propensity to metastasize to the lungs, bone, liver, and brain. RCC can be associated with von Hippel–Lindau disease. Unlike in adult RCC, local lymph node involvement is not a poor prognostic indicator in pediatric RCC. Nephrectomy alone may be adequate for early-stage RCC.

BIBLIOGRAPHY

Please visit the Nelson Textbook of Pediatrics *website at* *www.expertconsult.com* *for the complete bibliography.*

Chapter 494
Soft Tissue Sarcomas

Carola A.S. Arndt

The annual incidence of soft tissue sarcomas is 8.4 cases/million white children <14 yr of age. Rhabdomyosarcoma accounts for >50% of soft tissue sarcomas. The prognosis most strongly correlates with age and extent of disease at diagnosis, primary tumor site, and histology.

RHABDOMYOSARCOMA

Epidemiology

The most common pediatric soft tissue sarcoma, rhabdomyosarcoma, accounts for approximately 3.5% of childhood cancers. These tumors may occur at virtually any anatomic site but are usually found in the head and neck (25%), orbit (9%), genitourinary tract (24%), and extremities (19%); retroperitoneal and other sites account for the remainder of primary sites. The incidence at each anatomic site is related to both patient age and tumor type. Extremity lesions are more likely to occur in older children and to have alveolar histology. Rhabdomyosarcoma occurs with increased frequency in patients with neurofibromatosis and has been associated with maternal breast cancer in the Li-Fraumeni syndrome, suggesting a genetic influence.

Pathogenesis

Rhabdomyosarcoma is thought to arise from the same embryonic mesenchyme as striated skeletal muscle. On the basis of light microscopic appearance, it belongs to the general category of small round cell tumors that includes Ewing sarcoma, neuroblastoma, and non-Hodgkin lymphoma. Definitive diagnosis of a pathologic specimen requires immunohistochemical studies using antibodies to skeletal muscle (desmin, muscle-specific actin, myogenin) and reverse transcription polymerase chain reaction (RT-PCR) or fluorescent in situ hybridization (FISH) for PAX-FKHR (PAX-FOX01A) transcript in the case of alveolar tumors.

Determination of the specific histologic subtype is important in treatment planning and assessment of prognosis. There are four recognized histologic subtypes. The **embryonal type** accounts for about 60% of all cases and has an intermediate prognosis. The **botryoid type,** a variant of the embryonal form in which tumor cells and an edematous stroma project into a body cavity like a bunch of grapes, is found most often in the vagina, uterus, bladder, nasopharynx, and middle ear. The **alveolar type** accounts for about 25-40% of cases and often is characterized by 2;13 or 1;13 chromosomal translocations. The tumor cells tend to grow in nests that often have cleftlike spaces resembling alveoli. Alveolar tumors occur most often in the trunk and extremities and carry the poorest prognosis. The **pleomorphic type** (adult form) is rare in childhood, accounting for <1% of cases.

Clinical Manifestations

The most common presenting feature of rhabdomyosarcoma is a mass that may or may not be painful. Symptoms are caused by displacement or obstruction of normal structures (Table 494-1). Origin in the nasopharynx may be associated with nasal congestion, mouth breathing, epistaxis, and difficulty with swallowing and chewing. Regional extension into the cranium can produce cranial nerve paralysis, blindness, and signs of increased intracranial pressure with headache and vomiting. When the tumor develops in the face or cheek, there may be swelling, pain, trismus, and, as extension occurs, paralysis of cranial nerves. Tumors in the neck can produce progressive swelling with neurologic symptoms after regional extension. Orbital primary tumors are usually diagnosed early in their course because of associated proptosis, periorbital edema, ptosis, change in visual acuity, and local pain. When the tumor arises in the middle ear, the most common early signs are pain, hearing loss, chronic otorrhea, or a mass in the ear canal; extensions of tumor produce cranial nerve paralysis and signs of an intracranial mass on the involved side. An unremitting croupy cough and progressive stridor can accompany rhabdomyosarcoma of the larynx. Because most of these signs and symptoms also are associated with common childhood conditions, clinicians must be alert to the possibility of tumor.

Rhabdomyosarcoma of the trunk or extremities often is first noticed after trauma and initially may be regarded as a hematoma. If the swelling does not resolve or increases, malignancy should be suspected. Involvement of the genitourinary tract can produce hematuria, obstruction of the lower urinary tract, recurrent urinary tract infections, incontinence, or a mass detectable on abdominal or rectal examination. Paratesticular tumor usually manifests as a painless, rapidly growing mass in the scrotum. Vaginal rhabdomyosarcoma may manifest as a grapelike mass of tumor tissue bulging through the vaginal orifice, known as **sarcoma botryoides,** and can cause urinary tract or large bowel symptoms. Vaginal bleeding or obstruction of the urethra or rectum may occur. Similar findings can be noted with uterine primaries.

Tumors in any location may disseminate early and cause symptoms of pain or respiratory distress associated with pulmonary metastases. Extensive bone involvement can produce symptomatic hypercalcemia. In such cases, it may be difficult to identify the primary lesion.

Diagnosis

Early diagnosis of rhabdomyosarcoma requires a high index of suspicion. The microscopic appearance that of is of a small round blue cell tumor. Neuroblastoma, lymphoma, and Ewing sarcoma also are **small round blue cell tumors.** The differential diagnosis depends on the site of presentation. Definitive diagnosis is established by biopsy, microscopic appearance, and results of immunohistochemical stains. A lesion in an extremity may be thought to be a hematoma or hemangioma, an orbital lesion resulting in proptosis may be treated as an orbital cellulitis, or bladder-obstructive symptoms may be missed. Adolescents may ignore paratesticular lesions for a long time. Unfortunately, several months often elapse between the initial symptoms and biopsy. Diagnostic procedures are determined mainly by the area of involvement. CT or MRI is necessary for evaluation of the primary tumor site. With signs and symptoms in the head and neck area, radiographs should be examined for evidence of a tumor mass and for indications of bony erosion. MRI should be performed to identify intracranial extension or meningeal involvement and also to reveal bony involvement or erosion at the base of the skull. For abdominal and pelvic tumors, CT with a contrast agent or MRI can help delineate the tumor (Fig. 494-1). A radionuclide bone scan, chest CT, and bilateral bone marrow aspiration and biopsy should be performed to evaluate the patient for the presence of metastatic disease and to plan treatment. The most critical element of the diagnostic work-up is examination of tumor tissue, which includes the use of special histochemical stains and immunostains. Cytogenetics and molecular genetics may be helpful in detecting specific chromosomal translocations of fusion proteins present in alveolar rhabdomyosarcoma. Lymph nodes also should be sampled for presence of disease spread, especially in tumors of the extremities and in boys >10 yr of age with paratesticular tumors.

Table 494-1 COMMON CLINICAL SYMPTOMS OF RHABDOMYOSARCOMA

REGION	SYMPTOMS
Head and neck	Asymptomatic mass, may mimic enlarged lymph node
Orbit	Proptosis, chemosis, ocular paralysis, eyelid mass
Nasopharynx	Snoring, nasal voice, epistaxis, rhinorrhea, local pain, dysphagia, cranial nerve palsies
Paranasal sinuses	Swelling, pain, sinusitis, obstruction, epistaxis, cranial nerve palsies
Middle ear	Chronic otitis media, hemorrhagic discharge, cranial nerve palsies, extruding polypoid mass
Larynx	Hoarseness, irritating cough
Trunk	Asymptomatic mass (usually)
Biliary tract	Hepatomegaly, jaundice
Retroperitoneum	Painless mass, ascites, gastrointestinal or urinary tract obstruction, spinal cord symptoms
Bladder/prostate	Hematuria, urinary retention, abdominal mass, constipation
Female genital tract	Polypoid vaginal extrusion of mucosanguineous tissue, vulval nodule
Male genital tract	Painful or painless scrotal mass
Extremity	Painless mass, may be very small but with secondary lymph node involvement
Metastatic	Nonspecific symptoms, associated with the diagnosis of leukemia

From McDowell HP: Update on childhood rhabdomyosarcoma, *Arch Dis Child* 88:354–357, 2003.

Treatment

Patients with completely resected tumors have the best prognosis. Unfortunately, most rhabdomyosarcomas are not completely resectable. At the initial surgery, tumor margins should be carefully defined, and an appropriate search for regional or metastatic disease to adjacent structures or regional lymph nodes should be completed, even if the procedure is limited to biopsy. Treatment is based on the primary tumor location and disease stage, which defines the clinical group. Most patients are given preoperative chemotherapy in an attempt to reduce the extent of surgery required and to preserve vital organs, particularly of the genitourinary tract. Group I tumors are treated with complete local excision followed by chemotherapy to reduce the likelihood of subsequent metastases. Group II tumors (microscopic residual tumor) are treated with surgery followed by local irradiation and systemic chemotherapy. Group III tumors (gross residual tumor) are treated with systemic chemotherapy, irradiation, and possibly surgery. Group IV rhabdomyosarcoma (metastatic) is treated principally with systemic chemotherapy and irradiation. Standard chemotherapeutic agents include vincristine, dactinomycin, and cyclophosphamide (VAC). A trial in intermediate-risk

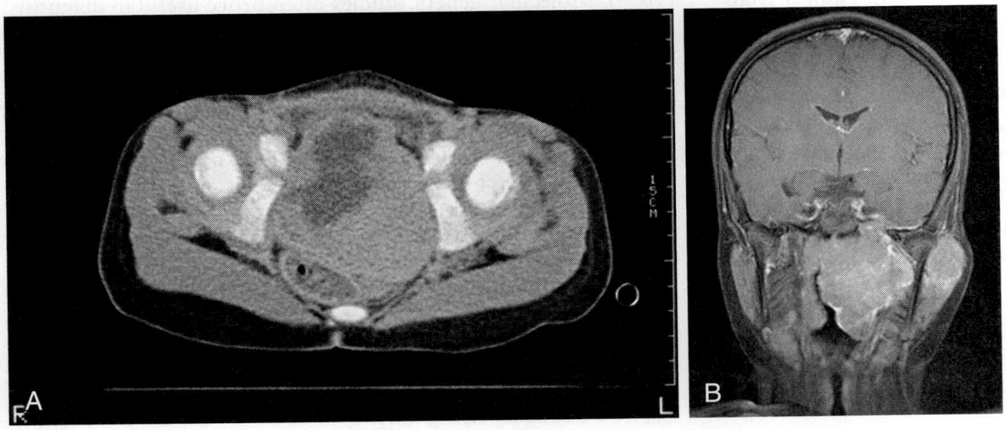

Figure 494-1 *A,* Pelvic CT scan of a child with a bladder rhabdomyosarcoma. *B,* MR image of a child with a parameningeal rhabdomyosarcoma.

Table 494-2 FEATURES OF MOST COMMON TYPES OF NON-RHABDOMYOCARCOMA SOFT TISSUE SARCOMAS

TISSUE TYPE	TUMOR	NATURAL HISTORY AND BIOLOGY
Adipose	Liposarcoma	A very rare tumor. Usually arises in the extremities or retroperitoneum; associated with a nonrandom translocation, t(12;16) (q13;p11). Tends to be locally invasive and rarely metastasizes; wide local excision is the treatment of choice. The role of radiation therapy and chemotherapy in treating gross residual or metastatic disease is not established.
Fibrous	Fibrosarcoma	Most common soft tissue sarcoma in children <1 yr. Congenital fibrosarcoma is a low-grade malignancy that commonly arises in the extremities or trunk and rarely metastasizes. Surgical excision is treatment of choice; dramatic responses to preoperative chemotherapy may occur. In children >4 yr, the natural history is similar to that in adults (a 5-yr survival rate of 60%); wide surgical excision and preoperative chemotherapy are commonly used. Associated with t(12;15) (p13;q25) or trisomy 11, also +8, +17, +20.
	Malignant fibrous histiocytoma	Most commonly arises in the trunk and extremities, deep in the subcutaneous layer. Histologically subdivided into storiform, giant cell, myxoid, and angiomatoid variants. The angiomatoid type tends to affect younger patients and is curable with surgical resection alone. Wide surgical excision is the treatment of choice. Chemotherapy has produced objective tumor regressions.
Vascular	Hemangiopericytoma	Often arises in the lower extremities or retroperitoneum; may manifest as hypoglycemia and hypophosphatemic rickets. Both benign and malignant histology. Nonrandom translocations t(12;19) (q13;q13) and t(13;22) (q22;q13.3) have been described. Complete surgical excision is the treatment of choice. Chemotherapy and radiation therapy may produce responses.
	Angiosarcoma	Rare in children; 33% arise in skin, 25% in soft tissue, and 25% in liver, breast, or bone. Associated with chronic lymphedema and exposure to vinyl chloride in adults. Survival rate is poor (12% at 5 yr) despite some responses to chemotherapy/radiation therapy.
	Hemangioendothelioma	Can occur in soft tissue, liver, and lung. Localized lesions have a favorable outcome; lesions in lung and liver often are multifocal and have a poor prognosis.
Peripheral nerves	Neurofibrosarcoma	Also known as the malignant peripheral nerve sheath tumor. Develops in up to 16% of patients with neurofibromatosis type 1 (NF1); almost 50% occur in patients with NF1. Deletions of chromosome 22q11-q13 or 17q11 and p53 mutations have been reported. Commonly arises in trunk and extremities and is usually locally invasive. Complete surgical excision is necessary for survival; response to chemotherapy is suboptimal.
Synovium	Synovial sarcoma	The most common non-rhabdomyosarcoma soft tissue sarcoma in some series. Often manifesting in the 3rd decade, but 33% of patients are <20 yr. Typically arises around the knee or thigh and is characterized by a nonrandom translocation t(X;18) (p11;q11). Wide surgical excision is necessary. Radiation therapy is effective in microscopic residual disease, and ifosfamide-based therapy is active in advanced disease.
Unknown	Alveolar soft part sarcoma	Slow-growing tumor; tends to recur or to metastasize to lung and brain years after diagnosis. Often arises in the extremities and head and neck. A myogenic origin has been proposed. Resection of primary and metastatic sites, when possible, is recommended.
Smooth muscle	Leiomyosarcoma	Often arises in the gastrointestinal tract and may be associated with a t(12;14) (q14;q23) translocation. Associated with Epstein-Barr virus in immunodeficiency syndromes (including AIDS). Complete surgical excision is the treatment of choice.

rhabdomyosarcoma randomized patients comparing VAC with VAC alternating with vincristine, topotecan, cyclophosphamide (VTC) and showed no improvement in outcome for patients treated with VAC/VTC over that of standard VAC therapy. Radiation therapy dosing was determined by response to second-look surgery, if performed. Irinotecan, another topoisomerase inhibitor, is currently being evaluated in patients with intermediate-risk. For patients with low-risk disease, clinical trials are investigating the reduction of therapy to maintain the same good outcome while decreasing late effects of treatment. More intensive approaches utilizing mulitagent chemotherapy in conjunction with biologic agents such as insulin-like growth factor inhibitors and other agents are being evaluated in clinical trials for the most high-risk disease.

Prognosis

Prognostic factors include age, stage, histology, and primary site. Among patients with resectable tumor and favorable histology, 80-90% have prolonged disease-free survival. Unresectable tumor localized to certain favorable sites, such as the orbit, also has a high likelihood of cure. About 65-70% of patients with incompletely resected tumor also achieve long-term disease-free survival. Patients with disseminated disease have a poor prognosis; only about 50% achieve remission, and fewer than 50% of these are cured. Older children have a poorer prognosis than younger children. For all patients, surveillance for late effects of cancer treatment (such as impaired bone growth secondary to irradiation, sterility from cyclophosphamide, and second malignancies) is important.

OTHER SOFT TISSUE SARCOMAS

The non-rhabdomyosarcoma soft tissue sarcomas (NRSTSs) constitute a heterogeneous group of tumors that account for 3% of all childhood malignancies (Table 494-2). Because they are relatively rare in children, much of the information about their natural history and treatment has been derived from studies in adult patients. In children, the median age at diagnosis is 12 yr, with a male:female ratio of 2.3:1. These tumors commonly arise in the trunk or lower extremities. The most common histologic types are synovial sarcoma (42%), fibrosarcoma (13%), malignant fibrous histiocytoma (12%), and neurogenic tumors (10%). Molecular genetic studies often prove useful in diagnosis, because several of these tumors have characteristic chromosomal translocations.

Surgery remains the mainstay of therapy, but a careful search for lung and bone metastases should be undertaken before surgical excision. Chemotherapy and radiation therapy should be considered for large, high-grade, and unresectable tumors. The role of chemotherapy for NRSTSs is not as well defined as for rhabdomyosarcoma. Patients with unresectable or metastatic disease are treated with multiagent chemotherapy in addition to irradiation and/or surgery. Tumor size, stage (clinical group), invasiveness, and histologic grade correlate with survival.

BIBLIOGRAPHY

Please visit the Nelson Textbook of Pediatrics *website at* *www.expertconsult.com* *for the complete bibliography.*

Chapter 495
Neoplasms of Bone

495.1 Malignant Tumors of Bone

Carola A.S. Arndt

The annual incidence of malignant bone tumors in the USA is approximately 7 cases/million white children <14 yr of age, with a slightly lower incidence in African-American children. Osteosarcoma is the most common primary malignant bone tumor in children and adolescents, followed by Ewing sarcoma (Table 495-1; Fig. 495-1). In children <10 yr of age, Ewing sarcoma is more common than osteosarcoma. Both tumor types are most likely to occur in the second decade of life.

OSTEOSARCOMA

Epidemiology

The annual incidence of osteosarcoma in the USA is 5.6 cases/million children <15 yr of age. The highest risk period for development of osteosarcoma is during the adolescent growth spurt, suggesting an association between rapid bone growth and malignant transformation. Patients with osteosarcoma are taller than their peers of similar age.

Pathogenesis

Although the cause of osteosarcoma is unknown, certain genetic or acquired conditions predispose patients to development of osteosarcoma. Patients with **hereditary retinoblastoma** have a significantly increased risk for development of osteosarcoma. The sites of osteosarcoma in these patients were initially thought to be located only in previously irradiated areas, but later studies have shown them to arise in sites far from the radiation field.

Table 495-1 COMPARISON OF FEATURES OF OSTEOSARCOMA AND THE EWING FAMILY OF TUMORS

FEATURE	OSTEOSARCOMA	EWING FAMILY OF TUMORS
Age	Second decade	Second decade
Race	All races	Primarily whites
Sex (M:F)	1.5:1	1.5:1
Cell	Spindle cell–producing osteoid	Undifferentiated small round cell, probably of neural origin
Predisposition	Retinoblastoma, Li-Fraumeni syndrome, Paget disease, radiotherapy	None known
Site	Metaphyses of long bones	Diaphyses of long bones, flat bones
Presentation	Local pain and swelling; often, history of injury	Local pain and swelling; fever
Radiographic findings	Sclerotic destruction (less commonly lytic); sunburst pattern	Primarily lytic, multilaminar periosteal reaction ("onion-skinning")
Differential diagnosis	Ewing sarcoma, osteomyelitis	Osteomyelitis, eosinophilic granuloma, lymphoma, neuroblastoma, rhabdomyosarcoma
Metastasis	Lungs, bones	Lungs, bones
Treatment	Chemotherapy	Chemotherapy
	Ablative surgery of primary tumor	Radiotherapy and/or surgery of primary tumor
Outcome	Without metastases, 70% cured; with metastases at diagnosis, ≤20% survival	Without metastases, 60% cured; with metastases at diagnosis, 20-30% survival

Predisposition to development of osteosarcoma in these patients may be related to loss of heterozygosity of the RB gene. Osteosarcoma also occurs in the **Li-Fraumeni syndrome,** which is a familial cancer syndrome associated with germline mutations of the p53 gene. Kindreds with **Li-Fraumeni syndrome** have a spectrum of malignancies in 1st-degree relatives, including carcinoma of the breast, soft tissue sarcomas, brain tumors, leukemia, adrenal cortical carcinoma, and other malignancies. **Rothmund-Thomson syndrome** is a rare syndrome associated with short stature, skin telangiectasia, small hands and feet, hypoplasticity or absence of the thumbs, and a high risk of osteosarcoma. Osteosarcoma also can be induced by irradiation for Ewing sarcoma, craniospinal irradiation for brain tumors, or high-dose irradiation for other malignancies. Other benign conditions that can be associated with malignant transformation to osteosarcoma include Paget disease, enchondromatosis, multiple hereditary exostoses, and fibrous dysplasia.

The pathologic diagnosis of osteosarcoma is made by demonstration of a highly malignant, pleomorphic, spindle cell neoplasm associated with the formation of malignant osteoid and bone. There are four pathologic subtypes of conventional high-grade osteosarcoma: osteoblastic, fibroblastic, chondroblastic, and telangiectatic. No significant differences in outcome are associated with the various subtypes, although the chondroblastic component of that subtype may not respond as well to chemotherapy. The role in prognosis of various genes such as drug resistance-related genes, tumor suppressor genes, and genes related to apoptosis is being evaluated.

Telangiectatic osteosarcoma may be confused with aneurysmal bone cyst because of its lytic appearance on radiography. High-grade osteosarcoma typically arises in the diaphyseal region of long bones and invades the medullary cavity. It also may be associated with a soft tissue mass. Two variants of osteosarcoma, parosteal and periosteal osteosarcoma, should be distinguished from conventional osteosarcoma because of their characteristic clinical features. **Parosteal osteosarcoma** is a low-grade, well-differentiated tumor that does not invade the medullary cavity and most commonly is found in the posterior aspect of the distal femur. Surgical resection alone often is curative in this lesion, which has a low propensity for metastatic spread. **Periosteal osteosarcoma** is a rare variant that arises on the surface of the bone but has a higher rate of metastatic spread than the parosteal type and an intermediate prognosis.

Clinical Manifestations

Pain, limp, and swelling are the most common presenting manifestations of osteosarcoma. Because these tumors occur most often in active adolescents, initial complaints may be attributed to a sports injury or sprain; any bone or joint pain not responding to conservative therapy within a reasonable time should be investigated thoroughly. Additional clinical findings may include limitation of motion, joint effusion, tenderness, and warmth. Results of routine laboratory tests, such as a complete blood cell count and chemistry panel, are usually normal, although alkaline phosphatase or lactic dehydrogenase values may be elevated.

Diagnosis

Bone tumor should be suspected in a patient who presents with deep bone pain often causing nighttime awakening in whom there is a palpable mass, and radiographs demonstrate a lesion. The lesion may be mixed lytic and blastic in appearance, but new bone formation is usually visible. The classic radiographic appearance of osteosarcoma is the **sunburst pattern** (Fig. 495-2). When osteosarcoma is suspected, the patient should be referred to a center with experience in managing bone tumors. The biopsy and the surgery should be performed by the same surgeon so that the incisional biopsy site can be placed in a manner that will not compromise the ultimate limb salvage procedure. Tissue

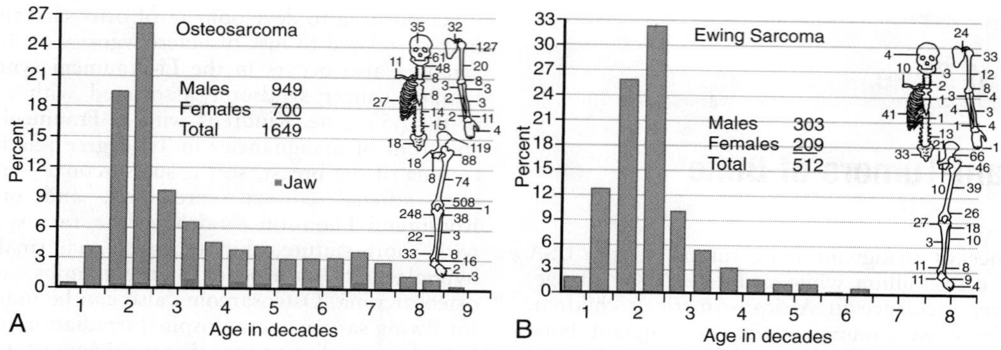

Figure 495-1 *A,* Age and skeletal distribution of 1,649 cases of osteosarcoma in the Mayo Clinic files. *B,* Age and skeletal distribution of 512 cases of Ewing sarcoma in the Mayo Clinic files. (From Unni KK, editor: *Dahlin's bone tumors: general aspects and data on 11,087 cases,* ed 5, Philadelphia, 1996, Lippincott-Raven. Reprinted by permission of the Mayo Foundation.)

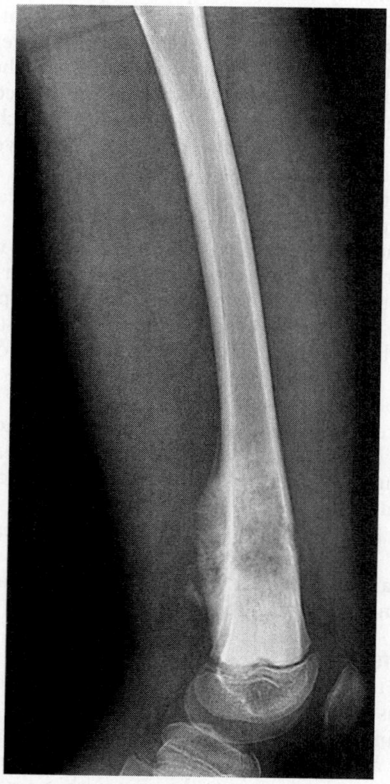

Figure 495-2 Radiograph of an osteosarcoma of the femur with typical "sunburst" appearance of bone formation.

usually is obtained for molecular and biologic studies at the time of the initial biopsy. Before biopsy, MRI of the primary lesion and the entire bone should be performed to evaluate the tumor for its proximity to nerves and blood vessels, soft tissue and joint extension, and skip lesions. The metastatic work-up, which should be performed before biopsy, includes CT of the chest and radionuclide bone scanning to evaluate for lung and bone metastases, respectively. The **differential diagnosis** of a lytic bone lesion includes histiocytosis, Ewing sarcoma, lymphoma, and bone cyst.

Treatment

With chemotherapy and surgery, the 5-yr disease-free survival rate of patients with nonmetastatic extremity osteosarcoma is 65-75%. Complete surgical resection of the tumor is important for cure. The current approach is to treat patients with preoperative chemotherapy in an attempt to facilitate limb salvage operations and to treat micrometastatic disease immediately. Up to 80% of patients are able to undergo limb salvage operations after initial chemotherapy. Some institutions use intra-arterial chemotherapy to infuse chemotherapy directly into an artery feeding the tumor, although this approach has not been shown to be better than conventional intravenous chemotherapy. It is important to resume chemotherapy as soon as possible after surgery. Lung metastases present at diagnosis should be resected by thoracotomies at some time during the course of treatment. Active agents currently in use in multidrug chemotherapy regimens for conventional osteosarcoma include doxorubicin, cisplatin, methotrexate, and ifosfamide.

One of the most important prognostic factors in osteosarcoma is the histologic response to chemotherapy. An international cooperative group is performing a randomized trial of the postoperative addition of high-dose ifosfamide with etoposide to standard three-drug therapy with cisplatin, doxorubicin, and methotrexate to improve the outcome of patients with a poor histologic response. Patients with good histologic response will be randomized to the addition of PEGylated interferon-α2b. For patients with metastatic disease, a new approach currently being investigated is the addition of zoledronic acid, a bisphosphonate, to intensive chemotherapy. After limb salvage surgery, intensive rehabilitation and physical therapy are necessary to ensure maximal functional outcome.

For patients who require amputation, early prosthetic fitting and gait training are essential to enable them to resume normal activities as soon as possible. Before definitive surgery, patients with tumors on weight-bearing bones should be instructed to use crutches to avoid stressing the weakened bones and causing pathologic fracture. The role of chemotherapy in parosteal and periosteal osteosarcomas is not well defined.

Prognosis

Surgical resection alone is curative only for patients with parosteal osteosarcoma. Conventional osteosarcoma requires multiagent chemotherapy. Up to 75% of patients with nonmetastatic extremity osteosarcoma are cured with current multiagent treatment protocols. The prognosis is not as favorable for patients with pelvic tumors as for those with primary tumors in extremities. Twenty percent to 30% of patients who have limited numbers of pulmonary metastases also can be cured with aggressive chemotherapy and resection of lung nodules. Patients with bone metastases and those with widespread lung metastases have an extremely poor prognosis. Long-term follow-up of patients with osteosarcoma is important to monitor for late effects of chemotherapy, such as cardiotoxicity from anthracycline. Patients in whom late, isolated lung metastases develop may be cured with surgical resection alone.

EWING SARCOMA

Epidemiology

The incidence of Ewing sarcoma in the USA is 2.1 cases/million children. It is rare among African-American children. Ewing sarcoma, an undifferentiated sarcoma of bone, also may arise from soft tissue. The term **Ewing sarcoma family of tumors** refers to a group of small, round cell, undifferentiated tumors thought to be of neural crest origin that generally carry the same chromosomal translocation. This family of tumors includes Ewing sarcoma of bone and soft tissue and peripheral **primitive neuroectodermal tumor.** Treatment protocols for these tumors are the same whether the tumors arise in bone or soft tissue. Anatomic sites of primary tumors arising in bone are distributed evenly between the extremities and the central axis (pelvis, spine, and chest wall). Primary tumors arising in the chest wall are often referred to as **Askin tumors.**

Pathogenesis

Immunohistochemical staining assists in the diagnosis of Ewing sarcoma to differentiate it from **small round blue cell tumors** such as lymphoma, rhabdomyosarcoma, and neuroblastoma. Histochemical stains may react positively with certain neural markers on tumor cells (neuron-specific enolase and S-100), especially in peripheral primitive neuroectodermal tumor. Reactivity with muscle markers (e.g., desmin, actin) is absent. Additionally, MIC-2 (CD99) staining is usually positive. A specific chromosomal translocation, t(11;22), or a variant thereof is found in most of the Ewing sarcoma family of tumors. Analysis for the translocation by routine cytogenetic or polymerase chain reaction analysis for the chimeric fusion gene products EWS/FLI1 or EWS/ERG can be helpful in confirming the diagnosis in extremely undifferentiated tumors.

Clinical Manifestations

Symptoms of Ewing sarcoma are similar to those of osteosarcoma. Pain, swelling, limitation of motion, and tenderness over the involved bone or soft tissue are common presenting symptoms. Patients with huge chest wall primary tumors may present with respiratory distress. Patients with paraspinal or vertebral primary tumors may present with symptoms of cord compression. Ewing sarcoma often is associated with **systemic manifestations,** such as fever and weight loss; patients may have undergone treatment for a presumptive diagnosis of osteomyelitis. Patients also may have a delay in diagnosis when their pain or swelling is attributed to a sports injury.

Diagnosis

The diagnosis of Ewing sarcoma should be suspected in a patient who presents with pain and swelling, with or without systemic symptoms, and with a radiographic appearance of a primarily lytic bone lesion with periosteal reaction, the characteristic **onion-skinning** (Fig. 495-3). A large associated soft tissue mass often is visualized on MRI or CT (Fig. 495-4). The **differential diagnosis** includes osteosarcoma, osteomyelitis, Langerhans cell histiocytosis, primary lymphoma of bone, metastatic neuroblastoma, or rhabdomyosarcoma in the case of a pure soft tissue lesion. Patients should be referred to a center with experience in managing bone tumors for evaluation and biopsy. Thorough evaluation for metastatic disease includes CT of the chest, radionuclide bone scan, and bone marrow aspiration and biopsy specimens from at least two sites. MRI of the tumor and the entire length of involved bone should be performed to determine the exact extension of the soft tissue and bony mass and the proximity of tumor to neurovascular structures. To avoid compromising an ultimate potential for limb salvage by a poorly planned biopsy incision, the same surgeon should perform the biopsy and the surgical procedure. CT-guided biopsy of the lesion often provides diagnostic tissue. It is important to

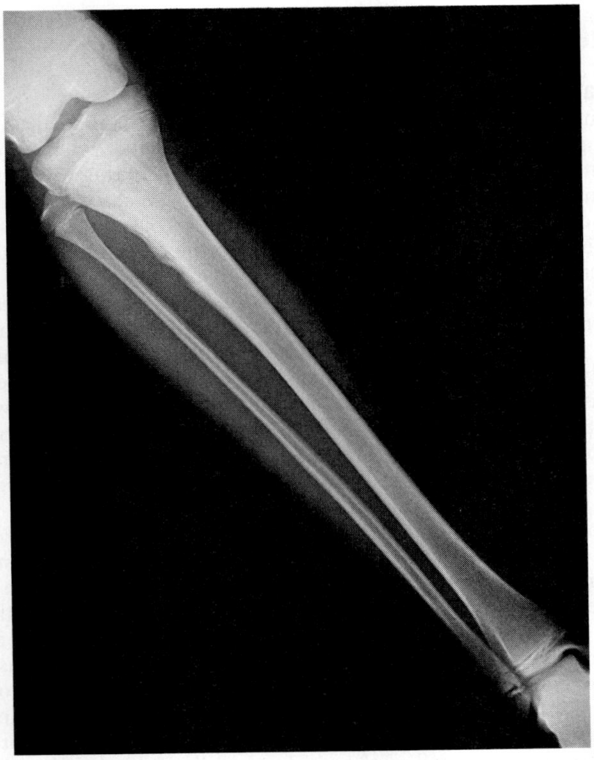

Figure 495-3 Radiograph of tibial Ewing sarcoma showing periosteal elevation or "onion-skinning."

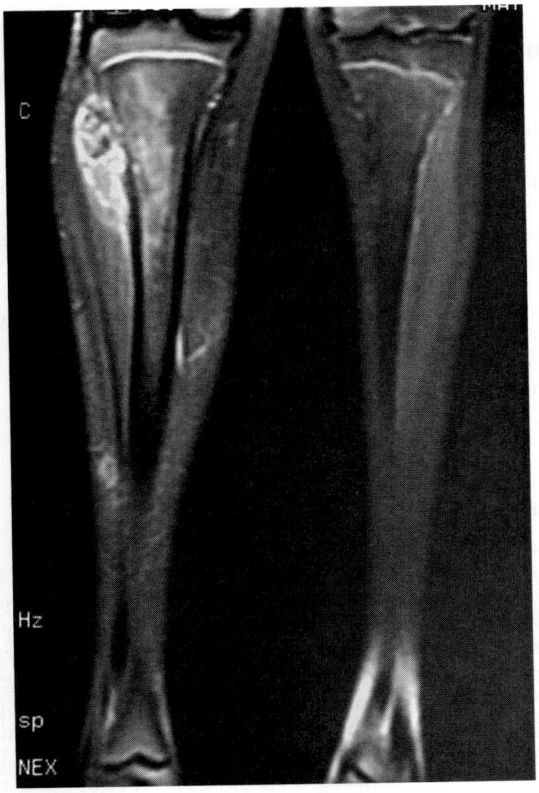

Figure 495-4 MR image of tibial Ewing sarcoma showing a large associated soft tissue mass.

obtain adequate tissue for special stains, cytogenetics, and molecular studies.

Treatment

Tumors of the Ewing sarcoma family are best managed with a comprehensive multidisciplinary approach in which the surgeon, chemotherapist, and radiation oncologist plan therapy. Multiagent chemotherapy is important because it can shrink the tumor rapidly and is usually given before local control is attempted. The addition of ifosfamide and etoposide to the conventional agents vincristine, doxorubicin, and cyclophosphamide improves the outcome for patients with nonmetastatic Ewing sarcoma. Chemotherapy usually causes dramatic shrinkage of the soft tissue mass and rapid, significant pain relief. One completed randomized study for patients with nonmetastatic Ewing sarcoma showed a statistically significantly better outcome when patients were treated on a 14-day schedule than on a 21-day schedule. Current studies are evaluating the addition of topoisomerase inhibitors to standard chemotherapy, and plans are under way to investigate the role of insulin-like growth factor receptor inhibitors for certain groups of patients. An international cooperative group trial is evaluating whether myeloablative chemotherapy and stem cell rescue is superior to chemotherapy with lung irradiation for patients with pulmonary metastases. Myeloablative chemotherapy for patients with extremely high risk disease (bone and marrow metastases) also is being studied, as are approaches using angiogenesis inhibitors on a standard chemotherapy backbone. Ewing sarcoma is considered a radiosensitive tumor, and local control may be achieved with irradiation or surgery. Radiation therapy is associated with a risk of radiation-induced second malignancies, especially osteosarcoma, as well as failure of bone growth in skeletally immature patients. Many centers prefer surgical resection, if possible, to achieve local control. It is important to provide the patient with crutches if the tumor is in a weight-bearing bone, to avoid a pathologic fracture before definitive local control. Chemotherapy should be resumed as soon as possible after surgery.

Prognosis

Patients with small, nonmetastatic, distally located extremity tumors have the best prognosis, with a cure rate of up to 75%. Patients with pelvic tumors have, until recently, had a much worse outcome. Patients with metastatic disease at diagnosis, especially bone or bone marrow metastases, have a poor prognosis, with <30% surviving long term. New approaches, such as very intensive chemotherapy with peripheral blood stem cell rescue, are being investigated in these patients.

Long-term follow-up of patients with Ewing sarcoma is important because of the potential for late effects of treatment, such as anthracycline cardiotoxicity; second malignancies, especially in the radiation field; and late relapses, even as long as 10 yr after initial diagnosis.

495.2 Benign Tumors and Tumor-like Processes of Bone

Carola A.S. Arndt

Benign bone lesions in children are common in comparison with the relatively rare malignant neoplasms of bone and present diagnostic challenges. Some, although histologically benign, can be life-threatening. No single element in the history or diagnostic test is sufficient to rule out malignancies or suggest nonneoplastic conditions. A broad range of diagnostic possibilities must be considered when confronted with an unknown bone lesion. Benign lesions may be painless or painful, especially if a pathologic fracture is impending. Night pain that awakens a child suggests malignancy; relief of such pain with aspirin is common with benign lesions such as osteoid osteomas. Rapidly enlarging lesions usually are associated with malignancy, but several benign lesions, such as aneurysmal bone cysts, can enlarge faster than most malignancies. Several conditions, such as osteomyelitis, can simulate the appearance of benign bone tumors.

Many benign bone tumors are diagnosed incidentally or after pathologic fracture. Management of these fractures is similar to that of nonpathologic fractures in the same location. It is unusual for benign bone tumors to interfere with fracture healing. Likewise, the fractures rarely result in changes or healing of these tumors, which usually are treated after the fracture has healed.

Radiographs of any suspected bone lesion should always be obtained in two planes. Additional studies may be necessary to help arrive at the correct diagnosis and to guide treatment. Although these lesions are benign, many do require intervention.

Osteochondroma (**exostosis**) is one of the most common benign bone tumors in children. Because many are completely asymptomatic and unrecognized, the true incidence of this lesion is unknown. Most osteochondromas develop in childhood, arising from the metaphysis of a long bone, particularly the distal femur, proximal humerus, and proximal tibia. The lesion enlarges with the child until skeletal maturity. Most are discovered at 5-15 yr of age, when the child or parent notices a bony, nonpainful mass. Some are discovered because they are irritated by pressure during athletic or other activities. Osteochondromas appear radiographically as stalks or broad-based projections from the surface of the bone, usually in a direction away from the adjacent joint. Invariably, the lesion is radiographically smaller than suggested by palpation because the cartilage cap covering the lesion is not seen. This cartilage cap may be up to 1 cm thick. Both the cortex of the bone and the marrow space of the involved bone are continuous with the lesion. Malignant degeneration of a chondrosarcoma is rare in children but occurs in as many as 1% of adults. Routine removal is not performed unless the lesion is large enough to cause symptoms or if the lesion grows rapidly.

Multiple hereditary exostoses is a related but rare condition characterized by the presence of multiple osteochondromas. Severely involved children can have short stature, limb-length inequality, premature partial physeal arrests, and deformity of both the upper and lower extremities. These children must be monitored carefully during growth.

Enchondroma is a benign lesion of hyaline cartilage that occurs centrally in the bone. Most of these lesions are asymptomatic and occur in the hands. Most are discovered incidentally, although pathologic fractures often lead to the diagnosis. Radiographically, the lesions occupy the medullary canal, are radiolucent, and are sharply marginated. Punctate or stippled calcification may be present within the lesion, but this is much more common in adults than in children. Almost all enchondromas are solitary. Most can simply be observed, with curettage and bone grafting reserved for lesions that are symptomatic or large enough to weaken the bone structurally. Multifocal involvement is referred to as **Ollier disease** and can result in bone dysplasia, short stature, limb-length inequality, and joint deformity. Surgery may be necessary to correct or prevent such deformities. When multiple enchondromas are associated with angiomas of the soft tissue, the condition is referred to as **Maffucci syndrome.** A high rate of malignant transformation has been reported in both of these multifocal conditions.

Chondroblastoma is a rare lesion usually found in the epiphysis of long bones. Most patients present in the second decade with complaints of mild to moderate pain in the adjacent joint. Common sites include the hip, shoulder, and knee. Muscle atrophy and local tenderness may be the only clinical findings. The lesion appears radiographically as a sharply marginated radiolucency within the epiphysis or apophysis, occasionally with metaphyseal extension across the physis. Proximity to the joint can cause deformity of the subchondral bone, an effusion, or erosion into the joint. Recognition is important because most lesions can be cured with curettage and bone grafting before joint destruction occurs.

Chondromyxoid fibroma is an uncommon benign bone tumor in children. This metaphyseal lesion usually causes pain and local tenderness. The lesion occasionally is asymptomatic. Chondromyxoid fibroma appears radiographically as eccentric, lobular, metaphyseal radiolucency with sharp, sclerotic, and scalloped margins. The lower extremity is involved most often. Treatment usually consists of curettage and bone grafting or en bloc resection.

Osteoid osteoma is a small benign bone tumor. Most of these tumors are diagnosed between 5-20 yr of age. The clinical pattern is characteristic, consisting of unremitting and gradually increasing pain that often is worst at night and is relieved by aspirin. Boys are affected more often than girls. Any bone can be involved, but the most common sites are the proximal femur and tibia. Vertebral lesions can cause scoliosis or symptoms that mimic a neurologic disorder. Examination can reveal a limp, atrophy, and weakness when the lower extremity is involved. Palpation and range of motion do not alter the discomfort. Radiographs are distinctive, showing a round or oval metaphyseal or diaphyseal lucency (0.5-1.0 cm diameter) surrounded by sclerotic bone. The central lucency, or nidus, shows intense uptake on bone scan. About 25% of osteoid osteomas are not visualized on plain radiographs but can be identified with CT. Because of the small size of the lesion and its location adjacent to thick cortical bone, MRI is poor at detecting osteoid osteomas. Treatment is directed at removing the lesion. This can involve en bloc excision, curettage, or percutaneous CT-guided ablation of the nidus. Patients with mild pain may be treated with salicylates. Some lesions resolve spontaneously after skeletal maturity.

Osteoblastoma is a locally destructive, progressively growing lesion of bone with a predilection for the vertebrae, although almost any bone may be involved. Most patients note the insidious onset of dull aching pain, which may be present for months before they seek medical attention. Spinal lesions can cause neurologic symptoms or deficits. The radiographic appearance is variable and less distinctive than that of other benign bone tumors. About 25% show features suggesting a malignant neoplasm, making biopsy necessary in many cases. Expansile spinal lesions often involve the posterior elements. Treatment involves curettage and bone grafting or en bloc excision, taking care to preserve nerve roots when treating spinal lesions. Surgical stabilization of the spine may be necessary.

Fibromas (nonossifying fibroma, fibrous cortical defect, metaphyseal fibrous defect) are fibrous lesions of bone that occur in 40% of children >2 yr of age. They most likely represent a defect in ossification rather than a neoplasm and usually are asymptomatic. Most are discovered incidentally when radiographs are taken for other reasons, usually to rule out a fracture after trauma. Occasional pathologic fractures can occur through rare large lesions. Physical examination usually is unrevealing. Radiographs show a sharply marginated eccentric lucency in the metaphyseal cortex. Lesions may be multilocular and expansile, with extension from the cortex into the medullary bone. The long axis of the lesion runs parallel to that of the bone. Approximately 50% are bilateral or multiple. Because of the characteristic radiographic appearance, most lesions do not require biopsy or treatment. Spontaneous regression can be expected after skeletal maturity. Curettage and bone grafting may be recommended for lesions occupying >50% of the bone diameter because of the risk of a pathologic fracture.

Unicameral bone cysts can occur at any age in childhood but are rare in children <3 yr of age and after skeletal maturity. The cause of these fluid-filled lesions is unknown. Some resolve spontaneously after skeletal maturity is reached. Most are asymptomatic until diagnosis, which usually follows a pathologic fracture. Such fractures can occur with relatively minor trauma, such as with throwing or catching a ball. Unicameral bone cysts appear radiographically as solitary, centrally located lesions within the medullary portion of the bone. These cysts are most common in the proximal humerus or femur. They often extend to (but not through) the physis and are sharply marginated. The cortex expands, but that does not exceed the width of the adjacent physis. Treatment involves allowing the pathologic fracture to heal, followed by aspiration and injection with methylprednisolone or bone marrow. Repeat injections, curettage, and bone grafting occasionally are necessary to treat recurrent lesions.

Aneurysmal bone cyst is a reactive lesion of bone seen in persons <20 yr of age. The lesion is characterized by cavernous spaces filled with blood and solid aggregates of tissue. Although the femur, tibia, and spine are most commonly involved, this progressively growing, expansile lesion develops in any bone. Pain and swelling are common. Spinal involvement can lead to cord or nerve root compression and associated neurologic symptoms, including paralysis. Radiographs show eccentric lytic destruction and expansion of the metaphysis surrounded by a thin sclerotic rim of bone. Posterior elements of the spine are involved more commonly than the vertebral body. Unlike most other benign bone tumors, which usually are confined to a single bone, aneurysmal bone cysts can involve adjacent vertebrae. Rapid growth is characteristic and can lead to confusion with malignant neoplasms. Treatment consists of curettage and bone grafting or excision. Spinal lesions can require stabilization after excision. As with other benign tumors, attempts are made to preserve nerve roots and other vital structures. Recurrence after surgical treatment occurs in 20-30% of patients, is more common in younger than older children, and usually occurs in the first 1-2 yr after treatment.

Fibrous dysplasia is a developmental abnormality characterized by fibrous replacement of cancellous bone. Lesions may be solitary or multifocal (polyostotic), relatively stable, or progressively more severe. Most children are asymptomatic, although those with skull involvement might have swelling or exophthalmos. Pain and limp are characteristic of proximal femoral involvement. Limb-length discrepancy, bowing of the tibia or femur, and pathologic fractures may be presenting complaints. The triad of polyostotic disease, precocious puberty, and cutaneous pigmentation is known as Albright syndrome. Radiographic features of fibrous dysplasia include a lytic or ground-glass expansile lesion of the metaphysis or diaphysis. The lesion is sharply marginated and often is surrounded by a thick rim of sclerotic bone. Bowing, especially of the proximal femur, may be present. Treatment usually involves observation. Surgery is indicated for patients with progressive deformity, pain, or impending pathologic fractures. Bone grafting is not as successful in the treatment of fibrous dysplasia as with other benign tumors because the lesion often recurs within the grafted bone. Reconstructive surgical techniques often are necessary to provide stability.

Osteofibrous dysplasia affects children 1-10 yr of age. This lesion usually involves the tibia. It is clinically, radiographically, and histologically distinct from fibrous dysplasia. Most children present with anterior swelling or enlargement of the leg. Progression is unlikely after 10 yr of age. Radiographs show solitary or multiple lucent cortical diaphyseal lesions surrounded by sclerosis. Anterior bowing of the tibia often is present. The radiographic appearance closely resembles that of adamantinoma, a malignant neoplasm, making biopsy more common than with other benign bone tumors. Treatment involves observation. Some lesions heal spontaneously. Excision and bone grafting should be delayed until the child is >10 yr of age because of a high recurrence rate before this age. Pathologic fractures heal with immobilization.

Eosinophilic granuloma is a monostotic or polyostotic disease with no extraskeletal involvement. This latter finding distinguishes eosinophilic granuloma from the other forms of

Langerhans' cell histiocytosis (Hand-Schüller-Christian or Letterer-Siwe variants), which can have a less favorable prognosis (Chapter 501). Eosinophilic granuloma usually occurs during the first 3 decades of life and is most common in boys 5-10 yr of age. The skull is most commonly affected, but any bone may be involved. Patients usually present with local pain and swelling. Marked tenderness and warmth often are present in the area of the involved bone. Spinal lesions can cause pain, stiffness, and occasional neurologic symptoms. The radiographic appearance of the skeletal lesions is similar in all forms of Langerhans' cell histiocytosis but is variable enough to mimic many other benign and malignant lesions of bone. The radiolucent lesions have well-defined or irregular margins with expansion of the involved bone and periosteal new bone formation. Spine involvement can cause uniform compression or flattening of the vertebral body. A skeletal survey is warranted because polyostotic involvement and the typical skull lesions strongly suggest the diagnosis of eosinophilic granuloma. Biopsy often is necessary to confirm the diagnosis because of the broad radiographic differential diagnosis. Treatment includes curettage and bone grafting, low-dose radiation therapy, or corticosteroid injection. Observation for symptomatic lesions is reasonable because most osseous lesions heal spontaneously and do not recur. Children with bone lesions should be evaluated for visceral involvement because treatment of Hand-Schüller-Christian disease and Letterer-Siwe disease is more complex and often systemic.

BIBLIOGRAPHY

Please visit the Nelson Textbook of Pediatrics *website at www.expertconsult.com for the complete bibliography.*

Chapter 496
Retinoblastoma

Peter E. Zage and Cynthia E. Herzog

Retinoblastoma is an embryonal malignancy of the retina and is the most common intraocular tumor in children. Although the survival rate of children in the USA and developed countries with retinoblastoma is extremely high, retinoblastoma progresses to metastatic disease and death in over 50% of children worldwide. Furthermore, the associated loss of vision and side effects of therapy are significant problems that remain to be addressed.

EPIDEMIOLOGY

Approximately 250-350 new cases of retinoblastoma are diagnosed each year in the USA, with no known racial or gender predilection. The cumulative lifetime incidence of retinoblastoma is approximately 1:20,000 live births, and retinoblastoma accounts for 4% of all pediatric malignancies. The median age at diagnosis is approximately 2 yr, and over 90% of cases are diagnosed in children under 5 yr of age. Overall, about two thirds to three quarters of children with retinoblastoma have unilateral tumors, with the remainder having bilateral retinoblastoma. Bilateral involvement is more common in younger children, particularly in those diagnosed under the age of 1 yr.

Retinoblastoma can be either hereditary or sporadic. Hereditary cases usually are diagnosed at a younger age and are multifocal and bilateral, while sporadic cases are usually diagnosed in older children who tend to have unilateral, unifocal involvement. The hereditary form is associated with loss of function of the **retinoblastoma gene *(RB1)*** via gene mutation or deletion. The *RB1* gene is located on chromosome 13q14 and encodes the **retinoblastoma protein (Rb)**, a tumor suppressor protein that controls cell-cycle phase transition and has roles in apoptosis and cell differentiation. Many different causative mutations have been identified, including translocations, deletions, insertions, point mutations, and epigenetic modifications such as gene methylation. The nature of the predisposing mutation can affect the penetrance and expressivity of retinoblastoma development.

According to Knudson's "two-hit" model of oncogenesis, two mutational events are required for retinoblastoma tumor development (Chapter 486). In the hereditary form of retinoblastoma, the first mutation in the *RB1* gene is inherited through germinal cells and a second mutation occurs subsequently in somatic retinal cells. Second mutations that lead to retinoblastoma often result in the loss of the normal allele and concomitant loss of heterozygosity. Most children with hereditary retinoblastoma have spontaneous new germinal mutations, and both parents have wild-type retinoblastoma genes. In the sporadic form of retinoblastoma, the two mutations occur in somatic retinal cells. Heterozygous carriers of oncogenic *RB1* mutations demonstrate variable phenotypic expression.

PATHOGENESIS

Histologically, retinoblastoma appears as a small round blue cell tumor with rosette formation (Flexner-Wintersteiner rosettes). It may arise in any of the nucleated layers of the retina and exhibit various degrees of differentiation. Retinoblastoma tumors tend to outgrow their blood supply, resulting in necrosis and calcification.

Endophytic tumors arise from the inner surface of the retina and grow into the vitreous, and can also grow as tumors suspended within the vitreous itself, known as **vitreous seeding.** Exophytic tumors grow from the outer retinal layer and can cause retinal detachment. Tumors can also be both endophytic and exophytic. These tumors can also spread by direct extension to the choroid or along the optic nerve beyond the lamina cribrosa, or by hematogenous or lymphatic spread to distant sites.

CLINICAL MANIFESTATIONS

Retinoblastoma classically presents with **leukocoria,** a white pupillary reflex (Fig. 496-1), which often is first noticed when a red reflex is not present at a routine newborn or well child

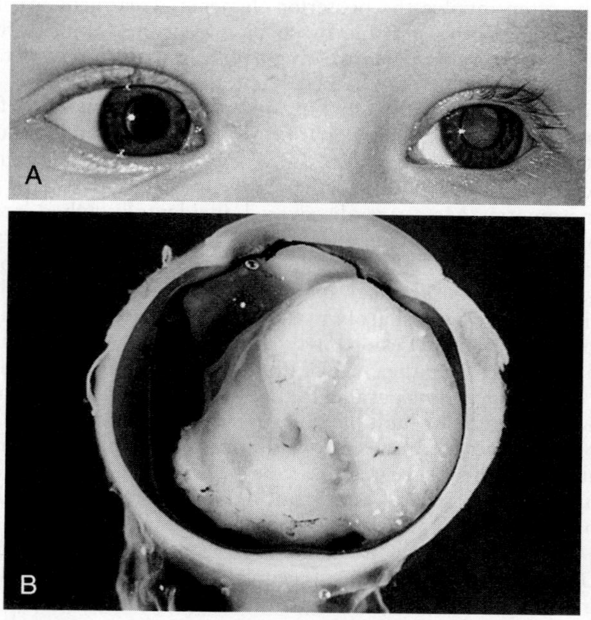

Figure 496-1 *A,* Leukocoria noted in the left eye of a child presenting with retinoblastoma. *B,* A large white tumor mass noted within the posterior chamber of the enucleated eye. (From Shields JA, Shields CL: Current management of retinoblastoma, *Mayo Clin Proc* 69:50–56, 1994.)

examination or in a flash photograph of the child. Strabismus often is an initial presenting complaint. Orbital inflammation, hyphema, and pupil irregularity can occur with advancing disease. Pain can occur if secondary glaucoma is present. Only about 10% of retinoblastoma cases are detected by routine ophthalmologic screening in the context of a positive family history.

DIAGNOSIS

The diagnosis is established by the characteristic ophthalmologic findings. Imaging studies are not diagnostic, and biopsies are contraindicated. Indirect ophthalmoscopy with slit-lamp evaluation can detect retinoblastoma tumors, but a complete evaluation requires an examination under general anesthesia by an experienced ophthalmologist to obtain complete visualization of both eyes, which also facilitates photographing and mapping of the tumors. Retinal detachment or vitreous hemorrhage can complicate the evaluation.

Orbital ultrasonography, CT, or MRI are used to evaluate the extent of intraocular disease and extraocular spread. Occasionally, a pineal area tumor is detected in a child with hereditary retinoblastoma, a phenomenon known as **trilateral retinoblastoma.** MRI allows for better evaluation of optic nerve involvement. Evaluation of the cerebrospinal fluid and bone marrow for tumor metastasis is required only if indicated by other clinical, laboratory, or imaging findings.

The **differential diagnosis** of retinoblastoma includes other causes of leukocoria, including persistent hyperplastic primary vitreous, Coats disease, cataract, endophthalmitis from *Toxocara canis*, choroidal coloboma, and retinopathy of prematurity.

TREATMENT

Treatment is determined by the size and location of the tumors and whether the child has hereditary or sporadic disease. The primary goal of treatment is always cure; the secondary goals include preserving vision and the eye itself. As newer modalities for local control of intraocular tumors and more effective systemic chemotherapy have emerged, primary enucleation is being performed less often.

Most unilateral disease presents with a solitary, large tumor. Enucleation is performed if there is no potential for the salvage of useful vision. With bilateral disease, chemoreduction in combination with **focal therapy** (laser photocoagulation or cryotherapy) has replaced the traditional approach of enucleation of the more severely affected eye and irradiation of the remaining eye. If feasible, small tumors can be treated with focal therapy with careful follow-up for recurrence or new tumor growth. Larger tumors often respond to multiagent chemotherapy including carboplatin, vincristine, and etoposide. If this approach fails, external-beam irradiation should be considered, although this approach may result in significant orbital deformity and increased incidence of second malignancies in patients with germ line *RB1* mutations. Brachytherapy, or episcleral plaque radiotherapy, is an alternative with less morbidity. Enucleation may be required for unresponsive or recurrent tumors. Alternative treatment options currently under investigation include other systemic chemotherapy agents such as topotecan and other sites of chemotherapy administration, including periocular and ophthalmic artery infusions.

All first-degree relatives of children with known or suspected hereditary retinoblastoma should have retinal examinations to identify retinomas or retinal scars, which may suggest hereditary retinoblastoma even though malignant retinoblastoma did not develop.

PROGNOSIS

Approximately 95% of children with retinoblastoma are cured with modern treatment in the USA. Current efforts using chemotherapy in combination with focal therapy are intended to preserve useful vision and avoid external-beam radiation or enucleation. Routine ophthalmologic examinations should continue until children are over age 7 yr. Unfortunately the diagnosis of retinoblastoma in many children from third-world countries is delayed, resulting in spread of the tumor outside of the orbit. The prognosis for these children with retinoblastoma that has spread outside of the eye is poor.

Children with germ line *RB1* mutations are at significant risk for development of second malignancies, especially osteosarcoma and also soft tissue sarcomas and malignant melanoma. The risk of second malignancies is further increased by the use of radiation therapy. Other radiation-related late adverse effects include cataracts, orbital growth deformities, lacrimal dysfunction, and late retinal vascular injury.

BIBLIOGRAPHY

Please visit the Nelson Textbook of Pediatrics *website at www.expertconsult.com for the complete bibliography.*

Chapter 497
Gonadal and Germ Cell Neoplasms

Cynthia E. Herzog and Winston W. Huh

EPIDEMIOLOGY

Malignant germ cell tumors (GCTs) and gonadal tumors are rare, with an incidence of 12 cases per million persons <20 yr of age. Most malignant tumors of the gonads in children are GCTs. The incidence varies according to age and sex. Sacrococcygeal tumors occur predominantly in infant girls. Testicular GCTs occur predominantly before age 4 yr and after puberty. Testicular GCTs occur much more often in whites than in blacks, whereas ovarian GCTs have a slight predominance in blacks. Klinefelter syndrome is associated with an increased risk of mediastinal GCTs; Down syndrome, undescended testes, infertility, testicular atrophy and inguinal hernias are associated with an increased risk of testicular cancer. The risk of testicular GCT is increased in first-degree relatives, and is highest among monozygotic twins.

PATHOGENESIS

The GCTs and non-GCTs arise from primordial germ cells and coelomic epithelium, respectively. Testicular and sacrococcygeal GCTs arising during early childhood characteristically have deletions at chromosome arms 1p and 6q and gains at 1q, and lack the isochromosome 12p that is highly characteristic of malignant GCTs of adults. Testicular GCT also may demonstrate loss of imprinting. Ovarian GCTs from older girls characteristically have deletions at 1p and gains at 1q and 21. Because GCTs may contain benign and mixed malignant elements in different areas of the tumor, extensive sectioning is essential to confirm the correct diagnosis. The many histologically distinct subtypes of GCTs include teratoma (mature and immature), endodermal sinus tumor, and embryonal carcinoma (Fig. 497-1). Non-GCTs of the ovary include epithelial (serous and mucinous) and sex cord–stromal tumors; non-GCTs of the testicle include sex cord/stromal tumors (e.g., Leydig cell, Sertoli cell).

CLINICAL MANIFESTATIONS AND DIAGNOSIS

The clinical presentation of germ cell neoplasms depends on location. Ovarian tumors often are quite large by the time they are diagnosed. Extragonadal GCTs occur in the midline, including the suprasellar region, pineal region, neck, mediastinum, and retroperitoneal and sacrococcygeal areas. Symptoms relate to

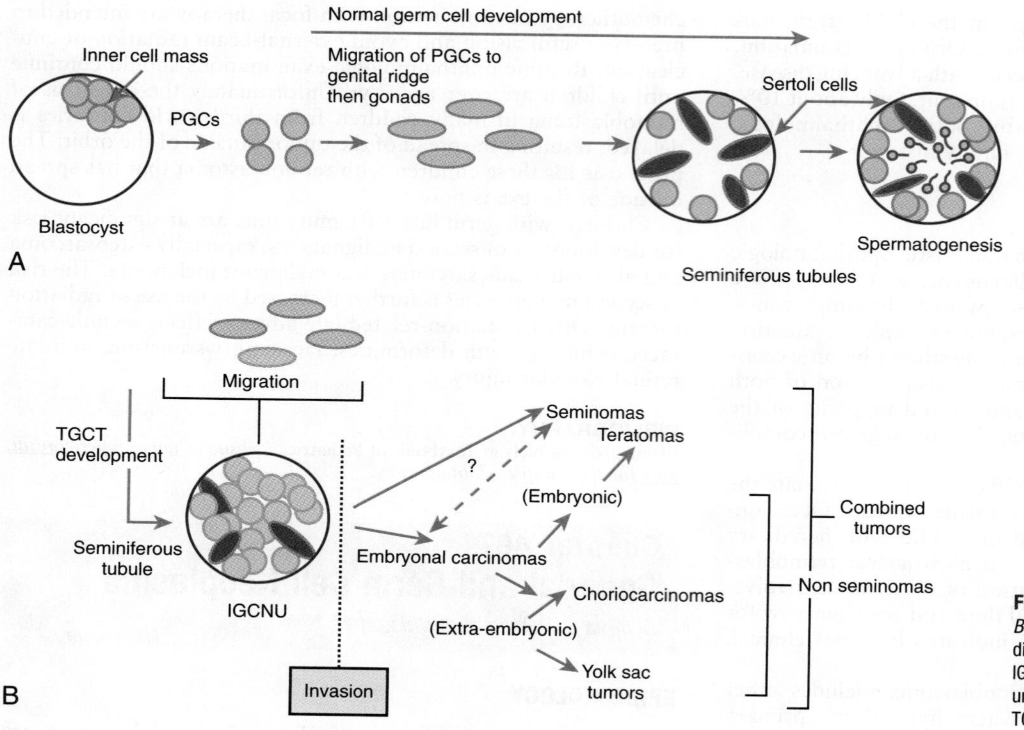

Figure 497-1 *A,* Normal germ cell development. *B,* Model for the origin and histogenesis of different subtypes of testicular germ cell tumors. IGCNU, intratubular germ cell neoplasia unclassified; PGC, primary germ cell; TGCT, testicular germ cell tumor(s).

mass effect, but the intracranial GCTs often present with anterior and posterior pituitary deficits (Chapter 491).

The **serum α-fetoprotein (AFP)** level is elevated with endodermal sinus tumors and may be minimally elevated with teratomas. Infants normally have higher levels of AFP, which fall to normal adult levels by about age 8 mo; therefore, high AFP levels must be interpreted with caution in this age group. Elevation of the β subunit of **human chorionic gonadotropin (β-hCG)**, which is secreted by syncytiotrophoblasts, is seen with choriocarcinoma and germinomas. Lactate dehydrogenase (LDH), although nonspecific, may be a useful marker. If elevated, these markers provide important confirmation of the diagnosis and provide a means to monitor the patient for tumor response and recurrence. Both serum and cerebrospinal fluid should be assayed for these markers in patients with intracranial lesions.

Diagnosis begins with physical examination and imaging studies, including plain radiographs of the chest and ultrasonography of the abdomen. CT or MRI can further delineate the primary tumor. If germ cell malignancy is strongly suggested, preoperative staging with CT of the chest and bone scan is appropriate. Primary surgical resection is indicated for tumors deemed resectable. Ovarian tumors also require detailed surgical evaluation including pelvic washings for cytologic analysis for peritoneal spread. Diagnosis of intracranial lesions can be established with imaging and AFP or β-hCG determinations of serum and cerebrospinal fluid.

Gonadoblastomas often occur in patients with gonadal dysgenesis and all or parts of a Y chromosome. Gonadal dysgenesis is characterized by failure to fully masculinize the external genitalia. If this syndrome is diagnosed, imaging of the gonad with ultrasonography or CT is performed, and surgical resection of the tumor usually is curative. Prophylactic resection of dysgenetic gonads at the time of diagnosis is recommended, because gonadoblastomas, some of which contain malignant germ cell tumor elements, often develop. Gonadoblastomas may produce abnormal amounts of estrogen.

Teratomas occur in many locations, presenting as masses. They are not associated with elevated markers unless malignancy is present. The sacrococcygeal region is the most common site for teratomas. Sacrococcygeal teratomas occur most commonly in infants and may be diagnosed in utero or at birth, with most found in girls. The rate of malignancy in this location varies, ranging from <10% in children <2 mo of age to >50% in children >4 mo of age.

Germinomas occur intracranially, in the mediastinum, and in the gonads. In the ovary, they are called **dysgerminomas;** in the testis, **seminomas.** They usually are tumor marker negative despite being malignant. Endodermal sinus or yolk sac tumor and choriocarcinoma appear highly malignant by histologic criteria. Both occur at gonadal and extragonadal sites. Embryonal carcinoma most often occurs in the testes. Choriocarcinoma and embryonal carcinoma rarely occur in the pure form and are usually found as part of a mixed malignant GCT.

Non–germ cell gonadal tumors are very uncommon in pediatrics and occur predominantly in the ovary. Epithelial carcinomas (usually an adult tumor), Sertoli-Leydig cell tumors, and granulosa cell tumors may occur in children. Carcinomas account for about one third of ovarian tumors in females <20 yr of age; most of these occur in older teens and are of the serous or mucinous subtype. Sertoli-Leydig cell tumors and granulosa cell tumors produce hormones that can cause virilization, feminization, or precocious puberty, depending on pubertal stage and the balance between Sertoli (estrogen production) and Leydig cells (androgen production). Diagnostic evaluation usually focuses on the chief complaint of inappropriate sex steroid effect and includes hormone measurements, which reflect gonadotropin-independent sex steroid production. Appropriate imaging also is performed to rule out a functioning gonadal tumor. Surgery usually is curative. No effective therapy for nonresectable disease has been found.

TREATMENT

Complete surgical excision of the tumor usually is indicated, except for patients with intracranial tumors, where the primary therapy consists of radiation therapy and chemotherapy. For testicular tumors, an inguinal approach is indicated. When complete excision cannot be accomplished, preoperative chemotherapy is indicated, with second-look surgery. For teratomas, both mature and immature, and completely resected malignant tumors, surgery alone is the treatment. Cisplatin-based chemotherapy regimens usually are curative in GCTs that cannot be completely resected, even if metastases are present. Except for GCTs of the central nervous system, radiation therapy is limited to those tumors that are not amenable to complete excision and are refractory to chemotherapy.

PROGNOSIS

The overall cure rate for children with GCTs is >80%. Age is the most predictive factor of survival for extragonadal GCTs. Children >12 yr of age have a 4-fold higher risk of death, and a 6-fold higher risk if the tumor is thoracic. Histology has little effect on prognosis. Nonresected extragonadal GCTs have a slightly worse prognosis.

BIBLIOGRAPHY

Please visit the Nelson Textbook of Pediatrics *website at www.expertconsult.com for the complete bibliography.*

Chapter 498
Neoplasms of the Liver

Cynthia E. Herzog

Hepatic tumors are rare in children. Primary tumors of the liver account for approximately 1% of malignancies in children, with an annual incidence of 1.6 cases per million children in the USA. Between 50-60% of hepatic tumors in children are malignant, with >65% of these malignancies being hepatoblastomas and most of the remainder, hepatocellular carcinomas. Rare hepatic malignancies include embryonal sarcoma, angiosarcoma, malignant germ cell tumor, rhabdomyosarcoma of the liver, and undifferentiated sarcoma. More common childhood malignancies such as neuroblastoma and lymphoma can metastasize to the liver. Benign liver tumors, which usually present in the first 6 mo of life, include hemangiomas, hamartomas, and hemangioendotheliomas.

HEPATOBLASTOMA

Epidemiology

Hepatoblastoma occurs predominantly in children <3 yr of age. The etiology is unknown. Hepatoblastomas are associated with familial adenomatous polyposis. Alterations in the antigen-presenting cell (APC)/β-catenin pathway have been found in most of the tumors evaluated. Hepatoblastoma also is associated with Beckwith-Wiedemann syndrome, which can show a similar loss of genomic imprinting of the insulin-like growth factor-2 gene. Low birthweight is associated with increased incidence of hepatoblastoma, with the risk increasing as birthweight decreases.

Pathogenesis

Hepatoblastoma can be epithelial type, containing fetal or embryonal malignant cells (either as a mixture or as pure elements), or the mixed type, containing mesenchymal and epithelial elements. Pure fetal histology predicts a more favorable outcome.

Clinical Manifestations

Hepatoblastoma usually presents as a large, asymptomatic abdominal mass. It arises from the right lobe 3 times more often than the left and usually is unifocal. As the disease progresses, weight loss, anorexia, vomiting, and abdominal pain may ensue.

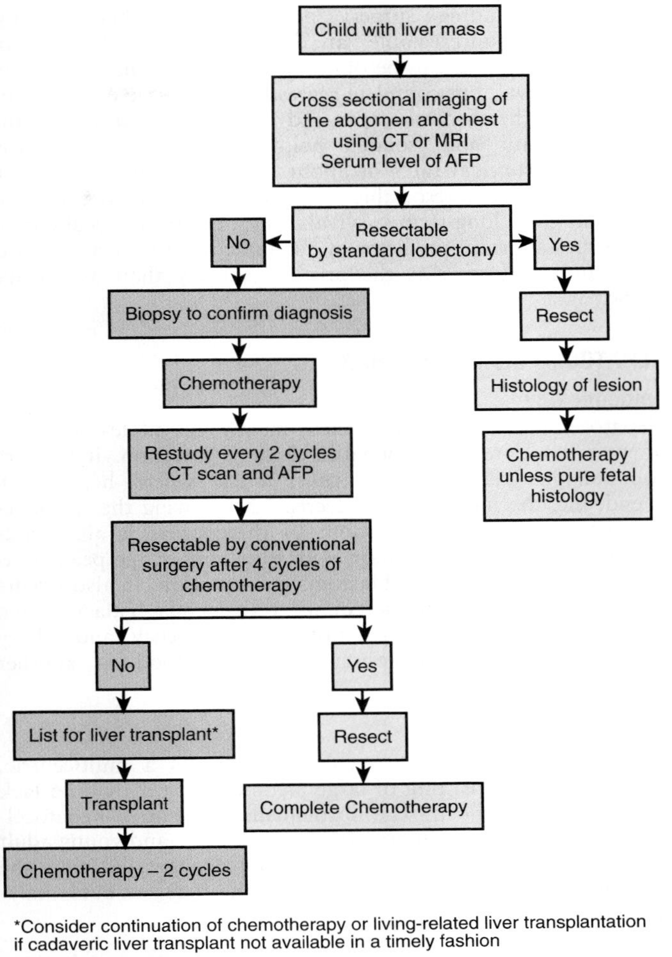

Figure 498-1 Algorithm for the management of a child who presents with a hepatoblastoma. AFP, α-fetoprotein. (From Tiao GM, Bobey N, Allen S, et al: The current management of hepatoblastoma: a combination of chemotherapy, conventional resection, and liver transplantation, *J Pediatr* 146:204–211, 2005.)

Metastatic spread of hepatoblastoma most commonly involves regional lymph nodes and the lungs.

A valuable serum tumor marker, **α-fetoprotein (AFP),** is used in the diagnosis and monitoring of hepatic tumors. AFP level is elevated in almost all hepatoblastomas. Bilirubin and liver enzymes usually are normal. Anemia is common, and thrombocytosis occurs in about 30% of patients. Hepatitis B and C serology should be obtained but usually are negative in hepatoblastoma.

Diagnostic imaging should include plain radiographs and ultrasonography of the abdomen to characterize the hepatic mass. Ultrasonography can differentiate malignant hepatic masses from benign vascular lesions. Either CT or MRI is an accurate method of defining the extent of intrahepatic tumor involvement and the potential for surgical resection. Evaluation for metastatic disease should include CT of the chest.

Treatment

In general, the cure of malignant hepatic tumors in children depends on complete resection of the primary tumor (Fig. 498-1). As much as 85% of the liver can be resected, with hepatic regeneration noted within 3-4 mo after surgery. Cisplatin in combination with vincristine and 5-fluorouracil or doxorubicin is effective treatment for hepatoblastoma and increases the chances of cure after complete surgical resection. In low-stage tumors, survival rates >90% can be achieved with multimodal treatment, including surgery and adjuvant chemotherapy. With tumors unresectable at diagnosis, survival rates of approximately 60% can be obtained. Metastatic disease further reduces survival, but complete regression of disease often can be obtained with chemotherapy and surgical resection of the primary tumor and isolated pulmonary metastatic disease, resulting in survival rates of about 25%. Liver transplant is a viable option for unresectable primary hepatic malignancies and results in good long-term survival. Pretransplant medical condition is an important predictor of outcome, and thus transplant is much more effective as the primary surgery than as salvage therapy.

HEPATOCELLULAR CARCINOMA

Epidemiology

Hepatocellular carcinoma occurs mostly in adolescents and often is associated with hepatitis B or C infection. It is more common in East Asia and other areas where hepatitis B is endemic, the incidence has decreased following the introduction of hepatitis B vaccination. In these areas it also tends to occur in a bimodal pattern, with the younger age peak overlapping the age of hepatoblastoma presentation. It also occurs in the chronic form of hereditary tyrosinemia, galactosemia, glycogen storage disease, α_1-antitrypsin deficiency, and biliary cirrhosis. Aflatoxin B contamination of food is another risk factor.

Pathogenesis

Hepatocellular carcinoma usually presents as a multicentric, invasive tumor consisting of large pleomorphic cells with a lack of underlying cirrhosis. The fibrolamellar variant of hepatocellular carcinoma occurs more often in adolescent and young adult patients. Although previous reports have suggested that the fibrolamellar type has a better prognosis, more recent data analysis refutes this.

Clinical Manifestations

Hepatocellular carcinoma usually presents as a hepatic mass, abdominal distention, and symptoms of anorexia, weight loss, and abdominal pain. Hepatocellular carcinoma can present as an acute abdominal crisis with rupture of the tumor and hemoperitoneum. The AFP level is elevated in approximately 60% of children with hepatocellular carcinoma. Evidence of hepatitis B and C infection usually is found in endemic areas but not in Western countries or with the fibrolamellar type. Bilirubin usually is normal, but liver enzymes may be abnormal.

Diagnostic imaging should include plain radiographs and ultrasonography of the abdomen to characterize the hepatic mass. Ultrasonography can differentiate malignant hepatic masses from benign vascular lesions. Either CT or MRI is an accurate method of defining the extent of intrahepatic tumor involvement and the potential for surgical resection. Evaluation for metastatic disease should include CT of the chest.

Treatment

Because of the multicentric origin of hepatocellular carcinoma, complete resection of this tumor is accomplished in only 30-40% of cases. Even with complete surgical resection, only 30% of children are long-term survivors. Chemotherapy, including cisplatin, doxorubicin, etoposide, and 5-fluorouracil, has shown some activity against this tumor, but improved long-term outcome has been difficult to achieve. Other techniques such as chemoembolization and liver transplantation are under study as therapy for hepatocellular carcinomas.

BIBLIOGRAPHY

Please visit the Nelson Textbook of Pediatrics *website at www.expertconsult.com for the complete bibliography.*

Chapter 499 Benign Vascular Tumors

499.1 Hemangiomas

Cynthia E. Herzog

Hemangiomas, the most common benign tumors of infancy, occur in about 5% of term infants (Chapter 642). The risk of hemangioma is 3-5 times higher in girls than boys. The risk is doubled in premature infants and 10 times higher in offspring of women who had chorionic villus sampling. Hemangiomas can be present at birth but usually arise shortly after birth and grow rapidly during the 1st yr of life, with slowing of growth in the next 5 yr and involution by 10-15 yr of age.

For the full continuation of this chapter, please visit the Nelson Textbook of Pediatrics *website at www.expertconsult.com.*

499.2 Lymphangiomas and Cystic Hygromas

Cynthia E. Herzog

Lymphatic malformations, including lymphangiomas and cystic hygromas, which arise in the embryonic lymph sac, are the 2nd most common benign vascular tumors in children. About half are located in the head and neck area. Approximately 50% are present at birth, with most presenting by 2 yr of age. There is no gender predisposition. Spontaneous regression has been reported but is not typical.

For the full continuation of this chapter, please visit the Nelson Textbook of Pediatrics *website at www.expertconsult.com.*

Chapter 500 Rare Tumors

500.1 Thyroid Tumors

Steven G. Waguespack

See Chapter 562.

BENIGN THYROID TUMORS

Benign thyroid tumors represent up to 80% of all thyroid nodules presenting in the pediatric population. The workup of a thyroid nodule includes the laboratory assessment of thyroid function, ultrasound (US) to assess the nodule and regional lymph node characteristics, and fine needle aspiration (usually under US guidance) for definitive diagnosis. Nuclear scintigraphy with ^{123}I or ^{99m}TC pertechnetate is generally not useful in the diagnostic evaluation, except in the event of a suppressed thyroid-stimulating hormone (TSH).

For the full continuation of this chapter, please visit the Nelson Textbook of Pediatrics *website at www.expertconsult.com.*

500.2 Melanoma

Cynthia E. Herzog

See Chapter 643.

The incidence of melanoma in persons <20 yr of age in the USA is 4.2 cases per million, with almost all of these cases occurring in adolescents (Chapter 643). Melanoma is more common among adolescent females than males. In the USA, incident rates of melanoma in younger age groups are increasing, although at a slower rate than in adults. Although sun exposure is a well-known risk factor for melanoma in adults, its role in pediatric melanoma is less clear. Pediatricians should counsel patients regarding avoidance of sun exposure to decrease the risk of later development of melanoma. Patients with fair skin and a family history of melanoma are at particularly high risk. Known risk factors for children are giant hairy nevus (>20 cm), dysplastic nevus syndrome, and xeroderma pigmentosum.

For the full continuation of this chapter, please visit the Nelson Textbook of Pediatrics *website at www.expertconsult.com.*

500.3 Nasopharyngeal Carcinoma

Cynthia E. Herzog

Nasopharyngeal carcinoma is rare in the pediatric population, but is one of the most common nasopharyngeal tumors in pediatric patients. In adults, the incidence is highest in South China, but it is also high among the Inuit people and in North Africa and Northeast India. In China, it is rare in the pediatric population, but in other populations a substantial proportion of cases occur in the pediatric age group, primarily in adolescents. It occurs in males twice as often as in females and is more common in blacks. In the pediatric population the tumors are more commonly of undifferentiated histology and associated with Epstein-Barr virus (EBV). Nasopharyngeal carcinoma has been associated with specific HLA types, and other genetic factors may play a role, especially in low incidence populations.

For the full continuation of this chapter, please visit the Nelson Textbook of Pediatrics *website at www.expertconsult.com.*

500.4 Adenocarcinoma of the Colon and Rectum

Cynthia E. Herzog

Colorectal carcinoma (CRC) is rare in the pediatric population. Even in patients with predisposing conditions, CRC usually does not present until adulthood. Hereditary nonpolyposis colon cancer (HNPCC) is an autosomal dominant disorder, with germline mutations in DNA mismatch repair genes *(MMR)* causing DNA repair errors and microsatellite instability. Familial adenomatous polyposis (FAP) and attenuated FAP (AFAP), are autosomal disorders, with germline mutations in the *APC* gene. In addition to CRC, patients with HNPCC, FAP, and AFAP are predisposed to a number of extracolonic cancers. *MYH*-associated polyposis (MAP), Peutz-Jeghers syndrome, and juvenile polyposis also predispose to CRC.

For the full continuation of this chapter, please visit the Nelson Textbook of Pediatrics *website at www.expertconsult.com.*

500.5 Adrenal Tumors

Steven G. Waguespack

See Chapter 575.

Adrenocortical tumors (ACT) arise from the outer adrenal cortex, whereas pheochromocytomas (PHEO) derive from the catecholamine-producing chromaffin cells of the adrenal medulla. The pathologic categorization of ACT in children as benign or malignant does not always correlate to the clinical behavior of these tumors, making it difficult to differentiate clinically significant adrenocortical carcinomas from those tumors that retain a good prognosis. ACT are very rare and tend to present at an age <5 yr. They have a female predominance and are functional tumors (producing androgens and/or glucocorticoids, typically) in >90% of cases. ACT may also present as an abdominal mass or pain. In children, ACT are associated with Li-Fraumeni syndrome (germ line inactivating mutations in the p53 tumor suppressor gene), Beckwith-Wiedemann syndrome (BWS), hemihypertrophy other than that seen as part of BWS, and rarely congenital adrenal hyperplasia. Other rare causes of nodular adrenocortical disease, which usually present with Cushing syndrome, include Carney complex and macronodular adrenal hyperplasia.

For the full continuation of this chapter, please visit the Nelson Textbook of Pediatrics *website at www.expertconsult.com.*

500.6 Desmoplastic Small Round Cell Tumor

Cynthia E. Herzog

Desmoplastic small round cell tumor (DSRCT) is a recently recognized tumor that occurs predominantly in adolescent males. It is associated with a translocation between the Ewing tumor gene and the Wilms tumor gene, t(11;22)(p13;q12). Patients typically present with diffuse abdominal disease with no definitive primary, although disease outside the abdomen is possible. Aggressive treatment with surgery, chemotherapy, and radiation has resulted in almost universally poor outcome.

For the full continuation of this chapter, please visit the Nelson Textbook of Pediatrics *website at www.expertconsult.com.*

Chapter 501 Histiocytosis Syndromes of Childhood

Stephan Ladisch

The childhood histiocytoses constitute a diverse group of disorders, which, although individually rare, may be severe in their clinical expression. These disorders are grouped together because they have in common a prominent proliferation or accumulation of cells of the monocyte-macrophage system of bone marrow origin. Although these disorders sometimes are difficult to distinguish clinically, accurate diagnosis is essential nevertheless for facilitating progress in treatment. A systematic classification of the childhood histiocytoses is based on histopathologic findings (Table 501-1). A thorough, comprehensive evaluation of a biopsy specimen obtained at the time of diagnosis is essential. This evaluation includes studies such as electron microscopy and immunsotaining that may require special sample processing.

CLASSIFICATION AND PATHOLOGY

Three classes of childhood histiocytosis are recognized, based on histopathologic findings. The most well-known childhood histiocytosis, previously known as **histiocytosis X,** constitutes class I and includes the clinical entities of eosinophilic granuloma, **Hand-Schüller-Christian disease,** and **Letterer-Siwe disease.** The name **Langerhans cell histiocytosis (LCH)** has been applied to the class I histiocytoses. The normal Langerhans cell is an antigen-presenting cell of the skin. The hallmark of LCH in all forms is the presence of a clonal proliferation of cells of the monocyte lineage containing the characteristic electron microscopic findings of a Langerhans cell. This is the **Birbeck granule,** a tennis racket–shaped bilamellar granule that, when seen in the cytoplasm of lesional cells in LCH, is diagnostic of the disease. The Birbeck granule expresses a newly characterized antigen, langerin (CD207), which is involved in antigen presentation to T lymphocytes. CD207 expression has been established to be uniformly present in LCH lesions and thus becomes an additional reliable diagnostic marker. The definitive diagnosis of LCH also can be

Table 501-1 CLASSIFICATION OF THE CHILDHOOD HISTIOCYTOSES

CLASS	DISEASE	CELLULAR CHARACTERISTICS OF LESIONS	TREATMENT
I	Langerhans cell histiocytosis	Langerhans cells (CD1a-positive, CD207-positive) with Birbeck granules	Local therapy for isolated lesions; chemotherapy for disseminated disease
II	Familial erythrophagocytic lymphohistiocytosis*	Morphologically normal reactive macrophages with prominent erythrophagocytosis, and CD8-positive T cells	Chemotherapy; allogeneic bone marrow transplantation
	Infection-associated hemophagocytic syndrome†		
III	Malignant histiocytosis	Neoplastic proliferation of cells with characteristics of monocytes/ macrophages or their precursors	Antineoplastic chemotherapy, including anthracyclines
	Acute monocytic leukemia‡	M5 by FAB classification	Antineoplastic chemotherapy

*Also called familial hemophagocytic lymphohistiocytosis (FHLH).
†Also called secondary hemophagocytic lymphohistiocytosis.
‡See Chapter 489.2.

established by demonstrating CD1a-positivity of lesional cells, which now can be done using fixed tissue. The lesions may contain various proportions of these Langerhans granule-containing cells, lymphocytes, granulocytes, monocytes, and eosinophils.

In contrast to the prominence of an antigen-presenting cell (the Langerhans cell) in the class I histiocytoses, the **class II histiocytoses** are nonmalignant proliferative disorders that are characterized by accumulation of antigen-processing cells (macrophages). **Hemophagocytic lymphohistiocytoses (HLH)** are the result of uncontrolled hemophagocytosis and uncontrolled activation (upregulation) of inflammatory cytokines similar to the macrophage activation syndrome (see Table 149-5). Tissue infiltration by activated CD8 T lymphocytes, activated macrophages, and hypercytokinemia are classic features. With the characteristic morphology of normal macrophages by light microscopy, these phagocytic cells are negative for the markers (Birbeck granules, CD1a-positivity, CD207-positivity) characteristic of the cells found in LCH. The 2 major diseases among the class II histiocytoses have indistinguishable pathologic findings. One is **familial hemophagocytic lymphohistiocytosis (FHLH),** previously called **familial erythrophagocytic lymphohistiocytosis (FEL),** which is the only inherited form of histiocytosis and is autosomal recessive. Some specific genes involved with FEL include mutations of perforin, Munc 13-4, and Syntaxin-11 and all are related to pathways of granule-mediated cellular cytotoxicity. The other is the **infection-associated hemophagocytic syndrome (IAHS),** also called secondary hemophagocytic lymphohistiocytosis (Table 501-2). Both diseases are characterized by disseminated lesions that involve many organ systems. The lesions are characterized by infiltration of the involved organ with activated phagocytic macrophages and lymphocytes, in which the lymphocyte (cytolytic pathway) defects are considered to be the primary abnormality. These diseases are grouped together under the term **hemophagocytic lymphohistiocytosis (HLH)** (Table 501-3).

The mixed cellular lesions of both the class I and class II histiocytoses are increasing believed to point to these as being disorders of immune regulation, resulting from either an unusual and unidentified antigenic stimulation or an abnormal and somehow defective cellular immune response. Mutations in the perforin (PRF1) gene or the Munc 13-4 gene cause defective function of the cytotoxic lymphocytes whose activity is inhibited in FHLH.

Table 501-2 INFECTIONS ASSOCIATED WITH HEMOPHAGOCYTIC SYNDROME

VIRAL
Adenovirus
Cytomegalovirus
Dengue virus
Epstein-Barr virus
Herpes simplex virus (HSV1, HSV2, HHV6, HHV8)
Human immunodeficiency virus
Parvovirus B19
Varicella-zoster virus
Hepatitis viruses
BACTERIAL
Babesia microti
Brucella abortus
Enteric gram-negative rods
Haemophilus influenzae
Mycoplasma pneumoniae
Staphylococcus aureus
Streptococcus pneumoniae
FUNGAL
Candida albicans
Cryptococcus neoformans
Histoplasma capsulatum
MYCOBACTERIAL
Mycobacterium tuberculosis
RICKETTSIAL
Coxiella brunetii
PARASITIC
Leishmania donovani

From Nathan DG, Orkin SH, Ginsburg D, et al, editors: *Nathan and Oski's hematology of infancy and childhood,* ed 6, Philadelphia, 2003, WB Saunders, p 1381.

The **class III histiocytoses,** in contrast, are unequivocal malignancies of cells of monocyte-macrophage lineage. By this definition, acute monocytic leukemia and true malignant histiocytosis are included among the class III histiocytoses (Chapter 489). The existence of neoplasms of Langerhans cells is controversial. Some cases of LCH demonstrate clonality.

BIBLIOGRAPHY

Please visit the Nelson Textbook of Pediatrics *website at* *www.expertconsult.com* *for the complete bibliography.*

501.1 Class I Histiocytoses

Stephan Ladisch

CLINICAL MANIFESTATIONS

LCH has an extremely variable presentation. The skeleton is involved in 80% of patients and may be the only affected site, especially in children >5 yr of age. Bone lesions may be single or multiple and are seen most commonly in the skull (Fig. 501-1). Other sites include the pelvis, femur, vertebra, maxilla, and mandible. They may be asymptomatic or associated with pain and local swelling. Involvement of the spine may result in collapse of the vertebral body, which can be seen radiographically, and may cause secondary compression of the spinal cord. In flat and long bones, osteolytic lesions with sharp borders occur and no evidence exists of reactive new bone formation until the lesions begin to heal. Lesions that involve weight-bearing long bones may result in pathologic fractures. Chronically draining, infected ears are commonly associated with destruction in the mastoid area. Bone destruction in the mandible and maxilla may result in

Table 501-3 DISTINGUISHING CHARACTERISTICS OF THE REACTIVE LYMPHOHISTIOCYTOSES

	GENETIC HISTORY	VIRUS INFECTION	CELLULAR IMMUNE FUNCTION	MISCELLANEOUS
HLH, genetic	Autosomal recessive	Possibly associated	$\downarrow$ CMI	Perforin deficiency
			$\downarrow$ NK cell activity	Hypertriglyceridemia, Perforin (PRF1),
			$\downarrow$ Monocyte killing	Munc 13-4 mutations
			$\downarrow$ CMI	
Secondary infection–associated	Sporadic	Yes	$\downarrow$ CMI	Coagulopathy early in the course of the disease
			NL or $\uparrow$ NK cell in instances associated with EBV	
			$\downarrow$ Anomalous EBV-related killing	
XLP	X-linked sporadic	EBV	NL or $\uparrow$ NK cell	*SH2DIA* mutation
			NL or $\uparrow$ anomalous EBV-related killing	Severe, often fatal hepatitis
SHML	Sporadic	?EBV	Not reported	Autoimmune phenomena
LG	Sporadic	EBV	$\downarrow$ CMI	Lymphoma development

CMI, cell-mediated immunity; EBV, Epstein-Barr virus; HLH, hemophagocytic lymphohistiocytosis; LG, lymphomatoid granulomatosis; NK, natural killer; NL, normal; SHML, sinus histiocytosis with massive lymphadenopathy; XLP, X-linked lymphoproliferative syndrome.
From Nathan DG, Orkin SH, Ginsburg D, et al, editors: *Nathan and Oski's hematology of infancy and childhood,* ed 6, Philadelphia, 2003, WB Saunders, p 1387.

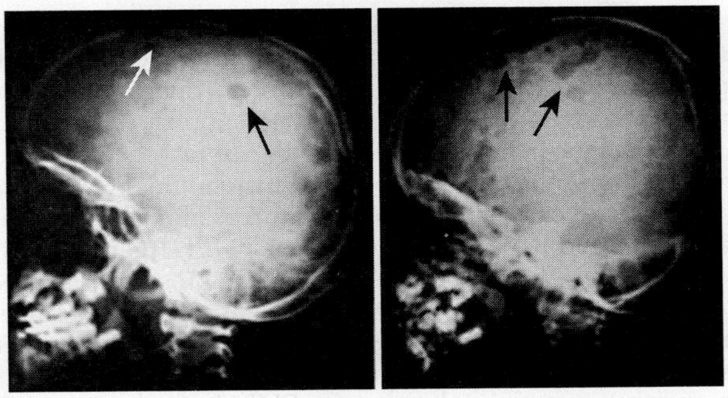

Figure 501-1 Two skull radiographs from patients with Langerhans cell histiocytosis (LCH). *Left,* The patient was >2 yr of age and had involvement limited to isolated bone lesions *(arrows).* She had a good recovery. *Right,* The patient was <2 yr of age and had extensive bone disease *(arrows),* a febrile course, anemia, severe skin eruption, generalized lymphadenopathy, hepatosplenomegaly, pulmonary infiltrates, and a fatal outcome despite antitumor chemotherapy. These patients represent opposite ends of the clinical spectrum of LCH.

teeth that, on radiographs, appear to be free floating. With response to therapy, healing may be complete.

About 50% of patients experience skin involvement at some time during the course of disease, usually as a hard-to-treat scaly, papular, seborrheic dermatitis of the scalp, diaper, axillary, or posterior auricular regions. The lesions may spread to involve the back, palms, and soles. The exanthem may be petechial or hemorrhagic, even in the absence of thrombocytopenia. Localized or disseminated lymphadenopathy is present in approximately 33% of patients. Hepatosplenomegaly occurs in approximately 20% of patients. Various degrees of hepatic malfunction may occur, including jaundice and ascites.

Exophthalmos, when present, often is bilateral and is caused by retro-orbital accumulation of granulomatous tissue. Gingival mucous membranes may be involved with infiltrative lesions that appear superficially like candidiasis. Otitis media is present in 30-40% of patients; deafness may follow destructive lesions of the middle ear. In 10-15% of patients, pulmonary infiltrates are found on radiography. The lesions may range from diffuse fibrosis and disseminated nodular infiltrates to diffuse cystic changes. Rarely, pneumothorax may be a complication. If the lungs are severely involved, tachypnea and progressive respiratory failure may result.

Pituitary dysfunction or hypothalamic involvement may result in growth retardation. In addition, patients may have diabetes insipidus; patients suspected of having LCH should demonstrate the ability to concentrate their urine before going to the operating room for a biopsy. Rarely, panhypopituitarism may occur. Primary hypothyroidism due to thyroid gland infiltration also may occur.

Patients with multisystem disease who are affected more severely may have systemic manifestations, including fever, weight loss, malaise, irritability, and failure to thrive. Bone marrow involvement may cause anemia and thrombocytopenia. Two uncommon but serious and unusual manifestations of LCH are hepatic involvement (leading to fibrosis and cirrhosis) and a peculiar central nervous system (CNS) involvement characterized by ataxia, dysarthria, and other neurologic symptoms. Hepatic involvement is associated with multisystem disease that is often already present at the time of diagnosis. In contrast, the CNS involvement, which is progressive and histopathologically characterized by gliosis, and for which no treatment is known, may be observed only many years after the initial diagnosis of LCH, which may have consisted only of mild bone disease. Neither of these manifestations evidences Langerhans cells or Birbeck granules, and both are suspected to be driven initially by cytokine abnormalities.

After tissue biopsy, which is diagnostic and is easiest to perform on skin or bone lesions, a thorough clinical and laboratory evaluation should be undertaken. This should include a series of studies in all patients (complete blood cell count, liver function tests, coagulation studies, skeletal survey, chest radiograph, and measurement of urine osmolality). In addition, detailed evaluation of any organ system that has been shown to be involved by physical examination or by these studies should be performed to establish the extent of disease before initiation of treatment.

TREATMENT AND PROGNOSIS

The clinical course of single-system disease (usually bone, lymph node, or skin) generally is benign, with a high chance of spontaneous remission. Therefore, treatment should be minimal and should be directed at arresting the progression of a bone lesion that could result in permanent damage before it resolves spontaneously. Curettage or, less often, low-dose local radiation therapy (5-6 Gy) may accomplish this goal. Multisystem disease, in contrast, should be treated with systemic multiagent chemotherapy. Several different regimens have been proposed, but a central element is the inclusion of either vinblastine or etoposide, both of which have been found to be very effective in treating LCH. Treatment of multisystem LCH includes therapy with multiple agents, designed to reduce reactivation of disease and long-term consequences. The response rate to therapy, contrary to previous belief, is high, and mortality in severe LCH has been substantially reduced by multiagent chemotherapy, especially if the diagnosis is made accurately and expeditiously. Experimental therapies, suggested only for unresponsive disease (often in very young children with multisystem disease and organ dysfunction who have not responded to multiagent initial treatment), include immunosuppressive therapy with cyclosporine/antithymocyte globulin and possibly certain new agents and modalities, such as imatinib, 2-chlorodeoxyadenosine, and stem cell transplantation. Late (fibrotic) complications, whether hepatic or pulmonary, are irreversible and require organ transplantation to be definitively treated. Current treatment approaches and experimental protocols for both class I and class II histiocytoses can be obtained at the website for the Histiocyte Society: www.histiocytesociety.org.

BIBLIOGRAPHY

Please visit the Nelson Textbook of Pediatrics *website at www.expertconsult.com for the complete bibliography.*

501.2 Class II Histiocytoses: Hemophagocytic Lymphohistiocytosis (HLH)

Stephan Ladisch

(**See earlier section,** Classification and Pathology.)

CLINICAL MANIFESTATIONS

The major forms of HLH, familial hemophagocytic lymphohistiocytosis (FHLF) and secondary HLH, have a remarkably similar presentation consisting of a generalized disease process, most often with fever, maculopapular and/or petechial rash, weight loss, and irritability (Tables 501-4 and 501-5). FHLH also is characterized by severe immunodeficiency. Children with FHLH frequently are <4 yr of age, and children with secondary HLH may present at an older age, but both forms are now recognized as presenting at any age. **Physical examination** often reveals hepatosplenomegaly, lymphadenopathy, respiratory distress, and symptoms of CNS involvement that are not unlike those of aseptic meningitis. The cerebrospinal fluid (CSF) in CNS involvement of FHLH is characterized by CSF cells that are the same phagocytic macrophages found in the peripheral blood or bone marrow. The definitive diagnosis is based on a set of criteria recently formulated by the Histiocyte Society: It can be made either on the basis of a molecular (genetic) defect (see later) or on the pathologic findings of hemophagocytosis in bone marrow biopsy and/or clinical findings of fever, splenomegaly, and associated laboratory findings (in both forms of HLH), including hyperlipidemia, hypofibrinogenemia, elevated levels of hepatic enzymes, extremely elevated levels of circulating soluble interleukin-2 receptors released by the activated lymphocytes, very high levels of serum ferritin (often >10,000), and cytopenias (especially pancytopenia from hemophagocytosis in the marrow). No absolute clinical or laboratory distinction can be made between FHLH and secondary HLH, although genetic markers for FHLH can complement a positive family history for other affected children. HLH may be present in the absence of genetic mutations of the perforin or Munc 13-4 genes, and can be diagnosed by the presence of 5 of the following: fever, splenomegaly, cytopenia of 2 cell lines, hypertriglyceridemia or hypofibrinogenemia, hyperferritinemia, elevated soluble CD25 (interleukin-2 receptor), reduced or absent NK cells, and bone marrow, CSF, or lymph node evidence of hemophagocytosis.

Table 501-4 DIAGNOSTIC GUIDELINES FOR HLH

The diagnosis of HLH is established by fulfilling 1 or 2 of the following criteria:

1. A molecular diagnosis consistent with HLH (e.g., *PRF* mutations, *SAP* mutations)

OR

2. Having 5 out of 8 of the following:
   - a. Fever
   - b. Splenomegaly
   - c. Cytopenia (affecting ≥2 cell lineages; hemoglobin ≤9 g/dL (or ≤10 g/dL for infants <4 wk of age, platelets <100,000/µL, neutrophils <1,000/µL)
   - d. Hypertriglyceridemia (≥265 mg/dL) and/or hypofibrinogenemia (≤150 mg/dL)
   - e. Hemophagocytosis in the bone marrow, spleen, or lymph nodes without evidence of malignancy
   - f. Low or absent NK cell cytotoxicity
   - g. Hyperferritinemia (≥500 ng/mL)
   - h. Elevated soluble CD25 (IL-2Rα chain; ≥2,400 U/mL)

(Note: Adapted from Treatment Protocol of the 2nd International HLH Study, 2004.)
From Verbsky JW, Grossman WJ: Hemophagocytic lymphohistiocytosis: diagnosis, pathophysiology, treatment, and future perspectives, *Ann Med* 38:20–31, 2006, p 21, Table 1.

TREATMENT AND PROGNOSIS

The diagnostic distinction between FHLH and secondary HLH sometimes can be based on the acute onset of secondary HLH in the presence of a documented infection. In this case, treatment of the underlying infection, coupled with supportive care, is critical. If the diagnosis is made in a setting of iatrogenic immunodeficiency, immunosuppressive treatment should be withdrawn and supportive care should be instituted along with specific therapy for underlying infection. When FHLH (gene mutations in perforin or Munc 13-4 proteins) is diagnosed or suspected and when an infection cannot be documented, therapy currently includes etoposide, corticosteroids, and intrathecal methotrexate. It should be stressed that pancytopenia is not a contraindication to cytotoxic therapy in FHLH. Some recommend antithymocyte globulin and cyclosporine for maintenance therapy. Nevertheless, even with chemotherapy, FHLH remains ultimately fatal, often after a relapse of the disease. Allogeneic **stem cell transplantation** is effective in curing approximately 60% of patients with FHLH.

In contrast, in secondary HLH, when an infection can be documented and effectively treated, the prognosis may be excellent without any other specific treatment. However, when a

Table 501-5 SPECTRUM OF DISEASES CHARACTERIZED BY HEMOPHAGOCYTOSIS

PRIMARY HLH
Familial HLH Chédiak-Higashi syndrome Griscelli syndrome X-linked lymphoproliferative (XLP) disease Wiskott-Aldrich syndrome (WAS)
SECONDARY HLH
Virus-associated HLH Herpes virus infection (EBV, CMV, HHV-6, HHV-8, VZV, HSV) HIV Parvovirus, adenovirus, hepatitis virus
INFECTION ASSOCIATED HLH
Numerous bacterial-, spirocetal-, and fungal-associated infections
MALIGNANCY ASSOCIATED HLH
MACROPHAGE ACTIVATION SYNDROME (MAS) ASSOCIATED WITH AUTOIMMUNE DISEASE
Systemic-onset juvenile rheumatoid arthritis (SOJRA) Others (systemic lupus erythematosus, enthesitis related arthritis), inflammatory bowel disease

CMV, cytomegalovirus; EBV, Epstein-Barr virus; HHV, human herpesvirus; VZV, Varicella-zoster virus.
From Verbsky JW, Grossman WJ: Hemophagocytic lymphohistiocytosis: diagnosis, pathophysiology, treatment, and future perspectives, *Ann Med* 38:20–31, 2006, p 22, Table 2.

treatable infection cannot be documented, which is the case in most patients presumed to have secondary HLH, the prognosis may be as poor as that of FHLH, and an identical chemotherapeutic approach, including etoposide, is recommended, even in the face of cytopenias. It is theorized that in both cases, by its cytotoxic effect on macrophages, etoposide interrupts cytokine production, the hemophagocytic process, and the accumulation of macrophages, all of which may contribute to the pathogenesis of IAHS. A broad spectrum of infectious agents, viruses (e.g., cytomegalovirus, Epstein-Barr virus, human herpesvirus 6), fungi, protozoa, and bacteria may trigger secondary HLH, usually in the setting of immunodeficiency (see Table 501-2). A thorough evaluation for infection should be undertaken in immunodeficient patients with hemophagocytosis. Rarely, the same syndrome may be identified in conjunction with a rheumatologic disorder (e.g., systemic lupus erythematosus, Kawasaki disease) or a neoplasm (leukemia); in this case, treatment of the underlying disease may cause resolution of the hemophagocytosis. In some patients, interferon and intravenous immunoglobulin have been effective.

BIBLIOGRAPHY

Please visit the Nelson Textbook of Pediatrics *website at www.expertconsult.com for the complete bibliography.*

501.3 Class III Histiocytoses

Stephan Ladisch

Acute monocytic leukemia and true malignant histiocytosis are included among the class III histiocytoses (Chapter 484), because they are unequivocal malignancies of the monocyte-macrophage lineage.

PART XXIII Nephrology

Section 1 GLOMERULAR DISEASE

Chapter 502 Introduction to Glomerular Diseases

502.1 Anatomy of the Glomerulus

Cynthia G. Pan and Ellis D. Avner

The kidneys lie in the retroperitoneal space slightly above the level of the umbilicus. They range in length and weight, respectively, from approximately 6 cm and 24 g in a full-term newborn to ≥12 cm and 150 g in an adult. The kidney (see Fig. 502-1 on the *Nelson Textbook of Pediatrics* website at www.expertconsult.com) has an outer layer, **the cortex**, which contains the glomeruli, proximal and distal convoluted tubules, and collecting ducts; and an inner layer, **the medulla**, that contains the straight portions of the tubules, the loops of Henle, the vasa recta, and the terminal collecting ducts (see Fig. 502-2 on the *Nelson Textbook of Pediatrics* website at www.expertconsult.com).

For the full continuation of this chapter, please visit the Nelson Textbook of Pediatrics *website at www.expertconsult.com.*

502.2 Glomerular Filtration

Cynthia G. Pan and Ellis D. Avner

As the blood passes through the glomerular capillaries, the plasma is filtered through the glomerular capillary walls. The ultrafiltrate, which is cell free, contains all of the substances in plasma (electrolytes, glucose, phosphate, urea, creatinine, peptides, low molecular weight proteins) except proteins having a molecular weight of ≥68 kd (such as albumin and globulins). The filtrate is collected in Bowman's space and enters the tubules, where its composition is modified by tightly regulated secretion and absorption of solute and fluid, until it leaves the kidney as urine.

For the full continuation of this chapter, please visit the Nelson Textbook of Pediatrics *website at www.expertconsult.com.*

502.3 Glomerular Diseases

Cynthia G. Pan and Ellis D. Avner

PATHOGENESIS

Glomerular injury may be a result of genetic, immunologic, perfusion, or coagulation disorders. Genetic disorders of the glomerulus result from mutations in the exons of DNA encoding proteins located within the glomerulus, interstitium, or tubular epithelium; mutations in the regulatory genes controlling DNA transcription; abnormal post-transcriptional modification of RNA transcripts; or abnormal post-translational modification of proteins. Immunologic injury to the glomerulus results in **glomerulonephritis,** which is a generic term for several diseases and a histopathologic term signifying inflammation of the glomerular capillaries. Evidence that glomerulonephritis is caused by immunologic injury includes morphologic and immunopathologic similarities to experimental immune-mediated glomerulonephritis; the demonstration of immune reactants (immunoglobulin, complement) in glomeruli; abnormalities in serum complement; and the finding of autoantibodies (anti-GBM) in some of these diseases (see Fig. 502-7 on the *Nelson Textbook of Pediatrics* website at www.expertconsult.com). There appear to be 2 major mechanisms of immunologic injury: glomerular deposition of circulating antigen-antibody immune complexes and interaction of antibody with local antigen in situ. In the latter circumstance, the antigen may be a normal component of the glomerulus (the noncollagenous domain [NC-1] of type IV collagen, a putative antigen in human anti-GBM nephritis) or an antigen that has been deposited in the glomerulus.

For the full continuation of this chapter, please visit the Nelson Textbook of Pediatrics *website at www.expertconsult.com.*

Section 2 CONDITIONS PARTICULARLY ASSOCIATED WITH HEMATURIA

Chapter 503 Clinical Evaluation of the Child with Hematuria

Cynthia G. Pan and Ellis D. Avner

Hematuria is defined as the presence of at least 5 red blood cells (RBCs) per microliter of urine and occurs with a prevalence of 0.5-2.0% among school-aged children. Quantitative studies demonstrate that normal children can excrete more than 500,000 RBCs per 12-hr period; this increases with fever and/or exercise. In the clinical setting, qualitative estimates are provided by a urinary dipstick that uses a very sensitive peroxidase chemical reaction between hemoglobin (or myoglobin) and a colorimetric chemical indicator impregnated on the dipstick. Chemstrip (Boehringer Mannheim), a common commercially available dipstick, is capable of detecting 3-5 RBCs/μL of unspun urine; significant hematuria is suggested by >50 RBCs/μL. False-negative results can occur in the presence of formalin (used as a urine preservative) or high urinary concentrations of ascorbic acid (i.e., in patients with vitamin C intake >2000 mg/ day). False-positive results may be seen in a child with an alkaline urine (pH > 9), or more commonly following contamination with oxidizing agents such as hydrogen peroxide used to clean the perineum before

Table 503-1 OTHER CAUSES OF RED URINE

HEME POSITIVE
Hemoglobin Myoglobin
HEME NEGATIVE **Drugs**
Chloroquine Deferoxamine Ibuprofen Iron sorbitol Metronidazole Nitrofurantoin Phenazopyridine (Pyridium) Phenolphthalein Phenothiazines Rifampin Salicylates Sulfasalazine
Dyes (Vegetable/Fruit)
Beets Blackberries Food coloring Rhubarb
Metabolites
Homogentisic acid Melanin Methemoglobin Porphyrin Tyrosinosis Urates

Table 503-2 CAUSES OF HEMATURIA IN CHILDREN

UPPER URINARY TRACT DISEASE
Isolated renal disease IgA nephropathy (Berger disease) Alport syndrome (hereditary nephritis) Thin glomerular basement membrane nephropathy Postinfectious GN (poststreptococcal GN)* Membranous nephropathy Membranoproliferative GN* Rapidly progressive GN Focal segmental glomerulosclerosis Antiglomerular basement membrane disease Multisystem disease Systemic lupus erythematosus nephritis* Henoch-Schönlein purpura nephritis Wegener granulomatosis Polyarteritis nodosa Goodpasture syndrome Hemolytic-uremic syndrome Sickle cell glomerulopathy HIV nephropathy Tubulointerstitial disease Pyelonephritis Interstitial nephritis Papillary necrosis Acute tubular necrosis Vascular Arterial or venous thrombosis Malformations (aneurysms, hemangiomas) Nutcracker syndrome Hemoglobinopathy (sickle cell trait/disease) Crystalluria Anatomic Hydronephrosis Cystic kidney disease Polycystic kidney disease Multicystic dysplasia Tumor (Wilms, rhabdomyosarcoma, angiomyolipoma) Trauma
LOWER URINARY TRACT DISEASE
Inflammation (infectious and noninfectious) Cystitis Urethritis Urolithiasis Trauma Coagulopathy Heavy exercise Bladder tumor Factitious syndrome, factitious syndrome by proxy[†]

*Denotes glomerulonephritides presenting with hypocomplementemia.
[†]Formerly Munchausen syndrome and Munchausen syndrome by proxy.
GN, glomerulonephritis.

obtaining a specimen. Microscopic analysis of 10-15 mL of freshly centrifuged urine is essential in confirming the presence of RBCs suggested by a positive dipstick.

Red urine **without** RBCs is seen in a number of conditions (Table 503-1). Heme-positive urine without RBCs is caused by the presence of either hemoglobin or myoglobin. Hemoglobinuria without hematuria can occur in the presence of hemolysis. Myoglobinuria without hematuria occurs in the presence of rhabdomyolysis resulting from skeletal muscle injury and is generally associated with a 5-fold increase in the plasma concentration of creatine kinase. Rhabdomyolysis can occur secondary to viral myositis, crush injury, severe electrolyte abnormalities (hypernatremia, hypophosphatemia), hypotension, disseminated intravascular coagulation, toxins (drugs, venom), metabolic disorders of muscles, and prolonged seizures. Heme-negative urine can appear red, cola colored, or burgundy, owing to ingestion of various drugs, foods (blackberries, beets), or food dyes, whereas dark brown (or black) urine can result from various urinary metabolites.

Evaluation of the child with hematuria begins with a careful history, physical examination, and urinalysis. This information is used to determine the level of hematuria (upper vs lower urinary tract) and to determine the urgency of the evaluation based on symptomatology. Special consideration needs to be given to family history, identification of anatomic abnormalities and malformation syndromes, presence of gross hematuria, and manifestations of hypertension, edema, or heart failure.

Causes of hematuria are listed in Table 503-2. Upper urinary tract sources of hematuria originate within the nephron (glomerulus, convoluted or collecting tubules, and interstitium). Lower urinary tract sources of hematuria originate from the pelvocalyceal system, ureter, bladder, or urethra. Hematuria from within the glomerulus is often associated with brown, cola or tea-colored, or burgundy urine, proteinuria >100 mg/dL via dipstick, urinary microscopic findings of RBC casts, and deformed urinary RBCs (particularly acanthocytes). Hematuria originating within the convoluted or collecting tubules may be associated with the presence of leukocytes or renal tubular epithelial cell casts. Lower urinary tract sources of hematuria may be associated with gross hematuria that is bright red or pink, terminal hematuria (gross hematuria occurring at the end of the urine stream), blood clots, normal urinary RBC morphology, and minimal proteinuria on dipstick (<100 mg/dL).

Patients with hematuria can present with a number of symptoms suggesting specific disorders. Tea- or cola-colored urine, facial or body edema, hypertension, and oliguria are classic symptoms of **acute nephritic syndrome.** Diseases commonly manifesting as acute nephritic syndrome include postinfectious glomerulonephritis, immunoglobulin A (IgA) nephropathy, membranoproliferative glomerulonephritis, Henoch-Schönlein purpura (HSP) nephritis, systemic lupus erythematosus (SLE) nephritis, Wegener granulomatosis, microscopic polyarteritis nodosa, Goodpasture syndrome, and hemolytic-uremic syndrome. A history of recent upper respiratory, skin, or gastrointestinal infection suggests postinfectious glomerulonephritis, hemolytic-uremic syndrome, or HSP nephritis. Rash and joint complaints suggest HSP nephritis or SLE nephritis. Hematuria associated with glomerulonephritis

Table 503-3 COMMON CAUSES OF GROSS HEMATURIA
Urinary tract infection
Meatal stenosis
Perineal irritation
Trauma
Urolithiasis
Hypercalciiuria
Coagulopathy
Tumor
Glomerular
Postinfectious glomerulonephritis
Henoch-Schönlein purpura nephritis
IgA nephropathy
Alport syndrome (hereditary nephritis)
Thin glomerular basement membrane disease
Systemic lupus erythematosus nephritis

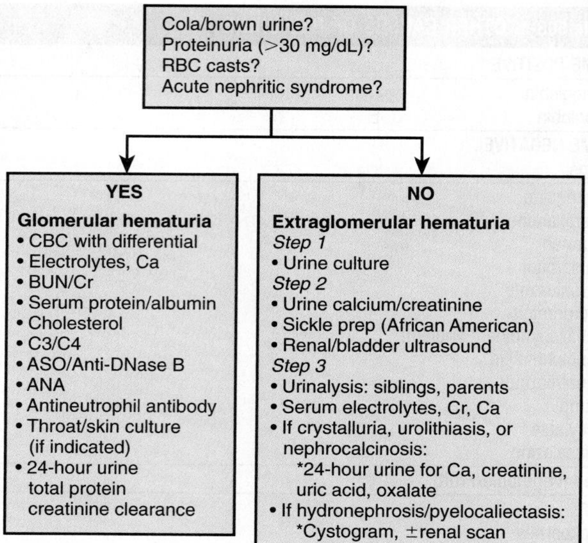

Figure 503-1 Algorithm of the general approach to the laboratory and radiologic evaluation of the patient with glomerular or extraglomerular hematuria. ANA, antinuclear antibody; ASO, antistreptolysin O; BUN, blood urea nitrogen; C3/C4, complement; CBC, complete blood cell count; Cr, creatinine; RBC, red blood cell.

is typically painless but it can be associated with flank pain. Frequency, dysuria, and unexplained fevers suggest a urinary tract infection, whereas renal colic suggests nephrolithiasis. A flank mass can signal hydronephrosis, renal cystic diseases, renal vein thrombosis, or tumor. Hematuria associated with headache, mental status changes, visual changes (diplopia), epistaxis, or heart failure suggests significant hypertension. Patients with a history of trauma require immediate evaluation (Chapter 66). Child abuse must always be suspected in the child presenting with unexplained perineal bruising and hematuria.

A careful family history is critical in the initial assessment of the child with hematuria in view of numerous genetic causes of renal disorders. Hereditary glomerular diseases include hereditary nephritis (Alport syndrome), thin glomerular basement membrane disease, SLE nephritis, and IgA nephropathy (Berger disease). Other hematuric renal disorders with a hereditary component include polycystic kidney disease (PKD) (both autosomal recessive [ARPKD] and autosomal dominant [ADPKD]), urolithiasis, and sickle cell disease/trait.

A complete physical examination is critical to assess the cause of hematuria. Hypertension, edema, or signs of heart failure suggest acute glomerulonephritis. Several malformation syndromes are associated with renal disease including VATER (*v*ertebral body anomalies, *a*nal atresia, *t*racheo*e*sophageal fistula, and *r*enal dysplasia) syndrome. Abdominal masses may be caused by bladder distention in posterior urethral valves, hydronephrosis in ureteropelvic junction obstruction, PKD, or Wilms tumor. Hematuria seen in patients with neurologic or cutaneous abnormalities may be the result of renal cystic disease or tumors associated with several syndromes, including tuberous sclerosis, von Hippel-Lindau syndrome, and Zellweger (cerebrohepatorenal) syndrome. Anatomic abnormalities of the external genitalia may be associated with hematuria and/or renal disease.

Patients with gross hematuria present additional challenges because of the associated parental anxiety. The most common cause of gross hematuria is bacterial urinary tract infection. Urethrorrhagia, which is urethral bleeding in the absence of urine, is associated with dysuria and blood spots on underwear after voiding. This condition, which often occurs in prepubertal boys at intervals several months apart, has a benign self-limited course. Less than 10% of patients have evidence of glomerulonephritis. Recurrent episodes of gross hematuria suggest IgA nephropathy, Alport syndrome, or thin glomerular basement membrane disease. Dysuria and abdominal or flank pain are symptoms of idiopathic hypercalciuria, or urolithiasis. Common causes of gross hematuria are listed in Table 503-3. A general approach to the laboratory and radiologic evaluation of the patient with glomerular or extraglomerular hematuria is outlined in Figure 503-1. Asymptomatic patients with isolated microscopic hematuria should not undergo extensive diagnostic evaluation because the hematuria is often transient and benign.

The child with asymptomatic isolated microscopic hematuria that persists on at least 3 urinalyses observed over a minimum of a 2-wk period poses a dilemma in regard to the degree of further diagnostic testing that should be performed. Significant disease of the urinary tract is uncommon with this clinical presentation. The initial evaluation of these children should include a urine culture followed by a spot urine for hypercalciuria with a calcium:creatinine ratio in culture-negative patients. In African-American patients, a sickle cell screen should be included. If these studies are normal, urinalysis of all first-degree relatives is indicated. Renal and bladder ultrasonography should be considered to rule out structural lesions such as tumor, cystic disease, hydronephrosis, or urolithiasis. Ultrasonography of the urinary tract is most informative in patients presenting with gross hematuria, abdominal pain, flank pain, or trauma. If these initial studies are normal, assessment of serum creatinine and electrolytes is recommended.

The finding of certain hematologic abnormalities can narrow the differential diagnosis. Anemia in this setting may be caused by intravascular dilution secondary to hypervolemia associated with acute renal failure; decreased RBC production in chronic renal failure; hemolysis from hemolytic-uremic syndrome or SLE; or blood loss from pulmonary hemorrhage, as seen in Goodpasture syndrome, or melena in patients with Henoch-Schönlein purpura or hemolytic-uremic syndrome. Inspection of the peripheral blood smear might reveal a microangiopathic process consistent with the hemolytic-uremic syndrome. The presence of autoantibodies in SLE can result in a positive Coombs test, the presence of antinuclear antibody, leukopenia, and multisystem disease. Thrombocytopenia can result from decreased platelet production (malignancies) or increased platelet consumption (SLE, idiopathic thrombocytopenic purpura, hemolytic-uremic syndrome, renal vein thrombosis). Although urinary RBC morphology may be normal with lower tract bleeding and dysmorphic from glomerular bleeding, cell morphology is not reliable to unequivocally delineate the site of hematuria. A bleeding diathesis is an unusual cause of hematuria. Coagulation studies are not routinely obtained unless personal or family history suggests a bleeding tendency.

A voiding cystourethrogram is only required in patients with a urinary tract infection, renal scarring, hydroureter, or pyelocaliectasis. Cystoscopy is an unnecessary and costly procedure in most pediatric patients with hematuria, and carries the associated risks of anesthesia. The diagnosis of "possible urethral stenosis" as an indication for cystoscopy should be viewed with a high degree of suspicion, because true urethral stenosis is quite rare. This procedure should be reserved for evaluating the rare child with a bladder mass noted on ultrasound, urethral abnormalities caused by trauma, posterior urethral valves, or tumor. The finding of unilateral gross hematuria localized by cystoscopy is rare, but it can indicate a vascular malformation or another anatomic abnormality.

Children with persistent asymptomatic isolated hematuria and a normal evaluation should have their blood pressure and urine checked every 3 months until the hematuria resolves. Referral to a pediatric nephrologist should be considered for patients with persistent asymptomatic hematuria greater than 1 yr's duration and is recommended for patients with nephritis (glomerulonephritis, tubulointerstitial nephritis), hypertension, renal insufficiency, urolithiasis or nephrocalcinosis, or a family history of renal disease such as PKD or hereditary nephritis. Renal biopsy is indicated for some children with persistent microscopic hematuria and most children with recurrent gross hematuria associated with decreased renal function, proteinuria, or hypertension.

BIBLIOGRAPHY

Please visit the Nelson Textbook of Pediatrics *website at www.expertconsult.com for the complete bibliography.*

Chapter 504

Isolated Glomerular Diseases with Recurrent Gross Hematuria

Cynthia G. Pan and Ellis D. Avner

Approximately 10% of children with gross hematuria have an acute or a chronic form of glomerulonephritis that may be associated with a systemic illness. The gross hematuria, which is usually characterized by brown or cola-colored urine, may be painless or associated with vague flank or abdominal pain. Presentation with gross hematuria is common within 1-2 days after the onset of an apparent viral upper respiratory tract infection in immunoglobulin A (IgA) nephropathy, and typically resolves within 5 days. This relatively short period contrasts to a latency period of 7-21 days occurring between the onset of a streptococcal pharyngitis or impetiginous skin infection and the development of poststreptococcal acute glomerulonephritis. Gross hematuria in these circumstances can last as long as 4-6 wk. Gross hematuria can also be seen in children with glomerular basement membrane (GBM) disorders such as hereditary nephritis (Alport syndrome [AS]) and thin GBM disease. These glomerular diseases can also manifest as microscopic hematuria and/or proteinuria without gross hematuria.

504.1 Immunoglobulin A Nephropathy (Berger Nephropathy)

Cynthia G. Pan and Ellis D. Avner

IgA nephropathy is the most common chronic glomerular disease. It is characterized by a predominance of IgA immunoglobulin within mesangial glomerular deposits in the absence of systemic disease (e.g., symptomatic systemic lupus erythematosus or Henoch-Schönlein purpura). Diagnosis requires renal biopsy, which is performed when clinical features warrant confirmation of the diagnosis or characterization of the histologic severity, which might affect therapeutic decisions.

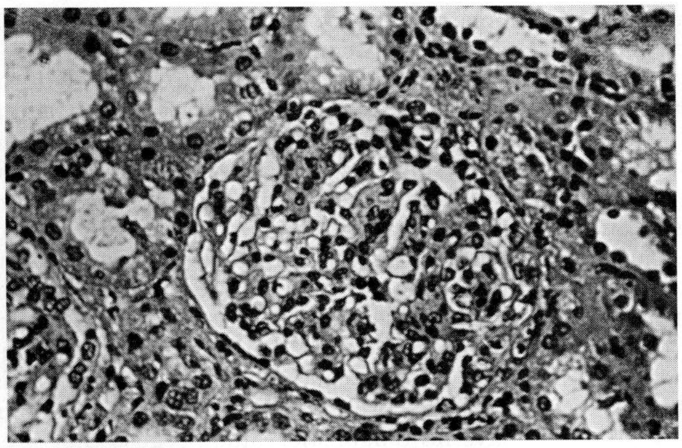

Figure 504-1 Light microscopy of immunoglobulin A nephropathy demonstrating segmental mesangial proliferation and increased matrix (×180).

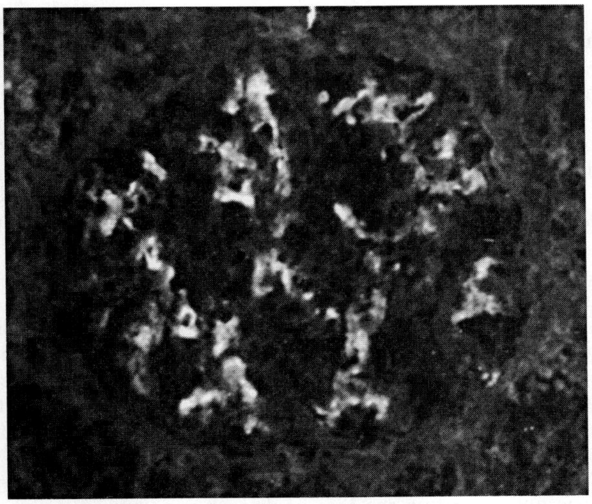

Figure 504-2 Immunofluorescence microscopy of the biopsy specimen from a child with episodes of gross hematuria demonstrating mesangial deposition of immunoglobulin A (×150).

PATHOLOGY AND PATHOLOGIC DIAGNOSIS

Focal and segmental mesangial proliferation and increased mesangial matrix are seen in the glomerulus (Fig. 504-1). Renal histology demonstrates mesangial proliferation that may be associated with epithelial cell crescent formation and sclerosis. IgA deposits in the mesangium are often accompanied by C3 complement (Fig. 504-2).

IgA nephropathy is an immune complex disease that appears to be caused by abnormalities in the IgA immune system. The abnormalities identified in the IgA immunoglobulin system have also been observed in patients with Henoch-Schönlein purpura and lends support to the hypothesis that these two diseases are part of the same disease spectrum. Familial clustering of IgA nephropathy cases suggests the importance of genetic factors. Genome-wide linkage analysis suggests the linkage of IgA nephropathy to 6q22-23 in multiplex IgA nephropathy kindreds.

CLINICAL AND LABORATORY MANIFESTATIONS

IgA nephropathy is seen more often in male than in female patients. Though there are rare cases of rapidly progressive forms of the disease, the clinical presentation of childhood IgA nephropathy is often benign in comparison to that of adults. IgA nephropathy is an uncommon cause of end-stage renal failure during childhood. A majority of children with IgA nephropathy in the

USA and Europe present with gross hematuria, whereas microscopic hematuria and/or proteinuria is a more common presentation in Japan. Other types of presentation include acute nephritic syndrome, nephrotic syndrome, or a combined nephritic-nephrotic picture. Gross hematuria often occurs within 1-2 days of onset of an upper respiratory or gastrointestinal infection, in contrast to the longer latency period observed in acute postinfectious glomerulonephritis, and may be associated with loin pain. Proteinuria is often <1000 mg/24 hr in patients with asymptomatic microscopic hematuria. Mild to moderate hypertension is most often seen in patients with nephritic or nephrotic syndrome but is rarely severe enough to result in hypertensive emergencies. Normal serum levels of C3 in IgA nephropathy help to distinguish this disorder from poststreptococcal glomerulonephritis. Serum IgA levels have no diagnostic value because they are elevated in only 15% of pediatric patients.

PROGNOSIS AND TREATMENT

Although IgA nephropathy does not lead to significant kidney damage in most children, progressive disease develops in 20-30% of patients 15-20 yr after disease onset. Therefore, most children with IgA nephropathy do not display progressive renal dysfunction until adulthood, prompting the need for careful long-term follow-up. Poor prognostic indicators at presentation or follow-up include persistent hypertension, diminished renal function, and heavy or prolonged proteinuria. A more-severe prognosis is correlated with histologic evidence of diffuse mesangial proliferation, extensive glomerular crescents, glomerulosclerosis, and diffuse tubulointerstitial changes, including inflammation and fibrosis.

The primary treatment of IgA nephropathy is appropriate blood pressure control. Fish oil, which contains anti-inflammatory omega-3 polyunsaturated fatty acids, decreases the rate of disease progression in adults. Immunosuppressive therapy with corticosteroids or more intensive multidrug regimens may be beneficial in some patients. Angiotensin-converting enzyme inhibitors and angiotensin II receptor antagonists are effective in reducing proteinuria and retarding the rate of disease progression when used as single agents or in combination. Tonsillectomy has been used as treatment for IgA nephropathy in many countries including Japan, but demonstration of its efficacy will require prospective controlled trials. Patients with IgA nephropathy may undergo successful kidney transplantation. Although recurrent disease is frequent, allograft loss caused by IgA nephropathy occurs in only 15-30% of patients.

BIBLIOGRAPHY

Please visit the Nelson Textbook of Pediatrics *website at www.expertconsult.com for the complete bibliography.*

504.2 Alport Syndrome

Cynthia G. Pan and Ellis D. Avner

AS, hereditary nephritis, is a genetically heterogeneous disease caused by mutations in the genes coding for type IV collagen, a major component of basement membranes. These genetic alterations are associated with marked variability in clinical presentation, natural history, and histologic abnormalities.

GENETICS

Approximately 85% of patients have X-linked disease caused by a mutation in the *COL4A5* gene encoding the α5 chain of type IV collagen. Patients with a subtype of X-linked AS and diffuse leiomyomatosis demonstrate a contiguous mutation within the *COL4A5* and *COL4A6* genes that encodes the α5 and α6 chains, respectively, of type IV collagen. Autosomal recessive forms of AS are caused by mutations in the *COL4A3* and *COL4A4* genes on chromosome 2 encoding the α3 and α4 chains, respectively, of type IV collagen. An autosomal dominant form of AS linked to the *COL4A3-COL4A4* gene locus occurs in 5% of cases.

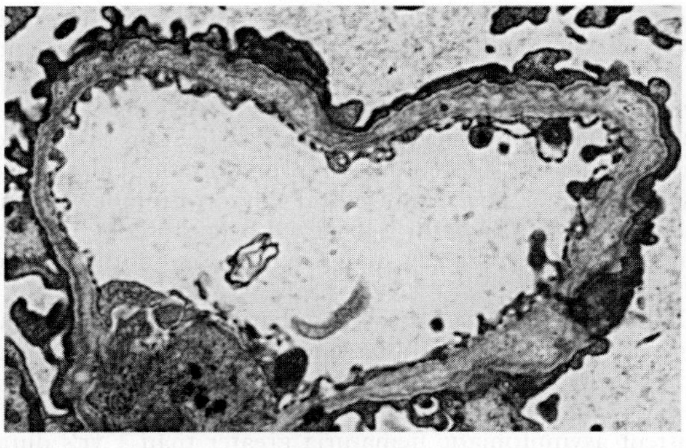

Figure 504-3 Electron micrograph of a biopsy specimen from a child with Alport syndrome depicting thickening, thinning, splitting, and layering of the glomerular basement membrane (×1,650). (From Yum M, Bergstein JM: Basement membrane nephropathy, *Hum Pathol* 14:996–1003, 1983.)

PATHOLOGY

Kidney biopsy specimens during the 1st decade of life might show few changes on light microscopy. Later, the glomeruli can develop mesangial proliferation and capillary wall thickening, leading to progressive glomerular sclerosis. Tubular atrophy, interstitial inflammation and fibrosis, and lipid-containing tubular or interstitial cells, called *foam cells,* develop as the disease progresses. Immunopathologic studies are usually nondiagnostic.

In most patients, electron microscopy reveals diffuse thickening, thinning, splitting, and layering of the glomerular and tubular basement membranes (Fig. 504-3). Ultrastructural analysis of the GBM in all genetic forms of AS may be completely normal, display nonspecific alterations, or demonstrate only uniform thinning.

CLINICAL MANIFESTATIONS

All patients with AS have asymptomatic microscopic hematuria, which may be intermittent in girls and younger boys. Single or recurrent episodes of gross hematuria commonly occurring 1-2 days after an upper respiratory infection are seen in approximately 50% of patients. Proteinuria is often seen in boys but may be absent, mild, or intermittent in girls. Progressive proteinuria, often exceeding 1 g/24 hr, is common by the 2nd decade of life and can be severe enough to cause nephrotic syndrome.

Bilateral sensorineural hearing loss, which is never congenital, occurs in 90% of hemizygous males with X-linked AS, 10% of heterozygous females with X-linked AS, and 67% of patients with autosomal recessive AS. This deficit begins in the high-frequency range but progresses to involve conversational speech, prompting the need for hearing aids. Ocular abnormalities, which occur in 30-40% of patients with X-linked AS, include anterior lenticonus (extrusion of the central portion of the lens into the anterior chamber), macular flecks, and corneal erosions. Leiomyomatosis of the esophagus, tracheobronchial tree, and female genitals in association with platelet abnormalities is rare.

DIAGNOSIS

A careful family history, a screening urinalysis of first-degree relatives, an audiogram, and an ophthalmologic examination are critical in making the diagnosis of AS. The presence of anterior lenticonus is pathognomonic. AS is highly likely in the patient who has hematuria and at least 2 of the following characteristic clinical features: macular flecks, recurrent corneal erosions, GBM thickening and thinning, or sensorineural deafness. Absence of epidermal basement membrane staining for the α5 chain of type IV collagen in male hemizygotes and discontinuous epidermal basement membrane staining in female heterozygotes is pathognomonic for X-linked AS and can preclude diagnostic renal biopsy. Mutation screening or linkage analysis is not readily available for routine clinical use. Prenatal diagnosis is available for families with members who have X-linked AS and who carry an identified mutation.

PROGNOSIS AND TREATMENT

The risk of progressive renal dysfunction leading to end-stage renal disease (ESRD) is highest among hemizygotes and autosomal recessive homozygotes. ESRD occurs before age 30 yr in approximately 75% of hemizygotes with X-linked AS. The risk of ESRD in X-linked heterozygotes is 12% by age 40 yr and 30% by age 60 yr. Risk factors for progression are gross hematuria during childhood, nephrotic syndrome, and prominent GBM thickening. Intrafamilial variation in phenotypic expression results in significant differences in the age of ESRD among family members. No specific therapy is available to treat AS, although angiotensin-converting enzyme inhibitors can slow the rate of progression. Careful management of renal failure complications such as hypertension, anemia, and electrolyte imbalance is critical. Patients with ESRD are treated with dialysis and kidney transplantation (Chapter 529). Approximately 5% of kidney transplant recipients develop anti-GBM nephritis, which occurs primarily in males with X-linked AS who develop ESRD before age 30 yr.

BIBLIOGRAPHY

Please visit the Nelson Textbook of Pediatrics *website at www.expertconsult.com for the complete bibliography.*

504.3 Thin Basement Membrane Disease

Cynthia G. Pan and Ellis D. Avner

Thin basement membrane disease (TBMD) is defined by the presence of persistent microscopic hematuria and isolated thinning of the glomerular basement membrane (GBM) (and occasionally tubular basement membranes) on electron microscopy. Microscopic hematuria is often initially observed during childhood and may be intermittent. Episodic gross hematuria can also be present, particularly after a respiratory illness. Isolated hematuria in multiple family members without renal dysfunction is referred to as **benign familial hematuria.** Although most of these patients will not undergo renal biopsy, it is often presumed that the underlying pathology is TBMD.

TBMD may be sporadic or transmitted as an autosomal dominant trait. Heterozygous mutations in the *COL4A3* and *COL4A4* genes, which encode the α3 and α4 chains of type IV collagen present in the GBM, result in TBMD. Rare cases of TBMD progress, and such patients develop significant proteinuria, hypertension, or renal insufficiency. Homozygous mutations in these same genes result in autosomal recessive Alport syndrome. Therefore, in these rare cases, the absence of a positive family history for renal insufficiency or deafness would not necessarily predict a benign outcome. Therefore, monitoring patients with benign familial hematuria for progressive proteinuria, hypertension, or renal insufficiency is important through childhood and young adulthood.

BIBLIOGRAPHY

Please visit the Nelson Textbook of Pediatrics *website at www.expertconsult.com for the complete bibliography.*

Chapter 505 Glomerulonephritis Associated with Infections

505.1 Acute Poststreptococcal Glomerulonephritis

Cynthia G. Pan and Ellis D. Avner

Group A β-hemolytic streptococcal (GAS) infections are common in children and can lead to the postinfectious complication of acute glomerulonephritis (GN). Acute poststreptococcal glomerulonephritis (APSGN) is a classic example of the **acute nephritic syndrome** characterized by the sudden onset of gross hematuria, edema, hypertension, and renal insufficiency. It is one of the most common glomerular causes of gross hematuria in children and is a major cause of morbidity in GAS infections.

ETIOLOGY AND EPIDEMIOLOGY

APSGN follows infection of the throat or skin by certain "nephritogenic" strains of GAS. Epidemics and clusters of household cases occur throughout the world, and 97% of cases occur in less-developed countries. The overall incidence has decreased in industrialized nations, presumably due to improved hygienic conditions. Poststreptococcal GN commonly follows streptococcal pharyngitis during cold-weather months and streptococcal skin infections or pyoderma during warm-weather months. Although epidemics of nephritis have been described in association with throat (serotype 12) and skin (serotype 49) infections, this disease is most commonly sporadic.

PATHOLOGY

The kidneys appear symmetrically enlarged. Glomeruli appear enlarged and relatively bloodless and show diffuse mesangial cell proliferation, with an increase in mesangial matrix (Fig. 505-1). Polymorphonuclear leukocyte infiltration is common in glomeruli during the early stage of the disease. Crescents and interstitial inflammation may be seen in severe cases, but these changes are not specific for poststreptococcal GN. Immunofluorescence microscopy reveals a pattern of "lumpy-bumpy" deposits of immunoglobulin and complement on the glomerular basement membrane (GBM) and in the mesangium. On electron microscopy, electron-dense deposits, or "humps," are observed on the epithelial side of the GBM (Fig. 505-2).

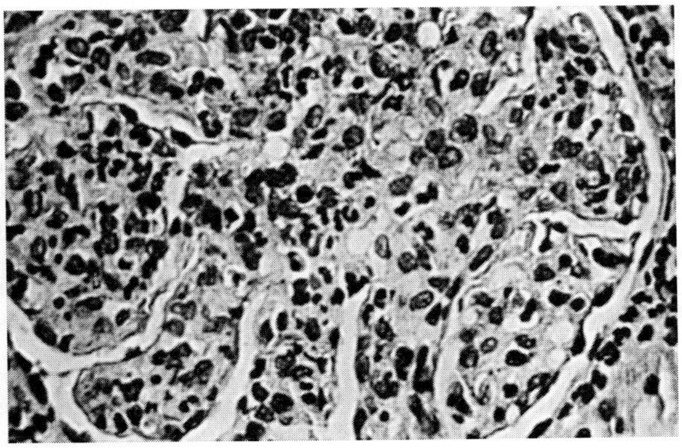

Figure 505-1 Glomerulus from a patient with poststreptococcal glomerulonephritis appears enlarged and relatively bloodless and shows mesangial proliferation and exudation of neutrophils (×400).

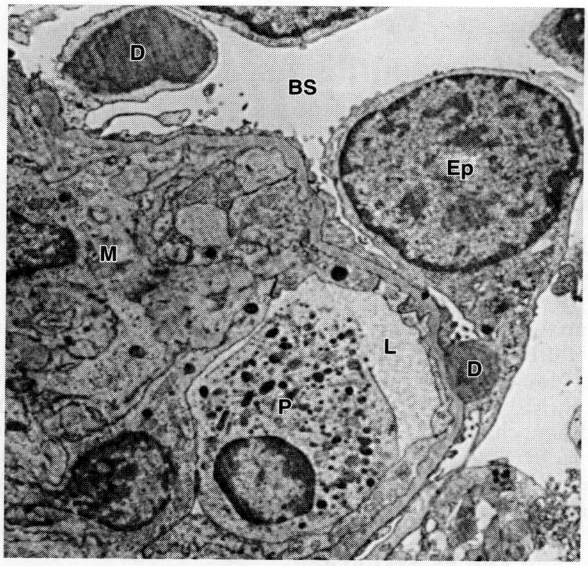

Figure 505-2 Electron micrograph in poststreptococcal glomerulonephritis demonstrating electron-dense deposits (D) on the epithelial cell (Ep) side of the glomerular basement membrane. A polymorphonuclear leukocyte (P) is present within the lumen (L) of the capillary. BS, Bowman space; M, mesangium.

PATHOGENESIS

Morphologic studies and a depression in the serum complement (C3) level provide strong evidence that ASPGN is mediated by immune complexes. Precise mechanisms by which nephritogenic streptococci induce immunologic injury continue to be elucidated. Several mechanisms of immune injury have been supported by experimental models and human studies and include circulating immune complex formation with streptococcal antigens and subsequent glomerular deposition, molecular mimicry whereby circulating antibodies elicited by streptococcal antigens react with normal glomerular antigens, in situ immune complex formation of antistreptococcal antibodies with glomerular deposited antigen, and complement activation by directly deposited streptococcal antigens.

Group A streptococci possess M proteins, and nephritogenic strains are related to the M protein serotype. The search for the precise nephritogenic antigen suggests that streptococcal pyogenic exotoxin (SPE B) and nephritis-associated streptococcal plasmin receptor (NAPlr) are promising candidates. Both have been identified in glomeruli of affected patients, and in 1 study, circulating antibodies to SPE B were found in all patients. Cross-reactivity of SPE B and other M proteins with various components of the glomerular basement membrane also give evidence for molecular mimicry.

CLINICAL MANIFESTATIONS

Poststreptococcal GN is most common in children aged 5-12 yr and uncommon before the age of 3 yr. The typical patient develops an acute nephritic syndrome 1-2 wk after an antecedent streptococcal pharyngitis or 3-6 wk after a streptococcal pyoderma. The history of a specific infection may be absent, because symptoms may have been mild or have resolved without patients receiving specific treatment or seeking the care of a medical provider.

The severity of kidney involvement varies from asymptomatic microscopic hematuria with normal renal function to gross hematuria with acute renal failure. Depending on the severity of renal involvement, patients can develop various degrees of edema, hypertension, and oliguria. Patients are at risk for developing encephalopathy and/or heart failure secondary to hypertension or hypervolemia. Hypertensive encephalopathy must be considered in patients with blurred vision, severe headaches, altered mental status, or new seizures. The effects of acute hypertension not only depend on the severity of hypertension but also the absolute change in comparison to the patient's baseline blood pressure and the rate at which it has risen. Encephalopathy can also result from the direct toxic effects of streptococcal antigens on the central nervous system. Respiratory distress, orthopnea, and cough may be symptoms of pulmonary edema and heart failure. Peripheral edema typically results from salt and water retention and is common; nephrotic syndrome develops in a minority (<5%) of childhood cases. Nonspecific symptoms such as malaise, lethargy, abdominal pain, or flank pain are common.

The acute phase generally resolves within 6-8 wk. Although urinary protein excretion and hypertension usually normalize by 4-6 wk after onset, persistent microscopic hematuria can persist for 1-2 yr after the initial presentation.

DIAGNOSIS

Urinalysis demonstrates red blood cells (RBCs), often in association with RBC casts, proteinuria, and polymorphonuclear leukocytes. A mild normochromic anemia may be present from hemodilution and low-grade hemolysis. The serum C3 level is significantly reduced in >90% of patients in the acute phase and returns to normal 6-8 wk after onset. Although serum CH50 is commonly depressed, C4 is most often normal in APSGN, or only mildly depressed.

Confirmation of the diagnosis requires clear evidence of a prior streptococcal infection. A positive throat culture report might support the diagnosis or might simply represent the carrier state. On the other hand, a rising antibody titer to streptococcal antigen(s) confirms a recent streptococcal infection. The anti-streptolysin O titer is commonly elevated after a pharyngeal infection but rarely increases after streptococcal skin infections. The best single antibody titer to document cutaneous streptococcal infection is the anti-deoxyribonuclease (DNase) B level. If available, a positive streptozyme screen (which measures multiple antibodies to different streptococcal antigens) is a valuable diagnostic tool. Serologic evidence for streptococcal infections is more sensitive than the history of recent infections and far more sensitive than positive bacterial cultures obtained at the time of onset of acute nephritis.

Magnetic resonance imaging of the brain is indicated in patients with severe neurologic symptoms and can demonstrate **reversible posterior leukoencephalopathy** in the parieto-occipital areas on T2-weighted images. Chest x-ray is indicated in those with signs of heart failure or respiratory distress, or physical exam findings of a heart gallop, decreased breath sounds, rales, or hypoxemia.

The clinical diagnosis of poststreptococcal GN is quite likely in a child presenting with acute nephritic syndrome, evidence of recent streptococcal infection, and a low C3 level. However, it is important to consider other diagnoses such as systemic lupus erythematosus and an acute exacerbation of chronic GN. Renal biopsy should be considered only in the presence of acute renal failure, nephrotic syndrome, absence of evidence of streptococcal infection, or normal complement levels. In addition, renal biopsy is considered when hematuria and proteinuria, diminished renal function, and/or a low C3 level persist more than 2 mo after onset. Persistent hypocomplementemia can indicate a chronic form of postinfectious GN or another disease such as membranoproliferative GN.

The differential diagnosis of poststreptococcal GN includes many of the causes of hematuria listed in Tables 503-2 and 505-1 and an algorithm to help with diagnosis is presented in Figure 505-3. Acute postinfectious GN can also follow other infections with coagulase-positive and coagulase-negative staphylococci, *Streptococcus pneumoniae,* and gram-negative bacteria. Bacterial

Table 505-1 SUMMARY OF PRIMARY RENAL DISEASES THAT MANIFEST AS ACUTE GLOMERULONEPHRITIS

DISEASES	POSTSTREPTOCOCCAL GLOMERULONEPHRITIS	IgA NEPHROPATHY	GOODPASTURE SYNDROME	IDIOPATHIC RAPIDLY PROGRESSIVE GLOMERULONEPHRITIS
CLINICAL MANIFESTATIONS				
Age and sex	All ages, mean 7 yr, 2:1 male	10-35 yr, 2:1 male	15-30 yr, 6:1 male	Adults, 2:1 male
Acute nephritic syndrome	90%	50%	90%	90%
Asymptomatic hematuria	Occasionally	50%	Rare	Rare
Nephrotic syndrome	10-20%	Rare	Rare	10-20%
Hypertension	70%	30-50%	Rare	25%
Acute renal failure	50% (transient)	Very rare	50%	60%
Other	Latent period of 1-3 wk	Follows viral syndromes	Pulmonary hemorrhage; iron deficiency anemia	None
Laboratory findings	↑ ASO titers (70%) Positive streptozyme (95%) ↓C3-C9; normal C1, C4	↑ Serum IgA (50%) IgA in dermal capillaries	Positive anti-GBM antibody	Positive ANCA in some
Immunogenetics	HLA-B12, D "EN" (9)*	HLA-Bw 35, DR4 (4)*	HLA-DR2 (16)*	None established
RENAL PATHOLOGY				
Light microscopy	Diffuse proliferation	Focal proliferation	Focal → diffuse proliferation with crescents	Crescentic GN
Immunofluorescence	Granular IgG, C3	Diffuse mesangial IgA	Linear IgG, C3	No immune deposits
Electron microscopy	Subepithelial humps	Mesangial deposits	No deposits	No deposits
Prognosis	95% resolve spontaneously 5% RPGN or slowly progressive	Slow progression in 25-50%	75% stabilize or improve if treated early	75% stabilize or improve if treated early
Treatment	Supportive	Uncertain (options include steroids, fish oil, and ACE inhibitors)	Plasma exchange, steroids, cyclophosphamide	Steroid pulse therapy

*Relative risk.
Ig, immunoglobulin; ASO, anti-streptolysin O; GBM, glomerular basement membrane; ANCA, antineutrophil cytoplasmic antibody; HLA, human leukocyte antigen; GN, glomerulonephritis; RPGN, idiopathic rapidly progressive glomerulonephritis; ACE, angiotensin-converting enzyme.
From Kliegman RM, Greenbaum LA, Lye PS: *Practical strategies in pediatric diagnosis and therapy,* ed 2, Philadelphia, 2004, Elsevier, p 427.

endocarditis can produce a hypocomplementemic GN with renal failure. Acute GN can occur after certain fungal, rickettsial, and viral diseases, particularly influenza.

COMPLICATIONS

Acute complications result from hypertension and acute renal dysfunction. Hypertension is seen in 60% of patients and is associated with hypertensive encephalopathy in 10% of cases. Although the neurologic sequelae are often reversible with appropriate management, severe prolonged hypertension can lead to intracranial bleeding. Other potential complications include heart failure, hyperkalemia, hyperphosphatemia, hypocalcemia, acidosis, seizures, and uremia. Acute renal failure can require treatment with dialysis.

PREVENTION

Early systemic antibiotic therapy for streptococcal throat and skin infections does not eliminate the risk of GN. Family members of patients with acute GN, especially young children, should be considered at risk and be cultured for group A β-hemolytic streptococci and treated if appropriate. Family pets, particularly dogs, have also been reported as carriers.

TREATMENT

Management is directed at treating the acute effects of renal insufficiency and hypertension (Chapter 529.1). Although a 10-day course of systemic antibiotic therapy with penicillin is recommended to limit the spread of the nephritogenic organisms, antibiotic therapy does not affect the natural history of GN. Sodium restriction, diuresis usually with intravenous furosemide, and pharmacotherapy with calcium channel antagonists, vasodilators, or angiotensin-converting enzyme inhibitors are standard therapies used to treat hypertension.

PROGNOSIS

Complete recovery occurs in >95% of children with APSGN. Recurrences are extremely rare. Mortality in the acute stage can be avoided by appropriate management of acute renal failure, cardiac failure, and hypertension. Infrequently, the acute phase is severe and leads to glomerulosclerosis and chronic renal disease in <2% of affected children. The true incidence of chronic renal disease that emerges later in adulthood as a result of childhood APSGN and reduction of functioning nephron number remains unknown.

BIBLIOGRAPHY

Please visit the Nelson Textbook of Pediatrics *website at www.expertconsult.com for the complete bibliography.*

505.2 Other Chronic Infections

Cynthia G. Pan and Ellis D. Avner

GN is a recognized complication of various chronic infections. Classic examples include bacterial endocarditis caused by viridans *Streptococcus* and other organisms, and ventriculoatrial shunts infected with *Staphylococcus epidermidis.* Other infections, observed less commonly in children than adults, include hepatitis B virus, hepatitis C virus, syphilis, and candidiasis. Parasitic infections associated with glomerular disease include malaria, schistosomiasis, leishmaniasis, filariasis, hydatid disease, trypanosomiasis, and toxoplasmosis. In each condition, the infecting organism has low virulence and the host is chronically infected with foreign antigen. In the presence of high levels of circulating antigen, the host's antibody response leads to formation of immune complexes that deposit in the kidneys and initiate glomerular inflammation. Foreign antigens can also stimulate an autoimmune response through the production of antibodies that

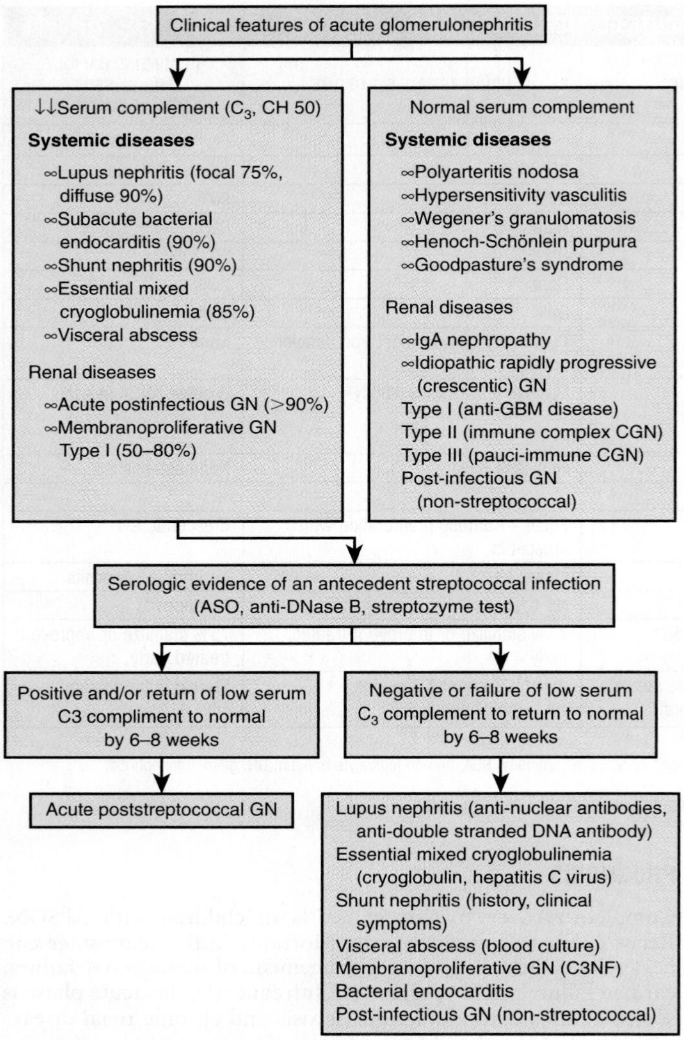

Figure 505-3 Differential diagnosis of acute glomerulonephritis (GN). ASO, antistreptolysin O; GBM, glomerular basement membrane. (Adapted from Sulyok E: Acute proliferative glomerulonephritis. In Avner ED, Harmon WE, Niaudet P, editors: *Pediatric nephrology,* ed 5, Philadelphia, 2004, Lippincott Williams & Wilkins, pp 601–613.)

cross react with such antigens incorrectly "recognized" as glomerular structural components.

The renal histopathology can resemble poststreptococcal GN, membranous GN, or membranoproliferative GN. The clinical manifestations are generally those of an acute nephritic or nephrotic syndrome. The serum C3 and CH50 complement levels are often decreased.

It has been demonstrated in HIV-associated nephropathy (HIVAN) that direct viral infection of nephrons can occur because renal cells express a variety of lymphocyte chemokine receptors that are essential for and facilitate viral invasion. The renal expression of HIV infection is quite variable and includes an immune complex injury and a direct cytopathic effect. The classic histopathologic lesion of HIVAN is focal segmental glomerulosclerosis.

Prompt eradication of any infection before severe glomerular injury occurs usually results in resolution of the GN. Progression to end-stage renal failure has been described but is uncommon. Spontaneous resolution of hepatitis B infection is common in children (30-50%) and results in remission of the glomerulopathy. Specific antivirals, interferon therapy, plasmapheresis, and immunosuppressive treatment have all been used successfully in adults with hepatitis C disease, but no controlled trials with any of these agents have been performed in pediatric patients.

BIBLIOGRAPHY

Please visit the Nelson Textbook of Pediatrics *website at* *www.expertconsult.com* *for the complete bibliography.*

Chapter 506
Membranous Glomerulopathy

Scott K. Van Why and Ellis D. Avner

Membranous glomerulopathy, now commonly called membranous nephropathy (MN), a common cause of nephrotic syndrome in adults, is a rare cause of nephrotic syndrome in children. MN is classified as the primary, idiopathic form, where there is isolated renal disease, or secondary MN, where nephropathy is associated with other identifiable systemic diseases or medications. In children, secondary MN is far more common than primary, idiopathic MN. The most common etiologies of secondary MN are systemic lupus erythematosus (SLE) or chronic infections. Among the latter, chronic hepatitis B infection and congenital syphilis are the best characterized and widely recognized causes of MN. However, other chronic infections have also been associated with MN, including malaria, which is the most common cause of MN worldwide. Certain medications, such as penicillamine and gold, can also cause MN. Rarely, tumors, such as neuroblastoma, or other idiopathic systemic diseases have been associated with MN. Identification of secondary causes of MN is critical, because removal of the offending agent or treatment of the causative disease often leads to resolution of the associated nephropathy and improves patient outcome.

PATHOLOGY

Glomeruli have diffuse thickening of the glomerular basement membrane (GBM), without significant cell proliferative changes. Immunofluorescence and electron microscopy typically demonstrate granular deposits of IgG and C3 located on the epithelial side of the GBM in a spikelike pattern. The GBM thickening presumably results from the production of membrane-like material in response to deposition of immune complexes.

PATHOGENESIS

MN is believed to be caused by in situ immune complex formation. Therefore, antigens from the infectious agents or medications associated with secondary MN directly contribute to the pathogenesis of the renal disease. The causative agents or antigens in the other secondary forms of MN have not been defined. Likewise, the causative antigen in idiopathic MN is not established, but the M-type phospholipase A2 receptor may be a target antigen in idiopathic MN. This receptor, present on normal podocytes, is found to be an antigen present in immune deposits extracted from glomeruli from patients with idiopathic MN. The majority of idiopathic MN patients also demonstrate circulating antibody against this antigen. Specific antigens trigger the onset of primary or secondary MN, but genetic factors significantly influence disease susceptibility and progression.

CLINICAL MANIFESTATIONS

In children, membranous glomerulopathy is most common in the 2nd decade of life, but it can occur at any age, including infancy. The disease usually manifests as nephrotic syndrome and accounts for 2-6% of all cases of childhood nephrotic syndrome. Most patients also have microscopic hematuria and only rarely present with gross hematuria. Approximately 20% of children have hypertension at presentation. A subset of patients with MN present with a major venous thrombosis, commonly renal vein thrombosis. This well-known complication of nephrotic syndrome (Chapter 521) is particularly common in patients with MN. Serum C3 and CH50 levels are normal, except in cases of SLE, where levels may be depressed (see Fig. 505-3).

DIAGNOSIS

Membranous glomerulopathy might be suspected on clinical grounds, particularly in the setting of known risk factors for secondary forms of the disease. The diagnosis can only be established by renal biopsy. No serologic test is specific for MN, but finding an active carrier state for hepatitis B or congenital syphilis would make the diagnosis probable in the appropriate clinical setting. Common indications for renal biopsy leading to the diagnosis of MN include presentation with nephrotic syndrome in a child >10 yr or unexplained persistent hematuria with significant proteinuria.

PROGNOSIS AND TREATMENT

The clinical course of idiopathic membranous glomerulopathy is variable. Children presenting with asymptomatic, low-grade proteinuria can enter remission spontaneously. Retrospective reports of children 1-15 yr after diagnosis, treated with a variety of regimens, indicate that 20% progress to chronic renal failure, 40% continue with active disease, and 40% achieve complete remission. Although no controlled trials have been performed in children, immunosuppressive therapy with an extended course of prednisone can be effective in promoting complete resolution of symptoms. The addition of chlorambucil or cyclophosphamide appears to provide further benefit to those not responding to steroids alone. For those unresponsive to immunosuppression, proteinuria can be reduced with angiotensin-converting enzyme inhibitors.

BIBLIOGRAPHY

Please visit the Nelson Textbook of Pediatrics *website at www.expertconsult.com for the complete bibliography.*

Chapter 507 Membranoproliferative Glomerulonephritis

Scott K. Van Why and Ellis D. Avner

Membranoproliferative glomerulonephritis (MPGN), also known as mesangiocapillary glomerulonephritis, most commonly occurs in children or young adults. MPGN can be classified into primary, idiopathic, and secondary forms of glomerular disease. Secondary forms of MPGN are most commonly associated with subacute and chronic infection, including hepatitis B and C, syphilis, subacute bacterial endocarditis, and infected shunts, especially ventriculoatrial shunts (shunt nephritis). MPGN can also be one of the glomerular lesions seen in lupus nephritis (Chapter 508).

PATHOLOGY

MPGN is defined by the histologic pattern of glomeruli as seen by light, immunofluorescence, and electron microscopy. Two subtypes have been defined on histologic criteria and are associated with different clinical phenotypes. **Type I MPGN** is most common. Glomeruli have an accentuated lobular pattern from diffuse mesangial expansion, endocapillary proliferation, and an increase in mesangial cells and matrix. The glomerular capillary walls are thickened, often with splitting from interposition of the mesangium. Crescents, if present, indicate a poor prognosis. Immunofluorescence microscopy reveals C3 and lesser amounts of immunoglobulin in the mesangium and along the peripheral capillary walls in a lobular pattern. Electron microscopy confirms numerous deposits in the mesangial and subendothelial regions.

Far less common is **type II MPGN,** also called dense deposit disease, which has similar light microscopic findings as type I MPGN. Differentiation from type I disease is by immunofluorescence and electron microscopy. In type II disease, C3 immunofluorescence typically is prominent without concomitant immunoglobulin. By electron microscopy, the lamina densa in the GBM undergoes a very dense transformation, without evident immune complex–type deposits.

PATHOGENESIS

Because the histology of **type I MPGN** produced by primary and secondary forms is indistinguishable, it appears that this form occurs because circulating immune complexes become trapped in the glomerular subendothelial space, which then causes injury, resulting in the characteristic proliferative response and mesangial expansion. Further evidence confirming this pathway to glomerular injury is the finding of complement activation through the classical pathway in as many as 50% of affected patients.

Type II MPGN appears to **not** be mediated by the immune complex. The pathogenesis of the disease is not known, but the characteristic finding of severely depressed serum complement levels suggests that deranged complement regulation might play a major role in disease. A typical finding is markedly depressed serum C3 complement levels, with normal levels of other complement components. In many patients with type II MPGN, **C3 nephritic factor** is present. This factor activates the alternative complement pathway. In unusual cases, patients with type II MPGN demonstrate an associated systemic disease called **partial lipodystrophy**, where there is diffuse loss of adipose tissue and decreased complement in the presence of C3 nephritic factor. Correlation among the presence of C3 nephritic factor, complement levels, and disease presence or severity is not uniform or tightly associated, indicating that the complement abnormalities alone are not sufficient to cause the disease.

CLINICAL MANIFESTATIONS

MPGN is most common in the 2nd decade of life. Systemic features could provide clues to which type of MPGN may be present in the secondary forms of the disease, but the 2 histologic types of idiopathic MPGN are indistinguishable on clinical grounds. Patients present in equal proportions with nephrotic syndrome, acute nephritic syndrome (hematuria, hypertension, and some level of renal insufficiency), or persistent asymptomatic microscopic hematuria and proteinuria. Serum C3 complement levels are low in the majority of cases (see Fig 505-3).

DIFFERENTIAL DIAGNOSIS

The differential diagnosis includes all forms of acute and chronic glomerulonephritis, including idiopathic and secondary forms, along with postinfectious glomerulonephritis. Postinfectious glomerulonephritis, far more common than MPGN, usually does not have nephrotic features but typically has hematuria, hypertension, renal insufficiency, and transient low C3 complement levels, all features that may be seen with MPGN. In contrast to MPGN, where C3 levels usually remain persistently low, C3 returns to normal within 2 months after the onset of postinfectious glomerulonephritis (Chapter 505 and Fig. 505-3). The diagnosis of MPGN is made by renal biopsy. Indications for biopsy include nephrotic syndrome in an older child, significant proteinuria with microscopic hematuria, and hypocomplementemia lasting >2 mo in a child with acute nephritis.

PROGNOSIS AND TREATMENT

It is important to determine whether MPGN is idiopathic or secondary to a systemic disease, particularly lupus or chronic infection, because treatment of the causative disease can result in resolution of MPGN. Untreated, idiopathic MPGN, regardless of type, has a poor prognosis. By 10 yr after onset, 50% of patients with MPGN have progressed to end-stage renal disease. By 20 yr after onset, up to 90% have lost renal function. Those with nephrotic syndrome at the time of presentation progress to renal failure more rapidly. No definitive therapy exists, but several reports, including a randomized, controlled trial, indicate that extended courses for years of alternate-day prednisone provide benefit. Some patients treated with steroids enter complete remission of their disease, but many have ongoing disease activity. Nevertheless, an extended course of prednisone is associated with significant preservation of renal function compared with patients receiving no such treatment.

BIBLIOGRAPHY
Please visit the Nelson Textbook of Pediatrics *website at www.expertconsult.com for the complete bibliography.*

Chapter 508
Glomerulonephritis Associated with Systemic Lupus Erythematosus

Cynthia G. Pan and Ellis D. Avner

Systemic lupus erythematosus (SLE) is characterized by fever, weight loss, dermatitis, hematologic abnormalities, arthritis, and involvement of the heart, lungs, central nervous system, and kidneys (Chapter 152). Glomerulonephritis is the most important cause of morbidity and mortality in SLE. Renal disease in childhood SLE is present in up 80% patients and is more active than that seen in adults. Occasionally, renal disease is the only presenting clinical manifestation.

PATHOGENESIS AND PATHOLOGY

The clinical manifestations of SLE are mediated by immune complexes. The classification of lupus nephritis of the World Health Organization (WHO) is based on a combination of light microscopy, immunofluorescence, and electron microscopy features. In patients with **WHO class I nephritis** (minimal mesangial lupus nephritis), no histologic abnormalities are detected on light microscopy but mesangial immune deposits are present on immunofluorescence or electron microscopy. In **WHO class II nephritis** (mesangial proliferative nephritis), light microscopy shows both mesangial hypercellularity and increased matrix along with mesangial deposits containing immunoglobulin and complement.

WHO class III nephritis and **WHO class IV** nephritis are interrelated lesions characterized by both mesangial and endocapillary lesions. Class III nephritis is defined by <50% glomeruli with involvement and class IV has ≥50% glomerular involvement. Immune deposits are present in both the mesangium and subendothelial areas. A subclassification scheme helps grade severity of the proliferative lesion based on whether the glomerular lesions are segmental (<50% glomerular tuft involved) or global (≥50% glomerular tuft involved). The WHO classification scheme also delineates whether there is a predominance of chronic disease versus active disease. Chronic injury results in glomerular sclerosis and is felt to be the consequence of significant proliferative disease seen in class III and IV. Other signs of active disease include capillary walls that are thickened secondary to subendothelial deposits (creating the wire-loop lesion), necrosis, and crescent formation. WHO class IV nephritis is associated with poorer outcomes but can be successfully treated with aggressive immunosuppressive therapy.

WHO class V nephritis (membranous lupus nephritis), is less commonly seen as an isolated lesion and resembles idiopathic membranous nephropathy with subepithelial immune deposits. This lesion is often seen in combination with class III or IV proliferative nephritis, and if the membranous lesion is present in >50% glomeruli, both classes are noted in designation. This classification scheme also identifies cases with combinations of mixed class III, IV, and V lesions, resulting in more appropriate treatment for such patients.

Transformation of the histologic lesion from one class to another is common. This is more likely to occur among inadequately treated patients and usually results in progression to a more severe histologic lesion.

CLINICAL MANIFESTATIONS

The majority of children with SLE are adolescent girls. The clinical findings in patients having milder forms of lupus nephritis (all class I-II, some class III) include hematuria, normal renal function, and proteinuria <1 g/24 hr. Some patients with class III and all patients with class IV nephritis have hematuria and proteinuria, reduced renal function, nephrotic syndrome, or acute renal failure. The urinalysis may be normal on rare occasions in patients with proliferative lupus nephritis. Patients with class V nephritis commonly present with nephrotic syndrome.

DIAGNOSIS

The diagnosis of SLE is confirmed by the detection of circulating antinuclear antibodies and by demonstrating antibodies that react with native double-stranded DNA. In most patients with active disease, C3 and C4 levels are depressed. In view of the lack of a clear correlation between the clinical manifestations and the severity of the renal involvement, renal biopsy should be performed in all patients with SLE. These results are used to guide the selection of immunosuppressive therapies.

TREATMENT

Children with SLE should be treated by pediatric specialists in medical centers where medical and psychologic support can be given to patients and their families. The goal of immunosuppressive therapy in lupus nephritis is producing a clinical and serologic remission, defined as normalization of anti-DNA antibody, C3, and C4 levels. Therapy is initiated in all patients with prednisone at a dose of 1-2 mg/kg/day in divided doses followed by a slow steroid taper over 4-6 mo beginning 4-6 wk after achieving a serologic remission. For patients having more severe forms of nephritis (WHO classes III and IV), 6 consecutive monthly intravenous infusions of cyclophosphamide at a dose of 500-1,000 mg/m^2 followed by additional infusions every 3 mo for 18 mo appears to reduce the risk of progressive renal dysfunction. Azathioprine at a single daily dose of 1.5-2.0 mg/kg may be used as a steroid-sparing agent in patients with WHO class I or II lupus nephritis. Single-center clinical trials also suggest the potential benefit of mycophenolate mofetil in patients with lupus nephritis, although results of long-term therapy, particularly compared with standard therapy, has not been systematically evaluated. Rituximab, a chimeric monoclonal antibody specific for human CD20, may be effective in patients with WHO type IV lupus nephritis resistant to conventional immunosuppressive therapies.

PROGNOSIS

Renal survival without the need for dialysis is seen in 80% of patients 10 years after the diagnosis of SLE nephritis. Patients with diffuse proliferative WHO class IV lupus nephritis exhibit the highest risk for progression to end-stage renal disease. Concerns regarding the side effects of chronic immunosuppressive therapy and the risk of recurrent disease are lifelong. Close monitoring for relapse of disease is imperative to ensure successful renal outcomes. Special care must be taken to minimize the risks of infection, osteoporosis, obesity, poor growth, hypertension, and diabetes mellitus associated with chronic steroid therapy. Patients require counseling regarding the risk of malignancy or infertility, which may be increased in those receiving a cumulative dose of >20 g of cyclophosphamide or other immunosuppressant therapies.

BIBLIOGRAPHY

Please visit the Nelson Textbook of Pediatrics *website at* *www.expertconsult.com* *for the complete bibliography.*

Chapter 509
Henoch-Schönlein Purpura Nephritis

Scott K. Van Why and Ellis D. Avner

Henoch-Schönlein purpura (HSP) is the most common small vessel vasculitis in childhood. It is characterized by a purpuric rash and commonly accompanied by arthritis and abdominal pain (Chapter 161.1). Approximately 50% of patients with HSP develop renal manifestations, which vary from asymptomatic microscopic hematuria to severe, progressive glomerulonephritis.

PATHOGENESIS AND PATHOLOGY

The pathogenesis of HSP nephritis appears to be mediated by the deposition of polymeric immunoglobulin A (IgA) in glomeruli. This is analogous to the same type of IgA deposits seen in systemic small vessels, primarily those of the skin and intestine. The glomerular findings can be indistinguishable from those of IgA nephropathy. IgA deposits are present by immunofluorescence, and a broad spectrum of glomerular lesions that can range from mild proliferation to necrotic and crescentic changes can be seen.

CLINICAL AND LABORATORY MANIFESTATIONS

The nephritis that can accompany HSP usually follows onset of the rash, often weeks or even months after the initial presentation of the disease. Nephritis can be manifest at initial presentation but only rarely before onset of the rash. Patients at presentation rarely display a severe combined acute nephritic and nephrotic picture (hematuria, hypertension, renal insufficiency, significant proteinuria, and nephrotic syndrome). Most patients have only mild renal manifestations, principally isolated microscopic hematuria without significant proteinuria. Initial mild renal involvement can progress to more severe nephritis despite resolution of all other features of HSP. The severity of the systemic manifestations does not correlate with the severity of the nephritis. Most patients who develop nephritis have urinary abnormalities by 1 month, and nearly all have abnormalities by 3 months after onset of HSP. Therefore, a urinalysis should be performed weekly in patients with HSP during the period of active clinical disease. Thereafter, a urinalysis should be performed once a month for up to 6 mo. If all urinalyses are normal, then nephritis is unlikely to develop. If proteinuria, renal insufficiency, or hypertension develops along with hematuria, consultation with a pediatric nephrologist is indicated.

PROGNOSIS AND TREATMENT

The prognosis of HSP nephritis for most patients is excellent. Spontaneous and complete resolution of the nephritis typically occurs in those with mild initial manifestations (isolated hematuria with insignificant proteinuria). However, such patients can progress to severe renal involvement, including development of chronic renal failure. Patients with acute nephritic or nephrotic syndrome at presentation have a guarded renal prognosis, especially if they are found to have concomitant necrosis or substantial crescentic changes on renal biopsy. Untreated, the risk of developing chronic kidney disease, including renal failure, is 2-5% in all patients with HSP but almost 50% in those with the most severe clinical and histologic features.

No studies have demonstrated whether short courses of oral corticosteroids administered promptly after onset of HSP have a significant favorable effect on the subsequent development or severity of subsequent HSP nephritis. Tonsillectomy has been proposed as an intervention for HSP nephritis, but it does not appear to have any measurable effect. Mild HSP nephritis does not require treatment because it usually resolves spontaneously.

Limited prospective controlled trials have been performed for severe HSP nephritis, and none have shown benefit from any therapy studied. Several uncontrolled studies have reported benefit from aggressive immunosuppression (high-dose and extended courses of corticosteroids with cyclophosphamide or azathioprine) in patients with poor prognostic features who might be expected to have a high risk of chronic renal failure. Aggressive therapy with careful monitoring may be reasonable in those with the most severe HSP nephritis (>50% crescents on biopsy).

BIBLIOGRAPHY

Please visit the Nelson Textbook of Pediatrics *website at* *www.expertconsult.com* *for the complete bibliography.*

Chapter 510
Rapidly Progressive (Crescentic) Glomerulonephritis

Scott K. Van Why and Ellis D. Avner

"Rapidly progressive" describes the clinical course of several forms of glomerulonephritis (RPGN) whose unifying feature is the histopathologic finding of crescents in the majority of glomeruli (Fig. 510-1). Therefore the terms *rapidly progressive glomerulonephritis* (RPGN) and *crescentic glomerulonephritis* (CGN) are synonymous. The natural history of most forms of CGN is rapid and relentless progression to end-stage renal failure.

CLASSIFICATION

CGN can be a severe manifestation of essentially every defined primary and secondary GN, but particular forms of GN are more likely to manifest as RPGN or evolve into CGN (Table 510-1). If no underlying cause is identified by systemic features, serologic testing, or histologic examination, the disease is classified as idiopathic CGN. The incidence of specific etiologies of CGN in children varies widely in reports from different centers; certain common themes are shared in all such reports. Patients with systemic vasculitis appear to be particularly prone to develop CGN. Patients with Henoch-Schönlein purpura (HSP), antineutrophil cytoplasmic antibody (ANCA)–mediated GN (microscopic polyangiitis and Wegener granulomatosis), and systemic lupus erythematosus (SLE) account for the majority of patients with CGN. Poststreptococcal GN rarely progresses to CGN, but because it is the most common form of GN in childhood it accounts for a significant percentage of patients with CGN in most reports. Membranoproliferative GN and idiopathic cases make up most of the remaining cases of CGN. Immunoglobulin (Ig)A nephropathy, a common GN, only rarely is rapidly progressive. Goodpasture

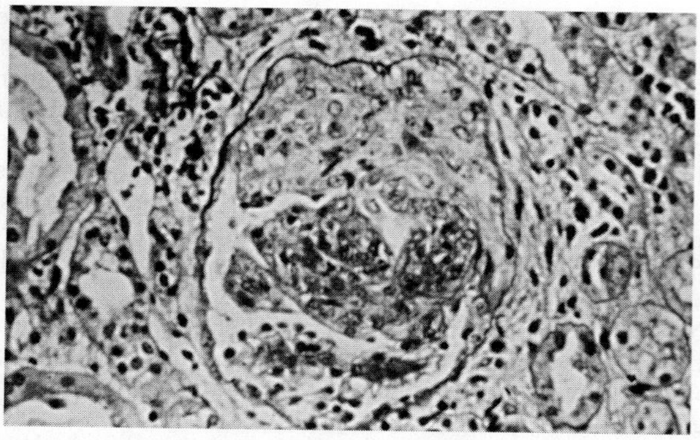

Figure 510-1 Light micrograph of a biopsy specimen from a child with Henoch-Schönlein purpura glomerulonephritis demonstrating a crescent overlying the glomerulus (×180).

Table 510-1 CLASSIFICATION OF RAPIDLY PROGRESSIVE (CRESCENTIC) GLOMERULONEPHRITIS

ANTI-GBM ANTIBODY-MEDIATED RPGN
Goodpasture syndrome Idiopathic anti-GBM nephritis Membranous nephropathy with crescents
RPGN ASSOCIATED WITH GRANULAR IMMUNE DEPOSITS
Postinfectious • Poststreptococcal glomerulonephritis • Bacterial endocarditis • Shunt nephritis • Visceral abscesses, other nonstreptococcal infections Noninfectious • Systemic lupus erythematosus • Henoch-Schönlein purpura • Mixed cryoglobulinemia • Solid tumors Primary renal disease • Membranoproliferative glomerulonephritis • IgA nephropathy • Idiopathic immune-complex nephritis
RPGN WITHOUT GLOMERULAR IMMUNE DEPOSITS
Vasculitis • Polyarteritis • Hypersensitivity vasculitis • Wegener granulomatosis Idiopathic RPGN

RPGN, rapidly progressive (crescentic) glomerulonephritis; GBM, glomerular basement membrane.

Modified from Kliegman RM, Greenbaum LA, Lye PS: *Practical strategies in pediatric diagnosis and therapy*, ed 2, Philadelphia, 2004, Saunders, p 426.

disease often has rapidly progressive GN as a component of the syndrome, but its rarity in childhood results in its making up only a small percentage of children with CGN.

PATHOLOGY AND PATHOGENESIS

The hallmark of CGN is the histopathologic finding of crescents in glomeruli (see Fig. 510-1). Crescent formation, through proliferation of parietal epithelial cells in Bowman's space, may be the final pathway of any severe inflammatory glomerular injury. Fibrin deposition and macrophage infiltration in the same areas suggest prominent involvement in the pathogenesis of the epithelial cell proliferation. Fibrous crescents, in which proliferative cellular crescents are replaced by collagen, are a late finding. The immunofluorescence findings, as well as the pattern of any deposits by electron microscopy (EM) can delineate the underlying glomerulopathy in CGN secondary to lupus, HSP nephritis, MPGN, postinfectious GN, IgA nephropathy or Goodpasture disease. Rare or absent findings by immunofluorescence and EM typify pauci-immune GN (Wegener disease and microscopic polyangiitis) and idiopathic crescentic GN.

CLINICAL MANIFESTATIONS

Most children present with acute nephritis (hematuria, some degree of renal insufficiency, and hypertension) and usually have concomitant proteinuria, often with nephrotic syndrome. Occasional patients present late in the course of disease with oliguric renal failure. Extrarenal manifestations, such as pulmonary involvement, joint symptoms, or skin lesions, can help lead to the diagnosis of the underlying systemic disease causing the CGN.

DIAGNOSIS AND DIFFERENTIAL DIAGNOSIS

The diagnosis of CGN is made by biopsy. Delineation of the underlying etiology is reached by a combination of additional biopsy findings (described earlier), extrarenal symptoms and signs, and serologic testing, including evaluation of antinuclear and anti-DNA antibodies, serum complement levels, and ANCA. If the patient has no extrarenal manifestations and a negative serologic evaluation, and if the biopsy has no immune or EM deposits, the diagnosis is idiopathic, rapidly progressive CGN.

PROGNOSIS AND TREATMENT

Although the outcome is not uniformly positive, children with rapidly progressive poststreptococcal GN and CGN can spontaneously recover. The natural course of the disease is far more severe in the setting of other etiologies, including the idiopathic category, and progression to end-stage renal failure within weeks to months from onset is common. Having a majority of fibrous crescents on the renal biopsy portends a poor prognosis, because the disease usually has progressed to irreversible injury. Although there are few controlled data, the consensus of most nephrologists is that the combination of high-dose corticosteroids and cyclophosphamide may be effective in preventing progressive renal failure in patients with SLE, HSP nephritis, Wegener granulomatosis, and IgA nephropathy if given early in the course when cellular crescents predominate. Although such therapy can also be effective in the other diseases causing RPGN, renal outcomes in those settings are less favorable. Progression to end-stage renal disease often occurs despite aggressive immunosuppressive therapy. In combination with immunosuppression, plasmapheresis has been reported to benefit patients with Goodpasture disease. However, the possible benefits of plasmapheresis in other forms of RPGN are unclear.

BIBLIOGRAPHY

Please visit the Nelson Textbook of Pediatrics *website at www.expertconsult.com for the complete bibliography.*

Chapter 511
Goodpasture Disease

Scott K. Van Why and Ellis D. Avner

Goodpasture disease is characterized by pulmonary hemorrhage and glomerulonephritis. The disease results from the attack of these normal organs by antibodies directed against specific epitopes of type IV collagen within the alveolar basement membrane in the lung and glomerular basement membrane (GBM) in the kidney. The etiology of these antibodies is unknown.

PATHOLOGY

Kidney biopsy shows crescentic glomerulonephritis in most patients. Immunofluorescence microscopy demonstrates continuous linear deposition of immunoglobulin G along the GBM (Fig. 511-1).

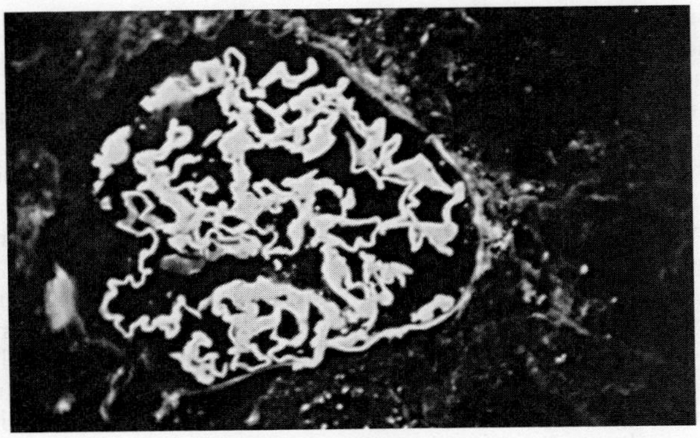

Figure 511-1 Immunofluorescence micrograph demonstrating the continuous linear staining of immunoglobulin G along the glomerular basement membrane in Goodpasture disease (×250).

CLINICAL MANIFESTATIONS

Goodpasture disease is rare in childhood. Patients usually present with hemoptysis from pulmonary hemorrhage that can be life-threatening. Concomitant renal manifestations include acute nephritic syndrome with hematuria, proteinuria, and hypertension, which usually follows a rapidly progressive course. Renal failure commonly develops within days to weeks of clinical presentation. Uncommonly, patients can have anti-GBM nephritis manifesting as isolated, rapidly progressive glomerulonephritis without pulmonary hemorrhage. In essentially all cases, serum anti-GBM antibody is present and complement C3 level is normal.

DIAGNOSIS AND DIFFERENTIAL DIAGNOSIS

The diagnosis is made by a combination of the clinical presentation of pulmonary hemorrhage with acute glomerulonephritis, the presence of serum antibodies directed against GBM (anti–type IV collagen in GBM), and characteristic renal biopsy findings. Other diseases that can cause a pulmonary-renal syndrome need to be considered and include systemic lupus erythematosus, Henoch-Schönlein purpura, Wegener granulomatosis, and microscopic polyangiitis. These diseases are ruled out by the absence of other characteristic clinical features, kidney biopsy findings, and negative serologic studies for antibodies against nuclear (ANA), DNA (A-DNase), and neutrophil cytoplasmic components (ANCA).

PROGNOSIS AND TREATMENT

Untreated, the prognosis of Goodpasture disease is poor. The combination of high-dose intravenous methylprednisolone, cyclophosphamide, and plasmapheresis appears to improve the possibility of survival. Nevertheless, patients who survive the pulmonary hemorrhage often progress to end-stage renal failure despite ongoing immunosuppressive therapy.

BIBLIOGRAPHY

Please visit the Nelson Textbook of Pediatrics *website at www.expertconsult.com for the complete bibliography.*

Chapter 512
Hemolytic-Uremic Syndrome

Scott K. Van Why and Ellis D. Avner

Hemolytic-uremic syndrome (HUS) is one of the most common causes of community-acquired acute kidney failure in young children. It is characterized by the triad of microangiopathic hemolytic anemia, thrombocytopenia, and renal insufficiency (Table 512-1). HUS has clinical features in common with thrombotic thrombocytopenic purpura (TTP). The etiology and pathophysiology of the more common forms of HUS clearly delineate childhood HUS as separate from idiopathic TTP.

Table 512-1 DEFINITION OF POSTDIARRHEAL HEMOLYTIC UREMIC SYNDROME: CENTERS FOR DISEASE CONTROL AND PREVENTION, 1996

CLINICAL DESCRIPTION
Hemolytic uremic syndrome (HUS) is characterized by the acute onset of microangiopathic hemolytic anemia, renal injury, and a low platelet count. Thrombotic thrombocytopenic purpura (TTP) also is characterized by these features but can include central nervous system (CNS) involvement and fever and can have a more gradual onset. Most cases of HUS (but few cases of TTP) occur after an acute gastrointestinal illness (usually diarrheal).
LABORATORY CRITERIA FOR DIAGNOSIS
The following are both present at some time during the illness: • Anemia (acute onset) with microangiopathic changes (i.e., schistocytes, burr cells, or helmet cells) on peripheral blood smear and • Renal injury (acute onset) evidenced by hematuria, proteinuria, or elevated creatinine level: ≥1.0 mg/dL in a child <13 yr or ≥1.5 mg/dL in a patient 13 yr or older or ≥50% increase over baseline. *Note:* A low platelet count can usually, but not always, be detected early in the illness, but it can then become normal or even high. If a platelet count obtained within 7 days after onset of the acute gastrointestinal illness is not <150,000/mm³, other diagnoses should be considered.
CASE CLASSIFICATION
Probable
• An acute illness diagnosed as HUS or TTP that meets the laboratory criteria in a patient who does not have a clear history of acute or bloody diarrhea in the preceding 3 wk, or • An acute illness diagnosed as HUS or TTP that (a) has onset within 3 wk after onset of an acute or bloody diarrhea and (b) meets the laboratory criteria except that microangiopathic changes are not confirmed.
Confirmed
• An acute illness diagnosed as HUS or TTP that both meets the laboratory criteria and began within 3 wk after onset of an episode of acute or bloody diarrhea
COMMENT
Some investigators consider HUS and TTP to be part of a continuum of disease. Therefore, criteria for diagnosing TTP on the basis of CNS involvement and fever are not provided because cases diagnosed clinically as postdiarrheal TTP also should meet the criteria for HUS. These cases are reported as postdiarrheal HUS.

From Elliott EJ, Robins-Browne RM: Hemolytic uremic syndrome, *Curr Probl Pediatr Adolesc Health Care* 35:305–344, 2005.

ETIOLOGY

The various etiologies of HUS allow classification into infection-induced, genetic, medication- induced, and HUS associated with systemic diseases characterized by microvascular injury (Tables 512-2 and 512-3). The most common form of HUS is caused by toxin-producing *Escherichia coli* that cause prodromal acute enteritis and is commonly termed *diarrhea-associated HUS*. In the subcontinent of Asia and southern Africa, the shiga toxin of *Shigella dysenteriae* type 1 is causative, whereas in Western countries verotoxin-producing *E. coli* (VTEC) are the usual causes.

Several serotypes of *E. coli* can produce verotoxin, and the O157:H7 type is most common in Europe and the Americas. The reservoir of VTEC is the intestinal tract of domestic animals, usually cows. Disease is usually transmitted by undercooked meat or unpasteurized milk or apple cider. Epidemics have followed ingestion of undercooked, contaminated hamburger at fast food restaurants. HUS outbreaks have also been associated with municipal water supply; petting farms; swimming in contaminated ponds, lakes, or pools; and consuming cheese, lettuce, or raw spinach contaminated with toxin (often by contact with meat on an unwashed cutting board). Less often, HUS has been spread by person-to-person contact within families or child care centers. A rare but distinct entity of infection-triggered HUS is related to neuraminidase-producing *Streptococcus pneumoniae*. HUS develops during acute infection with this organism, typically manifesting as pneumonia with empyema. A thrombotic microangiopathy, similar to HUS or TTP, also occurs in patients with untreated HIV infection.

Genetic forms of HUS compose the second major category of the disease that has become clearly defined (see Tables 512-2, 512-3). Inherited deficiencies of either von Willebrand factor–cleaving protease (ADAMTS 13) or complement factor H, I, or B and defects in vitamin B_{12} metabolism can cause HUS. There remain familial cases transmitted in autosomal dominant or recessive patterns in which a specific genetic defect has not yet been identified. Most of the genetic forms do not have a preceding diarrhea prodrome. Genetic forms of HUS can be indolent and unremitting once they become manifest, or they can have a relapsing pattern precipitated by an infectious illness. The latter feature likely explains the association of many infectious agents with HUS, particularly in reports published before the recognition of the unique pathophysiology of VTEC and neuraminidase- producing pneumococci in causing HUS.

HUS can be superimposed on any disease associated with microvascular injury, including malignant hypertension, systemic lupus erythematosus, and antiphospholipid syndrome. It can also occur following bone marrow or solid organ transplantation and may be triggered by the use of the calcineurin inhibitors cyclosporine and tacrolimus in that setting. Several other medications can also induce HUS (see Table 512-2).

Table 512-2 CLASSIFICATION OF HEMOLYTIC UREMIC SYNDROME

INFECTION INDUCED
Verotoxin-producing *Escherichia coli*
Shiga toxin-producing *Shigella dysentereriae* type 1
Neuraminidase-producing *Streptococcus pneumoniae*
Human immunodeficiency virus
GENETIC
von Willebrand factor-cleaving protease (ADAMTS 13) deficiency
Complement factor H (or related proteins) deficiency or mutation
Membrane cofactor protein (MCP) mutations
Thrombomodulin mutations
Complement factor I mutations
Vitamin B_{12} metabolism defects
Familial autosomal recessive of undefined etiology
Familial autosomal dominant of undefined etiology
Sporadic, recurrent, undefined etiology without diarrhea prodrome
OTHER DISEASES ASSOCIATED WITH MICROVASCULAR INJURY
Systemic lupus erythematosus
Antiphospholipid antibody syndrome
Following bone marrow transplantation
Malignant hypertension
Primary glomerulopathy
HELLP (*h*emolytic anemia, *e*levated *l*iver enzymes, *l*ow *p*latelet count) syndrome
MEDICATION-INDUCED
Calcineurin inhibitors (cyclosporine, tacrolimus)
Cytotoxic, chemotherapy agents (mitomycin C, cisplatin, gemcitabine)
Clopidogrel and ticlopidine
Quinine

PATHOLOGY

Kidney biopsies are only rarely performed in HUS because the diagnosis is made by clinical criteria. The risks of biopsy are significant during the active phase of the disease. Early glomerular changes include thickening of the capillary walls caused by swelling of endothelial cells and accumulation of fibrillar material between endothelial cells and underlying basement membrane, causing narrowing of the capillary lumens. Platelet-fibrin thrombi are often seen in glomerular capillaries. Thrombi are also seen in afferent arterioles and small arteries with fibrinoid necrosis of the arterial wall, leading to renal cortical necrosis from vascular occlusion. Late findings include glomerular sclerosis and obsolescence secondary to either severe direct glomerular involvement or glomerular ischemia from arteriolar involvement.

PATHOGENESIS

Microvascular injury with endothelial cell damage is characteristic of all forms of HUS. In the common, diarrhea-associated form of HUS, enteropathic organisms produce either Shiga toxin or the highly homologous Shiga-like verotoxin that directly cause endothelial cell damage. Shiga toxin can directly activate platelets to promote their aggregation. In pneumococcal-associated HUS, neuraminidase cleaves sialic acid on membranes of endothelial cells, red cells, and platelets to reveal the underlying cryptic

Table 512-3 GENETIC ABNORMALITIES AND CLINICAL OUTCOME IN PATIENTS WITH ATYPICAL HEMOLYTIC-UREMIC SYNDROME

GENE	PROTEIN AFFECTED	MAIN EFFECT	FREQUENCY (%)	RESPONSE TO SHORT-TERM PLASMA THERAPY*	LONG-TERM OUTCOME†	OUTCOME OF KIDNEY TRANSPLANTATION
CFH	Factor H	No binding to endothelium	20-30	Rate of remission: 60% (dose and timing dependent)	Rate of death or ESRD: 70-80%	Rate of recurrence: 80-90%‡
CFHR1/3	Factor HR1, R3	Anti-factor H antibodies	6	Rate of remission 70-80% (plasma exchange combined with immunosuppression)	Rate of ESRD: 30-40%	Rate of recurrence: 20%§
MCP	Membrane cofactor protein	No surface expression	10-15	No definitive indication for therapy	Rate of death or ESRD: <20%	Rate of recurrence: 15-20%§
CF1	Factor 1	Low level or low co-factor activity	4-10	Rate of remission: 30-40%	Rate of death or ESRD: 60-70%	Rate of recurrence: 70-80%‡
CFB	Factor B	C3 convertase stabilization	1-2	Rate of remission: 30%	Rate of death or ESRD: 70%	Recurrence in one case
C3	Complement C3	Resistance to C3b inactivation	5-10	Rate of remission: 40-50%	Rate of death or ESRD: 60%	Rate of recurrence: 40-50%
THBD	Thrombomodulin	Reduced C3b inactivation	5	Rate of remission: 60%	Rate of death or ESRD: 60%	Recurrence in 1 patient

ESRD, end-stage renal disease.
*Remission was defined as either complete remission or partial remission (i.e., hematologic remission with renal sequelae).
†The long-term outcome was defined as the outcome 5-10 yr after onset.
‡Patients in this category were eligible for combined liver and kidney transplantation.
§Patients in this category were eligible for single kidney transplantation.
From Norris M, Remuzzi G: Atypical hemolytic-uremic syndrome, *N Engl J Med* 361:1676–1687, 2009.

Thomsen-Friedenreich (T) antigen. Endogenous immunoglobulin M (IgM) recognizes the T antigen and triggers the microvascular angiopathy.

The familial recessive and dominant forms of HUS and the inherited deficiencies of ADAMTS 13 (usually TTP) and complement factor H probably predispose patients to developing HUS but do not cause the disease per se, because these patients might not develop HUS until later childhood or even adulthood. In such cases, HUS is often triggered by an inciting event such as an infectious disease. The absence of ADAMTS 13 impairs cleavage of von Willebrand factor multimers, which enhances platelet aggregation. Factor H plays a central role in complement regulation, primarily arresting amplification and propagation of complement activation. It may be that mild endothelial injury that would normally resolve instead evolves to an aggressive microangiopathy because of the inherited deficiencies of these factors.

In each form of HUS, capillary and arteriolar endothelial injury in the kidney leads to localized thrombosis, particularly in glomeruli, causing a direct decrease in glomerular filtration rate. Progressive platelet aggregation in the areas of microvascular injury results in consumptive thrombocytopenia. Microangiopathic hemolytic anemia results from mechanical damage to red blood cells as they pass through the damaged and thrombotic microvasculature.

CLINICAL MANIFESTATIONS

HUS is most common in preschool and school-aged children, but it can occur in adolescents. In HUS caused by exotoxin-producing *E. coli*, onset of HUS occurs a few days (as few as 3) after onset of gastroenteritis with fever, vomiting, abdominal pain, and diarrhea. The prodromal intestinal symptoms may be severe and require hospitalization, but they can be relatively mild and considered trivial. The diarrhea is often bloody, but not necessarily so, especially early in the illness. Following the prodromal illness, the sudden onset of pallor, irritability, weakness, and lethargy herald the onset of HUS. Oliguria can be present in early stages but may be masked by ongoing diarrhea because the prodromal enteritis often overlaps the onset of HUS. Thus, patients can present with HUS either with significant dehydration or volume overload, depending on whether the enteritis or renal insufficiency from HUS predominates and the amount of fluid that was administered.

Patients with pneumococcus-associated HUS usually are ill with pneumonia and empyema when they develop HUS. Onset can be insidious in patients with the genetic forms of HUS, with HUS triggered by a variety of illnesses, including mild, nonspecific gastroenteritis or respiratory tract infections.

HUS can be relatively mild or can progress to a severe, and even fatal, multisystem disease. Leukocytosis and severe prodromal enteritis portend a severe course, but no presenting features reliably predict the severity of HUS in any given patient. Patients with HUS who appear mildly affected at presentation can rapidly develop severe, multisystem, life-threatening complications. Renal insufficiency can be mild but also can rapidly evolve into severe oliguric or anuric renal failure. The combination of rapidly developing renal failure and severe hemolysis can result in life-threatening hyperkalemia. Volume overload, hypertension, and severe anemia can all develop soon after onset and together can precipitate heart failure. Direct cardiac involvement is rare, but pericarditis, myocardial dysfunction, or arrhythmias can occur without predisposing features of hypertension, volume overload, or electrolyte abnormalities.

The majority of patients with HUS have some central nervous system (CNS) involvement. Most have mild manifestations, with significant irritability, lethargy, and nonspecific encephalopathic features. Severe CNS involvement occurs in ≤20% of cases. Seizures and significant encephalopathy are the most common manifestations in those with severe CNS involvement and result from focal ischemia secondary to microvascular CNS thrombosis. Small infarctions in the basal ganglion and cerebral cortex have also been reported, but large strokes and intracranial hemorrhage are rare. Intestinal complications can be protean and include severe inflammatory colitis, ischemic enteritis, bowel perforation, intussusception, and pancreatitis. Patients can develop petechiae, but significant or severe bleeding is rare despite very low platelet counts.

DIAGNOSIS AND DIFFERENTIAL DIAGNOSIS

The diagnosis is made by the combination of microangiopathic hemolytic anemia with schistocytes, thrombocytopenia, and some degree of kidney involvement (see Table 512-1). The anemia, mild at presentation, rapidly progresses. Thrombocytopenia is an invariable finding in the acute phase, with platelet counts usually 20,000-100,000/mm^3. Partial thromboplastin and prothrombin times are usually normal. The Coombs test is negative, with the exception of pneumococci-induced HUS, where the Coombs test is usually positive. Leukocytosis is present and significant. Urinalysis typically shows microscopic hematuria and low-grade proteinuria. The renal insufficiency can vary from mild elevations in serum BUN and creatinine to acute, anuric kidney failure.

The etiology of HUS is often clear with the presence of a diarrheal prodrome or pneumococcal infection. The presence or absence of toxigenic, enteropathic organisms on stool culture has little role in making the diagnosis of diarrhea-associated, enteropathic HUS. Only a minority of patients infected with those organisms develops HUS, and the organisms that cause HUS may be rapidly cleared. Therefore the stool culture is often negative in patients who have diarrhea-associated HUS. If no history of diarrheal prodrome or pneumococcal infection is obtained, then evaluation for the genetic forms of HUS should be considered, because those patients are at risk for recurrence, have a severe prognosis, and can require different therapies.

Other causes of acute kidney failure associated with a microangiopathic hemolytic anemia and thrombocytopenia, such as systemic lupus erythematosus, malignant hypertension, and bilateral renal vein thrombosis, should be considered and excluded. A kidney biopsy is rarely indicated.

PROGNOSIS AND TREATMENT

The acute prognosis, with careful supportive care, for diarrhea-associated HUS has <5% mortality in most major medical centers. Half of the patients require dialysis support during the acute phase of the disease. Most recover renal function completely, but of surviving patients, 5% remain dependent on dialysis, and up to 20-30% are left with some level of chronic renal insufficiency. The prognosis for HUS not associated with diarrhea is more severe. Pneumococci-associated HUS causes increased patient morbidity, with mortality reported as 20%. The familial, genetic forms of HUS can be insidiously progressive or relapsing diseases and have a poor prognosis (see Table 512-3). Identification of specific factor deficiencies in some of these genetic forms provides opportunity for specific replacement therapy to improve outcomes.

The primary approach that has substantially improved acute outcome in HUS is early recognition of the disease, monitoring for potential complications, and meticulous supportive care. Supportive care includes careful management of fluid and electrolytes including correction of volume deficit, control of hypertension, and early institution of dialysis if the patient becomes anuric or significantly oliguric. Red cell transfusions are usually required because hemolysis can be brisk and recurrent until the active phase of the disease has resolved. In pneumococci-associated HUS, it is recommended that **any administered red cells be washed** before transfusion to remove residual plasma, because endogenous IgM directed against the revealed T antigen can play a pathogenic role. Platelets should generally not be administered, regardless of platelet count, to patients with HUS because they are almost immediately consumed by the active coagulation and can theoretically worsen the clinical course. Despite low platelet counts, serious bleeding is very rare in patients with HUS.

There is no evidence that any therapy directed at arresting the disease process of the most common, diarrhea-associated form of HUS provide benefit, and some can cause harm. Attempts have been made using anticoagulants, antiplatelets agents, fibrinolytic therapy, plasma therapy, immune globulin, and antibiotics. Anticoagulation, antiplatelet, and fibrinolytic therapy is specifically contraindicated because they increase the risk of serious hemorrhage. Antibiotic therapy to clear the toxigenic organisms can result in increased toxin release, potentially exacerbating the disease, and therefore is not recommended. Prompt treatment of any underlying pneumococcal infection is important. Attempts to bind Vero or Shiga toxin in the gut to prevent systemic absorption, and thereby prevent or ameliorate the course of HUS, have been unsuccessful in extensive controlled clinical trials.

Plasma infusion or plasmapheresis has been proposed for patients suffering severe manifestations of HUS, primarily serious CNS involvement. There are no controlled data demonstrating the effectiveness of this approach. Plasma therapy can be of substantial benefit to patients with identified deficits of ADAMTS 13 or factor H. It may also be considered in patients with other genetic forms of HUS, such as undefined familial (recessive or dominant) or sporadic but recurrent HUS.

Most patients with diarrhea-associated acquired forms of HUS recover completely with little risk of long-term sequelae. However, patients with hypertension, any level of renal insufficiency, or residual urinary abnormalities persisting a year after an episode of diarrhea-positive HUS require careful follow-up. Patients who have recovered completely, with no residual urinary abnormalities after a year, are unlikely to manifest long-term sequelae. Because of occasional reports of late sequelae in such patients, annual examinations with a primary physician are still warranted.

BIBLIOGRAPHY

Please visit the Nelson Textbook of Pediatrics *website at* *www.expertconsult.com* *for the complete bibliography.*

Chapter 513
Upper Urinary Tract Causes of Hematuria

513.1 Interstitial Nephritis

See Chapter 526.

513.2 Toxic Nephropathy

See Chapter 527.

513.3 Cortical Necrosis

See Chapter 528.

513.4 Pyelonephritis

See Chapter 532.

513.5 Nephrocalcinosis

See Chapter 541.

513.6 Vascular Abnormalities

Craig C. Porter and Ellis D. Avner

Hemangiomas, hemangiolymphangiomas, angiomyomas, and arteriovenous malformations of the kidneys and lower urinary tract are rare causes of hematuria. They can manifest with microscopic hematuria or gross hematuria with clots. Cutaneous vascular malformations, when present, can offer a clue to these underlying causes of hematuria. Renal colic can develop if the upper tract is involved. The diagnosis may be confirmed by angiography or endoscopy.

Unilateral bleeding of varicose veins of the left ureter, resulting from compression of the left renal vein between the aorta and superior mesenteric artery (mesoaortic compression), is referred to as the **nutcracker syndrome.** Patients with this syndrome typically present with persistent microscopic hematuria (occasionally, recurrent gross hematuria) that may be accompanied by proteinuria, lower abdominal pain, flank pain, or orthostatic hypotension. Diagnosis is confirmed by Doppler ultrasonography, CT, phlebography of the left renal vein, or magnetic resonance angiography.

BIBLIOGRAPHY

Please visit the Nelson Textbook of Pediatrics *website at* *www.expertconsult.com* *for the complete bibliography.*

513.7 Renal Vein Thrombosis

Craig C. Porter and Ellis D. Avner

EPIDEMIOLOGY

Renal vein thrombosis (RVT) occurs in 2 distinct clinical situations. In newborns and infants, RVT is commonly associated with asphyxia, dehydration, shock, sepsis, congenital hypercoagulable states, and maternal diabetes. In older children, RVT is seen in patients with nephrotic syndrome, cyanotic heart disease, inherited hypercoagulable states, and sepsis and following kidney transplantation and following exposure to angiographic contrast agents.

PATHOGENESIS

RVT begins in the intrarenal venous circulation and can spread to the main renal vein and inferior vena cava. Thrombus formation is mediated by endothelial cell injury resulting from hypoxia, endotoxin, or contrast media. Other contributing factors include hypercoagulability from either nephrotic syndrome or mutations in genes that encode clotting factors (i.e., factor V Leiden deficiency); hypovolemia and diminished vascular blood flow associated with septic shock, dehydration, or nephrotic syndrome; and intravascular sludging caused by polycythemia.

CLINICAL MANIFESTATIONS

The development of RVT is usually heralded by the sudden onset of gross hematuria and unilateral or bilateral flank masses. Patients can also present with microscopic hematuria, flank pain, hypertension, or oliguria. RVT is usually unilateral. Bilateral RVT results in acute kidney failure.

DIAGNOSIS

The diagnosis of RVT is suggested by the development of hematuria and flank masses in a patient with predisposing clinical factors. Patients can also have a microangiopathic hemolytic anemia and thrombocytopenia. Ultrasonography shows marked enlargement, and radionuclide studies reveal little or no renal function in the affected kidney(s). Doppler flow studies of the inferior vena cava and renal vein confirm the diagnosis. Contrast studies should be avoided to minimize the risk of further vascular damage.

DIFFERENTIAL DIAGNOSIS

The differential diagnosis of RVT includes other causes of hematuria that are associated with microangiopathic hemolytic anemia or enlargement of the kidneys. These include hemolytic-uremic syndrome, hydronephrosis, polycystic kidney disease, Wilms tumor, abscess, or hematoma. All patients should be evaluated for congenital and acquired hypercoagulable states.

TREATMENT

The primary treatment of RVT consists of supportive care, including correction of fluid and electrolyte imbalance and treatment of renal insufficiency. Treatment with anticoagulation (heparin) or thrombolytic agents including streptokinase, urokinase, or recombinant tissue plasminogen activator is common but remains controversial. Patients with thrombosis of the inferior vena cava can require surgical thrombectomy. Children with severe hypertension refractory to antihypertensive medications can require nephrectomy.

PROGNOSIS

Perinatal mortality from RVT has decreased significantly over the past 20 yr. Partial or complete renal atrophy is a common sequela of RVT in the neonate, leading to renal insufficiency, renal tubular dysfunction, and systemic hypertension. These complications are also seen in older children, although recovery of renal function is common in children with RVT resulting from nephrotic syndrome or cyanotic heart disease with correction of the underlying etiology.

BIBLIOGRAPHY
Please visit the Nelson Textbook of Pediatrics *website at www.expertconsult.com for the complete bibliography.*

513.8 Idiopathic Hypercalciuria

Craig C. Porter and Ellis D. Avner

Idiopathic hypercalciuria, which may be inherited as an autosomal dominant disorder, can manifest as recurrent gross hematuria, persistent microscopic hematuria, dysuria, or abdominal pain in the absence of stone formation. Hypercalciuria can also accompany conditions resulting in hypercalcemia, such as hyperparathyroidism, vitamin D intoxication, immobilization, and sarcoidosis. Hypercalciuria may be associated with Cushing syndrome, corticosteroid therapy, tubular dysfunction secondary to Fanconi syndrome (Wilson disease, oculocerebrorenal syndrome), Williams syndrome, distal renal tubular acidosis, or Bartter syndrome. Hypercalciuria may also be seen in patients with **Dent disease,** which is an X-linked form of nephrolithiasis associated with hypophosphatemic rickets. Although microcrystal formation and consequent tissue irritation are believed to mediate symptoms, the precise mechanism by which hypercalciuria causes hematuria or dysuria is unknown.

DIAGNOSIS

Hypercalciuria is diagnosed by a 24-hr urinary calcium excretion >4 mg/kg. A screening test for hypercalciuria in patients who cannot collect a timed urine specimen may be performed on a random urine specimen by measuring the calcium and creatinine concentrations. A spot urine calcium:creatinine ratio (mg/dL:mg/dL) >0.2 suggests hypercalciuria in an older child. Normal ratios may be as high as 0.8 in infants <7 mo of age.

TREATMENT

Left untreated, hypercalciuria leads to nephrolithiasis in approximately 15% of cases. Idiopathic hypercalciuria has been identified as a risk factor in 40% of children with kidney stones, and low urinary citrate level has been associated as a risk factor in approximately 38% of this group. Oral thiazide diuretics can normalize urinary calcium excretion by stimulating calcium reabsorption in the proximal and distal tubule. Such therapy can lead to resolution of gross hematuria or dysuria and can prevent nephrolithiasis. The precise indications for thiazide treatment remain controversial.

In patients with persistent gross hematuria or dysuria, therapy is initiated with hydrochlorothiazide at a dose of 1-2 mg/kg/24 hr as a single morning dose. The dose is titrated upward until the 24-hr urinary calcium excretion is <4 mg/kg and clinical manifestations resolve. After 1 yr of treatment, hydrochlorothiazide is usually discontinued but may be resumed if gross hematuria, nephrolithiasis, or dysuria recurs. During hydrochlorothiazide therapy, the serum potassium level should be monitored periodically to avoid hypokalemia. **Potassium citrate** at a dose of 1 mEq/kg/24 hr may also be beneficial, particularly in patients with low urinary citrate excretion and symptomatic dysuria.

Sodium restriction is important because calcium excretion parallels sodium excretion. Importantly, *dietary calcium restriction is not recommended* (except in children with massive calcium intake >250% of RDA by dietary history) because calcium is a critical requirement for growth and no evidence supports a relationship between decreased calcium intake and decreased urinary calcium levels. Reduced bone mineral density with evidence of bone resorption has been described in patients with hypercalciuria. In such patients, dietary calcium restriction is particularly contraindicated. Small-scale studies seem to support a role for bisphosphonate therapy, which leads to a reduction in urinary calcium excretion and improvement in bone mineral density. Controlled studies are necessary to establish a clear role for such therapy.

BIBLIOGRAPHY
Please visit the Nelson Textbook of Pediatrics *website at www.expertconsult.com for the complete bibliography.*

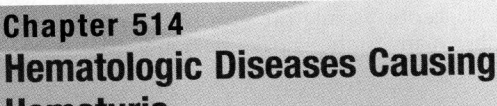

Chapter 514 Hematologic Diseases Causing Hematuria

514.1 Sickle Cell Nephropathy

Craig C. Porter and Ellis D. Avner

Gross or microscopic hematuria may be seen in children with sickle cell disease or sickle trait and tends to resolve spontaneously in the majority of children (Chapter 456.1). With the exception of the associated renal cell carcinoma, clinically apparent renal involvement occurs more commonly in patients with sickle cell disease than those with sickle cell trait.

ETIOLOGY

The renal manifestations of sickle cell nephropathy are generally related to microthrombosis secondary to sickling in the relatively hypoxic, acidic, hypertonic renal medulla where vascular stasis is present. Analgesic use, volume depletion with consequent prerenal failure, infectious complications, and iron-related hepatic disease are independent contributing factors.

PATHOLOGY

Ischemia, papillary necrosis, and interstitial fibrosis are present in the kidneys of these patients.

CLINICAL MANIFESTATIONS

Clinical manifestations of sickle cell nephropathy include polyuria caused by a urinary concentrating defect, renal tubular acidosis, and proteinuria associated with glomerular lesions resembling focal segmental glomerulosclerosis or membranoproliferative glomerulonephritis.

Approximately 20-30% of patients with sickle cell disease develop proteinuria. Nephrotic range proteinuria with or without clinically apparent nephrotic syndrome occurs less commonly and is often associated with progressive renal failure.

TREATMENT

Angiotensin-converting enzyme inhibitors, such as enalapril, can be used to achieve a significant reduction in urine protein excretion in patients with daily urine protein excretion exceeding 500 mg. Hydroxyurea can also be beneficial in reducing urinary protein excretion.

PROGNOSIS

Sickle cell nephropathy can eventually lead to hypertension, renal insufficiency, and progressive kidney failure. Dialysis and eventual kidney transplantation are successful treatment modalities when kidney failure is irreversible.

BIBLIOGRAPHY

Please visit the Nelson Textbook of Pediatrics *website at* *www.expertconsult.com* *for the complete bibliography.*

514.2 Coagulopathies and Thrombocytopenia

Craig C. Porter and Ellis D. Avner

Gross or microscopic hematuria may be associated with inherited or acquired disorders of coagulation (hemophilia, disseminated intravascular coagulation, thrombocytopenia). In these cases, however, hematuria is not usually the presenting complaint but develops after other manifestations (Chapters 469-478).

Chapter 515 Anatomic Abnormalities Associated with Hematuria

515.1 Congenital Anomalies

Craig C. Porter and Ellis D. Avner

Gross or microscopic hematuria may be associated with many types of different malformations of the urinary tract. The sudden onset of gross hematuria after minor trauma to the flank is often associated with ureteropelvic junction obstruction or cystic kidneys (see Chapter 531).

515.2 Autosomal Recessive Polycystic Kidney Disease

Craig C. Porter and Ellis D. Avner

Also known as **infantile polycystic disease,** autosomal recessive polycystic kidney disease (ARPKD) is an autosomal recessive disorder occurring with an incidence of 1:10,000 to 1:40,000. The gene for ARPKD *(PKHD1)* encodes fibrocystin, a large protein (>4,000 amino acids) with multiple isoforms.

PATHOLOGY

Both kidneys are markedly enlarged and grossly show innumerable cysts throughout the cortex and medulla. Microscopic studies demonstrate dilated, ectatic collecting ducts radiating from the medulla to the cortex, although transient proximal tubule cysts have been reported in the fetus. Development of progressive interstitial fibrosis and tubular atrophy during advanced stages of disease eventually leads to renal failure. Liver involvement is characterized by a basic ductal plate abnormality that leads to bile duct proliferation and ectasia, as well as hepatic fibrosis. This lesion is indistinguishable from congenital hepatic fibrosis or Caroli disease, and consequently ARPKD is increasingly referred to as ARPKD/CHF.

PATHOGENESIS

The function of fibrocystin in normal kidney development and the pathophysiology of its abnormal expression in ARPKD are largely unknown. Evolving information suggests that fibrocystin forms a multimeric complex with proteins of other primary genetic cystic diseases. It appears that altered intracellular signaling from these complexes, located at the apical cell surface, intercellular junction, and basolateral cell surface in association with the focal adhesion complex is a critical feature of disease pathophysiology.

Multiple mutations of *PKHD1* cause disease and their average detection rate is approximately 85%. Limited available information suggests some genotype-phenotype correlation: mutations that modify fibrocystin appear to cause less-severe disease than those that truncate fibrocystin.

CLINICAL MANIFESTATIONS

The typical child presents with bilateral flank masses during the neonatal period or early infancy. ARPKD may be associated with oligohydramnios, pulmonary hypoplasia, respiratory distress, and spontaneous pneumothorax in the neonatal period. Perinatal demise appears associated with truncating mutations. Components of the oligohydramnios complex including low-set ears, micrognathia, flattened nose, limb-positioning defects, and growth deficiency may be present. Hypertension is usually noted within the first few weeks of life and is often severe and difficult to control. Oliguria and acute renal failure are uncommonly seen, but transient hyponatremia, often in the presence of acute renal failure, often responds to diuresis. Renal function is usually impaired but may be initially normal in 20-30% of patients. Infrequently, ARPKD manifests beyond infancy, in young infants with a mixed clinical picture of renal and hepatic findings: variable degrees of portal hypertension (hepatosplenomegaly, gastroesophageal varices, prominent cutaneous periumbilical veins, reversal of portal vein flow, thrombocytopenia) and variable renal findings that range from asymptomatic abnormal

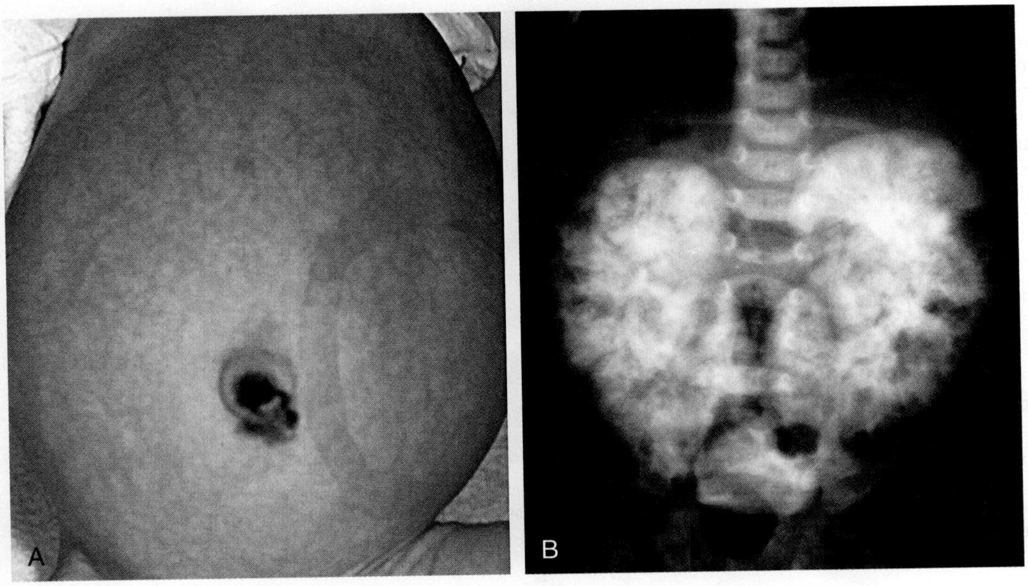

Figure 515-1 *A,* This infant with infantile polycystic kidney disease shows marked abdominal distention and bilaterally enlarged kidneys, as indicated by the *outlined area. B,* Intravenous pyelogram of the same patient shows the characteristic mottled nephrogram with brushlike medullary opacification secondary to retention of contrast material in dilated cortical and medullary collecting ducts. (From Zitelli BJ, Davis HW, editors: *Atlas of pediatric physical diagnosis,* ed 4, St Louis, 2002, Mosby, p 470.)

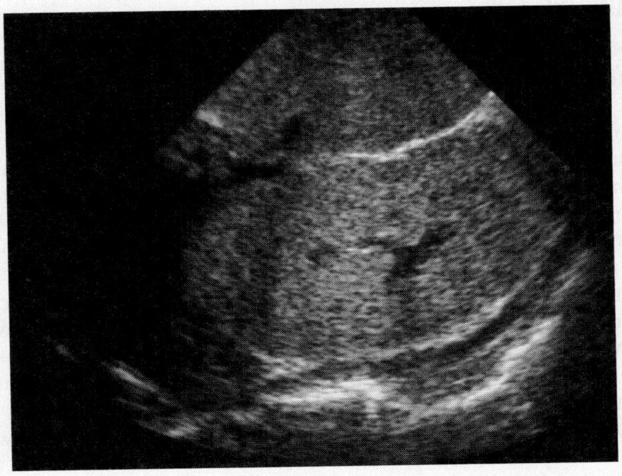

Figure 515-2 Ultrasound examination of a neonate with autosomal recessive polycystic kidney disease demonstrating renal enlargement (9 cm) and increased diffuse echogenicity with complete loss of corticomedullary differentiation resulting from multiple small cystic interfaces.

renal ultrasonography to systemic hypertension and renal insufficiency.

In the newborn, clinical evidence of liver disease by radiologic or clinical laboratory assessment is present in about 45% of children. It is believed to be universal by microscopic evaluation. Patients with ARPKD are at risk for developing ascending cholangitis, varices, and hypersplenism related to portal hypertension; they are also at risk for progressive liver fibrosis, which uncommonly leads to overt liver failure and cirrhosis. A subset of older children, and even young adults with ARPKD, present with prominent hepatosplenomegaly and display mild renal disease that is discovered incidentally during imaging studies of the abdomen.

DIAGNOSIS

The diagnosis of ARPKD is strongly suggested by bilateral palpable flank masses in an infant with pulmonary hypoplasia, oligohydramnios, and hypertension and the absence of renal cysts by sonography of the parents (Fig. 515-1). Markedly enlarged and uniformly hyperechogenic kidneys with poor corticomedullary differentiation are commonly seen on ultrasonography (Fig. 515-2). The diagnosis is supported by clinical and laboratory signs of hepatic fibrosis, pathologic findings of ductal plate abnormalities seen on liver biopsy, anatomic and pathologic proof of ARPKD in a sibling, or parental consanguinity. The differential diagnosis includes other causes of bilateral renal enlargement and/or cysts, such as multicystic dysplasia, hydronephrosis, Wilms tumor, and bilateral renal vein thrombosis (Table 515-1). Prenatal diagnostic testing using genetic linkage analysis or direct mutation analysis is available in families with ≥1 affected child.

Table 515-1 RENAL CYSTIC DISORDERS

Autosomal recessive polycystic kidney disease
Autosomal dominant polycystic kidney disease
Hereditary cystic disease with interstitial nephritis
Cerebello-ocular-renal syndromes
Cystic dysplastic kidneys
Joubert syndrome
Juvenile nephronophthisis
Meckel-Gruber syndrome
Autosomal dominant hereditary angiopathy with nephropathy
VATER syndrome
Trisomy 21, 18, 13
Tuberous sclerosis
von Hippel-Lindau syndrome
Orofacial digital syndrome
Bardet-Biedel syndrome
Simple benign cysts

TREATMENT

The treatment of ARPKD is supportive. Aggressive ventilatory support is often necessary in the neonatal period secondary to pulmonary hypoplasia, hypoventilation, and the many respiratory illnesses of prematurity (which are common). Careful management of hypertension, fluid and electrolyte abnormalities, and clinical manifestations of renal insufficiency is essential. Children with severe respiratory failure or feeding intolerance from enlarged kidneys can require unilateral or bilateral nephrectomies, prompting the need for renal replacement therapy. In families with a previous affected child, preimplantation genetic diagnosis coupled with in vitro fertilization is available in specialized centers and can lead to the birth of unaffected children in at-risk families.

PROGNOSIS

Mortality has improved dramatically, although approximately 30% of patients die in the neonatal period of complications from pulmonary hypoplasia. Neonatal respiratory support and renal replacement therapies have increased the 10-yr survival of children surviving beyond the 1st year of life to >80%. Fifteen-year survival is estimated at 70-80%. End-stage renal disease is seen in >50% of children and usually occurs during the 1st decade of life. As a result, dialysis and renal transplantation have become standard therapies for these children. Morbidity and mortality in the older child are related to complications from chronic renal failure and liver disease.

BIBLIOGRAPHY

Please visit the Nelson Textbook of Pediatrics *website at www.expertconsult.com for the complete bibliography.*

515.3 Autosomal Dominant Polycystic Kidney Disease

Craig C. Porter and Ellis D. Avner

Autosomal dominant polycystic kidney disease (ADPKD) is the most common hereditary human kidney disease, with an incidence of 1/500 to 1/1,000.

PATHOLOGY

Both kidneys are enlarged and show cortical and medullary cysts originating from all regions of the nephron.

PATHOGENESIS

Approximately 85% of patients with ADPKD have mutations that map to the *PKD1* gene on the short arm of chromosome 16, which encodes polycystin, a transmembrane glycoprotein. Another 10-15% of ADPKD mutations map to the *PKD2* gene on the long arm of chromosome 4, which encodes polycystin 2, a proposed nonselective cation channel. The majority of mutations appear to be unique to a given family. At present, a mutation can be found in 90% of patients with well-characterized disease. Mutations of *PKD1* are associated with more severe renal disease than mutations of *PKD2*. The pathophysiology of the disease appears to be related to disruption of normal multimeric cystoprotein complexes, with consequent abnormal intracellular signaling resulting in abnormal proliferation, tubular secretion, and cyst formation. Abnormal growth factor expression, coupled with low intracellular calcium and elevated cyclic adenosine monophosphate (cAMP), appear to be important features leading to formation of cysts and progressive enlargement.

CLINICAL PRESENTATION

The severity of renal disease and the clinical manifestations of ADPKD are highly variable. Although symptomatic ADPKD commonly occurs in the 4th or 5th decade of life, symptoms, including gross or microscopic hematuria, bilateral flank pain, abdominal masses, hypertension, and urinary tract infection, may be seen in children and neonates. Renal ultrasonography usually demonstrates multiple bilateral macrocysts in enlarged kidneys (Fig. 515-3), although normal kidney size and unilateral disease may be seen in the early phase of the disease.

ADPKD is a systemic disorder affecting many organ systems. Cysts may be present within the liver, pancreas, spleen, and ovaries and when present help confirm the diagnosis. **Intracranial aneurysms,** which appear to cluster within certain families, have an overall prevalence of 5% and are an important cause of mortality in adults but are rarely reported in children. Mitral valve prolapse is seen in approximately 12% of children. Hernias and intestinal diverticula can also occur in these children. Renal cell carcinoma has been reported in association with ADPKD.

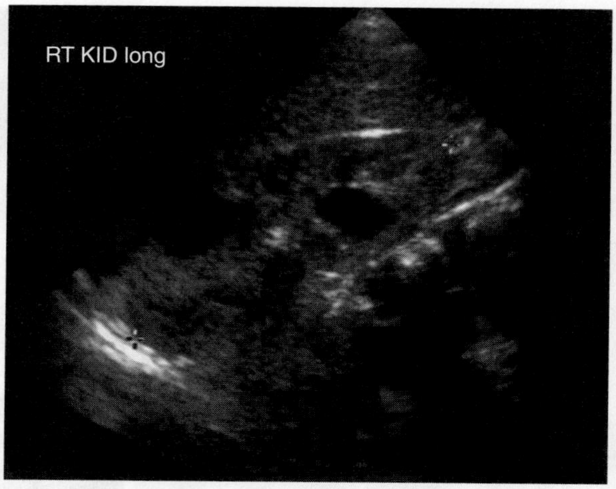

Figure 515-3 Ultrasound examination of an 18 mo old boy with autosomal dominant polycystic kidney disease demonstrating renal enlargement (10 cm) and two large cysts.

DIAGNOSIS

ADPKD is confirmed by the presence of enlarged kidneys with bilateral macrocysts in a patient with an affected first-degree relative. De novo mutations occur in 5-10% of patients with newly diagnosed disease. The diagnosis might be made in children before their affected parent, making parental renal sonography an important diagnostic test in families with no apparent family history. Among patients with genetically defined ADPKD, screening renal ultrasonography results may be normal in ≤20% by 20 yr of age and <5% by 30 yr of age.

Prenatal diagnosis is suggested from the presence of enlarged kidneys with or without cysts on ultrasonography in families with known ADPKD. Prenatal DNA testing is available in families with affected members whose disease is caused by identified mutations in the *PKD1* or *PKD2* genes.

The differential diagnosis includes renal cysts associated with glomerulocystic kidney disease, tuberous sclerosis, and von Hippel-Lindau disease, which may be inherited in an autosomal dominant pattern (see Table 515-1). The neonatal manifestations of ADPKD and ARPKD may be indistinguishable.

TREATMENT AND PROGNOSIS

Treatment of ADPKD is primarily supportive. Control of blood pressure is critical because the rate of disease progression in ADPKD correlates with the presence of hypertension. Angiotensin-converting enzyme inhibitors and/or angiotensin II receptor antagonists are agents of choice. Obesity, caffeine ingestion, smoking, multiple pregnancies, male sex, and possibly the use of calcium channel blockers appear to accelerate disease progression. Older patients with a family history of intracranial aneurysm rupture may be considered candidates for screening for aneurysms.

Although neonatal ADPKD may be fatal, long-term survival of the patient and the kidneys is possible for children surviving the neonatal period. ADPKD that occurs initially in older children has a favorable prognosis, with normal renal function during childhood seen in >80% of children.

An important resource for patients and their families worldwide is the Polycystic Kidney Disease Foundation (www.pkdcure.org).

BIBLIOGRAPHY

Please visit the Nelson Textbook of Pediatrics *website at www.expertconsult.com for the complete bibliography.*

515.4 Trauma

Craig C. Porter and Ellis D. Avner

Infants and children are more susceptible to renal injury following blunt or penetrating injury to the back or abdomen owing to their decreased muscle mass "protecting" the kidney. Gross or microscopic hematuria, flank pain, and abdominal rigidity can occur; associated injuries may be present (Chapter 66). In the absence of hemodynamic instability, most renal trauma can be managed nonoperatively. Urethral trauma can result from crush injury, often associated with a fractured pelvis or from direct injury. Such injury is suspected when gross blood appears at the external urethral meatus. Rhabdomyolysis and consequent renal failure is another complication of crush injury that can be ameliorated by vigorous fluid resuscitation.

BIBLIOGRAPHY
Please visit the Nelson Textbook of Pediatrics *website at www.expertconsult.com for the complete bibliography.*

515.5 Renal Tumors

See Chapters 492 and 493.

Chapter 516 Lower Urinary Tract Causes of Hematuria

516.1 Infectious Causes of Cystitis and Urethritis

Priya Pais and Ellis D. Avner

Gross or microscopic hematuria may be associated with bacterial, mycobacterial, or viral infections of the bladder (Chapter 532).

516.2 Hemorrhagic Cystitis

Priya Pais and Ellis D. Avner

Hemorrhagic cystitis is defined as acute or chronic bleeding of the bladder. Patients with hemorrhagic cystitis often present with gross hematuria and dysuria. In severe forms, bleeding can lead to a significant decrease in blood hemoglobin levels. Hemorrhagic cystitis can occur in response to chemical toxins (cyclophosphamide, penicillins, busulfan, thiotepa, dyes, insecticides), viruses (adenovirus types 11 and 21 (Chapter 254), and influenza A), radiation, and amyloidosis. The polyoma BK virus, present latently in immunocompetent hosts, has been recognized as playing an important role in the development of drug-induced cystitis in immunosuppressed patients.

For chemical irritation related to use of cyclophosphamide, hydration, and the use of mesna disulfide, which inactivates cyclophosphamide metabolites, helps to protect the bladder. Administration of oral cyclophosphamide in the morning followed by aggressive oral hydration throughout the remainder of the day is very effective in minimizing the risk of hemorrhagic cystitis. Bladder irrigation with saline, alum, silver nitrate, or aminocaproic acid may be necessary in more severe forms of this disorder regardless of etiology. Gross hematuria associated with viral hemorrhagic cystitis usually resolves within 1 wk.

BIBLIOGRAPHY
Please visit the Nelson Textbook of Pediatrics *website at www.expertconsult.com for the complete bibliography.*

516.3 Vigorous Exercise

Priya Pais and Ellis D. Avner

Gross or microscopic hematuria can follow vigorous exercise. Exercise hematuria is rare in girls and can be associated with dysuria. About 30-60% of runners completing marathons have dipstick-positive urine for blood. In limited follow-up, none appeared to have any significant urinary tract abnormalities. The color of the urine following vigorous exercise can vary from red to black. Blood clots may be present in the urine. Findings on urine culture, intravenous pyelography, voiding cystourethrography, and cystoscopy are normal in most patients. This seems to be a benign condition, and the hematuria generally resolves within 48 hr after cessation of exercise. The absence of red blood cell casts or evidence of renal disease and the presence of dysuria and blood clots in some patients suggest that the source of bleeding lies in the lower urinary tract. Rhabdomyolysis with myoglobinuria or hemoglobinuria must be considered in the differential diagnosis when associated with symptoms in the appropriate clinical context. Hydronephrosis or anatomic abnormalities must be considered in any child who presents with hematuria (particularly gross) after mild exercise or following mild trauma. Appropriate imaging studies are indicated in this setting.

BIBLIOGRAPHY
Please visit the Nelson Textbook of Pediatrics *website at www.expertconsult.com for the complete bibliography.*

Section 3 CONDITIONS PARTICULARLY ASSOCIATED WITH PROTEINURIA

Chapter 517 Introduction to the Child with Proteinuria

Priya Pais and Ellis D. Avner

The demonstration of proteinuria on a routine screening urinalysis is common; 10% of children aged 8-15 yr test positive for proteinuria by urinary dipstick at some time. The challenge is to differentiate the child with proteinuria related to renal disease from the otherwise healthy child with transient or other benign forms of proteinuria.

The urinary dipstick test offers a qualitative assessment of urinary protein excretion. Dipsticks primarily detect albuminuria and are less sensitive for other forms of proteinuria (low molecular weight proteins, Bence Jones protein, gamma globulins). Visual changes in the color of the dipstick are a semiquantitative measure of increasing urinary protein concentration. The dipstick is reported as negative, trace (10-20 mg/dL), 1+ (30 mg/dL), 2+ (100 mg/dL), 3+ (300 mg/dL), and 4+ (1000-2000 mg/dL).

False-negative test results can occur in patients with dilute urine (specific gravity <1.005) or in disease states in which the predominant urinary protein is not albumin. False-positive test results may be seen in patients with gross hematuria, contamination with antiseptic agents (chlorhexidine, benzalkonium chloride, hydrogen peroxide), urinary pH >7.0, or phenazopyridine therapy. The dipstick may also be falsely positive in patients with highly concentrated urine. A dipstick should be considered positive for protein if it registers >trace (10-29 mg/dL) in a urine sample in which the specific gravity is <1.010. If the specific gravity is >1.015, the dipstick must read ≥1+ to be considered clinically significant.

Because the dipstick reaction offers only a qualitative measurement of urinary protein excretion, children with persistent proteinuria should have proteinuria quantitated with the more precise spot urine protein:creatinine ratio (UPr:UCr). This ratio is calculated by dividing the UPr (mg/dL) concentration by the UCr (mg/dL) concentration and is best performed on a first morning voided urine specimen to eliminate the possibility of orthostatic (postural) proteinuria (Chapter 519). Ratios <0.5 in children <2 yr of age and <0.2 in children ≥2 yr of age suggest normal protein excretion. A ratio >2 suggests nephrotic-range proteinuria. UPr:UCr ratios have been shown to have a high correlation with protein excretion determinations in timed urine collection.

Timed (24-hr) urine collections offer more precise information regarding UPr excretion. A reasonable upper limit of normal protein excretion in healthy children is 150 mg/24 hr (0.15 g/24 hr). More specifically, normal protein excretion in children is defined as ≤4 mg/m^2/hr; abnormal is defined as 4-40 mg/m^2/hr; and nephrotic range is defined as >40 mg/m^2/hr. Timed urine collections are cumbersome to obtain, and accuracy depends on a complete collection. As a result, timed collections have largely been replaced by the spot protein:creatinine ratio.

Microalbuminuria is defined as the presence of albumin in the urine above the normal level but below the detectable range of conventional urine dipstick methods. In adults, microalbuminuria (defined as an albumin excretion of 30-300 mg/g creatinine) is widely accepted as predicting cardiovascular and renal disease. The mean level of albumin excretion has been shown fall between 8 and 10 mg/g creatinine in children >6 yr old. Similar to adults, microalbuminuria in children has been found to be associated with obesity and to predict, with reasonable specificity, the development of diabetic nephropathy in type 1 diabetes mellitus.

BIBLIOGRAPHY

Please visit the Nelson Textbook of Pediatrics *website at* *www.expertconsult.com* *for the complete bibliography.*

Chapter 518
Transient Proteinuria
Craig C. Porter and Ellis D. Avner

The majority of children found to have positive urinary dipstick values for protein have normal dipstick values on repeated measurements. Approximately 10% of children who undergo random urinalysis have proteinuria by a single dipstick measurement. Across the school-age spectrum this finding occurs more commonly in adolescents than in younger children. In most cases, serial testing of the patient's urine demonstrates resolution of the abnormality. This phenomenon defines **transient proteinuria,** and its cause remains elusive. Defined contributing factors include a temperature >38.3°C (101°F) (Chapter 169), exercise (Chapter 678), dehydration, cold exposure, heart failure, seizures, or stress. The proteinuria usually does not exceed 1-2+ on the dipstick. No evaluation or therapy is needed for children with this benign condition. Persistence of proteinuria, even if low grade, suggests the need for additional evaluation.

BIBLIOGRAPHY

Please visit the Nelson Textbook of Pediatrics *website at* *www.expertconsult.com* *for the complete bibliography.*

Chapter 519
Orthostatic (Postural) Proteinuria
Craig C. Porter and Ellis D. Avner

Orthostatic proteinuria is the most common cause of persistent proteinuria in school-aged children and adolescents, occurring in up to 60% of children with persistent proteinuria. Children with this condition are usually asymptomatic, and the condition is discovered on routine urinalysis. Patients with orthostatic proteinuria excrete normal or minimally increased amounts of protein in the supine position. In the upright position, urinary protein excretion may be increased 10-fold, up to 1,000 mg/24 hr (1 g/24 hr). Hematuria, hypertension, hypoalbuminemia, edema, and renal dysfunction are absent.

In a child with persistent asymptomatic proteinuria the initial evaluation should include an assessment for orthostatic proteinuria, a condition in which the 24-hr urinary protein excretion rarely exceeds 1 g. It begins with the collection of a first morning urine sample, with subsequent testing of any urinary abnormalities by a complete urinalysis and determination of a spot protein : creatinine (Pr : Cr) ratio. The correct collection of the first morning urine sample is critical. The child must fully empty the bladder before going to bed and then collect the first voided urine sample immediately upon arising in the morning. The absence of proteinuria (dipstick negative or trace for protein and urine Pr : Cr ratio <0.2) in the first morning urine sample for 3 consecutive days confirms the diagnosis of orthostatic proteinuria. No further evaluation is necessary, and the patient and family should be reassured of the benign nature of this condition. However, if there are other abnormalities of the urinalysis (e.g., hematuria) or the urine Pr : Cr ratio is >0.2, the patient should be referred to a pediatric nephrologist for a complete evaluation.

The cause of orthostatic proteinuria is unknown, although altered renal hemodynamics and partial renal vein obstruction in the upright position are possible causes. Long-term follow-up studies in young adults suggest that orthostatic proteinuria is a benign process, but similar data are not available for children. Therefore, long-term follow-up of children may be prudent to monitor patients for evidence of kidney disease, including hematuria, hypertension, edema, diminished renal function, or proteinuria exceeding 1,000 mg/24 hr.

BIBLIOGRAPHY

Please visit the Nelson Textbook of Pediatrics *website at* *www.expertconsult.com* *for the complete bibliography.*

Chapter 520
Fixed Proteinuria
Priya Pais and Ellis D. Avner

Persons found to have significant proteinuria on a first morning urine sample on 3 consecutive days (>1+ on dipstick with urine specific gravity >1.015 or protein : creatinine ratio >0.2) have fixed proteinuria. Fixed proteinuria indicates renal disease and may be caused by either glomerular or tubular disorders.

520.1 Glomerular Proteinuria

Priya Pais and Ellis D. Avner

The glomerular capillary wall consists of 3 layers: the fenestrated capillary endothelium, the glomerular basement membrane, and the podocytes (with foot processes and intercalated slit diaphragms). Glomerular proteinuria results from alterations in the permeability of any of the layers of the glomerular capillary wall to normally filtered proteins and occurs in a variety of renal diseases (Table 520-1). Glomerular proteinuria can range from <1 g to >30 g/24 hr.

Glomerular proteinuria should be suspected in any patient with a first morning urine protein : creatinine ratio >1.0, or proteinuria of any degree, accompanied by hypertension, hematuria, edema, or renal dysfunction. Disorders characterized primarily by proteinuria include idiopathic (minimal change) nephrotic syndrome, focal segmental glomerulosclerosis, mesangial proliferative glomerulonephritis, membranous nephropathy, membranoproliferative glomerulonephritis, amyloidosis, diabetic nephropathy, and obesity-related glomerulopathy. Other renal disorders that can include proteinuria as a prominent feature include acute postinfectious glomerulonephritis, immunoglobulin A nephropathy, lupus nephritis, Henoch-Schönlein purpura nephritis, and Alport syndrome.

Initial evaluation of a child with fixed proteinuria should include measurement of serum creatinine and electrolyte panel, first morning urine protein : creatinine ratio, serum albumin level, and complement levels. The child should be referred to a pediatric nephrologist for further evaluation and management. Renal biopsy is often necessary to establish a diagnosis and guide therapy.

In asymptomatic patients with low-grade proteinuria (protein : creatinine ratio 0.2-1.0) in whom all other findings are normal, renal biopsy might not be indicated because the underlying process may be transient or resolving or because specific pathologic features of a chronic kidney disease might not yet be apparent. Such patients should have periodic re-evaluation (every 4-6 mos *unless the patient is symptomatic*) consisting of a physical examination and blood pressure determination, urinalysis, and measurement of serum creatinine and first morning voided urine protein:creatinine ratio. Indications for renal biopsy include increasing proteinuria (protein:creatinine >1.0) and/or the development of hematuria, hypertension, or diminished renal function.

Table 520-1 CAUSES OF PROTEINURIA

TRANSIENT PROTEINURIA
Fever
Exercise
Dehydration
Cold exposure
Congestive heart failure
Seizure
Stress
ORTHOSTATIC (POSTURAL) PROTEINURIA
GLOMERULAR DISEASES CHARACTERIZED BY ISOLATED PROTEINURIA
Idiopatic (minimal change) nephrotic syndrome
Focal segmental glomerulosclerosis
Mesangial proliferative glomerulonephritis
Membranous nephropathy
Membranoproliferative glomerulonephritis
Amyloidosis
Diabetic nephropathy
Sickle cell nephropathy
GLOMERULAR DISEASES WITH PROTEINURIA AS A PROMINENT FEATURE
Acute postinfectious glomerulonephritis
Immunoglobulin A nephropathy
Henoch-Schönlein purpura nephritis
Lupus nephritis
Alport syndrome
TUBULAR DISEASES
Cystinosis
Wilson disease
Lowe syndrome
Dent disease (X-linked recessive nephrolithiasis)
Galactosemia
Tubulointerstitial nephritis
Heavy metal poisoning
Acute tubular necrosis
Renal dysplasia
Polycystic kidney disease
Reflux nephropathy

BIBLIOGRAPHY

Please visit the Nelson Textbook of Pediatrics *website at www.expertconsult.com for the complete bibliography.*

520.2 Tubular Proteinuria

Priya Pais and Ellis D. Avner

A variety of renal disorders that primarily involve the tubulointerstitial compartment of the kidney can cause low-grade fixed proteinuria (protein : creatinine ratio <1.0). In the healthy state, large amounts of proteins of lower molecular weight than albumin are filtered by the glomerulus and reabsorbed in the proximal tubule. Injury to the proximal tubules can result in diminished reabsorptive capacity and the loss of these low molecular weight proteins in the urine.

Tubular proteinuria (see Table 520-1) may be seen in acquired and inherited disorders and may be associated with other defects of proximal tubular function, such as the Fanconi syndrome (glycosuria, phosphaturia, bicarbonate wasting, and aminoaciduria). Tubular proteinuria is a consistent finding among patients with the X-linked tubular syndrome, Dent disease, caused by mutations of the renal chloride channel.

Asymptomatic patients having persistent proteinuria generally have glomerular rather than tubular proteinuria. In occult cases, glomerular and tubular proteinuria can be distinguished by electrophoresis of the urine. In tubular proteinuria, little or no albumin is detected, whereas in glomerular proteinuria the major protein is albumin.

BIBLIOGRAPHY

Please visit the Nelson Textbook of Pediatrics *website at www.expertconsult.com for the complete bibliography.*

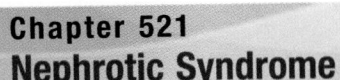

Chapter 521 Nephrotic Syndrome

Priya Pais and Ellis D. Avner

Nephrotic syndrome, a manifestation of glomerular disease, is characterized by nephrotic range proteinuria and the triad of clinical findings associated with large urinary losses of protein: hypoalbuminemia, edema, and hyperlipidemia. Nephrotic range proteinuria is defined as protein excretion of > 40 $mg/m^2/hr$ or a first morning protein : creatinine ratio of >2-3 : 1. The annual incidence is 2-3 cases per 100,000 children per year in most Western countries and higher in underdeveloped countries resulting predominantly from malaria. Though early referral to a pediatric nephrologist is recommended, once nephrotic syndrome has been diagnosed, management should be a collaborative effort between the nephrologist and primary care physician.

Table 521-1 CAUSES OF CHILDHOOD NEPHROTIC SYNDROME

GENETIC DISORDERS   **Nephrotic Syndrome (Typical)**
Finnish-type congenital nephrotic syndrome (absence of nephrin)   Focal segmental glomerulosclerosis (mutations in podocin, α-actinin 4, TRPC6)   Diffuse mesangial sclerosis (mutations in laminin β2 chain   Denys-Drash syndrome (mutations in WT1 transcription factor)
Proteinuria with or Without Nephrotic Syndrome
Nail-patella syndrome (mutation in LMX1B transcription factor)   Alport syndrome (mutation in collagen biosynthesis genes)
Multisystem Syndromes with or Without Nephrotic Syndrome
Galloway-Mowat syndrome   Charcot-Marie-Tooth disease   Jeune syndrome   Cockayne syndrome   Laurence-Moon-Biedl-Bardet syndrome
Metabolic Disorders with or Without Nephrotic Syndrome
Alagille syndrome α_1 Antitrypsin deficiency   Fabry disease   Glutaric acidemia   Glycogen storage disease   Hurler syndrome   Lipoprotein disorders   Mitochondrial cytopathies   Sickle cell disease
IDIOPATHIC NEPHROTIC SYNDROME
Minimal change disease   Focal segmental glomerulosclerosis   Membranous nephropathy
SECONDARY CAUSES   **Infections**
Hepatitis B, C   HIV-1   Malaria   Syphilis   Toxoplasmosis
Drugs
Penicillamine   Gold   Nonsteroidal anti-inflammatory drugs   Pamidronate   Interferon   Mercury   Heroin   Lithium
Immunologic or Allergic Disorders
Castleman disease   Kimura disease   Bee sting   Food allergens
Associated with Malignant Disease
Lymphoma   Leukemia
Glomerular Hyperfiltration
Oligomeganephronia   Morbid obesity   Adaptation to nephron reduction

Note: Childhood nephrotic syndrome can also be consequence of inflammatory glomerular disorders, normally associated with features of nephritis, e.g., vasculitis, lupus nephritis, membranoproliferative glomerulonephritis, IgA nephropathy.
From Eddy AA, Symons JM: Nephrotic syndrome in childhood, *Lancet* 362:629–638, 2003.

ETIOLOGY

Most children with nephrotic syndrome have a form of **primary** or idiopathic nephrotic syndrome (Table 521-1). Glomerular lesions associated with idiopathic nephrotic syndrome include minimal change disease (the most common), focal segmental glomerulosclerosis, membranoproliferative glomerulonephritis, membranous nephropathy and diffuse mesangial proliferation (Table 521-2). These etiologies have different age distributions (Fig. 521-1).

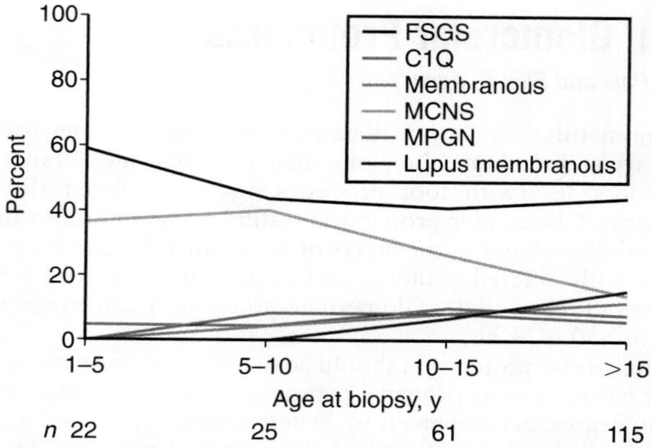

Figure 521-1 Kidney biopsy results from 223 children with proteinuria referred for diagnostic kidney biopsy (Glomerular Disease Collaborative Network, J. Charles Jennette, MD, Hyunsook Chin, MS, and D.S. Gipson, 2007). *n*, number of patients; C1Q, nephropathy; FSGS, focal segmental glomerulosclerosis; MCNS, minimal change nephrotic syndrome; MPGN, membranoproliferative glomerulonephritis. (From Gipson DS, Massengill SF, Yao L, et al: Management of childhood onset nephrotic syndrome, *Pediatrics* 124:747–757, 2009.)

Nephrotic syndrome may also be **secondary** to systemic diseases such as systemic lupus erythematosus, Henoch-Schönlein purpura, malignancy (lymphoma and leukemia), and infections (hepatitis, HIV, and malaria) (see Table 521-1).

A number of **hereditary** proteinuria syndromes are caused by mutations in genes that encode critical protein components of the glomerular filtration apparatus (Table 521-3).

PATHOPHYSIOLOGY

The underlying abnormality in nephrotic syndrome is an increased permeability of the glomerular capillary wall, which leads to massive proteinuria and hypoalbuminemia. On biopsy, the extensive effacement of podocyte foot processes (the hallmark of idiopathic nephrotic syndrome) suggests a pivotal role for the podocyte. Idiopathic nephrotic syndrome is associated with complex disturbances in the immune system, especially T cell–mediated immunity. In focal segmental glomerulosclerosis, a plasma factor, probably produced by a subset of activated lymphocytes, may be responsible for the increase in capillary wall permeability. Alternatively, mutations in podocyte proteins (podocin, α-actinin 4) and *MYH9* (podocyte gene) are associated with focal segmental glomerulosclerosis (see Table 521-3). Steroid-resistant nephrotic syndrome can be associated with mutations in *NPHS2* (podocin) and *WT1* genes, as well as other components of the glomerular filtration apparatus, such as the slit pore, and include nephrin, NEPH1, and CD-2 associated protein.

Although the mechanism of edema formation in nephrotic syndrome is incompletely understood, it seems likely that in most instances, massive urinary protein loss leads to hypoalbuminemia, which causes a decrease in plasma oncotic pressure and transudation of fluid from the intravascular compartment to the interstitial space. The reduction in intravascular volume decreases renal perfusion pressure, activating the renin-angiotensin-aldosterone system, which stimulates tubular reabsorption of sodium. The reduced intravascular volume also stimulates the release of antidiuretic hormone, which enhances the reabsorption of water in the collecting duct.

This theory does not apply to all patients with nephrotic syndrome because some patients actually have increased intravascular volume with diminished plasma levels of renin and aldosterone.

Table 521-2 SUMMARY OF PRIMARY RENAL DISEASES THAT MANIFEST AS IDIOPATHIC NEPHROTIC SYNDROME

Features	Minimal Change Nephrotic Syndrome	Focal Segmental Glomerulosclerosis	Membranous Nephropathy	MEMBRANOPROLIFERATIVE GLOMERULONEPHRITIS Type I	Type II
DEMOGRAPHICS					
Age (yr)	2-6, some adults	2-10, some adults	40-50	5-15	5-15
Sex	2:1 male	1.3:1 male	2:1 male	Male-female	Male-female
CLINICAL MANIFESTATIONS					
Nephrotic syndrome	100%	90%	80%	60%*	60%*
Asymptomatic proteinuria	0	10%	20%	40%	40%
Hematuria	10-20%	60-80%	60%	80%	80%
Hypertension	10%	20% early	Infrequent	35%	35%
Rate of progression to renal failure	Does not progress	10 yr	50% in 10-20 yr	10-20 yr	5-15 yr
Associated conditions	Allergy? Hodgkin disease, usually none	None	Renal vein thrombosis, cancer, SLE, hepatitis B	None	Partial lipodystrophy
LABORATORY FINDINGS					
	Manifestations of nephrotic syndrome ↑ BUN in 15-30%	Manifestations of nephrotic syndrome ↑ BUN in 20-40%	Manifestations of nephrotic syndrome	Low C1, C4, C3-C9	Normal C1, C4, low C3-C9
IMMUNOGENETICS					
	HLA-B8, B12 (3.5)†	Mutations in podocin, α-actinin-4, other genes	HLA-DRw3 (12-32)†	Not established	C3 nephritic factor Not established
RENAL PATHOLOGY					
Light microscopy	Normal	Focal sclerotic lesions	Thickened GBM, spikes	Thickened GBM, proliferation	Lobulation
Immunofluorescence	Negative	IgM, C3 in lesions	Fine granular IgG, C3	Granular IgG, C3	C3 only
Electron microscopy	Foot process fusion	Foot process fusion	Subepithelial deposits	Mesangial and subendothelial deposits	Dense deposits
RESPONSE TO STEROIDS					
	90%	15-20%	May be slow progression	Not established	Not established

*Approximate frequency as a cause of idiopathic nephrotic syndrome. About 10% of adult nephrotic syndrome is due to various diseases that usually manifest as acute glomerulonephritis.
†Relative risk.
SLE, systemic lupus erythematosus; ↑, elevated; BUN, blood urea nitrogen; C, complement; HLA, human leukocyte antigen; Ig, immunoglobulin; GBM, glomerular basement membrane.
Modified from Couser WG: Glomerular disorders. In Wyngaarden JB, Smith LH, Bennett JC, editors: *Cecil textbook of medicine,* ed 19, Philadelphia, 1992, WB Saunders, p 560.

Table 521-3 NEPHROTIC SYNDROME IN CHILDREN CAUSED BY GENETIC DISORDERS OF THE PODOCYTE

GENE	NAME	LOCATION	INHERITANCE	RENAL DISEASE
STEROID-RESISTANT NEPHROTIC SYNDROME				
NPHS1	Nephrin	19q13.1	Recessive	Finnish-type congenital nephrotic syndrome
NPHS2	Podocin	1q25	Recessive	FSGS
FSGS1	α-actinin-4 (αACTN4)	19q13	Dominant	FSGS
FSGS2	Unknown	11q21-22	Dominant	FSGS
WT1	Wilms tumor-suppressor gene	11p13	Dominant	Denys-Drash syndrome with diffuse mesangial sclerosis Frasier's syndrome with FSGS
LMX1B	LIM-homeodomain protein	9q34	Dominant	Nail-patella syndrome
SMARCAL1	SW1/SNF2-related, matrix-associated, actin-dependent regulator of chromatin, subfamily a-like 1	2q35	Recessive	Schimke immuno-osseous dysplasia with FSGS*
STEROID-RESPONSIVE NEPHROTIC SYNDROME				
Unknown	Unknown	Unknown	Recessive	MCNS

*Podocyte expression of *SMARCAL1* is presumptive but not yet established. Mutations in another protein, CD2-AP or NEPH1 (a novel protein structurally related to nephrin), cause congenital nephrotic syndrome in mice. A mutational variant in the *CD2AP* gene has been identified in a few patients with steroid-resistant nephrotic syndrome.
FSGS, focal segmental glomerulosclerosis; MCNS, minimal change nephrotic syndrome.
Modified from Eddy AA, Symons JM: Nephrotic syndrome in childhood, *Lancet* 362:629–638, 2003.

Therefore, other factors, including primary renal avidity for sodium and water, may be involved in the formation of edema in some patients with nephrotic syndrome.

In the nephrotic state, serum lipid levels (cholesterol, triglycerides) are elevated for 2 reasons. Hypoalbuminemia stimulates generalized hepatic protein synthesis, including synthesis of lipoproteins. This is also why a number of coagulation factors are increased, increasing the risk of thrombosis. In addition, lipid catabolism is diminished as a result of reduced plasma levels of lipoprotein lipase related to increased urinary losses of this enzyme.

Patients with nephrotic syndrome are at increased risk of infections (sepsis, peritonitis, pyelonephritis), especially with encapsulated organisms such as *Streptococcus pneumoniae* and *Haemophilus influenza*. Some reasons for this include loss of complement factor C3b, opsonins such as properdin factor B, and immunoglobulins in the urine. An additional risk factor is the use of immunosuppressive medications to treat nephrotic syndrome.

Nephrotic syndrome is a hypercoagulable state resulting from multiple factors: vascular stasis, an increase in hepatic production of fibrinogen and other clotting factors, decreased serum levels

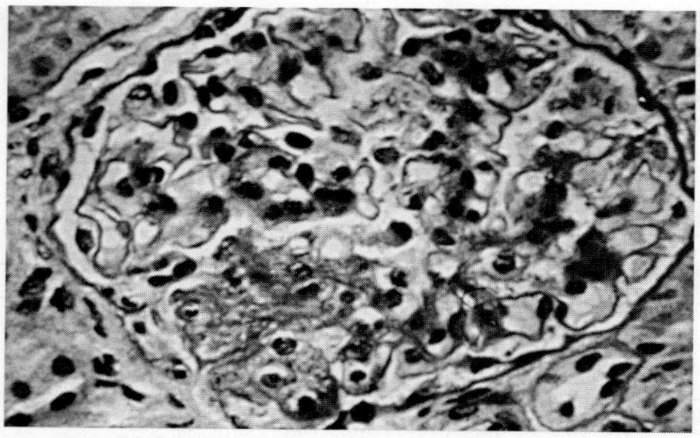

Figure 521-2 Glomerulus from a patient with steroid-resistant nephritic syndrome showing mesangial hypercellularity and an area of sclerosis in the lower portion (×250).

of anticoagulation factors, increased plasma platelet production (as an acute phase reactant), and increased platelet aggregation. The coagulopathy manifests with thromboembolic events.

BIBLIOGRAPHY

Please visit the Nelson Textbook of Pediatrics *website at* *www.expertconsult.com* *for the complete bibliography.*

521.1 Idiopathic Nephrotic Syndrome

Priya Pais and Ellis D. Avner

Approximately 90% of children with nephrotic syndrome have idiopathic nephrotic syndrome. Idiopathic nephrotic syndrome is associated with primary glomerular disease without evidence of a specific systemic cause. Idiopathic nephrotic syndrome includes multiple histologic types: minimal change disease, mesangial proliferation, focal segmental glomerulosclerosis, membranous nephropathy, and membranoproliferative glomerulonephritis.

PATHOLOGY

In **minimal change nephrotic syndrome (MCNS)** (about 85% of total cases of nephrotic syndrome in children), the glomeruli appear normal or show a minimal increase in mesangial cells and matrix. Findings on immunofluorescence microscopy are typically negative, and electron microscopy simply reveals effacement of the epithelial cell foot processes. More than 95% of children with minimal change disease respond to corticosteroid therapy.

Mesangial proliferation is characterized by a diffuse increase in mesangial cells and matrix on light microscopy. Immunofluorescence microscopy might reveal trace to 1+ mesangial IgM and/or IgA staining. Electron microscopy reveals increased numbers of mesangial cells and matrix as well as effacement of the epithelial cell foot processes. Approximately 50% of patients with this histologic lesion respond to corticosteroid therapy.

In **focal segmental glomerulosclerosis (FSGS)**, glomeruli show lesions that are both focal (present only in a proportion of glomeruli) and segmental (localized to ≥1 intraglomerular tufts). The lesions consist of mesangial cell proliferation segmental scarring on light microscopy (Fig. 521-2 and see Table 521-2). Immunofluorescence microscopy is positive for IgM and C3 staining in the areas of segmental sclerosis. Electron microscopy demonstrates segmental scarring of the glomerular tuft with obliteration of the glomerular capillary lumen. Similar lesions may be seen secondary to HIV infection, vesicoureteral reflux, and intravenous use of heroin and other drugs of abuse. Only 20% of patients with FSGS respond to prednisone. The disease is often progressive, ultimately involving all glomeruli, and ultimately leads to end-stage renal disease in most patients.

CLINICAL MANIFESTATIONS

The idiopathic nephrotic syndrome is more common in boys than in girls (2:1) and most commonly appears between the ages of 2 and 6 yr (see Fig. 521-1). However, it has been reported as early as 6 mo of age and throughout adulthood. MCNS is present in 85-90% of patients <6 yr of age. In contrast, only 20-30% of adolescents who present for the first time with nephrotic syndrome have MCNS. The more common cause of idiopathic nephrotic syndrome in this older age group is FSGS. The incidence of FSGS may be increasing; it may be more common in African-American, Hispanic, and Asian patients.

The initial episode of idiopathic nephrotic syndrome, as well as subsequent relapses, usually follows minor infections and, uncommonly, reactions to insect bites, bee stings, or poison ivy.

Children usually present with mild edema, which is initially noted around the eyes and in the lower extremities. Nephrotic syndrome can initially be misdiagnosed as an allergic disorder because of the periorbital swelling that decreases throughout the day. With time, the edema becomes generalized, with the development of ascites, pleural effusions, and genital edema. Anorexia, irritability, abdominal pain, and diarrhea are common. Important features of minimal change idiopathic nephrotic syndrome are the absence of hypertension and gross hematuria (previously termed *nephritic features*).

The differential diagnosis of the child with marked edema includes protein-losing enteropathy, hepatic failure, heart failure, acute or chronic glomerulonephritis, and protein malnutrition. A diagnosis other than MCNS should be considered in children <1 yr of age, a positive family history of nephrotic syndrome, presence of extrarenal findings (e.g., arthritis, rash, anemia), hypertension or pulmonary edema, acute or chronic renal insufficiency, and gross hematuria.

DIAGNOSIS

The urinalysis reveals 3+ or 4+ proteinuria, and microscopic hematuria is present in 20% of children. A spot urine protein:creatinine ratio exceeds 2.0, and urinary protein excretion exceeds 40 $mg/m^2/hr$. The serum creatinine value is usually normal, but it may be abnormally elevated if there is diminished renal perfusion from contraction of the intravascular volume. The serum albumin level is <2.5 g/dL, and serum cholesterol and triglyceride levels are elevated. Serum complement levels are normal. A renal biopsy is not routinely performed if the patient fits the standard clinical picture of MCNS.

TREATMENT

Children with their first episode of nephrotic syndrome and mild to moderate edema may be managed as outpatients. Such outpatient management is not practiced in all major centers, because the time required for successful education of the family regarding all aspects of the condition can require a short period of hospitalization. The pathophysiology and treatment of nephrotic syndrome must be carefully reviewed with the family to enhance understanding of their child's disease. The child's parents must be able to recognize the signs and symptoms of the complications of the disease and its treatment and must be taught how to use and interpret the results of urinary dipstick testing for protein.

Children with onset of uncomplicated nephrotic syndrome between 1 and 8 yr of age are likely to have steroid-responsive MCNS, and steroid therapy may be initiated without a diagnostic renal biopsy. Children with features that make MCNS less likely (gross hematuria, hypertension, renal insufficiency, hypocomplementemia, or age <1 yr or >8 yr) should be considered for renal biopsy before treatment.

In children with presumed MCNS, prednisone should be administered (after confirming a negative PPD test and administering the polyvalent pneumococcal vaccine) at a dose of 60 mg/m²/day (maximum daily dose, 80 mg) in a single daily dose for 4-6 consecutive wk. An initial 6-wk course of **daily** steroid treatment leads to a significantly lower relapse rate than previously recommended shorter courses of daily therapy. About 80-90% of children respond to steroid therapy (clinical remission, diuresis, and urine trace or negative for protein for 3 consecutive days) within 3 wk. The vast majority of children who respond to prednisone therapy do so within the first 5 wk of treatment.

After the initial 6-wk course, the prednisone dose should be tapered to 40 mg/m²/day given **every other day** as a single daily dose for at least 4 wk. The **alternate-day** dose is then slowly tapered and discontinued over the next 1-2 mo. There is evidence that both an increased dose of steroids and a prolonged duration of therapy are important factors in reducing the risk of relapse. While planning the duration of steroid therapy, the side effects of prolonged corticosteroid administration must be kept in mind.

Children with severe symptomatic edema, including large pleural effusions, ascites, or severe genital edema, should be hospitalized. In addition to sodium restriction, fluid restriction may be necessary if the child is hyponatremic. A swollen scrotum may be elevated with pillows to enhance fluid removal by gravity. Diuresis may be augmented by the administration of loop diuretics (furosemide), orally or intravenously, **although extreme caution should be exercised.** Aggressive diuresis can lead to intravascular volume depletion and a significantly increased risk of intravascular thrombosis.

When a patient has significant generalized edema with evidence of intravascular volume depletion (e.g., hemoconcentration), IV administration of 25% albumin (0.5-1.0 g albumin/kg), as a slow infusion followed by furosemide (1-2 mg/kg/dose IV) is sometimes necessary. Such therapy should be used only in collaboration with a pediatric nephrologist and mandates close monitoring of volume status, blood pressure, serum electrolyte balance, and renal function. Symptomatic volume overload, with hypertension, heart failure, and pulmonary edema is a potential complication of parenteral albumin therapy, particularly when administered as rapid infusions.

Children who continue to have proteinuria (2+ or greater) after 8 wk of steroid therapy are considered steroid resistant, and a diagnostic renal biopsy should be performed.

Children with nephrotic syndrome should attend school and participate in physical activities as tolerated. At the initial presentation and during relapse, a low-sodium diet should be followed. This restriction may be lifted once the child enters remission. Although there are no data to support their safety or efficacy, oral diuretics are used by many clinicians to control edema in children with nephrotic syndrome. Because of the increased risks of thromboembolic complications, **diuretic use should be reserved for patients with severe symptoms and must be closely monitored.**

Many children with nephrotic syndrome experience at least 1 relapse (3-4+ proteinuria plus edema). Although relapse rates of 60-80% have been noted in the past, the relapse rate in children treated with longer initial steroid courses may be as low as 30-40%.

Relapses should be treated with 60 mg/m²/day (80 mg daily max) in a single AM dose until the child enters remission (urine trace or negative for protein for 3 consecutive days). The prednisone dose is then changed to alternate-day dosing as noted with initial therapy, and gradually tapered over 4-8 wk.

A subset of patients relapse while on alternate-day steroid therapy or within 28 days of completing a successful course of prednisone therapy. Such patients are termed **steroid dependent.** Patients who respond well to prednisone therapy but relapse ≥4 times in a 12-mo period are termed **frequent relapsers.** Children who fail to respond to prednisone therapy within 8 wk of therapy are termed **steroid resistant.** Steroid-resistant nephrotic syndrome is usually caused by FSGS (80%), MCNS, or mesangial proliferative glomerulonephritis.

Steroid-dependent patients, frequent relapsers, and steroid-resistant patients are candidates for alternative therapies, particularly if the child has severe corticosteroid toxicity (cushingoid appearance, hypertension, cataracts, and/or growth failure). **Cyclophosphamide** prolongs the duration of remission and reduces the number of relapses in children with **frequently relapsing** and **steroid-dependent** nephrotic syndrome. The potential side effects of the drug (neutropenia, disseminated varicella, hemorrhagic cystitis, alopecia, sterility, increased risk of future malignancy) should be carefully reviewed with the family before initiating treatment. Cyclophosphamide (2 mg/kg) is given as a single oral dose for a total duration of 8-12 wk. Alternate-day prednisone therapy is often continued during the course of cyclophosphamide administration. During cyclophosphamide therapy, the white blood cell count must be monitored weekly and the drug should be withheld if the count falls below 5,000/mm³. The cumulative threshold dose above which oligo- or azoospermia occurs in boys is >250 mg/kg.

Cyclosporine or **tacrolimus** are also effective in inducing and maintaining prolonged remissions in children with steroid-resistant nephrotic syndrome and are useful as steroid-sparing agents. Children must be monitored for side effects, including hypertension, nephrotoxicity, hirsutism, and gingival hyperplasia. **Mycophenolate** can maintain remission in children with steroid-dependent or frequently relapsing nephrotic syndrome. **Levamisole**, an anthelmintic agent with immunomodulating effects that has been shown to reduce the risk of relapse in comparison to prednisone, is not available in the USA.

Most children who respond to cyclosporine, tacrolimus, or mycophenolate therapy tend to relapse when the medication is discontinued. Angiotensin-converting enzyme (ACE) inhibitors and angiotensin II blockers may be helpful as adjunct therapy to reduce proteinuria in steroid-resistant patients.

COMPLICATIONS

Infection is a major complication of nephrotic syndrome. Children in relapse have increased susceptibility to bacterial infections because of urinary losses of immunoglobulins and properdin factor B, defective cell-mediated immunity, their immunosuppressive therapy, malnutrition, and edema or ascites acting as a potential culture medium. **Spontaneous bacterial peritonitis** is a common infection, although sepsis, pneumonia, cellulitis, and urinary tract infections may also be seen. Although *Streptococcus pneumoniae* is the most common organism causing peritonitis, gram-negative bacteria such as *Escherichia coli* may also be encountered. The patient's caregivers should be counseled to seek medical attention if the child appears ill, has a fever, or complains of persistent abdominal pain. A high index of suspicion for bacterial peritonitis, prompt evaluation (including cultures of blood and peritoneal fluid), and early initiation of antibiotic therapy are critical.

Children with nephrotic syndrome should receive the 23-serotype pneumococcal vaccine (in addition to the 7-valent conjugate pneumococcal vaccine), given according to the routine childhood immunization schedule, ideally administered when the child is in remission and off daily prednisone therapy. Live virus vaccines should not be administered to children who are receiving daily or alternate-day high-dose steroids (≥2 mg/kg/day of prednisone or its equivalent, or ≥20 mg/day if the child weighs >10 kg). Vaccines can be administered after corticosteroid therapy has been discontinued for at least 1 mo. Nonimmune nephrotic children in relapse, if exposed to varicella, should receive varicella-zoster immunoglobulin (1 dose ≤96 hours after significant exposure). Influenza vaccine should be given on a yearly basis.

Children with nephrotic syndrome are also at increased risk of thromboembolic events. The incidence of this complication in

Table 521-4 MONITORING RECOMMENDATIONS FOR CHILDREN WITH NEPHROTIC SYNDROME

DISEASE AND TREATMENT	HOME URINE PROTEIN	WEIGHT, GROWTH, BMI	BLOOD PRESSURE	CREATININE	ELECTROLYTES	SERUM GLUCOSE	CBC	LIPID PROFILE	DRUG LEVELS	LIVER FUNCTION	URINALYSIS	CPK
DISEASE TYPE												
Mild (steroid responsive)	•	•	•								•	
Moderate (frequent relapsing, steroid dependent)	•	•	•	•				•			•	
Severe (steroid resistant)	•	•	•	•				•			•	
THERAPY												
Corticosteroids		•	•			•		•				
Cyclophosphamide				•			•				•	
Mycophenolate mofetil							•			•		
Calcineurin inhibitors			•	•	•	•		•	•			
ACE-Is/ARBs			•	•	•		•					
HMG-CoA reductase inhibitors								•		•		•

CBC, complete blood count; CPK, creatine kinase; ACEI, angiotensin-converting enzyme inhibitor; ARB, angiotensin II receptor blocker; HMG-CoA, 3-hydroxy-3-methylglutaryl coenzyme A.
From Gipson DS, Massengill SF, Yao L, et al: Management of childhood onset nephrotic syndrome, *Pediatrics* 124:747–757, 2009.

children is 2-5%, which represents a much lower risk than that of adults with nephrotic syndrome. Both arterial and venous thromboses may be seen, including renal vein thrombosis, pulmonary embolus, sagittal sinus thrombosis, and thrombosis of indwelling arterial and venous catheters. The risk of thrombosis is related to increased prothrombotic factors (fibrinogen, thrombocytosis, hemoconcentration, relative immobilization) and decreased fibrinolytic factors (urinary losses of antithrombin III, proteins C and S). Prophylactic anticoagulation is not recommended in children unless a previous thromboembolic event has occurred. To minimize the risk of thromboembolic complications, aggressive use of diuretics and the use of indwelling catheters should be avoided if possible. Hyperlipidemia, particularly in patients with complicated nephrotic syndrome, may be a risk factor for cardiovascular disease; myocardial infarction is a rare complication in children. It has been suggested that 3-hydroxy-3-methylglutaryl coenzyme A (HMG-CoA) reductase-inhibiting drugs should be used to treat the hyperlipidemia seen in persistent nephrotic syndrome, but controlled data regarding risks or benefits are not available.

Monitoring of children with nephrotic syndrome is noted in Table 521-4.

PROGNOSIS

Most children with steroid-responsive nephrotic syndrome have repeated relapses, which generally decrease in frequency as the child grows older. Although there is no proven way to predict an individual child's course, children who respond rapidly to steroids and those who have no relapses during the first 6 mo after diagnosis are likely to follow an infrequently relapsing course. It is important to indicate to the family that the child with steroid-responsive nephrotic syndrome is unlikely to develop chronic kidney disease, that the disease is rarely hereditary, and that the child (in the absence of prolonged cyclophosphamide therapy) will remain fertile. To minimize the psychologic effects of the condition and its therapy, children with idiopathic nephritic syndrome should not be considered chronically ill and should participate in all age-appropriate childhood activities and maintain an unrestricted diet when in remission.

Children with steroid-resistant nephrotic syndrome, most often caused by FSGS, generally have a much poorer prognosis. These children develop progressive renal insufficiency, ultimately leading to end-stage renal disease requiring dialysis or kidney transplantation. Recurrent nephrotic syndrome develops in 30-50% of transplant recipients with FSGS. There have not been adequate randomized clinical trials in this subset of patients to guide therapy. A large NIH sponsored multicenter, randomized clinical trial is comparing cyclosporine with mycophenolate mofetil in the treatment of focal segmental glomerulosclerosis.

BIBLIOGRAPHY

Please visit the Nelson Textbook of Pediatrics *website at* www.expertconsult.com *for the complete bibliography.*

521.2 Secondary Nephrotic Syndrome

Priya Pais and Ellis D. Avner

Nephrotic syndrome can occur as a secondary feature of many forms of glomerular disease. Membranous nephropathy, membranoproliferative glomerulonephritis, postinfectious glomerulonephritis, lupus nephritis, and Henoch-Schönlein purpura nephritis can all have a nephrotic component (see Tables 521-1 and 521-2). Secondary nephrotic syndrome should be suspected in patients >8 yr and those with hypertension, hematuria, renal dysfunction, extrarenal symptoms (rash, arthralgias, fever), or depressed serum complement levels.

In certain areas of the world, malaria and schistosomiasis are the leading causes of nephrotic syndrome. Other infectious agents associated with nephrotic syndrome include hepatitis B virus, hepatitis C virus, filaria, leprosy, and HIV.

Nephrotic syndrome has been associated with malignancy, particularly in the adult population. In patients with solid tumors, such as carcinomas of the lung and gastrointestinal tract, the renal pathology often resembles membranous glomerulopathy. Immune complexes composed of tumor antigens and tumor-specific antibodies presumably mediate the renal involvement. In patients with lymphomas, particularly Hodgkin lymphoma, the renal pathology most often resembles MCNS. The proposed mechanism of the nephrotic syndrome is that the lymphoma produces a lymphokine that increases permeability of the glomerular capillary wall. Nephrotic syndrome can develop before or after the malignancy is detected, resolve as the tumor regresses, and return if the tumor recurs.

Nephrotic syndrome has also developed during therapy with numerous drugs and chemicals. The histologic picture can resemble membranous glomerulopathy (penicillamine, captopril, gold, nonsteroidal anti-inflammatory drugs, mercury compounds), MCNS (probenecid, ethosuximide, methimazole, lithium), or proliferative glomerulonephritis (procainamide, chlorpropamide, phenytoin, trimethadione, paramethadione).

BIBLIOGRAPHY

Please visit the Nelson Textbook of Pediatrics *website at* www.expertconsult.com *for the complete bibliography.*

521.3 Congenital Nephrotic Syndrome

Priya Pais and Ellis D. Avner

Nephrotic syndrome (massive proteinuria, hypoalbuminemia, edema, and hypercholesterolemia) has a poorer prognosis when it occurs in the 1st yr of life, when compared to nephrotic syndrome manifesting in childhood. Congenital nephrotic syndrome is defined as nephrotic syndrome manifesting at birth or within the first 3 mo of life. Congenital nephrotic syndrome may be classified as primary or as secondary to a number of etiologies such as in-utero infections (cytomegalovirus, toxoplasmosis, syphilis, hepatitis B and C, HIV), infantile systemic lupus erythematosus, or mercury exposure.

Primary congenital nephrotic syndrome is due to a variety of syndromes inherited as autosomal recessive disorders (see Table 521-3). A number of structural and functional abnormalities of the glomerular filtration barrier causing congenital nephrotic syndrome have been elucidated. The glomerular filtration barrier, which is both size and charge selective, is composed of 3 layers: the fenestrated endothelium, the glomerular basement membrane, and the podocyte foot processes. The foot processes are interconnected by bridging structures, the slit diaphragms, which act as a size selective filter, whereas the glomerular basement membrane restricts molecules based on their ionic charge.

In a large European cohort of children with congenital nephrotic syndrome, 85% demonstrated disease, causing mutations in 4 genes (*NPHS1, NPHS2, WT1,* and *LAMB2*), the first 3 of which encode components of the glomerular filtration barrier. The Finnish type of congenital nephritic syndrome is caused by mutations in the *NPHS1* or *NPHS2* genes, which encode nephrin and podocin, critical components of the slit diaphragm. Affected infants most commonly present at birth with edema due to massive proteinuria, and they are typically delivered with an enlarged placenta (>25% of the infant's weight). Severe hypoalbuminemia, hyperlipidemia, and hypogammaglobulinemia result from loss of filtering selectivity at the glomerular filtration barrier. Prenatal diagnosis can be made by the presence of elevated maternal and amniotic α-fetoprotein levels.

Denys-Drash syndrome is caused by mutations in the *WT1* gene, which results in abnormal podocyte function. Patients present with early-onset nephrotic syndrome, progressive renal insufficiency, ambiguous genitalia, and Wilms' tumors.

Mutations in the *LAMB2* gene, seen in **Pierson syndrome,** lead to abnormalities of $\beta 2$ laminin, a critical component of glomerular and ocular basement membranes. In addition to congenital nephrotic syndrome, affected infants display bilateral microcoria (fixed narrowing of the pupil).

Regardless of the etiology of congenital nephrotic syndrome, diagnosis is made clinically in newborns or infants who demonstrate severe generalized edema, poor growth and nutrition with hypoalbuminemia, increased susceptibility to infections, hypothyroidism (due to urinary loss of thyroxin-binding globulin), and increased risk of thrombotic events. Most infants have progressive renal insufficiency.

Secondary congenital nephrotic syndrome can resolve with treatment of the underlying cause, such as syphilis (Table 521-5). The management of primary congenital nephrotic syndrome includes intensive supportive care with intravenous albumin and diuretics, regular administration of intravenous gamma-globulin, and aggressive nutritional support (often parenteral), while attempting to pharmacologically decrease urinary protein loss with angiotensin-converting enzyme inhibitors, angiotensin II receptor inhibitors, and prostaglandin synthesis inhibitors or even unilateral nephrectomy. If conservative management fails, and patients suffer from persistent anasarca or repeated severe infections, bilateral nephrectomies are performed and chronic dialysis is initiated. Renal transplantation is the definitive treatment of congenital nephrotic syndrome, though recurrence of the nephrotic syndrome has been reported to occur after transplantation.

Table 521-5 CAUSES OF NEPHROTIC SYNDROME IN INFANTS YOUNGER THAN 1 YEAR

SECONDARY CAUSES
Infections
Syphilis
Cytomegalovirus
Toxoplasmosis
Rubella
Hepatitis B
HIV
Malaria
Drug reactions
Toxins
Mercury
Systemic lupus erythematosus
Syndromes with associated renal disease
Nail-patella syndrome
Lowe syndrome
Nephropathy associated with congenital brain malformation
Denys-Drash syndrome: Wilms tumor
Hemolytic uremic syndrome
PRIMARY CAUSES
Congenital nephrotic syndrome
Diffuse mesangial sclerosis
Minimal change disease
Focal segmental sclerosis
Membranous nephropathy

From Kliegman RM, Greenbaum LA, Lye PS: *Practical strategies in pediatric diagnosis and therapy,* ed 2, Philadelphia, 2004, Saunders, p 418.

BIBLIOGRAPHY

Please visit the Nelson Textbook of Pediatrics *website at www.expertconsult.com for the complete bibliography.*

Section 4 TUBULAR DISORDERS

Chapter 522 Tubular Function

Rajasree Sreedharan and Ellis D. Avner

Water and electrolytes are freely filtered at the level of the glomerulus. Thus, the electrolyte content of ultrafiltrate at the beginning of the proximal tubule is similar to that of plasma. Carefully regulated processes of tubular reabsorption and/or tubular secretion determine final water content and electrolyte composition of urine. Bulk movement of solute tends to occur in the proximal portions of the nephron, and fine adjustments tend to occur distally (Chapter 52).

For the full continuation of this chapter, please visit the Nelson Textbook of Pediatrics *website at www.expertconsult.com.*

Chapter 523
Renal Tubular Acidosis

Rajasree Sreedharan and Ellis D. Avner

Renal tubular acidosis (RTA) is a disease state characterized by a normal anion gap (hyperchloremic) metabolic acidosis in the setting of normal or near-normal glomerular filtration rate. There are 4 main types: proximal (type II) RTA, classic distal (type I) RTA, hyperkalemic (type IV) RTA, and combined proximal and distal (type III). Proximal RTA results from impaired bicarbonate reabsorption and distal RTA from failure to secrete acid. Either of these defects may be inherited and persistent from birth or acquired, as is seen more commonly in clinical practice.

NORMAL URINARY ACIDIFICATION

Kidneys contribute to acid-base balance by reabsorption of filtered bicarbonate (HCO_3^-) and excretion of hydrogen ion (H^+) produced every day. Hydrogen ion secretion from tubule cells into the lumen is key in the reabsorption of HCO_3^-, formation of titratable acidity (H^+ bound to buffers such as HPO_4^{2-}), and formation of ammonium ions (NH_4^+). Because loss of filtered HCO_3^- is equivalent to addition of H^+ to the body, all filtered bicarbonate should be absorbed before dietary H^+ can be excreted. About 90% of filtered bicarbonate is absorbed in the proximal tubule and the remaining 10% in the distal segments, mostly thick ascending limb and outer medullary collecting tubule (CT) (Fig. 523-1). In the proximal tubule and thick ascending limb of the loop of Henle (TAL) H^+ from water is secreted by the Na^+-H^+ exchanger on the luminal membrane. H^+ combines with filtered bicarbonate resulting in the formation of H_2CO_3, which splits into water and CO_2 in the presence of carbonic anhydrase (CA) IV. CO_2 diffuses freely back into the cell, combines with OH^- (from H_2O) to form HCO_3^- in the presence of CA II, and returns to systemic circulation via the Na^+-$3HCO_3^-$ cotransporter situated at the basolateral membrane of the cell. In the CT, H^+ is secreted into lumen by H^+ATPase (adenosine triphosphatase) and H-CO_3^- is returned to systemic circulation by HCO_3^--Cl^- exchanger located on the basolateral membrane. The H^+ secreted proximally and distally in excess of the filtered HCO_3^- is excreted in the urine either as titratable acid or as NH_4^+.

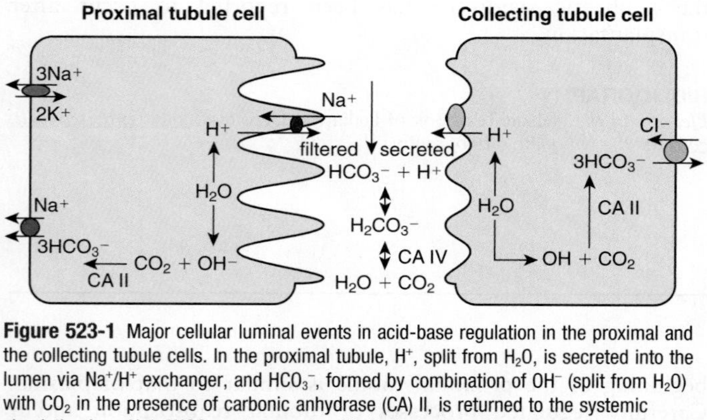

Figure 523-1 Major cellular luminal events in acid-base regulation in the proximal and the collecting tubule cells. In the proximal tubule, H^+, split from H_2O, is secreted into the lumen via Na^+/H^+ exchanger, and HCO_3^-, formed by combination of OH^- (split from H_2O) with CO_2 in the presence of carbonic anhydrase (CA) II, is returned to the systemic circulation by a Na^+-$3HCO_3^-$ cotransporter. Similarly, in the collecting tubule, H^+ is secreted into the lumen by an active H^+-ATPase (adenosine triphosphatase), and HCO_3^- is returned to the systemic circulation via a HCO_3^--Cl^- exchanger. H^+ secreted into the lumen combines with filtered HCO_3^- to form carbonic acid (H_2CO_3) and then CO_2 and H_2O in the presence of CA IV, which can be passively reabsorbed. (Modified from Rose BD, Post TW: *Clinical physiology of acid-base and electrolyte disorders,* ed 5, New York, 2001, McGraw-Hill.)

523.1 Proximal (Type II) Renal Tubular Acidosis

Rajasree Sreedharan and Ellis D. Avner

PATHOGENESIS

Proximal RTA can be inherited and persistent from birth or occur as a transient phenomenon during infancy. Although rare, it may be primary and isolated. Proximal RTA usually occurs as a component of global proximal tubular dysfunction or **Fanconi syndrome,** which is characterized by low molecular weight proteinuria, glycosuria, phosphaturia, aminoaciduria, and proximal RTA. The causes of proximal RTA and Fanconi syndrome are outlined in Table 523-1. Many of these causes are inherited disorders. In addition to **cystinosis** and **Lowe syndrome,** autosomal recessive and dominant pRTA are addressed further in this section. Other inherited forms of Fanconi syndrome include **galactosemia** (Chapter 81.2), **hereditary fructose intolerance** (Chapter 81.3), **tyrosinemia** (Chapter 79.2), and **Wilson disease** (Chapter 349.2). **Dent disease,** or X-linked nephrolithiasis, is discussed in Chapter 525.3. In children, an important form of secondary Fanconi syndrome is exposure to ifosfamide, a component of many treatment regimens for Wilms tumor and other solid tumors.

Autosomal Recessive Disease

Isolated **autosomal recessive pRTA** is caused by mutations in the gene encoding the sodium bicarbonate cotransporter NBC1. It manifests with ocular abnormalities (band keratopathy, cataracts, and glaucoma, often leading to blindness), short stature, enamel defects of the teeth, intellectual impairment, and occasionally basal ganglia calcification along with pRTA. Autosomal dominant pattern of inheritance has been identified in a single pedigree with nine members presenting with hyperchloremic metabolic acidosis, normal ability to acidify urine, normal renal function, and growth retardation.

Cystinosis

Cystinosis is a systemic disease caused by a defect in the metabolism of cystine, which results in accumulation of cystine crystals in most of the major organs of the body, notably the kidney, liver, eye, and brain. It occurs at an incidence of 1:100,000-1:200,000. In certain populations, such as French Canadians, the incidence is much higher. At least 3 clinical patterns have been described. Young children with the most severe form of the disease (*infantile* or *nephropathic cystinosis*) present in the first 2yr of life with severe tubular dysfunction and growth failure. If the disease is not treated, the children develop end-stage renal disease by the end of their 1st decade. A milder form of the disease manifests in adolescents and is characterized by less-severe tubular abnormalities and a slower progression to renal failure. A benign adult form with no renal involvement also exists.

Cystinosis is caused by mutations in the *CTNS* gene, which encodes a novel protein, cystinosin. Cystinosin is thought to be an H^+-driven lysosomal cystine transporter. Genotype-phenotype studies demonstrate that patients with severe nephropathic cystinosis carry mutations that lead to complete loss of cystinosin function. Patients with milder clinical disease have mutations that lead to expression of partially functional protein. Patients with nephropathic cystinosis present with **clinical manifestations** reflecting their pronounced tubular dysfunction and Fanconi syndrome, including polyuria and polydipsia, growth failure, and rickets. Fever, caused by dehydration or diminished sweat production, is common. Patients are typically fair skinned and blond because of diminished pigmentation. Ocular presentations include

Table 523-1 COMMON CAUSES OF RENAL TUBULAR ACIDOSIS

PROXIMAL RENAL TUBULAR ACIDOSIS **Primary**

Sporadic
Inherited
• Inherited renal disease (Idiopathic Fanconi)
  • Sporadic (most common)
  • Autosomal dominant
  • Autosomal recessive
  • X-linked (Dent disease)
• Inherited syndromes
  • Cystinosis
  • Tyrosinemia type 1
  • Galactosemia
  • Oculocerebral dystrophy (Lowe syndrome)
  • Wilson disease
  • Hereditary fructose intolerance

Secondary
Intrinsic renal disease • Autoimmune diseases (Sjögren's syndrome) • Hypokalemic nephropathy • Renal transplant rejection Hematologic disease • Myeloma Drugs • Gentamicin • Cisplatin • Ifosfamide • Sodium valproate Heavy metals • Lead • Cadmium • Mercury Organic compounds • Toluene Nutritional • Kwashiorkor Hormonal • Primary hyperparathyroidism
DISTAL RENAL TUBULAR ACIDOSIS **Primary**

Sporadic
Inherited
• Inherited renal diseases
  • Autosomal dominant
  • Autosomal recessive
  • Autosomal recessive with early-onset hearing loss
  • Autosomal recessive with later-onset hearing loss
• Inherited syndromes associated with type I renal tubular acidosis
  • Marfan syndrome
  • Wilson syndrome
  • Ehlers-Danlos syndrome
  • Familial hypercalciuria

DISTAL RENAL TUBULAR ACIDOSIS—cont'd **Secondary**
Intrinsic renal • Interstitial nephritis • Pyelonephritis • Transplant rejection • Sickle cell nephropathy • Lupus nephritis • Nephrocalcinosis • Medullary sponge kidney Urologic • Obstructive uropathy • Vesicoureteral reflux • Hepatic • Cirrhosis Toxins or medications • Amphotericin B • Lithium • Toluene • Cisplatin
HYPERKALEMIC RENAL TUBULAR ACIDOSIS **Primary**
Sporadic Genetic • Hypoaldosteronism • Addison disease • Congenital adrenal hyperplasia • Pseudohypoaldosteronism (type I or II)
Secondary
Urologic • Obstructive uropathy Intrinsic renal • Pyelonephritis • Interstitial nephritis Systemic • Diabetes mellitus • Sickle cell nephropathy Drugs • Trimethoprim/sulfamethoxazole • Angiotensin-converting enzyme inhibitors • Cyclosporine • Prolonged heparinization Addison disease

photophobia, retinopathy, and impaired visual acuity. Patients also can develop hypothyroidism, hepatosplenomegaly, and delayed sexual maturation. With progressive tubulointerstitial fibrosis, renal insufficiency is invariant.

The **diagnosis** of cystinosis is suggested by the detection of cystine crystals in the cornea and confirmed by measurement of increased leukocyte cystine content. Prenatal testing is available for at-risk families.

Treatment of cystinosis is directed at correcting the metabolic abnormalities associated with Fanconi syndrome or chronic renal failure. In addition, specific therapy is available with **cysteamine,** which binds to cystine and converts it to cysteine. This facilitates lysosomal transport and decreases tissue cystine. Oral cysteamine does not achieve adequate levels in ocular tissues, so additional therapy with cysteamine eyedrops is required. Early initiation of the drug can prevent or delay deterioration of renal function. Patients with growth failure that does not improve with cysteamine might benefit from treatment with growth hormone. Kidney transplantation is a viable option in patients with renal failure. With prolonged survival, additional complications may become evident, including central nervous system abnormalities, muscle weakness, swallowing dysfunction, and pancreatic insufficiency. It is unclear whether long-term cysteamine therapy decreases these complications.

Lowe Syndrome

Lowe syndrome *(oculocerebrorenal syndrome of Lowe)* is a rare X-linked disorder characterized by congenital cataracts, mental retardation, and Fanconi syndrome. The disease is caused by mutations in the *OCRL1* gene, which encodes the phosphatidylinositol polyphosphate 5-phosphatase protein. The abnormalities seen in Lowe syndrome are thought to be due to abnormal transport of vesicles within the Golgi apparatus. Kidneys show nonspecific tubulointerstitial changes. Thickening of glomerular basement membrane and changes in proximal tubule mitochondria are also seen.

Patients with Lowe syndrome typically present in infancy with cataracts, progressive growth failure, hypotonia, and Fanconi syndrome. Significant proteinuria is common. Blindness and renal insufficiency often develop. Characteristic behavioral abnormalities are also seen, including tantrums, stubbornness, stereotypy (repetitive behaviors), and obsessions. There is no specific therapy for the renal disease or neurologic deficits. Cataract removal is generally required.

CLINICAL MANIFESTATIONS OF PROXIMAL RTA AND FANCONI SYNDROME

Patients with isolated, sporadic, or inherited proximal RTA present with growth failure in the 1st year of life. Additional symptoms can include polyuria, dehydration (due to sodium loss), anorexia, vomiting, constipation, and hypotonia. Patients with primary Fanconi syndrome have additional symptoms, secondary to phosphate wasting, such as rickets. Those with systemic diseases present with additional signs and symptoms specific to their underlying disease. A non–anion gap metabolic acidosis is present. Urinalysis in patients with isolated proximal RTA is generally unremarkable. The urine pH is acidic (<5.5) because distal acidification mechanisms are intact in these patients. Urinary indices in patients with Fanconi syndrome demonstrate varying degrees of phosphaturia, aminoaciduria, glycosuria, uricosuria, and elevated urinary sodium or potassium. Depending on the nature of the underlying disorder, laboratory evidence of chronic renal insufficiency, including elevated serum creatinine, may be present.

523.2 Distal (Type I) Renal Tubular Acidosis

Rajasree Sreedharan and Ellis D. Avner

PATHOGENESIS

As with proximal RTA, distal RTA can be sporadic or inherited. It can also occur as a complication of inherited or acquired diseases of the distal tubules. Primary or secondary causes of distal RTA can result in damaged or impaired functioning of one or more transporters or proteins involved in the acidification process, including the H^+/ATPase, the HCO_3^-/Cl^- anion exchangers, or the components of the aldosterone pathway. Because of impaired hydrogen ion excretion, urine pH cannot be reduced to <5.5, despite the presence of severe metabolic acidosis. Loss of sodium bicarbonate distally, owing to lack of H^+ to bind to in the tubular lumen (see Fig. 523-1), results in increased chloride absorption and hyperchloremia. Inability to secrete H^+ is compensated by increased K^+ secretion distally, leading to hypokalemia. **Hypercalciuria** is usually present and can lead to nephrocalcinosis or nephrolithiasis. Chronic metabolic acidosis also impairs urinary citrate excretion. **Hypocitraturia** further increases the risk of calcium deposition in the tubules. Bone disease is common, resulting from mobilization of organic components from bone to serve as buffers to chronic acidosis.

CLINICAL MANIFESTATIONS

Distal RTA shares features with those of proximal RTA, including non–anion gap metabolic acidosis and growth failure. However, distinguishing features of distal RTA include nephrocalcinosis and hypercalciuria. The phosphate and massive bicarbonate wasting characteristic of proximal RTA is generally absent.

Causes of primary and secondary distal RTA are listed in Table 523-1. Although inherited forms are rare, 3 specific inherited forms of distal RTA have been identified, including an autosomal recessive form associated with sensorineural deafness.

Medullary sponge kidney is a relatively rare sporadic disorder in children, although not uncommon in adults. It is characterized by cystic dilatation of the terminal portions of the collecting ducts as they enter the renal pyramids. Ultrasonographically, patients often have medullary nephrocalcinosis. Although patients with this condition typically maintain normal renal function through adulthood, complications include nephrolithiasis, pyelonephritis, hyposthenuria (inability to concentrate urine), and distal RTA. Associations of medullary sponge kidney with Beckwith-Wiedemann syndrome or hemihypertrophy have been reported.

523.3 Hyperkalemic (Type IV) Renal Tubular Acidosis

Rajasree Sreedharan and Ellis D. Avner

PATHOGENESIS

Type IV RTA occurs as the result of impaired aldosterone production (hypoaldosteronism) or impaired renal responsiveness to aldosterone (pseudohypoaldosteronism). Acidosis results because aldosterone has a direct effect on the H^+/ATPase responsible for hydrogen secretion. In addition, aldosterone is a potent stimulant for potassium secretion in the collecting tubule; consequently, lack of aldosterone results in hyperkalemia. This further affects acid-base status by inhibiting ammoniagenesis and, thus, H^+ excretion. Aldosterone deficiency typically occurs as a result of adrenal gland disorders such as Addison disease or some forms of congenital adrenal hyperplasia. In children, aldosterone unresponsiveness is a more common cause of type IV RTA. This can occur transiently, during an episode of acute pyelonephritis or acute urinary obstruction, or chronically, particularly in infants and children with a history of obstructive uropathy. The latter patients can have significant hyperkalemia, even in instances when renal function is normal or only mildly impaired. Rare examples of inherited forms of type IV RTA have been identified.

CLINICAL MANIFESTATIONS

Patients with type IV RTA, like those with type I and II RTA, can present with growth failure in the first few years of life. Polyuria and dehydration (from salt wasting) are common. Rarely, patients (especially those with pseudohypoaldosteronism type 1) present with life-threatening hyperkalemia. Patients with obstructive uropathies can present acutely with signs and symptoms of pyelonephritis, such as fever, vomiting, and foul-smelling urine. Laboratory tests reveal a hyperkalemic non–anion gap metabolic acidosis. Urine may be alkaline or acidic. Elevated urinary sodium levels with inappropriately low urinary potassium levels reflect the absence of aldosterone effect.

DIAGNOSTIC APPROACH

The first step in the evaluation of a patient with suspected RTA is to confirm the presence of a normal anion gap metabolic acidosis, identify electrolyte abnormalities, assess renal function, and rule out other causes of bicarbonate loss such as diarrhea (Chapter 52). Metabolic acidosis associated with diarrheal dehydration is extremely common, and acidosis generally improves with correction of volume depletion. Patients with protracted diarrhea can deplete their total-body bicarbonate stores and can have persistent acidosis despite apparent restoration of volume status. In instances where a patient has a recent history of severe diarrhea, full evaluation for RTA should be delayed for several days to permit adequate time for reconstitution of total-body bicarbonate stores. If acidosis persists beyond a few days in this setting, additional studies are indicated.

Serum electrolytes, blood urea nitrogen, calcium, phosphorus, creatinine, and pH should be obtained by venous puncture. Traumatic blood draws (such as heel stick specimens), small volumes of blood in "adult-size" specimen collection tubes, or prolonged specimen transport time at room temperature can lead to falsely low bicarbonate levels, often in association with an elevated serum potassium value. True hyperkalemic acidosis is consistent with type IV RTA, whereas the finding of normal or low potassium suggests type I or II. The **blood anion gap** should be calculated using the formula $[Na^+] - [Cl^- + HCO_3^-]$. Values of <12 demonstrate the absence of an anion gap. Values of >20 are highly suggestive of the presence of an anion gap. If such an anion gap is found, then other diagnoses (lactic acidosis, inborn errors of metabolism, ingested toxins) should be investigated. If tachypnea is noted, evaluation of an arterial blood gas might help to rule out the possibility of a mixed acid-base disorder primarily involving respiratory and metabolic components. A detailed history, with particular attention to growth and development, recent or recurrent diarrheal illnesses, and family history of mental retardation, failure to thrive, end-stage renal disease, infant deaths, or miscarriages is essential. Physical examination should determine growth parameters and volume status as well as the presence of any dysmorphic features suggesting an underlying syndrome.

Once the presence of a non–anion gap metabolic acidosis is confirmed, urine pH can help distinguish distal from proximal causes. A urine pH <5.5 in the presence of acidosis suggests proximal RTA, whereas patients with distal RTA typically have a urine pH >6.0. The **urine anion gap** ([urine Na^+ + urine K^+] − urine Cl^-) is sometimes calculated to confirm the diagnosis of distal RTA. A positive gap suggests a deficiency of ammoniagenesis and, thus, the possibility of a distal RTA. A negative gap is consistent with proximal tubule bicarbonate wasting (gastrointestinal bicarbonate wasting). A urinalysis should also be obtained to determine the presence of glycosuria, proteinuria, or hematuria, suggesting more global tubular damage or dysfunction. Random or 24-hr urine calcium and creatinine measurements will identify hypercalciuria. Renal ultrasonography should be performed to identify underlying structural abnormalities such as obstructive uropathies as well as to determine the presence of nephrocalcinosis (Fig. 523-2).

TREATMENT AND PROGNOSIS

The mainstay of therapy in all forms of RTA is bicarbonate replacement. Patients with proximal RTA often require large quantities of bicarbonate, up to 20 mEq/kg/24 hr in the form of sodium bicarbonate or sodium citrate solution (Bicitra or Shohl's solution). The base requirement for distal RTAs is generally in the range of 2-4 mEq/kg/24 hr, although patients' requirements can vary. Patients with Fanconi syndrome usually require phosphate supplementation. Patients with distal RTA should be monitored for the development of hypercalciuria. Those with symptomatic hypercalciuria (recurrent episodes of gross hematuria), nephrocalcinosis, or nephrolithiasis can require thiazide diuretics to decrease urine calcium excretion. Patients with type IV RTA can require chronic treatment for hyperkalemia with sodium-potassium exchange resin (Kayexalate).

Prognosis depends to a large part on the nature of any underlying disease. Patients with treated isolated proximal or distal RTA generally demonstrate improvement in growth, provided serum bicarbonate levels can be maintained in the normal range. Patients with systemic illness and Fanconi syndrome can have ongoing morbidity with growth failure, rickets, and signs and symptoms related to their underlying disease.

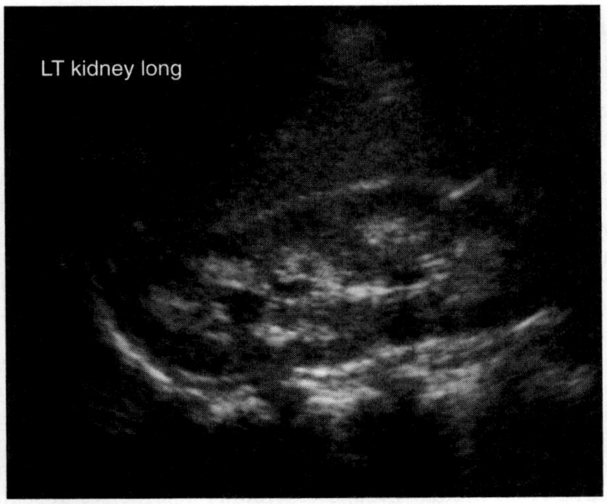

Figure 523-2 Ultrasound examination of a child with distal renal tubular acidosis demonstrating medullary nephrocalcinosis.

523.4 Rickets Associated with Renal Tubular Acidosis

Russell W. Chesney

Rickets may be present in primary RTA, particularly in type II or proximal RTA. Hypophosphatemia and phosphaturia are common in the renal tubular acidoses, which are also characterized by hyperchloremic metabolic acidosis, various degrees of bicarbonaturia, and, often, hypercalciuria and hyperkaluria. Bone demineralization without overt rickets usually is detected in type I and distal RTA. This metabolic bone disease may be characterized by bone pain, growth retardation, osteopenia, and, occasionally, pathologic fractures. Although acute metabolic acidosis in vitamin D–deficient animals can impair the conversion of 25-hydroxyvitamin D (25[OH]D) to 1,25-dihydroxyvitamin D ($1,25[OH]_2D$), resulting in reduced levels of this active metabolite, the circulating levels of $1,25(OH)_2D$ in patients with either type of RTA are normal. If patients with RTA have chronic renal insufficiency, serum $1,25(OH)_2D$ levels are reduced in relation to the degree of renal impairment.

Bone demineralization in distal RTA probably relates to dissolution of bone because the calcium carbonate in bone serves as a buffer against the metabolic acidosis due to the hydrogen ions retained by patients with RTA.

Administration of sufficient bicarbonate to reverse acidosis reverses bone dissolution and the hypercalciuria that is common in distal RTA. Proximal RTA is treated with both bicarbonate and oral phosphate supplements to heal rickets. Doses of phosphate similar to those used in familial hypophosphatemia or Fanconi syndrome may be indicated. Vitamin D is required to offset the secondary hyperparathyroidism that complicates oral phosphate therapy. Following therapy, growth in patients with type II (proximal) RTA is greater than in patients with primary Fanconi syndrome.

BIBLIOGRAPHY

Please visit the Nelson Textbook of Pediatrics *website at www.expertconsult.com for the complete bibliography.*

Chapter 524
Nephrogenic Diabetes Insipidus

Rajasree Sreedharan and Ellis D. Avner

Nephrogenic diabetes insipidus (NDI) is a rare congenital or, more commonly, acquired, disorder of water metabolism characterized by an inability to concentrate urine, even in the presence of antidiuretic hormone (ADH). The most common pattern of inheritance in congenital NDI is as an X-linked recessive disorder. Rarely, affected females are seen, presumably secondary to unfavorable X-chromosome inactivation. About 10% of cases of congenital NDI are inherited as autosomal dominant or recessive disorders, with males and females affected equally. The clinical phenotype of autosomal recessive forms is similar to that of the X-linked form. Secondary (acquired), either partial or complete, forms of NDI are not uncommon and may be seen in any disorder affecting renal tubular function including obstructive uropathies, acute or chronic renal failure, renal cystic diseases, interstitial nephritis, nephrocalcinosis, or toxic nephropathy due to hypokalemia, hypercalcemia, lithium, or amphotericin B.

PATHOGENESIS

The ability to concentrate urine (and thus absorb water) requires the presence of an intact concentrating gradient in the renal medulla and the ability to modulate water permeability in the collecting tubule. The latter is mediated by ADH (also called arginine vasopressin [AVP]), which is synthesized in the hypothalamus and stored in the posterior pituitary. Under basal situations, the collecting tubule is impermeable to water. However, in response to increased serum osmolarity (as detected by osmoreceptors in the hypothalamus) and/or severe volume depletion, ADH is released into the systemic circulation. It then binds to its receptor, vasopressin V_2 (AVPR2), on the basolateral membrane of the collecting tubule cell. Binding of the hormone to its receptor activates a cyclic adenosine monophosphate(cAMP)-dependent cascade that results in movement of preformed water channels (aquaporin 2 [AQP2]) to the luminal membrane of the collecting duct, rendering it permeable to water.

Defects in the *AVPR2* gene cause the more common X-linked form of NDI. Mutations in the *AQP2* gene have been identified in patients with the rarer autosomal dominant and recessive forms. Prenatal testing is available for families at risk for X-linked NDI. Patients with secondary forms of NDI can have ADH resistance owing to defective aquaporin expression (lithium intoxication). Secondary ADH resistance usually occurs as the result of loss of the hypertonic medullary gradient due to solute diuresis or tubular damage, resulting in the inability to absorb sodium or urea.

CLINICAL MANIFESTATIONS

Patients with congenital NDI typically present in the newborn period with massive polyuria, volume depletion, hypernatremia, and hyperthermia. Irritability and crying are common features. Constipation and poor weight gain are also seen. After multiple episodes of hypernatremic dehydration, patients can have developmental delay and mental retardation. Enuresis, caused by large urine volumes, is common. Because of the need to consume large volumes of water during the day, patients often have diminished appetite and poor food intake. However, even with adequate caloric supplementation, patients still exhibit growth abnormalities. Patients with congenital NDI also exhibit behavioral problems, including hyperactivity and short-term memory problems. Patients with the secondary form generally present later in life, primarily with hypernatremia and polyuria. Associated symptoms such as developmental delay and behavioral abnormalities are less common in this latter group.

DIAGNOSIS

The diagnosis is suggested in a male infant with polyuria, hypernatremia, and diluted urine. Simultaneous serum and urine osmolality measurements should be obtained. **If the serum osmolality value is 290 mOsm/kg or higher with a simultaneous urine osmolality value of <290 mOsm/kg, a formal water deprivation test is not necessary.** Because the differential diagnosis includes causes of **central diabetes insipidus,** the inability to respond to ADH (and thus the presence of NDI) should then be confirmed by the administration of vasopressin (10-20 µg intranasally) followed by serial urine and serum osmolality measurements hourly for 4 hr. In patients with possible "partial" or secondary diabetes insipidus, in whom the initial serum osmolality value may be <290 mOsm/kg, a water deprivation test should be considered. Fluids should be withheld and urine and serum osmolalities measured periodically until the serum osmolality value is >290 mOsm/kg; vasopressin is then given as before. Criteria for premature termination of a water deprivation test include a decrease in body weight of >3%. If NDI is confirmed or suspected, additional evaluation should include a detailed history to assess possible toxic exposures, determination of renal function by serum creatinine and blood urea nitrogen levels, and renal ultrasonography to identify obstructive uropathies or cystic disease. Because of massive urine output, patients with congenital NDI can have nonobstructive hydronephrosis of varying severity.

TREATMENT AND PROGNOSIS

Treatment of NDI includes maintenance of adequate fluid intake and access to free water, minimizing urine output by limiting solute load with a low-osmolar, low-sodium diet, and administering medications directed at decreasing urine output. For infants, human milk or a low-solute formula, such as Similac PM 60/40, is preferred. Most infants with congenital NDI require gastrostomy or nasogastric feedings to ensure adequate fluid administration throughout the day and night. Sodium intake in older patients should be <0.7 mEq/kg/24 hr. Thiazide diuretics (2-3 mg/kg/24 hr of hydrochlorothiazide) effectively induce sodium loss and stimulate proximal tubule reabsorption of water. Potassium-sparing diuretics, in particular, amiloride (0.3 mg/kg/24 hr in 3 divided doses), are often indicated. Patients who have an inadequate response to diuretics alone might benefit from the addition of indomethacin (2 mg/kg/24 hr), which has an additive effect in reducing water excretion in some patients. Renal function must be monitored closely in such patients because indomethacin can cause deterioration in renal function over time. Patients with secondary NDI might not require medications but should have access to free water. Such patients should have serum electrolytes and volume status monitored closely, particularly during periods of superimposed acute illnesses.

Prevention of recurrent dehydration and hypernatremia in patients with congenital NDI has significantly improved the neurodevelopmental outcome of these patients. However, behavioral issues remain a significant problem. In addition, chronic use of nonsteroidal anti-inflammatory drugs can predispose patients to renal insufficiency. Prognosis of patients with secondary NDI generally depends on the nature of the underlying disease.

BIBLIOGRAPHY

Please visit the Nelson Textbook of Pediatrics *website at www.expertconsult.com for the complete bibliography.*

Chapter 525 Bartter and Gitelman Syndromes and Other Inherited Tubular Transport Abnormalities

525.1 Bartter Syndrome

Rajasree Sreedharan and Ellis D. Avner

Bartter syndrome is a group of disorders characterized by hypokalemic metabolic alkalosis with hypercalciuria and salt wasting (Chapter 52) (Table 525-1). **Antenatal** Bartter syndrome (types I, II, IV) (also called hyperprostaglandin E syndrome) typically manifests in infancy and has a more-severe phenotype than classic Bartter syndrome (type III), including maternal polyhydramnios, neonatal salt wasting, and severe episodes of recurrent dehydration. The milder phenotype, **classic** Bartter syndrome, manifests in childhood with failure to thrive and a history of recurrent episodes of dehydration. A phenotypically related disease, Gitelman syndrome has a distinct genetic defect and is discussed in Chapter 525.2 (see Table 525-1). One distinct variant of antenatal Bartter syndrome is associated with sensorineural deafness (type IV).

PATHOGENESIS

The biochemical features of Bartter syndrome, including hypokalemic metabolic alkalosis with hypercalciuria, resemble those seen with chronic use of loop diuretics and reflect a defect in sodium, chloride, and potassium transport in the ascending loop of Henle. The loss of sodium and chloride, with resultant volume contraction, stimulates the renin-angiotensin II-aldosterone (RAA) axis. Aldosterone promotes sodium uptake and potassium secretion, exacerbating the hypokalemia. It also stimulates hydrogen ion secretion distally, worsening the metabolic alkalosis. Hypokalemia stimulates prostaglandin synthesis, which further activates the RAA axis. Bartter syndrome has been associated with 5 distinct genetic defects in loop of Henle transporters (see Table 525-1). Each contributes, in some manner, to sodium and chloride transport. Mutations in the genes that encode the $Na^+/K^+/2Cl^-$ transporter (NKCC2, the site of action of furosemide), the luminal potassium channel (ROMK), combined chloride channel (CLC-Ka, CLC-Kb), or subunit of chloride channels (barttin) cause neonatal Bartter syndrome. Isolated defects in the genes that produce the basolateral chloride channel ClC-Kb cause classic Bartter syndrome.

CLINICAL MANIFESTATIONS

A history of maternal polyhydramnios with or without prematurity may be elicited. Dysmorphic features, including triangular facies, protruding ears, large eyes with strabismus, and drooping mouth may be present on physical examination. Consanguinity suggests the presence of an autosomal recessive disorder. Older children can have a history of recurrent episodes of polyuria with dehydration, failure to thrive, and the classic biochemical abnormalities of a hypokalemic metabolic alkalosis. Urinary calcium levels are typically elevated, as are urinary potassium and sodium levels. Serum renin, aldosterone, and prostaglandin E levels are often markedly elevated, particularly in the more-severe antenatal form. Blood pressure is usually normal, although patients with the antenatal form can have severe salt wasting, resulting in dehydration and hypotension. Renal function is typically normal. Nephrocalcinosis, resulting from hypercalciuria, may be seen on ultrasound examination (types I, II, III, V).

DIAGNOSIS

The diagnosis is usually made based on clinical presentation and laboratory findings. The diagnosis in the neonate or infant is suggested by severe hypokalemia, usually <2.5 mmol/L, with metabolic alkalosis. Hypercalciuria is typical; hypomagnesemia is seen in a minority of patients but is more common in Gitelman syndrome. Because features of Bartter syndrome resemble chronic use of loop diuretics, diuretic abuse should be considered in the differential diagnosis, even in young children. Chronic vomiting can also give a similar clinical picture but can be distinguished by **measurement** of **urinary chloride,** which is elevated in Bartter syndrome and low in patients with chronic vomiting. Histologically, kidneys demonstrate hyperplasia of the juxtaglomerular apparatus. Renal biopsy is rarely performed to diagnose this condition.

TREATMENT AND PROGNOSIS

Treatment of Bartter syndrome is directed at preventing dehydration, maintaining nutritional status, and correcting hypokalemia. Potassium supplementation, often at very high doses, is required; potassium-sparing (aldosterone antagonists) diuretics may be of value. Even with appropriate therapy, serum potassium values might not normalize, particularly in patients with the neonatal form. Infants and young children require a high sodium diet and

Table 525-1 BARTTER AND GITELMAN SYNDROMES

	TYPE I BARTTER SYNDROME	TYPE II BARTTER SYNDROME	TYPE III BARTTER SYNDROME	TYPE IV BARTTER SYNDROME	TYPE V BARTTER SYNDROME	GITELMAN SYNDROME
Inheritance	AR	AR	AR	AR	AD	AR
Affected tubular region	TAL	TAL + CCD	TAL + DCT	TAL + DCT	TAL	DCT
Gene	*SLC12A1*	*KCNJ1*	*CLCBRK*	*BSND*	*CASR*	*SLC12A3*
Onset	Prenatal, postnatal	Prenatal, postnatal	Variable	Prenatal, postnatal	Variable	Adolescent, adult
Urine PGE2	Very high	Very high	Slightly elevated	Elevated	Elevated	Normal
Hypokalemic metabolic alkalosis	Present	Present	Present	Present	Present	Present
Features	Polyhydramnios, prematurity, nephrocalcinosis, dehydration, hyposthenuria, polyuria, failure to thrive	Same as type 1	Failure to thrive, dehydration, low serum magnesium in 20%, mildest form	Same as type I, with sensorineural hearing loss and no nephrocalcinosis	Hypocalcemia, low parathyroid hormone levels, hypercalciuria, uncommon cause of Bartter syndrome	Hypomagnesemia in 100%, mild dehydration, occasional growth retardation, tetany

AR, autosomal recessive; AD, autosomal dominant; TAL, thick ascending loop of Henle; CCD, cortisol collecting duct; DCT, descending convoluted tubule; PGE2, prostaglandin E2.

at times sodium supplementation. Indomethacin, a prostaglandin inhibitor, can also be effective. If hypomagnesemia is present, magnesium supplementation is required. With close attention to electrolyte balance, volume status, and growth, the long-term prognosis is generally good. In a minority of patients, chronic hypokalemia, nephrocalcinosis, and chronic indomethacin therapy can lead to chronic interstitial nephritis and chronic renal failure.

525.2 Gitelman Syndrome

Rajasree Sreedharan and Ellis D. Avner

Gitelman syndrome (often called a "Bartter syndrome variant") is a rare autosomal recessive cause of hypokalemic metabolic alkalosis, with distinct features of **hypocalciuria** and **hypomagnesemia.** Patients with Gitelman syndrome typically present in late childhood or early adulthood (see Table 525-1).

PATHOGENESIS

The biochemical features of Gitelman syndrome resemble those of chronic use of thiazide diuretics. Thiazides act on the sodium chloride co-transporter NCCT, present in the distal convoluted tubule. Through linkage analysis and mutational studies, defects in the gene encoding NCCT have been demonstrated in patients with Gitelman syndrome.

CLINICAL MANIFESTATIONS

Patients with Gitelman syndrome typically present at a later age than those with Bartter syndrome. Patients often have a history of recurrent muscle cramps and spasms, presumably caused by low serum magnesium levels. They usually do not have a history of recurrent episodes of dehydration. Biochemical abnormalities include hypokalemia, metabolic alkalosis, and hypomagnesemia. The urinary calcium level is usually very low (in contrast to the elevated urinary calcium level often seen in Bartter syndrome), and the urinary magnesium level is elevated. Renin and aldosterone levels are usually normal, and prostaglandin E secretion is not elevated. Growth failure is less prominent in Gitelman syndrome than in Bartter syndrome, but it may be present.

DIAGNOSIS

The diagnosis of Gitelman syndrome is suggested in an adolescent or adult presenting with hypokalemic metabolic alkalosis, hypomagnesemia, and hypocalciuria.

TREATMENT

Therapy is directed at correcting hypokalemia and hypomagnesemia with supplemental potassium and magnesium. Sodium supplementation or treatment with prostaglandin inhibitors is generally not necessary because patients typically do not have episodes of volume depletion or elevated prostaglandin E excretion.

525.3 Other Inherited Tubular Transport Abnormalities

Rajasree Sreedharan and Ellis D. Avner

Inherited abnormalities in distinct transporters in each segment of the nephron have now been identified and the molecular defects have been characterized. Renal tubular acidosis and nephrogenic diabetes insipidus are discussed in detail in Chapters 523 and 524, respectively. **Cystinuria** is an autosomal recessive disorder seen primarily in patients of Middle Eastern descent and is characterized by recurrent stone formation. The disease is caused by a defective high-affinity transporter for L-cystine and dibasic amino acids present in the proximal tubule.

Dent disease is an X-linked proximal tubulopathy with characteristic abnormalities that include low-molecular-weight (LMW) proteinuria, hypercalciuria, and other features of Fanconi syndrome, such as glycosuria, aminoaciduria, and phosphaturia. Although some patients develop nephrocalcinosis, nephrolithiasis, progressive renal failure, and hypophosphatemic rickets, patients with Dent disease typically do not have proximal renal tubular acidosis or extrarenal manifestations. Since the turn of the century, loss-of-function mutations of the *CLCN5* gene, which is located in Xp11.22 and encodes a renal Cl^-/H^+ antiporter (ClC-5), have been reported consistently in patients with Dent disease. Genetic heterogeneity of Dent disease in some patients who exhibit mutations in the gene for OCRL1 (responsible for Lowe syndrome) also meets Dent disease criteria:Dent-2 disease. Dent disease includes X-linked recessive nephrolithiasis with renal failure, X-linked recessive hypophosphatemic rickets, and idiopathic LMW proteinuria seen in Japanese children.

Mutations in an extracellular basolateral calcium sensing receptor (CASR), normally present in the loop of Henle can cause a dominant Bartter syndrome–like picture. These patients' predominant symptoms are hypocalcemic hypercalciuria, which differentiates them from patients with Bartter syndrome.

In the distal convoluted tubule, gain-of-function mutations in *WNK1* and loss-of-function mutations in *WNK4*, both serine threonine kinases, lead to excessive NCCT-mediated salt reabsorption with the clinical picture of pseudohypoaldosteronism type 2 (familial hyperkalemic hypertension [FHH], or **Gordon syndrome**).

In the collecting duct, gain-of-function mutations of the gene that encodes the epithelial sodium channel causes an inherited form of hypertension, **Liddle syndrome.** Patients with this disorder have constitutive sodium uptake in the collecting duct, with hypokalemia and suppressed aldosterone. Conversely, loss-of-function mutations cause pseudohypoaldosteronism, characterized by severe sodium wasting and hyperkalemia. A variant of the latter disorder is associated with systemic abnormalities, including defects in sweat chloride, and can resemble cystic fibrosis.

BIBLIOGRAPHY

Please visit the Nelson Textbook of Pediatrics *website at* *www.expertconsult.com* *for the complete bibliography.*

Chapter 526 Tubulointerstitial Nephritis

Craig C. Porter and Ellis D. Avner

Tubulointerstitial nephritis (TIN, also called interstitial nephritis) is the term applied to conditions characterized by tubulointerstitial inflammation and damage with relative sparing of glomeruli and vessels. Both acute and chronic primary forms exist. Interstitial nephritis can also be present with primary glomerular diseases as well as systemic diseases affecting the kidney.

ACUTE TUBULOINTERSTITIAL NEPHRITIS

Pathogenesis and Pathology

The hallmarks of acute TIN are lymphocytic infiltration of the tubulointerstitium, tubular edema, and varying degrees of tubular damage. Eosinophils may be present, especially in drug-induced TIN; occasionally, granulomas occur. The pathogenesis is not fully understood, but a T cell–mediated immune mechanism has been postulated. A large number of medications, especially antimicrobials, anticonvulsants, and analgesics, have been implicated as etiologic agents (Table 526-1). Other causes include infections, primary glomerular diseases, and systemic diseases such as systemic lupus erythematosus (SLE).

Clinical Manifestations

The classic presentation of acute TIN is fever, rash, and arthralgia in the setting of a rising serum creatinine. Although the full triad may be noted in drug-induced TIN, many patients with acute TIN do not have all the typical features. The rash can vary from maculopapular to urticarial and is often transient. Patients often have nonspecific constitutional symptoms of nausea, vomiting, fatigue, and weight loss. Flank pain may be present owing to stretching of the renal capsule from acute inflammatory enlargement of the kidney. If acute TIN is caused by a systemic disease such as SLE, the clinical presentation will be consistent with specific signs and symptoms of the underlying disease. Unlike the typical presentation of oliguric acute renal failure seen with glomerular diseases, 30-40% of patients with acute TIN are nonoliguric, and hypertension is less common. Peripheral eosinophilia can occur, especially with drug-induced TIN. Some degree of microscopic hematuria is invariably present, but significant hematuria or proteinuria >1.5 g/day is uncommon. One exception is patients whose TIN is caused by nonsteroidal anti-inflammatory drugs (NSAIDs), who can present with the nephrotic syndrome. Urinalysis can reveal white blood cells and granular or hyaline casts, but red blood cell casts, characteristic of glomerular disease, are not seen. The presence of urine eosinophils is neither sensitive nor specific.

Diagnosis

The diagnosis is usually made based on clinical presentation and laboratory findings. A renal biopsy will establish the correct diagnosis in cases where the etiology or clinical course confounds the diagnosis. A careful history of the timing of disease onset in relation to drug exposure is essential in suspected drug-induced TIN. Because of the immune-mediated nature of TIN, signs or symptoms generally appear in 1-2 wk after exposure. In children, antimicrobials are a common inciting agent. NSAIDs are an important cause of acute TIN in children, and volume depletion or underlying chronic renal disease can increase the risk of occurrence. Urinalysis and serial measurements of serum creatinine and electrolytes should be monitored. Renal ultrasonography is not diagnostic but can demonstrate enlarged, echogenic kidneys. Removal of a suspected offending agent followed by spontaneous improvement in renal function is highly suggestive of the diagnosis, and additional testing is generally not performed. In more severe cases, in which the cause is unclear or the patient's renal function deteriorates rapidly, a renal biopsy may be indicated.

Treatment and Prognosis

Treatment includes supportive care directed at addressing complications of acute renal failure such as hyperkalemia or volume overload. Corticosteroid administration within 2 wk of the discontinuation of certain offending agents (e.g., NSAIDs or antibiotics) can hasten recovery and improve long-term prognosis. Whether these data apply to other inciting agents is not clear. For patients with prolonged renal insufficiency, the prognosis remains guarded, and severe acute TIN from any cause can progress to chronic TIN.

CHRONIC TUBULOINTERSTITIAL NEPHRITIS

In children, chronic TIN most commonly occurs as the result of underlying congenital urologic renal disease, such as obstructive uropathy or vesicoureteral reflux, or an underlying metabolic disorder affecting the kidneys (see Table 526-1). Chronic TIN

Table 526-1 ETIOLOGY OF INTERSTITIAL NEPHRITIS

ACUTE
Drugs
• Antimicrobials
• Penicillin derivatives
• Cephalosporins
• Sulfonamides
• Trimethoprim-sulfamethoxazole
• Ciprofloxacin
• Tetracyclines
• Erythromycin derivatives
• Amphotericin B
• Anticonvulsants
• Carbamazepine
• Phenobarbital
• Phenytoin
• Sodium valproate
• Other drugs
• Allopurinol
• 5-Aminosalicylic acid
• Cimetidine
• Cyclosporine
• Diuretics
• Escitalopram
• Mesalazine
• Nonsteroidal anti-inflammatory drugs
• Protease inhibitors
• Proton pump inhibitors
Infections
• Adenovirus
• Bacteria associated with acute pyelonephritis
• BK virus
• Streptococcal species
• Cytomegalovirus
• Epstein-Barr virus
• Hepatitis B virus
• Histoplasmosis
• Human immunodeficiency virus
• Hantavirus
• Leptospirosis
• *Toxoplasma gondii*
Disease-associated
• Glomerulonephritis (e.g., systemic lupus erythematosus)
• Acute allograft rejection
• Tubulointerstitial nephritis and uveitis syndrome
Idiopathic
CHRONIC
Drugs and toxins
• Analgesics
• Cyclosporine
• Lithium
• Heavy metals
Infections (see Acute)
Disease-associated
• Metabolic and hereditary
• Cystinosis
• Oxalosis
• Fabry disease
• Wilson disease
• Sickle cell nephropathy
• Alport syndrome
• Juvenile nephronophthisis, medullary cystic disease
• Polycystic kidney disease
Immunologic
• Systemic lupus erythematosus
• Crohn disease
• Chronic allograft rejection
• Tubulointerstitial nephritis and uveitis syndrome
Urologic
• Posterior urethral valves
• Eagle-Barrett syndrome
• Ureteropelvic junction obstruction
• Vesicoureteral reflux
Miscellaneous
• Balkan nephropathy
• Chinese herb nephropathy
• Radiation
• Sarcoidosis
• Neoplasm
Idiopathic

can occur as an idiopathic disease, although this is more common in adults.

The juvenile nephronophthisis (JN)–medullary cystic kidney disease complex (MCKD) is a group of inherited cystic renal diseases that share a common histologic phenotype of chronic TIN. JN is generally inherited as an autosomal recessive trait. Although rare in the USA, JN causes 10-20% of pediatric end-stage renal disease (ESRD) in Europe. Patients with JN typically present with polyuria, growth failure, "unexplained" anemia, and chronic renal failure in late childhood or adolescence. Variants of JN with extrarenal involvement include **Senior-Løken syndrome** (retinitis pigmentosa), **Joubert syndrome,** and **oculomotor apraxia type Cogan. MCKD** is an autosomal dominant disease that typically manifests in adulthood. **Tubulointerstitial nephritis with uveitis** is a rare autoimmune syndrome of chronic TIN with anterior uveitis and bone marrow granulomas that occurs primarily in adolescent girls. Chronic TIN is seen in all forms of progressive renal disease, regardless of the underlying cause, and the severity of interstitial disease is the single most important factor predicting progression to ESRD.

Pathogenesis and Pathology

The pathophysiology of chronic TIN is undefined, but data suggest that it is immune-mediated. Cells making up the interstitial infiltrate appear to be a combination of native interstitial cells, inflammatory cells recruited from the circulation, and resident tubular cells that undergo epithelial-mesenchymal transformation. Grossly, kidneys can appear pale and small for age. Microscopically, tubular atrophy and "dropout" with interstitial fibrosis and a patchy lymphocytic interstitial inflammation are seen. Patients with JN often have characteristic small cysts in the corticomedullary region. In primary chronic TIN, glomeruli are relatively spared until late in the disease course. Patients with chronic TIN secondary to a primary glomerular disease have histologic evidence of the primary disease.

Clinical Manifestations

The clinical features of chronic TIN are often nonspecific and can reflect signs and symptoms of chronic renal insufficiency (Chapter 529). Fatigue, growth failure, polyuria, polydipsia, and enuresis are often present. Anemia that is seemingly disproportionate to the degree of renal insufficiency is common and is a particularly prominent feature of juvenile nephronophthisis. Because tubular damage often leads to renal salt wasting, significant hypertension is unusual. Fanconi syndrome, proximal renal tubular acidosis, distal renal tubular acidosis, and hyperkalemic distal renal tubular acidosis can occur.

Diagnosis

The diagnosis is suggested by signs or symptoms of renal tubular damage such as polyuria and an elevated serum creatinine value, coupled with a history suggestive of a chronic disease, such as long-standing enuresis or the presence of anemia resistant to iron therapy. Radiographic studies, in particular ultrasonography, can give additional evidence of chronicity, such as small, echogenic kidneys, corticomedullary microcysts suggesting JN, or findings of obstructive uropathy. A vesicocystourethrogram can demonstrate the presence of vesicoureteral reflux or bladder abnormalities. If JN is suspected, molecular diagnosis is available. In instances in which the cause is unclear, a renal biopsy may be performed. In cases of advanced disease, a renal biopsy might not be diagnostic. Many end-stage kidney diseases display a common histologic appearance of tubular fibrosis and inflammation.

Treatment and Prognosis

Therapy is directed at maintaining fluid and electrolyte balance and avoiding further exposure to nephrotoxic agents. Patients with obstructive uropathies can require salt supplementation and treatment with potassium-binding resin (Kayexalate). Prevention of infection by antibiotic prophylaxis can slow progression of renal damage in appropriate patients. Prognosis in patients with chronic TIN depends in large part on the nature of the underlying disease. Patients with obstructive uropathy or vesicoureteral reflux can have a variable degree of renal damage and thus a variable course. ESRD can develop over months to years. Patients with JN uniformly progress to ESRD by adolescence. Patients with metabolic disorders can benefit from treatment when available.

BIBLIOGRAPHY

Please visit the Nelson Textbook of Pediatrics *website at www.expertconsult.com for the complete bibliography.*

Section 5 TOXIC NEPHROPATHIES—RENAL FAILURE

Chapter 527 Toxic Nephropathy

Craig C. Porter and Ellis D. Avner

Aberrant renal function often results from purposeful or accidental exposure to any number of agents that are potential or actual nephrotoxins. Iodinated radiocontrast agents are generally well tolerated by most patients without significant adverse consequences. In volume-depleted patients or patients with underlying chronic kidney disease, their use poses a serious risk for the development of acute kidney injury with significant attendant morbidity and mortality. Biologic nephrotoxins include venomous exposures from insects, reptiles, amphibians, and a wide variety of sea-dwelling animals. The most common forms of toxic nephropathy unfortunately relate to the purposeful exposure of children to pharmacologic agents, accounting for close to 20% of episodes of acute kidney injury occurring in children and adolescents. Age, underlying medical condition including surgical exposure, genetics, exposure dose, and the concomitant use of other drugs all influence the likelihood of developing acute kidney injury.

Agents that commonly cause acute kidney injury and some of their clinical manifestations are summarized in Table 527-1. Mechanisms of injury often help to explain the presentation; multiple toxic exposures in patients with complicated clinical histories often limit the ability to clearly establish clinical cause and effect. For example, diminished urine output may be the clinical hallmark of tubular obstruction cause by agents such as methotrexate or agents that cause acute tubular necrosis such as amphotericin B or pentamidine. Alternatively, nephrogenic diabetes insipidus may be the critical clinical manifestation of agents that cause interstitial nephritis such as lithium or cisplatin. Nephrotoxicity is often reversible if the noxious agent is promptly removed.

Clinically necessary potential nephrotoxins should be used judiciously, not summarily avoided. Necessity of exposure, dosing parameters, and the use of drug levels or pharmacogenomic data, when available, should always be considered. Caution is particularly critical for patients with complex medical conditions that

Table 527-1 RENAL SYNDROMES PRODUCED BY NEPHROTOXINS

NEPHROTIC SYNDROME	**FANCONI SYNDROME**
Angiotensin-converting enzyme inhibitors Gold salts Interferon Mercury compounds Nonsteroidal anti-inflammatory drugs Penicillamine	Aminoglycosides Chinese herbs (aristolochic) Cisplatin Heavy metals (cadmium, lead, mercury, and uranium) Ifosfamide Lysol Outdated tetracycline
NEPHROGENIC DIABETES INSIPIDUS	**RENAL TUBULAR ACIDOSIS**
Amphotericin B Cisplatin Colchicine Demeclocycline Lithium Methoxyflurane Propoxyphene Vinblastine	Amphotericin B Lead Lithium Toluene
RENAL VASCULITIS	**INTERSTITIAL NEPHRITIS**
Hydralazine Isoniazid Penicillins Propylthiouracil Sulfonamides Numerous other drugs that can cause a hypersensitivity reaction	Amidopyrine *p*-Aminosalicylate Carbon tetrachloride Cephalosporins Cimetidine Cisplatin Colistin Copper Cyclosporine Ethylene glycol Foscarnet Gentamicin Gold salts Indomethacin Interferon-α Iron Kanamycin Lithium Mannitol Mercury salts Mitomycin C Neomycin Nonsteroidal anti-inflammatory drugs Penicillins (especially methicillin) Pentamidine Phenacetin Phenylbutazone Poisonous mushrooms Polymyxin B Radiocontrast agents Rifampin Salicylate Streptomycin Sulfonamides Tacrolimus Tetrachloroethylene Trimethoprim-sulfamethoxazole
THROMBOTIC MICROANGIOPATHY	
Cyclosporine A Oral contraceptive agents Mitomycin C	
NEPHROCALCINOSIS OR NEPHROLITHIASIS	
Allopurinol Bumetanide Ethylene glycol Furosemide Melamine Methoxyflurane Topiramate Vitamin D	
ACUTE RENAL FAILURE	
Acetaminophen Acyclovir Aminoglycosides Amphotericin B Angiotensin-converting enzyme inhibitors Biologic toxins (snake, spider, bee, wasp) Cisplatin Cyclosporine Ethylene glycol Halothane Heavy metals Ifosfamide Lithium Methoxyflurane Nonsteroidal anti-inflammatory drugs Radiocontrast agents Tacrolimus Vancomycin	
OBSTRUCTIVE UROPATHY	
Sulfonamides Acyclovir Methotrexate Protease inhibitors Ethylene glycol Methoxyflurane	

include pre-existing renal disease, cardiac disease, diabetes, and/or complicated surgeries. Alternative modalities of care provision should be also be considered when possible. Imaging modalities such as ultrasonography, radionuclide scanning, or magnetic resonance imaging may be preferable to contrast studies in some patients. Alternatively, judicious volume expansion with or without the administration of *N*-acetylcysteine might offer renoprotection when radioiodinated contrast studies are critical. Pharmacologic agents with no known renal effects can often be substituted for known nephrotoxins with equal clinical efficacy. In all cases, simultaneous use of known nephrotoxins should be avoided whenever necessary.

BIBLIOGRAPHY
Please visit the Nelson Textbook of Pediatrics *website at* *www.expertconsult.com* *for the complete bibliography.*

Chapter 528 Cortical Necrosis

Priya Pais and Ellis D. Avner

Renal cortical necrosis is a rare cause of acute renal failure occurring secondary to extensive ischemic damage of the renal cortex. It occurs most commonly in neonates and in adolescents of childbearing age.

ETIOLOGY

In newborns, cortical necrosis is most commonly associated with hypoxic or ischemic insults caused by perinatal asphyxia, placental abruption, and twin-twin or fetal-maternal transfusion. Other causes include renal vascular thrombosis and severe congenital heart disease. After the neonatal period, cortical necrosis is most commonly seen in children with septic shock or severe hemolytic-uremic syndrome. In adolescents and women, cortical necrosis occurs in association with obstetric complications including septic abortion and intrauterine fetal demise.

Less-common causes of cortical necrosis include extensive burns, snakebite, infectious endocarditis, and medications (e.g., nonsteroidal anti-inflammatory agents).

EPIDEMIOLOGY

Renal cortical necrosis is a rare disease entity accounting for only 2% of all cases of acute renal failure in developed countries. The incidence is higher in developing countries.

PATHOLOGY

Grossly, areas of necrosis are limited to the cortex of the kidney. Histologic findings consist of acute ischemic infarction. Intravascular and intraglomerular thromboses are present. These changes are bilateral and may be patchy or involve the whole cortex.

PATHOGENESIS

Cortical necrosis develops as a result of acute severe decreased renal arterial blood flow secondary to vascular spasm from ischemia or hypoxia or from endothelial cell injury from toxins or HUS. This leads to glomerular and arteriolar microthrombi and consequent cortical necrosis.

CLINICAL MANIFESTATIONS

Cortical necrosis manifests as acute renal failure in patients who have the previously mentioned predisposing causes. Urine output is diminished and gross and/or microscopic hematuria may be present. Hypertension is common, and thrombocytopenia may be present as a result of renal microvascular injury.

LABORATORY AND RADIOLOGIC FINDINGS

Laboratory results are consistent with acute renal failure: an elevated blood urea nitrogen (BUN) and creatinine, hyperkalemia, and metabolic acidosis. Anemia and thrombocytopenia are common. Urinalysis reveals hematuria and proteinuria.

Ultrasound examination with Doppler demonstrates decreased perfusion to both kidneys. A radionuclide renal scan shows decreased uptake with significantly delayed or absent function.

TREATMENT

It is important to treat the underlying cause, where possible. Therapy involves medical management of acute renal failure as well as the initiation of dialysis, where necessary. Management is otherwise supportive and involves volume repletion, correction of asphyxia, and treatment of sepsis.

PROGNOSIS

Untreated, renal cortical necrosis has a mortality rate >50%. Long-term recovery of renal function depends on the amount of surviving cortex. Children with partial recovery can require therapy for end-stage renal disease. All patients require continued follow-up for chronic kidney disease.

BIBLIOGRAPHY
Please visit the Nelson Textbook of Pediatrics *website at* *www.expertconsult.com* *for the complete bibliography.*

Chapter 529 Renal Failure

529.1 Acute Renal Failure

Rajasree Sreedharan and Ellis D. Avner

Acute renal failure (ARF), also termed *acute renal insufficiency*, is a clinical syndrome in which a sudden deterioration in renal function results in the inability of the kidneys to maintain fluid and electrolyte homeostasis. ARF occurs in 2-3% of children admitted to pediatric tertiary care centers and in as many as 8% of infants in neonatal intensive care units. A classification system has been proposed to standardize the definition of acute kidney injury in adults. These criteria of risk, injury, failure, loss, and end-stage renal disease were given the acronym of RIFLE. A modified RIFLE criteria (pRIFLE) has been developed to characterize the pattern of acute kidney injury in critically ill children (Table 529-1). Because RIFLE focuses on glomerular filtration rate (GFR), a modification (Acute Kidney Injury Network, AKIN) categorizes severity by rise in serum creatinine: stage 1 >150%, stage II >200%, stage III >300%.

PATHOGENESIS

ARF has been conventionally classified into 3 categories: prerenal, intrinsic renal, and postrenal (Table 529-2).

Prerenal ARF, also called *prerenal azotemia,* is characterized by diminished effective circulating arterial volume, which leads to inadequate renal perfusion and a decreased GFR. Evidence of kidney damage is absent. Common causes of prerenal ARF

Table 529-1 PEDIATRIC-MODIFIED RIFLE (PRIFLE) CRITERIA

CRITERIA	ESTIMATED CCl	URINE OUTPUT
Risk	eCCl decrease by 25%	<0.5 mL/kg/hr for 8 hr
Injury	eCCl decrease by 50%	<0.5 mL/kg/hr for 16 hr
Failure	eCCl decrease by 75% or eCCl <35 ml/min/1.73 m^2	<0.3 mL/kg/hr for 24 hr or anuric for 12 hr
Loss	Persistent failure >4 wk	
End-stage	End-stage renal disease (persistent failure >3 mo)	

eCCl, estimated creatinine clearance; pRIFLE, pediatric risk, injury, failure, loss and end-stage renal disease.

Table 529-2 COMMON CAUSES OF ACUTE RENAL FAILURE

PRERENAL
Dehydration Hemorrhage Sepsis Hypoalbuminemia Cardiac failure
INTRINSIC RENAL
Glomerulonephritis • Postinfectious/poststreptococcal • Lupus erythematosus • Henoch-Schönlein purpura • Membranoproliferative • Anti-glomerular basement membrane Hemolytic-uremic syndrome Acute tubular necrosis Cortical necrosis Renal vein thrombosis Rhabdomyolysis Acute interstitial nephritis Tumor infiltration Tumor lysis syndrome
POSTRENAL
Posterior urethral valves Ureteropelvic junction obstruction Ureterovesicular junction obstruction Ureterocele Tumor Urolithiasis Hemorrhagic cystitis Neurogenic bladder

include dehydration, sepsis, hemorrhage, severe hypoalbuminemia, and cardiac failure. If the underlying cause of the renal hypoperfusion is reversed promptly, renal function returns to normal. If hypoperfusion is sustained, intrinsic renal parenchymal damage can develop.

Intrinsic renal ARF includes a variety of disorders characterized by renal parenchymal damage, including sustained hypoperfusion and ischemia. Many forms of **glomerulonephritis,** including postinfectious glomerulonephritis, lupus nephritis, Henoch-Schönlein purpura nephritis, membranoproliferative glomerulonephritis, and anti-glomerular basement membrane nephritis, can cause ARF. **Hemolytic-uremic syndrome** (HUS) has been described as the most common cause of intrinsic ARF in the USA (Chapter 512).

Acute tubular necrosis (ATN) occurs most often in critically ill infants and children who have been exposed to nephrotoxic and/or perfusion insults. Sepsis, hypovolemic shock, and increased intra-abdominal pressure (abdominal compartment syndrome) are important causes of ATN. The typical pathologic process of ATN is tubular cell necrosis, although significant histologic changes are not consistently seen in patients with clinical ATN. The mechanisms of injury in ATN can include alterations in intrarenal hemodynamics, tubular obstruction, and passive backleak of the glomerular filtrate across injured tubular cells into the peritubular capillaries.

Tumor lysis syndrome is a specific form of ARF related to spontaneous or chemotherapy-induced cell lysis in patients with lymphoproliferative malignancies. This disorder is primarily caused by obstruction of the tubules by uric acid crystals (Chapters 489 and 490). **Acute interstitial nephritis** is an increasingly common cause of ARF and is usually a result of a hypersensitivity reaction to a therapeutic agent or various infectious agents (Chapter 526).

Postrenal ARF includes a variety of disorders characterized by obstruction of the urinary tract. In neonates and infants, congenital conditions such as posterior urethral valves and bilateral ureteropelvic junction obstruction account for the majority of cases of ARF. Other conditions such as urolithiasis, tumor (intra-abdominal or within the urinary tract), hemorrhagic cystitis, and neurogenic bladder can cause ARF in older children and adolescents. In a patient with 2 functioning kidneys, obstruction must be bilateral to result in ARF. Relief of the obstruction usually results in recovery of renal function except in patients with associated renal dysplasia or prolonged urinary tract obstruction.

CLINICAL MANIFESTATIONS AND DIAGNOSIS

A carefully taken history is critical in defining the cause of ARF. An infant with a 3-day history of vomiting and diarrhea most likely has prerenal ARF caused by volume depletion, but HUS must be a consideration. A 6 yr old child with a recent pharyngitis who presents with periorbital edema, hypertension, and gross hematuria most likely has intrinsic ARF related to acute postinfectious glomerulonephritis. A critically ill child with a history of protracted hypotension or with exposure to nephrotoxic medications most likely has ATN. A neonate with a history of hydronephrosis on prenatal ultrasound and a palpable bladder and prostate most likely has congenital urinary tract obstruction, probably related to posterior urethral valves.

The physical examination must be thorough, with careful attention to volume status. Tachycardia, dry mucous membranes, and poor peripheral perfusion suggest inadequate circulating volume and the possibility of prerenal ARF (Chapter 54). Peripheral edema, rales, and a cardiac gallop suggest volume overload and the possibility of intrinsic ARF from glomerulonephritis or ATN. The presence of a rash and arthritis might suggest systemic lupus erythematosus (SLE) or Henoch-Schönlein purpura nephritis. Palpable flank masses might suggest renal vein thrombosis, tumors, cystic disease, or urinary tract obstruction.

LABORATORY FINDINGS

Laboratory abnormalities can include anemia (the anemia is usually dilutional or hemolytic, as in SLE, renal vein thrombosis, HUS); leukopenia (SLE, sepsis); thrombocytopenia (SLE, renal vein thrombosis, sepsis, HUS); hyponatremia (dilutional); metabolic acidosis; elevated serum concentrations of blood urea nitrogen, creatinine, uric acid, potassium, and phosphate (diminished renal function); and hypocalcemia (hyperphosphatemia).

The serum C3 level may be depressed (postinfectious glomerulonephritis, SLE, or membranoproliferative glomerulonephritis), and antibodies may be detected in the serum to streptococcal (poststreptococcal glomerulonephritis), nuclear (SLE), neutrophil cytoplasmic (Wegener granulomatosis, microscopic polyarteritis), or glomerular basement membrane (Goodpasture disease) antigens.

The presence of hematuria, proteinuria, and red blood cell or granular urinary casts suggests intrinsic ARF, in particular glomerular disease. The presence of white blood cells and white blood cell casts, with low-grade hematuria and proteinuria, suggests tubulointerstitial disease. Urinary eosinophils may be present in children with drug-induced tubulointerstitial nephritis.

Urinary indices may be useful in differentiating prerenal ARF from intrinsic ARF (Table 529-3). Patients whose urine shows an elevated specific gravity (>1.020), elevated urine osmolality (UOsm > 500 mOsm/kg), low urine sodium (UNa < 20 mEq/L), and fractional excretion of sodium (FENa) <1% (<2.5% in neonates) most likely have prerenal ARF. Those with a specific gravity of <1.010, low urine osmolality (UOsm < 350 mOsm/kg), high urine sodium (UNa > 40 mEq/L), and FENa > 2% (>10% in neonates) most likely have intrinsic ARF.

Chest radiography may reveal cardiomegaly, pulmonary congestion (fluid overload) or pleural effusions. Renal ultrasonography can reveal hydronephrosis and/or hydroureter, which suggest urinary tract obstruction, or nephromegaly, suggesting

Table 529-3 URINALYSIS, URINE CHEMISTRIES, AND OSMOLALITY IN ACUTE RENAL FAILURE

	HYPOVOLEMIA	ACUTE TUBULAR NECROSIS	ACUTE INTERSTITIAL NEPHRITIS	GLOMERULONEPHRITIS	OBSTRUCTION
Sediment	Bland	Broad, brownish granular casts	White blood cells, eosinophils, cellular casts	Red blood cells, red blood cell casts	Bland or bloody
Protein	None or low	None or low	Minimal but may be increased with NSAIDs	Increased, >100 mg/dL	Low
Urine sodium, mEq/L*	<20	>30	>30	<20	<20 (acute) >40 (few days)
Urine osmolality, mOsm/kg	>400	<350	<350	>400	<350
Fractional excretion of sodium %†	<1	>1	Varies	<1	<1 (acute) >1 (few days)

*The sensitivity and specificity of urine sodium of <20 in differentiating prerenal azotemia from acute tubular necrosis are 90% and 82%, respectively.
†Fractional excretion of sodium is the urine:plasma (U/P) ratio of sodium divided by U/P of creatinine × 100. The sensitivity and specificity of fractional excretion of sodium of <1% in differentiating prerenal azotemia from acute tubular necrosis are 96% and 95%, respectively.
NSAIDs, nonsteroidal anti-inflammatory drugs.
From Singri N, Ahya SN, Levin ML: Acute renal failure, *JAMA* 289:747–751, 2003.

intrinsic renal disease. Renal biopsy can ultimately be required to determine the precise cause of ARF in patients who do not have clearly defined prerenal or postrenal ARF.

Though serum creatinine is used to measure kidney function, it is an insensitive and delayed measure of decreased kidney function following acute kidney injury. Other biomarkers under investigation include changes in plasma neutrophil gelatinase-associated lipocalin (NGAL) and cystatin C levels and urinary changes in NGAL, interleukin-18 (IL-18), and kidney injury molecule-1 (KIM-1).

TREATMENT

Medical Management

In infants and children with urinary tract obstruction, such as in a newborn with suspected posterior ureteral valves, a bladder catheter should be placed immediately to ensure adequate drainage of the urinary tract. The placement of a bladder catheter may also be considered in nonambulatory older children and adolescents to accurately monitor urine output during ARF.

Determination of the volume status is of critical importance when initially evaluating a patient with ARF. If there is no evidence of volume overload or cardiac failure, intravascular volume should be expanded by intravenous administration of isotonic saline, 20 mL/kg over 30 min. In the absence of blood loss or hypoproteinemia, colloid-containing solutions are not required for volume expansion. Severe hypovolemia may require additional fluid boluses (Chapters 53, 54, and 64). Determination of the central venous pressure may be helpful if adequacy of the blood volume is difficult to determine. After volume resuscitation, hypovolemic patients generally void within 2 hr; failure to do so points to intrinsic or postrenal ARF. Hypotension due to sepsis requires vigorous fluid resuscitation followed by a continuous infusion of norepinephrine.

Diuretic therapy should be considered only after the adequacy of the circulating blood volume has been established. Mannitol (0.5 g/kg) and furosemide (2-4 mg/kg) may be administered as a single IV dose. Bumetanide (0.1 mg/kg) may be given as an alternative to furosemide. If urine output is not improved, then a continuous diuretic infusion may be considered. To increase renal cortical blood flow, many clinicians administer dopamine (2-3 μg/kg/min) in conjunction with diuretic therapy, although no controlled data support this practice. There is little evidence that diuretics or dopamine can prevent ARF or hasten recovery. Mannitol may be effective in pigment (myoglobin, hemoglobin)-induced renal failure. Atrial natriuretic peptide may be of value in preventing or treating acute kidney injury; there is little pediatric evidence.

If there is no response to a diuretic challenge, diuretics should be discontinued and fluid restriction is essential. Patients with a relatively normal intravascular volume should initially be limited to 400 mL/m^2/24 hr (insensible losses) plus an amount of fluid equal to the urine output for that day. Extrarenal (blood, gastrointestinal [GI] tract) fluid losses should be replaced, milliliter for milliliter, with appropriate fluids. Markedly hypervolemic patients can require further fluid restriction, omitting the replacement of insensible fluid losses, urine output, and extrarenal losses to diminish the expanded intravascular volume. Fluid intake, urine and stool output, body weight, and serum chemistries should be monitored on a daily basis.

In ARF, rapid development of **hyperkalemia** (serum potassium level >6 mEq/L) can lead to cardiac arrhythmia, cardiac arrest, and death. The earliest electrocardiographic change seen in patients with developing hyperkalemia is the appearance of peaked T waves. This may be followed by widening of the QRS intervals, ST segment depression, ventricular arrhythmias, and cardiac arrest (Chapter 52.4). Procedures to deplete body potassium stores should be initiated when the serum potassium value rises to >6.0 mEq/L. Exogenous sources of potassium (dietary, intravenous fluids, total parenteral nutrition) should be eliminated. Sodium polystyrene sulfonate resin (Kayexalate), 1 g/kg, should be given orally or by retention enema. This resin exchanges sodium for potassium and can take several hours to take effect. A single dose of 1 g/kg can be expected to lower the serum potassium level by about 1 mEq/L. Resin therapy may be repeated every 2 hr, the frequency being limited primarily by the risk of sodium overload.

More-severe elevations in serum potassium (>7 mEq/L), especially if accompanied by electrocardiographic changes, require emergency measures in addition to Kayexalate. The following agents should be administered:

- Calcium gluconate 10% solution, 1.0 mL/kg IV, over 3-5 min
- Sodium bicarbonate, 1-2 mEq/kg IV, over 5-10 min
- Regular insulin, 0.1 U/kg, with glucose 50% solution, 1 mL/kg, over 1 hr

Calcium gluconate counteracts the potassium-induced increase in myocardial irritability but does not lower the serum potassium level. Administration of sodium bicarbonate, insulin, glucose lowers the serum potassium level by shifting potassium from the extracellular to the intracellular compartment. A similar effect has been reported with the acute administration of β-adrenergic agonists in adults, but there are no controlled data in pediatric patients. Because the duration of action of these emergency measures is just a few hours, persistent hyperkalemia should be managed by dialysis.

Mild **metabolic acidosis** is common in ARF because of retention of hydrogen ions, phosphate, and sulfate, but it rarely requires treatment. If acidosis is severe (arterial pH < 7.15; serum bicarbonate < 8 mEq/L) or contributes to hyperkalemia, treatment is required. The acidosis should be corrected partially by the intravenous route, generally giving enough bicarbonate to raise the arterial pH to 7.20 (which approximates a serum bicarbonate level of 12 mEq/L). The remainder of the correction may be accomplished by oral administration of sodium bicarbonate after normalization of the serum calcium and phosphorus levels. Correction of metabolic acidosis with intravenous bicarbonate can precipitate tetany in patients with renal failure as rapid correction of acidosis reduces the ionized calcium concentration (Chapter 52).

Hypocalcemia is primarily treated by lowering the serum phosphorus level. Calcium should not be given intravenously, except in cases of tetany, to avoid deposition of calcium salts into tissues. Patients should be instructed to follow a low-phosphorus diet, and phosphate binders should be orally administered to bind any ingested phosphate and increase GI phosphate excretion. Common agents include sevelamer (Renagel), calcium carbonate (Tums tablets or Titralac suspension), and calcium acetate (PhosLo). Aluminum-based binders, commonly employed in the past, should be avoided because of the established risk of aluminum toxicity.

Hyponatremia is most commonly a dilutional disturbance that must be corrected by fluid restriction rather than sodium chloride administration. Administration of hypertonic (3%) saline should be limited to patients with symptomatic hyponatremia (seizures, lethargy) or those with a serum sodium level <120 mEq/L. Acute correction of the serum sodium to 125 mEq/L (mmol/L) should be accomplished using the following formula:

$$\text{mEq NaCl required} = 0.6 \times \text{weight (kg)} \times [125 - \text{serum sodium (mEq/L)}]$$

ARF patients are predisposed to **GI bleeding** because of uremic platelet dysfunction, increased stress, and heparin exposure if on hemodialysis or continuous renal replacement therapy. Oral or intravenous H_2 blockers such as ranitidine are commonly administered to prevent this complication.

Hypertension can result from hyperreninemia associated with the primary disease process and/or expansion of the extracellular fluid volume and is most common in ARF patients with acute glomerulonephritis or HUS. Salt and water restriction is critical, and diuretic administration may be useful (Chapter 439). Isradipine (0.05-0.15 mg/kg/dose, maximum dose 5 mg qid) may be administered for relatively rapid reduction in blood pressure. Longer-acting agents such as calcium channel blockers (amlodipine, 0.1-0.6 mg/kg/24 hr qd or divided bid) or β-blockers (propranolol, 0.5-8 mg/kg/24 hr divided bid or tid; labetalol, 4-40 mg/kg/24 hr divided bid or tid) may be helpful in maintaining control of blood pressure. Children with severe symptomatic hypertension (hypertensive urgency or emergency) should be treated with continuous infusions of sodium nitroprusside (0.5-10 μg/kg/min), labetalol (0.25-3.0 mg/kg/hr), or esmolol (150-300 μg/kg/min) and converted to intermittently dosed antihypertensives when more stable.

Neurologic symptoms in ARF can include headache, seizures, lethargy, and confusion (encephalopathy). Potential etiologic factors include hyponatremia, hypocalcemia, hypertension, cerebral hemorrhage, cerebral vasculitis, and the uremic state. Diazepam is the most effective agent in controlling seizures, and therapy should be directed toward the precipitating cause.

The **anemia** of ARF is generally mild (hemoglobin 9-10 g/dL) and primarily results from volume expansion (hemodilution). Children with HUS, SLE, active bleeding, or prolonged ARF can require transfusion of packed red blood cells if their hemoglobin level falls below 7 g/dL. In hypervolemic patients, blood transfusion carries the risk of further volume expansion, which can precipitate hypertension, heart failure, and pulmonary edema. Slow (4-6 hr) transfusion with packed red blood cells (10 mL/kg) diminishes the risk of hypervolemia. The use of fresh washed red blood cells minimizes the risk of hyperkalemia. In the presence of severe hypervolemia or hyperkalemia, blood transfusions are most safely administered during dialysis or ultrafiltration.

Nutrition is of critical importance in children who develop ARF. In most cases, sodium, potassium, and phosphorus should be restricted. Protein intake should be restricted moderately while maximizing caloric intake to minimize the accumulation of nitrogenous wastes. In critically ill patients with ARF, parenteral hyperalimentation with essential amino acids should be considered.

Dialysis

Indications for dialysis in ARF include the following:

- Volume overload with evidence of hypertension and/or pulmonary edema refractory to diuretic therapy
- Persistent hyperkalemia
- Severe metabolic acidosis unresponsive to medical management
- Neurologic symptoms (altered mental status, seizures)
- Blood urea nitrogen >100-150 mg/dL (or lower if rapidly rising)
- Calcium:phosphorus imbalance, with hypocalcemic tetany

An additional indication for dialysis is the inability to provide adequate nutritional intake because of the need for severe fluid restriction. In patients with ARF, dialysis support may be necessary for days or for up to 12 wk. Many patients with ARF require dialysis support for 1-3 wk. The advantages and disadvantages of the 3 types of dialysis are shown in Table 529-4.

Intermittent hemodialysis is useful in patients with relatively stable hemodynamic status. This highly efficient process accomplishes both fluid and electrolyte removal in 3- to 4-hr sessions using a pump-driven extracorporeal circuit and large central venous catheter. Intermittent hemodialysis may be performed 3 to 7 times per week based on the patient's fluid and electrolyte balance.

Peritoneal dialysis is most commonly employed in neonates and infants with ARF, although this modality may be used in children and adolescents of all ages. Hyperosmolar dialysate is

Table 529-4 COMPARISON OF PERITONEAL DIALYSIS, INTERMITTENT HEMODIALYSIS, AND CONTINUAL RENAL REPLACEMENT THERAPY

	PD	IHC	CRRT
BENEFITS			
Fluid removal	+	++	++
Urea and creatinine clearance	+	++	+
Potassium clearance	++	++	+
Toxin clearance	+	++	+
COMPLICATIONS			
Abdominal pain	+	–	–
Bleeding	–	+	+
Dysequilibrium	–	+	–
Electrolyte imbalance	+	+	+
Need for heparinization	–	+	+
Hyperglycemia	+	–	–
Hypotension	+	++	+
Hypothermia	–	–	+
Central line infection	–	+	+
Inguinal or abdominal hernia	+	–	–
Peritonitis	+	–	–
Protein loss	+	–	–
Respiratory compromise	+	–	–
Vessel thrombosis	–	+	+

PD, peritoneal dialysis; IH, intermittent hemodialysis; CRRT, continual renal replacement therapy.

Adapted from Rogers MC: *Textbook of pediatric intensive care,* Baltimore, 1992, Williams & Wilkins.

infused into the peritoneal cavity via a surgically or percutaneously placed peritoneal dialysis catheter. The fluid is allowed to dwell for 45-60 min and is then drained from the patient by gravity (manually or with the use of a cycler machine), accomplishing fluid and electrolyte removal. Cycles are repeated for 8-24 hr/day based on the patient's fluid and electrolyte balance. Anticoagulation is not necessary. Peritoneal dialysis is contraindicated in patients with significant abdominal pathology.

Continuous renal replacement therapy (CRRT) is useful in patients with unstable hemodynamic status, concomitant sepsis, or multiorgan failure in the intensive care setting. CRRT is an extracorporeal therapy in which fluid, electrolytes, and small- and medium-sized solutes are continuously removed from the blood (24 hr/day) using a specialized pump-driven machine. Usually, a double-lumen catheter is placed into the subclavian, internal jugular, or femoral vein. The patient is then connected to the pump-driven CRRT circuit, which continuously passes the patient's blood across a highly permeable filter.

CRRT may be performed in 3 basic fashions. In continuous venovenous hemofiltration (CVVH), a large amount of fluid moves by pressure across the filter, bringing with it by convection other molecules such as urea, creatinine, phosphorus, and uric acid. The blood volume is reconstituted by IV infusion of a replacement fluid having a desirable electrolyte composition similar to that of blood. Continuous venovenous hemofiltration dialysis (CVVH-D) uses the principle of diffusion by circulating dialysate in a countercurrent direction on the ultrafiltrate side of the membrane. No replacement fluid is used. Continuous hemodiafiltration (CVVH-DF) employs both replacement fluid and dialysate, offering the most effective solute removal of all forms of CRRT.

Table 529-4 compares the relative risks and benefits of the various renal replacement therapies.

PROGNOSIS

The mortality rate in children with ARF is variable and depends entirely on the nature of the underlying disease process rather than on the renal failure itself. Children with ARF caused by a renal-limited condition such as postinfectious glomerulonephritis have a very low mortality rate (<1%); those with ARF related to multiorgan failure have a very high mortality rate (>90%).

The prognosis for recovery of renal function depends on the disorder that precipitated ARF. Recovery of renal function is likely after ARF resulting from prerenal causes, HUS, ATN, acute interstitial nephritis, or tumor lysis syndrome. Recovery of renal function is unusual when ARF results from most types of rapidly progressive glomerulonephritis, bilateral renal vein thrombosis, or bilateral cortical necrosis. Medical management may be necessary for a prolonged period to treat the sequelae of ARF, including chronic renal insufficiency, hypertension, renal tubular acidosis, and urinary concentrating defect.

BIBLIOGRAPHY

Please visit the Nelson Textbook of Pediatrics *website at www.expertconsult.com for the complete bibliography.*

529.2 Chronic Kidney Disease

Rajasree Sreedharan and Ellis D. Avner

Chronic kidney disease (CKD) is defined as renal injury (proteinuria) and/or a glomerular filtration rate <60 mL/min/1.73 m^2 for >3 mo. The prevalence of CKD in the pediatric population is approximately 18 per 1 million. The prognosis for the infant, child, or adolescent with CKD has improved dramatically since the 1970s because of improvements in medical management (aggressive nutritional support, recombinant erythropoietin, recombinant growth hormone [rGH]), dialysis techniques, and kidney transplantation.

ETIOLOGY

In children, CKD may be the result of congenital, acquired, inherited, or metabolic renal disease, and the underlying cause correlates closely with the age of the patient at the time when the CKD is first detected. CKD in children <5 yr old is most commonly a result of congenital abnormalities such as renal hypoplasia, dysplasia, or obstructive uropathy. Additional causes include congenital nephrotic syndrome, prune belly syndrome, cortical necrosis, focal segmental glomerulosclerosis, polycystic kidney disease, renal vein thrombosis, and hemolytic uremic syndrome.

After 5 yr of age, acquired diseases (various forms of glomerulonephritis including lupus nephritis) and inherited disorders (familial juvenile nephronophthisis, Alport syndrome) predominate. CKD related to metabolic disorders (cystinosis, hyperoxaluria) and certain inherited disorders (polycystic kidney disease) can occur throughout the childhood years.

PATHOGENESIS

In addition to progressive injury with ongoing structural or metabolic genetic diseases, renal injury can progress despite removal of the original insult.

Hyperfiltration injury may be an important final common pathway of glomerular destruction, independent of the underlying cause of renal injury. As nephrons are lost, the remaining nephrons undergo structural and functional hypertrophy characterized by an increase in glomerular blood flow. The driving force for glomerular filtration is thereby increased in the surviving nephrons. Although this compensatory hyperfiltration temporarily preserves total renal function, it can cause progressive damage to the surviving glomeruli, possibly by a direct effect of the elevated hydrostatic pressure on the integrity of the capillary wall and/or the toxic effect of increased protein traffic across the capillary wall. Over time, as the population of sclerosed nephrons increases, the surviving nephrons suffer an increased excretory burden, resulting in a vicious cycle of increasing glomerular blood flow and hyperfiltration injury.

Proteinuria itself can contribute to renal functional decline, as evidenced by studies that have shown a beneficial effect of reduction in proteinuria. Proteins that traverse the glomerular capillary wall can exert a direct toxic effect on tubular cells and recruit monocytes and macrophages, enhancing the process of glomerular sclerosis and tubulointerstitial fibrosis. Uncontrolled **hypertension** can exacerbate disease progression by causing arteriolar nephrosclerosis and by increasing the hyperfiltration injury.

Hyperphosphatemia can increase progression of disease by leading to calcium phosphate deposition in the renal interstitium and blood vessels. Hyperlipidemia, a common condition in CKD patients, can adversely affect glomerular function through oxidant-mediated injury.

CKD may be viewed as a continuum of disease, with increasing biochemical and clinical manifestations as renal function deteriorates. The pathophysiologic manifestations of CKD are outlined in Table 529-5. The terminology to describe the stages of chronic kidney disease is standardized (Table 529-6). End-stage renal disease (ESRD) is an administrative term in the USA, defining all patients treated with dialysis or kidney transplantation. Patients with ESRD are a subset of the patients with stage 5 CKD.

CLINICAL MANIFESTATIONS

The clinical presentation of CKD is varied and depends on the underlying renal disease. Children and adolescents with CKD

Table 529-5 PATHOPHYSIOLOGY OF CHRONIC KIDNEY DISEASE

MANIFESTATION	MECHANISMS
Accumulation of nitrogenous waste products	Decrease in glomerular filtration rate
Acidosis	Decreased ammonia synthesis Impaired bicarbonate reabsorption Decreased net acid excretion
Sodium retention	Excessive renin production Oliguria
Sodium wasting	Solute diuresis Tubular damage
Urinary concentrating defect	Solute diuresis Tubular damage
Hyperkalemia	Decrease in glomerular filtration rate Metabolic acidosis Excessive potassium intake Hyporeninemic hypoaldosteronism
Renal osteodystrophy	Impaired renal production of 1,25-dihydroxycholecalciferol Hyperphosphatemia Hypocalcemia Secondary hyperparathyroidism
Growth retardation	Inadequate caloric intake Renal osteodystrophy Metabolic acidosis Anemia Growth hormone resistance
Anemia	Decreased erythropoietin production Iron deficiency Folate deficiency Vitamin B_{12} deficiency Decreased erythrocyte survival
Bleeding tendency	Defective platelet function
Infection	Defective granulocyte function Impaired cellular immune functions Indwelling dialysis catheters
Neurologic symptoms (fatigue, poor concentration, headache, drowsiness, memory loss, seizures, peripheral neuropathy)	Uremic factor(s) Aluminum toxicity Hypertension
Gastrointestinal symptoms (feeding intolerance, abdominal pain)	Gastroesophageal reflux Decreased gastrointestinal motility
Hypertension	Volume overload Excessive renin production
Hyperlipidemia	Decreased plasma lipoprotein lipase activity
Pericarditis, cardiomyopathy	Uremic factor(s) Hypertension Fluid overload
Glucose intolerance	Tissue insulin resistance

Table 529-6 STANDARDIZED TERMINOLOGY FOR STAGES OF CHRONIC KIDNEY DISEASE

STAGE	DESCRIPTION	GFR (mL/min/1.73 m²)
1	Kidney damage with normal or increased GFR	>90
2	Kidney damage with mild decrease in GFR	60-89
3	Moderate decrease in GFR	30-59
4	Severe decrease in GFR	5-29
5	Kidney failure	<15 or on dialysis

GFR, glomerular filtration rate.

from chronic glomerulonephritis (membranoproliferative glomerulonephritis) can present with edema, hypertension, hematuria, and proteinuria. Infants and children with congenital disorders such as renal dysplasia and obstructive uropathy can present in the neonatal period with failure to thrive, polyuria dehydration, urinary tract infection, or overt renal insufficiency. Congenital kidney disease is diagnosed with prenatal ultrasonography in many infants, allowing early diagnostic and therapeutic intervention. Children with familial juvenile nephronophthisis can have a very subtle presentation with nonspecific complaints such as headache, fatigue, lethargy, anorexia, vomiting, polydipsia, polyuria, and growth failure over a number of years.

The physical examination in patients with CKD can reveal pallor and a sallow appearance. Patients with long-standing untreated CKD can have short stature and the bony abnormalities of renal osteodystrophy (Chapter 523.4). Children with CKD due to chronic glomerulonephritis (or children with advanced renal failure from any cause) can have edema, hypertension, and other signs of extracellular fluid volume overload.

LABORATORY FINDINGS

Laboratory findings can include elevations in blood urea nitrogen and serum creatinine. They can also reveal hyperkalemia, hyponatremia (if volume overloaded), acidosis, hypocalcemia, hyperphosphatemia, and an elevation in uric acid. Patients with heavy proteinuria can have hypoalbuminemia. A complete blood cell count shows a normochromic, normocytic anemia. Serum cholesterol and triglyceride levels are often elevated. In children with CKD caused by glomerulonephritis, the urinalysis shows hematuria and proteinuria. In children with CKD from congenital lesions such as renal dysplasia, the urinalysis usually has a low specific gravity and minimal abnormalities by dipstick or microscopy.

Inulin clearance is the gold standard to determine GFR, but it is not easy to measure. Endogenous creatinine clearance is the most widely used marker of GFR, but creatinine secretion falsely elevates the calculated GFR. Several other markers are under investigation to accurately determine GFR in children, such as cystatin C and iohexol. In children, the degree of renal dysfunction may be determined by applying the following formula, which provides an estimation of the patient's GFR:

$$\text{GFR (mL/min/1.73m}^2) = \frac{k \times \text{height (cm)}}{\text{serum creatinine (mg/dL)}}$$

where k is 0.33 for low-birthweight infants <1 yr old, 0.45 for term infants <1 yr old whose weight is appropriate for gestational age, 0.55 for children and adolescent girls, and 0.70 for adolescent boys.

TREATMENT

The treatment of CKD is aimed at replacing absent or diminished renal functions, which progressively deteriorate in parallel with the progressive loss of GFR, and slowing the progression of renal dysfunction. Children with CKD should be treated at a pediatric center capable of supplying multidisciplinary services, including medical, nursing, social service, nutritional, and psychological support.

The management of CKD requires close monitoring of a patient's clinical and laboratory status. Blood studies to be followed routinely include serum electrolytes, blood urea nitrogen, creatinine, calcium, phosphorus, albumin, alkaline phosphatase, and hemoglobin levels. Periodic measurement of intact parathyroid hormone (PTH) levels and roentgenographic studies of bone may be of value in detecting early evidence of renal osteodystrophy. Echocardiography should be performed periodically to identify left ventricular hypertrophy and cardiac dysfunction that can occur as a consequence of the complications of CKD.

Fluid and Electrolyte Management

Most children with CKD maintain normal sodium and water balance, with the sodium intake derived from an appropriate diet. Infants and children whose CKD is a consequence of renal dysplasia may be polyuric, with significant urinary sodium losses. These children can benefit from high-volume, low-caloric-density feedings with sodium supplementation. Children with high blood pressure, edema, or heart failure can require sodium restriction and diuretic therapy. Fluid restriction is rarely necessary in children with CKD until the development of end-stage renal disease (ESRD) requires the initiation of dialysis.

In most children with CKD, potassium balance is maintained until renal function deteriorates to the level at which dialysis is initiated. Hyperkalemia can develop, however, in patients with moderate renal insufficiency who have excessive dietary potassium intake, severe acidosis, or hyporeninemic hypoaldosteronism (related to destruction of the renin-secreting juxtaglomerular apparatus). Hyperkalemia may be treated by restriction of dietary potassium intake, administration of oral alkalinizing agents, and/or treatment with Kayexalate.

Acidosis

Metabolic acidosis develops in almost all children with CKD as a result of decreased net acid excretion by the failing kidneys. Either Bicitra (1 mEq sodium citrate/mL) or sodium bicarbonate tablets (650 mg = 8 mEq of base) may be used to maintain the serum bicarbonate level >22 mEq/L.

Nutrition

Patients with CKD usually require progressive restriction of various dietary components as their renal function declines. Dietary phosphorus, potassium, and sodium should be restricted according to the individual patient's laboratory studies and fluid balance. In infants with CKD, formulas containing a reduced amount of phosphate (Similac PM 60/40) are commonly employed.

The optimal caloric intake in patients with CKD is unknown, but it is recommended to provide at least the recommended dietary allowance of caloric intake for age. Protein intake should be 2.5 g/kg/24 hr and should consist of proteins of high biologic value that are metabolized primarily to usable amino acids rather than to nitrogenous wastes. The proteins of highest biologic value are those of eggs and milk, followed by meat, fish, and fowl.

Dietary intake should be adjusted according to response, optimally through consultation with a dietitian with expertise in childhood CKD. Caloric intake may be enhanced in infants by supplementing the formula with modular components of carbohydrates (Polycose), fat (medium chain triglyceride [MCT] oil), and protein (pro-Mod) as tolerated by the patient. In older children and adolescents, commercial enteral products (Boost) may be helpful. If oral caloric intake remains inadequate and/or weight gain and growth velocity are suboptimal, enteral tube feedings should be considered. Supplemental feedings may be provided via a nasogastric, gastrostomy, or gastrojejunal tube. Continuous overnight infusions with or without daytime bolus administrations are commonly employed.

Children with CKD can become deficient in water-soluble vitamins either because of inadequate dietary intake or dialysis losses. These should be routinely supplied, using preparations such as Nephrocaps (Fleming, Fenton, MO). Zinc and iron supplements should be added only if deficiencies are confirmed. Supplementation with fat-soluble vitamins A, E, and K is usually not required.

Growth

Short stature is a significant long-term sequela of childhood CKD. Children with CKD have an apparent growth hormone (GH)-resistant state, with elevated GH levels but decreased insulin-like growth factor 1 levels and major abnormalities of insulin-like growth factor–binding proteins.

Children with CKD who remain less than −2 SD for height despite optimal medical support (adequate caloric intake and effective treatment of renal osteodystrophy, anemia, and metabolic acidosis) might benefit from treatment with pharmacologic doses of recombinant human GH (rHuGH). Treatment may be initiated with rHuGH (0.05 mg/kg/24 hr) subcutaneously, with periodic adjustment in the dose to achieve a goal of normal height velocity for age.

Treatment with rHuGH continues until the patient reaches the 50th percentile for midparental height or achieves a final adult height or undergoes kidney transplantation. Long-term rHuGH treatment significantly improves final adult height and induces persistent catch-up growth; some patients achieve normal adult height.

Renal Osteodystrophy

The term *renal osteodystrophy* is used to indicate a spectrum of bone disorders seen in patients with CKD. The most common condition seen in children is high-turnover bone disease caused by secondary hyperparathyroidism. The skeletal pathologic finding in this condition is osteitis fibrosa cystica.

The **pathophysiology** of renal osteodystrophy is complex. Early in the course of CKD, when the GFR declines to approximately 50% of normal, the decrease in functional kidney mass leads to a decline in renal 1α-hydroxylase activity, with decreased production of activated vitamin D (1,25-dihydroxycholecalciferol). This deficiency in activated vitamin D results in decreased intestinal calcium absorption, hypocalcemia, and increased parathyroid gland activity. Excessive parathyroid hormone (PTH) secretion attempts to correct the hypocalcemia by effecting an increase in bone resorption. Later in the course of CKD, when the GFR declines to 20-25% of normal, compensatory mechanisms to enhance phosphate excretion become inadequate, resulting in hyperphosphatemia, which further promotes hypocalcemia and increased PTH secretion.

Clinical manifestations of renal osteodystrophy include muscle weakness, bone pain, and fractures with minor trauma. In growing children, rachitic changes, varus and valgus deformities of the long bones, and slipped capital femoral epiphyses may be seen. Laboratory studies can demonstrate a decreased serum calcium level, increased serum phosphorus level, increased alkaline phosphatase, and a normal PTH level. Radiographs of the hands, wrists, and knees show subperiosteal resorption of bone with widening of the metaphyses.

The goals of **treatment** are to prevent bone deformity and normalize growth velocity using both dietary and pharmacologic interventions. Children and adolescents should follow a low-phosphorus diet, and infants should be provided with a low-phosphorus formula such as Similac PM 60/40. It is impossible to fully restrict phosphorus intake, and so phosphate binders are used to enhance fecal phosphate excretion. Although calcium carbonate (Tums) and calcium acetate (PhosLo) have historically been the most commonly used phosphate binders, newer, non–calcium-based binders such as sevelamer (Renagel) are increasing in use, particularly in patients prone to hypercalcemia. Because aluminum may be absorbed from the GI tract and can lead to aluminum toxicity, aluminum-based binders should be avoided.

The cornerstone of therapy for renal osteodystrophy is vitamin D administration. **Vitamin D therapy** is indicated in patients with 25-hydroxy-vitamin D levels below the established goal range for the child's particular stage of CKD or in patients with PTH levels above the established goal range for CKD stage. Patients with low 25(OH)D (25-hydroxy-vitamin D) levels should be treated with ergocalciferol. Patients with a normal 25(OH)D level but elevated PTH level should be treated with 0.01-0.05 μg/kg/24 hr of calcitriol (Rocaltrol, 0.25-μg capsules or 1 μg/mL suspension). Newer activated vitamin D analogs such as paricalcitol and doxercalciferol are increasingly used, especially in patients predisposed to hypercalcemia. Phosphate binders and vitamin D should be adjusted to maintain the PTH level within the designated goal range and the serum calcium and phosphorus levels within the normal range for age. Many nephrologists also attempt to maintain the calcium/phosphorus product ($Ca \times PO_4$) at <55 to minimize the possibility of tissue deposition of calcium phosphorus salts.

Adynamic Bone Disease

Adynamic bone disease (low-turnover bone disease) has been recognized in children and adults with CKD. The pathologic finding is osteomalacia and is associated with oversuppression of PTH, perhaps related to the widespread use of calcium-containing phosphate binders and vitamin D analogs.

Anemia

Anemia in patients with CKD is primarily the result of inadequate erythropoietin production by the failing kidneys and usually becomes manifest in patients with stages 3-4 CKD.

Other possible contributory factors include iron deficiency, folic acid or vitamin B_{12} deficiency, and decreased erythrocyte survival. Recombinant human erythropoietin (rHuEPO) therapy has decreased the need for transfusion in patients with CKD. Erythropoietin is usually initiated when the patient's hemoglobin concentration falls below 10 g/dL, at a dose of 50-150 mg/kg/dose subcutaneously 1-3 times weekly. The dose is adjusted to maintain the hemoglobin concentration between 11 and 12 g/dL, not more than 13 g/dL. All patients receiving rHuEPO therapy should be provided with either oral or intravenous iron supplementation. Patients who appear to be resistant to rHuEPO should be evaluated for iron deficiency, occult blood loss, chronic infection or inflammatory state, vitamin B_{12} or folate deficiency, and bone marrow fibrosis related to secondary hyperparathyroidism. An alternative option is darbepoetin alfa (Aranesp), a longer-acting agent administered at a dose of 0.45 μg/kg/wk. The chief advantage of this agent is that it may be dosed once weekly to once monthly because of its extended duration of action.

Hypertension

Children with CKD can have sustained hypertension related to volume overload and/or excessive renin production related to glomerular disease. Hypertensive children with suspected volume overload should follow a salt-restricted diet (2-3 g/24 hr) and can benefit from diuretic therapy. Thiazide diuretics (hydrochlorothiazide 2 mg/kg/24 hr divided bid) are the initial diuretic class of choice for children with mild renal dysfunction (CKD stages 1-3). However, when a patient's estimated GFR falls into stage 4 CKD, thiazides are less effective and loop diuretics (furosemide 1-2 mg/kg/dose bid or tid) become the diuretic class of choice. **Angiotensin-converting enzyme (ACE) inhibitors** (enalapril, lisinopril) and angiotensin II blockers (losartan) are the antihypertensive medications of choice in all children with proteinuric renal disease because of their potential ability to slow the progression to ESRD. Extreme care must be used with these agents, however, to monitor renal function and electrolyte balance, particularly in children with advanced CKD. Calcium channel blockers (amlodipine), β-blockers (propranolol, atenolol), and centrally acting agents (clonidine) may be useful as adjunctive agents in children with CKD whose blood pressure cannot be controlled using dietary sodium restriction, diuretics, and ACE inhibitors.

Immunizations

Children with CKD should receive all standard immunizations according to the schedule used for healthy children. An exception must be made in withholding live vaccines from children with CKD related to glomerulonephritis during treatment with immunosuppressive medications. It is critical, however, to make every attempt to administer live virus vaccines for measles, mumps, and rubella (MMR) and varicella before kidney transplantation because these vaccines are not advised for use in immunosuppressed patients. All children with CKD should receive a yearly influenza vaccine. Data suggest that children with CKD might respond suboptimally to immunizations.

Adjustment In Drug Dose

Because many drugs are excreted by the kidneys, their dosing might need to be adjusted in patients with CKD to maximize effectiveness and minimize the risk of toxicity. Strategies in dosage adjustment include lengthening of the interval between doses, decreasing the absolute dose, or both.

Progression of Disease

Although there are no definitive treatments to improve renal function in children or adults with CKD, there are several strategies that may be effective in slowing the rate of progression of renal dysfunction. Optimal control of hypertension (maintaining the blood pressure at lower than the 75th percentile and perhaps even lower) is critical in all patients with CKD. ACE inhibitors or angiotensin II receptor blockers should be the antihypertensive drugs of choice in hypertensive children with chronic proteinuric renal disease. Such agents should also be strongly considered in children with CKD who have significant proteinuria, even in the absence of hypertension. Serum phosphorus should be maintained within the normal range for age and the calcium-phosphorus product <55 to minimize renal calcium-phosphorus deposition. Prompt treatment of infectious complications and episodes of dehydration can minimize additional loss of renal parenchyma.

Other potentially beneficial recommendations include correction of anemia with erythropoietin or darbepoetin alfa therapy, control of hyperlipidemia, avoidance of cigarette smoking, prevention of obesity, and minimization of use of nonsteroidal anti-inflammatory medications. Although dietary protein restriction has been shown to be useful in adults, this recommendation is generally not suggested for children with CKD because of the concern of adverse effects on growth and development.

BIBLIOGRAPHY

Please visit the Nelson Textbook of Pediatrics *website at www.expertconsult.com for the complete bibliography.*

529.3 End-Stage Renal Disease

Rajasree Sreedharan and Ellis D. Avner

ESRD represents the state in which a patient's renal dysfunction has progressed to the point at which homeostasis and survival can no longer be sustained with native kidney function and maximal medical management. At this point, renal replacement therapy (dialysis or renal transplantation) becomes necessary. The ultimate goal for children with ESRD is successful kidney transplantation (Chapter 530) because it provides the most normal lifestyle and possibility for rehabilitation for the child and family.

In the USA, 75% of children with ESRD require a period of dialysis before transplantation can be performed. It is recommended that plans for renal replacement therapy be initiated when a child reaches stage 4 CKD. The optimal time to actually initiate dialysis, however, is based on a combination of the biochemical and clinical characteristics of the patient including refractory fluid overload, electrolyte imbalance, acidosis, growth failure, or uremic symptoms, including fatigue, nausea, and impaired school performance. In general, most nephrologists attempt to initiate dialysis early enough to prevent the development of severe fluid and electrolyte abnormalities, malnutrition, and uremic symptoms. Pre-emptive transplantation before initiation of dialysis is increasingly being used.

The selection of dialysis modality must be individualized to fit the needs of each child. In the USA, ⅔ of children with ESRD are treated with peritoneal dialysis, whereas ⅓ are treated with hemodialysis. Age is a defining factor in dialysis modality selection: 88% of infants and children from birth to 5 yr of age are treated with peritoneal dialysis, and 54% of children >12 yr of age are treated with hemodialysis.

Table 529-7 MERITS OF PERITONEAL DIALYSIS IN PEDIATRIC PATIENTS WITH END-STAGE RENAL DISEASE
ADVANTAGES
Ability to perform dialysis treatment at home
Technically easier than hemodialysis, especially in infants
Ability to live a greater distance from medical center
Freedom to attend school and after-school activities
Less-restrictive diet
Less expensive than hemodialysis
Independence (adolescents)
DISADVANTAGES
Catheter malfunction
Catheter-related infections (peritonitis, exit site)
Impaired appetite (due to full peritoneal cavity)
Negative body image
Caregiver burnout

Peritoneal dialysis is a technique that employs the patient's peritoneal membrane as a dialyzer. Excess body water is removed by an osmotic gradient created by the high dextrose concentration in the dialysate; wastes are removed by diffusion from the peritoneal capillaries into the dialysate. Access to the peritoneal cavity is achieved by a surgically inserted, tunneled catheter.

Peritoneal dialysis may be provided either as continuous ambulatory peritoneal dialysis or as any of several forms of automated therapies using a cycler (continuous cyclic peritoneal dialysis, intermittent peritoneal dialysis, or nocturnal intermittent peritoneal dialysis). The majority of U.S. children treated with peritoneal dialysis use cycler-driven therapy, which allows the child and family to be free of dialysis demands during the waking hours. The exchanges are performed automatically during sleep by machine. This permits an uninterrupted day of activities, a reduction in the number of dialysis catheter connections and disconnections (which should decrease the risk of peritonitis), and a reduction in the time required by patients and parents to perform dialysis, reducing the risk of fatigue and burnout. Because peritoneal dialysis is not as efficient as hemodialysis, it must be performed daily rather than 3 times weekly as in hemodialysis. The merits of peritoneal dialysis are outlined in Table 529-7.

Hemodialysis, unlike peritoneal dialysis, is usually performed in a hospital setting. Children and adolescents typically have three 3- to 4-hr sessions per week during which fluid and solute wastes are removed. Access to the child's circulation is achieved by a surgically created arteriovenous fistula, graft, or indwelling subclavian or internal jugular catheter.

BIBLIOGRAPHY

Please visit the Nelson Textbook of Pediatrics *website at* *www.expertconsult.com* *for the complete bibliography.*

Chapter 530 Renal Transplantation

Minnie M. Sarwal and Cynthia J. Wong

Kidney transplantation is recognized as the optimal therapy for children with end-stage renal disease (ESRD). Five-yr survival rates in children who receive a kidney transplant are greater than survival rates of those who remain on hemodialysis or peritoneal dialysis according to U.S. Renal Data System (USRDS) data published in 2007. Children and adolescents with ESRD have special needs that differ from adults, including the need to achieve normal growth and cognitive development. Successful transplantation leads to improvement in their linear growth, allows them to attend school and be free of dietary restrictions. Immunosuppression protocols that employ steroid minimization or avoidance after transplantation demonstrate dramatic improvements in growth patterns for young children after transplantation. Improvements in surgical techniques and a reduction in the early complications in thrombosis have given young children the best long-term outcomes of all age groups among transplant recipients.

For the full continuation of this chapter, please visit the Nelson Textbook of Pediatrics *website at* *www.expertconsult.com.*

PART XXIV Urologic Disorders in Infants and Children

Chapter 531 Congenital Anomalies and Dysgenesis of the Kidneys

Jack S. Elder

EMBRYONIC DEVELOPMENT

For information on this topic, please visit the Nelson Textbook of Pediatrics *website at www.expertconsult.com.*

RENAL AGENESIS

Renal agenesis, or absent kidney development, can occur secondary to a defect of the wolffian duct, ureteric bud, or metanephric blastema. Unilateral renal agenesis has an incidence of 1/450-1,000 births. Unilateral renal agenesis often is discovered during the course of an evaluation for other congenital anomalies (VATER syndrome; e.g., Chapter 311). Its incidence is increased in newborns with a single umbilical artery. In true agenesis, the ureter and the ipsilateral bladder hemitrigone are absent. The contralateral kidney undergoes compensatory hypertrophy, to some degree prenatally but primarily after birth. Approximately 15% of these children have contralateral vesicoureteral reflux, and most males have an ipsilateral absent vas deferens because the wolffian duct is absent. Because the wolffian and müllerian ducts are contiguous, müllerian abnormalities in girls also are common. The **Mayer-Rokitansky-Kuster-Hauser** syndrome is a group of associated findings that includes unilateral renal agenesis or ectopia, ipsilateral müllerian defects, and vaginal agenesis (Chapter 548).

Renal agenesis is distinguished from aplasia, in which a nubbin of nonfunctioning tissue is seen capping a normal or abnormal ureter. This distinction may be difficult but usually is clinically insignificant. Unilateral renal agenesis is diagnosed in some patients based on the finding of an absent kidney on ultrasonography or excretory urography. Some of these patients actually were born with a hypoplastic kidney or a multicystic dysplastic kidney that underwent complete cyst regression. Although the specific diagnosis is not critical, if the finding of an absent kidney is based on an ultrasonogram, a functional imaging study such as an excretory urogram or renal scan should be performed because some of these patients have an ectopic kidney in the pelvis. If there is a normal contralateral kidney, long-term renal function should remain normal.

Bilateral renal agenesis is incompatible with extrauterine life and produces the **Potter syndrome.** Death occurs shortly after birth from pulmonary hypoplasia. The newborn has a characteristic facial appearance, termed *Potter facies* (Fig. 531-1). The eyes are widely separated with epicanthic folds, the ears are low set, the nose is broad and compressed flat, the chin is receding, and there are limb anomalies. Bilateral renal agenesis should be suspected when maternal ultrasonography demonstrates **oligohydramnios,** nonvisualization of the bladder, and absent kidneys. The incidence of this disorder is 1/3,000 births, with a male predominance, and represents 20% of newborns with the Potter phenotype. Other common causes of neonatal renal failure associated with the Potter phenotype include cystic renal dysplasia and obstructive uropathy. Less-common causes are autosomal recessive polycystic kidney disease (infantile), renal hypoplasia, and medullary dysplasia. Neonates with bilateral renal agenesis die of pulmonary insufficiency from pulmonary hypoplasia rather than renal failure (Chapter 95).

The term **familial renal adysplasia** describes families in which renal agenesis, renal dysplasia, multicystic kidney (dysplasia), or a combination, occurs in a single family. This disorder has an autosomal dominant inheritance pattern with a penetrance of 50-90% and variable expression. Because of this association, some clinicians advise screening first-degree relatives of persons who have renal agenesis or dysplasia, but this is not standard practice.

Whether persons with a solitary kidney should avoid contact sports such as football and karate is unresolved. The arguments favoring participation are that there are other solitary organs (spleen, liver, and brain) that do not preclude participation in contact sports, and there have been only a few reports of persons losing a kidney from sports injuries. The arguments against such participation are that the contralateral normal kidney is hypertrophic and not as well protected by the ribs, and a serious renal injury could have serious lifelong consequences. The American Academy of Pediatrics recommends an "individual assessment for contact, collision, and limited-contact sports."

RENAL DYSGENESIS: DYSPLASIA, HYPOPLASIA, AND CYSTIC ANOMALIES

Renal dysgenesis refers to maldevelopment of the kidney that affects its size, shape, or structure. The 3 principal types of dysgenesis are dysplastic, hypoplastic, and cystic. Although dysplasia always is accompanied by a decreased number of nephrons (hypoplasia), the converse is not true: Hypoplasia can occur in isolation. When both conditions are present, the term **hypodysplasia** is preferred. The term **dysplasia** is technically a histologic diagnosis and refers to focal, diffuse, or segmentally arranged primitive structures, specifically primitive ductal structures, resulting from abnormal metanephric differentiation. Nonrenal elements, such as cartilage, also may be present. The condition can affect all or only part of the kidney. If cysts are present, the condition is termed **cystic dysplasia.** If the entire kidney is dysplastic with a preponderance of cysts, the kidney is referred to as a **multicystic dysplastic kidney** (MCDK) (Fig. 531-2).

The pathogenesis of dysplasia is multifactorial. The "bud" theory proposes that if the ureteral bud arises in an abnormal location, such as an ectopic ureter, there is abnormal penetration and induction of the metanephric blastema, which causes abnormal kidney differentiation, resulting in dysplasia. Renal dysplasia also can occur with severe obstructive uropathy early in gestation, as with the most severe cases of posterior urethral valves or in an MCDK, in which a portion of the ureter is absent or atretic.

MCDK is a congenital condition in which the kidney is replaced by cysts and does not function; it can result from ureteral atresia. Kidney size is highly variable. The incidence is approximately 1/2,000. Some clinicians assume incorrectly that the terms *multicystic kidney* and *polycystic kidney* are synonymous. However, polycystic kidney disease is an inherited disorder that may be autosomal recessive or autosomal dominant and affects both kidneys (Chapter 515). MCDK usually is unilateral and generally is not inherited. Bilateral MCDKs are incompatible with life.

MCDK is the most common cause of an abdominal mass in the newborn, but the vast majority are nonpalpable at birth. In most cases it is discovered incidentally during prenatal sonography. In some patients, the cysts are identified prenatally, but the cysts regress in utero and no kidney is identified on imaging at birth. Contralateral hydronephrosis is present in 5-10% of patients. Sonography shows the characteristic appearance of a kidney replaced by multiple cysts of varying sizes that do not communicate, and no identifiable parenchyma is present; in most cases the diagnosis should be confirmed with a renal scan, which should demonstrate nonfunction. In some patients, usually boys, a small nonobstructing ureterocele is present in the bladder (Chapter 534). Although 15% have contralateral vesicoureteral reflux, obtaining a voiding cystourethrogram is optional, unless there is significant contralateral hydronephrosis. Management is controversial. Complete cyst regression occurs in nearly half of MCDKs by age 7 years. The risk of associated hypertension is 0.2-1.2%, and the risk of Wilms tumor arising from an MCDK is approximately 1/333. Because neoplasms arise from the stromal rather than the cystic component, even if the cysts regress completely, the likelihood that the kidney could develop a neoplasm is not altered.

Because of the occult nature of these potential problems, many clinicians advise annual follow-up with sonography and blood pressure measurement. The most important aspect of follow-up is being certain that the solitary kidney is functioning normally. If there is an abdominal mass, the cysts enlarge, the stromal core increases in size, or hypertension develops, nephrectomy is recommended. In lieu of follow-up screening, laparoscopic nephrectomy may be performed.

Renal hypoplasia refers to a small nondysplastic kidney that has fewer than the normal number of calyces and nephrons. The term encompasses a group of conditions with an abnormally small kidney and should be distinguished from aplasia, in which the kidney is rudimentary. If the condition is unilateral, the diagnosis usually is made incidentally during evaluation for another urinary tract problem or hypertension. Bilateral hypoplasia usually manifests with signs and symptoms of chronic renal failure and is a leading cause of end-stage renal disease during the 1st decade of life. A history of polyuria and polydipsia is common. Urinalysis results may be normal. In a rare form of bilateral hypoplasia called **oligomeganephronia,** the number of nephrons is markedly reduced and those present are markedly hypertrophied.

The **Ask-Upmark kidney,** also termed **segmental hypoplasia,** refers to small kidneys, usually weighing not more than 35 g, with one or more deep grooves on the lateral convexity, underneath which the parenchyma consists of tubules resembling those in the thyroid gland. It is unclear whether the lesion is congenital or acquired. Most patients are 10 yr or older at diagnosis and have severe hypertension. Nephrectomy usually controls the hypertension.

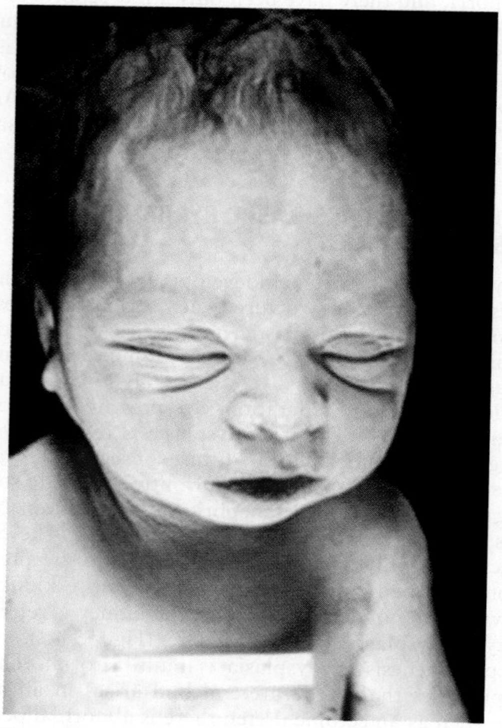

Figure 531-1 Stillborn infant with renal agenesis exhibiting characteristic Potter facies.

ANOMALIES IN SHAPE AND POSITION

During renal development the kidneys normally ascend from the pelvis into their normal position behind the ribs. The normal process of ascent and rotation of the kidney may be incomplete, resulting in renal ectopia or nonrotation. The ectopic kidney may be in a pelvic, iliac, thoracic, or contralateral position. If the ectopia is bilateral, in 90% of persons the two kidneys fuse. The incidence of renal ectopia is approximately 1 in 900 (Fig. 531-3).

Renal fusion anomalies are more common. The lower poles of the kidneys can fuse in the midline, resulting in a horseshoe kidney (Fig. 531-4); the fused portion is termed the *isthmus* and may be thick functioning parenchyma or a thin fibrous strand. Horseshoe kidneys occur in 1/400-500 births but are seen in 7% of patients with Turner syndrome. Horseshoe kidney is one of the many renal anomalies that occur in 30% of patients with Turner syndrome (Chapter 580). Wilms tumors are 4 times more common in children with horseshoe kidneys than in the general population. Stone disease and hydronephrosis secondary to ureteropelvic junction obstruction are other potential late complications. The incidence of MCDK affecting one of the 2 sides of a horseshoe kidney also appears to be increased. With crossed fused ectopia, one kidney crosses over to the other side and the

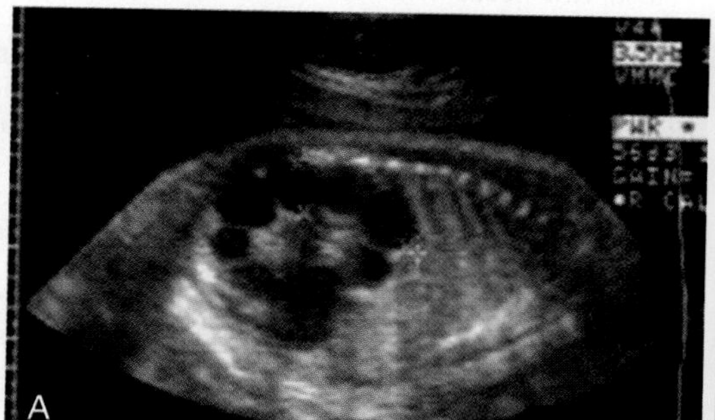

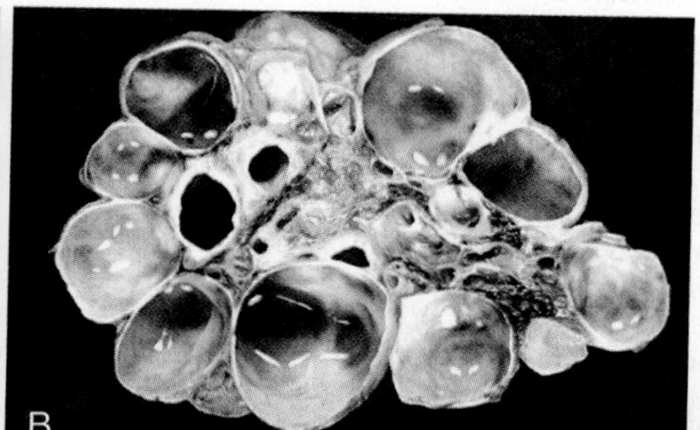

Figure 531-2 *A,* Prenatal sonogram demonstrating multicystic dysplastic kidney. *B,* Surgical specimen.

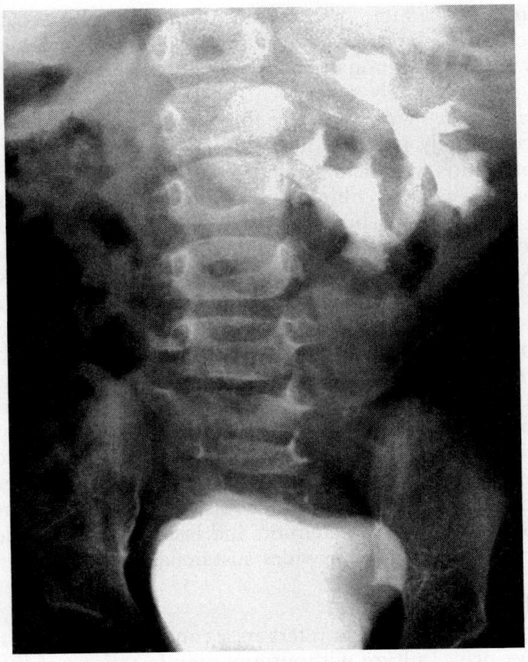

Figure 531-3 Crossed renal ectopia. Intravenous urography shows both renal collecting systems to the left of the spine. Segmentation anomalies of the sacrum, which are subtle in this child, are one of the skeletal anomalies associated with renal ectopia. (From Slovis T, editor: *Caffey's pediatric diagnostic imaging,* ed 11, vol 2, Philadelphia, 2008, Mosby, Fig 145-23A, p 2244.)

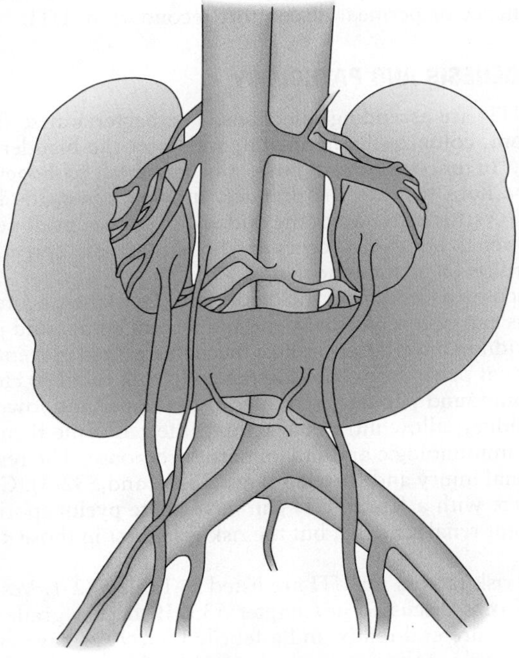

Figure 531-4 Horseshoe kidney.

parenchyma of the 2 kidneys is fused. Renal function usually is normal. In the most common finding, the left kidney may cross over and fuse with the lower pole of the right kidney. The insertion of the ureter to the bladder does not change, and the adrenal glands remain in their normal positions. The clinical significance of this anomaly is that if renal surgery is necessary, the blood supply is variable and can make partial nephrectomy more difficult.

ASSOCIATED PHYSICAL FINDINGS

Upper urinary tract anomalies are more common in children with certain physical findings. The incidence of renal anomalies is increased if there is a single umbilical artery and an abnormality of another organ system (congenital heart disease). External ear anomalies (particularly if the child has multiple congenital anomalies), imperforate anus, and scoliosis are associated with renal anomalies. Infants with these physical findings should undergo a renal sonogram.

BIBLIOGRAPHY

Please visit the Nelson Textbook of Pediatrics *website at* *www.expertconsult.com* *for the complete bibliography.*

Chapter 532
Urinary Tract Infections

Jack S. Elder

PREVALENCE AND ETIOLOGY

Urinary tract infections (UTIs) occur in 1-3% of girls and 1% of boys. In girls, the first UTI usually occurs by the age of 5 yr, with peaks during infancy and toilet training. In boys, most UTIs occur during the 1st yr of life; UTIs are much more common in uncircumcised boys, especially in the 1st year of life. The prevalence of UTIs varies with age. During the 1st yr of life, the male:female ratio is 2.8-5.4:1. Beyond 1-2 yr, there is a female preponderance, with a male:female ratio of 1:10.

UTIs are caused mainly by colonic bacteria. In girls, 75-90% of all infections are caused by *Escherichia coli* (Chapter 192), followed by *Klebsiella* spp and *Proteus* spp. Some series report that in boys >1 yr of age, *Proteus* is as common a cause as *E. coli;* others report a preponderance of gram-positive organisms in boys. *Staphylococcus saprophyticus* and enterococcus are pathogens in both sexes. Adenovirus and other viral infections also can occur, especially as a cause of cystitis.

Historically, UTIs have been considered a risk factor for the development of renal insufficiency or end-stage renal disease in children. Some researchers have questioned the importance of UTI as a risk factor, because only 2% of children with renal insufficiency report a history of UTI. This paradox may be secondary to better recognition of the risks of UTI and prompt diagnosis and therapy. Furthermore, many children receive antibiotics for fever without a focus (such as treating a questionable otitis media) resulting in a partially treated UTI.

CLINICAL MANIFESTATIONS AND CLASSIFICATION

The 3 basic forms of UTI are pyelonephritis, cystitis, and asymptomatic bacteriuria. Focal pyelonephritis (nephronia) and renal abscesses are less common.

Clinical Pyelonephritis

Clinical pyelonephritis is characterized by any or all of the following: abdominal, back, or flank pain; fever; malaise; nausea; vomiting; and, occasionally, diarrhea. *Fever may be the only manifestation.* Newborns can show nonspecific symptoms such as poor feeding, irritability, jaundice, and weight loss. Pyelonephritis is the most common serious bacterial infection in infants <24 mo of age who have fever without an obvious focus (Chapter 170). These symptoms are an indication that there is bacterial involvement of the upper urinary tract. Involvement of the renal parenchyma is termed *acute pyelonephritis,* whereas if there is no parenchymal involvement, the condition may be termed *pyelitis*. Acute pyelonephritis can result in renal injury, termed *pyelonephritic scarring*.

Acute lobar nephronia (acute lobar nephritis) is a renal mass caused by acute focal infection without liquefaction. It may be an early stage in the development of a renal abscess. Manifestations are identical to pyelonephritis; renal imaging demonstrates the abnormality (Fig. 532-1). *Renal abscess* can occur following a pyelonephritic infection due to the usual uropathogens or may be secondary to a primary bacteremia *(S. aureus)*. *Perinephric abscess* (see Fig. 532-4) can occur secondary to contiguous infection in the perirenal area (e.g., vertebral osteomyelitis, psoas abscess) or pyelonephritis that dissects to the renal capsule.

Xanthogranulomatous pyelonephritis is a rare type of renal infection characterized by granulomatous inflammation with giant cells and foamy histiocytes. It can manifest clinically as a renal mass or an acute or chronic infection. Renal calculi, obstruction, and infection with *Proteus* spp or *E. coli* contribute to the development of this lesion, which usually requires total or partial nephrectomy.

Cystitis

Cystitis indicates that there is bladder involvement; symptoms include dysuria, urgency, frequency, suprapubic pain, incontinence, and malodorous urine. Cystitis does not cause fever and does not result in renal injury. Malodorous urine is not specific for a UTI.

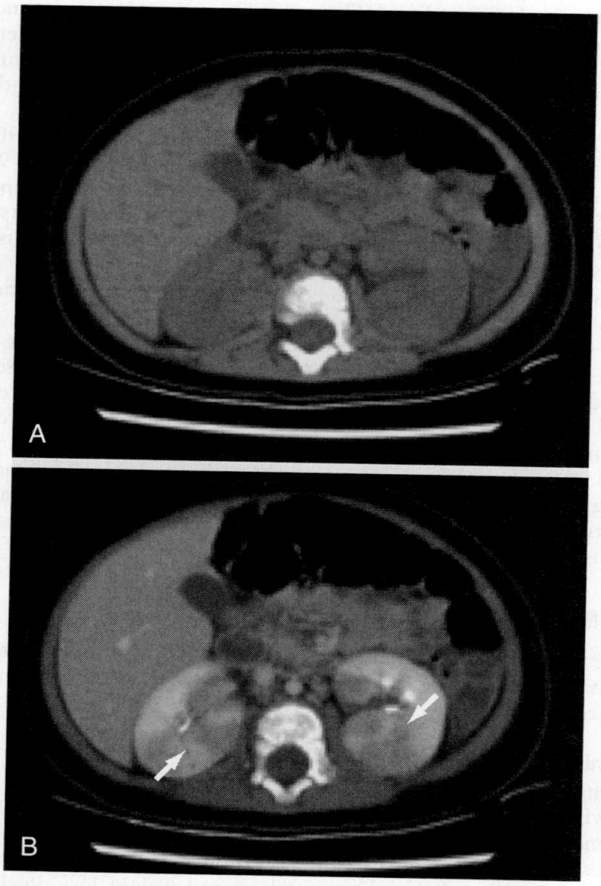

Figure 532-1 Characteristic precontrast *(A)* and contrast-enhanced *(B)* CT scans for an 8 mo old patient who had acute lobar nephronia and presented with severe bilateral nephromegaly but without a focal mass sonographically. No attenuation area is seen in the kidney before enhancement. (From Cheng CH, Tsau YK, Lin TY: Effective duration of antimicrobial therapy for the treatment of acute lobar nephronia, *Pediatrics* 117:e84–e89, 2006.)

Acute hemorrhagic cystitis often is caused by *E. coli;* it also has been attributed to adenovirus types 11 and 21. Adenovirus cystitis is more common in boys; it is self-limiting, with hematuria lasting approximately 4 days.

Eosinophilic cystitis is a rare form of cystitis of obscure origin that occasionally is found in children. The usual symptoms are those of cystitis with hematuria, ureteral dilation with occasional hydronephrosis, and filling defects in the bladder caused by masses that consist histologically of inflammatory infiltrates with eosinophils. Children with eosinophilic cystitis may have been exposed to an allergen. Bladder biopsy often is necessary to exclude a neoplastic process. Treatment usually includes antihistamines and nonsteroidal anti-inflammatory agents, but in some cases intravesical dimethyl sulfoxide instillation is necessary.

Interstitial cystitis is characterized by irritative voiding symptoms such as urgency, frequency, and dysuria, and bladder and pelvic pain relieved by voiding with a negative urine culture. The disorder is most likely to affect adolescent girls and is idiopathic (Chapter 513.1). Diagnosis is made by cystoscopic observation of mucosal ulcers with bladder distention. Treatments have included bladder hydrodistention and laser ablation of ulcerated areas, but no treatment provides sustained relief.

Asymptomatic Bacteriuria

Asymptomatic bacteriuria refers to a condition in which there is a positive urine culture without any manifestations of infection. It is most common in girls. The incidence is <1% in preschool and school-age girls and is rare in boys. The incidence declines with increasing age. This condition is benign and does not cause renal injury, except in pregnant women, in whom asymptomatic bacteriuria, if left untreated, can result in a symptomatic UTI. Some girls are mistakenly identified as having asymptomatic bacteriuria, whereas they actually are experiencing day or night incontinence or perineal discomfort secondary to UTI.

PATHOGENESIS AND PATHOLOGY

Most UTIs are ascending infections. The bacteria arise from the fecal flora, colonize the perineum, and enter the bladder via the urethra. In uncircumcised boys, the bacterial pathogens arise from the flora beneath the prepuce. In some cases, the bacteria causing cystitis ascend to the kidney to cause pyelonephritis. Rarely, renal infection occurs by hematogenous spread, as in endocarditis or in some neonates.

If bacteria ascend from the bladder to the kidney, acute pyelonephritis can occur. Normally the simple and compound papillae in the kidney have an antireflux mechanism that prevents urine in the renal pelvis from entering the collecting tubules. However, some compound papillae, typically in the upper and lower poles of the kidney, allow intrarenal reflux. Infected urine then stimulates an immunologic and inflammatory response. The result can cause renal injury and scarring (Figs. 532-2 and 532-3). Children of any age with a febrile UTI can have acute pyelonephritis and subsequent renal scarring, but the risk is highest in those <2 years of age.

Host risk factors for UTI are listed in Table 532-1. Vesicoureteral reflux is discussed in Chapter 533. If there is grade III, IV, or V vesicoureteral reflux and a febrile UTI, 90% have evidence of acute pyelonephritis on renal scintigraphy or other imaging studies. In girls, UTIs often occur at the onset of toilet training because of voiding dysfunction that occurs at that age. The child is trying to retain urine to stay dry, yet the bladder may have uninhibited contractions forcing urine out. The result may be high-pressure, turbulent urine flow or incomplete bladder emptying, both of which increase the likelihood of bacteriuria. Voiding dysfunction can occur in the toilet-trained child who voids infrequently. Similar problems can arise in school-age children who refuse to use the school bathroom. Obstructive uropathy resulting in hydronephrosis increases the risk of UTI because of urinary

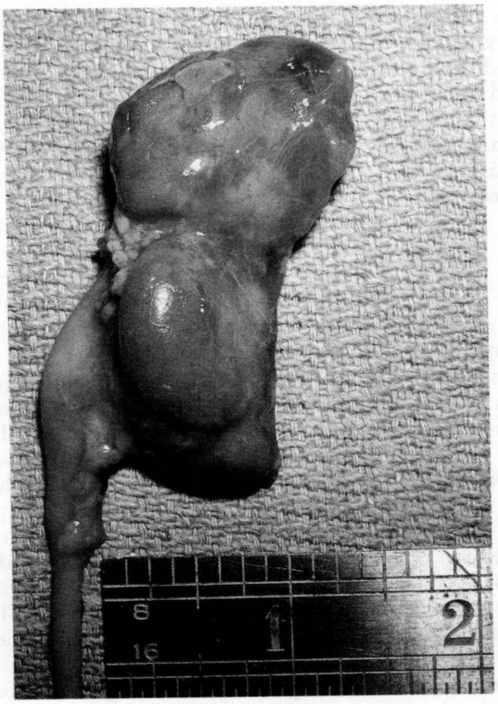

Figure 532-2 Scarred kidney from recurrent pyelonephritis.

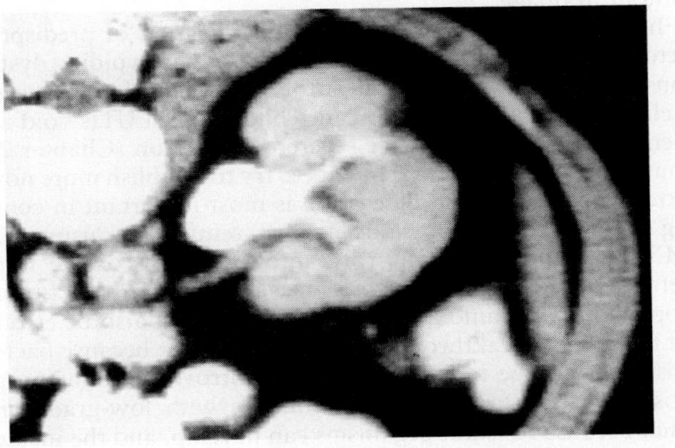

Figure 532-3 CT scan showing an area of parenchymal thinning corresponding to an underlying calyx, characteristic of pyelonephritic scarring or reflux nephropathy.

Table 532-1 RISK FACTORS FOR URINARY TRACT INFECTION

Female gender
Uncircumcised male
Vesicoureteral reflux*
Toilet training
Voiding dysfunction
Obstructive uropathy
Urethral instrumentation
Wiping from back to front in girls
Bubble bath?
Tight clothing (underwear)
Pinworm infestation
Constipation
Bacteria with P fimbriae
Anatomic abnormality (labial adhesion)
Neuropathic bladder
Sexual activity
Pregnancy

*Risk increased for clinical pyelonephritis, not cystitis.

stasis. Urethral catheterization for urine output monitoring or during a voiding cystourethrogram or nonsterile catheterization can infect the bladder with a pathogen. Constipation with fecal impaction can increase the risk of UTI because it can cause voiding dysfunction.

The pathogenesis of UTI is based in part on the presence of bacterial pili or fimbriae on the bacterial surface. There are two types of fimbriae, type I and type II. Type I fimbriae are found on most strains of *E. coli.* Because attachment to target cells can be blocked by D-mannose, these fimbriae are referred to as *mannose-sensitive.* They have no role in pyelonephritis. The attachment of type II fimbriae is not inhibited by mannose, and these are known as *mannose-resistant.* These fimbriae are expressed by only certain strains of *E. coli.* The receptor for type II fimbriae is a glycosphingolipid that is present on both the uroepithelial cell membrane and red blood cells. The Gal 1-4 Gal oligosaccharide fraction is the specific receptor. Because these fimbriae can agglutinate by P blood group erythrocytes, they are known as P fimbriae. Bacteria with P fimbriae are more likely to cause pyelonephritis. Between 76-94% of pyelonephritogenic strains of *E. coli* have P fimbriae, compared with 19-23% of cystitis strains.

Other host factors for UTI include anatomic abnormalities precluding normal micturition, such as a labial adhesion. This lesion acts as a barrier and causes vaginal voiding. A neuropathic bladder can predispose to UTIs if there is incomplete bladder emptying and/or detrusor-sphincter dyssynergia. Sexual activity is associated with UTIs in girls, in part because of incomplete bladder emptying. From 4-7% of pregnant women have asymptomatic bacteriuria, which can develop into a symptomatic UTI. The incidence of UTI in infants who are breast-fed is lower than in those fed with formula.

DIAGNOSIS

UTI may be suspected based on symptoms or findings on urinalysis, or both; *a urine culture is necessary for confirmation and appropriate therapy.* There are several ways to obtain a urine sample; some are more accurate than others. In toilet-trained children, a midstream urine sample usually is satisfactory; the introitus should be cleaned before obtaining the specimen. In uncircumcised boys, the prepuce must be retracted; if the prepuce is not retractable, a voided sample may be unreliable and contaminated with skin flora. In children who are not toilet trained, a catheterized urine sample should be obtained. Alternatively, the application of an adhesive, sealed, sterile collection bag after disinfection of the skin of the genitals can be useful only if the culture is negative or if a single uropathogen is identified. However, a positive culture can result from skin contamination, particularly in girls and uncircumcised boys. If treatment is planned immediately after obtaining the urine culture, a bagged specimen should not be the method because of a high rate of contamination often with mixed organisms. A suprapubic aspirate generally is unnecessary.

Pyuria (leukocytes in the urine) suggests infection, but infection can occur in the absence of pyuria; this finding is more confirmatory than diagnostic. Conversely, pyuria can be present without UTI.

Sterile pyuria (positive leukocytes, negative culture) occurs in partially treated bacterial UTIs, viral infections, renal tuberculosis, renal abscess, UTI in the presence of urinary obstruction, urethritis due to a sexually transmitted infection (STI) (Chapter 114), inflammation near the ureter or bladder (appendicitis, Crohn disease), and interstitial nephritis (eosinophils). Nitrites and leukocyte esterase usually are positive in infected urine. Microscopic hematuria is common in acute cystitis, but microhematuria alone does not suggest UTI. White blood cell casts in the urinary sediment suggest renal involvement, but in practice these are rarely seen. If the child is asymptomatic and the urinalysis result is normal, it is unlikely that there is a UTI. However, if the child is symptomatic, a UTI is possible, even if the urinalysis result is negative.

Prompt plating of the urine sample for culture is important, because if the urine sits at room temperature for more than 60 min, overgrowth of a minor contaminant can suggest a UTI when the urine might not be infected. Refrigeration is a reliable method of storing the urine until it can be cultured.

If the culture shows >100,000 colonies of a single pathogen, or if there are 10,000 colonies and the child is symptomatic, the child is considered to have a UTI. In a bag sample, if the urinalysis result is positive, the patient is symptomatic, and there is a single organism cultured with a colony count >100,000, there is a presumed UTI. If any of these criteria are not met, confirmation of infection with a catheterized sample is recommended.

With acute renal infection, leukocytosis, neutrophilia, and elevated serum erythrocyte sedimentation rate and C-reactive protein are common. The latter 2 are nonspecific markers of bacterial infection, and their elevation does not prove that the child has acute pyelonephritis. With a renal abscess, the white blood cell count is markedly elevated to >20,000-25,000/mm^3. Because sepsis is common in pyelonephritis, particularly in infants and in any child with obstructive uropathy, blood cultures should be considered before starting antibiotics if possible.

TREATMENT

Acute cystitis should be treated promptly to prevent possible progression to pyelonephritis. If the symptoms are severe, presumptive treatment is started pending results of the culture. If the symptoms are mild or the diagnosis is doubtful, treatment can be delayed until the results of culture are known, and the culture can be repeated if the results are uncertain. If treatment is initiated before the results of a culture and sensitivities are available, a 3- to 5-day course of therapy with trimethoprim-sulfamethoxazole (TMP-SMX) or trimethoprim is effective against most strains of *E. coli.* Nitrofurantoin (5-7 mg/kg/24 hr in 3-4 divided doses) also is effective and has the advantage of being active against *Klebsiella* and *Enterobacter* organisms. Amoxicillin (50 mg/kg/24 hr) also is effective as initial treatment but has no clear advantages over sulfonamides or nitrofurantoin.

In acute febrile infections suggesting **pyelonephritis,** a 10- to 14-day course of broad-spectrum antibiotics capable of reaching significant tissue levels is preferable. Children who are dehydrated, are vomiting, are unable to drink fluids, are ≤1mo of age, or in whom urosepsis is a possibility should be admitted to the hospital for IV rehydration and IV antibiotic therapy. Parenteral treatment with ceftriaxone (50-75 mg/kg/24 hr, not to exceed 2 g) or cefotaxime (100 mg/kg/24 hr), or ampicillin (100 mg/kg/24 hr) with an aminoglycoside such as gentamicin (3-5 mg/kg/24 hr in 1-3 divided doses) is preferable. The potential ototoxicity and nephrotoxicity of aminoglycosides should be considered, and serum creatinine and trough gentamicin levels must be obtained before initiating treatment, as well as daily thereafter as long as treatment continues. Treatment with aminoglycosides is particularly effective against *Pseudomonas* spp, and alkalinization of urine with sodium bicarbonate increases its effectiveness in the urinary tract.

Oral 3rd-generation cephalosporins such as cefixime are as effective as parenteral ceftriaxone against a variety of gram-negative organisms other than *Pseudomonas,* and these medications are considered by some authorities to be the treatment of choice for oral outpatient therapy. Nitrofurantoin should not be used routinely in children with a febrile UTI because it does not achieve significant renal tissue levels. The oral fluoroquinolone ciprofloxacin is an alternative agent for resistant microorganisms, particularly *Pseudomonas,* in patients >17 yr. It also has been used on occasion for short-course therapy in younger children with *Pseudomonas* UTI. However, the clinical use of fluoroquinolones in children should be restricted because of potential cartilage damage. In some children with a febrile UTI, intramuscular injection of a loading dose of ceftriaxone followed by oral therapy with a 3rd-generation cephalosporin is effective. A urine culture 1 wk after the termination of treatment of a UTI ensures that the urine is sterile but is not routinely needed. A urine culture during treatment almost invariably is negative.

Children with a renal or perirenal abscess or with infection in obstructed urinary tracts can require surgical or percutaneous drainage in addition to antibiotic therapy and other supportive measures (Fig. 532-4). Small abscesses may initially be treated without drainage.

In a child with recurrent UTIs, identification of predisposing factors is beneficial. Many school-aged girls have **voiding dysfunction** (Chapter 537); treatment of this condition often reduces the likelihood of recurrent UTI. Some children with UTIs void infrequently, and many also have severe constipation (Chapter 298). Counseling of parents and patients to try to establish more normal patterns of voiding and defecation is most important in controlling recurrences. Prophylaxis against reinfection, using TMP-SMX, trimethoprim, or nitrofurantoin at 30% of the normal therapeutic dose once a day, is one approach to this problem. Prophylaxis with amoxicillin or cephalexin can also be effective, but the risk of breakthrough UTI may be higher because bacterial resistance may be induced. There is controversy about prophylaxis against recurrent UTIs in children with low-grade or no reflux because resistant organisms can develop, and the incidence of recurrent infection might not consistently be reduced. Other more high risk conditions for recurrent UTIs that might need long-term prophylaxis include neurogenic bladder, urinary tract

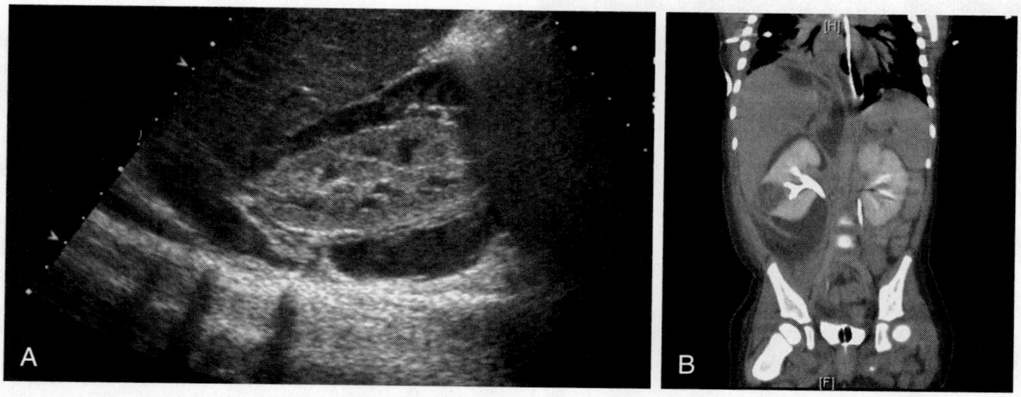

Figure 532-4 *A,* Renal sonogram, 19 mo old girl with perirenal abscess secondary to methicillin-resistant *Staphylococcus aureus. B,* CT scan demonstrates extensive perinephric and focal intrarenal abscess. Patient underwent incision and drainage.

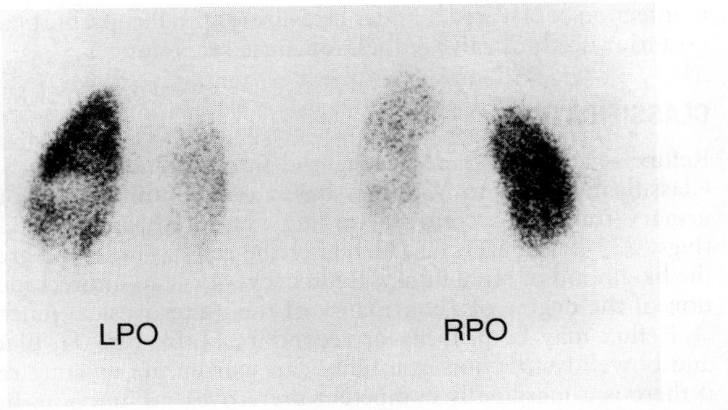

Figure 532-5 Dimercaptosuccinic acid renal scan showing bilateral photopenic areas indicating acute pyelonephritis and renal scarring. *LPO*, left posterior oblique; *RPO*, right posterior oblique.

stasis and obstruction, reflux, and calculi. There is interest in probiotic therapy, which replaces pathologic urogenital flora, and cranberry juice, which prevents bacterial adhesion and biofilm formation, but these agents have not proved beneficial in preventing UTI in children.

The main consequences of chronic renal damage caused by pyelonephritis are arterial hypertension and end-stage renal insufficiency; when they are found they should be treated appropriately (Chapters 439 and 529).

IMAGING STUDIES

The goal of imaging studies in children with a UTI is to identify anatomic abnormalities that predispose to infection, determine whether there is active renal involvement, and to assess whether renal function is normal or at risk.

Acute pyelonephritis, typically characterized by fever, malaise, abdominal or flank pain, and occasionally nausea and vomiting, is a significant risk factor for renal injury and scarring. Acute pyelonephritis may be imaged with a technetium-labeled dimercaptosuccinic acid (**DMSA**) renal scan. Typically, involved areas of the kidney are photopenic and the kidney is enlarged. Of children with a febrile UTI, approximately 50% have a positive DMSA scan. Of those with a positive scan, approximately 50% develop renal scarring in the areas of acute pyelonephritis, and in the remainder with acutely positive scans, the renal appearance will normalize. In children with dilating grades of reflux (III, IV, V), 80-90% with a febrile UTI have a DMSA scan consistent with acute pyelonephritis. Children with grades I and II reflux and those without reflux can also develop acute pyelonephritis. In longitudinal studies of children with grades I and II reflux and acute pyelonephritis, the reflux usually resolves. If the DMSA scan is normal during a febrile UTI, no scarring will result from that particular infection. CT is another diagnostic tool that can image acute pyelonephritis, but clinical experience with DMSA is much greater, and CT scans have more radiation.

In children with their 1st episode of clinical pyelonephritis—those with a febrile UTI, or, in infants, those with systemic illness—and a positive urine culture, irrespective of temperature, a sonogram of kidneys and bladder should be performed to assess kidney size, detect hydronephrosis and ureteral dilation, identify the duplicated urinary tract, and evaluate bladder anatomy. Next, a DMSA scan is performed to identify whether the child has acute pyelonephritis (Fig. 532-5). If the DMSA scan is positive and shows either acute pyelonephritis or renal scarring, a voiding cystourethrogram (VCUG) is performed (Fig. 532-6). If reflux is identified, treatment is based on the perceived long-term risk of the reflux to the child (Chapter 533). One limitation to this approach is that many hospitals caring for children with a febrile UTI might not have facilities for performing a DMSA scan in children. In these cases, a renal sonogram should be performed, and then the clinician needs to decide on whether to send the child to a facility with DMSA capability or instead do a VCUG.

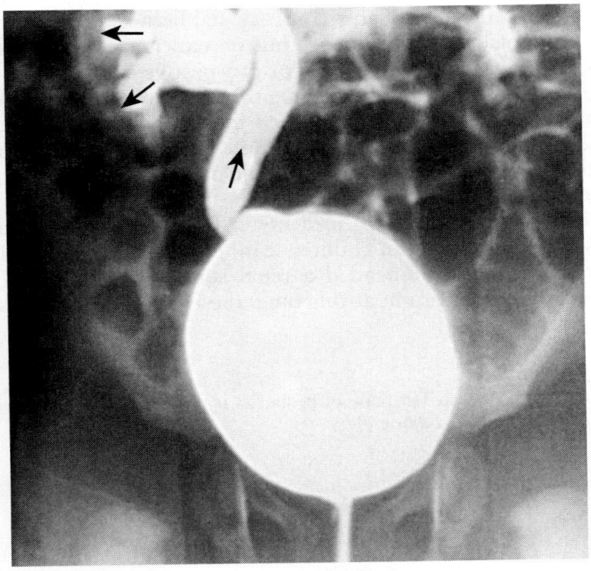

Figure 532-6 Intrarenal reflux. Voiding cystourethrogram in an infant boy with a past history of a urinary tract infection. Note the right vesicoureteral reflux with ureteral dilatation, with opacification of the renal parenchyma representing intrarenal reflux.

In some centers, the VCUG is delayed for 2-6 wk to allow inflammation in the bladder to resolve; however, the incidence of reflux is identical, regardless of whether the VCUG is obtained acutely at the time of treatment of the UTI or after 6 wk. Obtaining the VCUG before the child is discharged from the hospital is appropriate and ensures that the evaluation is complete. If available, a radionuclide VCUG rather than a contrast VCUG can be used in girls; this technique causes less radiation exposure to the gonads than does the contrast study. However, the radioisotope VCUG does not provide anatomic definition of the bladder, allow precise grading of reflux, demonstrate a paraureteral diverticulum, or show whether reflux is occurring into a duplicated collecting system or an ectopic ureter. In boys, VCUG definition of the urethra is important to detect posterior urethral values (Chapter 534).

In children with a second febrile UTI who previously had a negative upper tract evaluation, a VCUG is indicated, because low-grade reflux predisposes to clinical pyelonephritis.

In children with ≥1 infection of the lower urinary tract (dysuria, urgency, frequency, suprapubic pain), imaging is usually unnecessary. Instead, assessment and treatment of bladder and bowel dysfunction is important. If there are numerous lower urinary tract infections, then a renal sonogram is appropriate, but a VCUG rarely adds useful information.

ALTERNATIVE RECOMMENDATIONS FOR UTI

In 2007, the NICE (National Institute for Health and Clinical Excellence, UK) guidelines for diagnosis, management, and imaging after UTI were released. These recommendations divide children into those <6 mo, 6 mo to 3 yr, and >3 yr of age. The clinical categories are separated into those that respond to treatment within 48 hours, recurrent UTI, and atypical UTI (sepsis, non–*E. coli* UTI, suprapubic mass, elevated serum creatinine, hypertension). The recommendations include upper tract imaging with a renal sonogram and DMSA scan for all <6 mo with a UTI and all children <3 yr with an atypical or recurrent UTI. For children >3 yr, a DMSA scan is recommended only for recurrent UTI. A VCUG is recommended only in children <6 mo. These recommendations are highly controversial because the methodology was not based on evidence but on expert opinion. In addition, there was no retrospective or prospective assessment of the potential of this approach to identify significant uropathology. Coulthard and Tse have performed independent assessments of these recommendations and has found that a significant number of children with uropathology would not have been identified under these guidelines.

In 1999, the American Academy of Pediatrics released guidelines for management of children 2 m to 2 yr with a febrile UTI. This guideline recommended a renal sonogram and VCUG or radionuclide cystogram; at this time, these recommendations are being rewritten.

BIBLIOGRAPHY

Please visit the Nelson Textbook of Pediatrics *website at* *www.expertconsult.com* *for the complete bibliography.*

Chapter 533
Vesicoureteral Reflux

Jack S. Elder

Vesicoureteral reflux refers to the retrograde flow of urine from the bladder to the ureter and kidney. The ureteral attachment to the bladder normally is oblique, between the bladder mucosa and detrusor muscle, creating a flap-valve mechanism that prevents reflux (Fig. 533-1). Reflux occurs when the submucosal tunnel between the mucosa and detrusor muscle is short or absent. Reflux usually is congenital, occurs in families, and affects approximately 1% of children.

Reflux predisposes to infection of the kidney (pyelonephritis) by facilitating the transport of bacteria from the bladder to the upper urinary tract (Chapter 532). The inflammatory reaction caused by a pyelonephritic infection can result in renal injury or scarring, also termed **reflux-related renal injury** or **reflux nephropathy.** In children with a febrile urinary tract infection (UTI), those with reflux are 3 times more likely to develop renal injury compared to those without reflux. Extensive renal scarring impairs renal function and can result in renin-mediated hypertension (Chapter 439), renal insufficiency or end-stage renal disease (Chapter 529), impaired somatic growth, and morbidity during pregnancy.

Reflux nephropathy once accounted for as much as 15-20% of end-stage renal disease in children and young adults. With greater attention to the management of UTIs and a better understanding of reflux, end-stage renal disease secondary to reflux nephropathy is uncommon. Reflux nephropathy remains one of the most common causes of hypertension in children. Reflux in the absence of infection or elevated bladder pressure (e.g., neuropathic bladder, posterior urethral valves) does not cause renal injury.

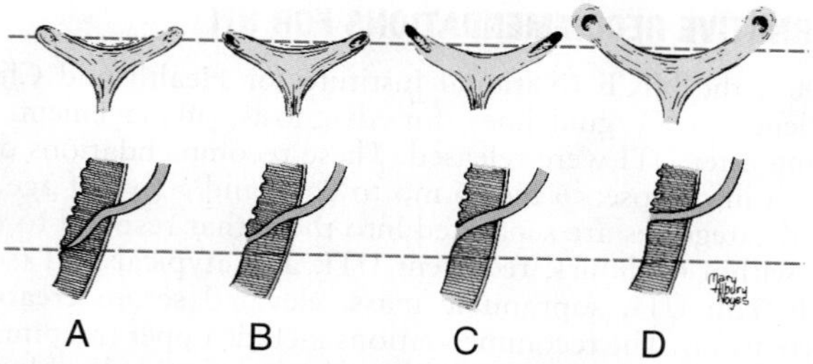

Figure 533-1 Normal and abnormal configuration of the ureteral orifices. Shown from *left* to *right,* progressive lateral displacement of the ureteral orifices and shortening of the intramural tunnels. *Top,* Endoscopic appearance. *Bottom,* Sagittal view through the intramural ureter.

CLASSIFICATION

Reflux severity is graded using the International Reflux Study Classification of I to V and is based on the appearance of the urinary tract on a contrast voiding cystourethrogram (VCUG) (Figs. 533-2 and 533-3). The higher the reflux grade, the greater the likelihood of renal injury. Reflux severity is an indirect indication of the degree of abnormality of the ureterovesical junction.

Reflux may be primary or secondary (Table 533-1). Bladder and bowel dysfunction instability can worsen pre-existing reflux if there is a marginally competent ureterovesical junction. In the most severe cases, there is such massive reflux into the upper tracts that the bladder becomes overdistended. This condition, the **megacystis-megaureter syndrome,** occurs primarily in boys and may be unilateral or bilateral (Fig. 533-4). Reimplantation of the ureters into the bladder to correct reflux resolves the condition.

Approximately 1/125 children have a **duplication** of the upper urinary tract in which 2 ureters rather than 1 drain the kidney.

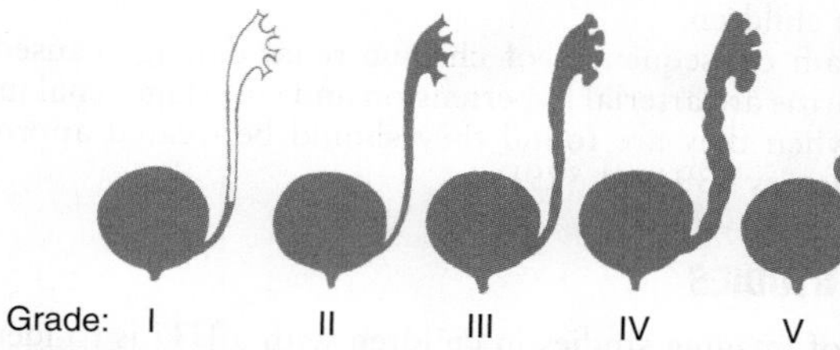

Figure 533-2 Grading of vesicoureteral reflux. Grade I: reflux into a nondilated ureter. Grade II: reflux into the upper collecting system without dilatation. Grade III: reflux into dilated ureter and/or blunting of calyceal fornices. Grade IV: reflux into a grossly dilated ureter. Grade V: massive reflux, with significant ureteral dilatation and tortuosity and loss of the papillary impression.

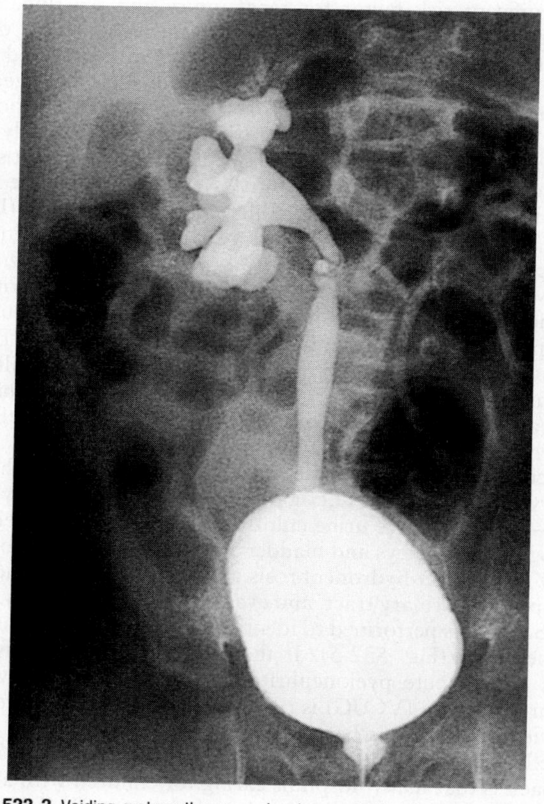

Figure 533-3 Voiding cystourethrogram showing grade IV right vesicoureteral reflux.

Table 533-1 CLASSIFICATION OF VESICOURETERAL REFLUX

TYPE	CAUSE
Primary	Congenital incompetence of the valvular mechanism of the vesicoureteral junction
Primary associated with other malformations of the ureterovesical junction	Ureteral duplication Ureterocele with duplication Ureteral ectopia Paraureteral diverticula
Secondary to increased intravesical pressure	Neuropathic bladder Non-neuropathic bladder dysfunction Bladder outlet obstruction
Secondary to inflammatory processes	Severe bacterial cystitis Foreign bodies Vesical calculi Clinical cystitis
Secondary to surgical procedures involving the ureterovesical junction	Surgery

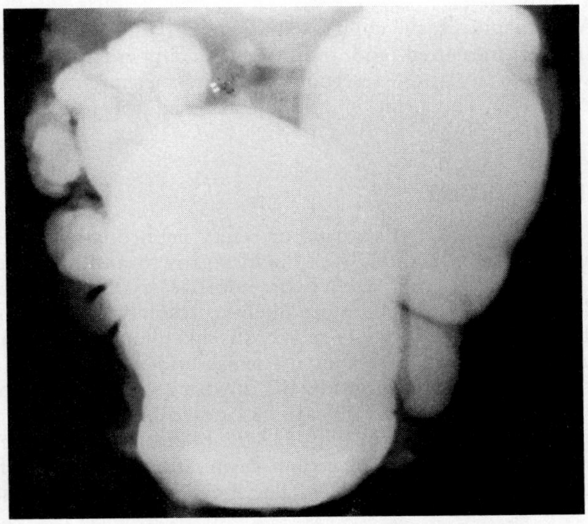

Figure 533-4 Voiding cystourethrogram in newborn boy with megacystis-megaureter syndrome. Note the massive ureteral dilatation due to high-grade vesicoureteral reflux. The bladder is very distended. There was no urethral obstruction or neuropathic dysfunction.

Duplication may be partial or complete. In partial duplication, the ureters join above the bladder and there is 1 ureteral orifice. In complete duplication, the attachment of the lower pole ureter to the bladder is superior and lateral to the upper pole ureter. The valve-like mechanism for the lower pole ureter often is marginal, and reflux into the lower ureter occurs in as many as 50% of cases. Reflux occurs into both the lower and upper systems in some persons (Fig. 533-5). With a duplication anomaly, some patients have an ectopic ureter, in which the upper pole ureter drains outside the bladder (Chapters 534 and 537 and see Figs. 537-6 and 537-7). If the ectopic ureter drains into the bladder neck, typically it is obstructed and refluxes. Duplication anomalies also are common in children with a ureterocele, which is a cystic swelling of the intramural portion of the distal ureter. These patients often have reflux into the associated lower pole ureter or the contralateral ureter. Generally reflux is present when the ureter enters a bladder diverticulum (Fig. 533-6).

Reflux is present at birth in 25% of children with **neuropathic bladder,** as occurs in myelomeningocele, sacral agenesis, and many cases of high imperforate anus. Reflux is seen in 50% of boys with posterior urethral valves. Reflux with increased intravesical pressure (as in detrusor-sphincter dyssynergia or bladder

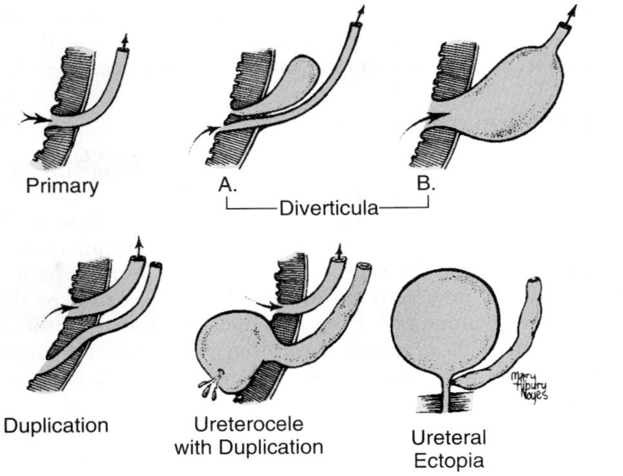

Figure 533-5 Various anatomic defects of the ureterovesical junction associated with vesicoureteral reflux.

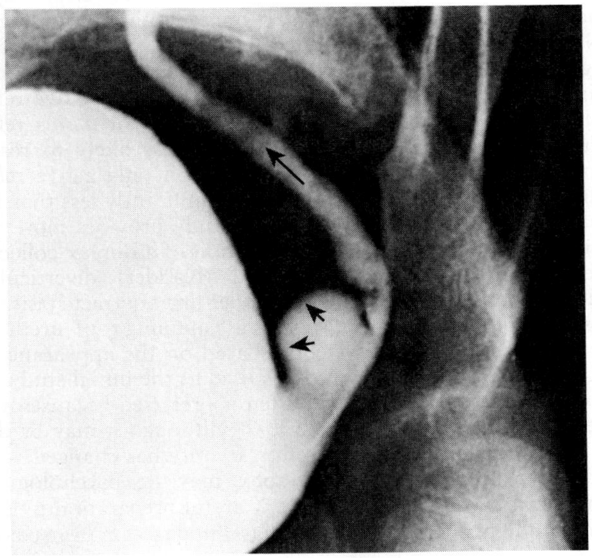

Figure 533-6 Reflux and bladder diverticulum. The voiding cystourethrogram demonstrates left vesicoureteral reflux and a paraureteral diverticulum.

outlet obstruction) can result in renal injury, even in the absence of infection.

Primary reflux occurs in association with several congenital urinary tract abnormalities. Of children with a multicystic dysplastic kidney or renal agenesis (Chapter 531), 15% have reflux into the contralateral kidney, and 10-15% of children with a ureteropelvic junction obstruction have reflux into either the hydronephrotic kidney or the contralateral kidney.

Reflux (idiopathic) appears to be an autosomal dominant inherited trait with variable penetrance. Approximately 35% of siblings of children with reflux also have reflux, and reflux is found in nearly half of newborn siblings. The likelihood of a sibling having reflux is independent of the grade of reflux or sex of the index child. Approximately 12% of asymptomatic siblings with reflux have evidence of renal scarring. In addition, 50% of children born to women with a history of reflux also have reflux. In 2010 the American Urological Association Vesicoureteral Reflux Guidelines Panel stated that, in siblings of individuals with reflux, a VCUG or radionuclide cystogram is recommended if there is evidence of renal cortical abnormalities or renal size asymmetry on sonography, or if the sibling has a history of UTI.

Otherwise, screening is optional. Reflux may be suggested on a prenatal ultrasound, which demonstrates dilated renal calyces. Primary reflux is less common in African-Americans.

CLINICAL MANIFESTATIONS

Reflux usually is discovered during evaluation for a UTI (Chapter 532). Among these children, 80% are female, and the average age at diagnosis is 2-3 yr. In other children, a VCUG is performed during evaluation of voiding dysfunction, renal insufficiency, hypertension, or other suspected pathologic process of the urinary tract. Primary reflux also may be discovered during evaluation for prenatal hydronephrosis. In this select population, 80% of affected children are male, and the reflux grade usually is higher than in girls whose reflux is diagnosed following a UTI.

DIAGNOSIS

Diagnosis of reflux requires catheterization of the bladder, instillation of a solution containing iodinated contrast or a radiopharmaceutical, and radiologic imaging of the lower and upper urinary tract: a contrast VCUG or radionuclide cystogram (RNC), respectively. The bladder and upper urinary tracts are imaged during bladder filling and voiding. Reflux occurring during bladder filling is termed *low-pressure* or *passive* reflux; reflux during voiding is termed *high-pressure* or *active* reflux. Reflux in children with passive reflux is less likely to resolve spontaneously than in children who exhibit only active reflux. Radiation exposure during an RNC is significantly less than that from a contrast VCUG. The contrast study provides more anatomic information, such as demonstration of a duplex collecting system, ectopic ureter, paraureteral (bladder) diverticulum, bladder outlet obstruction in boys, upper urinary tract stasis, and signs of voiding dysfunction, such as a "spinning top" urethra in girls. The reflux grading system is based on the appearance on VCUG. Consequently, the VCUG is used as the initial study. For follow-up evaluation, the RNC often is preferred because of the lower radiation exposure (Fig. 533-7), although it may be difficult to determine whether the reflux severity has changed.

Children undergoing cystography may be psychologically traumatized by the catheterization. Careful preparation by caregivers or administration of oral or nasal midazolam (for sedation and amnesia) or propofol before the study can result in a less-distressing experience.

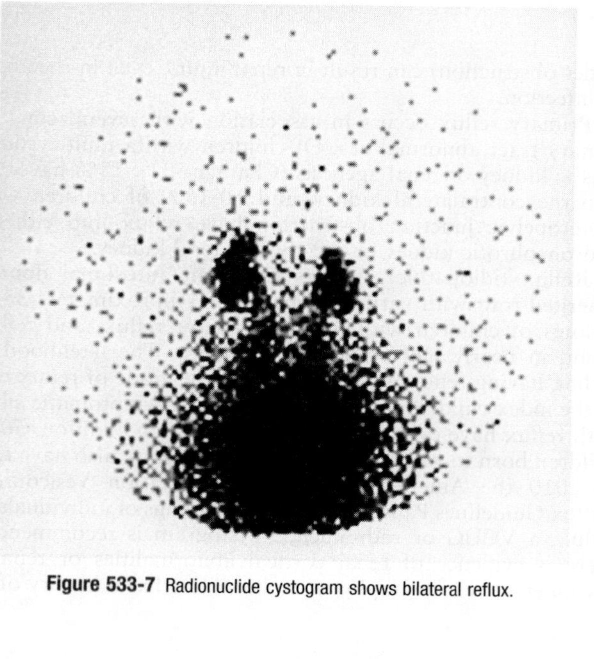

Figure 533-7 Radionuclide cystogram shows bilateral reflux.

Indirect cystography is a technique of detecting reflux without catheterization that involves injecting an intravenous radiopharmaceutical that is excreted by the kidneys, waiting for it to be excreted into the bladder, and imaging the lower urinary tract while the patient voids. This technique detects only 75% of reflux cases. Another technique, which avoids radiation exposure, involves instilling sonographic contrast medium through a urethral catheter. The kidneys are imaged sonographically. This technique is investigational.

After reflux is diagnosed, assessment of the upper urinary tract is important. The goal of upper tract imaging is to assess whether renal scarring and associated urinary tract anomalies are present. Renal imaging typically is performed with a renal sonogram or renal scintigraphy (Fig. 533-8; Chapter 532).

The child should be evaluated for bladder and bowel dysfunction, including urgency, frequency, diurnal incontinence, infrequent voiding, or a combination of these (Chapter 537). Children with an overactive bladder often undergo a regimen of behavioral modification with timed voiding, and, on occasion, anticholinergic therapy.

After diagnosis, the child's height, weight, and blood pressure should be measured and monitored. If upper tract imaging shows renal scarring, a serum creatinine measurement should be obtained. The urine should be assessed for infection and proteinuria.

NATURAL HISTORY

The incidence of renal scarring or reflux nephropathy increases with the grade of reflux. With bladder growth and maturation, the reflux grade can resolve or improve over time. Lower grades of reflux are much more likely to resolve than are higher grades. For grades I and II reflux, the likelihood of resolution is similar regardless of age at diagnosis and whether it is unilateral or bilateral. For grade III, a younger age at diagnosis and unilateral reflux usually are associated with a higher rate of spontaneous resolution (Fig. 533-9). Bilateral grade IV reflux is much less likely to resolve than is unilateral grade IV reflux. Grade V reflux rarely resolves. The mean age at reflux resolution is 6 yr.

Reflux does not usually cause renal injury in the absence of infection, but in situations with high-pressure reflux, as in children with posterior urethral valves, neuropathic bladder, and non-neurogenic neurogenic bladder (i.e., Hinman syndrome), sterile reflux can cause significant renal damage. Children with high-grade reflux who acquire a UTI are at significant risk for pyelonephritis and new renal scarring (see Fig. 533-8).

TREATMENT

The goals of treatment are to prevent pyelonephritis, reflux-related renal injury, and other complications of reflux. Medical therapy is based on the principle that reflux often resolves over time and that if UTI can be prevented, the morbidity or complications of reflux may be avoided without surgery. The basis for surgical therapy is that in selected children, ongoing reflux has caused or has significant potential for causing renal injury or other reflux-related complications and that elimination of reflux minimizes the likelihood of these problems.

In 1997, the American Urological Association (AUA) released treatment guidelines for vesicoureteral reflux.

Prophylaxis

Based on clinical series demonstrating the effectiveness of antibiotic prophylaxis, daily prophylaxis was recommended as initial therapy for most children with reflux. Drugs commonly used for prophylaxis include trimethoprim-sulfamethoxazole

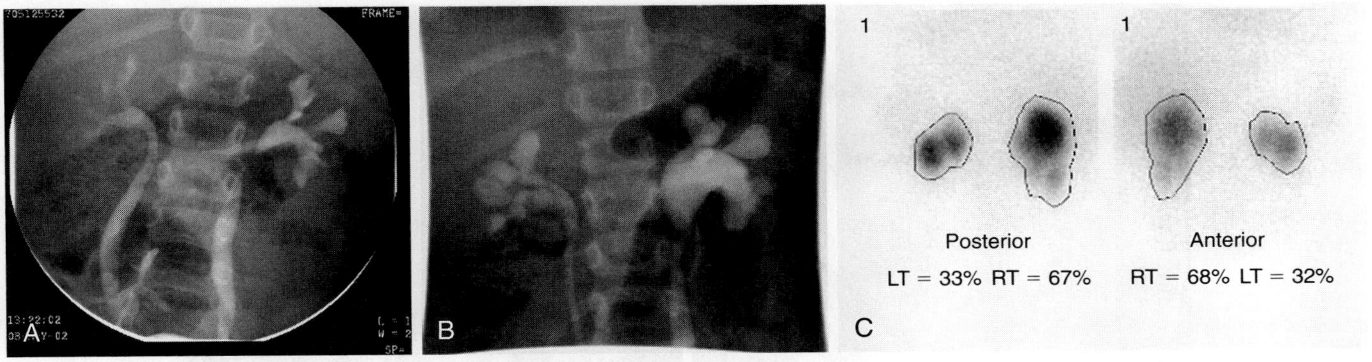

Figure 533-8 *A,* Voiding cystourethrogram (VCUG) in a 3 yr old girl with 2 febrile urinary tract infections shows bilateral grade III reflux. *B,* At 5 yr, repeat VCUG shows worsening reflux and calyceal clubbing, indicating renal scarring. *C,* At 11 yr, she has developed rennin-mediated hypertension. DMSA renal scan shows significant reflux-related renal scarring.

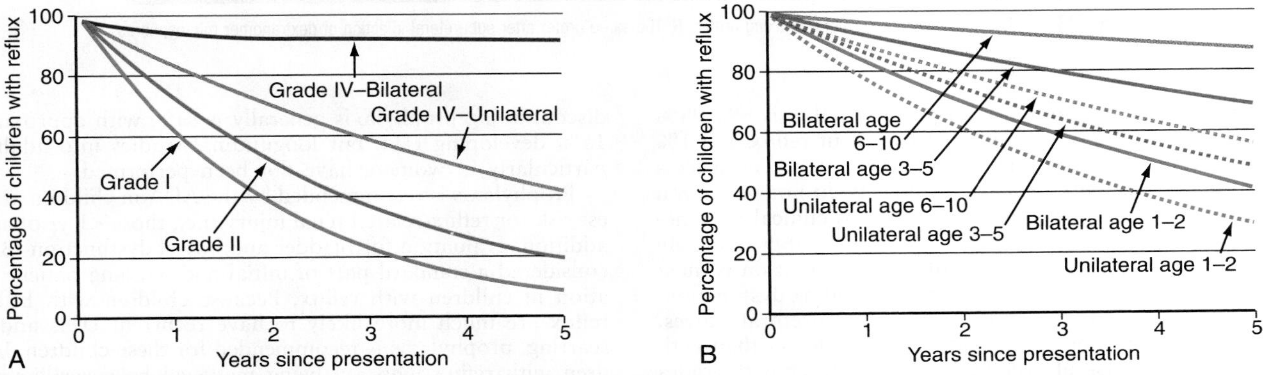

Figure 533-9 *A,* Percentage chance of reflux persistence, grades I, II, and IV, for 1-5 yr after presentation. *B,* Percentage chance of reflux persistence by age at presentation, grade III, for 1-5 yr after presentation. (From Elder JS, Peters CA, Arant BS Jr, et al: Pediatric Vesicoureteral Reflux Guidelines Panel summary report on the management of primary vesicoureteral reflux in children, *J Urol* 157:1846–1851, 1997.)

(TMP-SMX), trimethoprim, nitrofurantoin, or cephalexin, which are administered once daily at a dose of 25-30% of the dosage necessary to treat an acute infection. Prophylaxis was continued until reflux resolved or until the risk of reflux to the patient was considered to be low. Bladder and bowel dysfunction were aggressively treated (Chapter 537). A urine culture was recommended if there were symptoms or signs of a UTI. Children with renal scarring are at greatest risk for breakthrough febrile UTI. A VCUG or RNC and upper tract imaging were recommended every 12-18 mo. Annual assessment of the child's height, weight, and blood pressure was recommended.

Surgery

In children who fail medical management (breakthrough UTI, persistent reflux), or those with high reflux grades that are unlikely to resolve, the AUA recommended surgical therapy. The purpose of surgical therapy is to minimize the risks of ongoing reflux and nonsurgical therapy (prophylaxis and follow-up testing). Reflux can be corrected through a lower abdominal or inguinal incision, laparoscopically, or cystoscopically.

Open surgical management involves modifying the abnormal ureterovesical attachment to create a 4:1 to 5:1 ratio of intramural ureter length:ureteral diameter. The operation can be performed from either outside or inside the bladder. When reflux is associated with severe ureteral dilatation (i.e., megaureter) is corrected, the ureter must be tailored or narrowed to a more normal size to allow a normal length:width ratio for the intramural tunnel, and a corner of the bladder is attached to the psoas tendon, forming a *psoas hitch*. Most children can be discharged the day following surgery. If the refluxing kidney is poorly functioning, nephrectomy or nephroureterectomy is indicated. Laparoscopic reflux correction either through the bladder (termed *vesicoscopic*) or with an extravesical approach is being investigated.

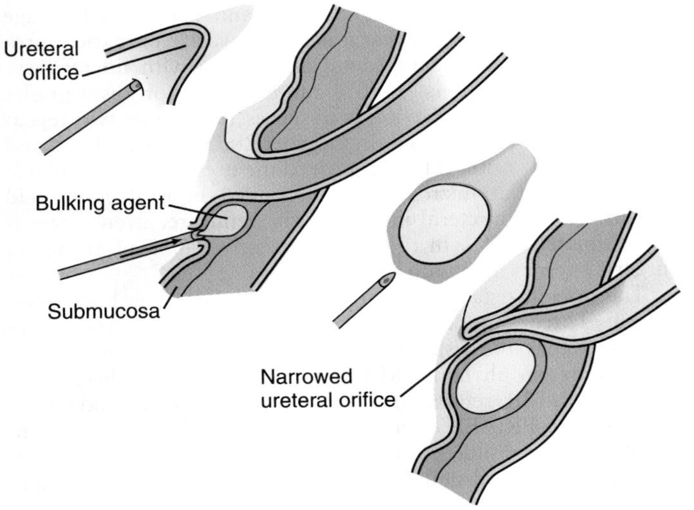

Figure 533-10 Endoscopic correction of reflux. Through a cystoscope, a needle is inserted into the submucosal plane deep to the ureteral orifice and bulking agent is injected, creating a flap-valve to prevent reflux. (Adapted from Ortenberg J: Endoscopic treatment of vesicoureteral reflux in children, *Urol Clin North Am* 25:151–156, 1998.)

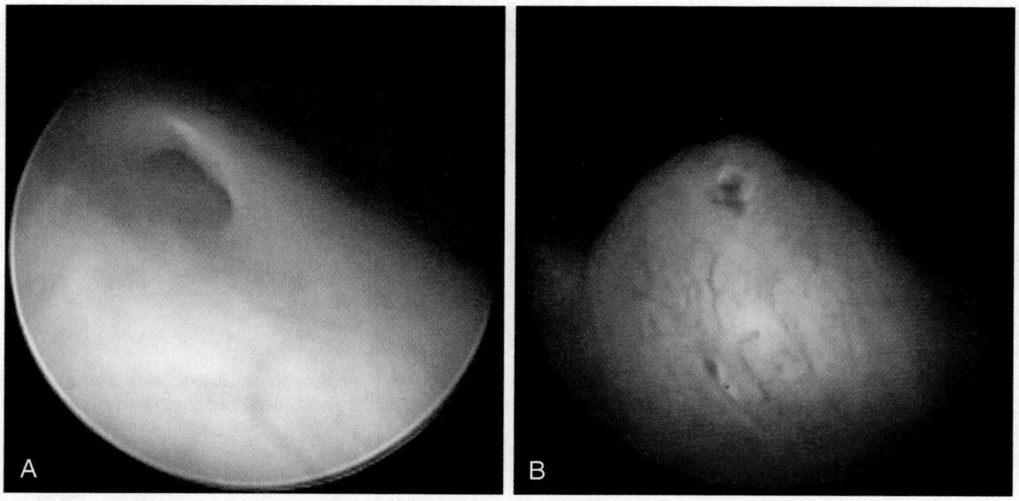

Figure 533-11 *A,* Endoscopic view of right refluxing ureter. *B,* The same ureter after subureteral injection of dextranomer microspheres.

The success rate in children with primary reflux is >95-98% for grades I-IV, with 2% experiencing persistent reflux and 1% having ureteral obstruction that requires correction. The success rate is so high that many pediatric urologists do not perform a postoperative VCUG unless the child develops clinical pyelonephritis. For grade V reflux, the success rate is approximately 80%. In lower grades of reflux, a failed reimplantation is most likely to occur in children with undiagnosed voiding dysfunction. In children with secondary reflux (posterior urethral valves, neuropathic bladder), the success rate is slightly lower than with primary reflux. The risk of pyelonephritis in children with grades III and IV reflux is significantly lower following open surgical correction. Surgical repair will not reverse renal scarring or cause improvement in renal function.

Endoscopic repair of reflux involves injection of a bulking agent through a cystoscope just beneath the ureteral orifice, creating an artificial flap-valve (Figs. 533-10 and 11). The advantage of subureteral injection is that it is a noninvasive outpatient procedure (performed under general anesthesia) with no recovery time. The success rate is 70-80% and is highest for lower grades of reflux. If the first injection is unsuccessful, one or two repeat injections can be performed. In October 2001, the U.S. Food and Drug Administration (FDA) approved the use of a biodegradable material, dextran microspheres suspended in hyaluronic acid (Deflux), for subureteral injection. The reflux recurrence rate is approximately 10%. In the USA, currently >40% of antireflux surgery is performed with this procedure.

The dogma regarding antibiotic prophylaxis has been questioned. Three randomized controlled prospective trials have suggested that the risk of UTI in children with reflux is not reduced by prophylaxis. Most of the children in these trials had grades I-III reflux, and few <1 yr old were studied. In contrast, the PRIVENT trial from Australia showed benefit to prophylaxis in children with reflux. The Swedish Reflux Trial in Children studied children <2 yr of age with grades III and IV reflux; they compared antibiotic prophylaxis to observation. In the surveillance group, there was a significantly higher incidence of febrile UTI and new renal scarring compared to the other treatment groups. In this series, trimethoprim was used for prophylaxis, whereas in the other trials TMP-SMX was the prophylactic medication. Consequently, further research is necessary. The National Institutes of Health (NIH) have instituted the Randomized Intervention for Vesicoureteral Reflux (RIVUR) trial to study the issue of prophylaxis. In children with persistent low-grade reflux and normal bladder function, several retrospective studies with short follow-up have demonstrated that discontinuing prophylaxis generally is safe, with approximately 15% developing UTI, but longitudinal studies into adulthood, particularly in women, have not been performed.

Prophylaxis is recommended by the AUA in children at greatest risk for reflux-related renal injury (i.e., those <1 yr of age). In addition, evaluation for bladder and bowel dysfunction (BBD) is considered a standard part of initial and ongoing patient evaluation in children with reflux. Because children with BBD and reflux are much more likely to have recurrent UTIs and renal scarring, prophylaxis is recommended for these children. In children with reflux who are being managed by surveillance, if a febrile UTI occurs, prophylaxis is recommended. The decision whether to recommend observation, medical therapy, or surgery is based on the risk of reflux to the patient, the likelihood of spontaneous resolution, and the parents' and patient's preferences, and the family should understand the risks and benefits of each treatment approach.

BIBLIOGRAPHY

Please visit the Nelson Textbook of Pediatrics *website at* *www.expertconsult.com* *for the complete bibliography.*

Chapter 534
Obstruction of the Urinary Tract
Jack S. Elder

Urinary tract obstruction can result from congenital (anatomic) lesions or can be caused by trauma, neoplasia, calculi, inflammatory processes, or surgical procedures, although most childhood obstructive lesions are congenital. Obstructive lesions occur at any level from the urethral meatus to the calyceal infundibula (Table 534-1). The pathophysiologic effects of obstruction depend on its level, the extent of involvement, the child's age at onset, and whether it is acute or chronic.

ETIOLOGY

Ureteral obstruction occurring early in fetal life results in renal dysplasia, ranging from multicystic kidney, which is associated with ureteral or pelvic atresia (see Fig. 531-2), to various degrees

Table 534-1 TYPES AND CAUSES OF URINARY TRACT OBSTRUCTION

LOCATION	CAUSE
Infundibula	Congenital Calculi Inflammatory (tuberculosis) Traumatic Postsurgical Neoplastic
Renal pelvis	Congenital (infundibulopelvic stenosis) Inflammatory (tuberculosis) Calculi Neoplasia (Wilms tumor, neuroblastoma)
Ureteropelvic junction	Congenital stenosis Calculi Neoplasia Inflammatory Postsurgical Traumatic
Ureter	Congenital obstructive megaureter Midureteral structure Ureteral ectopia Ureterocele Retrocaval ureter Ureteral fibroepithelial polyps Ureteral valves Calculi Postsurgical Extrinsic compression Neoplasia (neuroblastoma, lymphoma, and other retroperitoneal or pelvic tumors) Inflammatory (Crohn disease, chronic granulomatous disease) Hematoma, urinoma Lymphocele Retroperitoneal fibrosis
Bladder outlet and urethra	Neurogenic bladder dysfunction (functional obstruction) Posterior urethral valves Anterior urethral valves Diverticula Urethral strictures (congenital, traumatic, or iatrogenic) Urethral atresia Ectopic ureterocele Meatal stenosis (males) Calculi Foreign bodies Phimosis Extrinsic compression by tumors Urogenital sinus anomalies

of histologic renal cortical dysplasia that are seen with less severe obstruction. Chronic ureteral obstruction in late fetal life or after birth results in dilation of the ureter, renal pelvis, and calyces, with alterations of renal parenchyma ranging from minimal tubular changes to dilation of Bowman's space, glomerular fibrosis, and interstitial fibrosis. After birth, infections often complicate obstruction and can increase renal damage.

CLINICAL MANIFESTATIONS

Obstruction of the urinary tract generally causes **hydronephrosis,** which typically is asymptomatic in its early phases. An obstructed kidney secondary to a ureteropelvic junction (UPJ) or ureterovesical junction obstruction can manifest as a mass or cause upper abdominal or flank pain on the affected side. Pyelonephritis can occur because of urinary stasis. An upper urinary tract stone can occur, causing abdominal and flank pain and hematuria. With bladder outlet obstruction, the urinary stream may be weak; urinary tract infection (UTI; Chapter 532) is common.

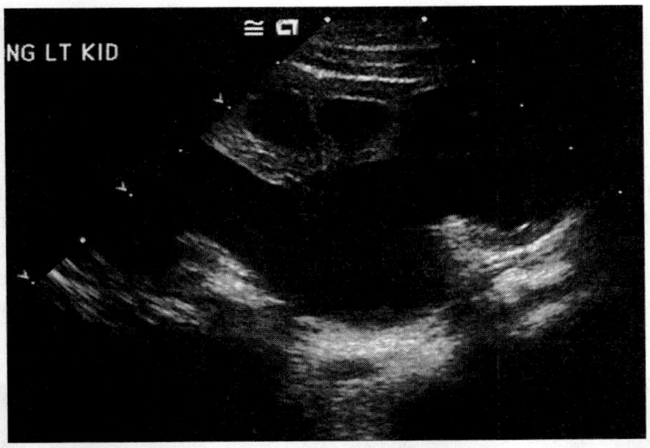

Figure 534-1 Ultrasonographic image of the kidney with marked pelvic and calyceal dilatation (grade 4 hydronephrosis) in a newborn with ureteropelvic junction obstruction.

Many of these lesions are identified by antenatal ultrasonography; an abnormality involving the genitourinary tract is suspected in as many as 1/100 fetuses.

Obstructive renal insufficiency can manifest itself by failure to thrive, vomiting, diarrhea, or other nonspecific signs and symptoms. In older children, *infravesical obstruction* can be associated with overflow urinary incontinence or a poor urine stream. *Acute ureteral obstruction* causes flank or abdominal pain; there may be nausea and vomiting. *Chronic ureteral obstruction* can be silent or can cause vague abdominal or typical flank pain with increased fluid intake.

DIAGNOSIS

Urinary tract obstruction may be diagnosed prenatally by ultrasonography, typically showing hydronephrosis. More complete evaluation, including imaging studies, should be undertaken in these children in the neonatal period.

Urinary tract obstruction is often silent. In the newborn infant, a palpable abdominal mass most commonly is a hydronephrotic or multicystic dysplastic kidney. With posterior urethral valves, which is an infravesical obstructive lesions in boys, a walnut-sized mass representing the bladder is palpable just above the pubic symphysis. A patent draining urachus also can suggest urethral obstruction. Urinary ascites in the newborn usually is caused by renal or bladder urinary extravasation secondary to posterior urethral valves. Infection and sepsis may be the first indications of an obstructive lesion of the urinary tract. The combination of infection and obstruction poses a serious threat to infants and children and generally requires parenteral administration of antibiotics and drainage of the obstructed kidney. Renal ultrasonography should be performed in all children during the acute stage of an initial febrile UTI.

Imaging Studies

RENAL ULTRASONOGRAPHY The presence of a dilated urinary tract is the most common characteristic of obstruction. Hydronephrosis is a common ultrasonographic finding (Fig. 534-1). Dilation is not diagnostic of obstruction and can persist after surgical correction of an obstructive lesion. Dilation can result from vesicoureteral reflux, or it may be a manifestation of abnormal development of the urinary tract, even when there is no obstruction. Renal length, degree of caliectasis and parenchymal thickness, and presence or absence of ureteral dilation should be assessed. Ideally, the severity of hydronephrosis should be graded from 1 to 4 using the Society for Fetal Urology grading scale (Table 534-2). The clinician should ascertain that the contralateral kidney is normal, and the bladder should be imaged to see whether the bladder wall is thickened, the lower ureter is dilated, and bladder emptying is complete. In acute or intermittent obstruction, the dilation of the collecting system may be minimal and ultrasonography may be misleading.

VOIDING CYSTOURETHROGRAM In all cases of congenital grade 3 or 4 hydronephrosis and in any child with ureteral dilatation, a contrast voiding cystourethrogram (VCUG) should be obtained, because the dilation is secondary to vesicoureteral reflux in 15% of cases. In boys, the VCUG also is performed to rule out urethral obstruction, particularly in cases of suspected posterior urethral valves. In infravesical obstruction in infants, the bladder may be palpable because of chronic distention and incomplete emptying.

Table 534-2 SOCIETY FOR FETAL UROLOGY GRADING SYSTEM FOR HYDRONEPHROSIS

GRADE OF HYDRONEPHROSIS	RENAL IMAGE: Central Renal Complex	RENAL IMAGE: Renal Parenchymal Thickness
0	Intact	Normal
1	Slight splitting	Normal
2	Evident splitting, complex confined within renal border	Normal
3	Wide splitting pelvis dilated outside renal border, calyces uniformly dilated	Normal
4	Further dilatation of pelvis and calyces (calyces may appear convex)	Thin

After Maizels M, Mitchell B, Kass E, et al: Outcome of nonspecific hydronephrosis in the infant: a report from the registry of the Society for Fetal Urology, *J Urol* 152:2324–2327, 1994.

In older children, the urinary flow rate can be measured noninvasively with a urinary flowmeter; decreased flow with a normal bladder contraction suggests infravesical obstruction. When the urethra cannot be catheterized to obtain a VCUG, the clinician should suspect a urethral stricture or an obstructive urethral lesion. Retrograde urethrography with contrast medium injected into the urethral meatus helps delineate the anatomy of the urethral obstruction.

RADIOISOTOPE STUDIES **Renal scintigraphy** is used to assess renal anatomy and function. The 2 most commonly used radiopharmaceuticals are mercaptoacetyl triglycine (MAG-3) and technetium-99m-labeled dimercaptosuccinic acid (DMSA). MAG-3, which is excreted by renal tubular secretion, is used to assess differential renal function, and when furosemide is administered, drainage also can be measured. An alternative to MAG-3 is diethylene tetrapentaacetic acid (DTPA), which is cleared by glomerular filtration. The background activity of DTPA is much higher than that of MAG-3. DMSA is a renal cortical imaging agent and is used to assess differential renal function and to demonstrate whether renal scarring is present. It is used infrequently in children with obstructive uropathy.

In a MAG-3 **diuretic renogram**, a small dose of technetium-labeled MAG-3 is injected intravenously (Figs. 534-2 and 534-3). During the first 2-3 min, renal parenchymal uptake is analyzed and compared, allowing computation of differential renal function. Subsequently, excretion is evaluated. After 20-30 min, furosemide 1 mg/kg is injected intravenously, and the rapidity and pattern of drainage from the kidneys to the bladder are analyzed. If no obstruction is present, half of the radionuclide should be cleared from the renal pelvis within 10-15 min, termed the

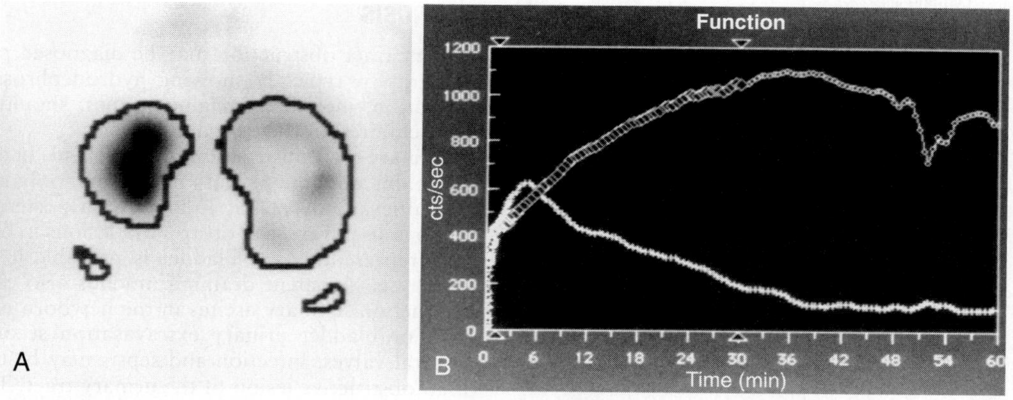

Figure 534-2 Same patient as in Figure 534-1. 6 wk old, MAG-3 diuretic renogram. The right kidney is on the *right* side of the image. *A,* Differential renal function: left kidney 70%, right kidney 30%. *B,* After administration of furosemide, drainage from the left kidney was normal and drainage from the right kidney was slow, consistent with right ureteropelvic junction obstruction. Pyeloplasty was performed on the right kidney.

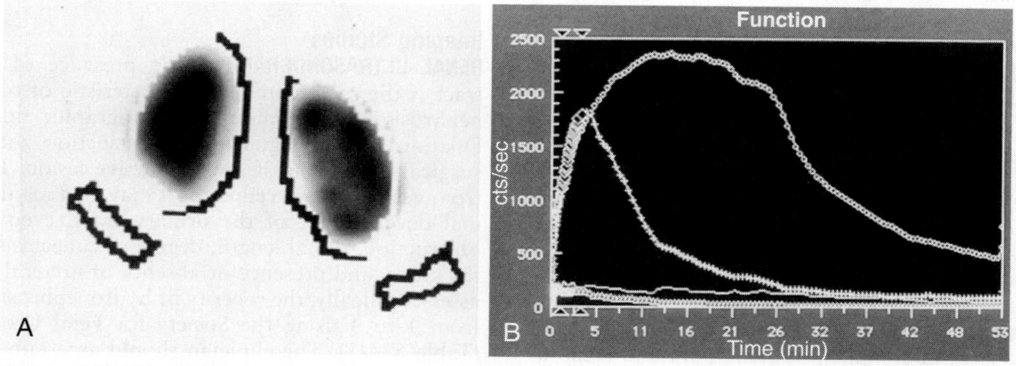

Figure 534-3 Same patient as in Figure 534-1. *A,* MAG-3 diuretic renogram at 14 mo of age shows equal function in the two kidneys. *B,* Prompt drainage after the administration of furosemide.

half-time ($t_{1/2}$). If there is significant upper tract obstruction, the $t_{1/2}$ usually is >20 min. A $t_{1/2}$ of 15-20 min is indeterminate. The images generated usually provide an accurate assessment of the site of obstruction. Numerous variables affect the outcome of the diuretic renogram. Newborn kidneys are functionally immature, and, in the first month of life, normal kidneys might not demonstrate normal drainage after diuretic administration. Dehydration prolongs parenchymal transit and can blunt the diuretic response. Giving an insufficient dose of furosemide can result in inadequate drainage. If vesicoureteral reflux is present, continuous bladder drainage is mandatory to prevent the radionuclide from refluxing from the bladder into the dilated upper tract, which would prolong the washout phase.

The MAG-3 diuretic renogram is considered superior to the excretory urogram in infants and children with hydronephrosis, because bowel gas and immaturity of renal function often cause the intravenous pyelogram (IVP) images to be suboptimal. The diuretic renogram provides an objective assessment of the relative function of each kidney.

EXCRETORY UROGRAM Excretory urogram is rarely used in assessing the pediatric urinary tract, although it may be useful in selected cases with indeterminate upper urinary tract obstruction or a suspected duplication anomaly.

MAGNETIC RESONANCE UROGRAPHY MR urography is also used to evaluate suspected upper urinary tract pathology. The child is hydrated and given intravenous furosemide. Gadolinium-DTPA is injected and routine T1-weighted and fat-suppressed fast spin-echo T2-weighted imaging is performed through the kidneys, ureters, and bladder. This study provides superb images of the pathology, and methodology permits assessment of differential renal function and drainage (Fig. 534-4). There is no radiation exposure; younger children need sedation or anesthesia. It is used primarily when renal sonography and nuclear imaging fail to delineate complex pathology.

COMPUTED TOMOGRAPHY In children with a suspected ureteral calculus, noncontrast spiral CT of the abdomen and pelvis is a standard method of demonstrating whether a calculus is present, its location, and whether there is significant proximal hydronephrosis. This study is the initial study of choice in many these patients. The disadvantage of CT is the significant radiation exposure, and it should be used only when the results will direct management decisions.

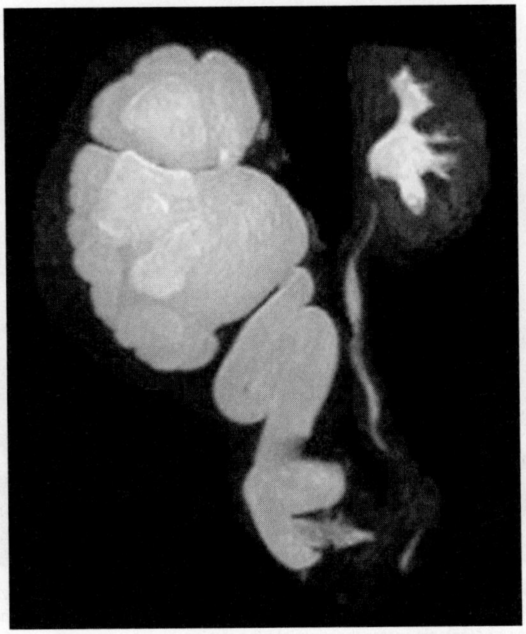

Figure 534-4 MR urogram in boy with distal ureterovesical obstruction.

Ancillary Studies

In unusual cases, an **antegrade pyelogram** (insertion of a percutaneous nephrostomy tube and injection of contrast agent), can be performed to assess the anatomy of the upper urinary tract. This procedure usually requires general anesthesia. In addition, an **antegrade pressure-perfusion flow study** (Whitaker test) may be performed, in which fluid is infused at a measured rate, usually 10 mL/min. The pressures in the renal pelvis and the bladder are monitored during this infusion, and pressure differences exceeding 20 cm H_2O suggest obstruction. In other cases, cystoscopy with retrograde pyelography provides excellent images of the upper urinary tract (Fig. 534-5).

SPECIFIC TYPES OF URINARY TRACT OBSTRUCTION AND THEIR TREATMENT

Hydrocalycosis

The term *hydrocalycosis* refers to a localized dilatation of the calyx caused by obstruction of its infundibulum, termed *infundibular stenosis*. Such obstruction can be developmental in origin or secondary to inflammatory processes, such as UTI. When the abnormality is not discovered by antenatal ultrasonography or incidentally, it usually is discovered during evaluation for pain or UTI. The diagnosis of infundibular stenosis is usually established by IVP or CT scan with contrast.

Ureteropelvic Junction Obstruction

Ureteropelvic junction (UPJ) obstruction is the most common obstructive lesion in childhood and usually is caused by intrinsic stenosis (see Figs. 534-1 to 534-4). An accessory artery to the lower pole of the kidney also can cause extrinsic obstruction. The typical appearance on ultrasonography is grade 3 or 4 hydronephrosis without a dilated ureter. UPJ obstruction most commonly manifests on antenatal sonography revealing fetal hydronephro-

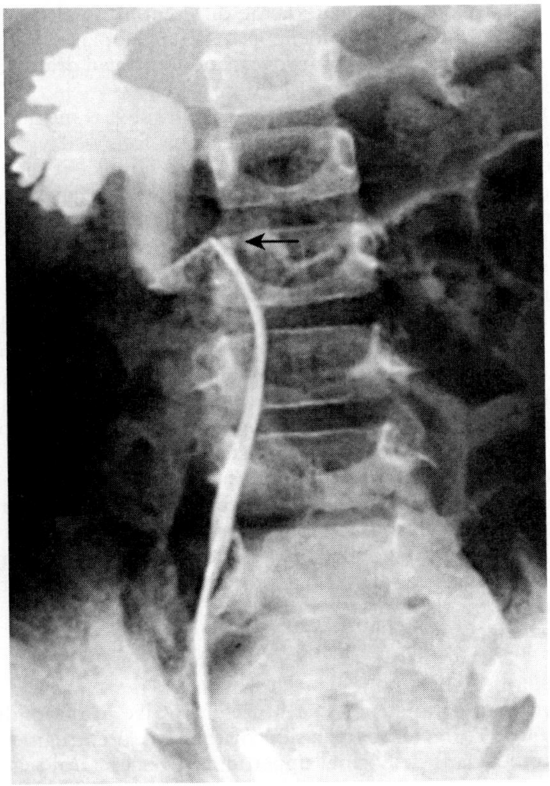

Figure 534-5 Retrograde pyelogram showing medial deviation of a dilated upper ureter to the level of the 3rd lumbar vertebra, characteristic of a retrocaval ureter.

sis; as a palpable renal mass in a newborn or infant; as abdominal, flank, or back pain; as a febrile UTI; or as hematuria after minimal trauma. Approximately 60% of cases occur on the left side, and the male:female ratio is 2:1. In 10% of cases, UPJ obstruction is bilateral. In kidneys with UPJ obstruction, renal function may be significantly impaired from pressure atrophy, but approximately half of affected kidneys have relatively normal function. The anomaly is corrected by performing a pyeloplasty, in which the stenotic segment is excised and the normal ureter and renal pelvis are reattached. Success rates are 91-98%. Pyeloplasty can be performed using laparoscopic techniques, often robotic-assisted using the da Vinci robot.

Lesser degrees of UPJ obstruction can cause mild hydronephrosis, which usually is nonobstructive, and typically these kidneys function normally. The spectrum of UPJ abnormalities has been referred to as *anomalous UPJ*. Another cause of mild hydronephrosis is fetal folds of the upper ureter, which also are nonobstructive.

The diagnosis can be difficult to establish in an asymptomatic infant in whom dilatation of the renal pelvis is found incidentally in a prenatal ultrasonogram. After birth, the sonographic study is repeated to confirm the prenatal finding. A VCUG is necessary because 10-15% of patients have ipsilateral vesicoureteral reflux. Because neonatal oliguria can cause temporary decompression of a dilated renal pelvis, it is ideal to perform the first postnatal sonogram after the 3rd day of life. Delaying the sonogram may be impractical. If no dilation is found on the initial sonogram, a repeat study should be performed at 1 mo of age. If the kidney shows grade 1 or 2 hydronephrosis and the renal parenchyma appears normal, a period of observation usually is appropriate, with sequential renal ultrasonograms to monitor the severity of hydronephrosis, and the hydronephrosis usually disappears. **Antibiotic prophylaxis** is not indicated for children with mild hydronephrosis. If the hydronephrosis is grade 3 or 4, spontaneous resolution is less likely and obstruction is more likely to be present, particularly if the renal pelvic diameter is 3 cm. A diuretic renogram with MAG-3 is performed at 4–6 wk of age. If there is poor upper tract drainage or the differential renal function is poor, pyeloplasty is recommended. After pyeloplasty the differential renal function often improves, and improved drainage with furosemide stimulation is expected.

If the differential function on renography is normal, and drainage is satisfactory, the infant can be followed with serial ultrasonograms, even with grade 4 hydronephrosis. If the hydronephrosis remains severe with no improvement, a repeat diuretic renogram after 6-12 mo can help in the decision between continued observation and surgical repair. Prompt surgical repair is indicated in infants with an abdominal mass, bilateral severe hydronephrosis, a solitary kidney, or diminished function in the involved kidney. In unusual cases in which the differential renal function is <10% but the kidney definitely has some function, insertion of a percutaneous nephrostomy tube allows drainage of the hydronephrotic kidney for a few weeks to allow reassessment of renal function. In older children who present with symptoms, the diagnosis of UPJ obstruction usually is established by ultrasonography and diuretic renography.

The following entities should be considered in the **differential diagnosis:** megacalycosis, a congenital nonobstructive dilatation of the calyces without pelvic or ureteric dilatation; vesicoureteral reflux with marked dilatation and kinking of the ureter; and midureteral or distal ureteral obstruction when the ureter is not well visualized on the urogram.

Midureteral Obstruction

Congenital ureteral stenosis or a ureteral valve in the midureter is rare. It is corrected by excision of the strictured segment and reanastomosis of the normal upper and lower ureteral segments. A **retrocaval ureter** is an anomaly in which the upper right ureter travels posterior to the inferior vena cava. In this anomaly, the vena cava can cause extrinsic compression and obstruction. An IVP shows the right ureter to be medially deviated at the level of the 3rd lumbar vertebra. The diagnosis may be confirmed by retrograde pyelography (see Fig. 534-5). Surgical treatment consists of transection of the upper ureter, moving it anterior to the vena cava, and reanastomosing the upper and lower segments. Repair is necessary only when obstruction is present. Retroperitoneal tumors, fibrosis caused by surgical procedures, inflammatory processes (as in chronic granulomatous disease), and radiation therapy can cause acquired midureteral obstruction.

Ectopic Ureter

A ureter that drains outside the bladder is referred to as an **ectopic ureter.** This anomaly is 3 times as common in girls as in boys and usually is detected prenatally. The ectopic ureter usually drains the upper pole of a duplex collecting system (2 ureters).

In girls, approximately 35% of these ureters enter the urethra at the bladder neck, 35% enter the urethrovaginal septum, 25% enter the vagina, and a few drain into the cervix, uterus, Gartner duct, or a urethral diverticulum. Often the terminal aspect of the ureter is narrowed, causing hydroureteronephrosis. With the exception of the ectopic ureter entering the bladder neck, in girls an ectopic ureter causes continuous urinary incontinence from the affected renal moiety. UTI is common because of urinary stasis.

In boys, ectopic ureters enter the posterior urethra (above the external sphincter) in 47%, the prostatic utricle in 10%, the seminal vesicle in 33%, the ejaculatory duct in 5%, and the vas deferens in 5%. Consequently, in boys, an ectopic ureter does not cause incontinence, and most patients present with a UTI or epididymitis.

Evaluation includes a renal sonogram, VCUG, and renal scan, which demonstrates whether the affected segment has significant function. The sonogram shows the affected hydronephrotic kidney or dilated upper pole and ureter down to the bladder (Fig. 534-6). If the ectopic ureter drains into the bladder neck (female), a VCUG usually shows reflux into the ureter. Otherwise, there is no reflux into the ectopic ureter, but there may be reflux into the ipsilateral lower pole ureter or contralateral collecting system.

Treatment depends on the status of the renal unit drained by the ectopic ureter. If there is satisfactory function, ureteral reimplantation into the bladder or ureteroureterostomy (anastomosing the ectopic upper pole ureter into the normally inserting lower

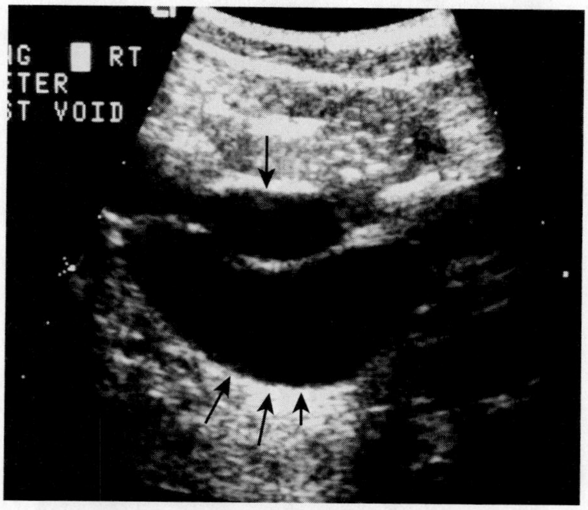

Figure 534-6 Ultrasonographic image of the right dilated ureter *(bottom arrows)* extending behind and caudal to a nearly empty bladder *(top arrow)* in a girl with urinary incontinence and ectopic ureter draining into the vagina.

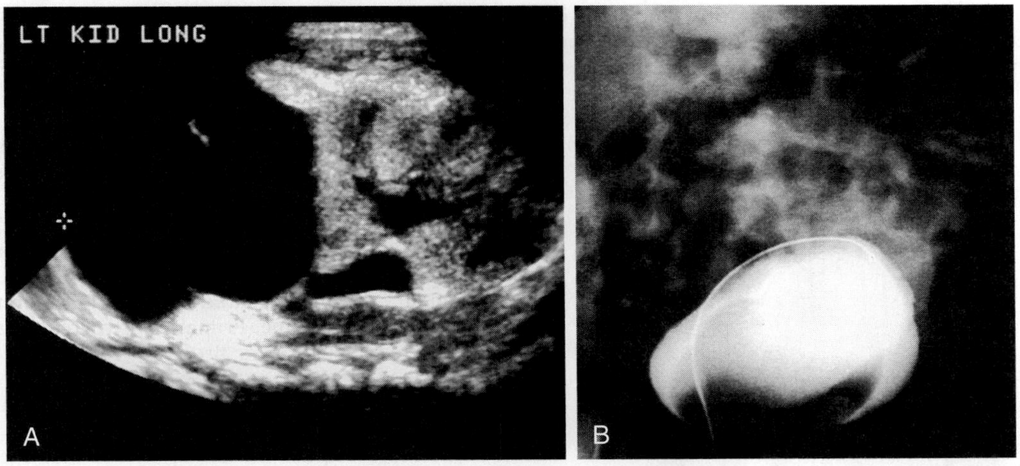

Figure 534-7 *A,* Infant with ectopic ureterocele. Sonogram of the left kidney shows massive dilation of the upper pole and a normal lower pole. *B,* Voiding cystourethrogram shows large ureterocele, draining the left upper pole, in the bladder. No reflux is present.

pole ureter) is indicated. If function is poor, partial or total nephrectomy is indicated. In many centers this procedure is done laparoscopically and often with robotic assistance using the da Vinci robot.

Ureterocele

A ureterocele is a cystic dilatation of the terminal ureter and is obstructive because of a pinpoint ureteral orifice. Ureteroceles are much more common in girls than in boys. Affected children usually are discovered by prenatal ultrasonography, but some present with a febrile UTI. Ureteroceles may be ectopic, in which case the cystic swelling extends through the bladder neck into the urethra, or orthotopic, in which case the ureterocele is entirely within the bladder. Both orthotopic and ectopic ureteroceles can be bilateral.

In girls, ureteroceles nearly always are associated with ureteral duplication (Fig. 534-7), whereas in 50% of affected boys there is only 1 ureter. When associated with a duplication anomaly, the ureterocele drains the upper renal moiety, which commonly functions poorly or is dysplastic because of congenital obstruction. The lower pole ureter drains into the bladder superior and lateral to the upper pole ureter and may reflux.

An **ectopic ureterocele** extends submucosally into the urethra. Rarely, large ectopic ureteroceles can cause bladder outlet obstruction and retention of urine with bilateral hydronephrosis. In girls, the ureterocele can prolapse from the urethral meatus. Ultrasonography is effective in demonstrating the ureterocele and whether the associated obstructed system is duplicated or single. VCUG usually shows a filling defect in the bladder, sometimes large, corresponding to the ureterocele, and it often shows reflux into the adjacent lower pole collecting system with typical findings of a "drooping lily" appearance to the kidney. Nuclear renal scintigraphy is most accurate in demonstrating whether the affected renal moiety has significant function.

Treatment of ectopic ureteroceles varies among different medical centers and depends on whether the upper pole functions on renal scan and whether there is reflux into the lower pole ureter. If there is nonfunction of the upper pole and there is no reflux, treatment usually involves laparoscopic, robotic, or open excision of the obstructed upper pole and most of the associated ureter. If there is function in the upper pole or significant reflux into the lower pole ureter, or if the patient is septic from infection of the hydronephrotic kidney, then transurethral incision with cautery or the holmium:YAG laser is appropriate initial therapy to decompress the ureterocele. However, reflux into the incised ureterocele is common, and subsequent excision of the ureterocele and ureteral reimplantation usually is necessary. An alternative method is to perform a upper-to-lower ureteroureterostomy, allowing the obstructed upper pole ureter to drain through the normal lower ureter; this procedure often is performed with minimally invasive laparoscopic (robotic) technique or through a small incision.

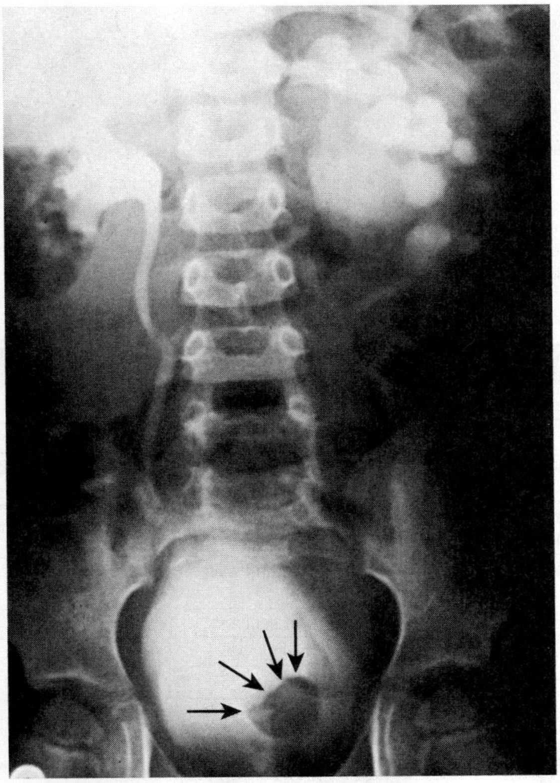

Figure 534-8 Simple intravesical ureterocele. The excretory urogram shows left hydronephrosis and a round filling defect on the left side of the bladder corresponding to a simple ureterocele causing left ureteral obstruction. This lesion was treated by transurethral incision and drainage of the ureterocele.

Orthotopic ureteroceles are associated with duplicated or single collecting systems, and the orifice is in the expected location in the bladder (Fig. 534-8). These anomalies usually are discovered during an investigation for prenatal hydronephrosis or a UTI. Ultrasonography is sensitive for detecting the ureterocele in the bladder and hydroureteronephrosis. IVP reveals varying degrees of ureteral and calyceal dilatation, and there is a round filling defect in the bladder. In delayed films, cystic dilatation of the ureter may be clearly visible and full of contrast material. Transurethral incision of the ureterocele effectively relieves the obstruction, but it can result in vesicoureteral reflux, necessitating ureteral reimplantation later. Some prefer open excision of the ureterocele and reimplantation as the initial form of treatment. Small, simple ureteroceles discovered incidentally without upper tract dilatation generally do not require treatment.

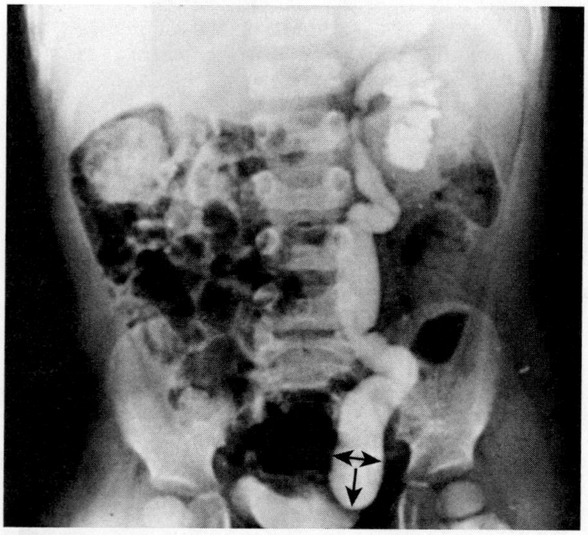

Figure 534-9 Obstructed nonrefluxing megaureter. Excretory urogram in a girl with a history of a febrile urinary tract infection. The right side is normal. The left side reveals hydroureteronephrosis with predominant dilatation of the distal ureter. Note the characteristic appearance of the distal ureter. There was no vesicoureteral reflux. The diagnosis of obstruction was confirmed by diuretic renography.

Megaureter

Table 534-3 presents a classification of megaureters (dilated ureter). Numerous disorders can cause ureteral dilation, and many are nonobstructive.

Megaureters usually are discovered during antenatal sonography, postnatal UTI, hematuria, or abdominal pain. A careful history, physical examination, and VCUG identify causes of secondary megaureters and refluxing megaureters as well as the prune-belly syndrome. Primary obstructed megaureters and nonobstructed megaureters probably represent varying degrees of severity of the same anomaly.

The primary obstructed nonrefluxing megaureter results from abnormal development of the distal ureter, with collagenous tissue replacing the muscle layer. Normal ureteral peristalsis is disrupted, and the proximal ureter widens. Usually there is not a true stricture. On IVP, the distal ureter is more dilated in its distal segment and tapers abruptly at or above the junction of the bladder (Fig. 534-9). The lesion may be unilateral or bilateral. Significant hydroureteronephrosis suggests obstruction. Megaureter predisposes to UTI, urinary stones, hematuria, and flank pain due to urinary stasis. In most cases, diuretic renography and sequential sonographic studies can reliably differentiate obstructed from nonobstructed megaureters. In most nonobstructed megaureters, the hydroureteronephrosis diminishes gradually (Fig. 534-10). Truly obstructed megaureters require surgical treatment, with excision of the narrowed segment, ureteral tapering, and reimplantation of the ureter. The results of surgical reconstruction usually are good, but the prognosis depends on preexisting renal function and whether complications develop.

Table 534-3 CLASSIFICATION OF MEGAURETER

REFLUXING		OBSTRUCTED		NONREFLUXING AND NONOBSTRUCTED	
Primary	**Secondary**	**Primary**	**Secondary**	**Primary**	**Secondary**
Primary reflux	Neuropathic bladder	Intrinsic (primary obstructed megaureter)	Neuropathic bladder	Nonrefluxing, nonobstructive	Diabetes insipidus
Megacystic-megaureter syndrome	Hinman syndrome	Ureteral valve	Hinman syndrome		Infection
Ectopic ureter	Posterior urethral valves	Ectopic ureter	Posterior urethral valves		Persistent after relief of obstruction
Prune-belly syndrome	Bladder diverticulum	Ectopic uretocele	Ureteral calculus		
	Postoperative		Extrinsic		
			Postoperative		

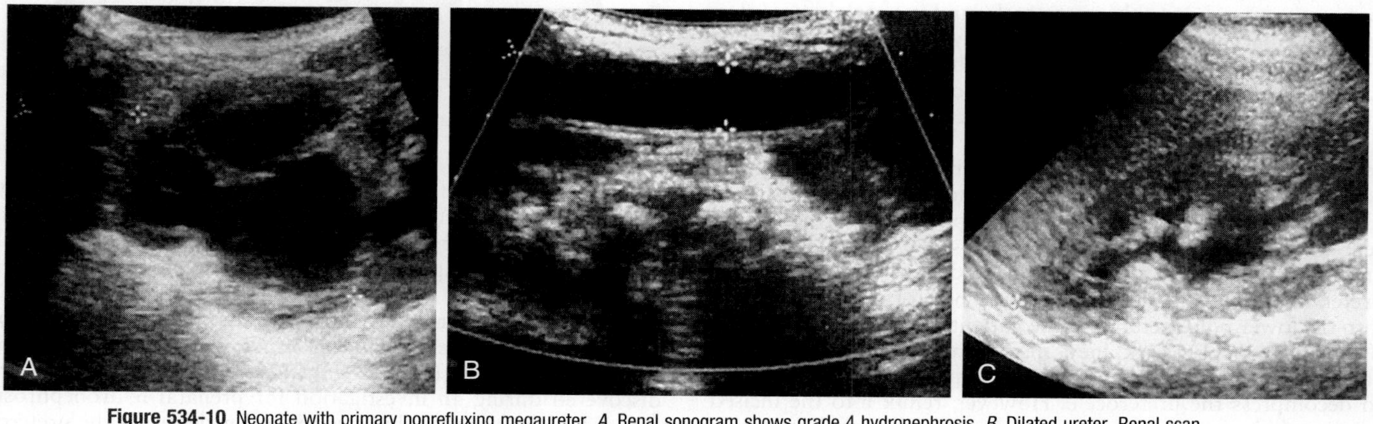

Figure 534-10 Neonate with primary nonrefluxing megaureter. *A,* Renal sonogram shows grade 4 hydronephrosis. *B,* Dilated ureter. Renal scan showed equal function with the contralateral kidney and satisfactory drainage with diuresis stimulation. *C,* Follow-up sonogram at 10 mo shows complete resolution of hydronephrosis.

If differential renal function is normal (>45%) and the child is asymptomatic, it is safe to follow the patient with serial ultrasonography and diuretic renography to monitor renal function and drainage. If there is grade 4 hydronephrosis, these children should receive prophylactic antimicrobial therapy. If renal function deteriorates, upper urinary tract drainage slows, or UTI occurs, ureteral reimplantation is recommended. Approximately 20% of children with a nonrefluxing megaureter undergo ureteral reimplantation.

Prune-Belly Syndrome

Prune-belly syndrome, also called **triad syndrome** or **Eagle-Barrett syndrome,** occurs in approximately 1 in 40,000 births; 95% of affected children are male. The characteristic association of deficient abdominal muscles, undescended testes, and urinary tract abnormalities probably results from severe urethral obstruction in fetal life (Fig. 534-11). Oligohydramnios and pulmonary hypoplasia are common complications in the perinatal period. Many affected infants are stillborn. Urinary tract abnormalities include massive dilatation of the ureters and upper tracts and a very large bladder, with a patent urachus or a urachal diverticulum. Most patients have vesicoureteral reflux. The prostatic urethra usually is dilated, and the prostate is hypoplastic. The anterior urethra may be dilated, resulting in a megalourethra. Rarely, there is urethral stenosis or atresia. The kidneys usually show various degrees of dysplasia, and the testes usually are intra-abdominal. Malrotation of the bowel often is present. Cardiac abnormalities occur in 10% of cases; >50% have abnormalities of the musculoskeletal system, including limb abnormalities and scoliosis. In girls, anomalies of the urethra, uterus, and vagina usually are present.

Many neonates with prune-belly syndrome have difficulty with effective bladder emptying because the bladder musculature is poorly developed, and the urethra may be narrowed. When no obstruction is present, the goal of treatment is the prevention of UTI with antibiotic prophylaxis. When obstruction of the ureters or urethra is demonstrated, temporary drainage procedures, such as a vesicostomy, can help to preserve renal function until the child is old enough for surgery. Some children with prune-belly syndrome have been found to have classic or atypical posterior urethral valves. UTIs occur often and should be treated promptly. Correction of the undescended testes by orchidopexy can be difficult in these children because the testes are located high in the abdomen and surgery is best accomplished in the first 6 mo of life. Reconstruction of the abdominal wall offers cosmetic and functional benefits.

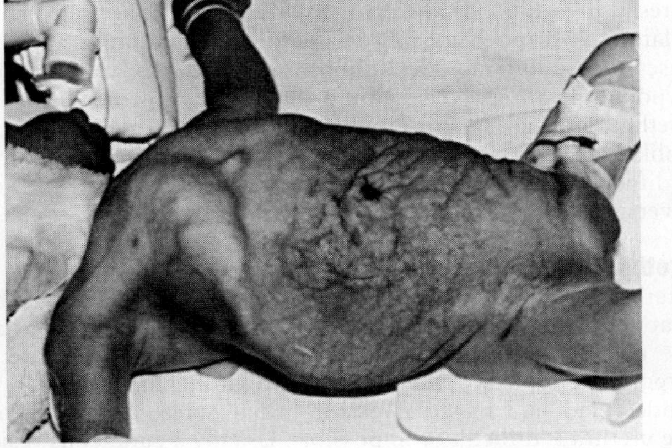

Figure 534-11 Photograph of a 1,600-g newborn with the prune-belly syndrome. Note the lack of tonicity of the abdominal wall and the wrinkled appearance of the skin.

The prognosis ultimately depends on the degree of pulmonary hypoplasia and renal dysplasia. One third of children with prune-belly syndrome are stillborn or die in the first few months of life because of pulmonary hypoplasia. As many as 30% of the long-term survivors develop end-stage renal disease from dysplasia or complications of infection or reflux and eventually require renal transplantation. Renal transplantation in these children offers good results.

Bladder Neck Obstruction

Bladder neck obstruction usually is secondary to ectopic ureterocele, bladder calculi, or a tumor of the prostate (rhabdomyosarcoma). The manifestations include difficulty voiding, urinary retention, UTI, and bladder distention with overflow incontinence. Apparent bladder neck obstruction is common in cases of posterior urethral valves, but it seldom has any functional significance. Primary bladder neck obstruction is extremely rare.

Posterior Urethral Valves

The most common cause of severe obstructive uropathy in children is posterior urethral valves, affecting 1 in 8,000 boys. The urethral valves are tissue leaflets fanning distally from the prostatic urethra to the external urinary sphincter. A slit-like opening usually separates the leaflets. Valves are of unclear embryologic origin and cause varying degrees of obstruction. Approximately 30% of patients experience end-stage renal disease or chronic renal insufficiency. The prostatic urethra dilates, and the bladder muscle undergoes hypertrophy. Vesicoureteral reflux occurs in 50% of patients, and distal ureteral obstruction can result from a chronically distended bladder or bladder muscle hypertrophy. The renal changes range from mild hydronephrosis to severe renal dysplasia; their severity probably depends on the severity of the obstruction and its time of onset during fetal development. As in other cases of obstruction or renal dysplasia, there may be oligohydramnios and pulmonary hypoplasia.

Affected boys with posterior urethral valves often are discovered prenatally when maternal ultrasonography reveals bilateral hydronephrosis, a distended bladder, and, if the obstruction is severe, oligohydramnios. Prenatal bladder decompression by percutaneous vesicoamniotic shunt or open fetal surgery has been reported. Experimental and clinical evidence of the possible benefits of fetal intervention is lacking, and few affected fetuses are candidates. Prenatally diagnosed posterior urethral valves, particularly when discovered in the 2nd trimester, carry a poorer prognosis than those detected after birth. In the male neonate, posterior urethral valves are suspected when there is a palpably **distended bladder** and the **urinary stream is weak.** If the obstruction is severe and goes unrecognized during the neonatal period, infants can present later in life with failure to thrive due to uremia or sepsis caused by infection in the obstructed urinary tract. With lesser degrees of obstruction, children present later in life with difficulty in achieving diurnal urinary continence or with UTI. The diagnosis is established with a VCUG (Fig. 534-12) or by perineal ultrasonography.

After the diagnosis is established, renal function and the anatomy of the upper urinary tract should be carefully evaluated. In the healthy neonate, a small polyethylene feeding tube (No. 5 or No. 8 French) is inserted in the bladder and left for several days. Passing the feeding tube may be difficult, because the tip of the tube can coil in the prostatic urethra. A sign of this problem is that urine drains around the catheter rather than through it. A Foley (balloon) catheter should not be used, because the balloon can cause severe bladder spasm, which can produce severe ureteral obstruction.

If the serum creatinine level remains normal or returns to normal, treatment consists of transurethral ablation of the valve leaflets, which is performed endoscopically under general

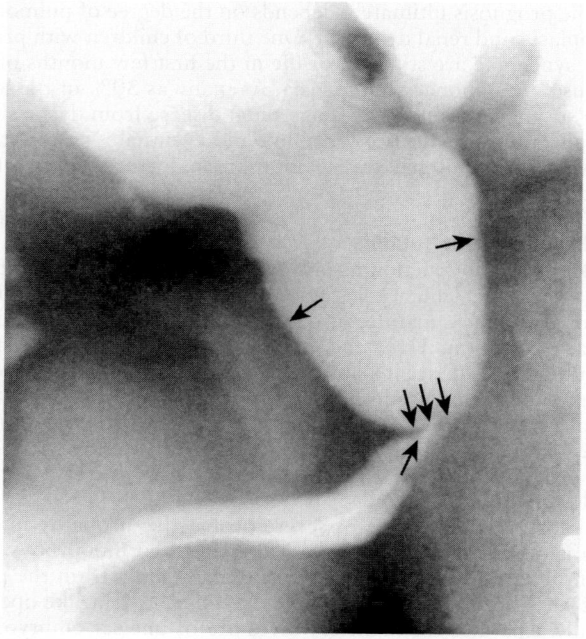

Figure 534-12 Voiding cystourethrogram in an infant with posterior urethral valves. Note the dilation of the prostatic urethra and the transverse linear filling defect corresponding to the valves.

anesthesia. If the urethra is too small for transurethral ablation, temporary vesicostomy is preferred, in which the dome of the bladder is exteriorized on the lower abdominal wall. When the child is older, the valves may be ablated and the vesicostomy closed.

If the serum creatinine level remains high or increases despite bladder drainage by a small catheter, secondary ureteral obstruction, irreversible renal damage, or renal dysplasia should be suspected. In such cases, a vesicostomy should be performed. Cutaneous pyelostomy rarely affords better drainage when compared with cutaneous vesicostomy, and the latter also allows continued bladder growth and gradual improvement in bladder wall compliance.

In the septic and uremic infant, lifesaving measures must include prompt correction of the electrolyte imbalance and control of the infection by appropriate antibiotics. Drainage of the upper tracts by percutaneous nephrostomy and hemodialysis may be necessary. After the patient's condition becomes stable, evaluation and treatment may be undertaken. Posterior valves are diagnosed in some older boys because of a poor stream, diurnal incontinence, or a UTI; these boys generally are treated by primary valve ablation.

Favorable prognostic factors include a normal prenatal ultrasonogram between 18 and 24 wk of gestation, a serum creatinine level <0.8-1.0 mg/dL after bladder decompression, and visualization of the corticomedullary junction on renal sonography. In several situations, a "popoff valve" can occur during urinary tract development, which preserves the integrity of one or both kidneys. For example, 15% of boys with posterior urethral valves have unilateral reflux into a nonfunctioning dysplastic kidney, termed the **VURD syndrome** (*v*alves, *u*nilateral *r*eflux, *d*ysplasia). In these boys, the high bladder pressure is dissipated into the nonfunctioning kidney, allowing normal development of the contralateral kidney. In newborn boys with urinary ascites, the urine generally leaks out from the obstructed collecting system through the renal fornices, allowing normal development of the kidneys. Unfavorable prognostic factors include the presence of oligohydramnios in utero, identification of hydronephrosis before 24 wk of gestation, a serum creatinine level >1.0 mg/dL after bladder decompression, identification of cortical cysts in both kidneys, and persistence of diurnal incontinence beyond 5 yr of age.

The prognosis in the newborn is related to the child's degree of pulmonary hypoplasia and potential for recovery of renal function. Severely affected infants often are stillborn. Of those who survive the neonatal period, approximately 30% eventually require kidney transplantation and 15% have renal insufficiency. In some series, kidney transplantation in children with posterior urethral valves has a lower success rate than does transplantation in children with normal bladders, presumably because of the adverse influence of altered bladder function on graft function and survival.

After valve ablation, antimicrobial prophylaxis is beneficial in preventing UTI, because hydronephrosis to some degree often persists for many years. These boys should be evaluated annually with a renal ultrasonogram, physical examination including assessment of somatic growth and blood pressure, urinalysis, and determination of serum levels of electrolytes. Many boys have significant polyuria resulting from a concentrating defect secondary to prolonged obstructive uropathy. If these children acquire a systemic illness with vomiting and/or diarrhea, urine output cannot be used to assess their hydration status. They can become dehydrated quickly, and there should be a low threshold for hospital admission for intravenous rehydration. Some of these patients have renal tubular acidosis, requiring oral bicarbonate therapy. If there is any significant degree of renal dysfunction, growth impairment, or hypertension, the child should be followed closely by a pediatric nephrologist. When vesicoureteral reflux is present, expectant treatment and prophylactic doses of antibacterial drugs are advisable. If breakthrough UTI occurs, surgical correction should be undertaken.

After treatment, boys with urethral valves often do not achieve diurnal urinary continence as early as other boys. Incontinence can result from a combination of factors, including uninhibited bladder contractions, poor bladder compliance, bladder atonia, bladder neck dyssynergia, or polyuria. Often these boys require urodynamic evaluation with urodynamics or videourodynamics to plan therapy. Boys with noncompliance are at significant risk for ongoing renal damage, even in the absence of infection. Overnight catheter drainage has been shown to be beneficial in boys with polyuria and can help preserve renal function. Urinary incontinence usually improves with age, particularly after puberty. Meticulous attention to bladder compliance, emptying, and infection can improve results in the future.

Urethral Atresia

The most severe form of obstructive uropathy in boys is urethral atresia, a rare condition. In utero there is a distended bladder, bilateral hydroureteronephrosis, and oligohydramnios. In most cases, these infants are stillborn or succumb to pulmonary hypoplasia. Some boys with prune-belly syndrome also have urethral atresia. If the urachus is patent, oligohydramnios is unlikely and the infant usually survives. Urethral reconstruction is difficult, and most patients are managed with continent urinary diversion.

Urethral Hypoplasia

Urethral hypoplasia is a rare form of obstructive uropathy in boys that is less severe than urethral atresia. In urethral hypoplasia, the urethral lumen is extremely small. Neonates with urethral hypoplasia typically have bilateral hydronephrosis and a distended bladder. Passage of a small pediatric feeding tube through the urethra is difficult or impossible. Usually a cutaneous vesicostomy must be performed to relieve upper urinary tract obstruction, and the severity of renal insufficiency is variable. The most severely affected boys have end-stage renal disease. Treatment includes urethral reconstruction, gradual urethral dilatation, or continent urinary diversion.

Urethral Strictures

Urethral strictures in boys usually result from urethral trauma, either iatrogenic (catheterization, endoscopic procedures, previous urethral reconstruction) or accidental (straddle injuries, pelvic fractures). Because these lesions can develop gradually, the decrease in force of the urinary stream is seldom noticed by the child or the parents. More commonly, the obstruction causes symptoms of bladder instability, hematuria, or dysuria. Catheterization of the bladder usually is impossible. The diagnosis is made by a voiding film obtained during intravenous urography or retrograde urethrography. Ultrasonography also has been used to diagnose urethral strictures. Endoscopy is confirmatory. Endoscopic treatment of short strictures by direct vision urethrotomy is often successful initially and results in a profoundly improved urinary stream, but often the stricture recurs and is found at long-term follow-up. Longer strictures surrounded by periurethral fibrosis often require urethroplasty. Repeated endoscopic procedures generally should be avoided, because they can cause additional urethral damage. Noninvasive measurement of the urinary flow rate and pattern is useful for diagnosis and follow-up.

In girls, true urethral strictures are rare because the female urethra is protected from trauma, particularly in childhood. In the past it was thought that a distal urethral ring commonly caused obstruction of the female urethra and UTI and that affected girls benefited from urethral dilatation. The diagnosis was suspected when a "spinning top" deformity of the urethra was found in the VCUG (see Fig. 537-3) and was confirmed by urethral calibration. There is no correlation between the radiologic appearance of the urethra in the VCUG and the urethral caliber and no significant difference in urethral caliber between girls with recurrent cystitis and normal age-matched controls. The finding usually is secondary to detrusor-sphincter dyssynergia. Consequently, urethral dilatation in girls rarely is indicated.

Anterior Urethral Valves and Urethral Diverticula in the Male

Anterior urethral valves are rare. The obstruction is not obstructing valve leaflets, as occurs in the posterior urethra. Rather, it is a urethral diverticulum in the penile urethra that expands during voiding. Distal extension of the diverticulum causes extrinsic compression of the distal penile urethra, causing urethral obstruction. Typically there is a soft mass on the ventral surface of the penis at the penoscrotal junction. In addition, the urinary stream often is weak, and the physical findings associated with posterior urethral valves often are present. The diverticulum may be small and minimally obstructive, or, in other cases, may be severely obstructive and cause renal insufficiency. The diagnosis is suspected on physical examination and is confirmed by the VCUG. Treatment involves open excision of the diverticulum or transurethral excision of the distal urethral cusp. Urethral diverticula occasionally occur after extensive hypospadias repair.

Fusiform dilatation of the urethra or **megalourethra** can result from underdevelopment of the corpus spongiosum and support structures of the urethra. This condition is commonly associated with the prune-belly syndrome.

Male Urethral Meatal Stenosis

See Chapter 538 for information on urethral meatal stenosis in males.

BIBLIOGRAPHY

Please visit the Nelson Textbook of Pediatrics *website at www.expertconsult.com for the complete bibliography.*

Chapter 535
Anomalies of the Bladder
Jack S. Elder

BLADDER EXSTROPHY

Classic exstrophy of the urinary bladder occurs in about 1/35,000-40,000 births. The male:female ratio is 2:1. The severity ranges from simple **epispadias** (in boys) to complete exstrophy of the cloaca involving exposure of the entire hindgut and the bladder (termed **cloacal exstrophy**).

For the full continuation of this chapter, please visit the Nelson Textbook of Pediatrics *website at www.expertconsult.com.*

Chapter 536
Neuropathic Bladder
Jack S. Elder

Neuropathic bladder dysfunction in children usually is congenital, generally resulting from neural tube defects or other spinal abnormalities. Acquired diseases and traumatic lesions of the spinal cord are less common. Central nervous system tumors, sacrococcygeal teratoma, spinal abnormalities associated with imperforate anus (Chapter 336), and spinal cord trauma also can result in abnormal innervation of the bladder and/or sphincter.

For the full continuation of this chapter, please visit the Nelson Textbook of Pediatrics *website at www.expertconsult.com.*

Chapter 537
Voiding Dysfunction
Jack S. Elder

NORMAL VOIDING AND TOILET TRAINING

The fetus voids by reflex bladder contraction in concert with simultaneous contraction of the bladder and relaxation of the sphincter. Urine storage consists of sympathetic and pudendal nerve-mediated inhibition of detrusor contractile activity accompanied by closure of the bladder neck and proximal urethra with increased activity of the external sphincter. The infant has coordinated reflex voiding as often as 15-20 times/day. Over time, bladder capacity increases. In children up to the age of 14 yr, the mean bladder capacity in ounces is equal to the age (in yrs) plus 2.

At 2-4 yr, the child is developmentally ready to begin toilet training. To achieve conscious bladder control, several conditions must be present: awareness of bladder filling; cortical inhibition (suprapontine modulation) of reflex (unstable) bladder contractions; ability to consciously tighten the external sphincter to prevent incontinence; normal bladder growth; and motivation by the child to stay dry. The transitional phase of voiding refers to the period when children are acquiring bladder control. Girls typically acquire bladder control before boys, and bowel control typically is achieved before bladder control.

DIURNAL INCONTINENCE

Daytime incontinence not secondary to neurologic abnormalities is common in children (Chapter 21.3). At age 5 yr, 95% have been dry during the day at some time and 92% are dry. At 7 yr, 96% are dry, although 15% have significant urgency at times. At 12 yr, 99% are dry during the day. The most common cause of daytime incontinence is an **overactive bladder**. Table 537-1 lists the causes of diurnal incontinence in children.

Important points in the history include the pattern of incontinence, including the frequency, the volume of urine lost during incontinent episodes, whether the incontinence is associated with urgency or giggling, whether it occurs after voiding, and whether the incontinence is continuous. The frequency of voiding and whether there is nocturnal enuresis, a strong, continuous urinary stream, or sensation of incomplete bladder emptying should be assessed. A diary of when the child voids and whether the child was wet or dry is helpful. Other urologic problems such as urinary tract infections (UTIs), reflux, neurologic disorders, or a family history of duplication anomalies should be assessed. Bowel habits also should be evaluated, because incontinence is common in children with constipation and/or encopresis. Diurnal incontinence can occur in girls with a history of sexual abuse. Physical examination is directed at identifying signs of organic causes of incontinence: short stature, hypertension, enlarged kidneys and/or bladder, constipation, labial adhesion, ureteral ectopy, back or sacral anomalies (see Fig. 536-4), and neurologic abnormalities.

Assessment tools include urinalysis, with culture if indicated; bladder diary (recorded times and volumes voided, whether wet or dry); postvoid residual urine volume (generally obtained by bladder scan); Dysfunctional Voiding Symptom Score (Fig. 537-1); Bristol Stool Form Score (Fig. 537-2); and uroflow with or without EMG (noninvasive assessment of urinary flow pattern and measurement of external sphincter activity). Imaging is performed in children who have significant physical findings, a family history of urinary tract anomalies or UTIs, and those who do not respond to therapy appropriately. A renal ultrasonogram with or without a voiding cystourethrogram (VCUG) is indicated. Urodynamics should be performed if there is evidence of neurologic disease and may be helpful if empirical therapy is ineffective.

Table 537-1 CAUSES OF URINARY INCONTINENCE IN CHILDHOOD

Overactive bladder
Infrequent voiding
Detrusor-sphincter dyssynergia
Non-neurogenic neurogenic bladder (Hinman syndrome)
Vaginal voiding
Giggle incontinence
Cystitis
Bladder outlet obstruction (posterior urethral valves)
Ectopic ureter and fistula
Sphincter abnormality (epispadias, exstrophy; urogenital sinus abnormality)
Neuropathic
Overflow incontinence
Traumatic
Iatrogenic
Behavioral
Combination

OVERACTIVE BLADDER

Children with an overactive bladder typically exhibit urinary frequency, urgency, and urge incontinence. Often a girl will squat down on her foot to try to prevent incontinence (termed *Vincent's curtsy*). The bladder in these children is functionally, but not anatomically, smaller than normal and exhibits strong uninhibited contractions. Approximately 25% of children with nocturnal enuresis also have symptoms of an overactive bladder. Many children indicate they do not feel the need to urinate, even just before they are incontinent. In girls, a history of recurrent UTI is common, but incontinence can persist long after infections are brought under control. It is not clear in these cases if the voiding dysfunction is a sequela of the UTIs or if the voiding dysfunction predisposes to recurrent UTIs. In girls, voiding cys-

Patient name:
Hospital number:
Reason for referral:
Date:

Over the last month	Almost never	Less than half the time	About half the time	Almost every time	Not available
1. I have had wet clothes or wet underwear during the day.	0	1	2	3	NA
2. When I wet myself, my underwear is soaked.	0	1	2	3	NA
3. I miss having a bowel movement every day.	0	1	2	3	NA
4. I have to push for my bowel movements to come out.	0	1	2	3	NA
5. I only go to the bathroom one or two times each day.	0	1	2	3	NA
6. I can hold onto my pee by crossing my legs, squatting or doing the "pee dance."	0	1	2	3	NA
7. When I have to pee, I cannot wait.					
8. I have to push to pee.	0	1	2	3	NA
9. When I pee it hurts.	0	1	2	3	NA
10. Parents to answer. Has your child experienced something stressful like the example below?	No (0)			Yes (3)	
Total*					

- New baby.
- New home.
- New school.
- School problems.
- Abuse (sexual/physical).
- Home problems (divorce/death).
- Special events (birthday).
- Accident/injury.
- Others.

*Females with a score ≥6 and males with a score ≥9 are most likely to have dysfunctional voiding.

Figure 537-1 Dysfunctional Voiding Score questionnaire. (From Farhat W, Bagli DJ, Capolicchio G, et al: The dysfunctional voiding scoring system: quantitative standardization of dysfunctional voiding symptoms in children, *J Urol* 164:1011–1015, 2000.)

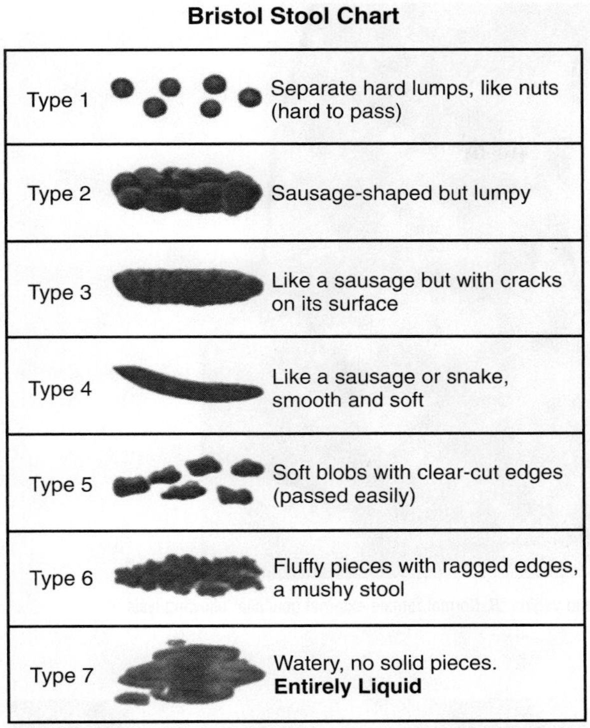
Bristol Stool Chart
Type 1
Separate hard lumps, like nuts (hard to pass)
Type 2
Sausage-shaped but lumpy
Type 3
Like a sausage but with cracks on its surface
Type 4
Like a sausage or snake, smooth and soft
Type 5
Soft blobs with clear-cut edges (passed easily)
Type 6
Fluffy pieces with ragged edges, a mushy stool
Type 7
Watery, no solid pieces.
Entirely Liquid

Figure 537-2 Bristol Stool Chart for evaluating bowel function.

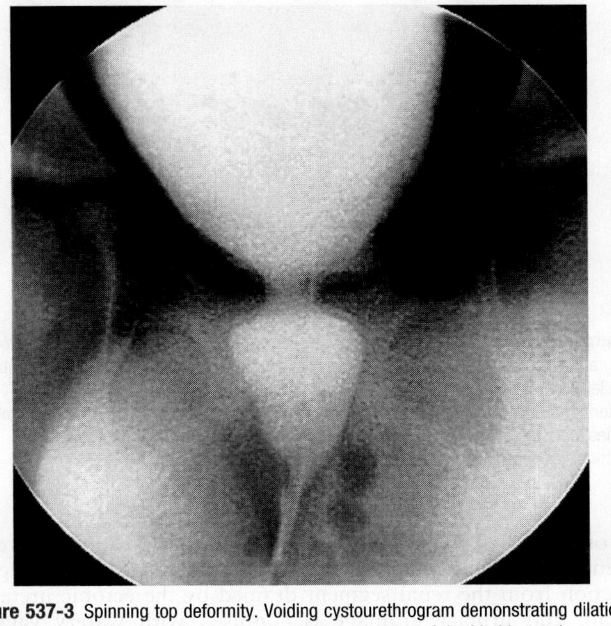

Figure 537-3 Spinning top deformity. Voiding cystourethrogram demonstrating dilation of the urethra with distal urethral narrowing and contraction of the bladder neck.

tourethrography often shows a dilated urethra ("spinning top deformity," Fig. 537-3) and narrowed bladder neck with bladder wall hypertrophy. The urethral finding results from inadequate relaxation of the external urinary sphincter. Constipation is common and should be treated, particularly with any child with Bristol Stool Score 1 or 2.

The overactive bladder nearly always resolves, but the time to resolution is highly variable, sometimes not until the teenage years. Initial therapy is timed voiding, every 1.5-2.0 hr. Treatment of constipation and UTIs is important. Another treatment

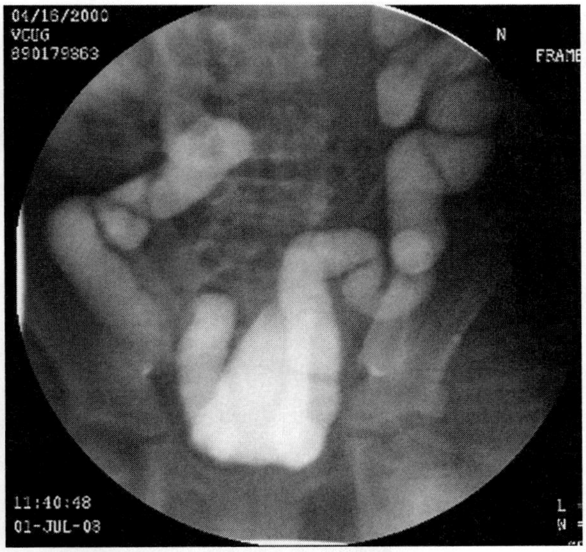

Figure 537-4 Voiding cystourethrogram demonstrating severe bladder trabeculation and vesicoureteral reflux in a 12-year-old boy with Hinman syndrome. The patient presented with day and night incontinence, had chronic renal failure, and underwent kidney transplantation.

is biofeedback, in which children are taught pelvic floor exercises (**Kegel exercises**), because there is evidence that daily performance of these exercises can reduce or eliminate unstable bladder contractions. Biofeedback also may include periodic uroflow studies with sphincter electromyography to be certain that the pelvic floor relaxes during voiding, and assessment of postvoid residual urine volume by sonography. Anticholinergic therapy with oxybutynin chloride, hyoscyamine, or tolterodine reduces bladder overactivity and may help the child achieve dryness. Treatment with an α-adrenergic blocker such as terazosin or doxazosin can aid in bladder emptying by promoting bladder neck relaxation; α-adrenergic blockers also have mild anticholinergic properties. If pharmacologic therapy is successful, the dosage should be tapered periodically to determine its continued need. Children who do not respond to therapy should be evaluated urodynamically to rule out other possible forms of bladder or sphincter dysfunction. In refractory cases, sacral nerve stimulation (Interstim) is a surgical procedure that has shown promise.

NON-NEUROGENIC NEUROGENIC BLADDER (HINMAN SYNDROME)

Hinman syndrome is a more serious but less common disorder involving failure of the external sphincter to relax during voiding in children without neurologic abnormalities. Children with this syndrome, also called **detrusor-sphincter dyssynergia**, typically exhibit a staccato stream, day and night wetting, recurrent UTIs, constipation, and encopresis. Evaluation of affected children often reveals vesicoureteral reflux, a trabeculated bladder, and a decreased urinary flow rate with an intermittent pattern (Fig. 537-4). In severe cases, hydronephrosis, renal insufficiency, and even end-stage renal disease can occur. The pathogenesis of this syndrome is thought to involve learning abnormal voiding habits during toilet training; the syndrome is rarely seen in infants. Urodynamic studies and magnetic resonance imaging of the spine are indicated to rule out a neurologic cause for the bladder dysfunction.

The treatment usually is complex and can include anticholinergic and α-adrenergic blocker therapy, timed voiding, treatment of constipation, behavioral modification, and encouragement of relaxation during voiding. Biofeedback has been used successfully in older children to teach relaxation of the external sphincter. In

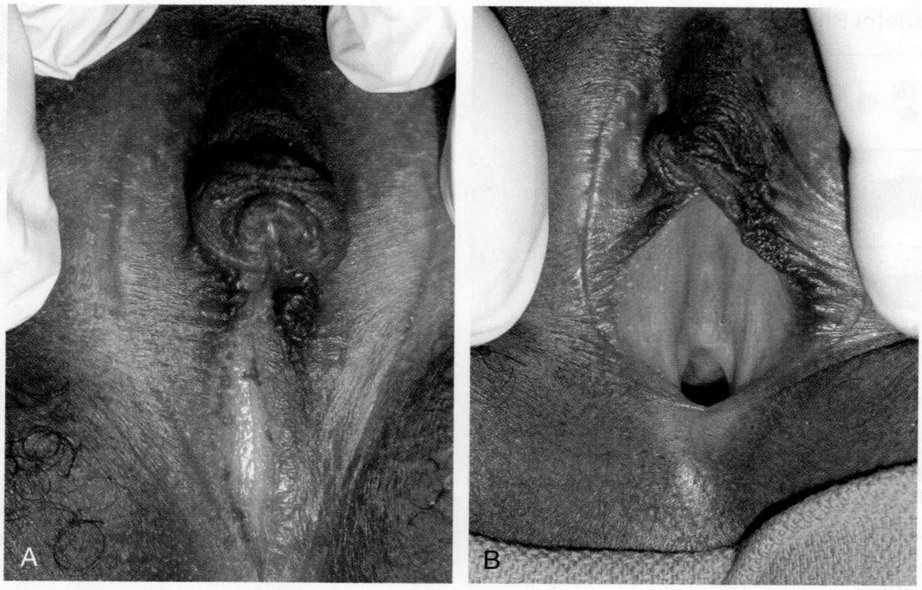

Figure 537-5 *A,* Labial adhesion. Note the inability to visualize the urethral meatus and vagina. *B,* Normal female external genitalia following lysis of labial adhesion.

some cases botulinum toxin (Botox) injection into the external sphincter can provide temporary sphincteric paralysis and thereby reduce outlet resistance. In severe cases, intermittent catheterization is necessary to ensure bladder emptying. In selected patients, external urinary diversion is necessary to protect the upper urinary tract. These children require long-term treatment and careful follow-up.

INFREQUENT VOIDING

Infrequent voiding is a common disorder of micturition, usually associated with UTIs. Affected children, usually girls, void only twice a day rather than the normal 4 to 7 times. With bladder overdistention and prolonged retention of urine, bacterial growth can lead to recurrent UTIs. Some of these children are constipated. Some also have occasional episodes of incontinence due to overflow or urgency. The disorder is behavioral. If the child has UTIs, treatment includes antibacterial prophylaxis and encouragement of frequent voiding and complete emptying of the bladder by double voiding until a normal pattern of micturition is re-established.

VAGINAL VOIDING

In girls with vaginal voiding, incontinence typically occurs after urination after the girl stands up. Usually the volume of urine is 5-10 mL. One of the most common causes is labial adhesion (see Fig. 537-5). This lesion is seen in young girls and can be managed either by topical application of estrogen cream to the adhesion or lysis in the office. Some girls experience vaginal voiding because they do not separate their legs widely during urination. These girls either are overweight or do not pull their underwear down to their ankles when they urinate. Management involves encouraging the girl to separate the legs as widely as possible during urination. The most effective way to do this is to have the child sit backward on the toilet seat during micturition.

OTHER CAUSES OF INCONTINENCE IN GIRLS

Ureteral ectopia, usually associated with a duplicated collecting system in girls, refers to a ureter that drains outside the bladder, often into the vagina or distal urethra. It can produce urinary incontinence characterized by constant urinary dripping all day, even though the child voids regularly. Sometimes the urine production from the renal segment drained by the ectopic ureter is small, and urinary drainage is confused with watery vaginal discharge. Children with a history of vaginal discharge or incontinence and an abnormal voiding pattern require careful study. The ectopic orifice usually is difficult to find. On ultrasonography or intravenous urography, one may suspect duplication of the collecting system (Fig. 537-6), but the upper collecting system drained by the ectopic ureter usually has poor or delayed function. CT scanning of the kidneys or an MR urogram should demonstrate subtle duplication anomalies. Examination under anesthesia for an ectopic ureteral orifice in the vestibule or the vagina may be necessary (Fig. 537-7). The treatment in these cases is either partial nephrectomy, with removal of the upper pole segment of the duplicated kidney and its ureter down to the pelvic brim, or ipsilateral ureteroureterostomy, in which the

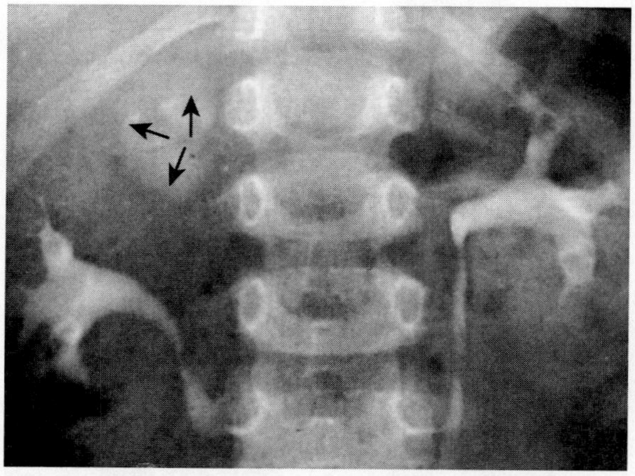

Figure 537-6 Duplication of the right collecting system with ectopic ureter. Excretory urogram in a girl presenting with a normal voiding pattern and constant urinary dribbling. The left kidney is normal, and the right side, well visualized, is the lower collecting system of a duplicated kidney. On the upper pole opposite the first and second vertebral bodies, note the accumulation of contrast material corresponding with a poorly functioning upper pole drained by a ureter opening in the vestibule.

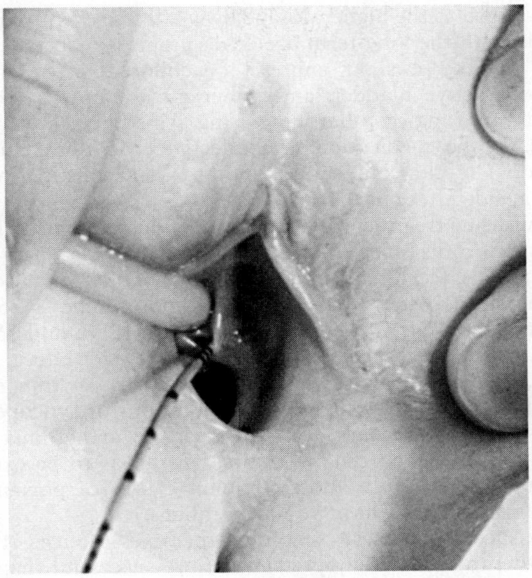

Figure 537-7 The photograph shows an ectopic ureter entering the vestibule next to the urethral meatus. The thin ureteral catheter with transverse marks has been introduced into this ectopic ureter. This girl had a normal voiding pattern and constant urinary dribbling.

upper pole ectopic ureter is anastomosed to the normally positioned lower pole ureter. These procedures often are performed by minimally invasive laparoscopy with or without robotic assistance.

Giggle incontinence typically affects girls 7-15 yr of age. The incontinence occurs suddenly during giggling, and the entire bladder volume is lost. The pathogenesis is thought to be sudden relaxation of the urinary sphincter. Anticholinergic medication and timed voiding occasionally are effective. The most effective treatment is low-dose methylphenidate.

Total incontinence in girls may be secondary to **epispadias** (Fig. 535-2). This condition, which affects only 1 of 480,000 females, is characterized by separation of the pubic symphysis, separation of the right and left sides of the clitoris, and a patulous urethra (Chapter 535). Treatment is bladder neck reconstruction or placement of an artificial urinary sphincter to repair the incompetent urethra.

A short, incompetent urethra may be associated with certain urogenital sinus malformations. The diagnosis of these malformations requires a high index of suspicion and a careful physical examination of all incontinent girls. In these cases, urethral and vaginal reconstruction often restores continence.

VOIDING DISORDERS WITHOUT INCONTINENCE

Some children have abrupt onset of severe urinary frequency, voiding as often as every 10-15 min during the day, without dysuria, UTI, daytime incontinence, or nocturia. The most common age for these symptoms to occur is 4-6 yr, after the child is toilet trained, and the vast majority are boys. This condition is termed the **daytime frequency syndrome of childhood** or **pollakiuria.** The condition is functional; no anatomic problem is detected. Often the symptoms occur just before a child starts kindergarten or if the child is having emotional family stress-related problems. These children should be checked for UTIs, and the clinician should ascertain that the child is emptying the bladder satisfactorily. Occasionally, pinworms cause these symptoms. The condition is self-limited, and symptoms generally resolve within 2-3 mo. Anticholinergic therapy rarely is effective.

Some children have the **dysuria-hematuria syndrome,** in which the child has dysuria without UTI and microscopic or gross hematuria. This condition affects children who are toilet-trained and is often secondary to hypercalciuria. A 24-hr urine sample should be obtained and calcium and creatinine excretion assessed. A 24-hr calcium excretion of >4 mg/kg is abnormal and deserves treatment with thiazides, because some of these children are at risk for urolithiasis.

Table 537-2 NOCTURNAL ENURESIS

CAUSES
Delayed maturation of the cortical mechanisms that allow voluntary control of the micturition reflex
Sleep disorders
"Deep sleeping" (no specific sleep pattern identified)
Reduced antidiuretic hormone production at night, resulting in an increased urine output
Genetic factors, with chromosomes 12 and 13q the likely sites of the gene for enuresis
Overactive bladder
Constipation
Organic factors, such as urinary tract infection or obstructive uropathy
Psychologic factors more often implicated in secondary enuresis
Sleep apnea (snoring) secondary to enlarged adenoids
OTHER FEATURES
Enuresis can occur in any stage of sleep
All children are most difficult to arouse in the 1st third of the night and easiest to awaken in the last third, but enuretic children are more difficult to arouse than those with normal bladder control
Enuretic children often are described as "soaking the bed"
Family history in enuretic children often positive for enuresis

NOCTURNAL ENURESIS

By 5 yr of age, 90-95% of children are nearly completely continent during the day, and 80-85% are continent at night. Nocturnal enuresis (Chapter 21.3) refers to the occurrence of involuntary voiding at night after 5 yr, the age when volitional control of micturition is expected. Enuresis may be primary (estimated 75-90% of children with enuresis; nocturnal urinary control never achieved) or secondary (10-25%; the child was dry at night for at least a few months and then enuresis developed). In addition, 75% of children with enuresis are wet only at night, and 25% are incontinent day and night. This distinction is important, because children with both forms are more likely to have an abnormality of the urinary tract.

Epidemiology

Approximately 60% of children with nocturnal enuresis are boys. Family history is positive in 50% of cases. Although primary nocturnal enuresis may be polygenetic, candidate genes have been localized to chromosomes 12 and 13. If one parent was enuretic, each child has a 44% risk of enuresis; if both parents were enuretic, each child has a 77% likelihood of enuresis. Nocturnal enuresis without overt daytime voiding symptoms affects up to 20% of children at the age of 5 yr; it ceases spontaneously in approximately 15% of involved children every year thereafter. Its frequency among adults is <1%.

Pathogenesis

The pathogenesis of nocturnal enuresis (normal daytime voiding habits) is multifactorial (Table 537-2).

Clinical Manifestations and Diagnosis

A careful history should be obtained, especially with respect to fluid intake at night and pattern of nocturnal enuresis. Children with diabetes insipidus (Chapter 552), diabetes mellitus (Chapter 583), and chronic renal disease (Chapter 529) can have a high obligatory urinary output and a compensatory polydipsia. The family should be asked whether the child snores loudly at night.

A complete physical examination should include palpation of the abdomen and rectal examination after voiding to assess the possibility of a chronically distended bladder. The child with nocturnal enuresis should be examined carefully for neurologic and spinal abnormalities. There is an increased incidence of bacteriuria in enuretic girls, and, if found, it should be investigated and treated (Chapter 532), although this does not always lead to resolution of bed-wetting. A urine sample should be obtained after an overnight fast and evaluated for specific gravity or osmolality to exclude polyuria as a cause of frequency and incontinence and to ascertain that the concentrating ability is normal. The absence of glycosuria should be confirmed. If there are no daytime symptoms, the physical examination and urinalysis are normal, and the urine culture is negative, further evaluation for urinary tract pathology generally is not warranted. A renal ultrasonogram is reasonable in an older child with enuresis or in children who do not respond appropriately to therapy.

Treatment

The best approach to treatment is to reassure the child and parents that the condition is self-limited and to avoid punitive measures that can affect the child's psychologic development adversely. Fluid intake should be restricted to 2 oz after 6 or 7 PM. The parents should be certain that the child voids at bedtime. Avoiding extraneous sugar and caffeine after 4 PM also is beneficial. If the child snores and the adenoids are enlarged, referral to an otolaryngologist should be considered, because adenoidectomy can cure the enuresis.

Active treatment should be avoided in children <6 yr of age, because enuresis is extremely common in younger children. Treatment is more likely to be successful in children approaching puberty compared with younger children.

The simplest initial measure is **motivational therapy** and includes a star chart for dry nights. Waking children a few hours after they go to sleep to have them void often allows them to awaken dry, although this measure is not curative. Some have recommended that children try holding their urine for longer periods during the day, but there is no evidence that this approach is beneficial. **Conditioning therapy** involves use of a loud auditory or vibratory alarm attached to a moisture sensor in the underwear. The alarm sounds when voiding occurs and is intended to awaken children and alert them to void. This form of therapy is considered curative and has a reported success of 30-60%, although the relapse rate is significant. Often the auditory alarm wakes up other family members and not the enuretic child; persistence for several months often is necessary. Conditioning therapy tends to be most effective in older children. Another form of therapy to which some children respond is self-hypnosis. The primary role of psychologic therapy is to help the child deal with enuresis psychologically and help motivate the child to void at night if he or she awakens with a full bladder.

Pharmacologic therapy is intended to treat the symptom of enuresis and thus is regarded as second-line and is not curative. Direct comparisons of the bell and bed with pharmacologic therapy favor the former because of lower relapse rates, although initial response rates are equivalent.

One form of treatment is desmopressin acetate, a synthetic analog of antidiuretic hormone that reduces urine production overnight. It is available as a tablet, with a dosage of 0.2-0.6 mg at bedtime. In the past a nasal spray was used, but some children have experienced hyponatremia and convulsions with this formulation and the nasal spray is no longer used for nocturnal enuresis. Hyponatremia has not been reported in children using the tablets. Fluid restriction at night is important, and the drug should not be used if the child has a systemic illness with vomiting or diarrhea or if the child has polydipsia. Desmopressin acetate is effective in as many as 40% of children. If effective, it should be used for 3-6 mo, and then an attempt should be made to taper the dosage. If tapering results in recurrent enuresis, the child should return to the higher dosage. Few adverse events have been reported with the long-term use of desmopressin acetate.

For therapy-resistant enuresis or children with symptoms of an overactive bladder, anticholinergic therapy is indicated. Oxybutynin 5 mg or tolterodine 2 mg at bedtime often are prescribed. If the medication is ineffective, the dosage may be doubled. The clinician should monitor for constipation as a potential side effect.

A third-line treatment is imipramine, which is a tricyclic antidepressant. This medication has mild anticholinergic and α-adrenergic effects, reduces urine output slightly, and also might alter the sleep pattern. The dosage of imipramine is 25 mg in children age 6-8 yr, 50 mg in children age 9-12 yr, and 75 mg in teenagers. Reported success rates are 30-60%. Side effects include anxiety, insomnia, and dry mouth, and heart rhythm may be affected. If there is any history of palpitations or syncope in the child, or sudden cardiac death or unstable arrhythmia in the family, long QT syndrome in the patient needs to be excluded. The drug is one of the most common causes of poisoning by prescription medication in younger siblings.

In unsuccessful cases, combining therapies often is effective. Alarm therapy plus desmopressin is more successful than either one alone. The combination of oxybutynin chloride and desmopressin is more successful than either one alone. Desmopressin and imipramine also may be combined.

BIBLIOGRAPHY

Please visit the Nelson Textbook of Pediatrics *website at* *www.expertconsult.com* *for the complete bibliography.*

Chapter 538
Anomalies of the Penis and Urethra

Jack S. Elder

HYPOSPADIAS

Hypospadias, a urethral opening that is on the ventral surface of the penile shaft, affects 1/250 male newborns, and its incidence may be increasing. Usually it is an isolated defect, but its incidence is increased in disorders of sexual differentiation (intersex), anorectal malformation, and congenital heart disease. Typically, there is incomplete development of the prepuce, called a **dorsal hood,** in which the foreskin is on the sides and dorsal aspect of the penile shaft and deficient or absent ventrally. Some boys with hypospadias, particularly those with proximal hypospadias, have **chordee,** in which there is ventral penile curvature during erection. It has been speculated that the incidence of hypospadias appears to be increasing, possibly because of in utero exposure to estrogenic or antiandrogenic endocrine-disrupting chemicals (e.g., polychlorobiphenyls, phytoestrogens).

Clinical Manifestations

Hypospadias is classified according to the position of the urethral meatus after taking into account whether chordee is present (Fig. 538-1). The deformity is described as glanular (on the glans penis), coronal, subcoronal, midpenile, penoscrotal, scrotal, or perineal. Approximately 60% of cases are distal, 25% are subcoronal or midpenile, and 15% are proximal. In the most severe cases, the scrotum is bifid and sometimes there is moderate penoscrotal transposition. As many as 15% of affected boys have a **megameatal variant,** in which the foreskin is developed normally (megameatus intact prepuce [MIP] variant), and there is either glanular or subcoronal hypospadias with a "fish mouth" meatus. These cases might not be diagnosed until after a circumcision is performed.

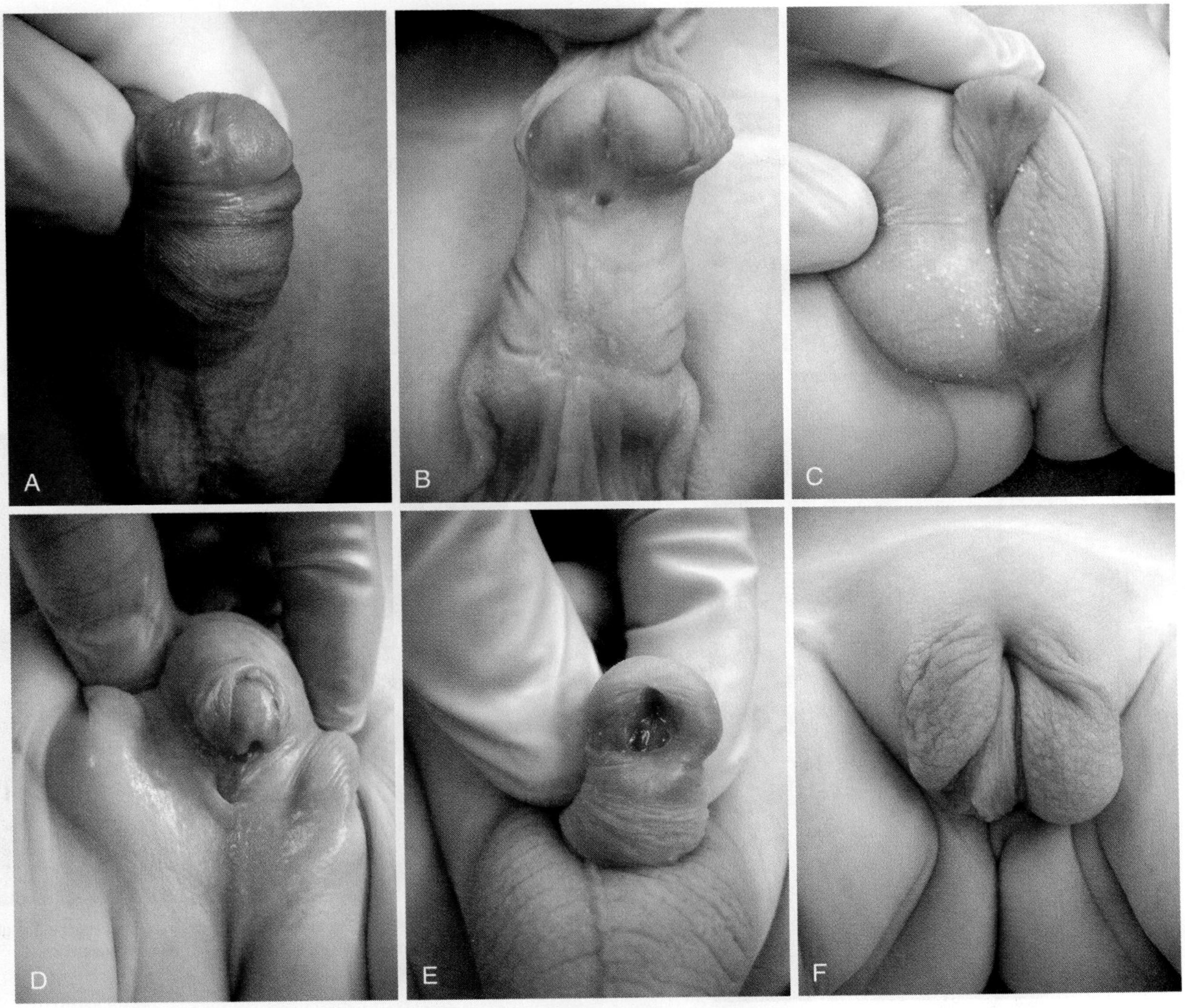

Figure 538-1 Varying forms of hypospadias. *A,* Glanular hypospadias. *B,* Subcoronal hypospadias. Note the dorsal hood of foreskin. *C,* Penoscrotal hypospadias with chordee. *D,* Perineal hypospadias with chordee and partial penoscrotal transposition. *E,* Megameatal variant of hypospadias diagnosed following circumcision; note absence of hooded foreskin. *F,* Complete penoscrotal transposition with scrotal hypospadias.

Approximately 10% of boys with hypospadias have an undescended testis; inguinal hernias also are common. In the newborn, the differential diagnosis of proximal hypospadias associated with an undescended testis should include forms of a disorder of sexual differentiation, particularly female virilization (congenital adrenal hyperplasia), mixed gonadal dysgenesis, partial androgen insensitivity, and true hermaphroditism. A karyotype should be obtained in patients with midpenile or proximal hypospadias and cryptorchidism (Chapter 577). In boys with penoscrotal hypospadias, a voiding cystourethrogram should be considered because 5-10% of these children have a dilated prostatic utricle, which is a remnant of the müllerian system (Chapter 548). The incidence of upper urinary tract abnormalities is low unless there are abnormalities of other organ systems.

Complications of untreated hypospadias include deformity of the urinary stream, typically ventral deflection or severe splaying; sexual dysfunction secondary to penile curvature; infertility if the urethral meatus is proximal; meatal stenosis (congenital), which is uncommon; and cosmetic appearance. The goal of hypospadias surgery is to correct the functional and cosmetic deformities. Whereas hypospadias repair is recommended for all boys with midpenile and proximal hypospadias, some boys with distal hypospadias have no functional abnormality and do not need any surgical correction.

Treatment

Management begins in the newborn period. Circumcision should be avoided, because the foreskin often is used in the repair in most cases. The ideal age for repair in a healthy infant is 6-12 mo, because the risk of general anesthesia at this age is similar to older children; penile growth over the next several years is slow; the child does not remember the surgical procedure; and postoperative analgesic needs are less than in older children. With the exception of proximal hypospadias, virtually all cases are repaired in a single operation on an ambulatory basis. The most common repair involves tubularization of the urethral plate distal to the urethral meatus, with coverage by a vascularized flap from the foreskin, termed a *tubularized incised plate* (TIP) repair. More proximal cases might require a 2-stage repair. The complication rate is low: 5% for distal hypospadias, 10% for midpenile hypospadias, and 15-20% for proximal hypospadias. The most common complications include urethrocutaneous fistula and meatal stenosis. Other complications include a deformed urinary stream, persistent penile curvature, and dehiscence of the

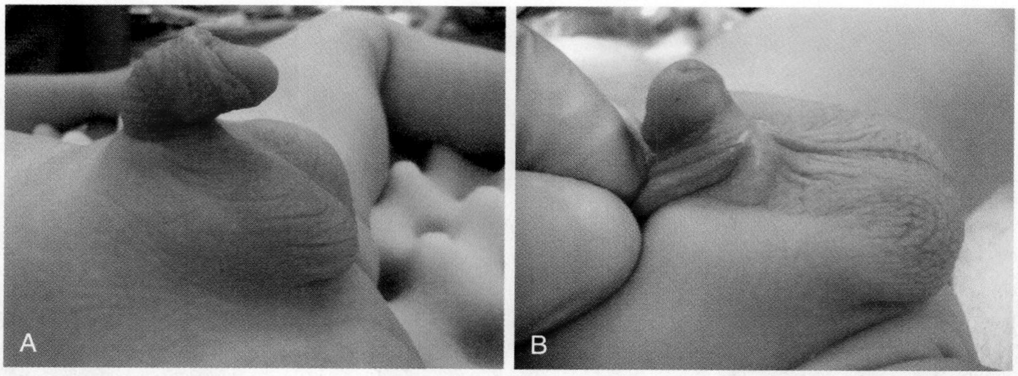

Figure 538-2 *A* and *B*, Two examples of chordee without hypospadias. Note hooded foreskin and normal location of urethral meatus.

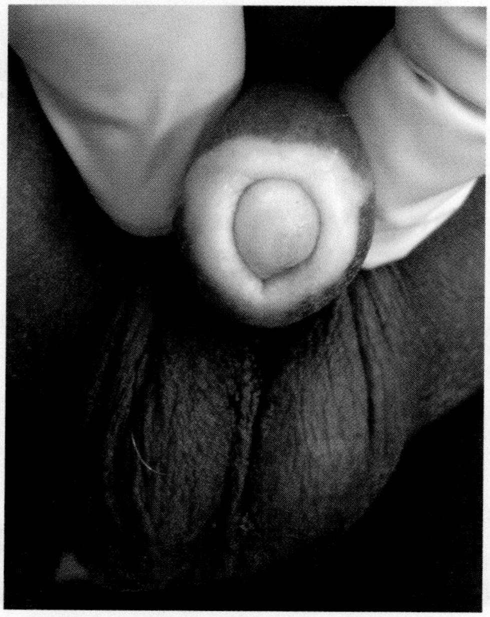

Figure 538-3 Balanitis xerotica obliterans. Note whitish cicatricial plaque.

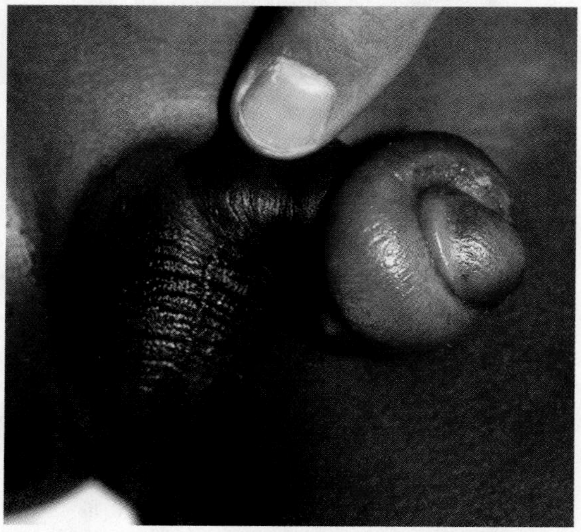

Figure 538-4 Paraphimosis. The foreskin has been retracted proximal to the glans penis and has become markedly swollen secondary to venous congestion.

hypospadias repair. Treatment of these complications generally is straightforward. In complex cases a buccal mucosa graft is used to create urethral mucosa. Repair of hypospadias is a technically demanding operation and should be performed by a surgeon with specialty training in pediatric urology and extensive experience.

CHORDEE WITHOUT HYPOSPADIAS

In some boys there is mild or moderate ventral penile curvature (**chordee**) and incomplete development of the foreskin (**dorsal hood**), but the urethral meatus is at the tip of the glans (Fig. 538-2). In most of these boys, the urethra is normal but there is insufficient ventral penile skin or prominent, inelastic ventral bands of dartos fascia that prevent a straight erection. In some cases, the urethra is hypoplastic, and a formal urethroplasty is necessary for repair. The only sign of this anomaly in the neonate may be the hooded foreskin, and delayed repair under general anesthesia at 6 mo of age is recommended.

PHIMOSIS AND PARAPHIMOSIS

Phimosis refers to the inability to retract the prepuce. At birth, phimosis is physiologic. Over time, the adhesions between the prepuce and glans lyse and the distal phimotic ring loosens. In 90% of uncircumcised boys the prepuce becomes fully retractable by 3 yr of age. Accumulation of epithelial debris under the infant's prepuce is physiologic and does not mandate circumcision. In older boys, phimosis may be physiologic, may be pathologic from inflammation and scarring at the tip of the foreskin (Fig. 538-3), or occurs after circumcision. The prepuce might have been retracted forcefully on 1 or 2 occasions in the past, which can result in a cicatricial scar that prevents subsequent retraction of the foreskin. In boys with persistent physiologic or pathologic phimosis, application of corticosteroid cream to the foreskin 3 times daily for 1 mo loosens the phimotic ring in 2/3 of cases. If there is ballooning of the foreskin during voiding or phimosis beyond 10 yr of age and topical corticosteroid therapy is ineffective, circumcision is recommended.

Paraphimosis occurs when the foreskin is retracted past the coronal sulcus and the prepuce cannot be pulled back over the glans (Fig. 538-4). Painful venous stasis in the retracted foreskin results, with edema leading to severe pain and inability to reduce the foreskin (pull it back over the glans). Treatment includes lubricating the foreskin and glans and then simultaneously compressing the glans and placing distal traction on the foreskin to try to push the phimotic ring past the coronal sulcus. In rare cases, emergency circumcision under general anesthesia is necessary.

CIRCUMCISION

Whether newborn boys should undergo circumcision is controversial. In the USA, circumcision usually is performed for cultural reasons. Reasons given in support of circumcision include reducing the risk of urinary tract infection (UTI) during infancy, reducing the risk of sexually transmitted infections, and preventing penile cancer, phimosis, HIV infection, and balanitis. Circumcision in men in Africa reduces the risk of HIV transmission from an infected partner. The Centers for Disease Control and Prevention (CDC) is considering whether to recommend routine circumcision for male newborns to reduce the risk of HIV transmission in the future. In 2010, the Royal Dutch Medical Association released a policy statement opposing nontherapeutic circumcision. When performing a neonatal circumcision, local analgesia, such as a dorsal nerve block or application of EMLA cream (lidocaine 2.5% and prilocaine 2.5%) is recommended.

UTIs are 10-15 times more common in uncircumcised infant boys than in circumcised infants, with the urinary pathogens arising from bacteria that colonize the space between the prepuce and glans. The risk of febrile UTI (Chapter 532) is highest between birth and 6 mo, but there is an increased risk of UTI until 5 yr of age. Many recommend circumcision in infants who are predisposed to UTI, such as those with congenital hydronephrosis and vesicoureteral reflux. Circumcision reduces the risk of sexually transmitted infections in adults (Chapter 114), in particular AIDS (Chapter 268). There have been only a handful of reports of men who were circumcised at birth and subsequently acquired penile carcinoma, but in Scandinavian countries, where few men are circumcised and hygiene is good, the incidence of penile cancer is low.

Complications after neonatal circumcision include bleeding, wound infection, meatal stenosis, secondary phimosis, removal of insufficient foreskin, and fibrous penile adhesions (skin bridge; Fig. 538-5); 0.2-3.0% of patients undergo a subsequent operative procedure. Boys with a large hydrocele or hernia are at particular risk for secondary phimosis because the scrotal swelling tends to displace the penile shaft skin over the glans. Potentially serious complications include sepsis, amputation of the distal part of the glans, removal of an excessive amount of foreskin, and urethrocutaneous fistula. Circumcision should not be performed in neonates with hypospadias, chordee without hypospadias, or a dorsal hood deformity (relative contraindication) or in those with a small penis (Fig. 538-6). In boys with a **wandering raphe**, in which the median raphe deviates to one side, there may be

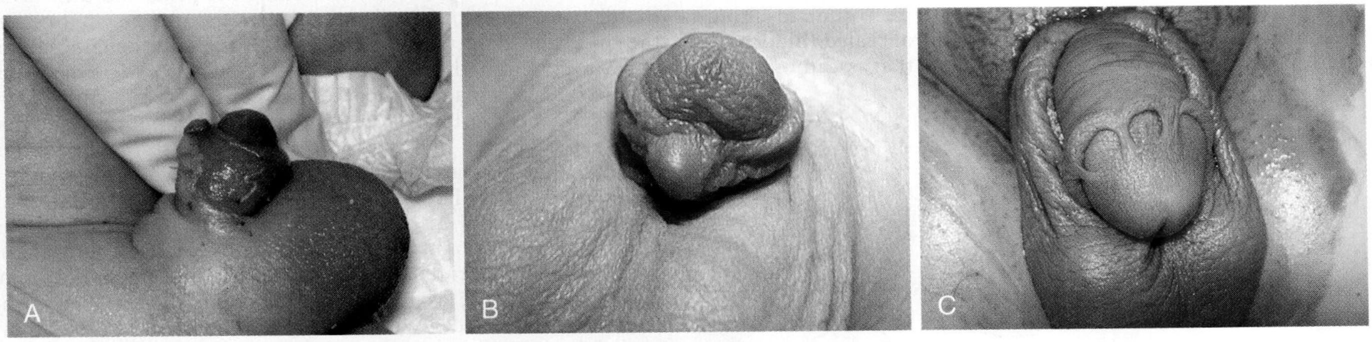

Figure 538-5 Complications of circumcision. *A,* Denuded penile shaft. With local care, the penis healed and appeared normal. *B,* Midline epithelial inclusion cyst. *C,* Fibrous penile skin bridges.

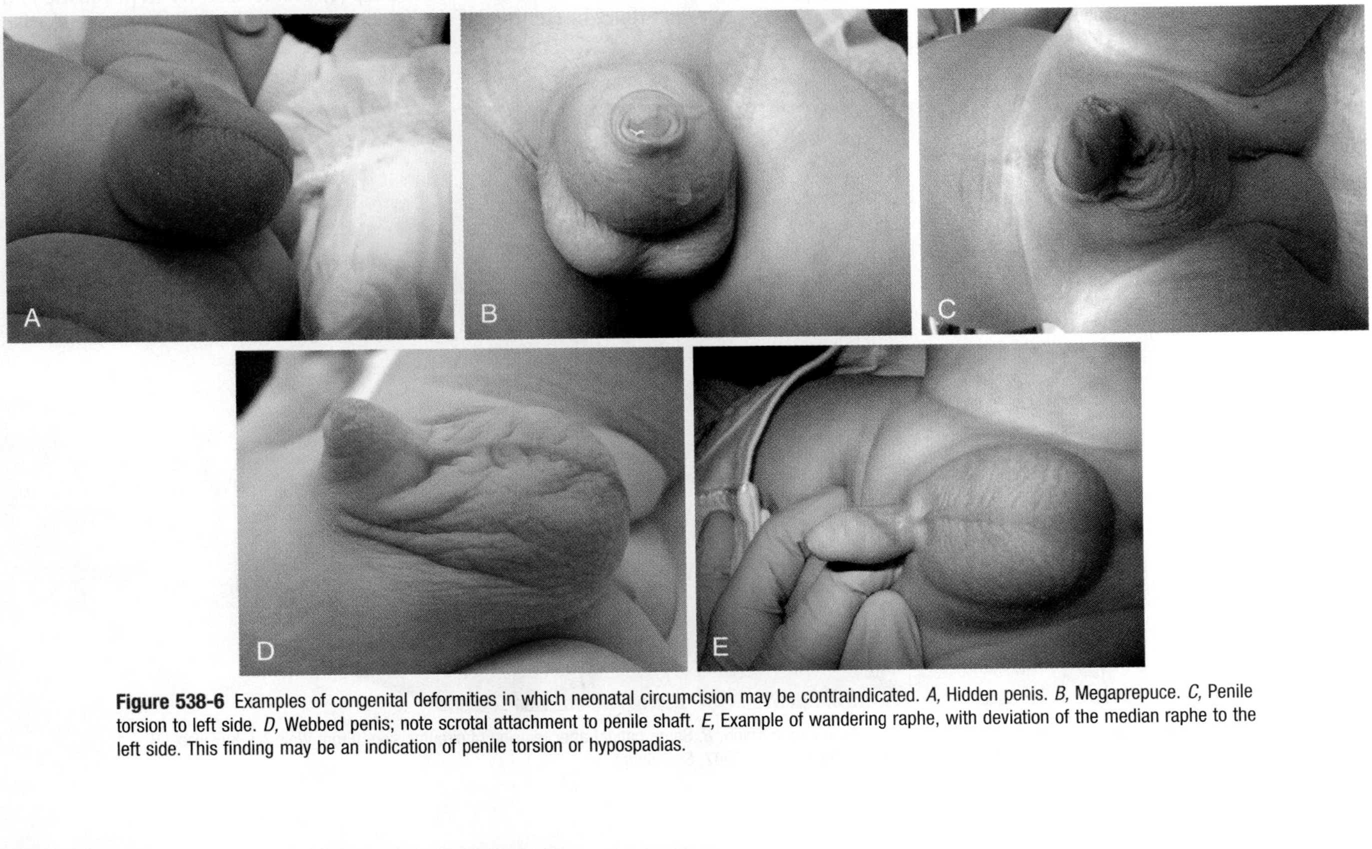

Figure 538-6 Examples of congenital deformities in which neonatal circumcision may be contraindicated. *A,* Hidden penis. *B,* Megaprepuce. *C,* Penile torsion to left side. *D,* Webbed penis; note scrotal attachment to penile shaft. *E,* Example of wandering raphe, with deviation of the median raphe to the left side. This finding may be an indication of penile torsion or hypospadias.

underlying penile torsion or hypospadias, and evaluation by a pediatric urologist is suggested before performing a circumcision.

PENILE TORSION

Penile torsion is a rotational defect of the penile shaft. It usually occurs in a counterclockwise direction, that is, to the left side (see Fig. 538-6). In most cases, penile development is normal, and the condition is unrecognized until circumcision is performed or the foreskin is retractable. In many cases the midline raphe of the penile shaft is deviated. Penile torsion also occurs in some boys with hypospadias. The defect has primarily cosmetic significance and correction is unnecessary if the rotation is <60 degrees from the midline.

INCONSPICUOUS PENIS

The term *inconspicuous penis* refers to a penis that appears to be small. A **webbed penis** is a condition in which the scrotal skin extends onto the ventral penile shaft. This deformity represents an abnormality of the attachment between the penis and scrotum. Although the deformity might appear mild, if a routine circumcision is performed, the penis can retract into the scrotum, resulting in secondary phimosis (**trapped penis**). The concealed (**hidden or buried**) penis is a normally developed penis that is camouflaged by the suprapubic fat pad (Fig. 538-7). This anomaly may be congenital, iatrogenic after circumcision, or a result of obesity. Surgical correction is indicated for cosmetic reasons or if there is a functional abnormality with a splayed stream.

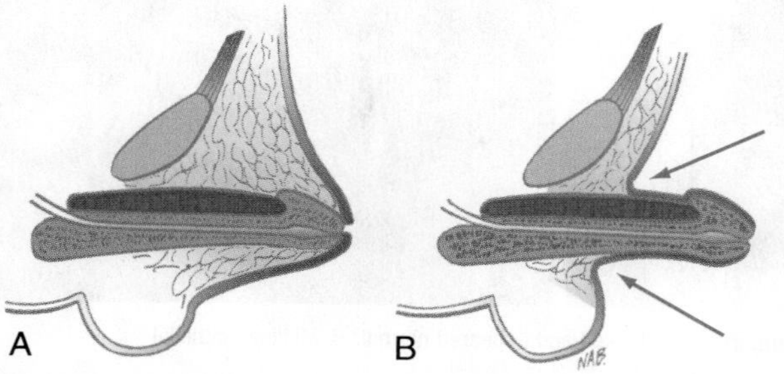

Figure 538-7 Concealed penis *(A),* which may be visualized by retracting skin lateral to penile shaft *(B).* (From Wein AJ, Kavoussi LR, Novick AC, et al, editors: *Campbell-Walsh urology,* ed 9, Philadelphia, 2007, Saunders.)

A **trapped penis** is an acquired form of inconspicuous penis and refers to a phallus that becomes embedded in the suprapubic fat pad after circumcision (Fig. 538-8). This deformity can occur after neonatal circumcision in an infant who has significant scrotal swelling from a large hydrocele or inguinal hernia or after routine circumcision in an infant with a webbed penis. This complication can predispose to UTIs and can cause urinary retention. Initial treatment of a trapped penis should include topical corticosteroid cream, which often loosens the phimotic ring. In some cases secondary repair is necessary at 6-9 mo.

MICROPENIS

Micropenis is defined as a normally formed penis that is at least 2.5 standard deviations below the mean in size (Fig. 538-9). Typically, the ratio of the length of the penile shaft to its circumference is normal. The pertinent measurement is the **stretched penile length,** which is measured by stretching the penis and measuring the distance from the penile base under the pubic symphysis to the tip of the glans. The mean length of the term newborn penis is 3.5 ± 0.7 cm and the diameter is 1.1 ± 0.2 cm. The diagnosis of micropenis is made if the stretched length is <1.9 cm.

Micropenis results from a hormonal abnormality that occurs after 14 wk of gestation. Common causes include hypogonadotropic hypogonadism, hypergonadotropic hypogonadism (primary testicular failure), and idiopathic micropenis. If growth hormone deficiency also is present, neonatal hypoglycemia can occur. The most common cause of micropenis is failure of the hypothalamus to produce an adequate amount of gonadotropin-releasing hormone, as typically occurs in Kallmann syndrome (Chapter 577), Prader-Willi syndrome (Chapter 102), and Lawrence-Moon-Biedl syndrome. In some cases, there is growth hormone deficiency. Primary testicular failure can result from gonadal dysgenesis or rudimentary testes syndrome and also occurs in **Robinow syndrome** (characterized by hypoplastic genitalia, shortening of the forearms, frontal bossing, hypertelorism,

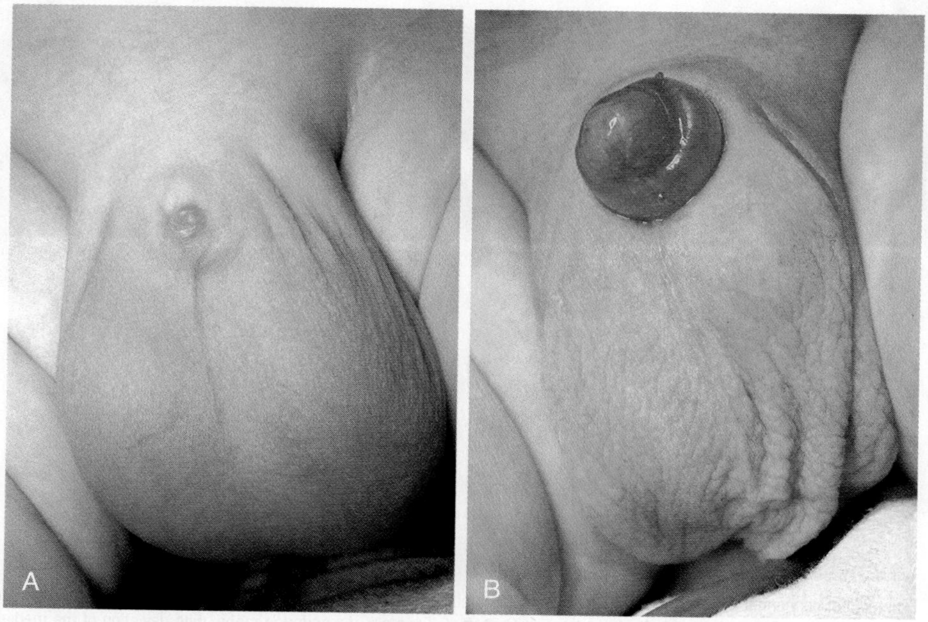

Figure 538-8 *A,* Trapped (concealed) penis resulting from circumcision. *B,* Same patient after revision of circumcision. (From Wein AJ, Kavoussi LR, Novick AC, et al, editors: *Campbell-Walsh urology,* ed 9, Philadelphia, 2007, Saunders.)

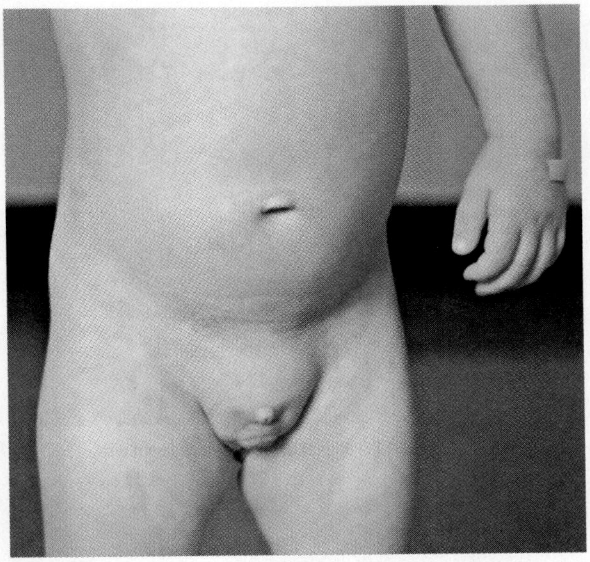

Figure 538-9 Micropenis secondary to hypopituitarism in an 8-year-old boy. (From Wein AJ, Kavoussi LR, Novick AC, et al, editors: *Campbell-Walsh urology,* ed 9, Philadelphia, 2007, Saunders.)

wide palpebral fissures, short broad nose, long philtrum, small chin, brachydactyly, and a normal karyotype).

A pediatric endocrinologist and pediatric urologist should examine all children with these syndromes. **Evaluation** includes a karyotype, assessment of anterior pituitary function and testicular function, and MRI to determine the anatomic integrity of the hypothalamus and the anterior pituitary gland as well as the midline structure of the brain. One of the difficult questions is whether androgen therapy is essential during childhood, because androgenic stimulation of penile growth in a prepubertal boy can limit the growth potential of the penis in puberty. Studies of small groups of men with micropenis suggest that many, although not all, have satisfactory sexual function. Consequently, a decision for gender reassignment is made infrequently.

PRIAPISM

Priapism is a persistent penile erection at least 4 hr in duration that continues beyond, or is unrelated to, sexual stimulation. Typically, only the corpora cavernosa are affected. There are 3 subtypes:

- Ischemic (veno-occlusive, low-flow) priapism is characterized by little or no cavernous blood flow, and cavernous blood gases are hypoxic, hypercapnic, and acidotic. The corpora are rigid and tender to palpation.
- Nonischemic (arterial, high-flow) priapism is caused by unregulated cavernous arterial inflow. Typically, the penis is neither fully rigid nor painful. There is often a history of antecedent trauma resulting in a cavernous artery–corpora cavernosa fistula.
- Stuttering (intermittent) priapism is a recurrent form of ischemic priapism with painful erections with intervening periods of detumescence.

The most common cause of priapism in children is sickle cell disease, which is characterized by predominance of sickle hemoglobin (Hb SS; Chapter 456.1). As many as 27.5% of children with sickle cell disease develop priapism. The priapism is generally related to a low-flow state, secondary to sickling of red blood cells within the sinusoids of the corpora cavernosa during normal erection, resulting in venous stasis. This situation results in decreased local oxygen tension and pH, which potentiates further stasis and sickling. Priapism typically occurs during sleep, when mild hypoventilatory acidosis depresses oxygen tension and pH in the corpora. There is typically significant corporal engorgement with sparing of the glans penis. If the spongiosum is involved, voiding may be impaired. Evaluation includes complete blood count and serum chemistry. If sickle cell status is unknown, hemoglobin electrophoresis should be performed. In some cases, corporal aspiration is performed to distinguish between a high-flow and low-flow state. Other causes of low-flow priapism include sildenafil ingestion and leukemia.

In priapism secondary to sickle cell disease, medical therapy includes exchange transfusion, hydration with hypotonic intravenous fluid, alkalinization, pain management with morphine, and oxygen. The American Urological Association guideline on priapism also recommends concurrent intracavernous treatment beginning with corporal aspiration and irrigation with a sympathomimetic agent, such as phenylephrine. If priapism has been present >48 hr, ischemia and acidosis impair the intracavernous smooth muscle response to sympathomimetics. If irrigation and medical therapy are unsuccessful, a corporoglanular shunt should be considered. For stuttering priapism, administration of an oral α-adrenergic agent (pseudoephedrine) once or twice daily is first-line therapy. If this treatment is unsuccessful, an oral β agonist (terbutaline) is recommended; a GnRH analog plus flutamide is recommended as third-line therapy. Long-term follow-up of adults treated for sickle cell disease as children shows that satisfactory erectile function is inversely related to the patient's age at onset of priapism and duration of priapism.

Nonischemic (high-flow) priapism most commonly follows perineal trauma, such as a straddle injury, that results in laceration of the cavernous artery. Typically, the aspirated blood is bright red, and the aspirate is similar to arterial blood. Color Doppler ultrasonography often demonstrates the fistula. The priapism can spontaneously resolve. If it does not, angiographic embolization is indicated.

OTHER PENILE ANOMALIES

Agenesis of the penis affects approximately 1 in 10 million boys. The karyotype is almost always 46,XY, and the usual appearance is that of a well-developed scrotum with descended testes and an absent penile shaft. Upper urinary tract abnormalities are common. In most cases, gender reassignment is recommended in the newborn period. **Diphallia** ranges from a small accessory penis to complete duplication. **Lateral penile curvature** usually is caused by overgrowth or hypoplasia of a corporal (erectile) body and usually is congenital. Surgical repair is recommended at age 6-12 mo.

MEATAL STENOSIS

Meatal stenosis is a condition that almost always is acquired and occurs after neonatal circumcision. It probably results from severe inflammation of the denuded glans. If the meatus is pinpoint, boys void with a forceful, fine stream that goes a great distance. These boys can experience dysuria, frequency, hematuria, or a combination of these conditions, typically at age 3-8 yr. UTI is uncommon. Other boys have dorsal deflection of the urinary stream. Although the meatus may be small, hydronephrosis or voiding difficulty is extremely rare unless there is associated **balanitis xerotica obliterans** (see Fig. 538-3; chronic dermatitis of unknown etiology, generally involving the glans and prepuce, occasionally extending into the urethra). **Treatment** is meatoplasty, in which the urethral meatus is opened surgically; this procedure can be performed either under anesthesia as an outpatient or in the office using local anesthesia (EMLA cream) with or without sedation. Routine cystoscopy is unnecessary.

OTHER MALE URETHRAL ANOMALIES

Parameatal urethral cyst manifests as an asymptomatic small cyst on one side of the urethral meatus. Treatment is excision under

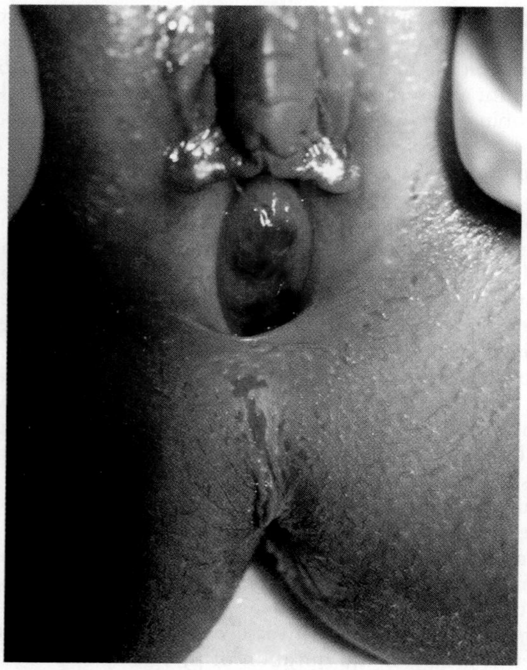

Figure 538-10 Urethral prolapse in a 4 yr old African-American girl who had bloody spotting on her underwear.

anesthesia. **Congenital urethral fistula** is a rare deformity in which a fistula is present from the penile urethra. It usually is an isolated abnormality. Treatment is fistula closure. **Megalourethra** is a large urethra that usually is associated with abnormal development of the corpus spongiosum. This condition is most commonly associated with prune-belly syndrome (Chapter 534). **Urethral duplication** is a rare condition in which the two urethral channels lie in the same sagittal plane. There are many variations with complete and incomplete urethral duplication. These boys often have a double stream. Most commonly the dorsal urethra is small and the ventral urethra is normal caliber. Treatment involves excision of the small urethra. **Urethral hypoplasia** is a rare condition in which the urethra is extremely small but patent. In some cases, a temporary cutaneous vesicostomy is necessary for satisfactory urinary drainage. Either gradual enlargement of the urethra or major urethroplasty is necessary. **Urethral atresia** refers to maldevelopment of the urethra and nearly always is fatal unless the urachus remains patent throughout gestation.

URETHRAL PROLAPSE (FEMALE)

Urethral prolapse is encountered predominantly in black girls 1-9 yr of age. The most common signs are bloody spotting on the underwear or diaper, although dysuria or perineal discomfort also can occur (Fig. 538-10). An inexperienced examiner can mistake the finding for sexual abuse. The usual therapy consists of application of estrogen cream 2-3 times daily for 3-4 wk and sitz baths. Surgical excision and reapproximation of the mucosal edges is curative.

OTHER FEMALE URETHRAL LESIONS

Paraurethral cyst results from retained secretions in the Skene glands secondary to ductal obstruction (Fig. 538-11). These lesions are present at birth, and most regress in size during the first 4-8 wk, although occasionally incision and drainage is necessary. A **prolapsed ectopic ureterocele** appears as a cystic mass protruding from the urethra and is a presenting symptom in 10% of girls with a ureterocele, which is a cystic swelling of the terminal ureter (Fig. 538-12). Ultrasonography should be performed to visualize the upper urinary tracts to confirm the diagnosis. Usually, either the ureterocele is incised or an upper urinary tract reconstructive procedure is necessary.

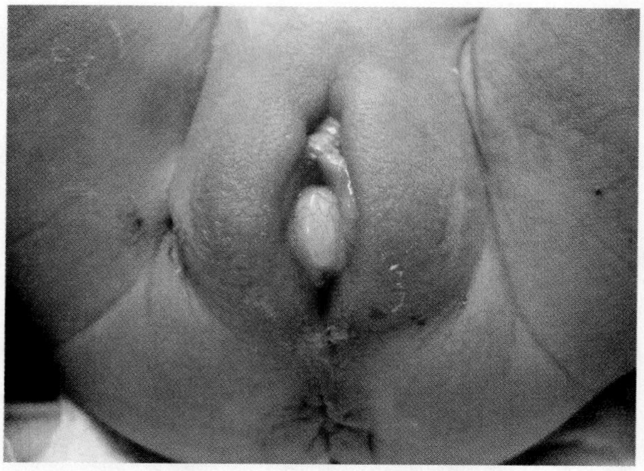

Figure 538-11 Paraurethral cyst in a newborn girl.

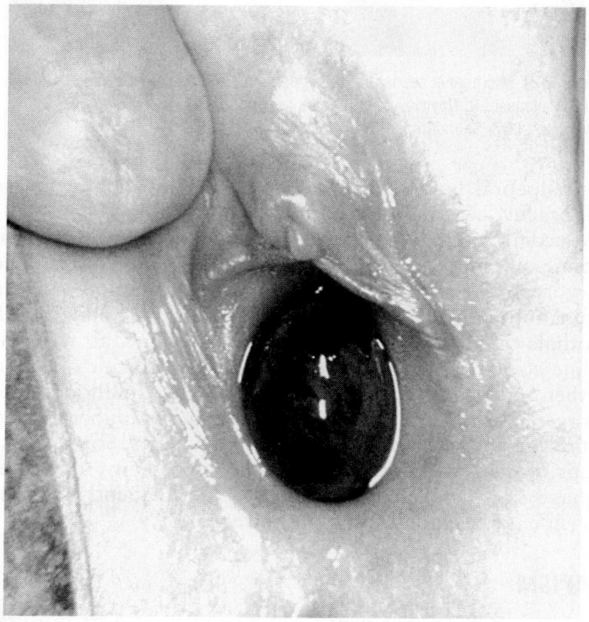

Figure 538-12 Prolapsed ectopic ureterocele in a female infant. She had a nonfunctioning upper pole collecting system connected to the ureterocele.

BIBLIOGRAPHY

Please visit the Nelson Textbook of Pediatrics *website at* *www.expertconsult.com* *for the complete bibliography.*

Chapter 539
Disorders and Anomalies of the Scrotal Contents

Jack S. Elder

UNDESCENDED TESTIS (CRYPTORCHIDISM)

Failure to find the testis in the scrotum indicates that the testis is undescended, absent, or retractile.

Epidemiology

An undescended (**cryptorchid**) testis is the most common disorder of sexual differentiation in boys. At birth, approximately 4.5% of boys have an undescended testis. Because testicular descent occurs at 7-8 mo of gestation, 30% of premature male infants have an undescended testis; the incidence is 3.4% at term. The majority of congenital undescended testes descend spontaneously during the first 3 mo of life, and by 6 mo the incidence decreases to 0.8%. If the testis has not descended by 4 mo, it will remain undescended. Cryptorchidism is bilateral in 10% of cases. There is some evidence that the incidence of cryptorchidism is increasing. Although cryptorchidism usually is considered to be congenital, an undescended testis is being diagnosed in an increasing number of older boys. Typically these boys have a scrotal testis that "ascends" to a low inguinal position, and therefore require an orchiopexy. Some boys have secondary cryptorchidism after repair of an inguinal hernia. This complication is most common in neonates and young infants and affects as many as 1-2% of patients undergoing hernia repair.

Pathogenesis

The process of testicular descent is regulated by an interaction between hormonal and mechanical factors, including testosterone, dihydrotestosterone, müllerian-inhibiting factor, the gubernaculum, intra-abdominal pressure, and the genitofemoral nerve. The testis develops at 7-8 wk of gestation. At 10-11 wk, the Leydig cells produce testosterone, which stimulates differentiation of the wolffian (mesonephric) duct into the epididymis, vas deferens, seminal vesicle, and ejaculatory duct. At 32-36 wk, the testis, which is anchored at the internal inguinal ring by the gubernaculum, begins its process of descent. The gubernaculum distends the inguinal canal and guides the testis into the scrotum. Following testicular descent, the patent processus vaginalis (hernia sac) normally involutes. A small percentage have Klinefelter syndrome or mutations in the insulin-like factor 3 receptor.

Clinical Manifestations

Undescended testes can be classified as **abdominal** (nonpalpable), **peeping** (abdominal but can be pushed into the upper part of the inguinal canal), **inguinal, gliding** (can be pushed into the scrotum but retracts immediately to the pubic tubercle), and **ectopic** (superficial inguinal pouch or, rarely, perineal). Most undescended testes are palpable just distal to the inguinal canal over the pubic tubercle.

A **disorder of sexual development** (**DSD;** aka intersex) should be suspected in a newborn phenotypic male with bilateral nonpalpable testes, as the child could be a virilized girl with congenital adrenal hyperplasia (Chapter 570). In a boy with midpenile or proximal hypospadias and a palpable undescended testis, DSD is present in 15%, and the risk is 50% if the testis is nonpalpable.

The **consequences of cryptorchidism** include infertility, testicular malignancy, associated hernia, torsion of the cryptorchid testis, and the possible psychologic effects of an empty scrotum.

The undescended testis is normal at birth histologically, but pathologic changes can be demonstrated by 6-12 mo. Delayed germ cell maturation, reduction in germ cell number, hyalinization of the seminiferous tubules, and reduced Leydig cell number are typical; these changes are progressive over time if the testis remains undescended. Similar, although less severe, changes are found in the contralateral descended testis after 4-7 yr. After treatment for a unilateral undescended testis, 85% of patients are fertile, which is slightly less than the 90% rate of fertility in an unselected population of men. In contrast, following bilateral orchiopexy, only 50-65% of patients are fertile.

The risk of a **germ cell malignancy** (Chapter 497) developing in an undescended testis is 2-4 times higher than that in the general population and is approximately 1/80 with a unilateral undescended testis and 1/40-50 for bilateral undescended testes. Testicular tumors are less common if the orchiopexy is performed before 10 yr of age, but they still occur, and adolescents should be instructed in testicular self-examination. The peak age for developing a testis tumor is 15-45 yr. The most common tumor developing in an undescended testis in an adolescent or adult is a **seminoma** (65%); after orchiopexy, seminomas represent only 30% of testis tumors. Orchiopexy seems to reduce the risk of seminoma. Whether early orchiopexy reduces the risk of developing cancer of the testis is controversial, but it is uncommon for testis tumors to occur after orchiopexy performed before the age of 2 yr. The contralateral scrotal testis is not at increased risk for malignancy.

An indirect inguinal hernia usually accompanies a congenital undescended testis but rarely is symptomatic. Torsion and infarction of the cryptorchid testis also are uncommon but can occur because of excessive mobility of undescended testes. Consequently, inguinal pain and/or swelling in a boy with an undescended testis should raise the suspicion of an incarcerated hernia or testicular torsion of the undescended testis.

"Acquired" or **ascending undescended testes** occurs when a boy has a descended testis at birth, but during childhood, usually between 4-10 yr of age, the testis does not remain in the scrotum. Such boys often have a history of a retractile testis. With testicular ascent, on physical examination the testis often can be manipulated into the scrotum, but there is obvious tension on the spermatic cord. This condition is speculated to result from incomplete involution of the processus vaginalis, restricting spermatic cord growth, resulting in the testis gradually moving out of its scrotal position.

Retractile testes may be misdiagnosed as undescended testes. Boys >1 yr often have a brisk cremasteric reflex, and if the child is anxious or ticklish during scrotal examination, the testis may be difficult to manipulate into the scrotum. Boys should be examined with their legs in a relaxed frog-leg position, and if the testis can be manipulated into the scrotum comfortably, it is probably retractile. It should be monitored every 6-12 mo with follow-up physical examinations, because it can become an acquired undescended testis. Overall, as many as one third of boys with a retractile testis develop an acquired undescended testis, and boys <7 yr of age at diagnosis of a retractile testis are at greatest risk. Most think that boys with a retractile testis are not at increased risk for infertility or malignancy.

A **nonpalpable testis** accounts for 10% of undescended testes. Of these, 50% are viable testes in the abdomen or high in the inguinal canal, and 50% are atrophic or absent, almost always in the scrotum, secondary to spermatic cord torsion in utero (**vanishing testis**). If the nonpalpable testis is abdominal, it will not descend after 3 mo of age. Although sonography often is performed to try to identify whether the testis is present, it rarely changes clinical management, because the abdominal testis and atrophic testis are not identified on sonography. CT scanning is relatively accurate in demonstrating the presence of the testis. MRI is even more accurate, but the disadvantage is that general anesthesia is necessary in most young children. Because imaging has not been proved to be 100% reliable in demonstrating whether the testis is present or absent, its routine use is discouraged.

On **physical examination** of the scrotum, the child should be entirely undressed, to help him relax. If the testis is nonpalpable, the "soap test" often is useful; soap is applied to the inguinal canal and the examiner's hand, significantly reducing friction and facilitating identification of an inguinal testis. In addition, pulling on the scrotum might make an inguinal testis palpable. One soft sign that a testis is absent is contralateral testicular hypertrophy, but this finding is not 100% diagnostic.

Treatment

The congenital undescended testis should be treated surgically no later than 9-15 mo of age. With anesthesia by a pediatric anesthesiologist, surgical correction at 6 mo is appropriate, because spontaneous descent of the testis will not occur after 4 mo of age. Most testes can be brought down to the scrotum with an orchiopexy, which involves an inguinal incision, mobilization of the testis and spermatic cord, and correction of the indirect inguinal hernia. The procedure is typically performed on an outpatient basis and has a success rate of 98%. In some boys with a testis that is close to the scrotum, a prescrotal orchiopexy can be performed. In this procedure, the entire operation is performed through an incision along the edge of the scrotum. Often the associated inguinal hernia also can be corrected with this incision. Advantages of this approach over the inguinal approach include shorter operative time and less postoperative discomfort.

Hormonal treatment is used infrequently. The theory is that because testicular descent is under androgenic regulation, human chorionic gonadotropin (HCG, which stimulates Leydig cell production of testosterone) or luteinizing hormone–releasing hormone (LHRH) may stimulate testicular descent. Although hormonal treatment has been used in Europe, randomized controlled trials have not shown either of these hormonal preparations to be effective in stimulating testicular descent. There has been some preliminary evidence that an LHRH analog, buserelin, may be helpful in increasing germ cell number and normalizing testicular histologic features.

In boys with a nonpalpable testis, diagnostic laparoscopy is performed in most centers. This procedure allows safe and rapid assessment of whether the testis is intra-abdominal. In most cases, orchiopexy of the intra-abdominal testis located immediately inside the internal inguinal ring is successful, but orchiectomy should be considered in more difficult cases or when the testis appears to be atrophic. A 2-stage orchiopexy sometimes is needed in boys with a high abdominal testis. Boys with abdominal testes are managed with laparoscopic techniques at many institutions. Testicular prostheses are available for older children and adolescents when the absence of the gonad in the scrotum might have an undesirable psychologic effect. The U.S. Food and Drug Administration (FDA) has approved a saline testicular implant. Solid silicone "carving block" implants also are used (Fig. 539-1). Placement of testicular prostheses early in childhood is recommended for boys with anorchia (absence of both testes).

SCROTAL SWELLING

Scrotal swelling may be acute or chronic and painful or painless. Abrupt onset of painful scrotal swelling necessitates prompt evaluation because some conditions, such as testicular torsion and incarcerated inguinal hernia, require emergency surgical management. The differential diagnosis is shown in Tables 539-1 and 539-2.

Clinical Manifestations

A detailed history is helpful in determining the cause of the swelling and includes onset of pain—with testicular torsion, the pain often is sudden in onset and may be associated with exercise or minor genital trauma; duration of pain; (3) radiation of pain—inguinal discomfort is common with testicular torsion, inguinal hernia, or epididymitis, and associated flank pain can occur with passage of a ureteral calculus; previous episodes of similar pain, which are common in boys with intermittent testicular torsion or inguinal hernia; nausea and vomiting, which are associated with

Table 539-1 DIFFERENTIAL DIAGNOSIS OF SCROTAL MASSES IN BOYS AND ADOLESCENTS

PAINFUL
Testicular torsion
Torsion of appendix testis
Epididymitis
Trauma: ruptured testis, hematocele
Inguinal hernia (incarcerated)
Mumps orchitis
PAINLESS
Hydrocele
Inguinal hernia*
Varicocele*
Spermatocele*
Testicular tumor*
Henoch-Schönlein purpura*
Idiopathic scrotal edema

*May be associated with discomfort.

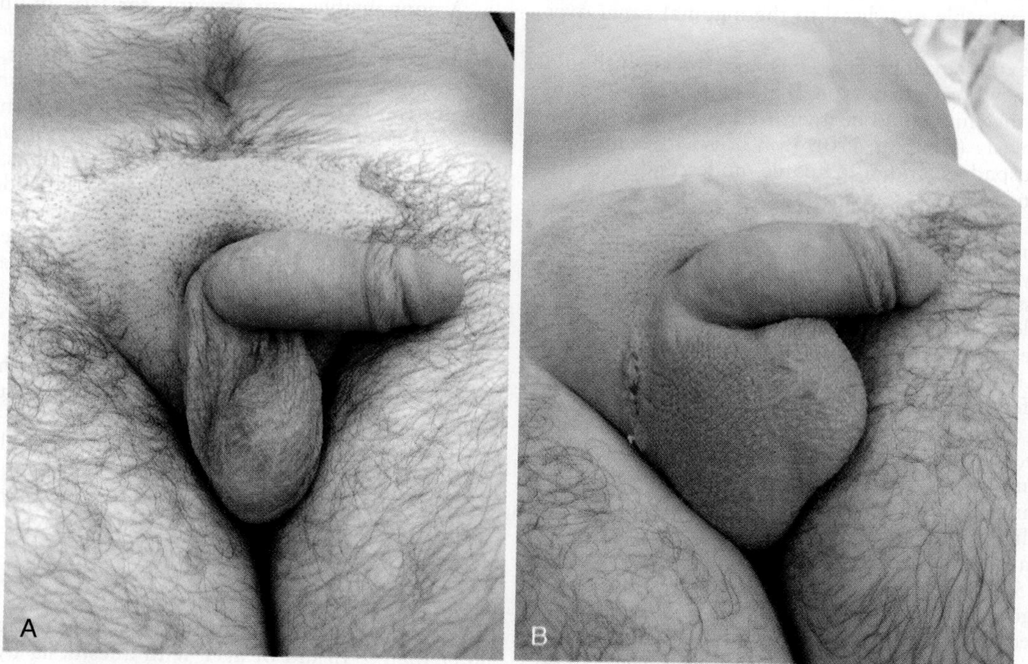

Figure 539-1 *A,* Adolescent with solitary left testis. *B,* Appearance following implantation of right testicular prosthesis.

testicular torsion and inguinal hernia; and irritative urinary symptoms, such as dysuria, urgency, and frequency, which indicate a urinary tract infection that can cause epididymitis. Boys with lower urinary tract pathology such as urethral stricture or neuropathic bladder may be prone to epididymitis.

Physical examination may be difficult in boys with a painful scrotum. Some have advocated performing a spermatic cord block or administering intravenous analgesia to facilitate the examination, but such measures usually are unnecessary. Scrotal wall erythema is common in testicular torsion, epididymitis, torsion of the appendix testis, and an incarcerated hernia. In boys with a normal cremasteric reflex, testicular torsion is unlikely. Absence of a cremasteric reflex is nondiagnostic.

Laboratory Findings and Diagnosis

Pertinent laboratory studies include a urinalysis and culture. A positive urinalysis suggests epididymitis. Serum studies are not helpful in establishing a diagnosis, unless a testicular malignancy is suspected. After initial evaluation, imaging studies may be helpful in establishing the diagnosis, because they assess whether testicular blood flow is normal, reduced, or increased. Imaging studies include color Doppler ultrasonography and a radionuclide testicular flow scan, although the latter is performed infrequently. If a hydrocele is present and the testis is nonpalpable, or if an abnormality of the testis is found, sonography is indicated. Imaging studies are not 100% accurate; they should not be used to decide whether a boy with testicular pain should be referred for urologic evaluation.

Color Doppler ultrasonography is performed most commonly and allows assessment of testicular blood flow and testicular morphologic features. Accuracy is 95% if the ultrasonographer is experienced. A false-negative study (demonstrates normal testicular blood flow) can occur in a boy with testicular torsion if the degree of torsion is <360 degrees and the duration of torsion is short, because there may be continued testicular perfusion. In prepubertal boys, blood flow may be difficult to demonstrate in 15% of normal testes.

Table 539-2 DIFFERENTIAL DIAGNOSIS OF SCROTAL SWELLING IN NEWBORN BOYS

Hydrocele
Inguinal hernia (reducible)
Inguinal hernia (incarcerated)*
Testicular torsion*
Scrotal hematoma
Testicular tumor
Meconium peritonitis
Epididymitis*

*May be associated with discomfort.

TESTICULAR (SPERMATIC CORD) TORSION

Etiology

Testicular torsion requires prompt diagnosis and treatment to salvage the testis. Torsion is the most common cause of testicular pain in boys 12 yr and older and is uncommon before age 10 yr. It is caused by inadequate fixation of the testis within the scrotum, resulting from a redundant tunica vaginalis, allowing excessive mobility of the testis. The abnormal attachment is termed a *bell clapper deformity* and often is bilateral. Shortly after torsion occurs, venous congestion begins and subsequently arterial flow is interrupted. The likelihood of testis survival depends on the duration and severity of torsion. Within 4-6 hr of absent blood flow to the testis, irreversible loss of spermatogenesis can occur.

Diagnosis

Testicular torsion produces acute pain and swelling of the scrotum. On examination, the scrotum is swollen, and the testis is exquisitely tender and often difficult to examine. The cremasteric reflex nearly always is absent. The condition can be differentiated from an incarcerated hernia because swelling in the inguinal area often is absent with torsion. If the pain duration is <4-6 hr, manual detorsion may be attempted. In 65% of cases the torsed testis rotates inward, so detorsion should be attempted in the opposite direction (e.g., the left testis is rotated clockwise). Successful manual detorsion results in dramatic pain relief.

Some adolescents experience *intermittent testicular torsion*. These boys report episodes of severe unilateral testicular pain that resolves spontaneously after 30-60 min. Treatment is elective bilateral scrotal orchiopexy (see later).

Treatment

Treatment is prompt surgical exploration and detorsion. If the testis is explored within 6 hr of torsion, up to 90% of the gonads survive. Testicular salvage decreases rapidly with a delay of >6 hr. If the degree of torsion is 360 degrees or less, the testis might have sufficient arterial flow to allow the gonad to survive, even after 24-48 hr. Following detorsion the testis is fixed in the scrotum with nonabsorbable sutures, termed *scrotal orchiopexy*, to prevent torsion in the future. The contralateral testis also should be fixed in the scrotum because the predisposing anatomic condition often is bilateral. If the testis appears nonviable, orchiectomy is performed (Fig. 539-2*A*). Some adolescents do not

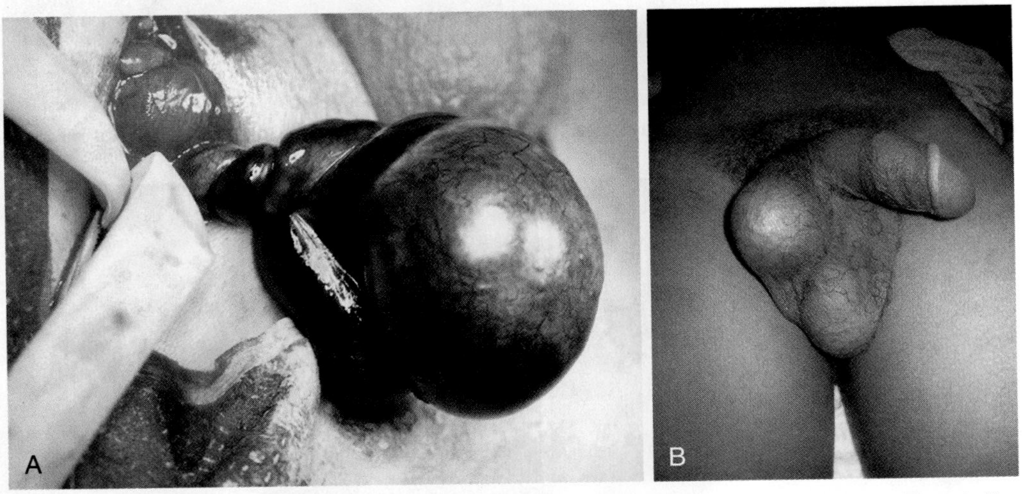

Figure 539-2 *A*, Left testicular torsion in adolescent with acute scrotum; the testis is necrotic. *B*, "Late phase torsion" in an adolescent with severe testicular pain 1 mo previously. Note absence of inflammation and high position of testis in scrotum.

undergo prompt evaluation and treatment and present with "late phase testicular torsion," in which the spermatic cord contracts and the testis is high in the scrotum and nontender (see Fig. 539-2*B*). Fertility is reduced in men with a history of spermatic cord torsion in adolescence, irrespective of whether detorsion or orchiectomy is performed.

Spermatic cord torsion also can occur in the fetus or neonate. This condition results from incomplete attachment of the tunica vaginalis to the scrotal wall and is "extravaginal." When torsion occurs in utero, the baby usually is born with a large, firm, nontender testis. Usually the ipsilateral hemiscrotum is ecchymotic (Fig. 539-3). In these cases, the testis rarely is viable because torsion was a remote event. However, the contralateral testis is at increased risk for torsion until 1 mo beyond term. Most pediatric urologists recommend exploration to establish the diagnosis, remove the necrotic testis, or rarely salvage a viable testis, and anchor the contralateral testis.

TORSION OF THE APPENDIX TESTIS

Torsion of the appendix testis is the most common cause of testicular pain in boys 2-10 yr but is rare in adolescents. The appendix testis is a stalk-like structure that is a vestigial embryonic remnant of the müllerian (paramesonephric) ductal system that is attached to the upper pole of the testis. When it undergoes torsion, progressive inflammation and swelling of the testis and epididymis occurs, resulting in testicular pain and scrotal erythema. The onset of pain usually is gradual. Palpation of the testis usually reveals a 3- to 5-mm tender indurated mass on the upper pole (Fig. 539-4*A*). In some cases, the appendage that has undergone torsion may be visible through the scrotal skin, in the "blue dot" sign. In some boys, distinguishing torsion of the appendix from testicular torsion is difficult. In such cases, a testicular flow scan or color Doppler ultrasonography is useful because testicular blood flow should be normal or increased. In such cases, the radiologist often recognizes epididymal enlargement and makes the diagnosis of epididymitis, reflecting the inflammatory reaction (see Fig. 539-4*B*).

The natural history of torsion of the appendix testis is for the inflammation to resolve in 3-10 days. Nonoperative treatment is recommended, including bed rest and analgesia with nonsteroidal anti-inflammatory medication for 5 days. If the diagnosis is uncertain, scrotal exploration is recommended.

EPIDIDYMITIS

Acute inflammation of the epididymis is an ascending retrograde infection from the urethra, through the vas into the epididymis. This condition causes acute scrotal pain, erythema, and swelling. It is rare before puberty and should raise the question of a congenital abnormality of the wolffian duct, such as an ectopic ureter entering the vas. In younger boys, the responsible organism often is *Escherichia coli* (Chapter 192). After puberty, bacterial epididymitis becomes progressively more common and is the principal cause of acute painful scrotal swelling in young sexually active men. Urinalysis usually reveals pyuria. Epididymitis can be infectious (usually gonococcus or chlamydia; Chapters 185 and 218), but often the organism remains undetermined.

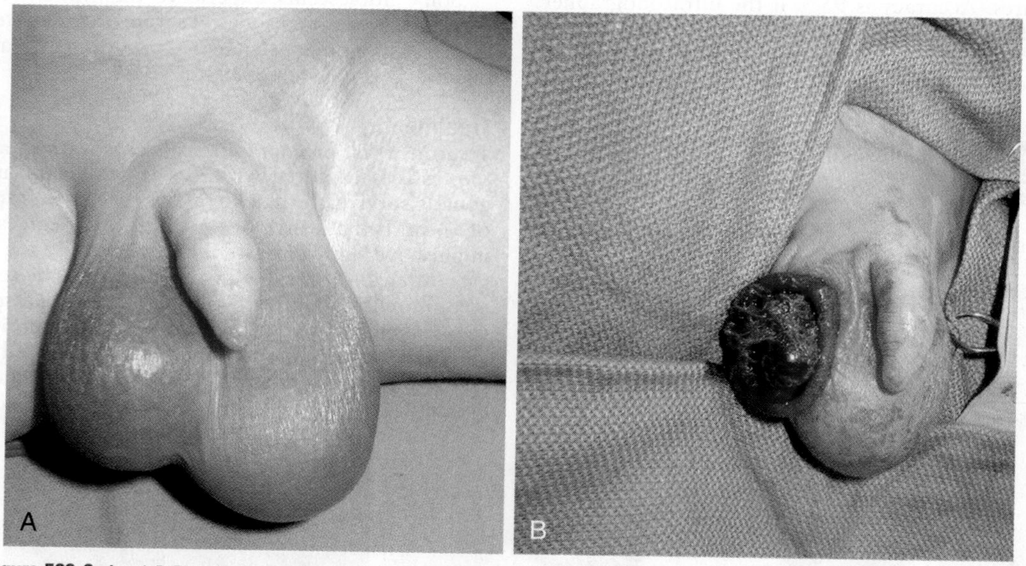

Figure 539-3 *A* and *B*, Right testicular torsion in a newborn. The right hemiscrotum is darker, and the testis was indurated and enlarged.

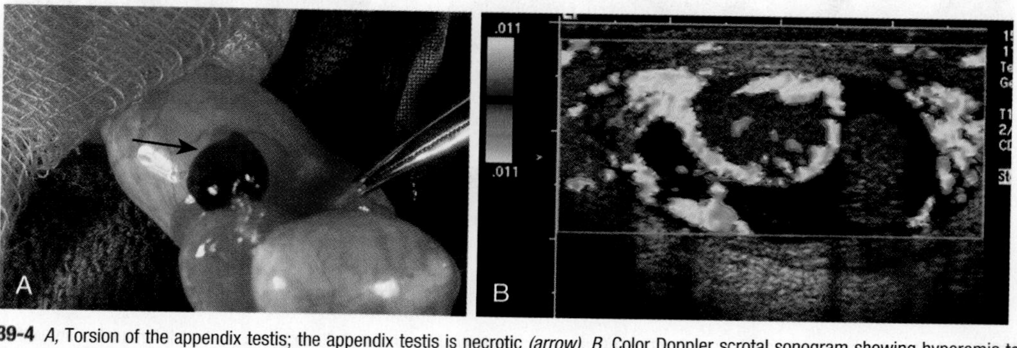

Figure 539-4 *A*, Torsion of the appendix testis; the appendix testis is necrotic *(arrow)*. *B*, Color Doppler scrotal sonogram showing hyperemia to the testis and absent flow to the appendix testis (right side). Symptoms resolved with medical therapy.

Additional etiologies include familial Mediterranean fever, enterovirus, and adenoviruses. Treatment consists of bed rest and antibiotics (Chapter 192). Differentiation from torsion can be difficult, and surgical exploration usually is required in children.

Henoch-Schönlein purpura (HSP; Chapter 478) is a systemic vasculitis that involves multiple organ systems and that can involve the kidney and spermatic cord. When the spermatic cord is involved, typically there is bilateral painful scrotal swelling with purpuric lesions involving the scrotum. Scrotal sonography should show normal testicular blood flow. Treatment is directed toward systemic treatment of the HSP.

VARICOCELE

A varicocele is a congenital condition in which there is abnormal dilation of the pampiniform plexus in the scrotum (Fig. 539-5). Dilation of the pampiniform venous plexus results from valvular incompetence of the internal spermatic vein. Approximately 15% of men have a varicocele; of these men, approximately 15% are subfertile. Varicocele is the most common (and virtually the only) surgically correctable cause of subfertility in men. A varicocele is found in 5-15% of adolescent boys, but it rarely is diagnosed in boys <10 yr old, because the varicocele becomes distended only after the increased blood flow associated with puberty occurs. Varicoceles occur predominantly on the left side, are bilateral in 2% of cases, and rarely involve the right side only. A varicocele in a boy <10 yr or one on the right side might indicate an abdominal or retroperitoneal mass; an abdominal sonogram or CT scan should be performed in such cases.

A varicocele typically is a painless paratesticular mass, often described as a "bag of worms." Occasionally patients describe a dull ache in the affected testis. Usually the varicocele is not apparent when the patient is supine because it is decompressed; in contrast, the varicocele becomes prominent when the patient is standing and enlarges with a Valsalva maneuver. Many pediatricians do not routinely screen adolescents for a varicocele. Varicoceles typically are graded from 1 to 3 with the boy standing: **grade 1** is palpable only with Valsalva; **grade 2** is palpable without Valsalva but is not visible on inspection; and **grade 3** is visible with inspection. Boys with a grade 3 varicocele are at greatest risk for testicular growth arrest. Testicular size should be documented with calipers, an orchiometer, or scrotal sonography, because if the affected left testis is significantly smaller than the right testis, spermatogenesis probably has been adversely affected.

The goal of varicocelectomy is to maximize chances for fertility. Surgical treatment of varicoceles is indicated in boys with a significant disparity in testicular size or pain in the affected testis or if the contralateral testis is diseased or absent. Typically the involved testis enlarges and catches up with the normal testis over the following 1-2 yr. Varicocelectomy should also be considered in boys with a large grade 3 varicocele, even if there is not a disparity in testicular size. Surgical repair is accomplished with a variety of techniques by ligation of the veins of the pampiniform plexus through an inguinal or subinguinal incision (with or without an operating microscope) or by ligating the internal spermatic vein in the retroperitoneum. Laparoscopic repair is becoming more popular. The operation is performed on an ambulatory basis.

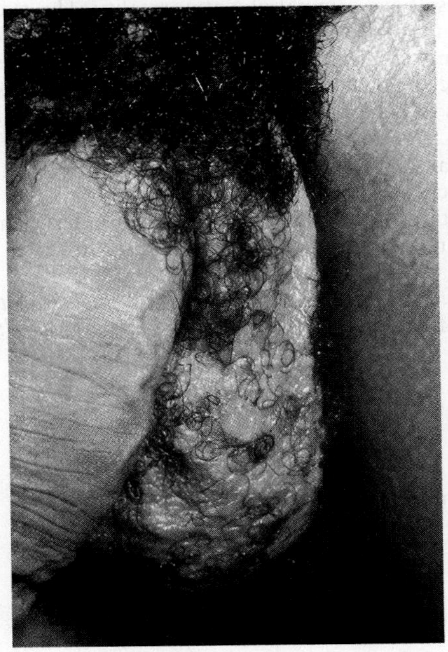

Figure 539-5 Left varicocele in an adolescent boy.

SPERMATOCELE

A spermatocele is a cystic lesion that contains sperm and is attached to the upper pole of the sexually mature testis. Spermatoceles usually are painless and are incidental findings on physical examination. Enlargement of the spermatocele or pain is an indication for removal.

HYDROCELE

Etiology

A hydrocele is an accumulation of fluid in the tunica vaginalis (Fig. 539-6). From 1-2% of neonates have a hydrocele. In most cases, the hydrocele is noncommunicating (the processus vaginalis was obliterated during development). In such cases, the hydrocele fluid disappears by 1 yr of age. If there is a persistently patent processus, the hydrocele persists and becomes progressively larger during the day and is small in the morning. A rare variant of a hydrocele is the abdominoscrotal hydrocele, in which there is a large, tense hydrocele that extends into the lower abdominal cavity. In some older boys, a noncommunicating hydrocele can result from an inflammatory condition within the scrotum, such as testicular torsion, torsion of the appendix testis, epididymitis, or testicular tumor. The long-term risk of a communicating hydrocele is the development of an inguinal hernia. Some older

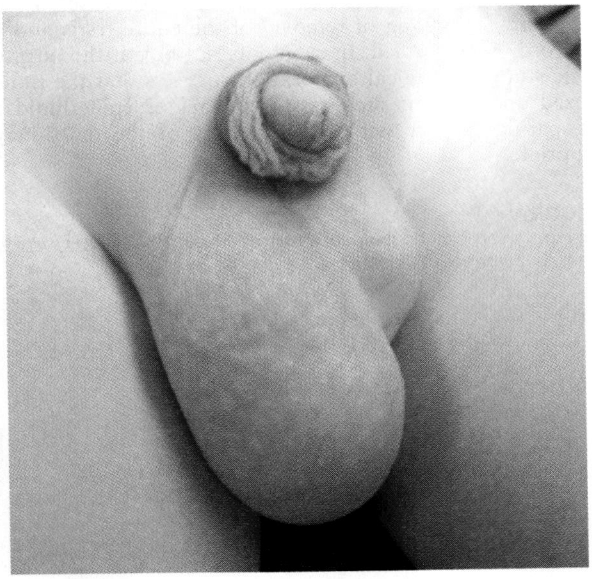

Figure 539-6 Newborn with large right hydrocele.

boys and adolescents also develop a hydrocele. In some cases hydrocele develop acutely after an episode of scrotal trauma or epididymo-orchitis, whereas others develop more insidiously.

Diagnosis

On examination, hydroceles are smooth and nontender. Transillumination of the scrotum confirms the fluid-filled nature of the mass. It is important to palpate the testis, because some young men develop a hydrocele in association with a testis tumor. If compression of the fluid-filled mass completely reduces the hydrocele, an inguinal hernia/hydrocele is the likely diagnosis.

Treatment

Most congenital hydroceles resolve by 12 mo of age following reabsorption of the hydrocele fluid. If the hydrocele is large and tense, however, early surgical correction should be considered, because it is difficult to verify that the child does not have a hernia, and large hydroceles rarely disappear spontaneously. Hydroceles persisting beyond 12-18 mo usually are communicating and should be repaired. Surgical correction is similar to a herniorrhaphy (Chapter 338). Through an inguinal incision, the spermatic cord is identified, the hydrocele fluid is drained, and a high ligation of the processus vaginalis is performed. If an older boy has a large hydrocele, often diagnostic laparoscopy can be performed to determine whether there is a patent processus vaginalis, and if the internal ring is closed, then the hydrocele may be corrected with a scrotal incision.

INGUINAL HERNIA

Inguinal hernia is discussed in Chapter 338.

TESTICULAR TUMOR

Testicular and paratesticular tumors can occur at any age, even in the newborn. Approximately 35% of prepubertal testis tumors are malignant; most commonly they are yolk sac tumors, although rhabdomyosarcoma and leukemia also can occur in this age group. In adolescents, 98% of painless solid testicular masses are malignant (Chapter 497). Most manifest as a painless, hard testicular mass that does not transilluminate. Scrotal ultrasonography should be performed to confirm the finding of a testicular mass and it can help to delineate the type of testis tumor. Serum tumor markers, including **α-fetoprotein** and β-HCG, should be drawn. Definitive therapy includes surgical exploration through an inguinal incision. In most cases, a radical orchiectomy, consisting of removal of the entire testis and spermatic cord, is performed. In a prepubertal boy, if the ultrasonographic study or surgical exploration suggests that the tumor is localized and benign, such as a teratoma or epidermoid cyst, testis-sparing surgery with removal only of the mass may be appropriate.

BIBLIOGRAPHY

Please visit the Nelson Textbook of Pediatrics *website at www.expertconsult.com for the complete bibliography.*

Chapter 540
Trauma to the Genitourinary Tract

Jack S. Elder

ETIOLOGY

Injuries to the genitourinary tract in children usually result from blunt trauma during falls, athletic activities, or motor vehicle accidents (Chapter 66). Children are at greater risk of blunt renal injury than are adults, because they have less body fat and because the kidneys are not located directly behind the ribs. Children with a pre-existing renal anomaly such as hydronephrosis secondary to a ureteropelvic junction obstruction, horseshoe kidney, or renal ectopia also are at increased risk for renal injury. Blunt abdominal or flank trauma often causes a renal injury. Falling can cause a deceleration injury that results in an injury to the renal pedicle, interrupting blood flow to the kidney. If the bladder is full, blunt lower abdominal trauma can cause a bladder rupture. Rupture of the membranous urethra occurs in 5% of pelvic fractures. Straddle injuries usually are associated with trauma to the bulbous urethra.

For the full continuation of this chapter, please visit the Nelson Textbook of Pediatrics *website at www.expertconsult.com.*

Chapter 541
Urinary Lithiasis

Jack S. Elder

Urinary lithiasis in children is less common in the USA than in other parts of the world. The wide geographic variation in the incidence of lithiasis in childhood is related to climatic, dietary, and socioeconomic factors. Approximately 7% of urinary calculi occur in children <16 yr of age. In the USA, many children with stone disease have a metabolic abnormality. The exceptions are patients with a neuropathic bladder (Chapter 536), who are prone to infection-initiated renal stones, and those who have urinary tract reconstruction with small or large intestine, which predisposes to bladder calculi. The incidence of metabolic stones is similar in boys and girls; they are most common in southeastern USA and are rare in African-Americans. In Southeast Asia, urinary calculi are endemic and are related to dietary factors. Contamination of formula with the organic base and unethical nitrogen-containing food additive melamine has been reported in China.

For the full continuation of this chapter, please visit the Nelson Textbook of Pediatrics *website at www.expertconsult.com.*

PART XXV Gynecologic Problems of Childhood

Chapter 542
History and Physical Examination

Kerith Lucco and Diane F. Merritt

HISTORY

With a preverbal or very young patient, clinicians obtain the majority of the history from a parent or caregiver, although even for the very young patient, developmentally appropriate social questions to the patient can put her at ease and help to develop cooperation and rapport that will facilitate a subsequent examination. Specific patient, caregiver, or provider concerns about vaginal discharge or bleeding, pruritus, external genital lesions, or abnormalities should direct a problem-focused history. In a patient presenting with vaginal bleeding, questions focus on recent growth and development, signs of puberty, trauma, vaginal discharge, medication exposure, and any history of foreign objects in the vagina. For complaints of vulvovaginal irritation, pruritus, or discharge, questions concentrate on perineal hygiene, the onset and duration of symptoms, the presence and quality of discharge, exposure to skin irritants, recent antibiotics, travel, presence of infections or medical conditions in the patient or family members, and other systemic illness or skin conditions. Clinicians may ask the patient about what has bothered her, any genital contact, and, if the complaint warrants, whether she ever placed something into her vagina. The patient should be encouraged to ask her own questions. Occasionally the child is brought to the clinician because she or her parents have concerns about anatomic findings, developmental changes, or congenital anomalies. It helps to understand the family's concerns and if a specific reason, event, or family history raised the issue.

For the full continuation of this chapter, please visit the Nelson Textbook of Pediatrics *website at www.expertconsult.com.*

Chapter 543
Vulvovaginitis

Diane F. Merritt

Vulvovaginitis is the most common gynecologic-based problem for prepubertal children. Poor or excessive hygiene and chemical irritants are the most common causes of vulvovaginitis. The condition is usually improved by hygiene measures and education of the caregivers and child.

ETIOLOGY

Vulvitis refers to external genital pruritus, burning, redness, or rash. **Vaginitis** implies inflammation of the vagina, which manifests as a discharge with or without an odor or bleeding. Vaginitis can cause vulvitis. When a child presents with vulvovaginitis, the history should include questions on hygiene (wiping from front to back) and information about possible chemical irritants (bath soaps, laundry detergents, swimming pools, or hot tubs). The caregiver can be asked about a history of diarrhea, perianal itching, or nighttime itching. The possibility of foreign objects being placed into the vagina should also be asked, although the young child is unlikely to remember or recall. Children are especially prone to nonspecific vulvovaginitis for a variety of reasons, including their nonestrogenized state, poor perianal hygiene, and the proximity of the anus to the vagina, which is without geographic barriers given the flattened labia and lack of pubic hair. Labial adhesions occur under similar conditions (Fig. 543-1 and Table 543-1).

EPIDEMIOLOGY

Infectious vulvovaginitis, where a specific pathogen is isolated as the cause of symptoms, may be caused by fecal or respiratory pathogens, and cultures might reveal *Escherichia coli* (Chapter 192), *Streptococcus pyogenes, Staphylococcus aureus* (Chapter 174), *Haemophilus influenzae* (Chapter 186), and, rarely, *Candida* spp. (Chapter 226). These organisms may be transmitted by the child using improper toilet hygiene and manually from the nasopharynx to the vagina. The children present with perianal redness, an inflamed introitus, and often a yellow-green or mildly bloody discharge. They may be observed to be grabbing their genital area or "digging" in their underwear, which is usually stained with yellow-brown discharge. Attempts to treat these bacterial etiologies with antifungal medication will fail; Table 543-2 gives specific recommendations.

Neisseria gonorrhoeae or *Chlamydia trachomatis* also are causes of specific infectious vulvovaginitis (Chapter 114). Management of children who have sexually transmitted infections (STIs) requires close cooperation between clinicians and child-protection authorities. Official investigations for sexual abuse, when indicated, should be initiated promptly (Chapter 371). If acquired after the neonatal period, some diseases (e.g., gonorrhea, syphilis, chlamydia) are 100% indicative of sexual contact. For other diseases (e.g., HPV infection and HSV), the association with sexual contact is not as clear. Although *Trichomonas vaginalis* can be transmitted vertically and can be seen in the newborn, it is an uncommon cause of specific infectious vulvovaginitis in the unestrogenized prepubertal girl.

Other causes of specific infectious vulvovaginitis include *Shigella* (often manifests with a blood-tinged purulent discharge) and *Yersinia enterocolitica*. *Candida* infections (yeast) commonly cause diaper rash, but they are unlikely to cause vaginitis in

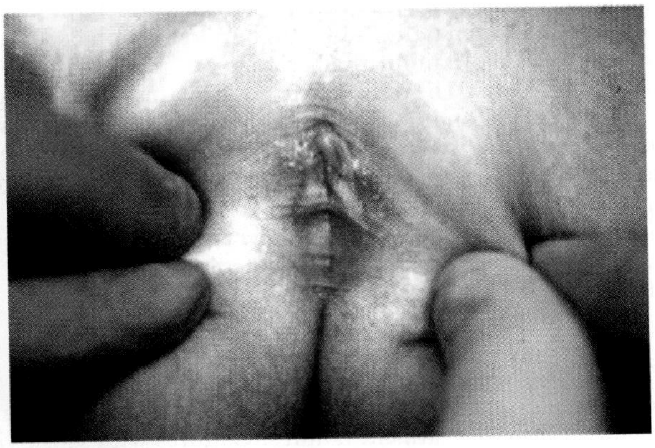

Figure 543-1 Labial adhesions. (Photo courtesy of Diane F. Merritt, MD.)

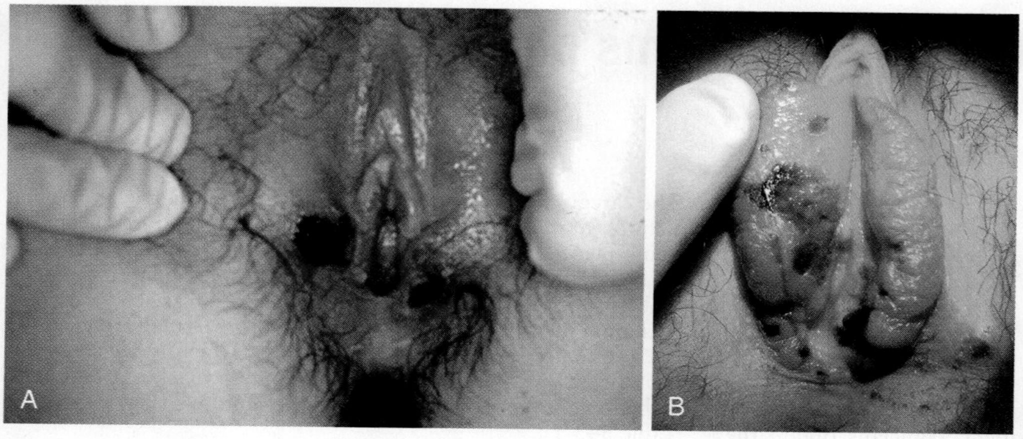

Figure 543-2 Apthous ulcers. (Photo courtesy of Diane F. Merritt, MD.)

children because the alkaline pH of the prepubertal vagina does not support fungal infections. Exceptions can occur in immunocompromised children or children on prolonged antibiotics. Pinworms are the most common helminthic infestation in the USA, with the highest rates in school-aged and preschool children. Perianal itching can lead to excoriation and, rarely, bleeding.

CLINICAL MANIFESTATIONS

Diaper Dermatitis

Diaper dermatitis is the most common dermatologic problem in infancy and occurs in half of all diaper-wearing infants and children. The moisture and contact with urine and feces irritates the skin, and colonization with *Candida* spp increases the severity of the dermatitis. First-line treatment includes hygiene measures such as increasing the frequency of diaper changes, allowing the infant to be diaper free, frequent bathing, and application of water-repellant barriers such as zinc oxide. If diaper dermatitis persists after these conservative measures, or if the classic satellite lesions of candida are present, treatment with an antifungal can decrease the inflammation.

Physiologic Leukorrhea

Neonates and peripubertal girls can present with a white discharge, which is a physiologic effect of estrogen. Some girls complain of the moisture and mucus, but an explanation should reassure the patient and her mother.

Genital Ulcers

Aphthous ulceration of the vulva (Fig. 543-2) in children and adolescents who are not sexually active is well described and can occur in association with oral aphthous ulcers or Epstein-Barr virus infection (Chapter 246). These lesions usually appear in the vestibule and begin as a painful red area that evolves into a sharply demarcated red-rimmed ulcer with a necrotic or eschar-like base. The time course is generally 7-14 days until remission occurs. The lesions are often so painful that urinary diversion with a Foley catheter is necessary. The only way to confirm this clinical diagnosis is to rule other conditions, including herpes, chancroid lesion, Crohn's disease, and syphilitic chancres. Treatment includes good hygiene, topical lidocaine, oral antibiotics to prevent superinfection, and short-term systemic steroids. The lesions can recur, and evaluation for Behçet's disease (Chapter 155) using the International Study Group diagnostic guidelines should be considered. See Table 543-1 for other common etiologies.

DIAGNOSIS AND DIFFERENTIAL DIAGNOSIS

Children with symptoms of vulvovaginitis often have had a previous evaluations and treatment failures. Cultures with sensitivities to test for specific pathogens may be obtained with cotton

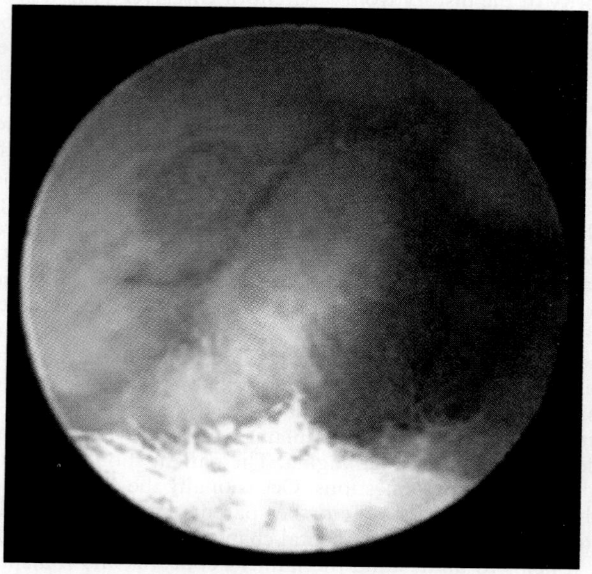

Figure 543-3 Vaginal foreign body as seen through vaginoscope. (Photo courtesy of Diane F. Merritt, MD.)

swabs or urethral (Calgiswabs) swabs moistened with nonbacteriostatic saline. Use of a swab can cause discomfort or, rarely, minimal bleeding. To distract the patient, the child can be asked to cough. A topical anesthetic can be applied before placing the swab into the vagina. The premoistened swab can be placed vertically between the labia minora to collect secretions. In this case, it is not necessary to place the swab into the vagina in the unanesthetized patient. If a discharge is present, an aerobic vaginal culture and gonorrhea and chlamydia testing may be done. Alternatively, a small feeding tube attached to a syringe with a small amount of saline for vaginal wash and aspiration can be used. This allows examination of the fluid under the microscope as well as sending the fluid off for culture. The minimal amount of normal saline should be used in order to not dilute the specimen. Testing for gonorrhea and chlamydia may be done by culture or by nucleic acid amplification testing, depending on institutional or state and Centers for Disease Control guidelines. Tests for shigella might require special media and collection procedures.

If pinworms (Chapter 286) are suspected, transparent adhesive tape or an anal swab should be applied to the anal region in the morning before defecation or bathing and then placed on a slide. Eggs seen on microscopic examination confirm the diagnosis, and sometimes the pinworms can be seen at the anal verge. Several samples may be required to detect the eggs, and false negative results still can occur.

If the vaginal discharge is serosanguineous, if a foul odor is present, or if the discharge fails to respond to hygiene measures, consider presence of a vaginal foreign body (Fig. 543-3). If inspection suggests presence of a foreign body, the vagina can be irrigated, or an examination under anesthesia may reveal the foreign body. Vaginoscopy is an excellent diagnostic tool and can be performed in an unsedated cooperative patient in an outpatient setting or under general anesthesia if necessary. Using a cystoscope with saline or water irrigation to gravity, insert the endoscopic device into the vagina, gently oppose the labia, the vagina will distend and the entire vaginal cavity and cervix may be easily assessed.

TREATMENT AND PREVENTION

The treatment of specific vulvovaginitis should be directed at the organism causing the symptoms (see Table 543-1). Treatment of nonspecific vulvovaginitis includes sitz baths and avoidance of irritating or harsh soaps and chemicals and tight clothing that abrades the perineum. External application of bland emollient barriers such as over-the-counter diaper rash medications and petroleum jelly may be helpful. Proper perineal hygiene is critical for long-term improvement. Younger children need supervised perineal hygiene, and caregivers should be advised to wipe the genital area from front to back. Use of a warm moistened washcloth or diaper wipe is helpful after initial wiping with toilet tissue. Little girls should wear cotton-only underwear and limit time spent in tights, leotards, and wet swimsuits. Soaking in warm clean bathwater for 15-minute intervals (no shampoo or bubble bath) is soothing and helps with cleaning the area. The parents should be counseled to avoid all scented, antiseptic and deodorant-based soaps and

Table 543-1 SPECIFIC VULVAR DISORDERS IN CHILDREN

ORGANISM	PRESENTATION	DIAGNOSIS	TREATMENT
Molluscum contagiosum (Fig. 543-4)	1- to 5-mm discrete, skin-colored, dome-shaped, umbilicated lesions with a central cheesy plug	Diagnosis usually is made by visual inspection	The disease generally is self-limited and the lesions can resolve spontaneously Treatment choices in children may include cryosurgery, application of topical anesthetic and curettage, and topical silver nitrate Use of topical 5% imiquimod cream has been reported
Condyloma accuminata	Skin-colored papules, some with a shaggy cauliflower-like appearance	Diagnosis usually is made by visual inspection. Biopsy should be reserved for when the diagnosis is in question. HPV DNA testing is not helpful	Destructive and excisional options, which can require general or local anesthesia, include topical trichloroacetic acid, local cryotherapy, electrocautery, excision by scalpel or scissors, and laser ablation Products not approved for children include provider application of podophyllin resin, and home application of imiquimod, and podophylox, and sinectechins (Veregen) ointment
Herpes simplex	Blisters that break, leaving tender ulcers	Visual inspection confirmed by culture from lesion	Infants: Acyclovir 20 mg/kg body weight IV q8 hr × 21 days for disseminated and CNS disease or × 14 days for disease limited to the skin and mucous membranes Children >2 yr may be treated with oral acyclovir 30-60 mg/kg/day × 10 days
Labial Agglutination (see Fig. 543-1)	The condition can cause urinary dribbling or be associated with vulvitis, urinary tract infection, or urethritis	Diagnosis is made by visual inspection of the adherent labia, often with a central semi-translucent line	This condition does not require treatment if the patient is asymptomatic Symptomatic patients: topical estrogen cream or bethamethosone ointment applied daily for 6 wk directly on the line of adhesions, using a cotton swab while applying gentle labial traction Estrogen must be discontinued if breast budding occurs Mechanical separation of the adhesions is rarely indicated The adhesions usually resolve in 6-12 wk, but unless good hygiene measures are followed, recurrence is common To decrease the risk of recurrence, an emollient (petroleum jelly, A&D ointment) should be applied to the inner labia for ≥1 mo at bedtime
Lichen sclerosus (Fig. 543-5)	A sclerotic, atrophic, parchment-like plaque with an hourglass or keyhole appearance of vulvar, perianal, or perineal skin, subepithelial hemorrhages may be misinterpreted as sexual abuse or trauma The patient can experience perineal itching, soreness, or dysuria	Diagnosis usually is made by visual inspection Biopsy should be reserved for when the diagnosis is in question	Ultrapotent topical corticosteroids is the first-line therapy (clobetasol propionate ointment 0.05%) once or twice a day for 4-8 wk Once symptoms are under control, the patient should be tapered off the drug unless therapy is required for a flare-up
Psoriasis	The classic extragenital psoriatic lesions are red plaques with well-demarcated silvery scales that are intensely pruritic	Diagnosis may be confirmed by locating other affected areas on the scalp or in nasolabial folds or behind the ears	Vulvar lesions may be treated with topical corticosteroids

Continued

Table 543-1 SPECIFIC VULVAR DISORDERS IN CHILDREN—cont'd

ORGANISM	PRESENTATION	DIAGNOSIS	TREATMENT
Atopic dermatitis	Chronic cases can result in crusty, weepy lesions that are accompanied by intense pruritus and erythema Scratching often results in excoriation of the lesions and secondary bacterial or candidal infection	It may be seen in the vulvar area but characteristically affects the face, neck, chest, and extremities	Children with this condition should avoid common irritants and use topical corticosteroids for flare-ups If dry skin is present, lotion or bath oil can be used to seal in moisture after bathing
Contact dermatitis	Erythematous, edematous, or weepy vulvar vesicles or pustules can result, but more often the skin appears inflamed	Associated with exposure to an irritant, such as perfumed soaps, bubble bath, talcum powder, lotions, elastic bands of undergarments, or disposable diaper components	Topical corticosteroids for flare-ups
Seborrheic dermatitis	Erythematous and greasy, yellowish scaling on vulva and labial crural folds associated with greasy dandruff-type rash of scalp, behind ears and face	Diagnosis usually is made by visual inspection	Gentle cleaning, topical clotrimazole with 1% hydrocortisone added

Table 543-2 ANTIBIOTIC RECOMMENDATIONS FOR SPECIFIC VULVOVAGINAL INFECTIONS

ETIOLOGY	TREATMENT
Streptococcus pyogenes *Streptococcus pneumoniae*	Penicillin V, 250 mg PO bid-tid ×10 days Amoxicillin 40 mg/kg/day (max 500 mg/dose) divided into 3 doses daily × 7 days Erythromycin ethyl succinate, 30-50 mg/kg/day (max 400 mg/dose) divided into 4 doses daily TMP-SMX 6-10 mg/kg/day (trimethoprim component) divided into 2 doses daily × 10 days Clarithromycin 7.5 mg/kg bid (max 1 g/day) × 5-10 days
Staphylococcus aureus	Cephalexin, 25-50 mg/kg/day PO × 7-10 days divided 16-12 hr Dicloxacillin, 25 mg/kg/d ayPO × 7-10 days divided q6 hr Amoxicillin-clavulanate, 20-40 mg/kg/d ay (of the amoxicillin) PO divided into 2 or 3 doses daily × 7-10 days Cefuroxime suspension 30 mg/kg/d ay divided twice daily (max 1 g) × 10 days (tabs: 250 mg bid) MRSA: TMP-SMX double strength 8-10 mg/kg/day; culture abscesses, incision and drainage
Haemophilus influenzae	Amoxicillin, 40 mg/kg/day divided into 3 doses daily × 7 days
Shigella	TMP-SMX 8-10 mg/kg/day (trimethoprim component) divided into 2 doses daily × 5 days or ampicillin 50-100 mg/kg/day divided into 4 doses daily (adult max 4 g/d) × 5 days For resistant organisms: ceftriaxone 50-75 mg/kg/day IV or IM divided into 1 or 2 doses (max 2 g/day)
Chlamydia trachomatis	TMP-SMX 8-10 mg/kg/day (trimethoprim component) divided into 2 doses daily × 5 days or ampicillin 50-100 mg/kg/day divided into 4 doses daily (adult max 4 g/d) × 5 days For resistant organisms: ceftriaxone 50-75 mg/kg/day IV or IM divided into 1 or 2 doses (max 2 g/day)
Neisseria gonorrhoeae	Children <45 kg: Ceftriaxone, 125 mg IM in a single dose (alternate: spectinomycin 40 mg/kg (maximum 2 g IM) once *plus* if chlamydial infection is not ruled out, prescribe for chlamydia as above Children ≥45 kg: Treat with adult regimen of cefixime, 400 mg PO in a single dose, or ceftriaxone, 125 mg IM in a single dose, *plus,* if chlamydial infection is not ruled out, azithromycin, 1 g PO in a single dose or doxycycline, 100 mg PO bid ×7 days Children with bacteremia or arthritis: Ceftriaxone, 50 mg/kg (max dose for children <45 kg: 1 g) IM or IV in a single dose daily × 7 days
Trichomonas	Metronidazole, 15 mg/kg/day tid (maximum 250 mg tid) × 7 days *or* Tinidazole 50 mg/kg (≤2 g) as a single dose for children >3 yr
Pinworms *(Enterobius vermicularis)*	Mebendazole (Vermox), 1 chewable 100 mg tablet, repeated in 2 wk or Albendazole, 100 mg for child <2 yr or 400 mg for older child, repeated in 2 w,

TMP-SMX, trimethoprim-sulfamethoxazole; MRSA, methicillin-resistant *Staphylococcus aureus.*

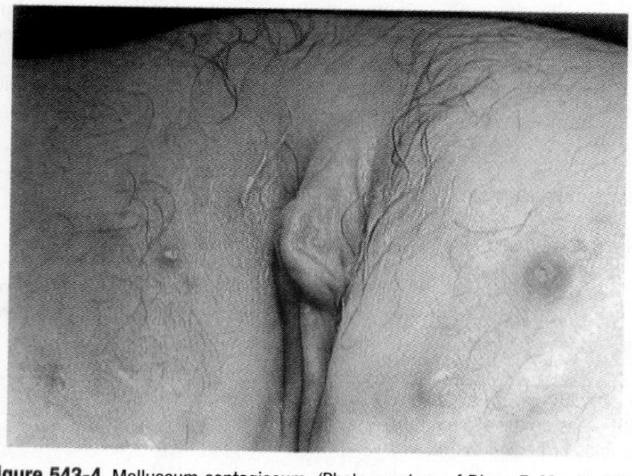

Figure 543-4 Molluscum contagiosum. (Photo courtesy of Diane F. Merritt, MD.)

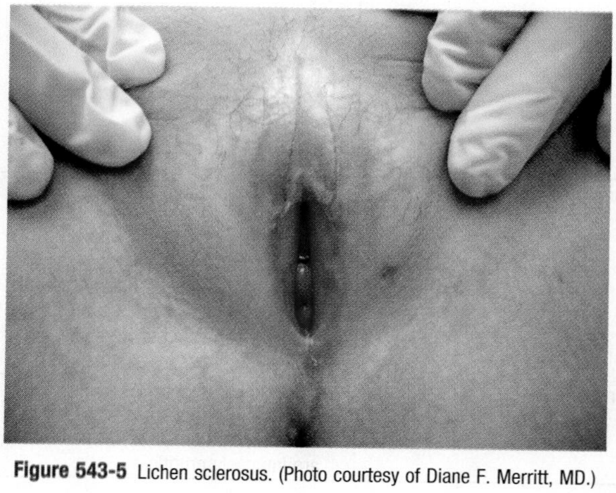

Figure 543-5 Lichen sclerosus. (Photo courtesy of Diane F. Merritt, MD.)

eliminate the use of fabric softeners or dryer sheets when laundering undergarments.

BIBLIOGRAPHY
Please visit the Nelson Textbook of Pediatrics *website at www.expertconsult.com for the complete bibliography.*

Chapter 544 Bleeding

Laura A. Parks and Diane F. Merritt

Vaginal bleeding in infants and prepubescent children is concerning for both the child and the parents and should always be evaluated. Bleeding can be seen as early as the 1st wk of life from maternal estrogen withdrawal until puberty when menstruation occurs. It can occur as light serosanguineous spotting to heavy bleeding with clots. A thorough history and physical must be obtained as the first step in diagnosing the problem. Common causes for vaginal bleeding in children are vulvovaginitis, foreign bodies, dermatologic conditions, and urethral prolapse; less common are endogenous or exogenous estrogenic effects; and, most worrisome, include neoplasms and trauma.

Vulvovaginitis may be caused by respiratory, oral and fecal pathogens, some of which produce a serosanguineous drainage (*Streptococcus* spp, *Shigella*) or cause vulvar bleeding due to irritation and excoriation of the skin. Prepubertal girls are at a higher risk for developing these irritations because the protective labia of pubertal girls are not fully developed and thus the vaginal opening and vagina are more exposed to irritants. Further, the mucosa is thin and the pH of the vagina is more alkaline than after menarche from low levels of estrogen. Hand-washing, improved perineal hygiene (wiping front to back, use of wet wipes after bowel movement), and avoidance of topical irritants, chemicals, and perfumed or deodorant soaps and bubble baths will reduce nonspecific vulvovaginitis. If hygiene does not result in improvement, a short course of antibiotics will be required to clear a recurrent or persistent infection (see Table 543-2). External application of bland emollient barriers such as over-the-counter diaper rash medications and petroleum jelly may be helpful.

A potential dermatologic reason for bleeding is **lichen sclerosus** (see Fig. 543-5 and Table 543-1). This condition is characterized by chronic inflammation, intense pruritus, and thinning and whitening of the vulvar and perianal skin in a keyhole fashion. Petechiae or blood blisters can arise and be mistaken as a sign of sexual abuse. Diagnosis is based on these classic clinical characteristics but may be confirmed by a tissue biopsy if necessary. Potent topical steroids are the first line of treatment and usually improve the appearance and symptoms of pruritus. The steroid should then be tapered and used for the shortest duration necessary; flare-ups can occur and require retreatment.

Foreign bodies are a common cause of vaginal bleeding, and children present with blood-stained and foul-smelling discharge. It can last from days to months until the correct diagnosis is made and the object is removed. The most common objects found are wadded up pieces of toilet paper. A physical exam in knee-chest or frog-leg position can sometimes reveal the object. Vaginal irrigation can then be done in the office using a small feeding tube and warm water. If the object is not visible on exam, irrigation is unlikely to remove it and exam under anesthesia and vaginoscopy are often required. Vaginoscopy not only allows removal of a foreign object but also can facilitate diagnosis of other causes of the bleeding.

Trauma to the vulva or vagina is especially concerning. Most of these injuries are accidental, but physical and sexual abuse must be ruled out (Chapter 37). Straddle injuries such as falling on the top bar of a bicycle or slipping in the bathtub may result in bruising, hematomas, and lacerations. Generally, if the trauma is accidental, the hymen is protected by the labia and defects are not seen. If there is a laceration of the hymen, especially posteriorly, abuse must be suspected. If the injury is penetrating, further exam and imaging are necessary to evaluate the urethra and anus and for internal injuries. General anesthesia may be needed to fully assess injuries and allow repair; minor lacerations can be repaired in a cooperative child under sedation or using local anesthesia. If the patient is able to void spontaneously, nonexpanding hematomas can be observed and treated with ice and with pain medications. Large expanding hematomas should be opened and drained, especially if the overlying skin is becoming ischemic. A Foley catheter should be placed for children who are having difficulty with voiding.

Urethral prolapse (Chapter 538) is another potential cause of bleeding in the prepubertal girl. It occurs when the distal end of the urethra prolapses either partially or completely. Patients may be asymptomatic or present with bleeding, dysuria, or difficulty with urination. Low estrogen state, trauma, chronic cough, and constipation are believed to be predisposing factors. Treatment is conservative, with application of estrogen cream at the area of prolapse twice daily for 2 wk and then, if prolapse is still present, continued use until the prolapse resolves. Surgical excision is very rarely necessary to remove necrotic tissue.

Neoplasms of the vulva and vagina are rare (Chapter 547). Of these, the most common in the prepubertal girl include hemangiomas, polyps, and sarcoma botryoides. The most obvious on exam is the cavernous hemangioma of the vulva. This is a benign growth of blood vessels that can cause bleeding from irritation to the skin from clothing overlying these vessels. Like hemangiomas found elsewhere on the body, these lesions are typically not seen at birth, increase in size over the 1st yr of life, and then begin to regress over the next several years. After this has occurred, there is rarely any evidence of the lesion with the exception of a discoloration of the skin that can sometimes be noted. Treatment is not necessary because these are self-limiting; however, a barrier cream can be applied if bleeding is a concern. Surgery is reserved for very severe cases causing heavy bleeding. Hemangiomas of the perineum may be associated with spinal dysraphism, so a neurologic assessment should be performed.

Like hemangiomas, hymenal polyps are also usually benign. If these polyps are noted at birth, they generally regress after maternal levels of estrogen decrease in the infant. Reassurance to the parents and expectant management are all that is needed. A barrier cream can be applied to the area until it resolves to decrease bleeding from friction with the diaper. Vaginal polyps, especially if they cause bleeding, should be removed and sent for pathologic evaluation.

Rhabdomyosarcoma (RMS) is a rare malignancy that affects <300 children a year in the USA. In children, the most common sites are the head and neck and genitourinary region (Chapter 494). Vaginal tumors tend to occur in young children and produce vaginal bleeding and discharge. The uterine tumors generally occur in older girls and may be extensive at the time of diagnosis. Treatment consists of a multimodal approach including surgery, radiation therapy, and chemotherapy. The survival rate is >90% when an early diagnosis is made.

Vaginal bleeding can be a presenting sign of **precocious puberty,** which is defined as pubertal development that is 2.5 to 3 standard deviations earlier than the average age. Guidelines for the evaluation of premature development state that pubic hair or breast development requires evaluation only when it occurs before age 7 yr in non–African-American girls and before age 6 yr in African-American girls (Chapters 555 and 556).

The most common etiology is gonadotropin-dependent or central **precocious puberty** (Chapter 556.1). Gonadotropin-independent and incomplete precocity are less common. A thorough physical exam must be done, looking for secondary sex characters. The child might require observation of progression from one stage of pubertal development to the next in <3-6 mo. Diagnostic studies include measurement of accelerated growth velocity demonstrated by growth charts and advanced bone age. Pelvic ultrasound might show presence of ovarian or adrenal pathology or uterine maturation. Serum estradiol levels >100 pg/mL may be associated with an ovarian cyst or tumor. The gold standard is measurement of gonadotropins after GnRH or GnRH-agonist stimulation. In all cases of central precocious puberty, MRI imaging of the brain is needed to determine if a tumor is present in the hypothalamus.

Another etiology for childhood vaginal bleeding is **exogenous exposures to estrogens.** These exposures can occur from ingestion of birth control pills, foods, beauty products, and plastics that contain estrogen or estrogen-like components. Several other studies have assessed the risk of bisphenol A (BPA) leaching from plastic cups and bottles. The importance of this is still being studied but BPA is known to have an estrogenic effect and thus could potentially be a cause for vaginal bleeding if ingested in high levels.

Vaginal bleeding in the prepubertal girl or infant can have many causes. A good history and physical must be done to identify the source of bleeding so that treatment can occur. Fortunately, most of these causes are easily treated and the patients do quite well.

BIBLIOGRAPHY

Please visit the Nelson Textbook of Pediatrics *website at www.expertconsult.com for the complete bibliography.*

Chapter 545

Breast Concerns

Nirupama K. DeSilva and Diane F. Merritt

Girls with breast disorders commonly present with questions about the development and appearance of their breasts, breast pain, nipple discharge, and concerns about the presence of a mass. Although children and adolescents are unlikely to have malignant or life-threatening breast problems, this population of patients should be referred to practitioners who have experience and familiarity with the immature and developing breast to avoid overtreatment with unnecessary diagnostic or surgical procedures.

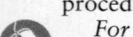

For the full continuation of this chapter, please visit the Nelson Textbook of Pediatrics *website at www.expertconsult.com.*

Chapter 546

Polycystic Ovary Syndrome and Hirsutism

Mark Gibson and Heather G. Huddleston

POLYCYSTIC OVARY SYNDROME

Etiology and Definition

Polycystic ovary syndrome (PCOS) is a common disorder of reproductive hormone dysfunction, often with associated metabolic abnormalities, that affects 5-8% of women of reproductive age. The disorder typically emerges in adolescence when a normal menstrual pattern is not established and there is clinical evidence of androgen excess. It is characterized by the triad of oligo-ovulation or anovulation, clinical or biochemical hyperandrogenism, and ovarian cysts (≥12 immature follicles) (the Rotterdam criteria). Various expert bodies prioritize these elements differently for establishing the diagnosis, and few require the presence of all 3. Hyperandrogenism with ovulatory dysfunction (with exclusion of other causes) is most often considered sufficient for diagnosis in the USA. Abnormalities commonly associated with PCOS include obesity, insulin resistance, and the metabolic syndrome, but the phenotype is variable (see Table 546-1 on the *Nelson Textbook of Pediatrics* website at www.expertconsult.com).

For the full continuation of this chapter, please visit the Nelson Textbook of Pediatrics *website at www.expertconsult.com.*

Chapter 547

Neoplasms and Adolescent Screening for Human Papilloma Virus

Nora T. Kizer and Diane F. Merritt

GYNECOLOGIC MALIGNANCIES

Cancer is the second most common cause of death in adolescents, after injuries. Although gynecologic malignancies are rare, they can be especially tragic given the emotional and psychologic impact associated with their diagnosis. Infertility, depression, and poor self-image may be lifelong issues for these patients.

The most common type of gynecologic malignancy found in children and adolescents is of ovarian origin and usually manifests as an abdominal mass, which must be distinguished from other organ-based tumors and ovarian functional, physiologic, inflammatory/infectious, or pregnancy-related processes. Ovarian neoplasms constitute 1% of all childhood malignancies, but account for 60-70% of all gynecologic malignancies in this age group. About 10-30% of all childhood or adolescent ovarian neoplasms are malignant. Less often, the vagina or cervix is a site of malignant lesions in children, with a few specific tumors having their greatest incidence within this population. Cervical dysplasia can occur in adolescents, and health care providers need to be aware of current screening guidelines as well as updates on preventive measures. Vulvar malignancies in children and adolescents are exceedingly rare.

IMPACT OF CANCER THERAPY ON FERTILITY

Chemotherapy and radiation therapy are associated with acute ovarian failure and premature menopause. Risk factors include older age, abdominal or spinal radiation, and certain chemotherapeutic drugs, such as alkylating agents (cyclophosphamide, busulfan). Uterine irradiation is associated with infertility, spontaneous pregnancy loss, and intrauterine growth restriction. Decreased uterine volume has been noted in girls who received abdominal radiation. The vagina, bladder, ureters, urethra, and rectum can also be injured by radiation. Vaginal shortening, vaginal stenosis, urinary tract fistulas, and diarrhea are important side effects of pelvic irradiation for pelvic cancers. Pregnancy outcomes appear to be influenced by prior chemotherapy and radiation treatment; 15% of childhood cancer survivors have infertility. Cancer survivors have an increased rate of spontaneous abortions, premature deliveries, and low-birthweight infants compared to their normal healthy siblings. No data support an increased incidence of congenital malformations in offspring.

Childhood cancer survivors require extensive counseling about these specific future health implications. As part of informed consent for cancer therapy, the possibility of infertility should be discussed with young patients and their families. Options for fertility preservation (pretreatment with GnRH analogs, harvesting and cryopreservation of oocytes and ovarian tissue) are at present experimental. Premature ovarian insufficiency is associated with an increased risk for cardiovascular complications, osteoporosis, and difficulties with sexual function. Risks and benefits of hormonal therapy need to be addressed.

OVARIES

Neonatal and Pediatric Ovarian Cysts

Normal follicles or physiologic ovarian cysts are seen by ultrasound examination of the ovaries in all healthy prepubertal girls. Most of these are <1 cm in diameter and not pathologic. In the neonatal period, physiologic follicular cysts due to maternal estrogen stimulation usually resolve spontaneously and may be followed with serial ultrasounds in the asymptomatic child. Children with an ovarian mass might have no symptoms and the mass may be detected incidentally or during a routine examination. Other children present with abdominal pain that may be accompanied by nausea, vomiting, or urinary frequency or retention. The cyst's most common complication, ovarian torsion, can result in loss of the ovary (autoamputation of the ovary has been documented to occur antenatally). Successful reports of antenatal aspiration and postnatal laparoscopic treatment exist. Large cysts (>4-5 cm), those with complex characteristics, or any ovarian cyst in premenarchal girls with associated signs or symptoms of hormonal stimulation deserve prompt evaluation. The incidence of ovarian cysts increases again with puberty.

Functional Cysts

Hemorrhagic cysts are an expected part of follicular development during the menstrual cycle. Normally, a dominant follicle forms and increases in size. Following ovulation, the dominant follicle becomes a corpus luteum that, if it bleeds, is termed a *hemorrhagic corpus luteum*. These can become symptomatic owing to size or peritoneal irritation from blood, and they have a characteristic complex appearance on ultrasound. Expectant management for a presumed functional or hemorrhagic cyst is appropriate. Physiologic cysts are usually no larger than 5 cm and resolve over the course of 6-8 wk during subsequent ultrasound imaging. Monophasic oral contraceptives can be used to suppress follicular development to prevent formation of additional cysts.

Teratomas

The most common neoplasm in adolescents is the *mature cystic teratoma (dermoid cyst)*. Most are benign and contain mature tissue of ectodermal (skin, hair, sebaceous glands), mesodermal, or endodermal origin. Occasionally well-formed teeth, cartilage, and bone are found. Calcification on an abdominal radiograph is often a hallmark of a benign teratoma. These tumors may be asymptomatic and found incidentally, or they can manifest as a mass or with abdominal pain (associated with torsion or rupture). If the major component of the dermoid is thyroid tissue (struma ovarii), hyperthyroidism can be the clinical presentation. Benign teratomas should be carefully resected, preserving as much normal ovarian tissue as possible. Oophorectomy (and salpingo-oophorectomy) for this benign lesion is excessive treatment. During surgery, both ovaries should be evaluated, and if there is any question about the nature of the lesion, the specimen should be evaluated by a pathologist. An association of dermoid tumors with neural elements and *anti-NMDA receptor encephalitis* has been reported. Excision of the ovarian tumor has led to improvement in neurologic symptoms in some patients.

Immature teratoma of the ovary is an uncommon tumor, accounting for less than 1% of ovarian teratomas. In contrast to the mature cystic teratoma, which is encountered most often during the reproductive years but occurs at all ages, the immature teratoma has a specific age incidence, occurring most commonly in the first 2 decades of life. By definition, an immature teratoma contains immature neural elements. Because the lesion is rarely bilateral in its ovarian involvement, the present method of therapy consists of unilateral salpingo-oophorectomy with wide sampling of peritoneal implants.

Cystadenomas

Serous and mucinous cystadenomas are the second most common benign ovarian tumor. These cystic lesions can become very large, yet with care, the tumor can be resected, preserving normal ovarian tissue for future reproductive potential.

Polycystic Ovarian Syndrome (PCOS)

See Chapter 546.

Endometriomas

Endometriosis is a syndrome defined by the presence of ectopic endometrial tissue usually located within the pelvis and abdomen. The principal clinical symptoms in adolescents consist of severe menstrual pain and pelvic pain. Endometriomas (chocolate cysts) form when the ovaries are involved and are collections of old blood and hemosiderin within an endometrium-lined cyst. They have a typical homogeneous echogenic appearance on ultrasound, and are more common in adults than in adolescents. Conservative management (suppressive therapy with ovulation suppression, and nonsteroidal anti-inflammatory drugs [NSAIDs]) and ovarian cystectomy with preservation of as much functioning ovary as possible is recommended for adolescents.

Pelvic Inflammatory Disease and Tubo-ovarian Abscess

Pelvic inflammatory disease complicated by a tubo-ovarian abscess should be considered in a sexually active adolescent with an adnexal mass and pain on examination (Chapter 114). These patients also typically exhibit fever with leukocytosis and cervical motion tenderness. Treatment consists of administration of intravenous antibiotics. If the lesion persists or is refractory to antibiotics, drainage of the pelvic abscess by interventional radiology should be considered.

Adnexal Torsion

Adnexal torsion of the ovary and/or fallopian tube can occur in children or adolescents with normal adnexa or those enlarged by cystic changes or ovarian neoplasms. When torsion occurs, the venous outflow is obstructed first, and the ovary swells and becomes hemorrhagic. Once the arterial flow is interrupted, necrosis begins. It is not known how long torsed adnexa will remain viable. When a female patient presents with lower abdominal pain, either episodic or constant, and if imaging studies shows unilateral enlargement of an adnexa, the diagnosis of adnexal torsion must be considered and acted upon. The sonographic presence of Doppler flow does not exclude the diagnosis of torsion. Prompt surgical intervention (by laparoscopy) is warranted if clinical suspicion is high. Detorsion of the adnexa and observation for viability is recommended, with excision only for obviously nonviable necrotic tissues. Oophoropexy (plication) of the affected and the contralateral adnexa remain controversial. Recovery of ovarian function after detorsion has been reported with identification of normal follicle development.

Ovarian Carcinoma

Ovarian cancer is very uncommon in children; only 2% of all ovarian cancers are diagnosed in patients <25 yr old. The SEER incidence rates are ≤0.8/100,000 at age 0-14 yr and 1.5/100,000 at ages 15-19 yr. Germ cell tumors are the most common and originate from primordial germ cells that then develop into a number of heterogeneous tumor types including dysgerminomas, malignant teratomas, endodermal sinus tumors, embryonal carcinomas, mixed cell neoplasms, and gonadoblastomas. Immature teratomas and endodermal sinus tumors are more aggressive malignancies than dysgerminomas and occur in a significantly higher proportion of younger girls (<10 yr of age). Sex-cord stromal tumors are more common among adolescents (Table 547-1). Tumor markers such as α-fetoprotein (AFP), carcinoembryonic antigen (CEA), and the antigen CA 125 are also used for diagnosis and treatment surveillance (Table 547-2).

Treatment is surgical excision followed by postoperative chemotherapy that usually consists of bleomycin, etoposide, and cisplatin (BEP). Radiotherapy is sometimes administered for disease recurrence in dysgerminomas, but it is otherwise not included in routine treatment. Staging at the beginning of therapy is of the utmost importance. In rare cases, a second-look laparotomy may be indicated for neoplasms with teratomatous elements or for those incompletely resected.

Epithelial ovarian cancers account for 19% of ovarian masses in the pediatric population, with a total of 16% being malignant. These tumors manifest almost exclusively after puberty. Common presenting symptoms include dysmenorrhea, abdominal pain, abdominal distention, nausea and vomiting, and vaginal discharge. Tumors of low malignant potential are common in adolescents and account for 30% of epithelial ovarian cancers in this age group. Given the young age of this population, although not the standard of care for adult patients, consideration may be given to conserving the contralateral ovary and uterus if they appear normal. Data suggest that in patients with early-stage disease, such an approach with appropriate surgical staging results in optimal outcomes. Overall 5-yr survival rates are approximately 73%. The number of term pregnancies and use of oral contraceptives decrease the risk of invasive epithelial ovarian cancer. Young women with a family history of ovarian cancer should seriously consider using long-term oral contraceptives for the preventive benefits when pregnancy is not being sought.

Table 547-1 MALIGNANT OVARIAN TUMORS IN ADOLESCENTS

TUMOR	OVERALL 5-YR SURVIVAL	CLINICAL FEATURES
GERM CELL TUMORS		
Dysgerminoma	85%	10-20% Bilateral Most common ovarian malignancy Gonadal dysgenesis/androgen insensitivity Sensitive to chemotherapy/radiation
Immature teratoma	97-100%	All 3 germ layers present
Endodermal sinus tumor	80%	Almost always large (>15 cm) Schiller-Duval bodies
Choriocarcinoma	30%	Rare Can mimic ectopic pregnancy
Embryonal carcinoma	25%	Endocrinologic symptoms (precocious puberty) Highly malignant
Gonadoblastoma	100%	Primary amenorrhea Virilization 45,X or 45,X/46,XY mosiacism
SEX CORD STROMAL TUMORS		
Juvenile granulosa stroma cell tumor	92%	Produce estrogen Menstrual irregularities Isosexual preccious pseudopuberty Call-Exner bodies rare
Sertoli-Leydig cell tumor	70-90%	Virilization in 40% Produce testosterone
Lipoid cell tumors		Heterologenous group with lipid-filled parenchyma
Gynandroblastoma		Low-grade mixed tumors that produce either estrogen or androgen

UTERUS

Rhabdomyosarcomas are the most common type of soft tissue sarcoma occurring in patients <20 yr of age (Chapter 494). They can develop in any organ or tissue within the body except bone, and roughly 3% originate from the uterus or vagina. Of the various histologic subtypes, embryonal rhabdomyosarcomas in the female patient most often occur in the genital tract of infants or young children. They are rapidly growing entities that can cause the tumor to be expelled through the cervix, with subsequent complications such as uterine inversion or large cervical polyps. Irregular vaginal bleeding may be another presenting clinical symptom. They are defined histologically by the presence of mesenchymal cells of skeletal muscle in various stages of differentiation intermixed with myxoid stroma. Treatment recommendations are based on protocols coordinated by the Intergroup Rhabdomyosarcoma Study Group and consist of a multimodal approach including surgery, radiation therapy, and chemotherapy. Vincrinstine, adriamycin, and cyclophosphamide with or without radiation therapy are the first line of treatment. Attitudes toward surgical management have changed dramatically, with resection rates decreasing from 100% in 1972 to 13% in 1996. Chemotherapy with restrictive surgery has enabled many patients to retain their uterus while achieving excellent long-term survival rates.

Table 547-2 SERUM TUMOR MARKERS

TUMOR	CA-125	AFP	hCG	LDH	E2	TESTOSTERONE	INHIBIN	MIS	VEGF	DHEA
Epithelial tumor	+									
Immature teratoma	+	+			+					+
Dysgerminoma			+	+	+					
Endodermal sinus tumor		+								
Embryonal carcinoma		+	+		+					
Choriocarcinoma			+							
Mixed germ cell		+	+	+						
Granulosa cell tumor	+				+		+	+		
Sertoli-Leydig						+	+			
Gonadoblastoma					+	+	+			+
Theca-fibroma									+	

CA-125, cancer antigen 125; AFP, Alfa-fetoprotein; hCG, human chorionic gonadotropin; LDH, lactate dehydrogenase; E2, estradiol; T, testosterone, MIS, müllerian inhibiting substance; VEGF, vascular endothelial growth factor; DHEA, dehydroepiandrostenedione.

Leiomyosarcomas and **leiomyomas** are extremely rare, occurring in <2/10 million individuals within the pediatric/adolescent age group. However, at least 13 cases in approximately 6,200 pediatric patients with AIDS have been reported. They usually involve the spleen, lung, or gastrointestinal tract, but they could also originate from uterine smooth muscle. Pathogenesis is thought to correlate with the Epstein-Barr virus (Chapter 246). Despite treatment that demands complete surgical resection (and chemotherapy for the sarcomas), they tend to recur frequently.

Endometrial stromal sarcoma and endometrial adenocarcinoma of the uterine corpus are extremely rare in children and adolescents, with only case reports noted in the literature. Vaginal bleeding not associated with sexual precocity is a common presenting sign. Treatment consists of hysterectomy, with removal of the ovaries, followed by adjunctive radiotherapy and/or chemotherapy, depending on the operative findings.

VAGINA

Sarcoma botryoides is a variant of embryonal rhabdomyosarcoma that occurs most commonly in the vagina of pediatric patients. Sarcoma botryoides tends to arise in the anterior wall of the vagina and manifests as a submucosal lesion that is grape-like in appearance; if located at the cervix it could resemble a cervical polyp or polypoid mass. These lesions were formerly treated with exenterative procedures; equal success has occurred with less-radical surgery (polypectomy, conization, and local excision) and adjuvant chemotherapy with or without radiotherapy. A combination of vincristine, dactinomycin, and cyclophosphamide appears to be effective. Outcomes depend on tumor size, extent of disease at time of diagnosis, and histologic subtype. The 5-year survival rates for patients with clinical stages I-IV were 83%, 70%, 52%, and 25%, respectively.

Vaginal adenosis can lead to the development of clear cell adenocarcinoma of the vagina in females exposed to diethylstilbestrol (DES) in utero. Pregnant women at risk for miscarriage are no longer exposed to DES, and thus fewer adolescent girls and young women are at risk for this unusual tumor.

A rare tumor occurring in the vagina of infants is the **endodermal sinus tumor**. This disease usually occurs in children <2 yr of age, and survival rates are poor. Combination surgery and chemotherapy are appropriate. Benign papillomas can arise in the vagina of children and result in vaginal bleeding. Rarely, vaginal bleeding is secondary to leukemia or a hemangioma.

VULVA

Any questionable vulvar lesion should be biopsied and submitted for histologic examination. Lipoma, liposarcoma, and malignant melanoma of the vulva have been reported in young patients. The most common lesion is likely condyloma acuminata, associated with the human papilloma virus (HPV) (Chapter 258). Diagnosis is usually made by visual inspection. Treatment consists of observation for spontaneous regression, topical trichloroacetic acid, local cryotherapy, electrocautery, excision, and laser ablation. Some products used to treat skin lesions in adults have not been approved for children, including provider application of podophyllin resin and home application of imiquimod, podophlox, and sinecatechin ointment.

CERVIX

Historically, cervical cancer screening has been cytology based using the Papanicolaou (Pap) test and Bethesda Classification System (Table 547-3). Advances in epidemiologic research and molecular techniques have allowed the identification of the integral role of HPV in development of cervical cancer. HPV has become an important factor in the interpretation of cytologic results and subsequent management. The discovery of HPV presents a unique target for cervical cancer prevention, with the pediatric and adolescent population at the forefront of its implementation. A vaccine is available against the 2 HPV strains most commonly associated with cervical cancer (HPV 16, HPV 18). It is thought to be 100% effective against these 2 subtypes and to prevent up to 70% of cervical cancers. The ACOG recommends vaccination for all girls and women aged 9-26 yr, and The Advisory Committee on Immunization Practices (*http://www.cdc.gov/vaccines/recs/acip/*) recommends routine vaccination of girls aged 11-12 yr with 3 doses of quadrivalent HPV vaccine, starting as early as 9 yr. Catch-up vaccination is indicated for girls and women aged 13-26 yr who have not been fully vaccinated. Female patients should be vaccinated even if sexually exposed; vaccination prior to exposure is ideal. Pap testing and screening for HPV DNA or HPV antibody is not required before vaccination. ACOG recommends that cervical cancer screening of women

Table 547-3 MANAGEMENT OF CYTOLOGIC ABNORMALITIES IN IMMUNOCOMPROMISED ADOLESCENTS (<20 YR)

CYTOLOGY RESULT	MANAGEMENT RECOMMENDATION	HPV TESTING?	COLPOSCOPY?
ASCUS	Repeat cytologic testing in 1 year	No	At 1 yr follow-up if HGSIL or greater result At 2 yr follow-up if persistent ASCUS or greater
LGSIL	Repeat cytologic testing in 1 year	No	At 1 yr follow-up if HGSIL or greater result At 2 yr follow-up if ASCUS or greater
HGSIL	If colposcopy is unsatisfactory: excisional procedure If colposcopy is satisfactory: • If no CIN 1-3: Pap and colposcopy q6mo until 2 are negative, or else for 2 yr and then treat • If CIN1: (ASCUS/LGSIL protocol) • If CIN2, CIN 2-3: Pap or colposcopy q6mo until 2 are negative, or else reboots at 1 yr, treat if persistent at 2 yr • If CIN 3: excisional procedure • **If persistent HGSIL without CIN 1-3 identified,** then excisional procedures at 2 yr	No	Yes, immediately
ASC-H or AGC	There are no specific recommendations in regard to adolescents; see ASCCP guidelines for adults Endometrial biopsy is *not* advised in adolescents	No	Yes, immediately

Note: Although the table states excisional procedure only, the ASCCP guidelines consider cryotherapy, laser ablation, and loop electrode excisional procedures (LEEP) to all be acceptable treatment options.
ASCUS, atypical squamous cell changes of undetermined significance; HGSIL, high-grade squamous intraepithelial dysplasia; LGSIL, low-grade squamous intraepithelial dysplasia; CIN, cervical dysplasia; Pap, Papanicolaou smear; ASC-H, atypical squamous cell changes, high grade; AGC, atypical glandular cells; ASCCP, American Society for Colposcopy and Cervical Pathology.

who have been immunized against HPV-16 and HPV-18 should not differ from that of nonimmunized women and should follow the exact same regimen.

The adolescent population presents a unique challenge to cervical cancer screening, because the prevalence of HPV is high. In adolescents aged 15-19 yr, HPV cumulative incidence rates after initiation of sexual activity have been reported as 17% at 1 yr and 35.7% at 3 yr. Correlating with the natural history of an HPV infection, >90% of low-grade intraepithelial lesions regress within this age group, giving the presence of HPV in this population little clinical significance. The overall incidence of a high-grade lesion on Pap test in the adolescent population remains low (0.7%); cervical cancer is uncommon in the age group. The SEER Cancer Statistics Review 1975-2006 published by the National Cancer Institute (NCI) reports an incidence of invasive cervical cancer as 0.1/100,000 in 15-19 yr olds, with no cases reported before the age of 15 yr; colposcopy for minor cytologic abnormalities within this age group should be highly discouraged, because it will result more often in harm than produce any clinical benefit.

The American Society for Colposcopy and Cervical Pathology and the American College of Obstetricians and Gynecologists guidelines recommend that adolescents should be managed conservatively and should not receive Pap smear screening until age 21 yr regardless of age of onset of sexual intercourse. If an HPV test is done, the results should be ignored. However, sexually active immunocompromised (HIV positive patients or organ transplant recipients) adolescents should undergo screening twice within the first year after diagnosis and annually thereafter. Table 547-3 demonstrates management recommendations for abnormal cytologic results within the adolescent population.

Clinic protocols that require teenagers to undergo Pap smears before prescribing contraceptives should be reconsidered in light of these recommendations.

BIBLIOGRAPHY

Please visit the Nelson Textbook of Pediatrics *website at www.expertconsult.com for the complete bibliography.*

Chapter 548
Vulvovaginal and Müllerian Anomalies

Amber R. Cooper and Diane F. Merritt

The sequence of events that occur in a developing embryo and early fetus to create a normal reproductive system includes cellular differentiation, duct elongation, fusion, resorption, canalization, and programmed cell death. Any of these processes can be interrupted during formation of the reproductive system, creating gonadal, müllerian, and/or vulvovaginal anomalies (see Table 548-1 on the *Nelson Textbook of Pediatrics* website at www.expertconsult.com). Genetic, epigenetic, enzymatic, and environmental factors all have some role in the process (see Table 548-2 on the *Nelson Textbook of Pediatrics* website at www.expertconsult.com). Most clinicians use the standard classification system adopted by the American Society for Reproductive Medicine (originally the American Fertility Society [AFS] classification). Others have proposed modified and more-detailed anatomic classification systems such as the modified AFS system or the VCUAM (vagina, cervix, uterus, and adnexa-associated malformation) system.

For the full continuation of this chapter, please visit the Nelson Textbook of Pediatrics *website at www.expertconsult.com.*

Chapter 549
Gynecologic Care for Girls with Special Needs

Elisabeth H. Quint

Adolescence is a challenging time for all children and their families, but especially for teens with special needs; the hormonal changes occurring and the start of menstrual cycles can profoundly affect the lives of teens and their families. In addition there may be concerns about sexual activity, safety and abuse, and unplanned pregnancies.

SEXUALITY AND SEXUAL EDUCATION

Adolescents with special needs can have physical and/or developmental disabilities. They are often seen by society, including their families and care providers, as asexual, and therefore sexual education might not have been provided or considered necessary. Physically disabled teens are as likely to be sexually active as nondisabled teens. The care provider needs to assess the teen's knowledge of anatomy and sexuality, her social knowledge of relationships, and her ability to consent to sexual activity. Education regarding HIV and other sexually transmitted infections (STIs), disease prevention, and contraception, including postcoital contraception, should be offered at a developmentally appropriate level. Teens with disabilities may be more at risk for isolation and depression during adolescence.

ABUSE

The risk for sexual abuse in teens with disabilities is difficult to estimate. Studies show that teens with physical disabilities are just as sexually active as their nondisabled counterparts but that more of their activity is nonvoluntary. Screening for abuse is mandatory. Abuse prevention education can include the No! Go! Tell! model. For teens with limited verbal capacity or developmental delay, abuse may be very hard to detect. The care provider needs to be vigilant in looking for signs on physical exam, such as unexplained bruises or scratches, or changes in behavior that may be indications of sexual abuse in those adolescents (Chapters 37.1 and 113).

PELVIC EXAMINATION

A pelvic exam is rarely indicated in teens who are not sexually active, unless they have vulvar issues such as discharge, irregular bleeding, suspicion for abuse, or foreign body and an external inspection can be performed. A speculum exam is not performed, and if the vagina or cervix needs to be visualized, an exam under anesthesia by a gynecologist should be considered. Testing for STIs can be accomplished by urine testing or vaginal swabs (Chapter 114).

MENSTRUATION

Irregular menstruation is common in teenagers, especially the first 5 years after menarche, due to immaturity of the hypothalamic-pituitary-ovarian (HPO) axis and subsequent anovulation (Chapter 110). Several conditions in teens with disabilities are associated with an even higher risk of irregular cycles. Teens with Down syndrome have a higher incidence of thyroid disease. There is a higher incidence of reproductive issues, including PCOS in teens with epilepsy and on certain antiepileptic drugs (AEDs) (Chapter 546). Antipsychotic medication can cause hyperprolactinemia, which can affect menstruation.

The main issue with menstrual cycles, whether they are regular, irregular or heavy, is the impact of menstruation on the patient's life and her normal activities. The history should focus on this aspect, and menstrual calendars may be helpful to document the cycles, behavior, and the impact of treatments. Most adolescents who self-toilet can learn to use menstrual hygiene products appropriately.

The evaluation for abnormal bleeding is the same as for all teens. Areas requiring particular attention for the child with special needs are the possible need for menstrual suppression for hygiene or cyclical behavioral issues, like crying, tantrums, or withdrawal, and a request for birth control, especially coming from a caregiver and not from the teen, which requires an evaluation of the teen's ability to consent and evaluate the safety of her environment.

Treatment

If after documenting the impact of the cycles on the patient's well-being (often through menstrual or behavioral charting for several months) the care provider, patient, and family decide on menstrual intervention, several options are available. Menstrual regulation is not different from that in the nondisabled teenager. Menstrual suppression leading to complete amenorrhea is usually difficult to obtain, so treatment goals should be set early on. Infrequent scheduled bleeds may be easier to manage than unpredictable spotting, a common side effect of treatment, for certain patients. Outcome goals can be to decrease the heaviness of flow, regulate cycles to predictable bleeding, relieve pain or cyclical behavior symptoms, provide contraception, and/or obtain amenorrhea.

After treatment has started, continue to monitor cycles, ideally with continued menstrual or behavior calendars. Guidelines for office follow-up include menses that are too heavy (in excess of 1 pad/hour), too long (>10 days), or too frequent (< 20 days from day 1 to the next cycle day 1).

If menorrhagia or dysmenorrhea (occasionally leading to cyclical behavior changes in nonverbal teens) is the main concern, the patient can be started on nonsteroidal anti-inflammatory drugs (NSAIDs). These can decrease the flow by up to 20% in adequate doses and can be used alone or in combination with other treatments.

CONTRACEPTION (CHAPTER 111)

Estrogen-Containing Methods

ORAL CONTRACEPTIVES Cyclical oral contraceptives usually lead to regular, lighter cycles. Extended cycling through the use of continuous use of oral contraceptives can suppress cycles, with amenorrhea rates improving with time. Some unpredictable spotting is usually unavoidable, and often teens with special needs prefer to have predictable cycles several times a year. A chewable oral contraceptive is available for those with swallowing issues.

CONTRACEPTIVE RING The contraceptive ring is usually used in a pattern of 3 weeks on and 1 week off, but it can be used in a continuous 4-week pattern, which can lead to less bleeding. However, the contraceptive ring may be difficult to use if the teen cannot place it herself, and help with placement has clear privacy issues.

CONTRACEPTIVE PATCH The patch can also be used in a continuous fashion. Some teens with developmental disabilities remove their patch erratically, and placement out of reach (e.g., on buttocks or shoulder) is advised. Pharmacologic data indicate that estrogen exposure is higher for the contraceptive patch than for oral contraceptives or the vaginal ring. It is unclear exactly how this might affect the risk of deep vein thrombosis (DVT), especially in nonmobile women.

ESTROGEN USE AND DEEP VEIN THROMBOSIS Immobility per se is not a contraindication to estrogen-containing contraceptives. However, there are minimal data on the risk of DVT in immobile teens in wheelchairs with or without extraneous estrogen. Obtain a thorough and extended family history for hypercoagulability before initiating estrogen therapy. Careful use of lower-dose estrogen preparations may be advisable, and 3rd-generation progestin combinations and the patch should only be used if other methods have failed.

Progesterone-Only Methods

INTRAMUSCULAR MEDROXYPROGESTERONE ACETATE Intramuscular medroxyprogesterone acetate (DMPA) has long been very useful in menstrual suppression. Two issues are particularly relevant to teens with disabilities. Studies on a decrease in bone density associated with longer-term use of DMPA and a black box warning by the FDA have raised concerns about use of these products in young women, although recent data indicate that the lowering of bone density improves after the medication is stopped. For teens with mobility issues or those with very low body weight who are already at risk for low bone density, this can be of more concern. The second issue is weight gain, especially in obese teens, which can lead to health and mobility issues. If long-term DMPA is considered for a specific patient, calcium and vitamin D supplementation is recommended and bone density could be measured after several years of use.

ORAL PROGESTINS Continuous oral progestins can also be very effective to obtain amenorrhea. These include the progesterone-only pill and other progestins used daily, such as norethindrone 2.5 mg or micronized progesterone 200 mg.

PROGESTERONE INTRAUTERINE DEVICE The progesterone IUD for off-label use of diminishing menstrual flow is not contraindicated in teens, but might require anesthesia to be inserted if the exam is very difficult due to contractures or a narrow vagina. Checking for strings in a clinic setting may be challenging; however, the IUD location can be confirmed by sonography. There may be a significant amount of irregular bleeding in the first several months, but there is 20% amenorrhea after insertion and 50% amenorrhea after 1 year of use.

IMPLANTS Progestin subdermal implants have relatively high rates of unscheduled bleeding and therefore might not be ideal for teens with special needs. They also require cooperation for insertion.

HORMONES AND ANTIEPILEPTIC DRUGS Certain enzyme-inducing seizure medications can interfere with oral contraceptives, change their effectiveness, and lead to intermittent bleeding. Higher estrogen dose or shorter injection intervals for DMPA may be considered.

Surgical Methods

Surgical procedures such as endometrial ablation and hysterectomy are available for treatment in adults, but they should only be used in very extreme situations for teenagers where all other methods have failed and the patient's health is severely compromised by her cycles. Ethical considerations and consent issues are difficult in these situations, and state law varies on this topic.

BIBLIOGRAPHY

Please visit the Nelson Textbook of Pediatrics *website at www.expertconsult.com for the complete bibliography.*

PART XXVI The Endocrine System

Section 1 DISORDERS OF THE HYPOTHALAMUS AND PITUITARY GLAND

Chapter 550
Hormones of the Hypothalamus and Pituitary

John S. Parks and Eric I. Felner

The pituitary gland is the major regulator of an elaborate hormonal system. The pituitary gland receives signals from the hypothalamus and responds by sending pituitary hormones to target glands. The target glands produce hormones that provide negative feedback at the level of the hypothalamus and pituitary. This feedback mechanism enables the pituitary to regulate the amount of hormone released into the bloodstream by the target glands. The pituitary's central role in this hormonal system and its ability to interpret and respond to a variety of signals has led to its designation as the "master gland."

For the full continuation of this chapter, please visit the Nelson Textbook of Pediatrics *website at www.expertconsult.com.*

Chapter 551
Hypopituitarism

John S. Parks and Eric I. Felner

Hypopituitarism denotes underproduction of growth hormone (GH) alone or in combination with deficiencies of other pituitary hormones. Affected children have postnatal growth impairment that is specifically corrected by replacement of GH. The incidence of congenital hypopituitarism is thought to be between 1 in 4,000 and 1 in 10,000 live births. With expanding knowledge of the genes that direct pituitary development or hormone production, an increasing proportion of cases can be attributed to specific genetic disorders. Mutations in 7 candidate genes account for 13% of isolated growth hormone deficiency (IGHD) and 20% of multiple pituitary hormone deficiency (MPHD) cases. The likelihood of finding mutations is increased by positive family histories and decreased in cases with adrenocorticotropin hormone (ACTH) deficiency. The genes, hormonal phenotypes, associated abnormalities and modes of transmission for such established genetic disorders are shown in Tables 551-1 and 551-2. Acquired hypopituitarism usually has a later onset and different causes (Table 551-3).

MULTIPLE PITUITARY HORMONE DEFICIENCY

Genetic Forms

Sequentially expressed transcriptional activation factors direct the differentiation and proliferation of anterior pituitary cell types. These proteins are members of a large family of DNA-binding proteins resembling homeobox genes. Mutations produce different forms of multiple pituitary hormone deficiency. *PROP1* and *POU1F1* genes are expressed fairly late in pituitary development and are expressed only in cells of the anterior pituitary. Mutations produce hypopituitarism without anomalies of other organ systems. The *HESX1, LHX3, LHX4,* and *PTX2* genes are expressed at earlier stages. They are also expressed in other organs. Mutations in these genes tend to produce phenotypes that extend beyond hypopituitarism to include abnormalities in other organs.

Table 551-1 ETIOLOGIC CLASSIFICATION OF MULTIPLE PITUITARY HORMONE DEFICIENCY

GENE OR LOCATION	PHENOTYPE	INHERITANCE
GENETIC FORMS		
POU1F1 (PIT1)	GH, TSH, PRL	R, D
PROP1	GH, TSH, PRL, LH, FSH, ±ACTH, variable AP	R
LHX3	GH, TSH, PRL, LH, FSH, variable AP, ±short neck	R
LHX4	GH, TSH, ACTH, small AP, EPP, ±Arnold Chiari	D
TPIT	ACTH, severe neonatal form	R
HESX1	GH, variable for others, small AP, EPP	R, D
SOX3	Variable deficiencies, ±MR, EPP, small AP and stalk	XL
PTX2	Rieger syndrome	D
GLI2	Holoprosencephaly, midline defects	D
GLI3	Hall-Pallister syndrome	D
SHH (Sonic hedgehog)	GH deficiency with single central incisor	D
ACQUIRED FORMS		
Idiopathic		
Irradiation	GH deficiency precedes other deficiencies	
Inflammation	Histiocytosis, sarcoidosis	
Autoimmune	Hypophysitis	
Post-surgical	Stalk section, vascular compromise	
Tumor	Craniopharyngioma, glioma, pinealoma	
Trauma	Battering, shaken baby, vehicular	
UNCERTAIN ETIOLOGY		
Idiopathic		
Congenital absence of pituitary		
Septo-optic dysplasia		
Birth trauma		

ACTH, adrenocorticotropic hormine; AP, anterior pituitary; D, dominant; EPP, ectopic posterior pituitary; FSH, follicle-stimulating hormone; GH, growth hormone; LH, luteinizing hormone; MR, mental retardation; PRL, prolactin; R, recessive; TSH, thyroid-stimulating hormone; XL, X-linked.

PROP1 *PROP1* is found in the nuclei of somatotropes, lactotropes, and thyrotropes. Its roles include turning on *POU1F1* expression, hence its name prophet of *PIT1*. Mutations of *PROP1* are the most common explanation for recessive MPHD and are 10 times as common as the combined total of mutations in other pituitary transcription factor genes. Deletions of 1 or 2 base pairs

Table 551-2 ETIOLOGIC CLASSIFICATION OF GROWTH HORMONE DEFICIENCY OR INSENSITIVITY

GENE OR LOCATION	PHENOTYPE		INHERITANCE
DEFICIENCY			
GHRH receptor	IGHD, small AP	Low GH, Low IGF-1	R
GH1	IGHD, small or normal AP	Low GH, Low IGF-1	R,D
GH1	Bioinactive GH	High GH, Low IGF-1	D
BTK (Xq21.3-q22)	IGHD, hypogammaglobulinemia	Low GH, Low IGF-1	XL
SOX3 (Xq27.1)	IGHD, MR	Low GH, Low IGF-1	XL
INSENSITIVITY			
GH receptor	Variable GHBP	High GH, Low IGF-1	R,D
STAT5b	Immunodeficiency	High GH, Low IGF-1	R
IGF-1	IUGR, MR, deafness	High GH, Low IGF-1	R
Acid-labile subunit	Mild short stature	Normal GH, Low IGF-1	R
IGF-1 receptor	IUGR	High GH, High IGF-1	R

AP, anterior pituitary; EPP, ectopic posterior pituitary; GH, growth hormone; GHBP, growth hormone–binding protein; GHRH, growth hormone–releasing hormone, IGHD, isolated growth hormone deficiency; IUGR, intrauterine growth restriction; MR, mental retardation; R, recessive; D, dominant; XL, X-linked.

Table 551-3 CAUSES OF ACQUIRED HYPOPITUITARISM

BRAIN DAMAGE*
Traumatic brain injury Subarachnoid hemorrhage Neurosurgery Irradiation Stroke
PITUITARY TUMORS*
Adenomas Others
NON-PITUITARY TUMORS
Craniopharyngiomas Meningiomas Gliomas Chordomas Ependymomas Metastases
INFECTION
Abscess Hypophysitis Meningitis Encephalitis
INFARCTION
Apoplexia Sheehan's syndrome
AUTOIMMUNE DISORDER
Lymphocytic hypophysitis
OTHER
Hemochromatosis, granulomatous diseases, histiocytosis Empty sella Perinatal insults

*Pituitary tumors are classically the most common cause of hypopituitarism. However, new findings imply that causes related to brain damage might outnumber pituitary adenomas in causing hypopituitarism.

From Schneider HJ, Aimaretti G, Kreitschmann-Andermahr I, et al: Hypopituitarism, *Lancet* 369:1461–1470, 2007.

in exon 2 are most common, followed by missense, nonsense, and splice-site mutations. Anterior pituitary hormone deficiencies are seldom evident in the neonatal period. Growth in the 1st yr of life is considerably better than with *POU1F1* defects. The median age at diagnosis of GH deficiency is around 6 yr. Recognition of thyroid-stimulating hormone (TSH) deficiency is delayed relative to recognition of GH deficiency. Basal and thyrotropin-releasing hormone (TRH)-stimulated prolactin (PRL) levels tend to be higher than in *POU1F1* mutations.

Most children with *PROP1* mutations develop deficiencies of luteinizing hormone (LH) and follicle-stimulating hormone (FSH). Some enter puberty spontaneously and then retreat from it. Girls experience secondary amenorrhea and boys show regression of testicular size and secondary sexual characteristics. Partial deficiency of ACTH develops over time in about 30% of patients with *PROP1* defects. Anterior pituitary size is small in most patients, but in others there is progressive enlargement of the pituitary. A central mass originates within the sella turcica but might extend above it. The cellular content of the mass during the active phase of enlargement is not known. With time, the contents of the mass appear to degenerate, with multiple cystic areas. The mass might persist as a nonenhancing structure or might disappear completely, leaving an empty sella turcica. At different stages, MRI findings can suggest a macroadenoma, microadenoma, craniopharyngioma, or a Rathke pouch cyst.

POU1F1 (PIT1) *POU1F1* (formerly *PIT1*) was identified as a nuclear protein that binds to the GH and PRL promoters. It is necessary for emergence and mature function of somatotropes, lactotropes, and thyrotropes. Dominant and recessive mutations in *POU1F1* are responsible for complete deficiencies of GH and PRL and variable TSH deficiency. Affected patients exhibit nearly normal fetal growth but experience severe growth failure in the 1st yr of life. With normal production of LH and FSH, puberty develops spontaneously, though at a later than normal age. These patients are not at risk for development of ACTH deficiency. Anterior pituitary size is normal to small.

HESX1 The *HESX1* gene is expressed in precursors of all 5 cell types of the anterior pituitary early in embryologic development. Mutations result in a complex phenotype with defects in development of the optic nerve. Heterozygotes for loss-of-function mutations show the combinations of isolated GH deficiency and optic nerve hypoplasia. Homozygotes can have full expression of septo-optic dysplasia (SOD). This condition combines incomplete development of the septum pellucidum with optic nerve hypoplasia and other midline abnormalities. Clinical observation of nystagmus and visual impairment in infancy leads to the discovery of optic nerve and brain abnormalities. SOD is associated with anterior and/or posterior pituitary hormone deficiencies in about 25% of the cases. These patients often show the triad of a small anterior pituitary gland, an attenuated pituitary stalk, and an ectopic posterior pituitary bright spot. The great majority of patients with SOD do not have *HESX1* mutations. The etiology might involve mutations in another gene or a nongenetic explanation (Chapters 585 and 623).

LHX3 *LHX3* activates the α-glycoprotein subunit (α-GSU) promoter and acts synergistically with *POU1F1* to increase transcription from the PRL, β-TSH, and POU1F1 promoters. The hormonal phenotype produced by recessive loss-of-function mutations in this gene resembles that produced by *PROP1* mutations. There are deficiencies of GH, PRL, TSH, LH, and FSH but not ACTH. It is not clear whether the deficiencies are present from birth or whether they appear later in childhood. Some affected persons show enlargement of the anterior pituitary. The 1st patients to be described had the unusual findings of a short neck and a rigid cervical spine. They were only able to rotate their necks about 90 degrees compared with the normal rotation of 150 to 180 degrees.

LHX4 Dominantly inherited mutations in the *LHX4* gene consistently produce GH deficiency, with the variable presence of

TSH and ACTH deficiencies. Additional findings can include a very small V-shaped pituitary fossa, Chiari I malformation, and an ectopic posterior pituitary.

PTX2 Rieger syndrome is a complex phenotype caused by mutations in the *PTX2* transcription factor gene. This gene is also referred to as *RIEG1*. It is expressed in multiple tissues, including the anterior pituitary gland. In addition to variable degrees of anterior pituitary hormone deficiency, children with Rieger syndrome have colobomas of the iris and abnormal development of the kidneys, gastrointestinal tract, and umbilicus.

Other Congenital Forms

Severe, early-onset MPHD including deficiency of ACTH is often associated with the triad of anterior pituitary hypoplasia, absence or attenuation of the pituitary stalk, and an ectopic posterior pituitary bright spot on MRI. Most cases are sporadic and there is a male predominance. Some are due to abnormalities of the *SOX3* gene, located on the X chromosome. As with septo-optic dysplasia, the majority of cases have not been explained at the genetic level.

Pituitary hypoplasia can occur as an isolated phenomenon or in association with more extensive developmental abnormalities such as anencephaly or holoprosencephaly. Midfacial anomalies (cleft lip, palate; Chapter 302) or the finding of a solitary maxillary central incisor indicate a high likelihood of GH or other anterior or posterior hormone deficiency. At least 12 genes have been implicated in the complex genetic etiology of holoprosencephaly (Chapter 585.7). In the Hall-Pallister syndrome, absence of the pituitary gland is associated with hypothalamic hamartoblastoma, postaxial polydactyly, nail dysplasia, bifid epiglottis, imperforate anus, and anomalies of the heart, lungs, and kidneys. The combination of anophthalmia and hypopituitarism has been associated with mutations in the *SIX6, SOX2*, and *OTX2* genes.

Acquired Forms

Any lesion that damages the hypothalamus, pituitary stalk, or anterior pituitary can cause pituitary hormone deficiency (see Table 551-3). Because such lesions are not selective, multiple hormonal deficiencies are usually observed. The most common lesion is the craniopharyngioma (Chapter 491). Central nervous system germinoma, eosinophilic granuloma (histiocytosis), tuberculosis, sarcoidosis, toxoplasmosis, meningitis, and aneurysms can also cause hypothalamic-hypophyseal destruction. Trauma, including shaken child syndrome (Chapter 37), motor vehicle accidents, traction at delivery, anoxia, and hemorrhagic infarction, can also damage the pituitary, its stalk, or the hypothalamus.

ISOLATED GROWTH HORMONE DEFICIENCY AND INSENSITIVITY

Genetic Forms of Growth Hormone Deficiency

Isolated GH deficiency (IGHD) is caused by abnormalities of the GH-releasing hormone (GHRH) receptor, growth hormone genes and by genes located on the X chromosome.

GHRH RECEPTOR Recessive loss-of-function mutations in the receptor for GHRH interfere with proliferation of somatotropes during pituitary development and disrupt the most important signals for release of GH. The anterior pituitary is small, in keeping with the observation that somatotropes normally account for >50% of pituitary volume. There is some compromise of fetal growth followed by severe compromise of postnatal growth.

GH1 The *GH1* gene is one of a cluster of five genes on chromosome 17q22-24. This cluster arose through successive duplications of an ancestral GH gene. Unequal crossing over at meiosis has produced a variety of gene deletions. Small deletions (<10 kb) remove only the *GH1* gene, whereas large deletions (45 kb) remove ≥1 of the adjacent genes *(CSL, CS1, GH2,* and *CS2)*. The growth phenotype is identical with deletion of *GH1* alone or *GH1* together with one or more of the adjacent genes. Loss of the *CS1, GH2,* and *CS2* genes without loss of *GH1* causes deficiency of chorionic somatomammotropin and placental GH in the maternal circulation, but it does not result in fetal or postnatal growth retardation. Children who are homozygous for *GH1* gene deletions respond very well to GH therapy.

Recessively transmitted mutations in the *GH1* gene produce a similar phenotype. Missense, nonsense, and frameshift mutations have been described. The most common involve the 4th and final intron of the gene. These mutations eliminate the normal splice donor site and foster use of an alternative site. The abnormal mRNA encodes a protein that is longer than normal and has no biologic activity.

Autosomal dominant IGHD is also caused by mutations in *GH1*. The mutations usually involve splice site errors in intron 3. There is overproduction of a 20-kd protein that lacks the amino acids normally encoded by exon 3. Accumulation of this protein interferes with the processing, storage, and secretion of the normal 22-kd GH protein. Additional deficiencies of TSH and/or ACTH have been recognized as late complications in patients with dominant mutations in GH1.

The existence of short stature owing to biologically inactive GH was proposed in 1978. Some patients with normal to high levels of circulating GH by immunoassay have lower levels of GH when assessed by cell-proliferation, receptor-binding, and receptor-activation assays. The best-documented example involves a child with homozygosity for a missense mutation of the *GH1* gene. Substitution of a glycine for the normal serine at position 53 prevents formation of a disulfide bridge between residues 53 and 165. The mutant molecule has subnormal activities in immunofunction, receptor binding, and activation of the Jak2/Stat5 signaling pathway. GH treatment produced increases in insulin-like growth factor–1 (IGF-1) levels and growth rate, and the patient attained a normal adult height.

X-LINKED ISOLATED GROWTH HORMONE DEFICIENCY Two loci on the X chromosome have been associated with hypopituitarism. The 1st lies at Xq21.3-q22 in the region of the Bruton thymidine kinase *(BTK)* gene. Mutations in this region produce hypogammaglobulinemia as well as IGHD. The second locus maps farther out on the long arm, at Xq24-q27.1, a region containing the *SOX2* transcription factor gene. Abnormalities in this locus have been linked to IGHD with mental retardation as well as to MPHD with the triad of pituitary hypoplasia, missing pituitary stalk, and ectopic posterior pituitary gland.

Acquired Forms

The GH axis is more susceptible to disruption by acquired conditions than are other hypothalamic-pituitary axes. Recognized causes of acquired GH deficiency include the use of radiotherapy for malignancy, meningitis, histiocytosis, and trauma.

Children who receive radiotherapy for CNS tumors or prevention of CNS malignancies (i.e., leukemia) are at risk for developing GH deficiency. Spinal irradiation contributes to disproportionately poor growth of the trunk. Growth typically slows during radiation therapy or chemotherapy, improves for 1-2 yr, and then declines with the development of GH deficiency. The dose and frequency of radiotherapy are important determinants of hypopituitarism. GH deficiency is almost universal 5 yr after therapy with a total dose ≥35 Gy. More subtle defects are seen with doses around 20 Gy. Deficiency of GH is the most common defect, but deficiencies of TSH and ACTH can also occur. In contrast to other forms of hypopituitarism, puberty tends to be early rather than delayed. The clinician is likely to encounter children in the 8-10 yr age range who are growing at rates that are normal for chronological age but subnormal for stage of pubertal development.

GROWTH HORMONE INSENSITIVITY

Abnormalities of the Growth Hormone Receptor

Growth hormone insensitivity is caused by disruption of pathways distal to production of GH. Laron syndrome involves mutations of the GH receptor. Children with this condition clinically resemble those with severe IGHD. Birth length tends to be about 1 standard deviation (SD) below the mean, and severe short stature with lengths >4 SD below the mean is present by 1 yr of age. Resting and stimulated GH levels tend to be high and IGF-1 levels are low. The GH receptor has an extracellular GH-binding domain, a transmembrane domain, and an intracellular signaling domain. Mutations in the extracellular domain interfere with binding of GH. Serum GH-binding protein (GHBP) activity, representing the circulating form of the membrane receptor for GH, is generally low. Mutations in the transmembrane domain can interfere with anchoring of the receptor to the plasma membrane. In these cases, circulating GHBP activity is normal or high. Mutations in the intracellular domain interfere with JAK/STAT signaling.

Post-Receptor Forms of Growth Hormone Insensitivity

Some children with severe growth failure, high GH and low IGF-1 levels, and normal GHBP levels have abnormalities distal to the GH binding and activation of the GH receptor. Several have been found to have mutations in the gene encoding signal transducer and activator of transcription 5b (STAT5b). Disruption of this key intermediate connecting receptor activation to gene transcription produces growth failure similar to that seen in Laron syndrome. These patients also suffer from chronic pulmonary infections, consistent with important roles for STAT5b in interleukin cytokine signaling.

IGF-1 GENE ABNORMALITIES Abnormalities of the IGF-1 gene produce severe prenatal and postnatal growth impairment. Microcephaly, mental retardation, and deafness are present in patients with exon deletion and a missense mutation. These patients can be expected to respond to recombinant IGF-1 treatment.

IGF BINDING PROTEIN ABNORMALITIES Mutation of the gene encoding the acid-labile subunit of the circulating 165-kd IGF-1, IGFBP3, ALS complex has been associated with short stature. Total IGF-1 levels were very low. The index case, with homozygosity for an ALS mutation, did not show an increase in IGF-1 levels or an increase in growth rate during GH treatment.

IGF-1 RECEPTOR GENE ABNORMALITIES Mutations of the IGF-1 receptor also compromise prenatal and postnatal growth. The phenotype does not appear to be as severe as that seen with absence of IGF-1. Adult heights are closer to the normal range, and affected patients do not have mental retardation or deafness.

CLINICAL MANIFESTATIONS

Congenital Hypopituitarism

The child with hypopituitarism is usually of normal size and weight at birth, although those with MPHD and genetic defects of the *GH1* or *GHR* gene have birth lengths that average 1 SD below the mean. Children with severe defects in GH production or action are more than 4 SD below the mean by 1 yr of age. Those with less-severe deficiencies grow at rates below the 25th percentile for age and gradually diverge from normal height percentiles. Delayed closure of the epiphyses permits growth beyond the normal age when growth should be complete.

Infants with congenital defects of the pituitary or hypothalamus usually present with neonatal emergencies such as apnea, cyanosis, or severe hypoglycemia with or without seizures. Microphallus in boys provides an additional diagnostic clue. Deficiency of GH may be accompanied by hypoadrenalism and hypothyroidism. Prolonged neonatal jaundice is common. It involves elevation of conjugated and unconjugated bilirubin and may be mistaken for neonatal hepatitis.

The head is round, and the face is short and broad. The frontal bone is prominent, and the bridge of the nose is depressed and saddle-shaped. The nose is small, and the nasolabial folds are well developed. The eyes are somewhat bulging. The mandible and the chin are underdeveloped, and the teeth, which erupt late, are often crowded. The neck is short and the larynx is small. The voice is high-pitched and remains high after puberty. The extremities are well proportioned, with small hands and feet. Weight for height is usually normal, but an excess of body fat and a deficiency of muscle mass contributes to a pudgy appearance. The genitals are usually small for age, and sexual maturation may be delayed or absent. Facial, axillary, and pubic hair usually is lacking, and the scalp hair is fine. Length is mainly affected, giving toddlers a pudgy appearance. Symptomatic hypoglycemia, usually after fasting, occurs in 10-15% of children with panhypopituitarism and those with IGHD. Intelligence is usually normal.

Acquired Hypopituitarism

The child is normal initially, and manifestations similar to those seen in idiopathic pituitary growth failure gradually appear and progress. When complete or almost complete destruction of the pituitary gland occurs, signs of pituitary insufficiency are present. Atrophy of the adrenal cortex, thyroid, and gonads results in loss of weight, asthenia, sensitivity to cold, mental torpor, and absence of sweating. Sexual maturation fails to take place or regresses if already present. There may be atrophy of the gonads and genital tract with amenorrhea and loss of pubic and axillary hair. There is a tendency to hypoglycemia. Growth slows dramatically. Diabetes insipidus (Chapter 552) may be present early but tends to improve spontaneously as the anterior pituitary is progressively destroyed.

If the lesion is an expanding tumor, symptoms such as headache, vomiting, visual disturbances, pathologic sleep patterns, decreased school performance, seizures, polyuria, and growth failure can occur (Chapter 491). Slowing of growth can antedate neurologic signs and symptoms, especially with craniopharyngiomas, but symptoms of hormonal deficit account for only 10% of presenting complaints. Evidence of pituitary insufficiency might first appear after surgical intervention. In children with craniopharyngiomas, visual field defects, optic atrophy, papilledema, and cranial nerve palsy are common.

LABORATORY FINDINGS

GH deficiency is suspected in children with moderate to severe postnatal growth failure. Criteria for growth failure include height below the 1st percentile for age and sex or height >2 SD below sex-adjusted mid-parent height. Acquired GH deficiency can occur at any age, and when it is of acute onset, height may be within the normal range. A strong clinical suspicion is important in establishing the diagnosis because laboratory measures of GH sufficiency lack specificity. Observation of low serum levels of IGF-1 and the GH-dependent IGF-BP3 can be helpful, but IGF-1 and IGF-BP3 levels should be matched to normal values for skeletal age rather than chronological age. Values in the upper part of the normal range for age effectively exclude GH deficiency. IGF-1 values in normally growing children and those with hypopituitarism overlap during infancy and early childhood.

Definitive diagnosis of GH deficiency traditionally requires demonstration of absent or low levels of GH in response to stimulation. A variety of provocative tests have been devised that rapidly increase the level of GH in normal children. These include administration of insulin, arginine, clonidine, or glucagon. In chronic GH deficiency, the demonstration of poor linear growth, a delayed skeletal age, and peak levels of GH (<10 ng/mL) in each of two provocative tests are compatible with GH deficiency. In acute GH deficiency, a high clinical suspicion of GH deficiency and low peak levels of GH (<10 ng/mL) in each of two provocative tests are compatible with GH deficiency. This rather arbitrary cutoff point is higher than the 3 or 5 ng/mL criteria used for diagnosis of adult GH deficiency. The frequency of negative GH responses to a single standard test in normally growing children is usually considered to approach 20%. Monoclonal antibody assays generally underestimate GH concentration compared to the earlier polyclonal antibody assays. There is no consensus regarding adoption of criteria that take into account age, sex, and GH assay characteristics. Stimulation with GHRH generally produces greater responses in children with GH deficiency caused by hypothalamic disorders and fails to elicit a response in those with GHRH receptor, *GH1, POU1F1, PROP1,* and *LHX3* mutations. One study suggests that a majority of normal prepubertal children fail to achieve GH values >10 ng/mL with two pharmacologic tests. The researchers suggest that 3 days of estrogen priming should be used before GH testing to achieve greater diagnostic specificity.

During the 3 decades in which hGH was obtained by extraction from human pituitary glands culled at autopsy, its supply was sharply limited and only patients with classic GH deficiency were treated. In addition, the question was raised whether rare patients treated with cadaveric hGH contracted Creutzfeldt-Jakob disease from this preparation. With the advent of an unlimited supply of recombinant GH, there has been a marked interest in redefining the criteria for GH deficiency to include children with lesser degrees of deficiency. It has become popular to evaluate the spontaneous secretion of GH by measuring its level every 20 min during a 24- or 12-hr (8 PM-8 AM) period. Some short children with normal levels of GH, when studied by provocative tests, show little spontaneous GH secretion. Such children are considered to have GH neurosecretory dysfunction. With the collection of more normative data, it is clear that frequent GH sampling also lacks diagnostic specificity. There is a wide range of spontaneous GH secretion in normally growing prepubertal children and considerable overlap with the values observed in children with classic GH deficiency. Although the clinical and laboratory criteria for GH deficiency in patients with severe (classic) hypopituitarism are well established, the diagnostic criteria are unsettled for short children with lesser degrees of GH deficiency.

In addition to establishing the diagnosis of GH deficiency, it is necessary to examine other pituitary functions. Levels of TSH, thyroxine (T_4), ACTH, cortisol, gonadotropins, and gonadal steroids might provide evidence of other pituitary hormonal deficiencies. The defect can be localized to the hypothalamus if there is a normal response to the administration of hypothalamic-releasing hormones for TSH, ACTH, or gonadotropins. When there is a deficiency of TSH, serum levels of T_4 and TSH are low. A normal increase in TSH and PRL after stimulation with TRH places the defect in the hypothalamus, and absence of such a response localizes the defect to the pituitary. An elevated level of plasma PRL taken at random in the patient with hypopituitarism is also strong evidence that the defect is in the hypothalamus rather than in the pituitary. Some children with craniopharyngiomas have elevated PRL levels before surgery, but after surgery, PRL deficiency occurs because of pituitary damage. Antidiuretic hormone deficiency may be established by appropriate studies.

RADIOLOGIC FINDINGS

Conventional x-ray films of the skull have been replaced by CT and, increasingly, by MRI. CT is appropriate for recognizing suprasellar calcification associated with craniopharyngiomas and bony changes accompanying histiocytosis. MRI provides a much more detailed view of hypothalamic and pituitary anatomy. Many cases of severe early-onset MPHD show the triad of a small anterior pituitary gland, a missing or attenuated pituitary stalk, and an ectopic posterior pituitary bright spot at the base of the hypothalamus. Subnormal anterior pituitary height, implying a small anterior pituitary, is common in genetic and idiopathic causes of IGHD. Craniopharyngiomas are common and pituitary adenomas are rare in children with hypopituitarism. Both hypoplastic and markedly enlarged anterior pituitary glands are seen in patients with *PROP1* or *LHX3* mutations.

Skeletal maturation is delayed in patients with IGHD and may be even more delayed when there is combined GH and TSH deficiency. Dual photon x-ray absorptiometry shows deficient bone mineralization, deficiencies in lean body mass, and a corresponding increase in adiposity.

DIFFERENTIAL DIAGNOSIS

The causes of growth disorders are legion. Systemic conditions such as inflammatory bowel disease, celiac disease, occult renal disease, and anemia must be considered. Patients with systemic conditions often have greater loss of weight than length. A few otherwise normal children are short (i.e., >3 SD below the mean for age) and grow 5 cm/yr or less but have normal levels of GH in response to provocative tests and normal spontaneous episodic secretion. Most of these children show increased rates of growth when treated with GH in doses comparable to those used to treat children with hypopituitarism. Plasma levels of IGF-1 in these patients may be normal or low. Several groups of treated children have achieved final or near-final adult heights. Different studies have found changes in adult height that range from −2.5 to +7.5 cm compared with pretreatment predictions. There are no methods that can reliably predict which of these children will become taller in adulthood as a result of GH treatment and which will have compromised adult height.

Diagnostic strategies for distinguishing between permanent GH deficiency and other causes of impaired growth are imperfect. Children with a combination of genetic short stature and constitutional delay of growth have short stature, below-average growth rates, and delayed bone ages. Many of these children exhibit minimal GH secretory responses to provocative stimuli. When children in whom idiopathic or acquired GH deficiency is diagnosed are treated with hGH and are retested as adults, the majority have peak GH levels within the normal range.

Constitutional Growth Delay

Constitutional growth delay is one of the variants of normal growth commonly encountered by the pediatrician. Length and weight measurements of affected children are normal at birth, and growth is normal for the 1st 4-12 mo of life. Height is sustained at a lower percentile during childhood. The pubertal growth spurt is delayed, so their growth rates continue to decline after their classmates have begun to accelerate. Detailed questioning often reveals other family members (often one or both parents) with histories of short stature in childhood, delayed puberty, and eventual normal stature. IGF-1 levels tend to be low for chronological age but within the normal range for bone age. GH responses to provocative testing tend to be lower than in children with a more typical timing of puberty. The prognosis for these children to achieve normal adult height is guarded. Predictions based on height and bone age tend to overestimate eventual height to a greater extent in boys than in girls. Boys with >2 yr of pubertal delay can benefit from a short course of testosterone therapy to hasten puberty after 14 yr of age. The cause of this variant of normal growth is thought to be persistence of the relatively hypogonadotropic state of childhood (Chapter 13).

Primary Hypothyroidism

Primary hypothyroidism (Chapter 559) is more common than GH deficiency. Low total or free T_4 and elevated TSH levels establish the diagnosis. Responses to GH provocative tests may be subnormal and the sella may be enlarged. Pituitary hyperplasia recedes during treatment with thyroid hormone. Because thyroid hormone is a necessary prerequisite for normal GH synthesis, it must always be assessed before GH evaluation.

Psychosocial Causes

Emotional deprivation is an important cause of retardation of growth and mimics hypopituitarism. The condition is known as *psychosocial dwarfism, maternal deprivation dwarfism*, or *hyperphagic short stature*. The mechanisms by which sensory and emotional deprivation interfere with growth are not fully understood. Functional hypopituitarism is indicated by low levels of IGF-1 and by inadequate responses of GH to provocative stimuli. Puberty may be normal or even premature. Appropriate history and careful observations reveal disturbed mother-child or family relations and provide clues to the diagnosis (Chapter 37). Proof may be difficult to establish because the parents or caregivers often hide the true family situation from professionals, and the children rarely divulge their plight. Emotionally deprived children often have perverted or voracious appetites, enuresis, encopresis, insomnia, crying spasms, and sudden tantrums. The subgroup of children with hyperphagia and a normal body mass index tends to show catch-up growth when placed in a less stressful environment.

TREATMENT

The Lawson Wilkins Pediatric Endocrine Society, the Academy of Pediatrics, and the GH Research Society have published guidelines for hGH treatment. In children with classic GH deficiency, treatment should be started as soon as possible to narrow the gap in height between patients and their classmates during childhood and to have the greatest effect on mature height. The recommended dose of hGH is 0.18-0.3 mg/kg/wk during childhood. Higher doses have been used during puberty. Recombinant GH is administered subcutaneously in 6 or 7 divided doses. Maximal response to GH occurs in the 1st yr of treatment. Growth velocity during this 1st yr is typically above the 95th percentile for age. With each successive yr of treatment, the growth rate tends to decrease. If growth rate drops below the 25th percentile, compliance should be evaluated before the dose is increased.

Concurrent treatment with GH and a gonadotropin-releasing hormone (GnRH) agonist has been used in the hope that interruption of puberty will delay epiphyseal fusion and prolong growth. This strategy can increase adult height. It can also increase the discrepancy in physical maturity between GH-deficient children and their age peers and can impair bone mineralization. There have also been attempts to forestall epiphyseal fusion in boys by giving drugs that inhibit aromatase, the enzyme responsible for converting androgens to estrogens. Therapy should be continued until near-final height is achieved. Criteria for stopping treatment include a decision by the patient that he or she is tall enough, a growth rate <1 inch/yr, and a bone age >14 yr in girls and >16 yr in boys.

Some patients develop either primary or central hypothyroidism while under treatment with GH. Similarly, there is a risk of developing adrenal insufficiency. If unrecognized, this can be fatal. Periodic evaluation of thyroid and adrenal function is indicated for all patients treated with GH.

Recombinant IGF-1 is approved for use in the United States. It is given subcutaneously twice a day. The risk of hypoglycemia is reduced by giving the injections concurrently with a meal or snack. In some situations its use is more efficacious than use of GH. These conditions include abnormalities of the GH receptor and *STAT5b* genes, as well as severe GH deficiency in patients who have developed antibodies to administered GH. Its utility in improving growth rate and adult stature in broader categories of short children is being explored.

The doses of GH used to treat children with classic GH deficiency usually enhance the growth of many non–GH-deficient children as well. Intensive investigation is in progress to determine the full spectrum of short children who may benefit from treatment with GH. GH is currently approved in the United States for treating children with growth failure as a result of Turner syndrome, end-stage renal failure before kidney transplantation, Prader-Willi syndrome, intrauterine growth retardation, and idiopathic short stature. The last indication specifies a height below the 1.2 percentile (−2.25 SD) for age and sex, a predicted height below the 5th percentile, and open epiphyses. Studies of the effect of GH treatment on adult height suggest a median gain of 2 to 3 inches, depending on dose and duration of treatment.

In children with MPHD, replacement should also be directed at other hormonal deficiencies. In TSH-deficient patients, thyroid hormone is given in full replacement doses. In ACTH-deficient patients, the optimal dose of hydrocortisone should not exceed 10 $mg/m^2/24$ hr. Increases are made during illness or in anticipation of surgical procedures. In patients with a deficiency of gonadotropins, gonadal steroids are given when bone age reaches the age at which puberty usually takes place. For infants with microphallus, 1 or 2 3-mo courses of monthly intramuscular injections of 25 mg of testosterone cypionate or testosterone enanthate can bring the penis to normal size without an inordinate effect on osseous maturation.

COMPLICATIONS AND ADVERSE EFFECTS OF GROWTH HORMONE TREATMENT

Some children treated with GH have developed leukemia. The increased risk is attributable to additional risk factors such as cranial irradiation. GH treatment does not increase the risk for recurrence of brain tumors or leukemia. Other reported side effects include pseudotumor cerebri, slipped capital femoral epiphysis, gynecomastia, and worsening of scoliosis. There is an increase in total body water during the 1st 2 wk of treatment. Fasting and postprandial insulin levels are characteristically low before treatment, and they normalize during GH replacement. Treatment does not increase risk of type 1 diabetes, but it might increase the risk of type 2 diabetes.

In the extracted pituitary GH treatment era, patients were at risk for Creutzfeldt-Jakob (CJ) disease for at least 10-20 yr after therapy and the development of antibodies to GH. Those developing antibodies to administered GH became resistant to treatment. Use of recombinant GH over the past 2 decades has eliminated the risk for CJ disease and for antibody formation during treatment.

BIBLIOGRAPHY

Please visit the Nelson Textbook of Pediatrics *website at* *www.expertconsult.com* *for the complete bibliography.*

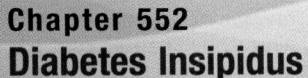

Chapter 552
Diabetes Insipidus

David T. Breault and Joseph A. Majzoub

Diabetes insipidus (DI) manifests clinically with polyuria and polydipsia and can result from either vasopressin deficiency (central DI) or vasopressin insensitivity at the level of the kidney (nephrogenic DI). Both central DI and nephrogenic DI can arise from inherited defects of congenital or neonatal onset or can be secondary to a variety of causes (Table 552-1).

PHYSIOLOGY OF WATER BALANCE

The control of extracellular tonicity (osmolality) and volume within a narrow range is critical for normal cellular structure and

Table 552-1 DIFFERENTIAL DIAGNOSIS OF POLYURIA AND POLYDIPSIA

Diabetes insipidus (DI)
• Central DI
Genetic (autosomal dominant)
Acquired
Trauma (surgical or accidental)
Congenital malformations
Neoplasms
Infiltrative, autoimmune, and infectious diseases
Drugs
• Nephrogenic DI
Genetic (X-linked, autosomal recessive, autosomal dominant)
Acquired
Hypercalcemia, hypokalemia
Drugs
Kidney disease
Primary polydipsia
Diabetes mellitus

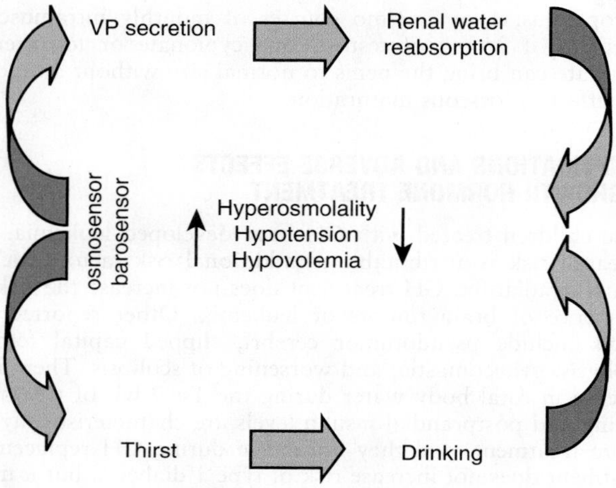

Figure 552-1 Regulation of vasopressin (VP) secretion and serum osmolality. Hyperosmolality, hypovolemia, and hypotension are sensed by osmosensors, volume sensors, and barosensors, respectively. These stimulate both VP secretion and thirst. VP, acting on the kidney, causes increased reabsorption of water (antidiuresis). Thirst causes increased water ingestion. The results of these dual negative feedback loops cause a reduction in hyperosmolality or in hypotension or hypovolemia. Additional stimuli for VP secretion include nausea, hypoglycemia, and pain. (From Muglia LJ, Majzoub JA: Disorders of the posterior pituitary. In Sperling MA, editor: *Pediatric endocrinology,* ed 2, Philadelphia, 2002, WB Saunders.)

function (Chapter 52). Extracellular fluid tonicity is regulated almost exclusively by water intake and excretion, whereas extracellular volume is regulated by sodium intake and excretion. The control of plasma tonicity and intravascular volume involves a complex integration of endocrine, neural, behavioral, and paracrine systems (Fig. 552-1). Vasopressin, secreted from the posterior pituitary, is the principal regulator of tonicity, with its release largely stimulated by increases in plasma tonicity. Volume homeostasis is largely regulated by the renin-angiotensin-aldosterone system, with contributions from both vasopressin and the natriuretic peptide family.

Vasopressin, a 9-amino-acid peptide, has both antidiuretic and vascular pressor activity and is synthesized in the paraventricular and supraoptic nuclei of the hypothalamus. It is transported to the posterior pituitary via axonal projections, where it is stored awaiting release into the systemic circulation. The half-life of vasopressin in the circulation is 5 min. In addition to responding to osmotic stimuli, vasopressin is secreted in response to significant decreases in intravascular volume and pressure (minimum of 8% decrement) via afferent baroreceptor pathways arising from the aortic arch (carotid sinus) and volume receptor pathways in the cardiac atria and pulmonary veins. Osmotic and hemodynamic stimuli interact synergistically.

The sensation of thirst is regulated by cortical as well as hypothalamic neurons. The thirst threshold is approximately 10 mOsm/kg higher (i.e., 293 mOsm/kg) than the osmotic threshold for vasopressin release. Therefore, under conditions of hyperosmolality, vasopressin is released before thirst is initiated, allowing ingested water to be retained. Chemoreceptors present in the oropharynx rapidly down-regulate vasopressin release following water ingestion.

Vasopressin exerts its principal effect on the kidney via V_2 receptors located primarily in the collecting tubule, the thick ascending limb of the loop of Henle, and the periglomerular tubules. The human V_2 receptor gene is located on the long arm of the X chromosome (Xq28) at the locus associated with **congenital, X-linked, vasopressin-resistant diabetes insipidus.** Activation of the V_2 receptor results in increases in intracellular cyclic adenosine monophosphate (cAMP), which leads to the insertion of the aquaporin-2 water channel into the apical (luminal) membrane. This allows water movement along its osmotic gradient into the hypertonic inner medullary interstitium from the tubule lumen and excretion of concentrated urine. In contrast to aquaporin-2, aquaporins-3 and -4 are expressed on the basolateral membrane of the collecting duct cells, and aquaporin-1 is expressed in the proximal tubule. These channels may also contribute to urinary concentrating ability.

Atrial natriuretic peptide (ANP), initially isolated from cardiac atrial muscle, has a number of important effects on salt and water balance, including stimulation of natriuresis, inhibition of sodium resorption, and inhibition of vasopressin secretion. ANP is expressed in endothelial cells and vascular smooth muscle, where it appears to regulate relaxation of arterial smooth muscle. ANP is also expressed in the brain, along with other natriuretic family members; the physiologic role of these factors has yet to be defined.

APPROACH TO THE PATIENT WITH POLYURIA, POLYDIPSIA, AND HYPERNATREMIA

The cause of pathologic polyuria or polydipsia (exceeding 2 L/m^2/24 hr) may be difficult to establish in children. Infants can present with irritability, failure to thrive, and intermittent fever. Patients with suspected DI should have a careful history taken, which should quantify the child's daily fluid intake and output and establish the voiding pattern, nocturia, and primary or secondary enuresis. A complete physical examination should establish the patient's hydration status, and the physician should search for evidence of visual and central nervous system dysfunction as well as other pituitary hormone deficiencies.

If pathologic polyuria or polydipsia is present, the following should be obtained: serum for osmolality, sodium, potassium, blood urea nitrogen, creatinine, glucose, and calcium; urine for osmolality, specific gravity, and glucose determination. The diagnosis of DI is established if the serum osmolality is >300 mOsm/kg and the urine osmolality is <300 mOsm/kg. DI is unlikely if the serum osmolality is <270 mOsm/kg or the urine osmolality is >600 mOsm/kg. If the patient's serum osmolality is <300 mOsm/kg (but >270 mOsm/kg) and pathologic polyuria and polydipsia are present, a water deprivation test is indicated to establish the diagnosis of DI and to differentiate central from nephrogenic causes.

In the inpatient postneurosurgical setting, central DI is likely if hyperosmolality (serum osmolality >300 mOsm/kg) is associated with urine osmolality less than serum osmolality. It is important to distinguish between polyuria resulting from postsurgical central DI and polyuria resulting from the normal diuresis of fluids received intraoperatively. Both cases may be associated with a large volume (>200 mL/m^2/hr) of dilute urine, although in patients with DI, the serum osmolality is high in comparison with patients undergoing postoperative diuresis.

CAUSES OF HYPERNATREMIA

Hypernatremia is discussed in Chapter 52.3.

Central Diabetes Insipidus

Central diabetes insipidus can result from multiple etiologies, including genetic mutations in the vasopressin gene; trauma (accidental or surgical) to vasopressin neurons; congenital malformations of the hypothalamus or pituitary; neoplasms; infiltrative, autoimmune, and infectious diseases affecting vasopressin neurons or fiber tracts; and increased metabolism of vasopressin. In approximately 10% of children with central DI, the etiology is idiopathic. Other pituitary hormone deficiencies may be present (Chapter 551).

Autosomal dominant central DI usually occurs within the first 5 yr of life and results from mutations in the vasopressin gene. A number of mutations can cause gene-processing defects in a subset of vasopressin-expressing neurons, which have been postulated to result in endoplasmic reticulum (ER) stress and cell death. **Wolfram syndrome,** which includes DI, diabetes mellitus, optic atrophy, and deafness, also results in vasopressin deficiency. Mutations in two genes, which give rise to ER proteins, have been associated with this condition. Congenital brain abnormalities (Chapter 585) such as **septo-optic dysplasia** with agenesis of the corpus callosum, the Niikawa-Kuroki syndrome, holoprosencephaly, and familial pituitary hypoplasia with absent stalk may be associated with central DI and defects in thirst perception. Empty sella syndrome, possibly resulting from unrecognized pituitary infarction, can be associated with DI in children.

Trauma to the base of the brain and neurosurgical intervention in the region of the hypothalamus or pituitary are common causes of central DI. The **triphasic response** following surgery refers to an initial phase of transient DI, lasting 12-48 hr, followed by a 2nd phase of syndrome of inappropriate antidiuretic hormone secretion (SIADH), lasting up to 10 days, which may be followed by permanent DI. The initial phase may be the result of local edema interfering with normal vasopressin secretion; the 2nd phase results from unregulated vasopressin release from dying neurons, whereas in the 3rd phase, permanent DI results if more than 90% of the neurons have been destroyed.

Given the anatomic distribution of vasopressin neurons over a large area within the hypothalamus, tumors that cause DI must either be very large and infiltrative or be strategically located near the base of the hypothalamus, where vasopressin axons converge before their entry into the posterior pituitary. Germinomas and pinealomas typically arise in this region and are among the most common primary brain tumors associated with DI. Germinomas can be very small and undetectable by MRI for several yr following the onset of polyuria. Quantitative measurement of the β-subunit of human chorionic gonadotropin, often secreted by germinomas and pinealomas, should be performed in children with idiopathic or unexplained DI in addition to serial MRI scans. Craniopharyngiomas and optic gliomas can also cause central DI when they are very large, although this is more often a postoperative complication of the treatment for these tumors (Chapter 491). Hematologic malignancies, as with acute myelocytic leukemia, can cause DI via infiltration of the pituitary stalk and sella.

Langerhans cell histiocytosis and lymphocytic hypophysitis are common types of infiltrative disorders causing central DI, with **hypophysitis** as the cause in 50% of cases of "idiopathic" central DI. Infections involving the base of the brain, including meningitis (meningococcal, cryptococcal, listerial, toxoplasmal), congenital cytomegalovirus infection, and nonspecific inflammatory diseases of the brain may give rise to central DI that is often transient. Drugs associated with the inhibition of vasopressin release include ethanol, phenytoin, opiate antagonists, halothane, and α-adrenergic agents.

Nephrogenic Diabetes Insipidus

Nephrogenic (vasopressin-insensitive) DI (NDI) can result from genetic or acquired causes. Genetic causes are less common but more severe than acquired forms of NDI. The polyuria and polydipsia associated with genetic NDI usually occurs within the first several weeks of life but might only become apparent after weaning or with longer periods of nighttime sleep. Many infants initially present with fever, vomiting, and dehydration. Failure to thrive may be secondary to the ingestion of large amounts of water, resulting in caloric malnutrition. Long-standing ingestion and excretion of large volumes of water can lead to nonobstructive hydronephrosis, hydroureter, and megabladder.

Congenital X-linked NDI results from inactivating mutations of the vasopressin V_2 receptor. **Congenital autosomal recessive NDI** results from defects in the aquaporin-2 gene. An **autosomal dominant form of NDI** is associated with processing mutations of the aquaporin-2 gene.

Acquired nephrogenic DI can result from hypercalcemia or hypokalemia and is associated with lithium, demeclocycline, foscarnet, clozapine, amphotericin, methicillin, and rifampin. Impaired renal concentrating ability can also be seen with ureteral obstruction, chronic renal failure, polycystic kidney disease, medullary cystic disease, Sjögren syndrome, and sickle cell disease. Decreased protein or sodium intake or excessive water intake, as in primary polydipsia, can lead to diminished tonicity of the renal medullary interstitium and nephrogenic DI.

TREATMENT OF CENTRAL DIABETES INSIPIDUS

Fluid Therapy

With an intact thirst mechanism and free access to oral fluids, a person with complete DI can maintain plasma osmolality and sodium in the high normal range, although at great inconvenience. Neonates and young infants are often best treated solely with fluid therapy, given their requirement for large volumes (3 L/m^2/24 hr) of nutritive fluid. The use of vasopressin analogs in patients with obligate high fluid intake is difficult given the risk of life-threatening hyponatremia. Although not FDA approved, the subcutaneous use of diluted parenteral long-acting vasopressin analog DDAVP (desmopressin) has been successfully administered to infants with central DI without causing severe hyponatremia.

VASOPRESSIN ANALOGS Treatment of central DI in older children is best accomplished with the use of DDAVP. DDAVP is available in an intranasal preparation (onset 5-10 min) and as tablets (onset 15-30 min). The intranasal preparation of DDAVP (10 μg/0.1 mL) can be administered by rhinal tube (allowing dose titration) or by nasal spray. Use of DDAVP oral tablets requires at least a 10-fold increase in the dosage compared with the intranasal preparation. Oral dosages of 25-300 μg every 8-12 hr are safe and effective in children. The appropriate dosage and route of administration is determined empirically based on the desired length of antidiuresis and patient preference. The use of DDAVP nasal spray (10 μg/mL, 0.1 mL) for the treatment of primary enuresis in older children should be regarded as a temporizing measure, given it does not affect the underlying condition, and should be used with great caution. To prevent water intoxication, patients should have at least 1 hr of urinary breakthrough between doses each day.

AQUEOUS VASOPRESSIN Central DI of acute onset following neurosurgery is best managed with continuous administration of synthetic aqueous vasopressin (pitressin). Under most circumstances, total fluid intake must be limited to 1 L/m^2/24 hr during antidiuresis. A typical dosage for intravenous vasopressin therapy is 1.5 mU/kg/hr, which results in a blood vasopressin concentration of approximately 10 pg/mL. On occasion, following hypothalamic (but not transsphenoidal) surgery, higher initial concentrations of vasopressin may be required to treat acute DI, which has been attributed to the release of a vasopressin inhibitory substance. Vasopressin concentrations >1,000 pg/mL should be avoided because they can cause cutaneous necrosis, rhabdomyolysis, cardiac rhythm disturbances, and hypertension. Post-neurosurgical patients treated with vasopressin infusion should be switched from intravenous to oral fluids as soon as possible to allow thirst sensation, if intact, to help regulate osmolality.

TREATMENT OF NEPHROGENIC DIABETES INSIPIDUS

The treatment of acquired NDI focuses on eliminating, if possible, the underlying disorder, such as offending drugs, hypercalcemia, hypokalemia, or ureteral obstruction. Congenital nephrogenic diabetes insipidus is often difficult to treat. The main goals are to ensure the intake of adequate calories for growth and to avoid severe dehydration. Foods with the highest ratio of caloric content to osmotic load (Na <1 mmol/kg/24 hr) should be ingested to maximize growth and to minimize the urine volume required to excrete the solute load. Even with the early institution of therapy, however, growth failure and mental retardation are common.

Pharmacologic approaches to the treatment of NDI include the use of thiazide diuretics and are intended to decrease the overall urine output. Thiazides appear to induce a state of mild volume depletion by enhancing sodium excretion at the expense of water and by causing a decrease in the glomerular filtration rate, which results in proximal tubular sodium and water reabsorption. Indomethacin and amiloride may be used in combination with thiazides to further reduce polyuria. High-dose DDAVP therapy, in combination with indomethacin, has been used in some subjects with NDI. This treatment could prove useful in patients with genetic defects in the V_2 receptor associated with a reduced binding affinity for vasopressin.

BIBLIOGRAPHY

Please visit the Nelson Textbook of Pediatrics *website at* *www.expertconsult.com* *for the complete bibliography.*

Chapter 553

Other Abnormalities of Arginine Vasopressin Metabolism and Action

David T. Breault and Joseph A. Majzoub

Hyponatremia (serum sodium <130 mEq/L) in children is usually associated with severe systemic disorders and is most often due to intravascular volume depletion, excessive salt loss, or hypotonic fluid overload, especially in infants (Chapter 52). The syndrome of inappropriate antidiuretic hormone secretion (SIADH) is an uncommon cause of hyponatremia in children.

The initial approach to the patient with hyponatremia begins with determination of the volume status. A careful review of the patient's history, physical examination, including changes in weight, and vital signs helps determine whether the patient is hypovolemic or hypervolemic. Supportive evidence includes laboratory data such as serum electrolytes, blood urea nitrogen, creatinine, uric acid, urine sodium, specific gravity, and osmolality (Chapter 52.3; Tables 553-1 and 553-2).

Table 553-1 DIFFERENTIAL DIAGNOSIS OF HYPONATREMIA

DISORDER	INTRAVASCULAR VOLUME STATUS	URINE SODIUM
Systemic dehydration	Low	Low
Decreased effective plasma volume	Low	Low
Primary salt loss (nonrenal)	Low	Low
Primary salt loss (renal)	Low	High
SIADH	High	High
Cerebral salt wasting	Low	Very high
Decreased free water clearance	Normal or high	Normal or high
Primary polydipsia	Normal or high	Normal
Runner's hyponatremia	Low	Low
NSIAD	High	High
Pseudohyponatremia	Normal	Normal
Factitious hyponatremia	Normal	Normal

NSIAD, nephrogenic syndrome of inappropriate antidiuresis; SIADH, syndrome of inappropriate antidiuretic hormone secretion.

Table 553-2 CLINICAL PARAMETERS TO DISTINGUISH AMONG SIADH, CEREBRAL SALT WASTING, AND CENTRAL DIABETES INSIPIDUS

CLINICAL PARAMETER	SIADH	CEREBRAL SALT WASTING	CENTRAL DI
Serum sodium	Low	Low	High
Urine output	Normal or low	High	High
Urine sodium	High	Very high	Low
Intravascular volume status	Normal or high	Low	Low
Vasopressin level	High	Low	Low

DI, diabetes insipidus; SIADH, syndrome of inappropriate antidiuretic hormone secretion.

CAUSES OF HYPONATREMIA

Syndrome of Inappropriate Antidiuretic Hormone Secretion

SIADH is characterized by hyponatremia, an inappropriately concentrated urine (>100 mOsm/kg), normal or slightly elevated plasma volume, normal-to-high urine sodium, and low serum uric acid. SIADH is uncommon in children, and most cases result from excessive administration of vasopressin in the treatment of central diabetes insipidus. It can also occur with encephalitis, brain tumors, head trauma, psychiatric disease, prolonged nausea, pneumonia, tuberculous meningitis, and AIDS and in the postictal phase following generalized seizures. SIADH is the cause of the hyponatremic second phase of the triphasic response seen after hypothalamic-pituitary surgery (Chapter 552). It is found in up to 35% of patients 1 wk after surgery and can result from retrograde neuronal degeneration with cell death and vasopressin release. Common drugs that have been shown to increase vasopressin secretion or mimic vasopressin action, resulting in hyponatremia, include oxcarbazepine, carbamazepine, oxcarbazepine, chlorpropamide, vinblastine, vincristine, and tricyclic antidepressants.

Nephrogenic Syndrome of Inappropriate Antidiuresis

Gain-of-function mutations in the V_2 vasopressin receptor gene have been described in male infants presenting with an SIADH-like clinical picture with undetectable vasopressin levels. Activating mutations in the aquaporin-2 gene might also give rise to the same syndrome but have not yet been described.

Systemic Dehydration

The initial manifestation of systemic dehydration is often hypernatremia and hyperosmolality, which subsequently lead to the activation of vasopressin secretion and a decrease in water excretion. As dehydration progresses, hypovolemia and/or hypotension becomes a major stimulus for vasopressin release, further decreasing free water clearance. Excessive free water intake with ongoing salt loss can also produce hyponatremia. Urinary sodium excretion is low (usually <10 mEq/L) owing to a low glomerular filtration rate and concomitant activation of the renin-angiotensin-aldosterone system, unless primary renal disease or diuretic therapy is present.

Primary Salt Loss
Hyponatremia can result from the primary loss of sodium chloride as seen in specific disorders of the kidney (congenital polycystic kidney disease, acute interstitial nephritis, chronic renal failure), gastrointestinal tract (gastroenteritis), and sweat glands (cystic fibrosis). The hyponatremia is not solely due to the salt loss, because the latter also causes hypovolemia, leading to an increase in vasopressin. Mineralocorticoid deficiency, pseudohypoaldosteronism (sometimes seen in children with urinary tract obstruction or infection), and diuretics can also result in loss of sodium chloride.

Decreased Effective Plasma Volume
Hyponatremia can result from decreased effective plasma volume, as found in congestive heart failure, cirrhosis, nephrotic syndrome, positive pressure mechanical ventilation, severe burns, bronchopulmonary dysplasia in neonates, cystic fibrosis with obstruction, and severe asthma. The resulting decrease in cardiac output leads to reduced water and salt excretion, as with systemic dehydration, and an increase in vasopressin secretion. In patients with impaired cardiac output and elevated atrial volume (congestive heart failure, lung disease), atrial natriuretic peptide concentrations are elevated further, leading to hyponatremia by promoting natriuresis. However, owing to the marked elevation of aldosterone in these patients, their urine sodium remains low (<20 mEq/L) despite this. Unlike dehydrated patients, these patients also have excess total body sodium from activation of the renin-angiotensin-aldosterone system and can demonstrate peripheral edema as well.

Primary Polydipsia (Increased Water Ingestion)
In patients with normal renal function, the kidney can excrete dilute urine with an osmolality as low as 50 mOsm/kg. To excrete a daily solute load of 500 mOsm/m^2, the kidney must produce 10 L/m^2 of urine per day. Therefore, to avoid hyponatremia, the maximum amount of water a person with normal renal function can consume is 10 L/m^2. Neonates, however, cannot dilute their urine to this degree, putting them at risk for water intoxication if water intake exceeds 4 L/m^2/day (approximately 60 mL/h in a newborn). Many infants develop transient but symptomatic hyponatremic seizures after being fed pure water without electrolytes rather than breast milk or formula.

Decreased Free Water Clearance
Hyponatremia due to decreased renal free water clearance, even in the absence of an increase in vasopressin secretion, can result from adrenal insufficiency or thyroid deficiency or can be related to a direct effect of drugs on the kidney. Both mineralocorticoids and glucocorticoids are required for normal free water clearance in a vasopressin-independent manner. In patients with unexplained hyponatremia, adrenal and thyroid insufficiency should be considered. In addition, patients with coexisting adrenal failure and diabetes insipidus might have no symptoms of the latter until glucocorticoid therapy unmasks the need for vasopressin replacement. Certain drugs can inhibit renal water excretion through direct effects on the nephron, thus causing hyponatremia; these drugs include high-dose cyclophosphamide, vinblastine, cisplatinum, carbamazepine, and oxcarbazepine.

Cerebral Salt Wasting
Cerebral salt wasting appears to be the result of hypersecretion of atrial natriuretic peptide and is seen primarily with central nervous system disorders including brain tumors, head trauma, hydrocephalus, neurosurgery, cerebrovascular accidents, and brain death. Hyponatremia is accompanied by elevated urinary sodium excretion (often >150 mEq/L), excessive urine output, hypovolemia, normal or high uric acid, suppressed vasopressin, and elevated atrial natriuretic peptide concentrations (>20 pmol/L). Thus, it is distinguished from SIADH, in which normal or decreased urine output, euvolemia, only modestly elevated urine sodium concentration, and an elevated vasopressin level occur. The distinction between cerebral salt wasting and SIADH is important because the treatment of the two disorders differs markedly. However, its existence has been questioned, because few patients with the suspected syndrome have documented hypovolemia and thus might truly have SIADH.

Runners' Hyponatremia
Excess fluid ingestion during long-distance running (e.g., marathon running) can result in severe hyponatremia due to hypovolemia-induced activation of AVP secretion coupled with excessive water ingestion and is correlated with weight gain, long racing time, and extremes of body mass index.

Pseudohyponatremia and Other Causes of Hyponatremia
Pseudohyponatremia can result from hypertriglyceridemia (Chapter 52). Elevated lipid levels result in a relative decrease in serum water content. As electrolytes are dissolved in the aqueous phase of the serum, they appear low when expressed as a fraction of the total serum volume. As a fraction of serum water, however, electrolyte content is normal. Modern laboratory methods that measure sodium concentration directly, independent of sample volume, do not cause this anomaly. Factitious hyponatremia can result from obtaining a blood sample proximal to the site of intravenous hypotonic fluid infusion.

Hyponatremia is also associated with hyperglycemia, which causes the influx of water into the intravascular space. Serum sodium decreases by 1.6 mEq/L for every 100 mg/dL increment in blood glucose >100 mg/dL. Glucose is not ordinarily an osmotically active agent and does not stimulate vasopressin release, probably because it can equilibrate freely across plasma membranes. In the presence of insulin deficiency and hyperglycemia, however, glucose acts as an osmotic agent, presumably because its normal intracellular access to osmosensor sites is prevented. Under these circumstances, an osmotic gradient exists, stimulating vasopressin release.

TREATMENT

Patients with systemic dehydration and hypovolemia should be rehydrated with salt-containing fluids such as normal saline or lactated Ringer solution. Because of activation of the renin-angiotensin-aldosterone system, the administered sodium is avidly conserved, and water diuresis quickly ensues as volume is restored and vasopressin concentrations decrease. Under these conditions, caution must be taken to prevent a too-rapid correction of hyponatremia, which can result in central pontine myelinolysis characterized by discrete regions of axonal demyelination and the potential for irreversible brain damage.

Hyponatremia due to a decrease in effective plasma volume caused by cardiac, hepatic, renal, or pulmonary dysfunction is more difficult to reverse. The most effective therapy is the least easily achieved: treatment of the underlying systemic disorder. For example, patients weaned from positive pressure ventilation undergo a prompt water diuresis and resolution of hyponatremia as cardiac output is restored and vasopressin concentrations decrease. AVP V_2 receptor antagonists (aquaretics) have been developed. One of these, conivaptan, has been approved in the United States for the intravenous treatment of hospitalized adults with hyponatremia due to congestive heart failure. The safety and effectiveness of conivaptan in pediatric patients have not been studied.

Patients with hyponatremia due to primary salt loss require supplementation with sodium chloride and fluids. Initially, intravenous replacement of urine volume with fluid containing sodium chloride, 150-450 mEq/L depending on the degree of salt loss, may be necessary; oral salt supplementation may be required subsequently. This treatment contrasts with that of SIADH, in which water restriction without sodium supplementation is the mainstay.

Emergency Treatment of Hyponatremia

The development of acute hyponatremia (onset <12 hr) or a serum sodium concentration <120 mEq/L may be associated with lethargy, psychosis, coma, or generalized seizures, especially in younger children. Acute hyponatremia can cause cell swelling and lead to neuronal dysfunction or to cerebral herniation. The emergency treatment of cerebral dysfunction resulting from acute hyponatremia includes water restriction and can require rapid correction with hypertonic 3% sodium chloride. If hypertonic saline treatment is undertaken, the serum sodium should be raised only high enough to cause an improvement in mental status, and in no case faster than 0.5 mEq/L/hr or 12 mEq/L/24 hr.

Treatment of SIADH

Chronic SIADH is best treated by oral fluid restriction. With full antidiuresis (urine osmolality of 1,000 mOsm/kg), a normal daily obligate renal solute load of 500 mOsm/m^2 would be excreted in 500 mL/m^2 water. This, plus a daily nonrenal water loss of 500 mL/m^2, would require that oral fluid intake be limited to 1,000 mL/m^2/24 hr to avoid hyponatremia. In young children, this degree of fluid restriction might not provide adequate calories for growth. In this situation, the creation of nephrogenic diabetes insipidus using demeclocycline therapy may be indicated to allow sufficient fluid intake for normal growth. Urea has also been safely used to induce an osmotic diuresis in infants and children.

Treatment of Cerebral Salt Wasting

Treatment of patients with cerebral salt wasting consists of restoring intravascular volume with sodium chloride and water, as for the treatment of other causes of systemic dehydration. The underlying cause of the disorder, which is usually due to acute brain injury, should also be treated if possible. Treatment involves the ongoing replacement of urine sodium losses volume for volume.

BIBLIOGRAPHY

Please visit the Nelson Textbook of Pediatrics *website at www.expertconsult.com for the complete bibliography.*

Chapter 554
Hyperpituitarism, Tall Stature, and Overgrowth Syndromes

Hidekazu Hosono and Pinchas Cohen

HYPERPITUITARISM

Primary hypersecretion of pituitary hormones rarely occurs in the pediatric population. Primary hyperpituitarism should be distinguished from **secondary hyperpituitarism,** which occurs in the setting of target hormone deficiencies resulting in decreased hormonal feedback, such as in hypogonadism, hypoadrenalism, or hypothyroidism. In some cases, chronic pituitary hypersecretion is accompanied by pituitary hyperplasia, which can enlarge and erode the sella, and, on rare occasions, increase intracranial pressure. Such enlargements should not be confused with primary pituitary tumors; they disappear when the underlying hormone deficiency is treated. The elevated pituitary hormone levels readily suppress to normal following replacement of end-organ hormones. Pituitary hyperplasia can also occur in response to stimulation by ectopic production of releasing hormones such as that seen occasionally in patients with Cushing syndrome secondary to corticotropin-releasing hormone excess or in children with acromegaly secondary to growth hormone-releasing hormone (GHRH) produced by a variety of systemic tumors.

For the full continuation of this chapter, please visit the Nelson Textbook of Pediatrics *website at www.expertconsult.com.*

Chapter 555
Physiology of Puberty

Luigi Garibaldi and Wassim Chemaitilly

Between early childhood and approximately 8-9 yr of age (prepubertal stage), the hypothalamic-pituitary-gonadal axis is dormant, as reflected by undetectable serum concentrations of luteinizing hormone (LH) and sex hormones (estradiol in girls, testosterone in boys). One to 3 yr before the onset of clinically evident puberty, low serum levels of LH during sleep become demonstrable (peripubertal period). This sleep-entrained LH secretion occurs in a pulsatile fashion and reflects endogenous episodic discharge of hypothalamic gonadotropin-releasing hormone (GnRH). Nocturnal pulses of LH continue to increase in amplitude and, to a lesser extent, in frequency as clinical puberty approaches. This pulsatile secretion of gonadotropins is responsible for enlargement and maturation of the gonads and the secretion of sex hormones. The appearance of the secondary sex characteristics in early puberty is the visible culmination of the sustained, active interaction occurring among hypothalamus, pituitary, and gonads in the peripubertal period. By mid-puberty, LH pulses become evident even during the daytime and occur at about 90- to 120-min intervals. A second critical event occurs in middle or late adolescence in girls, in whom cyclicity and ovulation occur. A positive feedback mechanism develops whereby increasing levels of estrogen in midcycle cause a distinct increase of LH.

For the full continuation of this chapter, please visit the Nelson Textbook of Pediatrics *website at www.expertconsult.com.*

Chapter 556
Disorders of Pubertal Development

Luigi Garibaldi and Wassim Chemaitilly

Precocious puberty is defined by the onset of secondary sexual characters before the age of 8 years in girls and 9 years in boys. The variation in the age of the onset of puberty in normal children, particularly of different ethnicities, makes this definition somewhat arbitrary. It remains in use by most clinicians.

Depending on the primary source of the hormonal production, precocious puberty may be classified as **central** (also known as **gonadotropin dependent,** or **true**) or **peripheral** (also known as **gonadotropin independent** or **precocious pseudopuberty**) (Table 556-1). **Central** precocious puberty is always isosexual and stems

Table 556-1 CONDITIONS CAUSING PRECOCIOUS PUBERTY

CENTRAL (GONADOTROPIN DEPENDENT, TRUE PRECOCIOUS PUBERTY)
Idiopathic
Organic brain lesions
Hypothalamic hamartoma
Brain tumors, hydrocephalus, severe head trauma, myelomeningocele
Hypothyroidism, prolonged and untreated*
COMBINED PERIPHERAL AND CENTRAL
Treated congenital adrenal hyperplasia
McCune-Albright syndrome, late
Familial male precocious puberty, late
PERIPHERAL (GONADOTROPIN INDEPENDENT, PRECOCIOUS PSEUDOPUBERTY)
Girls
Isosexual (feminizing) conditions
McCune-Albright syndrome
Autonomous ovarian cysts
Ovarian tumors
Granulosa-theca cell tumor associated with Ollier disease
Teratoma, chorionepithelioma
SCTAT associated with Peutz-Jeghers syndrome
Feminizing adrenocortical tumor
Exogenous estrogens
Heterosexual (masculinizing) conditions
Congenital adrenal hyperplasia
Adrenal tumors
Ovarian tumors
Glucocorticoid receptor defect
Exogenous androgens
Boys
Isosexual (masculinizing) conditions
Congenital adrenal hyperplasia
Adrenocortical tumor
Leydig cell tumor
Familial male precocious puberty
Isolated
Associated with pseudohypoparathyroidism
hCG-secreting tumors
Central nervous system
Hepatoblastoma
Mediastinal tumor associated with Klinefelter syndrome
Teratoma
Glucocorticoid receptor defect
Exogenous androgen
Heterosexual (feminizing) conditions
Feminizing adrenocortical tumor
SCTAT associated with Peutz-Jeghers syndrome
Exogenous estrogens
INCOMPLETE (PARTIAL) PRECOCIOUS PUBERTY
Premature thelarche
Premature adrenarche
Premature menarche

hCG, human chorionic gonadotropic; SCTAT, sex-cord tumor with annular tubules.
*Central without true gonadotropin dependency (see text).

from hypothalamic-pituitary-gonadal activation with ensuing sex hormone secretion and progressive sexual maturation. In **peripheral** precocious puberty, some of the secondary sex characters appear, but there is no activation of the normal hypothalamic-pituitary-gonadal interplay. In this latter group, the sex characteristics may be isosexual or heterosexual (contrasexual; Chapters 577-582).

Peripheral precocious puberty can induce maturation of the hypothalamic-pituitary-gonadal axis and trigger the onset of central puberty. This mixed type of precocious puberty occurs commonly in conditions such as congenital adrenal hyperplasia, McCune-Albright syndrome, and familial male-limited precocious puberty, when the bone age reaches the pubertal range (10.5-12.5 yr).

BIBLIOGRAPHY
Please visit the Nelson Textbook of Pediatrics *website at www.expertconsult.com for the complete bibliography.*

556.1 Central Precocious Puberty

Luigi Garibaldi and Wassim Chemaitilly

Central precocious puberty is defined by the onset of breast development before the age of 8 years in girls and by the onset of testicular development (volume ≥ 4 mL) before the age of 9 years in boys, as a result of the early activation of the hypothalamic-pituitary-gonadal axis. It occurs 5- to 10-fold more often in girls than in boys and is usually sporadic. A high prevalence of idiopathic central precocious puberty has been reported in girls adopted from developing countries, with the limitation that the exact date of birth may be uncertain.

Although approximately 90% of girls have an idiopathic form, a structural central nervous system (CNS) abnormality can be demonstrated in up to 75% of boys with central precocious puberty. Beyond its etiology, which thus needs to be specifically addressed, central precocious puberty can affect linear growth and the child's growth potential.

CLINICAL MANIFESTATIONS

Sexual development can begin at any age and generally follows the sequence observed in normal puberty. In girls, early menstrual cycles may be more irregular than they are with normal puberty. The initial cycles are usually anovulatory, but pregnancy has been reported as early as 5.5 yr of age (Fig. 556-1). In boys, testicular biopsies have shown stimulation of all elements of the testes, and spermatogenesis has been observed as early as 5-6 yr of age. In affected girls and boys, height, weight, and osseous maturation are advanced. The increased rate of bone maturation results in early closure of the epiphyses, and the ultimate stature is less than it would have been otherwise. Without treatment, approximately 30% of girls and an even larger percentage of boys achieve a height less than the 5th percentile as adults. Mental development is usually compatible with chronological age. Emotional behavior and mood swings are common, but serious psychological problems are rare.

Although the clinical course is variable, 3 main patterns of pubertal progression can be identified. Most girls (particularly those <6 yr of age at the onset) and a large majority of boys have rapidly progressive puberty, characterized by rapid physical and osseous maturation, leading to a loss of height potential. Some girls (>6 yr of age at the onset with an idiopathic form) have a slowly progressive variant, characterized by parallel advancement of osseous maturation and linear growth, with preserved height potential. A small percentage of girls have spontaneously regressive or unsustained central precocious puberty. This variability in the natural course of sexual precocity underscores the need for longitudinal observation at the onset of sexual development, before treatment is considered.

LABORATORY FINDINGS

Sex hormone concentrations are usually appropriate for the stage of puberty in both sexes. Serum estradiol concentrations in girls are low or undetectable in the early phase of sexual precocity, as they are in normal puberty. In boys, serum testosterone levels are detectable or clearly elevated by the time the parents seek medical attention, particularly if an early morning blood sample is obtained.

Sensitive immunometric (including immunoradiometric, immunofluorometric, and chemiluminescent) assays for luteinizing hormone (LH) have replaced the traditional LH radioimmunoassays and offer greater diagnostic sensitivity using random blood samples. With sensitive assays, serum LH concentrations are undetectable in prepubertal children but become detectable in 50-75% of girls and a higher percentage of boys with central sexual precocity. Measurement of LH in serial blood

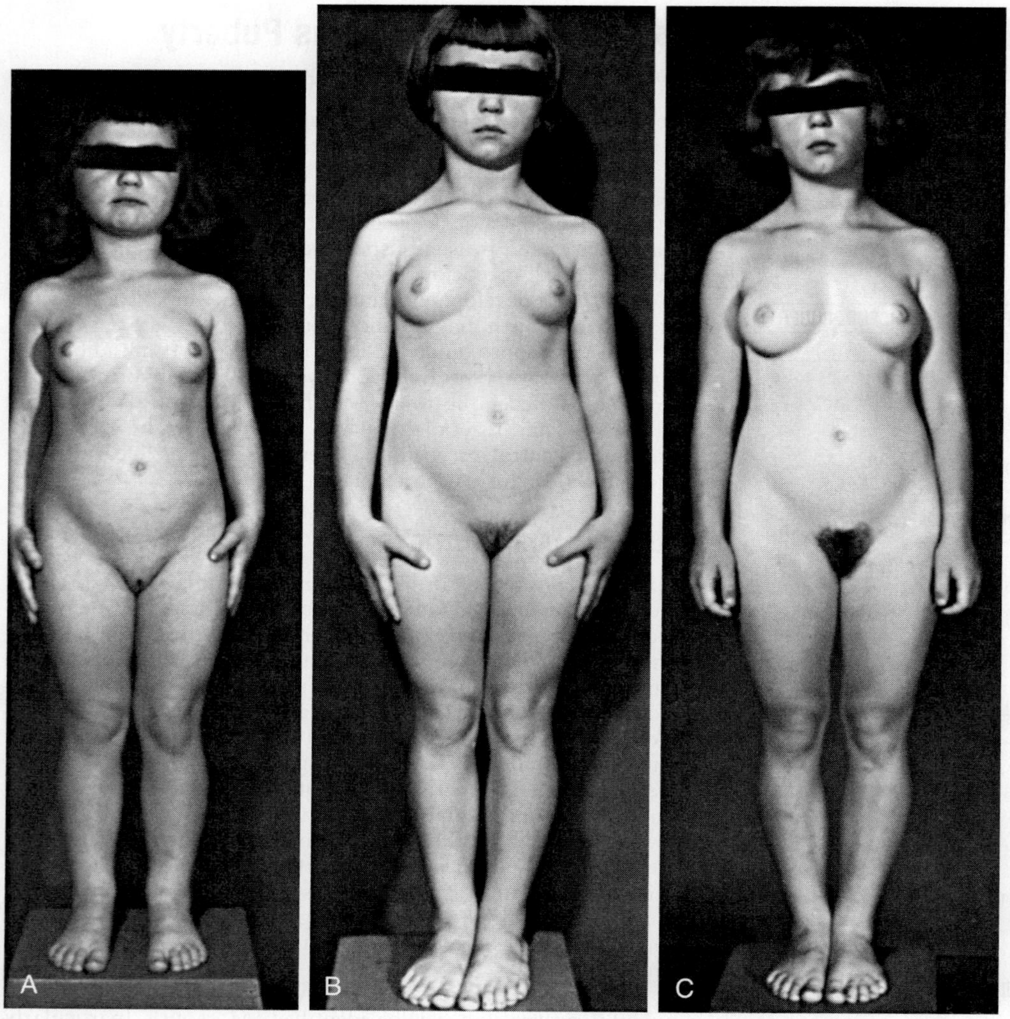

Figure 556-1 Natural course of idiopathic central precocious puberty. Patient *(A)* at $3\frac{1}{12}$, *(B)* at $5\frac{8}{12}$, and *(C)* at $8\frac{1}{2}$ yr of age. Breast development and vaginal bleeding began at $2\frac{1}{2}$ yr of age. Bone age was $7\frac{1}{2}$ yr at $3\frac{1}{12}$ and 14 yr at 8 yr of age. Intelligence and dental age were normal for chronological age. Growth was completed at 10 yr; ultimate height was 142 cm (56 in). No effective therapy was available at the time this patient sought medical attention.

samples obtained during sleep has greater diagnostic power than measurement in a single random sample, and it typically reveals a well-defined pulsatile secretion of LH.

Intravenous administration of gonadotropin-releasing hormone (GnRH stimulation test) or a GnRH agonist (leuprolide stimulation test) is a helpful diagnostic tool, particularly for boys, in whom a brisk LH response (LH peak >5-10 IU/L) with predominance of LH over follicle-stimulating hormone (FSH) tends to occur early in the course of precocious puberty. In girls with sexual precocity, however, the nocturnal LH secretion and the LH response to GnRH or GnRH agonist may be quite low at breast stages II to early III (immunometric LH peak <5IU/L), and the LH : FSH ratio can remain low until mid-puberty. In such girls with "low" LH response, the central nature of sexual precocity can be proved by detecting pubertal levels of estradiol (>50 pg/mL), 20-24 hr after stimulation with leuprolide.

Osseous maturation is variably advanced, often more than 2-3 standard deviations (SD). Pelvic ultrasonography in girls reveals progressive enlargement of the ovaries, followed by enlargement of the uterus to pubertal size. An MRI scan usually demonstrates physiologic enlargement of the pituitary gland, as seen in normal puberty; it may also reveal CNS pathology (Chapter 556.2).

DIFFERENTIAL DIAGNOSIS

Organic CNS causes of central sexual precocity should be ruled out by MRI scans. They are more likely in girls with rapid breast development, girls with estradiol >30 pg/mL, girls <6 yr of age, and in all boys, but specific criteria for ordering brain imaging are still lacking. Some authorities recommend MRI scans for all children with central precocious puberty.

Gonadotropin-independent causes of isosexual precocious puberty must be considered in the differential diagnosis (see Table 556-1). For girls, these include tumors of the ovaries, autonomously functioning ovarian cysts, feminizing adrenal tumors, McCune-Albright syndrome, and exogenous sources of estrogens. In boys, congenital adrenal hyperplasia, adrenal tumors, Leydig cell tumors, chorionic gonadotropin–producing tumors, and familial male precocious puberty should be considered.

TREATMENT

Virtually all boys and the large subgroup of girls with rapidly progressive precocious puberty are candidates for treatment. Girls with slowly progressive idiopathic central precocious puberty do not seem to benefit in terms of height prognosis from GnRH-agonist therapy. Children who were small for gestational age may be at greater risk of short stature as adults and can require more-aggressive treatment of precocious puberty, possibly in conjunction with human growth hormone (hGH) therapy. Certain patients require treatment solely for psychological or social reasons, including children with special needs and very young girls at risk of early menarche.

The observation that the pituitary gonadotropic cells require pulsatile, rather than continuous, stimulation by GnRH to maintain the ongoing release of gonadotropins provides the rationale for using GnRH agonists for treatment of central precocious puberty. By virtue of being more potent and having a longer duration of action than native GnRH, these GnRH agonists (after a brief period of stimulation) desensitize the gonadotropic cells of the pituitary to the stimulatory effect of endogenous GnRH and effectively halt the progression of central sexual precocity.

Long-acting formulations of GnRH agonists, which maintain fairly constant serum concentration of the drug for weeks or months, constitute the preparations of choice for treatment of central precocious puberty. In the USA, the most commonly used preparation is leuprolide acetate (Lupron Depot Ped), in a dose of 0.25-0.3 mg/kg (minimum, 7.5 mg) intramuscularly once every 4 wk. Other preparations (D-Trp6-GnRH [Decapeptyl], goserelin acetate [Zoladex]) are approved for treatment of precocious puberty in other countries. Recurrent sterile fluid collections at the sites of injections are the most troublesome local side effect and occur in <2-3% of treated patients. Alternatively, histrelin (Supprelin LA), a subcutaneous 50 mg implant with effects lasting 12 mo, is approved by the FDA for use in central precocious puberty. Other available treatment options include subcutaneous injections of aqueous leuprolide, given once or twice daily (total dose 60 µg/kg/24 hr), or intranasal administration of the GnRH agonist nafarelin (Synarel), 800 µg bid. The potential for irregular compliance with daily administration, as well as the variable absorption of the intranasal route for nafarelin, can limit the long-term benefit of the latter preparations on adult height. Preparations of depot-leuprolide with longer duration of action (90 days) are currently not FDA approved for treatment of central precocious puberty. GnRH antagonists are relatively new and have not been investigated sufficiently. Oral GnRH antagonists are also being investigated.

Treatment results in decrease of the growth rate, generally to age-appropriate values, and an even greater decrease of the rate of osseous maturation. Some children, particularly those with greatly advanced (pubertal) bone age, can show marked deceleration of their growth rate and a complete arrest in the rate of osseous maturation. Treatment results in enhancement of the predicted height, although the actual adult height of patients followed to epiphyseal closure is approximately 1 SD less than their mid-parental height.

In girls, breast development can regress in those with Tanner stage II-III development. Most commonly, the size of the breasts remains unchanged in girls with stage III-V development or even increases slightly because of progressive adipose tissue deposition. The amount of glandular tissue decreases. Pubic hair usually remains stable in girls or progresses slowly during treatment, reflecting the gradual increase in adrenal androgens. Menses, if present, cease. Pelvic sonography demonstrates a decrease of the ovarian and uterine size. In boys, there is decrease of testicular size, variable regression of pubic hair, and decrease in the frequency of erections.

Except for a reversible decrease in bone density (of uncertain clinical significance), no serious adverse effects of GnRH analogs have been reported in children treated for sexual precocity. If treatment is effective, the serum sex hormone concentrations decrease to prepubertal levels (testosterone, <10-20 ng/dL in boys; estradiol, <5-10 pg/mL in girls). The serum LH and FSH concentrations, as measured by sensitive immunometric assays, decrease to <1 IU/L in most patients, although almost never does the LH return to truly prepubertal levels (<0.1 IU/L). The incremental FSH and LH responses to GnRH stimulation decrease to <2-3 IU/L. Serum LH and sex hormone levels remain suppressed for as long as therapy is continued, but puberty resumes promptly when therapy is discontinued, typically at a "pubertal" chronological age. In girls, menarche and ovulatory cycles generally appear at an average of 18 mo (range 6-24 mo) of cessation of therapy. The addition of hGH to GnRH agonists has been used in children with precocious puberty, markedly advanced bone age, and prediction of short stature. The available data indicate that combined therapy can increase the adult height.

BIBLIOGRAPHY

Please visit the Nelson Textbook of Pediatrics *website at* *www.expertconsult.com* *for the complete bibliography.*

556.2 Precocious Puberty Resulting from Organic Brain Lesions

Luigi Garibaldi and Wassim Chemaitilly

ETIOLOGY

Hypothalamic hamartomas are the most common brain lesion causing central precocious puberty (Fig. 556-2). This congenital malformation consists of ectopically located neural tissue. Glial cells within the hamartoma have been shown to produce transforming growth factor β (TGF-β), which has the potential to activate the GnRH pulse generator. On MRI, it appears as a small pedunculated mass attached to the tuber cinereum or the floor of the third ventricle or, less often, as a sessile mass (Fig. 556-3) that remains static in size over years. Hypothalamic hamartomas,

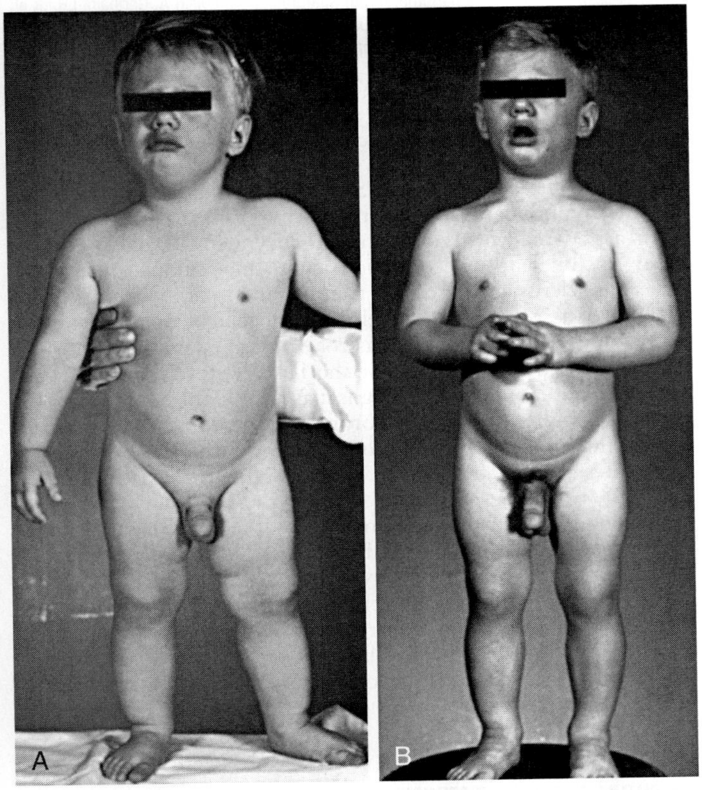

Figure 556-2 Natural course of precocious puberty with central nervous system lesion. Photographs at 1.5 *(A)* and 2.5 *(B)* yr of age. Accelerated growth, muscular development, osseous maturation, and testicular development were consistent with the degree of secondary sexual maturation. In early infancy, the patient began having frequent spells of rapid, purposeless motion; later in life, he had episodes of uncontrollable laughing with ocular movements. At 7 yr, he exhibited emotional lability, aggressive behavior, and destructive tendencies. Although a hypothalamic hamartoma had been suspected, it was not established until CT scanning became available when the patient was 23 yr of age. Epiphyses fused at 9 yr of age; final height was 142 cm (56 in). At 24 yr of age, he developed an embryonal cell carcinoma of the retroperitoneum.

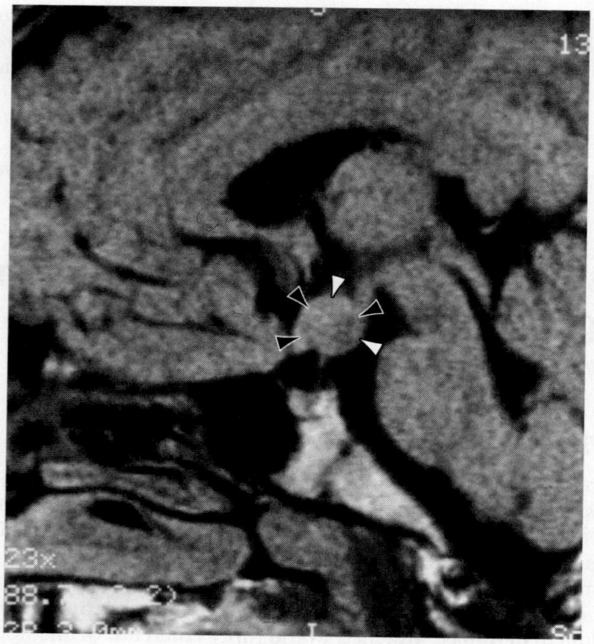

Figure 556-3 MRI of a central nervous system lesion in a child with central precocious puberty. A 6 yr old girl was referred for stage IV breast development and growth acceleration. Serum luteinizing hormone and estradiol concentrations were in the adult range. The midsagittal T1-weighted image shows an isointense hypothalamic mass *(arrowheads)*, typical of a hamartoma. (From Sharafuddin M, Luisiri A, Garibaldi LR, et al: MR imaging diagnosis of central precocious puberty: importance of changes in the shape and size of the pituitary gland, *Am J Roentgenol* 162:1167–1173, 1994.)

especially the sessile variant, can be associated with gelastic or psychomotor seizures.

A wide variety of other CNS lesions or insults, usually involving the hypothalamus by scarring, invasion, or pressure, have been associated with gonadotropin-dependent sexual precocity. They include postencephalitic scars, tuberculous meningitis, tuberous sclerosis, severe head trauma, and hydrocephalus, either isolated or associated with myelomeningocele. Neoplasms causing precocious puberty include astrocytomas, ependymomas, and optic tract tumors. Tumors of the latter type (typically slowly progressive or indolent optic gliomas) are highly prevalent (15-20%) in children with neurofibromatosis type 1 (NF-1) and constitute the main etiologic factor for the central sexual precocity encountered in a small subset (approximately 3%) of children with NF-1.

About 50% of the tumors in the pineal region are germinomas or astrocytomas; the remainder consists of a wide variety of histologically distinct tumor types. In boys, pineal or hypothalamic germinomas can cause central precocious puberty by secreting human chorionic gonadotropin (hCG), which stimulates the LH receptors in the Leydig cells of the testes. These same tumors usually do not produce precocious puberty in girls, presumably because complete ovarian function cannot occur without FSH priming.

CLINICAL MANIFESTATIONS

Some of these tumors or malformations (hypothalamic hamartomas) remain static in size or grow slowly, producing no signs other than precocious puberty. For lesions causing neurologic symptoms, the neuroendocrine manifestations may be present for 1-2 yr before the tumor can be detected radiologically. Hypothalamic signs or symptoms such as diabetes insipidus, adipsia, hyperthermia, unnatural crying or laughing (gelastic seizures), obesity, and cachexia should suggest the possibility of an intracranial lesion. Visual signs (proptosis, decreased visual acuity, visual field defects) may be the first manifestation of an optic glioma.

The sexual precocity is always isosexual, and the endocrine patterns are generally those found in children without demonstrable organic lesions. Rapidly progressive sexual precocity in very young children suggests the likelihood of a hypothalamic hamartoma. In conditions other than hypothalamic hamartoma, growth hormone deficiency can occur and may be masked by the growth-promoting effect of the increased sex hormone levels.

TREATMENT

Regardless of the cause, therapy with GnRH agonists is as effective in children with organic brain lesions causing central precocious puberty, and these analogs are the therapy of choice to halt premature sexual development. This includes patients with a hypothalamic hamartoma, if precocious puberty is its only manifestation. In patients with hypothalamic hamartoma and associated intractable gelastic or psychomotor seizures, however, stereotactic radiation therapy (gamma knife surgery) is effective and less risky than neurosurgical intervention. For other neurologic lesions, therapy depends on the nature and location of the pathologic process. Combined growth hormone therapy should be considered for patients with associated growth hormone deficiency.

BIBLIOGRAPHY

Please visit the Nelson Textbook of Pediatrics *website at* *www.expertconsult.com* *for the complete bibliography.*

556.3 Precocious Puberty Following Irradiation of the Brain

Luigi Garibaldi and Wassim Chemaitilly

Radiation therapy, generally for leukemia or intracranial tumors, increases the risk of precocious puberty considerably, whether the irradiation is directed to the hypothalamic area or to areas of the brain anatomically distant from the hypothalamus. Low-dose radiation (18-24 Gy) hastens the onset of puberty almost exclusively in girls. High-dose radiation (25-47 Gy), conversely, appears to trigger precocious sexual development in both sexes, and the risk of sexual precocity is inversely proportional to the age of the child at the time radiation was given.

This type of sexual precocity is often associated with growth hormone deficiency and may also be combined with other conditions (spinal irradiation, hypothyroidism) adversely affecting the prognosis for a reasonable adult height. Unless careful attention is paid to early signs of pubertal development in these children, the combination of growth hormone deficiency and the growth-promoting effect of sex steroids often results in a "normal" growth rate at the expense of a rapidly advancing bone age and impaired adult height potential.

TREATMENT

GnRH analogs are effective in arresting pubertal progression in this patient population. However, concomitant growth hormone deficiency (and/or thyroid hormone deficiency) should be diagnosed and treated promptly to improve the adult height prognosis.

Paradoxically, hypopituitarism with gonadotropin deficiency can subsequently develop as a late effect of high-dose CNS irradiation in patients with or without a history of precocious puberty, and it can require substitution therapy with sex steroids.

556.4 Syndrome of Precocious Puberty and Hypothyroidism

Luigi Garibaldi and Wassim Chemaitilly

In children with untreated hypothyroidism, the onset of puberty is usually delayed until epiphyseal maturation reaches 12-13 yr of age. Precocious puberty in a child with untreated hypothyroidism and a prepubertal bone age presents a strikingly unphysiologic association, yet it is common and occurs in as many as 50% of children with severe hypothyroidism of long duration. These children have the usual manifestations of hypothyroidism, including retardation of growth and of osseous maturation (Chapter 559). The cause of the hypothyroidism is usually Hashimoto thyroiditis, which often goes undiagnosed, especially in children with special needs such as those with trisomy 21, in whom the symptoms of profound hypothyroidism may be more difficult to recognize.

Sexual development in girls consists primarily of breast enlargement and menstrual bleeding; the latter can occur even in girls with minimal breast enlargement. Pelvic sonography can reveal large, multicystic ovaries. Boys have testicular enlargement associated with modest or no penile enlargement and no pubic hair development. Enlargement of the sella, which is typical of long-standing primary hypothyroidism, may be demonstrated by skull film or MRI.

Plasma levels of thyroid-stimulating hormone (TSH) are markedly elevated, often >500 µU/mL, and plasma levels of prolactin are mildly elevated. Although serum FSH is low and LH is undetectable, when measured by specific assays, the massively elevated concentrations of TSH appear to interact with the FSH receptor (specificity spillover), thus inducing FSH-like effects in the absence of LH effects on the gonads. As a consequence, unlike in central precocious puberty, testicular enlargement occurs without substantial testosterone secretion in boys. Thus, the precocious puberty associated with hypothyroidism behaves as an incomplete form of gonadotropin-dependent puberty.

Treatment of the hypothyroidism results in rapid return to normal of the biochemical and clinical manifestations. Rapid bone age advancement and possible progression to central puberty could occur in the months following the initiation of thyroid hormone replacement, a complication that justifies delaying puberty with GnRH analogs. Macroorchidism (testicular volume >30 mL) can persist in men despite adequate thyroxine therapy.

556.5 Gonadotropin-Secreting Tumors

Luigi Garibaldi and Wassim Chemaitilly

HEPATIC TUMORS

Isosexual precocious puberty is uncommonly associated with hepatoblastoma. All reported patients have been male, with the age of onset varying from 4 mo to 8 yr (average 2 yr). An enlarged liver or mass in the upper quadrant should suggest the diagnosis. The tumor cells produce hCG, which stimulates the LH receptors in the Leydig cells of the testes. The testicles are only minimally enlarged, and the testicular histology reveals interstitial cell hyperplasia and absence of spermatogenesis. Plasma levels of hCG and α-fetoprotein are usually markedly elevated; they serve as useful markers for following the effects of therapy. Plasma levels of testosterone are elevated, and the FSH and LH levels, as measured by specific immunometric assays, are low; in the past, LH levels were falsely elevated because of cross reaction with hCG on radioimmunoassay.

Treatment for these tumors is the same as that for other carcinomas of the liver; prognosis for survival beyond 1-2 yr from the time of diagnosis is poor.

OTHER TUMORS

Chorionic gonadotropin–secreting choriocarcinomas, teratocarcinomas, or teratomas (also called ectopic pinealomas or atypical teratomas), located in the CNS, mediastinum, gonads, or even adrenal glands, can cause precocious puberty, more commonly (10- to 20-fold) in boys than in girls. Affected patients often have marked elevations of hCG and α-fetoprotein. Mediastinal tumors, but not gonadal tumors, have been reported to cause precocious puberty in boys with Klinefelter syndrome.

PERIPHERAL PRECOCIOUS PUBERTY

The adrenal causes of pseudopuberty are discussed in Chapter 570, and the gonadal causes are discussed in Chapters 578 and 581.

556.6 McCune-Albright Syndrome (Precocious Puberty with Polyostotic Fibrous Dysplasia and Abnormal Pigmentation)

Luigi Garibaldi and Wassim Chemaitilly

The McCune-Albright syndrome is associated with patchy cutaneous pigmentation and fibrous dysplasia of the skeletal system. It is a rare condition with a prevalence between 1/100,000 and 1/1,000,000. A classic cause of peripheral precocious puberty, it can also induce pituitary, thyroid, and adrenal aberrations. It is characterized by autonomous hyperfunction of many glands and is caused by a missense mutation in the gene encoding the α-subunit of G_S, the G protein that stimulates cyclic adenosine monophosphate (cAMP) formation, resulting in the formation of the putative gsp oncoprotein. Activation of receptors (corticotropin [ACTH], TSH, FSH, and LH receptors) that operate via a cAMP-dependent mechanism, as well as cell proliferation, ensue. Because the mutation is somatic rather than genomic, it is expressed differently in different tissues, hence the variability of clinical expression.

Precocious puberty has been described predominantly in girls (Fig. 556-4). The average age at onset in affected girls is about 3 yr, but vaginal bleeding has occurred as early as 4 mo of age and secondary sex characters have occurred as early as 6 mo. Young girls have suppressed levels of LH and FSH, and there is no response to GnRH stimulation. Estradiol levels vary from normal to markedly elevated (>900 pg/mL), are often cyclic, and can correlate with the size of the cysts. In boys, precocious puberty is less common but has been reported in several instances. Unlike ovarian enlargement in girls, testicular enlargement in boys is fairly symmetric. It is followed by the appearance of phallic enlargement and pubic hair, as in normal puberty. Testicular histology has demonstrated large seminiferous tubules and no or minimal Leydig cell hyperplasia; these findings might simply reflect the fact that biopsy specimens were obtained at an early stage of pubertal development. In girls and boys, when the bone age reaches the usual pubertal age range, gonadotropin secretion begins, and the response to GnRH becomes pubertal. Central precocious puberty overrides the antecedent (gonadotropin-independent) precocious pseudopuberty. In girls, menses become more regular, but often not completely so, and fertility has been documented.

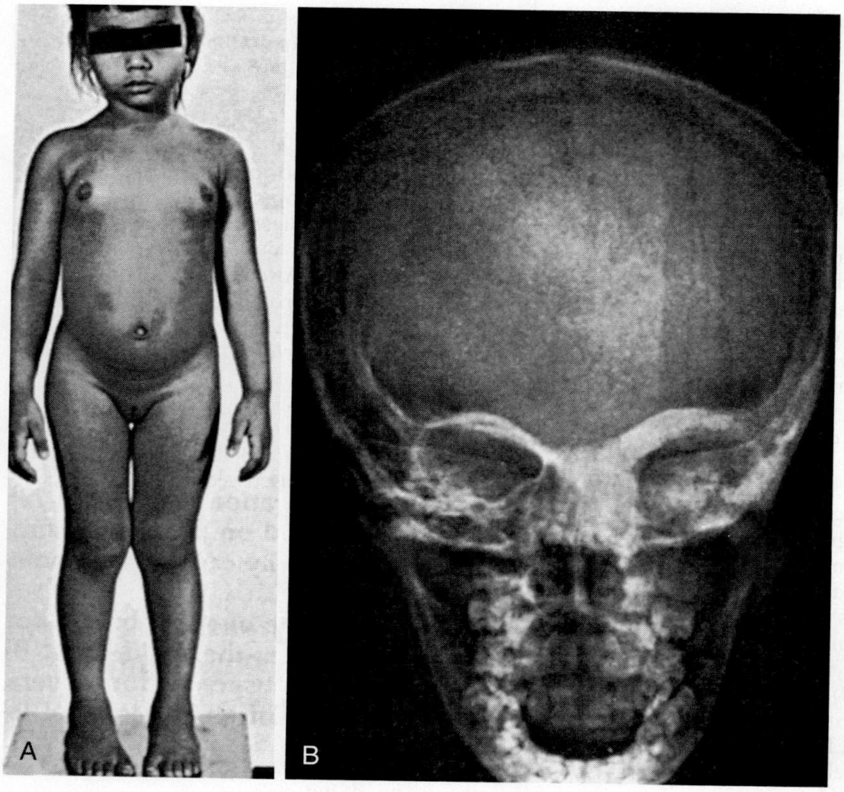

Figure 556-4 Precocious puberty associated with polyostotic fibrous dysplasia (McCune-Albright syndrome) in a girl 4.5 yr of age; at this time, her height age and bone age were normal. Menarche occurred at 4 yr of age. *A,* Note the bilateral breast development, hyperpigmented spots on the abdomen, and prominence of the left side of the face. *B,* Roentgenograms revealed fibrous dysplasia in the distal end of the left ulna and thickening of the bones about the left orbit and the maxillary portion of the frontal bones shown here.

Pubertal progression is variable in these patients. Functioning ovarian cysts often disappear spontaneously; aspiration or surgical excision of cysts is rarely indicated. For girls with persistent estradiol secretion, agents that interfere with the final step of estrogen biosynthesis, including aromatase inhibitors such as letrozole (1.25-2.5 mg/day orally) or antiestrogens (such as tamoxifen; fulvestrant is currently being investigated) limit, to a variable extent, the estrogen effects on pubertal and osseous maturation. The same compounds have also been used in boys, in combination with antiandrogens (such as spironolactone 50-100 mg bid, or flutamide 125-250 mg bid). These compounds are not approved by the FDA for this indication; tamoxifen and flutamide may be hepatotoxic, and high-dose spironolactone rarely causes hyperkalemia. Associated therapy with long-acting analogs of GnRH is indicated only for patients whose puberty has shifted from a gonadotropin-independent to a predominantly gonadotropin-dependent mechanism.

EXTRAGONADAL MANIFESTATIONS

The hyperthyroidism that occurs in this condition differs from that characteristic of Graves disease. There is an equal distribution between male and female patients; the goiters are multinodular. Clinical hyperthyroidism is uncommon in children, but goiters, mildly elevated triiodothyronine levels, suppressed TSH levels, and abnormalities on ultrasound have been reported. Thyroidectomy is rarely necessary.

In patients with associated Cushing syndrome, bilateral nodular adrenocortical hyperplasia has occurred in early infancy, antedating the sexual precocity. ACTH levels are low, and adrenal function is not suppressed by large doses of dexamethasone. Treatment is bilateral adrenalectomy.

Increased secretion of growth hormone occurs uncommonly and is manifested clinically by gigantism or acromegaly or by increased rates of growth even in the absence of precocious puberty. Girls and boys are equally affected. Serum levels of growth hormone are elevated and increase during sleep; they are augmented by thyrotropin (TRH) and poorly inhibited by oral glucose. Serum levels of prolactin are increased in most patients, but less than ½ of the patients have a demonstrable pituitary tumor. Octreotide or lanreotide, long-acting somatostatin analogs, can be used to treat the hypersomatotropism. The prognosis is favorable for longevity, but deformities, repeated fractures, pain, and occasional cranial nerve compression can result from the bony lesions.

Of the extraglandular manifestations, phosphaturia, leading to rickets or osteomalacia, is the most common. Cardiovascular and hepatic involvement is rare but may be life threatening (severe neonatal cholestasis).

BIBLIOGRAPHY

Please visit the Nelson Textbook of Pediatrics *website at* *www.expertconsult.com* *for the complete bibliography.*

556.7 Familial Male Gonadotropin-Independent Precocious Puberty

Luigi Garibaldi and Wassim Chemaitilly

Familial male gonadotropin-independent precocious puberty is a rare, autosomal dominant form of peripheral precocious puberty that is transmitted from affected male patients and unaffected female carriers of the gene to their male offspring. Signs of puberty appear by 2-3 yr of age. The testes are only slightly enlarged. Testicular biopsies show Leydig cell maturation and, sometimes, marked hyperplasia. Maturation of seminiferous tubules may be present. Testosterone levels are markedly elevated to the same range seen in boys with true precocious puberty; however, baseline levels of LH are prepubertal, pulsatile secretion of LH is absent, and LH does not respond to stimulation with GnRH or GnRH agonist. The cause for activation of Leydig cells independently of gonadotropin stimulation is a missense mutation of the LH receptor, leading to constitutive activation of cAMP production. Osseous maturation may be markedly advanced; when it reaches the pubertal age range, hypothalamic maturation shifts the mechanism of pubertal development to a gonadotropin-dependent one. This sequence of events is similar to that occurring in children with McCune-Albright syndrome (see earlier discussion) or in those with congenital adrenal hyperplasia (Chapter 570.1).

Gonadotropin-independent precocious puberty has been diagnosed in a few unrelated boys with type IA pseudohypoparathyroidism who had a single mutation of the $G_s\alpha$ protein. This mutation is inactivating at normal body temperature and causes pseudohypoparathyroidism, but in the cooler temperature of the testes, it is constitutionally activating, resulting in adenyl cyclase stimulation and production of testosterone. Although this mutation differs from the constitutive LH receptor mutation, which usually causes familial male gonadotropin-independent precocious puberty, the end result is the same.

TREATMENT

Young boys have been successfully treated with ketoconazole (600 mg/24 hr in divided doses every 8 hr), an antifungal drug that inhibits C-17,20-lyase and testosterone synthesis. Other investigators use a combination of antiandrogens (such as spironolactone 50-100 mg bid or flutamide 125-250 mg bid) and aromatase inhibitors (letrozole 2.5 mg/day, or anastrozole 1 mg/day), because estrogens derived from androgens stimulate bone maturation. These medications are unable to revert the serum testosterone to the normal (prepubertal) concentrations or completely offset the unfavorable effects of the elevated sex hormones. They slow down, but do not halt, the progression of puberty and might not improve the height prognosis. Boys whose GnRH pulse generator has matured require combined therapy with GnRH agonists.

BIBLIOGRAPHY

Please visit the Nelson Textbook of Pediatrics *website at www.expertconsult.com for the complete bibliography.*

556.8 Incomplete (Partial) Precocious Development

Luigi Garibaldi and Wassim Chemaitilly

Isolated manifestations of precocity without development of other signs of puberty are not unusual; development of the breasts in girls and growth of sexual hair in both sexes are the two most common forms.

PREMATURE THELARCHE

This term applies to a transient condition of isolated breast development that most often appears in the first 2 yr of life. In some girls, breast development is present at birth and persists. It may be unilateral or asymmetric and often fluctuates in degree. Growth and osseous maturation are normal or slightly advanced. The genitalia show no evidence of estrogenic stimulation. The condition is usually sporadic. Breast development might regress after 2 yr, often persists for 3-5 yr, and is rarely progressive. Menarche occurs at the expected age, and reproduction is normal. Basal serum levels of FSH and the FSH response to GnRH stimulation may be greater than that seen in normal girls. Plasma levels of LH and estradiol are consistently less than the limits of detection. Ultrasound examination of the ovaries reveals normal size, but a few small (<9 mm) cysts are not uncommon.

In some girls, breast development is associated with definite evidence of systemic estrogen effects, such as growth acceleration or bone age advancement. Pelvic sonography might reveal enlarged ovaries or uterus. This condition, referred to as **exaggerated or atypical thelarche,** differs from central precocious puberty because it spontaneously regresses. Leuprolide or GnRH stimulation elicits a robust FSH response, a low LH response, and (after leuprolide only) a moderate estradiol increment at 24 hr (average 60-90 pg/mL).

The pathogenesis of typical and exaggerated forms of thelarche is unclear; activating mutations of the *GNAS1* gene encoding the α-subunit of the G_S protein have been described in some patients without other signs of McCune-Albright syndrome (Chapter 556.6). Premature thelarche is a benign condition but may be the first sign of true or peripheral precocious puberty, or it may be caused by exogenous exposure to estrogens. In addition to a detailed history, a bone age should be obtained. The serum concentrations of FSH, LH, and estradiol are generally low and not diagnostic. Pelvic ultrasound examination is rarely indicated. Continued observation is important because the condition cannot be readily distinguished from true precocious puberty. Regression and recurrence suggest functioning follicular cysts. Occurrence of thelarche in children older than 3 yr most often is caused by a condition other than benign premature thelarche.

PREMATURE PUBARCHE (ADRENARCHE)

The term premature pubarche applies to the appearance of sexual hair before the age of 8 yr in girls or 9 yr in boys without other evidence of maturation. It is much more frequent in girls than in boys and might occur more commonly in African American girls than in others. Hair appears on the mons and labia majora in girls and in the perineal and scrotal area in boys; axillary hair generally appears later. Adult-type axillary odor is common. Affected children are slightly advanced in height and osseous maturation.

Premature adrenarche is an early maturational event of adrenal androgen production. This event coincides with precocious maturation of the zona reticularis, an associated decrease in 3β-hydroxysteroid dehydrogenase activity, and an increase in C-17,20-lyase activity. These enzymatic changes result in increased basal and ACTH-stimulated serum concentrations of the Δ^5-steroids (17-hydroxypregnenolone and dehydroepiandrosterone [DHEA]) and, to a lesser extent, of the Δ^4-steroids (particularly androstenedione) compared with age-matched control subjects. The levels of these steroids and of DHEA sulfate (DHEAS) are usually comparable to those of older children in the early stages of normal puberty.

Premature adrenarche is a slowly progressive condition that requires no therapy. However, a subset of patients with precocious pubarche have one or more features of systemic androgen effect, such as marked growth acceleration, clitoral (girls) or phallic (boys) enlargement, cystic acne, or advanced bone age (>2 SD above the mean for age). In these patients with **atypical premature adrenarche,** an ACTH stimulation test with measurement of steroid intermediates (mainly, serum 17-hydroxyprogesterone concentrations) is indicated to rule out nonclassical congenital adrenal hyperplasia due to 21-hydroxylase deficiency. Epidemiologic and molecular genetic studies have shown that the prevalence of nonclassic 21-hydroxylase deficiency is approximately 3-6% of unselected children with precocious pubarche; the prevalence of other enzyme defects (i.e., 3β-hydroxysteroid dehydrogenase or 11β-hydroxylase deficiencies) is extremely low.

Although idiopathic premature adrenarche has been considered a benign condition, longitudinal observations suggest that approximately 50% of girls with premature adrenarche are at high risk for **hyperandrogenism** and **polycystic ovary syndrome,** alone or more often in combination with other components of the metabolic syndrome (insulin resistance possibly progressing to type 2 diabetes mellitus, dyslipidemia, hypertension, increased abdominal fat) as adults. Whether the unfavorable progression to pubertal hyperandrogenism can be prevented by insulin-sensitizing agents (metformin 850-1000 mg/day) or lifestyle interventions (diet, exercise) remains to be proved in large studies. An increased risk of premature adrenarche and the metabolic syndrome has been documented in children born small for their gestational age. This appears to be associated with insulin resistance and decreased β-cell reserve, perhaps as a consequence of fetal undernutrition.

PREMATURE MENARCHE

Premature menarche is rare, much less common than premature thelarche or premature adrenarche, and is a diagnosis of exclusion. In girls with isolated vaginal bleeding in the absence of other secondary sexual characters, more common causes such as vulvovaginitis, a foreign body, or sexual abuse, and uncommon causes such as urethral prolapse and sarcoma botryoides must be carefully excluded. The majority of girls with idiopathic premature menarche have only 1-3 episodes of bleeding; puberty occurs at the usual time, and menstrual cycles are normal. Plasma levels of gonadotropins are normal, but estradiol levels may be elevated, probably owing to episodic ovarian estrogen secretion. Occasional patients are found to have ovarian follicular cysts on ultrasound.

BIBLIOGRAPHY

Please visit the Nelson Textbook of Pediatrics *website at www.expertconsult.com for the complete bibliography.*

556.9 Medicational Precocity

Luigi Garibaldi and Wassim Chemaitilly

A variety of medicaments can induce the appearance of secondary sexual characters that may be confused with precocious puberty. A careful history focused on exploring the possibility of accidental exposure to or ingestion of sex hormones is important. Peripheral precocious puberty has occurred in boys and girls from the accidental ingestion of estrogens (including contraceptive pills) and from the administration of anabolic steroids. Estrogens in cosmetics, hair creams, and breast augmentation creams have caused breast development in girls and gynecomastia in boys; estrogens are readily absorbed through the skin. The high prevalence of premature thelarche and peripheral precocious puberty in Puerto Rico has been attributed to contamination of meats, particularly chicken, with estrogens used in animal husbandry, but this has not been proved. Exogenous estrogens can produce a darkening of the areola that is not usually seen in endogenous types of precocity. The precocious changes disappear after cessation of exposure to the hormones. The use of testosterone gels or creams, which are applied to the skin for treatment of male hypogonadism, has resulted in virilization of children and women following skin contact at, and systemic absorption from, the area where the gel or cream was applied by their family member.

BIBLIOGRAPHY

Please visit the Nelson Textbook of Pediatrics *website at www.expertconsult.com for the complete bibliography.*

Section 2 DISORDERS OF THE THYROID GLAND

Chapter 557 Thyroid Development and Physiology

Stephen LaFranchi

FETAL DEVELOPMENT

The fetal thyroid bilobed shape is recognized by 7 wk of gestation, and characteristic thyroid follicle cell and colloid formation is seen by 10 wk. Thyroglobulin synthesis occurs from 4 wk, iodine trapping occurs by 8-10 wk, and thyroxine (T_4) and, to a lesser extent, triiodothyronine (T_3) synthesis and secretion occur from 12 wk of gestation. There is evidence that several transcription factors—TTF-1/NKX-2.1, TTF-2 (also termed FOXE1), NKX2.5, and PAX8—are important in thyroid gland morphogenesis and differentiation and possibly also in its caudal migration to its final location. These factors also bind to the promoters of thyroglobulin and thyroid peroxidase genes and so influence thyroid hormone production. Hypothalamic neurons synthesize thyrotropin-releasing hormone (TRH) by 6-8 wk, the pituitary portal vessel system begins development by 8-10 wk, and thyroid-stimulating hormone (TSH) secretion is evident by 12 wk of gestation. Maturation of the hypothalamic-pituitary-thyroid axis occurs over the 2nd half of gestation, but normal feedback relationships are not mature until approximately 3 mo of postnatal life. Another transcription factor, Pit-1, is important for differentiation and growth of thyrotrophs, along with somatotrophs and lactotrophs.

For the full continuation of this chapter, please visit the Nelson Textbook of Pediatrics *website at www.expertconsult.com.*

557.1 Thyroid Hormone Studies

Stephen LaFranchi

SERUM THYROID HORMONES

Methods are available to measure all the thyroid hormones in serum: T_4, free T_4, T_3, and free T_3. A metabolically inert T_3 (3,5′,3′-triiodothyronine), called reverse T_3, is also present in serum. Age must be considered in interpreting results, particularly in the neonate.

For the full continuation of this chapter, please visit the Nelson Textbook of Pediatrics *website at www.expertconsult.com.*

Chapter 558 Defects of Thyroxine-Binding Globulin

Stephen LaFranchi

Abnormalities in levels of thyroxine-binding globulin (TBG) are not associated with clinical disease and do not require treatment.

They are usually uncovered by a chance finding of abnormally low or high levels of thyroxine (T_4) and may be a source of confusion in the diagnosis of hypothyroidism or hyperthyroidism.

For the full continuation of this chapter, please visit the Nelson Textbook of Pediatrics *website at www.expertconsult.com.*

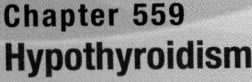

Chapter 559 Hypothyroidism

Stephen LeFranchi

Hypothyroidism results from deficient production of thyroid hormone, either from a defect in the gland itself (primary hypothyroidism) or a result of reduced thyroid-stimulating hormone (TSH) stimulation (central or hypopituitary hypothyroidism; Table 559-1). The disorder may be manifested from birth (congenital) or acquired. When symptoms appear after a period of apparently normal thyroid function, the disorder may be truly acquired or might only appear so as a result of one of a variety of congenital defects in which the manifestation of the deficiency is delayed. The term *cretinism,* although often used synonymously with endemic iodine deficiency and congenital hypothyroidism, is to be avoided.

Table 559-1 ETIOLOGIC CLASSIFICATION OF CONGENITAL HYPOTHYROIDISM

PRIMARY HYPOTHYROIDISM
Defect of fetal thyroid development (dysgenesis)
• Aplasia
• Hypoplasia
• Ectopia
Defect in thyroid hormone synthesis (dyshormonogenesis)
• Iodide transport defect: mutation in sodium-iodide symporter gene
• Thyroid organification, or coupling defect: mutation in thyroid peroxidase gene
• Defects in H_2O_2 generation: mutations in DUOXA2 maturation factor or *DUOX2* gene
• Thyroglobulin synthesis defect: mutation in thyroglobulin gene
• Deiodination defect: mutation in *DEHAL1* gene
TSH unresponsiveness
• $G_s\alpha$ mutation (e.g., type IA pseudohypoparathyroidism)
• Mutation in TSH receptor
Defect in thyroid hormone transport: mutation in monocarboxylate transporter 8 (*MCT8*) gene
Iodine deficiency (endemic goiter)
Maternal antibodies: thyrotropin receptor–blocking antibody (TRBAb, also termed *thyrotropin-binding inhibitor immunoglobulin*)
Maternal medications
• Iodides, amiodarone
• Propylthiouracil, methimazole
• Radioiodine
CENTRAL (HYPOPITUITARY) HYPOTHYROIDISM
PIT-1 mutations
• Deficiency of TSH
• Deficiency of growth hormone
• Deficiency of prolactin
PROP-1 mutations
• Deficiency of TSH
• Deficiency of growth hormone
• Deficiency of prolactin
• Deficiency of LH
• Deficiency of FSH
• ±Deficiency of ACTH
TSH deficiency: mutation in TSH β subunit gene (manifests as primary hypothyroidism with elevated TSH level)
Multiple pituitary deficiencies (e.g., craniopharyngioma)
TRH deficiency
• Isolated
• Multiple hypothalamic deficiencies (e.g., septo-optic dysplasia)
TRH unresponsiveness
Mutations in TRH receptor

ACTH, adrenocorticotropic hormone; FSH, follicle-stimulating hormone; LH, luteinizing hormone, TRH, thyroid-releasing hormone; TSH, thyroid-stimulating hormone.

CONGENITAL HYPOTHYROIDISM

Most cases of congenital hypothyroidism are not hereditary and result from thyroid dysgenesis. Some cases are familial; these are usually caused by one of the inborn errors of thyroid hormone synthesis and may be associated with a goiter. Most infants with congenital hypothyroidism are detected by newborn screening programs in the first few weeks after birth, before obvious clinical symptoms and signs develop. In infants born in areas with no screening program, severe cases manifest features in the first few weeks of life, but in cases of lesser deficiency, manifestations may be delayed for months.

Epidemiology

The prevalence of congenital hypothyroidism based on nationwide programs for neonatal screening is 1/3,000 infants worldwide; studies from the United States report that the prevalence is lower in black Americans and higher in Asian-Americans and Pacific islanders, Hispanics, and Native Americans. Twice as many girls as boys are affected.

Etiology

THYROID DYSGENESIS Some form of thyroid dysgenesis (aplasia, hypoplasia, or an ectopic gland) is the most common cause of congenital hypothyroidism, accounting for 80-85% of cases; 15% are caused by an inborn error of thyroxine synthesis (dyshormonogeneses), and 2% are the result of transplacental maternal thyrotropin-receptor blocking antibody (TRBAb). In about 33% of cases of dysgenesis, even sensitive radionuclide scans can find no remnants of thyroid tissue (aplasia). In the other 66% of infants, rudiments of thyroid tissue are found in an ectopic location, anywhere from the base of the tongue (lingual thyroid) to the normal position in the neck (hypoplasia).

The cause of thyroid dysgenesis is unknown in most cases. Thyroid dysgenesis occurs sporadically, but familial cases occasionally have been reported. The finding that thyroid developmental anomalies, such as thyroglossal duct cysts and hemiagenesis, are present in 8-10% of 1st-degree relatives of infants with thyroid dysgenesis supports an underlying genetic component.

Mutations in several transcription factors important for thyroid morphogenesis and differentiation (including TTF-1/NKX2.1, TTF-2 [also termed FOXE1] and PAX8) are monogenic causes of about 2% of the cases of thyroid dysgenesis. In addition, genetic defects leading to absent or ineffective thyrotropin action have been described.

The transcription factor TTF-1/NKX2.1 is expressed in the thyroid, lung, and central nervous system. Mutations in TTF-1/NKX2.1 have been reported to result in congenital hypothyroidism, respiratory distress, and persistent neurologic problems, including chorea and ataxia, despite early thyroid hormone treatment. NKX2.5 is expressed in the thyroid and heart. Mutations in *NKX2.5* are associated with congenital hypothyroidism and cardiac malformations. PAX-8 is expressed in the thyroid and kidney. Mutations in *PAX-8* are associated with congenital hypothyroidism and kidney and ureteral malformations.

The common finding of thyroid dysgenesis confined to only one of a pair of monozygotic twins suggests the operation of a deleterious factor during intrauterine life. Maternal antithyroid antibodies might be that factor. Although thyroid peroxidase (TPO) antibodies have been detected in some mother-infant pairs, there is little evidence of their pathogenicity. The demonstration of thyroid growth-blocking and cytotoxic antibodies in some infants with thyroid dysgenesis, as well as in their mothers, suggests a more likely pathogenetic mechanism.

DEFECTIVE SYNTHESIS OF THYROXINE (DYSHORMONOGENESIS) A variety of defects in the biosynthesis of thyroid hormone can result in congenital hypothyroidism; these account for 15% of cases detected by neonatal screening programs (1/30,000-1/50,000 live births). These defects are transmitted in an autosomal recessive manner. A **goiter** is almost always present. When the defect is incomplete, compensation occurs, and onset of hypothyroidism may be delayed for years.

DEFECT OF IODIDE TRANSPORT Defect of iodide transport is rare and involves mutations in the sodium-iodide symporter. Among the several cases now reported, it has been found in 9 related infants of the Hutterite sect, and about 50% of the cases are from Japan. Consanguinity is a factor in about 30% of the families.

In the past, clinical hypothyroidism, with or without a goiter, often developed in the first few months of life; the condition has been detected in neonatal screening programs. In Japan, however, untreated patients acquire goiter and hypothyroidism after 10 yr of age, perhaps because of the very high iodine content (often 19 mg/24 hr) of the Japanese diet.

The energy-dependent mechanisms for concentrating iodide are defective in the thyroid and salivary glands. In contrast to other defects of thyroid hormone synthesis, uptake of radioiodine and pertechnetate is low; a saliva to serum ratio of ^{123}I will establish the diagnosis. This condition responds to treatment with large doses of potassium iodide, but treatment with thyroxine (T_4) is preferable.

THYROID PEROXIDASE DEFECTS OF ORGANIFICATION AND COUPLING Thyroid peroxidase defects of organification and coupling are the most common of the T_4 synthetic defects. After iodide is trapped by the thyroid, it is rapidly oxidized to reactive iodine, which is then incorporated into tyrosine units on thyroglobulin. This process requires generation of H_2O_2, thyroid peroxidase, and hematin (an enzyme cofactor); defects can involve each of these components, and there is considerable clinical and biochemical heterogeneity. In the Dutch neonatal screening program, 23 infants were found with a complete organification defect (1/60,000), but its prevalence in other areas is unknown. A characteristic finding in all patients with this defect is a marked "discharge" of thyroid radioactivity when perchlorate or thiocyanate is administered 2 hr after administration of a test dose of radioiodine. In these patients, perchlorate discharges 40-90% of radioiodine compared with <10% in normal persons. Several mutations in the TPO gene have been reported in children with congenital hypothyroidism.

Dual oxidase maturation factor 2 (**DUOXA2**) is required to express **DUOX2** enzymatic activity, which is required for H_2O_2 generation, a crucial step in iodide oxidation. Biallelic DUOXA2 mutations produce permanent congenital hypothyroidism, whereas monoallelic mutations are associated with transient hypothyroidism. DUOX2 mutations can also cause permanent or transient congenital hypothyroidism. DUOX2 mutations are relatively common, present in 30% of cases of apparent dyshormonogenesis, whereas DUOXA2 are relatively rare, present in 2% of such cases.

Patients with **Pendred syndrome,** an autosomal recessive disorder comprising sensorineural deafness and goiter, also have impaired iodide organification and a positive perchlorate discharge. Pendred syndrome is due to a mutation in the chloride-iodide transport protein common to the thyroid gland and the cochlea.

DEFECTS OF THYROGLOBULIN SYNTHESIS Defects of thyroglobulin synthesis is a heterogeneous group of disorders characterized by goiter, elevated TSH, low T_4 levels, and absent or low levels of thyroglobulin (TG). It has been reported in approximately 100 patients. Molecular defects, primarily point mutations, have been described in several patients.

DEFECTS IN DEIODINATION Monoiodotyrosine and diiodotyrosine released from thyroglobulin are normally deiodinated within the thyroid or in peripheral tissues by a deiodinase. The liberated iodine is recycled in the synthesis of thyroid hormones. The *DEHAL1* gene encodes iodotyrosine deiodinase in the thyroid. *DEHAL1* mutations are relatively rare; patients with deiodinase deficiency experience severe iodine loss from the constant urinary excretion of nondeiodinated tyrosines, leading to hormonal deficiency and goiter. The deiodination defect may be limited to thyroid tissue only or to peripheral tissue only, or it may be universal.

DEFECTS IN THYROID HORMONE TRANSPORT Passage of thyroid hormone into the cell is facilitated by plasma membrane transporters. A mutation in one such transporter gene, monocarboxylate transporter 8 (MCT8), located on the X chromosome, has been reported in 5 boys with X-linked mental retardation. The defective transporter appears to impair passage of T_3 into neurons; this syndrome is characterized by elevated serum T_3 levels, low T_4 levels, normal or mildly elevated TSH levels, and psychomotor retardation.

THYROTROPIN RECEPTOR-BLOCKING ANTIBODY Maternal thyrotropin receptor-blocking antibody (TRBAb; often measured as thyrotropin-binding inhibitor immunoglobulin), is an unusual cause of transitory congenital hypothyroidism. Transplacental passage of maternal TRBAb inhibits binding of TSH to its receptor in the neonate. The incidence is approximately 1/50,000-100,000 infants. It should be suspected whenever there is a history of maternal autoimmune thyroid disease, including Hashimoto thyroiditis or Graves disease, maternal hypothyroidism on replacement therapy, or recurrent congenital hypothyroidism of a transient nature in subsequent siblings. In these situations, maternal levels of TRBAb should be measured during pregnancy. Affected infants and their mothers can also have thyrotropin receptor–stimulating antibodies (TRSAbs) and TPO antibodies. Technetium pertechnetate and ^{125}I scans might fail to detect any thyroid tissue, mimicking thyroid agenesis, but ultrasonography will show a thyroid gland. After the condition remits, a normal thyroid gland is demonstrable by scanning following discontinuation of replacement treatment. The half-life of the antibody is 21 days, and remission of the hypothyroidism occurs in about 3-6 mo. Correct diagnosis of this cause of congenital hypothyroidism prevents unnecessary protracted treatment, alerts the clinician to possible recurrences in future pregnancies, and allows a favorable prognosis.

RADIOIODINE ADMINISTRATION Hypothyroidism can occur as a result of inadvertent administration of radioiodine during pregnancy for treatment of Graves disease or cancer of the thyroid. The fetal thyroid is capable of trapping iodide by 70-75 days of gestation. Whenever radioiodine is administered to a woman of childbearing age, a pregnancy test must be performed before a therapeutic dose of ^{131}I is given, regardless of the menstrual history or putative history of contraception. Administration of radioactive iodine to lactating women also is contraindicated because it is readily excreted in milk.

THYROTROPIN AND THYROTROPIN-RELEASING HORMONE DEFICIENCY Deficiency of TSH and hypothyroidism can occur in any of the conditions associated with developmental defects of the pituitary or hypothalamus (Chapter 551). More often in these conditions, the deficiency of TSH is secondary to a deficiency of thyrotropin-releasing hormone (TRH). TSH-deficient hypothyroidism is found in 1/30,000-50,000 infants; most screening programs are designed to detect primary hypothyroidism, so most of these cases are not detected by neonatal thyroid screening. The majority of affected infants have multiple pituitary deficiencies and present with hypoglycemia, persistent jaundice, and micropenis in association with septo-optic dysplasia, midline cleft lip, midface hypoplasia, and other midline facial anomalies.

Mutations in genes coding for transcription factors essential to pituitary development, cell type differentiation, and hormone synthesis are associated with congenital TSH deficiency. *PIT-1* mutations include TSH deficiency associated with growth hormone (GH) and prolactin deficiency. Patients with *PROP-1* mutations ("prophet of pit-1") have not only TSH, GH, and prolactin deficiency but also LH and follicle-stimulating hormone (FSH) deficiency and variable ACTH deficiency. *HESX1* mutations are associated with TSH, GH, prolactin, and ACTH deficiencies and is found in some patients with optic nerve hypoplasia (septo-optic dysplasia syndrome).

Isolated deficiency of TSH is a rare autosomal recessive disorder that has been reported in several sibships. DNA studies in affected family members reveal defects in the TSH β subunit gene, including point mutations, frame shifts causing a stop codon, and splice site mutations. The diagnosis is usually delayed because the serum TSH level is not elevated, and so such patients are not detected by newborn screening programs.

THYROTROPIN HORMONE UNRESPONSIVENESS A mutation in the TSH-receptor gene is a relatively uncommon autosomal recessive cause of congenital hypothyroidism. Both homozygous and compound heterozygous mutations in the TSH receptor gene have been reported. Infants with a severe defect have elevated TSH levels and will be detected by newborn screening, whereas other patients with a mild defect remain euthyroid without treatment. A study of infants with congenital hypothyroidism detected by newborn screening from Tokyo reported TSH-receptor mutations in 4.3% of patients (1/118,000), with a founder mutation (p.R450H) accounting for 70% of gene defects.

Mild congenital hypothyroidism has been detected in newborn infants who subsequently proved to have **type Ia pseudohypoparathyroidism.** The molecular cause of resistance to TSH in these patients is the generalized impairment of cyclic adenosine monophosphate activation caused by genetic deficiency of the α subunit of the guanine nucleotide regulatory protein G_s (Chapter 566).

THYROTROPIN-RELEASING HORMONE RECEPTOR ABNORMALITY Mutations in the TRH receptor gene, a rare cause of congenital hypothyroidism, have now been reported in a few families. This condition, which results in isolated TSH deficiency and hypothyroidism, was suspected because of failure of both TSH and prolactin to respond to TRH stimulation.

Thyroid Hormone Unresponsiveness

This autosomal dominant disorder is caused by mutations in the thyroid hormone receptor. Most patients have a goiter, and levels of T_4, T_3, free T_4, and free T_3 are elevated. These findings often have led to the erroneous diagnosis of Graves disease, although most affected patients are clinically euthyroid. The unresponsiveness can vary among tissues. There may be subtle clinical features of hypothyroidism, including mild mental retardation, growth retardation, and delayed skeletal maturation. On the other hand, there may be clinical features compatible with hyperthyroidism, such as tachycardia and hyperreflexia. It is presumed that these patients have varying tissue resistance to thyroid hormone. One neurologic manifestation is an increased association of attention-deficit/hyperactivity disorder; the converse is not true because patients with attention-deficit/hyperactivity disorder do not have an increased risk of thyroid hormone resistance.

TSH levels are diagnostic in that they are not suppressed as in Graves disease but instead are moderately elevated or normal but inappropriate for the levels of T_4 and T_3. The failure of TSH suppression indicates that the resistance is generalized and affects the pituitary gland as well as peripheral tissues. More than 40 distinct point mutations in the hormone-binding domain of the β-thyroid receptor have been identified. Different phenotypes do not correlate with genotypes. The same mutation has been observed in patients with generalized or isolated pituitary resistance, even in different members of the same family. A child homozygous for the receptor mutation showed unusually severe resistance. These cases support the dominant negative effect of mutant receptors, in which the mutant receptor protein inhibits normal receptor action in heterozygotes. Elevated levels of T_4 on neonatal thyroid screening should suggest the possibility of this diagnosis. No treatment is usually required unless growth and skeletal retardation are present.

Two infants of consanguineous matings are known to have an autosomal recessive form of thyroid resistance. These infants had manifestations of hypothyroidism early in life, and genetic studies revealed a major deletion of the β-thyroid receptor in 1 of them. The resistance appears to be more severe in this form of the entity.

On rare occasions, resistance to thyroid hormone selectively affects the pituitary gland. Because the peripheral tissues are not resistant to thyroid hormones, the patient has a goiter and manifestations of hyperthyroidism. The laboratory findings are the same as those seen with generalized thyroid hormone resistance. This condition must be differentiated from a pituitary TSH-secreting tumor. Different treatments, including D-thyroxine, TRIAC (triiodothyroacetic acid), and TETRAC (tetraiodothyroacetic acid) have been successful in some patients. Bromocriptine administration, which interferes with TSH secretion, was reported to be successful in another patient. Whether isolated pituitary resistance to thyroid hormone exists as a distinct entity is controversial; it may be a variant of generalized resistance to thyroid hormone with varying tissue responsiveness.

IODINE EXPOSURE Congenital hypothyroidism can result from fetal exposure to excessive iodides. Perinatal exposure can occur with the use of iodine antiseptic to prepare the skin for caesarian section or painting of the cervix before delivery. It has also been reported in infants born to mothers in Japan who consumed large quantities of iodine-rich seaweed. These conditions are transitory and must not be mistaken for the other forms of hypothyroidism. In the neonate, topical iodine-containing antiseptics used in nurseries and by surgeons can also cause transient congenital hypothyroidism, especially in low-birthweight infants, and can lead to abnormal results on neonatal screening tests. In older children, the usual sources of iodides are proprietary preparations used to treat asthma. In a few instances, the cause of hypothyroidism was amiodarone, an antiarrhythmic drug with high iodine content. In most of these instances, goiter is present (Chapter 561.3).

IODINE-DEFICIENCY ENDEMIC GOITER Essentially unseen in the United States, iodine deficiency or endemic goiter is the most common cause of congenital hypothyroidism worldwide. Despite efforts at universal iodizination of salt in many countries, economic, political, and practical obstacles make achieving this objective difficult. Borderline iodine deficiency is more likely to cause problems in preterm infants who depend on a maternal source of iodine for normal thyroid hormone production.

Thyroid Function in Preterm Babies

Postnatal thyroid function in preterm babies is qualitatively similar but quantitatively reduced compared with that of term infants. The cord serum T_4 is decreased in proportion to gestational age and birthweight. The postnatal TSH surge is reduced, and infants with complications of prematurity, such as respiratory distress syndrome, actually experience a decrease in serum T_4 in the 1st wk of life. As these complications resolve, the serum T_4 gradually increases so that generally by 6 wk of life it enters the T_4 range seen in term infants. Serum free T_4 concentrations seem less affected, and when measured by equilibrium dialysis, these levels are often normal. Preterm babies also have a higher incidence of transient TSH elevations and apparent transient primary hypothyroidism. Premature infants <28 wk of gestation might have problems resulting from a combination of immaturity of the hypothalamic-pituitary-thyroid axis and loss of the maternal contribution of thyroid hormone and so may be candidates for temporary thyroid hormone replacement; further studies are needed.

Clinical Manifestations

Most infants with congenital hypothyroidism are asymptomatic at birth, even if there is complete agenesis of the thyroid gland. This situation is attributed to the transplacental passage of moderate amounts of maternal T_4, which provides fetal levels that are approximately 33% of normal at birth. Despite this maternal contribution of thyroxine, hypothyroid infants still have a low serum T_4 and elevated TSH level and so will be identified by newborn screening programs.

The clinician depends on neonatal screening tests for the diagnosis of congenital hypothyroidism. Laboratory errors occur, and awareness of early symptoms and signs must be maintained. Congenital hypothyroidism is twice as common in girls as in boys. Before neonatal screening programs, congenital hypothyroidism was rarely recognized in the newborn because the signs and symptoms are usually not sufficiently developed. It can be suspected and the diagnosis established during the early weeks of life if the initial but less characteristic manifestations are recognized. Birthweight and length are normal, but head size may be slightly increased because of myxedema of the brain. Prolongation of physiologic jaundice, caused by delayed maturation of glucuronide conjugation, may be the earliest sign. Feeding difficulties, especially sluggishness, lack of interest, somnolence, and choking spells during nursing, are often present during the 1st mo of life. Respiratory difficulties, due in part to the large tongue, include apneic episodes, noisy respirations, and nasal obstruction. Typically, respiratory distress syndrome also occurs. Affected infants cry little, sleep much, have poor appetites, and are generally sluggish. There may be constipation that does not usually respond to treatment. The abdomen is large, and an umbilical hernia is usually present. The temperature is subnormal, often <35°C (95°F), and the skin, particularly that of the extremities, may be cold and mottled. Edema of the genitals and extremities may be present. The pulse is slow, and heart murmurs, cardiomegaly, and asymptomatic pericardial effusion are common. Macrocytic anemia is often present and is refractory to treatment with hematinics. Because symptoms appear gradually, the clinical diagnosis is often delayed.

Approximately 10% of infants with congenital hypothyroidism have associated congenital anomalies. Cardiac anomalies are most common, but anomalies of the nervous system and eye have also been reported. Infants with congenital hypothyroidism may have associated hearing loss.

If congenital hypothyroidism goes undetected and untreated, these manifestations progress. Retardation of physical and mental development becomes greater during the following months, and by 3-6 mo of age the clinical picture is fully developed (Fig. 559-1). When there is only partial deficiency of thyroid hormone, the symptoms may be milder, the syndrome incomplete, and the onset delayed. Although breast milk contains significant amounts of thyroid hormones, particularly T_3, it is inadequate to protect the breast-fed infant who has congenital hypothyroidism, and it has no effect on neonatal thyroid screening tests.

The child's growth will be stunted, the extremities are short, and the head size is normal or even increased. The anterior and posterior fontanels are open widely; observation of this sign at birth can serve as an initial clue to the early recognition of congenital hypothyroidism. Only 3% of normal newborn infants have a posterior fontanel larger than 0.5 cm. The eyes appear far apart, and the bridge of the broad nose is depressed. The palpebral fissures are narrow and the eyelids are swollen. The mouth is kept open, and the thick, broad tongue protrudes. Dentition will be delayed. The neck is short and thick, and there may be deposits of fat above the clavicles and between the neck and shoulders. The hands are broad and the fingers are short. The skin is dry and scaly, and there is little perspiration. Myxedema is manifested, particularly in the skin of the eyelids, the back of the hands, and the external genitals. The skin shows general pallor with a sallow complexion. Carotenemia can cause a yellow discoloration of the skin, but the sclerae remain white. The scalp is thickened, and the hair is coarse, brittle, and scanty. The hairline reaches far down on the forehead, which usually appears wrinkled, especially when the infant cries.

Development is usually delayed. Hypothyroid infants appear lethargic and are late in learning to sit and stand. The voice is hoarse, and they do not learn to talk. The degree of physical and mental retardation increases with age. Sexual maturation may be delayed or might not take place at all.

The muscles are usually hypotonic, but in rare instances generalized muscular pseudohypertrophy occurs **(Kocher-Debré-**

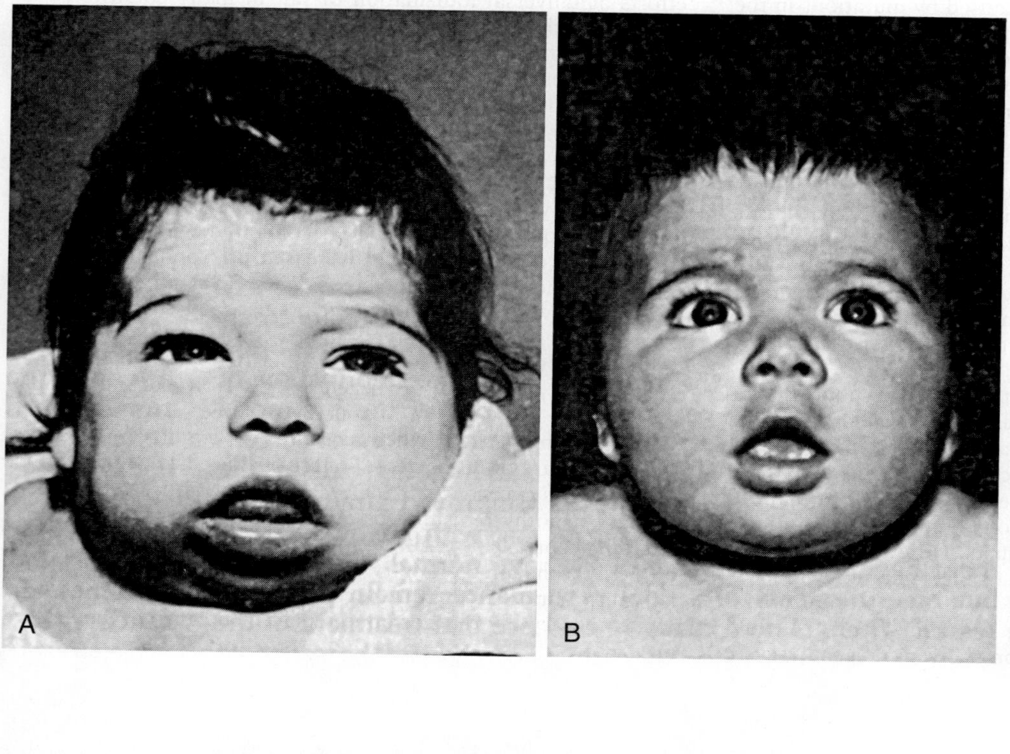

Figure 559-1 Congenital hypothyroidism in an infant 6 mo of age. The infant ate poorly in the neonatal period and was constipated. She had a persistent nasal discharge and a large tongue; she was very lethargic and had no social smile and no head control. *A,* Notice the puffy face, dull expression, and hirsute forehead. Tests revealed a negligible uptake of radioiodine. Osseous development was that of a newborn. *B,* Four months after treatment, note the decreased puffiness of the face, the decreased hirsutism of the forehead, and the alert appearance.

Sémélaigne syndrome). Affected older children can have an athletic appearance because of pseudohypertrophy, particularly in the calf muscles. Its pathogenesis is unknown; nonspecific histochemical and ultrastructural changes seen on muscle biopsy return to normal with treatment. Boys are more prone to development of the syndrome, which has been observed in siblings born from a consanguineous mating. Affected patients have hypothyroidism of longer duration and severity.

Some infants with mild congenital hypothyroidism have normal thyroid function at birth and so are not identified by newborn screening programs. In particular, some children with ectopic thyroid tissue (lingual, sublingual, subhyoid) produce adequate amounts of thyroid hormone for many years, or it eventually fails in early childhood. Affected children come to clinical attention because of a growing mass at the base of the tongue or in the midline of the neck, usually at the level of the hyoid. Occasionally, ectopia is associated with **thyroglossal duct cysts**. It can occur in siblings. Surgical removal of ectopic thyroid tissue from a euthyroid patient usually results in hypothyroidism, because most such patients have no other thyroid tissue.

Laboratory Findings

In developed countries, infants with congenital hypothyroidism are identified by newborn screening programs. Blood obtained by heel-prick between 2 and 5 days of life is placed on a filter paper card and sent to a central screening laboratory. Many newborn screening programs in North America and Europe measure levels of T_4, followed by measurement of TSH when T_4 is low. This approach identifies infants with primary hypothyroidism, some with hypothalamic or pituitary hypothyroidism, and infants with a delayed increase in TSH levels. Other neonatal screening programs in North America, Europe, Japan, Australia, and New Zealand are based on a primary measurement of TSH. This approach detects infants with primary hypothyroidism and can detect infants with subclinical hypothyroidism (normal T_4, elevated TSH), but it misses infants with delayed TSH elevation and with hypothalamic or pituitary hypothyroidism. With any of these tests, special care should be given to the normal range of values for age of the patient, particularly in the 1st weeks of life (Table 559-2). Regardless of the approach used for screening, some infants escape detection because of technical or human errors; clinicians must maintain their vigilance for clinical manifestations of hypothyroidism.

Serum levels of T_4 or free T_4 are low; serum levels of T_3 may be normal and are not helpful in the diagnosis. If the defect is primarily in the thyroid, levels of TSH are elevated, often to >100 mU/L. Serum levels of thyroglobulin are usually low in infants with thyroid agenesis or defects of thyroglobulin synthesis or secretion, whereas they are elevated with ectopic glands and other inborn errors of thyroxine synthesis, but there is a wide overlap of ranges.

Special attention should be paid to identical twins; in several reported cases, neonatal screening failed to detect the discordant twin with hypothyroidism, and the diagnosis was not made until the infants were 4-5 mo of age. Apparently, transfusion of euthyroid blood from the unaffected twin normalized the serum level of T_4 and TSH in the affected twin at the initial screening. Many newborn screening programs perform a routine second test in same-sex twins.

Retardation of osseous development can be shown radiographically at birth in about 60% of congenitally hypothyroid infants and indicates some deprivation of thyroid hormone during intrauterine life. The distal femoral epiphysis, normally present at birth, is often absent (Fig. 559-2*A*). In undetected and untreated patients, the discrepancy between chronologic age and osseous development increases. The epiphyses often have multiple foci of ossification (epiphyseal dysgenesis) (Fig. 559-2*B*); deformity ("beaking") of the 12th thoracic or 1st or 2nd lumbar vertebra is common. Roentgenograms of the skull show large fontanels and wide sutures;

Table 559-2 THYROID FUNCTION TESTS

AGE	US REFERENCE VALUE	CONVERSION FACTOR	SI REFERENCE VALUE
THYROID THYROGLOBULIN, SERUM			
Cord blood	14.7-101.1 ng/mL	×1	14.7-101.1 μg/L
Birth to 35 mo	10.6-92.0 ng/mL	×1	10.6-92.0 μg/L
3-11 yr	5.6-41.9 ng/mL	×1	5.6-41.9 μg/L
12-17 yr	2.7-21.9 ng/mL	×1	2.7-21.9 μg/L
THYROID STIMULATING HORMONE, SERUM			
Premature Infants (28-36 wk)			
1st wk of life	0.7-27.0 mIU/L	×1	0.7-27.0 mIU/L
Term Infants			
Birth to 4 days	1.0-38.9 mIU/L	×1	1.0-28.9 mIU/L
2-20 wk	1.7-9.1 mIU/L	×1	1.7-9.1 mIU/L
5 mo-20 yr	0.7-6.4 mIU/L	×1	0.7-6.4 mIU/L
THYROXINE BINDING GLOBULIN, SERUM			
Cord blood	1.4-94 mg/dL	×10	14-94 mg/L
1-4 wk	1.0-9.0 mg/dL	×10	10-90 mg/L
1-12 mo	2.0-7.6 mg/dL	×10	20-76 mg/L
1-5 yr	2.9-5.4 mg/dL	×10	29-54 mg/L
5-10 yr	2.5-5.0 mg/dL	×10	25-50 mg/L
10-15 yr	2.1-4.6 mg/dL	×10	21-46 mg/L
Adult	1.5-3.4 mg/dL	×10	15-34 mg/L
THYROXINE, TOTAL, SERUM			
Full-Term Infants			
1-3 days	8.2-19.9 μg/dL	×12.9	106-256 nmol/L
1 wk	6.0-15.9 μg/dL	×12.9	77-205 nmol/L
1-12 mo	6.1-14.9 μg/dL	×12.9	79-192 nmol/L
Prepubertal Children			
1-3 yr	6.8-13.5 μg/dL	×12.9	88-174 nmol/L
3-10 yr	5.5-12.8 μg/dL	×12.9	71-165 nmol/L
Pubertal Children and Adults			
>10 yr	4.2-13.0 μg/dL	×12.9	54-167 nmol/L
THYROXINE, FREE, SERUM			
Full-term (3 days)	2.0-4.9 ng/dL	×12.9	26-631 pmol/L
Infants	0.9-2.6 ng/dL	×12.9	12-33 pmol/L
Prepubertal children	0.8-2.2 ng/dL	×12.9	10-28 pmol/L
Pubertal children and adults	0.8-2.3 ng/dL	×12.9	10-30 pmol/L
THYROXINE, TOTAL, WHOLE BLOOD			
Newborn screen (filter paper)	6.2-22 μg/dL	×12.9	80-283 nmol/L
TRIIDOTHYRONINE, FREE, SERUM			
Cord blood	20-240 pg/dL	×0.01536	0.3-0.7 pmol/L
1-3 days	200-610 pg/dL	×0.01536	3.1-9.4 pmol/L
6 wk	240-560 pg/dL	×0.01536	3.7-8.6 pmol/L
Adult (20-50 yr)	230-660 pg/dL	×0.01536	3.5-10.0 pmol/L
TRIIODOTHYRONINE RESIN UPTAKE TEST (T3RU), SERUM			
Newborn	26-36%	×0.01	0.26-0.36 fractional uptake
Thereafter	26-35%	×0.01	0.26-0.35 fractional uptake
TRIIODOTHYRONINE, TOTAL, SERUM			
Cord blood	30-70 ng/dL	×0.0154	0.46-1.08 nmol/L
Newborn	75-260 ng/dL	×0.0154	1.16-4.00 nmol/L
1-5 yr	100-260 ng/dL	×0.0154	1.54-4.00 nmol/L
5-10 yr	90-240 ng/dL	×0.0154	1.39-3.70 nmol/L
10-15 yr	80-210 ng/dL	×0.0154	1.23-3.23 nmol/L
>15 yr	115-190 ng/dL	×0.0154	1.77-2.93 nmol/L

Adapted from Nicholson JF, Pesce MA: Reference ranges for laboratory tests and procedures. In Behrman RE, Kliegman RM, Jenson HB, editors: *Nelson textbook of pediatrics,* ed 17, Philadelphia, Saunders, 2004, pp 2412–2413.

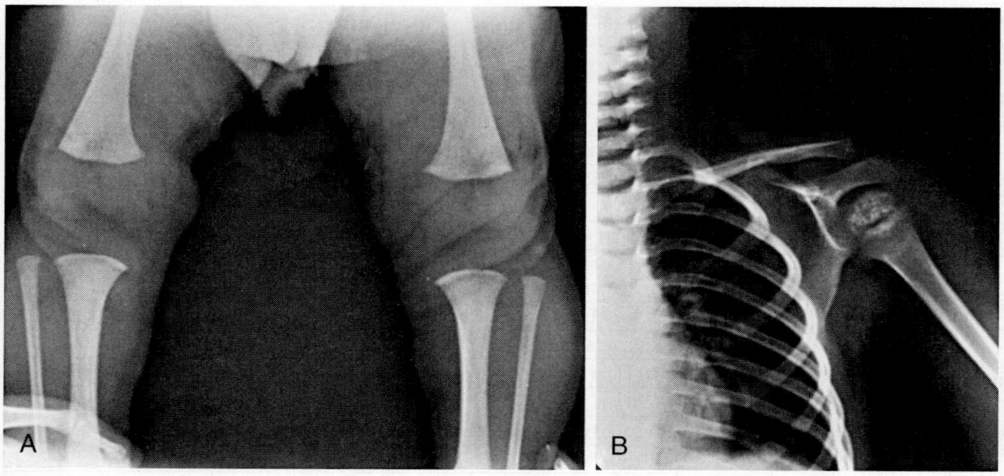

Figure 559-2 Congenital hypothyroidism. *A,* Absence of distal femoral epiphysis in a 3 mo old infant who was born at term. This is evidence for the onset of the hypothyroid state during fetal life. *B,* Epiphyseal dysgenesis in the head of the humerus in a 9 yr old girl who had been inadequately treated with thyroid hormone.

intersutural (wormian) bones are common. The sella turcica is often enlarged and round; in rare instances, there may be erosion and thinning. Formation and eruption of teeth can be delayed. Cardiac enlargement or pericardial effusion may be present.

Scintigraphy can help to pinpoint the underlying cause in infants with congenital hypothyroidism, but treatment should not be unduly delayed for this study. ^{123}I-sodium iodide is superior to ^{99m}Tc-sodium pertechnetate for this purpose. Ultrasonographic examination of the thyroid is helpful, but studies show it can miss some ectopic glands shown by scintigraphy. Demonstration of ectopic thyroid tissue is diagnostic of thyroid dysgenesis and establishes the need for lifelong treatment with T_4. Failure to demonstrate any thyroid tissue suggests thyroid aplasia, but this also occurs in neonates with TRBAb and in infants with the iodide-trapping defect. A normally situated thyroid gland with a normal or avid uptake of radionuclide indicates a defect in thyroid hormone biosynthesis. In the past, patients with goitrous hypothyroidism have required extensive evaluation, including radioiodine studies, perchlorate discharge tests, kinetic studies, chromatography, and studies of thyroid tissue, to determine the biochemical nature of the defect. Most can be evaluated by genetic studies looking for defects in the steps along the thyroxine biosynthetic pathway.

The electrocardiogram may show low-voltage P and T waves with diminished amplitude of QRS complexes and suggest poor left ventricular function and pericardial effusion. Echocardiography can confirm a pericardial effusion. The electroencephalogram often shows low voltage. In children >2 yr of age, the serum cholesterol level is usually elevated. Brain MRI before treatment is reportedly normal, although proton magnetic resonance spectroscopy shows high levels of choline-containing compounds, which can reflect blocks in myelin maturation.

Treatment

Levothyroxine given orally is the treatment of choice. Because 80% of circulating T_3 is formed by monodeiodination of T_4, serum levels of T_4 and T_3 in treated infants return to normal. This is also true in the brain, where 80% of required T_3 is produced locally from circulating T_4. The optimal dose of levothyroxine is controversial. Higher dosages can normalize T_4 more quickly and lead to improvement in cognitive scores, but there is some suggestion that children treated with these high doses are more likely to develop behavioral difficulties later on. In one study of neonates treated with dosages that ranged between 25 and 50 µg/day, infants treated with 50 µg/day attained normal thyroid function sooner, but there was no difference in rate of growth of length, weight, or head circumference between 3 and 18 mo of age as a function of levothyroxine dose. Currently, in neonates, the recommended initial starting dose is 10-15 µg/kg/day (totaling 37.5-50 µg/day). The starting dose can be tailored to the severity of hypothyroidism. Newborns with more severe hypothyroidism, as judged by a serum T_4 <5 µg/dL, should be started at the higher end of the dosage range. Thyroxine tablets should not be mixed with soy protein formulas, concentrated iron, or calcium, because these can bind T_4 and inhibit its absorption.

Levels of serum T_4 or free T_4 and TSH should be monitored at recommended intervals (approximately monthly in the first 6 mo of life, and then every 2-3 mo between 6 mo and 2 yr) and maintained in the normal range for age. The dose of levothyroxine on a weight basis gradually decreases with age. Children with hypothyroidism require about 4 µg/kg/24 hr, and adults require only 2 µg/kg/24 hr.

Later, confirmation of the diagnosis may be necessary for some infants to rule out the possibility of transient hypothyroidism. This is unnecessary in infants with proven thyroid ectopia or in those who manifest elevated levels of TSH after 6-12 mo of therapy because of poor compliance or an inadequate dose of T_4. Discontinuation of therapy at about 3 yr of age for 3-4 wk results in a marked increase in TSH levels in children with permanent hypothyroidism.

The only untoward effects of sodium-L-thyroxine are related to its dosage. Overtreatment can risk craniosynostosis and temperament problems.

Prognosis

Thyroid hormone is critical for normal cerebral development in the early postnatal months; biochemical diagnosis must be made soon after birth, and effective treatment must be initiated promptly to prevent irreversible brain damage. With the advent of neonatal screening programs for detection of congenital hypothyroidism, the prognosis for affected infants has improved dramatically. Early diagnosis and adequate treatment from the first weeks of life result in normal linear growth and intelligence comparable with that of unaffected siblings. Some screening programs report that the most severely affected infants, as judged by the lowest T_4 levels and retarded skeletal maturation, have reduced (5-10 points) IQs and other neuropsychological sequelae, such as incoordination, hypotonia or hypertonia, short attention span, and speech problems even with early diagnosis and adequate treatment. Psychometric testing can show problems with vocabulary and reading comprehension, arithmetic, and memory. Approximately 20% of children have a neurosensory hearing deficit.

Delay in diagnosis, failure to correct initial hypothyroxinemia rapidly, inadequate treatment, and poor compliance in the first 2-3 yr of life result in variable degrees of brain damage. Without treatment, affected infants are profoundly mentally deficient and growth retarded. When onset of hypothyroidism occurs after 2 yr of age, the outlook for normal development is much better even if diagnosis and treatment have been delayed, indicating how much more important thyroid hormone is to the rapidly growing brain of the infant.

ACQUIRED HYPOTHYROIDISM

Epidemiology

Studies of school-aged children report that hypothyroidism occurs in approximately 0.3% (1/333). Subclinical hypothyroidism (TSH >4.5 mU/L, normal T_4 or free T_4) is more common, occurring in approximately 2% of adolescents. Acquired hypothyroidism is most commonly a result of chronic lymphocytic thyroiditis; 6% of children aged 12-19 yr have evidence of autoimmune thyroid disease, which occurs with a 2:1 female:male preponderance.

Etiology

The most common cause of acquired hypothyroidism (Table 559-3) is chronic lymphocytic thyroiditis (Chapter 560). **Autoimmune thyroid disease** may be part of polyglandular syndromes; children with Down, Turner, and Klinefelter syndromes and celiac disease or diabetes are at higher risk for associated autoimmune thyroid disease (Chapter 560). In children with **Down syndrome**, anti-thyroid antibodies develop in approximately 30%, and subclinical or overt hypothyroidism occurs in approximately 15-20%. In girls with **Turner syndrome**, anti-thyroid antibodies develop in approximately 40%, and subclinical or overt hypothyroidism occurs in approximately 15-30%, rising with increasing age. In children with **type 1 diabetes mellitus**, approximately 20% develop anti-thyroid antibodies and 5% become hypothyroid. Additional autoimmune diseases with an increased risk of hypothyroidism include Sjögren syndrome, multiple sclerosis, pernicious anemia, Addison disease, and ovarian failure. Although typically seen in adolescence, it occurs as early as in the 1st yr of life. **Williams syndrome** is associated with subclinical hypothyroidism; this does not appear to be autoimmune, as anti-thyroid antibodies are negative.

Thyroidectomy for thyrotoxicosis or cancer results in hypothyroidism, as can removal of ectopic thyroid tissue. Thyroid tissue in a thyroglossal duct cyst usually constitutes the only source of thyroid hormone, and excision results in hypothyroidism. Because subhyoid glands usually mimic thyroglossal duct cysts, ultrasonographic examination or a radionuclide scan before surgery is indicated in these patients.

Irradiation of the area of thyroid that is incidental to the treatment of Hodgkin disease or other head and neck malignancies or that is administered before bone marrow transplantation often results in thyroid damage. About 30% of such children acquire elevated TSH levels within a yr after therapy, and another 15-20% progress to hypothyroidism within 5-7 yr. Some clinicians recommend periodic TSH measurements, but others recommend treatment of all exposed patients with doses of T_4 to suppress TSH.

Protracted ingestion of **medications** containing iodides—for example, expectorants—can cause hypothyroidism, usually accompanied by goiter (Chapter 561). Amiodarone, a drug used for cardiac arrhythmias and consisting of 37% iodine by weight, causes hypothyroidism in about 20% of treated children. It affects thyroid function directly by its high iodine content as well as by inhibition of 5′-deiodinase, which converts T_4 to T_3. Children treated with this drug should have serial measurements of T_4, T_3, and TSH. Children with Graves' disease treated with anti-thyroid drugs (methimazole or propylthiouracil) can develop hypothyroidism. Additional drugs that can produce hypothyroidism include lithium carbonate, interferon alpha, stavudine, thalidomide, valproate (subclinical), and aminoglutethimide.

Children with **nephropathic cystinosis,** a disorder characterized by intralysosomal storage of cystine in body tissues, acquire impaired thyroid function. Hypothyroidism may be overt, but subclinical forms are more common, and periodic assessment of TSH levels is indicated. By 13 yr of age, two thirds of these patients require T_4 replacement.

Histiocytic infiltration of the thyroid in children with Langerhans cell histiocytosis can result in hypothyroidism.

Children with chronic **hepatitis C infection** are at risk for subclinical hypothyroidism; this does not appear to be autoimmune, because anti-thyroid antibodies are negative.

Hypothyroidism can occur in children with large **hemangiomas** of the liver, because of increased type 3 deiodinase activity, which catalyzes conversion of T_4 to rT_3 and T_3 to T_2. Thyroid secretion is increased, but it is not sufficient to compensate for the large increase in degradation of T_4 to rT_3.

Some patients with congenital thyroid dysgenesis and residual thyroid function or with incomplete genetic defects in thyroid hormone synthesis do not display clinical manifestations until childhood and appear to have acquired hypothyroidism. Although these conditions are usually now detected by newborn screening programs, very mild defects can escape detection.

Any **hypothalamic** or **pituitary** disease can cause acquired central hypothyroidism (Chapter 551). TSH deficiency may be the result of a hypothalamic-pituitary tumor (craniopharyngioma most common in children) or a result of treatment for the tumor. Other causes include cranial radiation, head trauma, or diseases infiltrating the pituitary gland, such as Langerhans cell histiocytosis.

Table 559-3 ETIOLOGIC CLASSIFICATION OF ACQUIRED HYPOTHYROIDISM

Autoimmune (acquired hypothyroidism)
• Hashimoto thyroiditis
• Polyglandular autoimmune syndrome, types I and II
Iatrogenic
• Propylthiouracil, methimazole, iodides, lithium, amiodarone
• Irradiation
• Radioiodine
• Thyroidectomy
Systemic disease
• Cystinosis
• Langerhans cell histiocytosis
Hemangiomas (large) of the liver (type 3 iodothyronine deiodinase)
Hypothalamic-pituitary disease

Clinical Manifestations

Deceleration of growth is usually the first clinical manifestation, but this sign often goes unrecognized (Figs. 559-3 and 559-4). Goiter, which may be a presenting feature, typically is nontender and firm, with a rubbery consistency and a pebbly surface. Weight gain is mostly fluid retention (myxedema), not true obesity. Myxedematous changes of the skin, constipation, cold intolerance, decreased energy, and an increased need for sleep develop insidiously. Surprisingly, schoolwork and grades usually do not suffer, even in severely hypothyroid children. Additional features include bradycardia, muscle weakness or cramps, nerve entrapment, and ataxia. Osseous maturation is delayed, often strikingly, which is an indication of the duration of the hypothyroidism. Adolescents typically have delayed puberty; older adolescent girls manifest menometrorrhagia. Younger children might present with galactorrhea or pseudoprecocious puberty. Galactorrhea is a result of increased TRH stimulating prolactin secretion. The precocious puberty, characterized by breast development in girls and macroorchidism in boys, is thought to be the result of abnormally high TSH concentrations binding to the FSH, receptor with subsequent stimulation.

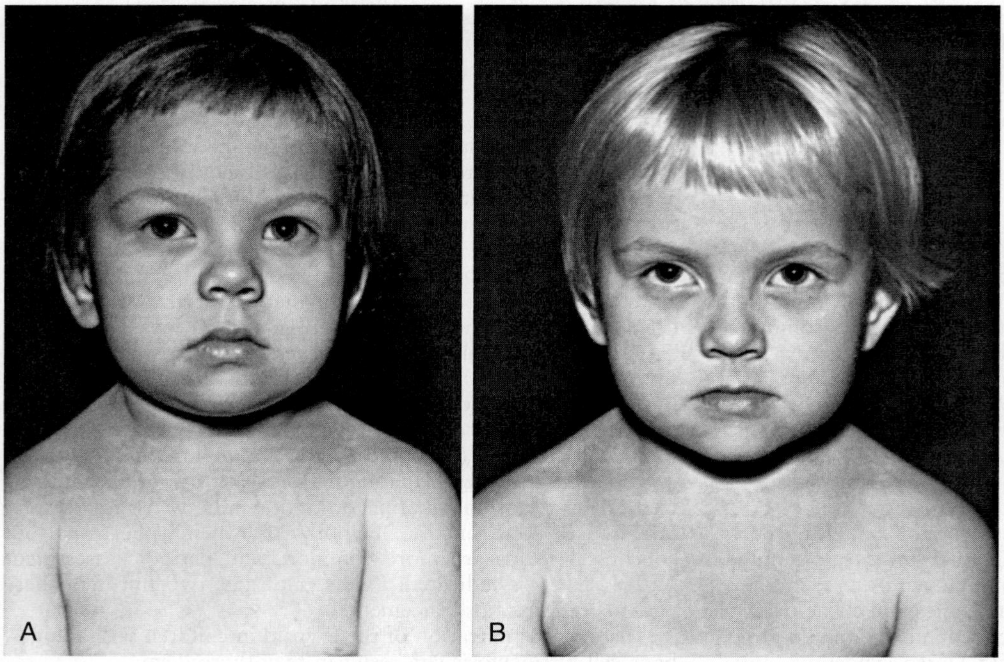

Figure 559-3 *A,* Acquired hypothyroidism in a girl 6 yr of age. She was treated with a wide variety of hematinics for refractory anemia for 3 yr. She had almost complete cessation of growth, constipation, and sluggishness for 3 yr. The height age was 3 yr; the bone age was 4 yr. She had a sallow complexion and immature facies with a poorly developed nasal bridge. Serum cholesterol, 501 mg/dL; radioiodine uptake, 7% at 24 hr; protein-bound iodine (PBI), 2.8 mg/dL. *B,* After therapy for 18 mo, note the nasal development, increased luster and decreased pigmentation of hair, and maturation of the face. The height age was 5.5 yr; the bone age was 7 yr. There was a decided improvement in her general condition. Menarche occurred at 14 yr. The ultimate height was 155 cm (61 in). She graduated from high school. The disorder was well controlled with sodium-L-thyroxine daily.

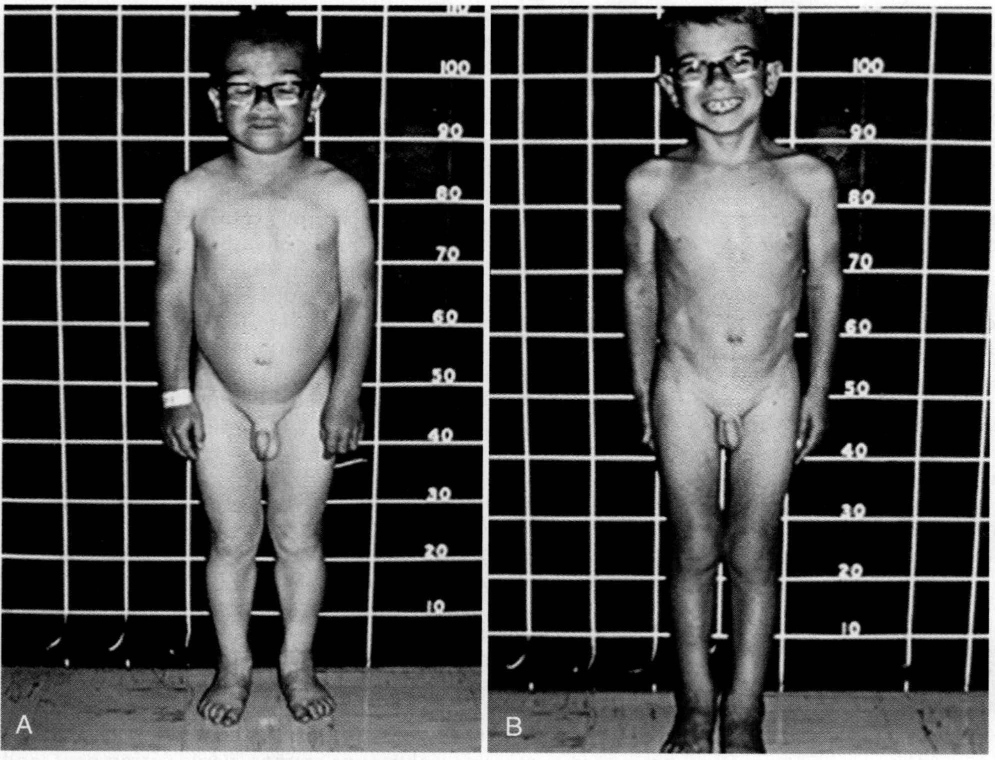

Figure 559-4 *A,* Short stature (108 cm, <3rd percentile), generalized myxedema, sleepy expression, protuberant abdomen, and coarse hair are signs of hypothyroidism in this 12-yr-old boy. Body proportions are immature for his age (1.25 : 1). *B,* Same boy 4 mo after treatment. His height increased by 4 cm; note the marked change in body habitus owing to loss of generalized myxedema, improved muscle tone, and bright facial expression. (From LaFranchi SH: Hypothyroidism, *Pediatr Clin North Am* 26:33–51, 1979.)

Some children have headaches and vision problems; they usually have hyperplastic enlargement of the pituitary gland, sometimes with suprasellar extension, after long-standing hypothyroidism; this condition, believed to be the result of thyrotroph hyperplasia, may be mistaken for a pituitary tumor (Chapter 551). Abnormal laboratory studies include hyponatremia, macrocytic anemia, hypercholesterolemia, and elevated CPK. Complications seen in severe hypothyroidism are noted in Table 559-4. All these changes return to normal with adequate replacement of T_4.

Diagnostic Studies

Children with suspected hypothyroidism should undergo measurement of serum free T_4 and TSH. Because the normal range for thyroid tests is slightly higher in children than adults, it is

Table 559-4 PATHOGENESIS OF GENERAL COMPLICATIONS IN MANAGEMENT OF COMPLICATED HYPOTHYROIDISM

COMPLICATION	PATHOGENESIS
Heart failure	Impaired ventricular systolic and diastolic functions and increased peripheral vascular resistance
Ventilatory failure	Blunted hypercapneic and hypoxic ventilatory drives
Hyponatremia	Impaired renal free water excretion and syndrome of inappropriate antidiuretic hormone secretion (SIADH)
Ileus	Bowel hypomotility
Medication sensitivity	Reduced clearance rate and increased sensitivity to sedative, analgesic, and anesthetic agents
Hypothermia and lack of febrile response to sepsis	Decreased calorigenesis
Delirium, dementia, seizure, stupor, and coma	Decreased central nervous system thyroid hormone actions, and encephalopathy due to hyponatremia and hypercapnia
Adrenal insufficiency	Associated intrinsic adrenal or pituitary disease, or reversible impairment of hypothalamic-pituitary-adrenal stress response
Coagulopathy	Acquired von Willebrand syndrome (type 1) and decreased factors VIII, VII, V, IX, and X

From Roberts CG, Landenson PW: Hypothyroidism, *Lancet* 363:793–803, 2004.

important to compare results to age-specific reference ranges. Measurement of antithyroglobulin and antiperoxidase (formerly, antimicrosomal) antibodies can pinpoint autoimmune thyroiditis as the cause. Generally, there is no indication for thyroid imaging. In cases with a goiter resulting from autoimmune thyroid disease, an ultrasound examination typically shows diffuse enlargement with scattered hypoechogenicity. Some children with acquired hypothyroidism and a goiter have a thyroid nodule discovered by palpation or neck sonography. Ultrasound examination is the most accurate method to follow nodule size and solid vs. cystic nature (Chapter 563.1). In children with a nodule and suppressed TSH, a radioactive iodine uptake and scan is indicated to determine if this is a "hot" or hyperfunctioning nodule. A bone age x-ray at diagnosis is useful, in that the degree of delay approximates duration and severity of hypothyroidism.

Treatment and Prognosis

Levothyroxine is the treatment of choice in children with hypothyroidism. The dose on a weight basis gradually decreases with age. For children 1-3 yr, the average L-T_4 dosage is 4-6 µg/kg/day; for 3-10 y4, 3-5 µg/kg/day; and for 10-16 yr, 2-4 µg/kg/day. Treatment should be monitored by measuring serum free T_4 and TSH every 4-6 mo as well as 6 wk after any change in dosage. In children with central hypothyroidism, where TSH levels are not helpful in monitoring treatment, the goal should be to maintain serum free T4 in the upper half of the normal reference range for age.

During the 1st yr of treatment, deterioration of schoolwork, poor sleeping habits, restlessness, short attention span, and behavioral problems might ensue, but these are transient; forewarning families about these manifestations enhances appropriate management. These may be partially ameliorated by starting at sub-replacement T_4 doses and advancing slowly. An occasional older child (8-13 yr) with acquired hypothyroidism may experience pseudotumor cerebri within the first 4 mo of treatment.

In older children, after catch-up growth is complete, the growth rate provides a good index of the adequacy of therapy. Periodic bone age x-rays are useful to monitor treatment and future growth potential. In children with long-standing hypothyroidism, catch-up growth may be incomplete (see Fig. 559-4). During the first 18 mo of treatment, skeletal maturation often exceeds expected linear growth, resulting in a loss of about 7 cm of predicted adult height; the cause is unknown.

BIBLIOGRAPHY

Please visit the Nelson Textbook of Pediatrics *website at www.expertconsult.com for the complete bibliography.*

Chapter 560 Thyroiditis

Stephen LaFranchi

LYMPHOCYTIC THYROIDITIS (HASHIMOTO THYROIDITIS, AUTOIMMUNE THYROIDITIS)

Lymphocytic thyroiditis is the most common cause of thyroid disease in children and adolescents and accounts for many of the enlarged thyroids formerly designated "adolescent" or "simple" goiter. It is also the most common cause of acquired hypothyroidism, with or without goiter.

One to 2% of younger school-aged children and 4-6% of adolescents have positive antithyroid antibodies as evidence of autoimmune thyroid disease.

Etiology

This typical organ-specific autoimmune disease is characterized histologically by lymphocytic infiltration of the thyroid. Early in the course of the disease, there may be hyperplasia only; this is followed by infiltration of lymphocytes and plasma cells between the follicles and by atrophy of the follicles. Lymphoid follicle formation with germinal centers is almost always present; the degree of atrophy and fibrosis of the follicles varies from mild to moderate.

Intrathyroidal lymphocyte subsets differ from those in blood. About 60% of infiltrating lymphoid cells are T cells, and about 30% express B-cell markers; the T-cell population is represented by helper ($CD4^+$) and cytotoxic ($CD8^+$) cells. The participation of cellular events in the pathogenesis is clear. Certain HLA haplotypes (HLA-DR4, HLA-DR5) are associated with an increased risk of goiter and thyroiditis, and others (HLA-DR3) are associated with the atrophic variant of thyroiditis.

A variety of different thyroid antigen autoantibodies are also involved. Thyroid antiperoxidase antibodies (TPOAbs; formerly called *antimicrosomal antibodies*) and antithyroglobulin antibodies are demonstrable in the sera of 90% of children with lymphocytic thyroiditis and in many patients with Graves disease. TPOAbs inhibit enzyme activity and stimulate natural killer cell cytotoxicity. Antithyroglobulin antibodies do not appear to play a role in the autoimmune destruction of the gland. Thyrotropin receptor–blocking antibodies are often present, especially in patients with hypothyroidism, and it is now believed that they are related to the development of hypothyroidism and thyroid atrophy in patients with autoimmune thyroiditis. Antibodies to pendrin, an apical protein on thyroid follicular cells, have been demonstrated in 80% of children with autoimmune thyroiditis.

Clinical Manifestations

The disorder is 2-4 times more common in girls than in boys. It can occur during the first 3 yr of life but becomes sharply more common after 6 yr of age and reaches a peak incidence during adolescence. The most common clinical manifestations are goiter and growth retardation. The goiter can appear insidiously and may be small or large. In most patients, the thyroid is diffusely enlarged, firm, and nontender. In about 30% of patients, the gland is lobular and can seem to be nodular. Most of the affected children are clinically euthyroid and asymptomatic; some may have symptoms of pressure in the neck, including difficulty swallowing and shortness of breath. Some children have clinical signs of hypothyroidism, but others who appear clinically euthyroid have laboratory evidence of hypothyroidism. A few children have manifestations suggesting hyperthyroidism, such as nervousness, irritability, increased sweating, and hyperactivity, but results of laboratory studies are not necessarily those of hyperthyroidism. Occasionally, the disorder coexists with Graves disease. Ophthalmopathy can occur in lymphocytic thyroiditis in the absence of Graves disease.

The clinical course is variable. The goiter might become smaller or might disappear spontaneously, or it might persist unchanged for years while the patient remains euthyroid. Most children who are euthyroid at presentation remain euthyroid, although a percentage of patients acquire hypothyroidism gradually within months or years. In children who initially have mild or subclinical hypothyroidism (elevated serum TSH, normal free T_4 level), over several years about 50% revert to euthyroidism, about 50% continue to have subclinical hypothyroidism, and a few develop overt hypothyroidism. Thyroiditis is the cause of most cases of nongoitrous (atrophic) hypothyroidism.

Familial clusters of lymphocytic thyroiditis are common; the incidence in siblings or parents of affected children may be as high as 25%. Autoantibodies to thyroglobulin and thyroid peroxidase in these families appear to be inherited in an autosomal dominant fashion, with reduced penetrance in males. The concurrence within families of patients with lymphocytic thyroiditis, "idiopathic" hypothyroidism, and Graves disease provides cogent evidence for a basic relationship among these 3 conditions.

The disorder has been associated with many other autoimmune disorders. Autoimmune thyroiditis occurs in 10% of patients with type I autoimmune polyglandular syndrome (APS-1), characterized by autoimmune polyendocrinopathy, candidiasis, and ectodermal dysplasia (APCED). APS-1 consists of 2 of the triad of hypoparathyroidism, Addison disease, and mucocutaneous candidiasis (HAM syndrome). This relatively rare autosomal recessive disorder occurs in childhood and is caused by mutations in the autoimmune regulatory *(AIRE)* gene on chromosome 21q22.3.

Autoimmune thyroiditis occurs in 70% of patients with APS-2 (Schmidt syndrome). APS-2 consists of the association of Addison disease with type 1 diabetes mellitus (T1DM) or autoimmune thyroid disease. The etiology is unknown, and it typically occurs in early adulthood. Autoimmune thyroid disease also tends to be associated with pernicious anemia, vitiligo, or alopecia. TPOAbs are found in approximately 20% of white and 4% of black children with T1DM. Autoimmune thyroid disease has an increased incidence in children with congenital rubella.

Lymphocytic thyroiditis is also associated with certain chromosomal disorders, particularly Turner syndrome and Down syndrome. In children with Down syndrome, one study reported that 28% had antithyroid antibodies (predominantly anti-TPOs), 7% had subclinical hypothyroidism, 7% had overt hypothyroidism, and 5% had hyperthyroidism. In a study of girls with Turner syndrome, 41% had antithyroid antibodies (again, predominantly anti-TPOs), 18% had goiter, and 8% had subclinical or overt hypothyroidism. Another study of 75 girls with Turner syndrome found that autoimmune thyroid disease increased from the 1st (15%) to the 3rd (30%) decade of life. Boys with Klinefelter syndrome are also at risk for autoimmune thyroid disease. The differential diagnosis is noted in Table 560-1.

Laboratory Findings

Thyroid function tests (free T_4 and TSH) are often normal, although the level of TSH may be slightly or even moderately elevated in some patients, termed *subclinical hypothyroidism.* The fact that many children with lymphocytic thyroiditis do not have elevated levels of TSH indicates that the goiter may be caused by the lymphocytic infiltrations or by thyroid growth-stimulating immunoglobulins. Young children with lymphocytic thyroiditis have serum antibody titers to TPO, but the antithyroglobulin test for thyroid antibodies is positive in <50%. Antibodies to TPO and thyroglobulin are found equally in adolescents with lymphocytic thyroiditis. When both tests are used, approximately 95% of patients with thyroid autoimmunity are detected. Levels in children and adolescents are lower than those in adults with lymphocytic thyroiditis, and repeated measurements are indicated in questionable instances because titers might increase later in the course of the disease.

Thyroid scans and ultrasonography usually are not needed. If they are done, thyroid scans reveal irregular and patchy distribution of the radioisotope, and in about 60% or more, the administration of perchlorate results in a >10% discharge of iodide from the thyroid gland. Thyroid ultrasonography shows scattered hypoechogenicity in most patients. The definitive diagnosis can be established by biopsy of the thyroid; this procedure is rarely clinically indicated.

Antithyroid antibodies may also be found in almost 50% of the siblings of affected patients and in a significant percentage of the mothers of children with Down syndrome or Turner syndrome without demonstrable thyroid disease. They are also

Table 560-1 CHARACTERISTICS OF THYROIDITIS SYNDROMES

CHARACTERISTIC	HASHIMOTO'S THYROIDITIS	PAINLESS POSTPARTUM THYROIDITIS	PAINLESS SPORADIC THYROIDITIS	PAINFUL SUBACUTE THYROIDITIS	ACUTE SUPPURATIVE THYROIDITIS	RIEDEL'S THYROIDITIS
Sex ratio (F:M)	8-9:1	—	2:1	5:1	1:1	3-4:1
Cause	Autoimmune	Autoimmune	Autoimmune	Unknown (Probably viral)	Infectious (Bacterial)	Unknown
Pathologic findings	Lymphocytic infiltration, germinal centers, fibrosis	Lymphocytic infiltration	Lymphocytic infiltration	Giant cells, granulomas	Abscess formation	Dense fibrosis
Thyroid function	Hypothyroidism	Thyrotoxicosis, hypothyroidism, or both	Thyrotoxicosis, hypothyroidism, or both	Thyrotoxicosis, hypothyroidism, or both	Usually euthyroidism	Usually euthyroidism
TPO antibodies	High titer, persistent	High titer, persistent	High titer, persistent	Low titer, or absent, or transient	Absent	Usually present
ESR	Normal	Normal	Normal	High	High	Normal
24-hour 123I uptake	Variable	<5%	<5%	<5%	Normal	Low or normal

ESR, erythrocyte sedimentation rate; ^{123}I, iodine 123; TPO, thyroid peroxidase.
From Pearce EN, Farwell AP, Braverman LE: Thyroiditis. *N Engl J Med* 348:2646–2654, 2003.

found in 20% of children with DM and in 23% of children with the congenital rubella syndrome.

Treatment

If there is evidence of hypothyroidism (overt or subclinical), replacement treatment with levothyroxine (at doses specific for size and age) is indicated. The goiter usually shows some decrease in size but can persist for years. In a euthyroid patient, treatment with suppressive doses of levothyroxine is unlikely to lead to a significant decrease in size of the goiter. Antibody levels fluctuate in both treated and untreated patients and persist for years. Because the disease is self-limited in some instances, the need for continued therapy requires periodic reevaluation. Untreated patients should also be checked periodically. Although there is some controversy about treating patients with subclinical hypothyroidism (normal T_4 or free T_4, elevated TSH), I prefer to treat such children until growth and puberty are complete, and then reevaluate their thyroid function.

Prominent **nodules**, i.e. >1.0 cm, that persist despite suppressive therapy should be examined histologically using fine needle aspiration (FNA), because thyroid carcinoma or lymphoma has occurred in patients with lymphocytic thyroiditis.

OTHER CAUSES OF THYROIDITIS

Acute suppurative thyroiditis is uncommon; it is usually preceded by a respiratory infection. The left lower lobe is affected predominantly. Abscess formation can occur. Anaerobic organisms, with or without aerobes, are the typical infectious agent. The most common organism is viridans streptococcus, followed by *Staphylococcus aureus* and pneumococcus. Recurrent episodes or detection of a mixed bacterial flora suggests that the infection arises from a **piriform sinus fistula** or, less commonly, from a **thyroglossal duct** remnant. Exquisite tenderness of the gland, swelling, erythema, dysphagia, and limitation of head motion are characteristic findings. Fever, chills, and sore throat are not uncommon, and leukocytosis is present. Scintigrams of the thyroid often reveal decreased uptake in the affected areas, and ultrasonography might show a complex echogenic mass. Thyroid function is usually normal, but thyrotoxicosis due to escape of thyroid hormone has been encountered in a child with suppurative thyroiditis resulting from *Aspergillus*. When abscesses form, incision and drainage and administration of parenteral antibiotics are indicated. After the infection subsides, a barium esophagram or CT scan with contrast is indicated to search for a fistulous tract; if one is found, surgical excision is indicated.

Subacute granulomatous thyroiditis (de Quervain disease) is rare in children. It is thought to have a viral cause and remits spontaneously. The disorder becomes manifested by an upper respiratory infection with vague tenderness over the thyroid and low-grade fever, followed by severe pain in the region of the thyroid gland. Inflammation results in leakage of preformed thyroid hormone from the gland into the circulation. Serum levels of T_4 and T_3 are elevated while TSH is suppressed, and mild symptoms of hyperthyroidism may be present, but radioiodine uptake is depressed. The erythrocyte sedimentation rate is increased. The course is variable but usually characterized by four phases: hyperthyroidism, usually followed by a euthyroid phase and then a hypothyroid phase, and remission usually occurring in several months, with recovery to euthyroidism.

Specific conditions such as tuberculosis, sarcoidosis, mumps, and cat-scratch disease are rare causes of thyroiditis in children. **Other forms of thyroiditis** seen in adults, such as painless sporadic thyroiditis and Riedel thyroiditis, are rare in children (see Table 560-1).

BIBLIOGRAPHY

Please visit the Nelson Textbook of Pediatrics *website at* *www.expertconsult.com* *for the complete bibliography.*

Chapter 561 Goiter

Stephen LaFranchi

A goiter is an enlargement of the thyroid gland. Persons with enlarged thyroids can have normal function of the gland (**euthyroidism**), thyroid deficiency (**hypothyroidism**), or overproduction of the hormones (**hyperthyroidism**). Goiter may be congenital or acquired, endemic, or sporadic.

The goiter often results from increased pituitary secretion of thyroid-stimulating hormone (TSH) in response to decreased circulating levels of thyroid hormones. Thyroid enlargement can also result from infiltrative processes that may be inflammatory or neoplastic. Goiter in patients with Graves disease and thyrotoxicosis is caused by thyrotropin receptor–stimulating antibodies (TRSAbs).

561.1 Congenital Goiter

Stephen LaFranchi

Congenital goiter is usually sporadic and can result from a fetal thyroxine (T_4) synthetic defect or from administration of antithyroid drugs or iodides during pregnancy for the treatment of maternal thyrotoxicosis. Goitrogenic drugs and iodides cross the placenta and at high doses can interfere with synthesis of thyroid hormone, resulting in goiter and hypothyroidism in the fetus. The concomitant administration of thyroid hormone with the goitrogen does not prevent this effect, because insufficient amounts of T_4 cross the placenta. Iodides are included in many proprietary cough preparations used to treat asthma; these preparations should be avoided during pregnancy because they have often been reported to cause congenital goiter. Amiodarone, an antiarrhythmic drug with 37% iodine content, has also caused congenital goiter with hypothyroidism. Even when the infant is clinically euthyroid, there may be retardation of osseous maturation, low levels of T_4, and elevated levels of TSH. In women with Graves disease receiving antithyroid drugs, these effects can occur when the mother takes propylthiouracil at only 100-200 mg/24 hr; all such infants should undergo thyroid studies at birth. Administration of thyroid hormone to affected infants may be indicated to treat clinical hypothyroidism, to hasten the disappearance of the goiter, and to prevent brain damage. Because the condition is rarely permanent, thyroid hormone may be safely discontinued after the antithyroid drug has been excreted by the neonate, usually after 1-2 wk.

Enlargement of the thyroid at birth may occasionally be sufficient to cause respiratory distress that interferes with nursing and can even cause death. The head may be maintained in extreme hyperextension. When respiratory obstruction is severe, partial thyroidectomy rather than tracheostomy is indicated (Fig. 561-1).

Goiter is almost always present in the infant with neonatal Graves' disease. These goiters usually are not large; the infant manifests clinical symptoms of hyperthyroidism. The mother often has a history of Graves disease, although discovery of neonatal hyperthyroidism can lead to the diagnosis of maternal Graves' disease. Thyroid enlargement results from transplacental passage of maternal thyroid-stimulating immunoglobulin (Chapter 562.1). TSH receptor-activating mutations are also a recognized cause of congenital goiter and hyperthyroidism.

When no causative factor is identifiable, a **defect in synthesis** of thyroid hormone should be suspected. Neonatal screening programs find congenital hypothyroidism caused by such a defect in 1/30,000-50,000 live births. It is advisable to treat immediately with thyroid hormone and to postpone more-detailed studies for later in life. If a specific defect is suspected, genetic tests to identify

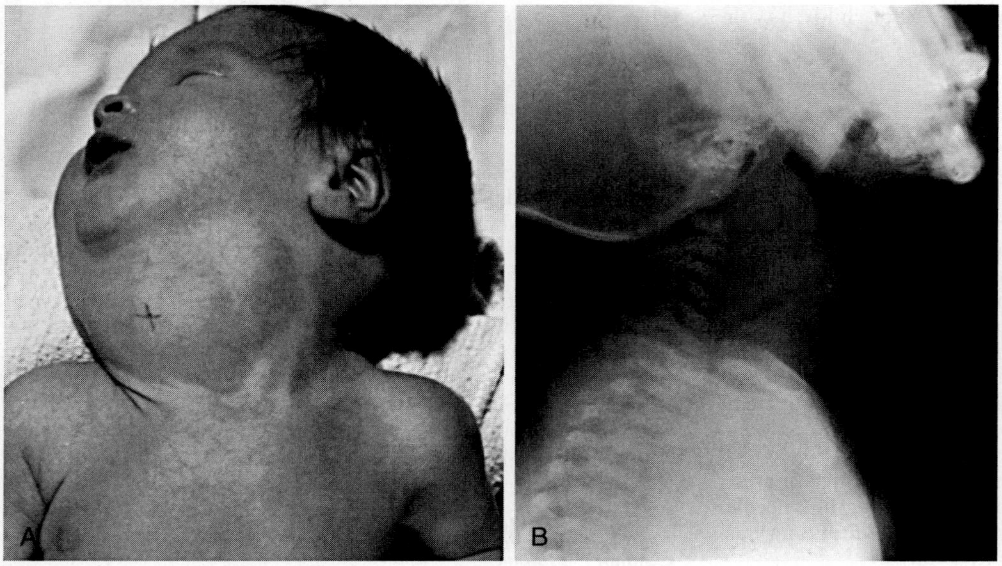

Figure 561-1 Congenital goiter in infancy. *A,* Large congenital goiter in an infant born to a mother with thyrotoxicosis who had been treated with iodides and methimazole during pregnancy. *B,* A different infant, 6 wk old, with increasing respiratory distress and cervical mass since birth. The operation revealed a large goiter that almost completely encircled the trachea. Notice the anterior deviation and posterior compression of the trachea. Partial thyroidectomy completely relieved the symptoms. It is apparent why a tracheostomy is not adequate treatment for these infants. The cause for the goiter was not found.

a mutation may be undertaken (Chapter 559). Because these defects are transmitted by recessive genes, a precise diagnosis is helpful for genetic counseling. Monitoring subsequent pregnancies with ultrasonography can be useful in detecting fetal goiters (Chapter 90).

Pendred's syndrome, characterized by familial goiter and neurosensory deafness, is caused by a mutation in the pendrin gene, which codes for a chloride-iodide transport protein present in the thyroid gland and cochlea. This defect results in abnormal iodide organification in the thyroid and can cause a goiter at birth. The more common presentation is a euthyroid goiter and deafness later in life.

Iodine deficiency as a cause of congenital goiter is rare in developed countries but persists in isolated endemic areas (see later). More important is the recognition that severe iodine deficiency early in pregnancy can cause neurologic damage during fetal development, even in the absence of goiter. The iodine deficiency can result in maternal and fetal hypothyroidism, preventing the partially protective transfer of maternal thyroid hormones.

When the "goiter" is lobulated, asymmetric, firm, or large to an unusual degree, a teratoma within or in the vicinity of the thyroid must be considered in the differential diagnosis (Chapter 563).

BIBLIOGRAPHY

Please visit the Nelson Textbook of Pediatrics *website at* *www.expertconsult.com* *for the complete bibliography.*

561.2 Intratracheal Goiter

Stephen LaFranchi

One of the many ectopic locations of thyroid tissue is within the trachea. The intraluminal thyroid lies beneath the tracheal mucosa and is often continuous with the normally situated extratracheal thyroid. The thyroid tissue is susceptible to goitrous enlargement, which involves the normally situated and the ectopic thyroid. When there is obstruction of the airway associated with a goiter, it must be ascertained whether the obstruction is extratracheal or endotracheal. If obstructive manifestations are mild, administration of sodium L-thyroxine usually causes the goiter to decrease in size. When symptoms are severe, surgical removal of the endotracheal goiter is indicated.

561.3 Endemic Goiter and Cretinism

Stephen LaFranchi

ETIOLOGY

The association between dietary deficiency of iodine and the prevalence of goiter or cretinism is well established. A moderate deficiency of iodine can be overcome by increased efficiency in the synthesis of thyroid hormone. Iodine liberated in the tissues is returned rapidly to the gland, which resynthesizes triiodothyronine (T_3) preferentially at a higher rate than normal. This increased activity is achieved by compensatory hypertrophy and hyperplasia (goiter), which satisfy the demands of the tissues for thyroid hormone. In geographic areas where deficiency of iodine is severe, decompensation and hypothyroidism can result. It is estimated that 1 billion persons in developing countries live in areas of iodine deficiency.

Seawater is rich in iodine; the iodine content of fish and shellfish is also high. Endemic goiter is therefore rare in populations living along the coast. Iodine is deficient in the water and native foods in the Pacific West and the Great Lakes areas of the United States. Deficiency of dietary iodine is even greater in certain Alpine valleys, the Himalayas, the Andes, the Congo, and the highlands of Papua New Guinea. In areas such as the United States, where iodine is provided in foods from other areas and in iodized salt, endemic goiter has disappeared. Iodized salt in the United States contains potassium iodide (100 µg/g), which provides excellent prophylaxis. Further iodine intake in the United States is contributed by iodates used in baking, iodine-containing coloring agents, and iodine-containing disinfectants used in the dairy industry. The recommended daily allowance of iodine is as follows:

- Newborn to 5 yr: 90 µg/day
- Ages 6-12 yr: 120 µg/day
- >12 yr and adults: 150 µg/day
- Pregnant and lactating women: 225 µg/day

The intake of iodine in adults in the United States decreased by approximately 50% from the 1970s to the 1990s, as reflected by a drop in median urinary iodine excretion from 320 µg/L to 145 µg/L. This decrease appears to have stabilized; the most recent NHANES (National Health and Nutrition Examination

Survey) from 2001-2002 reports median urinary iodine excretion of 167.8 μg/L. However, approximately 15% of women of reproductive age have iodine excretion <100 μg/L.

CLINICAL MANIFESTATIONS

If the deficiency of iodine is mild, thyroid enlargement does not become noticeable except when there is increased demand for the hormone during periods of rapid growth, as in adolescence and during pregnancy. In regions of moderate iodine deficiency, goiter observed in school children can disappear with maturity and reappear during pregnancy or lactation. Iodine-deficient goiters are more common in girls than in boys. In areas where iodine deficiency is severe, as in the hyperendemic highlands of Papua New Guinea, nearly half the population has large goiters, and endemic cretinism is common (Fig. 561-2).

Serum T_4 levels are often low in persons with endemic goiter, although clinical hypothyroidism is rare. This is true in New Guinea, the Congo, the Himalayas, and South America. Despite low serum T_4 levels, serum TSH concentrations are often normal or only moderately increased. In such patients, circulating levels of T_3 are elevated. Moreover, T_3 levels are also elevated in patients with normal T_4 levels, indicating a preferential secretion of T_3 by the thyroid in this disease.

Endemic cretinism is the most serious consequence of iodine deficiency; it occurs only in geographic association with endemic goiter. The term *endemic cretinism* includes 2 different but overlapping syndromes—a **neurologic type** and a **myxedematous type.** The incidence of the 2 types varies among different populations. In Papua New Guinea, the neurologic type occurs almost exclusively, whereas in the Congo, the myxedematous type predominates. Both types are found in all endemic areas, and some persons have intermediate or mixed features.

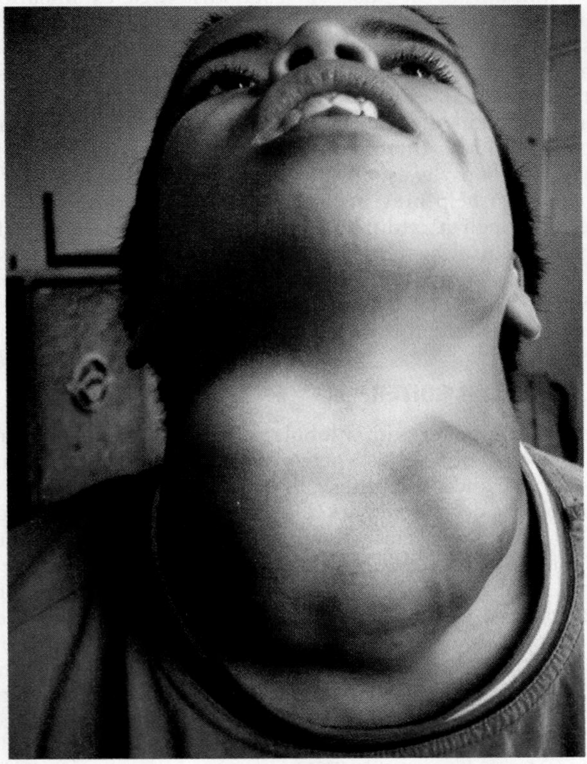

Figure 561-2 A 14 yr old boy with a large nodular goiter was seen in 2004, in an area of severe iodine-deficiency disorders in northern Morocco. He had tracheal and esophageal compression and hoarseness, probably due to damage to the recurrent laryngeal nerves. (From Zimmernamm MB, Jooste PL, Pandav CS: Iodine-deficiency disorders, *Lancet* 372:1251–1262, 2008.)

The **neurologic syndrome** is characterized by mental retardation, deaf-mutism, disturbances in standing and gait, and pyramidal signs such as clonus of the foot, the Babinski sign, and patellar hyperreflexia. Affected persons are goitrous but euthyroid, have normal pubertal development and adult stature, and have little or no impaired thyroid function. Persons with the **myxedematous syndrome** also are mentally retarded and deaf and have neurologic symptoms, but in contrast to the neurologic type they have delayed growth and sexual development, myxedema, and absence of goiter. Serum T_4 levels are low and TSH levels are markedly elevated. Delayed skeletal maturation may extend into the 3rd decade or later. Ultrasonographic examination shows thyroid atrophy.

PATHOGENESIS

The pathogenesis of the **neurologic syndrome** has been attributed to iodine deficiency and hypothyroxinemia during pregnancy, leading to fetal and postnatal hypothyroidism. Although some investigators have attributed brain damage to a direct effect of elemental iodine deficiency in the fetus, most believe the neurologic symptoms are caused by fetal and maternal hypothyroxinemia. There is evidence for the presence of thyroid hormone receptors in the fetal brain as early as 7 wk of gestation. Although the normal fetal thyroid gland does not begin to produce significant amounts of thyroid hormone until mid-gestation, there is measurable T_4 in the coelomic fluid as early as 6 weeks, almost certainly of maternal origin. These lines of evidence support a role for maternal thyroid hormone in fetal brain development in the first trimester. In addition, there is evidence of transplacental passage of maternal thyroid hormone into the fetus, which normally might ameliorate the effects of fetal hypothyroidism on the developing nervous system in the second half of pregnancy. Thus, iodine deficiency in the mother affects fetal brain development both in the first trimester and throughout pregnancy. Intake of iodine after birth is often sufficient for normal or only minimally impaired thyroid function.

The pathogenesis of the **myxedematous syndrome** leading to thyroid atrophy is more bewildering. Searches for additional environmental factors that might provoke continuing postnatal hypothyroidism have led to incrimination of selenium deficiency, goitrogenic foods, thiocyanates, and *Yersinia* (Table 561-1). Studies from western China suggest that thyroid autoimmunity might play a role. Children with myxedematous cretinism with thyroid atrophy, but not children with euthyroid cretinism, were found to have thyroid growth-blocking immunoglobulins of the kind found in infants with sporadic congenital hypothyroidism. Others are skeptical about any role of thyroid growth-blocking immunoglobulins to explain these findings.

TREATMENT

In many developing countries, administration of a single intramuscular injection of iodinated poppy seed oil to women prevents iodine deficiency during future pregnancies for about 5 yr. This form of therapy given to children younger than 4 yr of age with myxedematous cretinism results in a euthyroid state in 5 mo. Older children respond poorly and adults not at all to iodized oil injections, indicating an inability of the thyroid gland to synthesize hormone; these patients require treatment with T_4. Through the efforts of the World Health Organization and its program of universal salt iodization, endemic iodine deficiency worldwide has been reduced by approximately 50%. In the Xinjiang province of China, where the usual methods of iodine supplementation had failed, iodination of irrigation water has increased iodine levels in soil, animals, and human beings. In other countries, iodinated salt in school meal programs gives children the dietary iodine they need. Still, political, economic, and practical obstacles

Table 561-1 GOITROGENS AND THEIR MECHANISM

GOITROGEN	MECHANISM
FOODS	
Cassava, lima beans, linseed, sorghum, sweet potato	Contain cyanogenic glucosides that are metabolized to thiocyanates that compete with iodine for uptake by the thyroid
Cruciferous vegetables such as cabbage, kale, cauliflower, broccoli, turnips, rapeseed	Contain glucosinolates; metabolites compete with iodine for uptake by the thyroid
Soy, millet	Flavonoids impair thyroid peroxidase activity
INDUSTRIAL POLLUTANTS	
Perchlorate	Competitive inhibitor of the sodium-iodine symporter, decreasing iodine transport into the thyroid
Others (e.g., disulfides from coal processes)	Reduce thyroidal iodine uptake
Smoking	An important goitrogen; smoking during breast-feeding is associated with reduced iodine concentrations in breast milk; high serum concentration of thiocyanate due to smoking might compete with iodine for active transport into the secretory epithelium of the lactating breast
NUTRIENTS	
Selenium deficiency	Accumulated peroxides can damage the thyroid, and deiodinase deficiency impairs thyroid hormone synthesis
Iron deficiency	Reduces heme-dependent thyroperoxidase activity in the thyroid and might blunt the efficacy of iodine prophylaxis
Vitamin A deficiency	Increases TSH stimulation and goiter through decreased vitamin A–mediated suppression of the pituitary TSH-β gene

TSH, thyroid-stimulating hormone.
From Zimmernamm MB, Jooste PL, Pandav CS: Iodine-deficiency disorders, *Lancet* 372:1251–1262, 2008.

have limited penetration of iodized food into regular diets around the world.

BIBLIOGRAPHY

Please visit the Nelson Textbook of Pediatrics *website at* *www.expertconsult.com* *for the complete bibliography.*

561.4 Acquired Goiter

Stephen LaFranchi

Most acquired goiters are sporadic and develop from a variety of causes; patients are usually euthyroid but may be hypothyroid or hyperthyroid. The most common cause of acquired goiter is lymphocytic thyroiditis (Chapter 560). A rare cause in children is subacute thyroiditis (De Quervain disease) (Chapter 560). Other causes include excess iodide ingestion and certain drugs, including amiodarone and lithium. Intrinsic biochemical defects in the synthesis of thyroid hormone are almost always associated with goiter; milder defects occur later in childhood. The occurrence of the disorder in siblings, onset in early life, and possible association with hypothyroidism (goitrous hypothyroidism) are important clues to the diagnosis.

IODIDE GOITER

A small percentage of patients treated with iodide preparations for prolonged periods acquire goiters. Iodides are commonly included for their expectorant effect in cough medicines and in proprietary mixtures for asthma. Goiters resulting from iodide administration are firm and diffusely enlarged, and in some instances hypothyroidism develops. In normal persons, acute administration of large doses of iodide inhibits the organification of iodine and the synthesis of thyroid hormone (Wolff-Chaikoff effect). This effect is short-lived and does not lead to permanent hypothyroidism. When iodide administration continues, an autoregulatory mechanism in normal persons limits iodide trapping and permits the level of iodide in the thyroid to decrease and organification to proceed normally. In patients with iodide-induced goiter, this escape does not occur because of an underlying abnormality of biosynthesis of thyroid hormone. The persons most susceptible to the development of iodide goiter are those with lymphocytic thyroiditis or with a subclinical inborn error in thyroid hormone synthesis and those who have had a partial thyroidectomy.

Lithium carbonate, which is used to treat bipolar disorder, also causes goiters and mild hypothyroidism. Lithium competes with iodide, resulting in decreased T_4 and T_3 synthesis and release; the mechanism producing the goiter or hypothyroidism is similar to that described for iodide goiter. Lithium and iodide also act synergistically to produce goiter; their combined use should be avoided.

Amiodarone, a drug used to treat cardiac arrhythmias, can cause thyroid dysfunction with goiter because it is rich in iodine. It is also a potent inhibitor of 5′-deiodinase, preventing conversion of T_4 to T_3. It can cause hypothyroidism, particularly in patients with underlying autoimmune disease; in other patients, it can cause hyperthyroidism.

SIMPLE GOITER (COLLOID GOITER)

A few children with euthyroid goiters have simple goiters, a condition of unknown cause not associated with hypothyroidism or hyperthyroidism and not caused by inflammation or neoplasia. The condition predominates in girls and has a peak incidence before and during the pubertal years. Histologic examination of the thyroid either is normal or reveals variable follicular size, dense colloid, and flattened epithelium. The goiter may be small or large. It is firm in half the patients and occasionally is asymmetric or nodular. Levels of TSH are normal or low, scintiscans are normal, and thyroid antibodies are absent. Differentiation from lymphocytic thyroiditis might not be possible without a biopsy, but biopsy is usually not indicated. Therapy with thyroid hormone can help prevent progression to a large multinodular goiter, although it is difficult to separate any treatment effects from the natural history, which is for the goiter to decrease in size. Patients should be reevaluated periodically, because some have antibody-negative lymphocytic thyroiditis and therefore are at risk for changes in thyroid function (Chapter 560).

MULTINODULAR GOITER

Rarely, a firm goiter with a lobulated surface and single or multiple palpable nodules is encountered. Areas of cystic change, hemorrhage, and fibrosis may be present. The incidence of this condition has decreased markedly with the use of iodine-enriched salt. A mild goitrogenic stimulus, acting over a long time, is thought to be the cause. Ultrasonographic examination can reveal multiple echo-free and echogenic lesions that are nonfunctioning on scintiscans. Thyroid studies are usually normal. Some children with chronic lymphocytic thyroiditis develop multinodular goiter; TSH may be elevated, and thyroid antibodies may be present.

Children can develop toxic multinodular goiter, characterized by a suppressed TSH and hyperthyroidism. The condition occurs in children with **McCune-Albright syndrome** (usually resulting in hyperthyroidism), with **TSH receptor activating mutations,** and it has been described in 3 children (including 2 siblings) with digital anomalies and cystic kidney disease. Dominant nodules within a multinodular goiter, particularly those not suppressed by replacement therapy with T_4, may be an indication for evaluation by fine-needle aspiration because malignancy cannot readily be ruled out.

TOXIC GOITER (HYPERTHYROIDISM)

See Chapter 562.

BIBLIOGRAPHY
Please visit the Nelson Textbook of Pediatrics *website at www.expertconsult.com for the complete bibliography.*

Chapter 562
Hyperthyroidism
Stephen LaFranchi

Hyperthyroidism results from excessive secretion of thyroid hormone; during childhood, with few exceptions, it is due to Graves disease (Table 562-1). **Graves disease** is an autoimmune disorder; production of thyroid-stimulating immunoglobulin (TSI) results in diffuse toxic goiter. Germline mutations of the **thyroid-stimulating hormone (TSH) receptor** resulting in constitutively activating (gain-of-function) mutations are found in both familial (autosomal dominant) and sporadic cases of nonautoimmune hyperthyroidism. These patients, whose disease can appear in the neonatal period or in later childhood, have thyroid hyperplasia with goiter and suppressed levels of TSH. Different activating mutations have been identified in some cases of thyroid adenomas. Hyperthyroidism occurs in some patients with **McCune-Albright syndrome** as a result of an activating mutation of the α subunit of the G-protein; these patients tend to have a multinodular goiter. Other rare causes of hyperthyroidism that have been observed in children include toxic uninodular goiter (Plummer disease), hyperfunctioning thyroid carcinoma, thyrotoxicosis factitia, subacute thyroiditis, and acute suppurative thyroiditis.

Suppression of plasma TSH indicates that the hyperthyroidism is not pituitary in origin. Hyperthyroidism due to excess thyrotropin secretion is rare and, in most cases, is caused by pituitary resistance to thyroid hormone. TSH-secreting pituitary tumors have been reported only in adults. In infants born to mothers with Graves disease, hyperthyroidism is almost always a transitory phenomenon; classic Graves disease during the neonatal period is rare. Choriocarcinoma, hydatidiform mole, and struma ovarii have caused hyperthyroidism in adults but have not been recognized as causes in children.

Studies have examined the health and quality of life of subjects with subclinical hyperthyroidism (i.e., with TSH <0.1 mU/L) or who are euthyroid on antithyroid medication. These studies suggest that subclinical hyperthyroidism carries a risk of late-life atrial fibrillation and that treatment of hyperthyroidism with antithyroid medication does not reliably induce remission that is durable when medication is discontinued. There appears to be no difference in long-term quality of life among hyperthyroid patients treated with antithyroid medication, radioiodine ablation, or surgery. Quality of life was diminished relative to control subjects in all three cases (Chapter 562.1).

Table 562-1 CAUSES OF HYPERTHYROIDISM

CAUSES OF HYPERTHYROIDISM	PATHOPHYSIOLOGIC FEATURES	INCIDENCE
CIRCULATING THYROID STIMULATORS		
Graves disease	Thyroid-stimulating immunoglobulins	Common
Neonatal Graves disease	Thyroid-stimulating immunoglobulins	Rare
Thyrotropin-secreting tumor	Pituitary adenoma	Very rare
Choriocarcinoma	Human chorionic gonadatropin secretion	Rare
THYROIDAL AUTONOMY		
Toxic multinodular goiter	Activating mutations in thyrotropin receptor or G-protein	Common
Toxic solitary adenoma	Activating mutations in thyrotropin receptor or G-protein	Common
Congenital hyperthyroidism	Activating mutations in thyrotropin receptor	Very rare
Iodine-induced hyperthyroidism (Jod-Basedow)	Unknown; excess iodine results in unregulated thyroid hormone production	Uncommon in USA and other iodine-sufficient areas
DESTRUCTION OF THYROID FOLLICLES (THYROIDITIS)		
Subacute thyroiditis	Probable viral infection	Uncommon
Painless or postpartum thyroiditis	Autoimmune	Common
Amiodarone-induced thyroiditis	Direct toxic drug effects	Uncommon
Acute (infectious) thyroiditis	Thyroid infection (e.g., bacterial, fungal)	Uncommon
EXOGENOUS THYROID HORMONE		
Iatrogenic	Excess ingestion of thyroid hormone	Common
Factitious	Excess ingestion of thyroid hormone	Rare
Hamburger thyrotoxicosis	Thyroid gland included in ground beef	Probably rare
ECTOPIC THYROID TISSUE		
Struma ovarii	Ovarian teratoma containing thyroid tissue	Rare
Metastatic follicular thyroid cancer	Large tumor mass capable of secreting thyroid hormone autonomously	Rare
Pituitary resistance to thyroid hormone	Mutated thyroid hormone receptor with greater expression in the pituitary compared with peripheral tissues	Rare

Adapted from Cooper DS: Hyperthyroidism, *Lancet* 362:459–468, 2003.

562.1 Graves Disease
Stephen LaFranchi

EPIDEMIOLOGY

Graves disease occurs in approximately 0.02% of children (1:5,000). It has a peak incidence in the 11- to 15-yr old; there is a 5:1 female to male ratio. Most children with Graves disease have a positive family history of some form of autoimmune thyroid disease. In Japan, familial Graves disease, defined as Graves disease in a 1st-degree relative, occurs in 2-3% of cases.

ETIOLOGY

Enlargement of the thymus, splenomegaly, lymphadenopathy, infiltration of the thyroid gland and retro-orbital tissues with lymphocytes and plasma cells, and peripheral lymphocytosis are well-established findings in Graves disease. In the thyroid gland, T helper cells ($CD4^+$) predominate in dense lymphoid aggregates; in areas of lower cell density, cytotoxic T cells ($CD8^+$) predominate. The percentage of activated B lymphocytes infiltrating the thyroid is higher than in peripheral blood. A postulated failure of T suppressor cells allows expression of T helper cells, sensitized to the TSH antigen, which interact with B cells. These cells differentiate into plasma cells, which produce thyrotropin receptor–stimulating antibody (TRSAb). TRSAb binds to the receptor for TSH and stimulates cyclic adenosine monophosphate, resulting in thyroid hyperplasia and unregulated overproduction of thyroid hormone. In addition to TRSAb, thyrotropin receptor-blocking antibody (TRBAb) may also be produced, and the clinical course of the disease usually correlates with the ratio between the two antibodies.

The ophthalmopathy occurring in Graves disease appears to be caused by antibodies against antigens shared by the thyroid and eye muscle. TSH receptors have been identified in retro-orbital adipocytes and might represent a target for antibodies. The antibodies that bind to the extraocular muscles and orbital fibroblasts stimulate the synthesis of glycosaminoglycans by orbital fibroblasts and produce cytotoxic effects on muscle cells.

In whites, Graves disease is associated with HLA-B8 and HLA-DR3; the latter carries a 7-fold relative risk for Graves disease. Graves disease is also associated with other HLA-D3–related disorders such as Addison disease, type 1 diabetes mellitus, myasthenia gravis, and celiac disease. Systemic lupus erythematosus, rheumatoid arthritis, vitiligo, idiopathic thrombocytopenic purpura, and pernicious anemia have been described in children with Graves disease. In family clusters, the conditions associated most commonly with Graves disease are autoimmune lymphocytic thyroiditis and hypothyroidism. In Japanese children, Graves disease is associated with different HLA haplotypes: HLA-DRB1*0405 and HLA-DQB1*0401.

CLINICAL MANIFESTATIONS

About 5% of all patients with hyperthyroidism are <15 yr of age; the peak incidence in these children occurs during adolescence. Although rare, Graves disease has begun between 6 wk and 2 yr of age in children born to mothers without a history of hyperthyroidism. The incidence is about 5 times higher in girls than in boys.

The clinical course in children is highly variable but usually is not so fulminant as in many adults (Table 562-2). Symptoms develop gradually; the usual interval between onset and diagnosis is 6-12 mo and may be longer in prepubertal children compared with adolescents. The earliest signs in children may be emotional disturbances accompanied by motor hyperactivity. The children become irritable and excitable, and they cry easily because of emotional lability. They are restless sleepers and tend to kick their covers off. Their schoolwork suffers as a result of a short attention span and poor sleep. Tremor of the fingers can be noticed if the arm is extended. There may be a voracious appetite combined with loss of or no increase in weight. Recent height measurements might show an acceleration in growth velocity.

The size of the thyroid is variable. It may be so minimally enlarged that it initially escapes detection, but with careful examination, a diffuse goiter, soft with a smooth surface, is found in almost all patients. Exophthalmos is noticeable in most patients but is usually mild. Lagging of the upper eyelid as the eye looks downward, impairment of convergence, and retraction of the upper eyelid and infrequent blinking may be present (Figs. 562-1 and 562-2). Ocular manifestations can produce pain, lid erythema, chemosis, decreased extraocular muscle function, and decreased visual acuity (corneal or optic nerve involvement). The skin is smooth and flushed, with excessive sweating. Muscular weakness is uncommon but may be severe enough to result in clumsiness. Tachycardia, palpitations, dyspnea, and cardiac enlargement and insufficiency cause discomfort but rarely endanger the patient's life. Atrial fibrillation is a rare complication. Mitral regurgitation, probably resulting from papillary muscle dysfunction, is the cause of the apical systolic murmur present in some patients. The systolic blood pressure and the pulse pressure are increased. Reflexes are brisk, especially the return phase of the Achilles reflex. Many of the findings in Graves disease result from hyperactivity of the sympathetic nervous system.

Thyroid crisis, or **thyroid storm,** is a form of hyperthyroidism manifested by an acute onset, hyperthermia, severe tachycardia, heart failure, and restlessness. There may be rapid progression to delirium, coma, and death. Precipitating events include trauma, infection, radioactive iodine treatment, or surgery. **Apathetic, or masked, hyperthyroidism** is another variety of hyperthyroidism characterized by extreme listlessness, apathy, and cachexia. A combination of both forms can occur. These symptom complexes are rare in children.

Table 562-2 MAJOR SYMPTOMS AND SIGNS OF HYPERTHYROIDISM AND OF GRAVES DISEASE AND CONDITIONS ASSOCIATED WITH GRAVES DISEASE

MANIFESTATIONS OF HYPERTHYROIDISM
Symptoms
Hyperactivity, irritability, altered mood, insomnia, anxiety
Heat intolerance, increased sweating
Palpitations
Fatigue, weakness
Dyspnea
Weight loss with increased appetite (weight gain in 10% of patients)
Pruritus
Increased stool frequency
Thirst and polyuria
Oligomenorrhea or amenorrhea
Signs
Sinus tachycardia, atrial fibrillation (rare in children), supraventricular tachycardia
Fine tremor, hyperkinesis, hyperreflexia
Warm, moist skin
Palmar erythema, onycholysis
Hair loss
Osteoporosis
Muscle weakness and wasting
High-output heart failure
Chorea
Periodic (hypokalemic) paralysis (primarily in Asian men)
Psychosis (rare)
MANIFESTATIONS OF GRAVES DISEASE
Diffuse goiter
Ophthalmopathy
A feeling of grittiness and discomfort in the eye
Retrobulbar pressure or pain
Eyelid lag or retraction
Periorbital edema, chemosis, scleral injection
Exophthalmos (proptosis)
Extraocular muscle dysfunction
Exposure keratitis
Optic neuropathy
Localized dermopathy (rare in children)
Lymphoid hyperplasia
Thyroid acropachy (rare in children)
CONDITIONS ASSOCIATED WITH GRAVES DISEASE
Type 1 diabetes mellitus
Addison disease
Vitiligo
Pernicious anemia
Alopecia areata
Myasthenia gravis
Celiac disease

Adapted from Weetman AP: Graves disease, *N Engl J Med* 343:1236–1248, 2000.

LABORATORY FINDINGS

Serum levels of thyroxine (T_4), triiodothyronine (T_3), free T_4, and free T_3 are elevated. In some patients, levels of T_3 may be more elevated than those of T_4. Levels of TSH are suppressed to below

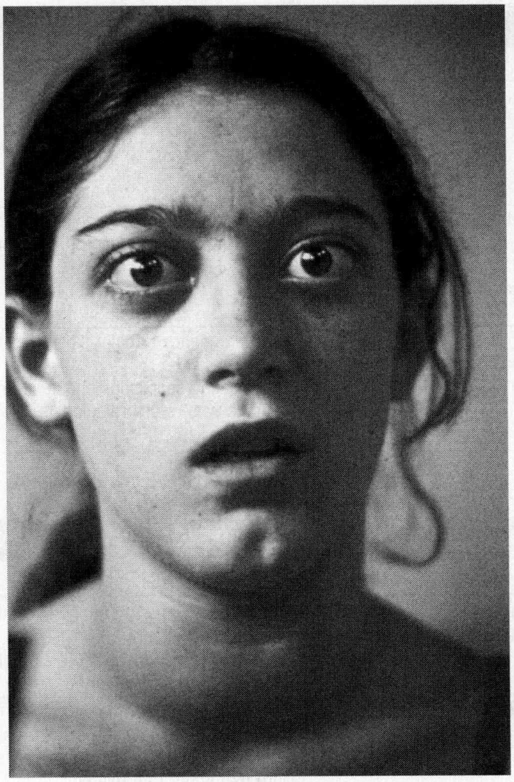

Figure 562-1 A 15 yr old girl with classic Graves disease. Clinical features include a goiter and exophthalmos. She was treated with antithyroid drugs, to which she had a good response.

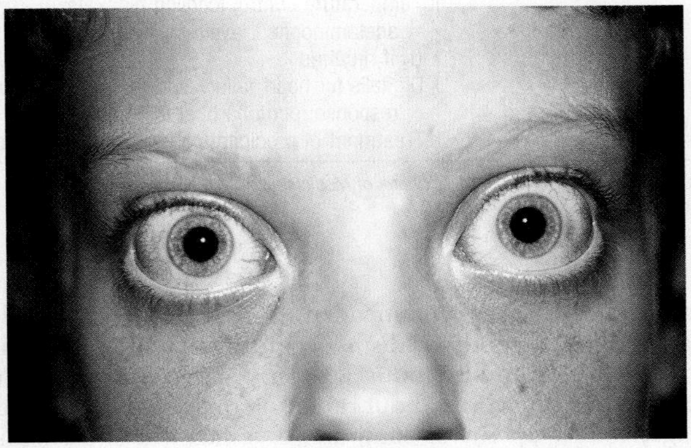

Figure 562-2 Retraction of upper eyelids in the primary gaze (Dalrymple sign). (From Kanski JJ: *Systemic diseases and the eye: signs and differential diagnosis,* London, 2001, Mosby.)

the lower range of normal. Antithyroid antibodies, including thyroid peroxidase antibodies, are often present. Most patients with newly diagnosed Graves disease have measurable TRSAb; the two methods to measure TRSAb are thyroid-stimulating immunoglobulin (TSI) or thyrotropin-binding inhibitor immunoglobulin (TBII). Measurement of TSI or TBII is useful in confirming the diagnosis of Graves disease. Radioiodine is rapidly and diffusely concentrated in the thyroid, but this study is rarely necessary. Children who experience an acceleration of growth might also have advanced skeletal maturation. Bone density may be reduced at diagnosis but returns to normal with treatment.

DIFFERENTIAL DIAGNOSIS

Diagnosis is rarely difficult once hyperthyroidism is considered. Elevated levels of T_4 or free T_4 and T_3 in association with suppressed levels of TSH are usually diagnostic (see Table 562-1). The presence of TRSAb establishes the cause as Graves disease.

Other causes of hyperthyroidism are uncommon. If a thyroid nodule is palpable, or if T_3 is preferentially elevated, a functional thyroid nodule must be considered. Radionuclide study is diagnostic, with uptake in the nodule and absent uptake in the rest of the gland (hot nodule). Children with a toxic multinodular goiter may have either a TSH receptor activating mutation or McCune-Albright syndrome. If precocious puberty, polyostotic fibrous dysplasia, or café-au-lait pigmentation is present, the autonomous thyroid disorder of McCune-Albright syndrome is likely. Hyperthyroidism associated with some form of thyroiditis, e.g., subacute thyroiditis, is relatively rare in childhood. Patients with generalized thyroid hormone resistance have elevated levels of free T_4, but levels of TSH are inappropriately elevated or normal. Patients with greater pituitary resistance to thyroid hormone than generalized thyroid hormone resistance also have clinical hyperthyroidism. They must be differentiated from patients with TSH-secreting pituitary tumors who have elevated serum levels of the TSH α chain. Most other causes of hyperthyroxinemia are uncommon but can result in erroneous diagnosis. Patients with elevated thyroxine-binding globulin (TBG) levels or familial dysalbuminemic hyperthyroxinemia have normal levels of free T_4 and TSH.

When hyperthyroxinemia is caused by **exogenous thyroid hormone,** levels of free T_4 and TSH are the same as those seen in Graves disease, but the level of thyroglobulin is very low, whereas in patients with Graves disease, it is elevated.

TREATMENT

Most pediatric endocrinologists recommend initial medical therapy using antithyroid drugs rather than radioiodine or subtotal thyroidectomy, although radioiodine is gaining acceptance as initial treatment in children >10 yr of age. All therapeutic options have advantages and disadvantages (Table 562-3). The 2 antithyroid drugs used historically are propylthiouracil (PTU) and methimazole (Tapazole). Both compounds inhibit incorporation of trapped inorganic iodide into organic compounds, and they might also suppress TRSAb levels by directly affecting intrathyroidal autoimmunity. However, there are important differences between the drugs. Methimazole is at least 10 times more potent than PTU on a weight basis and has a much longer serum half-life (6-8 hr vs 0.5 hr); PTU generally is administered 3 times daily, but methimazole can be given once daily. Unlike methimazole, PTU is heavily protein bound and has a lesser ability to cross the placenta and to pass into breast milk; theoretically, PTU is the preferred drug during pregnancy and for nursing mothers. Due to reports of **severe liver disease** in patients treated with **PTU,** with some patients requiring liver transplant or potentially suffering a fatal outcome, the consensus is to **use only methimazole** to treat children with Graves disease.

Adverse reactions occur with antithyroid drugs; most are mild, but some are life threatening. Minor adverse effects occur in approximately 10-20%, and more-severe adverse effects occur in 2-5% of children. Reactions are unpredictable and can occur after therapy of any duration. Transient granulocytopenia (<2,000/mm^3) is common; it is asymptomatic and is not a harbinger of agranulocytosis, and it usually is not a reason to discontinue treatment. Transient urticarial rashes are common. They may be managed by a short period off therapy, and then restarting the antithyroid drug. The most severe reactions are hypersensitive and include agranulocytosis (0.1-0.5%), hepatitis (0.2-1%), a lupus-like polyarthritis syndrome, glomerulonephritis, and an ANCA-positive vasculitis involving the skin and other organs. **Severe liver disease,** including liver failure requiring transplant, have been reported **exclusively with PTU.** The most common liver disease associated with methimazole is cholestatic jaundice, reversible when the drug is discontinued. Patients with severe

Table 562-3 TREATMENTS FOR HYPERTHYROIDISM CAUSED BY GRAVES DISEASE

TREATMENT	ADVANTAGE	DISADVANTAGE	COMMENT
Antithyroid drugs	Noninvasive Less initial cost Low risk of permanent hypothyroidism Possible remissions owing to immune effects	Cure rate 30-80% (average 40-50%) Adverse drug reactions Drug compliance required	First-line treatment in children and adolescents and in pregnancy Initial treatment in severe cases or preoperative preparation
Radioactive iodine (^{131}I)	Cure of hyperthyroidism Most cost effective	Permanent hypothyroidism is almost inevitable Might worsen ophthalmopathy Pregnancy must be deferred for 6-12 mo, mother cannot breast-feed; small potential risk of exacerbation of hyperthyroidism	No evidence for infertility, birth defects, cancer Best treatment for toxic nodules and toxic multinodular goiter
Surgery	Rapid, effective treatment especially in patients with large goiter	Most invasive therapy Potential complications (recurrent laryngeal nerve damage, hypoparathyroidism) Most costly therapy Permanent hypothyroidism; pain; scarring	Potential use in pregnancy if major side effect from antithyroid drugs Useful when coexisting suspicious nodule is present Option for patients who refuse radioiodine

From Cooper DS: Hyperthyroidism, *Lancet* 362:459–468, 2003.

adverse effects should be treated with radioiodine or thyroidectomy. Cases of congenital skin defects (aplasia cutis) have been seen in infants exposed in fetal life to methimazole, but this association does not appear to be a strong one.

The initial dosage of methimazole is 0.25-1.0 mg/kg/24 hr given once or twice daily. Smaller initial dosages should be used in early childhood. Careful surveillance is required after treatment is initiated. Rising serum levels of TSH to greater than normal indicates overtreatment and leads to increased size of the goiter. Clinical response becomes apparent in 3-6 wk, and adequate control is evident in 3-4 mo. The dose is decreased to the minimal level required to maintain a euthyroid state.

Most studies report a remission rate of approximately 25% after 2 years of antithyroid drug treatment in children. Some studies find that longer treatment is associated with higher remission rates, with one study reporting a 50% remission rate after 4.5 years of drug treatment. If a relapse occurs, it usually appears within 3 mo and almost always within 6 mo after therapy has been discontinued. Therapy may be resumed in case of relapse. Patients older than 13 yr of age, boys, those with a higher body mass index, and those with small goiters and modestly elevated T_3 levels appear to have earlier remissions.

A β-adrenergic blocking agent such as propranolol (0.5-2.0 mg/kg/24 hr orally, divided 3 times daily) or atenolol (1-2 mg/kg orally given once daily) is a useful supplement to antithyroid drugs in the management of severely toxic patients. Additional therapies for **thyroid storm** are listed in Table 562-4. Thyroid hormones potentiate the actions of catecholamines, including tachycardia, tremor, excessive sweating, lid lag, and stare. These symptoms abate with the use of propranolol, which does not, however, alter thyroid function or exophthalmos.

Radioiodine treatment or surgery is indicated when adequate cooperation for medical management is not possible, when adequate trial of medical management has failed to result in permanent remission, or when severe side effects preclude further use of antithyroid drugs. Either of these treatments may also be preferred by the patient or parent.

Radioiodine is an effective, relatively safe first or alternative therapy for Graves disease in children >10 yr of age. Pretreatment with antithyroid drugs is unnecessary; if a patient is taking them, they should be stopped a week before radioiodine administration. Many pediatric endocrinologists prefer to select a dose of radioiodine to ensure complete ablation of thyroid tissue. A dose of 300 μCi/g of thyroid tissue, or a total dose of approximately 15 mCi, will achieve this goal. Essentially all patients treated at this dose will become hypothyroid; the time course to hypothyroidism averages 11 wk, with a range of 9-28 wk. Because the full effects of treatment may not be complete for 1-6 mo, adjunctive therapy with a β-adrenergic antagonist and lower doses of

Table 562-4 MANAGEMENT OF THYROID STORM IN ADOLESCENTS

GOAL	TREATMENT
Inhibition of thyroid hormone formation and secretion	Propylthiouracil (PTU), 400 mg every 8 hr PO or by nasogastric tube Sodium iodide, 1 g IV in 24 hr, or saturated solution of KI, 5 drops every 8 hr
Sympathetic blockade	Propranolol, 20-40 mg every 4-6 hr, or 1.mg IV slowly (repeat doses until heart rate slows); not indicated in patients with asthma or heart failure that is not rate related
Glucocorticoid therapy	Hydrocortisone, 50-100 mg IV every 6 hr
Supportive therapy	Intravenous fluids (depending on indication: glucose, electrolytes, multivitamins) Temperature control (cooling blankets, acetaminophen; avoid salicylates) O_2 if required Digitalis for heart failure and to slow ventricular response; pentobarbital for sedation Treatment of precipitating event (e.g., infection)

From Goldman L, Ausiello D: *Cecil Textbook of Medicine,* ed 22, Philadelphia, 2004, WB Saunders, p 1401.

antithyroid drugs are recommended. With lower treatment doses of radioiodine, hypothyroidism occurs in 10-20% of patients after the 1st year and in about 3% per year thereafter. Although there have been concerns about radiation oncogenesis and genetic damage, follow-up for as long as 50 yr has not shown this in treated children. The use of lower doses of radioactive iodine (50-200 μCi/g) is associated with an increased risk of benign adenomas (0.6-1.9% in one study). Albeit second primary neoplasms are rare, a few studies report an increased risk of second primary neoplasms, including leukemia, in adult patients with Graves disease treated with radioactive iodine. Because children may be more susceptible to the effects of radioactive iodine, some cardiologists prefer surgery for children <10 yr of age who are candidates for a more definitive treatment.

Subtotal thyroidectomy, a safe procedure when performed by an experienced team, is done only after the patient has been brought to a euthyroid state. This may be accomplished with methimazole over 2-3 mo. After a euthyroid state has been attained, a saturated solution of potassium iodide, 5 drops/24 hr, are added to the regimen for 2 wk before surgery to decrease the vascularity of the gland. Complications of surgical treatment are rare and include hypoparathyroidism (transient or permanent) and paralysis of the vocal cords. The incidence of residual or recurrent hyperthyroidism or hypothyroidism depends on the extent of the surgery. Most recommend near-total thyroidectomy.

The incidence of recurrence is low, and most patients become hypothyroid.

The **ophthalmopathy** remits gradually and usually independently of the hyperthyroidism. Severe ophthalmopathy can require treatment with high-dose prednisone, orbital radiotherapy (of questionable value), or orbital decompression surgery. Cigarette smoking is a risk factor for thyroid eye disease and should be avoided or discontinued to avoid progression of eye involvement.

BIBLIOGRAPHY

Please visit the Nelson Textbook of Pediatrics *website at www.expertconsult.com for the complete bibliography.*

562.2 Congenital Hyperthyroidism

Stephen LaFranchi

ETIOLOGY AND PATHOGENESIS

Neonatal Graves disease is caused by transplacental passage of TRSAb, but the clinical onset, severity, and course may be modified by the concurrent presence of TRBAb and by the transplacental passage of antithyroid drugs taken by the mother. Very high levels of TRSAb usually result in classic neonatal hyperthyroidism, but if the infant has been exposed to antithyroid drugs, onset of symptoms is delayed by 3-4 days to allow degradation of the maternally derived antithyroid drug. If TRBAb is also present, onset of hyperthyroid symptoms may be delayed for several weeks. The mothers of these infants have active Graves disease, Graves disease in remission, a past history of Graves disease managed by radioactive iodine ablation or surgery, or rarely hypothyroidism and a history of lymphocytic thyroiditis.

Neonatal hyperthyroidism occurs in only about 2% of infants born to mothers with a history of Graves disease. The finding of very high levels of TRSAb in these mothers (usually >500% of normal) predicts the occurrence of an affected infant. Fetal tachycardia and goiter can allow prenatal diagnosis. Unlike Graves disease at all other ages, neonatal hyperthyroidism affects boys as often as girls. One would expect twins to be equally affected, but one case reported one twin to be hyperthyroid and the other twin to be hypothyroid. Both eventually recovered to euthyroidism.

The disorder usually remits spontaneously within 6-12 wk but can persist longer, depending on the levels of TRSAb. Mild asymptomatic hyperthyroxinemia also occurs. Rarely, classic neonatal Graves disease does not remit but persists for several years or longer. These children have impressive family histories of Graves disease. In these infants, TRSAb transfer from the mother apparently blends with the infantile onset of autonomous Graves disease.

CLINICAL MANIFESTATIONS

Many of the infants are premature and appear to have intrauterine growth restriction. Most have goiters. The infant is extremely restless, irritable, and hyperactive and appears anxious and unusually alert. Microcephaly and ventricular enlargement may be present. The eyes are opened widely and appear exophthalmic (Fig. 562-3). There may be extreme tachycardia and tachypnea, and the temperature is elevated. In severely affected infants, there is a progression of symptoms; weight loss occurs despite a ravenous appetite, hepatosplenomegaly increases, and jaundice can occur. Severe hypertension and cardiac decompensation can occur. The infant can die if therapy is not instituted promptly. The serum level of T_4 or free T_4 and T_3 are markedly elevated, and TSH is suppressed. Advanced bone age, frontal bossing with triangular facies, and cranial synostosis are common, especially in infants with persistent clinical manifestations of hyperthyroidism.

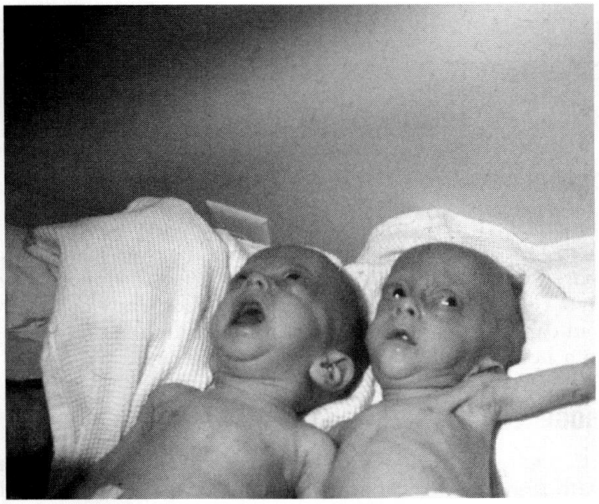

Figure 562-3 Twin boys with neonatal hyperthyroidism confirmed by abnormal thyroid function tests. Clinical features include lack of subcutaneous tissue owing to a hypermetabolic state and a wide-eyed, anxious stare. They were given the diagnosis of neonatal Graves disease, but in fact, their mother did not have Graves disease; they had persistent, not transient, hyperthyroidism. At age 8 yr, they were treated with radioiodine. They are now believed to have had some other form of neonatal hyperthyroidism, such as a constitutive activation of the thyroid-stimulating hormone (TSH) receptor.

TREATMENT

Treatment of the neonate consists of oral administration of propranolol (1-2 mg/kg/24 hr, orally in 3 divided doses) and methimazole (0.25-1.0 mg/kg/24 hr given every 12 hr); Lugol solution (1 drop every 8 hr) may be added. When propranolol is used during pregnancy to treat thyrotoxicosis, it crosses the placenta and can cause respiratory depression in the newborn infant. If the thyrotoxic state is severe, parenteral fluid therapy and corticosteroids may be indicated. If heart failure occurs, digitalization is indicated. After a euthyroid state is reached, only antithyroid drug treatment is necessary. The dose should be gradually tapered to keep the infant euthyroid. Most cases remit by 3-4 mo of age.

Occasionally, neonatal hyperthyroidism does not remit but persists into childhood. These patients can have an impressive family history of hyperthyroidism. Neonatal hyperthyroidism, without evidence for autoimmune disease in mother or infant, may be due to a mutation in the *TSHR* gene that produced constitutive activation of the receptor. Neonatal hyperthyroidism has also been reported in patients with McCune-Albright syndrome, a result of an activating mutation of the α subunit of the G-protein. Under these circumstances, hyperthyroidism recurs when antithyroid drugs are discontinued; these children eventually must be treated with radioiodine or surgery.

PROGNOSIS

Advanced osseous maturation, microcephaly, and mental retardation occur when treatment is delayed. Intellectual development is normal in most treated infants with neonatal Graves disease, though some manifest neurocognitive problems from in utero hyperthyroidism. In some infants, in utero hyperthyroidism appears to suppress the hypothalamic-pituitary-thyroid feedback mechanism, and they develop permanent central hypothyroidism, requiring lifelong thyroid hormone treatment.

BIBLIOGRAPHY

Please visit the Nelson Textbook of Pediatrics *website at www.expertconsult.com for the complete bibliography.*

Chapter 563
Carcinoma of the Thyroid

Stephen LaFranchi

EPIDEMIOLOGY

Carcinoma of the thyroid is rare in childhood; the annual incidence in children <15 yr of age is approximately 2/100,000 cases, compared with an annual incidence at all ages around the world of 4-10/100,000 cases. Despite being widespread at discovery, thyroid cancer in children usually has an indolent course, resulting in a better survival rate than in adults.

PATHOGENESIS

Genetic factors and radiation exposure are important factors in the pathogenesis of thyroid cancer. Rearrangements of the *RET* proto-oncogene are found in 3-33% of papillary carcinomas and 60-80% of those occurring after irradiation, as in children in Belarus exposed to radiation after the nuclear accident at Chernobyl or in those who were exposed to external therapeutic irradiation in childhood. Inactivating point mutations of the *p53* tumor-suppressor gene are rare in patients with differentiated thyroid carcinoma but are common in those with anaplastic thyroid cancer. Overall, 5-10% of cases of papillary thyroid carcinoma are familial and are usually inherited in an autosomal dominant manner.

The thyroid gland of children is unusually sensitive to exposure to external radiation. There probably is no threshold dose; 1 Gy results in a 7.7 relative risk of thyroid cancer. In the past, about 80% of children with cancer of the thyroid had received inappropriate therapeutic irradiation of the neck and adjacent areas during infancy for benign conditions such as "enlarged" thymus, hypertrophied tonsils and adenoids, hemangiomas, nevi, eczema, tinea capitis, and "cervical adenitis." With the discontinuation of irradiation for benign conditions, this cause of thyroid cancer has vanished. The long-term survival of children who have received appropriate therapeutic irradiation of areas of the neck for neoplastic disease has made this cause of thyroid cancer and nodules increasingly prevalent; increased dose, younger age at time of treatment, and female sex are factors that increase the risk of thyroid cancer. Long-term risk data for cancer are sparse, but 15-50% of children who have received irradiation and chemotherapy for Hodgkin disease, leukemia, bone marrow transplant, brain tumors, and other malignancies of the head and neck have elevated levels of thyroid-stimulating hormone (TSH) within the 1st yr of therapy, and 5-20% progress to hypothyroidism during the next 5-7 yr. Most large groups of treated children have a 10-30% incidence of benign thyroid nodules and an increased incidence of thyroid cancer. The latter begins to appear within 3-5 yr after radiation treatment and reaches a peak in 15-25 yr. It is unknown whether there is a period after which no more tumors develop. Administration of iodine-131 for diagnostic or therapeutic purposes does not increase the risk of thyroid cancer.

Differentiated thyroid carcinoma has been reported in patients with chronic lymphocytic thyroiditis; it is not clear whether there is an increased risk of thyroid cancer in children with autoimmune thyroid disease. Conversely, lymphocytic infiltration within the thyroid cancer carries a more favorable prognosis, perhaps as a sign of an immune response to the cancer. One retrospective study indicated that the prevalence of thyroid cancer among children with autoimmune thyroiditis may be as high as 3%. The clinical course of autoimmune thyroiditis patients with cancer was distinguished by lymphadenopathy, a lack of response to levothyroxine therapy, and a hypoechogenic thyroid nodule.

Thyroid cancer has been reported in children with thyroglossal duct cysts, and it also has been found in children with congenital goiter. In these patients, and also in children with autoimmune thyroiditis and hypothyroidism, chronic TSH stimulation appears to play a pathogenic role.

Histologically, the carcinomas are papillary or follicular variant of papillary carcinoma (88%), follicular (10%), medullary (2%), or mixed differentiated tumors. All of the thyroid cancers in a retrospective study of children with autoimmune thyroiditis were papillary carcinomas. Thyroid cancer in children is more likely to be multifocal, with spread to regional lymph nodes at presentation. The type of tumor and the natural course of disease in irradiated and nonirradiated patients are the same except that multicentricity is more common in irradiation-induced cancer. Undifferentiated (anaplastic) thyroid neoplasms are rare in children and usually have a rapidly fatal course. Lymphomas and teratomas of the thyroid are also reported in children.

CLINICAL MANIFESTATIONS

Girls are affected twice as often as boys. The average age at diagnosis is 9 yr, but the onset may be as early as the 1st yr of life. A painless nodule in the thyroid or in the neck is the usual initial evidence of disease. Rapid growth and large nodule size, firmness, fixation to adjacent tissues, hoarseness, dysphagia, and neck adenopathy are risk factors for thyroid cancer. Cervical lymph node involvement is often present at the time of initial diagnosis. Any unexplained cervical lymph node enlargement requires examination of the thyroid, which occasionally has a primary tumor too small to be felt; the diagnosis is based on biopsy results of the lymph node. The lungs are the most common site of metastases beyond the neck. There may be no clinical manifestations referable to them; radiologically, they appear as diffuse miliary or nodular infiltrations, principally in the basal portions. They may be mistaken for tuberculosis, histoplasmosis, or sarcoidosis. Other sites of metastasis include the mediastinum, axilla, long bones, skull, and brain. Almost all children are euthyroid, but rarely, the carcinoma is functional and produces symptoms of hyperthyroidism.

DIAGNOSIS

The most useful diagnostic test in the case of a solitary nodule is fine-needle aspiration (FNA). An ultrasonographic examination of the thyroid can provide information on the consistency of the nodule (solid vs cystic) and whether other nonpalpable nodules are present. A thyroid scan, preferably using ^{123}I or ^{99m}Tc-pertechnetate, can provide information on trapping function and whether the nodule is "cold," "warm," or "hot." The majority of cold nodules are benign. Neither ultrasound nor a thyroid scan can differentiate between a benign or malignant lesion. FNA specimens may be interpreted as benign, cancer, indeterminate (sometimes termed *follicular neoplasm*), or inadequate specimen. FNA experience in children shows a 5-10% false-negative rate and a 1-2% false-positive rate, with an overall diagnostic accuracy of 90-95%. Tests of thyroid function are normal, but Hashimoto's thyroiditis has been associated with thyroid cancer.

TREATMENT

Small (<1 cm) papillary carcinoma, the least-aggressive type, may be effectively treated by subtotal thyroidectomy and suppressive doses of thyroid hormone. However, because papillary carcinomas tend to be multicentric in children, and more than half have regional lymph node involvement at presentation, most patients should be managed by total thyroidectomy. For larger papillary carcinomas (>1.0 cm), and children with known follicular carcinoma, or with regional lymph node involvement, total thyroidectomy with excision of regional lymph nodes is the treatment of choice. There is no role for radical neck dissection. Thyroidectomy is usually followed by a dose (30-100 mCi) of ^{131}I to ablate residual thyroid tissue or persistent disease, discovered by post-treatment whole body scan. Only patients who have undergone total thyroidectomy can be monitored by whole body radioiodine scanning and serum thyroglobulin. Newer guidelines suggest that children with isolated (or "incidental") microcarcinomas (<1.0 cm) are cured by total thyroidectomy and therefore might not need radioactive iodine treatment.

After surgery, all patients should be treated with sodium L-thyroxine in doses sufficient to suppress TSH to the lower range of normal. Serum thyroglobulin (Tg) is an excellent marker for tumor recurrence, and periodic determinations of Tg levels should be performed. In patients who have undergone thyroid ablation, serum Tg level should be <1 ng/mL when thyroxine (T_4) suppressive therapy is being received. Elevation of serum Tg during periods of thyroid hormone withdrawal or with recombinant TSH stimulation might discover patients with elevated Tg levels. Patients with an elevated serum Tg should undergo whole-body radioactive iodine uptake and scan and ultrasound examination of the neck to locate the source of Tg and plan appropriate management.

PROGNOSIS

Although thyroid carcinoma is more widespread at discovery, the survival rate in children with thyroid carcinoma is better than in adults. The presence of regional lymph node spread does not affect survival in children. Even patients with recurrence of cancer or pulmonary metastases have survived many years. More than 95% of patients are alive 25 yr after initial treatment if the tumor was intrathyroid, <2 cm in diameter, and classified as grade 1. Greater tumor size, distant spread, and greater atypia are associated with increased cumulative mortality. Thyroid carcinomas that express telomerase and the IGF-1 receptor are more likely to show aggressive clinical features, and those that express the sodium-iodide symporter are associated with a lower risk of recurrence.

BIBLIOGRAPHY

Please visit the Nelson Textbook of Pediatrics *website at www.expertconsult.com for the complete bibliography.*

563.1 Solitary Thyroid Nodule

Stephen LaFranchi

Solitary nodules of the thyroid are common in children. They are found by palpation in approximately 2% of children aged 11-18 yr; ultrasound examination would likely show a higher prevalence, as it does in adults. Genetic factors play an etiologic role. Most thyroid nodules in children are benign, although several studies suggest that the proportion that are carcinomas is higher than in adults, varying from 2% to 40%. Considering the fact that thyroid nodules are common and thyroid cancer is rare, the true percentage of nodules that harbor cancer is probably closer to 2%. Children exposed to radiation have a high incidence of benign adenoma and carcinoma of the thyroid.

Benign disorders that can occur as solitary thyroid nodules include benign adenomas (follicular, embryonal, Hürthle cell), colloid (adenomatous) nodule, a simple cyst, lymphocytic thyroiditis, a thyroid abscess, and developmental anomalies such as thyroglossal duct cyst or hemiagenesis (Table 563-1). A suddenly appearing or rapidly enlarging thyroid mass can indicate hemorrhage into a cyst or benign adenoma. Ultrasonography is particularly useful in detecting cystic lesions. In most cases, the child is euthyroid, and thyroid function studies are normal. When lymphocytic thyroiditis is the cause of the nodule, thyroid antibodies are usually present. Ultrasonography shows diffuse hypoechogenicity. Radionuclide imaging reveals a moth-eaten appearance. Rarely, lymphocytic thyroiditis is associated with carcinoma of the thyroid.

Table 563-1 ETIOLOGIC CLASSIFICATION OF SOLITARY THYROID NODULES
Lymphoid follicle, as part of chronic lymphocytic thyroiditis
Thyroid developmental anomalies
Hemiagenesis
Intrathyroidal thyroglossal duct cyst
Thyroid abscess (acute suppurative thyroiditis)
Simple cyst
Neoplasms
Benign
Colloid (adenomatous) nodule
Follicular adenoma
Toxic adenoma
Nonthyroidal (e.g., lymphohemangioma)
Malignant
Papillary carcinoma
Follicular carcinoma
Mixed papillary-follicular carcinoma
Undifferentiated (anaplastic)
Medullary carcinoma
Nonthyroidal
Lymphoma
Teratoma

The diagnostic studies to delineate the underlying cause include serum thyroid function tests, antithyroid antibody determinations, ultrasonographic examination of the thyroid, and fine needle aspiration (FNA). Radioiodine uptake and scan are useful when a suppressed serum TSH suggests an autonomous "hot" nodule. Response to a trial of suppressive T_4 treatment to look for shrinkage of nodule size is not reliable. Although thyroid carcinomas generally occur as a solid, "cold" nodule, most "cold" nodules are benign lesions. FNA is useful in avoiding surgery for benign nodules. Surgery without delay is indicated when the nodule is hard or has grown rapidly, when there is evidence of tracheal or vocal cord involvement, and when there is enlargement of adjacent lymph nodes. All persons with a history of head or neck irradiation should have careful examinations of the thyroid at least every 2 yr and indefinitely.

Rarely, thyroid nodules are functional, producing hyperthyroidism (**Plummer disease**). These patients are discovered when thyroid function tests reveal a suppressed TSH, with T_3 more elevated than T_4 or free T_4 levels. The uptake of radionuclide is concentrated in the nodule ("hot" or "warm" nodule), with absent uptake in the rest of the gland. Such nodules are usually benign, but a few instances of carcinoma in such cases have been reported. Treatment consists of surgical removal of the nodule.

BIBLIOGRAPHY

Please visit the Nelson Textbook of Pediatrics *website at www.expertconsult.com for the complete bibliography.*

563.2 Medullary Thyroid Carcinoma

Stephen LaFranchi

Medullary thyroid carcinoma (MTC) arises from the parafollicular cells (C cells) of the thyroid and accounts for about 2% of thyroid malignancies in children. The majority of MTC cases are sporadic, but approximately 25% are familial, autosomal dominant disorders. Hereditary MTC is divided into three distinct syndromes: multiple endocrine neoplasia 2A (MEN2A), multiple endocrine neoplasia 2B (MEN2B), and familial MTC (FMTC). MTC is a result of mutations in the RET proto-oncogene on chromosome 10q11.2. Familial cases are associated with germ line mutations; most sporadic cases are caused by somatic cell mutations, but studies show that a small percentage, around 6-8%, are associated with germ line mutations and so can be passed on. Once an index case is diagnosed in a family, it is important to pinpoint the specific RET mutation and then screen all children in the family for the mutation. Thyroidectomy before the MTC has spread outside the gland represents the best chance for a cure.

The most common presentation of sporadic MTC is an asymptomatic, palpable thyroid nodule. When the tumor occurs sporadically, it is usually unicentric, but in the familial form, it is usually multicentric, and it begins as hyperplasia of parafollicular cells. X-rays can reveal dense, conglomerate, homogeneous calcification in the thyroid. Diagnosis of medullary carcinoma should lead to a careful search for associated tumors, particularly pheochromocytoma. No clinically recognizable manifestations result from the elevated serum levels of calcitonin or from the calcitonin gene-related peptide. Nonetheless, these tests are helpful in screening and monitoring therapy.

MULTIPLE ENDOCRINE NEOPLASIA, TYPE 2A

MEN 2A is an autosomal dominant disorder characterized by MTC, pheochromocytoma, and parathyroid hyperplasia. At least 19 different specific missense mutations of exon 10 or 11 of the extracellular domain of the *RET* gene have been described for MEN 2A and for cases of familial medullary thyroid carcinoma. DNA analysis permits unambiguous identification of carriers of the RET proto-oncogene mutation. Penetrance of MTC is close to 100%, but there is much variability in the other manifestations of MEN 2A. C-cell hyperplasia or MTC usually appears earlier than pheochromocytoma. Pheochromocytomas are often bilateral and may be multiple. Adrenal medullary hyperplasia is known to precede pheochromocytoma, but the detectable latent period is short. Hypercalcemia is a late manifestation and indicates hyperparathyroidism. The parathyroid glands might reveal chief-cell hyperplasia or only hypercellularity.

MULTIPLE ENDOCRINE NEOPLASIA, TYPE 2B

MEN 2B is an autosomal dominant disorder characterized by MTC and pheochromocytomas, but not hyperparathyroidism. The distinguishing feature of MEN 2B, also called the **mucosal neuroma syndrome,** is the occurrence of multiple neuromas and a characteristic phenotype. A missense mutation of the *RET* proto-oncogene in exon 16, the tyrosine catalytic domain of *RET,* is found in 93% of families; all patients have had the same point mutation.

The neuromas most often occur on the tongue, buccal mucosa, lips, and conjunctivae. Peripheral neurofibromas and café-au-lait patches may be present, and intestinal ganglioneuromatosis is common. Diffuse proliferation of nerves and ganglion cells is found in mucosal, submucosal, myenteric, and subserosal plexus involving the small and large bowel as well as the esophagus. The patients may be tall, with arachnodactyly and a Marfan-like appearance. Scoliosis, pectus excavatum, pes cavus, and muscular hypotonia are common. The eyelids may be thickened and everted, the lips patulous and blubbery, the jaw prognathic. Feeding difficulties, poor sucking, diarrhea, constipation, and failure to thrive can begin in infancy or early childhood, many years before the appearance of neuromas or endocrine symptoms.

TREATMENT

Total thyroidectomy is indicated for all children who are shown by genetic studies to carry the *RET* gene mutation. Recognition of familial forms of this tumor is critical to the early diagnosis in children at risk. MTC develops at an earlier age in patients with MEN2B and is more aggressive than in MEN2A. MTC has been seen in a 6 mo old child with MEN2B and in a 3-yr old child with MEN2A. In MEN2A, there is genotype-phenotype correlation between the specific mutation and the onset of C-cell hyperplasia or MTC. Codon 634 mutations occur at an early age, whereas mutations at codons 618, 620, and 804 tend to occur at a later age. In young children, mutation analysis might help individualize the age of total thyroidectomy. All these children should be screened for pheochromocytoma before surgery. Monitoring the levels of calcitonin is useful in following the course of the disease after operation and in detecting metastatic lesions. Periodic screening for the development of pheochromocytoma and hyperparathyroidism is indicated. Metastases to the regional lymph nodes and to the liver are common. Death can result, but long survival is common.

BIBLIOGRAPHY

Please visit the Nelson Textbook of Pediatrics *website at* *www.expertconsult.com* *for the complete bibliography.*

Section 3 DISORDERS OF THE PARATHYROID GLAND

Chapter 564 Hormones and Peptides of Calcium Homeostasis and Bone Metabolism

Daniel A. Doyle

Parathyroid hormone (PTH) and vitamin D are the principal regulators of calcium homeostasis (Chapters 48 and 694). Calcitonin and PTH-related peptide (PTHrP) are important primarily in the fetus.

For the full continuation of this chapter, please visit the Nelson Textbook of Pediatrics *website at* *www.expertconsult.com*.

Chapter 565 Hypoparathyroidism

Daniel A. Doyle

ETIOLOGY

Hypocalcemia is common between 12 and 72 hr of life, especially in premature infants, in infants with asphyxia, and in infants of diabetic mothers (early neonatal hypocalcemia) (Chapter 100) (Table 565-1). After the 2nd to 3rd day and during the 1st wk of life, the type of feeding also is a determinant of the level of serum calcium (late neonatal hypocalcemia). The role played by

Table 565-1 ETIOLOGIC CLASSIFICATION OF HYPOCALCEMIA

PARATHYROID HORMONE DEFICIENCY
Aplasia or hypoplasia of parathyroids • With 22q11 deletion DiGeorge syndrome Velocardiofacial syndrome Conotruncal-face syndrome • With 10p13 deletion • With maternal diabetes mellitus or retinoic acid embryopathy • With X-linked isolated hypoparathyroidism • With mutation of *GCMB* (glial cell missing B), autosomal recessive • With retardation and dysmorphism (Sanjad-Sakati syndrome), autosomal recessive • With deafness and renal dysplasia (*GATA3* mutation) • With osteosclerosis (Kenny-Caffey syndrome), *TBCE* mutation Suppression of neonatal PTH secretion due to maternal hyperparathyroidism Preproparathyroid hormone gene mutation • Autosomal dominant Ca^{2+}-sensing receptor activating mutation • Sporadic • Autosomal dominant Autoimmune parathyroiditis • Isolated • With type 1 autoimmune polyendocrinopathy, APECED Mutation of *AIRE* gene Infiltrative lesions • Hemosiderosis (treatment of thalassemia) • Copper deposition (Wilson disease)
PARATHYROID HORMONE RECEPTOR DEFECTS (PSEUDOHYPOPARATHYROIDISM)
Type 1a (inactivating mutation of $G_s\alpha$) • With gonadotropin-independent precocious puberty Type 1b (paternal imprinting of *GNAS1*) Type 2 (normal cAMP response)
MITOCHONDRIAL DNA MUTATIONS
Kearns-Sayre syndrome Pearson marrow pancreas syndrome Mutation of long-chain 3-hydroxyacylcoenzyme A dehydrogenase
MAGNESIUM DEFICIENCY
Renal magnesium loss (autosomal dominant) Magnesium malabsorption (autosomal recessive) Aminoglycoside therapy
EXOGENOUS INORGANIC PHOSPHATE EXCESS
Laxatives Soft drinks with phosphoric acid
VITAMIN D DEFICIENCY
Nutritional Vitamin D dependency (rickets) Mutation of 1α-(OH)ase (cytochrome P-450)

APECED, autoimmune polyendocrinopathy-candidiasis-ectodermal dystrophy; cAMP, cyclic adenosine monophosphate; PTH, parathyroid hormone.

the parathyroid glands in these hypocalcemic infants remains to be clarified, although functional immaturity of the parathyroid glands is invoked as one pathogenetic factor. In a group of infants with transient idiopathic hypocalcemia (1-8 wk of age), serum levels of parathyroid hormone (PTH) are significantly lower than those in normal infants. It is possible that the functional immaturity is a manifestation of a delay in development of the enzymes that convert glandular PTH to secreted PTH; other mechanisms are possible.

APLASIA OR HYPOPLASIA OF THE PARATHYROID GLANDS

Aplasia or hypoplasia of the parathyroid glands is often associated with the **DiGeorge/velocardiofacial syndrome** (see Fig. 564-1). This syndrome occurs in 1/4,000 newborns. In 90% of patients, the condition is caused by a deletion of chromosome 22q11.2. Approximately 25% of these patients inherit the chromosomal abnormality from a parent. Neonatal hypocalcemia occurs in 60% of affected patients, but it is transitory in the majority; hypocalcemia can recur or can have its onset later in life. Associated abnormalities of the 3rd and 4th pharyngeal pouches are common; these include conotruncal defects of the heart in 25%, velopharyngeal insufficiency in 32%, cleft palate in 9%, renal anomalies in 35%, and aplasia of the thymus with severe immunodeficiency in 1%. This syndrome has also been reported in a small number of patients with a deletion of chromosome 10p13, in infants of diabetic mothers, and in infants born to mothers treated with retinoic acid for acne early in pregnancy.

X-LINKED RECESSIVE HYPOPARATHYROIDISM

Familial clusters of hypoparathyroidism with various patterns of transmission have been described. In two large North American pedigrees, this disorder appears to be transmitted by an X-linked recessive gene located on Xq26-q27. In these families, the onset of afebrile seizures characteristically occurs in infants from 2 wk to 6 mo of age. The absence of parathyroid tissue after detailed examination of a boy with this condition suggests a defect in embryogenesis.

AUTOSOMAL RECESSIVE HYPOPARATHYROIDISM WITH DYSMORPHIC FEATURES

Autosomal recessive hypoparathyroidism with dysmorphic features has been described in Middle Eastern children. Parental consanguinity occurred for almost all of several dozen affected patients. Profound hypocalcemia occurs early in life, and dysmorphic features include microcephaly, deep-set eyes, beaked nose, micrognathia, and large floppy ears. Intrauterine and postnatal growth retardation are severe, and mental retardation is common. The putative gene is on chromosome 1q42-43. The autosomal recessive form of hypoparathyroidism that occurs with type I polyglandular autoimmune disease is described subsequently. In a few patients with autosomal recessive inheritance of isolated hypoparathyroidism, mutations of the *PTH* gene have been found.

HDR SYNDROME

Hypoparathyroidism, sensorineural deafness, and renal anomaly occur owing to mutations of the *GATA3* gene. The protein encoded by this gene is essential in the development of the parathyroids, auditory system, and kidneys. The *GATA3* gene is located at chromosome 10p14 and is nonoverlapping with the DiGeorge critical region at 10p13 (see Fig. 564-1).

SUPPRESSION OF NEONATAL PARATHYROID HORMONE SECRETION DUE TO MATERNAL HYPERPARATHYROIDISM

Neonatal PTH secretion can be suppressed by maternal hyperparathyroidism, resulting in transient hypocalcemia in the newborn infant. It appears that neonatal hypocalcemia results from suppression of the fetal parathyroid glands by exposure to elevated levels of calcium in maternal and hence fetal serum. Tetany usually develops within 3 wk but may be delayed by 1 mo or more if the infant is breast-fed. Hypocalcemia can persist for weeks or months. When the cause of hypocalcemia in an infant is unknown, measurements of calcium, phosphorus, and PTH should be obtained from the mother. Most affected mothers are asymptomatic, and the cause of their hyperparathyroidism is usually a parathyroid adenoma.

AUTOSOMAL DOMINANT HYPOPARATHYROIDISM

Patients with autosomal dominant hypoparathyroidism have an activating (gain-of-function) mutation of the Ca^{2+}-sensing receptor, forcing the receptor to an "on" state with subsequent depression of PTH secretion even during hypocalcemia. The patients have hypercalciuria. The hypocalcemia is usually mild and might not require treatment beyond childhood (see Fig. 564-1).

HYPOPARATHYROIDISM ASSOCIATED WITH MITOCHONDRIAL DISORDERS

Mitochondrial DNA mutations in Kearns-Sayre syndrome and in mitochondrial trifunctional protein have been associated with hypoparathyroidism. A diagnosis of mitochondrial cytopathy should be considered in patients with unexplained symptoms such as ophthalmoplegia, sensorineural hearing loss, cardiac conduction disturbances, and tetany (see Fig. 564-1).

SURGICAL HYPOPARATHYROIDISM

Removal or damage of the parathyroid glands can complicate thyroidectomy. Hypoparathyroidism has developed even when the parathyroid glands have been identified and left undisturbed at the time of operation. This may be the result of interference with the blood supply or of postoperative edema and fibrosis. Symptoms of tetany can occur abruptly postoperatively and may be temporary or permanent. In some instances, symptoms develop insidiously and go undetected until months after thyroidectomy. Occasionally, the first evidence of surgical hypoparathyroidism may be the development of cataract. The status of parathyroid function should be carefully monitored in all patients undergoing thyroidectomy.

Deposition of iron pigment or of copper in the parathyroid glands (thalassemia, Wilson disease) can produce hypoparathyroidism.

AUTOIMMUNE HYPOPARATHYROIDISM

An autoimmune mechanism for hypoparathyroidism is strongly suggested by the finding of parathyroid antibodies and by its frequent association with other autoimmune disorders or organ-specific antibodies. Autoimmune hypoparathyroidism is often associated with Addison disease and chronic mucocutaneous candidiasis. The association of at least 2 of these 3 conditions has been tentatively classified as **autoimmune polyglandular disease type I.** It is also known as autoimmune polyendocrinopathy, candidiasis, and ectodermal dystrophy (APCED). This syndrome is inherited in an autosomal recessive fashion and is not related to any single HLA-associated haplotype. One third of patients with this syndrome have all 3 components; 66% have only 2 of 3 conditions. The candidiasis almost always precedes the other disorders (70% of cases occur in children <5 yr of age); the hypoparathyroidism (90% after 3 yr of age) usually occurs before Addison disease (90% after 6 yr of age). A variety of other disorders occur at various times and include alopecia areata or totalis, malabsorption disorder, pernicious anemia, gonadal failure, chronic active hepatitis, vitiligo, and insulin-dependent diabetes. Some of these associations might not appear until adult life. Autoimmune thyroid disease is a rare concomitant finding.

Affected siblings can have the same or different constellations of disorders (hypoparathyroidism, Addison disease). The disorder is exceptionally prevalent among Finns and Iranian Jews. The gene for this disorder is designated *AIRE* (autoimmune regulator); it is located on chromosome 21q22. It appears to be a transcription factor that plays an essential role in the development of immunologic tolerance. Patients with Addison disease as part of polyendocrinopathy syndrome type I have demonstrated adrenal-specific autoantibody reactivity directed against the side-chain cleavage enzyme.

IDIOPATHIC HYPOPARATHYROIDISM

The term *idiopathic hypoparathyroidism* should be reserved for the small residuum of children with hypoparathyroidism for whom no causative mechanism can be defined. Most children in whom onset of hypoparathyroidism occurs after the first few years of life have an **autoimmune condition.** Autoantibodies to the extracellular domain of the calcium-sensing receptor have been identified in some patients with acquired hypoparathyroidism. One should always consider incomplete forms of DiGeorge syndrome or an activating calcium-sensing receptor mutation in the differential diagnosis.

Clinical Manifestations

There is a spectrum of parathyroid deficiencies with clinical manifestations varying from no symptoms to those of complete and long-standing deficiency. Mild deficiency may be revealed only by appropriate laboratory studies. Muscular pain and cramps are early manifestations; they progress to numbness, stiffness, and tingling of the hands and feet. There may be only a positive Chvostek or Trousseau sign or laryngeal and carpopedal spasms. Convulsions with or without loss of consciousness can occur at intervals of days, weeks, or months. These episodes can begin with abdominal pain, followed by tonic rigidity, retraction of the head, and cyanosis. Hypoparathyroidism is often mistaken for epilepsy. Headache, vomiting, increased intracranial pressure, and papilledema may be associated with convulsions and might suggest a brain tumor.

In patients with long-standing hypocalcemia, the teeth erupt late and irregularly. Enamel formation is irregular, and the teeth may be unusually soft. The skin may be dry and scaly, and the nails might have horizontal lines. Mucocutaneous candidiasis, when present, antedates the development of hypoparathyroidism; the candidal infection most often involves the nails, the oral mucosa, the angles of the mouth, and less often, the skin; it is difficult to treat.

Cataracts in patients with long-standing untreated disease are a direct consequence of hypoparathyroidism; other autoimmune ocular disorders such as keratoconjunctivitis can also occur. Manifestations of Addison disease, lymphocytic thyroiditis, pernicious anemia, alopecia areata or totalis, hepatitis, and primary gonadal insufficiency may also be associated with those of hypoparathyroidism.

Permanent physical and mental deterioration occur if initiation of treatment is long delayed.

Laboratory Findings

The serum calcium level is low (5-7 mg/dL), and the phosphorus level is elevated (7-12 mg/dL). Blood levels of ionized calcium (usually approximately 45% of the total) more nearly reflect physiologic adequacy but also are low. The serum level of alkaline phosphatase is normal or low, and the level of $1,25(OH)_2D_3$ is usually low, but high levels have been found in some children with severe hypocalcemia. The level of magnesium is normal but should always be checked in hypocalcemic patients. Levels of PTH are low when measured by immunometric assay. Radiographs of the bones occasionally reveal an increased density limited to the metaphyses, suggesting heavy metal poisoning, or an increased density of the lamina dura. Radiographs or CT scans of the skull can reveal calcifications in the basal ganglia. There is a prolongation of the QT interval on the electrocardiogram, which disappears when the hypocalcemia is corrected. The electroencephalogram usually reveals widespread slow activity; the tracing returns to normal after the serum calcium concentration has been within the normal range for a few weeks, unless irreversible brain damage has occurred or unless the parathyroid insufficiency is associated with epilepsy. When hypoparathyroidism occurs concurrently with Addison disease, the serum level of calcium may be normal, but hypocalcemia appears after effective treatment of the adrenal insufficiency.

Treatment

Emergency treatment of neonatal tetany consists of intravenous injections of 5-10 mL or 1-3 mg/kg of a 10% solution of calcium gluconate (elemental calcium 9.3 mg/mL) at the rate of 0.5-1 mL/min while the heart rate is monitored and a total dose not to exceed 20 mg of elemental calcium/kg. Additionally, 1,25-dihydroxycholecalciferol (calcitriol) should be given. The initial dosage is 0.25 μg/24 hr; the maintenance dosage ranges from 0.01-0.10 μg/kg/24 hr to a maximum of 1-2 μg/24 hr. Calcitriol has a short half-life and should be given in 2 equal divided doses; it has the advantages of rapid onset of effect (1-4 days) and rapid reversal of hypercalcemia after discontinuation in the event of overdosage (calcium levels begin to fall in 3-4 days). Calcitriol is supplied as an oral solution.

An adequate intake of calcium should be ensured. Supplemental calcium can be given in the form of calcium gluconate or calcium glubionate (Neo-Calglucon) to provide 800 mg of elemental calcium daily, but it is rarely essential. Foods with high phosphorus content such as milk, eggs, and cheese should be reduced in the diet.

Clinical evaluation of the patient and frequent determinations of the serum calcium levels are indicated in the early stages of treatment to determine the requirement for calcitriol or vitamin D_2. If hypercalcemia occurs, therapy should be discontinued and resumed at a lower dose after the serum calcium level has returned to normal. In long-standing cases of hypercalcemia, repair of cerebral and dental changes is not likely. Pigmentation, lowering of blood pressure, or weight loss can indicate adrenal insufficiency, which requires specific treatment. *Patients with autosomal dominant hypocalcemic hypercalciuria can develop nephrocalcinosis and renal impairment if treated with vitamin D.*

Differential Diagnosis

Magnesium deficiency must be considered in patients with unexplained hypocalcemia. Concentrations of serum magnesium <1.5 mg/dL (1.2 mEq/L) are usually abnormal. Familial hypomagnesemia with secondary hypocalcemia has been reported in about 50 patients, most of whom developed tetany and seizures at 2-6 wk of age. Administration of calcium is ineffective, but administration of magnesium promptly corrects both calcium and magnesium levels. Oral supplements of magnesium are necessary to maintain levels of magnesium in the normal range. Two genetic forms have been described. One is caused by an autosomal recessive gene on chromosome 9, resulting in a specific defect in absorption of magnesium. The other is caused by an autosomal dominant gene on chromosome 11q23, resulting in renal loss of magnesium.

Hypomagnesemia also occurs in malabsorption syndromes such as Crohn disease and cystic fibrosis. Patients with autoimmune polyglandular disease type I and hypoparathyroidism can also have concurrent steatorrhea and low magnesium levels. Therapy with aminoglycosides causes hypomagnesemia by increasing urinary losses.

It is not clear how low levels of magnesium lead to hypocalcemia. Evidence suggests that hypomagnesemia impairs release of PTH and induces resistance to the effects of the hormone, but other mechanisms also may be operative.

Poisoning with inorganic phosphate leads to hypocalcemia and tetany. Infants administered large doses of inorganic phosphates, either as laxatives or as sodium phosphate enemas, have had sudden onset of tetany, with serum calcium levels <5 mg/dL and markedly elevated levels of phosphate. Symptoms are quickly relieved by intravenous administration of calcium. The mechanism of the hypocalcemia is not clear (Chapter 52.6).

Hypocalcemia can occur early in the course of treatment of acute lymphoblastic leukemia. Hypocalcemia is usually associated with hyperphosphatemia resulting from destruction of lymphoblasts.

Episodic symptomatic hypocalcemia occurs in the **Kenny-Caffey syndrome,** which is characterized by medullary stenosis of the long bones, short stature, delayed closure of the fontanel, delayed bone age, and eye abnormalities. Idiopathic hypoparathyroidism and abnormal PTH levels have been found. Autosomal dominant and autosomal recessive modes of inheritance have been reported. Mutations of the *TBCE* gene (1q 43-44) perturb microtubule organization in diseased cells.

BIBLIOGRAPHY

Please visit the Nelson Textbook of Pediatrics *website at www.expertconsult.com for the complete bibliography.*

Chapter 566

Pseudohypoparathyroidism (Albright Hereditary Osteodystrophy)

Daniel A. Doyle

In contrast to the situation in hypoparathyroidism, in pseudohypoparathyroidism (PHP) the parathyroid glands are normal or hyperplastic and they can synthesize and secrete parathyroid hormone (PTH). Serum levels of immunoreactive PTH are elevated even when the patient is hypocalcemic and may be elevated when the patient is normocalcemic. Neither endogenous nor administered PTH raises the serum levels of calcium or lowers the levels of phosphorus. The genetic defects in the **hormone receptor adenylate cyclase system** are classified into various types depending on the phenotypic and biochemical findings.

TYPE IA

Type Ia accounts for the majority of patients with PHP. Affected patients have a genetic defect of the α subunit of the stimulatory guanine nucleotide-binding protein ($G_s\alpha$). This coupling factor is required for PTH bound to cell surface receptors to activate cyclic adenosine monophosphate (cAMP). Heterogeneous mutations of the $G_s\alpha$ gene have been documented; the gene is located on chromosome 20q13.2. Deficiency of the $G_s\alpha$ subunit is a generalized cellular defect and accounts for the association of other endocrine disorders with type Ia PHP. The defect is inherited as an autosomal dominant trait, and the paucity of father-to-son transmissions is thought to be due to decreased fertility in males.

Tetany is often the presenting sign. Affected children have a short, stocky build and a round face. Brachydactyly with dimpling of the dorsum of the hand is usually present. The 2nd metacarpal is involved least often. As a result, the index finger occasionally is longer than the middle finger. Likewise, the 2nd metatarsal is only rarely affected. There may be other skeletal abnormalities such as short and wide phalanges, bowing, exostoses, and thickening of the calvaria. These patients often have calcium deposits and metaplastic bone formation subcutaneously. Moderate degrees of mental retardation, calcification of the basal ganglia, and lenticular cataracts are common in patients whose disease is diagnosed late.

Some members of affected kindreds may have the usual anatomic stigmata of PHP, but serum levels of calcium and phosphorus are normal despite reduced $G_s\alpha$ activity; however, PTH levels may be slightly elevated. Such patients have been labeled as having **pseudopseudohypoparathyroidism.** Transition from normocalcemia to hypocalcemia often occurs with increasing age of the patient. These phenotypically similar but metabolically dissimilar patients may be in the same family and have the same mutations of $G_s\alpha$ protein. It is not known what other factors cause clinically overt hypocalcemia in some affected patients and not in others. There is some evidence to suggest that the $G_s\alpha$ mutation is paternally transmitted in pseudopseudohypoparathyroidism and maternally transmitted in patients with type Ia disease. The gene may be imprinted in a tissue-specific manner.

In addition to resistance to PTH, resistance to other G protein–coupled receptors for thyroid-stimulating hormone (TSH), gonadotropins, and glucagon can result in various metabolic effects. Clinical hypothyroidism is uncommon, but basal levels of TSH are elevated and thyrotropin-releasing hormone (TRH)-stimulated TSH responses are exaggerated. Moderately decreased levels of thyroxine and increased levels of TSH have been demonstrated by newborn thyroid-screening programs, leading to the detection of type Ia PHP in infancy. In adults, gonadal dysfunction is common, as manifested by sexual immaturity, amenorrhea, oligomenorrhea, and infertility. Each of these abnormalities can be related to deficient synthesis of cAMP secondary to a deficiency of $G_s\alpha$, but it is not clear why resistance to other G protein–dependent hormones (corticotropin, vasopressin) is much less affected.

Serum levels of calcium are low, and those of phosphorus and alkaline phosphatase are elevated. Clinical diagnosis can be confirmed by demonstration of a markedly attenuated response in urinary phosphate and cAMP after intravenous infusion of the synthetic 1-34 fragment of human PTH (teriparatide acetate). Definitive diagnosis is established by demonstration of the mutated G protein.

Type Ia with Precocious Puberty

Two boys have been reported with both type Ia PHP and gonadotropin-independent precocious puberty (Chapter 556.7). They were found to have a temperature-sensitive mutation of the G_s protein. Thus, at normal body temperature (37°C), the G_s is degraded, resulting in PHP, but in the cooler temperature of the testes (33°C) the G_s mutation results in constitutive activation of the luteinizing hormone receptor and precocious puberty.

TYPE IB

Affected patients have normal levels of G protein activity and a normal phenotypic appearance. These patients have tissue-specific resistance to PTH but not to other hormones. Serum levels of calcium, phosphorus, and immunoreactive PTH are the same as those in patients with type Ia PHP. These patients also show no rise in cAMP in response to exogenous administration of PTH. Bioactive PTH is not increased. The pathophysiology of the disorder in this group of patients is caused by paternal uniparental isodisomy of chromosome 20q and resulting *GNAS1* methylation. This, along with the loss of the maternal *GNAS1* gene, leads to PTH resistance in the proximal renal tubules, which leads to impaired mineral ion homeostasis.

TYPE II

Type II has been detected in only a few patients and differs from type I in that the urinary excretion of cAMP is elevated both in the basal state and after stimulation with PTH but phosphaturia does not increase. Phenotypically, patients are normal and hypocalcemia is present. The defect appears to be distal to cAMP because it is normally activated, but the cell is unable to respond to the signal.

BIBLIOGRAPHY

Please visit the Nelson Textbook of Pediatrics *website at* *www.expertconsult.com* *for the complete bibliography.*

Chapter 567
Hyperparathyroidism

Daniel A. Doyle

Excessive production of parathyroid hormone (PTH) can result from a primary defect of the parathyroid glands such as an adenoma or hyperplasia (**primary hyperparathyroidism**).

More often, the increased production of PTH is compensatory, usually aimed at correcting hypocalcemic states of diverse origins (**secondary hyperparathyroidism**). In vitamin D–deficient rickets and the malabsorption syndromes, intestinal absorption of calcium is deficient but hypocalcemia and tetany may be averted by increased activity of the parathyroid glands. In **pseudohypoparathyroidism,** PTH levels are elevated because a mutation in the $G_s\alpha$ protein interferes with response to PTH. Early in chronic renal disease, hyperphosphatemia results in a reciprocal fall in the calcium concentration with a consequent increase in PTH, but in advanced stages of renal failure, production of $1,25(OH)_2D_3$ is also decreased, leading to worsening hypocalcemia and further stimulation of PTH. In some instances, if stimulation of the parathyroid glands has been sufficiently intense and protracted, the glands continue to secrete increased levels of PTH for months or years after kidney transplantation, with resulting hypercalcemia.

ETIOLOGY

Childhood hyperparathyroidism is rare. Onset during childhood is usually the result of a single benign adenoma. It usually becomes manifested after 10 yr of age. There have been a number of kindreds in which multiple members have hyperparathyroidism transmitted in an autosomal dominant fashion. Most of the affected family members are adults, but children have been involved in about 30% of the pedigrees. Some affected patients in these families are asymptomatic, and disease is detected only by careful study. In other kindreds, hyperparathyroidism occurs as part of the constellation known as the **multiple endocrine neoplasia** (MEN) syndromes or of the hyperparathyroidism–jaw tumor syndrome.

Neonatal severe hyperparathyroidism is a rare disorder. Symptoms develop shortly after birth and consist of anorexia, irritability, lethargy, constipation, and failure to thrive. Radiographs reveal subperiosteal bone resorption, osteoporosis, and pathologic fractures. Symptoms may be mild, resolving without treatment, or can have a rapidly fatal course if diagnosis and treatment are delayed. Histologically, the parathyroid glands show diffuse hyperplasia. Affected siblings have been observed in some kindreds, and parental consanguinity has been reported in several kindreds. Most cases have occurred in kindreds with the clinical and biochemical features of **familial hypocalciuric hypercalcemia.** Infants with neonatal severe hyperparathyroidism may be homozygous or heterozygous for the mutation in the Ca^{2+}-sensing receptor gene, whereas most persons with 1 copy of this mutation exhibit autosomal dominant familial hypocalciuric hypercalcemia.

MEN type I is an autosomal dominant disorder characterized by hyperplasia or neoplasia of the endocrine pancreas (which secretes gastrin, insulin, pancreatic polypeptide, and occasionally glucagon), the anterior pituitary (which usually secretes prolactin), and the parathyroid glands. In most kindreds, hyperparathyroidism is usually the presenting manifestation, with a prevalence approaching 100% by 50 yr of age and occurring only rarely in children <18 yr of age. With appropriate DNA probes, it is possible to detect carriers of the gene with 99% accuracy at birth, avoiding unnecessary biochemical screening programs.

The gene for MEN type I is on chromosome 11q13; it appears to function as a tumor suppressor gene and follows the two-hit hypothesis of tumor development. The first mutation (germinal) is inherited and is recessive to the dominant allele; this does not result in tumor formation. A second mutation (somatic) is required to eliminate the normal allele, which then leads to tumor formation.

Hyperparathyroidism–jaw tumor syndrome is an autosomal dominant disorder characterized by parathyroid adenomas and fibro-osseous jaw tumors. Affected patients can also have polycystic kidney disease, renal hamartomas, and Wilms tumor. Although the condition affects adults primarily, it has been diagnosed as early as age 10 yr.

MEN type II may also be associated with hyperparathyroidism (Chapter 563.2).

Transient neonatal hyperparathyroidism has occurred in a few infants born to mothers with hypoparathyroidism (idiopathic or surgical) or with pseudohypoparathyroidism. In each case, the maternal disorder had been undiagnosed or inadequately treated during pregnancy. The cause of the condition is chronic intrauterine exposure to hypocalcemia with resultant hyperplasia of the fetal parathyroid glands. In the newborn, manifestations involve the bones primarily, and healing occurs between 4 and 7 mo of age.

CLINICAL MANIFESTATIONS

At all ages, the clinical manifestations of hypercalcemia of any cause include muscle weakness, fatigue, headache, anorexia, abdominal pain, nausea, vomiting, constipation, polydipsia, polyuria, weight loss, and fever. When hypercalcemia is of long duration, calcium may be deposited in the renal parenchyma (nephrocalcinosis), with progressively diminished renal function. Renal calculi can develop and can cause renal colic and hematuria. Osseous changes can produce pain in the back or extremities, disturbances of gait, genu valgum, fractures, and tumors. Height can decrease from compression of vertebrae; the patient can become bedridden. Detection of completely asymptomatic patients is increasing with the advent of automated panel assays that include serum calcium determinations.

Abdominal pain is occasionally prominent and may be associated with **acute pancreatitis.** Parathyroid crisis can occur, manifested by serum calcium levels >15 mg/dL and progressive oliguria, azotemia, stupor, and coma. In infants, failure to thrive, poor feeding, and hypotonia are common.

Mental retardation, convulsions, and blindness can occur as sequelae of long-standing hypercalcemia. Psychiatric manifestations include depression, confusion, dementia, stupor, and psychosis.

LABORATORY FINDINGS

The serum calcium level is elevated; 39 of 45 children with adenomas had levels >12 mg/dL. The hypercalcemia is more severe in infants with parathyroid hyperplasia; concentrations ranging from 15 to 20 mg/dL are common, and values as high as 30 mg/dL have been reported. Even when the total serum calcium level is borderline or only slightly elevated, ionized calcium levels are often increased. The serum phosphorus level is reduced to about 3 mg/dL or less, and the level of serum magnesium is low. The urine can have a low and fixed specific gravity, and serum levels of nonprotein nitrogen and uric acid may be elevated. In patients with adenomas who have skeletal involvement, serum phosphatase levels are elevated, but in infants with hyperplasia the levels of alkaline phosphatase may be normal even when there is extensive involvement of bone.

Serum levels of intact PTH are elevated, especially in relation to the level of calcium. Calcitonin levels are normal. Acute hypercalcemia can stimulate calcitonin release, but with prolonged hypercalcemia, hypercalcitoninemia does not occur.

The most consistent and characteristic radiographic finding is resorption of subperiosteal bone, best seen along the margins of the phalanges of the hands. In the skull, there may be gross trabeculation or a granular appearance resulting from focal rarefaction; the lamina dura may be absent. In more advanced disease, there may be generalized rarefaction, cysts, tumors, fractures, and deformities. About 10% of patients have radiographic signs of rickets. Radiographs of the abdomen can reveal renal calculi or nephrocalcinosis.

DIFFERENTIAL DIAGNOSIS

Other causes of hypercalcemia can result in a similar clinical pattern and must be differentiated from hyperparathyroidism (Table 567-1). A low serum phosphorus level with hypercalcemia is characteristic of primary hyperparathyroidism; elevated levels of PTH are also diagnostic. With hypercalcemia of any cause except hyperparathyroidism and familial hypocalciuric hypercalcemia, PTH levels are suppressed. Pharmacologic doses of corticosteroids lower the serum calcium level to normal in patients with hypercalcemia from other causes

Table 567-1 ETIOLOGIC CLASSIFICATION OF HYPERCALCEMIA

PARATHYROID HORMONE EXCESS (PRIMARY HYPERPARATHYROIDISM)

Adenoma
• Sporadic
• Autosomal dominant
• Hyperparathyroidism–jaw tumor syndrome
Hyperplasia or adenoma
• Multiple endocrine neoplasia type1
  Mutation in *MEN1* gene (11q13)
• Parathyroid hyperplasia of infancy
  Inactivating mutation of Ca^{2+}-sensing receptor
  Secondary to maternal hypoparathyroidism
Ectopic PTH production
• Nonendocrine malignancies

PARATHYROID HORMONE-RELATED PEPTIDE EXCESS
Nonendocrine malignancies Benign hypertrophy of breasts
Ca^{2+}-SENSING RECEPTOR INACTIVATING MUTATION
Heterozygous-familial hypocalciuric hypercalcemia Neonatal severe hyperparathyroidism
ACTIVATING MUTATION OF PTH/PTHrP RECEPTOR
Autosomal dominant Jansen-type metaphyseal chondrodysplasia
INACTIVATING MUTATION OF PTH/PTHrP RECEPTOR
Autosomal recessive Blomstrand chondrodysplasia
VITAMIN D EXCESS
Iatrogenic Ectopic production • Sarcoidosis • Tuberculosis • Granulomatous lesions • Subcutaneous fat necrosis Excessively fortified milk
UNKNOWN CAUSE
Williams syndrome (7q11.23 deletion)
OTHER
Hypophosphatasia • Mutation of tissue-nonspecific alkaline phosphatase gene Prolonged immobilization Thyrotoxicosis Hypervitaminosis A Leukemia Acquired hypocalciuric hypercalcemia (autoantibodies to calcium-sensing receptor)

PTH, parathyroid hormone; PTHrP, parathyroid hormone-related peptide.

but generally do not affect the calcium level in patients with hyperparathyroidism.

TREATMENT

Surgical exploration is indicated in all instances. All glands should be carefully inspected; if an adenoma is discovered, it should be removed; very few instances of carcinoma are known in children. Most neonates with severe hypercalcemia require total parathyroidectomy; less severe hypercalcemia remits spontaneously in others. A portion of a parathyroid gland may be autografted into the forearm. The patient should be carefully observed postoperatively for the development of hypocalcemia and tetany; intravenous administration of calcium gluconate may be required for a few days. The serum calcium level then gradually returns to normal, and, under ordinary circumstances, a diet high in calcium and phosphorus must be maintained for only several months after operation.

CT, real-time ultrasonography, and subtraction scintigraphy using sestamibi/Tc-pertechnetate alone and in combination have proved effective in localizing a single adenoma versus diffuse hyperplasia in 50-90% of adults. Parathyroid surgeons often rely on intraoperative selective venous sampling with intraoperative assay of PTH for localizing and removing the source of increased PTH secretion.

PROGNOSIS

The prognosis is good if the disease is recognized early and there is appropriate surgical treatment. When extensive osseous lesions are present, deformities may be permanent. A search for other affected family members is indicated.

567.1 Other Causes of Hypercalcemia

Daniel A. Doyle

FAMILIAL HYPOCALCIURIC HYPERCALCEMIA (FAMILIAL BENIGN HYPERCALCEMIA)

Patients with familial hypocalciuric hypercalcemia are usually asymptomatic, and the hypercalcemia is identified by chance during routine investigation for other conditions. The parathyroid glands are normal, PTH levels are inappropriately normal, and subtotal parathyroidectomy does not correct the hypercalcemia. Serum levels of magnesium are high normal or mildly elevated. The ratio of calcium:creatinine clearance is usually decreased despite hypercalcemia.

The disorder is inherited in an autosomal dominant manner and is caused by a mutant gene on chromosome 3q2. Penetrance is near 100%, and the disorder can be diagnosed early in childhood by serum and urinary calcium concentrations. Detection of other affected family members is important to avoid inappropriate parathyroid surgery. The defect is an inactivating mutation in the Ca^{2+}-sensing receptor gene. This G protein–coupled receptor senses the level of free Ca^{2+} in the blood and triggers the pathway to increase extracellular Ca^{2+} in the face of hypocalcemia. This receptor functions in the parathyroid and kidney to regulate calcium homeostasis; inactivating mutations lead to an increased set point with respect to serum Ca^{2+}, resulting in mild to moderate hypercalcemia in heterozygotes.

GRANULOMATOUS DISEASES

Hypercalcemia occurs in 30-50% of children with sarcoidosis and less often in patients with other granulomatous diseases such as tuberculosis. Levels of PTH are suppressed, and levels of $1,25(OH)_2D_3$ are elevated. The source of **ectopic $1,25(OH)_2D_3$** is the activated macrophage, through stimulation by interferon-α from T lymphocytes, which are present in abundance in granulomatous lesions. Unlike renal tubular cells, the 1α-hydroxylase in macrophages is unresponsive to homeostatic regulation. Oral administration of prednisone (2 mg/kg/24 hr) lowers serum levels of $1,25(OH)_2D_3$ to normal and corrects the hypercalcemia.

HYPERCALCEMIA OF MALIGNANCY

Hypercalcemia often occurs in adults with a wide variety of solid tumors but is identified much less often in children. It has been reported in infants with malignant rhabdoid tumors of the kidney or congenital mesoblastic nephroma and in children with neuroblastoma, medulloblastoma, leukemia, Burkitt lymphoma, dysgerminoma, and rhabdomyosarcoma. Serum levels of PTH are rarely elevated. In most patients, the hypercalcemia associated with malignancy is caused by elevated levels of parathyroid hormone-related peptide (PTHrP) and not PTH. Rarely, tumors produce $1,25(OH)_2D_3$ or PTH ectopically.

MISCELLANEOUS CAUSES OF HYPERCALCEMIA

Hypercalcemia can occur in infants with **subcutaneous fat necrosis.** Levels of PTH are normal. In one infant, the level of $1,25(OH)_2D_3$ was elevated and biopsy of the skin lesion revealed granulomatous infiltration, suggesting that the mechanism of the hypercalcemia was akin to that seen in patients with other granulomatous disease. In another infant, although the level of $1,25(OH)_2D_3$ was normal, PTH was suppressed, suggesting the hypercalcemia was not related to PTH. Treatment with prednisone is effective.

Hypophosphatasia, especially the severe infantile form, is usually associated with mild to moderate hypercalcemia (Chapter 696). Serum levels of phosphorus are normal, and those of alkaline phosphatase are subnormal. The bones exhibit rachitic-like lesions on radiographs. Urinary levels of phosphoethanolamine, inorganic pyrophosphate, and pyridoxal 5′-phosphate are elevated; each is a natural substrate to a tissue-nonspecific (liver, bone, kidney) alkaline phosphatase enzyme. Missense mutations of the tissue-nonspecific alkaline phosphatase enzyme gene result in an inactive enzyme in this autosomal recessive disorder.

Idiopathic hypercalcemia of infancy is manifested by failure to thrive and hypercalcemia during the 1st yr of life, followed by spontaneous remission. Serum levels of phosphorus and PTH are normal. The hypercalcemia results from increased absorption of calcium. Vitamin D may be involved in the pathogenesis. Both normal and elevated levels of $1,25(OH)_2D_3$ have been reported. An excessive rise in the level of $1,25(OH)_2D_3$ in response to PTH administration years after the hypercalcemic phase suggests that vitamin D has a role in the pathogenesis. A blunted calcitonin response to intravenous calcium has also been reported.

About 10% of patients with **Williams syndrome** also inconsistently exhibit associated infantile hypercalcemia. The phenotype consists of feeding difficulties, slow growth, elfin facies (small mandible, prominent maxilla, upturned nose), renovascular disorders, and a gregarious "cocktail party" personality. Cardiac lesions include supravalvular aortic stenosis, peripheral pulmonic stenosis, aortic hypoplasia, coronary artery stenosis, and atrial or ventricular septal defects. Nephrocalcinosis can develop if hypercalcemia persists. The IQ score of 50-70 is curiously accompanied by enhanced quantity and quality of vocabulary, auditory memory, and social use of language. A submicroscopic deletion at chromosome 7q11.23, which includes deletion of 1 elastin allele, occurs in 90% of patients and seems to account for the vascular problems. Definitive diagnosis can be established by specific fluorescence in situ hybridization. The hypercalcemia and central nervous system symptoms may be caused by deletion of adjacent genes. Hypercalcemia has been successfully controlled with either prednisone or calcitonin.

Hypervitaminosis D resulting in hypercalcemia from drinking milk that has been incorrectly fortified with excessive amounts of vitamin D has been reported. Not all patients with hypervitaminosis D develop hypercalcemia. Affected infants can manifest failure to thrive, nephrolithiasis, poor renal function, and osteosclerosis. Serum levels of 25(OH)D are a better indicator of hypervitaminosis D than levels of $1,25(OH)_2D_3$ because 25(OH) D has a longer half-life.

Prolonged immobilization can lead to hypercalcemia and occasionally to decreased renal function, hypertension, and encephalopathy. Children who have hypophosphatemic rickets and undergo surgery with subsequent long-term immobilization are at risk for hypercalcemia and should therefore have their vitamin D supplementation decreased or discontinued.

Jansen-type metaphyseal chondrodysplasia is a rare genetic disorder characterized by short-limbed dwarfism and severe but asymptomatic hypercalcemia (Chapter 695). Circulating levels of PTH and PTHrP are undetectable. These patients have an activating PTH-PTHrP receptor mutation that results in aberrant calcium homeostasis and abnormalities of the growth plate.

BIBLIOGRAPHY

Please visit the Nelson Textbook of Pediatrics *website at* *www.expertconsult.com* *for the complete bibliography.*

Section 4 DISORDERS OF THE ADRENAL GLAND

Chapter 568 Physiology of the Adrenal Gland

568.1 Histology and Embryology

Perrin C. White

The adrenal gland is composed of two endocrine tissues: the medulla and the cortex. The chromaffin cells of the adrenal medulla are derived from neuroectoderm, whereas the cells of the adrenal cortex are derived from mesoderm. Mesodermal cells also contribute to the development of the gonads. The adrenal glands and gonads have certain common enzymes involved in steroid synthesis; an inborn error in steroidogenesis in one tissue can also be present in the other.

For the full continuation of this chapter, please visit the Nelson Textbook of Pediatrics *website at* *www.expertconsult.com*.

568.2 Adrenal Steroid Biosynthesis

Perrin C. White

Cholesterol is the starting substrate for all steroid biosynthesis (see Fig. 568-1 on the *Nelson Textbook of Pediatrics* website at www.expertconsult.com). Although adrenal cortex cells can synthesize cholesterol de novo from acetate, circulating plasma lipoproteins provide most of the cholesterol for adrenal cortex hormone formation. Receptors for both low-density lipoprotein (LDL) and high-density lipoprotein (HDL) cholesterol are expressed on the surface of adrenocortical cells; the receptor is termed scavenger receptor class B, type I (SR-BI). Patients with familial hypercholesterolemia who lack LDL receptors have unimpaired adrenal steroidogenesis, suggesting that HDL is the more important source of cholesterol. Cholesterol is stored as cholesteryl esters in vesicles and subsequently hydrolyzed by cholesteryl ester hydrolases to liberate free cholesterol for steroid hormone synthesis.

For the full continuation of this chapter, please visit the Nelson Textbook of Pediatrics *website at* *www.expertconsult.com*.

568.3 Regulation of the Adrenal Cortex

Perrin C. White

REGULATION OF CORTISOL SECRETION

Glucocorticoid secretion is regulated mainly by adrenocorticotropic hormone (corticotropin, ACTH), a 39-amino-acid peptide that is produced in the anterior pituitary. It is synthesized as part of a larger-molecular-weight precursor peptide known as pro-opiomelanocortin (POMC). This precursor peptide is also the source of β-lipotropin (β-LPH). ACTH and β-LPH are cleaved further to yield α- and β-melanocyte-stimulating hormone, corticotropin-like intermediate lobe peptide (CLIP), γ-LPH, β- and γ-endorphin, and enkephalin (Chapter 550).

For the full continuation of this chapter, please visit the Nelson Textbook of Pediatrics *website at* *www.expertconsult.com*.

568.4 Adrenal Steroid Hormone Actions

Perrin C. White

Steroid hormones act through several distinct receptors corresponding to the known biologic activities of the steroid hormones: glucocorticoid, mineralocorticoid, progestin, estrogen, and androgen. These receptors belong to a larger superfamily of nuclear transcriptional factors that include, among others, thyroid hormone and retinoic acid receptors. They have a common structure that includes a carboxyterminal ligand-binding domain and a mid-region DNA-binding domain. The latter domain contains 2 zinc fingers, each of which consists of a loop of amino acids stabilized by 4 cysteine residues chelating a zinc ion.

For the full continuation of this chapter, please visit the Nelson Textbook of Pediatrics *website at* *www.expertconsult.com*.

568.5 Adrenal Medulla

Perrin C. White

The principal hormones of the adrenal medulla are the physiologically active catecholamines: dopamine, norepinephrine, and epinephrine (see Fig. 568-3 on the *Nelson Textbook of Pediatrics* website at www.expertconsult.com). Catecholamine synthesis also occurs in the brain, in sympathetic nerve endings, and in chromaffin tissue outside the adrenal medulla. Metabolites of catecholamines are excreted in the urine, principally 3-methoxy-4-hydroxymandelic acid (VMA), metanephrine, and normetanephrine. Urinary metanephrines and catecholamines are measured to detect pheochromocytomas of the adrenal medulla and sympathetic nervous system (Chapter 574).

For the full continuation of this chapter, please visit the Nelson Textbook of Pediatrics *website at www.expertconsult.com.*

Chapter 569
Adrenocortical Insufficiency

Perrin C. White

In primary adrenal insufficiency, congenital or acquired lesions of the adrenal cortex prevent production of cortisol and often aldosterone (Table 569-1). Acquired primary adrenal insufficiency is termed Addison disease. Dysfunction of the hypothalamus or anterior pituitary gland can cause a deficiency of corticotropin (ACTH) and lead to hypofunction of the adrenal cortex; this is termed secondary adrenal insufficiency (Table 569-2).

569.1 Primary Adrenal Insufficiency

Perrin C. White

Primary adrenal insufficiency may be caused by genetic conditions that are not always manifested in infancy and by acquired problems such as autoimmune conditions. Susceptibility to autoimmune conditions often has a genetic basis, and so these distinctions are not absolute.

INHERITED ETIOLOGIES

Inborn Defects of Steroidogenesis

The most common causes of adrenocortical insufficiency in infancy are the salt-losing forms of congenital adrenal hyperplasia (Chapter 570). Approximately 75% of infants with 21-hydroxylase deficiency, almost all infants with lipoid adrenal hyperplasia, and most infants with a deficiency of 3β-hydroxysteroid dehydrogenase manifest salt-losing symptoms in the newborn period because they are unable to synthesize either cortisol or aldosterone.

Adrenal Hypoplasia Congenita

Adrenal hypoplasia congenita (AHC) represents approximately half of cases of adrenal failure in boys that are not caused by congenital adrenal hyperplasia, autoimmune disease, or adrenoleukodystrophy. Hypoadrenalism usually occurs acutely in the neonatal period but may be delayed until later childhood or even adulthood with a more insidious onset. Histologic examination of the hypoplastic adrenal cortex reveals disorganization and cytomegaly. The disorder is caused by mutation of the *DAX1 (NR0B1)* gene, a member of the nuclear hormone receptor family, located on Xp21. Boys with AHC often do not undergo puberty owing to hypogonadotropic hypogonadism; both AHC and hypogonadotropic hypogonadism are caused by the same mutated *DAX1* gene. **Cryptorchidism,** often noted in these boys, is probably an early manifestation of hypogonadotropic hypogonadism.

AHC also occurs as part of a **contiguous gene deletion** syndrome together with Duchenne muscular dystrophy, glycerol kinase deficiency, mental retardation, or a combination of these conditions.

Other Genetic Causes of Adrenal Hypoplasia

The transcription factor SF-1 is required for adrenal and gonadal development (Chapter 568). Males with a heterozygous mutation in SF-1 *(NR5A1)* have impaired development of the testes despite the presence of a normal copy of the gene on the other chromosome and can appear to be female, similar to patients with lipoid adrenal hyperplasia (Chapter 570). Rarely, such patients have adrenal insufficiency as well.

Adrenal hypoplasia is also occasionally seen in patients with Palister-Hall syndrome caused by mutations in the GLI3 oncogene (Chapter 568).

Adrenoleukodystrophy

In adrenoleukodystrophy (ALD), adrenocortical deficiency is associated with demyelination in the central nervous system (Chapters 80 and 592.3). High levels of very long chain fatty acids are found in tissues and body fluids, resulting from their impaired β-oxidation in the peroxisomes.

The most common form of ALD is an X-linked disorder with various presentations. The most common clinical picture is of a degenerative neurologic disorder appearing in childhood or adolescence and progressing to severe dementia and deterioration of vision, hearing, speech, and gait, with death occurring within a few years. A milder form of X-linked ALD is adrenomyeloneuropathy (ALM), which begins in later adolescence or early adulthood. Many patients have evidence of adrenal insufficiency at the time of neurologic presentation, but Addison disease may be present without neurologic symptoms or can precede them by many years. X-linked adrenal leukodystrophy (X-ALD) is caused by mutations in the *ABCD1* gene located on Xq28. The gene encodes a transmembrane transporter involved in the importation of very long chain fatty acids into peroxisomes. More than 400 mutations have been described in patients with X-ALD; the majority of X-ALD families have a unique mutation. Clinical phenotypes can vary even within families, perhaps owing to modifier genes or other unknown factors. There is no correlation between the degree of neurologic impairment and severity of adrenal insufficiency. Prenatal diagnosis by DNA analysis and family screening by very long chain fatty acid assays and mutation analysis are available. Women who are heterozygous carriers of the X-ALD gene can develop symptoms in midlife or later; adrenal insufficiency is rare.

Neonatal ALD is a rare autosomal recessive disorder. Infants have neurologic deterioration and have or acquire evidence of adrenocortical dysfunction. Most patients have severe mental retardation and die before 5 yr of age. This disorder is a subset of Zellweger (cerebrohepatorenal) syndrome, in which peroxisomes do not develop at all owing to mutations in any of several genes controlling the development of this organelle.

Familial Glucocorticoid Deficiency

Familial glucocorticoid deficiency is a form of chronic adrenal insufficiency characterized by isolated deficiency of glucocorticoids, elevated levels of ACTH, and generally normal aldosterone production, although salt-losing manifestations as are present in most other forms of adrenal insufficiency occasionally occur. Patients mainly have hypoglycemia, seizures, and increased pigmentation during the 1st decade of life. The disorder affects both sexes equally and is inherited in an autosomal recessive manner. There is marked adrenocortical atrophy with relative sparing of the zona glomerulosa. Mutations in the gene for the ACTH receptor (*MCR2)* have been described in approximately 25% of these patients, most of which affect trafficking of receptor molecules from the endoplasmic reticulum to the cell surface.

Table 569-1 CAUSES OF PRIMARY ADRENAL INSUFFICIENCY

DIAGNOSIS	CLINICAL FEATURES IN ADDITION TO ADRENAL INSUFFICIENCY	PATHOGENESIS OR GENETICS
AUTOIMMUNE ADRENALITIS		
Isolated autoimmune adrenalitis	No other features	Associations with *HLA-DR, CTLA4*
Autoimmune adrenalitis as part of APS		
APS type 1 (APECED)	Hypoparathyroidism, chronic mucocutaneous candidiasis, other autoimmune disorders	Mutations in *AIRE*
APS type 2	Thyroid disease, type 1 diabetes mellitus, other autoimmune diseases (unusual in children)	Associations with *HLA-DR, CTLA4*
APS type 4	Other autoimmune diseases, excluding thyroid disease or diabetes (unusual in children)	Associations with *HLA-DR, CTLA4*
INFECTIOUS ADRENALITIS		
Tuberculous adrenalitis	Other organ manifestations of tuberculosis	Tuberculosis
AIDS	Other AIDS-associated diseases	HIV-1, cytomegalovirus
Fungal adrenalitis	Mostly in immunosuppressed patients	Cryptococcosis, histoplasmosis, coccidioidomycosis
GENETIC DISORDERS LEADING TO ADRENAL INSUFFICIENCY		
Adrenoleukodystrophy, adrenomyeloneuropathy	Demyelination of CNS (cerebral adrenoleukodystrophy), spinal cord, or peripheral nerves (adrenomyeloneuropathy)	Mutation in the *ABCD1* gene encoding a peroxisomal fatty acid transport protein
Congenital lipoid adrenal hypoplasia	XY sex reversal	Mutations in the *STAR* gene encoding steroidogenic acute regulatory protein; rare mutations in *CYP11A* encoding P-450scc
CYP oxidoreductase deficiency	Antley-Bixler syndrome	Mutations in *POR* encoding CYP oxidoreductase
Smith-Lemli-Opitz syndrome	Mental retardation, craniofacial malformations, growth failure	Mutations in *DHCR7* encoding 7-dehydrocholesterol reductase
Pallister-Hall syndrome	Hypothalamic hamartoblastoma, hypopituitarism, imperforate anus, postaxial polydactyly	Mutations in *GLI3*
IMAGe syndrome	Intrauterine growth retardation, metaphyseal dysplasia, adrenal insufficiency, genital anomalies	Unknown
Kearns-Sayre syndrome	External ophthalmoplegia, retinal degeneration, and cardiac conduction defects; other endocrinopathies	Mitochondrial DNA deletions
ACTH insensitivity syndromes (familial glucocorticoid deficiency)	Glucocorticoid deficiency, but no impairment of mineralocorticoid synthesis	
Type 1	Tall stature	Mutations in *MC2R* encoding the ACTH receptor
Type 2	No other features	Mutations in *MRAP*
Triple A syndrome (Allgrove's syndrome)	Alacrimia, achalasia; additional symptoms, including neurologic impairment, deafness, mental retardation, hyperkeratosis	Mutations in *AAAS*
Congenital Adrenal Hyperplasia		
21-Hydroxylase deficiency	Ambiguous genitalia in girls	Mutations in *CYP21A2*
11β-Hydroxylase deficiency	Ambiguous genitalia in girls and hypertension	Mutations in *CYP11B1*
3β-hydroxysteroid dehydrogenase deficiency	Ambiguous genitalia in boys, postnatal virilization in girls	Mutations in *HSD3B2*
17α-Hydroxylase deficiency	Ambiguous genitalia in boys, lack of puberty in both sexes, hypertension	Mutations in *CYP17*
Adrenal Hypoplasia Congenita		
X-linked	Hypogonadotropic hypogonadism	Mutations in *NR0B1 (DAX1)*
Xp21 contiguous gene syndrome	Duchenne muscular dystrophy and glycerol kinase deficiency (psychomotor retardation)	Deletion of the Duchenne muscular dystrophy, glycerol kinase, and *NR0B1 (DAX1)* genes
SF-1 linked	XY sex reversal	Mutations in *NR5A1 (SF1)*
OTHER CAUSES		
Bilateral adrenal hemorrhage	Symptoms of underlying disease	Septic shock, specifically meningococcal sepsis (Waterhouse-Friderichsen syndrome); primary antiphospholipid syndrome; anticoagulation
Adrenal infiltration	Symptoms of underlying disease	Adrenal metastases, primary adrenal lymphoma, sarcoidosis, amyloidosis, hemochromatosis
Bilateral adrenalectomy	Symptoms of underlying disease	
Drug-induced adrenal insufficiency	No other symptoms	Treatment with mitotane, aminoglutethimide, etomidate, ketoconazole, suramin, mifepristone, etomidate

ACTH, adrenocorticotropin hormone; APS, autoimmune polyendocrinopathy; CYP, cytochrome P-450; P-450scc, cytochrome P-450 side chain cleavage enzyme.
Adapted from Arlt W, Allolio B: Adrenal insufficiency, *Lancet* 361:1881–1892, 2003.

Another 20% of cases are caused by mutations in *MRAP,* which encodes a melanocyte receptor accessory protein required for this trafficking.

Another syndrome of ACTH resistance occurs in association with **achalasia** of the gastric cardia and **alacrima** (**triple A** or **Allgrove syndrome**). These patients often have a progressive neurologic disorder that includes autonomic dysfunction, mental retardation, deafness, and motor neuropathy. This syndrome is also inherited in an autosomal recessive fashion, and the *AAAS* gene has been mapped to chromosome 12q13. The encoded protein, aladin, might help regulate nucleocytoplasmic transport of other proteins.

Table 569-2 CAUSES OF SECONDARY ADRENAL INSUFFICIENCY

DIAGNOSIS	COMMENT
Pituitary tumors	Secondary adrenal insufficiency mostly as part of panhypopituitarism; additional symptoms (visual-field impairment): generally adenomas, carcinoma is a rarity; consequence of tumor growth, surgical treatment, or both
Other tumors of the hypothalamic-pituitary region	Craniopharyngioma, meningioma, ependymoma, germinoma, and intrasellar or suprasellar metastases
Pituitary irradiation	Craniospinal irradiation in leukemia, irradiation for tumors outside the hypothalamic-pituitary axis, irradiation of pituitary tumors
Lymphocytic hypophysitis	
Isolated	Autoimmune hypophysitis; most often in relation to pregnancy (80%); mostly hypopituitarism, but also isolated adrenocorticotropic hormone deficiency
As part of APS	Associated with autoimmune thyroid disease and, less often, with vitiligo, primary gonadal failure, type 1 diabetes, and pernicious anemia
Isolated congenital ACTH deficiency	Pro-opiomelanocortin cleavage enzyme defect?
Pro-opiomelanocortin-deficiency syndrome	Pro-opiomelanocortin gene mutations; clinical triad of adrenal insufficiency, early-onset obesity, and red hair pigmentation
Combined pituitary-hormone deficiency	Mutations in the gene encoding the pituitary transcription factor *PROP1* (Prophet of Pit1), progressive development of panhypopituitarism in the order GH, PRL, TSH, LH/FSH, (ACTH) Mutations in the homeobox gene *HESX1*, combined pituitary hormone deficiency, optic-nerve hypoplasia, and midline brain defects (septo-optic dysplasia)
Pituitary apoplexy (Sheehan's syndrome)	Onset mainly with abrupt severe headache, visual disturbance, and nausea or vomiting Histiocytosis syndromes, pituitary apoplexy or necrosis with peripartal onset, e.g., due to high blood loss or hypotension
Pituitary infiltration or granuloma	Tuberculosis, actinomycosis, sarcoidosis, Wegener granulomatosis
Head trauma	For example, pituitary stalk lesions
Previous chronic glucocorticoid excess	Exogenous glucocorticoid administration for >2 wk, endogenous glucocorticoid hypersecretion due to Cushing syndrome

ACTH, adrenocorticotropin hormone; APS, autoimmune polyendocrinopathy; FSH, follicle stimulating hormone; GH, growth hormone; LH, luteinizing hormone; PRL, prolactin; TSH, thyrotropin.
Adapted from Arlt W, Allolio B: Adrenal insufficiency, *Lancet* 361:1881–1892, 2003.

Type I Autoimmune Polyendocrinopathy

Although autoimmune Addison disease most often occurs sporadically (see later), it can occur as a component of 2 syndromes, each consisting of a constellation of autoimmune disorders (Chapter 560). **Type I autoimmune polyendocrinopathy (APS-1)**, also known as *autoimmune polyendocrinopathy–candidiasis–ectodermal dystrophy* (APECED) syndrome, is inherited in mendelian autosomal recessive manner, whereas APS-2 (described later) has complex inheritance. **Chronic mucocutaneous candidiasis** is most often the first manifestation of APS-1, followed by hypoparathyroidism and then by Addison disease, which typically develops in early adolescence. Other closely associated autoimmune disorders include gonadal failure, alopecia, vitiligo, keratopathy, enamel hypoplasia, nail dystrophy, intestinal malabsorption, and chronic active hepatitis. Hypothyroidism and type 1 diabetes mellitus occur in less than 10% of affected patients. Some components of the syndrome continue to develop as late as the 5th decade. The presence of antiadrenal antibodies and steroidal cell antibodies in these patients usually indicates a high likelihood of the development of Addison disease or, in female patients, ovarian failure. Adrenal failure can evolve rapidly in APS-1; death in patients with a previous diagnosis and unexplained deaths in siblings of patients with APS-1 have been reported, indicating the need to closely monitor patients with APS-1 and to thoroughly evaluate apparently unaffected siblings of patients with this disorder.

Autoantibodies to the cytochrome P-450 21 (CYP21), CYP17, and CYP11A1 enzymes have been reported in patients with APS-1. The gene affected in APS-1 is designated autoimmune regulator-1 *(AIRE1)*; it has been mapped to chromosome 21q22.3. The *AIRE1* gene encodes a protein that appears to be a transcription factor having an important role in immune response. Approximately 40 different mutations in the *AIRE1* gene have been described in patients with APS-1, with 2 mutations (R257X and a 3-bp deletion) being most common. There has been autosomal dominant transmission in 1 kindred owing to a specific missense mutation (G228W).

Disorders of Cholesterol Synthesis and Metabolism

Patients with disorders of cholesterol synthesis or metabolism, including abetalipoproteinemia with deficient lipoprotein B-containing lipoproteins, and familial hypercholesterolemia, with decreased or impaired LDL receptors, have been demonstrated to have limited adrenocortical function. Adrenal insufficiency has been reported in patients with **Smith-Lemli-Opitz syndrome** (SLOS), an autosomal recessive disorder manifesting with facial anomalies, microcephaly, limb anomalies, and developmental delay (Chapter 80.3). Mutations in the gene coding for sterol Δ^7-reductase, mapped to 11q12-q13, resulting in impairment of the final step in cholesterol synthesis with marked elevation of 7-dehydrocholesterol, abnormally low cholesterol, and adrenal insufficiency, have been identified in SLOS. **Wolman disease** is a rare autosomal recessive disorder caused by mutations in the gene encoding human lysosomal acid lipase on chromosome 10q23.2-23.3. Cholesteryl esters accumulate in lysosomes in most organ systems, leading to organ failure. Infants during the 1st or 2nd mo of life have hepatosplenomegaly, steatorrhea, abdominal distention, and failure to thrive. Adrenal insufficiency and bilateral adrenal calcification are present, and death usually occurs in the first year of life.

Corticosteroid-Binding Globulin Deficiency and Decreased Cortisol-Binding Affinity

Corticosteroid-binding globulin deficiency (CBG) and decreased cortisol-binding affinity result in low levels of plasma cortisol but normal urinary free cortisol and normal plasma ACTH levels. A high prevalence of hypotension and fatigue has been reported in some adults with abnormalities of CBG.

ACQUIRED ETIOLOGIES

Autoimmune Addison Disease

The most common cause of Addison disease is autoimmune destruction of the glands. The glands may be so small that they are not visible at autopsy, and only remnants of tissue are found in microscopic sections. Usually, the medulla is not destroyed, and there is marked lymphocytic infiltration in the area of the former cortex. In advanced disease, all adrenocortical function is lost, but early in the clinical course, isolated cortisol deficiency can occur. Most patients have **antiadrenal cytoplasmic antibodies** in their plasma; 21-hydroxylase (CYP 21) is the most commonly occurring autoantigen.

Addison disease can occur as a component of 2 autoimmune polyendocrinopathy syndromes. Type I (APS-1) was discussed previously. **Type II autoimmune polyendocrinopathy (APS-2)** consists of Addison disease associated with autoimmune thyroid disease (Schmidt syndrome) or type 1 diabetes

(Carpenter syndrome). Gonadal failure, vitiligo, alopecia, and chronic atrophic gastritis, with or without pernicious anemia, can occur. HLA-D3 and HLA-D4 are increased in these patients and appear to confer an increased risk for development of this disease; alleles at the major histocompatibility complex class I chain-related genes A and B *(MICA* and *MICB)* also have been associated with this disorder. The disorder is most common in middle-aged women and can occur in many generations of the same family. Antiadrenal antibodies, specifically antibodies to the CYP 21, CYP 17, and CYP 11A1 enzymes, are also found in these patients. Autoimmune adrenal insufficiency may also be seen in celiac disease (Chapter 330.2).

Infection

Tuberculosis was a common cause of adrenal destruction in the past but is much less prevalent now. The most common infectious etiology for adrenal insufficiency is meningococcemia (Chapter 184); adrenal crisis from this cause is referred to as the Waterhouse-Friderichsen syndrome. Patients with AIDS can have a variety of subclinical abnormalities in the hypothalamic-pituitary-adrenal axis, but frank adrenal insufficiency is rare. However, drugs used in the treatment of AIDS can affect adrenal hormone homeostasis.

Drugs

Ketoconazole, an antifungal drug, can cause adrenal insufficiency by inhibiting adrenal enzymes. Rifampicin and anticonvulsive drugs such as phenytoin and phenobarbital reduce the effectiveness and bioavailability of corticosteroid replacement therapy by inducing steroid-metabolizing enzymes in the liver. Mitotane (o,p′-DDD), used in the treatment of adrenal carcinoma and refractory Cushing syndrome (Chapters 571 and 574), is cytotoxic to the adrenal cortex and can also alter extra-adrenal cortisol metabolism. Signs of adrenal insufficiency occur in a substantial percentage of patients treated with mitotane. Etomidate, used in the induction and maintenance of general anesthesia, inhibits 11β-hydroxylase (CYP 11B1), and a single induction dose can block cortisol synthesis for 4-8 hr or longer. This may be problematic in severely stressed patients, particularly if repeated doses are used in a critical care setting.

Hemorrhage into Adrenal Glands

Hemorrhage into adrenal glands can occur in the neonatal period as a consequence of a difficult labor (especially breech presentation), or its etiology might not be apparent. An incidence rate of 3/100,000 live births has been suggested. The hemorrhage may be sufficiently extensive to result in death from exsanguination or hypoadrenalism. An abdominal mass, anemia, unexplained jaundice, or scrotal hematoma may be the presenting sign. Often, the hemorrhage is asymptomatic initially and is identified later by calcification of the adrenal gland. Fetal adrenal hemorrhage has also been reported. Postnatally, adrenal hemorrhage most often occurs in patients being treated with anticoagulants. It can also occur as a result of child abuse.

CLINICAL MANIFESTATIONS

Primary adrenal insufficiency leads to cortisol and often aldosterone deficiency. The signs and symptoms of adrenal insufficiency are most easily understood in the context of the normal actions of these hormones, which were discussed in Chapter 568.

Hypoglycemia is a prominent feature of adrenal insufficiency. It is often accompanied by ketosis as the body attempts to use fatty acids as an alternative energy source. Ketosis is aggravated by anorexia, nausea, and vomiting, all of which occur frequently.

Cortisol deficiency decreases cardiac output and vascular tone; moreover, catecholamines such as epinephrine have decreased inotropic and pressor effects in the absence of cortisol. These problems are initially manifested as orthostatic hypotension in older children and can progress to frank shock in patients of any age. They are exacerbated by aldosterone deficiency, which results in hypovolemia owing to decreased resorption of sodium in the distal nephron.

Hypotension and decreased cardiac output decrease glomerular filtration and thus decrease the ability of the kidney to excrete free water. Vasopressin (AVP) is secreted by the posterior pituitary in response to hypotension and also as a direct consequence of lack of inhibition by cortisol. These factors decrease plasma osmolality and lead in particular to hyponatremia. Hyponatremia is also caused by aldosterone deficiency and may be much worse when both cortisol and aldosterone are deficient.

In addition to hypovolemia and hyponatremia, aldosterone deficiency causes hyperkalemia by decreasing potassium excretion in the distal nephron. Cortisol deficiency alone does not cause hyperkalemia.

Cortisol deficiency decreases negative feedback on the hypothalamus and pituitary, leading to increased secretion of ACTH. Hyperpigmentation is caused by ACTH and other peptide hormones (γ-melanocyte-stimulating hormone) arising from the ACTH precursor pro-opiomelanocortin. In patients with a fair complexion, the skin can have a bronze cast. Pigmentation may be more prominent in skin creases, mucosa, and scars. In dark-skinned patients, it may be most readily appreciated in the gingival and buccal mucosa.

The clinical presentation of adrenal insufficiency depends on the age of the patient, whether both cortisol and aldosterone secretion are affected, and to some extent on the underlying etiology. The most common causes in early infancy are inborn errors of steroid biosynthesis, sepsis, adrenal hypoplasia congenita, and adrenal hemorrhage. Infants have a relatively greater requirement for aldosterone than do older children, possibly owing to immaturity of the kidney and also to the low sodium content of human breast milk and infant formula. Hyperkalemia, hyponatremia, and hypoglycemia are prominent presenting signs of adrenal insufficiency in infants. Ketosis is not consistently present because infants generate ketones less well than do older children. Hyperpigmentation is not usually seen because this takes weeks or months to develop, and orthostatic hypotension is obviously difficult to demonstrate in infants.

Infants can become ill very quickly. There may be only a few days of decreased activity, anorexia, and vomiting before critical electrolyte abnormalities develop.

In older children with Addison disease, symptoms include muscle weakness, malaise, anorexia, vomiting, weight loss, and orthostatic hypotension. These may be of insidious onset. It is not unusual to elicit, in retrospect, an episodic history spanning years with symptoms being noticeable only during intercurrent illnesses. Such patients can present with acute decompensation (**adrenal crisis**) during relatively minor infectious illnesses.

Hyperpigmentation is often but not necessarily present. Hypoglycemia and ketosis are common, as is hyponatremia. Hyperkalemia tends to occur later in the course of the disease in older children than in infants. Thus, the clinical presentation can be easily confused with gastroenteritis or other acute infections. Chronicity of symptoms can alert the clinician to the possibility of Addison disease, but this diagnosis should be considered in any child with orthostatic hypotension, hyponatremia, hypoglycemia, and ketosis.

Salt craving is seen in primary adrenal insufficiency with mineralocorticoid deficiency. Fatigue, myalgias, fever, eosinophilia, lymphocytosis, hypercalcemia, and anemia may be noted with glucocorticoid deficiency.

LABORATORY FINDINGS

Hypoglycemia, ketosis, hyponatremia, and hyperkalemia have been discussed. An electrocardiogram is useful for quickly detecting hyperkalemia in a critically ill child. Acidosis is often present, and the blood urea nitrogen level is elevated if the patient is dehydrated.

Cortisol levels are sometimes at the low end of the normal range but are invariably low when the patient's degree of illness is considered. ACTH levels are high in primary adrenal insufficiency but can take time to be reported by the laboratory. Similarly, aldosterone levels may be within the normal range but inappropriately low considering the patient's hyponatremia, hyperkalemia, and hypovolemia. Plasma renin activity is elevated. Blood eosinophils may be increased in number, but this is rarely useful diagnostically.

Urinary excretion of sodium and chloride are increased and urinary potassium is decreased, but these are difficult to assess on random urine samples. Accurate interpretation of urinary electrolytes requires more-prolonged (24 hr) urine collections and knowledge of the patient's sodium and potassium intake.

The **most definitive** test for adrenal insufficiency is measurement of serum levels of cortisol before and after administration of ACTH; resting levels are low and do not increase normally after administration of ACTH. Occasionally, normal resting levels that do not increase after administration of ACTH indicate an absence of adrenocortical reserve. A low initial level followed by a significant response to ACTH can indicate secondary adrenal insufficiency. Traditionally, this test has been performed by measuring cortisol levels before and 30 or 60 min after giving 0.250 mg of cosyntropin (ACTH 1-24) by rapid intravenous infusion. Aldosterone will transiently increase in response to this dose of ACTH and may also be measured. A low-dose test (1 µg ACTH 1-24/1.73 m^2) is a more sensitive test of pituitary-adrenal reserve but has somewhat lower specificity (more false-positive tests).

DIFFERENTIAL DIAGNOSIS

Upon presentation, Addison disease often needs to be distinguished from more acute illnesses such as gastroenteritis with dehydration or sepsis. Additional testing is directed at identifying the specific cause for adrenal insufficiency. When congenital adrenal hyperplasia is suspected, serum levels of cortisol precursors (17-hydroxyprogesterone) should be measured along with cortisol in an ACTH stimulation test (Chapter 570). Elevated levels of very long chain fatty acids are diagnostic of adrenoleukodystrophy. The presence of antiadrenal antibodies suggests an autoimmune pathogenesis. Patients with autoimmune Addison disease must be closely observed for the development of other autoimmune disorders. In children, hypoparathyroidism is the most commonly associated disorder, and it is suspected if hypocalcemia and elevated phosphate levels are present.

Ultrasonography, CT, or MRI can help define the size of the adrenal glands.

TREATMENT

Treatment of acute adrenal insufficiency must be immediate and vigorous. If the diagnosis of adrenal insufficiency has not been established, a blood sample should be obtained before therapy to determine electrolytes, glucose, ACTH, cortisol, aldosterone, and plasma renin activity. If the patient's condition permits, an ACTH stimulation test can be performed while initial fluid resuscitation is under way. An intravenous solution of 5% glucose in 0.9% saline should be administered to correct hypoglycemia, hypovolemia, and hyponatremia. Hypotonic fluids (e.g., 5% glucose in water or 0.2% saline) must be avoided because they can precipitate or exacerbate hyponatremia. If hyperkalemia is severe, it can require treatment with intravenous calcium and/or bicarbonate, intrarectal potassium-binding resin (Kayexalate), or intravenous infusion of glucose and insulin. A water-soluble form of hydrocortisone, such as hydrocortisone sodium succinate, should be given intravenously. As much as 10 mg for infants, 25 mg for toddlers, 50 mg for older children, and 100 mg for adolescents should be administered as a bolus and a similar total amount given in divided doses at 6-hr intervals for the first 24 hr. These doses may be reduced during the next 24 hr if progress is satisfactory. Adequate fluid and sodium repletion is achieved by intravenous saline administration, aided by the mineralocorticoid effect of high doses of hydrocortisone.

Particular caution should be exercised in the rare patient with concomitant adrenal insufficiency and hypothyroidism, because thyroxine can increase cortisol clearance. Thus, an adrenal crisis may be precipitated if hypothyroidism is treated without first ensuring adequate glucocorticoid replacement.

After the acute manifestations are under control, most patients require chronic replacement therapy for their cortisol and aldosterone deficiencies. Hydrocortisone (cortisol) may be given orally in daily doses of 10 mg/m^2/24 hr in 3 divided doses; some patients require 15 mg/m^2/24 hr to minimize fatigue, especially in the morning. Timed-release preparations of hydrocortisone are undergoing clinical trials but are not yet generally available. Equivalent doses (20-25% of the hydrocortisone dose) of prednisone or prednisolone may be used and divided and given twice daily. ACTH levels may be used to monitor adequacy of glucocorticoid replacement in primary adrenal insufficiency; in congenital adrenal hyperplasia, levels of precursor hormones are used instead (Chapter 570). Blood samples for monitoring should be obtained at a consistent time of day and in a consistent relation to (i.e., before or after) the hydrocortisone dose. Normalizing ACTH levels is unnecessary and can require excessive doses of hydrocortisone; generally morning ACTH levels high in the normal range to 2-3 times normal are satisfactory. Because untreated or severely undertreated patients can acutely decompensate during relatively minor illnesses, assessment of symptoms (or lack thereof) must not be used as a substitute for biochemical monitoring. During situations of stress, such as periods of infection or minor operative procedures, the dose of hydrocortisone should be increased 2- to 3-fold. Major surgery under general anesthesia requires high intravenous doses of hydrocortisone similar to those used for acute adrenal insufficiency.

If aldosterone deficiency is present, fludrocortisone (Florinef), a synthetic mineralocorticoid, is given orally in doses of 0.05-0.2 mg daily. Measurements of plasma renin activity are useful in monitoring the adequacy of mineralocorticoid replacement. Chronic overdosage with glucocorticoids leads to obesity, short stature, and osteoporosis, whereas overdosage with fludrocortisone results in tachycardia, hypertension, and occasionally hypokalemia.

Replacement of dehydroepiandrosterone (DHEA) in adults remains controversial; prepubertal children do not normally secrete large amounts of DHEA. Many adults with Addison disease complain of having decreased energy, and replacing DHEA can improve this problem, particularly in women in whom adrenal androgens represent approximately 50% of total androgen secretion.

Additional therapy might need to be directed at the underlying cause of the adrenal insufficiency in regard to infections and certain metabolic defects. Therapeutic approaches to adrenoleukodystrophy include administration of glycerol trioleate and glycerol trierucate (Lorenzo's oil), bone marrow transplantation, and lovastatin (Chapter 592.3).

BIBLIOGRAPHY

Please visit the Nelson Textbook of Pediatrics *website at* www.expertconsult.com *for the complete bibliography.*

569.2 Secondary Adrenal Insufficiency

Perrin C. White

ETIOLOGY

Abrupt Cessation of Administration of Corticosteroids

Secondary adrenal insufficiency most commonly occurs when the hypothalamic-pituitary-adrenal axis is suppressed by prolonged administration of high doses of a potent glucocorticoid and that agent is suddenly withdrawn or the dose is tapered too quickly. Patients at risk for this problem include those with leukemia, asthma (particularly when patients are transitioned from oral to inhaled corticosteroids), and collagen vascular disease or other autoimmune conditions and those who have undergone tissue transplants or neurosurgical procedures. The maximal duration and dosage of glucocorticoid that can be administered before encountering this problem is not known, but it is assumed that high-dose glucocorticoids (the equivalent of >10 times physiologic cortisol secretion) can be administered for at least 1 wk without requiring a subsequent taper of dose. On the other hand, when high doses of dexamethasone are given to children with leukemia, it can take up to 2 mo or longer after therapy is stopped before tests of adrenal function return to normal. Signs and symptoms of adrenal insufficiency are most likely in patients who are subsequently subjected to stresses such as severe infections or additional surgical procedures.

Corticotropin Deficiency

Pituitary or hypothalamic dysfunction can cause corticotropin deficiency (Chapter 551), usually associated with deficiencies of other pituitary hormones such as growth hormone and thyrotropin. Destructive lesions in the area of the pituitary, such as craniopharyngioma and germinoma, are the most common causes of corticotropin deficiency. In many cases the pituitary or hypothalamus is further damaged during surgical removal or radiotherapy of tumors in the midline of the brain. In rare instances, autoimmune hypophysitis is the cause of corticotropin deficiency.

Congenital lesions of the pituitary also occur. The pituitary alone may be affected, or additional midline structures may be involved, such as the optic nerves or septum pellucidum. The latter type of abnormality is termed **septo-optic dysplasia,** or de Morsier syndrome (Chapter 585.9). More-severe developmental anomalies of the brain, such as anencephaly and holoprosencephaly, can also affect the pituitary. These disorders are usually sporadic, although a few cases of autosomal recessive inheritance have occurred. Isolated deficiency of corticotropin has been reported, including in several sets of siblings. Patients with multiple pituitary hormone deficiencies caused by mutations in the *PROP1* gene have been described with progressive ACTH/cortisol deficiency. Isolated deficiency of corticotropin-releasing hormone has been documented in an Arab kindred as an autosomal recessive trait.

It has recently been recognized that up to 60% of children with **Prader-Willi syndrome** (Chapter 76) have some degree of secondary adrenal insufficiency as assessed by provocative testing with metyrapone (see later), although diurnal cortisol levels are normal. The clinical significance of this finding is uncertain, but it can contribute to the relatively high incidence of sudden death with infectious illness that occurs in this population. Although it is not yet a standard of care, some endocrinologists advocate treating patients who have Prader-Willi syndrome with hydrocortisone during febrile illness.

CLINICAL PRESENTATION

Aldosterone secretion is unaffected in secondary adrenal insufficiency because the adrenal gland is, by definition, intact and the renin-angiotensin system is not involved. Thus, signs and symptoms are those of cortisol deficiency. Newborns often have hypoglycemia. Older children can have orthostatic hypotension or weakness. Hyponatremia may be present.

When secondary adrenal insufficiency is due to an inborn or acquired anatomic defect involving the pituitary, there may be signs of associated deficiencies of other pituitary hormones. The penis may be small in male infants if gonadotropins are also deficient. Infants with secondary hypothyroidism are often jaundiced. Children with associated growth hormone deficiency grow poorly after the 1st yr of life.

Some children with pituitary abnormalities have hypoplasia of the midface. Children with optic nerve hypoplasia can have obvious visual impairment. They usually have a characteristic wandering nystagmus, but this is often not apparent until several months of age.

LABORATORY FINDINGS

Because the adrenal glands themselves are not directly affected, the diagnosis of secondary adrenal insufficiency is sometimes challenging. Historical gold standard dynamic tests include insulin-induced hypoglycemia, which provides a potent stress to the entire hypothalamic-pituitary-adrenal (HPA) axis. This test requires constant attendance by a physician and is considered by many endocrinologists to be too dangerous for routine use. A second gold standard test uses metyrapone, a specific inhibitor of steroid 11β-hydroxylase (CYP 11B1) to block cortisol synthesis, thus removing the normal negative feedback of cortisol on ACTH secretion. Although there a several protocols for this test, one version administers 30 mg/kg of metyrapone orally at midnight, with a blood sample obtained for cortisol and 11-deoxycortisol (the substrate for 11β-hydroxylase) at 8 AM. A low cortisol level (<5 µg/dL) demonstrates adequate suppression of cortisol synthesis, and an 11-deoxycortisol level >7 µg/dL indicates that ACTH has responded normally to the cortisol deficiency by stimulating the adrenal cortex. This test should be used with caution outside the research setting because it can precipitate adrenal crises in patients with marginal adrenal function; the drug is not available in all locales.

At present, the most commonly used test to diagnose secondary adrenal insufficiency is low-dose ACTH stimulation testing (1 µg/1.73 m^2 of cosyntropin given intravenously), the rationale being that there will be some degree of atrophy of the adrenal cortex if normal physiologic ACTH stimulation is lacking. Thus, this test may be falsely negative in cases of acute compromise of the pituitary (e.g., injury or surgery). Such circumstances rarely pose a diagnostic dilemma; in general, this test provides excellent sensitivity and specificity. Although assays vary somewhat, a threshold cortisol level of 18-20 µg/dL 30 minutes after cosyntropin administration may be used to dichotomize normal and abnormal responses.

At present, there seems to be little reason to use stimulation with corticotrophin-releasing hormone (CRH) instead of ACTH; although the CRH test has the theoretical advantage of testing the ability of the anterior pituitary to respond to this stimulus by secreting ACTH, in practice it doesn't provide improved sensitivity and specificity, and the agent is not as widely available.

TREATMENT

Iatrogenic secondary adrenal insufficiency (caused by chronic glucocorticoid administration) is best avoided by use of the smallest effective doses of systemic glucocorticoids for the shortest period of time. When a patient is thought to be at risk, tapering the dose rapidly to a level equivalent to or slightly less than physiologic replacement (~10 mg/m^2/24 hr of hydrocortisone) and further tapering over several wk can allow the adrenal cortex to recover without development of signs of adrenal insufficiency.

Patients with anatomic lesions of the pituitary should be treated indefinitely with glucocorticoids. Mineralocorticoid replacement is not required. In patients with panhypopituitarism, treating cortisol deficiency can increase free water excretion, thus unmasking central diabetes insipidus. Electrolytes must be monitored carefully when initiating cortisol therapy in panhypopituitary patients.

BIBLIOGRAPHY

Please visit the Nelson Textbook of Pediatrics *website at www.expertconsult.com for the complete bibliography.*

569.3 Adrenal Insufficiency in the Critical Care Setting

Perrin C. White

ETIOLOGY

Adrenal insufficiency in the context of critical illness is encountered in up to 20-50% of pediatric patients, often as a transient condition. In many cases, it is considered to be "functional" or "relative" in nature, meaning that cortisol levels are within normal limits but cannot increase sufficiently to meet the demands of critical illness. The causes are heterogeneous, and some were discussed in Chapter 569.1. They include adrenal hypoperfusion from shock, particularly septic shock, as is often seen in meningococcemia. Inflammatory mediators during septic shock, particularly interleukin-6, can suppress ACTH secretion, directly suppress cortisol secretion, or both. Etomidate, used as sedation for intubation, inhibits steroid 11β-hydroxylase and thus blocks cortisol biosynthesis. Neurosurgical patients with closed head trauma, or with tumors that involve the hypothalamus or pituitary, might have ACTH deficiency in the context of panhypopituitarism. Some children have been previously treated with systemic corticosteroids (e.g., children with leukemia) and have suppression of the hypothalamic-pituitary-adrenal axis for that reason. In the intensive care nursery, premature infants have not yet developed normal cortisol biosynthetic capacity (Chapter 568.2) and thus may not be able to secrete adequate amounts of this hormone when ill.

For the full continuation of this chapter, please visit the Nelson Textbook of Pediatrics *website at www.expertconsult.com.*

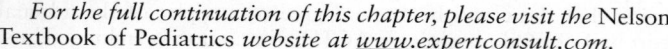

Chapter 570
Congenital Adrenal Hyperplasia and Related Disorders

Perrin C. White

Congenital adrenal hyperplasia (CAH) is a family of autosomal recessive disorders of cortisol biosynthesis (normal adrenal steroidogenesis is discussed in Chapter 568). Cortisol deficiency increases secretion of corticotropin (ACTH), which in turn leads to adrenocortical hyperplasia and overproduction of intermediate metabolites. Depending on the enzymatic step that is deficient, there may be signs, symptoms, and laboratory findings of mineralocorticoid deficiency or excess; incomplete virilization or premature puberty in affected males; and virilization or sexual infantilism in affected females (Figs. 570-1 and 570-2 and Table 570-1).

570.1 Congenital Adrenal Hyperplasia Due to 21-Hydroxylase Deficiency

Perrin C. White

ETIOLOGY

More than 90% of congenital adrenal hyperplasia (CAH) cases are caused by 21-hydroxylase deficiency. This P450 enzyme (CYP21, P450c21) hydroxylates progesterone and 17-hydroxyprogesterone (17-OHP) to yield 11-deoxycorticosterone (DOC) and 11-deoxycortisol, respectively (see Fig. 568-1). These conversions are required for synthesis of aldosterone and cortisol, respectively. Both hormones are deficient in the most severe, "salt-wasting" form of the disease. Slightly less severely affected patients are able to synthesize adequate amounts of aldosterone but have elevated levels of androgens of adrenal origin; this is termed *simple virilizing disease*. These 2 forms are collectively termed classical 21-hydroxylase deficiency. Patients with nonclassical disease have relatively mildly elevated levels of androgens and may have signs of androgen excess after birth.

EPIDEMIOLOGY

Classical 21-hydroxylase deficiency occurs in about 1 in 15,000-20,000 births in most populations. Approximately 70% of affected infants have the salt-losing form, whereas 30% have the simple virilizing form of the disorder. In the USA, CAH is less common in African-Americans compared with white children (1:42,000 vs 1:15,500). Nonclassical disease has a prevalence of about 1 in 1,000 in the general population but occurs more frequently in specific ethnic groups such as Ashkenazi Jews and Hispanics.

GENETICS

There are 2 steroid 21-hydroxylase genes—*CYP21P (CYP21A1P, CYP21A)* and *CYP21 (CYP21A2, CYP21B)*—which alternate in tandem with 2 genes for the 4th component of complement (C4A and C4B) in the human leukocyte antigen (HLA) major histocompatibility complex on chromosome 6p21.3 between the HLA-B and HLA-DR loci. Many other genes are located in this cluster. *CYP21* is the active gene; *CYP21P* is 98% identical in DNA sequence to *CYP21* but is a pseudogene due to 9 different mutations. More than 90% of mutations causing 21-hydroxylase deficiency are recombinations between *CYP21* and *CYP21P*. Approximately 20% are deletions generated by unequal meiotic crossing-over between *CYP21* and *CYP21P*, whereas the remainder is nonreciprocal transfers of deleterious mutations from *CYP21P* to *CYP21*, a phenomenon termed gene conversion.

The deleterious mutations in *CYP21P* have different effects on enzymatic activity when transferred to *CYP21*. Several mutations completely prevent synthesis of a functional protein, whereas others are missense mutations (they result in amino acid substitutions) that yield enzymes with 1-50% of normal activity. Disease severity correlates well with the mutations carried by an affected individual; for example, patients with salt-wasting disease usually carry mutations on both alleles that completely destroy enzymatic activity. Patients are frequently compound heterozygotes for different types of mutations (i.e., 1 allele is less severely affected than the other), in which case the severity of disease expression is largely determined by the activity of the less severely affected of the 2 alleles.

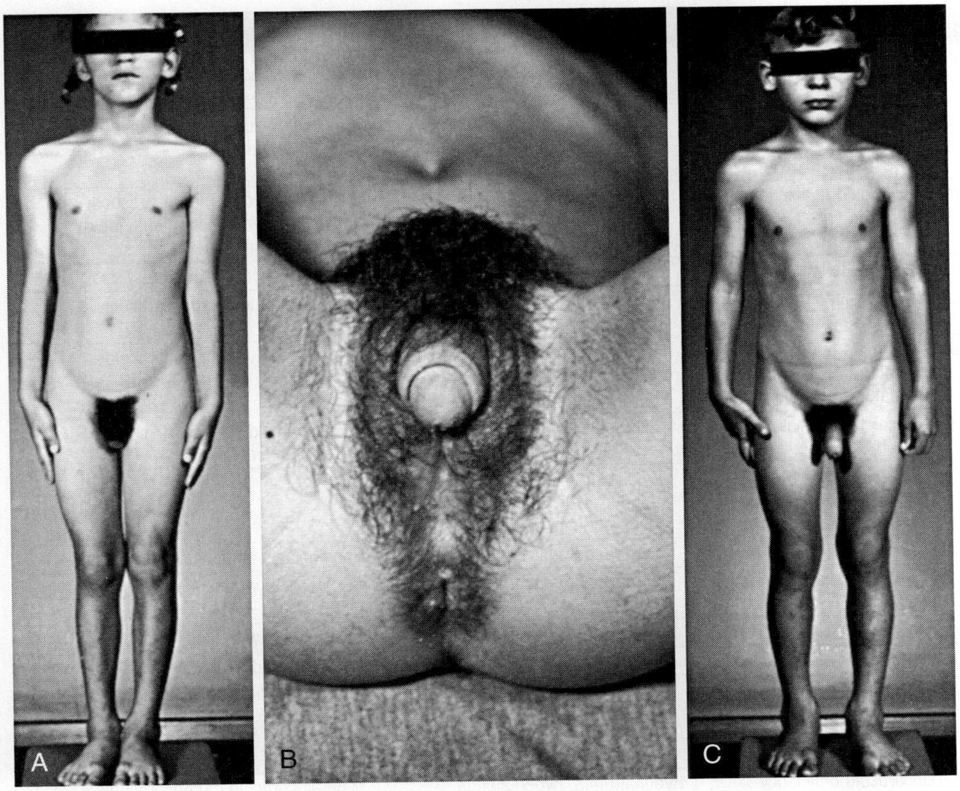

Figure 570-1 *A,* A 6-yr-old girl with congenital virilizing adrenal hyperplasia. The height age was 8.5 yr, and the bone age was 13 yr. *B,* Notice the clitoral enlargement and labial fusion. *C,* Her 5-yr-old brother was not considered to be abnormal by the parents. The height age was 8 yr, and the bone age was 12.5 yr.

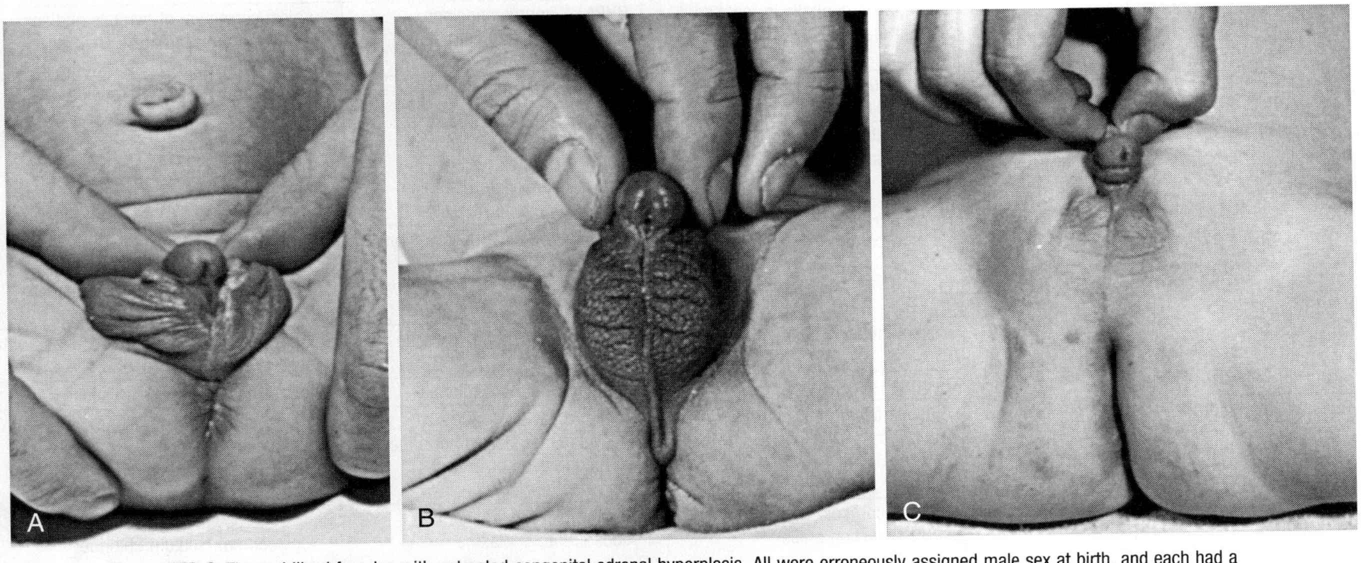

Figure 570-2 Three virilized females with untreated congenital adrenal hyperplasia. All were erroneously assigned male sex at birth, and each had a normal female sex-chromosome complement. Infants *A* and *B* had the salt-wasting form and received the diagnosis early in infancy. Infant *C* was referred at 1 yr of age because of bilateral cryptorchidism. Notice the completely penile urethra; such complete masculinization in females with adrenal hyperplasia is rare; most of these infants have the salt-wasting form.

PATHOGENESIS AND CLINICAL MANIFESTATIONS

Aldosterone and Cortisol Deficiency

Because both cortisol and aldosterone require 21-hydroxylation for their synthesis, both hormones are deficient in the most severe, salt-wasting form of the disease. This form constitutes about 70% of cases of classical 21-hydroxylase deficiency. The signs and symptoms of cortisol and aldosterone deficiency, and the pathophysiology underlying them, are essentially those described in Chapter 569. These include progressive weight loss, anorexia, vomiting, dehydration, weakness, hypotension, hypoglycemia, hyponatremia, and hyperkalemia. These problems typically 1st develop in affected infants at approximately 10-14 days of age. Without treatment, shock, cardiac arrhythmias, and death may occur within days or weeks.

CAH differs from other causes of primary adrenal insufficiency in that precursor steroids accumulate proximal to the blocked enzymatic conversion. Because cortisol is not synthesized

Table 570-1 DIAGNOSIS AND TREATMENT OF CONGENITAL ADRENAL HYPERPLASIA

DISORDER	AFFECTED GENE AND CHROMOSOME	SIGNS AND SYMPTOMS	LABORATORY FINDINGS	THERAPEUTIC MEASURES
21-Hydroxylase deficiency, classic form	*CYP21* 6p21.3	Glucocorticoid deficiency	↓ Cortisol, ↑ACTH ↑↑ Baseline and ACTH-stimulated 17-hydroxy-progesterone	Glucocorticoid (hydrocortisone) replacement
		Mineralocorticoid deficiency (salt-wasting crisis)	Hyponatremia, hyperkalemia ↑ Plasma renin	Mineralocorticoid (fludrocortisone) replacement; sodium chloride supplementation
		Ambiguous genitalia in females	↑ Serum androgens	Vaginoplasty and clitoral recession
		Postnatal virilization in males and females	↑ Serum androgens	Suppression with glucocorticoids
21-Hydroxylase deficiency, nonclassic form	*CYP21* 6p21.3	May be asymptomatic; precocious adrenarche, hirsutism, acne, menstrual irregularity, infertility	↑ Baseline and ACTH-stimulated 17-hydroxyprogesterone ↑ Serum androgens	Suppression with glucocorticoids
11β-Hydroxylase deficiency	*CYP11B1* 8q24.3	Glucocorticoid deficiency	↓ Cortisol, ↑ ACTH	Glucocorticoid (hydrocortisone) replacement
			↑↑ Baseline and ACTH-stimulated 11-deoxycortisol and deoxycorticosterone	
		Ambiguous genitalia in females	↑ Serum androgens	Vaginoplasty and clitoral recession
		Postnatal virilization in males and females	↑ Serum androgens	Suppression with glucocorticoids
		Hypertension	↓ Plasma renin, hypokalemia	Suppression with glucocorticoids
3β-Hydroxysteroid dehydrogenase deficiency, classical form	*HSD3B2* 1p13.1	Glucocorticoid deficiency	↓ Cortisol, ↑ ACTH ↑↑ Baseline and ACTH-stimulated Δ5 steroids (pregnenolone, 17-hydroxy pregnenolone, DHEA)	Glucocorticoid (hydrocortisone) replacement
		Mineralocorticoid deficiency (salt-wasting crisis)	Hyponatremia, hyperkalemia ↑ Plasma renin	Mineralocorticoid (fludrocortisone) replacement; sodium chloride supplementation
		Ambiguous genitalia in females and males	↑ DHEA, ↓ androstenedione, testosterone, and estradiol	Surgical correction of genitals and sex hormone replacement as necessary, consonant with sex of rearing
		Precocious adrenarche, disordered puberty	↑ DHEA, ↓ androstenedione, testosterone, and estradiol	Suppression with glucocorticoids
17α-Hydroxylase/17,20-lyase deficiency	*CYP17* 10q24.3	Cortisol deficiency (corticosterone is an adequate glucocorticoid)	↓ Cortisol, ↑ ACTH ↑ DOC, corticosterone Low 17α-hydroxylated steroids; poor response to ACTH	Glucocorticoid (hydrocortisone) administration
		Ambiguous genitalia in males	↓ Serum androgens; poor response to hCG	Orchidopexy or removal of intra-abdominal testes; sex hormone replacement consonant with sex of rearing
		Sexual infantilism	↓ Serum androgens or estrogens	Sex hormone replacement consonant with sex of rearing
		Hypertension	↓ Plasma renin; hypokalemia	Suppression with glucocorticoids
Congenital lipoid adrenal hyperplasia	*STAR* 8p11.2	Glucocorticoid deficiency	↑ ACTH Low levels of all steroid hormones, with decreased or absent response to ACTH	Glucocorticoid (hydrocortisone) replacement
		Mineralocorticoid deficiency (salt-wasting crisis)	Hyponatremia, hyperkalemia ↓ Aldosterone, ↑ plasma renin	Mineralocorticoid (fludrocortisone) replacement; sodium chloride supplementation
		Ambiguous genitalia in males	Decreased or absent response to hCG in males	Orchidopexy or removal of intra-abdominal testes; sex hormone replacement consonant with sex of rearing
		Poor pubertal development or premature ovarian failure in females	↑ FSH, ↑ LH, ↓ estradiol (after puberty)	Estrogen replacement
P450 oxidoreductase deficiency	*POR* 7q11.3	Glucocorticoid deficiency	↓ Cortisol, ↑ ACTH ↑ Pregnenolone, ↑ progesterone	Glucocorticoid (hydrocortisone) replacement
		Ambiguous genitalia in males and females	↑ Serum androgens prenatally, ↓ androgens and estrogens at puberty	Surgical correction of genitals and sex hormone replacement as necessary, consonant with sex of rearing
		Maternal virilization Antley-Bixler syndrome	Decreased ratio of estrogens to androgens	

efficiently, ACTH levels are high, leading to hyperplasia of the adrenal cortex and levels of precursor steroids that may be hundreds of times normal. In the case of 21-hydroxylase deficiency, these precursors include 17-hydroxyprogesterone and progesterone. Progesterone and perhaps other metabolites act as antagonists of the mineralocorticoid receptor and thus may exacerbate the effects of aldosterone deficiency in untreated patients.

Prenatal Androgen Excess

The most important problem caused by accumulation of steroid precursors is that 17-hydroxyprogesterone is shunted into the pathway for androgen biosynthesis, leading to high levels of androstenedione that are converted outside the adrenal gland to testosterone. This problem begins in affected fetuses by 8-10 wk of gestation and leads to abnormal genital development in females (see Figs. 570-1 and 570-2).

The external genitals of males and females normally appear identical early in gestation (Chapter 576). Affected females, who are exposed in utero to high levels of androgens of adrenal origin, have masculinized external genitalia (see Figs. 570-1 and 570-2). This is manifested by enlargement of the clitoris and by partial or complete labial fusion. The vagina usually has a common opening with the urethra (urogenital sinus). The clitoris may be so enlarged that it resembles a penis; because the urethra opens below this organ, some affected females may be mistakenly presumed to be males with hypospadias and cryptorchidism. The severity of virilization is usually greatest in females with the salt-losing form of 21-hydroxylase deficiency. The internal genital organs are normal, because affected females have normal ovaries and not testes and thus do not secrete antimüllerian hormone.

Prenatal exposure of the brain to high levels of androgens may influence subsequent sexually dimorphic behaviors in affected females. Girls tend to be interested in masculine toys such as cars and trucks and often show decreased interest in playing with dolls and demonstrate aggressive play behavior. Women may have decreased interest in maternal roles. There is an increased frequency of homosexuality in affected females. Nonetheless, most function heterosexually and do not have gender identity confusion or dysphoria. It is unusual for affected females to assign themselves a male role.

Male infants appear normal at birth. Thus, the diagnosis may not be made in boys until signs of adrenal insufficiency develop. Because patients with this condition can deteriorate quickly, infant boys are more likely to die than infant girls. For this reason, many states and countries have instituted newborn screening for this condition (see Newborn Screening, later).

Postnatal Androgen Excess

Untreated or inadequately treated children of both sexes develop additional signs of androgen excess after birth. Boys with the simple virilizing form of 21-hydroxylase deficiency often have delayed diagnosis because they appear normal and rarely develop adrenal insufficiency.

Signs of androgen excess include rapid somatic growth and accelerated skeletal maturation. Thus, affected patients are tall in childhood but premature closure of the epiphyses causes growth to stop relatively early, and adult stature is stunted (see Fig. 570-1). Muscular development may be excessive. Pubic and axillary hair may appear; and acne and a deep voice may develop. The penis, scrotum, and prostate may become enlarged in affected boys; however, the **testes are usually prepubertal** in size so that they appear relatively small in contrast to the enlarged penis. Occasionally, ectopic adrenocortical cells in the testes of patients become hyperplastic similarly to the adrenal glands, producing testicular adrenal rest tumors (Chapter 578). The clitoris may become further enlarged in affected females (see Fig. 570-1). Although the internal genital structures are female, breast development and menstruation may not occur unless the excessive production of androgens is suppressed by adequate treatment.

Similar but usually milder signs of androgen excess may occur in **nonclassical 21-hydroxylase deficiency.** In this attenuated form, cortisol and aldosterone levels are normal and affected females have normal genitals at birth. Males and females may present with precocious pubarche and early development of pubic and axillary hair. Hirsutism, acne, menstrual disorders, and infertility may develop later in life. However, many females and males are completely asymptomatic.

Adrenomedullary Dysfunction

Development of the adrenal medulla requires exposure to the extremely high cortisol levels normally present within the adrenal gland. Thus patients with classic CAH have abnormal adrenomedullary function, as evidenced by blunted epinephrine responses, decreased blood glucose and lower heart rates with exercise. Ability to exercise is unimpaired and the clinical significance of these findings is uncertain. Adrenomedullary dysfunction may exacerbate the cardiovascular effects of cortisol deficiency in untreated or undertreated patients.

LABORATORY FINDINGS (SEE TABLE 570-1)

Patients with salt-losing disease have typical laboratory findings associated with cortisol and aldosterone deficiency, including hyponatremia, hyperkalemia, metabolic acidosis, and often hypoglycemia, but these abnormalities can take 10-14 days or longer to develop after birth. Blood levels of **17-hydroxyprogesterone** are markedly elevated. However, levels of this hormone are high during the 1st 2-3 days of life, even in unaffected infants and especially if they are sick or premature. After infancy, once the circadian rhythm of cortisol is established, 17-hydroxyprogesterone levels vary in the same circadian pattern, being highest in the morning and lowest at night. Blood levels of cortisol are usually low in patients with the salt-losing type of disease. They are often normal in patients with simple virilizing disease but inappropriately low in relation to the ACTH and 17-hydroxyprogesterone levels. In addition to 17-hydroxyprogesterone, levels of androstenedione and testosterone are elevated in affected females; testosterone is not elevated in affected males because normal infant males have high testosterone levels compared with those seen later in childhood. Levels of urinary 17-ketosteroids and pregnanetriol are elevated but are now rarely used clinically because blood samples are easier to obtain than 24-hr urine collections. ACTH levels are elevated but have no diagnostic utility over 17-hydroxyprogesterone levels. Plasma levels of renin are elevated, and serum aldosterone is inappropriately low for the renin level. However, renin levels are high in normal infants in the 1st few weeks of life.

Diagnosis of 21-hydroxylase deficiency is most reliably established by measuring 17-hydroxyprogesterone before and 30 or 60 min after an intravenous bolus of 0.125-0.25 mg of cosyntropin (ACTH 1-24). Nomograms exist that readily distinguish normals and patients with nonclassical and classical 21-hydroxylase deficiency. Heterozygous carriers of this autosomal recessive disorder tend to have higher ACTH-stimulated 17-hydroxyprogesterone levels than genetically unaffected individuals, but there is significant overlap between subjects in these 2 categories. However, in infants with frank electrolyte abnormalities or circulatory instability, it may not be possible or necessary to delay treatment to perform this test, as levels of precursors will be sufficiently elevated on a random blood sample to make the diagnosis.

DIFFERENTIAL DIAGNOSIS

Intersex conditions are discussed more generally in Chapter 582. The initial step in evaluating an infant with ambiguous genitals is a thorough physical examination to define the anatomy of the genitals, locate the urethral meatus, palpate the scrotum or labia and the inguinal regions for testes (palpable gonads almost always indicate the presence of testicular tissue and thus that the infant is a genetic male), and look for any other anatomic abnormalities. Ultrasonography is helpful in demonstrating the presence or absence of a uterus and can often locate the gonads. A rapid karyotype (such as fluorescence in situ hybridization of interphase nuclei for X and Y chromosomes) can quickly determine the genetic sex of the infant. These results are all likely to be available before the results of hormonal testing and together allow the clinical team to advise the parents as to the genetic sex of the infant and the anatomy of internal reproductive structures. Injection of contrast medium into the urogenital sinus of female pseudohermaphrodites demonstrates a vagina and uterus, and most surgeons utilize this information to formulate a plan for surgical management.

PRENATAL DIAGNOSIS

Prenatal diagnosis of 21-hydroxylase is possible late in the 1st trimester by analysis of DNA obtained by chorionic villus sampling or during the 2nd trimester by amniocentesis. This is usually done because the parents already have an affected child. Most often, the *CYP21* gene is analyzed for frequently occurring mutations; more rare mutations may be detected by DNA sequencing.

NEWBORN SCREENING

Because 21-hydroxylase deficiency is often undiagnosed in affected males until they have severe adrenal insufficiency, all states in the USA and many other countries have instituted newborn screening programs. These programs analyze **17-hydroxyprogesterone** levels in dried blood obtained by heel-stick and absorbed on filter paper cards; the same cards are screened in parallel for other congenital conditions such as hypothyroidism and phenylketonuria. Potentially affected infants are typically quickly recalled for additional testing (electrolytes and repeat 17-hydroxyprogesterone determination) at approximately 2 wk of age. Infants with salt-wasting disease often have abnormal electrolytes by this age but are usually not severely ill. Thus, screening programs are effective in preventing many cases of adrenal crisis in affected males. The nonclassical form of the disease is not reliably detected by newborn screening, but this is of little clinical significance because adrenal insufficiency does not occur in this type of 21-hydroxylase deficiency.

The main difficulty with current newborn screening programs is that to reliably detect all affected infants, the cutoff 17-hydroxyprogesterone levels for recalls are set so low that there is a very high frequency of false-positive results (i.e., the test has a low positive predictive value of approximately 1%). This problem is worst in premature infants. Positive predictive value can be improved by using cutoff levels based on gestational age, and by utilizing more specific 2nd-tier screening methods such as liquid chromatography followed by tandem mass spectrometry (LC-MS/MS).

TREATMENT

Glucocorticoid Replacement

Cortisol deficiency is treated with glucocorticoids. Treatment also suppresses excessive production of androgens by the adrenal cortex and thus minimizes problems such as excessive growth and skeletal maturation and virilization. This often requires larger glucocorticoid doses than are needed in other forms of adrenal insufficiency, typically 15-20 mg/m^2/24 hr of hydrocortisone daily administered orally in 3 divided doses. Affected infants usually require dosing at the high end of this range. Double or triple doses are indicated during **periods of stress,** such as infection or surgery. Glucocorticoid treatment must be continued indefinitely in all patients with classical 21-hydroxylase deficiency but may not be necessary in patients with nonclassical disease unless signs of androgen excess are present. Therapy must be individualized. It is desirable to maintain linear growth along percentile lines; crossing to higher height percentiles may suggest undertreatment, whereas loss of height percentiles often indicates overtreatment with glucocorticoids. Overtreatment is also suggested by excessive weight gain. Pubertal development should be monitored by periodic examination, and skeletal maturation is evaluated by serial radiographs of the hand and wrist for bone age. Hormone levels, particularly 17-hydroxyprogesterone and androstenedione, should be measured early in the morning, before taking the morning medications, or at a consistent time in relation to medication dosing. In general, desirable 17-hydroxyprogesterone levels are in the high-normal range or several times normal; low-normal levels can usually be achieved only with excessive glucocorticoid doses.

Menarche occurs at the appropriate age in most girls in whom good control has been achieved; it may be delayed in girls with suboptimal control.

Children with simple virilizing disease, particularly males, are frequently not diagnosed until 3-7 yr of age, at which time skeletal maturation may be 5 yr or more in advance of chronological age. In some children, especially if the bone age is 12 yr or more, **spontaneous gonadotropin-dependent puberty** may occur when treatment is instituted, because therapy with hydrocortisone has suppressed production of adrenal androgens and stimulated release of pituitary gonadotropins if the appropriate level of hypothalamic maturation is present. This form of superimposed true precocious puberty may be treated with a gonadotropin hormone-releasing hormone analog such as leuprolide.

Males with 21-hydroxylase deficiency who have had inadequate corticosteroid therapy may develop adrenal rest testicular tumors, which usually regress with increased steroid dosage. Testicular MRI, ultrasonography, and color flow Doppler examination help define the character and extent of disease. Testis-sparing surgery for steroid-unresponsive tumors has been reported.

Mineralocorticoid Replacement

Patients with salt-wasting disease (i.e., aldosterone deficiency) require mineralocorticoid replacement with **fludrocortisone.** Infants may have very high mineralocorticoid requirements in the 1st few mo of life, usually 0.1-0.3 mg daily in 2 divided doses but occasionally up to 0.4 mg daily, and often require sodium supplementation (sodium chloride, 8 mmol/kg) in addition to the mineralocorticoid. Older infants and children are usually maintained with 0.05-0.1 mg daily of fludrocortisone. In some patients, simple virilizing disease may be easier to control with a low dose of fludrocortisone in addition to hydrocortisone even when these patients have normal aldosterone levels in the absence of mineralocorticoid replacement. Therapy is evaluated by monitoring of vital signs; tachycardia and hypertension are signs of overtreatment with mineralocorticoids. Serum electrolytes should be measured frequently in early infancy as therapy is adjusted. Plasma renin activity is a useful way to determine adequacy of therapy; it should be maintained in or near the normal range but not suppressed.

Additional approaches to improve outcome have been proposed but have not yet become the standard of care. These include an antiandrogen such as flutamide to block the effects of excessive androgen levels, and/or an aromatase inhibitor such as anastrozole, which blocks conversion of androgens to estrogen and thus retards skeletal maturation, a process that is sensitive to estrogens in both boys and girls. Aromatase inhibitors generally should not be used in pubertal girls because they will obviously retard normal puberty and may expose the ovaries to excessive levels of gonadotropins. Growth hormone, with or without LHRH agonists to retard skeletal maturation, has been suggested to improve adult height.

Surgical Management of Ambiguous Genitals

Significantly virilized females usually undergo surgery between 2-6 mo of age. If there is severe clitoromegaly, the clitoris is reduced in size, with partial excision of the corporal bodies and preservation of the neurovascular bundle; however, moderate clitoromegaly may become much less noticeable even without surgery as the patient grows. Vaginoplasty and correction of the urogenital sinus usually are performed at the time of clitoral surgery; revision in adolescence is often necessary.

Risks and benefits of surgery should be fully discussed with parents of affected females. There is limited long-term follow-up of functional outcomes in patients who have undergone **modern** surgical procedures, although it appears that there is frequent sexual dysfunction that increases in frequency and severity with the initial degree of genital virilization. Sex assignment of infants with **disorders of sexual differentiation** (including CAH) is usually based on expected sexual functioning and fertility in adulthood with early surgical correction of the external genitals to conform with the sex assignment. Confused psychosexual identity is not common with CAH. Lay and medical opponents of this practice for other intersex conditions state that it ignores any prenatally biased gender role predisposition and precludes the patient from having any decision as to his or her own preferred sexual identity and what surgical correction of the genitals should be performed. These individuals and groups say treatment should be aimed primarily at educating patient, family, and others about the medical condition, its treatment, and how to deal with the intersex condition. They propose that surgery should be delayed until the patient decides on what, if any, correction should be performed.

In adolescent and adult females with poorly controlled 21-hydroxylase deficiency (hirsutism, obesity, amenorrhea) bilateral laparoscopic adrenalectomy (with hormone replacement) may be an alternative to standard medical hormone replacement therapy, but patients treated in this way may be more susceptible to acute adrenal insufficiency if treatment is interrupted because the adrenal glands have been removed. Moreover, they may exhibit signs of elevated ACTH levels such as abnormal pigmentation.

Prenatal Treatment

Besides genetic counseling, the main goal of prenatal diagnosis is to facilitate appropriate prenatal treatment of affected females. Mothers with pregnancies at risk are given dexamethasone, a steroid that readily crosses the placenta, in an amount of 20 µg/kg prepregnancy maternal weight daily in 2 or 3 divided doses. This suppresses secretion of steroids by the fetal adrenal, including secretion of adrenal androgens. If started by 6 wk of gestation, it ameliorates virilization of the external genitals in affected females. Chorionic villus biopsy is then performed to determine the sex and genotype of the fetus; therapy is continued only if the fetus is an affected female. DNA analysis of fetal cells isolated from maternal plasma for sex determination and *CYP21* gene analysis may permit earlier identification of the affected female fetus. Children exposed to this therapy have slightly lower birthweights. Effects on personality or cognition, such as increased shyness, have been suggested but not consistently observed. At present there is insufficient information to determine whether there are any long-term risks, particularly in the males and unaffected females who derive no direct benefit from the treatment. Maternal side effects of prenatal treatment have included edema, excessive weight gain, hypertension, glucose intolerance, cushingoid facial features, and severe striae. Prenatal treatment is therefore carried out only under institutional protocols in some locales, but it is offered as an option outside the research setting by high-risk obstetricians in other communities.

BIBLIOGRAPHY

Please visit the Nelson Textbook of Pediatrics *website at* www.expertconsult.com *for the complete bibliography.*

570.2 Congenital Adrenal Hyperplasia Due to 11β-Hydroxylase Deficiency

Perrin C. White

ETIOLOGY

Deficiency of 11β-hydroxylase is due to a mutation in the *CYP11B1* gene located on chromosome 8q24. *CYP11B1* mediates 11-hydroxylation of 11-deoxycortisol to cortisol. Because 11-deoxycortisol is not converted to cortisol, levels of corticotropin are high. In consequence, precursors—particularly 11-deoxycortisol and deoxycorticosterone—accumulate and are shunted into androgen biosynthesis in the same manner as occurs in 21-hydroxylase deficiency. The adjacent *CYP11B2* gene encoding aldosterone synthase is generally unaffected in this disorder, so patients are able to synthesize aldosterone normally.

EPIDEMIOLOGY

11β-Hydroxylase deficiency accounts for approximately 5% of cases of adrenal hyperplasia; its incidence has been estimated as 1/250,000 to 1/100,000. More than 30 different mutations in *CYP11B1* have been identified. The disorder occurs relatively frequently in Israeli Jews of North African origin (1 in 15,000-17,000 live births); in this ethnic group almost all alleles carry an Arg448 to His (R448H) mutation. This disorder presents in a classical, severe form and very rarely in a nonclassical, milder form.

CLINICAL MANIFESTATIONS

Although cortisol is not synthesized efficiently, aldosterone synthetic capacity is normal, and some corticosterone is synthesized from progesterone by the intact aldosterone synthase enzyme. Thus, it is unusual for patients to manifest signs of adrenal insufficiency such as hypotension, hypoglycemia, hyponatremia, and hyperkalemia. Approximately 65% of patients become **hypertensive,** although this can take several years to develop. Hypertension is probably a consequence of elevated levels of deoxycorticosterone, which has mineralocorticoid activity. Infants may transiently develop signs of mineralocorticoid deficiency after treatment with hydrocortisone is instituted. This is presumably due to sudden suppression of deoxycorticosterone secretion in a patient with atrophy of the zona glomerulosa caused by chronic suppression of renin activity.

All signs and symptoms of androgen excess that are found in 21-hydroxylase deficiency may also occur in 11-hydroxylase deficiency.

LABORATORY FINDINGS

Plasma levels of 11-deoxycortisol and deoxycorticosterone are elevated. Because deoxycorticosterone and metabolites have mineralocorticoid activity, plasma renin activity is suppressed. Consequently, aldosterone levels are low even though the ability to synthesize aldosterone is intact. Hypokalemic alkalosis occasionally occurs.

TREATMENT

Patients are treated with hydrocortisone in doses similar to those used for 21-hydroxylase deficiency. Mineralocorticoid replacement is sometimes transiently required in infancy but is rarely necessary otherwise. Hypertension often resolves with glucocorticoid treatment but may require additional therapy if it is of long standing. Calcium channel blockers may be beneficial under these circumstances.

BIBLIOGRAPHY
Please visit the Nelson Textbook of Pediatrics *website at* *www.expertconsult.com* *for the complete bibliography.*

570.3 Congenital Adrenal Hyperplasia Due to 3β-Hydroxysteroid Dehydrogenase Deficiency

Perrin C. White

ETIOLOGY

Deficiency of 3β-hydroxysteroid dehydrogenase (3β-HSD) occurs in fewer than 2% of patients with adrenal hyperplasia. This enzyme is required for conversion of Δ5 steroids (pregnenolone, 17-hydroxypregnenolone, dehydroepiandrosterone [DHEA]) to Δ4 steroids (progesterone, 17-hydroxyprogesterone, and androstenedione). Thus, deficiency of the enzyme results in decreased synthesis of cortisol, aldosterone, and androstenedione but increased secretion of DHEA (see Fig. 568-1). The 3β-HSD enzyme expressed in the adrenal cortex and gonad is encoded by the *HSD3B2* gene located on chromosome 1p13.1. Over 30 mutations in the *HSD3B2* gene have been described in patients with 3β-HSD deficiency.

CLINICAL MANIFESTATIONS

Because cortisol and aldosterone are not synthesized in patients with the classical form of the disease, infants are prone to **salt-wasting crises.** Because androstenedione and testosterone are not synthesized, **boys are incompletely virilized.** Varying degrees of hypospadias may occur, with or without bifid scrotum or cryptorchidism. Because DHEA levels are elevated and this hormone is a weak androgen, girls are mildly virilized, with slight to moderate clitoral enlargement. Postnatally, continued excessive DHEA secretion can cause precocious adrenarche. During adolescence and adulthood, hirsutism, irregular menses, and polycystic ovarian disease occur in females. Males manifest variable degrees of hypogonadism, although appropriate male secondary sexual development may occur. A persistent defect of testicular 3β-HSD is demonstrated, however, by the high Δ5 to Δ4 steroid ratio in testicular effluent.

LABORATORY FINDINGS

The hallmark of this disorder is the marked elevation of the Δ5 steroids (such as 17-hydroxypregnenolone and DHEA) preceding the enzymatic block. Patients may also have elevated levels of 17-hydroxyprogesterone because of the extra-adrenal 3β-HSD activity that occurs in peripheral tissues; these patients may be mistaken for patients with 21-hydroxylase deficiency. The ratio of 17-hydroxypregnenolone to 17-hydroxyprogesterone is markedly elevated in 3β-HSD deficiency, in contrast to the decreased ratio in 21-hydroxylase deficiency. Plasma renin activity is elevated in the salt-wasting form.

DIFFERENTIAL DIAGNOSIS

It is not unusual for children with premature adrenarche, or women with signs of androgen excess, to have mild to moderate elevations in DHEA levels. It has been suggested that such individuals have "nonclassical 3β-HSD deficiency." Mutations in the *HSD3B2* gene are usually not found in such individuals, and a nonclassical form of this deficiency must actually be quite rare. The activity of 3β-HSD in the adrenal zonae fasciculata and reticularis, relative to CYP17 (17-hydroxylase/17,20-lyase) activity, normally decreases during adrenarche to facilitate DHEA synthesis, and so modest elevations in DHEA in preteenage children or women usually represent a normal variant.

TREATMENT

Patients require glucocorticoid and mineralocorticoid replacement with hydrocortisone and fludrocortisone, respectively, as in 21-hydroxylase deficiency. Incompletely virilized genetic males in whom a male sex of rearing is contemplated may benefit from several injections of a depot form of testosterone early in infancy to increase the size of the phallus. They may also require testosterone replacement at puberty.

BIBLIOGRAPHY
Please visit the Nelson Textbook of Pediatrics *website at* *www.expertconsult.com* *for the complete bibliography.*

570.4 Congenital Adrenal Hyperplasia Due to 17-Hydroxylase Deficiency

Perrin C. White

ETIOLOGY

Less than 1% of CAH cases are caused by 17-hydroxylase deficiency. A single polypeptide, CYP17, catalyzes 2 distinct reactions: 17-hydroxylation of pregnenolone and progesterone to 17-hydroxypregnenolone and 17-hydroxyprogesterone, respectively, and the 17,20-lyase reaction mediating conversion of 17-hydroxypregnenolone to DHEA and, to a lesser extent, 17-hydroxyprogesterone to Δ4-androstenedione. DHEA and androstenedione are steroid precursors of testosterone and estrogen (see Fig. 568-1). The enzyme is expressed in both the adrenal cortex and the gonads and is encoded by a gene on chromosome 10q24.3. Most mutations affect both the hydroxylase and lyase activities, but rare mutations can affect either activity alone.

CLINICAL MANIFESTATIONS AND LABORATORY FINDINGS

Patients with 17-hydroxylase deficiency cannot synthesize cortisol, but their ability to synthesize corticosterone is intact. Because corticosterone is an active glucocorticoid, patients do not develop adrenal insufficiency. Deoxycorticosterone, the immediate precursor of corticosterone, is synthesized in excess. This can cause **hypertension, hypokalemia,** and suppression of renin and aldosterone secretion, as occurs in 11-hydroxylase deficiency. In contrast to 11-hydroxylase deficiency, patients with 17-hydroxylase deficiency are unable to synthesize sex hormones. Affected **males are incompletely virilized** and present as phenotypic females (but gonads are usually palpable in the inguinal region or the labia) or with sexual ambiguity (male pseudohermaphroditism). Affected females usually present with **failure of sexual development** at the expected time of **puberty.** 17-Hydroxylase deficiency in females must be considered in the differential diagnosis of primary hypogonadism (Chapter 580). In addition to the increased DOC, suppressed renin and aldosterone, and decreased 17-hydroxylated steroids, cortisol, and sex steroids are unresponsive to stimulation with ACTH and human chorionic gonadotropin, respectively.

TREATMENT

Patients with 17-hydroxylase deficiency require cortisol replacement to suppress secretion of deoxycorticosterone and thus control hypertension. Additional antihypertensive medication may be required. Females require estrogen replacement at puberty. Genetic males may require either estrogen or androgen supplementation depending on the sex of rearing. Because of the possibility of malignant transformation of abdominal testes with androgen insensitivity syndrome (Chapter 577), genetic males with severe 17-hydroxylase deficiency being reared as females require gonadectomy at or before adolescence.

BIBLIOGRAPHY
Please visit the Nelson Textbook of Pediatrics *website at www.expertconsult.com for the complete bibliography.*

570.5 Lipoid Adrenal Hyperplasia

Perrin C. White

ETIOLOGY

Lipoid adrenal hyperplasia is a rare disorder, reported in fewer than 100 patients, the majority of whom are Japanese. In this disorder there is marked accumulation of cholesterol and lipids in the adrenal cortex and gonads, associated with severe impairment of all steroidogenesis. Lipoid adrenal hyperplasia is usually caused by mutations in the gene for steroidogenic acute regulatory protein (StAR), a mitochondrial protein that promotes the movement of cholesterol from the outer to the inner mitochondrial membrane. Mutations in the *CYP11A1* gene have been reported in 2 patients with lipoid adrenal hyperplasia.

Some cholesterol is able to enter mitochondria even in the absence of StAR, so it might be supposed that this disorder would not completely impair steroid biosynthesis. The accumulation of cholesterol in the cytoplasm is cytotoxic, eventually leading to death of all steroidogenic cells in which StAR is normally expressed. This occurs prenatally in the adrenals and testes. The ovaries do not normally synthesize steroids until puberty, so cholesterol does not accumulate and the ovaries can retain the capacity to synthesize estrogens until adolescence.

Although estrogens synthesized by the placenta are required to maintain pregnancy, the placenta does not require StAR for steroid biosynthesis. Thus, mutations of StAR are not prenatally lethal.

CLINICAL MANIFESTATIONS

Patients with lipoid adrenal hyperplasia are usually unable to synthesize any adrenal steroids. Thus, affected infants are likely to be confused with those with adrenal hypoplasia. Salt-losing manifestations are usual, and many infants die in early infancy. Genetic males are unable to synthesize androgens and thus are **phenotypically female** but with gonads. Genetic females appear normal at birth and may undergo feminization at puberty with menstrual bleeding. They too, progress to hypergonadotropic hypogonadism when accumulated cholesterol kills granulosa (i.e., steroid synthesizing) cells in the ovary.

LABORATORY FINDINGS

Adrenal and gonadal steroid hormone levels are low in lipoid adrenal hyperplasia, with a decreased or absent response to stimulation (ACTH, human chorionic gonadotropin). Plasma renin levels are increased.

Imaging studies of the adrenal gland demonstrating massive adrenal enlargement in the newborn help establish the diagnosis of lipoid adrenal hyperplasia.

TREATMENT

Patients require glucocorticoid and mineralocorticoid replacement. Genetic males are usually assigned a female sex of rearing; thus both genetic males and females require estrogen replacement at the expected age of puberty.

BIBLIOGRAPHY
Please visit the Nelson Textbook of Pediatrics *website at www.expertconsult.com for the complete bibliography.*

570.6 Deficiency of P450 Oxidoreductase (Antley-Bixler Syndrome)

Perrin C. White

ETIOLOGY, PATHOGENESIS, AND CLINICAL MANIFESTATIONS

P450 oxidoreductase (POR, gene located on chromosome 7q11.3) is required for the activity of all microsomal cytochrome P450 enzymes (Chapter 568) including the adrenal enzymes CYP17 and CYP21. Thus, complete POR deficiency abolishes all microsomal P450 activity. This is embryonically lethal in mice and presumably in humans as well. Patients with mutations that decrease but do not abolish POR activity have partial deficiencies of 17-hydroxylase and 21-hydroxylase activities in the adrenals. Deficiency of 17-hydroxylase leads to incomplete masculinization in males; 21-hydroxylase deficiency may lead to virilization in females. Additionally, aromatase (CYP19) activity in the placenta is decreased, leading to unopposed action of androgens produced by the fetal adrenal. This exacerbates virilization of female fetuses and may **virilize the mother** of an affected fetus as well. Although it is puzzling that affected females could be virilized despite a partial deficiency in CYP17 (which is required for androgen biosynthesis), an alternative biosynthetic pathway may be utilized in which 17-hydroxyprogesterone is converted to 5α-pregnane-3α,17α-diol-20-one, a metabolite that is a much better substrate for the 17,20-lyase activity of CYP17 than the usual substrate, 17-hydroxypregnenolone (Chapter 568). The metabolite is then converted in several enzymatic steps to dihydrotestosterone, a potent androgen.

Because many other P450 enzymes are affected, patients often (but not invariably) have other congenital anomalies collectively referred to as **Antley-Bixler syndrome.** These include craniosynostosis; brachycephaly; frontal bossing; severe midface hypoplasia with proptosis and choanal stenosis or atresia; humeroradial synostosis; medial bowing of ulnas; long, slender fingers with camptodactyly; narrow iliac wings; anterior bowing of femurs; and malformations of the heart and kidneys. Studies of mutant mice suggest that the metabolic defects responsible for these anomalies include defective metabolism of retinoic acid, leading to elevated levels of this teratogenic compound, and deficient biosynthesis of cholesterol.

EPIDEMIOLOGY

The prevalence is not known with certainty. It must be rare compared with 21-hydroxylase deficiency but might occur at similar frequencies to the other forms of CAH.

LABORATORY FINDINGS

Serum steroids that are not 17- or 21-hydroxylated are most increased, including pregnenolone and progesterone. 17-Hydroxy, 21-deoxy-steroids are also increased, including 17-hydroxypregnenolone, 17-hydroxyprogesterone, and 21-deoxycortisol. Urinary steroid metabolites may be determined by quantitative mass spectrometry. Metabolites excreted at increased levels include pregnanediol, pregnanetriol, pregnanetriolone, and corticosterone metabolites. Urinary cortisol metabolites are decreased. Genetic analysis demonstrates mutations in the *POR* gene.

DIFFERENTIAL DIAGNOSIS

This disorder must be distinguished from other forms of congenital adrenal hyperplasia, particularly 21-hydroxylase deficiency in females, which is far more common and has similar laboratory findings. Suspicion for *POR* deficiency may be raised if the mother is virilized or if the associated abnormalities of Antley-Bixler syndrome are present. Conversely, virilization of both the mother and her daughter can result from a luteoma of pregnancy, but in this case postnatal abnormalities of corticosteroid biosynthesis should not be observed. Antley-Bixler syndrome may also occur without abnormalities of steroid hormone biosynthesis, resulting from mutations in the fibroblast growth factor receptor, FGFR2.

BIBLIOGRAPHY

Please visit the Nelson Textbook of Pediatrics *website at www.expertconsult.com for the complete bibliography.*

570.7 Aldosterone Synthase Deficiency

Perrin C. White

ETIOLOGY

This is a rare autosomal recessive disorder in which conversion of corticosterone to aldosterone is impaired; a group of Iranian Jewish patients has been the most thoroughly studied. The majority of cases result from mutations in the *CYP11B2* gene coding for aldosterone synthase; however, linkage to *CYP11B2* has been excluded in other kindreds. When not due to *CYP11B2* mutations, the disorder has been termed familial hyperreninemic hypoaldosteronism type 2; the causative gene or genes have not yet been identified.

Aldosterone synthase mediates the 3 final steps in the synthesis of aldosterone from deoxycorticosterone (11-hydroxylation, 18-hydroxylation, and 18-oxidation). Although 11-hydroxylation is required to convert deoxycorticosterone to corticosterone, this conversion can also be catalyzed by the related enzyme, CYP11B1, located in the fasciculata, which is unaffected in this disorder. For the same reason, these patients have normal cortisol biosynthesis.

The disease has previously been classified into 2 types, termed corticosterone methyloxidase deficiency types I and II. They differ only in levels of the immediate precursor of aldosterone, 18-hydroxycorticosterone; levels are low in type I deficiency and elevated in type II deficiency. These differences do not correspond in a simple way to particular mutations and are of limited clinical importance.

CLINICAL MANIFESTATIONS

Infants with aldosterone synthase deficiency may have severe electrolyte abnormalities with **hyponatremia, hyperkalemia,** and **metabolic acidosis.** Because cortisol synthesis is unaffected, infants rarely become as ill as untreated infants with salt-losing forms of congenital adrenal hyperplasia such as 21-hydroxylase deficiency. Thus, some infants escape diagnosis. Later in infancy or in early childhood they may exhibit failure to thrive and poor growth. Adults often are asymptomatic, although they may develop electrolyte abnormalities when depleted of sodium through procedures such as bowel preparation for a barium enema.

LABORATORY FINDINGS

Infants have elevated plasma renin activity. Aldosterone levels are decreased; they may be at the lower end of the normal range but are always inappropriately low for the degree of hyperkalemia or hyperreninemia. Corticosterone levels are often elevated.

Some but not all patients have marked elevation of 18-hydroxycorticosterone, but low levels of this steroid do not exclude the diagnosis. In those kindreds that 18-hydroxycorticosterone levels are elevated in affected individuals, this biochemical abnormality persists in adults even when they have no electrolyte abnormalities.

DIFFERENTIAL DIAGNOSIS

It is important to distinguish aldosterone synthase deficiency from primary adrenal insufficiency in which both cortisol and aldosterone are affected (including salt-wasting forms of congenital adrenal hyperplasia) because the latter condition is usually associated with a much greater risk of shock and hyponatremia. This becomes apparent after the appropriate laboratory studies. **Pseudohypoaldosteronism** (Chapter 52) may have similar electrolyte abnormalities and hyperreninemia, but aldosterone levels are high, and this condition usually does not respond to fludrocortisone treatment.

TREATMENT

Treatment consists of giving enough fludrocortisone (0.05-0.3 mg daily), sodium chloride, or both to return plasma renin levels to normal. With increasing age, salt-losing signs usually improve and drug therapy can often be discontinued.

BIBLIOGRAPHY

Please visit the Nelson Textbook of Pediatrics *website at www.expertconsult.com for the complete bibliography.*

570.8 Glucocorticoid-Suppressible Hyperaldosteronism

Perrin C. White

ETIOLOGY

Glucocorticoid-suppressible aldosteronism (glucocorticoid-remediable aldosteronism, familial hyperaldosteronism type I) is an autosomal dominant form of **low-renin hypertension** in which hyperaldosteronism is rapidly suppressed by glucocorticoid administration. This unusual effect of glucocorticoids suggests that this disorder is regulated by ACTH aldosterone secretion instead of by the renin-angiotensin system. In addition to abnormally regulated secretion of aldosterone, there is marked overproduction of 18-hydroxycortisol and 18-oxocortisol. The synthesis of these steroids requires both 17-hydroxylase (CYP17) activity, which is expressed only in the zona fasciculata, and aldosterone synthase (CYP11B2) activity, which is normally expressed only in the zona glomerulosa. Together, these features imply that aldosterone synthase is being expressed in a manner similar to the closely related enzyme steroid 11-hydroxylase *(CYP11B1)*. The disorder is caused by unequal meiotic crossing over events between the *CYP11B1* and *CYP11B2* genes, which are closely linked on chromosome 8q24. An additional "hybrid" gene is produced, having regulatory sequences of *CYP11B1* juxtaposed with coding sequences of *CYP11B2*. This results in the inappropriate expression of a *CYP11B2*-like enzyme with aldosterone synthase activity in the adrenal fasciculata.

CLINICAL MANIFESTATIONS

Some affected children have no symptoms, the diagnosis being established after incidental discovery of moderate hypertension, typically about 30 mm Hg higher than unaffected family members of the same age. Others have more symptomatic hypertension with headache, dizziness, and visual disturbances. A strong family history of early-onset hypertension or early strokes may alert the clinician to the diagnosis. Some patients have chronic hypokalemia, but this is not a consistent finding and is usually mild.

LABORATORY FINDINGS

Patients have elevated plasma and urine levels of aldosterone and suppressed plasma renin activity. Hypokalemia is not consistently present. Urinary and plasma levels of 18-oxocortisol and 18-hydroxycortisol are markedly increased. The hybrid *CYP11B1/CYP11B2* gene can be readily detected by molecular genetic methods; these assays are not routinely available.

DIFFERENTIAL DIAGNOSIS

This condition should be distinguished from primary aldosteronism due to bilateral hyperplasia or an aldosterone-producing adenoma (Chapter 572). Most cases of primary aldosteronism are sporadic although rare affected kindreds have been reported. Patients with primary aldosteronism may also have elevated levels of 18-hydroxycortisol and 18-oxocortisol, and these biochemical tests should be used cautiously to distinguish primary and glucocorticoid-suppressible aldosteronism. A therapeutic trial of dexamethasone may be helpful if aldosterone secretion is suppressed, and genetic testing should identify the hybrid gene of glucocorticoid-suppressible hyperaldosteronism if it is present.

TREATMENT

Glucocorticoid-suppressible hyperaldosteronism is managed by daily administration of a glucocorticoid, usually dexamethasone, 25 μg/kg/day in divided doses. If necessary, effects of aldosterone can be blocked with a potassium-sparing diuretic such as spironolactone, eplerenone, or amiloride. Hypertension resolves in patients in whom the hypertension is not severe or of long standing. If hypertension is long standing, additional antihypertensive medication may be required, such as a calcium channel blocker.

GENETIC COUNSELING

Because of the autosomal dominant mode of inheritance, at-risk family members should be investigated for this easily treated cause of hypertension.

BIBLIOGRAPHY

Please visit the Nelson Textbook of Pediatrics *website at www.expertconsult.com for the complete bibliography.*

Chapter 571
Cushing Syndrome

Perrin C. White

Cushing syndrome is the result of abnormally high blood levels of cortisol or other glucocorticoids. This can be iatrogenic or the result of endogenous cortisol secretion, due either to an adrenal tumor or to hypersecretion of corticotropin (adrenocorticotropic hormone [ACTH]) by the pituitary (Cushing disease) or by a tumor (Table 571-1).

Table 571-1 ETIOLOGIC CLASSIFICATION OF ADRENOCORTICAL HYPERFUNCTION

EXCESS ANDROGEN
Congenital adrenal hyperplasia
21-Hydroxylase (P450c21) deficiency
11β-Hydroxylase (P450c11) deficiency
3β-Hydroxysteroid dehydrogenase defect (deficiency or dysregulation)
Tumor
EXCESS CORTISOL (CUSHING SYNDROME)
Bilateral adrenal hyperplasia
Hypersecretion of corticotropin (Cushing disease)
Ectopic secretion of corticotropin
Exogenous corticotropin
Adrenocortical nodular dysplasia
Pigmented nodular adrenocortical disease (Carney complex)
Tumor
EXCESS MINERALOCORTICOID
Primary hyperaldosteronism
Aldosterone-secreting adenoma
Bilateral micronodular adrenocortical hyperplasia
Glucocorticoid-suppressible aldosteronism
Tumor
Deoxycorticosterone excess
Congenital adrenal hyperplasia
11β-Hydroxylase (P450c11)
17α-Hydroxylase (P450c17)
Tumor
Apparent mineralocorticoid excess (deficiency of 11β-hydroxysteroid dehydrogenase type 2)
EXCESS ESTROGEN
Tumor

ETIOLOGY

The most common cause of Cushing syndrome is prolonged exogenous administration of glucocorticoid hormones, especially at the high doses used to treat lymphoproliferative disorders. This rarely represents a diagnostic challenge, but management of hyperglycemia, hypertension, weight gain, linear growth retardation, and osteoporosis often complicates therapy with corticosteroids.

Endogenous Cushing syndrome is most often caused in infants by a functioning adrenocortical tumor (Chapter 573). Patients with these tumors often exhibit signs of hypercortisolism along with signs of hypersecretion of other steroids such as androgens, estrogens, and aldosterone.

Although extremely rare in infants, the most common etiology of endogenous Cushing syndrome in children older than 7 yr of age is **Cushing disease,** in which excessive ACTH secreted by a pituitary adenoma causes bilateral adrenal hyperplasia. Such adenomas are often too small to detect by imaging techniques and are termed microadenomas. They consist principally of chromophobe cells and frequently show positive immunostaining for ACTH and its precursor, pro-opiomelanocortin (POMC).

ACTH-dependent Cushing syndrome may also result from ectopic production of ACTH, although this is uncommon in children. Ectopic ACTH secretion in children has been associated with islet cell carcinoma of the pancreas, neuroblastoma or ganglioneuroblastoma, hemangiopericytoma, Wilms tumor, and thymic carcinoid. Hypertension is more common in the ectopic ACTH syndrome than in other forms of Cushing syndrome, because very high cortisol levels may overwhelm 11β-hydroxysteroid dehydrogenase in the kidney (Chapter 568) and thus have an enhanced mineralocorticoid (salt-retaining) effect.

Several syndromes are associated with the development of multiple autonomously hyperfunctioning nodules of adrenocortical tissue, rather than single adenomas or carcinomas (which are discussed in Chapter 573). **Primary pigmented nodular**

adrenocortical disease (PPNAD) is a distinctive form of ACTH-independent Cushing syndrome. It may occur as an isolated event or, more commonly, as a familial disorder with other manifestations. The adrenal glands are small and have characteristic multiple, small (<4 mm in diameter), pigmented (black) nodules containing large cells with cytoplasm and lipofuscin; there is cortical atrophy between the nodules. This adrenal disorder occurs as a component of **Carney complex,** an autosomal dominant disorder also consisting of centrofacial lentigines and blue nevi; cardiac and cutaneous myxomas; pituitary, thyroid, and testicular tumors; and pigmented melanotic schwannomas. Carney complex is inherited in an autosomal dominant manner, although sporadic cases occur. Genetic loci for Carney complex have been mapped to the gene for the type 1α regulatory subunit of protein kinase A (PRKAR1A) on chromosome 17q22-24 and less frequently to chromosome 2p16. Patients with with Carney complex and PRKAR1A mutations generally develop PPNAD as adults, and those with the disorder mapping to chromosome 2 (and most sporadic cases) develop PPNAD less frequently and later. Conversely, children presenting with PPNAD as an isolated finding rarely have mutations in PRKAR1A, or subsequently develop other manifestations of Carney complex. Some patients with isolated PPNAD have mutations in the PDE8B or PDE11A genes encoding different phosphodiesterase isozymes.

ACTH-independent Cushing syndrome with nodular hyperplasia and adenoma formation occurs rarely in cases of **McCune-Albright syndrome,** with symptoms beginning in infancy or childhood. McCune-Albright syndrome is caused by a somatic mutation of the *GNAS* gene encoding the G protein, $G_s\alpha$, through which the ACTH receptor (MCR2) normally signals. This results in inhibition of guanosine triphosphatase activity and constitutive activation of adenylate cyclase, thus increasing levels of cyclic adenosine monophosphate (cAMP). When the mutation is present in adrenal tissue, cortisol and cell division are stimulated independently of ACTH. Other tissues in which activating mutations may occur are bone (producing fibrous dysplasia), gonads, thyroid, and pituitary. Clinical manifestations depend on which tissues are affected.

Where the genes causing nodular adrenocortical hyperplasia have been identified, they all produce overactivity of the ACTH signaling pathway either by constitutively activating $G_s\alpha$ (McCune-Albright syndrome), by reducing the breakdown of cAMP and thus increasing its intracellular levels (mutations of PDE8B or PDE11A), or by disrupting the regulation of the cAMP-dependent enzyme, protein kinase A (PRKAR1A mutations).

Additionally, adrenocortical lesions including diffuse hyperplasia, nodular hyperplasia, adenoma, and rarely carcinoma may occur as part of the multiple endocrine neoplasia type 1 syndrome, an autosomal dominant disorder, in which there is homozygous inactivation of the menin (**MEN1**) tumor suppressor gene on chromosome 11q13 (Chapter 567).

CLINICAL MANIFESTATIONS

Signs of Cushing syndrome have been recognized in infants younger than 1 yr of age. The disorder appears to be more severe and the clinical findings more flagrant in infants than in older children. The face is rounded, with prominent cheeks and a flushed appearance (moon facies). Generalized obesity is common in younger children. In children with adrenal tumors, signs of abnormal masculinization occur frequently; accordingly, there may be hirsutism on the face and trunk, pubic hair, acne, deepening of the voice, and enlargement of the clitoris in girls. Growth is impaired, with length falling below the 3rd percentile, except when significant virilization produces normal or even accelerated growth. Hypertension is common and may occasionally lead to heart failure. An increased susceptibility to infection may also lead to sepsis.

In older children, in addition to obesity, short stature is a common presenting feature. Gradual onset of obesity and deceleration or cessation of growth may be the only early manifestations. Older children most often have more severe obesity of the face and trunk compared with the extremities. Purplish striae on the hips, abdomen, and thighs are common. Pubertal development may be delayed, or amenorrhea may occur in girls past menarche. Weakness, headache, and emotional lability may be prominent. Hypertension and hyperglycemia usually occur; hyperglycemia may progress to frank diabetes. Osteoporosis is common and may cause pathologic fractures.

LABORATORY FINDINGS

Cortisol levels in blood are normally elevated at 8 AM and decrease to less than 50% by midnight except in infants and young children in whom a diurnal rhythm is not always established. In patients with Cushing syndrome this circadian rhythm is lost; midnight cortisol levels >4.4 μg/dL strongly suggest the diagnosis. It is difficult to obtain diurnal blood samples as part of an outpatient evaluation, but cortisol can be measured in saliva samples, which can be obtained at home at the appropriate times of day. Elevated nighttime salivary cortisol levels raise suspicion for Cushing syndrome.

Urinary excretion of free cortisol is increased. This is best measured in a 24-hr urine sample and is expressed as a ratio of micrograms of cortisol excreted per gram of creatinine. This ratio is independent of body size and completeness of the urine collection.

A single-dose dexamethasone suppression test is often helpful; a dose of 25-30 μg/kg (maximum of 2 mg) given at 11 PM results in a plasma cortisol level of less than 5 μg/dL at 8 AM the next morning in normal individuals but not in patients with Cushing syndrome. It is prudent to measure the dexamethasone level in the same blood sample to ensure adequacy of dosing.

A glucose tolerance test is often abnormal. Levels of serum electrolytes are usually normal, but potassium may be decreased, especially in patients with tumors that secrete ACTH ectopically.

After the diagnosis of Cushing syndrome has been established, it is necessary to determine whether it is caused by a pituitary adenoma, an ectopic ACTH-secreting tumor, or a cortisol-secreting adrenal tumor. ACTH concentrations are usually suppressed in patients with cortisol-secreting tumors, are very high in patients with ectopic ACTH-secreting tumors, but may be normal in patients with ACTH-secreting pituitary adenomas. After an intravenous bolus of corticotropin-releasing hormone (CRH), patients with ACTH-dependent Cushing syndrome have an exaggerated ACTH and cortisol response, whereas those with adrenal tumors show no increase in ACTH and cortisol. The 2-step dexamethasone suppression test consists of administration of dexamethasone, 30 and 120 μg/kg/24 hr in 4 divided doses, on consecutive days. In children with pituitary Cushing syndrome, the larger dose, but not the smaller dose, suppresses serum levels of cortisol. Typically, patients with ACTH-independent Cushing syndrome do not show suppressed cortisol levels with dexamethasone.

CT detects virtually all adrenal tumors larger than 1.5 cm in diameter. MRI may detect ACTH-secreting pituitary adenomas, but many are too small to be seen; the addition of gadolinium contrast increases the sensitivity of detection. Bilateral inferior petrosal blood sampling to measure concentrations of ACTH before and after CRH administration may be required to localize the tumor when a pituitary adenoma is not visualized; this is not routinely available in many centers.

DIFFERENTIAL DIAGNOSIS

Cushing syndrome is frequently suspected in children with obesity, particularly when striae and hypertension are present.

Children with simple obesity are usually tall, whereas those with Cushing syndrome are short or have a decelerating growth rate. Although urinary excretion of cortisol is often elevated in simple obesity, salivary nighttime levels of cortisol are normal and cortisol secretion is suppressed by oral administration of low doses of dexamethasone.

Elevated levels of cortisol and ACTH without clinical evidence of Cushing syndrome occur in patients with generalized glucocorticoid resistance. Affected patients may be asymptomatic or exhibit hypertension, hypokalemia, and precocious pseudopuberty; these manifestations are caused by increased mineralocorticoid and adrenal androgen secretion in response to elevated ACTH levels. Mutations in the glucocorticoid receptor have been identified.

TREATMENT

Transsphenoidal pituitary microsurgery is the treatment of choice in pituitary Cushing disease in children. The overall success rate with follow-up of less than 10 yr is 60-80%. Low postoperative serum or urinary cortisol concentrations predict long-term remission in the majority of cases. Relapses are treated with re-operation or pituitary irradiation.

Cyproheptadine, a centrally acting serotonin antagonist that blocks ACTH release, has been used to treat Cushing disease in adults; remissions are usually not sustained after discontinuation of therapy. This agent is rarely used in children. Inhibitors of adrenal steroidogenesis (metyrapone, ketoconazole, aminoglutethimide, etomidate) have been used preoperatively to normalize circulating cortisol levels and reduce perioperative morbidity and mortality.

If a pituitary adenoma does not respond to treatment or if ACTH is secreted by an ectopic metastatic tumor, the adrenal glands may need to be removed. This can often be accomplished laparoscopically. Adrenalectomy may lead to increased ACTH secretion by an unresected pituitary adenoma, evidenced mainly by marked hyperpigmentation; this condition is termed **Nelson Syndrome.**

Management of patients undergoing adrenalectomy requires adequate preoperative and postoperative replacement therapy with a corticosteroid. Tumors that produce corticosteroids usually lead to atrophy of the normal adrenal tissue, and replacement with cortisol (10 mg/m^2/24 hr in 3 divided doses after the immediate postoperative period) is required until there is recovery of the hypothalamic-pituitary-adrenal axis. Postoperative complications may include sepsis, pancreatitis, thrombosis, poor wound healing, and sudden collapse, particularly in infants with Cushing syndrome. Substantial catch-up growth, pubertal progress, and increased bone density occur, but bone density remains abnormal and adult height is often compromised. The management of adrenocortical tumors is discussed in Chapter 573.

BIBLIOGRAPHY
Please visit the Nelson Textbook of Pediatrics *website at* *www.expertconsult.com* *for the complete bibliography.*

Chapter 572 Primary Aldosteronism

Perrin C. White

Primary aldosteronism encompasses disorders caused by excessive aldosterone secretion independent of the renin-angiotensin system. These disorders are characterized by **hypertension, hypokalemia,** and suppression of the renin-angiotensin system.

For the full continuation of this chapter, please visit the Nelson Textbook of Pediatrics *website at* *www.expertconsult.com*.

Chapter 573 Adrenocortical Tumors

Perrin C. White

EPIDEMIOLOGY

Adrenocortical tumors are rare in childhood, with an incidence of 0.3-0.5 cases per million child-years. They occur in all age groups but most commonly in children younger than 6 yr of age, and are more frequent (1.6-fold) in girls. In 2-10% of cases, the tumors are bilateral. Symptoms of endocrine hyperfunction are present in more than 90% of children with adrenal tumors (see Table 571-1). Tumors may be associated with hemihypertrophy, usually occurring during the 1st few years of life. They are also associated with other congenital defects, particularly genitourinary tract and central nervous system abnormalities and hamartomatous defects.

For the full continuation of this chapter, please visit the Nelson Textbook of Pediatrics *website at* *www.expertconsult.com*.

573.1 Virilizing Adrenocortical and Feminizing Adrenal Tumors

Perrin C. White

CLINICAL MANIFESTATIONS

Virilization is the most common presenting symptom in children with adrenocortical tumors, occurring in 50-80%. In males, the clinical picture is similar to that of simple virilizing congenital adrenal hyperplasia: accelerated growth velocity and muscle development, acne, penile enlargement, and the precocious development of pubic and axillary hair. In females, virilizing tumors of the adrenal gland cause masculinization of a previously normal female with clitoral enlargement, growth acceleration, acne, deepening of the voice, and premature pubic and axillary hair development.

For the full continuation of this chapter, please visit the Nelson Textbook of Pediatrics *website at* *www.expertconsult.com*.

Chapter 574 Pheochromocytoma

Perrin C. White

Pheochromocytomas, catecholamine-secreting tumors, arise from chromaffin cells. The most common site of origin (approximately 90%) is the adrenal medulla; however, tumors may develop anywhere along the abdominal sympathetic chain and are likely to be located near the aorta at the level of the inferior mesenteric artery or at its bifurcation. They also appear in the peri-adrenal area, urinary bladder or ureteral walls, thoracic cavity, and cervical region. Ten percent occur in children, in whom they present most frequently between 6 and 14 yr of age. Tumors vary from 1 to 10 cm in diameter; they are found more often on the right side than on the left. In more than 20% of affected children, the adrenal tumors are bilateral; in 30-40% of children, tumors are found in both the adrenal and extra-adrenal areas or only in an extra-adrenal area.

Pheochromocytomas may be associated with genetic syndromes such as **von Hippel-Lindau disease,** as a component of **multiple endocrine neoplasia** (MEN) syndromes MEN-2A and MEN-2B, and more rarely in association with **neurofibromatosis.** The classic features of von Hippel–Landau syndrome, which occurs in 1:36,000 individuals, include retinal and central nervous system hemangioblastomas, renal clear cell carcinomas and pheochromocytomas, but kindreds differ in their propensity to develop pheochromocytoma; in some kindreds, pheochromocytoma is the only tumor to develop. Germline mutations in the *VHL* tumor suppressor gene on chromosome 3p25-26 have been identified patients with this syndrome. Mutations of the *RET* proto-oncogene on chromosome 10 (10q11.2) have been found in families with MEN-2A and MEN-2B. Patients with MEN-2 are at risk of developing medullary thyroid carcinoma and parathyroid tumors; approximately 50% develop pheochromocytoma, with patients carrying mutations at codon 634 of the *RET* gene being at particularly high risk. Mutations are present in the *NF1* gene on chromosome 17q11.2 in neurofibromatosis patients.

Pheochromocytomas may occur in kindreds along with paragangliomas, particularly at sites in the head and neck. Such families typically carry mutations in the *SDHB*, *SDHD*, and rarely the *SDHC* genes encoding subunits of the mitochondrial enzyme, succinate dehydrogenase.

Pheochromocytomas are also associated with tuberous sclerosis, Sturge-Weber syndrome, and ataxia-telangiectasia. Somatic mutations of the genes mentioned above, particularly *VHL*, have been found in some sporadic cases of pheochromocytoma (Chapter 589).

CLINICAL MANIFESTATIONS

Pheochromocytomas detected by surveillance of patients who are known carriers of mutations in tumor suppressor genes, such as those with von Hippel–Landau syndrome, may be asymptomatic. Otherwise, patients are detected due to hypertension, which results from excessive secretion of epinephrine and norepinephrine. All patients have hypertension at some time. Paroxysmal hypertension should particularly suggest pheochromocytoma as a diagnostic possibility. In contrast to adults, the hypertension in children is more often sustained rather than paroxysmal. When there are paroxysms of hypertension, the attacks are usually infrequent at first but become more frequent and eventually give way to a continuous hypertensive state. Between attacks of hypertension, the patient may be free of symptoms. During attacks, the patient complains of headache, palpitations, abdominal pain, and dizziness; pallor, vomiting, and sweating also occur. Convulsions and other manifestations of hypertensive encephalopathy may occur. In severe cases, precordial pains radiate into the arms; pulmonary edema and cardiac and hepatic enlargement may develop. Symptoms may be exacerbated by exercise, or with use of over-the-counter medications containing stimulants such as pseudoephedrine. The child has a good appetite but because of the hypermetabolic state does not gain weight, and severe cachexia may develop. Polyuria and polydipsia can be sufficiently severe to suggest diabetes insipidus. Growth failure may be striking. The blood pressure may range from 180 to 260 mm Hg systolic and from 120 to 210 mm Hg diastolic, and the heart may be enlarged. Ophthalmoscopic examination may reveal papilledema, hemorrhages, exudate, and arterial constriction.

LABORATORY FINDINGS

The urine may contain protein, a few casts, and occasionally glucose. Gross hematuria suggests that the tumor is in the bladder wall. Polycythemia is occasionally observed. The diagnosis is established by demonstration of elevated blood or urinary levels of catecholamines and their metabolites.

Pheochromocytomas produce norepinephrine and epinephrine. Normally, norepinephrine in plasma is derived from both the adrenal gland and adrenergic nerve endings, whereas epinephrine is derived primarily from the adrenal gland. In contrast to adults with pheochromocytoma in whom both norepinephrine and epinephrine are elevated, children with pheochromocytoma predominantly excrete norepinephrine. Total urinary catecholamine excretion usually exceeds 300 μg/24 hr. Urinary excretion of metanephrines (particularly normetanephrine) are also increased (see Fig. 568-2). Daily urinary excretion of these compounds by unaffected children increases with age. Although urinary excretion of vanillylmandelic acid (VMA, 3-methoxy-4-hydroxymandelic acid), the major metabolite of epinephrine and norepinephrine, is increased, vanilla-containing foods and fruits can produce falsely elevated levels of this compound, which therefore is no longer routinely measured.

Elevated levels of free catecholamines and metanephrines can also be detected in plasma. In children, the best sensitivity and specificity are obtained by measuring plasma normetanephrine, with plasma norepinephrine being next best. Plasma metanephrine and epinephrine are not reliably elevated in children. The best discrimination is obtained by using gender-specific pediatric reference ranges, rather than adult ranges. Additionally, the patient should be instructed to abstain from caffeinated drinks, and to avoid acetaminophen, which can interfere with plasma normetanephrine assays. If possible, the blood sample should be obtained from an indwelling IV catheter, to avoid acute stress associated with venipuncture.

Most tumors in the area of the adrenal gland are readily localized by CT or MRI, but extra-adrenal tumors may be difficult to detect. ^{131}I-metaiodobenzylguanidine (MBIG) is taken up by chromaffin tissue anywhere in the body and is useful for localizing small tumors. Venous catheterization with sampling of blood at different levels for catecholamine determinations is now only rarely necessary for localizing the tumor.

DIFFERENTIAL DIAGNOSIS

Various causes of hypertension in children must be considered, such as renal or renovascular disease; coarctation of the aorta; hyperthyroidism; Cushing syndrome; deficiencies of 11β-hydroxylase, 17α-hydroxylase, or 11β-hydroxysteroid dehydrogenase (type 2 isozyme); primary aldosteronism; adrenocortical tumors; and essential hypertension (Chapter 439). A nonfunctioning kidney may result from compression of a ureter or of a renal artery by a pheochromocytoma. Paroxysmal hypertension may be associated with porphyria or familial dysautonomia. Cerebral disorders, diabetes insipidus, diabetes mellitus, and hyperthyroidism must also be considered in the differential diagnosis. Hypertension in patients with neurofibromatosis may be caused by renal vascular involvement or by concurrent pheochromocytoma.

Neuroblastoma, ganglioneuroblastoma, and ganglioneuroma frequently produce catecholamines, but urinary levels of most catecholamines are higher in patients with pheochromocytoma, although levels of dopamine and homovanillic acid are usually higher in neuroblastoma. Secreting neurogenic tumors often produce hypertension, excessive sweating, flushing, pallor, rash, polyuria, and polydipsia. Chronic diarrhea may be associated with these tumors, particularly with ganglioneuroma, and at times may be sufficiently persistent to suggest celiac disease.

TREATMENT

These tumors must be removed surgically, but careful preoperative, intraoperative, and postoperative management is essential. Preoperative **α- and β-adrenergic blockade** and **fluid loading** are required. Because these tumors are often multiple in children, a thorough transabdominal exploration of all the usual sites offers the best opportunity to find them all. Appropriate choice of anesthesia and expansion of blood volume with appropriate fluids during surgery are critical to avoid a precipitous drop in blood pressure during operation or within 48 hr postoperatively. Manipulation and excision of these tumors result in marked increases in catecholamine secretion that increase blood pressure and heart rate. Surveillance must continue postoperatively.

Although these tumors often appear malignant histologically, the only accurate indicators of malignancy are the presence of metastatic disease, local invasiveness that precludes complete resection, or both. Approximately 10% of all adrenal pheochromocytomas are malignant. Such tumors are rare in childhood; pediatric malignant pheochromocytomas occur more frequently in extra-adrenal sites and are often associated with mutations in the *SDHB* gene encoding a subunit of succinate dehydrogenase. Prolonged follow-up is indicated because functioning tumors at other sites may be manifested many years after the initial operation. Examination of relatives of affected patients may reveal other individuals harboring unsuspected tumors that may be asymptomatic.

BIBLIOGRAPHY

Please visit the Nelson Textbook of Pediatrics *website at www.expertconsult.com for the complete bibliography.*

Chapter 575 Adrenal Masses

575.1 Adrenal Incidentaloma

Perrin C. White

Adrenal masses are discovered with increasing frequency in patients undergoing abdominal imaging for reasons unrelated to the adrenal gland. The rate of detection of single adrenal masses has ranged from less than 1% to more than 4% of abdominal CT examinations in adults. The unexpected discovery of such a mass presents the clinician with a dilemma in terms of diagnostic steps to undertake and treatment interventions to recommend. The differential diagnosis of adrenal incidentaloma includes benign lesions such as cysts, hemorrhagic cysts, hematomas, and myelolipomas. These lesions can usually be identified on CT or MRI. If the nature of the lesion is not readily apparent, additional evaluation is required. Included in the differential diagnosis of lesions requiring additional evaluation are benign adenomas, pheochromocytomas, adrenocortical carcinoma, and metastasis from an extra-adrenal primary carcinoma. Benign, hormonally inactive adrenocortical adenomas make up the majority of incidentalomas. Careful history, physical examination, and endocrine evaluation must be performed to seek evidence of autonomous cortisol, androgen, mineralocorticoid, or catecholamine secretion. Functional tumors require removal. If the adrenal mass is nonfunctional and larger than 4-6 cm, recommendations are to proceed with surgical resection of the mass. Lesions of 3 cm or less should be followed clinically with periodic re-imaging. Treatment must be individualized; nonsecreting adrenal incidentalomas may enlarge and become hyperfunctioning. Nuclear scan, and occasionally fine-needle aspiration, may be helpful in defining the mass.

575.2 Adrenal Calcification

Perrin C. White

Calcification within the adrenal glands may occur in a wide variety of situations, some serious and others of no obvious consequence. Adrenal calcifications are often detected as incidental findings in radiographic studies of the abdomen in infants and children. The physician may elicit a history of anoxia or trauma at birth. Hemorrhage into the adrenal gland at or immediately after birth is probably the most common factor that leads to subsequent calcification. Although it is advisable to assess the adrenocortical reserve of such patients, there is rarely any functional disorder.

For the full continuation of this chapter, please visit the Nelson Textbook of Pediatrics *website at www.expertconsult.com.*

Section 5 DISORDERS OF THE GONADS

Chapter 576 Development and Function of the Gonads

Patricia A. Donohoue

GENETIC CONTROL OF EMBRYONIC GONADAL DIFFERENTIATION

Gonadal differentiation is a complex, multistep process that requires the sequential action and interaction of multiple gene products.

For the full continuation of this chapter, please visit the Nelson Textbook of Pediatrics *website at www.expertconsult.com.*

Chapter 577 Hypofunction of the Testes

Omar Ali and Patricia A. Donohoue

Testicular hypofunction during fetal life can be a component of various disorders of sexual development (Chapter 582.2). Since prepubertal children normally do not produce significant amounts of testosterone and are not yet producing sperm, there are no discernible effects of testicular hypofunction in this age group. Testicular hypofunction from the age of puberty onward may lead to testosterone deficiency, infertility, or both. Such hypofunction may be primary in the testes (**primary hypogonadism**) or secondary to deficiency of pituitary gonadotropic hormones

Table 577-1 ETIOLOGIC CLASSIFICATION OF MALE HYPOGONADISM

HYPOGONADOTROPIC HYPOGONADISM
I. Hypothalamic
A. Genetic defects
1. X-linked Kallman syndrome (KAL-1 gene)
2. AD Kallman syndrome (FGFR1 gene), other Kallman syndrome genes (e.g., PROK2 and PROKR2)
3. Other genetic defects: leptin gene, leptin receptor, KiSS-1, GPCR54, DAX-1, SF-1
4. Inherited syndromes: Prader-Willi, Bardet-Biedl, Laurence-Moon-Biedl, Alström
5. Constitutional growth delay?
B. Acquired defects (reversible)
1. Anorexia nervosa
2. Drug use
3. Malnutrition
4. Chronic illness, esp. Crohn disease
5. Hyperprolactinemia
II. Pituitary
A. Genetic defects
1. Isolated hypogonadotropic hypogonadism at pituitary level (GnRH receptor, FSH and LH beta-subunit)
2. Septo-optic dysplasia (HESX-1 in some cases)
3. Disorders of pituitary organogenesis (PROP1, LHX3, LHX4, SOX-3, etc.)
B. Acquired defects
1. Pituitary tumors
2. Pituitary infarction
3. Infiltrative disorders (e.g., histiocytosis, sarcoidosis)
4. Hemosiderosis and hemochromatosis
5. Radiation
6. Unknown
HYPERGONADOTROPIC HYPOGONADISM: TESTES
I. Genetic defects
A. FSH and LH resistance
B. Mutations in steroid synthetic pathways
C. Gonadal dysgenesis
D. Klinefelter syndrome (47,XXY)
E. Noonan syndrome (PTPN-11 gene mutation in many cases)
F. Cystic fibrosis (infertility)
II. Acquired defects
A. Cryptorchidism (some cases)
B. Vanishing testes
C. Chemotherapy
D. Radiation
E. Infection (e.g., mumps)
F. Infarction (testicular torsion)
G. Trauma

(secondary hypogonadism). Both types may be due to inherited genetic defects or acquired causes, and in some cases the etiology may be unclear, but the level of the lesion (primary or secondary) is usually well defined; patients with primary hypogonadism have elevated levels of gonadotropins (hypergonadotropic); those with secondary hypogonadism have inappropriately low or absent levels (hypogonadotropic). Table 577-1 details the etiologic classification of male hypogonadism.

577.1 Hypergonadotropic Hypogonadism in the Male (Primary Hypogonadism)

Omar Ali and Patricia A. Donohoue

ETIOLOGY

Some degree of testicular function is essential in the development of phenotypically male infants. After sex differentiation has taken place, by the 14th wk of intrauterine life, hypogonadism may occur for a variety of reasons. Genetic or chromosomal anomalies may lead to testicular hypofunction that does not become apparent until the time of puberty, when these boys may have delayed or incomplete pubertal development. In other cases, normally developed testes may be compromised by infarction, trauma, radiation, chemotherapy, infections, infiltration, and other causes. In some cases, genetic defects may predispose to maldescent; torsion or infarction or may lead to progressive testicular damage and atrophy after a period of normal development. If testicular compromise is global, both testosterone secretion and fertility (sperm production) are likely to be effected. Even when the primary defect is in testosterone production, low levels of intratesticular testosterone will frequently lead to infertility. The reverse may not be true. Defects in sperm production and in the storage and transit of sperm may not be associated with low testosterone levels; infertility may thus be seen in patients with normal testosterone levels, normal libido, and normal secondary sexual characteristics.

Various degrees of primary hypogonadism also occur in a significant percentage of patients with chromosomal aberrations such as in **Klinefelter syndrome, males with more than 1 X chromosome** and **XX males.** These chromosomal anomalies are associated with other characteristic findings. Noonan syndrome is associated with cryptorchidism and infertility but other features dominate its clinical picture.

Congenital Anorchia: Boys in whom the external genitalia have developed normally (or near normally) and müllerian duct derivatives (uterus, fallopian tubes, etc.) are absent have obviously had testicular function for at least some part of gestation. If their testes cannot be palpated at birth, they are said to have **cryptorchidism.** In most such cases, the testes are undescended or retractile, but in a small number of cases, no testes are found in any location even after extensive investigation. This syndrome of absence of testes in a phenotypic male (indicating some period of testicular function in intrauterine life) is known as "vanishing testes," "congenital anorchia," or **"testicular regression syndrome."**

Congenital anorchia occurs in 0.6% of boys with nonpalpable testes (1/20,000 males). It is thought that many cases are due to infarction of the testes that occurs in late fetal life or at some point after birth. But the condition has been reported in monozygotic twins; familial occurrence also suggests a genetic etiology. Some cases are associated with micropenis and in these cases the testicular loss probably occurred after the 14th wk, but well before the time of birth, or this may indicate a pre-existing dysfunction of the male hormonal development. Low levels of testosterone (<10 ng/dL) and markedly elevated levels of luteinizing hormone (LH) and follicle-stimulating hormone (FSH) are found in the early postnatal months; thereafter, levels of gonadotropins tend to decrease even in agonadal children, rising to very high levels again as the pubertal years approach. Stimulation with human chorionic gonadotropin (hCG) fails to evoke an increase in the level of testosterone. Serum levels of antimüllerian hormone (AMH) are undetectable or low. All patients with undetectable testes should undergo these tests and if the results indicate that no testicular tissue is present, then the diagnosis of testicular regression syndrome is confirmed. If testosterone secretion is demonstrated, surgical exploration is indicated. Treatment of hypogonadism is discussed later. There is no possibility of normal fertility in these patients.

Chemotherapy and Radiation-Induced Hypogonadism: Testicular damage is a frequent consequence of **chemotherapy** and **radiotherapy** for cancer. The frequency and extent of damage depend on the agent used, total dose, duration of therapy, and post-therapy interval of observation. Another important variable is age at therapy; germ cells are less vulnerable in prepubertal than in pubertal and postpubertal boys. **Chemotherapy** is most damaging if more than 1 agent is used. The use of alkylating agents such as cyclophosphamide in prepubertal children does not impair pubertal development, even though there may be biopsy evidence of germ cell damage. High doses of cyclophosphamide and ifosfamide are associated with infertility. Cisplatin causes transient azoospermia or oligospermia at lower doses, while higher doses (400-600 mg/m^2) can cause permanent infertility. Interleukin-2 can depress Leydig cell function, whereas interferon-α does not seem to affect gonadal function. Most chemotherapeutic agents produce azoospermia and infertility; Leydig cell damage (leading to low testosterone levels) is less common. In many cases, the damage is transient and sperm counts recover after 12-24 mo. Both chemotherapy and radiotherapy are associated with increase in the percentage of abnormal gametes, but data concerning the outcomes of pregnancies after such therapy has NOT shown any increase in genetically mediated birth defects, possibly due to selection bias against abnormal sperm.

Radiation damage is dose dependent. Temporary oligospermia can be seen with doses as low as 0.1 Gy, with permanent azoospermia seen with doses greater than 2 Gy. Recovery of spermatogenesis can be seen as long as 5 yr (or more) after irradiation, with higher doses leading to slower recovery. Leydig cells are more resistant to irradiation. Mild damage as determined by elevated LH levels can be seen with up to 6 Gy; doses greater than 30 Gy cause hypogonadism in most. Whenever possible, testes should be shielded from irradiation. Testicular function should be carefully evaluated in adolescents after multimodal treatment for cancer in childhood. Replacement therapy with testosterone and counseling concerning fertility may be indicated. The storage of sperm prior to chemotherapy or radiation treatment in postpubertal males is an option. Even in those cases where sperm counts are abnormal, recovery is possible, though the chances of recovery decline with increasing dose of radiation. If sperm counts remain low, fertility is still possible with testicular sperm extraction and intracytoplasmic sperm injection.

Sertoli Cell–Only Syndrome: Small testes and azoospermia are seen in patients with the Sertoli cell–only syndrome (germ cell aplasia, or **Del Castillo syndrome**). These patients have no germ cells in the testes, but usually have normal testosterone production, and present as adults with the complaint of infertility. The cause is unknown.

Other Causes of Testicular Hypofunction: Atrophy of the testes may follow damage to the vascular supply as a result of manipulation of the testes during surgical procedures for correction of cryptorchidism or as a result of bilateral torsion of the testes. Acute orchitis in pubertal or adult males with mumps may occasionally damage the testes; though usually, only the reproductive function of the testes is impaired. The routine immunization of all prepubertal males with mumps vaccine may reduce the incidence of this complication. Autoimmune polyendocrinopathy may be associated with primary hypogonadism (associated with anti-P450scc antibodies) but this appears to be more common in females.

Testicular Dysgenesis Syndrome: The incidence of cryptorchidism, hypospadias, low sperm counts, and testicular cancer has increased in many developed societies. For example, 8% of all births in Europe are estimated to involve assisted reproductive techniques and 20% of Danish adult males have sperm counts below the World Health Organization standard of 20×10^6 per mL. Incidence of testicular cancer also appears to be rising and in some cases seems to parallel the higher incidence of hypofertility. There is evidence that the incidence of hypospadias and cryptorchidism has increased in several countries in the last few decades. It has been proposed that all these trends are linked by prenatal testicular dysgenesis. The hypothesis is that some degree of testicular dysgenesis develops in intrauterine life due to genetic as well as environmental factors, and is associated with increased risk of cryptorchidism, hypospadias, hypofertility, and testicular cancer. The environmental influences that have been implicated in this syndrome include environmental chemicals that act as endocrine disruptors, such as bisphenol A and phthalates (components of many types of plastics), several pesticides, phytoestrogens or mycoestrogens, and other chemicals. The fact that these lesions can be reproduced in some animal models by environmental chemicals has led to efforts to remove these chemicals from products used by infants and pregnant mothers, and from the environment in general. Nonetheless, the evidence is only suggestive and is not conclusive.

CLINICAL MANIFESTATIONS

Primary hypogonadism may be suspected at birth if the testes and penis are abnormally small. Normative data are available for different populations. The condition often is not noticed until puberty, when secondary sex characteristics fail to develop. Facial, pubic, and axillary hair is scant or absent; there is neither acne nor regression of scalp hair; and the voice remains high-pitched. The penis and scrotum remain infantile and may be almost obscured by pubic fat; the testes are small or not palpable. Fat accumulates in the region of the hips and buttocks and sometimes in the breasts and on the abdomen. The epiphyses close later than normal; therefore, extremities are long. The span may be several inches longer than the height, and the distance from the symphysis pubis to the soles of the feet (lower segment) is much greater than that from the symphysis to the vertex (upper segment). The proportions of the body are described as **eunuchoid.** The upper to lower segment ratio is considerably less than 0.9. Many individuals with milder degrees of hypogonadism may be detected only by appropriate studies of the pituitary-gonadal axis. Examination of the testes should be performed routinely by pediatricians; testicular volumes as determined by comparison with standard orchidometers or by measurement of linear dimensions should be recorded.

DIAGNOSIS

Levels of serum FSH and, to a lesser extent, of LH are elevated to greater than age-specific normal values in early infancy (when "minipuberty" normally occurs and the gonadotropins are normally disinhibited). This is followed by a period of time when even agonadal children may not exhibit significant elevation in gonadotropins, indicating that the gonadotropins are also suppressed at this stage by some mechanism independent of feedback inhibition by gonadal hormones. In the latter half of childhood and several years prior to onset of puberty, this inhibition is released and gonadotropin levels again rise above age-matched normals in subjects with primary hypogonadism. These elevated levels indicate that even in the prepubertal child there is an active hypothalamic-gonadal feedback relationship. After the age of 11 yr, FSH and LH levels rise significantly, reaching the castrate range. Measurements of random plasma testosterone levels in prepubertal boys are not helpful because they are ordinarily low in normal prepubertal children, rising during puberty to attain adult levels. During puberty, these levels correlate better with testicular size, stage of sexual maturity, and bone age than with chronological age. In patients with primary hypogonadism, testosterone levels remain low at all ages. There is an attenuated rise or no rise after administration of hCG, in contrast to normal males in whom hCG produces a significant rise in plasma testosterone at any stage of development.

AMH (antimüllerian hormone) is secreted by the Sertoli cells and this secretion is suppressed by testosterone. As a result, AMH levels are elevated in prepubertal boys and suppressed at onset of puberty. Boys with primary hypogonadism continue to have elevated AMH levels in puberty. Detection of AMH may be used in prepubertal years as an indicator of the presence of testicular tissue (e.g., in patients with bilateral cryptorchidism). Inhibin B is also secreted by the Sertoli cells, is present throughout childhood, and rises at onset of puberty (more in boys than in girls). It may be used as another marker of the presence of testicular tissue in bilateral cryptorchidism and as a marker of spermatogenesis (e.g., in delayed puberty, cancer survivors, and patients with Noonan syndrome). Bone age x-rays are useful to document delayed bone age in patients with constitutional growth delay as well as primary hypogonadism.

NOONAN SYNDROME

Etiology

The term Noonan Syndrome (NS) has been applied to males and females with normal karyotypes who have certain phenotypic features that occur also in females with Turner syndrome. Noonan syndrome occurs in 1 : 1,000-2,500 live births. About 20% of the cases are familial and exhibit autosomal dominant inheritance. Males and females are equally affected. Missense mutations in *PTPN11*—a gene on chromosome 12q24.1 encoding the nonreceptor protein tyrosine phosphatase SHP-2—are seen in about half the cases. It is now thought that several mutations in the RAS-MAPK pathway can cause Noonan syndrome and other related disorders. These include mutations in the *KRAS* gene and *SOS1* gene as well as duplications of the 12q24 region. Phenotypic features of NS therefore overlap with other syndromes involving the RAS-MAPK pathway, such as Leopard syndrome and cardio-facio-cutaneous syndrome.

Clinical Manifestations

The most common abnormalities are short stature, webbing of the neck, pectus carinatum or pectus excavatum, cubitus valgus, right-sided congenital heart disease, and characteristic facies. Hypertelorism, epicanthus, downward slanting palpebral fissures, ptosis, micrognathia, and ear abnormalities are common. Other abnormalities such as clinodactyly, hernias, and vertebral anomalies occur less frequently. The mean IQ of school-aged children with the condition is 86, with a range of 53 to 127. Verbal IQ tends to be better than performance IQ. High-frequency sensorineural hearing loss is common. The cardiac defect is most often pulmonary valvular stenosis, hypertrophic cardiomyopathy, or atrial septal defect. Hepatosplenomegaly and several hematologic diseases, including low clotting factors XI and XII, acute lymphoblastic leukemia, and chronic myelomonocytic leukemia, are noted. Noonan-like features can be part of the phenotypic variation of the NF1 (neurofibromatosis) gene mutation, possibly due to common involvement of the RAS-MAPK pathway in both diseases. Males frequently have cryptorchidism and small testes. Testosterone secretion may be low or normal, but spermatogenesis may be affected even in those with normal testosterone (and normal secondary sexual characteristics). Serum inhibin-B may be a useful marker of Sertoli cell function in these patients. Puberty is delayed and adult height is achieved by the end of the 2nd decade and usually reaches the lower limit of the normal population. Prenatal diagnosis should be suspected in fetuses with normal karyotype, edema, or hydrops and short femur length.

Treatment

Human growth hormone has resulted in improvement in growth velocity comparable to that seen in patients with Turner syndrome without adverse effects on cardiac ventricular wall thickness. Increased adult height after growth hormone treatment has been reported in a few patients. Patients with Noonan syndrome and demonstrable *PTNP11* mutations grow less well and are less responsive to growth hormone treatment than those without mutations. They have lower insulin-like growth factor-1 and higher growth hormone levels, suggesting the possibility of partial growth hormone resistance due to postreceptor signaling defects. Treatment of hypogonadism is discussed later.

KLINEFELTER SYNDROME (CHAPTER 76)

Etiology

Klinefelter syndrome (KS) is the most common sex chromosomal aneuploidy in males, with an incidence of 0.1 to 0.2% in the general population (1/500 to 1/1,000) and rising to 4% among infertile males and 10-11% in those with oligospermia or azoospermia. Approximately 80% of them have a 47,XXY chromosome complement, while mosaics and higher degrees of polyX are seen in the remaining 20%. Even with as many as 4 X chromosomes, the Y chromosome determines a male phenotype. The chromosomal aberration most often results from meiotic nondisjunction of an X chromosome during parental gametogenesis; the extra X chromosome is maternal in origin in 54% and paternal in origin in 46% of patients. A national study in Denmark revealed a prenatal prevalence of 213 per 100,000 male fetuses but in adult men, the prevalence was only 40/100,000, suggesting that only 1 in 4 of adult males with Klinefelter syndrome was diagnosed.

Clinical Manifestations

In patients who do not have a prenatal diagnosis, the diagnosis is rarely made before puberty because of the paucity or subtleness of clinical manifestations in childhood. Behavioral or psychiatric disorders may often be apparent long before defects in sexual development. These children tend to have learning disabilities and deficits in "executive function" (concept formation, problem solving, task switching, and planning), and the condition should be considered in boys with psychosocial, learning, or school adjustment problems. Affected children may be anxious, immature, or excessively shy and tend to have difficulty in social interactions throughout life. In a prospective study, a group of children with 47,XXY karyotypes identified at birth exhibited relatively mild deviations from normal during the 1st 5 yr of life. None had major physical, intellectual, or emotional disabilities; some were inactive, with poorly organized motor function and mild delay in language acquisition. Problems often first become apparent after the child begins school. Full-scale IQ scores may be normal, with verbal IQ being somewhat decreased. Verbal cognitive defects and underachievement in reading, spelling, and mathematics are common. By late adolescence, many boys with KS have generalized learning disabilities, most of which are language based. Despite these difficulties, most complete high school.

The patients tend to be tall, slim, and underweight and have a specific tendency to have long legs (out of proportion to the arms, and longer than those seen with other causes of hypogonadism), but body habitus can vary markedly. The testes tend to be small for age, but this sign may become apparent only after puberty, when normal testicular growth fails to occur. The phallus tends to be smaller than average, and cryptorchidism is more common than in the general population. Bone mineral density may be low in adults with KS and this correlates with lower testosterone levels.

Pubertal development may be delayed, although some children may undergo almost normal virilization. Despite normal testosterone levels, serum LH and FSH concentrations and their responses to gonadotropin-releasing hormone (GnRH) stimulation are elevated starting at around 13 yr of age. About 80% of adults have **gynecomastia;** they have sparser facial hair, most shaving less often than daily. The most common testicular lesions are spermatogenic arrest and Sertoli cell predominance. The sperm have a high incidence of sex chromosomal aneuploidy. Azoospermia and infertility are usual, although rare instances of fertility are known. It is now clear that germ cell numbers and sperm counts are higher in early puberty and decline with age. Testicular sperm extraction followed by intracytoplasmic sperm injection can result in the birth of healthy infants, with success rates declining with increasing age. In nonmosaic Klinefelter patients, most testicular sperm (94%) have a normal pattern of sex chromosome segregation, indicating that meiotic checkpoints can remove most aneuploid cells. Antisperm antibodies have been detected in 25% of tested specimens.

There is an increased incidence of pulmonary disease, varicose veins, and cancer of the breast. Among 93 unselected **male breast cancer** patients, 7.5% were found to have KS. Mediastinal germ cell tumors have been reported; some of these tumors produce hCG and cause precocious puberty in young boys. They may also be associated with leukemia, lymphoma, and other hematologic neoplasia. The highest cancer risk (relative risk 2.7) occurs in the 15-30 yr age group. A large cohort study in Britain demonstrated an overall significantly increased standardized mortality ratio (1.5), with particular increases in deaths due to diabetes, epilepsy, peripheral and intestinal vascular sufficiency, pulmonary embolism, and renal disease. Mortality from ischemic heart disease was decreased. In adults, structural brain abnormalities correlate with cognitive deficits.

In adults with XY/XXY mosaicism, the features of KS are decreased in severity and frequency. Children with mosaicism have a better prognosis for virilization, fertility, and psychosocial adjustment.

KLINEFELTER VARIANTS AND OTHER POLYX SYNDROMES When the number of X chromosomes exceeds 2, the clinical manifestations, including mental retardation and impairment of virilization, are more severe. Height decreases with increasing number of X chromosomes. The XXYY variant is the most common variant (1/18,000 to 1/40,000 male births). In most, mental retardation occurs with IQ scores between 60 and 80, but 10% have IQs greater than 110. The XXYY male phenotype is not distinctively different from that of the XXY patient, except that XXYY adults tend to be taller than the average XXY patient. The 49,XXXXY variant is sufficiently distinctive to be detected in childhood. Its incidence is estimated to be 1/80,000 to 1/100,000 male births. The disorder arises from sequential nondisjunction in meiosis. Affected patients are severely retarded and have short necks and typical coarse facies with wide-set eyes with a mild upward slant of the fissures, epicanthus, strabismus, a wide and flat upturned nose, a large open mouth, and large malformed ears. The testes are small and may be undescended, the scrotum is hypoplastic, and the penis is very small. Defects suggestive of Down syndrome (short, incurved terminal 5th phalanges, single palmar creases, and hypotonia) and other skeletal abnormalities (including defects in the carrying angle of the elbows and restricted supination) are common. The most frequent radiographic abnormalities are radioulnar synostosis or dislocation, elongated radius, pseudoepiphyses, scoliosis or kyphosis, coxa valga, and retarded osseous age. Most patients with such extensive changes have a 49,XXXXY chromosome karyotype; several mosaic patterns have also been observed: 48,XXXY/49,XXXXY, 48,XXXY/49,XXXXY/50,XXXXXY; and 48,XXXY/49,XXXXY/50,XXXXYY. Prenatal diagnosis of a 49,XXXXY infant has been reported. The fetus had intrauterine growth retardation, edema, and cystic hygroma colli.

The 48,XXXY variant is relatively rare. The characteristic features are generally less severe than those of patients with 49,XXXXY and more severe than those of 47,XXY patients. Mild mental retardation, delayed speech and motor development, and immature but passive and pleasant behavior are associated with this condition.

Very few patients have been described with 49,XYYY and 49,XXYYY karyotypes. Dysmorphic features and mental retardation are common to both.

Laboratory Findings

Most males with this condition go through life undiagnosed. The chromosomes should be examined in all patients suspected of having KS, particularly those attending child guidance, psychiatric, and mental retardation clinics. In infancy, inhibin B and AMH levels are normal but testosterone levels are lower than in controls. Before 10 yr of age, boys with 47,XXY KS have normal basal plasma levels of FSH and LH. Responses to gonadotropin-stimulating hormone and to hCG are normal. The testes show normal growth early in puberty, but by mid-puberty the testicular growth stops, gonadotropins become elevated, and testosterone levels are slightly low. Inhibin B levels are normal in early puberty, decrease in late puberty, and are low in adults with the syndrome. Elevated levels of estradiol, resulting in a high estradiol to testosterone ratio, account for the development of gynecomastia during puberty. SHBG levels are elevated, further decreasing free testosterone levels. Long androgen receptor polyglutamine (CAG) repeat length is associated with the more severe phenotype including gynecomastia, small testes, and short penile length.

Testicular biopsy before puberty may reveal only deficiency or absence of germinal cells. After puberty, the seminiferous tubular membranes are hyalinized, and there is adenomatous clumping of Leydig cells. Sertoli cells predominate. Azoospermia is characteristic, and infertility is the rule.

Treatment

Replacement therapy with a testosterone preparation depends on the age of the patient. It usually begins no later than 11-12 yr of age, when testosterone levels are found to be lower than the normal range. While testosterone treatment will normalize testosterone levels and stimulate the development of secondary sexual characteristics, it will NOT improve fertility (and will, in fact, suppress spermatogenesis). Either long-acting testosterone injections or daily application of testosterone gel may be used (testosterone patches have a high incidence of skin rash and are not frequently used in pediatrics). Testosterone enanthate ester may be used in a starting dose of 25-50 mg injected intramuscularly every 3-4 wk, with 50-mg increments every 6-9 mo until a maintenance dose for adults (200-250 mg every 3-4 wk) is achieved. At that time, testosterone patches or testosterone gel may be substituted for the injections. Depending on patient and physician preference, transdermal testosterone may be used as initial treatment instead of injections. For older boys, larger initial doses and increments can achieve more rapid virilization.

Gynecomastia may be treated with aromatase inhibitors (which will also increase endogenous testosterone levels) but medical treatment is not always successful. Fertility may not be an issue in the pediatric age group, but adults can father children using testicular sperm extraction (TSE) followed by intracytoplasmic sperm injection. Because sperm counts actually decrease with time, sperm banking is an option for older adolescents. HCG treatment may be used to stimulate sperm counts prior to TSE. Therapy, counseling and psychiatric services should be provided as needed for learning difficulties and psychosocial disabilities.

XX MALES

This disorder is thought to occur in 1 in 20,000 newborn males. Affected individuals have a male phenotype, small testes, a small phallus, and no evidence of ovarian or müllerian duct tissue. They appear, therefore, to be distinct from the ovotesticular disorder of sexual development. Undescended testes and hypospadias occur in a minority of patients. Infertility occurs in practically all cases and the histologic features of the testes are essentially the same as in Klinefelter syndrome. Patients with the condition usually come to medical attention in adult life because of hypogonadism, gynecomastia, or infertility. Hypergonadotropic hypogonadism occurs secondary to testicular failure. A few cases have been diagnosed perinatally as a result of discrepancies between prenatal ultrasonography and karyotype findings.

In 90% of XX males with normal male external genitals, 1 of the X chromosomes carries the *SRY* gene. The exchange from the Y to the X chromosome occurs during paternal meiosis, when the short arms of the Y and X chromosomes pair. XX males inherit 1 maternal X chromosome and 1 paternal X chromosome containing the translocated male-determining gene. A few cases of 46,XX males with 9P translocations were identified. Most XX males who are identified before puberty have hypospadias or micropenis; this group of patients may lack Y-specific sequences, suggesting other mechanisms for virilization. Fluorescent in situ hybridization and primed in situ labeling (PRINS) have been used to identify small *SRY* DNA segments. Yp fragment abnormalities may result in sexually ambiguous phenotypes.

45,X MALES

In a few male patients recognized with a 45,X karyotype, Yp sequences have been translocated to an autosomal chromosome. In 1 instance, the terminal short arm of the Y chromosome was translocated onto an X chromosome. In another, *SRY/autosomal* translocation was postulated. A male with 45,X karyotype and Leri-Weill dyschondrosteosis, *SHOX* gene loss, and SRY to Xp translocation was also described.

47,XXX MALES

A Japanese male with poor pubic hair development, hypoplastic scrotal testes (4 mL), normal penis and normal height, gynecomastia, and severe mental retardation had 47,XXX karyotype due to abnormal X-Y interchange during paternal meiosis and X-X nondisjunction during maternal meiosis.

BIBLIOGRAPHY

Please visit the Nelson Textbook of Pediatrics *website at* *www.expertconsult.com* *for the complete bibliography.*

577.2 Hypogonadotropic Hypogonadism in the Male (Secondary Hypogonadism)

Omar Ali and Patricia A. Donohoue

In hypogonadotropic hypogonadism, there is deficiency of 1 or both gonadotropins: follicle stimulating hormone (FSH) or luteinizing hormone (LH). The primary defect may lie either in the anterior pituitary or in the hypothalamus. Hypothalamic etiologies result in deficiency of gonadotropin-releasing hormone (GnRH), also known as *luteinizing hormone–releasing hormone* (LHRH). The testes are normal but remain in the prepubertal state because stimulation by gonadotropins is lacking. The disorder may be recognized in infancy, around the time of puberty, or rarely, in adulthood.

ETIOLOGY

Hypogonadotropic hypogonadism (HH) may be genetic or acquired. Several different genes can cause inherited forms of hypogonadotropic hypogonadism; the affected genes may be upstream of GnRH, at the level of GnRH receptors, or at the level of gonadotropin production. In addition, various genetic defects in transcription factors like POUF-1, LHX-3, LHX-4, and HESX-1 lead to defects in pituitary development and multiple pituitary hormone deficiencies, including deficiency of gonadotropins. Acquired pituitary gonadotropin deficiency may develop due to various lesions in the hypothalamic-pituitary region (e.g., tumors, infiltrative disease, autoimmune disease, trauma, stroke).

Isolated Gonadotropin Deficiency

Isolated gonadotropin deficiency is more likely to be due to defects in the secretion of GnRH from the hypothalamus rather than defects in gonadotropin synthesis in the pituitary. It affects about 1/10,000 males and 1/50,000 females and encompasses a heterogeneous group of entities. Many cases are associated with anosmia and this combination of anosmia and hypogonadotropic hypogonadism defines Kallman syndrome.

Kallmann syndrome is the commonest form of hypogonadotropic hypogonadism and is genetically heterogeneous, with autosomal recessive, X-linked and autosomal dominant forms of inheritance (see Table 76-7). Clinically, it is characterized by its association with **anosmia** or **hyposmia;** 85% of the cases are autosomal while 15% are X-linked. The X-linked form (KAL1) is caused by mutations of the *KAL1* gene at Xp22.3. This leads to failure of olfactory axons and GnRH-expressing neurons to migrate from their common origin in the olfactory placode to the brain. The *KAL* gene product anosmin-1, an extracellular 95 kDa matrix glycoprotein, facilitates neuronal growth and migration. The *KAL* gene is also expressed in various parts of the brain, facial mesenchyme, and mesonephros and metanephros, thus explaining some of the associated findings in patients with Kallmann syndrome, such as synkinesia (mirror movements), hearing loss, midfacial defects, and renal agenesis.

Some kindreds contain anosmic individuals with or without hypogonadism; others contain hypogonadal individuals who are anosmic. Cleft lip and palate, hypotelorism, median facial clefts, sensorineural hearing loss, unilateral renal aplasia, neurologic deficits, and other findings occur in some affected patients. When Kallmann syndrome is caused by terminal or interstitial deletions of the Xp22.3 region, it may be associated with other contiguous gene syndromes, such as steroid sulfatase deficiency, chondrodysplasia punctata, X-linked ichthyosis, or ocular albinism.

The autosomal dominant form of Kallman syndrome (KAL 2) occurs in up to 10% of patients, and is due to a loss of function mutation in the fibroblast growth factor receptor 1 (FGFR1) gene. Cleft lip and palate is associated with KAL2 but not with KAL1. Oligodontia and hearing loss may occur with both KAL1 and KAL2.

In a majority of patients with Kallman syndrome the affected gene remains undefined. Candidate genes include *CHD7* (responsible for CHARGE syndrome, which includes hypogonadism in its phenotype), *NELF* (another olfactory axonal outgrowth gene), and *PROK2* and its receptor *PROKR2* (may be responsible for up to 10% of Kallman Syndrome patients). Fibroblast growth factor 8 has also been implicated as a possible HH gene.

Hypogonadotropic Hypogonadism without Anosmia: Most cases of isolated HH without anosmia are idiopathic, but some genetic disorders leading to normosmic HH are now known. Several patients with HH have been found to have defects in G-protein coupled receptor 54 (GPCR 54) and its ligand kisspeptin (KiSS-1 gene). These patients have intact GnRH-secreting neurons and are able to produce GnRH, but fail to initiate GnRH secretion to start pubertal development. It appears that kisspeptin and GPCR54 play an important role in triggering puberty in humans and act downstream of the leptin receptor in this pathway. Rare cases of leptin deficiency and leptin receptor defects are also associated with HH. In addition, starvation and anorexia are associated with hypogonadism, most likely acting via the leptin pathway.

There are no known human mutations of the GnRH gene, but several families with mutations in the GnRH receptor have been described. These mutations account for 2-14% of idiopathic HH without anosmia. The severity of the defect is variable and many patients will respond to high dose GnRH with increased gonadotropin secretion, indicating that the receptor defect is partial and not complete.

Mutations in gonadotropin genes are extremely rare. Mutations in the common alpha subunit are not known in humans. Mutations in the LH-β subunit have been described in a few individuals and may lead to low, absent, or elevated LH levels, depending on the mutation. Defects in the FSH-β subunit may be the cause of azoospermia in a few rare cases.

Children with **X-linked congenital adrenal hypoplasia** have associated HH due to impaired GnRH secretion. In these patients, there is a mutation of the *DAX1* gene at Xp21.2-21.3. Conditions occasionally associated with these patients because of the **contiguous gene syndrome** include glycerol kinase deficiency, Duchenne muscular dystrophy, and ornithine transcarbamoyl transferase deficiency. Most boys with *DAX1* mutations develop HH in adolescence, although a patient with adult-onset adrenal insufficiency and partial HH and 2 females with HH and delayed puberty have also been described, the latter as part of extended families with males with classic HH. The *DAX1* gene defect is, however, rare in patients with delayed puberty or HH without at least a family history of adrenal failure (Chapter 570).

Other Disorders with HH

HH has been observed in a few patients with polyglandular autoimmune syndrome, in some with elevated melatonin levels, and in those with a variety of other syndromes such as Bardet-Biedl, Prader-Willi, multiple lentigines, and several ataxia syndromes. In rare cases, HH is associated with complex chromosomal abnormalities.

Hypogonadotropic Hypogonadism Associated with Other Pituitary Hormone Deficiencies

Defects in pituitary transcription factors such as PROP-1, HESX-1, LHX-4, SOX-3, and LHX-3 lead to multiple pituitary deficiencies, including HH. Most of these present with multiple pituitary hormone deficiency in infancy, but some cases (especially with PROP-1 mutations) may present with hypogonadism or hypoadrenalism in adult life. Growth hormone is almost always affected in multiple pituitary hormone deficiency, but TSH and adrenocorticotropic hormone (ACTH) may be spared in some cases. In patients with organic lesions in or near the pituitary, the gonadotropin deficiency is usually pituitary in origin. Microphallus (<2.5 cm) in the newborn male with growth hormone deficiency suggests the likelihood of gonadotropin deficiency.

DIAGNOSIS

Levels of gonadotropins and gonadal steroids are elevated for up to 6 mo after birth (minipuberty), and if the diagnosis of HH is suspected in early infancy these levels will be found to be inappropriately low. By the 2nd half of the 1st yr of life these levels normally decline to near zero and remain suppressed until late childhood. Therefore, routine lab tests cannot distinguish HH from this normal suppression of gonadotropins in this age group. At the normal age of puberty, these patients fail to show clinical signs of puberty or normal increase in LH and FSH levels. Children with constitutional delay of growth and puberty will have the same clinical picture and similar lab findings (and are far more common than true HH), and their differentiation from patients with HH is extremely difficult. Dynamic testing with GnRH or hCG may not be able to distinguish these groups in a reliable manner. A testosterone level greater than 50 ng/dL (1.7 nmol/L) generally indicates that normal puberty is likely, but a lower level does not reliably distinguish these groups. HH is likely if the patient has evidence of another pituitary deficiency, such as a deficiency of growth hormone, particularly if it is associated with ACTH deficiency. The presence of **anosmia** usually indicates permanent gonadotropin deficiency, but occasional instances of markedly delayed puberty (18-20 yr of age) have been observed in anosmic individuals. Although anosmia may be present in the family or in the patient from early childhood, its existence is rarely volunteered, and direct questioning is necessary in all patients with delayed puberty. **Hyperprolactinemia** is a known cause of delayed puberty and should be excluded by determination of serum prolactin levels.

In the absence of family history, it may not be possible to make the diagnosis of HH with certainty, but the diagnosis will become more and more likely as puberty is delayed further beyond the normal age. If pubertal delay persists beyond age 18 yr with low 8 AM testosterone level and inappropriately low gonadotropins (normal values are inappropriately low in this setting), then the patient can be presumptively diagnosed with HH. An MRI of the brain is indicated to look for tumors and other anomalies in the hypothalamic-pituitary region. Genetic testing for pituitary transcription factors and several of the genes involved in isolated HH is also available. Rarely, patients with inherited form of HH may go through puberty and may present with hypogonadism as adults.

Treatment

Constitutional delay of puberty should be ruled out before a diagnosis of HH is established and treatment is initiated. Testicular volume of less than 4 mL by 14 yr of age occurs in about 3% of boys, but true HH is a rare condition. Even relatively moderate delays in sexual development and growth may result in significant psychologic distress and require attention. Initially, an explanation of the variations characteristic of puberty and reassurance suffice for the majority of boys. If by 15 yr of age no clinical evidence of puberty is beginning and the testosterone level is less than 50 ng/dL, a brief course of testosterone may be recommended. Various regimens are used, including testosterone enanthate 100 mg intramuscularly once monthly for 4-6 mo or 150 mg once monthly for 3 mo. Some practitioners use oral oxandrolone, which may have the theoretical advantage that it is not aromatized and may have less effect on bone age advancement (though definitive evidence of advantage is lacking). Oral oxandrolone may cause hepatic dysfunction in some patients, and liver function tests should be monitored if it is used. Treatment is not necessary in all cases of constitutional delay, but if used, it is usually followed by normal progression through puberty and this may differentiate constitutional delay in puberty from isolated gonadotropin deficiency. The age of initiation of this treatment must be individualized.

Once a diagnosis of HH is made, 2 treatment options are available. Treatment with testosterone will induce secondary sexual characteristics but will NOT stimulate testicular growth or spermatogenesis. Treatment with gonadotropins (either as a combination of hCG and human menopausal gonadotropins [HMG] or using GnRH pulse therapy) will lead to testicular development, including spermatogenesis, but is much more complex to manage. If fertility is not desired, or complex treatment is not feasible, then testosterone treatment may be the best option. Either long-acting testosterone injections or daily application of testosterone gel may be used (testosterone patches have a high incidence of skin rash and are rarely used in pediatrics). Testosterone enanthate ester may be used in a starting dose of 25-50 mg injected intramuscularly every 3-4 wk, with 50-mg increments every 6-9 mo until a maintenance dose for adults (200-250 mg every 3-4 wk) is achieved. At that time, testosterone patches or testosterone gel may be substituted for the injections. Depending on patient and physician preference, transdermal testosterone may be used as initial treatment instead of injections. For older boys, larger initial doses and increments can achieve more rapid virilization.

Treatment with gonadotropins is more physiologic. If not feasible in adolescence, this treatment may also be attempted in adult life when fertility is desired. The treatment schedule varies from 1250-5000 IU hCG in combination with 12.5-150 IU hMG 3 times per wk intramuscularly. It may require up to 2 yr of treatment to achieve adequate spermatogenesis in adults. Recombinantly produced gonadotropins (LH and FSH) are also able to stimulate gonadal growth and function but are much more expensive. Treatment with GnRH (when available) is most physiologic, but requires the use of a subcutaneous infusion pump to deliver appropriately pulsed therapy since continuous exposure to GnRH will suppress gonadotropins rather than stimulating them. The rare patient with isolated LH deficiency can be treated effectively using hCG injections. Up to 10% of patients diagnosed with HH (with or without anosmia) exhibit spontaneous reversal of hypogonadism with sustained normal gonadal function off treatment; therefore, a brief trial of interruption of treatment is justified in patients with idiopathic HH.

BIBLIOGRAPHY

Please visit the Nelson Textbook of Pediatrics *website at www.expertconsult.com for the complete bibliography.*

Chapter 578
Pseudoprecocity Resulting from Tumors of the Testes

Omar Ali and Patricia A. Donohoue

Leydig cell tumors of the testes are rare causes of precocious pseudopuberty and cause asymmetric enlargement of the testes. Leydig cells are sparse before puberty and tumors derived from them are more common in the adult, but rare cases do occur in children and the youngest reported case was in a 1 yr old boy. These tumors are usually unilateral and benign; while up to 10% of adult tumors may be malignant, metastasizing malignant tumors have not been reported in children. Some tumors may be due to somatic activating mutations of the luteinizing hormone (LH) receptor.

For the full continuation of this chapter, please visit the Nelson Textbook of Pediatrics *website at www.expertconsult.com.*

Chapter 579
Gynecomastia

Omar Ali and Patricia A. Donohoue

Gynecomastia, the proliferation of mammary glandular tissue in the male, is a common condition. True gynecomastia (the presence of glandular breast tissue) needs to be distinguished from pseudogynecomastia due to accumulation of adipose tissue in the area of the breast that is commonly seen in overweight boys. True gynecomastia is characterized by the presence of a palpable fibroglandular mass at least 0.5 cm in diameter, located concentrically beneath the nipple and areaolar region.

Physiologic Forms of Gynecomastia: Gynecomastia occurs in many newborn males as a result of normal stimulation by maternal estrogen; the effect usually disappears in a few weeks. It is then extremely rare in prepubertal boys, in whom it should always be investigated to identify the cause. It is very common in puberty.

Neonatal Gynecomastia: Transient gynecomastia occurs in 60-90% of male newborns secondary to exposure to estrogens during pregnancy. Breast development may be asymmetrical and galactorrhea is seen in approximately 5%. Most cases resolve within 4-8 wk of birth, but a few can last as long as 12 mo.

Pubertal Gynecomastia: During early to mid-puberty, up to 65% of boys develop various degrees of subareolar hyperplasia of the breasts. Incidence peaks at 14 yr of age, at Tanner stage 3-4 and at a testicular volume of 5-10 mL. Physiologic pubertal gynecomastia may involve only 1 breast; it is not unusual for both breasts to enlarge at disproportionate rates or at different times. Tenderness of the breast is common but transitory. Spontaneous regression may occur within a few months; it rarely persists longer than 2 yr. Significant psychosocial distress may be present, especially in obese boys with relatively large breasts.

The cause is thought to be an imbalance between estrogen and androgen action at the level of breast tissue. Testing usually fails to reveal any significant difference in circulating estrogen and androgen levels between affected and unaffected males, but minor degrees of imbalance in free hormone levels may still be present. Other hormones including leptin and luteinizing hormone (LH) may directly stimulate breast development and may play an important role in pubertal gynecomastia. Some cases may be due to an increased sensitivity to estrogens and/or relative androgen resistance in the affected tissue. As androgen levels continue to rise in later puberty, most cases resolve.

Pathological Gynecomastia: Monogenic forms of gynecomastia are extremely rare, but do exist. Familial gynecomastia has occurred in several kindreds as an X-linked or autosomal dominant sex-limited trait. Some of these cases were found to be due to constitutive activation of the p450 aromatase enzyme (CYP19A1 gene), leading to increased peripheral conversion of C-19 steroids to estrogens (increased aromatization). A report of this syndrome in a father and his son and daughter suggests autosomal dominant inheritance. There was gynecomastia in the 9 yr old boy and macromastia and isosexual precocity in his 7½ yr old sister. Excess aromatase activity was shown in skin fibroblasts and transformed lymphocytes in vitro.

Exogenous sources of estrogens are an important cause of gynecomastia in prepubertal children. Very small amounts of estrogens can cause gynecomastia in male children and accidental exposure may occur by inhalation, percutaneous absorption, or ingestion. Common sources of estrogens include oral contraceptive pills, and oral and transdermal estrogen preparations. Gynecomastia has been reported in workers involved in the manufacture of estrogens and even in the children of such workers. Gynecomastia can also occur secondary to exposure to medications that decrease levels of androgens (especially free androgens), increase estradiol, or displace androgens from breast androgen receptors. Spironolactone, alkylating agents, anabolic steroids, human chorionic gonadotropin (hCG), ketoconazole, cimetidine, and androgen inhibitors such as flutamide are all associated with the occurrence of gynecomastia. Weaker associations are seen with a large number of other medications and drugs of abuse (opiates, alcohol) though the association with marijuana may not be as strong as previously thought. Lavender and certain tea oils have also been implicated as a cause of prepubertal gynecomastia.

Klinefelter syndrome and other causes of **hypergonadotropic hypogonadism** are strongly associated with gynecomastia. It is also seen in other conditions characterized by male undervirilization, including androgen insensitivity syndromes and 17-ketosteroid reductase deficiency. Gynecomastia has been observed in children with congenital virilizing adrenal hyperplasia (11β-hydroxylase deficiency) and may be associated with Leydig cell tumors of the testis or with feminizing tumors of the adrenal gland. Several boys with Peutz-Jeghers syndrome and gynecomastia had sex cord tumors of the testes. The testes may not be enlarged in these cases and the tumor is usually multifocal and bilateral. Excessive aromatase production accounts for the gynecomastia. When gynecomastia is associated with galactorrhea, a prolactinoma should be considered. Hyperthyroidism alters the androgen to estrogen ratio by increasing bound androgen and decreasing the free testosterone and may result in gynecomastia in up to 40% of cases. Gynecomastia is also seen in malnourished patients after restoration of normal nutrition (refeeding syndrome), in whom it may be due to hepatic dysfunction or abnormal activation of the gonadotropin axis.

Evaluation of Gynecomastia: In pubertal cases a detailed history and physical examination is all that is needed to exclude rare pathologic causes. Historical evaluation should include family history of male relatives with gynecomastia, history of liver or renal disease, use of medications or drugs of abuse, and exposure to herbal and cosmetic products that may contain phytoestrogens. Physical examination should include special attention to the breasts (looking for overlying skin changes, fixation, local lymphadenopathy, and nipple discharge) as well as a testicular exam. No laboratory evaluation is indicated in routine cases. All prepubertal cases, as well as pubertal cases with suspicious features should be investigated; initial laboratory evaluation should include thyroid function tests (to rule out hyperthyroidism), testosterone, estradiol, hCG and LH levels. If there is any evidence of galactorrhea, then prolactin level should also be obtained. Due to circadian variation, these levels should ideally be obtained in the morning. Other tests that may be indicated in selected cases include a karyotype, DHEAS, and liver and renal function tests.

Treatment in case of benign pubertal gynecomastia usually consists of reassuring the boy and his family of the physiologic and transient nature of the phenomenon. When the enlargement is striking and persistent and causes serious emotional disturbance to the patient, specific treatment may be justified. Unfortunately, medical treatment is generally ineffective in long standing cases. Early cases respond better to medical treatment but it is harder to justify treatment since most cases will resolve spontaneously. Agents that may be used for such treatment include androgens, aromatase inhibitors, and estrogen antagonists. The effectiveness of synthetic androgens is variable and side effects are a concern, so these are rarely used in pediatrics. Aromatase inhibitors make physiologic sense, but placebo-controlled trials have been disappointing. Estrogen antagonists like tamoxifen and raloxifene are more effective, with raloxifene being the superior agent in at least 1 well designed trial. Therefore, if medical treatment is attempted, it should be in early cases (less than 12 mo standing) using raloxifene (in a dose of 60 mg/day) or tamoxifen (10-20 mg/day) for 3-9 mo.

In those cases where breast development is excessive (Tanner stages 3-5), causes significant psychologic distress or fails to regress in 18-24 mo, surgical removal of the enlarged breast tissue is indicated. Various surgical approaches, including ultrasound assisted liposuction, are available.

BIBLIOGRAPHY

Please visit the Nelson Textbook of Pediatrics *website at www.expertconsult.com for the complete bibliography.*

Chapter 580 Hypofunction of the Ovaries

Alvina R. Kansra and Patricia A. Donohoue

Hypofunction of the ovaries can be either primary or central in etiology. It may be caused by congenital failure of development, postnatal destruction (primary or hypergonadotropic hypogonadism), or lack of central stimulation by the pituitary and/or hypothalamus (secondary or tertiary hypogonadotropic hypogonadism). Primary ovarian insufficiency (hypergonadotropic hypogonadism), which is also termed premature ovarian failure, is characterized by the arrest of normal ovarian function before the age of 40 yr. Mutations of certain genes could result in primary ovarian insufficiency. Hypofunction of the ovaries due to lack of central stimulation (hypogonadotropic hypogonadism) can be associated with other processes such as multiple pituitary hormone deficiencies and some chronic diseases. Table 580-1 details the etiologic classification of ovarian hypofunction.

Table 580-1 ETIOLOGIC CLASSIFICATION OF OVARIAN HYPOFUNCTION

HYPOGONADOTROPIC HYPOGONADISM
I. Hypothalamic
A. Genetic defects
1. Kallman syndrome
2. Other gene defects: leptin, leptin receptor, *KiSS-1*, *DAX-1*
3. Inherited syndromes: Prader-Willi, Bardet-Biedl, and others
4. Marked constitutional growth delay?
B. Acquired defects (reversible)
1. Anorexia nervosa
2. Drug use
3. Malnutrition
4. Chronic illness, esp. Crohn disease
5. Hyperprolactinemia
II. Pituitary
A. Genetic defects
1. Isolated gonadotropin deficiency (GnRH receptor, FSH, and LH beta subunit)
2. Septo-optic dysplasia (*HESX-1* in some cases)
3. Disorders of pituitary organogenesis (*PROP1, LHX3, LHX4, SOX-3,* etc.)
B. Acquired defects
1. Pituitary tumors
2. Pituitary infarction
3. Infiltrative disorders (histiocytosis, sarcoidosis)
4. Hemosiderosis and hemochromatosis
5. Radiation
HYPERGONDADOTROPIC HYPOGONADISM
I. Genetic
A. FSH and LH resistance
B. Mutations in steroidogenic pathways
C. 46,XX gonadal dysgenesis
D. Turner syndrome and its variants
E. Noonan syndrome (*PTPN-11* gene)
F. *SF-1* gene mutations
G. Galactosemia
H. Fragile X–associated disorders
I. Bloom syndrome
J. Werner syndrome
K. Ataxia-telangiectasia
L. Fanconi anemia
II. Acquired
A. Chemotherapy
B. Radiation
C. Autoimmune ovarian failure from autoimmune polyendocrine syndromes 1 and 2

580.1 Hypergonadotropic Hypogonadism in the Female (Primary Hypogonadism)

Alvina R. Kansra and Patricia A. Donohoue

Diagnosis of hypergonadotropic hypogonadism before puberty is difficult. Except in the case of Turner syndrome, most affected patients have no prepubertal clinical manifestations.

TURNER SYNDROME

Turner described a syndrome consisting of sexual infantilism, webbed neck, and cubitus valgus in adult females (Chapter 76). Ullrich described an 8 yr old girl with short stature and many of the same phenotypic features. The term Ullrich-Turner syndrome is frequently used in Europe but rarely used in the USA. The condition is defined as the combination of the characteristic phenotypic features accompanied by complete or partial absence of the second X chromosome with or without mosaicism.

Pathogenesis

Half the patients with Turner syndrome have a 45,X chromosomal complement. About 15% of patients are mosaics for 45,X and a normal cell line (45,X/46,XX). Other mosaics with isochromosomes, 45,X/46,X,i(Xq); with rings, 45,X/46,X,r(X); or with fragments, 45,X/46fra, occur less often. Mosaicism is detected most commonly when more than one tissue is examined. The single X is of maternal origin in nearly 80% of 45,X patients. The mechanism of chromosome loss is unknown, and the risk for the syndrome does not increase with maternal age. The genes involved in the Turner phenotype are X-linked genes that escape inactivation. A major locus involved in the control of linear growth has been mapped within the pseudoautosomal region of the X chromosome (PAR1). *SHOX*, a homeobox-containing gene of 170 kb of DNA within the PAR1, is thought to be important for controlling growth in children with Turner syndrome, Leri-Weill syndrome, and rarely in patients having idiopathic short stature. Genes for the control of normal ovarian function are postulated to be on Xp and perhaps two "supergenes" on Xq.

Turner syndrome occurs in about 1/1,500-2,500 live born females. The frequency of the 45,X karyotype at conception is about 3.0%, but 99% of these are spontaneously aborted, accounting for 5-10% of all abortuses. Mosaicism (45,X/46,XX) occurs in a proportion higher than that seen with any other aneuploid state, but the mosaic Turner constitution is rare among the abortuses; these findings indicate preferential survival for mosaic forms.

The normal fetal ovary contains about 7 million oocytes, but these begin to disappear rapidly after the 5th mo of gestation. At birth, there are only 2 million (1 million active follicles); by menarche, there are 400,000-500,000; and at menopause, 10,000 remain. In the absence of 1 X chromosome, this process is accelerated, and nearly all oocytes are gone by 2 yr of age. In aborted 45,X fetuses, the number of primordial germ cells in the gonadal ridge appears to be normal, suggesting that the normal process is accelerated in patients with Turner syndrome. Eventually, the ovaries are described as "streaks" and consist only of connective tissue, with only a few germ cells present.

Clinical Manifestations

Many patients with Turner syndrome are recognizable at birth because of a characteristic edema of the dorsa of the hands and feet and loose skinfolds at the nape of the neck. Low birthweight and decreased length are common (Chapter 76). Clinical manifestations in childhood include webbing of the neck, a low posterior hairline, small mandible, prominent ears, epicanthal folds, high arched palate, a broad chest presenting the illusion of widely spaced nipples, cubitus valgus, and hyperconvex fingernails. The diagnosis is often first suspected at puberty when breast development fails to occur.

Short stature, the cardinal finding in virtually all girls with Turner syndrome, may be present with little in the way of other clinical manifestations. The linear growth deceleration begins in infancy and young childhood, gets progressively more pronounced in later childhood and adolescence, and results in significant adult short stature. Sexual maturation fails to occur at the expected age. Among untreated patients with Turner syndrome, the mean adult height is 143-144 cm in the USA and most of northern Europe, but 140 cm in Argentina and 147 cm in Scandinavia (Fig. 580-1). The height is well correlated with the midparental height (average of the parents' heights). Specific growth curves for height have been developed for girls with Turner syndrome.

Associated cardiac defects are common. In the girls with Turner syndrome, life-threatening consequences of X-chromosome haploinsufficiency involve the cardiovascular system. There is a 4- to 5-fold increased rate of premature mortality secondary to congenital heart disease and premature coronary heart disease in adults with Turner syndrome. Clinically silent cardiac defects, mainly bicuspid aortic valve, but also ascending aortic dilation and partial anomalous pulmonary venous connections are present in patients with Turner syndrome. Regardless of the age, all patients with Turner syndrome at the time of diagnosis need comprehensive cardiovascular evaluation by a cardiologist specializing in congenital heart disease. Complete cardiologic evaluation, including echocardiography, reveals isolated nonstenotic bicuspid aortic valves in one third to one half of patients. In later life, bicuspid aortic valve disease can progress to dilatation of the aortic root. Less frequent defects include aortic coarctation (20%), aortic stenosis, mitral valve prolapse, and anomalous pulmonary venous drainage. In a study of 170/393 females with Turner syndrome in Denmark, 38% of patients with 45,X chromosomes had cardiovascular malformations compared with 11% of those with mosaic monosomy X; the most common were aortic valve abnormalities and aortic coarctation. Webbed neck in patients with or without recognized syndromes is associated with both flow-related and non–flow-related heart defects. Among patients with Turner syndrome, those with webbed neck have a much greater chance of having coarctation of the aorta than do those without webbed necks. Recent studies have suggested that in Turner syndrome there is a broader spectrum of cardiovascular abnormalities than previously recognized. Transthoracic echocardiogram in young girls is adequate if cardiac anatomy is clearly seen; otherwise magnetic resonance angiographic screening studies should be considered in asymptomatic individuals with Turner syndrome. During adolescence, and certainly before pregnancy is contemplated, repeat cardiac evaluation should be considered even in those without prior findings of cardiac abnormalities. Blood pressure should be routinely monitored even in the absence of cardiac or renal lesions and especially in

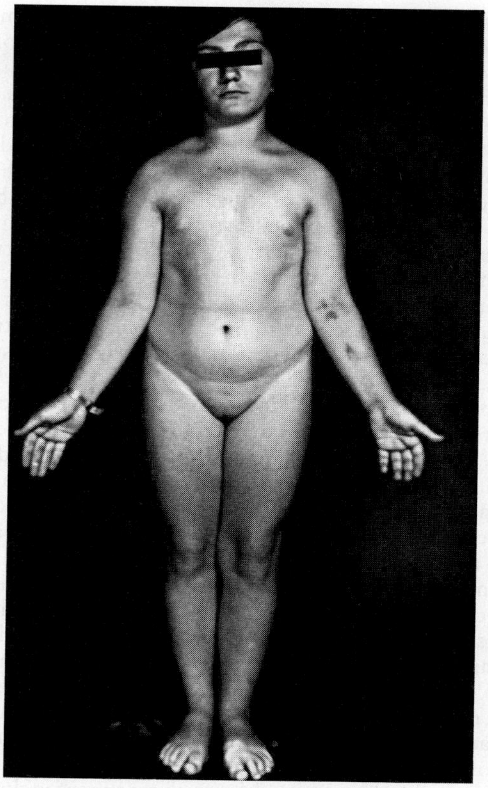

Figure 580-1 Turner syndrome in a 15 yr old girl exhibiting failure of sexual maturation, short stature, cubitus valgus, and a goiter. There is no webbing of the neck. Karyotyping revealed 45,X/46,XX chromosome complement.

those with suggestions of aortic root dilatation. Cardiac MRI is a valuable tool to detect and monitor aortic root dilation.

Renal ultrasound should be performed in all girls with Turner syndrome at diagnosis. One fourth to one third of patients have renal malformations on ultrasonographic examination (50% of those with 45,X karyotypes). The more serious defects include pelvic kidney, horseshoe kidney, double collecting system, complete absence of one kidney, and ureteropelvic junction obstruction. Some of the malformations may increase the risk of hypertension and urinary tract infection. Idiopathic hypertension is also common. Girls with Turner syndrome who had normal baseline renal ultrasound did not develop renal disease during a follow-up period averaging 6 yr.

When the ovaries were examined by ultrasonography, older studies found a significant decrease in percentage of detectable ovaries from infancy to later childhood. A subsequent report found no such age-related differences in a cross-sectional and longitudinal study conducted in Italy; 27-46% of patients had detectable ovaries at various ages; 76% of those with X mosaicism and 26% of those with 45,X karyotypes had detectable ovaries.

Sexual maturation usually fails to occur, but 10-20% of girls have spontaneous breast development, and a small percentage may have menstrual periods. Primary gonadal failure is associated with early onset of adrenarche (elevation in DHEA sulfate) but delayed pubarche (pubic hair development). Spontaneous pregnancies have been reported in menstruating patients with Turner syndrome. Premature menopause, increased risk of miscarriage, and offspring with increased risk of trisomy 21 have been reported in some of these women. A woman with a 45,X/46,X,r(X) karyotype treated with hormone replacement therapy had 3 pregnancies, resulting in a normal 46,XY male infant, a spontaneous abortion, and a healthy term female with Turner syndrome 45,X/46,Xr(X).

Antithyroid antibodies (thyroid peroxidase, and/or thyroglobulin antibodies) occur in 30-50% of patients. The prevalence increases with advancing age. Ten to 30% have **autoimmune thyroid disease,** with or without the presence of a goiter. Age-dependent abnormalities in carbohydrate metabolism characterized by abnormal glucose tolerance and insulin resistance and, only rarely, frank type 2 diabetes occur in patients with Turner syndrome. Impaired insulin secretion has been described in 45,X women. Cholesterol levels are elevated in adolescence, regardless of body mass index or karyotype.

Inflammatory bowel disease, both Crohn disease and ulcerative colitis; gastrointestinal bleeding due to abnormal mesenteric vasculature; and delayed gastric emptying time have all been reported. Screening for celiac disease is recommended by recent guidelines, since the risk of celiac disease is increased in Turner syndrome, with 4-6% of individuals affected. Although autoimmune diseases have been associated with Turner syndrome, the prevalence of type 1 diabetes with Turner syndrome is not very high.

Sternal malformations can be detected by lateral chest radiography. An increased carrying angle at the elbow is usually not clinically significant. Scoliosis occurs in about 10% of adolescent girls. Congenital hip dysplasia occurs more commonly than in the general population. Reported eye findings include anterior segment dysgenesis and keratoconus. Pigmented nevi become more prominent with age; melanocytic nevi are common. Essential hyperhidrosis, torus mandibularis, and alopecia areata occur rarely.

Recurrent bilateral otitis media develops in about 75% of patients. Sensorineural hearing deficits are common, and the frequency increases with age. Problems with gross and fine motor-sensory integration, failure to walk before 15 mo of age, and early language dysfunction often raise questions about developmental delay, but intelligence is normal in most patients. However, mental retardation does occur in patients with 45,X/46,X,r(X); the ring chromosome is unable to undergo inactivation and leads to 2 functional X chromosomes.

A special attention should be given to psychosocial development in girls with Turner syndrome. In general the behavior function is normal in girls with Turner syndrome, but they are at an increased risk for social isolation, immaturity, and anxiety. Other conditions such as dyslexia, nonverbal learning disability, and attention deficit disorder have been reported in girls with Turner syndrome. In adults, deficits in perceptual spatial skills are more common than they are in the general population. Some unconfirmed data suggest the existence of an imprinted X-linked locus that affects cognitive function such as verbal and higher-order executive function skills. These functions are apparently better when the X is paternal in origin.

The prevalence of mosaicism depends in large part on the techniques used for studying chromosomal patterns. The use of fluorescent in situ hybridization and reverse transcription–polymerase chain reaction (PCR) has increased the reported prevalence of mosaic patterns to as high as 60-74%.

Mosaicism involving the Y chromosome occurs in 5%. A population study of Danish women using PCR with 5 different primer sets found Y chromosome material in 12.2%. Gonadoblastoma among Y-positive patients occurred in 7-10%. Therefore, the current recommendation is that prophylactic gonadectomy should be performed even in the absence of MRI or CT evidence of tumors. The recommended timing of this procedure is at the time of diagnosis, but this may need to be re-evaluated in the future. The gonadoblastoma locus on the Y chromosome (GBY) maps close to the Y centromere. The presence of only the SRY (sex determining region on Y) locus is not sufficient to confer increased susceptibility for the development of gonadoblastoma. A careful study of 53 patients with Turner syndrome by nested PCR excluded low-level Y mosaicism in almost all cases. A 2nd round of PCR detected SRY on the distal short arm of the Y chromosome in only 2 subjects. Therefore, routine PCR for Y chromosome detection for the purpose of assigning gonadoblastoma risk does not seem indicated. High-throughput quantitative genotyping may provide an effective and inexpensive method for the identification of X chromosome abnormalities and Y chromosome material identification.

In patients with 45,X/46,XX mosaicism, the abnormalities are attenuated and fewer; short stature is as frequent as it is in the 45,X patient and may be the only manifestation of the condition other than ovarian failure (see Fig. 580-1).

Laboratory Findings

Chromosomal analysis must be considered routinely in short girls. In a systematic search, using Southern blot analysis of leukocyte DNA, Turner syndrome was detected in 4.8% of girls referred to an endocrinology service because of short stature. Patients with a marker chromosome in some or all cells should be tested for DNA sequences at or near the centromere of the Y chromosome for GBY.

Ultrasonography of the heart, kidneys, and ovaries is indicated after the diagnosis is established. The most common skeletal abnormalities are shortening of the 4th metatarsal and metacarpal bones, epiphyseal dysgenesis in the joints of the knees and elbows, Madelung deformity, scoliosis, and in older patients, inadequate osseous mineralization.

Plasma levels of gonadotropins, particularly follicle-stimulating hormone (FSH), are markedly elevated to greater than those of age-matched controls during infancy; at 2-3 yr of age, a progressive decrease in levels occurs until they reach a nadir at 6-8 yr of age, and by 10-11 yr, they rise to adult castrate levels.

Thyroid antiperoxidase antibodies should be checked periodically, and if positive, levels of thyroxine and thyroid-stimulating hormone should be obtained. Turner syndrome girls should be screened by measuring tissue transglutaminase (TGG) IgA antibodies for celiac disease. Initial testing should be done around age 4 yr and repeated every 2-5 yr. Extensive studies have failed to establish that growth hormone deficiency plays a primary role in the pathogenesis of the growth disorder. Defects in normal secretory patterns of growth hormone are seen in adolescents due to lack of gonadal steroids but not in younger girls with Turner syndrome. In vitro, monocytes and lymphocytes show decreased sensitivity to insulin-like growth factor-1 (IGF-1).

The American Academy of Pediatrics has published a comprehensive guide to the health supervision of children with Turner syndrome. A guide to the care of girls and women with Turner syndrome was published in 2007.

Treatment

Treatment with recombinant human growth hormone increases height velocity and ultimate stature in most but not all children. Many girls achieve heights of greater than 150 cm with early initiation of treatment. In a large, multicenter, placebo-controlled U.S. clinical trial, 99 patients with Turner syndrome who started receiving growth hormone at a mean age of 10.9 yr at doses between 0.27 and 0.36 mg/kg/wk achieved a mean height of 149 cm, with nearly one third reaching heights greater than 152.4 cm (60 in). In the Netherlands, higher doses of growth hormone (up to 0.63 mg/kg/wk in the 3rd yr of treatment) resulted in 85% of the subjects reaching adult heights in the normal range for the Dutch reference population. Growth hormone treatment should be initiated in early childhood and/or when there is evidence of height velocity attenuation on specific Turner syndrome growth curves. The starting dose of growth hormone is 0.375 mg/kg/wk. Growth hormone therapy does not significantly aggravate carbohydrate tolerance and does not result in marked adverse events in patients with Turner syndrome. Serum levels of IGF-1 should be monitored if the patient is receiving high doses of growth hormone.

Oxandrolone has also been used to treat the short stature associated with Turner syndrome, either alone or in combination with growth hormone. This synthetic anabolic steroid has weak androgenic effects, and patients should be monitored for signs of pubarche, as well as hepatotoxicity. The latter is rare.

Replacement therapy with estrogens is indicated, but there is little consensus about the optimal age at which to initiate treatment. The psychologic preparedness of the patient to accept therapy must be taken into account. The improved growth achieved by girls treated with growth hormone in childhood permits initiation of estrogen replacement at 12-13 yr. Delaying estrogen therapy to optimize height potential until 15 yr of age, as previously recommended, seems unwarranted. This change of starting early estrogen therapy was considered due to psychologic importance of age appropriate pubertal maturation. Also delaying estrogen therapy could be deleterious for bone health and other aspects of child's health. Low dose estrogen replacement at 12 yr of age permits a normal pace of puberty without interfering with the positive effect of growth hormone on the final adult height. Estrogen therapy improves verbal and nonverbal memory in girls with Turner syndrome. In young women with age-appropriate pubertal development who achieve normal height, health-related quality-of-life questionnaires have yielded normal results.

Although many forms of estrogen are available, oral estrogens have been mostly used. Both transdermal and injectable depot forms of estradiol may be more alternative physiological options. A conjugated estrogen (Premarin), 0.15-0.625 mg daily, or micronized estradiol (Estrace), 0.5 mg, given daily for 3-6 mo is usually effective in inducing puberty. The estrogen then is cycled (taken on days 1-23), and a progestin (Provera) is added (taken on days 10-23) in a dose of 5-10 mg daily. In the remainder of the calendar month, during which no treatment is given, withdrawal bleeding usually occurs.

Prenatal chromosome analysis for advanced maternal age has revealed a frequency of 45,X/46,XX that is 10 times higher than when diagnosed postnatally. Most of these patients have no clinical manifestations of Turner syndrome, and levels of gonadotropins are normal. Awareness of this mild phenotype is important in counseling patients.

Psychosocial support for these girls is an integral component of treatment. A comprehensive psychologic education evaluation is recommended either at the time of Turner syndrome diagnosis depending on the patient's age, or any of the components of behavior or cognition become obvious or immediately preceding school entry. The Turner Syndrome Society, which has local chapters in the USA, and similar groups in Canada and other countries provide a valuable support system for these patients and their families in addition to that given by the health care team.

Successful pregnancies have been carried to term using ovum donation and in vitro fertilization. Adolescents with few signs of spontaneous puberty may have ovaries with follicles. There remains a future possibility of using cryopreserved ovarian tissue with immature oocytes before the regression of the ovaries for the future pregnancies. In adult women with Turner syndrome, there seems to be a high prevalence of undiagnosed bone mineral density, lipid, and thyroid abnormalities. Glucose intolerance, diminished 1st-phase insulin response, elevated blood pressure, and lowered fat free mass are common. Glucose tolerance worsens, but fat free mass and blood pressure and general physical fitness improve with sex hormone replacement. The neurocognitive profile of adult women is unaffected by estrogen status.

XX GONADAL DYSGENESIS

Some phenotypically and genetically normal females have gonadal lesions identical to those in 45,X patients but without somatic features of Turner syndrome; their condition is termed pure gonadal dysgenesis or pure ovarian dysgenesis.

The disorder is rarely recognized in children because the external genitals are normal, no other abnormalities are visible, and growth is normal. At pubertal age, sexual maturation fails to take place. Plasma gonadotropin levels are elevated. Delay of epiphyseal fusion results in a **eunuchoid** habitus. Pelvic ultrasonography reveals streak ovaries.

Affected siblings, parental consanguinity, and failure to uncover mosaicism all point to female-limited autosomal recessive inheritance. The disorder appears to be especially frequent in Finland (1/8,300 liveborn girls). In this population, several mutations in the FSH receptor gene (on chromosome 2p) were demonstrated as the cause of the condition. FSH receptor gene mutations were not detected in Mexican women with 46,XX gonadal dysgenesis. In some patients, XX gonadal dysgenesis has been associated with sensorineural deafness (Perrault syndrome). A patient with this condition and concomitant growth hormone deficiency and virilization has also been reported. There may be distinct genetic forms of this disorder. **Müllerian agenesis,** or the **Mayer-Rokitansky-Küster-Hauser** syndrome, which is 2nd to gonadal dysgenesis as the most common cause of primary amenorrhea, occurring in 1:4,000 to 1:5,000 females, has been reported in association with 46,XX gonadal dysgenesis in a 17 yr old adolescent with primary amenorrhea and lack of breast development. One case of dysgerminoma with syncytiotrophoblastic giant cells was reported. An 18 yr old woman with primary amenorrhea and an absence of müllerian-derived structures, unilateral renal agenesis, and clinical signs of androgen excess—a phenotype resembling the Mayer-Rokitansky-Küster-Hauser syndrome was found to have a loss-of-function mutation in the *WNT4* gene. Treatment consists of estrogen replacement therapy.

45,X/46,XY GONADAL DYSGENESIS

45,X/46,XY gonadal dysgenesis, also called **mixed gonadal dysgenesis,** has extreme phenotypic variability postnatally that may extend from a Turner-like syndrome to a male phenotype with a penile urethra; it is possible to delineate 3 major clinical phenotypes. Short stature is a major finding in all affected children. Ninety percent of prenatally diagnosed cases have a normal male phenotype.

Some patients have no evidence of virilization; they have a female phenotype and often have the somatic signs of Turner syndrome. The condition is discovered prepubertally when chromosomal studies are made in short girls, or later when chromosomal studies are made because of failure of sexual maturation. Fallopian tubes and uterus are present. The gonads consist of intra-abdominal undifferentiated streaks; chromosomal study of the streak often reveals an XY cell line. The streak gonad differs somewhat from that in girls with Turner syndrome; in addition to wavy connective tissue, there are often tubular or cordlike structures, occasional clumps of granulosa cells, and frequently, mesonephric or hilar cells.

Some children have mild virilization manifested only by prepubertal clitorimegaly. Normal müllerian structures are present, but at puberty virilization occurs. These patients usually have an intra-abdominal testis, a contralateral streak gonad, and bilateral fallopian tubes.

Many children present with frank ambiguity of the genitals in infancy. A testis and vas deferens are found on one side in the labioscrotal fold, and a streak gonad is identified on the contralateral side. Despite the presence of a testis, fallopian tubes are often present bilaterally. An infantile or rudimentary uterus is almost always present.

Other genotypes and phenotypes have been described. About 25% of 200 analyzed patients have a dicentric Y chromosome (45,X/46,X,dic Y). In some patients, the Y chromosome may be represented by only a fragment (45,X/45,X +fra); application of Y-specific probes can establish the origin of the fragment. It is not clear why the same genotype (45,X/46,XY) can result in such diverse phenotypes. Mutations in the SRY gene have been described in some patients.

Children with a female phenotype present no problem in gender of rearing. Patients who are only slightly virilized are usually assigned a female gender of rearing before a diagnosis is established. Patients with ambiguity of the genitals are readily often clinically indistinguishable from patients with various types of 46,XY disorders of sex development (46,XY DSD). In many but not all instances, these children are best reared as females; the short stature, the ease of genital reconstruction, and the predisposition of the gonad to the development of malignancy may favor this choice. In some patients followed to adulthood, the putative normal testis proves to be dysgenetic with eventual loss of Leydig and Sertoli cell function (Chapter 577). In an analysis of 22 Australian patients with mixed gonadal dysgenesis, no significant associations or correlations were found between internal and external phenotypes or endocrine function and gonadal morphologic features. The sex of rearing was determined by the appearance of the external genitals. In 11 patients, basal and human chorionic gonadotropin–stimulated testosterone levels were lower than in control subjects.

Gonadal tumors, usually **gonadoblastomas,** occur in about 25% of these children. As described above, a gonadoblastoma locus has been localized to a region near the centromere of the Y chromosome (GBY). These germ cell tumors are preceded by the changes of carcinoma in situ. Accordingly, both gonads should be removed in all patients reared as girls, and the undifferentiated gonad should be removed in the patients reared as boys.

There is no correlation among the proportion of 45,X/46,XY cell lines in either blood or fibroblasts and phenotype. In the past, all patients came to clinical attention because of their abnormal phenotypes. However, 45,X/46,XY mosaicism is found in about 7% of fetuses with true chromosome mosaicism encountered prenatally. Of 76 infants with 45,X/46,XY mosaicism diagnosed prenatally, 72 had a normal male phenotype, 1 had a female phenotype, and only 3 males had hypospadias. Of 12 males whose gonads were examined, only 3 were abnormal. These data must be taken into account when counseling a family in which a 45,X/46,XY infant is discovered prenatally.

XXX, XXXX, AND XXXXX FEMALES

XXX Females

The 47,XXX (trisomy) chromosomal constitution is the most frequent extra–X chromosome abnormality in females, occurring in almost 1/1,000 liveborn females. In 68%, this condition is caused by maternal meiotic nondisjunction, but most 45,X and half of 47,XXY constitutions are caused by paternal sex chromosome errors. The phenotype is that of a normal female; affected infants and children are not recognized based on the genital appearance.

Sexual development and menarche are normal. Most pregnancies have resulted in normal infants. By 2 yr of age, delays in speech and language become evident and lack of coordination, poor academic performance, and immature behavior are seen in some. These girls tend to be tall and gangly, manifest behavior disorders, and are placed in special education classes. Using high-resolution MRI, 10 47,XXX subjects had lower amygdala volumes than 20 euploid controls; 10 47,XXY subjects had even lower amygdala volumes. In a review of 155 girls, 62% were physically normal. There is marked variability within the syndrome, and a small proportion of affected girls are well coordinated, socially outgoing, and academically superior.

XXXX and XXXXX Females

The great majority of females with these rare karyotypes have been mentally retarded. Commonly associated defects are epicanthal folds, hypertelorism, clinodactyly, transverse palmar creases, radioulnar synostosis, and congenital heart disease. Sexual maturation is often incomplete and may not occur at all. Nevertheless, 3 women with the tetra-X syndrome gave birth, but no pregnancies were reported in 49,XXXXX women. Most 48,XXXX women tend to be tall, with an average height of 169 cm, whereas short stature is a common feature of the 49,XXXXX phenotype.

NOONAN SYNDROME

Girls with Noonan syndrome show certain anomalies that also occur in girls with 45,X Turner syndrome, but they have normal 46,XX chromosomes. The most common abnormalities are the same as those described for males with Noonan syndrome (Chapter 577.1). The phenotype differs from Turner syndrome in several respects. Short stature is one of the cardinal signs of this syndrome. Mental retardation is often present, the cardiac defect is most often pulmonary valvular stenosis or an atrial septal defect rather than an aortic defect, normal sexual maturation usually occurs but is delayed by 2 yr on average, and premature ovarian failure has been reported. Growth hormone therapy is approved by the U.S. Food and Drug Administration for use in Noonan syndrome patients with short stature.

Other Ovarian Defects

Some young women with no chromosomal abnormality are found to have streak gonads that may contain only occasional or no germ cells. Gonadotropins are increased. Cytotoxic drugs, especially alkylating agents such as cyclophosphamide and busulfan, procarbazine, etoposide, and exposure of the ovaries to irradiation for the treatment of malignancy are frequent causes of ovarian failure. Young women with Hodgkin disease demonstrate that combination chemotherapy and pelvic irradiation may be more deleterious than either therapy alone. Teenagers are more likely than older women to retain or recover ovarian function after irradiation or combined chemotherapy; normal pregnancies have occurred after such treatment. Current treatment regimens may result in some ovarian damage in most girls treated for cancer. The LD_{50} for the human oocyte has been estimated to be about 4 Gy; doses as low as 6 Gy have produced primary amenorrhea. Ovarian transposition before abdominal and pelvic irradiation in childhood can preserve ovarian function by decreasing the ovarian exposure to less than 4-7 Gy.

Autoimmune ovarian failure occurs in 60% of children older than 13 yr of age with type I autoimmune polyendocrinopathy (Addison disease, hypoparathyroidism, candidiasis). This condition, also known as *polyglandular autoimmune disease* (PGAD) type 1 is rare worldwide but not in Finland, where, as a result of a founder gene effect, it occurs in 1:25,000 people. The gene for this disorder is located on chromosome 21 and is associated with HLA-DR5. In patients with PGAD-1 and ovarian failure, an association with HLA-A3 has been described. Affected girls may not develop sexually, or secondary amenorrhea may occur in young women. The ovaries may have lymphocytic infiltration or appear simply as streaks. Most affected patients have circulating steroid cell antibodies and autoantibodies to 21-hydroxylase. Among patients with polyglandular autoimmune syndromes, 5% were found to have hypogonadism.

The condition also occurs in young women as an isolated event or in association with other autoimmune disorders, leading to secondary amenorrhea (premature ovarian failure, POF). It occurs in 0.2-0.9% of women younger than 40 yr of age. Premature ovarian failure is a heterogeneous disorder with many causes: chromosomal, genetic, enzymatic, infectious, and iatrogenic. When associated with autoimmune adrenal disease, steroid cell autoantibodies are always present. These antibodies react with P450scc, 17α-OH, or 21-OH enzymes. When associated with an entire host of endocrine and nonendocrine autoimmune diseases and not adrenal autoimmunity, steroid cell autoantibodies are rarely found. A second autoimmune disorder, often subclinical, is found in 10-39% of adult patients with POF. One 17 yr old with idiopathic thrombocytopenic purpura and 47,XXX chromosomes had autoimmune POF. Patients with POF do not have the neurocognitive defects found in Turner syndrome patients.

Galactosemia, particularly the classical form of the disease, usually results in ovarian damage, beginning during intrauterine life. Levels of FSH and luteinizing hormone (LH) are elevated early in life. Ovarian damage may be due to deficient uridine diphosphate-galactose (Chapter 81). The **Denys-Drash syndrome,** caused by a *WT1* mutation, can result in ovarian dysgenesis.

Ataxia-telangiectasia may be associated with ovarian hypoplasia and elevated gonadotropins; the cause is unknown. Gonadoblastomas and dysgerminomas have occurred in a few girls.

Hypergonadotropic hypogonadism has been postulated to also occur because of the resistance of the ovary to both endogenous and exogenous gonadotropins (Savage syndrome). This condition occurs also in women with POF. Antiovarian antibodies or FSH receptor abnormalities may cause this condition. Mutation of the FSH receptor gene has been reported as an autosomal recessive condition (Chapter 576). A few females with 46,XX chromosomes presenting in primary amenorrhea with elevated gonadotropin levels were found to have inactivating mutations of the LH receptor gene. This suggests that LH action is needed for normal follicular development and ovulation. Other genetic defects associated with ovarian failure include mutations in *FOXL2, GNAS, CYP17,* and *CYP19*. Some data also suggest that mutations within the gene encoding transcription factor SF-1 are associated with early ovarian failure.

BIBLIOGRAPHY

Please visit the Nelson Textbook of Pediatrics *website at www.expertconsult.com for the complete bibliography.*

580.2 Hypogonadotropic Hypogonadism in the Female (Secondary Hypogonadism)

Alvina R. Kansra and Patricia A. Donohoue

Hypofunction of the ovaries can result from failure to secrete normal pulses of the gonadotropins LH (luteinizing hormone) and FSH (follicle stimulating hormone). Hypogonadotropic hypogonadism (HH) may occur if the hypothalamic-pituitary-gonadal axis is interrupted either at the hypothalamic or pituitary level. The mechanisms that result in HH include failure of the hypothalamic LHRH (luteinizing hormone–releasing hormone, also known as *GnRH* or *gonadotropin-releasing hormone*) pulse generator or inability of the pituitary to respond with secretion of LH and FSH. It is often difficult to distinguish between marked constitutional delay and hypogonadotropic hypogonadism.

ETIOLOGY

Hypopituitarism

Hypogonadotropic hypogonadism is most commonly seen with multiple pituitary hormone deficiencies resulting from malformations (e.g., septo-optic dysplasia, other midline defects), pituitary transcription factor defects such as in PROP-1, or lesions of the pituitary that are acquired postnatally. Familial isolated gonadotropin deficiency associated with anosmia was described in 1944. Many other genetic causes for hypogonadotropic hypogonadism have been identified. A gene important in LHRH secretion is named *KISS* (encoding the protein kisspeptin), which is suggested to play a significant role in the development of the LHRH secreting cells. Another set of genes recently implicated in hypogonadotrophic hypogonadism are the genes for neurokinin B *(TAC3)* and its receptor *(TAC3R)*.

In children with idiopathic hypopituitarism, the defect is usually found in the hypothalamus. In these patients, administration of gonadotropin-releasing hormone (GnRH) results in increased plasma levels of FSH and LH, establishing the integrity of the pituitary gland.

Hypogonadotropic hypogonadism is less common than hypergonadotropic hypogonadism. The latter condition underlies polycystic ovarian syndrome (PCOS; Stein-Leventhal syndrome; Chapter 546).

Isolated Deficiency of Gonadotropins

This heterogeneous group of disorders is sorted out with the help of the GnRH analog stimulation test. In most children, the pituitary is normal, with the defect residing in the hypothalamus. Patients with hyperprolactinemia, most often due to a pituitary prolactin-secreting adenoma, often have suppression of gonadotropin secretion. If breast development has occurred, then galactorrhea and amenorrhea are frequently seen.

Several sporadic instances of anosmia with hypogonadotropic hypogonadism have been reported. **Anosmic** hypogonadal females have also been reported in kindreds with Kallmann syndrome, but hypogonadism more frequently affects the males in these families. Mutations in the gene for the β-subunit of FSH and LH have been reported.

Some autosomal recessive disorders such as the Laurence-Moon-Biedl, multiple lentigines, and Carpenter syndromes appear in some instances to include gonadotropic hormone deficiency. Patients with Prader-Willi syndrome usually have some degree of hypogonadotropic hypogonadism. Girls with severe thalassemia may have gonadotropin deficiency from pituitary damage caused by chronic iron overload secondary to multiple transfusions. Anorexia nervosa frequently results in hypogonadotropic hypogonadism. The rare patients described with leptin deficiency or leptin receptor defects have failure of pubertal maturation due to gonadotropin deficiency.

DIAGNOSIS

The diagnosis may be apparent in patients with other deficiencies of pituitary tropic hormones, but, as in males, it is difficult to differentiate isolated hypogonadotropic hypogonadism from physiologic delay of puberty. Repeated measurements of FSH and LH, particularly during sleep, may reveal the rising levels that herald the onset of puberty. Stimulation testing with GnRH or one of its analogs may help establish the diagnosis. Morbidity for both men and women with hypogonadism includes infertility and an increased risk of osteoporosis.

BIBLIOGRAPHY

Please visit the Nelson Textbook of Pediatrics *website at www.expertconsult.com for the complete bibliography.*

Chapter 581
Pseudoprecocity Due to Lesions of the Ovary

Alvina R. Kansra and Patricia A. Donohoue

Ovarian tumors are rare in pediatrics, occurring at a rate of less than 3/100,000. Most ovarian masses are benign, but 10-30% may be malignant. Ovarian malignancies, the most common genital neoplasms in adolescence, account for only 1% of childhood cancers. More than 60% are germ cell tumors, most of which are dysgerminomas that can secrete tumor markers and hormones (Chapter 497). Five to 10% of them occur in phenotypic females with abnormal gonads associated with the presence of a Y chromosome. Next most common are epithelial cell tumors (20%), and nearly 10% are sex cord/stromal tumors (granulosa, Sertoli cell, and mesenchymal tumors). Multiple tumor markers can be seen in ovarian tumors, including α-fetoprotein, human chorionic gonadotropin (hCG), carcinoembryonic antigen, oncoproteins, p105, p53, *KRAS* mutations, cyclin D1, epidermal growth factor–related proteins and receptors, cathepsin B, and others. Variable levels of inhibin-activin subunit gene expression have been detected in ovarian tumors.

Functioning lesions of the ovary consist of benign cysts or malignant tumors. The majority synthesize estrogens; a few synthesize androgens. The most common estrogen producing ovarian tumor causing precocious puberty is the granulosa cell tumor. Other tumors that can cause precocious puberty are thecomas, luteomas, mixed types, theca-leutein and follicular cysts, and ovarian tumors (i.e., teratoma, choriocarcinoma, and dysgerminoma).

ESTROGENIC LESIONS OF THE OVARY

These lesions cause isosexual precocious sexual development but account for only a small percentage of all cases of precocity. Benign ovarian follicular cysts are the most common tumors associated with isosexual precocious puberty in girls; they may rarely be gonadotropin dependent.

Juvenile Granulosa Cell Tumor

In childhood, the most common neoplasm of the ovary with estrogenic manifestations is the granulosa cell tumor, although it makes up only 1-10% of all ovarian tumors. These tumors have distinctive histologic features that differ from those encountered in older women (adult granulosa cell tumor). The cells have high mitotic activity, follicles are often irregular, Call-Exner bodies are rare, and luteinization is frequent. The tumor may be solid or cystic, or both. It usually is benign. In a few instances, this tumor has been associated with multiple enchondromas (**Ollier disease**) and, in fewer still, with multiple subcutaneous hemangiomas (**Maffucci syndrome**).

Clinical Manifestations and Diagnosis

The tumor has been observed in newborns and may manifest with sexual precocity at 2 yr of age or younger; about half these tumors have occurred before 10 yr of age. The mean age at diagnosis is 7.5 yr. The tumors are almost always unilateral. The breasts become enlarged, rounded, and firm and the nipples prominent. The external genitals resemble those of a normal girl at puberty, and the uterus is enlarged. A white vaginal discharge is followed by irregular or cyclic menstruation. Ovulation, however, does not occur. The presenting manifestation may be abdominal pain or swelling. Pubic hair is usually absent unless there is mild virilization.

A mass is readily palpable in the lower portion of the abdomen in most children by the time sexual precocity is evident. The tumor may be small, however, and escape detection even on careful rectal and abdominal examination; the tumors may be detected by ultrasonography, but multidetector CT scans are most sensitive. Most such tumors (90%) are diagnosed at very early stages of malignancy (FIGO [International Federation of Gynecology and Obstetrics] stage I).

Plasma estradiol levels are markedly elevated. Plasma levels of gonadotropins are suppressed and do not respond to gonadotropin-releasing hormone (GnRH) analog stimulation. Levels of anti-müllerian hormone (AMH), inhibin B, and α-fetoprotein may be elevated. Activating mutations of GSα are seen in 30%, and GATA-4 expression is retained in the more aggressive tumors while AMH levels are inversely proportional to tumor size. Osseous development is moderately advanced. Several case reports showing the association of 45X/46XY karyotype and ambiguous genitalia with ovarian granulosa tumor have been published in literature.

Treatment and Prognosis

The tumor should be removed as soon as the diagnosis is established. Prognosis is excellent because fewer than 5% of these tumors in children are malignant. Advanced-stage tumors, however, behave aggressively and require difficult decisions regarding surgical approaches as well as the use of irradiation and chemotherapy. In adults with granulosa cell tumors, p53 expression is associated with unfavorable prognosis. Vaginal bleeding immediately after removal of the tumor is common. Signs of precocious puberty abate and may disappear within a few months after the operation. The secretion of estrogens returns to normal.

Sex cord tumor with annular tubules is a distinctive tumor, thought to arise from granulosa cells, that occurs primarily in patients with Peutz-Jeghers syndrome. These tumors are multifocal, bilateral, and usually benign. The presence of calcifications aids ultrasonographic detection. Increased aromatase production by these tumors results in gonadotropin-independent precocious puberty. Inhibin A and B levels are elevated and decrease after tumor removal. In 1 study, 9 of 13 sex cord/stromal tumors exhibited follicle-stimulating hormone (FSH) receptor mutations, suggesting a role for such mutation in the development of these tumors.

Chorioepithelioma has been reported only rarely. This highly malignant tumor is thought to arise from a pre-existing teratoma. The usually unilateral tumor produces large amounts of hCG, which stimulates the contralateral ovary to secrete estrogen. Elevated levels of hCG are diagnostic.

Follicular Cyst

Small ovarian cysts (<0.7 cm in diameter) are common in prepubertal children. At puberty and in girls with true isosexual precocious puberty, larger cysts (1-6 cm) are often seen; these are secondary to stimulation by gonadotropins. However, similar larger cysts occur occasionally in young girls with precocious puberty in the absence of LH and FSH. Because surgical removal or spontaneous involution of these cysts results in regression of pubertal changes, there is little doubt that they are its cause. The mechanism of production of these autonomously functioning cysts is unknown. Such cysts may form only once, or they may disappear and recur, resulting in waxing and waning of the signs of precocious puberty. They may be unilateral or bilateral. The sexual precocity that occurs in young girls with **McCune-Albright syndrome** is usually associated with autonomous follicular cysts caused by a somatic-activating mutation of the GSα-protein occurring early in development (Chapter 556.6). Gonadotropins are suppressed, and estradiol levels are often markedly elevated, but they may fluctuate widely and even temporarily may return to normal. GnRH analog stimulation fails to evoke an increase in gonadotropins. Ultrasonography is the method of choice for the detection and monitoring of such cysts. Aromatase inhibitors are shown to be the mainstay of the therapy in females with McCune-Albright Syndrome and persistent estradiol elevation. A short period of observation to ascertain the lack of spontaneous resolution is advisable before cyst aspiration or cystectomy is considered. Cystic neoplasms must be considered in the differential diagnosis.

ANDROGENIC LESIONS OF THE OVARY

Virilizing ovarian tumors are rare at all ages but particularly so in prepubertal girls. **Arrhenoblastoma** has been reported as early as 14 days of age, but few cases have been reported in girls younger than 16 yr of age.

The **Gonadoblastoma** occurs exclusively in dysgenetic gonads, particularly in phenotypic females who have a Y chromosome or a Y fragment in their genotype (46,XY; 45,X/46,XY; 45,X/46,X-fra). As noted above, there is a proposed gonadoblastoma locus on the Y chromosome (GBY). The tumors may be bilateral. Virilization occurs with some but not all tumors. The clinical features are the same as those seen in patients with virilizing adrenal tumors and include accelerated growth, acne, clitoral enlargement, and growth of sexual hair. A palpable, abdominal mass is found in about 50% of patients. Plasma levels of testosterone and androstenedione are elevated, and those of gonadotropins are suppressed. Ultrasonography, CT, and MRI usually localize the lesion. The dysgenetic gonad of phenotypic females with a Y chromosome or fragment of Y chromosome containing GBY should be removed prophylactically. When a unilateral tumor is removed, the contralateral dysgenetic gonad should also be removed. Association of gonadoblastoma and WAGR syndrome is also reported in the literature. In an immunohistochemical study of 2 gonadoblastomas, expressions of WT1, p53, and MIS as well as inhibin were all demonstrated.

Virilizing manifestations occur occasionally in girls with **juvenile granulosa cell tumors.** Adrenal rests and hilum cell tumors rarely lead to virilization. Activating mutations of G-protein genes have been described in ovarian (and testicular) tumors. *GSα* mutations, usually seen in gonadal tumors associated with **McCune-Albright syndrome,** were also noted in 4 of 6 Leydig cell tumors (3 ovarian, 1 testicular). Two granulosa cell tumors and 1 thecoma of 10 ovarian tumors studied were found to have *GIP-2* mutations.

Sertoli-Leydig cell tumors, rare sex cord/stromal neoplasms, constitute less than 1% of ovarian tumors. The average age at diagnosis is 25 yr; less than 5% of these tumors occur before puberty. AFP levels may be mildly elevated. In one 12 mo old with Sertoli-Leydig cell tumor presenting with isosexual precocity the only detectable tumor marker was the serum inhibin level, with elevations in both A and B subunits. Five-year survival rates are 70-90%.

Of 102 consecutive patients who underwent surgery because of ovarian masses over a 15 yr period, the presenting symptoms were acute abdominal pain in 56% and abdominal or pelvic mass in 22%. Of 9 children whose cause for surgery was presumed malignancy, 3 had dysgerminomas, 2 had teratomas, 2 had juvenile granulosa cell tumors, 1 had a Sertoli-Leydig cell tumor, and 1 had a yolk sac tumor.

BIBLIOGRAPHY

Please visit the Nelson Textbook of Pediatrics *website at www.expertconsult.com for the complete bibliography.*

Chapter 582
Disorders of Sex Development

Patricia A. Donohoue

SEXUAL DIFFERENTIATION (CHAPTER 576)

In normal differentiation, the final form of all sexual structures is consistent with normal sex chromosomes (either XX or XY). A 46,XX complement of chromosomes as well as genetic factors such as DAX1 and the signaling molecule WNT-4 are necessary for the development of normal ovaries. Development of the male phenotype is even more complex. It requires a Y chromosome and, specifically, an intact *SRY* gene, which, in association with other genes such as *SOX9, SF1,* and *WT1* and others (Chapter 576), directs the undifferentiated gonad to become a testis. Aberrant recombinations may result in X chromosomes carrying *SRY,* resulting in XX males, or Y chromosomes that have lost *SRY,* resulting in XY females.

Antimüllerian hormone (AMH) causes the müllerian ducts to regress; in its absence, they persist as the uterus, fallopian tubes, cervix, and upper vagina. AMH activation in the testes may require the *SF1* gene for activation. By about 8 wk of gestation, the Leydig cells of the testis begin to produce testosterone. During this critical period of male differentiation, testosterone secretion is stimulated by placental human chorionic gonadotropin (hCG), which peaks at 8-12 wk. In the latter half of pregnancy, lower levels of testosterone are maintained by luteinizing hormone secreted by the fetal pituitary. Testosterone produced locally initiates virilization of the ipsilateral Wolffian duct into the epididymis, vas deferens, and seminal vesicle. Development of the external genitals also requires dihydrotestosterone (DHT), an active metabolite of testosterone. DHT produced from circulating testosterone is necessary to fuse the genital folds to form the penis and scrotum. A functional androgen receptor, produced by an X-linked gene, is required for testosterone and DHT to induce these virilizing changes.

In the XX fetus with normal long and short arms of the X chromosome, the bipotential gonad develops into an ovary by about the 10th-11th wk. This occurs only in the absence of *SRY,* testosterone, and AMH and requires a normal gene in the DSS locus DAX1, and the WNT-4 molecule. A female phenotype develops in the absence of fetal gonads. However, the male phenotype development requires androgen production and action. Estrogen is unnecessary for normal prenatal sexual differentiation, as demonstrated by 46,XX patients with aromatase deficiency and by mice without estradiol receptors.

Chromosomal aberrations may result in ambiguity of the external genitalia. Conditions of aberrant sex differentiation may also occur with the XX or XY genotype. The appropriate term for what was previously called *intersex* is **disorders of sex development (DSD).** This term defines a condition "in which development of chromosomal, gonadal or anatomical sex is atypical." It is becoming more preferable to use the term "atypical genitalia"

Table 582-1 REVISED NOMENCLATURE

PREVIOUS	CURRENTLY ACCEPTED
Intersex	Disorders of sex development (DSD)
Male pseudohermaphrodite	46,XY DSD
Undervirilization of an XY male	46,XY DSD
Undermasculinization of an XY male	46,XY DSD
46,XY intersex	46,XY DSD
Female pseudohermaphrodite	46,XX DSD
Overvirilization of an XX female	46,XX DSD
Masculinization of an XX female	46,XX DSD
46,XX intersex	46,XX DSD
True hermaphrodite	Ovotesticular DSD
Gonadal intersex	Ovotesticular DSD
XX male or XX sex reversal	46,XX testicular DSD
XY sex reversal	46,XY complete gonadal dysgenesis

From Lee PA, Houk CP, Ahmed SF, et al: Consensus statement on management of intersex disorders, *Pediatrics* 118:e488–e500, 2006.

rather than "ambiguous genitalia." Comparison with the previous terms and a new etiologic classification are seen in Tables 582-1 and 582-2. Some of the genes involved in disorders of sex development are listed in Table 576-1.

The definition of atypical or ambiguous genitalia, in a broad sense, is any case in which the external genitalia do not appear completely male or completely female. Although there are standards for genital size dimensions, variations in size of these structures do not always constitute ambiguity.

Development of the external genitalia begins with the potential to be either male or female (Fig. 582-1). Virilization of a female, the most common form of DSD, results in varying phenotypes (Fig. 582-2), which start from the basic genital appearances of the embryo (see Fig. 582-1).

DIAGNOSTIC APPROACH TO THE PATIENT WITH ATYPICAL OR AMBIGUOUS GENITALIA

The appearance of the external genitalia is rarely diagnostic of a particular disorder, and thus does not often allow distinction among the various forms of DSD. The most common forms of 46,XX DSD are virilizing forms of congenital adrenal hyperplasia (CAH). It is important to note that in 46,XY DSD, the specific diagnosis is not found in up to 50% of cases. At 1 center with a large experience, the etiologies of DSD in 250 patients over 25 yr were compiled. The 6 most common diagnoses accounted for 50% of the cases. These included virilizing CAH (14%), androgen insensitivity syndrome (10%), mixed gonadal dysgenesis (8%), clitoral/labial anomalies (7%), hypogonadotropic hypogonadism (6%), and 46,XY small-for-gestational age males with hypospadias (6%).

This potential source of error in diagnosis and management emphasizes the need for careful diagnostic evaluation including biochemical characterization of possible steroidogenic enzymatic defects in each patient with genital ambiguity. The parents need counseling about the complex nature of the baby's condition, and guidance as to how to deal with their well-meaning but curious friends and family members. The evaluation and management should be carried out by a multidisciplinary team of experts that include pediatric endocrinology, pediatric surgery/urology, pediatric radiology, newborn medicine, genetics, and psychology. Once the sex of rearing has been agreed on by the family and team, treatment can be organized. Genetic counseling should be offered when the specific diagnosis is established.

After a complete history and physical exam, the common diagnostic approach includes multiple steps, described in the following outline. These steps are usually performed simultaneously rather than waiting for results of 1 test prior to performing another, due to the sensitive and sometimes urgent nature of the condition. Careful attention to the presence of physical features other than the genitalia is crucial, to determine if a diagnosis of a particular multisystem syndrome is possible. These are described in more detail in Chapters 582.1, 582.2, and 582.3. A summary of many features of commonly encountered causes of DSD is provided in Table 582-3.

Table 582-2 ETIOLOGIC CLASSIFICATION OF DISORDERS OF SEX DEVELOPMENT (DSD)

46,XX-DSD **Androgen Exposure**
Fetal/Fetoplacental Source 21-Hydroxylase (P450c21 or CYP21) deficiency 11β-Hydroxylase (P450c11 or CYP11B1) deficiency 3β-Hydroxysteroid dehydrogenase II (3β-HSD II) deficiency Cytochrome P450 oxidoreductase (POR) Aromatase (P450arom or CYP19) deficiency Glucocorticoid receptor gene mutation *Maternal Source* Virilizing ovarian tumor Virilizing adrenal tumor Androgenic drugs
Disorder of Ovarian Development
XX gonadal dysgenesis Testicular DSD (SRY+, SOX9 Duplication)
Undetermined Origin
Associated with genitourinary and gastrointestinal tract defects
46,XY DSD **Defects in Testicular Development**
Denys-Drash syndrome (mutation in *WT1* gene) WAGR syndrome (Wilms tumor, aniridia, genitourinary malformation, retardation) Deletion of 11p13 Campomelic syndrome (autosomal gene at 17q24.3-q25.1) and SOX9 mutation XY pure gonadal dysgenesis (Swyer syndrome) Mutation in SRY gene XY gonadal agenesis Unknown cause
Deficiency of Testicular Hormones
Leydig cell aplasia Mutation in LH receptor Lipoid adrenal hyperplasia (P450scc or CYP11A1) deficiency; mutation in StAR (steroidogenic acute regulatory protein) 3β-HSD II deficiency 17-Hydroxylase/17,20-lyase (P450c17 or CYP17) deficiency Persistent müllerian duct syndrome due to antimüllerian hormone gene mutations, or receptor defects for antimüllerian hormone
Defect in Androgen Action
5α-Reductase II mutations Androgen receptor defects: Complete androgen insensitivity syndrome Partial androgen insensitivity syndrome (Reifenstein and other syndromes) Smith-Lemli-Opitz syndrome (defect in conversion of 7-dehydrocholesterol to cholesterol, DHCR7)
Ovotesticular DSD
XX XY XX/XY chimeras
Sex Chromosome DSD
45,X (Turner syndrome and variants) 47,XXY (Klinefelter syndrome and variants) 45,X/46,XY (mixed gonadal dysgenesis, sometimes a cause of ovotesticular DSD) 46,XX/46,XY (chimeric, sometimes a cause of ovotesticular DSD)

From Lee PA, Houk CP, Ahmed SF, et al: Consensus statement on management of intersex disorders, *Pediatrics* 118:e488–e500, 2006.

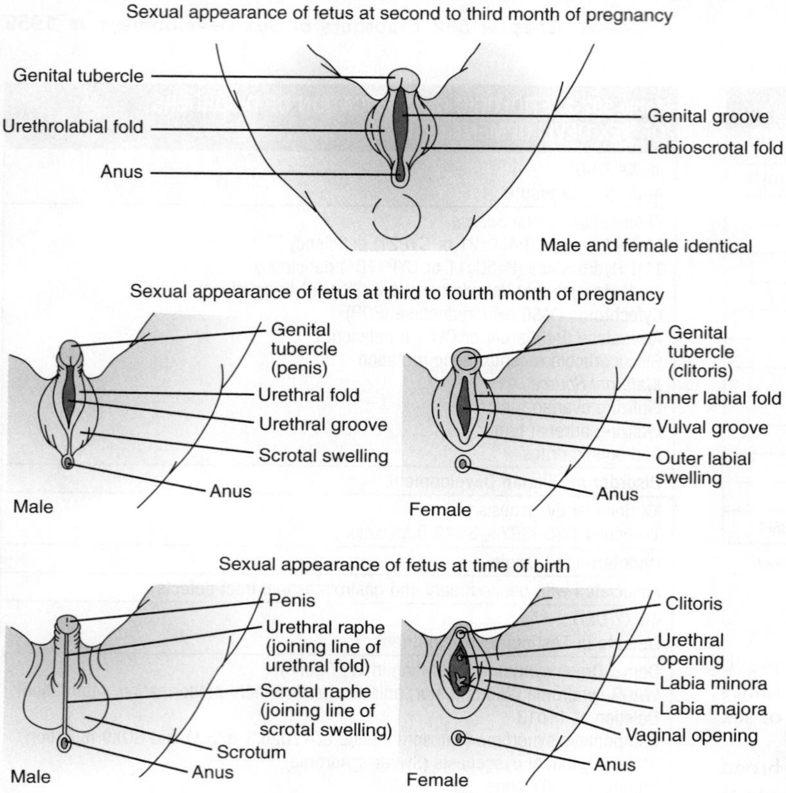

Figure 582-1 Schematic demonstration of differentiation of normal male and female genitalia during embryogenesis. (From Zitelli BJ, Davis HW: *Atlas of pediatric physical diagnosis,* ed 4, St Louis, 2002, Mosby, p 328.)

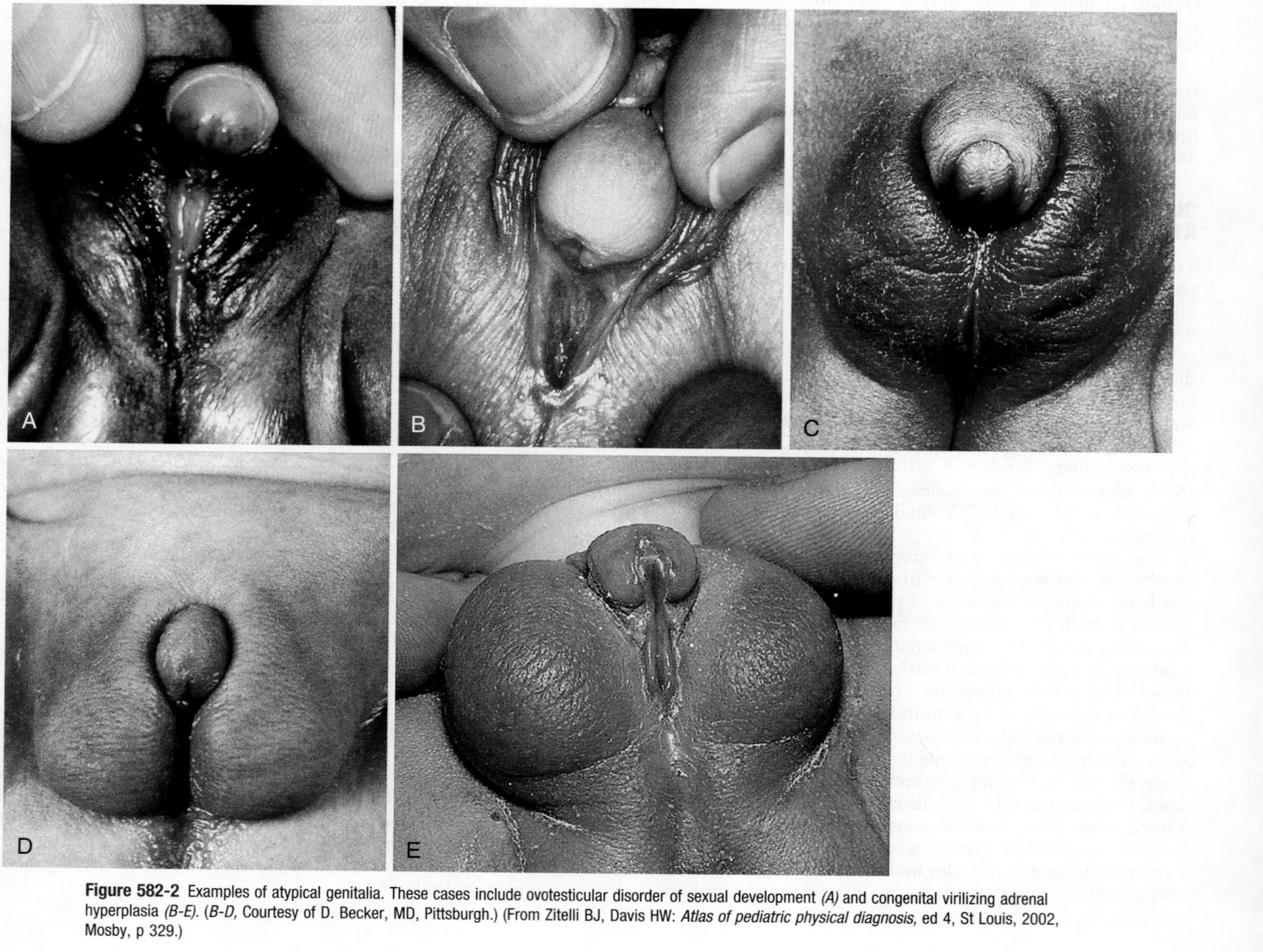

Figure 582-2 Examples of atypical genitalia. These cases include ovotesticular disorder of sexual development *(A)* and congenital virilizing adrenal hyperplasia *(B-E)*. (*B-D,* Courtesy of D. Becker, MD, Pittsburgh.) (From Zitelli BJ, Davis HW: *Atlas of pediatric physical diagnosis,* ed 4, St Louis, 2002, Mosby, p 329.)

Table 582-3 AMBIGUOUS GENITALIA: STEPS IN ESTABLISHING THE DIAGNOSIS

	21-OH DEFICIENCY*	GONADAL DYSGENESIS WITH Y CHROMOSOME	OVOTESTICULAR DSD	PARTIAL ANDROGEN INSENSITIVITY	BLOCK IN TESTOSTERONE SYNTHESIS
CLINICAL FEATURE					
Palpable gonad(s)	–	+/–	+/–	+	+
Uterus present†	+	+	Usually	–	–
Increased skin pigmentation	+/–	–	–	–	–
Sick baby	+/–	–	–	–	+/–
Dysmorphic features	–	+/–	–	–	–
DIAGNOSTIC CONSIDERATIONS					
Serum 17OHP	Elevated	Normal	Normal	Normal	Normal
Electrolytes	Possibly abnormal	Normal	Normal	Normal	Possibly abnormal
Karyotype	46,XX	45,X/46,XY or others	46,XX	46,XY	46,XY
Testosterone response to hCG	NA	Positive	Normal or reduced	Positive response	Reduced or absent
Gonadal biopsy	NA	Dysgenetic gonad	Ovotestis	Normal testis with +/–Leydig cell hyperplasia	Normal testis
Other testing				Genital skin fibroblast culture For AR‡ assay Or DNA screening for AR mutations in blood cells	Measure Testosterone Precursors

*21-Hydroxylase.
†As determined by ultrasound or rectal examination.
‡Androgen receptor.
NA, not applicable.
Adapted from Donohoue PA, Saenger PH: Ambiguous genitalia. In Finberg L, Kleinman RE, editors: *Saunders manual of pediatric practice*, Philadelphia, 2002, WB Saunders, p 874.

Diagnostic tests include the following:

1. Karyotype, with **rapid determination of sex chromosomes** (in many centers this is available within 24-48 hours)
2. Other blood tests
   a. Screen for congenital adrenal hyperplasia: cortisol biosynthetic precursors and adrenal androgens (particularly 17-hydroxyprogesterone and androstenedione for 21-hydroxylase deficiency, the most common form)
   b. Screen for androgens and their biosynthetic precursors
   c. Screen for gonadal response to gonadotropin in patients suspected of having testicular gonads: stimulation with injections of HCG; measure testosterone and dihydrotestosterone before and after HCG
   d. Molecular genetic analyses for SRY (sex-determining region of the Y chromosome) and other Y-specific loci
   e. Gonadotropin levels
3. The internal anatomy of patients with ambiguous genitalia can be defined with 1 or more of the following imaging studies:
   a. Voiding cystourethrogram (VCUG)
   b. Endoscopic examination of the genitourinary tract
   c. Pelvic ultrasound; renal and adrenal ultrasound
   d. Pelvic CT or MRI if needed

BIBLIOGRAPHY
Please visit the Nelson Textbook of Pediatrics *website at www.expertconsult.com for the complete bibliography.*

582.1 46,XX DSD

Patricia A. Donohoue

In this condition, the genotype is XX and the gonads are ovaries, but the external genitalia are virilized. Because there is no significant AMH production—the gonads are ovaries—the uterus, fallopian tubes, and cervix develop. The varieties and causes of this condition are relatively few. Most instances result from exposure of the female fetus to excessive exogenous or endogenous androgens during intrauterine life. The changes consist principally of virilization of the external genitalia (clitoral hypertrophy and labioscrotal fusion).

CONGENITAL ADRENAL HYPERPLASIA (CHAPTER 570.1)

This is the most common cause of genital ambiguity and of 46,XX DSD. Females with the 21-hydroxylase and 11-hydroxylase defects are the most highly virilized, although minimal virilization also occurs with the type II 3β-hydroxysteroid dehydrogenase defect (see Fig. 582-1). Salt losers tend to have greater degrees of virilization than do non–salt-losing patients. Masculinization may be so intense that a complete penile urethra results, and the condition may mimic a male with bilateral cryptorchidism.

AROMATASE DEFICIENCY

In genotypic females, the rare condition of aromatase deficiency during fetal life leads to 46,XX DSD and results in hypergonadotropic hypogonadism at puberty because of ovarian failure to synthesize estrogen (see Fig. 568-1).

Two 46,XX infants had enlargement of the clitoris and posterior labial fusion at birth. In 1 instance, maternal serum and urinary levels of estrogen were very low and serum levels of androgens were high. Cord serum levels of estrogen were also extremely low, but those of androgen were elevated. The 2nd patient also had virilization of unknown cause since birth, but the aromatase deficiency was not diagnosed until 14 yr of age, when she had further virilization and failed to go into puberty. At that time, she had elevated levels of gonadotropins and androgens but low estrogen levels, and ultrasonography revealed large ovarian cysts bilaterally. These 2 patients demonstrate the important role of aromatase in the conversion of androgens to estrogens. Additional female and male patients with aromatase deficiency due to mutations in the $P450_{arom}$ *(CYP19)* gene are known. Two siblings were described. The 28 yr old XY proband was 177.6 cm tall (+2.5 SD) after having received hormonal replacement therapy; her 24 yr old brother was 204 cm tall (+3.7 SD), and had a bone age of 14 yr. Low-dose estradiol replacement, carefully adjusted to maintain normal age-appropriate levels, may be indicated for affected females even prepubertally.

GLUCOCORTICOID RECEPTOR GENE MUTATION

A 9 yr old girl with 46,XX disorder of sexual development, thought to be due to 21-hydroxylase deficiency (congenital adrenal hyperplasia) since the age of 5 yr, had elevated cortisol levels both at baseline and after dexamethasone, hypertension, and hypokalemia, suggestive of the diagnosis of generalized glucocorticoid resistance. A novel homozygous mutation in exon 5 of the glucocorticoid receptor was demonstrated. In this Brazilian family, the condition was autosomal recessive.

POR, cytochrome P450 oxidoreductase, encoded by a gene on 7q11.2, is a cofactor implicated in combined P450C17 and P450C21 steroidogenic defects. Girls are born with ambiguous genitalia, but the virilization does not progress postnatally and androgen levels are normal or low. Boys may be born undervirilized. Both may exhibit bony abnormalities seen in **Antley-Bixler syndrome** (ABS). Conversely, in a series of ABS patients, those with ambiguous genitalia and disordered steroidogenesis had POR deficiency. Those without genital ambiguity with normal steroidogenesis had fibroblast growth factor receptor 2 *(FGFR2)* mutations. The cardinal features of ABS include craniosynostosis, severe midface hypoplasia, proptosis, choanal atresia/stenosis, frontal bossing, dysplastic ears, depressed nasal bridge, radiohumeral synostosis, long bone fractures and femoral bowing, and urogenital abnormalities.

VIRILIZING MATERNAL TUMORS

Rarely, the female fetus has been virilized during fetal life by a maternal androgen-producing tumor. In a few cases, the lesion was a benign adrenal adenoma, but all others were ovarian tumors, particularly androblastomas, luteomas, and Krukenberg tumors. **Maternal virilization** may be manifested by enlargement of the clitoris, acne, deepening of the voice, decreased lactation, hirsutism, and elevated levels of androgens. In the infant, there is enlargement of the clitoris of varying degrees, often with labial fusion. Mothers of children with unexplained 46,XX DSD should undergo physical examination and measurements of their own levels of plasma testosterone, dehydroepiandrosterone sulfate, and androstenedione.

ADMINISTRATION OF ANDROGENIC DRUGS TO WOMEN DURING PREGNANCY

Testosterone and 17-methyltestosterone have been reported to cause 46,XX DSD in some instances. The greatest number of cases has resulted from the use of certain progestational compounds for the treatment of threatened abortion. These progestins have been replaced by nonvirilizing ones.

Infants with virilization and 46,XX chromosomes and caudal anomalies have been reported for whom no virilizing agent could be identified. In such instances, the disorder is usually associated with other congenital defects, particularly of the urinary and gastrointestinal tracts. Y-specific DNA sequences, including SRY, are absent. In 1 case, a scrotal raphe and elevated testosterone levels were found, but the cause remains unknown.

BIBLIOGRAPHY

Please visit the Nelson Textbook of Pediatrics *website at* *www.expertconsult.com* *for the complete bibliography.*

582.2 46,XY DSD

Patricia A. Donohoue

In this condition, the genotype is XY, but the external genitalia are either not completely virilized, ambiguous (atypical), or completely female. When gonads can be found, they invariably contain testicular elements; their development ranges from rudimentary to normal. Because the process of normal virilization in the fetus is so complex, it is not surprising that there are many varieties and causes of 46,XY DSD.

DEFECTS IN TESTICULAR DIFFERENTIATION

The 1st step in male differentiation is conversion of the indifferent gonad into a testis. In the XY fetus, if there is a deletion of the short arm of the Y chromosome or of the *SRY* gene, male differentiation does not occur. The phenotype is female; müllerian ducts are well developed because of the absence of AMH, but gonads consist of undifferentiated streaks. By contrast, even extreme deletions of the long arm of the Y chromosome (Yq-) have been found in normally developed males, most of whom are azoospermic and have short stature. This indicates that the long arm of the Y chromosome normally has genes that prevent these manifestations. In many syndromes in which the testes fail to differentiate, Y chromosomes are morphologically normal.

Denys-Drash Syndrome

The constellation of nephropathy with ambiguous genitalia and **bilateral Wilms tumor** are the major characteristics of this syndrome. Most reported cases have been 46,XY. Müllerian ducts are often present, indicating a global deficiency of fetal testicular function. Patients with a 46,XX karyotype have normal external genitals. The onset of proteinuria in infancy progresses to **nephrotic syndrome** and end-stage renal failure by 3 yr of age, with focal or diffuse mesangial sclerosis being the most consistent histopathologic finding. Wilms tumor usually develops in children younger than 2 yr of age and is frequently bilateral. Gonadoblastomas have also been reported.

Several mutations of the Wilms tumor gene *(WT1),* located on chromosome 11p13, have been found. *WT1* functions as a tumor suppressor gene and a transcriptional factor, and is expressed in the genital ridge and fetal gonads. Nearly all reported mutations have been near or within the zinc finger–coding region. One report found a zinc finger domain mutation in the *WT1* alleles of a patient with no genitourinary abnormalities, suggesting that some cases of sporadic Wilms tumor may carry the *WT1* mutation. Different mutations of the *WT1* gene, constitutional heterozygote mutations at intron 9, have been described in **Fraser syndrome,** a condition of nonspecific focal and segmental glomerulosclerosis, 46,XY gonadal dysgenesis, and frequent gonadoblastoma, but **without** Wilms tumor.

WAGR Syndrome

This acronymic contiguous gene syndrome consists of Wilms tumor, aniridia, genitourinary malformations, and retardation. These children have a deletion of 1 copy of chromosome 11p13, which may be visible on karyotype analysis. The deleted region encompasses the aniridia gene *(PAX6)* and the Wilms tumor suppressor gene *(WT1).* Only the 46,XY males have genital abnormalities, ranging from cryptorchidism to severe deficiency of virilization. Gonadoblastomas have developed in the dysgenetic gonads. Wilms tumor usually occurs by 2 yr of age. Some cases also had unexplained obesity, raising the question of an obesity-associated gene in this region of chromosome 11 and naming the syndrome WAGRO.

Campomelic Syndrome (Chapter 695)

This form of **short-limbed dysplasia** is characterized by anterior bowing of the femur and tibia, small, bladeless scapulae, small thoracic cavities and 11 pairs of ribs, along with malformations of other organs. It is usually lethal in early infancy. About 75% of reported 46,XY patients exhibit a completely **female phenotype;** the external and internal genitalia are female. Some 46,XY patients have ambiguous genitals. The gonads appear to be ovaries but histologically may contain elements of both ovaries and testes.

The gene responsible for the condition is *SOX9* (SRY-related HMG-box gene) and is on 17q24-q25. This gene is structurally related to *SRY* and also directly regulates the type II collagen gene *(COL2A1)* development. The same mutations may result in different gonadal phenotypes. Gonadoblastoma was reported in a patient with this condition. The inheritance is autosomal dominant. Adrenal insufficiency and 46,XY gonadal dysgenesis has been described in patients with mutations of the *SF1* gene. In some of these patients, if the mother shares the *SF1* mutation she has premature ovarian insufficiency.

46,XY sex reversal has been described in patients with deletions of parts of autosomal loci on chromosomes 2q, 9p, and 10q.

XY Pure Gonadal Dysgenesis (Swyer Syndrome)

The designation "pure" distinguishes this condition from forms of gonadal dysgenesis that are of chromosomal origin and associated with somatic anomalies. Affected patients have normal stature and a **female phenotype,** including vagina, uterus, and fallopian tubes, but at pubertal age, breast development and menarche fail to occur. None of the defects associated with 45,X children is present. Patients present at puberty with hypergonadotropic primary amenorrhea. Familial cases suggest an X-linked or a sex-limited dominant autosomal transmission. Most of the patients examined have had mutations of the *SRY* gene. None had a *SOX9* gene mutation. The gonads consist of almost totally undifferentiated streaks despite the presence of a cytogenetically normal Y chromosome. The primitive gonad cannot accomplish any testicular function, including suppression of müllerian ducts. There may be hilar cells in the gonad capable of producing some androgens; accordingly, some virilization, such as clitoral enlargement, may occur at the age of puberty. The streak gonads may undergo neoplastic changes, such as gonadoblastomas and dysgerminomas, and should be removed shortly after diagnosis, regardless of age.

Pure gonadal dysgenesis also occurs in XX individuals (Chapter 580).

XY Gonadal Agenesis Syndrome (Embryonic Testicular Regression Syndrome)

In this rare syndrome, the external genitalia are slightly ambiguous but more nearly **female.** Hypoplasia of the labia; some degree of labioscrotal fusion; a small, clitoris-like phallus; and a perineal urethral opening are present. No uterus, no gonadal tissue, and usually no vagina can be found. At the age of puberty, no sexual development occurs and gonadotropin levels are elevated. Most children have been reared as females. In several patients with XY gonadal agenesis in whom no gonads could be found on exploration, significant rises in testosterone followed stimulation with hCG, indicating Leydig cell function somewhere. Siblings with the disorder are known.

It is presumed that testicular tissue was active long enough during fetal life for AMH to inhibit development of müllerian ducts but not long enough for testosterone production to result in virilization. In 1 patient, no deletion of the Y chromosome was found by means of Y-specific DNA probes. Testicular degeneration seems to occur between the 8th and the 12th fetal wk. Regression of the testis before the 8th wk of gestation results in Swyer syndrome; between the 14th and the 20th wk of gestation, it results in the rudimentary testis syndrome; and after the 20th wk, it results in anorchia.

In **bilateral anorchia,** testes are absent, but the **male phenotype** is complete; it is presumed that tissue with fetal testicular function was active during the critical period of genital differentiation but that sometime later it was damaged. Bilateral anorchia in identical twins and unilateral anorchia in identical twins and in siblings suggest a genetic predisposition. Coexistence of anorchia and the gonadal agenesis syndrome in a sibship is evidence for a relationship between the disorders. *SRY* defects have not yet been reported for patients with anorchia.

A retrospective review of urologic explorations revealed absent testes in 21% of 691 testes. Of those, 73% had blind-ending cord structures with the suggested site of the vanishing testes being the inguinal canal (59%), the abdomen (21%), superficial inguinal ring (18%), and scrotum (2%). It was suggested that the presence of cord structures on laparoscopy should prompt inguinal exploration because viable testicular tissue was found in 4 of these children. No hormonal data (hCG stimulation tests, AMH levels) were reported.

This condition is sometimes referred to as *vanishing testes syndrome*.

DEFECTS IN TESTICULAR HORMONES

Five genetic defects have been delineated in the enzymatic synthesis of testosterone by fetal testis, and a defect in Leydig cell differentiation has been described. These defects produce 46,XY males with inadequate masculinization (see Fig. 576-1). Because levels of testosterone are normally low before puberty, an hCG stimulation test may be needed in children to assess the ability of the testes to synthesize testosterone.

Leydig Cell Aplasia

Patients with aplasia or hypoplasia of the Leydig cells usually have **female phenotypes,** but there may be mild virilization. Testes, epididymis, and vas deferens are present; the uterus and fallopian tubes are absent due to normal production of MIS. There are no secondary sexual changes at puberty; but pubic hair may be normal. Plasma levels of testosterone are low and do not respond to hCG; luteinizing hormone (LH) levels are elevated. The Leydig cells of the testes are absent or markedly deficient. The defect may involve a lack of receptors for LH. In children, hCG stimulation is necessary to differentiate the condition from the androgen insensitivity syndromes (AISs). There is male-limited autosomal recessive inheritance. The human LH receptor is a member of the G-protein–coupled superfamily of receptors that contains 7 transmembrane domains. Several inactivating mutations of the LH receptor have been described in males with hypogonadism suspected of having Leydig cell hypoplasia or aplasia.

High serum LH and low follicle-stimulating hormone (FSH) were noted in 1 male with hypogonadism owing to a mutation in the gene for the β subunit of FSH (see Table 577-1).

Lipoid Adrenal Hyperplasia (Chapter 570)

The most severe form of congenital adrenal hyperplasia derives its name from the appearance of the enlarged adrenal glands resulting from accumulation of cholesterol and cholesterol esters. The rate-limiting process in steroidogenesis is the transport of free cholesterol through the cytosol to the inner mitochondrial membrane, where P450SCC (CYP11A1) acts. Cholesterol transport into mitochondria is mediated by the steroidogenetic acute regulatory protein (StAR) whose synthesis occurs via cAMP through a cyclic AMP response element–binding protein (CREB). StAR is a 30 kDa protein essential for steroidogenesis and is encoded by a gene on chromosome 8p11.2. The mitochondrial content of StAR increases between 1 and 5 hr after ACTH stimulation, long after the acute ACTH-induced increase in steroidogenesis. This has led some to suggest that extramitochondrial StAR might also be involved in the acute response to ACTH.

All serum steroid levels are low or undetectable, whereas corticotropin and plasma renin levels are quite elevated. The phenotype is female in both genetic females and males. Genetic males have no müllerian structures because the testes can produce normal AMH but no steroid hormones. These children present with acute adrenal crisis and salt wasting in infancy. Most patients are 46,XY. In a few patients, ovarian steroidogenesis is present at puberty.

The regulatory role of StAR-independent steroidogenesis is illustrated by 46,XX 4 mo old twins with lipoid adrenal hyperplasia. One died at 15 mo because of cardiac complications related to coarctation of the aorta. The adrenal glands had characteristic lipid deposits. The surviving twin had spontaneous puberty with feminization at 11.5 yr and menarche at 13.8 yr. When restudied at the age of 15 yr, a homozygous frameshift-inactivating mutation in her StAR gene was discovered. This and the fact that she survived as an infant until 4 mo of age without replacement therapy with detectable serum aldosterone levels supports the hypothesis that StAR-independent steroidogenesis was able to proceed until enough intracellular lipid accumulated to destroy steroidogenic activity. Partial defects in only partially virilized males and delayed onset of salt wasting have been described. Complete P450scc defects may be incompatible with life because only this enzyme can convert cholesterol to pregnenolone, which then becomes progesterone, a hormone essential for the maintenance of normal mammalian pregnancy. Heterozygous mutation in P450scc was described in a 4 yr old with 46,XY sex reversal and late-onset form of lipoid adrenal hyperplasia. At 6-7 wk of gestation, when maternal corpus luteum progesterone synthesis stops, the placenta, which does not express StAR, produces progesterone by StAR-independent steroidogenesis using the P450scc enzyme system.

3β-Hydroxysteroid Dehydrogenase Deficiency

Males with this form of congenital adrenal hyperplasia (Chapter 570) have various degrees of **hypospadias,** with or without bifid scrotum and cryptorchidism and, rarely, a complete female phenotype. Affected infants usually develop salt-losing manifestations shortly after birth. Incomplete defects, occasionally seen in boys with premature pubarche, as well as late-onset nonclassic forms have been reported. These children have point mutations of the gene for type II 3β-hydroxysteroid enzyme, resulting in impairment of steroidogenesis in the adrenals and gonads; the impairment may be unequal between adrenals and gonads. Normal pubertal changes in some boys could be explained by the normally present type I 3β-hydroxysteroid dehydrogenase present in many peripheral tissues. Infertility is frequent. There is no correlation between degree of salt wasting and degree of phenotypic abnormality.

Deficiency of 17-Hydroxylase/17,20 Lyase

A single enzyme (P450C17 or CYP17) encoded by a single gene on chromosome 10q24.3 has both 17-hydroxylase and 17,20 lyase activities in adrenal and gonadal tissues (Chapter 570). Many different genetic lesions have been reported. Genetic males usually have a complete female phenotype or, less often, various degrees of undervirilization from labioscrotal fusion to perineal hypospadias and cryptorchidism. Pubertal development fails to occur in both genetic sexes.

In the classical disorder, there is decreased synthesis of cortisol by the adrenals and of sex steroids by the adrenals and gonads. Levels of deoxycorticosterone (DOC) and corticosterone are markedly increased and lead to the hypertension and hypokalemia characteristic of this form of male DSD. Although levels of cortisol are low, the elevated corticotropin and corticosterone levels maintain a eucorticoid state. The renin-aldosterone axis is suppressed because of the strong mineralocorticoid effect of elevated DOC. Virilization does not occur at puberty; levels of testosterone are low, and those of gonadotropins are increased. Because fetal production of AMH is normal, no müllerian duct remnants are present. In phenotypic XY females, gonadectomy and replacement therapy with hydrocortisone and sex steroids are indicated.

The defect follows autosomal recessive inheritance. Affected XX females are usually not detected until young adult life, when they fail to experience normal pubertal changes and are found to have hypertension and hypokalemia. This condition should be suspected in patients presenting with primary amenorrhea and hypertension whose chromosomal complement is either 46,XX or 46,XY.

Deficiency of 17-Ketosteroid Reductase

This enzyme, also called *17β-hydroxysteroid dehydrogenase* (17β-HSD), catalizes the final step in testosterone biosynthesis. It is necessary to convert androstenedione to testosterone and also dehydroepiandrosterone to androstenediol and estrone to estradiol. Enzymatic defects in the fetal testis give rise to males with complete or near-complete female phenotype in 46,XY males. Müllerian ducts are absent, and a shallow vagina is present. The diagnosis is based on the ratio of androstenedione to testosterone; in prepubertal children, stimulation with hCG may be necessary to make the diagnosis.

The defect is inherited in an autosomal recessive fashion. At least 4 different types of 17β-HSD are recognized, each coded by a different gene or different chromosomes. Type III is the enzyme defect that is especially common in a highly inbred Arab population in Gaza. The gene for the disorder is at 9q22 and is expressed only in the testes, where it converts androstenedione to testosterone. Most patients are diagnosed at puberty because of the failure to menstruate and of virilization. Testosterone levels at puberty may approach normal, presumably as a result of peripheral conversion of androstenedione to testosterone; at this time, some patients spontaneously adopt a male gender role.

Type I 17β-HSD, encoded by a gene on chromosome 17q21, converts estrone to estradiol and is found in placenta, ovary, testis, liver, prostate, adipose tissue, and endometrium. Type II, whose gene is on chromosome 16q24, has activities that are opposite to those of types I and III (convert testosterone to androstenedione and estrone to estradiol). Type IV is similar in action to type II. A late-onset form of 17-ketosteroid reductase deficiency presents as gynecomastia in young adult males.

Persistent Müllerian Duct Syndrome

In this disorder, there is persistence of müllerian duct derivatives in otherwise completely virilized males. Cases have been reported in siblings and identical twins. **Cryptorchidism** is present in 80% of affected males; and during surgery for this or inguinal hernia, the condition is uncovered when a fallopian tube and uterus are found. The degree of müllerian development is variable and may be asymmetric. Testicular function is normal in most, but testicular degeneration has been reported. Some affected males acquire testicular tumors after puberty. In a study of 38 families, 16 families had defects in the AMH gene, located on the short arm of chromosome 19. They had low AMH levels. In 16 families with high AMH levels, the defect was in the AMH type II receptor gene, with 10/16 having identical 27-bp deletions on exon 10 in at least 1 allele.

Treatment consists of removal of as many of the müllerian structures as possible without causing damage to the testis, epididymis, or vas deferens.

DEFECTS IN ANDROGEN ACTION

In the following group of disorders, fetal synthesis of testosterone is normal and defective virilization results from inherited abnormalities in androgen action.

5α-Reductase Deficiency

Decreased production of dihydrotestosterone (DHT) in utero results in marked ambiguity of external genitalia of affected

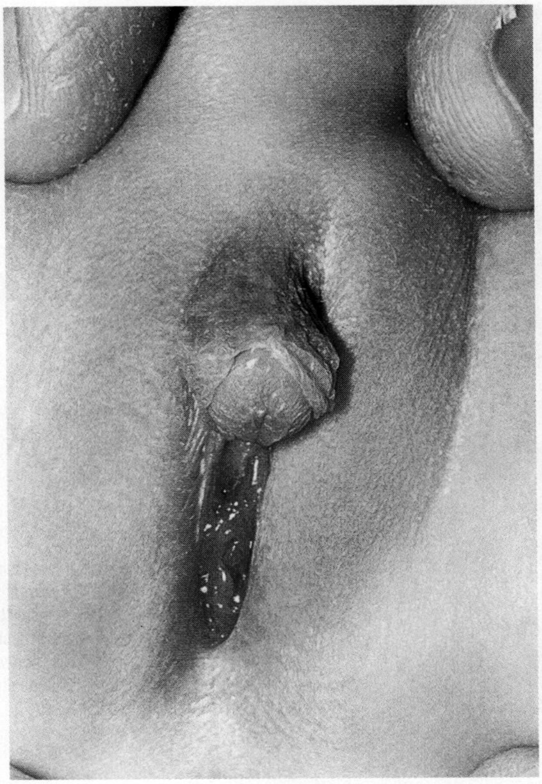

Figure 582-3 5α-Reductase deficiency. (From Wales JKH, Wit JM, Rogol AD: *Pediatric endocrinology and growth,* ed 2, Philadelphia, 2003, Elsevier/Saunders, p 165.)

males. Biosynthesis and peripheral action of testosterone are normal.

The phenotype most commonly associated with this condition results in boys who have a small phallus, bifid scrotum, urogenital sinus with perineal hypospadias, and a blind vaginal pouch (Fig. 582-3). Testes are in the inguinal canals or labioscrotal folds and are normal histologically. There are no müllerian structures. Wolffian structures—the vas deferens, epididymis, and seminal vesicles—are present. Most affected patients have been identified as females. At puberty, virilization occurs; the phallus enlarges, the testes descend and grow normally, and spermatogenesis occurs. There is no gynecomastia. Beard growth is scanty, acne is absent, the prostate is small, and recession of the temporal hairline fails to occur. Virilization of the Wolffian duct is caused by the action of testosterone itself, although masculinization of the urogenital sinus and external genitals depends on the action of DHT during the critical period of fetal masculinization. Growth of facial hair and of the prostate also appears to be DHT dependent.

The adult height reached is close to that of the father and other male siblings. There is significant phenotypic heterogeneity. This has led to a classification of such patients into 5 types of steroid 5α-reductase deficiency (SRD).

Several different gene defects leading to SRD have been identified in the 5α-reductase type 2 gene, located on the short arm of chromosome 2, in patients from throughout the world. Familial clusters have been reported from the Dominican Republic, Turkey, Papua New Guinea, Brazil, Mexico, and the Middle East. There is no reliable correlation between genotype and phenotype.

The disorder is inherited as an autosomal recessive trait but is limited to males; normal homozygous females with normal fertility indicate that in females DHT has no role in sexual differentiation or in ovarian function later in life. The clinical diagnosis should be made as early as possible in infancy. It is important to distinguish this from partial androgen insensitivity syndrome (PAIS), as patients with PAIS are far less sensitive to androgen than are patients with SRD. The biochemical diagnosis of SRD is based on finding normal serum testosterone levels, normal or low DHT levels with markedly increased basal and especially hCG-stimulated testosterone : DHT ratios (>17), and high ratios of urinary etiocholanolone to androsterone. Children with androgen insensitivity have normal hepatic 5α reduction and, thus, a normal ratio of tetrahydrocortisol to 5α-tetrahydrocortisol, as opposed to those with SRD.

It is important to note that most but not all children with SRD reared as females in childhood have changed to male around the time of puberty. It appears that exposures to testosterone in utero, neonatally, and at puberty have variable contributions to the formation of male gender identity. Much more needs to be learned about the influences of hormones such as androgens as well as the influences of cultural, social, psychologic, genetic, and other biologic factors in gender identity and behavior. Infants with this condition should be reared as boys whenever practical. Treatment of male infants with DHT results in phallic enlargement.

Androgen Insensitivity Syndromes

The AISs are the most common forms of male DSD, occurring with an estimated frequency of 1/20,000 genetic males. This group of heterogeneous X-linked recessive disorders is due to more than 150 different mutations in the androgen receptor gene, located on Xq11-12: single point mutations resulting in amino acid substitutions or premature stop codons, frameshift and premature terminations, gene deletions, and splice site mutations.

CLINICAL MANIFESTATIONS The clinical spectrum of patients with AISs, all of whom have a 46,XY chromosomal complement, range from phenotypic females (in complete AIS) to males with various forms of ambiguous genitalia and undervirilization (partial AIS, or clinical syndromes such as **Reifenstein syndrome**) to phenotypically normal-appearing males with infertility. In addition to normal 46,XY chromosomes, the presence of testes and normal or elevated testosterone and LH levels are common to all such children (Figs. 582-4 and 582-5).

In **complete AIS,** an extreme form of failure of virilization, genetic males appear female at birth and are invariably reared accordingly. The external genitalia are female. The vagina ends blindly in a pouch, and the uterus is absent due to the normal production and effect of AMH by the testes. In about one third of patients, unilateral or bilateral fallopian tube remnants are found. The testes are usually intra-abdominal but may descend into the inguinal canal; they consist largely of seminiferous tubules. At puberty, there is normal development of breasts, and the habitus is female, but menstruation does not occur and sexual hair is absent. Adult heights of these women are commensurate with those of normal males despite profound congenital deficiency of androgenic effects.

The testes of affected adult patients produce normal male levels of testosterone and DHT. Failure of normal male differentiation during fetal life reflects defective response to androgens at that time. The absence of androgenic effects is caused by a striking resistance to the action of endogenous or exogenous testosterone at the cellular level.

Prepubertal children with this disorder are often detected when inguinal masses prove to be testes or when a testis is unexpectedly found during herniorrhaphy in a phenotypic female. About 1-2% of girls with an inguinal hernia prove to have this disorder. In infants, elevated gonadotropin levels should suggest the diagnosis. In adults, **amenorrhea** is the usual presenting symptom. In prepubertal children, the condition must be differentiated from other types of XY under virilized males in which there is complete feminization. These include XY gonadal dysgenesis (Swyer syndrome), true agonadism, Leydig cell aplasia including LH receptor defects, and 17-ketosteroid reductase deficiency; all these conditions, unlike complete AIS, are

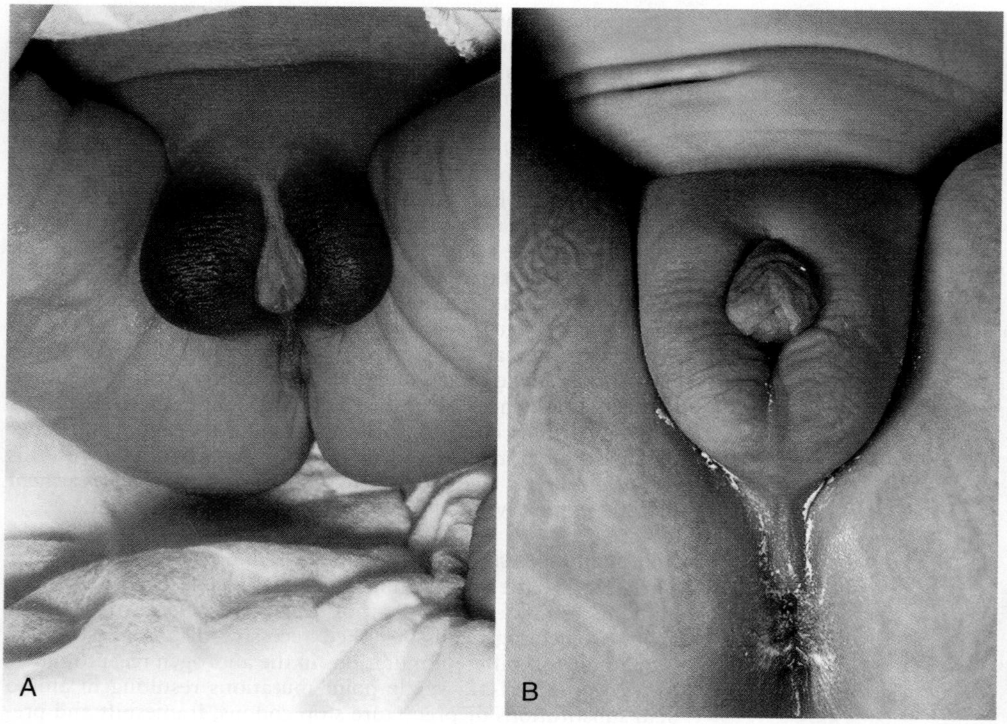

Figure 582-4 *A,* Partial androgen insensitivity with descended testes in bifid labioscrotal folds. *B,* Less severe partial androgen insensitivity with severe hypospadias and maldescent of testes. (From Wales JKH, Wit JM, Rogol AD: *Pediatric endocrinology and growth,* ed 2, Philadelphia, 2003, Elsevier/Saunders, p 165.)

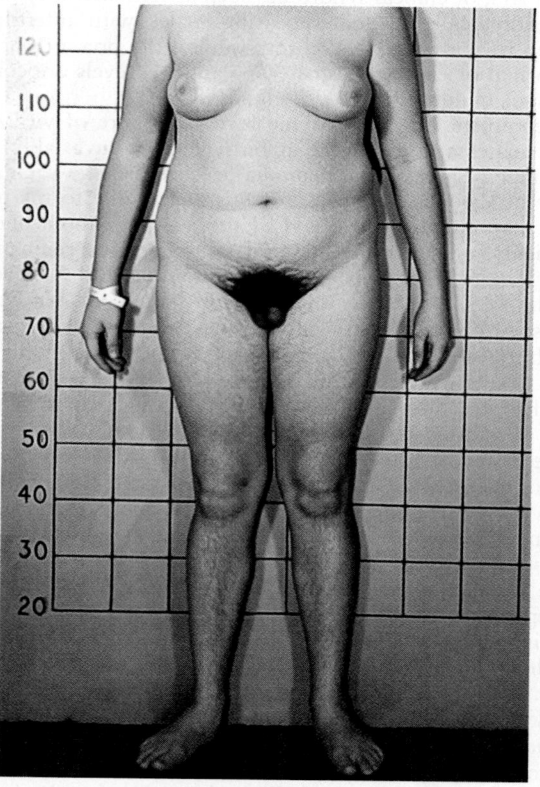

Figure 582-5 Partial androgen insensitivity syndrome at adolescence, male sex of rearing. Note gynecomastia from peripheral aromatase conversion of testosterone to estrogen. Abundant pubic hair implies only partial resistance. (From Wales JKH, Wit JM, Rogol AD: *Pediatric endocrinology and growth,* ed 2, 2003, Philadelphia, Elsevier/Saunders, p 165.)

characterized by **low levels of testosterone** as neonates and during adult life and by failure to respond to hCG during the prepubertal years. Although patients with complete AIS have unambiguously female external genitals at birth, those with **partial AIS** have a wide variety of phenotypic presentations ranging from **perineoscrotal hypospadias,** bifid scrotum, and cryptorchidism to extreme under virilization appearing as clitoromegaly and labial fusion. Some forms of partial AIS have been known as specific syndromes. Patients with **Reifenstein syndrome** have incomplete virilization characterized by hypogonadism, severe hypospadias, and gynecomastia (see Fig. 582-5). **Gilbert-Dreyfus** and **Lubs** are additional syndromes classified as partial AIS. In all cases, abnormalities in the androgen receptor gene have been identified.

DIAGNOSIS The diagnosis of patients with partial AIS may be particularly difficult in infancy. The postnatal surge in testosterone and LH is diminished in those with complete AIS (CAIS) but not in those with partial AIS (PAIS). In some, especially those sufficiently virilized in infancy, the diagnosis is not suspected until puberty when there is inadequate virilization with lack of facial hair or voice change and the appearance of gynecomastia. Azoospermia and infertility are common. Increasingly, androgen receptor defects are being recognized in adults who have a small phallus and testes and infertility. A single-amino-acid substitution in the androgen receptor was reported in a large Chinese family in whom some affected members were fertile while others had gynecomastia and/or hypospadias. IGF2 and IGFBP2 but not IGFBP3 production by genital skin fibroblasts is decreased in CAIS compared with normal genital skin fibroblasts, suggesting a possible role for the IGF system in modulating androgen action.

TREATMENT AND PROGNOSIS In patients with CAIS whose sexual orientation is unambiguously female, the testes should be removed as soon as they are discovered. Laparoscopic removal of Y chromosome–bearing gonads has been performed in patients with AIS and in those with gonadal dysgenesis. In one third of patients, malignant tumors, usually seminomas, develop by 50 yr of age. Several teenage girls have acquired seminomas. Replacement therapy with estrogens is indicated at the age of puberty.

Normal breasts develop in affected girls who have not had their testes removed by the age of puberty. In these individuals, production of estradiol results from aromatase activity on testicular testosterone. The absence of androgenic activity also contributes to the feminization of these women.

The psychosexual and surgical management of patients with partial AIS is extremely complex and depends in large part on the presenting phenotype. Osteopenia is recognized as a late feature of AIS.

Molecular analyses have suggested that phenotype may depend in part on somatic mosaicism of the androgen receptor gene. This was based on the case of a 46,XY patient who had a premature stop codon in exon 1 of the AR gene but who also had evidence of virilization (pubic hair and clitoral enlargement) explained by the discovery of the wild-type alleles on careful examination of the sequencing gel. The presence of mosaicism shifts the phenotype to a higher degree of virilization than expected from the genotype of the mutant allele alone.

Genetic counseling is difficult in families with androgen receptor gene mutation. In addition to lack of genotype-phenotype correlations, there is a high rate (27%) of de novo mutations in families.

Sex hormone–binding globulin reduction after exogenous androgen administration (stanozolol) has been shown to correlate with the severity of the receptor defect and may become a useful clinical tool. Successful therapy with supplemental androgens has been reported in patients with partial AIS and various mutations of the androgen receptor in the DNA-binding domain and the ligand-binding domain.

Mutated androgen receptors are also reported in patients with spinal and bulbar muscular atrophy in whom clinical manifestations including testicular atrophy, infertility, gynecomastia, and elevated LH, FSH, and estradiol levels usually manifest between the 3rd and 5th decades of life. Androgen receptor mutations have also been described in patients with prostate cancer.

UNDETERMINED CAUSES

Other XY undervirilized males display great variability of the external and internal genitalia and various degrees of phallic and müllerian development. Testes may be histologically normal or rudimentary, or there may only be 1. Even the newer techniques may find no recognized cause in a up to 50% of children with 46,XY DSD. Some ambiguity of the genitalia is associated with a wide variety of chromosomal aberrations, which must always be considered in the differential diagnosis, the most common being the 45,X/46,XY syndrome (Chapter 580.1). It may be necessary to karyotype several tissues to establish mosaicism. Other complex genetic syndromes, many resulting from single gene mutations, are associated with varying degrees of ambiguity of the genitalia, particularly in the male. These entities must be identified on the basis of the associated extragenital malformations.

Smith-Lemli-Opitz syndrome is an autosomal recessive disorder caused by mutations in the sterol Δ7-reductase gene located on chromosome 11q12-q13. It is characterized by prenatal and postnatal growth retardation, microcephaly, ptosis, anteverted nares, broad alveolar ridges, syndactyly of the 2nd-3rd toes, and severe mental retardation (Chapter 80.3). Its incidence is 1/20,000 to 1/60,000; 70% are male. Genotypic males usually have genital ambiguity and, occasionally, partial sex reversal with female genital ambiguity or complete sex reversal with female external genitals. Müllerian duct derivatives are usually absent. Affected 46,XX patients have normal genitalia. Two types of Smith-Lemli-Opitz syndrome have been recognized. The **classical form** (type I) described earlier and the acrodysgenital syndrome, which is usually lethal within 1 yr and is associated with severe malformations, postaxial polydactyly, and extremely abnormal external genitalia (type II). Pyloric stenosis is associated with Smith-Lemli-Opitz syndrome type I and Hirschsprung disease with type II. Cleft palate, skeletal abnormalities, and 1 case of a lipoma of the pituitary gland have been seen in **type II** cases. Some authors believe in a spectrum of disease severity rather than in the above classification. Low plasma cholesterol with elevated 7-dehydrocholesterol, its precursor, are found in types 1 and 2, and the levels do not correlate with severity. Maternal apolipoprotein E values do seem to correlate with severity. The most common prenatal expression of Smith-Lemli-Opitz syndrome is intrauterine growth retardation (see Chapter 80.3 for treatment).

46,XY DSD subjects also have been described in siblings with the α-thalassemia/mental retardation syndrome.

BIBLIOGRAPHY

Please visit the Nelson Textbook of Pediatrics *website at* *www.expertconsult.com* *for the complete bibliography.*

582.3 Ovotesticular DSD

Patricia A. Donohoue

In ovotesticular DSD, both ovarian and testicular tissues are present, either in the same or in opposite gonads. Affected patients have ambiguous genitalia, varying from normal female with only slight enlargement of the clitoris to almost normal male external genitalia (see Fig. 582-2*A*).

About 70% of all patients have a 46,XX karyotype. Ninety-seven percent of affected patients of African descent are 46,XX. Fewer than 10% of persons with ovotesticular DSD are 46,XY. About 20% have 46,XX/46,XY mosaicism. Half of these are derived from more than 1 zygote and are chimeras (chi 46,XX/46,XY). The presence of paternal and both maternal alleles for some blood groups is demonstrated. An ovotesticular DSD chimera, 46,XX/46,XY, was reported as resulting from embryo amalgamation after in vitro fertilization. Each embryo was derived from an independent, separately fertilized ovum.

Examination of 46,XX ovotesticular DSD patients with Y-specific probes has detected fewer than 10% with a portion of the Y chromosome including the *SRY* gene. Ovotesticular DSD is usually sporadic, but a number of siblings have been reported. The cause of most cases of ovotesticular DSD is unknown.

The most frequently encountered gonad in ovotesticular DSD is an ovotestis, which may be bilateral. If unilateral, the contralateral gonad is usually an ovary but may be a testis. The ovarian tissue is normal, but the testicular tissue is dysgenetic. The presence and function of testicular tissue can be determined by measuring basal and hCG-stimulated testosterone levels as well as AMH levels. Patients who are highly virilized and have had adequate testicular function with no uterus are usually reared as males. If a uterus exists, virilization is often mild and testicular function minimal; assignment of female sex may be indicated. Selective removal of gonadal tissue inconsistent with sex of rearing may be indicated. In a few families, 46,XY ovotesticular DSD subjects and 44,XX males have been described in the same sibship.

Pregnancies with living offspring have been reported in 46,XX ovotesticular DSD individuals reared as females, but very few males with ovotesticular DSD have fathered children. About 5% of patients will develop gonadoblastomas, dysgerminomas, or seminomas.

DIAGNOSIS AND MANAGEMENT

In the neonate, ambiguity of the genitals requires immediate attention to decide on the sex of rearing as early in life as possible.

The family of the infant needs to be informed of the child's condition as early, completely, compassionately, and honestly as possible. Caution must be used to avoid feelings of guilt, shame, and discomfort. Guidance needs to be provided to alleviate both short-term and long-term concerns and to allow the child to grow up in a completely supportive environment. The initial care is best provided by a team of professionals that include neonatologists and pediatric specialists, endocrinologists, radiologists, urologists, psychologists, and geneticists, all of whom remain focused foremost on the needs of the child. Management of the potential psychologic upheaval that these disorders can generate in the child or the family is of paramount importance and requires physicians and other health care professionals with sensitivity, training, and experience in this field.

While awaiting the results of chromosomal analysis, pelvic ultrasonography is indicated to determine the presence of a uterus and ovaries. Presence of a uterus and absence of palpable gonads usually suggests a virilized XX female. A search for the source of virilization should be undertaken; this includes studies of adrenal hormones to rule out varieties of congenital adrenal hyperplasia, and studies of androgens and estrogens occasionally may be necessary to rule out aromatase deficiency. Virilized XX females are generally (but not always) reared as females even when highly virilized.

The absence of a uterus, with or without palpable gonads, almost always indicates an under virilized male and an XY karyotype. Measurements of levels of gonadotropins, testosterone, AMH, and DHT are necessary to determine whether testicular production of androgen is normal. Under virilized males who are totally feminized may be reared as females. Certain significantly feminized infants, such as those with 5α-reductase deficiency, may be reared as males because these children virilize normally at puberty. Sixty percent of individuals with 5α-reductase deficiency assigned as female in infancy live as males. An infant with a comparable degree of feminization resulting from an androgen receptor defect, such as CAIS, is best reared as a female.

When receptor disorders are suspected in the XY male with a small phallus (micropenis), a course of 3 monthly intramuscular injections of testosterone enanthate (25-50 mg) may assist in the differential diagnosis of androgen insensitivity, as well as in treatment.

In some mammals, the female exposed to androgens prenatally or in early postnatal life exhibits nontraditional sexual behavior in adult life. Most, but not all, girls who have undergone fetal masculinization from congenital adrenal hyperplasia or from maternal progestin therapy have female sexual identity, although during childhood they may appear to prefer male playmates and activities over female playmates and feminine play with dolls in mothering roles.

In the past it was thought that surgical treatment of ambiguous genitalia to create a female appearance, particularly when a vagina is present, was more successful than construction of male genitalia. Considerable controversy exists regarding these decisions. Sexual functioning is to a large extent more dependent on neurohormonal and behavioral factors than the physical appearance and functional ability of the genitalia. Similarly, controversy exists regarding the timing of the performance of invasive and definitive procedures, such as surgery. Whenever possible without endangering the physical or psychologic health of the child, an expert multidisciplinary team should consider deferring elective surgical repairs and gonadectomies until the child can participate in the informed consent for the procedure. One study (n = 59 boys and 18 girls) with gender dysphoria but without documentation of genomic or enzymologic abnormalities indicated that most of these children no longer have gender dysphoria after completion of puberty. Among those who do, homosexuality and bisexuality are the most frequent diagnoses.

The pediatrician, pediatric endocrinologist, and psychologist, along with the appropriate additional specialists, should provide ongoing compassionate, supportive care to the patient and the patient's family throughout childhood, adolescence, and adulthood. Support groups are available for families and patients with many of the conditions discussed.

BIBLIOGRAPHY

Please visit the Nelson Textbook of Pediatrics *website at www.expertconsult.com for the complete bibliography.*

Section 6 DIABETES MELLITUS IN CHILDREN

Chapter 583 Diabetes Mellitus

583.1 Introduction and Classification

Ramin Alemzadeh and Omar Ali

Diabetes mellitus (DM) is a common, chronic, metabolic syndrome characterized by hyperglycemia as a cardinal biochemical feature. The major forms of diabetes are classified according to those caused by deficiency of insulin secretion due to pancreatic β-cell damage (type 1 DM, or T1DM) and those that are a consequence of insulin resistance occurring at the level of skeletal muscle, liver, and adipose tissue, with various degrees of β-cell impairment (type 2 DM, or T2DM). T1DM is the most common endocrine-metabolic disorder of childhood and adolescence, with important consequences for physical and emotional development. Individuals with T1DM confront serious lifestyle alterations that include an absolute daily requirement for exogenous insulin, the need to monitor their own glucose level, and the need to pay attention to dietary intake. Morbidity and mortality stem from acute metabolic derangements and from long-term **complications** (usually in adulthood) that affect small and large vessels resulting in retinopathy, nephropathy, neuropathy, ischemic heart disease, and arterial obstruction with gangrene of the extremities. The acute clinical manifestations are due to hypoinsulinemic hyperglycemic ketoacidosis. Autoimmune mechanisms are factors in the genesis of T1DM; the long-term complications are related to metabolic disturbances (hyperglycemia).

For the full continuation of this chapter, please visit the Nelson Textbook of Pediatrics *website at www.expertconsult.com.*

583.2 Type 1 Diabetes Mellitus (Immune Mediated)

Ramin Alemzadeh and Omar Ali

EPIDEMIOLOGY

T1DM accounts for about 10% of all diabetes, affecting 1.4 million in the USA and over 15 million in the world. While it accounts for most cases of diabetes in childhood, it is not limited to this age group; new cases continue to occur in adult life and approximately 50% of individuals with T1DM present as adults. The incidence of T1DM is highly variable among different ethnic groups. The overall age-adjusted incidence of type 1 DM varies from 0.7/100,000 per year in Karachi (Pakistan) to over 40/100,000 per year in Finland (Fig. 583-1). This represents a more than 400-fold variation in the incidence among 100 populations. The incidence of T1DM is increasing in most (but not all) populations and this increase appears to be most marked in populations where the incidence of autoimmune diseases was historically low. Data from Western European diabetes centers suggest that the annual rate of increase in T1DM incidence is 2-5%, whereas some central and eastern European countries demonstrate an even more rapid increase. The rate of increase is greatest among the youngest children. In the USA, the overall prevalence of diabetes among school-aged children is about 1.9/1,000, increasing from a prevalence of 1/1,430 children at 5 yr of age to 1/360 children at 16 yr. Among African Americans, the occurrence of T1DM is 30-60% of that seen in American whites. The annual incidence of new cases in the USA is about 14.9/100,000 of the child population. It is estimated that 30,000 new cases occur each year in the USA, affecting 1 in 300 children and as many as 1 in 100 adults during the lifespan. Rates are similar or higher in most Western European countries and significantly lower in Asia and Africa. But while incidence rates are much higher in European populations, the absolute number of new cases is almost equal in Asia and Europe because the population base is so much larger in Asia. Thus it is estimated that of the 400,000 total new cases of type 1 diabetes occurring annually in all children under age 14 yr in the world, about half are in Asia even though the incidence rates in that continent are much lower, because the total number of children in Asia is larger.

Girls and boys are almost equally affected but there is a modest female preponderance in some low-risk populations (e.g., the Japanese); there is no apparent correlation with socioeconomic status. Peaks of presentation occur in 2 age groups: at 5-7 yr of age and at the time of puberty. The 1st peak may correspond to the time of increased exposure to infectious agents coincident with the beginning of school; the 2nd peak may correspond to the pubertal growth spurt induced by gonadal steroids and the increased pubertal growth hormone secretion (which antagonizes insulin). These possible cause-and-effect relationships remain to be proved. A growing number of cases are presenting between 1 and 2 yr of age, especially in high-risk groups; the average age of presentation is older in low-risk populations. Low-risk groups that migrate to a high-risk country seem to acquire an increased risk; for example, the children of Pakistani immigrants in the United Kingdom (UK) have an incidence rate similar to the local English population and 20 fold higher than the rates in Pakistan. On the other hand, there can be marked differences in incidence rates in various ethnic groups within the same country; for example, incidence rates in the 10-14 yr age group in the USA range from a low of 7.1 in Native Americans, to 17.6 in Hispanics, 19.2 in African-Americans, and

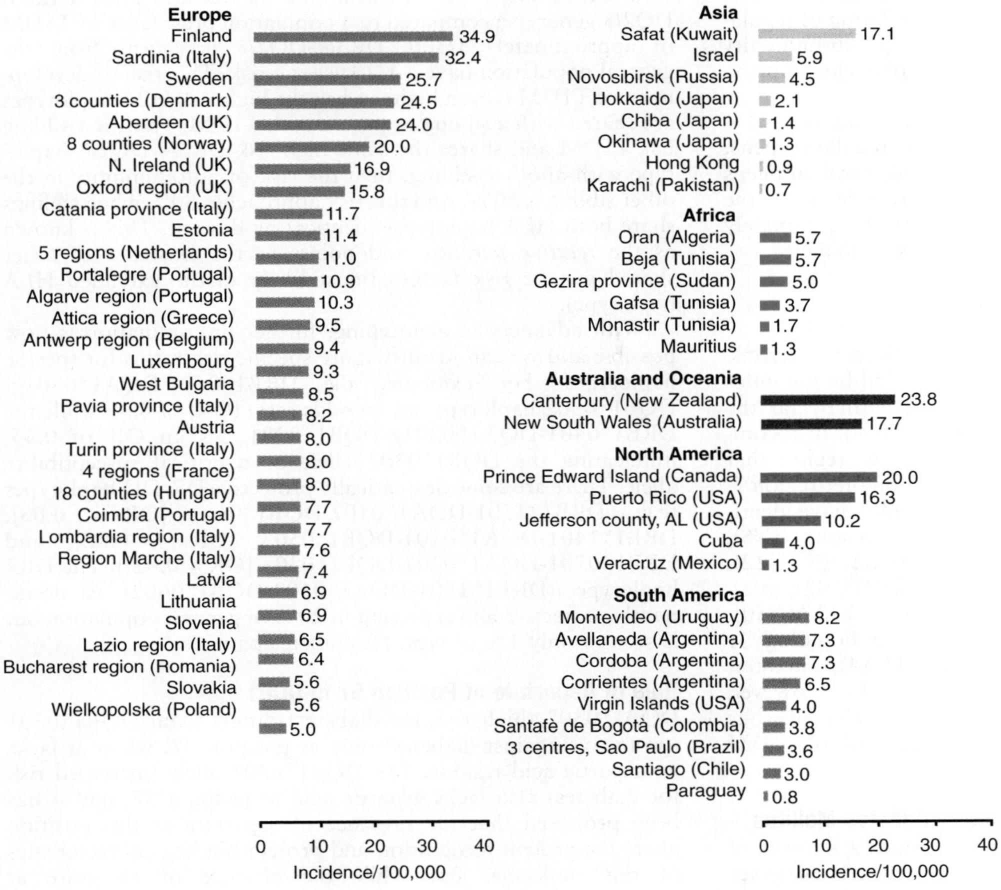

Figure 583-1 Incidence rates of type 1 diabetes mellitus by region and country. (From Karvonen M, Viik-Kajander M, Moltchanova E, et al: Incidence of type I diabetes worldwide. Diabetes Mondiale (DiaMond) Project Group, *Diabetes Care* 23:1516–1526, 2000.)

32.9 in whites. These variations also remain unexplained at this time.

GENETICS

There is a clear familial clustering of T1DM, with prevalence in siblings approaching 6% while the prevalence in the general population in the USA is only 0.4%. Risk of diabetes is also increased when a parent has diabetes and this risk differs between the 2 parents; the risk is 2% if the mother has diabetes, but 7% when the father has diabetes. In monozygotic twins, the concordance rate ranges from 30-65%, whereas dizygotic twins have a concordance rate of 6-10%. Since the concordance rate of dizygotic twins is higher than the sibling risk, factors other than the shared genotypes (for example the shared intrauterine environment) may play a role in increasing the risk in dizygotic twins. Furthermore, the genetic susceptibility for T1DM in the parents of a child with diabetes is estimated at 3%. It should be kept in mind that although there is a large genetic component in T1DM, 85% of newly diagnosed type 1 diabetic patients do not have a family member with T1DM. Thus, we cannot rely on family history to identify patients who may be at risk for the future development of T1DM as most cases will develop in individuals with no such family history.

Monogenic Type 1 Diabetes Mellitus

Classic single gene defects are an extremely rare cause of type 1 diabetes, but they are not unknown. In 2 rare syndromes (IPEX and APS-1) the genetic susceptibility that leads to diabetes is due to a classic single gene defect. The IPEX (immune dysfunction, polyendocrinopathy, enteropathy, X-linked) syndrome is caused by mutations of the FOXP3 gene. The FOXP3 (forkhead box P3) is a gene involved in immune system responses. A member of the FOX protein family, FOXP3 appears to function as the master regulator in the development and function of regulatory T cells. These mutations lead to the lack of a major population of regulatory T lymphocytes with resulting overwhelming autoimmunity and development of diabetes (as early as 2 days of age) in approximately 80% of the children with this disorder.

APS-I (autoimmune polyendocrinopathy syndrome type 1) is caused by mutations of the AIRE (autoimmune regulator) gene, leading to abnormalities in expression of peripheral antigens within the thymus and/or abnormalities of negative selection in the thymus. This results in widespread autoimmunity. Approximately 18% of children with this syndrome develop type 1a diabetes.

Genes Altering the Risk of Autoimmune Type 1 Diabetes Mellitus

Most patients with T1DM do not have single gene defects. Instead, their risk of developing T1DM is modified by the influence of several risk loci. The genomic region with by far the greatest contribution to the risk of T1DM is the major histocompatibility complex on chromosome 6. One other region that consistently shows up in genetic studies is the promoter region 5′ of the insulin gene on chromosome 11. Other studies have identified several other risk loci. These loci include insulin (INS), protein tyrosine phosphatase nonreceptor type 22 (PTPN22), protein tyrosine phosphatase nonreceptor type 2 (PTPN2), interleukin (IL)-2 receptor (CD25), a lectin-like gene (KIAA0350), v-erb-b2 erythroblastic leukemia viral oncogene homolog 3e (ERBB3e), cytotoxic T-lymphocyte antigen 4 (CTLA4), and interferon-induced with helicase C domain 1 (IFIH1). However, except for PTPN22, their contribution is relatively small, thus making them less useful for predicting the genetic risk of T1DM in a given individual.

MHC/HLA Encoded Susceptibility to Type 1 Diabetes Mellitus

The MHC is a large genomic region that contains a number of genes related to immune system function in humans. These genes are further divided into HLA class I, II, III, and IV genes. Class II genes are the ones most strongly associated with risk of T1DM, but as genetic studies become more detailed it is becoming apparent that some of the risk associated with various HLA types is due to variation in genes in HLA classes other than class II. Overall, genetic variation in the HLA region can explain 40-50% of the genetic risk of T1DM (Fig 583-2).

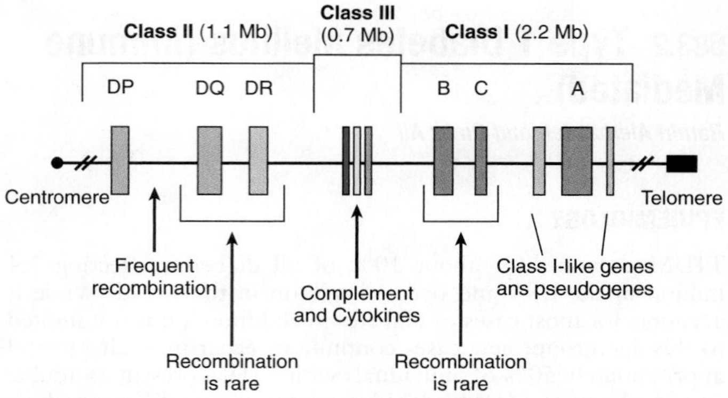

Figure 583-2 The human leukocyte antigen (HLA) complex (6p21.31). Graphic representation of the HLA complex, showing the relative locations the 3 classes of HLA genes. (Courtesy of Dr. George Eisenbarth.)

Initially, much of the risk associated with diabetes appeared to be linked to DR3 and DR4 alleles, but the genes of the HLA locus display strong linkage disequilibrium and it is now known that some of the earlier identified risk alleles (like DR3/DR4) confer much of their increased risk because of their linkage with other alleles in the DQ region with which they are tightly linked with relatively low recombination rates.

Some of the known associations include the HLA DR3/4-DQ2/8 genotype; compared to a population prevalence of T1DM of approximately 1/300, DR3/4-DQ2/8 newborns from the general population have a 1/20 genetic risk. This risk of development of T1DM is even higher when the high-risk HLA haplotypes are shared with a sibling or parent with T1DM. Thus, if 1 sibling has T1DM and shares the same high-risk DR3/4-DQ2/8 haplotype with another sibling, then the risk of autoimmunity in the other sibling is 50%. And this risk approaches 80% when siblings share both HLA haplotypes identical by descent. This is known as the *relative paradox* and points to the existence of other shared genetic risk factors (most likely in the extended HLA haplotype).

With advances in genotyping, further discrimination is now possible and we can identify more specific risk ratios for specific haplotypes. For example, the DRB1*0401-DQA1*0301g-DQB1*0302 haplotype has an odds ratio (OR) of 8.39 while the DRB1*0401-DQA1*0301g-DQB1*0301 has an OR of 0.35, implicating the DQB1*0302 allele as a critical susceptibility allele. There are some dramatically protective DR-DQ haplotypes (e.g., DRB1*1501-DQA1*0102-DQB1*0602 [OR = 0.03], DRB1*1401-DQA1*0101-DQB1*0503 [OR = 0.02], and DRB1*0701-DQA1*0201-DQB1*0303 [OR = 0.02]). The DR2 haplotype (DRB1*1501-DQA1*0102-DQB1*0602) is dominantly protective and is present in 20% of general population but is seen in only 1% of type 1A diabetes patients.

Role of Aspartate at Position 57 in DQB1

DQB1*0302 (high risk for diabetes) differs from DQB1*0301 (protective against diabetes) only at position 57, where it lacks an aspartic acid residue. The DQB1*0201 allele (increased risk for diabetes) also lacks aspartic acid at position 57, and it has been proposed that the presence of aspartate at this position alters the protein recognition and protein binding characteristics of this molecule. But while the absence of aspartate at this position appears to be important in most studies on white individuals, it does not have the same role in Korean and Japanese populations. Moreover, certain low-risk DQB1 genotypes also lack aspartic acid at position 57, including DQB1*0302/DQB1*0201 (DR7), and DQB1*0201 (DR3)/DQB1*0201 (DR7). Thus, the presence of aspartate at this position is usually, but not always, protective in white populations, but not necessarily in other populations.

Role of HLA Class I

While the alleles of class II HLA genes appear to have the strongest associations with diabetes, recent genotyping studies and analyses of pooled data have identified associations with other elements in the HLA complex, especially HLA-A and HLA-B. The most significant association is with HLA-B39, which confers high risk for type 1A diabetes in 3 different populations, makes up the majority of the signal from HLA-B, and is associated with a lower age of onset of the disease.

Insulin Gene Locus, *IDDM2*

The 2nd locus found to be associated with risk of T1DM was labeled IDDM2 and has been localized to a region upstream of the insulin gene (5′ of the insulin gene). It is estimated that this locus accounts for about 10% of the familial risk of T1DM. Susceptibility in this region has been primarily mapped to a variable number of tandem repeats (VNTR) about 500 bp upstream of the insulin gene. This highly polymorphic region consists of anywhere from 30 to several hundred repeats of a 14-15 bp unit sequence (ACAGGGGTCTGGGG). Shorter number of repeats is associated with increased risk of T1DM.

PTPN22 (Lymphoid Tyrosine Phosphatase)

A single-nucleotide polymorphism (SNP) in the PTPN22 gene on chromosome 1p13 that encodes lymphoid tyrosine phosphatase (Lyp) correlates strongly with the incidence of T1DM in 2 independent populations. Since then, this discovery had been replicated in several populations and the gene has been found to have association with several other autoimmune diseases.

CTLA-4

The cytotoxic T lymphocyte–antigen 4 (CTLA-4) gene is located on chromosome 2q33 and has been found to be associated with type 1 diabetes risk as well as the risk of other autoimmune disorders in several studies. This gene is a negative regulator of T-cell activation and therefore is a good biologic candidate for type 1 diabetes risk modification.

Interleukin-2 (IL-2) Receptor

SNPs in or near the gene for the IL-2 receptor have been found to have an association with T1DM risk.

Interleukin-1 (IL-1) Receptor

IL-1 receptor activation and chemokines involved in monocyte/macrophage and neutrophil chemotaxis, have been also identified as critical steps in nitric oxide (NO)-induced islet necrosis and subsequent apoptosis. Indeed, inhibition of the activation of IL-1β–dependent inflammatory pathways by an IL-1 receptor antagonist in cultured rat islets exposed to NO prevented necrosis and apoptosis supporting evaluation in human islets in vitro and potentially as a post-transplant therapy.

Interferon-Induced Helicase

Another gene identified as having a modest effect on the risk of type 1 diabetes is the interferon-induced helicase (IFIH1) gene. This gene is thought to play a role in protecting the host from viral infections and given the specificity of different helicases for different RNA viruses, it is possible that knowledge of this gene locus will help to narrow down the list of viral pathogens that may have a role in type 1 diabetes.

CYP27B1

Cytochrome p450, subfamily 27, polypeptide 1 gene encodes vitamin D 1α-hydroxylase. Because of the known role of vitamin D in immune regulation and because of epidemiologic evidence that vitamin D may play a role in T1DM, this gene was examined as a candidate gene and 2 SNPs were found to be associated.

Other Genes

Several other genes (e.g., protein tyrosine phosphatase nonreceptor type 2 [PTPN-2]) and linkage blocks, including 2 linkage blocks on chromosome 12 (12q13 and 12q24) and blocks on 16p13, 18p11 and 18q22 have been found to be significant in genome-wide association studies and further fine mapping and functional studies of genes in these regions are pending.

ENVIRONMENTAL FACTORS

The fact that 50% or so of monozygotic twins are discordant for T1DM, the variation seen in urban and rural areas populated by the same ethnic group, the change in incidence that occurs with migration, the increase in incidence that has been seen in almost all populations in the last few decades, and the occurrence of seasonality all provide evidence that environmental factors also play a significant role in the causation of T1DM.

Viral Infections

It is possible that various viruses do play a role in the pathogenesis of T1DM, but no single virus, and no single pathogenic mechanism, stands out in the environmental etiology of T1DM. Instead, a variety of viruses and mechanisms may contribute to the development of diabetes in genetically susceptible hosts.

Congenital Rubella Syndrome

The clearest evidence of a role for viral infection in human T1DM is seen in congenital rubella syndrome (CRS). Prenatal infection with rubella is associated with β-cell autoimmunity in up to 70%, with development of T1DM in up to 40% of infected children. The time lag between infection and development of diabetes may be as high as 20 yr. Type 1 diabetes after congenital rubella is more likely in patients that carry the higher risk genotypes. Interestingly, there appears to be no increase in risk of diabetes when rubella infection develops after birth, or when live-virus rubella immunization is used. Exactly how rubella infection leads to diabetes and why it is pathogenic only if infection occurs prenatally, remains unknown.

Enteroviruses

Studies have shown an increase in evidence of enteroviral infection in patients with T1DM and an increased prevalence of enteroviral RNA in prenatal blood samples from children who subsequently developed T1DM. In addition, there are case reports of association between enteroviral infection and subsequent T1DM. But the true significance of these infections remains unknown at this time.

Mumps Virus

It has been observed that mumps infection leads to the development of β-cell autoimmunity with high frequency and to T1DM in some cases. It has also been noted that there is an uptick in the incidence of T1DM 2-4 yr after an epidemic of mumps infection. But a large European study did not find any association between mumps infection and subsequent development of diabetes. Mumps vaccination, on the other hand, appears to be protective against diabetes. But while mumps may play a role in some cases of diabetes, the fact that T1DM diabetes incidence has increased steadily in several countries after universal mumps vaccination was introduced, and that incidence is extremely low in several populations where mumps is still prevalent, indicates that mumps is not an important causal factor in diabetes.

Role of Childhood Immunizations

Several large-scale well-designed studies have conclusively shown that routine childhood immunizations do NOT increase the risk of T1DM. On the contrary, immunization against mumps and pertussis has been shown to decrease the risk of T1DM.

The Hygiene Hypothesis: Possible Protective Role of Infections

While some viral infections may increase the risk of T1DM, infectious agents may also play a protective role against diabetes. The hygiene hypothesis states that lack of exposure to childhood infections may somehow increase an individual's chances of developing autoimmune diseases, including T1DM. Epidemiologic patterns suggest that this may indeed be the case. Rates of T1DM and other autoimmune disorders are generally lower in underdeveloped nations with high prevalence of childhood infections, and tend to increase as these countries become more developed. The incidence of T1DM differs almost 6-fold between Russian Karelia and Finland even though both are populated by a genetically related population and are located next to each other at the same latitude. The incidence of autoimmunity in the 2 populations varies inversely with IgE antibody levels, and IgE is involved in the response to parasitic infestation. All these observations indicate that decreased exposure to certain parasites and other microbes in early childhood may lead to an increased risk of autoimmunity in later life, including autoimmune diabetes. On the other hand, retrospective case-control studies have been equivocal at best and direct evidence of protection by childhood infections is still lacking.

Diet

Breast-feeding may lower the risk of T1DM, either directly or by delaying exposure to cow's milk protein. Early introduction of cow's milk protein and early exposure to gluten have both been implicated in the development of autoimmunity and it has been suggested that this is due to the "leakiness" of the immature gut to protein antigens. Antigens that have been implicated include β-lactoglobulin, a major lipocalin protein in bovine milk, which is homologous to the human protein glycodelin (PP14), a T-cell modulator. Other studies have focused on bovine serum albumin as the inciting antigen, but the data are contradictory and not yet conclusive.

Other dietary factors that have been suggested at various times as playing a role in diabetes risk include omega-3 fatty acids, vitamin D, ascorbic acid, zinc, and vitamin E. Vitamin D is biologically plausible (it has a role in immune regulation), deficiency is more common in northern countries like Finland, and there is some epidemiologic evidence that decreased vitamin D levels in pregnancy or early childhood may be associated with diabetes risk; but the evidence is not yet conclusive and it is hoped that ongoing studies like TEDDY (The Environmental Determinants of Diabetes in the Young) will help to resolve some of the uncertainties in this area.

Psychologic Stress

Several studies show an increased prevalence of stressful psychologic situations among children who subsequently developed T1DM. Whether these stresses only aggravate pre-existing autoimmunity or whether they can actually trigger autoimmunity, remains unknown.

Role of Insulin Resistance: The Accelerator Hypothesis

The accelerator hypothesis proposes that T1DM and T2DM are the same disorder of insulin resistance, set against different genetic backgrounds. This "strong statement" of the accelerator hypothesis has been criticized as ignoring the abundant genetic and clinical evidence that the 2 diseases are distinct. Still, the hypothesis has focused attention on the role of insulin resistance and obesity in T1DM and there is evidence that the incidence of T1DM is indeed higher in children who exhibit more rapid weight gain. Whether this is simply another factor that stresses the β cell in the course of a primarily autoimmune disorder, or whether T1DM and T2DM can really be regarded as the same disease, is still open to question.

PATHOGENESIS AND NATURAL HISTORY OF TYPE 1 DIABETES MELLITUS

In type 1A diabetes mellitus, a genetically susceptible host develops autoimmunity against his or her own β cells. What triggers this autoimmune response remains unclear at this time. In some (but not all) patients, this autoimmune process results in progressive destruction of β cells until a critical mass of β cells is lost and insulin deficiency develops. Insulin deficiency in turn leads to the onset of clinical signs and symptoms of T1DM. At the time of diagnosis, some viable β cells are still present and these may produce enough insulin to lead to a partial remission of the disease (honeymoon period) but over time, almost all β cells are destroyed and the patient becomes totally dependent on exogenous insulin for survival (Fig. 583-3). Over time, some of these patients develop secondary complications of diabetes that appear to be related to how well-controlled the diabetes has been. Thus, the natural history of T1DM involves some or all of the following stages:

1. Initiation of autoimmunity
2. Preclinical autoimmunity with progressive loss of β-cell function
3. Onset of clinical disease
4. Transient remission
5. Established disease
6. Development of complications

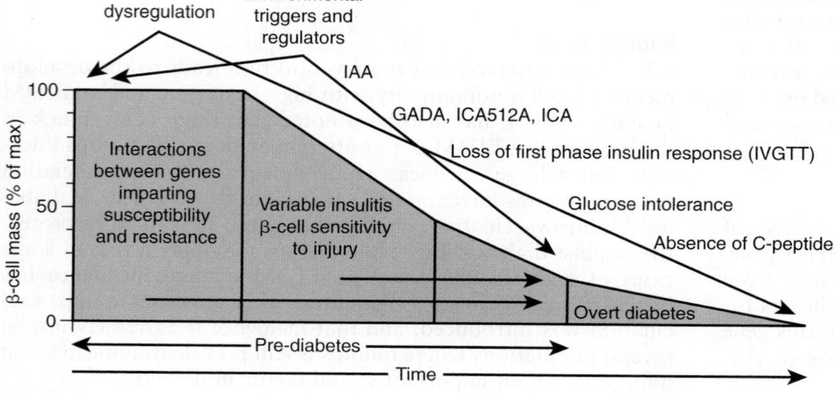

Figure 583-3 Proposed model of the pathogenesis and natural history of type 1 diabetes mellitus. IAA, insulin autoantibodies; GADA, glutamic acid decarboxylase antibody; ICA, islet cell antibody; IVGTT, intravenous glucose tolerance test. (Adapted from Atkinson MA, Eisenbarth GS: Type 1 diabetes: new perspectives on disease pathogenesis and treatment, *Lancet* 358:221–229, 2001.)

Initiation of Autoimmunity

Genetic susceptibility to T1DM is determined by several genes (see section on genetics), with the largest contribution coming from variants in the HLA system. But it is important to keep in mind that even with the highest risk haplotypes, most carriers will NOT develop T1DM. Even in monozygotic twins, the concordance is 30-65%. A number of factors including prenatal influences, diet in infancy, viral infections, lack of exposure to certain infections, even psychologic stress, have been implicated in the pathogenesis of T1DM, but their exact role and the mechanism by which they trigger or aggravate autoimmunity remains uncertain (Fig. 583-4). What is clear is that markers of autoimmunity are much more prevalent than clinical T1DM, indicating that initiation of autoimmunity is a necessary but not a sufficient condition for T1DM. Whatever the triggering factor, it seems that in most cases of T1DM that are diagnosed in childhood, the onset of autoimmunity occurs very early in life. In a majority of the children diagnosed before age 10 yr, the 1st signs of autoimmunity appear before age 2 yr. Development of autoimmunity is associated with the appearance of several autoantibodies. Insulin associated antibodies (IAA) are usually the 1st to appear in young children, followed by glutamic acid decarboxylase 65 kd (GAD65) and tyrosine phosphatase insulinoma-associated 2 (IA-2) antibodies. The earliest antibodies are predominantly of the IgG1 subclass. Not only is there "spreading" of autoimmunity to more antigens (IAA, and then GAD 65 and IA-2) but there is also epitope spreading within 1 antigen. Initial GAD65 antibodies tend to be against the middle region or the carboxyl-terminal region, while amino-terminal antibodies usually appear later and are less common in children.

Preclinical Autoimmunity with Progressive Loss of β-Cell Function

In some, but not all patients, the appearance of autoimmunity is followed by progressive destruction of β cells. Antibodies are a marker for the presence of autoimmunity, but the actual damage to the β cells is primarily T-cell mediated (Fig. 583-5). Histologic analysis of the pancreas from patients with recent-onset T1DM reveals insulitis, with an infiltration of the islets of Langerhans by mononuclear cells, including T and B lymphocytes, monocytes/macrophages, and natural killer (NK) cells. In the NOD mouse, a similar cellular infiltrate is followed by linear loss of β cells until they completely disappear. But it appears that the process in human T1DM is not necessarily linear and there may be an undulating downhill course in the development of T1DM.

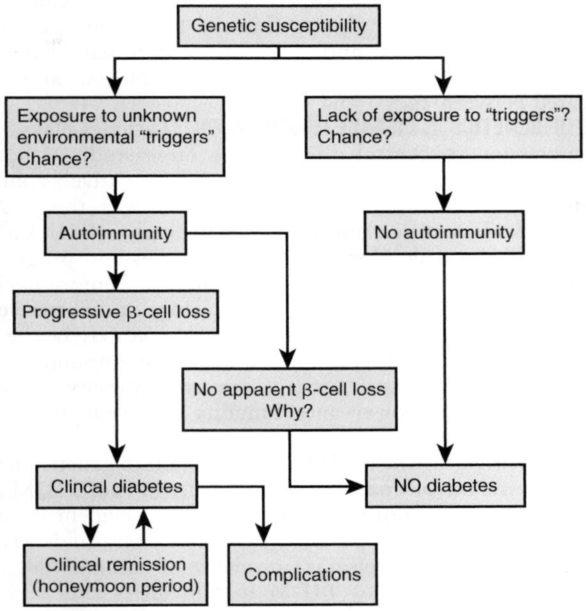

Figure 583-4 Schematic representation of the natural history of type 1 diabetes mellitus. Unknown triggers act upon a genetically susceptible host to trigger autoimmunity. Some proportion of those with autoimmunity develop progressive β-Cell loss that eventually leads to clinical diabetes. This is followed by temporary clinical remission (honeymoon period) in most patients. Over time, insulin secretion is almost completely lost and complications may develop in some patients (in direct proportion to the occurrence of hyperglycemia).

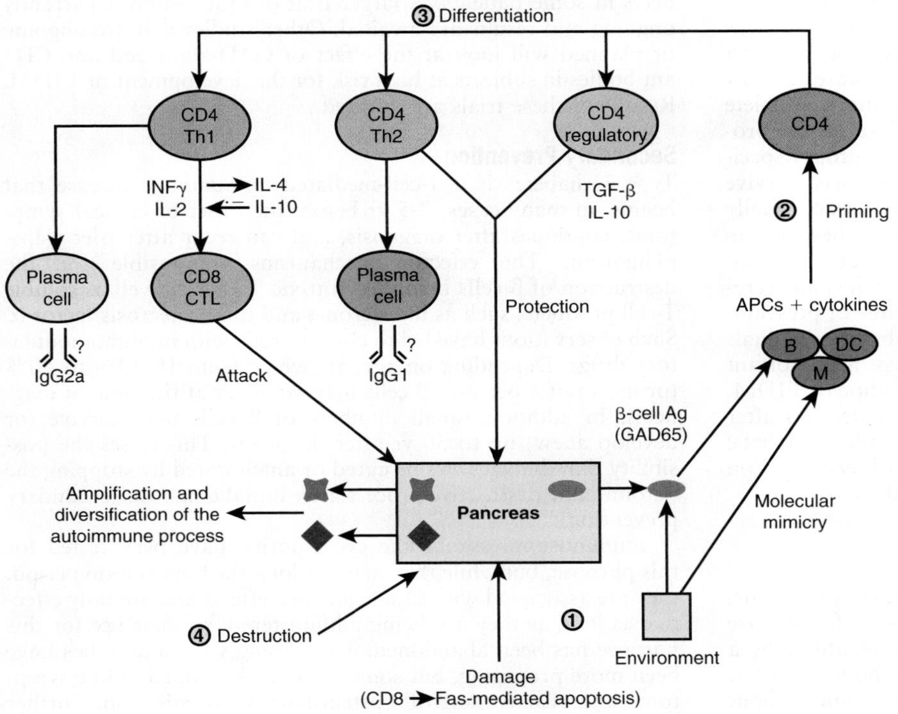

Figure 583-5 Schematic representation of the autoimmune response against pancreatic β cells. An insult to the pancreas leads to the release of β-cell antigens (GAD65), which are taken up by antigen-presenting cells (APCs) and the epitopes presented to the CD4 T cells. Type and stages of activation of APCs as well as the cytokine environment, in which the CD4 T cell priming takes place, dictate the differentiation of autoreactive T cells toward diabetogenic T helper-1 (Th1) cells, Th2 cells, or antigen-specific regulatory T cells. A predominant Th1 autoimmune response results in the recruitment and differentiation of cytotoxic CD8 cells, which attack the pancreatic β cells, leading to a massive release of β-cell antigens (Ag), epitope spreading, and destruction of the pancreatic islets. B, B lymphocyte; DC, dendritic cell; M, macrophage; CTL, cytotoxic cell; TGF-β, tumor growth factor-β; INFγ, interferon-γ; IL, interleukin. (Adapted from Casares S, Brumeanu TD: Insights into the pathogenesis of T1DM: a hint for novel immunospecific therapies, *Curr Mol Med* 1:357–378, 2001.)

ROLE OF AUTOANTIBODIES The risk of developing clinical disease increases dramatically with an increase in the number of antibodies; only 30% of children with 1 antibody will progress to diabetes, but this risk increases to 70% when 2 antibodies are present and 90% when 3 are present. The risk of progression also varies with the intensity of the antibody response and those with higher antibody titers are more likely to progress to clinical disease. Another factor that appears to influence progression of β-cell damage is the age at which autoimmunity develops; children in whom IAAs appeared within the 1st 2 yr of life rapidly developed anti–islet cell antibodies and progressed to diabetes more frequently than children in whom the 1st antibodies appeared between ages 5 and 8 yr.

ROLE OF GENETICS IN DISEASE PROGRESSION Genetics plays a role in progression to clinical disease. In a large study of healthy children, the appearance of single antibodies is relatively common and usually transient, and does not correlate with the presence of high-risk HLA alleles, but those carrying high-risk HLA alleles are more likely to develop multiple antibodies and progress to disease. Similarly, the appearance of antibodies is more likely to predict diabetes in those with a family history of diabetes versus those with no family history of T1DM. Thus, it may be the case that environmental factors can induce transient autoimmunity in many children, but those with genetic susceptibility are more likely to see progression of autoimmunity and eventual development of diabetes.

ROLE OF ENVIRONMENTAL FACTORS In addition to genetic factors, environmental factors may also act as accelerators of T1DM after the initial appearance of autoimmunity. This is evident from the fact that the incidence of T1DM can vary severalfold between populations that have the same prevalence of autoimmunity. For instance, the incidence of T1DM in Finland is almost 4-fold higher than in Lithuania, but the incidence of autoimmunity is similar in both countries.

The fact that all children with evidence of autoimmunity do not progress to diabetes indicates that there are "checkpoints" at which the autoimmune process can be halted or reversed before it progresses to full-blown diabetes. This has raised the possibility of preventing T1DM by intervening in the preclinical stage.

Onset of Clinical Disease

Patients with progressive β-cell destruction will eventually present with clinical T1DM. It was thought that 90% of the total β-cell mass is destroyed by the time clinical disease develops, but later studies have revealed that this is not always the case. It now appears that β-cell destruction is more rapid and more complete in younger children, while in older children and adults the proportion of surviving β cells is greater (10-20% in autopsy specimens) and some β cells (about 1% of the normal mass) survive up to 30 yr after the onset of diabetes. Since autopsies are usually done on patients who died of diabetic ketoacidosis, these figures may underestimate the actual β-cell mass present at diagnosis. Functional studies indicate that up to 40% of the insulin secretory capacity may be preserved in adults at the time of presentation of T1DM. The fact that newly diagnosed diabetic individuals may still have significant surviving β-cell mass is important because it raises the possibility of secondary prevention of T1DM. Similarly, the existence of viable β cells years or decades after initial presentation indicates that even longstanding diabetic patients may be able to exhibit some recovery of β-cell function if the autoimmune destructive process can be halted.

PREDICTION AND PREVENTION

Autoimmunity precedes clinical T1DM, and indicators of maturing autoimmune responses may be useful markers for disease prediction. Individuals at risk for T1DM can be identified by a combination of genetic, immunologic, and metabolic markers. The most informative genetic locus, HLA class II, confers about half of the total genetic risk but has a low positive predictive value (PPV) when used in the general population. Autoantibodies provide a practical readout of β-cell autoimmunity, are easily sampled in venous blood, and have become the mainstay of T1DM prediction efforts. In the first-degree relatives of patients with T1DM, the number of positive d-aab can help estimate the risk of developing T1DM: low risk (single d-aab: PPV of 2-6%), moderate risk (2 d-aab: PPV of 21-40%), and high risk (>2 d-aab: PPV of 59-80%) over a 5 yr period. In children carrying the T1DM highest-risk genotype (HLA-DQB1*0201-DQA1*05/DQB1*0302-DQA1*03), insulitis is almost 10 times more frequent (PPV 21%) than in children with other genotypes (PPV 2.2%). But while autoantibodies are useful for detecting developing T1DM in close relatives of diabetic patients, most cases are sporadic rather than familial, necessitating general population screening. This has been difficult, in part, because the observed autoantibody prevalence greatly exceeds the low disease prevalence in nonrelatives, leading to high false-positive rates.

Primary Prevention of Type 1 Diabetes Mellitus

A safe, effective, inexpensive, and easily administered intervention could theoretically be targeted at all newborns, but no such universally effective intervention is yet available. Delaying the introduction of cow's milk protein, delaying introduction of cereals, and increasing the duration of breast-feeding are all potentially beneficial and trials of these interventions are ongoing. But the fact that the disease has continued to increase in incidence in Northern Europe while breast-feeding has increased indicates that these interventions may not be sufficient to reverse the epidemic. Other dietary interventions that are being tested, or may be tested in high-risk subjects, include supplementing omega-3 fatty acids and vitamin D, and taking cod liver oil during pregnancy. In all these cases, there are some hints of possible benefit but nothing has been conclusively proven at this point.

In high-risk populations (relatives of individuals with T1DM, especially those with high-risk genotypes), it is feasible to test more targeted interventions. One of the 1st interventions to be tested in a high-risk population was the use of nicotinamide supplementation, but this failed to prevent T1DM. Parenteral insulin and nasal insulin proved similarly ineffective in preventing diabetes, but oral insulin appeared to delay the incidence of diabetes in some patients. A larger trial of oral insulin is currently ongoing and results are awaited. Other studies that are ongoing or planned will look at the effect of GAD-alum and anti-CD3 antibodies in subjects at high risk for the development of T1DM. Results of these trials are awaited.

Secondary Prevention

Type 1 diabetes is a T-cell-mediated autoimmune disease that begins, in many cases, 3-5 yr before the onset of clinical symptoms, continues after diagnosis, and can recur after islet transplantation. The effector mechanisms responsible for the destruction of β cells involve cytotoxic T cells as well as soluble T-cell products, such as interferon-γ and tumor necrosis factor-α. Such observations have led to clinical trials with immunomodulatory drugs. Depending on age, anywhere from 10-20% to 40% (or more) of a person's β cells may be intact at the time of diagnosis. In addition, small numbers of β cells may survive (or develop anew) up to 30 yr after diagnosis. This raises the possibility that diabetes can be cured or ameliorated by stopping the autoimmune destructive process after initial diagnosis (secondary prevention).

Immunosuppressants like cyclosporine have been tested for this purpose, but while they may prolong the honeymoon period, they are associated with significant side effects and are only effective as long as they are being administered, so their use for this purpose has been abandoned. Trials using CD3 antibodies have been more promising, but some patients developed flulike symptoms and reactivation of Epstein-Barr virus infection. Further trials of this therapy and other therapies targeted at various components of T cells and β cells are planned or ongoing.

The possibility of using glucagon-like peptide (GLP-1) agonists (e.g., exenatide) alone or in combination with immunomodulatory therapies is also being explored as these agents are capable of increasing β cell mass in animals.

PATHOPHYSIOLOGY

Insulin performs a critical role in the storage and retrieval of cellular fuel. Its secretion in response to feeding is exquisitely modulated by the interplay of neural, hormonal, and substrate-related mechanisms to permit controlled disposition of ingested foodstuff as energy for immediate or future use. Insulin levels must be lowered to then mobilize stored energy during the fasted state. Thus, in normal metabolism, there are regular swings between the postprandial, high-insulin anabolic state and the fasted, low-insulin catabolic state that affect liver, muscle, and adipose tissue (Table 583-1). T1DM is a progressive low-insulin catabolic state in which feeding does not reverse but rather exaggerates these catabolic processes. With moderate insulinopenia, glucose utilization by muscle and fat decreases and postprandial hyperglycemia appears. At even lower insulin levels, the liver produces excessive glucose via glycogenolysis and gluconeogenesis, and fasting hyperglycemia begins. Hyperglycemia produces an osmotic diuresis (glycosuria) when the renal threshold is exceeded (180 mg/dL; 10 mmol/L). The resulting loss of calories and electrolytes, as well as the persistent dehydration, produce a physiologic stress with hypersecretion of stress hormones (epinephrine, cortisol, growth hormone, and glucagon). These hormones, in turn, contribute to the metabolic decompensation by further impairing insulin secretion (epinephrine), by antagonizing its action (epinephrine, cortisol, growth hormone), and by promoting glycogenolysis, gluconeogenesis, lipolysis, and ketogenesis (glucagon, epinephrine, growth hormone, and cortisol) while decreasing glucose utilization and glucose clearance (epinephrine, growth hormone, cortisol).

The combination of insulin deficiency and elevated plasma values of the counter-regulatory hormones is also responsible for accelerated lipolysis and impaired lipid synthesis, with resulting increased plasma concentrations of total lipids, cholesterol, triglycerides, and free fatty acids. The hormonal interplay of insulin deficiency and glucagon excess shunts the free fatty acids into ketone body formation; the rate of formation of these ketone bodies, principally β-hydroxybutyrate and acetoacetate, exceeds the capacity for peripheral utilization and renal excretion. Accumulation of these keto acids results in metabolic acidosis (diabetic ketoacidosis, DKA) and compensatory rapid deep breathing in an attempt to excrete excess CO_2 (Kussmaul respiration). Acetone, formed by nonenzymatic conversion of acetoacetate, is responsible for the characteristic fruity odor of the breath. Ketones are excreted in the urine in association with cations and thus further increase losses of water and electrolyte. With progressive dehydration, acidosis, hyperosmolality, and diminished cerebral oxygen utilization, consciousness becomes impaired, and the patient ultimately becomes comatose.

TABLE 583-1 INFLUENCE OF FEEDING (HIGH INSULIN) OR OF FASTING (LOW INSULIN) ON SOME METABOLIC PROCESSES IN LIVER, MUSCLE, AND ADIPOSE TISSUE*

	HIGH PLASMA INSULIN (POSTPRANDIAL STATE)	LOW PLASMA INSULIN (FASTED STATE)
Liver	Glucose uptake	Glucose production
	Glycogen synthesis	Glycogenolysis
	Absence of gluconeogenesis	Gluconeogenesis
	Lipogenesis	Absence of lipogenesis
	Absence of ketogenesis	Ketogenesis
Muscle	Glucose uptake	Absence of glucose uptake
	Glucose oxidation	Fatty acid and ketone oxidation
	Glycogen synthesis	Glycogenolysis
	Protein synthesis	Proteolysis and amino acid release
Adipose tissue	Glucose uptake	Absence of glucose uptake
	Lipid synthesis	Lipolysis and fatty acid release
	Triglyceride uptake	Absence of triglyceride uptake

*Insulin is considered to be the major factor governing these metabolic processes. Diabetes mellitus may be viewed as a permanent low-insulin state that, untreated, results in exaggerated fasting.

CLINICAL MANIFESTATIONS

As diabetes develops, symptoms steadily increase, reflecting the decreasing β-cell mass, worsening insulinopenia, progressive hyperglycemia, and eventual ketoacidosis. Initially, when only insulin reserve is limited, occasional hyperglycemia occurs. When the serum glucose increases above the renal threshold, intermittent polyuria or nocturia begins. With further β-cell loss, chronic hyperglycemia causes a more persistent diuresis, often with nocturnal enuresis, and polydipsia becomes more apparent. Female patients may develop monilial vaginitis due to the chronic glycosuria. Calories are lost in the urine (glycosuria), triggering a compensatory hyperphagia. If this hyperphagia does not keep pace with the glycosuria, loss of body fat ensues, with clinical weight loss and diminished subcutaneous fat stores. An average, healthy 10 yr old child consumes about 50% of 2,000 daily calories as carbohydrate. As that child becomes diabetic, daily losses of water and glucose may be 5 L and 250 g, respectively, representing 1,000 calories, or 50%, of the average daily caloric intake. Despite the child's compensatory increased intake of food, the body starves because unused calories are lost in the urine.

When extremely low insulin levels are reached, keto acids accumulate. At this point, the child quickly deteriorates. Keto acids produce abdominal discomfort, nausea, and emesis, preventing oral replacement of urinary water losses. Dehydration accelerates, causing weakness or orthostasis—but polyuria persists. As in any hyperosmotic state, the degree of dehydration may be clinically underestimated because intravascular volume is conserved at the expense of intracellular volume. Ketoacidosis exacerbates prior symptoms and leads to Kussmaul respirations (deep, heavy, rapid breathing), fruity breath odor (acetone), prolonged corrected Q-T interval (QTc), diminished neurocognitive function, and possible coma. About 20-40% of children with new-onset diabetes progress to DKA before diagnosis.

This entire progression happens much more quickly (over a few weeks) in younger children, probably owing to more aggressive autoimmune destruction of β cells. In infants, most of the weight loss is acute water loss because they will not have had prolonged caloriuria at diagnosis, and there will be an increased incidence of DKA at diagnosis. In adolescents, the course is usually more prolonged (over months), and most of the weight loss represents fat loss due to prolonged starvation. Additional weight loss due to acute dehydration may occur just before diagnosis. In any child, the progression of symptoms may be accelerated by the stress of an intercurrent illness or trauma, when counter-regulatory (stress) hormones overwhelm the limited insulin secretory capacity.

DIAGNOSIS

The diagnosis of T1DM is usually straightforward. Although most symptoms are nonspecific, the most important clue is an inappropriate polyuria in any child with dehydration, poor weight gain, or "the flu." Hyperglycemia, glycosuria, and ketonuria can be determined quickly. Nonfasting blood glucose greater than 200 mg/dL (11.1 mmol/L) with typical symptoms is diagnostic with or without ketonuria. In the obese child, T2DM must be considered (see Type 2 Diabetes Mellitus, later). Once hyperglycemia is confirmed, it is prudent to determine whether DKA is present (especially if ketonuria is found) and to evaluate electrolyte abnormalities—even if signs of dehydration are minimal. A baseline hemoglobin A_{1C} (HbA_{1c}) allows an estimate of the duration of hyperglycemia and provides an initial value by which to compare the effectiveness of subsequent therapy.

In the nonobese child, testing for autoimmunity to β cells is not necessary. Other autoimmunities associated with T1DM should be sought, including celiac disease (by tissue transglutaminase IgA and total IgA) and thyroiditis (by antithyroid peroxidase and antithyroglobulin antibodies). Because significant physiologic distress can disrupt the pituitary-thyroid axis, free thyroxine (T_4) and thyroid-stimulating hormone (TSH) levels should be checked after the child is stable for a few weeks.

Rarely, a child has transient hyperglycemia with glycosuria while under substantial physical stress. This usually resolves permanently during recovery from the stressors. Stress-produced hyperglycemia can reflect a limited insulin reserve temporarily revealed by counter-regulatory hormones. A child with temporary hyperglycemia should therefore be monitored for the development of symptoms of persistent hyperglycemia and tested if such symptoms occur. Formal testing in a child who remains clinically asymptomatic is not necessary.

Routine screening procedures, such as postprandial determinations of blood glucose or screening oral glucose tolerance tests, have yielded low detection rates in healthy, asymptomatic children, even among those considered at risk, such as siblings of diabetic children. Accordingly, such screening procedures are not recommended in children.

Diabetic Ketoacidosis

DKA is the end result of the metabolic abnormalities resulting from a severe deficiency of insulin or insulin effectiveness. The latter occurs during stress as counter-regulatory hormones block insulin action. DKA occurs in 20-40% of children with new-onset diabetes and in children with known diabetes who omit insulin doses or who do not successfully manage an intercurrent illness. DKA may be arbitrarily classified as mild, moderate, or severe (Table 583-2), and the range of symptoms depends on the depth of ketoacidosis. There is a large amount of ketonuria, an increased ion gap, a decreased serum bicarbonate (or total CO_2) and pH, and an elevated effective serum osmolality, indicating hypertonic dehydration.

TREATMENT

Therapy is tailored to the degree of insulinopenia at presentation. Most children with new diabetes (60-80%) have mild to moderate symptoms, have minimal dehydration with no history of emesis, and have not progressed to ketoacidosis. Once DKA has resolved in the newly diagnosed child, therapy is transitioned to that described for children with nonketotic onset. Children with previously diagnosed diabetes who develop DKA are usually transitioned to their previous insulin regimen.

Table 583-2 CLASSIFICATION OF DIABETIC KETOACIDOSIS

	NORMAL	MILD	MODERATE	SEVERE†
CO_2 (mEq/L, venous)*	20-28	16-20	10-15	<10
pH (venous)*	7.35-7.45	7.25-7.35	7.15-7.25	<7.15
Clinical	No change	Oriented, alert but fatigued	Kussmaul respirations; oriented but sleepy; arousable	Kussmaul or depressed respirations; sleepy to depressed sensorium to coma

*CO_2 and pH measurement are method dependent; normal ranges may vary.
†Severe hypernatremia (corrected Na >150 mEq/L) would also be classified as severe diabetic ketoacidosis.

New-Onset Diabetes without Ketoacidosis

Excellent diabetes control involves many goals: to maintain a balance between tight glucose control and avoiding hypoglycemia, to eliminate polyuria and nocturia, to prevent ketoacidosis, and to permit normal growth and development with minimal effect on lifestyle. Therapy encompasses initiation and adjustment of insulin, extensive teaching of the child and caretakers, and reestablishment of the life routines. Each aspect should be addressed early in the overall care. Ideally, therapy can begin in the outpatient setting, with complete team staffing by a pediatric endocrinologist, experienced nursing staff, dietitians with training as diabetes educators, and a social worker. Close contact between the diabetes team and family must be assured. Otherwise, initial therapy should be done in the hospital setting.

Insulin Therapy

Several factors influence the initial daily insulin dose per kilogram of body weight. The dose is usually higher in pubertal children. It is higher in those who have to restore greater deficits of body glycogen, protein, and fat stores and who, therefore, have higher initial caloric capacity. On the other hand, most children with new-onset diabetes have some residual β-cell function (the honeymoon period), which reduces exogenous insulin needs. Children with long-standing diabetes and no insulin reserve require about 0.7 U/kg/day if prepubertal, 1.0 U/kg/day at midpuberty, and 1.2 U/kg/day by the end of puberty. A reasonable dose in the newly diagnosed child, then, is about 60-70% of the full replacement dose based on pubertal status. The optimal insulin dose can only be determined empirically, with frequent self-monitored blood glucose levels and insulin adjustment by the diabetes team. Residual β-cell function usually fades within a few months and is reflected as a steady increase in insulin requirements and wider glucose excursions.

The initial insulin schedule should be directed toward the optimal degree of glucose control in an attempt to duplicate the activity of the β cell. There are inherent limits to our ability to mimic the β cell. Exogenous insulin does not have a 1st pass to the liver, whereas 50% of pancreatic portal insulin is taken up by the liver, a key organ for the disposal of glucose; absorption of an exogenous dose continues despite hypoglycemia, whereas endogenous insulin release ceases and serum levels quickly lower with a normally rapid clearance; and absorption rate from an injection varies by injection site and patient activity level, whereas endogenous insulin is secreted directly into the portal circulation. Despite these fundamental physiologic differences, acceptable glucose control can be obtained with new insulin analogs used in a basal-bolus regimen, that is, with slow-onset, long-duration background insulin for between-meal glucose control and rapid-onset insulin at each meal.

All preanalog insulins form hexamers, which must dissociate into monomers subcutaneously before being absorbed into the circulation. Thus, a detectable effect for regular (R) insulin is delayed by 30-60 min after injection. This, in turn, requires delaying the meal 30-60 min after the injection for optimal effect—a delay rarely attained in a busy child's life. R has a wide peak and a long tail for bolus insulin (Figs. 583-6 and 583-7). This profile limits postprandial glucose control, produces prolonged peaks with excessive hypoglycemic effects between meals, and increases the risk of nighttime hypoglycemia. These unwanted between-meal effects often necessitate "feeding the insulin" with snacks and limiting the overall degree of blood glucose control. NPH and Lente insulins also have inherent limits because they do not create a peakless background insulin level (see Fig. 583-7*C-E*). This produces significant hypoglycemic effect during the

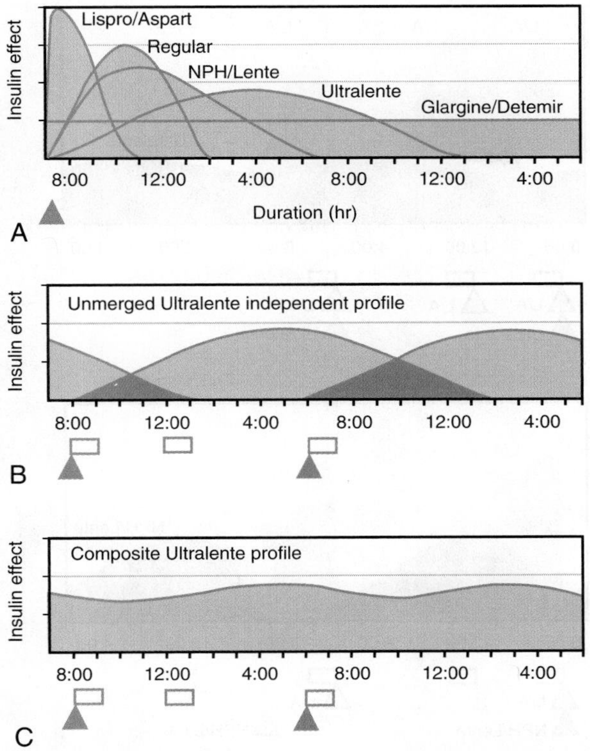

Figure 583-6 Approximate insulin effect profiles. Meals are shown as rectangles below time axis. *A*, The following relative peak effect and duration units are used: lispro/aspart, peak 20 for 4 hr; regular, peak 15 for 7 hr; NPH/Lente, peak 12 for 12 hr; Ultralente, peak 9 for 18 hr; glargine, peak 5 for 24 hr. Though Lente and Ultralente are no longer manufactured, they are shown to give historical comparison to newer insulin analogs. ▲, Injection time. *B*, Two Ultralente injections given at breakfast and supper. Note overlap of profiles. *C*, Composite curve showing approximate cumulative insulin effect for the 2 Ultralente injections. This composite view is much more useful to the patient, parents, and medical personnel because it shows important combined effects of multiple insulin injections with variable absorption characteristics and overlapping durations.

midrange of their duration. Thus, it is often difficult to predict their interaction with fast-acting insulins. When R is combined with NPH or Lente (see Fig. 583-7*E*), the composite insulin profile poorly mimics normal endogenous insulin secretion. There are broad areas of excessive insulin effect alternating with insufficient effect throughout the day and night. Lente and Ultralente insulins have been discontinued and are no longer available.

Lispro (L) and aspart (A), insulin analogs, are absorbed much quicker because they do not form hexamers. They provide discrete pulses with little if any overlap and short tail effect. This allows better control of post-meal glucose increase and reduces between-meal or nighttime hypoglycemia (see Fig. 583-7*A*). The long-acting analog glargine (G) creates a much flatter 24-hr profile, making it easier to predict the combined effect of a rapid bolus (L or A) on top of the basal insulin, producing a more physiologic pattern of insulin effect (see Fig. 583-7*A*). Postprandial glucose elevations are better controlled, and between-meal and nighttime hypoglycemia are reduced.

Ultralente (UL) given twice a day provided a reasonable basal profile (see Fig. 593-6C) and was quite effective when used with lispro or aspart (see Fig. 583-7*B*). Since UL is no longer available, G may be given every 12 hr in young children if a single daily dose of G does not produce complete 24-hr basal coverage. The basal insulin glargine should be 25-30% of the total dose in toddlers and 40-50% in older children. The remaining portion of the total daily dose is divided evenly as bolus injections for the 3 meals. A simple 3- or 4-step dosing schedule is begun based on the blood glucose level (Table 583-3). As soon as the family is taught to calculate the carbohydrate content of meals, bolus insulin can be more accurately dosed by both the carbohydrate content of the meal as well as the ambient glucose (see Table 583-3).

Frequent blood glucose monitoring and insulin adjustment are necessary in the 1st weeks as the child returns to routine activities and adapts to a new nutritional schedule, and as the total daily insulin requirements are determined. The major physiologic limit to tight control is hypoglycemia. Intensive control dramatically reduces the risk of long-term vascular complications; it is associated with a 3-fold increase in severe hypoglycemia. Use of insulin analogs moderates but does not eliminate this problem.

Some families may be unable to administer 4 daily injections. In these cases, a compromise may be needed. A 3-injection regimen combining NPH with a rapid analog bolus at breakfast, a rapid-acting analog bolus at supper, and NPH at bedtime may provide fair glucose control. Further compromise to a 2-injection regimen (NPH and rapid analog at breakfast and supper) may occasionally be needed. However, such a schedule would provide poor coverage for lunch and early morning, and would increase the risk of hypoglycemia at midmorning and early night.

Insulin Pump Therapy

Continuous subcutaneous insulin infusion (CSII) via battery-powered pumps provides a closer approximation of normal plasma insulin profiles and increased flexibility regarding timing of meals and snacks compared with conventional insulin injection regimens. Insulin pump models can be programmed with a patient's personal insulin dose algorithms, including the insulin to carbohydrate ratio and the correction scale for pre-meal glucose levels. The patient can enter his or her blood glucose level and the carbohydrate content of the meal, and the pump computer will calculate the proper insulin bolus dose. Insulin pump therapy in adolescents with T1DM is associated with improved metabolic control and reduced risk of severe hypoglycemia without affecting psychosocial outcomes. The use of overnight CSII improves the metabolic control in children aged 7-10 yr. CSII has also been useful in toddlers. CSII may not always improve metabolic control. Some studies show improvement in less than one half and worsening control (higher HbA_{1c}) in one fifth of patients. It is likely that the degree of glycemic control is mainly dependent on how closely patients adhere to the principles of diabetes self-care, regardless of the type of intensive insulin regimen. One benefit of pump therapy may be a reduction in severe hypoglycemia and associated seizures. Randomized trials comparing multiple daily insulin (MDI) regimen using glargine insulin and CSII in children with T1DM demonstrate similar metabolic control and frequency of hypoglycemic events.

It is anticipated that existing subcutaneous glucose sensors and external insulin pumps can be linked with an insulin delivery algorithm to create a completely automated closed-loop system. The development of a closed-loop insulin pump technology is currently being evaluated and has been an active area of research over the past several years. The development of such a system, with particular emphasis on creating a system mimicking the physiologic properties of the β cell is highly desirable. Closed-loop glucose control using an external sensor and insulin pump provided a means to achieve near-normal glucose concentrations in youth with T1DM during the overnight period. The addition of small manual priming bolus doses of insulin, given 15 min before meals, improved postprandial glycemic excursions.

Inhaled and Oral Insulin Therapies

Preprandial inhaled insulin is being evaluated in adults with T1DM and T2DM. The preliminary metabolic data are promising. Patients taking pre-meal inhaled insulin in combination with once daily bedtime long-acting insulin (Ultralente) injection achieved similar metabolic control compared with patients taking 2-3 daily injections of insulin. There was no significant difference

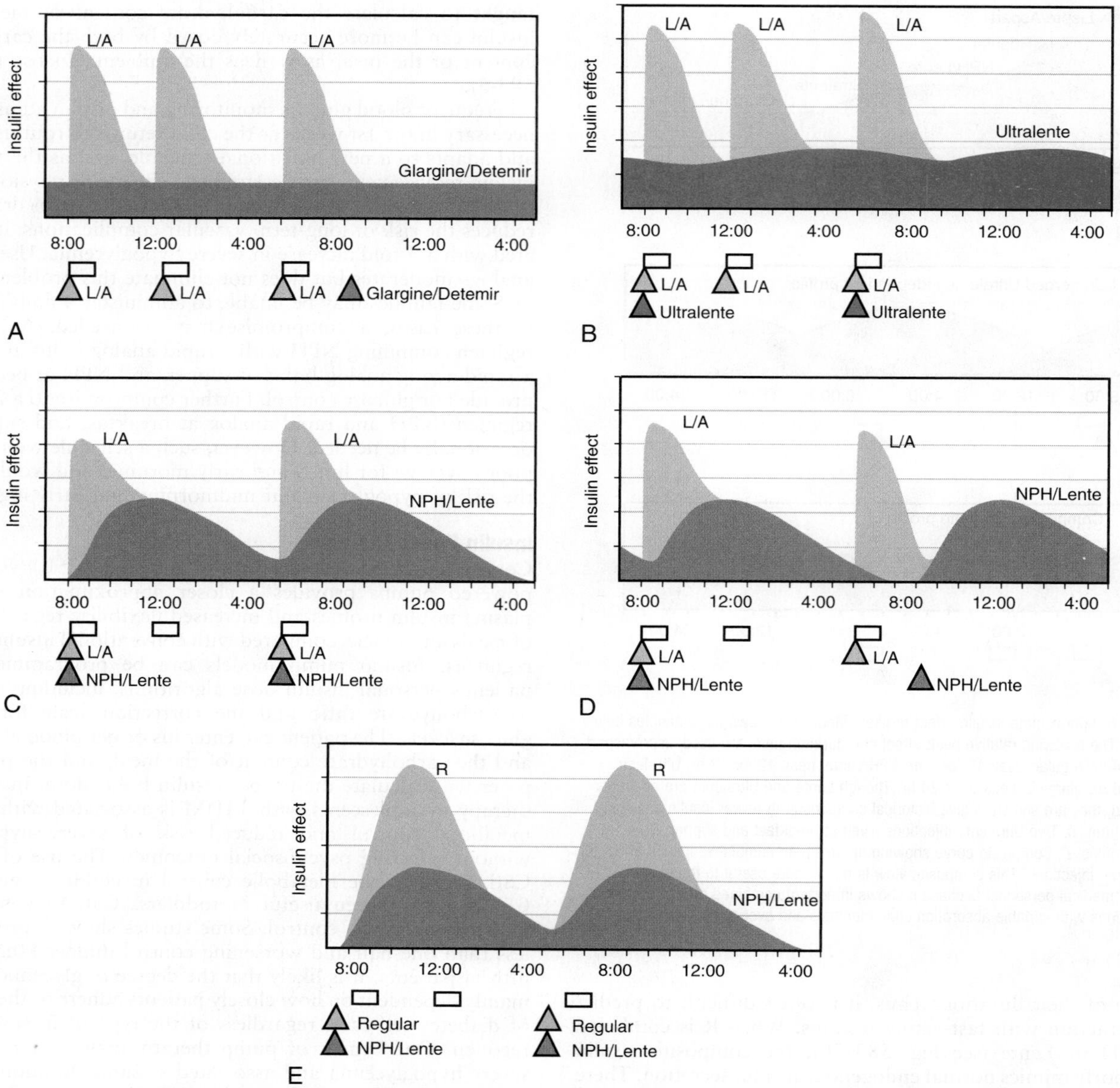

Figure 583-7 Approximate composite insulin effect profiles. Meals are shown as *rectangles* below time axis. Injections are shown as labeled *triangles*. L/A, lispro or aspart. Even though the fast- and long-acting insulins are shaded differently to show the addition of 1 insulin effect to another, the profile is changed to show the combined effect. For example, in the breakfast injection in *C*, the quick decline of L/A effect is blunted by the rising NPH/Lente effect, producing a broad tail, which slowly declines to baseline at supper. All profiles are idealized using average absorption and clearance rates. In typical clinical situations, these profiles vary among patients. A given patient has varying rates of absorption depending on the injection site, physical activity, and other variables. *A,* L or A pre-meal; glargine at bedtime. The rapid onset and short duration of L or A reduce overlap between pre-meal injections, and there is no extended nighttime action. This reduces the risk of hypoglycemia. Glargine provides a steady basal profile that simplifies prediction of bolus insulin effect. *B,* L or A pre-meal; Ultralente at breakfast and supper. Ultralente produces a basal profile similar to that seen with glargine. Some excessive insulin effect, however, is seen before supper and at nighttime. *C,* L or A pre-meal; NPH or Lente at breakfast and supper. The broad peak of NPH or Lente produces substantial risk of hypoglycemia before lunch and during the early hours of the night. The waning insulin effect before supper and breakfast may also allow breakthrough hyperglycemia. *D,* L or A pre-meal; NPH or Lente at breakfast and bedtime. Moving the evening long-acting insulin helps to cover the pre-breakfast hours, but the risk of nighttime lows persists. *E,* Regular and NPH or Lente at breakfast and supper. This produces the least physiologic profile, with large excesses before lunch and during the early night, combined with poor coverage before supper and breakfast. Though Lente and Ultralente are no longer manufactured, they are shown to give historical comparison to newer insulin analogs.

in the frequency of hypoglycemic episodes between the 2 groups. There have been reports of pulmonary fibrosis in a small number of patients, necessitating further monitoring and evaluation of patients taking inhaled insulin before this route of insulin administration is deemed safe. Bioavailability of inhaled insulin is increased with smoking and reduced with asthma.

Pre-meal oral insulin (Oralin) has been evaluated in comparison with oral hypoglycemic agents, mostly in patients with T2DM. The clinical data appear promising, but further evaluation of efficacy in T1DM is needed. In addition, pre-meal inhaled insulin (Exubera), a powder form of recombinant human insulin, has been evaluated for use in individuals with T1DM and T2DM. Although Exubera insulin was shown to be effective and safe in long-term clinical initial trials with minor risk of lung fibrosis and cancer in smokers, it was discontinued by Pfizer Pharmaceuticals in 2008 due to high cost to patients compared to subcutaneous insulin. Currently, other formulations of inhaled insulin are under investigations in clinical trials in patients with T1DM and T2DM.

Amylin-Based Adjunct Therapy

Pramlintide acetate, a synthetic analog of amylin, may be of therapeutic value combined with insulin therapy. In adolescents it has been shown to decrease postprandial hyperglycemia, insulin dosage, gastric emptying, and HbA_{1c} levels. It is given as a subcutaneous dose before meals.

Basic and Advanced Diabetes Education

Therapy consists not only of initiation and adjustment of insulin dose but also of education of the patient and family. Teaching is most efficiently provided by experienced diabetes educators and nutritionists. In the acute phase, the family must learn the "basics," which includes monitoring the child's blood glucose and urine ketones, preparing and injecting the correct insulin dose subcutaneously at the proper time, recognizing and treating low blood glucose reactions, and having a basic meal plan. Most families are trying to adjust psychologically to the new diagnosis of diabetes in their child and thus have a limited ability to retain new information. Written materials covering these basic topics help the family during the 1st few days.

Children and their families are also required to complete advanced self-management classes in order to facilitate implementation of flexible insulin management. These educational classes will help patients and their families acquire skills for managing diabetes during athletic activities and sick days.

Table 583-3 SUBCUTANEOUS INSULIN DOSING

AGE (yr)	TARGET GLUCOSE (mg/dL)	TOTAL DAILY INSULIN (U/kg/day)*	BASAL INSULIN, % OF TOTAL DAILY DOSE	BOLUS† INSULIN Units Added per 100 mg/dL Above Target	BOLUS† INSULIN Units Added per 15 g at Meal
0-5	100-200	0.6-0.7	25-30	0.50	0.50
5-12	80-150	0.7-1.0	40-50	0.75	0.75
12-18	80-130	1.0-1.2	40-50	1.0-2.0‡	1.0-2.0

*Newly diagnosed children in the "honeymoon" may only need 60-70% of a full replacement dose. Total daily dose per kg increases with puberty.
†Newly diagnosed children who do not use carbohydrate dosing should divide the nonbasal portion of the daily insulin dose into equal doses for each meal. A dosing scale is then added for each dose. For example: a 6 yr old child who weighs 20 kg needs about (0.7 U/kg/24 hr × 20 kg) = 14 U/24 hr with 7 U (50%) as basal and 7 U as total daily bolus. Give basal as glargine at bedtime. Give 2 U lispro or aspart before each meal if the blood glucose is within target; subtract 1 U if below target; add 0.75 U for each 100 mg/dL above target (round the dose to the nearest 0.5 U).
‡For finer control, extra insulin may be added in 50-mg/dL increments.

Ketoacidosis

Severe insulinopenia (or lack of effective insulin action) results in a physiologic cascade of events in 3 general pathways:

1. Excessive glucose production coupled with reduced glucose utilization raises serum glucose. This produces an osmotic diuresis, with loss of fluid and electrolytes, dehydration, and activation of the renin-angiotensin-aldosterone axis with accelerated potassium loss. If glucose elevation and dehydration are severe and persist for several hours, the risk of cerebral edema increases.
2. Increased catabolic processes result in cellular losses of sodium, potassium, and phosphate.
3. Increased release of free fatty acids from peripheral fat stores supplies substrate for hepatic keto acid production. When keto acids accumulate, buffer systems are depleted and a metabolic acidosis ensues. Therapy must address both the initiating event in this cascade (insulinopenia) and the subsequent physiologic disruptions.

Reversal of DKA is associated with inherent risks that include hypoglycemia, hypokalemia, and cerebral edema. Any protocol must be used with caution and close monitoring of the patient. Adjustments based on sound medical judgment may be necessary for any given level of DKA (Table 583-4).

Hyperglycemia and Dehydration

Insulin must be given at the beginning of therapy to accelerate movement of glucose into cells, to subdue hepatic glucose production, and to halt the movement of fatty acids from the periphery to the liver. An initial insulin bolus does not speed recovery and may increase the risk of hypokalemia and hypoglycemia. Therefore, insulin infusion is begun **without** a bolus at a rate of 0.1 U/kg/hr. This approximates maximal insulin output in normal subjects during an oral glucose tolerance test. Rehydration also lowers glucose levels by improving renal perfusion and enhancing renal excretion. The combination of these therapies usually causes a rapid initial decline in serum glucose levels. Once glucose goes below 180 mg/dL (10 mmol/L), the osmotic diuresis stops and rehydration accelerates without further increase in the infusion rate.

Repair of hyperglycemia occurs well before correction of acidosis. Therefore, insulin is still needed to control fatty acid release after normal glucose levels are reached. To continue the insulin infusion without causing hypoglycemia, glucose must be added to the infusion, usually as a 5% solution. Glucose should be added when the serum glucose has decreased to about 250 mg/dL (14 mmol/L) so that there is sufficient time to adjust the

Table 583-4 DIABETIC KETOACIDOSIS (DKA) TREATMENT PROTOCOL

TIME	THERAPY	COMMENTS
1st hr	10-20 mL/kg IV bolus 0.9% NaCl or LR Insulin drip at 0.05 to 0.10 µ/kg/hr	Quick volume expansion; may be repeated. NPO. Monitor I/O, neurologic status. Use flow sheet. Have mannitol at bedside; 1g/kg IV push for cerebral edema.
2nd hr until DKA resolution	0.45% NaCl: plus continue insulin drip 20 mEq/L KPhos and 20 mEq/L KAc 5% glucose if blood sugar >250 mg/dL (14 mmol/L)	$\text{IV rate} = \frac{85\text{ mL/kg} + \text{maintenance} - \text{bolus}}{23\text{ hr}}$
		If K <3 mEq/L, give 0.5 to 1.0 mEq/kg as oral K solution OR increase IV K to 80 mEq/L
Variable	Oral intake with subcutaneous insulin	No emesis; CO_2 ≥16 mEq/L; normal electrolytes
Note that the initial IV bolus is considered part of the total fluid allowed in the 1st 24 hr and is subtracted before calculating the IV rate.		
Maintenance (24 hr) = 100 mL/kg (for the 1st 10 kg) + 50 mL/kg (for the 2nd 10 kg) + 25 mL/kg (for all remaining kg)		
Sample calculation for a 30-kg child:		
1st hr = 300 mL IV bolus 0.9% NaCl or LR		
$\text{2nd and subsequent hours} = \frac{(85\text{ mL} \times 30) + 1750\text{ mL} - 300\text{ mL}}{23\text{ hr}} = \frac{175\text{ mL}}{\text{hr}}$ (0.45% NaCl with 20 mEq/L Kphos and 20 mEq/LKAC)		

I/O, input and output (urine, emesis); KAc, potassium acetate; KPhos, potassium phosphate; LR, lactated Ringer solution; NaCl, sodium chloride.

infusion before the serum glucose falls further. The insulin infusion can also be lowered from the initial maximal rate once hyperglycemia has resolved.

Repair of fluid deficits must be tempered by the potential risk of cerebral edema. It is prudent to approach any child in any hyperosmotic state with cautious rehydration. The effective serum osmolality ($E_{osm} = 2 \times [Na_{uncorrected}] + [glucose]$) is an accurate index of tonicity of the body fluids, reflecting intracellular and extracellular hydration better than measured plasma osmolality. It is calculated with sodium and glucose in mmol/L. This value is usually elevated at the beginning of therapy and should steadily normalize. A rapid decline, or a slow decline to a subnormal range, may indicate an excess of free water entering the vascular space and an increasing risk of cerebral edema. Therefore, patients should not be allowed oral fluids until rehydration is well progressed and significant electrolyte shifts are no longer likely. Limited ice chips may be given as a minimal oral intake. All fluid intake and output should be closely monitored.

Calculation of fluid deficits using clinical signs is difficult in children with DKA because intravascular volume is better maintained in the hypertonic state. For any degree of tachycardia, delayed capillary refill, decreased skin temperature, or orthostatic blood pressure change, the child with DKA will be more dehydrated than the child with a normotonic fluid deficit. The protocol in Table 583-4 corrects a deficit of 85 mL/kg (8.5% dehydration) for all patients in the 1st 24 hr. Children with mild DKA rehydrate earlier and can be switched to oral intake, whereas those with severe DKA and a greater volume deficit require 30-36 hr with this protocol. This more gradual rehydration of the child with severe DKA is an inherent safety feature. The initial intravenous bolus (20 mL/kg of glucose-free isotonic sodium salt solution such as Ringer lactate or 0.9% sodium chloride) for all patients ensures a quick volume expansion and may be repeated if clinical improvement is not quickly seen. This bolus is given as isotonic saline because the patient is inevitably hypertonic, keeping most of the initial infusion in the intravascular space. Subsequent fluid is hypotonic to repair the free water deficit, to allow intracellular rehydration, and to allow a more appropriate replacement of ongoing hypotonic urine losses.

The initial serum sodium is usually normal or low because of the osmolar dilution of hyperglycemia and the effect of an elevated sodium-free lipid fraction. An estimate of the reconstituted, or "true," serum sodium for any given glucose level above 100 mg/dL (5.6 mmol/L) is calculated as follows:

$$\frac{[Na^+] + \text{glucose} - \mathit{100} \times 1.6}{100}$$

where glucose is in mg/dL, or

$$\frac{[Na^+] + \text{glucose} - \mathit{5.6} \times 1.6}{5.6}$$

where glucose is in mmol/L.

The sodium should increase by about 1.6 mmol/L for each 100 mg/dL decline in the glucose. The corrected sodium is usually normal or slightly elevated and indicates moderate hypernatremic dehydration. If the corrected value is greater than 150 mmol/L, severe hypernatremic dehydration may be present and may require slower fluid replacement. The sodium should steadily increase with therapy. *Declining sodium may indicate excessive free water accumulation and the risk of cerebral edema.*

Catabolic Losses

Both the metabolic shift to a catabolic predominance and the acidosis move potassium and phosphate from the cell to the serum. The osmotic diuresis, the kaliuretic effect of the hyperaldosteronism, and the ketonuria then accelerate renal losses of potassium and phosphate. Sodium is also lost with the diuresis, but free water losses are greater than isotonic losses. With prolonged illness and severe DKA, total body losses can approach 10-13 mEq/kg of sodium, 5-6 mEq/kg of potassium, and 4-5 mEq/kg of phosphate. These losses continue for several hours during therapy until the catabolic state is reversed and the diuresis is controlled. For example, 50% of infused sodium may be lost in the urine during IV therapy. Even though the sodium deficit may be repaired within 24 hr, intracellular potassium and phosphate may not be completely restored for several days.

Although patients with DKA have a total body potassium deficit, the initial serum level is often normal or elevated. This is due to the movement of potassium from the intracellular space to the serum, both as part of the keto acid buffering process and as part of the catabolic shift. These effects are reversed with therapy, and potassium returns to the cell. Improved hydration increases renal blood flow, allowing for increased excretion of potassium in the elevated aldosterone state. The net effect is often a dramatic decline in serum potassium levels, especially in severe DKA, and can precipitate changes in cardiac conductivity, flattening of T waves, and prolongation of the QRS complex and can cause skeletal muscle weakness or ileus. The risk of myocardial dysfunction is increased with shock and acidosis. Potassium levels must be closely followed and electrocardiographic monitoring continued until DKA is substantially resolved. If needed, the parenteral potassium can be increased to 80 mEq/L or an oral supplement can be given if there is no emesis. Rarely, the IV insulin must be temporarily stopped.

It is unclear whether phosphate deficits contribute to symptoms of DKA such as generalized muscle weakness. In pediatric patients, a deficit has not been shown to compromise oxygen delivery via a deficiency of 2,3-diphosphoglycerate (2,3-DPG). Because the patient will receive an excess of chloride, which may aggravate acidosis, it is prudent to use potassium phosphate rather than potassium chloride as a potassium source. Potassium acetate is also used, because it provides an additional buffer.

Pancreatitis is occasionally seen with DKA, especially if prolonged abdominal distress is present; serum amylase may be elevated. If the serum lipase is not elevated, the amylase is likely nonspecific or salivary in origin. Serum creatinine adjusted for age may be falsely elevated owing to interference by ketones in the autoanalyzer methodology. An initial elevated value rarely indicates renal failure and should be rechecked when the child is less ketonemic. Blood urea nitrogen (BUN) may be elevated with prerenal azotemia and should be rechecked as the child is rehydrated. Mildly elevated creatine or BUN is not a reason to withhold potassium therapy if good urinary output is present.

Keto Acid Accumulation

Low insulin infusion rates (0.02-0.05 U/kg/hr) are usually sufficient to stop peripheral release of fatty acids, thereby eliminating the flow of substrate for ketogenesis. Therefore, the initial infusion rate may be decreased if blood glucose levels go below 150 mg/dL (8 mmol/L) despite the addition of glucose to the infusion. Ketogenesis continues until fatty acid substrates already in the liver are depleted, but this production declines much more quickly without new substrate inflow. Bicarbonate buffers, regenerated by the distal renal tubule and by metabolism of ketone bodies, steadily repair the acidosis once keto acid production is controlled. *Bicarbonate therapy is rarely necessary and may even increase the risk of hypokalemia and cerebral edema.*

There should be a steady increase in pH and serum bicarbonate as therapy progresses. Kussmaul respirations should abate and abdominal pain resolve. Persistent acidosis may indicate inadequate insulin or fluid therapy, infection, or rarely lactic acidosis. Urine ketones may be positive long after ketoacidosis has resolved because the nitroprusside reaction routinely used to measure urine ketones by dipstick measures only acetoacetate. During DKA, most excess ketones are β-hydroxybutyrate, which increases the normal ratio to acetoacetate from 3 : 1 to as high as

8:1. With resolution of the acidosis, β-hydroxybutyrate converts to acetoacetate, which is excreted into the urine and detected by the dipstick test. Therefore, persistent ketonuria may not accurately reflect the degree of clinical improvement and should not be relied on as an indicator of therapeutic failure.

All patients with DKA should be checked for initiating events that may have triggered the metabolic decompensation.

DKA Protocol (See Table 583-4)

Even though DKA can be of variable severity, a common approach to all cases simplifies the therapeutic regimen and can be safely used for most children. Fluids are best calculated based on weight, not body surface area (m^2), because heights are rarely available for the calculation. The Milwaukee protocol has been used for more than 20 yr in a large clinic setting with no deaths and no neurologic sequelae in any child treated initially with this protocol. It can be used for children of all ages and with all degrees of DKA. It is designed to restore most electrolyte deficits, to reverse the acidosis, and to rehydrate the moderately ill child in about 24 hr. A standard water deficit (85 mL/kg) is assumed. This amount, when added to maintenance, yields about 4 L/m^2 for children of all sizes. Children with milder DKA recover in 10-20 hr (and need less total IV fluid before switching to oral intake), whereas those with more severe DKA require 30-36 hr with this protocol. Any child can be easily transitioned to oral intake and subcutaneous insulin when DKA has essentially resolved (total CO_2 >15 mEq/L; pH >7.30; sodium stable between 135 and 145 mEq/L; no emesis). The IV is capped, and the 1st dose of subcutaneous insulin is given with a meal. Children with mild DKA often can be discharged after a few hours of therapy in the emergency department if adequate follow-up is provided.

A flow sheet is mandatory for accurate monitoring of changes in acidosis, electrolytes, fluid balance, and clinical status, especially if the patient is transferred from the emergency department to an inpatient setting with new caretakers. This flow sheet is best implemented by a central computer system, which allows for rapid update and wide availability of results, as well as rule-driven highlighting of critical values. A paper flow sheet suffices if it stays with the patient, is kept current, and is reviewed frequently by the physician. Any flow sheet should include columns for serial electrolytes, pH, glucose, and fluid balance. Blood testing should occur every 1-2 hr for children with severe DKA and every 3-4 hr for those with mild to moderate DKA.

Cerebral Edema

Cerebral edema complicating DKA remains the major cause of morbidity and mortality in children and adolescents with T1DM. However, its etiology remains unknown. A case-control study of DKA, suggested that baseline acidosis and abnormalities of sodium, potassium, and BUN concentrations were important predictors of risk of cerebral edema. Early administration of insulin and high volumes of fluid were also identified as risk factors. The incidence of cerebral in children with DKA has not changed over the past 15-20 yr, despite the widespread introduction of gradual rehydration protocols during this interval. This study confirmed the previously published observation that radiographic imaging is frequently unhelpful in making the diagnosis of cerebral edema immediately after presentation of symptoms. Even though this protocol has a long safety record, each patient must be closely monitored. For all but the mildest cases, this includes frequent neurologic checks for any signs of increasing intracranial pressure, such as a change of consciousness, depressed respiration, worsening headache, bradycardia, apnea, pupillary changes, papilledema, posturing, and seizures. Mannitol must be readily available for use at the earliest sign of cerebral edema. The physician must also keep informed of the laboratory changes; hypokalemia or hypoglycemia can occur rapidly. Children with moderate to severe DKA have a higher overall risk and should be treated in an intensive care environment. This protocol may not be appropriate for some patients such as the severely hypernatremic child (corrected sodium >150 mEq/L), who may need slower rehydration with a longer duration of isotonic fluids.

Some residual β-cell function is seen even in children with DKA. This function may improve as the child recovers from the effects of hyperglycemia and elevated counter-regulatory hormones. This residual secretion may necessitate a reduction in the initial total subcutaneous insulin dose used in the 1st few days of therapy.

Nonketotic Hyperosmolar Coma

This syndrome is characterized by severe hyperglycemia (blood glucose >800 mg/dL), absence of or only slight ketosis, nonketotic acidosis, severe dehydration, depressed sensorium or frank coma, and various neurologic signs that may include grand mal seizures, hyperthermia, hemiparesis, and positive Babinski signs. Respirations are usually shallow, but coexistent metabolic (lactic) acidosis may be manifested by Kussmaul breathing. Serum osmolarity is commonly 350 mOsm/kg or greater. This condition is uncommon in children; among adults, mortality rates have been high, possibly in part because of delays in recognition and institution of appropriate therapy. In children, there has been a high incidence of pre-existing neurologic damage. Profound hyperglycemia may develop over a period of days and, initially, the obligatory osmotic polyuria and dehydration may be partially compensated for by increasing fluid intake. With progression of disease, thirst becomes impaired, possibly because of alteration of the hypothalamic thirst center by hyperosmolarity and, in some instances, because of a pre-existing defect in the hypothalamic osmoregulating mechanism.

The low production of ketones is attributed mainly to the hyperosmolarity, which in vitro blunts the lipolytic effect of epinephrine and the antilipolytic effect of residual insulin; blunting of lipolysis by the therapeutic use of β-adrenergic blockers may contribute to the syndrome. Depression of consciousness is closely correlated with the degree of hyperosmolarity in this condition as well as in DKA. Hemoconcentration may also predispose to cerebral arterial and venous thromboses.

Treatment of nonketotic hyperosmolar coma is directed at rapid repletion of the vascular volume deficit and very slow correction of the hyperosmolar state. One half isotonic saline (0.45% NaCl; some use normal saline) is administered at a rate estimated to replace 50% of the volume deficit in the 1st 12 hr, and the remainder is administered during the ensuing 24 hr. The rate of infusion and the saline concentration are titrated to result in a slow decline of serum osmolality. When the blood glucose concentration approaches 300 mg/dL, the hydrating fluid should be changed to 5% dextrose in 0.2 normal (N) saline. Approximately 20 mEq/L of potassium chloride should be added to each of these fluids to prevent hypokalemia. Serum potassium and plasma glucose concentrations should be monitored at 2 hr intervals for the 1st 12 hr and at 4 hr intervals for the next 24 hr to permit appropriate adjustments of administered potassium and insulin.

Insulin can be given by continuous IV infusion beginning with the 2nd hr of fluid therapy. Blood glucose may decrease dramatically with fluid therapy alone. The IV insulin dosage should be 0.05 U/kg/hr of regular (fast-acting) rather than 0.1 U/kg/hr as advocated for patients with DKA.

Nutritional Management

Nutrition plays an essential role in the management of patients with T1DM. This is of critical importance during childhood and adolescence, when appropriate energy intake is required to meet the needs for energy expenditure, growth, and pubertal development. Nutritional treatment alone or in combination with appropriate insulin therapy averts or relieves symptoms of hyperglycemia in diabetic patients. Moreover, nutritional practices may influence the development of long-term complications of diabetes (diabetic nephropathy). There are no special nutritional requirements for

Table 583-5 CALORIE NEEDS FOR CHILDREN AND YOUNG ADULTS

AGE	kcal REQUIRED/kg BODY WEIGHT*
CHILDREN	
0-12 mo	120
1-10 yr	100-75
YOUNG WOMEN	
11-15 yr	35
≥16 yr	30
YOUNG MEN	
11-15 yr	80-55 (65)
16-20 yr	
Average activity	40
Very physically active	50
Sedentary	30

Numbers in parentheses are means.
*Gradual decline in calories per unit weight as age increases.
From *Nutrition guide for professionals: diabetes education and meal planning,* Alexandria, VA, and Chicago, IL, 1988, The American Diabetes Association and The American Dietetic Association.

Table 583-6 SUMMARY OF NUTRITION GUIDELINES FOR CHILDREN AND/OR ADOLESCENTS WITH TYPE 1 DIABETES MELLITUS

NUTRITION CARE PLAN		
Promotes optimal compliance.		
Incorporates goals of management: normal growth and development, control of blood glucose, maintenance of optimal nutritional status, and prevention of complications. Uses staged approach.		
NUTRIENT RECOMMENDATIONS AND DISTRIBUTION		
NUTRIENT	**(%) of CALORIES**	**RECOMMENDED DAILY INTAKE**
Carbohydrate	Will vary	High fiber, especially soluble fiber; optimal amount unknown
Fiber	>20g per day	
Protein	12-20	
Fat	<30	
Saturated	<10	
Polyunsaturated	6-8	
Monounsaturated	Remainder of fat allowance	
Cholesterol		300 mg
Sodium		Avoid excessive; limit to 3,000-4,000 mg if hypertensive
ADDITIONAL RECOMMENDATIONS		
Energy: If using measured diet, reevaluate prescribed energy level at least every 3 mo.		
Protein: High-protein intakes may contribute to diabetic nephropathy. Low intakes may reverse preclinical nephropathy. Therefore, 12-20% of energy is recommended; lower end of range is preferred. In guiding toward the end of the range, a staged approach is useful.		
Alcohol: Safe use of moderate alcohol consumption should be taught as routine anticipatory guidance as early as junior high school.		
Snacks: Snacks vary according to individual needs (generally 3 snacks per day for children; midafternoon and bedtime snacks for junior high children or teens).		
Alternative sweeteners: Use of a variety of sweeteners is suggested.		
Educational techniques: No single technique is superior. Choice of educational method used should be based on patient needs. Knowledge of variety of techniques is important. Follow-up education and support are required.		
Eating disorders: Best treatment is prevention. Unexplained poor control or severe hypoglycemia may indicate a potential eating disorder.		
Exercise: Education is vital to prevent delayed or immediate hypoglycemia and to prevent worsened hyperglycemia and ketosis.		

From Connell JE, Thomas-Doberson D: Nutritional management of children and adolescents with insulin-dependent diabetes mellitus: a review by the Diabetes Care and Education Dietetic Practice Group, *J Am Diet Assoc* 91:1556, 1991.

the diabetic child other than those for optimal growth and development. In outlining nutritional requirements for the child on the basis of age, sex, weight, and activity, food preferences, including cultural and ethnic ones, must be considered.

Total recommended caloric intake is based on size or surface area and can be obtained from standard tables (Tables 583-5 and 583-6). The caloric mixture should comprise approximately 55% carbohydrate, 30% fat, and 15% protein. Approximately 70% of the carbohydrate content should be derived from complex carbohydrates such as starch; intake of sucrose and highly refined sugars should be limited. Complex carbohydrates require prolonged digestion and absorption so that plasma glucose levels increase slowly, whereas glucose from refined sugars, including carbonated beverages, is rapidly absorbed and may cause wide swings in the metabolic pattern; carbonated beverages should be sugar free. Priority should be given to total calories and total carbohydrate consumed rather than its source. Carbohydrate counting has become a mainstay in the nutrition education and management of patients with DM. Each carbohydrate exchange unit is 15 g. Patients and their families are provided with information regarding the carbohydrate contents of different foods and food label reading. This allows patients to adjust their insulin dosage to their mealtime carbohydrate intake. The use of carbohydrate counting and insulin to carbohydrate ratios and the use of fast-acting insulin analogs and long-acting basal insulin (detemir and glargine) provide many children with less rigid meal planning. Flexibility in the use of insulin in relation to carbohydrate content of food improves the quality of life.

Although in children there is concern about the potential cumulative effect of saccharin, available data do not support an association of moderate amounts with bladder cancer. Other nonnutritive sweeteners such as aspartame are used in a variety of products. Sorbitol and xylitol should not be used as artificial sweeteners; they are products of the polyol pathway and are implicated in some of the complications of diabetes.

Diets with high fiber content are useful in improving control of blood glucose. Moderate amounts of sucrose consumed with fiber-rich foods such as whole-meal bread may have no more glycemic effect than their low-fiber, sugar-free equivalents. The concept of biologic equivalence or of a "glycemic index" of foods is under investigation.

The intake of fat is adjusted so that the polyunsaturated : saturated ratio is increased to about 1.2 : 1.0, in contrast to the estimated American average of 0.3 : 1.0. Dietary fats derived from animal sources are, therefore, reduced and replaced by polyunsaturated fats from vegetable sources. Substituting margarine for butter, vegetable oil for animal oils in cooking, and lean cuts of meat, poultry, and fish for fatty meats, such as bacon, is advisable. The intake of cholesterol is also reduced by these measures and by limiting the number of egg yolks consumed. These simple measures reduce serum low-density lipoprotein cholesterol, a predisposing factor to atherosclerotic disease. Less than 10% of calories should be derived from saturated fats, up to 10% from polyunsaturated fats, and the remaining fat-derived calories from monounsaturated fats. Table 583-6 summarizes current nutritional guidelines.

The total daily caloric intake is divided to provide 20% at breakfast, 20% at lunch, and 30% at dinner, leaving 10% for each of the midmorning, midafternoon, and evening snacks, if they are desired. In older children, the midmorning snack may be omitted and its caloric equivalent added to lunch. Special brochures and pamphlets describing sample meal plans for children are usually available from regional diabetes associations; their use should be encouraged as part of the educational process. Meal plans are often based on groups of food exchanges; within each of the exchange lists of the foods that are principal sources of carbohydrates, proteins, and fats, there is a wide variety of foods that can be substituted or exchanged. There are few restrictions so that each child can select a diet based on personal taste or preferences with the help of the physician or dietitian (or both). Emphasis should be placed on regularity of food intake and on constancy of carbohydrate intake. Occasional excesses for birthdays and other parties are permissible and tolerated to not foster rebellion and stealth in obtaining desired food. Cakes and even candies are permissible on special occasions as long as the food exchange value and carbohydrate content are adjusted in the meal plan. Adjustments in meal planning must constantly be made to meet the needs as well as the desires of each child although a consistent eating pattern with appropriate supplements for exercise, the pubertal growth spurt, and pregnancy in a diabetic adolescent are important for metabolic control.

The prevalence of overweight children and adolescents with T1DM has tripled over the past 20 yr, which appears to correspond to the increasing prevalence of obesity in the general population. The authors have observed that among our patients with T1DM, normal-weight preschool children have better glycemic control than age-matched overweight children. This may mean that excess body weight status may impede achievement of therapeutic goals in this group of patients. There is also an increased frequency of eating disorders among young women with diabetes. Thus, expectations and educational advice regarding nutrition must be dealt with in a sensitive, careful manner, especially in adolescents.

Monitoring

Success in the daily management of the diabetic child can be measured by the competence acquired by the family, and subsequently by the child, in assuming responsibility for daily "diabetic care." Their initial and ongoing instruction in conjunction with their supervised experience can lead to a sense of confidence in making intermittent adjustments in insulin dosage for dietary deviations, for unusual physical activity, and even for some minor intercurrent illnesses, as well as for otherwise unexplained repeated hypoglycemic reactions and excessive glycosuria. Such acceptance of responsibility should make them relatively independent of the physician for their ordinary care. The physician must maintain ongoing interested supervision and shared responsibility with the family and the child.

Self-monitoring of blood glucose (SMBG) is an essential component of managing diabetes. Monitoring often also needs to include insulin dose, unusual physical activity, dietary changes, hypoglycemia, intercurrent illness, and other items that may influence the blood glucose. These items may be valuable in interpreting the SMBG record, prescribing appropriate adjustments in insulin doses, and teaching the family. If there are discrepancies in the SMBG and other measures of glycemic control (such as the HbA_{1c}), the clinician should attempt to clarify the situation in a manner that does not undermine their mutual confidence.

Daily blood glucose monitoring has been markedly enhanced by the availability of strips impregnated with glucose oxidase that permit blood glucose measurement from a drop of blood. A portable calibrated reflectance meter can approximate the blood glucose concentration accurately. Many meters contain a memory "chip" enabling recall of each measurement, its average over a given interval, and the ability to display the pattern on a computer screen. Such information is a useful educational tool for verifying degree of control and modifying recommended regimens. A small, spring-loaded device that automates capillary bloodletting (lancing device) in a relatively painless fashion is commercially available. Parents and patients should be taught to use these devices and measure blood glucose at least 4 times daily—before breakfast, lunch, and supper and at bedtime. When insulin therapy is initiated and when adjustments are made that may affect the overnight glucose levels, SMBG should also be performed at 12 A.M. and 3 A.M. to detect nocturnal hypoglycemia. Ideally, the blood glucose concentration should range from approximately 80 mg/dL in the fasting state to 140 mg/dL after meals. In practice, however, a range of 60-220 mg/dL is acceptable, based on age of the patient (Table 583-7). Blood glucose measurements that are consistently at or outside these limits, in the absence of an identifiable cause such as exercise or dietary indiscretion, are an indication for a change in the insulin dose. If the fasting blood glucose is high, the evening dose of long-acting insulin is increased by 10-15% and/or additional fast-acting insulin (lispro or aspart) coverage for bedtime snack may be considered. If the noon glucose level exceeds set limits, the morning fast-acting insulin (lispro or aspart) is increased by 10-15%. If the pre-supper glucose is high, the noon dose of fast-acting insulin is increased by 10-15%. If the pre-bedtime glucose is high, the pre-supper dose of fast-acting insulin is increased by 10-15%. Similarly, reductions in the insulin type and dose should be made if the corresponding blood glucose measurements are consistently below desirable limits.

Table 583-7 TARGET PRE-MEAL AND 30-DAY AVERAGE BLOOD GLUCOSE RANGES AND THE CORRESPONDING HEMOGLOBIN A_{1C} FOR EACH AGE GROUP

AGE GROUP (yr)	TARGET PRE-MEAL BG RANGE (mg/dL)	30-DAY AVERAGE BG RANGE (mg/dL)	TARGET HBA_{1C} (%)
<5	100-200	180-250	7.5-9.0
5-11	80-150	150-200	6.5-8.0
12-15	80-130	120-180	6.0-7.5
16-18	70-120	100-150	5.5-7.0

In our laboratory, the nondiabetic reference range for HbA_{1c} is 4.5-5.7% (95% confidence interval).
BG, blood glucose; HbA_{1c}, hemoglobin A_{1c}.

A minimum of 4 daily blood glucose measurements should be performed. However, some children and adolescents may need to have more frequent blood glucose monitoring based on their level of physical activity and history of frequent hypoglycemic reactions. Families should be encouraged to become sufficiently knowledgeable about managing diabetes. They can maintain near-normal glycemia for prolonged periods by self-monitoring of blood glucose levels before and 2 hr after meals, and in conjunction with multiple daily injections of insulin, adjusted as necessary.

A continuous glucose monitoring system (CGMS) records data obtained from a subcutaneous sensor every 5 min for up to 72 hr and provides the clinician with a continuous profile of tissue glucose levels. The interstitial glucose levels lag 13 min behind the blood glucose values at any given level. The CGMS values tend to have a high correlation coefficient for blood glucose values ranging between 40 and 400 mg/dL. CGMS is minimally invasive and entails the placement of a small, subcutaneous catheter that can be easily worn by adults and children. The system provides information that allows the patient and health care team to adjust the insulin regimen and the nutrition plan to improve glycemic control. CGMS can be helpful in detecting asymptomatic nocturnal hypoglycemia as well as in lowering HbA_{1c} values without increasing the risk for severe hypoglycemia. While there are potential pitfalls in CGMS use, including suboptimal compliance, human error, incorrect technique, and sensor failure, the implementation of CGMS in ambulatory diabetes practice allows the clinician to diagnose abnormal glycemic patterns in a more precise manner.

Real-Time CGM (RT-CGM)

Real-time continuous glucose monitoring (RT-CGM) is an evolving technology with the potential of transforming current concepts of glycemic control and optimal diabetes management. Newer generations of continuous glucose monitors not only display real-time glucose data but also the alarm can be set at below or above predetermined blood glucose thresholds. The latter safety feature can assist parents of young children to guard against nocturnal hypoglycemia. In addition, CGM shows the rate and direction of glucose change and alerting patients to trends that could lead to dangerous hypoglycemia or hyperglycemia. However, the use of CGM without clinical decision-making algorithms and guidelines has not been proven to be very effective in improving glycemic control. Currently, available RT-CGM devices are not accompanied by any diabetes management tools or guidelines aimed at patients or clinicians especially in pediatric and adolescent age group.

Glycosylated Hemoglobin (HbA_{1c})

A reliable index of long-term glycemic control is provided by measurement of glycosylated hemoglobin. HbA_{1c} represents the fraction of hemoglobin to which glucose has been nonenzymatically attached in the bloodstream. The formation of HbA_{1c} is a slow reaction that is dependent on the prevailing concentration of blood glucose; it continues irreversibly throughout the red blood cell's life span of approximately 120 days. The higher the blood glucose concentration and the longer the red blood cell's exposure to it, the higher is the fraction of HbA_{1c}, which is expressed as a percentage of total hemoglobin. Because a blood sample at any given time contains a mixture of red blood cells of varying ages, exposed for varying times to varying blood glucose concentrations, an HbA_{1c} measurement reflects the average blood glucose concentration from the preceding 2-3 mo. When measured by standardized methods to remove labile forms, the fraction of HbA_{1c} is not influenced by an isolated episode of hyperglycemia. Consequently, as an index of long-term glycemic control, a measurement of HbA_{1c} is superior to measurements of glycosuria or even multiple blood glucose determinations. (The latter can reveal important fluctuations but may not accurately reflect the average overall glycemic control.) It is recommended that HbA_{1c} measurements be obtained 3-4 times per yr to obtain a profile of long-term glycemic control. The more consistently lower the HbA_{1c} level, and hence the better the metabolic control, the more likely it is that microvascular complications such as retinopathy and nephropathy will be less severe, delayed in appearance, or even avoided altogether. Depending on the method used for determination, HbA_{1c} values may be spuriously elevated in thalassemia (or other conditions with elevated hemoglobin F) and spuriously lower in sickle cell disease (or other conditions with high red blood cell turnover). Although values of HbA_{1c} may vary according to the method used for measurement, in nondiabetic individuals, the HbA_{1c} fraction is usually less than 6%; in diabetics, values of 6-7.9% represent good metabolic control, values of 8.0-9.9%, fair control, and values of 10% or higher, poor control. Adjustments in target HbA_{1c} should be made for younger children (see Table 583-7).

Exercise

No form of exercise, including competitive sports, should be forbidden to the diabetic child. A major complication of exercise in diabetic patients is the presence of a hypoglycemic reaction during or within hours after exercise. If hypoglycemia does not occur with exercise, adjustments in diet or insulin are not necessary, and glucoregulation is likely to be improved through the increased utilization of glucose by muscles. The major contributing factor to hypoglycemia with exercise is an increased rate of absorption of insulin from its injection site. Higher insulin levels dampen hepatic glucose production so that it is inadequate to meet the increased glucose utilization of exercising muscle. Regular exercise also improves glucoregulation by increasing insulin receptor number. In patients who are in poor metabolic control, vigorous exercise may precipitate ketoacidosis because of the exercise-induced increase in the counter-regulatory hormones.

In anticipation of vigorous exercise, 1 additional carbohydrate exchange may be taken before exercise, and glucose from orange juice, a carbonated nondietetic beverage, or candy should be available during and after exercise. With experience and trial and error, each patient, guided by the physician, should develop an appropriate regimen for regularly planned exercise that is frequently associated with hypoglycemia; in such instances, the total dose of insulin may be reduced by about 10-15% on the day of the scheduled exercise. Prolonged exercise, such as long-distance running, may require reduction of as much as 50% or more of the usual insulin dose. It is also important to watch for delayed hypoglycemia several hours after exercise.

Benefits of Improved Glycemic Control

The Diabetes Control and Complications Trial (DCCT) established conclusively the association between higher glucose levels and long-term microvascular complications. Intensive management produced dramatic reductions of retinopathy, nephropathy, and neuropathy by 47-76%. The data from the adolescent cohort demonstrated the same degree of improvement and the same relationship between the outcome measures of microvascular complications. Adolescents gained more weight and experienced significantly more frequent episodes of severe hypoglycemia and ketoacidosis than did adults. Other studies of children and adolescents have not documented increased frequency or severity of hypoglycemia.

The beneficial effect of intensified treatment was determined by the degree of blood glucose normalization, independently of the type of intensified treatment used. Frequent blood glucose monitoring was considered an important factor in achieving better glycemic control for the intensively treated adolescents and adults. Patients who were intensively treated had individualized glucose targets, frequent adjustments based on ongoing capillary blood glucose monitoring, and a team approach that focused on the person with diabetes as the prime initiator of ambulatory care. Care was constantly adjusted toward reaching normal or near-normal glycemic goals while avoiding or minimizing severe episodes of hypoglycemia. Teaching emphasized a preventive approach to blood glucose fluctuations with constant readjustment to counterbalance any high or low blood glucose readings. Target blood glucose goals were adjusted upward if hypoglycemia could not be prevented.

Total duration of diabetes contributes to development and severity of complications. Nonetheless, many professionals have concerns about applying the results of the DCCT to preschool-aged children, who often have hypoglycemia unawareness with unique safety issues, and to prepubertal school-aged children, who were not included in the DCCT. When the DCCT ended in 1993, researchers continued to study more than 90% of participants. The follow-up study, called Epidemiology of Diabetes Interventions and Complications (EDIC), was assessing the incidence and predictors of cardiovascular disease events such as heart attack, stroke, or needed heart surgery, as well as diabetic complications related to the eye, kidney, and nerves. The EDIC demonstrated that **intensive blood glucose control reduced risk of** any cardiovascular disease event by 42%. In addition, intensive therapy reduced risk of nonfatal heart attack, stroke, or death from cardiovascular causes by 57%.

Current Intensive Insulin Replacement Regimens

The goal of physiologic insulin replacement for T1DM is accomplished with short-acting insulins that more closely mimic the sharp increase and short duration of pancreatic insulin secreted with nutrient intake. The rapid-acting insulin analog lispro has superior pharmacokinetic properties for the control of postprandial glucose. Improved postprandial glucose responses occur with twice-daily injections (conventional insulin, CI), multiple daily insulin (MDI), or CSII. The use of lispro or aspart insulin reduces the frequency of between-meal hypoglycemic events, especially when it is carefully balanced with the carbohydrate content of meal. This has improved how insulin is given to toddlers as well as how to manage a flexible meal plan.

The carbohydrate content of food does not influence glycemic control if pre-meal rapid-acting insulin (bolus) is adjusted to the carbohydrate content of meal. Wide variations in carbohydrate intake do not modify long-acting (detemir or glargine) or basal insulin requirements. Insulin replacement strategies stress the importance of administering smaller doses of insulin throughout the day. This approach allows insulin doses to be changed as needed to correct hyperglycemia, supplement for additional anticipated carbohydrate intake, or subtract for exercise. Indeed, bolus-basal treatment with multiple injections is better adapted to the physiologic profiles of insulin and glucose and can therefore provide better glycemic control than the conventional 2- to 3-dose regimen. Age-adjusted and individualized insulin to carbohydrate ratios and insulin dosage adjustment algorithms have been developed to normalize elevated blood glucose levels and to compensate for alterations in carbohydrate intake. The use of flexible multiple daily injections (FMDIs) and CSII in children with T1DM improves glycemic control without an increase in the incidence of severe hypoglycemia.

Hypoglycemic Reactions

Hypoglycemia is the major limitation to tight control of glucose levels. Once injected, insulin absorption and action are independent of the glucose level, thus creating a unique risk of hypoglycemia from an unbalanced insulin effect. Insulin analogs may help reduce but cannot eliminate this risk. Most children with T1DM can expect mild hypoglycemia each week, moderate hypoglycemia a few times each year, and severe hypoglycemia every few years. These episodes are usually not predictable, although exercise, delayed meals or snacks, and wide swings in glucose levels increase the risk. Infants and toddlers are at higher risk because they have more variable meals and activity levels, are unable to recognize early signs of hypoglycemia, and are limited in their ability to seek a source of oral glucose to reverse the hypoglycemia. The very young have an increased risk of permanently reduced cognitive function as a long-term sequela of severe hypoglycemia. For this reason, a more relaxed degree of glucose control is necessary until the child matures (see Table 583-7).

Hypoglycemia can occur at any time of day or night. Early symptoms and signs (mild hypoglycemia) may occur with a sudden decrease in blood glucose to levels that do not meet standard criteria for hypoglycemia in nondiabetic children (Chapter 86). The child may show pallor, sweating, apprehension or fussiness, hunger, tremor, and tachycardia, all due to the surge in catecholamines as the body attempts to counter the excessive insulin effect. Behavioral changes such as tearfulness, irritability, aggression, and naughtiness are more prevalent in children. As glucose levels decline further, cerebral glucopenia occurs with drowsiness, personality changes, mental confusion, and impaired judgment (moderate hypoglycemia), progressing to inability to seek help and seizures or coma (severe hypoglycemia). Prolonged severe hypoglycemia can result in a depressed sensorium or strokelike focal motor deficits that persist after the hypoglycemia has resolved. Although permanent sequelae are rare, severe hypoglycemia is frightening for the child and family and can result in significant reluctance to attempt even moderate glycemic control afterward.

Important counter-regulatory hormones in children include growth hormone, cortisol, epinephrine, and glucagon. The latter 2 seem more critical in the older child. Many older patients with long-standing T1DM lose their ability to secrete glucagon in response to hypoglycemia. In the young adult, epinephrine deficiency may also develop as part of a general autonomic neuropathy. This substantially increases the risk of hypoglycemia because the early warning signals of a declining glucose level are due to catecholamine release. Recurrent hypoglycemic episodes associated with tight metabolic control may aggravate partial counter-regulatory deficiencies, producing a syndrome of hypoglycemia unawareness and reduced ability to restore euglycemia (hypoglycemia-associated autonomic failure). Avoidance of hypoglycemia allows some recovery from this unawareness syndrome.

The most important factors in the management of hypoglycemia are an understanding by the patient and family of the symptoms and signs of the reaction and an anticipation of known precipitating factors such as gym or sports activities. Tighter glucose control increases the risk. Families should be taught to look for typical hypoglycemic scenarios or patterns in the home blood glucose log, so that they may adjust the insulin dose and avert predictable episodes. A source of emergency glucose should be available at all times and places, including at school and during visits to friends. If possible, it is initially important to document the hypoglycemia before treating, because some symptoms may not always be due to hypoglycemia. Most families and children develop a good sense for true hypoglycemic episodes and can institute treatment before testing. Any child suspected of having a moderate to severe hypoglycemic episode should also be treated before testing. It is important not to give too much glucose; 5-10 g should be given as juice or a sugar-containing carbonated beverage or candy, and the blood glucose checked 15-20 minutes later. Patients, parents, and teachers should also be instructed in the administration of glucagon when the child cannot take glucose orally. An injection kit should be kept at home and school. The intramuscular dose is 0.5 mg if the child weighs less than 20 kg and 1.0 mg if more than 20 kg. This produces a brief release of glucose from the liver. Glucagon often causes emesis, which precludes giving oral supplementation if the blood glucose declines after the glucagon effects have waned. Caretakers must then be prepared to take the child to the hospital for IV glucose administration, if necessary. Mini-dose glucagon (10 µg/yr of age up to a maximum of 150 µg subcutaneously) is effective in treating hypoglycemia in children with blood glucose less than 60 mg/dL who failed to respond to oral glucose and remained symptomatic.

Somogyi Phenomenon, Dawn Phenomenon, and Brittle Diabetes

There are several reasons that blood glucose levels increase in the early morning hours before breakfast. The most common is a simple decline in insulin levels and is seen in many children using NPH or Lente as the basal insulin at supper or bedtime. This usually results in routinely elevated morning glucose. The **dawn phenomenon** is thought to be due mainly to overnight growth hormone secretion and increased insulin clearance. It is a normal physiologic process seen in most nondiabetic adolescents, who compensate with more insulin output. A child with T1DM cannot compensate and may actually have declining insulin levels if using evening NPH or Lente. The dawn phenomenon is usually recurrent and modestly elevates most morning glucose levels.

Rarely, high morning glucose is due to the **Somogyi phenomenon,** a theoretical rebound from late night or early morning hypoglycemia, thought to be due to an exaggerated counter-regulatory response. It is unlikely to be a common cause, in that most children remain hypoglycemic (do not rebound) once nighttime glucose levels decline. Continuous glucose monitoring systems may help clarify ambiguously elevated morning glucose levels.

The term **brittle diabetes** has been used to describe the child, usually an adolescent female, with unexplained wide fluctuations in blood glucose, often with recurrent DKA, who is taking large doses of insulin. An inherent physiologic abnormality is rarely present because these children usually show normal insulin responsiveness when in the hospital environment. Psychosocial or psychiatric problems, including eating disorders, and dysfunctional family dynamics are usually present, which preclude effective diabetes therapy. Hospitalization is usually needed to confirm the environmental effect, and aggressive psychosocial or psychiatric evaluation is essential. Therefore, clinicians should refrain from using "brittle diabetes" as a diagnostic term.

Behavioral/Psychologic Aspects and Eating Disorders

Diabetes in a child affects the lifestyle and interpersonal relationships of the entire family. Feelings of anxiety and guilt are common in parents. Similar feelings, coupled with denial and rejection, are equally common in children, particularly during the rebellious teenage years. Family conflict has been associated with poor treatment adherence and poor metabolic control among youths with T1DM. On the other hand, it has been shown that shared responsibility is consistently associated with better psychologic health, good self-care behavior, and good metabolic control, whereas child and parent responsibility were not. In some cases, links of shared responsibility to health outcomes were stronger among older adolescents. However, no specific personality disorder or psychopathology is characteristic of diabetes; similar feelings are observed in families with other chronic disorders.

COGNITIVE FUNCTION

There is increasing agreement that children with T1DM are at higher risk of developing cognitive difficulties than healthy age-matched peers. Evidence suggests that early-onset diabetes (younger than 7 yr) is associated with cognitive difficulties compared to late-onset diabetes and healthy controls. These cognitive difficulties were primarily observed learning and memory skills (both verbal and visual) and attention/executive function skills. It is likely that impact of diabetes on pediatric cognition appears shortly after diagnosis. Indeed, it has been observed that early-onset diabetes and longer duration of diabetes in children with diabetes adversely affects their school performance and educational achievements.

COPING STYLES

Children and adolescents with T1DM are faced with a complex set of developmental changes as well as shifting burdens of the disease. Adjustment problems might affect psychologic well-being and the course of the disease by contributing to poor self-management and poor metabolic control. Coping styles refer to typical habitual preferences for ways of approaching problems and might be regarded as strategies that people generally use to cope across a wide range of stressors. Problem-focused coping refers to efforts directed toward rational management of a problem, and it is aimed at changing the situation causing distress. On the other hand, emotion-focused coping implies efforts to reduce emotional distress caused by the stressful event and to manage or regulate emotions that might accompany or result from the stressor. In adolescents with diabetes, avoidance coping and venting emotions have been found to predict poor illness-specific self-care behavior and poor metabolic control. Patients who use more mature defenses and exhibit greater adaptive capacity are more likely to adhere to their regimen. Coping strategies seem to be age dependent, with adolescents using more avoidance coping than younger children with diabetes.

NONADHERENCE

Family conflict, denial, and feelings of anxiety find expression in nonadherence to instructions regarding nutritional and insulin therapy and in noncompliance with self-monitoring. The presence of youth perceptions of critical parenting and youth externalizing behavior problems may interfere with adherence, leading to deterioration of glycemic control. In addition, deliberate overdosage with insulin, resulting in hypoglycemia, or omission of insulin, often in association with excesses in nutritional intake and resulting in ketoacidosis, may be pleas for psychologic help or manipulative attempts to escape an environment perceived as undesirable or intolerable; occasionally, they may be manifestations of suicidal intent. Frequent admissions to the hospital for ketoacidosis or hypoglycemia should arouse suspicion of an underlying emotional conflict. Overprotection on the part of parents is common and often is not in the best interest of the patient. Feelings of being different or of being alone, or both, are common and may be justified in view of the restrictive schedules imposed by testing of urine and blood, administration of insulin, and nutritional limitations. Furthermore, concern about the likelihood of complications developing and the decreased life span of patients with diabetes fosters anxiety. Unfortunately, misinformation abounds about the risks of the development of diabetes in siblings or offspring and of pregnancy in young diabetic women. Even appropriate information may cause further anxiety.

Many of these problems can be averted through continued empathic counseling based on correct information and attempts to build attitudes of normality in the patient and a feeling of being a productive member of society. Recognizing the potential impact of these problems, peer discussion groups have been organized in many locales; feelings of isolation and frustration tend to be lessened by the sharing of common problems. Summer camps for diabetic children afford an excellent opportunity for learning and sharing under expert supervision. Education about the pathophysiology of diabetes, insulin dose, technique of administration, nutrition, exercise, and hypoglycemic reactions can be reinforced by medical and paramedical personnel. The presence of numerous peers with similar problems offers new insights to the diabetic child. Residential treatment for children and adolescents with difficult to manage T1DM is an option available only in some centers.

ANXIETY AND DEPRESSION

It has been shown that there are significant correlations between poor metabolic control and depressive symptoms, a high level of anxiety, or a previous psychiatric diagnosis. In a similar way, poor metabolic control is related to higher levels of personal, social, school maladjustment, or family environment dissatisfaction. It is estimated that 20-26% of adolescent patients may develop major depressive disorder (MDD), which is similar to the occurrence rate of MDD in nondiabetic adolescents. The course characteristics of MDD in young diabetic subjects and psychiatric control subjects appear to be similar; however, eventual propensity of diabetic youths for more protracted depressions is greater and there is higher risk of recurrence among young diabetic females. Therefore, the health care providers managing a child or adolescent with diabetes should be aware of their pivotal role as counselor and advisor and should closely monitor the mental health of patients with diabetes.

FEAR OF SELF-INJECTING AND SELF-TESTING

Extreme fear of self-injecting (FSI) insulin (injection phobia) is likely to compromise glycemic control as well as emotional well-being. Likewise, fear of finger pricks can be a source of distress and may seriously hamper self-management. Children and adolescents may either omit insulin dosing or refuse to rotate their injection sites because repeated injection in the same site is associated with less pain sensation. Failure to rotate injection sites results in subcutaneous scar formation (lipohypertrophy). Insulin injection into the lipohypertrophic skin is usually associated with poor insulin absorption and/or insulin leakage with resultant suboptimal glycemic control.

EATING DISORDERS

Treatment of T1DM involves constant monitoring of food intake. In addition, improved glycemic control is commonly associated with increased weight gain. In adolescent females, these 2 factors, along with individual, familial, and socioeconomic factors, can lead to an increased incidence of both nonspecific and specific eating disorders, which can disrupt glycemic control and increase the risk of long-term complications. Eating disorders and subthreshold eating disorders are almost twice as common in adolescent females with T1DM as in their nondiabetic peers. The reports of the frequencies of specific (anorexia or bulimia nervosa) eating disorders vary from 1% to 6.9% among female patients with T1DM. The prevalence of nonspecific and subthreshold eating disorders is 9% and 14%, respectively. About 11% of T1DM adolescent females take less insulin than prescribed in order to lose weight. Among adolescent females with an eating disorder, about 42% of patients misuse insulin, whereas the estimates of insulin misuse prevalence in subthreshold and nondisordered eating groups are 18% and 6%, respectively. While there is little information regarding the prevalence of eating disorders among male adolescents with T1DM, available data suggest normal eating attitudes in most. Among healthy adolescent males who participate in wrestling, however, the drive to lose weight has led to the seasonal, transient development of abnormal eating attitudes and behaviors, which may lead to insulin dose omission in order to lose weight.

When behavioral/psychologic problems and/or eating disorders are assumed to be responsible for poor compliance with the medical regimen, referral for psychologic evaluation and management is indicated. Children and adolescents with injection phobia and fear of self-testing can be counseled by a trained behavioral therapist and benefit from such techniques as desensitization and biofeedback to attenuate pain sensation and psychologic distress associated these procedures. Behavioral therapists and psychologists usually form part of the pediatric diabetes team in most centers and can help assess and manage emotional and behavioral disorders in diabetic children. Evaluation of nurse-delivered motivational enhancement with and without cognitive behavior therapy in adults revealed the combined therapy resulted in modest improvement in glycemic control. However, motivational enhancement therapy alone did not improve glycemic control. While in some studies the effect of therapist-delivered motivational enhancement therapy on glycemic control in adolescents with T1DM lasted as long as intensive individualized counseling continued, in other studies, motivational interviewing was shown to be an effective method of facilitating changes in teenager's behavior with T1DM with corresponding improvement in glycemic control.

Management During Infections

Although infections are no more common in diabetic children than in nondiabetic ones, they can often disrupt glucose control and may precipitate DKA. In addition, the diabetic child is at increased risk of dehydration if hyperglycemia causes an osmotic diuresis or if ketosis causes emesis. Counter-regulatory hormones associated with stress blunt insulin action and elevate glucose levels. If anorexia occurs, however, lack of caloric intake increases the risk of hypoglycemia. Although children younger than 3 yr tend to become hypoglycemic and older children tend toward hyperglycemia, the overall effect is unpredictable. Therefore, frequent blood glucose monitoring and adjustment of insulin doses are essential elements of sick day guidelines (Table 583-8).

The overall goals are to maintain hydration, control glucose levels, and avoid ketoacidosis. This can usually be done at home if proper sick day guidelines are followed and with telephone contact with health care providers. The family should seek advice if home treatment does not control ketonuria, hyperglycemia, or hypoglycemia, or if the child shows signs of dehydration. A child with large ketonuria and emesis should be seen in the emergency department for a general examination, to evaluate hydration, and to determine whether ketoacidosis is present by checking serum electrolytes, glucose, pH, and total CO_2. A child whose blood glucose declines to less than 50-60 mg/dL (2.8-3.3 mmol/L) and who cannot maintain oral intake may need IV glucose, especially if further insulin is needed to control ketonemia.

Table 583-8 GUIDELINES FOR SICK DAY MANAGEMENT

URINE KETONE STATUS	GLUCOSE TESTING AND EXTRA RAPID-ACTING INSULIN		COMMENT
	Insulin	Correction Doses*	
Negative or small†	q2 hr	q2 hr for glucose >250 mg/dL	Check ketones every other void
Moderate to large‡	q1 hr	q1 hr for glucose >250 mg/dL	Check ketones each void. Go to hospital if emesis occurs.

Basal insulin: glargine or detemir basal insulin should be given at the usual dose and time. NPH and Lente should be reduced by one half if blood glucose <150 mg/dL and the oral intake is limited.
Oral fluids: sugar-free if blood glucose >250 mg/dL (14 mmol/L); sugar-containing if blood glucose <250 mg/dL.
Call physician or nurse if blood glucose remains elevated after 3 extra doses; if blood glucose remains less than 70 mg/dL and child cannot take oral supplement; if dehydration occurs.
*Give insulin based on individualized dosing schedule. Also give usual dose for carbohydrate intake if glucose >150 mg/dL.
†For home serum ketones <1.5 mmol/L per commercial kit.
‡For home serum ketones >1.5 mmol/L.

Table 583-9 GUIDELINES FOR INTRAVENOUS INSULIN COVERAGE DURING SURGERY

BLOOD GLUCOSE LEVEL (mg/dL)	INSULIN INFUSION (U/kg/hr)	BLOOD GLUCOSE MONITORING
<120	0.00	1 hr
121-200	0.03	2 hr
200-300	0.06	2 hr
300-400	0.08	1 hr†
400	0.10	1 hr†

An infusion of 5% glucose and 0.45% saline solution with 20 mEq/L of potassium acetate is given at 1.5 times maintenance rate.
†Check urine ketones.

Management During Surgery

Surgery can disrupt glucose control in the same way as can intercurrent infections. Stress hormones associated with the underlying condition as well as with surgery itself decrease insulin sensitivity. This increases glucose levels, exacerbates fluid losses, and may initiate DKA. On the other hand, caloric intake is usually restricted, which decreases glucose levels. The net effect is as difficult to predict as during an infection. Vigilant monitoring and frequent insulin adjustments are required to maintain euglycemia and avoid ketosis.

Maintaining glucose control and avoiding DKA are best accomplished with IV insulin and fluids. A simple insulin adjustment scale based on the patient's weight and blood glucose level can be used in most situations (Table 583-9). The IV insulin is continued after surgery as the child begins to take oral fluids; the IV fluids can be steadily decreased as oral intake increases. When full oral intake is achieved, the IV may be capped and subcutaneous insulin begun. When surgery is elective, it is best performed early in the day, allowing the patient maximal recovery time to restart oral intake and subcutaneous insulin therapy. When elective surgery is brief (less than 1 hr) and full oral intake is expected shortly afterward, one may simply monitor the blood glucose hourly and give a dose of insulin analog according to the child's home glucose correction scale. If glargine or detemir is used as the basal insulin, a full dose is given the evening before planned surgery. If NPH or Lente is used, one half of the morning dose is given before surgery. The child should not be discharged until blood glucose levels are stable and oral intake is tolerated.

LONG-TERM COMPLICATIONS: RELATION TO GLYCEMIC CONTROL

The increasingly prolonged survival of the diabetic child is associated with an increasing prevalence of complications. Complications of DM can be divided into 3 major categories—(1) microvascular complications, specifically, retinopathy and nephropathy; (2) macrovascular complications, particularly accelerated coronary artery disease, cerebrovascular disease, and peripheral vascular disease; and (3) neuropathies, both peripheral and autonomic, affecting a variety of organs and systems (Table 583-10). In addition, cataracts may occur more frequently.

Diabetic retinopathy is the leading cause of blindness in the USA in adults aged 20-65 yr. The risk of diabetic retinopathy after 15 yr duration of diabetes is 98% for individuals with T1DM and 78% for those with T2DM. Lens opacities (due to glycation of tissue proteins and activation of the polyol pathway) are present in at least 5% of those younger than 19 yr. Although the metabolic control has an impact on the development of this complication, genetic factors also have a role, because only 50% of patients develop proliferative retinopathy. The earliest clinically apparent manifestations of diabetic retinopathy are classified as nonproliferative or background diabetic retinopathy—microaneurysms, dot and blot hemorrhages, hard and soft exudates, venous dilation and beading, and intraretinal microvascular abnormalities. These changes do not impair vision. The more severe form is proliferative diabetic retinopathy—manifested by neovascularization, fibrous proliferation, and preretinal and vitreous hemorrhages. Proliferative retinopathy, if not treated, is relentlessly progressive and impairs vision, leading to blindness. The mainstay of treatment is panretinal laser photocoagulation. In advanced diabetic eye disease—manifested by severe vitreous hemorrhage or fibrosis, often with retinal detachment—vitrectomy is an important therapeutic modality. Eventually, the eye disease becomes quiescent, a stage termed involutional retinopathy. A separate subtype of retinopathy is diabetic maculopathy, which is manifested by severe macular edema impairing central vision, for which focal laser photocoagulation may be effective.

Guidelines suggest that diabetic patients have an initial dilated and comprehensive examination by an ophthalmologist shortly after the diagnosis of diabetes is made in patients with T2DM, and within 3-5 yr after the onset of T1DM (but not before age 10 yr). Any patients with visual symptoms or abnormalities should be referred for ophthalmologic evaluation. Subsequent evaluations for both T1DM and T2DM patients should be repeated annually by an ophthalmologist who is experienced in diagnosing the presence of diabetic retinopathy and is knowledgeable about its management (see Table 583-10).

Diabetic nephropathy is the leading known cause of end-stage renal disease (ESRD) in the USA. Most ESRD from diabetic nephropathy is preventable. Diabetic nephropathy affects 20-30% of patients with T1DM and 15-20% of T2DM patients 20 yr after onset. The mean 5-yr life expectancy for patients with diabetes-related ESRD is less than 20%. The increased mortality risk in long-term T1DM may be due to nephropathy, which may account for about 50% of deaths. The risk of nephropathy increases with duration of diabetes (up until 25-30 yr duration, after which this complication rarely begins), degree of metabolic control, and genetic predisposition to essential hypertension. Only 30-40% of patients affected by T1DM eventually experience ESRD. The glycation of tissue proteins results in glomerular basement membrane thickening. The course of diabetic nephropathy is slow. An increased urinary albumin excretion rate (AER) of 30-300 mg/24 hr (20-200 μg/min)—*microalbuminuria*—can be detected and constitutes an early stage of nephropathy from intermittent to persistent (incipient), which is commonly associated with glomerular hyperfiltration and blood pressure elevation. As nephropathy evolves to early overt stage with proteinuria (AER >300 mg/24 hr, or >200 μg/min), it is accompanied by hypertension. Advanced stage nephropathy is defined by a progressive decline in renal function (declining glomerular filtration rate and elevation of serum blood urea and creatinine), progressive proteinuria, and hypertension. Progression to ESRD is recognized by the appearance of uremia, the nephritic syndrome, and the need for renal replacement (transplantation or dialysis).

Screening for diabetic nephropathy is a routine aspect of diabetes care (see Table 583-10). The American Diabetes Association (ADA) recommends yearly screening for individuals with T2DM and yearly screening for those with T1DM after 5 yr duration of disease (but not before puberty). Twenty-four hour AER (urinary albumin and creatinine) or timed (overnight) urinary AER are acceptable techniques. Positive results should be confirmed by a 2nd measurement of AER because of the high variability of albumin excretion in patients with diabetes. Short-term hyperglycemia, exercise, urinary tract infections, marked hypertension, heart failure, and acute febrile illness can cause transient elevation urinary albumin excretion. There is marked day-to-day variability in albumin excretion, so at least 2 of 3 collections done in a 3- to 6-mo period should show elevated levels before microalbuminuria is diagnosed and treatment is started. Once albuminuria is diagnosed, a number of factors attenuate the effect of hyperfiltration on kidneys: (1) meticulous control of

Table 583-10 SCREENING GUIDELINES

	WHEN TO COMMENCE SCREENING	FREQUENCY	PREFERRED METHOD OF SCREENING	OTHER SCREENING METHODS	POTENTIAL INTERVENTION
Retinopathy	After 5 yr duration in prepubertal children, after 2 yr in pubertal children	1-2 yearly	Fundal photography	Fluorescein angiography, mydriatic ophthalmoscopy	Improved glycemic control, laser therapy
Nephropathy	After 5 yr duration in prepubertal children, after 2 yr in pubertal children	Annually	Overnight timed urine excretion of albumin	24-hr excretion of albumin, urinary albumin/creatinine ratio	Improved glycemic control, blood pressure control, ACE inhibitors
Neuropathy	Unclear	Unclear	Physical examination	Nerve conduction, thermal and vibration threshold, pupillometry, cardiovascular reflexes	Improved glycemic control
Macrovascular disease	After age 2 yr	Every 5 yr	Lipids	Blood pressure	Statins for hyperlipidemia Blood pressure control
Thyroid disease	At diagnosis	Every 2-3 yr	TSH	Thyroid peroxidase antibody	Thyroxine
Celiac disease	At diagnosis	Every 2-3 yr	Tissue transglutaminase, endomysial antibody	Antigliadin antibodies	Gluten-free diet

From Glastras SJ, Mohsin F, Donaghue KC: Complications of diabetes mellitus in childhood, *Pediatr Clin North Am* 52:1735–1753, 2005.

hyperglycemia, (2) aggressive control of systemic blood pressure, (3) selective control of arteriolar dilation by use of angiotensin-converting enzyme (ACE) inhibitors (thus decreasing transglomerular capillary pressure), and (4) dietary protein restriction (because high protein intake increases renal perfusion rate). Tight glycemic control will delay the progression of microalbuminuria and slow the progression of diabetic nephropathy. Previous extensive therapy of diabetes has a persistent benefit for 7-8 yr and may delay or prevent the development of diabetic nephropathy.

DIABETIC NEUROPATHY

Both the peripheral and autonomic nervous systems can be involved, and adolescents with diabetes can show early evidence of neuropathy. This complication can be traced to the metabolic effects of hyperglycemia and/or other effects of insulin deficiency on the various constituents of the peripheral nerve. The polyol pathway, nonenzymatic glycation, and/or disturbances of myo-inositol metabolism affecting 1 or more cell types in the multicellular constituents of the peripheral nerve appear likely to have an inciting role. The role of other factors, such as possible direct neurotrophic effects of insulin, insulin-related growth factors, nitric oxide, and stress proteins, seems to be relevant. Peripheral neuropathy may first present in some adolescents with long-standing history of diabetes. Using quantitative sensory testing (QST), abnormal cutaneous thermal perception is a common finding in both upper and lower limbs in neurologically asymptomatic young diabetic patients. Heat-induced pain threshold in the hand is correlated with the duration of the diabetes. There is no correlation between QST scores and metabolic control. Subclinical motor nerve impairment as manifested by reduced sensory nerve conduction velocity and sensory nerve action potential amplitude can be detected during late puberty and after puberty in about 10% of adolescents. Poor metabolic control during puberty appears to induce deteriorating peripheral neural function in young patients. An early sign of autonomic neuropathy such as decreased heart rate variability may present in adolescents with a history of long-standing disease and poor metabolic control. A number of therapeutic strategies have been attempted with variable results. These treatment modalities include (1) improvement in metabolic control, (2) use of aldose reductase inhibitors to reduce byproducts of the polyol pathway, (3) use of α-lipoic acid (an antioxidant) that enhances tissue nitric oxide and its metabolites, and (4) use of anticonvulsants (e.g., lorazepam, valproate, carbamazepine, tiagabine, and topiramate) for treatment of neuropathic pain.

Other complications in diabetic children include dwarfism associated with a glycogen-laden enlarged liver (**Mauriac syndrome**), osteopenia, and a syndrome of limited joint mobility associated with tight, waxy skin; growth impairment; and maturational delay. The Mauriac syndrome is related to underinsulinization; it is much less common since longer-acting insulins have become available. Clinical features of Mauriac syndrome include moon face, protuberant abdomen, proximal muscle wasting, and enlarged liver due to fat and glycogen infiltration. The syndrome of limited joint mobility is frequently associated with the early development of diabetic microvascular complications, such as retinopathy and nephropathy, which may appear before 18 yr of age.

PROGNOSIS

T1DM is a serious, chronic disease. It has been estimated that the average life span of individuals with diabetes is about 10 yr shorter than that of the nondiabetic population. Although diabetic children eventually attain a height within the normal adult range, puberty may be delayed, and the final height may be less than the genetic potential. From studies in identical twins, it is apparent that despite seemingly satisfactory control, the diabetic twin manifests delayed puberty and a substantial reduction in height when onset of disease occurs before puberty. These observations indicate that, in the past, conventional criteria for judging control were inadequate and that adequate control of T1DM was almost never achieved by routine means.

The introduction of portable devices (insulin pumps) that can be programmed to provide CSII with meal-related pulses is 1 approach to the resolution of these long-term problems. In selected individuals, nearly normal patterns of blood glucose and other indices of metabolic control, including HbA_{1C}, have been maintained for several years. This approach, however, should be reserved for highly motivated persons committed to rigorous self-monitoring of blood glucose who are alert to the potential complications, such as mechanical failure of the infusion device causing hyperglycemia or hypoglycemia and to infection at the site of catheter insertion.

The changing pattern of metabolic control is having a profound influence on reducing the incidence and the severity of certain complications. For example, after 20 yr of diabetes, there is a decline in the incidence of nephropathy in T1DM in Sweden among children whose disease was diagnosed in 1971-1975 compared with in the preceding decade. In addition, in most patients with microalbuminuria in whom it was possible to obtain good glycemic control, microalbuminuria disappeared. This improved prognosis is directly related to metabolic control.

PANCREAS AND ISLET TRANSPLANTATION AND REGENERATION

In an attempt to cure T1DM, transplantation of a segment of the pancreas or of isolated islets has been performed. These procedures are both technically demanding and associated with the risks of disease recurrence and complications of rejection or its treatment by immunosuppression. Complications of immunosuppression include the development of malignancy. Some antirejection drugs, notably cyclosporine and tacrolimus, are toxic to the islets of Langerhans, impairing insulin secretion and even causing diabetes. Hence, segmental pancreas transplantation is generally only performed in association with transplantation of a kidney for a patient with ESRD due to diabetic nephropathy in which the immunosuppressive regimen is indicated for the renal transplantation. Several thousand such transplants have been performed in adults. With experience and newer immunosuppressive agents, functional survival of the pancreatic graft may be achieved for up to several years, during which time patients may be in metabolic control with no or minimal exogenous insulin and reversal of some of the microvascular complications. However, because children and adolescents with DM are not likely to have ESRD from their diabetes, pancreas transplantation as a primary treatment in children cannot be recommended.

Attempts to transplant isolated islets have been equally challenging because of rejection. Research continues to improve techniques for the yield, viability, and reduction of immunogenicity of the islets of Langerhans for transplantation. An islet transplantation strategy (**Edmonton protocol**) infuses isolated pancreatic islets into the portal vein of a group of adults with T1DM. This therapeutic strategy also involves the use of a new generation of immunosuppressive medications that apparently have lower side-effect profiles than do other drugs. Of 36 consecutive patients with at least 2 yr of follow-up after the initial transplant, 5 (14%) were insulin independent at 2 yr. Although patients experienced minimal side effects from immunosuppressive medications, some complications associated with islet transplantation procedures were observed that included portal vein thrombosis, bleeding related to the percutaneous portal vein access, an expanding intrahepatic and subscapular hemorrhage on anticoagulation (requiring transfusion and surgery). Elevated liver function test results were found in 46% of subjects but resolved in all. However, only half of the patients remained insulin free at 2 yr. It has been suggested that positive long-term clinical outcome is dependent on islet graft composition, especially the presence of high numbers of islet progenitor (ductal-epithelial) cells. There is improved islet engraftment by the peritransplant administration of immunosuppressants, antithymocyte globulin, and etanercept. Long-term monitoring will be needed before the success of these techniques can be assessed.

Regeneration of islets is an approach that could potentially cure T1DM. It is classified into 3 categories:

1. In vitro therapy using transplanted cultured cells, including embryonic stem cells, pancreatic stem cells, and β-cell lines, in conjunction with immunosuppressive therapy or immunoisolation.
2. Ex vivo regeneration therapy, in which patients' own cells, such as bone marrow stem cells, which are transiently removed and induced to differentiate into β cells in vitro. Although some investigators have reported successful transdifferentiation of embryonic stem cells into pancreatic β cells after transplantation of bone marrow cells into rodents, others have failed to observe such effects. Therefore, insulin-producing cells cannot be generated from bone marrow stem cells consistently at this time.
3. In vivo regeneration therapy, in which impaired tissues regenerate from patients' own cells in vivo. β-cell neogenesis from non–β cells and β-cell proliferation in vivo has been considered, particularly as regeneration therapies for T2DM.

High-dose immunosuppression and autologous nonmyeloablative hematopoietic stem cell transplantation (AHST) in 11 out of 15 (73.3%) newly diagnosed T1DM patients (aged 14-31 yr) became insulin-free for at least 6 mo, whereas only 4 out of 15 (26.6%) were insulin-free for 21 mo. Subsequently, 8 additional patients were included with mean follow-up period of 28.9 mo. This pilot study demonstrated that with AHST, β-cell function was increased significantly and majority of patients achieved insulin independence with good glycemic control.

583.3 Type 2 Diabetes Mellitus

Ramin Alemzadeh and Omar Ali

Formerly known as non–insulin dependent diabetes or adult-onset diabetes, T2DM is a heterogeneous disorder, characterized by peripheral insulin resistance and failure of the β cell to keep up with increasing insulin demand. These patients have relative rather than absolute insulin deficiency. Generally, they are not ketosis prone, but ketoacidosis may develop in some circumstances. The specific etiology is not known, but these patients do not have autoimmune destruction of β cells, nor do they have any of the known causes of secondary diabetes.

NATURAL HISTORY

T2DM is considered a polygenic disease aggravated by environmental factors, such as low physical activity and excessive caloric intake. Most patients are obese, though the disease can occasionally be seen in normal weight individuals. Asians in particular appear to be at risk for T2DM at lower degrees of total adiposity. Some patients may not necessarily meet overweight or obese criteria for age and gender despite abnormally high percentage of body fat in the abdominal region. Obesity, in particular, central obesity, is associated with the development of insulin resistance. In addition, patients who are at risk for developing T2DM exhibit decreased glucose-induced insulin secretion. Obesity does not lead to the same degree of insulin resistance in all individuals and even those who develop insulin resistance do not necessarily exhibit impaired β-cell function. Thus, many obese individuals have some degree of insulin resistance, but compensate for it by increasing insulin secretion. But those who are unable to adequately compensate for insulin resistance by increasing insulin secretion, develop impaired glucose tolerance and impaired fasting glucose (usually, thought not always, in that order). Hepatic insulin resistance leads to excessive hepatic glucose output (failure of insulin to suppress hepatic glucose output), while skeletal muscle insulin resistance leads to decreased glucose uptake in a major site of glucose disposal. Over time hyperglycemia worsens, a phenomenon that has been attributed to the deleterious effect of chronic hyperglycemia (glucotoxicity) or chronic hyperlipidemia (lipotoxicity) on β-cell function and is often accompanied by increased triglyceride content and decreased insulin gene expression. At some point, blood glucose elevation meets the criteria for diagnosis of T2DM (see Web Table 583-2 on the *Nelson Textbook of Pediatrics* website at www.expertconsult.com), but most patients with T2DM remain asymptomatic for months to years after this point because hyperglycemia is moderate and symptoms are not as dramatic as the polyuria and weight loss accompanying T1DM. Even weight gain may continue. The prolonged hyperglycemia may be accompanied by the development of microvascular and macrovascular complications. In time, β-cell function can decrease to the point that the patient has absolute insulin deficiency and becomes dependent on exogenous insulin. In T2DM, insulin deficiency is rarely absolute, so patients usually do not need insulin to survive. Nevertheless, glycemic control can be improved by exogenous insulin. DKA is uncommon in patients with T2DM, but may occur and is usually associated with the stress of another illness such as severe infection and may resolve when the stressful illness resolves. DKA tends to be more common in African-American patients than in other ethnic groups. Although it is generally believed that autoimmune destruction of pancreatic β cells does not occur in T2DM, autoimmune markers of T1DM—namely, GAD65, ICA512, and IAA—may be positive in up to one third of the cases of adolescent T2DM. The presence of these autoimmune markers does not rule out T2DM in children and adolescents. At the same time, due to the general increase in obesity, the presence of obesity does not preclude the diagnosis of T1DM. While the majority of newly diagnosed diabetics can be confidently assigned a diagnosis of T1DM or T2DM, a few exhibit features of both types and are difficult to classify.

EPIDEMIOLOGY

The latest NHANES data (from 1999-2002) shows that the prevalence of T2DM in 12-19 yr olds in the USA is 1.46/1000. The SEARCH study found that the prevalence of type 2 diabetes in the 10-19 yr old age group in the USA was 15% in 2001 and it is likely that this proportion has increased over time. Certain ethnic groups appear to be at higher risk; for example, Native Americans, Hispanic Americans, and African Americans (in that order) have higher incidence rates than white Americans. While a majority of children presenting with diabetes still have T1DM, the percentage of children presenting with T2DM is increasing and represents up to 50% of the new diabetics in some centers. We, at Children's Hospital of Wisconsin (Milwaukee), have observed a more than 10-fold increase in incidence of T2DM (from less than 2% to about 22% of new cases of DM) in children aged 10-18 yr in the past decade. Prevalence in the rest of the world varies widely and accurate data are not available for many countries, but it is clear that the prevalence is increasing in every part of the world. Asians in general seem to develop T2DM at lower BMI levels than Europeans. In conjunction with their low incidence of type 1 diabetes, this means that T2DM accounts for a higher proportion of childhood diabetics in many Asian countries.

The epidemic of T2DM in children and adolescents parallels the emergence of the obesity epidemic (Chapter 44). Although obesity itself is associated with insulin resistance, diabetes does not develop until there is some degree of failure of insulin secretion. Thus, when measured, insulin secretion in response to glucose or other stimuli is always lower in persons with T2DM than in control subjects matched for age, sex, weight, and equivalent glucose concentration.

GENETICS

T2DM has a strong genetic component; concordance rates among identical twins are in the 60-90% range. But it should be kept in mind that twinning itself increases the risk of T2DM (due to intrauterine growth retardation [IUGR]) and this may distort estimates of genetic risk. In at least 1 study from Denmark, both monozygotic and dizygotic twins have a lifetime concordance of T2DM of around 70%, indicating that shared environmental factors (including the prenatal environment) may play a large role in the development of T2DM. The genetic basis for T2DM is complex and incompletely defined; no single identified defect predominates as does the HLA association with T1DM. Genome-wide association studies have now identified certain genetic polymorphisms that are associated with increased T2DM risk in most populations studied; the most consistently identified are variants of the TCF7L2 (transcription factor 7–like 2) gene, which may have a role in β-cell function. Other identified risk alleles include variants in PPARG and KCNJ11 and at least 18 other genes and the list is growing longer by the day. In addition, other variants increase diabetes risk by increasing the risk of obesity (for example, variants in the FTO gene). But to date, all these identified variants explain only a small portion (probably less than 20%) of the population risk of diabetes and in many cases the mechanism by which these polymorphisms confer risk of T2DM is not clear.

EPIGENETICS AND FETAL PROGRAMMING

Low birthweight and IUGR are associated with increased risk of T2DM and this risk appears to be higher in low-birthweight infants who gain weight more rapidly in the 1st few years of life. These findings have led to the formulation of the "thrifty phenotype" hypothesis, which postulates that poor fetal nutrition somehow programs these children to maximize storage of nutrients and makes them more prone to future weight gain and development of diabetes. Epigenetic modifications may play a role in this phenomenon, but the detailed molecular mechanisms involved are yet to be determined. But whatever the exact mechanism, prenatal and early childhood environments play an important role in the pathogenesis of T2DM and may do so by epigenetic modification of the genetic code (in addition to other factors).

ENVIRONMENTAL AND LIFESTYLE-RELATED RISK FACTORS

Obesity is the most important lifestyle factor associated with development of diabetes. This in turn is associated with the intake of high-energy foods, physical inactivity, TV viewing ("screen time") and low socioeconomic status (in developed countries). Maternal smoking also increases the risk of diabetes and obesity in the offspring. Interestingly, smoking by young adults also increases their own risk of diabetes by as yet unknown mechanisms. In addition, sleep deprivation and psychosocial stress are associated with increased risk of obesity in childhood and with impaired glucose tolerance in adults, possibly via overactivation of the hypothalamic-pituitary-adrenal axis. Many antipsychotics (especially the atypical antipsychotics like olanzapine and quetiapine) and antidepressants (both tricyclic antidepressants and newer antidepressants like fluoxetine and paroxetine) induce weight gain. In addition to the risk conferred by increased obesity, some of these medications may also have a direct role in causing insulin resistance, β-cell dysfunction, leptin resistance, and activation of inflammatory pathways. To complicate matters further, there is evidence that schizophrenia and depression themselves increase the risk of T2DM and the metabolic syndrome, independent of the risk conferred by drug treatment. As a result, both obesity and T2DM are more prevalent in this population and with increasing use of antipsychotics and antidepressants in the pediatric population, this association is likely to become stronger.

CLINICAL FEATURES

In the USA, T2DM in children is more likely to be diagnosed in Native American, Hispanic American, and African American youth, with the highest incidence being reported in Pima Indian youth, where its prevalence in the 15-19 yr age group is 5%. While cases may be seen as young as 6 yr of age, most are diagnosed in adolescence and incidence increases with increasing age. Family history of T2DM is present in practically all cases. Typically, these patients are obese and present with mild symptoms of polyuria and polydipsia, or are asymptomatic and detected on screening tests. But presentation with diabetic ketoacidosis occurs in up to 10% of cases and may be higher in African Americans. Physical examination frequently reveals the presence of acanthosis nigricans, most commonly on the neck and in other flexural areas. Other findings may include striae and an increased waist-hip ratio. Laboratory testing reveals elevated HbA_{1c} levels and HbA_{1c} values are higher at diagnosis among minority youth. Hyperlipidemia characterized by elevated triglycerides and low-density lipoprotein (LDL) cholesterol levels are commonly seen in patients with T2DM at diagnosis. Therefore lipid screening is indicated in all new cases of T2DM. Since hyperglycemia develops slowly and patients may be asymptomatic for months or years after they develop T2DM, screening for T2DM is recommended in high-risk children (Table 583-11) and many patients are diagnosed upon routine screening. The ADA recommends that all youth who are overweight and have at least 2 other risk factors be tested for T2DM beginning at age 10 yr or at the onset of puberty and every 2 yr after that. These risk factors include family history of T2DM in first- or second-degree relatives, history of gestational diabetes in the mother, belonging to certain ethnic groups (i.e., Native Americans, African American, Hispanic, or Asian/Pacific Islander) and having signs of insulin resistance (e.g., acanthosis nigricans, hypertension, dyslipidemia, or polycystic ovary syndrome). The current recommendation is to use fasting blood glucose as a screening test, but some authorities now recommend that HbA_{1c} be used as a screening tool and it has the advantage that a fasting sample is not required. In borderline or asymptomatic cases, the diagnosis may be confirmed

Table 583-11 TESTING FOR TYPE 2 DIABETES IN CHILDREN

Criteria*
• Overweight (BMI >85th percentile for age and sex, weight for height >85th percentile, or weight >120% of ideal for height)
Plus
Any 2 of the following risk factors:
• Family history of type 2 diabetes in 1st- or 2nd-degree relative
• Race/ethnicity (American Indian, African American, Hispanic, Asian/Pacific Islander)
Signs of insulin resistance or conditions associated with insulin resistance (acanthosis nigricans, hypertension, dyslipidemia, polycystic ovary syndrome)
Age of initiation: Age 10 yr or at onset of puberty if puberty occurs at a younger age
Frequency: Every 2 yr
Test: Fasting plasma glucose preferred

*Clinical judgment should be used to test for diabetes in high-risk patients who do not meet these criteria.

From American Diabetes Association: Type 2 diabetes in children and adolescents, *Diabetes Care* 23:386, 2000. Reproduced by permission.

using a standard glucose tolerance test, but this test is not required if typical symptoms are present or fasting plasma glucose is clearly elevated on 2 separate occasions.

TREATMENT

Type 2 diabetes is a progressive syndrome that gradually leads to complete insulin deficiency during the patient's life. A systematic approach for treatment of T2DM should be implemented according to the natural course of the disease, including adding insulin when hypoglycemic oral agent failure occurs. Nevertheless, lifestyle modification (diet and exercise) is an essential part of the treatment regimen and consultation with a dietitian is usually necessary. There is no particular dietary or exercise regimen that has been conclusively shown to be superior but most centers recommend a low-calorie, low-fat diet and 30-60 minutes of physical activity at least 5 times per week. Screen time should be limited to 1-2 hr per day. These children often come from a household environment with a poor understanding of healthy eating habits. Commonly observed behaviors include skipping meals, heavy snacking, and excessive daily television viewing, video game playing, and computer use. Adolescents engage in non–appetite-based eating (i.e., emotional eating, television-cued eating, boredom) and cyclic dieting ("yo-yo" dieting). Treatment in these cases is frequently challenging and may not be successful unless the entire family buys into the need to change their unhealthy lifestyle.

When lifestyle interventions fail to normalize blood glucose, oral hypoglycemic agents are introduced for management of persistent hyperglycemia (Table 583-12). Patients who present with DKA or with markedly elevated HbA_{1c} (>9.0%) will require treatment with insulin using protocols similar to those used for treating T1DM. Once blood glucose levels are under control most cases can be managed with oral hypoglycemic agents and lifestyle changes, but some patients will continue to require insulin therapy.

The most commonly used oral agent is metformin. Renal function must be assessed before starting metformin as impaired renal function has been associated with potentially fatal lactic acidosis in adults. Significant hepatic dysfunction is also a contraindication, though mild elevations in liver enzymes may not be an absolute contraindication. The usual starting dose is 500 mg bid and this may be increased to a maximum dose of 2,500 mg per day. Abdominal symptoms are common early in the course of treatment, but in most cases will resolve with time.

Other agents like thiazolidinediones (TZDs), sulfonylureas, acarbose, pramlintide, and incretin mimetics are being used routinely in adults, but in pediatrics they constitute 2nd-line agents at this time. Sulfonylureas are widely used in adults, but experience in pediatrics is limited. Sulfonylureas cause insulin release by closing the potassium channel (K_{ATP}) on β cells. They are occasionally used when metformin monotherapy is unsuccessful or contraindicated for some reason (use in certain forms of neonatal diabetes is discussed in the section on neonatal diabetes). TZDs are not yet approved for use in pediatrics but are occasionally used as insulin sensitizers in patients who are not candidates for metformin treatment for any reason. Pramlintide (Symlin) is an analog of IAPP (islet amyloid polypeptide), which is a peptide that is co-secreted with insulin by the β cells and acts to delay gastric emptying, suppress glucagon, and possibly suppress food

Table 583-12 ORAL HYPOGLYCEMIC AGENTS

DRUG	MECHANISM OF ACTION	DURATION OF BIOLOGIC EFFECT (hr)	USUAL DAILY DOSE (mg)	DOSES/DAY	SIDE EFFECTS	CAUTION
Biguanide	Insulin sensitizer				Gastrointestinal disturbance, lactic acidosis	Avoid in hepatic or renal impairment
Metformin			1500-2500	2-3		
Sulfonylureas						
1st generation						
Acetohexamide		12-18	500-750	1 or divided		
Chlorpropamide		27-72	250-500	1		
Tolbutamide		14-16	1000-2000	1 or divided		
2nd generation						
Glipizide		14-16	2.5-10	1 or divided		
			XL: 5-10	1		
Glyburide		20-24+	2.5-10	1 or divided		
Glimepride		24+	2-4	1		
Glitinides	Promote insulin secretion					Titrate carefully in renal or hepatic dysfunction
Repaglinide		≤24	2-16	3		
Nateglinide		4	360	3		
α-Glucosidase inhibitors	Slow hydrolysis and absorption		150-300	3 (with meals)	Transient gastrointestinal disturbances	
Acarbose	of complex carbohydrates		150-300	3 (with meals)		
Miglitol						
Thiazolidinedione	Peripheral insulin sensitizer				Upper respiratory tract infection,	
Rosiglitazone			4-8	1 or divided	headache, edema, weight gain	
Pioglitazone			15-45	1		
Sitagliptin	GLP-1 receptor agonist	24	50-100	1	Upper respiratory tract infection, sore throat, diarrhea	No data in children or adolescents

From Jacobson-Dickman E, Levistky L: Oral agents in managing diabetes mellitus in children and adolescents, *Pediatr Clin North Am* 52:1689–1703, 2005.

intake. It is not yet approved for pediatric use. Incretins are gut-derived peptides like GLP-1 (glucagon like peptide-1), GLP-2, and GIP (glucose-dependent insulinotropic peptide, previously known as gastric inhibitory protein) that are secreted in response to meals and act to enhance insulin secretion and action, suppress glucagon production and delay gastric emptying (among other actions). GLP-1 analogs (e.g., exenatide) and agents that prolong endogenous GLP-1 action (e.g., sitagliptin) are now available for use in adults but are not yet approved for use in children and their use in pediatrics remains experimental at this time.

COMPLICATIONS

In the SEARCH study of diabetes in youth, 92% of the patients with T2DM had 2 or more elements of the metabolic syndrome (hypertension, hypertriglyceridemia, decreased HDL, increased waist circumference), including 70% with hypertension. In addition, the incidence of microalbuminuria and diabetic retinopathy appears to be higher in T2DM than it is in T1DM. In the SEARCH study, the incidence of microalbuminuria among patients who had T2DM of LESS than 5 yr duration was 7-22%, while retinopathy was present in 18.3%. Thus, all adolescents with T2DM should be screened for hypertension and lipid abnormalities and screening for microalbuminuria and retinopathy may be indicated even earlier than it is in T1DM. Sleep apnea and fatty liver disease are being diagnosed with increasing frequency and may necessitate referral to the appropriate specialists. Complications associated with all forms of diabetes and recommendations for screening are noted in Table 583-10 while Table 583-13 lists additional conditions particularly associated with T2DM.

PREVENTION

The difficulties in achieving good glucose control and preventing diabetes complications make prevention a compelling strategy. This is particularly true for T2DM, which is clearly linked to modifiable risk factors (obesity, a sedentary lifestyle). The Diabetes Prevention Program (DPP) was designed to prevent or delay the development of T2DM in adult individuals at high risk by virtue of impaired glucose tolerance (IGT). DPP results demonstrated that intensified lifestyle or drug intervention in individuals with IGT prevented or delayed the onset of T2DM. The results were striking. Lifestyle intervention reduced diabetes incidence by 58%; metformin reduced the incidence by 31% compared with placebo. The effects were similar for men and women and for all racial and ethnic groups. Lifestyle interventions are believed to have similar beneficial effects in obese adolescents with IGT. Screening is indicated for at-risk patients (see Table 583-11).

Table 583-13 MONITORING FOR COMPLICATIONS AND CO-MORBIDITIES

CONDITION	SCREENING TEST	COMMENT
Hypertension	Blood pressure	
Fatty liver	AST, ALT, possibly liver ultrasound	
Polycystic ovary syndrome	Menstrual history, assessment for androgen excess with free/total testosterone, DHEA	
Microalbuminuria	Urine albumin concentration and albumin/creatinine ratios	
Dyslipidemia	Fasting lipid profile (total, LDL, HDL cholesterol, triglycerides)	Obtain at diagnosis and every 2 yr
Sleep apnea	Sleep study to assess overnight oxygen saturation	

From Liu L, Hironaka K, Pihoker C: Type 2 diabetes in youth, *Curr Probl Pediatr Adolesc Health Care* 34:249–280, 2004.

IMPAIRED GLUCOSE TOLERANCE

The term impaired glucose tolerance (IGT) is suggested as a replacement for terms such as asymptomatic diabetes, chemical diabetes, subclinical diabetes, borderline diabetes, and latent diabetes in order to avoid the stigma associated with the term diabetes mellitus. Such diagnostic labels may influence the choice of vocation, eligibility for health or life insurance, and self-image. Although IGT represents a biochemical intermediate between normal glucose metabolism and that of diabetes, experience has shown that few children with IGT go on to acquire diabetes; estimates range from zero to 10%. There is disagreement about whether the degree of glucose intolerance is useful as a prognostic index of the likelihood of progression, but there is evidence that among the few instances of progression, the insulin response during glucose tolerance testing is severely impaired. Islet cell or insulin autoantibodies as well as the HLA-DR3 or HLA-DR4 haplotype are commonly found in those who go on to develop clinical diabetes. In most obese children with IGT, insulin responses during oral glucose tolerance tests are higher than the mean for age-adjusted but not weight-adjusted control subjects; these individuals have some resistance to the effects of insulin rather than a total inability to secrete it.

In healthy nondiabetic children, the glucose response during an oral glucose tolerance test is similar at all ages. In contrast, plasma insulin responses during the test increase progressively within the age span of about 3-15 yr and are significantly higher during puberty so that interpretation of these responses requires comparison with age- and puberty-adjusted responses.

The performance of the glucose tolerance test should be standardized according to currently accepted criteria. These include at least 3 days of a well-balanced diet containing approximately 50% of calories from carbohydrates, fasting from midnight until the time of the test in the morning, and a dose of glucose for the test of 1.75 g/kg but not more than 75 g. Plasma samples are obtained before ingestion of the glucose and at 1, 2, and 3 hr thereafter. The arbitrarily designated response to the test that identifies IGT is a fasting plasma glucose value of less than 126 mg/dL and a value at 2 hr of more than 140 mg/dL but less than 200 mg/dL (see Web Table 583-2 on the *Nelson Textbook of Pediatrics* website at www.expertconsult.com). Determination of serum insulin responses during the glucose tolerance test is not a prerequisite for reaching a diagnosis; the magnitude of the response, however, may have prognostic value.

In children with IGT but without fasting hyperglycemia, repeated oral glucose tolerance tests are not recommended. Investigations in such children indicate that the degree of impaired glucose tolerance tends to remain stable or may actually improve over a period of years, except in patients with markedly subnormal insulin responses. Consequently, apart from reduction in weight for the obese child, no therapy is indicated. At this time, the use of oral hypoglycemic agents should be considered investigational.

583.4 Other Specific Types of Diabetes

Ramin Alemzadeh and Omar Ali

Most cases of diabetes in children as well as adults fall into the 2 broad categories of type 1 and type 2 diabetes, but up to 1-4 % of cases are due to single gene disorders. These disorders include hereditary defects of β-cell function and insulin action, as well as rare forms of mitochondrial diabetes.

GENETIC DEFECTS OF β-CELL FUNCTION

Maturity-Onset Diabetes of Youth

Several forms of diabetes are associated with monogenic defects in β-cell function. Before these genetic defects were identified, this subset of diabetics was diagnosed on clinical grounds and described by the term MODY or maturity-onset diabetes of youth. This subtype of DM consists of a group of heterogeneous clinical entities that are characterized by onset between the ages of 9 and 25 yr, autosomal dominant (AD) inheritance, and a primary defect in insulin secretion. Strict criteria for the diagnosis of MODY include diabetes in at least 3 generations with AD transmission and diagnosis before age 25 yr in at least 1 affected subject. Now that the genetic basis and mechanism of these disorders is better understood, the term MODY is used for dominantly inherited monogenic defects of insulin secretion. The ADA groups these disorders together under the broader category of "genetic defects of β-cell function." Six of these defects typically meet the clinical criteria for the diagnosis of MODY and are listed in Table 583-14. Just 2 of them (MODY2 and MODY3) account for 80% of the cases in this category in European populations, but the distribution may be different in other ethnic groups. Except for MODY2 (which is due to mutations in the enzyme glucokinase), all other forms are due to genetic defects in various transcription factors (see Table 583-14).

MODY2 This is the 2nd most common form of MODY and accounts for about 15% of all patients diagnosed with MODY. Glucokinase plays an essential role in β-cell glucose sensing and heterozygous mutations in this gene lead to mild reductions in pancreatic β-cell response to glucose. Homozygotes with the same mutations are completely unable to secrete insulin in response to glucose and develop a form of permanent neonatal diabetes. Patients with heterozygous mutations have a higher threshold for insulin release but are able to secrete insulin adequately once blood glucose rises above 7 mmol/L. This results in a relatively mild form of diabetes (HbA_{1c} is usually less than 7%), with mild fasting hyperglycemia and IGT in the majority of patients. Some of these patients may be misdiagnosed as type 1 diabetes if diagnosed in childhood, as gestational diabetes in pregnancy, and as well controlled type 2 diabetes in adults. An accurate diagnosis is important because most cases are not progressive, and except for gestational diabetes, may not require treatment. When needed, they can usually be treated with small doses of exogenously administered insulin. Treatment with oral agents (sulfonylureas and related drugs) can be successful and may be more acceptable to many patients.

Table 583-14 SUMMARY OF MODY TYPES AND SPECIAL CLINICAL CHARACTERISTICS

	GENE MUTATED	FUNCTION	SPECIAL FEATURE
MODY1	HNF4α	Transcription factor	Decreased levels of triglycerides, apolipoproteins apoAII and apoCIII
MODY2	Glucokinase (GCK)	Enzyme, glucose sensor	Hyperglycemia of early onset but mild and nonprogressive
MODY3	HNF-1α	Transcription factor	Decreased renal absorption of glucose and consequent glycosuria
MODY4	IPF-1	Necessary for pancreatic development	Homozygous mutation causes pancreatic agenesis
MODY5	HNF-1β	Transcription factor	Nonhyperglycemic renal disease; associated with uterine abnormalities, hypospadias, joint laxity, and learning difficulties
MODY6	NEUROD1	Differentiation factor in the development of pancreatic islets	Extremely rare

MODY, maturity-onset diabetes of the young.
From Nakhla M, Polychronakos C: Monogenic and other unusual causes of diabetes mellitus, *Pediatr Clin North Am* 52:1637–1650, 2005.

MODY3 Patients affected with mutations in the transcription factor HNF-1α (hepatocyte nuclear factor 1 alpha) show abnormalities of carbohydrate metabolism varying from impaired glucose tolerance to severe diabetes and often progressing from a mild to a severe form over time. They are also prone to the development of vascular complications. This is the most common MODY subtype and accounts for 65% of all cases. These patients are very sensitive to the action of sulfonylureas and can usually be treated with relatively low doses of these oral agents, at least in the early stages of the disease. In children, this form of MODY is sometimes misclassified as type 1 and treated with insulin. Evaluation of autoimmune markers may assist in classification, and in doubtful cases genetic testing for this form of MODY is now available and is indicated in patients with relatively mild diabetes and a family history suggestive of AD inheritance. On the other hand, even patients with relatively mild and gradual onset of diabetes may have T1DM, and in the absence of a family history suggestive of AD inheritance, the diagnosis of MODY is not warranted. Accurate diagnosis can lead to avoidance of unnecessary insulin treatment and specific genetic counseling.

HNF 4α (MODY1), IPF-1/PDF-1 (MODY4), HNF 1β/TCF2 (MODY5), and NeuroD1 (MODY6) are all transcription factors that are involved in β-cell development and function and mutations in these lead to various rare forms of MODY. In addition to diabetes they can also have specific findings unrelated to hyperglycemia; for example, MODY1 is associated with low triglyceride and lipoprotein levels and MODY5 is associated with renal cysts and renal dysfunction. In terms of treatment, MODY1 and MODY4 may respond to oral sulfonylureas, but MODY5 does not respond to oral agents and requires treatment with insulin. NeuroD1 defects are extremely rare and not much is known about their natural history.

Primary or secondary defects in the glucose transporter-2 (GLUT-2), which is an insulin-independent glucose transporter, may also be associated with diabetes. Diabetes may also be a manifestation of a polymorphism in the glycogen synthase gene. This enzyme is crucially important for storage of glucose as glycogen in muscle. Patients with this defect are notable for marked insulin resistance and hypertension, as well as a strong family history of diabetes.

Mitochondrial Gene Defects

MIDD (MATERNALLY INHERITED DIABETES AND DEAFNESS) Point mutations in mitochondrial DNA are sometimes associated with maternally inherited DM and deafness. The most common mutation in these cases is the point mutation m.3243A>G. This mutation is identical to the mutation in MELAS (myopathy, encephalopathy, lactic acidosis, and strokelike syndrome), but this syndrome is not associated with diabetes; the phenotypic expression of the same defect varies. Diabetes in most of these cases presents insidiously but approximately 20% of patients have an acute presentation resembling T1DM. The mean age of diagnosis of diabetes is 37 yr but cases have been reported as young as 11 yr. This mutation has been estimated to be present in 1.5% of Japanese diabetics, which may be higher than the prevalence in other ethnic groups. Metformin should be avoided in these patients because of the theoretical risk of severe lactic acidosis in the presence of mitochondrial dysfunction.

Another form of IDDM, sometimes associated with mitochondrial mutations, is the Wolfram syndrome. Wolfram syndrome is characterized by diabetes insipidus, DM, optic atrophy, and deafness—thus, the acronym DIDMOAD. Some patients with diabetes appear to have severe insulinopenia, whereas others have significant insulin secretion as judged by C-peptide. The overall prevalence is 1/770,000. The sequence of appearance of the stigmata is as follows: nonautoimmune IDDM in the 1st decade, central diabetes insipidus and sensorineural deafness in two thirds to three fourths of the patients in the 2nd decade, renal tract anomalies in about one half of the patients in the 3rd decade, and neurologic complications such as cerebellar ataxia and myoclonus in one half to two thirds of the patients in the 4th decade. Other features include primary gonadal atrophy in the majority of males and a progressive neurodegenerative course with neurorespiratory death at a median age of 30 yr. Some (but not all) cases are due to mutations in the WFS-1 (wolframin) gene on chromosome 4p.

DIABETES MELLITUS OF THE NEWBORN

Neonatal diabetes mellitus is rare, with an estimated incidence of 1 per 100,000 newborns. Onset of classic autoimmune T1DM before the age of 6 mo is most unusual and most cases of diabetes in this age range are caused by genetic mutations.

Transient Neonatal Diabetes Mellitus (TNDM)

Neonatal diabetes is transient in about 50% of cases, but after an interim period of normal glucose tolerance, 50-60% of these patients develop permanent diabetes (at an average age of 14 yr). There are also reports of patients with classic T1DM who formerly had transient diabetes of the newborn. It remains to be determined whether this association of transient diabetes in the newborn followed much later in life by classic T1DM is a chance occurrence or causally related.

The syndrome of transient DM in the newborn infant has its onset in the 1st wk of life and persists several weeks to months before spontaneous resolution. Median duration is 12 wk. It occurs most often in infants who are small for gestational age and is characterized by hyperglycemia and pronounced glycosuria, resulting in severe dehydration and, at times, metabolic acidosis, but with only minimal or no ketonemia or ketonuria. Insulin responses to glucose or tolbutamide are low to absent; basal plasma insulin concentrations are normal. After spontaneous recovery, the insulin responses to these same stimuli are brisk and normal, implying a functional delay in β-cell maturation with spontaneous resolution. Occurrence of the syndrome in consecutive siblings has been reported. About 70% of cases are due to a**bnormalities of chromosome 6q24**, resulting in overexpression of paternally expressed genes such as pleomorphic adenoma gene–like 1 (PLAGL1/ZAC) and hydatidiform mole associated and imprinted (HYMAI). Most of the remaining cases are due to mutations in K_{ATP} channels. Mutations in K_{ATP} channels also cause many cases of permanent neonatal diabetes, but there is practically no overlap between the mutations that lead to TNDM and those causing permanent neonatal diabetes mellitus (PNDM). This syndrome of TNDM should be distinguished from the severe hyperglycemia that may occur in hypertonic dehydration; that usually occurs in infants beyond the newborn period and responds promptly to rehydration with minimal or no requirement for insulin.

Administration of insulin is mandatory during the active phase of DM in the newborn. One to 2 U/kg/24 hr of an intermediate-acting insulin in 2 divided doses usually results in dramatic improvement and accelerated growth and gain in weight. Attempts at gradually reducing the dose of insulin may be made as soon as recurrent hypoglycemia becomes manifested or after 2 mo of age. Genetic testing is now available for 6q24 abnormalities as well as potassium channel defects and should be obtained on all patients.

Permanent Neonatal Diabetes Mellitus (PNDM)

Permanent DM in the newborn period is caused in approximately 50% of the cases by mutations in the *KCNJ11* (potassium inwardly-rectifying channel J, member 11) and *ABCC8* (ATP-binding cassette, subfamily C, member 8) genes. These genes code for the Kir6.2 and SUR1 subunits of the ATP-sensitive potassium channel, which is involved in an essential step in insulin secretion by the β cell. Some cases are caused by pancreatic agenesis due to homozygous mutations in the IPF-1 gene (where heterozygous mutations cause MODY4); homozygous mutations in the glucokinase gene (where heterozygous mutations cause MODY2) and mutations in the insulin gene. Almost all these infants are small at birth because of the role of insulin as an intrauterine growth factor. Instances of affected twins and families with more than 1 affected infant have been reported. Infants with permanent neonatal DM may be initially euglycemic and typically present between birth and 6 mo of life (mean age of presentation is 5 wk). There is a spectrum of severity and up to 20% have neurologic features. The most severely affected patients have the syndrome of *D*evelopmental delay, *E*pilepsy and *N*eonatal *D*iabetes (DEND syndrome). Less severe forms of DEND are labeled intermediate DEND or i-DEND.

Activating mutations in the *KCNJ11* gene (encoding the ATP-sensitive potassium channel subunit Kir6.2) are associated with both TNDM and PNDM, with particular mutations being associated with each phenotype. More than 90% of these patients respond to sulfonylureas (at higher doses than those used in T2DM) but patients with severe neurologic disease may be less responsive. Mutations in the *ABCC8* gene (encoding the SUR1 subunit of this potassium channel) were thought to be less likely to respond to sulfonylureas (because this is the subunit that binds sulfonylurea drugs) but some of these mutations have now been reported to respond and have been successfully switched from insulin to oral therapy. Several protocols for switching the patient from insulin to glibenclamide are available and patients are usually stabilized on doses ranging from 0.4-1 mg/kg/day. Because approximately 50% of neonatal diabetics have K-channel mutations that can be switched to sulfonylurea therapy, with dramatic improvement in glycemic control and quality of life, ALL patients with diabetes diagnosed before 6 mo of age (and perhaps even those diagnosed before 12 mo of age) should now be screened for these mutations by genetic testing.

IPEX Syndrome: Mutations in the FOXP3 (Forkhead box P3) gene lead to severe immune dysregulation and rampant autoimmunity. Autoimmune diabetes develops in >90% of cases, usually within the 1st few weeks of life and is accompanied by enteropathy, failure to thrive and other autoimmune disorders (Chapter 120.5).

Abnormalities of the Insulin Gene

Diabetes of variable degrees may also result from defects in the insulin gene that lead to various amino acid substitutions that impair the effectiveness of insulin at the receptor level. Insulin gene defects are exceedingly rare and may be associated with relatively mild diabetes or even normal glucose tolerance. Diabetes may also develop in patients with faulty processing of proinsulin to insulin (an autosomal dominant defect). These defects are notable for the high concentration of insulin as measured by radioimmunoassay, whereas MODY and GLUT-2 defects are characterized by relative or absolute deficiency of insulin secretion for the prevailing glucose concentrations.

GENETIC DEFECTS OF INSULIN ACTION

Various genetic mutations in the insulin receptor (IR) can impair the action of insulin at the IR or impair postreceptor signaling, leading to insulin resistance.

The mildest form of the syndrome with mutations in the IR was previously known as *type A insulin resistance*. This is associated with hirsutism, hyperandrogenism, and cystic ovaries in females, without obesity. Acanthosis nigricans may be present and life expectancy is not significantly impaired. More severe forms of insulin resistance are seen in 2 mutations in the insulin receptor gene that cause the pediatric syndromes of leprechaunism and Rabson-Mendenhall syndrome.

Leprechaunism

This is a syndrome characterized by IUGR, fasting hypoglycemia, and postprandial hyperglycemia in association with profound resistance to insulin, whose serum concentrations may be 100-fold that of comparable age-matched infants during an oral glucose tolerance test. Various defects of the insulin receptor have been described, thereby attesting to the important role of insulin and its receptor in fetal growth and possibly in morphogenesis. Most of these patients die in the 1st yr of life.

Rabson-Mendenhall Syndrome

This entity is defined by clinical manifestations that appear to be intermediate between those of acanthosis nigricans with insulin resistance type A and leprechaunism. The features include extreme insulin resistance, acanthosis nigricans, abnormalities of the teeth and nails, and pineal hyperplasia. It is not clear whether this syndrome is entirely distinct from leprechaunism; however, patients with Rabson-Mendenhall tend to live significantly longer than patients with leprechaunism.

Lipoatrophic Diabetes: Various forms of lipodystrophy are associated with insulin resistance and diabetes. Familial partial lipoatrophy is associated with mutations in the LMNA gene, encoding nuclear envelope proteins lamin A and C. Severe generalized lipoatrophy is associated with mutations in the seipin and AGPAT2 genes, but the mechanism by which these mutations lead to insulin resistance and diabetes is not known.

Stiff-Person Syndrome: This is an extremely rare autoimmune CNS disorder that is characterized by progressive stiffness and painful spasms of the axial muscles and very high titers of GAD-65 antibodies. About one third of the patients also develop T1DM.

SLE: In rare cases, patients with systemic lupus erythematosus (SLE) may develop autoantibodies to the insulin receptor, leading to insulin resistance and diabetes.

CYSTIC FIBROSIS-RELATED DIABETES (CHAPTER 395)

As patients with cystic fibrosis (CF) live longer, an increasing number are being diagnosed with cystic fibrosis-related diabetes (CFRD). Females appear to have a somewhat higher risk of CFRD than males and prevalence increases with increasing age until age 40 yr (there is a decline in prevalence after that, presumably because only the healthiest CF patients survive beyond that age). There is an association with pancreatic insufficiency and there may be higher risk in patients with class I and class II cystic fibrosis transmembrane conductance regulator (CFTR) mutations. A large multi-center study in the USA reported prevalence (in all ages) of 17% in females and 12% in males. Cross sectional studies indicate that the prevalence of impaired glucose tolerance may be significantly higher than this and up to 65% of children with CF have diminished 1st phase insulin secretion, even when they have normal glucose tolerance. In Denmark, oral glucose tolerance screening of the entire CF population demonstrated no diabetes in patients younger than 10 yr, 12% diabetes in patients aged 10-19 yr, and 48% diabetes in adults aged 20 yr and older. At a Midwestern center where routine annual oral glucose tolerance screening is performed, only about one half of children and one fourth of adults have normal glucose tolerance. The care of these patients is very different from that of patients with T1DM or T2DM, because CFRD patients have distinct pathophysiologic and complicated nutritional and medical problems.

Patients with CFRD have features of both T1DM and T2DM. In the pancreas, exocrine tissue is replaced by fibrosis and fat and many of the pancreatic islets are destroyed. The remaining islets demonstrate diminished numbers of β-, α-, and pancreatic polypeptide-secreting cells. Secretion of the islet hormones insulin, glucagon, and pancreatic polypeptide is impaired in patients with CF in response to a variety of secretagogues. This pancreatic damage leads to slowly progressive insulin deficiency, of which the earliest manifestation is an impaired 1st phase insulin response. As patients age, this response becomes progressively delayed and less robust than normal. At the same time, these patients develop insulin resistance due to chronic inflammation and the use of steroids. Insulin deficiency and insulin resistance lead to a very gradual onset of impaired glucose tolerance that eventually evolves into diabetes. In some cases, diabetes may wax and wane with disease exacerbations and the use of corticosteroids. The clinical presentation is similar to that of T2DM in that the onset of the disease is insidious and the occurrence of ketoacidosis is rare. Islet antibody titers are negative. Microvascular complications do develop, but may do so at a slower rate than in typical T1DM or T2DM. Macrovascular complications do not appear to be of concern in CFRD, perhaps because of the shortened life span of these patients. Several factors unique to CF influence the onset and the course of diabetes. For example: (1) frequent infections are associated with waxing and waning of insulin resistance; (2) energy needs are increased because of infection and pulmonary disease; (3) malabsorption is common, despite enzyme supplementation; (4) nutrient absorption is altered by abnormal intestinal transit time; (5) liver disease is frequently present; (6) anorexia and nausea are common; (7) there is a wide variation in daily food intake based on the patient's acute health status; and (8) both insulin and glucagon secretion are impaired (in contrast to autoimmune diabetes, in which only insulin secretion is affected).

Impaired glucose tolerance and CFRD are associated with poor weight gain and there is evidence that treatment with insulin improves weight gain and slows the rate of pulmonary deterioration. Because of these observations, the CF foundation recommends routine diabetes screening of all children with CF, starting at age 12 yr. There is some debate over the ideal screening modality; fasting blood glucose is easier to perform but will miss some cases as postprandial glucose may be abnormal before fasting glucose becomes elevated. A 2 hr glucose tolerance test is therefore recommended, though it is possible that simply obtaining a single 2 hr postprandial glucose value may be sufficient. When hyperglycemia develops, the accompanying metabolic derangements are usually mild, and relatively low doses of insulin usually suffice for adequate management. Basal insulin may be started initially, but basal-bolus therapy similar to that used in T1DM will eventually be needed. Some centers also use oral agents (sulfonylureas as well as metformin) but consensus guidelines have not been developed regarding the use of oral agents. Dietary restrictions are minimal as increased energy needs are present and weight gain is usually desired. Ketoacidosis is uncommon but may occur with progressive deterioration of islet cell function. Impaired glucose tolerance is not necessarily an indication for treatment, but patients who have poor growth and inadequate weight gain may benefit from the addition of basal insulin even if they do not meet the criteria for diagnosis of diabetes.

AUTOIMMUNE DISEASES

Chronic lymphocytic thyroiditis (Hashimoto thyroiditis) is frequently associated with T1DM in children (Chapter 560). As many as 1 in 5 insulin-dependent diabetic patients have thyroid antibodies in their serum; the prevalence is 2-20 times greater than in control populations. Only a small proportion of these patients, however, acquire clinical hypothyroidism; the interval between diagnosis of diabetes and thyroid disease averages about 5 yr. Periodic palpation of the thyroid gland is indicated in all diabetic children; if the gland feels firm or enlarged, serum measurements of thyroid antibodies and thyroid-stimulating hormone (TSH) should be obtained. A confirmed TSH level of greater than 10 µU/mL indicates existing or incipient thyroid dysfunction that warrants replacement with thyroid hormone. Deceleration in the rate of growth may also be due to thyroid failure and is, in itself, a reason for securing serum measurements of thyroxine and TSH concentrations.

When diabetes and thyroid disease coexist, the possibility of autoimmune adrenal insufficiency should be considered. It may be heralded by decreasing insulin requirements, increasing pigmentation of the skin and buccal mucosa, salt craving, weakness, asthenia and postural hypotension, or even frank Addisonian crisis. This syndrome is most unusual in the 1st decade of life, but it may become apparent in the 2nd decade or later.

Celiac disease, which is due to hypersensitivity to dietary gluten, is another autoimmune disorder that occurs with significant frequency in children with T1DM (Chapter 330.2). It is estimated that about 7% of children with T1DM develop celiac disease within the 1st 6 yr of diagnosis, and the incidence of celiac disease is significantly higher in children under 4 yr of age and in girls. Young children with T1DM and celiac disease usually present with gastrointestinal symptoms (abdominal cramping, diarrhea, and gastroesophageal reflux), growth failure due to suboptimal weight gain, and unexplained hypoglycemic reactions due to nutrient malabsorption; adolescents may remain asymptomatic. The diagnosis of celiac disease is considered if serum antiendomysial and/or tissue transglutaminase antibody titers are positive in the presence of normal serum total IgA level. The diagnosis is confirmed on endoscopic evaluation and biopsy of small bowel revealing characteristic atrophy of intestinal villi. Therapy consists of a gluten-free diet, which will alleviate gastrointestinal symptoms and may reduce glycemic excursions.

Circulating antibodies to gastric parietal cells and to intrinsic factor are 2-3 times more common in patients with T1DM than in control subjects. The presence of antibodies to gastric parietal cells is correlated with atrophic gastritis and antibodies to intrinsic factor are associated with malabsorption of vitamin B_{12}. However, megaloblastic anemia is rare in children with T1DM.

A variant of the multiple endocrine deficiency syndrome is characterized by T1DM, idiopathic intestinal mucosal atrophy with associated inflammation and severe malabsorption, IgA deficiency, and circulating antibodies to multiple endocrine organs including the thyroid, adrenal, pancreas, parathyroid, and gonads. In addition, nondiabetic family members have an increased frequency of vitiligo, Graves disease, and multiple sclerosis as well as low complement levels and antibodies to endocrine tissues.

ENDOCRINOPATHIES

The endocrinopathies listed in Web Table 583-1 on the *Nelson Textbook of Pediatrics* website at www.expertconsult.com are only rarely encountered as a cause of diabetes in childhood. They may accelerate the manifestations of diabetes in those with inherited or acquired defects in insulin secretion or action.

DRUGS

High-dose oral or parenteral steroid therapy usually results in significant insulin resistance leading to glucose intolerance and overt diabetes. The immunosuppressive agents cyclosporin and tacrolimus are toxic to β cells, causing IDDM in a significant proportion of patients treated with these agents. Their toxicity to pancreatic β cells was 1 of the factors that limited their usefulness in arresting ongoing autoimmune destruction of β cells. Streptozotocin and the rodenticide Vacor are also toxic to β cells, causing diabetes.

There are no consensus guidelines regarding treatment of steroid-induced hyperglycemia in children. Many patients on high-dose steroids have elevated blood glucose during the day and evening but become normoglycemic late at night and early in the morning. In general, significant hyperglycemia in an inpatient setting is treated with short acting insulin on an as-needed basis. Basal insulin may be added when fasting hyperglycemia is significant. Outpatient treatment can be more difficult, but when treatment is needed, protocols similar to the basal-bolus regimens used in T1DM are used.

GENETIC SYNDROMES ASSOCIATED WITH DIABETES MELLITUS

A number of rare genetic syndromes associated with IDDM or carbohydrate intolerance have been described (see Web Table 583-1 on the *Nelson Textbook of Pediatrics* website at www.expertconsult.com). These syndromes represent a broad spectrum of diseases ranging from premature cellular aging, as in the Werner and Cockayne syndromes (Chapter 84) to excessive obesity associated with hyperinsulinism, resistance to insulin action, and carbohydrate intolerance, as in the Prader-Willi syndrome (Chapters 75 and 76). Some of these syndromes are characterized by primary disturbances in the insulin receptor or in antibodies to the insulin receptor without any impairment in insulin secretion. Although rare, these syndromes provide unique models to understand the multiple causes of disturbed carbohydrate metabolism from defective insulin secretion or from defective insulin action at the cell receptor or postreceptor level.

BIBLIOGRAPHY

Please visit the Nelson Textbook of Pediatrics *website at www.expertconsult.com for the complete bibliography.*

PART XXVII The Nervous System

Chapter 584
Neurologic Evaluation

Rebecca K. Lehman and Nina F. Schor

A comprehensive neurologic evaluation—including history, physical examination, and the judicious use of ancillary studies—allows the clinician to localize and determine the etiology of central and peripheral nervous system pathology.

For the full continuation of this chapter, please visit the Nelson Textbook of Pediatrics *website at www.expertconsult.com.*

Chapter 585
Congenital Anomalies of the Central Nervous System

Stephen L. Kinsman and Michael V. Johnston

Central nervous system (CNS) malformations are grouped into neural tube defects and associated spinal cord malformations; encephaloceles; disorders of structure specification (gray matter structures, neuronal migration disorders, disorders of connectivity, and commissure and tract formation); disorders of the posterior fossa, brainstem, and cerebellum; disorders of brain growth and size; and disorders of skull growth and shape. Classification of these conditions into syndromic, nonsyndromic, and single-gene etiologies is also important. These disorders can also be seen as isolated findings or as being a consequence of environmental exposures. Elucidation of single-gene causes has outpaced our understanding of epigenetic and environmental mechanisms.

These disorders are heterogeneous in their presentation. Common presentations and clinical problems include disorders of head size and/or shape; hydrocephalus; fetal ultrasonographic brain abnormalities; neonatal encephalopathy; developmental delay, cognitive impairment, and mental retardation; hypotonia, motor impairment, and cerebral palsy; seizures, epilepsy, and drug-resistant epilepsy; cranial nerve dysfunction; and spinal cord dysfunction.

BIBLIOGRAPHY

Please visit the Nelson Textbook of Pediatrics *website at www.expertconsult.com for the complete bibliography.*

585.1 Neural Tube Defects

Stephen L. Kinsman and Michael V. Johnston

Neural tube defects (NTDs) account for the largest proportion of congenital anomalies of the CNS and result from failure of the neural tube to close spontaneously between the 3rd and 4th wk of in utero development. Although the precise cause of NTDs remains unknown, evidence suggests that many factors, including hyperthermia, drugs (valproic acid), malnutrition, chemicals, maternal obesity or diabetes, and genetic determinants (mutations in folate-responsive or folate-dependent enzyme pathways) can adversely affect normal development of the CNS from the time of conception. In some cases, an abnormal maternal nutritional state or exposure to radiation before conception increases the likelihood of a congenital CNS malformation. The major NTDs include spina bifida occulta, meningocele, myelomeningocele, encephalocele, anencephaly, caudal regression syndrome, dermal sinus, tethered cord, syringomyelia, diastematomyelia, and lipoma involving the conus medullaris and/or filum terminale and the rare condition iniencephaly.

The human nervous system originates from the primitive ectoderm that also develops into the epidermis. The ectoderm, endoderm, and mesoderm form the three primary germ layers that are developed by the 3rd wk. The endoderm, particularly the notochordal plate and the intraembryonic mesoderm, induces the overlying ectoderm to develop the neural plate in the 3rd wk of development (Fig. 585-1*A*). Failure of normal induction is responsible for most of the NTDs, as well as disorders of prosencephalic development. Rapid growth of cells within the neural plate causes further invagination of the neural groove and differentiation of a conglomerate of cells, the neural crest, which migrate laterally on the surface of the neural tube (see Fig. 585-1*B*). The notochordal plate becomes the centrally placed notochord, which acts as a foundation around which the vertebral column ultimately develops. With formation of the vertebral column, the notochord undergoes involution and becomes the nucleus pulposus of the intervertebral disks. The neural crest cells differentiate to form the peripheral nervous system, including the spinal and autonomic ganglia and the ganglia of cranial nerves V, VII, VIII, IX, and X. In addition, the neural crest forms the leptomeninges, as well as Schwann cells, which are responsible for myelination of the peripheral nervous system. The dura is thought to arise from the paraxial mesoderm. In the region of the embryo destined to become the head, similar patterns exist. In this region, the notocord is replaced by the precordal mesoderm.

In the 3rd wk of embryonic development, invagination of the neural groove is completed and the neural tube is formed by separation from the overlying surface ectoderm (see Fig. 585-1*C*). Initial closure of the neural tube is accomplished in the area corresponding to the future junction of the spinal cord and medulla and moves rapidly both caudally and rostrally. For a brief period, the neural tube is open at both ends, and the neural canal communicates freely with the amniotic cavity (see Fig. 585-1*D*). Failure of closure of the neural tube allows excretion of fetal substances (α-fetoprotein [AFP], acetylcholinesterase) into the amniotic fluid, serving as biochemical markers for a NTD. Prenatal screening of maternal serum for AFP in the 16th-18th wk of gestation is an effective method for identifying pregnancies at risk for fetuses with NTDs in utero. Normally, the rostral end of the neural tube closes on the 23rd day and the caudal neuropore closes by a process of secondary neurulation by the 27th day of development, before the time that many women realize they are pregnant.

The embryonic neural tube consists of three zones: ventricular, mantle, and marginal (see Fig. 585-1*E*). The ependymal layer consists of pluripotential, pseudostratified, columnar neuroepithelial cells. Specific neuroepithelial cells differentiate into primitive neurons or neuroblasts that form the mantle layer. The marginal zone is formed from cells in the outer layer of the neuroepithelium, which ultimately becomes the white matter. Glioblasts, which act as the primitive supportive cells of the CNS, also arise from the neuroepithelial cells in the ependymal zone. They migrate to the mantle and marginal zones and become future astrocytes and oligodendrocytes. The importance of other pathways of progenitor cell generation and migration are also being elucidated. It is likely that microglia originate from

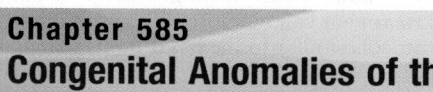

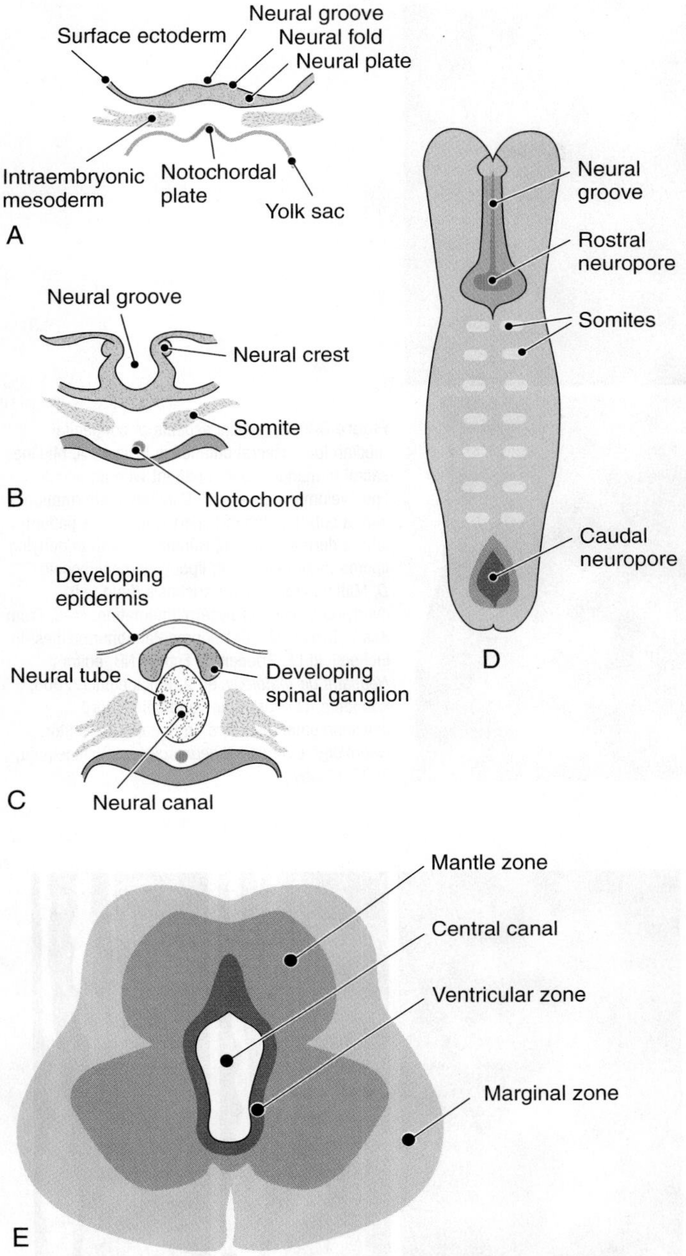

Figure 585-1 Diagrammatic illustration of the developing nervous system. *A*, Transverse sections of the neural plate during the 3rd wk. *B*, Formation of the neural groove and the neural crest. *C*, The neural tube is developed. *D*, Longitudinal drawing showing the initial closure of the neural tube in the central region. *E*, Cross-sectional drawing of the embryonic neural tube (primitive spinal cord).

mesenchymal cells at a later stage of fetal development when blood vessels begin to penetrate the developing nervous system.

585.2 Spina Bifida Occulta (Occult Spinal Dysraphism)

Stephen L. Kinsman and Michael V. Johnston

Spina bifida occulta is a common anomaly consisting of a midline defect of the vertebral bodies without protrusion of the spinal cord or meninges. Most patients are asymptomatic and lack neurologic signs, and the condition is usually of no consequence. Some consider the term *spina bifida occulta* to denote merely a posterior vertebral body fusion defect. This simple defect does not have an associated spinal cord malformation. Other clinically more significant forms of this closed spinal cord malformation are more correctly termed *occult spinal dysraphism.* In most of these cases, there are cutaneous manifestations such as a hemangioma, discoloration of the skin, pit, lump, dermal sinus, or hairy patch (Fig. 585-2). A spine roentgenogram in simple spina bifida occulta shows a defect in closure of the posterior vertebral arches and laminae, typically involving L5 and S1; there is no abnormality of the meninges, spinal cord, or nerve roots. Occult spinal dysraphism is often associated with more significant developmental abnormalities of the spinal cord, including syringomyelia, diastematomyelia, and/or a tethered cord. A spine roentgenogram in these cases might show bone defects or may be normal. All cases of occult spinal dysraphism are best investigated with MRI (Fig. 585-3). Initial screening in the neonate may include ultrasonography.

A dermoid sinus usually forms a small skin opening, which leads into a narrow duct, sometimes indicated by protruding hairs, a hairy patch, or a vascular nevus. Dermoid sinuses occur in the midline at the sites where meningoceles or encephaloceles can occur: the lumbosacral region or occiput, respectively. Dermoid sinus tracts can pass through the dura, acting as a conduit for the spread of infection. Recurrent meningitis of occult origin should prompt careful examination for a small sinus tract in the posterior midline region, including the back of the head. Lower back sinuses are usually above the gluteal fold and are directed cephalad. Tethered spinal cord syndrome may also be an associated problem. Diastematomyelia commonly has bony abnormalities that require surgical intervention along with untethering of the spinal cord.

An approach to imaging of the spine in patients with cutaneous lesions is noted in Table 585-1.

585.3 Meningocele

Stephen L. Kinsman and Michael V. Johnston

A meningocele is formed when the meninges herniate through a defect in the posterior vertebral arches or the anterior sacrum. The spinal cord is usually normal and assumes a normal position in the spinal canal, although there may be tethering, syringomyelia, or diastematomyelia. A fluctuant midline mass that might transilluminate occurs along the vertebral column, usually in the lower back. Most meningoceles are well covered with skin and pose no immediate threat to the patient. Careful neurologic examination is mandatory. Orthopedic and urologic examination should also be considered. In asymptomatic children with normal neurologic findings and full-thickness skin covering the meningocele, surgery may be delayed or sometimes not performed.

Before surgical correction of the defect, the patient must be thoroughly examined with the use of plain x-rays, ultrasonography, and MRI to determine the extent of neural tissue involvement, if any, and associated anomalies, including diastematomyelia, lipoma, and possible clinically significant tethered spinal cord. Urologic evaluation, usually including cystometrogram (CMG), identifies children with neurogenic bladder who are at risk for renal deterioration. Patients with leaking cerebrospinal fluid (CSF) or a thin skin covering should undergo immediate surgical treatment to prevent meningitis. A CT scan or MRI of the head is recommended for children with a meningocele because of the association with hydrocephalus in some cases. An anterior meningocele projects into the pelvis through a defect in the sacrum. Symptoms of constipation and bladder dysfunction develop due to the increasing size of the lesion. Female patients might have associated anomalies of the genital tract, including a rectovaginal fistula and vaginal septa. Plain x-rays demonstrate a defect in the sacrum, and CT scanning or MRI outlines the extent of the meningocele and any associated anomalies.

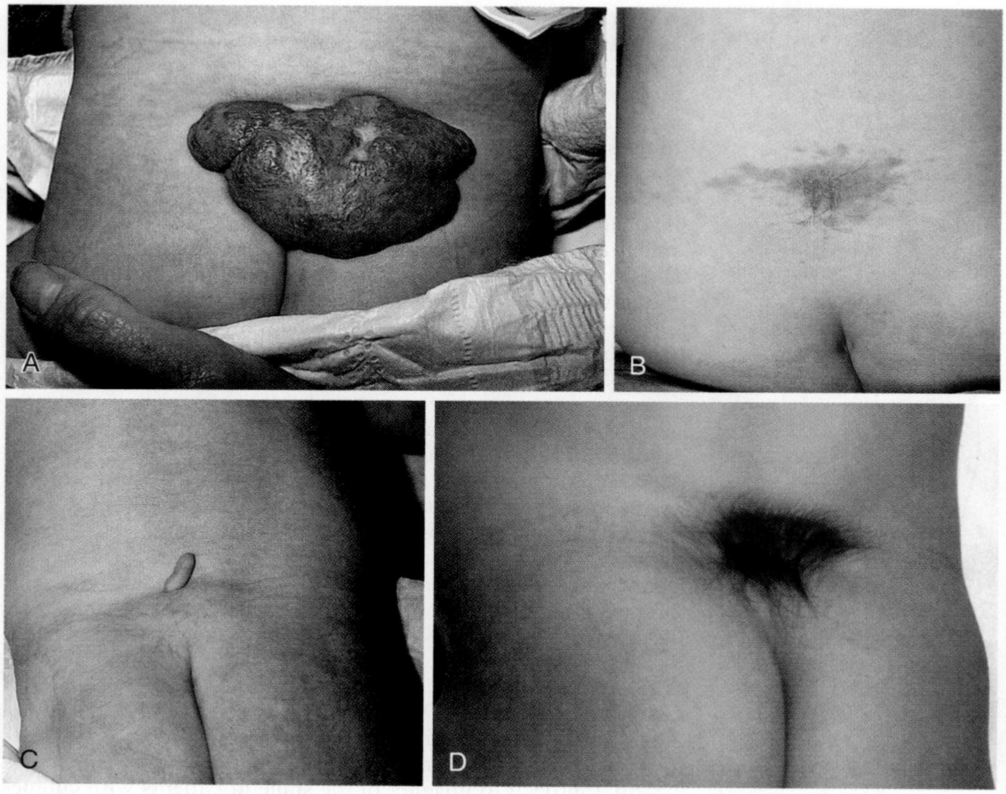

Figure 585-2 Clinical aspects of congenital median lumbosacral cutaneous lesions. *A,* Midline sacral hemangioma in a patient with an occult lipomyelomeningocele. *B,* Capillary malformation with a subtle patch of hypertrichosis in a patient with a dermal sinus. *C,* Human tail with underlying lipoma in an infant with lipomyelomeningocele. *D,* Midline area of hypertrichosis (faun tail) overlying a patch of hyperpigmentation. (*A-C,* From Kos L, Drolet BA: Developmental abnormalities. In Eichenfield LF, Frieden IJ, Esterly NB, editors: *Neonatal dermatology,* ed 2, Philadelphia, 2008, Saunders. *D,* From Spine and spinal cord: developmental disorders. In Schapira A, editor: *Neurology and clinical neuroscience,* Philadelphia, 2007, Mosby.)

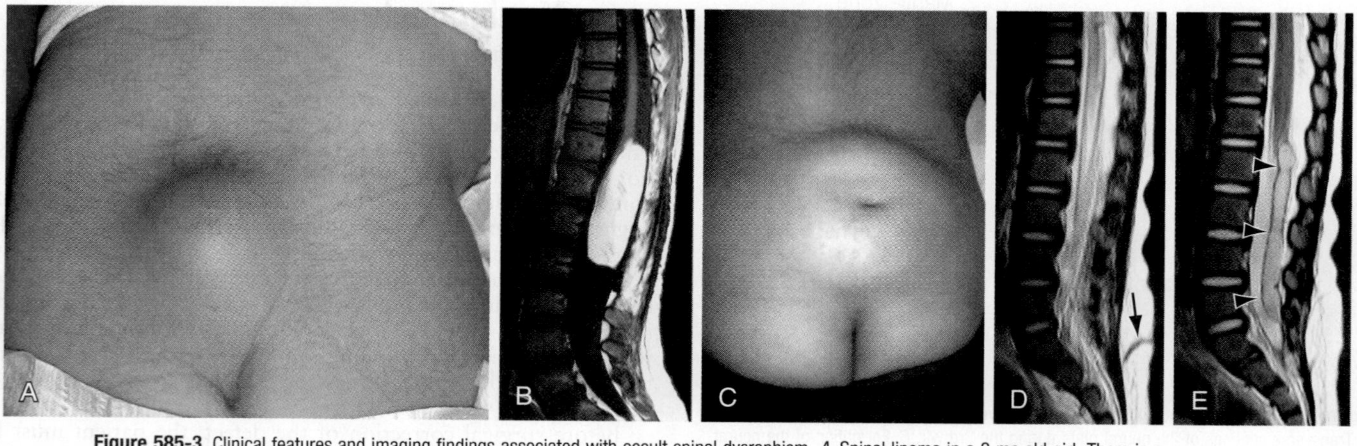

Figure 585-3 Clinical features and imaging findings associated with occult spinal dysraphism. *A,* Spinal lipoma in a 2 mo old girl. There is a skin-covered lumbosacral mass above the intergluteal cleft in the midline, surrounded by overgrowing hair. *B,* Sagittal T1-weighted image shows huge intradural lipoma, merging with the conus medullaris superiorly. *C,* Lipoma and central dermal sinus. *D* and *E,* Dermal sinus with dermoid, 8 yr old girl. Slightly parasagittal T2-weighted image shows sacral dermal sinus coursing obliquely downward in subcutaneous fat (*arrow*) *(D).* Midsagittal T2-weighted image shows huge dermoid in the thecal sac (*arrowheads*), extending upward to the tip of the conus medullaris *(E).* The mass gives a slightly lower signal than cerebrospinal fluid and is outlined by a thin low-signal rim. (*A,* From Rossi A: Spinal dysraphism. In Raybaud C, Naidich TP, editors: *Pediatric neuroimaging,* Philadelphia, Elsevier, in press. *B, D,* and *E,* From Rossi A, Biancheri R, Cama A, et al: Imaging in spine and spinal cord malformations, *Eur J Radiol* 50(2):177–200, 2004, Fig 9a. *C,* From Jaiswal AK, Garg A, Mahapatra AK: Spinal ossifying lipoma, *J Clin Neurosci* 12:714–717, 2005, Fig 1.)

585.4 Myelomeningocele

Stephen L. Kinsman and Michael V. Johnston

Myelomeningocele represents the most severe form of dysraphism, a so-called aperta or open form, involving the vertebral column and spinal cord, which occurs with an incidence of approximately 1/4,000 live births.

ETIOLOGY

The cause of myelomeningocele is unknown, but as with all neural tube closure defects including anencephaly, a genetic predisposition exists; the risk of recurrence after one affected child is 3-4% and increases to 10% with 2 prior affected children. Both epidemiologic evidence and the presence of substantial familial aggregation of anencephaly, myelomeningocele, and

Table 585-1 CUTANEOUS LESIONS ASSOCIATED WITH OCCULT SPINAL DYSRAPHISM

IMAGING INDICATED
Subcutaneous mass or lipoma Hairy patch Dermal sinus Atypical dimples (deep, >5 mm, >25 mm from anal verge) Vascular lesion, e.g., hemangioma or telangiectasia Skin appendages or polypoid lesions, e.g., skin tags, tail-like appendages Scarlike lesions
IMAGING UNCERTAIN
Hyperpigmented patches Deviation of the gluteal fold
IMAGING NOT REQUIRED
Simple dimples (<5 mm, <25 mm from anal verge) Coccygeal pits

From Williams H: Spinal sinuses, dimples, pits and patches: what lies beneath? *Arch Dis Child Educ Pract Ed* 91:ep75–ep80, 2006.

craniorachischisis indicate heredity, on a polygenic basis, as a significant contributor to the etiology of NTDs. Nutritional and environmental factors have a role in the etiology of myelomeningocele as well.

Folate is intricately involved in the prevention and etiology of NTDs. Folate functions in single-carbon transfer reactions and exists in many chemical forms. Folic acid (pteroylmonoglutamic acid), which is the most oxidized and stable form of folate, occurs rarely in food but is the form used in vitamin supplements and in fortified food products, particularly flour. Most naturally occurring folates (food folate) are pteroylpolyglutamates, which contain 1-6 additional glutamate molecules joined in a peptide linkage to the γ-carboxyl of glutamate. Folate coenzymes are involved in DNA synthesis, purine synthesis, generation of formate into the formate pool, and amino acid interconversion; the conversion of homocysteine to methionine provides methionine for the synthesis of *S*-adenosyl-methionine (SAM-e, an agent important for in vivo methylation). Mutations in the genes encoding the enzymes involved in homocysteine metabolism include 5,10 methylenetetrahydrofolate reductase (MTHFR), cystathionine β-synthase, and methionine synthase. An association between a thermolabile variant of MTHFR and mothers of children with NTDs might account for up to 15% of preventable NTDs. Maternal periconceptional use of folic acid supplementation reduces the incidence of NTDs in pregnancies at risk by at least 50%. To be effective, folic acid supplementation should be initiated before conception and continued until at least the 12th wk of gestation, when neurulation is complete. The mechanisms by which folic acid prevents NTDs remain poorly understood.

PREVENTION

The U.S. Public Health Service has recommended that all women of childbearing age and who are capable of becoming pregnant take 0.4 mg of folic acid daily. If, however, a pregnancy is planned in high-risk women (previously affected child), supplementation should be started with 4 mg of folic acid daily, beginning 1 mo before the time of the planned conception. The modern diet provides about half the daily requirement of folic acid. To increase folic acid intake, fortification of flour, pasta, rice, and cornmeal with 0.15 mg folic acid per 100 g was mandated in the United States and Canada in 1998. The added folic acid will be insufficient to maximize the prevention of preventable NTDs. Therefore, informative educational programs and folic acid vitamin supplementation remain essential for women planning a pregnancy and possibly for all women of childbearing age. In addition, women should also strive to consume food folate from a varied diet. Certain drugs, including drugs that antagonize folic acid, such as trimethoprim and the anticonvulsants carbamazepine, phenytoin, phenobarbital, and primidone, increase the risk of myelomeningocele. The anticonvulsant valproic acid causes NTDs in approximately 1-2% of pregnancies when administered during pregnancy. Some epilepsy clinicians recommend that all female patients of childbearing potential who take anticonvulsant medications also receive folic acid supplements.

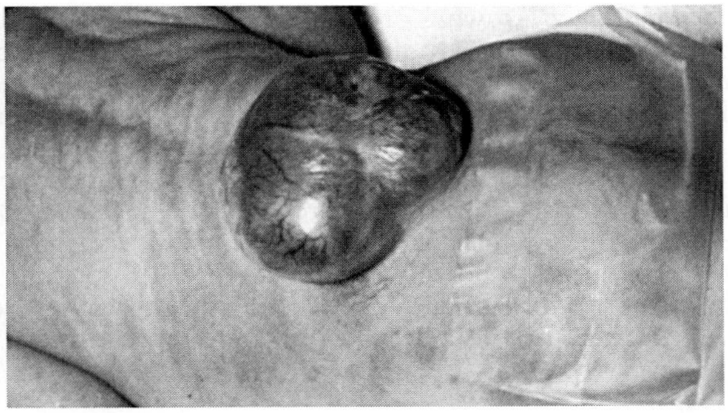

Figure 585-4 A lumbar myelomeningocele is covered by a thin layer of skin.

CLINICAL MANIFESTATIONS

Myelomeningocele produces dysfunction of many organs and structures, including the skeleton, skin, and gastrointestinal and genitourinary tracts, in addition to the peripheral nervous system and the CNS. A myelomeningocele may be located anywhere along the neuraxis, but the lumbosacral region accounts for at least 75% of the cases. The extent and degree of the neurologic deficit depend on the location of the myelomeningocele and the associated lesions. A lesion in the low sacral region causes bowel and bladder incontinence associated with anesthesia in the perineal area but with no impairment of motor function. Newborns with a defect in the midlumbar or high lumbothoracic region typically have either a saclike cystic structure covered by a thin layer of partially epithelialized tissue (Fig. 585-4) or an exposed flat neural placode without overlying tissues. When a cyst or membrane is present, remnants of neural tissue are visible beneath the membrane, which occasionally ruptures and leaks CSF, whereas the placode is composed of neural tissue.

Examination of the infant shows a flaccid paralysis of the lower extremities, an absence of deep tendon reflexes, a lack of response to touch and pain, and a high incidence of lower extremity deformities (clubfeet, ankle and/or knee contractures, and subluxation of the hips). Some children have constant urinary dribbling and a relaxed anal sphincter. Other children do not leak urine and in fact have a high-pressure bladder and sphincter dyssynergy. Thus, a myelomeningocele above the midlumbar region tends to produce lower motor neuron signs due to abnormalities and disruption of the conus medullaris and above spinal cord structures.

Infants with myelomeningocele typically have an increasing neurologic deficit as the myelomeningocele extends higher into the thoracic region. These infants sometimes have an associated kyphotic gibbus that requires neonatal orthopedic correction. Patients with a myelomeningocele in the upper thoracic or cervical region usually have a very minimal neurologic deficit and, in most cases, do not have hydrocephalus. They can have neurogenic bladder and bowel.

Hydrocephalus in association with a type II Chiari malformation develops in at least 80% of patients with myelomeningocele. Generally, the lower the deformity is in the neuraxis (sacrum), the less likely is the risk of hydrocephalus. The possibility of hydrocephalus developing should always be considered, no matter what the spinal level. Ventricular enlargement may be indolent and slow growing or may be rapid causing a bulging anterior fontanel, dilated scalp veins, setting-sun appearance of the eyes, irritability, and vomiting associated with an increased head circumference. About 15% of infants with hydrocephalus and Chiari II malformation develop symptoms of hindbrain dysfunction, including difficulty feeding, choking, stridor, apnea, vocal cord paralysis, pooling of secretions, and spasticity of the upper extremities, which, if untreated, can lead to death. This Chiari crisis is due to downward herniation of the medulla and cerebellar tonsils through the foramen magnum as well is endogenous malformations in the cerebellum and brainstem.

TREATMENT

Management and supervision of a child and family with a myelomeningocele require a multidisciplinary team approach, including surgeons, physicians, and therapists, with one individual (often a pediatrician) acting as the advocate and coordinator of the treatment program. The news that a newborn child has a devastating condition such as myelomeningocele causes parents to feel considerable grief and anger. They need time to learn about the handicap and the associated complications and to reflect on the various procedures and treatment plans. A knowledgeable individual in an unhurried and nonthreatening setting must give the parents the facts, along with general prognostic information and management strategies and timelines. If possible, discussions with other parents of children with NTDs are helpful in resolving important questions and issues.

Surgery is often done within a day or so of birth but can be delayed for several days (except when there is a CSF leak) to allow the parents time to begin to adjust to the shock and to prepare for the multiple procedures and inevitable problems that lie ahead. Evaluation of other congenital anomalies and renal function can also be initiated before surgery. Most pediatric centers aggressively treat the majority of infants with myelomeningocele. After repair of a myelomeningocele, most infants require a shunting procedure for hydrocephalus. If symptoms or signs of hindbrain dysfunction appear, early surgical decompression of the posterior fossa is indicated. Clubfeet can require taping or casting, and dislocated hips can require operative procedures.

Careful evaluation and reassessment of the genitourinary system are some of the most important components of the management. Teaching the parents, and ultimately the patient, to regularly catheterize a neurogenic bladder is a crucial step in maintaining a low residual volume and bladder pressure that prevents urinary tract infections and reflux leading to pyelonephritis, hydronephrosis, and bladder damage. Latex-free catheters and gloves must be used to prevent development of latex allergy. Periodic urine cultures and assessment of renal function, including serum electrolytes and creatinine as well as renal scans, vesiculourethrograms (VCUGs), renal ultrasonography, and cystometrograms (CMGs), are obtained according to the risk status and progress of the patient and the results of the physical examination. This approach to urinary tract management has greatly reduced the need for urologic diversionary procedures and significantly decreased the morbidity and mortality associated with progressive renal disease in these patients. Some children can become continent with surgical implantation of an artificial urinary sphincter (these are used less often) or bladder augmentation at a later age.

Although incontinence of fecal matter is common and is socially unacceptable during the school years, it does not pose the same organ-damaging risks as urinary dysfunction, but occasionally fecal impaction and/or megacolon develop. Many children can be bowel-trained with a regimen of timed enemas or suppositories that allows evacuation at a predetermined time once or twice a day. Special attention to low anorectal tone and enema administration and retention is often required. Appendicostomy for antegrade enemas may also be helpful (Chapter 21.4).

Functional ambulation is the wish of each child and parent and may be possible, depending on the level of the lesion and on intact function of the iliopsoas muscles. Almost every child with a sacral or lumbosacral lesion obtains functional ambulation; approximately half the children with higher defects ambulate with the use of braces, other orthotic devices, and canes. Ambulation is often more difficult as adolescence approaches and body mass increases. Deterioration of ambulatory function, particularly during earlier years, should prompt referral for evaluation of tethered spinal cord and other neurosurgical issues.

In utero surgical closure of a spinal lesion has been successful in a few centers. Preliminary reports suggest a lower incidence of hindbrain abnormalities and hydrocephalus (fewer shunts) as well as improved motor outcomes. This suggests that the defects may be progressive in utero and that prenatal closure might prevent the development of further loss of function. In utero diagnosis is facilitated by maternal serum α-fetoprotein screening and by fetal ultrasonography (Chapter 90).

PROGNOSIS

For a child who is born with a myelomeningocele and who is treated aggressively, the mortality rate is 10-15%, and most deaths occur before age 4 yr, although life-threatening complications occur at all ages. At least 70% of survivors have normal intelligence, but learning problems and seizure disorders are more common than in the general population. Previous episodes of meningitis or ventriculitis adversely affect intellectual and cognitive function. Because myelomeningocele is a chronic disabling condition, periodic multidisciplinary follow-up is required for life. Renal dysfunction is one of the most important determinants of mortality.

BIBLIOGRAPHY

Please visit the Nelson Textbook of Pediatrics *website at www.expertconsult.com for the complete bibliography.*

585.5 Encephalocele

Stephen L. Kinsman and Michael V. Johnston

Two major forms of dysraphism affect the skull, resulting in protrusion of tissue through a bony midline defect, called cranium bifidum. A cranial meningocele consists of a CSF-filled meningeal sac only, and a cranial encephalocele contains the sac plus cerebral cortex, cerebellum, or portions of the brainstem. Microscopic examination of the neural tissue within an encephalocele often reveals abnormalities. The cranial defect occurs most commonly in the occipital region at or below the inion, but in certain parts of the world, frontal or nasofrontal encephaloceles are more prominent. These abnormalities are one tenth as common as neural tube closure defects involving the spine. The etiology is presumed to be similar to that for anencephaly and myelomeningocele; examples of each are reported in the same family.

Infants with a cranial encephalocele are at increased risk for developing hydrocephalus due to **aqueductal stenosis, Chiari malformation**, or the **Dandy-Walker syndrome**. Examination might show a small sac with a pedunculated stalk or a large cystlike structure that can exceed the size of the cranium. The lesion may be completely covered with skin, but areas of denuded lesion can occur and require urgent surgical management. Transillumination of the sac can indicate the presence of neural tissue. A plain x-ray of the skull and cervical spine is indicated to define the anatomy of the vertebrae. Ultrasonography is most helpful in determining the contents of the sac. MRI or CT further helps define the spectrum of the lesion. Children with a cranial meningocele generally have a good prognosis, whereas patients with an encephalocele are at risk for vision problems, microcephaly, mental retardation, and seizures. Generally, children with neural tissue within the sac and associated hydrocephalus have the poorest prognosis.

Cranial encephalocele is often part of a syndrome. Meckel-Gruber syndrome is a rare autosomal recessive condition that is characterized by an occipital encephalocele, cleft lip or palate, microcephaly, microphthalmia, abnormal genitalia, polycystic kidneys, and polydactyly. Determination of maternal serum α-fetoprotein levels and ultrasound measurement of the biparietal diameter as well as identification of the encephalocele itself can diagnose encephaloceles in utero. Fetal MRI can help define the extent of associated CNS anomalies and the degree of brain herniated into the encephalocele.

BIBLIOGRAPHY

Please visit the Nelson Textbook of Pediatrics *website at www.expertconsult.com for the complete bibliography.*

585.6 Anencephaly

Stephen L. Kinsman and Michael V. Johnston

An anencephalic infant presents a distinctive appearance with a large defect of the calvarium, meninges, and scalp associated with a rudimentary brain, which results from failure of closure of the rostral neuropore, the opening of the anterior neural tube. The primitive brain consists of portions of connective tissue, vessels, and neuroglia. The cerebral hemispheres and cerebellum are usually absent, and only a residue of the brainstem can be identified. The pituitary gland is hypoplastic, and the spinal cord pyramidal tracts are missing owing to the absence of the cerebral cortex. Additional anomalies include folding of the ears, cleft palate, and congenital heart defects in 10-20% of cases. Most anencephalic infants die within several days of birth.

The incidence of anencephaly approximates 1/1,000 live births; the greatest incidence is in Ireland, Wales, and Northern China. The recurrence risk is approximately 4% and increases to 10% if a couple has had two previously affected pregnancies. Many factors in addition to genetics have been implicated as the cause of anencephaly, including low socioeconomic status, nutritional and vitamin deficiencies, and a large number of environmental and toxic factors. It is very likely that several noxious stimuli interact on a genetically susceptible host to produce anencephaly. The incidence of anencephaly has been decreasing in the past 2 decades. Approximately 50% of cases of anencephaly have associated polyhydramnios. Couples who have had an anencephalic infant should have successive pregnancies monitored, including amniocentesis, determination of AFP levels, and ultrasound examination between the 14th and 16th wk of gestation.

585.7 Disorders of Neuronal Migration

Stephen L. Kinsman and Michael V. Johnston

Disorders of neuronal migration can result in minor abnormalities with little or no clinical consequence (small heterotopia of neurons) or devastating abnormalities of CNS structure and/or function (mental retardation, seizures, lissencephaly, and schizencephaly, particularly the open-lip form) (Fig. 585-5). One of the most important mechanisms in the control of neuronal migration is the radial glial fiber system that guides neurons to their proper site. Migrating neurons attach to the radial glial fiber and then disembark at predetermined sites to form, ultimately, the precisely designed six-layered cerebral cortex. Another important mechanism is the tangential migration of progenitor neurons destined to become cortical interneurons. The severity and the extent of the disorder are related to numerous factors, including the timing of a particular insult and a host of environmental and genetic contributors.

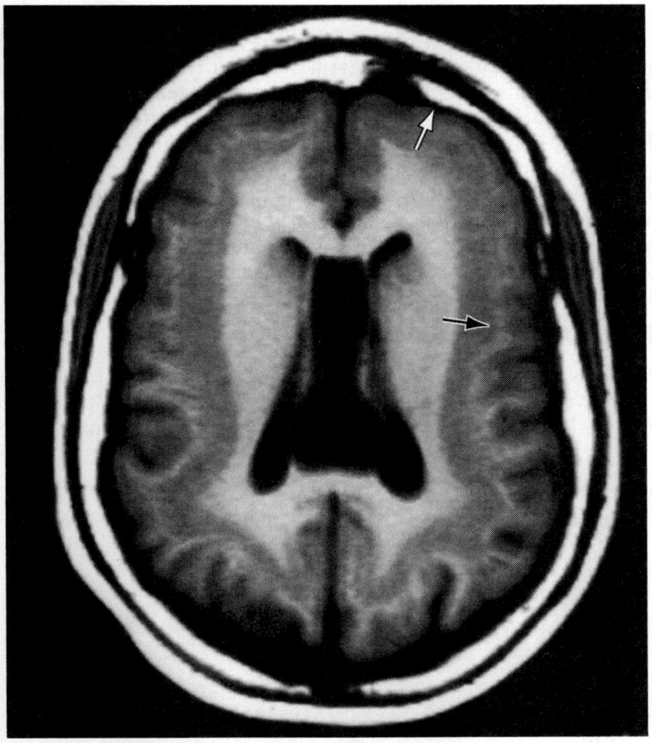

Figure 585-5 T1-weighted MRI scan demonstrating band heterotopia. A thin layer of white matter *(black arrow)* lies between the band of heterotopic gray matter and the cortical surface. Failure of cortical organization with lissencephaly is present in both frontal lobes *(white arrow)*.

LISSENCEPHALY

Lissencephaly, or agyria, is a rare disorder that is characterized by the absence of cerebral convolutions and a poorly formed sylvian fissure, giving the appearance of a 3-4 mo fetal brain. The condition is probably a result of faulty neuroblast migration during early embryonic life and is usually associated with enlarged lateral ventricles and heterotopias in the white matter. In some forms, there is a four-layered cortex, rather than the usual six-layered one, with a thin rim of periventricular white matter and numerous gray heterotopias visible by microscopic examination.

These infants present with failure to thrive, microcephaly, marked developmental delay, and a severe seizure disorder. Ocular abnormalities are common, including hypoplasia of the optic nerve and microphthalmia. Lissencephaly can occur as an isolated finding, but it is associated with Miller-Dieker syndrome (MDS) in about 15% of cases. These children have characteristic facies, including a prominent forehead, bitemporal hollowing, anteverted nostrils, a prominent upper lip, and micrognathia. About 90% of children with MDS have visible or submicroscopic chromosomal deletions of 17p13.3.

The gene *LIS*-1 (lissencephaly 1) that maps to chromosome region 17p13.3 is deleted in patients with MDS. CT and MRI scans typically show a smooth brain with an absence of sulci (Fig. 585-6). *Doublecortin* is an X chromosome gene that causes lissencephaly when mutated in males and subcortical band heterotopia when mutated in females. Other important forms of lissencephaly include the Walker-Warburg variant and other cobblestone cortical malformations.

SCHIZENCEPHALY

Schizencephaly is the presence of unilateral or bilateral clefts within the cerebral hemispheres owing to an abnormality of morphogenesis (Fig. 585-7). The cleft may be fused or unfused and, if unilateral and large, may be confused with a porencephalic cyst. Not infrequently, the borders of the cleft are surrounded by abnormal brain, particularly microgyria. MRI is the study of choice for elucidating schizencephaly and associated malformations.

Many patients are severely mentally retarded, with seizures that are difficult to control, and microcephalic, with spastic quadriparesis when the clefts are bilateral. Some cases of bilateral schizencephaly are associated with septo-optic dysplasia and endocrinologic disorders. Unilateral schizencephaly is a common cause of congenital hemiparesis. It remains controversial whether genetic causes of schizencephaly exist.

NEURONAL HETEROTOPIAS

Subtypes of neuronal heterotopias include periventricular nodular heterotopias, subcortical heterotopia (including band-type), and marginal glioneuronal heterotopias. Intractable seizures are a common feature. Several genes have been identified that are a cause of these conditions.

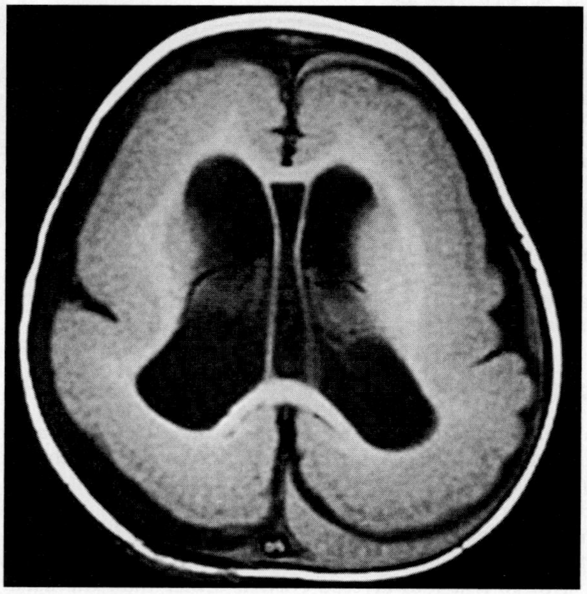

Figure 585-6 MRI of an infant with lissencephaly. Note the absence of cerebral sulci and the maldeveloped sylvian fissures associated with enlarged ventricles.

POLYMICROGYRIAS

Polymicrogyria is characterized by an augmentation of small convolutions separated by shallow enlarged sulci. Epilepsy, including drug-resistant forms, is a common feature. Several genes have been identified that cause several of the forms of this condition.

FOCAL CORTICAL DYSPLASIAS

Focal cortical dysplasias consist of abnormal cortical lamination in a discrete area of cortex. High-resolution, thin-section MRI can reveal these areas sometimes in the setting of drug-resistant epilepsy.

PORENCEPHALY

Porencephaly is the presence of cysts or cavities within the brain that result from developmental defects or acquired lesions, including infarction of tissue. True porencephalic cysts are most commonly located in the region of the sylvian fissure and typically communicate with the subarachnoid space, the ventricular system, or both. They represent developmental abnormalities of cell migration and are often associated with other malformations of the brain, including microcephaly, abnormal patterns of adjacent gyri, and encephalocele. Affected infants tend to have many problems, including mental retardation, spastic hemiparesis or quadriparesis, optic atrophy, and seizures.

Several risk factors for porencephalic cyst formation have been identified including: hemorrhagic venous infarctions, various thrombophilias such as protein C deficiency and factor V Leiden mutations, perinatal alloimmune thrombocytopenia, von Willebrand's disease, maternal warfarin use, maternal cocaine use, congenital infections, trauma such as amniocentesis, and maternal abdominal trauma. Mutations in the *COL4A1* gene have been described in cases of familial porencephaly.

Pseudoporencephalic cysts characteristically develop during the perinatal or postnatal period and result from abnormalities (infarction, hemorrhage) of arterial or venous circulation. These cysts tend to be unilateral, do not communicate with a fluid-filled cavity, and are not associated with abnormalities of cell migration or CNS malformations. Infants with pseudoporencephalic cysts

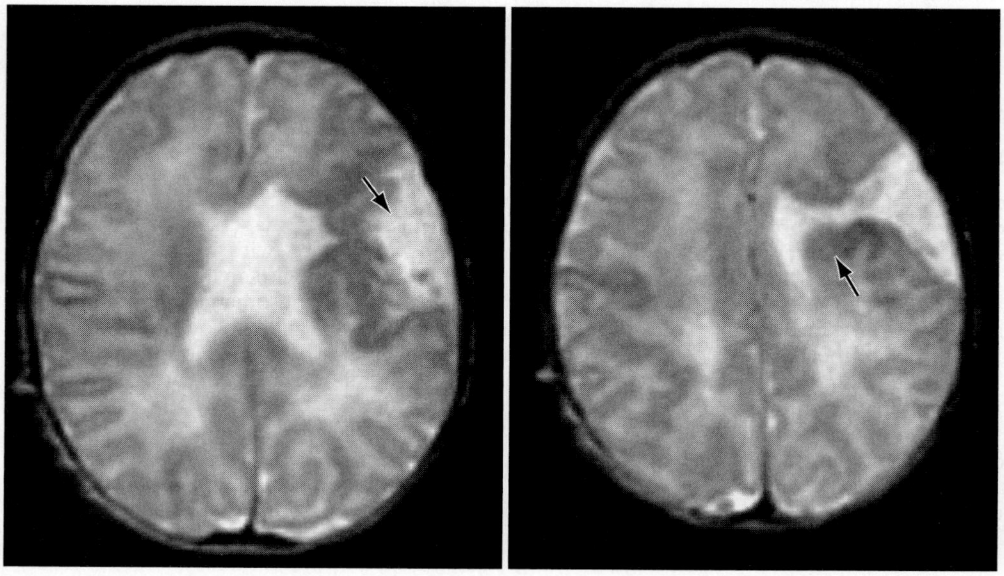

Figure 585-7 Unilateral schizencephaly shown on axial MR images of the brain. Example of an open-lip schizencephaly with a cleft communicating between the ventricle and the extra-axial cranial space (*arrow* on left panel). Many of these clefts are lined with abnormal gray matter (*arrow* on right panel).

present with hemiparesis and focal seizures in the 1st year of life and sometimes present with neonatal encephalopathy or as a floppy newborn or infant.

BIBLIOGRAPHY

Please visit the Nelson Textbook of Pediatrics *website at www.expertconsult.com for the complete bibliography.*

585.8 Agenesis of the Corpus Callosum

Stephen L. Kinsman and Michael V. Johnston

Agenesis of the corpus callosum consists of a heterogeneous group of disorders that vary in expression from severe intellectual and neurologic abnormalities to the asymptomatic and normally intelligent patient (Fig. 585-8). The corpus callosum develops from the commissural plate that lies in proximity to the anterior neuropore. Either a direct insult to the commissural plate or disruption of the genetic signaling that specifies and organizes this area during early embryogenesis causes agenesis of the corpus callosum.

It is often said that the outcome of agenesis of the corpus callosum is dictated by "the company it keeps." When agenesis of the corpus callosum is an isolated phenomenon, the patient may be normal. When it is accompanied by brain anomalies due to cell migration defects, such as heterotopias, microgyria, and pachygyria (broad, wide gyri), patients often have significant neurologic abnormalities, including mental retardation, microcephaly, hemiparesis, diplegia, and seizures.

The anatomic features of agenesis of the corpus callosum are best depicted on MRI or CT scan and include widely separated frontal horns with an abnormally high position of the third ventricle between the lateral ventricles. MRI precisely outlines the extent of the corpus callosum defect.

Absence of the corpus callosum may be inherited as an X-linked recessive trait or as an autosomal dominant trait and on occasion as an autosomal recessive trait. The condition may be associated with specific chromosomal disorders, particularly trisomy 8 and trisomy 18. Single-gene mutations have also been identified, usually in association with other anomalies. Agenesis of the corpus callosum is also seen in metabolic disorders.

Aicardi syndrome represents a complex disorder that affects many systems and is typically associated with agenesis of the corpus callosum, distinctive chorioretinal lacunae, and infantile spasms. Patients are almost all female, suggesting a genetic abnormality of the X chromosome (it may be lethal in males during fetal life). Seizures become evident during the 1st few months and are typically resistant to anticonvulsants. An electroencephalogram (EEG) shows independent activity recorded from both hemispheres as a result of the absent corpus callosum and often hemi-hypsarrhythmia. All patients have severe mental retardation and can have abnormal vertebrae that may be fused or only partially developed (hemivertebra). Abnormalities of the retina, including circumscribed pits or lacunae and coloboma of the optic disc, are the most characteristic findings of Aicardi syndrome.

Colpocephaly refers to an abnormal enlargement of the occipital horns of the ventricular system and can be identified as early as the fetal period. It is often associated with agenesis of the corpus callosum, but it can occur in isolation. It is also associated with microcephaly. It can also be seen in anatomic megalencephaly such as in Sotos syndrome.

HOLOPROSENCEPHALY

Holoprosencephaly is a developmental disorder of the brain that results from defective formation of the prosencephalon and inadequate induction of forebrain structures. The abnormality, which represents a spectrum of severity, is classified into 3 groups: alobar, semilobar, and lobar, depending on the degree of the cleavage abnormality (Fig. 585-9). A fourth type, the middle interhemispheric fusion (MIHF) variant or syntelencephaly, involves a segmental area of noncleavage, actually a nonseparation, of the posterior frontal and parietal lobes. Facial abnormalities including cyclopia, synophthalmia, cebocephaly, single nostril, solitary central incisor tooth, and premaxillary agenesis are common in severe cases, because the prechordal mesoderm that induces the ventral prosencephalon is also responsible for induction of the median facial structures. Alobar holoprosencephaly is characterized by a single ventricle, an absent falx, and nonseparated deep cerebral nuclei. Care must be taken not to overdiagnose holoprosencephaly based on ventricular abnormalities alone. Evidence of nonseparated midline deep brain structures such as caudate, putamen, globus pallidus, and hypothalamus is the critical element for diagnosis.

Affected children with the alobar type have high mortality rates, but some live for years. Mortality and morbidity with milder types are more variable, and morbidity is less severe. Care must be taken not to prognosticate severe outcomes in all cases. The incidence of holoprosencephaly ranges from 1/5,000 to 1/16,000. A prenatal diagnosis can be confirmed by ultrasonography after the 10th wk of gestation for more severe types, but fetal MRI at later gestational ages gives far greater anatomic precision.

The cause of holoprosencephaly is often not identified. There appears to be an association with maternal diabetes. Chromosomal abnormalities, including deletions of chromosomes 7q and 3p, 21q, 2p, 18p, and 13q, as well as trisomy 13 and 18, account for upwards of 50% of all cases. Mutations in the sonic hedgehog

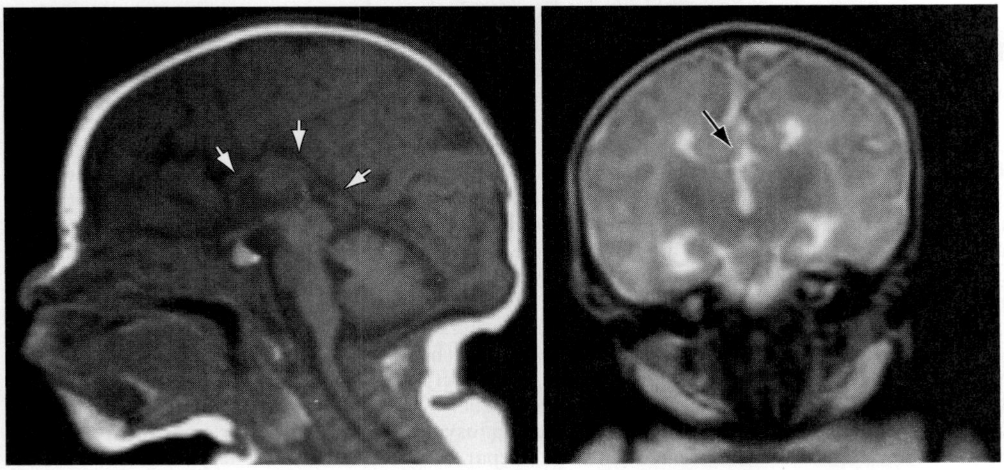

Figure 585-8 Agenesis of the corpus callosum shown on MR images of the brain. Sagittal *(left panel)* and coronal *(right panel)* views of an infant show the total absence of a midsagittal white matter structure *(left panel, arrows)*. The coronal view *(right panel)* demonstrates (despite some motion artifact) the absence of a structure bridging the two hemispheres (area under *arrow*).

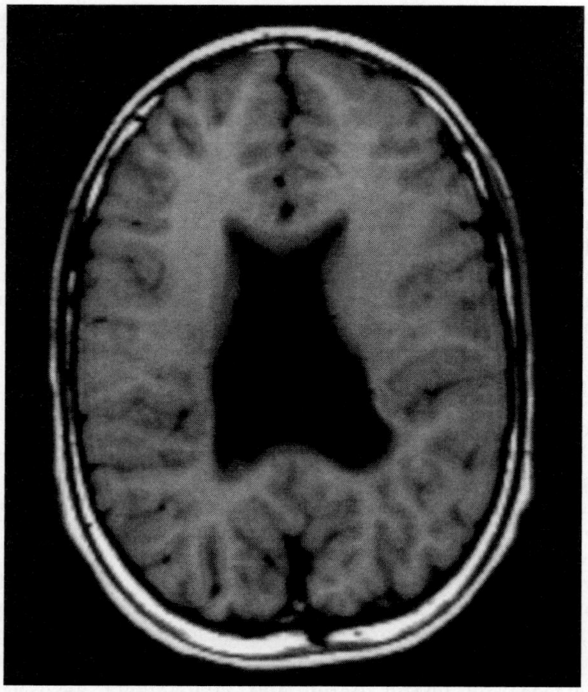

Figure 585-9 Lobar holoprosencephaly. T1-weighted MRI scan demonstrates failure of separation of the hemispheres and a persistent fused ventricle.

gene at 7q have been shown to cause holoprosencephaly. OMIM lists 10 loci and 6 single-gene causes. Clinically, it is important to look for associated anomalies, because many syndromes are associated with holoprosencephaly.

BIBLIOGRAPHY

Please visit the Nelson Textbook of Pediatrics *website at www.expertconsult.com for the complete bibliography.*

585.9 Agenesis of the Cranial Nerves and Dysgenesis of the Posterior Fossa

Stephen L. Kinsman and Michael V. Johnston

Classification of disorders of cranial nerve, brainstem, and cerebellum development remains anatomic, but future classification systems will likely be based on the molecular biology of brain development based on the genes involved and the roles they play in orchestrating brain architecture.

CONGENITAL CRANIAL DYSINNERVATION DISORDERS

Absence of the cranial nerves or the corresponding central nuclei has been described in several conditions and includes the optic nerve, congenital ptosis, Marcus Gunn phenomenon (sucking jaw movements causing simultaneous eyelid blinking; this congenital synkinesis results from abnormal innervation of the trigeminal and oculomotor nerves), the trigeminal and auditory nerves, and cranial nerves IX, X, XI, and XII. Increased understanding of these disorders and their genetic causes has led to the term *congenital cranial dysinnervation disorders* (CCDD).

Optic nerve hypoplasia can occur in isolation or as part of the septo-optic dysplasia complex (De Morsier syndrome). Septo-optic dysplasia can be caused by a mutation in the *HESX1* gene.

Möbius syndrome is characterized by bilateral facial weakness, which is often associated with paralysis of the abducens nerve. Hypoplasia or agenesis of brainstem nuclei as well as absent or decreased numbers of muscle fibers has been reported. Affected infants present in the newborn period with facial weakness, causing feeding difficulties owing to a poor suck. The immobile, dull facies might give the incorrect impression of mental retardation; the prognosis for normal development is excellent in most cases. The facial appearance of Möbius syndrome has been improved by facial surgery.

Duane retraction syndrome is characterized by congenital limitation of horizontal globe movement and some globe retraction on attempted adduction and is believed to be the result of abnormal innervations by the oculomotor nerve of the lateral rectus muscle. Abnormalities of cranial nerve development have been demonstrated in this condition.

Less common than Duane retraction syndrome and Möbius syndrome are the group of disorders known as **congenital fibrosis of the extraocular muscles** (CFEOM). CFEOM is characterized by severe restriction of eye movements and ptosis from abnormal oculomotor and trochlear nerve development and/or from abnormalities of extraocular muscle innervations.

BRAINSTEM AND CEREBELLAR DISORDERS

Disorders of the posterior fossa structures include abnormalities of not only the brainstem and cerebellum but also the cerebrospinal fluid spaces. Commonly encountered malformations include Chiari malformation, Dandy-Walker malformation, arachnoid cysts, mega cistern magna, persisting Blake pouch, Joubert syndrome, rhombencephalosynapsis, Lhermitte-Duclos disease, and pontocerebellar hypoplasias.

Chiari malformation is the most common malformation of the posterior fossa and hindbrain. It consists of herniation of the cerebellar tonsils though the foramen magnum. There is also an associated developmental abnormality of the bones of the skull base leading to a small posterior fossa. Cases are either asymptomatic or symptomatic. When symptoms develop, they often do not do so until late childhood. Symptoms include headaches that are worse with straining and other maneuvers that increase intracranial pressure. Symptoms of brainstem compression such as diplopia, oropharyngeal dysfunction, tinnitus, and vertigo can occur. Obstructive hydrocephalus and/or syringomyelia can also occur.

Dandy-Walker malformation is part of a continuum of posterior fossa anomalies that include cystic dilatation of the fourth ventricle, hypoplasia of the cerebellar vermis, hydrocephalus, and an enlarged posterior fossa with elevation of the lateral venous sinuses and the tentorium. Extracranial anomalies are also seen. Variable degrees of neurologic impairment are usually present. The etiology of Dandy-Walker malformation includes chromosomal abnormalities, single gene disorders, and exposure to teratogens.

Arachnoid cysts of the posterior fossa can be associated with hydrocephalus. Mega cistern magna is characterized by an enlarged CSF space inferior and dorsal to the cerebellar vermis and when present in isolation may be considered a normal variant. Persisting Blake pouch is a cyst that obstructs the subarachnoid space and is associated with hydrocephalus.

Joubert syndrome is an autosomal recessive disorder with significant genetic heterogeneity that is associated with cerebellar vermis hypoplasia and the pontomesencephalic molar tooth sign (a deepening of the interpeduncular fossa with thick and straight superior cerebellar peduncles). It is associated with hypotonia, ataxia, characteristic breathing abnormalities including episodic apnea and hyperpnea, global developmental delay, nystagmus, strabismus, and oculomotor apraxia. There can be many associated systemic features including progressive retinal dysplasia, coloboma, congenital heart disease, microcystic kidney disease, liver fibrosis, polydactyly, tongue protrusion, and soft tissue tumors of the tongue.

Rhombencephalosynapsis is an absent or small vermis associated with a nonseparation or fusion of the deep midline cerebellar structures. Ventriculomegaly or hydrocephalus is often seen. There is variable clinical presentation from normal to cognitive and language impairments, epilepsy, and spasticity. **Lhermitte-Duclos** disease is a dysplastic gangliocytoma of the cerebellum leading to focal enlargement of the cerebellum and macrocephaly, cerebellar signs, and seizures.

Pontocerebellar hypoplasias are a group of disorders characterized by impairment of cerebellar and pontine development together with histopathologic features of neuronal death and glial replacement. Clinical features tend to be nonspecific and include hypotonia, feeding difficulties, developmental delay, and breathing difficulties. Causes include type I (with features of anterior horn cell involvement), type II (with extrapyramidal features, seizures, and acquired microcephaly), Walker-Warburg syndrome, muscle-eye-brain disease, congenital disorders of glycosylation type 1A, mitochondrial cytopathies, teratogen exposure, congenital cytomegalovirus (CMV) infection, 3-methylglutaconic aciduria, PEHO syndrome (progressive encephalopathy with edema, hypsarrhythmia, and optic atrophy), autosomal recessive cerebellar hypoplasia in the Hutterite population, lissencephaly with cerebellar hypoplasia, and other subtypes of pontocerebellar hypoplasia.

BIBLIOGRAPHY

Please visit the Nelson Textbook of Pediatrics *website at www.expertconsult.com for the complete bibliography.*

585.10 Microcephaly

Stephen L. Kinsman and Michael V. Johnston

Microcephaly is defined as a head circumference that measures more than 3 standard deviations below the mean for age and sex. This condition is relatively common, particularly among developmentally delayed children. Although there are many causes of microcephaly, abnormalities in neuronal migration during fetal development, including heterotopias of neuronal cells and cytoarchitectural derangements, are often found. Microcephaly may be subdivided into 2 main groups: primary (genetic) microcephaly and secondary (nongenetic) microcephaly. A precise diagnosis is important for genetic counseling and for prediction for future pregnancies.

ETIOLOGY

Primary microcephaly refers to a group of conditions that usually have no associated malformations and follow a mendelian pattern of inheritance or are associated with a specific genetic syndrome. Affected infants are usually identified at birth because of a small head circumference. The more common types include familial and autosomal dominant microcephaly and a series of chromosomal syndromes that are summarized in Table 585-2. Primary microcephaly is also associated with at least 7 loci, and 4 single etiologic genes have been identified. It is known as autosomal recessive primary microcephaly (MCPH) and has autosomal inheritance. Many X-linked causes of microcephaly are caused by gene mutations that lead to severe structural brain malformations such as lissencephaly, and these should be sought on MRI. Secondary microcephaly results from a large number of noxious agents that can affect a fetus in utero or an infant during periods of rapid brain growth, particularly the 1st 2 yr of life.

Acquired microcephaly can be seen in conditions such as Rett syndrome and in genetic conditions known also to cause primary microcephaly.

CLINICAL MANIFESTATIONS AND DIAGNOSIS

A thorough family history should be taken, seeking additional cases of microcephaly or disorders affecting the nervous system.

Table 585-2 CAUSES OF MICROCEPHALY

CAUSES	CHARACTERISTIC FINDINGS
PRIMARY (GENETIC)	
Familial (autosomal recessive)	Incidence 1/40,000 births Typical appearance with slanted forehead, prominent nose and ears; severe mental retardation and prominent seizures; surface convolutional markings of the brain, poorly differentiated and disorganized cytoarchitecture
Autosomal dominant	Nondistinctive facies, upslanting palpebral fissures, mild forehead slanting, and prominent ears Normal linear growth, seizures readily controlled, and mild or borderline mental retardation
Syndromes	
Down (trisomy 21)	Incidence 1/800 Abnormal rounding of occipital and frontal lobes and a small cerebellum; narrow superior temporal gyrus, propensity for Alzheimer neurofibrillary alterations, ultrastructure abnormalities of cerebral cortex
Edward (trisomy 18)	Incidence 1/6,500 Low birthweight, microstomia, micrognathia, low-set malformed ears, prominent occiput, rocker-bottom feet, flexion deformities of fingers, congenital heart disease, increased gyri, heterotopias of neurons
Cri-du-chat (5 p-)	Incidence 1/50,000 Round facies, prominent epicanthic folds, low-set ears, hypertelorism, characteristic cry No specific neuropathology
Cornelia de Lange	Prenatal and postnatal growth delay, synophrys, thin downturning upper lip Proximally placed thumb
Rubinstein-Taybi	Beaked nose, downward slanting of palpebral fissures, epicanthic folds, short stature, broad thumbs and toes
Smith-Lemli-Opitz	Ptosis, scaphocephaly, inner epicanthic folds, anteverted nostrils Low birthweight, marked feeding problems
SECONDARY (NONGENETIC) **Congenital Infections**	
Cytomegalovirus	Small for dates, petechial rash, hepatosplenomegaly, chorioretinitis, deafness, mental retardation, seizures Central nervous system calcification and microgyria
Rubella	Growth retardation, purpura, thrombocytopenia, hepatosplenomegaly, congenital heart disease, chorioretinitis, cataracts, deafness Perivascular necrotic areas, polymicrogyria, heterotopias, subependymal cavitations
Toxoplasmosis	Purpura, hepatosplenomegaly, jaundice, convulsions, hydrocephalus, chorioretinitis, cerebral calcification
Drugs	
Fetal alcohol	Growth retardation, ptosis, absent philtrum and hypoplastic upper lip, congenital heart disease, feeding problems, neuroglial heterotopia, disorganization of neurons
Fetal hydantoin	Growth delay, hypoplasia of distal phalanges, inner epicanthic folds, broad nasal ridge, anteverted nostrils
Other Causes	
Radiation	Microcephaly and mental retardation most severe with exposure before 15th wk of gestation
Meningitis/ encephalitis	Cerebral infarcts, cystic cavitation, diffuse loss of neurons
Malnutrition	Controversial cause of microcephaly
Metabolic	Maternal diabetes mellitus and maternal hyperphenylalaninemia
Hyperthermia	Significant fever during 1st 4-6 wk has been reported to cause microcephaly, seizures, and facial anomalies Pathologic studies show neuronal heterotopias Further studies showed no abnormalities with maternal fever
Hypoxic-ischemic encephalopathy	Initially diffuse cerebral edema; late stages characterized by cerebral atrophy and abnormal signals on MR imaging

It is important to measure a patient's head circumference at birth to diagnose microcephaly as early as possible. A very small head circumference implies a process that began early in embryonic or fetal development. An insult to the brain that occurs later in life, particularly beyond the age of 2 yr, is less likely to produce severe microcephaly. Serial head circumference measurements are more meaningful than a single determination, particularly when the abnormality is minimal. The head circumference of each parent and sibling should be recorded.

Laboratory investigation of a microcephalic child is determined by the history and physical examination. If the cause of the microcephaly is unknown, the mother's serum phenylalanine level should be determined. High phenylalanine serum levels in an asymptomatic mother can produce marked brain damage in an otherwise normal nonphenylketonuric infant. A karyotype and/or array-comparative genomic hybridization (array-CGH) study is obtained if a chromosomal syndrome is suspected or if the child has abnormal facies, short stature, and additional congenital anomalies. MRI is useful in identifying structural abnormalities of the brain such as lissencephaly, pachygyria, and polymicrogyria, and CT scanning is useful to detect intracerebral calcification. Additional studies include a fasting plasma and urine amino acid analysis; serum ammonia determination; *to*xoplasmosis, *r*ubella, *c*ytomegalovirus, and *h*erpes simplex (TORCH) titers as well as HIV testing of the mother and child; and a urine sample for the culture of cytomegalovirus. Single gene mutations as a cause of both primary microcephaly and syndromic microcephaly are being increasingly identified.

TREATMENT

Once the cause of microcephaly has been established, the physician must provide accurate and supportive genetic and family counseling. Because many children with microcephaly are also mentally retarded, the physician must assist with placement in an appropriate program that will provide for maximal development of the child (Chapter 33).

BIBLIOGRAPHY

Please visit the Nelson Textbook of Pediatrics *website at* *www.expertconsult.com* *for the complete bibliography.*

585.11 Hydrocephalus

Stephen L. Kinsman and Michael V. Johnston

Hydrocephalus is not a specific disease; it represents a diverse group of conditions that result from impaired circulation and absorption of CSF or, in rare circumstances, from increased production of CSF by a choroid plexus papilloma (Table 585-3). Because megalencephaly is often discovered as part of an evaluation for hydrocephalus in children with macrocephaly, it is included in this section.

Table 585-3 CAUSES OF HYDROCEPHALUS

COMMUNICATING
Achondroplasia
Basilar impression
Benign enlargement of subarachnoid space
Choroid plexus papilloma
Meningeal malignancy
Meningitis
Posthemorrhagic
NONCOMMUNICATING
Aqueductal stenosis
Infectious*
X-linked
Mitochondrial
Autosomal recessive
Autosomal dominant
L1CAM mutations
Chiari malformation
Dandy-Walker malformation
Klippel-Feil syndrome
Mass lesions
Abscess
Hematoma
Tumors and neurocutaneous disorders
Vein of Galen malformation
Walker-Warburg syndrome
HYDRANENCEPHALY
Holoprosencephaly
Massive hydrocephalus
Porencephaly

*Toxoplasmosis, neurocysticercosis mumps.
From Fenichel GM: *Clinical pediatric neurology,* ed 5, Philadelphia, 2005, Elsevier, p 354.

PHYSIOLOGY

The CSF is formed primarily in the ventricular system by the choroid plexus, which is situated in the lateral, 3rd, and 4th ventricles. Although most CSF is produced in the lateral ventricles, approximately 25% originates from extrachoroidal sources, including the capillary endothelium within the brain parenchyma. There is active neurogenic control of CSF formation because adrenergic and cholinergic nerves innervate the choroid plexus. Stimulation of the adrenergic system diminishes CSF production, whereas excitation of the cholinergic nerves can double the normal CSF production rate. In a normal child, about 20 mL/hr of CSF is produced. The total volume of CSF approximates 50 mL in an infant and 150 mL in an adult. Most of the CSF is extraventricular. The choroid plexus forms CSF in several stages; through a series of intricate steps, a plasma ultrafiltrate is ultimately processed into a secretion, the CSF.

CSF flow results from the pressure gradient that exists between the ventricular system and venous channels. Intraventricular pressure may be as high as 180 mm H_2O in the normal state, whereas the pressure in the superior sagittal sinus is in the range of 90 mm H_2O. Normally, CSF flows from the lateral ventricles through the foramina of Monro into the 3rd ventricle. It then traverses the narrow aqueduct of Sylvius, which is about 3 mm long and 2 mm in diameter in a child, to enter the 4th ventricle. The CSF exits the 4th ventricle through the paired lateral foramina of Luschka and the midline foramen of Magendie into the cisterns at the base of the brain. Hydrocephalus resulting from obstruction within the ventricular system is called obstructive or noncommunicating hydrocephalus. The CSF then circulates from the basal cisterns posteriorly through the cistern system and over the convexities of the cerebral hemispheres. CSF is absorbed primarily by the arachnoid villi through tight junctions of their endothelium by the pressure forces that were noted earlier. CSF is absorbed to a much lesser extent by the lymphatic channels directed to the paranasal sinuses, along nerve root sleeves, and by the choroid plexus itself. Hydrocephalus resulting from obliteration of the subarachnoid cisterns or malfunction of the arachnoid villi is called nonobstructive or communicating hydrocephalus.

PATHOPHYSIOLOGY AND ETIOLOGY

Obstructive or noncommunicating hydrocephalus develops most commonly in children because of an abnormality of the aqueduct or a lesion in the 4th ventricle. Aqueductal stenosis results from an abnormally narrow aqueduct of Sylvius that is often associated with branching or forking. In a small percentage of cases, aqueductal stenosis is inherited as a sex-linked recessive trait. These patients occasionally have minor neural tube closure defects, including spina bifida occulta. Rarely, aqueductal stenosis is associated with neurofibromatosis. Aqueductal gliosis can also give rise to hydrocephalus. As a result of neonatal meningitis or a subarachnoid hemorrhage in a premature infant, the ependymal lining of the aqueduct is interrupted and a brisk glial response results in complete obstruction. Intrauterine viral infections can also produce aqueductal stenosis followed by hydrocephalus, and mumps meningoencephalitis has been reported as a cause in a child. A vein of Galen malformation can expand to become large and, because of its midline position, obstruct the flow of CSF. Lesions or malformations of the posterior fossa are prominent causes of hydrocephalus, including posterior fossa brain tumors, Chiari malformation, and the Dandy-Walker syndrome.

Nonobstructive or communicating hydrocephalus most commonly follows a subarachnoid hemorrhage, which is usually a result of intraventricular hemorrhage in a premature infant. Blood in the subarachnoid spaces can cause obliteration of the cisterns or arachnoid villi and obstruction of CSF flow. Pneumococcal and tuberculous meningitis have a propensity to produce a thick, tenacious exudate that obstructs the basal cisterns, and intrauterine infections can also destroy the CSF pathways. Leukemic infiltrates can seed the subarachnoid space and produce communicating hydrocephalus.

CLINICAL MANIFESTATIONS

The clinical presentation of hydrocephalus is variable and depends on many factors, including the age at onset, the nature of the lesion causing obstruction, and the duration and rate of increase of the intracranial pressure (ICP). In an infant, an accelerated rate of enlargement of the head is the most prominent sign. In addition, the anterior fontanel is wide open and bulging, and the scalp veins are dilated. The forehead is broad, and the eyes might deviate downward because of impingement of the dilated suprapineal recess on the tectum, producing the setting-sun eye sign. Long-tract signs including brisk tendon reflexes, spasticity, clonus (particularly in the lower extremities), and Babinski sign are common owing to stretching and disruption of the corticospinal fibers originating from the leg region of the motor cortex. In an older child, the cranial sutures are partially closed so that the signs of hydrocephalus may be subtler. Irritability, lethargy, poor appetite, and vomiting are common to both age groups, and headache is a prominent symptom in older patients. A gradual change in personality and deterioration in academic productivity suggest a slowly progressive form of hydrocephalus. With regard to other clinical signs, serial measurements of the head circumference often indicate an increased velocity of growth. Percussion of the skull might produce a cracked pot sound or MacEwen's sign, indicating separation of the sutures. A foreshortened occiput suggests Chiari malformation, and a prominent occiput suggests the Dandy-Walker malformation. Papilledema, abducens nerve palsies, and pyramidal tract signs, which are most evident in the lower extremities, are apparent in many cases.

Chiari malformation consists of two major subgroups. Type I typically produces symptoms during adolescence or adult life and is usually not associated with hydrocephalus. Patients complain of recurrent headache, neck pain, urinary frequency, and progressive lower extremity spasticity. The deformity consists of displacement of the cerebellar tonsils into the cervical canal (Fig. 585-10). Although the pathogenesis is unknown, a prevailing theory suggests that obstruction of the caudal portion of the 4th ventricle during fetal development is responsible. Other theories include tethering of the cord or additional anomalies (syrinx).

The type II Chiari malformation is characterized by progressive hydrocephalus with a myelomeningocele. This lesion represents an anomaly of the hindbrain, probably owing to a failure of pontine flexure during embryogenesis, and results in elongation of the 4th ventricle and kinking of the brainstem, with displacement of the inferior vermis, pons, and medulla into the cervical canal (Fig. 585-11). Approximately 10% of type II malformations produce symptoms during infancy, consisting of stridor, weak cry, and apnea, which may be relieved by shunting or by decompression of the posterior fossa. A more indolent form consists of abnormalities of gait, spasticity, and increasing incoordination during childhood.

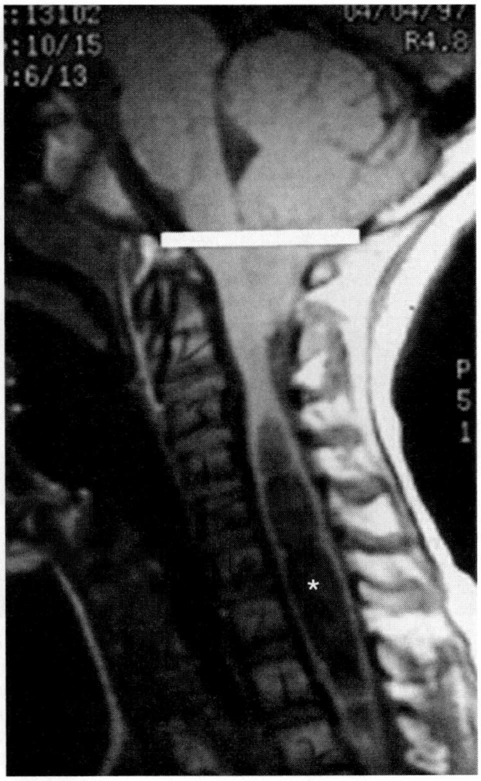

Figure 585-10 Sagittal MR scan of a patient with Chiari malformation type I. Cerebellar tonsils are displaced through the foramen magnum *(white bar)* to the lower aspect of C2 with clear crowding at the foramen. A syrinx *(white asterisk)* is visible extending from C3 to T2. (From Yassari R, Frim D: Evaluation and management of the Chiari malformation type 1 for the primary care pediatrician, *Pediatr Clin North Am* 51:477–490, 2004.)

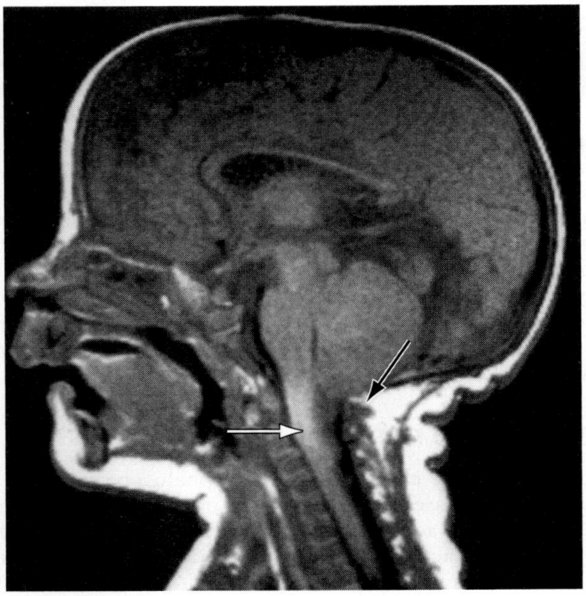

Figure 585-11 A midsagittal T1-weighted MRI of a patient with type II Chiari malformation. The cerebellar tonsils *(white arrow)* have descended below the foramen magnum *(black arrow)*. Note the small, slitlike 4th ventricle, which has been pulled into a vertical position.

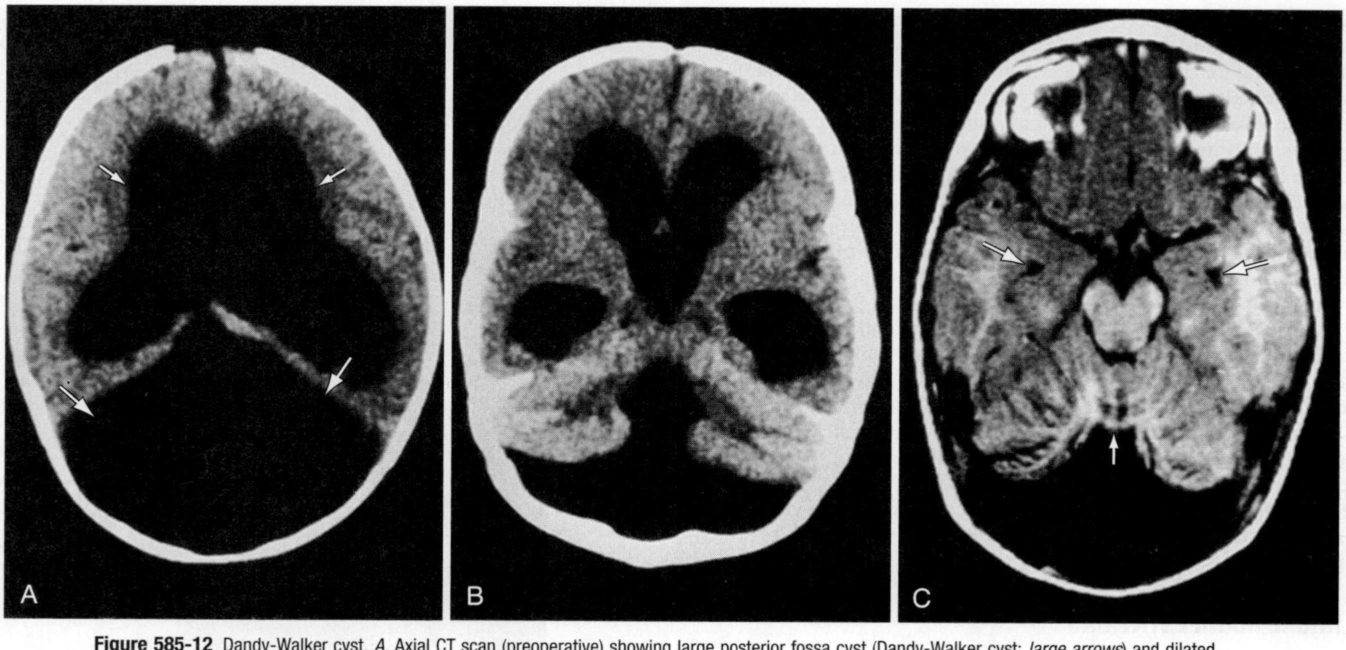

Figure 585-12 Dandy-Walker cyst. *A,* Axial CT scan (preoperative) showing large posterior fossa cyst (Dandy-Walker cyst; *large arrows*) and dilated lateral ventricles *(small arrows)*, a complication secondary to cerebrospinal fluid (CSF) pathway obstruction at the 4th ventricular outlet. *B,* Same patient, with a lower axial CT scan showing splaying of the cerebellar hemispheres by the dilated 4th ventricle (Dandy-Walker cyst). The dilated ventricles proximal to the 4th ventricle again show CSF obstruction caused by the Dandy-Walker cyst. *C,* MRI of the same patient showing decreased size of the Dandy-Walker cyst and temporal horns *(arrows)* after shunting. The incomplete vermis *(small arrow)* now becomes recognizable.

Plain skull radiographs show a small posterior fossa and a widened cervical canal. CT scanning with contrast and MRI display the cerebellar tonsils protruding downward into the cervical canal and the hindbrain abnormalities. The anomaly is treated by surgical decompression, but asymptomatic or mildly symptomatic patients may be managed conservatively.

The Dandy-Walker malformation consists of a cystic expansion of the 4th ventricle in the posterior fossa and midline cerebellar hypoplasia, which results from a developmental failure of the roof of the 4th ventricle during embryogenesis (Fig. 585-12). Approximately 90% of patients have hydrocephalus, and a significant number of children have associated anomalies, including agenesis of the posterior cerebellar vermis and corpus callosum. Infants present with a rapid increase in head size and a prominent occiput. Transillumination of the skull may be positive. Most children have evidence of long-tract signs, cerebellar ataxia, and delayed motor and cognitive milestones, probably due to the associated structural anomalies. The Dandy-Walker malformation is managed by shunting the cystic cavity (and on occasion the ventricles as well) in the presence of hydrocephalus.

DIAGNOSIS AND DIFFERENTIAL DIAGNOSIS

Investigation of a child with hydrocephalus begins with the history. Familial cases suggest X-linked or autosomal hydrocephalus secondary to aqueductal stenosis. A past history of prematurity with intracranial hemorrhage, meningitis, or mumps encephalitis is important to ascertain. Multiple café-au-lait spots and other clinical features of neurofibromatosis point to aqueductal stenosis as the cause of hydrocephalus.

Examination includes careful inspection, palpation, and auscultation of the skull and spine. The occipitofrontal head circumference is recorded and compared with previous measurements. The size and configuration of the anterior fontanel are noted, and the back is inspected for abnormal midline skin lesions, including tufts of hair, lipoma, or angioma that might suggest spinal dysraphism. The presence of a prominent forehead or abnormalities in the shape of the occiput can suggest the pathogenesis of the hydrocephalus. A cranial bruit is audible in association with many cases of vein of Galen arteriovenous malformation. Transillumination of the skull is positive with massive dilatation of the ventricular system or in the Dandy-Walker syndrome. Inspection of the eyegrounds is mandatory because the finding of chorioretinitis suggests an intrauterine infection, such as toxoplasmosis, as a cause of the hydrocephalus. Papilledema is observed in older children but is rarely present in infants because the cranial sutures separate as a result of the increased pressure.

Plain skull films typically show separation of the sutures, erosion of the posterior clinoids in an older child, and an increase in convolutional markings (beaten-silver appearance) with long-standing increased ICP. The CT scan and/or MRI along with ultrasonography in an infant are the most important studies to identify the specific cause and severity of hydrocephalus.

The head might appear enlarged and can be confused with hydrocephalus secondary to a thickened cranium resulting from chronic anemia, rickets, osteogenesis imperfecta, and epiphyseal dysplasia. Chronic subdural collections can produce bilateral parietal bone prominence. Various metabolic and degenerative disorders of the CNS produce megalencephaly due to abnormal storage of substances within the brain parenchyma. These disorders include lysosomal diseases (Tay-Sachs, gangliosidosis, and the mucopolysaccharidoses), the aminoacidurias (maple syrup urine disease), and the leukodystrophies (metachromatic leukodystrophy, Alexander disease, Canavan disease). In addition, cerebral gigantism and neurofibromatosis are characterized by increased brain mass. Familial megalencephaly is inherited as an autosomal dominant trait and is characterized by delayed motor milestones and hypotonia but normal or near-normal intelligence. Measurement of parents' head circumferences is necessary to establish the diagnosis.

MEGALENCEPHALY

Megalencephaly is an anatomic disorder of brain growth defined as a brain weight:volume ratio >98th percentile for age (or ≥2 standard deviations [SD] above the mean) that is usually accompanied by macrocephaly (an occipitofrontal circumference [OFC] >98th percentile). Various storage and degenerative diseases are associated with megalencephaly, but anatomic and genetic causes exist as well. The most common cause of anatomic megalencephaly is benign familial megalencephaly. This condition is easily diagnosed by careful family history and measurement of the parents' head circumferences (OFCs). On the other hand, in >100 syndromes macrocephaly a known feature.

Anatomic megalencephaly is usually apparent at birth, and head growth continues to run parallel to the upper percentiles. Sometimes, in some syndromes, increased OFC is the presenting sign. Neuroimaging is critical in identifying the various structural and gyral abnormalities seen in syndromic macrocephaly and determining whether anatomic megalencephaly exists.

Common megalencephaly-associated macrocephaly syndromes include syndromes with prenatal and/or postnatal somatic overgrowth such as Sotos, Simpson-Golabi-Behmel, fragile X, Weaver, M-CMTC, and Bannayan-Ruvalcaba-Riley syndromes and syndromes without somatic overgrowth such as FG, Greig cephalopolysyndactyly, acrocallosal, and Gorlin syndromes.

Sotos syndrome (cerebral gigantism) is the most common megalencephalic syndrome, with 50% of patients having prenatal macrocephaly and 100% of patients having macrocephaly by age 1 yr. Early postnatal overgrowth normalizes by adulthood. Facial features include high forehead with frontal bossing, sparse hair in the frontoparietal region, downslanting palpebral fissures, apparent hypertelorism, long narrow face, prominent mandible, and malar flushing. Hypotonia, poor coordination, and speech delay are common. Most children show mental retardation, ranging from mild to severe.

HYDRANENCEPHALY

Hydranencephaly may be confused with hydrocephalus. The cerebral hemispheres are absent or represented by membranous sacs with remnants of frontal, temporal, or occipital cortex dispersed over the membrane. The midbrain and brainstem are relatively intact (Fig. 585-13). The cause of hydranencephaly is unknown, but bilateral occlusion of the internal carotid arteries during early fetal development would explain most of the pathologic abnormalities. Affected infants can have a normal or enlarged head circumference at birth that grows at an excessive rate postnatally. Transillumination shows an absence of the cerebral hemispheres. The child is irritable, feeds poorly, develops seizures and spastic quadriparesis, and has little or no cognitive development. A ventriculoperitoneal shunt prevents massive enlargement of the cranium.

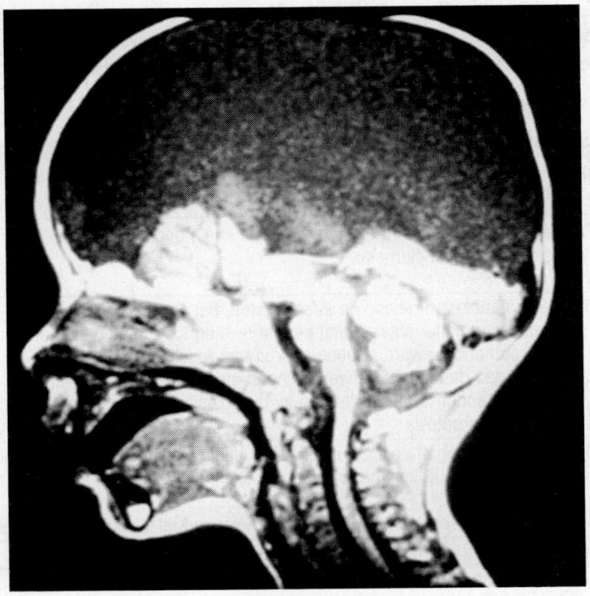

Figure 585-13 Hydranencephaly. MRI scan showing the brainstem and spinal cord with remnants of the cerebellum and the cerebral cortex. The remainder of the cranium is filled with cerebrospinal fluid.

TREATMENT

Therapy for hydrocephalus depends on the cause. Medical management, including the use of acetazolamide and furosemide, can provide temporary relief by reducing the rate of CSF production, but long-term results have been disappointing. Most cases of hydrocephalus require extracranial shunts, particularly a ventriculoperitoneal shunt. Endoscopic third ventriculostomy (ETV) has evolved as a viable approach and criteria have been developed for its use, but the procedure might need to be repeated to be effective. Ventricular shunting may be avoided with this approach. The major complications of shunting are occlusion (characterized by headache, papilledema, emesis, mental status changes) and bacterial infection (fever, headache, meningismus), usually due to *Staphylococcus epidermidis*. With meticulous preparation, the shunt infection rate can be reduced to <5%. The results of intrauterine surgical management of fetal hydrocephalus have been poor, possibly because of the high rate of associated cerebral malformations in addition to the hydrocephalus, except for some promise in cases of hydrocephalus associated with fetal meningomyelocele.

PROGNOSIS

Prognosis depends on the cause of the dilated ventricles and not on the size of the cortical mantle at the time of operative intervention, except in cases in which the cortical mantle has been severely compressed and stretched. Hydrocephalic children are at increased risk for various developmental disabilities. The mean intelligence quotient is reduced compared with the general population, particularly for performance tasks as compared with verbal abilities. Many children have abnormalities in memory function. Vision problems are common, including strabismus, visuospatial abnormalities, visual field defects, and optic atrophy with decreased acuity secondary to increased ICP. The visual-evoked potential latencies are delayed and take some time to recover after correction of the hydrocephalus. Although most hydrocephalic children are pleasant and mild mannered, some children show aggressive and delinquent behavior. Accelerated pubertal development in patients with shunted hydrocephalus or myelomeningocele is relatively common, possibly because of increased gonadotropin secretion in response to increased ICP. It is imperative that hydrocephalic children receive long-term follow-up in a multidisciplinary setting.

BIBLIOGRAPHY

Please visit the Nelson Textbook of Pediatrics *website at www.expertconsult.com for the complete bibliography.*

585.12 Craniosynostosis

Stephen L. Kinsman and Michael V. Johnston

Craniosynostosis is defined as premature closure of the cranial sutures and is classified as primary or secondary. It is associated with varying types of abnormal skull shape. Primary craniosynostosis refers to closure of one or more sutures owing to abnormalities of skull development, whereas secondary craniosynostosis results from failure of brain growth and expansion and is not discussed here. The incidence of primary craniosynostosis approximates 1/2,000 births. The cause is unknown in the majority of children; however, genetic syndromes account for 10-20%

of cases. Deformational forces appear important in occipital and frontal plagiocephaly in many cases. Early detection of posterior skull shape is critical and allows successful intervention to be offered in the form of physical therapy for torticollis and other positional asymmetries that lead to plagiocephaly.

DEVELOPMENT AND ETIOLOGY

The bones of the cranium are well developed by the 5th mo of gestation (frontal, parietal, temporal, and occipital) and are separated by sutures and fontanels. The brain grows rapidly in the 1st several years of life and is normally not impeded because of equivalent growth along the suture lines. The cause of craniosynostosis is unknown, but the prevailing hypothesis suggests that abnormal development of the base of the skull creates exaggerated forces on the dura that act to disrupt normal cranial suture development. Genetic factors have been identified for some isolated and for many syndromic causes of craniosynostosis (Table 585-4).

Table 585-4 COMMONLY USED CLINICAL GENETIC CLASSIFICATIONS OF CRANIOSYNOSTOSES

DISORDER	CAUSE
ISOLATED CRANIOSYNOSTOSIS	
Morphologically described	Unknown, uterine constraint, or *FGFR3* mutation
SYNDROMIC CRANIOSYNOSTOSIS	
Antler-Bixler syndrome	Unknown
Apert syndrome	Usually one of two mutations in *FGFR2*
Baere-Stevenson syndrome	Mutation in *GFGR2* or *FGFR3*
Bailler-Gerold syndrome	Mutation in *TWIST* heterogenous
Carpenter syndrome	Unknown
Craniofrontonasal dysplasia	Unknown gene at Xp22
Crouzon syndrome	Numerous different mutations at *FGFR2*
Crouzonomesodermoskeletal syndrome	Mutation in *FGFR3*
Jackson-Weiss syndrome	Mutation in *FGFR2*
Muenke syndrome	Mutation in *FGFR3*
Pfeiffer syndrome	Mutation in *FGFR1* or numerous mutation in *FGFR2*
Saethre-Chotzen syndrome	Mutation in *TWIST*
Shprintzen-Goldberg syndrome	Mutation in *FBEN1*

From Ridgway EB, Weiner HL: Skull deformaties, *Pediatr Clin North Am* 51:359–387, 2004.

CLINICAL MANIFESTATIONS AND TREATMENT

Most cases of craniosynostosis are evident at birth and are characterized by a skull deformity that is a direct result of premature suture fusion. Palpation of the suture reveals a prominent bony ridge, and fusion of the suture may be confirmed by plain skull roentgenograms, CT scan or bone scan in ambiguous cases (Table 585-5).

Premature closure of the sagittal suture produces a long and narrow skull, or **scaphocephaly,** the most common form of craniosynostosis. Scaphocephaly is associated with a prominent occiput, a broad forehead, and a small or absent anterior fontanel. The condition is sporadic, is more common in males, and often causes difficulties during labor because of cephalopelvic disproportion. Scaphocephaly does not produce increased ICP or hydrocephalus, and results of neurologic examination of affected patients are normal.

Frontal plagiocephaly is the next most common form of craniosynostosis and is characterized by unilateral flattening of the forehead, elevation of the ipsilateral orbit and eyebrow, and a prominent ear on the corresponding side. The condition is more common in females and is the result of premature fusion of a coronal and sphenofrontal suture. Surgical intervention produces a cosmetically pleasing result. When imaging does not reveal a closed suture, positional factors are of primary importance.

Occipital plagiocephaly is most often a result of positioning during infancy and is more common in an immobile child or a child with a disability, but fusion or sclerosis of the lambdoid suture can cause unilateral occipital flattening and bulging of the ipsilateral frontal bone. **Trigonocephaly** is a rare form of craniosynostosis caused by premature fusion of the metopic suture. These children have a keel-shaped forehead and hypotelorism and are at risk for associated developmental abnormalities of the forebrain. Milder forms of metopic ridging are more common. **Turricephaly** refers to a cone-shaped head due to premature fusion of the coronal and often sphenofrontal and frontoethmoidal sutures. The **kleeblattschädel deformity** is a peculiarly shaped skull that resembles a cloverleaf. Affected children have very prominent temporal bones, and the remainder of the cranium is constricted. Hydrocephalus is a common complication.

Premature fusion of only one suture rarely causes a neurologic deficit. In this situation, the sole indication for surgery is to enhance the child's cosmetic appearance, and the prognosis depends on the suture involved and on the degree of

Table 585-5 EPIDEMIOLOGY AND CLINICAL CHARACTERISTICS OF THE COMMON CRANIOSYNOSTOSES

TYPE	EPIDEMIOLOGY	SKULL DEFORMITY	CLINICAL PRESENTATION
Sagittal	Most common CSO affecting a single suture, 80% male	Dolicocephaly or scaphocephaly (boat-shaped)	Frontal bossing, prominent occiput, palpable keel ridge. OFC normal and reduced biparietal diameter
Coronal	18% of CSO, more common in girls Associated with Apert syndrome (with syndactly) and Crouzon disease, which includes abnormal sphenoid, orbital, and facial bones (hypoplasia of the midface)	Unilateral: plagiocephaly Bilateral: brachycephaly, acrocephaly	Unilateral: flattened forehead on affected side, flat checks, nose deviation on normal side; higher supraorbital margin leading to harlequin sign on radiograph and outward rotation of orbit can result in amblyopia Bilateral: broad, flattened forehead. In Apert syndrome accompanied by syndactyly and in Crouzon disease by hypoplasia of the midface and progressive proptosis
Lambdoid	10-20% of CSO, M:F ratio 4:1	Lambdoid/occipital plagiocephaly; right side affected in 70% of cases	Unilateral: flattening of occiput, indentation along synostotic suture, bulging of ipsilateral forehead leading to rhomboid skull, ipsilateral ear is anterior and inferior Bilateral: brachycephaly with bilateral anteriorly and inferiorly displaced ears
Metopic	Association with 19p chromosome abnormality	Trigoncephaly	Pointed forehead and midline ridge, hypotelorism
Multiple		Oxycephaly	Tower skull with undeveloped sinuses and shallow orbits, and elevated intercranial pressure

CSO, craniosynostosis; OFC, occipital-frontal circumference.
From Ridgway EB, Weiner HL: Skull deformities, *Pediatr Clin North Am* 51:359–387, 2004.

disfigurement. Neurologic complications, including hydrocephalus and increased ICP, are more likely to occur when two or more sutures are prematurely fused, in which case operative intervention is essential. The role of early repositioning efforts and therapy for torticollis and the use of cranial molding devices are beyond the scope of this review.

The most prevalent genetic disorders associated with craniosynostosis include Crouzon, Apert, Carpenter, Chotzen, and Pfeiffer syndromes. Crouzon syndrome is characterized by premature craniosynostosis and is inherited as an autosomal dominant trait. The shape of the head depends on the timing and order of suture fusion but most often is a compressed back-to-front diameter or brachycephaly due to bilateral closure of the coronal sutures. The orbits are underdeveloped, and ocular proptosis is prominent. Hypoplasia of the maxilla and orbital hypertelorism are typical facial features.

Apert syndrome has many features in common with Crouzon syndrome. Apert syndrome is usually a sporadic condition, although autosomal dominant inheritance can occur. It is associated with premature fusion of multiple sutures, including the coronal, sagittal, squamosal, and lambdoid sutures. The facies tend to be asymmetric, and the eyes are less proptotic than in Crouzon syndrome. Apert syndrome is characterized by syndactyly of the 2nd, 3rd, and 4th fingers, which may be joined to the thumb and the 5th finger. Similar abnormalities often occur in the feet. All patients have progressive calcification and fusion of the bones of the hands, feet, and cervical spine.

Carpenter syndrome is inherited as an autosomal recessive condition, and the many fusions of sutures tend to produce the kleeblattschädel skull deformity. Soft tissue syndactyly of the hands and feet is always present, and mental retardation is common. Additional but less common abnormalities include congenital heart disease, corneal opacities, coxa valga, and genu valgum.

Chotzen syndrome is characterized by asymmetric craniosynostosis and plagiocephaly. The condition is the most prevalent of the genetic syndromes and is inherited as an autosomal dominant trait. It is associated with facial asymmetry, ptosis of the eyelids, shortened fingers, and soft tissue syndactyly of the 2nd and 3rd fingers.

Pfeiffer syndrome is most often associated with turricephaly. The eyes are prominent and widely spaced, and the thumbs and great toes are short and broad. Partial soft tissue syndactyly may be evident. Most cases appear to be sporadic, but autosomal dominant inheritance has been reported.

Mutations of the fibroblast growth factor receptor (FGFR) gene family have been shown to be associated with phenotypically specific types of craniosynostosis. Mutations of the *FGFR1* gene located on chromosome 8 result in Pfeiffer syndrome; a similar mutation of the *FGFR2* gene causes Apert syndrome. Identical mutations of the *FGFR2* gene can result in both Pfeiffer and Crouzon phenotypes.

Each of the genetic syndromes poses a risk of additional anomalies, including hydrocephalus, increased ICP, papilledema, optic atrophy resulting from abnormalities of the optic foramina, respiratory problems secondary to a deviated nasal septum or choanal atresia, and disorders of speech and deafness. Craniectomy is mandatory for management of increased ICP, and a multidisciplinary craniofacial team is essential for the long-term follow-up of affected children. Craniosynostosis may be surgically corrected with good outcomes and relatively low morbidity and mortality, especially for nonsyndromic infants.

BIBLIOGRAPHY

Please visit the Nelson Textbook of Pediatrics *website at www.expertconsult.com for the complete bibliography.*

Chapter 586
Seizures in Childhood

Mohamad A. Mikati

A seizure is a transient occurrence of signs and/or symptoms resulting from abnormal excessive or synchronous neuronal activity in the brain. The International Classification of Epileptic Seizures divides epileptic seizures into 2 large categories: In **focal (partial) seizures,** the first clinical and electroencephalographic (EEG) changes suggest initial activation of a system of neurons limited to part of one cerebral hemisphere; in **generalized seizures,** the first clinical and EEG changes indicate synchronous involvement of all of both hemispheres (Table 586-1). Approximately 30% of patients who have a first afebrile seizure have later epilepsy; the risk is about 20% if neurologic exam, EEG, and neuroimaging are normal. **Febrile seizures** are a special category. **Acute symptomatic seizures** occur secondary to an acute problem affecting brain excitability such as electrolyte imbalance or meningitis. Most children with these types of seizures do well, but sometimes such seizures signify major structural, inflammatory, or metabolic disorders of the brain, such as meningitis, encephalitis, acute stroke, or brain tumor; the prognosis depends on the underlying disorder, including its reversibility or treatability and the likelihood of developing epilepsy from it. **Unprovoked seizure** is not an acute symptomatic seizure. **Remote symptomatic seizure** is thought to be secondary to a distant brain injury such as an old stroke.

Epilepsy is a disorder of the brain characterized by an enduring predisposition to generate seizures and by the neurobiologic, cognitive, psychological, and social consequences of this condition. The clinical diagnosis of epilepsy usually requires the occurrence of at least 1 unprovoked epileptic seizure with either a second such seizure or enough EEG and clinical information to convincingly demonstrate an enduring predisposition to develop recurrences. For epidemiologic purposes epilepsy is considered to be present when ≥2 unprovoked seizures occur in a time frame of >24 hr. Approximately 4-10% of children experience at least 1 seizure in the first 16 yr of life. The cumulative lifetime incidence of epilepsy is 3%, and more than half of the cases start in childhood. The annual prevalence is 0.5-1%. Thus, the occurrence of a single seizure or of febrile seizures does not necessarily imply the diagnosis of epilepsy. **Seizure disorder** is a general term that is usually used to include any one of several disorders including epilepsy, febrile seizures, and possibly single seizures and seizures secondary to metabolic, infectious, or other etiologies (e.g., hypocalcemia, meningitis).

An **epileptic syndrome** is a disorder that manifests one or more specific seizure types and has a specific age of onset and a specific prognosis. Several types of epileptic syndromes can be distinguished (Tables 586-2 to 586-4). This classification has to be distinguished from the classification of epileptic seizures that refers to single events rather than to clinical syndromes. In general, seizure type is the primary determinant of the type of medications the patient is likely to respond to, and the epilepsy syndrome determines the type of prognosis one could expect. An **epileptic encephalopathy** is an epilepsy syndrome in which the severe EEG abnormality is thought to result in cognitive and other impairments in the patient. Idiopathic **epilepsy** is an epilepsy syndrome that is genetic or presumed genetic and in which there is no underlying disorder affecting development or other neurologic function (e.g., petit mal epilepsy). Symptomatic **epilepsy** is an epilepsy syndrome caused by an underlying brain disorder (e.g., epilepsy secondary to tuberous sclerosis). A **cryptogenic epilepsy** (also termed **presumed symptomatic epilepsy**) is an epilepsy syndrome in which there is a presumed underlying brain disorder causing the epilepsy and affecting neurologic function, but the underlying disorder is not known.

Table 586-1 TYPES OF EPILEPTIC SEIZURES

SELF-LIMITED SEIZURE TYPES	CONTINUOUS SEIZURE TYPES
Focal Seizures	**Generalized Status Epilepticus**
Focal sensory seizures • With elementary sensory symptoms (e.g., occipital and parietal lobe seizures) • With experiential sensory symptoms (e.g., temporo-parieto-occipital junction seizures) Focal motor seizures • With elementary clonic motor signs • With asymmetrical tonic motor seizures (e.g., supplementary motor seizures) • With typical (temporal lobe) automatisms (e.g., mesial temporal lobe seizures) • With hyperkinetic automatisms • With focal negative myoclonus • With inhibitory motor seizures Gelastic seizures Hemiclonic seizures Secondarily generalized seizures Reflex seizures in focal epilepsy syndromes	Generalized tonic-clonic status epilepticus Clonic status epilepticus Absence status epilepticus Tonic status epilepticus Myoclonic status epilepticus **Focal Status Epilepticus** Epilepsia partialis continua of Kojevnikov Aura continua Limbic status epilepticus (psychomotor status) Hemiconvulsive status with hemiparesis
Generalized Seizures	**PRECIPITATING STIMULI FOR REFLEX SEIZURES**
Tonic-clonic seizures (includes variations beginning with a clonic or myoclonic phase) Clonic seizures • Without tonic features • With tonic features Typical absence seizures Atypical absence seizures Myoclonic absence seizures Tonic seizures Spasms Myoclonic seizures Eyelid myoclonia • Without absences • With absences Myoclonic atonic seizures Negative myoclonus Atonic seizures Reflex seizures in generalized epilepsy syndromes	Visual stimuli • Flickering light—color to be specified when possible • Patterns • Other visual stimuli Thinking Music Eating Praxis Somatosensory Proprioceptive Reading Hot water Startle

From International League Against Epilepsy: *Epileptic seizure types and precipitating stimuli for reflex seizures* (website), May 13, 2009. http://www.ilae-epilepsy.org/Visitors/Centre/ctf/seizure_types.cfm. Accessed October 8, 2010.

Table 586-2 CLASSIFICATION FOR EPILEPSY SYNDROMES WITH AN INDICATION OF AGE OF ONSET, DURATION OF ACTIVE EPILEPSY, PROGNOSIS, AND THERAPEUTIC OPTIONS

SPECIFIC SYNDROMES	AGE AT ONSET	AGE AT REMISSION	PROGNOSIS	MONOTHERAPY OR ADD-ON	POSSIBLE ADD-ON	SURGERY
IDIOPATHIC FOCAL EPILEPSIES OF INFANCY AND CHILDHOOD						
Benign infantile seizures (nonfamilial)	Infant	Infant	Good	PB	—	No
Benign childhood epilepsy with centrotemporal spikes	3-13 yr	16 yr	Good	OXC, VPA, CBZ, LEV	—	No
Early and late onset idiopathic occipital epilepsy	2-8 yr; 6-17 yr	12 yr or earlier; 18 yr	Good	OXC, VPA, CBZ, LEV	—	No
FAMILIAL (AUTOSOMAL DOMINANT) EPILEPSIES						
Benign familial neonatal convulsions	Newborn to young infant	Newborn to young infant	Good	PB	—	No
Benign familial infantile convulsions	Infant	Infant	Good	CBZ, PB	—	No
Autosomal dominant nocturnal frontal lobe epilepsy	Childhood	Unclear	Variable	CBZ, OXC, TPM, PHT, GBP	LEV, PHT, PB, CLB	No
Familial lateral temporal lobe epilepsy	Childhood to adolescence	Unclear	Variable	CBZ, OXC, VPA, TPM, PHT, GBP	LEV, PHT, PB, CLB	No
Generalized epilepsies with febrile seizures plus	Childhood to adolescence	Unclear	Variable	VPA, ESM, TPM, LTG	CLB, LEV	No
SYMPTOMATIC (OR PROBABLY SYMPTOMATIC) FOCAL EPILEPSIES						
Limbic Epilepsy						
Mesial temporal lobe epilepsy with hippocampal sclerosis	School age or earlier	Long lasting	Variable	CBZ, VPA, OXC, TPM, PHT, GBP	LEV, PHT, PB, CLB	Temporal resection
Mesial temporal lobe epilepsy defined by specific causes	Variable	Long lasting	Variable	CBZ, VPA, OXC, TPM, PHT, GBP	LEV, PHT, PB, CLB	Temporal resection
Other types defined by location and causes	Variable	Long lasting	Variable	CBZ, VPA, OXC, TPM, PHT, GBP	LEV, PHT, PB, CLB	Lesionectomy ± cortical resection

Table 586-2 CLASSIFICATION FOR EPILEPSY SYNDROMES WITH AN INDICATION OF AGE OF ONSET, DURATION OF ACTIVE EPILEPSY, PROGNOSIS, AND THERAPEUTIC OPTIONS—cont'd

SPECIFIC SYNDROMES	AGE AT ONSET	AGE AT REMISSION	PROGNOSIS	MONOTHERAPY OR ADD-ON	POSSIBLE ADD-ON	SURGERY
Neocortical Epilepsies						
Rasmussen syndrome	6-12 yr	Progressive	Ominous	Plasmapheresis, immunoglobulins	PHT, CBZ, PB, TPM, CLB	Functional hemispherectomy
Hemiconvulsion-hemiplegia syndrome	1-5 yr	Chronic	Severe	CBZ, VPA, OXC, TPM, PHT, GBP	LEV, PHT, PB, CLB	Functional hemispherectomy
Other types defined by location and cause	Variable	Long lasting	Variable	CBZ, VPA, OXC, TPM, PHT, GBP	LEV, PHT, PB, CLB	Lesionectomy ± cortical resection
Migrating partial seizures of early infancy	Infant	No remission	Ominous	PB, PHT, CBZ, TPM, VPA	BDZ	No
IDIOPATHIC GENERALIZED EPILEPSIES						
Benign myoclonic epilepsy in infancy	3 mo-3 yr	3-5 yr	Variable	VPA, TPM, LEV	BDZ	No
Epilepsy with myoclonic astatic seizures	3-5 yr	Variable	Variable	VPA, ESM, TPM	BDZ, LTG, LEV	No
Childhood absence epilepsy	5-6 yr	10-12 yr	Good	VPA, ESM, LTG	—	No
Epilepsy with myoclonic absences	1-12 yr	Variable	Guarded	VPA, ESM	BDZ	No
IDIOPATHIC GENERALIZED EPILEPSIES WITH VARIABLE PHENOTYPES						
Juvenile absence epilepsy	10-12 yr	Usually lifelong	Good	VPA, ESM, LTG	BDZ	No
Juvenile myoclonic epilepsy	12-18 yr	Usually lifelong	Good	VPA, TPM, LEV	BDZ, PRM, PB, LTG	No
Epilepsy with generalized tonic-clonic seizures only	12-18 yr	Usually lifelong	Good	VPA, LTG, TPM, CBZ	BDZ, LEV	No
REFLEX EPILEPSIES						
Idiopathic photosensitive occipital lobe epilepsy	10-12 yr	Unclear	Variable	VPA	LEV, BDZ	No
Other visual sensitive epilepsies	2-5 yr	Unclear	Variable	VPA	LEV, BDZ	No
Startle epilepsy	Variable	Long-lasting	Guarded	CBZ, VPA, OXC, TPM, PHT, GBP	LEV, PHT, PB, CLB	Lesionectomy ± cortical resection
EPILEPTIC ENCEPHALOPATHIES						
Early myoclonic encephalopathy and Ohtahara syndrome	Newborn-infant	No remission	Ominous	Steroids, PB	BDZ, VGB	No
West syndrome	Infant	Variable	Variable	Steoids, VGB	BDZ, TPM, IVIG	Lesionectomy ± cortical resection
Dravet's syndrome (severe myoclonic epilepsy in infancy)	Infant	No remission	Severe	Stiripentol-CLB, VPA, TPM	BDZ, TPM	No
Lennox-Gastaut syndrome	3-10 yr	No remission	Severe	—	BDZ, IVIG	Callosotomy
Landau-Kleffner syndrome	3-6 yr	8-12 yr	Guarded	VPA, ESM, steroids	BDZ, LTG, IVIG	Multiple subpial transections
Epilepsy with continuous spike waves during slow-wave sleep	4-7 yr	8-12 yr	Guarded	VPA, ESM, steroids	BDZ, LTG, IVIG	No
PROGRESSIVE MYOCLONUS EPILEPSIES						
Unverricht-Lundborg, lafora, ceroidolipofuscinoses, etc.	Late infant to adolescent	Progressive	Ominous	VPA, TPM	BDZ, PB	No
SEIZURES NOT NECESSARILY NEEDING A DIAGNOSIS OF EPILEPSY						
Benign neonatal seizures	Newborn	Newborn	Good	PB	—	No
Febrile seizures	3-5 yr	3-6 yr	Good	VPA if repeated and prolonged	—	No
Reflex seizures	Variable	n/a		—	—	No
Drug or other chemically induced seizures	Variable	n/a		—	—	No
Immediate and early post-traumatic seizures	Variable	n/a		—	—	No

BDZ, benzodiazepine; CBZ, carbamazepine; CLB, clobazam; ESM, ethosuximide; GBP, gabapentin; IVIG, intravenous immunoglobulin; LEV, levetiracetam; LTG, lamotrigine; OXC: oxcarbazepine; PB, phenobarbital; PHT, phenytoin; PRM, primidone; TPM, topiramate; VGB: vigabatrin; VPA, valproic acid.
Adapted from Guerrini R: Epilepsy in children, *Lancet* 367:499–524, 2006.

EVALUATION OF THE FIRST SEIZURE

Initial evaluation of an infant or child during or shortly after a suspected seizure should include an assessment of the adequacy of the airway, ventilation, and cardiac function as well as measurement of temperature, blood pressure, and glucose concentration. For acute evaluation of the 1st seizure, the physician should search for potentially life-threatening causes of seizures such as meningitis, systemic sepsis, unintentional and intentional head trauma, and ingestion of drugs of abuse and other toxins. The history should attempt to define factors that might have promoted the convulsion and to provide a detailed description of the seizure and the child's postictal state. Most parents vividly recall their child's initial convulsion and can describe it in detail.

The 1st step in an evaluation is to determine whether the seizure has a focal onset or is generalized. **Focal seizures** may be

Table 586-3 IDENTIFIED GENES FOR EPILEPSY

GENE		FUNCTION	LOCUS	EPILEPSY SYNDROME	SEIZURE TYPES
GABRA1	$GABA_A$ α1 receptor subunit	Partial inhibition of GABA-activated currents	5q34	AD JME	TCS, myoclonic, absence
GABRG2	$GABA_A$ receptor γ2 subunit	Rapid inhibition of GABAergic neurons	5q31	FS, CAE, GEFS+	Febrile, absence, TCS, myoclonic, clonic, partial
GABRD	$GABA_A$ receptor δ2 subunit	Decreased GABAA receptor current amplitudes	1p36	GEFS+	Febrile and afebrile seizures
SCN2A	Sodium channel α2 subunit	Fast sodium influx initiation and propagation of action potential	2q24	GEFS+ BFNIC	Febrile, afebrile generalized tonic, and TCS
SCN1A	Sodium channel α1 subunit	Somatodendritic sodium influx	2q24	GEFS+ SMEI	Febrile, absence, myoclonic, TCS, partial
SCN1B	Sodium channel β1 subunit	Coadjuvate and modulate β subunit	19q13	GEFS+	Febrile, absence, tonic clonic, myoclonic
KCNQ2	Potassium channel	M current interacts with KCNQ3	20q13	BFNC	Neonatal convulsions
KCNQ3		M current interacts with KCNQ2	8q24	BFNC	Neonatal convulsions
ATP1A2	Na^+,K^+-ATPase pump	Dysfunction of ion transportation	1q23	BFNIC and familial hemiplegic migraine	Infantile convulsions
CHRNA4	Acetylcholine receptor α4 subunit	Nicotinic current modulation; interacts with β2 subunit	20q13	ADNFLE	Sleep-related focal seizures
CHRNB2	Acetylcholine receptor β2 subunit	Nicotinic current modulation; interacts with α4 subunit	1p21	ADNFLE	Sleep-related focal seizures
LGI1	Leucine-rich, glioma activated	Disregulates homeostasis, interactions between neurons and glia?	10q24	ADPEAF	Partial seizures with auditory or visual hallucinations
CLCN2	Voltage-gated chloride channel	Neuronal chloride efflux	3q26	IGE	TCS, myoclonic, absence
EFHC1	Protein with an EF-hand motif	Reduced mouse hippocampal induced apoptosis	6p12-p11	JME	TCS, myoclonic
BRD2 (RING3)	Nuclear transcriptional regulator	?	6p21	JME	TCS, myoclonic

AD, autosomal dominant; ADNFLE, autosomal dominant nocturnal frontal lobe epilepsy; ADPEAF, autosomal dominant partial epilepsy with auditory features; BFNC, benign familial neonatal convulsions; BFNIC, benign familial neonatal-infantile convulsion; $GEFS^+$, generalized epilepsy with febrile seizures plus; JME, juvenile myoclonic epilepsy; SMEI, severe myolconic epilepsy of infancy; TCS, tonic-clonic seizures.
Adapted from Guerrini R: Epilepsy in children, *Lancet* 367:499–524, 2006.

Table 586-4 CHILDHOOD EPILEPTIC SYNDROMES WITH GENERALLY GOOD PROGNOSIS

SYNDROME	COMMENT
Benign neonatal familial convulsions	Dominant, may be severe and resistant during a few days Febrile or afebrile seizures (benign) occur later in a minority
Infantile familial convulsions	Dominant, seizures often in clusters (overlap with benign partial complex epilepsy of infancy)
Febrile convulsions plus syndromes (see Table 586-2)	In some families, febrile and afebrile convulsions occur in different members, GEFS+ The old dichotomy between febrile convulsions or epilepsy does not always hold
Benign myoclonic epilepsy of infancy	Often seizures during sleep, one rare variety with reflex myoclonic seizures (touch, noise)
Partial idiopathic epilepsy with rolandic spikes	Seizures with falling asleep or on awakening; focal sharp waves with centrotemporal location on EEG; genetic
Idiopathic occipital partial epilepsy	Early childhood form with seizures during sleep and ictal vomiting; can occur as status epilepticus Later forms with migrainous symptoms; not always benign
Petit mal absence epilepsy	Cases with absences only, some have generalized seizures. 60-80% full remission In most cases, absences disappear on therapy but there are resistant cases (unpredictable)
Juvenile myoclonic epilepsy	Adolescence onset, with early morning myoclonic seizures and generalized seizures during sleep; often history of absences in childhood

EEG, electroencephalogram; GEFS+, generalized epilepsy with febrile seizures plus.
From Deonna T: Management of epilepsy, *Arch Dis Child* 90:5–9, 2005.

characterized by motor or sensory symptoms and include forceful turning of the head and eyes to one side, unilateral clonic movements beginning in the face or extremities, or a sensory disturbance such as paresthesias or pain localized to a specific area. Focal seizures in an adolescent or adult usually indicate a localized lesion, but investigation of focal seizures during childhood may be nondiagnostic. Focal seizures in a neonate may be seen in perinatal stroke. Motor seizures may be focal or generalized and tonic-clonic, tonic, clonic, myoclonic, or atonic. **Tonic seizures** are characterized by increased tone or rigidity, and **atonic seizures** are characterized by flaccidity or lack of movement during a convulsion. **Clonic seizures** consist of rhythmic muscle contraction and relaxation; **myoclonus** is most accurately described as shocklike contraction of a muscle. The duration of the seizure and state of consciousness (retained or impaired) should be documented. The history should determine whether an **aura** preceded the convulsion and the behavior of the child immediately preceding the seizure. The most common aura experienced by children consists of epigastric discomfort or pain and a feeling of fear. The posture of the patient, presence and distribution of cyanosis, vocalizations, loss of sphincter control (particularly of the urinary bladder), and postictal state (including sleep, headache, and hemiparesis) should be noted.

In addition to the assessment of cardiorespiratory and metabolic status described, examination of a child with a seizure disorder should be geared toward the search for an organic cause. The child's head circumference, length, and weight are plotted on a growth chart and compared with previous measurements. A careful general and neurologic examination should be performed. The **eyegrounds** must be examined for the presence of papilledema, retinal hemorrhages, chorioretinitis, coloboma, or macular changes, as well as retinal phakoma. The finding of unusual facial features or associated physical findings such as hepatosplenomegaly point to an underlying metabolic or storage disease as the cause of the neurologic disorder. Positive results of a search for vitiliginous lesions of tuberous sclerosis using an ultraviolet light source and examination for adenoma sebaceum, shagreen patch, multiple café-au-lait spots, a nevus flammeus, and the presence of retinal phakoma could indicate a **neurocutaneous** disorder as the cause of the seizure.

Localizing neurologic signs such as a subtle **hemiparesis** with hyperreflexia, an equivocal Babinski sign, and a downward-drifting extended arm with eyes closed might suggest a contralateral hemispheric structural lesion, such as a slow-growing temporal lobe glioma, as the cause of the seizure disorder. Unilateral growth arrest of the thumbnail, hand, or extremity in a child with a focal seizure disorder suggests a chronic condition such as a porencephalic cyst, arteriovenous malformation, or cortical atrophy in the opposite hemisphere.

586.1 Febrile Seizures

Mohamad A. Mikati

Febrile seizures are seizures that occur between the age of 6 and 60 mo with a temperature of 38°C or higher, that are not the result of central nervous system infection or any metabolic imbalance, and that occur in the absence of a history of prior afebrile seizures. A **simple febrile seizure** is a primary generalized, usually tonic-clonic, attack associated with fever, lasting for a maximum of 15 min, and not recurrent within a 24-hour period. A **complex febrile seizure** is more prolonged (>15 min), is focal, and/or recurs within 24 hr. **Febrile status epilepticus** is a febrile seizure lasting >30 min.

Between 2% and 5% of neurologically healthy infants and children experience at least 1, usually simple, febrile seizure. Simple febrile seizures do not have an increased risk of mortality even though they are concerning to the parents. Complex febrile seizures may have an approximately 2-fold long-term increase in mortality, as compared to the general population over the subsequent 2 yr, probably secondary to coexisting pathology. There are no long-term adverse effects of having ≥1 simple febrile seizures. Specifically, recurrent simple febrile seizures do not damage the brain. Compared with age-matched controls, patients with febrile seizures do not have any increase in incidence of abnormalities of behavior, scholastic performance, neurocognitive function, or attention. Children who develop later epilepsy might experience such difficulties. Febrile seizures recur in approximately 30% of those experiencing a first episode, in 50% after 2 or more episodes, and in 50% of infants <1 yr old at febrile seizure onset. Several factors affect recurrence risk (Table 586-5). Although about 15% of children with epilepsy have had febrile seizures, only 2-7% of children who experience febrile seizures proceed to develop epilepsy later in life. There are several predictors of epilepsy after febrile seizures (Table 586-6).

GENETIC FACTORS

The genetic contribution to incidence of febrile seizures is manifested by a positive family history for febrile seizures. In many families the disorder is inherited as an autosomal dominant trait, and multiple single genes causing the disorder have been identified. In most cases the disorder appears polygenic, and the genes predisposing to it remain to be identified. Identified single genes include *FEB 1, 2, 3, 4, 5, 6,* and *7* genes on chromosomes 8q13-q21, 19p13.3, 2q24, 5q14-q15, 6q22-24, 18p11.2, and 21q22. Only the function of *FEB 2* is known: it is a sodium channel gene, SCN1A.

Almost any type of epilepsy can be preceded by febrile seizures, and a few epilepsy syndromes typically start with febrile seizures. These are **generalized epilepsy with febrile seizures plus** (GEFS+), **severe myoclonic epilepsy of infancy** (SMEI, also called Dravet syndrome), and, in many patients, temporal lobe epilepsy secondary to mesial temporal sclerosis.

GEFS+ is an autosomal dominant syndrome with a highly variable phenotype. Onset is usually in early childhood and remission is usually in mid-childhood. It is characterized by multiple febrile seizures and several types of afebrile generalized seizures, including generalized tonic-clonic, absence, myoclonic, atonic, or myoclonic astatic seizures with variable degrees of severity.

Dravet syndrome is considered to be the most severe of the phenotypic spectrum of febrile seizures plus. It constitutes a distinctive separate entity that is one of the most severe forms of epilepsy starting in infancy. Its onset is in the 1st yr of life, characterized by febrile and afebrile unilateral clonic seizures recurring every 1 or 2 mo. These early seizures are typically induced by fever, but they differ from the usual febrile convulsions in that they are more prolonged, are more frequent, and come in clusters. Seizures subsequently start to occur with lower fevers and then without fever. During the 2nd yr of life, myoclonus, atypical absences, and partial seizures occur frequently and developmental delay usually follows. This syndrome is usually caused by a new mutation, although rarely it is inherited in an autosomal dominant manner. The mutated gene is located on 2q24-31 and encodes for SCN1A, the same gene mutated in GEFS+ spectrum. However, in Dravet syndrome the mutations lead to loss of function and thus to a more severe phenotype.

The majority of patients who had had prolonged febrile seizures and encephalopathy after vaccination and who had been presumed to have suffered from **vaccine encephalopathy (seizures and psychomotor regression occurring after vaccination and presumed to be caused by it)** have Dravet syndrome mutations, indicating that their disease is due to the mutation and not secondary to the vaccine. This has raised doubts about the very existence of the entity termed *vaccine encephalopathy.*

WORK-UP

The general approach the patient with febrile seizures is delineated in Figure 586-1. Each child who presents with a febrile seizure requires a detailed history and a thorough general and neurologic examination. These are the cornerstones of the evaluation. Febrile seizures often occur in the context of otitis media, roseola and human herpesvirus 6 (HHV6) infection, shigella, or similar infections, making the evaluation more demanding. Several investigations need to be considered.

Table 586-5 RISK FACTORS FOR RECURRENCE OF FEBRILE SEIZURES

MAJOR
Age <1 yr Duration of fever <24 hr Fever 38-39°C
MINOR
Family history of febrile seizures Family history of epilepsy Complex febrile seizure Day care Male gender Lower serum sodium

Having no risk factors carries a recurrence risk of about 12%; 1 risk factor, 25-50%; 2 risk factors, 50-59%; 3 or more, 73-100%.
Modified from Mikati MA, Rahi A: Febrile seizures: from molecular biology to clinical practice, *Neurosciences* 10:14–22, 2004.

Table 586-6 RISK FACTORS FOR OCCURRENCE OF SUBSEQUENT EPILEPSY

RISK FACTOR	RISK FOR SUBSEQUENT EPILEPSY
Simple febrile seizure	1%
Neurodevelopmental abnormalities	33%
Focal complex febrile seizure	29%
Family history of epilepsy	18%
Fever <1 hr before febrile seizure	11%
Complex febrile seizure, any type	6%
Recurrent febrile seizures	4%

Modified from Mikati MA, Rahi A: Febrile seizures: from molecular biology to clinical practice, *Neurosciences* 10:14–22, 2004.

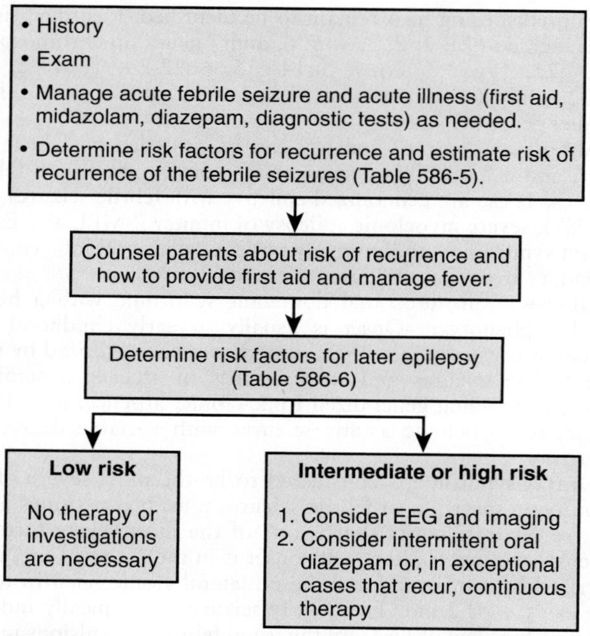

• History
• Exam
• Manage acute febrile seizure and acute illness (first aid, midazolam, diazepam, diagnostic tests) as needed.
• Determine risk factors for recurrence and estimate risk of recurrence of the febrile seizures (Table 586-5).
Counsel parents about risk of recurrence and how to provide first aid and manage fever.
Determine risk factors for later epilepsy (Table 586-6)
Low risk
No therapy or investigations are necessary
Intermediate or high risk
1. Consider EEG and imaging
2. Consider intermittent oral diazepam or, in exceptional cases that recur, continuous therapy

Figure 586-1 Management of febrile seizures. (Modified from Mikati MA, Rahi A: Febrile seizures: from molecular biology to clinical practice, *Neurosciences* 10:14–22, 2004.)

Lumbar Puncture

Lumbar puncture is recommended in children <12 mo of age after their first febrile seizure to rule out meningitis. It is especially important to consider if the child has received prior antibiotics that would mask the clinical symptoms of the meningitis. The presence of an identified source of fever, such as otitis media, does not eliminate the possibility of meningitis. Seizures are the major sign of meningitis in 13-15% of children presenting with this disease, and 30-35% of such children have no other meningeal signs. According to the American Academy of Pediatrics (AAP) practice parameter, it is strongly recommended in infants <1 yr of age because other signs of the infection might not be present. A child between 12 and 18 mo of age should also be considered for lumbar puncture because the clinical symptoms of meningitis may be subtle in this age group. For the well-appearing child after a febrile seizure, the yield of lumbar puncture is very low. For children >18 mo of age, a lumbar puncture is indicated in the presence of clinical signs and symptoms of meningitis (e.g., neck stiffness, Kernig sign, Brudzinski sign) or if the history and/or physical examination otherwise suggest intracranial infection.

Electroencephalogram

If the child is presenting with his or her first simple febrile seizure and is otherwise neurologically healthy, an EEG need not normally be performed as part of the evaluation. An EEG would not predict the future recurrence of febrile seizures or epilepsy even if the result is abnormal. Spikes during drowsiness are often seen in children with febrile seizures, particularly those >4 yr old, and these do not predict later epilepsy. EEGs performed within 2 wk of a febrile seizure often have nonspecific slowing, usually posteriorly. Thus, in many cases, if an EEG is indicated, it is delayed until or repeated after >2 wk have passed. EEG should therefore generally be restricted to special cases in which epilepsy is highly suspected, and it should be used to delineate the type of epilepsy rather than to predict its occurrence. If an EEG is done, it should be performed for at least 30 min in wakefulness and in sleep according to international guidelines to avoid misinterpretation and drawing of erroneous conclusions. At times, if the patient does not recover immediately from a seizure, then EEG can help distinguish between ongoing seizure activity and a prolonged postictal period sometimes termed a **nonepileptic twilight state (NETS)**.

Blood Studies

Blood studies (serum electrolytes, calcium, phosphorus, magnesium, and complete blood count [CBC]) are not routinely recommended in the work-up of a child with a first simple febrile seizure. Blood glucose should be determined only in children with prolonged postictal obtundation or those with poor oral intake (prolonged fasting). Serum electrolyte values may be abnormal in children after a febrile seizure, but this should be suggested by precipitating or predisposing conditions elicited in the history and reflected in abnormalities of the physical examination. If clinically indicated (e.g., in a history or physical examination suggesting dehydration) these tests are indicated.

Neuroimaging

According to the AAP practice parameter, a CT or MRI is not recommended in evaluating the child after a first simple febrile seizure.

The work-up of children with complex febrile seizures needs to be individualized. This can include EEG and neuroimaging, particularly if the child is neurologically abnormal. Patients with febrile status epilepticus have been reported to have swelling of their hippocampus acutely and subsequent long-term hippocampal atrophy. These patients may be candidates for neuroimaging, because they may be at risk for later temporal lobe epilepsy.

TREATMENT

In general, antiepileptic therapy, continuous or intermittent, is not recommended for children with one or more simple febrile seizures. Parents should be counseled about the relative risks of recurrence of febrile seizures and recurrence of epilepsy, educated on how to handle a seizure acutely, and given emotional support. If the seizure lasts for >5 min, then acute treatment with diazepam, lorazepam, or midazolam is needed (see Chapter 586.8 for acute management of seizures and status epilepticus). Rectal diazepam is often prescribed to be given at the time of recurrence of febrile seizure lasting >5 min (see Table 586-12 for dosing). Alternatively, buccal or intranasal midazolam may be used and is often preferred by parents. Intravenous benzodiazepines, phenobarbital, phenytoin, or valproate may be needed in the case of febrile status epilepticus. If the parents are very anxious concerning their child's seizures, intermittent oral diazepam can be given during febrile illnesses (0.33 mg/kg every 8 hr during fever) to help reduce the risk of seizures in children known to have had febrile seizures with previous illnesses. Intermittent oral nitrazepam, clobazam, and clonazepam (0.1 mg/kg/day) have also been used. Other therapies have included intermittent diazepam prophylaxis (0.5 mg/kg administered as a rectal suppository every 8 hr), phenobarbital (4-5 mg/kg/day in 1 or 2 divided doses), and valproate (20-30 mg/kg/day in 2 or 3 divided doses). In the vast majority of cases it is not justified to use these medications owing to the risk of side effects and lack of demonstrated long-term benefits, even if the recurrence rate of febrile seizures is expected to be decreased by these drugs. Other antiepileptic drugs (AEDs) have not been shown to be effective.

Antipyretics can decrease the discomfort of the child but do not reduce the risk of having a recurrent febrile seizure, probably because the seizure often occurs as the temperature is rising or falling. Chronic antiepileptic therapy may be considered for children with a high risk for later epilepsy. Currently available data indicate that the possibility of future epilepsy does not change with or without antiepileptic therapy. Iron deficiency has been shown to be associated with an increased risk of febrile seizures, and thus screening for that problem and treating it appears appropriate.

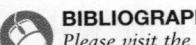

BIBLIOGRAPHY
Please visit the Nelson Textbook of Pediatrics *website at* *www.expertconsult.com* *for the complete bibliography.*

586.2 Unprovoked Seizures

Mohamad A. Mikati

HISTORY AND EXAMINATION

Acute evaluation of a first seizure includes evaluation of vital signs and respiratory and cardiac function and institution of measures to normalize and stabilize them as needed. Signs of head trauma, abuse, drug intoxication, poisoning, meningitis, sepsis, focal abnormalities, increased intracranial pressure, herniation, neurocutaneous stigmata, brain stem dysfunction, and/or focal weakness should all be sought because they could suggest an underlying etiology for the seizure.

The **history** should also include details of the seizure manifestations, particularly those that occurred at its initial onset. These could give clues to the type and brain localization of the seizure. One should question whether there were other previous signs or symptoms that might signify the occurrence of seizures that the parents overlooked or did not report. In some instances, if the events have been going on for a time and there is a question about their nature (e.g., sleep myoclonus versus seizures), then the family can video record the patient and make the video available to the health care provider. Having the parents imitate the seizure can also be helpful. Seizure patterns (e.g., clustering), precipitating conditions (e.g., sleep or sleep deprivation, television, visual patterns, mental activity, stress), exacerbating conditions (e.g., menstrual cycle, medications), frequency, duration, time of occurrence, and other characteristics need to be carefully documented. Parents often overlook, do not report, or underreport absence, complex partial, or myoclonic seizures. A history of personality change or symptoms of increased intracranial pressure can suggest an intracranial tumor. Similarly, a history of cognitive regression can suggest a degenerative or metabolic disease. Certain medications such as stimulants or antihistamines can precipitate seizures. A history of prenatal or perinatal distress or of developmental delay can suggest etiologic congenital or perinatal brain dysfunction. Details of the spells can suggest nonepileptic paroxysmal disorders that mimic seizures (Chapter 587).

DIFFERENTIAL DIAGNOSIS

The various types of seizures, as classified by the International League Against Epilepsy (ILAE), are enumerated in Table 586-1. Some seizures might begin with an aura. **Auras** are sensory experiences reported by the patient and not observed externally. These can take the form of visual (e.g., flashing lights or seeing colors or complex visual hallucinations), somatosensory (tingling), olfactory, auditory, vestibular, or experiential (e.g., déjà vu, déjà vécu feelings) sensations, depending upon the precise localization of the origin of the seizures.

Motor seizures can be **tonic** (sustained contraction), **clonic** (rhythmic contractions), **myoclonic** (rapid shocklike contractions, usually <50 msec in duration, that may be isolated or may repeat but usually are not rhythmic), **atonic**, or **astatic**. **Astatic** seizures often follow myoclonic seizures and cause a very momentary loss of tone with a sudden fall. **Atonic** seizures, on the other hand, are usually longer and the loss of tone often develops more slowly. Sometimes it is difficult to distinguish among tonic, myoclonic, atonic, or astatic seizures based on the history alone when the family reports only that the patient "falls"; in such cases, the seizure may be described as a **drop attack.** A mechanistically similar seizure can involve the tone of only the head and neck; this seizure morphology is referred to as a **head drop**. Tonic, clonic, myoclonic, and atonic seizures can be focal (including one limb or one side only), focal with secondary generalization, or primary generalized. **Spasms** (axial spasms) consist of flexion or extension of truncal and extremity musculature that is sustained for 1-2 sec, shorter than what is seen in tonic seizures, which last >2 sec. Focal motor seizures are usually clonic and/or myoclonic. These seizures sometimes persist for days, months, or even longer. This phenomenon is termed **epilepsia partialis continua.**

Absence seizures are generalized seizures consisting of staring, unresponsiveness, and eye flutter lasting usually for few seconds. **Typical absences** are associated with 3 Hz spike–and–slow wave discharges and with petit mal epilepsy, which has a good prognosis. **Atypical absences** are associated with 1-2 Hz spike–and–slow wave discharges, with head atony and myoclonus during the seizures and with Lennox-Gastaut syndrome, which has a poor prognosis. Seizure type together with the other nonseizure clinical manifestations helps determine the type of **epilepsy syndrome** with which a particular patient is afflicted (Table 586-7; Chapters 586.3 and 586.4).

Family history of epilepsy can suggest a specific one of the known familial epilepsy syndromes. More often, different members of a family with a positive history of epilepsy have different types of seizures and of epilepsy. Head circumference can indicate the presence of microcephaly or of macrocephaly. Eye exam could show papilledema, retinal hemorrhages, chororetinitis, colobomata (associated with brain malformations), a cherry red spot, optic atrophy, macular changes (associated with genetic neurodegenerative and storage diseases) or phakomas (associated with tuberous sclerosis). Skin exam could show a trigeminal V-1 distribution capillary hemangioma (associated with Sturge-Weber syndrome), hypopigmented lesions (sometimes associated with tuberous sclerosis and detected more reliably by viewing the skin under UV light), or other neurocutaneous manifestations such as Shagreen patches and adenoma sebaceum (associated with tuberous sclerosis), or whorl-like hypopigmented areas (hypomelanosis of Ito, associated with hemimegalencephaly). Subtle asymmetries on the exam such as drift of one of the extended arms, posturing of an arm on stress gait, slowness in rapid alternating movements, small hand or thumb and thumb nail on one side, or difficulty in hopping on one leg relative to the other can signify a subtle hemiparesis associated with a lesion on the contralateral side of the brain.

Guidelines on the evaluation and treatment of a **first unprovoked nonfebrile** seizure include a careful history and physical examination and brain imaging by head CT or MRI. Emergency head CT in the child presenting with a first unprovoked nonfebrile seizure is often useful for acute management of the patient. Laboratory studies are recommended in specific clinical situations: Spinal tap is considered in patients with suspected meningitis or encephalitis, in children without brain swelling or papilledema, and in children in whom a history of intracranial bleeding is suspected without evidence of such on head CT. In the second of these, examination of the CSF for xanthochromia is essential. CSF tests can also confirm with the appropriate clinical setup the diagnosis of glucose transporter deficiency, cerebral folate deficiency, pyridoxine dependency, pyridoxal dependency, mitochondrial disorders, nonketotic hyperglycemia, and neurotransmitter deficiencies. Electrocardiography (ECG) to rule out long QT or other cardiac dysrhythmias and other tests directed at disorders that could mimic seizures may be needed (Chapter 587).

Patients with **recurrent seizures** with 2 seizures spaced apart by >24 hr warrant further work-up directed at the underlying etiology. Often, particularly in infants, a full metabolic work-up including amino acids, organic acids, biotinidase, and CSF studies is needed. In infants who do not respond immediately to antiepileptic therapy, vitamin B_6 (100 mg intravenously) is given as a

Table 586-7 SELECTED EPILEPSY SYNDROMES BY AGE OF ONSET

NEONATAL PERIOD
Benign familial neonatal seizures (BFNS) Early myoclonic encephalopathy (EME) Ohtahara syndrome
INFANCY
Migrating partial seizures of infancy West syndrome Myoclonic epilepsy in infancy (MEI) Benign infantile seizures Dravet syndrome Myoclonic encephalopathy in nonprogressive disorders
CHILDHOOD
Early-onset benign childhood occipital epilepsy (Panayiotopoulos type) Epilepsy with myoclonic astatic seizures Benign childhood epilepsy with centrotemporal spikes (BCECTS) Late-onset childhood occipital epilepsy (Gastaut type) Epilepsy with myoclonic absences Lennox-Gastaut syndrome Epileptic encephalopathy with continuous spike-and-wave during sleep (CSWS), including Landau-Kleffner syndrome Childhood absence epilepsy (CAE)
ADOLESCENCE
Juvenile absence epilepsy (JAE) Juvenile myoclonic epilepsy (JME) Epilepsy with generalized tonic-clonic seizures only Progressive myoclonus epilepsies (PME)
AGE-RELATED (AGE OF ONSET LESS SPECIFIC)
Autosomal dominant nocturnal frontal lobe epilepsy (ADNFLE) Familial temporal lobe epilepsies Autosomal dominant partial epilepsy with auditory features Generalized epilepsies with febrile seizures plus (GEFS+) Familial focal epilepsy with variable foci Reflex epilepsies Idiopathic photosensitive occipital lobe epilepsy Visual sensitive epilepsies Primary reading epilepsy Startle epilepsy
SEIZURE DISORDERS THAT ARE NOT TRADITIONALLY GIVEN THE DIAGNOSIS OF EPILEPSY
Benign neonatal seizures (BNS) Febrile seizures (FS)
EPILEPTIC ENCEPHALOPATHIES
Early myoclonic encephalopathy (EME) Ohtahara syndrome Migrating partial seizures of infancy West syndrome Dravet syndrome Myoclonic encephalopathy in nonprogressive disorders Epilepsy with myoclonic astatic seizures Lennox-Gastaut syndrome Epileptic encephalopathy with continuous spike-and-wave during sleep (CSWS) including Landau-Kleffner syndrome
OTHER SECONDARY GENERALIZED EPILEPSIES
Generalized epilepsy secondary to neurodegenerative disease Progressive myoclonus epilepsies

Lists from International League Against Epilepsy: *Table 1: genetic and developmental epilepsy syndromes by age of onset* (website). http://www.ilae.org/Visitors/Centre/ctf/CTFtable1.cfm. Accessed October 26, 2010; and International League Against Epilepsy: *Table 2. epileptic encephalopathies and other forms of secondary generalized epilepsies* (website). http://www.ilae.org/Visitors/Centre/ctf/CTFtable2.cfm. Accessed October 26, 2010.

therapeutic trial to rule out pyridoxine-responsive seizures, with precautions to guard against possible apnea. The trial is best done with continuous EEG monitoring, including a preadministration baseline recording period. Prior to the B_6 trial, a pipecolic acid level can be drawn, because it is often elevated in this rare syndrome. Pyridoxal phosphate given orally up to 50 mg/kg and folinic acid (up to 3 mg/kg) over several weeks can change pyridoxal dependency and cerebral folate deficiency.

Table 586-8 PROPOSED DIAGNOSTIC SCHEME FOR PEOPLE WITH EPILEPTIC SEIZURES AND WITH EPILEPSY

Epileptic seizures and epilepsy syndromes are to be described and categorized according to a system that uses standardized terminology and that is sufficiently flexible to take into account the following practical and dynamic aspects of epilepsy diagnosis:

1. Some patients cannot be given a recognized syndromic diagnosis.
2. Seizure types and syndromes change as new information is obtained.
3. Complete and detailed descriptions of ictal phenomenology are not always necessary.
4. Multiple classification schemes can, and should, be designed for specific purposes (e.g., communication and teaching; therapeutic trials; epidemiologic investigations; selection of surgical candidates; basic research; genetic characterizations).

This diagnostic scheme is divided into five parts, or axes, organized to facilitate a logical clinical approach to the development of hypotheses necessary to determine the diagnostic studies and therapeutic strategies to be undertaken in individual patients:

Axis 1: Ictal phenomenology, from the Glossary of Descriptive Ictal Terminology, can be used to describe ictal events with any degree of detail needed.

Axis 2: Seizure type, from the List of Epileptic Seizures. Localization within the brain and precipitating stimuli for reflex seizures should be specified when appropriate.

Axis 3: Syndrome, from the List of Epilepsy Syndromes, with the understanding that a syndromic diagnosis may not always be possible.

Axis 4: Etiology, from a Classification of Diseases Frequently Associated with Epileptic Seizures or Epilepsy Syndromes when possible, genetic defects, or specific pathologic substrates for symptomatic focal epilepsies.

Axis 5: Impairment, this is an optional, but often useful, additional diagnostic parameter that can be derived from an impairment classification adapted from the WHO ICIDH-2.

From International League Against Epilepsy: *Table 2: proposed diagnostic scheme for people with epileptic seizures and with epilepsy* (website). http://www.ilae-epilepsy.org/Visitors/Centre/ctf/table2.cfm. Accessed October 26, 2010.

APPROACH TO THE PATIENT AND ADDITIONAL TESTING

The approach to the patient with epilepsy is based on the diagnostic scheme proposed by the ILAE Task Force on Classification and Terminology, presented in Table 586-8. This emphasizes the total approach to the patient, including identification, if possible, of the underlying etiology of the epilepsy and the impairments that result from it. The impairments are very often just as important as, if not more important than, the seizures themselves. There are now many epilepsy syndromes that have been associated with specific gene mutations (see Table 586-2). Different mutations of the same gene can result in different epilepsy syndromes, and mutations of different genes can cause the same epilepsy syndrome phenotype. The clinical use of gene testing in the diagnosis and management of childhood epilepsy has been limited to patients manifesting specific underlying malformational, metabolic, or degenerative disorders, patients with severe named epilepsy syndromes (such as West and Dravet syndromes and progressive myoclonic epilepsies), and, rarely, patients with familial syndromes (see Table 586-2).

Additional testing in infants and children with recurrent seizures, depending on the clinical findings, can include measurement of serum lactate, pyruvate, acyl carnitine profile, creatine, very long chain fatty acids, and guanidino-acetic acid. Blood and serum are tested for white blood cell lysosomal enzymes, serum coenzyme Q levels, and serum copper and ceruloplasmin levels (for Menkes syndrome). Serum isoelectric focusing is performed for carbohydrate deficient transferrin.

CSF glucose testing looks for glucose transporter deficiency, and CSF can be examined for cells and proteins (for parainfectious and postinfectious syndromes, and for Aicardi Goutieres syndrome which also shows cerebral calcifications). Other laboratory studies include immunoglobulin G (IgG) index, NMDA (*N*-methyl-D-aspartate) receptor antibodies, and measles titers.

Urine is tested for urinary sulfite indicating molybdenum cofactor deficiency and for oligosaccharides and mucopolysaccharides.

MR spectroscopy is performed for lactate and creatine peaks.

Gene testing looks for specific disorders that can manifest with seizures, including *SCN1A* mutations in Dravet syndrome; *ARX* gene for infantile spasms in boys; *MECP2, CDKL5,* and protocadeherin 19 for Rett syndrome and similar presentations; syntaxin binding protein for Ohtahara syndrome; and polymerase G for infantile spasms and other seizures in infants. Gene testing can also be performed for other dysmorphic or metabolic syndromes.

Other tests include neurotransmitter metabolites for neurotransmitter disorders including pyridoxal-responsive seizures, cerebral folate deficiency, adenylsuccinate lyase deficiency, and specific neurotransmitter disorders. Muscle biopsy can be performed for mitochondrial enzymes, and skin biopsy for inclusion bodies seen in neuronal ceroid lipofuschinosis and Lafora body disease is sometimes needed.

Most patients do not require a work-up anywhere near this extensive. The pace and extent of the work-up must depend critically upon the clinical nonepileptic features that accompany the seizures, the family and antecedent personal history of the patient, the medication responsiveness of the seizures, the likelihood of identifying a treatable or palliable condition, and the wishes of the family to assign a specific diagnosis to the child's illness.

BIBLIOGRAPHY

Please visit the Nelson Textbook of Pediatrics *website at* *www.expertconsult.com* *for the complete bibliography.*

586.3 Partial Seizures and Related Epilepsy Syndromes

Mohamad A. Mikati

Partial seizures account for approximately 40% of seizures in children and can be divided into **simple partial** seizures, in which consciousness is not impaired and **complex partial** seizures, in which consciousness is affected. Simple and complex partial seizures can each occur in isolation, one can temporally lead to the other (usually simple to complex), or each can progress into **secondary generalized seizures** (tonic, clonic, atonic, or most often tonic-clonic).

SIMPLE PARTIAL SEIZURES

These can take the form of sensory seizures (auras) or brief motor seizures, the specific nature of which gives clues as to the location of the seizure focus, as described earlier. Brief motor seizures are the most common and include (focal tonic, clonic or atonic seizures. Often there is a motor (Jacksonian) march from face to arm to leg, adversive head and eye movements to the contralateral side, or postictal (Todd's) paralysis that can last minutes or hours, and sometimes longer. Unlike tics, motor seizures are not under partial voluntary control; seizures are more often stereotyped and less likely than tics to manifest different types in a given patient.

COMPLEX PARTIAL SEIZURES

Complex partial seizures usually last 1-2 min and are often preceded by an **aura**, such as a rising abdominal feeling, déjà vu or déjà vécu, a sense of fear, complex visual hallucinations, micropsia or macropsia (temporal lobe), generalized difficult-to-characterize sensations (frontal lobe), focal sensations (parietal lobe), or simple visual experiences (occipital lobe). Children <7 yr old are less likely than older children to report auras, but parents might observe unusual preictal behaviors that suggest the experiencing of auras. Subsequent manifestations consist of decreased responsiveness, staring, looking around seemingly purposelessly, and automatisms. **Automatisms** are automatic semipurposeful movements of the mouth (oral, alimentary such as chewing) or of the extremities (manual, such as manipulating the sheets; leg automatisms such as shuffling, walking). Often there is salivation, dilation of the pupils, and flushing or color change. The patient might appear to react to some of the stimulation around him or her but does not later recall the epileptic event. At times, walking and/or marked limb flailing and agitation occur, particularly in patients with frontal lobe seizures. Frontal lobe seizures often occur at night and can be very numerous and brief, but other complex partial seizures from other areas in the brain can also occur at night. There is often contralateral dystonic posturing of the arm and, in some cases, unilateral or bilateral tonic arm stiffening. Some seizures have these manifestations with minimal or no automatisms. Others consist of altered consciousness with contralateral motor, usually clonic, manifestations. After the seizure, the patient can have postictal automatisms, sleepiness, and/or other transient focal deficits such as weakness or aphasia.

SECONDARY GENERALIZED SEIZURES

Secondary generalized seizures can start with generalized clinical phenomena (due to rapid spread of the discharge from the initial focus), or as simple or complex partial seizures with subsequent clinical generalization. There is often adversive eye and head deviation to the contralateral side followed by generalized tonic, clonic, or tonic-clonic activity. Tongue biting, urinary and stool incontinence, vomiting with risk of aspiration, and cyanosis are common. Fractures of the vertebrae or humerus are rare complications. Most such seizures last 1-2 min. Tonic focal or secondary generalized seizures often manifest adversive head deviation to the contralateral side, or fencing, hemi- or full figure-of-four arm, or Statue of Liberty postures. These postures often suggest frontal origin, particularly when consciousness is preserved during them, indicating that the seizure originated from the medial frontal supplementary motor area.

EEG in patients with partial seizures usually shows focal spikes or sharp waves in the lobe where the seizure originates. A sleep-deprived EEG with recording during sleep increases the diagnostic yield and is advisable in all patients whenever possible (Fig. 586-2). Despite that, about 15% of children with epilepsy initially have normal EEGs because the discharges are relatively infrequent or the focus is deep. If repeating the test does not detect paroxysmal findings, then 24-hour video EEG monitoring may be helpful and can allow visualization of the clinical events and the corresponding EEG tracing.

Brain imaging is critical in patients with focal seizures. In general, MRI is preferable to CT and can show pathologies such as changes due to previous strokes or hypoxic injury, malformations, medial temporal sclerosis, arteriovenous malformations, or tumors (Fig. 586-3).

BENIGN EPILEPSY SYNDROMES WITH PARTIAL SEIZURES

The most common such syndrome is **benign childhood epilepsy with centrotemporal spikes** (**BECTS**) which typically starts during childhood and is outgrown in adolescence. The child typically wakes up at night owing to a simple partial seizure causing buccal and throat tingling and tonic or clonic contractions of one side of the face, with drooling and inability to speak but with preserved consciousness and comprehension. Complex partial and secondary generalized seizures can also occur. EEG shows typical broad-based centrotemporal spikes that are markedly increased in frequency during drowsiness and sleep. MRI is normal. Patients respond very well to AEDs such as carbamazepine. In some patients who only have rare and mild seizures treatment might not be needed.

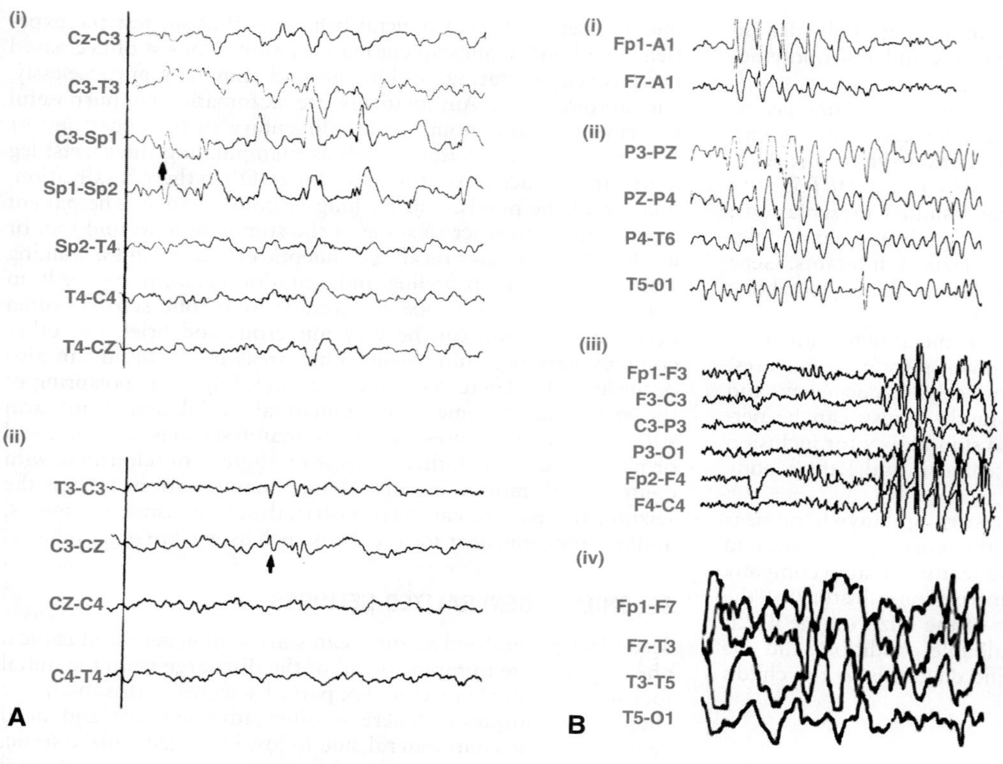

Figure 586-2 *A,* An EEG of partial seizures: (i) spike discharges from the left temporal lobe *(arrow)* in a patient with complex partial seizures; (ii) left parietal central spikes *(arrow)* characteristic of benign partial epilepsy with centrotemporal spikes. *B,* Representative EEGs of generalized seizures: (i) 3/sec spike-and-wave discharge of absence seizures with normal background activity; (ii) complex myoclonic epilepsy (Lennox-Gastaut syndrome) with interictal slow spike waves; (iii) juvenile myoclonic epilepsy showing 4-6/sec spike and waves enhanced by photic stimulation; (iv) hypsarrhythmia with an irregular high-voltage spike and wave activity.

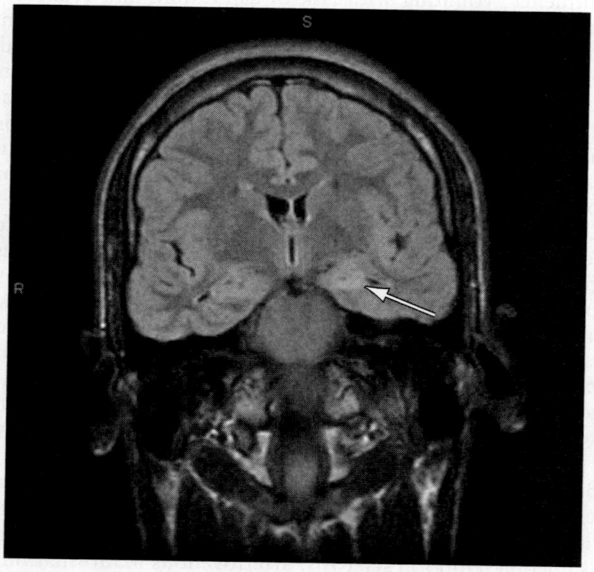

Figure 586-3 Coronal fluid-attenuated inversion-recovery (FLAIR) MRI scan of a 13 yr old with intractable seizures and mesial temporal sclerosis (MTS). The *arrow* points at the hippocampus with the high-intensity signal characteristic of MTS. (From Lee JYK, Adelson PD: Neurosurgical management of pediatric epilepsy, *Pediatr Clin North Am* 51:441–456, 2004.)

Benign epilepsy with occipital spikes can occur in early childhood (Panayiotopoulos type) and manifests with complex partial seizures with ictal vomiting or they appear in later childhood (Gastaut type) with complex partial seizures, visual auras, and migraine headaches. Both are typically outgrown in a few years.

In infants, several less-common **benign infantile familial convulsion syndromes** have been reported. For some of these, the corresponding gene mutation and its function are known (see Tables 586-2 and 586-4), but for others, the genetic underpinnings are yet to be determined. Specific syndromes include benign infantile familial convulsions with parieto-occipital foci linked to chromosomal loci 19q and 2q, benign familial infantile convulsions with associated choreoathetosis linked to chromosomal locus 16p12-q12, and benign infantile familial convulsions with hemiplegic migraine linked to chromosome 1. A number of **benign infantile nonfamilial syndromes** have been reported, including complex partial seizures with temporal foci, secondary generalized tonic-clonic seizures with variable foci, tonic seizures with midline foci, and partial seizures in association with mild gastroenteritis. All of these have a good prognosis and respond to treatment promptly, often necessitating only short-term (e.g., 6 mo), if any, therapy. **Nocturnal autosomal dominant frontal lobe epilepsy** has been linked to acetylcholine-receptor gene mutations and manifests with nocturnal seizures with dystonic posturing that respond promptly to carbamazepine. Several other less-frequent familial benign epilepsy syndromes with different localizations have also been described, some of which occur exclusively or predominantly in adults (see Table 586-2).

SEVERE EPILEPSY SYNDROMES WITH PARTIAL SEIZURES

Symptomatic epilepsy secondary to focal brain lesions has a higher chance of being severe and refractory to therapy than idiopathic epilepsy. In infants this is often due to severe metabolic problems, hypoxic-ischemic injury, or congenital malformations. In addition, in this age group, a syndrome of multifocal severe partial seizures with progressive mental regression and cerebral atrophy called **migrating partial epilepsy** of infancy has been described. In infants and older children, several types of lesions, which can occur in any lobe, can cause intractable epilepsy and seizures. These include focal cortical dysplasia, hemimegalencephaly, Sturge-Weber hemangioma, tuberous sclerosis, and congenital tumors such as ganglioglioma, and dysembroyplastic neuroepithelial tumors (DNET), as well as others. The intractable seizures can be simple partial, complex partial, secondary generalized, or combinations thereof. If secondary generalized seizures predominate and take the form of absence-like seizures and drop attacks, the clinical picture can mimic the generalized epilepsy syndrome of Lennox-Gastaut syndrome and has been termed by some **pseudo Lennox-Gastaut syndrome.**

Temporal lobe epilepsy can be caused by any temporal lobe lesion. A common cause is **mesial (also termed medial) temporal sclerosis,** a condition often preceded by febrile seizures and, rarely, genetic in origin. Pathologically, these patients have atrophy and gliosis of the hippocampus and, in some, of the amygdala. It is the most common cause of surgically remediable partial epilepsy in adolescents and adults. Occasionally, in patients with other symptomatic or cryptogenic partial or generalized epilepsies, the focal discharges are so continuous that they cause an epileptic encephalopathy. Activation of temporal discharges in sleep can lead to loss of speech and verbal auditory agnosia (**Landau-Kleffner epileptic aphasia syndrome**). Activation of frontal and secondary generalized discharges in sleep leads to more global delay secondary to the **syndrome of continuous spike waves in slow-wave sleep** (>85% of slow-wave sleep recording dominated by discharges).

The syndrome of **Rasmussen's encephalitis** is a form of chronic encephalitis that manifests with unilateral intractable partial seizures, epilepsia partialis continua, and progressive hemiparesis of the affected side, with progressive atrophy of the contralateral hemisphere. The etiology is usually unknown. Some cases have been attributed to cytomegalovirus and others to anti-NMDA receptor autoantibodies.

586.4 Generalized Seizures and Related Epilepsy Syndromes

Mohamad A. Mikati

ABSENCE SEIZURES

Typical absence seizures usually start at 5-8 yr of age and are often, owing to their brevity, overlooked by parents for many months even though they can occur up to hundreds of times per day. Unlike complex partial seizures they do not have an aura, usually last for only a few seconds, and are accompanied by flutter or upward rolling of the eyes but typically not by automatisms of the complex partial seizure type (absence seizures can have simple automatisms like lip-smacking or picking at clothing and the head can minimally fall forward). Absence seizures do not have a postictal period and are characterized by immediate resumption of what the patient was doing before the seizure. Hyperventilation for 3-5 min can precipitate the seizures and the accompanying 3 Hz spike–and–slow wave discharges. The presence of periorbital, lid, perioral or limb myoclonic jerks with the typical absence usually predicts difficulty in controlling the seizures with medication.

Atypical absence seizures have associated myoclonic components and tone changes of the head and body and are also usually more difficult to treat. They are precipitated by drowsiness and are usually accompanied by 1-2 Hz spike–and–slow wave discharges.

Juvenile absence seizures are similar to typical absences but occur at a later age and are accompanied by 4-6 Hz spike–and–slow wave and polyspike–and–slow wave discharges. These are usually associated with juvenile myoclonic epilepsy (see later).

GENERALIZED MOTOR SEIZURE

The most common generalized motor seizures are generalized tonic-clonic seizures that can be either primarily generalized (bilateral) or secondarily generalized (as described in Chapter 586.3) from a unilateral focus. If there is no partial component then the seizure usually starts with loss of consciousness and at times with a sudden cry, upward rolling of the eyes, and a generalized tonic contraction with falling, apnea, and cyanosis. In some, a clonic or myoclonic component precedes the tonic stiffening. The tonic phase is followed by a clonic phase that, as the seizure progresses, shows slowing of the rhythmic contractions until the seizure stops usually 1-2 min later. Incontinence and a postictal period often follow. The latter usually lasts for 30 min to several hours with semicoma or obtundation and postictal sleepiness, ataxia, hyper- or hyporeflexia, and headaches. There is a risk of aspiration and injury. First aid measures include positioning the patient on his or her side, clearing the mouth if it is open, loosening tight clothes or jewelry, and gently extending the head and, if possible, insertion of an airway by a trained professional. The mouth should not be forced open with a foreign object (this could dislodge teeth, causing aspiration) or with a finger in the mouth (this could result in serious injury to the examiner's finger). Many patients have single **idiopathic generalized tonic-clonic seizures** that may be associated with intercurrent illness or with a cause that cannot be ascertained (Chapter 586.2). Generalized tonic, atonic, and astatic seizures often occur in severe pediatric epilepsies. Generalized myoclonic seizures can occur in either benign or difficult-to-control epilepsies.

BENIGN GENERALIZED EPILEPSIES

Petit mal epilepsy typically starts in mid-childhood, and most patients outgrow it before adulthood. Approximately 25% of patients also develop generalized tonic-clonic seizures, half before and half after the onset of absences. **Benign myoclonic epilepsy of infancy** consists of the onset of myoclonic and other seizures during the 1st yr of life, with generalized 3 Hz spike–and–slow wave discharges. Often it is initially difficult to distinguish this type from more-severe syndromes, but follow-up clarifies the diagnosis. **Febrile seizures plus syndrome** manifests febrile seizures and multiple types of generalized seizures in multiple family members, and at times different individuals within the same family manifest different generalized and febrile seizure types (Chapter 586.1).

Juvenile myoclonic epilepsy (Janz syndrome) is the most common generalized epilepsy in young adults, accounting for 5% of all epilepsies. It has been linked to mutations in many genes including *CACNB4; CLNC2; EJM2, 3,* and *4; GABRA1; GABRD;* and *Myoclonin1/EFHC1* (see Table 586-2). Typically, it starts in early adolescence with one or more of the following manifestations: myoclonic jerks in the morning, often causing the patient to drop things; generalized tonic clonic or clonic-tonic-clonic seizures upon awakening; and juvenile absences. Sleep deprivation, alcohol (in older patients), and photic stimulation or, rarely, certain cognitive activities can act as precipitants. The EEG usually shows generalized 4-5 Hz polyspike–and–slow wave discharges. There are other forms of generalized epilepsies such as **photoparoxysmal epilepsy,** in which occipital, generalized tonic clonic, absence or myoclonic generalized seizures are precipitated by photic stimuli such as flipping through TV channels and viewing video games. Other forms of reflex (i.e., stimulus-provoked) epilepsy can occur; associated seizures are usually generalized, although some may be focal (see Table 586-1).

SEVERE GENERALIZED EPILEPSIES

Severe generalized epilepsies are associated with intractable seizures and developmental delay. **Early myoclonic infantile encephalopathy (EMIE)** starts during the first 2 mo of life with severe myoclonic seizures and burst suppression pattern on EEG. It is usually caused by inborn errors of metabolism. **Early epileptic infantile encephalopathy (EEIE, Ohtahara syndrome)** has similar age of onset and EEG but manifests tonic seizures and is usually caused by brain malformations or syntaxin binding protein 1 mutations. Severe myoclonic epilepsy of infancy (Dravet syndrome) starts as focal febrile status epilepticus and later manifests myoclonic and other seizure types (Chapter 586.1).

West syndrome starts between the ages of 2 and 12 mo and consists of a triad of infantile spasms that usually occur in clusters (particularly in drowsiness or upon arousal), developmental regression, and a typical EEG picture called **hypsarrhythmia** (see Fig. 586-2); hypsarrhythmia is a high-voltage, slow, chaotic background with multifocal spikes. Patients with cryptogenic (sometimes called idiopathic) disease have normal development before onset, and symptomatic patients have preceding developmental delay owing to perinatal encephalopathies, malformations, underlying metabolic disorders, or other etiologies (Chapter 586.2). In boys, West syndrome can also be caused by *ARX* gene mutations (often associated with ambiguous genitalia). Recognizing West syndrome, especially in cryptogenic cases, is a medical emergency because diagnosis delayed for 3 wk or longer can affect long-term prognosis. The spasms are often overlooked by parents and by physicians, being mistaken for startles due to colic or for other benign paroxysmal syndromes (Chapter 587).

Many patients start with Ohtahara syndrome, develop West syndrome, and then progress to **Lennox-Gastaut syndrome**. Lennox-Gastaut syndrome typically starts between the age of 2 and 10 yr and consists of a triad of developmental delay, multiple seizure types that as a rule include atypical absences, and myoclonic, astatic, and tonic seizures. The tonic seizures occur either in wakefulness (causing falls and injuries) or also, typically, in sleep. The third component is the EEG findings (see Fig. 586-2): 1-2 Hz spike–and-slow waves, polyspike bursts in sleep, and a slow background in wakefulness. Patients commonly have myoclonic, atonic, and other seizure types, and most are left with long-term mental retardation and intractable seizures despite multiple therapies. **Myoclonic astatic epilepsy** is a syndrome similar to but milder than Lennox-Gastaut syndrome that usually does not have tonic seizures or polyspike bursts in sleep. The prognosis is more favorable than that for Lennox Gastaut syndrome.

Progressive myoclonic epilepsies are a group of epilepsies characterized by progressive dementia and worsening myoclonic and other seizures. **Type I or Unvericht Lundborg disease** (secondary to a cystatin B mutation) is more slowly progressive than the other types and usually starts in adolescence. **Type II or Lafora body disease** can have an early childhood onset but usually starts in adolescence, is more quickly progressive, and is usually fatal within the second or third decade. It can be associated with photosensitivity, manifests periodic acid–Schiff (PAS)-positive Lafora inclusions on muscle or skin biopsy (in eccrine sweat gland cells), and has been shown to be due to laforin *(EPM2A)* or malin *(EPM2B)* gene mutations. Other causes of progressive myoclonic epilepsy include myoclonic epilepsy with ragged red fibers (MERRF), sialidosis type I, neuronal ceroid lipofuschinosis, juvenile neuropathic Gaucher disease, dentatorubral-pallidoluysian atrophy, and juvenile neuroaxonal dystrophy.

Myoclonic encephalopathy in nonprogressive disorders is an epileptic encephalopathy that occurs in some congenital disorders affecting the brain, such as Anglemann syndrome, and consists of almost continuous and difficult-to-treat myoclonic and, at times, other seizures.

Landau-Kleffner syndrome is a rare condition of unknown cause. It is more common in boys and has a mean onset of 5½ yr. It is often confused with autism, in that both conditions are associated with a loss of language function. Landau-Kleffner syndrome is characterized by loss of language skills in a previously normal child. At least 70% have an associated seizure disorder. The **aphasia** may be primarily receptive or expressive, and auditory agnosia may be so severe that the child is oblivious to everyday sounds. Hearing is normal, but behavioral problems, including irritability and poor attention span, are particularly common.

The seizures are of several types, including focal or generalized tonic-clonic, atypical absence, partial complex, and, occasionally, myoclonic. High-amplitude spike and wave discharges predominate and tend to be bitemporal. In the evolutionary stages of the condition, the EEG findings may be normal. The spike discharges are always more apparent during non–rapid eye movement (NREM) sleep; thus, a child in whom Landau-Kleffner syndrome is suspected should have an EEG during sleep, particularly if the awake record is normal. If the sleep EEG is normal but Landau-Kleffner syndrome continues to be suspected, the child should be referred to a tertiary pediatric epilepsy center for prolonged EEG recordings. CT and MRI studies typically yield normal results, and positron emission tomography (PET) scans have demonstrated either unilateral or bilateral hypometabolism or hypermetabolism. In the related but clinically distinct epilepsy syndrome with continuous spike waves in slow wave sleep, the discharges are more likely to be frontal or generalized and the delay is likely to be global. The approach and therapy to the two syndromes are similar.

Valproic acid is the anticonvulsant of choice; some children require a combination of valproic acid and clobazam. Levetiracetam is also helpful as is nocturnal diazepam therapy (0.2-0.5 mg/kg PO at bedtime for several months). If the seizures and aphasia persist, a trial of steroids should be considered; oral prednisone is started at 2 mg/kg/24 hr for 1 mo and tapered to 1 mg/kg/24 hr for an additional month. With clinical improvement, the prednisone is reduced further to 0.5 mg/kg/24 hr for up to 6-12 mo. It is imperative to initiate speech therapy and maintain treatment for several years, because improvement in language function occurs over a prolonged period. Some centers advocate an operative procedure—subpial transection—when medical management fails. Methylphenidate should be considered for patients with severe hyperactivity and inattention. Seizures, if poorly controlled, may be potentiated by methylphenidate; anticonvulsants are usually protective. Intravenous immunoglobulin may be helpful in Landau-Kleffner syndrome.

Some children experience a recurrence of aphasia and seizures after apparent recovery. Most children with Landau-Kleffner syndrome have a significant abnormality of speech function in adulthood. The onset of Landau-Kleffner syndrome at an early age (<2 yr) uniformly tends to be associated with a poor prognosis for recovery of speech.

586.5 Mechanisms of Seizures

Mohamad A. Mikati

One can distinguish in the pathophysiology of epilepsy four distinct, often sequential, mechanistic processes. First is the **underlying etiology,** which is any process that can disrupt neuronal function and connectivity and that eventually leads to the process of making the brain epileptic (epileptogenesis). The underlying etiologies of epilepsy are diverse and include, among other things, brain tumors, strokes, scarring, or mutations of specific genes. These mutations can involve voltage-gated channels (Na^+, K^+, Ca^{2+}, Cl^- and HCN), ligand-gated channels (nicotinic acetylcholine and γ-aminobutyric acid A receptors [$GABA_A$]) or miscellaneous proteins. In some but not in all such mutations the molecular and cellular deficits caused by the mutations have been identified. For example, in Dravet syndrome, the loss of function mutation in the *SCN1A* gene causes decreased excitability in inhibitory GABAergic interneurons, leading to increased excitability and epilepsy. In human cortical dysplasia, the expression of the NR2B subunit of the NMDA receptor is increased, leading to excessive depolarizing current. In many other epileptic conditions, a clear etiology is still lacking and in others the etiology may be known, but it is still not known how the identified underlying genetic etiology or brain insult results in epilepsy.

Second, **epileptogenesis** is the mechanism during which the brain turns epileptic. **Kindling** is an animal model for human temporal lobe epilepsy in which repeated electrical stimulation of selected areas of the brain with a low-intensity current initially causes no apparent changes but with repeated stimulation results in epilepsy. This repetitive stimulation leads to epilepsy through activation of metabotropic and ionotropic glutamate receptors (by glutamate) as well as the tropomyosin-related kinase B (TrkB) receptor (by brain-derived neurotrophic factor [BDNF] and neurotrophin 4 [NT-4]). This leads to an increase in the intraneuronal calcium, which in turn activates calcium calmodulin-dependent protein kinase (CaMKII) and calcineurin, a phosphatase, resulting eventually in calcium-dependent epileptogenic gene expression (e.g., c-fos) and promoting mossy fiber sprouting. **Mossy fibers** are fibers that connect the granule cells to the CA3 region within the hippocampus and have been shown to underlie increased excitability in medial temporal lobe epilepsy resulting from mesial temporal sclerosis in humans and in animal models. The cell loss in the CA3 region associated with the sclerosis (presumably resulting from an original insult such as a prolonged febrile status epilepticus episode or hypoxia) leads to a pathologic attempt at compensation by sprouting of the excitatory mossy fibers. Mossy fiber sprouting leads to increased excitability and to epilepsy. Presumably other, possibly similar, epileptogenesis mechanisms underlie other epilepsies.

The third process is the resultant **epileptic state of increased excitability** that is present in all patients irrespective of the underlying etiology or mechanism of epileptogenesis. In a seizure focus, each neuron has a stereotypic synchronized response called **paroxysmal depolarization shift (PDS)** that consists of a sudden depolarization phase, resulting from glutamate and calcium channel activation, with a series of action potentials at its peak followed by an afterhyperpolarization phase, resulting from activation of potassium channels and GABA receptors. When the afterhyperpolarization is disrupted in a sufficient number of GABAergic interneurons, the inhibitory surround is lost and a population of neurons fires at the same rate and time, resulting in a seizure focus. In childhood absence epilepsy, the discharging neurons also develop a PDS similar to the one found in partial epilepsy. However, the mechanism of PDS generation is different because it involves thalamocortical connections bilaterally. T-type calcium channels on thalamic relay neurons are activated during hyperpolarization by GABAergic interneurons in the reticular thalamic nucleus, which results in the typical generalized spike-wave pattern. In tumor-related epilepsy, particularly in that related to oligodendroglioma, the voltage-gated sodium channels are present on the surface of tumor cells at a higher density than on normal cells, and their inactivation is impaired by the alkaline pH present in this condition. In hypothalamic hamartoma causing gelastic seizures, clusters of GABAergic interneurons spontaneously fire, thus synchronizing the output of the hypothalamic hamartoma neurons projecting to the hippocampus.

The fourth process is **seizure-related neuronal injury** as demonstrated by MRI in patients after prolonged febrile and afebrile status epilepticus. Many such patients show acute swelling in the hippocampus and long-term hippocampal atrophy with sclerosis on MRI. In experimental models, the mechanisms of such injuries have been shown to involve both apoptosis and necrosis of neurons in the involved regions. There is evidence from surgically resected epileptic tissue that apoptotic pathways are activated in foci of intractable epilepsy.

BIBLIOGRAPHY

Please visit the Nelson Textbook of Pediatrics *website at* *www.expertconsult.com* *for the complete bibliography.*

586.6 Treatment of Seizures and Epilepsy

Mohamad A. Mikati

DECIDING ON LONG-TERM THERAPY

After a first seizure, if the risk of recurrence is low and the patient has normal neurodevelopmental status, EEG, and MRI (risk about 20%), then treatment is usually not started. If the patient has abnormal EEG, MRI, development, and/or neurologic exam and/or a positive family history of epilepsy, then the risk is higher and often treatment is started. Other considerations are also important, such as motor vehicle driving status and type of employment in older patients or the parents' ability to deal with recurrences or AED drug therapy in children. The decision is therefore always individualized. All aspects of this decision-making process should be discussed with the family. An overview of the approach to the treatment of seizures and epilepsy is presented in Figure 586-4.

COUNSELING

An important part of the management of a patient with epilepsy is educating the family and the child about the disease, its management, and the limitations it might impose and how to deal with them. It is important to establish a successful therapeutic alliance. Some restrictions on driving (in adolescents) and on swimming are usually necessary (Table 586-9). In most states, the physician is not required to report the epileptic patient to the motor vehicle registry; this is the responsibility of the patient. Also in most states, a seizure-free period of 6 mo, and in some states longer, is required before driving is allowed. Often swimming in rivers, lakes, or sea, and underwater diving are prohibited but swimming in swimming pools may be allowable. When swimming, patients with epilepsy, even if the epilepsy is under excellent control, should be under the continuous supervision of an observer who is aware of their condition and capable of lifeguard-level rescue.

The American Academy of Pediatrics recommends that the physician, parents, and child jointly evaluate the risk of involvement in athletic activities. To participate in athletics, proper medical management, good seizure control, and proper supervision are crucial to avoid significant risks. Any activity where a seizure might cause a dangerous fall should be avoided; these activities include rope climbing, use of the parallel bars, and high diving. Participation in collision or contact sports depends on the patient's condition. Epileptic children should not automatically be banned from participating in hockey, baseball, basketball, football, or wrestling. Rather, individual consideration should be based on the child's specific case (see Table 586-9).

Counseling is helpful to support the family and to educate them about the resources available in the community. Educational and, in some cases, psychological evaluation may be necessary to evaluate for possible learning disabilities or abnormal behavioral patterns that might coexist with the epilepsy. Epilepsy does carry risk of increased mortality (2 or more times the standardized mortality rates of the general population) and of sudden unexpected death. This is mostly related to the conditions associated with or underlying the epilepsy (e.g., metabolic diseases), to poor seizure control (e.g., in patients with severe epileptic encephalopathies), and to poor compliance with prescribed therapies. Thus, family members can be usually be informed about this increased risk without inappropriately increasing their anxiety. Many family members feel they need to observe the patient continuously in wakefulness and sleep and have the patient sleep in the parent's rooms to detect seizures. This has never been shown to improve outcome and should generally be discouraged because it will affect the psychology of the child with no proven benefits. Education about what to do in case of seizures, the choices of treatment or no treatment and of medications and their side effects, and potential complications of epilepsy should be provided to the parents and, if he or she is old enough, to the child.

MECHANISMS OF ACTION OF ANTIEPILEPTIC DRUGS

Current AEDs reduce excitability by interfering with the sodium or calcium ion channels, by reducing glutamate induced

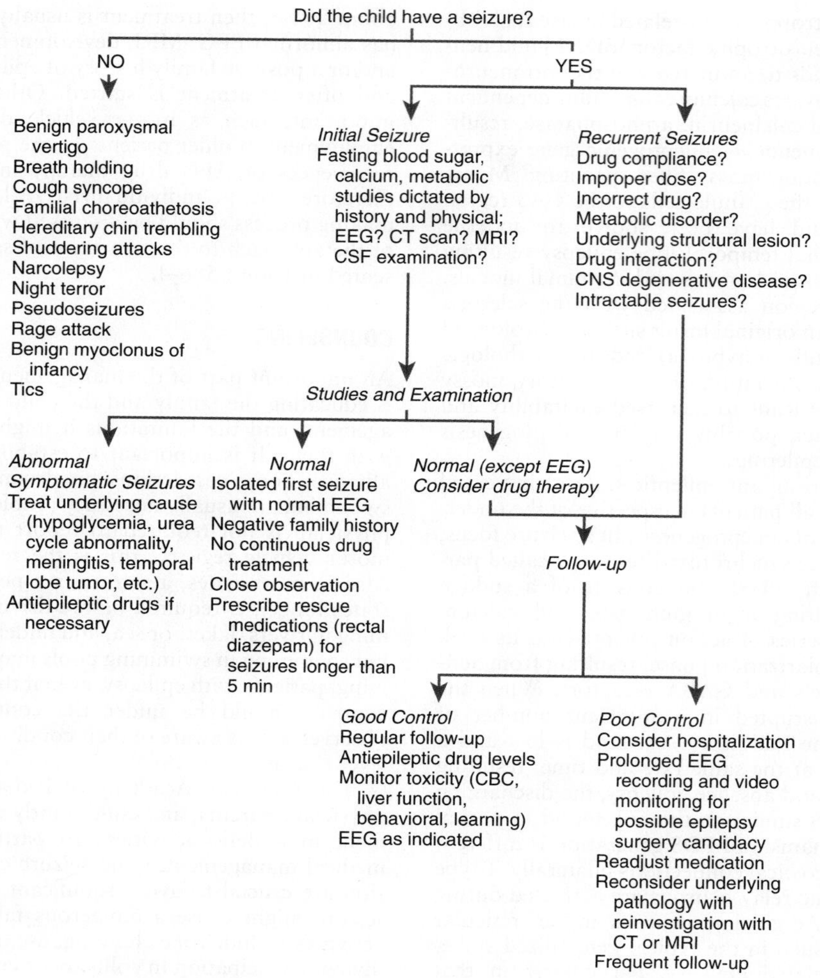

Figure 586-4 An approach to the child with a suspected convulsive disorder.

Table 586-9 SPORTS AND SPECIAL CONSIDERATIONS FOR THE CHILD WITH EPILEPSY*

SPORTS TYPE	SPECIAL CONSIDERATIONS
Body contact sports	If there are more than occasional seizures, physician evaluation of benefits and risks of participation should be made based on the child's condition
Noncontact sports	Anxiety and fatigue can cause a problem in some children Individualization based on clinical history must be the rule
Gymnastics	A fall can result if the child experiences a sudden seizure, especially with trampolines, parallel bars, and rope climbing, which therefore should be avoided Individual consideration remains the basic determinant
Swimming	The child should always be under supervision, and competitive underwater swimming should be discouraged

*Specific advice should be individualized depending on the patient's clinical condition. Many patients actually have fewer seizures when they are active than when they are idle.
Based on Committee on Children with Handicaps: The epileptic child and competitive school athletics, *Pediatrics* 42:700–702, 1968.

excitatory function, or by enhancing GABAergic inhibition. Most medications have multiple mechanisms of action, and the exact mechanism responsible for their activity in human epilepsy is usually not fully understood. Often, medications acting on sodium channels are effective against partial seizures, and medications acting on T-type calcium channels are effective against absence seizures. Voltage-gated sodium channels are blocked by felbamate, valproate, topiramate, carbamazepine, oxcarbazepine, lamotrigine, phenytoin, rufinamide, lacosamide, and zonisamide. T-type calcium channels, found in the thalamic area, are blocked by valproate, zonisamide, and ethosuximide. Voltage-gated calcium channels are inhibited by lamotrigine, felbamate, gabapentin and pregabalin. N-type calcium channels are inhibited by levetiracetam.

$GABA_A$ receptors are activated by phenobarbital, benzodiazepines, topiramate, felbamate, and levetiracetam. Tiagabine, by virtue of its binding to GABA transporters 1 (GAT-1) and 3 (GAT-3), is a GABA reuptake inhibitor. GABA levels are increased by vigabatrin via its irreversible inhibition of GABA transaminases, and valproate inhibits GABA transaminases, acts on $GABA_B$ presynaptic receptors (also done by gabapentin), and activates glutamic acid decarboxylase (the enzyme that forms GABA).

Glutaminergic transmission is decreased by felbamate that blocks NMDA and AMPA (α-amino-3-hydroxy-5-methyl-4-isoxazole-propionic acid)/kainate receptors. Topiramate also blocks AMPA/kainate receptors. Levetiracetam binds to the presynaptic vesicle protein SV2A found in all neurotransmitter vesicles and possibly results in inhibition of presynaptic neurotransmitter release in a use-dependent manner.

CHOICE OF DRUG ACCORDING TO SEIZURE TYPE AND EPILEPSY SYNDROME

Drug therapy should be based on the type of seizure and the epilepsy syndrome. In general, the **drugs of first choice** for focal

Table 586-10 COMPARISON OF RECOMMENDATIONS FOR THE TREATMENT OF PEDIATRIC EPILEPSY

SEIZURE TYPE OR EPILEPSY SYNDROME	FDA APPROVED	SIGN (2003)	NICE (2004)	AAN (2004)	ILAE (2006)*	PEDIATRIC EXPERT CONSENSUS SURVEY (NORTH AMERICA-2005)	PEDIATRIC EXPERT CONSENSUS SURVEY (EUROPE-2007)
Partial-onset	PB, PHT, CBZ, OXC, TPM, LTG, LEV	PHT, VPA, CBZ, LTG, TPM, OXC, VGB, CLB	CBZ, VPA LTG, OXC, TPM	OXC, CBZ, LTG (men)	A: OXC B: none C: CBZ, PB, PHT TPM,VPA	OXC, CBZ	OXC, CBZ
BCECT	None	Not specifically mentioned	CBZ, OXC, LTG, VPA	Not surveyed	A, B: none C: CBZ, VPA	OXC, CBZ	VPA
Childhood absence epilepsy	ESM, VPA	VPA, ESM, LTG	VPA, LTG	VPA, LTG	A,B: none C:ESM, LTG, VPA	ESM	VPA
Juvenile myoclonic epilepsy	TPM, LEV, LTG	VPA, LTG, TPM	VPA, LTG	VPA, LTG	A, B, C: none	VPA, LTG	VPA
Lennox-Gastaut syndrome	FLB, TPM, LTG	Not specifically mentioned	LTG, VPA, TPM	Not surveyed	Not reviewed	VPA, TPM	VPA
Infantile spasms	None	Not specifically mentioned	VGB, cortico-steroids	ACTH, VGB	Not reviewed	VGB, ACTH	VGB

*ILAE recommendations are listed according to levels of evidence supporting the efficacy of the options. Level A: ≥1 class I randomized controlled trial (RCT) or ≥2 class II RCTs; Level B: 1 class II RCT; Level C: ≥2 class III RCTs.
AAN: American Academy of Neurology; ACTH: adrenocorticotropic hormone; BCECT: benign childhood epilepsy with centrotemporal spikes; CBZ: carbamazepine; CLB: clobazam; ESM: ethosuximide; FDA: Food and Drug Administration; FLB: felbamate; ILAE: International League against Epilepsy; LEV, levetiracetam; LTG: lamotrigine; NICE: National Institute for Clinical Excellence; OXC: oxcarbazepine; PB: phenobarbital; PHT: phenytoin; SIGN: Scottish Intercollegiate Guidelines Network; TPM: topiramate; VGB: vigabatrin; VPA: valproic acid.
Adapted from Wheless JW, Clarke DF, Arzimanoglou A, et al: Treatment of pediatric epilepsy: European expert opinion, *Epileptic Disord* 9:353–412, 2007.

seizures and epilepsies are oxcarbazepine and carbamazepine; for absence seizures, ethosuximide; for juvenile myoclonic epilepsy, valproate and lamotrigine; for Lennox-Gastaut syndrome, valproate, topiramate, lamotrigine, and, most recently, as add on, rufinamide; and for infantile spasms, adrenocorticotropic hormone (ACTH). Lamotrigine has been shown to be effective for partial seizures, and valproate has been shown to be effective for generalized and unclassified epilepsies. There is significant controversy about these choices, and therapy should always be individualized (see the next section and Table 586-10).

West syndrome is best treated with adrenocorticotropic hormone (ACTH). There are several protocols that range in dose from high to intermediate to low. The increase in price of ACTH gel in the USA has led many physicians to use the lowest dose even though a better response usually occurs with the higher doses. The initial ACTH dose in one high-dose protocol is 150 IU/m^2/day of ACTH gel intramuscularly in 2 divided doses for 1 wk. During the 2nd wk, the dose is 75 IU/m^2/day in 1 daily dose for 1 wk. For the 3rd wk, the dose is 75 IU/m^2 every other day for 1 wk. ACTH is gradually tapered over the next 9 wk. The lot number of the ACTH gel is recorded. Response is usually observed within the first 7 days; however, if no response is observed within 2 wk, the lot is changed. During the tapering period, and especially in symptomatic patients, relapse can occur. Remediation entails increasing the dose to the previously effective dose for 2 wk and then beginning the taper again. If seizures persist after this, the dose is increased to 150 IU/m^2/day and the protocol is initiated again. Synthetic ACTH has also been used: Synacthen Depot intramuscular 0.25 mg/mL or 1 mg/mL is used; 1 mg is considered to have the potency of 100 IU in stimulating the adrenal. Other protocols include the use of 110 IU/m^2 per day for 3 wk with a subsequent taper over 6 wk. A third protocol is to use 20 IU/day (low dose) and to taper and discontinue therapy immediately after achieving a response.

Awake and asleep EEG is often done 1, 2, and 4 wk after the initiation of ACTH to monitor the patient's response. Side effects, more common with the higher doses, include hypertension, electrolyte imbalance, infections, hyperglycemia and/or glycosuria, and gastric ulcers. All should be carefully monitored for. ACTH is generally thought to offer an added advantage over prednisone or other steroids alone. There is often amelioration of the seizures and of the EEG findings. The majority of patients have a poor prognosis despite ACTH. Cryptogenic cases have a better chance for a response.

In August 2009, vigabatrin was approved by the FDA for use in children with infantile spasms. Where available, it is considered by some as an alternative to ACTH as the drug of first choice. Its principal side effect is its retinal toxicity, with resultant visual field defects that can persist despite withdrawal of the drug. The level of evidence for its efficacy is weaker than that for ACTH and stronger than that of other alternative medications, including valproate, benzodiazepines like nitrazepam, and clonazepam, topiramate, lamotrigine, zonisamide, pyridoxine, ketogenic diet, and intravenous gamma globulin (IVIG). None of these alternative drugs offers uniformly satisfactory results. However, they are useful for decreasing the frequency and severity of seizures in patients with symptomatic infantile spasms and as adjunctive therapy in patients with cryptogenic infantile spasms who do not respond completely to ACTH or vigabatrin.

Lennox-Gastaut syndrome is another difficult-to-treat epilepsy syndrome. Treatment of seizures in Lennox-Gastaut syndrome varies according to the preponderant seizure type. For drop attacks (tonic, atonic, or myoclonic astatic seizures), valproate, lamotrigine, or topiramate have been found to be especially effective. These drugs might control other types of seizures (partial, generalized tonic-clonic, atypical absence, other tonic, myoclonic), as well. For patients who have a preponderance of atypical absence seizures, lamotrigine or ethosuximide are often suitable drugs to try because they are relatively less toxic than many of the alternative drugs. Lamotrigine or valproate should be used if other seizures coexist with absences. Clonazepam and other benzodiazepines are also often helpful for all seizure types but produce significant sedation and often tolerance to their antiepileptic effects develops in a few months. In resistant cases of Lennox-Gastaut syndrome and related epilepsies, rufinamide, zonisamide, felbamate, levetiracetam, acetazolamide, methsuximide, corticosteroids, ketogenic diet, or IVIG can be used.

Dravet syndrome is usually treated with valproate and benzodiazepines such as clonazepam; the ketogenic diet can also be useful in patients with this syndrome. In some countries clobazam and stiripentol are available, and these appear to result more commonly in successes, particularly if used in combination with valproate. Other medications include zonisamide and topiramate. Lamotrigine has been reported to exacerbate seizures in Dravet syndrome and other myoclonic epilepsies.

Very rare cases of patients who have neonatal, infantile, or early childhood epilepsy who have **pyridoxine-dependent epilepsy** (demonstrated to be due to antiquitin gene mutation) respond to pyridoxine 10-100 mg/day orally (up to 600 mg/day has been used) within 3-7 days of the initiation of oral therapy and almost immediately if given parenterally. Seizure types include myoclonic, partial, or generalized seizures. Some patients have seizures that are intractable from onset, but other seizures show an initial but transient response to traditional AEDs. Some of these patients also require concurrent folinic acid (5-15 mg/day). Rarely, patients require the active form of vitamin B_6, specifically, pyridoxal phosphate (50 mg/day initial dose that can be increased gradually up to 15 mg/kg every 6 hr) owing to the patient's deficiency of **pyridoxamine phosphate oxidase (PNPO)**. In both the PNPO-deficient/pyridoxal phosphate-dependent and the pyridoxine-dependent forms, hypotonia and hypopnea can occur after initiation of vitamin therapy. Pyridoxine has also been used by some, specifically in Japan, early in the treatment of West syndrome. Patients with **cerebral folate deficiency** can respond to folinic acid supplementation (usually started at low doses of 0.5-1 mg/kg/day). Traditionally these entities have been diagnosed by giving the vitamin B_6 or folinic acid in therapeutic trials. There are biologic markers for the different forms of the disorder. One is elevation of pipecolic acid and of α-amino adipic semialdehyde (AASA) in vitamin B_6–dependent epilepsy due to a defect in the enzyme AASA dehydrogenase; another is abnormal metabolites in the CSF of patients with cerebral folate deficiency and PNPO deficiency.

Absence seizures are most often initially treated with ethosuximide, which is as effective as and less toxic than valproate and more effective than lamotrigine. Alternative drugs of first choice are lamotrigine and valproate, especially if generalized tonic-clonic seizures coexist with absence seizures. Patients resistant to ethosuximide might still respond to valproate or to lamotrigine. In absence seizures, the EEG is usually helpful in monitoring the response to therapy and is often more sensitive than the parents' observations in detecting these seizures. The EEG often normalizes when complete seizure control is achieved. This is usually not true for partial epilepsies. Other medications that could be used for absence seizures include acetazolamide, zonisamide, or clonazepam.

Benign myoclonic epilepsies are often best treated with valproate, particularly when patients have associated generalized tonic-clonic and absence seizures. Benzodiazepines, clonazepam, lamotrigine, and topiramate are alternatives for the treatment of benign myoclonic epilepsy. Severe myoclonic epilepsies and Dravet syndrome (see earlier) are treated with topiramate, clobazam, valproate, and stiripentol.

Partial and secondary generalized tonic and clonic seizures can be treated with oxcarbazepine, carbamazepine, phenobarbital, topiramate, valproic acid, lamotrigine, clobazam, clonazepam, or levetiracetam (see Table 586-8). Oxcarbazepine, levetiracetam, carbamazepine (USA) or valproate (Europe) are often used first. One study favored lamotrigine as initial monotherapy for partial seizures and valproate for generalized seizures. Almost any of these medications has been used as first or second choice depending on the individualization of the therapy.

CHOICE OF DRUG: OTHER CONSIDERATIONS

Because there are many options for each patient, the choice of which drug to use is always an individualized decision based on comparative effectiveness data from randomized controlled trials and several other considerations.

Comparative effectiveness and **potential for paradoxical seizure aggravation** by some AEDs (e.g., precipitation of absence seizures and myoclonic seizures by carbamazepine and tiagabine) must be considered (see Table 586-10).

Comparative tolerability: Adverse effects can vary according to the profile of the patient. The most prominent example is the increased risk of liver toxicity for valproate therapy in children <2 yr of age, on polytherapy, and or with metabolic disorders. Thus, if metabolic disorders are suspected, other drugs should be considered first and, in any case, valproate should not be started until these are ruled out by normal amino acids, organic acids, acylcarnitine profile, lactate, pyruvate, liver function tests, and perhaps other tests. The choice of an AED can also be influenced by the likelihood of occurrence of nuisance side effects such as weight gain (valproate, carbamazepine), gingival hyperplasia (phenytoin), alopecia (valproate), hyperactivity (benzodiazepines, barbiturates, valproate, gabapentin), and others. Children with behavior problems and/or with attention deficit disorder can become particularly hyperactive with GABAergic drugs such as benzodiazepines and barbiturates or even valproate. This often affects the choice of medications.

Cost and availability: The cost of the newer AEDs often precludes their use, particularly in developing countries where cost is a major issue. Also, many drugs are not available in many countries either because they are too expensive, because, paradoxically, they are too inexpensive, or because of regulatory restrictions. In general, AEDs have a narrow therapeutic range, and thus switching from brand name to generic formulations or from one generic to another can result in changes in levels that could result in breakthrough seizures or side effects. Thus, generic substitution is generally best avoided if a brand name drug has already proved efficacious.

Ease of initiation of the AED: Medications that are started very gradually such as lamotrigine and topiramate may not be chosen in situations when there is a need to achieve a therapeutic level quickly. In such situations, medications that have intravenous preparations or that can be started and titrated more quickly such as valproate, phenytoin, or levetiracetam may be chosen instead.

Drug interactions and presence of background medications: An example is the potential interference of enzyme-inducing drugs with many chemotherapeutic agents. In those cases, medications like gabapentin or levetiracetam are used. Also, valproate inhibits the metabolism and increases the levels of lamotrigine, phenobarbital, and felbamate. It also displaces protein-bound phenytoin from protein-binding sites, increasing the free fraction, and thus the free and not the total level needs to be checked when both medications are being used together. Enzyme inducers like phenobarbital, carbamazepine, phenytoin, and primidone reduce levels of lamotrigine, valproate, and, to a lesser extent, topiramate and zonisamide. Medications exclusively excreted by the kidney like levetiracetam and gabapentin are not subject to such interactions.

The presence of comorbid conditions: For example, the presence of migraine in a patient with epilepsy can lead to the choice of a medication that is effective against both conditions such as valproate or topiramate. In an obese patient, a medication such as valproate might be avoided, and a medication that decreases appetite such as topiramate might be used instead. In adolescent girls of child-bearing potential, enzyme-inducing AEDs should be avoided because they can interfere with birth control pills; other AEDs, particularly valproate, can increase risks for fetal malformations (see Table 586-9).

Coexisting seizures: In a patient with both absence and generalized tonic-clonic seizures, a drug that has a broad spectrum of antiseizure effects such as lamotrigine or valproate could be used rather than medications that have a narrow spectrum of efficacy, such as phenytoin.

History of prior response to specific AEDs: For example, if a patient or a family member with the same problem had previously responded to carbamazepine, carbamazepine could be a desirable choice.

Mechanism of drug actions: At present, the understanding of the pathophysiology of epilepsy does not allow specific choice of AEDs based on the assumed pathophysiology of the epilepsy. However, in general, it is believed that it is better to avoid combining medications that have similar mechanisms of action, such as phenytoin and carbamazepine (both work on sodium channels). A number of medications, such as lamotrigine and valproate or topiramate and lamotrigine, have been reported to have synergistic effects, possibly because they have different mechanisms of action.

Ease of use: Medications that are given once or twice a day are easier to use than medications that are given 3 or 4 times a day. Availability of a pediatric liquid preparation, particularly if such a preparation is palatable, also plays a role.

Ability to monitor the medication and adjust the dose: Some medications are difficult to adjust and to follow, requiring frequent blood levels. The prototype of such medications is phenytoin, but many of the older medications require blood level monitoring. This helps physicians gauge efficacy and avoid potential toxicity. However, monitoring in itself can represent a practical or patient satisfaction disadvantage as compared to the newer AEDs, which generally do not require blood level monitoring.

Patient's and family's preferences: All things being equal, the choice between two or more acceptable alternative AEDs might also depend on the patient's or family's preferences. For example, some patients might want to avoid gingival hyperplasia and hirsutism as side effects but might tolerate weight loss, or vice versa.

Genetics and genetic testing: A genetic predisposition to developing AED-induced side effects is another factor that may be a consideration. For example, there is a strong association between the human leukocyte antigen HLA-B*1502 allele and severe cutaneous reactions induced by carbamazepine, phenytoin, or lamotrigine in Chinese patients; hence these AEDs should be avoided in genetically susceptible persons. Mutations of the *SCN1A* sodium channel gene indicating Dravet syndrome could also lead to avoiding lamotrigine because it can exacerbate seizures in this syndrome.

Teratogenic profiles: Some AEDs, including valproate and to a lesser extent carbamazepine, phenobarbital, and phenytoin, are associated with teratogenic effects (Table 586-11).

Some of these considerations can be addressed by resorting to expert opinion surveys (see Table 586-10) or to guidelines developed by concerned societies such as the ILAE, National Institute for Clinical Excellence (NICE) in England, Scottish Intercollegiate Guidelines Network (SIGN), or the American Academy of Neurology (AAN). Some guidelines are totally evidence based (AAN, ILAE), and others (NICE, SIGN) incorporate other considerations as well. However, no guideline is able to incorporate all the considerations relevant to each patient. Thus, the process of choosing an AED involves incorporating the evidence from randomized controlled trials, guidelines, expert opinion surveys, and all of the other considerations inherent in individualizing therapy and in tailoring therapy to the patient's specific condition.

INITIATING AND MONITORING THERAPY

In nonemergency situations or when loading is not necessary, the maintenance dose of the chosen AED is started (Table 586-12). With some medications (e.g., carbamazepine and topiramate), in many cases even smaller doses are initially started then **gradually increased** up to the maintenance dose to build tolerance to adverse effects such as sedation. For example, the starting dose of carbamazepine is usually 5-10 mg/kg/day. Increments of 5 mg/kg/day can be added every 3 days until a therapeutic level is achieved and a therapeutic response is established or until unacceptable adverse effects occur. With other medications such as zonisamide, phenobarbital, phenytoin, or valproate, starting at the maintenance dose is usually tolerated. With some, such as levetiracetam and gabapentin, either approach can be used. Patients should be counseled about potential adverse effects, and these should be monitored during follow-up visits (Table 586-13).

Table 586-11 TERATOGENESIS AND PERINATAL OUTCOMES OF ANTIEPILEPTIC DRUGS

FINDING	RECOMMENDATION	LEVEL OF EVIDENCE
VPA as part of polytherapy and possibly monotherapy probably contributes to the development of major congenital malformations and adverse cognitive outcome	If possible, avoidance of valproate polytherapy during the first trimester of pregnancy should be considered so as to decrease the risk of major congenital malformations and adverse cognitive outcome	B
AED polytherapy, as compared to monotherapy, regimens probably contribute to the development of major congenital malformations and to adverse cognitive outcomes	If possible, avoidance of AED polytherapy during the first trimester of pregnancy should be considered to decrease the risk of major congenital malformations and adverse cognitive outcome	B
Monotherapy exposure to phenytoin or phenobarbital possibly increases the likelihood of adverse cognitive outcomes	If possible, avoidance of phenytoin and phenobarbital during pregnancy may be considered to prevent adverse cognitive outcomes	C
Neonates of women with epilepsy taking AEDs probably have an increased risk of being small for gestational age and possibly have an increased risk of a 1-min Apgar score of <7	Pregnancy risk stratification should reflect that the offspring of women with epilepsy taking AEDs are probably at increased risk for being small for gestational age (level B) and possibly at increased risk of 1-min Apgar scores of <7	C

Levels of recommendation: A: strongest recommendation; based on Class 1 data, B and C: lower levels of recommendations.
Types of malformations: Prior studies had reported the occurrence of spina bifida with valproate and carbamazepine therapy, and of cardiac malformation and cleft palate after carbamazepine phenytoin and phenobarbital exposure. There is variability from study to study. However, in general the relative incidence of major malformations of about 10% for valproate monotherapy, higher with valproate polytherapy, and in the range of 5% for monotherapy with the other above three AEDs and higher with polytherapy.
FDA categories: Valproate, phenobarbital, carbamazepine, and phenytoin are classified by the FDA as category D. Ethosuximide, felbamate, gabapentin, lamotrigine, levetiracetam, oxcarbazepine, tiagabine, topiramate, and zonisamide are category C. Category C: Animal studies have shown an adverse effect and there are no adequate and well-controlled studies in pregnant women or no animal studies have been conducted and there are no adequate and well-controlled studies in pregnant women. Category D: Studies, adequate well-controlled or observational, in pregnant women have demonstrated a risk to the fetus. However, the benefits of therapy might outweigh the potential risk.
AED, antiepileptic drug; VPA, valproate.
Data from Harden CI, Meador KJ, Pennell PB, et al: Practice parameter update: management issues for women with epilepsy—focus on pregnancy (an evidence-based review): teratogenesis and perinatal outcomes. Report of the Quality Standards Subcommittee and Therapeutics and Technology Subcommittee of the American Academy of Neurology and American Epilepsy Society, *Neurology* 73(2):133–141, 2009.

Titration

Levels of many AEDs should usually be determined after initiation to ensure compliance and therapeutic concentrations. Monitoring is most helpful for the older AEDs such as phenytoin, carbamazepine, valproate, phenobarbital, and ethosuximide. After starting the maintenance dosage or after any change in the dosage, a steady state is not reached until 5 half-lives have elapsed which, for most AEDs, is 2-7 days (half-life, 6-24 hr). For phenobarbital, it is 2-4 wk (mean half-life, 69 hr). For zonisamide it is 14 days during monotherapy and less than that during polytherapy with enzyme inducers (half-life, 63 hr in monotherapy and 27-38 hr during combination therapy with enzyme inducers). If a therapeutic level needs to be achieved faster, a **loading dose** may be used, loading with a single dose that is twice the usual maintenance dose per half-life. For valproate it is 25 mg/kg, for phenytoin it is 20 mg/kg, and for phenobarbital it is 10-20 mg/kg. A lower dosage of phenobarbital is sometimes given in older

Table 586-12 DOSAGES OF SELECTED ANTIEPILEPTIC DRUGS

MEDICATION	MAINTENANCE ORAL DOSAGE (mg/kg/day) UNLESS OTHERWISE SPECIFIED	USUAL DOSING	THERAPEUTIC LEVELS	PREPARATIONS
Acetazolamide	1-12 mo; 10 <1 yr: 20-30	bid or tid		125, 250 and 500 mg tabs
Bromide	50-100	bid or qd	10-15 mEq/L	Supplied as triple bromide soln (240 mg/mL of bromide salt)
Carbamazepine*	10-20	tid or qid SR usually bid	3-12 mg/L	150 and 300 mg ER caps 100, 200, 400 mg ER tabs 100 mg chewable tabs 200 mg tabs 100 mg/5 mL susp
Clobazam†	10-20 mg/day	bid or tid	60-200 µg/L	5 mg caps 10 mg tabs
Clonazepam†	0.01-0.02	bid or tid	25-85 µg/L	0.5, 1 and 2 mg tabs 0.125, 0.25, 0.5 mg orally disintegrating tabs
Diazepam	0.25-1.5 0.01-0.25 IV 0.2-0.5 mg/kg rectal (according to age; see Table 586-15)	bid or tid	100-700 µg/L	2, 5, 10 mg tabs 5 mg/mL, 5 mg/5 mL soln Rectal gel that can be dialed to dispense 2.5, 5, 7.5, 10, 12.5, 15, 17.5, 20 mg
Ethosuximide	20-30	bid or tid	40-100 mg/L	250 mg caps 250 mg/5 mL syrup, soln
Felbamate	15-45	bid or tid	50-110 mg/L	400, 600 mg tabs 600 mg/5 mL susp
Gabapentin‡	30-60	tid	2-20 mg/L	100, 300, and 400 mg caps, 600 and 800 mg tabs
Lamotrigine	5-15§ 1-5¶	tid bid	1-15 mg/L	25, 100, 150, 200 mg tabs 5, 25 mg chewable dispersible tabs
Levetiracetam†	20-40	bid or tid	6-20 mg/L	250, 500, 750 mg tabs 100 mg/mL soln 500, 750 mg SR (XR) tabs
Lorazepam	0.03	bid or tid	20-30 µg/L	0.5, 1, 2 mg tabs 2 mg/mL soln
Methsuximide (normethsuximide)	10-30	bid or tid	10-50 mg/L	150, 300 mg caps
Nitrazepam	0.25-1	bid or tid	<200 µg/L	5 mg tabs
Oxcarbazepine*	20-40	bid	13-28 mg/L	150, 300, 600 mg tabs 300 mg/5 mL susp
Phenobarbital	<5 yr, 3-5 >5 yr, 2-3	bid or qd	10-40 mg/L	15, 30, 60, 90, 100 mg tabs 4 mg/mL soln
Phenytoin	<3 yr, 8-10 >3 yr, 4-7	tabs, susp: tid caps: qd	5-20 mg/L	50 mg tabs 30 ,100 mg caps 125 mg/5 mL susp
Primidone	10-20	bid or tid	4-13 mg/L	50, 250 mg tabs, susp
Rufinamide†	30-45	bid		200, 400 mg tabs
Sulthiame	5-15	bid or tid	1.5-20 µg/mL	50, 200 mg caps Not available in all countries
Tiagabine	0.5-2	bid, tid, qid	80-450 µg/L	2, 4, 12, 16 mg tabs
Topiramate†	3-9, slow titration	bid or tid	2-25 mg/L	25, 100, 200 mg tabs 15, 25 mg sprinkle caps
Valproate	15-40. Higher doses are used if the patient is on enzyme inducers (up to 60 kg/day)	Sprinkle caps: bid Soln: tid	50-100 mg/L	250 mg caps 125 mg sprinkle caps 125, 250, 500 mg tabs 250 mg/5 mL soln
Zonisamide	4-8	bid or qd	10-40 mg/L	100-mg caps

*Usually start by ¼ maintenance dose and increase by ¼ every 2-3 days to full dose.
†Usually start with ¼ maintenance dose and increase by ¼ every 7 days to full dose.
‡Usually start with ¼ maintenance dose and increase by ¼ every day to full dose.
¶Child on valproate.
§Child on enzyme inducers.
Unless specified otherwise, as above, one would usually target the lower range of therapeutic dose then adjust as needed depending on response and/or levels. Dosing schedule (e.g., bid or tid) can depend on if a sustained release preparation is available and if the patient is on enzyme inducers (e.g., carbamazepine) or inhibitors (e.g., valproic acid) that could affect that drug (as indicated in the dosing in the table and in the text).
cap, capsule; ER, extended release; soln, solution; SR, sustained release; susp, suspension; tab, tablet.

children (5 mg/kg, which may be repeated once or more in 24 hr), to avoid excessive sedation.

Only one drug should be used initially and the dose increased until complete control is achieved or until side effects prohibit further increases. Then, and only then, may another drug be added and the initial one subsequently tapered. Control with 1 drug (**monotherapy**) should be the goal, although some patients eventually need to take multiple drugs. When appropriate, levels should also be checked upon addition (or discontinuation) of a second drug because of potential drug interactions. During follow-up, repeating the EEG every few months may be helpful to evaluate changes in the predisposition to seizures. This is

Table 586-13 SOME COMMON ADVERSE EFFECTS OF ANTIEPILEPTIC DRUGS

ANTIEPILEPTIC DRUG	SIDE EFFECT(S)
Acetazolamide	Nuisance: Dizziness, polyuria, electrolyte imbalance Serious: Stevens-Johnson syndrome
Benzodiazepines	Nuisance: Dose-related neurotoxicity (drowsiness, sedation, ataxia), hyperactivity, drooling, increased secretions Serious: Apnea
Bromide	Nuisance: Irritability, spurious hyperchloremia (falsely high chloride owing to bromide) Serious: Psychosis, rash, toxicity developing slowly owing to the very long half-life
Carbamazepine	Nuisance: Tics, transient leukopenia; hyponatremia, weight gain, nausea; dizziness Serious: Stevens-Johnson syndrome, agranulocytosis, aplastic anemia, liver toxicity
Felbamate	Nuisance: Anorexia, vomiting, insomnia, hyperactivity, dizziness Serious: Major risks for liver and hematologic toxicity requiring close monitoring (1 : 500)
Gabapentin	In children: Acute onset of aggression, hyperactivity In adults: Euphoria and behavioral disinhibiting, weight gain
Lamotrigine	Nuisance: CNS side effects: headache, ataxia, dizziness, tremor, but usually less than other AEDs Serious: Stevens-Johnson syndrome, rarely liver toxicity
Levetiracetam	CNS adverse events: Somnolence, asthenia, dizziness, but usually less than other AEDs In adults: Depressive mood; in children behavioral symptoms are common
Oxcarbazepine	Somnolence, headache, dizziness, nausea, apathy, rash, hypertrichosis, gingival hypertrophy, hyponatremia
Phenobarbital and other barbiturates	Neurotoxicity, insomnia, hyperactivity, signs of distractibility, fluctuation of mood, aggressive outbursts Serious: Liver toxicity, Stevens-Johnson syndrome
Phenytoin and other hydantoins	Nuisance: Gingival hyperplasia, coarsening of the facies, hirsutism, cerebellovestibular symptoms (nystagmus and ataxia) Serious: Stevens-Johnson syndrome, liver toxicity
Primidone	Nuisance: CNS toxicity (dizziness, slurred speech, giddiness, drowsiness, depression) Serious: Liver toxicity, Stevens-Johnson syndrome
Rufinamide	Nuisance: Somnolence, vomiting Serious: Contraindicated in familial short QT interval
Succinimides	Nuisance: Nausea, abdominal discomfort, anorexia, hiccups Serious: Stevens-Johnson syndrome, drug-induced lupus
Tiagabine	Nuisance: Dizziness, somnolence, asthenia, headache and tremor, precipitation of absence or myoclonic seizures Serious: Precipitation of nonconvulsive status epilepticus
Topiramate	Nuisance: Cognitive dysfunction; weight loss; renal calculi; hypohydrosis, fever Serious: precipitation of glaucoma
Valproic acid	Nuisance: Weight gain; hyperammonemia tremor, alopecia, menstrual irregularities Serious: Hepatic and pancreatic toxicity
Vigabatrin	Nuisance: Hyperactivity Serious: Irreversible visual field deficits, retinopathy
Zonisamide	Fatigue, dizziness, anorexia, psychomotor slowing, ataxia, rarely hallucinations, hypohydrosis and fever

Essentially all AEDs can cause CNS toxicity and potentially rashes and serious allergic reactions. Lacosamide has recently been approved as add-on therapy for partial seizures for patients ≥17 yr of age and requires a baseline EEG before starting it.
AED, antiepileptic drug; CNS, central nervous system; EEG, electroencephalogram.

especially true in situations where tapering off of medication is contemplated because a particular epilepsy syndrome is sometimes outgrown. This is necessary, for example, in absence seizures and in benign rolandic epilepsy, and it is useful but less important in most forms of partial epilepsy.

Monitoring

For the older AEDs, before starting treatment, **baseline laboratory studies** including CBC, platelets, liver enzymes, and possibly kidney function tests and urinalysis are often obtained and repeated periodically. Laboratory monitoring is more relevant early on, because idiosyncratic adverse effects such as allergic hepatitis and agranulocytosis are more likely to occur in the first 3-6 mo of therapy. These laboratory studies are usually initially checked once or twice during the first month, then every 3 to 4 mo thereafter. Serious concerns have been raised about the real usefulness of routine monitoring (in the absence of clinical signs) because the yield of significant adverse effects is low and the costs may be high. There are currently many advocates of less-frequent routine monitoring.

It is not uncommon (in ~10% of patients) to encounter reversible dose-related leukopenia in patients on carbamazepine or on phenytoin. This adverse effect responds to decreasing the dose or to stopping the medication and should be distinguished from the much less common idiosyncratic aplastic anemia or agranulocytosis. One exception requiring frequent (even weekly) monitoring of liver function and of blood counts throughout the therapy is felbamate, owing to the high incidence of liver and hematologic toxicity (1:500). Gum hyperplasia seen with phenytoin necessitates good oral hygiene (brushing teeth at least twice per day and rinsing the mouth after taking the phenytoin); in a few cases it may be severe enough to warrant surgical reduction and/or change of medication. Allergic rash can occur with any medication but is probably most common with lamotrigine, carbamazepine, and phenytoin.

Side Effects

During follow-up the patient should be monitored for **side effects**. Occasionally, a Stevens-Johnson–like syndrome develops; it has been found to be particularly common in Chinese patients who have the allele HLA-B*1502 and are taking carbamazepine.

Other potential side effects are rickets from phenytoin, phenobarbital, primidone, and carbamazepine (enzyme inducers that reduce 25-hyrdroxy-vitamin D level by inducing its metabolism) and hyperammonemia from valproate. Skeletal monitoring is warranted in patients on chronic AED therapy. Chronic AED therapy is often associated with vitamin D abnormalities (low bone density, rickets and hypocalcemia) in children and adults, particularly those on enzyme-inducing medications. Thus, counseling the patient about sun exposure and vitamin D intake, monitoring its levels, and, in some cases, vitamin D supplementation are recommended. There is currently no consensus on the dose to be used for supplementation or prophylaxis, but doses of 400-2000 IU/day have been used.

Irreversible hepatic injury and death are particularly feared in young children (<2 yr old) who are on valproate in combination with other AEDs particularly those who might have inborn errors of metabolism such as acidopathies and mitochondrial disease. Virtually all AEDs can produce sleepiness, ataxia, nystagmus, and slurred speech with toxic levels.

The FDA has determined that the use of AEDs may be associated with an increased risk of suicidal ideation and action and has recommended counseling about this side effect before starting these medications. This is obviously more applicable to adolescents and adults and those who use AEDs for purposes other than the treatment of epilepsy (e.g., chronic pain).

When adding a new AED, the doses used are often affected by the background medications. For example, if the patient is on enzyme inducers, the doses needed of valproate and lamotrigine are often double the usual maintenance doses. On the other hand, if the patient is on valproate, the doses of phenobarbital or lamotrigine are approximately half of what is usually needed. Genetic variability in enzymes that metabolize AEDs, **pharmacogenomics**, might account for some of the variation among individuals in responding to certain AEDs. Although numerous variants of the cytochrome P-450 (CYP) enzymes have been characterized, the use of this new knowledge is currently largely restricted to research investigations, and it has yet to be applied in routine clinical practice.

Additional Treatment

The principles of monotherapy indicate that a second medication needs to be considered after the first either is pushed as high as tolerated and still does not control the seizures or results in intolerable adverse effects. In those cases, a second drug is started and the first is tapered and then discontinued. The second drug is then again pushed to the dose that controls the seizure or that results in intolerable side effects. If the second drug fails, monotherapy with a third drug or **dual (combination) therapy** is considered.

Patients with **drug resistance** (at times also referred to as intractable or refractory) **epilepsy** warrant a careful diagnostic reevaluation to look for degenerative, metabolic or inflammatory underlying disorders (e.g., mitochondrial disease, Rasmussen's encephalitis, Chapter 586.2). Treatable metabolic disorders that can manifest as intractable epilepsy include pyridoxine-dependent and pyridoxal-responsive epilepsy, folinic acid–responsive seizures (recently demonstrated to be the same disorder as pyridoxine-dependent epilepsy), cerebral folate deficiency, neurotransmitter disorders, biotinidase deficiency, glucose transporter 1 deficiency (responds to the ketogenic diet), serine synthesis defects, creatine deficiency syndromes, and untreated phenylketonuria. Often patients who do not respond to antiepileptic drugs are candidates for steroids, intravenous gamma globulin, or the ketogenic diet.

Steroids, usually given as ACTH (see the earlier discussion of West syndrome) or as prednisone 2 mg/kg/day (or equivalent), are often used in epileptic encephalopathies such as West, Lennox-Gastaut, myoclonic astatic, continuous spike-waves in slow-wave sleep, and Landau-Kleffner syndromes. The course usually is for 2-3 mo with a taper over a similar period. Relapses occur commonly during tapering; in Landau-Kleffner syndrome, therapy for >1 yr is sometimes needed.

Intravenous gamma globulin (IVIG) has also been reported to be similarly effective in nonimmune-deficient patients with West, Lennox Gastaut, Landau-Kleffner, and continuous spike-waves in slow-wave sleep syndromes and possibly in partial seizures. One should check the IgA levels before starting the infusions (to assess the risk for allergic reactions, because these are increased in patients with IgA deficiency) and guard against allergic reactions during the infusion. The usual regimen is 2 g/kg divided over 4 consecutive days followed by 1 g/kg once a month for 6 mo. The mechanism of action of steroids and of IVIG are not known but is presumed to be anti-inflammatory, because it has been demonstrated that seizures increase cytokines and that these, in turn, increase neuronal excitability by several mechanisms, including activation of glutamate receptors. Steroids and ACTH might also stimulate brain neurosteroid receptors that enhance GABA activity and might reduce corticotrophin-releasing hormone, which is known to be epileptogenic.

The **ketogenic diet** is believed to be effective in glucose transporter protein 1 (GLUT-1) deficiency, pyruvate dehydrogenase deficiency, myoclonic-astatic epilepsy, tuberous sclerosis complex, Rett syndrome, severe myoclonic epilepsy of infancy (Dravet syndrome), and infantile spasms. There is also suggestion of possible efficacy in selected mitochondrial disorders, glycogenosis type V, Landau-Kleffner syndrome, Lafora body disease, and subacute sclerosing panencephalitis. The diet is absolutely contraindicated carnitine deficiency (primary), carnitine palmitoyltransferase I or II deficiency, carnitine translocase deficiency, β-oxidation defects, medium-chain acyl dehydrogenase deficiency, long-chain acyl dehydrogenase deficiency, short-chain acyl dehydrogenase deficiency, long-chain 3-hydroxyacyl-CoA deficiency, medium-chain 3-hydroxyacyl-CoA deficiency, pyruvate carboxylase deficiency, and porphyrias. Thus, an appropriate metabolic work-up, depending on the clinical picture, might need to be performed before starting the diet (e.g., acyl carnitine profile). The diet has been used for refractory seizures of various types (partial or generalized) and consists of an initial period of fasting followed by a diet with a 3 : 1 or 4 : 1 fat:nonfat ratio, with fats consisting of animal fat, vegetable oils, or medium chain triglycerides. Many patients do not tolerate it owing to diarrhea, vomiting, hypoglycemia, dehydration, or lack of palatability. Diets such as the low-glycemic-index diet and the Atkins diet are easier to institute and do not require hospitalization, but it is not known yet if they are as effective as the classic diet.

APPROACH TO EPILEPSY SURGERY

If a patient has failed 3 drugs, the chance of achieving seizure freedom using AEDs is generally <10%. Therefore, proper evaluation for surgery is necessary as soon as patients fail 2 or 3 AEDs, usually within 2 yr of the onset of epilepsy and often sooner than 2 yr. Performing epilepsy surgery in children at an earlier stage (e.g., <5 yr) allows transfer of function in the developing brain. Candidacy for epilepsy surgery requires proof of resistance to AEDs used at maximum, tolerably nontoxic doses; absence of expected unacceptable adverse consequences of surgery, and a properly defined **epileptogenic zone** (area that needs to be resected to achieve seizure freedom). The epileptogenic zone can be identified by seizure semiology, interictal EEG, video-EEG long-term monitoring, and MRI. Other techniques such as invasive EEG (depth electrodes, subdurals), single photon emission CT (SPECT), magnetoencephalography (MEG), and positron emission tomography (PET) are used when the epileptogenic zone is difficult to localize or when it is close to eloquent cortex. To avoid resection of eloquent cortex, several techniques can be used including the **Wada test.** In this test, intracarotid infusion of amobarbital is used to anesthetize one hemisphere to lateralize memory and speech by testing them during that unilateral anesthesia. Other tests to localize function include functional MRI, MEG, or subdural electrodes with cortical stimulation. Developmental delay or psychiatric diseases need to be considered in assessing the potential impact of surgery on the patient. The usual minimal presurgical evaluation includes EEG monitoring, imaging, and age-specific neuropsychologic assessment.

Epilepsy surgery is often used to treat refractory epilepsy of a number of etiologies including cortical dysplasia, tuberous sclerosis, polymicrogyria, hypothalamic hamartoma, and hemispheric syndromes, such as Sturge-Weber syndrome, hemimegalencephaly, Rasmussen encephalitis, and Landau-Kleffner syndrome. Patients with intractable epilepsy resulting from metabolic or degenerative problems are not candidates for resective epilepsy surgery. **Focal resection** of the epileptogenic zone is the most common procedure. **Hemispherectomy** is used for diffuse hemispheric lesions; **multiple subpial transection**, a surgical technique in which the connections of the epileptic focus are partially cut without resecting it, is sometimes used for unresectable foci located in eloquent cortex. In Lennox-Gastaut syndrome, **corpus callosotomy** is used for drop attacks. **Vagal nerve stimulation** (VNS) is often used for intractable epilepsies of various types and for seizures of diffuse or multifocal anatomic origin that do not yield themselves to resective surgery. Focal resection and hemispherectomy result in a high rate (50-80%) of seizure freedom. Corpus callosotomy and VNS result in lower rates (5-10%) of seizure freedom; however, these procedures do result in significant reductions in the frequency and severity of seizures, decrease in medication requirements, and meaningful improvements in the patient's quality of life in approximately half or more of eligible patients.

DISCONTINUATION OF THERAPY

Discontinuation of AEDs is usually indicated when children are free of seizures for at least 2 yr. In more-severe syndromes such as temporal lobe epilepsy secondary to mesial temporal sclerosis, Lennox-Gastaut syndrome, or severe myoclonic epilepsy, a prolonged period of seizure freedom on treatment is often warranted before AEDs are withdrawn, if withdrawal is attempted at all. In benign epilepsy syndromes, the duration of therapy can often be as short as 6 mo.

Many factors should be considered before discontinuing medication, including the likelihood of remaining seizure free after drug withdrawal based on the type of epilepsy syndrome and etiology, the risk of injury in case of seizure recurrence (e.g., if the patient drives), and the adverse effects of AED therapy. Most children who have not had a seizure for ≥2 yr and who have a normal EEG when AED withdrawal is initiated remain free of seizures after discontinuing medication, and most relapses occur within the first 6 mo.

Certain risk factors can help the clinician predict the prognosis after AED withdrawal. The most important risk factor for seizure relapse is an abnormal EEG before medication is discontinued. Children who have remote symptomatic epilepsy are less likely to be able to stop AEDs than children who have idiopathic epilepsy. In patients with absences or in those treated with valproate for primary generalized epilepsy, the risk of relapse might still be high despite a normal EEG because valproate can normalize EEGs with generalized spike-wave abnormalities. Thus, in these patients, repeating the EEG during drug withdrawal can help identify recurrence of the EEG abnormality and associated seizure risk before clinical seizures recur. Older age of epilepsy onset, longer duration of epilepsy, presence of multiple seizure types, and need to use >1 AED are all factors associated with a higher risk of seizure relapse after AED withdrawal.

AED therapy should be discontinued gradually, often over a period of 3-6 mo. Abrupt discontinuation can result in withdrawal seizures or status epilepticus. Withdrawal seizures are especially common with phenobarbital and benzodiazepines; therefore, special attention must be given to a prolonged tapering schedule during the withdrawal of these AEDs. Seizures that occur >2 to 3 mo after AEDs are completely discontinued indicate relapse, and resumption of treatment is usually warranted.

The decision to attempt AED withdrawal must be assessed mutually among the clinician, the parents, and the child. Risk factors should be identified and precautionary measures should be anticipated in case of seizure relapse. The patient and family should be counseled fully on what to expect, what precautions to take (including cessation of driving for a period of time), and what to do in case of relapse. A prescription for rectal diazepam to be given at the time of seizures that might occur during and after tapering may be warranted (see Table 586-12 for dosing).

BIBLIOGRAPHY

Please visit the Nelson Textbook of Pediatrics *website at* *www.expertconsult.com* *for the complete bibliography.*

586.7 Neonatal Seizures

Mohamad A. Mikati

Seizures are the most important and common indicator of significant neurologic dysfunction in the neonatal period. Seizure incidence is higher during this period than in any other period in life: 57.5/1,000 in infants with birth weights <1,500 g and 2.8/1,000 in infants weighing between 2,500 and 3,999 g have seizures.

PATHOPHYSIOLOGY

The immature brain has many differences from the mature brain that render it more excitable and more likely to develop seizures. Based predominantly on animal studies, these are delay in Na^+, K^+-ATPase maturation and increased NMDA and AMPA receptor density. In addition, the specific types of these receptors that are increased are those that are permeable to calcium (GLUR2 AMPA receptors). This contributes to increased excitability and to the long-term consequences associated with seizures, particularly those resulting from perinatal hypoxia. Medications that block AMPA receptors such as topiramate may thus prove useful in this clinical setup.

Another difference is delay in the development of inhibitory GABAergic transmission. In fact, GABA in the immature brain has an excitatory function as the chloride gradient is reversed relative to the mature brain, with higher concentrations of chloride being present intracellularly than extracellularly. Thus, opening of the chloride channels in the immature brain results in depolarizing the cell and not in hyperpolarizing it. This phenomenon appears to be more prominent in male neonates, perhaps explaining their greater predisposition to seizures. The reason for this is that the Cl^- transporter, NKCC1, is predominantly expressed in the neonatal period, leading to transport of Cl^- into the cell, and to cellular depolarization upon activation of $GABA_A$ receptors. This is important for neuronal development but renders the neonatal brain hyperexcitable. With maturation, expression of NCCK1 decreases and KCC2 increases. KCC2 transports Cl^- out of the cell, resulting in reduction of intracellular chloride concentration so that when $GABA_A$ receptors are activated, Cl^- influx and hyperpolarization occur. Bumetanide, a diuretic that blocks NKCC1, can prevent excessive GABA depolarization and avert the neuronal hyperexcitability underlying neonatal seizures.

Although it is susceptible to developing seizures, the immature brain appears to be more resistant to the deleterious effects of seizures than the mature brain, as a result of increases in calcium binding proteins that buffer injury-related increases in calcium, increased extracellular space, decreased levels of the second messenger inositol triphosphate, and the immature brain's ability to tolerate hypoxic conditions by resorting to anaerobic energy metabolism.

Whether seizures are injurious to the immature brain is controversial. Many animal studies indicate that seizures are detrimental to the immature brain. Human studies also suggest harmful effects of seizures as shown by MRI and by the association of worse prognosis in neonates with seizures even when correcting for confounding factors. Even electrographic seizures without clinical correlates have been shown to be associated with worse prognosis. However, it is difficult in most models and in human studies to distinguish effects of seizures, the underlying disease responsible for the seizures, and, in the case of expedient treatment, the AEDs used to stop the seizures. Most physicians currently believe that it is favorable to control clinical as well as electrographic seizures, but not at the expense of causing severe systemic toxicity from AEDs.

TYPES OF NEONATAL SEIZURES

There are 5 main neonatal seizure types: subtle, clonic, tonic, spasms, and myoclonic. Spasms, focal clonic or tonic, and generalized myoclonic seizures are, as a rule, associated with electrographic discharges (epileptic seizures), whereas the subtle, generalized tonic and other myoclonic seizures are usually not associated with discharges and thus are thought to usually represent release phenomena with abnormal movements secondary to brain injury rather than true epileptic seizures. To determine clinically whether such manifestations are seizures or release phenomena is often difficult, but precipitation of such manifestations by stimulation and aborting them by restraint or manipulation would suggest that they are not seizures. Performing such maneuvers at the bedside is often helpful. In addition, continuous bedside EEG monitoring helps make this distinction. Thus, such monitoring is the standard of care in many nurseries.

Subtle Seizures

Subtle seizures include transient eye deviations, nystagmus, blinking, mouthing, abnormal extremity movements (rowing, swimming, bicycling, pedaling, and stepping), fluctuations in heart rate, hypertension episodes, and apnea. Subtle seizures occur more commonly in premature than in full-term infants.

Clonic Seizures

Clonic seizures can be focal or multifocal. Multifocal clonic seizures incorporate several body parts and are migratory in nature. The migration follows a non-Jacksonian trend; for example, jerking of the left arm can be associated with jerking of the right leg. Generalized clonic seizures, which are bilateral, symmetrical, and synchronous, are uncommon in the neonatal period presumably due to decreased connectivity associated with incomplete myelination at this age.

Tonic Seizures

Tonic seizures can be focal or generalized (generalized are more common). Focal tonic seizures include persistent posturing of a limb or posturing of trunk or neck in an asymmetric way often with persistent horizontal eye deviation. Generalized tonic seizures are bilateral tonic limb extension or tonic flexion of upper extremities often associated with tonic extension of lower extremities.

Spasms

Spasms are sudden generalized jerks lasting 1-2 sec that are distinguished from generalized tonic spells by their shorter duration and by the fact that spasms are usually associated with a single, very brief, generalized discharge.

Myoclonic Seizures

Myoclonic seizures are divided into focal, multifocal, and generalized types. Myoclonic seizures can be distinguished from clonic seizures by the rapidity of the jerks and by their lack of rhythmicity. Focal myoclonic seizures characteristically affect the flexor muscles of the upper extremities and are sometimes associated with seizure activity on EEG. Multifocal myoclonic movements involve asynchronous twitching of several parts of the body and are not commonly associated with seizure discharges on EEG. Generalized myoclonic seizures involve bilateral jerking associated with flexion of upper and occasionally lower extremities. The latter type of myoclonic jerks is more commonly correlated with EEG abnormalities than the other types.

Seizures vs. Jitteriness

Jitteriness can be defined as rapid motor activities, such as a tremor or shake, that can be ended by flexion or holding the limb. Seizures, on the other hand, generally do not end with tactile or motor suppression. Jitteriness, unlike most seizures, is usually induced by a stimulus. Also unlike jitteriness, seizures often involve eye deviation and autonomic changes.

ETIOLOGY

Causes of neonatal seizures are shown in Table 586-14.

Hypoxic-Ischemic Encephalopathy

This is the most common cause of neonatal seizures, accounting for 50-60% of patients. Seizures secondary to this encephalopathy occur within 12 hr of birth.

Vascular Events

These include intracranial bleeds and ischemic strokes and account for 10-20% of patients. Three types of hemorrhage can be distinguished: primary subarachnoid hemorrhage, germinal matrix–intraventricular hemorrhage, and subdural hemorrhage. Patients with arterial strokes or venous sinus thrombosis can present with seizure and these can be diagnosed by neuroimaging. Venous sinus thrombosis could be missed unless MR or CT venography studies are requested.

Intracranial Infections

Bacterial and nonbacterial infections account for 5-10% of the cases of neonatal seizures and include bacterial meningitis, TORCH (*t*oxoplasmosis, *o*ther infections, *r*ubella, *c*ytomegalovirus, *h*erpes simplex virus) infections, particularly herpes simplex encephalitis.

Brain Malformations

Brain malformations account for 5-10% of neonatal seizure cases. An example is Aicardi syndrome, which affects girls and consists of retinal lacunae, agenesis of the corpus callosum, and severe seizures including subsequent infantile spasms with hypsarrhythmia that is sometimes initially unilateral on EEG.

Metabolic Disturbances

Metabolic disturbances include disturbances in glucose, calcium, magnesium, other electrolytes, amino acids, or organic acids and pyridoxine dependency.

Hypoglycemia can cause neurologic disturbances and is very common in small neonates and neonates whose mothers are diabetic or prediabetic. The duration of hypoglycemia is very critical in determining the incidence of neurologic symptoms.

Hypocalcemia occurs at two peaks. The first peak corresponds to low-birthweight infants and is evident in the first 2-3 days of life. The second peak occurs later in neonatal life and often involves large, full-term babies who consume milk that has an unfavorable ratio of phosphorus to calcium and phosphorus to magnesium. **Hypomagnesemia** is often associated with hypocalcemia. **Hyponatremia** can cause seizures and is often secondary to inappropriate antidiuretic hormone secretion.

Local anesthetic intoxication seizures can result from neonatal intoxication with local anesthetics administered into the infant's scalp.

Neonatal seizures can also result from disturbances in **amino acid or organic acid** metabolism. These are usually associated with acidosis and/or hyperammonemia. However, even in the absence of these findings, if a cause of the seizures is not immediately evident, then ruling out metabolic causes requires a full metabolic work-up (Chapter 586.2) including examination of

Table 586-14 CAUSES OF NEONATAL SEIZURES

AGES 1-4 DAYS

Hypoxic-ischemic encephalopathy
Drug withdrawal, maternal drug use of narcotic or barbiturates
Drug toxicity: lidocaine, penicillin
Intraventricular hemorrhage
Acute metabolic disorders
• Hypocalcemia
  • Perinatal asphyxia, small for gestational age
  • Sepsis
  • Maternal diabetes, hyperthyroidism, or hypoparathyroidism
• Hypoglycemia
  • Perinatal insults, prematurity, small for gestational age
  • Maternal diabetes
  • Hyperinsulinemic hypoglycemia
  • Sepsis
• Hypomagnesemia
• Hyponatremia or hypernatremia
  • Iatrogenic or inappropriate antidiuretic hormone secretion
Inborn errors of metabolism
• Galactosemia
• Hyperglycinemia
• Urea cycle disorders
Pyridoxine deficiency (must be considered at any age)

AGES 4-14 DAYS

Infection
• Meningitis (bacterial)
• Encephalitis (enteroviral, herpes simplex)
Metabolic disorders
• Hypocalcemia
  • Diet, milk formula
• Hypoglycemia, persistent
  • Inherited disorders of metabolism
  • Galactosemia
  • Fructosemia
  • Leucine sensitivity
  • Hyperinsulinemic hypoglycemia, hyperinsulinism, hyperammonemia syndrome
  • Anterior pituitary hypoplasia, pancreatic islet cell tumor
  • Beckwith syndrome
Drug withdrawal, maternal drug use of narcotics or barbiturates
Benign neonatal convulsions, familial and nonfamilial
Kernicterus, hyperbilirubinemia
Developmental delay, epilepsy, neonatal diabetes (DEND) syndrome

AGES 2-8 WK
Infection • Herpes simplex or enteroviral encephalitis • Bacterial meningitis Head injury • Subdural hematoma • Child abuse Inherited disorders of metabolism • Aminoacidurias • Urea cycle defects • Organic acidurias • Neonatal adrenoleukodystrophy Malformations of cortical development • Lissencephaly • Focal cortical dysplasia Tuberous sclerosis Sturge-Weber syndrome

From Kliegman RM, Greenbaum LA, Lye PS: *Practical strategies in pediatric diagnosis and therapy*, ed 2, Philadelphia, 2004, Elsevier, p 681.

serum amino acids, acyl carnitine profile, lactate, pyruvate, and ammonia, examination of urine for amino acids and organic acids, and examination of CSF for glucose, protein, cells, amino acids, very long chain fatty acids (for neonatal adrenoleukodystropy and Zellweger syndrome), lactate, pyruvate, and perhaps other tests. This is because many inborn errors of metabolism such as nonketotic hyperglycinemia can manifest with neonatal seizures (often mistaken initially for hiccups) and can be detected only by performing these tests. Definitive diagnosis of **nonketotic hyperglycinemia**, for example, requires measuring the ratio of CSF glycine to plasma glycine.

Pyridoxine and pyridoxal dependency, which are malfunctions of pyridoxine metabolism, can cause severe seizures. These seizures, which are often multifocal clonic, usually start during the first hours of life. Mental retardation is often associated if therapy is delayed (Chapter 586.6).

Drug Withdrawal

Seizures can rarely be caused by the neonate's passive addiction and then drug withdrawal. Such drugs include narcotic analgesics, sedative-hypnotics, and others. The associated seizures appear during the first 3 days of life.

Neonatal Seizure Syndromes

Seizure syndromes include **benign idiopathic neonatal seizures (fifth day fits)**, which are usually apneic and focal motor seizures that start around the fifth day of life. Interictal EEG shows a distinctive pattern called *theta pointu alternant* (runs sharp 4-7 Hz activity), and ictal EEG shows multifocal electrographic seizures. Patients have a good response to medications and a good prognosis. Autosomal dominant **benign familial neonatal seizures** have onset at 2-4 days of age and usually remit at 2-15 wk of age. The seizures consist of ocular deviation, tonic posturing, clonic jerks, and, at times, motor automatisms. Interictal EEG is usually normal. These have been shown to be due to mutations in the *KCNQ2* and *KCNQ3* genes. Approximately 16% of patients develop later epilepsy. **Early myoclonic encephalopathy** and **early infantile epileptic encephalopathy (Ohtahara syndrome)** are discussed in Chapter 586.4.

Miscellaneous Conditions

Miscellaneous conditions include benign neonatal sleep myoclonus and hyperekplexia, which are nonepileptic conditions (Chapter 587).

DIAGNOSIS

Some cases can be correctly diagnosed by simply taking the prenatal and postnatal history and performing an adequate physical examination. Depending on the case, additional tests or procedures can be performed. EEG is considered the main tool for diagnosis. It can show paroxysmal activity (e.g., sharp waves) in between the seizures and electrographic seizure activity if a seizure is captured. However, some neonatal seizures might not be associated with EEG abnormalities as noted above either because they are "release phenomena" or alternatively because the discharge is deep and is not detected by the scalp EEG. Additionally, electrographic seizures can occur without observed clinical signs (**electroclinical dissociation**). This is presumed to be due to the immaturity of cortical connections resulting in many cases in no or minimal motor manifestations. Continuously monitoring the EEG at the bedside in the neonatal intensive care unit (NICU) for neonates at risk for neonatal seizures and brain injury has become part of routine clinical practice in many centers, providing real-time measurements of the brain's electrical activity and identifying seizure activity. Some centers apply EEG monitoring to at-risk babies even before seizures develop; others monitor patients who have manifested or are suspected of having seizures. In addition, there are currently attempts to develop methods for continuous monitoring of cerebral activity with automated detection and background analysis of neonatal seizures, similar to the continuous ECG monitoring in intensive care facilities.

Careful neurologic examination of the infant might uncover the cause of the seizure disorder. Examination of the **retina** might show the presence of chorioretinitis, suggesting a congenital TORCH infection, in which case titers of mother and infant are indicated. The **Aicardi syndrome**, which occurs exclusively in infant girls, is associated with coloboma of the iris and retinal lacunae, refractory seizures, and absence of the corpus callosum. Inspection of the **skin** might show hypopigmented lesions characteristic of tuberous sclerosis or the typical crusted vesicular lesions of incontinentia pigmenti; both neurocutaneous syndromes are associated with generalized myoclonic seizures beginning early in life. An unusual body odor suggests an inborn error of metabolism.

Blood should be obtained for determinations of glucose, calcium, magnesium, electrolytes, and blood urea nitrogen. If hypoglycemia is a possibility, serum glucose testing is indicated so that treatment can be initiated immediately. Hypocalcemia can occur in isolation or in association with hypomagnesemia. A lowered serum calcium level is often associated with birth trauma or a CNS insult in the perinatal period. Additional causes include maternal diabetes, prematurity, DiGeorge syndrome, and high-phosphate feedings. Hypomagnesemia (<1.5 mg/dL) is often associated with hypocalcemia and occurs particularly in infants of malnourished mothers. In this situation, the seizures are resistant to calcium therapy but respond to intramuscular magnesium, 0.2 mL/kg of a 50% solution of $MgSO_4$. Serum electrolyte measurement can indicate significant hyponatremia (serum sodium <135 mEq/L) or hypernatremia (serum sodium >150 mEq/L) as a cause of the seizure disorder.

A **lumbar puncture** is indicated in virtually all neonates with seizures, unless the cause is obviously related to a metabolic disorder such as hypoglycemia or hypocalcemia secondary to feeding of high concentrations of phosphate. The latter infants are normally alert interictally and usually respond promptly to appropriate therapy. The CSF findings can indicate a bacterial meningitis or aseptic encephalitis. Prompt diagnosis and appropriate therapy improve the outcome for these infants. Bloody CSF indicates a traumatic tap or a subarachnoid or intraventricular bleed. Immediate centrifugation of the specimen can assist in differentiating the two disorders. A clear supernatant suggests a traumatic tap, and a xanthochromic color suggests a subarachnoid bleed. Mildly jaundiced normal infants can have a yellowish discoloration of the CSF that makes inspection of the supernatant less reliable in the newborn period.

Many **inborn errors of metabolism** cause generalized convulsions in the newborn period. Because these conditions are often inherited in an autosomal recessive or X-linked recessive fashion, it is imperative that a careful family history be obtained to determine whether siblings or close relatives developed seizures or died at an early age. Serum ammonia determination is useful for screening for the hypoglycemic hyperammonemia syndrome and for suspected urea cycle abnormalities. In addition to having generalized clonic seizures, these latter infants present during the 1st few days of life with increasing lethargy progressing to coma, anorexia and vomiting, and a bulging fontanel. If the blood gases show an anion gap and a metabolic acidosis with hyperammonemia, urine organic acids should be immediately determined to investigate the possibility of methylmalonic or propionic acidemia.

Maple syrup urine disease (MSUD) should be suspected when a metabolic acidosis occurs in association with generalized clonic seizures, vomiting, bulging fontanel, and muscle rigidity during the 1st wk of life. The result of a rapid screening test using 2,4-dinitrophenylhydrazine that identifies keto derivatives in the urine is positive in MSUD.

Additional metabolic causes of neonatal seizures include nonketotic hyperglycinemia, a lethal condition characterized by markedly elevated plasma and CSF glycine levels, persistent generalized seizures, and lethargy rapidly leading to coma; ketotic hyperglycinemia in which seizures are associated with vomiting, fluid and electrolyte disturbances, and a metabolic acidosis; and Leigh disease suggested by elevated levels of serum and CSF lactate or an increased lactate:pyruvate ratio. Biotinidase deficiency should also be considered. A comprehensive description of the diagnosis and management of these metabolic diseases is discussed in Part XI.

Unintentional **injection of a local anesthetic** into a fetus during labor can produce intense tonic seizures. These infants are often thought to have had a traumatic delivery because they are flaccid at birth, have abnormal brainstem reflexes, and show signs of respiratory depression that sometimes requires ventilation. Examination may show a needle puncture of the skin or a perforation or laceration of the scalp. An elevated serum anesthetic level confirms the diagnosis. The treatment consists of supportive measures and promotion of urine output by administering intravenous fluids with appropriate monitoring to prevent fluid overload.

Benign familial neonatal seizures, an autosomal dominant condition, begins on the 2nd-3rd day of life, with a seizure frequency of 10-20/day. Patients are normal between seizures, which stop in 1-6 mo. **Fifth-day fits** occur on day 5 of life (4-6 days) in normal-appearing neonates. The seizures are multifocal and are often present for <24 hr. The diagnosis requires exclusion of other causes of seizures. The prognosis is good.

Pyridoxine dependency, a rare disorder, must be considered when generalized clonic seizures begin shortly after birth with signs of fetal distress in utero. These seizures are particularly resistant to conventional anticonvulsants such as phenobarbital or phenytoin. The history may suggest that similar seizures occurred in utero. Some cases of pyridoxine dependency are reported to begin later in infancy or in early childhood. This condition is inherited as an autosomal recessive trait. In affected infants, large amounts of pyridoxine are required to maintain adequate production of GABA. When pyridoxine-dependent seizures are suspected, 100-200 mg of pyridoxine or pyridoxal phosphate should be administered intravenously during the EEG, which should be promptly performed once the diagnosis is considered. The seizures abruptly cease, and the EEG normalizes in the next few hours. Not all cases of pyridoxine dependency respond dramatically to the initial bolus of IV pyridoxine. Therefore, a 6-wk trial of oral pyridoxine (10-20 mg/day) or preferably pyridoxal phosphate (as pyridoxine does not help infants with the related but distinct syndrome of pyridoxal dependency) is recommended for infants in whom a high index of suspicion continues after a negative response to IV pyridoxine. Measurement of serum pipecolic acid (elevated) and CSF pyridoxal-5-phosphate (decreased) might prove to be the more precise method of confirming the diagnosis of pyridoxine dependency. These children require lifelong supplementation of oral pyridoxine 10 mg/day. Generally, the earlier the diagnosis and therapy with pyridoxine, the more favorable the outcome. Untreated children have persistent seizures and are uniformly severely mentally retarded.

Drug-withdrawal seizures can occur in the newborn nursery but can take several weeks to develop because of prolonged excretion of the drug by the neonate. The incriminated drugs include barbiturates, benzodiazepines, heroin, and methadone. The infant may be jittery, irritable, and lethargic and can have myoclonus or frank clonic seizures. The mother might deny the use of drugs; a serum or urine analysis can identify the responsible agent.

Infants with focal seizures, suspected stroke or intracranial hemorrhage, and severe **cytoarchitectural abnormalities** of the brain (including lissencephaly and schizencephaly) who clinically may appear normal or microcephalic should undergo MRI or CT scan. Indeed, it is appropriate to recommend imaging of all neonates with seizures unexplained by serum glucose, calcium, or electrolyte disorders. Infants with chromosome abnormalities and adrenoleukodystrophy are also at risk for seizures and should be evaluated with investigation of a karyotype and serum long-chain fatty acids, respectively.

PROGNOSIS

Over the last few decades, prognosis of neonatal seizures has become better owing to improvement and advancement of obstetric care and intensive neonatal care. Mortality from neonatal seizures has decreased from 40 to 20%. The correlation between EEG and prognosis is very clear. Although neonatal EEG interpretation is very difficult, EEG was found to be highly associated with the outcome in premature and full-term infants. An abnormal background is a powerful predictor of less-favorable later outcome. In addition, prolonged electrographic seizures (>10 min/hour), multifocal periodic electrographic discharges, and spread of the electrographic seizures to the contralateral hemisphere also correlate with poorer outcome. The underlying etiology of the seizures is the main determinant of outcome. For example, patients with seizures secondary to hypoxic-ischemic encephalopathy have a 50% chance of developing normally, whereas those with seizures due to primary subarachnoid hemorrhage or hypocalcemia have a much better prognosis.

TREATMENT

A mainstay in the therapy of neonatal seizures is the diagnosis and treatment of the underlying etiology (e.g., hypoglycemia, hypocalcemia, meningitis, drug withdrawal, trauma), whenever one can be identified. There are conflicting approaches regarding the control of neonatal seizures. Proponents of the first approach argue that complete control of clinical as well as all electrographic seizures is needed. Others would only treat clinical seizures. Most centers favor the first approach but not at the expense of systemic toxicity. An important consideration before starting anticonvulsants is deciding if the patient needs to receive intravenous therapy and loading with an initial bolus or can simply be started on maintenance doses of a long-acting drug. Patients often require assisted ventilation after receiving intravenous or oral loading doses of AEDs, and thus precautions for observations and needed interventions are necessary.

Phenobarbital

Phenobarbital is considered by many to be the drug of first choice in neonatal seizures. The usual loading dose of is 20 mg/kg. If this dosage is not effective, then additional doses of 5 to 10 mg/kg can be given until a dose of 40 mg/kg is reached. Twenty-four hours after starting the loading dose, maintenance dosing can be started at 3-6 mg/kg/day usually administered in 2 separate doses. Phenobarbital is metabolized in the liver and is excreted through kidneys. Thus, any abnormality in the function of these organs alters the drug's metabolism and can result in toxicity. In infants with acidosis or critical illness that might alter serum protein content, free (i.e., not protein bound) levels of the drug should be followed carefully.

Phenytoin and Fosphenytoin

If a total loading dose of 40 mg/kg of phenobarbital was not effective, then a loading dose of 15-20 mg/kg of phenytoin can be administered intravenously. The rate at which the dose should be given must not exceed 0.5-1 mg/kg/min in order to prevent cardiac problems, and the medication needs to be avoided in patients with significant heart disease. Heart rate should be monitored while administrating the drug. It is not possible to mix phenytoin or fosphenytoin with dextrose solutions. Owing to its reduced solubility, potentially severe local cutaneous reactions, interaction with other drugs and possible cardiac toxicity, intravenous phenytoin is not widely used.

Fosphenytoin, which is a phosphate ester prodrug, is preferable. It is highly soluble in water and can be administered very safely intravenously and intramuscularly, without causing injury to tissues. Fosphenytoin is administered in phenytoin equivalents (PE). The usual loading dose of fosphenytoin is 15-20 PE/kg administered over 30 min. Maintenance doses of 4-8 PE/kg/day can be given. As is the case for phenobarbital, free levels of the drug should be monitored in neonates whose serum pH or protein content might not be normal.

Lorazepam

The initial drug used to control acute seizures is usually lorazepam. This can be used either as the initial drug or as second-line treatment in a newborn who did not respond to treatment with phenobarbital and phenytoin (15-40% of cases). Lorazepam is distributed to the brain very quickly and exerts its anticonvulsant effect in <5 min. It is not very lipophilic and does not clear out from the brain very rapidly. Its action can last 6-24 hr. Usually, it does not cause hypotension or respiratory depression. The dose is 0.05 mg/kg (range, 0.02-0.10 mg/kg) every 4-8 hr.

Diazepam and Midazolam

Diazepam is highly lipophilic, so it distributes very rapidly into the brain and then is cleared very quickly out, carrying the risk of recurrence of seizures. Like other intravenous benzodiazepines, it carries a risk of apnea and hypotension, particularly if the patient is also on a barbiturate, so patients need to be observed for 3-8 hr after administration. The usual dose is 0.1-0.3 mg/kg IV over 3-5 min, given every 15-30 min to a maximum total dose of 2 mg. However, because of the respiratory and blood pressure limitations and because the intravenous preparation contains sodium benzoate and benzoic acid, it is currently not recommended as a first-line agent. There is increasing experience with midazolam use in neonates. The doses used have been in the range of 0.05-0.1 mg/kg IV, with a continuous infusion of 0.5-1 μg/kg/min IV that can be gradually titrated upward every 5 min to about 2 μg/kg/min to achieve seizure control.

Other Medications

Primidone, lidocaine, carbamazepine, valproate, lamotrigine, topiramate, and levetiracetam have been used. However, many of these drugs are potentially toxic, and some, including valproate, are more likely to be toxic in children <2 yr of age than in older children. On the other hand, despite the absence of data on neonatal kinetics of either drug, topiramate and levetiracetam have been reported to be the drugs of second and third choice for approximately half of surveyed pediatric neurologists. The dosages used were up to 20 mg/kg/day of topiramate and 10-30 mg/kg/day of levetiracetam.

Duration of Therapy

Duration of therapy is related to the risk of developing later epilepsy in infants suffering from neonatal seizures, which ranges from 10-30% and depends on the individual neurologic examination, the etiology of seizures, and the EEG at the time of discharge from the hospital. In general, if the EEG at the time of discharge is not paroxysmal, then medications are usually tapered. If the EEG remains paroxysmal, then the decision is usually delayed for several months after discharge.

BIBLIOGRAPHY

Please visit the Nelson Textbook of Pediatrics *website at* *www.expertconsult.com* *for the complete bibliography.*

586.8 Status Epilepticus

Mohamad A. Mikati

Status epilepticus is a medical emergency that should be anticipated in any patient who presents with an acute seizure. It is defined as continuous seizure activity or recurrent seizure activity without regaining of consciousness lasting for >30 min. Some have advocated 5 min (rather than 30) as the time limit, but others have suggested using the term **impending status epilepticus** for seizures between 5 and 30 min. The measures used to treat status epilepticus need to be started in any patient with acute seizures that do not stop within a few minutes. The most common type is **convulsive status epilepticus** (generalized tonic, clonic, or tonic-clonic), but other types do occur, including nonconvulsive status (complex partial, absence), myoclonic status, epilepsia partialis continua, and neonatal status epilepticus. About 30% of patients presenting with status epilepticus are having their first seizure, and approximately 40% of these later develop epilepsy. Febrile status epilepticus is the most common type of status epilepticus in children. In the 1950s and 1960s, mortality rates of 6-18% were reported after status epilepticus; currently, with the recognition of status epilepticus as a medical emergency, a lower mortality rate of 4-5% is observed, most of it secondary to the underlying etiology rather than to the seizures. Status epilepticus carries an approximately 14% risk of new neurologic deficits, most of this (12.5%) secondary to the underlying pathology.

Nonconvulsive status epilepticus manifests as a confusional state, dementia, hyperactivity with behavioral problems, fluctuating impairment of consciousness with at times unsteady sitting or walking (absence status), fluctuating mental status, confusional state, hallucinations, paranoia, aggressiveness catatonia, and psychotic symptoms. Epilepsia partialis continua has been defined previously and can be caused by tumor, vascular etiologies, mitochondrial disease (MELAS), and Rasmussen encephalitis.

Refractory status epilepticus is status epilepticus that has failed to respond to therapy, usually with at least 2 (although some have specified 3) medications. Whether there should be a minimum duration has not been agreed upon, as authors have variably cited 30-min, 60-min, or 2-hr durations. **New-onset refractory status epilepticus** (NORSE) has been identified as a distinct entity that can be caused by almost any of the causes of status epilepticus in a patient without prior epilepsy. It also is often of unknown etiology, presumed to be encephalitic or post-encephalitic, can last several weeks or longer, and often has a poor prognosis.

ETIOLOGY

Etiologies include new-onset epilepsy of any type, drug intoxication (e.g., tricyclic antidepressants) in children and drug and alcohol abuse in adolescents, drug withdrawal or overdose in patients on AEDs, hypoglycemia, electrolyte imbalance (hypocalcemia, hyponatremia, hypomagnesemia), acute head trauma, encephalitis, meningitis, ischemic (arterial or venous) stroke, intracranial hemorrhage, pyridoxine, folinic acid and pyridoxal phosphate dependency, inborn errors of metabolism (Chapter 586.2) such as nonketotic hyperglycinemia in neonates and mitochondrial encephalopathy with lactic acidosis (MELAS) in children and adolescents, hypoxic-ischemic injury (e.g., after cardiac arrest), systemic conditions (such as hypertensive encephalopathy, renal or hepatic encephalopathy), brain tumors, and any other disorders that can cause epilepsy (such as brain malformations, neurodegenerative disorders, different types of progressive myoclonic epilepsy, storage diseases).

A rare condition called **hemiconvulsion, hemiplegia, epilepsy (HHE) syndrome** consists of prolonged febrile status epilepticus presumably due to focal acute encephalitis with resultant atrophy in the involved hemisphere, contralateral hemiplegia, and chronic epilepsy and needs to be suspected early on to attempt to control the seizures as early as possible. A somewhat similar condition in older children presenting as fever-induced refractory epileptic encephalopathy (FIRES) has been reported. Rasmussen encephalitis often causes epilepsia partialis continua (Chapter 586.3) and sometimes convulsive status epilepticus. Several types of infections are more likely to cause encephalitis with status epilepticus such as herpes simplex (complex partial and convulsive status), *Bartonella* (particularly nonconvulsive status), Epstein-Barr virus, and mycoplasma (postinfections encephalomyelitis with any type of status epilepticus). Postinfectious encephalitis and acute disseminated encephalomyelitis are common causes of status epilepticus including refractory status epilepticus.

MECHANISMS

The mechanisms leading to the establishment of sustained seizure activity seen in status epilepticus appear to involve failure of desensitization of AMPA glutamate receptors, thus persistence of increased excitability, and reduction of GABA-mediated inhibition due to intracellular internalization of $GABA_A$ receptors. This might explain the clinical observations that status epilepticus is often less likely to stop in the next specific period of time the longer the seizure has lasted and why benzodiazepines appear to be decreasingly effective the longer seizure activity lasts. During status epilepticus there is increased cerebral metabolic rate and a compensatory increase in cerebral blood flow that, after about half an hour, is not able to keep up with the increases in cerebral metabolic rate. This leads to a transition from adequate to inadequate cerebral oxygen tensions and, together with other factors, contributes to neuronal injury resulting from status epilepticus. Status epilepticus can cause both neuronal necrosis and apoptosis. The mechanisms of apoptosis are thought to be related to increases in intracellular calcium and pro-apoptotic factors such as ceramide, Bax, and apoptosis-inducing factor.

THERAPY

Status epilepticus is a medical emergency that requires initial and continuous attention to securing airway breathing, and circulation (with continuous monitoring of vital signs including ECG) and determination and management of the underlying etiology (e.g., hypoglycemia). Laboratory studies including glucose and sodium, calcium, or other electrolytes, are abnormal in about 6% and are generally ordered as routine practice. Blood and spinal fluid cultures, toxic screens, and tests for inborn errors of metabolism are often needed, and AED levels need to be determined in known epileptic children already taking these drugs. EEG is often helpful in ruling out **pseudo–status epilepticus** (psychological conversion reaction mimicking status epilepticus) and in identifying the type of status epilepticus (generalized versus focal), which can guide further testing for the underlying etiology and further therapy. EEG can also help distinguish between postictal depression and later stages of status epilepticus in which the clinical manifestations are subtle (e.g., minimal myoclonic jerks) or absent (electroclinical dissociation) and can help in monitoring the therapy, particularly in patients who are paralyzed and intubated. Neuroimaging needs to be considered after the child has been stabilized, especially if it is indicated by the clinical manifestations or asymmetric or focal nature of the EEG abnormalities or if the seizure etiology is unknown. The EEG manifestations of status epilepticus show several stages that consist of initial distinct electrographic seizures (stage I) followed by waxing and waning electrographic seizures (stage II), continuous electrographic seizures (stage III; many patients start with this directly), continuous ictal discharges punctuated by flat periods (stage IV) and periodic epileptiform discharges on flat background (stage V). The last 2 stages are often associated with subtle clinical manifestations.

The initial therapy usually involves intravenous lorazepam, which is at least as effective as intravenous diazepam but has fewer side effects (Table 586-15). In infants, a trial of pyridoxine is often warranted. If intravenous access is not available, buccal midazolam or intranasal lorazepam are 2 effective options. With all options, respiratory depression is a potential side effect for which the patient should be monitored and managed as needed. Nasal midazolam and rectal diazepam have also been used, but there is less evidence to support their use in status epilepticus as compared to the other options.

After the initial benzodiazepine, the next medication is usually fosphenytoin, and the loading dose is usually 15-20 PE/kg. A level is usually taken 2 hr later to ensure achievement of a therapeutic concentration. Depending on the level maintenance dose, it can be started right away or, more commonly, in 6 hr. With

Table 586-15 DOSES OF COMMONLY USED ANTIEPILEPTIC DRUGS IN STATUS EPILEPTICUS

DRUG	ROUTE	DOSAGE (mg/kg)
Lorazepam	Intravenous	0.05-0.1
	Intranasal	0.1
Midazolam	Intravenous	0.2 loading 0.08-0.23/hr maintenance
	Intramuscular	0.1-0.5
	Intranasal	0.2-0.3
	Buccal	0.2-0.5
Diazepam	Intravenous	0.2-0.5
	Rectal	2-5 yr: 0.5
		6-11 yr: 0.3
		≥12 yr: 0.2
Phosphenytoin	Intravenous	15-20 PE, then 3-6/24 hr
Paraldehyde	Intramuscular	0.2 mL/kg
	Rectal	0.4 mL/kg + same volume of olive oil
Phenobarbital		5-20
Pentobarbital coma		13.0, then 1-5/hr
Propofol		1 (bolus), then 1-15/hr (infusion)
Thiopental		5/1st hour, then 1-2/hr
Valproate	Intravenous	Loading: 25, then 30-60/24 hr

phenytoin and phenobarbital, each 1 mg/kg (1 PE/kg for fosphenytoin) increases the serum concentration by about 1 µg/mL; for valproate, each 1 mg/kg increases the serum concentration by approximately 4 µg/mL. Precautions about the rate of infusion of fosphenytoin and phenytoin (not >0.5-1 mg/kg/min) and the other medications need to be followed because side effects often depend on infusion rate.

The subsequent medication is often phenobarbital. The dose used in neonates is usually 20 mg/kg loading dose, but in infants and children often the dose is 5-10 mg/kg (to avoid respiratory depression), with the dose repeated if there is not an adequate response. There is some evidence to support the use of intravenous valproate as a third-line medication. The place of intravenous levetiracetam awaits further study.

After the second or third medication is given, and sometimes before that, the patient might need to be intubated. All patients with status, even the ones who respond, need to be admitted to the ICU for completion of therapy and monitoring. For refractory status epilepticus, an intravenous bolus of midazolam, propofol, pentobarbital, or thiopental is usually initially used with maintenance of a corresponding continuous intravenous drip. This is done in the ICU. Subsequent boluses and adjustment of the rate of the infusion are usually made depending on clinical and EEG response. Because most of these patients need to be intubated and paralyzed, the EEG becomes the method of choice by which to follow them. The goal is to stop electrographic seizure activity before reducing the therapy. Usually this implies achievement of complete flattening of the EEG. Some consider that achieving a burst suppression pattern may be enough, and the periods of flattening in such a case need to be >5 sec. However, this is an area that is in need of further study.

Patients on these therapies require careful attention to blood pressure and to systemic complications, and some develop multiorgan failure. It is not unusual for patients put into pentobarbital coma to have to be on multiple pressors to maintain their blood pressure during therapy.

The choice among options to treat refractory status epilepticus often depends on the experience of the specific center. Midazolam probably has fewer side effects but is less effective, and barbiturate coma is more effective but carries a higher risk of side effects. On propofol, some patients develop a propofol infusion syndrome with lactic acidosis, hemodynamic instability, and rhabdomyolysis with higher infusion rates (>67 µg/kg/min). Thus electrolytes, creatine phosphokinase, and organ function studies need to be monitored. Often, barbiturate coma and similar therapies are maintained for 1 or more days before it is possible to gradually taper the therapy, usually over a few days. However, in some cases, including cases of new onset refractory status epilepticus (NORSE), such therapies need to be maintained for several weeks or even months. Even though the prognosis in NORSE cases is often poor and many patients do not survive, meaningful recovery despite a prolonged course is still possible. Occasionally, inhalational anesthetics are useful. Probably isoflorane is preferable because halothane can increase intracranial pressure and enflurane can induce seizures.

For nonconvulsive status epilepticus and epilepsia partialis continua, therapy needs to be tailored according to the clinical manifestations and often consists of trials of sequential oral or sometimes parenteral AEDs without resorting to barbiturate coma or overmedication that could result in respiratory compromise. The approach to complex partial status epilepticus is sometimes similar to the approach to convulsive status epilepticus and sometimes intermediate between the approach for epilepsia partialis and that for convulsive status, depending on severity. Long-term consequences after complex partial status epilepticus have been reported, but the complications might also be less severe than those after convulsive status epilepticus. Prolonged nonconvulsive complex partial status epilepticus can last for as much as 4-12 wk, with patients manifesting psychotic symptoms and confusional states. These cases can be resistant to therapy. Despite that, patients still can have a full recovery. Some of these cases appear to improve with the use of steroids or intravenous gamma globulin, which are used if an autoimmune, parainfectious etiology is suspected. Potential therapies under study for convulsive status epilepticus include induction of acidosis (e.g., by hypercapnia), which reduces neuronal excitability and hypothermia. A ketogenic diet has been advocated by some for selected cases of status epilepticus, such as children suffering from FIRES.

BIBLIOGRAPHY

Please visit the Nelson Textbook of Pediatrics *website at www.expertconsult.com for the complete bibliography.*

Chapter 587
Conditions That Mimic Seizures

Mohamad A. Mikati and Makram Obeid

The misdiagnosis of epilepsy has been estimated to be as high as 5-40%, implying that many patients may be subjected to unnecessary therapy and tests. Often all that is needed to differentiate nonepileptic paroxysmal disorders from epilepsy is a careful history and thorough exam; but sometimes, more advanced testing may be necessary. Nonepileptic paroxysmal disorders can be classified according to the age of presentation and the clinical manifestations: (1) generalized paroxysms, (2) abnormal movements and postures, (3) oculomotor abnormalities, and (4) sleep-related disorders (see Table 587-1 on the *Nelson Textbook of Pediatrics* website at www.expertconsult.com).

For the full continuation of this chapter, please visit the Nelson Textbook of Pediatrics *website at www.expertconsult.com.*

Chapter 588
Headaches

Andrew D. Hershey

Headache is a common complaint in children and teenagers. Headaches can be a primary problem themselves or represent a symptom of another disorder and therefore represent a secondary headache. Recognizing this difference is essential for choosing the appropriate evaluation and treatment to ensure successful management of the headache. Primary headaches are most often recurrent, episodic headaches and for most children are sporadic in their presentation.

The most common forms of primary headaches of childhood are migraine and tension-type headaches with other forms of primary headaches including the trigeminal autonomic cephalalgias occurring much less commonly. The primary headaches can progress to very frequent headaches with chronic migraine and chronic tension-type headaches being increasingly recognized. These more frequent headaches can have an enormous impact on the life of the child and adolescent, as reflected in school absences and decreased school performance, social withdrawal, and changes in family interactions. To reduce this impact, a treatment strategy that incorporates acute treatments, preventive treatments, and biobehavioral therapies must be implemented.

Secondary headaches are headaches that are a symptom of an underlying illness. The underlying illness should be clearly present as a direct cause of the headaches. This is often difficult when 2 or more common conditions occur in close temporal association. This frequently leads to the misdiagnosis of a primary headache as a secondary headache. This is frequently the case when migraine is misdiagnosed as a sinus headache. In general, the key components of a secondary headache are the likely direct cause and effect relationship between the headache and the precipitating condition, and the lower likelihood in this specific patient and circumstance of the headaches being the result of a recurrent headache disorder. In addition, once the underlying suspected cause is treated, the secondary headache should resolve. If this does not occur, either the diagnosis must be re-evaluated or the effectiveness of the treatment reassessed. One key clue that additional investigation is warranted is the presence of an abnormal neurologic examination or unusual neurologic symptoms.

588.1 Migraine

Andrew D. Hershey

Migraine is the most frequent type of recurrent headache that is brought to the attention of parents and primary care providers. Migraine is characterized by episodic headaches that may be moderate to severe in intensity, focal in location on the head, have a throbbing quality, and may be associated with nausea, vomiting, light sensitivity, and sound sensitivity. Migraine can also be associated with an aura that may be typical (visual, sensory, or dysphasic) or atypical (i.e., hemiplegic, Alice in Wonderland syndrome). In addition, a number of migraine variants have been described and, in children, include abdominal related symptoms without headaches and components of the periodic syndromes of childhood. Treatment of migraine requires the incorporation of an acute treatment plan, a preventive treatment plan if the migraine occurs frequently or is disabling, and a biobehavioral plan to help cope with both the acute attacks and frequent or persistent attacks if present.

EPIDEMIOLOGY

Up to 75% of children report having a significant headache (migraine) by the time they are 15 yr old. Recurrent headaches are less common, but remain highly frequent. Migraine has been reported to occur in up to 10.6% of children between the ages of 5 and 15 yr, and up to 28% of older adolescents. When the headaches become frequent, they convert into chronic daily headaches in up to 1.0% of children.

There are small differences in incidence geographically, but migraine remains common across all areas of the world. Indeed, migraine remains one of the most frequently encountered afflictions of childhood.

Migraine can impact a patient's life through school absences, limitation of home activities, and restriction of social activities. As headaches become more frequent, their negative impact increases in magnitude. This can lead to further complications including anxiety and school avoidance, requiring a more extensive treatment plan.

CLASSIFICATION AND CLINICAL MANIFESTATIONS

Criteria have been established to guide the clinical and scientific study of headaches; these are summarized in *The International Classification of Headache Disorders,* 2nd edition (ICHD-II). The different clinical types of migraine are contrasted in Table 588-1. The specific criteria for migraine without aura and migraine with aura are listed in Table 588-2.

Migraine without Aura

Migraine without aura is the most common form of migraine in both children and adults. The ICHD-II (see Table 588-2) requires this to be recurrent (at least 5 headaches that meet the criteria, but there is no time limit over which this must occur). The recurrent episodic nature helps differentiate this from a secondary headache, as well as separates migraine from tension-type headache, but may limit the diagnosis in children as they may just be beginning to have headaches.

The duration of the headache is defined as 4-72 hr for adults. It has been recognized that children may have shorter duration headaches, so an allowance has been made to reduce this duration to 2-72 hr or 1-72 hr with diary confirmation. Note that this duration is for the untreated or unsuccessfully treated headache. Furthermore, if the child falls asleep with the headache, the entire sleep period is considered part of the duration. These duration limits help differentiate migraine from both short duration headaches, including the trigeminal autonomic cephalalgias, and prolonged headaches, like those due to pseudotumor cerebri. Some prolonged headaches may still be migraine, but a migraine that

Table 588-1 INTERNATIONAL CLASSIFICATION OF HEADACHE DISORDERS, 2ND EDITION*

MIGRAINE	ICHD-II CODE
Migraine without aura	1.1
Migraine with aura	1.2
Typical aura with migraine headache	1.2.1
Typical migraine with nonmigraine headache	1.2.2
Typical aura without headache	1.2.3
Familial hemiplegic migraine	1.2.4
Sporadic hemiplegic migraine	1.2.5
Basilar-type migraine	1.2.6
Childhood periodic syndromes that are commonly precursors of migraine	1.3
Cyclic vomiting	1.3.1
Abdominal migraine	1.3.2
Benign paroxysmal vertigo of childhood	1.3.3
Retinal migraine	1.4
Complications of migraine	1.5
Chronic migraine	1.5.1
Status migrainosus	1.5.2
Persistent aura without infarction	1.5.3
Migrainous infarction	1.5.4
Probable migraine	1.6

*Headache Classification Subcommittee of the International Headache Society: The International Classification of Headache Disorders: 2nd edition, *Cephalalgia* 24(Suppl 1):9–160, 2004.

Table 588-2 ICHD-II CRITERIA FOR MIGRAINE WITHOUT AURA AND MIGRAINE WITH AURA*

MIGRAINE WITHOUT AURA (ICHD-II, 1.1)
I. At least 5 attacks fulfilling B-D
II. Headaches lasting 4-72 hr (untreated or unsuccessfully treated)
III. Headaches with at least two characteristics
A. Unilateral location
B. Pulsating quality
C. Moderate of severe pain intensity
D. Aggravation by or causing avoidance of routine physical activity
IV. During the headache have at least 1 of the following:
A. Nausea and/or vomiting
B. Photophobia and phonophobia
V. Not attributed to another disorder
MIGRAINE WITH AURA, TYPICAL (ICHD-II, 1.2.1)
I. At least 2 attacks fulfilling criteria II-IV
II. Aura consists of at least 1 of the following, but no motor weakness
A. Fully reversible visual symptoms
B. Fully reversible sensory symptoms
C. Fully reversible dysphasic speech disturbance
III. At least 2 of the following
A. Homonymous visual symptoms and/or unilateral sensory symptoms
B. At least 1 aura symptom develops gradually over ≧5 min and/or different aura symptoms occur in succession over ≧5 min
C. Each symptom lasts ≧5 and ≦60 min
IV. Headache fulfilling criteria II-IV for migraine without aura begins during the aura or follows within 60 min
V. Not attributed to another disorder

persists beyond 72 hr is classified as a variant termed **status migrainosus.**

The quality of migraine pain is often, but not always, throbbing or pounding. This may be difficult to elicit in young children and drawings or demonstrations may help confirm the throbbing quality.

The location of the pain has classically been described as **unilateral (hemicrania)**; in children it is more commonly bilateral. A more appropriate way to think of the location would therefore be focal in location to differentiate it from the diffuse location of tension-type headaches. Of particular concern is the exclusively occipital headache as, although these can be migraines, they are more frequently secondary to another, more proximate etiology.

Migraine, when allowed to fully develop, often worsens in the face of and secondarily results in altered activity level. This has been classically identified in adults as resulting from worsening of pain when, for example, going up or down stairs. This history is often not elicited in children. A change in the child's activity pattern, however, can be easily observed by a reduction in play or physical activity. For older children, sports or exercise may be limited or restricted during a headache attack.

Migraine may have a variety of associated symptoms. In younger children, nausea and vomiting may be the most obvious symptoms and often outweigh the headache itself. This often leads to the overlap with several of the gastrointestinal periodic diseases, including recurrent abdominal pain, recurrent vomiting, cyclic vomiting, and abdominal migraine. The commonality of all of these related conditions is an increased propensity for the later development of migraine. Oftentimes, early childhood recurrent vomiting may in fact be migraine, but the child is not asked about headache pain or is unable to describe headache pain. Once this becomes clear, the earlier diagnosis of a gastrointestinal disorder is no longer appropriate. When headache is present, vomiting raises the concern of a secondary headache, particularly related to increased intracranial pressure. One of the red flags for this is the daily or near daily early morning vomiting that increases in intensity as the intracranial pressure continues to build. When the headache with vomiting episodes are episodic and not worsening, it is more likely that the diagnosis is migraine. Vomiting and headache due to increased intracranial pressure are frequently present on first awakening and remit with maintenance of upright posture. In contrast, if a migraine is present on first awakening *(a relatively infrequent occurrence in children)*, getting up and going about normal, upright activities usually makes the headache and vomiting worse.

As the child ages, light and sound sensitivity (**photophobia and phonophobia**) may become more apparent. This is either by direct report of the patient, or the interpretation by the parents of the child's activity. These symptoms are likely a component of the hypersensitivity that develops during an acute migraine attack and may also include smell sensitivity (osmophobia) and touch sensitivity (cutaneous allodynia with central sensitization). Although only the photophobia and phonophobia are components of the ICHD-II criteria, these other symptoms are helpful in confirming the diagnosis and may be helpful in understanding the underlying pathophysiology and determining the response to treatment.

The final ICHD-II requirement is the exclusion of causes of secondary headaches, and this should be an integral component of the headache history.

Although not part of the ICHD-II criteria, it has been recognized migraine typically runs in families with reports up to 90% of children having a first- or second-degree relative with recurrent headaches. Given the underdiagnosis and misdiagnosis in adults, this is often not recognized by the family and a headache family history is required. When a family history is not identified, this may be due to either unawareness of migraine within the family or an underlying secondary headache in the child. Any child whose family, upon close and both direct and indirect questioning, does not include individuals with migraine or related syndromes (e.g., motion sickness, cyclic vomiting, menstrual headache), should have an imaging procedure performed to look for anatomic etiologies for headache.

In addition to the classifying features, there may additional markers of a migraine disorder. These include such things as triggers (skipping meals, inadequate or irregular sleep, dehydration and weather changes are the most common), pattern recognition (associated with menstrual periods in adolescents or Monday morning headaches due to change in sleep patterns over the weekend and nonphysiologic early waking on Monday mornings for school), and prodromes (a feeling of irritability, tiredness, and food cravings prior to the start of the headache). Although these additional features may not be consistent, they do raise the index of suspicion for migraine and provide a potential mechanism of intervention. In the past, food triggers were considered widely common, but the majority of these have either been discredited with scientific study or represent such a small number of patients that they only need to be addressed when consistently triggering the headache.

Migraine with Aura

The aura associated with migraine is a neurologic warning that a migraine is going to occur. In the common forms this can be the start of a typical migraine or a headache without migraine, or it may even occur in isolation. For a typical aura, the aura needs to be visual, sensory, or dysphasic, lasting longer than 5 min and less than 60 min with the headache starting within 60 min (see Table 588-2). The importance of the aura lasting longer than 5 min is to differentiate the migraine aura from a seizure with a postictal headache, while the 60 min maximal duration is to separate migraine aura from the possibility of a more prolonged neurologic event such as a transient ischemic attack.

The most common type of visual aura in children and adolescents is **photopsia** (flashes of light or light bulbs going off everywhere). These photopsias are often multiple colored and when gone, the child may report not being able to see where the flash occurred. Less likely in children are the typical adult auras including fortification spectra (brilliant white zigzag lines resembling a starred pattern castle) or shimmering scotoma (sometimes described as a shining spot that grows or a sequined curtain closing). In adults the auras typically involve only half the visual field, while in children they may be randomly dispersed. Blurred vision is often confused as an aura, but is difficult to separate from photophobia or difficulty concentrating during the pain of the headache.

Sensory auras are less common. They typically occur unilaterally. Many children describe this sensation as insects are worms crawling from their hand, up their arm to their face with a numbness following this sensation. Once the numbness occurs, the child may have difficulty using the arm as they have lost sensory input, and a misdiagnosis of hemiplegic migraine may be made.

Dysphasic auras are the least common type of typical aura and have been described as an inability or difficulty to respond verbally. The patient afterwards will describe an ability to understand what is being asked, but cannot answer back. This may be the basis of what in the past has been referred to a confusional migraine and special attention needs to be paid to asking the child about this possibility and their degree of understanding during the initial phases of the attack.

Much less commonly, atypical forms of aura can occur, including hemiplegia (true weakness, not numbness, and may be familial), vertigo or lower cranial nerve symptoms (basilar-type, formerly thought to be due to basilar artery dysfunction, now thought to be more brainstem based), and distortion (Alice in Wonderland syndrome). Whenever these rarer forms of aura are present, further investigation is warranted.

Hemiplegic migraine is one of the better known forms of rare auras. This transient unilateral weakness usually lasts only a few hours, but may persist for days. Both familial and sporadic forms have been described. The familial hemiplegic migraine (FHM) is an autosomal dominant disorder with mutations described in 3 separate genes: (1) *CACNA1A,* (2) *ATP1A2,* and (3) *SCN1A.* Multiple polymorphisms have been described for these genes.

Basilar-type migraine was formerly considered a disease of the basilar artery as many of the unique symptoms were attributed to dysfunction in this area of the brainstem. Some of the symptoms described include vertigo, tinnitus, diplopia, blurred vision, scotoma, ataxia, and an occipital headache. The pupils may be dilated, and ptosis may be evident.

HaNDL (transient headache with neurologic deficits, CSF pleocytosis) is considered a pseudomigraine syndrome.

Childhood periodic syndromes are a group of potentially related symptoms that occur in increased frequency in children with migraine. The hallmark of these symptoms is the recurrent episodic nature of the events. Some of these have included gastrointestinal-related symptoms (motion sickness, recurrent abdominal pain, recurrent vomiting including cyclic vomiting, and abdominal migraine), sleep disorders (sleepwalking, sleep-talking, and night terrors), unexplained recurrent fevers, and even seizures.

The gastrointestinal symptoms span the spectrum from the relatively mild (motion sickness on occasional long car rides) to severe episodes of uncontrollable vomiting that may lead to dehydration and the need for hospital admission to receive fluids. These latter episodes may occur on a predictable time schedule and hence have been called **cyclic vomiting.** During these attacks, the child may appear pale and frightened but does not lose consciousness. After a period of deep sleep, the child awakens and resumes normal play and eating habits as if the vomiting had not occurred. Many children with cyclic vomiting have a positive family history of migraine, and as they grow older have a high association with the development of migraine. Cyclic vomiting may be responsive to migraine-specific therapies with careful attention to fluid replacement if the vomiting is excessive. Cyclic vomiting of migraine must be differentiated from gastrointestinal disorders including intestinal obstruction (malrotation, intermittent volvulus, duodenal web, duplication cysts, superior mesenteric artery compression, internal hernias), peptic ulcer, gastritis, giardiasis, chronic pancreatitis, and Crohn disease. Abnormal gastrointestinal motility and pelviureteric junction obstruction can also cause cyclic vomiting. Metabolic causes include disorders of amino acid metabolism (heterozygote ornithine transcarbamylase deficiency), organic acidurias (propionic acidemia, methylmalonic acidemia), fatty acid oxidation defects (medium-chain acyl-CoA dehydrogenase deficiency), disorders of carbohydrate metabolism (hereditary fructose intolerance), acute intermittent porphyria, and structural central nervous system (CNS) lesions (posterior fossa brain tumors, subdural hematoma or effusions).

The diagnosis of **abdominal migraine** can be confusing, but can be thought of as a migraine without the headache. Like a migraine, it is an episodic disorder characterized by mid-abdominal pain with pain-free periods between attacks. At times this pain can be associated with nausea and vomiting (thus crossing into the recurrent abdominal pain or cyclic vomiting spectrum). The pain is usually described as "dull" and may be moderate to severe. The pain may persist from 1 to 72 hr and, although usually midline, may be periumbilical or poorly localized by the child. To meet the criteria of abdominal migraine, the child must complain at the time of the abdominal pain of at least 2 of the following: anorexia, nausea, vomiting, or pallor. As with cyclic vomiting, a thorough history and physical examination with appropriate laboratory studies must be completed to rule out an underlying gastrointestinal disorder as a cause of the abdominal pain. Careful questioning about the presence of headache or head pain needs to be addressed directly with the child, as many times this is truly a migraine, but in the child's mind (as well as the parents' observation) the abdominal symptoms are paramount.

DIAGNOSIS AND DIFFERENTIAL DIAGNOSIS

A thorough history and physical examination including a neurologic examination with special focus on headache has been shown to be the most sensitive indicator of an underlying etiology. The history needs to include a thorough evaluation of the prodromic symptoms, any potential triggering events or timing of the headaches, associated neurologic symptoms, and a detailed characterization of the headache attacks, including frequency, severity, duration, associated symptoms, use of medication, and disability. The disability assessment should include the impact on school, home, and social activities and can easily be assessed with tools such as PedMIDAS. Family history of headaches and any other neurologic, psychiatric, and general health conditions is also important both for identification of migraine within the family as well as the identification of possible secondary headache disorders. The familial penetrance of migraine is so robust that the absence of a family history of migraine or its equivalent phenomena should trigger obtaining of an imaging procedure. When headaches are refractory, a history of potential co-morbid conditions that may influence adherence and acceptability of the treatment plan may also need to be addressed.

Neuroimaging is warranted when the neurologic examination is abnormal or unusual neurologic features occur during the migraine; when the child has headaches that awaken him or her from sleep or that are present on first awakening and remit with upright posture; when the child has brief headaches that only occur with cough or bending over; and when the child has migrainous headache with an absolutely negative family history of migraine or its equivalent (e.g., motion sickness, cyclic vomiting) (Table 588-3). In this case, an MRI is the imaging of choice as it provides the highest sensitivity of detecting posterior fossa lesions and does not expose the child to radiation. The greatest concern in younger children is sedation for the MRI. Special attention should be paid if the location of the pain is exclusively occipital as this has been associated with a higher risk of an underlying pathologic process.

When the presentation is atypical, as in the child with a headache that is instantaneously at its worst at onset, further

Table 588-3 INDICATIONS FOR NEUROIMAGING IN A CHILD WITH HEADACHES
Abnormal neurologic examination
Abnormal or focal neurologic signs or symptoms
• Focal neurologic symptoms or signs developing during a headache (i.e., complicated migraine)
• Focal neurologic symptoms or signs (except classic visual symptoms of migraine) develop during the aura, with fixed laterality; focal signs of the aura persisting or recurring in the headache phase
Seizures or very brief auras (<5 min)
Unusual headaches in children
• Atypical auras including basilar-type, hemiplegic
• Trigeminal autonomic cephalalgia including cluster headaches in child or adolescent
• An acute secondary headache (i.e., headache with known underlying illness or insult)
Headache in children <6 yr old or any child that cannot adequately describe their headache
Brief cough headache in a child or adolescent
Headache worst on first awakening or that awakens the child from sleep
Migrainous headache in the child with no family history of migraine or its equivalent

investigation may be warranted. This should be directed to the underlying suspected secondary cause. For example, the child with the "thunderclap" headache should have a CT scan looking for blood and, if it is negative, a lumbar puncture looking especially for xanthochromia of the cerebrospinal fluid. There is no evidence that laboratory studies or electroencephalogram are beneficial in a typical migraine without aura or migraine with aura.

TREATMENT (TABLE 588-4)

The American Academy of Neurology established useful practice guidelines for the management of migraine as follows:

1. Reduction of headache frequency, severity, duration, and disability
2. Reduction of reliance on poorly tolerated, ineffective, or unwanted acute pharmacotherapies
3. Improvement in quality of life
4. Avoidance of acute headache medication escalation
5. Education and enabling of patients to manage their disease to enhance personal control of their migraine
6. Reduction of headache-related distress and psychologic symptoms

In order to accomplish these goals, 3 components need to be incorporated into the treatment plan:

1. An acute treatment strategy should be developed for stopping a headache attack on a consistent basis with return to function.
2. A preventive treatment strategy should be considered when the headaches are frequent (1/wk or more) and disabling.
3. Biobehavioral therapy should be started, including a discussion of adherence, elimination of barriers to treatment, and healthy habit management.

Acute Treatment

Management of an acute attack is to provide headache freedom as quickly as possible with return to normal function. This mainly includes 2 groups of medicines: nonsteroidal antiinflammatory drugs (NSAIDs) and triptans. Most migraine headaches in children will respond to appropriate doses of NSAIDs when administered at the onset of the headache attack. Ibuprofen has been the most well documented at a dose of 7.5-10 mg/kg. Special concerns for the use of ibuprofen or other NSAIDs is ensuring that the children can recognize and respond to onset of the headache. This includes discussing the importance of telling the teacher when the headache starts at school and ensuring that proper dosing guidelines and permission have been provided to the school. In addition, overuse needs to be avoided, limiting the NSAID (or any combination of over-the-counter [OTC] analgesics) to not more that 2-3 times per week. If ibuprofen is not effective, naproxen sodium may also be tried in similar doses, and for older children (>15 yr old) aspirin may be effective. The goal of the primary acute medication should be headache relief within 1 hr with return to function in 10 out of 10 headaches.

When a migraine is especially severe, NSAIDs alone may not be sufficient. In this case a triptan may be considered. Currently, only almotriptan has been approved by the U.S. Food and Drug Administration (FDA) for the treatment of acute migraine in adolescents (age 12-17 yr). There have been multiple studies that have demonstrated their effectiveness and tolerability. The difficulty with these studies was that effectiveness of the triptans was the same as in adults, but the placebo effectiveness rate was higher than in studies with an "adult design." For most adolescents, dosing is the same as for adults; a reduction in dose is made for small adolescents or younger children. The triptans vary by rapidity of onset and biologic half-life. This is related to both their variable lipophilicity and dose. Clinically, 60-70% of patients respond to the 1st triptan tried, with 60-70% of the patients that did not respond to the 1st triptan responding to the next triptan. Therefore, in the patient who does not respond to the 1st triptan in the desired way (rapid reproducible response without relapse or side effects), it is worthwhile to try a different triptan. The most common side effects of the triptans are due to their mechanism of action—tightness in the jaw, chest, and fingers due to vascular constriction and a subsequent feeling of grogginess and fatigue due to the central serotonin effect. The vascular constriction symptoms can be alleviated through adequate fluid hydration during an attack.

The most effective way to administer the NSAIDs and triptans is to use the NSAIDs first, restricting their use to fewer than 2-3 times per wk, and adding the triptan for moderate to severe attacks, restricting their use to not more than 4-6 times per mo.

As vascular dilatation is a common feature of migraine that may be responsible for some of the facial flushing followed by paleness and the lightheaded feeling accompanying the attacks, fluid hydration should be integrated into the acute treatment plan. For oral hydration this can include the sports drinks that combine electrolytes and sugar to provide the intravascular rehydration.

In the past, antiemetics were used for acute treatment of the nausea and vomiting. Further study has identified that their unique mechanism of effectiveness in headache treatment is related to their antagonism of dopaminergic neurotransmission. Therefore, the antiemetics with the most robust dopamine antagonism (i.e., prochlorperazine and metoclopramide) have the best efficacy. These can be very effective for status migrainosus or a migraine that is unresponsive to the NSAIDs and triptans. They require intravenous administration, as other forms of administration of these drugs are less effective than the NSAIDs or triptans. When combined with ketorolac and intravenous fluids in the emergency department or an acute infusion center, intravenous antiemetics can be very effective. When they are not effective, further inpatient treatment may be required using dihydroergotomine (DHE).

Preventive Therapy

When the headaches are frequent (≧1/wk) or disabling (missing school, home, or social activities, or a PedMIDAS score above 20), preventive or **prophylactic therapy** is warranted. The goal of this therapy should to be to reduce frequency (1-2 headaches or fewer per mo) and disability (PedMIDAS <10). Prophylactic agents should be given for at least 4-6 mo at an adequate dose and then weaned over several weeks' time. Evidence in adult studies has begun to demonstrate that persistent frequent headaches foreshadow an increased risk of progression with decreased

Table 588-4 DRUGS USED IN THE MANAGEMENT OF MIGRAINE HEADACHES IN CHILDREN

DRUG	DOSE	MECHANISM	SIDE EFFECTS	COMMENTS
ACUTE MIGRAINE				
Analgesics				
Acetaminophen	15 mg/kg/dose	Analgesic effects	Overdose, fatal hepatic necrosis	Effectiveness limited in migraine
Ibuprofen	7.5-10 mg/kg/dose	Antiinflammatory and analgesic	GI bleeding stomach upset, kidney injury	Avoid overuse (2-3 times per wk)
Triptans (Only Almotriptan Approved for Use for Adolescents)				
Almotriptan	12.5 mg	5-HT1b/1d agonist	Vascular constriction, serotonin symptoms	Avoid overuse (more than 4-6 times per mo)
Eletriptan	40 mg	Same	Same	Avoid overuse (more than 4-6 times per mo)
Frovatriptan	2.5 mg	Same	Same	May be effective for menstrual migraine prevention Avoid overuse (more than 4-6 times per mo)
Naratriptan	2.5 mg	Same	Same	May be effective for menstrual migraine prevention Avoid overuse (more than 4-6 times per mo)
Rizatriptan	5 mg, 10 mg	Same	Same	Available in tablets and melts Avoid overuse (more than 4-6 times per mo)
Sumatriptan	Oral: 25 mg, 50 mg, 100 mg Nasal: 10 mg Subcutaneous: 6 mg	Same	Same	Avoid overuse (more than 4-6 times per mo)
Zolmitriptan	Oral: 2.5 mg, 5 mg Nasal: 5 mg	Same	Same	Available in tablets and melts Avoid overuse (more than 4-6 times per mo)
PROPHYLAXIS (NONE APPROVED BY FDA FOR CHILDREN)				
Calcium Channel Blockers				
Flunarizine*	5 mg hs	Calcium channel blocking agent	Headache, lethargy, dizziness	May ↑ to 10 mg hs
Anticonvulsants				
Valproic acid	20 mg/kg/24 hr (begin 5 mg/kg/24 hr)	↑ brain GABA	Nausea, pancreatitis, fatal hepatotoxicity	↑ 5 mg/kg every 2 wk
Topiramate	100-200 mg divided BID	↑ activity of GABA	Fatigue, nervousness	Increase slowly over 12-16 wk
Levatiracetam	20-60 mg/kg divided BID	Unknown	Irritability, fatigue	Increase every 2 wk starting at 20 mg/kg divided BID
Gabapentin	900-1800 mg divided BID	Unknown	Somnolence, fatigue aggression, weight gain	Begin 300 mg, ↑ 300 mg/wk
Antidepressants				
Amitriptyline	1.0 mg/kg/day	↑ CNS serotonin and norepinephrine	Cardiac conduction, abnormalities and dry mouth, constipation, drowsiness, confusion	Increase by 0.25 mg/kg every 2 wk Morning sleepiness reduced by administration at dinnertime
Antihistamines				
Cyproheptadine	0.2-0.4 mg/kg divided BID	H_1-receptor and serotonin agonist	Drowsiness, thick bronchial secretions	Max 0.5 mg/kg/24 hr
Antihypertensive				
Propranolol (contraindicated in asthma and depression)	10-20 mg tid	Nonselective β-adrenergic blocking agent	Dizziness, lethargy	Begin 10 mg/24 hr ↑ 10 mg/wk
SEVERE INTRACTABLE				
Prochlorperazine	0.15 mg/kg/IV	Dopamine antagonist	Agitation, muscle stiffness	May have increased effectiveness when combined with ketolorac and fluid hydration

*Not available in USA.
GABA, γ-aminobutyric acid; GI, gastrointestinal; hs, at night; SC, subcutaneous.

responsiveness and increased risk of refractoriness in the future. It is unclear if this also occurs in children and/or adolescents and if early treatment of headache in childhood prevents development of refractory headache in adulthood.

Multiple preventive medications have been utilized for migraine prophylaxis in children. When analyzed as part of a practice parameter, only one medication—flunarizine—was demonstrated to reach a level of effectiveness viewed as substantial and it is not available in the USA. Flunarizine is typically dosed at 5 mg orally daily and increased after 1 mo to 10 mg orally daily, with a month off of drug every 4-6 mo.

The most commonly used preventive therapy for headache and migraine is amitriptyline. It was first used for this purpose in the 1970s and has subsequently been used worldwide as one of the first-line preventive agents. Typically a dose of 1 mg/kg daily at dinner or in the evening is effective. However, this dose needs to be reached slowly (i.e., over weeks) to minimize side effects and improve tolerability. The most common side effects are those related to amitriptyline's anticholinergic activity and sleepiness. Weight gain has been observed in adults using amitriptyline but is less frequent in children. Amitriptyline does have the potential to exacerbate prolonged QT syndrome, so it should be avoided in patients with this diagnosis and looked for in patients on the drug who complain of rapid or irregular heart rate.

Antiepileptic medications are more recently commonly used for migraine prophylaxis, with topiramate, valproic acid, and levetiracetam having been demonstrated to be effective in adults. There are limited studies in children for migraine prevention, but all of these medications have been assessed for safety and tolerability in children with epilepsy.

Topiramate has become widely used for migraine prophylaxis in adults. Topiramate has also been demonstrated to be effective in an adolescent study. This study demonstrated that a 25-mg dose twice a day was equivalent to placebo, while a 50-mg dose twice a day was superior. Thus it appears that the adult dosing schedule is also effective in adolescents with an effective dosage range or 50 mg twice a day to 100 mg twice a day. This dose needs to be reached slowly to minimize the cognitive slowing associated with topiramate use. Additional side effects include weight loss, paresthesias, kidney stones, lowered bicarbonate levels, decreased sweating, and rarely glaucoma and changes in serum transaminases. In addition, in adolescent girls taking birth control pills the lowering of the effectiveness of the birth control by topiramate needs to be discussed.

Valproic acid has long been used for epilepsy in children and has been demonstrated to be effective in migraine prophylaxis in adults. The effective dose in children appears to be 10 mg/kg orally twice a day. Side effects of weight gain, ovarian cysts, and changes in serum transaminases and platelet counts need to be monitored.

Other antiepileptics including lamotrigine, levetiracetam, zonisamide, gabapentin, and pregabalin have also been used for migraine prevention.

β-Blockers have also been used for migraine prevention. The studies on β-blockers have a mixed response pattern with variability both between β-blockers and between patients with a given β-blocker. Propranolol has been the best studied for pediatric migraine prevention with unequivocally positive results. The contraindication for use of propranolol in children with asthma or allergic disorders or diabetes and the increased incidence of depression in adolescents using propranolol limit its use somewhat. It may be very effective for a mixed subtype of migraine (basilar-type migraine with postural orthostatic tachycardia syndrome [BAM-POTS]). This syndrome has been reported to be responsive to propranolol.

In very young children, cyproheptadine may be effective in prevention of migraine or the related variants. Young children tend to tolerate the increased appetite induced by the cyproheptadine and tend not to be subject to the lethargy seen in older children and adults; the weight gain is limiting once children start to enter puberty. Typical dosing is 0.1 to 0.2 mg/kg orally twice a day.

Biobehavioral Therapy

Biobehavioral evaluation and therapy is essential for effective migraine management. This includes identification of behavioral barriers to treatment, like a child's shyness or limitation in notifying a teacher of the start of a migraine or a teacher's unwillingness to accept the need for treatment. Additional barriers include a lack of recognition of the significance of their headache problem and reverting to "bad habits" once the headaches have responded to treatment. Adherence is equally important for acute and preventive treatment. The need to have a sustained response for long enough to prevent relapse (i.e., to stay on preventive medication) is often difficult when the child starts to feel better. Having a defined end-point and duration (1-2 or fewer headaches per mo for 4-6 mo) helps with acceptance.

As many of the potential triggers for frequent migraines (skipping meals, dehydration, decreased or altered sleep) are related to a child's daily routine, a discussion of healthy habits is a component of biobehavioral therapy. This should include adequate fluid intake without caffeine, regular exercise, not skipping meals and making healthy food choices, and adequate (8-9 hr) sleep on a regular basis. Sleep is often difficult in adolescents, as middle and high schools often have very early start times, and the adolescent's sleep architecture features a shift to later sleep onset and waking. This has been one of the explanations for worsening headaches during the school years in general and at the beginning of the school year and week.

Biofeedback-assisted relaxation therapy has been demonstrated to be effective for both acute and preventive therapy and may be incorporated into this multiple treatment strategy. This provides the child with a degree of self-control over the headaches and may further help the child cope with frequent headaches.

BIBLIOGRAPHY

Please visit the Nelson Textbook of Pediatrics *website at www.expertconsult.com for the complete bibliography.*

588.2 Secondary Headaches

Andrew D. Hershey

Headaches can be a common symptom of other underlying illnesses. In recognition of this, the ICHD-II has classified the potential secondary headaches (Table 588-5). The key to the diagnosis of a secondary headache is to recognize the underlying cause and demonstrate a direct cause and effect. Until this has been demonstrated the diagnosis is speculative. This is especially true when the suspected etiology is common.

Common causes or suspected causes of secondary headaches in children include the sequelae of head trauma and sinusitis. Post-traumatic headaches often occur in children who have not had a prior history of headaches and are temporally related to the initiating head injury. Frequently, though, these children have a family history of migraine or its equivalent. The head injury may be minor or major and the subsequent headache may be acute (resolves within 3 mo, most typically within 10 days) or chronic (>15 days per mo for more than 3 mo). Bed rest appears to be the most effective treatment for acute post-traumatic headache ("house arrest"), while magnesium supplementation and migraine prophylaxis may also be effective. When a child has a history of episodic headaches, the head trauma or the overuse of daily medications may lead to status migrainosus or chronic migraine and the diagnosis may be difficult to sort out.

Sinus headache is the most overdiagnosed form of recurrent headaches. Although no studies have evaluated the frequency of misdiagnosis of an underlying migraine as a sinus headache in

Table 588-5 SECONDARY HEADACHES WITH SELECTIVE SUBTYPES

DIAGNOSIS	ICHD-II CODE
Headache attributed to head and/or neck trauma	5
Acute post-traumatic headache	5.1
Chronic post-traumatic headache	5.2
Headache attributed to cranial or cervical vascular disorder	6
Headache attributed to nonvascular intracranial disorder	7
Headache attributed to high cerebrospinal fluid pressure	7.1
Headache attributed to low cerebrospinal fluid pressure	7.2
Headache attributed to intracranial neoplasm	7.4
Headache attributed to epileptic seizure	7.6
Headache attributed to a substance or its withdrawal	8
Medication-overuse headaches	8.2
Headache attributed to infection	9
Headache attributed to disorder of homeostasis	10
Headache of facial pain attributed to disorder of cranium, neck, eyes, ears, nose, sinuses, teeth, mouth, or other facial or cranial structures	11
Headache attributed to rhinosinusitis	11.5
Headache attributed to psychiatric disorder	12

children, in adults, it has been found that up to 90% of adults diagnosed as having a sinus headache by either themselves or their physician appear to have migraine. When headaches are recurrent and respond within hours to analgesics, migraine should be considered first. In the absence of purulent nasal discharge, fever, or chronic cough, the diagnosis of sinus headache should not be made.

Medication overuse headaches frequently complicate primary and secondary headaches. Some of the signs that should raise suspicion of medication overuse are the increasing use of analgesics (OTC or prescription) with either decreased effectiveness or frequently wearing off (i.e., analgesic rebound). This can be worsened by using ineffective medications and underdosing or misdiagnosing the headache. Patients should be cautioned against the frequent use of analgesic or antimigraine medication.

Serious causes of secondary headaches are likely to be related to increased intracranial pressure. This can be due to a mass (tumor, vascular malformation, cystic structure) or an instrinsic increase in pressure (benign intracranial hypertension [BIH] or pseudotumor cerebri). In the former case, the headache is due to the mass effect and local pressure on the dura; in the latter case, the headache is due to diffuse pressure on the dura. The etiology of BIH may be the intake of excessive amounts of fat soluble compounds (e.g., vitamin A, retinoic acid, minocycline), hormonal changes (increased incidence in females) or blockage of venous drainage (as with inflammation of the transverse venous sinus from mastoiditis). When increased pressure is suspected, either by historical suspicion or the presence of papilledema, an MRI with magnetic resonance angiography and magnetic resonance venography should be performed, followed by a lumbar puncture if no mass or vascular anomaly is noted. The lumbar puncture can be diagnostic and therapeutic of BIH, but must be performed with the patient in a relaxed recumbent position with legs extended, as abdominal pressure can artificially raise intracranial pressure (ICP). If headache persists or there are visual field changes, pharmaceutical treatment with a carbonic anhydrase inhibitor, optic nerve fenestration, or a shunt needs to be considered.

Additional causes of secondary headaches in children that may not be associated with increased ICP include arteriovenous malformations, berry aneurysm, collagen vascular diseases affecting the CNS, hypertensive encephalopathy, acute subarachnoid hemorrhage, and stroke. The management of secondary headache depends on the cause. Helpful laboratory tests and neuroradiologic procedures depend on the clues provided by the history and physical examination. By definition, a secondary headache has a specific cause and should resolve once this cause is treated. If the headache persists, the diagnosis and treatment should be questioned because either the diagnosis may be incorrect, the headache may be a primary headache, and/or the treatment chosen may have been incorrect.

BIBLIOGRAPHY

Please visit the Nelson Textbook of Pediatrics *website at* *www.expertconsult.com* *for the complete bibliography.*

588.3 Tension-Type Headaches

Andrew D. Hershey

Tension-type headaches (TTH) may be very common in children and adolescents, but due to their mild to moderate nature, relative lack of associated symptoms and lower degree of associated disability they are often ignored or have a minimal impact. The ICHD-II subclassifies TTH as infrequent (<12 times per yr), frequent (1-15 times per mo), and chronic (>15 headaches per mo). They can further be separated into headaches with or without pericranial muscle tightness. The classification of TTH can be likened to the opposite of migraine. Whereas migraine are typically moderate to severe, are focal in location, are worsened by physical activity or limit physical activity, and have a throbbing quality, TTH are mild to moderate in severity, are diffuse in location, are not affected by activity (although the patient may not feel like being active), and are nonthrobbing (often described as a constant pressure). TTH is much less frequently associated with nausea, photophobia, or phonophobia and is never associated with more than 1 of these at a time or with vomiting. Like migraine, TTH must be recurrent, but at least 10 headaches are required and the duration can be 30 min to 7 days. Also, as in migraine, secondary headaches with other underlying etiologies must be ruled out.

Evaluation of patients with suspected TTH requires a detailed headache history and complete general and neurologic examination. This is to establish the diagnosis and ensure exclusion of secondary etiologies. When secondary headaches are suspected, further, directed evaluation is indicated.

Treatment of TTH can require acute therapy to stop attacks, preventive therapy when frequent or chronic and behavioral therapy. It is often suspected that there may be underlying psychologic stressors (hence the misnomer as a "stress" headache), but this is often difficult to identify in children, and although it may be suspected by the parents, it cannot be confirmed in the child. Studies of and conclusive evidence to guide the treatment of TTH in children are lacking, but the same general principles and medications used in migraine can be applied to children with TTH (see Chapter 588.1). Oftentimes, simple analgesics (ibuprofen or acetaminophen) can be effective for acute treatment. Amitriptyline has the most evidence of effective prevention of TTH, while biobehavioral intervention, including biofeedback-assisted relaxation training and coping skills training may also be beneficial.

BIBLIOGRAPHY

Please visit the Nelson Textbook of Pediatrics *website at* *www.expertconsult.com* *for the complete bibliography.*

Chapter 589
Neurocutaneous Syndromes

Mustafa Sahin

The neurocutaneous syndromes include a heterogeneous group of disorders characterized by abnormalities of both the integument and central nervous system (CNS). Most disorders are familial and believed to arise from a defect in differentiation of the primitive ectoderm. Disorders classified as neurocutaneous syndromes include neurofibromatosis, tuberous sclerosis, Sturge-Weber syndrome, von Hippel–Lindau disease, PHACE syndrome, ataxia telangiectasia, linear nevus syndrome, hypomelanosis of Ito, and incontinentia pigmenti.

589.1 Neurofibromatosis

Mustafa Sahin

Neurofibromatoses are autosomal dominant disorders that cause tumors to grow on nerves and result in other abnormalities such as skin changes and bone deformities. It was previously thought that there were 2 types of neurofibromatosis (type 1 and type 2); it is recognized that they are clinically and genetically distinct diseases and should be considered separate entities: neurofibromatosis 1 (NF-1) and neurofibromatosis 2 (NF-2).

CLINICAL MANIFESTATIONS AND DIAGNOSIS

NF-1 is the most prevalent type, with an incidence of 1/3,000, and is diagnosed when any 2 of the following 7 features are

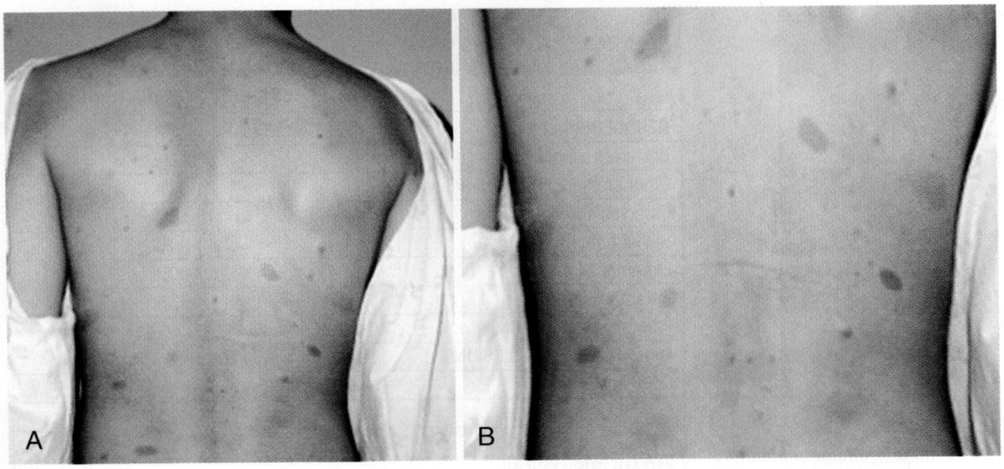

Figure 589-1 *A* and *B,* Multiple café-au-lait spots over the back. Note the dermal neurofibromas below the right scapula and right side of the lower back. (From Hersh JH, Committee on Genetics: Health supervision for children with neurofibromatosis, *Pediatrics* 121:633–642, 2008, Fig 1.)

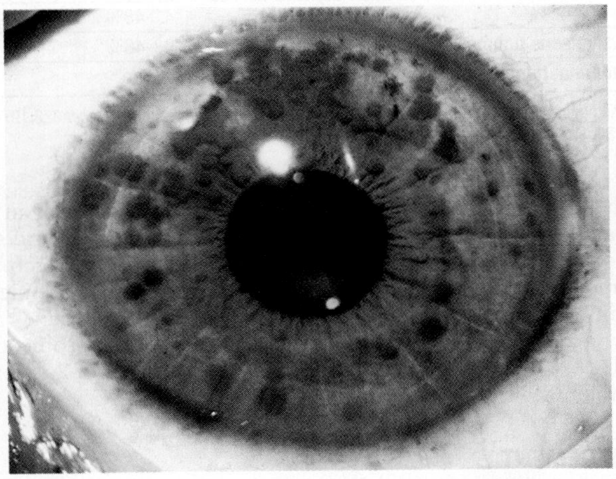

Figure 589-2 Neurofibromatosis 1. Pigmented hamartomas of the iris (Lisch nodules). (From Zitelli BJ, Davis HW: *Atlas of pediatric physical diagnosis,* ed 4, St Louis, 2002, Mosby, p 507.)

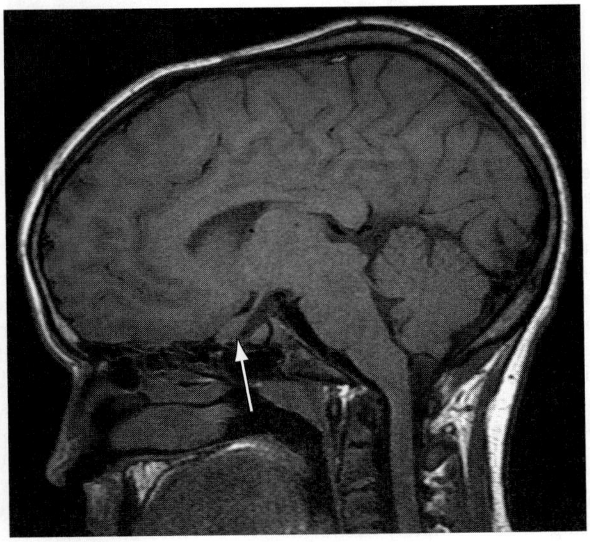

Figure 589-3 Optic glioma. Sagittal T1-weighted MRI scan of a patient with neurofibromatosis 1 shows thickening of the optic nerve *(arrow).*

present: (1) Six or more café-au-lait macules over 5 mm in greatest diameter in prepubertal individuals and over 15 mm in greatest diameter in postpubertal individuals. Café-au-lait spots are the hallmark of neurofibromatosis and are present in almost 100% of patients. They are present at birth but increase in size, number, and pigmentation, especially during the first few yrs of life (Fig. 589-1). The spots are scattered over the body surface, with predilection for the trunk and extremities but sparing the face. (2) Axillary or inguinal freckling consisting of multiple hyperpigmented areas 2-3 mm in diameter. Skinfold freckling usually appears between 3 and 5 yr of age. The frequency of axillary and inguinal freckling has been reported to be greater than 80% by 6 yr of age. (3) Two or more iris Lisch nodules. Lisch nodules are hamartomas located within the iris and are best identified by a slit-lamp examination (Fig. 589-2). They are present in >74% of patients with NF-1 but are not a component of NF-2. The prevalence of Lisch nodules increases with age, from only 5% of children <3 yr of age, to 42% among children 3-4 yr of age, and virtually 100% of adults ≥21 yr of age. (4) Two or more neurofibromas or 1 plexiform neurofibroma. Neurofibromas typically involve the skin, but they may be situated along peripheral nerves and blood vessels and within viscera including the gastrointestinal tract. These lesions appear characteristically during adolescence or pregnancy, suggesting a hormonal influence. They are usually small, rubbery lesions with a slight purplish discoloration of the overlying skin. Plexiform neurofibromas are usually evident at birth and result from diffuse thickening of nerve trunks that are frequently located in the orbital or temporal region of the face. The skin overlying a plexiform neurofibroma may be hyperpigmented to a greater degree than a café-au-lait spot. Plexiform neurofibromas may produce overgrowth of an extremity and a deformity of the corresponding bone. (5) A distinctive osseous lesion such as sphenoid dysplasia (which may cause pulsating exophthalmos) or cortical thinning of long bones (e.g., of the tibia) with or without pseudoarthrosis. (6) Optic gliomas are present in approximately 15% of patients with NF-1 and represent mostly low-grade astrocytomas. They are the main CNS tumor with a marked increased frequency in NF-1. Because of their growth, it is recommended that all children age 10 yr or younger with NF-1 undergo annual ophthalmologic examinations. When they progress, visual symptoms are produced because the tumors enlarge and put pressure on the optic nerves and chiasm resulting in impaired visual acuity and visual fields. Extension into the hypothalamus can lead to endocrine deficiencies or failure to thrive. The MRI findings of an optic glioma include diffuse thickening, localized enlargement, or a distinct focal mass originating from the optic nerve or chiasm (Fig. 589-3). (7) A first-degree relative with NF-1 whose diagnosis was based on the aforementioned criteria.

Children with NF-1 are susceptible to **neurologic complications.** MRI studies of selected children have shown abnormal hyperintense T2 weighted signals in the optic tracts, brainstem,

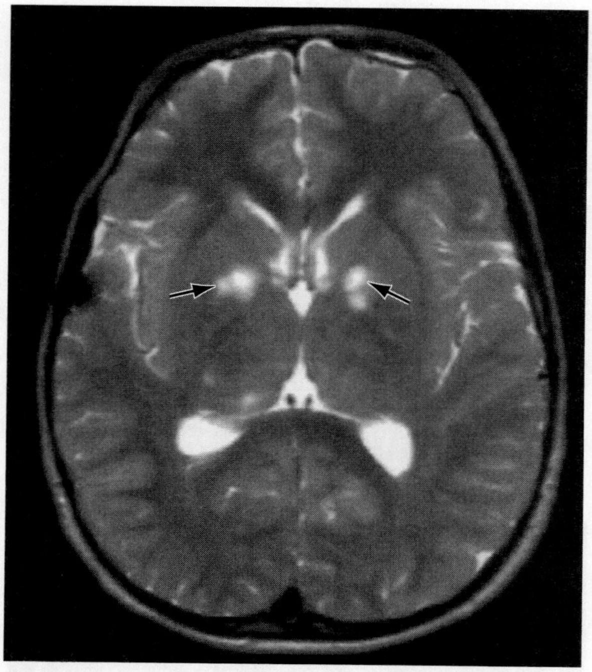

Figure 589-4 T2-weighted MRI scan of a patient with neurofibromatosis 1. Note the high-signal areas (unidentified bright objects) in the basal ganglia *(arrows)*.

Table 589-1 FREQUENCY OF LESIONS ASSOCIATED WITH NEUROFIBROMATOSIS TYPE 2

	FREQUENCY OF ASSOCIATION WITH NF2
NEUROLOGIC LESIONS	
Bilateral vestibular schwannomas	90-95%
Other cranial nerve schwannomas	24-51%
Intracranial meningiomas	45-58%
Spinal tumors	63-90%
Extramedullary	55-90%
Intramedullary	18-53%
Peripheral neuropathy	Up to 66%
OPHTHALMOLOGIC LESIONS	
Cataracts	60-81%
Epiretinal membranes	12-40%
Retinal hamartomas	6-22%
CUTANEOUS LESIONS	
Skin tumors	59-68%
Skin plaques	41-48%
Subcutaneous tumors	43-48%
Intradermal tumors	Rare

From Asthagiri AR, Parry DM, Butman JA, et al: Neurofibromatosis type 2, *Lancet* 373:1974–1984, 2009, Table 1.)

globus pallidus, thalamus, internal capsule, and cerebellum (Fig. 589-4). These signals, **"unidentified bright objects (UBOs),"** tend to disappear with age; most have disappeared by 30 yr of age. It is unclear what the UBOs represent pathologically, and there is disagreement as to the presence and number of UBOs and their relationship to learning disabilities, attention deficit disorders, behavioral and psychosocial problems, and abnormalities of speech among affected children. Therefore, imaging studies such as brain MRIs should be reserved only for patients with clinical symptoms.

One of the most common complications is learning disability affecting approximately 30% of NF-1 children. Seizures are observed in approximately 8% of NF-1 patients. The cerebral vessels may develop aneurysms, or stenosis resulting in moyamoya disease (Chapter 594.1). Neurologic sequelae of these vascular abnormalities include transient cerebrovascular ischemic attacks, hemiparesis, and cognitive defects. Precocious puberty may become evident in the presence or absence of lesions of the optic chiasm and hypothalamus. Malignant neoplasms are also a significant problem in patients with NF-1, affecting approximately 3% of patients. A neurofibroma occasionally differentiates into a malignant peripheral nerve sheath tumor (MPNST). The incidence of pheochromocytoma, rhabdomyosarcoma, leukemia, and Wilms tumor is higher than in the general population. Scoliosis is a common complication found in about 10% of the patients. Patients with NF-1 are at risk for hypertension, which may result from renal vascular stenosis or a pheochromocytoma.

NF-2 is a rarer condition, with an incidence of 1/25,000, and may be diagnosed when 1 of the following 4 features is present: (1) bilateral vestibular schwannomas; (2) a parent, sibling, or child with NF-2 and either unilateral vestibular schwannoma or any 2 of the following: meningioma, schwannoma, glioma, neurofibroma, or posterior subcapsular lenticular opacities; (3) unilateral vestibular schwannoma and any 2 of the following: meningioma, schwannoma, glioma, neurofibroma, or posterior subcapsular lenticular opacities; (4) multiple meningiomas (2 or more) and unilateral vestibular schwannoma or any 2 of the following: schwannoma, glioma, neurofibroma, or cataract. Symptoms of tinnitus, hearing loss, facial weakness, headache, or unsteadiness may appear during childhood, although signs of a cerebellopontine angle mass are more commonly present in the 2nd and 3rd decades of life. Although café-au-lait spots and skin neurofibromas are classic findings in NF-1, they are much less common in NF-2. Posterior subcapsular lens opacities are identified in about 50% of patients with NF-2. The *NF2* gene (also known as merlin or schwannomin) is located on chromosome 22q1.11. The frequency of lesions associated with NF-2 is noted in Table 589-1.

MANAGEMENT

Because of the diverse and unpredictable complications associated with NF-1, close multidisciplinary follow-up is necessary. Patients with NF-1 should have regular clinical assessments at least yearly, focusing the history and examination on the potential problems for which they are at increased risk. These assessments include yearly ophthalmologic examination, neurologic assessment, blood pressure monitoring, and scoliosis evaluation. Neuropsychologic and educational testing should be considered as needed. The NIH Consensus Development Conference has advised against routine imaging studies of the brain and optic tracts because treatment in these asymptomatic NF-1 children is rarely required. All symptomatic cases (i.e., those with visual disturbance, proptosis, or increased intracranial pressure) must be studied without delay.

GENETIC COUNSELING

While NF-1 is an autosomal dominant disorder, over half the cases are sporadic, representing de novo mutations. The *NF1* gene on chromosome region 17q11.2 encodes a protein also known as neurofibromin. Neurofibromin acts as an inhibitor of the oncogene *ras*. The diagnosis of NF-1 is based on the clinical features. However, molecular testing for the *NF1* gene is available and can be useful in a number of cases. Scenarios in which genetic testing is helpful include patients who have only 1 of the criteria for clinical diagnosis, those with unusually severe disease, and those seeking prenatal/pre-implantation diagnosis.

BIBLIOGRAPHY

Please visit the Nelson Textbook of Pediatrics *website at* www.expertconsult.com *for the complete bibliography.*

589.2 Tuberous Sclerosis

Mustafa Sahin

Tuberous sclerosis complex (TSC) is inherited as an autosomal dominant trait with variable expression and a prevalence of 1/6,000 newborns. Spontaneous genetic mutations occur in ⅔ of the cases. Molecular genetic studies have identified 2 foci for TSC: the *TSC1* gene is located on chromosome 9q34, and the *TSC2* gene is on chromosome 16p13. The *TSC1* gene encodes a protein called *hamartin*. The *TSC2* gene encodes the protein *tuberin*. Within a cell, these 2 proteins bind to one another and work together. That is why a mutation in the *TSC1* gene and a mutation in the *TSC2* gene result in a similar disease in people. The loss of either tuberin or hamartin results in the formation of numerous benign tumors (hamartomas). Thus, the *TSC1* and *TSC2* genes are tumor suppressor genes. Tuberin and hamartin are involved in a key pathway in the cell that regulates protein synthesis and cell size. One of the ways cells regulate their growth is by controlling the rate of protein synthesis. A protein called mTOR was identified as 1 of the master regulators of cell growth. mTOR, in turn, is controlled by rheb, a small cytoplasmic GTPase. When rheb is activated, the protein synthesis machinery is turned on, most likely via mTOR, and the cell grows in size.

TSC is an extremely heterogeneous disease with a wide clinical spectrum varying from severe mental retardation and incapacitating seizures to normal intelligence and a lack of seizures, often within the same family. The disease affects many organ systems other than the skin and brain, including the heart, kidney, eyes, lungs, and bone.

CLINICAL MANIFESTATIONS AND DIAGNOSIS

Definite TSC is diagnosed when at least 2 major or 1 major plus 2 minor features are present see Tables 589-2 and 589-3 for major and minor features, respectively).

The hallmark of TSC is the involvement of the CNS (Fig. 589-5). Retinal lesions consist of 2 types: hamartomas (elevated mulberry lesions or plaquelike lesions) and white depigmented patches (similar to the hypopigmented skin lesions) (Fig. 589-6). The characteristic brain lesion is a cortical tuber (see Fig. 589-5). Brain MRI is the best way of identifying cortical tubers. Based on fetal MRI studies, we know that cortical tubers are formed while in utero. Subependymal nodules are lesions found along the wall of the lateral ventricles where they undergo calcification and project into the ventricular cavity, producing a candle-dripping appearance. These lesions do not cause any problems; in 5-10% of cases, these benign lesions can grow into subependymal giant cell astrocytomas (SEGAs). These tumors can grow and block the circulation of cerebrospinal fluid (CSF) around the brain and cause hydrocephalus, which requires immediate neurosurgical intervention.

The most common neurologic manifestations of TSC consist of epilepsy, cognitive impairment, and autism spectrum disorders. TSC may present during infancy with infantile spasms and a hypsarrhythmic electroencephalogram (EEG) pattern. It is important to remember that you can have hypsarrhythmia without infantile spasms and infantile spasms without hypsarrhythmia especially in TSC patients. The seizures may be difficult to control and, at a later age, they may develop into myoclonic epilepsy (Chapter 586). In Europe and Canada, infantile spasms associated with TSC are treated with vigabatrin (rather than ACTH) with good results. In the USA, ACTH had been the drug of choice

Table 589-2 MAJOR FEATURES OF TUBEROUS SCLEROSIS COMPLEX

Cortical tuber
Subependymal nodule
Subependymal giant cell astrocytoma
Facial angiofibroma or forehead plaque
Ungual or periungual fibroma (nontraumatic)
Hypomelanotic macules (>3)
Shagreen patch
Multiple retinal hamartomas
Cardiac rhabdomyoma
Renal angiomyolipoma
Pulmonary lymphangioleiomyomatosis

Table 589-3 MINOR FEATURES OF TUBEROUS SCLEROSIS COMPLEX

Cerebral white matter migration lines
Multiple dental pits
Gingival fibromas
Bone cysts
Retinal achromatic patch
Confetti skin lesions
Nonrenal hamartomas
Multiple renal cysts
Hamartomatous rectal polyps

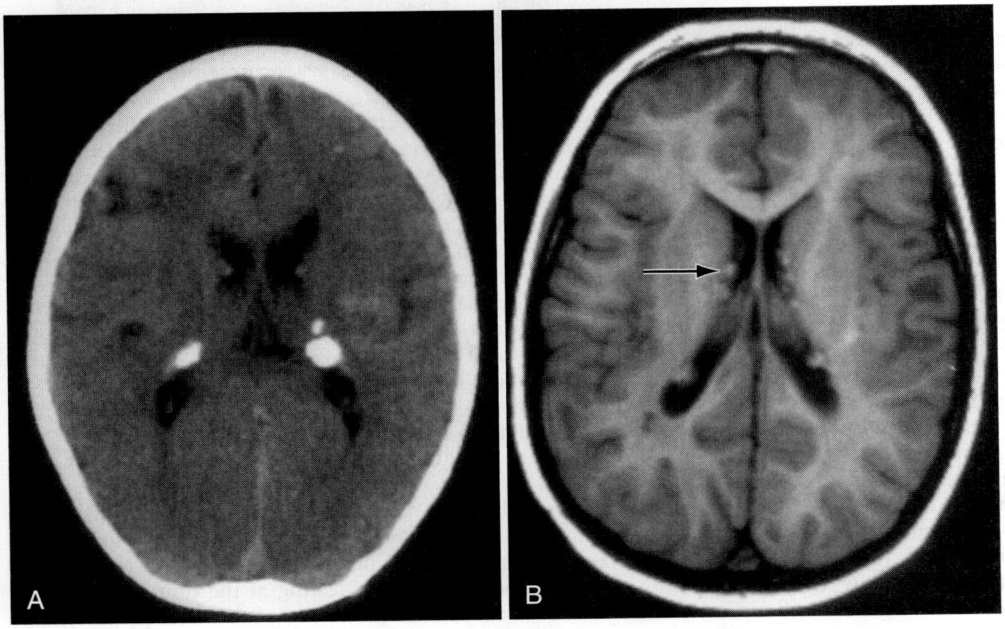

Figure 589-5 Tuberous sclerosis. *A,* CT scan with subependymal calcifications characteristic of tuberous sclerosis. *B,* The MRI demonstrates multiple subependymal nodules in the same patient *(arrow).* Parenchymal tubers are also visible on both the CT and the MRI scan as low-density areas in the brain parenchyma.

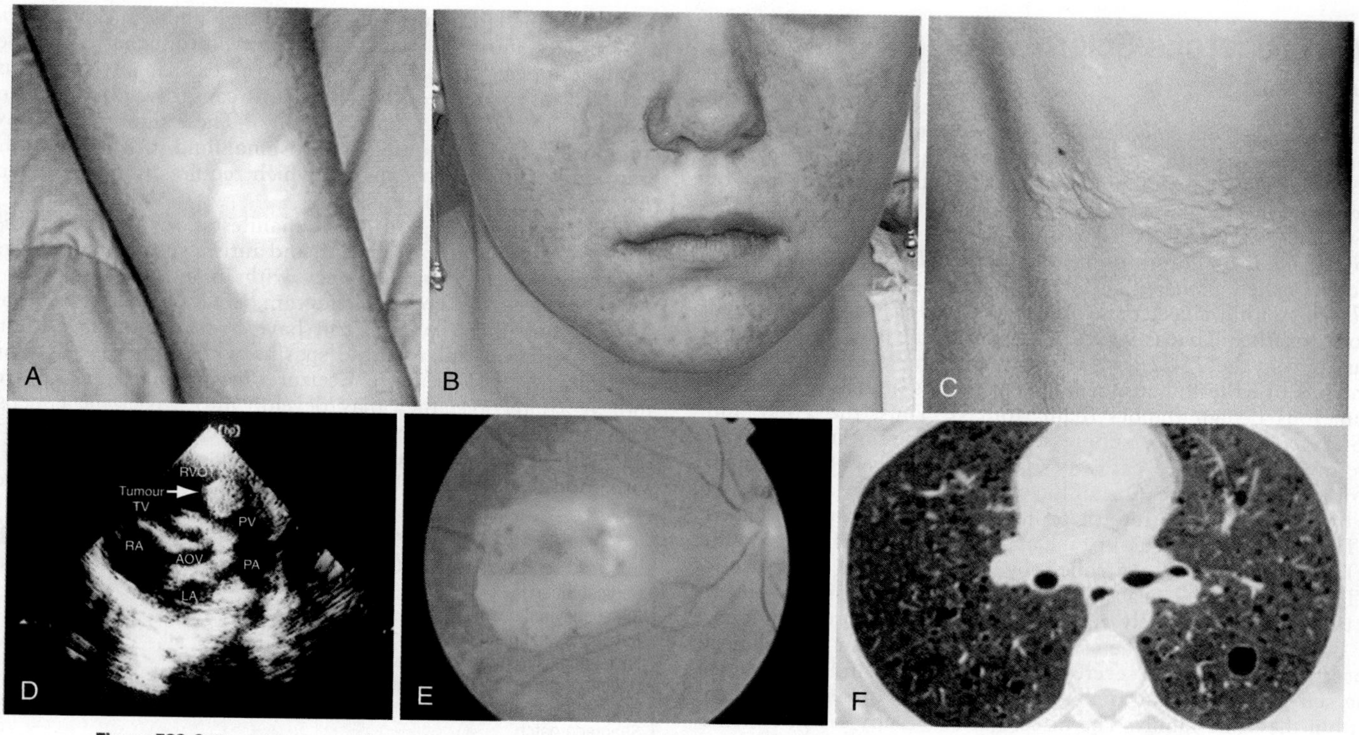

Figure 589-6 Dermatological, cardiac, and pulmonary manifestations of tuberous sclerosis. Hypomelanotic macules *(A)*. Facial angiofibromas *(B)*. Shagreen patch *(C)*. Hyperechoic rhabdomyoma detected by echocardiography *(D)*. Retinal hamartoma *(E)*. Lymphangioleiomyomatosis *(F)*. (From Curatolo P, Bombardieri R, Jozwiak S: Tuberous sclerosis, *Lancet* 372:657–668, 2008, Fig 7.)

until vigabatrin was approved by the U.S. Food and Drug Administration (FDA) for use in infantile spasms. Many patients with TSC have normal intelligence and few, if any, neurologic abnormalities.

SKIN LESIONS

More than 90% of cases show the typical hypomelanotic macules that have been likened to an ash leaf on the trunk and extremities. Visualization of the hypomelanotic macule is enhanced by the use of a Wood ultraviolet lamp (Chapter 645). To count as a major feature, at least 3 hypomelanotic macules must be present (see Fig. 589-6). Facial angiofibromas develop between 4 and 6 yr of age; they appear as tiny red nodules over the nose and cheeks and are sometimes confused with acne (see Fig. 589-6). Later, they enlarge, coalesce, and assume a fleshy appearance. A *shagreen patch* is also characteristic of TSC and consists of a roughened, raised lesion with an orange-peel consistency located primarily in the lumbosacral region. During adolescence or later, small fibromas or nodules of skin may form around fingernails or toenails in 15-20% of the TSC patients (Fig. 589-7).

OTHER ORGAN INVOLVEMENT

Approximately 50% of children with TSC have cardiac rhabdomyomas, which may be detected in a fetus at risk by an echocardiogram. The rhabdomyomas may be numerous or located at the apex of the left ventricle, and although they can cause congestive heart failure and arrhythmias, they tend to slowly resolve spontaneously. The kidneys in 75-80% of patients >10 yr of age have angiomyolipomas that are usually benign tumors. Angiomyolipomas begin in childhood in many individuals with TSC, but they may not be problematic until young adulthood. By the 3rd decade of life, they may cause lumbar pain and hematuria from slow bleeding, and rarely, they may result in sudden retroperitoneal bleeding. The current recommendation is to follow them by yearly imaging, and when the lesion becomes larger than 4 cm,

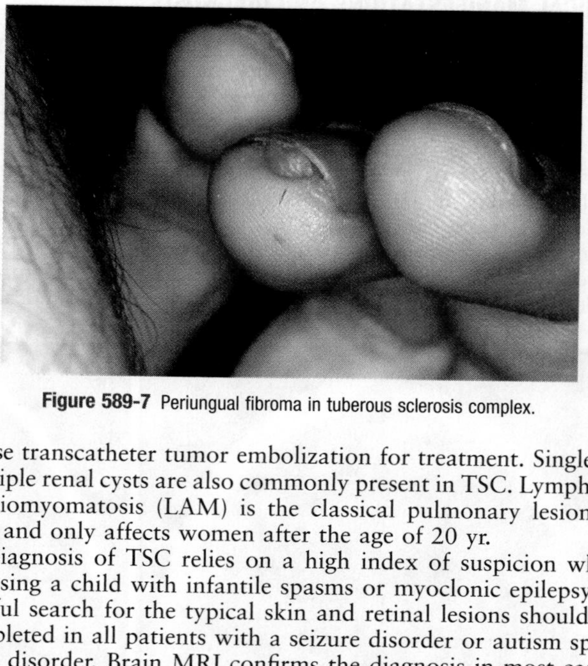

Figure 589-7 Periungual fibroma in tuberous sclerosis complex.

to use transcatheter tumor embolization for treatment. Single or multiple renal cysts are also commonly present in TSC. Lymphangioleiomyomatosis (LAM) is the classical pulmonary lesion in TSC and only affects women after the age of 20 yr.

Diagnosis of TSC relies on a high index of suspicion when assessing a child with infantile spasms or myoclonic epilepsy. A careful search for the typical skin and retinal lesions should be completed in all patients with a seizure disorder or autism spectrum disorder. Brain MRI confirms the diagnosis in most cases. Genetic testing for *TSC1* and *TSC2* mutations is available and may be considered when the individual patient does not meet all the clinical criteria. Prenatal testing may be offered when a known TSC mutation exists in that family.

Management

As for routine follow-up of individuals with TSC, the following are recommended in addition to physical examination: brain MRI every 1-3 yr, renal imaging (ultrasound, CT, or MRI) every 1-3 yr, and neurodevelopmental testing at the time of beginning 1st grade. Based on the complications of the disease, additional follow-up testing may be required for each individual. Symptoms and signs of increased intracranial pressure suggest obstruction of the foramen of Monro by a SEGA and warrant immediate investigation and surgical intervention. For treatment of SEGAs in TSC patients, who are not candidates for surgical resection, the FDA approved everolimus in November 2010.

BIBLIOGRAPHY

Please visit the Nelson Textbook of Pediatrics *website at www.expertconsult.com for the complete bibliography.*

589.3 Sturge-Weber Syndrome

Mustafa Sahin

Sturge-Weber syndrome (SWS) is a sporadic vascular disorder and consists of a constellation of symptoms and signs including a facial capillary malformation (**port-wine stain**), abnormal blood vessels of the brain (leptomeningeal angioma), and abnormal blood vessels of the eye leading to glaucoma. Patients present with seizures, hemiparesis, strokelike episodes, headaches and developmental delay. An estimated frequency of approximately 1 per 50,000 live births have SWS.

ETIOLOGY

The etiology remains unclear. The sporadic incidence and focal nature of SWS suggest the presence of somatic mutations, but this has not been demonstrated to date. The condition is thought to result from anomalous development of the embryonic vascular bed in the early stages of facial and cerebral development. There are hypotheses about aberrant sympathetic innervation, increased vascular growth factors and defects in extracellular matrix, but these remain to be tested. Low flow angiomatosis of the leptomeninges appears to result in a chronic hypoxic state leading to cortical atrophy and calcifications.

CLINICAL MANIFESTATIONS

The facial port-wine stain is present at birth, tends to be unilateral, and always involves the upper face and eyelid, in a distribution consistent with the ophthalmic division of the trigeminal nerve. The capillary malformation may also be evident over the lower face, trunk, and in the mucosa of the mouth and pharynx. It is important to note that not all children with facial port-wine stain have SWS. In fact, the overall incidence of SWS has been reported to be 8-33% in those with a port-wine stain. Buphthalmos and glaucoma of the ipsilateral eye are common complications. The incidence of epilepsy in patients with SWS is 75-90%, and seizures develop in most patients in the 1st yr of life. They are typically focal tonic-clonic and contralateral to the side of the facial capillary malformation. The seizures may become refractory to anticonvulsants and are associated with a slowly progressive hemiparesis in many cases. Transient strokelike episodes or visual defects persisting for several days and unrelated to seizure activity are common and probably result from thrombosis of cortical veins in the affected region. Although neurodevelopment appears to be normal in the 1st yr of life, mental retardation or severe learning disabilities are present in at least 50% in later childhood, probably the result of intractable epilepsy and increasing cerebral atrophy.

DIAGNOSIS

MRI with contrast is the imaging modality of choice for demonstrating the leptomeningeal angioma in SWS (Figure 589-8). White matter abnormalities are common and are thought to be a result of chronic hypoxia. Often, atrophy is noted ipsilateral to the leptomeningeal angiomatosis. Calcifications can be seen best with a head CT (Fig. 589-9). Ophthalmologic evaluation for

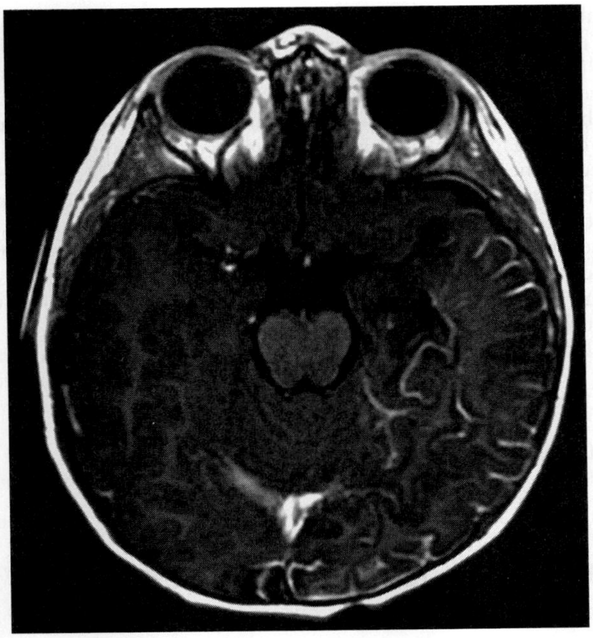

Figure 589-8 Gadolinium-enhanced axial T1 FLAIR image of a 15 mo old with Sturge-Weber syndrome shows leptomeningeal enhancement in the left hemisphere.

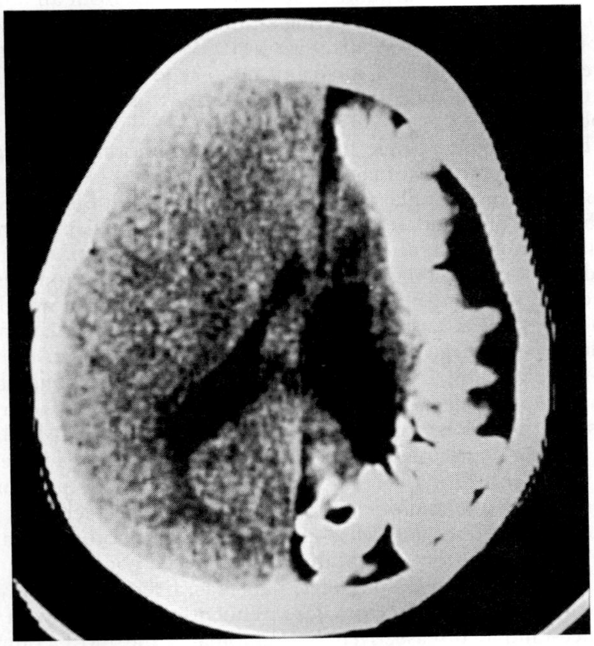

Figure 589-9 CT scan of a patient with Sturge-Weber syndrome showing unilateral calcification and underlying atrophy of a cerebral hemisphere.

glaucoma is also necessary. Based on the involvement of the brain and the face, there are 3 types according to the Roach Scale:

1. Type I: Both facial and leptomeningeal angiomas; may have glaucoma
2. Type II: Facial angioma alone (no CNS involvement); may have glaucoma
3. Type III: Isolated leptomeningeal angiomas; usually no glaucoma

MANAGEMENT

Management of SWS is symptomatic and multidisciplinary, but not well studied prospectively. It is aimed at controlling seizures, treating headaches, preventing strokelike episodes, monitoring for glaucoma, and using laser therapy for the cutaneous capillary malformations. Seizures beginning in infancy are not always associated with a poor neurodevelopmental outcome. For patients with well-controlled seizures and normal or near-normal development, management consists of anticonvulsants and surveillance for complications including glaucoma, buphthalmos, and behavioral abnormalities. If the seizures are refractory to anticonvulsant therapy, especially in infancy and the 1st 1-2 yr of life, and arise primarily from 1 hemisphere, most centers advise a hemispherectomy. Because of the risk of glaucoma, regular measurement of intraocular pressure is indicated. The facial port-wine stain is often a target of ridicule by classmates, leading to psychologic trauma. Pulsed dye laser therapy often provides excellent clearing of the port-wine stain, particularly if it is located on the forehead.

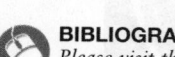

BIBLIOGRAPHY

Please visit the Nelson Textbook of Pediatrics *website at www.expertconsult.com for the complete bibliography.*

589.4 Von Hippel–Lindau Disease

Mustafa Sahin

Von Hippel–Lindau (VHL) disease affects many organs, including the cerebellum, spinal cord, retina, kidney, pancreas, and epididymis. Its incidence is around 1 : 36,000. It results from an autosomal dominant mutation affecting a tumor suppressor gene, *VHL*. Around 80% of individuals with VHL disease have an affected parent, and around 20% have a de novo gene mutation. Molecular testing is available and detects mutations in almost 100% of probands.

The major neurologic features of the condition include cerebellar hemangioblastomas and retinal angiomas. Patients with cerebellar hemangioblastoma present in early adult life or beyond with symptoms and signs of increased intracranial pressure. A smaller number of patients have hemangioblastoma of the spinal cord, producing abnormalities of proprioception and disturbances of gait and bladder dysfunction. The CT scan and MRI typically show a cystic cerebellar lesion with a vascular mural nodule. Total surgical removal of the tumor is curative.

Approximately 25% of patients with cerebellar hemangioblastoma have retinal angiomas. Retinal angiomas are characterized by small masses of thin-walled capillaries that are fed by large and tortuous arterioles and venules. They are usually located in the peripheral retina so that vision is unaffected. Exudation in the region of the angiomas may lead to retinal detachment and visual loss. Retinal angiomas are treated with photocoagulation and cryocoagulation, and both have produced good results.

Cystic lesions of the kidneys, pancreas, liver, and epididymis as well as pheochromocytoma are frequently associated with von Hippel–Lindau disease. Renal carcinoma is the most common cause of death. Regular follow-up and appropriate imaging studies are necessary to identify lesions that may be treated at an early stage.

BIBLIOGRAPHY

Please visit the Nelson Textbook of Pediatrics *website at www.expertconsult.com for the complete bibliography.*

589.5 Linear Nevus Syndrome

Mustafa Sahin

This sporadic condition is characterized by a facial nevus and neurodevelopmental abnormalities. The nevus is located on the forehead and nose and tends to be midline in its distribution. It may be quite faint during infancy but later becomes hyperkeratotic, with a yellow-brown appearance. Two thirds of patients with linear nevus syndrome demonstrate associated neurologic findings, including cortical dysplasia, glial hamartomas, and low-grade gliomas. Cerebral and cranial anomalies, predominantly hemimegalencephaly and enlargement of the lateral ventricles, were reported in 72% of cases. Incidence of epilepsy has been reported as high as 75% and mental retardation as high as 60%. Focal neurologic signs including hemiparesis and homonymous hemianopia may also be seen.

BIBLIOGRAPHY

Please visit the Nelson Textbook of Pediatrics *website at www.expertconsult.com for the complete bibliography.*

589.6 PHACE Syndrome

Mustafa Sahin

The syndrome denotes *p*osterior fossa malformations, *h*emangiomas, *a*rterial anomalies, *c*oarctation of the aorta and other cardiac defects, and *e*ye abnormalities. It is also referred to as *PHACES syndrome* when ventral developmental defects including sternal clefting and/or a supraumbilical raphe are present. Large facial hemangiomas may be associated with a Dandy-Walker malformation, vascular anomalies (coarctation of aorta, aplasia or hypoplastic carotid arteries, aneurysmal carotid dilation, aberrant left subclavian artery), glaucoma, cataracts, microphthalmia, optic nerve hypoplasia, and ventral defects (sternal clefts). The facial hemangioma is typically ipsilateral to the aortic arch. The Dandy-Walker malformation is the most common developmental abnormality of the brain. Other anomalies included hypoplasia or agenesis of the cerebellum, cerebellar vermis, corpus callosum, cerebrum, and septum pellucidum. Cerebrovascular anomalies can result in acquired, progressive vessel stenosis and acute ischemic stroke. There is a female predominance. The underlying pathogenesis of PHACE syndrome remains unknown.

BIBLIOGRAPHY

Please visit the Nelson Textbook of Pediatrics *website at www.expertconsult.com for the complete bibliography.*

589.7 Incontinentia Pigmenti

Mustafa Sahin

This rare, heritable, multisystem ectodermal disorder features dermatologic, dental, and ocular abnormalities. The phenotype is produced by functional mosaicism caused by random X-inactivation of an X-linked dominant gene that is lethal in males (*IKK-gamma/NEMO* gene). The paucity of affected males, the occurrence of female-to-female transmission, and an increased frequency of spontaneous abortions in carrier females support this supposition.

CLINICAL MANIFESTATIONS AND DIAGNOSIS

This disease has 4 phases, not all of which may occur in a given patient. The **1st phase** is evident at birth or in the 1st few weeks of life and consists of erythematous linear streaks and plaques of vesicles (Fig. 589-10) that are most pronounced on the limbs and circumferentially on the trunk. The lesions may be confused with those of herpes simplex, bullous impetigo, or mastocytosis, but the linear configuration is unique. Histopathologically, epidermal edema and eosinophil-filled intraepidermal vesicles are present. Eosinophils also infiltrate the adjacent epidermis and dermis. Blood eosinophilia as high as 65% of the white blood cell count is common. The 1st stage generally resolves by 4 mo of age, but mild, short-lived recurrences of blisters may develop during febrile illnesses. In the **2nd phase,** as blisters on the distal limbs

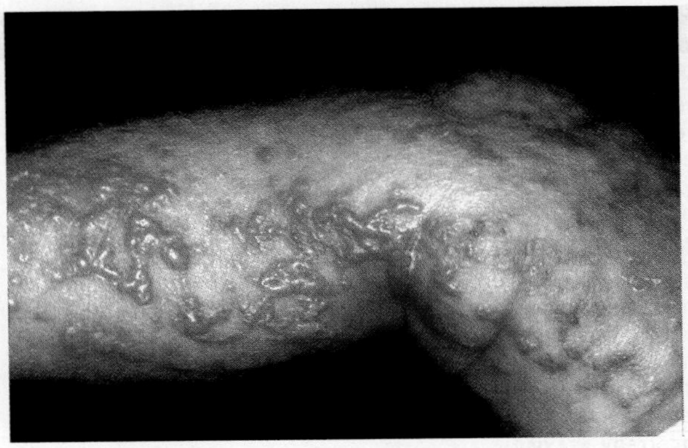

Figure 589-10 Whorled vesicular phase of incontinentia pigmenti.

resolve, they become dry and hyperkeratotic, forming verrucous plaques. The verrucous plaques rarely affect the trunk or face and generally involute within 6 mo. Epidermal hyperplasia, hyperkeratosis, and papillomatosis are characteristic. The **3rd or pigmentary stage** is the hallmark of incontinentia pigmenti. It generally develops over weeks to months and may overlap the earlier phases, be evident at birth, or, more commonly, begin to appear in the 1st few weeks of life. Hyperpigmentation is more often apparent on the trunk than the limbs and is distributed in macular whorls, reticulated patches, flecks, and linear streaks that follow Blaschko lines. The axillae and groin are invariably affected. The sites of involvement are not necessarily those of the preceding vesicular and warty lesions. The pigmented lesions, once present, persist throughout childhood. They generally begin to fade by early adolescence and often disappear by age 16 yr. Occasionally, the pigmentation remains permanently, particularly in the groin. The lesion, histopathologically, shows vacuolar degeneration of the epidermal basal cells and melanin in melanophages of the upper dermis as a result of incontinence of pigment. In the **4th stage,** hairless, anhidrotic, hypopigmented patches or streaks occur as a late manifestation of incontinentia pigmenti; they may develop, however, before the hyperpigmentation of stage 3 has resolved. The lesions develop mainly on the flexor aspect of the lower legs and less often on the arms and trunk.

Approximately 80% of affected children have other defects. Alopecia, which may be scarring and patchy or diffuse, is most common on the vertex and occurs in up to 40% of patients. Hair may be lusterless, wiry, and coarse. Dental anomalies, which are present in up to 80% of patients and are persistent throughout life, consist of late dentition, hypodontia, conical teeth, and impaction. CNS manifestations, including motor and cognitive developmental retardation, seizures, microcephaly, spasticity, and paralysis, are found in up to ⅓ of affected children. Ocular anomalies, such as neovascularization, microphthalmos, strabismus, optic nerve atrophy, cataracts, and retrolenticular masses, occur in >30% of children. Nonetheless, >90% of patients have normal vision. Less common abnormalities include dystrophy of nails (ridging, pitting) and skeletal defects.

Diagnosis of incontinentia pigmenti is made on clinical grounds, although major and minor criteria have been established to aid in diagnosis. Wood lamp examination may be useful in older children and adolescents to highlight pigmentary abnormalities. Clinical molecular testing is available, and in 80% of the affected patients a deletion that removes exons 4 through 10 of *NEMO* can be detected. Differential diagnosis includes hypomelanosis of Ito, which presents with similar skin manifestations and is often associated with chromosomal mosaicism.

MANAGEMENT

The choice of investigative studies and the plan of management depend on the occurrence of particular noncutaneous abnormalities since the skin lesions are benign. The high incidence of associated major anomalies warrants genetic counseling.

BIBLIOGRAPHY

Please visit the Nelson Textbook of Pediatrics *website at www.expertconsult.com for the complete bibliography.*

Chapter 590
Movement Disorders

Erika F. Augustine and Jonathan W. Mink

Movement disorders are characterized by abnormal or excessive involuntary movements that may result in abnormalities in posture, tone, balance, or fine motor control. Most movement disorders in children are characterized by involuntary movements. These involuntary movements can represent the sole disease manifestation, or they may be one of many symptoms and signs.

Evaluation of movement disorders, like all neurologic symptoms, begins with a comprehensive history. Because it can be difficult to describe the quality of movement, careful neurologic examination and observation of the movements are critical. There is no specific diagnostic test to differentiate among movement disorders. The category of movement assists in localizing the pathologic process, whereas the onset, age, and degree of abnormal motor activity and associated neurologic findings help organize the investigation.

When considering the type of movement disorder, the following questions concerning the history and examination of the movement are helpful.

- Distribution?
- Symmetry?
- Speed of movement—fast (excessive movement, hyperkinetic) or slow (paucity of movement, hypokinetic)?
- Presence at rest? With action?
- Relation to certain postures or positions?
- Task specificity?
- Ability to suppress?
- Stereotyped?
- Rhythmic?
- Continuous? Intermittent? Occurring in discrete episodes?
- Association with an urge?
- Persistence during sleep?
- Association with functional motor impairment?
- Aggravating/alleviating factors?

In the event of intermittent movements that do not occur in the setting of an office visit, home video can be invaluable. With the decreasing cost of home video cameras as well as video capability on many cellular phones, obtaining a short video is a reasonable request for most families. Resources are available to guide families in gathering useful video data.

Once the category of movement disorder is recognized, etiology can be considered. Clinical history, including birth history, medication/toxin exposure, trauma, infections, family history, progression of the involuntary movements, developmental progress, and behavior should be explored as the underlying cause is established. Hyperkinetic movement disorders are more common than akinetic-rigid syndromes in childhood (Table 590-1).

590.1 Ataxias

Denia Ramirez-Montealegre and Jonathan W. Mink

Ataxia is the inability to make smooth, accurate, and coordinated movements, usually due to a dysfunction of the cerebellum, its inputs or outputs, sensory pathways in the posterior columns of

Table 590-1 SELECTED TYPES OF INVOLUNTARY MOVEMENT IN CHILDHOOD

HYPOKINETIC
Parkinsonism (akinetic-rigid)
HYPERKINETIC
Stereotypies Tics Tremor Dystonia Chorea Athetosis Myoclonus Ballism Restless legs syndrome

Table 590-2 ACUTE OR RECURRENT ATAXIA

Brain tumor
Conversion reaction
Drug ingestion
Encephalitis (brainstem)
Genetic disorders
Dominant recurrent ataxia
Episodic ataxia type 1
Episodic ataxia type 2
Hartnup disease
Maple syrup urine disease
Pyruvate dehydrogenase deficiency
Migraine
Basilar
Benign paroxysmal vertigo
Postinfectious/immune
Acute disseminated encephalomyelitis
Acute postinfectious cerebellitis (varicella)
Miller Fisher syndrome
Multiple sclerosis
Myoclonic encephalopathy/neuroblastoma
Pseudoataxia (epileptic)
Trauma
Hematoma
Postconcussion
Vertebrobasilar occlusion
Vascular disorders
Cerebellar hemorrhage
Kawasaki disease

the spinal cord, or a combination of these. Ataxias may be generalized or primarily affect gait or the hands and arms; they may be acute (Table 590-2) or chronic (Table 590-3). **Congenital anomalies** of the posterior fossa, including the Dandy-Walker syndrome, Chiari malformation, and encephalocele, are prominently associated with ataxia because of their destruction or replacement of the cerebellum (Chapters 585.9 and 585.11). **Agenesis of the cerebellar vermis** presents in infancy with generalized hypotonia and decreased deep tendon reflexes. Delayed motor milestones and truncal ataxia are typical. **Joubert syndrome** is an autosomal recessive disorder marked by agenesis of the cerebellar vermis, ataxia, hypotonia, oculomotor apraxia, neonatal breathing problems, and mental retardation. Mutations have been identified in the *AHI1* gene on chromosome 6, encoding the Jouberin protein. This gene is strongly expressed in embryonic hindbrain, especially in neurons that give rise to the axons of the corticospinal tract and superior cerebellar peduncles, which fail to cross properly in Joubert syndrome. MRI is the method of choice for investigating congenital abnormalities of the cerebellum, vermis, and related structures. In Joubert syndrome, MRI reveals enlargement of the 4th ventricle at the junction between the midbrain and medulla, creating the "molar tooth sign."

Table 590-3 CHRONIC OR PROGRESSIVE ATAXIA

BRAIN TUMORS
Cerebellar astrocytoma Cerebellar hemangioblastoma (von Hippel–Lindau disease) Ependymoma Medulloblastoma Supratentorial tumors
CONGENITAL MALFORMATIONS
Basilar impression Cerebellar aplasias Cerebellar hemisphere aplasia Dandy-Walker malformation Vermal aplasia Chiari malformation
HEREDITARY ATAXIAS
Autosomal dominant inheritance
Autosomal recessive inheritance
Abetalipoproteinemia
Ataxia-telangiectasia
Ataxia without oculomotor apraxia
Ataxia with episodic dystonia
Friedreich ataxia
Hartnup disease
Juvenile GM_2 gangliosidosis
Juvenile sulfatide lipidoses
Maple syrup urine disease
Marinesco-Sjögren syndrome
Pyruvate dehydrogenase deficiency
Ramsay Hunt syndrome
Refsum disease (HSMN IV)
Respiratory chain disorders
X-linked inheritance
Adrenoleukodystrophy
Leber optic neuropathy
With adult-onset dementia
With deafness
With deafness and loss of vision

From Fenichel GM: *Clinical pediatric neurology*, ed 5, Philadelphia, 2005, Elsevier, p 220.

The major **infectious causes of ataxia** include cerebellar abscess, acute labyrinthitis, and acute cerebellar ataxia. **Acute cerebellar ataxia** occurs primarily in children 1-3 yr of age and is a diagnosis of exclusion. The condition often follows a viral illness, such as varicella, coxsackievirus, or echovirus infection by 2-3 wk and is thought to represent an autoimmune response to the viral agent affecting the cerebellum (Chapters 242, 245, and 595). The onset is sudden, and the truncal ataxia can be so severe that the child is unable to stand or sit. Vomiting may occur initially, but fever and nuchal rigidity are absent. Horizontal nystagmus is evident in approximately 50% of cases and, if the child is able to speak, dysarthria may be impressive. Examination of the cerebrospinal fluid (CSF) is typically normal at the onset of ataxia; a pleocytosis of lymphocytes (10-30/mm^3) is not unusual. Later in the course, the CSF protein undergoes a moderate elevation. The ataxia begins to improve in a few weeks but may persist for as long as 2 mo. The incidence of acute cerebellar ataxia appears to have declined with increased rates of vaccination against varicella. The prognosis for complete recovery is excellent; a small number have long-term sequelae, including behavioral and speech disorders as well as ataxia and incoordination. **Acute labyrinthitis** may be difficult to differentiate from acute cerebellar ataxia in a toddler. The condition is associated with middle-ear infections and intense vertigo, vomiting, and abnormalities in labyrinthine function, particularly ice water caloric testing.

Toxic causes of ataxia include alcohol, thallium (which is used occasionally in homes as a pesticide), and the anticonvulsants, particularly phenytoin when serum levels reach or exceed 30 μg/mL (120 μmol/L).

Brain tumors, including tumors of the cerebellum and frontal lobe, as well as peripheral nervous system neuroblastoma, may present with ataxia. Frontal lobe tumors may cause ataxia due to destruction of the association fibers connecting the frontal lobe with the cerebellum or due to increased intracranial pressure. Neuroblastoma may be associated with a paraneoplastic encephalopathy characterized by progressive ataxia, myoclonic jerks, and opsoclonus (nonrhythmic, conjugate horizontal and vertical oscillations of the eyes).

Several **metabolic disorders** are characterized by ataxia, including abetalipoproteinemia, arginosuccinic aciduria, and Hartnup disease. **Abetalipoproteinemia** (Bassen-Kornzweig disease) begins in childhood with steatorrhea and failure to thrive (Chapter 592). A blood smear shows acanthocytosis and decreased serum levels of cholesterol and triglycerides, and the serum β-lipoproteins are absent. Neurologic signs become evident by late childhood and consist of ataxia, retinitis pigmentosa, peripheral neuritis, abnormalities in position and vibration sense, muscle weakness, and mental retardation. Vitamin E is undetectable in the serum of patients with neurologic symptoms.

Degenerative diseases of the central nervous system (CNS) represent an important group of ataxic disorders of childhood because of the genetic consequences and poor prognosis. **Ataxia-telangiectasia,** an autosomal recessive condition, is the most common of the degenerative ataxias and is heralded by ataxia beginning at about age 2 yr and progressing to loss of ambulation by adolescence (Chapter 589). Ataxia-telangiectasia is caused by mutations in the *ATM* gene located at 11q22-q23. ATM is a phosphytidylinositol-3 kinase that phosphorylates proteins involved in DNA repair and cell cycle control. Oculomotor apraxia of horizontal gaze, defined as having difficulty fixating smoothly on an object and therefore overshooting the target with lateral movement of the head, followed by refixating the eyes, is a frequent finding, as is strabismus, hypometric saccade pursuit abnormalities, and nystagmus. Ataxia-telangiectasia may present with chorea rather than ataxia. The telangiectasia becomes evident by mid-childhood and is found on the bulbar conjunctiva, over the bridge of the nose, and on the ears and exposed surfaces of the extremities. Examination of the skin shows a loss of elasticity. Abnormalities of immunologic function that lead to frequent sinopulmonary infections include decreased serum and secretory IgA as well as diminished IgG_2, IgG_4, and IgE levels in more than 50% of patients. Children with ataxia-telangiectasia have a 50- to 100-fold greater chance over the normal population of developing lymphoreticular tumors (lymphoma, leukemia, and Hodgkin disease) as well as brain tumors. Additional laboratory abnormalities include an increased incidence of chromosome breaks, particularly of chromosome 14, and elevated levels of α-fetoprotein. Death results from infection or tumor dissemination.

Friedreich ataxia is inherited as an autosomal recessive disorder involving the spinocerebellar tracts, dorsal columns in the spinal cord, the pyramidal tracts, and the cerebellum and medulla. The majority of patients are homozygous for a GAA repeat expansion in the noncoding region of the gene coding for the mitochondrial protein frataxin. Mutations cause oxidative injury associated with excessive iron deposits in mitochondria. The onset of ataxia is somewhat later than in ataxia-telangiectasia but usually occurs before age 10 yr. The ataxia is slowly progressive and involves the lower extremities to a greater degree than the upper extremities. The Romberg test result is positive; the deep tendon reflexes are absent (particularly the Achilles), and the plantar response is extensor. Patients develop a characteristic explosive, dysarthric speech, and nystagmus is present in most children. Although patients may appear apathetic, their intelligence is preserved. They may have significant weakness of the distal musculature of the hands and feet. Typically noted is a marked loss of vibration and position sense caused by degeneration of the posterior columns and indistinct sensory changes in the distal extremities. Friedreich ataxia is also characterized by skeletal abnormalities, including high-arched feet (pes cavus) and hammertoes, as well as progressive kyphoscoliosis. Results of electrophysiologic studies including visual, auditory brainstem, and somatosensory-evoked potentials are often abnormal. Hypertrophic cardiomyopathy with progression to intractable congestive heart failure is the cause of death for most patients. Antioxidant therapy with coenzyme Q10 and vitamin E has been reported to slow progression in some patients.

Several forms of **spinocerebellar ataxia** are similar to Friedreich ataxia. **Roussy-Levy disease** has, in addition, atrophy of the muscles of the lower extremity with a similar pattern of wasting observed in Charcot-Marie-Tooth disease; **Ramsay Hunt syndrome** has an associated myoclonic epilepsy. There are also more than 20 dominantly inherited spinocerebellar ataxias, some of which present in childhood. These include those associated with CAG (polyglutamine) repeats and noncoding microsatellite expansions. Dominantly inherited episodic ataxias caused by potassium or calcium channel dysfunction present as episodes of ataxia and muscle weakness. Some of these disorders may respond to acetazolamide. The dominantly inherited **olivopontocerebellar atrophies** (OPCA) include ataxia, cranial nerve palsies, and abnormal sensory findings in the 2nd or 3rd decade, but can present in children with rapidly progressive ataxia, nystagmus, dysarthria, and seizures.

Additional degenerative ataxias include **Pelizaeus-Merzbacher disease, neuronal ceroid lipofuscinoses,** and late-onset **GM_2 gangliosidosis** (Chapter 592). Rare forms of progressive cerebellar ataxia have been described in association with **vitamin E deficiency.** A number of autosomal dominant progressive spinocerebellar ataxias have been defined at the molecular level, including those caused by unstable trinucleotide repeat expansions.

BIBLIOGRAPHY

Please visit the Nelson Textbook of Pediatrics *website at* *www.expertconsult.com* *for the complete bibliography.*

590.2 Chorea, Athetosis, Tremor

Denia Ramirez-Montealegre and Jonathan W. Mink

Chorea, meaning "dance-like" in Greek, refers to rapid, chaotic movements that seem to flow from one body part to another. Affected individuals exhibit motor impersistence, with difficulty keeping the tongue protruded ("darting tongue") or maintaining grip ("milkmaid grip"). Chorea tends to occur both at rest and with action. Patients often attempt to incorporate the involuntary movements into more purposeful movements, making them appear fidgety. *Chorea increases with stress and disappears in sleep.* Chorea can be divided into primary (i.e., disorders in which chorea is the dominant symptom and the etiology is presumed to be genetic) and secondary forms, with the vast majority of pediatric cases falling into the latter category (Tables 590-4 and 590-5).

Sydenham chorea (SC, St. Vitus dance) is the most common acquired chorea of childhood. It occurs in 10% to 20% of patients with **acute rheumatic fever,** typically weeks to months after a group A β-hemolytic streptococcal infection (Chapter 176.1). Peak incidence is at age 8 to 9 yr, with a female predominance of 2:1.

Pathophysiologically, there is good evidence that group A streptococci promote the generation of cross-reactive or polyreactive antibodies through molecular mimicry between streptococcal and host antigens. Specifically, antibodies against the *N*-acetyl-β-D-glucosamine epitope (GlcNAc) of streptococcal group A carbohydrate have been shown to target intracellular β-tubulin and extracellular lysoganglioside G_{M1} in human caudate-putamen preparations. These antibodies are also capable of directing calcium/calmodulin–dependent protein kinase II activation, which may cause the neurologic manifestations of SC by increasing dopamine release into the synapse.

Table 590-4 ETIOLOGICAL CLASSIFICATION OF CHOREIC SYNDROMES

GENETIC CHOREAS
Huntington disease (rarely presents with chorea in childhood)
Huntington disease–like 2 and other HD-like syndromes
Dentatorubropallidoluysian atrophy
Neuroacanthocytosis
Ataxia telangiectasia
Benign hereditary chorea
Spinocerebellar ataxia (types 2, 3, or 17)
Paroxysmal kinesigenic choreoathetosis
STRUCTURAL BASAL-GANGLIA LESIONS
Vascular chorea in stroke
Mass lesions (e.g., CNS lymphoma, metastatic brain tumors)
Multiple sclerosis plaques
Extrapontine myelinolysis
PARAINFECTIOUS AND AUTOIMMUNE DISORDERS
Sydenham chorea
Systemic lupus erythematosus
Chorea gravidarum
Antiphospholipid antibody syndrome
Postinfectious or postvaccinal encephalitis
Paraneoplastic choreas
INFECTIOUS CHOREA
HIV encephalopathy
Toxoplasmosis
Cysticercosis
Diphtheria
Bacterial endocarditis
Neurosyphilis
Scarlet fever
Viral encephalitis (mumps, measles, varicella)
METABOLIC OR TOXIC ENCEPHALOPATHIES
Acute intermittent porphyria
Hypo/hypernatremia
Hypocalcemia
Hyperthyroidism
Hypoparathyroidism
Hepatic/renal failure
Carbon monoxide poisoning
Manganese poisoning
Mercury poisoning
Organophosphate poisoning
DRUG-INDUCED CHOREA (SEE TABLE 590-6)

From Cardoso F, Seppi K, Mair KJ, et al: Seminar on choreas, *Lancet* 5:589–602, 2006.

The clinical hallmarks of SC are chorea, hypotonia, and emotional lability. Onset of the chorea is usually insidious but may be abrupt. Most patients have generalized chorea. However, the majority has asymmetric chorea and up to 20% of patients have hemichorea. Hypotonia manifests with the "pronator sign" (arms and palms turn outward when held overhead) and the "choreic hand" (spooning of the extended hand by flexion of the wrist and extension of the fingers). When chorea and hypotonia are severe, the child may be incapable of feeding, dressing, or walking. Speech is often involved, sometimes to the point of being unintelligible. Periods of uncontrollable crying and extreme mood swings are characteristic and may precede the onset of the movement disorder.

Sydenham chorea is a clinical diagnosis; however, a combination of acute *and* convalescent serum antistreptolysin O titers may help to confirm an acute streptococcal infection. Negative titers do not exclude the diagnosis. All patients with SC should be evaluated for carditis and started on long-term antibiotic prophylaxis (e.g., penicillin G benzathine 1.2 million units IM every 2-3 weeks) to decrease the risk of rheumatic heart disease. For patients with chorea that is impairing, treatment options include valproate, carbamazepine, and/or dopamine receptor antagonists. Although phenothiazines, haloperidol, and pimozide are also effective, their side effects limit their utility. Historically, there have been conflicting data regarding the efficacy of prednisone, intravenous immunoglobulin, and other immunomodulatory agents in SC, making it difficult to recommend their routine use. Recently, a randomized, double-blinded study of 37 children with SC compared high-dose prednisone (2 mg/kg/day, max. 60 mg) for 4 wk versus a placebo and found that steroids significantly reduced time to remission (54.3 days versus 119.9 days in controls).

Sydenham chorea usually resolves spontaneously within 6 to 9 mo, though it can persist for up to 2 yr and, in rare cases, can remain a lifelong condition. Relapse in the 1st few years is relatively common, occurring in 37.9% of patients in 1 series. Remote recurrence of chorea is rare but may be provoked by streptococcal infections, pregnancy (**chorea gravidarum**), or oral contraceptive use.

Though much rarer than SC, **systemic lupus erythematosus** (SLE) is a well-known cause of chorea in children. In some cases, chorea may be the presenting sign of SLE. A recent retrospective study of a large pediatric lupus cohort examined the prevalence of antiphosolipid antibodies and evaluated their association with neuropsychiatric symptoms. There was a statistically significant association between a persistently positive lupus anticoagulant and chorea ($p = .02$); however, only 2 of the 137 patients in the cohort had chorea. Regardless, any child with chorea of unknown cause should be investigated for the presence of antiphospholipid antibodies.

Additional causes of secondary chorea include metabolic (hyperthyroidism, hypoparathyroidism), infectious (Lyme disease), immune-mediated (systemic lupus erythematosus), vascular (stroke, moyamoya disease), heredodegenerative disorders (Wilson disease), and drugs (Table 590-6). Although chorea is a hallmark of Huntington disease in adults, children who develop Huntington disease tend to present with rigidity and bradykinesia (**Westphal variant**) or dystonia rather than chorea.

Athetosis is characterized by slow, continuous, writhing movements that repeatedly involve the same body part(s), usually the distal extremities, face, neck, or trunk. Like chorea, athetosis may occur at rest and is often worsened by voluntary movement. Because athetosis tends to co-occur with other movement disorders, such as chorea (**choreoathetosis**) and dystonia, it is often difficult to distinguish as a discrete entity. Choreoathetosis is associated with cerebral palsy, kernicterus, and other forms of basal ganglia injury; therefore, it is often seen in conjunction with **rigidity**—increased muscle tone that is equal in the flexors and extensors in all directions of passive movement regardless of the velocity of the movement. This is to be differentiated from **spasticity**, a velocity-dependent ("clasp-knife") form of hypertonia that is seen with upper motor neuron dysfunction. As with chorea, athetosis/choreoathetosis can also be seen with hypoxic-ischemic injury and dopamine-blocking drugs.

Tremor is a rhythmic, oscillatory movement around a central point or plane, which results from the action of antagonist muscles. Tremor can affect the extremities, head, trunk, or voice and can be classified by both its frequency (slow [4 Hz], intermediate [4-7 Hz], and fast [>7 Hz]) and by the context in which it is most pronounced. **Rest tremor** is maximal when the affected body part is inactive and supported against gravity, whereas **postural tremor** is most notable when the patient sustains a position against gravity. **Action tremor** occurs with performance of a voluntary activity and can be subclassified into **simple kinetic tremor**, which occurs with limb movement, and **intention tremor**, which occurs as the patient's limb approaches a target and is a feature of cerebellar disease.

Essential tremor (ET) is the most common movement disorder in adults, and 50% of persons diagnosed with ET report an onset in childhood; thus ET may be more common in the pediatric population than the literature would suggest. ET is an autosomal dominant condition with variable expressivity but complete penetrance by the age of 60 yr. Although the genetics of ET are not

Table 590-5 GENETIC CHOREAS

	MODE OF INHERITANCE	GENE, LOCATION	PROTEIN PRODUCT	USUAL AGE AT ONSET (YR)	CLINICAL SIGNS
HDL2*	AD†	JPH3, 16q	Junctophilin-3	20-40	Huntington disease phenotype, sometimes acanthocytosis; almost exclusively African ethnicity
SCA17	AD†	TBP, 6q	TBP	10-30	Cerebellar ataxia, chorea, dystonia, hyperreflexia, cognitive decline
DRPLA	AD†	DRPLA, 12p	Atrophin-1	About 20	Variable phenotypic picture including chorea, ataxia, seizures, psychiatric disturbances, dementia; more common in Japan than in Europe or USA
SCA3/MJD	AD†	MJD, 14q	Ataxin-3	35-40	Wide phenotypic variability with cerebellar ataxia, protruded eyes, chorea, dystonia, parkinsonian features, neuropathy, pyramidal tract features
SCA2	AD†	Ataxin-2, 12q	Ataxin-2	30-35	Cerebellar ataxia, chorea, markedly reduced velocity of saccadic eye movements, hyporeflexia
Chorea-acanthocytosis	AR	VPS13A (formerly CHAC), 9q	Chorein	20-50	Orofacial self-mutilation, dystonia, neuropathy, myopathy, seizures, acanthocytosis
McLeod syndrome	X-linked, recessive	XK, Xp	XK-protein	40-70	Dystonia, neuropathy, myopathy, cardiomyopathy, seizures, acanthocytosis, raised creatine kinase, weak expression of Kell antigen
Neuroferritinopathy	AD	FTL, 19q	FTL	20-55	Chorea, dystonia, parkinsonian features; usually reduced serum ferritin; MR abnormalities with cyst formation and increased T2 signal in globus pallidus and putamen
AT and ATLD	AR	ATM, 11q (AT) MRE11, 11q (ATLD)	ATM (AT) MRE11 (ATLD)	Childhood	Ataxia, neuropathy, oculomotor apraxia, other extrapyramidal manifestations including chorea, dystonia, and myoclonus In AT: oculocutaneous telangiectasias; predisposition to malignancies, IgA and IgG deficiency, high α-fetoprotein in serum and high concentrations of carcinoembryogenic antigen
AOA 1 and 2	AR	APTX, 9p (AOA 1) SETX, 9q (AOA 2)	Aprataxin (AOA 1) Senataxin (AOA 2)	Childhood or adolescence (later onset in AOA 2)	Ataxia, neuropathy, oculomotor apraxia, other extrapyramidal manifestations including chorea and dystonia; ataxia with oculomotor apraxia type 1: hypoalbuminemia and hypercholesterolemia; ataxia with oculomotor apraxia type 2: raised α-fetoprotein in serum
Pantothenate kinase associated neurodegeneration (formerly Hallervorden-Spatz syndrome)	AR	PANK2, 20p	Pantothenate kinase 2	Childhood, but also adult-onset subtype	Chorea, dystonia, parkinsonian features, pyramidal tract features; MR abnormalities with decreased T2 signal in the globus pallidus and substantia nigra, "eye of the tiger" sign (hyperintense area within the hypointense area); sometimes acanthocytosis, abnormal cytosomes in lymphocytes
Lesch-Nyhan syndrome	X-linked, recessive	HPRT, Xq	Hypoxanthine-guanine phosphoribosyl-transferase	Childhood	Chorea, dystonia, hypotonia, self-injurious behavior with biting of fingers and lips, mental retardation; short stature, renal calculi, hyperuricemia
Wilson disease	AR	ATP7B, 13q	Copper transporting P-type ATPase	<40	Parkinsonian features, dystonia, tremor, rarely chorea, behavioral and cognitive change, corneal Kayser-Fleischer rings, liver disease
PKC syndrome and ICCA syndrome	AD	Unknown, 16p	Unknown	<1-40	Paroxysmal movement disorders presenting with recurrent brief episodes of abnormal involuntary movements with dramatic response to low dose carbamazepine (PKC); recurrent brief episodes of abnormal involuntary movements in association with infantile convulsions (ICCA)
Benign hereditary chorea	AD	TITF-1, 14q; other	Thyroid transcription factor 1	Childhood	Chorea, mild ataxia; genetically heterogeneous

*HDL1, HDL3, and HDL4 are very rare conditions (only 1 family known) and therefore not included in the table.
†Disorders based on expanded CAG repeats (HDL2 based on CAG/CTG repeats; SCA 17 based on CAG/CAA repeats); age of symptom onset inversely related to repeat size.
AD, autosomal dominant; AOA, ataxia with oculomotor apraxia (types 1 or 2); AR, autosomal recessive; AT, ataxia telangiectasia; ATLD, ataxia telangiectasia–like disorder; DRPLA, dentatorubropallidoluysian atrophy; ICCA, infantile convulsions and paroxysmal choreoathetosis syndrome; MJD, Machado-Joseph disease; PKC, paroxysmal kinesigenic choreoathetosis; SCA, spinocerebellar ataxia (types 2, 3, or 17).
Modified from Cardoso F, Seppi K, Mair KJ, et al: Seminar on choreas, *Lancet Neurol* 5:589–602, 2006, p 593.

fully understood, at least 3 different loci—*EMT1* on chromosome 3q13, *EMT2* on chromosome 2p22-25, and a locus on 6p23—have been linked to the condition. Based on functional imaging studies, the defect is thought to localize to cerebellar circuits.

Essential tremor is characterized by a slowly progressive, bilateral, 4-9 Hz postural tremor that involves the upper extremities and occurs in the absence of other known causes of tremor. Mild asymmetry is common, but ET is rarely unilateral. ET may be worsened by actions, such as trying to pour water from cup to cup, and affected adults may report a history of ethanol responsiveness. Most young children present to care because a parent, teacher, or physician has noticed the tremor,

Table 590-6 DRUGS THAT CAN INDUCE CHOREA
DOPAMINE RECEPTOR BLOCKING AGENTS
Phenothiazines Butyrophenones Benzamides
ANTIPARKINSONIAN DRUGS
L-Dopa Dopamine agonists Anticholinergics
ANTIEPILEPTIC DRUGS
Phenytoin Carbamazepine Valproic acid
PSYCHOSTIMULANTS
Amphetamines Pemoline Cocaine
CALCIUM CHANNEL BLOCKERS
Cinnarizine Flunarizine Verapamil
OTHERS
Lithium Baclofen Digoxin Tricyclic antidepressants Cyclosporine Steroids/oral contraceptives Theophylline

From Cardoso F, Seppi K, Mair KJ, et al: Seminar on choreas, *Lancet* 5:589–602, 2006.

Table 590-7 SELECTED CAUSES OF TREMOR IN CHILDREN
BENIGN
Enhanced physiologic tremor Shuddering attacks Jitteriness Spasmus nutans
STATIC INJURY/STRUCTURAL
Cerebellar malformation Stroke (particularly in the midbrain or cerebellum) Multiple sclerosis
HEREDITARY/DEGENERATIVE
Familial essential tremor Fragile X premutation Wilson disease Huntington disease Juvenile parkinsonism (tremor is rare) Pallidonigral degeneration
METABOLIC
Hyperthyroidism Hyperadrenergic state (including pheochromocytoma and neuroblastoma) Hypomagnesemia Hypocalcemia Hypoglycemia Hepatic encephalopathy Vitamin B_{12} deficiency Inborn errors of metabolism Mitochondrial disorders
DRUGS/TOXINS
Valproate, phenytoin, carbamazepine, lamotrigine, gabapentin, lithium, tricyclic antidepressants, stimulants (cocaine, amphetamine, caffeine, thyroxine, bronchodilators), neuroleptics, cyclosporin, toluene, mercury, thallium, amiodarone, nicotine, lead, manganese, arsenic, cyanide, naphthalene, ethanol, lindane, serotonin reuptake inhibitors
PERIPHERAL NEUROPATHIES
PSYCHOGENIC

rather than because the tremor is causing impairment. That being the case, most children with ET do not require pharmacologic intervention. If they are having difficulty with their handwriting or self-feeding, an occupational therapy evaluation and/or assistive devices, such as wrist weights and weighted silverware, may be helpful. Teenagers tend to report more impairment from ET; however, it is unclear whether this is due to actual or subjective progression of the tremor. Teenagers who do require pharmacotherapy usually respond to the same medications that are used in adults—propranolol and primidone. Propranolol, which is generally considered the first-line treatment, can be started at 30 mg daily and then titrated to effect, with most patients responding to doses of 60-80 mg/day. Propranolol should not be used in patients with reactive airway disease. Primidone can be started at 12.5-25 mg at bedtime and increased gradually in a twice daily schedule. Most patients respond to doses of 50-200 mg/day. Other treatments options for ET reported in the adult literature include sotalol, atenolol, gabapentin, topiramate, and alprazolam. Botulinum toxin A may be effective for treating limb tremor, though it causes nonpermanent, dose-dependent limb weakness. Surgical treatments, which include deep brain stimulation of the thalamus and unilateral thalamotomy, are generally reserved for adults.

While ET is the most common primary etiology of tremor in children, there are numerous secondary etiologies (Table 590-7). **Holmes tremor,** previously referred to as midbrain or rubral tremor, is characterized by a slow frequency, high amplitude tremor that is present at rest and with intention. It is a symptomatic tremor, which usually results from lesions of the brainstem, cerebellum, or thalamus. **Psychogenic tremor** is distinguished by its variable appearance, abrupt onset and remission, nonprogressive course, and association with selective but not task-specific disabilities. In some cases, tremor may even occur as a manifestation of another movement disorder, as is seen with position- or task-specific tremor (e.g., writing tremor), dystonic tremor, and myoclonic tremor.

When evaluating a child with tremor, it is important to screen for common metabolic disturbances, including electrolyte abnormalities and thyroid disease, assess the child's caffeine intake, and review the child's medication list for known tremor-inducing agents. It is also critical to exclude Wilson disease, which has a characteristic "wing-beating" tremor, as this is a treatable condition.

BIBLIOGRAPHY

Please visit the Nelson Textbook of Pediatrics *website at* *www.expertconsult.com* *for the complete bibliography.*

590.3 Dystonia

Denia Ramirez-Montealegre and Jonathan W. Mink

Dystonia is a disorder of movement characterized by sustained muscle contraction, frequently causing twisting and repetitive movements or abnormal postures. Major causes of dystonia include primary generalized dystonia, medications, metabolic disorders, and perinatal asphyxia. In this section, we will provide an overview of major causes of dystonia, organized by etiologic category.

INHERITED PRIMARY DYSTONIAS

Primary generalized dystonia, also referred to as primary torsion dystonia or *dystonia musculorum deformans*, is caused by a group of genetic disorders with onset in childhood. One form, which occurs more commonly in the Ashkenazi Jewish population, is caused by a dominant mutation in the ***DYT1*** gene coding for the adenosine triphosphate (ATP) binding protein Torsin A.

The initial manifestation of DYT1 dystonia is often intermittent unilateral posturing of a lower extremity, which assumes an extended and rotated position. Ultimately, all 4 extremities and the axial musculature can be affected. Although cranial involvement can occur, it is more common in non-DYT1 dystonias. There is a wide clinical spectrum, varying even within families. If a family history of dystonia is absent, the diagnosis should still be considered, given the intrafamilial variability in clinical expression.

More than a dozen loci for genes for torsion dystonia have been identified (DYT1-DYT20). One is the autosomal dominant disorder **dopa-responsive dystonia (DRD, *DYT5a*)**, also called Segawa syndrome. The gene for DRD codes for GTP cyclohydrolase 1, the rate-limiting enzyme for tetrahydrobiopterin synthesis, which is a cofactor for synthesis of the neurotransmitters dopamine and serotonin. Thus, the genetic mutation results in dopamine deficiency. The hallmark of the disorder is diurnal variation; symptoms worsen as the day progresses and may transiently improve with sleep. Early-onset patients, who tend to present with delayed or abnormal gait due to dystonia of a lower extremity, can easily be confused with patients with dyskinetic cerebral palsy. It should be noted that in the presence of a progressive dystonia, diurnal fluctuation, or if loss of previously achieved motor skills occurs, a prior diagnosis of cerebral palsy should be re-examined. DRD responds dramatically to very small daily doses of levodopa. The responsiveness to levodopa is a sustained benefit, even if the diagnosis is delayed several years, as long as contractures have not developed.

Myoclonus dystonia (DYT11), due to mutations in the epsilon-sarcoglycan (SCGE) gene, is characterized by dystonia involving the upper extremities, head, and/or neck as well as myoclonic movements in these regions. Although a combination of myoclonus and dystonia typically occurs, each manifestation can present in isolation. When repetitive, the myoclonus may take on a tremor-like appearance, termed dystonic tremor. Improvement in symptoms following alcohol ingestion, reported by affected adult family members, may be a helpful clue to this diagnosis.

Common to the inherited dystonias, there is considerable intrafamilial variability in clinical manifestations, distribution, and severity of dystonia. In primary dystonias, although the main clinical features are motor, there may be an increased risk for major depression. Anxiety, obsessive-compulsive disorder, and depression have all been reported in the myoclonus-dystonia syndrome. Screening for psychiatric co-morbidities cannot be overlooked in this population.

DRUG-INDUCED DYSTONIAS

A number of medications are capable of inducing involuntary movements, drug-induced movement disorders (DIMD), in children and adults. Dopamine-blocking agents, including antipsychotics (e.g., haloperidol) and antiemetics (e.g., metoclopramide, prochlorperazine), as well as atypical antipsychotics (e.g., risperidone) can produce acute dystonic reactions or delayed (tardive) DIMD. **Acute dystonic reactions**, occurring in the 1st days of exposure, typically involve the face and neck, manifesting as torticollis, retrocollis, oculogyric crisis, or tongue protrusion. Life-threatening presentations with laryngospasm and airway compromise can also occur, requiring prompt recognition and treatment of this entity. Intravenous diphenhydramine, 1-2 mg/kg/dose, may rapidly reverse the drug-related dystonia. High potency of the dopamine blocker, young age, and prior dystonic reactions may be predisposing factors. Acute dystonic reactions have also been described with cetirizine.

Severe rigidity combined with high fever, autonomic symptoms (tachycardia, diaphoresis), delirium, and dystonia are signs of **neuroleptic malignant syndrome** (NMS) which typically occurs a few days after starting or increasing the dose of a neuroleptic drug, or in the setting of withdrawal from a dopaminergic agent. In contrast to acute dystonic reactions, which take place within days, NMS occurs within a month of medication initiation or dose increase.

Delayed onset involuntary movements, **tardive dyskinesias**, develop in the setting of chronic neuroleptic use, at least 3 mo in duration. Involvement of the face, particularly the mouth, lips, and/or jaw with chewing or tongue thrusting is characteristic. The risk of tardive dyskinesia, which is much less frequent in children compared to adults, increases as medication dose and duration of treatment increase. There are data to suggest that children with autism spectrum disorders may also be at increased risk for this DIMD. Unlike acute dystonic reactions and neuroleptic malignant syndrome, discontinuation of the offending agent may not result in clinical improvement. In these patients, use of dopamine-depletors such as reserpine or tetrabenazine may prove helpful.

Therapeutic doses of phenytoin or carbamazepine rarely cause progressive dystonia in children with epilepsy, particularly in those who have an underlying structural abnormality of the brain.

During evaluation of new onset dystonia, a careful history of prescriptions and potential medication exposures is critical.

CEREBRAL PALSY

Of children with cerebral palsy (CP), 10-15% have a dyskinetic form characterized largely by involuntary movements such as dystonia or chorea, rather than predominant spasticity. Dyskinetic CP is a more common presentation in term infants who suffer from perinatal asphyxia, as compared to premature infants who are more likely to develop spastic CP. Typically, these signs develop during infancy; though rarely, the onset of dystonia can be delayed by several years. In patients with delayed-onset dystonia, involvement of the neck spreading to an upper limb or hemidystonia (involvement of the arm and leg on 1 side of the body) may be the initial presentation, which differs from the typical presentation of other childhood-onset dystonias. Review of birth history remains an important component of the evaluation of new onset dystonia, even in adolescence, when evidence of prior mild motor deficits exists. Birth injury, kernicterus, stroke, encephalitis, and head trauma are all potential causes of delayed-onset dystonia.

METABOLIC DISORDERS

Disorders of monamine neurotransmitter metabolism, of which DRD is 1, present in infancy and early childhood with dystonia, hypotonia, oculogyric crises and/or autonomic symptoms. The more common disorders among this group of rare diseases include DRD, tyrosine hydroxylase deficiency, and aromatic amino acid decarboxylase deficiency. Detailed discussion is beyond the scope of this chapter, however reviews are available for reference.

Wilson disease is an autosomal recessive inborn error of copper transport characterized by cirrhosis of the liver and degenerative changes in the CNS, particularly the basal ganglia (Chapter 349.2). It has been determined that there are multiple mutations in the Wilson disease gene (WND), accounting for the variability in presentation of the condition. The neurologic manifestations of Wilson disease rarely appear before age 10 yr, and the initial sign is often progressive dystonia. Tremors of the extremities develop, unilaterally at first, but they eventually become coarse, generalized, and incapacitating. Other neurologic signs of Wilson disease relate to progressive basal ganglia disease, such as parkinsonism, dysarthria, dysphonia, and choreoathetosis. Less frequent are ataxia, and pyramidal signs. The MRI or CT scan shows ventricular dilatation in advanced cases with atrophy of the cerebrum, cerebellum, and/or brainstem along with signal intensity change in the basal ganglia, thalamus, and/or brainstem, particularly the midbrain.

Table 590-8 SELECTED CAUSES OF PRIMARY AND SECONDARY DYSTONIA IN CHILDHOOD

DIAGNOSIS	ADDITIONAL CLINICAL FEATURES
Aicardi-Goutieres syndrome	Encephalopathy, developmental regression Acquired microcephaly Sterile pyrexias Lesions on the digits, ears (chilblain) Epilepsy CT: calcification of the basal ganglia
Alternating hemiplegia of childhood	Episodic hemiplegia/quadriplegia Abnormal ocular movements Autonomic symptoms Epilepsy Global developmental impairment Environmental triggers for spells
Aromatic amino acid decarboxylase deficiency (AADC)	Developmental delay Oculogyric crises Autonomic dysfunction Hypotonia
ARX gene mutation (X-linked)	Male Cognitive impairment Infantile spasms, epilepsy Brain malformation
Benign paroxysmal torticollis of infancy	Episodic Cervical dystonia only Family history of migraine
Complex regional pain syndrome	Lower limb involvement Prominent pain
Dopa-responsive dystonia (DRD)	Diurnal variation
Drug-induced dystonia	
Dystonia-deafness optic neuropathy syndrome	Sensorineural hearing loss in early childhood Psychosis Optic atrophy in adolescence
DYT1 dystonia	Lower limb onset followed by generalization
Glutaric aciduria type 1	Macrocephaly Encephalopathic crises MRI: striatal necrosis
GM1 gangliosidosis type 3	Short stature, skeletal dysplasia Orofacial dystonia Speech/swallowing disturbance Parkinsonism MRI: putaminal hyperintensity
Huntington disease (HD)	Parkinsonism Epilepsy Family history of HD
Kernicterus	Jaundice in infancy Hearing loss Impaired upgaze Enamel dysplasia MRI: hyperintense lesions in the globus pallidus
Leigh syndrome	Motor delays, weakness, hypotonia Ataxia, tremor Elevated lactate MRI: bilateral symmetric hyperintense lesions in the basal ganglia or thalamus
Lesch-Nyhan syndrome (X-linked)	Male Self-injurious behavior Hypotonia Oromandibular dystonia, inspiratory stridor Oculomotor apraxia Cognitive impairment Elevated uric acid
Myoclonus dystonia	Myoclonus Head, upper limb involvement
Niemann-Pick type C	Hepatosplenomegaly Hypotonia Supranuclear gaze palsy Ataxia, dysarthria Epilepsy Psychiatric symptoms
Neuroacanthocytosis	Oromandibular and lingual dystonia
Neurodegeneration with brain iron accumulation	Cognitive impairment Retinal pigmentary degeneration, optic atrophy
Rapid onset dystonia parkinsonism (DYT12)	Acute onset Distribution face>arm>leg Prominent bulbar signs
Rett syndrome	Female Developmental regression following a period of normal development Stereotypic hand movements Acquired microcephaly Epilepsy
Spinocerebellar ataxia 17 (SCA17)	Ataxia Dementia, psychiatric symptoms Parkinsonism
Tics	Stereotyped movements Premonitory urge, suppressible
Tyrosine hydroxylase deficiency	Infantile encephalopathy, hypotonia Oculogyric crises, ptosis Autonomic symptoms Less diurnal fluctuation than DRD

Pantothenate kinase associated neurodegeneration (**PKAN**, *Hallervorden-Spatz disease*) is a rare autosomal recessive neurodegenerative disorder. Many patients have mutations in pantothenate kinase 2 (PANK2) localized to mitochondria in neurons. The condition usually begins before 6 yr of age and is characterized by rapidly progressive dystonia, rigidity, and choreoathetosis. Spasticity, extensor plantar responses, dysarthria, and intellectual deterioration become evident during adolescence, and death usually occurs by early adulthood. MRI shows lesions of the globus pallidus, including low signal intensity in T2 weighted images (corresponding to iron pigments) and an anteromedial area of high signal intensity (tissue necrosis and edema), or "eye-of-the-tiger" sign. Neuropathologic examination indicates excessive accumulation of iron-containing pigments in the globus pallidus and substantia nigra. More recently, similar disorders of high brain iron content without PANK2 mutations, including infantile neuroaxonal dystrophy, neuroferritinopathy, and aceruloplasminemia, have been grouped as disorders of neurodegeneration with brain iron accumulation (**NBIA**). Patterns of iron deposition visualized by brain MRI have shown utility in differentiating these disorders.

Although dystonia may present in isolation as the 1st sign of a metabolic or neurodegenerative disorder, this group of diseases should be considered mainly in those who demonstrate signs of systemic disease, (e.g., organomegaly, short stature, hearing loss, vision impairment, epilepsy), those with episodes of severe illness, evidence of regression, or cognitive impairment. Additional features suggestive of specific disorders are outlined in Table 590-8.

OTHER DISORDERS

Although uncommon, movement disorders, including dystonia, may be part of the presenting symptoms of **complex regional pain syndrome** (CPRS). Onset of involuntary movements within 1 yr of the traumatic event, affected lower limb, pain out of proportion to inciting event, and changes in the overlying skin and blood flow to the affected area suggest CPRS. Although sustained dystonia can produce pain or discomfort, CPRS should be considered in those who have a prominent component of pain and recent history of trauma to the affected limb.

There are disorders unique to childhood that warrant exploration in this section. **Benign paroxysmal torticollis of infancy** is characterized by recurrent episodes of cervical dystonia beginning in the 1st months of life. The torticollis may alternate sides from 1 episode to the next and may also persist during sleep. Associated signs and symptoms include irritability, pallor, vomiting, vertigo, ataxia, and occasionally limb dystonia. Family history is often notable for migraine and/or motion sickness in first-degree relatives. Despite the high frequency of spells, imaging studies are normal, and the outcome is uniformly benign with resolution by 3 yr of age.

In **alternating hemiplegia of childhood** (AHC), episodic hemiplegia affecting either side of the body is the hallmark of the disorder. However, patients are also affected by episodes of dystonia, ranging from minutes to days in duration. On average, both features of the disorder commence at approximately 6 mo of age. Episodic abnormal eye movements are observed in a large proportion of patients (93%) with onset as early as the 1st week of life. Thought to represent a migraine variant, AHC can similarly be triggered by fluctuations in temperature, certain foods, or water exposure. Over time, epilepsy and cognitive impairment emerge, and the involuntary movements change from episodic to constant. Infantile onset and the paroxysmal nature of symptoms early in the disease course are key features to this diagnosis.

Finally, although a diagnosis of exclusion, the presence of odd movements or selective disability may indicate a psychogenic dystonia in older children. There is considerable overlap in features of organic and **psychogenic movement disorders,** making the diagnosis difficult to establish. For instance, both organic and psychogenic movement disorders have the potential to worsen in the setting of stress and may dissipate with relaxation or sleep. History should include review of recent stressors, psychiatric symptoms, and exposure to others with similar disorders. On examination, a changing movement disorder, inconsistent motor or sensory exam, or response to suggestion are supportive of a possible psychogenic movement disorder. Early recognition of this disorder may lessen morbidity caused by unnecessary diagnostic and interventional procedures.

TREATMENT

Children with generalized dystonia, including those with involvement of the muscles of swallowing, may respond to the anticholinergic agent trihexyphenidyl (Artane). Titration occurs slowly over the course of months in an effort to limit untoward side effects, such as urinary retention, mental confusion, or blurred vision. Additional drugs that have been effective include levodopa, and diazepam. Segmental dystonia such as torticollis often responds well to botulinum toxin injections. Intrathecal baclofen delivered through implantable constant infusion pump may be helpful in some patients. Deep brain stimulation (DBS) with leads implanted in the globus pallidus is most helpful for children with severe primary generalized dystonia. Recent data suggests, however, that DBS may also be of benefit in children with secondary dystonias, such as cerebral palsy.

In the case of drug-induced dystonias, removal of the offending agent and treatment with intravenous diphenhydramine typically suffice. For neuroleptic malignant syndrome, dantrolene may be indicated.

BIBLIOGRAPHY

Please visit the Nelson Textbook of Pediatrics *website at* *www.expertconsult.com* *for the complete bibliography.*

Chapter 591
Encephalopathies

Michael V. Johnston

Encephalopathy is a generalized disorder of cerebral function that may be acute or chronic, progressive or static. The etiologies of the encephalopathies in children include infectious, toxic (carbon monoxide, drugs, lead), metabolic, genetic and ischemic causes. Hypoxic-ischemic encephalopathy is discussed in Chapter 93.5.

591.1 Cerebral Palsy

Michael V. Johnston

See Chapters 33 and 91.2.

Cerebral palsy (CP) is a diagnostic term used to describe a group of permanent disorders of movement and posture causing activity limitation, that are attributed to nonprogressive disturbances in the in the developing fetal or infant brain. The motor disorders are often accompanied by disturbances of sensation, perception, cognition, communication, and behavior as well as by epilepsy and secondary musculoskeletal problems. CP is caused by a broad group of developmental, genetic, metabolic, ischemic, infectious, and other acquired etiologies that produce a common group of neurologic phenotypes. CP has historically been considered a static encephalopathy, but some of the neurologic features of CP, such as movement disorders and orthopedic complications including scoliosis and hip dislocation, can change or progress over time. Many children and adults with CP function at a high educational and vocational level, without any sign of cognitive dysfunction.

EPIDEMIOLOGY AND ETIOLOGY

CP is the most common and costly form of chronic motor disability that begins in childhood, and recent data from the Centers for Disease Control and Prevention indicate that the incidence is 3.6/1000 with a male/female ratio of 1.4/1. The Collaborative Perinatal Project (CPP), in which approximately 45,000 children were regularly monitored from in utero to the age of 7 yr, found that most children with CP had been born at term with uncomplicated labors and deliveries. In 80% of cases, features were identified pointing to antenatal factors causing abnormal brain development. A substantial number of children with CP had congenital anomalies external to the central nervous system (CNS). Fewer than 10% of children with CP had evidence of intrapartum asphyxia. Intrauterine exposure to maternal infection (chorioamnionitis, inflammation of placental membranes, umbilical cord inflammation, foul-smelling amniotic fluid, maternal sepsis, temperature >38°C during labor, urinary tract infection) was associated with a significant increase in the risk of CP in normal birthweight infants. Elevated levels of inflammatory cytokines have been reported in heelstick blood collected at birth from children who later were identified with CP. Genetic factors may contribute to the inflammatory cytokine response, and a functional polymorphism in the interleukin-6 gene has recently been associated with a higher rate of CP in term infants.

The prevalence of CP has increased somewhat due to the enhanced survival of very premature infants weighing <1,000 g, who go on to develop CP at a rate of approximately 15/100. However, the gestational age at birth-adjusted prevalence of CP among 2 yr old former premature infants born at 20-27 wk of gestation has decreased over the past decade. The major lesions that contribute to CP in this group are **intracerebral hemorrhage** and **periventricular leukomalacia** (PVL). Although the incidence of intracerebral hemorrhage has declined significantly, PVL remains a major problem. PVL reflects the enhanced vulnerability of immature oligodendroglia in premature infants to oxidative stress caused by ischemia or infectious/inflammatory insults. White matter abnormalities (loss of volume of periventricular white matter, extent of cystic changes, ventricular dilatation, thinning of the corpus callosum) present on MRI at 40 wk of gestational age among former preterm infants are a predictor of later CP.

In 2006, the European Cerebral Palsy Study examined prenatal and perinatal factors as well as clinical findings and results of MRI in a contemporary cohort of more than 400 children with CP. In agreement with the CPP study, more than half the children with CP in this study were born at term, and less than 20% had clinical or brain imaging indicators of possible intrapartum factors such as asphyxia. The contribution of intrapartum factors to CP is higher in some underdeveloped regions of the world. Also in agreement with earlier data, antenatal infection was strongly associated with CP and 39.5% of mothers of children with CP reported having an infection during the pregnancy, with 19% having evidence of a urinary tract infection and 11.5% reporting taking antibiotics. Multiple pregnancy was also associated with a higher incidence of CP and 12% of the cases in the European CP study resulted from a multiple pregnancy, in contrast to a 1.5% incidence of multiple pregnancy in the study. Other studies have also documented a relationship between multiple births and CP, with a rate in twins that is 5-8 times greater than in singleton pregnancies and a rate in triplets that is 20-47 times greater. Death of a twin in utero carries an even greater risk of CP that is 8 times that of a pregnancy in which both twins survive and approximately 60 times the risk in a singleton pregnancy. Infertility treatments are also associated with a higher rate of CP, probably because these treatments are often associated with multiple pregnancies. Among children from multiple pregnancies, 24% were from pregnancies after infertility treatment compared with 3.4% of the singleton pregnancies in the study. CP is more common and more severe in boys compared to girls and this effect is enhanced at the extremes of body weight. Male infants with intrauterine growth retardation and a birthweight less than the 3rd percentile are 16 times more likely to have CP than males with optimal growth, and infants with weights above the 97th percentile are 4 times more likely to have CP.

CLINICAL MANIFESTATIONS

CP is generally divided into several major motor syndromes that differ according to the pattern of neurologic involvement, neuropathology, and etiology (Table 591-1). The physiologic classification identifies the major motor abnormality, whereas the topographic taxonomy indicates the involved extremities. CP is also commonly associated with a spectrum of developmental disabilities, including mental retardation, epilepsy, and visual, hearing, speech, cognitive, and behavioral abnormalities. The motor handicap may be the least of the child's problems.

Infants with **spastic hemiplegia** have decreased spontaneous movements on the affected side and show hand preference at a very early age. The arm is often more involved than the leg and difficulty in hand manipulation is obvious by 1 yr of age. Walking is usually delayed until 18-24 mo, and a circumductive gait is apparent. Examination of the extremities may show growth arrest, particularly in the hand and thumbnail, especially if the contralateral parietal lobe is abnormal, because extremity growth is influenced by this area of the brain. Spasticity refers to the quality of increased muscle tone which increases with the speed of passive muscle stretching and is greatest in antigravity muscles. It is apparent in the affected extremities, particularly at the ankle, causing an equinovarus deformity of the foot. An affected child often walks on tiptoe because of the increased tone in the antigravity gastrocnemius muscles, and the affected upper extremity assumes a flexed posture when the child runs. Ankle clonus and a Babinski sign may be present, the deep tendon reflexes are increased, and weakness of the hand and foot dorsiflexors is evident. About one third of patients with spastic hemiplegia have a seizure disorder that usually develops in the 1st yr or 2; approximately 25% have cognitive abnormalities including mental retardation. MRI is far more sensitive than CT for most lesions seen with CP, although a CT scan may be useful for detecting calcifications associated with congenital infections. In the European CP study, 34% of children with hemiplegia had injury to the white matter that probably dated to the in utero period and 27% had a focal lesion that may have resulted from a stroke. Other children with hemiplegic CP had had malformations from multiple causes including infections (e.g., cytomegalovirus), lissencephaly, polymicrogyria, schizencephaly, or cortical dysplasia. Focal cerebral infarction (stroke) secondary to intrauterine or perinatal thromboembolism related to thrombophilic disorders, like the presence of anticardiolipin antibodies, is an important cause of hemiplegic CP (Chapter 594). Family histories suggestive of thrombosis and inherited clotting disorders, such as factor V Leiden mutation, may be present and evaluation of the mother may provide information valuable for future pregnancies and other family members.

Spastic diplegia is bilateral spasticity of the legs that is greater than in the arms. Spastic diplegia is strongly associated with damage to the immature white matter during the vulnerable period of immature oligodendroglia between 20-34 wk of

Table 591-1 CLASSIFICATION OF CEREBRAL PALSY AND MAJOR CAUSES

MOTOR SYNDROME (APPROX % OF CP)	NEUROPATHOLOGY/MRI	MAJOR CAUSES
Spastic diplegia (35%)	Periventricular leukomalacia Periventricular cysts or scars in White matter, enlargement of ventricles, squared of posterior ventricles	Prematurity Ischemia Infection Endocrine/metabolic (e.g., thyroid)
Spastic quadriplegia (20%)	Periventricular leukomalacia	Ischemia, infection
	Multicystic encephalomalacia Cortical malformations	Endocrine/metabolic, genetic/developmental
Hemiplegia (25%)	Stroke: in utero or neonatal Focal infarct or cortical, subcortical damage Cortical malformations	Thrombophilic disorders Infection Genetic/developmental Periventricular hemorrhagic infarction
Extrapyramidal (athetoid, dyskinetic) (15%)	Asphyxia: symmetric scars in putamen and thalamus Kernicterus: scars in globus pallidus, hippocampus Mitochondrial: scaring globus pallidus, caudate, putamen, brainstem No lesions: ? dopa-responsive dystonia	Asphyxia Kernicterus Mitochondrial Genetic/metabolic

gestation. However, about 15% of cases of spastic diplegia result from in utero lesions in infants who go on to delivery at term. The 1st clinical indication of spastic diplegia is often noted when an affected infant begins to crawl. The child uses the arms in a normal reciprocal fashion but tends to drag the legs behind more as a rudder (commando crawl) rather than using the normal four-limbed crawling movement. If the spasticity is severe, application of a diaper is difficult because of the excessive adduction of the hips. If there is paraspinal muscle involvement, the child may be unable to sit. Examination of the child reveals spasticity in the legs with brisk reflexes, ankle clonus, and a bilateral Babinski sign. When the child is suspended by the axillae, a scissoring posture of the lower extremities is maintained. Walking is significantly delayed, the feet are held in a position of equinovarus, and the child walks on tiptoe. Severe spastic diplegia is characterized by disuse atrophy and impaired growth of the lower extremities and by disproportionate growth with normal development of the upper torso. The prognosis for normal intellectual development for these patients is good, and the likelihood of seizures is minimal. Such children often have learning disabilities and deficits in other abilities, such as vision, due to disruption of multiple white matter pathways that carry sensory as well as motor information.

The most common neuropathologic finding in children with spastic diplegia is PVL, which is visualized on MRI in more than 70% of cases. MRI typically shows scarring and shrinkage in the periventricular white matter with compensatory enlargement of the cerebral ventricles. However, neuropathology has also demonstrated a reduction in oligodendroglia in more widespread subcortical regions beyond the periventricular zones, and these subcortical lesions may contribute to the learning problems these patients can have. MRI with diffusion tensor imaging (DTI) is being used to map white matter tracks more precisely in patients with spastic diplegia, and this technique has shown that thalamocortical sensory pathways are often injured as severely as motor corticospinal pathways (Fig 591-1). These observations have led to greater interest in the importance of sensory deficits in these patients, which may be important for designing rehabilitative techniques.

Spastic quadriplegia is the most severe form of CP because of marked motor impairment of all extremities and the high association with mental retardation and seizures. Swallowing difficulties are common as a result of supranuclear bulbar palsies, often leading to aspiration pneumonia. The most common lesions seen on pathologic examination or on MRI scanning are severe PVL and multicystic cortical encephalomalacia. Neurologic examination shows increased tone and spasticity in all extremities, decreased spontaneous movements, brisk reflexes, and plantar extensor responses. Flexion contractures of the knees and elbows are often present by late childhood. Associated developmental disabilities, including speech and visual abnormalities, are particularly prevalent in this group of children. Children with spastic quadriparesis often have evidence of athetosis and may be classified as having mixed CP.

Athetoid CP, also called **choreoathetoid, extrapyramidal, or dyskinetic** CP, is less common than spastic cerebral palsy and makes up about 15-20% of patients with CP. Affected infants are characteristically hypotonic with poor head control and marked head lag and develop variably increased tone with rigidity and dystonia over several years. The term dystonia refers to the abnormality in tone in which muscles are rigid throughout their range of motion and involuntary contractions can occur in both flexors and extensors leading to limb positioning in fixed postures. Unlike spastic diplegia, the upper extremities are generally more affected than the lower extremities in extrapyramidal CP. Feeding may be difficult, and tongue thrust and drooling may be prominent. Speech is typically affected because the oropharyngeal muscles are involved. Speech may be absent or sentences are slurred, and voice modulation is impaired. Generally, upper motor neuron signs are not present, seizures are uncommon, and intellect is preserved in many patients. This form of CP is also referred to in Europe as dyskinetic CP and is the type most likely to be associated with **birth asphyxia.** In the European CP study, 76% of patients with this form of CP had lesions in the basal

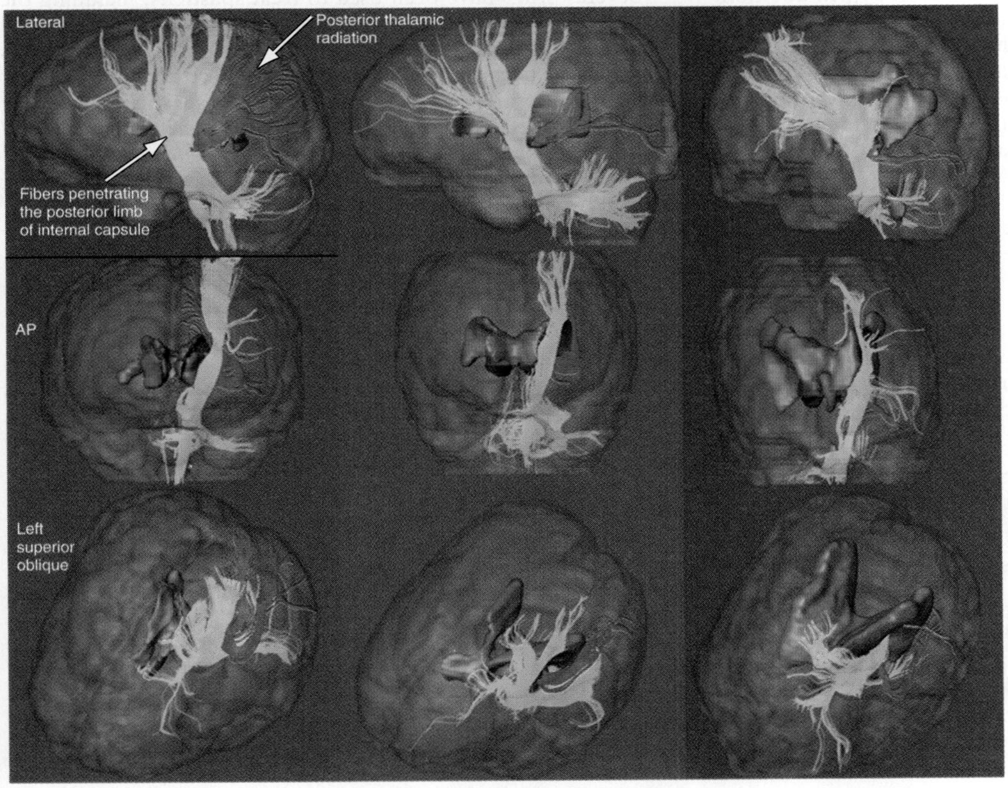

Figure 591-1 Diffusion tensor image of white matter pathways in the brains of 2 patients with spastic diplegia on the right compared to a normal child on the far left. Yellow fibers are corticospinal pathways projected from the motor cerebral cortex at the top downward into the brainstem, while the red fibers are thalamocortical sensory fibers projected from the thalamus upward to the cortex. In the children with spastic diplegia, both the corticospinal and thalamocortical pathways are reduced in size, but the ascending thalamocortical pathways are more affected. (From Nagae LM, Hoon AH Jr, Stashinko E, et al: Diffusion tensor imaging in children with periventricular leukomalacia: variability of injuries to white matter tracts, *AJNR Am J Neuroradiol* 28:1213–1222, 2007.)

ganglia and thalamus. Extrapyramidal CP secondary to acute intrapartum near-total asphyxia is associated with bilaterally symmetric lesions in the posterior putamen and ventrolateral thalamus. These lesions appear to be the correlate of the neuropathologic lesion called *status marmoratus* in the basal ganglia. Athetoid CP can also be caused by **kernicterus** secondary to high levels of bilirubin, and in this case the MRI scan shows lesions in the globus pallidus bilaterally. Extrapyramidal CP can also be associated with lesions in the basal ganglia and thalamus caused by metabolic genetic disorders such as mitochondrial disorders and glutaric aciduria. MRI scanning and possibly metabolic testing are important in the evaluation of children with extrapyramidal CP to make a correct etiologic diagnosis. In patients with dystonia who have a normal MRI, it is important to have a high level of suspicion for dihydroxyphenylalanine (DOPA)-responsive dystonia (Segawa disease), which causes prominent dystonia that can resemble CP. These patients typically have diurnal variation in their signs with worsening dystonia in the legs during the day; however this may not be prominent. These patients can be tested for a response to small doses of L-dopa and/or cerebrospinal fluid can be sent for neurotransmitter analysis.

DIAGNOSIS

A thorough history and physical examination should preclude a **progressive disorder** of the CNS, including degenerative diseases, metabolic disorders, spinal cord tumor, or muscular dystrophy. The possibility of anomalies at the base of the skull or other disorders affecting the cervical spinal cord needs to be considered in patients with little involvement of the arms or cranial nerves. An MRI scan of the brain is indicated to determine the location and extent of structural lesions or associated congenital malformations; an MRI scan of the spinal cord is indicated if there is any question about spinal cord pathology. Additional studies may include tests of hearing and visual function. Genetic evaluation should be considered in patients with congenital malformations (chromosomes) or evidence of metabolic disorders (e.g., amino acids, organic acids, MR spectroscopy). In addition to the genetic disorders mentioned earlier that can present as CP, the urea cycle disorder arginase deficiency is a rare cause of spastic diplegia and a deficiency of sulfite oxidase or molybdenum cofactor can present as CP caused by perinatal asphyxia. Tests to detect inherited thrombophilic disorders may be indicated in patients in which an in utero or neonatal stroke is suspected as the cause of CP.

Because CP is usually associated with a wide spectrum of developmental disorders, a multidisciplinary approach is most helpful in the assessment and treatment of such children.

TREATMENT

Ultimately, the treatment of CP must be prevention before it occurs. The variable and often cryptic etiology of CP is problematic in this regard. However, a recent study indicates that prenatal treatment of the mothers with magnesium lowers the prevalence of CP in their children at a corrected age of 2 yr.

A team of physicians from various specialties, as well as occupational and physical therapists, speech pathologists, social workers, educators, and developmental psychologists provide important contributions to the treatment of those children who develop CP. Parents should be taught how to work with their child in daily activities such as feeding, carrying, dressing, bathing, and playing in ways that limit the effects of abnormal muscle tone. They also need to be instructed in the supervision of a series of exercises designed to prevent the development of contractures, especially a tight Achilles tendon. Physical and occupational therapies are useful for promoting mobility and the use of the upper extremities for activities of daily living. Speech language pathologists promote acquisition of a functional means of communications. These therapists help children to achieve their potential, and often recommend further evaluations and adaptive equipment.

Children with spastic diplegia are treated initially with the assistance of adaptive equipment, such as walkers, poles, and standing frames. If a patient has marked spasticity of the lower extremities or evidence of hip dislocation, consideration should be given to performing surgical soft tissue procedures that reduce muscle spasm around the hip girdle, including an adductor tenotomy or psoas transfer and release. A rhizotomy procedure in which the roots of the spinal nerves are divided produces considerable improvement in selected patients with severe spastic diplegia (Fig. 591-2). A tight heel cord in a child with spastic hemiplegia may be treated surgically by tenotomy of the Achilles tendon. Quadriplegia is managed with motorized wheelchairs, special feeding devices, modified typewriters, and customized seating arrangements. The function of the affected extremities in children with **hemiplegic CP** can often be improved by therapy in which movement of the good side is constrained with casts while the impaired extremities perform exercises which induce improved hand and arm functioning. This constraint-induced movement therapy is effective in patients of all ages.

Several drugs have been used to **treat spasticity,** including the benzodiazepines and baclofen. These medications have beneficial effects in some patients, but can also cause side effects such as sedation for benzodiazepines and lowered seizure threshold for baclofen. Several drugs can be used to **treat spasticity,** including oral diazepam (0.5-7.5 mg/dose, BID or QID), baclofen (0.2-2 mg/kg/day, BID or TID) or dantrolene (0.5-10/kg/day, BID). Small doses of levodopa (0.5-2 mg/kg/day) can be used to treat dystonia or DOPA-responsive dystonia. Artane (trihexyphenidyl, 0.25 mg/day, BID or TID and titrated upward) is sometimes useful for treating dystonia and can increase use of the upper extremities and vocalizations. Reserpine (0.01 µg/kg/day, BID) or tetrabenzine (12.5-25 mg, BID or TID) can be useful for hyperkinetic movement disorders including athetosis or chorea.

Intrathecal baclofen delivered with an implanted pump has been used successfully in many children with severe spasticity,

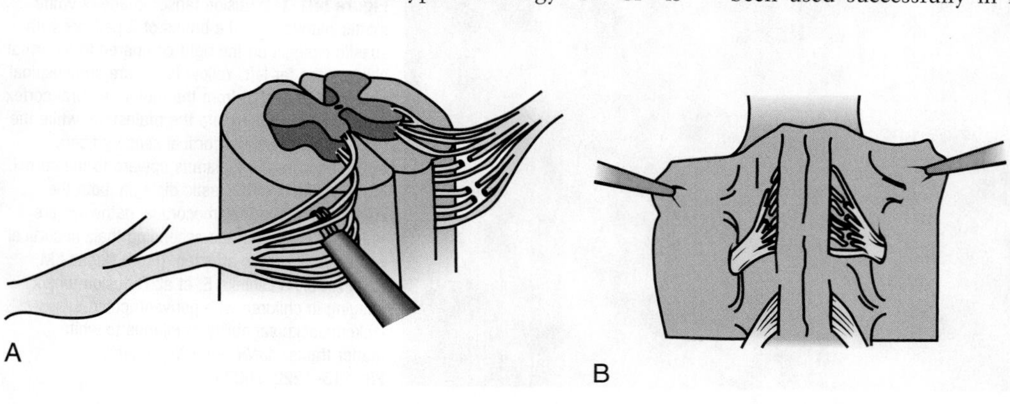

Figure 591-2 Schematic representation of the technique of selected dorsal rhizotomy. *A,* After laminectomy, the dura is opened and the dorsal spinal rootlets are exposed. The rootlets are stimulated so that abnormal rootlet activity can be identified. *B,* A proportion of rootlets are transected. (From Koman LA, Smith BP, Shilt JS: Cerebral palsy, *Lancet* 363:1619–1631, 2004. Reproduced with permission from Wake Forest University Orthopaedic Press.)

and can be useful because it delivers the drug directly around the spinal cord where it reduces neurotransmission of afferent nerve fibers. Direct delivery to the spinal cord overcomes the problem of CNS side effects caused by the large oral doses needed to penetrate the blood brain barrier. This therapy requires a team approach and constant follow-up for complications of the infusion pumping mechanism and infection. **Botulinum toxin** injected into specific muscle groups for the management of spasticity shows a very positive response in many patients. Botulism toxin injected into salivary glands may also help reduce the severity of drooling, which is seen in 10-30% of patients with CP and has been traditionally treated with anticholinergic agents. Patients with rigidity, dystonia, and spastic quadriparesis sometimes respond to levodopa, and children with dystonia may benefit from carbamazepine or trihexyphenidyl. Hyperbaric oxygen has not been shown to improve the condition of children with CP.

Communication skills may be enhanced by the use of Bliss symbols, talking typewriters, electronic speech generating devices, and specially adapted computers including artificial intelligence computers to augment motor and language function. Significant behavior problems may substantially interfere with the development of a child with CP; their early identification and management are important, and the assistance of a psychologist or psychiatrist may be necessary. Learning and attention deficit disorders and mental retardation are assessed and managed by a psychologist and educator. Strabismus, nystagmus, and optic atrophy are common in children with CP; an ophthalmologist should be included in the initial assessment. Lower urinary tract dysfunction should receive prompt assessment and treatment.

BIBLIOGRAPHY

Please visit the Nelson Textbook of Pediatrics *website at* *www.expertconsult.com* *for the complete bibliography.*

591.2 Mitochondrial Encephalomyopathies

Michael V. Johnston

See Chapters 81.4 and 603.4.

Mitochondrial encephalomyopathies are a heterogeneous group of clinical syndromes caused by genetic lesions that impair energy production through oxidative phosphorylation. The signs and symptoms of these disorders reflect the vulnerability of the nervous system, muscles and other organs to energy deficiency. Signs of brain and muscle dysfunction (seizures, weakness, ptosis, external ophthalmoplegia, psychomotor regression, hearing loss, movement disorders, and ataxia) in association with lactic acidosis are prominent features of mitochondrial disorders. Cardiomyopathy and diabetes mellitus can also result from mitochondrial disorders.

Children with mitochondrial disorders often have multifocal signs that are intermittent or relapsing-remitting, often in association with intercurrent illness. Many of these disorders were described as clinical syndromes before their genetics were understood. Children with mitochondrial encephalomyopathy with lactic acidosis and strokelike episodes (MELAS) present with developmental delay, weakness and headaches as well as focal signs that suggest a stroke. Brain imaging indicates that injury does not fit within the usual vascular territories. Children with myoclonic epilepsy with ragged red fibers (MERRF) present with myoclonus and myoclonic seizures as well as intermittent muscle weakness. The ragged red fibers referred to in the name of this disorder are clumps of abnormal mitochondria seen within muscle fibers in sections from a muscle biopsy stained with Gomori trichrome stain. NARP syndrome (neuropathy, ataxia and retinitis pigmentosa), Kearn-Sayre syndrome (KSS) (ptosis, ophthalmoplegia, heart block, Leigh disease (subacute necrotizing encephalomyelopathy), and Leber hereditary optic neuropathy (LHON) have also been defined as relatively homogeneous clinical subgroups (Table 591-2). It is important to keep in mind that mitochondrial disorders can be difficult to diagnose. They

Table 591-2 CLINICAL MANIFESTATIONS OF MITOCHONDRIAL ENCEPHALOMYOPATHIES

TISSUE	SYMPTOMS/SIGNS	MELAS	MERRF	NARP	KSS	LEIGH	LHON
CNS	Regression	+	+		+	+	
	Seizures	+	+				
	Ataxia	+	+	+	+		
	Cortical blindness	+					
	Deafness	+		+			
	Migraine	+					
	Hemiparesis	+					
	Myoclonus	+	+				
	Movement disorder	+					+
Nerve	Peripheral neuropathy	+	+	+	+		
Muscle	Ophthalmoplegia				+		
	Weakness	+	+	+	+	+	
	RRF on muscle biopsy	+	+		+		
	Ptosis				+		
Eye	Pigmentary retinopathy			+	+		
	Optic atrophy				+	+	+
	Cataracts						
Heart	Conduction block				+		+
	Cardiomyopathy				+		
Blood	Anemia	+					
	Lactic acidosis		+		+	+	
Endocrine	Diabetes mellitus				+		
	Short stature	+	+		+		
Kidney	Fanconi syndrome	+	+		+		

KSS, Kearn-Sayre syndrome; LHON, Leber hereditary optic neuropathy; MELAS, mitochondrial myopathy, encephalopathy, lactic acidosis, and strokelike episodes; MERRF, myoclonic epilepsy with ragged red fibers; NARP, neuropathy, ataxia and retinitis pigmentosa; RRF, ragged red fibers.

often present with novel combinations of signs and symptoms due to high mutation rates for mitochondrial DNA (mtDNA), and the severity of disease varies from person to person.

Mitochondrial diseases can be caused by mutations of nuclear DNA (nDNA) or mtDNA (Chapters 75, 80, and 81). Oxidative phosphorylation in the respiratory chain is mediated by 5 intramitochondrial enzyme complexes (complexes I-V) and 2 mobile electron carriers (coenzyme Q and cytochrome c) that are responsible for producing the adenosine triphosphate (ATP) required for normal cellular function. The maintenance of oxidative phosphorylation requires coordinated regulation of nuclear DNA and mitochondrial DNA genes. Human mtDNA is a small (16.6 kb), circular, double-stranded molecule that has been completely sequenced and encodes 13 structural proteins, all of which are subunits of the respiratory chain complexes, as well as 2 ribosomal RNAs and 22 tRNAs needed for translation. The nuclear DNA is responsible for synthesizing approximately 70 subunits, transporting them to the mitochondria via chaperone proteins, ensuring their passage across the inner mitochondrial membrane, and coordinating their correct processing and assembly. Diseases of mitochondrial oxidative phosphorylation can be divided into 3 groups: (1) defects of mtDNA, (2) defects of nDNA, and (3) defects of communication between the nuclear and mitochondrial genome.

mtDNA is distinct from nDNA for the following reasons: (1) its genetic code differs from nDNA, (2) it is tightly packed with information because it contains no introns, (3) it is subject to spontaneous mutations at a higher rate than nDNA, (4) it has less efficient repair mechanisms, and (5) it is present in hundreds or thousands of copies per cell and is transmitted by maternal inheritance. mtDNA is contributed only by the oocyte in the formation of the zygote. If a mutation in mtDNA occurs in the ovum or zygote, it may be passed on randomly to subsequent generations of cells. Some receive few or no mutant genomes (**normal** or **wild-type homoplasmy**), while others receive a mixed population of **mutant** and **wild-type** mtDNAs (**heteroplasmy**), and still others receive primarily or exclusively **mutant** genomes (**mutant homoplasmy**). The important implications of maternal inheritance and heteroplasmy are as follows: (1) inheritance of the disease is maternal, but both sexes are equally affected; (2) phenotypic expression of an mtDNA mutation depends on the relative proportions of mutant and wild-type genomes, with a minimum critical number of mutant genomes being necessary for expression (threshold effect); (3) at cell division, the proportional distribution may shift between daughter cells (mitotic segregation), leading to a corresponding phenotypic change; and (4) subsequent generations are affected at a higher rate than in autosomal dominant diseases. The critical number of mutant mtDNAs required for the threshold effect may vary, depending on the vulnerability of the tissue to impairments of oxidative metabolism as well as on the vulnerability of the same tissue over time that may increase with aging. In contrast to maternally inherited disorders due to mutations in mtDNA, diseases resulting from defects in nDNA follow mendelian inheritance. Mitochondrial diseases caused by defects in nDNA include defects in substrate transport (plasmalemmal carnitine transporter, carnitine palmitoyltransferase I and II, carnitine acylcarnitine translocase defects), defects in substrate oxidation (pyruvate dehydrogenase complex, pyruvate carboxylase, intramitochondrial fatty acid oxidation defects), defects in the Krebs cycle (α-ketoglutarate dehydrogenase, fumarase, aconitase defects), and defects in the respiratory chain (complexes I-V) including defects of oxidation/phosphorylation coupling (Luft syndrome) and defects in mitochondrial protein transport.

Diseases caused by defects in mtDNA can be divided into those associated with point mutations that are maternally inherited (e.g., LHON, MELAS, MERRF, and NARP syndromes) and those due to deletions or duplications of mtDNA that reflect altered communication between the nucleus and the mitochondria (KSS; Pearson syndrome, a rare severe encephalopathy with anemia and pancreatic dysfunction; and progressive external ophthalmoplegia [PEO]). These disorders can be inherited by sporadic, autosomal dominant, or recessive mechanisms and mutations in multiple genes, including mitochondrial mtDNA polymerase γ catalytic subunit (POLG) have been identified. POLG mutations have also been identified in patients with Alpers-Huttenlocher syndrome which causes a refractory seizure disorder and hepatic failure. Other genes that regulate the supply of nucleotides for mtDNA synthesis have been associated with severe encephalopathy and liver disease, and new disorders are being identified that result from defects in the interactions between mitochondria and their milieu in the cell.

MITOCHONDRIAL MYOPATHY, ENCEPHALOPATHY, LACTIC ACIDOSIS, AND STROKELIKE EPISODES (MELAS)

Children with MELAS may be normal for the 1st several years, but they gradually display delayed motor and cognitive development and short stature. The clinical syndrome is characterized by (1) recurrent strokelike episodes of hemiparesis or other focal neurologic signs with lesions most commonly seen in the posterior temporal, parietal, and occipital lobes (CT or MRI evidence of focal brain abnormalities); (2) lactic acidosis, ragged red fibers (RRF), or both; and (3) at least 2 of the following: focal or generalized seizures, dementia, recurrent migraine headaches, and vomiting. In 1 series, onset was before age 15 yr in 62% of patients, and hemianopia or cortical blindness was the most common manifestation. Cerebrospinal fluid protein is often increased. The MELAS 3243 mutation on mtDNA can also be associated with different combinations of exercise intolerance, myopathy, ophthalmoplegia, pigmentary retinopathy, hypertrophic or dilated cardiomyopathy, cardiac conduction defects, deafness, endocrinopathy (diabetes mellitus), and proximal renal tubular dysfunction. Two patients have also been described with bilateral rolandic lesions and epilepsia partialis continua associated with mitochondrial DNA mutations at 10158T>C and 10191T>C. MELAS is a progressive disorder that has been reported in siblings. It is punctuated with episodes of stroke leading to dementia (Chapter 603.4).

Regional cerebral hypoperfusion can be detected by single-photon emission CT (SPECT) studies and MR spectroscopy can detect focal areas of lactic acidosis in the brain. Neuropathology may show cortical atrophy with infarct-like lesions in both cortical and subcortical structures, basal ganglia calcifications, and ventricular dilatation. Muscle biopsy specimens usually show RRF. Mitochondrial accumulations and abnormalities have been shown in smooth muscle cells of intramuscular vessels and of brain arterioles and in the epithelial cells and blood vessels of the choroid plexus, producing a mitochondrial angiopathy. Muscle biochemistry shows complex I deficiency in many cases; however, multiple defects have also been documented involving complexes I, III, and IV. Targeted molecular testing for specific mutations or sequence analysis and mutation scanning are generally used to make a diagnosis of MELAS when clinical evaluation suggests the diagnosis. Because the number of mutant genomes is lower in blood than in muscle, muscle is the preferable tissue for examination. Inheritance is maternal, and there is a highly specific, although not exclusive, point mutation at nt 3243 in the $tRNA^{Leu(UUR)}$ gene of mtDNA in ≈80% of patients. An additional 7.5% have a point mutation at nt 3271 in the $tRNA^{Leu(UUR)}$ gene. A 3rd mutation has been identified at nt 3252 in the $tRNA^{Leu(UUR)}$ gene. The prognosis in patients with the full syndrome is poor. Therapeutic trials reporting some benefit have included corticosteroids, coenzyme Q10, nicotinamide, riboflavin, and L-arginine and preclinical studies reported some success with resveratrol.

REVERSIBLE INFANTILE CYTOCHROME C OXIDASE DEFICIENCY MYOPATHY

A reversible form of severe neuromuscular weakness and hypotonia in infants was recently characterized and found to be due to a maternally inherited homoplasmic m.14674T>C mt-tRNA^{Glu} mutation associated with a deficiency of cytochrome c oxidase (COX) in 17 patients from 12 families. Affected children presented within the 1st few weeks of life with hypotonia, severe muscle weakness and very elevated serum lactate levels, and they often required mechanical ventilation. However, feeding and psychomotor development were not affected. Muscle biopsies taken from these children in the neonatal period show ragged red fibers and deficient COX activity, but these findings disappeared within 5-20 mo when the infants recovered spontaneously. It was difficult to distinguish these infants from those with lethal mitochondrial disorders without waiting for them to improve. The mechanism for this recovery has not been established, but it may reflect a developmental switch in mitochondrial RNAs later in infancy. This reversible disorder has been observed only in COX deficiency associated with the 14674T>C mt-tRNA^{Glu} mutation, so it has been suggested that infants with this type of severe weakness in the neonatal period be tested for this mutation to help with prognosis.

MYOCLONUS EPILEPSY AND RAGGED RED FIBERS (MERRF)

This syndrome is characterized by progressive myoclonic epilepsy, mitochondrial myopathy, and cerebellar ataxia with dysarthria and nystagmus. Onset may be in childhood or in adult life, and the course may be slowly progressive or rapidly downhill. Other features include dementia, sensorineural hearing loss, optic atrophy, peripheral neuropathy, and spasticity. Because some patients have abnormalities of deep sensation and pes cavus, the condition may be confused with Friedreich ataxia. A significant number of patients have a positive family history and short stature. This condition is maternally inherited.

Pathologic findings include elevated serum lactate concentrations, RRF on muscle biopsy, and marked neuronal loss and gliosis affecting, in particular, the dentate nucleus and inferior olivary complex with some dropout of Purkinje cells and neurons of the red nucleus. Pallor of the posterior columns of the spinal cord and degeneration of the gracile and cuneate nuclei occur. Muscle biochemistry has shown variable defects of complex III, complexes II and IV, complexes I and IV, or complex IV alone. More than 80% of cases are caused by a heteroplasmic G to A point mutation at nt 8344 of the tRNA^{Lys} gene of mtDNA. Additional patients have been reported with a T to C mutation at nt 8356 in the tRNA^{Lys} gene. Targeted mutation analysis or mutation analysis after sequencing of the mitochondrial genome are used to diagnosis MERRF.

There is no specific therapy, although coenzyme Q10 appeared to be beneficial in a mother and daughter with the MERRF mutation. The anticonvulsant levetiracetam has been reported to help reduce myoclonus and myoclonic seizures in this disorder.

LEIGH DISEASE (SUBACUTE NECROTIZING ENCEPHALOMYOPATHY)

There are several known genetically determined causes of Leigh disease: pyruvate dehydrogenase complex deficiency, complex I or II deficiency, complex IV (COX) deficiency, complex V (ATPase) deficiency, and deficiency of coenzyme Q10. These defects may occur sporadically or be inherited by autosomal recessive transmission, as in the case of COX deficiency; by X-linked transmission, as in the case of pyruvate dehydrogenase $E_1\alpha$ deficiency; or by maternal transmission, as in complex V (ATPase 6 nt 8993 mutation) deficiency. About 30% of cases are due to mutations in mtDNA. Leigh disease is a progressive degenerative disorder, and most cases become apparent during infancy with feeding and swallowing problems, vomiting, and failure to thrive. Delayed motor and language milestones may be evident, and generalized seizures, weakness, hypotonia, ataxia, tremor, pyramidal signs, and nystagmus are prominent findings. Intermittent respirations with associated sighing or sobbing are characteristic and suggest brainstem dysfunction. Some patients have external ophthalmoplegia, ptosis, retinitis pigmentosa, optic atrophy, and decreased visual acuity. Abnormal results on CT or MRI scan consist of bilaterally symmetric areas of low attenuation in the basal ganglia and brainstem as well as elevated lactic acid on MR spectroscopy. Pathologic changes consist of focal symmetric areas of necrosis in the thalamus, basal ganglia, tegmental gray matter, periventricular and periaqueductal regions of the brainstem, and posterior columns of the spinal cord. Microscopically, these spongiform lesions show cystic cavitation with neuronal loss, demyelination, and vascular proliferation. Elevations in serum lactate levels are characteristic and hypertrophic cardiomyopathy, hepatic failure and rental tubular dysfunction can occur. The overall outlook is poor, but a few patients experience prolonged periods of remission. There is no definitive treatment for the underlying disorder, but a range of vitamins including riboflavin, thiamine, and coenzyme Q are often given to try to improve mitochondrial function. Biotin, creatine, succinate, and idebenone as well as a high-fat diet have also been used, but phenobarbital and valproic acid should be avoided due to their inhibitory effect on the mitochondrial respiratory chain.

NARP SYNDROME

This maternally inherited disorder presents with either Leigh syndrome or with neurogenic weakness and neuropathy, ataxia, and retinitis pigmentosa (NARP syndrome) as well as seizures. It is due to a point mutation at nt 8993 within the ATPase subunit 6 gene. The severity of the disease presentation appears to have close correlation with the percentage of mutant mtDNA in leukocytes. There is no treatment.

LEBER HEREDITARY OPTIC NEUROPATHY (LHON)

LHON is characterized by onset usually between the ages of 18 and 30 yr of acute or subacute visual loss caused by severe bilateral optic atrophy, although children as young as 5 yr have been reported to have LHON. At least 85% of patients are young men. An X-linked factor may modulate the expression of the mitochondrial DNA point mutation. The classic ophthalmologic features include circumpapillary telangiectatic microangiopathy and pseudoedema of the optic disc. Variable features may include cerebellar ataxia, hyperreflexia, Babinski sign, psychiatric symptoms, peripheral neuropathy, or cardiac conduction abnormalities (pre-excitation syndrome). Some cases have been associated with widespread white matter lesions as seen with multiple sclerosis. Lactic acidosis and RRF tend to be conspicuously absent in LHON. More than 11 mtDNA point mutations have been described, including a usually homoplasmic G to A transition at nt 11,778 of the ND4 subunit gene of complex I. The latter leads to replacement of a highly conserved arginine residue by histidine at the 340th amino acid and accounts for 50-70% of cases in Europe and >90% of cases in Japan. Certain LHON pedigrees with other point mutations are associated with complex neurologic disorders and may have features in common with MELAS syndrome and with infantile bilateral striatal necrosis. One family has been reported with pediatric onset of progressive generalized dystonia with bilateral striatal necrosis associated with a homoplasmic G14459A mutation in the mtDNA ND6 gene, which has also been associated with LHON alone and LHON with dystonia.

KEARNS-SAYRE SYNDROME (KSS)

The criteria for KSS include a triad of (1) onset before age 20 yr, (2) progressive external ophthalmoplegia (PEO) with ptosis, and (3) pigmentary retinopathy. There must also be at least 1 of the following: heart block, cerebellar syndrome, or cerebrospinal fluid protein >100 mg/dL. Other nonspecific but common features include dementia, sensorineural hearing loss, and multiple endocrine abnormalities, including short stature, diabetes mellitus, and hypoparathyroidism. The prognosis is guarded, despite placement of a pacemaker, and progressively downhill, with death resulting by the 3rd or 4th decade. Unusual clinical presentations can include renal tubular acidosis and Lowe syndrome. There are also a few overlap cases of children with KSS and strokelike episodes. Muscle biopsy shows RRF and variable COX-negative fibers. Most patients have mtDNA deletions, and some have duplications. These may be new mutations accounting for the generally sporadic nature of KSS. A few pedigrees have shown autosomal dominant transmission. Patients should be monitored closely for endocrine abnormalities, which can be treated. Coenzyme Q has been reported anecdotally to have some beneficial effect and positive effects of folinic acid for low folate levels has been reported. A report of positive effects of a cochlear implant for deafness has also appeared.

Sporadic PEO with RRF is a clinically benign condition characterized by adolescent or young adult–onset ophthalmoplegia, ptosis, and proximal limb girdle weakness. It is slowly progressive and compatible with a relatively normal life. The muscle biopsy material demonstrates RRF and COX-negative fibers. Approximately 50% of patients with PEO have mtDNA deletions, and there is no family history.

REYE SYNDROME

This encephalopathy, which has become uncommon, is associated with pathologic features characterized by fatty degeneration of the viscera (microvesicular steatosis) and mitochondrial abnormalities and biochemical features consistent with a disturbance of mitochondrial metabolism (Chapter 353).

Recurrent Reye-like syndrome is encountered in children with genetic defects of fatty acid oxidation, such as deficiencies of the plasmalemmal carnitine transporter, carnitine palmitoyltransferase I and II, carnitine acylcarnitine translocase, medium- and long-chain acyl-CoA dehydrogenase, multiple acyl-CoA dehydrogenase, and long-chain L-3 hydroxyacyl-CoA dehydrogenase or trifunctional protein. These disorders are manifested by recurrent hypoglycemic and hypoketotic encephalopathy, and they are inherited in an autosomal recessive pattern. Other potential inborn errors of metabolism presenting with Reye syndrome include urea cycle defects (ornithine transcarbamylase, carbamyl phosphate synthetase) and certain of the organic acidurias (glutaric aciduria type I), respiratory chain defects, and defects of carbohydrate metabolism (fructose intolerance).

BIBLIOGRAPHY

Please visit the Nelson Textbook of Pediatrics *website at www.expertconsult.com for the complete bibliography.*

591.3 Other Encephalopathies

Michael V. Johnston

HIV ENCEPHALOPATHY

Encephalopathy is an unfortunate and common manifestation in infants and children with HIV infection (Chapter 268). Neurologic signs in congenitally infected patients may appear during early infancy or may be delayed to as late as 5 yr of age. The primary features of HIV encephalopathy include an arrest in brain growth, evidence of developmental delay, and the evolution of neurologic signs including weakness with pyramidal tract signs, ataxia, myoclonus, pseudobulbar palsy, and seizures. However, the introduction of highly active antiretroviral therapy (HAART) and CNS-penetrating antiretroviral regimens for perinatally infected children has been associated with a 10-fold decrease in the incidence of HIV encephalopathy starting in 1996. Introduction of HAART for children has also resulted in an increase in CD4 T-cell count and a reduction in opportunistic infections and organ-specific diseases including wasting syndrome, thrombocytopenia, cardiomyopathy, and lymphoid interstitial pneumonia. High CNS-penetrating regimens are associated with 74% reduction in the risk of death in children with a diagnosis of HIV encephalopathy compared to low CNS-penetrating drugs.

LEAD ENCEPHALOPATHY

See Chapter 702.

BURN ENCEPHALOPATHY

An encephalopathy develops in about 5% of children with significant burns in the 1st several weeks of hospitalization (Chapter 68). There is no single cause of burn encephalopathy but rather a combination of factors that include anoxia (smoke inhalation, carbon monoxide poisoning, laryngospasm), electrolyte abnormalities, bacteremia and sepsis, cortical vein thrombosis, a concomitant head injury, cerebral edema, drug reactions, and emotional distress. Seizures are the most common clinical manifestation of burn encephalopathy, but altered states of consciousness, hallucinations, and coma may also occur. Management of burn encephalopathy is directed to a search for the underlying cause and treatment of hypoxemia, seizures, specific electrolyte abnormalities, or cerebral edema. The prognosis for complete neurologic recovery is generally excellent, particularly if seizures are the primary abnormality.

HYPERTENSIVE ENCEPHALOPATHY

Hypertensive encephalopathy is most commonly associated with renal disease in children, including acute glomerulonephritis, chronic pyelonephritis, and end-stage renal disease (Chapters 439 and 529). In some cases, hypertensive encephalopathy is the initial manifestation of underlying renal disease. Marked systemic hypertension produces vasoconstriction of the cerebral vessels, which leads to vascular permeability, causing areas of focal cerebral edema and hemorrhage. The onset may be acute, with seizures and coma, or more indolent, with headache, drowsiness and lethargy, nausea and vomiting, blurred vision, transient cortical blindness, and hemiparesis. Examination of the eyegrounds may be nondiagnostic in children, but papilledema and retinal hemorrhages may occur. MRI often shows increased signal intensity in the occipital lobes on T2 weighted images, which is known as **posterior reversible leukoencephalopathy (PRES)** and may be confused with cerebral infarctions. These high signal areas may appear in other regions of the brain as well. Treatment is directed at restoration of a normotensive state and control of seizures with appropriate anticonvulsants.

AUTOIMMUNE ENCEPHALITIS

Limbic encephalitis is an inflammatory syndrome manifested by memory loss, temporal lobe seizures, and affective symptoms. Neuronal antibodies (VGKC, GAD) that may be paraneoplastic (neuroblastoma) or idiopathic are present. The outcome is poor.

Anti-NMDAR (N-methyl-D aspartate receptor) encephalitis is manifested by mood, personality and behavioral changes, and seizures, dyskinesias, and sleep disturbances. Ovarian teratomas or idiopathic mechanisms may be present.

RADIATION ENCEPHALOPATHY

Acute radiation encephalopathy is most likely to develop in young patients who have received large daily doses of radiation.

Excessive radiation injures vessel endothelium, resulting in enhanced vascular permeability, cerebral edema, and numerous hemorrhages. The child may suddenly become irritable and lethargic, complain of headache, or present with focal neurologic signs and seizures. Patients occasionally develop hemiparesis due to an infarct secondary to vascular occlusion of the cerebral vessels. Steroids are often beneficial in reducing the cerebral edema and reversing the neurologic signs. Late radiation encephalopathy is characterized by headaches and slowly progressive focal neurologic signs, including hemiparesis and seizures. Exposure of the brain to radiation for treatment of childhood cancer increases the risk of later cerebrovascular disease, including stroke, moyamoya disease, aneurysm, vascular malformations, mineralizing microangiopathy and strokelike migraines. Some children with acute lymphocytic leukemia treated with a combination of intrathecal methotrexate and cranial irradiation develop neurologic signs months or years later; signs consist of increasing lethargy, loss of cognitive abilities, dementia, and focal neurologic signs and seizures (Chapter 488). The CT scan shows calcifications in the white matter, and the postmortem examination demonstrates a necrotizing encephalopathy. This devastating complication of the treatment of leukemia has prompted reevaluation and reduction in the use of cranial radiation in the treatment of these children.

ZELLWEGER SYNDROME (CEREBROHEPATORENAL SYNDROME [CHRS])

This rare, lethal disorder is inherited as an autosomal recessive trait. It represents the prototype of a group of peroxisomal disorders that have overlapping symptoms, signs, and biochemical abnormalities (Chapter 80.2). The cause of the severe neurologic abnormalities is related to an arrest of migrating neuroblasts during early development, resulting in cerebral pachygyria with neuronal heterotopia (Chapter 585.7).

BIBLIOGRAPHY

Please visit the Nelson Textbook of Pediatrics *website at www.expertconsult.com for the complete bibliography.*

Chapter 592 Neurodegenerative Disorders of Childhood

Jennifer M. Kwon

Neurodegenerative disorders of childhood encompass a large, heterogeneous group of diseases that result from specific genetic and biochemical defects, chronic viral infections, and varied unknown causes. Children with suspected neurodegenerative disorders were once subjected to brain and rectal (neural) biopsies, but with modern neuroimaging techniques and specific biochemical and molecular diagnostic tests, these invasive procedures are rarely necessary. The most important component of the diagnostic investigation continues to be a thorough history and physical examination. The hallmark of a neurodegenerative disease is **regression and progressive deterioration** of neurologic function with loss of speech, vision, hearing, or locomotion, often associated with seizures, feeding difficulties, and impairment of intellect. The age of onset, rate of progression, and principal neurologic findings determine whether the disease affects primarily the white or the gray matter. Upper motor neuron signs and progressive spasticity are the hallmarks of white matter disorders; convulsions, intellectual, and visual impairment that occur early in the disease course are the hallmarks of grey matter disorders. A precise history confirms regression of developmental milestones, and the neurologic examination localizes the process within the nervous system. Although the outcome of a neurodegenerative condition is usually fatal and available therapies are often limited in effect, it is important to make the correct diagnosis so that genetic counseling may be offered and prevention strategies can be implemented. Bone marrow transplantation and other novel therapies may prevent the progression of disease in certain presymptomatic individuals. For all conditions in which the specific enzyme defect is known, prevention by prenatal diagnosis (chorionic villus sampling or amniocentesis) is possible. Carrier detection is also often possible by enzyme assay. Table 592-1 summarizes selected inherited neurodegenerative and metabolic disorders by their age of onset.

592.1 Sphingolipidoses

Jennifer M. Kwon

The sphingolipidoses are characterized by intracellular storage of lipid substrates resulting from defective catabolism of the sphingolipids comprising cellular membranes (Fig. 592-1). The sphingolipidoses are subclassified into 6 categories: Niemann-Pick disease, Gaucher disease, GM_1 gangliosidosis, GM_2 gangliosidosis, Krabbe disease, and metachromatic leukodystrophy. Niemann-Pick disease and Gaucher disease are discussed in Chapter 80.4.

GANGLIOSIDOSES (CHAPTER 80.4)

Gangliosides are glycosphingolipids, normal constituents of the neuronal and synaptic membranes. The basic structure of GM_1 ganglioside consists of an oligosaccharide chain attached to a hydroxyl group of ceramide and sialic acid bound to galactose. The gangliosides are catabolized by sequential cleavage of the sugar molecules by specific exoglycosidases. Abnormalities in catabolism result in an accumulation of the ganglioside within the cell. Defects in ganglioside degradation can be classified into 2 groups: the GM_1 gangliosidoses and the GM_2 gangliosidoses.

GM_1 Gangliosidoses

The 3 subtypes of GM_1 gangliosidoses are classified according to age at presentation: infantile (type 1), juvenile (type 2), and adult (type 3). The condition is inherited as an autosomal recessive trait and results from a marked deficiency of acid β-galactosidase. This enzyme may be assayed in leukocytes and cultured fibroblasts. The acid β-galactosidase gene has been mapped to chromosome 3p14.2. Prenatal diagnosis is possible by measurement of acid β-galactosidase in cultured amniotic cells.

Infantile GM_1 gangliosidosis presents at birth or during the neonatal period with anorexia, poor sucking, and inadequate weight gain. Development is globally retarded, and generalized seizures are prominent. The phenotype is striking and shares many characteristics with Hurler syndrome. The facial features are coarse, the forehead is prominent, the nasal bridge is depressed, the tongue is large (macroglossia), and the gums are hypertrophied. Hepatosplenomegaly is present early in the course as a result of accumulation of foamy histiocytes, and kyphoscoliosis is evident because of anterior beaking of the vertebral bodies. The neurologic examination is dominated by apathy, progressive blindness, deafness, spastic quadriplegia, and decerebrate rigidity. A cherry red spot in the macular region is visualized in approximately 50% of cases. The **cherry red spot** is characterized by an opaque ring (sphingolipid-laden retinal ganglion cells) encircling the normal red fovea (Fig. 592-2). Children rarely survive beyond age 2-3 yr, and death is due to aspiration pneumonia.

Juvenile GM_1 gangliosidosis has a delayed onset beginning about 1 yr of age. The initial symptoms consist of incoordination, weakness, ataxia, and regression of language. Thereafter,

Table 592-1 NEUROMETABOLIC CONDITIONS ASSOCIATED WITH DEVELOPMENTAL REGRESSION

AGE AT ONSET (yr)	CONDITIONS	COMMENTS
<2, with hepatomegaly	Fructose intolerance	Vomiting, hypoglycemia, poor feeding, failure to thrive (when given fructose)
	Galactosemia	Lethargy, hypotonia, icterus, cataract, hypoglycemia (when given lactose)
	Glycogenosis (glycogen storage disease) types I-IV	Hypoglycemia, cardiomegaly (type II)
	Mucopolysaccharidosis types I and II	Coarse facies, stiff joints
	Niemann-Pick disease, infantile type	Gray matter disease, failure to thrive
	Tay-Sachs disease	Seizures, cherry red macula, edema, coarse facies
	Zellweger syndrome	Hypotonia, high forehead, flat facies
	Gaucher disease (neuronopathic form)	Extensor posturing, irritability
	Carbohydrate-deficient glycoprotein syndromes	Dysmyelination, cerebellar hypoplasia
<2, without hepatomegaly	Krabbe disease	Irritability, extensor posturing, optic atrophy and blindness
	Rett syndrome	Girls with deceleration of head growth, loss of hand skills, hand wringing, impaired language skills, gait apraxia
	Maple syrup urine disease	Poor feeding, tremors, myoclonus, opisthotonos
	Phenylketonuria	Light pigmentation, eczema, seizures
	Menkes kinky hair disease	Hypertonia, irritability, seizures, abnormal hair
	Subacute necrotizing encephalopathy of Leigh	White matter disease
	Canavan disease	White matter disease, macrocephaly
	Neurodegeneration with brain iron accumulation disease	White matter disease, movement disorder
2-5	Niemann-Pick disease types III and IV	Hepatosplenomegaly, gait difficulty
	Wilson disease	Liver disease, Kayser-Fleischer ring; deterioration of cognition is late
	Gangliosidosis type II	Gray matter disease
	Neuronal ceroid lipofuscinosis	Gray matter disease
	Mitochondrial encephalopathies (e.g., myoclonic epilepsy with ragged red fibers [MERRF])	Gray matter disease
	Ataxia-telangiectasia	Basal ganglia disease
	Huntington disease (chorea)	Basal ganglia disease
	Neurodegeneration with brain iron accumulation syndrome	Basal ganglia disease
	Metachromatic leukodystrophy	White matter disease
	Adrenoleukodystrophy	White matter disease, behavior problems, deteriorating school performance, quadriparesis
5-15	Adrenoleukodystrophy	Same as for adrenoleukodystrophy in 2 to 5 yr olds
	Multiple sclerosis	White matter disease
	Neuronal ceroid lipofuscinosis, juvenile and adult (Spielmeyer-Vogt and Kufs disease)	Gray matter disease
	Schilder disease	White matter disease, focal neurologic symptoms
	Refsum disease	Peripheral neuropathy, ataxia, retinitis pigmentosa
	Sialidosis II, juvenile form	Cherry red macula, myoclonus, ataxia, coarse facies
	Subacute sclerosing panencephalitis	Diffuse encephalopathy, myoclonus; may occur years after measles

From Kliegman RM, Greenbaum LA, Lye PS: *Practical strategies in pediatric diagnosis and therapy*, ed 2, Philadelphia, 2004, Elsevier/Saunders, p 542.

convulsions, spasticity, decerebrate rigidity, and blindness are the major findings. Unlike the infantile type, this type is not usually marked by coarse facial features and hepatosplenomegaly. Radiographic examination of the lumbar vertebrae may show minor beaking. Children rarely survive beyond 10 yr of age. ***Adult GM$_1$ gangliosidosis*** is a slowly progressive disease consisting of spasticity, ataxia, dysarthria, and a gradual loss of cognitive function.

GM$_2$ Gangliosidoses

The GM$_2$ gangliosidoses are a heterogeneous group of autosomal recessive inherited disorders that consist of several subtypes, including Tay-Sachs disease (TSD), Sandhoff disease, juvenile GM$_2$ gangliosidosis, and adult GM$_2$ gangliosidosis. **Tay-Sachs disease** is most prevalent in the Ashkenazi Jewish population and has an approximate carrier rate of 1/30. TSD is due to mutations in the *HEXA* gene located on chromosome 15q23-q24. Affected infants appear normal until ≈6 mo of age, except for a marked startle reaction to noise that is evident soon after birth. Affected children then begin to lag in developmental milestones and, by 1 yr of age, they lose the ability to stand, sit, and vocalize. Early hypotonia develops into progressive spasticity, and relentless deterioration follows, with convulsions, blindness, deafness, and cherry red spots in almost all patients (see Fig. 592-2). Macrocephaly becomes apparent by 1 yr of age and results from the 200- to 300-fold normal content of GM$_2$ ganglioside deposited in the brain. Few children live beyond 3-4 yr of age, and death is usually associated with aspiration or bronchopneumonia. A deficiency of the isoenzyme hexosaminidase A is found in tissues of patients with TSD. Mass screening for prenatal diagnosis of TSD is a reliable and cost-effective method of prevention because the condition occurs most frequently in a defined population (Ashkenazi Jews). Targeted screening is responsible for the fact that currently, the rare children with TSD born in the USA are most commonly born to non-Jewish parents who are not routinely screened. An accurate and inexpensive carrier detection test is available (serum or leukocyte hexosaminidase A), and the disease can be reliably diagnosed by chorionic villus sampling in the 1st trimester of pregnancy in couples at risk (heterozygote parents).

Sandhoff disease is very similar to TSD in the mode of presentation, including progressive loss of motor and language

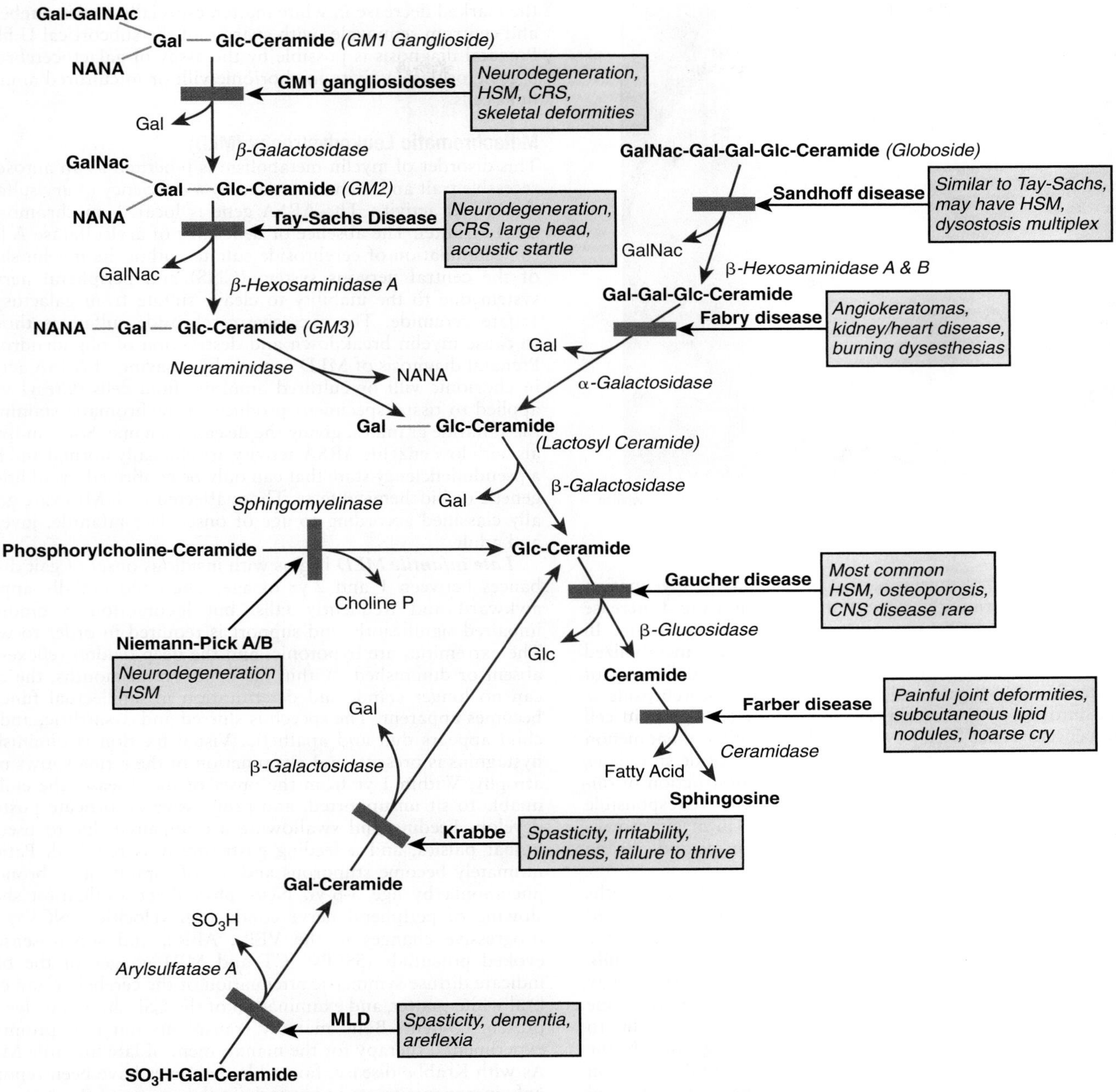

Figure 592-1 Sphingolipid degradation pathway showing the sites of enzyme deficiencies and their associated disorders. Sphingolipids are composed of a ceramide backbone with oligosaccharide side chains.

milestones beginning at 6 mo of age. Seizures, cherry red spots, macrocephaly, and doll-like facies are present in most patients; however, children with Sandhoff disease may also have splenomegaly. The visual-evoked potentials (VEPs) are normal early in the course of Sandhoff disease and TSD but become abnormal or absent as the disease progresses. The auditory brainstem responses (ABRs) show prolonged latencies. The diagnosis of Sandhoff disease is established by finding deficient levels of hexosaminidase A and B in serum and leukocytes. Children usually die by 3 yr of age. Sandhoff disease is due to mutations in the *HEXB* gene located on chromosome 5q13.

Juvenile GM_2 gangliosidosis develops in mid-childhood, initially with clumsiness followed by ataxia. Signs of spasticity, athetosis, loss of language, and seizures gradually develop. Progressive visual loss is associated with optic atrophy, but cherry red spots rarely occur in juvenile GM_2 gangliosidosis. A deficiency of hexosaminidase is variable (total deficiency to near normal) in these patients. Death occurs around 15 yr of age.

Adult GM_2 gangliosidosis is characterized by a myriad neurologic signs, including slowly progressive gait ataxia, spasticity, dystonia, proximal muscle atrophy, and dysarthria. Generally, visual acuity and intellectual function are unimpaired. Hexosaminidase A activity alone or hexosaminidase A and B activity is reduced significantly in the serum and leukocytes.

Krabbe Disease (Globoid Cell Leukodystrophy)

Krabbe disease (KD) is a rare autosomal recessive neurodegenerative disorder characterized by severe myelin loss and the presence of globoid bodies in the white matter. The gene for KD *(GALC)* is located on chromosome 14q24.3-q32.1. The disease results from a marked deficiency of the lysosomal enzyme galactocerebroside β-galactosidase. KD is a disorder of myelin destruction

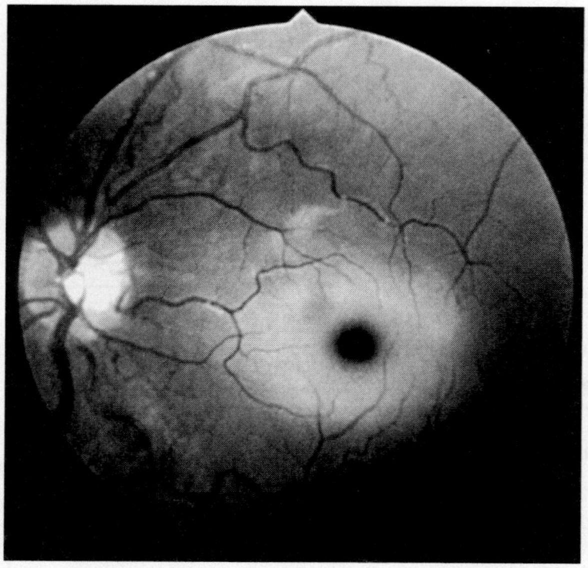

Figure 592-2 A cherry red spot in a patient with GM_1 gangliosidosis. Note the whitish ring of sphingolipid-laden ganglion cells surrounding the fovea.

rather than abnormal myelin formation. Normally, myelination begins in the 3rd trimester, corresponding with a rapid increase of galactocerebroside β-galactosidase activity in the brain. In patients with KD, galactocerebroside cannot be metabolized during the normal turnover of myelin because of deficiency of galactocerebroside β-galactosidase. When galactocerebroside is injected into the brains of experimental animals, a globoid cell reaction ensues. It has been postulated that a similar phenomenon occurs in humans; nonmetabolized galactocerebroside stimulates the formation of globoid cells that reflect the destruction of oligodendroglial cells. Because oligodendroglial cells are responsible for the elaboration of myelin, their loss results in myelin breakdown, thus producing additional galactocerebroside and causing a vicious circle of myelin destruction.

The symptoms of KD become evident in the 1st few months of life and include excessive irritability and crying, unexplained episodes of hyperpyrexia, vomiting, and difficulty feeding. In the initial stage of KD, children are often treated for colic or "milk allergy" with frequent formula changes. Generalized seizures may appear early in the course of the disease. Alterations in body tone with rigidity and opisthotonos and visual inattentiveness due to optic atrophy become apparent as the disease progresses. In the later stages of the illness, blindness, deafness, absent deep tendon reflexes, and decerebrate rigidity constitute the major physical findings. Most patients die by 2 yr of age. MRI and magnetic resonance spectroscopy are useful for evaluating the extent of demyelination in Krabbe disease. Umbilical cord blood (stem cell) transplantation from unrelated donors in asymptomatic babies may favorably alter the natural history but will not help patients who already have neurologic symptoms.

Late-onset KD has been described beginning in childhood or adolescence. Patients present with optic atrophy and cortical blindness, and their condition may be confused with adrenoleukodystrophy. Slowly progressive gait disturbances, including spasticity and ataxia, are prominent. As with classic KD, globoid cells are abundant in the white matter, and leukocytes are deficient in galactocerebroside β-galactosidase. An examination of the cerebrospinal fluid (CSF) shows an elevated protein content, and the nerve conduction velocities are markedly delayed due to segmental demyelination of the peripheral nerves. The VEPs decrease gradually in amplitude with no response in the late stages of the disease, and the ABRs are characterized by the presence of only waves I and II. CT scans and MRI studies highlight the marked decrease in white matter, especially of the cerebellum and centrum semiovale, with sparing of the subcortical U fibers. Prenatal diagnosis is possible by the assay of galactocerebroside β-galactosidase activity in chorionic villi or in cultured amniotic fluid cells.

Metachromatic Leukodystrophy (MLD)

This disorder of myelin metabolism is inherited as an autosomal recessive trait and is characterized by a deficiency of arylsulfatase A (ARSA) activity. The ARSA gene is located on chromosome 22q13-13qter. The absence or deficiency of arylsulfatase A leads to accumulation of cerebroside sulfate within the myelin sheath of the central nervous system (CNS) and peripheral nervous system due to the inability to cleave sulfate from galactosyl-3-sulfate ceramide. The excessive cerebroside sulfate is thought to cause myelin breakdown and destruction of oligodendroglia. Prenatal diagnosis of MLD is made by assaying of ARSA activity in chorionic villi or cultured amniotic fluid cells. Cresyl violet applied to tissue specimens produces metachromatic staining of the sulfatide granules, giving the disease its name. Some individuals with low enzyme ARSA activity are clinically normal and have a pseudodeficiency state that can only be confirmed by additional genetic or biochemical tests. Those affected with MLD are generally classified according to age of onset: late infantile, juvenile, and adult.

Late infantile MLD begins with insidious onset of gait disturbances between 1 and 2 yr of age. The child initially appears awkward and frequently falls, but locomotion is gradually impaired significantly and support is required in order to walk. The extremities are hypotonic, and the deep tendon reflexes are absent or diminished. Within the next several months, the child can no longer stand, and deterioration in intellectual function becomes apparent. The speech is slurred and dysarthric, and the child appears dull and apathetic. Visual fixation is diminished, nystagmus is present, and examination of the retina shows optic atrophy. Within 1 yr from the onset of the disease, the child is unable to sit unsupported, and progressive decorticate postures develop. Feeding and swallowing are impaired due to pseudobulbar palsies, and a feeding gastrostomy is required. Patients ultimately become stuporous and die of aspiration or bronchopneumonia by age 5-6 yr. Neurophysiologic evaluation shows slowing of peripheral nerve conduction velocities (NCVs) and progressive changes in the VEPs, ABRs, and somatosensory-evoked potentials (SSEPs). CT and MRI images of the brain indicate diffuse symmetric attenuation of the cerebellar and cerebral white matter, and examination of the CSF shows an elevated protein content. Bone marrow transplantation is a promising experimental therapy for the management of late infantile MLD. As with Krabbe disease, favorable outcomes have been reported only in patients treated very early in the course of the disease.

Juvenile MLD has many features in common with late infantile MLD, but the onset of symptoms is delayed to 5-10 yr of age. Deterioration in school performance and alterations in personality may herald the onset of the disease. This is followed by incoordination of gait, urinary incontinence, and dysarthria. Muscle tone becomes increased, and ataxia, dystonia, or tremor may be present. In the terminal stages, generalized tonic-clonic convulsions are prominent and are difficult to control. Patients rarely live beyond mid-adolescence.

Adult MLD occurs from the 2nd to 6th decade. Abnormalities in memory, psychiatric disturbances, and personality changes are prominent features. Slowly progressive neurologic signs, including spasticity, dystonia, optic atrophy, and generalized convulsions, lead eventually to a bedridden state characterized by decorticate postures and unresponsiveness.

BIBLIOGRAPHY

Please visit the Nelson Textbook of Pediatrics *website at www.expertconsult.com for the complete bibliography.*

592.2 Neuronal Ceroid Lipofuscinoses

Jennifer M. Kwon

The neuronal ceroid lipofuscinoses (NCLs) are a group of inherited, neurodegenerative, lysosomal storage disorders characterized by visual loss, progressive dementia, seizures, motor deterioration, and early death. The NCLs are so named because of the intracellular accumulation of fluorescent lipopigments, ceroid and lipofuscin. They comprise a genetically and phenotypically heterogeneous group of disorders (the current number of NCL types is 10) that have traditionally been subclassified by age of onset, among other clinical features. They differ from one another in the associated ultrastructural patterns of the inclusions as seen by electron microscopy. Evaluation of neuronal biopsies (either brain, rectal, conjunctival, or skin) was once required for diagnosis (see Table 592-1). With the advent of enzymatic and molecular testing methods, clinicians can make specific NCL diagnoses using less invasive methods (Table 592-2).

Infantile type (INCL, Haltia-Santavuori) begins in the 1st yr of life with myoclonic seizures, intellectual deterioration, and blindness. Optic atrophy and brownish discoloration of the macula are evident on examination of the retina, and cerebellar ataxia is prominent. The electroretinogram (ERG) typically shows small-amplitude or absent waveforms. Death occurs during childhood. The infantile form is caused by recessive mutations of the gene for the lysosomal enzyme palmitoyl-protein thioesterase-1 (PPT1) on chromosome 1p32. A number of cell types in INCL patients show characteristic intracellular fine granular osmiophile deposits (GRODs) discernible by electron microscopy.

A subset of children with PPT1 enzyme deficiency has a much less severe course with clinical features resembling those of the juvenile-onset NCL patients. Clinically, these "variant INCL" patients have a course that is often quite distinct from the typical, classic rapidly degenerating infantile form. Yet they have PPT1 deficiency and GRODs on pathology. There is no clear *CLN1* genotype that predicts severity of phenotype.

Late infantile type (LINCL, Jansky-Bielschowsky) generally presents with myoclonic seizures beginning between 2 and 4 yr of age in a previously normal child. Dementia and ataxia are combined with a progressive loss of visual acuity and microcephaly. Examination of the retina shows marked attenuation of vessels, peripheral black "bone spicule" pigmentary abnormalities, optic atrophy, and a subtle brown pigment in the macular region. The ERG and VEP are abnormal early in the course of disease. The autofluorescent material is deposited in neurons, fibroblasts, and secretory cells. Electron microscopic examination of the storage material in skin or conjunctival biopsy material typically shows curvilinear profiles. LINCL can be caused by autosomal recessive mutations of several different genes: *CLN2* gene, which codes for a tripeptidyl peptidase-1 (TPP1) that is essential for the degradation of cholecystokinin-8, as well as the *CLN5*, *CLN6*, and *CLN8* genes that code for membrane proteins that have not been completely characterized. *CLN8* is also known as the locus of Northern epilepsy syndrome, which is often called progressive epilepsy with mental retardation (EPMR).

Juvenile type (JNCL, Spielmeyer-Vogt or Batten disease) is the most common form of NCL disease and is generally caused by autosomal recessive mutations in *CLN3*. (Patients who present clinically with JNCL but have PPT1 or TPP1 deficiency are said to have variant INCL or LINCL, respectively.) Children affected with JNCL tend to develop normally for the 1st 5 yr of life. Their initial symptom is usually progressive visual loss and their retinal pigmentary changes often results in an initial diagnosis of retinitis pigmentosa. The funduscopic changes are similar to those for the late infantile type. After disease onset, there may be rapid decline with changes in cognition and personality, motor incoordination, and seizures. Myoclonic seizures are not as prominent as in LINCL, but parkinsonism can develop and impair ambulation. Patients die in their late twenties to early thirties. In JNCL caused by *CLN3*, the electron microscopy of tissues show deposits called "fingerprint profiles," and routine light microscopy of a peripheral blood smear may show lymphocyte vacuoles.

BIBLIOGRAPHY

Please visit the Nelson Textbook of Pediatrics *website at* *www.expertconsult.com* *for the complete bibliography.*

592.3 Adrenoleukodystrophy

Jennifer M. Kwon

See Chapter 80.2.

The adrenoleukodystrophies consist of a group of CNS degenerative disorders that are often associated with adrenal cortical insufficiency and are inherited by X-linked recessive transmission. *Classic adrenoleukodystrophy* (ALD), also called cerebral ALD (CERALD) is considered to be the most common leukodystrophy. Boys present between 5 and 15 yr of age with evidence of academic difficulties, behavioral disturbances, and gait abnormalities. ALD is caused by accumulation of very long chain fatty acids in neural tissue and adrenals due to mutations in the *ABCD1* gene coding for the ALD protein, an adenosine triphosphate (ATP)-binding cassette half transporter on Xq28.

The incidence of ALD approximates 1/20,000 boys. In 40% of male hemizygotes, the disease presents in its classic form,

Table 592-2 CLINICAL AND GENETIC CHARACTERISTICS OF THE NCLs*

NCL TYPE	GENE†	PROTEIN‡	AGE OF ONSET	CLINICAL PRESENTATION
Congenital	*CLN10*	Cathepsin‡	Birth (but can present later)	Severe seizures, blindness, rigidity, early death Can also present similar to late infantile forms
Infantile	*CLN1*	Palmitoyl-protein thioesterase-1 (PPT1)‡	6-24 months	Early onset, often rapid progression of seizures; cognitive and motor decline with visual loss
Variant infantile	*CLN1*		3 years to adulthood	Chronic course Initial visual loss followed then by slow mental and motor decline and seizures
Late infantile	*CLN2*	Tripeptidyl peptidase-1 (TPP1)‡	2-8 years	Seizures, often severe and intractable; cognitive and motor decline; and visual loss
	CLN5	Partially soluble protein		
	CLN6	Membrane protein		
	CLN8	Membrane protein	5-10 years	Severe epilepsy, progressive with mental retardation (EPMR)
Juvenile	*CLN3*	Membrane protein	4-10 years	Visual loss is usually the initial presenting complaint Also have mental, motor disorder and seizures

*Note that all the NCL genes have the prefix *CLN*. The adult form (also called Kufs disease, with locus *CLN4*) is not well characterized and is not included.
†Direct genetic testing is available.
‡Enzyme testing available.

CERALD, as an inflammatory demyelinating disease. Generalized seizures are common in the early stages. Upper motor neuron signs include spastic quadriparesis and contractures, ataxia, and marked swallowing disturbances secondary to pseudobulbar palsy. These dominate the terminal stages of the illness. Hypoadrenalism is present in approximately 50% of cases, and adrenal insufficiency characterized by abnormal skin pigmentation (tanning without exposure to sun) may precede the onset of neurologic symptoms. CT scans and MRI studies of patients indicate periventricular demyelination beginning posteriorly; this advances progressively to the anterior regions of the cerebral white matter. ABRs, VEPs, and SSEPs may be normal initially but ultimately show prolonged latencies and abnormal waveforms. Death occurs within 10 yr of the onset of the neurologic signs.

Bone marrow transplant can prevent the progression of the disease when done at an early stage before clinical signs develop. Lorenzo's oil (LO), a mixture of glyceryl trioleate and glyceryl trierucate, lowers very long chain fatty acid (VLCFA) levels by inhibiting synthesis. While LO has not been shown to effectively reverse or slow neurologic deterioration in CERALD boys, it may be effective in slowing onset of cerebral disease when given to asymptomatic boys with no clinical or MRI findings.

Adrenomyeloneuropathy occurs in another 40% of boys with X-linked ALD and presents as a more chronic disorder of the spinal cord and peripheral nerves. It begins with a slowly progressive spastic paraparesis, urinary incontinence, and onset of impotence during the 3rd or 4th decade, even though adrenal insufficiency may have been present since childhood. Cases of typical ALD have occurred in relatives of those with adrenomyeloneuropathy. One of the most difficult problems in the management of X-linked ALD is the common observation that affected individuals in the same family may have quite different clinical courses. For example, in 1 family, 1 affected boy had severe classic ALD culminating in death by age 10 yr; another affected male (a brother) had late-onset adrenomyeloneuropathy, and a 3rd had no symptoms at all. A panel of brain neuroimaging studies, which can provide quantitative information about the progression of adrenoleukodystrophies, aids the selection of patients for bone marrow therapy, and has improved counseling for these disorders.

Neonatal ALD is characterized by marked hypotonia, severe psychomotor retardation, and early onset of seizures. It is inherited as an autosomal recessive condition. Visual inattention is secondary to optic atrophy. Results of adrenal function tests are normal, but adrenal atrophy is evident postmortem. Correction of adrenal insufficiency is ineffective in halting neurologic deterioration.

The diagnosis of ALD is frequently made on the basis of characteristic clinical features that raise suspicion; an MRI that demonstrates posterior leukoencephalopathy; and serum studies that demonstrate abnormally elevated very long chain fatty acids. In classical and late-onset ALD, the male child is affected, but the carrier mother may show spasticity of spinal cord origin.

592.4 Sialidosis

Jennifer M. Kwon

Sialidosis is the result of lysosomal sialidase deficiency, secondary to autosomal recessive mutations in the sialidase (α-neuraminidase, *NEU1*) gene on chromosome 6p21.3. The accumulation of sialic acid–oligosaccharides with markedly increased urinary excretion of sialic acid–containing oligosaccharides is associated with clinical presentations that range from the milder sialidosis type I to the more severe sialidosis type II associated with both neurologic and somatic features.

Sialidosis type I, the **cherry red spot myoclonus syndrome** (CRSM), usually presents in the 2nd decade of life, when a patient complains of visual deterioration. Inspection of the retina shows a cherry red spot, but, unlike patients with TSD, visual acuity declines slowly in individuals with CRSM. Myoclonus of the extremities is gradually progressive and often debilitating and eventually renders patients nonambulatory. The myoclonus is triggered by voluntary movement, touch, and sound and is not controlled with anticonvulsants. Generalized convulsions responsive to antiepileptic drugs occur in most patients.

Sialidosis type II patients present at a younger age and have cherry red spots and myoclonus, as well as somatic involvement, including coarse facial features, corneal clouding (rarely), and dysostosis multiplex, producing anterior beaking of the lumbar vertebrae. Type II patients may be further subclassified into congenital and infantile (childhood) forms, depending on the age at presentation. Examination of lymphocytes shows vacuoles in the cytoplasm, biopsy of the liver demonstrates cytoplasmic vacuoles in Kupffer cells, and membrane-bound vacuoles are found in Schwann cell cytoplasm, all attesting to the multiorgan nature of sialidosis type II. No distinctive neuroimaging findings or abnormalities in electrophysiologic studies are noted in this group of disorders. Patients with sialidosis have been reported to live beyond the 5th decade.

Some cases of what appears to be sialidosis type II are the result of combined deficiencies of β-galactosidase and α-neuraminidase due to deficiency of "protective protein/cathepsin A" (PPCA) that prevents premature intracellular degradation of these two enzymes. These patients have galactosialidosis and they are clinically indistinguishable from those with sialidosis type II. Therefore patients who have features of sialidosis type II with marked urinary excretion of oligosaccharides should be tested for PPCA deficiency as well as sialidase deficiency.

592.5 Miscellaneous Disorders

Jennifer M. Kwon

PELIZAEUS-MERZBACHER DISEASE

Pelizaeus-Merzbacher disease (PMD) is an X-linked recessive disorder characterized by nystagmus and abnormalities of myelin. PMD is caused by mutations in the proteolipid protein *(PLP1)* gene, on chromosome Xq22, which is essential for CNS myelin formation and oligodendrocyte differentiation. Mutations in the same gene can cause familial spastic paraparesis (progressive spastic paraparesis type 2, SPG2). *PLP1* mutations causing disease include point mutations, deletions, gene duplications, and other gene dosage changes.

Clinically, classic PMD is recognized by nystagmus and roving eye movements with head nodding during infancy. Developmental milestones are delayed; ataxia, choreoathetosis, and spasticity ultimately develop. Optic atrophy and dysarthria are associated findings, and death occurs in the 2nd or 3rd decade. The major pathologic finding is a loss of myelin with intact axons, suggesting a defect in the function of oligodendroglia. An MRI scan shows a symmetric pattern of delayed myelination. Multimodal-evoked potential studies demonstrate early in the course a pattern consisting of loss of waves III-V on the ABR. This finding is useful in the investigation of nystagmus in infant boys. VEPs show prolonged latencies, and SSEPs show absent cortical responses or delayed latencies. It is now recognized that a broad spectrum of phenotypes, including SPG2 and peripheral nerve abnormalities, can also result from mutations in the *PLP1* gene.

Recently, individuals with a clinical and radiologic phenotype like PMD including hypomyelinating leukodystrophy, have been identified with autosomal recessive mutations of gap junction protein alpha 12 (GJA12, or connexin 47).

ALEXANDER DISEASE

This is a rare disorder that causes progressive macrocephaly and leukodystrophy. Alexander disease is caused by dominant mutations in the glial fibrillary acidic protein (GFAP) gene, on chromosome 17q21 and cases are usually sporadic in their families. Pathologic examination of the brain discloses deposition of eosinophilic hyaline bodies called Rosenthal fibers in astrocyte processes. These accumulate in a perivascular distribution throughout the brain. In the classic infantile form of Alexander disease, degeneration of white matter is most prominent frontally. Affected children develop progressive loss of intellect, spasticity, and unresponsive seizures causing death by 5 yr of age. However, there are milder forms that present later in life and that may not have the characteristic frontal predominance or megalencephaly.

CANAVAN SPONGY DEGENERATION

See Chapter 79.15.

OTHER LEUKODYSTROPHIES

Metabolic and degenerative disorders can present with significant cerebral white matter changes, such as some mitochondrial disorders (Chapters 80.1 and 591.2) and glutaric aciduria type 1 (Chapter 79). In addition, the broader use of MRI has brought to light new leukodystrophies. One example is vanishing white matter disease or childhood ataxia with central nervous system hypomyelination (VWM/CACH) characterized by ataxia and spasticity. Some patients also have optic atrophy, seizures, and cognitive deterioration. The age of presentation and the rapidity of decline can be quite variable. In the early-onset forms, decline is usually rapid and followed quickly by death; in the later-onset forms, mental decline is usually slower and milder. Interestingly, acute demyelination in these disorders can be triggered by fever or fright. The diagnosis of VWM/CACH is based on clinical findings, characteristic abnormalities on cranial MRI, and autosomal recessive mutations in 1 of 5 causative genes (*EIF2B1, EIF2B2, EIF2B3, EIF2B4,* and *EIF2B5*) encoding the 5 subunits of the eucaryotic translation initiation factor, eIF2B.

MENKES DISEASE

Menkes disease (kinky hair disease) is a progressive neurodegenerative condition inherited as a X-linked recessive trait. The Menkes gene codes for a copper-transporting, P-type ATPase, and mutations in the protein are associated with low serum copper and ceruloplasmin levels as well as a defect in intestinal copper absorption and transport. Symptoms begin in the 1st few months of life and include hypothermia, hypotonia, and generalized myoclonic seizures. The facies are distinctive, with chubby, rosy cheeks and kinky, colorless, friable hair. Microscopic examination of the hair shows several abnormalities, including trichorrhexis nodosa (fractures along the hair shaft) and pili torti (twisted hair). Feeding difficulties are prominent and lead to failure to thrive. Severe mental retardation and optic atrophy are constant features of the disease. Neuropathologic changes include tortuous degeneration of the gray matter and marked changes in the cerebellum with loss of the internal granule cell layer and necrosis of the Purkinje cells. Death occurs by 3 yr of age in untreated patients.

Copper-histidine therapy may be effective in preventing neurologic deterioration in some patients with Menkes disease, particularly when treatment is begun in the neonatal period or, preferably, with the fetus. These presymptomatic children are currently identified because of a family history of an affected brother. Copper is essential in the early stages of CNS development, and its absence probably accounts for the neuropathologic changes. In presymptomatic neonatally diagnosed patients the dosage regimen is copper histidine, 250 µg by subcutaneous injection twice daily to 1 yr of age and 250 µg once daily thereafter. Optimal response to copper-injection treatment appears to occur only in patients who are identified in the newborn period and whose mutations permit residual copper-transport activity.

The **occipital horn syndrome,** a skeletal dysplasia caused by different mutations in the same gene as that involved in Menkes disease, is a relatively mild disease. The 2 diseases are often confused, because the biochemical abnormalities are identical. Resolution of the uncertainty about treatment of patients with Menkes disease will require careful genotype-phenotype correlation, along with further clinical trials of copper therapy.

RETT SYNDROME (RS)

This syndrome is not strictly speaking a degenerative disease, but a disorder of early brain development marked by a period of developmental regression and deceleration of brain growth after a relatively normal neonatal course. It occurs predominantly in girls. The frequency is ≈1/15,000-1/22,000. RS is caused by mutations in *MeCP2,* a transcription factor that binds to methylated CpG islands and silences transcription. Development may proceed normally until 1 yr of age, when regression of language and motor milestones and acquired microcephaly become apparent. An ataxic gait or fine tremor of hand movements is an early neurologic finding. Most children develop peculiar sighing respirations with intermittent periods of apnea that may be associated with cyanosis. The hallmark of Rett syndrome is repetitive hand-wringing movements and a loss of purposeful and spontaneous use of the hands; these features may not appear until 2-3 yr of age. Autistic behavior is a typical finding in all patients. Generalized tonic-clonic convulsions occur in the majority and are usually well controlled by anticonvulsants. Feeding disorders and poor weight gain are common. After the initial period of neurologic regression, the disease process appears to plateau, with persistence of the autistic behavior. Cardiac arrhythmias may result in sudden, unexpected death at a rate that is higher than the general population. Generally girls survive into adulthood.

Postmortem studies show significantly reduced brain weight (60-80% of normal) with a decrease in the number of synapses, associated with a decrease in dendritic length and branching. The phenotype may be related to failure to suppress expression of genes that are normally silent in the early phases of postnatal development. Although very few males survive with the classic RS phenotype, genotyping of boys without the classic RS phenotype but with mental retardation and other atypical neurologic features has detected a significant number with mutations in *MeCP2.* Mutations in *MeCP2* have been demonstrated in normal female carriers, females with Angelman syndrome, and in males with fatal encephalopathy, Klinefelter (47 XXY) syndrome, and familial X-linked mental retardation.

Some girls have an atypical Rett phenotype associated with severe myoclonic seizures in infancy, slowing of head growth, and developmental arrest and have mutations in another X-linked gene encoding for cyclin-dependent kinase–like 5 (CDKL5), which may interact with MeCP2 and other proteins regulating gene expression.

SUBACUTE SCLEROSING PANENCEPHALITIS

This is a rare, progressive neurologic disorder caused by persistent measles virus infection of the CNS (Chapter 238). The number of reported cases has decreased dramatically to 0.06 cases/million population, paralleling the decline in reported measles cases. The initial clinical manifestations include personality changes, aggressive behavior, and impaired cognitive function in individuals who have been exposed to natural measles virus in early childhood. Myoclonic seizures soon dominate the clinical picture. Later, generalized tonic-clonic convulsions, hypertonia, and choreoathetosis become evident, followed by progressive bulbar palsy, hyperthermia, and decerebrate postures. Funduscopic examination early in the course of the disease reveals papilledema in approximately 20% of the cases. Optic atrophy, chorioretinitis, and macular pigmentation are observed in most patients. The diagnosis is established by the typical clinical course and 1 of the following: (1) measles antibody detected in the CSF, (2) a characteristic electroencephalogram consisting of bursts of high-voltage slow waves interspersed with a normal background that occur with a constant periodicity in the early stages of the disease, and (3) typical histologic findings in the brain biopsy or postmortem specimen. Treatment with a series of antiviral agents has been attempted without success. Death occurs usually within 1-2 yr from the onset of symptoms.

BIBLIOGRAPHY

Please visit the Nelson Textbook of Pediatrics *website at* www.expertconsult.com *for the complete bibliography.*

Chapter 593
Demyelinating Disorders of the CNS

Jayne Ness

Demyelinating disorders of the central nervous system (CNS) cause acute or relapsing-remitting encephalopathy and other multifocal signs of brain, brainstem, and spinal cord dysfunction. They affect white matter, which is formed by myelin contained within oligodendrocytes, providing electrical insulation for neurons and neuronal connections. In contrast to genetically determined leukodystrophies (sometimes called dysmyelinating disorders) that also produce disrupted white matter, demyelinating disorders generally target normally formed white matter through immune-mediated mechanisms. Major demyelinating disorders in childhood include multiple sclerosis (MS) and acute disseminated encephalomyelitis (ADEM). The rare macrophage activating syndromes and isolated angiitis of the CNS can sometimes be confused with ADEM (Table 593-1).

Table 593-1 SUMMARY OF CONSENSUS DEFINITIONS FOR PEDIATRIC CENTRAL NERVOUS SYSTEM INFLAMMATORY DEMYELINATION

MONOPHASIC CNS INFLAMMATORY DEMYELINATION	
ADEM	Clinical event must include encephalopathy (behavioral change and/or altered consciousness)
	New symptoms or signs within 3 months are considered part of same ADEM event
CIS	Clinical event that can be monofocal (e.g., isolated optic neuritis) or polyfocal, but cannot include encephalopathy
NMO	Must have optic neuritis and transverse myelitis as major criteria. Must have spinal MRI lesion extending over 3 or more segments or be NMO-IgG positive
RELAPSING CNS INFLAMMATORY DEMYELINATION	
Recurrent ADEM	New event of ADEM (must have encephalopathy) with recurrence of initial ADEM symptoms and signs 3 or more months after initial event and not related to withdrawal of steroids
Multiphasic ADEM	ADEM followed by new clinical event also meeting criteria for ADEM, but involving new CNS lesions (clinically and radiologically)
Relapsing NMO	Relapse of NMO as described above. Additional clinical and radiologic features extrinsic to optic nerve and spinal cord are well described and acceptable for diagnosis
Pediatric MS	Two or more events separated in time (4 or more weeks) and space. First episode cannot be ADEM. If 1st episode is ADEM, 2 or more non-ADEM events are required for diagnosis of MS. New MRI lesions 3 months or longer after the initial clinical event can be used to satisfy criteria for dissemination in time

All events must include compatible MRI features of CNS inflammatory demyelination and exclude alternative causes.
ADEM, acute disseminated encephalomyelitis; CIS, clinically isolated syndrome; CNS, central nervous system; MS, multiple sclerosis; NMO, neuromyelitis optica.
(Data from Krupp LB, Banwell B, Tenembaum S: Consensus definitions proposed for pediatric multiple sclerosis and related disorders, *Neurology* 68[16 Suppl 2]:S7–S12, 2007.)

593.1 Multiple Sclerosis

Jayne Ness

Multiple sclerosis (MS) is a chronic demyelinating disorder of the brain, spinal cord and optic nerves characterized by a relapsing-remitting course of neurologic episodes separated in time and space.

EPIDEMIOLOGY

Pediatric MS is rare, with an estimated 2-5% of MS patients experiencing their 1st symptoms before age 18 yr. Pediatric MS has a slight male predominance when disease onset is before age 6 yr, but by age 12 yr, females outnumber males 2 : 1.

PATHOGENESIS

A complex interplay of environmental, infectious, and genetic factors influence MS susceptibility. Immune system dysregulation involving T and B lymphocytes triggers inflammation, axonal demyelination, axonal loss, and regeneration within both white and gray matter. Inflammatory infiltrates within actively demyelinating lesions of relapsing-remitting MS are targets for disease modifying therapy (DMT). Neurodegenerative changes predominate in progressive forms of MS.

CLINICAL MANIFESTATIONS

Presenting symptoms in pediatric MS include hemiparesis or paraparesis, unilateral or bilateral optic neuritis, focal sensory loss, ataxia, diplopia, dysarthria, or bowel/bladder dysfunction (Table 593-2). Polyregional symptoms are reported in 30% of patients. Encephalopathy is less common and suggests consideration of acute disseminated encephalomyelitis (ADEM).

LABORATORY FINDINGS

Cranial MRI exhibits discrete T2 lesions in cerebral white matter, particularly periventricular regions as well as brainstem, cerebellum, and juxtacortical and deep gray matter. Alternatively, tumefactive T2 lesions are also seen. Spine MRI typically shows partial-width cord lesions restricted to 1-2 spine segments. CSF may be normal or exhibit mild pleocytosis, particularly in younger children. Abnormal MS profiles (increased IgG index, and/or CSF oligoclonal bands) increase likelihood of MS but may be negative in 10-60% of pediatric MS patients, particularly prepubertal children (Fig. 593-1). Abnormal evoked potential studies can localize disruptions in visual, auditory, or somatosensory pathways.

DIAGNOSIS AND DIFFERENTIAL DIAGNOSIS

Like adult MS, pediatric MS can be diagnosed following 2 demyelinating episodes localizing to distinct CNS regions, lasting >24 hr and separated by >30 days, provided no other plausible explanation exists. Alternatively, accumulation of T2 or gadolinium-enhancing lesions in the brain or spine >3 mo later can demonstrate dissemination in time, enabling MS diagnosis after the 1st event. Challenges arise in distinguishing pediatric MS from other demyelinating syndromes such as acute disseminated encephalomyelitis (ADEM) or neuromyelitis optica (NMO), ADEM is a self-limited syndrome characterized by encephalopathy, polyregional neurologic deficits, and diffuse multifocal MRI

Table 593-2 SYMPTOMS AND SIGNS OF MULTIPLE SCLEROSIS BY SITE

	SYMPTOMS	SIGNS
Cerebrum	Cognitive impairment	Deficits in attention, reasoning, and executive function (early); dementia (late)
	Hemisensory and motor	Upper motor neuron signs
	Affective (mainly depression)	
	Epilepsy (rare)	
	Focal cortical deficits (rare)	
Optic nerve	Unilateral painful loss of vision	Scotoma, reduced visual acuity, color vision, and relative afferent papillary defect
Cerebellum and cerebellar pathways	Tremor	Postural and action tremor, dysarthria
	Clumsiness and poor balance	Limb incoordination and gait ataxia
Brainstem	Diplopia, oscillopsia	Nystagmus, internuclear and other complex ophthalmoplegias
	Vertigo	
	Impaired swallowing	Dysarthria
	Impaired speech and emotional lability	Pseudobulbar palsy
	Paroxysmal symptoms	
Spinal cord	Weakness	Upper motor neuron signs
	Stiffness and painful spasms	Spasticity
	Bladder dysfunction	
	Erectile impotence	
	Constipation	
Other	Pain	
	Fatigue	
	Temperature sensitivity and exercise intolerance	

Modified from Compston A, Coles A: Multiple sclerosis, *Lancet* 372:1502–1517, 2008, p 1503.

T2 abnormalities followed by subsequent clinical improvement and resolution of MRI T2 lesions (see Tables 593-1 and 593-3). However, a subset of pediatric MS patients (10-25%) present with an ADEM phenotype and then experience multiple relapses with accumulation of MRI T2 lesions. NMO, traditionally a combined myelitis and optic neuritis with normal brain MRI, now has a broader phenotype with the recent identification of the NMO antibody against the CNS water channel aquaporin-4. The NMO spectrum now includes isolated bilateral ON or longitudinally extensive transverse myelitis even in the presence of brain MRI abnormalities or encephalopathy.

COMPLICATIONS

Similar to adults with MS, pediatric MS patients can acquire fixed neurologic deficits affecting vision and other cranial nerves, motor and sensory function, balance, and bowel/bladder function. Cognitive impairment can impede academic achievement.

TREATMENT

Relapses causing functional disability may be treated with methylprednisolone, 20-30 mg/kg/day (maximum 1,000 mg/day) for 3-5 days, with or without prednisone taper. Injectable DMT (interferon-beta1α or interferon-beta1β; glatiramer acetate) reduces relapse frequency and lowers MRI T2 lesion load in adult MS, especially with early institution of therapy. Although not yet approved by the U.S. Food and Drug Administration for pediatric MS, injectable DMT use has been reported in >1,000 children and adolescents with MS. Pediatric experience is limited with intravenously infused DMT, natalizumab, and mitoxantrone. Drugs that target lymphocyte subtypes (cladribine, alemtuzumab) or interfere with lymphocyte myelin interaction (fingolimod, natalizumab) are promising agents in trials in adult patients with MS. Natalizumab therapy has been associated with the risk of developing progressive multifocal encephalopathy (CNS infection with human polyomavirus JC).

PROGNOSIS

Retrospective studies of patients diagnosed with MS prior to widespread DMT use suggest slower disease progression in pediatric MS patients compared to adults. Despite a longer time to irreversible disability (20-30 yr), pediatric MS patients acquire irreversible disability at a younger age than adults.

BIBLIOGRAPHY

Please visit the Nelson Textbook of Pediatrics *website at www.expertconsult.com for the complete bibliography.*

593.2 Neuromyelitis Optica

Nina F. Schor

Neuromyelitis optica (NMO) (Devic disease) is a demyelinating disorder characterized by monophasic or polyphasic episodes of optic neuritis and/or transverse myelitis. It was once thought that NMO was a variant of MS; most authorities believe that NMO is a distinct disorder.

EPIDEMIOLOGY

NMO has an age of onset of 31.2 ± 11 yr. In 1 study, in monophasic patients, the range of age of onset was 1-54 yr; in polyphasic patients, the range was 6-72 yr. NMO is more common in women and girls than in men and boys; 65% of monophasic and 80-85% of polyphasic NMO patients are female. It is also more common in Asians than in blacks or whites and appears to have a higher mortality rate in individuals of African descent than in others.

PATHOGENESIS

NMO is associated with IgG antibodies to the aquaporin-4 water channel. It is not clear why the attack on and depletion of spinal cord and optic nerve aquaporin-4 results in disruption of the myelin sheath in these parts of the CNS, but pathologic examination of autopsy specimens reveals both anti–aquaporin-4 IgG deposits and B cells in the spinal cord and optic nerves of NMO patients. Although most cases of NMO are idiopathic and only occasional familial cases have been reported, there have been reports of postinfectious NMO. HIV, syphilis, chlamydia, varicella, cytomegalovirus, and Epstein-Barr virus have been associated with subsequent development of NMO.

CLINICAL MANIFESTATIONS

NMO presents with either optic neuritis or transverse myelitis or both. Visual field defects and color desaturation are common. The symptoms and signs of transverse myelitis depend on the spinal level and completeness of the inflammatory changes. NMO differs from MS in that other parts of the nervous system are generally not involved either symptomatically or on imaging studies; recovery of visual and spinal cord function is generally not as complete after each episode; optic neuritis is

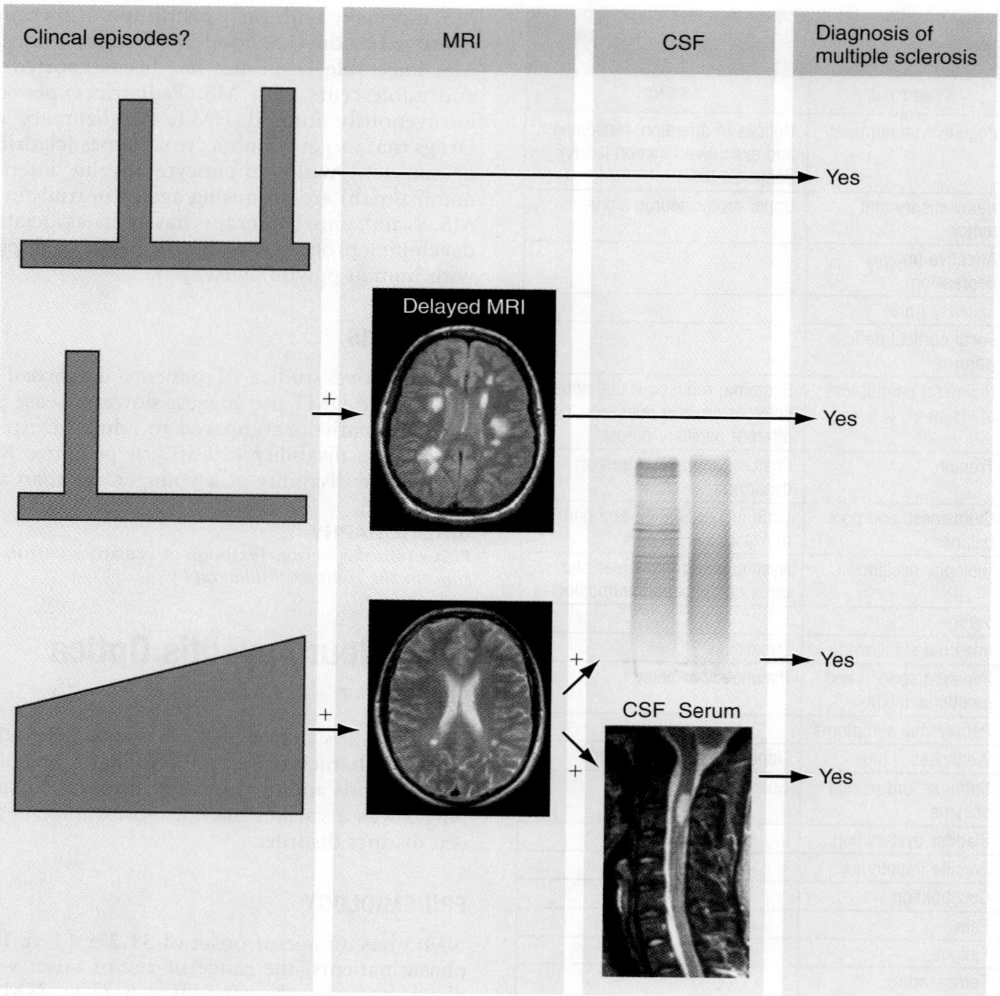

Figure 593-1 Criteria for the diagnosis of multiple sclerosis (MS). The principle is to establish dissemination in time and place of lesions, meaning that episodes affecting separate sites within the central nervous system have occurred at least 30 days apart. MRI can substitute for 1 of these clinical episodes. Dissemination in time of magnetic resonance lesions requires: 1 gadolinium-enhancing lesion at least 3 mo after the onset of the clinical event; or a new T2 lesion compared with a reference scan done at least 30 days after onset of the clinical event. In the case of recurrent stereotyped clinical episodes at the same neurologic site, criteria for MRI definition of dissemination in space are 3 features from the following: (1) 1 gadolinium-enhancing lesion or 9 T2 MRI lesions; (2) 1 or more infratentorial lesions; (3) 1 or more juxtacortical lesions; or (4) 3 or more periventricular lesions (a spinal cord lesion can replace some of these brain lesions). Primary progressive MS can be diagnosed after 1 yr of a progressive deficit and 2 of the following: (1) a positive brain MRI; (2) a positive spinal cord MRI; and (3) positive oligoclonal bands. Patients having an appropriate clinical presentation but who do not meet all of the diagnostic criteria can be classified as having possible MS. CSF, cerebrospinal fluid. (From Compston A, Coles A: Multiple sclerosis, *Lancet* 372:1502–1517, 2008, Fig 1, p 1504.)

more frequently bilateral in NMO than in MS; and NMO is more frequently fatal than MS.

LABORATORY FINDINGS

CSF in patients with NMO often has 50 or more WBC/µL. Unlike MS, it is devoid of oligoclonal bands. Serum positivity for anti–aquaporin-4 antibodies (so-called NMO antibodies) has a sensitivity of 73% and a specificity of 91% for NMO. Neuroimaging studies may show small, asymptomatic lesions in the white matter of the brainstem or hemispheres, but not the large (>3 mm), oval lesions in the periventricular white matter seen in MS.

DIAGNOSIS AND DIFFERENTIAL DIAGNOSIS

Clinical criteria for the diagnosis of NMO include finding at least 2 of the following: normal brain MRI, spinal cord widening and cavitation involving at least 3 spinal segments, decreased serum/CSF albumin ratio with normal IgG synthesis rate and the absence of oligoclonal bands, and acute episode(s) of spinal cord and/or optic nerve involvement separated by months or years without any other systemic or neurologic features. The differential diagnosis includes MS; ADEM (Chapter 593.3); rheumatologic etiologies of transverse myelitis and/or optic neuritis including systemic lupus erythematosus, Behçet disease, and neurosarcoidosis (usually accompanied by other nonneurologic manifestations); idiopathic transverse myelitis, tropical spastic paraparesis, and viral encephalomyelitis (none of which have NMO antibodies in the serum or CSF); and metabolic and idiopathic causes of isolated optic neuritis or other acute monocular or binocular visual loss (Chapter 623).

COMPLICATIONS

Similar to adults with NMO, pediatric NMO patients often are left with fixed neurologic deficits affecting visual acuity, visual fields, color vision, motor and sensory function, balance, and bowel/bladder function.

TREATMENT

Initial episodes and relapses may be treated acutely with methylprednisolone, 20-30 mg/kg/day (maximum 1,000 mg/day) for 3-5 days, followed by a slow prednisone taper. It is not yet known whether injectable DMT (interferon-beta1α or interferon-beta1β; glatiramer acetate) reduces relapse frequency in NMO. However, agents like rituximab that reduce B cell number and function have shown promise in this regard in early studies.

PROGNOSIS

The prognosis in NMO is generally poor for patients with NMO. In 1 study, approximately 20% remained functionally blind (i.e., 20/200 vision or worse) in at least 1 eye and 31% had permanent monoplegia or paraplegia. Five-year survival of the patients with paraplegia is approximately 90%.

BIBLIOGRAPHY

Please visit the Nelson Textbook of Pediatrics *website at* www.expertconsult.com *for the complete bibliography.*

593.3 Acute Disseminated Encephalomyelitis (ADEM)

Nina F. Schor

ADEM is an initial inflammatory, demyelinating event with multifocal neurologic deficits, typically accompanied by encephalopathy.

EPIDEMIOLOGY

ADEM can occur at any age but most series report a mean age between 5 and 8 yr with a slight male predominance. Reported incidence ranges from 0.07-0.4 per 100,000 per yr in the pediatric population.

PATHOGENESIS

Molecular mimicry induced by infectious exposure or vaccine may trigger production of CNS autoantigens. Many patients experience a transient febrile illness in the month prior to ADEM onset. Preceding infections associated with ADEM include influenza, Epstein-Barr virus, cytomegalovirus, varicella, enterovirus, measles, mumps, rubella, herpes simplex, and *Mycoplasma pneumoniae.* Postvaccination ADEM has been reported following immunizations for rabies, smallpox, measles, mumps, rubella, Japanese encephalitis B, pertussis, diphtheria-polio-tetanus, and influenza.

CLINICAL MANIFESTATIONS

Initial symptoms of ADEM may include lethargy, fever, headache, vomiting, meningeal signs, and seizure, including status epilepticus. Encephalopathy is a hallmark of ADEM, ranging from ongoing confusion to persistent irritability to coma. Focal neurologic deficits can be difficult to ascertain in the obtunded or very young child but common neurologic signs in ADEM include visual loss, cranial neuropathies, ataxia, motor and sensory deficits, plus bladder/bowel dysfunction with concurrent spinal cord demyelination.

NEUROIMAGING

Head CT may be normal or show hypodense regions. Cranial MRI, the imaging study of choice, typically exhibits large, multifocal and sometimes confluent or tumefactive T2 lesions with variable enhancement within white and often gray matter of the cerebral hemispheres, cerebellum, and brainstem (Fig. 593-2).

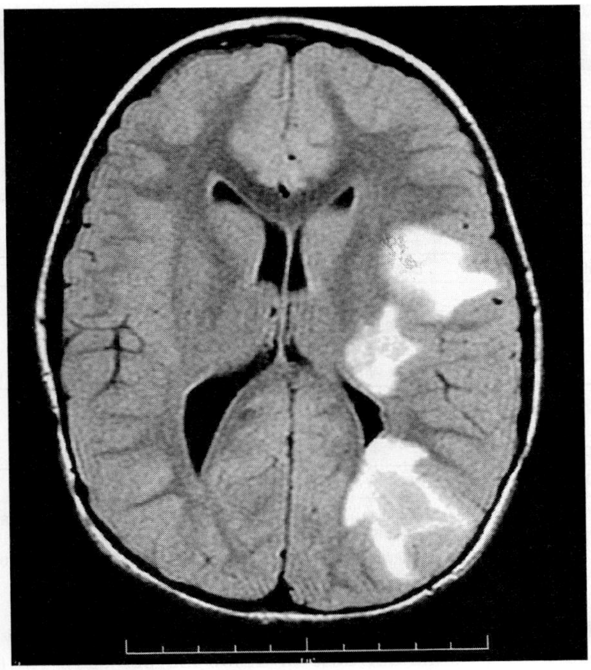

Figure 593-2 Axial T2-weighted FLAIR MRI of the brain in a child with acute disseminated encephalomyelitis (ADEM). High signal *(white)* lesions in the T2-weighted image reflect areas of demyelination and edema in deep subcortical and periventricular white matter as well as the basal ganglia and thalamus on the left side.

Deep gray matter structures (thalami, basal ganglia) are often involved although this may not be specific to ADEM. Spinal cord may have abnormal T2 signal or enhancement, with or without clinical signs of myelitis. MRI lesions of ADEM typically appear to be of similar age but their evolution may lag behind the clinical presentation. Serial MRI imaging 3-12 mo following ADEM shows improvement and often complete resolution of T2 abnormalities although residual gliosis may remain.

LABORATORY FINDINGS

There is no biologic marker for ADEM and laboratory findings can vary widely. CSF studies often exhibit pleocytosis with lymphocytic or monocytic predominance. CSF protein can be elevated, especially in repeat studies. Up to 10% of ADEM have oligoclonal bands in the CSF and/or elevated CSF immune globulin production. Electroencephalograms (EEG) often show generalized slowing, consistent with encephalopathy, although polyregional demyelination of ADEM can also cause focal slowing or epileptiform discharges.

DIFFERENTIAL DIAGNOSIS

The differential diagnosis for ADEM is broad but can be narrowed by careful history, appropriate laboratory evaluations, and MRI. Empirical antibiotic and antiviral treatment should be considered while infectious evaluations are pending. Follow-up MRI examinations 3-12 mo after ADEM should show improvement; new or enlarging T2 lesions should prompt re-evaluation for other etiologies such as MS, leukodystrophies, tumor, vasculitis, or mitochondrial, metabolic, or rheumatologic disorders (see Table 593-3).

TREATMENT

Although there are no randomized controlled trials to compare acute treatments for ADEM or other demyelinating disorders of childhood, high dose intravenous steroids are commonly

Table 593-3 CLINICAL AND MRI FEATURES THAT MAY DISTINGUISH ADEM FROM FIRST ATTACK OF MS

	ADEM	MS
Age	<10 yr	>10 yr
Stupor/coma	+	–
Fever/vomiting	+	–
Family history	No	20%
Sensory complaints	+	+
Optic neuritis	Bilateral	Unilateral
Manifestations	Polysymptomatic	Monosymptomatic
MRI imaging	Widespread lesions: basal ganglia, thalamus, cortical gray-white junction	Isolated lesions: periventricular white matter, corpus callosum
CSF	Pleocytosis (lymphocytosis)	Oligoclonal bands
Response to steroids	+	+
Follow-up	No new lesions	New lesions

Some features that may help distinguish an initial acute episode of demyelination from a 1st attack of MS in children. Final diagnosis of MS is based on follow-up evaluation and possibly MRI. ADEM, acute disseminated encephalomyelitis; CSF, cerebrospinal fluid; MS, multiple sclerosis; +, more likely to be present; –, less likely to be present.

employed (typically methylprednisolone 20-30 mg/kg per day for 5 days with a maximum dose of 1,000 mg per day). An oral prednisone taper over 1 mo may prevent relapse. Other treatment options include intravenous immune globulin (IVIG; usually 2 g/kg administered over 2-5 days) or plasmapheresis (typically 5-7 exchanges administered every other day). There is no consensus about timing of these treatments for ADEM.

PROGNOSIS

Many children experience full recovery after ADEM but some are left with residual motor and/or cognitive deficits. ADEM is usually a monophasic illness but demyelinating symptoms can fluctuate for several months. Repeated bouts of demyelination more than 3 mo after ADEM later raise the question of MS versus repeated ADEM.

BIBLIOGRAPHY

Please visit the Nelson Textbook of Pediatrics *website at www.expertconsult.com for the complete bibliography.*

Chapter 594
Pediatric Stroke Syndromes

Adam Kirton and Gabrielle deVeber

Stroke has emerged as an important cause of acquired brain injury in newborns and children. The ischemic varieties of arterial ischemic stroke (AIS) and cerebral sinovenous thrombosis (CSVT) are more common than brain malignancy (incidence ~5/100,000/yr) and affect 1 in 2,000 newborns. A similar number suffer from hemorrhagic stroke (HS) and other forms of cerebrovascular disease. Diagnosis is challenging and pathophysiology and risk factors are poorly understood. The frequent adverse neurologic outcomes suffered by most children who have strokes can be reduced by increasing pediatric physician awareness, facilitating early recognition, diagnosis, and specific treatment.

594.1 Arterial Ischemic Stroke (AIS)

Adam Kirton and Gabrielle deVeber

Arterial blood reaches the brain via the anterior (internal carotid) and posterior (vertebrobasilar) circulations, converging at the circle of Willis. Strokes involve the middle cerebral artery (MCA) territory more frequently than either the anterior or posterior cerebral arteries. AIS is the focal brain infarction that results from occlusion of these arteries or their branches. AIS is a leading cause of acquired brain injury in children, with the perinatal period carrying the highest risk (see later).

In children the diagnosis of stroke is frequently delayed or missed. This is due to subtle and nonspecific clinical presentations, a complicated differential diagnosis (Chapter 594.4) and a lack of awareness by primary care pediatric physicians. ***The acute onset of a focal neurologic deficit in a child is stroke until proven otherwise.*** The most common focal presentation is hemiparesis but acute visual, speech, sensory, or balance deficits also occur. Children with these presentations require urgent neuroimaging and consultation with a child neurologist as emergency interventions may be indicated. AIS is a clinical and radiographic diagnosis. CT imaging can demonstrate larger mature AIS and exclude hemorrhage, however MRI identifies early and small infarcts and is therefore required to exclude ischemic stroke. **Diffusion weighted MRI** (DWI) can demonstrate AIS within minutes of onset, and MR angiography can confirm vascular occlusion and suggest arteriopathy as the underlying cause (Fig. 594-1).

Most etiologies for AIS are well-established; some represent only potential associations (Tables 594-1 and 594-2). AIS often remains idiopathic although most children have identifiable, frequently multiple risk factors. Three main categories of etiology should be considered: **arteriopathic, cardiac, and hematological;** full investigation often reveals multiple risk factors in a given individual.

Arteriopathy refers to disorders of the cerebral arteries and has emerged as the leading cause of childhood AIS, present in >50% of children. Idiopathic arterial stenosis has been termed **focal cerebral arteriopathy** (FCA), and may be more specfically identified as transient cerebral arteriopathy (TCA) or postvaricella angiopathy (PVA). These diseases likely represent focal, localized, unilateral vasculitis. More diffuse or bilateral **vasculitis** may be primary or associated with systemic inflammatory conditions (Table 594-3). **Arterial dissection** can be spontaneous or post-traumatic and can affect extracranial internal carotid or vertebral arteries, or intracranial arteries. **Moyamoya disease** may be idiopathic or associated with other conditions (NF-1, trisomy 21, sickle cell anemia, radiation therapy) and demonstrates progressive occlusion of the distal internal carotid arteries (Table 594-4, Fig. 594-2). Congenital malformations of the craniocervical arteries, including PHACES syndrome, may predispose to AIS.

Cardioembolic stroke comprises about 25% of childhood AIS with embolism occurring either spontaneously, or during catheterization or surgical repair. AIS complicates 1 in 185 pediatric cardiac surgeries, and re-operation increases the risk. **Complex congenital heart diseases** are the most frequent cause for AIS, however acquired conditions including arrhythmia, cardiomyopathy, and infective endocarditis should also be considered. The presence of a patent foramen ovale provides the possibility of paradoxical venous thromboembolism. All children with suspected AIS require thorough cardiovascular examination, electrocardiogram, and echocardiogram.

Hematologic disorders include **iron deficiency anemia and sickle cell anemia (SCA).** In SCA the risk of AIS is increased 400-fold. Coagulation disorders are also frequently identified in AIS. They include hereditary (e.g., factor V Leiden) and acquired (e.g., antiphospholipid antibodies) **prothrombotic states** and **prothrombotic medications,** including oral contraceptives and asparaginase chemotherapy. Additional AIS risk factors include migraine, acute childhood illnesses, chronic systemic illnesses, illicit drugs and toxins, and rare inborn errors of metabolism.

Treatment of childhood AIS is multifaceted and 3 consensus-based guidelines are now available. Emergency thrombolysis is not yet established for children as there are no safety data

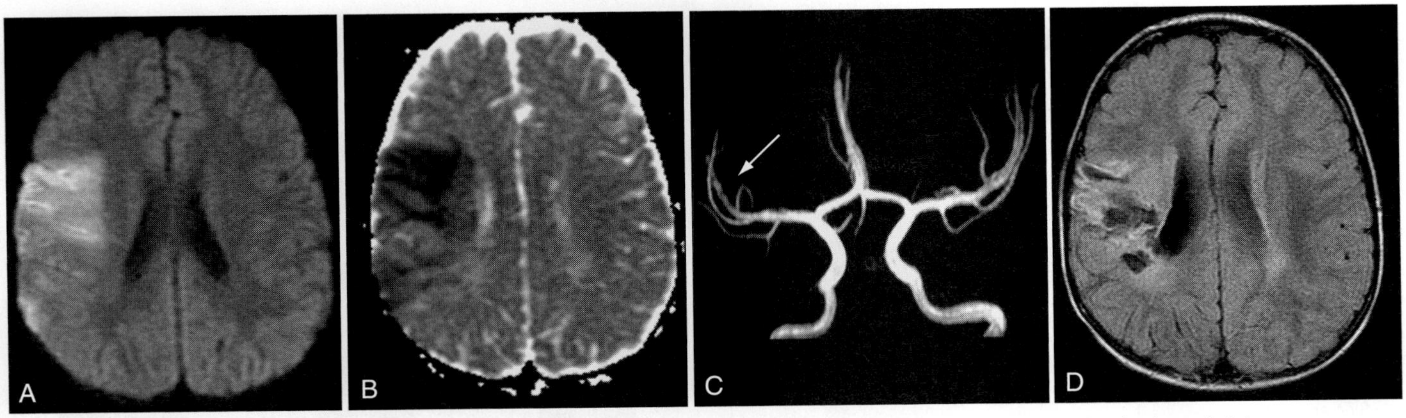

Figure 594-1 Arterial ischemic stroke. A healthy 3 yr old boy experienced the sudden onset of left-sided weakness. Examination also demonstrated left-sided hemisensory loss and neglect. Diffusion weighted MRI shows focal increased signal in the right temporal-parietal region in the territory of the middle cerebral artery (MCA, *A*). Apparent diffusion coefficient map confirms restricted diffusion consistent with infarction (ischemic stroke) *(B)*. MR angiogram shows no occlusion or stenosis and decreased flow in the MCA *(C)*. Follow-up MRI at 3 mo shows atrophy and gliosis in the same region *(D)*.

Table 594-1 COMMON RISK FACTORS FOR ARTERIAL ISCHEMIC STROKE IN CHILDREN

MAJOR CATEGORY	EXAMPLES
Arteriopathic	Focal cerebral arteriopathy (FCA) Postvaricella angiopathy (PVA) Transient cerebral arteriopathy (TCA) Childhood primary angiitis of the CNS (cPACNS) Systemic/secondary vasculitis (e.g., Takayasu arteritis) Craniocervical arterial dissection Moyamoya disease/syndrome Arterial infection (e.g., bacterial meningitis, tuberculosis) Fibromuscular dysplasia Vasospasm (e.g., Call-Fleming syndrome) Migraine (migrainous infarction)? Congenital arterial abnormalities (e.g., PHACES syndrome)
Cardiac	Complex congenital heart diseases (cyanotic >> acyanotic) Cardiac catheterization/procedure (e.g., balloon atrial septostomy) Cardiac surgery Arrhythmia Valvular heart disease Endocarditis Cardiomyopathy, severe ventricular dysfunction Intracardiac lesions (e.g., atrial myxoma) Patent foramen ovale (and possible paradoxical emboli)
Hematologic	Sickle cell anemia Iron deficiency anemia Inherited prothrombotic (e.g., factor V Leiden, prothrombin gene mutation 20210A) Acquired prothrombotic (e.g., protein C/S deficiency, antithrombin III deficiency, lipoprotein [a], antiphospholipid antibodies, oral contraceptives, pregnancy)
Other	Acute systemic illness (e.g., dehydration, sepsis, diabetic ketoacidosis) Chronic systemic illness (e.g., systemic lupus erythematosus, leukemia) Illicit drugs and toxins (e.g., cocaine) Extracorporeal membrane oxygenation (ECMO) Inborn errors of metabolism (e.g., Fabry disease, homocystinuria) See also strokelike events (Chapter 594.4)

Table 594-2 MISCELLANEOUS AND GENETIC RISK FACTORS FOR STROKE

Hereditary dyslipoproteinemia
Familial hypoalphalipoproteinemia
Familial hypercholesterolemia
Type IV, type III hyperlipoproteinemia
Tangier disease
Progeria
Heritable disorders of connective tissue
Ehlers-Danlos syndrome (type IV)
Marfan syndrome
Pseudoxanthoma elasticum
Homocystinuria (cystathionine β-synthase deficiency, or 5,20-MTHFR)
Menkes syndrome
Organic acidemias
Methylmalonic acidemia
Propionic acidemia
Isovaleric acidemia
Glutaric aciduria type II
Mitochondrial encephalomyopathies
MELAS
MERRF
MERRF/MELAS overlap syndrome
Kearns-Sayre syndrome
Fabry disease (α-galactosidase A deficiency)
Subacute necrotizing encephalomyelopathy (Leigh disease)
Sulfite oxidase deficiency
11-β-ketoreductase deficiency
17-α-hydroxylase deficiency
Purine nucleoside phosphorylase deficiency
Ornithine transcarbamylase deficiency
Neurofibromatosis type 1
HERNS

HERNS, hereditary endotheliopathy with retinopathy, nephropathy, and stroke; MELAS, mitochondrial myopathy, encephalopathy, lactic acidosis, and strokelike episodes; MERRF, myoclonic epilepsy with ragged red fibers.
From Roach ES, Golomb MR, Adams R, et al: Management of stroke in infants and children, *Stroke* 39:2644–2691, 2008, Table 2, p 6.

available. **Antithrombotic strategies** depend on the suspected cause but include anticoagulation with heparins or antiplatelet strategies such as aspirin. **Neuroprotective strategies** are essential to prevent progressive ischemic brain injury. These include careful control of blood glucose, temperature, and seizures and aggressive maintenance of cerebral perfusion pressure, with systolic blood pressures maintained in the high normal range. Malignant cerebral edema in the initial 72 hr is life-threatening and more common in children; emergency surgical decompression can be lifesaving. Disease-specific treatments include transfusion therapy in SCA, immunosuppression in vasculitis, and revascularization surgery in moyamoya disease. Long-term treatment goals include **secondary stroke prevention**, including antiplatelet therapy or, for cardiogenic causes, anticoagulation. Multimodal, family-centered **rehabilitation** programs are required for most survivors targeting motor deficits, language and intellectual impairments, behavioral and social disabilities, and epilepsy. Long term attention to

Table 594-3 CLASSIFICATION OF CEREBRAL VASCULITIS

Infectious vasculitis
Bacterial, fungal, parasitic
Spirochetal (syphilis, Lyme disease, leptospirosis)
Viral, rickettsial, mycobacterial, free-living amebae, cysticercosis, other helminths
Necrotizing vasculitides
Classic polyarteritis nodosa
Wegener granulomatosis
Allergic angiitis and granulomatosis (Churg-Strauss syndrome)
Necrotizing systemic vasculitis overlap syndrome
Lymphomatoid granulomatosis
Vasculitis associated with collagen vascular disease
Systemic lupus erythematosus
Rheumatoid arthritis
Scleroderma
Sjögren syndrome
Vasculitis associated with other systemic diseases
Behçet disease
Ulcerative colitis
Sarcoidosis
Relapsing polychondritis
Kohlmeier-Degos disease
Takayasu arteritis
Hypersensitivity vasculitides
Henoch-Schönlein purpura
Drug-induced vasculitides
Chemical vasculitides
Essential mixed cryoglobulinemia
Miscellaneous
Vasculitis associated with neoplasia
Vasculitis associated with radiation
Cogan syndrome
Dermatomyositis-polymyositis
X-linked lymphoproliferative syndrome
Kawasaki disease
Primary CNS vasculitis

From Roach ES, Golomb MR, Adams R, et al: Management of stroke in infants and children, *Stroke* 39:2644–2691, 2008, Table 5, p 8.

Table 594-4 RISK FACTORS FOR MOYAMOYA DISEASE

	PATIENTS (*n*)
No associated conditions (idiopathic)	66
Neurofibromatosis type 1	16
Asian heritage	16
Cranial therapeutic radiation	15
Hypothalamic-optic system glioma	8
Craniopharyngioma	4
Medulloblastoma, with Gorlin syndrome	1
Acute lymphocytic leukemia, intrathecal chemotherapy	2
Down syndrome	10
Congenital cardiac anomaly, previously operated	7
Renal artery stenosis	4
Hemoglobinopathy (2 sickle cell anemia, 1 "Bryn Mawr")	3
Other (hematologic: 1 spherocytosis, 1 idiopathic thrombocytopenic purpura)	2
Giant cervicofacial hemangiomas	3
Shunted hydrocephalus	3
Idiopathic hypertension requiring medication	3
Hyperthyroidism (1 with Graves syndrome)	2

Other syndromes, 1 patient each: Reye (remote), Williams, Alagille, cloacal exstrophy, renal artery fibromuscular dysplasia, and congenital cytomegalic inclusion virus infection (remote). Two patients had unclassified syndromic presentations. There were 4 blacks, 2 of whom had sickle cell disease.
From Roach ES, Golomb MR, Adams R, et al: Management of stroke in infants and children, *Stroke* 39:2644–2691, 2008, Table 6, p 11.

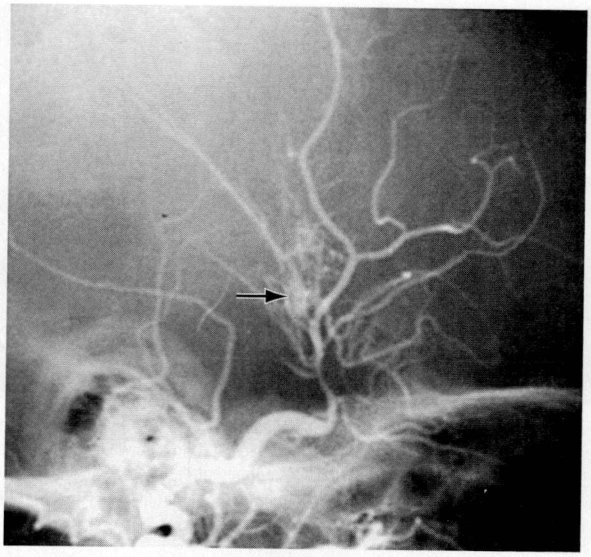

Figure 594-2 Cerebral angiogram showing idiopathic supraclinoid–internal carotid arteriopathy with classic moyamoya collaterals *(arrow)*.

arterial health lifestyle factors (avoiding obesity and smoking) is also important. Outcomes after childhood stroke include death in 6-10%, neurological deficits in 60-70%, and seizure disorders in 15%.

Perinatal stroke, the leading cause of term-born cerebral palsy (congenital hemiplegia), requires separate consideration. Acute neonatal stroke typically presents with seizures alone. Presumed perinatal ischemic stroke presents with gradual evolution of hemiparesis in later infancy and remote AIS on neuroimaging. Etiologies for both include cardiac and prothrombotic conditions discussed earlier, but additional maternal, prenatal, perinatal, placental, and neonatal factors must also be considered. Acute neonatal AIS requires neuroprotective treatment, but antithrombotic agents are only provided for cardiogenic embolism. Long-term morbidity is present in most children and requires comprehensive rehabilitation, as deficits continue to emerge with maturation.

BIBLIOGRAPHY

Please visit the Nelson Textbook of Pediatrics *website at www.expertconsult.com for the complete bibliography.*

594.2 Cerebral Sinovenous Thrombosis (CSVT)

Adam Kirton and Gabrielle deVeber

Cerebral venous drainage occurs via superficial (cortical veins, superior sagittal sinus) and deep (internal cerebral veins, straight sinus) systems that converge at the torcula to exit via the paired transverse and sigmoid sinuses and jugular veins. In CSVT, thrombotic occlusion of these venous structures can create increased intracranial pressure, cerebral edema, and, in 50% of cases, venous infarction (stroke). CSVT may be more common in children than in adults, and risk is greatest risk in the neonatal period.

Clinical presentations are often more gradual, variable, and nonspecific compared to AIS. Neonates typically present with diffuse neurologic signs and seizures. Children may present with progressive headache, papilledema, diplopia secondary to 6th nerve palsies (frequently misdiagnosed as idiopathic intracranial hypertension), or acute focal deficits. Seizures, lethargy, and

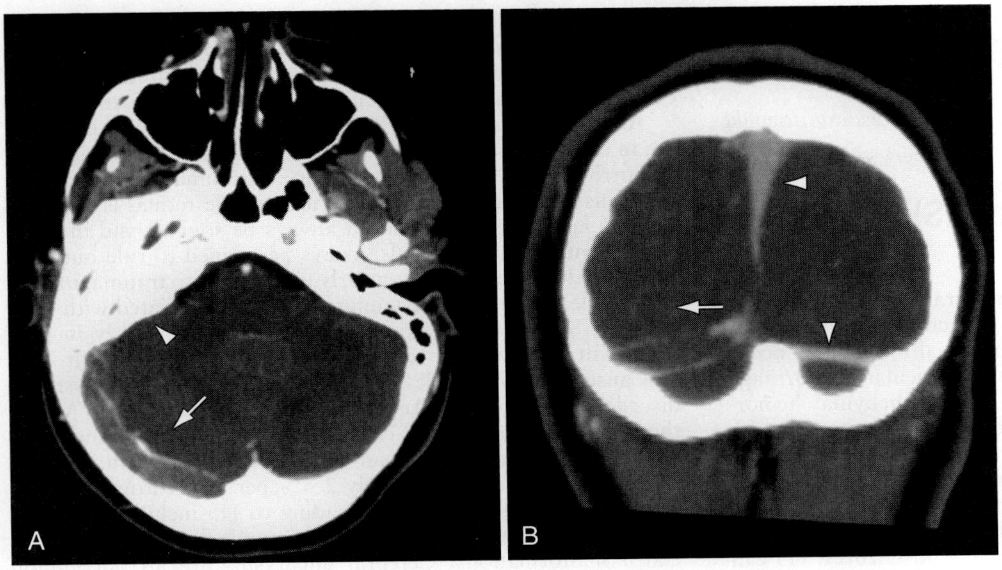

Figure 594-3 Cerebral sinovenous thrombosis. A 9 yr old girl presented with fever and progressive right-sided headache. She complained of double vision and had papilledema on examination. Axial *(A)* and coronal *(B)* CT venography demonstrates a large thrombus in the right transverse sinus that fails to opacify with contrast *(arrows)*. Note normal filling superior sagittal and left transverse sinuses *(arrowheads in B)* and opacification of the mastoid air cells *(arrowhead in A)*. Cause was otitis media/mastoiditis with septic thrombophlebitis of transverse sinus.

confusion are common. Diagnosis requires a high clinical suspicion and purposeful imaging of the cerebral venous system. Nonenhanced CT is very insensitive for CSVT, and contrast **CT venography (CTV)** is usually necessary to demonstrate filling defects in the cerebral venous system (Fig. 594-3). However MRI includes diffusion imaging of the brain parenchyma and modern MR venography (MRV) can be comparable to CTV in accuracy. Intraventricular hemorrhage in term infants suggests CSVT.

The Virchow triad is helpful in understanding the risk factors for CSVT (Table 594-5). Hypercoagulable states are frequently associated with childhood venous thrombosis including CSVT. **Prothrombotic states** frequently detected in childhood CSVT include inherited (e.g., prothrombin gene 20210A mutation) and acquired (e.g., antiphospholipid antibodies) conditions, prothrombotic medications (asparaginase, oral contraceptives), and common childhood illnesses, including iron deficiency anemia and severe **dehydration. Systemic diseases** associated with increased CSVT risk include leukemia, inflammatory bowel disease, and nephrotic syndrome.

Head and neck disorders can directly involve cerebral veins and sinuses causing CSVT. Common **infections** including meningitis, otitis media, and mastoiditis can cause **septic thrombophlebitis** of venous channels. CSVT can complicate head **trauma** especially adjacent to skull fractures. Neurosurgical procedures in proximity to cerebral venous structures may lead to injury and CSVT. Finally, obstruction of the cervical jugular veins and proximal stasis may result in CSVT. In neonates the unfused status of cranial sutures enables compression of underlying venous sinuses during delivery, or postnatally during supine lying when the occipital bone can compress the posterior sagittal sinus, possibly predisposing to CSVT.

Anticoagulation therapy plays an important role in childhood CSVT treatment. Despite no randomized trials, substantial indirect evidence has led to consensus across published guidelines which uniformly recommend anticoagulation with unfractionated or low molecular weight heparins in most children. Hemorrhagic transformation of venous infarcts is not an absolute contraindication to anticoagulation. Treatment is often continued for 3 mo at which time re-imaging either confirms recanalization (treatment usually discontinued) or persistent thrombus (treatment usually extended to 6 mo). However anticoagulation of neonates is more controversial and guidelines differ. New evidence suggests that protocol-based anticoagulants are safe in neonatal CSVT. About 30% of untreated neonates will extend their thrombosis in the 1st week postdiagnosis and additional

Table 594-5 COMMON RISK FACTORS FOR CEREBRAL SINOVENOUS THROMBOSIS IN CHILDREN

MAJOR CATEGORIES (VIRCHOW TRIAD)	EXAMPLES
Blood coagulation	Prothrombotic conditions Factor V Leiden, prothrombin gene mutation 20210A, protein C deficiency, protein S deficiency, antithrombin III deficiency, lipoprotein (a), antiphospholipid antibodies (lupus anticoagulant, anticardiolipin antibodies), pregnancy/puerperium Dehydration (e.g., gastroenteritis, neonatal failure to thrive) Iron deficiency anemia Drugs and toxins (e.g., L-aspariginase, oral contraceptives) Acute systemic illness (e.g., sepsis, disseminated intravascular coagulation) Chronic systemic illness (e.g., inflammatory bowel disease, leukemia) Nephrotic syndrome Inborn errors of metabolism (e.g., homocystinuria)
Blood vessel	Infection Otitis media, mastoiditis, bacterial meningitis Lemierre syndrome (human necrobacillosis) Trauma: skull fractures Compression: birth, occipital bone compression in neonates Iatrogenic: neurosurgery, jugular lines, extracorporeal membrane oxygenation Venous malformations (e.g., dural arteriovenous fistulas)

venous infarction can result. Therefore if anticoagulation is withheld, early repeat venous imaging is paramount. Protocols supporting initial anticoagulation recommend shorter treatment durations in neonates (i.e., 6 weeks, 3 mo). Children with persistent risk factors carry risk for recurrence and may require long-term anticoagulation. **Neuroprotective** and supportive interventions include aggressive management of infection, maintenance of hydration, and neuroprotective measures (normothermia, normotension, seizure control). **Optic neuropathy** secondary to increased intracranial pressure is an important and often overlooked complication of CSVT. Regular fundoscopic examination by an ophthalmologist and measures to reduce intracranial pressure (e.g., acetazolamide, serial lumbar puncture) may be required. Most neurologic morbidity is suffered by those incurring venous infarction, and children with bilateral injuries can be devastated. Consistent with other forms of childhood stroke, a comprehensive neurorehabilitation program is required for children with venous infarction.

BIBLIOGRAPHY

Please visit the Nelson Textbook of Pediatrics *website at* *www.expertconsult.com* *for the complete bibliography.*

594.3 Hemorrhagic Stroke (HS)

Adam Kirton and Gabrielle deVeber

Hemorrhagic stroke (HS) includes nontraumatic intracranial hemorrhage and is classified by the intracranial compartment containing the hemorrhage. Intraparenchymal bleeds may occur in any location within the brain. Intraventricular hemorrhage may be primary or an extension of intraparenchymal hemorrhage. Bleeding outside the brain may occur in the subarachnoid, subdural, or epidural spaces.

Clinical presentations vary according to location, cause, and rate of bleeding. Acute hemorrhages may feature instantaneous or **thunderclap headache,** loss of consciousness, and nuchal rigidity in addition to focal neurologic deficits and seizures. HS can be rapidly fatal. In bleeds associated with vascular malformations, pulsatile tinnitus, cranial bruit, macrocephaly, and high-output heart failure may be present. Diagnosis relies on imaging, and CT is highly sensitive to acute HS. However lumbar puncture may be required to exclude subarachnoid hemorrhage. Modern MRI is highly sensitive to even small amounts of acute hemorrhage and it images residual blood products long-term following most parenchymal bleeds (Fig. 594-4). **Angiography** by CT, MR, or conventional means is often required to exclude underlying vascular abnormalities (e.g., vascular malformations, aneurysms).

Abusive (nonaccidental) head trauma with intracranial bleeding in children may present as primary subdural or parenchymal hemorrhage with no apparent history of trauma. Subtle scalp or ear bruising, retinal hemorrhages in multiple retinal layers, and chronic failure to thrive should always be sought, and in small infants with subdural bleeds, x-rays performed to rule out fractures. Epidural hematoma is nearly always due to trauma, including middle meningeal artery injury typically associated with skull fracture. Subdural hematoma can occur spontaneously in children with brain atrophy due to stretching of bridging veins.

Causes of HS include vascular malformations and systemic disorders (Table 594-6). **Arteriovenous malformations** (AVM) are the most common cause of childhood subarachnoid and intraparenchymal HS and may occur anywhere in the brain. Risk of AVM bleeding is approximately 2-4% per year throughout life. Other vascular malformations leading to HS include cavernous angiomas (**cavernomas**), dural arteriovenous fistulas, and vein of Galen malformations. Cerebral **aneurysms** are an uncommon cause of subarachnoid hemorrhage in children and may suggest an underlying disorder (e.g., polycystic kidney disease, infective endocarditis). A common cause for HS is bleeding from a preexisting brain tumor. Arterial diseases that usually cause ischemic stroke can also predispose to HS including the central nervous system (CNS) vasculitides and moyamoya disease. Additional

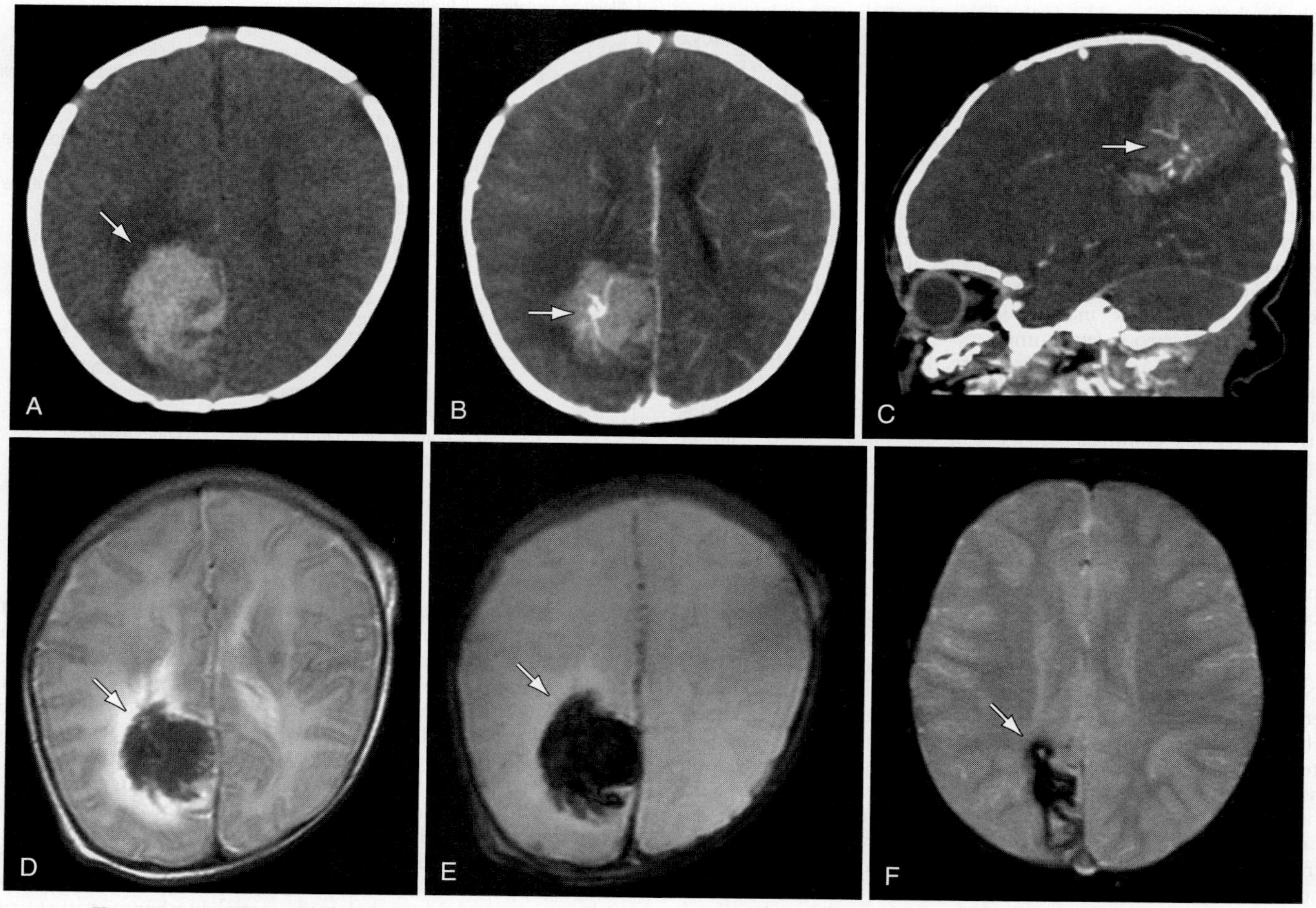

Figure 594-4 Hemorrhagic stroke due to vascular malformation. A healthy 1 mo old presented with sudden onset irritability followed by focal left body seizures. Plain CT head demonstrates a large hyperdense lesion in the right parietal region with surrounding edema consistent with acute hemorrhage *(A).* Axial *(B)* and sagittal *(C)* contrast CT scans suggest an abnormal cluster of vessels in the center of the hemorrhage. T2-weighted MRI differentiates the acute hemorrhage from surrounding edema *(D).* Gradient ECHO MRI, both acutely *(E)* and at 3 mo *(F),* demonstrates the presence of blood product.

Table 594-6 POTENTIAL RISK FACTORS FOR HEMORRHAGIC STROKE IN CHILDREN

MAJOR CATEGORIES	EXAMPLES
Vascular disorder	Arteriovenous malformations Cavernous malformations (cavernomas) Venous angiomas Hereditary hemorrhagic telangiectasia Intracranial aneurysm Choroid plexus angiomas (pure intraventricular hemorrhage) Moyamoya disease/syndrome Inflammatory vasculitis (Chapter 611) Neoplastic lesions with unstable vasculature Drugs/toxins (cocaine, amphetamine)
Blood disorder	Idiopathic thrombocytopenic purpura Hemolytic uremic syndrome Hepatic disease/failure coagulopathy Vitamin K deficiency (hemorrhagic disease of the newborn) Disseminated intravascular coagulation
Trauma	Middle meningeal artery injury (epidural hematoma) Bridging vein injury (subdural hematoma) Subarachnoid hemorrhage Hemorrhagic contusions (coup and contrecoup) Nonaccidental trauma (subdural hematomas of different ages) Iatrogenic (neurosurgical procedures, angiography)

causes of parenchymal HS include hypertensive hemorrhage and **hematologic disorders** such as thrombocytopenic purpura, hemophilia, acquired coagulopathies (e.g., disseminated intravascular coagulation, liver failure), anticoagulant therapy (e.g., warfarin), or illicit drug use. Ischemic infarcts may undergo hemorrhagic transformation, particularly in CSVT, and can be difficult to differentiate from primary HS.

Management of childhood HS may include emergent neurosurgical intervention for large or rapidly expanding lesions. The same principles of **neuroprotection** for vulnerable brain suggested in the ischemic stroke sections also apply to HS. Reversal of anticoagulant therapy may be required (e.g., vitamin K, fresh frozen plasma) but the role of other medical interventions such as factor VII are unstudied in children. Recurrence risk for those with structural lesions is significant and serial imaging may be required. Outcomes from childhood HS are not well studied but likely depend on lesion size, location, and etiology. Compared with ischemic stroke, death is more frequent in HS, however greater degrees of recovery from the initial deficit can be expected.

Neonatal hemorrhagic strokes are different. Cranial ultrasound can detect most significant neonatal bleeds. In the preterm infant, germinal matrix bleeding and intraventricular hemorrhage are common (Chapter 93.3). Subarachnoid and subdural blood may be imaged in up to 25% of normal term newborns. Term HS is poorly studied and includes the etiologies listed earlier, but may be idiopathic in >50% of cases. Term intraventricular bleeding is often secondary to either deep CSVT or choroid plexus angiomas.

BIBLIOGRAPHY

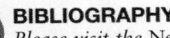

Please visit the Nelson Textbook of Pediatrics *website at www.expertconsult.com for the complete bibliography.*

594.4 Differential Diagnosis of Strokelike Events

Adam Kirton and Gabrielle deVeber

The diagnosis of stroke in childhood requires a high index of suspicion, balanced with awareness of the differential diagnosis. Acute onset of a focal neurologic deficit or in neonates, seizures, should be considered stroke until proven otherwise and assessed with neuroimaging. Pediatric stroke must be differentiated from other strokelike disorders (Table 594-7) that may require their own urgent specific treatment.

MIGRAINE

Careful history and examination can often suggest migraine as the cause of acute focal deficits. Migraine auras should last between 5 and 60 min and resolve completely. The neurologic deficit representing the aura of migraine typically evolves slowly compared with stroke, with sensory disturbance or weakness "marching" from distal to proximal limb over minutes. Evolution into a migrainous headache is expected, however headache may also accompany acute infarction. A group of uncommon migraine subtypes can more closely mimic stroke in children, including familial hemiplegic migraine, basilar migraine, and migraine aura without headache. Migraine can rarely cause a stroke, referred to as migrainous infarction.

SEIZURE

Prolonged focal seizure activity is frequently followed by a period of focal neurologic deficit (Todd paralysis) which typically resolves within an hour. Very rarely, focal seizures can manifest with only negative symptoms producing acute onset, focal neurologic deficits. A history of jerks or tonic posturing at onset, a known past history of seizures, and EEG findings may be helpful. Imaging is required in all new cases of seizure with persisting Todd paralysis because stroke in children frequently is associated with seizures at onset.

INFECTION

Life-threatening and treatable brain infections can be mistaken for stroke including bacterial meningitis and herpes encephalitis. However, symptom onset in primary CNS infection is typically more gradual and less focal with fever as a consistent feature. Children with bacterial meningitis are at risk for both venous and arterial stroke.

DEMYELINATION

Acute disseminated encephalomyelitis (ADEM), clinically isolated syndrome (CIS), multiple sclerosis, and other demyelinating conditions can present with acute focal neurological deficits. Symptom onset and initial progression is more gradual (over hours or days) compared with stroke onset (over minutes). Multifocal deficits, or concurrent encephalopathy in the case of ADEM, would decrease the probability of stroke.

HYPOGLYCEMIA

Acute drops in blood glucose can produce focal deficits mimicking stroke. New onset hypoglycemia in otherwise healthy children is rare, but predisposing conditions include insulin-dependent diabetes, adrenal insufficiency and steroid withdrawal, hypopituitarism, and ketogenic diet.

GLOBAL HYPOXIC-ISCHEMIC ENCEPHALOPATHY (HIE)

Generalized decreases in cerebral perfusion can produce focal areas of watershed brain infarction which can mimic stroke. Watershed ischemic injury should be accompanied by recognized hypotension or conditions predisposing to low cerebral perfusion such as sepsis, dehydration, or cardiac dysfunction. Clinical presentations would involve more generalized and bilateral cerebral dysfunction compared to stroke and the anatomic location of the infarct is in typical bilateral watershed zones rather than a single arterial territory.

Table 594-7 DIFFERENTIAL DIAGNOSIS OF STROKELIKE EPISODES IN CHILDREN

DISORDER	CLINICAL DISTINCTION FROM STROKE	IMAGING DISTINCTION FROM STROKE
Migraine	Evolving or "marching" symptoms, short duration, complete resolution, headache, personal or family history of migraine	Typically normal Migrainous infarction is rare
Seizure	Positive symptoms, Todd paralysis is postseizure and limited	Normal or may identify source of seizures (e.g., malformation, old injury)
Infection	Fever, encephalopathy, gradual onset, meningismus	Normal or signs of encephalitis/cerebritis, which are typically diffuse and bilateral AIS and CSVT can occur in bacterial meningitis
Demyelination	Gradual onset, multifocal symptoms, encephalopathy Accompanying optic neuritis or transverse myelitis	Multifocal lesions, typical appearance (e.g., patchy in ADEM, ovoid in MS), typical locations (e.g., pericallosal in MS), less likely to show restricted diffusion
Hypoglycemia	Risk factor (e.g., insulin therapy), related to meals, additional systemic symptoms	Bilateral, symmetric May see restricted diffusion Posterior dominant pattern
Watershed infarction due to global HIE	Risk factor (e.g., hypotension, sepsis, heart disease), bilateral deficits	Bilateral, symmetric restricted diffusion in border zones between major arteries (watersheds)
Hypertensive encephalopathy (PRES)	Documented hypertension, bilateral visual symptoms, encephalopathy	Posterior dominant, bilateral, patchy lesions involving gray and white matter; usually no restricted diffusion
Inborn errors of metabolism	Pre-existing delays/regression, multisystem disease, abnormal biochemical profiles	May have restricted diffusion lesions but bilateral, symmetrical, not within vascular territories MR spectroscopy changes (e.g., high lactate in MELAS)
Vestibulopathy	Symptoms limited to vertigo, imbalance (i.e., no weakness) Gradual onset	Normal
Acute cerebellar ataxia	Sudden onset bilaterally symmetric ataxia postviral	Normal
Channelopathy	Syndromic cluster of symptoms not localizing to single lesion Gradual onset, progressive evolution	Normal
Alternating hemiplegia	History contralateral events Choreoathetosis/dystonia	Normal

ADEM, acute disseminated encephalomyelitis; AIS, arterial ischemic stroke; CSVT, cerebral sinovenous thrombosis; HIE, hypoxic-ischemic encephalopathy; MELAS, mitochondrial myopathy, encephalopathy, lactic acidosis, and strokelike episodes; MR, magnetic resonance; MS, multiple sclerosis; PRES, posterior reversible leukoencephalopathy syndrome.

HYPERTENSIVE ENCEPHALOPATHY (PRES)

Posterior reversible leukoencephalopathy syndrome (PRES) is seen in children with hypertension, often in the context of an acute rise in blood pressure. Posterior regions are selectively involved, typically resulting in symptoms of bilateral cortical visual dysfunction in addition to encephalopathy and seizures.

INBORN ERRORS OF METABOLISM

Mitochondrial myopathy, encephalopathy, lactic acidosis, and strokelike episodes (MELAS; Chapter 591.2) is the classic example, though other mitochondrial disease can mimic stroke. Features favoring MELAS would include a history of developmental regression, posterior (and often bilateral) lesions not respecting vascular territories on MRI, and elevated serum or cerebrospinal fluid lactate (MR spectroscopy). In contrast to these types of "metabolic infarction," children with Fabry disease and homocystinuria are at risk of true ischemic stroke.

VESTIBULOPATHY/ATAXIA

Acute onset vertigo and/or ataxia can be confused with brainstem or cerebellar stroke. Simple bedside tests of vestibular function with otherwise intact brainstem functions are reassuring. This differential diagnosis includes acute vestibular neuronopathy, viral labyrinthitis, and the benign paroxysmal vertigos as well as acute cerebellar ataxia and episodic ataxias.

CHANNELOPATHIES

An increasing number of nervous system ion channel mutations are described that feature sudden focal neurologic deficits, thereby mimicking stroke. These include the migraine syndromes mentioned earlier as well as a growing list of episodic ataxias. A strong family history raises suspicion but most require additional investigation.

ALTERNATING HEMIPLEGIA OF CHILDHOOD (AHC)

AHC typically presents in infancy with acute intermittent episodes of hemiplegia lasting hours (range minute to weeks) that alternate from 1 side of the body to the other. The hemiplegia persists for minutes to weeks and then resolves spontaneously. Choreoathetosis and dystonic movements are commonly observed in the hemiparetic extremity. Signs spontaneously regress with sleep but recur with awakening. Neuroimaging including MR angiography should be completed to exclude moyamoya disease. AHC has been linked to mutations in certain ion channels.

Chapter 595
Central Nervous System Infections

Charles G. Prober and LauraLe Dyner

Infection of the central nervous system (CNS) is the most common cause of fever associated with signs and symptoms of CNS disease in children. Many microorganisms can cause infection. Nonetheless, specific pathogens are identifiable and are influenced by the age and immune status of the host and the epidemiology of the pathogen. In general, viral infections of the CNS are much more common than bacterial infections, which, in turn, are more common than fungal and parasitic infections. Infections caused by rickettsiae (Rocky Mountain spotted fever, *Ehrlichia*) are relatively uncommon but assume important roles under certain epidemiologic circumstances. *Mycoplasma* spp. can also cause infections of the CNS, although their precise contribution is often difficult to determine.

Regardless of etiology, most patients with CNS infection have similar clinical manifestations. **Common symptoms** include headache, nausea, vomiting, anorexia, restlessness, altered state of consciousness, and irritability; most of these symptoms are nonspecific. **Common signs** of CNS infection, in addition to fever, include photophobia, neck pain and rigidity, obtundation, stupor, coma, seizures, and focal neurologic deficits. The severity and constellation of signs are determined by the specific pathogen, the host, and the area of the CNS affected.

Infection of the CNS may be diffuse or focal. Meningitis and encephalitis are examples of diffuse infection. Meningitis implies primary involvement of the meninges, whereas encephalitis indicates brain parenchymal involvement. Because these anatomic boundaries are often not distinct, many patients have evidence of both meningeal and parenchymal involvement and should be considered to have meningoencephalitis. Brain abscess is the best example of a focal infection of the CNS. The neurologic expression of this infection is determined by the site and extent of the abscess(es) (Chapter 596).

The diagnosis of diffuse CNS infections depends on examination of cerebrospinal fluid (CSF) obtained by lumbar puncture (LP). Table 595-1 provides an overview of the expected CSF abnormalities with various CNS disorders.

595.1 Acute Bacterial Meningitis Beyond the Neonatal Period

Charles G. Prober and LauraLe Dyner

Bacterial meningitis is one of the most potentially serious infections occurring in infants and older children. This infection is associated with a high rate of acute complications and risk of long-term morbidity. The incidence of bacterial meningitis is sufficiently high in febrile infants that it should be included in the differential diagnosis of those with altered mental status and other evidence of neurologic dysfunction.

ETIOLOGY

The most common cause of bacterial meningitis in children 1 mo to 12 yr of age in the USA is *Neisseria meningitidis*. Bacterial meningitis caused by *Streptococcus pneumoniae* and *Haemophilus influenzae* type b has become much less common in developed countries since the introduction of universal immunization against these pathogens beginning at 2 mo of age. Demonstrating the importance of vaccination, invasive *H. influenzae* disease was reported in Minnesota in 2008 in 5 children with no relationship to one another and who were partially or not immunized. It is the largest number of children with invasive *H. influenzae* in Minnesota since 1992. Infection caused by *S. pneumoniae* or *H. influenzae* type b must be considered in incompletely vaccinated individuals or those in developing countries. Those with certain underlying immunologic (HIV infection, IgG subclass deficiency) or anatomic (splenic dysfunction, cochlear defects or implants) disorders also may be at increased risk of infection caused by these bacteria.

Alterations of host defense due to anatomic defects or immune deficits also increase the risk of meningitis from less common pathogens such as *Pseudomonas aeruginosa, Staphylococcus aureus*, coagulase-negative staphylococci, *Salmonella* spp., and *Listeria monocytogenes*.

EPIDEMIOLOGY

A major risk factor for meningitis is the lack of immunity to specific pathogens associated with young age. Additional risks include recent colonization with pathogenic bacteria, close contact (household, daycare centers, college dormitories, military barracks) with individuals having invasive disease caused by *N. meningitidis* and *H. influenzae* type b, crowding, poverty, black or Native American race, and male gender. The mode of transmission is probably person-to-person contact through respiratory tract secretions or droplets. The risk of meningitis is increased among infants and young children with occult bacteremia; the odds ratio is greater for meningococcus (85 times) and *H. influenzae* type b (12 times) relative to that for pneumococcus.

Specific host defense defects due to altered immunoglobulin production in response to encapsulated pathogens may be responsible for the increased risk of bacterial meningitis in Native Americans and Eskimos. Defects of the complement system (C5-C8) have been associated with recurrent meningococcal infection, and defects of the properdin system have been associated with a significant risk of lethal meningococcal disease. Splenic dysfunction (sickle cell anemia) or asplenia (due to trauma, or congenital defect) is associated with an increased risk of pneumococcal, *H. influenzae* type b (to some extent), and, rarely, meningococcal sepsis and meningitis. T-lymphocyte defects (congenital or acquired by chemotherapy, AIDS, or malignancy) are associated with an increased risk of *L. monocytogenes* infections of the CNS.

Congenital or acquired CSF leak across a mucocutaneous barrier, such as cranial or midline facial defects (cribriform plate) and middle ear (stapedial foot plate) or inner ear fistulas (oval window, internal auditory canal, cochlear aqueduct), or CSF leakage through a rupture of the meninges due to a basal skull fracture into the cribriform plate or paranasal sinus, is associated with an increased risk of pneumococcal meningitis. The risk of bacterial meningitis, caused by *S. pneumoniae,* in children with cochlear implants, used for the treatment of hearing loss, is more than 30 times the risk in the general U.S. population. Lumbosacral dermal sinus and meningomyelocele are associated with staphylococcal and gram-negative enteric bacterial meningitis. CSF shunt infections increase the risk of meningitis due to staphylococci (especially coagulase-negative species) and other low virulence bacteria that typically colonize the skin.

STREPTOCOCCUS PNEUMONIAE (CHAPTER 181)

The epidemiology of infections caused by *S. pneumoniae* has been dramatically altered by the widespread use of the 7-valent pneumococcal protein-polysaccharide conjugate vaccine (serotypes 4, 6B, 9V, 14, 18C, 19F, 23F), licensed in the USA in February 2000. The vaccine has led to a dramatic decrease in rates of pneumococcal meningitis, accompanied by a slight increase in meningitis caused by some nonvaccine serotypes. This vaccine is recommended for routine administration to all children 23 mo of age and younger at 2, 4, 6, and 12-15 mo of age. Immunization targets this population because the incidence of invasive pneumococcal infections peaks in the 1st 2 yr of life, reaching rates of 228/100,000 in children 6-12 mo of age. Children with anatomic or functional asplenia secondary to sickle cell disease and those infected with HIV have infection rates that are 20- to 100-fold higher than in those of healthy children in the 1st 5 yr of life. Additional risk factors for contracting pneumococcal meningitis include otitis media, sinusitis, pneumonia, CSF otorrhea or rhinorrhea, the presence of a cochlear implant, and chronic graft versus host disease following bone marrow transplantation. The 7-valent pneumococcal vaccine has been replaced by the 13-valent pneumococcal vaccine, which includes additional serotypes 1, 3, 5, 6A, 7F, and 19A.

NEISSERIA MENINGITIDIS (CHAPTER 184)

Five serogroups of meningococcus, A, B, C, Y, and W-135, are responsible for disease. Meningococcal meningitis may be sporadic or may occur in epidemics. In the USA, serogroups B, C, and Y each account for ≈30% of cases, although serogroup

Table 595-1 CEREBROSPINAL FLUID FINDINGS IN CENTRAL NERVOUS SYSTEM DISORDERS

CONDITION Normal	PRESSURE (mm H_2O) 50-80	LEUKOCYTES (mm³) <5, ≥75% Lymphocytes	PROTEIN (mg/dL) 20-45	GLUCOSE (mg/dL) >50 (or 75% Serum Glucose)	COMMENTS
COMMON FORMS OF MENINGITIS					
Acute bacterial meningitis	Usually elevated (100-300)	100-10,000 or more; usually 300-2,000; PMNs predominate	Usually 100-500	Decreased, usually <40 (or <50% serum glucose)	Organisms usually seen on Gram stain and recovered by culture
Partially treated bacterial meningitis	Normal or elevated	5-10,000; PMNs usual but mononuclear cells may predominate if pretreated for extended period of time	Usually 100-500	Normal or decreased	Organisms may be seen on Gram stain Pretreatment may render CSF sterile. Antigen may be detected by agglutination test
Viral meningitis or meningoencephalitis	Normal or slightly elevated (80-150)	Rarely >1,000 cells. Eastern equine encephalitis and lymphocytic choriomeningitis (LCM) may have cell counts of several thousand. PMNs early but mononuclear cells predominate through most of the course	Usually 50-200	Generally normal; may be decreased to <40 in some viral diseases, particularly mumps (15-20% of cases)	HSV encephalitis is suggested by focal seizures or by focal findings on CT or MRI scans or EEG. Enteroviruses and HSV infrequently recovered from CSF. HSV and enteroviruses may be detected by PCR of CSF
UNCOMMON FORMS OF MENINGITIS					
Tuberculous meningitis	Usually elevated	10-500; PMNs early, but lymphocytes predominate through most of the course	100-3,000; may be higher in presence of block	<50 in most cases; decreases with time if treatment is not provided	Acid-fast organisms almost never seen on smear. Organisms may be recovered in culture of large volumes of CSF. *Mycobacterium tuberculosis* may be detected by PCR of CSF
Fungal meningitis	Usually elevated	5-500; PMNs early but mononuclear cells predominate through most of the course. Cryptococcal meningitis may have no cellular inflammatory response	25-500	<50; decreases with time if treatment is not provided	Budding yeast may be seen. Organisms may be recovered in culture. Cryptococcal antigen (CSF and serum) may be positive in cryptococcal infection
Syphilis (acute) and leptospirosis	Usually elevated	50-500; lymphocytes predominate	50-200	Usually normal	Positive CSF serology. Spirochetes not demonstrable by usual techniques of smear or culture; dark-field examination may be positive
Amebic *(Naegleria)* meningoencephalitis	Elevated	1,000-10,000 or more; PMNs predominate	50-500	Normal or slightly decreased	Mobile amebae may be seen by hanging-drop examination of CSF at room temperature
BRAIN ABSCESSES AND PARAMENINGEAL FOCUS					
Brain abscess	Usually elevated (100-300)	5-200; CSF rarely acellular; lymphocytes predominate; if abscess ruptures into ventricle, PMNs predominate and cell count may reach >100,000	75-500	Normal unless abscess ruptures into ventricular system	No organisms on smear or culture unless abscess ruptures into ventricular system
Subdural empyema	Usually elevated (100-300)	100-5,000; PMNs predominate	100-500	Normal	No organisms on smear or culture of CSF unless meningitis also present; organisms found on tap of subdural fluid
Cerebral epidural abscess	Normal to slightly elevated	10-500; lymphocytes predominate	50-200	Normal	No organisms on smear or culture of CSF
Spinal epidural abscess	Usually low, with spinal block	10-100; lymphocytes predominate	50-400	Normal	No organisms on smear or culture of CSF
Chemical (drugs, dermoid cysts, myelography dye)	Usually elevated	100-1,000 or more; PMNs predominate	50-100	Normal or slightly decreased	Epithelial cells may be seen within CSF by use of polarized light in some children with dermoids
NONINFECTIOUS CAUSES					
Sarcoidosis	Normal or elevated slightly	0-100; mononuclear	40-100	Normal	No specific findings
Systemic lupus erythematosus with CNS involvement	Slightly elevated	0-500; PMNs usually predominate; lymphocytes may be present	100	Normal or slightly decreased	No organisms on smear or culture. Positive neuronal and ribosomal P protein antibodies in CSF
Tumor, leukemia	Slightly elevated to very high	0-100 or more; mononuclear or blast cells	50-1,000	Normal to decreased (20-40)	Cytology may be positive

CSF, cerebrospinal fluid; EEG, electroencephalogram; HSV, herpes simplex virus; PCR, polymerase chain reaction; PMN, polymorphonuclear neutrophils.

distribution varies by location and time. Epidemic disease, especially in developing countries, is usually caused by serogroup A. Cases occur throughout the year but may be more common in the winter and spring and following influenza virus infections. Nasopharyngeal carriage of *N. meningitidis* occurs in 1-15% of adults. Colonization may last weeks to months; recent colonization places nonimmune younger children at greatest risk for meningitis. The incidence of disease occurring in association with an index case in the family is 1%, a rate that is 1,000-fold the risk in the general population. The risk of secondary cases occurring in contacts at daycare centers is about 1/1,000. Most infections of children are acquired from a contact in a daycare facility, a colonized adult family member, or an ill patient with meningococcal disease. Children younger than 5 yr have the highest rates of meningococcal infection. A 2nd peak in incidence occurs in persons between 15 and 24 yr of age. College freshmen living in dormitories have an increased incidence of infection compared to non–college-attending, age-matched controls.

The Centers for Disease Control and Prevention (CDC) recommends vaccination against meningococcus with 1 dose of a quadrivalent conjugate meningococcal vaccine between the ages of 11 and 18 yr and for persons 2-10 yr who are at increased risk for meningococcal disease. College freshmen living in dormitories who have not been previously vaccinated should also be vaccinated with MCV4.

HAEMOPHILUS INFLUENZAE TYPE B (CHAPTER 186)

Before universal *H. influenzae* type b vaccination in the USA, about 70% of cases of bacterial meningitis occurring in the 1st 5 yr of life were caused by this pathogen. Invasive infections occurred primarily in infants 2 mo to 2 yr of age; peak incidence was at 6-9 mo of age, and 50% of cases occurred in the 1st yr of life. The risk to children was markedly increased among family or daycare center contacts of patients with *H. influenzae* type b disease. Incompletely vaccinated individuals, those in underdeveloped countries who are not vaccinated, and those with blunted immunologic responses to vaccine (children with HIV infection) remain at risk for *H. influenzae* type b meningitis.

PATHOLOGY AND PATHOPHYSIOLOGY

A meningeal purulent exudate of varying thickness may be distributed around the cerebral veins, venous sinuses, convexity of the brain, and cerebellum and in the sulci, sylvian fissures, basal cisterns, and spinal cord. Ventriculitis with bacteria and inflammatory cells in ventricular fluid may be present (more often in neonates), as may subdural effusions and, rarely, empyema. Perivascular inflammatory infiltrates also may be present, and the ependymal membrane may be disrupted. Vascular and parenchymal cerebral changes characterized by polymorphonuclear infiltrates extending to the subintimal region of the small arteries and veins, vasculitis, thrombosis of small cortical veins, occlusion of major venous sinuses, necrotizing arteritis producing subarachnoid hemorrhage, and, rarely, cerebral cortical necrosis in the absence of identifiable thrombosis have been described at autopsy. **Cerebral infarction,** resulting from vascular occlusion due to inflammation, vasospasm, and thrombosis, is a frequent sequela. Infarct size ranges from microscopic to involvement of an entire hemisphere.

Inflammation of spinal nerves and roots produces meningeal signs, and inflammation of the cranial nerves produces cranial neuropathies of optic, oculomotor, facial, and auditory nerves. Increased intracranial pressure (ICP) also produces oculomotor nerve palsy due to the presence of temporal lobe compression of the nerve during tentorial herniation. Abducens nerve palsy may be a nonlocalizing sign of elevated ICP.

Increased ICP is due to cell death (cytotoxic cerebral edema), cytokine-induced increased capillary vascular permeability (vasogenic cerebral edema), and, possibly, increased hydrostatic pressure (interstitial cerebral edema) after obstructed reabsorption of CSF in the arachnoid villus or obstruction of the flow of fluid from the ventricles. ICP may exceed 300 mm H_2O; cerebral perfusion may be further compromised if the cerebral perfusion pressure (mean arterial pressure minus ICP) is <50 cm H_2O due to systemic hypotension with reduced cerebral blood flow. The syndrome of inappropriate antidiuretic hormone secretion (SIADH) may produce excessive water retention and potentially increase the risk of elevated ICP (Chapter 553). Hypotonicity of brain extracellular spaces may cause cytotoxic edema after cell swelling and lysis. Tentorial, falx, or cerebellar herniation does not usually occur because the increased ICP is transmitted to the entire subarachnoid space and there is little structural displacement. Furthermore, if the fontanels are still patent, increased ICP is not always dissipated.

Hydrocephalus can occur as an acute complication of bacterial meningitis. It most often takes the form of a communicating hydrocephalus due to adhesive thickening of the arachnoid villi around the cisterns at the base of the brain. Thus, there is interference with the normal resorption of CSF. Less often, obstructive hydrocephalus develops after fibrosis and gliosis of the aqueduct of Sylvius or the foramina of Magendie and Luschka.

Raised CSF protein levels are due in part to increased vascular permeability of the blood-brain barrier and the loss of albumin-rich fluid from the capillaries and veins traversing the subdural space. Continued transudation may result in subdural effusions, usually found in the later phase of acute bacterial meningitis. **Hypoglycorrhachia** (reduced CSF glucose levels) is due to decreased glucose transport by the cerebral tissue.

Damage to the cerebral cortex may be due to the focal or diffuse effects of vascular occlusion (infarction, necrosis, lactic acidosis), hypoxia, bacterial invasion (cerebritis), toxic encephalopathy (bacterial toxins), elevated ICP, ventriculitis, and transudation (subdural effusions). These pathologic factors result in the clinical manifestations of impaired consciousness, seizures, cranial nerve deficits, motor and sensory deficits, and later psychomotor retardation.

PATHOGENESIS

Bacterial meningitis most commonly results from hematogenous dissemination of microorganisms from a distant site of infection; **bacteremia** usually precedes meningitis or occurs concomitantly. Bacterial colonization of the nasopharynx with a potentially pathogenic microorganism is the usual source of the bacteremia. There may be prolonged carriage of the colonizing organisms without disease or, more likely, rapid invasion after recent colonization. Prior or concurrent viral upper respiratory tract infection may enhance the pathogenicity of bacteria producing meningitis.

N. meningitidis and *H. influenzae* type b attach to mucosal epithelial cell receptors by pili. After attachment to epithelial cells, bacteria breach the mucosa and enter the circulation. *N. meningitidis* may be transported across the mucosal surface within a phagocytic vacuole after ingestion by the epithelial cell. Bacterial survival in the bloodstream is enhanced by large bacterial capsules that interfere with opsonic phagocytosis and are associated with increased virulence. Host-related developmental defects in bacterial opsonic phagocytosis also contribute to the bacteremia. In young, nonimmune hosts, the defect may be due to an absence of preformed IgM or IgG anticapsular antibodies, whereas in immunodeficient patients, various deficiencies of components of the complement or properdin system may interfere with effective opsonic phagocytosis. Splenic dysfunction may also reduce opsonic phagocytosis by the reticuloendothelial system.

Bacteria gain entry to the CSF through the choroid plexus of the lateral ventricles and the meninges and then circulate to the extracerebral CSF and subarachnoid space. Bacteria rapidly multiply because the CSF concentrations of complement and antibody are inadequate to contain bacterial proliferation. Chemotactic factors then incite a local inflammatory response characterized by polymorphonuclear cell infiltration. The presence of bacterial cell wall lipopolysaccharide (endotoxin) of gram-negative bacteria (*H. influenzae* type b, *N. meningitidis*) and of pneumococcal cell wall components (teichoic acid, peptidoglycan) stimulates a marked inflammatory response, with local production of tumor necrosis factor, interleukin 1, prostaglandin E, and other inflammatory mediators. The subsequent inflammatory response is characterized by neutrophilic infiltration, increased vascular permeability, alterations of the blood-brain barrier, and vascular thrombosis. Meningitis-associated brain injury is not simply caused by viable bacteria but occurs as a consequence of the host reaction to the inflammatory cascade initiated by bacterial components.

Rarely, meningitis may follow bacterial invasion from a contiguous focus of infection such as paranasal sinusitis, otitis media, mastoiditis, orbital cellulitis, or cranial or vertebral osteomyelitis or may occur after introduction of bacteria via penetrating cranial trauma, dermal sinus tracts, or meningomyeloceles.

CLINICAL MANIFESTATIONS

The onset of acute meningitis has 2 predominant patterns. The more dramatic and, fortunately, less common presentation is sudden onset with rapidly progressive manifestations of shock, purpura, disseminated intravascular coagulation (DIC), and reduced levels of consciousness often resulting in progression to coma or death within 24 hr. More often, meningitis is preceded by several days of fever accompanied by upper respiratory tract or gastrointestinal symptoms, followed by nonspecific signs of CNS infection such as increasing lethargy and irritability.

The signs and symptoms of meningitis are related to the nonspecific findings associated with a systemic infection and to manifestations of meningeal irritation. Nonspecific findings include fever, anorexia and poor feeding, headache, symptoms of upper respiratory tract infection, myalgias, arthralgias, tachycardia, hypotension, and various cutaneous signs, such as petechiae, purpura, or an erythematous macular rash. Meningeal irritation is manifested as nuchal rigidity, back pain, **Kernig sign** (flexion of the hip 90 degrees with subsequent pain with extension of the leg), and **Brudzinski sign** (involuntary flexion of the knees and hips after passive flexion of the neck while supine). In some children, particularly in those younger than 12-18 mo, Kernig and Brudzinski signs are not consistently present. Indeed fever, headache, and nuchal rigidity are present in only 40% of adults with bacterial meningitis. Increased ICP is suggested by headache, emesis, bulging fontanel or diastasis (widening) of the sutures, oculomotor (anisocoria, ptosis) or abducens nerve paralysis, hypertension with bradycardia, apnea or hyperventilation, decorticate or decerebrate posturing, stupor, coma, or signs of herniation. Papilledema is uncommon in uncomplicated meningitis and should suggest a more chronic process, such as the presence of an intracranial abscess, subdural empyema, or occlusion of a dural venous sinus. Focal neurologic signs usually are due to vascular occlusion. Cranial neuropathies of the ocular, oculomotor, abducens, facial, and auditory nerves may also be due to focal inflammation. Overall, about 10-20% of children with bacterial meningitis have focal neurologic signs.

Seizures (focal or generalized) due to cerebritis, infarction, or electrolyte disturbances occur in 20-30% of patients with meningitis. Seizures that occur on presentation or within the 1st 4 days of onset are usually of no prognostic significance. Seizures that persist after the 4th day of illness and those that are difficult to treat may be associated with a poor prognosis.

Alterations of mental status are common among patients with meningitis and may be due to increased ICP, cerebritis, or hypotension; manifestations include irritability, lethargy, stupor, obtundation, and coma. Comatose patients have a poor prognosis. Additional manifestations of meningitis include photophobia and tache cérébrale, which is elicited by stroking the skin with a blunt object and observing a raised red streak within 30-60 sec.

DIAGNOSIS

The diagnosis of acute pyogenic meningitis is confirmed by analysis of the CSF, which typically reveals microorganisms on Gram stain and culture, a neutrophilic pleocytosis, elevated protein, and reduced glucose concentrations (see Table 595-1). LP should be performed when bacterial meningitis is suspected. **Contraindications** for an immediate LP include (1) evidence of increased ICP (other than a bulging fontanel), such as 3rd or 6th cranial nerve palsy with a depressed level of consciousness, or hypertension and bradycardia with respiratory abnormalities (Chapter 584); (2) severe cardiopulmonary compromise requiring prompt resuscitative measures for shock or in patients in whom positioning for the LP would further compromise cardiopulmonary function; and (3) infection of the skin overlying the site of the LP. Thrombocytopenia is a relative contraindication for LP. If an LP is delayed, empirical antibiotic therapy should be initiated. CT scanning for evidence of a brain abscess or increased ICP should not delay therapy. LP may be performed after increased ICP has been treated or a brain abscess has been excluded.

Blood cultures should be performed in all patients with suspected meningitis. Blood cultures reveal the responsible bacteria in up to 80-90% of cases of meningitis.

Lumbar Puncture (Chapter 584)

The CSF leukocyte count in bacterial meningitis usually is elevated to >1,000/mm^3 and, typically, there is a neutrophilic predominance (75-95%). Turbid CSF is present when the CSF leukocyte count exceeds 200-400/mm^3. Normal healthy neonates may have as many as 30 leukocytes/mm^3 (usually <10), but older children without viral or bacterial meningitis have <5 leukocytes/mm^3 in the CSF; in both age groups there is a predominance of lymphocytes or monocytes.

A CSF leukocyte count <250/mm^3 may be present in as many as 20% of patients with acute bacterial meningitis; pleocytosis may be absent in patients with severe overwhelming sepsis and meningitis and is a poor prognostic sign. Pleocytosis with a lymphocyte predominance may be present during the early stage of acute bacterial meningitis; conversely, neutrophilic pleocytosis may be present in patients in the early stages of acute viral meningitis. The shift to lymphocytic-monocytic predominance in viral meningitis invariably occurs within 8 to 24 hr of the initial LP. The Gram stain is positive in 70-90% of patients with untreated bacterial meningitis.

A diagnostic conundrum in the evaluation of children with suspected bacterial meningitis is the analysis of CSF obtained from children already receiving antibiotic (usually oral) therapy. This is an important issue, because 25-50% of children being evaluated for bacterial meningitis are receiving oral antibiotics when their CSF is obtained. CSF obtained from children with bacterial meningitis, after the initiation of antibiotics, may be negative on Gram stain and culture. Pleocytosis with a predominance of neutrophils, elevated protein level, and a reduced concentration of CSF glucose usually persist for several days after the administration of appropriate intravenous antibiotics. Therefore, despite negative cultures, the presumptive diagnosis of bacterial meningitis can be made. Some clinicians test CSF for the presence of bacterial antigens if the child has been pretreated with antibiotics and the diagnosis of bacterial meningitis is in doubt. These tests have technical limitations.

A traumatic LP may complicate the diagnosis of meningitis. Repeat LP at a higher interspace may produce less hemorrhagic fluid, but this fluid usually also contains red blood cells.

Interpretation of CSF leukocytes and protein concentration are affected by LPs that are traumatic, although the Gram stain, culture, and glucose level may not be influenced. Although methods for correcting for the presence of red blood cells have been proposed, it is prudent to rely on the bacteriologic results rather than attempt to interpret the CSF leukocyte and protein results of a traumatic LP.

Differential Diagnosis

In addition to *S. pneumoniae, N. meningitidis,* and *H. influenzae* type b, many other microorganisms can cause generalized infection of the CNS with similar clinical manifestations. These organisms include less typical bacteria, such as *Mycobacterium tuberculosis, Nocardia* spp., *Treponema pallidum* (syphilis), and *Borrelia burgdorferi* (Lyme disease); fungi, such as those endemic to specific geographic areas (*Coccidioides, Histoplasma,* and *Blastomyces*) and those responsible for infections in compromised hosts (*Candida, Cryptococcus,* and *Aspergillus*); parasites, such as *Toxoplasma gondii* and those that cause cysticercosis and, most frequently, viruses (Chapter 595.2) (Table 595-2). Focal infections of the CNS including brain abscess and parameningeal abscess (subdural empyema, cranial and spinal epidural abscess) may also be confused with meningitis. In addition, noninfectious illnesses can cause generalized inflammation of the CNS. Relative to infections, these disorders are uncommon and include malignancy, collagen vascular syndromes, and exposure to toxins (see Table 595-2).

Determining the specific cause of CNS infection is facilitated by careful examination of the CSF with specific stains (Kinyoun carbol fuchsin for mycobacteria, India ink for fungi), cytology, antigen detection *(Cryptococcus),* serology (syphilis, West Nile virus, arboviruses), viral culture (enterovirus), and polymerase chain reaction (herpes simplex, enterovirus, and others). Other potentially valuable diagnostic tests include blood cultures, CT or MRI of the brain, serologic tests, and, rarely, brain biopsy.

Acute viral meningoencephalitis is the most likely infection to be confused with bacterial meningitis (Tables 595-2 and 595-3). Although, in general, children with viral meningoencephalitis appear less ill than those with bacterial meningitis, both types of infection have a spectrum of severity. Some children with bacterial meningitis may have relatively mild signs and symptoms, whereas some with viral meningoencephalitis may be critically ill. Although classic CSF profiles associated with bacterial versus viral infection tend to be distinct (see Table 595-1), specific test results may have considerable overlap.

TREATMENT

The therapeutic approach to patients with presumed bacterial meningitis depends on the nature of the initial manifestations of the illness. A child with rapidly progressing disease of less than 24 hr duration, in the absence of increased ICP, should receive antibiotics as soon as possible after an LP is performed. If there are signs of increased ICP or focal neurologic findings, antibiotics should be given without performing an LP and before obtaining a CT scan. Increased ICP should be treated simultaneously (Chapter 63). Immediate treatment of associated multiple organ system failure, shock (Chapter 64), and acute respiratory distress syndrome (Chapter 65) is also indicated.

Patients who have a more protracted subacute course and become ill over a 4-7 day period should also be evaluated for signs of increased ICP and focal neurologic deficits. Unilateral headache, papilledema, and other signs of increased ICP suggest a focal lesion such as a brain or epidural abscess, or subdural empyema. Under these circumstances, antibiotic therapy should be initiated before LP and CT scanning. If signs of increased ICP and/or focal neurologic signs are present, CT scanning should be performed first to determine the safety of performing an LP.

Initial Antibiotic Therapy

The initial (empirical) choice of therapy for meningitis in immunocompetent infants and children is primarily influenced by the antibiotic susceptibilities (Table 595-4) of *S. pneumoniae.* Selected antibiotics should achieve bactericidal levels in the CSF. Although there are substantial geographic differences in the frequency of resistance of *S. pneumoniae* to antibiotics, rates are increasing throughout the world. In the USA, 25-50% of strains of *S. pneumoniae* are currently resistant to penicillin; relative resistance (MIC = 0.1-1.0 μg/mL) is more common than high-level resistance (MIC = 2.0 μg/mL). Resistance to cefotaxime and ceftriaxone is also evident in up to 25% of isolates. In contrast, most strains of *N. meningitidis* are sensitive to penicillin and cephalosporins, although rare resistant isolates have been reported. Approximately 30-40% of isolates of *H. influenzae* type b produce β-lactamases and, therefore, are resistant to ampicillin. These β-lactamase–producing strains are sensitive to the extended-spectrum cephalosporins.

Based on the substantial rate of resistance of *S. pneumoniae* to β-lactam drugs, vancomycin (60 mg/kg/24 hr, given every 6 hr) is recommended as part of initial empirical therapy. Because of the efficacy of 3rd-generation cephalosporins in the therapy of meningitis caused by sensitive *S. pneumoniae, N. meningitidis,* and *H. influenzae* type b, cefotaxime (200 mg/kg/24 hr, given every 6 hr) or ceftriaxone (100 mg/kg/24 hr administered once per day or 50 mg/kg/dose, given every 12 hr) should also be used in initial empirical therapy. Patients allergic to β-lactam antibiotics and >1 mo of age can be treated with chloramphenicol, 100 mg/kg/24 hr, given every 6 hr. Alternatively, patients can be desensitized to the antibiotic (Chapter 146).

If *L. monocytogenes* infection is suspected, as in young infants or those with a T-lymphocyte deficiency, ampicillin (200 mg/kg/24 hr, given every 6 hr) also should also be given because cephalosporins are inactive against *L. monocytogenes.* Intravenous trimethoprim-sulfamethoxazole is an alternative treatment for *L. monocytogenes.*

If a patient is immunocompromised and gram-negative bacterial meningitis is suspected, initial therapy might include ceftazidime and an aminoglycoside.

DURATION OF ANTIBIOTIC THERAPY

Therapy for uncomplicated penicillin-sensitive *S. pneumoniae* meningitis should be completed with 10 to 14 days with a 3rd-generation cephalosporin or intravenous penicillin (400,000 U/kg/24 hr, given every 4-6 hr). If the isolate is resistant to penicillin and the 3rd-generation cephalosporin, therapy should be completed with vancomycin. Intravenous penicillin (400,000 U/kg/24 hr) for 5-7 days is the treatment of choice for uncomplicated *N. meningitidis* meningitis. Uncomplicated *H. influenzae* type b meningitis should be treated for 7-10 days. Patients who receive intravenous or oral antibiotics before LP and who do not have an identifiable pathogen but do have evidence of an acute bacterial infection on the basis of their CSF profile should continue to receive therapy with ceftriaxone or cefotaxime for 7-10 days. If focal signs are present or the child does not respond to treatment, a parameningeal focus may be present and a CT or MRI scan should be performed.

A routine repeat LP is not indicated in patients with uncomplicated meningitis due to antibiotic-sensitive *S. pneumoniae, N. meningitidis,* or *H. influenzae* type b. Repeat examination of CSF is indicated in some neonates, in patients with gram-negative bacillary meningitis, or in infection caused by a β-lactam–resistant *S. pneumoniae.* The CSF should be sterile within 24-48 hr of initiation of appropriate antibiotic therapy.

Meningitis due to *Escherichia coli* or *P. aeruginosa* requires therapy with a 3rd-generation cephalosporin active against the isolate in vitro. Most isolates of *E. coli* are sensitive to cefotaxime or ceftriaxone, and most isolates of *P. aeruginosa* are sensitive to

Table 595-2 CLINICAL CONDITIONS AND INFECTIOUS AGENTS ASSOCIATED WITH ASEPTIC MENINGITIS

VIRUSES
Enteroviruses (coxsackievirus, echovirus, poliovirus, enterovirus)
Arboviruses: Eastern equine, Western equine, Venezuelan equine, St. Louis encephalitis, Powassan and California encephalitis, West Nile virus, Colorado tick fever
Herpes simplex (types 1, 2)
Human herpesvirus type 6
Varicella-zoster virus
Epstein-Barr virus
Parvovirus B19
Cytomegalovirus
Adenovirus
Variola (smallpox)
Measles
Mumps
Rubella
Influenza A and B
Parainfluenza
Rhinovirus
Rabies
Lymphocytic choriomeningitis
Rotaviruses
Coronaviruses
Human immunodeficiency virus type 1
BACTERIA
Mycobacterium tuberculosis
Leptospira species (leptospirosis)
Treponema pallidum (syphilis)
Borrelia species (relapsing fever)
Borrelia burgdorferi (Lyme disease)
Nocardia species (nocardiosis)
Brucella species
Bartonella species (cat-scratch disease)
Rickettsia rickettsii (Rocky Mountain spotted fever)
Rickettsia prowazekii (typhus)
Ehrlichia canis
Coxiella burnetii
Mycoplasma pneumoniae
Mycoplasma hominis
Chlamydia trachomatis
Chlamydia psittaci
Chlamydia pneumoniae
Partially treated bacterial meningitis
BACTERIAL PARAMENINGEAL FOCUS
Sinusitis
Mastoiditis
Brain abscess
Subdural-epidural empyema
Cranial osteomyelitis
FUNGI
Coccidioides immitis (coccidioidomycosis)
Blastomyces dermatitidis (blastomycosis)
Cryptococcus neoformans (cryptococcosis)
Histoplasma capsulatum (histoplasmosis)
Candida species
Other fungi (*Alternaria, Aspergillus, Cephalosporium, Cladosporium, Drechslera hawaiiensis, Paracoccidioides brasiliensis, Petriellidium boydii, Sporotrichum schenckii, Ustilago* species, *Zygomycetes*)
PARASITES (EOSINOPHILIC)
Angiostrongylus cantonensis
Gnathostoma spinigerum
Baylisascaris procyonis
Strongyloides stercoralis
Trichinella spiralis
Toxocara canis
Taenia solium (cysticercosis)
Paragonimus westermani
Schistosoma species
Fasciola species
PARASITES (NONEOSINOPHILIC)
Toxoplasma gondii (toxoplasmosis)
Acanthamoeba species
Naegleria fowleri
Malaria
POSTINFECTIOUS
Vaccines: rabies, influenza, measles, poliovirus
Demyelinating or allergic encephalitis
SYSTEMIC OR IMMUNOLOGICALLY MEDIATED
Bacterial endocarditis
Kawasaki disease
Systemic lupus erythematosus
Vasculitis, including polyarteritis nodosa
Sjögren syndrome
Mixed connective tissue disease
Rheumatoid arthritis
Behçet syndrome
Wegener granulomatosis
Lymphomatoid granulomatosis
Granulomatous arteritis
Sarcoidosis
Familial Mediterranean fever
Vogt-Koyanagi-Harada syndrome
MALIGNANCY
Leukemia
Lymphoma
Metastatic carcinoma
Central nervous system tumor (e.g., craniopharyngioma, glioma, ependymoma, astrocytoma, medulloblastoma, teratoma)
DRUGS
Intrathecal infections (contrast media, serum, antibiotics, antineoplastic agents)
Nonsteroidal antiinflammatory agents
OKT3 monoclonal antibodies
Carbamazepine
Azathioprine
Intravenous immune globulins
Antibiotics (trimethoprim-sulfamethoxazole, sulfasalazine, ciprofloxacin, isoniazid)
MISCELLANEOUS
Heavy metal poisoning (lead, arsenic)
Foreign bodies (shunt, reservoir)
Subarachnoid hemorrhage
Postictal state
Postmigraine state
Mollaret syndrome (recurrent)
Intraventricular hemorrhage (neonate)
Familial hemophagocytic syndrome
Post neurosurgery
Dermoid-epidermoid cyst
Headache, neurologic deficits
CSF lymphocytosis (HANDL)

Compiled from Cherry JD: Aseptic meningitis and viral meningitis. In Feigin RD, Cherry JD, editors: *Textbook of pediatric infectious diseases,* ed 4, Philadelphia, 1998, WB Saunders, p 450; Davis LE: Aseptic and viral meningitis. In Long SS, Pickering LK, Prober CG, editors: *Principles and practice of pediatric infectious disease*, New York, 1997, Churchill Livingstone, p 329; Kliegman RM, Greenbaum LA, Lye PS: *Practical strategies in pediatric diagnosis therapy,* ed 2, Philadelphia, 2004, Elsevier, p 961.

ceftazidime. Gram-negative bacillary meningitis should be treated for 3 wk or for at least 2 wk after CSF sterilization, which may occur after 2-10 days of treatment.

Side effects of antibiotic therapy of meningitis include phlebitis, drug fever, rash, emesis, oral candidiasis, and diarrhea. Ceftriaxone may cause reversible gallbladder pseudolithiasis, detectable by abdominal ultrasonography. This is usually asymptomatic but may be associated with emesis and upper right quadrant pain.

Corticosteroids

Rapid killing of bacteria in the CSF effectively sterilizes the meningeal infection but releases toxic cell products after cell lysis (cell wall endotoxin) that precipitate the cytokine-mediated

Table 595-3 CLASSIFICATION OF ENCEPHALITIS BY CAUSE AND SOURCE

I. INFECTIONS: VIRAL
- A. Spread: person to person only
  1. Mumps: frequent in an unimmunized population; often mild
  2. Measles: may have serious sequelae
  3. Enteroviruses: frequent at all ages; more serious in newborns
  4. Rubella: uncommon; sequelae rare except in congenital rubella
  5. Herpesvirus group
     - a. Herpes simplex (types 1 and 2, possibly 6): relatively common; sequelae frequent; devastating in newborns
     - b. Varicella-zoster virus: uncommon; serious sequelae not rare
     - c. Cytomegalovirus, congenital or acquired: may have delayed sequelae in congenital type
     - d. Epstein-Barr virus (infectious mononucleosis): not common
  6. Pox group
     - a. Vaccinia and variola: uncommon, but serious CNS damage occurs
  7. Parvovirus (erythema infectiosum): not common
  8. Influenza A and B
  9. Adenovirus
  10. Other: reoviruses, respiratory syncytial, parainfluenza, hepatitis B
- B. Arthropod-borne agents

  Arboviruses: spread to humans by mosquitoes or ticks; seasonal epidemics depend on ecology of the insect vector; the following occur in the USA:

Eastern equine	California
Western equine	Powassan
Venezuelan equine	Dengue
St. Louis	Colorado tick fever
West Nile	
- C. Spread by warm-blooded mammals
  1. Rabies: saliva of many domestic and wild mammalian species
  2. Herpesvirus simiae ("B" virus): monkeys' saliva
  3. Lymphocytic choriomeningitis: rodents' excreta

II. INFECTIONS: NONVIRAL
- A. Rickettsial: in Rocky Mountain spotted fever and typhus; encephalitic component from cerebral vasculitis
- B. *Mycoplasma pneumoniae:* interval of some days between respiratory and CNS symptoms
- C. Bacterial: tuberculous and other bacterial meningitis; often has encephalitic component
- D. Spirochetal: syphilis, congenital or acquired; leptospirosis; Lyme disease
- E. Cat-scratch disease
- F. Fungal: immunologically compromised patients at special risk: cryptococcosis; histoplasmosis; aspergillosis; mucormycosis; candidosis; coccidioidomycosis
- G. Protozoal: *Plasmodium, Trypanosoma, Naegleria,* and *Acanthamoeba* species*; Toxoplasma gondii*
- H. Metazoal: trichinosis; echinococcosis; cysticercosis; schistosomiasis

III. PARAINFECTIOUS: POSTINFECTIOUS, ALLERGIC, AUTOIMMUNE

Patients in whom an infectious agent or 1 of its components plays a contributory role in etiology, but the intact infectious agent is not isolated in vitro from the nervous system; it is postulated that in this group, the influence of cell-mediated antigen-antibody complexes plus complement is especially important in producing the observed tissue damage
- A. Associated with specific diseases (these agents may also cause direct CNS damage; see I and II

Measles	Rickettsial infections
Rubella	Influenza A and B
Mumps	Varicella-zoster
Mycoplasma pneumoniae	
- B. Associated with vaccines

Rabies	Measles
Vaccinia	Yellow fever
- C. Autoimmune
  - Paraneoplastic
  - Idiopathic

IV. HUMAN SLOW-VIRUS DISEASES

Accumulating evidence that viruses frequently acquired earlier in life, not necessarily with detectable acute illness, participate in later chronic neurologic disease (similar events also known to occur in animals)
- A. Subacute sclerosing panencephalitis; measles; rubella?
- B. Creutzfeldt-Jakob disease (spongiform encephalopathy)
- C. Progressive multifocal leukoencephalopathy
- D. Kuru (Fore tribe in New Guinea only)
- E. Human immunodeficiency virus

V. UNKNOWN: COMPLEX GROUP

This group constitutes more than two thirds of the cases of encephalitis reported to the Centers for Disease Control and Prevention, Atlanta, Georgia; the yearly epidemic curve of these undiagnosed cases suggests that the majority are probably caused by enteroviruses and/or arboviruses.

There is also a miscellaneous group that is based on clinical criteria: Reye syndrome is 1 current example; others include the extinct von Economo encephalitis (epidemic during 1918-1928); myoclonic encephalopathy of infancy; retinomeningoencephalitis with papilledema and retinal hemorrhage; recurrent encephalomyelitis (? allergic or autoimmune); pseudotumor cerebri; and epidemic neuromyasthenia (Iceland disease).

An encephalitic clinical pattern may follow ingestion or absorption of a number of known and unknown toxic substances; these include ingestion of lead and mercury, and percutaneous absorption of hexachlorophene as a skin disinfectant and gamma benzene hexachloride as a scabicide.

CNS, central nervous system.

Modified from Behrman RE, editor: *Nelson textbook of pediatrics,* ed 14, Philadelphia, 1992, WB Saunders, p 667. From Kliegman RM, Greenbaum LA, Lye PS: *Practical strategies in pediatric diagnosis and therapy,* ed 2, Philadelphia, 2004, Elsevier, p 967.

Table 595-4 ANTIBIOTICS USED FOR THE TREATMENT OF BACTERIAL MENINGITIS*

DRUG	NEONATES		INFANTS AND CHILDREN
	0-7 Days	8-28 Days	
Amikacin[†‡]	15-20 divided q12h	20-30 divided q8h	20-30 divided q8h
Ampicillin	200-300 divided q8h	300 divided q6h	300 divided q4h or q6h
Cefotaxime	100 divided q12h	150-200 divided q8h or q6h	225-300 divided q8h or q6h
Ceftriaxone[§]	—	—	100 divided q12h or q24h
Ceftazidime	150 divided q12h	150 divided q8h	150 divided q8h
Gentamicin[†‡]	5 divided q12h	7.5 divided q8h	7.5 divided q8h
Meropenem	—	—	120 divided q8h
Nafcillin	100-150 divided q8h or q12h	150-200 divided q8h or q6h	150-200 divided q4h or q6h
Penicillin G	150,000 divided q8h	200,000 divided q6h	400,000 divided q4h or q6h
Rifampin	—	10-20 divided q12h	20 divided q12h or q24h
Tobramycin[†‡]	5 divided q12h	7.5 divided q8h	7.5 divided q8h
Vancomycin[†‡]	30 divided q12h	30-45 divided q8h	60 divided q6h

*Dosages in mg/kg (U/kg for penicillin G) per day.

†Smaller doses and longer dosing intervals, especially for aminoglycosides and vancomycin for very low birthweight neonates, may be advisable.

‡Monitoring of serum levels is recommended to ensure safe and therapeutic values.

§Use in neonates is not recommended because of inadequate experience in neonatal meningitis.

Modified from Klein JO: Antimicrobial treatment and prevention of meningitis, *Pediatr Ann* 23:76, 1994; and from Kliegman RM, Greenbaum LA, Lye PS: *Practical strategies in pediatric diagnosis and therapy,* ed 2, Philadelphia, 2004, Elsevier, p 963.

inflammatory cascade. The resultant edema formation and neutrophilic infiltration may produce additional neurologic injury with worsening of CNS signs and symptoms. Therefore, agents that limit production of inflammatory mediators may be of benefit to patients with bacterial meningitis.

Data support the use of intravenous dexamethasone, 0.15 mg/kg/dose given every 6 hr for 2 days, in the treatment of children older than 6 wk with acute bacterial meningitis caused by *H. influenzae* type b. Among children with meningitis due to *H. influenzae* type b, corticosteroid recipients have a shorter duration of fever, lower CSF protein and lactate levels, and a reduction in sensorineural hearing loss. Data in children regarding benefits, if any, of corticosteroids in the treatment of meningitis caused by other bacteria are inconclusive. Early treatment of adults with bacterial meningitis, especially those with pneumococcal meningitis, results in improved outcome.

Corticosteroids appear to have maximum benefit if given 1-2 hr before antibiotics are initiated. They also may be effective if given concurrently with or soon after the 1st dose of antibiotics. Complications of corticosteroids include gastrointestinal bleeding, hypertension, hyperglycemia, leukocytosis, and rebound fever after the last dose.

Glycerol

Glycerol increases plasma osmolality, reducing CNS edema and enhancing cerebral circulation. In one study conducted in Latin America, glycerol appeared to reduce the incidence of severe neurologic sequelae, including blindness, hydrocephalus requiring shunt placement, severe psychomotor retardation, quadriparesis, and quadriplegia, in children with bacterial meningitis. Because it is safe, inexpensive, available, easy to store, and has oral administration, it may be helpful in resource-poor areas; however more data are necessary before this intervention is standardized.

Supportive Care

Repeated medical and neurologic assessments of patients with bacterial meningitis are essential to identify early signs of cardiovascular, CNS, and metabolic complications. Pulse rate, blood pressure, and respiratory rate should be monitored frequently. Neurologic assessment, including pupillary reflexes, level of consciousness, motor strength, cranial nerve signs, and evaluation for seizures, should be made frequently in the 1st 72 hr, when the risk of neurologic complications is greatest. Important laboratory studies include an assessment of blood urea nitrogen; serum sodium, chloride, potassium, and bicarbonate levels; urine output and specific gravity; complete blood and platelet counts; and, in the presence of petechiae, purpura, or abnormal bleeding, measures of coagulation function (fibrinogen, prothrombin, and partial thromboplastin times).

Patients should initially receive nothing by mouth. If a patient is judged to be normovolemic, with normal blood pressure, intravenous fluid administration should be restricted to one half to two thirds of maintenance, or 800-1,000 mL/m^2/24 hr, until it can be established that increased ICP or SIADH is not present. Fluid administration may be returned to normal (1,500-1,700 mL/m^2/24 hr) when serum sodium levels are normal. Fluid restriction is not appropriate in the presence of systemic hypotension because reduced blood pressure may result in reduced cerebral perfusion pressure and CNS ischemia. Therefore, shock must be treated aggressively to prevent brain and other organ dysfunction (acute tubular necrosis, acute respiratory distress syndrome). Patients with shock, a markedly elevated ICP, coma, and refractory seizures require intensive monitoring with central arterial and venous access and frequent vital signs, necessitating admission to a pediatric intensive care unit. Patients with septic shock may require fluid resuscitation and therapy with vasoactive agents such as dopamine and epinephrine. The goal of such therapy in patients with meningitis is to avoid excessive increases in ICP without compromising blood flow and oxygen delivery to vital organs.

Neurologic complications include increased ICP with subsequent herniation, seizures, and an enlarging head circumference due to a subdural effusion or hydrocephalus. Signs of increased ICP should be treated emergently with endotracheal intubation and hyperventilation (to maintain the pCO_2 at approximately 25 mm Hg). In addition, intravenous furosemide (Lasix, 1 mg/kg) and mannitol (0.5-1.0 g/kg) osmotherapy may reduce ICP (Chapter 63). Furosemide reduces brain swelling by venodilation and diuresis without increasing intracranial blood volume, whereas mannitol produces an osmolar gradient between the brain and plasma, thus shifting fluid from the CNS to the plasma, with subsequent excretion during an osmotic diuresis.

Seizures are common during the course of bacterial meningitis. Immediate therapy for seizures includes intravenous diazepam (0.1-0.2 mg/kg/dose) or lorazepam (0.05-0.10 mg/kg/dose), and careful attention paid to the risk of respiratory suppression. Serum glucose, calcium, and sodium levels should be monitored. After immediate management of seizures, patients should receive phenytoin (15-20 mg/kg loading dose, 5 mg/kg/24 hr maintenance) to reduce the likelihood of recurrence. Phenytoin is preferred to phenobarbital because it produces less CNS depression and permits assessment of a patient's level of consciousness. Serum phenytoin levels should be monitored to maintain them in the therapeutic range (10-20 μg/mL).

COMPLICATIONS

During the treatment of meningitis, acute CNS complications can include seizures, increased ICP, cranial nerve palsies, stroke, cerebral or cerebellar herniation, and thrombosis of the dural venous sinuses.

Collections of fluid in the subdural space develop in 10-30% of patients with meningitis and are asymptomatic in 85-90% of patients. **Subdural effusions** are especially common in infants. Symptomatic subdural effusions may result in a bulging fontanel, diastasis of sutures, enlarging head circumference, emesis, seizures, fever, and abnormal results of cranial transillumination. CT or MRI scanning confirms the presence of a subdural effusion. In the presence of increased ICP or a depressed level of consciousness, symptomatic subdural effusion should be treated by aspiration through the open fontanel (Chapters 63 and 584). Fever alone is not an indication for aspiration.

SIADH occurs in some patients with meningitis, resulting in hyponatremia and reduced serum osmolality. This may exacerbate cerebral edema or result in hyponatremic seizures (Chapter 52).

Fever associated with bacterial meningitis usually resolves within 5-7 days of the onset of therapy. **Prolonged fever** (>10 days) is noted in about 10% of patients. Prolonged fever is usually due to intercurrent viral infection, nosocomial or secondary bacterial infection, thrombophlebitis, or drug reaction. Secondary fever refers to the recrudescence of elevated temperature after an afebrile interval. Nosocomial infections are especially important to consider in the evaluation of these patients. Pericarditis or arthritis may occur in patients being treated for meningitis, especially that caused by *N. meningitidis.* Involvement of these sites may result either from bacterial dissemination or from immune complex deposition. In general, infectious pericarditis or arthritis occurs earlier in the course of treatment than does immune-mediated disease.

Thrombocytosis, eosinophilia, and anemia may develop during therapy for meningitis. Anemia may be due to hemolysis or bone marrow suppression. DIC is most often associated with the rapidly progressive pattern of presentation and is noted most commonly in patients with shock and purpura. The combination of endotoxemia and severe hypotension initiates the coagulation cascade; the coexistence of ongoing thrombosis may produce symmetric peripheral gangrene.

PROGNOSIS

Appropriate antibiotic therapy and supportive care have reduced the mortality of bacterial meningitis after the neonatal period to <10%. The highest mortality rates are observed with pneumococcal meningitis. Severe neurodevelopmental sequelae may occur in 10-20% of patients recovering from bacterial meningitis, and as many as 50% have some, albeit subtle, neurobehavioral morbidity. The prognosis is poorest among infants younger than 6 mo and in those with high concentrations of bacteria/bacterial products in their CSF. Those with seizures occurring more than 4 days into therapy or with coma or focal neurologic signs on presentation have an increased risk of long-term sequelae. There does not appear to be a correlation between duration of symptoms before diagnosis of meningitis and outcome.

The most common neurologic sequelae include hearing loss, mental retardation, recurrent seizures, delay in acquisition of language, visual impairment, and behavioral problems. **Sensorineural hearing** loss is the most common sequela of bacterial meningitis and, usually, is already present at the time of initial presentation. It is due to cochlear infection and occurs in as many as 30% of patients with pneumococcal meningitis, 10% with meningococcal, and 5-20% of those with *H. influenzae* type b meningitis. Hearing loss may also be due to direct inflammation of the auditory nerve. All patients with bacterial meningitis should undergo careful audiologic assessment before or soon after discharge from the hospital. Frequent reassessment on an outpatient basis is indicated for patients who have a hearing deficit.

PREVENTION

Vaccination and antibiotic prophylaxis of susceptible at-risk contacts represent the 2 available means of reducing the likelihood of bacterial meningitis. The availability and application of each of these approaches depend on the specific infecting bacteria.

Neisseria meningitidis

Chemoprophylaxis is recommended for all close contacts of patients with meningococcal meningitis regardless of age or immunization status. Close contacts should be treated with rifampin 10 mg/kg/dose every 12 hr (maximum dose of 600 mg) for 2 days as soon as possible after identification of a case of suspected meningococcal meningitis or sepsis. Close contacts include household, daycare center, and nursery school contacts and health care workers who have direct exposure to oral secretions (mouth-to-mouth resuscitation, suctioning, intubation). Exposed contacts should be treated immediately on suspicion of infection in the index patient; bacteriologic confirmation of infection should not be awaited. In addition, all contacts should be educated about the early signs of meningococcal disease and the need to seek prompt medical attention if these signs develop.

Two quadrivalent (A, C, Y, W-135), conjugated vaccines (MCV-4; Menactra and Menueo) are licensed by the U.S. Food and Drug Administration. The Advisory Committee on Immunization Practices (ACIP) to the CDC recommends routine administration of this vaccine to 11-12 yr old adolescents. Meningococcal vaccine is also recommended for high-risk children older than 2 yr. High-risk patients include those with anatomic or functional asplenia or deficiencies of terminal complement proteins. Use of meningococcal vaccine should be considered for college freshmen, especially those who live in dormitories, because of an observed increased risk of invasive meningococcal infections compared to the risk in non–college-attending, age-matched controls. In the United Kingdom and Canada, a novel tetravalent meningococcal glycoconjugate vaccine (MenACWY) has been shown to be immunogenic in infancy. The vaccine also may be used as an adjunct with chemoprophylaxis for exposed contacts and during epidemics of meningococcal disease.

Haemophilus influenzae Type B

Rifampin prophylaxis should be given to all household contacts of patients with invasive disease caused by *H. influenzae* type b, if any close family member younger than 48 mo has not been fully immunized or if an immunocompromised person, of any age, resides in the household. A household contact is one who lives in the residence of the index case or who has spent a minimum of 4 hr with the index case for at least 5 of the 7 days preceding the patient's hospitalization. Family members should receive rifampin prophylaxis immediately after the diagnosis is suspected in the index case because >50% of secondary family cases occur in the 1st wk after the index patient has been hospitalized.

The dose of rifampin is 20 mg/kg/24 hr (maximum dose of 600 mg) given once each day for 4 days. Rifampin colors the urine and perspiration red-orange, stains contact lenses, and reduces the serum concentrations of some drugs, including oral contraceptives. Rifampin is contraindicated during pregnancy.

The most striking advance in the prevention of childhood bacterial meningitis followed the development and licensure of conjugated vaccines against *H. influenzae* type b. Four conjugate vaccines are licensed in the USA. Although each vaccine elicits different profiles of antibody response in infants immunized at 2-6 mo of age, all result in protective levels of antibody with efficacy rates against invasive infections ranging from 70-100%. Efficacy is not as consistent in Native American populations, a group recognized as having an especially high incidence of disease. All children should be immunized with *H. influenzae* type b conjugate vaccine beginning at 2 mo of age (Chapter 165).

Streptococcus Pneumoniae

Routine administration of conjugate vaccine against *S. pneumoniae* is recommended for children younger than 2 yr of age. The initial dose is given at about 2 mo of age. Children who are at high risk of invasive pneumococcal infections, including those with functional or anatomic asplenia and those with underlying immunodeficiency (such as infection with HIV, primary immunodeficiency, and those receiving immunosuppressive therapy) should also receive the vaccine.

BIBLIOGRAPHY

Please visit the Nelson Textbook of Pediatrics *website at* *www.expertconsult.com* *for the complete bibliography.*

595.2 Viral Meningoencephalitis

Charles G. Prober and LauraLe Dyner

Viral meningoencephalitis is an acute inflammatory process involving the meninges and, to a variable degree, brain tissue. These infections are relatively common and may be caused by a number of different agents. The CSF is characterized by pleocytosis and the absence of microorganisms on Gram stain and routine bacterial culture. In most instances, the infections are self-limited. In some cases, substantial morbidity and mortality occur.

ETIOLOGY

Enteroviruses are the most common cause of viral meningoencephalitis. To date, more than 80 serotypes of these small RNA viruses have been identified. The severity of infection caused by enteroviruses ranges from mild, self-limited illness with primarily meningeal involvement to severe encephalitis resulting in death or significant sequelae.

Arboviruses are arthropod-borne agents, responsible for some cases of meningoencephalitis during summer months. Mosquitoes and ticks are the most common vectors, spreading disease to humans and other vertebrates, such as horses, after biting infected birds or small animals. Encephalitis in horses ("blind staggers") may be the 1st indication of an incipient epidemic. Although rural exposure is most common, urban and suburban outbreaks also are frequent. The most common arboviruses responsible for CNS infection in the USA are West Nile virus (WNV) and St. Louis and California encephalitis viruses (Chapter 259). West Nile virus made its appearance in the Western hemisphere in 1999. It has gradually made its way from the east to the west coast over successive summers. Cumulatively, from 1999 through 2005, a total of 46 states reported roughly 19,000 human infections caused by WNV. WNV may also be transmitted by blood transfusion, organ transplantation, or vertically across the placenta. Most children with WNV are either asymptomatic or have a nonspecific viral-like illness. Approximately 1% develop CNS disease; adults are more severely affected than children.

Several members of the **herpes family** of viruses can cause meningoencephalitis. Herpes simplex virus type 1 (HSV-1) is an important cause of severe, sporadic encephalitis in children and adults. Brain involvement usually is focal; progression to coma and death occurs in 70% of cases without antiviral therapy. Severe encephalitis with diffuse brain involvement is caused by herpes simplex virus type 2 (HSV-2) in neonates who usually contract the virus from their mothers at delivery. A mild transient form of meningoencephalitis may accompany genital herpes infection in sexually active adolescents; most of these infections are caused by HSV-2. Varicella-zoster virus (VZV) may cause CNS infection in close temporal relationship with chickenpox. The most common manifestation of CNS involvement is cerebellar ataxia, and the most severe is acute encephalitis. After primary infection, VZV becomes latent in spinal and cranial nerve roots and ganglia, expressing itself later as herpes zoster, sometimes with accompanying mild meningoencephalitis. Cytomegalovirus (CMV) infection of the CNS may be part of congenital infection or disseminated disease in immunocompromised hosts, but it does not cause meningoencephalitis in normal infants and children. Epstein-Barr virus (EBV) has been associated with myriad CNS syndromes (Chapter 246). Human herpes virus 6 (HHV-6) can cause encephalitis, especially among immunocompromised hosts.

Mumps is a common pathogen in regions where mumps vaccine is not widely used. Mumps meningoencephalitis is mild, but deafness due to damage of the 8th cranial nerve may be a sequela. Meningoencephalitis is caused occasionally by respiratory viruses (adenovirus, influenza virus, parainfluenza virus), rubeola, rubella, or rabies; it may follow live virus vaccinations against polio, measles, mumps, or rubella.

EPIDEMIOLOGY

The epidemiologic pattern of viral meningoencephalitis is primarily determined by the prevalence of enteroviruses, the most common etiology. Infection with enteroviruses is spread directly from person to person, with a usual incubation period of 4-6 days. Most cases in temperate climates occur in the summer and fall. Epidemiologic considerations in aseptic meningitis due to agents other than enteroviruses also include season, geography, climatic conditions, animal exposures, and factors related to the specific pathogen.

PATHOGENESIS AND PATHOLOGY

Neurologic damage is caused by direct invasion and destruction of neural tissues by actively multiplying viruses or by a host reaction to viral antigens. Tissue sections of the brain generally are characterized by meningeal congestion and mononuclear infiltration, perivascular cuffs of lymphocytes and plasma cells, some perivascular tissue necrosis with myelin breakdown, and neuronal disruption in various stages, including, ultimately, neuronophagia and endothelial proliferation or necrosis. A marked degree of demyelination with preservation of neurons and their axons is considered to represent predominantly "postinfectious" or "allergic" encephalitis.

The cerebral cortex, especially the temporal lobe, is often severely affected by HSV; the arboviruses tend to affect the entire brain; rabies has a predilection for the basal structures. Involvement of the spinal cord, nerve roots, and peripheral nerves is variable.

CLINICAL MANIFESTATIONS

The progression and severity of disease are determined by the relative degree of meningeal and parenchymal involvement, which, in part, is determined by the specific etiology. The clinical course resulting from infection with the same pathogen varies widely. Some children may appear to be mildly affected initially, only to lapse into coma and die suddenly. In others, the illness may be ushered in by high fever, violent convulsions interspersed with bizarre movements, and hallucinations alternating with brief periods of clarity, followed by complete recovery.

The onset of illness is generally acute, although CNS signs and symptoms are often preceded by a nonspecific febrile illness of a few days' duration. The presenting manifestations in older children are headache and hyperesthesia, and in infants, irritability and lethargy. Headache is most often frontal or generalized; adolescents frequently complain of retrobulbar pain. Fever, nausea and vomiting, photophobia, and pain in the neck, back, and legs are common. As body temperature increases, there may be mental dullness, progressing to stupor in combination with bizarre movements and convulsions. Focal neurologic signs may be stationary, progressive, or fluctuating. West Nile virus and nonpolio enteroviruses may cause anterior horn cell injury and a flaccid paralysis. Loss of bowel and bladder control and unprovoked emotional outbursts may occur.

Exanthems often precede or accompany the CNS signs, especially with echoviruses, coxsackieviruses, VZV, measles, rubella, and, occasionally, West Nile virus. Examination often reveals nuchal rigidity without significant localizing neurologic changes, at least at the onset.

Specific forms or complicating manifestations of CNS viral infection include Guillain-Barré syndrome, transverse myelitis, hemiplegia, and cerebellar ataxia.

DIAGNOSIS

The diagnosis of viral encephalitis is usually made on the basis of the clinical presentation of nonspecific prodrome followed by progressive CNS symptoms. The diagnosis is supported by examination of the CSF, which usually shows a mild mononuclear predominance (see Table 595-1). Other tests of potential value in the evaluation of patients with suspected viral meningoencephalitis include an electroencephalogram (EEG) and neuroimaging studies. The EEG typically shows diffuse slow-wave activity, usually without focal changes. Neuroimaging studies (CT or MRI) may show swelling of the brain parenchyma. Focal seizures or focal findings on EEG, CT, or MRI, especially involving the temporal lobes, suggest HSV encephalitis.

Differential Diagnosis

A number of clinical conditions that cause CNS inflammation mimic viral meningoencephalitis (see Table 595-2). The most important group of alternative infectious agents to consider is bacteria. Most children with acute bacterial meningitis appear more critically ill than those with CNS viral infection. Parameningeal bacterial infections, such as brain abscess or subdural or epidural empyema, may have features similar to viral CNS infections. Infections caused by *M. tuberculosis, T. pallidum* (syphilis), *B. burgdorferi* (Lyme disease), and *Bartonella henselae,* the bacillus associated with cat scratch disease, tend to result in indolent courses. Analysis of CSF and appropriate serologic tests are necessary to differentiate these various pathogens.

Infections due to fungi, rickettsiae, mycoplasma, protozoa, and other parasites may also need to be included in the differential diagnosis. Consideration of these agents usually arises as a result of accompanying symptoms, geographic locality of infection, or host immune factors.

Various noninfectious disorders may be associated with CNS inflammation and have manifestations overlapping with those associated with viral meningoencephalitis. Some of these disorders include malignancy, collagen vascular diseases, intracranial hemorrhage, and exposure to certain drugs or toxins. Attention to history and other organ involvement usually allows elimination of these diagnostic possibilities.

Laboratory Findings

The CSF contains from a few to several thousand cells per cubic millimeter. Early in the disease, the cells are often polymorphonuclear; later, mononuclear cells predominate. This change in cellular type is often demonstrated in CSF samples obtained as little as 8-12 hr apart. The protein concentration in CSF tends to be normal or slightly elevated, but concentrations may be very high if brain destruction is extensive, such as that accompanying HSV encephalitis. The glucose level is usually normal, although with certain viruses, for example, mumps, a substantial depression of CSF glucose concentrations may be observed.

The CSF should be cultured for viruses, bacteria, fungi, and mycobacteria; in some instances, special examinations are indicated for protozoa, mycoplasma, and other pathogens. The success of isolating viruses from the CSF of children with viral meningoencephalitis is determined by the time in the clinical course that the specimen is obtained, the specific etiologic agent, whether the infection is a meningitic as opposed to a localized encephalitic process, and the skill of the diagnostic laboratory staff. Isolating a virus is most likely early in the illness, and the enteroviruses tend to be the easiest to isolate, although recovery of these agents from the CSF rarely exceeds 70%. To increase the likelihood of identifying the putative viral pathogen, specimens for culture should also be obtained from nasopharyngeal swabs, feces, and urine. Although isolating a virus from 1 or more of these sites does not prove causality, it is highly suggestive. Detection of viral DNA or RNA by polymerase chain reaction may be useful in the diagnosis of CNS infection caused by HSV and enteroviruses, respectively. CSF serology is the diagnostic test of choice for WNV.

A serum specimen should be obtained early in the course of illness and, if viral cultures are not diagnostic, again 2-3 wk later for serologic studies. Serologic methods are not practical for diagnosing CNS infections caused by the enteroviruses because there are too many serotypes. This approach may be useful in confirming that a case is caused by a known circulating serotype. Serologic tests may also be of value in determining the etiology of nonenteroviral CNS infection, such as arboviral infection.

TREATMENT

With the exception of the use of acyclovir for HSV encephalitis (Chapter 244), treatment of viral meningoencephalitis is supportive. Treatment of mild disease may require only symptomatic relief. Headache and hyperesthesia are treated with rest, non–aspirin-containing analgesics, and a reduction in room light, noise, and visitors. Acetaminophen is recommended for fever. Codeine, morphine, and medications to reduce nausea may be useful, but if possible, their use in children should be minimized because they may induce misleading signs and symptoms. Intravenous fluids are occasionally necessary because of poor oral intake. More severe disease may require hospitalization and intensive care.

It is important to monitor patients with severe encephalitis closely for convulsions, cerebral edema, inadequate respiratory exchange, disturbed fluid and electrolyte balance, aspiration and asphyxia, and cardiac or respiratory arrest of central origin. In patients with evidence of increased ICP, placement of a pressure transducer in the epidural space may be indicated. The risks of cardiac and respiratory failure or arrest are high with severe disease. All fluids, electrolytes, and medications are initially given parenterally. In prolonged states of coma, parenteral alimentation is indicated. SIADH is common in acute CNS disorders; monitoring of serum sodium concentrations is required for early detection (Chapter 553). Normal blood levels of glucose, magnesium, and calcium must be maintained to minimize the likelihood of convulsions. If cerebral edema or seizures become evident, vigorous treatment should be instituted.

PROGNOSIS

Supportive and rehabilitative efforts are very important after patients recover. Motor incoordination, convulsive disorders, total or partial deafness, and behavioral disturbances may follow viral CNS infections. Visual disturbances due to chorioretinopathy and perceptual amblyopia may also occur. Special facilities and, at times, institutional placement may become necessary. Some sequelae of infection may be very subtle. Therefore, neurodevelopmental and audiologic evaluations should be part of the routine follow-up of children who have recovered from viral meningoencephalitis.

Most children completely recover from viral infections of the CNS, although the prognosis depends on the severity of the clinical illness, the specific cause, and the age of the child. If the clinical illness is severe and substantial parenchymal involvement is evident, the prognosis is poor, with potential deficits being intellectual, motor, psychiatric, epileptic, visual, or auditory in nature. Severe sequelae should also be anticipated in those with infection caused by HSV. Although some literature suggests that infants who contract viral meningoencephalitis have a poorer long-term outcome than older children, most other data refute this observation. Approximately 10% of children younger than 2 yr with enteroviral CNS infections suffer an acute complication such as seizures, increased ICP, or coma. Almost all have favorable long-term neurologic outcomes.

PREVENTION

Widespread use of effective viral vaccines for polio, measles, mumps, rubella, and varicella has almost eliminated CNS complications from these diseases in the USA. The availability of domestic animal vaccine programs against rabies has reduced the frequency of rabies encephalitis. Control of encephalitis due to arboviruses has been less successful because specific vaccines for the arboviral diseases that occur in North America are not available. Control of insect vectors by suitable spraying methods and eradication of insect breeding sites, however, reduces the incidence of these infections. Furthermore, minimizing mosquito bites through the application of DEET-containing insect repellents on exposed skin and wearing long-sleeved shirts, long pants, and socks when outdoors, especially at dawn and dusk, reduces the risk of arboviral infection.

BIBLIOGRAPHY
Please visit the Nelson Textbook of Pediatrics *website at* *www.expertconsult.com* *for the complete bibliography.*

595.3 Eosinophilic Meningitis

Charles G. Prober and LauraLe Dyner

Eosinophilic meningitis is defined as 10 or more eosinophils/mm^3 of CSF. The most common cause worldwide of eosinophilic pleocytosis is CNS infection with helminthic parasites. In countries such as the USA, where helminthic infestation is uncommon, however, the differential diagnosis of CSF eosinophilic pleocytosis is broad.

ETIOLOGY

Although any tissue-migrating helminth may cause eosinophilic meningitis, the most common cause is human infection with the rat lungworm, *Angiostrongylus cantonensis* (Chapter 289). Other parasites that can cause eosinophilic meningitis include *Gnathostoma spinigerum* (dog and cat roundworm) (Chapter 289), *Baylisascaris procyonis* (raccoon roundworm), *Ascaris lumbricoides* (human roundworm), *Trichinella spiralis, Toxocara canis, T. gondii, Paragonimus westermani, Echinococcus granulosus, Schistosoma japonicum, Onchocerca volvulus,* and *Taenia solium.* Eosinophilic meningitis may also occur as an unusual manifestation of more common viral, bacterial, or fungal infections of the CNS. Noninfectious causes of eosinophilic meningitis include multiple sclerosis, malignancy, hypereosinophilic syndrome, or a reaction to medications or a ventriculoperitoneal shunt.

EPIDEMIOLOGY

A. cantonensis is found in Southeast Asia, the South Pacific, Japan, Taiwan, Egypt, Ivory Coast, and Cuba. Infection is acquired by eating raw or undercooked freshwater snails, slugs, prawns, or crabs containing infectious 3rd-stage larvae. *Gnathostoma* infections are found in Japan, China, India, Bangladesh, and Southeast Asia. Gnathostomiasis is acquired by eating undercooked or raw fish, frog, bird, or snake meat.

CLINICAL MANIFESTATIONS

When eosinophilic meningitis results from helminthic infestation, patients become ill 1-3 wk after exposure, because the parasites migrate from the gastrointestinal tract to the CNS. Common concomitant findings include fever, peripheral eosinophilia, vomiting, abdominal pain, creeping skin eruptions, or pleurisy. Neurologic symptoms may include headache, meningismus, ataxia, cranial nerve palsies, and paresthesias. Paraparesis or incontinence can result from radiculitis or myelitis.

DIAGNOSIS

The presumptive diagnosis of helminth-induced eosinophilic meningitis is made by travel and exposure history in the presence of typical clinical and laboratory findings.

TREATMENT

Treatment is supportive, because infection is self-limited and anthelmintic drugs do not appear to influence the outcome of infection. Analgesics should be given for headache and radiculitis, and CSF removal or shunting should be performed to relieve hydrocephalus, if present. Steroids may decrease the duration of headaches in adults with eosinophilic meningitis.

PROGNOSIS

The prognosis is good; 70% of patients improve sufficiently to leave the hospital in 1-2 wk. Mortality associated with eosinophilic meningitis is <1%.

BIBLIOGRAPHY

Please visit the Nelson Textbook of Pediatrics *website at www.expertconsult.com for the complete bibliography.*

Chapter 596
Brain Abscess

Charles G. Prober and LauraLe Dyner

Brain abscesses can occur in children of any age but are most common in children between 4 and 8 yr and neonates. The causes of brain abscess include embolization due to congenital heart disease with right-to-left shunts (especially tetralogy of Fallot), meningitis, chronic otitis media and mastoiditis, sinusitis, soft tissue infection of the face or scalp, orbital cellulitis, dental infections, penetrating head injuries, immunodeficiency states, and infection of ventriculoperitoneal shunts.

PATHOLOGY

Cerebral abscesses are evenly distributed between the 2 hemispheres, and 80% of cases are divided equally between the frontal, parietal, and temporal lobes. Brain abscesses in the occipital lobe, cerebellum, and brainstem account for about 20% of the cases. Most brain abscesses are single, but 30% are multiple and may involve more than 1 lobe. The pathogenesis is undetermined in 10-15% of cases. An abscess in the frontal lobe is often caused by extension from sinusitis or orbital cellulitis, whereas abscesses located in the temporal lobe or cerebellum are frequently associated with chronic otitis media and mastoiditis. Abscesses resulting from penetrating injuries tend to be singular and caused by *Staphylococcus aureus,* whereas those resulting from septic emboli, congenital heart disease, or meningitis often have several causal organisms.

ETIOLOGY

The responsible bacteria include streptococci (*Streptococcus milleri, Streptococcus pyogenes* group A or B, *Streptococcus pneumoniae, Enterococcus faecalis*), anaerobic organisms (gram-positive cocci, *Bacteroides* spp., *Fusobacterium* spp., *Prevotella* spp., *Actinomyces* spp.), and gram-negative aerobic bacilli (*Haemophilus aphrophilus, Haemophilus parainfluenzae, Haemophilus influenzae, Enterobacter, Escherichia coli, Proteus* spp.). *Citrobacter* is most common in neonates. One organism is cultured in 70% of abscesses, 2 in 20%, and 3 or more in 10% of cases. Abscesses associated with mucosal infections (sinusitis) frequently have anaerobic bacteria. Fungal abscesses *(Aspergillus, Candida)* are more common in immunosuppressed patients.

CLINICAL MANIFESTATIONS

The early stages of cerebritis and abscess formation are associated with nonspecific symptoms, including low-grade fever, headache, and lethargy. The significance of these symptoms is generally not recognized, and an oral antibiotic is often prescribed with resultant transient relief. As the inflammatory process proceeds, vomiting, severe headache, seizures, papilledema, focal neurologic signs (hemiparesis), and coma may develop. A cerebellar abscess is characterized by nystagmus, ipsilateral ataxia and dysmetria, vomiting, and headache. If the abscess ruptures into the ventricular cavity, overwhelming shock and death usually ensue.

DIAGNOSIS

The peripheral white blood cell count can be normal or elevated, and the blood culture is positive in 10% of cases. Examination of the cerebrospinal fluid (CSF) shows variable results; the white blood cells and protein may be minimally elevated or normal, and the glucose level may be low. CSF cultures are rarely positive; aspiration of the abscess is much more likely to establish a bacteriologic diagnosis. Molecular diagnostics with PCR are being

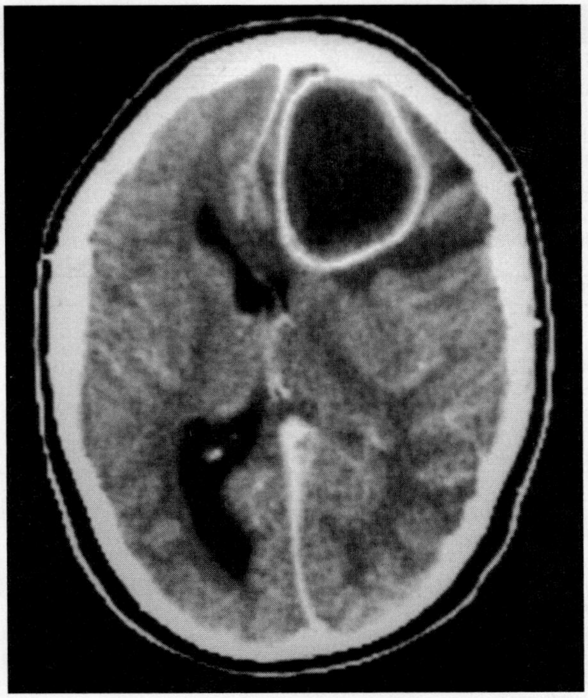

Figure 596-1 CT with contrast. Note the large, wall-enhancing abscess in the left frontal lobe causing a shift of the brain to the right. The patient had no neurologic signs until just before the CT scan because the abscess is located in the frontal lobe, a "silent" area of the brain.

evaluated to establish a bacterial etiology in aspirates from brain abscesses. Because examination of the CSF is seldom useful and a lumbar puncture may cause herniation of the cerebellar tonsils, the procedure should not be undertaken in a child suspected of having a brain abscess. The electroencephalogram (EEG) shows corresponding focal slowing, and the radionuclide brain scan indicates an area of enhancement due to disruption of the blood-brain barrier in >80% of cases. CT with contrast and MRI are the most reliable methods of demonstrating cerebritis and abscess formation (Fig. 596-1). MRI is the diagnostic test of choice. The CT findings of cerebritis are characterized by a parenchymal low-density lesion, and MRI T2 weighted images indicate increased signal intensity. An abscess cavity shows a ring-enhancing lesion by contrast CT, and the MRI also demonstrates an abscess capsule with gadolinium administration.

TREATMENT

The initial management of a brain abscess includes prompt diagnosis and institution of an antibiotic regimen that is based on the probable pathogenesis and the most likely organism. When the cause is unknown, the combination of vancomycin, a 3rd-generation cephalosporin, and metronidazole is commonly used. The same regimen is initiated when otitis media, sinusitis, or mastoiditis is the likely cause. If there is a history of penetrating head injury, head trauma, or neurosurgery, vancomycin plus a 3rd-generation cephalosporin is appropriate. When cyanotic congenital heart disease is the predisposing factor, ampicillin-sulbactam alone or a 3rd-generation cephalosporin plus metronidazole may be used. Meropenem has good activity against gram-negative bacilli, anaerobes, staphylococci, and streptococci, including most antibiotic-resistant pneumococci, and may be used alone to replace the combination of metronidazole and a β-lactam in the previous regimens. Notably, meropenem does not provide activity against methicillin-resistant *S. aureus* and may have decreased activity against penicillin-resistant strains of *S. pneumoniae,* indicating that vancomycin should remain a part of the initial regimen when these organisms are suspected. Abscesses secondary to an infected ventriculoperitoneal shunt may be initially treated with vancomycin and ceftazidime. When *Citrobacter* meningitis (often in neonates) leads to abscess formation, a 3rd-generation cephalosporin is used, typically in combination with an aminoglycoside. *Listeria monocytogenes* may cause a brain abscess in the neonate and if suspected, ampicillin should be added to the cephalosporin. In immunocompromised patients, broad-spectrum antibiotic coverage is used, and amphotericin B therapy should be considered.

A brain abscess can be treated with antibiotics without surgery if the abscess is <2 cm in diameter, the illness is of short duration (<2 wk), there are no signs of increased intracranial pressure, and the child is neurologically intact. If the decision is made to treat with antibiotics alone, the child should have follow-up neuroimaging studies to ensure the abscess is decreasing in size. An encapsulated abscess, particularly if the lesion is causing a mass effect or increased intracranial pressure, should be treated with a combination of antibiotics and aspiration. Surgical excision of an abscess is rarely required, because the procedure may be associated with greater morbidity compared with aspiration of a cavity. Surgery is indicated when the abscess is >2.5 cm in diameter, gas is present in the abscess, the lesion is multiloculated, the lesion is located in the posterior fossa, or a fungus is identified. Associated infectious processes, such as mastoiditis, sinusitis, or a periorbital abscess, may require surgical drainage. The duration of antibiotic therapy depends on the organism and response to treatment, but is usually 4-6 wk.

PROGNOSIS

Mortality rate associated with brain abscess has decreased significantly to 15-20% with the use of CT or MRI and prompt antibiotic and surgical management. Factors associated with high mortality rate at the time of admission include age <1 yr, multiple abscesses and coma. Long-term sequelae occur in at least 50% of survivors and include hemiparesis, seizures, hydrocephalus, cranial nerve abnormalities, and behavior and learning problems.

BIBLIOGRAPHY

Please visit the Nelson Textbook of Pediatrics *website at* *www.expertconsult.com* *for the complete bibliography.*

Chapter 597
Pseudotumor Cerebri

Misha L. Pless

Pseudotumor cerebri, also known as idiopathic intracranial hypertension, is a clinical syndrome that mimics brain tumors and is characterized by increased intracranial pressure (ICP; >200 mm H_2O in infants and >250 mm H_2O in children), with a normal cerebrospinal fluid (CSF) cell count and protein content and normal ventricular size, anatomy, and position documented by MRI. Papilledema is universally present in children old enough to have a closed fontanel.

ETIOLOGY

Table 597-1 lists the many causes of pseudotumor cerebri. There are many explanations for the development of pseudotumor cerebri, including alterations in CSF absorption and production, cerebral edema, abnormalities in vasomotor control and cerebral blood flow, and venous obstruction. The causes of pseudotumor are numerous and include metabolic disorders (galactosemia,

Table 597-1 ETIOLOGY OF CHILDHOOD PSEUDOTUMOR CEREBRI

HEMATOLOGIC	Wiskott-Aldrich syndrome Iron deficiency anemia Aplastic anemia Sickle cell disease Polycythemia? Bone marrow transplant? Prothrombotic states?
INFECTIONS	Acute sinusitis Otitis media Mastoiditis Tonsillitis Measles Roseola Varicella Lyme disease? HIV?
DRUGS	Tetracyclines Sulfonamides Nalidixic acid Corticosteroid therapy and withdrawal Nitrofurantoin Cytarabine Cyclosporine Phenytoin Mesalamine Amiodarone? DDAVP? Lithium? Levonorgestrel implants?
RENAL	Nephrotic syndrome Chronic renal insufficiency? Post–renal transplant? Peritoneal dialysis?
NUTRITIONAL	Hypovitaminosis A Vitamin A intoxication Hyperalimentation in malnourished patient Vitamin D–dependent rickets
CONNECTIVE TISSUE DISORDERS	Antiphospholipid antibody syndrome Systemic lupus erythematosus? Behçet disease
ENDOCRINE	Menarche Polycystic ovarian syndrome Thyroxine replacement Hypoparathyroidism/hyperparathyroidism Congenital adrenal hyperplasia Addison disease Recombinant growth hormone
OTHER	Dural sinus thrombosis Obesity (in pubertal patients) Head trauma Superior vena cava syndrome Arteriovenous malformation Sleep apnea Guillain-Barré syndrome Crohn disease Turner syndrome
POSSIBLE ASSOCIATIONS	Cystic fibrosis Cystinosis Down syndrome Hypomagenesemia-hypercalciuria Galactokinase deficiency Galactosemia Atrial septal defect repair Moebius syndrome Sarcoidosis?

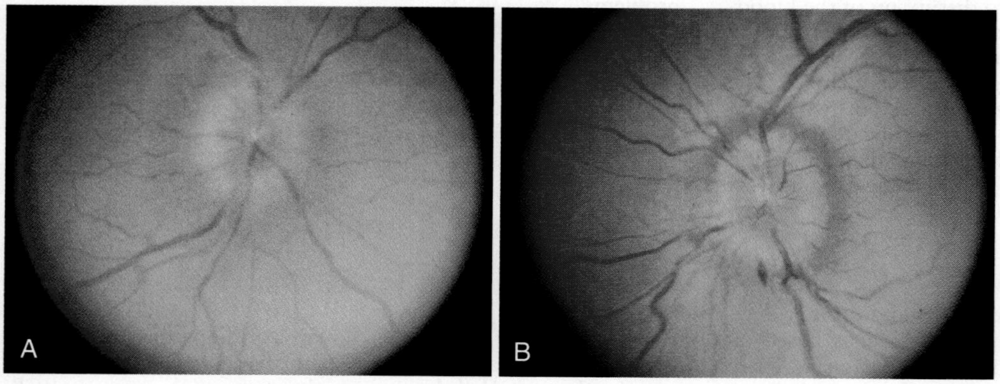

Figure 597-1 Moderate papilledema in the optic nerves (*A*, OD; *B*, OS) of a 3 yr old boy with severe iron deficiency anemia resulting in pseudotumor cerebri. Note mild pallor in OD optic nerve and a flame hemorrhage in OS optic nerve.

hypoparathyroidism, pseudohypoparathyroidism, hypophosphatasia, prolonged corticosteroid therapy or rapid corticosteroid withdrawal, possibly growth hormone treatment, refeeding of a significantly malnourished child, hypervitaminosis A, severe vitamin A deficiency, Addison disease, obesity, menarche, oral contraceptives, and pregnancy), infections (roseola infantum, sinusitis, chronic otitis media and mastoiditis, Guillain-Barré syndrome), drugs (nalidixic acid, doxycycline, minocycline, tetracycline, nitrofurantoin), isotretinoin used for acne therapy especially when combined with tetracycline, hematologic disorders (polycythemia, hemolytic and iron-deficiency anemias [Fig. 597-1], Wiskott-Aldrich syndrome), obstruction of intracranial drainage by venous thrombosis (lateral sinus or posterior sagittal sinus thrombosis), head injury, and obstruction of the superior vena cava. When a cause is not identified, the condition is classified as idiopathic intracranial hypertension.

CLINICAL MANIFESTATIONS

The most frequent symptom is headache, and although vomiting also occurs; the vomiting is rarely as persistent and insidious as that associated with a posterior fossa tumor. Transient visual obscuration and diplopia (secondary to dysfunction of the abducens nerve) may also occur. Most patients are alert and lack constitutional symptoms. Examination of the infant with pseudotumor cerebri characteristically reveals a bulging fontanel and a "cracked pot sound" or MacEwen sign (percussion of the skull produces a resonant sound) due to separation of the cranial sutures. **Papilledema** with an enlarged blind spot is the most consistent sign in a child beyond infancy. Papilledema may be absent or mild in infants with pseudotumor cerebri because high CSF pressure may be transmitted to the soft fontanels earlier than the optic nerves. Early optic nerve edema may be noted with orbit ultrasonography. An inferior nasal visual field defect may be detected on formal tangent screen testing. The presence of focal neurologic signs should prompt an investigation to uncover a process other than pseudotumor cerebri. Any patient suspected of pseudotumor cerebri should undergo an MRI. MRA/MRV should be considered in patients suspected of dural sinus thrombosis.

TREATMENT

The key objective in management is recognition and treatment of the underlying cause. There are no randomized clinical trials to guide the treatment of pseudotumor cerebri. Pseudotumor cerebri can be a self-limited condition, but optic atrophy and blindness are the most significant complications of untreated pseudotumor cerebri. The obese patient should be treated with a weight loss regimen, and if a drug is thought to be responsible, it should be discontinued. For most patients old enough to participate in such testing, serial monitoring of visual function is required. Serial determination of visual acuity, color vision, and visual fields is critical in this disease. Serial optic nerve examination is essential as well. Serial visual-evoked potentials are useful if the visual acuity cannot be reliably documented. The initial lumbar tap that follows a CT or MRI scan is diagnostic and may be therapeutic. The spinal needle produces a small rent in the dura that allows CSF to escape the subarachnoid space, thus reducing the ICP. Several additional lumbar taps and the removal of sufficient CSF to reduce the opening pressure by 50% occasionally lead to resolution of the process. Acetazolamide, 10-30 mg/kg/24 hr, is an effective regimen. Corticosteroids are not routinely administered, although they may be used in a patient with severe ICP elevation who is at risk of losing visual function and is awaiting a surgical decompression. Sinus thrombosis is typically addressed by anticoagulation therapy. Rarely, a ventriculoperitoneal shunt or subtemporal decompression is necessary, if the aforementioned approaches are unsuccessful and optic nerve atrophy supervenes. Some centers perform optic nerve sheath fenestration to prevent visual loss. Any patient whose ICP proves to be refractory to treatment warrants consideration for repeat neuroradiologic studies. A **slow-growing tumor** or **obstruction of a venous sinus** may become evident by the time of reinvestigation.

BIBLIOGRAPHY

Please visit the Nelson Textbook of Pediatrics *website at* *www.expertconsult.com* *for the complete bibliography.*

Chapter 598
Spinal Cord Disorders

598.1 Tethered Cord

Harold L. Rekate

Beyond infancy the spinal cord in humans ends in the conus medullaris at about the level of L1. The position of the conus below L2 is consistent with a congenital tethered spinal cord. For normal humans as the spine flexes and extends, the spinal cord is free to move up and down within the spinal canal. If the spinal cord is fixed at any point, this movement is restricted and the spinal cord and associated nerve roots become stretched. This

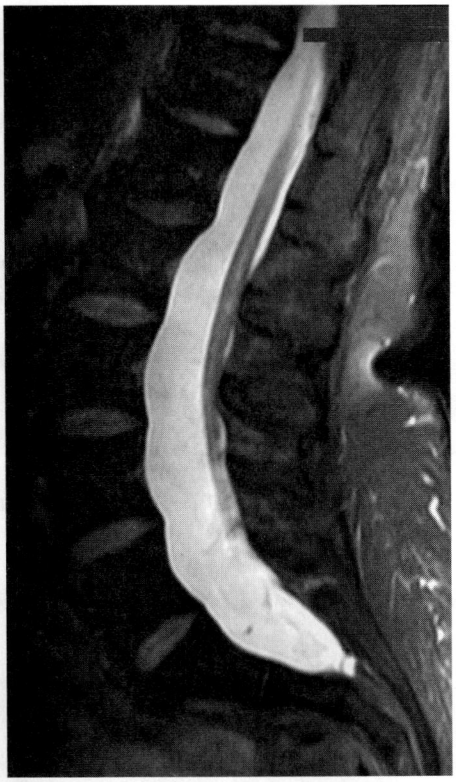

Figure 598-1 Sagittal MRI showing thickening of the filum terminale in a patient with a symptomatic tethered spinal cord. (Used with permission from Barrow Neurological Institute.)

fixing of the spinal cord, regardless of the underlying cause of the fixation, is called a tethered cord. When severe pain or neurologic deterioration occurs in response to the fixation, it is called the **tethered cord syndrome.**

In its simplest form the tethered cord syndrome results from a thickened filum terminale, which normally extends as a thin, very mobile structure from the tip of the conus to the sacrococcygeal region where it attaches. When this structure is thickened and shortened, the conus is found to end at levels below L2. This stretching between 2 points is likely to cause symptoms later in life. Fatty infiltration is often seen in the thickened filum (Fig. 598-1).

Any condition that fixes the spinal cord can be the cause of the tethered cord syndrome. Conditions that are well established to cause symptomatic tethering include various forms of occult dysraphism such as lipomyelomeningocele, myelocystocele, and diastematomyelia. These conditions are associated with cutaneous manifestations such as midline lipomas often with asymmetry of the gluteal fold (Fig. 598-2), and hairy patches called hypertrichosis (Fig. 598-3). Probably the most common type of symptomatic tethered cord involves patients who had previously undergone closure of an open myelomeningocele and later become symptomatic with pain or neurologic deterioration. Tethered cord syndrome can also be associated with attachment of the spinal cord in patients who undergo surgical procedures that disrupt the pial surface of the spinal cord.

CLINICAL MANIFESTATIONS

Patients at risk for the subsequent development of the tethered cord syndrome can often be identified at birth by the presence of an open myelomeningocele or by cutaneous manifestations of dysraphism. It is important to examine the back of the newborn for cutaneous midline lesions (lipoma, dermal sinus, tail, hair patch, hemangioma, port-wine stain) that may signal an

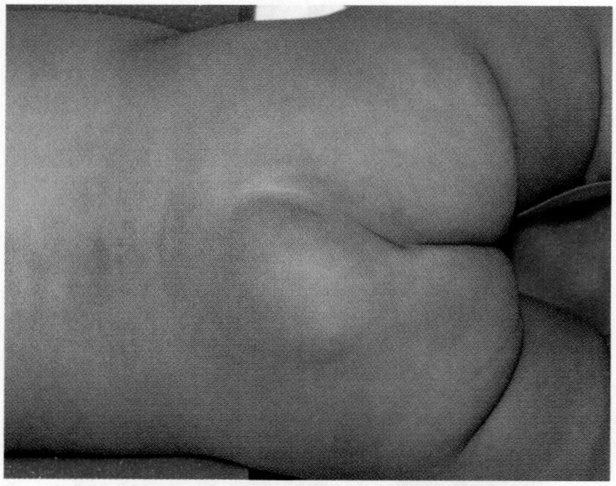

Figure 598-2 Child with a lipomyelomeningocele demonstrating an extraspinal mass and an asymmetry of the gluteal fold indicative of underlying occult dysraphism. (Used with permission from Barrow Neurological Institute.)

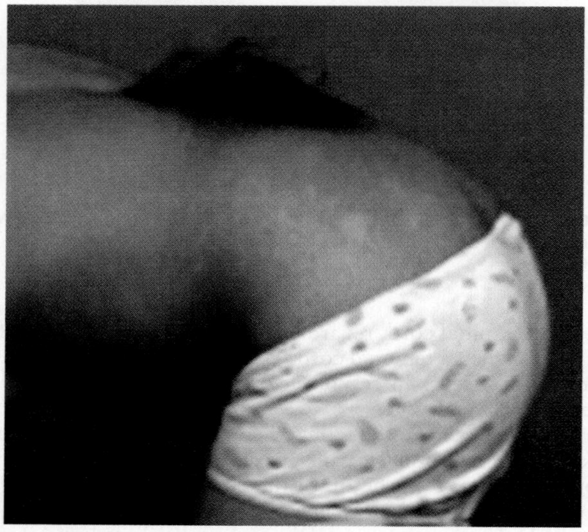

Figure 598-3 Hairy patch or hypertrichosis usually associated with diastematomyelia. (Used with permission from Barrow Neurological Institute.)

underlying form of occult dysraphism. Dermal sinuses are usually located above the gluteal fold. Cutaneous abnormalities are not found in patients with an isolated thickened filum terminale. Patients who become symptomatic later in life often exhibit an asymmetry of the feet (i.e., one is smaller than the other). The smaller foot will show a high arch and clawing of the toes (Fig. 598-4). Characteristically, there is no ankle jerk on the involved side and the calf is atrophied. This condition is termed the neuro-orthopedic syndrome.

Three clinical syndromes can occur at the time of deterioration. The most likely clinical presentation is increasing urinary urgency and, finally, incontinence. Deterioration of motor and sensory function in the lower extremities is a compelling reason for intervention. Finally, severe generalized back pain, often radiating into the lower extremities, can occur, particularly in older adolescents and adults.

DIAGNOSTIC EVALUATION

When patients present with symptoms related to the tethered cord syndrome, a thorough motor and sensory examination of the patient must be documented. Assessment of bladder function

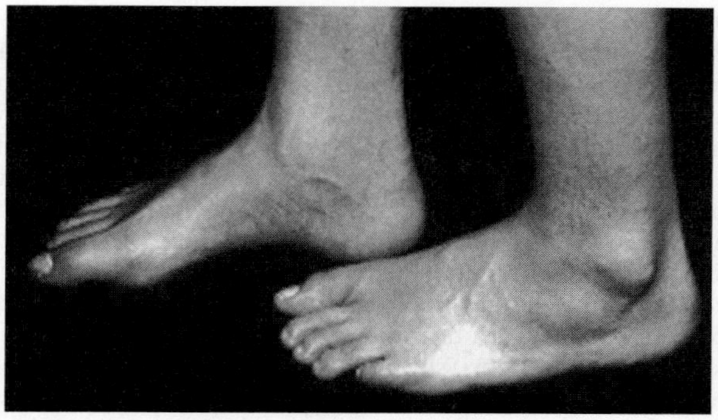

Figure 598-4 Example of the neuro-orthopedic syndrome involving a larger left foot than right foot, a high arch, and absent ankle jerk frequently associated with tethered cord regardless of the etiology. (Used with permission from Barrow Neurological Institute.)

with an ultrasound of the bladder and urodynamic studies is useful in analyzing bladder innervation. MRI is the diagnostic study of choice to reflect the anatomy of the tethering lesion and to provide information about the risks of surgical intervention.

TREATMENT

There are no nonsurgical options for the management of tethered cord syndrome. Because the presence of tethering is most likely to be at least suspected in the newborn, prophylactic surgery to prevent late deterioration has been advocated by some neurosurgeons. This strategy remains controversial and depends to some extent on a careful assessment of the risks compared to the benefits. If surgical intervention is chosen, microsurgical dissection with release of the spinal cord attachment to the overlying dura is the goal of treatment.

OUTCOME

The outcome of releasing a thickened filum terminale or detethering of patients with diastematomyelia is routinely good, and the chance of recurrent symptoms is very low. Patients with symptomatic tethered cord who undergo repair of a myelomeningocele or a lipomyelomeningocele have a significant possibility of recurrent tethering and recurrent symptoms.

BIBLIOGRAPHY

Please visit the Nelson Textbook of Pediatrics *website at* *www.expertconsult.com* *for the complete bibliography.*

598.2 Diastematomyelia

Harold L. Rekate

DIASTEMATOMYELIA: SPLIT CORD MALFORMATION

Diastematomyelia is a relatively rare form of occult dysraphism in which the spinal cord is divided into 2 halves. In type 1 split cord malformation, there are 2 spinal cords, each in its own dural tube and separated by a spicule of bone and cartilage (Fig. 598-5*A*). In a type 2 split cord malformation, the 2 spinal cords are enclosed in a single dural sac with a fibrous septum between the 2 spinal segments (Fig. 598-5*B*). In both cases the anatomy of the outer half of the spinal cord is essentially normal while the medial half is extremely underdeveloped. Undeveloped nerve roots and dentate ligaments terminate medially into the medial dural tube in type 1 cases and terminate in the membranous septum in type 2 cases. Both types have an associated defect in the bony spinal segment. In the case of type 2 lesions, this defect can be quite subtle.

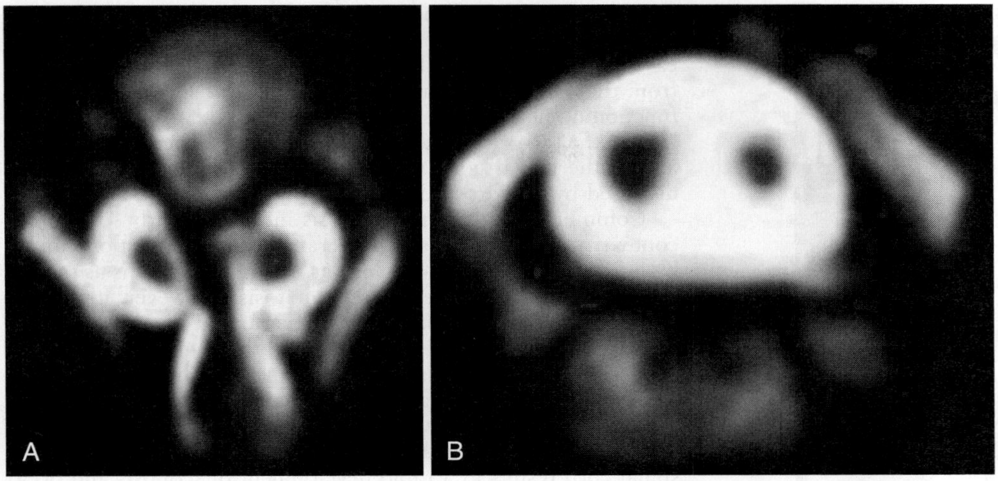

Figure 598-5 *A,* T2-weighted axial MRI of a type 1 split cord malformation showing the 2 spinal cords within 2 separate dural compartments. *B,* Type two split cord malformation with two spinal cords sharing a single dural compartment. (*A* and *B* used with permission from Barrow Neurological Institute.)

CLINICAL MANIFESTATIONS

Patients with both type 1 and type 2 split cord malformations may have subtle signs of neurologic involvement such as unilateral calf atrophy and a high arch to one or both feet early in life, but they are more likely to be neurologically normal. These patients are tethered by the adherence of the spinal cord to the median membrane or dural sac. Later they may develop progressive loss of bowel and bladder function and sensory and motor difficulties in the lower extremities. Back pain is a common symptom in adolescents and adults with split cord malformation but is uncommon in small children.

Cutaneous manifestations of dysraphism are present in 90% of patients with split cord malformations. Large hairy midline patches called hypertrichosis, the most common cutaneous manifestations, are present in about 60% of the cases.

DIAGNOSTIC EVALUATION

MRI, the study of choice, shows the 2 spinal cords. The frequent association of bony abnormalities in this condition may require further evaluation with radiography or computed tomography.

TREATMENT

The treatment of split cord malformations is surgical. This abnormality is a form of tethered cord syndrome, and its treatment is to release the spinal cord to move freely with movement of the spine. In type 1 split cord malformations, the 2 half cords are in separate dural sacs with medial attachment to the dura and bony septum. In this case the dura needs to be opened, the bony septum removed, the medial attachments to the dura lysed, and a single dural tube created. For type 2 lesions, the membranous septum should be lysed. An attachment of this membrane to the anterior dura should be explored and lysed as well. Retethering of this type is rare as there is no reason to disrupt the pial layer of the spinal cord.

BIBLIOGRAPHY

Please visit the Nelson Textbook of Pediatrics *website at www.expertconsult.com for the complete bibliography.*

598.3 Syringomyelia

Harold L. Rekate

Syringomyelia is a cystic distension of the spinal cord caused by obstruction of the flow of spinal fluid from within the spinal cord to its point of absorption. There are 3 recognized forms of syringomyelia depending on the underlying cause. Communicating syringomyelia implies that cerebrospinal fluid (CSF) from within the ventricles communicates with the fluid within the spinal cord and is assumed to be the source of the CSF that distends the spinal cord. Noncommunicating syringomyelia implies that ventricular CSF does not communicate with the fluid within the spinal cord. It primarily occurs in the context of intramedullary tumors and obstructive lesions. In the final form of syringomyelia, that is, post-traumatic syringomyelia, spinal cord injury results in damage and subsequent softening of the spinal cord. This softening, combined with the scarring of the surrounding spinal cord tissue, results in progressive distension of the cyst.

CLINICAL MANIFESTATIONS

Signs and symptoms of syringomyelia develop insidiously over years or decades. The classic presentation is the **central cord syndrome.** In this situation the patient develops numbness beginning in the shoulder in a capelike distribution followed by the development of atrophy and weakness in the upper extremities. Trophic ulcers of the hands are characteristic of advanced cases. The central cord syndrome results from damage to the central spinal cord and the orientation of spinal tracts from proximal to distal leading to selective involvement of the upper rather than the lower extremities.

Other forms of presentation include scoliosis that may be rapidly progressive and often can be presumed from the absence of superficial abdominal reflexes. Urgency and bladder dysfunction as well as lower extremity spasticity also may be part of the presentation.

In patients with syringomyelia related to spinal cord injury, the presentation is usually severe pain in the area of the spinal cord distension above the level of the initial injury. There is also an ascending level of motor and sensory dysfunction.

DIAGNOSTIC EVALUATION

MRI is the radiologic study of choice (Figs. 598-6 and 598-7). The study should include the entire spine and should include gadolinium-enhanced sequences. Specific attention should be paid to the craniovertebral junction due to the frequent association of syringomyelia with Chiari I and II malformations. Obstruction to the flow of CSF from the 4th ventricle can cause syringomyelia; therefore, most patients also should undergo imaging of the brain.

TREATMENT

The treatment of syringomyelia should be tailored to the underlying cause. If that cause can be removed or ameliorated, the syrinx

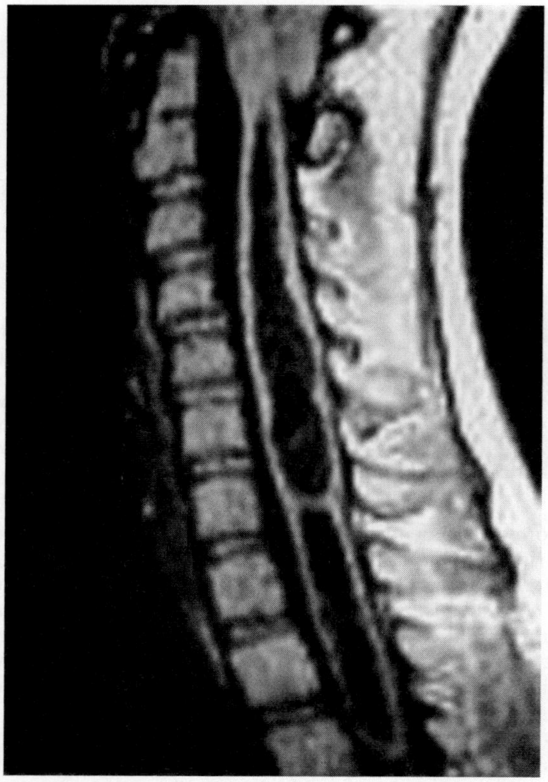

Figure 598-6 Sagittal MRI of patient with a Chiari I malformation and a holocord syrinx. (Used with permission from Barrow Neurological Institute.)

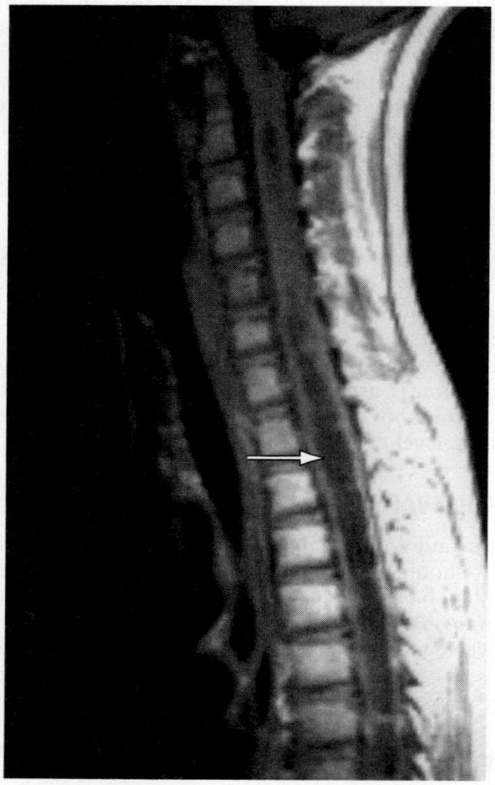

Figure 598-7 T1-weighted MRI scan of upper spinal cord showing an extensive syringomyelia *(arrow).*

should improve. Traumatic syrinxes are treated by preventing distension of the spinal cord by transecting the spinal cord in cases of complete spinal cord injury. Doing so drains the fluid from the spinal cord. In cases of incomplete spinal cord injury, functioning neurologic elements must be protected. Microscopic lysis of the scar surrounding the spinal cord at the point of injury allows the spinal cord to collapse and prevents it from being distorted by a hydrostatic column.

Communicating syringomyelia is most frequently seen in the context of abnormalities at the craniovertebral junction caused by inflammatory conditions such as chronic meningitis as seen in tuberculosis or meningeal carcinomatosis. However, it is most often associated with hindbrain herniation as in Chiari malformations. In such cases decompression of the craniovertebral junction is usually effective in the management of the syringomyelia. In the context of the Chiari II malformation associated with spina bifida, syringomyelia usually results from an insidious failure of the shunt used to treat the hydrocephalus. This distension of the spinal cord results in a rapid development of scoliosis and occasionally spasticity in the lower extremities. Repair of the shunt is effective treatment.

Noncommunicating syringomyelia results from blocking the flow of spinal cord extracellular fluid or CSF within the central canal by an intramedullary spinal cord tumor or severe external compression of the spinal cord. In such cases management should be directed to tumor resection or to decompression of constricting elements.

Drainage procedures can result in symptomatic and radiographic improvement. Syrinx-to-subarachnoid shunting with a small piece of shunt tubing is 1 form of treatment. Syrinx-to-pleural or syrinx-to-peritoneal shunting is more likely to result in improvement in the radiographic appearance of the syrinx. In patients with syringomyelia that extends to the conus medullaris, remnants of the central canal can be found in the filum terminale. Lysis of this structure near the conus can provide effective drainage.

BIBLIOGRAPHY

Please visit the Nelson Textbook of Pediatrics *website at www.expertconsult.com for the complete bibliography.*

598.4 Spinal Cord Tumors

Harold L. Rekate

Tumors of the spine and spinal cord are rare in children. Different types of tumors have different relationships with the spinal cord, meninges, and bony elements of the spine (Fig. 598-8). Intramedullary spinal cord tumors arise within the substance of the spinal cord itself (Fig. 598-9). They represent between 5% and 15% of primary central nervous system tumors. This percentage may well reflect the total volume of spinal cord as opposed to brain. About 10% of intramedullary spinal cord tumors are malignant astrocytic tumors, but most are World Health Organization grade I or II tumors of glial or ependymal origin. In children, low-grade astrocytomas and gangliogliomas represent the most common tumor types with ependymomas being less common than in adults. Ependymomas in children are frequently associated with neurofibromatosis (NF 2).

Except in the context of NF 1 and NF 2, intradural extramedullary tumors are extremely rare in children. Most are nerve sheath tumors, either schwannomas or, in the case of NF 2, neurofibromas. Intraspinal meningiomas in children are essentially found only in patients with NF 2. The intradural extramedullary compartment is also a site for metastatic tumors from primary cancers such as leukemia or primitive neuroectodermal tumors.

Extradural spinal tumors characteristically begin in the bones of the spine. Primary tumors in this location include aneurysmal bone cysts, Langerhans cell histiocytosis (formerly called

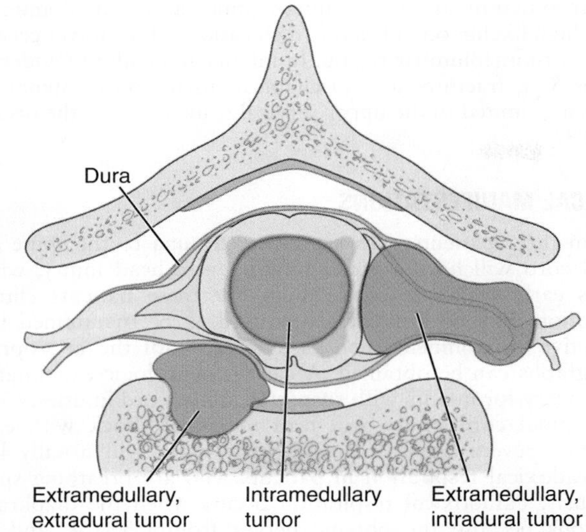

Figure 598-8 Diagram of the relationship of various tumors to the spine, nerve roots, and spinal cord. (Used with permission from Barrow Neurological Institute.)

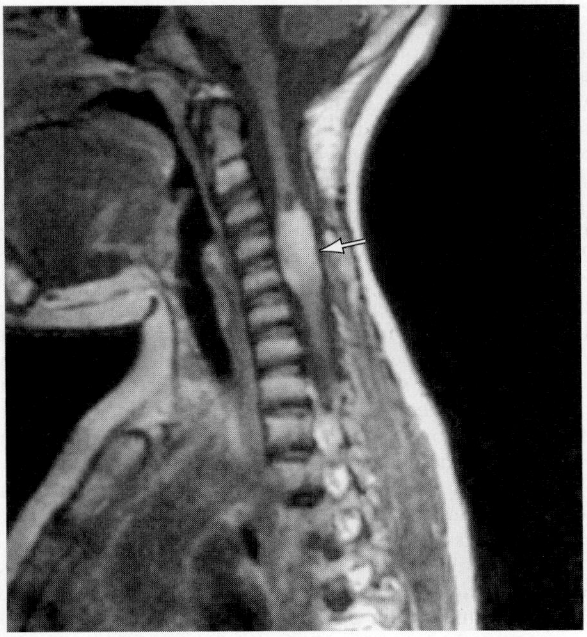

Figure 598-9 T1-weighted MRI scan of a spinal cord tumor *(arrow)*. The fusiform expansion of the cervical cord enhances after intravenous gadolinium injection.

eosinophilic granuloma), and giant cell tumors. In infants the extradural space is often the site of neuroblastomas or ganglioneuroblastomas, which tend to be present in the epidural space and in the paraspinous tissue through the intervertebral foramen. In older patients the bones of the spine may be the site of multiple myeloma and metastases from common malignant tumors.

CLINICAL MANIFESTATIONS

With the exception of the uncommon malignant glial tumors of the spinal cord, which tend to present precipitously, intramedullary spinal cord tumors present in a very insidious manner. Back pain related to the level of the tumor is a common presenting complaint. It is likely that this pain will awaken the child from sleep and improve as the day progresses. Before the use of MRI became routine, the time from the 1st onset of symptoms to diagnosis of the tumor could be as long as 9 yr. Weakness, gait disturbance, and sensory deficits are usually minor and are often found when formal neurologic examinations are performed. Scoliosis, urinary urgency, and incontinence may be the presenting complaints associated with intramedullary spinal cord tumors.

Extramedullary extradural tumors have a propensity to cause an acute block of the CSF pathways owing to rapid growth within a confined space. Such children present with a flaccid paraplegia, urinary retention, and a patulous anus. Some extramedullary tumors produce the *Brown-Séquard syndrome,* which consists of ipsilateral weakness, spasticity, and ataxia, with contralateral loss of pain and temperature sensation. Papilledema is observed in a few patients, usually in association with markedly elevated CSF protein levels that presumably interfere with normal CSF flow dynamics.

Nerve sheath tumors primarily arise from the sensory rootlet of the exiting spinal nerve. They are very slow-growing tumors and present with symptoms and signs relative to the nerve root involved. Pain in a bandlike distribution around the chest or into an extremity is the most common presenting complaint. Tumor growth eventually leads to spinal cord compression and involvement of adjacent nerve roots.

Tumors rarely arise in the fat of the epidural space; most epidural tumors arise in the bony compartment of the spine. They can present abruptly with severe pain and neurologic deficit at the time of pathologic fracture of the vertebral body. Benign tumors such as giant cell tumors and aneurysmal bone cysts present more insidiously as the tumor slowly grows and begins to compress neural structures.

DIAGNOSTIC EVALUATION

MRI with and without gadolinium enhancement of the spinal cord is the diagnostic study of choice and is essential in the diagnosis of spinal cord tumors, especially intramedullary spinal cord tumors. Most astrocytic tumors of the spinal cord and most ependymomas show diffuse enhancement and will distend the spinal cord focally. These tumors may involve the entire length of the spinal cord (holocord astrocytomas). MRI also shows the relationship between the normal spinal cord and tumor embedded within spinal cord tissue. These tumors are frequently associated with a syrinx, which is usually distal to the tumor. Nerve sheath tumors characteristically enhance and are focal. They may exit through the neural foramen and distend the canal as can be seen on MRI. They also may be visualized on plain radiographs of the affected area of the spine.

Plain radiographs of the spine are helpful in defining the relationship of extradural tumors to the bony spine and in documenting evidence of instability in the case of pathologic compression fractures. When a pathologic fracture occurs, CT is essential to determine the effect of the tumor on the bone. Because many of these tumors occur as metastatic lesions, a general staging of the extent of disease is essential. In the case of Langerhans cell histiocytosis, a thorough bone survey should be conducted to look for other lesions. Radionucleotide bone scanning is also useful in determining the extent of the disease.

TREATMENT

The primary treatment of both intramedullary and extramedullary intradural tumors is surgical removal. For both low-grade astrocytomas and ependymomas, microsurgical removal with the intent of total removal is the treatment of choice. This goal should be attainable in all patients with ependymomas and in most patients with low-grade astrocytomas and gangliogliomas. Adjunctive treatment of these tumors is unwarranted in patients treated with adequate surgical resection. Likewise, schwannomas should be resectable. Occasionally, however, the nerve root must be resected. Doing so is of no consequence in the thoracic spinal cord, but an attempt to remove the tumor while salvaging the motor root in the cervical and thoracic region is critical to preserve movement. Malignant astrocytic tumors cannot be resected without major morbidity and, in any case care, carry an extremely poor prognosis. In the case of grade III and IV astrocytomas of the spinal cord, decompression and biopsy followed by radiation therapy and possibly chemotherapy are utilized.

The diagnosis and treatment of extramedullary spinal cord tumors must be individualized. Patients with distension of the vertebral body or with unstable pathologic fractures benefit from extensive resection of the involved vertebral bodies and will likely need fusion. For extramedullary tumors with soft tissue components such as neuroblastomas, treatment is determined by the nature of the tumor and degree of spinal cord compression, and directed following needle biopsy of the lesion. In the absence of significant neurologic compression, surgical intervention is rarely indicated.

OUTCOME

The prognosis for patients with benign intramedullary spinal cord tumors depends, to some extent, on the patient's condition at the time of surgical intervention. It is very unlikely that nonambulatory patients will improve after surgery. If, however, patients are ambulatory at the time of surgery, they may experience increased weakness after surgery. They are likely to recover at least their preoperative level of function. Malignant spinal cord tumors are usually lethal with death resulting from diffuse metastases via the CSF pathways. Successful resection of nerve sheath tumors should be curative. In the context of neurofibromatosis, however, many more tumors can be found at other levels or can be expected to develop later in life. Surgical intervention in the context of neurofibromatoses should be performed only on clearly symptomatic lesions.

The outcome of treatment of extramedullary tumors depends on the cell type and, in most cases, on the efficacy of nonsurgical, adjunctive therapies. For aneurysmal bone cysts and giant cell tumors, resection of the tumor and fusion of the spine are the treatments of choice.

BIBLIOGRAPHY

Please visit the Nelson Textbook of Pediatrics *website at www.expertconsult.com for the complete bibliography.*

598.5 Spinal Cord Injuries in Children

Harold L. Rekate

Spine and spinal cord injuries are very rare in children, particularly in young children. The spine of a small child is very mobile, and fractures of the spine are exceedingly rare. This increased mobility is not always a positive feature. Transfer of energy leading to spinal distortion can maintain the structural integrity of the spine but lead to significant injuries of the spinal cord. Spinal cord injury without radiographic bone (vertebral) abnormalities, called **SCIWORA,** is more common in children than adults. There seem to be 2 distinct forms. The infantile form involves severe injury of the cervical or thoracic spine. These patients have a poor likelihood of complete recovery. In older children and adolescents, SCIWORA is more likely to cause a less severe injury and the likelihood of complete recovery over time is high. The adolescent form is assumed to be a spinal cord concussion or mild contusion as opposed to the severe spinal cord injury related to the mobility of the spine in small children.

Although the mechanisms of spinal cord injury in children include birth trauma, falls, and child abuse, the major cause of morbidity and mortality remains motor vehicle injuries. While the mechanisms of injury and diagnosis are distinct in very small children, adolescents incur spinal cord injuries with epidemiology similar to that of adults, including significant male predominance and a high likelihood of fracture dislocations of the lower cervical spine or thoracolumbar region. In infants and children under the age of 5 yr, fractures and mechanical disruption of spinal elements are limited to the upper cervical spine between the occiput and C3.

CLINICAL MANIFESTATIONS

One in three patients with significant trauma to the spine and spinal cord will have a concomitant severe head injury, which makes early diagnosis challenging. For these patients clinical evaluation may be difficult. They need to be maintained in a protective environment such as a collar until the appropriate radiographs can be obtained. A careful neurologic examination is necessary for infants with suspected spinal cord injuries. Complete spinal cord injury will lead to **spinal shock** with early areflexia. Severe cervical spinal cord injuries will usually lead to paradoxical respiration in patients who are breathing spontaneously. Paradoxical respiration occurs when the diaphragm functions because the phrenic nerves from C3, C4, and C5 are functioning normally but the intercostal musculature innervated by the thoracic spinal cord is paralyzed. In this situation, inspiration fails to expand of the chest wall but distends the abdomen.

The *mildest injury* to the spinal cord is transient quadriparesis evident for seconds or minutes with complete recovery in 24 hr. This injury follows a concussion of the cord.

A transverse injury in the high cervical cord level (C1-C2) causes respiratory arrest and death in the absence of ventilatory support. *Fracture dislocations at the C5-C6 level* resulting in spinal cord injuries are characterized by flaccid quadriparesis, loss of sphincter function, and a sensory level corresponding to the upper sternum. Fractures or dislocations in the low thoracic (T12-L1) region may produce the **conus medullaris syndrome,** which includes a loss of urinary and rectal sphincter control, flaccid weakness, and sensory disturbances of the legs. A **central cord lesion** may result from contusion and hemorrhage and typically involves the upper extremities to a greater degree than the legs. There are lower motor neuron signs in the upper extremities and upper motor neuron signs in the legs, bladder dysfunction, and loss of sensation caudal to the lesion. There may be considerable recovery, particularly in the lower extremities.

Thoracolumbar injuries are usually fracture-dislocations such as occur in severe motor vehicle accidents when children are wearing lap belts but not shoulder harnesses. These injuries lead to a conus medullaris syndrome. These patients exhibit a loss of bowel and bladder function and lower motor neuron injuries involving the innervation of the lower extremities.

TREATMENT

The initial management of spine and spinal cord injuries in children is similar to that in adults. The cervical spine should be immobilized in the field by the emergency medical technicians. In cases of acute spinal cord injury, some data support the acute infusion of a bolus of high-dose (30 mg/kg) methylprednisolone followed by a 23-hr infusion (5.4 mg/kg/hr). The data for this treatment in children are controversial. Imaging studies, including lateral cervical spine x-rays, should be performed in the emergency room. If instability is recognized, precautions such as fixation with a collar or halo device should be instituted. In patients with documented neurologic dysfunction, MRI should be performed, including imaging of soft tissue to look for ligamentous instability.

Surgical management of unstable spinal injuries must be tailored to the patient's age. For occipitocervical dislocations, early surgery with fusion from the occiput to C2 or C3 should be performed, even in babies older than 6 mo. Fixation of the subaxial spine must be tailored to the size of the pedicles and other osseus structures of the developing axial skeleton.

PREVENTION

The most important aspect of the care of spinal cord injuries in children relates to injury prevention. In this regard, the use of appropriate child restraints in automobiles is the most important precaution. In older children and adolescents, rules against spear tackling in football and the "Feet First, First Time Program" from the Think First Foundation aimed at adolescents diving into swimming pools and natural water areas are important ways to help prevent severe cervical spinal cord injuries.

BIBLIOGRAPHY

Please visit the Nelson Textbook of Pediatrics *website at www.expertconsult.com for the complete bibliography.*

598.6 Transverse Myelitis

Harold L. Rekate

Transverse myelitis is a condition characterized by rapid development of both motor and sensory deficits (Table 598-1). It has multiple causes and tends to occur in 2 distinct contexts. Small children, 3 yr of age and younger, develop spinal cord dysfunction over hours to a few days. They have a history of an infectious disease, usually of viral origin, or of an immunization within the few weeks preceding the 1st development of their neurologic difficulties. The clinical loss of function is often severe and may seem complete. Although a slow recovery is common in these cases, it is likely to be incomplete. The likelihood of independent ambulation in these small children is about 40%. The pathologic findings of perivascular infiltration with mononuclear cells imply an infectious or inflammatory basis. Overt necrosis of spinal cord can be seen.

In older children, the syndrome is somewhat different. Although the onset is also rapid with a nadir in neurologic function occurring between 2 days and 2 wk, recovery is more rapid and more likely to be complete. Pathologic or imaging examination shows acute demyelination.

CLINICAL MANIFESTATIONS

In both forms the patient shows or complains of discomfort or overt pain in the neck or back, depending on the level of the lesion. Depending on its severity, the condition progresses to numbness, anesthesia, and weakness in the truncal and appendicular musculature. Paralysis begins as flaccidity, but over a few weeks spasticity develops. Urinary retention is an early finding; incontinence occurs later in the course.

Table 598-1 DIAGNOSTIC CRITERIA FOR TRANSVERSE MYELITIS*

Bilateral (not necessarily symmetric) sensorimotor and autonomic spinal cord dysfunction
Clearly defined sensory level
Progression to nadir of clinical deficits between 4 hours and 21 days after symptom onset
Demonstration of spinal cord inflammation: cerebrospinal fluid pleocytosis or elevated IgG index,† or MRI revealing a gadolinium-enhancing cord lesion
Exclusion of compressive, postradiation, neoplastic, and vascular causes

*Clinical events that are consistent with transverse myelitis but that are not associated with cerebrospinal fluid abnormalities or abnormalities detected on MRI and that have no identifiable underlying cause are categorized as possible idiopathic transverse myelitis.

†The IgG index is a measure of intrathecal synthesis of immunoglobulin and is calculated with the use of the following formula: (CSF IgG ÷ serum IgG) ÷ (CSF albumin ÷ serum albumin), where CSF denotes cerebrospinal fluid.

From Frohman EM, Wingerchuk DM: Transverse myelitis, *N Engl J Med* 363:564–572, 2010, Table 1, p 565.

The differential diagnosis includes demyelination disorders, overt meningitis, spinal cord infarction, or mass lesions such as bony distortion, abscess, and spine and spinal cord tumors.

DIAGNOSTIC EVALUATION

MRI with and without contrast enhancement is essential to rule out a mass lesion requiring neurosurgical intervention. In both conditions, T1 weighted images of the spine at the anatomic level of involvement may be normal or may show distension of the spinal cord. In the infantile form, T2 weighted images show high signal intensity that extends over multiple segments. In the adolescent form, the high signal intensity will likely be limited to 1 or 2 segments. A limited degree of contrast enhancement after the administration of gadolinium is expected, especially in the infantile form, and denotes an inflammatory condition. MRI of the brain is also indicated and shows evidence of other foci of demyelination in at least 30% of patients similar to the adult population.

After a mass lesion associated with spinal cord compression or complete subarachnoid column block from spinal cord swelling have been ruled out, a lumbar puncture is indicated. In both forms of disease, the number of mononuclear cells is usually elevated minimally. The level of CSF protein is elevated mildly. CSF should be analyzed for myelin basic protein and immunoglobulin levels, which are usually elevated in transverse myelitis. The presence of inflammatory cells is essential for the diagnosis of transverse myelitis.

Because one of the most important possibilities for this condition is neuromyelitis optica (NMO; Devic syndrome) the serum of all patients should be analyzed for the NMO antigen. This test is positive in 60% of patients with Devic syndrome which, as opposed to a presenting syndrome for multiple sclerosis, is likely to be a monophasic condition. As in adults with transverse myelitis, older children with the condition should have serum studies sent for autoimmune disorders, especially systemic lupus erythematosus.

TREATMENT

There are no standards for the treatment of transverse myelitis. Available evidence suggests that modulation of the immune response may be effective in decreasing the severity and length of the condition. In the absence of open clinical trials, the use of high-dose steroids, particularly methylprednisolone, is a reasonable approach to treatment of both the early and late childhood forms of this condition.

BIBLIOGRAPHY

Please visit the Nelson Textbook of Pediatrics *website at www.expertconsult.com for the complete bibliography.*

598.7 Spinal Arteriovenous Malformations

Harold L. Rekate

Arteriovenous malformations of the spinal cord are rare lesions in children. Only about 60 patients under the age of 18 yr are treated in the USA each year. These lesions are complex. Despite their rarity there are multiple subtypes, which require different treatment strategies. Patients commonly present with back or neck pain, depending on the segments of the spinal cord involved, and they may experience the insidious onset of motor and sensory disturbances. Sudden onset of paraplegia secondary to hemorrhage has been reported. Occasionally, patients present with subarachnoid hemorrhage without overt neurologic deficits, similar to the presentation associated with cerebral aneurysms. In some cases, bruits are audible upon auscultation over the bony spine.

DIAGNOSTIC EVALUATION

When a spinal arteriovenous malformation is suspected, MRI of the spinal cord is 1st needed to make the diagnosis and to obtain a general idea of the location of the lesion. MR angiography or CT angiography may provide further information, but formal catheter angiography of the spinal cord is needed to obtain an adequate understanding of the complex anatomy of the lesion and to plan the intervention.

TREATMENT

Open microsurgery had been the mainstay of treatment for spinal cord arteriovenous fistulae and arteriovenous malformations. With the rapid development of interventional techniques, the percentage of patients undergoing microsurgery has decreased from 70% to about 30%. Stereotactic radiosurgery may be used adjunctively. Treatment of these complex lesions requires the commitment of an organized neurovascular treatment program.

PART XXVIII Neuromuscular Disorders

Chapter 599 Evaluation and Investigation

Harvey B. Sarnat

The term **neuromuscular disease** defines disorders of the motor unit and excludes influences on muscular function from the brain, such as spasticity. The motor unit has 4 components: a motor neuron in the brainstem or ventral horn of the spinal cord; its axon, which, together with other axons, forms the peripheral nerve; the neuromuscular junction; and all muscle fibers innervated by a single motor neuron. The size of the motor unit varies among different muscles and with the precision of muscular function required. In large muscles, such as the glutei and quadriceps femoris, hundreds of muscle fibers are innervated by a single motor neuron; in small, finely tuned muscles, such as the stapedius or the extraocular muscles, a 1:1 ratio can prevail. The motor unit is influenced by suprasegmental or upper motor neuron control that alters properties of muscle tone, precision of movement, reciprocal inhibition of antagonistic muscles during movement, and sequencing of muscle contractions to achieve smooth, coordinated movements. Suprasegmental impulses also augment or inhibit the monosynaptic stretch reflex; the corticospinal tract is inhibitory upon this reflex.

Diseases of the motor unit are common in children. These neuromuscular diseases may be genetically determined, congenital or acquired, acute or chronic, and progressive or static. Because specific therapy is available for many diseases and because of genetic and prognostic implications, precise diagnosis is important; laboratory confirmation is required for most diseases because of overlapping clinical manifestations.

Many chromosomal loci have been identified with specific neuromuscular diseases as a result of genetic linkage studies and the isolation and cloning of a few specific genes. In some cases, such as Duchenne muscular dystrophy, the genetic defect has been shown to be a deletion of nucleotide sequences and is associated with a defective protein product, dystrophin; in other cases, such as myotonic muscular dystrophy, the genetic defect is an expansion or repetition, rather than a deletion, in a codon (a set of three consecutive nucleotide repeats that encodes for a single amino acid), with many copies of a particular codon, in this example also associated with abnormal mRNA. Some diseases manifest as autosomal dominant and autosomal recessive traits in different pedigrees; these distinct mendelian genotypes can result from different genetic mutations on different chromosomes (nemaline rod myopathy) or may be small differences in the same gene at the same chromosomal locus (myotonia congenita), despite many common phenotypic features and shared histopathologic findings in a muscle biopsy specimen. Among the several clinically defined mitochondrial myopathies, specific mtDNA deletions and tRNA point mutations are recognized. The inheritance patterns and chromosomal and mitochondrial loci of common neuromuscular diseases affecting infants and children are summarized in Table 600-1.

CLINICAL MANIFESTATIONS

Examination of the neuromuscular system includes an assessment of muscle bulk, tone, and strength. Tone and strength should not be confused: **Passive tone** is range of motion around a joint; **active tone** is physiologic resistance to movement. Head lag when an infant is pulled to a sitting position from supine is a sign of weakness, not of low tone. Hypotonia may be associated with normal strength or with weakness; enlarged muscles may be weak or strong; thin, wasted muscles may be weak or have unexpectedly normal strength. The distribution of these components is of diagnostic importance. In general, myopathies follow a proximal distribution of weakness and muscle wasting (with the notable exception of myotonic muscular dystrophy); neuropathies are generally distal in distribution (with the notable exception of juvenile spinal muscular atrophy; Table 599-1). Involvement of the face, tongue, palate, and extraocular muscles provides an important distinction in the differential diagnosis. **Tendon stretch reflexes** are generally lost in neuropathies and in motor neuron diseases and are diminished but preserved in myopathies (see Table 599-1). A few specific clinical features are important in the diagnosis of some neuromuscular diseases. **Fasciculations** of muscle, which are often best seen in the tongue, are a sign of denervation. Sensory abnormalities indicate neuropathy. Fatigable weakness is characteristic of neuromuscular junctional disorders. Myotonia is specific for a few myopathies.

Some features do not distinguish myopathy from neuropathy. Muscle pain or **myalgias** are associated with acute disease of either myopathic or neurogenic origin. Acute dermatomyositis and acute polyneuropathy (Guillain-Barré syndrome) are characterized by myalgias. Muscular dystrophies and spinal muscular atrophies are not associated with muscle pain. Myalgias also occur in several metabolic diseases of muscle and in ischemic myopathy, including vascular diseases such as dermatomyositis. Myalgias denote the acuity, rather than the nature, of the process, so that progressive but chronic diseases, such as muscular dystrophy and spinal muscular atrophy, are not painful, but acute stages of inflammatory myopathies and acute denervation of muscle often do present muscular pain and tenderness to palpation. **Contractures** of muscles, whether present at birth or developing later in the course of an illness, occur in both myopathic and neurogenic diseases.

Infant boys who are weak in late fetal life and in the neonatal period often have **undescended testes**. The testes are actively pulled into the scrotum from the anterior abdominal wall by a pair of cords that consist of smooth and striated muscle called the gubernaculum. The gubernaculum is weakened in many congenital neuromuscular diseases, including spinal muscular atrophy, myotonic muscular dystrophy, and many congenital myopathies.

The thorax of infants with congenital neuromuscular disease often has a funnel shape, and the ribs are thin and radiolucent as a result of intercostal muscle weakness during intrauterine growth. This phenomenon is characteristically found in infantile spinal muscular atrophy but also occurs in myotubular myopathy, neonatal myotonic dystrophy, and other disorders (Fig. 599-1). Because of the small muscle mass, birth weight may be low for gestational age.

Generalized hypotonia and motor developmental delay are the most common presenting manifestations of neuromuscular disease in infants and young children (Table 599-2). These features can also be expressions of neurologic disease, endocrine and systemic metabolic diseases, and Down syndrome, or they may be nonspecific neuromuscular expressions of malnutrition or chronic systemic illness (Table 599-3). A prenatal history of decreased fetal movements and intrauterine growth retardation is often found in patients who are symptomatic at birth. Developmental disorders tend to be of slow onset and are progressive.

Acute flaccid paralysis in older infants and children has a different differential diagnosis (Table 599-4).

LABORATORY FINDINGS

Serum Enzymes

Several lysosomal enzymes are released by damaged or degenerating muscle fibers and may be measured in serum. The most useful of these enzymes is **creatine kinase (CK)**, which is found in only 3 organs and may be separated into corresponding isozymes: MM for skeletal muscle, MB for cardiac muscle, and BB for brain. Serum CK determination is not a universal screening test for neuromuscular disease because many diseases of the motor unit are not associated with elevated enzymes. The CK level is characteristically elevated in certain diseases, such as Duchenne muscular dystrophy, and the magnitude of increase is characteristic for particular diseases.

Molecular Genetic Markers

Many DNA markers of hereditary myopathies and neuropathies are available from blood samples. If the clinical manifestations suggest a particular disease, these tests can provide a definitive diagnosis and not subject the child to more-invasive procedures, such as muscle biopsy. Other molecular markers are available only in muscle biopsy tissue.

Nerve Conduction Velocity

Motor and sensory nerve conduction velocity (NCV) may be measured electrophysiologically by using surface electrodes. Neuropathies of various types are detected by decreased conduction.

Table 599-1 DISTINGUISHING FEATURES OF DISORDERS OF THE MOTOR SYSTEM

LOCUS OF LESION	WEAKNESS: Face	Arms	Legs	Proximal-Distal	DEEP TENDON REFLEXES	ELECTROMYOGRAPHY	MUSCLE BIOPSY	OTHER
Central	0	+	+	> or =	Normal or ↑	Normal	Normal	Seizures, hemiparesis, and delayed development
Ventral horn cell	Late	++++	++++	> or =	0	Fasciculations and fibrillations	Denervation pattern	Fasciculations (tongue)
Peripheral nerve	0	+++	+++	<	↓	Fibrillations	Denervation pattern	Sensory deficit, elevated cerebrospinal fluid protein, depressed nerve biopsy
Neuromuscular junction	+++	+++	+++	=	Normal	Decremental response (myasthenia); incremental response and BSAP (botulism)	Normal	Response to neostigmine or edrophonium (myasthenia); constipation and fixed pupils (botulism)
Muscle	Variable (+ to ++++)	++	+	>	↓	Short duration, small-amplitude motor unit potentials and myopathic polyphasic potentials	Myopathic pattern*	Elevated muscle enzyme levels (variable)

+ to ++++, varying degrees of severity; BSAP, brief duration, small amplitude, overly abundant motor unit potentials.
*Can also show unique features, such as in central core disease, nemaline myopathy, myotubular myopathy, and congenital fiber type disproportion.
From Volpe J: *Neurology of the newborn,* ed 4, Philadelphia, 2001, WB Saunders, p 706.

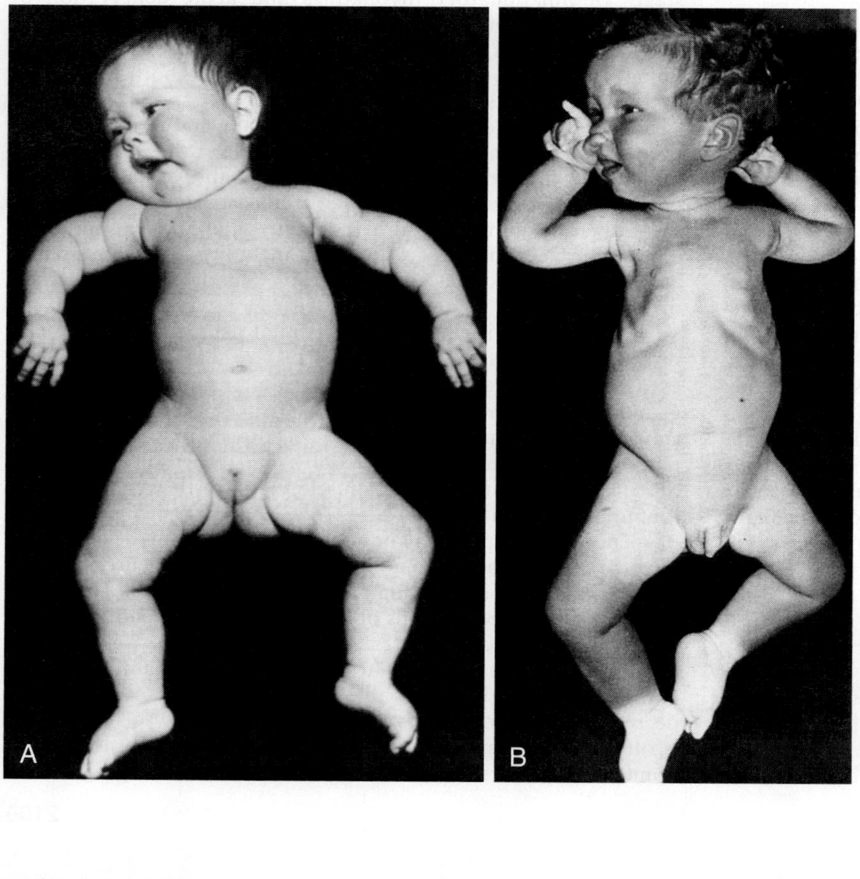

Figure 599-1 Type 1 spinal muscular atrophy (Werdnig-Hoffmann disease). Characteristic postures in 6 wk old *(A)* and 1 yr old *(B)* infants with severe weakness and hypotonia from birth. Note the frog-leg posture of the lower limbs and internal rotation ("jug handle") *(A)* or external rotation *(B)* at the shoulders. Note also intercostal recession, especially evident in *B,* and normal facial expressions. (From Volpe J: *Neurology of the newborn,* ed 4, Philadelphia, 2001, WB Saunders, p 645.)

Table 599-2 PATTERN OF WEAKNESS AND LOCALIZATION IN THE FLOPPY INFANT

ANATOMIC REGION OF HYPOTONIA	CORRESPONDING DISORDERS	PATTERN OF WEAKNESS AND INVOLVEMENT
Central nervous system	Chromosomal disorders Inborn errors of metabolism Cerebral dysgenesis Cerebral, spinal cord trauma	Central hypotonia Axial hypotonia more prominent Hyperactive reflexes
Motor neuron	Spinal muscular atrophy	Generalized weakness; often spares the diaphragm, facial muscles, pelvis, and sphincters
Nerve	Peripheral neuropathies	Distal muscle groups involved Weakness with wasting
Neuromuscular junction	Myasthenia syndromes Infantile botulism	Bulbar, oculomotor muscles exhibit greater degree of involvement
Muscle	Congenital myopathies Metabolic myopathies CMD Congenital myotonic dystrophy	Weakness is prominent Proximal musculature Hypoactive reflexes Joint contractures

CMD, congenital muscular dystrophy.
From Prasad AN, Prasad C: The floppy infant: contribution of genetic and metabolic disorders, *Brain Dev* 27:457–476, 2003.

The site of a traumatic nerve injury may also be localized. The nerve conduction at birth is about half of the mature value achieved by age 2 yr. Tables are available for normal values at various ages in infancy, including for preterm infants. Because the NCV study measures only the fastest conducting fibers in a nerve, 80% of the total nerve fibers must be involved before slowing in conduction is detected.

Electromyography

Electromyography (EMG) requires insertion of a needle into the belly of a muscle and recording the electric potentials in various states of contraction. It is less useful in pediatrics than in adult medicine, in part because of technical difficulties in recording these potentials in young children and in part because the best results require the patient's cooperation for full relaxation and maximal voluntary contraction of a muscle. Many children are too frightened to provide such cooperation. Characteristic EMG patterns distinguish denervation from myopathic involvement. The specific type of myopathy is not usually definitively diagnosed, but certain specialized myopathic conditions, such as myotonia, may be demonstrated. An EMG can transiently raise the serum CK level.

EMG combined with repetitive electrical stimulation of a motor nerve supplying a muscle to produce tetany is useful in demonstrating myasthenic decremental responses. Small muscles, such as the abductor digiti quinti of the hypothenar eminence, are used for such studies.

Imaging of Muscle

Ultrasonography, CT scans, and, more often, MRI are used to image muscle in many neuromuscular diseases. Although these methods are not always definitively diagnostic, in experienced hands, they provide a supplementary means of following the progression of disease over time. MRI is quite useful in identifying inflammatory myopathies of immune (dermatomyositis) or infectious (viral, bacterial, parasitic) origin. MRI is the study of choice to image the spinal cord or nerve roots and plexus (e.g., brachial plexus).

Muscle Biopsy

The muscle biopsy is the most important and specific diagnostic study of most neuromuscular disorders, if the definitive diagnosis of a hereditary disease is not provided by molecular genetic testing in blood. Not only are neurogenic and myopathic processes distinguished, but also the type of myopathy and specific enzymatic deficiencies may be determined. The vastus lateralis (quadriceps femoris) is the muscle that is most commonly sampled. The deltoid muscle should be avoided in most cases because it normally has a 60-80% predominance of type I fibers so that the distribution patterns of fiber types are difficult to recognize. Muscle biopsy is a simple outpatient procedure that may be performed under local anesthesia with or without femoral

Table 599-3 DIFFERENTIAL DIAGNOSIS OF INFANTILE HYPOTONIA

Cerebral hypotonia
- Benign congenital hypotonia
- Chromosome disorders
  - Prader-Willi syndrome
  - Trisomy
- Chronic nonprogressive encephalopathy
  - Cerebral malformation
  - Perinatal distress
  - Postnatal disorders
- Peroxisomal disorders
  - Cerebrohepatorenal syndrome (Zellweger syndrome)
  - Neonatal adrenoleukodystrophy
- Other genetic defects
  - Familial dysautonomia
  - Oculocerebrorenal syndrome (Lowe syndrome)
- Other metabolic defects
  - Acid maltase deficiency (see "Metabolic Myopathies")
  - Infantile G_{M_1} gangliodisosis

Spinal cord disorders

Spinal muscular atrophies
- Acute infantile
  - Autosomal dominant
  - Autosomal recessive
  - Cytochrome-*c* oxidase deficiency
  - X-linked
- Chronic infantile
  - Autosomal dominant
  - Autosomal recessive
  - Congenital cervical spinal muscular atrophy
  - Infantile neuronal degeneration
  - Neurogenic arthrogryposis

Polyneuropathies
- Congenital hypomyelinating neuropathy
- Giant axonal neuropathy
- Hereditary motor-sensory neuropathies

Disorders of neuromuscular transmission
- Familial infantile myasthenia
- Infantile botulism
- Transitory myasthenia gravis

Fiber-type disproportion myopathies
- Central core disease
- Congenital fiber-type disproportion myopathy
- Myotubular (centronuclear) myopathy
  - Acute
  - Chronic
- Nemaline (rode) myopathy
  - Autosomal dominant
  - Autosomal recessive

Metabolic myopathies
- Acid maltase deficiency
- Cytochrome-*c* oxidase deficiency

Muscular dystrophies
- Bethlem myopathy
- Congenital dystrophinopathy
- Congenital muscular dystrophy
  - Merosin deficiency primary
  - Merosin deficiency secondary
  - Merosin positive
- Congenital myotonic dystrophy

From Fenichel GM: The hypotonic infant. In *Clinical pediatric neurology: a signs and symptoms approach*, ed 5, Philadelphia, 2005, Saunders, p. 150.

Table 599-4 DIFFERENTIAL DIAGNOSIS OF ACUTE FLACCID PARALYSIS

Brainstem stroke
Brainstem encephalitis
Acute anterior poliomyelitis
• Caused by poliovirus
• Caused by other neurotropic viruses
Acute myelopathy
• Space-occupying lesions
• Acute transverse myelitis
Peripheral neuropathy
• Guillain-Barré syndrome
• Post–rabies vaccine neuropathy
• Diphtheritic neuropathy
• Heavy metals, biologic toxins, or drug intoxication
• Acute intermittent porphyria
• Vasculitic neuropathy
• Critical illness neuropathy
• Lymphomatous neuropathy
Disorders of neuromuscular transmission
• Myasthenia gravis
• Biologic or industrial toxins
• Tic paralysis
Disorders of muscle
• Hypokalemia
• Hypophosphatemia
• Inflammatory myopathy
• Acute rhabdomyolysis
• Trichinosis
• Periodic paralyses

From Hughes RAC, Camblath DR: Guillain-Barré syndrome, *Lancet* 366:1653–1666, 2005.

nerve block. Needle biopsies are preferred in some centers, but are not percutaneous and require an incision in the skin similar to open biopsy; numerous samples must be taken to conduct an adequate examination of the tissue, and they provide inferior specimens. The volume of tissue from a needle biopsy is usually not adequate for all required studies, including supplementary biochemical studies, such as mitochondrial respiratory chain enzymes; a small, clean, open biopsy is therefore advantageous.

Histochemical studies of frozen sections of the muscle are obligatory in all pediatric muscle biopsies because many congenital and metabolic myopathies cannot be diagnosed from paraffin sections using conventional histologic stains. Immunohistochemistry is a useful supplement in some cases, such as for demonstrating dystrophin in suspected Duchenne muscular dystrophy or merosin in congenital muscular dystrophy. A portion of the biopsy specimen should be fixed for potential electron microscopy, but ultrastructure has additional diagnostic value only in selected cases. Interpretation of muscle biopsy samples is complex and should be performed by an experienced pathologist. A portion of frozen muscle tissue should also be routinely saved for possible biochemical analysis (mitochondrial cytopathies, carnitine palmityltransferase, acid maltase).

Nerve Biopsy

The most commonly sampled nerve is the sural nerve, a pure sensory nerve that supplies a small area of skin on the lateral surface of the foot. Whole or fascicular biopsy specimens of this nerve may be taken. When the sural nerve is severed behind the lateral malleolus of the ankle, regeneration of the nerve occurs in >90% of cases, so that permanent sensory loss is not experienced. The sural nerve is often involved in many neuropathies whose clinical manifestations are predominantly motor.

Electron microscopy is performed on most nerve biopsy specimens because many morphologic alterations cannot be appreciated at the resolution of a light microscope. Teased fiber preparations are sometimes useful in demonstrating segmental demyelination, axonal swellings, and other specific abnormalities, but this time-consuming procedure is not done routinely. Special stains may be applied to ordinary frozen or paraffin sections of nerve biopsy material to demonstrate myelin, axoplasm, and metabolic products.

Electrocardiography

Cardiac evaluation is important if myopathy is suspected because of involvement of the heart in muscular dystrophies and in inflammatory and metabolic myopathies. Electrocardiography (ECG) often detects early cardiomyopathy or conduction defects that are clinically asymptomatic. At times, a more complete cardiac work-up, including echocardiography and consultation with a pediatric cardiologist, is indicated. Serial pulmonary function tests also should be performed in muscular dystrophies and in other chronic or progressive diseases of the motor unit.

BIBLIOGRAPHY

Please visit the Nelson Textbook of Pediatrics *website at* www.expertconsult.com *for the complete bibliography.*

Chapter 600
Developmental Disorders of Muscle

Harvey B. Sarnat

A heterogeneous group of congenital neuromuscular disorders is known as the **congenital myopathies,** but in some of these disorders, the assumption that the pathogenesis is primarily myopathic is unjustified. Most congenital myopathies are nonprogressive conditions, but some patients show slow clinical deterioration accompanied by additional changes in their muscle histology. Most of the diseases in the category of congenital myopathies are hereditary; others are sporadic. Although clinical features, including phenotype, can raise a strong suspicion of a congenital myopathy, the definitive diagnosis is determined by the histopathologic findings in the muscle biopsy specimen. In conditions for which the defective gene has been identified, the diagnosis may be established by the specific molecular analysis of the suspected gene expressed in lymphocytes. The morphologic and histochemical abnormalities differ considerably from those of the muscular dystrophies, spinal muscular atrophies, and neuropathies. Many are reminiscent of the embryologic development of muscle, thus suggesting possible defects in the genetic regulation of muscle development.

MYOGENIC REGULATORY GENES AND GENETIC LOCI OF INHERITED DISEASES OF MUSCLE

A family of four myogenic regulatory genes shares encoding transcription factors of "basic helix-loop-helix" (bHLH) proteins associated with common DNA nucleotide sequences (Table 600-1). These genes direct the differentiation of striated muscle from any undifferentiated mesodermal cell. The earliest bHLH gene to program the differentiation of myoblasts is myogenic factor 5 *(Myf5).* The second gene, *myogenin,* promotes fusion of myoblasts to form myotubes. *Herculin* (also known as *MYF6*) and *MYOD1* are the other two myogenic genes. *Myf5* cannot support myogenic differentiation without myogenin, *MyoD,* and *MYF6.* Each of these four genes can activate the expression of at least one other and, under certain circumstances, can autoactivate as well. The expression of *MYF5* and of *herculin* is transient in early ontogenesis but returns later in fetal life and persists into adult life. The human locus of the *MYOD1* gene is on chromosome 11, very near to the domain associated with embryonal rhabdomyosarcoma. The genes encoding *Myf5* and *herculin* are on chromosome 12 and that for *myogenin* is on chromosome 1.

The myogenic genes are activated during muscle regeneration, recapitulating the developmental process; *MyoD* in particular is required for myogenic stem cell (satellite cell) activation in adult

Table 600-1 INHERITANCE PATTERNS AND CHROMOSOMAL OR MITOCHONDRIAL LOCI OF NEUROMUSCULAR DISEASES AFFECTING THE PEDIATRIC AGE GROUP

DISEASE	TRANSMISSION	LOCUS
Duchenne and Becker muscular dystrophy	XR	Xp21.2
Emery-Dreifuss muscular dystrophy	XR	Xq28
Myotonic muscular dystrophy (Steinert)	AD	19q13
Facioscapulohumeral muscular dystrophy	AD	4q35
Limb-girdle muscular dystrophy	AD	5q
Limb-girdle muscular dystrophy	AR	15q
Congenital muscular dystrophy with merosin deficiency	AR	6q2
Congenital muscular dystrophy (Fukuyama)	AR	8q31-33
Myotubular myopathy	XR	Xq28
Myotubular myopathy	AR	Unknown
Nemaline rod myopathy (NEM1)	AD	1q21-q23
Nemaline rod myopathy (NEM2)	AR	2q21.2-q22
Nemaline rod myopathy (NEM3)	AD, AR	1q42.1
Nemaline rod myopathy (NEM4)	AD	9q13
Nemaline rod myopathy (NEM5)	AR	19q13
Congenital muscle fiber-type disproportion	AR, X-linked R	19p13.2, Xp23.12-p11.4, Xq13.1-q22.1; t(10; 17); sporadic
Central core disease	AD	19q13.1
Myotonia congenita (Thomsen)	AD	7q35
Myotonia congenita (Becker)	AR	7q35
Paramyotonia congenita	AD	17q13.1-13.3
Hyperkalemic periodic paralysis	AD	17q13.1-13.3
Hyperkalemic periodic paralysis	AD	1q31-q32
Glycogenosis II (Pompe; acid maltase deficiency)	AR	17q23
Glycogenosis V (McArdle; myophosphorylase deficiency)	AR	11q13
Glycogenosis VII (Tarui; phosphofructokinase deficiency)	AR	1cenq32
Glycogenosis IX (phosphoglycerate kinase deficiency)	XR	Xq13
Glycogenosis X (phosphoglycerate mutase deficiency)	AR	7p12-p13
Glycogenosis XI (lactate dehydrogenase deficiency)	AR	11p15.4
Muscle carnitine deficiency	AR	Unknown
Muscle carnitine palmityltransferase deficiency 2	AR	1p32
Spinal muscular atrophy (Werdnig-Hoffmann; Kugelberg-Welander)	AR	5q11-q13
Familial dysautonomia (Riley-Day)	AR	9q31-33
Hereditary motor-sensory neuropathy (Charcot-Marie-Tooth; Dejerine-Sottas)	AD	17p11.2
Hereditary motor-sensory neuropathy (axonal type)	AD	1p35-p36
Hereditary motor-sensory neuropathy (Charcot-Marie-Tooth-X)	XR	Xq13.1
Mitochondrial myopathy (Kearns-Sayre)	Maternal; sporadic	Single large mtDNA deletion
Mitochondrial myopathy (MERRF)	Maternal	tRNA point mutation at position 8344
Mitochondrial myopathy (MELAS)	Maternal	tRNA point mutation at positions 3243 and 3271

AD, autosomal dominant; AR, autosomal recessive; MELAS, mitochondrial encephalopathy lactic acidosis, and stroke; MERRF, myoclonic epilepsy with ragged-red fibers; mtDNA, mitochondrial deoxyribonucleic acid; tRNA, transfer ribonucleic acid; XR, X-linked recessive.

muscle. *PAX3* and *PAX7* genes also play an important role in myogenesis and interact with each of the four basic genes mentioned above. Another gene, *myostatin,* is a negative regulator of muscle development by preventing myocytes from differentiating. The precise role of the myogenic genes in developmental myopathies is not yet fully defined.

Satellite cells in mature muscle that mediate regeneration have the same somitic origin as embryonic muscle progenitor cells, but the genes that regulate them differ. *Pax3* and *Pax7* mediate the migration of primitive myoblast progenitors from the myotomes of the somites to their peripheral muscle sites in the embryo, but only one of two *Pax7* genes continues to act postnatally for satellite cell survival. Then it, too, no longer is required after the juvenile period for muscle satellite (i.e., stem) cells to become activated for muscle regeneration.

BIBLIOGRAPHY

Please visit the Nelson Textbook of Pediatrics *website at www.expertconsult.com for the complete bibliography.*

600.1 Myotubular Myopathy

Harvey B. Sarnat

The term **myotubular myopathy** implies a maturational arrest of fetal muscle during the myotubular stage of development at 8-15 wk of gestation. It is based on the morphologic appearance of myofibers: A row of central nuclei lies within a core of cytoplasm; contractile myofibrils form a cylinder around this core (Fig. 600-1). Many challenge this interpretation and use the more neutral term **centronuclear myopathy** when referring to this myopathy. This term is nonspecific because internal nuclei occur in many unrelated myopathies.

PATHOGENESIS

The molecular mechanism appears similar in the X-linked recessive and autosomal recessive forms of myotubular myopathy. The common pathogenesis involves loss of myotubularin protein,

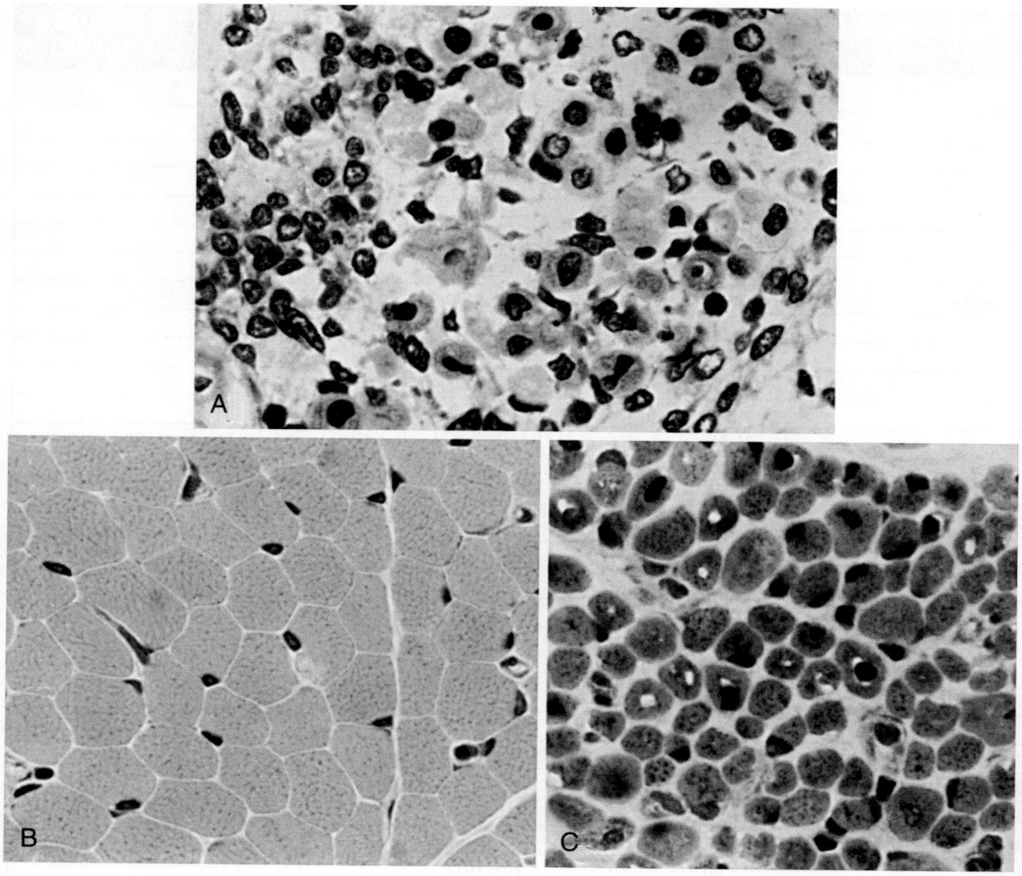

Figure 600-1 Cross section of muscle from a 14 wk old human fetus *(A),* a normal full-term neonate *(B),* and a term neonate with X-linked recessive myotubular myopathy *(C).* Myofibers have large central nuclei in the fetus and in myotubular myopathy, and nuclei are at the periphery of the muscle fiber in the term neonate as in the adult (H&E, ×500).

leading to structural and functional abnormalities in the organization of T-tubules and sarcoplasmic reticulum and defective excitation-contraction coupling. This pathogenesis also provides a link to central core and multicore and minicore myopathies to at least partially explain the clinical and histopathologic similarities of these different congenital myopathies.

Persistently high fetal concentrations of vimentin and desmin are demonstrated in myofibers of infants with myotubular myopathy, although not reproduced in cultured myocytes of patients. These intermediate filament proteins serve as cytoskeletal elements in fetal myotubes, attaching nuclei and mitochondria to the sarcolemmal membranes to preserve their central positions. As intracellular organization changes with maturation, the nuclei move to the periphery and mitochondria are redistributed between myofibrils. At the same time, vimentin and desmin diminish. Vimentin disappears altogether by term, and desmin remains only in trace amounts. Persistent fetal vimentin and desmin in muscle fibers may be one mechanism of "maturational arrest." A secondary myasthenia-like defect in neuromuscular transmission also occurs in some infants with myotubular myopathy. Myocytes of patients co-cultured with nerve in vitro develop normal innervation and mature normally, not reproducing the in vivo pathologic changes.

The defective gene of the X-linked form and 3 genes of the autosomal recessive form are known.

CLINICAL MANIFESTATIONS

Fetal movements can decrease in late gestation. Polyhydramnios is a common complication because of pharyngeal weakness of the fetus and inability to swallow amniotic fluid.

At birth, affected infants have a thin muscle mass involving axial, limb girdle, and distal muscles; severe generalized hypotonia; and diffuse weakness. Respiratory efforts may be ineffective, requiring ventilatory support. Gavage feeding may be required because of weakness of the muscles of sucking and deglutition. The testes are often undescended. Facial muscles may be weak, but infants do not have the characteristic facies of myotonic dystrophy. Ptosis may be a prominent feature. Ophthalmoplegia is observed in a few cases. The palate may be high. The tongue is thin, but fasciculations are not seen. Tendon stretch reflexes are weak or absent.

Myotubular myopathy is not associated with cardiomyopathy (mature cardiac muscle fibers normally have central nuclei), but one report describes complete AV block without cardiomyopathy in a patient with confirmed X-linked myotubular myopathy. Congenital anomalies of the central nervous system or of other systems are not associated. A single patient with progressive dementia was reported, who had a mutation removing the start signal of exon 2.

Older children and adults can develop centronuclear myopathy with variable weakness. The relation of this disorder to the severe neonatal disease is uncertain.

LABORATORY FINDINGS

Serum levels of creatine kinase (CK) are normal. Electromyography (EMG) does not show evidence of denervation; results are usually normal or show minimal nonspecific myopathic features in early infancy. Nerve conduction velocity may be slow but is usually normal. The electrocardiogram (ECG) appears normal. Chest radiographs show no cardiomegaly; the ribs may be thin.

DIAGNOSIS

The muscle biopsy findings are diagnostic at birth, even in premature infants. More than 90% of muscle fibers are small and have centrally placed, large vesicular nuclei in a single row. Spaces between nuclei are filled with sarcoplasm containing

Table 600-2 SPECIFIC CONGENITAL MYOPATHIES: DISTINGUISHING CLINICAL FEATURES

MYOPATHY	NEONATAL HYPOTONIA AND WEAKNESS	SEVERE FORM WITH NEONATAL DEATH	FACIAL WEAKNESS	PTOSIS	EXTRAOCULAR MUSCULAR WEAKNESS
Central core disease	+	0	±	0	0
Nemaline myopathy	+	+	+	0	0
Myotubular myopathy	+	+	+	+	+
Congenital fiber type disproportion	+	±	±	0	+

+, often a prominent feature; ±, variably a prominent feature; 0, not a prominent feature.
From Volpe JJ: *Neurology of the newborn,* ed 5, Philadelphia, 2008, Elsevier Saunders, p 820.

mitochondria. Histochemical stains for oxidative enzymatic activity and glycogen reveal a central distribution as in fetal myotubes. The cylinder of myofibrils shows mature histochemical differentiation with adenosine triphosphatase stains. The connective tissue of muscle spindles, blood vessels, intramuscular nerves, and motor end plates are mature. Ultrastructural features in neonatal myotubular myopathy, other than those that define the disease, are also mature. Vimentin and desmin show strong immunoreactivity in muscle fibers in myotubular myopathy and no demonstrable activity in normal term neonatal muscle. The molecular genetic marker in blood is available and is useful not only for confirming the diagnosis but also for early prenatal diagnosis. The differentiation from other forms of congenital myopathy is noted in Table 600-2.

GENETICS

X-linked recessive inheritance is the most common trait in this disease affecting boys. The mothers of affected infants are clinically asymptomatic, but their muscle biopsy specimens show minor alterations. Genetic linkage on the X chromosome has been localized to the Xq28 site, a locus different from the Xp21 gene of Duchenne and Becker muscular dystrophies. A deletion in the responsible *MTM1* gene has been identified. It encodes a protein called myotubularin. This gene belongs to a family of similar genes encoding enzymatically active and inactive forms of phosphatidylinositol-3-phosphatases that form dimers. The pathogenesis is in the regulation of enzymatic activity and binding to other proteins induced by dimer interactions. Although only a single gene is involved, 5 distinct point mutations of the *MTM1* gene out of 242 known mutations account for only 27% of cases; many different alleles can produce the same clinical disease. Other **rarer centronuclear myopathies** also are known, some being autosomal dominant or recessive and affecting both sexes and others being sporadic and of unknown genetics. The recessive forms are sometimes divided into an early-onset form with or without ophthalmoplegia and a late-onset form without ophthalmoplegia. Autosomal dominant forms are usually mild and might not manifest clinically until adult life as diffuse, slowly progressive weakness and generalized muscular pseudohypertrophy.

TREATMENT

Only supportive and palliative treatment is available. Progressive scoliosis may be treated by long posterior fusion.

PROGNOSIS

About 75% of severely affected neonates die within the first few weeks or months of life. Survivors do not experience a progressive course but have major physical handicaps, rarely walk, and remain severely hypotonic.

BIBLIOGRAPHY
Please visit the Nelson Textbook of Pediatrics *website at* www.expertconsult.com *for the complete bibliography.*

600.2 Congenital Muscle Fiber-Type Disproportion

Harvey B. Sarnat

Congenital muscle fiber-type disproportion (CMFTD) occurs as an isolated congenital myopathy but also develops in association with various unrelated disorders that include nemaline rod disease, Krabbe disease (globoid cell leukodystrophy) early in the course before expression of the neuropathy, cerebellar hypoplasia and certain other brain malformations, fetal alcohol syndrome, some glycogenoses, multiple sulfatase deficiency, Lowe syndrome, rigid spine myopathy, and some infantile cases of myotonic muscular dystrophy. CMFTD should therefore be regarded as a syndrome, unless a specific genetic mutation is confirmed.

PATHOGENESIS

The association of CMFTD with cerebellar hypoplasia suggests that the pathogenesis may be an abnormal suprasegmental influence on the developing motor unit during the stage of histochemical differentiation of muscle between 20 and 28 wk of gestation. Muscle fiber types and growth are determined by innervation and are mutable even in adults. Although CMFTD does not actually correspond with any normal stage of development, it appears to be an embryologic disturbance of fiber type differentiation and growth.

CLINICAL MANIFESTATIONS

As an isolated condition not associated with other diseases, CMFTD is a nonprogressive disorder present at birth. Patients have generalized hypotonia and weakness, but the weakness is usually not severe and respiratory distress and dysphagia are rare. Contractures are present at birth in 25% of patients. Poor head control and developmental delay for gross motor skills are common in infancy. Walking is usually delayed until 18-24 mo but is eventually achieved. Because of the hypotonia, subluxation of the hips can occur. Muscle bulk is reduced. The muscle wasting and hypotonia are proportionately greater than the weakness, and the child may be stronger than expected during examination. Cardiomyopathy is a rare complication.

The facies of children with CMFTD often raise suspicion, especially if the child is referred for assessment of developmental delay and hypotonia. The head is dolichocephalic, and facial weakness is present. The palate is usually high arched. Thin muscles of the trunk and extremities give a thin, wasted appearance. The phenotype is very similar to that of nemaline myopathy that also includes CMFTD as part of the pathological picture. Patients do not complain of myalgias. The clinical course is nonprogressive.

LABORATORY FINDINGS

Serum CK, ECG, EMG, and nerve conduction velocity results are normal in simple CMFTD. If other diseases are associated, laboratory investigation of those conditions discloses the specific features.

DIAGNOSIS

CMFTD is diagnosed by muscle biopsy that shows disproportion in size and relative ratios of histochemical fiber types: Type I fibers are uniformly small, and type II fibers are hypertrophic; type I fibers are more numerous than type II fibers. Degeneration of myofibers and other primary myopathic features are absent. The biopsy is diagnostic at birth. Differentiating features from other congenital myopathies are noted in Table 600-2.

GENETICS

Many cases of simple CMFTD are sporadic, although autosomal recessive inheritance is well documented in some families and an autosomal dominant trait is suspected in others. The genetic basis is heterogeneous in hereditary forms; a mutation in the insulin receptor gene at 19p13.2 is reported. Translocation t(10;17) was seen in one family. X-linked transmission with linkage to Xp23.12-p11.4 and Xq13.1-q22.1 also is described. In 3 unrelated families with CMFTD, a heterozygous missense mutation of the skeletal muscle α-actin gene (*ACTA1*) was demonstrated, but this genetic defect represents a minority; mutations in *TPM3* is a more common genetic mutation. Whether these genes affect striated muscle directly or they mediate their expression through motor neurons remains uncertain. In CMFTD associated with cerebellar hypoplasia, the genetic effect is on cerebellar development and the muscular expression is secondary.

TREATMENT

No drug therapy is available. Physiotherapy may be helpful for some patients in strengthening muscles that do not receive sufficient exercise in daily activities. Mild congenital contractures often respond well to gentle range-of-motion exercises and rarely require plaster casting or surgery.

BIBLIOGRAPHY

Please visit the Nelson Textbook of Pediatrics *website at www.expertconsult.com for the complete bibliography.*

600.3 Nemaline Rod Myopathy

Harvey B. Sarnat

Nemaline rods (derived from the Greek *nema,* meaning "thread") are rod-shaped, inclusion-like abnormal structures within muscle fibers. They are difficult to demonstrate histologically with conventional hematoxylin-eosin stain but are easily seen with special stains. They are not foreign inclusion bodies but rather consist of excessive Z-band material with a similar ultrastructure (Fig. 600-2). Chemically, the rods are composed of actin, α-actinin, tropomyosin-3, and the protein nebulin. Nemaline rod formation may be an unusual reaction of muscle fibers to injury because these rod structures have rarely been found in other diseases. They are most abundant in the congenital myopathy known as *nemaline rod disease.* Most rods are within the myofibrils (cytoplasmic), but intranuclear rods are occasionally demonstrated by electron microscopy.

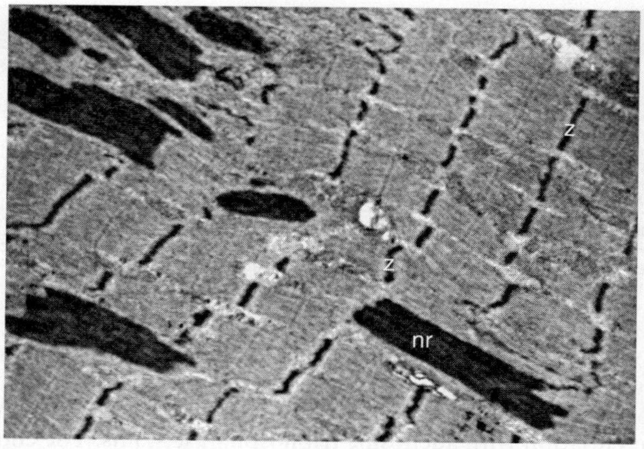

Figure 600-2 Electron micrograph of the muscle from a patient shown in Figure 600-4. Nemaline rods *(nr)* are seen within many myofibrils. They are identical in composition to the normal Z bands *(z)* (×6,000).

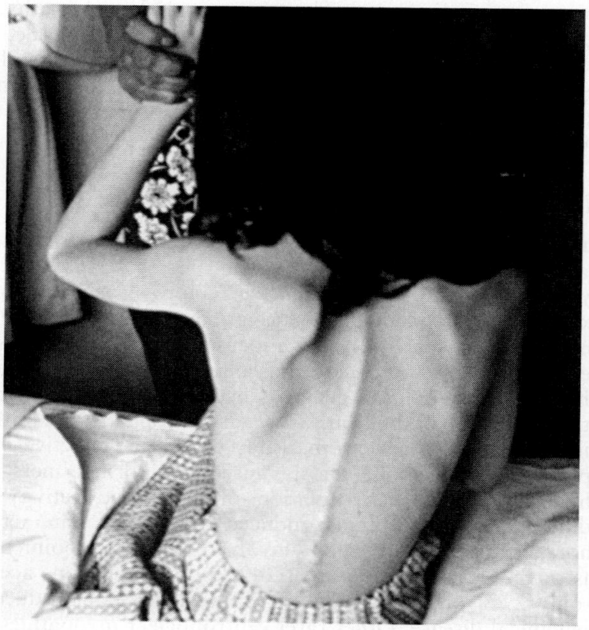

Figure 600-3 Back of a 13 yr old girl with the juvenile form of nemaline rod disease. The paraspinal muscles are very thin, and winging of the scapulas is evident. The muscle mass of the extremities is also greatly reduced proximally and distally.

CLINICAL MANIFESTATIONS

Neonatal, infantile, and juvenile forms of the disease are known. The neonatal form is severe and usually fatal because of respiratory failure since birth. In the infantile form, generalized hypotonia and weakness, which can include bulbar-innervated and respiratory muscles, and a very thin muscle mass are characteristic (Fig. 600-3). The head is dolichocephalic, and the palate high arched or even cleft. Muscles of the jaw may be too weak to hold it closed (Fig. 600-4). Decreased fetal movements are reported by the mother, and neonates suffer from hypoxia and dysphagia; arthrogryposis may be present. Infants with severe neonatal and infantile nemaline myopathy have facies and phenotype that are nearly indistinguishable from those of neonatal myotonic dystrophy, but their mothers have normal facies. The juvenile form is the mildest and is not associated with respiratory failure, but the phenotype, including facial involvement, is similar.

LABORATORY FINDINGS

Serum CK level is normal or mildly elevated. The muscle biopsy is diagnostic. In addition to the characteristic nemaline rods, it also shows CMFTD or at least fiber type I predominance. In some patients, uniform type I fibers are seen with few or no type II fibers. Focal myofibrillar degeneration and an increase in lysosomal enzymes have been found in a few severe cases

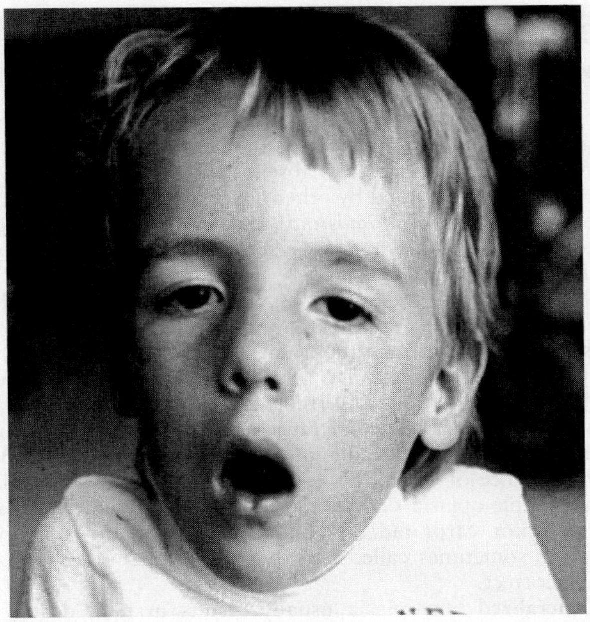

Figure 600-4 Infantile form of nemaline rod disease in a 6 yr old boy. Facial weakness and generalized muscle wasting are severe. The head is dolichocephalic. The mouth is usually open because the masseters are too weak to lift the mandible against gravity for more than a few seconds.

associated with progressive symptoms. Intranuclear nemaline rods correlate with the most severe clinical manifestations. They are demonstrated by electron microscopy. Because nemaline bodies can occur in other myopathies, their presence in the muscle biopsy is not pathognomonic in the absence of the supportive clinical manifestations. Adult-onset cases may be associated with monoclonal gammopathy.

GENETICS

Autosomal dominant and autosomal recessive forms of nemaline rod disease occur, and an X-linked dominant form in girls also can occur. Five genes are associated with this condition. One autosomal dominant nemaline rod myopathy (NEM1) has been mapped to the 1q21-23 locus; the responsible *TPM3* gene produces defective α-tropomyosin. Another genetic mutation (NEM2) at the 2q21.2-q22 locus produces *nebulin,* a large molecule also needed for Z-band integrity, and is transmitted as an autosomal recessive trait, particularly in Ashkenazi Jews. Nebulin defects account for half the total cases of nemaline myopathy. NEM3 is due to an α-actin defect and both autosomal dominant and recessive varieties occur at the same 1q42.1 locus. NEM4 is an autosomal dominantly inherited defect of β-tropomyosin at 9q13. The α- and β-tropomyosin defects are rare and account for only 3% of patients with nemaline myopathy. NEM5 is an autosomal recessive troponin-T defect at 19q13, but it has been found only in the Amish population; in the Amish community the incidence of nemaline myopathy is as high as 1:500, whereas in Australia it is estimated at 1:500,000. The myopathy occurs in all ethnic groups.

TREATMENT AND PROGNOSIS

Therapy is supportive. Survivors are confined to an electric wheelchair and are usually unable to overcome gravity. Both proximal and distal muscles are involved. Congenital arthrogryposis can occur and predicts a poor prognosis. Gastrostomy may be needed for chronic dysphagia. In the juvenile form, patients are ambulatory and are able to perform most tasks of daily living. Weakness is not usually progressive, but some patients have more difficulty over time or enter a phase of progressive weakness. Cardiomyopathy is an uncommon complication. Death usually results from respiratory insufficiency, with or without superimposed pneumonia.

BIBLIOGRAPHY

Please visit the Nelson Textbook of Pediatrics *website at www.expertconsult.com for the complete bibliography.*

600.4 Central Core, Minicore, and Multicore Myopathies

Harvey B. Sarnat

Central core myopathies are transmitted as either an autosomal dominant or recessive trait and are caused by the same abnormal gene at the 19q13.1 locus. The gene programs the ryanodine receptor *(RYR1),* a tetramere receptor to a non–voltage-gated calcium channel in the sarcoplasmic reticulum. Mutations in this gene are also the cause of malignant hyperthermia. Infantile hypotonia, proximal weakness, muscle wasting, and involvement of facial muscles and neck flexors are the typical features in both the dominant and recessive forms. Contractures of the knees, hips, and other joints are common, and kyphoscoliosis and pes cavus often develop, even without much axial or distal muscle weakness. There is a high incidence of cardiac abnormalities. The course is not progressive, except for the contractures.

The disease is characterized pathologically by central cores within muscle fibers in which only amorphous, granular cytoplasm is found with an absence of myofibrils and organelles. Histochemical stains show a lack of enzymatic activities of all types within these cores. The serum CK value is normal in central core disease except during crises of malignant hyperthermia (Chapter 603.2). Central core disease is consistently associated with malignant hyperthermia, which can precede the diagnosis of central core disease. All patients should have special precautions with pretreatment by dantrolene before an anesthetic agent is administered.

Variants of central cores, called *minicores* and *multicores,* are described in some families, but minicore myopathy is a different genetic disease without gender bias. Cases with a similar mutation in the *RYR1* gene are reported; others have a defective selenoprotein-N *(SEPN1)* gene, the latter also implicated in rigid spine myopathy, but together these 2 genes account for only half of patients genetically tested. Children with this disorder are hypotonic in early infancy and have a benign course but often develop progressive kyphoscoliosis or a rigid spine in adolescence. Distal joint hypermobility is another finding, particularly in ryanodine-mediated minicore myopathy. In one variant, external ophthalmoplegia also is present. Rare cases of minicore myopathy also show hypertrophic cardiomyopathy associated with short chain acyl-CoA dehydrogenase deficiency.

Preliminary trials of salbutamol therapy for central core and minicore myopathy suggest a potentially effective treatment.

BIBLIOGRAPHY

Please visit the Nelson Textbook of Pediatrics *website at www.expertconsult.com for the complete bibliography.*

600.5 Myofibrillar Myopathies

Harvey B. Sarnat

Most myofibrillar myopathies are not symptomatic in childhood, but occasionally older children and adolescents show early symptoms of nonspecific proximal and distal weakness. An infantile form also occurs and can cause mild neonatal hypotonia and weakness with disproportionately severe dysphagia and

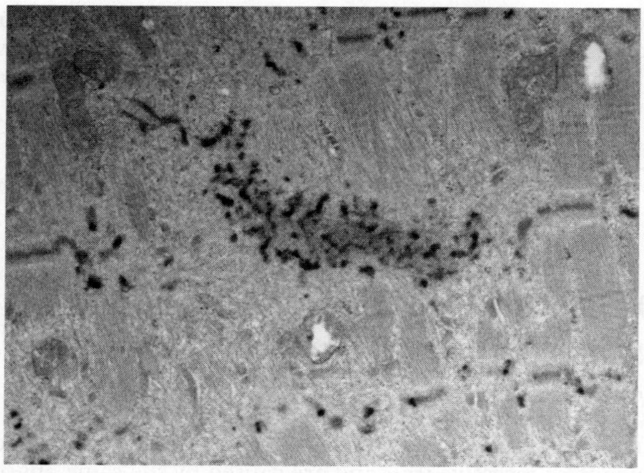

Figure 600-5 Electron micrograph (EM) of quadriceps femoris muscle biopsy of a 1-month-old native girl with Cree myofibrillar myopathy. Within the same myofiber, some sarcomeres are well formed and others exhibit disarray of the thick and thin myofilaments and fragmentation of Z-bands. Mitochondria appear normal (×21,400).

respiratory insufficiency, at times leading to early death. It is not progressive, however, and some patients show improvement in later infancy and early childhood, acquiring the ability to swallow by 3 yr of age. Cardiomyopathy is a complication in a minority. The diagnosis is by muscle biopsy: some sarcomeres of myofibers have disorganization or dissolution of myofibrils adjacent to other areas of normal sarcomeres within the same fiber. These zones are associated with streaming of the Z-bands and focally increased desmin intermediate filaments, myotilin, and αB-crystallin. Immunocytochemical and ultrastructural study of the muscle biopsy tissue is required. Mutation in the desmin gene is implicated as the etiology. An associated mitochondrial defect is detected in some patients.

A unique autosomal recessive myopathy in Cree native infants is characterized by severe generalized muscular hypertonia that is not relieved by neuromuscular blockade, hence is myopathic in origin. Most die in infancy of respiratory insufficiency due to diaphragmatic involvement. The muscle biopsy shows findings similar to many other myofibrillar myopathies (Fig. 600-5).

600.6 Brain Malformations and Muscle Development

Harvey B. Sarnat

Infants with **cerebellar hypoplasia** are hypotonic and developmentally delayed, especially in gross motor skills. Muscle biopsy is sometimes performed to exclude a congenital myopathy. A biopsy specimen can show delayed maturation of muscle, fiber-type predominance, or CMFTD. Other malformations of the brain may also be associated with abnormal histochemical patterns, but supratentorial lesions are less likely than brainstem or cerebellar lesions to alter muscle development. Abnormal descending impulses along bulbospinal pathways probably alter discharge patterns of lower motor neurons that determine the histochemical differentiation of muscle at 20-28 wk of gestation. The corticospinal tract does not participate because it is not yet functional during this period of fetal life. In several congenital muscular dystrophies, including the Walker-Warburg syndrome, Fukuyama disease, and muscle-eye-brain disease of Santavuori, major cerebral malformations, such as pachygyria and lissencephaly, are present.

BIBLIOGRAPHY

Please visit the Nelson Textbook of Pediatrics *website at* *www.expertconsult.com* *for the complete bibliography.*

600.7 Amyoplasia

Harvey B. Sarnat

Congenital absence of individual muscles is common and is often asymmetric. A common aplasia is the *palmaris longus muscle* of the ventral forearm, which is absent in 30% of normal subjects and is fully compensated by other flexors of the wrist. Unilateral absence of a *sternocleidomastoid muscle* is one cause of congenital torticollis. Absence of one *pectoralis major muscle* is part of the **Poland anomalad.**

When innervation does not develop, as in the lower limbs in severe cases of *myelomeningocele,* muscles can fail to develop. In *sacral agenesis,* the abnormal somites that fail to form bony vertebrae can also fail to form muscles from the same defective mesodermal plate, a disorder of induction resulting in segmental amyoplasia. Skeletal muscles of the extremities fail to differentiate from embryonic myomeres if the long bones do not form. Absence of 1 long bone, such as the radius, is associated with variable aplasia or hypoplasia of associated muscles, such as the flexor carpi radialis. End-stage neurogenic atrophy of muscle is sometimes called **amyoplasia,** but this use is semantically incorrect.

Generalized amyoplasia usually results in fetal death, and liveborn neonates rarely survive. A mutation in 1 of the myogenic genes is the suspected etiology because of genetic knockout studies in mice, but it has not been proven in humans.

600.8 Muscular Dysgenesis (Proteus Syndrome Myopathy)

Harvey B. Sarnat

Proteus syndrome is a disturbance of cellular growth involving ectodermal and mesodermal tissues. The cause is unknown, but it is not a mendelian trait. It manifests as asymmetric overgrowth of the extremities, verrucous cutaneous lesions, angiomas of various types, thickening of bones, syndromic hemimegalencephaly, and excessive growth of muscles without weakness. Severe seizures, beginning in neonates, are uncommon. Histologically, the muscle demonstrates a unique *muscular dysgenesis.* Abnormal zones are adjacent to zones of normal muscle formation and do not follow anatomic boundaries.

600.9 Benign Congenital Hypotonia

Harvey B. Sarnat

Benign congenital hypotonia is not a disease, but it is a descriptive term for infants or children with nonprogressive hypotonia of unknown origin. The hypotonia is not usually associated with weakness or developmental delay, although some children acquire gross motor skills more slowly than normal. Tendon stretch reflexes are normal or hypoactive. There are no cranial nerve abnormalities, and intelligence is normal.

The **diagnosis** is one of exclusion after results of laboratory studies, including muscle biopsy and imaging of the brain with special attention to the cerebellum, are normal (see Table 599-2). No known molecular genetic basis for this syndrome has been identified. The differential diagnosis is noted in Table 599-3.

The **prognosis** is generally good; no specific therapy is required. Contractures do not develop. Physical therapy might help achieve motor milestones (walking) sooner than expected. Hypotonia persists into adult life. The disorder is not always as "benign" as its name implies because a common complication is recurrent dislocation of joints, especially the shoulders. Excessive motility of the spine can result in stretch injury, compression, or vascular compromise of nerve roots or of the spinal cord. These are particular hazards for patients who perform gymnastics or who become circus performers because of agility of joints without weakness or pain.

BIBLIOGRAPHY
Please visit the Nelson Textbook of Pediatrics *website at www.expertconsult.com for the complete bibliography.*

600.10 Arthrogryposis

Harvey B. Sarnat

Arthrogryposis multiplex congenita is not a disease but is a descriptive term that signifies numerous congenital contractures (Chapter 674).

Chapter 601 Muscular Dystrophies

Harvey B. Sarnat

The term dystrophy means abnormal growth, derived from the Greek *trophe,* meaning "nourishment." A muscular dystrophy is distinguished from all other neuromuscular diseases by four obligatory criteria: It is a primary myopathy, it has a genetic basis, the course is progressive, and degeneration and death of muscle fibers occur at some stage in the disease. This definition excludes neurogenic diseases such as spinal muscular atrophy, nonhereditary myopathies such as dermatomyositis, nonprogressive, and non-necrotizing congenital myopathies such as congenital muscle fiber-type disproportion (CMFTD), and nonprogressive inherited metabolic myopathies. Some metabolic myopathies can fulfill the definition of a progressive muscular dystrophy but are not traditionally classified as dystrophies (muscle carnitine deficiency).

All muscular dystrophies might eventually be reclassified as metabolic myopathies once the biochemical defects are better defined. Muscular dystrophies are a group of unrelated diseases, each transmitted by a different genetic trait and each differing in its clinical course and expression. Some are severe diseases at birth that lead to early death; others follow very slow progressive courses over many decades, may be compatible with normal longevity, and might not even become symptomatic until late adult life. Some categories of dystrophies, such as limb-girdle muscular dystrophy (LGMD), are not homogeneous diseases but rather syndromes encompassing several distinct myopathies. Relationships among the various muscular dystrophies are resolved by molecular genetics rather than by similarities or differences in clinical and histopathologic features.

BIBLIOGRAPHY
Please visit the Nelson Textbook of Pediatrics *website at www.expertconsult.com for the complete bibliography.*

601.1 Duchenne and Becker Muscular Dystrophies

Harvey B. Sarnat

Duchenne muscular dystrophy (DMD) is the most common hereditary neuromuscular disease affecting all races and ethnic groups. Its characteristic clinical features are progressive weakness, intellectual impairment, hypertrophy of the calves, and proliferation of connective tissue in muscle. The incidence is 1:3,600 liveborn infant boys. This disease is inherited as an X-linked recessive trait. The abnormal gene is at the Xp21 locus and is one of the largest genes. **Becker muscular dystrophy** (BMD) is a fundamentally similar disease as DMD, with a genetic defect at the same locus, but clinically it follows a milder and more protracted course.

CLINICAL MANIFESTATIONS

Infant boys are only rarely symptomatic at birth or in early infancy, although some are mildly hypotonic. Early gross motor skills, such as rolling over, sitting, and standing, are usually achieved at the appropriate ages or may be mildly delayed. Poor head control in infancy may be the first sign of weakness. Distinctive facies are not an early feature because facial muscle weakness is a late event; in later childhood, a "transverse" or horizontal smile may be seen. Walking is often accomplished at the normal age of about 12 mo, but hip girdle weakness may be seen in subtle form as early as the 2nd year. Toddlers might assume a lordotic posture when standing to compensate for gluteal weakness. An early Gowers sign is often evident by age 3 yr and is fully expressed by age 5 or 6 yr (see Fig. 584-5). A Trendelenburg gait, or hip waddle, appears at this time. Common presentations in toddlers include delayed walking, falling, toe walking and trouble running or walking upstairs, developmental delay, and, less often, malignant hyperthermia after anesthesia.

The length of time a patient remains ambulatory varies greatly. Some patients are confined to a wheelchair by 7 yr of age; most patients continue to walk with increasing difficulty until age 10 yr without orthopedic intervention. With orthotic bracing, physiotherapy, and sometimes minor surgery (Achilles tendon lengthening), most are able to walk until age 12 yr. Ambulation is important not only for postponing the psychologic depression that accompanies the loss of an aspect of personal independence but also because scoliosis usually does not become a major complication as long as a patient remains ambulatory, even for as little as 1 hr per day; scoliosis often becomes rapidly progressive after confinement to a wheelchair.

The relentless progression of **weakness** continues into the 2nd decade. The function of distal muscles is usually relatively well enough preserved, allowing the child to continue to use eating utensils, a pencil, and a computer keyboard. Respiratory muscle involvement is expressed as a weak and ineffective cough, frequent pulmonary infections, and decreasing respiratory reserve. Pharyngeal weakness can lead to episodes of aspiration, nasal regurgitation of liquids, and an airy or nasal voice quality. The function of the extraocular muscles remains well preserved. Incontinence due to anal and urethral sphincter weakness is an uncommon and very late event.

Contractures most often involve the ankles, knees, hips, and elbows. **Scoliosis** is common. The thoracic deformity further compromises pulmonary capacity and compresses the heart. Scoliosis usually progresses more rapidly after the child becomes nonambulatory and may be uncomfortable or painful. Enlargement of the calves (pseudohypertrophy) and wasting of thigh muscles are classic features. The enlargement is caused by hypertrophy of some muscle fibers, infiltration of muscle by fat, and proliferation of collagen. After the calves, the next most common site of muscular hypertrophy is the tongue, followed by muscles of the forearm. Fasciculations of the tongue do not occur. The voluntary sphincter muscles rarely become involved.

Unless ankle contractures are severe, ankle deep tendon reflexes remain well preserved until terminal stages. The knee deep tendon reflexes may be present until about 6 yr of age but are less brisk than the ankle jerks and are eventually lost. In the upper extremities, the brachioradialis reflex is usually stronger than the biceps or triceps brachii reflexes.

Cardiomyopathy, including persistent tachycardia and myocardial failure, is seen in 50-80% of patients with this disease. The severity of cardiac involvement does not necessarily correlate with the degree of skeletal muscle weakness. Some patients die early of severe cardiomyopathy while still ambulatory; others in terminal stages of the disease have well-compensated cardiac function. Smooth muscle dysfunction, particularly of the gastrointestinal (GI) tract, is a minor, but often overlooked, feature.

Intellectual impairment occurs in all patients, although only 20-30% have an IQ <70. The majority have learning disabilities that still allow them to function in a regular classroom, particularly with remedial help. A few patients are profoundly mentally retarded, but there is no correlation with the severity of the myopathy. Epilepsy is slightly more common than in the general pediatric population. Dystrophin is expressed in brain and retina, as well as in striated and cardiac muscle, though the level is lower in brain than in muscle. This distribution might explain some of the central nervous system (CNS) manifestations. Abnormalities in cortical architecture and of dendritic arborization may be detected neuropathologically; cerebral atrophy is demonstrated by MRI late in the clinical course. The degenerative changes and fibrosis of muscle constitute a painless process. Myalgias and muscle spasms do not occur. Calcinosis of muscle is rare.

Death occurs usually at about 18-20 yr of age. The causes of death are respiratory failure in sleep, intractable heart failure, pneumonia, or occasionally aspiration and airway obstruction.

In **Becker muscular dystrophy,** boys remain ambulatory until late adolescence or early adult life. Calf pseudohypertrophy, cardiomyopathy, and elevated serum levels of creatine kinase (CK) are similar to those of patients with DMD. Learning disabilities are less common. The onset of weakness is later in Becker than in DMD. Death often occurs in the mid to late 20s; fewer than half of patients are still alive by age 40 yr; these survivors are severely disabled.

LABORATORY FINDINGS

The serum CK level is consistently greatly elevated in DMD, even in presymptomatic stages, including at birth. The usual serum concentration is 15,000-35,000 IU/L (normal <160 IU/L). A normal serum CK level is incompatible with the diagnosis of DMD, although in terminal stages of the disease, the serum CK value may be considerably lower than it was a few years earlier because there is less muscle to degenerate. Other lysosomal enzymes present in muscle, such as aldolase and aspartate aminotransferase, are also increased but are less specific.

Cardiac assessment by echocardiography, electrocardiography (ECG), and radiography of the chest is essential and should be repeated periodically. After the diagnosis is established, patients should be referred to a pediatric cardiologist for long-term cardiac care.

Electromyography (EMG) shows characteristic myopathic features but is not specific for DMD. No evidence of denervation is found. Motor and sensory nerve conduction velocities are normal.

DIAGNOSIS

Polymerase chain reaction (PCR) for the dystrophin gene mutation is the primary test, if the clinical features and serum CK are consistent with the diagnosis. If the blood PCR is diagnostic, muscle biopsy may be deferred, but if it is normal and clinical suspicion is high, the more specific dystrophin immunocytochemistry performed on muscle biopsy sections detects the 30% of cases that do not show a PCR abnormality. Immunohistochemical staining of frozen sections of muscle biopsy tissue detects differences in the rod domain, the carboxyl-terminus (that attaches to the sarcolemma), and the amino-terminus (that attaches to the actin myofilaments) of the large dystrophin molecule, and may be prognostic of the clinical course as Duchenne or Becker disease. More severe weakness occurs with truncation of the dystrophin molecule at the carboxyl-terminus than at the amino-terminus. The diagnosis should be confirmed by blood PCR or muscle biopsy in every case. Dystroglycans and other sarcolemmal regional proteins, such as merosin and sarcoglycans, also can be measured because they may be secondarily decreased.

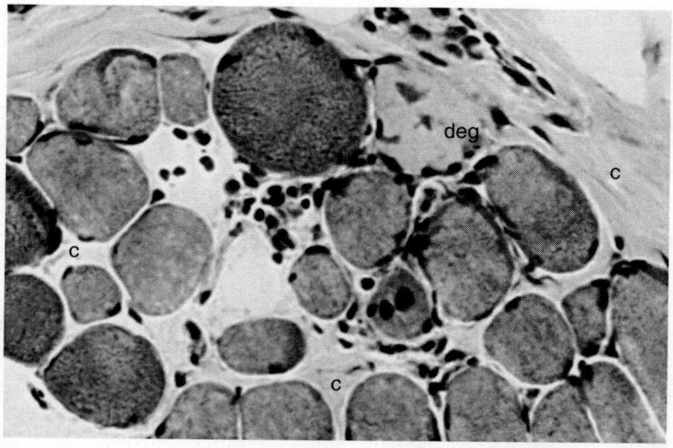

Figure 601-1 Muscle biopsy of a 4 yr old boy with Duchenne muscular dystrophy. Both atrophic and hypertrophic muscle fibers are seen, and some fibers are degenerating *(deg).* Connective tissue *(c)* between muscle fibers is increased (H&E, ×400).

The **muscle biopsy** is diagnostic and shows characteristic changes (Figs. 601-1 and 601-2). Myopathic changes include endomysial connective tissue proliferation, scattered degenerating and regenerating myofibers, foci of mononuclear inflammatory cell infiltrates as a reaction to muscle fiber necrosis, mild architectural changes in still-functional muscle fibers, and many dense fibers. These hypercontracted fibers probably result from segmental necrosis at another level, allowing calcium to enter the site of breakdown of the sarcolemmal membrane and trigger a contraction of the whole length of the muscle fiber. Calcifications within myofibers are correlated with secondary β-dystroglycan deficiency.

The decision about whether muscle biopsy should be performed to establish the diagnosis sometimes presents problems. If there is a family history of the disease, particularly in the case of an involved brother whose diagnosis has been confirmed, a patient with typical clinical features of DMD and high concentrations of serum CK probably does not need to undergo biopsy. The result of the PCR might also influence whether to perform a muscle biopsy. A first case in a family, even if the clinical features are typical, should have the diagnosis confirmed to ensure that another myopathy is not masquerading as DMD. The most common muscles sampled are the vastus lateralis (quadriceps femoris) and the gastrocnemius.

GENETIC ETIOLOGY AND PATHOGENESIS

Despite the X-linked recessive inheritance in DMD, about 30% of cases are new mutations, and the mother is not a carrier. The female carrier state usually shows no muscle weakness or any clinical expression of the disease, but affected girls are occasionally encountered, usually having much milder weakness than boys. These symptomatic girls are explained by the Lyon hypothesis in which the normal X chromosome becomes inactivated and the one with the gene deletion is active (Chapter 75). The full clinical picture of DMD has occurred in several girls with Turner syndrome in whom the single X chromosome must have had the Xp21 gene deletion.

The asymptomatic carrier state of DMD is associated with elevated serum CK values in 80% of cases. The level of increase is usually in the magnitude of hundreds or a few thousand but does not have the extreme values noted in affected males. Prepubertal girls who are carriers of the dystrophy also have increased serum CK values, with highest levels at 8-12 yr of age.

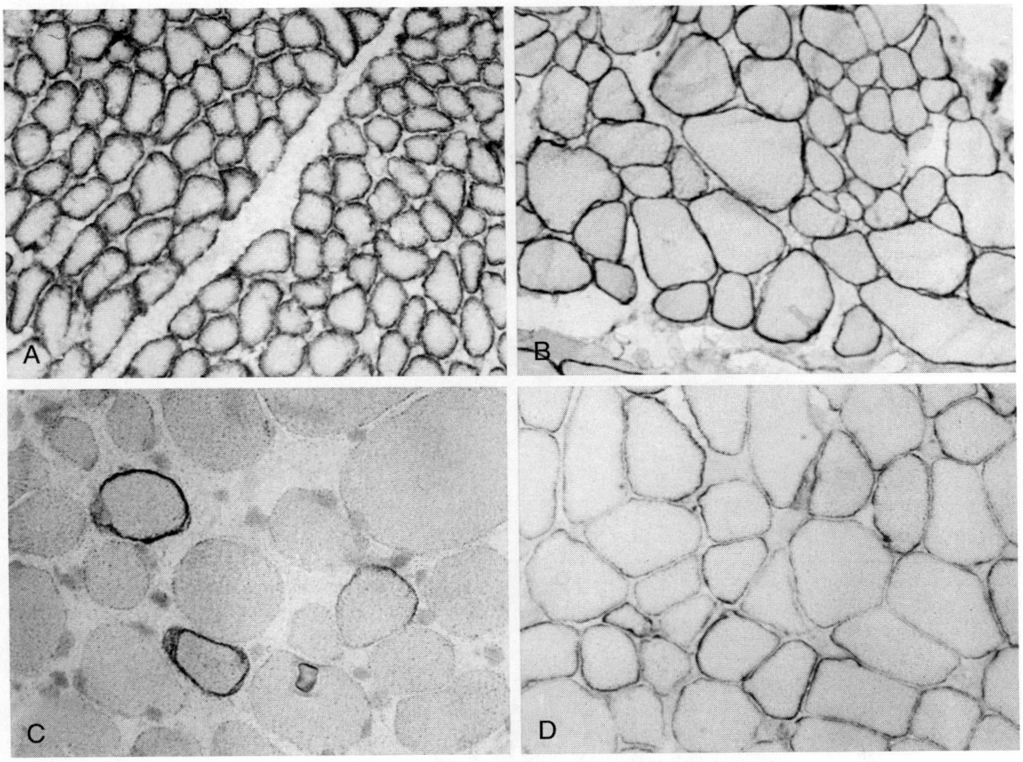

Figure 601-2 Dystrophin is demonstrated by immunohistochemical reactivity in the muscle biopsies of a normal term male neonate *(A)*, a 10 yr old boy with limb-girdle muscular dystrophy *(B)*, a 6 yr old boy with Duchenne muscular dystrophy *(C)*, and a 10 yr old boy with Becker muscular dystrophy *(D)*. In the normal condition and also in non–X-linked muscular dystrophies in which dystrophin is not affected, the sacrolemmal membrane of every fiber is strongly stained, including atrophic and hypertrophic fibers. In Duchenne dystrophy, most myofibers express no detectable dystrophin, but a few scattered fibers known as *revertant fibers* show near-normal immunoreactivity. In Becker muscular dystrophy, the abnormal dystrophin molecule is expressed as thin, with pale staining of the sarcolemma, in which reactivity varies not only between myofibers but also along the circumference of individual fibers (×250).

Approximately 20% of carriers have normal serum CK values. If the mother of an affected boy has normal CK levels, it is unlikely that her daughter can be identified as a carrier by measuring CK. Muscle biopsy of suspected female carriers can detect an additional 10% in whom serum CK is not elevated; a specific genetic diagnosis using PCR on peripheral blood is definitive. Some female carriers suffer cardiomyopathy without weakness of striated muscles.

A 427-kd cytoskeletal protein known as *dystrophin* is encoded by the gene at the Xp21.2 locus. This gene contains 79 exons of coding sequence and 2.5 Mb of DNA, 10 times larger than the next largest gene yet identified. This subsarcolemmal protein attaches to the sarcolemmal membrane overlying the A and M bands of the myofibrils and consists of 4 distinct regions or domains: the amino-terminus contains 250 amino acids and is related to the *N*-actin binding site of α-actinin; the second domain is the largest, with 2,800 amino acids, and contains many repeats, giving it a characteristic rod shape; a 3rd, cysteine-rich, domain is related to the carboxyl-terminus of α-actinin; and the final carboxyl-terminal domain of 400 amino acids is unique to dystrophin and to a dystrophin-related protein encoded by chromosome 6. Dystrophin deficiency at the sarcolemma disrupts the membrane cytoskeleton and leads to loss secondarily of other components of the cytoskeleton.

The molecular defects in the dystrophinopathies vary and include intragenic deletions, duplications, or point mutations of nucleotides. About 65% of patients have deletions, and only 7% exhibit duplications. The site or size of the intragenic abnormality does not always correlate well with the phenotypic severity; in both Duchenne and Becker forms the mutations are mainly near the middle of the gene, involving deletions of exons 46-51. Phenotypic or clinical variations are explained by the alteration of the translational reading frame of mRNA, which results in unstable, truncated dystrophin molecules and severe, classic DMD; mutations that preserve the reading frame still permit translation of coding sequences further downstream on the gene and produce a semifunctional dystrophin, expressed clinically as BMD. An even milder form of adult-onset disease, formerly known as **quadriceps myopathy,** is also caused by an abnormal dystrophin molecule. The clinical spectrum of the dystrophinopathies not only includes the classic Duchenne and Becker forms but also ranges from a severe neonatal muscular dystrophy to asymptomatic children with persistent elevation of serum CK levels >1,000 IU/L.

Analysis of the dystrophin protein requires a muscle biopsy and is demonstrated by Western blot analysis or in tissue sections by immunohistochemical methods using either fluorescence or light microscopy of antidystrophin antisera (see Fig. 601-2). In classic DMD, levels of <3% of normal are found; in BMD, the molecular weight of dystrophin is reduced to 20-90% of normal in 80% of patients, but in 15% of patients the dystrophin is of normal size but reduced in quantity, and 5% of patients have an abnormally large protein caused by excessive duplications or repeats of codons. Selective immunoreactivity of different parts of the dystrophin molecule in sections of muscle biopsy material distinguishes the Duchenne and Becker forms (Fig. 601-3). The demonstration of deletions and duplications also can be made from blood samples by the more rapid PCR, which identifies as many as 98% of deletions by amplifying 18 exons but cannot detect duplications. The diagnosis can thus be confirmed at the molecular genetic level from either the muscle biopsy material or from peripheral blood, although as many as 30% of boys with DMD or BMD have a false-normal blood PCR; all cases of dystrophinopathy are detected by muscle biopsy.

The same methods of DNA analysis from blood samples may be applied for carrier detection in female relatives at risk, such as sisters and cousins, and to determine whether the mother is a carrier or whether a new mutation occurred in the embryo. Prenatal diagnosis is possible as early as the 12th wk of gestation by sampling chorionic villi for DNA analysis by Southern blot or PCR and is confirmed in aborted fetuses with DMD by immunohistochemistry for dystrophin in muscle.

TREATMENT

There is neither a medical cure for this disease nor a method of slowing its progression. Much can be done to treat complications

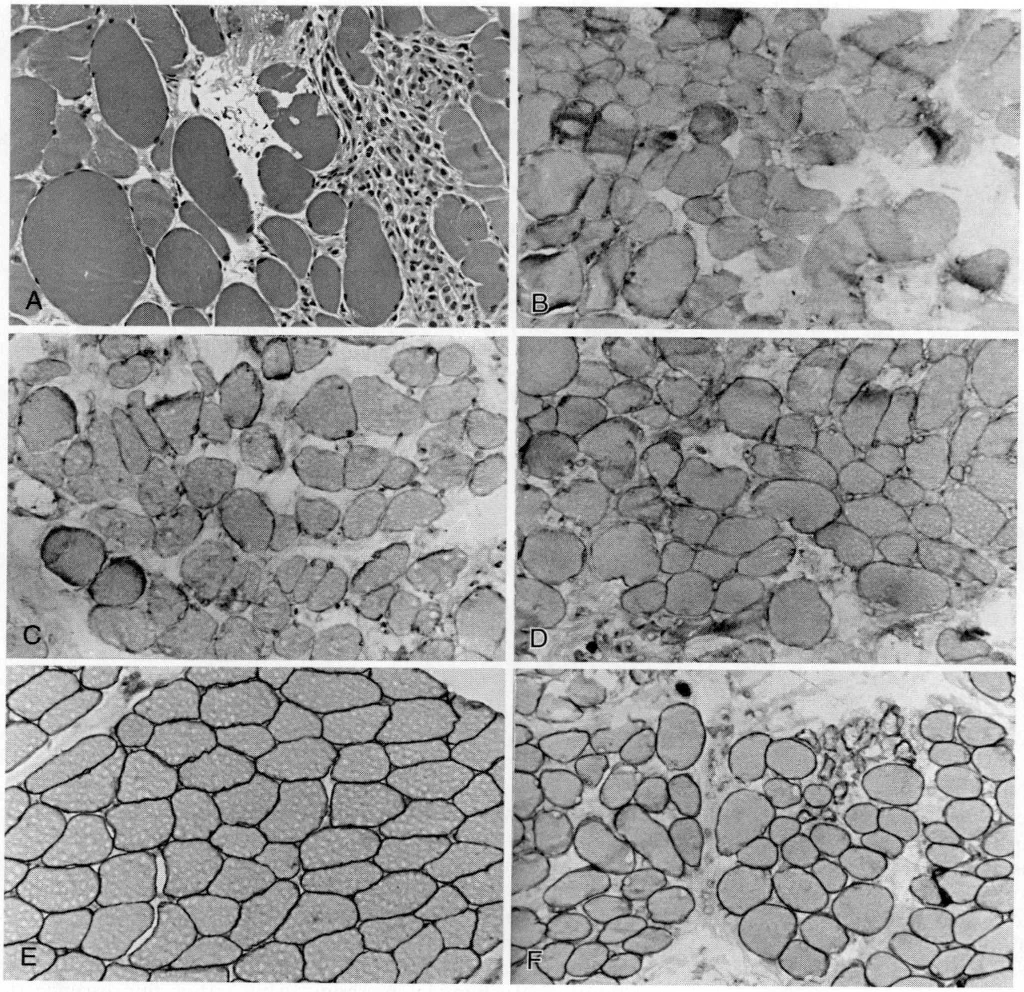

Figure 601-3 Quadriceps femoris muscle biopsy specimens from a 4 yr old boy with Becker muscular dystrophy. *A,* Myofibers vary greatly in size, with both atrophic and hypertrophic forms; at the *right* is a zone of degeneration and necrosis infiltrated by macrophages, similar to Duchenne muscular dystrophy (H&E, ×250). Immunoreactivity using antibodies against the dystrophin molecule in the rod domain *(B),* carboxyl-terminus *(C),* and amino-terminus *(D)* all show deficient but not totally absent dystrophin expression; most fibers of all sizes retain some dystrophin in parts of the sarcolemma but not around the entire circumference in cross section. Alternatively, the prominence of dystrophin is less, appearing weak, when compared with the simultaneously incubated normal control from another child of similar age *(E). F,* Merosin expression is normal in this patient with Becker dystrophy, in both large and small myofibers, and is lacking only in frankly necrotic fibers. Compare with classic Duchenne muscular dystrophy illustrated in Figure 601-2*C* and with Figure 601-5.

and to improve the quality of life of affected children. **Cardiac decompensation** often responds initially well to digoxin. **Pulmonary infections** should be promptly treated. Patients should avoid contact with children who have obvious respiratory or other contagious illnesses. Immunizations for influenza virus and other routine vaccinations are indicated.

Preservation of a good **nutritional state** is important. DMD is not a vitamin-deficiency disease, and excessive doses of vitamins should be avoided. Adequate calcium intake is important to minimize osteoporosis in boys confined to a wheelchair, and fluoride supplements may also be given, particularly if the local drinking water is not fluoridated. Because sedentary children burn fewer calories than active children and because depression is an additional factor, these children tend to eat excessively and gain weight. Obesity makes a patient with myopathy even less functional because part of the limited reserve muscle strength is dissipated in lifting the weight of excess subcutaneous adipose tissue. Dietary restrictions with supervision may be needed.

Physiotherapy delays but does not always prevent contractures. At times, contractures are actually useful in functional rehabilitation. If contractures prevent extension of the elbow beyond 90 degrees and the muscles of the upper limb no longer are strong enough to overcome gravity, the elbow contractures are functionally beneficial in fixing an otherwise flail arm and in allowing the patient to eat and write. Surgical correction of the elbow contracture may be technically feasible, but the result may be deleterious. Physiotherapy contributes little to muscle strengthening because patients usually are already using their entire reserve for daily function, and exercise cannot further strengthen involved muscles. Excessive exercise can actually accelerate the process of muscle fiber degeneration.

Other treatment of patients with DMD involves the use of prednisone, prednisolone, deflazacort, or other steroids. Glucocorticoids decrease the rate of apoptosis or programmed cell death of myotubes during ontogenesis and can decelerate the myofiber necrosis in muscular dystrophy. Strength usually improves initially, but the long-term complications of chronic steroid therapy, including considerable weight gain and osteoporosis, can offset this advantage or even result in greater weakness than might have occurred in the natural course of the disease. Nevertheless, some patients with DMD treated early with steroids appear to have an improved long-term prognosis as well as the short-term improvement, and steroids can help keep patients ambulatory for more years than expected without treatment. One protocol gives prednisone (0.75 mg/kg/day) for the first 10 days of each month to avoid chronic complications. Fluorinated steroids, such as dexamethasone or triamcinolone, should be avoided because they induce myopathy by altering the myotube abundance of ceramide. The American Academy of Neurology and the Child Neurology Society recommend administering corticosteroids during the ambulatory stage of the disease.

Another potential treatment still under investigation is the intramuscular injection of antisense oligonucleotide drugs that induce exon skipping during mRNA splicing to restore the open reading frame in the DMD gene. Stem cell implantation or activation in muscle was theoretically plausible but has not proved practical.

BIBLIOGRAPHY
Please visit the Nelson Textbook of Pediatrics *website at www.expertconsult.com for the complete bibliography.*

601.2 Emery-Dreifuss Muscular Dystrophy

Harvey B. Sarnat

Emery-Dreifuss muscular dystrophy, also known as **scapuloperoneal or scapulohumeral muscular dystrophy,** is a rare X-linked recessive dystrophy. The locus is on the long arm within the large Xq28 region that includes other mutations that cause myotubular myopathy, neonatal adrenoleukodystrophy, and the Bloch-Sulzberger type of incontinentia pigmenti; it is far from the gene for DMD on the short arm of the X chromosome. Another, rarer form of Emery-Dreifuss dystrophy is transmitted as an autosomal dominant trait and is localized at 1q. This form can manifest quite late, in adolescence or early adult life, although the muscular and cardiac symptoms and signs are similar, and sudden death from ventricular fibrillation is a risk.

Clinical manifestations begin at between 5 and 15 yr of age, but many patients survive to late adult life because of the slow progression of its course. A rarer severe infantile presentation also is documented. Muscles do not hypertrophy. Contractures of elbows and ankles develop early, and muscle becomes wasted in a scapulohumeroperoneal distribution. Facial weakness does not occur; this disease is thus distinguished clinically from autosomal dominant scapulohumeral and scapuloperoneal syndromes of neurogenic origin. Myotonia is absent. Intellectual function is normal. Cardiomyopathy is severe and is often the cause of death, more commonly from conduction defects and sudden ventricular fibrillation than from intractable myocardial failure. The serum CK value is only mildly elevated, further distinguishing this disease from other X-linked recessive muscular dystrophies.

Nonspecific myofiber necrosis and endomysial fibrosis are seen in the muscle biopsy. Many centronuclear fibers and selective histochemical type I muscle fiber atrophy can cause confusion with myotonic dystrophy. The defective gene in the X-linked form is called emerin and, unlike other dystrophies in which the defective gene is expressed at the sarcolemmal membrane, emerin is expressed at the inner nuclear membrane; this protein stabilizes the nuclear membrane against the mechanical stresses that occur during muscular contraction. It interacts with *Nesprin-1* and *Nesprin-2* genes, also critical for nuclear membrane integrity. Desmin protein also may be mutated and abnormally expressed. Emerin and desmin may be demonstrated immunocytochemically in the muscle biopsy for definitive diagnosis. Emerin also may be tested as a genetic marker in blood. The defective protein in the autosomal dominant form is called lamin-A/C, proteins that constitute part of the nuclear lamina, a fibrous layer on the inner nuclear membrane. Several subtypes and different mutations are demonstrated. Homozygous nonsense mutations in these *lamin A/C* genes are lethal owing to cardiomyopathy and conduction disturbances.

Treatment should be supportive, with special attention to cardiac conduction defects, and can require medications or a pacemaker. Implantable cardioverter-defibrillators are now available and have prevented sudden death in patients with Emery-Dreifuss muscular dystrophy.

BIBLIOGRAPHY
Please visit the Nelson Textbook of Pediatrics *website at www.expertconsult.com for the complete bibliography.*

601.3 Myotonic Muscular Dystrophy

Harvey B. Sarnat

Myotonic dystrophy (Steinert disease) is the second most common muscular dystrophy in North America, Europe, and Australia, having an incidence varying from 1:100,000 to 1:30,000 in the general population. It is inherited as an autosomal dominant trait. Classic myotonic dystrophy (DM1) is caused by a CTG trinucleotide expansion on chromosome 19q13.3 in the 3′ untranslated region of *DMPK,* the gene that encodes a serine-threonine protein kinase. A second form (DM2) is associated with unstable CTG repeat expansion on chromosome 3q21 of an intron of the zinc finger 9 protein gene. A third, late, form (DM3) is identified, at locus 15q21-q24.

Myotonic dystrophy is an example of a genetic defect causing dysfunction in multiple organ systems. Not only is striated muscle severely affected, but smooth muscle of the alimentary tract and uterus is also involved, cardiac function is altered, and patients have multiple and variable endocrinopathies, immunologic deficiencies, cataracts, dysmorphic facies, intellectual impairment, and other neurologic abnormalities.

CLINICAL MANIFESTATIONS

In the usual clinical course, **excluding the severe neonatal** form, infants can appear almost normal at birth, or facial wasting and hypotonia can already be early expressions of the disease. The facial appearance is characteristic, consisting of an inverted V-shaped upper lip, thin cheeks, and scalloped, concave temporalis muscles (Fig. 601-4). The head may be narrow, and the palate is high and arched because the weak temporal and pterygoid muscles in late fetal life do not exert sufficient lateral forces on the developing head and face.

Weakness is mild in the first few years. Progressive wasting of distal muscles becomes increasingly evident, particularly involving intrinsic muscles of the hands. The thenar and hypothenar eminences are flattened, and the atrophic dorsal interossei leave deep grooves between the fingers. The dorsal forearm muscles and anterior compartment muscles of the lower legs also become wasted. The tongue is thin and atrophic. Wasting of the sternocleidomastoids gives the neck a long, thin, cylindrical contour. Proximal muscles also eventually undergo atrophy, and scapular winging appears. Difficulty with climbing stairs and Gowers sign are progressive. Tendon stretch reflexes are usually preserved.

The distal distribution of muscle wasting in myotonic dystrophy is an *exception* to the general rule of myopathies having proximal and neuropathies having distal distribution patterns. The muscular atrophy and weakness in myotonic dystrophy

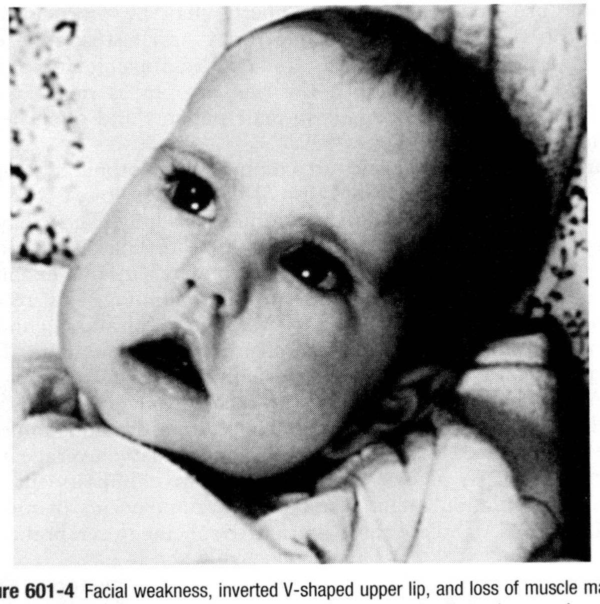

Figure 601-4 Facial weakness, inverted V-shaped upper lip, and loss of muscle mass in the temporal fossae are characteristic of myotonic muscular dystrophy, even in infancy, as seen in this 8 mo old girl.

are slowly progressive throughout childhood and adolescence and continue into adulthood. It is rare for patients with myotonic dystrophy to lose the ability to walk even in late adult life, although splints or bracing may be required to stabilize the ankles.

Myotonia, a characteristic feature shared by few other myopathies, does not occur in infancy and is usually not clinically or even electromyographically evident until about age 5 yr. Exceptional patients develop it as early as age 3 yr. Myotonia is a very slow relaxation of muscle after contraction, regardless of whether that contraction was voluntary or was induced by a stretch reflex or electrical stimulation. During physical examination, myotonia may be demonstrated by asking the patient to make tight fists and then to quickly open the hands. It may be induced by striking the thenar eminence with a rubber percussion hammer, and it may be detected by watching the involuntary drawing of the thumb across the palm. Myotonia can also be demonstrated in the tongue by pressing the edge of a wooden tongue blade against its dorsal surface and by observing a deep furrow that disappears slowly. The severity of myotonia does not necessarily parallel the degree of weakness, and the weakest muscles often have only minimal myotonia. *Myotonia is not a painful muscle spasm.* Myalgias do not occur in myotonic dystrophy.

The **speech** of patients with myotonic dystrophy is often articulated poorly and is slurred because of the involvement of the muscles of the face, tongue, and pharynx. Difficulties with swallowing sometimes occur. Aspiration pneumonia is a risk in severely involved children. Incomplete external ophthalmoplegia sometimes results from extraocular muscle weakness.

Smooth muscle involvement of the **gastrointestinal tract** results in slow gastric emptying, poor peristalsis, and constipation. Some patients have encopresis associated with anal sphincter weakness. Women with myotonic dystrophy can have ineffective or abnormal uterine contractions during labor and delivery.

Cardiac involvement is usually manifested as heart block in the Purkinje conduction system and arrhythmias rather than as cardiomyopathy, unlike most other muscular dystrophies.

Endocrine abnormalities involve many glands and appear at any time during the course of the disease so that endocrine status must be re-evaluated annually. Hypothyroidism is common; hyperthyroidism occurs rarely. Adrenocortical insufficiency can lead to an addisonian crisis even in infancy. Diabetes mellitus is common in patients with myotonic dystrophy; some children have a disorder of insulin release rather than defective insulin production. Onset of puberty may be precocious or, more often, delayed. Testicular atrophy and testosterone deficiency are common in adults and are responsible for a high incidence of male infertility. Ovarian atrophy is rare. Frontal baldness is also characteristic in male patients and often begins in adolescence.

Immunologic deficiencies are common in myotonic dystrophy. The plasma immunoglobulin (Ig)G level is often low.

Cataracts often occur in myotonic dystrophy. They may be congenital, or they can begin at any time during childhood or adult life. Early cataracts are detected only by slit-lamp examination; periodic examination by an ophthalmologist is recommended. Visual evoked potentials are often abnormal in children with myotonic dystrophy and are unrelated to cataracts. They are not usually accompanied by visual impairment.

About half of the patients with myotonic dystrophy are **intellectually impaired,** but severe mental retardation is unusual. The remainder are of average or occasionally above-average intelligence. Epilepsy is not common. Cognitive impairment and mental retardation might result from accumulations of mutant *DMPK* mRNA and aberrant alternative splicing in cerebral cortical neurons.

A severe **congenital form** of myotonic dystrophy appears in a minority of involved infants born to mothers with symptomatic myotonic dystrophy. All patients with this severe congenital disease to date have had the DM1 form. Clubfoot deformities alone or more extensive congenital contractures of many joints can involve all extremities and even the cervical spine. Generalized hypotonia and weakness are present at birth. Facial wasting is prominent. Infants can require gavage feeding or ventilator support for respiratory muscle weakness or apnea. Those requiring ventilation for <30 days often survive, and those with prolonged ventilation have an infant mortality of 25%. Children ventilated for <30 days have better motor, language, and daily activity skills than those requiring prolonged ventilation. One or both leaves of the diaphragm may be nonfunctional. The abdomen becomes distended with gas in the stomach and intestine because of poor peristalsis from smooth muscle weakness. The distention further compromises respiration. Inability to empty the rectum can compound the problem.

LABORATORY FINDINGS

The classic myotonic electromyogram is not found in infants but can appear in toddlers or children in the early school years. The levels of serum CK and other serum enzymes from muscle may be normal or only mildly elevated in the hundreds (never the thousands).

ECG should be performed annually in early childhood. Ultrasound imaging of the abdomen may be indicated in affected infants to determine diaphragmatic function. Radiographs of the chest and abdomen and contrast studies of GI motility may be needed.

Endocrine assessment should be undertaken to determine thyroid and adrenal cortical function and to verify carbohydrate metabolism (glucose tolerance test). Immunoglobulins should be examined, and, if needed, more extensive immunologic studies should be performed.

DIAGNOSIS

The primary diagnostic test is a DNA analysis of blood to demonstrate the abnormal expansion of the CTG repeat. Prenatal diagnosis also is feasible. The muscle biopsy specimen in older children shows many muscle fibers with central nuclei and selective atrophy of histochemical type I fibers, but degenerating fibers are usually few and widely scattered, and there is little or no fibrosis of muscle. Intrafusal fibers of muscle spindles are also abnormal. In young children with the common form of the disease, the biopsy specimen can even appear normal or at least not show myofiber necroses, which is a striking contrast with DMD. In the severe neonatal form of myotonic dystrophy, the muscle biopsy reveals maturational arrest in various stages of development in some and congenital muscle fiber-type disproportion in others. It is likely that the sarcolemmal membrane of muscle fibers not only has abnormal properties of electrical polarization but is also incapable of responding to trophic influences of the motor neuron. Muscle biopsy is not usually required for diagnosis, which in typical cases can be based on the clinical manifestations including family history. **Neonatal myotonic dystrophy** must be distinguished from amyoplasia, congenital muscular dystrophy with or without merosin expression, congenital myasthenia gravis, spinal muscular atrophy, and arthrogryposis secondary to oligohydramnios.

GENETICS

The genetic defect in myotonic muscular dystrophy is on chromosome 19 at the 19q13 locus. It consists of an expansion of the *DM* gene that encodes a serine-threonine kinase *(DMPK),* with numerous repeats of the CTG codon. Expansions range from 50 to >2,000, with the normal alleles of this gene ranging in size from 5-37; the larger the expansion, the more severe the clinical expression, with the largest expansions seen in the severe neonatal form. Rarely, the disease is associated with no detectable repeats, perhaps a spontaneous correction of a previous expansion but a phenomenon still incompletely understood. Another myotonic dystrophy (PROMM) is a clinical entity linked to at least 2 different chromosomal loci than classic myotonic dystrophy but 1 that shares a common unique pathogenesis in being mediated by a mutant mRNA. Defects in RNA splicing explain the insulin resistance in myotonic dystrophies as well as the myotonia.

Clinical and genetic expression can vary between siblings or between an affected parent and child. In the severe neonatal form of the disease, the mother is the transmitting parent in 94% of cases, a fact not explained by increased male infertility alone. Several cases of paternal transmission have been reported. Genetic analysis reveals that symptomatic neonates usually have many more repeats of the CTG codon than do patients with the more classic form of the disease, regardless of which parent is affected. Myotonic dystrophy often exhibits a pattern of **anticipation** in which each successive generation has a tendency to be more severely involved than the previous generation. Prenatal genetic diagnosis of myotonic dystrophy is available.

TREATMENT

There is no specific medical treatment, but the cardiac, endocrine, GI, and ocular complications can often be treated. Physiotherapy and orthopedic treatment of contractures in the neonatal form of the disease may be beneficial.

Myotonia may be diminished, and function may be restored by drugs that raise the depolarization threshold of muscle membranes, such as mexiletine, phenytoin, carbamazepine, procainamide, and quinidine sulfate. These drugs also have cardiotropic effects; thus, cardiac evaluation is important before prescribing them. Phenytoin and carbamazepine are used in doses similar to their use as anticonvulsants (Chapter 586.6); serum concentrations of 10-20 µg/mL for phenytoin and 5-12 µg/mL for carbamazepine should be maintained. If a patient's disability is caused mainly by weakness rather than by myotonia, these drugs will be of no value.

OTHER MYOTONIC SYNDROMES

Most patients with myotonia have myotonic dystrophy. However, myotonia is not specific for this disease and occurs in several rarer conditions.

Myotonic chondrodystrophy (Schwartz-Jampel disease) is a rare congenital disease characterized by generalized muscle hypertrophy and weakness. Dysmorphic phenotypical features and the radiographic appearance of long bones are reminiscent of Morquio disease (Chapter 82), but abnormal mucopolysaccharides are not found. Dwarfism, joint abnormalities, and blepharophimosis are present. Several patients have been the products of consanguinity, suggesting autosomal recessive inheritance. The muscle protein perlecan, encoded by the *SJS1* gene, a large heparan sulfate proteoglycan of basement membranes and cartilage, is defective in some cases of Schwartz-Jampel disease and explains both the muscular hyperexcitability and the chondrodysplasia.

EMG reveals continuous electrical activity in muscle fibers closely resembling or identical to myotonia. Muscle biopsy reveals nonspecific myopathic features, which are minimal in some cases and pronounced in others. The sarcotubular system is dilated.

Myotonia congenita (Thomsen disease) is a channelopathy (Table 601-1) and is characterized by weakness and generalized muscular hypertrophy so that affected children resemble bodybuilders. Myotonia is prominent and can develop at age 2-3 yr, earlier than in myotonic dystrophy. The disease is clinically stable and is apparently not progressive for many years. Muscle biopsy specimens show minimal pathologic changes, and the EMG demonstrates myotonia. Various families are described as showing either autosomal dominant (Thomsen disease) or recessive (Becker disease, not to be confused with BMD or DMD) inheritance. Rarely, myotonic dystrophy and myotonia congenita coexist in the same family. The autosomal dominant and autosomal recessive forms of myotonia congenita have been mapped to the same 7q35 locus. This gene is important for the integrity of chloride channels of the sarcolemmal and T-tubular membranes.

Table 601-1 CHANNELOPATHIES AND RELATED DISORDERS

DISORDER	PATTERN OF CLINICAL FEATURES	INHERITANCE	CHROMOSOME	GENE
CHLORIDE CHANNELOPATHIES				
Myotonia Congenita				
Thomsen disease	Myotonia	Autosomal dominant	7q35	*CLC1*
Becker disease	Myotonia and weakness	Autosomal recessive	7q35	*CLC1*
SODIUM CHANNELOPATHIES				
Paramyotonia congenita	Paramyotonia	Autosomal dominant	17q13.1-13.3	*SCNA4A*
Hyperkalemic periodic paralysis	Periodic paralysis with myotonia and paramyotonia	Autosomal dominant	17q13.1-13.3	*CNA4A*
Hypokalemic periodic paralysis	Periodic paralysis	Autosomal dominant	17q13.1-13.3	*SCNA4A*
POTASSIUM-AGGRAVATED MYOTONIAS				
Myotonia fluctuans	Myotonia	Autosomal dominant	17q13.1-13.3	*SCNA4A*
Myotonia permanens	Myotonia	Autosomal dominant	17q13.1-13.3	*SCNA4A*
Acetazolamide-responsive myotonia	Myotonia	Autosomal dominant	17q13.1-13.3	*SCNA4A*
CALCIUM CHANNELOPATHIES				
Hypokalemic periodic paralysis	Periodic paralysis	Autosomal dominant	1q31-32	Dihydropyridine receptor
Schwartz-Jampel syndrome (chondrodystrophic myotonia)	Myotonia; dysmorphic	Autosomal recessive	1q34.1-36.1	Perlecan
Rippling muscle disease	Muscle mounding, stiffness	Autosomal dominant	1q41	Caveolin-3
Anderson syndrome	Periodic paralysis, cardiac arrhythmia, distinctive facies	Autosomal dominant	17q23	KCNJ2-Kir2.1
Brody disease	Delayed relaxation, no EMG myotonia	Autosomal recessive	16p12	Calcium ATPase
Malignant hyperthermia	Anesthetic-induced delayed relaxation	Autosomal dominant	19q13.1	Ryanodine receptor

ATPase, adenosine triphosphatase; EMG, electromyogram.
From Goldman L, Ausiello D: *Cecil textbook of medicine,* ed 22, Philadelphia, 2004, WB Saunders.

Paramyotonia is a temperature-related myotonia that is aggravated by cold and alleviated by warm external temperatures. Patients have difficulty when swimming in cold water or if they are dressed inadequately in cold weather. *Paramyotonia congenita* (Eulenburg disease) is a defect in a gene at the 17q13.1-13.3 locus, the identical locus identified in hyperkalemic periodic paralysis. By contrast with myotonia congenita, paramyotonia is a disorder of the voltage-gated sodium channel caused by a mutation in the α subunit. Myotonic dystrophy also is a sodium channelopathy (see Table 601-1).

In sodium channelopathies, exercise produces increasing myotonia, whereas in chloride channelopathies, exercise reduces the myotonia. This is easily tested during examination by asking patients to close the eyes forcefully and open them repeatedly; it becomes progressively more difficult in sodium channel disorders and progressively easier in chloride channel disorders.

BIBLIOGRAPHY

Please visit the Nelson Textbook of Pediatrics *website at* *www.expertconsult.com* *for the complete bibliography.*

601.4 Limb-Girdle Muscular Dystrophies

Harvey B. Sarnat

Limb-girdle muscular dystrophies encompass a group of progressive hereditary myopathies that mainly affect muscles of the hip and shoulder girdles (Table 601-2). Distal muscles also eventually become atrophic and weak. Hypertrophy of the calves and ankle contractures develop in some forms, causing potential confusion with BMD. Sixteen genetic forms of LGMD are now described, each at a different chromosomal locus and expressing different protein defects. Some include diseases classified with other traditional groups, such as the lamin-A/C defects of the nuclear membrane (see Emery-Dreifuss muscular dystrophy, earlier), and some forms of congenital muscular dystrophy.

The initial **clinical manifestations** rarely appear before middle or late childhood or may be delayed until early adult life. Low back pain may be a presenting complaint because of the lordotic posture resulting from gluteal muscle weakness. Confinement to a wheelchair usually becomes obligatory at about 30 yr of age. The rate of progression varies from one pedigree to another but is uniform within a kindred. Although weakness of neck flexors and extensors is universal, facial, lingual, and other bulbar-innervated muscles are rarely involved. As weakness and muscle wasting progress, tendon stretch reflexes become diminished. Cardiac involvement is unusual. Intellectual function is generally normal. The clinical **differential diagnosis** of LGMD includes juvenile spinal muscular atrophy (Kugelberg-Welander disease), myasthenia gravis, and metabolic myopathies.

Most cases of LGMD are of autosomal recessive inheritance, but some families express an autosomal dominant trait. The latter often follows a benign course with little functional impairment.

The EMG and muscle biopsy show confirmatory evidence of muscular dystrophy, but none of the findings is specific enough to make the definitive **diagnosis** without additional clinical criteria. In some cases, α-sarcoglycan (formerly known as *adhalen*), a dystrophin-related glycoprotein of the sarcolemma, is deficient; this specific defect may be demonstrated in the muscle biopsy by immunocytochemistry. Increased serum CK level is usual, but the magnitude of elevation varies among families. The ECG is usually unaltered.

In one autosomal dominant form of LGMD, a genetic defect has been localized to the long arm of chromosome 5. In the autosomal recessive disease, it is on the long arm of chromosome 15. A mutated dystrophin-associated protein in the sarcoglycan complex (sarcoglycanopathy; LGMD types 2C,E,F) is responsible for some cases of autosomal recessive LGMD. Most sarcoglycanopathies result from a mutation in α-sarcoglycan; other LGMD resulting from deficiencies in β-, γ-, and δ-sarcoglycan also occur. In normal smooth muscle, α-sarcoglycan is replaced by ε-sarcoglycan, and the others are the same.

Another group of LGMDs (type 2B) are caused by allelic mutations of the dysferlin *(DYSF)* gene, another gene expressing a protein essential to structural integrity of the sarcolemma, though not associated with the dystrophin-glycoprotein complex. *DYSF* interacts with caveolin-3 or calpain-3, and *DYSF* deficiency may be secondary to defects in these other gene products. Primary calpain-3 defect (type 2A) is reported in Amish families and in families from French Reunion Island and from Brazil. Autosomal recessive (Miyoshi myopathy) and autosomal dominant traits are documented. Both are slowly progressive myopathies with onset in adolescence or young adult life and can affect distal as well as proximal muscles. Cardiomyopathy is rare. Chronically elevated serum CK in the thousands is found in dysferlinopathies. Ultrastructure shows a thickened basal lamina over defects in the sarcolemma and replacement of the sarcolemma by multiple layers of small vesicles. Regenerating myofibers outnumber degenerating myofibers. These disorders were formerly called *hyperCKemia* and *rippling muscle disease,* the latter sometimes confused with myotonia. There is overlap of the group of LGMDs with the congenital muscular dystrophies, such as Walker-Warburg syndrome with a *POMT* and Fukuyama muscular dystrophy with *FKRP* genetic defects and Ullrich muscular dystrophy of collagen VI subunits.

BIBLIOGRAPHY

Please visit the Nelson Textbook of Pediatrics *website at* *www.expertconsult.com* *for the complete bibliography.*

601.5 Facioscapulohumeral Muscular Dystrophy

Harvey B. Sarnat

Facioscapulohumeral muscular dystrophy, also known as **Landouzy-Dejerine disease,** is probably not a single disease entity but a group of diseases with similar clinical manifestations. Autosomal dominant inheritance is the rule; genetic anticipation is often found within several generations of a family, the succeeding more severely involved at an earlier age than the preceding. The

Table 601-2 AUTOSOMAL RECESSIVE LIMB-GIRDLE MUSCULAR DYSTROPHIES

TYPE	LOCATION	GENE PRODUCT	CLINICAL FEATURES
LGMD2A	15q	Calpain 3	Onset at 8-15 yr, progression variable
LGMD2B	2p13-16	Dysferlin	Onset at adolescence, mild weakness; gene site is the same as for Miyoshi myopathy
LGMD2C	13q12	Sarcoglycan	Duchenne-like, severe childhood autosomal recessive muscular dystrophy (SCARMD1)
LGMD2D	17q12	α-Sarcoglycan (adhalin)	Duchenne-like, severe childhood autosomal recessive muscular dystrophy (SCARMD2)
LGMD2E	4q12	β-Sarcoglycan	Phenotype between Duchenne and Becker muscular dystrophies
LGMD2F	5q33-34	Sarcoglycan	Slowly progressive, growth retardation

LGMD, limb-girdle muscular dystrophy.

From Fenichel GM: *Clinical pediatric neurology: a signs and symptoms approach,* ed 5, Philadelphia, 2005, Elsevier Saunders, p 176, Table 7-5.

frequency is 1:20,000. The genetic mechanism in autosomal dominant facioscapulohumeral dystrophy involves integral deletions of a 3.3-kb tandem repeat (D4Z4) in the subtelomeric region at the 4q35 locus. A closely homologous 3.3-kb repeat array at the subtelomeric locus 10q26, with chromosomal translocation or sequence conversion between these 2 regions, possibly predisposes to the DNA rearrangement causing facioscapulohumeral dystrophy. About 10% of families with this phenotype do not map to the 4q35 locus.

CLINICAL MANIFESTATIONS

Facioscapulohumeral dystrophy shows the earliest and most severe weakness in facial and shoulder girdle muscles. The facial weakness differs from that of myotonic dystrophy; rather than an inverted V-shaped upper lip, the mouth in facioscapulohumeral dystrophy is rounded and appears puckered because the lips protrude. Inability to close the eyes completely in sleep is a common expression of upper facial weakness; some patients have extraocular muscle weakness, although ophthalmoplegia is rarely complete. Facioscapulohumeral dystrophy has been associated with Möbius syndrome on rare occasions. Pharyngeal and tongue weakness may be absent and are never as severe as the facial involvement. Hearing loss, which may be subclinical, and retinal vasculopathy (indistinguishable from Coats disease) are associated features, particularly in severe cases of facioscapulohumeral dystrophy with early childhood onset.

Scapular winging is prominent, often even in infants. Flattening or even concavity of the deltoid contour is seen, and the biceps and triceps brachii muscles are wasted and weak. Muscles of the hip girdle and thighs also eventually lose strength and undergo atrophy, and Gowers sign and a Trendelenburg gait appear. Contractures of the extremities are rare. Finger and wrist weakness occasionally is the first symptom. Weakness of the anterior tibial and peroneal muscles can lead to footdrop; this complication usually occurs only in advanced cases with severe weakness. Lumbar lordosis and kyphoscoliosis are common complications of axial muscle involvement. Calf pseudohypertrophy is not a usual feature but is described rarely.

Facioscapulohumeral muscular dystrophy can also be a mild disease causing minimal disability. Clinical manifestations might not be expressed in childhood and are delayed into middle adult life. Unlike most other muscular dystrophies, asymmetry of weakness is common. About 30% of affected patients are asymptomatic or show only mild scapular winging and decreased tendon stretch reflexes, of which they were unaware until formal neurologic examination was performed.

LABORATORY FINDINGS

Serum levels of CK and other enzymes vary greatly, ranging from normal or near normal to elevations of several thousand. ECG should be performed, although the anticipated findings are usually normal. EMG reveals nonspecific myopathic muscle potentials. Diagnostic molecular testing in individual cases and within families is indicated for prediction.

DIAGNOSIS AND DIFFERENTIAL DIAGNOSIS

Muscle biopsy distinguishes more than one form of facioscapulohumeral dystrophy, consistent with clinical evidence that several distinct diseases are embraced by the term *FSH dystrophy.* Muscle biopsy and EMG also distinguish the primary myopathy from a neurogenic disease with a similar distribution of muscular involvement. The general histopathologic findings in the muscle biopsy material are extensive proliferation of connective tissue between muscle fibers, extreme variation in fiber size with many hypertrophic as well as atrophic myofibers, and scattered degenerating and regenerating fibers. An "inflammatory" type of facioscapulohumeral muscular dystrophy is also distinguished, characterized by extensive lymphocytic infiltrates within muscle fascicles. Despite the resemblance of this form to inflammatory myopathies, such as polymyositis, there is no evidence of autoimmune disease, and steroids and immunosuppressive drugs do not alter the clinical course. A precise histopathologic diagnosis has important therapeutic implications. Mononuclear cell "inflammation" in a muscle biopsy sample of infants <2 yr old is usually facioscapulohumeral dystrophy or, less often, a congenital muscular dystrophy.

TREATMENT

Physiotherapy is of no value in regaining strength or in retarding progressive weakness or muscle wasting. Foot drop and scoliosis may be treated by orthopedic measures. In selected cases, surgical wiring of the scapulas to the thoracic wall provides improved shoulder stability and abduction of the arm, but brachial plexopathy, frozen shoulder, and scapular fractures are reported complications. Cosmetic improvement of the facial muscles of expression may be achieved by reconstructive surgery, which grafts a fascia lata to the zygomatic muscle and to the zygomatic head of the quadratus labiae superioris muscle. Exercise of facial muscles can help minimize secondary disuse atrophy. No effective pharmacologic treatment is available.

BIBLIOGRAPHY

Please visit the Nelson Textbook of Pediatrics *website at www.expertconsult.com for the complete bibliography.*

601.6 Congenital Muscular Dystrophy

Harvey B. Sarnat

The term *congenital muscular dystrophy* is misleading because all muscular dystrophies are genetically determined. It is used to encompass several distinct diseases with a common characteristic of severe involvement at birth but that ironically usually follow a benign clinical course. Autosomal recessive inheritance is the rule.

CLINICAL MANIFESTATIONS

Infants often have contractures or arthrogryposis at birth and are diffusely hypotonic. The muscle mass is thin in the trunk and extremities. Head control is poor. Facial muscles may be mildly involved, but ophthalmoplegia, pharyngeal weakness, and weak sucking are not common. A minority have severe dysphagia and require gavage or gastrostomy. Tendon stretch reflexes may be hypoactive or absent. Arthrogryposis is common in all forms of congenital muscular dystrophy (Chapter 600.10). Congenital contractures of the elbows have a high association with the Ullrich type of congenital muscular dystrophy owing to a defect in 1 or more of the 3 collagen VI genes, each at a different locus.

The **Fukuyama type** of congenital muscular dystrophy is the second most common muscular dystrophy in Japan (after DMD); it has also been reported in children of Dutch, German, Scandinavian, and Turkish ethnic backgrounds. In the Fukuyama variety, severe cardiomyopathy and malformations of the brain usually accompany the skeletal muscle involvement. Signs and symptoms related to these organs are prominent: cardiomegaly and heart failure, mental retardation, seizures, microcephaly, and failure to thrive. The genetic defect in Fukuyama congenital muscular dystrophy has been identified at the 8q31-33 locus in Japanese patients.

Central neurologic disease can accompany forms of congenital muscular dystrophy other than Fukuyama disease. Mental and neurologic status are the most variable features; an apparently normal brain and normal intelligence do not preclude the diagnosis if other manifestations indicate this myopathy. The cerebral malformations that occur are not consistently of one type and vary from severe dysplasias (holoprosencephaly, lissencephaly) to milder conditions (agenesis of the corpus callosum, focal heterotopia of the cerebral cortex and subcortical white matter, cerebellar hypoplasia).

Congenital muscular dystrophy is a consistent association with cerebral dysgenesis in the **Walker-Warburg syndrome** and **in muscle-eye-brain disease of Santavuori.** The neuropathologic findings are those of neuroblast migratory abnormalities in the cerebral cortex, cerebellum, and brainstem. Mutations in genes of O-mannosylation of α-dystroglycan (*POMT1* and *POMGnT1)*, essential for neuroblast migration in the fetal brain, have been demonstrated. Studies indicate considerably more genetic overlap between Walker-Warburg, Fukuyama, and muscle-eye-brain forms of congenital muscular dystrophy that explain mixed and transitional phenotypes, so that, for example, the *Fukutin* (*FKRP*) gene can cause a Walker-Warburg or muscle-eye-brain presentation, or *POMGnT1* also can produce phenotypes other than classic Walker-Warburg disease.

Another separate form of congenital muscular dystrophy is characterized by microcephaly and mental retardation.

LABORATORY FINDINGS

Serum CK level is usually moderately elevated from several hundred to many thousand IU/L; only marginal increases are sometimes found. EMG shows nonspecific myopathic features. Investigation of all forms of congenital muscular dystrophy should include cardiac assessment and an imaging study of the brain. Muscle biopsy is essential for the diagnosis.

DIAGNOSIS

Muscle biopsy is diagnostic in the neonatal period or thereafter. An extensive proliferation of endomysial collagen envelops individual muscle fibers even at birth, also causing them to be rounded in cross-sectional contour by acting as a rigid sleeve, especially during contraction. The perimysial connective tissue and fat are also increased, and the fascicular organization of the muscle may be disrupted by the fibrosis. Tissue cultures of intramuscular fibroblasts exhibit increased collagen synthesis, but the structure of the collagen is normal. Muscle fibers vary in diameter, and many show central nuclei, myofibrillar splitting, and other cytoarchitectural alterations. Scattered degenerating and regenerating fibers are seen. No inflammation or abnormal inclusions are found.

Immunocytochemical reactivity for merosin (α_2 chain of laminin) at the sarcolemmal region is absent in about 40% of cases and normally expressed in the others (Figs. 601-5 and 601-6). Merosin is a protein that binds the sarcolemmal membrane of the myofiber to the basal lamina or basement membrane. Its defect is a mutation of the *LAMA2* gene at the 6q22-q23 locus. Merosin also is expressed in brain and in Schwann cells. The

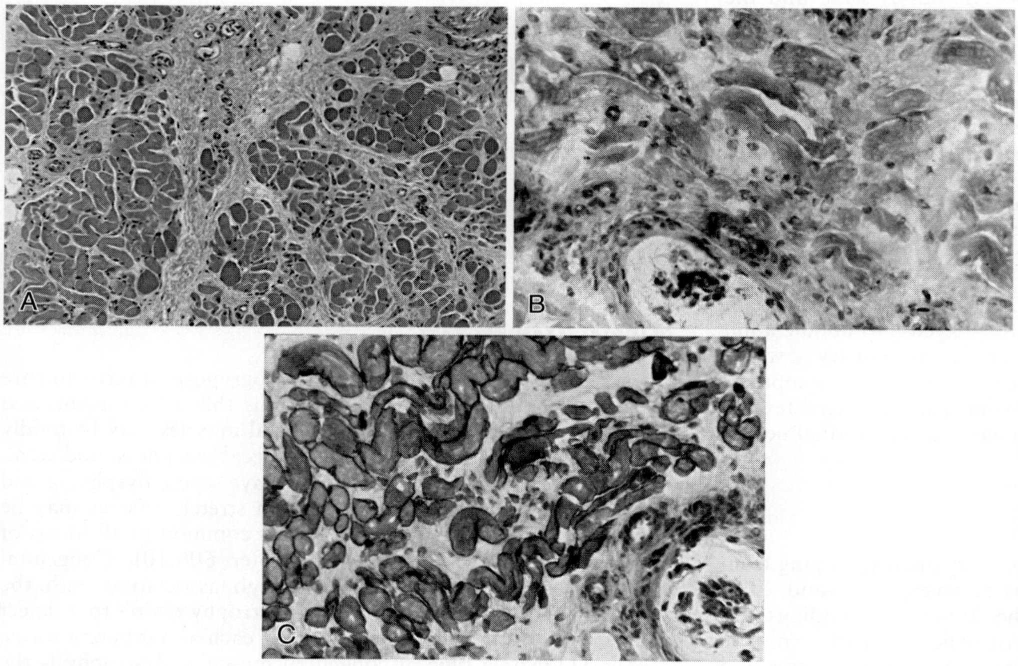

Figure 601-5 Quadriceps femoris muscle biopsy of a 6 mo old girl with congenital muscular dystrophy associated with merosin (α_2-laminin) deficiency. *A,* Histologically, the muscle is infiltrated by a great proliferation of collagenous connective tissue; myofibers vary in diameter, but necrotic fibers are rare. *B,* Immunocytochemical reactivity for merosin (α_2-laminin) is absent in all fibers, including the intrafusal myofibers of a muscle spindle seen at bottom. *C,* Dystrophin expression (rod domain) is normal. Compare with Figures 601-2, 601-3, and 601-6.

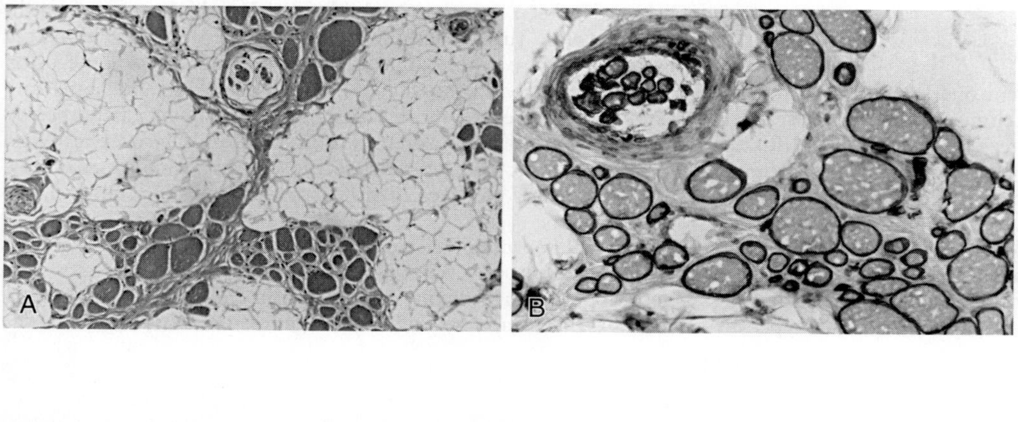

Figure 601-6 Quadriceps femoris muscle biopsy specimen of a 2 yr old girl with congenital muscular dystrophy. *A,* The fascicular architecture of the muscle is severely disrupted, and muscle is replaced by fat and connective tissue; the remaining small groups of myofibers of variable size are seen, including a muscle spindle at top. *B,* Merosin expression is normal in both extrafusal fibers of all sizes and in intrafusal spindle fibers. The severity of the myopathy does not relate to the presence or absence of merosin in congenital muscular dystrophy. Compare with Figure 601-5.

presence or absence of merosin does not always correlate with the severity of the myopathy or predict its course, but cases with merosin deficiency tend to have more severe cerebral involvement and myopathy. Adhalen (α-dystroglycan) may be secondarily reduced in some cases. Collagen VI is selectively reduced or absent in Ullrich disease because of a mutation in the *COL6A* gene. Mitochondrial dysfunction may be a secondary defect.

TREATMENT

Only supportive therapy is available in general. Cyclosporin A might correct the mitochondrial dysfunction and muscular apoptosis in collagen VI myopathy.

BIBLIOGRAPHY

Please visit the Nelson Textbook of Pediatrics *website at* www.expertconsult.com *for the complete bibliography.*

Chapter 602
Endocrine and Toxic Myopathies

Harvey B. Sarnat

THYROID MYOPATHIES (SEE ALSO CHAPTERS 557-562)

Thyrotoxicosis causes proximal weakness and wasting accompanied by myopathic electromyographic changes. Thyroxine binds to myofibrils and, if in excess, impairs contractile function. **Hyperthyroidism** can also induce myasthenia gravis and hypokalemic periodic paralysis.

Hypothyroidism, whether congenital or acquired, consistently produces hypotonia and a proximal distribution of weakness. Although muscle wasting is most characteristic, one form of cretinism, the Kocher-Debré-Sémélaigne syndrome, is characterized by generalized pseudohypertrophy of weak muscles. Infants can have a Herculean appearance reminiscent of myotonia congenita. The serum creatine kinase (CK) level is elevated in hypothyroid myopathy and returns to normal after thyroid replacement therapy.

Results of muscle biopsy in hypothyroidism reveal acute myopathic changes, including myofiber necrosis and sometimes central cores. In hyperthyroidism, the muscle biopsy specimen shows only mild, nonspecific myopathic changes without necrosis of myofibers.

The clinical and pathologic features of hyperthyroid myopathy and hypothyroid myopathy resolve after appropriate treatment of the thyroid disorder. Many of the systemic symptoms of hyperthyroidism, including myopathic weakness and ophthalmoparesis, improve with the administration of β-blockers.

Most patients with primary **hyperparathyroidism** (Chapter 567) develop weakness, fatigability, fasciculations, and muscle wasting that is reversible after removal of the parathyroid adenoma. The serum CK and muscle biopsy remain normal, but the electromyography can show nonspecific myopathic features. A minority of patients develop myotonia that could be confused with myotonic dystrophy.

STEROID-INDUCED MYOPATHY

Natural Cushing disease and iatrogenic Cushing syndrome due to exogenous corticosteroid administration can cause painless, symmetrical, progressive proximal weakness, increased serum CK levels, and a myopathic electromyogram and muscle biopsy specimen (Chapter 571). Myosin filaments may be selectively lost. The 9α-fluorinated steroids, such as dexamethasone, betamethasone, and triamcinolone, are the most likely to produce *steroid myopathy.* Dexamethasone alters the abundance of ceramides in myotubes in developing muscle. In patients with dermatomyositis or other myopathies treated with steroids, it is sometimes difficult to distinguish refractoriness of the disease from steroid-induced weakness, especially after long-term steroid administration. All patients who have been taking steroids for long periods develop reversible type II myofiber atrophy; this is a *steroid effect* but is not steroid myopathy unless it progresses to become a necrotizing myopathy. At greatest risk in the pediatric age group are children requiring long-term steroid therapy for asthma, rheumatoid arthritis, dermatomyositis, lupus, and other autoimmune or inflammatory diseases and in the treatment of leukemia and other hematologic diseases. In addition to steroids, acute or chronic toxic myopathies can occur from other drugs (Table 602-1).

Hyperaldosteronism (Conn syndrome) is accompanied by episodic and reversible weakness similar to that of periodic paralysis. The proximal myopathy can become irreversible in chronic cases. Elevated CK levels and even myoglobinuria sometimes occur during acute attacks.

Chronic growth hormone excess (sometimes illicitly acquired by adolescent athletes or seen in acromegaly) produces atrophy

Table 602-1 TOXIC MYOPATHIES

INFLAMMATORY
Cimetidine
D-Penicillamine
Procainamide
L-Tryptoplan
L-Dopa
NONINFLAMMATORY NECROTIZING OR VACUOLAR
Cholesterol-lowering agents
Chloroquine
Colchicine
Emetine
ε-Aminocaproic acid
Labetalol
Cyclosporine and tacrolimus
Isoretinoic acid (vitamin A analog)
Vincristine
Alcohol
RHABDOMYOLYSIS AND MYOGLOBINURIA
Cholesterol-lowering drugs
Alcohol
Heroin
Amphetamine
Toluene
Cocaine
ε-Aminocaproic acid
Pentazocine
Phencyclidine
MALIGNANT HYPERTHERMIA
Halothane
Ethylene
Diethyl ether
Methoxyflurane
Ethyl chloride
Trichloroethylene
Gallamine
Succinylcholine
MITOCHONDRIAL
Zidovudine
MYOTONIA
2,4-*d*-Chlorophenoxyacetic acid
Anthracene-9-carboxycyclic acid
Cholesterol-lowering drugs
Chloroquine
Cyclosporine
MYOSIN LOSS
Nondepolarizing neuromuscular blocking agents
Intravenous glucocorticoids

From Goldman L, Ausiello D: *Cecil textbook of medicine,* ed 22, Philadelphia, 2004, Saunders, p 2399.

of some myofibers and hypertrophy of others, and scattered myofiber degeneration. Despite the augmented protein synthesis induced by growth hormone, it impairs myofibrillar adenosine triphosphatase (ATPase) activity and reduces sarcolemmal excitability, with resultant diminished, rather than increased, strength corresponding to the larger muscle mass.

BIBLIOGRAPHY

Please visit the Nelson Textbook of Pediatrics *website at* *www.expertconsult.com* *for the complete bibliography.*

Chapter 603
Metabolic Myopathies

Harvey B. Sarnat

The differential diagnosis of metabolic myopathies is noted in Table 603-1.

603.1 Periodic Paralyses (Potassium-Related)

Harvey B. Sarnat

Episodic, reversible weakness or paralysis known as **periodic paralysis** is associated with transient alterations in serum potassium levels, usually hypokalemia but occasionally hyperkalemia. All familial forms of periodic paralysis are caused by mutations in genes encoding voltage-gated ion channels in muscle: sodium, calcium, and potassium (see Table 603-1). During attacks, myofibers are electrically inexcitable, although the contractile apparatus can respond normally to calcium. The disorder is inherited as an autosomal dominant trait. It is precipitated in some patients by a heavy carbohydrate meal, insulin, epinephrine including that induced by emotional stress, hyperaldosteronism or hyperthyroidism, administration of amphotericin B, or ingestion of licorice. The defective genes are at the 17q13.1-13.3 locus in **hyperkalemic periodic paralysis,** the same as in paramyotonia congenita, and at the 1q31-32 locus in **hypokalemic periodic paralysis.**

Table 603-1 METABOLIC AND MITOCHONDRIAL MYOPATHIES

GLYCOGEN METABOLISM DEFICIENCIES
Type II α-1,4 Glucosidase (acid maltase)
Type III Debranching
Type IV Branching
Type V Phosphorylase (McArdle disease)*
Type VII Phosphofructokinase (Tarui disease)*
Type VIII Phosphorylase B kinase*
Type IX Phosphoglycerate kinase*
Type X Phosphoglycerate mutase*
Type XI Lactate dehydrogenase*
LIPID METABOLISM DEFICIENCIES
Carnitine palmitoyl transferase*
Primary systemic/muscle carnitine deficiency
Secondary carnitine deficiency
β-Oxidation defects
Medications (valproic acid)
PURINE METABOLISM DEFICIENCIES
Myoadenylate deaminase deficiency*
MITOCHONDRIAL MYOPATHIES
Pyruvate dehydrogenase complex deficiencies (including Leigh syndrome)
Progressive external ophthalmoplegia
Autosomal dominant with multiple mitochondrial DNA deletions
Adenine nucleotide translocator 1
TWINKLE (C10ORF2)
Polymerase gamma
Kearns-Sayre syndrome
Mitochondrial encephalopathy, lactic acidosis, and stroke
Myoclonic epilepsy with ragged-red fibers
Mitochondrial neurogastrointestinal encephalomyopathy
Mitochondrial depletion syndrome
Leigh syndrome and neuropathy, ataxia, retinitis pigmentosa
Succinate dehydrogenase deficiency*

*Deficiency can produce exercise intolerance and myoglobinuria.
From Goldman L, Ausiello D: *Cecil textbook of medicine*, ed 22, Philadelphia, 2004, WB Saunders, p 2392.

Attacks often begin in infancy, particularly in the hyperkalemic form, and the disease is nearly always symptomatic by 10 yr of age, affecting both sexes equally. Late childhood or adolescence is the more typical age of onset of the hypokalemic form, Andersen-Tawil syndrome (see later) and paramyotonia congenita. Periodic paralysis is an episodic event; patients are unable to move after awakening and gradually recover muscle strength during the next few minutes or hours. Muscles that remain active in sleep, such as the diaphragm and cardiac muscle, are not affected. Patients are normal between attacks, but in adult life the attacks become more frequent, and the disorder causes progressive myopathy with permanent weakness even between attacks. The usual frequency of attacks in childhood is once a week. The differential diagnosis includes thyrotoxic periodic paralysis, myotonia congenita, and paramyotonia congenita. A triad of periodic paralysis, potentially fatal cardiac ventricular ectopy (due to a defect in Kir2.1 channels for terminal repolarization), and characteristic physical features is known as *Andersen-Tawil syndrome.*

Alterations in serum potassium level occur only during acute episodes and are accompanied by T-wave changes in the electrocardiogram. Hypokalemia may be due to alterations in calcium gradients. The creatine kinase (CK) level may be mildly elevated at those times. Plasma phosphate levels often decrease during symptomatic periods. Muscle biopsy findings are often normal between attacks, but during an attack a vacuolar myopathy is demonstrated. Pathologic changes in the periodic paralyses are similar whether the disease is due to a sodium or a potassium channel defect, suggesting that they might result from the recurrent paralytic state rather than the specific channelopathy. The vacuoles are dilated sarcoplasmic reticulum and invaginations of the extracellular space into the cytoplasm, and they may be filled with glycogen. Hypoglycemia does not occur. Loci for the majority of periodic paralyses have been demonstrated and the genes at least partially characterized, but many patients with the same clinical phenotype exhibit no mutations in the identified genes.

TREATMENT

Paralytic attacks of hypokalemic periodic paralysis are best treated by the oral administration of potassium or even fruit juices that contains potassium. A low sodium intake and the administration of acetazolamide, 125-250 mg bid or tid in school-age children, often is effective in abolishing attacks or at least reducing their frequency and severity. Spironolactone, in a dose of 100-200 mg/day PO in school-aged children, may be beneficial as well.

BIBLIOGRAPHY

Please visit the Nelson Textbook of Pediatrics *website at* *www.expertconsult.com* *for the complete bibliography.*

603.2 Malignant Hyperthermia

Harvey B. Sarnat

(See also Chapters 70 and 600.4.)

This syndrome is usually inherited as an autosomal dominant trait. It occurs in all patients with central core disease but is not limited to that particular myopathy. The gene is at the 19q13.1 locus in both central core disease and malignant hyperthermia without this specific myopathy. At least 15 separate mutations in this gene are associated with malignant hyperthermia. The gene programs the ryanodine receptor, a tetrameric calcium release channel in the sarcoplasmic reticulum, in apposition to the voltage-gated calcium channel of the transverse tubule. It occurs rarely in Duchenne and other muscular dystrophies, in various other myopathies, in some children with scoliosis, and in an isolated syndrome not associated with other muscle disease. Affected children sometimes have peculiar facies. All ages are affected, including premature infants whose mothers underwent general anesthesia for cesarean section.

Acute episodes are precipitated by exposure to general anesthetics and occasionally to local anesthetic drugs. Patients suddenly develop extreme fever, rigidity of muscles, and metabolic and respiratory acidosis; the serum CK level rises to as high as 35,000 IU/L. Myoglobinuria can result in tubular necrosis and acute renal failure.

The muscle biopsy specimen obtained during an episode of malignant hyperthermia or shortly afterward shows widely scattered necrosis of muscle fibers known as *rhabdomyolysis*. Between attacks, the muscle biopsy specimen is normal unless there is an underlying chronic myopathy.

It is important to recognize patients at risk of malignant hyperthermia because the attacks may be prevented by administering dantrolene sodium before an anesthetic is given. Patients at risk, such as siblings, are identified by the caffeine contracture test: A portion of fresh muscle biopsy tissue in a saline bath is attached to a strain gauge and exposed to caffeine and other drugs; an abnormal spasm is diagnostic. The syndrome receptor also may be demonstrated by immunochemistry in frozen sections of the muscle biopsy. The gene defect of the ryanodine receptor is present in 50% of patients; gene testing is available only for this genetic group. This receptor also may be seen in the muscle biopsy by immunoreactivity. Another candidate gene is at the 1q31 locus.

Apart from the genetic disorder of malignant hyperthermia, some drugs can induce acute rhabdomyolysis with myoglobinuria and potential renal failure, but this usually occurs in patients who are predisposed by some other metabolic disease (mitochondrial myopathies). Valproic acid can induce this process in children with mitochondrial cytopathies or with carnitine palmitoyltransferase deficiency.

603.3 Glycogenoses

Harvey B. Sarnat

(See also Chapter 81.1.)

Glycogenosis I (von Gierke disease) is not a true myopathy because the deficient liver enzyme glucose-6-phosphatase is not normally present in muscle. Nevertheless, children with this disease are hypotonic and mildly weak for unknown reasons.

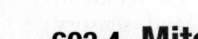

For the full continuation of this chapter, please visit the Nelson Textbook of Pediatrics *website at* *www.expertconsult.com*.

603.4 Mitochondrial Myopathies

Harvey B. Sarnat

(See also Chapters 81.4 and 591.2.)

Several diseases involving muscle, brain, and other organs are associated with structural and functional abnormalities of mitochondria, producing defects in aerobic cellular metabolism, the electron transport chain, and the Krebs cycle. The structural aberrations are best demonstrated by electron microscopy of the muscle biopsy sample, revealing a proliferation of abnormally shaped cristae including stacked or whorled cristae that fuse to form paracrystalline structures. Histochemical study of the muscle biopsy specimen reveals abnormal clumping of oxidative enzymatic activity and scattered myofibers, with loss of cytochrome-c oxidase activity and with increased neutral lipids within myofibers and/or ragged-red muscle fibers in some mitochondrial myopathies, with accumulations of membranous material beneath the muscle fiber membrane, best demonstrated by special stains.

These characteristic histochemical and ultrastructural changes are most consistently seen with point mutation in mitochondrial transfer RNA. The large mitochondrial DNA (mtDNA) deletions of 5 or 7.4 kb (the single mitochondrial chromosome has 16.5 kb) are associated with defects in mitochondrial respiratory oxidative enzyme complexes, if as few as 2% of the mitochondria are affected, but minimal or no morphologic or histochemical changes may be noted in the muscle biopsy specimen, even by electron microscopy; hence, quantitative biochemical studies of the muscle tissue are needed to confirm the diagnosis. Because most of the subunits of the respiratory chain complexes are encoded by nuclear DNA (nDNA) rather than mtDNA, mendelian autosomal inheritance is possible rather than maternal transmission as with pure mtDNA point mutations. Serum lactate is elevated in some diseases, and cerebrospinal fluid (CSF) lactate is more consistently elevated, even if serum concentrations are normal.

Several distinct mitochondrial diseases that primarily affect striated muscle or muscle and brain are identified. These can be divided into the ragged red fiber diseases and non–ragged fiber diseases. The ragged red fiber diseases include Kearns-Sayre, MELAS (*m*itochondrial *e*ncephalopathy, *l*actic *a*cidosis, and *s*troke) syndrome, MERRF (*m*yoclonic *e*pilepsy with *r*agged-*r*ed *f*ibers) syndrome, and progressive external ophthalmoplegia syndromes, which are associated with a combined defect in respiratory chain complexes I and IV. The non–ragged fiber diseases include Leigh encephalopathy and Leber hereditary optic atrophy; they involve complex I or IV alone or, in children, the common combination of defective complexes III and V. ***Kearns-Sayre syndrome*** is characterized by the triad of progressive external ophthalmoplegia, pigmentary degeneration of the retina, and onset before age 20 yr. Heart block, cerebellar deficits, and high CSF protein content are often associated. Visual evoked potentials are abnormal. Patients usually do not experience weakness of the trunk or extremities or dysphagia. Most cases are sporadic.

Chronic progressive external ophthalmoplegia may be isolated or accompanied by limb muscle weakness, dysphagia, and dysarthria. A few patients described as having *ophthalmoplegia plus* have additional central nervous system (CNS) involvement. Autosomal dominant inheritance is found in some pedigrees, but most cases are sporadic.

MERRF and ***MELAS syndromes*** are other mitochondrial disorders affecting children. The latter is characterized by stunted growth, episodic vomiting, seizures, and recurrent cerebral insults causing hemiparesis, hemianopia or even cortical blindness, and dementia. The disease behaves as a degenerative disorder, and children die within a few years.

Other "degenerative" diseases of the CNS that also involve myopathy with mitochondrial abnormalities include **Leigh subacute necrotizing encephalopathy** (Chapter 81.4) and **cerebrohepatorenal (Zellweger) disease** (Chapter 80.2). Another recognized mitochondrial myopathy is **cytochrome-c oxidase deficiency. Oculopharyngeal muscular dystrophy** is also fundamentally a mitochondrial myopathy. ***Mitochondrial depletion syndrome of early infancy*** is characterized by severely decreased oxidative enzymatic activities in all 5 of the complexes; in addition to diffuse muscle weakness, neonates and young infants can show multisystemic involvement, with failure of liver, kidney, and heart functions; encephalopathy; and sometimes bullous skin lesions or generalized edema. Many other rare diseases with only a few case reports are suspected of being mitochondrial disorders. It is also now recognized that secondary mitochondrial defects occur in a wide range of non-mitochondrial diseases, including inflammatory autoimmune myopathies, Pompe disease, and some cerebral malformations, and also may be induced by certain drugs and toxins, so that interpretation of mitochondrial abnormalities as primary defects must be approached with caution.

mtDNA is distinct from the DNA of the cell nucleus and is inherited exclusively from the mother; mitochondria are present in the cytoplasm of the ovum but not in the head of the sperm, the only part that enters the ovum at fertilization. The rate of mutation of mtDNA is 10 times higher than that of nDNA. The mitochondrial respiratory enzyme complexes each have subunits encoded either in mtDNA or nDNA. Complex II (succinate dehydrogenase, a Krebs cycle enzyme) has 4 subunits, all encoded in nDNA; complex III (ubiquinol or cytochrome-b oxidase) has 9 subunits, only 1 of which is encoded by mtDNA and 8 of which are programmed by nDNA; complex IV (cytochrome-c oxidase) has 13 subunits, only 3 of which are encoded by mtDNA. For this reason, mitochondrial diseases of muscle may be transmitted as autosomal recessive traits rather than by strict maternal transmission, even though all mitochondria are inherited from the mother.

In Kearns-Sayre syndrome, a single large mtDNA deletion has been identified, but other genetic variants are known; in MERRF and MELAS syndromes of mitochondrial myopathy, point mutations occur in transfer RNA (see Table 600-1).

Investigation for mitochondrial cytopathies includes serum and sometimes CSF lactate, cardiac evaluation, and molecular markers in blood for the common diseases with known mtDNA point mutations. The muscle biopsy provides the best evidence of all mitochondrial myopathies and should include histochemistry for oxidative enzymes, electron microscopy, and quantitative biochemical assay of respiratory chain enzymes complexes and coenzyme-Q10; muscle tissue also can be analyzed for mtDNA.

There is no effective treatment of mitochondrial cytopathies, but various "cocktails" are often used empirically to try to overcome the metabolic deficits. These include oral carnitine supplements, riboflavin, coenzyme-Q_{10}, ascorbic acid (vitamin C), vitamin E, and other antioxidants. Although some anecdotal reports are encouraging, no controlled studies that prove efficacy have been published.

BIBLIOGRAPHY

Please visit the Nelson Textbook of Pediatrics *website at www.expertconsult.com for the complete bibliography.*

603.5 Lipid Myopathies

Harvey B. Sarnat

(See Chapter 80.4.)

Considered as metabolic organs, skeletal muscles are the most important sites in the body for long-chain fatty acid metabolism because of their large mass and their rich density of mitochondria where fatty acids are metabolized. Hereditary disorders of lipid metabolism that cause progressive myopathy are an important, relatively common, and often treatable group of muscle diseases. Increased lipid within myofibers is seen in the muscle biopsy of some mitochondrial myopathies and is a constant, rather than an unpredictable, feature of specific diseases. Among the ragged red fiber diseases, Kearns-Sayre syndrome always shows increased neutral lipid, whereas MERRF and MELAS syndromes do not, a useful diagnostic marker for the pathologist.

For the full continuation of this chapter, please visit the Nelson Textbook of Pediatrics *website at www.expertconsult.com.*

603.6 Vitamin E Deficiency Myopathy

Harvey B. Sarnat

In experimental animals, deficiency of vitamin E (α-tocopherol, an antioxidant also important in mitochondrial superoxide generation) produces a progressive myopathy closely resembling a muscular dystrophy. Myopathy and neuropathy are recognized in humans who lack adequate intake of this antioxidant. Patients with chronic malabsorption, those undergoing long-term dialysis, and premature infants who do not receive vitamin E supplements are particularly vulnerable. Treatment with high doses of vitamin E can reverse the deficiency. Myopathy due to chronic hypervitaminosis E also occurs.

BIBLIOGRAPHY

Please visit the Nelson Textbook of Pediatrics *website at www.expertconsult.com for the complete bibliography.*

Chapter 604
Disorders of Neuromuscular Transmission and of Motor Neurons

604.1 Myasthenia Gravis

Harvey B. Sarnat

Myasthenia gravis is a chronic disease characterized by rapid fatigability of striated muscle. The most common cause is an immune-mediated neuromuscular blockade. The release of acetylcholine (ACh) into the synaptic cleft by the axonal terminal is normal, but the postsynaptic muscle membrane or *motor endplate* is less responsive than normal. A decreased number of available ACh receptors is due to circulating receptor-binding antibodies in most cases of acquired myasthenia. The disease is generally not hereditary and is an autoimmune disorder. A rare familial myasthenia gravis is probably an autosomal recessive trait and is not associated with plasma anti-ACh antibodies. One familial form is a deficiency of motor endplate acetylcholinesterase (AChE). Infants born to myasthenic mothers can have a transient neonatal myasthenic syndrome secondary to placentally transferred anti-ACh receptor antibodies, distinct from congenital myasthenia gravis (Table 604-1).

CLINICAL MANIFESTATIONS

Three clinical varieties are distinguished in childhood: juvenile myasthenia gravis in late infancy and childhood, congenital myasthenia, and transient neonatal myasthenia. In the juvenile form, ptosis and some degree of extraocular muscle weakness are the earliest and most constant signs. Older children might complain of diplopia, and young children might hold open their eyes with their fingers or thumbs if the ptosis is severe enough to obstruct vision. The pupillary responses to light are preserved. Dysphagia and facial weakness are also common, and in early infancy, feeding difficulties are often the cardinal sign of myasthenia. Poor head control because of weakness of the neck flexors is also prominent. Involvement may be limited to bulbar-innervated muscles, but the disease is systemic and weakness involves limb-girdle muscles and distal muscles of the hands in most cases. Fasciculations of muscle, myalgias, and sensory symptoms do not occur. Tendon stretch reflexes may be diminished but rarely are lost.

Rapid fatigue of muscles is a characteristic feature of myasthenia gravis that distinguishes it from most other neuromuscular diseases. Ptosis increases progressively as patients are asked to sustain an upward gaze for 30-90 sec. Holding the head up from the surface of the examining table while lying supine is very difficult, and gravity cannot be overcome for more than a few seconds. Repetitive opening and closing of the fists produces rapid fatigue of hand muscles, and patients cannot elevate their arms for more than 1-2 min because of fatigue of the deltoids.

Table 604-1 CLINICAL, PATHOLOGIC, AND NEUROPHYSIOLOGIC CHARACTERISTICS OF VARIOUS CONGENITAL MYASTHENIC SYNDROMES

	LEMS	CMS-EA	ENDPLATE AChE DEFICIENCY	SLOW CHANNEL SYNDROMES	FAST CHANNEL SYNDROME	ACh RECEPTOR DEFICIENCY
Mode of inheritance	AR-sporadic	AR	AR	AD	AR	AR
Gene location		17pter	3p24.2 (for type 1c)	2q24-q32, 17p11-p12 & 17p13	17p13	17p13
Gene product		FIM	COLQ	CHRNA, CHRNB1 & CHRNE	CHRNE	CHRNE
Pathogenesis/defect	Autoimmune	Presynaptic	Synaptic	Postsynaptic	Postsynaptic	Postsynaptic
Contractures	–	+	–	–	–	–
Tendon reflexes	–	+	±	±	±	±
Early manifestations	+	+	+	Variable	–	Variable
Episodic crises	±	+	–	–	–	–
Response to ACh inhibitors	–	+	–	–	+	+
Response to 3,4-DAP	Sometimes	–	–	–	Mild response	+
Response to quinidine	–	–	–	+	–	–
Low-frequency RS	Decrement	Decrement	Decrement	Decrement	Decrement	Decrement
High-frequency RS	Increment	Decrement	Decrement	Decrement	Decrement	Decrement
Repetitive CMAP	–	–	+	+	–	–
Low-amplitude baseline CMAP	+	–	–	–	–	–
Small MUP in electromyography	–	–	+	+	+	+
Muscle biopsy	Normal	Normal	Abnormal	Abnormal	Normal	Abnormal

AChE, acetycholinesterase; AD, autosomal dominant; AR, Autosomal recessive; CHRNA, acetylcholine receptor α subunit; CHRNB1, acetylcholine receptor β subunit; CHRNE, acetylcholine receptor e subunit; CMAP, compound muscle action potential; CMS-EA, congenital myasthenic syndrome with episodic apnea; COLQ, collagen Q; 3,4-DAP, 3,4-diaminopyridine; FIM, familial infantile myasthenia; LEMS, Lambert-Eaton myasthenic syndrome; MUP, motor unit potential; RS, repetitive stimulation; +, present; –, absent; ±, equivocal.
From Zafeiriou DI, Pitt M, de Sousa C: Clinical and neurophysiological characteristics of congenital myasthenic syndromes presenting in early infancy. *Brain Dev* 26:47–52, 2004.

Patients are more symptomatic late in the day or when tired. Dysphagia can interfere with eating, and the muscles of the jaw soon tire when an affected child chews.

Left untreated, myasthenia gravis is usually progressive and can become life threatening because of respiratory muscle involvement and the risk of aspiration, particularly at times when the child is otherwise unwell with an upper respiratory tract infection. Familial myasthenia gravis usually is not progressive.

Infants born to myasthenic mothers can have respiratory insufficiency, inability to suck or swallow, and generalized hypotonia and weakness. They might show little spontaneous motor activity for several days to weeks. Some require ventilatory support and feeding by gavage during this period. After the abnormal antibodies disappear from the blood and muscle tissue, these infants regain normal strength and are not at increased risk of developing myasthenia gravis in later childhood.

The syndrome of *transient neonatal myasthenia gravis* is to be distinguished from a rare and often hereditary **congenital myasthenia gravis** not related to maternal myasthenia that is nearly always a permanent disorder without spontaneous remission (see Table 604-1). Several distinct genetic forms are recognized, all with onset at birth or in early infancy with hypotonia, ophthalmoplegia, ptosis, dysphagia, weak cry, facial weakness, easy muscle fatigue generally, and sometimes respiratory insufficiency or failure, the last often precipitated by a minor respiratory infection. Cholinesterase inhibitors have a favorable effect in most, but in some forms the symptoms and signs are actually worsened. Most congenital myasthenic syndromes are transmitted as autosomal recessive traits, but the slow channel syndrome is autosomal dominant. Five defective postsynaptic molecules have been identified in the pathogenesis of congenital myasthenia gravis and account for 85% of cases; rapsyn may be the most common. Acetylcholine receptor deficiencies have >60 identified genetic mutations. Anti-AChR and anti-MuSK antibodies are absent in serum, unlike autoimmune forms of myasthenia gravis affecting older children and adults.

Three **presynaptic congenital myasthenic syndromes** are recognized, all as autosomal recessive traits; some of these have anti-MuSK antibodies. These children exhibit weakness of extraocular, pharyngeal, and respiratory muscles and later show shoulder girdle weakness as well. Episodic **apnea** is a problem in congenital myasthenia gravis. Another synaptic form is caused by absence or marked deficiency of motor endplate AChE in the synaptic basal lamina, and postsynaptic forms of congenital myasthenia are caused by mutations in ACh receptor subunit genes that alter the synaptic response to ACh. An abnormality of the ACh receptor channels appearing as high conductance and excessively fast closure may be the result of a point mutation in a subunit of the receptor affecting a single amino acid residue. Children with congenital myasthenia gravis do not experience myasthenic crises and rarely exhibit elevations of anti-ACh antibodies in plasma.

Myasthenia gravis is occasionally associated with hypothyroidism, usually due to **Hashimoto thyroiditis.** Other collagen vascular diseases may also be associated. Thymomas, noted in some adults, rarely coexist with myasthenia gravis in children, nor do carcinomas of the lung occur, which produce a unique form of myasthenia in adults called **Eaton-Lambert syndrome.** Postinfectious myasthenia gravis in children is transitory and usually follows a varicella-zoster infection by 2-5 wk as an immune response.

LABORATORY FINDINGS AND DIAGNOSIS

Myasthenia gravis is one of the few neuromuscular diseases in which electromyography (EMG) is more specifically diagnostic than a muscle biopsy. A decremental response is seen to repetitive nerve stimulation; the muscle potentials diminish rapidly in amplitude until the muscle becomes refractory to further stimulation. Motor nerve conduction velocity remains normal. This unique EMG pattern is the electrophysiologic correlate of the fatigable weakness observed clinically and is reversed after a cholinesterase inhibitor is administered. A myasthenic decrement may be absent or difficult to demonstrate in muscles that are not involved clinically. This feature may be confusing in early cases or in patients showing only weakness of extraocular muscles. Microelectrode studies of endplate potentials and currents reveal whether the transmission defect is presynaptic or postsynaptic. Special electrophysiologic studies are required in the classification of congenital myasthenic syndromes and involve estimating the number of ACh receptors per endplate and in vitro study of endplate function. These special studies and patch-clamp recordings of kinetic properties of channels are performed on special biopsy samples of intercostal muscle strips that include both origin and insertion of the muscle but are only performed in specialized centers. If myasthenia is limited to the extraocular muscles, levator palpebrae, and pharyngeal muscles, evoked-potential EMG of the muscles of the extremities and spine, diagnostic in the generalized disease, usually is normal.

Anti-ACh antibodies should be assayed in the plasma but are inconsistently demonstrated. About 30% of affected adolescents show elevations, but anti-ACh receptor antibodies are only occasionally demonstrated in the plasma of prepubertal children. Many juvenile myasthenics who show no anti-ACh antibodies in serum have antibodies against the receptor tyrosine kinase (MuSK), which also is localized at the neuromuscular junction and appears essential to fetal development of this junction. Many cases of congenital myasthenia gravis do not result from a refractory postsynaptic membrane at the neuromuscular junction as in juvenile and adult myasthenia but rather result from failure to synthesize or release ACh at the presynaptic membrane. In some cases, the gene that mediates the enzyme choline acetyltransferase for the synthesis of ACh is mutated. In others, there is a defect in the quantal release of vesicles containing ACh. The treatment of such patients with cholinesterase inhibitors is futile. Assay of anti-rapsyn antibody will become commercially available in the near future.

Other serologic tests of autoimmune disease, such as antinuclear antibodies and abnormal immune complexes, should also be sought. If these are positive, more extensive autoimmune disease involving vasculitis or tissues other than muscle is likely. A thyroid profile should always be examined. The serum creatine kinase (CK) level is normal in myasthenia gravis.

The heart is not involved, and electrocardiographic findings remain normal. Radiographs of the chest often reveal an enlarged thymus, but the hypertrophy is not a thymoma. It may be further defined by tomography or by CT scanning of the anterior mediastinum.

The role of conventional muscle biopsy in myasthenia gravis is limited. It is not required in most cases, but about 17% of patients show inflammatory changes, sometimes called *lymphorrhages,* that are interpreted by some physicians as a mixed myasthenia-polymyositis immune disorder. Muscle biopsy tissue in myasthenia gravis shows nonspecific type II muscle fiber atrophy, similar to that seen with disuse atrophy, steroid effects on muscle, polymyalgia rheumatica, and many other conditions. The ultrastructure of motor endplates shows simplification of the membrane folds; the ACh receptors are located in these postsynaptic folds, as shown by bungarotoxin (snake venom), which binds specifically to the ACh receptors.

A **clinical test for myasthenia gravis** is administration of a short-acting cholinesterase inhibitor, usually edrophonium chloride. Ptosis and ophthalmoplegia improve within a few seconds, and fatigability of other muscles decreases.

Recommendations on the Use of Cholinesterase Inhibitors as a Diagnostic Test for Myasthenia Gravis in Infants and Children

CHILDREN 2 YEARS AND OLDER

- The child should have a specific fatigable weakness that can be measured, such as ptosis of the eyelids, dysphagia, or inability of the cervical muscles to support the head. Nonspecific generalized weakness without cranial nerve motor deficits is not a criterion.
- An IV infusion should be started to enable the administration of medications in the event of an adverse reaction.
- Electrocardiographic monitoring is recommended during the test.
- A dose of atropine sulfate (0.01 mg/kg) should be available in a syringe, ready for IV administration at the bedside during the edrophonium test, to block acute muscarinic effects of the cholinesterase inhibitor, mainly abdominal cramps and/or sudden diarrhea from increased peristalsis, profuse bronchotracheal secretions that can obstruct the airway, or, rarely, cardiac arrhythmias. Some physicians pretreat all patients with atropine before administering edrophonium, but this is not recommended unless there is a history of reaction to tests. Atropine can cause the pupils to be dilated and fixed for as long as 14 days after a single dose, and the pupillary effects of homatropine can last 4-7 days.
- Edrophonium chloride (Tensilon) is administered IV. Initially, a test dose of 0.04 mg/kg is given to ensure that the patient does not have an allergic reaction or is otherwise very sensitive to muscarinic side effects. If this test dose is well tolerated, the diagnostic dose administered is 0.1-0.2 mg/kg; the maximum single dose is 10 mg regardless of weight. In children weighing <30 kg, 2 mg is the maximum dose; a typical dose for a 3-5 yr old child is 5 mg. These doses may be given IM or subcutaneously, but these routes are not recommended because the results are much more variable owing to unpredictable absorption, and the test may be ambiguous or falsely negative.
- Effects should be seen within 10 sec and disappear within 120 sec. Weakness is measured as, for example, distance between upper and lower eyelids before and after administration, degree of external ophthalmoplegia, or ability to swallow a sip of water.
- Long-acting cholinesterase inhibitors, such as pyridostigmine (Mestinon), are generally not as useful for the acute assessment of myasthenic weakness. The prostigmine test may be used (as outlined later) but might not be as definitively diagnostic as the edrophonium test.

FOR CHILDREN YOUNGER THAN 2 YEARS

- Infants ideally should have a specific fatigable weakness that can be measured, such as ptosis of the eyelids, dysphagia, and inability of cervical muscles to support the head. Nonspecific generalized weakness without cranial nerve motor deficits makes it less easy to assess results but may be a criterion at times.
- An IV infusion should be started as a rapid route for medications in the event of an adverse effect of the test medication.
- Electrocardiographic monitoring is recommended during the test.
- Pretreatment with atropine sulfate to block the muscarinic effects of the test medication is not recommended but it should be available at the bedside in a prepared syringe. If needed, it should be administered IV in a dose of 0.1 mg/kg.
- Edrophonium is not recommended for use in infants; its effect is too brief for objective assessment and an increased incidence of acute cardiac arrhythmias is reported in infants, especially neonates, with this drug.
- Prostigmine methylsulfate (Neostigmine) is administered IM at a dose of 0.04 mg/kg. If the result is negative or equivocal, another dose of 0.04 mg/kg may be administered 4 hr after the first dose (a typical dose is 0.5-1.5 mg). The peak effect is seen in 20-40 min. IV prostigmine is contraindicated because of the risk of cardiac arrhythmias, including fatal ventricular fibrillation, especially in young infants.
- Long-acting cholinesterase inhibitors administered orally, such as pyridostigmine (Mestinon), are generally not as useful for the acute assessment of myasthenic weakness because onset and duration are less predictable.

The test should be performed in the emergency department, hospital ward, or, intensive care unit; the important issue is preparation for potential complications such as cardiac arrhythmia or cholinergic crisis, as outlined.

TREATMENT

Some patients with mild myasthenia gravis require no treatment. **Cholinesterase-inhibiting drugs** are the primary therapeutic agents. Neostigmine methylsulfate (0.04 mg/kg) may be given IM every 4-6 hr, but most patients tolerate oral neostigmine bromide, 0.4 mg/kg every 4-6 hr. If dysphagia is a major problem, the drug should be given about 30 min before meals to improve swallowing. Pyridostigmine is an alternative; the dose required is about 4 times greater than that of neostigmine, but it may be slightly longer acting. Overdoses of cholinesterase inhibitors produce cholinergic crises; atropine blocks the muscarinic effects but does not block the nicotinic effects that produce additional skeletal muscle weakness. In the rare familial myasthenia gravis caused by absence of endplate AChE, cholinesterase inhibitors are not helpful and often cause increased weakness; these patients can be treated with ephedrine or diaminopyridine, both of which increase ACh release from terminal axons.

Because of the autoimmune basis of the disease, long-term **steroid treatment** with prednisone may be effective. **Thymectomy** should be considered and might provide a cure. Thymectomy is most effective in patients who have high titers of anti-ACh receptor antibodies in the plasma and who have been symptomatic for <2 yr. Thymectomy is ineffective in congenital and familial forms of myasthenia gravis. Treatment of hypothyroidism usually abolishes an associated myasthenia without the use of cholinesterase inhibitors or steroids.

Plasmapheresis is effective treatment in some children, particularly those who do not respond to steroids, but plasma exchange therapy provides only temporary remission. **IV immunoglobulin** (IVIG) is beneficial and should be tried before plasmapheresis because it is less invasive. Plasmapheresis and IVIG appear to be most effective in patients with high circulating levels of anti-ACh receptor antibodies. Refractory patients might respond to rituximab, a monoclonal antibody to the B-cell CD20 antigen.

Neonates with transient maternally transmitted myasthenia gravis require cholinesterase inhibitors for only a few days or occasionally for a few weeks, especially to allow feeding. No other treatment is usually necessary. In non–maternally transmitted congenital myasthenia gravis, identification of the specific molecular defect is important for treatment; specific therapies for each type are summarized in Table 604-2.

Table 604-2 POTENTIAL THERAPIES IN CONGENITAL MYASTHENIC SYNDROMES

AChE	Ephedrine 3 mg/kg/day in 3 divided doses; begin with 1 mg/kg; not obtainable in several countries If ephedrine is not obtainable, 3,4-DAP 1 mg/kg/day in 4 divided doses, up to 60 mg/day in adults Avoid AChE inhibitors
AChR deficiency	AChE inhibitors: pyridostigmine bromide (Mestinon) 4-5 mg/kg/day in 4-6 divided doses If necessary add 3,4-DAP 1 mg/kg/day in 4 divided doses, up to 60 mg/day in adults
AChR fast channel	AChE inhibitors: pyridostigmine bromide (Mestinon) 4-5 mg/kg/day in 4-6 divided doses If necessary add 3,4-DAP 1 mg/kg/day in 4 divided doses, up to 60 mg/day in adults
AChR slow channel	Quinidine sulfate • Adults: Begin for 1 wk with 200 mg tid; gradual increase to maintain a serum level of 1-25 µg/mL • Children: 15-60 mg/kg/day in 4-6 divided doses; not available in several countries If quinidine sulfate is not available, fluoxetine 80-100 mg/day in adults Avoid AChE inhibitors
ChAT	AChE inhibitors: pyridostigmine bromide (Mestinon) 4-5 mg/kg/day in 4-6 divided doses If necessary add 3,4-DAP 1 mg/kg/day in 4 divided doses, up to 60 mg/day in adults
Dok7	Ephedrine 3 mg/kg/day in 3 divided doses; begin with 1 mg/kg; not obtainable in several countries If ephedrine is not obtainable, 3,4-DAP 1 mg/kg/day in 4 divided doses, up to 60 mg/day in adults Avoid AChE inhibitors
Laminin β2	Ephedrine 3 mg/kg/day in 3 divided doses; begin with 1 mg/kg; not obtainable in several countries Avoid AChE inhibitors
MuSK	AChE inhibitors: pyridostigmine bromide (Mestinon) 4-5 mg/kg/day in 4-6 divided doses 3,4-DAP 1 mg/kg/day in 4 divided doses, up to 60 mg/day in adults
Rapsyn	AChE inhibitors: pyridostigmine bromide (Mestinon) 4-5 mg/kg/day in 4-6 divided doses If necessary add 3,4-DAP 1 mg/kg/day in 4 divided doses, up to 60 mg/day in adults

Modified from Eyemard B, Hantai D, Estounet B: Congenital myasthenic syndromes. In Dulac O, Sarnat HB, Lassonde M, editors: *Handbook of clinical neurology: paediatric neurology,* vol 2, Philadelphia, Elsevier, in press.

COMPLICATIONS

Children with myasthenia gravis do not tolerate neuromuscular-blocking drugs, such as succinylcholine and pancuronium, and may be paralyzed for weeks after a single dose. An anesthesiologist should carefully review myasthenic patients who require a surgical anesthetic. Also, certain antibiotics can potentiate myasthenia and should be avoided; these include the aminoglycosides (gentamicin and others).

PROGNOSIS

Some patients experience spontaneous remission after a period of months or years; others have a permanent disease extending into adult life. Immunosuppression, thymectomy, and treatment of associated hypothyroidism might provide a cure.

OTHER CAUSES OF NEUROMUSCULAR BLOCKADE

Organophosphate chemicals, commonly used as insecticides, can cause a myasthenia-like syndrome in children exposed to these toxins (Chapter 58).

Botulism results from ingestion of food containing the toxin of *Clostridium botulinum,* a gram-positive, spore-bearing, anaerobic bacillus (Chapter 202). Honey is a common source of contamination. The incubation period is short, only a few hours, and symptoms begin with nausea, vomiting, and diarrhea. Cranial nerve involvement soon follows, with diplopia, dysphagia, weak suck, facial weakness, and absent gag reflex. Generalized hypotonia and weakness then develop and can progress to respiratory failure. Neuromuscular blockade is documented by EMG with repetitive nerve stimulation. Respiratory support may be required for days or weeks until the toxin is cleared from the body. No specific antitoxin is available. Guanidine, 35 mg/kg/24 hr, may be effective for extraocular and limb muscle weakness but not for respiratory muscle involvement.

Tick paralysis is a disorder of ACh release from axonal terminals due to a neurotoxin that blocks depolarization. It also affects large myelinated motor and sensory nerve fibers. This toxin is produced by the wood tick or dog tick, insects common in the Appalachian and Rocky Mountains of North America. The tick embeds its head into the skin, usually the scalp, and neurotoxin production is maximal about 5-6 days later. Motor symptoms include weakness, loss of coordination, and sometimes an ascending paralysis resembling Guillain-Barré syndrome. Tendon reflexes are lost. Sensory symptoms of tingling paresthesias can occur in the face and extremities. The diagnosis is confirmed by EMG and nerve conduction studies and by identifying the tick. The tick must be removed completely and the buried head not left beneath the skin. Patients then recover completely within hours or days.

BIBLIOGRAPHY

Please visit the Nelson Textbook of Pediatrics *website at* *www.expertconsult.com* *for the complete bibliography.*

604.2 Spinal Muscular Atrophies

Harvey B. Sarnat

Spinal muscular atrophies (SMAs) are degenerative diseases of motor neurons that begin in fetal life and continue to be progressive in infancy and childhood. The progressive denervation of muscle is compensated in part by reinnervation from an adjacent motor unit, but giant motor units are thus created with subsequent atrophy of muscle fibers when the reinnervating motor neuron eventually becomes involved. Upper motor neurons remain normal.

SMA is classified into a severe infantile form, also known as **Werdnig-Hoffmann disease** or SMA type 1; a late infantile and more slowly progressive form, SMA type 2; and a more chronic or juvenile form, also called **Kugelberg-Welander disease,** or SMA type 3. A severe fetal form that is usually fatal in the perinatal period has been described as SMA type 0, with motor neuron degeneration demonstrated in the spinal cord as early as midgestation. These distinctions of types are clinical and are based on age at onset, severity of weakness, and clinical course; muscle biopsy does not distinguish types 1 and 2, although type 3 shows a more adult than perinatal pattern of denervation and reinnervation. Type 0 can show biopsy features more similar to myotubular myopathy because of maturational arrest; scattered myotubes and other immature fetal fibers also are demonstrated in the muscle biopsies of patients with types 1 and 2, but do not predominate. About 25% of patients have type 1, 50% type 2, and 25% type 3; type 0 is rare and accounts for <1%. Some patients are transitional between types 1 and 2 or between types 2 and 3 in terms of clinical function. A variant of SMA, **Fazio-Londe disease,** is a progressive bulbar palsy resulting from motor neuron degeneration more in the brainstem than the spinal cord. Other variants are noted in Table 604-3.

Table 604-3 SPINAL MUSCULAR ATROPHY VARIANTS: PROGRESSIVE OR SEVERE NEONATAL ANTERIOR HORN CELL DISEASE NOT LINKED TO *SMN*

VARIANT	MAJOR FEATURES
SMA with respiratory distress type 1 (SMARD1)	Mild hypotonia, weak cry, distal contractures initially Respiratory distress from diaphragmatic paralysis 1-6 mo, progressive distal weakness Autosomal recessive, locus 11q13.2, gene: immunoglobulin mu-binding protein 2 *(IGHMBP2)*
Pontocerebellar hypoplasia type 1	Arthrogryposis, hypotonia, weakness, bulbar deficits early; later, microcephaly, extraocular defects, cognitive deficits: pontocerebellar hypoplasia Molecular defect unknown Likely autosomal recessive
X-linked infantile SMA with bone fractures	Arthrogryposis, hypotonia, weakness, congenital bone fractures, respiratory failure Lethal course as in severe type 1 SMA Most cases X-linked (X9/11.3-q11.2), a few cases likely autosomal recessive
Congenital SMA with predominant lower limb involvement	Arthrogyposis, hypotonia, weakness, especially distal lower limbs early Nonprogressive but severe disability Autosomal dominant or sporadic; locus 12q23-24

SMA, spinal muscular atrophy.
From Vole JJ: *Neurology of the newborn,* ed 5, Philadelphia, 2008, Saunders Elsevier, p 775.

ETIOLOGY

The cause of SMA is a pathologic continuation of a process of programmed cell death (apoptosis) that is normal in embryonic life. A surplus of motor neuroblasts and other neurons is generated from primitive neuroectoderm, but only about half survive and mature to become neurons; the excess cells have a limited life cycle and degenerate. If the process that arrests physiologic cell death fails to intervene by a certain stage, neuronal death can continue in late fetal life and postnatally. The survivor motor neuron gene *(SMN)* arrests apoptosis of motor neuroblasts. Unlike most genes that are highly conserved in evolution, *SMN* is a uniquely mammalian gene. An additional function of SMN, both centrally and peripherally, is to transport RNA binding proteins to the axonal growth cone to ensure an adequate amount of protein-encoding transcripts essential for growth cone mobility both during fetal development and in postnatal synaptic remodeling.

CLINICAL MANIFESTATIONS

The cardinal features of **SMA type 1** are severe hypotonia (Fig. 604-1); generalized weakness; thin muscle mass; absent tendon stretch reflexes; involvement of the tongue, face, and jaw muscles; and sparing of extraocular muscles and sphincters. Diaphragmatic involvement is late. Infants who are symptomatic at birth can have respiratory distress and are unable to feed. Congenital contractures, ranging from simple clubfoot to generalized arthrogryposis, occur in about 10% of severely involved neonates. Infants lie flaccid with little movement, unable to overcome gravity (see Fig. 599-1). They lack head control. More than 65% of children die by 2 yr of age, and many die early in infancy.

In **type 2 SMA,** affected infants are usually able to suck and swallow, and respiration is adequate in early infancy. These children show progressive weakness, but many survive into the school years or beyond, although confined to an electric wheelchair and severely handicapped. Nasal speech and problems with deglutition develop later. Scoliosis becomes a major complication in many patients with long survival.

Kugelberg-Welander disease is the mildest **SMA (type 3)**, and patients can appear normal in infancy. The progressive weakness is proximal in distribution, particularly involving shoulder girdle muscles. Patients are ambulatory. Symptoms of bulbar muscle weakness are rare. About 25% of patients with this form of SMA have muscular hypertrophy rather than atrophy, and it may easily be confused with a muscular dystrophy. Longevity can extend well into middle adult life. Fasciculations are a specific clinical sign of denervation of muscle. In thin children, they may be seen in the deltoid, biceps brachii, and occasionally the quadriceps femoris muscles, but the continuous, involuntary, wormlike movements may be masked by a thick pad of subcutaneous fat. Fasciculations are best observed in the tongue, where almost no subcutaneous connective tissue separates the muscular layer from the epithelium. If the intrinsic lingual muscles are contracted, such as in crying or when the tongue protrudes, fasciculations are more difficult to see than when the tongue is relaxed.

The outstretched fingers of children with SMA often show a characteristic tremor owing to fasciculations and weakness. It should not be confused with a cerebellar tremor. *Myalgias are not a feature of SMA.*

The heart is not involved in SMA. Intelligence is normal, and children often appear brighter than their normal peers because the effort they cannot put into physical activities is redirected to intellectual development, and they are often exposed to adult speech more than to juvenile language because of the social repercussions of the disease.

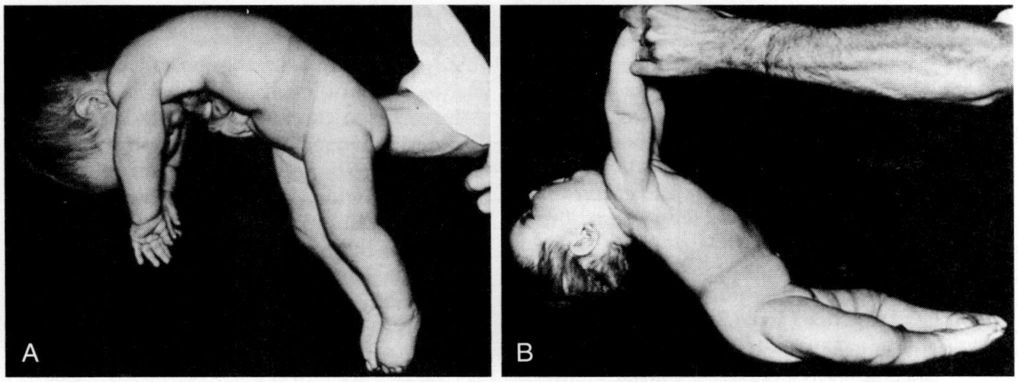

Figure 604-1 Type 1 spinal muscular atrophy (Werdnig-Hoffmann disease). Clinical manifestations of weakness of limb and axial musculature in a 6 wk old infant with severe weakness and hypotonia from birth. Note the marked weakness of the limbs and trunk on ventral suspension *(A)* and of neck on pull to sit *(B)* (From Volpe J: *Neurology of the newborn,* ed 4, Philadelphia, 2001, WB Saunders, p 644).

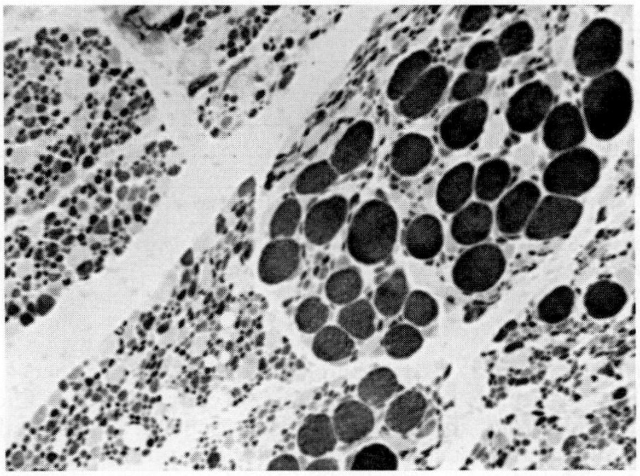

Figure 604-2 Muscle biopsy of neonate with infantile spinal muscular atrophy. Groups of giant type I (darkly stained) fibers are seen within muscle fascicles of severely atrophic fibers of both histochemical types. This is the characteristic pattern of perinatal denervation of muscle. Myofibrillar ATPase, preincubated at pH 4.6 (×400).

LABORATORY FINDINGS

The serum CK level may be normal but more commonly is mildly elevated in the hundreds. A CK level of several thousand is rare. Results of motor nerve conduction studies are normal, except for mild slowing in terminal stages of the disease, an important feature distinguishing SMA from peripheral neuropathy. EMG shows fibrillation potentials and other signs of denervation of muscle. A secondary mtDNA depletion is sometimes demonstrated in the muscle biopsy of infants with SMA.

DIAGNOSIS

The simplest, most definitive diagnostic test is a molecular genetic marker in blood for the *SMN* gene. Muscle biopsy reveals a characteristic pattern of perinatal denervation that is unlike that of mature muscle. Groups of giant type I fibers are mixed with fascicles of severely atrophic fibers of both histochemical types (Fig. 604-2). Scattered immature myofibers resembling myotubes also are demonstrated. In juvenile SMA, the pattern may be more similar to adult muscle that has undergone many cycles of denervation and reinnervation. Neurogenic changes in muscle also may be demonstrated by EMG, but the results are less definitive than by muscle biopsy in infancy. Sural nerve biopsy sometimes shows mild sensory neuropathic changes, and sensory nerve conduction velocity may be slowed; hypertrophy of unmyelinated axons also is seen. At autopsy, mild degenerative changes are seen in sensory neurons of dorsal root ganglia and in somatosensory nuclei of the thalamus, but these alterations are not perceived clinically as sensory loss or paresthesias. The most pronounced neuropathologic lesions are the extensive neuronal degeneration and gliosis in the ventral horns of the spinal cord and brainstem motor nuclei, especially the hypoglossal nucleus.

GENETICS

Molecular genetic diagnosis by DNA probes in blood samples or in muscle biopsy or chorionic villi tissues is available for diagnosis of suspected cases and for prenatal diagnosis. Most cases are inherited as an autosomal recessive trait. The incidence of SMA is 10-15/100,000 live births, affecting all ethnic groups; it is the 2nd most common neuromuscular disease, following Duchenne muscular dystrophy. The incidence of heterozygosity for autosomal recessive SMA is 1:50.

The genetic locus for all 3 of the common forms of SMA is on chromosome 5, a deletion at the 5q11-q13 locus, indicating that they are variants of the same disease rather than different diseases. The affected *SMN* gene contains 8 exons that span 20 kb, telomeric and centromeric exons that differ only by 5bp and produce a transcript encoding 294 amino acids. Another gene, the *neuronal apoptosis inhibitory gene (NAIP),* is located next to the *SMN* gene and in many cases there is an inverted duplication with 2 copies, telomeric and centromeric, of both genes; isolated mutations or deletions of *NAIP* do not produce clinical SMA and generate a mostly nonfunctional isoform lacking the carboxy-terminus amino acids encoded by exon 7. Milder forms of SMA have more than 2 copies of *SMN2*, and in late-onset patients with homozygous deletion of the *SMN1* gene, there are 4 copies of *SMN2*. An additional gene mapped to 11q13-q21 in SMA may help explain early respiratory failure in some patients. Nucleotide expansions account for only 5-10% of cases of SMA, and deletions or splicing out of exons 7 and 8 are the genetic mechanism in the great majority of cases. Another pair of genes adjacent to the *SMN1* and *SMN2* genes, *SERF1* and *SERF2*, also may play a secondary role.

Infrequent families with autosomal dominant inheritance are described, and a rare X-linked recessive form also occurs. Carrier testing by dose analysis is available.

TREATMENT

No medical treatment is able to delay the progression. Supportive therapy includes orthopedic care with particular attention to scoliosis and joint contractures, mild physiotherapy, and mechanical aids for assisting the child to eat and to be as functionally independent as possible. Most children learn to use a computer keyboard with great skill but cannot use a pencil easily. Valproic acid is sometimes administered because it increases SMN2 protein, and gabapentin and oral phenylbutyrate also may slow the progression, but these treatments do not alter the course in all patients. A benefit of antioxidants is unproved. Gene replacement and protein replacement, including lentiviral, therapies are theoretical and experimental at this time.

BIBLIOGRAPHY
Please visit the Nelson Textbook of Pediatrics *website at* *www.expertconsult.com* *for the complete bibliography.*

604.3 Other Motor Neuron Diseases

Harvey B. Sarnat

Motor neuron diseases other than SMA are rare in children. *Poliomyelitis* used to be a major cause of chronic disability, but since the routine use of polio vaccine, this viral infection is now rare (Chapter 241). Other enteroviruses, such as coxsackievirus and echovirus, or the live polio vaccine virus can also cause an acute infection of motor neurons with symptoms and signs similar to poliomyelitis, although usually milder. Specific polymerase chain reaction tests and viral cultures of cerebrospinal fluid are diagnostic. Motor neuron infection with the West Nile virus also occurs.

A **juvenile form of amyotrophic lateral sclerosis** is rare. Upper and lower motor neuron loss is evident clinically, unlike in SMA. The course is progressive and ultimately fatal.

Pena-Shokeir and **Marden-Walker syndromes** are progressive motor neuron degenerations associated with severe arthrogryposis and congenital anomalies of many organ systems. **Pontocerebellar hypoplasias** are progressive degenerative diseases of the central nervous system that begin in fetal life; one form also involves motor neuron degeneration resembling an SMA, but the *SMN* gene on chromosome 5 is normal.

Motor neurons become involved in several metabolic diseases of the nervous system, such as gangliosidosis (Tay-Sachs disease), ceroid lipofuscinosis (Batten disease), and glycogenosis II (Pompe disease), but the signs of denervation may be minor or obscured by the more prominent involvement of other parts of the central nervous system or of muscle.

Chapter 605
Hereditary Motor-Sensory Neuropathies

Harvey B. Sarnat

The hereditary motor-sensory neuropathies (HMSNs) are a group of progressive diseases of peripheral nerves. Motor components generally dominate the clinical picture, but sensory and autonomic involvement is expressed later.

605.1 Peroneal Muscular Atrophy (Charcot-Marie-Tooth Disease; HMSN Type I)

Harvey B. Sarnat

Charcot-Marie-Tooth disease is the most common genetically determined neuropathy and has an overall prevalence of 3.8/100,000. It is transmitted as an autosomal dominant trait with 83% expressivity; the 17p11.2 locus is the site of the abnormal gene. Autosomal recessive transmission also is described but is rarer. The gene product is peripheral myelin protein 22 (PMP22). A much rarer X-linked HMSN type I results from a defect at the Xq13.l locus, causing mutations in the gap junction protein connexin-32. Other forms have been reported (Table 605-1).

Table 605-1 CHARCOT-MARIE-TOOTH (CMT) DISEASE

DISEASE	INHERITANCE	LOCUS	PRODUCT
CMT1A	AD	17p11	Peripheral myelin protein
CMT1B	AD	1q22	Myelin P0 protein
CMT1C	AD	16p13.1.1-p12.3	
CMT1D	AD	10q21.1-22.1	Early growth response protein 2
CMT2A	AD	1p36	Kinosin-like protein, mitofusin 2
CMT2B	AD	3q21	Ras-related protein
CMT2C	AD	12q23-24	Unknown
CMT2D	AD	7p15	Clycyl-tRNA synthetase
CMT2E	AD	8p21	Neurofilament triplet L protein
CMT2G	AD	2q12-13	Unknown
CMT2L	AD	12q24	Unknown
CMT4A	AR	8q13-q21	Ganglioside-induced differentiation
CMT4B1	AR	11q22	Myotubularin-related protein 2
CMT4B2	AR	11q15	Myotubularin-related protein 13
CMT4C	AR	5q32	Unknown
CMT4D	AR	8q24.3	NDRG1 protein
CMT4E	AR	10q21	Early growth response protein 2
CMTX	XLD	Xq13.1	Connexin 32

Modified from Bird TD: *Charcot-Marie-Tooth hereditary neuropathy overview* (database online). www.geneclinics.org. Accessed April 12, 2010.

CLINICAL MANIFESTATIONS

Most patients are asymptomatic until late childhood or early adolescence, but young children sometimes manifest gait disturbance as early as the 2nd year of life. The peroneal and tibial nerves are the earliest and most severely affected. Children with the disorder are often described as being clumsy, falling easily, or tripping over their own feet. The onset of symptoms may be delayed until after the 5th decade.

Muscles of the anterior compartment of the lower legs become wasted, and the legs have a characteristic stork-like contour. The muscular atrophy is accompanied by progressive weakness of dorsiflexion of the ankle and eventual footdrop. The process is bilateral but may be slightly asymmetric. Pes cavus deformities invariably develop due to denervation of intrinsic foot muscles, further destabilizing the gait. Atrophy of muscles of the forearms and hands is usually not as severe as that of the lower extremities, but in advanced cases contractures of the wrists and fingers produce a claw hand. Proximal muscle weakness is a late manifestation and is usually mild. Axial muscles are not involved.

The disease is slowly progressive throughout life, but patients occasionally show accelerated deterioration of function over a few years. Most patients remain ambulatory and have normal longevity, although orthotic appliances are required to stabilize the ankles.

Sensory involvement mainly affects large myelinated nerve fibers that convey proprioceptive information and vibratory sense, but the threshold for pain and temperature can also increase. Some children complain of tingling or burning sensations of the feet, but pain is rare. Because the muscle mass is reduced, the nerves are more vulnerable to trauma or compression. Autonomic manifestations may be expressed as poor vasomotor control with blotching or pallor of the skin of the feet and inappropriately cold feet.

Nerves often become palpably enlarged. Tendon stretch reflexes are lost distally. Cranial nerves are not affected. Sphincter control remains well preserved. Autonomic neuropathy does not affect the heart, gastrointestinal tract, or bladder. Intelligence is normal. A unique point mutation in *PMP22* causes progressive auditory nerve deafness in addition, but this is usually later in onset than the peripheral neuropathy.

Davidenkow syndrome is a variant of HMSN type I with a scapuloperoneal distribution.

LABORATORY FINDINGS AND DIAGNOSIS

Motor and sensory nerve conduction velocities are greatly reduced, sometimes as slow as 20% of normal conduction time. In new cases without a family history, both parents should be examined, and nerve conduction studies should be performed.

Electromyography (EMG) and muscle biopsy are not usually required for diagnosis, but they show evidence of many cycles of denervation and reinnervation. Serum creatine kinase level is normal. Cerebrospinal fluid (CSF) protein may be elevated, but no cells appear in the CSF.

Sural nerve biopsy is diagnostic. Large- and medium-sized myelinated fibers are reduced in number, collagen is increased, and characteristic **onion bulb formations** of proliferated Schwann cell cytoplasm surround axons. This pathologic finding is called **interstitial hypertrophic neuropathy.** Extensive segmental demyelination and remyelination also occur.

The definitive molecular genetic diagnosis may be made in blood.

TREATMENT

Stabilization of the ankles is a primary concern. In early stages, stiff boots that extend to the mid-calf often suffice, particularly when patients walk on uneven surfaces such as ice and snow or stones. As the dorsiflexors of the ankles weaken further, lightweight plastic splints may be custom made to extend beneath the foot and around the back of the ankle. They are worn inside the socks and are not visible, reducing self-consciousness. External short-leg braces may be required when footdrop becomes complete. Surgical fusion of the ankle may be considered in some cases.

The leg should be protected from traumatic injury. In advanced cases, compression neuropathy during sleep may be prevented by placing soft pillows beneath or between the lower legs. Burning paresthesias of the feet are not common but are often abolished by phenytoin or carbamazepine. No medical treatment is available to arrest or slow the progression.

605.2 Peroneal Muscular Atrophy (Axonal Type)

Harvey B. Sarnat

Peroneal muscular atrophy is clinically similar to HMSN type I, but the rate of progression is slower and the disability is less. EMG shows denervation of muscle. Sural nerve biopsy reveals axonal degeneration rather than the demyelination and whorls of Schwann cell processes typical in type I. The locus is on chromosome 1 at 1p35-p36; this is a different disease than HMSN type I, although both are transmitted as autosomal dominant traits. An autosomal recessive infantile motor axonal neuropathy can closely mimic infantile spinal muscular atrophy.

605.3 Déjerine-Sottas Disease (HMSN Type III)

Harvey B. Sarnat

Déjerine-Sottas disease is an interstitial hypertrophic neuropathy of autosomal dominant transmission. It is similar to HMSN type I but is more severe. Symptoms develop in early infancy and are rapidly progressive. Pupillary abnormalities, such as lack of reaction to light and *Argyll Robertson pupil,* are common. Kyphoscoliosis and pes cavus deformities complicate about 35% of cases. Nerves become palpably enlarged at an early age.

For the full continuation of this chapter, please visit the Nelson Textbook of Pediatrics *website at www.expertconsult.com.*

605.4 Roussy-Lévy Syndrome

Harvey B. Sarnat

Roussy-Lévy syndrome is defined as a combination of HMSN type I and cerebellar deficit resembling Friedreich ataxia, but it does not have cardiomyopathy.

605.5 Refsum Disease

Harvey B. Sarnat

(See Chapter 80.2.)

Refsum disease is a rare autosomal recessive disease caused by an enzymatic block in β-oxidation of phytanic acid to pristanic acid. Phytanic acid is a branched-chain fatty acid that is derived mainly from dietary sources: spinach, nuts, and coffee. Levels of phytanic acid are greatly elevated in plasma, CSF, and brain tissue. The CSF shows an albuminocytologic dissociation, with a protein concentration of 100-600 mg/dL. Genetic linkage studies identify 2 distinct loci at 10p13 and 6q22-q24 with *PHYH* and *PEX7* genetic mutations, respectively.

For the full continuation of this chapter, please visit the Nelson Textbook of Pediatrics *website at www.expertconsult.com.*

605.6 Fabry Disease

Harvey B. Sarnat

(See Chapter 80.4.)

Fabry disease, a rare X-linked recessive trait, results in storage of ceramide trihexose due to deficiency of the enzyme ceramide trihexosidase, which cleaves the terminal galactose from ceramide trihexose (ceramide-glucose-galactose-galactose), resulting in tissue accumulation of this trihexose lipid in central nervous system (CNS) neurons, Schwann cells and perineurial cells, ganglion cells of the myenteric plexus, skin, kidneys, blood vessel endothelial and smooth muscle cells, heart, sweat glands, cornea, and bone marrow. It results from a missense mutation disrupting the crystallographic structure of α-galactosidase A.

CLINICAL MANIFESTATIONS

The presentation is in late childhood or adolescence, with recurrent episodes of burning pain and paresthesias of the feet and lower legs so severe that patients are unable to walk. These episodes are often precipitated by fever or by physical activity. Objective sensory and motor deficits are not demonstrated on neurologic examination, and reflexes are preserved. Characteristic skin lesions are seen in the perineal region, scrotum, buttocks, and periumbilical zone as flat or raised red-black telangiectases known as **angiokeratoma corporis diffusum.** Hypohidrosis may be present. Corneal opacities, cataracts, and necrosis of the femoral heads are inconstant features. Tortuosity of retinal vessels and of the vertebral and basilar arteries can occur. The disease is progressive. Hypertension and renal failure are usually delayed until early adult life. Recurrent strokes result from vascular wall involvement. Death often occurs in the 5th decade owing to cerebral infarction or renal insufficiency, but a significant morbidity already occurs in childhood despite the absence of major organ failure. Heterozygous female carriers may be asymptomatic or, rarely, are as affected as males; corneal opacities involve 70-80%, though cataracts are rare.

LABORATORY FINDINGS

Motor and sensory nerve conduction velocities are normal to only mildly slow, showing preservation of large myelinated nerve fibers. CSF protein is normal. Proteinuria is present early in the course.

Pathologic features are usually first detected in skin or sural nerve biopsy specimens. Crystalline glycosphingolipids appear as *zebra bodies* in lysosomes of endothelial cells, in smooth myocytes of arterioles, and in Schwann cells, best demonstrated by electron microscopy. Nerves show a selective loss of small myelinated fibers and relative preservation of large and medium-sized axons, contrasting to most axonal neuropathies in which large myelinated fibers are most involved.

Assay for the deficient enzyme, α-galactosidase-A, may be performed from skin fibroblasts, leukocytes, and other tissues. This test permits detection of the female carrier state and provides a reliable means of prenatal diagnosis.

TREATMENT

(See Chapter 80.4 for specific therapy of Fabry disease, including enzyme replacement.)

Medical therapy of painful neuropathies includes management of the initiating disease and therapy directed to the neuropathic pain independent of etiology. Pain may be burning or associated with paresthesias, hyperalgesia (abnormal response to noxious stimuli), or allodynia (induced by non-noxious stimuli; Chapter 71). Neuropathic pain is often successfully managed by tricyclic antidepressants; selective serotonin reuptake inhibitors are less effective. Anticonvulsants (carbamazepine, phenytoin, gabapentin, lamotrigine) are effective, as are narcotic and non-narcotic analgesics. Enzyme replacement therapy has improved the short and long term prognosis.

605.7 Giant Axonal Neuropathy

Harvey B. Sarnat

Giant axonal neuropathy is a rare autosomal recessive disease with onset in early childhood. It is a progressive mixed peripheral neuropathy and degeneration of central white matter, similar to the leukodystrophies. Ataxia and nystagmus are accompanied by signs of progressive peripheral neuropathy. A large majority of affected children have frizzy hair, which microscopically shows variation in diameter of the shaft and twisting, similar to that in Menkes disease; hence, microscopic examination of a few scalp hairs provides a simple screening tool in suspected cases. Focal axonal enlargements are seen in both the peripheral nervous system and the CNS, but the myelin sheath is intact. The disease is a general proliferation of intermediate filaments, including neurofilaments in axons, glial filaments (i.e., Rosenthal fibers) in brain, cytokeratin in hair, and vimentin in Schwann cells and fibroblasts.

For the full continuation of this chapter, please visit the Nelson Textbook of Pediatrics *website at www.expertconsult.com.*

605.8 Congenital Hypomyelinating Neuropathy

Harvey B. Sarnat

Congenital hypomyelinating neuropathy is a lack of normal myelination of motor and sensory peripheral nerves but not of CNS white matter. It is not a degeneration or loss of previously formed myelin, thus differentiating it from a leukodystrophy. Schwann cells are preserved, and axons are normal. Cases in siblings suggest autosomal recessive inheritance. Mutations in the *MTMR2, PMP22, EGR2,* and *MPZ* genes have been demonstrated in various children with this neuropathy; hence, it is a syndrome rather than a single disease.

For the full continuation of this chapter, please visit the Nelson Textbook of Pediatrics *website at www.expertconsult.com.*

605.9 Tomaculous (Hypermyelinating) Neuropathy; Hereditary Neuropathy with Liability to Pressure Palsies

Harvey B. Sarnat

This hereditary neuropathy is characterized by redundant overproduction of myelin around each axon in an irregular segmental fashion so that tomaculous (sausage-shaped) bulges occur in the individual myelinated nerve fibers. Other sections of the same nerve can show loss of myelin. Such nerves are particularly prone to pressure palsies, and patients, usually beginning in adolescence, present with recurrent or intermittent mononeuropathies secondary to minor trauma or entrapment neuropathies, such as carpal tunnel syndrome, peroneal palsies, and even "writer's cramp." It is transmitted as an autosomal dominant trait, with loci identified at 17p11.2 and 17p12, deletion of exons in the *PMP22* gene. Duplication of the same 17p12 locus leads to Charcot-Marie-Tooth disease type 1A, myelin protein zero *(MPZ)* gene mutation. Sural nerve biopsy is diagnostic, but special teased fiber preparations should be made to demonstrate the myelin abnormalities most clearly. Skin or conjunctival biopsies also may be diagnostic. Electrophysiologic nerve conduction studies are abnormal but nonspecific. Genetic studies are definitive.

Treatment is supportive and includes avoiding trauma and prolonged nerve compression, including postures when sitting or lying. Surgical release of entrapped nerves is indicated at times.

605.10 Leukodystrophies

Harvey B. Sarnat

Several hereditary degenerative diseases of white matter of the CNS also cause peripheral neuropathy. The most important are Krabbe disease (globoid cell leukodystrophy), metachromatic leukodystrophy, and adrenoleukodystrophy (see Chapters 80 and 592).

BIBLIOGRAPHY

Please visit the Nelson Textbook of Pediatrics *website at www.expertconsult.com for the complete bibliography.*

Chapter 606
Toxic Neuropathies

Harvey B. Sarnat

Many chemicals (organophosphates), toxins, and drugs can cause peripheral neuropathy (Table 606-1). Heavy metals are well-known neurotoxins. Lead poisoning, especially if chronic, causes mainly a motor neuropathy selectively involving large nerves, such as the common peroneal, radial, and median nerves, a condition known as **mononeuritis multiplex** (Chapter 702). Arsenic produces painful burning paresthesias and motor polyneuropathy. Exposure to industrial and agricultural chemicals is a less common cause of toxic neuropathy in children than in adults, but insecticides are neurotoxins for both insects and humans, and if they are used as sprays in closed spaces, they may be inhaled and induce lethargy, vomiting, seizures, and neuropathy, particularly with recurrent or long-term exposure. Working adolescents and children in developing countries are also at risk. Puffer fish poisoning, usually by ingestion of even cooked fish meat contaminated with the venom, produces a Guillain-Barré–like syndrome.

Antimetabolic and immunosuppressive drugs, such as vincristine, cisplatin, and paclitaxel, produce polyneuropathies as complications of chemotherapy for neoplasms. This iatrogenic cause is the most common etiology of toxic neuropathies in children. It is usually an axonal degeneration rather than primary demyelination, unlike autoimmune neuropathies.

Chronic uremia is associated with toxic neuropathy and myopathy. The neuropathy is caused by excessive levels of circulating parathyroid hormone. Reduction in serum parathyroid hormone levels is accompanied by clinical improvement and a return to normal of nerve conduction velocity.

Biologic neurotoxins are associated with tick paralysis, diphtheria, botulism, and the variants of paralytic shellfish poisoning. Lyme disease, West Nile virus, leprosy, herpes viruses (Bell palsy), and rabies also produce peripheral nerve– or ventral horn cell–induced weakness or paralysis. Various inborn errors of metabolism are also associated with peripheral neuropathy from metabolite toxicity or deficiencies (Part XI and Table 606-1).

Table 606-1 TOXIC AND METABOLIC NEUROPATHIES

METALS
Arsenic (insecticide, herbicide)
Lead (paint, batteries, pottery)
Mercury (metallic, vapor)
Thallium (rodenticides)
Gold
OCCUPATIONAL OR INDUSTRIAL CHEMICALS
Acrylamide (grouting, flocculation)
Carbon disulfide (solvent)
Cyanide
Dichlorophenoxyacetate
Dimethylaminopropionitrite
Ethylene oxide (gas sterilization)
Hexacarbons (glue, solvents)
Organophosphates (insecticides, petroleum additive)
Polychlorinated biphenyls
Tetrachlorbiphenyl
Trichloroethylene
DRUGS
Amiodarone
Chloramphenicol
Chloroquine
Cisplatin
Colchicine
Dapsone
Ethambutol
Ethanol
Gold
Hydralazine
Isoniazid
Metronidazole
Nitrofurantoin
Nitrous oxide
Nucleosides (antiretroviral agents ddC, ddI, d4T, others)
Penicillamine
Pentamidine
Phenytoin
Pyridoxine (excessive)
Statins
Stilbamidine
Suramin
Taxanes (paclitaxel, docetaxal)
Thalidomide
Tryptophan (eosinophilia-myalgia syndrome)
Vincristine
METABOLIC DISORDERS
Fabry disease
Krabbe disease
Leukodystrophies
Porphyria
Tangier disease
Tyrosinemia
Uremia

Chapter 607 Autonomic Neuropathies

Harvey B. Sarnat

Involvement of small, lightly, or unmyelinated autonomic nerve fibers may be seen in many peripheral neuropathies; the autonomic manifestations are usually mild or subclinical. Certain autonomic neuropathies are more symptomatic and demonstrate varying degrees of involvement of the autonomic nervous system regulation of the cardiovascular, gastrointestinal (GI), genitourinary, thermoregulatory, sudomotor, and pupillomotor systems.

The differential diagnosis is noted in Table 607-1. Autonomic nervous system functional tests are noted in Table 607-2. The general treatment of acquired autonomic dysfunction includes treating the primary disorder (systemic lupus erythematosus, diabetes) and long-term management of specific organ system manifestations (Table 607-3). Acute fluctuations of autonomic symptoms may be seen in Guillain-Barré syndrome. Rapid fluctuations of hypertension or tachycardia changing to hypotension or bradycardia should be managed carefully and with very short-acting medications.

607.1 Familial Dysautonomia

Harvey B. Sarnat

Familial dysautonomia (Riley-Day syndrome) is an autosomal recessive disorder that is common in Eastern European Jews, among whom the incidence is 1/10,000-20,000, and the carrier state is estimated to be 1%. It is rare in other ethnic groups. The defective gene is at the 9q31-q33 locus. The familial dysautonomia gene is identified as *IKBKAP* (IκB kinase–associated protein), with aberrant splicing and a truncated protein. This and other autonomic neuropathies are often regarded as **neurocristopathies** because the abnormal target tissues are largely derived from neural crest.

Table 607-1 AUTONOMIC NEUROPATHIES

Guillain-Barré syndrome (Chapter 608)
Non–Guillain-Barré syndrome autoimmunity
• Paraneoplastic (type I antineuronal nuclear antibody)
• Lambert-Eaton syndrome
• Antibodies to neuronal nicotinc acetylcholine receptors
• Antibodies to P/Q type calcium channels
• Other autoantibodies
• Systemic lupus erythematosus
Hereditary
• Type I autosomal dominant
• Type II autosomal recessive (Morvan disease)
• Type III autosomal recessive (Riley-Day)
• Type IV autosomal recessive (congenital insensitivity to pain with anhidrosis)
• Type V absence of pain
Metabolic
• Fabry disease
• Diabetes mellitus
• Tangier disease
• Porphyria
Infectious
• HIV
• Chagas' disease
• Botulism
• Leprosy
• Diphtheria
Other
• Triple A (Allgrove) syndrome
• Navajo Indian neuropathy
• Multiple endocrine neoplasia type 2b
Toxins (see Table 606-1)

Table 607-2 AUTONOMIC FUNCTION TESTING

Sympathetic and parasympathetic divisions of the autonomic nervous system are involved in all tests of autonomic function
CARDIAC PARASYMPATHETIC NERVOUS SYSTEM FUNCTION
Heart rate variability with deep respiration (respiratory sinus arrhythmia); time-domain and frequency-domain assessments Heart rate response to Valsalva maneuver Heart rate response to standing
SYMPATHETIC ADRENERGIC FUNCTION
Blood pressure response to upright posture (standing or tilt table) Blood pressure response to Valsalva maneuver Microneurography
SYMPATHETIC CHOLINERGIC FUNCTION
Thermoregulatory sweat testing Quantitative sudomotor-axon reflex test Sweat imprint methods Sympathetic skin response

From Freeman R: Autonomic peripheral neuropathy, *Lancet* 365:1259–1270, 2005.

Table 607-3 MANAGEMENT OF AUTONOMIC NEUROPATHIES

PROBLEM	TREATMENT
Orthostatic hypotension	Volume and salt supplements Fluorohydrocortisone (mineralocorticoid) Midodrine (α agonist)
Gastroparesis	Prokinetic agents (metaclopramide, domperidone, erythromycin)
Hypomotility	Fiber, laxatives
Urinary dysfunction	Timed voiding; bladder catheterization
Hyperhidrosis	Anticholinergic agents (glycopyrrolate, propanthdine) Intracutaneous botulism toxin

PATHOLOGY

This disease of the peripheral nervous system is characterized pathologically by a reduced number of small unmyelinated nerve fibers that carry pain, temperature, and taste sensations and that mediate autonomic functions. Large myelinated afferent nerve fibers that relay impulses from muscle spindles and Golgi tendon organs also are deficient. The degree of demonstrable anatomic change in peripheral and especially autonomic nerves is variable. Fungiform papillae of the tongue (taste buds) are absent or reduced in number. The number of parasympathetic ganglion cells in the myenteric plexuses is reduced. There is terminal vessel hyperperfusion in tissues, despite an overall hypoperfusion of organs and extremities.

CLINICAL MANIFESTATIONS

The disease is expressed in infancy by poor sucking and swallowing. Aspiration pneumonia can occur. Feeding difficulties remain a major symptom throughout childhood. Vomiting crises can occur. Apart from dysphagia, esophageal dysmotility can contribute to these symptoms. Episodic somnolence can occur in infants. Excessive sweating and blotchy erythema of the skin are common, especially at mealtime or when the child is excited. Infants are vulnerable to heatstroke. Episodic hyperhidrosis is due to chemical hypersensitivity of the remaining reduced number of sudomotor axons rather than of the sweat gland secretory cells. Breath-holding spells followed by syncope are common in the first 5 years of life.

As affected children become older, insensitivity to pain becomes evident and traumatic injuries are frequent. Corneal ulcerations are common. Newly erupting teeth cause tongue ulcerations. Walking is delayed or clumsy or appears ataxic because of poor sensory feedback from muscle spindles. The ataxia is probably related more to deficient muscle spindle feedback and to vestibular nerve dysfunction than to cerebellar involvement. Tendon stretch reflexes are absent. Scoliosis is a serious complication in the majority of patients and usually is progressive. Overflow tearing with crying does not normally develop until 2-3 mo of age but fails to develop after that time or is severely reduced in children with familial dysautonomia. There is an increased incidence of urinary incontinence. Bradycardia and other cardiac arrhythmias can occur, and some patients require a cardiac pacemaker.

About 40% of patients have generalized major motor seizures, some of which are associated with acute hypoxia during breath holding, some with extreme fevers, but most without an apparent precipitating event. Body temperature is poorly controlled; both hypothermia and extreme fevers occur. Impaired intellectual function is not secondary to epilepsy. Emotional lability and learning disabilities are common in school-age children with the disorder. Puberty is often delayed, especially in girls. Short stature can occur, but growth velocity can be accelerated by treatment with growth hormone. Speech is often slurred or nasal.

After 3 yr of age, autonomic crises begin, usually with attacks of cyclic vomiting lasting 24-72 hr or even several days. Retching and vomiting occur every 15-20 min and are associated with hypertension, profuse sweating, blotching of the skin, apprehension, and irritability. Prominent gastric distention can occur, causing abdominal pain and even respiratory distress. Hematemesis can complicate pernicious vomiting.

Allgrove syndrome is a clinical variant, involving alacrima, achalasia, autonomic dysfunction with orthostatic hypotension and altered heart rate variability, and sensorimotor polyneuropathy, usually manifesting in adolescence. Cholinergic dysfunction may be demonstrated.

LABORATORY FINDINGS

Electrocardiography discloses prolonged correcting QT intervals with lack of appropriate shortening with exercise, a reflection of the aberration in autonomic regulation of cardiac conduction. Chest radiographs show atelectasis and pulmonary changes resembling cystic fibrosis. Urinary vanillylmandelic acid level is decreased, and homovanillic acid level is increased. Plasma level of dopamine β-hydroxylase (the enzyme that converts dopamine to epinephrine) is diminished. Sural nerve biopsy shows a decreased number of unmyelinated fibers. Electroencephalography is useful for evaluating seizures.

DIAGNOSIS

Slow IV infusion of norepinephrine produces an exaggerated pressor response. The hypotensive response to infusion of methacholine is increased. Intradermal injection of 1 : 1,000 histamine phosphate fails to produce a normal axon flare, and local pain is absent or diminished. Because the skin of a normal infant reacts more intensely to histamine, a 1 : 10,000 dilution should be used. Instillation of 2.5% methacholine into the conjunctival sac produces miosis in patients with familial dysautonomia and no detectable effect on a normal pupil; this is a nonspecific sign of parasympathetic denervation due to any cause. Methacholine is applied to only 1 eye in this test, with the other eye serving as a control; the pupils are compared at 5-min intervals for 20 min. A test for the genetic marker in blood is available in selected centers around the USA and Israel for definitive diagnostic testing.

TREATMENT

Symptomatic treatment includes special attention to the respiratory and GI systems to prevent aspiration and malnutrition, methylcellulose eye drops or topical ocular lubricants to replace tears and prevent corneal ulceration, orthopedic management of scoliosis and joint problems, and appropriate anticonvulsants for epilepsy. Chlorpromazine is an effective antiemetic and may be given as rectal suppositories during autonomic crises. It also reduces apprehension and lowers the blood pressure. Diazepam also is effective in some cases. Dehydration and electrolyte disturbances should be anticipated. Bethanechol may be an alternative drug for cyclic vomiting. It is also useful for enuresis, another common complication, and augments tear production. Protection from injuries is important because of the lack of pain as a protective mechanism. Scoliosis often requires surgical treatment. Antiepileptic drugs may be required. A cardiac pacemaker may be required by some children. Blood pressure monitoring may be important in some cases. A promising genetic approach to treatment, which corrects the splicing defect, is the use of oral kinetin to regulate the expression of *IKBKAP* transcripts. Tocotrienols also have a theoretical value in treating familial dysautonomia.

PROGNOSIS

Sixty percent of patients die in childhood before the age of 20 yr, usually of chronic pulmonary failure or aspiration. Treatment in a center familiar with the diverse complications greatly extends the life expectancy; some have survived by age 40 yr. Prevention of aspiration with fundoplication, gastrostomy, and tube feeding reduces the risk of aspiration.

BIBLIOGRAPHY

Please visit the Nelson Textbook of Pediatrics *website at* *www.expertconsult.com* *for the complete bibliography.*

607.2 Other Autonomic Neuropathies

Harvey B. Sarnat

MYENTERIC PLEXUS NEUROPATHIES

Aganglionic megacolon (Hirschsprung disease) is a failure of embryonic development of parasympathetic neurons in the submucosal and myenteric plexuses of segments of the colon and rectum. Nerves between the longitudinal and circular layers of smooth muscle of the gut wall are hypertrophic; ganglion cells are absent (Chapter 324).

CONGENITAL INSENSITIVITY TO PAIN AND ANHIDROSIS

Congenital insensitivity to pain and anhidrosis is a hereditary disorder of uncertain genetic transmission. It affects many more boys than girls and manifests in early infancy. Patients have episodes of high fever related to warm environmental temperatures because they do not perspire. Frequent burns and traumatic injuries result from apparent lack of pain perception. Intelligence is normal. Nerve biopsy reveals an almost total absence of unmyelinated nerve fibers that convey impulses of pain, temperature, and autonomic functions. Some cases of hypomyelinating neuropathy manifest clinically as congenital insensitivity to pain (Chapter 605.8). The sympathetic skin response as an electrophysiologic study is a reliable diagnostic test in cases associated with a mutation at the TrKA receptor for nerve growth factor.

REFLEX SYMPATHETIC DYSTROPHY

Reflex sympathetic dystrophy is a form of local causalgia, usually involving a hand or foot but not corresponding to the anatomic distribution of a peripheral nerve (Chapter 162.2). A continuous burning pain and hyperesthesia are associated with vasomotor instability in the affected zone, resulting in increased skin temperature, erythema, and edema due to vasodilatation and hyperhidrosis. In the chronic state, atrophy of skin appendages, cool and clammy skin, and disuse atrophy of underlying muscle and bone occur. More than 1 extremity is occasionally involved. The pain is disabling and is exacerbated by the movement of an associated joint, although no objective signs of arthritis are seen; immobilization provides some relief. The most common preceding event is local trauma in the form of a contusion, laceration, sprain, or fracture that occurred days or weeks earlier.

Several theories of pathogenesis have been proposed to explain this phenomenon. The most widely accepted is reflexive overactivity of autonomic nerves in response to injury, and regional sympathetic blockade often affords temporary relief. Physiotherapy also is helpful. Some cases resolve spontaneously after weeks or months, but others continue to be symptomatic and require sympathectomy. A psychogenic component is suspected in some cases but is difficult to prove.

BIBLIOGRAPHY

Please visit the Nelson Textbook of Pediatrics *website at* *www.expertconsult.com* *for the complete bibliography.*

Chapter 608
Guillain-Barré Syndrome

Harvey B. Sarnat

Guillain-Barré syndrome is a postinfectious polyneuropathy involving mainly motor but sometimes also sensory and autonomic nerves. This syndrome affects people of all ages and is not hereditary. Most patients have a demyelinating neuropathy, but primarily axonal degeneration is documented in some cases mainly in China and Japan.

CLINICAL MANIFESTATIONS

The paralysis usually follows a nonspecific viral infection by about 10 days. The original infection might have caused only gastrointestinal (especially *Campylobacter jejuni,* but also *Helicobacter pylori*) or respiratory tract (especially *Mycoplasma pneumoniae*) symptoms. West Nile virus also can cause Guillain-Barré-like syndrome, but more often it causes motor neuron disease similar to poliomyelitis. Guillain-Barré syndrome is reported following administration of vaccines against rabies, influenza, and poliomyelitis (oral) and following administration of conjugated meningococcal vaccine, particularly serogroup C.

Weakness usually begins in the lower extremities and progressively involves the trunk, the upper limbs, and finally the bulbar muscles, a pattern known as **Landry ascending paralysis.** Proximal and distal muscles are involved relatively symmetrically, but asymmetry is found in 9% of patients. The onset is gradual and progresses over days or weeks. Particularly in cases with an abrupt onset, tenderness on palpation and pain in muscles is common in the initial stages. Affected children are irritable. Weakness can progress to inability or refusal to walk and later to flaccid tetraplegia. Paresthesias occur in some cases. The differential diagnosis of acute weakness is noted in Table 599-3 and of Guillain Barré syndrome in Table 608-1.

Bulbar involvement occurs in about half of cases. Respiratory insufficiency can result. Dysphagia and facial weakness are often impending signs of respiratory failure. They interfere with eating and increase the risk of aspiration. The facial nerves may be involved. Some young patients exhibit symptoms of viral meningitis or meningoencephalitis. Extraocular muscle involvement is rare, but in an uncommon variant, oculomotor and other cranial neuropathies are severe early in the course. **Miller-Fisher syndrome** consists of acute external ophthalmoplegia, ataxia, and areflexia. Papilledema is found in some cases, although visual impairment is not clinically evident. Urinary incontinence or retention of urine is a complication in about 20% of cases but is

Table 608-1 DIFFERENTIAL DIAGNOSIS OF CHILDHOOD GUILLAIN-BARRÉ SYNDROME

SPINAL CORD LESIONS
Acute transverse myelitis Epidural abscess Tumors Poliomyelitis Hopkins syndrome Vascular malformations Cord infarction Fibrocartilaginous embolism Cord compression from vertebral subluxation related to congenital abnormalities or trauma Acute disseminated encephalomyelitis
PERIPHERAL NEUROPATHIES
Toxic • Vincristine • Glue sniffing • Heavy metal • Organophosphate pesticides Infections • HIV • Diphtheria • Lyme disease Inborn errors of metabolism • Leigh disease • Tangier disease • Porphyria Critical illness: polyneuropathy/myopathy
NEUROMUSCULAR JUNCTION DISORDERS
Tick paralysis, myasthenia gravis, botulism, hypercalcemia Myopathies Periodic paralyses, dermatomyositis, critical illness myopathy/polyneuropathy

From Agrawal S, Peake D, Whitehouse WP: Management of children with Guillain Barré syndrome, *Arch Dis Child Edu Pract Ed* 92:161–168, 2007.

Table 608-2 CLASSIFICATION OF GUILLAIN-BARRÉ SYNDROME AND RELATED DISORDERS AND TYPICAL ANTIGANGLIOSIDE ANTIBODIES BY PATHOLOGY

DISORDER	ANTIBODIES
Acute inflammatory demyelinating polyradiculoneuropathy	Unknown
Acute motor and sensory axonal neuropathy	GM1, GM1b, GD1a
Acute motor axonal neuropathy	GM1, GM1b, GD1a, GalNac-GD1a
Acute sensory neuronopathy	GD1b
ACUTE PANDYSAUTONOMIA	
Regional Variants	
Fisher syndrome	GQ1b, GT1a
Oropharyngeal	GT1a
Overlap	
Fisher/Guillain-Barré overlap syndrome	GQ1b, GM1, GM1b, GD1a, GalNac-GD1a

From Hughes RAC: Treatment of Guillain-Barré syndrome with corticosteroids: lack of benefit? *Lancet* 363:181–182, 2004.

usually transient. Miller-Fisher syndrome overlaps with Bickerstaff brainstem encephalitis, which also shares many features with Guillain-Barré syndrome with lower motor neuron involvement and might indeed be the same basic disease.

Tendon reflexes are lost, usually early in the course, but are sometimes preserved until later. This variability can cause confusion when attempting early diagnosis. The autonomic nervous system is also involved in some cases. Lability of blood pressure and cardiac rate, postural hypotension, episodes of profound bradycardia, and occasional asystole occur. Cardiovascular monitoring is important. A few patients require insertion of a temporary venous cardiac pacemaker.

Chronic inflammatory demyelinating polyradiculoneuropathies (CIDP, sometimes called *chronic inflammatory relapsing polyneuritis* or *chronic unremitting polyradiculoneuropathy*) are chronic varieties of Guillain-Barré syndrome that recur intermittently or do not improve or progress slowly and relentlessly for periods of months to years. About 7% of children with Guillain-Barré syndrome suffer an acute relapse. Patients are usually severely weak and can have a flaccid tetraplegia with or without bulbar and respiratory muscle involvement. Hyporeflexia or areflexia are almost universal. Motor deficits occur in 94% of cases, sensory paresthesias in 64%, and cranial nerve involvement in less than a third of patients. Autonomic and micturitional involvement is variable. CSF shows no pleocytosis and protein is variably normal or mildly elevated. Nerve conduction velocity (NCV) studies and sural nerve biopsy are abnormal. Polymorphic nucleotide repeats in the *SH2D2A* gene has been associated with a predisposition to CIDP.

Congenital Guillain-Barré syndrome is described rarely, manifesting as generalized hypotonia, weakness, and areflexia in an affected neonate, fulfilling all electrophysiologic and cerebrospinal fluid (CSF) criteria and in the absence of maternal neuromuscular disease. Treatment might not be required, and there is gradual improvement over the first few months and no evidence of residual disease by 1 yr of age. In 1 case, the mother had ulcerative colitis treated with prednisone and mesalamine from the 7th mo of gestation until delivery at term.

LABORATORY FINDINGS AND DIAGNOSIS

CSF studies are essential for diagnosis. The CSF protein is elevated to more than twice the upper limit of normal, glucose level is normal, and there is no pleocytosis. Fewer than 10 white blood cells/mm^3 are found. The results of bacterial cultures are negative, and viral cultures rarely isolate specific viruses. The dissociation between high CSF protein and a lack of cellular response in a patient with an acute or subacute polyneuropathy is diagnostic of Guillain-Barré syndrome. MRI of the spinal cord may be indicated to rule out disorders in Table 608-1. MRI findings include thickening of the cauda equina and intrathecal nerve roots with gadolinium enhancement. These finds are fairly sensitive and are present in >90% of patients (Fig. 608-1). Imaging in CIDP is similar but demonstrates greater enhancement of spinal nerve roots (Fig. 608-2).

Motor NCVs are greatly reduced, and sensory nerve conduction time is often slow. Electromyography (EMG) shows evidence of acute denervation of muscle. Serum creatine kinase (CK) level may be mildly elevated or normal. Antiganglioside antibodies, mainly against G_{M1} and G_{D1}, are sometimes elevated in the serum in Guillain-Barré syndrome, particularly in cases with primarily axonal rather than demyelinating neuropathy, and suggest that they might play a role in disease propagation and/or recovery in some cases (Table 608-1). Muscle biopsy is not usually required for diagnosis; specimens appear normal in early stages and show evidence of denervation atrophy in chronic stages. Sural nerve biopsy tissue shows segmental demyelination, focal inflammation, and wallerian degeneration but also is usually not required for diagnosis.

Serologic testing for *Campylobacter* and *Helicobacter* infections helps establish the cause if results are positive but does not alter the course of treatment. Results of stool cultures are rarely positive because the infection is self-limited and only occurs for about 3 days, and the neuropathy follows the acute gastroenteritis.

TREATMENT

Patients in early stages of this acute disease should be admitted to the hospital for observation because the ascending paralysis can rapidly involve respiratory muscles during the next 24 hr.

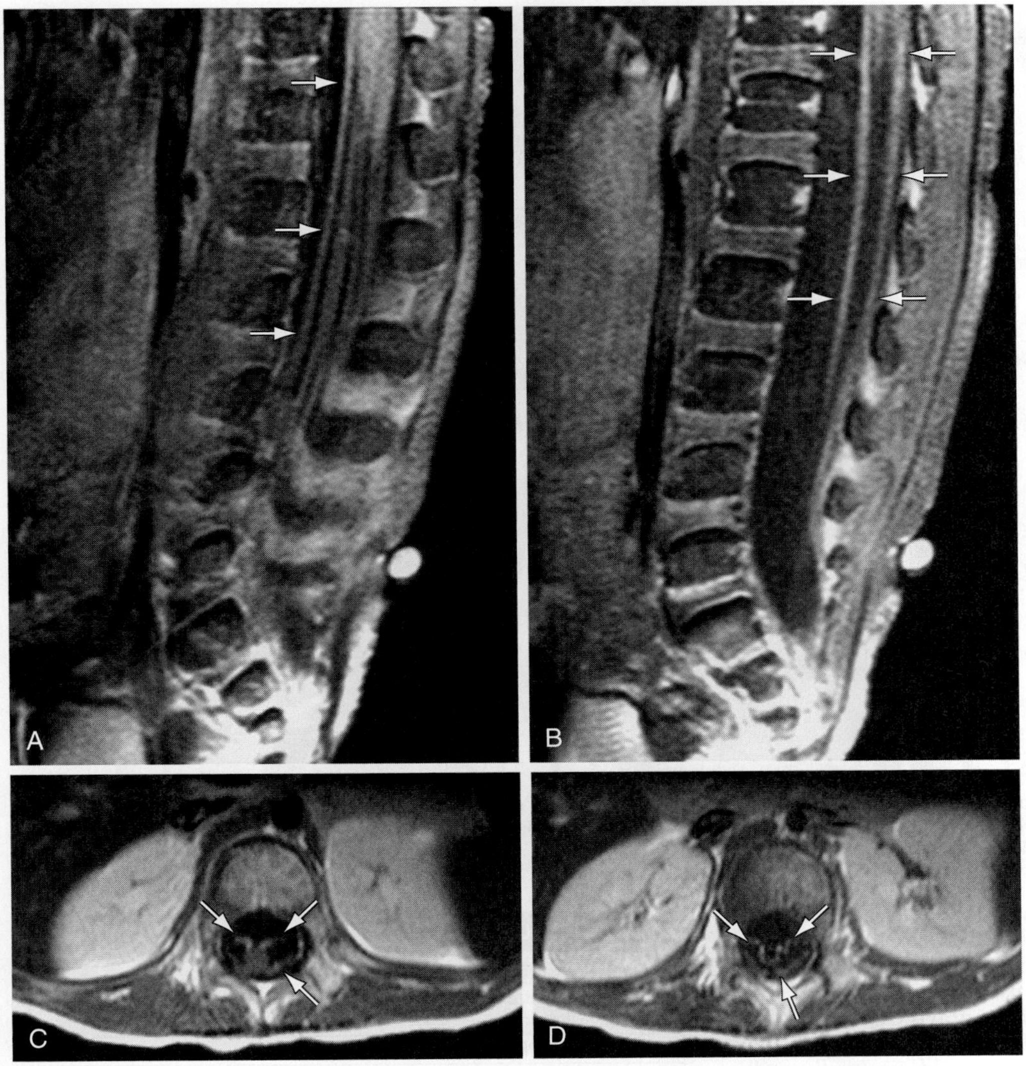

Figure 608-1 Guillain-Barré syndrome. Sagittal off-midline *(A)* and midline *(B)* postgadolinium T1-weighted fat-saturated images through the lumbar spine of a patient who could not ambulate. *C* and *D,* Axial postcontrast T1-weighted images through the conus medullaris and proximal lumbar nerve roots respectively. The images show extensive contrast enhancement of nerve roots *(arrows* in *A-D),* in keeping with changes of Guillain-Barré. (From Slovis TL, editor: *Caffey's pediatric diagnostic imaging,* ed 11, vol 1, Philadelphia, 2008, Mosby Elsevier, p 991.)

Respiratory effort (negative inspiratory force, spirometry) must be monitored to prevent respiratory failure and respiratory arrest. Patients with slow progression might simply be observed for stabilization and spontaneous remission without treatment. Rapidly progressive ascending paralysis is treated with intravenous immunoglobulin (IVIG), administered for 2, 3, or 5 days. A commonly recommended protocol is IVIG 0.4 g/kg/day for 5 consecutive days. Plasmapheresis and/or immunosuppressive drugs are alternatives if IVIG is ineffective. Steroids are not effective. Combined administration of immunoglobulin and interferon is effective in some patients. Supportive care, such as respiratory support, prevention of decubiti in children with flaccid tetraplegia, and treatment of secondary bacterial infections, is important.

CIDPs, whether relapsing-remitting or unremitting, also are treated with oral or pulsed steroids or with IVIG. Subcutaneous immunoglobulin infusion may be an alternative to the intravenous route. Plasma exchange, sometimes requiring as many as 10 exchanges daily, is an alternative. Remission in these cases may be sustained, but relapses can occur within days, weeks, or even after many months; relapses usually respond to another course of plasmapheresis. Steroid and immunosuppressive drugs are another alternative, but their effectiveness is less predictable. High-dose pulsed methylprednisolone given intravenously is successful in some cases. The prognosis in chronic forms of the Guillain-Barré syndrome is more guarded than in the acute form, and many patients are left with major residual handicaps.

Even if *C. jejuni* infection is documented by stool culture or serologic tests, treatment of the infection is not necessary because it is self-limited, and the use of antibiotics does not alter the course of the polyneuropathy.

For the treatment of chronic neuropathic pain following Guillain-Barré syndrome, gabapentin is more effective than carbamazepine, and the requirement for fentanyl is reduced.

PROGNOSIS

The clinical course is usually benign, and spontaneous recovery begins within 2-3 wk. Most patients regain full muscular strength, although some are left with residual weakness. The tendon reflexes are usually the last function to recover. Improvement usually follows a gradient opposite the direction of involvement: bulbar function recovering first, and lower extremity weakness resolving last. Bulbar and respiratory muscle involvement can lead to death if the syndrome is not recognized and treated. Although prognosis is generally good and the majority of children recover completely, 3 clinical features are predictive of poor outcome with sequelae: cranial nerve involvement, intubation, and maximum disability at the time of presentation. The electrophysiologic features of conduction block are predictive of good outcome. Long-term follow-up studies of patients who recover

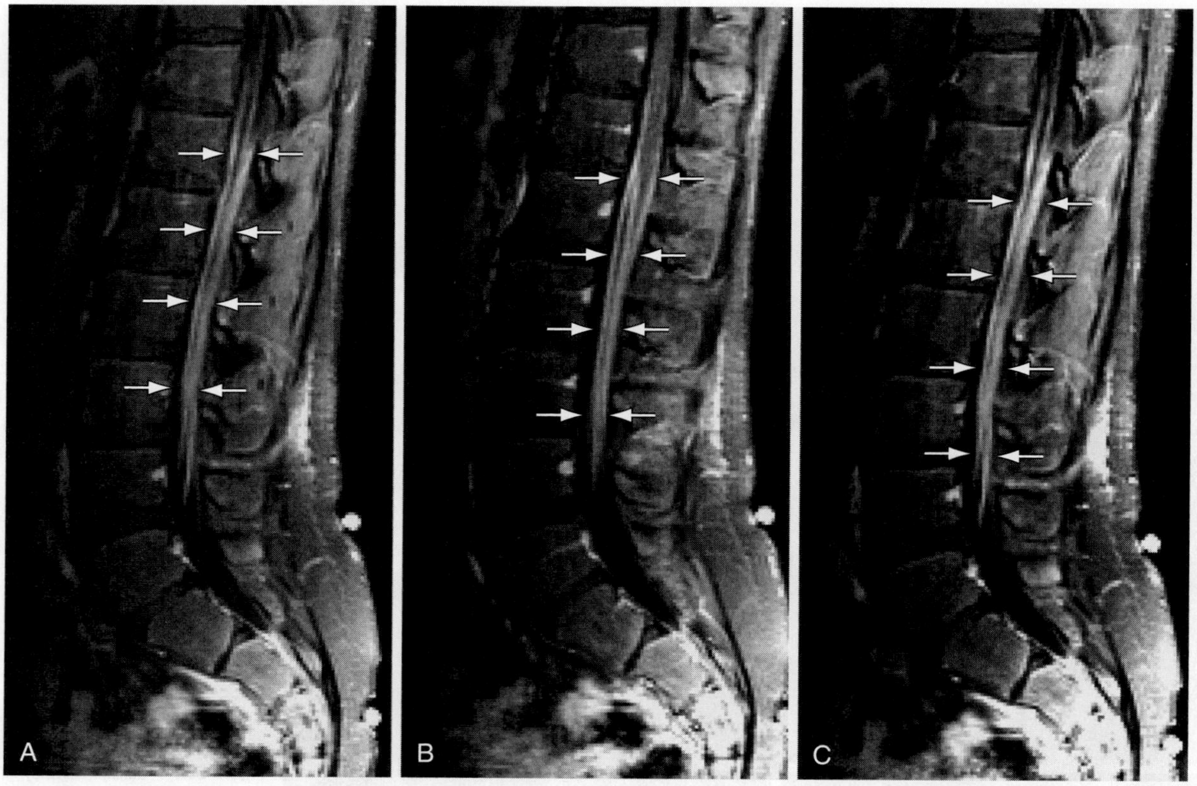

Figure 608-2 Chronic inflammatory demyelinating polyneuropathy (CIDP) in a 13-year-old boy with peripheral neuropathy and gait disturbance. Sagittal fat-saturated T1-weighted images off the midline to the right *(A)*, at the midline *(B)*, and off the midline to the left *(C)*. (From Slovis TL, editor: *Caffey's pediatric diagnostic imaging,* ed 11, vol 1, Philadelphia, 2008, Mosby Elsevier, p 992.)

from an attack of Guillain-Barré syndrome reveal that many do have some permanent axonal loss, with or without residual clinical signs of chronic neuropathy. Easy fatigue is one of the most common chronic symptoms, but it is not the rapid fatigability of muscles seen in myasthenia gravis. Among patients with the axonal form of Guillain-Barré syndrome, most who had slow recovery over the first 6 mo could eventually walk, although some required years to recover. EMG and NCV electrophysiologic studies do not necessarily predict the long-term outcome.

BIBLIOGRAPHY

Please visit the Nelson Textbook of Pediatrics *website at www.expertconsult.com for the complete bibliography.*

Chapter 609
Bell Palsy
Harvey B. Sarnat

Bell palsy is an acute unilateral facial nerve palsy that is not associated with other cranial neuropathies or brainstem dysfunction. It is a common disorder at all ages from infancy through adolescence and usually develops abruptly about 2 wk after a systemic viral infection. The preceding infection is caused by the herpes simplex virus, varicella-zoster virus, Epstein-Barr virus, Lyme disease, mumps virus, or *Mycoplasma* (Table 609-1). Active or reactivation of herpes simplex or varicella-zoster virus may be the most common cause of Bell palsy (Fig. 609-1). The disease is occasionally a postinfectious allergic or immune demyelinating facial neuritis. It also may be a focal toxic or inflammatory neuropathy and has been associated with ribavirin and interferon-α therapy for hepatitis C.

Table 609-1 ETIOLOGIES OF ACUTE PERIPHERAL FACIAL PALSY

COMMON
Herpes simplex virus type 1*
Varicella-zoster virus*
LESS COMMON INFECTIONS
Otitis media ± cholesteatoma
Lyme disease
Epstein-Barr virus
Cytomegalovirus
Mumps
Human herpesvirus 6
Intranasal influenza vaccine
Mycoplasma
OTHER LESS COMMON CONDITIONS
Trauma
Tumor
Hypertension
Guillain-Barré syndrome
Sarcoidosis
Melkersson-Rosenthal syndrome†
Ribavirin
Interferon

*Implicated in idiopathic Bell palsy.
†Noncaseating granulomas with facial (lips, eyelids) edema, recurrent alternating facial paralysis, family history, migraines, or headaches.

CLINICAL MANIFESTATIONS

The upper and lower portions of the face are paretic, and the corner of the mouth droops. Patients are unable to close the eye on the involved side and can develop an exposure keratitis at night. Taste on the anterior 2/3 of the tongue is lost on the involved side in about 50% of cases; this finding helps to establish the anatomic limits of the lesion as being proximal or distal to

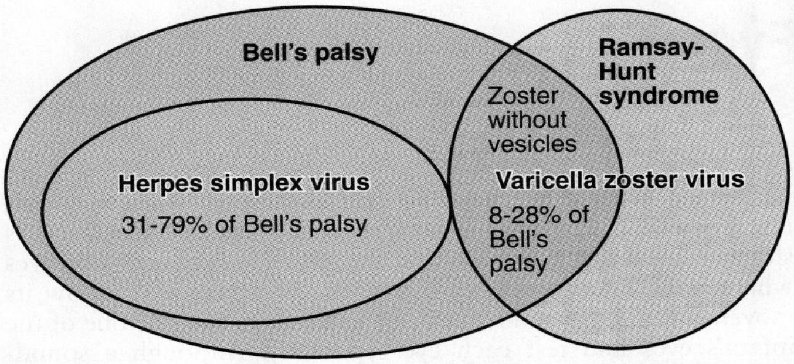

Figure 609-1 Involvement of herpes simplex and varicella zoster viruses in acute facial palsy. (From Hato N, Murakami S. Gyo K: Steroid and antiviral treatment for Bell's palsy, *Lancet* 371:1818–1820, 2008.)

the chorda tympani branch of the facial nerve. Numbness and paresthesias do not usually occur, but ipsilateral numbness of the face is reported in a few cases and probably is due to viral (especially herpes) or postviral immunologic impairment of the trigeminal and the facial nerves. Several grading systems have been devised for Bell palsy, including the Sunnybrook, House-Brackmann, and Yanagihara systems.

TREATMENT

Oral prednisone (1 mg/kg/day for 1 wk, followed by a 1-wk taper) started within the first 3-5 days results in improved outcome and is a traditional treatment. Because of the recovery of herpes simplex virus in the neural fluid of the 7th nerve, some also recommend adding oral acyclovir or valacyclovir to the prednisone therapy. Alone, antiviral agents are not effective in reducing adverse sequelae (synkinesis, autonomic dysfunction) but added to prednisone may be associated with an additional small benefit for a complete recovery. Surgical decompression of the facial canal, theoretically to provide more space for the swollen facial nerve, is not of value. Physiotherapy to the facial muscles is recommended in some chronic cases with poor recovery, but the efficacy of this treatment is uncertain. Protection of the cornea with methylcellulose eyedrops or an ocular lubricant is especially important at night. Some plastic surgeons use botulinum toxin to treat chronic unilateral ptosis, but this has little application in pediatric patients.

PROGNOSIS

The prognosis is excellent. More than 85% of patients recover spontaneously with no residual facial weakness. Another 10% have mild facial weakness as a sequela, and only 5% are left with permanent severe facial weakness. In patients who do not recover within a few weeks (chronic), electrophysiologic examination of the facial nerve helps to determine the degree of neuropathy and regeneration. In chronic cases, other causes of facial neuropathy should be considered, including facial nerve tumors such as schwannomas and neurofibromas, infiltration of the facial nerve by leukemic cells or by a rhabdomyosarcoma of the middle ear, brainstem infarcts or tumors, and traumatic injury of the facial nerve.

FACIAL PALSY AT BIRTH

Facial palsy at birth is usually a compression neuropathy from forceps application during delivery and recovers spontaneously in a few days or weeks in most cases. Congenital absence of the depressor angularis oris muscle causes facial asymmetry, especially when an affected infant cries, and is often associated with other congenital anomalies, especially of the heart. It is not a facial nerve lesion but is a cosmetic defect that does not interfere with feeding. Infants with Möbius syndrome can have bilateral or, less commonly, unilateral facial palsy; this syndrome is usually caused by symmetric calcified infarcts in the tegmentum of the pons and medulla oblongata during mid-gestation or late fetal life, although it rarely is a developmental anomaly of the brainstem.

BIBLIOGRAPHY

Please visit the Nelson Textbook of Pediatrics *website at www.expertconsult.com for the complete bibliography.*

PART XXIX Disorders of the Eye

Chapter 610
Growth and Development

Scott E. Olitsky, Denise Hug, Laura S. Plummer, and Merrill Stass-Isern

The eye of a normal full-term infant at birth is approximately 65% of adult size. Postnatal growth is maximal during the 1st yr, proceeds at a rapid but decelerating rate until the 3rd yr, and continues at a slower rate thereafter until puberty, after which little change occurs. The anterior structures of the eye are relatively large at birth but thereafter grow proportionately less than the posterior structures. This results in a progressive change in the shape of the globe; it becomes more spherical.

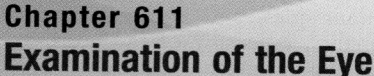

For the full continuation of this chapter, please visit the Nelson Textbook of Pediatrics *website at www.expertconsult.com.*

Chapter 611
Examination of the Eye

Scott E. Olitsky, Denise Hug, Laura S. Plummer, and Merrill Stass-Isern

Examination of the eyes is a routine part of the periodic pediatric assessment beginning in the newborn period. The primary care physician is very important in detecting both obvious and insidious asymptomatic eye diseases. Screening by lay persons in schools and community programs can also be effective in detecting problems early. The best method of screening (ages 3-5 yrs) is currently being investigated. The American Academy of Ophthalmology recommend preschool vision screening as a means of reducing preventable visual loss (Table 611-1). This testing should also be done by pediatricians during well child visits. Children should be examined by an ophthalmologist whenever a significant ocular abnormality or vision defect is noted or suspected. Children who are at high risk of ophthalmologic problems, such as genetically inherited ocular conditions and various systemic disorders, should also be examined by an ophthalmologist.

Basic examination, whether done by a pediatrician or an ophthalmologist, must include evaluation of visual acuity and the visual fields, assessment of the pupils, ocular motility and alignment, a general external examination, and an ophthalmoscopic examination of the media and fundi. When indicated, biomicroscopy (slit-lamp examination), cycloplegic refraction, and tonometry are performed by an ophthalmologist. Special diagnostic procedures, such as ultrasonic examination, fluorescein angiography, electroretinography, or visual evoked response (VER) testing, are also indicated for specific conditions.

VISUAL ACUITY

There are many tests of visual acuity. Which test is used depends on a child's age and ability to cooperate, as well as a clinician's preference and experience with each test. The most common visual acuity test in infants is an assessment of their ability to fixate and follow a target. If appropriate targets are used, this reflex can be demonstrated by about 6 weeks of age. The test is performed by seating the child comfortably in the caretaker's lap. The object of visual interest, usually a bright-colored toy, is slowly moved to the right and to the left. The examiner observes whether the infant's eyes turn toward the object and follow its movements. The examiner can use a thumb to occlude one of the infant's eyes and test each eye separately. Although a sound-producing object might compromise the purity of the visual stimulus, in practice, toys that squeak or rattle heighten an infant's awareness and interest in the test.

The human face is a better target than test objects. The examiner can exploit this by moving his or her face slowly in front of the infant's face. If the appropriate following movements are not elicited, the test should be repeated with the caretaker's face as the test stimulus. It should be remembered that even children with poor vision can follow a large object without apparent difficulty, especially if only one eye is affected.

An objective measurement of visual acuity is usually possible when children reach 2.5-3 years of age. Children this age are tested using a schematic picture or other illiterate eye chart. Each eye should be tested separately. It is essential to prevent peeking. The examiner should hold the occluder in place and observe the child throughout the test. The child should be reassured and encouraged throughout the test because many children are intimidated by the procedure and fear a "bad grade" or punishment for errors.

The **E test,** in which a child points in the direction of the letter, is the most widely used visual acuity test for preschool children. Right-left presentations are more confusing than up-down presentations. With pretest practice, this test can be performed by most children 3-4 years of age.

An adult-type **Snellen acuity chart** can be used at about 5 or 6 years of age if the child knows letters. An acuity of 20/40 is generally accepted as normal for 3 yr old children. At 4 yr of age, 20/30 is typical. By 5 or 6 years of age, most children attain 20/20 vision.

Optokinetic nystagmus (the response to a sequence of moving targets; "railroad" nystagmus) can also be used to assess vision; this can be calibrated by targets of various sizes (stripes or dots) or by a rotating drum at specified distances. The VER, an electrophysiologic method of evaluating the response to light and special visual stimuli, such as calibrated stripes or a checkerboard pattern, can also be used to study visual function in selected cases. Preferential looking tests are also used for evaluating vision in infants and children who cannot respond to standard acuity tests. This is a behavioral technique based on the observation that given a choice, an infant prefers to look at patterned rather than unpatterned stimuli. Because these tests require the presence of a skilled examiner, their use is often limited to research protocols involving preverbal children.

VISUAL FIELD ASSESSMENT

Like visual acuity testing, visual field assessment must be geared to a child's age and abilities. Formal visual field examination (perimetry and scotometry) can often be accomplished in school-aged children. The examiner must often rely on confrontation techniques and finger counting in quadrants of the visual field. In many children, only testing by attraction can be accomplished; the examiner observes a child's response to familiar objects brought into each of the four quadrants of the visual field of each eye in turn. The child's bottle, a favorite toy, and lollipops are particularly effective attention-getting items. These gross methods

Table 611-1 VISION SCREENING GUIDELINES*

FUNCTION	RECOMMENDED TESTS	REFERRAL CRITERIA	COMMENTS
AGES 3-5 YEARS			
Distance visual acuity	Snellen letters Snellen numbers Tumbling E test HOTV test Picture tests: Allen figures, Lea symbols	<4 of 6 correct on 20-ft line with either eye tested at 10 ft monocularly (i.e., <10/20 or 20/40) *or* Two-line difference between eyes, even within the passing range (i.e., 10/12.5 and 10/20 or 20/25 and 20/40)	Tests are listed in decreasing order of cognitive difficulty The highest test that the child is capable of performing should be used In general, use the tumbling E or the HOTV test for ages 3-5 yr and Snellen letters or numbers for ages ≥6 yr Testing distance of 3 m (10 ft) is recommended for all visual acuity tests A line of figures is preferred over single figures The nontested eye should be covered by an occluder held by the examiner or by an adhesive occluder patch applied to eye; the examiner must ensure that it is not possible to peek with the nontested eye
Ocular alignment	Cross cover test at 3 m (10 ft)	Any eye movement	
	Random dot E stereo test at 40 cm (630 sec of arc)	<4 of 6 correct	
	Simultaneous red reflex test (Bruckner test)	Any asymmetry of pupil color, size, brightness	Direct ophthalmoscope used to view both red reflexes simultaneously in a darkened room from 2-3 ft away Detects asymmetric refractive errors as well
Ocular media clarity (e.g., cataracts, tumors)	Red reflex	White pupil, dark spots, absent reflex	Direct ophthalmoscope, darkened room View eyes separately at 12-18 in; white reflex indicates possible retinoblastoma
AGES 6 YEARS AND OLDER			
Distance visual acuity	Snellen letters Snellen numbers Tumbling E test HOTV test Picture tests: Allen figures, Lea symbols	<4 of 6 correct on 20-ft line with either eye tested at 10 ft monocularly (i.e., <10/15 or 20/30) *or* Two-line difference between eyes, even within the passing range (i.e., 10/10 and 10/15 or 20/20 and 20/30)	Tests are listed in decreasing order of cognitive difficulty The highest test that the child is capable of performing should be used In general, use the tumbling E or the HOTV test for ages 3-5 yr and Snellen letters or numbers for ages ≥6 yr Testing distance of 3 m (10 ft) is recommended for all visual acuity tests A line of figures is preferred over single figures The nontested eye should be covered by an occluder held by the examiner or by an adhesive occluder patch applied to eye; the examiner must ensure that it is not possible to peek with the nontested eye
Ocular alignment	Cross cover test at 3 m (10 ft)	Any eye movement	
	Random dot E stereo test at 40 cm (630 sec of arc)	<4 of 6 correct	
	Simultaneous red reflex test (Bruckner test)	Any asymmetry of pupil color, size, brightness	Direct ophthalmoscope used to view both red reflexes simultaneously in a darkened room from 2-3 ft away Detects asymmetric refractive errors as well
Ocular media clarity (e.g., cataracts, tumors)	Red reflex	White pupil, dark spots, absent reflex	Direct ophthalmoscope, darkened room View eyes separately at 12-18 in; white reflex indicates possible retinoblastoma

Assessing visual acuity (vision screening) represents one of the most sensitive techniques for detecting eye abnormalities in children. The American Academy of Pediatrics Section on Ophthalmology, in cooperation with the American Association for Pediatric Ophthalmology and Strabismus and the American Academy of Ophthalmology, has developed these guidelines to be used by physicians, nurses, educational institutions, public health departments, and other professionals who perform vision evaluation services.

*Vision screening guidelines were developed by the AAP Section on Ophthalmology Executive Committee, 1991-1992; Robert D. Gross, MBA, MD, Chairman; Walter M. Fierson, MD, Jane D. Kivlin, MD, I. Matthew Rabinowicz, MD, David R. Stager, MD, Mark S. Ruttum, MD, AAPOS; and Earl R. Crouch, Jr., MD, American Academy of Ophthalmology.

Committee on Practice and Ambulatory Medicine, Section on Ophthalmology; American Association of Certified Orthoptists; American Association for Pediatric Ophthalmology and Strabismus; American Academy of Ophthalmology: Eye examination in infants, children, and young adults by pediatricians, *Pediatrics* 111:902–907, 2003.

can often detect diagnostically significant field changes such as the bitemporal hemianopia of a chiasmal lesion or the homonymous hemianopia of a cerebral lesion.

COLOR VISION TESTING

Color vision testing can be accomplished whenever a child is able to name or trace the test symbols; these may be numbers, Xs, Os, triangles, or other symbols. Color vision testing is not often necessary in young children, but parents sometimes request it, particularly if their child seems to be slow in learning colors. Parents are often reassured to know that "color-deficient" children do not misname colors and that true "color blindness" is very rare and not compatible with normal vision. Defective color vision is common in male patients but is rare in female patients. Achromatopsia, a total color vision defect with subnormal visual acuity, nystagmus, and photophobia, is encountered occasionally. A change in color discrimination can be a sign of optic nerve or retinal disease.

PUPILLARY EXAMINATION

Examination of the pupils includes evaluation of both, the direct and consensual reactions to light, the reaction on near gaze, and the response to reduced illumination, noting the size and symmetry of the pupils under all conditions. Special care must be taken to differentiate the reaction to light from the reaction to near gaze. A child's natural tendency is to look directly at the approaching light, inducing the near gaze reflex when one is attempting to test only the reaction to light; accordingly, every effort must be made to control fixation. The swinging flashlight test is especially useful for detecting unilateral or asymmetric prechiasmatic afferent defects in children (see "Marcus Gunn Pupil" section in Chapter 614).

OCULAR MOTILITY

Ocular motility is tested by having a child follow an object into the various positions of gaze. Movements of each eye individually (ductions) and of the two eyes together (versions, conjugate movements, and convergence) are assessed. Alignment is judged by the symmetry of the corneal light reflexes and by the response to alternate occlusion of each eye (see discussion on cover tests for strabismus in Chapter 615).

BINOCULAR VISION

A determination of the degree of binocular vision is commonly performed by an ophthalmologist. The Titmus test is probably the most commonly used test; a series of three-dimensional images are shown to the child while he or she wears a set of Polaroid glasses. The level of difficulty with which these images can be detected correlates with the degree of binocular vision that is present. Other tests may also be used to detect the presence of abnormal binocular adaptations secondary to poor vision or strabismus.

EXTERNAL EXAMINATION

The external examination begins with general inspection in good illumination noting size, shape, and symmetry of the orbits; position and movement of the lids; and position and symmetry of the globes. Viewing the eyes and lids from above aids in detecting orbital asymmetry, lid masses, proptosis (**exophthalmos**), and abnormal pulsations. Palpation is also important in detecting orbital and lid masses.

The lacrimal apparatus is assessed by looking for evidence of tear deficiency, overflow of tears (**epiphora**), erythema, and swelling in the region of the tear sac or gland. The sac is massaged to check for reflux when obstruction is suspected. The presence and position of the puncta are also checked.

The lids and conjunctivae are specifically examined for focal lesions, foreign bodies, and inflammatory signs; loss and maldirection of lashes should also be noted. When necessary, the lids can be everted in the following manner: (1) instruct the patient to look down; (2) grasp the lashes of the patient's upper lid between the thumb and index finger of one hand; (3) place a probe, a cotton-tipped applicator, or the thumb of the other hand at the upper margin of the tarsal plate; and (4) pull the lid down and outward, everting it over the probe, using the instrument as a fulcrum. Foreign bodies commonly lodge in the concavity just above the lid margin and are exposed only by fully everting the lid.

The anterior segment of the eye is then evaluated with oblique focal illumination, noting the luster and clarity of the cornea, the depth and clarity of the anterior chamber, and the features of the iris. Transillumination of the anterior segment aids in detecting opacities and in demonstrating atrophy or hypopigmentation of the iris; these latter signs are important when ocular albinism is suspected. When necessary, fluorescein dye can be used to aid in diagnosing abrasions, ulcerations, and foreign bodies.

BIOMICROSCOPY (SLIT-LAMP EXAMINATION)

The slit-lamp examination provides a highly magnified view of the various structures of the eye and an optical section through the media of the eye—the cornea, aqueous humor, lens, and vitreous. Lesions can be identified and localized according to their depth within the eye; the resolution is sufficient to detect individual inflammatory cells in the aqueous and vitreous. With the addition of special lenses and prisms, the angle of the anterior chamber and regions of the fundus also can be examined with a slit lamp. Biomicroscopy is often crucial in trauma and in examining for iritis. It is also helpful in diagnosing many metabolic diseases of childhood.

FUNDUS EXAMINATION (OPHTHALMOSCOPY)

Ophthalmoscopy is best done with the pupil dilated unless there are neurologic or other contraindications. Tropicamide (Mydriacyl) 0.5-1% and phenylephrine (Neo-Synephrine) 2.5% are recommended as mydriatics of short duration. These are safe for most children, but the possibility of adverse systemic effects must be recognized. For very small infants, more-dilute preparations may be advisable. Beginning with posterior landmarks, the disc and the macula, the four quadrants are systematically examined by following each of the major vessel groups to the periphery. More of the fundus can be seen if a child is directed to look up and down and to the right and left. Even with care, only a limited amount of the fundus can be seen with a direct or hand-held ophthalmoscope. For examination of the far periphery, an indirect ophthalmoscope is used, and full dilation of the pupil is essential.

REFRACTION

A test of refraction determines the refractive state of the eye: the degree of nearsightedness, farsightedness, or astigmatism. Retinoscopy provides an objective determination of the amount of correction needed and can be performed at any age. In young children, it is best done with cycloplegia. Subjective refinement of refraction involves asking patients for preferences in the strength and axis of corrective lenses; it can be accomplished in many school-aged children. Refraction and determination of visual acuity with appropriate corrective lenses in place are essential steps in deciding whether a patient has a visual defect or amblyopia. Photoscreening cameras aid ancillary medical personnel in screening for abnormal refractive errors in preverbal children. The accuracy and practical usefulness of these devices are still being investigated.

TONOMETRY

Tonometry measures intraocular pressure; it may be performed with a portable, stand-alone instrument or by the applanation method with the slit lamp. Alternative methods are pneumatic, electronic, or rebound tonometry. When accurate measurement of the pressure is necessary in a child who cannot cooperate, it may be performed with sedation or general anesthesia. A gross estimate of pressure can be made by palpating the globe with the index fingers placed side by side on the upper lid above the tarsal plate.

BIBLIOGRAPHY

Please visit the Nelson Textbook of Pediatrics *website at www.expertconsult.com for the complete bibliography.*

Chapter 612
Abnormalities of Refraction and Accommodation

Scott E. Olitsky, Denise Hug, Laura S. Plummer, and Merrill Stass-Isern

Emmetropia is the state in which parallel rays of light come to focus on the retina with the eye at rest (nonaccommodating). Although such an ideal optical state is common, the opposite condition, ametropia, often occurs. Three principal types of **ametropia** exist: **hyperopia** (farsightedness), **myopia** (nearsightedness), and **astigmatism.** The majority of children are physiologically hyperopic at birth, but a significant number, especially those born prematurely, are myopic and often have some degree of astigmatism. With growth, the refractive state tends to change and should be evaluated periodically.

Measurement of the refractive state of the eye (refraction) can be accomplished both objectively and subjectively. The objective method involves directing a beam of light from a retinoscope onto a patient's retina. Based on the way the light behaves with movement of the retinoscope and manipulation with lenses of various strengths held in front of the eye, a precise refraction can be performed. An objective refraction can be carried out at any age because it requires no response from the patient. In infants and children, it is generally more accurate to perform a refraction after instilling eyedrops that produce mydriasis (dilatation of the pupil) and cycloplegia (paralysis of accommodation); those used most commonly are tropicamide (Mydriacyl), cyclopentolate (Cyclogyl), and atropine sulfate.

A subjective refraction involves placing lenses in front of the eye and having the patient report which lenses provide the clearest image of the letters on a chart. This method depends on a patient's ability to discriminate and communicate, but it can be used for some children and can be helpful in determining the best refractive correction for children who are developmentally capable.

HYPEROPIA

If parallel rays of light come to focus posterior to the retina with the eye in a state of rest, hyperopia or **farsightedness** exists. This can result because the anteroposterior diameter of the eye is too short or the refractive power of the cornea or lens is less than normal.

In hyperopia, accommodation is used to bring objects into focus for both far and near gaze. If the accommodative effort required is not too great, the child has clear vision and is comfortable with both distant and close work. In high degrees of hyperopia requiring greater accommodative effort, vision may be blurred, and the child might complain of eyestrain, headaches, or fatigue. Squinting, eye rubbing, and lack of interest in reading are common manifestations. If the induced discomfort is great enough, a child might not make an effort to see well and can develop bilateral amblyopia (ametropic amblyopia). Esotropia may also be associated (see the discussion of convergent strabismus, accommodative esotropia in Chapter 615).

Convex lenses (spectacles or contact lenses) of sufficient strength to provide clear vision and comfort are prescribed when indicated. Even children who have high degrees of hyperopia but who have good vision will happily wear glasses because they provide comfort by eliminating the excessive accommodation required to see well. Preverbal children should also be given glasses for high levels of hyperopia to prevent the development of esotropia or amblyopia. Children with normal levels of hyperopia do not require correction in the majority of cases.

MYOPIA

In myopia, parallel rays of light come to focus anterior to the retina. This can result because the anteroposterior diameter of the eye is too long or the refractive power of the cornea or lens is greater than normal. The principal symptom is blurred vision for distant objects. The far point of clear vision varies inversely with the degree of myopia; as the myopia increases, the far point of clear vision moves closer to the eye. With myopia of 1 diopter, for example, the far point of clear focus is 1 m from the eye; with myopia of 3 diopters, the far point of clear vision is only ⅓ m from the eye. Thus, myopic children tend to hold objects and reading matter close, prefer to be close to the blackboard, and may be uninterested in distant activities. Squinting is common because the visual acuity is improved when the lid aperture is reduced, also known as the *pinhole effect*.

Myopia is uncommon in infants and preschool-aged children. It is more common in infants with a history of **retinopathy of prematurity.** A hereditary tendency to myopia is also observed, and children of myopic parents should be examined at an early age. The incidence of myopia increases during the school years, especially during the preteen and teen years. The degree of myopia also increases with age during the growing years.

Concave lenses (spectacles or contact lenses) of appropriate strength to provide clear vision and comfort are prescribed. Changes are usually needed periodically, sometimes in every year or 2, sometimes every few months. Excessive accommodation during near work has been considered by some to lead to progression of myopia. Based on this philosophy, some practitioners advocate the use of cycloplegic agents, bifocals, intentional undercorrection of myopic refractive errors, or mandatory removal of myopic glasses for near work in an effort to retard the progression of myopia. The value of such treatment has not been scientifically proved.

Excimer laser correction for myopia has been approved for adults since 1995. The LASIK (laser-assisted in situ keratomileusis) procedure uses either a microkeratome or a femtosecond laser that produces an epithelial-stromal flap, permitting the underlying corneal tissue to be ablated to correct vision; the flap then re-covers the area of the cornea. Correction of vision is usually excellent and stable over time. Risks are greatest with high degrees of myopia (>10 diopters) and include starbursts, halos, and distorted images or multiple images (usually at night). Refractive surgery is currently not approved for pediatric patients but its use is being studied, especially for the treatment of some forms of amblyopia.

In most cases, myopia is not a result of pathologic alteration of the eye and is referred to as simple or physiologic myopia. Some children have pathologic myopia, a rare condition caused by a pathologically abnormal axial length of the eye; this is usually associated with thinning of the sclera, choroid, and retina and often with some degree of uncorrectable visual impairment. Tears or breaks in the retina can occur as it becomes increasingly thin, leading to the development of retinal detachments. Myopia can also occur as a result of other ocular abnormalities, such as keratoconus, ectopia lentis, congenital stationary night blindness, and glaucoma. Myopia is also a major feature of Stickler syndrome.

ASTIGMATISM

In astigmatism, the refractive power of the various meridians of the eye differs. Most cases are caused by irregularity in the curvature of the cornea; some astigmatism results from changes in the lens. Mild degrees of astigmatism are common and might produce no symptoms. With greater degrees, there may be distortion of vision. To achieve a clearer image, a person with astigmatism uses accommodation or squints to obtain a pinhole effect. Symptoms include eyestrain, headache, and fatigue. Cylindric or spherocylindric lenses are used to provide optical correction when indicated. Glasses may be needed constantly or only part time, depending on the degree of astigmatism and the severity of the attendant symptoms. In some cases, contact lenses are used.

Infants and children with corneal irregularity resulting from injury, periorbital and eyelid hemangiomas, and ptosis are at increased risk of astigmatism and attendant amblyopia.

ANISOMETROPIA

When the refractive state of one eye is significantly different from the refractive state of the other eye, anisometropia exists. If the condition remains uncorrected, one eye might always be out of focus, leading to the development of amblyopia. Early detection and correction are essential if normal visual development in both eyes is to be achieved.

ACCOMMODATION

During accommodation, the ciliary muscle contracts, the suspensory fibers of the lens relax, and the lens assumes a more rounded shape to bring rays of light into focus on the retina. The amplitude of accommodation is greatest during childhood and gradually diminishes with age. The physiologic decrease in accommodative ability that occurs with age is called *presbyopia.*

Disorders of accommodation in children are relatively rare. Premature presbyopia is occasionally encountered in young children. The most common cause of paralysis of accommodation in children is intentional or inadvertent use of cycloplegic substances, topically or systemically; included are all the anticholinergic drugs and poisons, as well as plants and plant substances having these effects. Neurogenic causes of accommodative paralysis include lesions affecting the oculomotor nerve (cranial nerve III) in any part of its course.

Differential diagnosis includes tumors, degenerative diseases, vascular lesions, trauma, and infectious diseases. Systemic disorders that can cause impairment of accommodation include botulism, diphtheria, Wilson disease, diabetes mellitus, and syphilis. **Adie tonic pupil** can also lead to a deficiency of accommodation after some viral illnesses (Chapter 614). An apparent defect in accommodation may be psychogenic in origin; it is common for a child to feign inability to read when it can be demonstrated that visual acuity and ability to focus are normal.

BIBLIOGRAPHY

Please visit the Nelson Textbook of Pediatrics *website at www.expertconsult.com for the complete bibliography.*

Chapter 613
Disorders of Vision

Scott E. Olitsky, Denise Hug, Laura S. Plummer, and Merrill Stass-Isern

Severe visual impairment (corrected vision poorer than **6/60**) and blindness in children have many etiologies and may be due to multiple defects affecting any structure or function along the visual pathways (Table 613-1). The overall incidence is approximately 2.5 per 100,000 children; the incidence is higher in developing countries, in low birthweight infants, and in the first year of life. The most common causes occur during the prenatal and perinatal time periods; the cerebral-visual pathways, optic nerve, and retinal sites are most often affected. Important prenatal causes include autosomal recessive (most common), autosomal dominant, and X-linked genetic disorders as well as hypoxia and chromosomal syndromes. Perinatal and neonatal causes include retinopathy of prematurity, hypoxia-ischemia, and infection. Severe visual impairment starting in older children can result from central nervous system or retinal tumors, infections, hypoxia-ischemia, injuries, neurodegenerative disorders, or juvenile rheumatoid arthritis.

AMBLYOPIA

Amblyopia is a decrease in visual acuity, unilateral or bilateral, that occurs in visually immature children as a result of a lack of a clear image projecting onto the retina. The unformed retinal image can occur secondary to a deviated eye (**strabismic amblyopia**), an unequal need for vision correction between the eyes (**anisometropic amblyopia**), a high refractive error in both eyes (**ametropic amblyopia**), or a media opacity within the visual axis (**deprivation amblyopia**).

The development of visual acuity normally proceeds rapidly in infancy and early childhood. Anything that interferes with the formation of a clear retinal image during this early developmental period can produce amblyopia. Amblyopia may occur only during the critical period of development, before the cortex has become visually mature, within the first decade of life. The younger the child, the more susceptible he or she is to the development of amblyopia.

The **diagnosis** of amblyopia is confirmed when a complete ophthalmologic examination reveals reduced acuity that is unexplained by an organic abnormality. If the history and ophthalmologic examination do not support the diagnosis of amblyopia in a child with poor vision, other causes (neurologic, psychologic) must be considered. Amblyopia is usually asymptomatic and detected only by screening programs. Screening is easier in older children. Just as amblyopia is less likely to occur in an older child, it is also more resistant to treatment at an older age. Amblyopia is reversed more rapidly in younger children whose visual system is less mature. The key to the successful treatment of amblyopia is early detection and prompt intervention.

Treatment generally first consists of removing any media opacity or prescribing appropriate glasses, if needed, so that a well-focused retinal image can be produced in each eye. The sound eye is then covered (occlusion therapy) or blurred with glasses or drops (penalization therapy) to stimulate proper visual development of the more severely affected eye. Occlusion therapy can provide a speedier improvement in vision, but some children better tolerate atropine penalization. The best treatment for any one patient should be selected on an individual basis. The goals of treatment should be thoroughly understood, and the treatment must be carefully supervised. Close monitoring of amblyopia therapy by an ophthalmologist is essential, especially in the very young, to avoid deprivation amblyopia in the good eye. Many families need reassurance and support throughout the trying course of treatment. Although full-time occlusion has historically been considered the best way to treat children with amblyopia, a series of prospective studies have shown that some children can achieve similar results with less patching or through the use of atropine drops. In the past it was generally thought that older children would not respond to amblyopia therapy, but this has been shown to be untrue. Studies now suggest that treatment should be offered to children who previously were deemed visually mature and thus thought to have no hope of improving their vision.

DIPLOPIA

Diplopia, or double vision, is generally a result of a misalignment of the visual axes. Occluding either eye relieves the diplopia if it is binocular in origin; affected children commonly squint, cover one eye with a hand, or assume an abnormal head posture (a face turn or head tilt) to alleviate the bothersome sensation. These mannerisms, especially in preverbal children, are important clues to diplopia. The onset of diplopia in any child warrants prompt evaluation; it may signal the onset of a serious problem such as increased intracranial pressure, a brain tumor, or an orbital mass.

Monocular diplopia results from dislocation of the lens, cataract, or some defect in the media or macula. With this type of diplopia, occluding the nondiplopic eye will not relieve the symptoms.

SUPPRESSION

In the presence of strabismus, diplopia occurs secondary to the same image falling on different regions of the retina in each eye. In a visually immature child, a process can occur in the cortex that eliminates the disability of seeing double. This is an active process and is termed *suppression.* It develops only in children. Although suppression eliminates the annoying symptom of diplopia, it is the potential awareness of a second image that tends to keep our eyes properly aligned. Once suppression develops, it can allow an intermittent strabismus to become constant or

Table 613-1 CAUSES OF CHILDHOOD SEVERE VISUAL IMPAIRMENT OR BLINDNESS

CONGENITAL	Optic nerve hypoplasia or aplasia Septo-optic dysplasia Optic coloboma Congenital hydrocephalus Hydranencephaly Porencephaly Micrencephaly Encephalocele, particularly occipital Morning glory disc Aniridia Microphthalmia/anophthalmia Peters anomaly Reiger's anomaly Persistent pupillary membrane Glaucoma Cataracts Persistent hyperplastic primary vitreous
PHAKOMATOSES	Tuberous sclerosis Neurofibromatosis (special association with optic glioma) Sturge-Weber syndrome von Hippel-Lindau disease
TUMORS	Retinoblastoma Optic glioma Perioptic meningioma Craniopharyngioma Cerebral glioma Astrocytoma Posterior and intraventricular tumors when complicated by hydrocephalus Pseudotumor cerebri
NEURODEGENERATIVE DISEASES	Cerebral storage disease Gangliosidoses, particularly Tay-Sachs disease, Sandhoff variant, generalized gangliosidosis Other lipidoses and ceroid lipofuscinoses, particularly the late-onset disorders such as those of Jansky-Bielschowsky and of Batten-Mayou-Spielmeyer-Vogt Mucopolysaccharidoses, particularly Hurler syndrome and Hunter syndrome Leukodystrophies (dysmyelination disorders), particularly metachromatic leukodystrophy and Canavan disease Demyelinating sclerosis (myelinoclastic diseases), especially Schilder disease and Devic neuromyelitis optica Special types: Dawson disease, Leigh disease, the Bassen-Kornzweig syndrome, Refsum disease Retinal degenerations: retinitis pigmentosa and its variants and Leber congenital type Optic atrophies: congenital autosomal recessive type, infantile and congenital autosomal dominant types, Leber disease, and atrophies associated with hereditary ataxias—the types of Behr, of Marie, and of Sanger-Brown
INFECTIOUS AND INFLAMMATORY PROCESSES	Encephalitis, especially in the prenatal infection syndromes due to *Toxoplasma gondii*, cytomegalovirus, rubella virus, *Treponema pallidum*, herpes simplex virus Meningitis; arachnoiditis Chorioretinitis Endophthalmitis Trachoma Keratitis Uveitis
HEMATOLOGIC DISORDERS	Leukemia with central nervous system involvement
VASCULAR AND CIRCULATORY DISORDERS	Collagen vascular diseases Arteriovenous malformations: intracerebral hemorrhage, subarachnoid hemorrhage Central retinal occlusion
TRAUMA	Contusion or avulsion of optic nerves, chiasm, globe, cornea Cerebral contusion or laceration Intracerebral, subarachnoid, or subdural hemorrhage Retinal detachment
DRUGS AND TOXINS	Quinine Ethambutol Methanol Many others
OTHER	Retinopathy of prematurity Sclerocornea Conversion reaction Optic neuritis Osteopetrosis

Modified from Kliegman R: *Practical strategies in pediatric diagnosis and therapy,* Philadelphia, 1996, WB Saunders.

strabismus to redevelop later in life, even after successful treatment during childhood.

AMAUROSIS

Amaurosis is partial or total loss of vision; the term is usually reserved for profound impairment, blindness, or near blindness. When amaurosis exists from birth, primary consideration in the differential diagnosis must be given to developmental malformations, damage consequent to gestational or perinatal infection, anoxia or hypoxia, perinatal trauma, and the genetically determined diseases that can affect the eye itself or the visual pathways. Often, the reason for amaurosis can be readily determined by objective ophthalmic examination; examples are severe microphthalmia, corneal opacification, dense cataracts, chorioretinal scars, macular defects, retinal dysplasia, and severe optic nerve hypoplasia. In other cases, an intrinsic retinal disease might not be apparent on initial ophthalmoscopic examination or the defect might involve the brain and not the eye. Neuroradiologic (CT or MRI) and electrophysiologic (electroretinography) evaluation may be especially helpful in these cases.

Amaurosis that develops in a child who once had useful vision has different implications. In the absence of obvious ocular disease (cataract, chorioretinitis, retinoblastoma, retinitis pigmentosa), consideration must be given to many neurologic and systemic disorders that can affect the visual pathways. Amaurosis of rather rapid onset can indicate an encephalopathy (hypertension), infectious or parainfectious processes, vasculitis, migraine, leukemia, toxins, or trauma. It may be caused by acute demyelinating disease affecting the optic nerves, chiasm, or cerebrum. In some cases, precipitous loss of vision is a result of increased intracranial pressure, rapidly progressive hydrocephalus, or dysfunction of a shunt. More slowly progressive visual loss suggests tumor or neurodegenerative disease. Gliomas of the optic nerve and chiasm and craniopharyngiomas are primary diagnostic considerations in children who show progressive loss of vision.

Clinical manifestations of impairment of vision vary with the age and abilities of a child, the mode of onset, and the laterality and severity of the deficit. The first clue to amaurosis in an infant may be **nystagmus** or **strabismus,** with the vision deficit itself passing undetected for some time. Timidity, clumsiness, or behavioral change may be the initial clues in the very young. Deterioration in school progress and indifference to school activities are common signs in an older child. School-aged children often try to hide their disability and, in the case of very slowly progressive disorders, might not themselves realize the severity of the problem; some detect and promptly report small changes in their vision.

Any evidence of loss of vision requires prompt and thorough ophthalmic evaluation. Complete delineation of childhood amaurosis and its cause can require extensive investigation involving neurologic evaluation, electrophysiologic tests, neuroradiologic procedures, and sometimes metabolic and genetic studies. Furthermore, attendant special educational, social, and emotional needs must be met.

NYCTALOPIA

Nyctalopia, or **night blindness**, is vision that is defective in reduced illumination. It generally implies impairment in function of the rods, particularly in dark adaptation time and perceptual threshold. Stationary congenital night blindness can occur as an autosomal dominant, autosomal recessive, or X-linked recessive condition. It may be associated with myopia and nystagmus. Children can have excessive problems going to sleep in a dark room, which may be mistaken for a behavioral problem. Progressive night blindness usually indicates primary or secondary retinal, choroidal, or vitreoretinal degeneration (Chapter 622); it occurs also in vitamin A deficiency or as a result of retinotoxic drugs such as quinine.

PSYCHOGENIC DISTURBANCES

Vision problems of psychogenic origin are common in school-aged children. Both conversion reactions and willful feigning are encountered. The usual manifestation is a report of reduced visual acuity in one or both eyes. Another common manifestation is constriction of the visual field. In some cases, the symptom is diplopia or polyopia (Chapters 20 and 23).

Important clues to the diagnosis are inappropriate affect, excessive grimacing, inconsistency in performance, and suggestibility. A thorough ophthalmologic examination is essential to differentiate organic from functional visual disorders.

Affected children usually fare well with reassurance and positive suggestions. In some cases, psychiatric care is indicated. In all cases, the approach must be supportive and nonpunitive.

DYSLEXIA

Dyslexia is the inability to develop the capability to read at an expected level despite an otherwise normal intellect. The terms *reading disability* and *dyslexia* are often used interchangeably. Most dyslexic persons also display poor writing ability. Dyslexia is a primary reading disorder and should be differentiated from secondary reading difficulties due to mental retardation, environmental or educational deprivation, and physical or organic diseases. Because there is no one standard test for dyslexia, the diagnosis is usually made by comparing reading ability with intelligence and standard reading expectations. Dyslexia is a language-based disorder and is not caused by any defect in the eye or visual acuity per se, nor is it attributable to a defect in ocular motility or binocular alignment. Although ophthalmologic evaluation of children with a reading problem is recommended to diagnose and correct any concurrent ocular problems such as a refractive error, amblyopia, or strabismus, treatment directed to the eyes themselves cannot be expected to correct developmental dyslexia (Chapter 31).

BIBLIOGRAPHY

Please visit the Nelson Textbook of Pediatrics *website at www.expertconsult.com for the complete bibliography.*

Chapter 614
Abnormalities of Pupil and Iris

Scott E. Olitsky, Denise Hug, Laura S. Plummer, and Merrill Stass-Isern

ANIRIDIA

The term *aniridia* is a misnomer because iris tissue is usually present, although it is hypoplastic (Fig. 614-1). Two thirds of the cases are dominantly transmitted with a high degree of penetrance. The other 30% of cases are sporadic and are considered to be new mutations. The condition is bilateral in 98% of all patients, regardless of the means of transmission, and is found in approximately 1/50,000 persons.

Aniridia is a panocular disorder and should not be thought of as an isolated iris defect. Macular and optic nerve hypoplasias are commonly present and lead to decreased vision and sensory nystagmus. The visual acuity is measured as 20/200 in most patients, although the vision occasionally is better. Other ocular deformities are common and can involve the lens and cornea. The cornea may be small, and a cellular infiltrate (pannus) occasionally develops in the superficial layers of the peripheral cornea. Clinically, this appears as a gray opacification. The pannus results from a stem cell deficiency and therefore must be treated with keratolimbal stem cell transplantation rather than cornea transplantation. Lens abnormalities include cataract formation and partial or total lens dislocation. **Glaucoma** develops in as many as 75% of patients with aniridia.

Aniridia is caused by a defect in the *PAX6* gene on chromosome 11p13. The *PAX6* gene is the master control gene for eye morphogenesis. Aniridia can be sporadic or familial. The familial form is autosomal dominant with complete penetrance but variable expressivity. Sporadic aniridia is associated with Wilms

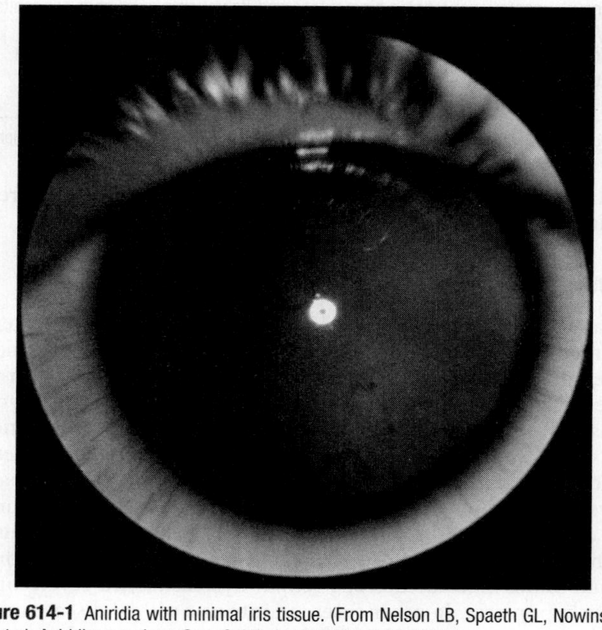

Figure 614-1 Aniridia with minimal iris tissue. (From Nelson LB, Spaeth GL, Nowinski TS, et al: Aniridia: a review, *Surv Ophthalmol* 28:621–642, 1984.)

tumor in as many as 30% of cases (Chapter 493.1). The combination of aniridia and Wilms tumor represents a contiguous gene syndrome in which the adjacent *PAX6* and Wilms tumor *(WT1)* genes are both deleted. Some deletions create the WAGR complex of Wilms tumor, *a*niridia, genitourinary malformations, and mental *r*etardation. All children with sporadic aniridia should undergo chromosomal deletional analysis to exclude the possibility of Wilms tumor formation. Children who test positive for the deletion should undergo repeated abdominal ultrasonographic and clinical examinations. Wilms tumor has also been reported in patients with familial aniridia. Therefore, these patients should also undergo chromosomal analysis.

COLOBOMA OF THE IRIS

Coloboma of the iris is a developmental defect that can occur as a defect in a sector of the iris, a hole in the substance of the iris, or a notch in the pupil's margin. Simple colobomas are often transmitted as an autosomal dominant trait and can occur alone or in association with other anomalies. A coloboma is formed when the embryonic fissure fails to close completely. Because of the anatomic location of the embryonic fissure, an iris coloboma is always located inferiorly, giving the iris a keyhole appearance. An iris coloboma may be the only externally visible part of an extensive malclosure of the embryonic fissure that also involves the fundus and optic nerve. When this occurs, vision is likely to be severely affected. Therefore, all children with an iris coloboma should undergo a full ophthalmologic examination.

MICROCORIA

Microcoria (congenital miosis) appears as a small pupil that does not react to light or accommodation and that dilates poorly, if at all, with medication. The condition may be unilateral or bilateral. In bilateral cases, the degree of miosis may be different in each eye. The eye may be otherwise normal or may demonstrate other abnormalities of the anterior segment. Congenital microcoria is usually transmitted as an autosomal dominant trait, although it can occur sporadically.

CONGENITAL MYDRIASIS

In congenital mydriasis, the pupils appear dilated, do not constrict significantly to light or near gaze, and respond minimally to miotic agents. The iris is otherwise normal, and affected children are usually healthy. Trauma, pharmacologic mydriasis, and neurologic disorders should be considered. Many apparent cases of congenital mydriasis show abnormalities of the central iris structures and may be considered a form of aniridia.

DYSCORIA AND CORECTOPIA

Dyscoria is abnormal shape of the pupil, and corectopia is abnormal position of the pupil. They can occur together or independently as congenital or acquired anomalies.

Congenital corectopia is usually bilateral and symmetric and rarely occurs as an isolated anomaly; it is usually accompanied by dislocation of the lens (ectopia lentis et pupillae), and the lens and pupil are commonly dislocated in opposite directions. Ectopia lentis et pupillae is transmitted as an autosomal recessive disorder; consanguinity is common.

When these are acquired, distortion and displacement of the pupil are often a result of trauma or intraocular inflammation. Prolapse of the iris after perforating injuries of the eye leads to peaking of the pupil in the direction of the perforation. Posterior synechiae (adhesions of the iris to the lens) are commonly seen when inflammation due to any cause occurs in the anterior segment.

ANISOCORIA

This is inequality of the pupils. The difference in size may be due to local or neurologic disorders. As a rule, if the inequality is more pronounced in the presence of bright focal illumination or on near gaze, there is a defect in pupillary constriction and the larger pupil is abnormal. If the anisocoria is worse in reduced illumination, a defect in dilation exists and the smaller pupil is abnormal. Neurologic causes of anisocoria (parasympathetic or sympathetic lesions) must be differentiated from local causes such as synechiae (adhesions), congenital iris defects (colobomas, aniridia), and pharmacologic effects. Simple central anisocoria can occur in otherwise healthy children. The combination of anisocoria and ptosis may be seen in Horner syndrome.

HORNER SYNDROME

The principal signs of **oculosympathetic paresis** (Horner syndrome) are homolateral miosis, mild ptosis, and apparent enophthalmos with slight elevation of the lower lid. Patients may also have decreased facial sweating, increased amplitude of accommodation, and transient decrease in intraocular pressure. If paralysis of the ocular sympathetic fibers occurs before the age of 2 yr, iris heterochromia with hypopigmentation of the iris can occur on the affected side but can take time to develop.

Oculosympathetic paralysis may be caused by a lesion in the midbrain, brainstem, upper spinal cord, neck, middle fossa, or orbit. Congenital oculosympathetic paresis, often as part of Klumpke brachial palsy, is common, although the ocular signs, particularly the anisocoria, can pass undetected for years. Horner syndrome is also seen in some children after thoracic surgery, such as for congenital heart disease. Congenital Horner syndrome can occur in association with vertebral anomalies and with enterogenous cysts. In some infants and children, Horner syndrome is the presenting sign of tumor in the mediastinal or cervical region, particularly neuroblastoma.

The diagnosis of Horner syndrome can be confirmed with the use of topical cocaine or apraclonidine drops. A normal pupil dilates within 20-45 min after instillation of 1 or 2 drops of 4% cocaine, whereas the miotic pupil of an oculosympathetic paresis dilates poorly, if at all, with cocaine. Apraclonidine causes reversal of the anisocoria with dilation of the affected (smaller) pupil and no effect on the normal pupil. It should be used in caution in young children because it can cause excessive sedation owing to its CNS side effects. Pharmacologic testing might not be needed in the presence of typical clinical findings.

Horner's syndrome in children can result from trauma, surgery, or the presence of neuroblastoma affecting the sympathetic chain in the chest. Evaluation of acquired Horner syndrome in a child without a history of trauma or surgery that could explain the anisocoria should include imaging studies of the brain, neck, and chest. Examining old photographs and old records is sometimes helpful in establishing the age at onset of Horner syndrome.

DILATED FIXED PUPIL

Differential diagnosis of a dilated unreactive pupil includes internal ophthalmoplegia caused by a central or peripheral lesion, Hutchinson pupil of transtentorial herniation, tonic pupil, pharmacologic blockade, and iridoplegia secondary to ocular trauma.

The most common cause of a dilated unreactive pupil is purposeful or accidental instillation of a cycloplegic agent, particularly atropine and related substances. Central nervous system lesions, such as a pinealoma, can cause internal ophthalmoplegia in children. Because the external surface of the oculomotor nerve carries the fibers responsible for pupillary constriction, compression of the nerve along its intracranial course may be associated with internal ophthalmoplegia, even before the development of ptosis or an ocular motility deficit. Although ophthalmoplegic migraine is a common cause of a 3rd nerve palsy with pupillary involvement in children, an intracranial aneurysm must also be considered in the differential diagnosis. The **blown pupil** of transtentorial herniation, occurring with increasing intracranial pressure, is generally unilateral, and patients usually are obviously ill. The pilocarpine test can help differentiate neurologic iridoplegia from pharmacologic blockade. In the case of neurologic iridoplegia, the dilated pupil constricts within minutes after instillation of 1 or 2 drops of 0.5-1% pilocarpine; if the pupil has been dilated with atropine, pilocarpine has no effect. Because pilocarpine is a long-acting drug, this test is not to be used in acute situations in which pupillary signs must be carefully monitored. Because of the consensual pupil response to light, even complete uniocular blindness does not cause a unilaterally dilated pupil.

TONIC PUPIL

Tonic pupil is typically a large pupil that reacts poorly to light (the reaction may be very slow or essentially nil), reacts poorly and slowly to accommodation, and redilates in a slow, tonic manner. The features of tonic pupil are explained by cholinergic supersensitivity of the sphincter after peripheral (postganglionic) denervation and imperfect reinnervation. A distinctive feature of a tonic pupil is its sensitivity to dilute cholinergic agents. Instillation of 0.125% pilocarpine causes significant constriction of the involved pupil and has little or no effect on the unaffected side. The condition is usually unilateral.

Tonic pupil can develop after the acute stage of a partial or complete iridoplegia. It can be seen after trauma to the eye or orbit and can occur in association with toxic or infectious conditions. For those in the pediatric age group, tonic pupil is uncommon. Infectious processes (primarily viral syndromes) and trauma are the primary causes. Features of tonic pupil may also be seen in infants and children with familial dysautonomia (Riley-Day syndrome), although the significance of these findings has been questioned. Tonic pupil has also been reported in young children with Charcot-Marie-Tooth disease. The occurrence of tonic pupil in association with decreased deep tendon reflexes in young women is referred to as **Adie syndrome.**

MARCUS GUNN PUPIL

This relative afferent pupillary defect indicates an asymmetric, prechiasmatic, afferent conduction defect. It is best demonstrated by the swinging flashlight test; this allows comparison of the direct and consensual pupillary responses in both eyes. With patients fixing on a distant target (to control accommodation), a bright focal light is directed alternately into each eye in turn. In the presence of an afferent lesion, both the direct response to light in the affected eye and the consensual response in the other eye are subnormal. Swinging the light to the better or normal eye causes both pupils to react (constrict) normally. Swinging the light back to the affected eye causes both pupils to redilate to some degree, reflecting the defective conduction. This is a very sensitive and useful test for detecting and confirming optic nerve and retinal disease. This test is only abnormal if there is a "relative" difference in the conduction properties of the optic nerves. Therefore, patients with bilateral and symmetric optic nerve disease do not demonstrate an afferent pupillary defect. A subtle relative afferent defect is found in some children with amblyopia.

PARADOXICAL PUPIL REACTION

Some children exhibit paradoxical constriction of the pupils to darkness. An initial brisk constriction of the pupils occurs when the light is turned off, followed by slow redilatation of the pupils. The response to direct light stimulation and the near response are normal. The mechanism is not clear, but paradoxical constriction of the pupils in reduced light can be a sign of retinal or optic nerve abnormalities. The phenomenon has been observed in children with congenital stationary night blindness, albinism, retinitis pigmentosa, Leber congenital retinal amaurosis, and Best disease. It has also been observed in those with optic nerve anomalies, optic neuritis, optic atrophy, and possibly amblyopia.

PERSISTENT PUPILLARY MEMBRANE

Involution of the pupillary membrane and anterior vascular capsule of the lens is usually completed during the 5th-6th mo of fetal development. It is common to see some remnants of the pupillary membrane in newborns, particularly in premature infants. These membranes are nonpigmented strands of obliterated vessels that cross the pupil and can secondarily attach to the lens or cornea. The remnants tend to atrophy in time and usually present no problem. In some children, however, significant remnants that remain obscure the pupil and interfere with vision. Rarely, there is patency of the vascular elements; hyphema can result from rupture of persistent vessels.

Intervention must be considered to minimize amblyopia in infants with extensive persistent pupillary membrane of sufficient degree to interfere with vision in the early months of life. In some cases, mydriatics and occlusion therapy are effective, but in others, surgery is needed to provide an adequate pupillary aperture.

HETEROCHROMIA

In heterochromia, the two irides are of different color (heterochromia iridium) or a portion of an iris differs in color from the remainder (heterochromia iridis). Simple heterochromia can occur as an autosomal dominant characteristic. Congenital heterochromia is also a feature of **Waardenburg syndrome**, an autosomal dominant condition characterized principally by lateral displacement of the inner canthi and puncta, pigmentary disturbances (usually a median white forelock and patches of hypopigmentation of the skin), and defective hearing. The color of the iris can change as a result of trauma, hemorrhage, intraocular inflammation (iridocyclitis, uveitis), intraocular tumor (especially retinoblastoma), intraocular foreign body, glaucoma, iris atrophy, oculosympathetic palsy (Horner syndrome), melanosis oculi, previous intraocular surgery, and some glaucoma medications.

OTHER IRIS LESIONS

Discrete nodules of the iris, referred to as **Lisch nodules,** are commonly seen in patients with neurofibromatosis. Lisch nodules represent melanocytic hamartomas of the iris and vary from slightly elevated pigmented areas to distinct ball-like excrescences. Lisch nodules are found in 92-100% of patients >5 yr of age who have neurofibromatosis. Slit-lamp identification of these nodules can help to fulfill the criteria required to confirm the diagnosis of neurofibromatosis.

In leukemia, there may be infiltration of the iris, sometimes with **hypopyon,** an accumulation of white blood cells in the anterior chamber, which can herald relapse or involvement of the central nervous system.

The lesion of **juvenile xanthogranuloma** (nevoxanthoendothelioma) can occur in the eye as a yellowish fleshy mass or plaque of the iris. Spontaneous hyphema (blood in the anterior chamber), glaucoma, or a red eye with signs of uveitis may be associated. A search for the skin lesions of xanthogranuloma (Chapter 80.3) should be made in any infant or young child with spontaneous hyphema. In many cases, the ocular lesion responds to topical corticosteroid therapy.

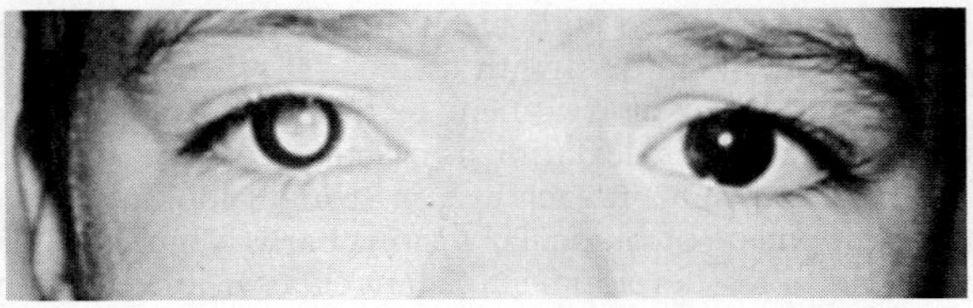

Figure 614-2 Leukocoria. White pupillary reflex in a child with retinoblastoma.

LEUKOCORIA

Leukocoria includes any white pupillary reflex, also called cat eye reflex. Primary diagnostic considerations in any child with leukocoria are cataract, persistent hyperplastic primary vitreous, cicatricial retinopathy of prematurity, retinal detachment and retinoschisis, larval granulomatosis, and retinoblastoma (Fig. 614-2). Also to be considered are endophthalmitis, organized vitreous hemorrhage, leukemic ophthalmopathy, exudative retinopathy (as in Coats disease), and less-common conditions such as medulloepithelioma, massive retinal gliosis, the retinal pseudotumor of Norrie disease, the pseudoglioma of the Bloch-Sulzberger syndrome, retinal dysplasia, and the retinal lesions of the phakomatoses. A white reflex might also be seen with fundus coloboma, large atrophic chorioretinal scars, and ectopic medullation of retinal nerve fibers. Leukocoria is an indication for prompt and thorough evaluation.

The diagnosis can often be made by direct examination of the eye by ophthalmoscopy and biomicroscopy. Ultrasonographic and radiologic examinations are often helpful. In some cases, the final diagnosis rests with a pathologist.

BIBLIOGRAPHY

Please visit the Nelson Textbook of Pediatrics *website at www.expertconsult.com for the complete bibliography.*

Chapter 615
Disorders of Eye Movement and Alignment

Scott E. Olitsky, Denise Hug, Laura S. Plummer, and Merrill Stass-Isern

STRABISMUS

Strabismus, or misalignment of the eyes, is one of the most common eye problems encountered in children, affecting approximately 4% of children <6 yr of age. Strabismus can result in vision loss (amblyopia) and can have significant psychologic effects. Early detection and treatment of strabismus is essential to prevent permanent visual impairment. Of children with strabismus, 30-50% develop amblyopia. Restoration of proper alignment of the visual axis must occur at an early stage of vision development to allow these children a chance to develop normal binocular vision.

Strabismus means "to squint or to look obliquely." Many terms are used in discussing and characterizing strabismus.

Orthophoria is the ideal condition of exact ocular balance. It implies that the oculomotor apparatus is in perfect equilibrium so that the eyes remain coordinated and aligned in all positions of gaze and at all distances. Even when binocular vision is interrupted, as by occlusion of one eye, truly orthophoric persons maintain perfect alignment. Orthophoria is seldom encountered because most people have a small latent deviation (heterophoria).

Heterophoria is a latent tendency for the eyes to deviate. This latent deviation is normally controlled by fusional mechanisms that provide binocular vision or avoid diplopia (double vision). The eye deviates only under certain conditions, such as fatigue, illness, or stress, or during tests that interfere with maintenance of these normal fusional abilities (such as covering one eye). If the amount of heterophoria is large, it can give rise to bothersome symptoms, such as transient diplopia (double vision), headaches, or asthenopia (eyestrain). Some degree of heterophoria is found in normal persons; it is usually asymptomatic.

Heterotropia is a misalignment of the eyes that is constant. It occurs because of an inability of the fusional mechanism to control the deviation. Tropias can be alternating, involving both eyes, or unilateral. In an alternating tropia, there is no preference for fixation of either eye, and both eyes drift with equal frequency. Because each eye is used periodically, vision usually develops normally. A unilateral tropia is a more serious situation because only one eye is constantly misaligned. The undeviated eye becomes the preferred eye, resulting in loss of vision or amblyopia of the deviated eye.

It is common in ocular misalignments to describe the type of deviation. This helps to make decisions on the cause and treatment of the strabismus. The prefixes *eso-*, *exo-*, *hyper-*, and *hypo-* are added to the terms *-phoria* and *-tropia* to further delineate the type of strabismus. Esophorias and esotropias are inward or convergent deviations of the eyes, commonly known as crossed eyes. Exophorias and exotropias are divergent or outward-facing eye deviations, *walleye* being the lay term. Hyperdeviations and hypodeviations are upward or downward, respectively, deviations of an eye. In cases of unilateral strabismus, the deviating eye is often part of the description of the misalignment (left esotropia).

Diagnosis

Many techniques are used to assess ocular alignment and movement of the eyes to aid in diagnosing strabismic disorders. In a child with strabismus or any other ocular disorder, assessment of visual acuity is mandatory. Decreased vision in one eye requires evaluation for strabismus or other ocular abnormalities, which may be difficult to discern on a brief screening evaluation. Even strabismic deviations of only a few degrees in magnitude, too small to be evident by gross inspection, can lead to amblyopia and devastating vision loss.

Corneal light reflex tests are perhaps the most rapid and easily performed diagnostic tests for strabismus. They are particularly useful in children who are uncooperative and in those who have poor ocular fixation. To perform the **Hirschberg corneal reflex test,** the examiner projects a light source onto the cornea of both eyes simultaneously as a child looks directly at the light. Comparison should then be made of the placement of the corneal light reflex in each eye. In straight eyes, the light reflection appears symmetric and, because of the relationship between the cornea and the macula, slightly nasal to the center of each pupil. If strabismus is present, the reflected light is asymmetric and appears displaced in one eye. The Krimsky method of the corneal reflex test uses prisms placed over one or both eyes to align the light reflections. The amount of prism needed to align the reflections is used to measure the degree of deviation. Although it is a useful screening test, corneal light reflex testing might not detect a small angle or an intermittent strabismus.

Cover tests for strabismus require a child's attention and cooperation, good eye movement capability, and reasonably good vision in each eye. If any of these are lacking, the results of these tests might not be valid. These tests consist of the cover-uncover test and the alternate cover test. In the cover-uncover test, a child looks at an object in the distance, preferably 6 m away. An eye chart is commonly used for fixation in children >3 yr of age. For younger children, a noise-making toy or movie helps hold their attention for the test. As the child looks at the distant object, the examiner covers one eye and watches for movement of the uncovered eye. If no movement occurs, there is no apparent misalignment of that eye. After one eye is tested, the same procedure is repeated on the other eye. When performing the alternate cover test, the examiner rapidly covers and uncovers each eye, shifting back and forth from one eye to another. If the child has an ocular deviation, the eye rapidly moves as the cover is shifted to the other eye. Both the cover-uncover test and the alternate cover test should be performed at both distance and near fixation. The cover-uncover test differentiates tropias, or manifest deviations, from latent deviations, or phorias.

Clinical Manifestations and Treatment

The etiologic classification of strabismus is complex, and the causative types must be distinguished; there are comitant and noncomitant forms of strabismus.

COMITANT STRABISMUS Comitant strabismus is the most common type of strabismus. The individual extraocular muscles usually have no defect. The amount of deviation is constant, or relatively constant, in the various directions of gaze.

Pseudostrabismus (pseudoesotropia) is one of the most common reasons a pediatric ophthalmologist is asked to evaluate an infant. This condition is characterized by the false appearance of strabismus when the visual axes are aligned accurately. This appearance may be caused by a flat, broad nasal bridge, prominent epicanthal folds, or a narrow interpupillary distance. The observer might see less white sclera nasally than would be expected, and the impression is that the eye is turned in toward the nose, especially when the child gazes to either side. Parents often comment that when their child looks to the side, the eye almost disappears from view. Pseudoesotropia can be differentiated from a true misalignment of the eyes when the corneal light reflex is centered in both eyes and when the cover-uncover test shows no refixation movement. Once pseudoesotropia has been confirmed, parents can be reassured that the child will outgrow the appearance of esotropia. As the child grows, the bridge of the nose becomes more prominent and displaces the epicanthal folds, and the medial sclera becomes proportional to the amount visible on the lateral aspect. It is the appearance of crossing that the child will outgrow. Some parents of children with pseudoesotropia erroneously believe that their child has an actual esotropia that will resolve on its own. Because true esotropia can develop later in children with pseudoesotropia, parents and pediatricians should be cautioned that reassessment is required if the apparent deviation does not improve.

Esodeviations are the most common type of ocular misalignment in children and represent >50% of all ocular deviations. *Congenital esotropia* is a confusing term. Few children who have this disorder are actually born with an esotropia. Most reports in the literature have therefore considered infants with confirmed onset earlier than 6 mo as having the same condition, which some observers have designated *infantile esotropia.*

The characteristic angle of congenital esodeviations is large and constant (Fig. 615-1). Because of the large deviation, cross-fixation is often encountered. This is a condition in which the child looks to the right with the left eye and to the left with the right eye. With cross-fixation, there is no need for the eye to turn away from the nose (abduction) because the adducting eye is used in side gaze; this condition simulates a 6th nerve palsy. Abduction can be demonstrated by the doll's head maneuver or by patching 1 eye for a short time. Children with congenital esotropia tend to have refractive errors similar to those of normal children of the same age. This contrasts with the characteristic high level of farsightedness associated with accommodative esotropia. **Amblyopia** is common in children with congenital esotropia.

The primary goal of treatment in congenital esotropia is to eliminate or reduce the deviation as much as possible. Ideally, this results in normal sight in each eye, in straight-looking eyes, and in the development of binocular vision. Early treatment is more likely to lead to the development of binocular vision, which helps to maintain long-term ocular alignment. Once any associated amblyopia is treated, surgery is performed to align the eyes. Even with successful surgical alignment, it is common for vertical deviations to develop in children with a history of congenital esotropia. The two most common forms of vertical deviations to develop are inferior oblique muscle overaction and dissociated vertical deviation. In inferior oblique muscle overaction, the overactive inferior oblique muscle produces an upshoot of the eye closest to the nose when the patient looks to the side (Fig. 615-2). In dissociated vertical deviation, 1 eye drifts up slowly, with no movement of the other eye. Surgery may be necessary to treat either or both of these conditions.

It is important that parents realize that early successful surgical alignment is only the beginning of the treatment process. Because many children redevelop strabismus or amblyopia, they need to be monitored closely during the visually immature period of life.

Accommodative esotropia is defined as a "convergent deviation of the eyes associated with activation of the accommodative (focusing) reflex." It usually occurs in a child who is between 2 and 3 yr of age and who has a history of acquired intermittent or constant crossing. Amblyopia occurs in the majority of cases.

The mechanism of accommodative esotropia involves uncorrected hyperopia, accommodation, and accommodative convergence. The image entering a hyperopic (farsighted) eye is blurred. If the amount of hyperopia is not significant, the blurred image can be sharpened by accommodating (focusing of the lens of the eye). Accommodation is closely linked with convergence (eyes turning inward). If a child's hyperopic refractive error is large or if the amount of convergence that occurs in response to each unit of accommodative effort is great, esotropia can develop.

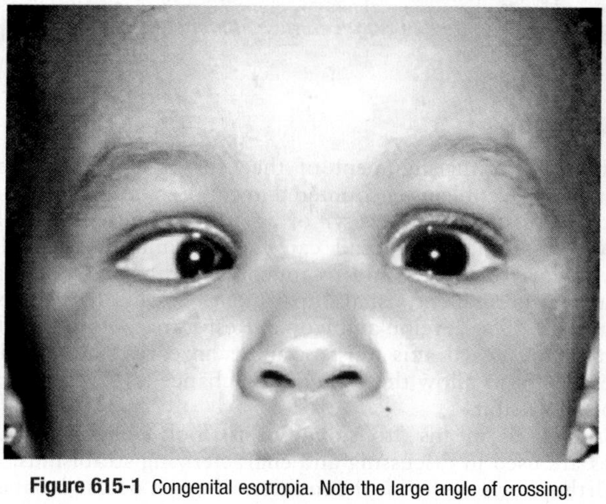

Figure 615-1 Congenital esotropia. Note the large angle of crossing.

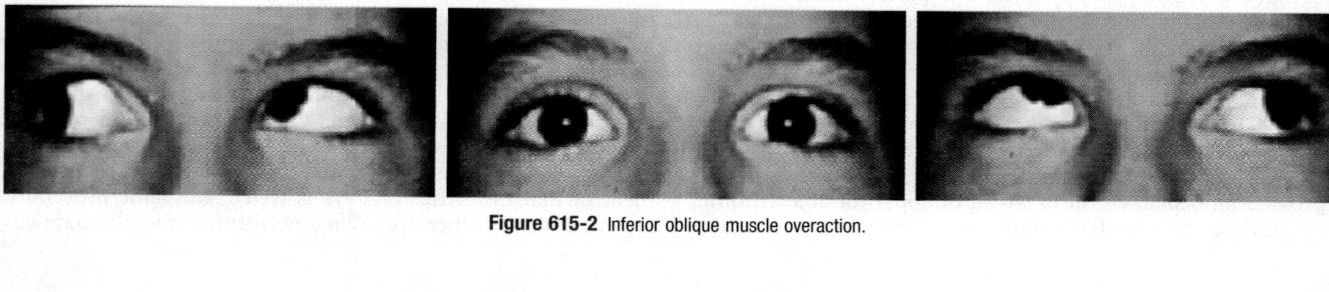

Figure 615-2 Inferior oblique muscle overaction.

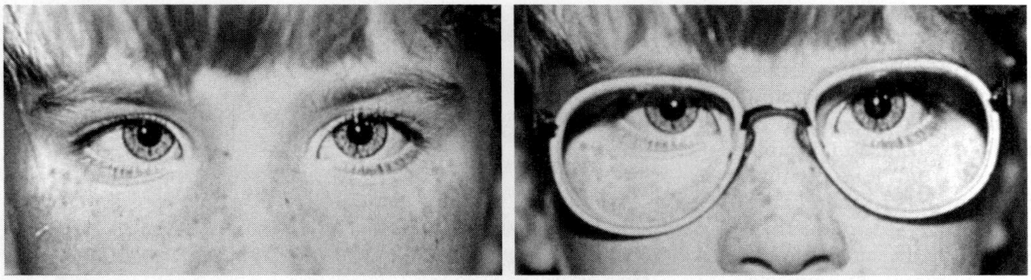

Figure 615-3 Accommodative esotropia; control of deviation with corrective lenses.

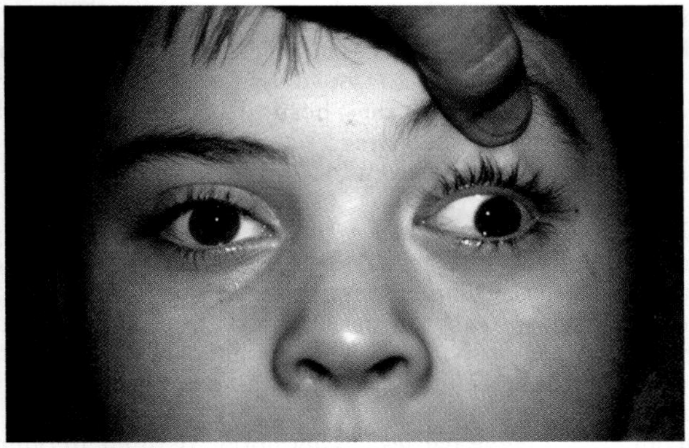

Figure 615-4 Third cranial nerve palsy of the left eye.

To treat accommodative esotropia, the full hyperopic (farsighted) correction is initially prescribed. These glasses eliminate a child's need to accommodate and therefore correct the esotropia (Fig. 615-3). Although many parents are initially concerned that their child will not want to wear glasses, the benefits of binocular vision and the decrease in the focusing effort required to see clearly provide a strong stimulus to wear glasses, and they are generally accepted well. The full hyperopic correction sometimes straightens the eye position at distance fixation but leaves a residual deviation at near fixation; this may be observed or treated with bifocal lenses, antiaccommodative drops, or surgery.

It is important to warn parents of children with accommodative esotropia that the esodeviation might appear to increase without glasses after the initial correction is worn. Parents often state that before wearing glasses, their child had a small esodeviation, whereas after removing the glasses, the esodeviation becomes quite large. Parents often blame the increased esodeviation on the glasses. This apparent increase is due to a child's using the appropriate amount of accommodative effort after the glasses have been worn. When these children remove their glasses, they continue to use an accommodative effort to bring objects into proper focus and increase the esodeviation.

Most children maintain straight eyes once initially treated. Because hyperopia generally decreases with age, many patients outgrow the need to wear glasses to maintain alignment. In some patients, a residual esodeviation persists even when wearing their glasses. This condition commonly occurs when there is a delay between the onset of accommodative esotropia and treatment. In others, the esotropia may initially be eliminated with glasses but crossing redevelops and is not correctable with glasses. The crossing that is no longer correctable with glasses is the deteriorated or nonaccommodative portion. Surgery for this portion of the crossing may be indicated to restore binocular vision.

Exodeviations are the second most common type of misalignment. The divergent deviation may be intermittent or constant. Intermittent exotropia is the most common exodeviation in childhood. It is characterized by outward drifting of one eye, which usually occurs when a child is fixating at distance. The deviation is generally more common with fatigue or illness. Exposure to bright light can cause reflex closure of the exotropic eye. Because the eyes initially can be kept straight most of the time, visual acuity tends to be good in both eyes and binocular vision is initially normal.

The age at onset of intermittent exotropia varies but is often between ages 6 mo and 4 yr. The decision to perform eye muscle surgery is based on the amount and frequency of the deviation. If the deviation is small and infrequent, it is reasonable to observe the child. If the exotropia is large or increasing in frequency, surgery is indicated to maintain normal binocular vision.

Constant exotropia may rarely be congenital. Congenital exotropia may be associated with neurologic disease or abnormalities of the bony orbit, as in Crouzon syndrome. Exotropia that occurs later in life might represent a deterioration of an intermittent exotropia that was present in childhood. Surgery can restore binocular vision even in long-standing cases.

NONCOMITANT STRABISMUS When an eye muscle is paretic, palsied, or restricted, a muscle imbalance occurs in which the deviation of the eye varies according to the direction of gaze. Recent onset of paresis can be suggested by the symptom of double vision that increases in one direction, the findings of an ocular deviation that increases in the field of action of the paretic muscle, and an increase in the deviation when the child fixates with the paretic eye. It is important to differentiate a noncomitant strabismus from a comitant deviation because noncomitant forms of strabismus are often associated with trauma, systemic disorders, or neurologic abnormalities.

THIRD NERVE PALSY In the pediatric population, 3rd nerve palsies are usually congenital. The congenital form is often associated with a developmental anomaly or birth trauma. Acquired 3rd nerve palsies in children can be an ominous sign and can indicate a neurologic abnormality such as an intracranial neoplasm or an aneurysm. Other less-serious causes include an inflammatory or infectious lesion, head trauma, postviral syndromes, and migraines.

A 3rd nerve palsy, whether congenital or acquired, usually results in an exotropia and a hypotropia, or downward deviation of the affected eye, as well as complete or partial ptosis of the upper lid (Fig. 615-4). This characteristic strabismus results from the action of the normal, unopposed muscles, the lateral rectus muscle, and the superior oblique muscle. If the internal branch of the 3rd nerve is involved, pupillary dilation may be noted as well. Eye movements are usually limited nasally in elevation and in depression. In addition, clinical findings and treatment may be complicated in congenital and traumatic cases of 3rd nerve palsy owing to misdirection of regenerating nerve fibers, referred to as aberrant regeneration. This results in anomalous and paradoxical eyelid, eye, and pupil movement such as elevation of the eyelid, constriction of the pupil, or depression of the globe on attempted medial gaze.

FOURTH NERVE PALSY Fourth nerve palsies can be congenital or acquired. Because the 4th nerve has a long intracranial course, it is susceptible to damage resulting from head trauma. In children, however, 4th nerve palsies are more commonly congenital than traumatic. A palsied 4th nerve results in weakness in the superior oblique muscle, which causes an upward deviation of the eye, a hypertropia. Because the antagonist muscle, the inferior oblique, is relatively unopposed, the affected eye demonstrates an upshoot when looking toward the nose. Children typically present with a head tilt to the shoulder opposite the affected eye, their chin down, and their face turned away from the affected side. This head position places the eye away from the area of greatest action of the affected muscle and therefore minimizes the deviation and the associated double vision. Long-standing head tilts can lead to facial asymmetry. Because the abnormal head posture maintains the child's ocular alignment, amblyopia is uncommon. Because no abnormality exists in the neck muscles, attempts to correct the head tilt by exercises and neck muscle surgery are ineffective. Recognition of a superior oblique paresis can be difficult because deviation of the head and the eye may be minimal. Eye muscle surgery can be performed to improve the ocular alignment and eliminate the abnormal head posture.

SIXTH NERVE PALSY Sixth nerve palsies produce markedly crossed eyes with limited ability to move the afflicted eye laterally. Children often present with their head turned toward the palsied muscle, a position that helps preserve binocular vision. The esotropia is largest when the eye is moved toward the affected muscle.

Congenital 6th nerve palsies are rare. Decreased lateral gaze in infants is often associated with other disorders, such as congenital esotropia or Duane retraction syndrome (Chapter 585.9). In neonates, a transient 6th nerve paresis can occur; it usually clears spontaneously by 6 wk. It is thought that increased intracranial pressure associated with labor and delivery is the contributing factor.

Acquired 6th nerve palsies in childhood are often an ominous sign because the 6th nerve is susceptible to increased intracranial pressure associated with hydrocephalous and intracranial tumors. Other causes of 6th nerve defects in children include trauma, vascular malformations, meningitis, and Gradenigo syndrome. A benign 6th nerve palsy, which is painless and acquired, can be noted in infants and older children. This is often preceded by a febrile illness or upper respiratory tract infection and may be recurrent. Complete resolution of the palsy is usual. Although not uncommon, other causes of an acute 6th nerve palsy should be eliminated before this diagnosis is made.

Strabismus Syndromes

Special types of strabismus have unusual clinical features. Most of these disorders are caused by structural anomalies of the extraocular muscles or adjacent tissues. Most strabismus syndromes produce noncomitant misalignments.

MONOCULAR ELEVATION DEFICIENCY A monocular elevation deficiency is an inability to elevate the eye in both adduction and abduction. It can represent a paresis of both elevators, the superior rectus and inferior oblique muscles, or a possible restriction to elevation from a fibrotic inferior rectus muscle. When an affected child fixates with the nonparetic eye, the paretic eye is hypotropic and the ipsilateral upper eyelid can appear ptotic. Fixation with the paretic eye causes a hypertropia of the nonparetic eye and a disappearance of the ptosis (Fig. 615-5). Because the apparent ptosis is actually secondary to the strabismus, correction of the hypotropia treats the pseudoptosis.

DUANE SYNDROME Duane syndrome (Chapter 585.9) is a congenital disorder of ocular motility characterized by retraction of the globe on adduction. This is attributed to the absence of the 6th nerve nucleus and anomalous innervation of the lateral rectus muscle, which results in co-contraction of the medial and lateral rectus muscles on attempted adduction of the affected eye. Within the spectrum of Duane syndrome, patients can exhibit impairment of abduction, impairment of adduction, or upshoot or downshoot of the involved eye on adduction. They can have esotropia, exotropia, or relatively straight eyes. Many exhibit a compensatory head posture to maintain single vision. Some develop amblyopia. Surgery to improve alignment or to reduce a noticeable face turn can be helpful in selected cases.

Duane syndrome usually occurs sporadically. It is sometimes inherited as an autosomal dominant trait. It usually occurs as an isolated condition but can occur in association with various other ocular and systemic anomalies.

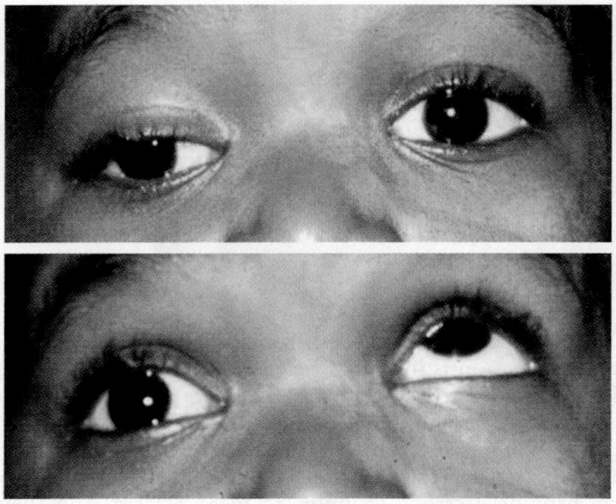

Figure 615-5 Double elevator palsy of the right eye. Note the disappearance of the apparent ptosis when fixating with the involved eye.

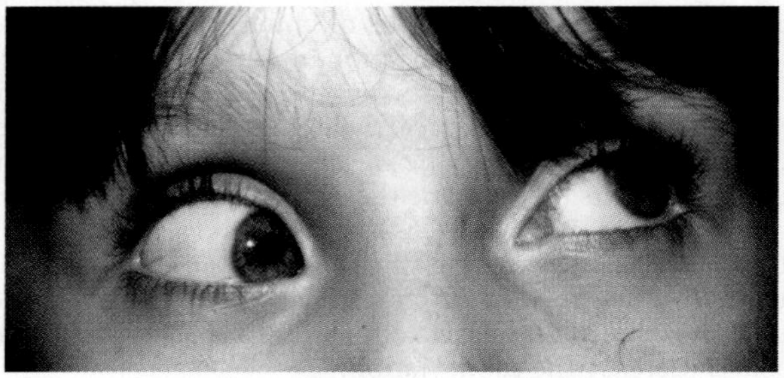

Figure 615-6 Brown syndrome of the right eye.

MÖBIUS SYNDROME The distinctive features of Möbius syndrome (Chapter 585.9) are congenital facial paresis and abduction weakness. The facial palsy is commonly bilateral, often asymmetric, and often incomplete, tending to spare the lower face and platysma. Ectropion, epiphora, and exposure keratopathy can develop. The abduction defect may be unilateral or bilateral. Esotropia is common. The cause is unknown. Whether the primary defect is maldevelopment of cranial nerve nuclei, hypoplasia of the muscles, or a combination of central and peripheral factors is unclear. Some familial cases have been reported. Associated developmental defects include ptosis, palatal and lingual palsy, hearing loss, pectoral and lingual muscle defects, micrognathia, syndactyly, supernumerary digits, and the absence of hands, feet, fingers, or toes. Surgical correction of the esotropia is indicated, and any attendant amblyopia should be treated.

BROWN SYNDROME In Brown syndrome, elevation of the eye in the adducted position is restricted (Fig. 615-6). An associated downward deviation of the affected eye in adduction can also occur. A compensatory head posture may be evident.

Various causes have been described. Some cases have been attributed to structural abnormalities such as a tight superior oblique tendon, congenital shortening or thickening of the superior oblique tendon sheath, or connective tissue trabeculae between the superior oblique tendon and the trochlea. Acquired Brown syndrome can follow trauma to the orbit involving the region of the trochlea or sinus surgery. It can also occur with inflammatory processes, particularly sinusitis and juvenile rheumatoid arthritis.

Acquired inflammatory Brown syndrome might respond to treatment with either nonsteroidal medications or corticosteroids. Surgery may be helpful for children with true congenital Brown syndrome.

PARINAUD SYNDROME Parinaud syndrome is a palsy of vertical gaze, isolated or associated with pupillary or nuclear oculomotor (3rd cranial nerve) paresis. It indicates a lesion affecting the mesencephalic tegmentum. The ophthalmic signs of midbrain disease include vertical gaze palsy, dissociation of the pupillary responses to light and to near focus, general pupillomotor paralysis, corectopia, dyscoria, accommodative disturbances, pathologic lid retraction, ptosis, extraocular muscle paresis, and convergence paralysis. Some patients have associated spasms of convergence, convergent retraction nystagmus, and vertical nystagmus, particularly on attempted vertical gaze. Combinations of these signs are referred to as the *sylvian aqueduct syndrome.*

A principal cause of vertical gaze palsy and associated mesencephalic signs in children is tumor of the pineal gland or 3rd ventricle. Differential diagnosis includes trauma and demyelinating disease. In children with hydrocephalus, impairment of vertical gaze and pathologic lid retraction are referred to as the *setting-sun sign.* A transient supranuclear disorder of gaze is sometimes seen in healthy neonates.

CONGENITAL OCULAR MOTOR APRAXIA

Congenital ocular motor apraxia is a congenital disorder of conjugate gaze characterized by a defect in voluntary horizontal gaze, compensatory jerking movement of the head, and retention of slow pursuit and reflexive eye movements (Chapter 590.1). Additional features are absence of the fast (refixation) phase of optokinetic nystagmus and obligate contraversive deviation of the eyes on rotation of the body. Affected children typically are unable to look quickly to either side voluntarily in response to a command or in response to an eccentrically presented object but may be able to follow a slowly moving target to either side. To compensate for the defect in purposive lateral eye movements, children jerk their head to bring the eyes into the desired position and might also blink repetitively in an attempt to change fixation. The signs tend to become less conspicuous with age.

The pathogenesis of congenital ocular motor apraxia is unknown. It may be a result of delayed myelination of the ocular motor pathways. Structural abnormalities of the central nervous system have been found in a few patients, including agenesis of the corpus callosum and cerebellar vermis, porencephaly, hamartoma of the foramen of Monro, and macrocephaly. Many children with congenital ocular motor apraxia show delayed motor and cognitive development.

NYSTAGMUS

Nystagmus (rhythmic oscillations of one or both eyes) may be caused by an abnormality in any one of the three basic mechanisms that regulate position and movement of the eyes: the fixation, conjugate gaze, or vestibular mechanisms. In addition, physiologic nystagmus may be elicited by appropriate stimuli (Table 615-1 and Chapter 590.1).

Congenital sensory nystagmus is generally associated with ocular abnormalities that lead to decreased visual acuity; common disorders that lead to early-onset nystagmus include albinism, aniridia, achromatopsia, congenital cataracts, congenital macular lesions, and congenital optic atrophy. In some instances, nystagmus occurs as a dominant or X-linked characteristic without obvious ocular abnormalities.

Congenital idiopathic motor nystagmus is characterized by horizontal jerky oscillations with gaze preponderance; the nystagmus is coarser in one direction of gaze than in the other, with the jerk toward the direction of gaze. There are no ocular anatomic defects that cause the nystagmus, and the visual acuity is generally near normal. There may be a null point in which the nystagmus lessens and the vision improves; a compensatory head posture develops that places the eyes into the position of least nystagmus. The cause of congenital idiopathic motor nystagmus is unknown; in some instances, it is familial. Eye muscle surgery may be performed to eliminate an abnormal head posture by bringing the point of best vision into straight-ahead gaze. Recent evidence also suggests that surgery might help to improve the quality of vision in these patients.

Acquired nystagmus requires prompt and thorough evaluation. Worrisome pathologic types are the gaze-paretic or gaze-evoked oscillations of cerebellar, brainstem, or cerebral disease.

Nystagmus retractorius or **convergent nystagmus** is repetitive jerking of the eyes into the orbit or toward each other. It is usually seen with vertical gaze palsy as a feature of Parinaud (sylvian aqueduct) syndrome. The causal condition may be neoplastic, vascular, or inflammatory. In children, nystagmus retractorius suggests particularly the presence of pinealoma or hydrocephalus.

A diagnostic approach to nystagmus is noted in Figure 615-7.

Spasmus nutans is a special type of acquired nystagmus in childhood (Table 590-6). In its complete form, it is characterized by the **triad** of pendular nystagmus, head nodding, and torticollis. The nystagmus is characteristically very fine, very rapid, horizontal, and pendular; it is often asymmetric, sometimes unilateral. Signs usually develop within the 1st yr or 2 of life. Components

Table 615-1 SPECIFIC PATTERNS OF NYSTAGMUS

PATTERN	DESCRIPTION	ASSOCIATED CONDITIONS
Latent nystagmus	Conjugate jerk nystagmus toward viewing eye	Congenital vision defects, occurs with occlusion of eye
Manifest latent nystagmus	Fast jerk to viewing eye	Strabismus, congenital idiopathic nystagmus
Periodic alternating	Cycles of horizontal or horizontal-rotary that change direction	Caused by both visual and neurologic conditions
See-saw nystagmus	One eye rises and intorts as the other eye falls and extorts	Usually associated with optic chiasm defects
Nystagmus retractorius	Eyes jerk back into orbit or toward each other	Caused by pressure on mesencephalic tegmentum (Parinaud syndrome)
Gaze-evoked nystagmus	Jerk nystagmus in direction of gaze	Caused by medications, brainstem lesion, or labyrinthine dysfunction
Gaze-paretic nystagmus	Eyes jerk back to maintain eccentric gaze	Cerebellar disease
Downbeat nystagmus	Fast phase beating downward	Posterior fossa disease, drugs
Upbeat nystagmus	Fast phase beating upward	Brainstem and cerebellar disease; some visual conditions
Vestibular nystagmus	Horizontal-torsional or horizontal jerks	Vestibular system dysfunction
Asymmetric or monocular nystagmus	Pendular vertical nystagmus	Disease of retina and visual pathways
Spasmus nutans	Fine, rapid, pendular nystagmus	Torticollis, head nodding; idiopathic or gliomas of visual pathways

From Kliegman R: *Practical strategies in pediatric diagnosis and therapy,* Philadelphia, 1996, WB Saunders.

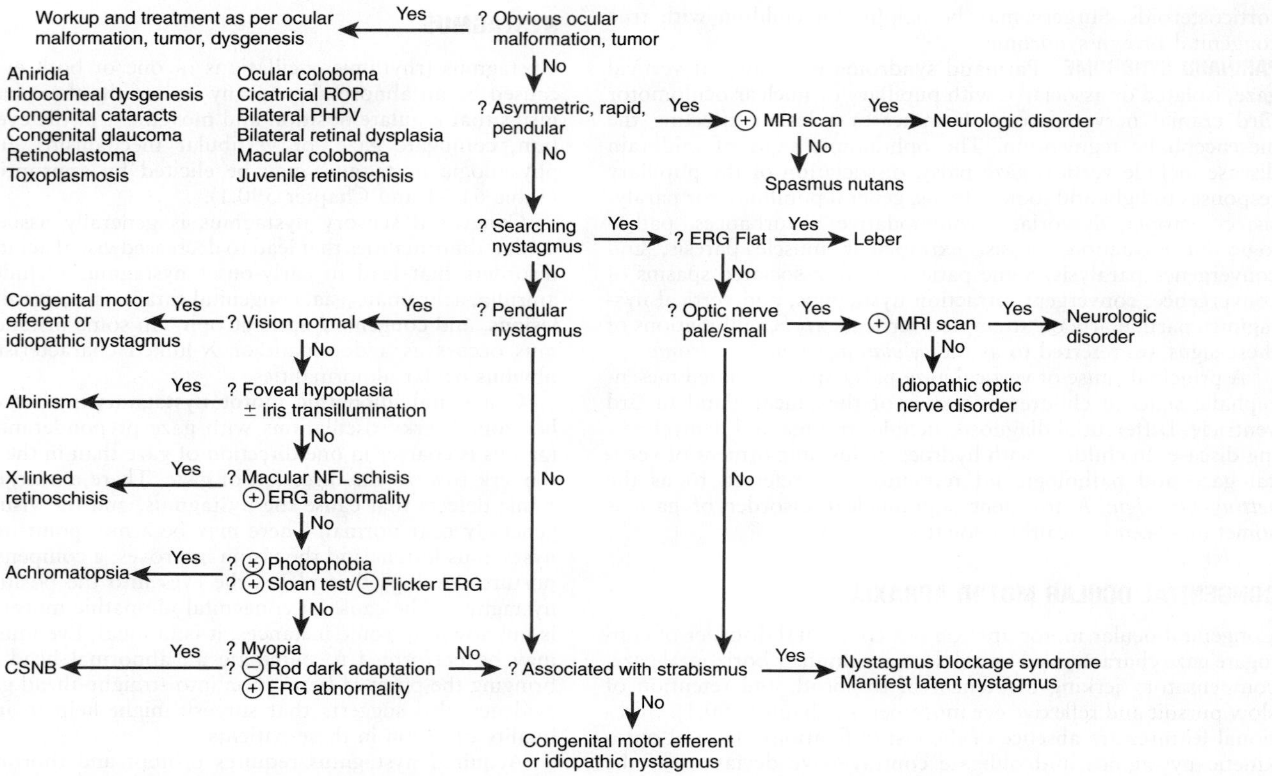

Figure 615-7 Algorithm for the work-up of an infant with nystagmus. ⊕, positive; ⊖, negative; CNNB, congenital stationary night blindness; ERG, electroretinogram; NFL, nerve fiber layer; PHPV, persistent hyperplastic primary vitreous; ROP, retinopathy of prematurity. (From Nelson LB: *Harley's pediatric ophthalmology,* ed 4, Philadelphia, 1998, WB Saunders, p 470.)

Table 615-2 SPECIFIC PATTERNS OF NON-NYSTAGMUS EYE MOVEMENTS

PATTERN	DESCRIPTION	ASSOCIATED CONDITIONS
Opsoclonus	Multidirectional conjugate movements of varying rate and amplitude	Hydrocephalus, diseases of brainstem and cerebellum, neuroblastoma
Ocular dysmetria	Overshoot of eyes on rapid fixation	Cerebellar dysfunction
Ocular flutter	Horizontal oscillations with forward gaze and sometimes with blinking	Cerebellar disease, hydrocephalus, or central nervous system neoplasm
Ocular bobbing	Downward jerk from primary gaze, remain for a few seconds, then drift back	Pontine disease
Ocular myoclonus	Rhythmic to-and-fro pendular oscillations of the eyes, with synchronous nonocular muscle movement	Damage to red nucleus, inferior olivary nucleus, and ipsilateral dentate nucleus

From Kliegman R: *Practical strategies in pediatric diagnosis and therapy,* Philadelphia, 1996, WB Saunders.

of the triad can develop at various times. In many cases, the condition is benign and self-limited, usually lasting a few months, sometimes years. The cause of this classic type of spasmus nutans, which usually resolves spontaneously, is unknown. Some children exhibiting signs resembling those of spasmus nutans have underlying brain tumors, particularly hypothalamic and chiasmal optic gliomas. Appropriate neurologic and neuroradiologic evaluation and careful monitoring of infants and children with nystagmus are therefore recommended.

OTHER ABNORMAL EYE MOVEMENTS

To be differentiated from true nystagmus are certain special types of abnormal eye movements, particularly opsoclonus, ocular dysmetria, and flutter (Table 615-2 and Chapter 590.1).

Opsoclonus

Opsoclonus and ataxic conjugate movements are spontaneous, nonrhythmic, multidirectional, chaotic movements of the eyes. The eyes appear to be in agitation, with bursts of conjugate movement of varying amplitude in varying directions. Opsoclonus is most often associated with encephalitis. It may be the first sign of neuroblastoma (Chapter 492).

Ocular Motor Dysmetria

Ocular motor dysmetria is analogous to dysmetria of the limbs. Affected persons show a lack of precision in performing movements of refixation, characterized by an overshoot (or undershoot) of the eyes with several corrective to-and-fro oscillations on looking from one point to another. Ocular motor dysmetria is a sign of cerebellar or cerebellar pathway disease.

Flutter-like Oscillations

Flutter-like oscillations are intermittent to-and-fro horizontal oscillations of the eyes that can occur spontaneously or on change of fixation. They are characteristic of cerebellar disease.

BIBLIOGRAPHY

Please visit the Nelson Textbook of Pediatrics *website at www.expertconsult.com for the complete bibliography.*

Chapter 616
Abnormalities of the Lids

Scott E. Olitsky, Denise Hug, Laura S. Plummer, and Merrill Stass-Isern

PTOSIS

In blepharoptosis, the upper eyelid droops below its normal level. Congenital ptosis is usually a result of a localized dystrophy of the levator muscle in which the striated muscle fibers are replaced with fibrous tissue. The condition may be unilateral or bilateral and can be transmitted as a dominant trait.

Parents often comment that the eye looks smaller because of the drooping eyelid. The lid crease is decreased or absent where the levator muscle would normally insert below the skin surface. Because the levator is replaced by fibrous tissue, the lid does not move downward fully in downgaze (lid lag). If the ptosis is severe, affected children often attempt to raise the lid by lifting their brow or adapting a chin-up head posture to maintain binocular vision. **Marcus Gunn jaw-winking ptosis** accounts for 5% of ptosis in children. In this syndrome, an abnormal synkinesis exists between the 5th and 3rd cranial nerves; this causes the eyelid to elevate with movement of the jaw. The wink is produced by chewing or sucking and may be more noticeable than the ptosis itself.

Although ptosis in children is often an isolated finding, it may occur in association with other ocular or systemic disorders. Systemic disorders include myasthenia gravis, muscular dystrophy, and botulism. Ocular disorders include mechanical ptosis secondary to lid tumors, blepharophimosis syndrome, congenital fibrosis syndrome, combined levator/superior rectus maldevelopment, and congenital or acquired 3rd nerve palsy. A small degree of ptosis is seen in Horner syndrome (Chapter 614). A complete ophthalmic and systemic examination is therefore important in the evaluation of a child with ptosis.

Amblyopia may occur in children with ptosis. The amblyopia may be secondary to the lid's covering the visual axis (deprivation) or induced astigmatism (anisometropia). When amblyopia occurs, it should generally be treated before treating the ptosis.

Treatment of ptosis in a child is indicated for elimination of an abnormal head posture, improvement in the visual field, prevention of amblyopia, and restoration of a normal eyelid appearance. The timing of surgery depends on the degree of ptosis, its cosmetic and functional severity, the presence or absence of compensatory posturing, the wishes of the parents, and the discretion of the surgeon. Surgical treatment is determined by the amount of levator function that is present. A levator resection may be used in children with moderate to good function. In patients with poor or absent function, a frontalis suspension procedure may be necessary. This technique requires that a suspension material be placed between the frontalis muscle and the tarsus of the eyelid. It allows patients to use their brow and frontalis muscle more effectively to raise their eyelid. Amblyopia remains a concern even after surgical correction and should be monitored closely.

EPICANTHAL FOLDS

These vertical or oblique folds of skin extend on either side of the bridge of the nose from the brow or lid area, covering the inner canthal region. They are present to some degree in most young children and become less apparent with age. The folds may be sufficiently broad to cover the medial aspect of the eye, making the eyes appear crossed (pseudoesotropia). Epicanthal folds are a common feature of many syndromes, including chromosomal aberrations (trisomies) and disorders of single genes.

LAGOPHTHALMOS

This is a condition in which complete closure of the lids over the globe is difficult or impossible. It may be paralytic because of a facial palsy involving the orbicularis muscle, or spastic, as in thyrotoxicosis. It may be structural when retraction or shortening of the lids results from scarring or atrophy consequent to injury (burns) or disease. For example, children with various craniosynostosis syndromes can have problematic lagophthalmos. Infants with collodion membrane may have temporary lagophthalmos caused by the restrictive effect of the membrane on the lids. Lagophthalmos may accompany proptosis or buphthalmos (enlarged cornea due to elevated intraocular pressure) when the lids, although normal, cannot effectively cover the enlarged or protuberant eye. A degree of physiologic lagophthalmos may occur normally during sleep, but functional lagophthalmos in an unconscious or debilitated patient can be a problem.

In patients with lagophthalmos, exposure of the eye may lead to drying, infection, corneal ulceration, or perforation of the cornea; the result may be loss of vision, even loss of the eye. In lagophthalmos, protection of the eye by artificial tear preparations, ophthalmic ointment, or moisture chambers is essential. Gauze pads are to be avoided because the gauze may abrade the cornea. In some cases, surgical closure of the lids (tarsorrhaphy) may be necessary for long-term protection of the eye.

LID RETRACTIONS

Pathologic retraction of the lid may be myogenic or neurogenic. Myogenic retraction of the upper lid occurs in thyrotoxicosis, in which it is associated with 3 classic signs: a staring appearance (Dalrymple sign), infrequent blinking (Stellwag sign), and lag of the upper lid on downward gaze (von Graefe sign).

Neurogenic retraction of the lids may occur in conditions affecting the anterior mesencephalon. Lid retraction is a feature of the syndrome of the sylvian aqueduct. In children, it is commonly a sign of hydrocephalus. It may occur with meningitis. Paradoxical retraction of the lid is seen in the Marcus Gunn jaw-winking syndrome. It may also be seen with attempted eye movement after recovery from a 3rd nerve palsy, if aberrant regeneration of the oculomotor nerve fibers has occurred.

Simple staring and the physiologic or reflexive lid retraction ("eye popping"), in contrast to pathologic lid retractions, occur in infants in response to a sudden reduction in illumination or as a startle reaction.

ECTROPION, ENTROPION, AND EPIBLEPHARON

Ectropion is eversion of the lid margin; it may lead to overflow of tears (epiphora) and subsequent maceration of the skin of the lid, inflammation of exposed conjunctiva, or superficial exposure keratopathy. Common causes are scarring consequent to inflammation, burns, or trauma, or weakness of the orbicularis muscle as a result of facial palsy; these forms may be corrected surgically. Protection of the cornea is essential. Ectropion is also seen in certain children who have faulty development of the lateral canthal ligament; this may occur in Down syndrome.

Entropion is inversion of the lid margin, which may cause discomfort and corneal damage because of the inward turning of the lashes (trichiasis). A principal cause is scarring secondary to inflammation such as occurs in trachoma or as a sequela of Stevens-Johnson syndrome. There is also a rare congenital form. Surgical correction is effective in many cases.

Epiblepharon is commonly seen in childhood and may be confused with entropion. In epiblepharon, a roll of skin beneath the lower eyelid lashes causes the lashes to be directed vertically and to touch the cornea (Fig. 616-1). Unlike entropion, the eyelid margin itself is not rotated toward the cornea. Epiblepharon

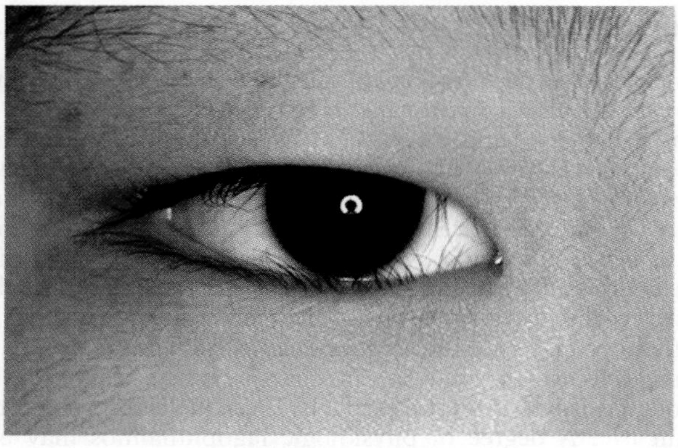

Figure 616-1 Epiblepharon.

usually resolves spontaneously. If corneal scarring begins to occur, surgical correction may be necessary.

BLEPHAROSPASM

This spastic or repetitive closure of the lids may be caused by irritative disease of the cornea, conjunctiva, or facial nerve; fatigue or uncorrected refractive error; or common tic. Thorough ophthalmic examination for pathologic causes, such as trichiasis, keratitis, conjunctivitis, or foreign body, is indicated. Local injection of botulinum toxin may give relief but frequently must be repeated.

BLEPHARITIS

This inflammation of the lid margins is characterized by erythema and crusting or scaling; the usual symptoms are irritation, burning, and itching. The condition is commonly bilateral and chronic or recurrent. The two main types are **staphylococcal** and **seborrheic.** In staphylococcal blepharitis, ulceration of the lid margin is common, the lashes tend to fall out, and conjunctivitis and superficial keratitis are often associated. In seborrheic blepharitis, the scales tend to be greasy, the lid margins are less red, and ulceration usually does not occur. The blepharitis is often of mixed type.

Thorough daily cleansing of the lid margins with a cloth or moistened cotton applicator to remove scales and crusts is important in the **treatment** of both forms. Staphylococcal blepharitis is treated with an antistaphylococcal antibiotic applied directly to the lid margins. When a child also has seborrhea, concurrent treatment of the scalp is important.

Pediculosis of the eyelashes may produce a clinical picture of blepharitis. The lice can be smothered with ophthalmic-grade petrolatum ointment applied to the lid margin and lashes. Nits should be mechanically removed from the lashes. It should be remembered that pediculosis represents a sexually transmitted disease.

HORDEOLUM

Infection of the glands of the lid may be acute or subacute; tender focal swelling and redness are noted. The usual agent is *Staphylococcus aureus.* When the meibomian glands are involved, the lesion is referred to as an internal hordeolum; the abscess tends to be large and may point through either the skin or the conjunctival surface. When the infection involves the glands of Zeis or Moll, the abscess tends to be smaller and more superficial and points at the lid margin; it is then referred to as an external hordeolum or stye.

Treatment is frequent warm compresses and, if necessary, surgical incision and drainage. In addition, topical antibiotic preparations are often used. Untreated, the infection may progress to cellulitis of the lid or orbit, requiring the use of systemic antibiotics.

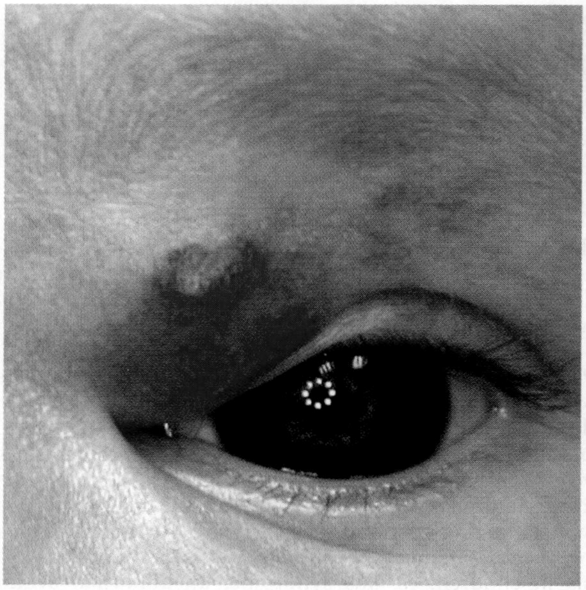

Figure 616-2 Capillary hemangioma of the eyelid. (Courtesy of Amy Nopper, MD, and Brandon Newell, MD.)

CHALAZION

A chalazion is a granulomatous inflammation of a meibomian gland characterized by a firm, nontender nodule in the upper or lower lid. This lesion tends to be chronic and differs from internal hordeolum in the absence of acute inflammatory signs. Although many chalazia subside spontaneously, excision may be necessary if they become large enough to distort vision (by inducing astigmatism by exerting pressure on the globe) or to be a cosmetic blemish. Patients who experience frequent chalazia formation, or those who have significant corneal changes secondary to the underlying blepharitis, may benefit from systemic, low dose erythromycin or azithromycin treatment.

COLOBOMA OF THE EYELID

This cleftlike deformity may vary from a small indentation or notch of the free margin of the lid to a large defect involving almost the entire lid. If the gap is extensive, ulceration and corneal opacities may result from exposure. Early surgical correction of the lid defect is recommended. Other deformities frequently associated with lid colobomas include dermoid cysts or dermolipomas on the globe; they often occur in a position corresponding to the site of the lid defect. Lid colobomas may also be associated with extensive facial malformation, as in mandibulofacial dysostosis (Franceschetti or Treacher Collins syndrome).

TUMORS OF THE LID

A number of lid tumors arise from surface structures (the epithelium and sebaceous glands). Nevi may appear in early childhood; most are junctional. Compound nevi tend to develop in the prepubertal years and dermal nevi at puberty. Malignant epithelial tumors (basal cell carcinoma, squamous cell carcinoma) are rare in children, but the basal cell nevus syndrome and the malignant lesions of xeroderma pigmentosum and of Rothmund-Thomson syndrome may develop in childhood.

Other lid tumors arise from deeper structures (the neural, vascular, and connective tissues). Capillary hemangiomas are especially common in children (Fig. 616-2). Many tend to regress spontaneously, although they may show alarmingly rapid growth in infancy. In many cases, the best management of such hemangiomas is patient observation, allowing spontaneous regression to occur (Chapter 642). In the case of a rapidly expanding lesion, which may cause amblyopia by obstructing the visual axis or inducing astigmatism, corticosteroid, interferon, or surgical treatment should be considered. Recently, systemic propranalol has shown benefit as well. Nevus flammeus (port-wine stain), a noninvoluting hemangioma, occurs as an isolated lesion or in association with other signs of Sturge-Weber syndrome. Affected patients should be monitored for the development of glaucoma. Lymphangiomas of the lid appear as firm masses at or soon after birth and tend to enlarge slowly during the growing years. Associated conjunctival involvement, appearing as a clear, cystic, sinuous conjunctival mass, may provide a clue to the diagnosis. In some cases, there is also orbital involvement. The **treatment** is surgical excision.

Plexiform neuromas of the lids occur in children with neurofibromatosis, often with ptosis as the first sign. The lid may take on an S-shaped configuration. The lids may also be involved by other tumors, such as retinoblastoma, neuroblastoma, and rhabdomyosarcoma of the orbit; these conditions are discussed elsewhere.

BIBLIOGRAPHY

Please visit the Nelson Textbook of Pediatrics *website at* *www.expertconsult.com* *for the complete bibliography.*

Chapter 617
Disorders of the Lacrimal System

Scott E. Olitsky, Denise Hug, Laura S. Plummer, and Merrill Stass-Isern

THE TEAR FILM

This film, which bathes the eye, is actually a complex structure composed of 3 layers. The innermost mucin layer is secreted by the goblet and epithelial cells of the conjunctiva and the acinar cells of the lacrimal gland. It adds stability and provides an attachment for the tear film to the conjunctiva and cornea. The middle aqueous layer constitutes 98% of the tear film and is produced by the main lacrimal gland and accessory lacrimal glands. It contains various electrolytes and proteins as well as antibodies. The outermost lipid layer is produced largely from the sebaceous meibomian glands of the eyelid and retards evaporation of the tear film. Tears drain medially into the punctal openings of the lid margin and flow through the canaliculi into the lacrimal sac and then through the nasolacrimal duct into the nose. Preterm infants have reduced tear secretion. This may mask the diagnosis of a nasolacrimal duct obstruction and concentrate topically applied medications. Tear production reaches adult levels near term.

DACRYOSTENOSIS

Congenital nasolacrimal duct obstruction (CNLDO), or dacryostenosis, is the most common disorder of the lacrimal system, occurring in up to 6% of newborn infants. It is usually caused by a failure of canalization of the epithelial cells that form the nasolacrimal duct as it enters the nose (valve of Hasner). Signs of CNLDO may be present at the time of birth, although the condition may not become evident until normal tear production develops. Signs of CNLDO include an excessive tear lake, overflow of tears onto the lid and cheek, and reflux of mucoid material that is produced in the lacrimal sac. Erythema or maceration of the skin may result from irritation and rubbing produced by dripping of tears and discharge. If the blockage is complete, these signs may be severe and continuous. If obstruction is only partial, the nasolacrimal duct may be capable of draining the basal tear film that is produced. However, under periods of increased tear production (exposure to cold, wind, sunlight) or increased closure of the distal end of the nasolacrimal duct (nasal mucosal edema), tear overflow may become evident or may increase.

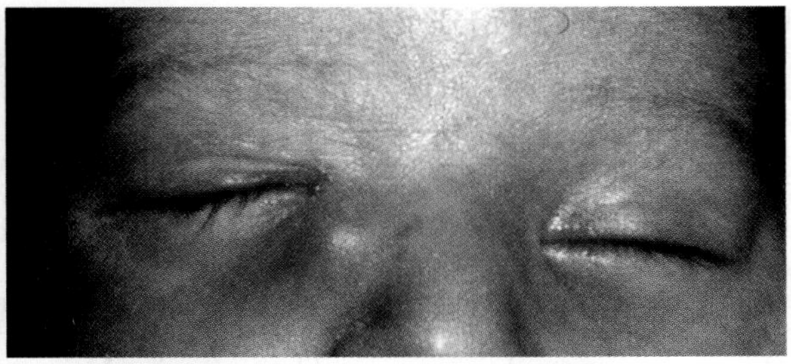

Figure 617-1 Dacryocystocele below inner canthus of the right eye.

Infants with CNLDO may develop acute infection and inflammation of the nasolacrimal sac (**dacryocystitis**), inflammation of the surrounding tissues (**pericystitis**), or rarely periorbital cellulitis. With dacryocystitis, the sac area is swollen, red, and tender, and patients may have systemic signs of infection such as fever and irritability.

The primary **treatment** of uncomplicated nasolacrimal duct obstruction is a regimen of nasolacrimal massage, usually 2-3 times daily, accompanied by cleansing of the lids with warm water. Topical antibiotics are used for control of mucopurulent drainage. A bland ophthalmic ointment may be used on eyelids if the skin is macerated. Most cases of CNLDO resolve spontaneously; 96% before 1 yr of age. For cases that do not resolve by 1 yr, the nasolacrimal duct may be probed, with a cure rate of approximately 80%. Some ophthalmologists intubate the nasolacrimal system at the same time because this has been shown to improve the outcome of the procedure.

Acute dacryocystitis or cellulitis requires prompt treatment with systemic antibiotics. In such cases, some form of definitive surgical intervention is usually indicated.

A **dacryocystocele** (mucocele) is an unusual presentation of a nonpatent nasolacrimal sac that is obstructed both proximally and distally. Dacryocystoceles can be seen at birth or shortly after birth as a bluish subcutaneous mass just below the medial canthal tendon (Fig. 617-1). Initial treatment of dacryocystocele is usually conservative, involving massage/digital decompression of the lacrimal sac. If resolution of the dacryocystocele is not achieved with conservative management, the surgical probing may be beneficial. At times, the intranasal portion of the nasolacrimal duct becomes distended causing respiratory compromise. In a recent study, 9.5% of infants with dacryocystocele had related respiratory compromise. These infants benefit from early probing. Another associated complication of dacryocystocele is that of dacryocystitis/cellulitis. This requires systemic antibiotics, often with hospitalization. In the aforementioned study, 65% of infants with dacryocystocele developed dacryocystitis/cellulitis. Once the cellulitis has improved, the nasolacrimal system should be probed if spontaneous resolution has not occurred.

Not all tearing in infants and children is caused by nasolacrimal obstruction. Tearing may also be a sign of glaucoma, intraocular inflammation, or external irritation, such as that from a corneal abrasion or foreign body.

ALACRIMA AND "DRY EYE"

Alacrima refers to a wide spectrum of disorders with reduced or absent tear secretion. Occasionally, normal basal tearing occurs with an absence of emotional tearing. Etiologies can be divided into syndromes, pathologic association or inherited. Associated syndromes include familial dysautonomia (Riley-Day syndrome), anhidrotic ectodermal dysplasia, triple-A syndrome (Allgrove syndrome). Examples of pathologic association include aplasia of cranial nerve nuclei and lacrimal gland aplasia/hypoplasia. Both autosomal recessive and autosomal dominant inheritance has been reported in isolated congenital alacrima. The patients with alacrima have variable presentation including no symptoms, photophobia, foreign body sensation, eye pain, and decreased vision. The symptoms, if present, often occur early in life. Because the dryness can be severe, damage to the cornea and subsequently loss of vision may occur. The goal of treatment is to minimize corneal irritation, corneal scarring, and loss of vision. Aggressive ocular lubrication is used to prevent these sequelae.

An acquired abnormality of any layer of the tear film may produce a dry eye. Commonly acquired disorders that may lead to a decreased or unstable tear film include Sjögren syndrome, Stevens-Johnson syndrome, vitamin A deficiency, ocular pemphigoid, trachoma, chemical burns, irradiation, and meibomian gland dysfunction. Any tear deficiency can lead to corneal ulceration, scarring, or infection. **Treatment** includes correction of the underlying disorder when possible and frequent instillation of an ocular lubricant. In some cases, occlusion of the lacrimal puncta is helpful. In severe cases, tarsorrhaphy may be necessary to protect the cornea.

BIBLIOGRAPHY

Please visit the Nelson Textbook of Pediatrics *website at* *www.expertconsult.com* *for the complete bibliography.*

Chapter 618
Disorders of the Conjunctiva

Scott E. Olitsky, Denise Hug, Laura S. Plummer, and Merrill Stass-Isern

CONJUNCTIVITIS

The conjunctiva reacts to a wide range of bacterial and viral agents, allergens, irritants, toxins, and systemic diseases. Conjunctivitis is common in childhood and may be infectious or noninfectious. The differential diagnosis of a red-appearing eye includes conjunctival as well as other ocular sites (Table 618-1).

Ophthalmia Neonatorum

This form of conjunctivitis, occurring in infants younger than 4 wk of age, is the most common eye disease of newborns. Its many different causal agents vary greatly in their virulence and outcome. Silver nitrate instillation may result in a mild self-limited chemical conjunctivitis, whereas *Neisseria gonorrhoeae* and *Pseudomonas* are capable of causing corneal perforation, blindness, and death. The risk of conjunctivitis in newborns depends on frequencies of maternal infections, prophylactic measures, circumstances during labor and delivery, and postdelivery exposure to microorganisms.

EPIDEMIOLOGY Conjunctivitis during the neonatal period is usually acquired during vaginal delivery and reflects the sexually transmitted infections prevalent in the community. In 1880, 10% of European children developed gonococcal conjunctivitis at birth. Ophthalmia neonatorum was the leading cause of blindness during that period. The epidemiology of this condition changed dramatically in 1881, when Crede reported that 2% silver nitrate solution instilled in the eyes of newborns reduced the incidence of gonococcal ophthalmia from 10% to 0.3%.

During the 20th century, the incidence of gonococcal ophthalmia neonatorum decreased in industrialized countries secondary to widespread use of silver nitrate prophylaxis and prenatal screening and treatment of maternal gonorrhea. Gonococcal ophthalmia neonatorum has an incidence of 0.3/1,000 live births in the USA. In comparison, *Chlamydia trachomatis* is the most common organism causing ophthalmia neonatorum in the USA, with an incidence of 8.2/1,000 births.

CLINICAL MANIFESTATIONS The clinical manifestations of the various forms of ophthalmia neonatorum are not specific enough to allow an accurate diagnosis. Although the timing and character of the signs are somewhat typical for each cause of this condition, there is considerable overlap and physicians should not rely solely on clinical findings. Regardless of its cause, ophthalmia neonatorum is characterized by redness and chemosis (swelling) of the conjunctiva, edema of the eyelids, and discharge, which may be purulent.

Neonatal conjunctivitis is a potentially blinding condition. The infection may also have associated systemic manifestations that require treatment. Therefore, any newborn infant who develops signs of conjunctivitis needs a prompt and comprehensive systemic and ocular evaluation to determine the agent causing the infection and the appropriate treatment.

The onset of inflammation caused by silver nitrate drops usually occurs within 6-12 hr after birth, with clearing by 24-48 hr. The usual incubation period for conjunctivitis due to *N. gonorrhoeae* is 2-5 days, and for that due to *C. trachomatis*, it is 5-14 days. Gonococcal infection may be present at birth or be delayed beyond 5 days of life owing to partial suppression by ocular prophylaxis. Gonococcal conjunctivitis may also begin in infancy after inoculation by the contaminated fingers of adults. The time of onset of disease with other bacteria is highly variable.

Gonococcal conjunctivitis begins with mild inflammation and a serosanguineous discharge. Within 24 hr, the discharge becomes thick and purulent, and tense edema of the eyelids with marked chemosis occurs. If proper treatment is delayed, the infection may spread to involve the deeper layers of the conjunctivae and the cornea. Complications include corneal ulceration and perforation, iridocyclitis, anterior synechiae, and rarely panophthalmitis. Conjunctivitis caused by *C. trachomatis* (inclusion blennorrhea) may vary from mild inflammation to severe swelling of the eyelids with copious purulent discharge. The process involves mainly the tarsal conjunctivae; the corneas are rarely affected. Conjunctivitis due to *Staphylococcus aureus* or other organisms is similar to that produced by *C. trachomatis*. Conjunctivitis due to *Pseudomonas aeruginosa* is uncommon, acquired in the nursery, and a potentially serious process. It is characterized by the appearance on days 5-18 of edema, erythema of the lids, purulent discharge, pannus formation, endophthalmitis, sepsis, shock, and death.

DIAGNOSIS Conjunctivitis appearing after 48 hr should be evaluated for a possibly infectious cause. Gram stain of the purulent discharge should be performed and the material cultured. If a viral cause is suspected, a swab should be submitted in tissue culture media for virus isolation. In chlamydial conjunctivitis, the diagnosis is made by examining Giemsa-stained epithelial cells scraped from the tarsal conjunctivae for the characteristic intracytoplasmic inclusions, by isolating the organisms from a conjunctival swab using special tissue culture techniques, by immunofluorescent staining of conjunctival scrapings for chlamydial inclusions, or by tests for chlamydial antigen or DNA. The differential diagnosis of ophthalmia neonatorum includes dacryocystitis caused by congenital nasolacrimal duct obstruction with lacrimal sac distention (dacryocystocele).

Treatment

Treatment of infants in whom gonococcal ophthalmia is suspected and the Gram stain shows the characteristic intracellular gram-negative diplococci should be initiated immediately with ceftriaxone, 50 mg/kg/24 hr for 1 dose, not to exceed 125 mg. The eye should also be irrigated initially with saline every 10-30 min, gradually increasing to 2-hr intervals until the purulent discharge has cleared. An alternative regimen includes cefotaxime (100 mg/kg/24 hr given IV or IM every 12 hr for 7 days or 100 mg/kg as a single dose). Treatment is extended if sepsis or other extraocular

Table 618-1 THE RED EYE

CONDITION	ETIOLOGY	SIGNS AND SYMPTOMS	TREATMENT
Bacterial conjunctivitis	*Haemophilus influenzae, Haemophilus aegyptius, Streptococcus pneumoniae*	Mucopurulent unilateral or bilateral discharge, normal vision, photophobia	Topical antibiotics, parenteral ceftriaxone for gonococcus, *H. influenzae*
	Neisseria gonorrhoeae	Conjunctival injection and edema (chemosis); gritty sensation	
Viral conjunctivitis	Adenovirus, ECHO virus, coxsackievirus	As above; may be hemorrhagic, unilateral	Self-limited
Neonatal conjunctivitis	*Chlamydia trachomatis*, gonococcus, chemical (silver nitrate), *Staphylococcus aureus*	Palpebral conjunctival follicle or papillae; as above	Ceftriaxone for gonococcus and erythromycin for *C. trachomatis*
Allergic conjunctivitis	Seasonal pollens or allergen exposure	Itching, incidence of bilateral chemosis (edema) greater than that of erythema, tarsal papillae	Antihistamines, topical mast cell stabilizers or prostaglandin inhibitors, steroids
Keratitis	Herpes simplex virus, adenovirus, *S. pneumoniae, S. aureus, Pseudomonas, Acanthamoeba*, chemicals	Severe pain, corneal swelling, clouding, limbus erythema, hypopyon, cataracts; contact lens history with amebic infection	Specific antibiotics for bacterial/fungal infections; keratoplasty, acyclovir for herpes
Endophthalmitis	*S. aureus, S. pneumoniae, Candida albicans*, associated surgery or trauma	Acute onset, pain, loss of vision, swelling, chemosis, redness; hypopyon and vitreous haze	Antibiotics
Anterior uveitis (iridocyclitis)	JRA, postinfectious with arthritis and rash, sarcoidosis, Behçet disease, Kawasaki disease, inflammatory bowel disease	Unilateral/bilateral; erythema, ciliary flush, irregular pupil, iris adhesions; pain, photophobia, small pupil, poor vision	Topical steroids, plus therapy for primary disease
Posterior uveitis (choroiditis)	Toxoplasmosis, histoplasmosis, *Toxocara canis*	No signs of erythema, decreased vision	Specific therapy for pathogen
Episcleritis/scleritis	Idiopathic autoimmune disease (e.g., SLE, Henoch-Schönlein purpura)	Localized pain, intense erythema, unilateral; blood vessels bigger than in conjunctivitis; scleritis may cause globe perforation	Episcleritis is self-limiting; topical steroids for fast relief
Foreign body	Occupational exposure	Unilateral, gritty feeling; visible or microscopic size	Irrigation, removal; check for ulceration
Blepharitis	*S. aureus, Staphylococcus epidermidis*, seborrheic, blocked lacrimal duct; rarely molluscum contagiosum, *Phthirus pubis, Pediculus capitis*	Bilateral, irritation, itching, hyperemia, crusting, affecting lid margins	Topical antibiotics, warm compresses, lid hygiene
Dacryocystitis	Obstructed lacrimal sac: *S. aureus, H. influenzae*, pneumococcus	Pain, tenderness, erythema and exudates in area of lacrimal sac (inferomedial to inner canthus); tearing (epiphora); possible orbital cellulites	Systemic, topical antibiotics; surgical drainage
Dacryoadenitis	*S. aureus, Streptococcus*, CMV, measles, EBV, enteroviruses; trauma, sarcoidosis, leukemia	Pain, tenderness, edema, erythema over gland area (upper temporal lid); fever, leukocytosis	Systemic antibiotics; drainage of orbital abscesses
Orbital cellulitis (postseptal cellulitis)	Paranasal sinusitis: *H. influenzae, S. aureus, S. pneumoniae*, streptococci Trauma: *S. aureus* Fungi: *Aspergillus, Mucor* spp. if immunodeficient	Rhinorrhea, chemosis, vision loss, painful extraocular motion, proptosis, ophthalmoplegia, fever, lid edema, leukocytosis	Systemic antibiotics, drainage of orbital abscesses
Periorbital cellulitis (preseptal cellulitis)	Trauma: *S. aureus*, streptococci Bacteremia: pneumococcus, streptococci, *H. influenzae*	Cutaneous erythema, warmth, normal vision, minimal involvement of orbit; fever, leukocytosis, toxic appearance	Systemic antibiotics

CMV, cytomegalovirus; EBV, Epstein-Barr virus; ECHO, enteric cytopathic human orphan; JRA, juvenile rheumatoid arthritis; SLE, systemic lupus erythematosus.
From Behrman R, Kliegman R: *Nelson's essentials of pediatrics*, ed 3, Philadelphia, 1998, WB Saunders.

sites are involved (meningitis, arthritis). Neonatal conjunctivitis secondary to *Chlamydia* is treated with oral erythromycin (50 mg/kg/24 hr in 4 divided doses) for 2 wk. This cures conjunctivitis and may prevent subsequent chlamydial pneumonia. *Pseudomonas* neonatal conjunctivitis is treated with systemic antibiotics, including an aminoglycoside, plus local saline irrigation and gentamicin ophthalmic ointment. Staphylococcal conjunctivitis is treated with parenteral methicillin and local saline irrigation.

Prognosis and Prevention

Before the institution of topical ophthalmic prophylaxis at birth, gonococcal ophthalmia was a common cause of blindness or permanent eye damage. If properly applied, this form of prophylaxis is highly effective unless infection is present at birth. Drops of 0.5% erythromycin or 1% silver nitrate are instilled directly into the open eyes at birth using wax or plastic single-dose containers. Saline irrigation after silver nitrate application is unnecessary. Silver nitrate is ineffective against active infection and may have limited use against *Chlamydia*. Povidone-iodine (2% solution) may also be an effective prophylactic agent.

Identification of maternal gonococcal infection and appropriate treatment has become a standard element of routine prenatal care. An infant born to a woman who has untreated gonococcal infection should receive a single dose of ceftriaxone, 50 mg/kg (maximum 125 mg) IV or IM, in addition to topical prophylaxis. The dose should be reduced for premature infants. Penicillin (50,000 U) should be used if the mother's gonococcal isolate is known to be penicillin sensitive.

Neither topical prophylaxis nor topical treatment prevents the afebrile pneumonia that occurs in 10-20% of infants exposed to *C. trachomatis*. Although chlamydial conjunctivitis is often a self-limiting disease, chlamydial pneumonia may have serious consequences. It is important that infants with chlamydial disease receive systemic treatment. Treatment of colonized pregnant women with erythromycin may prevent neonatal disease.

Acute Purulent Conjunctivitis

This is characterized by more or less generalized conjunctival hyperemia, edema, mucopurulent exudate, glued eyes (lids stuck together after sleeping), and various degrees of ocular pain and discomfort. It is usually a result of bacterial infection. The most frequent causes are nontypeable *Haemophilus influenzae* (associated with ipsilateral otitis media), pneumococci, staphylococci, and streptococci. Bacterial purulent conjunctivitis, especially due to pneumococcus or *H. influenzae* may occur in epidemics. Conjunctival smear and culture are helpful in differentiating specific types. These common forms of acute purulent conjunctivitis usually respond well to warm compresses and frequent topical instillation of antibiotic drops. Brazilian purpuric fever due to *Haemophilus aegyptius* manifests as conjunctivitis and sepsis. *N. gonorrhoeae* and *Chlamydia* are relatively common causes of acute purulent conjunctivitis in children beyond the newborn period, especially in adolescents. These infections require specific testing and treatment. Patients with a low risk of bacterial conjunctivitis have been characterized as >6 yr of age, becoming ill between April and November, having minimal or a watery discharge, and not having morning glue eye.

Viral Conjunctivitis

This is generally characterized by a watery discharge. Follicular changes (small aggregates of lymphocytes) are often found in the palpebral conjunctiva. Conjunctivitis resulting from adenovirus infection is relatively common, sometimes with corneal involvement as well as pharyngitis or pneumonia. Outbreaks of conjunctivitis caused by enterovirus are also encountered; this type may be hemorrhagic. Acute hemorrhagic conjunctivitis may be epidemic due to enterovirus CA24 or 70 and is characterized by red, swollen, and painful eyes with a hemorrhagic watery discharge. Conjunctivitis is commonly associated with such systemic viral infections as the childhood exanthems, particularly measles. Viral conjunctivitis is usually self-limited.

Epidemic Keratoconjunctivitis

This is caused by adenovirus type 8 and is transmitted by direct contact. It initially presents as a sensation of a foreign body beneath the lids, with itching and burning. Edema and photophobia develop rapidly, and large oval follicles appear within the conjunctiva. Preauricular adenopathy and a pseudomembrane on the conjunctival surface occur frequently. Subepithelial corneal infiltrates may develop and may cause blurring of vision; these usually disappear but may permanently reduce visual acuity. Corneal complications are less common in children than in adults. Children may have associated upper respiratory tract infection and pharyngitis. No specific medical therapy is available to decrease the symptoms or shorten the course of the disease. Emphasis must be placed on prevention of spread of the disease. Replicating virus is present in 95% of patients 10 days after the appearance of symptoms.

Membranous and Pseudomembranous Conjunctivitis

These types of conjunctivitis can be encountered in a number of diseases. The classic membranous conjunctivitis is that of diphtheria, accompanied by a fibrin-rich exudate that forms on the conjunctival surface and permeates the epithelium; the membrane is removed with difficulty and leaves raw bleeding areas. In pseudomembranous conjunctivitis, the layer of fibrin-rich exudate is superficial and can often be stripped easily, leaving the surface smooth. This type occurs with many bacterial and viral infections, including staphylococcal, pneumococcal, streptococcal, or chlamydial conjunctivitis, and in epidemic keratoconjunctivitis. It is also found in vernal conjunctivitis and in Stevens-Johnson disease.

Allergic Conjunctivitis

This is usually accompanied by intense itching, clear watery discharge, and conjunctival edema. It is commonly seasonal. Cold compresses and decongestant drops give symptomatic relief. Topical mast cell stabilizers or prostaglandin inhibitors may also help. In selected cases, topical corticosteroids are used under an ophthalmologist's supervision.

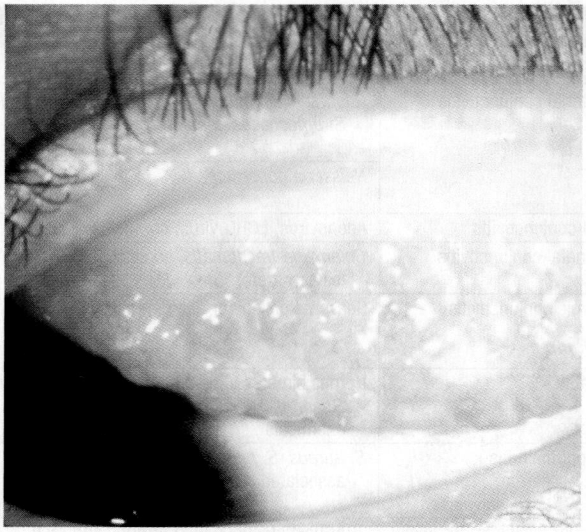

Figure 618-1 Vernal conjunctivitis.

Vernal Conjunctivitis

This usually begins in the prepubertal years and may recur for many years. Atopy appears to have a role in its origin, but the pathogenesis is uncertain. Extreme itching and tearing are the usual complaints. Large, flattened, cobblestone-like papillary lesions of the palpebral conjunctivae are characteristic (Fig. 618-1). A stringy exudate and a milky conjunctival pseudomembrane are frequently present. Small elevated lesions of the bulbar conjunctiva adjacent to the limbus (limbal form) may be found. Smear of the conjunctival exudate reveals many eosinophils. Topical corticosteroid therapy and cold compresses afford some relief. Topical mast cell stabilizers or prostaglandin inhibitors are useful when long-term control is needed. The long-term use of corticosteroids should be avoided.

Parinaud Oculoglandular Syndrome

This represents a form of cat-scratch disease and is caused by *Bartonella henselae*, which is transmitted from cat to cat by fleas (Chapter 201). Kittens are more likely than adult cats to be infected. Humans can become infected when they are scratched by a cat. In addition, bacteria may pass from a cat's saliva to its fur during grooming. The bacteria can then be deposited on the conjunctiva after rubbing one's eyes after handling the cat. Lymphadenopathy and conjunctivitis are hallmarks of the disease. Conjunctival granulomas may develop (Fig. 618-2). The course is generally self-limited, but antibiotics may be used in some cases.

Chemical Conjunctivitis

This can result when an irritating substance enters the conjunctival sac (as in the acute but benign conjunctivitis caused by silver nitrate in newborns). Other common offenders are household cleaning substances, sprays, smoke, smog, and industrial pollutants. Alkalis tend to linger in the conjunctival tissues and continue to inflict damage for hours or days. Acids precipitate the proteins in tissues and so produce their effect immediately. In either case, prompt, thorough, and copious irrigation is crucial. Extensive tissue damage, even loss of the eye, can result, especially if the offending agent is an alkali.

Other Conjunctival Disorders

Subconjunctival hemorrhage is manifested by bright or dark red patches in the bulbar conjunctiva and may result from injury or

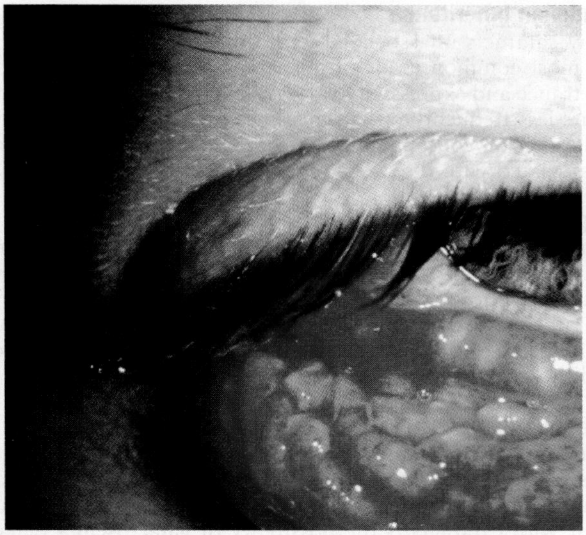

Figure 618-2 Conjunctival granulomas in Parinaud oculoglandular syndrome.

inflammation. It commonly occurs spontaneously. It may occasionally result from severe sneezing or coughing. Rarely, it may be a manifestation of a blood dyscrasia. Subconjunctival hemorrhages are self-limiting and require no treatment.

Pinguecula is a yellowish-white, slightly elevated mass on the bulbar conjunctiva, usually in the interpalpebral region. It represents elastic and hyaline degenerative changes of the conjunctiva. No treatment is required except for cosmetic reasons, in which case simple excision suffices.

Pterygium is a fleshy triangular conjunctival lesion that may encroach on the cornea. It typically occurs in the nasal interpalpebral region. The pathologic findings are similar to those of a pinguecula. The development of pterygia is related to exposure to ultraviolet light, and it therefore is more commonly found among people who live near the equator. Removal is suggested when the lesion encroaches far onto the cornea. Recurrence after removal is common.

Dermoid cyst and dermolipoma are benign lesions, clinically similar in appearance. They are smooth, elevated, round to oval lesions of various sizes. The color varies from yellowish white to fleshy pink. The most frequent site is the upper outer quadrant of the globe; they also commonly occur near or straddling the limbus. Dermolipoma is composed of adipose and connective tissue. Dermoid cysts may also contain glandular tissue, hair follicles, and hair shafts. Excision for cosmetic reasons is feasible. Dermolipomas are often connected to the extraocular muscles, making their complete removal impossible without sacrificing ocular motility.

Conjunctival nevus is a small, slightly elevated lesion that may vary in pigmentation from pale salmon to dark brown. It is usually benign, but careful observation for progressive growth or changes suggestive of malignancy is advised.

Symblepharon is a cicatricial adhesion between the conjunctiva of the lid and the globe; the lower lid is usually affected. It follows operation or injuries, especially burns from lye, acids, or molten metals. It is a serious complication of Stevens-Johnson syndrome. It may interfere with motion of the eyeball and may cause diplopia. The adhesions should be separated and the raw surfaces kept from uniting during healing. Grafts of oral mucous membrane may be necessary.

BIBLIOGRAPHY

Please visit the Nelson Textbook of Pediatrics *website at www.expertconsult.com for the complete bibliography.*

Chapter 619
Abnormalities of the Cornea

Scott E. Olitsky, Denise Hug, Laura S. Plummer, and Merrill Stass-Isern

MEGALOCORNEA

This is a nonprogressive symmetric condition characterized by an enlarged cornea (>12 mm in diameter) and an anterior segment in which there is no evidence of previous or concurrent ocular hypertension. High myopia is frequently present and may lead to reduced vision. A frequent complication is the development of lens opacities in adult life. All modes of inheritance have been described, although X-linked recessive is the most common; therefore, this disorder more commonly affects males. Systemic abnormalities that may be associated with megalocornea include Marfan syndrome, craniosynostosis, and Alport syndrome. The cause of the enlargement of the cornea and the anterior segment is unknown, but possible explanations include a defect in the growth of the optic cup and an arrest of congenital glaucoma. The region on the X chromosome responsible for this disorder has been identified.

For the full continuation of this chapter, please visit the Nelson Textbook of Pediatrics *website at www.expertconsult.com.*

Chapter 620
Abnormalities of the Lens

Scott E. Olitsky, Denise Hug, Laura S. Plummer, and Merrill Stass-Isern

CATARACTS

A cataract is any opacity of the lens (Fig. 620-1). Some are clinically unimportant; others significantly affect visual function. The incidence of infantile cataracts is approximately 2-13/10,000 live births. An epidemiologic study of infantile cataracts published in 2003 suggests that approximately 60% of cataracts are an isolated defect; 22% are part of a syndrome; and the remainder is associated with other unrelated major birth defects. Cataracts are more common in low birthweight infants. Infants at or below 2,500 g have a 3- to 4-fold increased odds of developing infantile cataracts. Some cataracts are associated with other ocular or systemic disease.

Differential Diagnosis

The differential diagnosis of cataracts in infants and children includes a wide range of developmental disorders, infectious and inflammatory processes, metabolic diseases, and toxic and traumatic insults (Table 620-1). Cataracts may also develop secondary to intraocular processes, such as retinopathy of prematurity, persistent hyperplastic primary vitreous, retinal detachment, retinitis pigmentosa, and uveitis. A portion of cataracts in children are inherited (Fig. 620-2).

Developmental Variants

Early developmental processes may lead to various congenital lens opacities. Discrete dots or white plaquelike opacities of the lens capsule are common and sometimes involve the contiguous subcapsular region. Small opacities of the posterior capsule may be associated with persistent remnants of the primitive hyaloid vascular system (the common Mittendorf dot), whereas those of the anterior capsule may be associated with persistent strands of the pupillary membrane or vascular sheath of the lens. Congenital cataracts of this type are usually stationary and rarely interfere with vision; in some, progression occurs.

Prematurity

A special type of lens change seen in some preterm newborn infants is the so-called cataract of prematurity. The appearance is of a cluster of tiny vacuoles in the distribution of the Y sutures of the lens. They can be visualized with an ophthalmoscope and are best seen with the pupil well dilated. The pathogenesis is unclear. In most cases, the opacities disappear spontaneously, often within a few weeks.

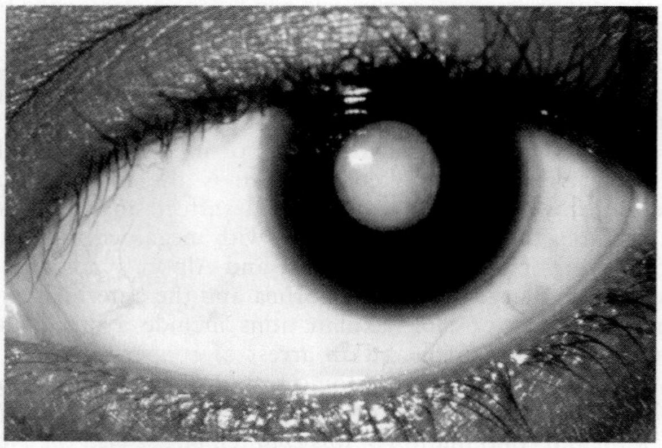

Figure 620-1 Leukocoria secondary to cataract.

Mendelian Inheritance

Many cataracts unassociated with other diseases are hereditary. The most common mode of inheritance is autosomal dominant. Penetrance and expressivity vary. Autosomal recessive inheritance occurs less frequently; it is sometimes found in populations with high rates of consanguinity. X-linked inheritance of cataracts unassociated with disease is relatively rare.

Congenital Infection Syndrome

Cataracts in infants and children can be a result of prenatal infection. Lens opacity may occur in any of the major congenital infection syndromes (e.g., toxoplasmosis, cytomegalovirus, syphilis, rubella, herpes simplex virus). Cataracts may also occur secondary to other perinatal infections, including measles, poliomyelitis, influenza, varicella-zoster, and vaccinia.

Metabolic Disorders

Cataracts are a prominent manifestation of many metabolic diseases, particularly certain disorders of carbohydrate, amino acid, calcium, and copper metabolism. A primary consideration in any infant with cataracts is the possibility of **galactosemia** (Chapter 81.2). In classic infantile galactosemia, galactose-1-phosphate uridyl transferase deficiency, the cataract is typically of the zonular type, with haziness or opacification of 1 or more of the perinuclear layers of the lens Haziness or clouding of the nucleus also often occurs. In its early stages, the cataract generally has a

Table 620-1 DIFFERENTIAL DIAGNOSIS OF CATARACTS

DEVELOPMENTAL VARIANTS
Prematurity (Y-suture vacuoles) with or without retinopathy of prematurity
GENETIC DISORDERS
Simple Mendelian Inheritance
Autosomal dominant (most common)
Autosomal recessive
X-linked
Major Chromosomal Defects
Trisomy disorders (13, 18, 21)
Turner syndrome (45X)
Deletion syndromes (11p13, 18p, 18q)
Duplication syndromes (3q, 20p, 10q)
Multisystem Genetic Disorders
Alport syndrome (hearing loss, renal disease)
Alström syndrome (nerve deafness, diabetes mellitus)
Apert disease (craniosynostosis, syndactyly)
Cockayne syndrome (premature senility, skin photosensitivity)
Conradi disease (chondrodysplasia punctata)
Crouzon disease (dysostosis craniofacialis)
Hallermann-Streiff syndrome (microphthalmia, small pinched nose, skin atrophy, and hypotrichosis)
Hypohidrotic ectodermal dysplasia (anomalous dentition, hypohidrosis, hypotrichosis)
Ichthyosis (keratinizing disorder with thick, scaly skin)
Incontinentia pigmenti (dental anomalies, mental retardation, cutaneous lesions)
Lowe syndrome (oculocerebrorenal syndrome: hypotonia, renal disease)
Marfan syndrome
Meckel-Gruber syndrome (renal dysplasia, encephalocele)
Myotonic dystrophy
Nail-patella syndrome (renal dysfunction, dysplastic nails, hypoplastic patella)
Marinesco-Sjögren syndrome (cerebellar ataxia, hypotonia)
Nevoid basal cell carcinoma syndrome (autosomal dominant, basal cell carcinoma erupts in childhood)
Peters anomaly (corneal opacifications with iris-corneal dysgenesis)
Reiger syndrome (iris dysplasia, myotonic dystrophy)
Rothmund-Thomson syndrome (poikiloderma: skin atrophy)
Rubinstein-Taybi syndrome (broad great toe, mental retardation)
Smith-Lemli-Opitz syndrome (toe syndactyly, hypospadias, mental retardation)
Sotos syndrome (cerebral gigantism)
Spondyloepiphyseal dysplasia (dwarfism, short trunk)
Werner syndrome (premature aging in 2nd decade of life)
Inborn Errors of Metabolism
Abetalipoproteinemia (absent chylomicrons, retinal degeneration)
Fabry disease (α-galactosidase A deficiency)
Galactokinase deficiency
Galactosemia (galactose-1-phosphate uridyl transferase deficiency)
Homocystinemia (subluxation of lens, mental retardation)
Mannosidosis (acid α-mannosidase deficiency)
Niemann-Pick disease (sphingomyelinase deficiency)
Refsum disease (phytanic acid α-hydrolase deficiency)
Wilson disease (accumulation of copper leads to cirrhosis and neurologic symptoms)
ENDOCRINOPATHIES
Hypocalcemia (hypoparathyroidism)
Hypoglycemia
Diabetes mellitus
CONGENITAL INFECTIONS
Toxoplasmosis
Cytomegalovirus infection
Syphilis
Rubella
Perinatal herpes simplex infection
Measles (rubeola)
Poliomyelitis
Influenza
Varicella-zoster
OCULAR ANOMALIES
Microphthalmia
Coloboma
Aniridia
Mesodermal dysgenesis
Persistent pupillary membrane
Posterior lenticonus
Persistent hyperplastic primary vitreous
Primitive hyaloid vascular system
MISCELLANEOUS DISORDERS
Atopic dermatitis
Drugs (corticosteroids)
Radiation
Trauma
IDIOPATHIC

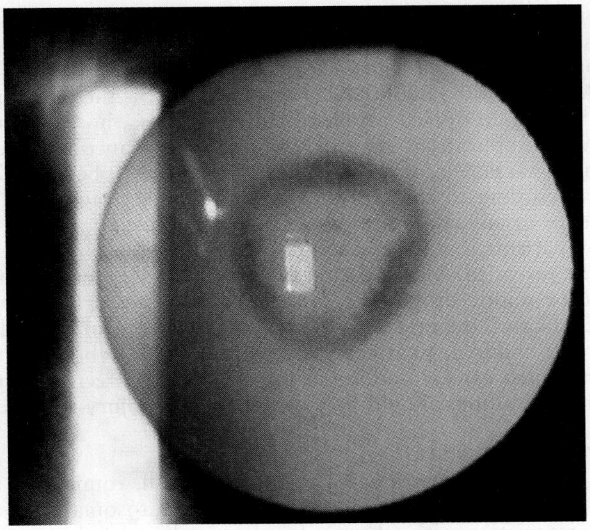

Figure 620-2 Central lamellar cataract.

distinctive oil droplet appearance and is best detected with the pupil fully dilated. Progression to complete opacification of the lens may occur within weeks. With early treatment (galactose-free diet), the lens changes may be reversible.

In **galactokinase deficiency,** cataracts are the sole clinical manifestation. The cataracts are usually zonular and may appear in the 1st months of life, 1st years of life, or later in childhood.

In children with juvenile-onset diabetes mellitus, lens changes are uncommon. Some develop snowflake-like white opacities and vacuoles of the lens. Others develop cataracts that may progress and mature rapidly, sometimes in a matter of days, especially during adolescence. An antecedent event may be the sudden development of myopia caused by changes in the optical density of the lens.

Congenital lens opacities may be seen in children of diabetic and prediabetic mothers. Hypoglycemia in neonates can also be associated with early development of cataracts. Ketotic hypoglycemia is also associated with cataracts.

An association between cataracts and hypocalcemia is well established. Various lens opacities may be seen in patients with hypoparathyroidism.

The **oculocerebral renal syndrome of Lowe** is associated with cataracts in infants. Affected male children frequently have dense bilateral cataracts at birth, often in association with glaucoma and miotic pupils. Punctate lens opacities are frequently present in heterozygous females.

The distinctive sunflower cataract of **Wilson disease** is not commonly seen in children. Various lens opacities may be seen in children with certain of the sphingolipidoses, mucopolysaccharidoses, and mucolipidoses, particularly Niemann-Pick disease, mucosulfatidosis, Fabry disease, and aspartylglycosaminuria (Chapters 80 and 82).

Chromosomal Defects

Lens opacities of various types may occur in association with chromosomal defects, including trisomies 13, 18, and 21; Turner syndrome; and a number of deletion (11p13, 18p, 18q) and duplication (3q, 20p, 10q) syndromes (Chapter 76).

Drugs, Toxic Agents, and Trauma

Of the various drugs and toxic agents that may produce cataracts, corticosteroids are of major importance in the pediatric age group. Steroid-related cataracts characteristically are posterior subcapsular lens opacities. The incidence and severity vary. The relative significance of dose, mode of administration, duration of treatment, and individual susceptibility is controversial, and the pathogenesis of steroid-induced cataracts is unclear. The effect on vision depends on the extent and density of the opacity. In many cases, the acuity is only minimally or moderately impaired. Reversibility of steroid-induced cataracts may occur in some cases. All children receiving long-term steroid treatment should have periodic eye examinations.

Trauma to the eye is a major cause of cataracts in children. Opacification of the lens may result from contusion or penetrating injury. Cataracts are an important manifestation of child abuse.

Cataract formation after exposure to radiation is dose and duration dependent. Adult research shows 50% occurrence in lens dose of 15 Gy. Delayed onset is the rule.

Miscellaneous Disorders

The list of multisystem syndromes and diseases associated with lens opacities and other eye anomalies is extensive (see Table 620-1).

TREATMENT The treatment of cataracts that significantly interfere with vision includes the following: (1) surgical removal of lens material to provide an optically clear visual axis; (2) correction of the resultant aphakic refractive error with spectacles, contact lenses, or intraocular lens implantation; and (3) correction of any associated sensory deprivation amblyopia. Because the use of spectacles may not be possible in children after cataract removal, the use of contact lenses for visual rehabilitation is sometimes a medical necessity. Intraocular lens implantation has become a mainstay for visual rehabilitation in older children. Patients are currently being recruited into a multicenter trial to help determine visual outcomes with contact lenses versus intraocular lens implants in very young children. Treatment of the amblyopia may be the most demanding and difficult step in the visual rehabilitation of infants or children with cataracts. Not all cataracts require surgical intervention. Cataracts that are not visually significant should be monitored for change and the child should be monitored for development of amblyopia.

PROGNOSIS Prognosis depends on many factors, including the nature of the cataract, the underlying disease, age at onset, age at intervention, duration and severity of any attendant amblyopia, and presence of any associated ocular abnormalities (e.g., microphthalmia, retinal lesions, optic atrophy, glaucoma, nystagmus, and strabismus). Persistent amblyopia is the most common cause of poor visual recovery after cataract surgery in children. Secondary conditions and complications may develop in children who have had cataract surgery, including inflammatory sequelae, secondary membranes, glaucoma, retinal detachment, and changes in the axial length of the eye. All these should be considered in planning treatment.

Ectopia Lentis

Normally, the lens is suspended in place behind the iris diaphragm by the zonular fibers of the ciliary body. Abnormalities of the suspensory system resulting from a developmental defect, disease, or trauma may result in instability or displacement of the lens. Displacement of the lens is classified as luxation (dislocation–complete displacement of the lens) (Fig. 620-3) or as subluxation (partial displacement–shifting or tilting of the lens) (Fig. 620-4). Symptoms include blurring of vision, which is often the result of refractive changes such as myopia, astigmatism, or aphakic hyperopia. Some patients experience diplopia (double vision). An important sign of displacement is iridodonesis, a tremulousness of the iris caused by the loss of its usual support. Also, the anterior chamber may appear deeper than normal. Sometimes the equatorial region ("edge") of the displaced lens may be visible in the pupillary aperture. On ophthalmoscopy, this may appear as a black crescent. Also, the difference between the phakic and aphakic portions can be appreciated when focusing on the fundus.

DIFFERENTIAL DIAGNOSIS A major cause of lens displacement is trauma. Displacement may also occur as a result of ocular disease

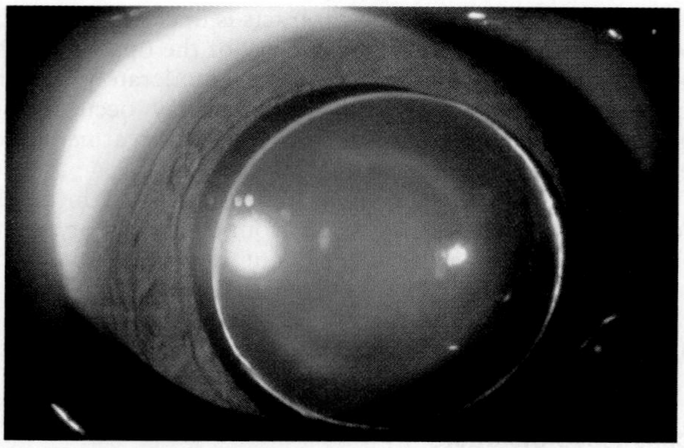

Figure 620-3 Complete dislocation of lens into the anterior chamber seen in Weill-Marchesani syndrome.

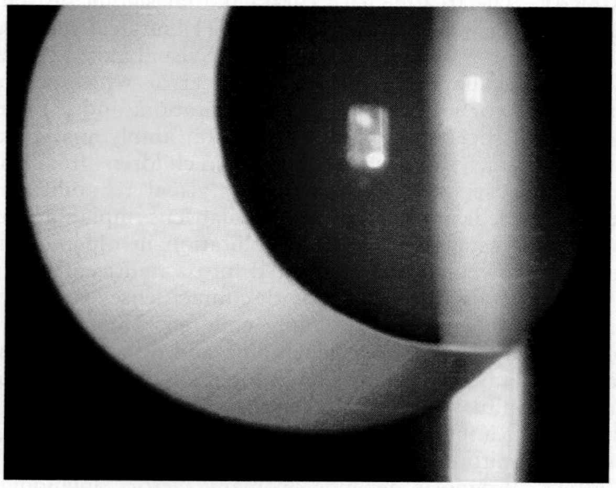

Figure 620-4 Subluxation of the lens in Marfan syndrome.

such as uveitis, intraocular tumor, congenital glaucoma, high myopia, megalocornea, aniridia, or in association with cataract. Ectopia lentis may also be inherited or associated with systemic disease.

Displacement of the lens occurring as a heritable ocular condition unassociated with systemic abnormalities is referred to as simple ectopia lentis. Simple ectopia lentis is usually transmitted as an autosomal dominant condition. The lens is generally displaced upward and temporally. The ectopia may be present at birth or may appear later in life. Another form of heritable dislocation is ectopia lentis et pupillae. In this condition, both the lens and pupil are displaced, usually in opposite directions. This condition is generally bilateral, with 1 eye being almost a mirror image of the other. Ectopia lentis et pupillae is a recessive condition, although variable expression with some intermingling with simple ectopia lentis has been reported.

Systemic disorders associated with displacement of the lens include Marfan syndrome, homocystinuria, Weill-Marchesani syndrome, and sulfite oxidase deficiency (Chapter 79). Ectopia lentis occurs in approximately 80% of patients with Marfan syndrome, and in about 50% of patients; the ectopia is evident by the age of 5 yr. In most cases, the lens is displaced superiorly and temporally; it is almost always bilateral and relatively symmetric. In homocystinuria, the lens is usually displaced inferiorly and somewhat nasally. It occurs early in life and is often evident by 5 yr of age. In Weill-Marchesani syndrome, the displacement of the lens is often downward and forward, and the lens tends to be small and round.

Ectopia lentis is also associated occasionally with other conditions, including Ehlers-Danlos, Sturge-Weber, Crouzon, and Klippel-Feil syndromes; oxycephaly; and mandibulofacial dysostosis. A syndrome of dominantly inherited blepharoptosis, high myopia, and ectopia lentis has also been described.

TREATMENT AND PROGNOSIS Displacement of the lens often results only in optical problems. In some cases, however, more serious complications may develop, such as glaucoma, uveitis, retinal detachment, or cataract. Management must be individualized according to the type of displacement, its cause, and the presence of any complicating ocular or systemic conditions. For many patients, optical correction by spectacles or contact lenses can be provided. Manipulation of the iris diaphragm with mydriatic or miotic drops may sometimes help improve vision. In selected cases, the best treatment is surgical removal of the lens. In many children, treatment of any associated amblyopia must be instituted early. In addition, for children with ectopia lentis, safety precautions should be taken to prevent injury to the eye.

Microspherophakia

The term *microspherophakia* refers to a small, round lens that may occur as an isolated anomaly (probably autosomal recessive) or in association with other ocular abnormalities, such as ectopia lentis, myopia, or retinal detachment (possibly autosomal dominant). Microspherophakia may also occur in association with various systemic disorders, including Marfan syndrome, Weill-Marchesani syndrome, Alport syndrome, mandibulofacial dysostosis, and Klinefelter syndrome.

Anterior Lenticonus

Anterior lenticonus is a rare bilateral condition in which the anterior surface of the lens bulges centrally. It may be accompanied by lens opacities or other eye anomalies and is a prominent feature of Alport syndrome. The increased curvature of the central area may cause high myopia.

Rupture of the anterior capsule may occur, requiring prompt surgical intervention.

Posterior Lenticonus

Posterior lenticonus, which occurs more commonly than anterior lenticonus, is characterized by a circumscribed round or oval bulge of the posterior lens capsule and cortex, restricted to the 2-7 mm central region. In the early stages, by the red reflex test, this may look like an oil droplet. It occurs in infants and young children and tends to increase with age. Usually the lens material within and surrounding the capsular bulge eventually becomes opacified. Posterior lenticonus usually occurs as an isolated ocular anomaly. It is generally unilateral but may be bilateral. It is believed to be sporadic, although autosomal dominant and X-linked inheritance has been suggested in some cases. Infants or children with posterior lenticonus may require optical correction, amblyopia treatment, and surgery for progressive cataract.

BIBLIOGRAPHY

Please visit the Nelson Textbook of Pediatrics *website at www.expertconsult.com for the complete bibliography.*

Chapter 621
Disorders of the Uveal Tract

Scott E. Olitsky, Denise Hug, Laura S. Plummer, and Merrill Stass-Isern

UVEITIS (IRITIS, CYCLITIS, CHORIORETINITIS)

The uveal tract (the inner vascular coat of the eye, consisting of the iris, ciliary body, and choroid) is subject to inflammatory involvement in a number of systemic diseases, both infectious and noninfectious, and in response to exogenous factors, including trauma and toxic agents (Table 621-1). Inflammation

Table 621-1 UVEITIS IN CHILDHOOD

ANTERIOR UVEITIS
Juvenile rheumatoid arthritis (pauciarticular)
Sarcoidosis
Trauma
Tuberculosis
Kawasaki disease
Ulcerative colitis
Post infectious (enteric or genital) with arthritis and rash
Spirochetal (syphilis, leptospiral)
Heterochromic iridocyclitis (Fuchs)
Viral (herpes simplex, herpes zoster)
Ankylosing spondylitis
Stevens-Johnson syndrome
Idiopathic
Drugs
POSTERIOR UVEITIS (CHOROIDITIS—MAY INVOLVE RETINA)
Toxoplasmosis
Parasites (toxocariasis)
Sarcoidosis
Tuberculosis
Viral (rubella, herpes simplex, HIV, cytomegalovirus)
Subacute sclerosing panencephalitis
Idiopathic
ANTERIOR AND/OR POSTERIOR UVEITIS
Sympathetic ophthalmia (trauma to other eye)
Vogt-Koyanagi-Harada syndrome (uveo-otocutaneous syndrome: poliosis, vitiligo, deafness, tinnitus, uveitis, aseptic meningitis, retinitis)
Behçet syndrome
Lyme disease

Table 621-2 EXAMINATION SCHEDULE FOR CHILDREN WITH JRA WITHOUT KNOWN IRIDOCYCLITIS

JRA SUBTYPE	AGE AT ONSET	
	<7 Years	≥7 Years
PAUCIARTICULAR		
Positive ANA		
Less than 4 years' duration	Every 3-4 mo	Every 6 mo
4-7 years duration	Every 6 mo	Annually
More than 7 years' duration	Annually	Annually
Negative ANA		
Less than 4 years' duration	Every 6 mo	Every 6 mo
4-7 years duration	Every 6 mo	Annually
More than 7 years' duration	Annually	Annually
POLYARTICULAR		
Positive ANA		
Less than 4 years' duration	Every 3-4 mo	Every 6 mo
4-7 years duration	Every 6 mo	Annually
More than 7 years' duration	Annually	Annually
Negative ANA		
Less than 4 years' duration	Every 6 mo	Every 6 mo
4-7 years duration	Every 6 mo	Annually
More than 7 years' duration	Annually	Annually
SYSTEMIC	Annually, regardless of duration	Annually, regardless of duration

ANA, antinuclear antibody; JRA, juvenile rheumatoid arthritis.

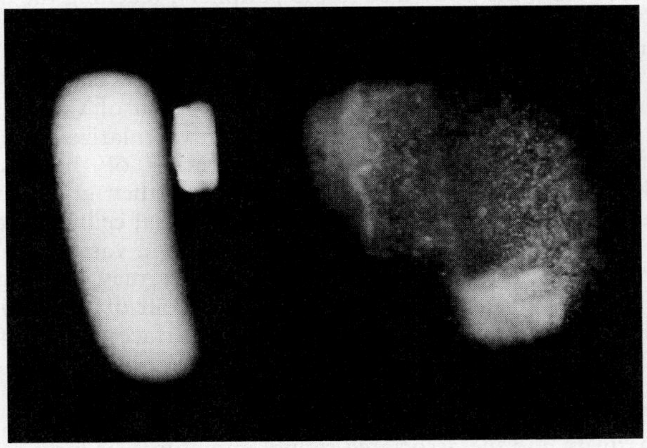

Figure 621-1 Cell and flare in the anterior chamber. The flare represents protein leakage. (Courtesy of Peter Buch, CRA.)

may affect any 1 portion of the uveal tract preferentially or all parts together.

Iritis may occur alone or in conjunction with inflammation of the ciliary body as iridocyclitis or in association with pars planitis. Pain, photophobia, and lacrimation are the characteristic symptoms of acute anterior uveitis, but the inflammation may develop insidiously without disturbing symptoms. Signs of anterior uveitis include conjunctival hyperemia, particularly in the perilimbal region (ciliary flush), and cells and protein ("flare") in the aqueous humor (Fig. 621-1). Inflammatory deposits on the posterior surface of the cornea (keratic precipitates) and congestion of the iris may also be seen. More chronic cases may show degenerative changes of the cornea (band keratopathy), lenticular opacities (cataract), development of glaucoma, and impairment of vision. The cause of anterior uveitis is often obscure; primary considerations in children are rheumatoid disease, particularly pauciarticular rheumatoid arthritis, Kawasaki disease, reactive arthritis (postinfectious), and sarcoidosis. Iritis may be secondary to corneal disease, such as herpetic keratitis or a bacterial or fungal corneal ulcer, or to a corneal abrasion or foreign body. Traumatic iritis and iridocyclitis are especially common in children.

Iridocyclitis that occurs in children with arthritis deserves special mention. Unlike most forms of anterior uveitis, it rarely creates pain, photophobia, or conjunctival hyperemia. Loss of vision may not be noticed until severe and irreversible damage has occurred. Because of the lack of symptoms and the high incidence of uveitis in these children, routine periodic screening is necessary. Ophthalmic screening guidelines are based on 3 factors that predispose children with arthritis to uveitis:

1. Type of arthritis
2. Age of onset of arthritis
3. Antinuclear antibody status

Table 621-2 has been developed by the American Academy of Pediatrics for children with juvenile rheumatoid arthritis without known iridocyclitis.

Choroiditis, inflammation of the posterior portion of the uveal tract, invariably also involves the retina; when both are obviously affected, the condition is termed chorioretinitis. The causes of posterior uveitis are numerous; the more common are toxoplasmosis, histoplasmosis, cytomegalic inclusion disease, sarcoidosis, syphilis, tuberculosis, and toxocariasis (Fig. 621-2). Depending on the etiology, the inflammatory signs may be diffuse or focal. Vitreous reaction often occurs as well. With many types, the result is atrophic chorioretinal scarring demarcated by pigmentation, often with visual impairment. Secondary complications include retinal detachment, glaucoma, and phthisis.

Panophthalmitis is inflammation involving all parts of the eye. It is frequently suppurative, most often as a result of a perforating injury or of septicemia. It produces severe pain, marked congestion of the eye, inflammation of the adjacent orbital tissues and eyelids, and loss of vision. In many cases, the eye is lost despite intensive treatment of the infection and inflammation. Enucleation of the eye or evisceration of the orbit may be necessary.

Sympathetic ophthalmia is a rare type of inflammatory response that affects the uninjured eye after a perforating injury. It may occur weeks, months, or even years after the injury. A hypersensitivity phenomenon is the most probable cause. Loss of

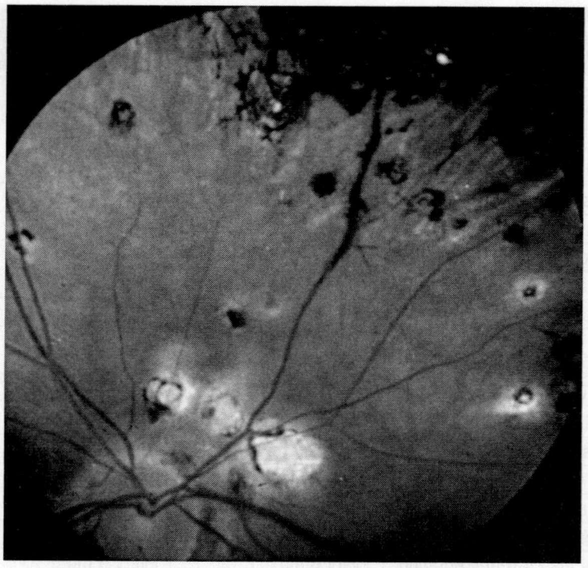

Figure 621-2 Focal atrophic and pigmented scars of chorioretinitis.

vision in the uninjured (sympathizing) eye may result. Removal of the injured eye prevents the development of sympathetic ophthalmia but does not stop the progression of the disease once it has occurred. Therefore, early enucleation should be considered if there is no hope of visual recovery after a severe injury.

Treatment

The various forms of intraocular inflammation are treated according to their causal factors. When infection is proved or suspected, appropriate systemic antimicrobial or antiviral therapy is used. In some cases, intravitreal injection is indicated.

Elimination of the intraocular inflammation is important to reduce the risk of severe, and often permanent, vision loss. Untreated, the inflammatory process may lead to the development of band keratopathy (calcium deposition in the cornea), cataracts, glaucoma, and irreversible retinal damage. Anterior inflammation may respond well to topical corticosteroid treatment. Posterior cases often require systemic therapy. The use of topical and systemic corticosteroids can lead to the development of glaucoma and cataracts. To reduce the need for topical and systemic corticosteroids, systemic immunosuppression is often used in patients requiring long-term treatment. Commonly used immunosuppressive agents include methotrexate, cyclosporine, and tumor necrosis factor inhibitors. Multiple agents may be needed in recalcitrant cases. Cycloplegic agents, particularly atropine, are also used to reduce inflammation and to prevent adhesion of the iris to the lens (posterior synechiae), especially in anterior uveitis. Extensive posterior synechiae formation can lead to acute angle closure glaucoma.

Surgery may be required for patients who develop glaucoma due to the underlying disease process or the need for corticosteroid treatment. Cataract surgery should be delayed until the inflammation has been under control for a period of time. Cataract surgery in children with a history of prolonged uveitis can carry significant risk. There is no universal agreement concerning the use of intraocular lenses in these patients.

Pars planitis is an uncommon idiopathic form of intermediate uveitis characterized by anterior chamber involvement, anterior vitreous cells and condensations and peripheral retinal vasculitis. The average age of onset is 9 yr. It is predominately bilateral and seen more frequently in males. Painless decreased vision is the usual presenting sign. The prognosis is good when adequate medical treatment is sought early in the course of the disease.

Masquerade syndromes can sometimes mimic intraocular inflammation. Retinoblastoma, leukemia, retained intraocular foreign body, juvenile xanthogranuloma, and peripheral retinal detachments may produce signs similar to those seen in uveitis. These syndromes should be kept in mind when evaluating a patient with suspected uveitis or if a patient does not respond as anticipated to antiinflammatory treatment.

BIBLIOGRAPHY

Please visit the Nelson Textbook of Pediatrics *website at www.expertconsult.com for the complete bibliography.*

Chapter 622
Disorders of the Retina and Vitreous

Scott E. Olitsky, Denise Hug, Laura S. Plummer, and Merrill Stass-Isern

RETINOPATHY OF PREMATURITY

Retinopathy of prematurity (ROP) is a complex disease of the developing retinal vasculature in premature infants. It may be acute (early stages) or chronic (late stages). Clinical manifestations range from mild, usually transient changes of the peripheral retina to severe progressive vasoproliferation, scarring, and potentially blinding retinal detachment. ROP includes all stages of the disease and its sequelae. Retrolental fibroplasia, the previous name for this disease, described only the cicatricial stages.

Pathogenesis

Beginning at 16 wk of gestation, retinal angiogenesis normally proceeds from the optic disc to the periphery, reaching the outer rim of the retina (ora serrata) nasally at about 36 wk and extending temporally by approximately 40 wk. Injury to this process results in various pathologic and clinical changes. The first observation in the acute phase is cessation of vasculogenesis. Rather than a gradual transition from vascularized to avascular retina, there is an abrupt termination of the vessels, marked by a line in the retina. The line can then grow into a ridge composed of mesenchymal and endothelial cells. Cell division and differentiation might later resume, and vascularization of the retina can proceed. Alternatively, there may be progression to an abnormal proliferation of vessels out of the plane of the retina, into the vitreous, and over the surface of the retina. Cicatrization and traction on the retina can follow, leading to retinal detachment.

The risk factors associated with ROP are not fully known, but prematurity and the associated retinal immaturity at birth represent the major factors. Oxygenation, respiratory distress, apnea, bradycardia, heart disease, infection, hypercarbia, acidosis, anemia, and the need for transfusion are thought by some to be contributory factors. Generally, the lower the gestational age, the lower the birthweight, and the sicker the infant, the greater the risk is for ROP.

The basic pathogenesis of ROP is still unknown. Exposure to the extrauterine environment including the necessarily high inspired oxygen concentrations produces cellular damage, perhaps mediated by free radicals. Later in the course of the disease, peripheral hypoxia develops and vascular endothelial growth factors (VEGFs) are produced in the nonvascularized retina. These growth factors stimulate abnormal vasculogenesis, and neovascularization can occur. Because of poor pulmonary function, a state of relative retinal hypoxia occurs. This causes upregulation of VEGF, which, in susceptible infants, can cause abnormal fibrovascular growth. This neovascularization can then lead to scarring and vision loss.

Classification

The currently used international classification of ROP describes the location, extent, and severity of the disease. To delineate

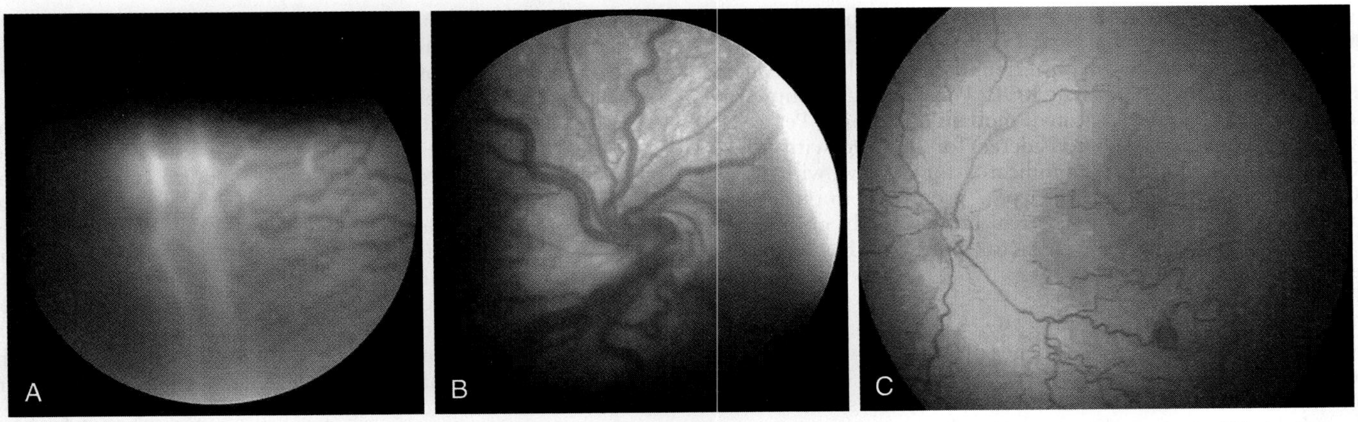

Figure 622-1 Retinopathy of prematurity (ROP). *A,* In stage 3, there is a ridge and extraretinal vascular tissue. *B,* Retinal vessels are dilated and tortuous in active ROP plus disease. *C,* Zone 1, stage ROP with plus disease.

location, the retina is divided into three concentric zones, centered on the optic disc. Zone I, the posterior or inner zone, extends twice the disc-macular distance, or 30 degrees in all directions from the optic disc. Zone II, the middle zone, extends from the outer edge of zone I to the ora serrata nasally and to the anatomic equator temporally. Zone III, the outer zone, is the residual crescent that extends from the outer border of zone II to the ora serrata temporally. The extent of involvement is described by the number of circumferential clock hours involved.

The phases and severity of the disease process are classified into 5 stages. Stage 1 is characterized by a demarcation line that separates vascularized from avascular retina. This line lies within the plane of the retina and appears relatively flat and white. Often noted is abnormal branching or arcading of the retinal vessels that lead into the line. Stage 2 is characterized by a ridge; the demarcation line has grown, acquiring height, width, and volume and extending up and out of the plane of the retina. Stage 3 is characterized by the presence of a ridge and by the development of extraretinal fibrovascular tissue (Fig. 622-1*A*). Stage 4 is characterized by subtotal retinal detachment caused by traction from the proliferating tissue in the vitreous or on the retina. Stage 4 is subdivided into 2 phases: (a) subtotal retinal detachment not involving the macula and (b) subtotal retinal detachment involving the macula. Stage 5 is total retinal detachment.

When signs of posterior retinal vascular changes accompany the active stages of ROP, the term *plus disease* is used (see Fig. 622-1*B,C*). Patients reaching the point of dilatation and tortuosity of the retinal vessels also often demonstrate the associated findings of engorgement of the iris, pupillary rigidity, and vitreous haze.

Clinical Manifestations and Prognosis

In >90% of at-risk infants, the course is one of spontaneous arrest and regression, with little or no residual effects or visual disability. Less than 10% of infants progress to severe disease, with significant extraretinal vasoproliferation, cicatrization, detachment of the retina, and impairment of vision.

Some children with arrested or regressed ROP are left with demarcation lines, undervascularization of the peripheral retina, or abnormal branching, tortuosity, or straightening of the retinal vessels. Some are left with retinal pigmentary changes, dragging of the retina (dragged disc), ectopia of the macula, retinal folds, or retinal breaks. Others proceed to total retinal detachment, which commonly assumes a funnel-like configuration. The clinical picture is often that of a retrolental membrane, producing leukocoria (a white reflex in the pupil). Some patients develop cataracts, glaucoma, and signs of inflammation. The end stage is often a painful blind eye or a degenerated phthisical eye. The spectrum of ROP also includes myopia, which is often progressive and of significant degree in infancy. The incidence of anisometropia, strabismus, amblyopia, and nystagmus may also be increased.

Table 622-1 TIMING OF FIRST EYE EXAMINATION BASED ON GESTATIONAL AGE AT BIRTH

GESTATIONAL AGE AT BIRTH (wk)	AGE AT INITIAL EXAMINATION (WK) Postmenstrual	Chronologic
22	31	9
23	31	8
24	31	7
25	31	6
26	31	5
27	31	4
28	32	4
29	33	4
30	34	4
31	35	4
32	36	4

Diagnosis

Systematic serial ophthalmologic examinations of infants at risk are recommended. In 2006 the American Academy of Pediatrics (AAP) published new screening guidelines for ROP. Infants with a birth weight of <1,500 g or gestational age of ≤32 wk and selected infants with a birth weight between 1,500 and 2,000 g or gestational age of >32 wk with an unstable clinical course, including those requiring cardiorespiratory support and who are believed by their attending pediatrician or neonatologist to be at high risk, should have retinal screening examinations. The timing of the initial screening exam is based on the infant's age. Table 622-1 was developed from an evidence-based analysis of the Mutlicenter Trial of Cryotherapy for ROP. The examination can be stressful to fragile preterm infants, and the dilating drops can have untoward side effects. Infants must be carefully monitored during and after the examination. Some neonatologists and ophthalmologists advocate the use of topical tetracaine and/or oral sucrose to reduce the discomfort and stress to the infant. Follow-up is based on the initial findings and risk factors but is usually at 2 wk or less.

Treatment

In selected cases, cryotherapy or laser photocoagulation of the avascular retina reduces the more-severe complications of progressive ROP. Advances in vitreoretinal surgical techniques have led to limited success in reattaching the retina in infants with total retinal detachment (stage 5 ROP), but the visual results are often disappointing. The Early Treatment for Retinopathy of Prematurity cooperative study demonstrated the importance of plus disease and the presence of posterior retinal involvement in the determination of when to treat ROP. This study also supported the fact that **laser is the treatment modality of choice.** Peripheral retinal ablation should be considered for any eye with type 1 ROP. Serial examinations are indicated for any eye with type 2 ROP; treatment is considered if type 2 progresses to type 1 or if threshold ROP develops. Intravitreal bevacizumab, an inhibitor of vascular endothelial growth factor, may also have a role in treatment.

Prevention

Prevention of ROP ultimately depends on prevention of premature birth and its attendant problems. The association between ROP and oxygen saturation has been studied for decades. More-recent research has focused on keeping severely premature infants at lower oxygen saturation (85-92%) at age <34 wk and maintaining them at higher oxygen saturation (92-97%) at age >34 wk. This reduction in oxygen saturation early in the infant's life effectively reduces the phase I hyperoxia and can stimulate the retina to develop normally. The reversal of the hypoxic phase II by elevating the oxygen saturation might ultimately decrease the incidence of severe ROP by down-regulating the secretion of VEGF. Most likely, a multicenter, prospective, randomized study will need to be performed to answer this question. Some investigators have suggested supplemental vitamin E for its antioxidant properties in infants at risk for ROP. Its efficacy has not been proved; at certain dosage levels, it can produce untoward side effects (Chapter 91.2).

PERSISTENT FETAL VASCULATURE

Persistent fetal vasculature (PFV), formerly called *persistent hyperplastic primary vitreous,* includes a spectrum of manifestations caused by the persistence of various portions of the fetal hyaloid vascular system and associated fibrovascular tissue.

Pathogenesis

During development of the eye, the hyaloid artery extends from the optic disc to the posterior aspect of the lens; it sends branches into the vitreous and ramifies to form the posterior portion of the vascular capsule of the lens. The posterior portion of the hyaloid system normally regresses by the 7th fetal mo and the anterior portion regresses by the 8th fetal mo. Small remnants of the system, such as a tuft of tissue at the disc (Bergmeister papilla) or a tag of tissue on the posterior capsule of the lens (Mittendorf dot), are common findings in healthy persons. More-extensive remnants and associated complications constitute PFV. Two major forms are described, anterior PFV and posterior PFV. Variability is great, and mixed or intermediate forms occur.

Clinical Manifestations

The usual clinical feature of anterior PFV is the presence of a vascularized plaque of tissue on the back surface of the lens in an eye that is microphthalmic or slightly smaller than normal. The condition is usually unilateral and can occur in infants with no other abnormalities and no history of prematurity. The fibrovascular tissue tends to undergo gradual contracture. The ciliary processes become elongated, and the anterior chamber can become shallow. The lens usually is smaller than normal and may be clear but often develops cataracts and can swell or absorb fluid. Large or anomalous vessels of the iris may be present. The anterior chamber angle can have abnormalities. In time, the cornea can become cloudy.

Anterior PFV is usually noted in the 1st wk or mo of life. The most common presenting signs are leukocoria (white pupillary reflex), strabismus, and nystagmus. The course is usually progressive and the outcome poor. Major complications are spontaneous intraocular hemorrhage, swelling of the lens caused by rupture of the posterior capsule, and glaucoma. The eye might eventually deteriorate. The spectrum of posterior PFV includes fibroglial veils around the disc and macula, vitreous membranes and stalks containing hyaloid artery remnants projecting from the disc, and meridional retinal folds. Traction detachment of the retina can occur. Vision may be impaired, but the eye is usually retained.

Treatment

Surgery is performed in an effort to prevent complications, to preserve the eye and a reasonably good cosmetic appearance, and, in some cases, to salvage vision. Surgical treatment usually involves aspirating the lens and excising the abnormal tissue. If useful vision is to be attained, refractive correction and aggressive amblyopia therapy are required. In some cases, the affected eye is enucleated because distinguishing between this white mass and retinoblastoma can be difficult. Ultrasonography and CT are valuable diagnostic aids.

RETINOBLASTOMA

Retinoblastoma (Fig. 622-2, Chapter 496) is the most common primary malignant intraocular tumor of childhood. It occurs in approximately 1/15,000 live births; 250-300 new cases are diagnosed in the United States annually. Hereditary and nonhereditary patterns of transmission occur; there is no gender or race predilection. The hereditary form is usually bilateral and multifocal, whereas the nonhereditary form is generally unilateral and unifocal. About 15% of unilateral cases are hereditary. Bilateral cases often manifest earlier than unilateral cases. Unilateral tumors are often large by the time they are discovered. The average age at diagnosis is 15 mo for bilateral cases, compared with 25 mo for unilateral cases. It is unusual for a child to present

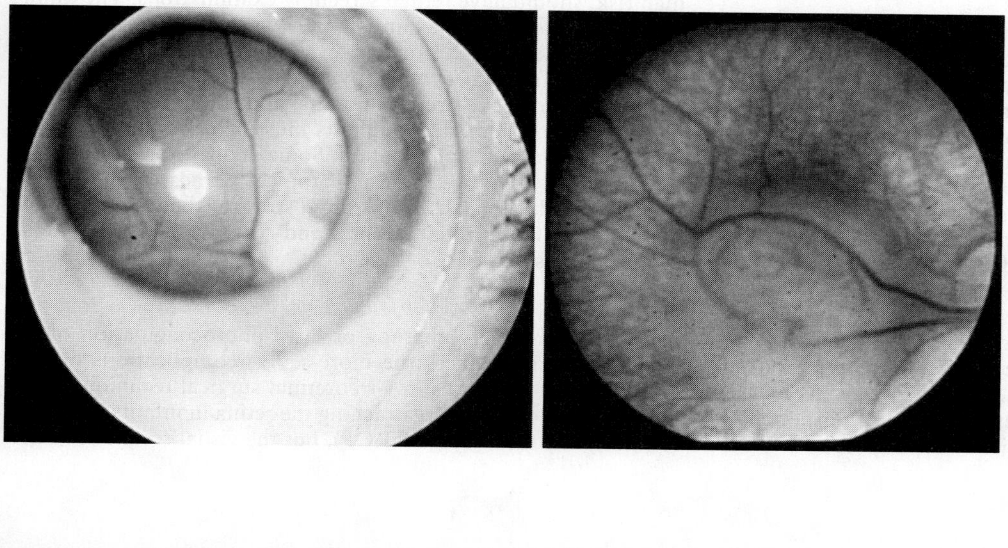

Figure 622-2 Retinoblastoma.

with a retinoblastoma after 3 yr of age. Rarely, the tumor is discovered at birth, during adolescence, or even in early adulthood.

Clinical Manifestations

The clinical manifestations of retinoblastoma vary, depending on the stage at which the tumor is detected. The initial sign in the majority of patients is a white pupillary reflex (leukocoria). Leukocoria results because of the reflection of light off the white tumor. The second most common initial sign of retinoblastoma is strabismus. Less-common presenting signs include pseudohypopyon (tumor cells layered inferiorly in front of the iris) caused by tumor seeding in the anterior chamber of the eye, hyphema (blood layered in front of the iris) secondary to iris neovascularization, vitreous hemorrhage, and signs of orbital cellulitis. On examination, the tumor appears as a white mass, sometimes small and relatively flat, sometimes large and protuberant. It might appear nodular. Vitreous haze or tumor seeding may be evident.

The retinoblastoma gene is a recessive suppressor gene located on chromosome 13 at the 13q14 region. Because of the hereditary nature of retinoblastoma, family members of affected children should undergo a complete ophthalmologic examination and genetic counseling. Newborn siblings and children of affected patients should be referred to an ophthalmologist shortly after birth, when the peripheral retina can be evaluated without the need for an examination under anesthesia.

Diagnosis

Diagnosis is made by direct observation by an experienced ophthalmologist. Ancillary testing such as CT or ultrasonography can help to confirm the diagnosis and demonstrate calcification within the mass. MRI can better detect the presence of an associated pinealblastoma (trilateral retinoblastoma). A definitive diagnosis occasionally cannot be made, and removal of the eye must be considered to avoid the possibility of lethal metastasis of the tumor. Because a biopsy can lead to spread of the tumor, histologic confirmation before enucleation is not possible in most cases. Therefore, removal of a blind eye in which the diagnosis of retinoblastoma is likely may be appropriate.

Treatment

Therapy varies, depending on the size and location of the tumor as well as whether it is unilateral or bilateral. Advanced tumors may be treated by enucleation. Other treatment modalities include external beam irradiation, radiation plaque therapy, laser or cryotherapy, and chemotherapy. Since the turn of the century there has been a dramatic shift in the treatment of retinoblastomas. Chemoreduction (systemic chemotherapy) followed by local therapies (laser, cryotherapy, and brachytherapy) have markedly reduced the use of external beam radiation and is a more vision-sparing technique. Children who are irradiated during their 1st year of life are 2-8 times more likely to develop second cancers as those irradiated after 1 yr of age. Patients treated with radiation tend to develop brain tumors and sarcomas of the head and neck. Secondary cataracts can also develop from radiation.

Nonocular secondary tumors are common in patients with germinal mutations estimated to occur with an incidence of 1% per year of life. The most common secondary tumors are osteogenic sarcoma of the skull and long bones.

The prognosis for children with retinoblastoma depends on the size and extension of the tumor. When confined to the eye, most tumors can be cured. The prognosis for long-term survival is poor when the tumor has extended into the orbit or along the optic nerve.

RETINITIS PIGMENTOSA

Retinitis pigmentosa (RP) is a progressive retinal degeneration characterized by pigmentary changes, arteriolar attenuation, usually some degree of optic atrophy, and progressive impairment of visual function. Dispersion and aggregation of the retinal pigment produce various ophthalmoscopically visible changes, ranging from granularity or mottling of the retinal pigment pattern to distinctive focal pigment aggregates with the configuration of bone spicules (Fig. 622-3). Other ocular findings include subcapsular cataract, glaucoma, and keratoconus.

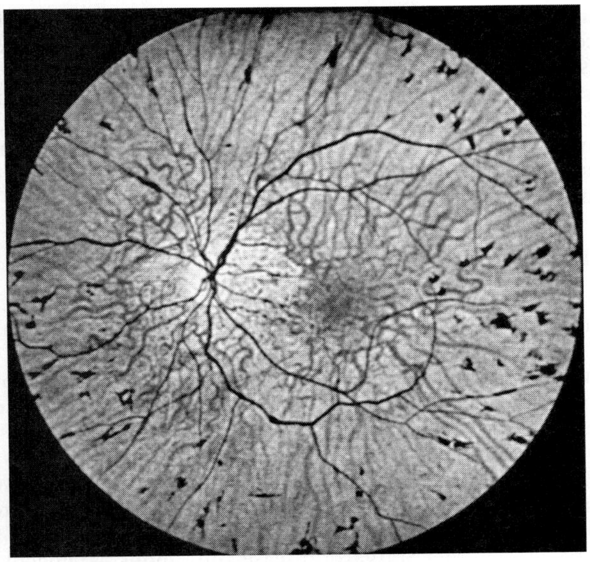

Figure 622-3 Retinitis pigmentosa.

Impairment of night vision or dark adaptation is often the first clinical manifestation noted in adolescents. Progressive loss of peripheral vision, often in the form of an expanding ring scotoma or concentric contraction of the field, is usual. There may be loss of central vision. Retinal function, as measured by electroretinography (ERG), is characteristically reduced. The disorder may be autosomal recessive, autosomal dominant, or X linked. There are >45 identified genes that account for only 60% of patients. These genes are involved in the phototransduction cascade, vitamin A metabolism, cytoskeletal structure, signaling or synaptic pathways, trafficking of intracellular proteins, maintenance of cilia, pH regulation, and phagocytosis. Children with autosomal recessive RP are more likely to become symptomatic at an earlier age (median age, 10.7 yr). Those with autosomal dominant RP are more likely to present in their 20s. Only supportive treatment is available. Vitamin A palmitate and omega-3–rich fish oil might slow disease progression.

A special form of RP is **Leber congenital retinal amaurosis (LCA)**, in which the retinal changes tend to be pleomorphic, with various degrees of pigment disorder, arteriolar attenuation, and optic atrophy. The retina can appear normal during infancy. Vision impairment, nystagmus, and poor pupillary reaction is usually evident soon after birth, and the ERG findings are abnormal early and confirm the diagnosis. LCA is caused by mutations in at least 13 genes. Type 2 LCA is seen in approximately 6% of patients and is due to a mutation in the *RPE65* gene, which produces 11-*cis*-retinal from all-*trans*-retinyl esters. Gene replacement therapy (subretinal injection) currently shows early promise for children affected with LCA type 2.

Clinically similar secondary pigmentary retinal degenerations that need to be differentiated from RP occur in a wide variety of metabolic diseases, neurodegenerative processes, and multifaceted syndromes. Examples include the progressive retinal changes of the mucopolysaccharidoses (particularly Hurler, Hunter, Scheie, and Sanfilippo syndromes) and certain of the late-onset gangliosidoses (Batten-Mayou, Spielmeyer-Vogt, and Jansky-Bielschowsky diseases), the progressive retinal degeneration that is associated with progressive external ophthalmoplegia

(Kearns-Sayre syndrome), and the RP-like changes in the Laurence-Moon and Bardet-Biedl syndromes. The retinal manifestations of abetalipoproteinemia (Bassen-Kornzweig syndrome) and Refsum disease are also similar to those found in RP. The diagnosis of these latter two disorders in a patient with presumed RP is important because treatment is possible. There is also an association of RP and congenital hearing loss, as in Usher syndrome (Chapters 80 and 82).

STARGARDT DISEASE (FUNDUS FLAVIMACULATUS)

Stargardt disease is an autosomal recessive retinal disorder characterized by slowly progressive bilateral macular degeneration and vision impairment. It usually appears at 8-14 yr of age and is often initially misdiagnosed as functional visual loss. The foveal reflex becomes obtunded or appears grayish, pigment spots develop in the macular area, and macular depigmentation and chorioretinal atrophy eventually occur. Macular hemorrhages can develop. Some patients also have white or yellow spots beyond the macula or pigmentary changes in the periphery; the term fundus flavimaculatus is commonly used for this condition. It is now recognized that Stargardt disease and fundus flavimaculatus represent different parts on the spectrum of the same disease. Central visual acuity is reduced, often to 20/200, but total loss of vision does not occur. ERG findings vary. The condition is not associated with central nervous system abnormalities and is to be differentiated from the macular changes of many progressive metabolic neurodegenerative diseases. The genetic mutation responsible for Stargardt macular dystrophy has been identified.

BEST VITELLIFORM DEGENERATION

Best vitelliform degeneration is a macular dystrophy characterized by a distinctive yellow or orange discoid subretinal lesion in the macula, resembling the intact yolk of a fried egg. Diagnosis is usually made at 3-15 yr of age, with a mean age of presentation of 6 yr. Vision is usually normal at this stage. The condition may be progressive; the yolklike lesion can eventually degenerate ("scramble") and result in pigmentation, chorioretinal atrophy, and vision impairment. The condition is usually bilateral. There is no association with systemic abnormalities. Inheritance is usually autosomal dominant. The vitelliform macular dystrophy gene *(VMD2)* has been identified and DNA testing is available. In vitelliform macular degeneration, the ERG response is normal. Electro-oculographic findings are abnormal in affected patients and carriers, and this test is useful in diagnosis and in genetic counseling.

CHERRY RED SPOT

Because of the special histologic features of the macula, certain pathologic processes affecting the retina produce an ophthalmoscopically visible sign referred to as a cherry red spot, a bright to dull red spot at the center of the macula surrounded and accentuated by a grayish-white or yellowish halo. The halo is a result of a loss of transparency of the retinal ganglion cell layer secondary to edema, lipid accumulation, or both. Because ganglion cells are not present in the fovea, the retina surrounding the fovea is opacified but the fovea transmits the normal underlying choroidal color (red), accounting for the presence of the cherry red spot. A cherry red spot typically occurs in certain sphingolipidoses, principally in Tay-Sachs disease (GM_2 type 1), in the Sandhoff variant (GM_2 type 2), and in generalized gangliosidosis (GM_1 type 1). Similar but less-distinctive macular changes occur in some cases of metachromatic leukodystrophy (sulfatide lipidosis), in some forms of neuronopathic Niemann-Pick disease, and in certain mucolipidoses (Chapters 80.4 and 80.5). The cherry red spot that characteristically occurs as a result of retinal ischemia secondary to vasospasm, ocular contusion, or occlusion of the central retinal artery must be differentiated from the cherry red spot of neurodegenerative disease.

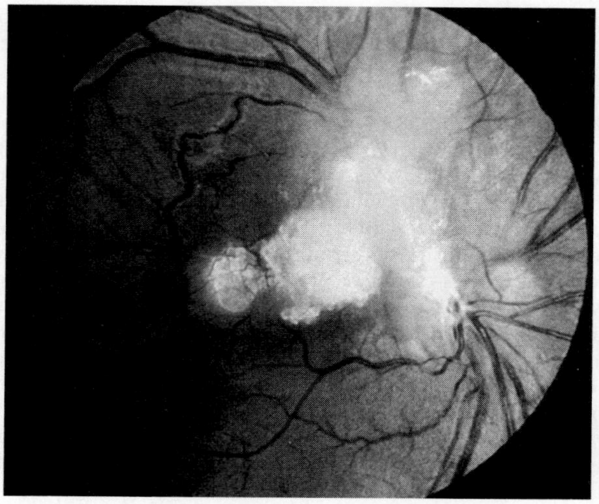

Figure 622-4 Retinal phakoma of tuberous sclerosis.

PHAKOMAS

Phakomas (Chapter 589) are the herald lesions of the hamartomatous disorders. In Bourneville disease (tuberous sclerosis), the distinctive ocular lesion is a refractile, yellowish, multinodular cystic lesion arising from the disc or retina; the appearance of this typical lesion is often compared with that of an unripe mulberry (Fig. 622-4). Equally characteristic and more common in tuberous sclerosis are flatter, yellow to whitish retinal lesions, varying in size from minute dots to large lesions approaching the size of the disc. These lesions are benign astrocytic proliferations. Rarely, similar retinal phakomas occur in von Recklinghausen disease (neurofibromatosis). In von Hippel-Lindau disease (angiomatosis of the retina and cerebellum), the distinctive fundus lesion is a hemangioblastoma; this vascular lesion usually appears as a reddish globular mass with large paired arteries and veins passing to and from the lesion. In Sturge-Weber syndrome (encephalofacial angiomatosis), the fundus abnormality is a choroidal hemangioma; the hemangioma can impart a dark color to the affected area of the fundus, but the lesion is best seen with fluorescein angiography.

RETINOSCHISIS

Congenital hereditary retinoschisis, also referred to as juvenile X-linked retinoschisis, is a bilateral vitreoretinal dystrophy that has a bimodal age of presentation. The first group presents with strabismus and nystagmus at a mean age of 1.5-2 yr and is the most severely affected group. The second group presents at 6-7 yr with poor vision. It is characterized by splitting of the retina into inner and outer layers. The usual ophthalmoscopic finding in affected boys is an elevation of the inner layer of the retina, most commonly in the inferotemporal quadrant of the fundus, often with round or oval holes visible in the inner layer. Schisis of the fovea is virtually pathognomonic and is found in almost 100% of patients. Ophthalmoscopically, this appears in early stages as small, fine striae in the internal limiting membrane. These striae radiate outward in a petaloid or spoke-wheel configuration. In some cases, frank retinal detachment or vitreous hemorrhage occurs.

Vision impairment varies from mild to severe; visual acuity can worsen with age, but good vision is often retained. Carrier females are asymptomatic, but linkage studies may be useful to help detect carriers.

RETINAL DETACHMENT

A retinal detachment is a separation of the outer layers of the retina from the underlying retinal pigment epithelium (RPE). During embryogenesis, the retina and RPE are initially separated. During ocular development, they join and are held in apposition to each other by various physiologic mechanisms. Pathologic events leading to a retinal detachment return the retina-RPE to its former separated state. The detachment can occur as a congenital anomaly but more commonly arises secondary to other ocular abnormalities or trauma.

Three types of detachment are described; each can occur in children. Rhegmatogenous detachments result from a break in the retina that allows fluid to enter the subretinal space. In children, these are usually a result of trauma (such as child abuse) but can occur secondary to myopia or ROP or after congenital cataract surgery. Tractional retinal detachments result when vitreoretinal membranes pull on the retina. They can occur in diabetes, sickle cell disease, and ROP. Exudative retinal detachments result when exudation exceeds absorption. This can be seen in Coats disease, retinoblastoma, and ocular inflammation.

The presenting sign of retinal detachment in an infant or child may be loss of vision, secondary strabismus or nystagmus, or leukocoria (white pupillary reflex). In addition to direct examination of the eye, special diagnostic studies such as ultrasonography and neuroimaging (CT, MRI) may be necessary to establish the cause of the detachment and the appropriate treatment. Prompt treatment is essential if vision is to be salvaged.

COATS DISEASE

Coats disease is an exudative retinopathy of unknown cause characterized by telangiectasia of retinal vessels with leakage of plasma to form intraretinal and subretinal exudates and by retinal hemorrhages and detachment (Fig. 622-5). The condition is usually unilateral. It predominantly affects boys, usually appearing in the 1st decade. The condition is nonfamilial and for the most part occurs in otherwise healthy children. The most common presenting signs are blurring of vision, leukocoria, and strabismus. Rubeosis of the iris, glaucoma, and cataract can develop. **Treatment** with photocoagulation or cryotherapy may be helpful.

FAMILIAL EXUDATIVE VITREORETINOPATHY

Familial exudative vitreoretinopathy (FEVR) is a progressive retinal vascular disorder of unknown cause, but clinical and angiographic findings suggest an aberration of vascular development. Avascularity of the peripheral temporal retina is a significant finding in most cases, with abrupt cessation of the retinal capillary network in the region of the equator. The avascular zone often has a wedge- or V-shaped pattern in the temporal meridian. Glial proliferation or well-marked retinochoroidal atrophy may be found in the avascular zone. Excessive branching of retinal arteries and veins, dilatation of the capillaries, arteriovenous shunt formation, neovascularization, and leakage from retinal vessels of the farthest vascularized retina occur. Vitreoretinal adhesions are usually present at the peripheral margin of the vascularized retina. Traction, retinal dragging and temporal displacement of the macula, falciform retinal folds, and retinal detachment are common. Intraretinal or subretinal exudation, retinal hemorrhage, and recurrent vitreous hemorrhages can develop. Patients can also develop cataracts and glaucoma. Vision impairment of varying severity occurs. The condition is usually bilateral. FEVR is usually an autosomal dominant condition with incomplete penetrance. Asymptomatic family members often display a zone of avascular peripheral retina.

The findings in FEVR can resemble those of ROP in the cicatricial stages, but unlike ROP, the neovascularization of FEVR seems to develop years after birth and most patients with FEVR have no history of prematurity, oxygen therapy, prenatal or postnatal injury or infection, or developmental abnormalities. FEVR is also to be differentiated from Coats disease, angiomatosis of the retina, peripheral uveitis, and other disorders of the posterior segment.

HYPERTENSIVE RETINOPATHY

In the early stages of hypertension, no retinal changes may be observable. Generalized constriction and irregular narrowing of the arterioles are usually the first signs in the fundus. Other alterations include retinal edema, flame-shaped hemorrhages, cotton-wool spots (retinal nerve fiber layer infarcts), and papilledema (Fig. 622-6). These changes are reversible if the hypertension can be controlled in the early stages, but in long-standing hypertension, changes may be irreversible. Thickening of the vessel wall can produce a silver- or copper-wire appearance. Hypertensive retinal changes in a child should alert the physician to renal disease, pheochromocytoma, collagen disease, and cardiovascular disorders, particularly coarctation of the aorta.

DIABETIC RETINOPATHY

The retinal changes of diabetes mellitus are classified as nonproliferative or proliferative. Nonproliferative diabetic retinopathy

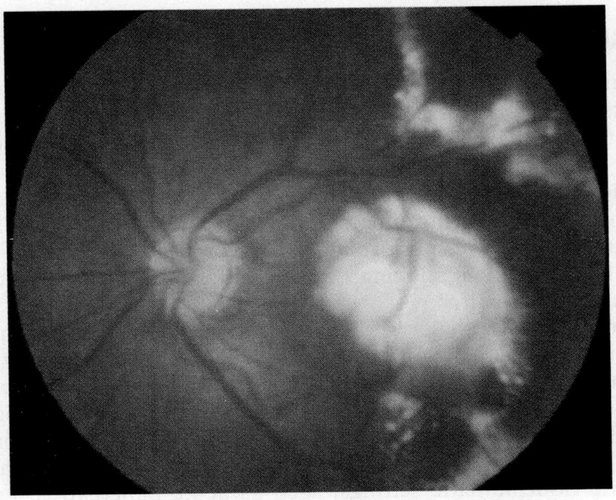

Figure 622-5 Coats disease with massive retinal exudation.

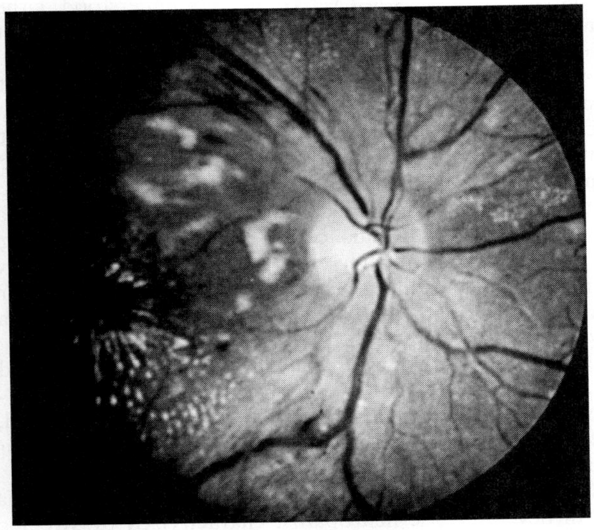

Figure 622-6 Hypertensive retinopathy.

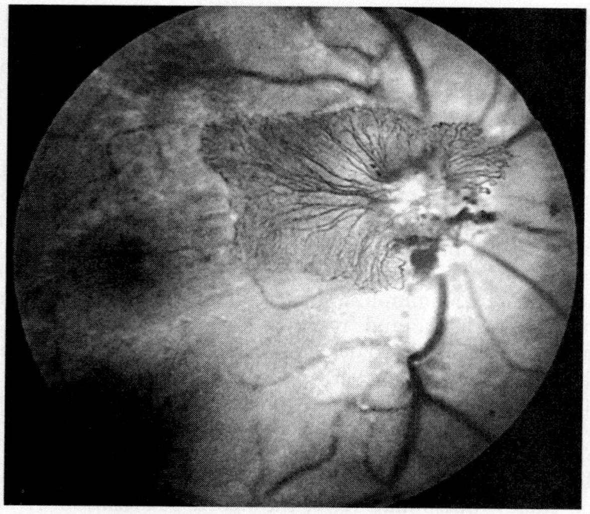

Figure 622-7 Proliferative diabetic retinopathy with neovascularization of the disc.

is characterized by retinal microaneurysms, venous dilatation, retinal hemorrhages, and exudates. The microaneurysms appear as tiny red dots. The hemorrhages may be of both the dot and blot type, representing deep intraretinal bleeding, and the splinter or flame-shaped type, involving the superficial nerve fiber layer. The exudates tend to be deep and to appear waxy. There may also be superficial nerve fiber infarcts called cytoid bodies or cotton-wool spots, as well as retinal edema. These signs may wax and wane. They are seen primarily in the posterior pole, around the disc and macula, well within the range of direct ophthalmoscopy. Involvement of the macula can lead to decreased vision.

Proliferative retinopathy, the more serious form, is characterized by neovascularization and proliferation of fibrovascular tissue on the retina, extending into the vitreous. Neovascularization can occur on the optic disc (NVD), elsewhere on the retina (NVE), or on the iris and in the anterior chamber angle (NVI, or rubeosis irides) (Fig. 622-7). Traction on these new vessels leads to hemorrhage and eventually scarring. The vision-threatening complications of proliferative diabetic retinopathy are retinal and vitreous hemorrhages, cicatrization, traction, and retinal detachment. Neovascularization of the iris can lead to secondary glaucoma if not treated promptly.

Diabetic retinopathy involves the alteration and nonperfusion of retinal capillaries, retinal ischemia, and neovascularization, but its pathogenesis is not yet completely understood, either in terms of location of the primary pathogenetic mechanism (retinal vessels vs surrounding neuronal or glial tissue) or the specific biochemical factors involved. The better the degree of long-term metabolic control, the lower the risk of diabetic retinopathy.

Clinically, the prevalence and course of retinopathy relate to a patient's age and to disease duration. Detectable microvascular changes are rare in prepubertal children, with the prevalence of retinopathy increasing significantly after puberty, especially after the age of 15 yr. The incidence of retinopathy is low during the first 5 yr of disease and increases progressively thereafter, with the incidence of proliferative retinopathy becoming substantial after 10 yr and with increased risk of visual impairment after 15 yr or more.

Ophthalmic examination guidelines have been proposed by the AAP. An initial exam is recommended at age 9 yr if the diabetes is poorly controlled. If the diabetes is well controlled, an initial exam 3 years after puberty with annual follow-up is recommended.

In addition to retinopathy, patients with juvenile-onset diabetes can develop optic neuropathy, characterized by swelling of the disc and blurring of vision. Patients with diabetes can also develop cataracts, even at an early age, sometimes with rapid progression.

Treatment

Macular edema is the leading cause of visual loss in diabetic persons. Photocoagulation may be used to decrease the risk of continued vision loss in patients with macular edema.

Proliferative retinopathy causes the most-severe vision loss and can lead to total loss of vision and even loss of the eye. Patients who have proliferative disease and who display certain high-risk characteristics should undergo panretinal photocoagulation to preserve their central vision. Neovascularization of the iris is also treated with panretinal photocoagulation to stop the development of neovascular glaucoma.

Vitrectomy and other intraocular surgery may be necessary in patients with nonresolving vitreous hemorrhage or traction retinal detachment. The value of technologic advances, such as insulin infusion pumps and pancreatic transplants, in preventing ocular complications is under investigation (Chapter 583).

SUBACUTE BACTERIAL ENDOCARDITIS

At some time during the course of the disease, retinopathy is present in approximately 40% of cases of subacute bacterial endocarditis. The lesions include hemorrhages, hemorrhages with white centers (Roth spots), papilledema, and, rarely, embolic occlusion of the central retinal artery.

BLOOD DISORDERS

In primary and secondary anemias, retinopathy in the form of hemorrhages and cotton-wool patches can occur. Vision can be affected if hemorrhage occurs in the macular area. The hemorrhages may be light and feathery or dense and preretinal. In polycythemia vera, the retinal veins are dark, dilated, and tortuous. Retinal hemorrhages, retinal edema, and papilledema may be observed. In leukemia, the veins are characteristically dilated, with sausage-shaped constrictions; hemorrhages, particularly white-centered hemorrhages and exudates, are common during the acute stage. In the sickling disorders, fundus changes include vascular tortuosity, arterial and venous occlusions, salmon patches, refractile deposits, pigmented lesions, arteriolar-venous anastomoses, and neovascularization (with sea-fan formations), sometimes leading to vitreous hemorrhage and retinal detachment. Patients with HbSC and HbS-β-thalassemia hemoglobinopathies are at a higher risk for developing retinopathy than are those with HbSS disease. It is thought that the more anemic state of patients with SS disease offers protection from vascular occlusions in the retina.

TRAUMA-RELATED RETINOPATHY

Retinal changes can occur in patients who suffer trauma to other parts of the body. The occurrence of retinal hemorrhages in infants who have been physically abused is well documented (Fig. 622-8; Chapter 37). Retinal, subretinal, subhyaloid, and vitreous hemorrhages have been described in infants and young children with inflicted neurotrauma. Often there are no signs of direct trauma to the eye, periocular region, or head. Such cases can result from violent shaking of an infant, and permanent retinal damage can result.

In patients with severe head or chest compressive trauma, a traumatic retinal angiopathy known as **Purtscher retinopathy** can occur. This is characterized by retinal hemorrhage, cotton-wool spots, possible disc swelling, and decreased vision. The pathogenesis is unclear, but there is evidence of arteriolar obstruction in this condition. A Purtscher-like fundus picture can also occur in several nontraumatic settings, such as acute pancreatitis, lupus erythematosus, and childbirth.

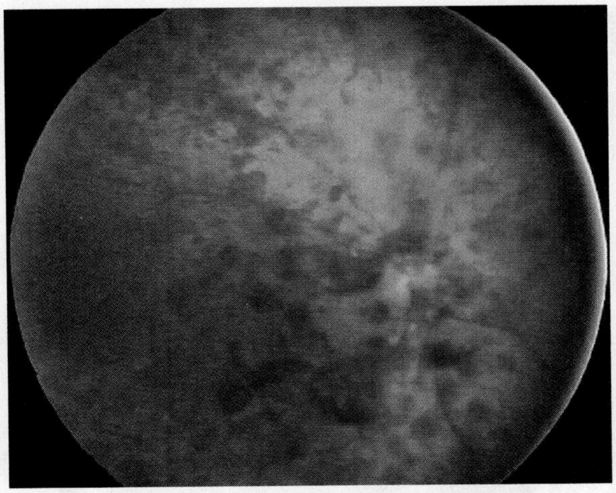

Figure 622-8 Shaken baby syndrome (inflicted neurotrauma). Retinal hemorrhages in multiple layers too numerous to count into far periphery.

MYELINATED NERVE FIBERS

Myelination of the optic nerve fibers normally terminates at the level of the disc, but in some children, ectopic myelination extends to nerve fibers of the retina. The condition is most commonly seen adjacent to the disc, although more peripheral areas of the retina may be involved. The characteristic ophthalmoscopic picture is a focal white patch with a feathered edge or brush-stroke appearance. Because the macula is generally unaffected, the visual prognosis is good. A relative or absolute visual field defect corresponding to areas of ectopic myelination is usually the only associated ocular abnormality. Extensive unilateral involvement, however, has been associated with ipsilateral myopia, amblyopia, and strabismus. If unilateral high myopia and amblyopia are present, appropriate optical correction and occlusion therapy should be instituted. For unknown reasons, the disorder is more commonly encountered in patients with craniofacial dysostosis, oxycephaly, neurofibromatosis, and Down syndrome.

COLOBOMA OF THE FUNDUS

The term *coloboma* describes a defect such as a gap, notch, fissure, or hole. The typical fundus coloboma is a result of malclosure of the embryonic fissure, which leaves a gap in the retina, RPE, and choroid, thus baring the underlying sclera. The defect may be extensive, involving the optic nerve, ciliary body, iris, and even lens, or it may be localized to 1 or more portions of the fissure. The usual appearance is of a well-circumscribed, wedge-shaped white area extending inferonasally below the disc, sometimes involving or engulfing the disc. In some cases, there is ectasia or cyst formation in the area of the defect. Less-extensive colobomatous defects might appear as only single or multiple focal punched-out chorioretinal defects or anomalous pigmentation of the fundus in the line of the embryonic fissure. Colobomas can occur in 1 or both eyes. A visual field defect usually corresponds to the chorioretinal defect. Visual acuity may be impaired, particularly if the defect involves the disc or macula.

Fundus colobomas can occur in isolation as sporadic defects or as an inherited condition. Isolated colobomatous anomalies are commonly inherited in an autosomal dominant manner with highly variable penetrance and expressivity. Family members of affected patients should receive appropriate genetic counseling. Colobomas may also be associated with such abnormalities as microphthalmia, glioneuroma of the eye, cyclopia, or encephale. They occur in children with various chromosomal disorders, including trisomies 13 and 18, triploidy, cat-eye syndrome, and 4p-. Ocular colobomas also occur in many multisystem disorders, including the CHARGE association (*c*oloboma, *h*eart disease, *a*tresia choanae, *r*etarded growth and development and/or central nervous system anomalies, *g*enetic anomalies and/or hypogonadism, *e*ar anomalies and/or deafness); Joubert, Aicardi, Meckel, Warburg, and Rubinstein-Taybi syndromes; linear sebaceous nevus; Goldenhar and Lenz microphthalmia syndromes; and Goltz focal dermal hypoplasia.

BIBLIOGRAPHY

Please visit the Nelson Textbook of Pediatrics *website at www.expertconsult.com for the complete bibliography.*

Chapter 623
Abnormalities of the Optic Nerve

Scott E. Olitsky, Denise Hug, Laura S. Plummer, and Merrill Stass-Isern

OPTIC NERVE APLASIA

Optic nerve aplasia is a rare congenital anomaly and is typically unilateral. The optic nerve, retinal ganglion cells, and retinal blood vessels are absent. A vestigial dural sheath usually connects with the sclera in a normal position, but no neural tissue is present within this sheath. Optic nerve aplasia typically occurs sporadically in an otherwise healthy person. A wide variety of ocular abnormalities can occur, but colobomas are the most common associated finding.

For the full continuation of this chapter, please visit the Nelson Textbook of Pediatrics *website at www.expertconsult.com.*

Chapter 624
Childhood Glaucoma

Scott E. Olitsky, Denise Hug, Laura S. Plummer, and Merrill Stass-Isern

Glaucoma is a general term used to indicate damage to the optic nerve with visual field loss that is caused by or related to elevated pressure within the eye. It is classified according to the age of the patient at presentation and the association of other ocular or systemic conditions. Glaucoma that begins within the first 3 yr of life is called *infantile* (congenital); glaucoma that begins between the ages of 3 and 30 yr is called *juvenile*.

Primary glaucoma indicates that the cause is an isolated anomaly of the drainage apparatus of the eye (trabecular meshwork). More than 50% of infantile glaucoma is primary. In secondary glaucoma, other ocular or systemic abnormalities are associated, even if a similar developmental defect of the trabecular meshwork is also present. Primary infantile glaucoma occurs with an incidence of 0.03% (see Table 624-1 on the *Nelson Textbook of pediatrics* website at www.expertconsult.com).

For the full continuation of this chapter, please visit the Nelson Textbook of Pediatrics *website at www.expertconsult.com.*

Chapter 625
Orbital Abnormalities

Scott E. Olitsky, Denise Hug, Laura S. Plummer, and Merrill Stass-Isern

HYPERTELORISM AND HYPOTELORISM

Hypertelorism is wide separation of the eyes or an increased interorbital distance, which can occur as a morphogenetic variant, a primary deformity, or a secondary phenomenon in association with developmental abnormalities, such as frontal meningocele or encephalocele or the persistence of a facial cleft. Often associated are strabismus, generally exotropia, and sometimes optic atrophy.

Hypotelorism refers to narrowness of the interorbital distance, which can occur as a morphogenetic variant alone or in association with other anomalies, such as epicanthus or holoprosencephaly or secondary to a cranial dystrophy, such as scaphocephaly.

EXOPHTHALMOS AND ENOPHTHALMOS

Protrusion of the eye is referred to as *exophthalmos* or proptosis and is a common indicator of orbital disease. It may be caused by shallowness of the orbits, as in many craniofacial malformations, or by increased tissue mass within the orbit, as with neoplastic, vascular, and inflammatory disorders. Ocular complications include exposure keratopathy, ocular motor disturbances, and optic atrophy with loss of vision.

Posterior displacement or sinking of the eye back into the orbit is referred to as *enophthalmos.* This can occur with orbital fracture or with atrophy of orbital tissue.

ORBITAL INFLAMMATION

Inflammatory disease involving the orbit may be primary or secondary to systemic disease. Idiopathic orbital inflammation (**orbital pseudotumor**) represents a wide spectrum of clinical entities. Symptoms at the time of presentation can include pain, eyelid swelling, proptosis, a red eye, and fever. The inflammation can involve a single extraocular muscle (myositis) or the entire orbit. Orbital apex syndrome is a serious condition that can also involve the cavernous sinus and can compress or displace the optic nerve. Confusion with orbital cellulitis is common but can be differentiated by the lack of associated sinus disease, its appearance on CT scan, and lack of improvement with systemic antibiotics. Orbital pseudotumor is associated with systemic lupus erythematosus, Crohn disease, myasthenia gravis, and lymphoma. **Treatment** includes the use of high-dose systemic corticosteroids. Often, the symptoms improve dramatically shortly after treatment is initiated. Bilateral involvement, associated uveitis, disc edema, and recurrence of inflammation are not uncommon in the pediatric population. Immunotherapy or radiation treatment may be necessary for resistant or recurrent cases.

Thyroid-related ophthalmopathy is thought to be secondary to an immune mechanism, leading to inflammation and deposition of mucopolysaccharides and collagen in the extraocular muscles and orbital fat. Involvement of the extraocular muscles can lead to a restrictive strabismus. Lid retraction and exophthalmos can cause corneal exposure and infection or perforation. Involvement of the posterior orbit can compress the optic nerve. Treatment of thyroid-related ophthalmopathy may include the use of systemic corticosteroids, radiation of the orbit, eyelid surgery, strabismus surgery, or orbital decompression to eliminate symptoms and protect vision. The degree of orbital involvement is often independent of the status of the systemic disease (Chapter 562).

Other systemic disorders that can cause inflammatory disease within the orbit include lymphoma, sarcoidosis, amyloidosis, polyarteritis nodosa, systemic lupus erythematosus, dermatomyositis, Wegener granulomatosis, and juvenile xanthogranuloma.

TUMORS OF THE ORBIT

Various tumors occur in and about the orbit in childhood. Among benign tumors, the most common are vascular lesions (principally hemangiomas) (Fig. 625-1) and dermoids. Among malignant neoplasms, rhabdomyosarcoma, lymphosarcoma, and metastatic neuroblastoma are the most common. Optic nerve gliomas are most often seen in patients with neurofibromatosis and can manifest with poor vision or proptosis. Retinoblastoma can extend into the orbit if it is discovered late or if it goes untreated. Teratomas are rare tumors that typically grow rapidly after birth and exhibit explosive proptosis.

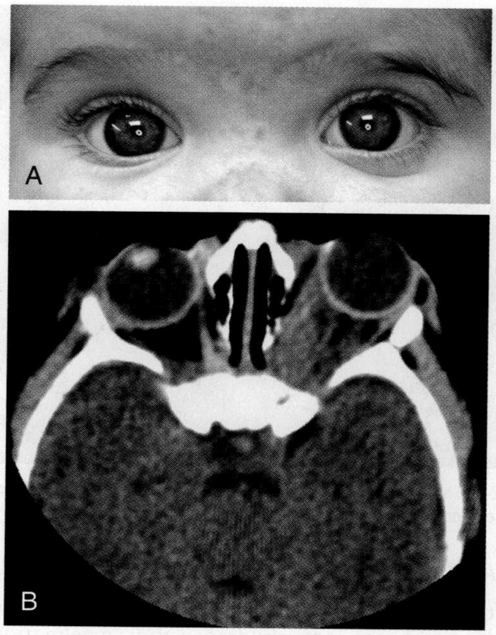

Figure 625-1 Orbital hemangioma. *A,* Note the proptosis. *B,* CT scan. (Courtesy of Amy Nopper, MD, and Brandon Newell, MD.)

The effects of orbital tumors vary with their locations and growth patterns. The principal signs are proptosis, resistance to retroplacement of the eye, and impairment of eye movement. A palpable mass may be found. Other significant signs are ptosis, optic nerve head congestion, optic atrophy, and loss of vision. Bruit and visible pulsation of the globe are important clues to vascular lesions.

Evaluation of orbital tumors includes ultrasonography, MRI, and CT. Pseudotumor of the orbit also must be considered in children with signs of a mass lesion. In selected cases, an incisional or excisional biopsy of the lesion may be warranted.

BIBLIOGRAPHY

Please visit the Nelson Textbook of Pediatrics *website at* *www.expertconsult.com* *for the complete bibliography.*

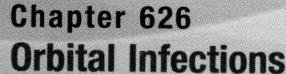

Chapter 626
Orbital Infections

Scott E. Olitsky, Denise Hug, Laura S. Plummer, and Merrill Stass-Isern

Orbital infections are common in children. It is important to be able to distinguish the different forms of infection that occur in the orbital region to allow rapid diagnosis and treatment to prevent loss of vision or spread of the infection to the nearby intracranial structures (see Table 618-1).

DACRYOADENITIS

Dacryoadenitis, or inflammation of the lacrimal gland, is uncommon in childhood. It can occur with mumps (in which case it is usually acute and bilateral, subsiding in a few days or weeks) or with infectious mononucleosis. *Staphylococcus aureus* can produce a suppurative dacryoadenitis. Chronic dacryoadenitis is associated with certain systemic diseases, particularly sarcoidosis, tuberculosis, and syphilis. Some systemic diseases produce enlargement of the lacrimal and salivary glands (Mikulicz syndrome).

DACRYOCYSTITIS

Dacryocystitis is an infection of the lacrimal sac. Dacryocystitis generally requires obstruction of the nasolacrimal system to allow its development. Acute dacryocystitis manifests with redness and swelling over the region of the lacrimal sac. It is treated with warm compresses and systemic antibiotics. This will help to control the infection, but the obstruction usually requires definitive treatment to reduce the risk of recurrence.

Dacryocystitis can occur in newborns as a complication of a congenital dacryocystocele. Systemic antibiotics and digital pressure for decompression are recommended. The obstruction of the nasolacrimal system can resolve once the infection clears. If spontaneous resolution does not occur, probing should be considered within a short time. An intranasal cyst may be present in conjunction with the dacryocystocele. If this occurs, marsupialization of the cyst may be needed at the time of the probing.

PRESEPTAL CELLULITIS

Inflammation of the lids and periorbital tissues without signs of true orbital involvement (such as proptosis or limitation of eye movement) is generally referred to as periorbital or preseptal cellulitis and is a form of facial cellulitis. This is common in young children and may be caused by bacteremia, trauma, an infected wound, or an abscess of the lid or periorbital region (pyoderma, hordeolum, conjunctivitis, dacryocystitis, insect bite). Patients present with eyelid swelling; the edema may be so intense as to make it difficult to evaluate the globe. Prior to the *Haemophilus influenzae* type B vaccine, the most common cause of pediatric preseptal (facial) cellulitis was bacteremia due to *H. influenzae* type B. Group A streptococcal infection a common is cause. Clinical examination shows lack of proptosis, normal ocular movement, and normal pupil function. CT examination demonstrates edema of the lids and subcutaneous tissues anterior to the orbital septum (Fig. 626-1). Antibiotic therapy and careful monitoring for signs of sepsis and local progression are essential.

ORBITAL CELLULITIS

Orbital cellulitis is a condition involving inflammation of the tissues of the orbit, with proptosis, limitation of movement of the eye, edema of the conjunctiva (chemosis), and inflammation and swelling of the eyelids with potentially decreased visual acuity. The mean age is about 7 yr but the range is 10 mo-18 yr. Patients often feel ill with general symptoms of toxicity, fever, and leukocytosis.

Orbital cellulitis can follow direct infection of the orbit from a wound, metastatic deposition of organisms during bacteremia, or **more often** direct extension or venous spread of infection from contiguous sites such as the lids, conjunctiva, globe, lacrimal gland, nasolacrimal sac, or **more commonly** the paranasal (ethmoid) sinuses (Table 626-1). In some cases, primary or metastatic tumor in the orbit can produce the clinical picture of orbital cellulitis. The most common cause of orbital cellulitis in children is paranasal sinusitis. The spread of infection to the orbit from the sinuses is more prevalent in children because of their thinner bony septa and sinus wall, greater porosity of bones, open suture lines, and larger vascular foramina. The spread of infection is also facilitated by the venous and lymphatic communication between the sinuses and surrounding structures, which allow flow in either direction, facilitating retrograde thrombophlebitis. Common pathogenic organisms include *Staphylococcus* species, including methicillin-resistant *S. aureus* (MRSA), *Streptococcus* species, and *Haemophilus* species.

The potential for complications is great. Vision loss can occur secondary to an increase in orbital pressure that causes retinal artery occlusion or optic neuritis. This is more likely to occur in the presence of an orbital abscess. Extension of infection from the orbit into the cranial cavity can lead to cavernous sinus thrombosis or meningitis, epidural or subdural empyema, or brain abscesses (see Table 626-1).

Orbital cellulitis must be recognized promptly and treated aggressively. Hospitalization and systemic antibiotic therapy are usually indicated. All patients require CT imaging of the orbit (including the surrounding CNS), preferably with intravenous contrast to detect a subperiosteal abscess, orbital abscess, or intracranial extension. Parenteral antibiotics must be started immediately. Antimicrobial agents that generally provide coverage for methicillin-sensitive *S. aureus* as well as aerobic and anaerobic sinus-derived bacteria include vancomycin and a third-generation cephalosporin (cefotaxime, ceftriaxone), and amoxicillin or ticarcillin combined with a β-lactamase inhibitor (clavulanic acid). Metronidazole may be administered in

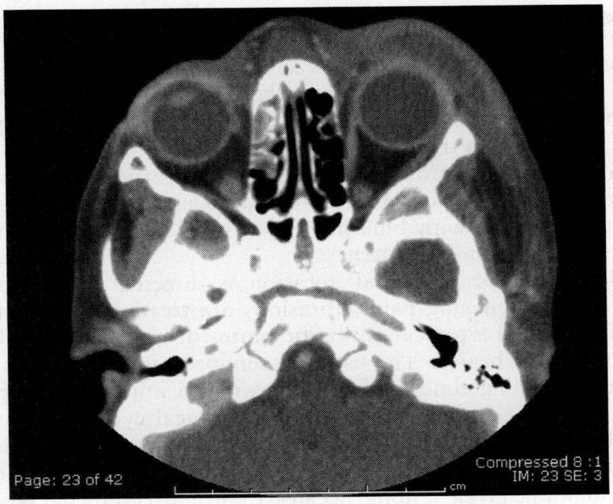

Figure 626-1 CT scan of a patient with preseptal cellulitis.

Table 626-1 CHANDLER CLASSIFICATION OF ORBITAL COMPLICATIONS OF SINUSITIS, A CLINICAL DESCRIPTION

CHANDLER CLASS	STAGE	CLINICAL DESCRIPTION AND DEFINITION
I	Inflammatory edema	Eyelid edema and erythema
		Normal extraocular movement
		Normal visual acuity
II	Orbital cellulitis	Diffuse edema of orbital contents without discrete abscess formation
III	Subperiosteal abscess	Collection of purulent exudate* beneath periosteum of lamina papyracea
		Displacement of globe downward/laterally
IV	Orbital abscess	Purulent collection within orbit*
		Proptosis
		Chemosis
		Ophthalmoplegia
		Decreased vision
V	Cavernous sinus thrombosis	Bilateral eye findings
		Prostration
		Meningismus

*The radiographic correlation of a subperiosteal or orbital abscess seen with CT is a contrast-enhancing mass in the extraconal or intraconal space, possibly with areas of cavitation, because purulence cannot be determined with CT scanning.

From Rudloe TF, Harper M, Prabhu SP, et al: Acute periorbital infections: who needs emergent imaging? *Pediatrics* 125:e719–e726, 2010.

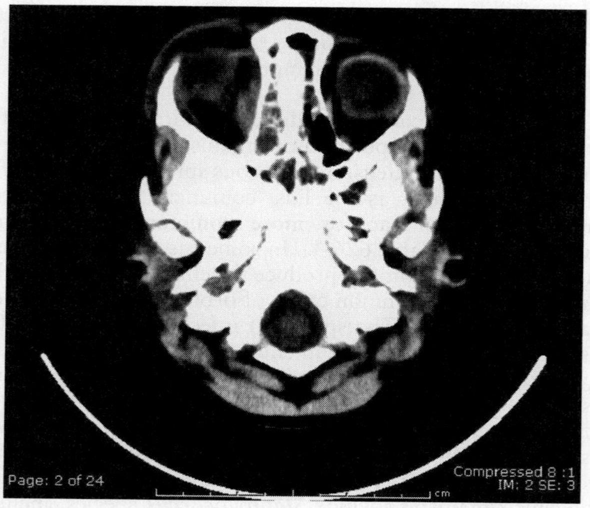

Figure 626-2 CT scan demonstrating a subperiosteal abscess along the medial wall of the orbit.

combination with an agent effective against aerobic or facultative streptococci and *S. aureus* if anaerobes are suspected or in the presence of intracranial extension. If there is no evidence of improvement or if there are signs of progression, sinus drainage may be required. An orbital or subperiosteal abscess (Fig. 626-2) can require urgent drainage of the orbit. The clinical presentation and course of each individual patient should dictate the need and timing of abscess drainage. The use of adjunctive corticosteroids and anticoagulation for cavernous venous thrombosis and or superior ophthalmic vein thrombosis is controversial.

BIBLIOGRAPHY

Please visit the Nelson Textbook of Pediatrics *website at* *www.expertconsult.com* *for the complete bibliography.*

Chapter 627

Injuries to the Eye

Scott E. Olitsky, Denise Hug, Laura S. Plummer, and Merrill Stass-Isern

About 30% of all blindness in children results from trauma. Children and adolescents account for a disproportionate number of episodes of ocular trauma. Boys ages 11-15 yr are the most vulnerable; their injuries outnumber those in girls by a ratio of about 4 : 1. The majority of injuries are related to sports, toy darts, other projectiles, sticks, stones, fireworks, paint balls, and air-powered BB guns. The last causes particularly devastating ocular and orbital injuries. Much of the trauma is avoidable (Chapter 5.1). Any part of the orbit or globe may be affected (Fig. 627-1).

ECCHYMOSIS AND SWELLING OF THE EYELIDS

Ecchymosis and edema of the eyelids is common after blunt trauma. These are self-limiting, absorb spontaneously, and can be treated with iced compresses and analgesics. Periorbital ecchymosis should prompt careful examination of the eye and surrounding structures for more-serious injury such as orbital bone fracture, intraocular hemorrhage, or rupture of the globe.

LACERATIONS OF THE EYELIDS

Eyelid lacerations can vary from simple to complex. When evaluating an eyelid laceration, key findings include depth of the laceration, its location, and whether there is involvement of the canaliculus. Most superficial eyelid lacerations may be closed by the primary caregiver, but if it is deep, involves the lid margin, or involves the canaliculus the laceration should be evaluated by an ophthalmologist. The levator muscle is responsible for elevation of the eyelid and runs deep to the skin and orbicularis oculi muscle. If the levator muscle is compromised and this is not recognized at initial repair, ptosis will occur. Therefore, if orbital fat is visible in the laceration, the laceration has compromised the skin, orbicularis oculi, levator, and orbital septum and must be meticulously repaired to prevent ptosis. Eyelid margin involvement also requires careful repair to avoid lid malpostition and notch formation. These can lead to ocular surface problems in the future, resulting in corneal scarring and loss of vision. Lacerations involving the canaliculus require intubation of the nasolacrimal system in addition to repair of the laceration to prevent future tearing problems. Proper primary repair of eyelid lacerations often achieves an outcome superior to secondary repair at a later date. As with any eyelid injury, careful examination of the eye and surrounding tissue is required.

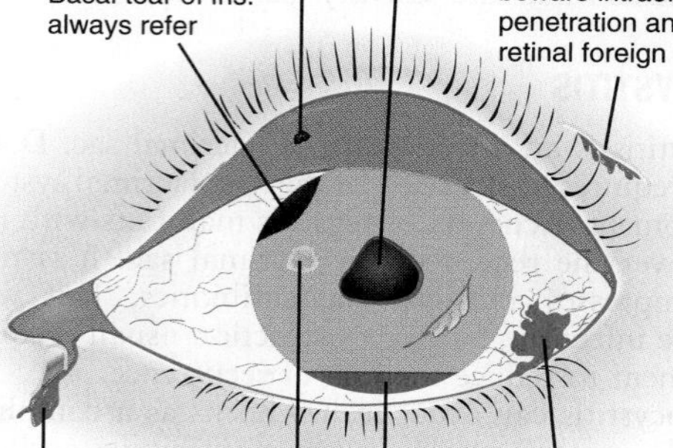

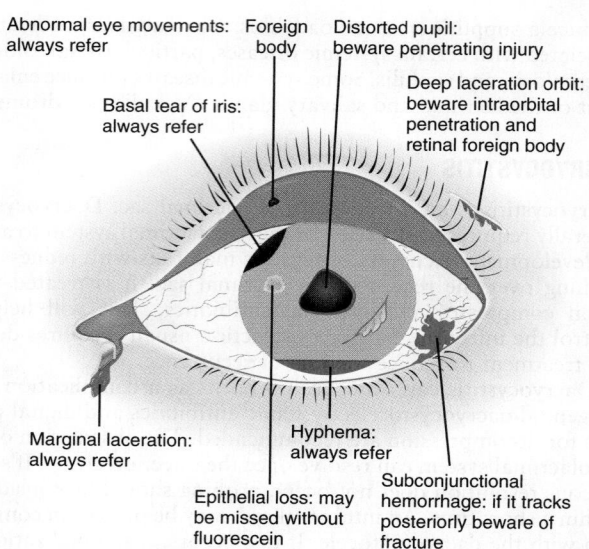

Figure 627-1 The injured eye. (From Khaw PT, Shah P, Elkington AR: Injury to the eye, *BMJ* 328:36–38, 2004.)

SUPERFICIAL ABRASIONS OF THE CORNEA

When the corneal epithelium is scratched, abraded, or denuded, it exposes the underlying epithelial basement layer and superficial corneal nerves. This is accompanied by pain, tearing, photophobia, and decreased vision. Corneal abrasions are detected by instilling fluorescein dye and inspecting the cornea using a blue-filtered light. A slit lamp is ideal for this examination, but a direct ophthalmoscope with blue filter or a hand-held Wood lamp is adequate for young children.

Treatment of a corneal abrasion is directed at promoting healing and relieving pain. Abrasions are treated with frequent applications of a topical antibiotic ointment until the epithelium is completely healed. The use of a semipressure patch does not improve healing time or decrease pain. An improperly applied patch can itself abrade the cornea. A topical cycloplegic agent (cyclopentolate hydrochloride 1%) can relieve the pain from ciliary spasm in patients with large abrasions. Topical anesthetics should not be given at home because they retard epithelial healing and inhibit the natural blinking reflex.

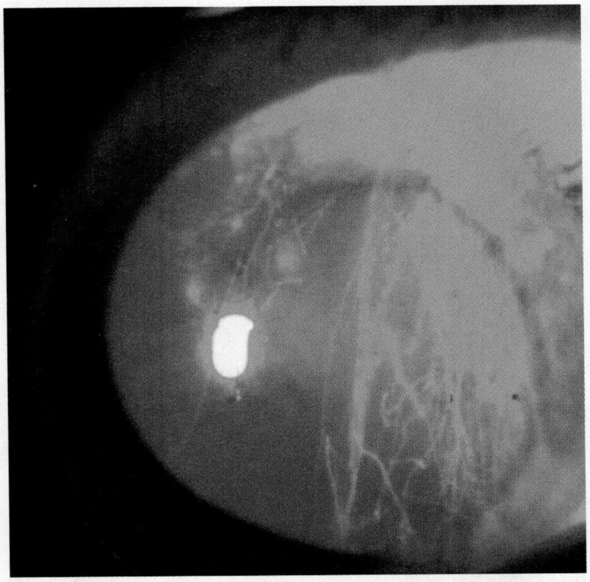

Figure 627-2 Vertically oriented linear corneal abrasions secondary to a foreign body underneath the upper eyelid.

FOREIGN BODY INVOLVING THE OCULAR SURFACE

A foreign body usually produces acute discomfort, lacrimation, and inflammation. Most foreign bodies can be detected by examination in good light with the aid of magnification or a direct ophthalmoscope set on a high plus lens (+10 or +12). In many cases, slit-lamp examination is necessary, especially if the particle is deep or metallic. Some conjunctival foreign bodies tend to lodge under the upper eyelid, causing the sensation of corneal foreign body as they come into contact with the globe on eyelid movement; they can also produce vertically oriented linear corneal abrasions (Fig. 627-2). Finding these abrasions should lead to a suspicion of such a foreign body, and eversion of the lid may be necessary (Chapter 611). If a foreign body is suspected but not found, further examination is indicated. If the history suggests injury with a high-velocity particle, radiologic examination of the eye may be needed to explore the possibility of an intraocular foreign body.

Removal of a foreign body can be facilitated by instillation of a drop of topical anesthetic. Many foreign bodies can be removed by irrigating or by gently wiping them away with a moistened cotton-tipped applicator. Embedded foreign bodies or foreign bodies in the central cornea should be treated by an ophthalmologist. Removal of corneal foreign bodies can leave epithelial defects, which are treated as corneal abrasions. Metallic foreign bodies can cause rust to form in the corneal tissues; examination by an ophthalmologist 1 or 2 days after removal of a foreign body is recommended because a rust ring might require further treatment (curettage).

HYPHEMA

Hyphema is the presence of blood in the anterior chamber of the eye. It can occur with either a blunt or perforating injury and represents a potential vision-threatening situation. Hyphema appears as a bright or dark red fluid level between the cornea and iris or as a diffuse murkiness of the aqueous humor. Children with hyphema present with acute loss of vision and pain.

The treatment of hyphema involves efforts to minimize the vision-threatening sequelae such as rebleeding, glaucoma, and corneal blood staining. The patient is put on bed rest with elevation of the head of the bed to 30 degrees. A shield is placed on the affected eye, and a cycloplegic agent is used to immobilize the iris. Additionally, topical or systemic steroids are used to minimize intraocular inflammation. Antiemetics should be considered if the patient is experiencing nausea. All nonsteroidal anti-inflammatories and aspirin must be avoided. Rarely, hospitalization and sedation are necessary to ensure compliance in some children. If the intraocular pressure is elevated, topical and systemic pressure lowering medications are used. If the pressure is not controllable by such measures, then surgical evacuation of the clot may be required to minimize the risk of permanent vision loss.

Patients with sickle cell disease or trait are at higher risk of acute loss of vision secondary to elevated intraocular pressure or optic nerve infarction and can require more-aggressive intervention. Patients with a history of traumatic hyphema have an increased incidence of glaucoma later in life and should be monitored on a regular basis throughout their life.

OPEN GLOBE

A penetrating, perforating, or blunt injury resulting in compromise of the cornea or sclera of the eye is one of the most sight-threatening injuries that can be sustained. This is known as an *open globe*. An open globe is a true ophthalmologic emergency that requires prompt, careful evaluation and immediate repair to minimize vision loss. Permanent vision loss can result from corneal scarring, loss of intraocular contents, or infection. Evaluation involves careful history including time and mechanism of the injury, as well as tests of visual acuity and inspection of the eye. A full-thickness corneal wound often has prolapse of iris tissue though the wound. If this is not immediately evident, a peaked or irregular pupil may be seen. Scleral compromise may be more difficult to identify because of overlying structures. The thinnest part of the sclera is at the corneoscleral junction (the limbus) and just posterior to the insertion of the rectus muscles. When an open globe is caused by blunt force injury, these are the 2 areas most likely involved. The overlying conjunctiva might not be compromised but a subconjunctival hemorrhage may be present, obscuring the view. In these cases, look for a shallow anterior chamber, low intraocular pressure, or pigment within the involved area. If an open globe is diagnosed, the examination should be stopped, an eye shield should be placed immediately, and the ophthalmologist should be contacted to minimize further ocular compromise.

OPTIC NERVE TRAUMA

The optic nerve may be injured in penetrating of blunt trauma. The injury can occur at any point between the globe and the chiasm. Traumatic injury to the optic nerve, regardless of cause or location, results in reduced vision and a pupillary defect. Direct trauma to the intraorbital optic nerve can cause transection, partial transection, or optic sheath hemorrhage. Fractures involving the skull base can cause injury to the intracranial portions of the optic nerve. Treatment decisions are difficult because there are no universally accepted guidelines, and prognosis for good visual outcome is often poor.

Medical management involves observation and using high-dose corticosteroids, although corticosteroids have not been shown to improve visual outcomes. Surgical intervention involves optic nerve sheath decompression for nerve sheath hemorrhages. If compression of optic nerve is secondary to orbital hemorrhage, prompt lateral canthotomy and cantholysis should be performed to relieve intraorbital pressure. Decompression of the optic canal may be performed if there is compression of the optic nerve by bone fragment. Optic canal decompression is controversial in the absence of direct bone decompression.

CHEMICAL INJURIES

Chemical burns of the cornea and adnexal tissue are among the most urgent of ocular emergencies. Alkali burns are usually more destructive than acid burns because they react with fats to form soaps, which damage cell membranes, allowing further penetration of the alkali into the eye. Acids generally cause less-severe, more-localized tissue damage. The corneal epithelium offers moderate protection against weak acids, and little damage occurs unless the pH is 2.5 or less. Most stronger acids precipitate tissue proteins, creating a physical barrier against their further penetration.

Mild acid or alkali burns are characterized by conjunctival injection and swelling and mild corneal epithelial erosions. The corneal stroma may be mildly edematous, and the anterior chamber can have mild to moderate cell and flare reactions. With strong acids, the cornea and conjunctiva rapidly become white and opaque. The corneal epithelium can slough, leaving a relatively clear stroma; this appearance can initially mask the severity of the burn. Severe alkali burns are characterized by corneal opacification.

Emergency treatment of a chemical burn begins with copious immediate irrigation with water or saline. Local debridement and removal of foreign particles should be performed while still irrigating. If the nature of the chemical injury is unknown, the use of pH test paper is helpful in determining whether the agent was basic or acidic. Irrigation should continue for at least 30 min or until 2 L of irrigant has been instilled in mild cases and for 2-4 hr or until 10 L of irrigant has been instilled in severe cases. At the end of irrigation, the pH should be within a normal range (7.3-7.7). The pH should be checked again approximately 30 min after irrigation to ensure that it has not changed. The goal of treatment is to minimize vision-threatening sequelae such as conjunctival scarring, corneal scarring and opacification, glaucoma, cataract, vision loss, and phthisis.

ORBITAL FRACTURES

The orbit is the bony structure surrounding the eye. Any of these bones can fracture in a traumatic incident. Superior and lateral wall fractures are the least common of the fracture sites, but superior orbital fracture is the most significant because of the potential of intracranial injury. The medial wall of the orbit is very susceptible to fracture because of the thin nature of the lamina papyracea. Perhaps the most common site of fracture from blunt trauma is the orbital floor. This is often referred to as *blow-out fracture*. At times, the fracture acts as a trapdoor, entrapping orbital contents within the fracture site.

The patient often presents with recent history of periorbital trauma and pain. Diplopia, eyelid swelling, eye movement restriction, and hypesthesia might or might not be present. A complete ophthalmic exam including history of injury, visual acuity, pupils, ocular alignment and motility, anterior segment, and fundus is required because there are often accompanying ocular injuries. Fracture is suspected if the eye is misaligned, movement is restricted, or the eye is sunken. The diagnosis is verified by orbital CT scan.

Medical management includes iced compresses to the orbit and elevation for the head of the bed for the first 24-48 hr. Broad-spectrum antibiotics are sometimes recommended for 14 days because of the exposure of the orbital contents to the sinus cavity. In medial wall fractures, the patient should be instructed not to blow the nose so as to prevent orbital emphysema and subsequent optic nerve compression.

Consider neurosurgical consultation in orbital roof fractures. Indications for surgical repair of orbital fractures are diplopia in primary or downgaze that persists for 2 weeks, enophthalmos, or fracture of the orbital floor involving >50% of the floor. Extraocular muscle entrapment often requires prompt surgical repair because these patients have significant pain, nausea, and vomiting that is difficult to control. Rarely, extraocular muscle entrapment can cause the activation of the oculocardiac reflex, requiring urgent fracture repair.

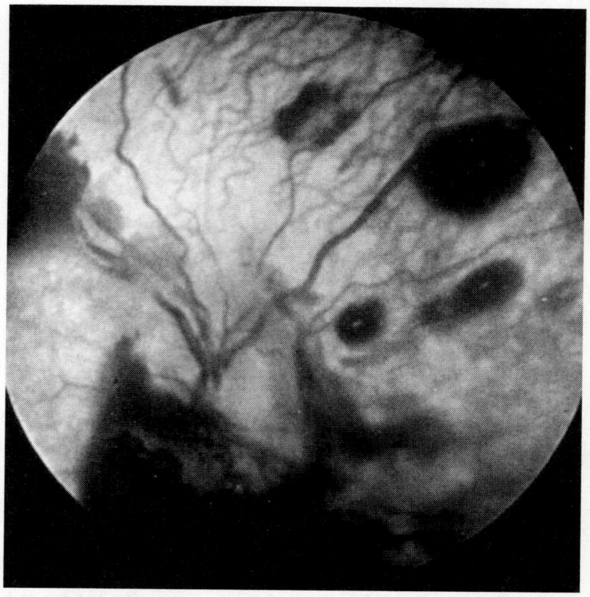

Figure 627-3 Retinal hemorrhages in an abused child with subdural hematoma.

PENETRATING WOUNDS OF THE ORBIT

Penetrating wounds demand careful evaluation for possible damage to the eye, the optic nerve, or the brain. Examination should include investigation for retained foreign body. Orbital hemorrhage and infection are common with penetrating wounds of the orbit; such injuries must be treated as emergencies.

CHILD ABUSE

Child abuse (Chapter 37) is a major cause of injuries to the eye and orbital region. The possibility of nonaccidental trauma must be considered in any child with ecchymosis or laceration of the lids, hemorrhage in or about the eye, cataract or dislocated lens, retinal detachment, or fracture of the orbit. Inflicted childhood neurotrauma (shaken baby syndrome) occurs secondary to violent, nonaccidental, repetitive, unrestrained acceleration-deceleration head and neck movements, with or without blunt head trauma, in children typically <3 yr of age. Inflicted childhood neurotrauma accounts for approximately 10% of all cases of child abuse and carries a mortality rate of up to 25%. Detection of abuse is not only important in order to treat the pathology that is discovered but also to prevent further abuse or even death. The ocular manifestations are numerous and can have a prominent role in recognition of this syndrome. Retinal hemorrhage is the most common ophthalmic finding and occurs at all levels of the retina. The pattern of hemorrhage helps to distinguish this disorder from other causes of retinal hemorrhage or from accidental injuries (Fig. 627-3). Retinal hemorrhages can occur without associated intracranial pathology.

FIREWORKS-RELATED INJURIES

Injuries related to the use of fireworks can be the most devastating of all ocular traumas that occur in children. At least 20% of emergency department visits for fireworks-related injuries are for ocular trauma. In the United States, a majority of these injuries take place around Independence Day, and most occur despite adult supervision.

SPORTS-RELATED OCULAR INJURIES AND THEIR PREVENTION

Although sports injuries occur in all age groups, far more children and adolescents participate in high-risk sports than do adults.

The greater number of participating children, their athletic immaturity, and the increased likelihood of their using inadequate or improper eye protection account for their disproportionate share of sports-related eye injuries (Chapters 680 and 684).

The sports with the highest risk of eye injury are those in which no eye protection can be worn, including boxing, wrestling, and martial arts. High-risk sports include those that use a rapidly moving ball or puck, bat, stick, racquet, or arrow (baseball, hockey, lacrosse, racquet sports, and archery) or involve aggressive body contact (football and basketball). Related to both risk and frequency of participation, the highest percentage of eye injuries are in basketball and baseball.

Protective eyewear, designed for a specific activity, is available for most sports. For basketball, racquet sports, and other recreational activities that do not require a helmet or face mask, molded polycarbonate sports goggles that are secured to the head by an elastic strap are suggested. For hockey, football, lacrosse, and baseball (batter), specific helmets with polycarbonate face shields and guards are available. Children should also wear sports goggles under the helmets. For baseball, goggles and helmets should be worn for batting, catching, and base running; goggles alone are usually sufficient for other positions.

BIBLIOGRAPHY

Please visit the Nelson Textbook of Pediatrics *website at* *www.expertconsult.com* *for the complete bibliography.*

PART XXX The Ear

Chapter 628
General Considerations and Evaluation
Joseph Haddad, Jr.

CLINICAL MANIFESTATIONS

Diseases of the ear and temporal bone commonly manifest with one or more of eight clinical signs and symptoms.

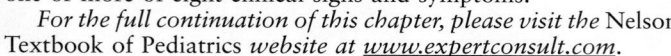

For the full continuation of this chapter, please visit the Nelson Textbook of Pediatrics *website at www.expertconsult.com.*

Chapter 629
Hearing Loss
Joseph Haddad, Jr.

INCIDENCE AND PREVALENCE

Bilateral neural hearing loss is categorized as mild (20-30 dB), moderate (30-50 dB), severe (50-70 dB), or profound (>70 dB). An estimated 278 million people worldwide have moderate or worse hearing loss; an additional 364 million people have mild hearing loss. In the USA, the average incidence of neonatal hearing loss is 1.1/1,000 infants; the rate by state varies from 0.22 to 3.61/1,000. Among children and adolescents, the rate of mild or greater hearing loss is 3.1% and is higher among Latin Americans, African Americans, and persons from lower-income families.

The onset of hearing loss can occur at any time in childhood. When less severe hearing loss or the transient hearing loss that commonly accompanies middle-ear disease in young children is considered, the number of affected children increases substantially.

TYPES OF HEARING LOSS

Hearing loss can be peripheral or central in origin. Peripheral hearing loss can be conductive, sensorineural, or mixed. **conductive hearing loss (CHL)** commonly is caused by dysfunction in the transmission of sound through the external or middle ear or by abnormal transduction of sound energy into neural activity in the inner ear and the 8th nerve. CHL is the most common type of hearing loss in children and occurs when sound transmission is physically impeded in the external and/or middle ear. Common causes of CHL in the *ear canal* include atresia or stenosis, impacted cerumen, or foreign bodies. In the *middle ear*, perforation of the tympanic membrane (TM), discontinuity or fixation of the ossicular chain, otitis media (OM) with effusion, otosclerosis, and cholesteatoma can cause CHL.

Damage to or maldevelopment of structures in the inner ear can cause **sensorineural hearing loss (SNHL).** Causes include hair cell destruction from noise, disease, or ototoxic agents; cochlear malformation; perilymphatic fistula of the round or oval window membrane; and lesions of the acoustic division of the 8th nerve. A combination of CHL and SNHL is considered a **mixed hearing loss.**

An auditory deficit originating along the central auditory nervous system pathways from the proximal 8th nerve to the cerebral cortex usually is considered **central** (or **retrocochlear) hearing loss.** Tumors or demyelinating disease of the 8th nerve and cerebellopontine angle can cause hearing deficits but spare the outer, middle, and inner ear. These causes of hearing loss are rare in children. Other forms of central auditory deficits, known as **central auditory processing disorders,** include those that make it difficult even for children with normal hearing to listen selectively in the presence of noise, to combine information from the two ears properly, to process speech when it is slightly degraded, and to integrate auditory information when it is delivered faster although they can process it when delivered at a slow rate. These deficits can manifest as poor attention or as academic or behavior problems in school. Strategies for coping with such disorders are available for older children, and identification and documentation of the central auditory processing disorder often is valuable so that parents and teachers can make appropriate accommodations to enhance learning.

ETIOLOGY

The etiology of a hearing impairment depends on whether the hearing loss is conductive or sensorineural. Most CHL is acquired, with middle ear fluid the most common cause. Congenital causes include anomalies of the pinna, external ear canal, TM, and ossicles. Rarely, congenital cholesteatoma or other masses in the middle ear manifest as CHL. TM perforation (e.g., trauma, OM), ossicular discontinuity (e.g., infection, cholesteatoma, trauma), tympanosclerosis, acquired cholesteatoma, or masses in the ear canal or middle ear (e.g., Langerhans' cell histiocytosis, salivary gland tumors, glomus tumors, rhabdomyosarcoma) also can manifest as CHL. Uncommon diseases that affect the middle ear and temporal bone and can manifest with CHL include otosclerosis, osteopetrosis, fibrous dysplasia, and osteogenesis imperfecta.

SNHL may be congenital or acquired. Acquired SNHL may be caused by genetic, infectious, autoimmune, anatomic, traumatic, ototoxic, and idiopathic factors (Tables 629-1, 629-2, 629-3, and 629-4). The recognized risk factors account for about 50% of cases of moderate to profound SNHL.

Sudden SNHL in a previously healthy child is uncommon but may be due to otitis media or other middle ear pathologies. Usually these causes are obvious from the history and physical examination. Sudden loss of hearing in the absence of obvious causes often is the result of a vascular event affecting the cochlear apparatus or nerve, such as embolism or thrombosis (secondary to prothrombotic conditions). Additional causes include perilymph fistula, drugs, trauma, and the first episode of Ménière syndrome. In adults, sudden SNHL is often idiopathic and unilateral; it may be associated with tinnitus and vertigo. Identifiable causes of sudden SNHL include infections (Epstein-Barr virus, varicella zoster virus, herpes simplex virus), vascular injury to the cochlea, endolymphatic hydrops, and inflammatory diseases.

Infectious Causes

The most common infectious cause of congenital SNHL is **cytomegalovirus (CMV)**, which infects 1/100 newborns in the USA (Chapters 247 and 630). Of these, 6,000-8,000 infants each year have clinical manifestations, including approximately 75% with SNHL. Congenital CMV warrants special attention because it is associated with hearing loss in its symptomatic and asymptomatic forms, and the hearing loss may be progressive. Some children with congenital CMV have suddenly lost residual hearing at 4-5 yr of age. Much less common congenital infectious causes of

Table 629-1 INDICATORS ASSOCIATED WITH HEARING LOSS

INDICATORS ASSOCIATED WITH SENSORINEURAL AND/OR CONDUCTIVE HEARING LOSS
Neonates (Birth to 28 Days) When Universal Screening Is Not Available
Family history of hereditary childhood sensorineural hearing loss In utero infection, such as cytomegalovirus, rubella, syphilis, herpes simplex, or toxoplasmosis Craniofacial anomalies, including those with morphologic abnormalities of the pinna, ear canal, ear tags, ear pits, and temporal bone anomalies. Birth weight <1500 g (3.3 lb) Hyperbilirubinemia at a serum level requiring exchange transfusion Ototoxic medications, including but not limited to the aminoglycosides, used in multiple courses or in combination with loop diuretics Bacterial meningitis Apgar scores of 0-4 at 1 min or 0-6 at 5 min Mechanical ventilation lasting ≥5 days; ECMO Stigmata or other findings associated with a syndrome known to include a sensorineural and/or conductive hearing loss; white forelock
Infants and Toddlers (Age 29 Days to 2 Yr) When Certain Health Conditions Develop that Require Rescreening
Parent or caregiver concern regarding hearing, speech, language, and/or developmental delay Bacterial meningitis and other infections associated with sensorineural hearing loss Head trauma associated with loss of consciousness or skull fracture Stigmata or other findings associated with a syndrome known to include a sensorineural and/or conductive hearing loss; neurofibromatosis, osteopetrosis, and Usher Hunter, Waardenburg, Alport, Pendred, or Jervell and Lange-Nielson syndromes Ototoxic medications, including but not limited to chemotherapeutic agents or aminoglycosides used in multiple courses or in combination with loop diuretics Recurrent or persistent otitis media with effusion for ≥3 mo
Infants and Toddlers (Age 29 Days to 3 Yr) Who Require Periodic Monitoring of Hearing
Some newborns and infants pass initial hearing screening but require periodic monitoring of hearing to detect delayed-onset sensorineural and/or conductive hearing loss. Infants with these indicators require hearing evaluation at least every 6 mo until age 3 yr, and at appropriate intervals thereafter.
INDICATORS ASSOCIATED WITH DELAYED-ONSET SENSORINEURAL HEARING LOSS
Family history of hereditary childhood hearing loss In utero infection, such as cytomegalovirus, rubella, syphilis, herpes simplex, or toxoplasmosis Neurofibromatosis type 2 and neurodegenerative disorders
INDICATORS ASSOCIATED WITH CONDUCTIVE HEARING LOSS
Recurrent or persistent otitis media with effusion Anatomic deformities and other disorders that affect eustachian tube function Neurodegenerative disorders

Note: At all ages, parents' concern about hearing loss must be taken seriously even in the absence of risk factors.
ECMO, extracorporeal membrane oxygenation.
Adapted from American Academy of Pediatrics, Joint Committee on Infant Hearing: Joint Committee on Infant Hearing 1994 position statement, *Pediatrics* 95:152, 1995.

SNHL include toxoplasmosis and syphilis. Congenital CMV, toxoplasmosis, and syphilis also can manifest with delayed onset of SNHL months to years after birth. Rubella, once the most common viral cause of congenital SNHL, is very uncommon because of effective vaccination programs. In utero infection with herpes simplex virus is rare, and hearing loss is not an isolated manifestation.

Other postnatal infectious causes of SNHL include neonatal group B streptococcal sepsis and bacterial meningitis at any age. *Streptococcus pneumoniae* is the most common cause of bacterial meningitis that results in SNHL after the neonatal period and has become less common with the routine administration of pneumococcal conjugate vaccine. *Haemophilus influenzae* type b, once the most common cause of meningitis resulting in SNHL, is rare owing to the Hib conjugate vaccine. Uncommon infectious causes of SNHL include Lyme disease, parvovirus B19, and varicella. Mumps, rubella, and rubeola, all once common causes of SNHL in children, are rare owing to vaccination programs.

Genetic Causes

Genetic causes of SNHL probably are responsible for as many as 50% of SNHL cases (see Tables 629-2 and 629-3). These disorders may be associated with other abnormalities, may be part of a named syndrome, or can exist in isolation. SNHL often occurs with abnormalities of the ear and eye and with disorders of the metabolic, musculoskeletal, integumentary, renal, and nervous systems.

Autosomal dominant hearing losses account for about 10% of all cases of childhood SNHL. Waardenburg (types I and II) and branchio-otorenal syndromes represent 2 of the most common autosomal dominant syndromic types of SNHL. Types of SNHL are coded with a 4-letter code and a number, as follows: **DFN** = deafness, A = dominant, B = recessive, and number = order of discovery, for example DFNA 13. Autosomal dominant conditions in addition to those just discussed include DFNA 1-11, 13, 15, 17, 20, 22, 28, 36, 48 and mutations in the crystallin gene *(CRYM)*.

Autosomal recessive genetic SNHL, both syndromic and nonsyndromic, accounts for about 80% of all childhood cases of SNHL. Usher syndrome (types 1, 2, and 3), Pendred syndrome, and the Jervell and Lange-Nielsen syndrome (one form of the long Q-T syndrome) are 3 of the most common syndromic recessive types of SNHL. Other autosomal recessive conditions include Alström syndrome, type 4 Bartter syndrome, biotinidase deficiency and DFNB1-4, 6-9, 12, 16, 18, 21-23, 28-31, 36, 37, 67.

Unlike children with an easily identified syndrome or with anomalies of the outer ear, who may be identified as being at risk for hearing loss and consequently monitored adequately, children with nonsyndromic hearing loss present greater diagnostic difficulty. Mutations of the connexin-26 and -30 genes have been identified in autosomal recessive (DNFB 1) and autosomal dominant (DNFA 3) SNHL and in sporadic patients with nonsyndromic SNHL; up to 50% of nonsyndromic SNHL may be related to a mutation of connexin-26. Mutations of the *GJB2* gene co-localize with DFNA 3 and DFNB 1 loci on chromosome 13, are associated with autosomal nonsyndromic susceptibility to deafness, and are associated with as many as 30% of cases of sporadic severe to profound congenital deafness and 50% of cases of autosomal recessive nonsyndromic deafness. Sex-linked disorders associated with SNHL, thought to account for 1-2% of SNHL, include Norrie disease, the otopalatal digital syndrome, Nance deafness, and Alport syndrome. Chromosomal abnormalities such as trisomy 13-15, trisomy 18, and trisomy 21 also can be accompanied by hearing impairment. Patients with Turner syndrome have monosomy for all or part of 1 X chromosome and can have CHL, SNHL, or mixed hearing loss. The hearing loss may be progressive. Mitochondrial genetic abnormalities also can result in SNHL (see Table 629-2).

Many genetically determined causes of hearing impairment, both syndromic and nonsyndromic, do not express themselves until some time after birth. Alport, Alström, and Down syndromes, von Recklinghausen disease, and Hunter-Hurler syndrome are genetic diseases that can have SNHL as a late manifestation.

Physical Causes

Agenesis or malformation of cochlear structures including the Scheibe, Mondini (Fig. 629-1), Alexander, and Michel anomalies; enlarged vestibular aqueducts (which may be associated with Pendred Syndrome); and semicircular canal anomalies may be genetic. These anomalies probably occur before the 8th wk of gestation and result from arrest in normal development, aberrant development, or both. Many of these anomalies also have been described in association with other congenital conditions such as intrauterine CMV and rubella infections. These abnormalities are

Table 629-2 COMMON TYPES OF HEREDITARY NONSYNDROMIC SENSORINEURAL HEARING LOSS

LOCUS	GENE	AUDIO PHENOTYPE
DFN3	*POU3F4*	Conductive hearing loss due to stapes fixation mimicking otosclerosis; superimposed progressive SNHL
DFNA1	*DIAPH1*	Low-frequency loss beginning in the 1st decade and progressing to all frequencies to produce a flat audio profile with profound losses throughout the auditory range
DFNA2	*KCNQ4*	Symmetrical high-frequency sensorineural loss beginning in the 1st decade and progressing over all frequencies
	GJB3	Symmetrical high-frequency sensorineural loss beginning in the 3rd decade
DFNA 6/14/38	*WFS1*	Early-onset low-frequency sensorinerual loss; about 75% of families dominantly segregating this audio profile carry missense mutations in the C-terminal domain of wolframin.
DFNA10	*EYA4*	Progressive loss beginning in the 2nd decade as a flat to gently sloping audio profile that becomes steeply sloping with age
DFNA13	*COL11A2*	Congenital mid-frequency sensorineural loss that shows age-related progression across the auditory range
DFNA15	*POU4F3*	Bilateral progressive sensorineural loss beginning in the 2nd decade
DFNA20/26	*ACTG1*	Bilateral progressive sensorineural loss beginning in the 2nd decade; with age, the loss increases with threshold shifts in all frequencies, although a sloping configuration is maintained in most cases
DFNB1	*GJB2, GJB6*	Hearing loss varies from mild to profound. The most common genotype, 35delG/35delG, is associated with severe to profound SNHL in about 90% of affected children; severe to profound deafness is observed in only 60% of children who are compound heterozygotes carrying 1 35delG allele and any other *GJB2* SNHL-causing allele variant; in children carrying 2 *GJB2* SNHL-causing missense mutations, severe to profound deafness is not observed.
DFNB4	*SLC26A4*	DFNB4 and Pendred syndrome (see Table 629-3) are allelic. DFNB4 hearing loss is associated with dilatation of the vestibular aqueduct and can be unilateral or bilateral. In the high frequencies, the loss is severe to profound; in the low frequencies, the degree of loss varies widely. Onset can be congenital (prelingual), but progressive postlingual loss also is common.
mtDNA 1555A > G	*12S rRNA*	Degree of hearing loss varies from mild to profound but usually is symmetrical; high frequencies are preferentially affected; precipitous loss in hearing can occur after aminoglycoside therapy.

SNHL, sensorineural hearing loss.
From Smith RJH, Bale JF Jr, White KR: Sensorineural hearing loss in children, *Lancet* 365:879–890, 2005.

Table 629-3 COMMON TYPES OF SYNDROMIC SENSORINEURAL HEARING LOSS

SYNDROME	GENE	PHENOTYPE
DOMINANT		
Waardenberg (WS1)	*PAX3*	Major diagnostic criteria include dystopia canthorum, congenital hearing loss, heterochromic irises, white forelock, and an affected first-degree relative. About 60% of affected children have congenital hearing loss; in 90%, the loss is bilateral.
Waardenberg (WS2)	*MITF*, others	Major diagnostic criteria are as for WS1 but without dystopia canthorum. About 80% of affected children have congenital hearing loss; in 90%, the loss is bilateral.
Branchio-otorenal	*EYA1*	Diagnostic criteria include hearing loss (98%), preauricular pits (85%), and branchial (70%), renal (40%), and external-ear (30%) abnormalities. The hearing loss can be conductive, sensorineural, or mixed, and mild to profound in degree.
RECESSIVE		
Pendred syndrome	*SLC26A4*	Diagnostic criteria include sensorineural hearing loss that is congenital, nonprogressive, and severe to profound in many cases, but can be late-onset and progressive; bilateral dilation of the vestibular aqueduct with or without cochlear hypoplasia; and an abnormal perchlorate discharge test or goiter.
Usher syndrome type 1 (USH1)	*USH1A, MYO7A, USH1C, CDH23, USH1E, PCDH15, USH1G*	Diagnostic criteria include congenital, bilateral, and profound hearing loss, vestibular areflexia, and retinitis pigmentosa (commonly not diagnosed until tunnel vision and nyctalopia become severe enough to be noticeable).
Usher syndrome type 2 (USH2)	*USH2A, USH2B, USH2C*, others	Diagnostic criteria include mild to severe, congenital, bilateral hearing loss and retinitis pigmentosa; hearing loss may be perceived as progressing over time because speech perception decreases as diminishing vision interferes with subconscious lip reading.
Usher syndrome type 3 (USH3)	*USH3*	Diagnostic criteria include postlingual, progressive sensorineural hearing loss, late-onset retinitis pigmentosa, and variable impairment of vestibular function.

From Smith RJH, Bale JF Jr, White KR: Sensorineural hearing loss in children, *Lancet* 365:879–890, 2005.

quite common; in as many as 20% of children with SNHL, obvious or subtle temporal bone abnormalities are seen on high-resolution CT scanning or MRI.

Conditions, diseases, or syndromes that include craniofacial abnormalities may be associated with conductive hearing loss and possibly with SNHL. Pierre Robin, Treacher Collins, Klippel-Feil, Crouzon, and branchio-otorenal syndromes and osteogenesis imperfecta often are associated with hearing loss. Congenital anomalies causing CHL include malformations of the ossicles and middle-ear structures and atresia of the external auditory canal.

SNHL also can occur secondary to exposure to toxins, chemicals, and antimicrobials. Early in pregnancy, the embryo is particularly vulnerable to the effects of toxic substances. Ototoxic drugs, including aminoglycosides, loop diuretics, and chemotherapeutic agents (cisplatin) also can cause SNHL. Congenital SNHL can occur secondary to exposure to these drugs as well as to thalidomide and retinoids. Certain chemicals, such as quinine, lead, and arsenic, can cause hearing loss both pre- and postnatally.

Trauma, including temporal bone fractures, inner ear concussion, head trauma, iatrogenic trauma (e.g., surgery, extracorporeal membrane oxygenation [ECMO]), radiation exposure, and noise, also can cause SNHL. Other uncommon causes of SNHL in children include immune disease (systemic or limited to the inner ear), metabolic abnormalities, and neoplasms of the temporal bone.

EFFECTS OF HEARING IMPAIRMENT

The effects of hearing impairment depend on the nature and degree of the hearing loss and on the individual characteristics of the child. Hearing loss may be unilateral or bilateral, conductive, sensorineural, or mixed; mild, moderate, severe, or profound; of sudden or gradual onset; stable, progressive, or fluctuating; and affecting a part or all of the audible spectrum. Other factors, such as intelligence, medical or physical condition (including accompanying syndromes), family support, age at onset, age at time of identification, and promptness of intervention, also affect the impact of hearing loss on a child.

Most hearing-impaired children have some usable hearing. Only 6% of those in the hearing-impaired population have bilateral profound hearing loss. Hearing loss very early in life can affect the development of speech and language, social and emotional development, behavior, attention, and academic achievement. Some cases of hearing impairment are misdiagnosed because affected children have sufficient hearing to respond to environmental sounds and can learn some speech and language but when challenged in the classroom cannot perform to full potential.

Even mild or unilateral hearing loss can have a detrimental effect on the development of a young child and on school performance. Children with such hearing impairments have greater difficulty when listening conditions are unfavorable (e.g., background noise and poor acoustics), as can occur in a classroom. The fact that schools are auditory-verbal environments is unappreciated by those who minimize the impact of hearing impairment on learning. Hearing loss should be considered in any child with speech and language difficulties or below-par performance, poor behavior, or inattention in school (Table 629-5).

Table 629-4 INFECTIOUS PATHOGENS IMPLICATED IN SENSORINEURAL HEARING LOSS IN CHILDREN

CONGENITAL INFECTIONS
Cytomegalovirus
Lymphocytic choriomeningitis virus
Rubella virus
Toxoplasma gondii
Treponema pallidum
ACQUIRED INFECTIONS
Borrelia burgdorferi
Epstein-Barr virus
Haemophilus influenzae
Lassa virus
Measles virus
Mumps virus
Neisseria meningitidis
Non-polio enteroviruses
Plasmodium falciparum
Streptococcus pneumoniae
Varicella zoster virus

From Smith RJH, Bale JF Jr, White KR: Sensorineural hearing loss in children, *Lancet* 365:879–890, 2005.

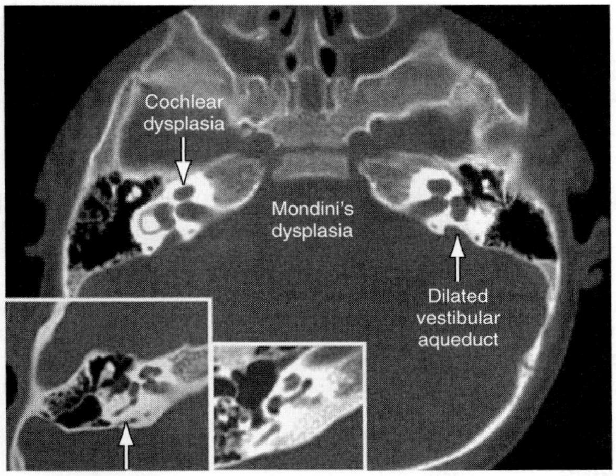

Figure 629-1 Mondini's dysplasia shown by CT of the temporal bone in a child with Pendred syndrome. Both dilatation of the vestibular aqueduct and cochlear dysplasia are present in this section. In the larger of the two inset images of a normal temporal bone, the vestibular aqueduct is visible but much smaller *(arrow)*. The cochlea appears normal, and in the smaller inset image of a more inferior axial section, the expected number of cochlear turns can be clearly counted. *Internal auditory canal. (From Smith RJH, Bale JF Jr, White KR: Sensorineural hearing loss in children, *Lancet* 365:879–890, 2005.)

Table 629-5 HEARING HANDICAP AS A FUNCTION OF AVERAGE HEARING THRESHOLD LEVEL OF THE BETTER EAR

AVERAGE THRESHOLD LEVEL (dB) AT 500-2,000 Hz (ANSI)	DESCRIPTION	COMMON CAUSES	WHAT CAN BE HEARD WITHOUT AMPLIFICATION	DEGREE OF HANDICAP (IF NOT TREATED IN 1ST YR OF LIFE)	PROBABLE NEEDS
0-15	Normal range	Conductive hearing loss	All speech sounds	None	None
16-25	Slight hearing loss	Otitis media, TM perforation, tympanosclerosis; eustachian tube dysfunction; some SNHL	Vowel sounds heard clearly, may miss unvoiced consonant sounds	Mild auditory dysfunction in language learning Difficulty in perceiving some speech sounds	Consideration of need for hearing aid, speech reading, auditory training, speech therapy, appropriate surgery, preferential seating
26-30	Mild	Otitis media, TM perforation, tympanosclerosis, severe eustachian dysfunction, SNHL	Hears only some speech sounds, the louder voiced sounds	Auditory learning dysfunction Mild language retardation Mild speech problems Inattention	Hearing aid Lip reading Auditory training Speech therapy Appropriate surgery
31-50	Moderate hearing loss	Chronic otitis, ear canal/ middle ear anomaly, SNHL	Misses most speech sounds at normal conversational level	Speech problems Language retardation Learning dysfunction Inattention	All of the above, plus consideration of special classroom situation
51-70	Severe hearing loss	SNHL or mixed loss due to a combination of middle-ear disease and sensorineural involvement	Hears no speech sound of normal conversations	Severe speech problems Language retardation Learning dysfunction Inattention	All of the above; probable assignment to special classes
71+	Profound hearing loss	SNHL or mixed	Hears no speech or other sounds	Severe speech problems Language retardation Learning dysfunction Inattention	All of the above; probable assignment to special classes or schools

ANSI, American National Standards Institute; SNHL, sensorineural hearing loss; TM, tympanic membrane.
Modified from Northern JL, Downs MP: *Hearing in children,* 4th ed, Baltimore, 1991, Williams & Wilkins.

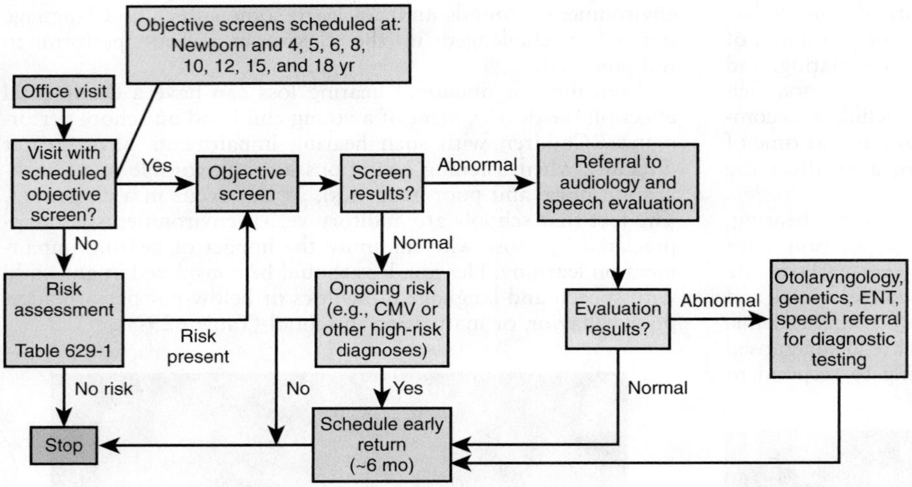

Figure 629-2 Hearing-assessment algorithm within an office visit. CMV, cytomegalovirus; ENT, ear, nose, and throat. Modified from Harlor AD Jr, Bower C: Clinical report—hearing assessment in infants and children: recommendations beyond neonatal screening, *Pediatrics* 124:1252–1263, 2009.)

Children with moderate, severe, or profound hearing impairment and those with other handicapping conditions often are educated in classes or schools for children with special needs. The auditory management and choices regarding modes of communication and education for children with hearing handicaps must be individualized, because these children are not a homogeneous group. A team approach to individual case management is essential, because each child and family unit has unique needs and abilities.

HEARING SCREENING

Hearing impairment can have a major impact on a child's development, and because early identification improves prognosis, screening programs have been widely and strongly advocated. The National Center for Hearing Assessment and Management estimates that the detection and treatment at birth of hearing loss saves $400,000 per child in special education costs; screening costs approximately $8-50/child. Data from the Colorado newborn screening program suggest that if hearing-impaired infants are identified and treated by age 6 mo, these children (with the exception of those with bilateral profound impairment) should develop the same level of language as their age-matched peers who are not hearing impaired. This is compelling support for the establishment of mandated newborn hearing screening programs for all children. The American Academy of Pediatrics endorses the goal of universal detection of hearing loss in infants before 3 mo of age, with appropriate intervention no later than 6 mo of age. Currently, hearing screening has been mandated in 39 states in the USA, plus the District of Columbia and Puerto Rico.

Until mandated screening programs are established universally, many hospitals will continue to use other criteria to screen for hearing loss. Some use the high-risk criteria (see Table 629-1) to decide which infants to screen; some screen all infants who require intensive care; and some do both. The problem with using high-risk criteria to screen is that 50% of cases of hearing impairment will be missed, either because the infants are hearing impaired but do not meet any of the high-risk criteria or because they develop hearing loss after the neonatal period.

The recommended hearing screening techniques are either otoacoustic emissions (OAE) testing or auditory brainstem evoked responses (ABR). The ABR test, an auditory evoked electrophysiologic response that correlates highly with hearing, has been used successfully and cost-effectively to screen newborns and to identify further the degree and type of hearing loss. OAE tests, used successfully in most universal newborn screening programs, are quick, easy to administer, and inexpensive, and they provide a sensitive indication of the presence of hearing loss. Results are relatively easy to interpret. OAE tests elicit no response if hearing is worse than 30-40 dB, no matter what the cause; children who fail OAE tests undergo an ABR for a more definitive evaluation. Screening methods such as observing behavioral responses to uncalibrated noisemakers or using automated systems such as the Crib-o-gram (Canon) or the auditory response cradle (in which movement of the infant in response to sound is recorded by motion sensors) are not recommended.

Many children become hearing impaired after the neonatal period and therefore are not identified by newborn-screening programs. Often it is not until children are in preschool or kindergarten that further hearing screening takes place. Primary care physicians and pediatricians should be alert to the signs and symptoms of childhood hearing impairment, so that children with hearing impairment who have not been screened formally can be identified as early as possible. Recommendations for post-neonatal screening are noted in Figure 629-2.

IDENTIFICATION OF HEARING IMPAIRMENT

The impact of hearing impairment is greatest on an infant who has yet to develop language; therefore, identification, diagnosis, description, and treatment should begin as soon as possible. In general, infants with a prenatal or perinatal history that puts them at risk (see Table 629-2) or those who have failed a formal hearing screening should be monitored closely by an experienced clinical audiologist until a reliable assessment of auditory function has been obtained. Pediatricians should encourage families to cooperate with the follow-up plan. Infants who are born at risk but who were not screened as neonates (often because of transfer from one hospital to another) should have a hearing screening by age 3 mo.

Hearing-impaired infants, who are born at risk or are screened for hearing loss in a neonatal hearing screening program, account for only a portion of hearing-impaired children. Children who are congenitally deaf because of autosomal recessive inheritance or subclinical congenital infection often are not identified until 1-3 yr of age. Usually, those with more severe hearing loss are identified at an earlier age, but identification often occurs later than the age at which intervention can provide an optimal outcome. Children who hear normally develop an extensive language by 3-4 yr of age (Table 629-6) and exhibit behavior reflecting normal auditory function (Table 629-7). Failure to fulfill these criteria should be the reason for an audiologic evaluation. Parents' concern about hearing and any delayed development of speech and language should alert the pediatrician, because parents' concern usually precedes formal identification and diagnosis of hearing impairment by 6 mo to 1 yr of age.

Table 629-6 CRITERIA FOR REFERRAL FOR AUDIOLOGIC ASSESSMENT

AGE (mo)	REFERRAL GUIDELINES FOR CHILDREN WITH "SPEECH" DELAY
12	No differentiated babbling or vocal imitation
18	No use of single words
24	Single-word vocabulary of ≤10 words
30	<100 words; no evidence of 2-word combinations; unintelligible
36	<200 words; no use of telegraphic sentences; clarity <50%
48	<600 words; no use of simple sentences clarity ≤80%

From Matkin ND: Early recognition and referral of hearing-impaired children, *Pediatr Rev* 6:151–156, 1984. Reproduced by permission of *Pediatrics*.

Table 629-7 GUIDELINES FOR REFERRAL OF CHILDREN WITH SUSPECTED HEARING LOSS

AGE (mo)	NORMAL DEVELOPMENT
0-4	Should startle to loud sounds, quiet to mother's voice, momentarily cease activity when sound is presented at a conversational level
5-6	Should correctly localize to sound presented in a horizontal plane, begin to imitate sounds in own speech repertoire or at least reciprocally vocalize with an adult
7-12	Should correctly localize to sound presented in any plane Should respond to name, even when spoken quietly
13-15	Should point toward an unexpected sound or to familiar objects or persons when asked
16-18	Should follow simple directions without gestural or other visual cues; can be trained to reach toward an interesting toy at midline when a sound is presented
19-24	Should point to body parts when asked; by 21-24 mo, can be trained to perform play audiometry

From Matkin ND: Early recognition and referral of hearing-impaired children, *Pediatr Rev* 6:151–156, 1984. Reproduced by permission of *Pediatrics*.

CLINICAL AUDIOLOGIC EVALUATION

Even the youngest infants can be evaluated for auditory function. When hearing impairment is suspected in a young child, reliable and valid estimates of auditory function can be obtained. Successful treatment strategies for hearing-impaired children rely on prompt identification and ongoing assessment to define the dimensions of auditory function. Cooperation among the pediatrician and specialists in areas such as audiology, speech and language pathology, education, and child development is necessary to optimize auditory-verbal development. Therapy for hearing-impaired children includes considering and often fitting an amplification device, using an FM system in the classroom, monitoring hearing and auditory skills, counseling parents and families, advising teachers, and dealing with public agencies.

Audiometry

The technique of the audiologic evaluation varies as a function of the age or developmental level of the child, the reason for the evaluation, and the child's otologic condition or history. An audiogram provides the fundamental description of hearing sensitivity (Fig. 629-3). Hearing thresholds are assessed as a function of frequency using pure tones (sine waves) at octave intervals from 250-8,000 Hz. Earphones typically are used when age-appropriate, and hearing is assessed independently for each ear. **Air-conducted signals** are presented through earphones (or loudspeakers) and are used to provide information about the sensitivity of the auditory system. These same test sounds can be delivered to the ear through an oscillator that is placed on the head, usually on the mastoid. Such signals are considered bone-conducted because the bones of the skull transmit vibrations as sound energy directly to the inner ear, essentially bypassing the outer and middle ears. In a normal ear, and also in children with SNHL, the air- and bone-conduction thresholds are the same. In those

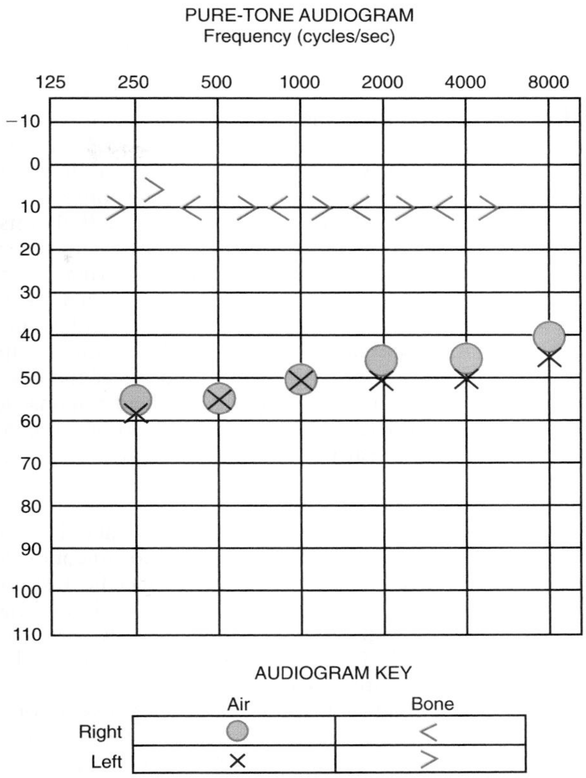

Figure 629-3 Audiogram showing bilateral conductive hearing loss.

with CHL, the air- and bone-conduction thresholds differ. This is called the **air-bone gap,** which indicates the amount of hearing loss attributable to dysfunction in the outer and/or middle ear. With mixed hearing loss, both the bone- and air-conduction thresholds are abnormal, and there is an air-bone gap.

Speech-Recognition Threshold

Another measure useful for describing auditory function is the speech-recognition threshold (SRT), which is the lowest intensity level at which a score of approximately 50% correct is obtained on a task of recognizing spondee words. Spondee words are 2-syllable words or phrases that have equal stress on each syllable, such as baseball, hotdog, and pancake. Listeners must be familiar with all the words for a valid test result to be obtained. The SRT should correspond to the average of pure-tone thresholds at 500, 1,000, and 2,000 Hz, the pure-tone average (PTA). The SRT is relevant as an indicator of a child's potential for development and use of speech and language; it also serves as a check of the validity of a test because children with nonorganic hearing loss (malingerers) might show a discrepancy between the PTA and SRT.

The basic battery of hearing tests concludes with an assessment of a child's ability to understand monosyllabic words when presented at a comfortable listening level. Performance on such word intelligibility tests assists in the differential diagnosis of hearing impairment and provides a measure of how well a child performs when speech is presented at loudness levels similar to those encountered in the environment.

Play Audiometry

Hearing testing is age-dependent. For children at or above the developmental level of a 5-6 yr old, conventional test methods can be used. For children 30 mo to 5 yr of age, play audiometry can be used. Responses in play audiometry usually are conditioned motor activities associated with a game, such as dropping blocks in a bucket, placing rings on a peg, or completing a puzzle. The technique can be used to obtain a reliable audiogram for a preschool child. For those who will not or cannot repeat words clearly for the SRT and word intelligibility tasks, pictures can be used with a pointing response.

Visual Reinforcement Audiometry

For children between the ages of about 6 mo and 30 mo, visual reinforcement audiometry (VRA) commonly is used. In this technique, the child is observed for a head-turning response on activation of an animated (mechanical) toy reinforcer. If infants are properly conditioned, by giving sounds associated with the visual toy cue, VRA can provide reliable estimates of hearing sensitivity for tones and speech sounds. In most applications of VRA, sounds are presented by loudspeakers in a sound field, so no *ear-specific* information is obtained. Assessment of an infant often is designed to rule out hearing loss that would affect the development of speech and language. Normal sound-field response levels of infants indicate sufficient hearing for this purpose despite the possibility of different hearing levels in the 2 ears.

Behavioral Observation Audiometry

Used as a screening device for infants <5 mo of age, behavioral observation audiometry (BOA) is limited to unconditioned, reflexive responses to complex (not frequency-specific) test sounds such as noise, speech, or music presented using calibrated signals from a loudspeaker or uncalibrated noisemakers. Response levels can vary widely within and among infants and usually do not provide a reliable estimate of sensitivity.

Assessment of a child with suspected hearing loss is not complete until pure-tone hearing thresholds and SRTs (a reliable audiogram) have been obtained in each ear. BOA and VRA in sound-field testing give estimates of hearing responsivity in the *better-hearing ear*.

Acoustic Immittance Testing

Acoustic immittance testing is a standard part of the clinical audiologic test battery and includes tympanometry. It is a useful objective assessment technique that provides information about the status of the middle ear. Tympanometry can be performed in a physician's office and is helpful in the diagnosis and management of OM with effusion, a common cause of mild to moderate hearing loss in young children.

TYMPANOMETRY Tympanometry provides a graph of the middle ear's ability to transmit sound energy (admittance, or compliance) or impede sound energy (impedance) as a function of air pressure in the external ear canal. Because most immittance test instruments measure acoustic admittance, the term *admittance* is used here. The principles apply to whatever units of measurement are used.

A probe is inserted into the entrance of the external ear canal so that an airtight seal is obtained. The probe varies air pressure, presents a tone, and measures sound pressure level in the ear canal through the probe assembly. The sound pressure measured in the ear canal relative to the known intensity of the probe signal is used to estimate the acoustic admittance of the ear canal and middle-ear system. Admittance can be expressed in a unit called a millimho (mmho) or as a volume of air (mL) with equivalent acoustic admittance. The test is performed so that an estimate can be made of the volume of air enclosed between the probe tip and TM. The acoustic admittance of this volume of air is deducted from the overall admittance measure to obtain a measure of the admittance of the middle-ear system alone. Estimating ear canal volume also has a diagnostic benefit, because an abnormally large value is consistent with the presence of an opening in the TM (perforation or tube).

Once the admittance of the air mass in the external auditory canal has been eliminated, it is assumed that the remaining admittance measure accurately reflects the admittance of the entire middle-ear system. Its value is controlled largely by the dynamics of the TM. Abnormalities of the TM can dictate the shape of tympanograms, thus obscuring abnormalities medial to the TM. In addition, the frequency of the probe tone, the speed and direction of the air pressure change, and the air pressure at which the tympanogram is initiated can all influence the outcome.

When air pressure in the ear canal is equal to that in the middle ear, the middle-ear system is functioning optimally. Therefore, the ear canal pressure at which there is the greatest flow of energy (admittance) should be a reasonable estimate of the air pressure in the middle-ear space. This pressure is determined by finding the maximum or **peak admittance** on the tympanogram and obtaining its value on the x-axis. The value on the y-axis at the tympanogram peak is an estimate of peak admittance based on admittance tympanometry (Table 629-8). This peak measure sometimes is referred to as **static acoustic admittance,** even though it is estimated from a dynamic measure (Fig. 632-4A).

TYMPANOMETRY IN OTITIS MEDIA WITH EFFUSION Children who have OM with effusion often have reduced peak admittance or high negative tympanometric peak pressures (see Fig. 632-4C). However, in the diagnosis of effusion, the tympanometric measure

Table 629-8 NORMS FOR PEAK (STATIC) ADMITTANCE USING A 226-HZ PROBE TONE FOR CHILDREN AND ADULTS

AGE GROUP	ADMITTANCE (mL)	SPEED OF AIR PRESSURE SWEEP ≤50 daPa/sec*	200 daPa/sec†
Children (3-5 yr)	Lower limit	0.30	0.36
	Median	0.55	0.61
	Upper limit	0.90	1.06
Adults	Lower limit	0.56	0.27
	Median	0.85	0.72
	Upper limit	1.36	1.38

*Ear canal volume measurement based on admittance at lowest tail of tympanogram.
†Ear canal measurement based on admittance at lowest tail of tympanogram for children and at +200 daPa for adults.
daPa, decaPascals.
Adapted from Margolis RH, Shanks JE: Tympanometry: basic principles of clinical application. In Rintelman WS, editor: *Hearing assessment*, ed 2, Austin, 1991, PRODED, pp 179–245.

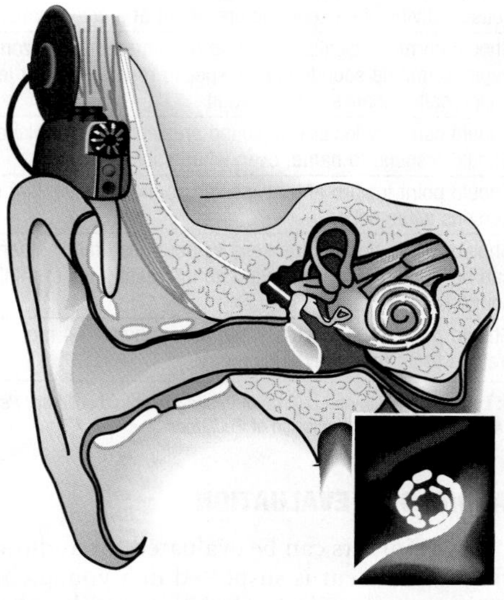

Figure 629-4 All cochlear implants share key components, including a microphone, speech processor, and transmitter coil, shown in a behind-the-ear position in this diagram. The microphone and speech processor picks up environmental sounds and digitizes them into coded signals. The signals are sent to the transmitter coil and relayed through the skin to the internal device imbedded in the skull. The internal device converts the code to electronic signals, which are transmitted to the electrode array wrapping around the cochlea. The inset shows the radiographic appearance of the stimulating electrode array. Reproduced with permission from MED-EL Corporation, Innsbruck, Austria. (From Smith RJH, Bale JF Jr, White KR: Sensorineural hearing loss in children, *Lancet* 365:879–890, 2005.)

with the greatest sensitivity and specificity is the shape of the tympanogram rather than its peak pressure or admittance. This shape sometimes is referred to as the tympanometric gradient or width; it measures the degree of roundness or **peakedness** of the tympanogram. The more rounded the peak (or, in an absent peak, a flat tympanogram), the higher is the probability that an effusion is present (see Fig. 632-4*B*). It is important to know which instrument is used, because some compute gradient automatically but others do not.

ACOUSTIC REFLEX TEST The acoustic reflex test (ART) also is part of the immittance test battery. With a properly functioning middle-ear system, admittance at the TM changes on activation of the stapedius and tensor tympani muscles. In healthy ears, the stapedial reflex occurs after exposure to loud sounds. Admittance instruments are designed to present reflex activating signals (pure tones of various frequencies or noise), either to the same or the contralateral ear, while monitoring admittance. Very small admittance changes that are time-locked to presentations of the signal are considered to be a result of middle-ear muscle reflexes. Admittance changes may be absent when the hearing loss is sufficient to prevent the signal from reaching the loudness level necessary to elicit the reflex or when a middle-ear condition affects the ear's ability to monitor a small admittance change. Reflexes usually are absent in patients with CHL due to the presence of an abnormal transfer system; thus, the ART is useful in the differential diagnosis of hearing impairment. The ART also is used in the assessment of SNHL and the integrity of the neurologic components of the reflex arc, including cranial nerves VII and VIII.

Auditory Brainstem Response

The ABR test is used to screen newborn hearing, confirm hearing loss in young children, obtain ear-specific information in young children, and test children who cannot, for whatever reason, cooperate with behavioral test methods. It also is important in the diagnosis of auditory dysfunction and of disorders of the auditory nervous system. The ABR test is a far-field recording of minute electrical discharges from numerous neurons. The stimulus, therefore, must be able to cause simultaneous discharge of the large numbers of neurons involved. Stimuli with very rapid onset, such as clicks or tone bursts, must be used. Unfortunately, the rapid onset required to create a measurable ABR also causes energy to be spread in the frequency domain, reducing the frequency-specificity of the response.

The ABR result is not affected by sedation or general anesthesia. Infants and children from about 4 mo to 4 yr of age routinely are sedated to minimize electrical interference caused by muscle activity during testing. The ABR also can be performed in the operating room when a child is anesthetized for another procedure. Children <4 mo of age might sleep for a long enough period of time after feeding to allow an ABR to be done.

The ABR is recorded as 5-7 waves. Waves I, III, and V can be obtained consistently in all age groups; waves II and IV appear less consistently. The latency of each wave (time of occurrence of the wave peak after stimulus onset) increases, and the amplitude decreases with reductions in stimulus intensity or loudness; latency also decreases with increasing age, with the earliest waves reaching mature latency values earlier in life than the later waves.

The ABR test has two major uses in a pediatric setting. As an audiometric test, it provides information on the ability of the peripheral auditory system to transmit information to the auditory nerve and beyond. It also is used in the differential diagnosis or monitoring of central nervous system pathology. For audiometry, the goal is to find the minimum stimulus intensity that yields an observable ABR. Plotting latency versus intensity for various waves also aids in the differential diagnosis of hearing impairment. A major advantage of auditory assessment using the ABR test is that ear-specific threshold estimates can be obtained on infants or patients who are difficult to test. ABR thresholds using click stimuli correlate best with behavioral hearing thresholds in the higher frequencies (1,000-4,000 Hz); responsivity in the low frequencies requires different stimuli (tone bursts or filtered clicks) or the use of masking, neither of which isolates the low-frequency region of the cochlea in all cases, and this can affect interpretation.

The ABR test does not assess "hearing." It reflects auditory neuronal electric responses that can be correlated to behavioral hearing thresholds, but a normal ABR result only suggests that the auditory system, up to the level of the midbrain, is responsive to the stimulus used. Conversely, a failure to elicit an ABR indicates an impairment of the system's synchronous response but does not necessarily mean that there is no "hearing." The behavioral response to sound sometimes is normal when no ABR can be elicited, such as in neurologic demyelinating disease. The ABR test may be used to infer whether and at what level of the auditory system impairment exists.

Hearing losses that are sudden, progressive, or unilateral are indications for ABR testing. Although it is believed that the different waves of the ABR reflect activity in increasingly rostral levels of the auditory system, the neural generators of the response have not been precisely determined. Each ABR wave beyond the earliest waves probably is the result of neural firing at many levels of the system, and each level of the system probably contributes to several ABR waves. High-intensity click stimuli are used for the neurologic application. The morphology of the response and wave and interwave latencies are examined in respect to age-appropriate forms. Delayed or missing waves in the ABR result often have diagnostic significance.

The ABR and other electrical responses are extremely complex and difficult to interpret. A number of factors, including instrumentation design and settings, environment, degree and configuration of hearing loss, and patients' characteristics, can influence the quality of the recording. Therefore, testing and interpretation of electrophysiologic activity as it possibly relates to hearing should be carried out by trained audiologists to avoid the risk that unreliable or erroneous conclusions will affect a patient's care.

Otoacoustic Emissions

During normal hearing, OAEs originate from the hair cells in the cochlea and are detected by sensitive amplifying processes. They travel from the cochlea through the middle ear to the external auditory canal, where they can be detected using miniature microphones. Transient evoked OAEs (TEOAEs) may be used to check the integrity of the cochlea. In the neonatal period, detection of OAEs can be accomplished during natural sleep, and TEOAEs can be used as screening tests in infants and children for hearing at the 30 dB level of hearing loss. They are less time-consuming and elaborate than ABR and are more sensitive than behavioral tests in young children. TEOAEs are reduced or absent owing to various dysfunctions in the middle and inner ears. They are absent in patients with >30 dB of hearing loss and are not used to determine hearing threshold; rather, they provide a screen for whether hearing is present at >30-40 dB. Diseases such as OM or congenitally abnormal middle ear structures reduce the transfer of TEOAEs and may incorrectly indicate a cochlear hearing disorder. If a hearing loss is suspected based on the absence of OAE, the ears should be examined for evidence of pathology, and then ABR testing should be used for confirmation and identification of the type, degree, and laterality of hearing loss.

Acoustic Reflectometry

In acoustic reflectometry, a hand-held instrument is placed next to the opening of a child's ear canal and 80-dB sound is delivered that varies in frequency from 2,000-4,500 Hz in a 100-msec period. The instrument measures the total level of reflected and transmitted sound. Some physicians have found this device useful to help gauge the presence or absence of middle-ear fluid, and a

Table 629-9 RECOMMENDED PNEUMOCOCCAL VACCINATION SCHEDULE FOR PERSONS WITH COCHLEAR IMPLANTS

AGE AT FIRST PCV13 DOSE (mo)*	PCV12 PRIMARY SERIES	PCV13 ADDITIONAL DOSE	PPV23 DOSE
2-6	3 doses, 2 mo apart[†]	1 dose at 12-15 mo of age[‡]	Indicated at ≥24 mo of age[§]
7-11	2 doses, 2 mo apart[†]	1 dose at 12-15 mo of age[‡]	Indicated at ≥24 mo of age[§]
12-23	2 doses, 2 mo apart[¶]	Not indicated	Indicated at ≥24 mo of age[§]
24-59	2 doses, 2 mo apart[¶]	Not indicated	Indicated[§]
≥60	Not indicated[‖]	Not indicated[‖]	Indicated

*A schedule with a reduced number of total 13-valent pneumococcal conjugate vaccine (PCV13) doses is indicated if children start late or are incompletely vaccinated. Children with a lapse in vaccination should be vaccinated according to the catch-up schedule (Chapter 175).
†For children vaccinated at age <1 yr, minimum interval between doses is 4 wk.
‡The additional dose should be administered ≥8 wk after the primary series has been completed.
§Children aged <5 yr should complete the PCV13 series first; 23-valent pneumococcal polysaccharide vaccine (PPV23) should be administered to children aged ≥24 mo ≥8 wk after the last dose of PCV13 (Chapter 175). (Centers for Disease Control and Prevention Advisory Committee on Immunization Practices: Preventing pneumococcal disease among infants and young children: Recommendations of the Advisory Committee on Immunization Practices (ACIP), *MMWR Recomm Rep* 49[RR-9]:1–35, 2000.)
¶Minimum interval between doses is 8 wk.
‖PCV13 is not recommended generally for children aged ≥5 yr.
From Centers for Disease Control and Prevention Advisory Committee on Immunization Practices: Pneumococcal vaccination for cochlear implant candidates and recipients: Updated recommendations of the Advisory Committee on Immunization Practices, *MMWR* 52:739–740, 2003.

commercial version is marketed to parents as a way to monitor ear fluid. The instrument does not provide any information about hearing; if the presence of chronic fluid is suggested, audiometric evaluation should be obtained.

TREATMENT

With the use of universal hearing screening in the majority of states within the USA, the early diagnosis and treatment of children with hearing loss is common. Testing for hearing loss is possible even in very young children, and it should be done if parents suspect a problem. Any child with a known risk factor for hearing loss should be evaluated in the 1st 6 mo of life.

Once a hearing loss is identified, a full developmental and speech and language evaluation is needed. Counseling and involvement of parents are required in all stages of the evaluation and treatment or rehabilitation. A conductive hearing loss often can be corrected through treatment of a middle-ear effusion (i.e., ear tube placement) or surgical correction of the abnormal sound-conducting mechanism. Children with SNHL should be evaluated for possible hearing aid use by a pediatric audiologist. Hearing aids may be fitted for children as young as 2 mo of age. Compelling evidence from the hearing screening program in Colorado shows that identification and amplification before age 6 mo makes a very significant difference in the speech and language abilities of affected children, compared with cases identified and amplified after the age of 6 mo. In these children, repeat audiologic testing is needed to reliably identify the degree of hearing loss and to fine tune the use of hearing aids.

Infants and young children with profound congenital or prelingual onset of deafness have benefited from **multichannel cochlear implants** (see Fig. 629-4). These implants bypass injury to the organ of Corti and provide neural stimulation by way of an external microphone and a signal processor that digitizes auditory stimuli into digital radiofrequency impulses. Cochlear implantation before age 2 yr (and even 1 yr) improves hearing and speech, enabling more than 90% of children to be in mainstream education. Most develop age-appropriate auditory perception and oral language skills.

A serious complication of cochlear implants is an excessively high incidence of pneumococcal meningitis. All children receiving a cochlear implant must be vaccinated with the PCV-13 vaccine (Table 629-9).

The best approach to the education of children with significant hearing loss is a subject of ongoing controversy. Because we live in a predominantly speaking world, some have advocated a pure auditory and oral approach to hearing therapy. However, because affected children often are slow to develop communication skills, many advocate a total communication approach; depending on the individual child's needs, this technique uses a mixture of sign language, lip-reading, hearing aids, and speech. The appropriate program for each child depends on the patient, family, and available resources.

GENETIC COUNSELING

Families of children with the diagnosis of SNHL, or a syndrome associated with SNHL and/or CHL, should consider genetic counseling, which will allow a discussion of the likelihood of similar diagnoses in future pregnancies. The geneticist also can help in the evaluation and further testing of the patient with hearing loss to establish a diagnosis.

BIBLIOGRAPHY

Please visit the Nelson Textbook of Pediatrics *website at www.expertconsult.com for the complete bibliography.*

Chapter 630 Congenital Malformations

Joseph Haddad, Jr.

The external and middle ears, derived from the 1st and 2nd branchial arches and grooves, grow throughout puberty, but the inner ear, which develops from the otocyst, reaches adult size and shape by mid-fetal development. The ossicles are derived from the 1st and 2nd arches (malleus and incus), and the stapes arises from the 2nd arch and the otic capsule. The malleus and incus achieve adult size and shape by the 15th wk of gestation, and the stapes achieves adult size and shape by the 18th wk of gestation. Although the pinna, ear canal, and tympanic membrane (TM) continue to grow after birth, congenital abnormalities of these structures develop during the 1st half of gestation. Malformed external and middle ears may be associated with serious renal anomalies, mandibulofacial dysostosis, hemifacial microsomia, and other craniofacial malformations. Facial nerve abnormalities may be associated with any of the congenital abnormalities of the ear and temporal bone. Malformations of the external and middle ears also may be associated with abnormalities of the inner ear and both conductive (CHL) and sensorineural hearing loss (SNHL).

For the full continuation of this chapter, please visit the Nelson Textbook of Pediatrics *website at www.expertconsult.com.*

Chapter 631 External Otitis (Otitis Externa)

Joseph Haddad, Jr.

In an infant, the outer two thirds of the ear canal is cartilaginous and the inner one third is bony. In an older child and adult only the outer one third is cartilaginous. The epithelium is thinner in the bony portion than in the cartilaginous portion, there is no subcutaneous tissue, and epithelium is tightly applied to the underlying periosteum; hair follicles, sebaceous glands, and apocrine glands are scarce or absent. The skin in the cartilaginous area has well-developed dermis and subcutaneous tissue and contains hair follicles, sebaceous glands, and apocrine glands. The highly viscid secretions of the sebaceous glands and the watery, pigmented secretions of the apocrine glands in the outer portion of the canal combine with exfoliated surface cells of the skin to form **cerumen**, a protective, waxy, water-repellent coating.

The normal flora of the external canal consists mainly of aerobic bacteria and includes coagulase-negative staphylococci, *Corynebacterium* (diphtheroids), *Micrococcus,* and, occasionally, *Staphylococcus aureus,* viridans streptococci, and *Pseudomonas aeruginosa.* Excessive wetness (swimming, bathing, increased environmental humidity), dryness (dry canal skin and lack of cerumen), the presence of other skin pathology (previous infection, eczema, or other forms of dermatitis), and trauma (digital or foreign body, cotton tip applicators [Q-tips]) make the skin of the canal vulnerable to infection by the normal flora or exogenous bacteria.

ETIOLOGY

External otitis (**swimmer's ear,** although it can occur without swimming) is caused most commonly by *P. aeruginosa,* but *S. aureus, Enterobacter aerogenes, Proteus mirabilis, Klebsiella pneumoniae,* streptococci, coagulase-negative staphylococci, diphtheroids, and fungi such as *Candida* and *Aspergillus* also may be isolated. External otitis results from chronic irritation and maceration from excessive moisture in the canal. The loss of protective cerumen may play a role, as may trauma, but cerumen impaction with trapping of water also can cause infection. Inflammation of the ear canal due to herpesvirus, varicella-zoster, other skin exanthems, and eczema also may predispose to external otitis.

CLINICAL MANIFESTATIONS

The predominant symptom is acute ear pain, often severe, accentuated by manipulation of the pinna or by pressure on the tragus and by jaw motion. The severity of the pain and tenderness may be disproportionate to the degree of inflammation, because the skin of the external ear canal is tightly adherent to the underlying perichondrium and periosteum. Itching often is a precursor of pain and usually is characteristic of chronic inflammation of the canal or resolving acute otitis externa. Conductive hearing loss may result from edema of the skin and tympanic membrane (TM), serous or purulent secretions, or the canal skin thickening associated with chronic external otitis.

Edema of the ear canal, erythema, and thick, clumpy otorrhea are prominent signs of the acute disease. The cerumen usually is white and soft in consistency, as opposed to its usual yellow color and firmer consistency. The canal often is so tender and swollen that the entire ear canal and TM cannot be adequately visualized, and complete otoscopic examination may be delayed until the acute swelling subsides. If the TM can be visualized, it may appear either normal or opaque. TM mobility may be normal or, if thickened, reduced in response to positive and negative pressure.

Other physical findings may include palpable and tender lymph nodes in the periauricular region, and erythema and swelling of the pinna and periauricular skin. Rarely, facial paralysis, other cranial nerve abnormalities, vertigo, and/or sensorineural hearing loss are present. If these occur, **necrotizing (malignant) otitis externa** is probable. This invasive infection of the temporal bone and skull base requires immediate culture, intravenous antibiotics, and imaging studies to evaluate the extent of the disease. Surgical intervention to obtain cultures or debride devitalized tissue may be necessary. *P. aeruginosa* is the most common causative organism of necrotizing otitis externa. Fortunately, this disease is rare in children and is seen only in association with immunocompromise or severe malnourishment. In adults it is associated with diabetes mellitus.

DIAGNOSIS

Diffuse external otitis may be confused with furunculosis, **otitis media (OM),** and mastoiditis. **Furuncles** occur in the lateral hair-bearing part of the ear canal; furunculosis usually causes a localized swelling of the canal limited to 1 quadrant, whereas external otitis is associated with concentric swelling and involves the entire ear canal. In OM, the TM may be perforated, severely retracted, or bulging and immobile; hearing usually is impaired. If the middle ear is draining through a perforated TM or tympanostomy tube, secondary external otitis may occur; if the TM is not visible owing to drainage or ear canal swelling, it may be difficult to distinguish acute OM with drainage from an acute external otitis. Pain on manipulation of the auricle and significant lymphadenitis are not common features of OM, and these findings assist in the differential diagnosis. In some patients with external otitis, the periauricular edema is so extensive that the auricle is pushed forward, creating a condition that may be confused with acute mastoiditis and a subperiosteal abscess; in **mastoiditis,** the postauricular fold is obliterated, whereas in external otitis the fold is usually better preserved. In acute mastoiditis, a history of OM and hearing loss is usual; tenderness is noted over the mastoid and not on movement of the auricle; and otoscopic examination may show sagging of the posterior canal wall.

Referred otalgia may come from disease in the paranasal sinuses, teeth, pharynx, parotid gland, neck and thyroid, and cranial nerves (trigeminal neuralgia) (herpes simplex virus, varicella zoster virus).

TREATMENT

Topical otic preparations containing neomycin (active against gram-positive organisms and some gram-negative organisms, notably *Proteus* spp.) with either colistin or polymyxin (active against gram-negative bacilli, notably *Pseudomonas* spp.) and corticosteroids are highly effective in treating most forms of acute external otitis. Newer preparations of eardrops (e.g., ofloxacin, ciprofloxacin) are preferable and do not contain potentially ototoxic antibiotics. If canal edema is marked, the patient may need referral to a specialist for cleaning and possible wick placement. An otic antibiotic and corticosteroid eardrop is often recommended. A wick can be inserted into the ear canal and topical antibiotics applied to the wick 3 times a day for 24-48 hr. The wick can be removed after 2-3 days, at which time the edema of the ear canal usually is markedly improved, and the ear canal and TM are better seen. Topical antibiotics are then continued by direct instillation. When the pain is severe, oral analgesics (e.g., ibuprofen, codeine) may be necessary for a few days. Careful evaluation for underlying conditions should be undertaken in patients with severe or recurrent otitis externa. An approach to management is noted in Figure 631-1.

As the inflammatory process subsides, cleaning the canal with a suction or cotton-tipped applicator to remove the debris enhances the effectiveness of the topical medications. In subacute and chronic infections, periodic cleansing of the canal is essential. In severe, acute external otitis associated with fever and lymphadenitis, oral or parenteral antibiotics may be indicated; an ear canal culture should be done, and empiric antibiotic treatment can then be modified if necessary, based on susceptibility of the organism cultured. A fungal infection of the external auditory canal, or **otomycosis,** is characterized by fluffy white debris, sometimes with black spores seen; treatment includes cleaning and application of antifungal solutions such as clotrimazole or

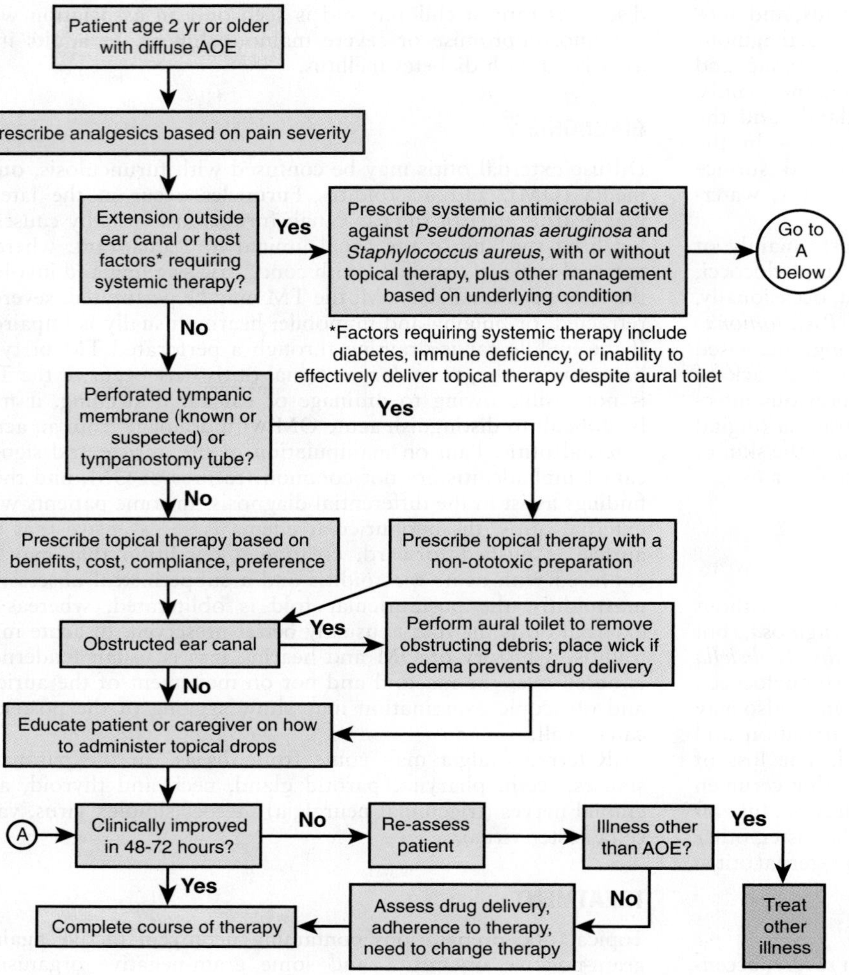

Figure 631-1 Flowchart for managing acute otitis externa (AOE). (From Rosenfeld RM, Brown L, Cannon CR, et al: Clinical practice guideline: acute otitis externa, *Otolaryngol Head Neck Surg* 134:S4–S23, 2006.© 2006 American Academy of Otolaryngology-Head and Neck Surgery Foundation, Inc.)

nystatin; other antifungal agents include m-cresyl acetate 25%, gentian violet 2%, and thimerosal 1:1,000.

PREVENTION

Preventing external otitis may be necessary for individuals susceptible to recurrences, especially children who swim. The most effective prophylaxis is instillation of dilute alcohol or acetic acid (2%) immediately after swimming or bathing. During an acute episode of otitis externa, patients should not swim and the ears should be protected from excessive water during bathing. A hair dryer may be used to clear moisture from the ear after swimming as a method of prevention.

OTHER DISEASES OF THE EXTERNAL EAR

Furunculosis

Furunculosis is caused by *S. aureus* and affects only the hair-containing outer third of the ear canal. Mild forms are treated with oral antibiotics active against *S. aureus*. If an abscess develops, incision and drainage may be necessary.

Acute Cellulitis

Acute cellulitis of the auricle and external auditory canal usually is caused by group A streptococcus and occasionally by *S. aureus*. The skin is red, hot, and indurated, without a sharply defined border. Fever may be present with little or no exudate in the canal. Parenteral administration of penicillin G or a penicillinase-resistant penicillin is the therapy of choice.

Perichondritis and Chondritis

Perichondritis is an infection involving the skin and perichondrium of the auricular cartilage; extension of infection to the cartilage is termed **chondritis**. The ear canal, especially the lateral aspect, also may be involved. Early perichondritis may be difficult to differentiate from cellulitis because both are characterized by skin that is red, edematous, and tender. The main cause of perichondritis/chondritis and cellulitis is trauma (accidental or iatrogenic, laceration or contusion), including ear piercing, especially when done through the cartilage. The most commonly isolated organism in perichondritis and chondritis is *P. aeruginosa*, although other gram-negative and, occasionally, gram-positive organisms may be found. Treatment involves systemic, often parenteral, antibiotics; surgery to drain an abscess or remove nonviable skin or cartilage may also be needed. Removal of all ear jewelry is mandatory in the presence of infection.

Dermatoses

Various dermatoses (seborrheic, contact, infectious eczematoid, or neurodermatoid) are common causes of inflammation of the external canal; scratching and the introduction of infecting organisms cause acute external otitis in these conditions.

Seborrheic dermatitis is characterized by greasy scales that flake and crumble as they are detached from the epidermis; associated changes in the scalp, forehead, cheeks, brow, postauricular areas, and concha are usual.

Contact dermatitis of the auricle or canal may be caused by earrings, or by topical otic medications such as neomycin, which may produce erythema, vesiculation, edema, and weeping. Poison ivy, oak, and sumac also may produce contact dermatitis. Hair care products have been implicated in sensitive individuals.

Infectious eczematoid dermatitis is caused by a purulent infection of the external canal, middle ear, or mastoid; the purulent drainage infects the skin of the canal, auricle, or both. The lesion is weeping, erythematous, or crusted.

Atopic dermatitis occurs in children with a familial or personal history of allergy; the auricle, particularly the postauricular fold, becomes thickened, scaly, and excoriated.

Neurodermatitis is recognized by intense itching and erythematous, thickened epidermis localized to the concha and orifice of the meatus.

Treatment of these dermatoses depends on the type but should include application of an appropriate topical medication, elimination of the source of infection or contact when identified, and management of any underlying dermatologic problem. In addition to topical antibiotics (or antifungals), topical steroids are helpful if contact dermatitis, atopic dermatitis, or eczematoid dermatitis is suspected.

Herpes Simplex Virus

Herpes simplex virus may appear as vesicles on the auricle and lips. The lesions eventually become encrusted and dry and may be confused with impetigo. Topical application of a 10% solution of carbamide peroxide in anhydrous glycerol is symptomatically helpful. The **Ramsay Hunt syndrome** (herpes zoster oticus with facial paralysis) may present with herpes vesicles in the ear canal and on the pinna and with facial paralysis and pain. Other cranial nerves may be affected as well, especially the 8th nerve. The current recommended treatment of herpes zoster oticus includes systemic antiviral agents, such as acyclovir, and corticosteroids. As many as 50% of patients with Ramsay Hunt syndrome do not completely recover their facial nerve function.

Bullous Myringitis

Commonly associated with an acute upper respiratory tract infection, bullous myringitis presents as an ear infection with more severe pain than usual. On examination, hemorrhagic or serous blisters (bullas) may be seen on the TM. The disease sometimes is difficult to differentiate from acute OM, because a large bulla may be confused with a bulging TM. The organisms involved are the same as those that cause acute OM, including both bacteria and viruses. Treatment consists of empiric antibiotic therapy and pain medications. In addition to ibuprofen or codeine for severe pain, a topical anesthetic eardrop may also provide some relief. Incision of the bullae, although not necessary, promptly relieves the pain.

Exostoses and Osteomas

Exostoses represent benign hyperplasia of the perichondrium and underlying bone (Chapter 495.2). Those involving the auditory canal tend to be found in people who swim often in cold water. Exostoses are broad-based, often multiple, and bilateral. Osteomas are benign bony growths in the ear canal of uncertain cause (Chapter 495.2). They usually are solitary and attached by a narrow pedicle to the tympanosquamous or tympanomastoid suture line. Both are more common in males; exostoses are more common than osteomas. Surgical treatment is recommended when large masses cause cerumen impaction, ear canal obstruction, or hearing loss.

BIBLIOGRAPHY

Please visit the Nelson Textbook of Pediatrics *website at* *www.expertconsult.com* *for the complete bibliography.*

Chapter 632
Otitis Media

Joseph E. Kerschner

Over 80% of children will have experienced at least one episode of otitis media (OM) by the age of 3 yr. The peak incidence and prevalence of OM is during the 1st 2 yr of life. OM is the leading reason for physician visits and for use of antibiotics and figures importantly in the differential diagnosis of fever. OM is the most common reason for prescribing antimicrobial drugs to children, often serves as the sole or the main basis for undertaking the most frequently performed operations in infants and young children: myringotomy with insertion of tympanostomy tubes and adenoidectomy. It is the most common cause of hearing loss in children. An important characteristic of OM is its propensity to become chronic and recur. The earlier in life a child experiences the 1st episode, the greater the degree of subsequent difficulty he or she is likely to experience in terms of frequency of recurrence, severity, and persistence of middle-ear effusion.

Accurate diagnosis of OM in infants and young children may be difficult (Table 632-1). Symptoms may not be apparent, especially in early infancy and in chronic stages of the disease. The eardrum may be obscured by cerumen, removal of which may be arduous and time-consuming. Abnormalities of the eardrum may be subtle and difficult to appreciate. In the face of these difficulties, both underdiagnosis and overdiagnosis occur. Once a diagnosis of OM has been established, its significance to the child's health and well-being and its optimal method of management remain open to question and the subjects of continuing controversy. There is lack of consensus among authorities concerning benefit-risk ratios of available medical and surgical treatments; while OM can be responsible for serious infectious complications, middle- and inner-ear damage, hearing impairment, and indirect impairments of speech, language, cognitive, and psychosocial development, most cases of OM are not severe and are self-limiting.

The term **otitis media** has 2 main categories: acute infection, which is termed **suppurative** or **acute otitis media (AOM);** and inflammation accompanied by effusion, termed **nonsuppurative** or **secretory OM,** or **otitis media with effusion (OME)**. These 2 main types of OM are interrelated: acute infection usually is succeeded by residual inflammation and effusion that, in turn, predispose children to recurrent infection. **Middle-ear effusion** (MEE) is a feature both of AOM and of OME and is an expression of the underlying middle-ear mucosal inflammation. In children with OM, mucosal inflammation is also present in the mastoid air cells, which are in continuity with the middle-ear

Table 632-1 DEFINITION OF ACUTE OTITIS MEDIA

A diagnosis of AOM requires (1) a history of acute onset of signs and symptoms, (2) the presence of MEE, and (3) signs and symptoms of middle-ear inflammation.
The definition of AOM includes:
Recent, usually abrupt, onset of signs and symptoms of middle-ear inflammation and MEE
The presence of MEE, indicated by any of the following:
Bulging of the TM
Limited or absent mobility of the TM
Air-fluid level behind the TM
Otorrhea
Signs or symptoms of middle-ear inflammation, indicated by either
Distinct erythema of the TM, *or*
Distinct otalgia (discomfort clearly referable to the ear[s] that results in interference with or precludes normal activity or sleep)

AOM, acute otitis media; MEE, middle-ear effusion; TM, tympanic membrane.
From Subcommittee on Management of Acute Otitis Media: Diagnosis and management of acute otitis media, *Pediatrics* 113:1451–1465, 2004.

cavity. It is this MEE that results in the conductive hearing loss associated with OM. The hearing loss is of a variable degree ranging from none to as much as 50 decibels hearing level (dB HL). Losses of 21-30 dB HL are usual. Although most individual episodes of OM subside within several weeks, MEE persists for 3 mo or longer in approximately 10-25% of cases.

EPIDEMIOLOGY

Factors believed to affect the occurrence of OM include age, gender, race, genetic background, socioeconomic status, type of milk used in infant feeding, degree of exposure to tobacco smoke, degree of exposure to other children, presence or absence of respiratory allergy, season of the year, and vaccination status. Children with certain types of congenital craniofacial anomalies are particularly prone to OM.

Age

Although prevalence by age may be somewhat affected by socioeconomic status, the development of at least 1 episode of OM has been reported as 63-85% by 12 mo and 66-99% by 24 mo of age. The percentage of days with MEE has been reported as 5-27% during the 1st yr of life and 6-18% during the 2nd yr of life. Across groups, rates were highest during 6-20 mo of age. After the age of 2 yr, the incidence and prevalence of OM decline progressively, although the disease remains relatively common into the early school-age years. The most likely reasons for the higher rates in infants and younger children include less well-developed immunologic defenses and less favorable eustachian tubal factors involving both the structure and function of the tube.

The age of onset of OM has been demonstrated to be an important predictor of the development of recurrent and chronic OM, with earlier age of onset having an increased risk for exhibiting these difficulties later in life.

Gender

Although some studies have found no gender-related differences in the occurrence of OM, epidemiologic data taken as a whole would suggest an incidence greater in boys than in girls. Supporting a greater predilection for the disease in boys, and also suggesting greater severity in boys, are the facts that boys have predominated in most reported studies of the treatment of OM, and, compared with girls, consistently had higher rates of operations aimed at relieving the effects or reducing the occurrence of OM, namely, tympanostomy tube insertion and adenoidectomy.

Race

OM is especially prevalent and severe among Native American, Inuit, and Indigenous Australian children. Studies comparing the occurrence of OM in white children and black children have given conflicting results. Most of the studies have reported higher rates in white children.

Genetic Background

That middle-ear disease tends to run in families is a commonplace observation suggesting that OM has a heritable component. The degree of concordance for the occurrence of OM is much greater among monozygotic than among dizygotic twins. OM may be associated with genetic polymorphisms of host inflammatory response mechanisms.

Socioeconomic Status

Poverty has long been considered an important contributing factor to both the development and the severity of OM. Elements contributing to this relationship include crowding, limited hygienic facilities, suboptimal nutritional status, limited access to medical care, and limited resources for complying with prescribed medical regimens.

Breast Milk Compared to Formula Feeding

In general, studies have found a protective effect of breast milk feeding against OM. This protective effect is probably relatively limited, but may be greater in socioeconomically disadvantaged than in more advantaged children. The protective effect is attributable to the milk itself rather than to the mechanics of breastfeeding.

Exposure to Tobacco Smoke

Studies that have used objective measures to determine infant exposure to second-hand tobacco smoke, such as cotinine levels, have more consistently identified a significant linkage between tobacco smoke and OM. This evidence would suggest that exposure to tobacco smoke should be considered an important preventable risk factor in the development of OM.

Exposure to Other Children

Many studies have established that a strong, positive relationship exists between the occurrence of OM and the extent of repeated exposure to other children—measured mainly by the number of other children involved—whether at home or in out-of-home group daycare. Together, but independently, family socioeconomic status and the extent of exposure to other children appear to constitute 2 of the most important identifiable risk factors for developing OM.

Season

In temperate climates, in keeping with the pattern of occurrence of upper respiratory tract infections in general, highest rates of occurrence of OM are observed during cold weather months and lowest rates during warm weather months. In OM, it is likely that these findings strongly depend on the significant association of OM to viral respiratory illnesses.

Congenital Anomalies

OM is universal among infants with unrepaired palatal clefts, and is also highly prevalent among children with submucous cleft palate, other craniofacial anomalies, and Down syndrome (Chapter 76). The common feature in these congenital anomalies is a deficiency in the functioning of the eustachian tubes, which predisposes these children to middle ear disease.

Vaccination Status

Streptococcus pneumoniae (Chapter 175) has historically been the most common pathogen identified in patients with acute OM. Vaccination of infants with a conjugated pneumococcal vaccine has a modest effect, lowering visits to physicians and antibiotic prescriptions for OM by only 6-8%. Vaccination does appear to have a somewhat more protective effect in limiting frequent OM episodes and the need for surgical intervention with tympanostomy tubes. Pneumococcal vaccination has decreased the overall rate of episodes of OM associated with pneumococcus and increased quality of life (Fig. 632-1). Annual influenza virus vaccination also results in a decrease in OM incidence.

Other Factors

Pacifier use is linked with an increased incidence of OM and recurrence of OM, although the effect is small. Neither maternal age nor birthweight nor season of birth appears to influence the occurrence of OM once other demographic factors are taken into account. Very limited data is available regarding the association of OM to bottle feeding in the recumbent position.

Understanding the epidemiology of OM can be important in making clinical decisions. Patients that have craniofacial abnormalities should be considered as prone to otitis. Children that have high exposure rates to other children through daycare, lower socioeconomic status, tobacco exposure, strong family history of OM, and early age of 1st onset of OM should be considered as being more prone to OM. Identifying these factors

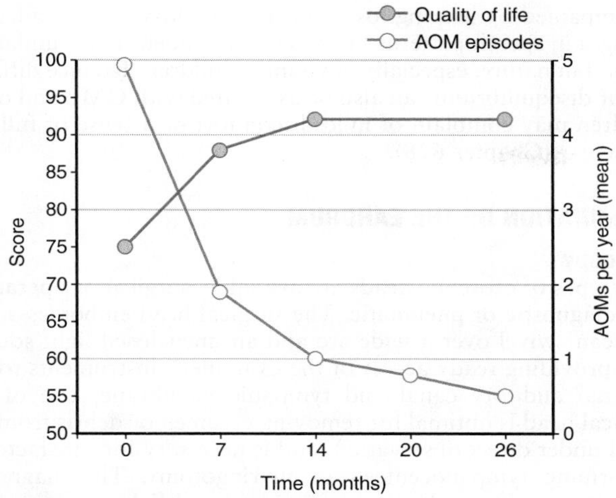

Figure 632-1 Quality of life and frequency of acute otitis media (AOM). (From Brouwer AR, Maillé M, Rovers R, et al: Effect of pneumococcal vaccination on quality of life in children with recurrent otitis media: a randomized, controlled trial, *Pediatrics* 115:273–279, 2005, Fig 2.)

may be important in counseling caregivers, assisting with changing risk behaviors and making decisions for referral for surgical management with tympanostomy tube placement.

ETIOLOGY

Acute Otitis Media (AOM)

Pathogenic bacteria can be isolated by standard culture techniques from middle-ear fluid in a majority of well-documented AOM. A high percentage of cases have cultures with either no growth or the presence of organisms generally considered nonpathogenic. Three pathogens predominate in AOM: *Streptococcus pneumoniae*, nontypeable *Haemophilus influenzae*, and *Moraxella catarrhalis*. The overall incidence of these organisms has changed with the widespread use of the conjugate pneumococcal vaccine. In countries where this vaccine is employed, nontypeable *H. influenzae* has overtaken *S. pneumoniae* as the most common pathogen; found in 40-50% of cases. *S. pneumoniae* still represents a common pathogen found in 30-50% of cases with *M. catarrhalis* representing the majority of the remaining cases. Other pathogens include group A streptococcus, *Staphylococcus aureus*, and gram-negative organisms. *S. aureus* and gram-negative organisms are found most commonly in neonates and very young infants who are hospitalized; in outpatient settings, the distribution of pathogens in these young infants is similar to that in older infants. Molecular techniques to identify bacterial pathogens have suggested the importance of other bacterial species such as *Alloiococcus otitidis*.

Evidence of respiratory viruses also may be found in middle-ear exudates of children with AOM, either alone or, more commonly, in association with pathogenic bacteria. Of these viruses, rhinovirus and respiratory syncytial virus (RSV) are found most often. AOM is a known complication of bronchiolitis; middle ear aspirates in children with bronchiolitis regularly contain bacterial pathogens, suggesting that RSV is rarely, if ever, the sole cause of their AOM. Using more precise measures of viable bacteria than standard culture techniques, such as polymerase chain reaction assays, a much higher rate of bacterial pathogens can be demonstrated. It remains uncertain whether viruses alone can cause AOM, or whether, their role is limited to setting the stage for bacterial invasion, and perhaps also to amplifying the inflammatory process and interfering with resolution of the bacterial infection. Viral pathogens have a negative impact on eustachian tube function, can impair local immune function, increase bacterial adherence and change pharmacokinetics reducing the efficacy of antimicrobial medications.

Otitis Media with Effusion (OME)

Using standard culture techniques, the pathogens typically found in AOM are recoverable in only 30% of children with OME. However, in studies of children with OME using PCR assays, middle-ear effusions have been found to contain evidence of bacterial DNA and viral RNA in much larger proportions of these children. These studies suggest that these patients do not have sterile effusions as previously thought.

PATHOGENESIS

Anatomic Factors

Patients with significant craniofacial abnormalities affecting the eustachian tube function have an increased incidence of OM. In addition, during the pathogenesis of OM the eustachian tube demonstrates decreased effectiveness in ventilating the middle-ear space.

Under usual circumstances the eustachian tube is passively closed and is opened by contraction of the tensor veli palatini muscle. In relation to the middle ear, the tube has 3 main functions: ventilation, protection, and clearance. The middle-ear mucosa depends on a continuing supply of air from the nasopharynx delivered by way of the eustachian tube. Interruption of this ventilatory process by tubal obstruction initiates an inflammatory response that includes secretory metaplasia, compromise of the mucociliary transport system, and effusion of liquid into the tympanic cavity. Measurements of eustachian tube function have demonstrated that the tubal function is suboptimal during the events of OM with increased opening pressures.

Eustachian tube obstruction may result from extraluminal blockage via hypertrophied nasopharyngeal adenoid tissue or tumor, or may result from intraluminal obstruction via inflammatory edema of the tubal mucosa, most commonly as a consequence of a viral upper respiratory tract infection. Progressive reduction in tubal wall compliance with increasing age may explain the progressive decline in the occurrence of OM as children grow older. The protection and clearance functions of the eustachian tube may also be involved in the pathogenesis of OM. Thus, if the eustachian tube is patulous or excessively compliant, it may fail to protect the middle ear from reflux of infective nasopharyngeal secretions, whereas impairment of the mucociliary clearance function of the tube might contribute to both the establishment and persistence of infection. The shorter and more horizontal orientation of the tube in infants and young children may increase the likelihood of reflux from the nasopharynx and impair passive gravitational drainage through the eustachian tube.

In special patient populations with craniofacial abnormalities there exists an increased incidence of OM that has been associated with the abnormal eustachian tube function. In children with cleft palate, where OM is a universal finding, the main factor underlying the chronic middle-ear inflammation appears to be impairment of the opening mechanism of the eustachian tube, due perhaps to greater-than-normal compliance of the tubal wall. Another possible factor is defective velopharyngeal valving, which may result in disturbed aerodynamic and hydrodynamic relationships in the nasopharynx and proximal portions of the eustachian tubes. In children with other craniofacial anomalies and with Down syndrome, the high prevalence of OM has also been attributed to structural and/or functional eustachian tubal abnormalities.

Host Factors

The effectiveness of a child's immune system in response to the bacterial and viral insults of the upper airway and middle ear during early childhood probably is the most important factor in determining which children are otitis prone. The maturation of this immune system during early childhood is most likely the primary event leading to the decrease in incidence of OM as children move through childhood. IgA deficiency is found in some children with recurrent AOM but the significance is questionable, inasmuch as IgA deficiency is also found not infrequently in children without recurrent AOM. Selective IgG subclass deficiencies (despite normal total serum IgG) may be found in children with recurrent AOM in association with recurrent sinopulmonary infection, and these deficiencies probably underlie the susceptibility to infection. Children with recurrent OM that is not associated with recurrent infection at other sites rarely have a readily identifiable immunologic deficiency. Nonetheless, evidence that subtle immune deficits play a role in the pathogenesis of recurrent AOM is provided by studies involving antibody responses to various types of infection and immunization; by the observation that breast milk feeding, as opposed to formula feeding, confers limited protection against the occurrence of OM in infants with cleft palate; and by studies in which young children with recurrent AOM achieved a measure of protection from intramuscularly administered bacterial polysaccharide immune globulin or intravenously administered polyclonal immunoglobulin. This evidence, along with the documented decrease incidence of upper respiratory tract infections and OM as children's immune systems develop and mature is indicative of the importance of a child's innate immune system in the pathogenesis of OM (Chapter 118).

Viral Pathogens

Although OM may develop and certainly may persist in the absence of apparent respiratory tract infection, many, if not most, episodes are initiated by viral or bacterial upper respiratory tract infection. In a study of children in group daycare, AOM was observed in approximately 30-40% of children with respiratory illness caused by RSV (Chapter 252), influenza viruses (Chapter 250), or adenoviruses (Chapter 254), and in approximately 10-15% of children with respiratory illness caused by parainfluenza viruses, rhinoviruses, or enteroviruses. Viral infection of the upper respiratory tract results in release of cytokines and inflammatory mediators, some of which may cause eustachian tube dysfunction. Respiratory viruses also may enhance nasopharyngeal bacterial colonization and adherence and impair host immune defenses against bacterial infection.

Allergy

Evidence that respiratory allergy is a primary etiologic agent in OM is not convincing; however, in children with both conditions it is possible that the otitis is aggravated by the allergy.

Risk profile and host-pathogen interactions have increasingly become recognized as playing important roles in the pathogenesis of otitis media. Such events as alterations in mucociliary clearance through repeated viral exposure experienced in daycare settings or through exposure to tobacco smoke may tip the balance of pathogenesis in less virulent OM pathogens in their favor. Children with frequent exposure to other children have an increased risk of both nasopharyngeal colonization and acute OM pathology with bacterial types with multiple antimicrobial resistances making treatment more difficult and prolonged pathology more likely.

CLINICAL MANIFESTATIONS

Symptoms of AOM are variable, especially in infants and young children. In young children, evidence of ear pain may be manifested by irritability or a change in sleeping or eating habits and occasionally, holding or tugging at the ear (see Table 632-1). Pulling at the ear has a low sensitivity and specificity. Fever may also be present. Rupture of the tympanic membrane with purulent otorrhea is uncommon. Systemic symptoms and symptoms associated with upper respiratory tract infections also occur; occasionally there may be no symptoms, the disease having been discovered at a routine health examination. OME often is not accompanied by overt complaints of the child but can be accompanied by hearing loss. This hearing loss may manifest as changes in speech patterns but often goes undetected if unilateral or mild in nature, especially in younger children. Balance difficulties or disequilibrium can also be associated with OME and older children may complain of mild discomfort or a sense of fullness in the ear (Chapter 628).

EXAMINATION OF THE EARDRUM

Otoscopy

Two types of otoscope heads are available: **surgical** or **operating**, and **diagnostic** or **pneumatic**. The surgical head embodies a lens that can swivel over a wide arc and an unenclosed light source, thus providing ready access of the examiner's instruments to the external auditory canal and tympanic membrane. Use of the surgical head is optimal for removing cerumen or debris from the canal under direct observation, and is necessary for satisfactorily performing tympanocentesis or myringotomy. The diagnostic head incorporates a larger lens, an enclosed light source, and a nipple for the attachment of a rubber bulb and tubing. When an attached speculum is fitted snugly into the external auditory canal, an airtight chamber is created comprising the vault of the otoscope head, the bulb and tubing, the speculum, and the proximal portion of the external canal. Although examination of the ear in young children is a relatively invasive procedure that is often met with lack of cooperation by the patient, this task can be enhanced if done with as little pain as possible. The outer portion of the ear canal contains hair-bearing skin and subcutaneous fat and cartilage that allow a speculum to be placed with relatively little discomfort. Closer to the tympanic membrane the ear canal is made of bone and is lined only with skin and no adnexal structures or subcutaneous fat; a speculum pushed too far forward and placed in this area often causes skin abrasion and pain. Using a rubber-tipped speculum or adding a small sleeve of rubber tubing to the tip of the plastic speculum may serve to minimize patient discomfort and enhance the ability to achieve a proper fit and an airtight seal.

Learning to perform pneumatic otoscopy is a critical skill in being able to assess a child's ear and in making an accurate diagnosis of OM. By observing as the bulb is alternately squeezed gently and released, the degree of tympanic membrane mobility in response to both positive and negative pressure can be estimated providing a critical assessment of middle ear fluid which is a hallmark sign of both AOM and OME. With both types of otoscope heads, bright illumination is also critical for adequate visualization of the tympanic membrane.

Clearing the External Auditory Canal

If the tympanic membrane is obscured by cerumen, the cerumen may be removed under direct observation through the surgical head of the otoscope, using a Buck curette (N-400-0, Storz Instrument Co). Remaining bits can then be wiped away using a Farrell applicator (N-2001A, Storz Instrument Co), with its tip (triangular in cross section) wrapped with a bit of dry or alcohol-moistened cotton to create a dry or wet "mop." Alternatively, gentle suction may be applied, using a No. 5 or 7 French ear suction tube. During this procedure it may be most advantageous to restrain the infant or young child in the prone position, turning the child's head to the left or right as each ear is cleared. One adult, usually a parent, can place one hand on each of the child's buttocks and brace the child's hips against the examining table, using his or her own weight for additional bracing if necessary. Another adult can restrain the child's head with one hand and the child's free arm with the other, changing hands for the opposite ear. In children old enough to cooperate, usually beginning at about 5 yr of age, clearing of the external canal may be achieved more easily and safely and less traumatically by lavage than by mechanical removal, provided one can be certain that a tympanic membrane perforation is not present. In general, many

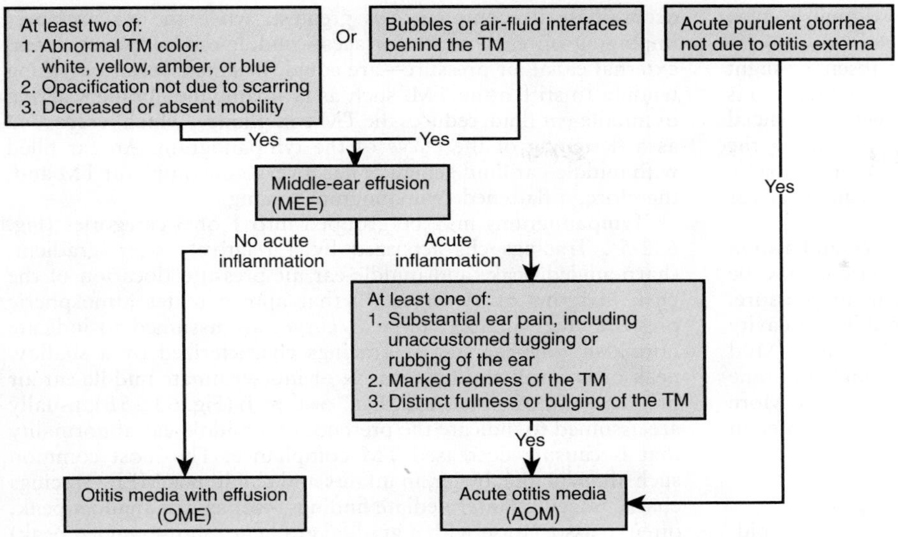

Figure 632-2 Algorithm for distinguishing between acute otitis media and otitis media with effusion. TM, tympanic membrane.

children's ears are "self-cleaning" due to squamous migration of ear canal skin, and parental cleaning of cerumen with cotton swabs often complicates cerumen impaction by pushing cerumen deeper into the canal and compacting it.

Tympanic Membrane Findings

Important characteristics of the tympanic membrane consist of contour, color, translucence, structural changes if any, and mobility. Normally the contour of the membrane is **slightly concave;** abnormalities consist of fullness or bulging, or conversely, extreme retraction. The normal color of the tympanic membrane is **pearly gray.** Erythema may be a sign of inflammation or infection, but unless intense, erythema alone may result from crying or vascular flushing. Abnormal whiteness of the membrane may result from either scarring or the presence of liquid in the middle-ear cavity; liquid also may impart an amber, pale yellow, or, rarely, bluish color. Normally, the membrane is translucent, although some degree of opacity may be normal in the 1st few mo of life; later, opacification denotes either scarring, or more commonly, underlying effusion. Structural changes include scars, perforations, retraction pockets, and a more severe complication of OM, cholesteatoma formation. Of all the visible characteristics of the tympanic membrane, mobility is the most sensitive and specific in determining the presence or absence of MEE. Mobility is not an all-or-none phenomenon; although total absence of mobility, in the absence of a tympanic membrane perforation, is virtually always indicative of MEE, substantial impairment of mobility is the more common finding.

Diagnosis

A certain diagnosis of OM should contain all of the following elements: (1) recent and usually acute onset of illness, (2) presence of MEE, and (3) signs and symptoms of middle-ear inflammation including erythema of the tympanic membrane or otalgia (see Table 632-1). A simplified differentiating schema establishes a diagnosis of AOM when, in addition to having MEE, a child gives evidence of recent, clinically important ear pain or the tympanic membrane shows marked redness or distinct fullness or bulging.

Distinguishing between AOM and OME on clinical grounds is straightforward in most cases, although each condition may evolve into the other without any clearly differentiating physical findings; any schema for distinguishing between them is to some extent arbitrary. In an era of increasing bacterial resistance, distinguishing between AOM and OME is important in determining treatment, because OME in the absence of acute infection does not require antimicrobial therapy. Purulent otorrhea of recent onset is indicative of AOM; thus, difficulty in distinguishing clinically between AOM and OME is limited to circumstances in which purulent otorrhea is not present. Both AOM without otorrhea and OME are accompanied by physical signs of MEE, namely, the presence of at least 2 of 3 tympanic membrane abnormalities: white, yellow, amber, or (rarely) blue discoloration; opacification other than that due to scarring; and decreased or absent mobility. Alternatively in OME, either air-fluid levels or air bubbles outlined by small amounts of fluid may be visible behind the tympanic membrane, a condition often indicative of impending resolution (Fig. 632-2).

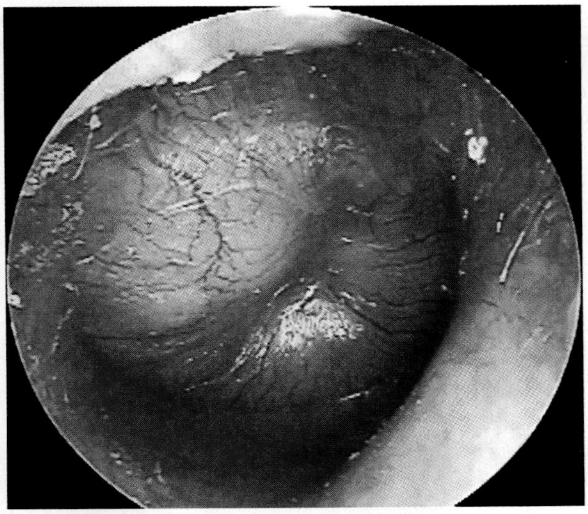

Figure 632-3 Tympanic membrane in acute otitis media.

To support a diagnosis of AOM instead of OME in a child with MEE, distinct fullness or bulging of the tympanic membrane may be present, with or without accompanying erythema; or, at minimum, MEE should be accompanied by ear pain that appears clinically important. Unless intense, erythema alone is insufficient because erythema, without other abnormalities, may result from crying or vascular flushing. In AOM the malleus may be obscured, and the tympanic membrane may resemble a bagel without a hole but with a central depression (Fig. 632-3). Rarely the tympanic membrane may be obscured by surface bullae, or may have a cobblestone appearance. **Bullous myringitis** is a physical manifestation of AOM and not an etiologically discrete entity. Within days after onset, fullness of the membrane may diminish, even though infection may still be present.

In OME, bulging of the tympanic membrane is absent or slight or the membrane may be retracted (Fig. 632-4); erythema also is absent or slight, but may increase with crying or with superficial trauma to the external auditory canal incurred in clearing the canal of cerumen. In children with MEE but without tympanic membrane fullness or bulging, the presence of unequivocal ear pain is usually indicative of AOM.

Commonly, both before and after episodes of OM and also in the absence of otitis media, the tympanic membrane may be retracted as a consequence of negative middle-ear air pressure. The presumed cause is diffusion of air from the middle-ear cavity more rapidly than it is replaced via the eustachian tube. Mild retraction cannot be considered pathologic, although in some children it is accompanied by mild conductive hearing loss. More extreme retraction, however, is of concern, as discussed later in the section on sequelae of OM.

Tympanometry

Tympanometry, or **acoustic immittance testing,** is a simple, rapid, atraumatic test that, when performed correctly, offers objective evidence of the presence or absence of MEE. The tympanogram provides information about tympanic membrane (TM) **compliance** in electroacoustic terms that can be thought of as roughly equivalent to TM mobility as perceived visually during pneumatic otoscopy. The absorption of sound by the TM varies inversely with its stiffness. The stiffness of the membrane is least, and accordingly its compliance is greatest, when the air pressures impinging on each of its surfaces—middle-ear air pressure and external canal air pressure—are equal. In simple terms, anything tending to stiffen the TM, such as tympanic membrane scarring or middle-ear fluid, reduces the TM compliance, which is recorded as a flattening of the curve of the tympanogram. An ear filled with middle-ear fluid generally has a very noncompliant TM and, therefore, a flattened tympanogram tracing.

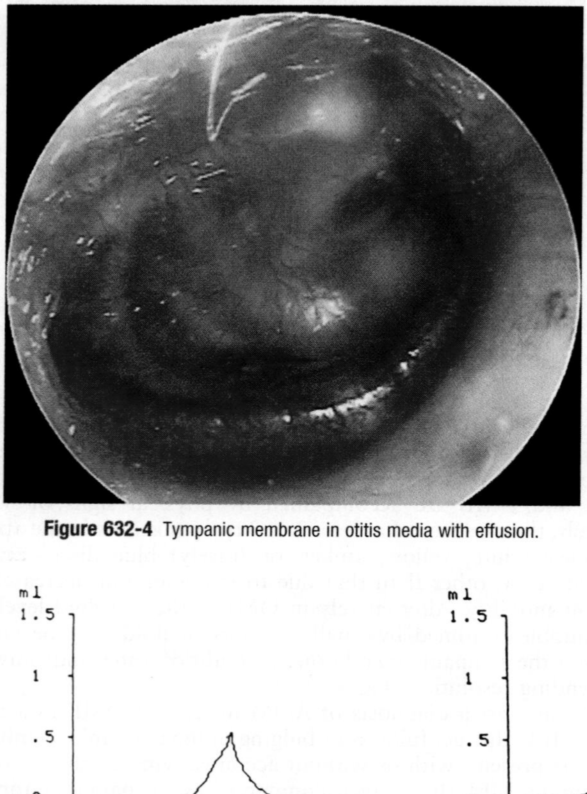

Figure 632-4 Tympanic membrane in otitis media with effusion.

Tympanograms may be grouped into 1 of 3 categories (Fig. 632-5). Tracings characterized by a relatively steep gradient, sharp-angled peak, and middle-ear air pressure (location of the peak in terms of air pressure) that approximates atmospheric pressure (Fig. 632-5*A*) (type A curve) are assumed to indicate normal middle-ear status. Tracings characterized by a shallow peak or no peak and by negative or indeterminate middle-ear air pressure, and often termed "flat" or type B (Fig. 632-5*B*), usually are assumed to indicate the presence of a middle-ear abnormality that is causing decreased TM compliance. The most common such abnormality, by far, in infants and children is MEE. Tracings characterized by intermediate findings—somewhat shallow peak, often in association with a gradual gradient (obtuse-angled peak) or negative middle-ear air pressure, or combinations of these features (Fig. 632-5*C*)—may or may not be associated with MEE, and must be considered nondiagnostic or equivocal. In general, the shallower the peak, the more gradual the gradient, and the more negative the middle-ear air pressure, the greater the likelihood of MEE.

When reading a tympanogram it is important to look at the volume measurement also provided. A patient with a tympanic membrane perforation or patent tympanostomy tube will have a flat type B tympanogram and a "high volume." The tympanometer measures and records the volume of the external auditory canal, and if a tympanic membrane perforation or a patent tympanostomy tube is present, the volume of the middle ear and mastoid air cells as well. A volume reading >1.0 mL should suggest the presence of either a perforation or a patent tympanostomy tube. Therefore, in a child with a tympanostomy tube present, a flat tympanogram with a volume <1.0 mL would suggest a plugged or nonfunctioning tube and middle-ear fluid, while a flat tympanogram with a volume >1.0 mL would suggest a patent tympanostomy tube.

Although tympanometry is quite sensitive in detecting MEE, it can be limited by patient cooperation, the skill of the individual administering the test, and the age of the child, with less reliable results in very young children. Use of tympanometry may be helpful in office screening, by obviating the need for routine otoscopic examination in difficult-to-examine patients whose tympanic membranes have been visualized previously, who are asymptomatic, and whose tympanograms are classified as normal, and by identifying patients who require further attention because their tympanograms are abnormal. Tympanometry also may be

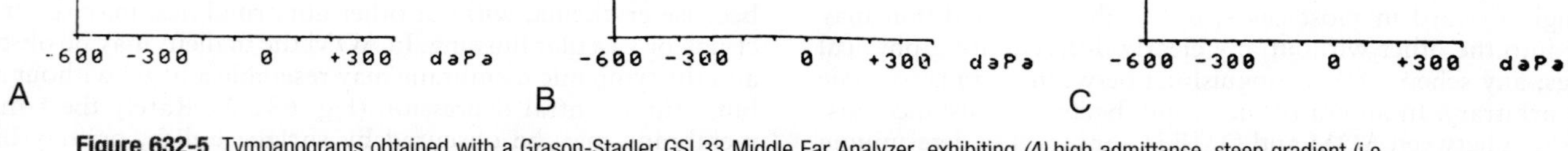

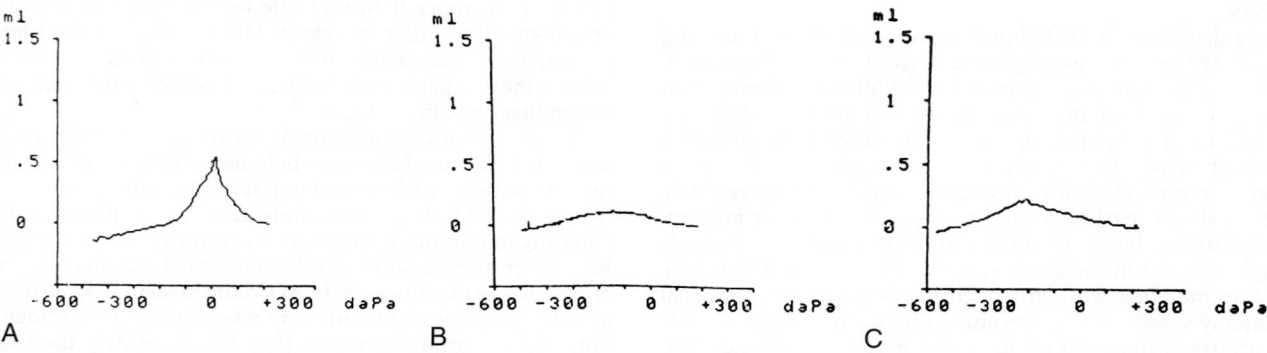

Figure 632-5 Tympanograms obtained with a Grason-Stadler GSI 33 Middle Ear Analyzer, exhibiting *(A)* high admittance, steep gradient (i.e., sharp-angled peak), and middle-ear air pressure approximating atmospheric pressure (0 decaPascals [daPa]); *(B)* low admittance and indeterminate middle-ear air pressure; and *(C)* somewhat low admittance, gradual gradient, and markedly negative middle-ear air pressure.

used to help confirm, refine, or clarify questionable otoscopic findings; to objectify the follow-up evaluation of patients with known middle-ear disease; and to validate otoscopic diagnoses of MEE. Importantly, even though tympanometry can predict the probability of MEE, it cannot distinguish the effusion of OME from that of AOM.

Conjunctivitis Otitis Media Syndrome

Simultaneous appearance of purulent and erythematous conjunctivitis with an ipsilateral OM is a well-recognized syndrome, due in most children to nontypeable *H. influenzae* (Chapter 186). The disease often is present in multiple family members and affects young children and infants. Topical ocular antibiotics are ineffective; therapy includes oral antibiotics (see later) effective against nontypeable *H. influenzae*.

TREATMENT

Management of Acute Otitis Media

Individual episodes of AOM have customarily been treated with antimicrobial drugs. Concern about increasing bacterial resistance has prompted some clinicians to recommend withholding antimicrobial treatment in some or most cases unless symptoms persist for 2 or 3 days, or worsen (Table 632-2). Three factors argue in favor of routinely prescribing antimicrobial therapy for children who have documented AOM using the diagnostic criteria outlined previously (see Table 632-1 and Fig. 632-3). First, pathogenic bacteria cause a large majority of cases. Second, symptomatic improvement and resolution of infection occur more promptly and more consistently with antimicrobial treatment than without, even though most untreated cases eventually resolve. Third, prompt and adequate antimicrobial treatment may prevent the development of suppurative complications. The sharp decline in such complications during the last half-century seems likely attributable, at least in part, to the widespread routine use of antimicrobials for AOM. In the Netherlands, where initial antibiotic treatment is routinely withheld from most children older than 6 mo of age, and where only approximately 30% of children with AOM receive antibiotics at all, the incidence of acute mastoiditis, although low (in children <14 yr, 3.8 per 100,000 person years), appears slightly higher than rates in other countries with higher antibiotic prescription rates by about 1-2 episodes per 100,000 person years. It is also the case that follow-up of children in the Netherlands may be generally more assiduous than is customary in other countries including the USA, where failure to improve or worsening symptoms might not be detected as promptly.

These considerations in treating AOM with antimicrobial therapy must be balanced against the continued increasing rates of bacterial antimicrobial resistance. In countries such as the Netherlands where use of antibiotics for OM is much less common, the antimicrobial resistance rates for the major pathogens in OM are substantially lower than those in countries that routinely treat AOM with antibiotics. Given that most episodes of OM will spontaneously resolve, consensus guidelines have been published by the American Academy of Pediatrics to assist clinicians who wish to consider a period of "watchful waiting" or observation prior to treating AOM with antibiotics (Tables 632-2 and 632-3; Fig. 632-6). The most important aspect of these guidelines is that close follow-up of the patient must be ensured to assess for lack of spontaneous resolution or worsening of symptoms and that patients should be provided with adequate analgesic medications (acetaminophen, ibuprofen) during the period of observation. When pursuing the practice of watchful waiting in patients with AOM, the certainty of the diagnosis, the patient's age, and the severity of the disease should be considered. For younger patients, <2 yr of age, it is recommended to treat all confirmed diagnoses of AOM. In very young patients, <6 mo, even presumed episodes of AOM should be treated due to the increased potential of significant morbidity from infectious complications. In children between 6 and 24 mo who have a questionable diagnosis of OM but severe disease, defined as temperature of >102°F (>39°C), significant otalgia, or toxic appearance, antibiotic therapy is also recommended. Children in this age group with a questionable diagnosis and nonsevere disease can be observed for a period of 2-3 days with close follow-up. In children older than 2 yr of age, observation might be considered in all episodes of nonsevere OM or episodes of questionable diagnosis, while antibiotic therapy is reserved for confirmed, severe episodes of AOM.

Table 632-2 CRITERIA FOR INITIAL ANTIBACTERIAL-AGENT TREATMENT OR OBSERVATION IN CHILDREN WITH AOM

AGE	CERTAIN DIAGNOSIS	UNCERTAIN DIAGNOSIS
<6 mo	Antibacterial therapy	Antibacterial therapy
6 mo-2 yr	Antibacterial therapy	Antibacterial therapy if severe illness; observation option* if nonsevere illness
≥2 yr	Antibacterial therapy if severe illness; observation option* if nonsevere illness	Observation option*

This table was modified with permission from the New York State Department of Health and the New York Region Otitis Project Committee.

*Observation is an appropriate option only when follow-up can be ensured and antibacterial agents started if symptoms persist or worsen. Nonsevere illness is mild otalgia and fever <39°C in the past 24 hr. Severe illness is moderate to severe otalgia or fever ≥39°C. A certain diagnosis of AOM meets all 3 criteria: (1) rapid onset; (2) signs of MEE; and (3) signs and symptoms of middle-ear inflammation.

From Subcommittee on Management of Acute Otitis Media: Diagnosis and management of acute otitis media, *Pediatrics* 113:1451–1465, 2004.

Bacterial Resistance

Persons at greatest risk of harboring resistant bacteria are those who are <2 yr of age; are in regular contact with large groups of other children, especially in daycare settings; or who recently have received antimicrobial treatment. Bacterial resistance is a particular problem in relation to OM. The development of resistant bacterial strains and their rapid spread have been fostered and facilitated by selective pressure resulting from extensive use of antimicrobial drugs, the most common target of which, in children, is OM. Many strains of each of the pathogenic bacteria that commonly cause AOM are resistant to commonly used antimicrobial drugs.

Although antimicrobial resistance rates vary between countries, in the USA approximately 40% of strains of nontypeable *H. influenzae* and almost all strains of *M. catarrhalis* are resistant to aminopenicillins (e.g., ampicillin and amoxicillin). In most cases the resistance is attributable to production of β-lactamase, and can be overcome by combining amoxicillin with a β-lactamase inhibitor (clavulanate), or by using a β-lactamase–stable antibiotic. Occasional strains of nontypeable *H. influenzae* that do not produce β-lactamase are resistant to aminopenicillins and other β-lactam antibiotics by virtue of alterations in their penicillin-binding proteins.

In the USA, approximately 50% of strains of *S. pneumoniae* are penicillin-nonsusceptible, divided approximately equally between penicillin-intermediate and, even more difficult to treat, penicillin-resistant strains. A much higher incidence of resistance is seen in children attending daycare. Resistance by *S. pneumoniae* to the penicillins and other β-lactam antibiotics is mediated not by β-lactamase production, but by alterations in penicillin-binding proteins. There are at least 6 known penicillin-binding proteins, and the degree of resistance increases in response to the number of alterations in these proteins. This mechanism of resistance can be overcome if higher concentrations of β-lactam antibiotics at the site of infection can be achieved for a sufficient time interval. Many penicillin-resistant strains of *S. pneumoniae* are also resistant to other antimicrobial drugs, including sulfonamides, macrolides, and cephalosporins. In general, as penicillin resistance increases, so also does resistance to other antimicrobial classes. Resistance to macrolides, including azithromycin and clarithromycin, by *S. pneumoniae* has increased rapidly, rendering theses antimicrobials far less effective in treating AOM. Two mechanisms of macrolide resistance have been identified: one, mediated by the mef(A) gene, involves an efflux pump that decreases intracellular accumulation of macrolides and results in low-level resistance; the other mechanism, mediated by the erm(B) gene, involves production of ribosomal methylases that modify ribosomal RNA and result in high-level resistance. The latter mechanism also results in resistance to clindamycin, which otherwise is generally effective against resistant strains of *S. pneumoniae*. Unlike resistance to β-lactam antibiotics, macrolide resistance cannot be overcome by increasing the dose. Although vancomycin was previously a fail-safe antimicrobial in treating *S. pneumoniae*, clinical cases of vancomycin-tolerant *S. pneumoniae* have been identified, further raising the importance and hazard of antimicrobial resistance.

First-Line Antimicrobial Treatment

Amoxicillin remains the drug of 1st choice for uncomplicated AOM under most circumstances because of its excellent record of safety, relative efficacy, palatability, and low cost (see Table 632-3). In particular, amoxicillin is the most efficacious of available oral antimicrobial drugs against both penicillin-susceptible and penicillin-nonsusceptible strains of *S. pneumoniae*. Increasing the dose from the traditional 40-45 mg/kg/24 hr to 80-90 mg/kg/24 hr will generally provide efficacy against penicillin-intermediate and some penicillin-resistant strains. This higher dose should be used particularly in children <2 yr of age, in children who have recently received treatment with β-lactam drugs, and in children who are exposed to large numbers of other children due to their increased likelihood of an infection with a nonsusceptible strain of *S. pneumoniae*. A limitation of amoxicillin is that it may be inactivated by the β-lactamases produced by many strains of nontypeable *H. influenzae* and most strains of *M. catarrhalis*. This factor has become increasingly important with data demonstrating an overall increase in frequency of *H. influenzae* as the primary pathogen in AOM secondary to widespread utilization of the conjugated pneumococcal vaccine in young children. Episodes of AOM caused by these pathogens often resolve spontaneously. Allergies to penicillin antibiotics should be categorized into type I hypersensitivity, consisting of urticaria or anaphylaxis, and those that fall short of type I reactions, such as rash formation. For children with a non–type I

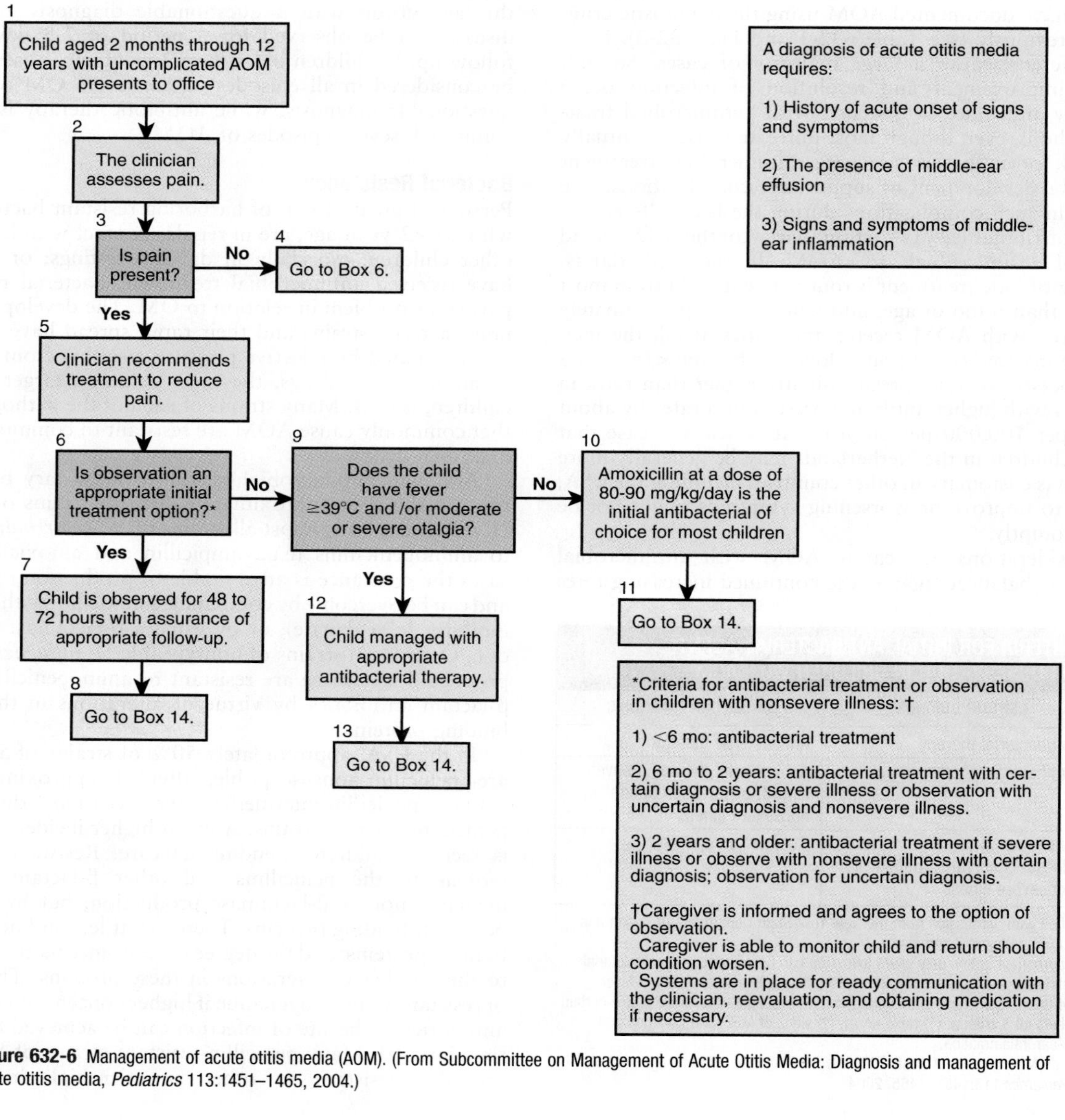

Figure 632-6 Management of acute otitis media (AOM). (From Subcommittee on Management of Acute Otitis Media: Diagnosis and management of acute otitis media, *Pediatrics* 113:1451–1465, 2004.)

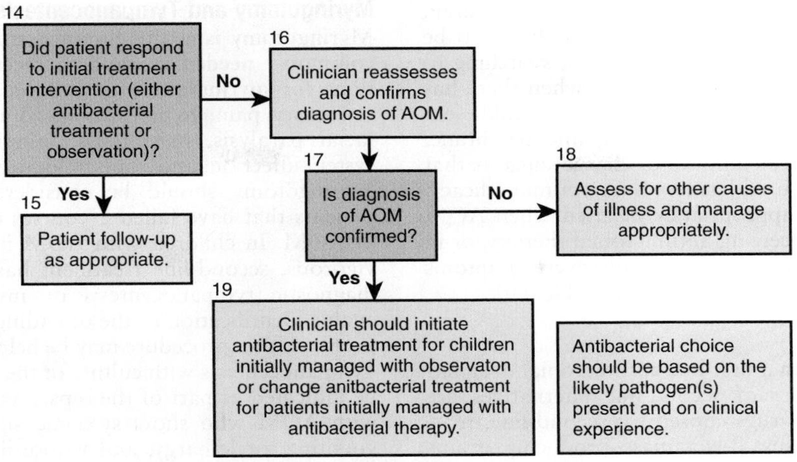

Figure 632-6, cont'd For legend, see opposite page.

Table 632-3 RECOMMENDED ANTIBACTERIAL AGENTS FOR PATIENTS WHO ARE BEING TREATED INITIALLY WITH ANTIBACTERIAL AGENTS OR HAVE FAILED 48 TO 72 HOURS OF OBSERVATION OR INITIAL MANAGEMENT WITH ANTIBACTERIAL AGENTS

TEMPERATURE ≥39°C AND/OR SEVERE OTALGIA	AT DIAGNOSIS FOR PATIENTS BEING TREATED INITIALLY WITH ANTIBACTERIAL AGENTS		CLINICALLY DEFINED TREATMENT FAILURE AT 48-72 HR AFTER INITIAL MANAGEMENT WITH OBSERVATION OPTION		CLINICALLY DEFINED TREATMENT FAILURE AT 48-72 HR AFTER INITIAL MANAGEMENT WITH ANTIBACTERIAL AGENTS	
	Recommended	Alternative for Penicillin Allergy	Recommended	Alternative for Penicillin Allergy	Recommended	Alternative for Penicillin Allergy
No	Amoxicillin, 80-90 mg/kg per day	Non–type 1: cefdinir, cefuroxime, cefpodoxime; type 1: azithromycin, clarithromycin	Amoxicillin, 80-90 mg/kg per day	Non–type 1: cefdinir, cefuroxime, cefpodoxime; type 1: azithromycin, clarithromycin	Amoxicillin-clavulanate, 90 mg/kg per day of amoxicillin component, with 6.4 mg/kg per day of clavulanate	Non–type 1: ceftriaxone, 3 days; type 1: clindamycin
Yes	Amoxicillin-clavulanate, 90 mg/kg per day of amoxicillin, with 6.4 mg/kg per day of clavulanate	Ceftriaxon, 1 or 3 days	Amoxicillin, clavulanate, 90 mg/kg per day of amoxicillin, with 6.4 mg/kg per day of clavulanate	Ceftriaxon, 1 or 3 days	Ceftriaxone, 3 days	Tympanocentesis, clindamycin

From Subcommittee on Management of Acute Otitis Media: Diagnosis and management of acute otitis media, *Pediatrics* 113:1451–1465, 2004.

reaction in which cross reactivity with cephalosporins is less of a concern, first-line therapy with cefdinir would be an appropriate choice. In children with a type I reaction or known sensitivity to cephalosporin antibiotics, or in whom palatability or convenience of administration are of overriding importance, azithromycin is an appropriate alternative first-line drug. Resistance to trimethoprim-sulfamethoxazole (TMP-SMZ), by many strains of both *H. influenzae* and *S. pneumoniae* and a reported high clinical failure rate in children with AOM treated initially with this antimicrobial argue against its use as first-line treatment.

Duration of Treatment

The duration of treatment of AOM has historically been set at 10 days and most efficacy studies examining antimicrobial treatment in AOM have utilized this duration as a benchmark. However, 10 days may be unduly long for some children while not long enough for others. Studies comparing shorter with longer durations of treatment suggest that short-course treatment will often prove inadequate in children <6 yr of age, and particularly in children <2 yr of age. Thus, for most episodes in most children, treatment that provides tissue concentrations of an antimicrobial for at least 10 days would seem advisable. Treatment for shorter periods, of 3-5 days, may be appropriate for older children with mild episodes who improve quickly; in these cases, simple observation without antimicrobial therapy may often be the preferred intervention. Treatment for longer than 10 days may be required for children who are very young or are having severe episodes or whose previous experience with OM has been problematic.

Follow-Up

The principal goals of follow-up are to assess the outcome of treatment and to differentiate between inadequate response to treatment and early recurrence. The appropriate interval for follow-up should be individualized. Follow-up within days is advisable in the young infant with a severe episode or in a child of any age with continuing pain. Follow-up within 2 wk is appropriate for the infant or young child who has apparently been having frequent recurrences. At that point, the tympanic membrane is not likely to have returned to normal, but substantial improvement in its appearance should be evident. In the child with only a sporadic episode of AOM and prompt symptomatic improvement, follow-up 1 mo after initial examination is early enough, or in older children, no follow-up may be necessary. The continuing presence of MEE alone following an episode of AOM is not an indication for additional or second-line antimicrobial treatment.

Unsatisfactory Response to First-Line Treatment

AOM is essentially a closed-space infection and its resolution depends both on eradication of the offending organism and restoration of middle-ear ventilation. Factors contributing to unsatisfactory response to first-line treatment, in addition to inadequate antimicrobial efficacy, include poor compliance with treatment regimens, concurrent or intercurrent viral infection, persistent eustachian tube dysfunction and middle-ear under-aeration, re-infection from other sites or from incompletely eradicated middle ear pathogens, and immature or impaired host defenses. The identification of biofilm formation in the middle ear of children with chronic OM also indicates that, in some children, eradication with standard antimicrobial therapy is likely to be unsuccessful. Despite these many potential factors, switching to an alternative or second-line drug is reasonable when there has been inadequate improvement in symptoms or in middle-ear status as reflected in the appearance of the tympanic membrane, or when the persistence of purulent nasal discharge suggests that the antimicrobial drug being used has less than optimal efficacy. Second-line drugs may also appropriately be used when AOM develops in a child already receiving antimicrobial therapy, or in an immunocompromised child, or in a child with severe symptoms whose previous experience with OM has been problematic.

Second-Line Treatment

When treatment of AOM with a first-line antimicrobial drug has proven inadequate, a number of second-line alternatives are available (see Table 632-3). Drugs chosen for second-line treatment should be effective against β-lactamase–producing strains of *H. influenzae* and *M. catarrhalis* and against susceptible and most nonsusceptible strains of *S. pneumoniae*. Only 4 antimicrobial agents meet these requirements: amoxicillin-clavulanate, cefdinir, cefuroxime axetil, and intramuscular ceftriaxone. Because high-dose amoxicillin (80-90 mg/kg/24 hr) is effective against most strains of *S. pneumoniae* and because the addition of clavulanate extends the effective antibacterial spectrum of amoxicillin to include β-lactamase–producing bacteria, high-dose amoxicillin-clavulanate is particularly well-suited as a second-line drug for treating AOM. The 14:1 amoxicillin-clavulanate formulation contains twice as much amoxicillin as the previously available 7:1 formulation. Diarrhea, especially in infants and young children, is a common adverse effect, but may be ameliorated in some cases by feeding yogurt, and usually is not severe enough to require cessation of treatment. Cefdinir has demonstrated broad efficacy in treatment, is generally well tolerated with respect to taste and can be given as a once-daily regimen. The ability to also utilize cefdinir in children with mild type 1 hypersensitivity reactions has further added to its favorable selection as a second-line agent. Both cefuroxime axetil and intramuscular ceftriaxone have important limitations for use in young children. The currently available suspension of cefuroxime axetil is not palatable and its acceptance is low. Ceftriaxone treatment entails both the pain of intramuscular injection and substantial cost, and the injection may need to be repeated once or twice at 2-day intervals to achieve the desired degree of effectiveness. Nonetheless, use of ceftriaxone is appropriate in severe cases of AOM when oral treatment is not feasible, or in highly selected cases after treatment failure using orally administered second-line antimicrobials (i.e., amoxicillin-clavulanate or cefuroxime axetil), or when highly resistant *S. pneumoniae* is found in aspirates obtained from diagnostic tympanocentesis.

Clarithromycin and azithromycin have only limited activity against nonsusceptible strains of *S. pneumoniae* and against β-lactamase–producing strains of *H. influenzae*. Macrolide use also appears to be a major factor in causing increases in rates of resistance to macrolides by group A streptococcus and *S. pneumoniae*. Clindamycin is active against most strains of *S. pneumoniae,* including resistant strains, but is not active against *H. influenzae* or *M. catarrhalis*. It should therefore be reserved for patients known to have infection caused by penicillin-nonsusceptible pneumococci.

The remaining antimicrobial agents that have been traditionally utilized in the management of AOM have such significant lack of effectiveness against resistant organisms that employment seldom outweighs the potential side effects or complications possible from the medications. This includes, cefprozil, cefaclor, loracarbef, cefixime, TMP-SMZ, and erythromycin-sulfisoxazole. Cefpodoxime has demonstrated reasonable effectiveness in some investigations but is generally poorly tolerated due to its taste.

Myringotomy and Tympanocentesis

Myringotomy is a time-honored treatment for AOM but is not commonly needed in children receiving antimicrobials. **Indications for myringotomy** in children with AOM include severe, refractory pain; hyperpyrexia; complications of AOM such as facial paralysis, mastoiditis, labyrinthitis, or central nervous system infection; and immunologic compromise from any source. Myringotomy should be considered as third-line therapy in patients that have failed 2 courses of antibiotics for an episode of AOM. In children with AOM in whom clinical response to vigorous, second-line treatment has been unsatisfactory, either diagnostic tympanocentesis or myringotomy is indicated to enable identification of the offending organism and its sensitivity profile. Either procedure may be helpful in effecting relief of pain. Tympanocentesis with culture of the middle-ear aspirate may also be indicated as part of the sepsis work-up in very young infants with AOM who show systemic signs of illness such as fever, vomiting, or lethargy, and whose illness accordingly cannot be presumed to be limited to infection of the middle ear. Performing tympanocentesis can be facilitated by use of a specially designed tympanocentesis aspirator. Many primary care physicians do not feel comfortable performing this procedure and referral to an otolaryngologist may be appropriate. Many parents view this procedure as traumatic. Often children requiring this intervention have a strong enough history of recurrent OM to warrant the consideration of ventilation tube placement allowing the procedure to be performed under general anesthesia.

Early Recurrence after Treatment

Recurrence of AOM after apparent resolution may be due either to incomplete eradication of infection in the middle ear or upper respiratory tract re-infection by the same or a different bacteria or bacterial strain. Recent antibiotic therapy predisposes patients to an increased incidence of resistant organisms, which should also be considered in choosing therapy and, generally, initiating therapy with a second-line agent is advisable.

Myringotomy and Insertion of Tympanostomy Tubes

When AOM is recurrent, despite appropriate medical therapy, consideration of surgical management of AOM with tympanostomy tube insertion is warranted. This procedure has been shown to be highly effective in reducing the rate of AOM in patients with recurrent OM and to significantly improve the quality of life in patients with recurrent AOM. Individual patient factors including risk-profile, severity of AOM episodes, the child's development and age, the presence of a history of adverse drug reactions, concurrent medical problems, and the parental wishes will impact when a decision is made to consider referral for this procedure. When a patient requires 3-4 courses of antibiotics for episodes of AOM in a 6-mo period or 5-6 episodes in a 12-mo period, potential surgical management of the child's AOM should be discussed with the parents.

Tube Otorrhea

Although tympanostomy tubes generally greatly reduce the incidence of AOM in most children, patients with tympanostomy tubes may still develop AOM. One advantage of tympanostomy tubes in children with recurrent AOM is that if they do develop an episode of AOM with a functioning tube in place these patients will manifest purulent drainage from the tube. By definition, children with functioning tympanostomy tubes without otorrhea do not have AOM as a cause for a presentation of fever or behavioral changes. If tympanostomy tube otorrhea develops, **ototopical** treatment should be considered as first-line therapy. With a functioning tube in place, the infection is able to drain, and the possibility of developing a serious complication from an episode of AOM is negligible The current quinolone otic drops approved by the U.S. Food and Drug Administration for use in the middle-ear space in children are formulated with ciprofloxacin/

dexamethasone (Ciprodex) and ofloxacin (Floxin). The topical delivery of these otic drops allows them to utilize a higher concentration than would be tolerated orally and have excellent coverage of even the most resistant strains of common middle-ear pathogens as well as coverage of *S. aureus* and *P. aeruginosa*. The high rate of success of these topical preparations, their broad coverage, the lower likelihood of their contributing to the development of resistant organisms, the relative ease of administration, the lack of significant side effects and their lack of ototoxicity makes them the 1st choice for tube otorrhea. Oral antibiotic therapy should generally be reserved for cases of tube otorrhea that have other associated systemic symptoms, patients that have difficulty in tolerating the use of topical preparations, or, possibly, in patients that have failed an attempt at topical otic drops. Due to the relative ease in obtaining fluid for culture, and the possibility of other pathogens not covered by topical agents, such as a fungal infection, patients that fail topical therapy should also have culture performed if initial treatment fails. Other otic preparations are available; although these either have some risk of ototoxicity or have not received approval for use in the middle ear, many of these preparations were widely used prior to the development of the current quinolone drops and were generally considered reasonably safe and effective. In all cases of tube otorrhea, attention to aural toilet (e.g., cleansing the external auditory canal of secretions, and avoidance of external ear water contamination) is important. In some cases with very thick, tenacious discharge, topical therapy may be inhibited due to lack of delivery of the medication to the site of infection. Suctioning and removal of the secretions, often done through referral to an otolaryngologist, may be quite helpful. When children with tube otorrhea fail to improve satisfactorily with conventional outpatient management, they may require tube removal, or hospitalization to receive parenteral antibiotic treatment, or both.

MANAGEMENT OF OTITIS MEDIA WITH EFFUSION (OME)

To distinguish between persistence and recurrence, examination should be conducted monthly until resolution; hearing should be assessed if effusion has been present for >3 mo (see Fig. 632-4). Management of OME depends on an understanding of its natural history and its possible complications and sequelae. Most cases of OME resolve without treatment within 3 mo. When MEE persists longer than 3 mo, consideration of surgical management with tympanostomy tubes is appropriate. In considering the decision to refer the patient for consultation the clinician should attempt to determine the impact of the OME on the child. Although hearing loss may be of primary concern, OME causes a number of other difficulties in children that should also be considered. These include predisposition to recurring AOM, pain, disturbance of balance, and tinnitus. In addition, long-term sequelae that have been demonstrated to be associated with OME include pathologic middle-ear changes; atelectasis of the tympanic membrane and retraction pocket formation; adhesive OM; cholesteatoma formation and ossicular discontinuity; and conductive and sensorineural hearing loss. Long-term adverse effects on speech, language, cognitive, and psychosocial development have also been demonstrated, although some studies have demonstrated that the long-term adverse impact of OME on development may be small. In considering the impact of OME on development, it is especially important to take into consideration the overall presentation of the child. Although it is unlikely that OME causing unilateral hearing loss in the mild range will have long-term negative effects on an otherwise healthy and developmentally normal child, even a mild hearing loss in a child with other developmental or speech delays certainly has the potential to compound this child's difficulties (Table 632-4). At a minimum, children with OME persisting >3 mo deserve close monitoring of their hearing levels with skilled audiologic evaluation; frequent assessment of developmental milestones, including speech and language assessment; and attention paid to their rate of recurrent AOM.

Table 632-4 SENSORY, PHYSICAL, COGNITIVE, OR BEHAVIORAL FACTORS THAT PLACE CHILDREN WHO HAVE OME AT AN INCREASED RISK FOR DEVELOPMENTAL DIFFICULTIES (DELAY OR DISORDER)

Permanent hearing loss independent of OME
Suspected or diagnosed speech and language delay or disorder
Autism-spectrum disorder and other pervasive developmental disorders
Syndromes (e.g., Down) or craniofacial disorders that include cognitive, speech, and language delays
Blindness or uncorrectable visual impairment
Cleft palate with or without associated syndrome
Developmental delay

From American Academy of Family Physicians; American Academy of Otolaryngology-Head and Neck Surgery; American Academy of Pediatrics Subcommittee on Otitis Media with Effusion: Otitis media with effusion, *Pediatrics* 113(5):1412–1429, 2004, Table 3, p 1416.

Variables Influencing OME Management Decisions

Patient-related variables that affect decisions on how to manage OME include the child's age; the frequency and severity of previous episodes of AOM and the interval since the last episode; the child's current speech and language development; the presence of a history of adverse drug reactions, concurrent medical problems, or risk factors such as daycare attendance; and the parental wishes. In considering surgical management of OME with tympanostomy tubes, particular benefit is seen in patients with persisting OME punctuated by episodes of AOM, as the tubes generally provide resolution of both conditions. Disease-related variables to consider in the treatment of OME include whether the effusion is unilateral or bilateral; the apparent quantity of effusion; the duration, if known; the degree of hearing impairment; the presence or absence of other possibly related symptoms, such as tinnitus, vertigo, or disturbance of balance; and the presence or absence of mucopurulent or purulent rhinorrhea, which, if sustained for >2 wk, would suggest that concurrent nasopharyngeal or paranasal sinus infection is contributing to continuing compromise of middle-ear ventilation.

Medical Treatment

Antimicrobials have some efficacy in resolving OME, presumably because they help eradicate nasopharyngeal infection or unapparent middle-ear infection or both. However, mainly because of the short-term nature of their benefit and because of the contribution of antimicrobial usage to the development of bacterial resistance, routine antimicrobial treatment of OME is generally not recommended. Instead, treatment should be limited to cases in which there is evidence of associated bacterial upper respiratory tract infection or untreated middle ear infection. For this purpose, the most broadly effective drug available should be used as recommended for AOM.

The efficacy of corticosteroids in the treatment of OME is probably short-term. The risk : benefit ratio for steroids would argue against their use. Antihistamine-decongestant combinations are not effective in treating children with OME. Antihistamines alone, decongestants alone, and mucolytic agents are unlikely to be effective. Allergic management, including antihistamine therapy, might prove helpful in children with problematic OME who also have evidence of environmental allergies, although supporting data specifically analyzing this patient population is not conclusive. Inflation of the eustachian tube by the Valsalva maneuver or other means has no proven long-term efficacy.

Myringotomy and Insertion of Tympanostomy Tubes

When OME persists despite an ample period of watchful waiting, generally 3-6 mo or perhaps longer in children with unilateral effusion, consideration of surgical intervention with tympanostomy tubes is appropriate. Myringotomy alone, without tympanostomy tube insertion, permits evacuation of middle-ear

Table 632-5 DIFFERENTIAL DIAGNOSIS OF POSTAURICULAR INVOLVEMENT OF ACUTE MASTOIDITIS WITH PERIOSTEITIS/ABSCESS

DISEASE	POSTAURICULAR SIGNS AND SYMPTOMS				EXTERNAL CANAL INFECTION	MIDDLE-EAR EFFUSION
	Crease*	Erythema	Mass	Tenderness		
Acute mastoiditis with periosteitis	May be absent	Yes	No	Usually	No	Usually
Acute mastoiditis with subperiosteal abscess	Absent	Maybe	Yes	Yes	No	Usually
Periosteitis of pinna with postauricular extension	Intact	Yes	No	Usually	No	No
External otitis with postauricular extension	Intact	Yes	No	Usually	Yes	No
Postauricular lymphadenitis	Intact	No	Yes (Circumscribed)	Maybe	No	No

*Postauricular crease (fold) between pinna and postauricular area.
From Bluestone CD, Klein JO, editors: *Otitis media in infants and children,* ed 3, Philadelphia, 2001, WB Saunders, p 333.

effusion and may sometimes be effective; but often the incision heals before the middle ear mucosa returns to normal and the effusion soon re-accumulates. Inserting a tympanostomy tube offers the likelihood that middle-ear ventilation will be sustained for at least as long as the tube remains in place and functional, about 12-16 mo on average and nearly uniformly reverses the conductive hearing loss associated with OME. Occasional episodes of obstruction of the tube lumen and premature tube extrusion may limit the effectiveness of tympanostomy tubes, and tubes can also be associated with otorrhea. However, placement of tympanostomy tubes is generally quite effective in providing resolution of OME in children. Sequelae following tube extrusion include residual perforation of the eardrum, tympanosclerosis, localized or diffuse atrophic scarring of the eardrum that may predispose to the development of atelectasis or a retraction pocket or both, residual conductive hearing loss, and cholesteatoma. The more serious of these sequelae are quite infrequent. Recurrence of middle-ear effusion following the extrusion of tubes does develop, especially in younger children; most children without underlying craniofacial abnormalities only require one set of tympanostomy tubes with developmental changes providing improved middle ear health and resolution of their chronic OME by the time of tube extrusion. Because even previously persistent OME often clears spontaneously during the summer months, watchful waiting through the summer season is also advisable in most children with OME who are otherwise well. In considering surgical management of OME in children, primarily in those with bilateral disease and hearing loss, it has been demonstrated that placement of tympanostomy tubes has a significant improvement in their quality of life.

Complications of Acute Otitis Media

Most complications of AOM consist of the spread of infection to adjoining or nearby structures or the development of chronicity, or both. Suppurative complications are relatively uncommon in children in developed countries, but occur not infrequently in disadvantaged children whose medical care is limited. The complications of AOM may be classified as either intratemporal or intracranial.

INTRATEMPORAL COMPLICATIONS Direct but limited extension of AOM leads to complications within the temporal bone. These complications include dermatitis, tympanic membrane perforation, chronic suppurative OM (CSOM), mastoiditis, hearing loss, facial nerve paralysis, cholesteatoma formation, and labyrinthitis.

INFECTIOUS DERMATITIS This is an infection of the skin of the external auditory canal resulting from contamination by purulent discharge from the middle ear. The skin is often erythematous, edematous, and tender. Management consists of proper hygiene combined with systemic antimicrobials and ototopical drops as appropriate for treating AOM and tube otorrhea.

TYMPANIC MEMBRANE PERFORATION Rupture of the tympanic membrane can occur with episodes of either AOM or OME. Although damage to the tympanic membrane from these episodes generally heals spontaneously, chronic perforations can develop in a small number of cases and require further surgical intervention in the future.

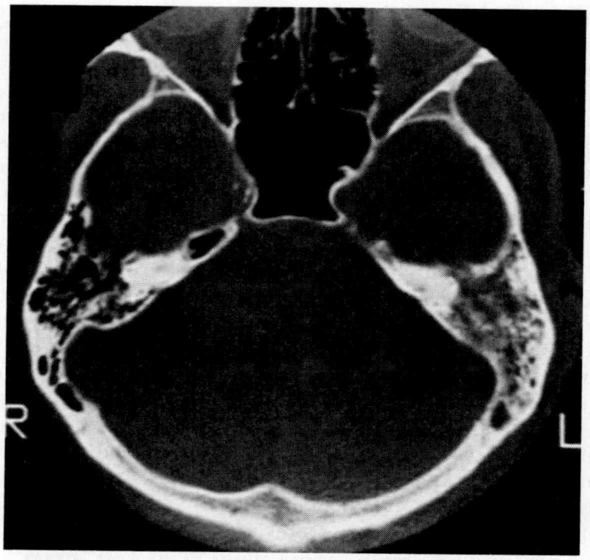

Figure 632-7 CT scan of temporal bones showing left acute osteitis with loss of septa between the mastoid air cells, which has been termed acute coalescent mastoiditis; right mastoid is normal. Mastoid surgery was performed in this case. (From Bluestone CD, Klein JO, editors: *Otitis media in infants and children,* ed 3, Philadelphia, 2001, WB Saunders, p 337.)

CHRONIC SUPPURATIVE OTITIS MEDIA (CSOM) CSOM consists of persistent middle-ear infection with discharge through a tympanic membrane perforation. The disease is initiated by an episode of AOM with rupture of the membrane. The mastoid air cells are invariably involved. The most common etiologic organisms are *P. aeruginosa* and *S. aureus;* however, the typical AOM bacterial pathogens may also be the cause. Treatment is guided by the results of microbiologic investigation. If an associated cholesteatoma is not present, parenteral antimicrobial treatment combined with assiduous aural cleansing is likely to be successful in clearing the infection, but in refractory cases, tympanomastoidectomy can be required.

ACUTE MASTOIDITIS Technically, all cases of AOM are accompanied by mastoiditis by virtue of the associated inflammation of the mastoid air cells. However, early in the course of the disease, no signs or symptoms of mastoid infection are present, and the inflammatory process usually is readily reversible, along with the AOM, in response to antimicrobial treatment. Spread of the infection to the overlying periosteum, but without involvement of bone, constitutes **acute mastoiditis with periosteitis.** In such cases, signs of mastoiditis are usually present, including inflammation in the postauricular area, often with displacement of the pinna inferiorly and anteriorly (Table 632-5). Treatment with myringotomy and parenteral antibiotics, if instituted promptly, usually provides satisfactory resolution.

In acute mastoid osteitis, or **coalescent mastoiditis,** infection has progressed further to cause destruction of the bony trabeculae of the mastoid (Fig. 632-7). Frank signs and symptoms of mastoiditis are usually, but not always, present. In acute **petrositis,** infection has extended further to involve the petrous portion of the temporal bone. Eye pain is a prominent symptom, due to irritation of the ophthalmic branch of cranial nerve V. Cranial nerve VI palsy is a later finding suggesting further extension of the infectious process along the cranial base. **Gradenigo syndrome** is the triad of suppurative OM, paralysis of the external rectus muscle, and pain in the ipsilateral orbit. Rarely, mastoid infection spreads external to the temporal bone into the neck musculature that attaches to the mastoid tip, resulting in an abscess in the neck, termed a **Bezold abscess.**

When mastoiditis is suspected or diagnosed clinically, CT scanning of the temporal bones should be carried out to further clarify the nature and extent of the disease (see Fig. 632-7). Bony destruction of the mastoid must be differentiated from the simple clouding of mastoid air cells that is found often in uncomplicated cases of OM. The most common causative organisms in all variants of acute mastoiditis are *S. pneumoniae* and nontypeable *H. influenzae*. *P. aeruginosa* is also a causative agent, primarily in patients with CSOM. Children with acute mastoid osteitis generally require intravenous antimicrobial treatment and mastoidectomy, with the extent of the surgery dependent on the extent of the disease process. As imaging techniques have become more commonly employed in assessing children, early cases of mastoid osteitis are more frequently identified and may respond to myringotomy and parenteral antibiotics. Insofar as possible, choice of the antimicrobial regimen should be guided by the findings of microbiologic examination.

Each of the variants of mastoiditis may also occur in subacute or chronic form. Symptoms are correspondingly less prominent. Chronic mastoiditis is always accompanied by CSOM, and occasionally will respond to the conservative regimen recommended for that condition. In most cases, mastoidectomy also is required.

FACIAL PARALYSIS The facial nerve, as it traverses the middle ear and mastoid bone, may be affected by adjacent infection. Facial paralysis occurring as a complication of AOM is uncommon, and often resolves after myringotomy and parenteral antibiotic treatment. However, facial paralysis in the presence of AOM requires urgent attention as prolonged infection can result in the development of permanent facial paralysis, which, when it occurs, can have a devastating effect on a child. If facial paralysis develops in a child with mastoid osteitis or with chronic suppurative otitis media, mastoidectomy should be undertaken urgently.

ACQUIRED CHOLESTEATOMA Cholesteatoma is a cystlike growth originating in the middle ear, lined by keratinized, stratified squamous epithelium and containing desquamated epithelium and/or keratin (Chapter 630) (Fig. 632-8). Acquired cholesteatoma develops most often as a complication of long-standing chronic OM. The condition also may develop from a deep retraction pocket of the tympanic membrane or as a consequence of epithelial implantation in the middle-ear cavity from traumatic perforation of the tympanic membrane or insertion of a tympanostomy tube. Cholesteatomas tend to expand progressively, causing bony resorption, often extend into the mastoid cavity, and may extend intracranially with potentially life-threatening consequences. Cholesteatoma commonly presents as a chronically draining ear in a patient with a history of previous ear disease. Cholesteatoma should be suspected if otoscopy demonstrates an area of TM retraction or perforation with white, caseous debris persistently overlying this area. Along with otorrhea from this area, granulation tissue or polyp formation identified in conjunction with this history and presentation should prompt suspicion of cholesteatoma. The most common location for cholesteatoma development is in the superior portion of the TM, also called the *pars flaccida*. Most patients also present with conductive hearing loss on audiologic evaluation. When cholesteatoma is suspected, otolaryngology consultation should be sought immediately. Delay in recognition and treatment can have significant long-term consequences, including the need for more extensive surgical treatment, permanent hearing loss, facial nerve injury, labyrinthine damage with loss of balance function, and intracranial extension. The required treatment for cholesteatoma is tympanomastoid surgery.

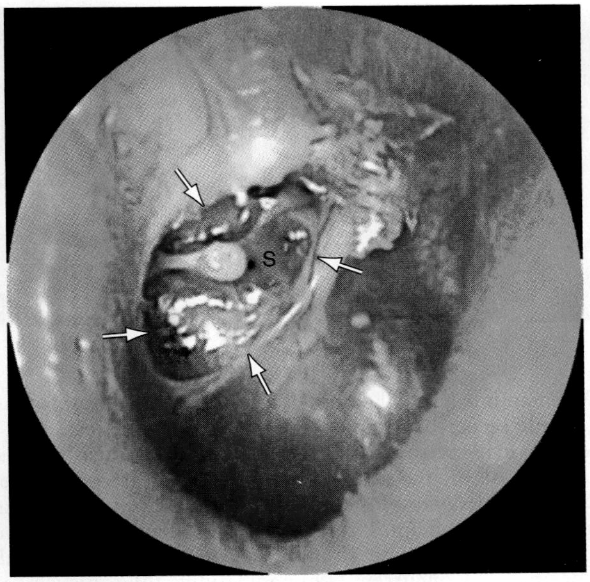

Figure 632-8 A retraction-pocket cholesteatoma of the posterosuperior quadrant. The incus long process is eroded, which leaves the drum adherent to the stapes head (S). An effusion is present in the middle ear, and squamous debris emanates from the attic. (From Isaacson G: Diagnosis of pediatric cholesteatoma, *Pediatrics* 120:603–608, 2007, Fig 9, p 607.)

CONGENITAL CHOLESTEATOMA Congenital cholesteatoma is an uncommon condition generally identified in younger patients (Fig. 632-9). The etiology of congenital cholesteatoma is thought to be a result of epithelial implantation in the middle ear space during otologic development in utero. Congenital cholesteatoma most commonly presents in the anterior superior quadrant of the TM but can be found elsewhere. Congenital cholesteatoma appears as a discrete, white opacity in the middle ear space on otoscopy. Unlike patients with acquired cholesteatoma, there is generally not a strong history of OM or chronic ear disease, history of otorrhea, or changes in the TM anatomy such as perforation or retraction. Similar to acquired cholesteatoma many patients do have some degree of abnormal findings on audiologic evaluation, unless identified very early. Congenital cholesteatoma also requires surgical resection.

LABYRINTHITIS This occurs uncommonly as a result of the spread of infection from the middle ear and/or mastoid to the inner ear. Cholesteatoma or CSOM is the usual source. Symptoms and signs include vertigo, tinnitus, nausea, vomiting, hearing loss, nystagmus, and clumsiness. Treatment is directed at the underlying condition and must be undertaken promptly to preserve inner ear function and prevent the spread of infection.

INTRACRANIAL COMPLICATIONS

Meningitis, epidural abscess, subdural abscess, focal encephalitis, brain abscess, sigmoid sinus thrombosis (also called *lateral sinus thrombosis*), and otitic hydrocephalus each may develop as a complication of acute or chronic middle-ear or mastoid infection, through direct extension, hematogenous spread, or thrombophlebitis. Bony destruction adjacent to the dura is often involved, and a cholesteatoma may be present. In a child with middle-ear or mastoid infection, the presence of any systemic symptom, such as high spiking fevers, headache, lethargy of extreme degree, a finding of meningismus or of any central nervous system sign on physical examination should prompt suspicion of an intracranial complication.

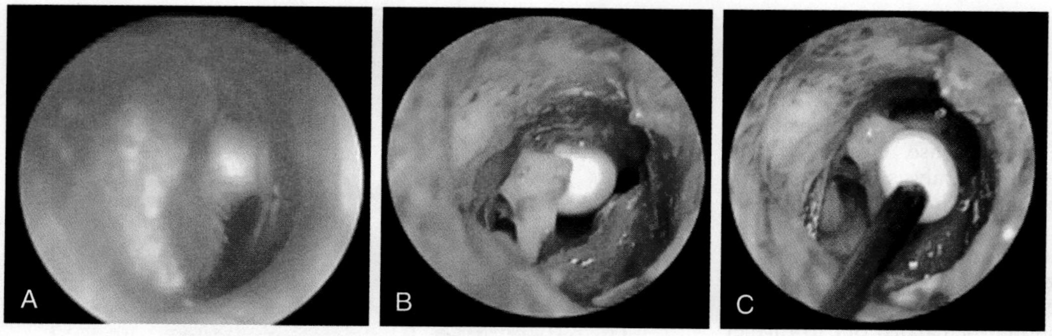

Figure 632-9 *A,* Congenital cholesteatoma of the anterosuperior quadrant. *B,* The eardrum is reflected downward to reveal a white spherical lesion. *C,* Removal of the lesion. (From Isaacson G: Diagnosis of pediatric cholesteatoma, *Pediatrics* 120:603–608, 2007, Fig 3, p 605.)

When an intracranial complication is suspected, lumbar puncture should be performed only after imaging studies establish that there is no evidence of mass effect or hydrocephalus. In addition to examination of the cerebrospinal fluid, culture of middle ear exudate obtained via tympanocentesis may identify the causative organism, thereby helping guide the choice of antimicrobial medications, and myringotomy should be performed to permit middle-ear drainage. Concurrent tympanostomy tube placement is preferable to allow for continued decompression of the "infection under pressure" that is the causative event leading to intracranial spread of the infection.

Treatment of intracranial complications of OM requires urgent, otolaryngologic, and often, neurosurgical consultation, intravenous antibiotic therapy, drainage of any abscess formation, and tympanomastoidectomy in patients with coalescent mastoiditis.

Sigmoid sinus thrombosis may be complicated by dissemination of infected thrombi with resultant development of septic infarcts in various organs. With prompt recognition and wide availability of MRI, which facilitates diagnosis, this complication is exceedingly rare. Mastoidectomy may be required even in the absence of osteitis or coalescent mastoiditis, especially in the case of propagation or embolization of infected thrombi. In the absence of coalescent mastoiditis, sinus thrombosis can often be treated with tympanostomy tube placement and intravenous antibiotics. Anticoagulation therapy may also be considered in the treatment of sigmoid sinus thrombosis; however, otolaryngology consultation should be obtained before initiating this therapy to coordinate the possible need for surgical intervention prior to anticoagulation.

Otitic hydrocephalus, a form of **pseudotumor cerebri,** is an uncommon condition that consists of increased intracranial pressure without dilatation of the cerebral ventricles, occurring in association with acute or chronic OM or mastoiditis (Chapter 597). The condition is commonly also associated with lateral sinus thrombosis, and the pathophysiology is thought to involve obstruction by thrombus of intracranial venous drainage into the neck, producing a rise in cerebral venous pressure and a consequent increase in cerebrospinal fluid pressure. Symptoms are those of increased intracranial pressure. Signs may include, in addition to evidence of OM, paralysis of 1 or both lateral rectus muscles and papilledema. MRI can confirm the diagnosis. Treatment measures include the use of antimicrobials and medications such as acetazolamide or furosemide to reduce intracranial pressure, mastoidectomy, repeated lumbar puncture, lumboperitoneal shunt, and ventriculoperitoneal shunt. If left untreated, otitic hydrocephalus may result in loss of vision secondary to optic atrophy.

PHYSICAL SEQUELAE

The physical sequelae of OM consist of structural middle-ear abnormalities resulting from long-standing middle-ear inflammation. In most instances, these sequelae are consequences of severe and/or chronic infection, but some may also result from the noninfective inflammation of long-standing OME. The various sequelae may occur singly, or interrelatedly in various combinations.

Tympanosclerosis consists of whitish plaques in the TM and nodular deposits in the submucosal layers of the middle ear. The changes involve hyalinization with deposition of calcium and phosphate crystals. Uncommonly, there may be associated conductive hearing loss. In developed countries, probably the most common cause of tympanosclerosis is tympanostomy tube insertion.

Atelectasis of the TM is a descriptive term applied to either severe retraction of the TM caused by high negative middle-ear pressure or loss of stiffness and medial prolapse of the membrane as a consequence of long-standing retraction or severe or chronic inflammation. A **retraction pocket** is a localized area of atelectasis. Atelectasis is often transient and usually unaccompanied by symptoms, but a deep retraction pocket may lead to erosion of the ossicles and adhesive otitis, and may serve as the nidus of a cholesteatoma. For a deep retraction pocket, and for the unusual instance in which atelectasis is accompanied by symptoms such as otalgia, tinnitus, or conductive hearing loss, the required treatment is tympanostomy tube insertion and, at times, tympanoplasty. Patients with persisting atelectasis and retraction pockets should have referral to an otolaryngologist.

Adhesive OM consists of proliferation of fibrous tissue in the middle-ear mucosa, which may, in turn, result in severe TM retraction, conductive hearing loss, impaired movement of the ossicles, ossicular discontinuity, and cholesteatoma. The hearing loss may be amenable to surgical correction.

Cholesterol granuloma is an uncommon condition in which the TM may appear to be dark blue secondary to middle-ear fluid of this color. Cholesterol granulomas are rare, benign cysts that occur in the temporal bone. They are expanding masses that contain fluids, lipids, and cholesterol crystals surrounded by a fibrous lining and generally require surgical removal. Tympanostomy tube placement will not provide satisfactory relief. This lesion requires differentiation from bluish middle ear fluid, which can also rarely develop in patients with the more common OME.

Chronic perforation may rarely develop after spontaneous rupture of the tympanic membrane during an episode of AOM or from acute trauma, but more commonly results as a sequelae of CSOM or as a result of failure of closure of the tympanic membrane following extrusion of a tympanostomy tube. Chronic perforations are generally accompanied by conductive hearing loss. Surgical repair of a TM perforation is recommended to restore hearing, prevent infection from water contamination in the middle-ear space and prevent cholesteatoma formation. Chronic perforations are almost always amenable to surgical repair, usually after the child has been free of OM for an extended period.

Permanent **conductive hearing loss** may result from any of the conditions just described. Rarely, permanent sensorineural hearing loss may occur in association with acute or chronic OM, secondary to spread of infection or products of inflammation through the round window membrane, or as a consequence of suppurative labyrinthitis.

POSSIBLE DEVELOPMENTAL SEQUELAE

Permanent hearing loss in children has a significant negative impact on development, particularly in speech and language. The degree to which OM impacts long-term development in children is difficult to assess and there have been conflicting studies examining this question. Developmental impact is most likely to be significant in children that have greater levels of hearing loss, hearing loss that is sustained for longer periods of time, hearing loss that is bilateral and in those children that have other developmental difficulties or risk factors for developmental delay (see Table 632-4).

PREVENTION

General measures to prevent OM consist of breast-feeding; avoiding, insofar as possible, exposure to individuals with respiratory infection; avoiding environmental tobacco smoke; and getting pneumococcal vaccination.

IMMUNOPROPHYLAXIS

Heptavalent pneumococcal conjugate vaccine reduced the overall number of episodes of AOM by only 6-8% but with a 57% reduction in serotype-specific episodes. Reductions of 9-23% are seen in children with histories of frequent episodes, and a 20% reduction is seen in the number of children undergoing tympanostomy tube insertion. The further development of vaccines against the pathogens that cause AOM offers promise of improved overall protection. Influenza vaccine may also provide a measure of protection against OM, however, the relatively limited exposure time of this virus to individuals and even communities limits it effectiveness to broadly reduce the incidence of OM. Passive immunization by exogenously administered immunoglobulin is not practicable because of the discomfort, risks, cost, and inconvenience entailed.

ANTIMICROBIAL PROPHYLAXIS

In children who have developed frequent episodes of AOM, antimicrobial prophylaxis with subtherapeutic doses of an aminopenicillin or a sulfonamide has been utilized in the past to provide protection against recurrences of AOM (although not of OME). However, because of the increased incidence of resistant organisms and the contribution of antimicrobial usage to bacterial resistance, the risks of sustained antimicrobial prophylaxis now appear to outweigh the likely benefits, particularly for children in daycare who are at increased risk of colonization with multiply resistant *S. pneumoniae*.

MYRINGOTOMY AND INSERTION OF TYMPANOSTOMY TUBES

In children with persistent OME, several studies have shown tympanostomy tube insertion to be effective in reducing the children's subsequent proportion of time with MEE, improving their hearing levels, and also reducing their recurrence rate of AOM. In children with AOM, studies have demonstrated that tympanostomy tubes are quite effective in reducing the rate of recurrent AOM in patients. Importantly, in both children with OME and AOM, quality of life studies have demonstrated a significant improvement in quality of life in children that have undergone surgical management with tympanostomy tube placement.

How best to manage the individual child who is severely affected with recurrent AOM must remain a matter of individual judgment and depends on a number of factors including the severity of the episodes, risk factor profile, tolerance of antimicrobial therapy, hearing assessment, parental preferences, and the child's overall health and development. Reasonable interventions include continued reliance on episodic treatment with antimicrobial therapy, watchful waiting in episodes of AOM to attempt to reduce the overall use of antibiotics, or referral for tympanostomy tube placement.

ADENOIDECTOMY

Adenoidectomy is efficacious to some extent in reducing the risk of subsequent recurrences of both AOM and OME in children who have undergone tube insertion and in whom, after extrusion of tubes, OM continues to be a problem. Efficacy appears to be independent of adenoid size, and probably derives from removal of the focus of infection in the nasopharynx as a site of biofilm formation, chronic inflammation impacting eustachian tube function, and recurrent seeding of the middle ear via the eustachian tube. In younger children with recurrent AOM who have not previously undergone tube insertion, however, adenoidectomy is usually not recommended along with tube insertion, unless significant nasal airway obstruction or recurrent rhinosinusitis is associated, in which case, performing adenoidectomy might be considered.

BIBLIOGRAPHY

Please visit the Nelson Textbook of Pediatrics *website at www.expertconsult.com for the complete bibliography.*

Chapter 633
The Inner Ear and Diseases of the Bony Labyrinth

Joseph Haddad, Jr.

Genetic factors can affect the anatomy and function of the inner ear. Infectious agents, including viruses, bacteria, and protozoa, also can cause abnormal function, most commonly as sequelae of congenital infection or bacterial meningitis. Other acquired diseases of the labyrinthine capsule include otosclerosis, osteopetrosis, Langerhans' cell histiocytosis, fibrous dysplasia, and other types of bony dysplasia. All of these can cause both conductive and sensorineural hearing loss as well as vestibular dysfunction. Use of currently available vaccines reduces the risk for bacterial meningitis and the associated sensorineural hearing loss.

For the full continuation of this chapter, please visit the Nelson Textbook of Pediatrics *website at www.expertconsult.com.*

Chapter 634
Traumatic Injuries of the Ear and Temporal Bone

Joseph Haddad, Jr.

AURICLE AND EXTERNAL AUDITORY CANAL

Auricle trauma is common in certain sports, and quick drainage of a hematoma can prevent irreversible damage. Hematoma, with accumulation of blood between the perichondrium and the cartilage, can follow trauma to the pinna and is especially common in teenagers related to wrestling or boxing. Immediate needle aspiration or, when the hematoma is extensive or recurrent, incision and drainage and a pressure dressing are necessary to prevent perichondritis, which can result in cartilage loss and a cauliflower ear deformity. Sports helmets should be worn when appropriate during activities when head trauma is possible.

For the full continuation of this chapter, please visit the Nelson Textbook of Pediatrics *website at* *www.expertconsult.com*.

Chapter 635
Tumors of the Ear and Temporal Bone

Joseph Haddad, Jr.

Benign tumors of the external canal include osteomas and monostotic and polyostotic fibrous dysplasia. Osteomas manifest as bony masses in the canal and require removal only if hearing is impaired or external otitis results; osteomas may be confused clinically with exostoses (Chapter 495.2). Masses occurring over the mastoid bone, such as first branchial cysts, dermoid cysts, and lipomas, may be confused with primary mastoid tumors; imaging can help with the diagnosis and treatment plan.

For the full continuation of this chapter, please visit the Nelson Textbook of Pediatrics *website at* *www.expertconsult.com*.

PART XXXI The Skin

Chapter 636
Morphology of the Skin
Joseph G. Morelli

EPIDERMIS

The mature epidermis is a stratified epithelial tissue composed predominantly of keratinocytes. The function of the epidermis is protection of the organism from the external environment and the prevention of water loss. The process of epidermal differentiation results in the formation of a functional barrier to the external world. Keratinocytes are composed largely of keratin filaments. These proteins are members of the family of intermediate filaments. The predominant keratins expressed within the keratinocytes change with cellular differentiation. The epidermis comprises four histologically recognizable layers. The first or basal layer consists of columnar cells that rest on the dermal-epidermal junction. Basal keratinocytes are connected to the dermal-epidermal junction by hemidesmosomes. Basal keratinocytes are attached to themselves and to the cells in the spinous layer by desmosomal, tight, gap, and adherens junctions. The role of the basal keratinocyte is to serve as a continuing supply of keratinocytes for the normally differentiating epidermis as well as a reservoir of cells to repair epidermal damage. The second layer consists of 3 to 4 rows of spinous cells. Their role is to begin formation of the epidermal barrier and to initiate vitamin D synthesis. The third layer consists of 2 to 3 rows of granular appearing cells. Granular cells continue the process of epidermal barrier formation and prepare for the formation of the fourth layer or stratum corneum, which is composed of multiple layers of dead, highly compacted cells. The dead cells are composed mainly of disulfide-bonded keratins cross-linked by filaggrins. The intercellular spaces are composed of hydrophobic lipids, predominantly ceramides. As the stratum corneum is replenished, the old stratum corneum is shed in a highly regulated process. The normal process of epidermal differentiation from basal cell to shedding of stratum corneum takes 28 days.

For the full continuation of this chapter, please visit the Nelson Textbook of Pediatrics *website at www.expertconsult.com.*

Chapter 637
Evaluation of the Patient
Joseph G. Morelli

HISTORY AND PHYSICAL EXAMINATION

Although many skin disorders are easily recognized by simple inspection, the history and physical examination are often necessary for accurate assessment. The entire body surface, all mucous membranes, conjunctiva, hair, and nails should always be examined thoroughly under adequate illumination. The color, turgor, texture, temperature, and moisture of the skin and the growth, texture, caliber, and luster of the hair and nails should be noted. Skin lesions should be palpated, inspected, and classified on the bases of morphology, size, color, texture, firmness, configuration, location, and distribution. One must also decide whether the changes are those of the *primary* lesion itself or whether the clinical pattern has been altered by a *secondary* factor such as infection, trauma, or therapy.

For the full continuation of this chapter, please visit the Nelson Textbook of Pediatrics *website at www.expertconsult.com.*

637.1 Cutaneous Manifestations of Systemic Diseases
Joseph G. Morelli

Selected diseases have signature skin findings, often as the presenting signs of illness, that can facilitate the assessment of patients with complex medical status (see Table 637-2 on the *Nelson Textbook of Pediatrics* website at www.expertconsult.com).

For the full continuation of this chapter, please visit the Nelson Textbook of Pediatrics *website at www.expertconsult.com.*

637.2 Multisystem Medication Reactions
Joseph G. Morelli

See also Chapter 146.

Most cutaneous reactions that result from the use of systemic medications are confined to the skin and resolve without sequelae after discontinuation of the offending agent (see Table 637-3 on the *Nelson Textbook of Pediatrics* website at www.expertconsult.com). More severe drug eruptions may be life-threatening, making rapid recognition vital (Chapter 646).

For the full continuation of this chapter, please visit the Nelson Textbook of Pediatrics *website at www.expertconsult.com.*

Chapter 638
Principles of Therapy
Joseph G. Morelli

Competent skin care requires an appreciation of primary versus secondary lesions, a specific diagnosis, and knowledge of the natural course of the disease. If the diagnosis is uncertain, it is better to err on the side of less rather than more aggressive treatment.

In the use of topical medication, consideration of vehicle is as important as the specific therapeutic agent. Acute **weeping lesions** respond best to wet compresses, followed by lotions or creams. For **dry, thickened,** scaly skin or for treatment of a contact allergic reaction possibly due to a component of a topical medication, an ointment base is preferable. Gels and solutions are most useful for the scalp and other hairy areas. The site of involvement is of considerable importance because the most desirable vehicle may not be cosmetically or functionally appropriate, such as an ointment on the face or hands. A patient's preference should also play a part in the choice of vehicle because compliance is poor if a medication is not acceptable to a patient. Cosmetically acceptable foam delivery systems have been developed, and the number of products available is increasing.

Most **lotions** are mixtures of water and oil that can be poured. After the water evaporates, the small amount of remaining oil covers the skin. Some shake lotions are a suspension of water and insoluble powder; as the water evaporates, cooling the skin, a thin film of powder covers the skin. **Creams** are emulsions of oil and water that are viscous and do not pour (more oil than in lotions). **Ointments** have oils and a small amount of water or no water at all; they feel greasy, lubricate dry skin, trap water, and may be occlusive. Ointments without water usually require no preservatives because microorganisms require water to survive.

Therapy should be kept as simple as possible, and specific written instructions about the frequency and duration of application should be provided. Physicians should become familiar with one or two preparations in each category and should learn to use them appropriately. Prescribing nonspecific proprietary medications that may contain sensitizing agents should be avoided. Certain preparations, such as topical antihistamines and sensitizing anesthetics, are never indicated.

WET DRESSINGS

Wet dressings cool and dry the skin by evaporation and cleanse it by removing crusts and exudate, which would cause further irritation if permitted to remain. The dressings decrease pruritus, burning, and stinging sensations, and are indicated for acutely inflamed moist or oozing dermatitis. Although various astringent and antiseptic substances may be added to the solution, cool or tepid tap water compresses are just as effective. Dressings of multiple layers of Kerlix, gauze, or soft cotton material may be saturated with water and remoistened as often as necessary. Compresses should be applied for 10-20 min at least every 4 hr and should usually be continued for 24-48 hr.

Alternatively, cotton long johns can be soaked in water and then wrung as dry as possible. These are placed on the child and covered with dry pajamas, preferably sleeper pajamas with feet. The child should sleep in these overnight. This type of dressing can be used nightly for up to 1 wk.

BATH OILS, COLLOIDS, SOAPS

Bath oil has little benefit in the treatment of children. It offers little moisturizing effect but increases the risk of injury during a bath. Bath oil may lubricate the surface of the bathtub, causing an adult or child to fall when stepping into the tub. Tar bath solutions can be prescribed and may be helpful for psoriasis and atopic dermatitis. Colloids such as starch powder and colloidal oatmeal are soothing and antipruritic for some patients when added to the bathwater. Oilated colloidal oatmeal contains mineral oil and lanolin derivatives for lubrication if the skin is dry. These can also lubricate the bathtub surface. Ordinary bath soaps may be irritating and drying if patients have dry skin or dermatitis. Synthetic soaps are much less irritating. When skin is acutely inflamed, avoidance of soap is advised. Some patients find that lipid-free cleansers containing cetyl alcohol are soothing.

LUBRICANTS

Lubricants, such as lotions, creams, and ointments, can be used as emollients for dry skin and as vehicles for topical agents such as corticosteroids and keratolytics. In general, ointments are the most effective emollients. Numerous commercial preparations are available. Some patients do not tolerate ointments, and some may be sensitized to a component of the lubricant; some preservatives of creams are also sensitizers. These preparations can be applied several times a day if necessary. Maximal effect is achieved when they are applied to dry skin 2 or 3 times daily. Lotions containing menthol and camphor in an emollient vehicle can be used to help control pruritus and dryness.

SHAMPOOS

Special shampoos containing sulfur, salicylic acid, zinc, and selenium sulfide are useful for conditions in which there is scaling of the scalp. Most shampoos also contain surfactants and detergents. Tar-containing shampoos are useful for psoriasis and severe seborrheic dermatitis. They should be used as frequently as necessary to control scaling. Patients should be instructed to leave the lathered shampoo in contact with the scalp for 5-10 min.

SHAKE LOTIONS

Shake lotions are useful antipruritic agents; they consist of a suspension of powder in a liquid vehicle. Water-dispersible oil may be added for lubrication. These preparations can be used effectively in combination with wet dressings for exudative dermatitis. Cooling occurs as the lotion evaporates and the powder deposited on the skin absorbs moisture.

POWDERS

Powders are hygroscopic and serve as absorptive agents in areas of excessive moisture. When dry, powders decrease friction between 2 surfaces. They are most useful in the intertriginous areas and between the toes, where maceration and abrasion may result from friction on movement. Coarse powders may cake; therefore, they should be of fine particle size and inert, unless medication has been incorporated in the formulation.

PASTES

Pastes contain fine powder in ointment vehicles and are not often prescribed in current dermatologic therapy; in certain situations, however, they can be used effectively to protect vulnerable or damaged skin. A stiff zinc oxide paste is bland and inert and can be applied to the diaper area to prevent further irritation due to diaper dermatitis. Zinc oxide paste should be applied in a thick layer completely obscuring the skin and is removed more easily with mineral oil than with soap and water.

KERATOLYTIC AGENTS

Urea-containing agents are hydrophilic; they hydrate the stratum corneum and make the skin more pliable. In addition, because urea dissolves hydrogen bonds and epidermal keratin, it is effective in treating scaling disorders. Concentrations of 10-40% are available in several commercial lotions and creams, which can be applied once or twice daily as tolerated. Salicylic acid is an effective keratolytic agent and can be incorporated into various vehicles in concentrations up to 6% to be applied 2 or 3 times daily. Salicylic acid preparations should not be used in treating small infants or on large surface areas or denuded skin; percutaneous absorption may result in salicylism. The α-hydroxy acids, particularly lactic acid and glycolic acid, are available in commercial preparations or can be incorporated in an ointment vehicle in concentrations up to 12%. Some creams contain both urea and lactic acid. The α-hydroxy acid preparations are useful for the treatment of keratinizing disorders and may be applied once or twice daily. Some patients complain of burning with their use; in such cases, the frequency of application should be decreased.

TAR COMPOUNDS

Tars are obtained from bituminous coal, shale, petrolatum (coal tars), and wood. They are antipruritic and astringent and appear to promote normal keratinization. They may be useful for chronic eczema and psoriasis, and their efficacy may be increased if the affected area is exposed to ultraviolet (UV) light after the tar has been removed. Tars should not be used for acute inflammatory lesions. Tars are often messy and unacceptable because they may stain and they have an odor. They may be incorporated into shampoos, bath oils, lotions, and ointments. A useful preparation for pediatric patients is liquor carbonis detergens 2-5% in a cream or ointment vehicle. Tar gel and tar in light body oil are relatively pleasant cosmetic preparations that cause minimal staining of skin and fabrics. Tars can also be incorporated into a vehicle with a topical corticosteroid. The frequency of application varies from 1 to 3 times daily, according to tolerance. Many children refuse to use tar preparations because of their odor and staining characteristics.

ANTIFUNGAL AGENTS

Antifungal agents are available as powders, lotions, creams, and ointments for the treatment of dermatophyte and yeast infections. Nystatin, naftifine, and amphotericin B are specific for *Candida albicans* and are ineffective in other fungal disorders. Tolnaftate is effective against dermatophytes but not against yeast. The spectrum for ciclopirox olamine includes the dermatophytes, *Malassezia furfur,* and *Candida albicans*. The azoles clotrimazole, econazole, ketoconazole, miconazole, oxiconazole, and sulconazole have a similar broad spectrum. Butenafine has a similar broad spectrum and also has anti-inflammatory properties. Terbinafine has greater activity against dermatophytes but poorer activity against yeasts than the azoles. The topical antifungal agents should be applied 1 to 2 times a day for most fungal infections. All have low sensitizing potential; additives such as preservatives and stabilizers in the vehicles may cause allergic contact dermatitis. Ointments containing 6% benzoic acid and 3% salicylic acid are potent keratolytic agents that have also been used for the treatment of dermatophyte infections. Irritant reactions are common.

TOPICAL ANTIBIOTICS

Topical antibiotics have been used for many years to treat local cutaneous infections, although their efficacy, with the exception of mupirocin, fusidic acid and retapamulin, has been questioned. Ointments are the preferred vehicles (except in the treatment of acne vulgaris; Chapter 661) and combinations with other topical agents such as corticosteroids are, in general, inadvisable. Whenever possible, the etiologic agent should be identified and treated specifically. Antibiotics in wide use as systemic preparations should be avoided because of the risk of bacterial resistance. The sensitizing potential of certain topical antibiotics, such as neomycin and nitrofurazone, should be kept in mind. Mupirocin, fusidic acid, and retapamulin are the most effective topical agents currently available and are as effective as oral erythromycin in treatment of mild to moderate impetigo. Polysporin and bacitracin are not as effective.

TOPICAL CORTICOSTEROIDS

Topical corticosteroids are potent anti-inflammatory agents and effective antipruritic agents. Successful therapeutic results are achieved in a wide variety of skin conditions. Corticosteroids can be divided into 7 different categories on the basis of strength (Table 638-1), but for practical purposes 4 categories can be used: low, moderate, high, and super. Low-potency preparations include hydrocortisone, desonide, and hydrocortisone butyrate. Medium-potency compounds include amcinonide, betamethasone, flurandrenolide, fluocinolone, mometasone furoate, and triamcinolone. High-potency topical steroids include fluocinonide and halcinonide. Betamethasone dipropionate and clobetasol propionate are superpotent preparations and should be prescribed with care. Some of these compounds are formulated in several strengths according to clinical efficacy and degree of vasoconstriction. Physicians using topical steroids should become familiar with preparations within each class.

Table 638-1 POTENCY OF TOPICAL GLUCOCORTICOSTEROIDS

CLASS 1—SUPERPOTENT
Betamethasone dipropionate, 0.05% gel, ointment Clobetasol propionate cream, ointment, 0.05%
CLASS 2—POTENT
Betamethasone dipropionate cream 0.05% Desoximetasone cream, ointment, gel 0.05% and 0.25% Fluocinonide cream, ointment, gel, 0.05%
CLASS 3—UPPER MID-STRENGTH
Betamethasone dipropionate cream, 0.05% Betamethasone valerate ointment, 0.1% Fluticasone propionate ointment, 0.005% Mometasone furoate ointment, 0.1% Triamcinolone acetonide cream, 0.5%
CLASS 4—MID-STRENGTH
Desoximetasone cream, 0.05% Fluocinolone acetonide ointment, 0.025% Triamcinolone acetonide ointment, 0.1%
CLASS 5—LOWER MID-STRENGTH
Betamethasone valerate cream/lotion, 0.1% Fluocinolone acetonide cream, 0.025% Fluticasone propionate cream, 0.05% Triamcinolone acetonide cream/lotion, 0.1%
CLASS 6—MILD STRENGTH
Desonide cream, 0.05%
CLASS 7—LEAST POTENT
Topicals with hydrocortisone, dexamethasone, flumethasone, methylprednisolone, and prednisolone

From Weston WL, Lane AT, Morelli JG: *Color textbook of pediatric dermatology,* ed 4, St Louis, 2007, Mosby/Elsevier, p 418.

All corticosteroids can be obtained in various vehicles, including creams, ointments, solutions, gels, and aerosols. Some are available in a foam vehicle. Absorption is enhanced by an ointment or gel vehicle, but the vehicle should be selected on the basis of the type of disorder and the site of involvement. Frequency of application should be determined by the potency of the preparation and the severity of the eruption. Applying a thin film 2 times daily usually suffices. Adverse local effects include cutaneous atrophy, striae, telangiectasia, acneiform eruptions, purpura, hypopigmentation, and increased hair growth. Systemic adverse effects of high-potency and superpotent topical steroids occur with long-term use and include poor growth, cataracts, and suppression of adrenal function.

In selected circumstances, corticosteroids may be administered by intralesional injection (acne cysts, keloids, psoriatic plaques, alopecia areata, persistent insect bite reactions). Only experienced physicians should use this method of administration.

TOPICAL NONSTEROIDAL ANTI-INFLAMMATORY AGENTS

Calcineurin-inhibiting anti-inflammatory agents that inhibit T-cell activation may be used instead of topical steroids for the treatment of atopic dermatitis and other inflammatory conditions. These agents are pimecrolimus and tacrolimus. They do not have the adverse local effects seen with topical steroid. Stinging with application is the most common complaint. These agents are only as strong as medium-potency topical steroids. They should be used with caution owing to evidence from animal experiments and case reports of an increased risk of lymphoma.

SUNSCREENS

Sunscreens are of 2 general types: (1) those, such as zinc oxide and titanium dioxide, that absorb all wavelengths of the UV and visible spectrums; and (2) a heterogeneous group of chemicals that selectively absorb energy of various wavelengths within the UV spectrum. In addition to the spectrum of light that is blocked, other factors to be considered include cosmetic acceptance, sensitizing potential, retention on skin while swimming or sweating, required frequency of application, and cost. Sunscreen ingredients include para-aminobenzoic acid (PABA) with ethanol, PABA esters, cinnamates, and benzophenone. These block transmission of the majority of solar UVB and some UVA wavelengths. Avobenzone and ecamsule are more effective in blocking UVA. Antioxidants may also be found in some sunscreens. Lip protectants that absorb in the UVB range are also available. Sunscreens are designated by sun protection factor (SPF). The SPF is defined as the amount of time to develop a mild sunburn with the sunscreen compared with the amount of time without the sunscreen. A minimum SPF factor of 15 is required for most fair-skinned individuals to prevent sunburn. The higher the SPF, the better the protection is against UVB rays. Sunscreens do not include any measurement of the efficacy in blocking UVA. The efficacy of these agents depends on careful attention to instructions for use. Chemical sunscreens should be applied at least 30 min before sun exposure to permit penetration into the epidermis and then again on arrival at the destination. Most patients with photosensitivity eruptions require protection by agents that absorb both UVB and UVA wavelengths (Chapters 147 and 648).

Although sunscreens do confer photoprotection and may decrease the development of nevi, protection is incomplete against all harmful UV light. Midday (10 AM to 3 PM) sun avoidance is the primary method of photoprotection. Clothing, hats, and staying in the shade offer additional sun protection.

LASER THERAPY

The vascular-specific pulsed dye laser therapy is used mainly for the treatment of port-wine stains. Spider telangiectasia, small facial pyogenic granulomas, superficial and ulcerated hemangioma, and warts may also be treated. Vascular-specific pulsed dye lasers produce light that is readily absorbed by oxyhemoglobin, producing selective photothermolysis.

BIBLIOGRAPHY

Please visit the Nelson Textbook of Pediatrics *website at www.expertconsult.com for the complete bibliography.*

Chapter 639
Diseases of the Neonate

Joseph G. Morelli

Minor evanescent lesions of newborn infants, particularly when florid, may cause undue concern. Most of the entities are relatively common, benign, and transient and do not require therapy.

SEBACEOUS HYPERPLASIA

Minute, profuse, yellow-white papules are frequently found on the forehead, nose, upper lip, and cheeks of a term infant; they represent hyperplastic sebaceous glands (Fig. 639-1). These tiny papules diminish gradually in size and disappear entirely within the first few weeks of life.

MILIA

Milia are superficial epidermal inclusion cysts that contain laminated keratinized material. The lesion is a firm cyst, 1-2 mm in diameter, and pearly, opalescent white. Milia may occur at any age but in neonates are most frequently scattered over the face and gingivae and on the midline of the palate, where they are called **Epstein pearls**. Milia exfoliate spontaneously in most infants and may be ignored; those that appear in scars or sites of trauma in older children may be gently unroofed and the contents extracted with a fine-gauge needle.

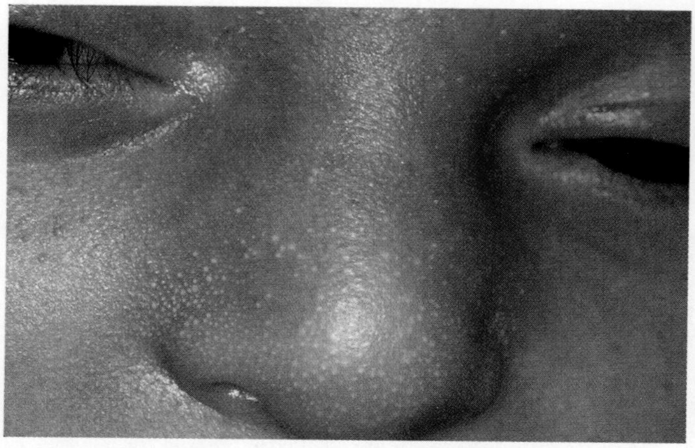

Figure 639-1 Sebaceous hyperplasia. Minute white-yellow papules on the nose of a newborn.

SUCKING BLISTERS

Solitary or scattered superficial bullae present at birth on the upper limbs of infants at birth are presumably induced by vigorous sucking on the affected part in utero. Common sites are the radial aspect of the forearm, thumb, and index finger. These bullae resolve rapidly without sequelae and should be distinguished from sucking pads (calluses), which are found on the lips in the first few months and are due to combined intracellular edema and hyperkeratosis. The diagnosis can be confirmed by observing the neonate sucking the affected area.

CUTIS MARMORATA

When a newborn infant is exposed to low environmental temperatures, an evanescent, lacy, reticulated red and/or blue cutaneous vascular pattern appears over most of the body surface. This vascular change represents an accentuated physiologic vasomotor response that disappears with increasing age, although it is sometimes discernible even in older children. Cutis marmorata telangiectatica congenita is clinically similar, but the lesions are more intense, may be segmental, are persistent, and may be associated with loss of dermal tissue, epidermal atrophy, and ulceration.

HARLEQUIN COLOR CHANGE

A rare but dramatic vascular event, harlequin color change occurs in the immediate newborn period and is most common in low birthweight (LBW) infants. It probably reflects an imbalance in the autonomic vascular regulatory mechanism. When the infant is placed on one side, the body is bisected longitudinally into a pale upper half and a deep red dependent half. The color change lasts only for a few minutes and occasionally affects only a portion of the trunk or face. Changing the infant's position may reverse the pattern. Muscular activity causes generalized flushing and obliterates the color differential. Repeated episodes may occur but do not indicate permanent autonomic imbalance.

SALMON PATCH (NEVUS SIMPLEX)

Salmon patches are small, pale pink, ill-defined, vascular macules that occur most commonly on the glabella, eyelids, upper lip, and

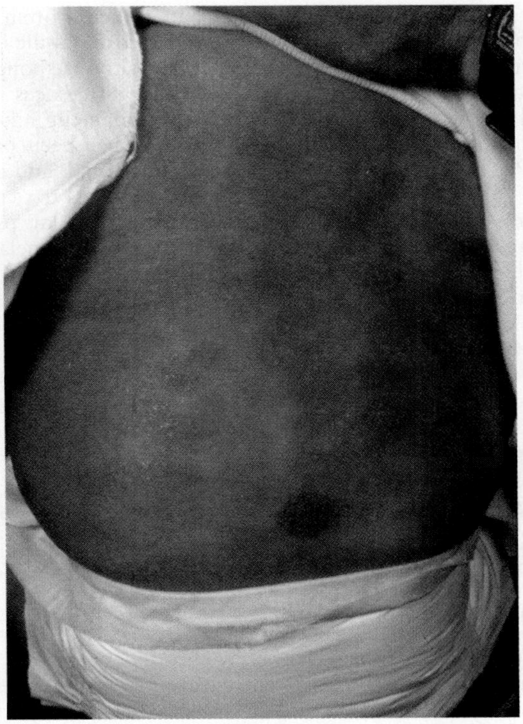

Figure 639-2 Extensive Mongolian spot on the back of a newborn. (Courtesy of Fitzsimons Army Medical Center teaching file.)

nuchal area of 30-40% of normal newborn infants. These lesions, which represent localized **vascular ectasia,** persist for several months and may become more visible during crying or changes in environmental temperature. Most lesions on the face eventually fade and disappear completely, although lesions occupying the entire central forehead often do not. Those on the posterior neck and occipital areas usually persist. The facial lesion should not be confused with a port-wine stain, which is a permanent lesion. The salmon patch is usually symmetric, with lesions on both eyelids or on both sides of midline. Port-wine stains are often larger and unilateral, and they usually end along the midline (Chapter 642).

MONGOLIAN SPOTS

Mongolian spots, which are blue or slate-gray macular lesions, have variably defined margins; they occur most commonly in the presacral area but may be found over the posterior thighs, legs, back, and shoulders (Fig. 639-2). They may be solitary or numerous and often involve large areas. More than 80% of black, Asian, and East Indian infants have these lesions, whereas the incidence in white infants is <10%. The peculiar hue of these macules is due to the dermal location of melanin-containing melanocytes (mid-dermal melanocytosis) that are presumably arrested in their migration from neural crest to epidermis. Mongolian spots usually fade during the first few years of life as a result of darkening of the overlying skin. Malignant degeneration does not occur. The characteristic appearance and congenital onset distinguish these spots from the bruises of child abuse.

ERYTHEMA TOXICUM

A benign, self-limited, evanescent eruption, erythema toxicum occurs in ≈ 50% of full-term infants; preterm infants are affected less commonly. The lesions are firm, yellow-white, 1- to 2-mm papules or pustules with a surrounding erythematous flare (Fig. 639-3). At times, splotchy erythema is the only manifestation.

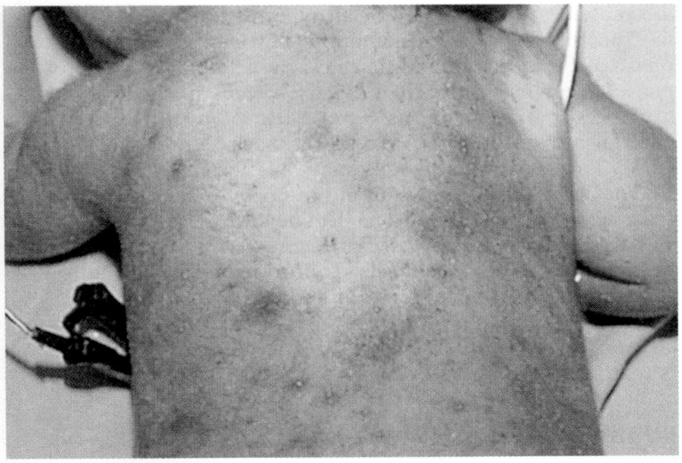

Figure 639-3 Erythema toxicum on the trunk of a newborn infant.

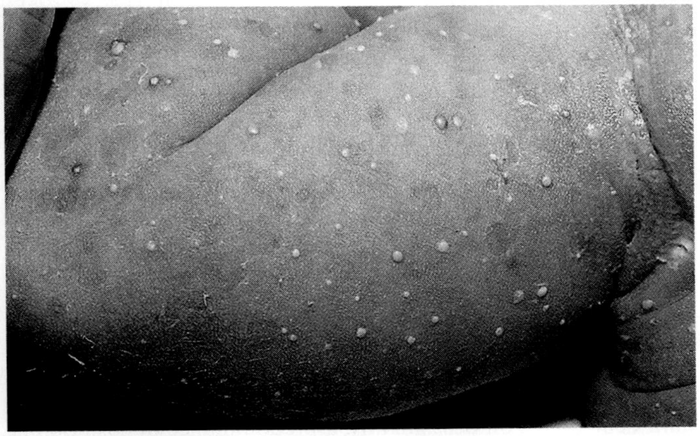

Figure 639-4 Transient neonatal pustular melanosis. Multiple papules present at birth on the arm of an infant. (From Weston WL, Lane AT, Morelli JG, editors: *Color textbook of pediatric dermatology,* ed 3, Philadelphia, 2002, Mosby, p 331.)

Lesions may be sparse or numerous and either clustered in several sites or widely dispersed over much of the body surface. The palms and soles are usually spared. Peak incidence occurs on the 2nd day of life, but new lesions may erupt during the 1st few days as the rash waxes and wanes. Onset may occasionally be delayed for a few days to weeks in premature infants. The pustules form below the stratum corneum or deeper in the epidermis and represent collections of eosinophils that also accumulate around the upper portion of the pilosebaceous follicle. The **eosinophils** can be demonstrated in Wright-stained smears of the intralesional contents. Cultures are sterile.

The cause of erythema toxicum is unknown. The lesions can mimic pyoderma, candidosis, herpes simplex, transient neonatal pustular melanosis, and miliaria but can be differentiated by the characteristic infiltrate of eosinophils and the absence of organisms on a stained smear. The course is brief, and no therapy is required. Incontinentia pigmenti and eosinophilic pustular folliculitis also have eosinophilic infiltration but can be distinguished by their distribution, histologic type, and chronicity.

TRANSIENT NEONATAL PUSTULAR MELANOSIS

Pustular melanosis, which is more common among black than among white infants, is a transient, benign, self-limited dermatosis of unknown cause that is characterized by 3 types of lesions: (1) evanescent superficial pustules, (2) ruptured pustules with a collarette of fine scale, at times with a central hyperpigmented macule, and (3) hyperpigmented macules (Fig. 639-4). Lesions are present at birth, and 1 or all types of lesions may be found in a profuse or sparse distribution. Pustules represent the early phase of the disorder, and macules, the late phase. The pustular phase rarely lasts more than 2-3 days; hyperpigmented macules may persist for as long as 3 mo. Sites of predilection are the anterior neck, forehead, and lower back, although the scalp, trunk, limbs, palms, and soles may be affected.

The active phase shows an intracorneal or subcorneal pustule filled with **polymorphonuclear leukocytes,** debris, and an occasional eosinophil. The macules are characterized only by increased melanization of epidermal cells. Cultures and smears can be used to distinguish these pustules from those of erythema toxicum and pyoderma, because the lesions of pustular melanosis do not contain bacteria or dense aggregates of eosinophils. No therapy is required.

INFANTILE ACROPUSTULOSIS

Onset of infantile acropustulosis generally occurs at 2-10 mo of age; lesions are occasionally noted at birth. Black males have a predisposition, but infants of both sexes and all races may be affected. The cause is unknown.

The lesions are initially discrete erythematous papules that become vesiculopustular within 24 hr and subsequently crust before healing. They are intensely pruritic. Preferred sites are the palms of the hands and the soles and sides of the feet, where the lesions may develop in profusion. A less dense eruption may be found on the dorsum of the hands and feet, ankles, and wrists. Pustules occasionally occur elsewhere on the body. Each episode lasts 7-14 days, during which time pustules continue to appear in crops. After a 2- to 4-wk remission, a new outbreak follows. This cyclic pattern continues for about 2 yr; permanent resolution is often preceded by longer intervals of remission between periods of activity. Infants with acropustulosis are otherwise well.

Wright-stained smears of intralesional contents show abundant neutrophils or, occasionally, a predominance of eosinophils. Histologically, well-circumscribed, subcorneal, neutrophilic pustules, with or without eosinophils, are noted.

The **differential diagnosis** in neonates includes transient neonatal pustular melanosis, erythema toxicum, milia, cutaneous candidosis, and staphylococcal pustulosis. In older infants and toddlers, additional diagnostic considerations include scabies; dyshidrotic eczema; pustular psoriasis; subcorneal pustular dermatosis; and hand-foot-and-mouth disease. A therapeutic trial of a scabicide is warranted in equivocal cases.

Therapy is directed at minimizing discomfort for infants. Topical corticosteroid preparations and/or oral antihistamines decrease the severity of the pruritus and an infant's irritability. Dapsone 2 mg/kg/24 hr taken orally twice daily has been effective but has potentially serious side effects—notably, hemolytic anemia and methemoglobinemia—and should be used with caution.

EOSINOPHILIC PUSTULAR FOLLICULITIS

Eosinophilic pustular folliculitis (EPF) is defined as recurrent crops of pruritic, coalescing, follicular papulopustules on the face, trunk, and extremities. Fifty percent of patients have peripheral eosinophilia with eosinophil counts exceeding 5%, and about 30% have leukocytosis (>10,000 leukocytes/mm^3).

Infants account for <10% of all cases of EPF. The clinical and histologic appearances of this disorder in infants closely resemble those in immunocompetent adults, with minor exceptions. In infants, the lesions are most prominent on the scalp, although they also occur on the trunk and extremities and occasionally are found on the palms and soles. The classic annular and polycyclic appearance with centrifugal enlargement is not seen in infants. Adults have an eosinophilic infiltrate that invades sebaceous glands and the outer root sheath of hair follicles, often leading to spongiosis in the outer root sheath. The eosinophilic infiltrate in most infants, however, is perifollicular, without spongiosis in the outer root sheath. Because of the slight differences between clinical findings and course in immunocompetent adults and those in infants and patients with AIDS, it has been proposed that EPF) be **subclassified** into classic, HIV-related, and infantile forms. The **differential diagnosis** includes erythema toxicum neonatorum, infantile acropustulosis, localized pustular psoriasis, pustular folliculitis, and transient neonatal pustular melanosis.

High-potency or superpotent topical corticosteroids are the most effective treatment (see Table 638-1).

BIBLIOGRAPHY

Please visit the Nelson Textbook of Pediatrics *website at www.expertconsult.com for the complete bibliography.*

Chapter 640
Cutaneous Defects

Joseph G. Morelli

SKIN DIMPLES

Cutaneous depressions over bony prominences and in the acral area, at times associated with pits and creases, may occur in normal children and in association with dysmorphologic syndromes. Skin dimples may develop in utero as a result of interposition of tissue between a sharp bony point and the uterine wall, which leads to decreased subcutaneous tissue formation.

Dimples may also be present overlying an area of bone hypoplasia. Bilateral acromial skin dimples are usually an isolated finding, but they are also seen in association with deletion of the long arm of chromosome 18. Dimples tend to occur over the patella in congenital rubella, over the lateral aspects of the knees and elbows in prune-belly syndrome, on the pretibial surface in campomelic dwarfs, and in the shape of an H on the chin in whistling-face syndrome.

Sacral dimples are common and usually are isolated findings. They may be seen in multiple syndromes or in association with spina bifida occulta and diastomyelia. Association with a mass or other cutaneous stigma (hair, aplasia cutis, hemangioma) should increase concern for underlying **spinal dysraphism** (Chapter 585). Ultrasonography during the first 3 mo of life, before ossification of the posterior elements of the lower spine, may provide a cost-effective, noninvasive method of assessing any associated lumbosacral spine abnormalities.

REDUNDANT SKIN

Loose folds of skin must be differentiated from a congenital defect of elastic tissue or collagen such as cutis laxa, Ehlers-Danlos syndrome, or pseudoxanthoma elasticum. Redundant skin over the posterior part of the neck is common in the Turner, Noonan, Down, and Klippel-Feil syndromes and monosomy 1p36; more generalized folds of skin occur in infants with trisomy 18 and short-limbed dwarfism.

AMNIOTIC CONSTRICTION BANDS

Partial or complete constriction bands that produce defects in extremities and digits are found in 1/10,000-1/45,000 otherwise normal infants. Constrictive tissue bands are caused by primary amniotic rupture, with subsequent entanglement of fetal parts, particularly limbs, in shriveled fibrotic amniotic strands. This event is probably sporadic, with negligible risk of recurrence. Formation of constrictive tissue bands is associated with abdominal

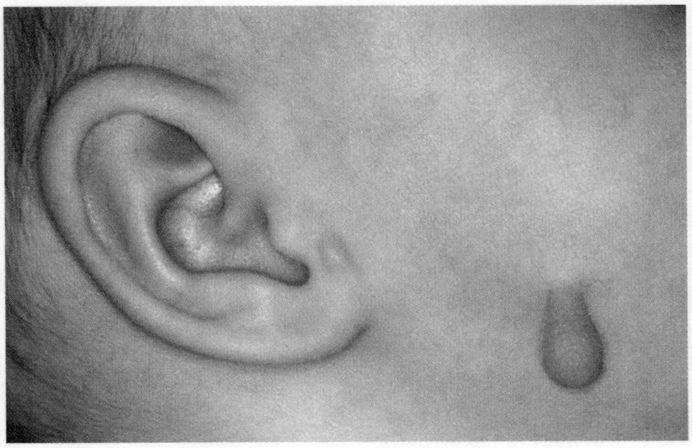

Figure 640-1 Accessory tragus on cheek along jaw line.

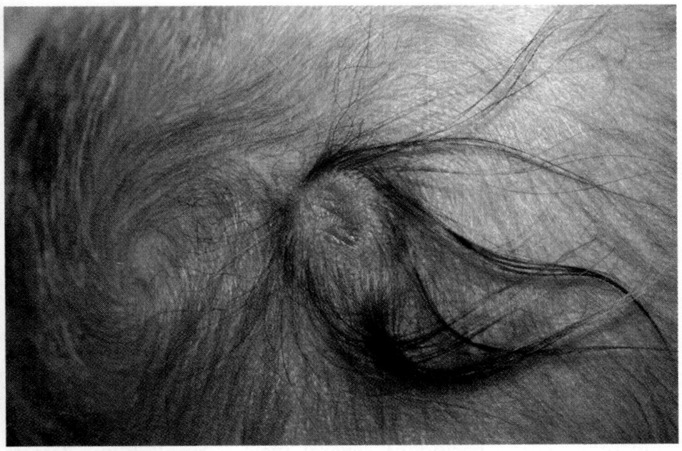

Figure 640-2 Solitary scalp vertex lesion of aplasia cutis congenita with hair collar.

trauma, amniocentesis, and hereditary defects of collagen such as Ehlers-Danlos syndrome and osteogenesis imperfecta.

Adhesive bands involve the craniofacial area and are associated with severe defects such as encephalocele and facial clefts. Adhesive bands result from broad fusion between disrupted fetal parts and an intact amniotic membrane. The craniofacial defects appear not to be caused by constrictive amniotic bands but to result from a vascular disruption sequence with or without cephaloamniotic adhesion (Chapter 102).

The **limb–body wall complex** (**LBWC**) involves vascular disruption early in development, affecting several embryonic structures; it includes at least 2 of the following 3 characteristics: exencephaly or encephalocele with facial clefts, thoracoschisis and/or abdominoschisis, and limb defects.

PREAURICULAR SINUSES AND PITS

Pits and sinus tracts anterior to the pinna may be a result of imperfect fusion of the tubercles of the 1st and 2nd branchial arches. These anomalies may be unilateral or bilateral, may be familial, are more common among females and blacks, and at times are associated with other anomalies of the ears and face. Preauricular pits are present in **branchio-otorenal dysplasia 1 syndrome** (*EYA*-1 gene), an autosomal dominant disorder that consists of external ear malformations, branchial fistulas, hearing loss, and renal anomalies. When the tracts become chronically infected, retention cysts may form and drain intermittently; such lesions may require excision.

ACCESSORY TRAGI

An accessory tragus typically appears as a single pedunculated, flesh-colored papule in the preauricular region anterior to the tragus. Less commonly, accessory tragi are multiple or bilateral, and may be located in the preauricular area, on the cheek along the line of the mandible (Fig. 640-1), or on the lateral aspect of the neck anterior to the sternocleidomastoid muscle. In contrast to the rest of the pinna, which develops from the 2nd branchial arch, the tragus and accessory tragi derive from the 1st branchial arch. Accessory tragi may occur as isolated defects or in chromosomal 1st branchial arch syndromes that include anomalies of the ears and face, such as cleft lip, cleft palate, and mandibular hypoplasia. An accessory tragus is consistently found in **oculo-auriculo-vertebral syndrome** (Goldenhar syndrome). Surgical excision is appropriate.

BRANCHIAL CLEFT AND THYROGLOSSAL CYSTS AND SINUSES

Cysts and sinuses in the neck may be formed along the course of the 1st, 2nd, 3rd, or 4th branchial clefts as a result of improper closure during embryonic life. Second branchial cleft cysts are the most common. The lesions may be unilateral or bilateral (2-3%) and may open onto the cutaneous surface or drain into the pharynx. Secondary infection is an indication for systemic antibiotic therapy. These anomalies may be inherited as autosomal dominant traits.

Thyroglossal cysts and fistulas are similar defects located in or near the midline of the neck; they may extend to the base of the tongue. A pathognomonic sign is vertical motion of the mass with swallowing and tongue protrusion. In nearly 50% of affected children, the cyst or fistula manifests as an infected midline upper neck mass. Cysts in the tongue base may be differentiated from an undescended lingual thyroid by radionuclide scanning. Unlike branchial cysts, a thyroglossal duct cyst often appears after an upper respiratory infection (Chapter 557).

SUPERNUMERARY NIPPLES

Solitary or multiple accessory nipples may occur in a unilateral or bilateral distribution along a line from the anterior axillary fold to the inguinal area. They are more common among black (3.5%) than white (0.6%) children. Accessory nipples may or may not have areolae and may be mistaken for congenital nevi. They may be excised for cosmetic reasons. Renal or urinary tract anomalies and hematologic abnormalities may occur in children with this finding (Chapter 545).

APLASIA CUTIS CONGENITA (CONGENITAL ABSENCE OF SKIN)

Developmental absence of skin is usually noted on the scalp as multiple or solitary (70%), noninflammatory, well-demarcated, oval or circular 1- to 2-cm ulcers. The appearance of lesions varies, depending on when they occurred during intrauterine development. Those that form early in gestation may heal before delivery and appear as atrophic, fibrotic scars with associated alopecia, whereas more recent defects may manifest as ulcerations. Most occur at the vertex just lateral to the midline, but similar defects may also occur on the face, trunk, and limbs, where they are often symmetric. The depth of the ulcer varies. Only the epidermis and upper dermis may be involved, resulting in minimal scarring or hair loss, or the defect may extend to the deep dermis, to the subcutaneous tissue, and, rarely, to the periosteum, skull, and dura. Lesions may be surrounded by a collar of hair (Fig. 640-2).

Diagnosis is made on the basis of physical findings indicative of in utero disruption of skin development. Lesions are sometimes mistakenly attributed to scalp electrodes or obstetric trauma.

Although most individuals with aplasia cutis congenita have no other abnormalities, these lesions may be associated with isolated physical anomalies or with malformation syndromes, including Opitz, Adams-Oliver, oculocerebrocutaneous, Johanson-Blizzard, and 4p(-), X-p22 microdeletion syndromes, trisomy 13-15, and chromosome 16-18 defects. Aplasia cutis congenita may also be found in association with an overt or underlying embryologic malformation, such as meningomyelocele, gastroschisis, omphalocele, or spinal dysraphism. Aplasia cutis congenita in association with fetus papyraceus is apparently due to ischemic or thrombotic events in the placenta and fetus. Blistering or skin fragility and/or absence or deformity of nails in association with aplasia cutis congenita is a well-recognized manifestation of **epidermolysis bullosa.** Aplasia cutis may be confused with traumatic skin injury from monitoring devices and spontaneous atrophic patches (anetoderma) of prematurity.

Major complications are hemorrhage, secondary local infection, and meningitis. If the defect is small, recovery is uneventful, with gradual epithelialization and formation of a hairless atrophic scar over a period of several weeks. Small bony defects usually close spontaneously in the 1st year of life. Large or numerous scalp defects may require excision. Truncal and limb defects, despite being large, usually epithelialize and form atrophic scars, which can later be revised.

FOCAL FACIAL ECTODERMAL DYSPLASIA (BITEMPORAL APLASIA CUTIS CONGENITA, ECTODERMAL DYSPLASIA OF THE FACE)

The rare disorder known as focal facial ectodermal dysplasia is characterized by congenital atrophic scar–like lesions on the temples. Sweating is absent over the defects, the lateral third of the eyebrows is sparse, and linear vertical wrinkles are present on the forehead. Autosomal dominant and autosomal recessive inheritances have been documented; patients with both types lack associated facial anomalies. Patients with **Setleis syndrome** have bitemporal scarring in association with leonine facies, nasal bridge abnormalities, low frontal hairline, and normal growth and development.

FOCAL DERMAL HYPOPLASIA (GOLTZ SYNDROME)

A rare congenital mesoectodermal and ectodermal disorder, focal dermal hypoplasia is characterized by dysplasia of connective tissue in the skin and skeleton. This disorder is an X-linked dominant disorder caused by mutations in the *PORCN* gene. It manifests as numerous soft tan papillomas. Other cutaneous findings include linear atrophic lesions; reticulated hypopigmentation and hyperpigmentation; telangiectasias; congenital absence of skin; angiofibromas presenting as verrucous excrescences; and papillomas of the lips, tongue, circumoral region, vulva, anus, and the inguinal, axillary, and periumbilical areas. Partial alopecia, sweating disorders, and dystrophic nails are additional, less common ectodermal anomalies. The most frequent skeletal defects are syndactyly, clinodactyly, polydactyly, and scoliosis. **Osteopathia striata** are fine parallel vertical stripes noted on radiographs in the metaphyses of long bones of patients with this disorder; these are highly characteristic of focal dermal hypoplasia but are not pathognomonic. Many ocular abnormalities, the most common of which are colobomas, strabismus, nystagmus, and microphthalmia, are also characteristic. Small stature, dental defects, soft tissue anomalies, and peculiar dermatoglyphic patterns are also common. Mental deficiency occurs occasionally.

DYSKERATOSIS CONGENITA (ZINSSER-ENGMAN-COLE SYNDROME)

Dyskeratosis congenita, a rare familial syndrome, consists classically of the triad of reticulated hyperpigmentation of the skin (Fig. 640-3), dystrophic nails, and mucous membrane leukoplakia in association with immunologic and hematologic abnormalities. Patients with dyskeratosis congenita also show signs of premature aging and increased occurrence of cancer, especially squamous cell carcinoma. Dyskeratosis congenita may be X-linked recessive (*DKC-1* gene), autosomal dominant (*hTERC* and *TINF2* genes), or autosomal recessive (*NOLA3* gene). Onset occurs in childhood, most commonly as **nail dystrophy.** The nails become atrophic and ridged longitudinally with progression to pterygia and complete nail loss. Skin changes usually appear after onset of nail changes and consist of reticulated gray-brown pigmentation, atrophy, and telangiectasia, especially on the neck, face, and chest. Hyperhidrosis and hyperkeratosis of the palms and soles, sparse scalp hair, and easy blistering of the hands and feet are also characteristic. Blepharitis, ectropion, and excessive tearing due to atresia of the lacrimal ducts are occasional manifestations. Oral leukokeratosis may give rise to squamous cell carcinoma. Other mucous membranes, including conjunctival, urethral, and genital, may be involved. Infection, malignancy, and bone marrow failure are common, and death before age 40 yr is typical (Chapter 462).

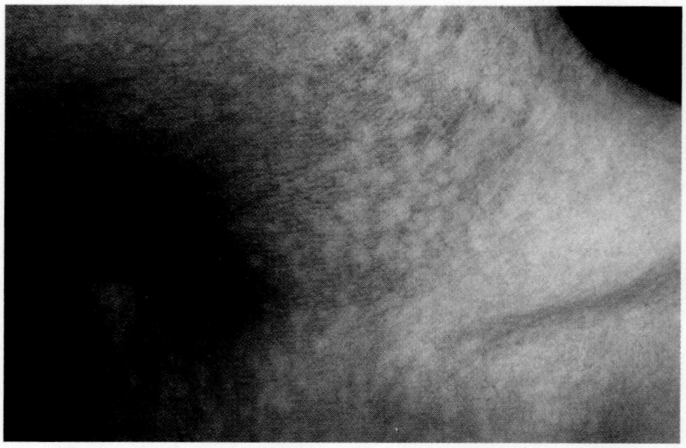

Figure 640-3 Reticulated dyspigmentation on neck of patient with dyskeratosis congenita.

CUTIS VERTICIS GYRATA

Cutis verticis gyrata, an unusual alteration of the scalp that is more common in males, may be present from birth or may develop during adolescence. The scalp is characterized by convoluted elevated folds, 1-2 cm in thickness, usually in the fronto-occipital axis. Unlike the lax skin of other disorders, the convolutions cannot generally be flattened by traction. Primary cutis gyrata may be associated with mental retardation, retinitis pigmentosa, sensorineural deafness, and thyroid aplasia. Secondary cutis gyrata may be due to chronic inflammatory diseases, tumors, nevi, and acromegaly.

BIBLIOGRAPHY
Please visit the Nelson Textbook of Pediatrics *website at www.expertconsult.com for the complete bibliography.*

Chapter 641
Ectodermal Dysplasias

Joseph G. Morelli

Ectodermal dysplasia (ED) is a heterogeneous group of disorders characterized by a constellation of findings involving defects of 2 or more of the following: teeth, skin, and appendageal structures including hair, nails, and eccrine and sebaceous glands.

Table 641-1 FOUR RECOGNIZED TYPES OF ANHIDROTIC ECTODERMAL DYSPLASIA

TYPE	INHERITANCE	GENE DEFECT
ED-1	X-linked recessive	Ectodysplasin A (EDA)
ED-anhidrotic	Autosomal recessive	Ectodyplasin A anhidrotic receptor (EDAR)
		EDAR-associated death gene (EDARADD)
ED-3	Autosomal dominant	EDAR
ED-anhidrotic with immune deficiency	X-linked recessive Autosomal Dominant	IκK-gamma (NEMO) NFκB-IA

Although more than 150 ectodermal dysplasias have been described, the majority are rare and most have not been genetically defined.

ANHIDROTIC (HYPOHIDROTIC) ECTODERMAL DYSPLASIA

The syndrome known as anhidrotic ectodermal dysplasia manifests as a triad of defects: partial absence (hypohidrosis) or complete absence of sweat glands, anomalous dentition, and hypotrichosis. There are 4 recognized types of anhidrotic ectodermal dysplasia (Table 641-1). The X-linked form is most common.

In ED-1, affected males are unable to sweat and may experience episodes of high fever in warm environments, which may be mistakenly considered to be fevers of unknown origin. This error is particularly common in infancy, when the facial changes are not easily appreciated. Diagnosis at this time may be made using the starch-iodine test or palmar or scalp biopsy. Scalp biopsy is the most sensitive and is 100% specific. The typical facies is characterized by frontal bossing; malar hypoplasia; a flattened nasal bridge; recessed columella; thick, everted lips; wrinkled, hyperpigmented periorbital skin; and prominent, low-set ears (Fig. 641-1). The skin over the entire body is dry, finely wrinkled, and hypopigmented, often with a prominent venous pattern. Extensive peeling of the skin is a clinical clue to diagnosis in the newborn period. The paucity of sebaceous glands may account for the dry skin. The scalp hair is sparse, fine, and lightly pigmented, and eyebrows and lashes are sparse or absent. Other body hair is also sparse or absent. Sexual hair growth is normal. Anodontia or hypodontia with widely spaced, conical teeth is a consistent feature (see Fig. 641-1). Otolaryngeal and ophthalmologic abnormalities secondary to decreased saliva and tear production are seen. The incidence of atopic diseases in children with ED-1 is high. Gastroesophageal reflux is common and may play a role in failure to thrive, which is seen in 20% of cases. Sexual development is usually normal. Historically, the infant mortality rate has been 30%. Carrier females have no or variable clinical manifestations.

The clinical findings in autosomal recessive anhidrotic ectodermal dysplasia are identical to those of the X-linked recessive disorder, except that females are affected to the same degree as males. The clinical findings in the autosomal dominant form are also seen in both sexes and are similar to the X-linked recessive form but much milder. Hypohidrotic ED with immune deficiencies causes similar findings in sweating and hair and nail development, in association with a **dysgammaglobulinemia.** Significant mortality is seen from recurrent infections.

Treatment of children with hypohidrotic ED includes protecting them from exposure to high ambient temperatures. Early dental evaluation is necessary so that prostheses can be provided for cosmetic reasons and for adequate nutrition. The use of artificial tears prevents damage to the cornea in patients with defective lacrimation. Alopecia may necessitate the wearing of a wig to improve appearance.

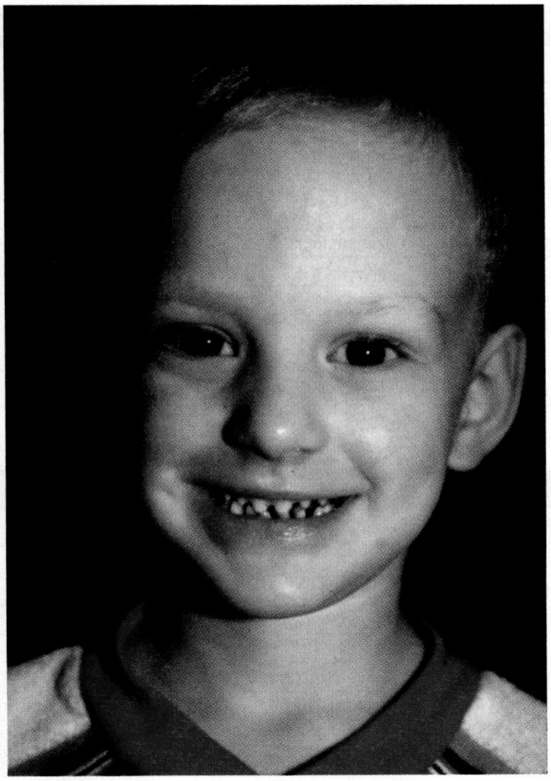

Figure 641-1 Hypohidrotic ectodermal dysplasia is characterized by pointed ears, fine hair, periorbital hyperpigmentation, midfacial hypoplasia, and pegged teeth. (Courtesy of the Fitzsimons Army Medical Center teaching file.)

HIDROTIC ECTODERMAL DYSPLASIA (CLOUSTON SYNDROME)

The salient features of the autosomal dominant disorder hidrotic ED are dystrophic, hypoplastic, or absent nails; sparse hair; and hyperkeratosis of the palms and soles. Conjunctivitis and blepharitis are common. The dentition and sweating are always normal. Absence of eyebrows and eyelashes and hyperpigmentation over the knees, elbows, and knuckles have been noted in some affected individuals. Mutations in the *GJB6* gene encoding the gap junction protein connexin 30 are responsible for this disorder. A similar disorder associated with deafness has been described with mutations in the *GJB2* gene encoding the connexin 26 protein.

BIBLIOGRAPHY

Please visit the Nelson Textbook of Pediatrics *website at www.expertconsult.com for the complete bibliography.*

Chapter 642 Vascular Disorders

Joseph G. Morelli

Vascular lesions of childhood may be divided into vascular birthmarks (malformations and tumors), benign acquired disorders, and genetic diseases. Familial disorders may involve arterial, capillary, lymph, or venous malformations (Table 642-1).

VASCULAR BIRTHMARK

Vascular birthmarks consist of malformations that are present at birth and tumors, which usually arise in the 1st 2 mo of life.

Table 642-1 FAMILIAL VASCULAR ANOMALIES WITH IDENTIFIED GENETIC MUTATIONS

DISORDER	CHROMOSOME	GENE	FUNCTION
Hereditary hemorrhagic telangiectasia	Type 1 9q34.1	Endoglin activin receptor–like kinase 1 (*ALK-1*)	TGF-β binding proteins
	Type 2 12q11-q14	Activin A receptor type II-like 1 (*ACVRL1*)	TGF-β binding proteins
Cerebral cavernous malformations	CCM-1 7q11.2-q21 (Hispanic)	*KRIT 1*	RapIA GTPase signal transdution pathway
	CCM-2 7p13	*CCM2*	
	CCM-3 3q26.1	*PDCD10*	
Disseminated cutaneous glomangioma	1p21-22	Glomulin	
Familial lymphedema	5q35.3	*VEGFR3* (*FLT4*)	Lymphatic development
Familial venous malformation	9p21	Tie-2	Endothelial cell/smooth muscle cell interaction
Familial hemangioma	4q12 2p13.1	*VEGFR* *TEM8*	

GTPase, guanosine triphosphate; TGF, transforming growth factor.
From Blei F: Vascular anomalies: from bedside to bench and back again, *Curr Prob Pediatr Adolesc Health* 32:72–93, 2002.

Table 642-2 VASCULAR MALFORMATIONS

TYPE	EXAMPLE(S)
Capillary	Port-wine stain
Venous	Venous malformation
	Angiokeratoma circumscriptum (hyperkeratotic venule)
	Cutis marmorata telangiectasia congenita (congenital phlebectasia)
Arterial	Arteriovenous malformation
Lymphatic	Superficial lymphatic malformation (lymphangioma circumscriptum)
	Deep lymphatic malformation with macrocysts and/or microcysts (cystic hygroma)

VASCULAR MALFORMATION

Vascular malformations are developmental errors in blood vessel formation. Malformations do not regress but slowly enlarge. They should be named after the predominant blood vessel forming the lesion (Table 642-2). Table 642-3 helps differentiate vascular malformations from true hemangiomas.

CAPILLARY MALFORMATION (PORT-WINE STAIN)

Port-wine stains are present at birth. These vascular malformations consist of mature dilated dermal capillaries. The lesions are macular, sharply circumscribed, pink to purple, and tremendously varied in size (Fig. 642-1). The head and neck region is the most common site of predilection; most lesions are unilateral. The mucous membranes can be involved. As a child matures into adulthood, the port-wine stain may become darker in color and pebbly in consistency; it may occasionally develop elevated areas that bleed spontaneously.

True port-wine stains should be distinguished from the most common vascular malformation, the salmon patch of neonates, which, in contrast, is a relatively transient lesion (Chapter 639). When a port-wine stain is localized to the trigeminal area of the face, specifically around the eyelids, the diagnosis of **Sturge-Weber syndrome** (glaucoma, leptomeningeal venous angioma, seizures, hemiparesis contralateral to the facial lesion, intracranial calcification) must be considered (Chapter 589.3). Early screening for glaucoma is important to prevent additional damage to the eye. Port-wine stains also occur as a component of Klippel-Trenaunay syndrome and with moderate frequency in other syndromes, including Cobb (spinal arteriovenous malformation, port-wine stain), Proteus, Beckwith-Wiedemann, and Bonnet-Dechaume-Blanc syndromes. In the absence of associated anomalies, morbidity from these lesions may include a poor self-image, hypertrophy of underlying structures, and traumatic bleeding.

The most effective **treatment** for port-wine stains is with the pulsed dye laser (PDL). This therapy is targeted to hemoglobin within the lesion and avoids thermal injury to the surrounding normal tissue. After such treatment, the texture and pigmentation of the skin are generally normal without scarring. Therapy can begin in infancy, when the surface area of involvement is smaller; there may be advantages to treating within the 1st year of life. Although this approach is quite effective, redarkening of the stain may occur 10 yr after therapy. Masking cosmetics may also be used.

VENOUS MALFORMATION

Venous malformations include vein-only malformation, angiokeratomas (hyperkeratotic venule), and cutis marmorata telangiectasia congenita.

Malformations consisting of veins only run the gamut from nodules containing a mass of venules (Fig. 642-2) to diffuse large vein abnormalities that may consist of either a superficial component resembling varicose veins, deeper venous malformations, or both. Nodular venous malformations are frequently confused with hemangiomas. Venous malformations may be differentiated by their presence at birth, lack of rapid growth phase, and no tendency toward regression. The treatment of choice for superficial nodular vascular malformations is surgical excision. Treatment of larger vein malformations is at best difficult and often impossible. Percutaneous sclerotherapy with direct injection of polidocanol microfoam, with color Doppler ultrasonographic guidance, is helpful in many patients, including those with Klippel-Trenaunay syndrome.

Angiokeratoma Circumscriptum

Several forms of angiokeratoma have been described. Angiokeratomas, characterized by ectasia of superficial dermal vessels and hyperkeratosis of the overlying epidermis, look like flat hemangiomas with a verrucous, irregular surface. Angiokeratoma circumscriptum is a rare disorder consisting of a solitary lesion or multiple lesions that manifest as a plaque or plaques of blue-red papules or nodules with a verrucous surface. The limbs are the sites of predilection. If therapy is desired, surgical excision is the treatment of choice.

Cutis Marmorata Telangiectatica Congenita (Congenital Phlebectasia)

Cutis marmorata telangiectatica congenita is benign vascular anomaly that represents dilatation of superficial capillaries and veins and is apparent at birth. Involved areas of skin have a reticulated red or purple hue that resembles physiologic cutis marmorata but is more pronounced and relatively unvarying (Fig. 642-3). The lesions may be restricted to a single limb and a portion of the trunk or may be more widespread. Port-wine stain may also be associated. The lesions become more pronounced during changes in environmental temperature, physical activity, or crying. In some cases, the underlying subcutaneous tissue is

Table 642-3 MAJOR DIFFERENCES BETWEEN HEMANGIOMAS AND VASCULAR MALFORMATIONS

	HEMANGIOMAS	VASCULAR MALFORMATIONS (CAPILLARY, VENOUS, LYMPHATIC, ARTERIAL, AND ARTERIOVENOUS, PURE, OR COMPLEX-COMBINED)
Clinical	Variably visible at birth	Usually visible at birth (AVMs may be quiescent)
	Subsequent rapid growth	Growth proportionate to the skin's growth (or slow progression); present lifelong
	Slow, spontaneous involution	
Sex ratio F:M	3:1 to 5:1; 7:1 in severe cases	1:1
Pathology	Proliferating stage: hyperplasia of endothelial cells and smooth muscle cell actin–positive cells	Flat endothelium
	Multilaminated basement membrane	Thin basement membrane
	Higher mast cell content in involution	Often irregularly attenuated walls (VM, LM)
Radiology	Fast-flow lesion on Doppler sonography	Slow flow (CM, LM, VM) or fast flow (AVM) on Doppler ultrasonography
	Tumoral mass with flow voids on MRI	MRI: Hyperintense signal on T2-weighted images when slow-flow (LM, VM); flow voids on T1- and T2-weighted images when fast-flow (AVM)
	Lobular tumor on arteriogram	Arteriography of AVM demonstrates AV shunting
Bone changes	Rarely mass effect with distortion but no invasion	*Slow-flow VM:* distortion of bones, thinning, underdevelopment
		Slow-flow CM: hypertrophy
		Slow-flow LM: distortion, hypertrophy, and invasion of bones
		High-flow AVM: destruction, rarely extensive lytic lesions
		Combined malformations (e.g., slow-flow [capillary lymphatic venous malformation, Klippel-Trenaunay syndrome] or fast-flow [capillary arteriovenous malformation Parkes-Weber syndrome]): overgrowth of limb bones, gigantism
Immunohistochemistry on tissue samples	*Proliferating hemangioma:* high expression of PCNA, type IV collagenase, VEGF, urokinase, and bFGF, Glucose transporter-1	Lack expression of PCNA, type IV collagenase, urokinase, VEGF, and bFGF One familial (rare) form of VM linked to a mutated gene on 9p (*VMCM1*)
	Involuting hemangioma: high levels of tissue inhibitor of metalloproteinase-1, bFGF	
Hematology	No coagulopathy (Kasabach-Merritt syndrome is a complication of other vascular tumors of infancy, e.g., kaposiform hemangioendothelioma and tufted angioma)	Slow-flow VM, LM, or LVM may have an associated localized intravascular coagulopathy with risk of bleeding (disseminated intravascular coagulation)

AVM, Arteriovenous malformation; bFGF, basic fibroblast growth factor; CM, capillary malformation/port-wine stain; LM, lymphatic malformation; LVM, lymphovenous malformation; PCNA, proliferating cell nuclear antigen; VEGF, vascular endothelial growth factor; VM, venous malformation.
From Eichenfield LF, Frieden IJ, Esterly NB: *Textbook of neonatal dermatology,* Philadelphia, 2001, WB Saunders, p 337.

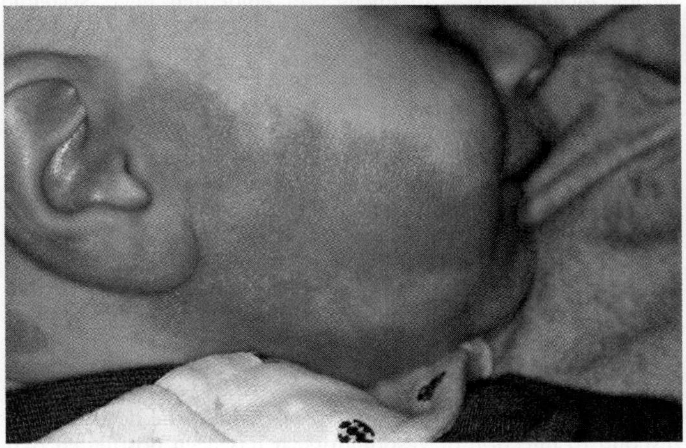

Figure 642-1 Capillary malformation. Pink macule on the cheek of an infant.

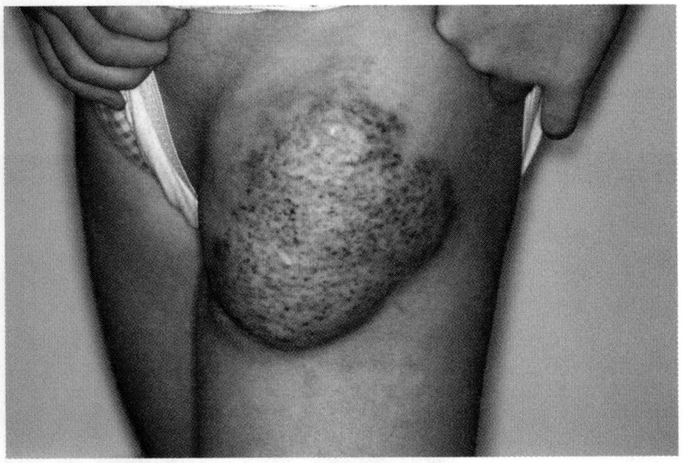

Figure 642-2 Nodular venous malformation on the leg of an adolescent.

underdeveloped, and ulceration may occur within the reticulated bands. Rarely, defective growth of bone and other congenital abnormalities may be present. No specific therapy is indicated. Mild vascular-only cases may show gradual improvement. Adams-Oliver syndrome and cutis marmorata telangiectatica congenita–macrocephaly syndrome are rarely associated disorders.

ARTERIOVENOUS MALFORMATION

Arteriovenous malformations (AVMs) are direct connections of artery to vein that bypass the capillary bed (Fig. 642-4). AVMs of the skin are very rare. They are diagnosed from their obvious arterial palpation. Many physicians mistakenly call all vascular malformations AVMs.

LYMPHATIC MALFORMATIONS

See Chapter 483.

KLIPPEL-TRENAUNAY AND KLIPPEL-TRENAUNAY-WEBER SYNDROMES

Klippel-Trenaunay syndrome (KT) is a cutaneous vascular malformation that, in combination with bony and soft tissue

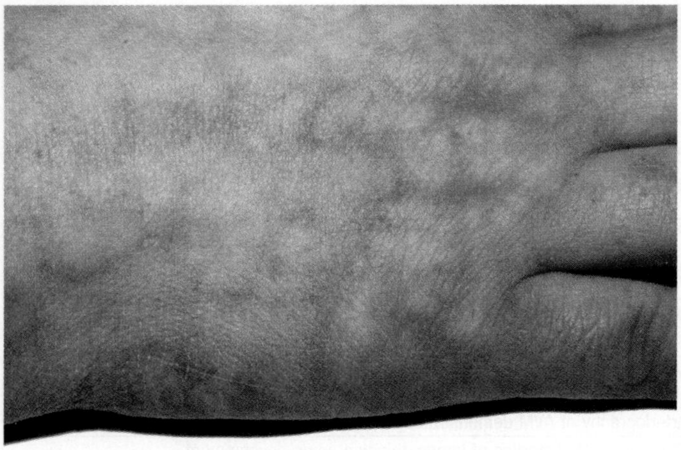

Figure 642-3 Mottled pattern of cutis marmorata telangiectatica congenita on the right hand.

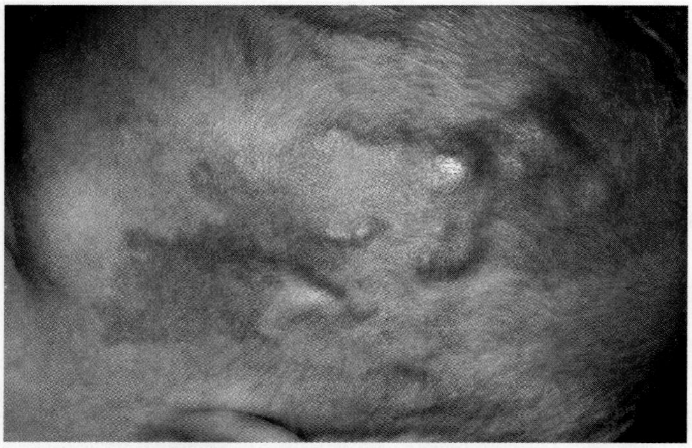

Figure 642-4 Arteriovenous malformation (AVM) in conjunction with a port-wine stain of the scalp of a newborn.

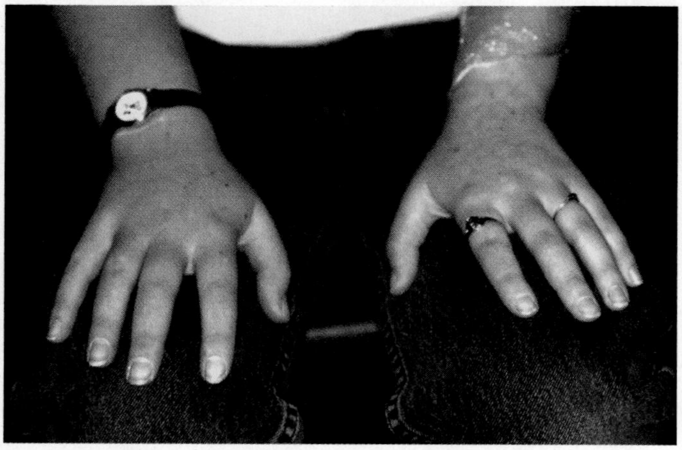

Figure 642-5 Overgrowth of the right arm and hand in and adolescent with Klippel-Trenaunay syndrome.

hypertrophy and venous abnormalities, constitutes the triad of defects of this nonheritable disorder (Fig. 642-5). The anomaly is present at birth and usually involves a lower limb but may involve more than one as well as portions of the trunk or face. Enlargement of the soft tissues may be gradual and may involve the entire extremity, a portion of it, or selected digits. The vascular lesion most often is a capillary malformation, generally localized to the hypertrophied area. The deep venous system may be absent or hypoplastic. Venous blebs and/or vesicular lymphatic lesions may be present on the malformation's surface. Thick-walled venous varicosities typically become apparent ipsilateral to the vascular malformation after the child begins to ambulate. If there is an associated AVM, the disorder is called Klippel-Trenaunay-Weber syndrome (KTW).

These disorders can be confused with Maffucci syndrome or, if the surface vascular lesion is minimal, with Milroy disease. Pain, limb swelling, and cellulitis may occur. Thrombophlebitis, dislocations of joints, gangrene of the affected extremity, heart failure, hematuria secondary to angiomatous involvement of the urinary tract, rectal bleeding from lesions of the gastrointestinal tract, pulmonary lesions, and malformations of the lymphatic vessels are infrequent complications. Arteriograms, venograms, and CT or MRI may delineate the extent of the anomaly, but surgical correction or palliation is often difficult. Percutaneous sclerotherapy guided by color echo Doppler ultrasonography is of benefit when a venous component is the dominant vessel in the malformation. The indications for radiologic studies of viscera and bones are best determined by clinical evaluation. Supportive care includes compression bandages for varicosities; surgical treatment may help carefully selected patients. Leg-length differences should be treated with orthotic devices to prevent the development of spinal deformities. Corrective bone surgery may eventually be needed to treat significant leg-length discrepancy.

PHAKOMATOSIS PIGMENTOVASCULARIS

Phakomatosis pigmentovascularis is a rare disorder characterized by the association of a capillary malformation and melanocytic lesions. Typically, the capillary malformation is extensive, and associated pigmentary lesions may include dermal melanocytosis (mongolian spots), café-au-lait macules, or a nevus spilus (speckled nevus). Nonpigmented skin lesions that may occur in this setting include nevus anemicus and epidermal nevi. Systemic anomalies are seen in rare cases.

NEVUS ANEMICUS

Although present at birth, nevus anemicus may not be detectable until early childhood. The nevus consists of solitary or numerous, sharply delineated pale macules that are most often on the trunk but may also occur on the neck or limbs. These nevi may simulate plaques of vitiligo, leukoderma, or nevoid pigmentary defects, but they can be readily distinguished because of their response to firm stroking. Stroking evokes an erythematous line and flare in normal surrounding skin, but the skin of a nevus anemicus does not redden. They can also be diagnosed by diascopy, in which pressure of the skin with a glass slide will obscure the borders of a nevus anemicus. Although the cutaneous vasculature appears normal histologically, the blood vessels within the nevus do not respond to injection of vasodilators. It has been postulated that the persistent pallor may represent a sustained localized adrenergic vasoconstriction.

VASCULAR TUMOR

Vascular tumors include hemangiomas (the most common tumor of childhood), tufted angiomas, kaposiform hemangioendotheliomas, rapidly involuting congenital hemangiomas (RICHs), and non-involuting congenital hemangiomas (NICHs).

Hemangioma

Hemangiomas are proliferative hamartomas of vascular endothelium that may be present at birth or, more commonly, may become apparent in the 1st 2 mo of life, predictably enlarge, and then spontaneously involute. Hemangiomas are the most common

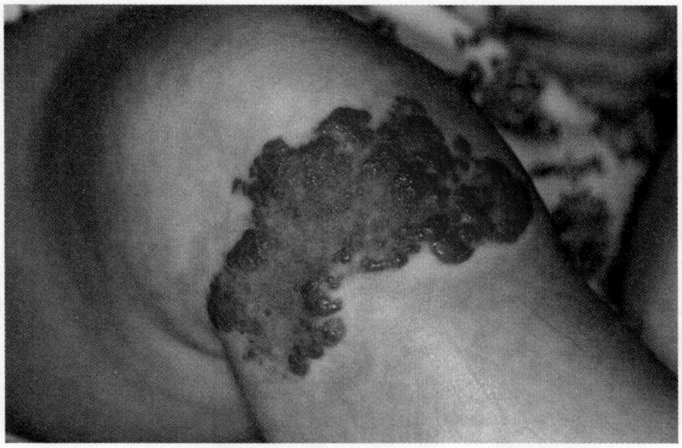

Figure 642-6 Superficial hemangioma on the right knee.

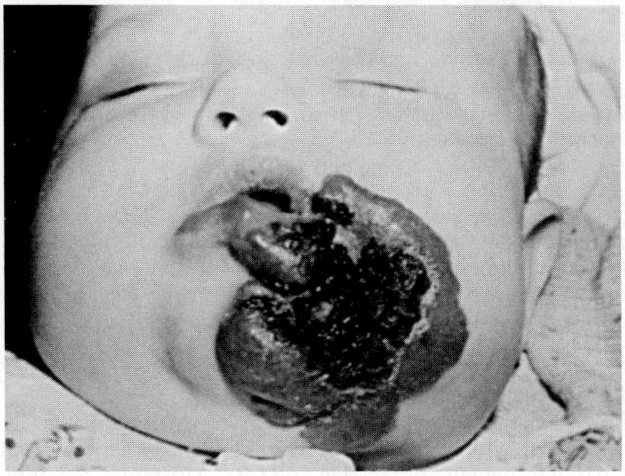

Figure 642-7 Large hemangioma with central crusted ulcer.

tumor of infancy, occurring in 1-2% of newborns (higher in preterm infants) and 10% of white infants in the 1st year of life. Hemangiomas should be classified as superficial, deep, or mixed. The terms *strawberry* and *cavernous* should not be used to describe hemangiomas. The immunohistochemical marker GLUT-1 separates hemangiomas from the other vascular tumors of infancy. Superficial hemangiomas are bright red, protuberant, compressible, sharply demarcated lesions that may occur on any area of the body (Figs. 642-6 and 642-7). Although sometimes present at birth, they more often appear in the 1st two months of life and are heralded by an erythematous or blue mark or an area of pallor, which subsequently develops a fine telangiectatic pattern before the phase of expansion. The presenting sign may occasionally be an ulceration of the perineum or lip. Girls are affected more often than boys. Favored sites are the face, scalp, back, and anterior chest; lesions may be solitary or multiple. Patterns of facial involvement include frontotemporal, maxillary, mandibular, and frontonasal regions. Hemangiomas that are more deeply situated are more diffuse and are less defined than superficial hemangiomas. The lesions are cystic, firm, or compressible, and the overlying skin may appear normal in color or may have a bluish hue (Fig. 642-8).

Most hemangiomas are mixed, having both superficial and deep components. Hemangiomas undergo a phase of rapid expansion, followed by a stationary period and finally by spontaneous involution. Regression may be anticipated when the lesion develops blanched or pale gray areas that indicate fibrosis. The course of a particular lesion is unpredictable, but ≈ 60% of these lesions reach maximal involution by 5 yr of age, and 90-95% by 9 yr. Spontaneous involution cannot be correlated with size or site of involvement, but lip lesions seem to persist most often. Complications include ulceration, secondary infection, and, rarely, hemorrhage (Table 642-4). The location of a lesion may interfere with a vital function (e.g., on eyelid interfering with vision, on urethra with urination, on airway with respiration). Hemangiomas in a "beard" distribution may be associated with upper airway or subglottic involvement. Respiratory symptoms should suggest a tracheobronchial lesion. Large hemangiomas may be complicated by coexistent hypothyroidism due to type 3 iodothyronine deiodinase, and symptoms may be difficult to detect in this age group. Other concerning features are listed in Table 642-5.

In the usual patient with a hemangioma who has no serious complications or extensive growth resulting in tissue destruction and severe disfigurement, treatment consists of expectant observation. Because almost all lesions regress spontaneously, therapy is rarely indicated and may cause further harm. Parents require repeated reassurance and support. After spontaneous involution, many patients are left with small cosmetic defects, such as telangiectasia, hypopigmentation, fibrofatty deposits, and scars if the lesion has ulcerated. Residual telangiectasias may be treated with

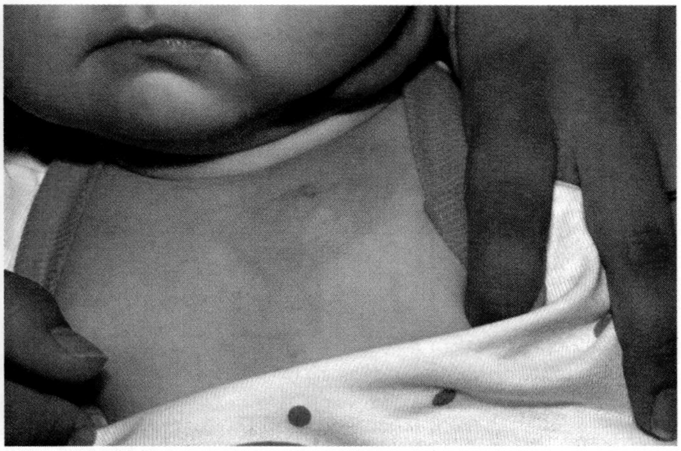

Figure 642-8 Deep hemangioma of the chest.

Table 642-4 COMPLICATIONS OF HEMANGIOMA AND THEIR TREATMENT

CLINICAL FINDING	RECOMMENDED TREATMENT
Severe ulceration/ maceration	Encourage twice-daily cleansing regimen
	Dilute sodium bicarbonate soaks
	± Flashlamp pulsed dye laser
	± Oral corticosteroids or propranolol
	± Culture-directed systemic antibiotics for infection
Bleeding (not KMP)	Gelfoam or Surgifoam or propranolol
	Compression therapy ± embolization
Hemangioma with ophthalmologic sequelae	Patching therapy as directed by ophthalmologist
	Intralesional vs oral corticosteroids vs propranolol
Subglottic hemangioma	Oral corticosteroids ± potassium titanyl phosphate (KtP) laser
	Tracheotomy if required
KMP	Corticosteroids, aminocaproic acid, vincristine, interferon-α ± embolization
High-flow hepatic hemangioma	Corticosteroids or interferon ± embolization

KMP, Kasabach-Merritt phenomenon.
From Blei F: Vascular anomalies: from bedside to bench and back again, *Curr Prob Pediatr Adolesc Health* 32:72–93, 2002.

Table 642-5 CLINICAL "RED FLAGS" ASSOCIATED WITH HEMANGIOMAS

CLINICAL FINDING	RECOMMENDED EVALUATION
Facial hemangioma involving significant area of face	Evaluate for PHACES (posterior fossa abnormalities, hemangioma, and arterial, cardiac, eye, and sternal abnormalities): MRI for orbital hemangioma ± posterior fossa malformation
	Cardiac, ophthalmologic evaluation
	Evaluate for midline abnormality: supraumbilical raphe, sternal atresia, cleft palate, thyroid abnormality
Cutaneous hemangiomas in *beard* distribution	Evaluate for airway hemangioma, especially if manifesting with stridor
Periocular hemangioma	MRI of orbit Ophthalmologic evaluation
Paraspinal midline vascular lesion	Ultrasonography or MRI to evaluate for occult spinal dysraphism
Hemangiomatosis (multiple small cutaneous hemangiomas)	Evaluate for parenchymal hemangiomas, especially hepatic/central nervous system Guaiac stool test
Large hemangioma, especially hepatic	Ultrasonongraphy with Doppler flow study
	MRI
	Thyroid function studies
Thrill and/or bruit associated with hemangioma	Consider cardiac evaluation and echocardiography to rule out diastolic reversal of flow in aorta
	MRI to evaluate extent and flow characteristics
Head tilting	Evaluate appropriately for specific site of lesion, and consider physical therapy evaluation
Delayed milestones	Consider side effect of corticosteroids (myopathy, weight-related)
	Consider side effect of interferon (especially spastic diplegia)

From Blei F: Vascular anomalies: from bedside to bench and back again, *Curr Prob Pediatr Adolesc Health* 32:67–102, 2002.

PDL therapy. Other defects can be treated or minimized by judicious plastic repair if desired.

In the rare case in which intervention is required, if the lesion is very superficial, early therapy with PDL may be beneficial in decreasing growth of the hemangioma. PDL is also useful for the treatment of small (<4-5 cm) ulcerated hemangiomas. Elastic bandages may reduce the amount of tissue distortion resulting from rapid growth, but they are appropriate only in selected patients with large hemangiomas. Rarely, these lesions impinge on vital structures; interfere with functions such as vision, breathing, defecation, urination, or feeding; or cause grotesque disfigurement because of rapid growth.

If further treatment becomes necessary, a course of prednisolone (2-3 mg/kg/24 hr) is effective in most infants. Termination of growth and sometimes regression may be evident after ≈ 2-4 wk of therapy. When a response is obtained, the dose should be decreased gradually. Intralesional corticosteroid injection in the hands of an experienced physician can also induce rapid involution of a localized hemangioma. Propranolol (2 mg/kg) has been used for hemangiomas unresponsive to corticosteroid therapy. Results have been excellent, but exact indications for usage, dosage, length of treatment, and long-term sequelae have not been thoroughly investigated. Hypoglycemia may be a complication of propranolol therapy. Vincristine is used by some oncologists to treat significant hemangiomas. Interferon-α (IFN-α) therapy may also be effective, but spastic diplegia is seen in 10% of cases.

Syndromes associated with hemangiomas include **PHACES** (**p**osterior fossa brain defects such as Dandy-Walker malformation or cerebellar hypoplasia, large plaquelike facial **h**emangioma, **a**rterial cerebrovascular abnormalities such as aneurysms and stroke, **c**oarctation of the aorta, **e**ye abnormalities, and **s**ternal raphe defects such as pits, scars, or supraumbilical raphe), **Gorham** (cutaneous hemangiomas with massive osteolysis), and **Bannayan-Riley-Ruvalcaba** (macrocephaly lipomas, hemangiomas of autosomal dominant inheritance).

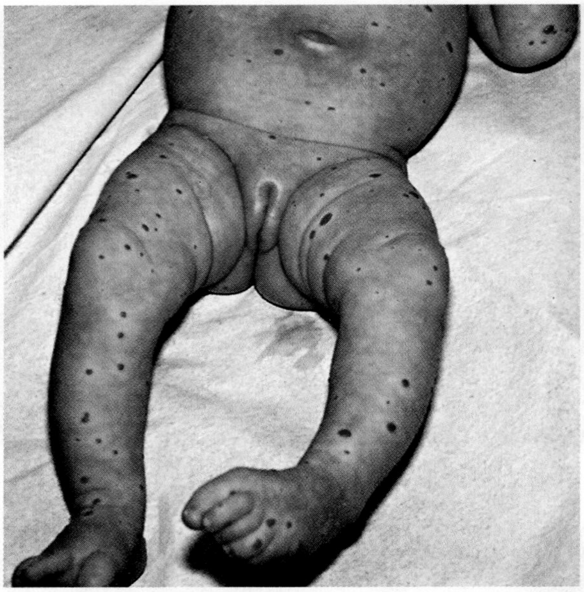

Figure 642-9 Disseminated cutaneous (and liver) neonatal hemangiomatosis. (From Eichenfield LF, Frieden IJ, Esterly NB: *Textbook of neonatal dermatology,* ed 2, Philadelphia, 2008, Saunders, p 359.)

Diffuse Hemangiomatosis

Diffuse hemangiomatosis is a condition in which numerous hemangiomas are widely distributed. The skin usually has many small red papular hemangiomas (Fig. 642-9). Most affected infants have benign neonatal hemangiomatosis, with widespread cutaneous hemangiomas in the absence of apparent visceral involvement. Diffuse neonatal hemangiomatosis is the association of multiple cutaneous hemangiomas of the skin with similar lesions in internal organs. The internal hemangiomas may involve any of the viscera; the liver, gastrointestinal tract, central nervous system, and lungs are the most common sites. In cases of *benign* neonatal hemangiomatosis, spontaneous regression of the lesions without complications is probable. Infants with *diffuse* neonatal hemangiomatosis are usually ill at birth. In these cases, ultrasonography and CT are indicated to determine the extent of visceral or neural involvement. The disorder is often fatal because of high-output cardiac failure, visceral hemorrhage, obstruction of the respiratory tract, or compression of central neural tissue. Treatment consists of systemic corticosteroid therapy alone or in combination with vincristine, IFN-α, surgery, or irradiation and support with blood products for erythrocyte, platelet, and coagulation factor consumption.

Tufted Angioma

Tufted angiomas are defined histologically by discrete "cannonball-like" tufts of dermal blood vessels. Two clinical patterns are seen. The classic, more common type is a slowly expanding dusky reddish-blue plaque with satellite lesions. More than 50% of these lesions occur on the head and neck. Regression is not expected. A less common form manifests as a solitary vascular nodule (Fig. 642-10). Clinical differentiation of tufted angioma from a nodular venous malformation is difficult; spontaneous regression of this type of lesion has been reported.

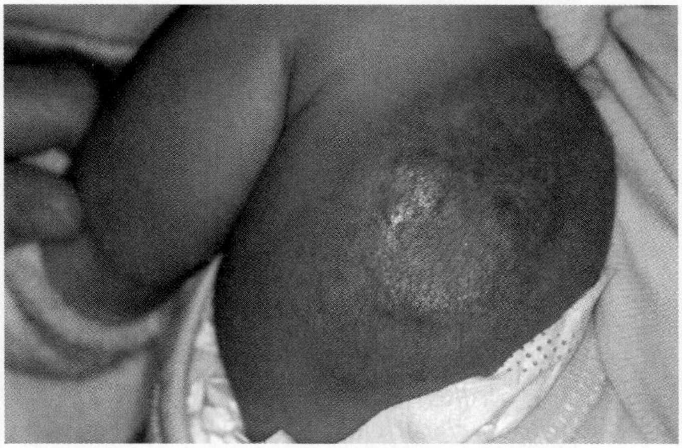

Figure 642-10 Nodular tufted angioma on the left thigh.

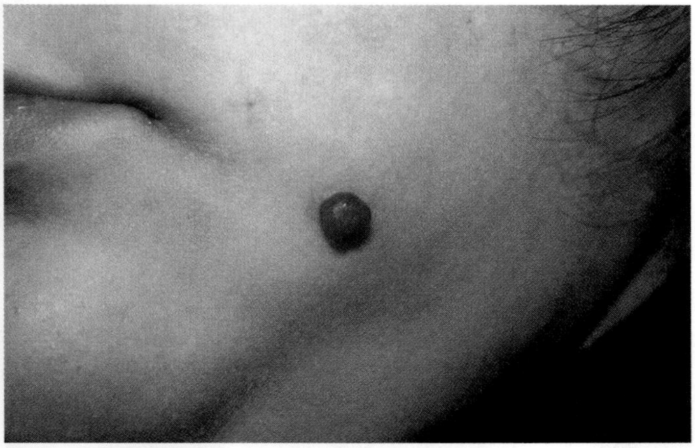

Figure 642-11 Pyogenic granuloma on the left cheek.

Kaposiform Hemangioendothelioma

Kaposiform hemangioendotheliomas are very aggressive locally and, although not malignant, may be fatal. Lesions are usually solitary, firm, and deep purple in color. They do not spontaneously regress.

Both tufted angiomas and Kaposiform hemangioendotheliomas are difficult to treat. All treatments used for hemangiomas have been tried, and results are extremely variable. Kasabach-Merritt syndrome is seen almost exclusively in patients with tufted angiomas and Kaposiform hemangioendotheliomas.

Kasabach-Merritt Syndrome

Kasabach-Merritt syndrome is a life-threatening combination of a rapidly enlarging tufted angioma or kaposiform hemangioendothelioma, thrombocytopenia, microangiopathic hemolytic anemia, and an acute or chronic consumption coagulopathy. The clinical manifestations are usually evident during early infancy. The vascular lesion is usually cutaneous and is only rarely located in viscera. The associated thrombocytopenia may lead to precipitous hemorrhage accompanied by ecchymoses, petechiae, and a rapid increase in the size of the vascular lesion. Severe anemia due to hemorrhage or microangiopathic hemolysis may ensue. The platelet count is depressed, but the bone marrow contains increased numbers of normal or immature megakaryocytes. The thrombocytopenia has been attributed to sequestration or increased destruction of platelets within the lesion. Hypofibrinogenemia and decreased levels of consumable clotting factors are relatively common (Chapter 478.6).

Treatment involves management of thrombocytopenia, anemia, and consumptive coagulopathy by administration of platelets and by transfusion of red blood cells and fresh frozen plasma. The use of heparinization in this syndrome is controversial but has benefited some patients when combined with transfusions. Treatment of Kasabach-Merritt syndrome includes surgical excision of small lesions, systemic steroids, embolization, radiation therapy, vincristine, aminocaproic acid, cyclophosphamide, pentoxifylline, or recombinant IFN-α. The mortality rate is significant.

Rapidly Involuting Congenital Hemangioma

RICHs, by definition, are present at birth. They manifest as raised violaceous nodules with ectatic veins, as grayish nodules with overlying telangiectasias surrounded by pale rims of vasoconstriction, or as flat infiltrative lesions with violaceous skin. They do not undergo a rapid growth phase, and they involute spontaneously by 1 yr of age.

Noninvoluting Congenital Hemangioma

Like RICHs, the solitary vascular lesions known as NICHs are present at birth. They are round to oval plaques with central or peripheral pallor and coarse overlying telangiectasias. They also do not undergo a rapid growth phase, but they do not spontaneously involute. They are probably better classified as vascular malformations than as tumors.

Benign Acquired Vascular Disorders

PYOGENIC GRANULOMA (LOBULAR CAPILLARY HEMANGIOMA) A pyogenic granuloma is a small red, glistening, sessile, or pedunculated papule that often has a discernible epithelial collarette (Fig. 642-11). The surface may be weeping and crusted or completely epithelialized. Pyogenic granulomas initially grow rapidly, may ulcerate, and bleed easily when traumatized because they consist of exuberant granulation tissue. They are relatively common in children, particularly on the face, arms, and hands. Such a lesion located on a finger or hand may appear as a subcutaneous nodule. Pyogenic granulomas may arise at sites of injury, but a history of trauma often cannot be elicited. Clinically, they resemble and are often indistinguishable from small hemangiomas. Microscopically, an early pyogenic lesion resembles an early capillary hemangioma. Collarette formation at the base of the tumor and edema of the stroma may allow differentiation from a capillary hemangioma.

Pyogenic granulomas are benign but a nuisance because they bleed easily with trauma and may recur if incompletely removed. Numerous satellite papules have developed after surgical excision of pyogenic granulomas from the back, particularly in the interscapular region. Small lesions may regress after cauterization with silver nitrate; larger lesions require excision and electrodesiccation of the base of the granuloma. Small (< 5 mm) lesions may be treated successfully with the flashlamp pumped PDL.

ANGIOKERATOMA OF MIBELLI Angiokeratoma of Mibelli is characterized by 1- to 8-mm red, purple, or black scaly, verrucous, occasionally crusted papules and nodules that appear on the dorsum of the fingers and toes and on the knees and the elbows. Less commonly, palms, soles, and ears may be affected. In many patients, onset has followed frostbite or chilblains. These nodules bleed freely after injury and may involute in response to trauma. They may be effectively eradicated by cryotherapy, electrofulguration, excision, or laser ablation.

SPIDER ANGIOMA A vascular spider (nevus araneus) consists of a central feeder artery with many dilated radiating vessels and a surrounding erythematous flush, varying from a few millimeters to several centimeters in diameter (Fig. 642-12). Pressure over the central vessel causes blanching; pulsations visible in larger nevi are evidence for the arterial source of the lesion. Spider angiomas are associated with conditions in which there are increased levels of circulating estrogens, such as cirrhosis and pregnancy, but they also occur in up to 15% of normal preschool-aged children and 45% of school-aged children. Sites of predilection in children are

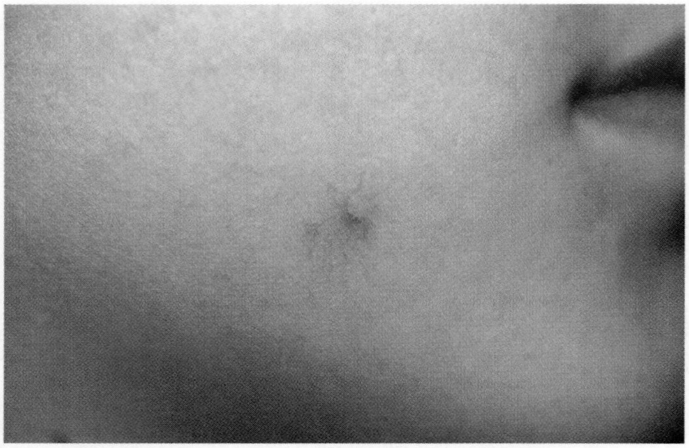

Figure 642-12 Spider telangiectasia with visible central arteriole component.

the dorsum of the hand, forearm, face, and ears. Lesions often regress spontaneously after puberty. If removal is desired, PDL is the mode of choice; resolution is achieved in 90% of cases with a single treatment.

GENERALIZED ESSENTIAL TELANGIECTASIA A rare and presumably nevoid anomaly of unknown cause, essential telangiectasia may have its onset in childhood or adulthood. Mild expression consists of patchy retiform telangiectases, particularly on the limbs, with occasional progression to involve large areas of the body surface. The condition must be distinguished from the secondary telangiectasias of connective tissue diseases, xeroderma pigmentosum, poikiloderma, and ataxia-telangiectasia. Treatment with PDL is effective.

UNILATERAL NEVOID TELANGIECTASIA An unusual entity, unilateral nevoid telangiectasia is characterized by the appearance of telangiectasia in a unilateral distribution, primarily on the face, neck, chest, and arms. The acquired form occurs most commonly in females at onset of menses or during pregnancy. When initiated by pregnancy, the telangiectasia may fade or disappear postpartum.

Genetic Disorders

BLUE RUBBER BLEB NEVUS Blue rubber bleb nevus is a syndrome consisting of numerous venous malformations of the skin, mucous membranes, and gastrointestinal tract. Typical lesions are blue-purple and rubbery in consistency; they vary in size from a few millimeters to a few centimeters in diameter. They are sometimes painful or tender. The nodules occasionally are present at birth but usually appear in childhood. New lesions may continue to develop throughout life. Large disfiguring and irregular blue marks may also occur. The lesions, which can rarely be located in the liver, spleen, and central nervous system in addition to the skin and gastrointestinal tract, do not involute spontaneously. Recurrent gastrointestinal hemorrhage due to nevi in the gastrointestinal tract may lead to severe anemia. Palliation can be achieved by excision of involved bowel.

MAFFUCCI SYNDROME The association of numerous vascular and, occasionally, lymphatic malformations with **nodular enchondromas** in the metaphyseal or diaphyseal portion of long bones is known as Maffucci syndrome. Mutations in the PTH/PTHRP type 1 receptor have been identified in the enchondromatoses. Vascular lesions are typically soft, compressible, asymptomatic blue to purple subcutaneous masses that grow in proportion to a child's growth and stabilize by adulthood. Mucous membranes or viscera may also be involved. Onset occurs during childhood. Bone lesions may produce limb deformities and pathologic fractures. Malignant transformation of enchondromas (chondrosarcoma, angiosarcoma) or primary malignancies (ovarian, fibrosarcoma, glioma, pancreatic) may be a complication (Chapter 495).

HEREDITARY HEMORRHAGIC TELANGIECTASIA (OSLER-WEBER-RENDU DISEASE) Hereditary hemorrhagic telangiectasia (HHT), which is inherited as an autosomal dominant trait, occurs in two types. The gene in HHT-1 encodes endoglin, a membrane glycoprotein on endothelial cells that binds transforming growth factor-β. HHT-2 is caused by mutations in the *ACVRL1* gene and is associated with increased risk for hepatic involvement and pulmonary hypertension. Affected children may experience recurrent epistaxis before detection of the characteristic skin and mucous membrane lesions. The mucocutaneous lesions, which usually develop at puberty, are 1- to 4-mm, sharply demarcated red to purple macules, papules, or spider-like projections, each composed of a tightly woven mat of tortuous telangiectatic vessels. The nasal mucosa, lips, and tongue are usually involved; less commonly, cutaneous lesions occur on the face, ears, palms, and nail beds. Vascular ectasias may also arise in the conjunctivae, larynx, pharynx, gastrointestinal tract, bladder, vagina, bronchi, brain, and liver.

Massive hemorrhage is the most serious complication of HHT and may result in severe anemia. Bleeding may occur from the nose, mouth, gastrointestinal tract, genitourinary tract, or lungs; epistaxis is often the only complaint, however, occurring in 80% of patients. Approximately 15-20% of patients with AVMs in the lungs present with stroke due to embolic abscesses. Persons with HHT have normal levels of clotting factors and an intact clotting mechanism. In the absence of serious complications, lifespan of a person with HHT is normal. Local lesions may be ablated temporarily with chemical cautery or electrocoagulation. More drastic surgical measures may be required for lesions in critical sites, such as the lung or gastrointestinal tract. Anemia should be treated with iron.

HEREDITARY BENIGN TELANGIECTASIA A rare disorder, hereditary benign telangiectasia is inherited as an autosomal dominant trait and develops during childhood. The face, upper trunk, and arms are the areas of predilection. The condition is progressive but remains limited to the skin.

ATAXIA-TELANGIECTASIA (CHAPTER 590.1) Ataxia-telangiectasia is transmitted as an autosomal recessive trait because of a mutation in the *ATM* gene. The characteristic telangiectasias develop at about 3 yr of age, first on the bulbar conjunctivae and later on the nasal bridge, malar areas, external ears, hard palate, upper anterior chest, and antecubital and popliteal fossae. Additional cutaneous stigmata include café-au-lait spots, premature graying of the hair, and sclerodermatous changes. Progressive cerebellar ataxia, neurologic deterioration, sinopulmonary infections, and malignancies are also seen.

ANGIOKERATOMA CORPORIS DIFFUSUM (FABRY DISEASE) (CHAPTER 80.4) An inborn error of glycolipid metabolism (α-galactosidase), angiokeratoma corporis diffusum is an X-linked recessive disorder that is fully penetrant in males and is of variable penetrance in carrier females. Angiokeratomas appear before puberty and occur in profusion over the genitalia, hips, buttocks, and thighs and in the umbilical and inguinal regions. They consist of 0.1- to 3-mm red to blue-black papules that may have a hyperkeratotic surface. Telangiectasias are seen in the mucosa and conjunctiva. On light microscopy, these angiokeratomas appear as blood-filled, dilated, endothelium-lined vascular spaces. Granular lipid deposits are demonstrable in dermal macrophages, fibrocytes, and endothelial cells.

Additional clinical manifestations include recurrent episodes of fever and agonizing pain, cyanosis and flushing of the acral limb areas, paresthesias of the hands and feet, corneal opacities detectable on slit-lamp examination, and hypohidrosis. Renal involvement and cardiac involvement are the usual causes of death. The biochemical defect is a deficiency of the lysosomal enzyme α-galactosidase, with accumulation of ceramide trihexoside in tissues, particularly vascular endothelium, and excretion in urine (see Chapter 80.4 for therapy). Similar cutaneous lesions have also been described in another lysosomal enzyme disorder, α-L-fucosidase deficiency, and in sialidosis, a storage disease with neuraminidase deficiency.

BIBLIOGRAPHY

Please visit the Nelson Textbook of Pediatrics *website at www.expertconsult.com for the complete bibliography.*

Chapter 643
Cutaneous Nevi

Joseph G. Morelli

Nevus skin lesions are characterized histopathologically by collections of well-differentiated cell types normally found in the skin. Vascular nevi are described in Chapter 642. Melanocytic nevi are subdivided into 2 broad categories: those that appear after birth (acquired nevi) and those that are present at birth (congenital nevi).

ACQUIRED MELANOCYTIC NEVUS

Melanocytic nevus is a benign cluster of melanocytic nevus cells that arises as a result of alteration and proliferation of melanocytes at the epidermal-dermal junction.

Epidemiology

The number of acquired melanocytic nevi increases gradually during childhood and more slowly in early adulthood. The number reaches a plateau in the 3rd or 4th decade and then slowly decreases thereafter. The mean number of melanocytic nevi in an adult varies depending on genetics, skin color, and sun exposure. The greater the number of nevi present, the greater is the risk for development of **melanoma.** Sun exposure during childhood, particularly intermittent, intense exposure of an individual with light skin, and a propensity to burn and freckle rather than tan are important determinants of the number of melanocytic nevi that develop. Red-haired children, despite their light skin and propensity to freckle and sunburn, have fewer nevi than other children. Increased numbers of nevi are also associated with immunosuppression and administration of chemotherapy.

Clinical Manifestations

Nevocellular nevi have a well-defined life history and are classified as **junctional, compound,** or **dermal** in accordance with the location of the nevus cells in the skin. In childhood, > 90% of nevi are junctional; melanocyte proliferation occurs at the junction of the epidermis and dermis to form nests of cells. Junctional nevi appear anywhere on the body in various shades of brown; they are relatively small, discrete, flat, and variable in shape. The melanized nevus cells are cuboidal or epithelioid in configuration and occur in nests on the epidermal side of the basement membrane. Although some nevi, particularly those on the palms, soles, and genitalia, remain junctional throughout life, most become compound as melanocytes migrate into the papillary dermis to form nests at both the epidermal-dermal junction and within the dermis. If the junctional melanocytes stop proliferating, nests of melanocytes remain only within the dermis, forming an intradermal nevus. With maturation, compound and intradermal nevi may become raised, dome-shaped, verrucous, or pedunculated. Slightly elevated lesions are usually compound. Distinctly elevated lesions are usually intradermal. With age, the dermal melanocytic nests regress and the nevi gradually disappear.

Prognosis and Treatment

Acquired pigmented nevi are benign, but a very small percentage undergoes malignant transformation. Suspicious changes are indications for excision and histopathologic evaluation; they include rapid increase in size; development of satellite lesions; variegation of color, particularly with shades of red, brown, gray, black, and blue; pigmentary incontinence; notching or irregularity of the borders; changes in texture such as scaling, erosion, ulceration, and induration; and regional lymphadenopathy. Most of these changes are due to irritation, infection, or maturation; darkening and gradual increase in size and elevation normally occur during adolescence and should not be cause for concern. Two common benign changes are clonal nevi (fried-egg moles) and rim nevi. A clonal nevus is light brown with a dark raised center representing a clonal change of a subset of nevus cells within the lesion. Rim nevi are flat and light brown with dark brown rims. They are seen primarily in the scalp (Fig. 643-1). Consideration should be given to the presence of risk factors for development of melanoma and the patient's parents' wishes about removal of the nevus. If doubt remains about the benign nature of a nevus, excision is a safe and simple outpatient procedure that may be justified to allay anxiety.

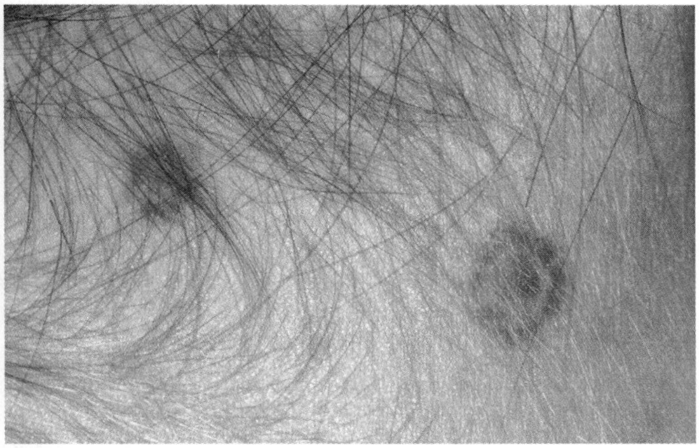

Figure 643-1 Rim moles in the scalp.

ATYPICAL MELANOCYTIC NEVUS

Atypical melanocytic nevi occur both in an autosomal dominant familial melanoma-prone setting (familial mole–melanoma syndrome, dysplastic nevus syndrome, BK mole syndrome) and as a sporadic event. Only 2% of all pediatric melanomas occur in individuals with this familial syndrome; melanoma develops before age 20 yr in 10% of individuals with the syndrome. Malignant melanoma has been reported in children with the dysplastic nevus syndrome as young as 10 yr. Risk for development of melanoma is essentially 100% in individuals with dysplastic nevus syndrome who have 2 family members who have had melanomas. The term atypical mole syndrome describes lesions in those individuals without an autosomal dominant familial history of melanoma but with > 50 nevi, some of which are atypical. The lifetime risk of melanoma associated with dysplastic nevi in this context is estimated to be 5-10%.

Atypical nevi tend to be large (5-15 mm) and round to oval. They have irregular margins and variegated color, and portions of them are elevated. These nevi are most common on the posterior trunk, suggesting that intermittent, intense sun exposure has a role in their genesis. They may also occur in sun-protected areas such as the breasts, buttocks, and scalp. Atypical nevi do not usually develop until puberty, although scalp lesions may be present earlier. Atypical nevi demonstrate disordered proliferation of atypical intraepidermal melanocytes, lymphocytic infiltration, fibroplasia, and angiogenesis. It may be helpful to obtain histopathologic documentation of dysplastic change by biopsy to identify these individuals. It is prudent to excise borderline atypical nevi in immunocompromised children or in those treated with irradiation or chemotherapeutic agents. Although chemotherapy has been associated with the development of a greater number of melanocytic nevi, it has not been directly linked to increased risk for development of melanoma. The threshold for removal of clinically atypical nevi is also lower at sites that are difficult to observe, such as the scalp. Children with atypical nevi should undergo a complete skin examination every 6-12 mo. In these children, photographic mole mapping serves as a useful adjunct in following nevus change. Parents must be counseled about the importance of sun protection and avoidance and should be instructed to look for early signs of melanoma on a regular basis, approximately every 3-4 mo.

CONGENITAL MELANOCYTIC NEVUS

Congenital melanocytic nevi are present in ≈1% of newborn infants. These nevi have been categorized by size: giant congenital nevi are >20 cm in diameter (adult size) or >5% of the body surface, small congenital nevi are <2 cm in diameter, and intermediate nevi are in between these dimensions. Congenital nevi are characterized by the presence of nevus cells in the lower reticular dermis; between collagen bundles; surrounding cutaneous appendages, nerves, and vessels in the lower dermis; and occasionally extending to the subcuticular fat. Identification is often uncertain, however, because they may have the histologic features of ordinary junctional, compound, or intradermal nevi. Some nevi that were not present at birth display histopathologic features of congenital nevi; these should not be considered congenital. Furthermore, congenital nevi may be difficult to distinguish clinically from other types of pigmented lesions, adding to the difficulty that parents may have in identifying nevi that were present at birth. The clinical differential diagnosis includes mongolian spots, café-au-lait spots, smooth muscle hamartoma, and dermal melanocytosis (nevi of Ota and Ito).

Sites of predilection for small congenital nevi are the lower trunk, upper back, shoulders, chest, and proximal limbs. The lesions may be flat, elevated, verrucous, or nodular and may be various shades of brown, blue, or black. Given the difficulty in identifying small congenital nevi with certainty, data regarding their malignant potential are controversial and likely overstated. The true incidence of melanoma in congenital nevi, especially small and medium-sized lesions, is unknown. Removal of all small congenital nevi is not warranted because the development of melanoma in a small congenital nevus is an exceedingly rare event before puberty. A number of factors must be weighed in the decision about whether or not to remove a nevus, including its location, the ability to be monitor it clinically, the potential for scarring, the presence of other risk factors for melanoma, and the presence of atypical clinical features.

Giant congenital pigmented nevi (<1/20,000 births) occur most commonly on the posterior trunk (Fig. 643-2) but may also appear on the head or extremities. These nevi are of special significance because of their association with leptomeningeal melanocytosis (neurocutaneous melanocytosis) and their predisposition for development of malignant melanoma. Leptomeningeal involvement occurs most often when the nevus is located on the head or midline on the trunk, particularly when associated with multiple "satellite" melanocytic nevi (>20 lesions). Nevus cells within the leptomeninges and brain parenchyma may cause increased intracranial pressure, hydrocephalus, seizures, retardation, and motor deficits and may result in melanoma. Malignancy can be identified by careful cytologic examination of the cerebrospinal fluid for melanin-containing cells. MRI demonstrates asymptomatic leptomeningeal melanosis in ≈ 30% of individuals with giant congenital nevus of the type described above. The overall incidence of malignant melanoma arising in a giant congenital nevus has been estimated to be ≈ 5-10% but is more likely to be approximately 1-2%. The median age at diagnosis of the melanomas that arise within a giant congenital nevus is 7 yr. The mortality rate approaches 100%. The risk of melanoma is greater in patients in whom the predicted adult size of the nevus is > 40 cm. Management of giant congenital nevi remains controversial and should involve the parents, pediatrician, dermatologist, and plastic surgeon. If the nevus lies over the head or spine, MRI may allow detection of neural melanosis, the presence of which makes gross removal of a nevus from the skin a futile effort. In the absence of neural melanosis, early excision and repair aided by tissue expanders or grafting may reduce the burden of nevus cells and thus the potential for development of melanoma, but at the cost of many potentially disfiguring operations. Nevus cells deep within subcutaneous tissues may evade excision. Random biopsies of the nevus are not helpful, but biopsy of newly expanding nodules is indicated. Follow-up every 6 mo for 5 yr and every 12 mo thereafter is recommended. Serial photographs of the nevus may aid in detecting changes.

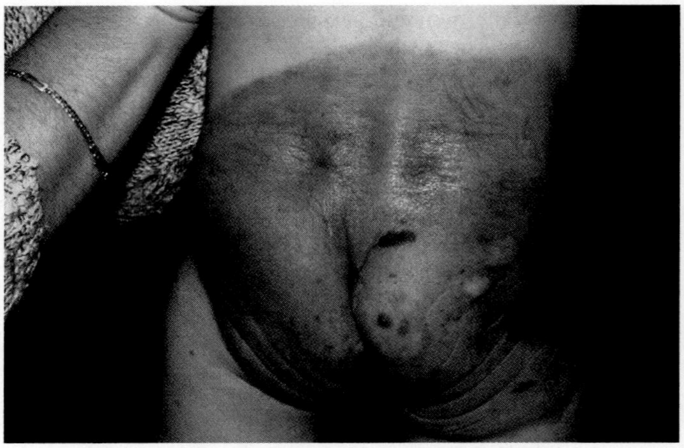

Figure 643-2 "Bathing suit" large congenital melanocytic nevus.

MELANOMA

Malignant melanoma accounts for 1-3% of all pediatric malignancies, and approximately 2% of all melanomas occur before age 20 yr. The incidence of melanoma continues to increase. Melanoma is 7 times more frequent in the 2nd decade of life than in the 1st decade of life. Melanoma develops primarily in white individuals, on the head and trunk in males, and on the extremities in females. Risk factors for development of melanoma include the presence of the familial atypical mole–melanoma syndrome or xeroderma pigmentosum; an increased number of acquired melanocytic nevi, or atypical nevi; fair complexion; excessive sun exposure, especially intermittent exposure to intense sunlight; a personal or family (first-degree relative) history of a previous melanoma, giant congenital nevus, and immunosuppression. In previously well children, ultraviolet (UV) radiation is responsible for most melanomas. Fewer than 5% of childhood melanomas develop within giant congenital nevi or in individuals with the familial atypical mole–melanoma syndrome. Approximately 40-50% of the time, melanoma develops at a site where there was no apparent nevus. The mortality rate from melanoma is related primarily to tumor thickness and the level of invasion into the skin. The overall mortality rate reaches ≈ 40%, regardless of whether the tumor arises in a child or adult.

Given the lack of effective therapy for melanoma, prevention and early detection are the most effective measures. Emphasis should be given to avoidance of intense midday sun exposure between 10 AM and 3 PM; wearing of protective clothing such as a hat, long sleeves, and pants; and use of sunscreen. Early detection includes frequent clinical and photographic examinations of patients at risk (dysplastic nevus syndrome) and prompt response to rapid changes in nevi (size, shape, color, inflammation, bleeding or crusting, and sensation). The **ABCD rule** (asymmetry, border

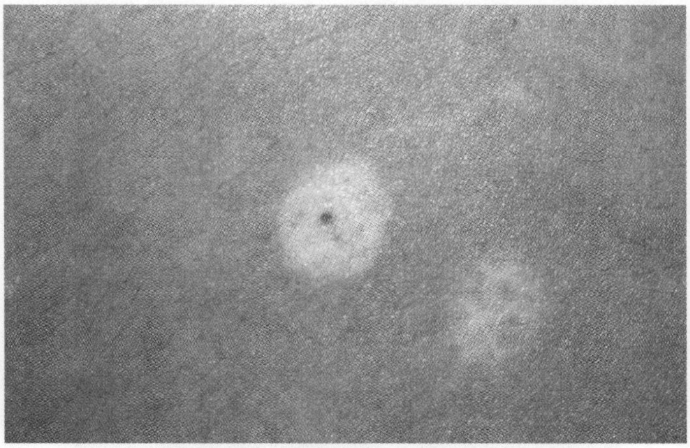

Figure 643-3 Well-developed halo nevus.

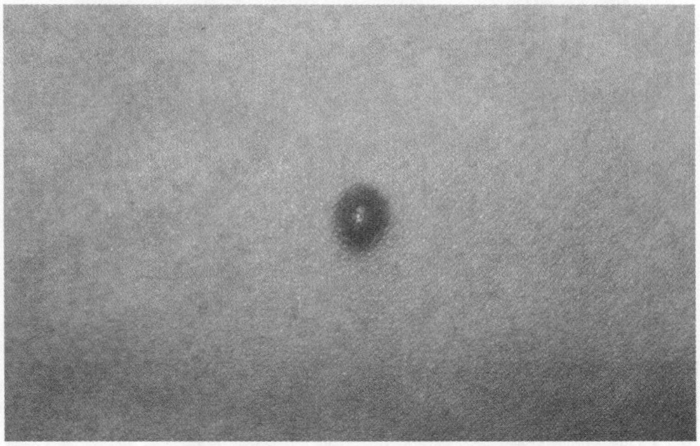

Figure 643-4 Dome-shaped red Spitz nevus.

irregularities, color variability, diameter >6 mm), which is a useful screening tool for adults, may not be as effective for children.

HALO NEVUS

Halo nevi occur primarily in children and young adults, most commonly on the back (Fig. 643-3). Development of the lesion may coincide with puberty or pregnancy. Several pigmented nevi frequently develop halos simultaneously. Subsequent disappearance of the central nevus over several months is the usual outcome, and the depigmented area usually repigments. Excision and histopathologic examination of the lesion is indicated only when the nature of the central lesion is in question. An acquired melanocytic nevus occasionally develops a peripheral zone of depigmentation over a period of days to weeks. There is a dense inflammatory infiltrate of lymphocytes and histiocytes in addition to the nevus cells. The pale halo reflects disappearance of the melanocytes. This phenomenon is associated with congenital nevi, blue nevi, Spitz nevi, dysplastic nevi, neurofibromas, and primary and secondary malignant melanoma, and occasionally with poliosis, Vogt-Koyanagi-Harada syndrome, and pernicious anemia. Patients with vitiligo have an increased incidence of halo nevi. Individuals with halo nevi have circulating antibodies against the cytoplasm of melanocytes and nevus cells.

SPITZ NEVUS (SPINDLE AND EPITHELIOID CELL NEVUS)

Spitz nevus manifests most commonly in the 1st 2 decades of life as a pink to red, smooth, dome-shaped, firm, hairless papule on the face, shoulder, or upper limb (Fig. 643-4). Most are <1 cm in

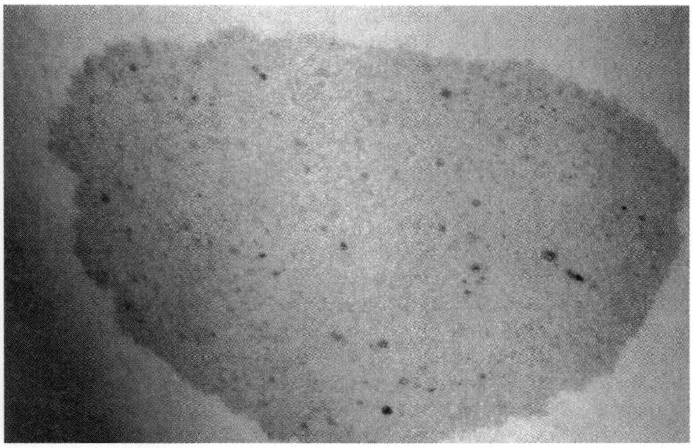

Figure 643-5 Nevus spilus.

diameter, but they can achieve a size of 3 cm. Rarely, they occur as numerous grouped lesions. Visually similar lesions include pyogenic granuloma, hemangioma, nevocellular nevus, juvenile xanthogranuloma, and basal cell carcinoma, but these entities are histologically distinguishable. Spitz nevus may be difficult to distinguish histopathologically from malignant melanoma because nuclear atypia is a common feature, particularly after local recurrence of the nevus. Difficulty arises in the fact that many other clinical types of melanocytic nevi have a similar histologic appearance. Local recurrence after excision may occur up to 5% of the time. If a nevus arouses clinical suspicion that it may be a melanoma, an excisional biopsy of the entire lesion is recommended. If the margins of excision of a Spitz nevus are positive, re-excision of the site is prudent to avoid difficulties in histopathologic interpretation of the lesion in the future.

ZOSTERIFORM LENTIGINOUS NEVUS (AGMINATED LENTIGINE)

Zosteriform lentiginous nevus is a unilateral, linear, bandlike collection of numerous 2- to 10-mm brown or black macules on the face, trunk, or limbs. The nevus may be present at birth or may develop during childhood. There are higher numbers of melanocytes in elongated rete ridges of the epidermis.

NEVUS SPILUS (SPECKLED LENTIGINOUS NEVUS)

Nevus spilus is a flat brown patch within which are darker flat or raised brown melanocytic elements (Fig. 643-5). It varies considerably in size and can occur anywhere on the body. The color of the macular component may vary from light to dark brown, and the number of darker lesions may be low or high. Nevus spilus is rare at birth and is commonly acquired in late infancy or early childhood. Dark elements within the nevus are usually present initially and tend to increase in number gradually over time. The darker macules represent nevus cells in a junctional or dermal location; the patch has increased numbers of melanocytes in a lentiginous epidermal pattern. The malignant potential of these nevi is uncertain; nevus spilus is found more commonly in individuals with melanoma than in matched control subjects. The nevi need not be excised, unless atypical features or recent clinical changes are noted.

NEVUS OF OTA AND NEVUS OF ITO

Nevus of Ota is more common among females, Asian, and black patients. This nevus consists of a permanent patch composed of partially confluent blue, black, and brown macules. Enlargement and darkening may occur with time. Occasionally, some areas of the nevus are raised. The macular nevi resemble mongolian spots in color and occur unilaterally in the areas supplied by the 1st and 2nd divisions of the trigeminal nerve. Nevus of Ota differs from a mongolian spot, not only by its distribution but also by having a speckled rather than a uniform appearance. Both are forms of mid-dermal melanocytosis. Nevus of Ota also has a greater concentration of elongated, dendritic dermal melanocytes located in the upper rather than the lower portion of the dermis. This nevus is sometimes present at birth; in other cases, it may arise during the 1st or 2nd decade of life. Patchy involvement of the conjunctiva, hard palate, pharynx, nasal mucosa, buccal mucosa, or tympanic membrane occurs in some patients. Malignant change is exceedingly rare. Laser therapy may effectively decrease the pigmentation.

Nevus of Ito is localized to the supraclavicular, scapular, and deltoid regions. This nevus tends to be more diffuse in its distribution and less mottled than nevus of Ota. It is also a form of mid-dermal melanocytosis. The only available treatments are masking with cosmetics and laser therapy.

BLUE NEVI

The common blue nevus is a solitary, asymptomatic, smooth, dome-shaped, blue to blue-gray papule <10 mm in diameter on the dorsal aspect of the hands and feet. Rarely, common blue nevi form large plaques. Blue nevus is nearly always acquired, often during childhood and more commonly in females. Microscopically, it is characterized by groups of intensely pigmented spindle-shaped melanocytes in the dermis. This nevus is benign.

The cellular blue nevus is typically 1-3 cm in diameter and occurs most frequently on the buttocks and in the sacrococcygeal area. In addition to collections of deeply pigmented dermal dendritic melanocytes, cellular islands composed of large spindle-shaped cells are noted in the dermis and may extend into the subcutaneous fat. A histologic continuum may be seen from blue nevi to cellular blue nevi. A combined nevus is the association of a blue nevus with an overlying melanocytic nevus.

The blue-gray that is characteristic of these nevi is an optical effect caused by dermal melanin. Longer wavelengths of visible light penetrate to the deep dermis and are absorbed there by melanin; shorter-wavelength blue light cannot penetrate deeply but instead is reflected back to the observer.

NEVUS DEPIGMENTOSUS (ACHROMIC NEVUS)

Nevi depigmentosi are usually present at birth; they are localized macular hypopigmented patches or streaks, often with bizarre, irregular borders (Fig. 643-6). They can resemble hypomelanosis of Ito clinically, except that they are more localized and often unilateral. Small lesions may also resemble the ash leaf macules of tuberous sclerosis. Nevi depigmentosi appear to represent a focal defect in transfer of melanosomes to keratinocytes.

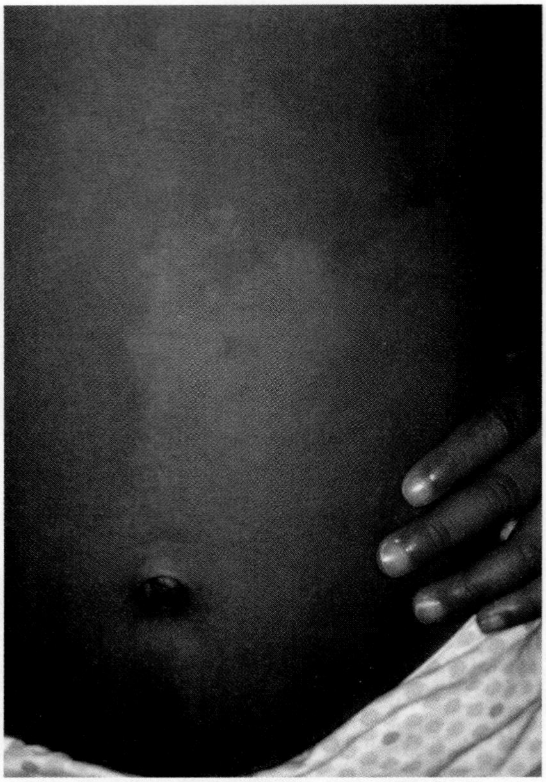

Figure 643-6 Large nevus depigmentosus of the abdomen.

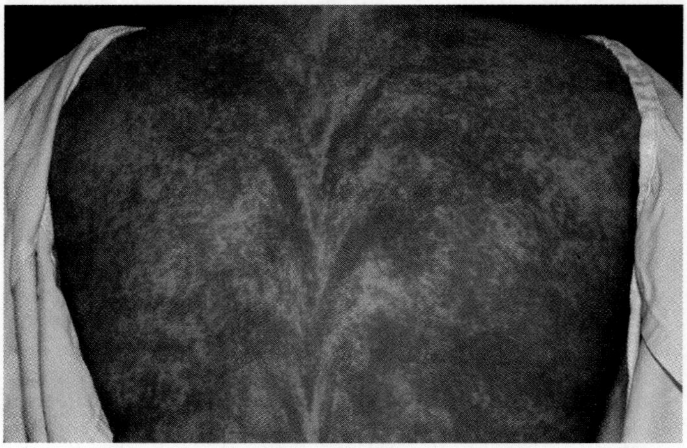

Figure 643-7 Epidermal nevus (ichthyosis hystrix type).

EPIDERMAL NEVI

Epidermal nevi may be visible at birth or may develop in the first months or years of life. They affect both sexes equally and usually occur sporadically. Epidermal nevi are hamartomatous lesions characterized by hyperplasia of the epidermis and/or adnexal structures in a focal area of the skin.

Epidermal nevi are classified into a number of variants, depending on the morphology and extent of the individual nevus and the predominant epidermal structure. An epidermal nevus may appear initially as a discolored, slightly scaly patch that, with maturation, becomes more linear, thickened, verrucous, and hyperpigmented. *Systematized* refers to a diffuse or extensive distribution of lesions, and *ichthyosis hystrix* indicates that the distribution is extensive and bilateral (Fig. 643-7). Morphologic types include pigmented papillomas, often in a linear distribution; unilateral hyperkeratotic streaks involving a limb and perhaps a portion of the trunk; velvety hyperpigmented plaques; and whorled or marbled hyperkeratotic lesions in localized plaques or over extensive areas of the body along Blaschko lines. An inflammatory linear verrucous variant is markedly pruritic and tends to become erythematous, scaling, and crusted.

The histologic pattern evolves as an epidermal nevus matures, but epidermal hyperplasia of some degree is apparent in all stages of development. One or another dermal appendage may predominate in a particular lesion. These nevi must be distinguished from lichen striatus, lymphangioma circumscriptum, shagreen patch of tuberous sclerosis, congenital hairy nevi, linear porokeratosis, linear lichen planus, linear psoriasis, the verrucous stage of incontinentia pigmenti, and nevus sebaceus (Jadassohn). Keratolytic agents such as retinoic acid and salicylic acid may be moderately effective in reducing scaling and controlling pruritus, but definitive treatment requires full-thickness excision; recurrence is usual

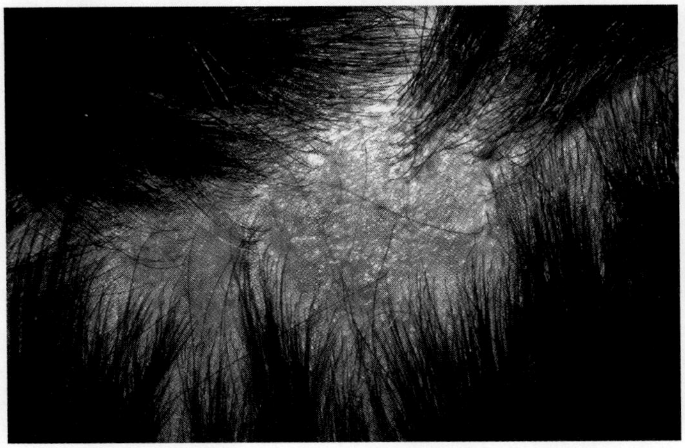

Figure 643-8 Orange-yellow nevus sebaceus of the scalp.

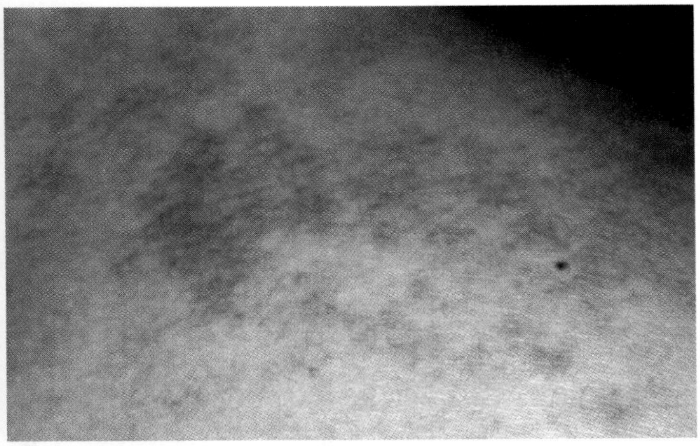

Figure 643-9 Becker nevus on the shoulder of an adolescent male.

if more superficial removal is attempted. Alternatively, the nevus may be left intact. Epidermal nevi are occasionally associated with other abnormalities of the skin and soft tissues, eyes, and nervous, cardiovascular, musculoskeletal, and urogenital systems. In these instances, the disorder is referred to as epidermal nevus syndrome, and a mosaic phenotype is expressed. This syndrome, however, is not a distinct clinical entity. The well-established syndromes that involve a type of epidermal nevus and distinct birth defects include the **proteus** and **CHILD** (congenital hemidysplasia with ichthyosiform erythroderma and limb defects) syndromes.

Nevus Sebaceus (Jadassohn)

A relatively small, sharply demarcated, oval or linear, elevated yellow-orange plaque that is usually devoid of hair, nevus sebaceus occurs on the head and neck of infants (Fig. 643-8). It may occur occasionally on the trunk. Although the lesion is characterized histopathologically by an abundance of sebaceous glands, all elements of the skin are represented. It is frequently flat and inconspicuous in early childhood. With maturity, usually during adolescence, the lesions become verrucous and studded with large rubbery nodules. The changing clinical appearance reflects the histologic pattern, which is characterized by a variable degree of hyperkeratosis, hyperplasia of the epidermis, malformed hair follicles, and often a profusion of sebaceous glands and the presence of ectopic apocrine glands. It is believed that these nevi form from pluripotential primary epithelial germ cells, which can dedifferentiate into various **epithelial tumors.** Consequently, during adulthood, these nevi are frequently complicated by secondary malignancies and benign adnexal tumors, most commonly basal cell carcinoma or syringocystadenoma papilliferum. Deletions in the *PTCH* gene, the putative gene defect in basal cell carcinoma, have been found in sebaceus nevi. The **treatment of choice** is total excision before adolescence. Sebaceus nevi associated with central nervous system, skeletal, and ocular defects represent a variant of the epidermal nevus syndrome.

Becker Nevus (Becker Melanosis)

Becker nevus develops predominantly in males, during childhood or adolescence, initially as a hyperpigmented patch. The lesion commonly develops hypertrichosis, limited to the area of hyperpigmentation, and evolves into a unilateral, slightly thickened, irregular, hyperpigmented plaque. The most common sites are the upper torso and upper arm (Fig. 643-9). The nevus shows an increased number of basal melanocytes and variable epidermal hyperplasia. Becker melanosis is commonly associated with a smooth muscle hamartoma, which may appear as slight perifollicular papular elevations or slight induration. Stroking of such a lesion may induce smooth muscle contraction and make the hairs stand up. The nevus is benign, has no risk for malignant change, and is rarely associated with other anomalies.

NEVUS COMEDONICUS

An uncommon organoid nevus of epithelial origin, nevus comedonicus consists of linear plaques of plugged follicles that simulate comedones; they may be present at birth or may appear during childhood. The horny plugs represent keratinous debris within dilated, malformed pilosebaceous follicles. The lesions are most often unilateral and may develop at any site. Rarely, they are associated with other congenital malformations, including skeletal defects, cerebral anomalies, and cataracts. Although these lesions are often asymptomatic, some affected individuals experience recurrent inflammation, resulting in cyst formation, fistulas, and scarring. There is no effective treatment except full-thickness excision; palliation of larger lesions may be achieved by regular applications of a retinoic acid preparation.

CONNECTIVE TISSUE NEVUS

Connective tissue nevus is a hamartoma of collagen, elastin, and/or glycosaminoglycans of the dermal extracellular matrix. It may occur as a solitary defect or as a manifestation of an associated disorder. These nevi may occur at any site but are most common on the back, buttocks, arms, and thighs. They are skin-colored, ivory, or yellow plaques, 2-15 cm in diameter, composed of many tiny papules or grouped nodules that are frequently difficult to appreciate visually because of the subtle color changes. The plaques have a rubbery or cobblestone consistency on palpation. Biopsy findings are variable and include increased amounts and/or degeneration or fragmentation of dermal collagen, elastic tissue, or ground substance. Similar lesions occurring with tuberous sclerosis are called shagreen patches; however, shagreen patches consist only of excessive amounts of collagen. The association of many small papular connective tissue nevi with osteopoikilosis is called dermatofibrosis lenticularis disseminata (**Buschke-Ollendorf syndrome**).

SMOOTH MUSCLE HAMARTOMA

Smooth muscle hamartoma is a developmental anomaly resulting from hyperplasia of the smooth muscle (arrector pili) associated with hair follicles. It is usually evident at birth or shortly thereafter as a flesh-colored or lightly pigmented plaque with overlying hypertrichosis on the trunk or limbs (Fig. 643-10). Transient elevation or a rippling movement of the lesion, caused by contraction of the muscle bundles, can sometimes be elicited by stroking of the surface. Smooth muscle hamartoma can be mistaken for

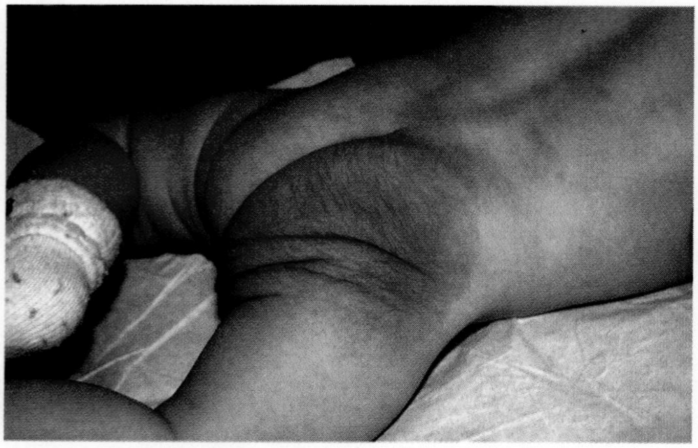

Figure 643-10 Large smooth muscle hamartoma of the buttock.

congenital pigmented nevus, but the distinction is important because the former has no risk for malignant melanoma and need not be removed.

BIBLIOGRAPHY

Please visit the Nelson Textbook of Pediatrics *website at www.expertconsult.com for the complete bibliography.*

Chapter 644
Hyperpigmented Lesions

Joseph G. Morelli

DISORDERS OF PIGMENT

Normal pigmentation requires migration of melanoblasts from the neural crest to the dermal-epidermal junction, enzymatic processes to form pigment, structural components to contain the pigment (melanosomes), and transfer of pigment to the surrounding keratinocytes. Increased skin color may be generalized or localized and may result from various defects in any of these requirements. Some of these aberrations are a manifestation of systemic disease, others represent generalized or focal developmental or genetic defects, and still others may be nonspecific and the result of cutaneous inflammation.

EPHELIDES (FRECKLES)

Ephelides are light or dark brown macules usually <3 mm in diameter, with a poorly defined margin, that occur in sun-exposed areas such as the face, upper back, arms, and hands. They are induced by exposure to sun, particularly during the summer, and may fade or disappear during the winter. They are more common in redheads and fair-haired individuals and first appear in the preschool years. Histologically, they are marked by increased melanin pigment in epidermal basal cells, which have more numerous and larger dendritic processes than the melanocytes of the surrounding paler skin. The lack of melanocytic proliferation or elongation of epidermal rete ridges distinguishes them from lentigines. Freckles have been identified as a risk factor for melanoma independent of melanocytic nevi.

LENTIGINES

Lentigines, often mistaken for freckles or junctional nevi, are small (<3 cm), round, dark brown macules that can appear anywhere on the body. They are unrelated to sun exposure and remain permanently. Histologically, they have elongated, club-shaped, epidermal rete ridges with increased numbers of melanocytes and dense epidermal deposits of melanin. No nests of melanocytes are found. The lesions are benign and, when few, may be viewed as a normal occurrence and are seen most commonly on the lower lip.

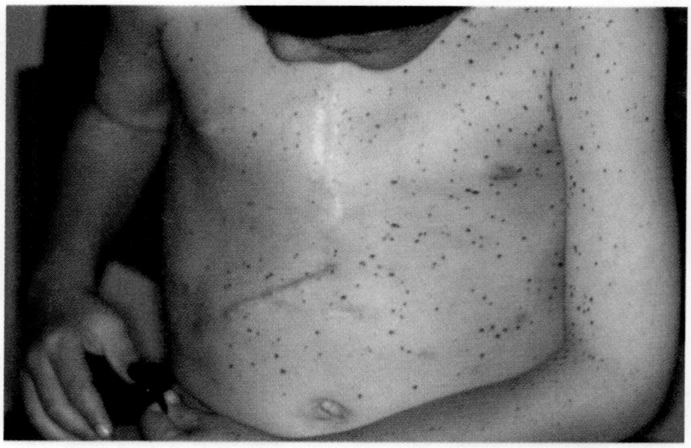

Figure 644-1 Multiple lentigines in LEOPARD (*l*entigines in association with *e*lectrocardiogram *a*bnormalities, *o*cular hypertelorism, *p*ulmonary stenosis, *a*bnormal genitals [cryptorchidism, hypogonadism, hypospadias], growth *r*etardation, and sensorineural *d*eafness) syndrome.

Lentiginosis profusa involves innumerable small, pigmented macules that are present at birth or appear during childhood. There are no associated abnormalities, and mucous membranes are spared. **LAMB syndrome** (Carney complex), a multiple endocrine neoplasia syndrome, consists of *l*entigines of the face and vulva, *a*trial myxoma, *m*ucocutaneous myxomas, and *b*lue nevi (type 1, *PRKAR1* gene; type 2, gene map locus 2p16-gene as yet to be identified). The Carney complex variant is associated with distal arthrogryposis (*MYH8* gene). The multiple lentigines **(LEOPARD) syndrome** is an autosomal dominant entity consisting of a generalized, symmetric distribution of *l*entigines (Fig. 644-1) in association with *e*lectrocardiogram *a*bnormalities, *o*cular hypertelorism, *p*ulmonary stenosis, *a*bnormal genitals (cryptorchidism, hypogonadism, hypospadias), growth *r*etardation, and sensorineural *d*eafness (type 1, *PTPN11* gene; type 2, *RAF1* gene). Other features include hypertrophic obstructive cardiomyopathy and pectus excavatum or carinatum.

The **Peutz-Jeghers syndrome** is characterized by melanotic macules on the lips and mucous membranes and by gastrointestinal (GI) polyposis. It is inherited as an autosomal dominant trait (*STK11* gene). Onset is noted in infancy and early childhood when pigmented macules appear on the lips and buccal mucosa. The macules are usually a few millimeters in size but may be as large as 1-2 cm. Macules also appear occasionally on the palate, gums, tongue, and vaginal mucosa. Cutaneous lesions may develop on the nose, hands, and feet; around the mouth, eyes, and umbilicus; and as longitudinal bands or diffuse hyperpigmentation of the nails. Pigmented macules often fade from the lips and skin during puberty and adulthood but generally do not disappear from mucosal surfaces. Buccal mucosal macules are the most constant feature of the disorder; in some families, occasional members may be affected only with the pigmentary changes. Indistinguishable pigmentary changes beginning in adult life, without intestinal involvement, also occur sporadically in individuals.

Polyposis usually involves the jejunum and ileum but may also occur in the stomach, duodenum, colon, and rectum (Chapter 337). Episodic abdominal pain, diarrhea, melena, and intussusception are frequent complications. Patients have a significantly increased risk of GI tract and non–GI tract tumors at a young age. GI cancer has been reported in ≈ 2-3% of patients; the lifetime relative risk for GI malignancy is 13. The relative risk

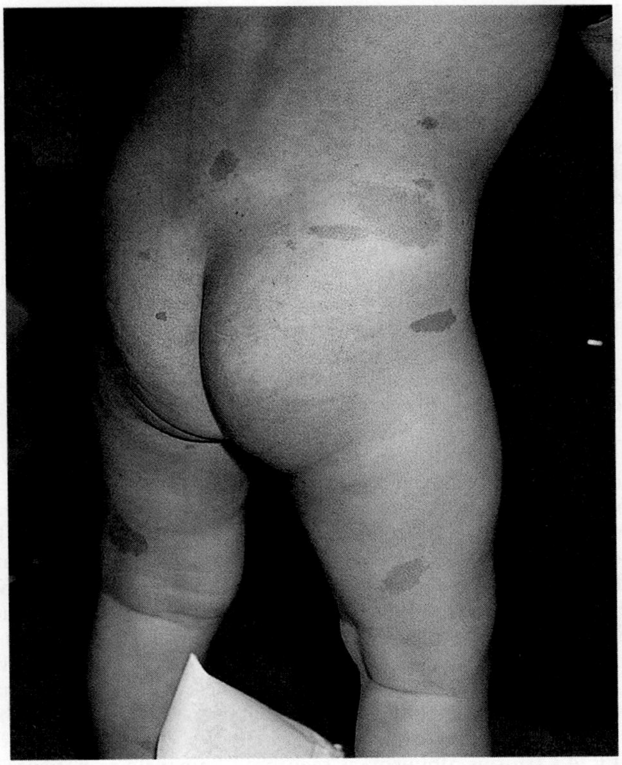

Figure 644-2 Multiple café au lait macules on a child with neurofibromatosis type 1. (From Eichenfield LF, Frieden IJ, Esterly NB: *Textbook of neonatal dermatology,* Philadelphia, 2001, WB Saunders, p 372.)

of non–GI tract malignancies, including ovarian, cervical, and testicular tumors, is 9. Peutz-Jeghers syndrome must be differentiated from other syndromes associated with multiple lentigines (Laugier-Hunziker syndrome), from ordinary freckling, from Gardner syndrome, and from Cronkhite-Canada syndrome, a disorder characterized by GI polyposis, alopecia, onychodystrophy, and diffuse pigmentation of the palms, volar aspects of the fingers, and dorsal hands. **Treatment** of Peutz-Jeghers melanotic macules with multiple different lasers has been successful, in some cases.

CAFÉ-AU-LAIT SPOTS

Café-au-lait spots are uniformly hyperpigmented, sharply demarcated macular lesions, the hues of which vary with the normal degree of pigmentation of the individual: They are tan or light brown in white individuals and may be dark brown in black children (Figs. 644-2 and 644-3). Café-au-lait spots vary tremendously in size and may be large, covering a significant portion of the trunk or limb. Generally the borders are smooth, but some have exceedingly irregular borders. The lesions are characterized by increased numbers of melanocytes and melanin in the epidermis but lack the clubbed rete ridges that typify lentigines. One to 3 café-au-lait spots are common in normal children; ≈ 10% of normal children have café-au-lait macules. The spots may be present at birth or may develop during childhood.

Large, often asymmetric café-au-lait spots with irregular borders are characteristic of patients with McCune-Albright syndrome (*GNAS1* gene) (Chapter 556.6). This disorder includes polyostotic fibrous dysplasia of bone, leading to pathologic fractures; precocious puberty; and numerous hyperfunctional endocrinopathies. The macular hyperpigmentation may be present at birth or may develop late in childhood (see Fig. 644-3). Cutaneous pigmentation is typically most extensive on the side showing the most severe bone involvement.

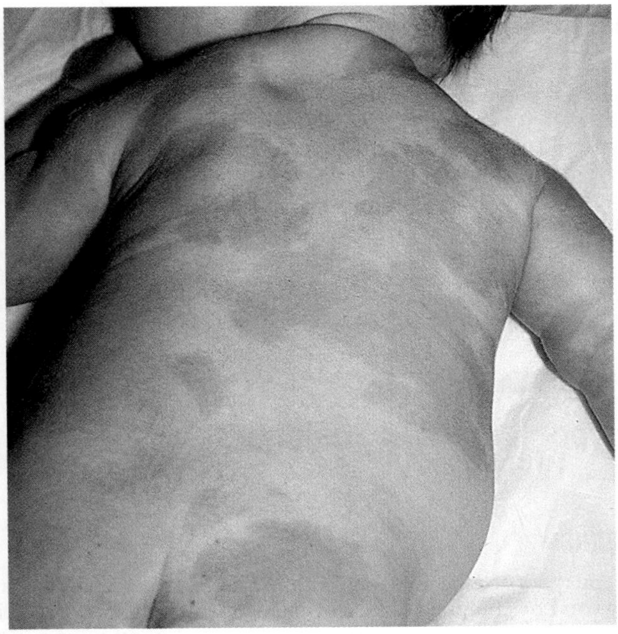

Figure 644-3 Multiple patterned café-au-lait spots in a child with McCune-Albright syndrome. (From Eichenfield LF, Frieden IJ, Esterly NB: *Textbook of neonatal dermatology,* Philadelphia, 2001, WB Saunders, p 373.)

Table 644-1 DISORDERS WITH CAFÉ-AU-LAIT SPOTS

Neurofibromatosis types 1 and 2
McCune-Albright syndrome
Russell-Silver syndrome
Ataxia-telangiectasia
Fanconi anemia
Tuberous sclerosis
Bloom syndrome
Basal cell nevus syndrome
Gaucher disease
Chédiak-Higashi syndrome
Hunter syndrome
Maffucci syndrome
Multiple mucosal neuroma syndrome
Watson syndrome
Proteus syndrome
Turner syndrome
Ring chromosome syndrome
Jaffe-Campanacci syndrome

Neurofibromatosis Type 1 (Von Recklinghausen Disease)

The café-au-lait spot is the most familiar cutaneous hallmark of the autosomal dominant neurocutaneous syndrome known as neurofibromatosis type 1 (neurofibromin gene) (see Fig. 644-2 and Chapter 589.1). The lesions also occur with certain other disorders, including other types of neurofibromatosis, but in these disorders the café-au-lait spots are not a major feature of the disorder and do not aid in diagnosis (Table 644-1). Included in the criteria for this diagnosis is the presence of 5 or more café-au-lait spots >5 mm in diameter in prepubertal patients or 6 or more café-au-lait spots >15 mm in diameter in postpubertal patients. Multiple café-au-lait macules commonly produce a freckled appearance of non–sun-exposed areas such as the axillae (Crowe sign), the inguinal and inframammary regions, and under the chin.

INCONTINENTIA PIGMENTI (BLOCH-SULZBERGER DISEASE)

See Chapter 589.7 for a full discussion of this condition.

POSTINFLAMMATORY PIGMENTARY CHANGES

Either hyperpigmentation or hypopigmentation can occur as a result of cutaneous inflammation. Alteration in pigmentation usually follows a severe inflammatory reaction but may result from mild dermatitis. Dark-skinned children are more likely to show these changes than fair-skinned ones. Although altered pigmentation may persist for weeks to months, patients can be reassured that these lesions are usually temporary.

BIBLIOGRAPHY

Please visit the Nelson Textbook of Pediatrics *website at www.expertconsult.com for the complete bibliography.*

Chapter 645
Hypopigmented Lesions

Joseph G. Morelli

ALBINISM

Several types of congenital oculocutaneous albinism (OCA) consist of partial or complete failure of melanin production in the skin, hair, and eyes despite the presence of normal number, structure, and distribution of melanocytes. They may be divided into two major classes: those with abnormal protein function involved in the formation and transfer of melanin, and those with defects in melanosomes (Table 645-1). Tyrosinase is the copper-containing enzyme that catalyzes at multiple steps in melanin biosynthesis (Chapter 79.2). Tyrosinase-positive variants are characterized by darkening of the hair bulb on incubation with tyrosine.

Table 645-1 GENES ASSOCIATED WITH HYPOPIGMENTATION

DISORDER	GENE DEFECT
Oculocutaneous albinism:	
OCA1	Tyrosinase
OCA2	P protein
OCA3	*TRP-1*
OCA4	*MATP*
Hermansky-Pudlak:	
Type 1	HPS-1 Mouse (pale ear)
Type 2	HPS-2 b3A subunit of AP3
Type 3	HPS-3 Mouse (cocoa)
Type 4	HPS-4 Mouse (light ear)
Type 5	HPS-5 KIAA107
Type 6	HPS-6 Mouse (ruby eye)
Type 7	HPS-7 DTNBP1
Type 8	HPS-8 Bloc153
Chédiak-Higashi	*CHS1/LYST*
Piebaldism	C-KIT receptor
	Heterozygous SLUG
Waardenburg:	
Type 1	Heterozygous PAX-3
Type 2a	*MITF*
Type 2b	Chromosome 1p
Type 2c	Chromosome 8p23
Type 2d	*SNAIL*
Type 2e	*Sox 10*
Type 3	Homozygous PAX-3
Type 4	*SOX 10*
	Endothelin 3
	Endothelin B receptor

Oculocutaneous albinism type 1 (OCA1) is characterized by great reduction in or absence of tyrosinase activity. OCA1A, the most severe form, is characterized by a lack of visible pigment in hair, skin, and eyes (Fig. 645-1). This manifests as photophobia, nystagmus, defective visual acuity, white hair, and white skin. The irises are blue-gray in oblique light and prominent pink in reflected light. OCA1B, or yellow mutant albinism, manifests at birth as white hair, pink skin, and gray eyes. This type is particularly prevalent in Amish communities. Progressively the hair becomes yellow-red, the skin tans lightly on exposure to the sun, and the irises may accumulate some brown pigment, with a resultant improvement in visual acuity. Photophobia and nystagmus are present but mild. OCATS is a temperature-sensitive type of albinism. The abnormal tyrosinase has decreased activity at 35-37°C. Therefore, cooler regions of the body such as the limbs and head pigment to some degree, whereas other areas remain depigmented.

OCA2 ranges from nearly normal to closely resembling type 1 albinism. This is the most common form of albinism seen worldwide. Little or no melanin is present at birth, but pigment, particularly red-yellow pigment, may accumulate during childhood to produce straw-colored or light brown skin in white individuals. Pigmented nevi may develop. Progressive improvement in visual acuity and nystagmus occurs with aging. Black individuals may have yellow-brown skin, dark-brown freckles in sun-exposed areas, and brown coloration of the irises. **Brown OCA** is an allelic variant of OCA2. Prader-Willi and Angelman syndromes, which include hypopigmentation, have deletions that include the gene involved in OCA2.

OCA3 (rufous albinism) is seen predominantly in patients of African descent. It is characterized by red hair, reddish brown skin, pigmented nevi, freckles, reddish brown to brown eyes, nystagmus, photophobia, and decreased visual acuity.

OCA4 is a rare OCA with clinical findings similar to those in OCA2.

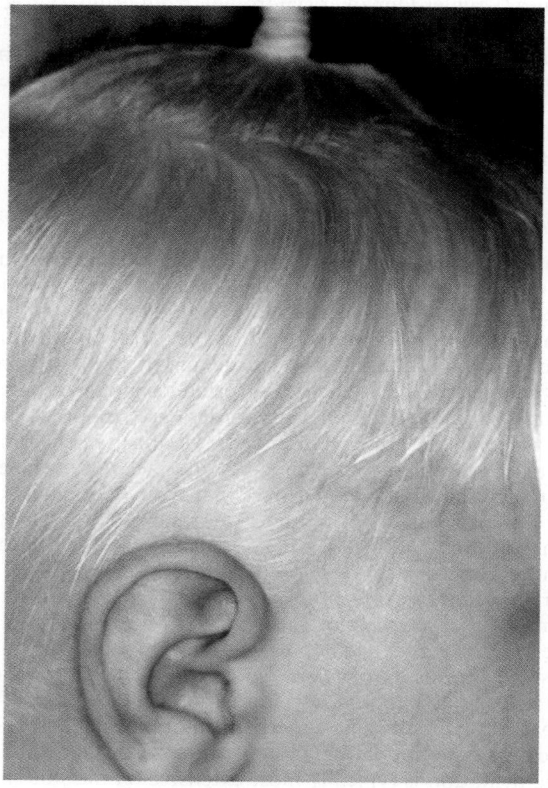

Figure 645-1 White hair and skin in oculocutaneous albinism type 1 (OCA1).

The **Cross-McKusick-Breen syndrome** consists of tyrosinase-positive albinism with ocular abnormalities, retardation, spasticity, and athetosis. The genetic defect is unidentified.

Because of the absence of normal protection by adequate amounts of epidermal melanin, persons with albinism are predisposed to development of actinic keratoses and cutaneous carcinoma secondary to skin damage by ultraviolet light. Protective clothing and a broad-spectrum sunscreen preparation (Chapter 648) should be worn during exposure to sunlight.

Oculocutaneous Albinism with Melanosomal Abnormalities (See Table 645-1)

Hermansky-Pudlak syndrome is a collection of autosomal recessive genetic disorders characterized by oculocutaneous albinism, ceroid accumulation in lysosomes, and prolonged bleeding time. In mice, 16 distinct genetic loci that produce coat color mutant phenotypes associated with platelet deficiencies are recognized; eight have been identified in humans.

Chédiak-Higashi syndrome (CHS; Chapter 124) is another genetic abnormality associated with dysfunction of lysosome-related organelles. Patients with CHS have hypopigmentation of the skin, eyes, and hair; prolonged bleeding times and easy bruising; recurrent infections; abnormal natural killer cell function; and peripheral neuropathy. CHS is caused by mutations in the *CHS1/LYST* gene, which is a lysosomal trafficking regulatory gene.

MELANOBLAST MIGRATION ABNORMALITIES (SEE TABLE 645-1)

Piebaldism

A congenital autosomal dominant disorder, piebaldism is characterized by sharply demarcated amelanotic patches that occur most frequently on the forehead, anterior scalp (producing a white forelock), ventral trunk, elbows, and knees. Islands of normal or darker than normal pigmentation may be present within the amelanotic areas (Fig. 645-2). The plaques are a result of a permanent localized absence of melanocytes. The pattern of depigmentation arises from defective melanoblast migration from the neural crest during development. The reason that piebaldism is a localized and not a generalized process remains unknown. Piebaldism must be differentiated from vitiligo, which may be progressive and is not usually congenital, nevus depigmentosus, and Waardenburg syndrome.

Waardenburg Syndrome

Waardenburg syndrome also manifests at birth as localized areas of depigmented skin and hair. There are four types of Waardenburg syndrome. The hallmark of Waardenburg type 1 is the white forelock, which is seen in 20-60% of patients. Only 15% of patients have areas of depigmented skin. Deafness occurs in 9-37%, heterochromia irides in 20%, and unibrow (synophrys) in 17-69% of those affected. Dystopia canthorum (i.e., telecanthus) is seen in all patients with Waardenburg type 1. Waardenburg type 2 is similar to type 1, except that patients with type 2 lack dystopia canthorum, but they also have a higher incidence of deafness. Waardenburg type 3 is similar to Waardenburg type 1, except that patients also have limb abnormalities. It is also called the Klein-Waardenburg syndrome. Waardenburg type 4 is also called the Shah-Waardenburg syndrome. Patients with this type all have Hirschsprung disease. Dystopia canthorum is seldom seen in these patients.

Tuberous Sclerosis Complex (*TSC1, TSC2* Genes)

See Chapter 589.2 for a discussion of this complex.

Hypomelanosis of Ito

Hypomelanosis of Ito is a congenital skin disorder affecting children of both sexes and frequently associated with defects in several organ systems. There is no evidence for genetic transmission; chromosomal mosaicism and chromosomal translocations have been reported. Hypomelanosis of Ito is currently a descriptive rather than definitive diagnosis. Blaschkoid hypomelanosis is a better descriptive term.

The skin lesions of hypomelanosis of Ito are generally present at birth but may be acquired in the first 2 years of life. The lesions are similar to a negative image of those present in incontinentia pigmenti, consisting of bizarre, patterned, hypopigmented macules arranged over the body surface in sharply demarcated whorls, streaks, and patches that follow the lines of Blaschko (Fig. 645-3). The palms, soles, and mucous membranes are spared. The hypopigmentation remains unchanged throughout childhood but fades during adulthood. The degree of depigmentation varies from hypopigmented to achromic. Neither inflammatory nor vesicular lesions precede the development of the pigmentary changes as in incontinentia pigmenti. The hypopigmented areas demonstrate fewer and smaller melanocytes and a decreased number of melanin granules in the basal cell layer than normal. Inflammatory cells and pigment incontinence are lacking.

The most commonly associated abnormalities involve the nervous system, including mental retardation (70%), seizures (40%), microcephaly (25%), and muscular hypotonia (15%). The musculoskeletal system is the second most frequently involved system, affected by scoliosis and thoracic and limb deformities. Minor ophthalmologic defects (strabismus, nystagmus) are present in 25% of patients, and 10% have cardiac defects. These frequencies are likely to be overestimated because patients with

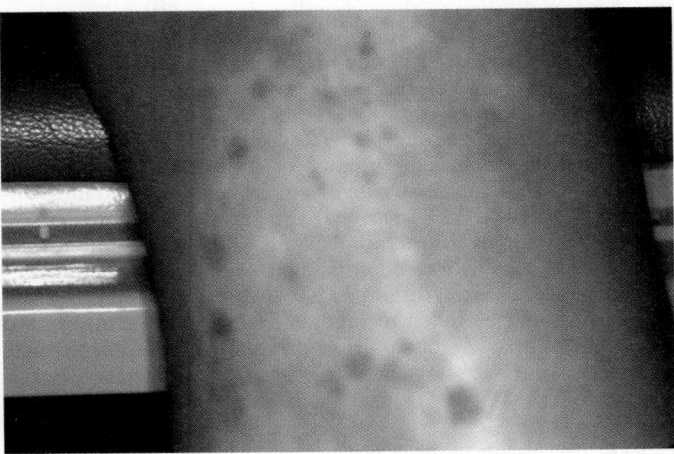

Figure 645-2 Depigmented macule with islands of hyperpigmentation in piebaldism.

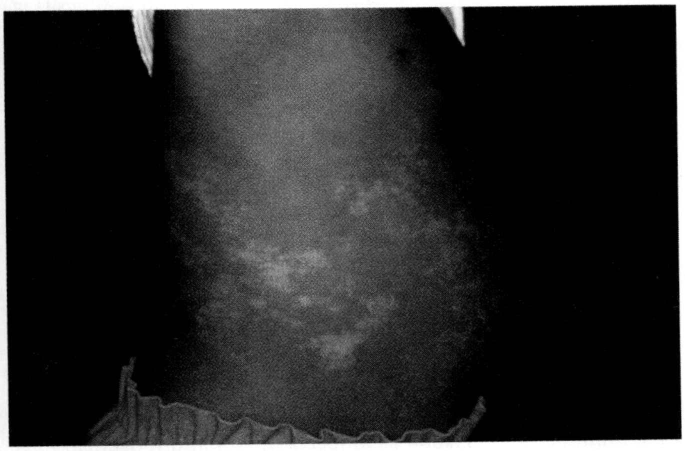

Figure 645-3 Marbled hypopigmented streaks on the abdomen in hypomelanosis of Ito.

isolated skin disease often do not seek further evaluation. The differential diagnosis includes systematized nevus depigmentosus, which is a stable leukoderma not associated with systemic manifestations. Differentiation from incontinentia pigmenti, particularly the hypopigmented fourth stage, is critical for genetic counseling because incontinentia pigmenti, unlike hypomelanosis of Ito, is inherited.

Vitiligo

EPIDEMIOLOGY AND ETIOLOGY Vitiligo is macular depigmentation associated with the destruction of melanocytes. The disorder represents a clinical end-point resulting from a complex interaction of environmental, genetic, and immunologic factors. Autoimmune, genetic, autocytotoxic, and neural theories have been postulated. The prevalence is 0.5% of most populations.

There is definitely an autoimmune component to vitiligo. Eighty percent of patients with active disease have an antibody to a surface antigen on pigmented melanoma cells. These antibodies appear to be cytotoxic for melanocytes. There is also a correlation between disease activity and the titer of serum antimelanocyte antibody. Melanocyte-specific CD8+ T lymphocytes are also involved in the pathogenesis of vitiligo. These antibodies and T cells recognize a variety of melanocyte enzymatic and structural proteins.

The genetic epidemiology of vitiligo is part of a broader genetically determined autoimmune and autoinflammatory diathesis. Fifteen percent to 20% of patients with generalized vitiligo have one or more affected first-degree relatives. In these families the genetic pattern is suggestive of polygenic, multifactorial inheritance. In the other patients, the disease occurs sporadically.

Many authorities believe that the cause of melanocyte destruction in vitiligo is an endogenous cellular abnormality. It has been suggested that melanocytes are destroyed because of the accumulation of a toxic melanin synthesis intermediate and/or lack of protection from hydrogen peroxide and other oxygen radicals. There is in vitro evidence that some of these metabolites may be lethal to melanocytes. Others believe that neurochemical factors damage melanocytes and cause depigmentation. This possibility would explain the pattern of involvement in segmental vitiligo that runs roughly along the course of a dermatome.

CLINICAL MANIFESTATIONS There are two subtypes of vitiligo, generalized (nonsegmental) and segmental, which probably are distinctly different diseases (Table 645-2). Generalized vitiligo (85-90% of cases) may be divided into widespread (type A) and localized (type B). About 50% of all patients with vitiligo have onset before 18 yr of age, and 25% demonstrate depigmentation before age 8. Most children have the generalized form, but the segmental type is more common among children than among adults. Patients with the generalized form usually present with a remarkably symmetric pattern of white macules and patches (Fig. 645-4); the margins may be somewhat hyperpigmented. The patches tend to be acral and/or periorificial. Occasionally, almost the entire skin surface becomes depigmented.

There are several varieties of localized vitiligo. A form of localized vitiligo is the halo nevus phenomenon, whereby benign moles develop depigmented rings at the periphery. Premature graying of scalp hair (canities) has also been considered a form of localized vitiligo. In segmental vitiligo, depigmented areas are limited to a quasidermatomal distribution. This type of vitiligo has a rapid onset and progression in a localized area without the development of depigmentation in other areas.

A number of **autoimmune diseases** occur in patients with vitiligo, including Addison disease, Hashimoto thyroiditis, pernicious anemia, diabetes mellitus, hypoparathyroidism, and polyglandular autoimmune syndrome with selective immunoglobulin (Ig) A deficiency. In addition, other diseases with possible immune defects, such as alopecia areata and morphea, have been seen in patients with vitiligo.

Table 645-2 TYPICAL FEATURES OF SEGMENTAL AND NONSEGMENTAL VITILIGO

SEGMENTAL VITILIGO	NONSEGMENTAL VITILIGO
Often begins in childhood	Can begin in childhood, but later onset is more common
Has rapid onset and stabilizes	Is progressive, with flare-ups
Involves hair compartment soon after onset	Involves hair compartment in later stages
Is usually not accompanied by other autoimmune diseases	Is often associated with personal or family history of auto-immunity
Often occurs in the face	Commonly occurs at sites sensitive to pressure and friction and prone to trauma
Is usually responsive to autologous grafting, with stable repigmentation	Frequently relapses in situ after autologous grafting
Can be difficult to distinguish from nevus depigmentosus, especially in cases with early onset	

From Taïeb A, Picardo M: Vitiligo, *N Engl J Med* 360:160–168, 2009.

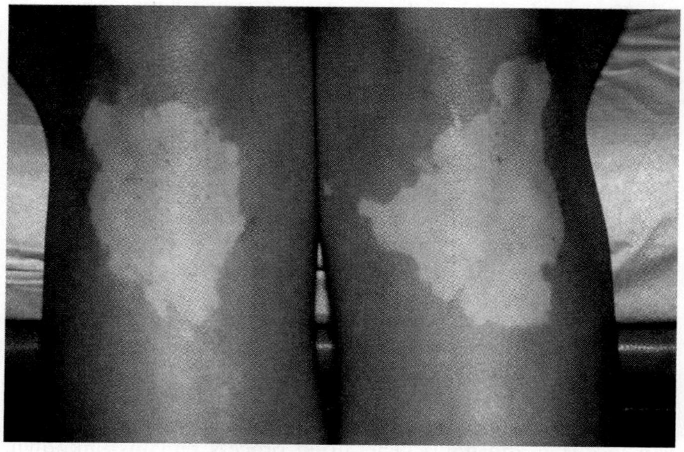

Figure 645-4 Sharply demarcated, symmetric, depigmented areas of vitiligo.

Vogt-Koyanagi-Harada syndrome is vitiligo associated with uveitis, dysacusia, meningoencephalitis, and depigmentation of the skin, scalp hair, eyebrows, and eyelashes. In the **Alezzandrini syndrome**, vitiligo is associated with tapetoretinal degeneration and deafness.

Light microscopic examination of early lesions shows mild inflammatory change. Over time, degenerative changes occur in melanocytes, leading to their complete disappearance.

The differential diagnosis of vitiligo includes other causes of widespread acquired leukoderma. The two most common problem diagnoses are tinea versicolor and postinflammatory hypopigmentation.

TREATMENT Localized areas of vitiligo may respond to potent topical steroid, topical tacrolimus, or topical pimecrolimus. In patients with more extensive involvement, narrow-band ultraviolet light B (UVB) [UVB311] is the treatment of choice. In all forms of vitiligo, response to therapy is slow, taking many months to years. For those not interested in treatment, cover-up cosmetics may be used. All areas of vitiligo are susceptible to sun damage, and care should be taken to minimize sun exposure of affected areas. Spontaneous remission may be seen in a small percentage of cases.

BIBLIOGRAPHY

Please visit the Nelson Textbook of Pediatrics *website at www.expertconsult.com for the complete bibliography.*

Chapter 646 Vesiculobullous Disorders

Joseph G. Morelli

Many diseases are characterized by vesiculobullous lesions; they vary considerably in cause, age of onset, and pattern. The morphology of the blister often provides a visual clue to the location of the lesion within the skin. Blisters localized to the **epidermal layers** are thin-walled, relatively flaccid, and easily ruptured. **Subepidermal blisters** are tense, thick-walled, and more durable. Biopsies of blisters can be diagnostic because the level of cleavage within the skin and associated findings, such as the nature of the inflammatory infiltrate, are characteristic for a particular disorder. Other diagnostic procedures, such as immunofluorescence and electron microscopy, can often help distinguish vesiculobullous disorders that have nearly identical histopathologic findings (Table 646-1).

646.1 Erythema Multiforme

Joseph G. Morelli

ETIOLOGY

Among the numerous factors implicated in the etiology of erythema multiforme (EM), infection with herpes simplex virus (HSV) is the most common. HSV labialis and, less commonly, HSV genitalis have been implicated in 60% of episodes of EM and are believed to trigger nearly all episodes of recurrent EM, frequently in association with sun exposure. HSV antigens and DNA are present in skin lesions of EM but are absent in nonlesional skin. Presence of the human leukocyte antigens A33, B62, B35, DQB1*0301, and DR53 is associated with an increased risk of HSV-induced EM, particularly the recurrent form. Most patients experience a single self-limited episode of EM. Lesions of HSV-induced recurrent EM (HA-EM) typically develop 10-14 days after onset of recurrent HSV eruptions, have a similar appearance from episode to episode, but may vary in frequency and duration in a given patient. Not all episodes of recurrent HSV evolve into EM in susceptible patients.

CLINICAL MANIFESTATIONS

EM has numerous morphologic manifestations on the skin, varying from erythematous macules, papules, vesicles, bullae, or urticaria-appearing plaques to patches of confluent erythema. The eruption appears most commonly in patients between the ages of 10 and 40 yr and usually is asymptomatic, although a burning sensation or pruritus may be present. The diagnosis of EM is established by finding the classic lesion: doughnut-shaped, target-like (iris or bull's-eye) papules with an erythematous outer border, an inner pale ring, and a dusky purple to necrotic center (Figs. 646-1 and 646-2).

EM is characterized by an abrupt, symmetric cutaneous eruption, most commonly on the extensor upper extremities; lesions are relatively sparse on the face, trunk, and legs. The eruption often appears initially as red macules or urticarial plaques that expand centrifugally to form lesions up to 2 cm in diameter with a dusky to necrotic center. Lesions of a particular episode typically appear within 72 hr and remain fixed in place. Oral lesions may occur with a predilection for the vermilion border of the lips and the buccal mucosa, but other mucosal surfaces are spared. Prodromal symptoms are generally absent. Lesions typically resolve without sequelae in about 2 wk; progression to Stevens-Johnson syndrome does not occur. EM may manifest initially as urticarial lesions, but unlike urticaria, a given lesion of EM does not fade within 24 hr.

Table 646-1 SITES OF BLISTER FORMATION AND DIAGNOSTIC STUDIES FOR THE VESICULOBULLOUS DISORDERS

DISORDER	BLISTER CLEAVAGE SITE	DIAGNOSTIC STUDIES
Acrodermatitis enteropathica	IE	Zn level
Bullous impetigo	GL	Smear, culture
Bullous pemphigoid	SE (junctional)	Direct and indirect immunofluorescence studies
Candidosis	SC	KOH preparation, culture
Dermatitis herpetiformis	SE	Direct immunofluorescence studies
Dermatophytosis	IE	KOH preparation, culture
Dyshidrotic eczema	IE	Routine histopathology
EB—simplex	IE	Electron microscopy; immunofluorescence mapping
EB of the hands and feet	IE	Electron microscopy; immunofluorescence mapping
Junctional EB (letalis)	SE (junctional)	Electron microscopy; immunofluorescence mapping
Recessive dystrophic EB	SE	Electron microscopy; immunofluorescence mapping
Dominant dystrophic EB	SE	Electron microscopy; immunofluorescence mapping
Epidermolytic hyperkeratosis	IE	Routine histopathology
Erythema multiforme	SE	Routine histopathology
Erythema toxicum	SC, IE	Smear for eosinophils
Incontinentia pigmenti	IE	Smear for eosinophils Routine histopathology
Insect bites	IE	Routine histopathology
Linear IgA dermatosis	SE	Direct immunofluorescence studies
Mastocytosis	SE	Routine histopathology
Miliaria crystallina	IC	Routine histopathology
Neonatal pustular melanosis	SC, IE	Smear for cells
Pemphigus foliaceus	GL	Direct and indirect immunofluorescence studies Tzanck smear
Pemphigus vulgaris	Suprabasal	Direct and indirect immunofluorescence studies Tzanck smear
Scabies	IE	Scraping
Staphylococcal scalded skin syndrome	GL	Routine histopathology
Toxic epidermal necrolysis	SE	Routine histopathology
Viral blisters	IE	Tzanck smear for herpesvirus infections Direct immunofluorescence for herpes simplex virus and varicella-zoster virus Culture Routine histopathology

EB, epidermolysis bullosa; GL, granular layer; IC, intracorneal; IE, intraepidermal; KOH, potassium hydroxide; SC, subcorneal; SE, subepidermal.

Pathogenesis

The pathogenesis of EM is unclear, but it may be a host-specific, cell-mediated immune response to an antigenic stimulus, resulting in damage to keratinocytes. HSV *Pol1* gene expressed in HA-EM lesions upregulates/activates the transcription factor SP1 and inflammatory cytokines. These cytokines, released by activated mononuclear cells and keratinocytes, may contribute to epidermal cell death and constitutional symptoms.

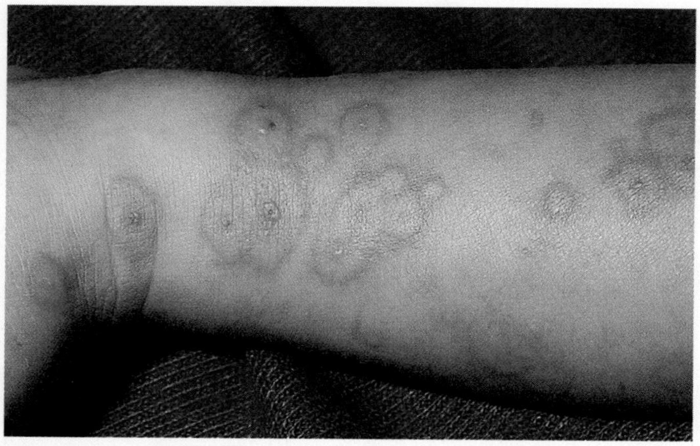

Figure 646-1 Early fixed papules with a central dusky zone on the dorsum of the hand of a child with erythema multiforme due to herpes simplex virus. (From Weston WL, Lane AT, Morelli J: *Color textbook of pediatric dermatology,* ed 3, St Louis, 2002, Mosby, p 156.)

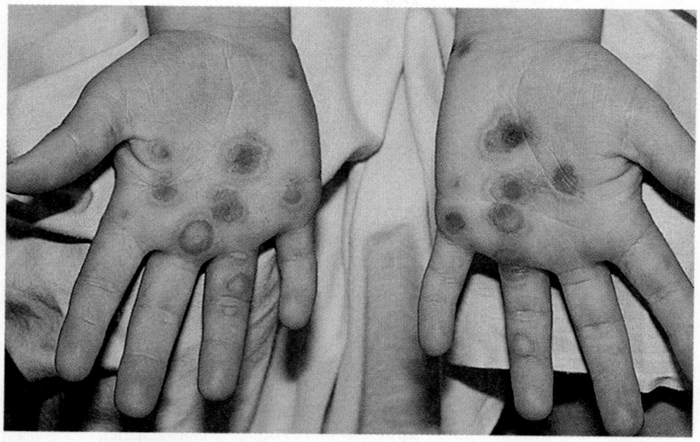

Figure 646-2 "Target" or "iris" lesions with characteristic central dusky zone on palms of a child with erythema multiforme due to herpes simplex virus. (From Weston WL, Lane AT, Morelli J: *Color textbook of pediatric dermatology,* ed 3, St Louis, 2002, Mosby, p 156.)

Pathology

Microscopic findings in EM are variable but may aid in diagnosis. Early lesions typically show slight intercellular edema, rare dyskeratotic keratinocytes, and basal vacuolation in the epidermis and a perivascular lymphohistiocytic infiltrate with edema in the upper dermis. More mature lesions show an accentuation of these characteristics and the development of lymphocytic exocytosis and an intense, perivascular, and interstitial mononuclear infiltrate in the upper third of the dermis. In severe cases, the entire epidermis becomes necrotic.

Differential Diagnosis

The **differential diagnosis** of EM also includes bullous pemphigoid, pemphigus, linear immunoglobulin (Ig) A dermatosis, graft versus host disease, bullous drug eruption, urticaria, viral infections such as HSV, reactive arthritis syndromes, Kawasaki disease, Behçet disease, allergic vasculitis, erythema annulare centrifugum, and periarteritis nodosa. EM that primarily involves the oral mucosa may be confused with bullous pemphigoid, pemphigus vulgaris, vesiculobullous or erosive lichen planus, Behçet syndrome, recurrent aphthous stomatitis, and primary herpetic gingivostomatitis. Serum sickness-like reaction (SSLR) to cefaclor may also manifest as EM-like lesions; the lesions may develop a dusky to purple center, but in most cases, the eruption of cefaclor-induced SSLR is pruritic, transient, and migratory and is probably urticarial rather than true EM.

Treatment

Treatment of EM is supportive. Topical emollients, systemic antihistamines, and nonsteroidal anti-inflammatory agents do not alter the course of the disease but may provide symptomatic relief. No controlled, prospective studies support the use of corticosteroids in the management of EM. Rather, glucocorticoid therapy may be permissive of HSV replication and make EM episodes more frequent or continuous. Prophylactic oral acyclovir given for 6 mo may be effective in controlling recurrent episodes of HSV-associated EM. On discontinuation of acyclovir, both HSV and EM may recur, although episodes may be less frequent and milder.

BIBLIOGRAPHY

Please visit the Nelson Textbook of Pediatrics *website at www.expertconsult.com for the complete bibliography.*

646.2 Stevens-Johnson Syndrome

Joseph G. Morelli

ETIOLOGY

Mycoplasma pneumoniae is the most convincingly demonstrated infectious cause of Stevens-Johnson syndrome. Drugs, particularly sulfonamides, nonsteroidal anti-inflammatory agents, antibiotics, and anticonvulsants, are the most common precipitants of Stevens-Johnson syndrome and toxic epidermal necrolysis. HLA-B*1502 and HLA-B*5801 have been implicated in the development of these two disorders in Han Chinese patients receiving carbamazepine and in Japanese patients receiving allopurinol, respectively.

Clinical Manifestations

Cutaneous lesions in Stevens-Johnson syndrome generally consist initially of erythematous macules that rapidly and variably develop central necrosis to form vesicles, bullae, and areas of denudation on the face, trunk, and extremities. The skin lesions are typically more widespread than in EM and are accompanied by involvement of **two or more mucosal surfaces,** namely the eyes, oral cavity, upper airway or esophagus, gastrointestinal tract, or anogenital mucosa (Fig. 646-3). A burning sensation, edema, and erythema of the lips and buccal mucosa are often the presenting signs, followed by development of bullae, ulceration, and hemorrhagic crusting. Lesions may be preceded by a flu-like upper respiratory illness. Pain from mucosal ulceration is often severe, but skin tenderness is minimal to absent in Stevens-Johnson syndrome, in contrast to pain in toxic epidermal necrolysis. Corneal ulceration, anterior uveitis, panophthalmitis, bronchitis, pneumonitis, myocarditis, hepatitis, enterocolitis, polyarthritis, hematuria, and acute tubular necrosis leading to renal failure may occur. Disseminated cutaneous bullae and erosions may result in increased insensible fluid loss and a high risk of bacterial superinfection and sepsis. New lesions occur in crops, and complete healing may take 4-6 wk; ocular scarring, visual impairment, and strictures of the esophagus, bronchi, vagina, urethra, or anus may remain. Nonspecific laboratory abnormalities in Stevens-Johnson syndrome include leukocytosis, elevated erythrocyte sedimentation rate, and, occasionally, increased liver transaminase levels and decreased serum albumin values. **Toxic epidermal necrolysis** is the most severe disorder in the clinical spectrum of the disease, involving considerable constitutional toxicity and extensive necrolysis of the mucous membranes and > 30% of the body surface area (Fig. 646-4).

Pathogenesis

Pathogenesis is related to drug-specific CD8+ cytotoxic T cells, with perforin/granzyme B and granulysin triggering keratinocyte apoptosis. This process is followed by expanded enactment of

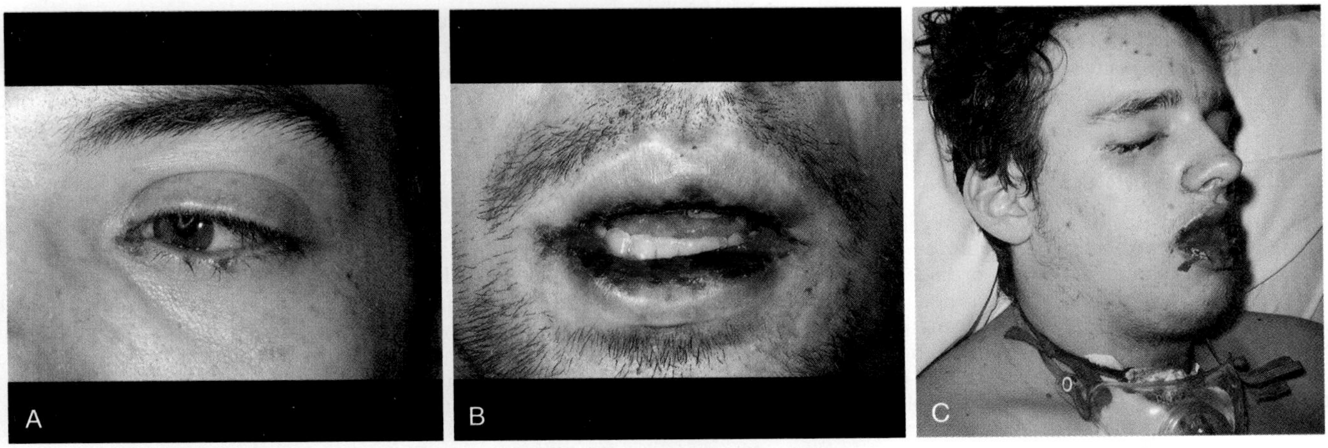

Figure 646-3 Bullae are present on the conjunctivae *(A)* and in the mouth *(B)* with Stevens-Johnson syndrome. Sloughing, ulceration, and necrosis in the oral cavity interfere with eating *(C)*. Genital lesions cause dysuria and interfere with voiding. (From Habif TP, editor: *Clinical dermatology,* ed 4, Philadelphia, 2004, Mosby, p 631.)

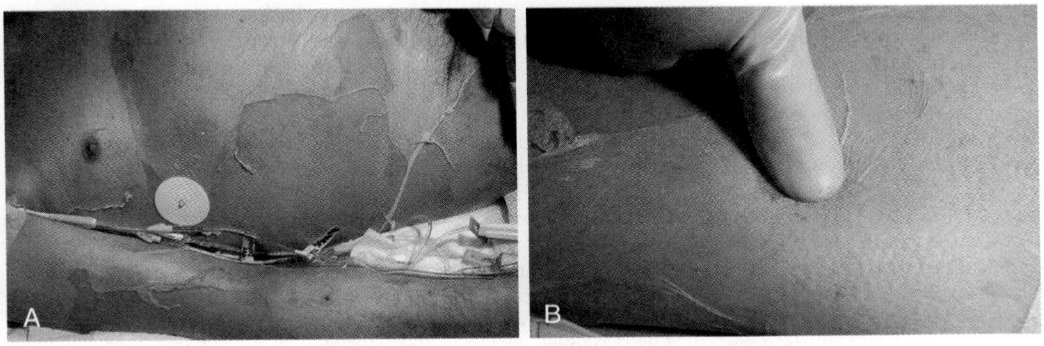

Figure 646-4 *A,* Large sheets of full-thickness epidermis are shed. *B,* Toxic epidermal necrolysis begins with diffuse, hot erythema. In hours the skin becomes painful, and with slight thumb pressure, the skin wrinkles, slides laterally, and separates from the dermis (Nikolsky sign). (From Habif TP, editor: *Clinical dermatology,* ed 4, Philadelphia, 2004, Mosby, p 633.)

apoptosis involving the interaction of soluble Fas ligand with Fas receptor.

Differential Diagnosis

The differential diagnosis of Stevens-Johnson syndrome includes toxic epidermal necrolysis, urticaria, DRESS (drug rash [or reaction] with eosinophilia and systemic symptoms) syndrome (Chapter 637.2) and other drug eruptions and viral exanthems, including Kawasaki disease.

Treatment

Management of Stevens-Johnson syndrome is supportive and symptomatic. Potentially offending drugs must be discontinued as soon as possible. Ophthalmologic consultation is mandatory because ocular sequelae such as corneal scarring can lead to vision loss. Application of cryopreserved amniotic membrane to the ocular surface during the acute phase of the disease limits the destructive and long-term sequelae. Oral lesions should be managed with mouthwashes and glycerin swabs. Vaginal lesions should be observed closely and treated to prevent vaginal stricture or fusion. Topical anesthetics (diphenhydramine, dyclonine, viscous lidocaine) may provide relief from pain, particularly when applied before eating. Denuded skin lesions can be cleansed with saline or Burrow solution compresses. Antibiotic therapy is appropriate for documented secondary bacterial infection. Treatment may require admission to an intensive care unit; intravenous (IV) fluids; nutritional support; sheepskin or air-fluid bedding; daily saline or Burow solution compresses; paraffin gauze or colloidal gel (Hydrogel) dressing of denuded areas; saline compresses on the eyelids, lips, or nose; analgesics; and urinary catheterization (when needed). A daily examination for infection and ocular lesions, which constitute the major cause of long-term morbidity, is essential. Systemic antibiotics are indicated for documented urinary or cutaneous infections and for suspected bacteremia (due to *S. aureus* or *P. aeruginosa*) because infection is the leading cause of death. Prophylactic systemic antibiotics are not necessary. Although corticosteroids are sometimes advocated in early, severe cases of Stevens-Johnson syndrome, no prospective double-blind studies evaluating their efficacy have been reported. Most authorities discourage their use because of reports of increased morbidity and mortality (sepsis) with their administration. IV immunoglobulin (IVIG) (1.5-2.0 g/kg/day × 3 days) should be considered in early disease.

Two severe cases of toxic epidermal necrolysis have been treated successfully with etanercept.

BIBLIOGRAPHY

Please visit the Nelson Textbook of Pediatrics *website at* *www.expertconsult.com* *for the complete bibliography.*

646.3 Toxic Epidermal Necrolysis

Joseph G. Morelli

EPIDEMIOLOGY AND ETIOLOGY

The pathogenesis of toxic epidermal necrolysis is not proved but may involve a hypersensitivity phenomenon that results in damage primarily to the basal cell layer of the epidermis. Epidermal damage appears to result from keratinocyte apoptosis (Chapter 646.2). This condition is triggered by many of the same factors that are thought to be responsible for Stevens-Johnson syndrome, principally drugs such as the sulfonamides, amoxicillin, phenobarbital, hydantoin, butazones, and allopurinol. Toxic epidermal necrolysis is defined by (1) widespread blister formation and morbilliform or confluent erythema, associated with skin tenderness; (2) absence of target lesions; (3) sudden onset and generalization within 24-48 hr; (4) histologic findings of full-thickness epidermal necrosis and a minimal to absent dermal infiltrate. These criteria categorize toxic epidermal necrolysis as a separate entity from EM.

CLINICAL MANIFESTATIONS

The prodrome consists of fever, malaise, localized skin tenderness, and diffuse erythema. Inflammation of the eyelids, conjunctivae, mouth, and genitals may precede skin lesions. Flaccid bullae may develop, although this is not a prominent feature. Characteristically, full-thickness epidermis is lost in large sheets (see Fig. 646-4). **Nikolsky sign** (denudation of the skin with gentle tangential pressure) is present but only in the areas of erythema (see Fig. 646-4). Healing takes place over 14 or more days. Scarring, particularly of the eyes, may result in corneal opacity. The course may be relentlessly progressive, complicated by severe dehydration, electrolyte imbalance, shock, and secondary localized infection and septicemia. Loss of nails and hair may also occur. Long-term morbidity includes alterations in skin pigmentation, eye problems (lack of tears, conjunctival scarring, loss of lashes), and strictures of mucosal surfaces. The **differential diagnosis** includes staphylococcal scalded skin syndrome, in which the blister cleavage plane is intraepidermal; graft versus host disease; chemical burns; drug eruptions; toxic shock syndrome; and pemphigus.

Anticonvulsant hypersensitivity syndrome (DRESS syndrome; Chapter 637.2) is a multisystem reaction that appears approximately 4 wk to 3 mo after the start of therapy with phenytoin, carbamazepine, phenobarbitone, primidone, or other drugs, most commonly antibiotics. The mucocutaneous eruption may be identical to that of EM, Stevens-Johnson syndrome, or toxic epidermal necrolysis, but the reaction also typically includes lymphadenopathy as well as fever, hepatic, renal and pulmonary disease, eosinophilia, atypical lymphocytosis, and leukocytosis.

TREATMENT

Appreciation of the specific etiologic factor is crucial. When the disorder is drug induced, administration of the drug must be discontinued as soon as possible. Management is similar to that for severe burns and may be best accomplished in a burn unit (Chapter 68). It may include strict reverse isolation, meticulous fluid and electrolyte therapy, use of an air-fluid bed, and daily cultures. Systemic antibiotic therapy is indicated when secondary infection is evident or suspected. Skin care consists of cleansing with isotonic saline or Burow solution. Biologic or colloid gel (Hydrogel) dressings alleviate pain and reduce fluid loss. Narcotics are often required for pain relief. Mouth and eye care, as for EM major, may be necessary. Because of an immune mechanism, systemic glucocorticosteroids and IVIG have been used with apparent success. Nonetheless, this treatment remains controversial.

BIBLIOGRAPHY

Please visit the Nelson Textbook of Pediatrics *website at www.expertconsult.com for the complete bibliography.*

646.4 Mechanobullous Disorders

Joseph G. Morelli

EPIDERMOLYSIS BULLOSA

Diseases categorized under the general term epidermolysis bullosa (EB) are a heterogeneous group of congenital, hereditary blistering disorders. They differ in severity and prognosis, clinical and histologic features, and inheritance patterns, but are all characterized by induction of blisters by trauma and exacerbation of blistering in warm weather. The disorders can be categorized under 3 major headings with multiple subgroupings: epidermolysis bullosa simplex (EBS), junctional epidermolysis bullosa (JEB), and dystrophic epidermolysis bullosa (DEB) (Table 646-2). **Kindler syndrome** (Kindlin-1 gene), which includes poikiloderma and photosensitivity as well as easy blistering, is also considered a separate form of EB.

Epidermolysis Bullosa Simplex

EBS is a nonscarring, autosomal dominant disorder. The defect in most common types of EBS is in keratin 5 or 14, which makes up intermediate filaments of the basal keratinocytes. The intraepidermal bullae result from cytolysis of the basal cells. There are multiple other rare variants with defects that also result in intraepidermal blistering.

In **EBS—generalized other (formerly Koebner)**, blisters are usually present at birth or during the neonatal period. Sites of predilection are the hands, feet, elbows, knees, legs, and scalp. Intraoral lesions are minimal, nails rarely become dystrophic and usually regrow even when they are shed, and dentition is normal. Bullae heal with minimal to no scar or milia formation. Secondary infection is the primary complication. The propensity to blister decreases with age, and the long-term prognosis is good. Blisters should be drained by puncturing, but the blister top should be left intact to protect the underlying skin. Erosions may be covered with a semipermeable dressing.

EBS—localized (formerly Weber-Cockayne) predominantly affects the hands and feet and often manifests when a child begins to walk; onset may be delayed until puberty or early adulthood, when heavy shoes are worn or the feet are subjected to increased trauma. Bullae are usually restricted to the hands and feet (Fig. 646-5); rarely, they occur elsewhere, such as the dorsal aspect of the arms and the shins. The disorder ranges from mildly incapacitating to crippling at times of severe exacerbations.

EBS—Dowling-Meara (herpetiformis) is characterized by grouped blisters resembling those of herpes simplex (Fig. 646-6). During infancy, blistering may be severe and extensive, may involve mucous membranes, and may result in shedding of nails, formation of milia, and mild pigmentary changes, without scarring. After the first few months of life, warm temperatures do not appear to exacerbate blistering. Hyperkeratosis and hyperhidrosis of the palms and soles may develop, but generally, the condition improves with age.

JUNCTIONAL EPIDERMOLYSIS BULLOSA

JEB—Herlitz is an autosomal recessive condition that is life threatening. Blisters appear at birth or develop during the neonatal period, particularly on the perioral area, scalp, legs, diaper area, and thorax. Nails eventually become dystrophic and then often permanently lost. Mucous membrane involvement may be severe, and ulceration of the respiratory, gastrointestinal, and genitourinary epithelium has been documented in many affected children, although less frequently than in severe recessive dystrophic epidermolysis bullosa (RDEB). Healing is delayed, and vegetating granulomas may persist for a long time. Large, moist, erosive plaques (Fig. 646-7) may provide a portal of entry for bacteria, and septicemia is a frequent cause of death. Mild atrophy may be seen in areas of recurrent blistering. Defective dentition with early loss of teeth as a result of rampant caries is characteristic. Growth retardation and recalcitrant anemia are almost invariable. In addition to infection, cachexia and circulatory failure are common causes of death. Most patients die within the first 3 yr of life.

JEB—non-Herlitz is a heterogeneous group of disorders. Blistering may be severe in the neonatal period, making

Table 646-2 CLINICAL PRESENTATION AND DIAGNOSIS OF SELECTED EPIDERMOLYSIS BULLOSA SUBTYPES IN THE NEONATAL PERIOD

EB SUBTYPE (USUAL INHERITANCE)	CLINICAL FEATURES Cutaneous	Extracutaneous	DIAGNOSIS
EB simplex—generalized (AD)	Mild to moderate blistering, often generalized	Occasional mucosal blistering	EM: Intrabasal layer split; IF: BPAG1 (BP230), BP-180 (BPAG2, collagen XVII), α6β4 integrin, laminin 1, laminin 332, type IV collagen, type VII collagen (EBA antigen) at base of blister
	Rare scarring, milia		
EB simplex—localized (AD)	Mild blistering, often localized, sometimes in first 24 mo, but often not until later infancy or childhood	Rare mucosal involvement	EM: Intrastratum basale split IF: Same as for EB simplex—generalized
	Rare scarring, milia		
EB simplex—Dowling-Meara (AD)	Moderate to severe blistering, which starts generalized, then is grouped (herpetiform); milia; nail dystrophy, shedding	Mild mucosal blistering	EM: Intrastratum basale split; clumped keratin filaments IF: Same as for EB simplex—generalized
Junctional EB—non-Herlitz (AR)	Moderate blistering; atrophic scars; nail dystrophy	Mild mucosal blistering; enamel hypoplasia	EM: Intralamina lucida cleavage; variable reduction in hemidesmosomes IF: Absence of staining with 19-DEJ-1 (uncein); variable staining with GB3 and other laminin 332 antibodies, including 46 and K140; BPAG1 (BP230) BP180 (BPAG2, collagen XVII), α6β4 integrin in blister roof; laminin 1, type IV collagen, type VII collagen (EBA antigen) at base of blister
Junctional EB—Herlitz (AR)	Severe generalized blistering that heals poorly; granulation tissue; scarring; nail dystrophy	Severe mucosal blistering; GI involvement common; laryngeal involvement with airway obstruction; urologic involvement	EM: Cleavage intralamina lucida; markedly reduced or no hemidesmosomes; absence of sub-basal dense plates IF: Absence of staining with 19-DEJ-1 (uncein) and GB3 (laminin 332) and of staining with other laminin 332 antibodies, including 46 and K140; BPAG1 (BP230) and BP180 (BPAG2, type XVII collagen) in blister roof; laminin-1, type IV collagen and type VII collagen at base of blister
Junctional EB—pyloric atresia (AR)	Severe blistering	Polyhydramnios; pyloric atresia; urologic involvement: uretovesicular obstruction, hydronephrosis	EM: Cleavage intralamina lucida and intraplasma membrane; small hemidesmosomes IF: BPAG1 (BP230) and BP180 (BPAG2, type XVII collagen) in blister roof;laminin-1, type IV collagen and type VII collagen at base of blister; Absence of 19-DEJ-1(uncein), α6β4 integrin absent or reduced
Dominant dystrophic EB (AD)	Mild to moderate blistering (but may be more severe in newborn period) Milia, scarring	Mild mucosal blistering	EM: Cleavage sublamina densa; variable reduction in anchoring fibrils IF: BPAG1 (BP230), BP-180 (BPAG2, collagen XVII), α6β4 integrin, laminin 1, type IV collagen at top of blister
			Staining for type VII collagen (EBA antigen) is normal, variable, or absent
	Nail dystrophy		
Recessive dystrophic EB—Hallopeau-Siemens (AR)	Severe blistering Milia, scarring	Severe mucosal blistering; GI involvement common; urologic involvement	EM: Cleavage sublamina densa; absence of anchoring fibrils IF: BPAG1 (BP230), BP-180 (BPAG2, collagen XVII), α6β4 integrin, laminin 1, type IV collagen at top of blister Variability or absence of staining for type VII collagen (EBA antigen)

AD, autosomal dominant; AR, autosomal recessive; EB, epidermolysis bullosa; EM, electron microscopy; GI, gastrointestinal; IF, immunohistochemical, and immunofluorescence antigen mapping findings.
Modified from Eichenfield LF, Frieden IJ, Esterly NB: *Textbook of neonatal dermatology*, Philadelphia, 2001, WB Saunders, p 159.

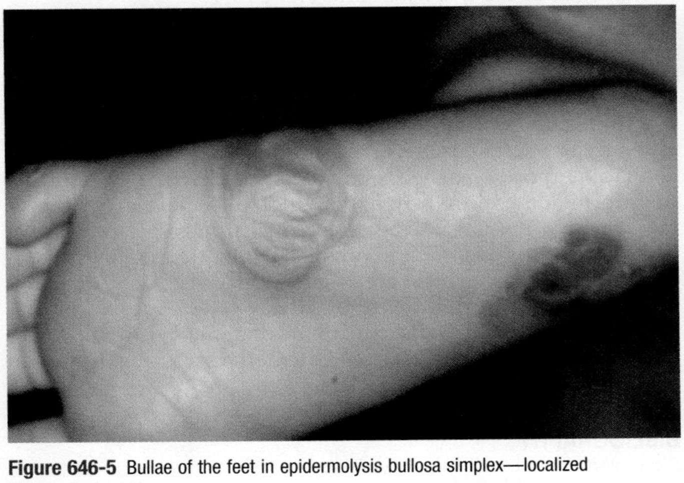

Figure 646-5 Bullae of the feet in epidermolysis bullosa simplex—localized (Weber-Cockayne).

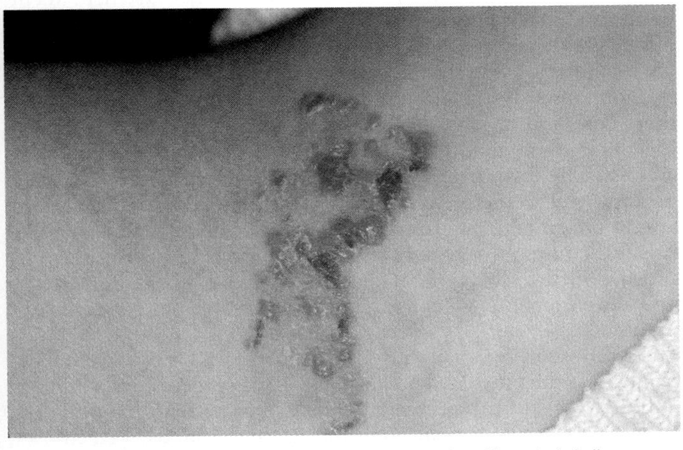

Figure 646-6 Grouped vesicle on an erythematous base in epidermolysis bullosa simplex—Dowling-Meara.

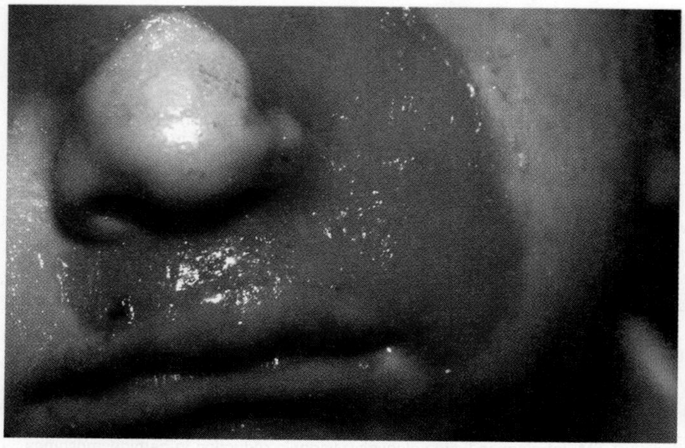

Figure 646-7 Nonhealing granulation tissue in junctional epidermolysis bullosa.

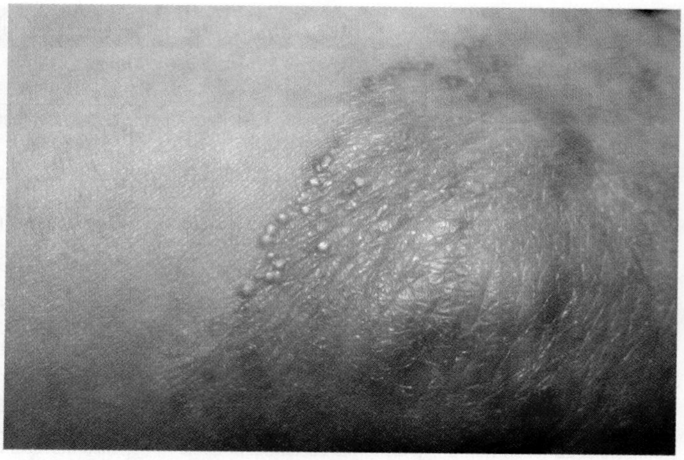

Figure 646-8 Scarring with milia formation over the knee in dominant dystrophic epidermolysis bullosa.

differentiation from the Herlitz type difficult. All conditions associated with the Herlitz type may be seen but are usually milder. **JEB—non-Herlitz generalized (formerly generalized atrophic benign epidermolysis bullosa)** is included as a variant of non-Herlitz JEB. Another variant of non-Herlitz JEB is associated with **pyloric atresia.**

In all types of JEB, a subepidermal blister is found on light microscopic examination, and electron microscopy demonstrates a cleavage plane in the lamina lucida, between the plasma membranes of the basal cells and the basal lamina. Absence or a great reduction of hemidesmosomes is seen on electron micrographs in **JEB—Herlitz** and some cases of **JEB—non-Herlitz.** The defect is in laminin 332 (formerly laminin 5), a glycoprotein associated with anchoring filaments beneath the hemidesmosomes. In JEB—non-Herlitz, defects have also been described in other hemidesmosomal components, such as Col17A1. In **JEB—pyloric atresia,** the defect is in the $\alpha6\beta4$ integrin.

Treatment for junctional epidermolysis bullosa is supportive. The diet should provide adequate calories and supplemental iron. Infections should be treated promptly. Transfusions of packed red blood cells may be required if the patient shows no response to iron and erythropoietin therapy. Tissue-engineered skin grafts (artificial skin derived from human keratinocytes and fibroblasts) may be beneficial.

DYSTROPHIC EPIDERMOLYSIS BULLOSA

All forms of DEB result from mutations in collagen VII, a major component of anchoring fibrils that tether the basement membrane and overlying epidermis to its dermal foundation. The blister is subepidermal in all types of DEB. The type and location of the mutation dictate the severity of the phenotype.

Dominant dystrophic epidermolysis bullosa (DDEB) is the most common type of DEB. The spectrum of DDEB is varied. Blisters may be manifest at birth and are often limited and characteristically form over acral bony prominences. The lesions heal promptly, with the formation of soft, wrinkled scars, milia, and alterations in pigmentation (Fig. 646-8). Abnormal nails and nail loss are common. In many cases, the blistering process is mild, causing little restriction of activity and not impairing growth and development. Mucous membrane involvement tends to be minimal.

RDEB—severe generalized (formerly RDEB—Hallopeau-Siemens) is the most incapacitating form of epidermolysis bullosa, although the clinical spectrum is wide. Some patients have blisters, scarring, and milia formation primarily on the hands, feet, elbows, and knees (Fig. 646-9). Others have extensive erosions and blister formation at birth that seriously impedes their care and feeding.

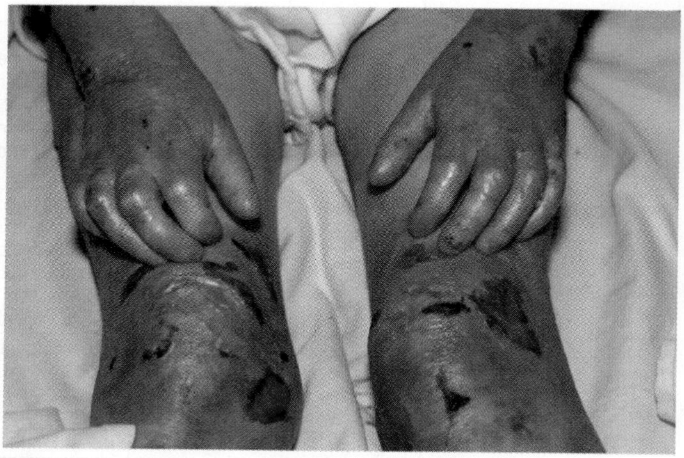

Figure 646-9 Severe scarring of the hands and knees in recessive dystrophic epidermolysis bullosa.

Mucous membrane lesions are common and may cause severe nutritional deprivation, even in older children, whose growth may be retarded. During childhood, esophageal erosions and strictures, scarring of the buccal mucosa, flexion contractures of joints secondary to scarring of the integument, development of cutaneous carcinomas, and the development of digital fusion may significantly limit the quality of life (Fig. 646-10).

Although the skin becomes less sensitive to trauma with aging in patients with RDEB, the progressive and permanent deformities complicate management, and the overall prognosis is poor. Foods that traumatize the buccal or esophageal mucosa should be avoided. If esophageal scarring develops, a semiliquid diet and esophageal dilatations may be required. Stricture excision or colonic interposition may be needed to relieve esophageal obstruction. In infants, severe oropharyngeal involvement may necessitate the use of special feeding devices such as a gastrostomy tube. Iron therapy for anemia, intermittent antibiotic therapy for secondary infections, which are a common cause of death, and periodic surgery for release of digits may reduce morbidity. Tissue-engineered skin grafts containing keratinocytes and fibroblasts are of some benefit. Allogeneic bone marrow transplantation may also be beneficial.

BIBLIOGRAPHY

Please visit the Nelson Textbook of Pediatrics *website at www.expertconsult.com for the complete bibliography.*

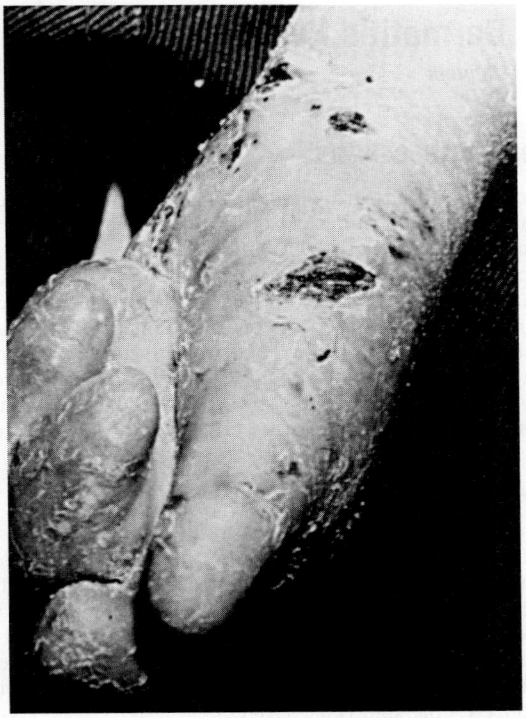

Figure 646-10 Mitten-hand deformity of recessive dystrophic epidermolysis bullosa.

646.5 Pemphigus

Joseph G. Morelli

PEMPHIGUS VULGARIS

Etiology/Pathogenesis

Pemphigus vulgaris (PV) is caused by circulating antibodies to desmoglein III that result in suprabasal cleaving with consequent blister formation. Desmoglein III is a 30-kd glycoprotein that is complexed with plakoglobin, a plaque protein of desmosomes. The desmogleins are a subfamily of the cadherin family of cell adhesion molecules.

Clinical Manifestations

PV usually first appears as painful oral ulcers, which may be the only evidence of the disease for weeks or months. Subsequently, large, flaccid bullae emerge on nonerythematous skin, most commonly on the face, trunk, pressure points, groin, and axillae. **Nikolsky sign** is present. The lesions rupture and enlarge peripherally, producing painful, raw, denuded areas that have little tendency to heal. When healing occurs, it is without scarring, but hyperpigmentation is common. Malodorous, verrucous, and granulomatous lesions may develop at sites of ruptured bullae, particularly in the skinfolds; as this pattern becomes more pronounced, the condition may be more properly referred to as *pemphigus vegetans*. Because the course may rapidly lead to debility, malnutrition, and death, prompt diagnosis is essential. **Neonatal PV** develops in utero as a result of placental transfer of maternal antidesmoglein antibodies from women who have active PV, although it may occur when the mother is in remission. High antepartum maternal titers of PV antibodies and increased maternal disease activity correlate with a poor fetal outcome, including demise.

Pathology

Biopsy of a fresh small blister reveals a suprabasal (intraepidermal) blister containing loose, acantholytic epidermal cells that have lost their intercellular bridges and thus their contact with one another. Immunofluorescence staining (IF) with an IgG antibody produces a characteristic pattern on direct immunofluorescence preparations of both involved and uninvolved skin of essentially all patients. Serum IgG antibody titers to desmoglein correlate with the clinical course in many patients; thus, serial determinations may have predictive value.

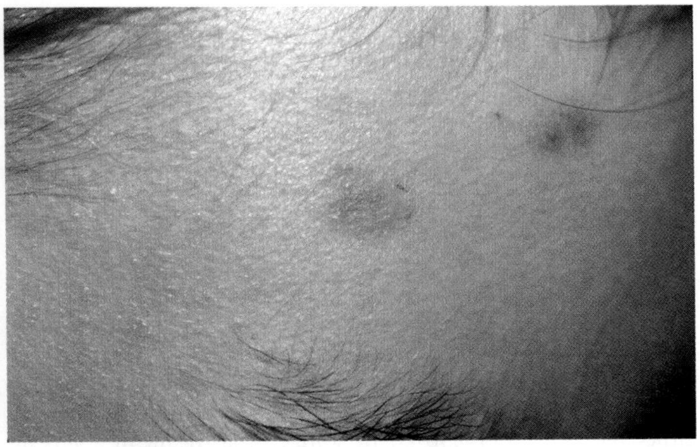

Figure 646-11 Superficial erosions in pemphigus foliaceus.

Differential Diagnosis

PV must be differentiated from EM, bullous pemphigoid, Stevens-Johnson syndrome, and toxic epidermal necrolysis.

Treatment

The disease is best treated initially with systemic methylprednisolone 1-2 mg/kg/day. Azathioprine, cyclophosphamide, and methotrexate therapy all have been useful in maintenance regimens. IVIG given in cycles may be beneficial to patients whose disease does not respond to steroids. Rituximab with IVIG replacement has been effective in the management of severe pemphigus. Excellent control of the disease may be obtained, but relapse is common.

PEMPHIGUS FOLIACEUS

Etiology/Pathogenesis

Pemphigus foliaceus is caused by circulating antibodies to a 50-kd portion of the 160-kd desmosomal glycoprotein desmoglein I, which result in subcorneal cleavage leading to superficial erosions. This extremely rare disorder is characterized by subcorneal blistering; the site of cleavage is high in the epidermis rather than suprabasal as in PV.

Clinical Manifestations

The superficial blisters rupture quickly, leaving erosions surrounded by erythema that heal with crusting and scaling (Fig. 646-11). **Nikolsky sign** is present. Focal lesions are usually localized to the scalp, face, neck, and upper trunk. Mucous membrane lesions are minimal or absent. Pruritus, pain, and a burning sensation are frequent complaints. The clinical course varies but is generally more benign than that of PV. **Fogo selvagem,** which is endemic in certain areas of Brazil, is identical clinically, histopathologically, and immunologically to pemphigus foliaceus.

Pathology

An intraepidermal acantholytic bulla high in the epidermis is diagnostic. It is imperative to select an early lesion for biopsy. Immunofluorescent staining with an IgG antibody reveals a characteristic intercellular staining pattern similar to that of PV but higher in the epidermis.

Differential Diagnosis

When generalized, the eruption may resemble exfoliative dermatitis or any of the chronic blistering disorders; localized erythematous plaques simulate seborrheic dermatitis, psoriasis, impetigo, eczema, and systemic lupus erythematosus.

For localized disease, superpotent topical steroids used twice a day may be all that is needed for control until remission. For more generalized disease, long-term remission is usual after suppression of the disease by systemic methylprednisolone (1 mg/kg/day) therapy. Dapsone (25-100 mg/day) also may be used.

BULLOUS PEMPHIGOID

Etiology/Pathogenesis

Bullous pemphigoid (BP) is caused by circulating antigens to either the 180-kd or 230-kd BP antigen that result in a subepidermal blister. The 230-kd protein is part of the hemidesmosome, whereas the 180-kd antigen localizes to both the hemidesmosome and the upper lamina lucida and is a transmembrane collagenous protein.

Clinical Manifestations

The blisters of BP typically arise in crops on a normal, erythematous, eczematous, or urticarial base. Bullae appear predominantly on the flexural aspects of the extremities, in the axillae, and on the groin and central abdomen. Infants have involvement of the palms, soles, and face more frequently than older children. Individual lesions vary greatly in size, are tense, and are filled with serous fluid that may become hemorrhagic or turbid. Oral lesions occur less frequently and are less severe than in PV. Pruritus, a burning sensation, and subcutaneous edema may accompany the eruption, but constitutional symptoms are not prominent.

Pathology

Biopsy material should be taken from an early bulla arising on an erythematous base. A subepidermal bulla and a dermal inflammatory infiltrate, predominantly of eosinophils, can be identified histopathologically. In sections of a blister or perilesional skin, a band of immunoglobulin (usually IgG) and C3 can be demonstrated in the basement membrane zone by direct immunofluorescence. Indirect immunofluorescence studies of serum have positive results in ≈ 70% of cases for IgG antibodies to the basement membrane zone; the titers, however, do not correlate well with the clinical course.

Diagnosis and Differential Diagnoses

BP rarely occurs in children but must be considered in the differential diagnosis of any chronic blistering disorder. The **differential diagnosis** includes bullous erythema multiforme, pemphigus, linear IgA dermatosis, bullous drug eruption, dermatitis herpetiformis, herpes simplex infection, and bullous impetigo, which can be differentiated by histologic examination, immunofluorescence studies, and cultures. The large, tense bullae of BP can generally be distinguished from the smaller, flaccid bullae of PV.

Treatment

Localized bullous pemphigoid can be successfully suppressed with superpotent topical twice a day. Generalized disease usually requires systemic methylprednisolone (1 mg/kg/day) therapy. Rarely are other immunosuppressive treatments necessary. Ultimately, the condition usually remits permanently.

BIBLIOGRAPHY

Please visit the Nelson Textbook of Pediatrics *website at* www.expertconsult.com *for the complete bibliography.*

646.6 Dermatitis Herpetiformis

Joseph G. Morelli

ETIOLOGY/PATHOGENESIS

In dermatitis herpetiformis (DH), IgA antibodies are directed at epidermal transglutaminase. Gluten-sensitive enteropathy is found in all patients with DH, although the majority are asymptomatic or have minimal gastrointestinal symptoms (Chapter 330.2). The severity of the skin disease and the responsiveness to gluten restriction do not correlate with the severity of the intestinal inflammation. An antibody to smooth muscle endomysium is found in 70-90% of patients with DH. Ninety percent of patients with the disease express HLA DQ2. HLA DQ2–negative patients with DH usually express HLA DQ8.

CLINICAL MANIFESTATIONS

DH is characterized by symmetric, grouped, small, tense, erythematous, stinging, intensely pruritic papules and vesicles. The eruption is pleomorphic, including erythematous, urticarial, papular, vesicular, and bullous lesions. Sites of predilection are the knees, elbows, shoulders, buttocks, and scalp; mucous membranes are usually spared. Hemorrhagic lesions may develop on the palms and soles. When pruritus is severe, excoriations may be the only visible sign (Fig. 646-12).

PATHOLOGY

Subepidermal blisters composed predominantly of neutrophils are found in dermal papillae. The presence of granular IgA in the dermal papillary tips is diagnostic.

DIFFERENTIAL DIAGNOSIS

DH may mimic other chronic blistering diseases and may also resemble scabies, papular urticaria, insect bites, contact dermatitis, and papular eczema.

TREATMENT

Patients with DH show response within weeks to months to a gluten-free diet. Alternatively, oral administration of dapsone (0.5-2.0 mg/kg/day divided qd or bid) provides immediate relief from the intense pruritus but must be used with caution because of possible serious side effects (methemoglobinemia, hemolysis, and hypersensitivity syndrome [sulfone syndrome]).

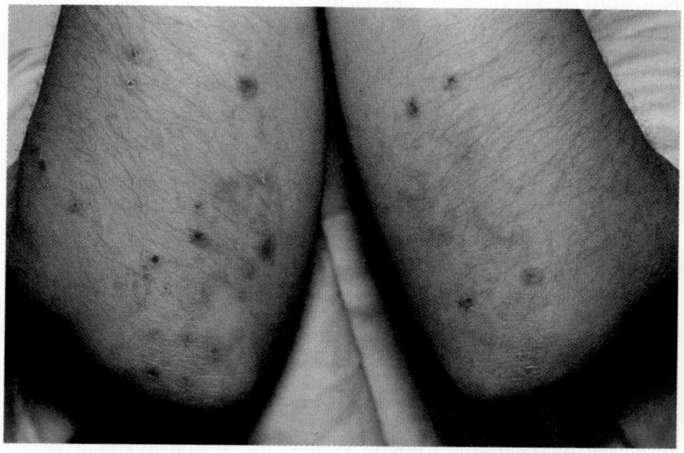

Figure 646-12 Multiple excoriations around the elbows in dermatitis herpetiformis.

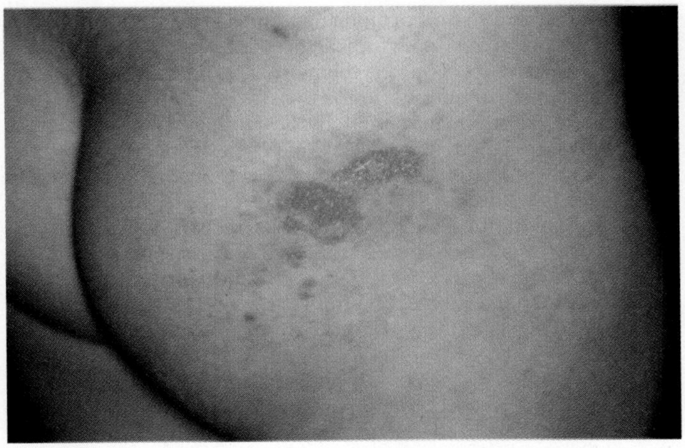

Figure 646-13 Erosion on an erythematous base post loss of blister roof in linear IgA dermatosis.

Local antipruritic measures may also be useful. Jejunal biopsy is indicated to diagnose gluten-sensitive enteropathy, because cutaneous manifestations may precede malabsorption. The disease is chronic and either a gluten-free diet or dapsone must be continued indefinitely to prevent relapse.

BIBLIOGRAPHY

Please visit the Nelson Textbook of Pediatrics *website at www.expertconsult.com for the complete bibliography.*

646.7 Linear IgA Dermatosis (Chronic Bullous Dermatosis of Childhood)

Joseph G. Morelli

ETIOLOGY/PATHOGENESIS

Linear IgA dermatosis is a heterogeneous autoimmune disorder with antibodies targeting multiple antigens. It is caused by circulating IgA antibodies, most commonly to LABD97 and LAD-1, which are degradation proteins of BP180 (type 17 collagen). Linear IgA dermatosis may also be seen as a drug eruption. Most cases of drug-induced linear IgA dermatosis are related to vancomycin, although anticonvulsants, ampicillin, cyclosporine, and captopril have been implicated.

CLINICAL MANIFESTATIONS

This rare dermatosis is most common in the 1st decade of life, with a peak incidence during the preschool years. The eruption consists of many large, tense bullae filled with clear or hemorrhagic fluid that develop on a normal or erythematous, urticarial base. Areas of predilection are the genitals and buttocks (Fig. 646-13), the perioral region, and the scalp. Sausage-shaped bullae may be arranged in an annular or rosette-like fashion around a central crust (Fig. 646-14). Erythematous plaques with gyrate margins bordered by intact bullae may develop over larger areas. Pruritus may be absent or very intense, and systemic signs or symptoms are absent.

PATHOLOGY

The subepidermal bullae are infiltrated with a mixture of inflammatory cells. Neutrophilic abscesses may be noted in the dermal papillary tips, indistinguishable from those of dermatitis herpetiformis. The infiltrate may also be largely eosinophilic, resembling that in BP. Therefore, direct immunofluorescence studies are required for a definitive diagnosis of linear IgA dermatosis; perilesional skin demonstrates linear deposition of IgA and sometimes IgG and C3 at the dermal-epidermal junction. Immunoelectron microscopy has localized the immunoreactants to the sublamina densa, although a combined sublamina densa and lamina lucida pattern has also been seen.

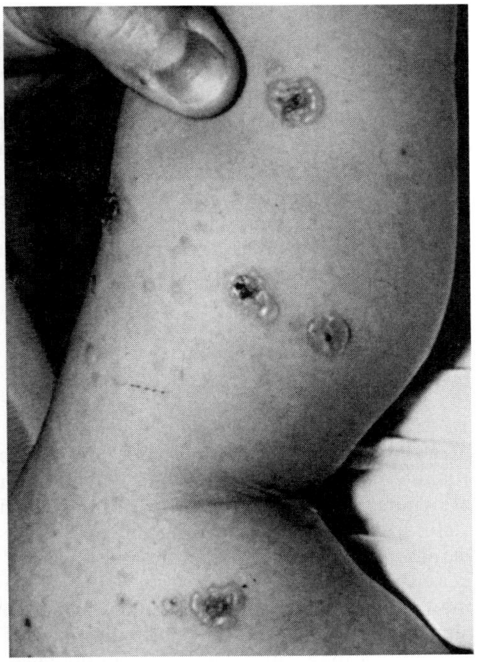

Figure 646-14 Rosette-like blisters around a central crust typical of linear IgA dermatosis (chronic bullous dermatosis of childhood).

DIFFERENTIAL DIAGNOSIS

The eruption can be distinguished by histopathologic and immunofluorescence studies from pemphigus, BP, DH, and EM. Gram stain and culture preclude the diagnosis of bullous impetigo.

TREATMENT

Many cases of linear IgA dermatosis respond favorably to oral dapsone (see treatment of DH). Children who show no response to dapsone may benefit from oral therapy with a methylprednisolone (1 mg/kg/day) or a combination of these drugs. The usual course is 2-4 yr, although some children have persistent or recurrent disease; there are no long-term sequelae.

BIBLIOGRAPHY

Please visit the Nelson Textbook of Pediatrics *website at www.expertconsult.com for the complete bibliography.*

Chapter 647 Eczematous Disorders

Joseph G. Morelli

Eczematous skin disorders are characterized by exudation, lichenification, and pruritus. Acute eczematous lesions demonstrate erythema, weeping, oozing, and the formation of microvesicles within the epidermis. Chronic lesions are generally thickened, dry, and scaly, with coarse skin markings (lichenification) and altered pigmentation. Many types of eczema occur in children;

the most common is **atopic dermatitis** (Chapter 139), although seborrheic dermatitis, allergic and irritant contact dermatitis, nummular eczema, and vesicular hand and foot dermatitis (dyshidrosis) are also relatively common in childhood.

Once the diagnosis of eczema has been established, it is important to classify the eruption more specifically for proper management. Pertinent historical data often provide the clue. In some instances, the subsequent course and character of the eruption permit classification. Histologic changes are relatively nonspecific, but all types of eczematous dermatitis are characterized by intraepidermal edema known as spongiosis.

647.1 Contact Dermatitis

Joseph G. Morelli

The form of eczema known as contact dermatitis can be subdivided into irritant dermatitis, resulting from nonspecific injury to the skin, and allergic contact dermatitis, in which the mechanism is a delayed hypersensitivity reaction. Irritant dermatitis is more frequent in children, particularly during the early years of life.

Irritant contact dermatitis can result from prolonged or repetitive contact with various substances that include saliva, citrus juices, bubble bath, detergents, abrasive materials, strong soaps, and proprietary medications. Saliva is probably one of the most common offenders; it may cause dermatitis on the face and in the neck folds of a drooling infant or a retarded child. In older children who habitually lick their lips because of dryness, frequently without being aware, a striking, sharply demarcated perioral rash may develop (Fig. 647-1). Among the exogenous irritants, citrus juices, proprietary medications, and bubble bath preparations are relatively common. Excessive accumulation of sweat and moisture as a result of wearing occlusive shoes may also cause irritant dermatitis.

Irritant contact dermatitis may be indistinguishable from atopic dermatitis or allergic contact dermatitis. A detailed history and consideration of the sites of involvement, the age of the child, and contactants usually provide clues to the etiologic agent. The propensity for development of irritant dermatitis varies considerably among children; some may respond to minimal injury, making it difficult to identify the offending agent through history. Irritant contact dermatitis usually clears after removal of the stimulus and temporary treatment with a topical corticosteroid preparation (Chapter 638). Education of patients and parents about the causes of contact dermatitis is crucial to successful therapy.

Diaper dermatitis can be regarded as the prototype of irritant contact dermatitis. As a reaction to overhydration of the skin, friction, maceration, and prolonged contact with urine and feces, retained diaper soaps, and topical preparations, the skin of the diaper area may become erythematous and scaly, often with papulovesicular or bullous lesions, fissures, and erosions (Fig. 647-2). The eruption can be patchy or confluent, but the genitocrural folds are often spared. Chronic hypertrophic, flat-topped papules and infiltrative nodules may occur. Secondary infection with yeast is common. Discomfort may be marked because of intense inflammation. Allergic contact dermatitis, seborrheic dermatitis, psoriasis, candidosis, atopic dermatitis, and rare disorders such as Langerhans cell histiocytosis (histiocytosis X) and acrodermatitis enteropathica should be considered when the eruption is persistent or is recalcitrant to simple therapeutic measures.

Diaper dermatitis often responds to simple measures; some infants are predisposed to diaper dermatitis, and management may be difficult. The damaging effects of overhydration of the skin and prolonged contact with feces and urine can be obviated by frequent changing of the diapers. Over-washing should be avoided because it leads to chapping and a worsening of the dermatitis. Disposable diapers containing a superabsorbent material may help maintain a relatively dry environment. Frequent topical applications of a bland protective barrier agent (petrolatum or zinc oxide paste) may suffice to prevent dermatitis. **Candidal infection** is signified by red-pink tender skin that has numerous 1- to 2-mm pustules and papules at the periphery of the dermatitis. Treatment with a topical anticandidal agent may be helpful.

Juvenile plantar dermatosis is a common form of irritant contact dermatitis occurring mainly in prepubertal children. The dermatitis characteristically involves the weight-bearing surfaces, may be pruritic or painful, and causes a glazed appearance of the plantar skin (Fig. 647-3). Fissuring may become extensive, producing considerable discomfort. The dermatitis results from alternating excessive hydration and rapid moisture loss, which cause chapping of the skin and cracking of the stratum corneum. Affected children often have hyperhidrosis, wear occlusive synthetic footwear, and subject their feet to rapid drying without moisturization. Immediate application of a thick emollient when socks and shoes are removed or immediately after swimming

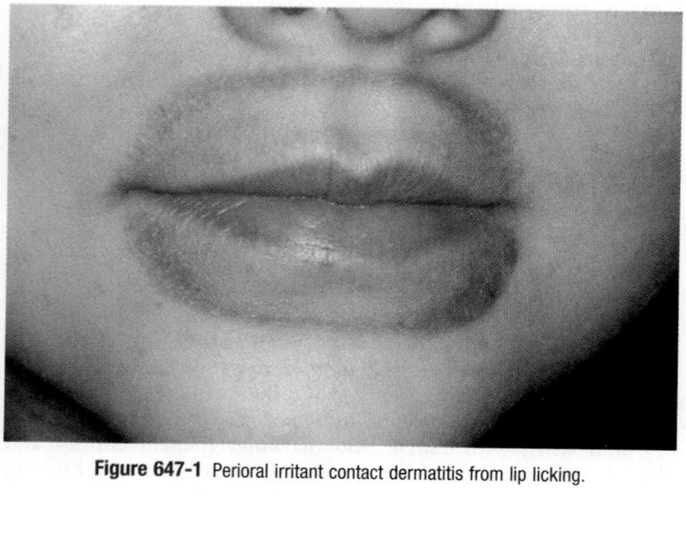

Figure 647-1 Perioral irritant contact dermatitis from lip licking.

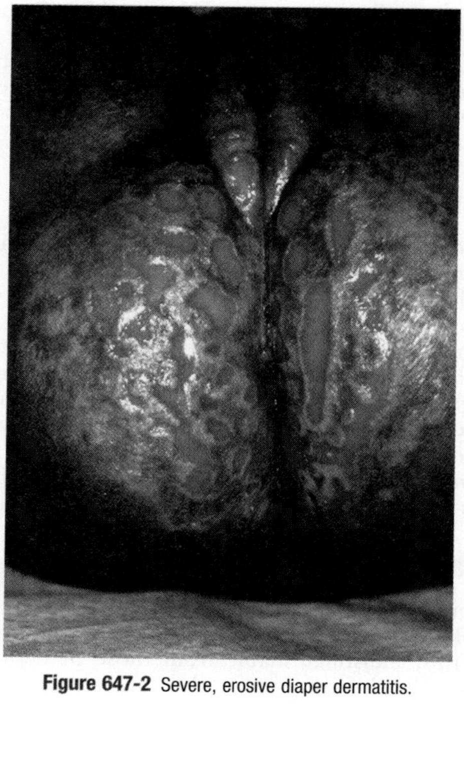

Figure 647-2 Severe, erosive diaper dermatitis.

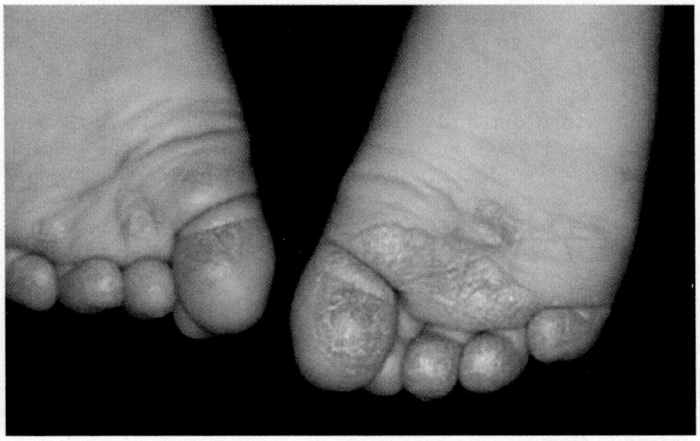

Figure 647-3 Red, scaly juvenile plantar dermatosis.

usually minimizes this condition. Severe inflammatory cases may require short-term (1-2 wk) application of a medium- to high-potency topical steroid.

Allergic contact dermatitis is a T cell–mediated hypersensitivity reaction that is provoked by application of an antigen to the skin surface. The antigen penetrates the skin, where it is conjugated with a cutaneous protein, and the hapten-protein complex is transported to the regional lymph nodes by antigen-presenting Langerhans cells. A primary immunologic response occurs locally in the nodes and becomes generalized, presumably because of dissemination of sensitized T cells. Sensitization requires several days and, when followed by a fresh antigenic challenge, manifests as allergic contact dermatitis. Generalized distribution may also occur if enough antigen finds its way into the circulation. Once sensitization has occurred, each new antigenic challenge may provoke an inflammatory reaction within 8-12 hr; sensitization to a particular antigen usually persists for many years.

Acute allergic contact dermatitis is an erythematous, intensely pruritic, eczematous dermatitis, which, if severe, may be edematous and vesiculobullous. The chronic condition has the features of long-standing eczema: lichenification, scaling, fissuring, and pigmentary change. The distribution of the eruption often provides a clue to the diagnosis. Volatile sensitizers usually affect exposed areas, such as the face and arms. Jewelry, topical agents, shoes, clothing, henna tattoo dyes, and plants cause dermatitis at points of contact.

Rhus dermatitis (poison ivy, poison sumac, poison oak) is often vesiculobullous and may be distinguished by linear streaks of vesicles where the plant leaves have brushed against the skin (Fig. 647-4). Fluid from ruptured cutaneous vesicles does not spread the eruption; antigen retained on the skin, under the fingernails, and on clothing initiates new plaques of dermatitis if not removed by washing with soap and water. Antigen may also be carried by animals on their fur. **Black spot poison ivy** is a rare variant that manifests as small discrete black lacquer-like glossy papules with surrounding erythema and edema. The saplike allergen (oleoresin) is present on live and dead leaves, and sensitization to one plant produces cross reactions with the others.

Nickel dermatitis usually develops from contact with jewelry or metal closures on clothing and is seen most frequently on the earlobes, such as when earring posts of nickel-containing metal rather than nonmetallic materials or stainless steel are used to keep a pierced tract open. Metal closures on pants frequently cause periumbilical dermatitis (Fig. 647-5). Some children are exquisitely sensitive to nickel, with even the trace amounts found in gold jewelry provoking eruptions.

Shoe dermatitis typically affects the dorsum of the feet and toes, sparing the interdigital spaces; it is usually symmetric. Other

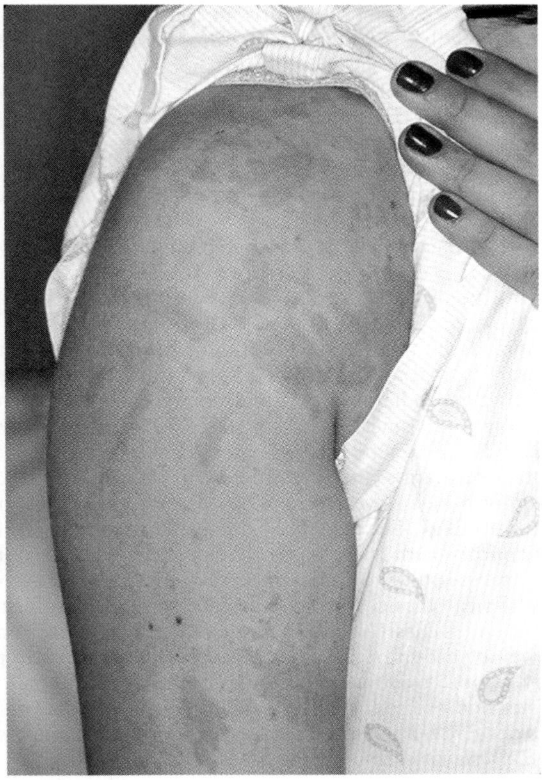

Figure 647-4 Linear lesions in poison ivy.

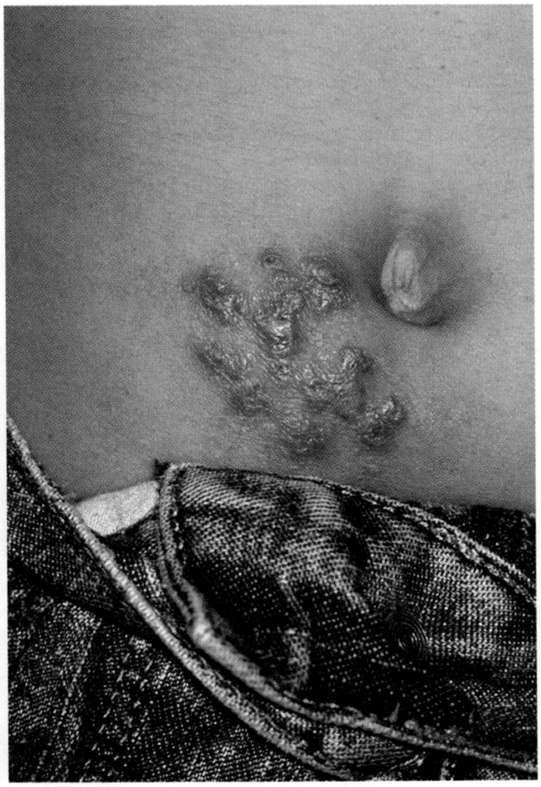

Figure 647-5 Chronic periumbilical nickel dermatitis.

forms of allergic contact dermatitis, in contrast to irritant dermatitis, rarely involve the palms and soles. Common allergens are the antioxidants and accelerators in shoe rubber and the chromium salts in tanned leather or shoe dyes. Excessive sweating often leaches these substances from their source.

Wearing apparel contains a number of sensitizers, including dyes, mordants, fabric finishes, fibers, resins, and cleaning solutions. Dye may be poorly fixed to clothing and so may be leached out with sweating, as are the partially cured formaldehyde resins. The elastic in garments is also a frequent cause of clothing dermatitis.

Topical medications and cosmetics may be unsuspected as allergens, particularly if a medication is being used for a pre-existing dermatitis. The most common offenders are neomycin, thimerosal, topical antihistamines, topical anesthetics, preservatives, and ethylenediamine, a stabilizer present in many medications. All types of cosmetics can cause facial dermatitis; involvement of the eyelids is characteristic for nail polish sensitivity.

Contact dermatitis can be confused with other types of eczema, dermatophytoses, and vesiculobullous diseases. Patch testing may clarify the etiology. The essential principle in **treatment** is elimination of contact with the allergen. Acute dermatitis responds to cool compresses and topical application of a medium- to high-potency topical corticosteroid ointment. An oral antihistamine may be useful. Massive acute bullous reactions or reactions that cause swelling around the eyes or genitals, such as those to poison ivy, may require treatment with a 2-wk tapering course of oral corticosteroids beginning with 1 mg/kg/day. If secondary infection has occurred, appropriate systemic antibiotic therapy should be given. Desensitization therapy is rarely indicated.

BIBLIOGRAPHY

Please visit the Nelson Textbook of Pediatrics *website at www.expertconsult.com for the complete bibliography.*

647.2 Nummular Eczema

Joseph G. Morelli

Nummular eczema is unrelated to other types of eczema and is characterized by more or less coin-shaped eczematous plaques. Common sites are the extensor surfaces of the extremities (Fig. 647-6), buttocks, and shoulders. The plaques are relatively discrete, boggy, vesicular, severely pruritic, and exudative; when chronic, they often become thickened and lichenified. The cause is unknown. Most frequently, these lesions are mistaken for tinea corporis, but plaques of nummular eczema are distinguished by the lack of a raised, sharply circumscribed border; the lack of fungal organisms on a potassium hydroxide (KOH) preparation; and frequent weeping or bleeding when scraped. Control of pruritus and inflammation is usually achieved with a potent topical corticosteroid preparation. Steroid-impregnated tapes may simultaneously treat and provide barrier protection to these circumscribed eczematous plaques. An antihistamine may be helpful, particularly at night. Antibiotics are indicated for secondary infection.

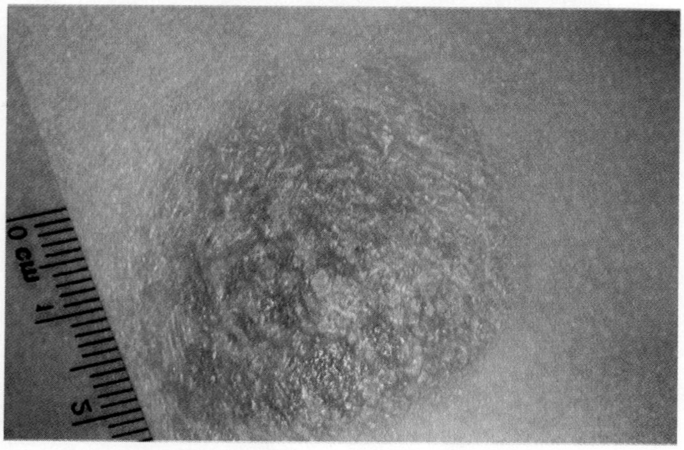

Figure 647-6 Discrete, boggy plaque of nummular dermatitis.

BIBLIOGRAPHY

Please visit the Nelson Textbook of Pediatrics *website at www.expertconsult.com for the complete bibliography.*

647.3 Pityriasis Alba

Joseph G. Morelli

Pityriasis alba occurs mainly in children; the lesions are hypopigmented, round or oval, macular or slightly elevated patches with fine adherent scale (Fig. 647-7). They may be mildly erythematous and relatively well defined but lack a sharply marginated border. Lesions occur on the face, neck, upper trunk, and proximal portions of the arms. Itching is minimal or absent. The cause is unknown, but the eruption appears to be exacerbated by dryness and is often regarded as a mild form of eczema. Pityriasis alba is frequently misdiagnosed as vitiligo, tinea versicolor, or tinea corporis. The lesions wax and wane but eventually disappear. Application of a lubricant may ameliorate the condition; if pruritus is troublesome, a low-potency topical steroid may used. Normal pigmentation often takes months to return.

647.4 Lichen Simplex Chronicus

Joseph G. Morelli

Lichen simplex chronicus is characterized by a chronic pruritic, eczematous, circumscribed, solitary plaque that is usually lichenified and hyperpigmented (Fig. 647-8). The most common sites are the posterior aspect of the neck, the dorsum of the feet, the wrists, and the ankles. Although the initiating event may be a transient lesion such as an insect bite, trauma from rubbing and scratching accounts for persistence of the plaque. Pruritus must be controlled to permit healing. A topical fluorinated corticosteroid preparation is often helpful, but constant irritation of the skin must be avoided. A covering to prevent scratching may be necessary.

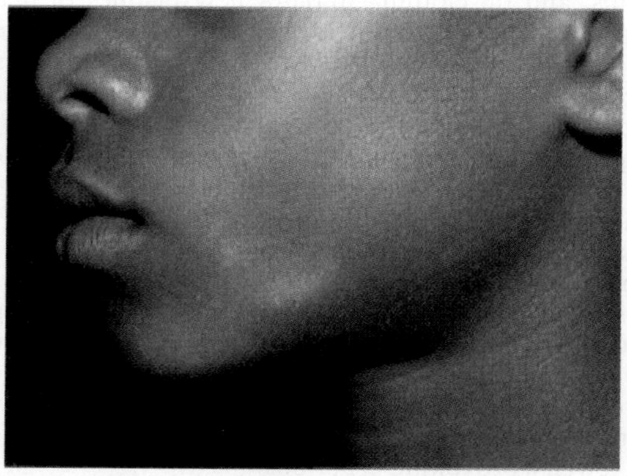

Figure 647-7 Patchy hypopigmented lesions with diffuse borders characteristic of pityriasis alba.

647.5 Vesicular Hand and Foot Dermatitis (Dyshidrotic Eczema, Dyshidrosis, Pompholyx)

Joseph G. Morelli

A recurrent, sometimes seasonal, blistering disorder of the hands and feet, vesicular hand and foot dermatitis occurs in all age groups but is uncommon in infancy. The pathogenesis is unknown; no genetic factor has been identified, although an increased incidence of atopy has been recorded in affected patients and their relatives. The disease is characterized by recurrent crops of small, intensely pruritic vesicles on the hands and feet. Sites of predilection are the palms, soles, and lateral aspects of the fingers and toes. Primary lesions are noninflammatory and are filled with clear fluid, which, unlike sweat, has a physiologic pH and contains protein. Larger vesicles and bullae may occur (Fig. 647-9), and maceration and secondary infection are frequent because of scratching. The chronic phase is characterized by thickened, fissured plaques that may cause considerable discomfort. Hyperhidrosis is common in many patients, but the association may be fortuitous. The diagnosis is made clinically. The disorder may be confused with allergic contact dermatitis, which usually affects the dorsal rather than the volar surfaces, and with dermatophytosis, which can be distinguished by a KOH preparation of the roof of a vesicle and by appropriate cultures.

Vesicular hand and foot dermatitis responds to wet dressings, followed by a potent topical corticosteroid preparation during the acute phase. Control of the chronic stage is difficult; lubricants containing mild keratolytic agents in conjunction with a potent topical fluorinated corticosteroid preparation may be indicated. Secondary bacterial infection should be treated systemically with an appropriate antibiotic. Patients should be told to expect recurrence and should protect their hands and feet from the damaging effects of excessive sweating, chemicals, harsh soaps, and adverse weather. Unfortunately, it is impossible to prevent recurrence or to predict its frequency.

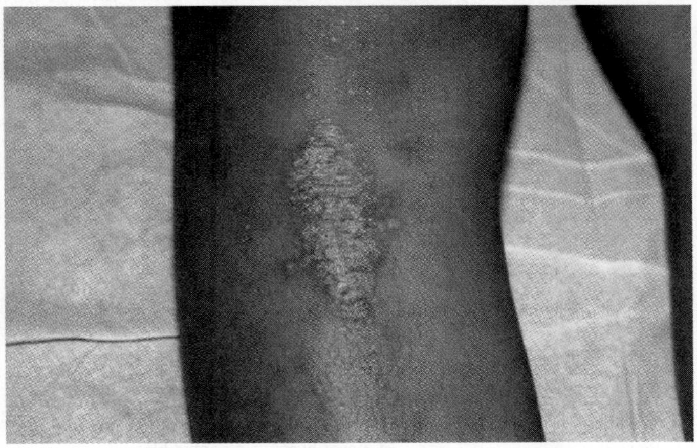

Figure 647-8 Thickened plaque of lichen simplex chronicus.

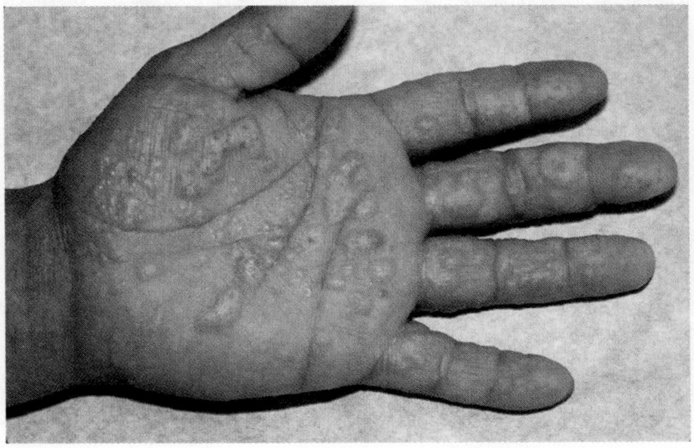

Figure 647-9 Vesicular palmar lesions of dyshidrotic eczema with large bullae.

647.6 Seborrheic Dermatitis

Joseph G. Morelli

ETIOLOGY

Seborrheic dermatitis is a chronic inflammatory disease most common in infancy and adolescence that parallels the distribution, size, and activity of the sebaceous glands. The cause is unknown, as is the role of the sebaceous glands in the disease. *Malassezia furfur* has been implicated as a causative agent, although its role in the etiology of infantile seborrheic dermatitis is unclear.

It is also unknown whether infantile seborrheic dermatitis and adolescent seborrheic dermatitis are the same or different entities. There is no evidence that children with infantile seborrheic dermatitis will experience seborrheic dermatitis as adolescents. A generalized eruption with features of seborrheic dermatitis is common in HIV-infected children and adolescents.

CLINICAL MANIFESTATIONS

The disorder may begin in the 1st mo of life and may be most troublesome in the 1st yr. Diffuse or focal scaling and crusting of the scalp, sometimes called cradle cap (Fig. 647-10), may be the initial and at times the only manifestation. A greasy, scaly, erythematous papular dermatitis, which is usually nonpruritic, may involve the face, neck, retroauricular areas, axillae, and diaper area. The dermatitis may be patchy and focal or may spread to involve almost the entire body (Fig. 647-11). Postinflammatory pigmentary changes are common, particularly in black infants. When the scaling becomes pronounced, the condition may resemble psoriasis and, at times, can be distinguished only with difficulty. The possibility of coexistent atopic dermatitis must be considered when there is an acute weeping dermatitis with pruritus, and the two are often clinically inseparable at an early age. An intractable seborrhea-like dermatitis with chronic diarrhea and failure to thrive may reflect systemic dysfunction of the immune system. A chronic seborrhea-like pattern, which responds

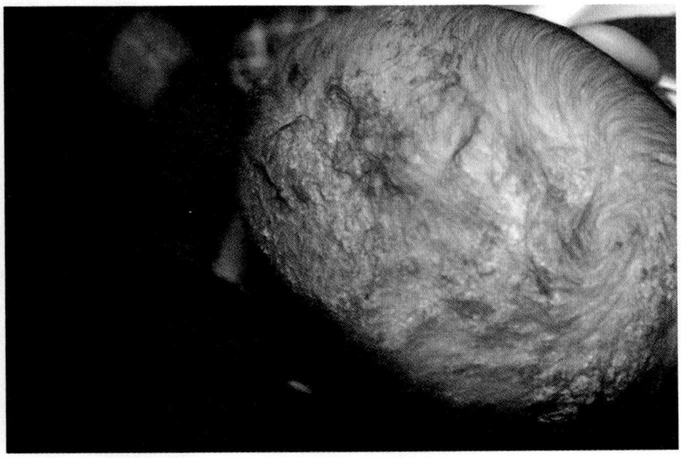

Figure 647-10 Cradle cap in an infant.

poorly to treatment, may also result from cutaneous histiocytic infiltrates in infants with **Langerhans cell histiocytosis**. Seborrheic dermatitis is a common cutaneous manifestation of **AIDS** in young adults and is characterized by thick, greasy scales on the scalp and large hyperkeratotic erythematous plaques on the face, chest, and genitals.

During adolescence, seborrheic dermatitis is more localized and may be confined to the scalp and intertriginous areas. Also noted may be marginal blepharitis and involvement of the external auditory canal. Scalp changes may vary from diffuse, brawny scaling to focal areas of thick, oily, yellow crusts with underlying erythema. Loss of hair is common, and pruritus may be absent to marked. When the dermatitis is severe, erythema and scaling may occur at the frontal hairline, the medial aspects of the eyebrows, and in the nasolabial and retroauricular folds. Red, scaly plaques may appear in the axillae, inguinal region, gluteal cleft, and umbilicus. On the extremities, seborrheic plaques may be more eczematous and less erythematous and demarcated.

DIFFERENTIAL DIAGNOSIS

The differential diagnosis of seborrheic dermatitis includes psoriasis, atopic dermatitis, dermatophytosis, histiocytic disorders, and candidosis. Secondary bacterial infections and superimposed candidosis are common.

TREATMENT

Scalp lesions should be controlled with an antiseborrheic shampoo (selenium sulfide, sulfur, salicylic acid, zinc pyrithione, tar), used daily if necessary. Inflamed lesions usually respond promptly to low- to medium-potency topical corticosteroid therapy. Topical immunomodulatory agents (tacrolimus, pimecrolimus) approved for the treatment of atopic dermatitis in children ≥2 yr of age (Chapter 139) may have a role in the treatment of other eczematous disorders such as seborrheic dermatitis. Concerns for systemic absorption and potential immunosuppression are higher in the younger patient population typically afflicted with seborrheic dermatitis. Topical antifungal agents (ketoconazole, ciclopirox, bifonazole) effective against *Malassezia* have been advocated. These are available as gels, creams, foams, and shampoos. The efficacy of antifungal agents is well documented in controlled trials in adults. Wet compresses should be applied to the moist or fissured lesions before application of the steroid ointment. Many patients require continued use of an antiseborrheic shampoo. Response to therapy is usually rapid unless there are complicating factors or the diagnosis is in error.

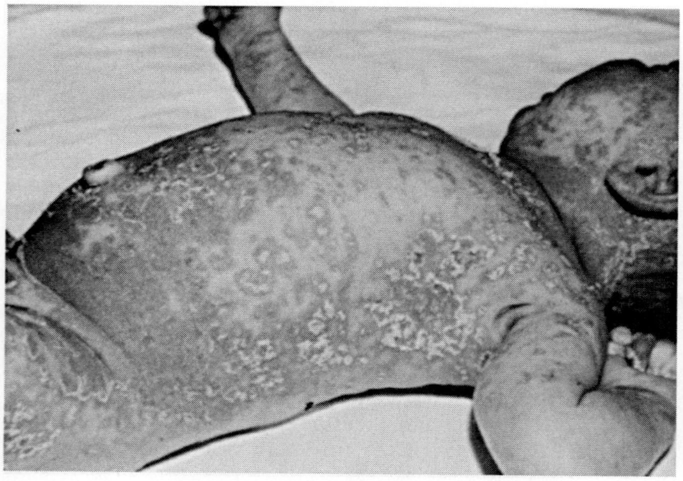

Figure 647-11 Widespread seborrheic dermatitis.

BIBLIOGRAPHY

Please visit the Nelson Textbook of Pediatrics *website at www.expertconsult.com for the complete bibliography.*

Chapter 648
Photosensitivity

Joseph G. Morelli

Photosensitivity denotes a qualitatively or quantitatively abnormal cutaneous reaction to sunlight or artificial light.

ACUTE SUNBURN REACTION

The most common photosensitive reaction seen in children is acute sunburn. Sunburn is caused mainly by ultraviolet (UV) B radiation (290-320 nm wavelength). Sunlight contains many times more UVA (320-400 nm) than UVB radiation, but UVA must be encountered in much larger quantities than UVB radiation to produce sunburn.

Pathophysiology and Clinical Manifestations

Transmitted radiation <300 nm is largely absorbed in the epidermis, whereas that >300 nm is mostly transmitted to the dermis after variable epidermal melanin absorption. Children vary in susceptibility to UV radiation, depending on their skin type (amount of pigment) (Table 648-1). Immediate pigment darkening is due to UVA radiation–induced photo-oxidative darkening of existing melanin and its transfer from melanocytes to keratinocytes. This effect generally lasts for a few hours and is not photoprotective. UVB-induced effects appear 6-12 hr after initial exposure and reach a peak in 24 hr. Effects include redness, tenderness, edema, and blistering (Fig. 648-1). Reactive oxidation species generated by UVB induce keratinocyte membrane damage and are involved in the pathogenesis of sunburn. A portion of

Table 648-1 SUN-REACTIVE SKIN TYPES

TYPE AND DEMOGRAPHICS	SUNBURN, TANNING HISTORY
I Red hair, freckles, Celtic origin	Always burns easily, no tanning
II Fair skin, fair-haired, blue-eyed, white	Usually burns, minimal tanning
III Darker-skinned white	Sometimes burns, gradual light brown tan
IV Mediterranean background	Minimal to no burning, always tans
V Middle Eastern white, Mexican	Rarely burns, tans profusely dark brown
VI Black	Never burns, pigmented black

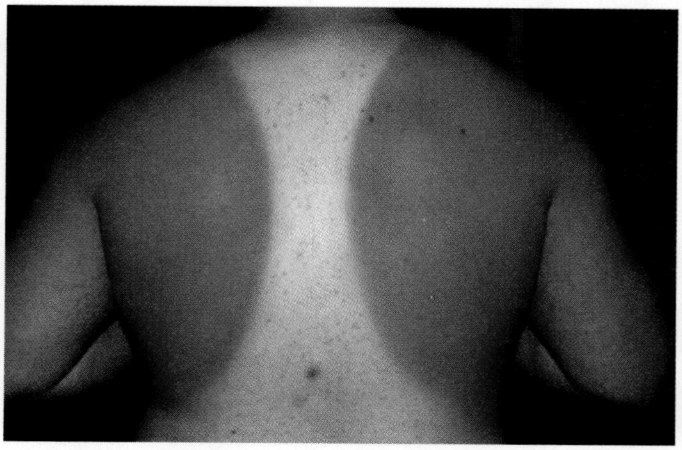

Figure 648-1 Sunburn. Well-demarcated, severe erythema.

Table 648-2 CUTANEOUS REACTIONS TO SUNLIGHT

Sunburn
Photoallergic drug eruptions:
- Systemic drugs include tetracyclines, psoralens, chlorthiazides, sulfonamides, barbiturates, griseofulvin, thiazides, quinidine, phenothiazines
- Topical agents include coal tar derivatives, psoralens, halogenated salicylanilides (soaps), perfume oils (e.g., oil of bergamot), sunscreens (e.g., PABA, cinnamates, benzophenones)

Phototoxic drug eruptions:
- High doses of agents causing photoallergic eruptions; nalidixic acid, 5-fluorouracil, psoralens, furosemide, nonsteroidal anti-inflammatory agents (naproxen, piroxicam), sulfonamides, tetracyclines, phenothiazines, furocoumarins (e.g., lime, lemon, carrot, celery, dill, parsnip, parsley)

Genetic disorders with photosensitivity:
- Xeroderma pigmentosum
- Bloom syndrome
- Cockayne syndrome
- Rothmund-Thomson syndrome

Inborn errors of metabolism:
- Porphyrias
- Hartnup disease

Infectious diseases associated with photosensitivity:
- Recurrent herpes simplex infection
- Viral exanthems (accentuated photodistribution; e.g., varicella)

Skin disease exacerbated or precipitated by light:
- Lichen planus
- Darier disease
- Lupus erythematosus
- Dermatomyositis
- Scleroderma
- Granuloma annulare
- Psoriasis
- Erythema multiforme
- Sarcoid
- Atopic dermatitis
- Hailey-Hailey disease
- Pemphigus
- Acne rosacea
- Bullous pemphigoid

Deficient protection due to lack of pigment:
- Vitiligo
- Oculocutaneous albinism
- Phenylketonuria
- Chédiak-Higashi syndrome
- Hermansky-Pudlak syndrome
- Waardenburg syndrome
- Piebaldism

the vasodilatation seen in UVB-induced erythema is mediated by prostaglandins E_2 and F_2. Delayed melanogenesis as a result of UVB radiation begins in 2-3 days and lasts several days to a few weeks. Manufacture of new melanin in melanocytes, transfer of melanin from melanocytes to keratinocytes, increase in size and arborization of melanocytes, and activation of quiescent melanocytes produce delayed melanogenesis. This effect reduces skin sensitivity to development of UV-induced erythema. The amount of protection afforded depends on the skin type of the patient. Additional effects and possible complications of sun exposure include increased thickness of the stratum corneum, recurrence or exacerbation of herpes simplex labialis, lupus erythematosus, and many other conditions (Table 648-2).

Treatment

Acute severe sunburn should be managed with cool compresses. Topical corticosteroids and oral prostaglandin inhibitors such as ibuprofen and indomethacin may decrease erythema and pain but must be administered preradiation or early in the course of the sunburn. Once peak erythema has been reached, little help is afforded by these medications. Proprietary preparations containing topical anesthetics are relatively ineffective and potentially hazardous because of their propensity to cause contact dermatitis. A bland emollient is effective in the desquamative phase.

Prognosis and Prevention of Sequelae

The long-term sequelae of chronic and intense sun exposure are not often seen in children, but most individuals receive >50% of their lifetime UV dose by age 20 yr. Therefore, pediatricians have a pivotal role in educating patients and their parents about the harmful effects, potential malignancy risks, and irreversible skin damage that result from unduly prolonged exposure to the sun and tanning lights. Premature aging, senile elastosis, actinic keratoses, squamous and basal cell carcinomas, and melanomas all occur with greater frequency in sun-damaged skin. In particular, blistering sunburns in childhood and adolescence significantly increase the risk for development of malignant melanoma. Sun protection is best achieved by sun avoidance, which includes minimizing time in the midday sun (10 AM to 3 PM), staying in the shade, and wearing protective clothing including wide-brimmed hats. Protection is enhanced by a wide variety of sunscreen agents. Physical opaque sunscreens (zinc oxide, titanium dioxide) block UV light, whereas chemical sunscreens (para-aminobenzoic acid [PABA], PABA esters, salicylates, benzophenones, dibenzoylmethanes [avobenzone], cinnamates, terephthalylidene dicamphor sulfonic acid [ecamsule]) absorb damaging radiation. The benzophenones and dibenzoylmethanes provide protection in both the UVA and UVB ranges. Stabilizers such as octocrylene and diethyl 2,6-naphthalate increase the time of function of the dibenzoylmethanes. Ecamsule and drometrizole trisiloxane are UVA sunscreens. Vitamins C and E added to sunscreen may also be beneficial in reduction of the formation of reactive oxygen species. Children with skin types I to III (see Table 648-1) require sunscreens with a sun protection factor (SPF) of at least 15, although the higher SPF, the more protection. SPF is defined as the minimal dose of sunlight required to produce cutaneous erythema after application of a sunscreen, divided by the dose required with no use of sunscreen. SPF applies only to UVB protection. UVA rating of sunscreens should be available in the near future.

PHOTOSENSITIVE REACTIONS

Photosensitizers in combination with a particular wavelength of light cause dermatitis that can be classified as a phototoxic or a photoallergic reaction. Contact of the skin with the photosensitizer may occur externally, internally by enteral or parenteral administration, or through host synthesis of photosensitizers in response to an administered drug.

Photoallergic reactions occur in only a small percentage of persons exposed to photosensitizers and light and require a time interval for sensitization to take place. Thereafter, dermatitis appears within ≈ 24 hr of re-exposure to the photosensitizer and light. Photoallergic dermatitis is a T cell–mediated delayed hypersensitivity reaction in which the drug, acting as a hapten, may combine with a skin protein to form the antigenic substance. Photoallergic reactions vary in morphology and may occur on partially covered and on light-exposed skin. Some of the important classes of drugs and chemicals responsible for photosensitivity reactions are listed in Table 648-2.

Phototoxic reactions occur in all individuals who accumulate adequate amounts of a photosensitizing drug or chemical within the skin. Prior sensitization is not required. Dermatitis develops within hours after exposure to radiation in the range of 285-450 nm. The eruption is confined to light-exposed areas and often resembles exaggerated sunburn, but it may be urticarial or bullous. It results in postinflammatory hyperpigmentation. All the drugs that cause photoallergic reactions may also cause a phototoxic dermatitis if given in sufficiently high doses. Several additional drugs and contactants cause phototoxic reactions, notably the plant-derived furocoumarins (see Table 648-2). Differentiation from contact dermatitis due to poison ivy or poison oak may be difficult, but itching is prominent in contact dermatitis. In phytophotodermatitis, burning is prominent and is confined to sun-exposed areas, sparing the upper eyelids, beneath the nose and chin, and the retroauricular areas. Postinflammatory hyperpigmentation develops rapidly and is usually the presenting sign.

Although photodermatitis caused by drugs or chemicals may be diagnosed by photopatch testing, facilities for this diagnostic procedure are not widely available. A high index of suspicion combined with an appreciation of the distribution pattern of the eruption and a history of application or ingestion of a known photosensitizing agent is all that is required to make a diagnosis. Discontinuation of the offending medication or avoidance of sun exposure, oral administration of an antihistamine, and application of a topical corticosteroid to alleviate pruritus are appropriate therapeutic measures. Severe reactions may necessitate systemic corticosteroid therapy for a brief time.

PORPHYRIAS (CHAPTER 85)

Porphyrias are acquired or inborn disorders due to abnormalities of specific enzyme mutations in the heme biosynthetic pathway. Two in particular occur in children and have photosensitivity as a consistent feature. Signs and symptoms may be negligible during the winter, when sun exposure is minimal.

Congenital erythropoietic porphyria (Günther disease) is a rare autosomal recessive disorder. It manifests in the first few months of life as exquisite sensitivity to light, which may induce repeated severe bullous eruptions that result in mutilating scars (Fig. 648-2). **Hyperpigmentation,** hyperkeratosis, vesiculation, and fragility of skin develop in light-exposed areas. **Hirsutism** in areas of mild involvement, scarring **alopecia** in severely affected areas, pink to red urine, brown teeth, hemolytic anemia, splenomegaly, and increased amounts of uroporphyrin I in urine, plasma, and erythrocytes and of coproporphyrin I in feces are additional characteristic manifestations. Urine from affected patients fluoresces reddish pink under a Wood light. Total protection from sunlight is the treatment of choice.

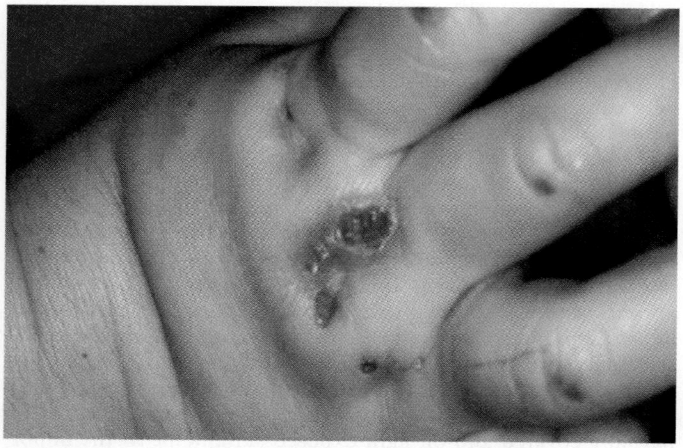

Figure 648-2 Crusted ulcerations in an infant with congenital erythropoietic porphyria.

Erythropoietic protoporphyria, an autosomal dominant trait, becomes apparent in early childhood and manifests as pain, tingling, and a burning sensation within ≈ 30 min of sun exposure, followed by erythema, edema, urticaria, and, rarely, vesicles on light-exposed areas. Nail changes consist of opacification of the nail plate, onycholysis, pain, and tenderness. Mild systemic symptoms such as malaise, chills, and fever may accompany the acute skin reaction. Recurrent sun exposure produces a chronic eczematous dermatitis with thickened, lichenified skin, especially over the finger joints (Fig. 648-3A), and persistent violaceous erythema, ulcers, and pitted or linear, crusted atrophic scars on the face (Fig. 648-3B) and rims of the ears. Pigmentation, hypertrichosis, skin fragility, and mutilation are uncommon. Liver disease is uncommon and generally mild, with only 3% of patients demonstrating severe disease.

The wavelengths of light mainly responsible for eliciting cutaneous reactions in porphyria are in the region of 400 nm. Window glass, which transmits wavelengths >320 nm, is not protective, and artificial lights of a certain wavelength may be pathogenic. Patients must avoid direct sunlight, wear protective clothing, and use a sunscreen agent that effectively blocks wavelengths in the region of 400 nm. Administration of beta-carotene (Solatene) 120-180 mg/day to achieve a level of 11-15 μmol/L is often effective in reducing symptoms.

COLLOID MILIUM

Colloid milium is a rare, asymptomatic disorder that occurs on the face (nose, upper lip, upper cheeks) and may extend to the dorsum of the hands and the neck as a profuse eruption of tiny, ivory to yellow, firm, grouped papules. Lesions appear before puberty on otherwise normal skin, unlike the adult variant that develops on sun-damaged skin. Onset may follow an acute sunburn or long-term sun exposure. Most cases reach maximal severity within ≈ 3 yr and remain unchanged thereafter, although the condition may remit spontaneously after puberty. Histopathologic changes include well-circumscribed accumulations of fissured eosinophilic material, primarily in the upper dermis in contact with the epidermis. Treatment options include dermabrasion and ablative lasers.

HYDROA VACCINIFORME

A vesiculobullous disorder, hydroa vacciniforme is more common in boys than in girls, begins in early childhood, but may remit at puberty. The peak incidence is in the spring and summer. Erythematous, pruritic macules develop symmetrically within hours of sun exposure over the ears, nose, lips, cheeks, and dorsal surfaces of the hands and forearms. Lesions progress to stinging tender papules and hemorrhagic vesicles and bullae. Severe lesions of hydroa vacciniforme resemble the vesicles of chickenpox. They become umbilicated, ulcerated, and crusted

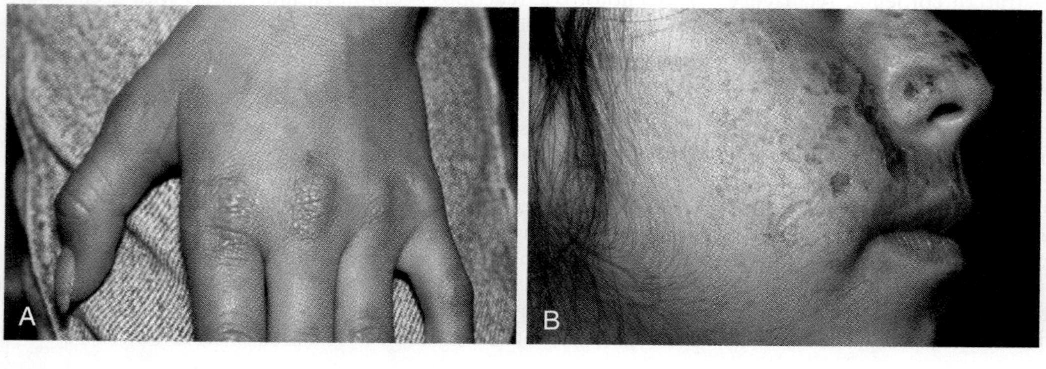

Figure 648-3 Erythropoietic porphyria. *A,* Erythematous thickening over the metacarpal phalangeal joints. *B,* Linear crusts and scarring.

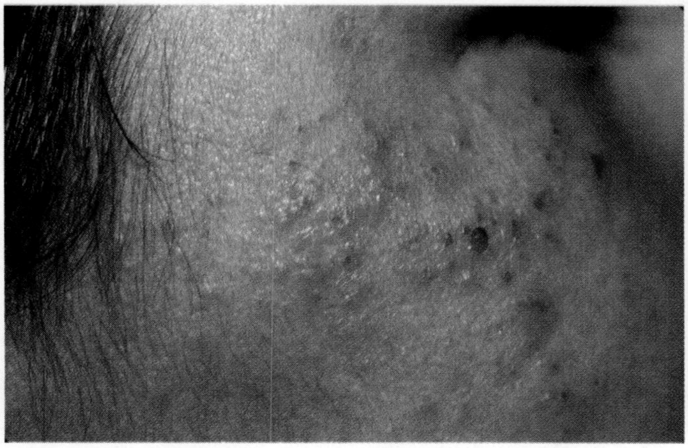

Figure 648-4 Erythematous, excoriated papules in actinic prurigo.

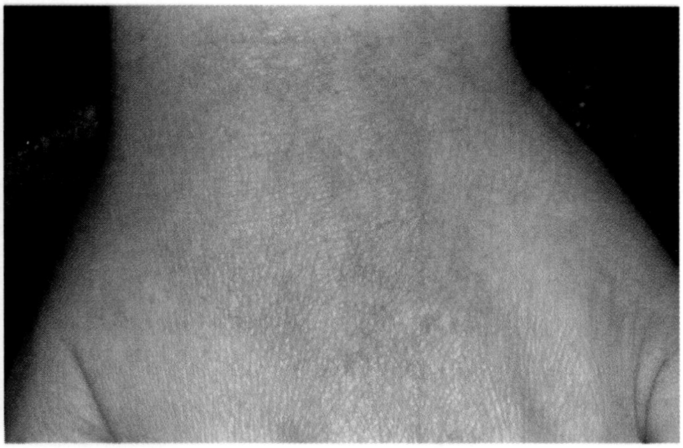

Figure 648-5 Urticaria after 5-min exposure to artificial ultraviolet A radiation.

and heal with pitted scars and telangiectasias. Fever and malaise are noted occasionally during the acute phase. Histopathologically, lesions show intraepidermal multilocular vesicles, leading to focal epidermal and dermal necrosis. Noted early is a dermal perivascular mononuclear cell infiltrate, which later surrounds areas of necrosis. This eruption should be distinguished from erythropoietic protoporphyria, which rarely shows vesicles. Pathogenesis of hydroa vacciniforme is related to latent Epstein-Barr virus infections. Typical lesions have been reproduced with repeated doses of UVA or UVB light. A **mid-potency topical corticosteroid** may be useful for the inflammatory phase of the eruption. Sun avoidance and broad-spectrum sunscreens may also be helpful, as may low-dose courses of narrow-band UVB (NB-UVB) therapy or psoralen with UVA (PUVA) therapy (hardening).

ACTINIC PRURIGO

A chronic familial photodermatitis, actinic prurigo is inherited as an autosomal dominant trait among the Native Americans of North and South America. HLA DRB1*0407 (60-70%) and HLA DRB1*0401 (20%) are strongly associated with actinic prurigo. The first episode generally occurs in early childhood, several hours to 2 days after intense sun exposure. Most patients are female and are sensitive to UVA radiation. Lesions are intensely pruritic, erythematous papules on the face (Fig. 648-4), lower lip, distal extremities, and, in severe cases, buttocks. Facial lesions may heal with minute pitted or linear scarring. Lesions often become chronic, without periods of total clearing, merging into eczematous plaques that lichenify and may become secondarily infected. Associated features that distinguish this disorder from other photoeruptions and atopic dermatitis include cheilitis, conjunctivitis, and traumatic alopecia of the outer half of the eyebrows. Actinic prurigo is a chronic condition that generally persists into adult life, although it may improve spontaneously in the late teenage years. Sun avoidance, protective clothing, and broad-spectrum sunscreens may be helpful in preventing the eruption. **Mid- to high-potency topical corticosteroids** and **antihistamines** palliate the pruritus and inflammation. **Thalidomide 50-100 mg/day** is very effective, but its use is limited by toxicity.

SOLAR URTICARIA

Solar urticaria is a rare disorder induced by UV or visible irradiation. The disorder is mediated by immunoglobulin (Ig) E antibodies to either an abnormal chromophore (type I) or a normal chromophore (type II), leading to mast cell degranulation and histamine release. This reaction occurs within 5-10 min of sun exposure, fades within 1-2 hr, and is characterized by widespread severe wheal formation (Fig. 648-5), which may lead to faintness, headache, nausea, syncope, or bronchospasm. H_1-blocking antihistamines may be useful to prevent or abate the eruption.

POLYMORPHOUS LIGHT ERUPTION

Polymorphous light eruption develops most commonly in females younger than 30 yr. The first eruption typically appears after prolonged sun exposure during the spring or summer. Onset of the eruption is delayed by hours to days after sun exposure and lasts for days to sometimes weeks. Areas of involvement tend to be symmetric and are characteristic for a given patient, including some but not all of the exposed or lightly covered skin on the face, neck, upper chest, and distal extremities. Lesions have various morphologies but most commonly are pruritic, 2- to 5-mm, grouped erythematous papules or papulovesicles or edematous plaques that are > 5 cm in diameter. Most cases involve sensitivity to UVA radiation, although some are UVB induced. **Therapeutic** approaches include sun avoidance, protective clothing, broad-spectrum sunscreens, mid- to high-potency topical or systemic corticosteroids, or prophylactic NB-UVB or PUVA phototherapy (hardening).

COCKAYNE SYNDROME

Onset of Cockayne syndrome, an autosomal recessive disorder, is characterized by the appearance, at ≈ 1 yr of age, of facial erythema in a butterfly distribution after sun exposure, followed by loss of adipose tissue and development of thin, atrophic, hyperpigmented skin, particularly over the face. Associated features include dwarfism; mental retardation; large, protuberant ears; long limbs; disproportionately large hands and feet, which are sometimes cool and cyanotic; pinched nose; carious teeth; unsteady gait with tremor; limitation of joint mobility; progressive deafness; cataracts; retinal degeneration; optic atrophy; decreased sweating and tearing; and premature graying of the hair. Diffuse extensive demyelination of the peripheral and central nervous systems ensues, and patients generally die of atheromatous vascular disease before the third decade. There are 2 types of Cockayne syndrome. Type I (CSA gene) is less severe than type II (CSB gene). Xeroderma pigmentosum–Cockayne syndrome (XP-CS) demonstrates complementation with xeroderma pigmentosa groups B, D, or G. Patients with XP-CS are phenotypically more like patients with Cockayne syndrome. Photosensitivity is due to deficient rates of repair of UV-induced damage, specifically within actively transcribing regions of DNA (transcription-coupled DNA repair). The syndrome is distinguished from progeria (Chapter 84) by the

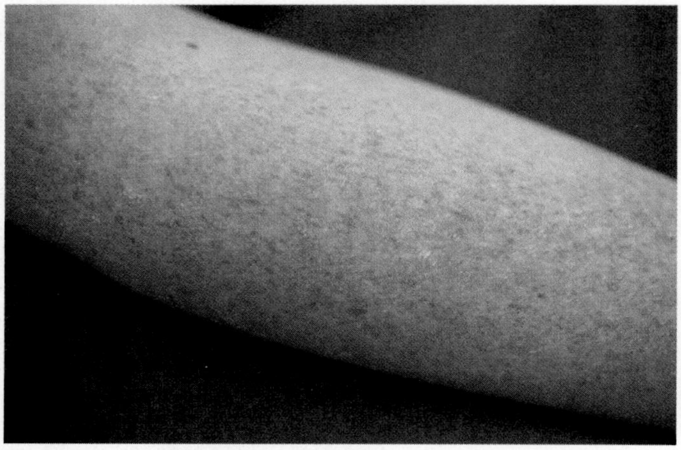

Figure 648-6 Dyspigmentation and actinic keratoses in child with xeroderma pigmentosum.

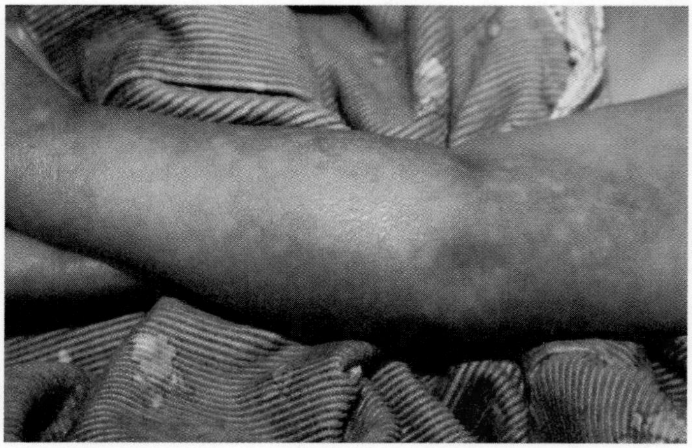

Figure 648-7 Poikiloderma on the arm of an infant with Rothmund-Thomson syndrome.

presence in Cockayne syndrome of photosensitivity and the ocular abnormalities.

XERODERMA PIGMENTOSUM

Xeroderma pigmentosum is a rare autosomal recessive disorder that results from a defect in nucleotide excision repair. Seven complementation groups have been recognized, on the basis of each group's separate defect in ability to repair damaged DNA. Xeroderma pigmentosum variant is caused by mutations in the DNA polymerase *ETA* gene (*POLH*), which lead to a defect in the conversion of newly synthesized DNA after UV radiation. The wavelength of light that induces the DNA damage ranges from 280 to 340 nm. Skin changes are first noted during infancy or early childhood in sun-exposed areas such as the face, neck, hands, and arms; lesions may occur, however, at other sites, including the scalp. The skin lesions consist of erythema, scaling, bullae, crusting, ephelides, telangiectasia, keratoses (Fig. 648-6), basal and squamous cell carcinomas, and malignant melanomas. Ocular manifestations include photophobia, lacrimation, blepharitis, symblepharon, keratitis, corneal opacities, tumors of the lids, and possible eventual blindness. Neurologic abnormalities such as mental deterioration and sensorineural deafness may develop in ≈ 20% of patients.

This disease is a serious mutilating disorder, and the life span of an affected patient is often brief. Affected families should have genetic counseling. Xeroderma pigmentosum is detectable in cells cultured from amniotic fluid. Affected children should be totally protected from sun exposure; protective clothing, eyeglasses, and opaque broad-spectrum sunscreens should be used even for mildly affected children. Light from unshielded fluorescent bulbs and sunlight passing through glass windows are also harmful. Early detection and removal of malignancies is mandatory.

ROTHMUND-THOMSON SYNDROME

Rothmund-Thomson syndrome is also known as poikiloderma congenitale because of the striking skin changes (Fig. 648-7). It is inherited as an autosomal recessive trait. Mutations in the *RECQL4* gene are found in approximately 65% of the patients. The other mutations causing Rothmund-Thomson syndrome are unknown. Skin changes are noted as early as 3 mo of age. Plaques of erythema and edema appear on the cheeks, forehead, ears, neck, dorsal portions of the hands, extensor surfaces of the arms, and buttocks and are replaced gradually by reticulated, atrophic, hyperpigmented, telangiectatic plaques. Light sensitivity is present in many cases, and exposure to the sun may provoke formation of bullae. Areas of involvement, however, are not strictly photodistributed. Short stature; small hands and feet; sparse eyebrows, eyelashes, and pubic and axillary hair, and sparse, fine, prematurely gray scalp hair or alopecia; bony defects; and hypogenitalism are common. Cataracts may also occur at an early age. Most patients have normal mental development. Keratoses and later squamous cell carcinomas may develop on exposed skin. The most worrisome association is that with osteosarcoma, which occurs only in those patients with Rothmund-Thomson syndrome and *RECQL4* mutations.

BLOOM SYNDROME

The defect in Bloom syndrome (*BLM/RECQL3* gene) is inherited in an autosomal recessive manner. Patients are sensitive to UV radiation, and their rate of chromosomal breaks and sister chromatid exchanges is markedly increased. Erythema and telangiectasia develop during infancy in a butterfly distribution on the face after exposure to sunlight. A bullous eruption on the lips and telangiectatic erythema on the hands and forearms may develop. Café-au-lait spots and hypopigmented macules may be present. Prenatal and postnatal short stature and a distinctive facies consisting of a prominent nose and ears and a small, narrow face are generally found. Intellect is average to low average. Immunodeficiency is seen in all patients, manifesting as recurrent ear and pulmonary infections. Gastrointestinal malabsorption is common. Affected children have an unusual tendency to experience both solid tumors and lymphoreticular malignancies.

HARTNUP DISEASE (CHAPTER 79.5)

Hartnup disease is a rare inborn error of metabolism with autosomal recessive inheritance. Neutral amino acids, including tryptophan, are not transported across the brush border epithelium of the intestine and kidneys, resulting in deficiency of synthesis of nicotinamide and causing a photo-induced **pellagra-like syndrome.** The urine contains increased amounts of monoamine monocarboxylic amino acids. Cutaneous signs, which precede neurologic manifestations, initially develop during the early months of life, consisting of an eczematous, occasionally vesiculobullous eruption noted on the face and extremities in a glove-and-stocking photodistribution. Hyperpigmentation and hyperkeratosis may supervene and are intensified by further exposure to sunlight. Episodic flares may be precipitated by febrile illness, sun exposure, emotional stress, and poor nutrition. In most cases, mental development is normal, but some patients display emotional instability and episodic cerebellar ataxia. Neurologic symptoms are fully reversible. Administration of nicotinamide and protection from sunlight results in improvement of both cutaneous and neurologic manifestations.

BIBLIOGRAPHY

Please visit the Nelson Textbook of Pediatrics *website at www.expertconsult.com for the complete bibliography.*

Chapter 649 Diseases of the Epidermis

649.1 Psoriasis

Joseph G. Morelli

ETIOLOGY/PATHOGENESIS

Psoriasis is characterized by proliferation and abnormal differentiation of keratinocytes and inflammatory cell infiltration of the epidermis and dermis secondary to a primary T-cell abnormality. Psoriasis has a complex multifactorial genetic basis. The major psoriasis-susceptibility gene (*PSORS1*) is HLA-CW*0602. Numerous other psoriasis susceptibility genes have been identified (*PSORS2-PSORS9*). Interleukins IL12B and IL23R are the most compelling gene products involved in the pathogenesis of psoriasis.

CLINICAL MANIFESTATIONS

This common, chronic skin disorder is first evident in ≈ 30% of affected individuals within the first 2 decades of life. The lesions consist of erythematous papules that coalesce to form plaques with sharply demarcated, irregular borders. If they are unaltered by treatment, a thick silvery or yellow-white scale (resembling mica) develops (Fig. 649-1*A*). Removal of the scale may result in pinpoint bleeding (**Auspitz sign**). The **Koebner,** or isomorphic, response, in which new lesions appear at sites of trauma, is a valuable diagnostic feature. Lesions may occur anywhere, but preferred sites are the scalp, knees, elbows, umbilicus, superior intergluteal fold, and genitals. Small raindrop-like lesions on the face are common. Nail involvement, a valuable diagnostic sign, is characterized by pitting of the nail plate, detachment of the plate (onycholysis), yellowish brown subungual discoloration, and accumulation of subungual debris (Fig. 649-1*B*).

Psoriasis is rare in neonates but may be severe and recalcitrant and may pose a diagnostic problem. Other rare forms include psoriatic erythroderma, localized or generalized pustular psoriasis, and linear psoriasis.

Guttate psoriasis, a variant that occurs predominantly in children, is characterized by an explosive eruption of profuse, small, oval or round lesions that morphologically are identical to the larger plaques of psoriasis (Fig. 649-1*C*). Sites of predilection are the trunk, face, and proximal portions of the limbs. The onset frequently follows a **streptococcal** infection; a culture of the throat and serologic titers should be obtained. Guttate psoriasis has also been observed after perianal streptococcal infection, viral infections, sunburn, and withdrawal of systemic corticosteroid therapy.

DIFFERENTIAL DIAGNOSIS

Psoriasis is a clinical diagnosis. The differential diagnosis of plaque-type psoriasis includes nummular dermatitis, tinea corporis, seborrheic dermatitis, postinfectious arthritis syndromes, pityriasis rosea, pityriasis lichenoides, and pityriasis rubra pilaris.

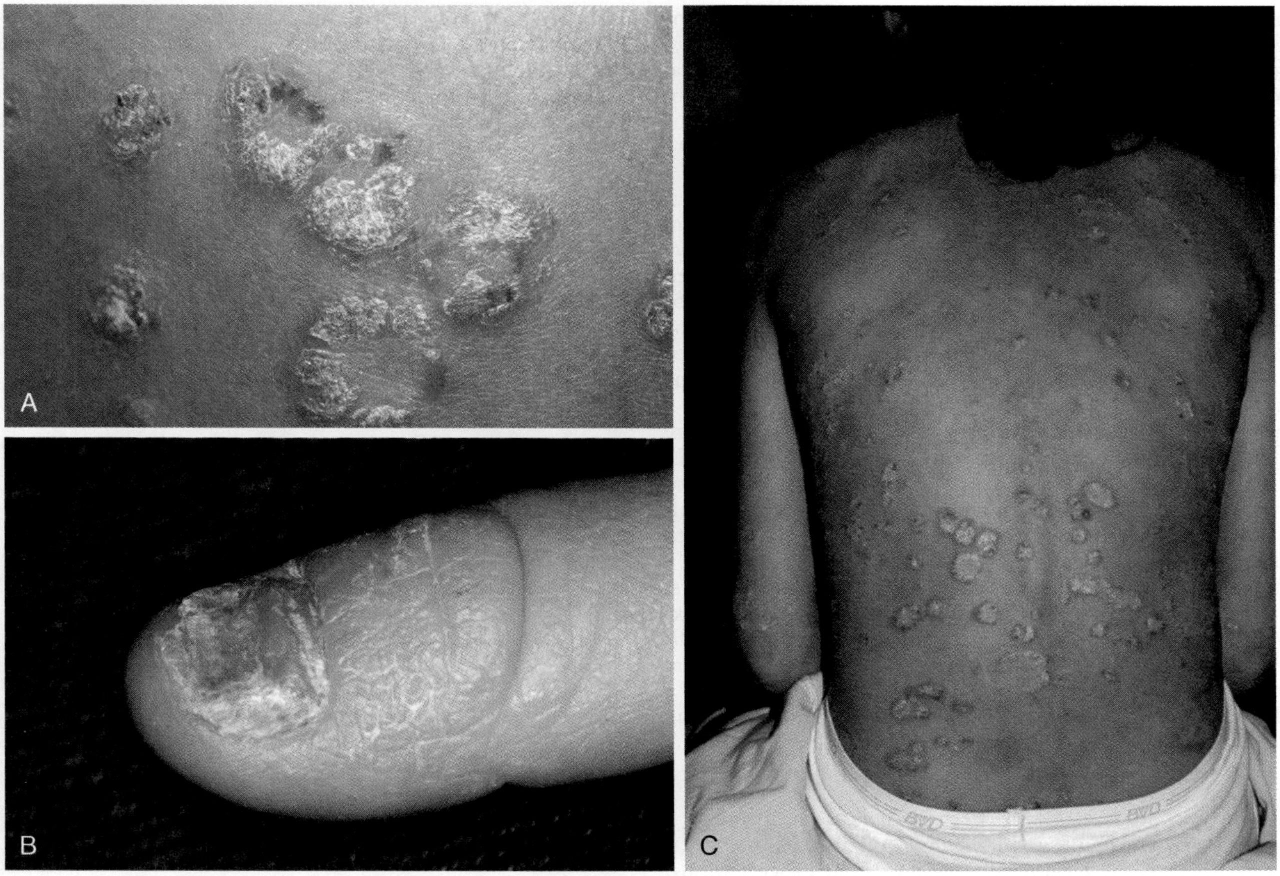

Figure 649-1 *A,* Chronic psoriatic plaques. *B,* Psoriatic nail dystrophy. *C,* Guttate psoriasis in widespread distribution over the trunk.

Scalp lesions may be confused with seborrheic dermatitis, atopic dermatitis, or tinea capitis. Diaper area psoriasis may mimic seborrheic dermatitis, eczematous diaper dermatitis, perianal streptococcal disease, or candidosis. Guttate psoriasis can be confused with viral exanthems, secondary syphilis, pityriasis rosea, pityriasis rubra pilaris, and pityriasis lichenoides chronica (PLC). Nail psoriasis must be differentiated from onychomycosis, lichen planus, and onychodystrophy.

PATHOLOGY

When the diagnosis is in doubt, histopathologic examination of an untreated lesion reveals characteristic changes of psoriasis, demonstrating hyperkeratosis, parakeratosis, acanthosis, elongated rete ridges, neutrophilic infiltrate in the epidermis, and lymphocytic infiltrate in the dermis.

TREATMENT

The therapeutic approach varies with the age of the child, type of psoriasis, sites of involvement, and extent of the disease. Physical and chemical trauma to the skin should be avoided as much as possible (see previous discussion of Koebner response).

The treatment of psoriasis should be viewed as a 4-tier process. The **1st tier** is **topical therapy.** Topical corticosteroid preparations are effective. Mid-potency or stronger topical steroids are necessary (Chapter 638). The preparation that is least potent but effective should be applied twice a day. The topical vitamin D analog calcipotriene is also effective. Calcipotriene can burn and sting, limiting its usefulness in children. One commonly used strategy is to use calcipotriene twice a day on weekdays and a high- to super-potency topical steroid twice a day on weekends. Tazarotene, a topical retinoid, is also useful. It may be used alone or in combination with other topical modalities. Tar preparation and anthralin may also be used. For scalp lesions, applications of a phenol and saline solution (e.g., Baker Cummins P & S Liquid) followed by a tar shampoo are effective in the removal of scales. A high- to super-potency corticosteroid in a foam, solution, lotion, or gel base may be applied when the scaling is diminished. Nail lesions are difficult to treat but may respond to topical tazarotene.

The **2nd tier** of therapy is **phototherapy.** Narrow-band ultraviolet B (UVB 311 nm; NB-UVB) irradiation is the primary form of UVB therapy used in childhood. It is as or nearly as effective as psoralen with UVA (PUVA), without the side effects associated with psoralen. If available, phototherapy should be used for children with extensive disease in whom topical therapy has failed. Excimer (308-nm) laser UVB irradiation may be used for localized treatment-resistant plaques. These treatments are time consuming and available only at limited locations.

The **3rd tier** is **systemic therapy.** A few children with severe psoriasis require systemic therapy. Methotrexate (0.2 to 0.4 mL/kg once a week), oral retinoids (0.3 to 1.0 mg/kg/day), and cyclosporine (3-5 mg/kg/day) are used for the rare severe and generalized forms of psoriasis. Oral retinoids may be combined with phototherapy.

The **4th tier** of therapy is the biologic response modifiers, including the tumor necrosis factor inhibitors etanercept, infliximab, and adalimumab and the T-cell function inhibitors efalizumab and alefacept. Ustekinumab, a human monoclonal antibody that prevents interactions between interleukins IL-12 and IL-23 and their cell surface receptor, has efficacy in treating moderate to severe chronic psoriasis and psoriatic arthritis.

PROGNOSIS

Prognosis is best for children with limited disease. Psoriasis is a lifelong disease characterized by remissions and exacerbations. Arthritis may be an extracutaneous complication.

BIBLIOGRAPHY

Please visit the Nelson Textbook of Pediatrics *website at* *www.expertconsult.com* *for the complete bibliography.*

649.2 Pityriasis Lichenoides

Joseph G. Morelli

Pityriasis lichenoides encompasses pityriasis lichenoides acuta (PLA; pityriasis lichenoides et varioliformis acuta [PLEVA] and Mucha-Habermann disease) and PLC. The designation of pityriasis lichenoides as acute or chronic refers to the morphologic appearance of the lesions rather than to the duration of the disease. No correlation is found between the type of lesion at the onset of the eruption and the duration of the disease. Many patients have both acute and chronic lesions simultaneously, and transition of lesions from one form into another occurs occasionally. A rare variant, acute febrile ulcernecrotic Mucha-Habermann disease, is also included in the spectrum of pityriasis lichenoides.

ETIOLOGY/PATHOGENESIS

Two main theories exist for the etiology of pityriasis lichenoides. The first is that it arises in a genetically susceptible individual from an atypical immune response to a foreign antigen. The second is that it represents a monoclonal T-cell lymphocytic proliferation on the pathway to cutaneous T-cell dyscrasia.

CLINICAL MANIFESTATIONS

Pityriasis lichenoides most commonly manifests in the second and third decades of life; 30% of cases manifest before age 20 yr.

PLC manifests as generalized, multiple, 3- to 5-mm brown-red papules that are covered by a fine grayish scale (Fig. 649-2). Lesions may be asymptomatic or may cause minimal pruritus and occasionally become vesicular, hemorrhagic, crusted, or superinfected. Individual papules become flat and brownish in 2-6 wk, ultimately leaving a hyperpigmented or hypopigmented macule. Scarring is unusual. Lesions are most common on the trunk and extremities and generally spare the face, palmoplantar surfaces, scalp, and mucous membranes.

PLA manifests as an abrupt eruption of numerous papules that have a vesiculopustular and then a purpuric center, are covered by a dark adherent crust, and are surrounded by an erythematous halo (Fig. 649-3). Constitutional symptoms such as fever, malaise, headache, and arthralgias may be present for 2-3 days after the initial outbreak. Lesions are distributed diffusely on the trunk and extremities, as in PLC. Individual lesions heal within a few

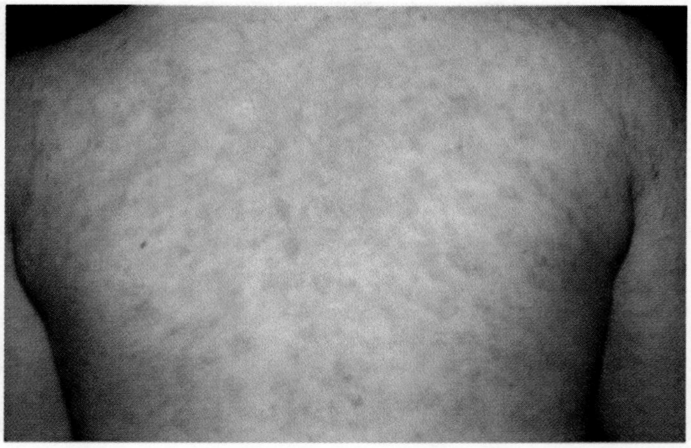

Figure 649-2 Widespread plaques with fine scale in pityriasis lichenoides chronica.

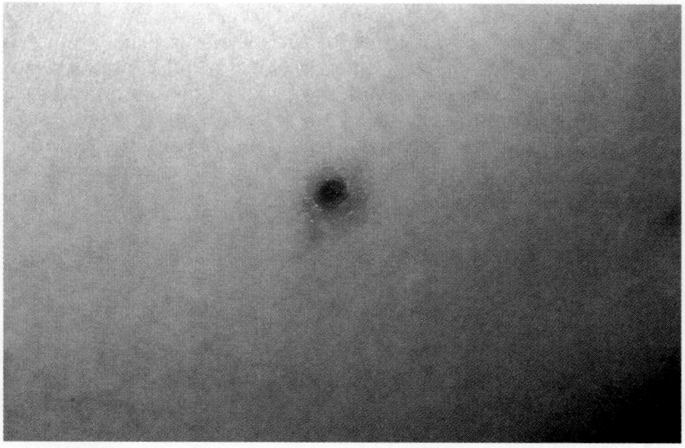

Figure 649-3 Necrotic lesion with erythematous halo in pityriasis lichenoides acuta.

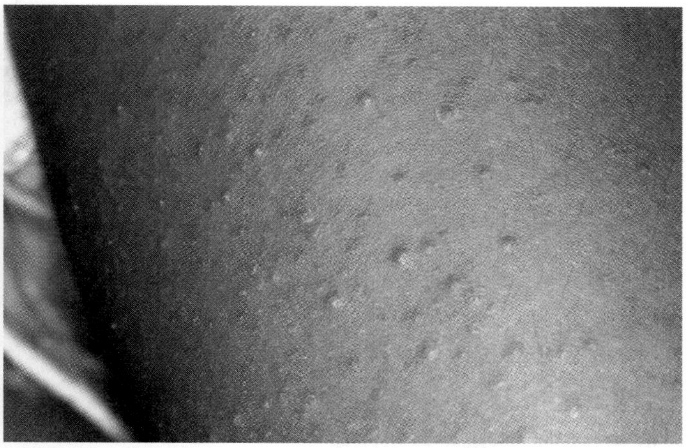

Figure 649-4 Keratotic follicular plugs with surrounding erythema in keratosis pilaris.

weeks, sometimes leaving a varioliform scar, and successive crops of papules produce the characteristic polymorphous appearance of the eruption, with lesions in various stages of evolution. The overall eruption persists for months to years.

Acute febrile ulceronecrotic Mucha-Habermann disease manifests as fever and ulceronecrotic plaques up to 1 cm in diameter, which are most common on the anterior trunk and flexors of the proximal upper extremities. Arthritis and superinfection of cutaneous lesions with *Staphylococcus aureus* may also develop. The ulceronecrotic lesions heal with hypopigmented scarring in a few weeks.

PATHOLOGY

PLC histologically shows a parakeratotic, thickened corneal layer; epidermal spongiosis; a superficial perivascular infiltrate of macrophages and predominantly CD8 lymphocytes that may extend into the epidermis; and small numbers of extravasated erythrocytes in the papillary dermis.

The histopathologic changes of PLA reflect its more severe nature. Intercellular and intracellular edema in the epidermis may lead to degeneration of keratinocytes. A dense perivascular mononuclear cell infiltrate that extends upward into the epidermis and downward into the reticular dermis, endothelial cell swelling, and extravasation of erythrocytes into the epidermis and dermis are additional characteristic features. The histology of acute febrile ulceronecrotic Mucha-Habermann disease is similar to that of PLA, with leukocytoclastic vasculitis occasionally seen.

DIFFERENTIAL DIAGNOSIS

The differential diagnosis of pityriasis lichenoides includes guttate psoriasis, pityriasis rosea, drug eruptions, secondary syphilis, viral exanthems, and lichen planus. The chronicity of pityriasis lichenoides helps preclude pityriasis rosea, viral exanthems, and some drug eruptions. A skin biopsy helps distinguish pityriasis lichenoides from other entities in the differential diagnosis.

TREATMENT

In general, pityriasis lichenoides should be considered a benign condition that does not alter the health of the child. A lubricant to remove excessive scaling may be all that is necessary if the patient is asymptomatic. Topical steroids may help the pruritus but do not alter the course of the disease. Some children may benefit from treatment with erythromycin (30-50 mg/kg/24hr for 2 mo). Natural sunlight is also helpful. NB-UVB is the **treatment of choice** for **widespread,** pruritic disease. The rare febrile ulceronecrotic form may require systemic corticosteroids, other systemic immunosuppressives or anti–tumor necrosis factor or anti–T cell biologic response modifiers.

BIBLIOGRAPHY

Please visit the Nelson Textbook of Pediatrics *website at* *www.expertconsult.com for the complete bibliography.*

649.3 Keratosis Pilaris

Joseph G. Morelli

Keratosis pilaris is a common papular eruption that may vary in extent from sparse lesions over the extensor aspects of the limbs to involvement of most of the body surface; typical areas of involvement include the upper extensor surface of the arms and the thighs, cheeks, and buttocks. The lesions may resemble gooseflesh; they are noninflammatory, scaly, follicular papules that do not coalesce. Irritation of the follicular plugs occasionally causes erythema surrounding the keratotic papules (Fig. 649-4). A subset of patients have keratosis pilaris associated with facial telangiectasia and ulerythema ophryogenes, a rare cutaneous disorder characterized by inflammatory keratotic facial papules that may result in scars, atrophy, and alopecia. Because the lesions of keratosis pilaris are associated with and accentuated by dry skin, they are often more prominent during the winter. They are more frequent in patients with atopic dermatitis and are most common during childhood and early adulthood, tending to subside in the 3rd decade of life. Mild or localized eruptions are **treated** with lubrication with a bland emollient; more pronounced or widespread lesions require regular applications of a 10-40% urea cream or an α-hydroxy acid preparation such as 12% lactic acid cream or lotion. Therapy may improve the condition but does not cure it.

BIBLIOGRAPHY

Please visit the Nelson Textbook of Pediatrics *website at* *www.expertconsult.com for the complete bibliography.*

649.4 Lichen Spinulosus

Joseph G. Morelli

Lichen spinulosus is an uncommon disorder that occurs principally in children and more frequently in boys. The cause is unknown. The lesions consist of sharply circumscribed irregular plaques of spiny, keratinous projections that protrude from the orifices of the pilosebaceous canals. Plaques may occur anywhere on the body and are often distributed symmetrically on the trunk, elbows, knees, and extensor surfaces of the limbs. Although sometimes erythematous, the lesions are usually skin colored. They are readily palpable and represent keratotic follicular plugs. Lichen spinulosus is easily differentiated from keratosis pilaris because the latter lesions are never grouped to form plaques. More commonly, lichen spinulosus is confused with papular eczema.

Treatment is usually unnecessary. For patients who regard the eruption as a cosmetic defect, urea-containing lubricants (10-40%) are often effective in flattening the projections. Tretinoin gel and hydroactive adhesives may also be used. The plaques usually disappear spontaneously after several months or years.

BIBLIOGRAPHY

Please visit the Nelson Textbook of Pediatrics *website at www.expertconsult.com for the complete bibliography.*

649.5 Pityriasis Rosea

Joseph G. Morelli

ETIOLOGY/PATHOGENESIS

The cause of pityriasis rosea is unknown; a viral agent is suspected, and there is debate over the role of human herpesviruses 6 and 7 in this condition.

CLINICAL MANIFESTATIONS

This benign, common eruption occurs most frequently in children and young adults. Although a prodrome of fever, malaise, arthralgia, and pharyngitis may precede the eruption, children rarely complain of such symptoms. A **herald patch**, a solitary, round or oval lesion that may occur anywhere on the body and is often but not always identifiable from its large size, usually precedes the generalized eruption. Herald patches vary from 1 to 10 cm in diameter; they are annular in configuration and have a raised border with fine, adherent scales. Approximately 5-10 days after the appearance of the herald patch, a widespread, symmetric eruption involving mainly the trunk and proximal limbs becomes evident (Fig. 649-5). When the disease is extensive, the face, scalp, and distal limbs may be involved; in the inverse form of pityriasis rosea, only those sites may be affected. Lesions may appear in crops for several days. Typical lesions are oval or round, <1 cm in diameter, slightly raised, and pink to brown. The developed lesion is covered by a fine scale, which gives the skin a crinkly appearance. Some lesions clear centrally and produce a collarette of scale that is attached only at the periphery. Papular, vesicular, urticarial, hemorrhagic, and large annular lesions are unusual variants. The long axis of each lesion is usually aligned with the cutaneous cleavage lines, a feature that creates the so-called **Christmas tree pattern** on the back. Conformation to skin lines is often more discernible in the anterior and posterior axillary folds and supraclavicular areas. Duration of the eruption varies from 2 to 12 wk. The lesions may be asymptomatic or mildly to severely pruritic.

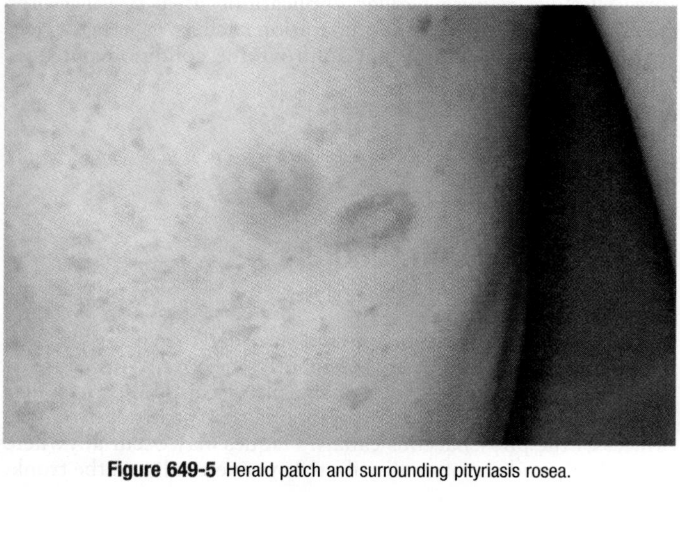

Figure 649-5 Herald patch and surrounding pityriasis rosea.

DIFFERENTIAL DIAGNOSIS

The herald patch may be mistaken for tinea corporis, a pitfall that can be avoided if microscopic evaluation of a potassium hydroxide preparation of scrapings of the lesion is performed. The generalized eruption resembles a number of other diseases; secondary syphilis is the most important. Drug eruptions, viral exanthems, guttate psoriasis, PLC, and nummular dermatitis can also be confused with pityriasis rosea.

TREATMENT

Therapy is unnecessary for asymptomatic patients with pityriasis rosea. If scaling is prominent, a bland emollient may suffice. Pruritus may be suppressed by a lubricating lotion containing menthol and camphor or by an oral antihistamine for sedation, particularly at night, when itching may be troublesome. Occasionally, a mid-potency topical corticosteroid preparation may be necessary to alleviate pruritus. After the eruption has resolved, postinflammatory hypopigmentation or hyperpigmentation may be pronounced, particularly in dark-skinned patients. These changes disappear in subsequent weeks to months.

BIBLIOGRAPHY

Please visit the Nelson Textbook of Pediatrics *website at www.expertconsult.com for the complete bibliography.*

649.6 Pityriasis Rubra Pilaris

Joseph G. Morelli

ETIOLOGY

The cause of pityriasis rubra pilaris is unknown. Although a genetic form with autosomal dominant transmission may account for some cases in childhood, most cases are sporadic.

CLINICAL MANIFESTATIONS

This rare chronic dermatosis often has an insidious onset with diffuse scaling and erythema of the scalp, which is indistinguishable from the findings in seborrheic dermatitis, and with thick hyperkeratosis of the palms and soles (Fig. 649-6A). Lesions over the elbows and knees are also common (Fig. 649-6B). The characteristic primary lesion is a firm, dome-shaped, tiny, acuminate papule, which is pink to red and has a central keratotic plug pierced by a vellus hair. Masses of these papules coalesce to form large, erythematous, sharply demarcated orangish plaques, within which islands of normal skin can be distinguished, creating a bizarre effect. Typical papules on the dorsum of the proximal phalanges are readily palpated. Gray plaques or papules resembling lichen planus may be found in the oral cavity. Dystrophic changes in the nails may occur and mimic those of psoriasis.

DIFFERENTIAL DIAGNOSIS

Differential diagnosis includes ichthyosis, seborrheic dermatitis, keratoderma of the palms and soles, and psoriasis.

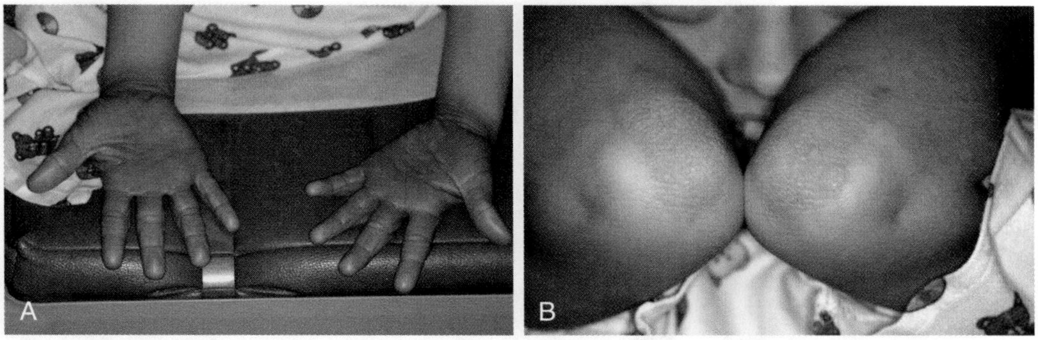

Figure 649-6 Pityriasis rubra pilaris, *A,* Orange palmar hyperkeratosis. *B,* Elbow lesions.

HISTOLOGY

Skin biopsy revealing follicular plugging, parakeratotic, perifollicular shoulder, and checkerboard pattern of orthokeratosis and hypogranulosis may differentiate this condition from psoriasis and seborrheic dermatitis.

TREATMENT

The numerous therapeutic regimens recommended are difficult to evaluate because pityriasis rubra pilaris has a capricious course with exacerbations and remissions. Lubrication alone is useful in mild cases. Topical and oral retinoids (1 mg/kg/day) have been used most frequently. In childhood, the prognosis for eventual resolution is relatively good.

BIBLIOGRAPHY

Please visit the Nelson Textbook of Pediatrics *website at www.expertconsult.com for the complete bibliography.*

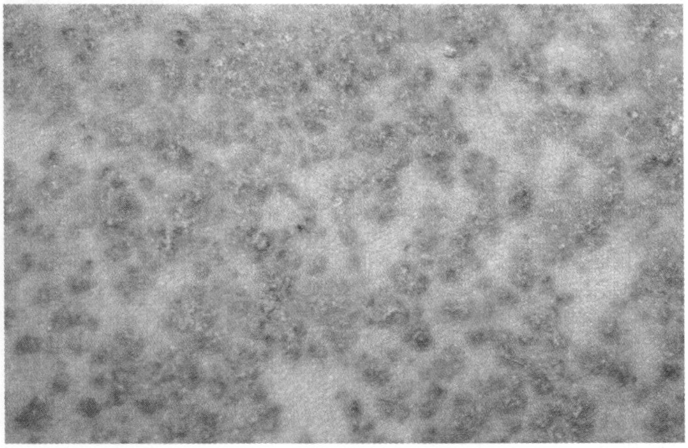

Figure 649-7 Papules coalescing into large plaque on the back of a patient with Darier disease.

649.7 Darier Disease (Keratosis Follicularis)

Joseph G. Morelli

ETIOLOGY

A rare genetic disorder, Darier disease is inherited as an autosomal dominant trait (*ATP2A2* gene).

CLINICAL MANIFESTATIONS

Onset usually occurs in late childhood. Typical lesions are small, firm, skin-colored papules that are not always follicular in location. The lesions eventually acquire yellow malodorous crusts; coalesce to form large, gray-brown, vegetative plaques (Fig. 649-7); and usually involve the face, neck, shoulders, chest, back, and limb flexures in a symmetric distribution. Papules, fissures, crusts, and ulcers may appear on the mucous membranes of the lips, tongue, buccal mucosa, pharynx, larynx, and vulva. Hyperkeratosis of the palms and soles and nail dystrophy with subungual hyperkeratosis are variable features. Severe pruritus, secondary infection, offensive odor, and aggravation of the dermatosis on exposure to sunlight may occur.

HISTOLOGY

Histologic changes seen in Darier disease are diagnostic: hyperkeratosis, intraepidermal separation with formation of suprabasal clefts, and dyskeratotic epidermal cells are characteristic features.

DIFFERENTIAL DIAGNOSIS

Darier disease is most likely to be confused with seborrheic dermatitis or flat warts.

TREATMENT

Treatment is nonspecific. Some cases respond to topical retinoic acid, with or without occlusive dressings. Severe disease may be controlled with oral retinoids (1 mg/kg/day). Secondary infection may require local cleansing and systemically administered antibiotics. Affected individuals usually suffer more during the summer.

BIBLIOGRAPHY

Please visit the Nelson Textbook of Pediatrics *website at www.expertconsult.com for the complete bibliography.*

649.8 Lichen Nitidus

Joseph G. Morelli

ETIOLOGY

The etiology of lichen nitidus is unknown.

CLINICAL MANIFESTATIONS

This chronic, benign, papular eruption is characterized by minute (1-2 mm), flat-topped, shiny, firm papules of uniform size. The papules are most often skin colored but may be pink or red. In

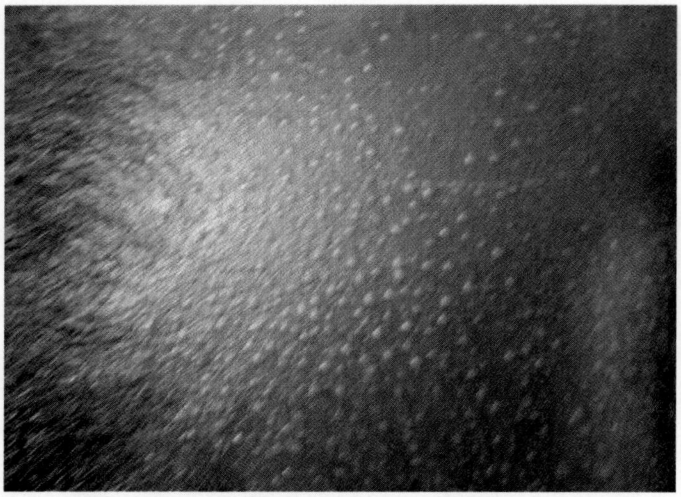

Figure 649-8 Slightly hypopigmented, uniform papules of lichen nitidus.

black individuals, they are usually hypopigmented (Fig. 649-8). Sites of predilection are the genitals, abdomen, chest, forearms, wrists, and inner aspects of the thighs. The lesions may be sparse or numerous and may form large plaques; careful examination usually discloses linear papules in a line of scratch (Koebner phenomenon), a valuable clue to the diagnosis because it occurs in only a few diseases. Lichen nitidus occurs in all age groups. The cause is unknown. Patients with lichen nitidus are usually asymptomatic and constitutionally well, although pruritus may be severe. The lesions may be confused with those of lichen planus and rarely coexist with them.

DIFFERENTIAL DIAGNOSIS

Widespread keratosis pilaris can also be confused with lichen nitidus, but the follicular localization of the papules and the absence of Koebner phenomenon in the former distinguish them. Verruca plana (flat warts) if small and uniform in size may occasionally resemble lichen nitidus.

HISTOLOGY

Although the diagnosis can be made clinically, a biopsy is occasionally indicated. The lichen nitidus papule consists of sharply circumscribed nests of lymphocytes and histiocytes in the upper dermis enclosed by clawlike epidermal rete ridges.

TREATMENT

The course of lichen nitidus spans months to years, but the lesions eventually involute completely. Mid- to high-potency topical steroids may be effective treatment, especially for pruritus.

BIBLIOGRAPHY

Please visit the Nelson Textbook of Pediatrics *website at www.expertconsult.com for the complete bibliography.*

649.9 Lichen Striatus

Joseph G. Morelli

ETIOLOGY

The cause and explanation for the linear distribution of lichen striatus are unknown.

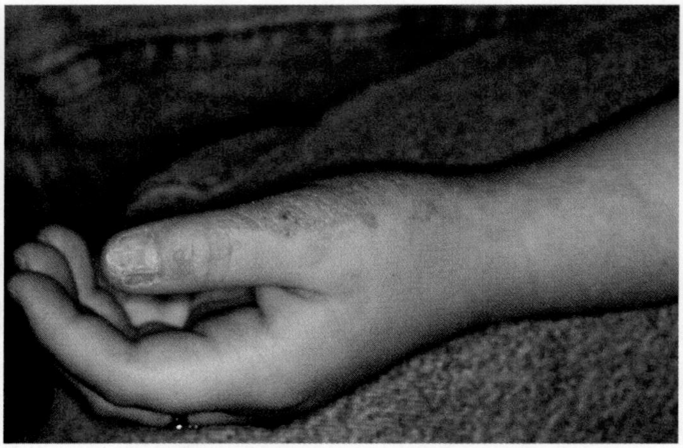

Figure 649-9 Lichen striatus with nail dystrophy.

CLINICAL MANIFESTATIONS

A benign, self-limited eruption, lichen striatus consists of a continuous or discontinuous linear band of papules in a Blaschkoid distribution. The primary lesion is a flat-topped, red to violaceous papule covered with fine scale. Aggregates of these papules form multiple bands or plaques. In black patients, the lesions may be hypopigmented. The eruption evolves over a period of days or weeks in an otherwise healthy child, remains stationary for weeks to months, and finally remits without sequelae usually within 2 years. Symptoms are usually absent, although some children complain of itching. Nail dystrophy may occur when the eruption involves the posterior nail fold and matrix (Fig. 649-9).

DIFFERENTIAL DIAGNOSIS

Lichen striatus is occasionally confused with other disorders. The initial plaque may resemble papular eczema or lichen nitidus until the linear configuration becomes apparent. Linear lichen planus and linear psoriasis are usually associated with typical individual lesions elsewhere on the body. Linear epidermal nevi are permanent lesions that often become more hyperkeratotic and hyperpigmented than those of lichen striatus.

TREATMENT

A mid-potency topical corticosteroid preparation provides sufficient relief when pruritus is a problem in a patient with lichen striatus.

BIBLIOGRAPHY

Please visit the Nelson Textbook of Pediatrics *website at www.expertconsult.com for the complete bibliography.*

649.10 Lichen Planus

Joseph G. Morelli

ETIOLOGY

Lichen planus is the result of an attack on the skin by cytotoxic T cells. The cause is unknown, but granzyme B and granulysin are markedly increased in skin involved with lichen planus.

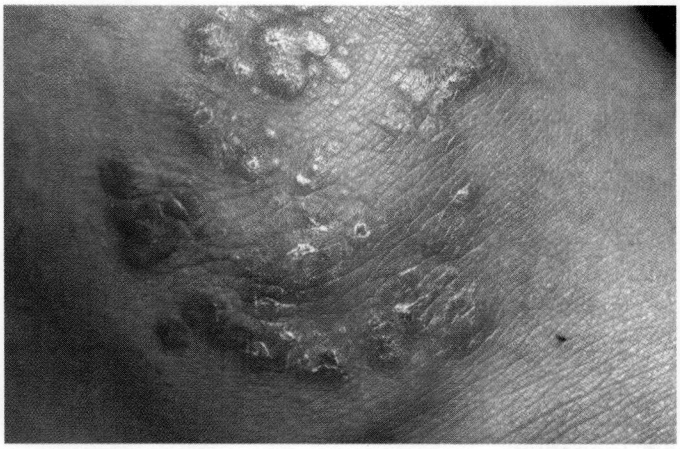

Figure 649-10 Flat-topped, purple polygonal papules of lichen planus.

CLINICAL MANIFESTATIONS

This is a rare disorder in young children and uncommon in older ones. It is more often seen in children from the Indian subcontinent. The primary lesion is a violaceous, sharply demarcated, polygonal papule with fine lines or thin white scales on the surface. Papules may coalesce to form large plaques (Fig. 649-10). The papules are intensely pruritic, and additional papules are often induced by scratching (Koebner phenomenon) so that lines of them are often detected. Sites of predilection are the flexor surfaces of the wrists, the forearms, and the inner aspects of the thighs. Characteristic lesions of mucous membranes consist of pinhead-sized white papules that coalesce to form reticulated and lacy patterns on the oral mucosa and sometimes on the lips and tongue.

Acute eruptive lichen planus is probably the most common form in children. The lesions erupt in an explosive fashion, much like a viral exanthem, and spread to involve most of the body surface. Hypertrophic, linear, bullous, atrophic, annular, follicular, erosive, and ulcerative forms of lichen planus may also occur. Nail involvement may develop in the chronic forms but is rarely evident in children. The disorder may persist for months to years, but the acute eruptive form is most likely to involute permanently. Intense hyperpigmentation frequently persists for a long time after the resolution of lesions.

HISTOLOGY

The histopathologic findings in lichen planus are specific, consisting of irregular acanthosis, wedge-shaped hypergranulosis, and basal cell degeneration with a bandlike lymphocytic infiltrate at the epidermal-dermal junction. Pigment incontinence is frequently seen. Biopsy is indicated if the diagnosis is unclear.

TREATMENT

Treatment is directed at alleviation of the intense pruritus and amelioration of the skin lesions. Oral antihistamines are often helpful. The skin lesions respond best to regular applications of a high potency topical corticosteroid preparation. Rarely, systemic corticosteroid therapy is necessary to gain control of widespread, intractable lesions. Phototherapy has also been used for extensive disease.

BIBLIOGRAPHY

Please visit the Nelson Textbook of Pediatrics *website at* *www.expertconsult.com* *for the complete bibliography.*

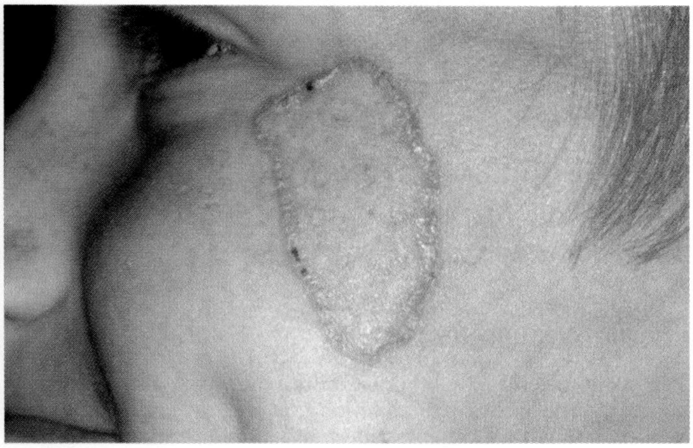

Figure 649-11 Large plaque of porokeratosis of Mibelli with raised border and depressed center.

649.11 Porokeratosis

Joseph G. Morelli

ETIOLOGY

Porokeratosis is a disorder of epidermal keratinization. The etiology is unknown except for the disseminated actinic form, which is secondary to chronic sun exposure.

CLINICAL MANIFESTATIONS

Porokeratosis is a rare, chronic, progressive disease. Several forms have been delineated: solitary plaques, linear porokeratosis, hyperkeratotic lesions of the palms and soles, disseminated eruptive lesions, and superficial actinic porokeratosis. Other types of porokeratosis are more common in males and begin in childhood. Sites of predilection are the limbs, face, neck, and genitals. The primary lesion is a small, keratotic papule that enlarges peripherally so that the center becomes depressed, with the edge forming an elevated wall or collar (Fig. 649-11). The configuration of the plaque may be round, oval, or gyrate. The elevated border is split by a thin groove from which minute cornified projections protrude. The enclosed central area is yellow, gray, or tan and sclerotic, smooth, and dry, whereas the hyperkeratotic border is a darker gray, brown, or black. The disease is slowly progressive but relatively asymptomatic. Malignant degeneration to **squamous cell carcinoma** has been reported in long-standing cases.

HISTOLOGY

A skin biopsy discloses the characteristic cornoid lamella (plug of stratum corneum cells with retained nuclei), which is responsible for the invariable linear ridge of the lesion.

DIFFERENTIAL DIAGNOSIS

The differential diagnosis of porokeratosis includes warts, epidermal nevi, lichen planus, granuloma annulare, and elastosis perforans serpiginosa.

TREATMENT

No treatment is uniformly successful. Treatments with liquid nitrogen, laser, topical retinoids, 5-fluorouracil (5-FU), and the immune response modifier imiquimod have been employed.

BIBLIOGRAPHY
Please visit the Nelson Textbook of Pediatrics *website at www.expertconsult.com for the complete bibliography.*

649.12 Papular Acrodermatitis of Childhood (Gianotti-Crosti Syndrome)

Joseph G. Morelli

ETIOLOGY/PATHOGENESIS

The pathogenesis of Gianotti-Crosti syndrome, also known as papular acrodermatitis of childhood, is unclear, but an immunologic reaction to viral infections and immunizations has been postulated. In an Italian cohort, this eruption was initially associated with primary liver infection by hepatitis B virus. The disease is usually benign and, in the USA, is rarely associated with hepatitis. This eruption has been seen in children after immunizations (hepatitis A, others) and in patients infected with Epstein-Barr virus (most common association), coxsackievirus A16, parainfluenza virus, and other viral infections.

CLINICAL MANIFESTATIONS

This distinctive eruption is occasionally associated with malaise and low-grade fever but few other constitutional symptoms. The incidence peaks in early childhood. Occurrences are usually sporadic, but epidemics have been recorded. The skin lesion is a monomorphous, usually nonpruritic, flat-topped, firm, dusky, or coppery red papule ranging in size from 1 to 10 mm (Fig. 649-12), although there is considerable variation in lesion type between patients. The papules appear in crops and may become profuse but remain discrete, forming a symmetric eruption on the face, buttocks, and limbs, including the palms and soles. The papules often have the appearance of vesicles; when opened, however, no fluid is obtained. The papules sometimes become hemorrhagic. Lines of papules (**Koebner phenomenon**) may be noted on the extremities. The trunk is relatively spared, as are the scalp and mucous membranes. Generalized lymphadenopathy and hepatomegaly (in patients with hepatitis B viremia) constitute the only other abnormal physical findings. The eruption resolves spontaneously in 15-60 days. Lymphadenopathy and hepatomegaly, if present, may persist for several months. Elevation of serum transaminase and alkaline phosphatase values without concomitant hyperbilirubinemia is usual.

HISTOLOGY

Skin biopsy in Gianotti-Crosti syndrome is not specific, being characterized by a perivascular mononuclear cell infiltrate and capillary endothelial swelling.

DIFFERENTIAL DIAGNOSIS

Papular acrodermatitis can be confused with lichen planus, erythema multiforme, histiocytosis X, and Henoch-Schönlein purpura.

TREATMENT

The lesions resolve spontaneously, and pruritus may be relieved by a mid-potency topical steroid.

BIBLIOGRAPHY
Please visit the Nelson Textbook of Pediatrics *website at www.expertconsult.com for the complete bibliography.*

649.13 Acanthosis Nigricans

Joseph G. Morelli

See also Chapter 44.

ETIOLOGY

The skin lesions of acanthosis nigricans appear to be a manifestation of insulin resistance or mutations in fibroblast growth factor receptor genes. The clinical severity and histopathologic features of acanthosis nigricans correlate positively with the degree of hyperinsulinism. Insulin resistance with compensatory hyperinsulinism may lead to insulin binding to and activation of insulin-like growth factor receptors, promoting epidermal growth. In the paraneoplastic form in adults, tumor-secreted growth factors and resultant hyperinsulinemia may be the proximate etiology of acanthosis nigricans. In familial cases, acanthosis nigricans is inherited as an autosomal dominant trait.

CLINICAL MANIFESTATIONS

Acanthosis nigricans is characterized by hyperpigmented velvety, hyperkeratotic, plaques that are most often localized to the neck, axillae (Fig. 649-13), inframammary areas, groin, inner thighs, and anogenital region. Acanthosis nigricans has classically been associated with obesity; drugs such as nicotinic acid;

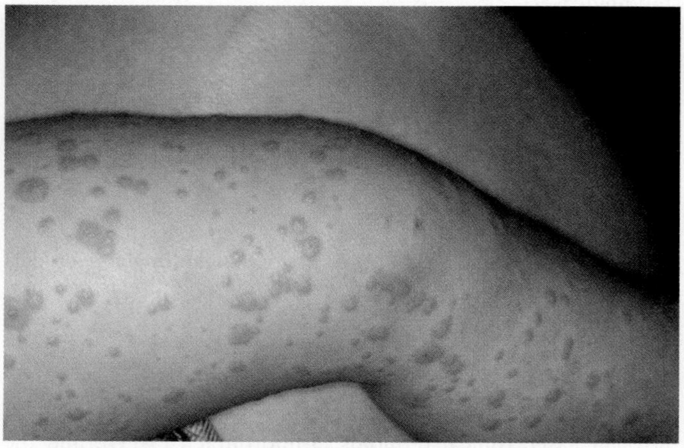

Figure 649-12 Numerous, flat-topped, red papules in Gianotti-Crosti syndrome.

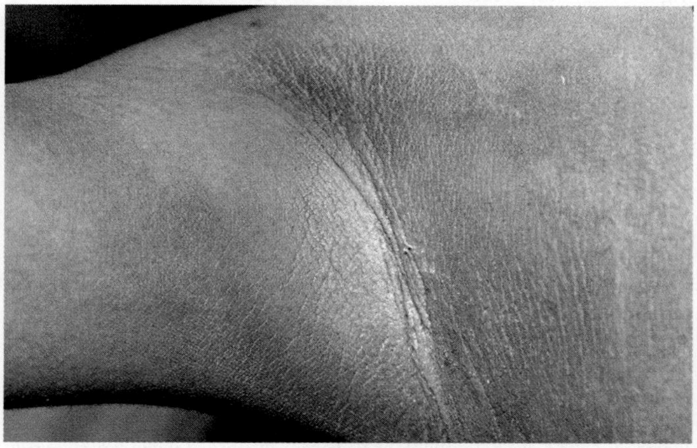

Figure 649-13 Velvety hyperpigmentation of the axilla in acanthosis nigricans.

endocrinopathies, most commonly, diabetes mellitus and hyperandrogenic or hypogonadal syndromes; and genetic disorders caused by mutation in fibroblast growth factor receptor genes. Acanthosis nigricans is found more commonly in African-American and Hispanic children. It is seen in >60% of children with a body mass index >98%. Although acanthosis nigricans is associated with malignancy in adults, this is rare in childhood.

HISTOLOGY

The histologic changes are those of papillomatosis and hyperkeratosis rather than acanthosis or excessive pigment formation.

TREATMENT

This skin disorder is extremely difficult to treat but may be improved by palliation of the underlying disorder. Acanthosis nigricans in the obese child is associated with risk factors for glucose homeostasis abnormalities, and counseling families on its causes and consequences may motivate them to make healthy lifestyle changes that can decrease the risk for development of cardiac disease and diabetes mellitus. In children with obesity-related acanthosis nigricans, weight loss should be the primary goal. In all children with acanthosis nigricans, treatment with 40% urea cream may be helpful.

BIBLIOGRAPHY

Please visit the Nelson Textbook of Pediatrics *website at* *www.expertconsult.com* *for the complete bibliography.*

Chapter 650 Disorders of Keratinization

Joseph G. Morelli

DISORDERS OF CORNIFICATION

Disorders of cornification (**ichthyoses**) are a primary group of inherited conditions characterized clinically by patterns of scaling and histopathologically by hyperkeratosis. They are usually distinguishable on the basis of inheritance patterns, clinical features, associated defects, and histopathologic changes (Table 650-1).

Harlequin Ichthyosis

ETIOLOGY/PATHOGENESIS Harlequin ichthyosis is caused by mutations in the *ABCA12* gene. Mutation in the gene leads to defective lipid transport and *ABCA12* activity is required for the generation of long-chain ceramides that are essential for the development of the normal skin barrier.

CLINICAL MANIFESTATIONS At birth, markedly thickened, ridged, and cracked skin forms horny plates over the entire body, disfiguring the facial features and constricting the digits. Severe ectropion and chemosis obscure the orbits, the nose and ears are flattened, and the lips are everted and gaping. Nails and hair may be absent. Joint mobility is restricted, and the hands and feet appear fixed and ischemic. Affected neonates have respiratory difficulty, suck poorly, and are subject to severe cutaneous infection. Most die within the first days to weeks of life, but patients occasionally survive beyond infancy and have severe ichthyosis usually resembling lamellar ichthyosis or congenital ichthyosiform erythroderma.

HISTOLOGY Common morphologic abnormalities include hyperkeratosis, accumulation of lipid droplets within corneocytes, and absence of normal lamellar granules.

TREATMENT Initial treatment includes high fluid intake to avoid dehydration from transepidermal water loss and use of a humidified heated incubator, emulsifying ointments, careful attention to hygiene, and oral retinoids (1 mg/kg/day). Prenatal diagnosis has been accomplished by fetoscopy, fetal skin biopsy, and microscopic examination of cells from amniotic fluid.

Collodion Baby

ETIOLOGY Collodion baby is not a single entity but a newborn phenotype that is most often seen in babies who will eventually demonstrate lamellar ichthyosis or congenital ichthyosiform erythroderma. Less commonly, collodion babies evolve into babies with other forms of ichthyosis or Gaucher disease. A small subset become otherwise healthy babies without chronic skin disease.

CLINICAL MANIFESTATIONS Collodion babies are covered at birth by a thick, taut membrane resembling oiled parchment or collodion (Fig. 650-1), which is subsequently shed. Affected neonates have ectropion, flattening of the ears and nose, and fixation of the lips in an O-shaped configuration. Hair may be absent or may perforate the abnormal covering. The membrane cracks with initial respiratory efforts and, shortly after birth, begins to desquamate in large sheets. Complete shedding may take several weeks, and a new membrane may occasionally form in localized areas.

Neonatal morbidity and mortality may be due to cutaneous infection, aspiration pneumonia (squamous material), hypothermia, or hypernatremic dehydration from excessive transcutaneous fluid losses as a result of increased skin permeability. The outcome is uncertain, and accurate prognosis is impossible with respect to the subsequent development of ichthyosis.

HISTOLOGY Biopsy reveals a thickened stratum corneum with compact orthokeratotic hyperkeratosis.

TREATMENT A high-humidity environment and application of nonocclusive lubricants facilitates shedding of the membrane.

Lamellar Ichthyosis and Congenital Ichthyosiform Erythroderma (Nonbullous Congenital Ichthyosiform Erythroderma)

Lamellar ichthyosis and congenital ichthyosiform erythroderma (nonbullous congenital ichthyosiform erythroderma) are the most common types of autosomal recessively inherited ichthyosis. Both forms are present soon or shortly after birth. Most infants with these forms of ichthyosis present with erythroderma and scaling; but among collodion babies, most turn out to have one of these ichthyosis variants.

ETIOLOGY/PATHOGENESIS Three genes have been identified that cause **lamellar ichthyosis** (LI). These are *LI1* (*TGM1*), *LI2* (*ABCA12*), and *LI3* (*CYP4F22*). Other genes have also been linked to LI, but they have not yet been identified. Transglutaminase mutations lead to abnormalities in the cornified envelope, whereas defects in *ABCA12* cause abnormal lipid transport and those in *CYP4F22* produce abnormal lamellar granules.

Three mutations have also been identified as the causes of **congenital ichthyosiform** erythroderma. These are *TGM1*, *ALOX12B*, and *ALOX3*. The *ALOX* genes encode for lipoxygenases the function of which is not definitively known. These lipoxygenases are likely to play a role in epidermal barrier formation by affecting lipid metabolism.

Mutations in the gene encoding ichthyn may cause either lamellar ichthyosis or congenital ichthyosiform erythroderma. The function of icthyn is unknown.

CLINICAL MANIFESTATIONS After shedding of the collodion membrane, if present, lamellar ichthyosis evolves into large, quadrilateral, dark scales that are free at the edges and adherent at the center. Scaling is often pronounced and involves the entire body surface, including flexural surfaces (Fig. 650-2). The face is often markedly involved, including ectropion and small, crumpled ears. The palms and soles are generally hyperkeratotic. The hair may be sparse and fine, but the teeth and mucosal surfaces are normal. Unlike in congenital ichthyosiform erythroderma, there is little erythema.

Table 650-1 DISORDERS OF CORNIFICATION THAT USUALLY MANIFEST IN THE FIRST WEEKS OF LIFE

DISORDER	INHERITANCE	CLINICAL FEATURES	MUTATION	VISUAL METHOD OF DIAGNOSIS
Harlequin ichthyosis	AR	Thick, armor-like scale with fissuring	ABCA12	Clinical
Collodion baby	Usually AR	Shiny collodion membrane	Various	Clinical
Recessive X-linked ichthyosis	Recessive X-linked	Collodion membrane May have genital anomalies	Steroid sulfatase	Plasma cholesterol sulfate
Lamellar ichthyosis	Usually AR	Collodion membrane	Transglutaminase I	Clinical
			ABCA12	
			CYP4F22	
Congenital ichthyosiform erythroderma	AR	Collodion membrane	Transglutaminase 1	Clinical
			ALOX12B	
			ALOXE3	
Epidermolytic hyperkeratosis	AD	Scaling and blistering	Keratins 1, 10, 2e	Clinical and histologic
Ichthyosis hystrix	AD	Plaques of hyperkeratosis	Keratin 1, GJB2	Clinical
Familial peeling skin	AR	Superficial peeling	Unknown	Clinical and histologic
Sjögren-Larsson syndrome	AR	Variable skin thickening	FAD	Clinical and fibroblast cultures for FAD
		Mental, developmental retardation		
		Spastic diplegia		
		Seizures		
		"Glistening dots"		
Neutral lipid storage disease	AR	Collodion membrane or ichthyosiform erythroderma	CGI58	Blood smear for vacuolated polymorphonuclear leukocytes
Netherton syndrome	AR	Ichthyosiform erythroderma	*SPINK 5*	Clinical; hair exam later in infancy
		Scant hair, often failure to thrive	Unknown	Clinical and hair microscopy; hair sulfur content
Trichothiodystrophy	AR	Collodion membrane	XPB	
		Broken hair	XPD	
KID (keratitis with ichthyosis and deafness) syndrome	May be AD, AR	Erythrokeratodermatous or thick, leathery skin with stippled papules	GJB2	Clinical; auditory evoked potentials
CHILD (congenital hemidysplasia with ichthyosiform erythroderma and limb defects) syndrome	X-linked dominant	Alopecia	NSDHL	Clinical
		Unilateral waxy yellow, scaling		
		Hemidysplasia		
		Limb defects		
Conradi-Hünermann syndrome	X-linked dominant	Thick, psoriasiform scale over erythroderma, patterned along Blaschko lines	ARSE	Clinical
		Proximal limb shortening		
Ichthyosis follicularis	Usually X-linked recessive	Prominent follicular hyperkeratoses	MBTPS2	Clinical
		Alopecia		
		Photophobia		
CHIME (colobomas of the eyes, heart defects, ichthyosiform dermatosis, mental retardation, and ear abnormalities) syndrome	AR	Ichthyotic erythematous plaques	Unknown	Clinical
		Cardiac defects; typical facies		
		Retinal colobomas		
Gaucher disease	AR	Collodion membrane	β-Glucocerebrosidase	Clinical; fibroblast cultures
		Hepatosplenomegaly		

AD, autosomal dominant; AR, autosomal recessive.; FAD, fatty aldehyde
From Eichenfield LF, Frieden IJ, Esterly NB: *Textbook of neonatal dermatology*, Philadephia, 2001, WB Saunders, p 277.

In congenital ichthyosiform erythroderma, erythroderma tends to be persistent, and scales, although they are generalized, are finer and whiter than in lamellar ichthyosis (Fig. 650-3). Hyperkeratosis is particularly noticeable around the knees, elbows, and ankles. Palms and soles are uniformly hyperkeratotic. Patients have sparse hair, cicatricial alopecia, and nail dystrophy. Neither form includes blistering.

HISTOLOGY A markedly thickened stratum corneum and mild, irregular epidermal thickening characterize lamellar ichthyosis. Congenital ichthyosiform erythroderma involves more epidermal thickening with parakeratosis but less hyperkeratosis and hypergranulosis than in lamellar ichthyosis.

TREATMENT Pruritus may be severe and responds minimally to antipruritic therapy. The unattractive appearance of the child and the bad odor from bacterial colonization of macerated scales may create serious psychological problems. A high-humidity environment in winter and air conditioning in summer reduce discomfort. Generous and frequent applications of emollients and keratolytic agents such as lactic or glycolic acid (5-12%), urea (10-40%), tazarotene (0.1% gel), and retinoic acid (0.1% cream) may lessen the scaling to some extent, although these agents produce stinging if applied to fissured skin. Oral retinoids (1 mg/kg/day) have a beneficial effect in these conditions but do not alter the underlying defect and, therefore, must be administered indefinitely. The long-term risks of these compounds (teratogenic effects and toxicity to bone) may limit their usefulness. Ectropion requires ophthalmologic care and, at times, plastic surgical procedures.

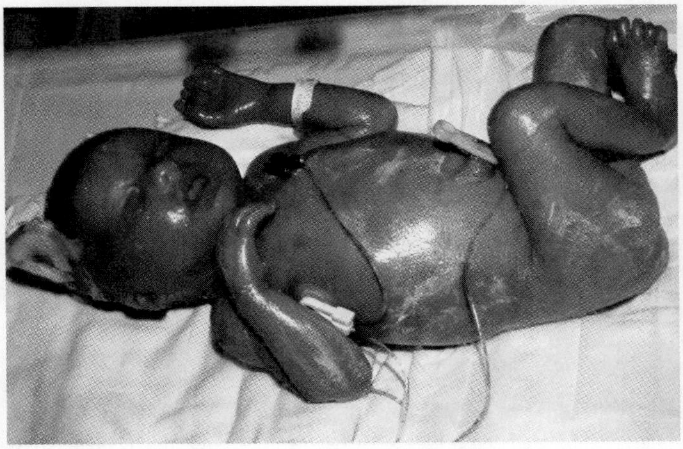

Figure 650-1 Typical appearance of a collodion baby.

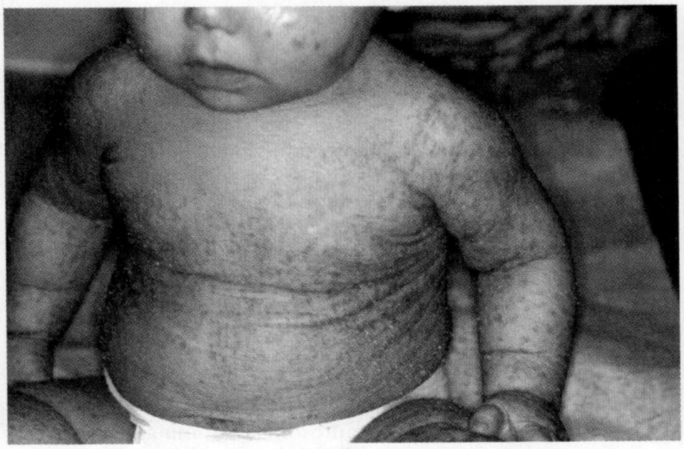

Figure 650-2 Generalized scaling of lamellar ichthyosis.

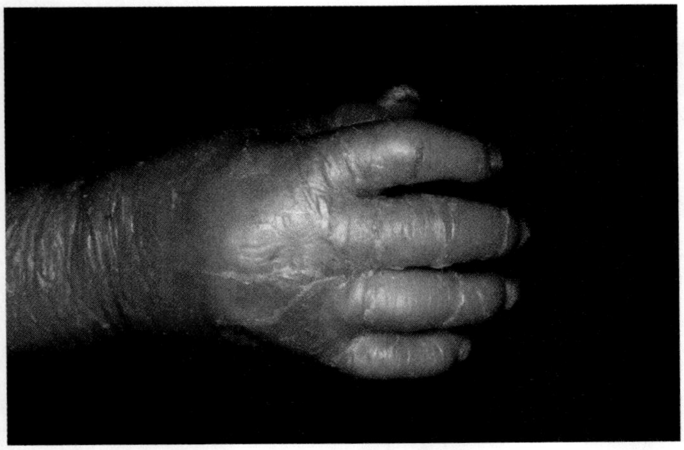

Figure 650-3 Prominent erythema and scale in congenital ichthyosiform erythroderma.

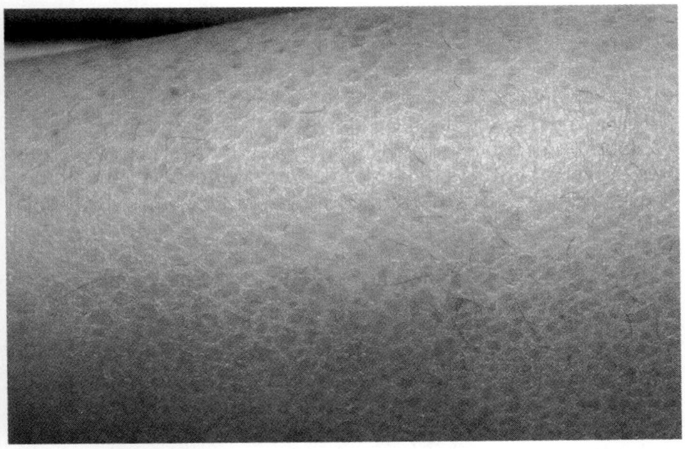

Figure 650-4 Scale over the shin in ichthyosis vulgaris.

Ichthyosis Vulgaris

ETIOLOGY/PATHOGENESIS Autosomal dominant or recessive mutations in the filaggrin gene cause ichthyosis vulgaris. Filaggrin is a filament-aggregating protein that assembles the keratin filament cytoskeleton, causing collapse of the granular cells into classic flattened squamous cell shape. Mutations in filaggrin lead to absence or marked reductions in keratohyalin granules.

CLINICAL MANIFESTATIONS Ichthyosis vulgaris is the **most common** of the disorders of keratinization, with an incidence of 1/250 live births. Onset generally occurs in the 1st yr of life. In most cases, it is trivial, consisting only of slight roughening of the skin surface. Scaling is most prominent on the extensor aspects of the extremities, particularly the legs (Fig. 650-4). Flexural surfaces are spared, and the abdomen, neck, and face are relatively uninvolved. Keratosis pilaris, particularly on the upper arms and thighs, accentuated markings, and hyperkeratosis on the palms and soles, and atopy are relatively common. Scaling is most pronounced during the winter months and may abate completely during warm weather. There is no accompanying disorder of hair, teeth, mucosal surfaces, or other organ systems.

HISTOLOGY The histopathologic changes in ichthyosis vulgaris differ from those of other types of ichthyosis in that the hyperkeratosis is associated with a decrease or absence of the granular layer. Abnormally small and crumbly keratohyalin granules are found in epidermal cells on electron microscopy.

TREATMENT Scaling may be diminished by daily applications of an emollient or a lubricant containing urea (10-40%), salicylic acid, or an α-hydroxy acid such as lactic acid (5-12%).

X-Linked Ichthyosis

ETIOLOGY/PATHOGENESIS X-linked ichthyosis involves a deficiency of steroid sulfatase, which hydrolyzes cholesterol sulfate and other sulfated steroids to cholesterol. Cholesterol sulfate accumulates in the stratum corneum and plasma. In the epidermis this accumulation causes malformation of intercellular lipid layers, leading to barrier defects and delay of corneodesmosome degradation, resulting in corneocyte retention.

CLINICAL MANIFESTATIONS Skin peeling may be present at birth but typically begins at 3-6 mo of life. Scaling is most pronounced on the sides of the neck, lower face, preauricular areas, anterior trunk, and the limbs, particularly the legs. The elbow (Fig. 650-5) and knee flexures are generally spared but may be mildly involved. The palms and soles may be slightly thickened but are also usually spared. The condition gradually worsens in severity and extent. Keratosis pilaris is not present, and there is no increased incidence of atopy. Deep corneal opacities that do not interfere with vision develop in late childhood or adolescence and are a useful marker for the disease because they may also be present in carrier females. Some patients have larger deletions on the X chromosome that encompass neighboring genes, generating *contiguous gene deletion syndromes*. These include **Kallmann syndrome** (*KAL1* gene), which consists of hypogonadotrophic hypogonadism and anosmia, **X-linked chondroplasia punctata** (*ARSE* gene), **short stature,** and **ocular albinism**. The rate of testicular cancer may be increased in patients with coexistent Kallmann syndrome. There is also an increased risk of attention deficit hyperactivity disorder and autism owing to a contiguous gene defect in neuroglin 4.

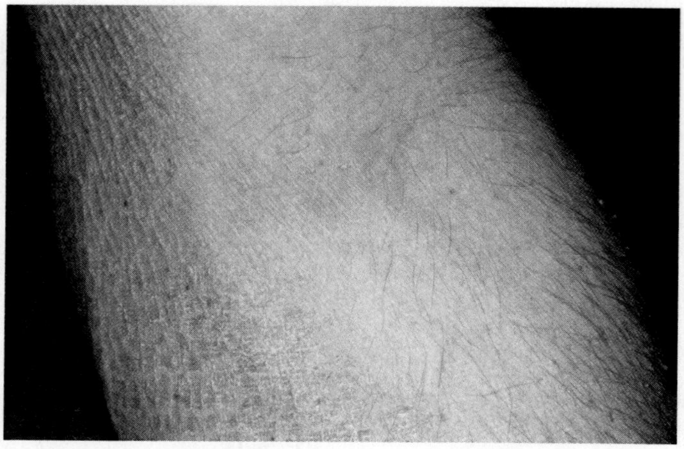

Figure 650-5 Sparing of the antecubital fossa in X-linked ichthyosis.

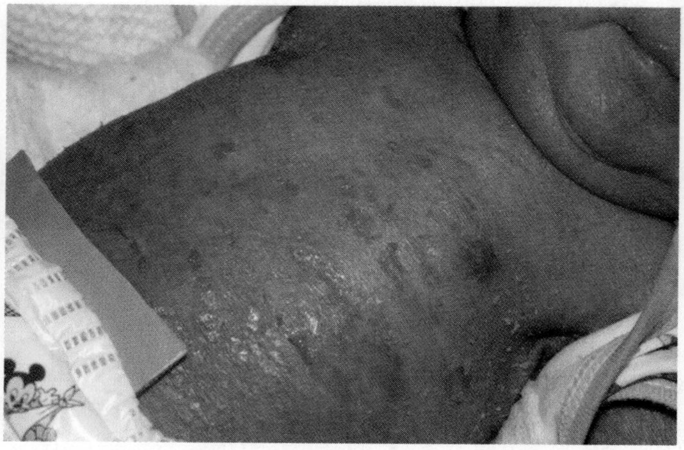

Figure 650-6 Superficial erosions and hyperkeratosis in epidermolytic hyperkeratosis.

Reduced steroid sulfatase enzyme activity can be detected in fibroblasts, keratinocytes, and leukocytes and, prenatally, in amniocytes or chorionic villus cells. In affected families, an affected male can be detected by restriction enzyme analysis of cultured chorionic villus cell DNA or amniocytes or by in situ hybridization, which identifies steroid sulfatase gene deletions prenatally in chorionic villus cells. A placental steroid sulfatase deficiency in carrier mothers may result in low urinary and serum estriol values, prolonged labor, and insensitivity of the uterus to oxytocin and prostaglandins.

HISTOLOGY Histologic findings in X-linked ichthyosis consist of hyperkeratosis of the stratum corneum, a well-developed granular layer, and a hyperplastic epidermis.

TREATMENT Daily application of emollients and a urea-containing lubricant (10-40%) are usually effective. Glycolic or lactic acid (5-12%) in an emollient base and propylene glycol (40-60%) in water with occlusion overnight are alternative forms of therapy.

Epidermolytic Hyperkeratosis (Bullous Congenital Ichthyosiform Erythroderma)

ETIOLOGY/PATHOGENESIS Epidermolytic hyperkeratosis is an autosomal dominant trait that has been shown to be due to defects in either keratin 1 or keratin 10. These keratins are required to form the keratin-intermediate filaments in cells of the suprabasilar layers of the epidermis.

CLINICAL MANIFESTATIONS The clinical manifestations are initially characterized by the onset at birth of widespread blisters and erosions on a background of generalized erythroderma (Fig. 650-6). Recurrent blistering may be widespread in neonates and may cause diagnostic confusion with other blistering disorders. With time, the blister formation ceases, erythema decreases, and generalized hyperkeratosis develops. The scales are small, hard, and verrucous. Distinctive, parallel hyperkeratotic ridges develop over the joint flexures, including the axillary, popliteal, and antecubital fossae, and on the neck and hips. Palmoplantar keratoderma is associated with keratin 1 defects. The hair, nails, mucosa, and sweat glands are normal. Malodorous secondary bacterial infection is common and requires appropriate antibiotic therapy.

PATHOLOGY The histopathology is diagnostic of epidermolytic hyperkeratosis, consisting of hyperkeratosis, degeneration of the epidermal granular layer with an increased number of keratohyalin granules, clear spaces around nuclei, and indistinct cellular boundaries of cells in the upper epidermis. On electron microscopic examination, keratin-intermediate filaments are clumped, and many desmosomes are attached to only one keratinocyte instead of connecting neighboring keratinocytes. Localized forms of the disease may resemble epidermal nevi or keratoderma of the palms and soles but share the distinctive histopathologic changes of epidermolytic hyperkeratosis.

TREATMENT Treatment of epidermolytic hyperkeratosis is difficult. Morbidity is increased in the neonatal period as a result of prematurity, sepsis, and fluid and electrolyte imbalance. Bacterial colonization of macerated scales produces a distinctive bad odor that can be controlled somewhat by use of an antibacterial cleanser. Intermittent oral antibiotics are generally necessary. Keratolytic agents are often poorly tolerated. Oral retinoids (1 mg/kg/day) may produce significant improvement. Prenatal diagnosis for affected families is possible by examination of DNA extracts from chorionic villus cells or amniocytes, provided that the specific mutation in the affected parent is known.

Erythrokeratoderma Variabilis

ETIOLOGY/PATHOGENESIS An autosomal dominant disorder, erythrokeratoderma variabilis (EKV) is caused by mutations in connexins 31 and 30.3. Connexins are proteins that form gap junctions between cells that allow for transport and signaling between neighboring epidermal cells.

CLINICAL MANIFESTATIONS EKV usually manifests in the early months of life, progresses in childhood, and stabilizes in adolescence. It is characterized by two distinctive manifestations: sharply demarcated, hyperkeratotic plaques (Fig. 650-7*A*) and transient figurate erythema (Fig. 650-7*B*). The distribution is generalized but sparse; sites of predilection are the face, buttocks, axillae, and extensor surfaces of the limbs. The palms and soles may be thickened, but hair, teeth, and nails are normal.

HISTOLOGY Histopathology demonstrates hyperkeratosis, papillomatosis, and irregular hyperplasia of the epidermis.

TREATMENT There are case reports that topical tazarotene gel 0.1% and oral retinoids (1 mg/kg/day) are effective for treatment of EKV.

Symmetric Progressive Erythrokeratoderma

ETIOLOGY/PATHOGENESIS Symmetric progressive erythrokeratoderma is an autosomal dominant disorder caused by mutations in the gene encoding loricrin. Loricrin is a major component of the epidermal cornified cell envelope.

CLINICAL MANIFESTATIONS The disorder manifests in childhood as large, fixed, geographic and symmetric, fine, scaling, hyperkeratotic, erythematous plaques primarily on the extremities, buttocks, face, ankles, and wrists. The primary feature distinguishing this disorder from EKV is the lack of variable erythema seen in the latter condition.

HISTOLOGY There is papillated epidermal hyperplasia with hypergranulosis, parakeratosis and orthokeratosis.

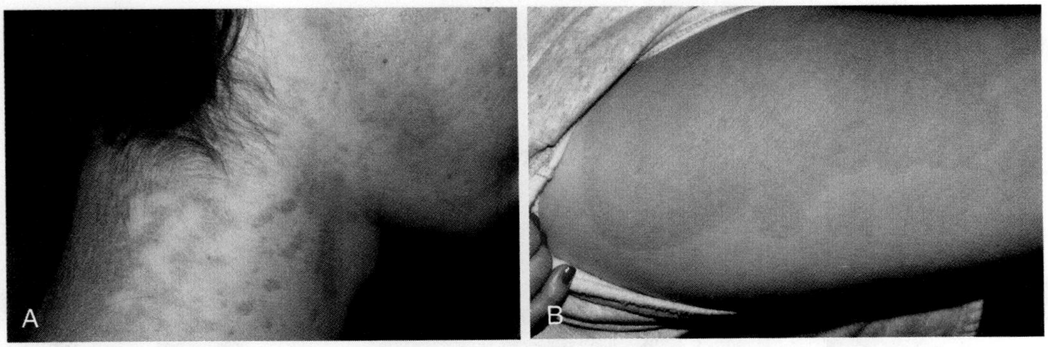

Figure 650-7 Erythrokeratoderma variabilis. *A,* Fixed, hyperkeratotic plaques, *B,* Migratory, erythematous lesion.

TREATMENT Symmetric progressive erythrokeratoderma is a very rare disorder, but reports of response to topical and oral retinoids (1 mg/kg/day) exist.

Ichthyosiform Dermatoses

Several rare and distinct syndromes include ichthyosis as a constant feature.

SJÖGREN-LARSSON SYNDROME

Etiology/Pathogenesis The autosomal recessive inborn error of metabolism known as Sjögren-Larsson syndrome is an abnormality of fatty alcohol oxidation that results from a deficiency of fatty aldehyde dehydrogenase (*ALDH3A2*), a component of the fatty alcohol–nicotinamide adenine dinucleotide oxidoreductase enzyme complex.

Clinical Manifestations The clinical picture of Sjögren-Larsson syndrome consists of ichthyosis, mental retardation, and spasticity. The ichthyosis is generalized but is accentuated on the flexures and the lower abdomen and consists of erythroderma, fine scaling, larger platelike scales, and dark hyperkeratosis. The degree of scale varies markedly from patient to patient. Most individuals have palmoplantar hyperkeratosis. The skin changes may be identical to the other forms of ichthyosis, and diagnosis is often delayed until the onset of neurologic symptoms. Pruritus is severe and hypohidrosis is common. Glistening dots in the foveal area are a cardinal ophthalmologic sign. About half the patients have primary retinal degeneration. Motor and speech developmental delays are usually noted before 1yr of age, and spastic diplegia or tetraplegia, epilepsy, and mental retardation generally become evident in the first 3 yr of life. Some patients may walk with the aid of braces, but most are confined to wheelchairs. This deficiency can be demonstrated in cultured skin fibroblasts of affected patients and carriers and, prenatally, in cultured chorionic villus cells and amniocytes from affected fetuses. Elevation of urinary leukotriene B4 (LTB4) may provide an easier approach to diagnosis.

Treatment Treatment is similar to that for the other forms of ichthyosis; 5-lipoxygenase inhibitors have been used to decrease pruritus.

NETHERTON SYNDROME

Etiology/Pathogenesis A rare autosomal recessive disorder, Netherton syndrome is caused by mutations in the *SPINK 5* gene, which encodes a serine protease inhibitor (LEKT1).

Clinical Manifestations Netherton syndrome is characterized by ichthyosis (usually ichthyosis linearis circumflexa but occasionally the lamellar or congenital types of ichthyosiform erythroderma), trichorrhexis invaginata and other hair shaft anomalies, and atopic diathesis. The disorder manifests at birth or in the first few months of life as generalized erythema and scaling. The trunk and limbs have diffuse erythema and superimposed migratory, polycyclic, and serpiginous hyperkeratotic lesions (Fig. 650-8), some with a distinctive double-edged margin of scale. Lichenification or hyperkeratosis tends to persist in the antecubital and popliteal fossae. The face and scalp may remain erythematous and scaling. Many hair shaft deformities, most notably, trichorrhexis invaginata, have been described in most patients with Netherton syndrome.

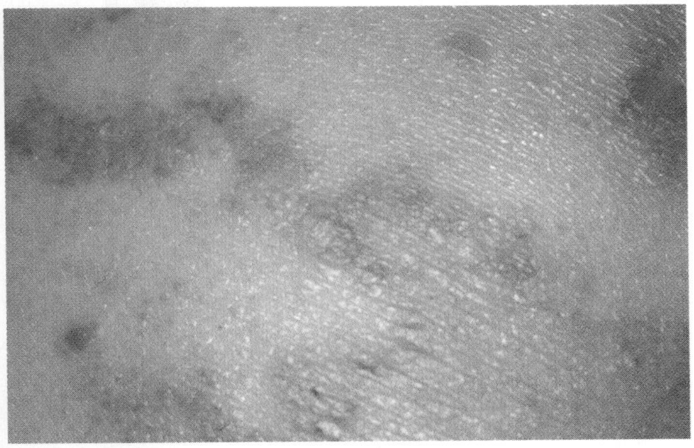

Figure 650-8 Serpiginous, erythematous, hyperkeratotic lesions of ichthyosis linearis circumflexa.

The ichthyosis is present in the first 10 days of life and may be especially marked around the eyes, mouth, and perineal area. The erythroderma is often intensified after infection. Infants may suffer from failure to thrive, recurrent bacterial and candidal infections, elevated serum immunoglobulin (Ig) E values, and marked hypernatremic dehydration. The most frequent allergic manifestations are urticaria, angioedema, atopic dermatitis, and asthma. Scalp hair is sparse and short and fractures easily (Fig. 650-9); eyebrows, eyelashes, and body hair are also abnormal. The characteristic hair abnormality can be identified with light microscopy; in the newborn, it may best be identified in eyebrow hair.

Histology Nonspecific psoriasiform changes are found on histopathologic examination.

Treatment Owing to the inflammatory nature of the skin disease, oral antihistamines and topical steroids, as used in the treatment of atopic dermatitis, are helpful for Netherton syndrome.

REFSUM SYNDROME (CHAPTERS 80.2 AND 605.5)

Etiology/Pathogenesis There are 2 types of Refsum syndrome. The classic form is autosomal recessive and caused by mutations in the *PAHX* gene that result in an increase in phytanic acid. A novel Refsum-like disorder has been mapped to chromosome 20 (20p11.21-q12), but the gene remains unidentified. The infantile forms of Refsum syndrome are also autosomal recessive and caused by mutations in the *PEX1*, *PEX2*, or *PEX26* genes. These are peroxisomal abnormalities that lead to an increase in very long chain fatty acids, di- and tri-hydroxycholestanoic acid, and pipecolic acid as well as phytanic acid.

Clinical Manifestations Refsum syndrome is a multisystem disorder that becomes symptomatic in the 2nd or 3rd decade of life. The ichthyosis may be generalized, is relatively mild, and

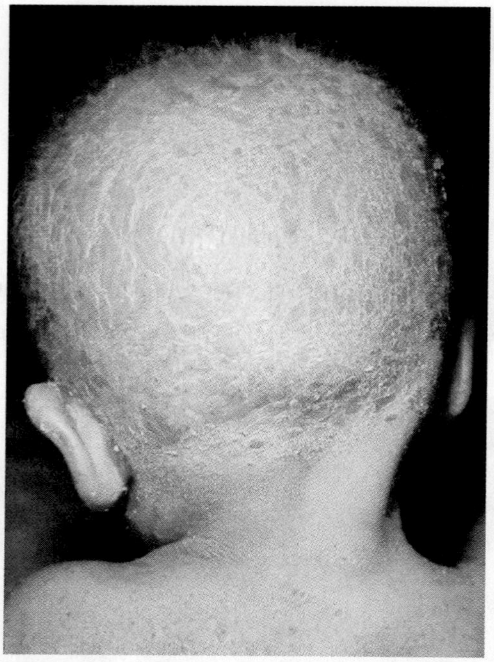

Figure 650-9 Very short scalp hair and thick scale in Netherton syndrome.

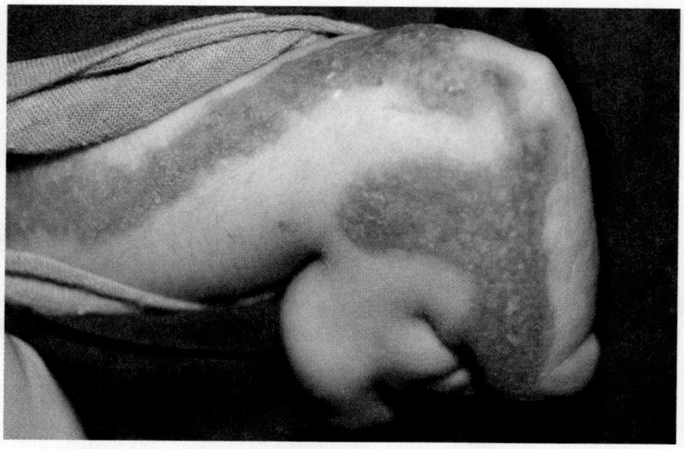

Figure 650-10 Limb dysplasia and ichthyosiform eruption in CHILD (congenital hemidysplasia with ichthyosiform erythroderma and limb defects) syndrome.

resembles ichthyosis vulgaris. The ichthyosis may also be localized to the palms and soles. Chronic polyneuritis with progressive paralysis and ataxia, retinitis pigmentosa, anosmia, deafness, bony abnormalities, and electrocardiographic changes are the most characteristic features. The condition is diagnosed through lipid analysis of the blood or skin, which shows elevated phytanic acid values.

The infantile form begins, as suggested by the name, early in life, and in addition to the changes seen in the classic form, affected patients have hepatomegaly, abnormal bile acid profiles, developmental delay, and mental retardation.

Treatment Phytanic acid is exclusively derived from dietary chlorophyll. Lifelong dietary avoidance of phytanic acid–containing produces clinical improvement in classic Refsum syndrome.

CHONDRODYSPLASIA PUNCTATA (CHAPTER 80.2)

Etiology/Pathogenesis Chondrodysplasia punctata (CPD) is a clinically and genetically heterogeneous condition. X-linked dominant CPD, also known as Conradi-Hünermann syndrome, is the best-characterized form. There is also an X-linked recessive form caused by mutation in the *ARSE* gene. Rhizomelic chondrodysplasia punctata type 1 is an autosomal recessive disorder caused by mutations in the *PEX7* gene, which encodes the peroxisomal type 2 targeting signal (*PTS2*) receptor. CPD can also be caused by maternal vitamin K deficiency or warfarin teratogenicity.

Clinical Manifestations These heterogeneous disorders are marked by ichthyosis and bone changes. Nearly all patients with the X-linked dominant form and approximately 25% of those with the recessive type have cutaneous lesions, ranging from severe, generalized erythema and scaling to mild hyperkeratosis. **Rhizomelic chondrodysplasia punctata** is associated with cataracts, hypertelorism, optic nerve atrophy, disproportionate shortening of the proximal extremities, psychomotor retardation, failure to thrive, and spasticity; most affected patients die in infancy. Patients with the X-linked dominant form have asymmetric, variable shortening of the limbs and a distinctive ichthyosiform eruption at birth. Thick, yellow, tightly adherent, keratinized plaques are distributed in a whorled pattern over the entire body. The eruption typically resolves in infancy and may be superseded by a follicular atrophoderma and patchy alopecia.

Additional features in all variants include cataracts and abnormal facies with saddle nose and frontal bossing. The pathognomonic defect, termed **chondrodysplasia punctata**, is stippled epiphyses in the cartilaginous skeleton. This defect, which is seen in various settings and inherited disorders, often in association with peroxisomal deficiency and disturbance of cholesterol biosynthesis, disappears by 3-4 yr of age.

OTHER SYNDROMES WITH ICHTHYOSIS A number of other rare syndromes with ichthyosis as a consistent feature include the following: keratitis with ichthyosis and deafness (**KID syndrome**, *connexin 26 gene*), ichthyosis with defective hair having a banded pattern under polarized light and a low sulfur content (**trichothiodystrophy**), multiple sulfatase deficiency, neutral lipid storage disease with ichthyosis (**Chanarin-Dorfman syndrome**/*CGI58 gene*), and **CHILD syndrome** (Fig. 650-10; congenital hemidysplasia with ichthyosiform erythroderma and limb defects; *NSDHL* gene).

PALMOPLANTAR KERATODERMAS

Excessive hyperkeratosis of the palms and soles may occur as a manifestation of a focal or generalized congenital hereditary skin disorder or may result from such chronic skin diseases as psoriasis, eczema, pityriasis rubra pilaris, lupus erythematosus, or postinfectious arthritis syndrome.

Diffuse Hyperkeratosis of Palms and Soles (Unna-Thost, Vorner)

Unna-Thost and Vorner type palmoplantar keratodermas (PPKs), although clinically inseparable, were thought to be separate entities. They were separated histologically by the presence (Vorner) or absence (Unna-Thost) of epidermolytic hyperkeratosis. They represent the clinical spectrum of the same disease caused by mutations in keratin (*KRT1* and *KRT9* genes). This autosomal dominant disorder manifests in the first few months of life as erythema that gradually progresses to sharply demarcated, hyperkeratotic, scaling plaques over the palms (Fig. 650-11) and soles. The margins of the plaques often remain red; plaques may extend along the lateral aspects of the hands and feet and onto the volar wrists and the heels. Hyperhidrosis is usually present, but hair, teeth, and nails are usually normal. Striate (*DSG1*, *DSP*, *KRT1* genes) and punctate forms of palmar and plantar hyperkeratosis represent distinct entities.

Mal de Meleda (*SLURP-1* Gene)

A rare, progressive autosomal recessive condition, mal de Meleda is characterized by erythema and thick scales on the palms, fingers, soles, and flexor aspects of the wrists, knees, and elbows. Hyperhidrosis, nail thickening or koilonychia, and eczema may also occur.

Vohwinkel Palmoplantar Keratoderma (Mutilating Keratoderma)

Vohwinkel PPK is a progressive autosomal dominant disease consisting of honeycombed hyperkeratosis of palms and soles, sparing the arches; starfish-like and linear keratoses on the dorsum of the hands, fingers, feet, and knees; and ainhum-like constriction of the digits that sometimes leads to autoamputation. Varying degrees of alopecia may be seen. Two forms have been identified. Vohwinkel PPK with ichthyosis is caused by mutations in the loricrin gene, and Vohwinkel PPK with deafness by mutations in connexin 26.

Papillon-Lefèvre Syndrome (Cathepsin C Gene)

An autosomal recessive erythematous hyperkeratosis of the palms and soles, Papillon-Lefèvre syndrome sometimes extends to the dorsal hands and feet, elbows, and knees later in childhood. The PPK may be either diffuse, striate, or punctuate. This syndrome is characterized by periodontal inflammation, leading to loss of teeth by age 4-5 yr if untreated.

Other Syndromes

Keratoderma of palms and soles also occurs as a feature of some forms of ichthyosis and ectodermal dysplasia. **Richner-Hanhart syndrome** is an autosomal recessive palmoplantar keratoderma with corneal ulcers, progressive mental impairment, and a deficiency of tyrosine aminotransferase, which leads to tyrosinemia. **Pachyonychia congenita** is transmitted as an autosomal dominant trait with variable expressivity. The classic type I form (**Jadassohn-Lewandowski syndrome**) is due to mutations in the gene for keratin 16. Major features of the syndrome are onychogryphosis; palmoplantar keratoderma; follicular hyperkeratosis, especially of the elbows and knees; and oral leukokeratosis. The nail dystrophy is the most striking feature and may be present at birth or develop early in life. The nails are thickened and tubular, projecting upward at the free edge to form a conical roof over a mass of subungual keratotic debris. Repeated paronychial inflammation may result in shedding of the nails. The feature seen most consistently among patients with this condition is keratoderma of the palms and soles. Additional associated features include hyperhidrosis of the palms and soles, and bullae and erosions on the palms and soles. Some patients have shown a selective cell-mediated defect in recognition and processing of *Candida*. Surgical removal of the nails and excision of the nail matrix have been helpful in some patients.

Treatment

Treatment for PPK is the same no matter what its cause. In mild cases, emollient therapy may suffice. Keratolytic agents such as salicylic acid, lactic acid, and urea creams may be required. Oral retinoids are the treatment of choice for severe cases unresponsive to topical therapy.

BIBLIOGRAPHY

Please visit the Nelson Textbook of Pediatrics *website at* *www.expertconsult.com* *for the complete bibliography.*

Chapter 651
Diseases of the Dermis

Joseph G. Morelli

KELOID

Etiology/Pathogenesis

Keloids are usually induced by trauma and commonly follow ear piercing, burns, scalds, and surgical procedures. Certain individuals are predisposed to keloid formation; a familial tendency (recessive or dominant inheritance) or the presence of foreign material in the wound may have a pathogenic role. Keloids are a rare feature of Ehlers-Danlos syndrome, Rubinstein-Taybi syndrome, and pachydermoperiostosis. Keloids result from an abnormal fibrous wound healing response in which tissue repair and regeneration-regulation control mechanisms are lost. Collagen production is 20 times that seen in normal scars and the type I/type III collagen ratio is abnormally high. In keloids, tissue values of tumor growth factor-β (TGF-β) and platelet-derived growth factor (PDGF) are elevated; fibroblasts are more sensitive to their effects, and their degradation rate is decreased.

Clinical Manifestations

A *keloid* is a sharply demarcated, benign, dense growth of connective tissue that forms in the dermis after trauma. The lesions are firm, raised, pink, and rubbery; they may be tender or pruritic. Sites of predilection are the face, earlobes (Fig. 651-1), neck, shoulders, upper trunk, sternum, and lower legs. In both keloids and hypertrophic scars, new collagen forms over a much longer period than in wounds that heal normally.

Histology

A keloid consists of whorled and interlaced hyalinized collagen fibers.

Differential Diagnosis

Keloids should be differentiated from *hypertrophic scars*, which remain confined to the site of injury and gradually involute over time.

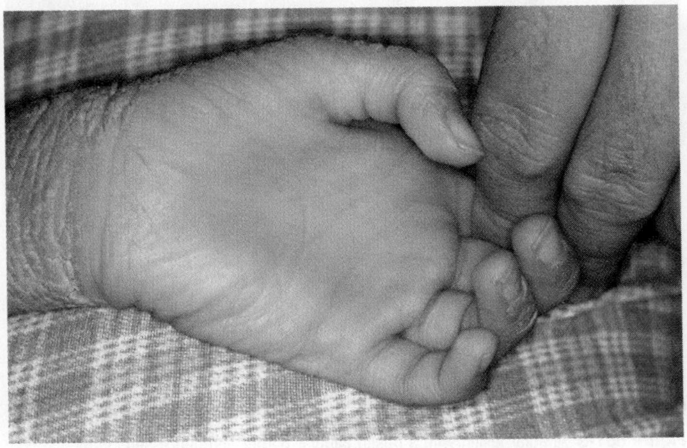

Figure 650-11 Palmar keratoderma with epidermolytic changes seen on biopsy.

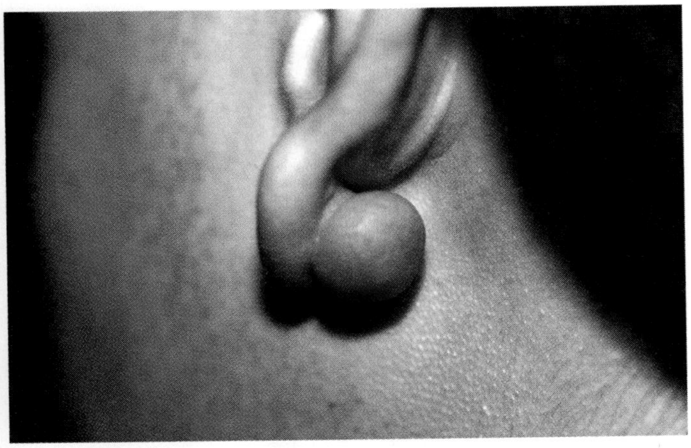

Figure 651-1 Keloid of ear lobe after piercing.

Treatment
Young keloids may diminish in size if injected intralesionally at 4-wk intervals with triamcinolone suspension (10-40 mg/mL). At times, a more concentrated suspension is required. Large or old keloids may require surgical excision followed by intralesional injections of corticosteroid. The risk of recurrence at the same site argues against surgical excision alone, although ear lobe keloids respond well to surgical excision, pressure dressings, and intralesional steroids. Placement of topical silicon gel sheeting over the keloid for several hours per day for several weeks may help in some patients.

STRIAE CUTIS DISTENSAE (STRETCH MARKS)

Etiology/Pathogenesis
Striae formation is common in adolescence. The most frequent causes are rapid growth, pregnancy, obesity, Cushing disease, and prolonged corticosteroid therapy. The pathogenesis is unknown, but the occurrence of alterations in elastic fibers is thought to be the primary process.

Clinical Manifestations
These thinned, depressed, erythematous bands of atrophic skin eventually become silvery, opalescent, and smooth. They occur most frequently in areas that have been subject to distention, such as the lower back (Fig. 651-2), buttocks, thighs, breasts, abdomen, and shoulders.

Differential Diagnosis
Striae distensae resemble atrophic scars.

Treatment
Controlled trials of treatments for striae are lacking; however, striae tend to spontaneously become less conspicuous with time.

CORTICOSTEROID-INDUCED ATROPHY

Etiology/Pathogenesis
Both topical and systemic corticosteroid treatment can result in cutaneous atrophy. This is particularly common when a potent or superpotent topical corticosteroid is applied under occlusion or to an intertriginous area for a prolonged period. Keratinocyte growth is decreased, but epidermal maturation is accelerated, resulting in a thinning of the epidermis and stratum corneum. Fibroblast growth and function are also decreased, leading to the dermal changes. The mechanism involves inhibition of synthesis of collagen type I, noncollagenous proteins, and total protein content of the skin, along with progressive reduction of dermal proteoglycans and glycosaminoglycans.

Clinical Manifestations
Affected skin is thin, fragile, smooth, and semitransparent, with telangiectasias and loss of normal skin markings.

Histology
Histopathologically, one sees thinning of the epidermis. Spaces between dermal collagen and elastic fibers are small, producing a more compact but thin dermis.

Treatment
Optimal treatment is prevention by proper use of topical steroids to avoid side effects.

GRANULOMA ANNULARE

Etiology/Pathogenesis
The cause of granuloma annulare is unknown. Some cases of granuloma annulare, particularly the generalized form, may be associated with diabetes mellitus or with anterior uveitis. However, most cases are seen in healthy children.

Clinical Manifestations
This common dermatosis occurs predominantly in children and young adults. Affected children are usually healthy. Typical lesions begin as firm, smooth, erythematous papules. They gradually enlarge to form annular plaques with a papular border and a normal, slightly atrophic or discolored central area up to several centimeters in size. Lesions may occur anywhere on the body, but mucous membranes are spared. Favored sites include the dorsum of the hands (Fig. 651-3) and feet. The disseminated papular form is rare in children. Subcutaneous granuloma annulare tends to develop on the scalp and limbs, particularly in the pretibial area. These lesions are firm, usually nontender, skin-colored nodules. Perforating granuloma annulare is characterized by the development of a yellowish center in some of the superficial papular lesions as a result of transepidermal elimination of altered collagen.

Differential Diagnosis
Annular lesions are often mistaken for tinea corporis because of the elevated advancing border. They differ in that they are not scaly. Papular lesions, another variant, may simulate rheumatoid nodules, particularly when grouped on the fingers and elbows.

Histology
The lesion of granuloma annulare consists of a granuloma with a central area of necrotic collagen; mucin deposition; and a peripheral palisading infiltrate of lymphocytes, histiocytes, and

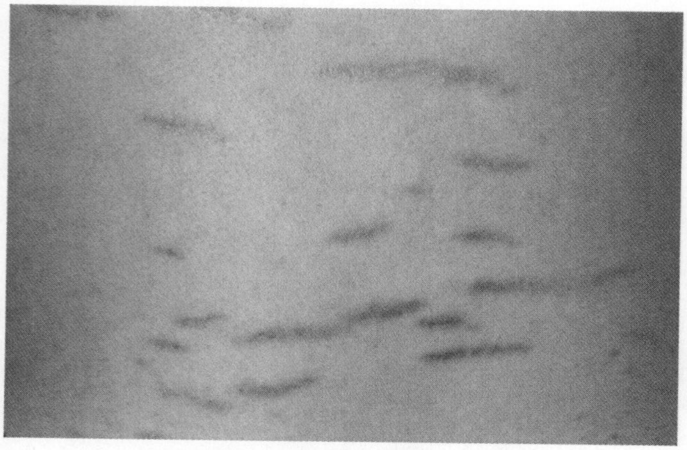

Figure 651-2 Striae on the back of an adolescent.

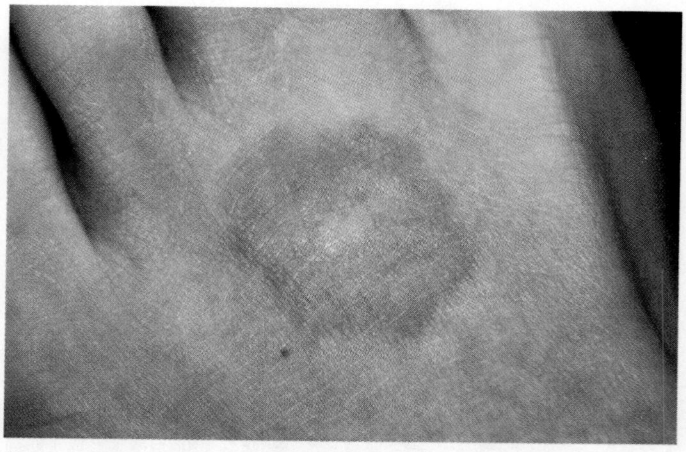

Figure 651-3 Annular lesion with a raised papular border and depressed center, characteristic of granuloma annulare.

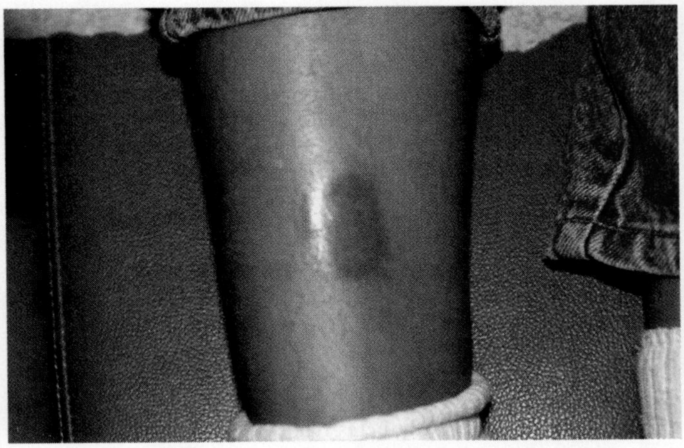

Figure 651-4 Yellow sclerotic plaque of necrobiosis lipoidica on the shin.

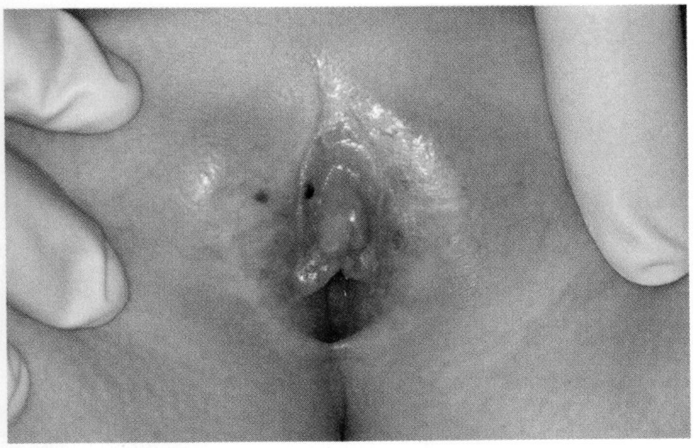

Figure 651-5 Ivory-colored perivaginal plaque with hemorrhage.

foreign body giant cells. The pattern resembles that of necrobiosis lipoidica and rheumatoid nodule, but subtle histologic differences usually permit differentiation.

Treatment

The eruption persists for months to years, but spontaneous resolution without residual change is usual; 50% of lesions clear within 2 years. Application of a potent or superpotent topical corticosteroid preparation or intralesional injections (5-10 mg/mL) of corticosteroid may hasten involution, but nonintervention is usual.

NECROBIOSIS LIPOIDICA

Etiology/Pathogenesis

The cause of necrobiosis lipoidica is unknown, but 50-75% of patients have **diabetes mellitus**; necrobiosis lipoidica occurs in 0.3% of all diabetic patients.

Clinical Manifestations

This disorder manifests as erythematous papules that evolve into irregularly shaped, sharply demarcated, yellow, sclerotic plaques with central telangiectasia and a violaceous border. Scaling, crusting, and ulceration are frequent. Lesions develop most commonly on the shins (Fig. 651-4). Slow extension of a given lesion over the years is usual, but long periods of quiescence or complete healing with scarring may occur.

Histology

Poorly defined areas of necrobiotic collagen are seen throughout, but primarily low in the dermis, associated with mucin deposition. Surrounding the necrobiotic, disordered areas of collagen is a palisading lymphohistiocytic granulomatous infiltrate. Some lesions are more characteristically granulomatous, with limited necrobiosis of collagen.

Differential Diagnosis

Necrobiosis lipoidica must be differentiated clinically from xanthomas, morphea, granuloma annulare, erythema nodosum, and pretibial myxedema.

Treatment

The lesions persist despite good control of the diabetes but may improve minimally after applications of high-potency topical steroids or local injection of a corticosteroid. Pentoxifylline (400 mg 3×/day) has also been used.

LICHEN SCLEROSUS

Etiology/Pathogenesis

The cause of lichen sclerosis is unknown.

Clinical Manifestations

Lichen sclerosus manifests initially as shiny, indurated, ivory-colored papules, often with a violaceous halo. The surface shows prominent dilated pilosebaceous or sweat duct orifices that often contain yellow or brown plugs. The papules coalesce to form irregular plaques of variable size, which may develop hemorrhagic bullae in their margins. In the later stages, atrophy results in a depressed plaque with a wrinkled surface. This disorder occurs more commonly in girls than in boys. Sites of predilection in girls are the vulvar (Fig. 651-5), perianal, and perineal skin. Extensive involvement may produce a sclerotic, atrophic plaque of hourglass configuration; shrinkage of the labia and stenosis of the introitus may result. Vaginal discharge precedes vulvar lesions in approximately 20% of patients. In boys, the prepuce and glans penis are often involved, usually in association with phimosis; most boys with the disorder were not circumcised early in life. Sites elsewhere on the body that are most commonly involved include the upper trunk, the neck, the axillae, the flexor surfaces of wrists, and the areas around the umbilicus and the eyes. Pruritus may be severe.

Differential Diagnosis

In children, lichen sclerosus is most frequently confused with focal morphea (Chapter 154), with which it may coexist. In the genital area, it may be mistakenly attributed to sexual abuse.

Histology

Biopsy is diagnostic, revealing hyperkeratosis with follicular plugging, hydropic degeneration of basal cells, a bandlike dermal lymphocytic infiltrate, homogenized collagen, and thinned elastic fibers in the upper dermis.

Treatment

Vulvar lichen sclerosus in childhood usually improves with puberty but does not usually resolve, and symptoms can recur throughout life. Long-term observation for the development of squamous cell carcinoma is necessary. Superpotent topical corticosteroids provide relief from pruritus and produce clearing of lesions, including those in the genital area. Topical tacrolimus and pimecrolimus have also been used. It is not known how response to treatment affects long-term cancer risk.

MORPHEA

Etiology/Pathogenesis

Morphea is a sclerosing condition of the dermis and subcutaneous tissue of unknown etiology.

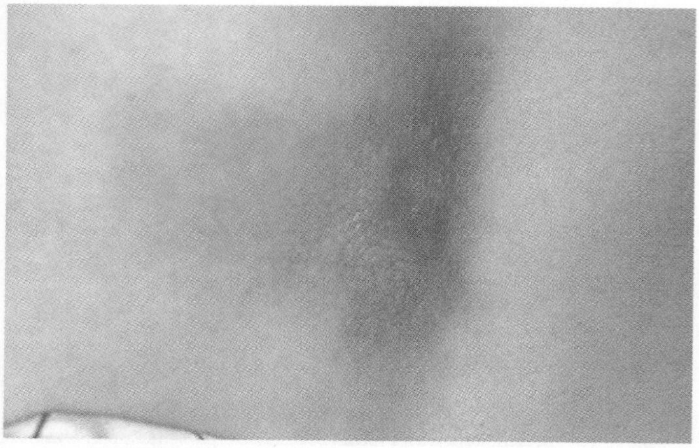

Figure 651-6 Erythematous, hyperpigmented plaque of early morphea.

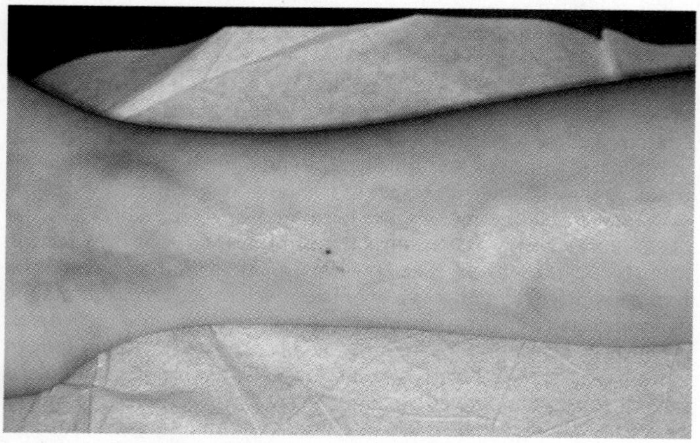

Figure 651-7 Linear morphea with involvement over the ankle.

Clinical Manifestations

Morphea is characterized by solitary, multiple or linear circumscribed areas of erythema that evolve into indurated, sclerotic, atrophic plaques (Fig. 651-6), later healing, or "burning out" with pigment change. It is seen more commonly in females. The most common types of morphea are plaque and linear. Morphea can affect any area of skin. When confined to the frontal scalp, forehead, and midface in a linear band, it is referred to as **en coup de sabre**. When located on one side of the face, it is called **progressive hemifacial atrophy**. These forms of morphea carry a poorer prognosis because of the associated underlying musculoskeletal atrophy that can be cosmetically disfiguring. Linear morphea over a joint may lead to restriction of mobility (Fig. 651-7). Pansclerotic morphea is a rare severe disabling variant.

Differential Diagnosis

The differential diagnosis of morphea includes granuloma annulare, necrobiosis lipoidica, lichen sclerosis, and late-stage Lyme disease (acrodermatitis chronica atrophicans).

Histology

Thickening or sclerosis of the dermis with collagen degeneration is seen in morphea.

Treatment

Morphea tends to persist, with gradual outward expansion on the skin for 3-5 yr until spontaneous cessation of the inflammatory phase occurs. Topical calcipotriene alone or in combination with high- to super-potency topical steroids or topical tacrolimus have been used for less severe disease. For the various forms of linear morphea and for severe plaque morphea, ultraviolet A-1 (UVA-1) phototherapy, methotrexate 0.3-0.5 mg/kg/week, and glucocorticosteroids 1 mg/kg/day may halt progression and help shorten the disease course. There are no comparison studies to suggest which therapy is optimal. Physical therapy is needed in linear morphea over a joint to maintain mobility. Significant postinflammatory pigment alteration may persist for years.

SCLEREDEMA (SCLEREDEMA ADULTORUM, SCLEREDEMA OF BUSCHKE)

Etiology/Pathogenesis

The cause of scleredema is unknown. There are 3 types. Type I (55% of cases) is preceded by a febrile illness. Type 2 (25%) is associated with paraproteinemias, including multiple myeloma. Type 3 (20%) is seen in diabetes mellitus.

Clinical Manifestations

Fifty percent of patient with scleredema are younger than 20 yr and almost always have type 1. Onset of type 1 is sudden, with brawny edema of the face and neck that spreads rapidly to involve the thorax and arms in a sweater distribution; the abdomen and legs are usually spared. The face acquires a waxy, masklike appearance. The involved areas feel indurated and woody, are nonpitting, and are not sharply demarcated from normal skin. The overlying skin is normal in color and is not atrophic.

Onset in patients with type 2 and type 3 scleredema may occur insidiously. Systemic involvement, which is uncommon and usually associated with types 2 and 3, is marked by thickening of the tongue; dysarthria; dysphagia; restriction of eye and joint movements; and pleural, pericardial, and peritoneal effusions. Electrocardiographic changes may also be observed. Laboratory data are not helpful.

Differential Diagnosis

Scleredema must be differentiated from scleroderma (Chapter 154), morphea, myxedema, trichinosis, dermatomyositis, sclerema neonatorum, and subcutaneous fat necrosis.

Histology

Skin biopsy demonstrates an increase in dermal thickness as a result of swelling and homogenization of the collagen bundles, which are separated by large interfibrous spaces. Special stains can identify increased amounts of mucopolysaccharides in the dermis of patients with scleredema.

Treatment

In type 1 scleredema, the active phase of the disease persists for 2-8 wk; spontaneous and complete resolution usually occurs in 6 mo to 2 yr. Recurrent attacks are unusual. In type 2 and 3, disease is slowly progressive. There is no specific therapy.

LIPOID PROTEINOSIS (URBACH-WIETHE DISEASE, HYALINOSIS CUTIS ET MUCOSAE)

Etiology/Pathogenesis

Lipoid proteinosis, an autosomal recessive disorder, is caused by mutations in the *ECM-1* gene, which encodes the ECM-1 protein. ECM-1 (extracellular matrix protein) has a functional role in the structural organization of the dermis by binding to perlecan, matrix metalloproteinase (MMP) 9, and fibulin. Pathogenesis involves infiltration of hyaline material into the skin, oral cavity, larynx, and internal organs.

Clinical Manifestations

Lipoid proteinosis may be noted initially in early infancy as hoarseness. Skin lesions appear during childhood and consist of yellowish papules and nodules that may coalesce to form plaques. The classic sign is beaded papules on the eyelids. Lesions also occur on the face, forearms, neck, genitals, dorsum of the fingers, and scalp, where they result in patchy alopecia. Similar deposits are found on the lips, undersurface of the tongue, fauces, uvula, epiglottis, and vocal cords. The tongue becomes enlarged and feels firm on palpation. The patient may be unable to protrude the tongue. Pocklike atrophic scars may develop on the face. Hypertrophic, hyperkeratotic nodules occur at sites of friction, such as the elbows and knees; the palms may be diffusely thickened. The disease progresses until early adult life, but the prognosis is good. Symmetric ossification lateral to the sella turcica in the medial temporal region, identifiable roentgenographically, is pathognomonic but is not always present. Involvement of the larynx can lead to respiratory compromise, particularly in infancy, necessitating tracheostomy. Associated anomalies include dental abnormalities, epilepsy, and recurrent parotitis as a result of infiltrates in the Stensen duct. Virtually any organ can be involved.

Histology
The distinctive histologic pattern in lipoid proteinosis includes dilatation of dermal blood vessels and infiltration of homogeneous eosinophilic extracellular hyaline material along capillary walls and around sweat glands. Hyaline material in homogeneous bundles, diffusely arranged in the upper dermis, produces a thickened dermis. The infiltrates appear to contain both lipid and mucopolysaccharide substances.

Treatment
There is no specific treatment for lipoid proteinosis.

MACULAR ATROPHY (ANETODERMA)

Etiology/Pathogenesis
Anetoderma is characterized by circumscribed areas of slack skin associated with loss of dermal substance. This disorder may have no associated underlying disease (primary macular atrophy) or may develop after an inflammatory skin condition. Secondary macular atrophy may be due to direct destruction of dermal elastin or elastolysis on an immunologic basis, especially the presence of antiphospholipid antibodies, which are related to autoimmune disorders. The elastolysis may then be due to release of elastase from inflammatory cells.

Clinical Manifestations
Lesions vary from 0.5 to 1 cm in diameter and, if inflammatory, may initially be erythematous. They subsequently become thin, wrinkled, and blue-white or hypopigmented. The lesions often protrude as small outpouchings that, on palpation, may be readily indented into the subcutaneous tissue because of the dermal atrophy. Sites of predilection include the trunk, thighs, upper arms, and, less commonly, the neck and face. Lesions remain unchanged for life; new lesions often continue to develop for years.

Histology
All types of macular atrophy show focal loss of elastic tissue on histopathologic examination, a change that may not be recognized unless special stains are used.

Differential Diagnosis
Lesions of anetoderma occasionally resemble morphea, lichen sclerosus, focal dermal hypoplasia, atrophic scars, or end-stage lesions of chronic bullous dermatoses.

Treatment
There is no effective therapy for macular atrophy.

CUTIS LAXA (DERMATOMEGALY, GENERALIZED ELASTOLYSIS)

Etiology/Pathogenesis
Cutis laxa is a heterogenous group of disorders related to abnormalities in elastic tissue. It may be autosomal recessive (type I—*fibulin 5* and *fibulin* 4 genes, type II—*ATP6V0A2* gene), autosomal dominant (*elastin* and *fibulin* 5 genes), X-linked (*Cu (2+)-transporting ATPase, alpha polypeptide*), or acquired. Acquired cutis laxa has developed after a febrile illness, inflammatory skin diseases such as lupus erythematosus or erythema multiforme, amyloidosis, urticaria, angioedema, and hypersensitivity reactions to penicillin, and in infants born to women who were taking penicillamine.

Clinical Manifestations
There may be widespread folds of lax skin, or changes may be mild and limited in extent, resembling anetoderma. Patients with severe cutis laxa have characteristic facial features, including an aged appearance with sagging jowls (bloodhound appearance) (Fig. 651-8), a hooked nose with everted nostrils, a short columella, a long upper lip, and everted lower eyelids. The skin is also lax elsewhere on the body and may resemble an ill-fitting suit. Hyperelasticity and hypermobility of the joints are not present as they are in the Ehlers-Danlos syndrome. Many infants have a hoarse cry, probably as a result of laxity of the vocal cords. Tensile strength of the skin is normal.

The dominant form of cutis laxa may develop at any age and is generally benign. When it manifests in infancy, it may be associated with intrauterine growth restriction, ligamentous laxity, and delayed closure of the fontanels. Pulmonary emphysema and mild cardiovascular manifestations may also occur. Patients with the more *common recessive* form of the disease are susceptible to severe complications, such as multiple hernias, rectal prolapse, diaphragmatic atony, diverticula of the gastrointestinal and genitourinary tracts, cor pulmonale, emphysema, pneumothoraces, peripheral pulmonary artery stenosis, and aortic dilatation. Characteristic facial features include downward-slanting palpebral fissures, a broad, flat nose, and large ears. Skeletal anomalies, dental caries, growth retardation, and developmental delay also occur. Such patients often have a shortened life span.

Cutis laxa–like skin changes may also be seen in association with multiple other syndromes, including De Barsy syndrome, Lenz-Majewski syndrome, hyperostotic dwarfism, SCARF (skeletal abnormalities, cutis laxa craniostenosis, ambiguous genitalia, retardation, facial abnormalities) syndrome, wrinkling skin syndrome, and Costello syndrome.

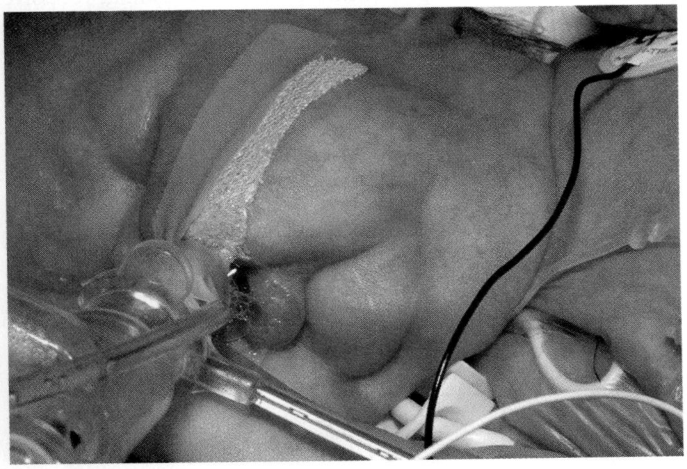

Figure 651-8 Pendulous folds of skin of an infant with cutis laxa.

Histology
Histologically, elastic tissue is reduced throughout the dermis, with fragmentation, distention, and clumping of the elastic fibers.

Treatment
Treatment for cutis laxa is supportive.

EHLERS-DANLOS SYNDROME
Ehlers-Danlos syndrome (EDS) is a group of genetically heterogeneous connective tissue disorders. Affected children appear normal at birth, but skin hyperelasticity, fragility of the skin and blood vessels, delayed wound healing, and joint hypermobility (Fig. 651-9) develop. The essential defect is a quantitative deficiency of fibrillar collagen.

Classification
Ehlers-Danlos syndrome has been reclassified into 6 clinical forms.

CLASSIC (*COL5A1, COL5A2, COL1A1* GENES; PREVIOUSLY EDS TYPE I—GRAVIS, EDS TYPE II—MITIS) This autosomal dominant disorder is characterized by premature birth caused by rupture of membranes, skin hyperelasticity and fragility, easy bruising, generalized and severe joint hypermobility, scoliosis, and mitral valve prolapse. Insignificant lacerations may form gaping wounds that leave broad, atrophic, papyraceous scars. Additional cutaneous manifestations include molluscoid pseudotumors over pressure points from accumulations of connective tissue. Life expectancy is not reduced.

HYPERMOBILE (*COL3A1* GENE; PREVIOUSLY EDS TYPE III) This disorder has autosomal dominant inheritance and manifests as generalized severe joint hypermobility and minimal skin manifestations. Musculoskeletal pain is common, and osteoarthritis may develop prematurely.

VASCULAR (*COL3A1* GENE; PREVIOUSLY EDS TYPE IV—ARTERIAL ECCHYMOTIC) This autosomal dominant disorder shows the most pronounced dermal thinning of all. Consequently, the underlying venous network is prominent. The skin has minimal hyperextensibility, and the joints are not hypermobile, except perhaps during childhood. Premature birth, extensive ecchymoses from trauma, a high incidence of keloids, rupture of the bowel (especially the colon), uterine rupture during pregnancy, rupture of the great vessels, dissecting aortic aneurysm, and stroke all contribute to the increased morbidity and shortened life span. Patients should be advised to avoid becoming pregnant, avoid activities that raise intracranial pressure as a result of a Valsalva maneuver, such as trumpet playing, and minimize trauma to the skin. Celiprolol, a β_1 antagonist and a β_2 agonist (vasodilates), may reduce vascular events.

KYPHOSCOLIOSIS (LYSYL HYDROXYLASE [*PLOD* GENE] DEFICIENCY; PREVIOUSLY EDS TYPE VI) Patients with this autosomal recessive type have joint hyperextensibility, hypotonia, kyphoscoliosis, fragile cornea, keratoconus, skin hyperelasticity, and fragile bones. Prenatal diagnosis is available through measurement of lysyl hydroxylase activity in amniocytes. The diagnosis can also be confirmed by detection of decreased lysyl hydroxylase activity in cultured dermal fibroblasts.

ARTHROCHALASIA (*COLA1A* GENE, TYPE A; *COL1A2* GENE, TYPE B; PREVIOUSLY EDS TYPES VIIA AND B—ARTHROCHALASIS MULTIPLEX CONGENITA) The A type is an autosomal dominant disorder characterized by short stature, marked joint hyperextensibility and dislocation, and moderate hyperelasticity and bruisability of skin. The B type is autosomal dominant and is characterized by skin hyperelasticity and marked joint hypermobility.

DERMATOSPRAXIS (TYPE 1 COLLAGEN *N*-PEPTIDASE; PREVIOUSLY EDS TYPE VIIC) This autosomal recessive condition that includes premature rupture of membranes; delayed closure of fontanels; skin fragility and laxity; easy bruisability; growth retardation; short limbs; umbilical hernia; and characteristic facies with micrognathia, jowls, and prominent, puffy eyelids.

Differential Diagnosis
Ehlers-Danlos syndrome has been confused with cutis laxa, but the features of the two disorders differ considerably. The skin of patients with cutis laxa hangs in redundant folds, whereas the skin of those with Ehlers-Danlos syndrome is hyperextensible and snaps back into place when stretched. Because of the marked skin fragility in Ehlers-Danlos syndrome, minor trauma results in ecchymoses, bleeding, and poor healing with atrophic cigarette-paper scars, which are most prominent on the forehead and lower legs and over pressure points. Surgical procedures are fraught with risk; dehiscence of wounds is common.

PSEUDOXANTHOMA ELASTICUM

Etiology/Pathogenesis
Pseudoxanthoma elasticum (PXE) is a primary disorder of elastic tissue. The overwhelming majority of cases are due to mutations in the *ABCC6* gene. The primary abnormality seen in PXE is an accumulation of mineralized tissue in the skin, Bruch membrane in the retina, and vessel walls. Although other forms of PXE have been postulated, their existence is now debated.

Clinical Manifestations
Onset of skin manifestations often occurs during childhood, but the changes produced by early lesions are subtle and may not be recognized. The characteristic **pebbly, "plucked chicken skin" cutaneous lesions** are 1-2 mm, asymptomatic, yellow papules that are arranged in a linear or reticulated pattern or in confluent plaques. Preferred sites are the flexural neck (Fig. 651-10),

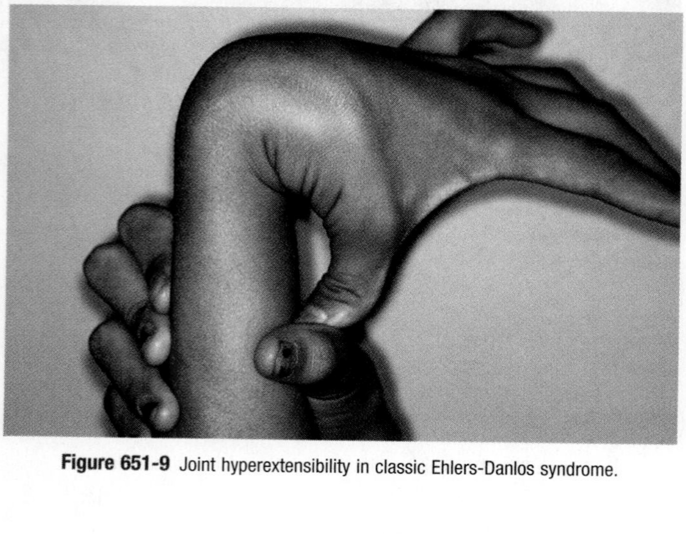

Figure 651-9 Joint hyperextensibility in classic Ehlers-Danlos syndrome.

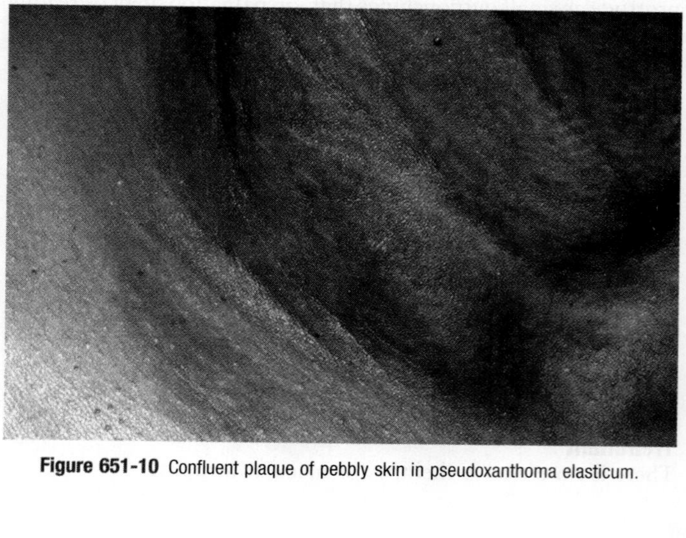

Figure 651-10 Confluent plaque of pebbly skin in pseudoxanthoma elasticum.

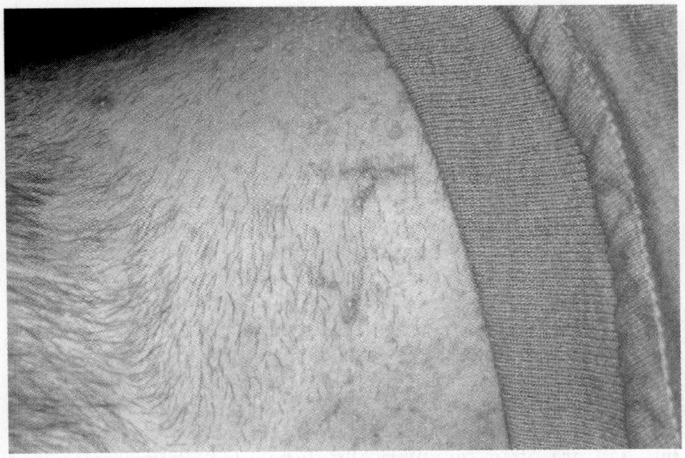

Figure 651-11 Arcuate keratotic papule of elastosis perforans serpiginosa.

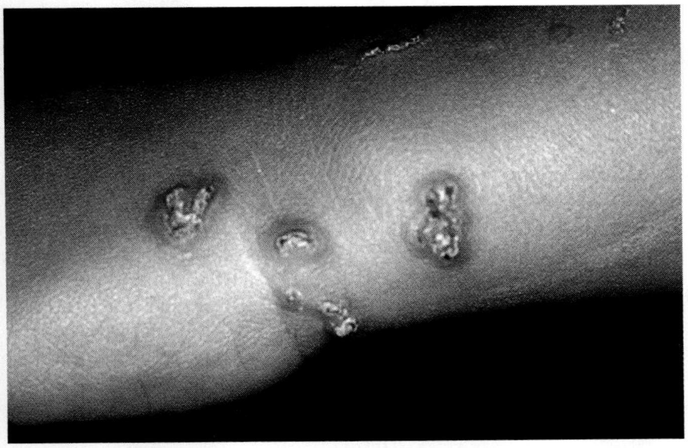

Figure 651-12 Hyperkeratotic papules in reactive perforating collagenosis.

axillary and inguinal folds, umbilicus, thighs, and antecubital and popliteal fossae. As the lesions become more pronounced, the skin acquires a velvety texture and droops in lax, inelastic folds. The face is usually spared. Mucous membrane lesions may involve the lips, buccal cavity, rectum, and vagina. There is involvement of the connective tissue of the media, and intima of blood vessels, Bruch membrane of the eye, and endocardium or pericardium may result in visual disturbances, angioid streaks in Bruch membrane, intermittent claudication, cerebral and coronary occlusion, hypertension, and hemorrhage from the gastrointestinal tract, uterus, or mucosal surfaces. Women with PXE have an increased risk of miscarriage in the 1st trimester. Arterial involvement generally manifests in adulthood, but claudication and angina have occurred in early childhood.

Pathology
Histopathologic examination shows fragmented, swollen, and clumped elastic fibers in the middle and lower third of the dermis. The fibers stain positively for calcium. Collagen in the vicinity of the altered elastic fibers is reduced in amount and is split into small fibers. Aberrant calcification of the elastic fibers of the internal elastic lamina of arteries in PXE leads to narrowing of vessel lumina.

Treatment
There is no effective treatment for PXE, although laser therapy may help prevent retinal hemorrhage.

ELASTOSIS PERFORANS SERPIGINOSA

Etiology/Pathogenesis
Elastosis perforans serpiginosa (EPS) is characterized by the extrusion of altered elastic fibers through the epidermis. The primary abnormality is probably in the dermal elastin, which provokes a cellular response that ultimately leads to extrusion of the abnormal elastic tissue.

Clinical Manifestations
This is an unusual skin disorder in which 1- to 3-mm, firm, skin-colored, keratotic papules tend to cluster in arcuate and annular patterns on the posterolateral neck and limbs (Fig. 651-11) and, occasionally, on the face and trunk. Onset usually occurs in childhood or adolescence. A papule consists of a circumscribed area of epidermal hyperplasia that communicates with the underlying dermis by a narrow channel. There is a great increase in the amount and size of elastic fibers in the upper dermis, particularly in the dermal papillae. Approximately 30% occur in association with osteogenesis imperfecta, Marfan syndrome, pseudoxanthoma elasticum, Ehlers-Danlos syndrome, Rothmund-Thomson syndrome, scleroderma, acrogeria, and Down syndrome. EPS has also occurred in association with penicillamine therapy.

Histology
Histopathology reveals a hyperplastic epidermis with extrusion of abnormal elastic fibers and a lymphocytic superficial infiltrate.

Differential Diagnosis
Differential diagnosis of EPS includes tinea corporis, perforating granuloma annulare, reactive perforating collagenosis, lichen planus, creeping eruption, and porokeratosis of Mibelli.

Treatment
Treatment of EPS is ineffective; however, the lesions are asymptomatic and may disappear spontaneously.

REACTIVE PERFORATING COLLAGENOSIS

Etiology/Pathogenesis
The primary process in reactive perforating collagenosis (RPC) represents transepidermal elimination of altered collagen. A familial autosomal recessive form has been described.

Clinical Manifestations
RPC usually manifests in early childhood as small papules on the dorsal areas of the hands and forearms, elbows, knees, and, sometimes, face and trunk. Over a period of several weeks, the papules enlarge to 5-10 mm, become umbilicated, and develop keratotic plugs in their centers (Fig. 651-12). Individual lesions resolve spontaneously in 2-4 mo, leaving hypopigmented macules or scars. Lesions may recur in crops; may undergo a linear Koebner phenomenon; and may form in response to cold temperatures or superficial trauma such as abrasions, insect bites, and acne lesions.

Histology
Collagen in the papillary dermis is engulfed within a cup-shaped perforation in the epidermis. The central crater contains pyknotic inflammatory cells and keratinous debris.

Differential Diagnosis
EPS and Kyle disease may mimic RPC.

Treatment
RPC resolves spontaneously in 6-8 wk. Topical retinoic acid enhances the resolution.

XANTHOMAS

See Chapter 80.

FABRY DISEASE

See Chapter 80.

MUCOPOLYSACCHARIDOSES (CHAPTER 82)

In several of the mucopolysaccharidoses, thick, rough, inelastic skin, particularly on the extremities, and generalized hirsutism are characteristic but nonspecific features. Telangiectasias on the face, forearms, trunk, and legs have been observed in Scheie and Morquio syndromes. In some patients with Hunter syndrome, ivory-colored, distinctive firm papulonodules with a corrugated surface texture are grouped into symmetric plaques on the upper trunk (Fig. 651-13), arms, and thighs. Onset of these unusual lesions occurs in the 1st decade of life, and spontaneous disappearance has been noted.

MASTOCYTOSIS

Etiology/Pathogenesis

Mastocytosis encompasses a spectrum of disorders that range from solitary cutaneous nodules to diffuse infiltration of skin associated with involvement of other organs (Table 651-1). All of the disorders are characterized by aggregates of mast cells in the dermis. There are 4 types of mastocytoses: solitary mastocytoma; urticaria pigmentosa (2 forms); diffuse cutaneous mastocytosis; and telangiectasia macularis eruptiva perstans. The 2 forms of urticaria pigmentosa are the childhood variant, which resolves without sequelae, and the form that may start in either childhood or adult life and is associated with a mutation (most commonly the *D816V* mutation) in the stem cell factor gene. Stem cell factor (mast cell growth factor), which can be secreted by keratinocytes, stimulates the proliferation of mast cells and increases the production of melanin by melanocytes. The local and systemic manifestations of the disease are due, at least in part, to release of histamine and heparin from mast cell granules; although heparin is present in significant amounts in mast cells, coagulation disturbances occur only rarely. The vasodilator prostaglandin D_2 or its metabolite appears to exacerbate the flushing response. Serum tryptase values are often elevated.

Clinical Manifestations

Solitary mastocytomas are 1-5 cm in diameter. Lesions may be present at birth or may arise in early infancy at any site. The lesions may manifest as recurrent, evanescent wheals or bullae; in time, an infiltrated, pink, yellow, or tan, rubbery plaque develops at the site of whealing or blistering (Fig. 651-14). The surface acquires a pebbly, orange peel–like texture, and hyperpigmentation may become prominent. Stroking or trauma to the nodule may lead to urtication (Darier sign) as a result of local histamine release; rarely, systemic signs of histamine release become apparent.

Urticaria pigmentosa is the most common form of mastocytosis. In the first type of urticaria pigmentosa, the classic infantile type, lesions may be present at birth but more often erupt in crops in the first several months to 2 yr of age. New lesions seldom arise after age 3-4 yr. In some cases, early bullous or urticarial lesions fade, only to recur at the same site, ultimately becoming fixed and hyperpigmented. In others, the initial lesions are hyperpigmented. Vesiculation usually abates by 2 yr of age. Individual lesions range in size from a few millimeters to several centimeters and may be macular, papular, or nodular. They range in color from yellow-tan to chocolate brown and often have ill-defined borders (Fig. 651-15). Larger nodular lesions, like mastocytomas, may have a characteristic orange peel texture. Lesions of urticaria pigmentosa may be sparse or numerous and are often symmetrically distributed. Palms, soles, and face are sometimes spared, as are the mucous membranes. The rapid appearance of erythema and whealing in response to vigorous stroking of a lesion can usually be elicited; dermographism of intervening normal skin is also common. Affected children can have intense pruritus. Systemic signs of histamine

Table 651-1 MASTOCYTOSIS CLASSIFICATION*

Cutaneous mastocytosis:
1. Urticaria pigmentosa:
Classic infantile type
Chronic with stem cell factor mutations
2. Diffuse cutaneous mastocytosis
3. Mastocytoma of the skin
4. Telangiectasia macularis eruptive perstans
Systemic mastocytosis (without an associated hematologic non–mast cell disorder or leukemic mast cell disease):
1. Systemic indolent mastocytosis
2. Systemic smoldering mastocytosis
Systemic mastocytosis with an associated hematologic non–mast cell disorder:
1. Myeloproliferative syndrome
2. Myelodysplastic syndrome
3. Acute myeloid leukemia
4. Non-Hodgkin lymphoma
Systemic aggressive mastocytosis
Mast cell leukemia
Mast cell sarcoma
Extracutaneous mastocytoma

*Classification adopted from World Health Organization classification.
Adapted from Carter MC, Metcalfe DD: Paediatric mastocytosis, *Arch Dis Child* 86:315-319, 2002.

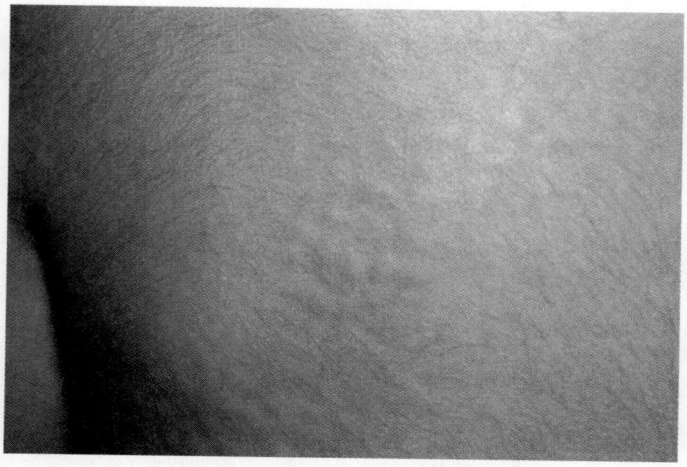

Figure 651-13 Ivory-colored papules on the upper back in Hunter syndrome.

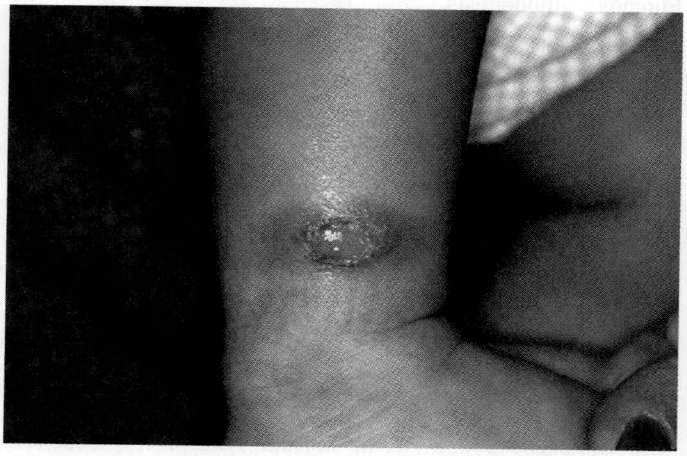

Figure 651-14 Solitary mastocytoma that is partially blistered.

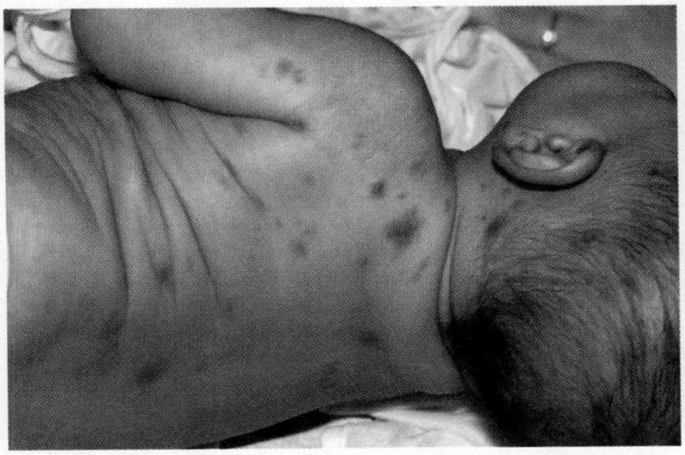

Figure 651-15 Hyperpigmented papular lesions of urticaria pigmentosa.

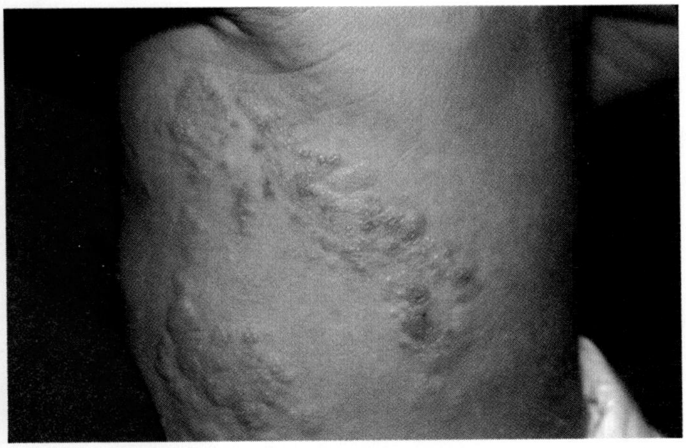

Figure 651-16 Severe blistering in diffuse cutaneous mastocytosis.

release, such as hypotension, syncope, headache, episodic flushing, tachycardia, wheezing, colic, and diarrhea, occur most frequently in the more severe types of mastocytosis. Flushing is by far the most common symptom seen.

The second type of urticaria pigmentosa may begin any time from infancy to adulthood. This type does not resolve, and new lesions continue to develop throughout life. It is associated with mutations in the stem cell factor gene. Patients with this type of mastocytosis are the population in whom systemic involvement may develop. The only way to tell whether urticaria pigmentosa in a child will progress to the adult form is to identify the mutated form of stem cell factor.

Systemic mastocytosis is marked by an abnormal increase in the number of mast cells in other than cutaneous tissues. It occurs in approximately 5-10% of patients with mutant stem cell factor–related mastocytosis and is more common in adults than in children. Bone lesions may be silent but are detectable radiologically as osteoporotic or osteosclerotic areas, principally in the axial skeleton. Gastrointestinal tract involvement may produce complaints of abdominal pain, nausea, vomiting, diarrhea, steatorrhea, and bloating. Mucosal infiltrates may be detectable by barium studies or by small bowel biopsy. Peptic ulcers also occur. Hepatosplenomegaly as a result of mast cell infiltrates and fibrosis has been described, as has mast cell proliferation in lymph nodes, kidneys, periadrenal fat, and bone marrow. Abnormalities in the peripheral blood, such as anemia, leukocytosis, and eosinophilia, are noted in approximately 30% of patients. Mast cell leukemia may occur.

Diffuse cutaneous mastocytosis is characterized by diffuse involvement of the skin rather than discrete hyperpigmented lesions. Affected patients are usually normal at birth and demonstrate features of the disorder after the first few months of life. Rarely, the condition may present with intense generalized pruritus in the absence of visible skin changes. The skin usually appears thickened and pink to yellow and may have a doughy feel and a texture resembling an orange peel. Surface changes are accentuated in flexural areas. Recurrent bullae (Fig. 651-16), intractable pruritus, and flushing attacks are common, as is systemic involvement.

Telangiectasia macularis eruptiva perstans is another variant that consists of telangiectatic hyperpigmented macules that are usually localized to the trunk. These lesions do not urticate when stroked. This form of the disease is seen primarily in adolescents and adults.

Differential Diagnosis

The differential diagnosis of solitary mastocytomas includes recurrent bullous impetigo, herpes simplex, congenital melanocytic nevi, and juvenile xanthogranuloma.

Table 651-2 PHARMACOLOGIC AGENTS AND PHYSICAL STIMULI THAT MAY EXACERBATE MAST CELL MEDIATOR RELEASE IN PATIENTS WITH MASTOCYTOSIS

IMMUNOLOGIC STIMULI
Venoms (immunoglobulin E–mediated bee venom)
Complement-derived anaphylatoxins
Biologic peptides (substance P, somatostatin)
Polymers (dextran)
NONIMMUNOLOGIC STIMULI
Physical stimuli (extreme temperature, friction, sunlight)
Drugs
Acetylsalicylic acid and related nonsteroidal analgesics*
Thiamine
Ketorolac tromethamine
Alcohol
Narcotics (codeine, morphine)*
Radiographic dyes (iodine containing)

*Appears to be a problem in <10% of patients.
From Carter MC, Metcalfe DD: Paediatric mastocytosis, *Arch Dis Child* 86:315-319, 2002.

Urticaria pigmentosa can be confused with drug eruptions, postinflammatory pigmentary change, juvenile xanthogranuloma, pigmented nevi, ephelides, xanthomas, chronic urticaria, insect bites, and bullous impetigo.

Diffuse cutaneous mastocytoma may be confused with epidermolytic hyperkeratosis.

Telangiectasia macularis eruptiva perstans must be differential from other causes of telangiectasia.

Prognosis

Spontaneous involution occurs in all patients with solitary mastocytomas and classic infantile urticaria pigmentosa. The incidence of systemic manifestations in these patients is very low. The continued development of lesions past the age of 4 yr implies likely chronic disease with stem cell factor gene mutation and a higher risk for systemic involvement.

Treatment

Solitary mastocytomas usually do not require treatment. Lesions that blister may be treated with a 2-wk course of a superpotent topical steroid following each blistering episode.

In urticaria pigmentosa, flushing can be precipitated by excessively hot baths, vigorous rubbing of the skin, and certain drugs, such as codeine, aspirin, morphine, atropine, ketorolac, alcohol, tubocurarine, iodine-containing radiographic dyes, and polymyxin B (Table 651-2). Avoidance of these triggering factors is advisable; it is notable that general anesthesia may be safely performed with appropriate precautions.

For patients who are symptomatic, oral antihistamines may be palliative. H_1 receptor antagonists (hydroxyzine) are the initial drugs of choice for systemic signs of histamine release. If H_1 antagonists are unsuccessful, H_2 receptor antagonists may be helpful in controlling pruritus or gastric hypersecretion. Superpotent topical steroids are of benefit in controlling skin urtication and blistering. Oral mast cell–stabilizing agents, such as cromolyn sodium or ketotifen, may also be effective for diarrhea or abdominal cramping and some systemic symptoms such as headache or muscle pain.

For patients with diffuse cutaneous mastocytosis, the treatment is the same as for urticaria pigmentosa, although in early life. Phototherapy with narrow-band ultraviolet (UVB or UVA-1) or psoralen with UVA (PUVA) treatment may be required to control symptoms.

Lesions of telangiectasia macularis eruptiva perstans may be cautiously treated with vascular pulsed dye lasers.

BIBLIOGRAPHY

Please visit the Nelson Textbook of Pediatrics *website at www.expertconsult.com for the complete bibliography.*

Chapter 652 Diseases of Subcutaneous Tissue

Joseph G. Morelli

Diseases involving the subcutis are usually characterized by necrosis and/or inflammation; they may occur either as a primary event or as a secondary response to various stimuli or disease processes. The principal diagnostic criteria relates to the appearance and distribution of the lesions, associated symptoms, results of laboratory studies, histopathology, and natural history and exogenous provocative factors of these conditions.

CORTICOSTEROID-INDUCED ATROPHY

Intradermal injection of a corticosteroid can produce deep atrophy accompanied by surface pigmentary changes and telangiectasia (Fig. 652-1). These changes occur approximately 2 wk after injection and may last for months.

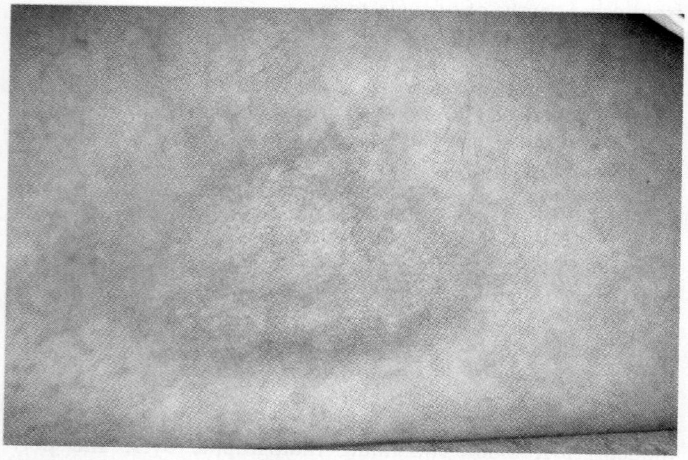

Figure 652-1 Localized fat atrophy with overlying erythema after steroid injection.

652.1 Panniculitis and Erythema Nodosum

Joseph G. Morelli

Inflammation of fibrofatty subcutaneous tissue may primarily involve the fat lobule or, alternatively, the fibrous septum that compartmentalizes the fatty lobules. Lobular panniculitis that spares the subcutaneous vasculature includes post-steroid panniculitis, lupus erythematosus profundus, pancreatic panniculitis, α_1-antitrypsin deficiency, subcutaneous fat necrosis of the newborn, sclerema neonatorum, cold panniculitis, subcutaneous sarcoidosis, and factitial panniculitis. Lobar panniculitis with vasculitis occurs in erythema induratum and, occasionally, as a feature of Crohn disease (Chapter 328.2). Inflammation predominantly within the septum, sparing the vasculature, may be seen in erythema nodosum (Table 652-1 and Fig. 652-2), necrobiosis

Table 652-1 ETIOLOGY OF ERYTHEMA NODOSUM

VIRUSES
Epstein-Barr, hepatitis B, mumps
FUNGI
Coccidioidomycosis, histoplasmosis, blastomycosis, sporotrichosis
BACTERIA AND OTHER INFECTIOUS AGENTS
Group A streptococcus,* tuberculosis,* *Yersinia*, cat-scratch disease, leprosy, leptospirosis, tularemia, mycoplasma, Whipple disease, lymphogranuloma venereum, psittacosis, brucellosis
OTHER
Sarcoidosis, inflammatory bowel disease,* estrogen-containing oral contraceptives,* systemic lupus erythematosus, Behçet syndrome, severe acne, Hodgkin disease, lymphoma, sulfonamides, bromides, Sweet syndrome, pregnancy, idiopathic*

*Common.

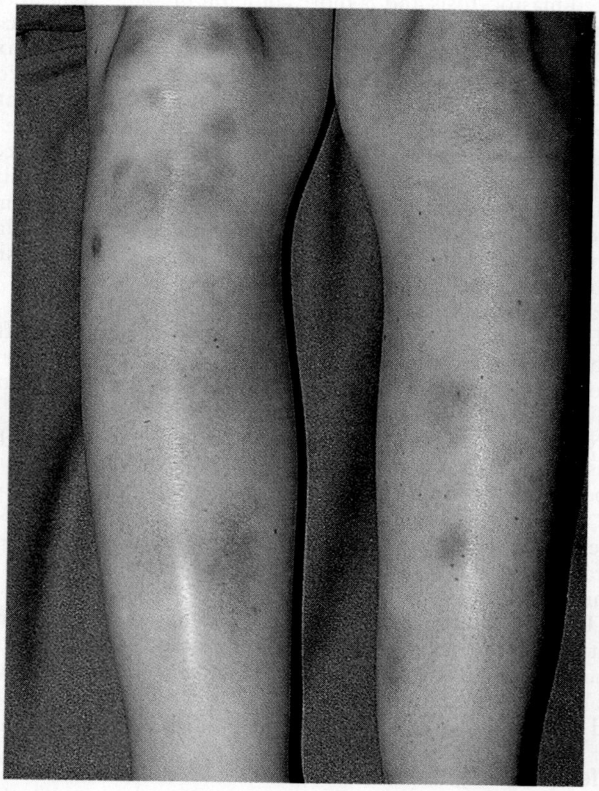

Figure 652-2 Tender red nodules with indistinct borders in a teenage girl with erythema nodosum. (From Weston AL, Lane AT, Morelli JG: *Color textbook of pediatric dermatology*, ed 3, St Louis, 2002, Mosby, p 212.)

lipoidica, progressive systemic sclerosis (Chapter 154), and subcutaneous granuloma annulare (Chapter 649). Septal panniculitis that includes inflammation of the vessels is found primarily in leukocytoclastic vasculitis and polyarteritis nodosa (Chapter 161).

ERYTHEMA NODOSUM

Erythema nodosum is a nodular, erythematous hypersensitivity reaction that typically appears with multiple lesions on the exterior surfaces of the arms and legs in the pretibial area (more common) and less often in other cutaneous areas containing subcutaneous fat. The lesions vary in size from 1 to 6 cm, are symmetric, and are oval with the longer axis parallel to the extremity. They initially appear bright or dull red but progress to a brown or purple; they are tense and painful and usually do not ulcerate (see Fig. 652-2). Initial lesions may resolve in 1-2 wk, but new lesions may continue to appear for 2-6 wk. Repeat episodes may occur weeks to months later. Prior to or immediately at the onset of lesions, there may be systemic manifestations that include fever, malaise, arthralgias (50-90%) and rheumatoid factor negative arthritis.

The etiology is unknown in 30-50% of pediatric cases of erythema nodosum; other etiologies are noted in Table 652-1. Group A streptococcal infection and inflammatory disorders (inflammatory bowel disease) are common etiologies in children; sarcoidosis should be considered in young adults.

Treatment includes that of the underlying disease as well as symptomatic relief with nonsteroidal antiinflammatory agents. Salicylates, supersaturated solution of potassium iodide (oral), colchicine, intraintestinal injections of steroidsand, in severe, persistent, or recurrent lesions, oral steroids have been employed. The idiopathic form is a self-limited disorder.

POST-STEROID PANNICULITIS

Etiology/Pathogenesis

The mechanism of the inflammatory reaction in the fat in post-steroid panniculitis is unknown.

Clinical Manifestations

Fewer than 20 cases of post-steroid panniculitis have been reported, with most of these being in children. The disorder occurs in children who have received high-dose corticosteroids. In 1-2 wk after discontinuation of the drug, multiple subcutaneous nodules usually appear on the cheeks, although other areas may be involved. Nodules range in size from 0.5 to 4 cm, are erythematous or skin colored, and may be pruritic.

Histology

A lobular panniculitis with a mixed infiltrate of lymphocytes, histiocytes, and neutrophils is seen. Scattered swollen adipocytes with eosinophilic, needle-shaped crystals are also seen. The epidermis, dermis, and fibrous septa of the fat are normal. Vasculitis is not seen.

Treatment

Treatment of post-steroid panniculitis is unnecessary because the lesions remit spontaneously over a period of months without scarring.

LUPUS ERYTHEMATOSUS PROFUNDUS (LUPUS ERYTHEMATOSUS PANNICULITIS)

Etiology/Pathogenesis

It is unknown what separates those patients in whom lupus erythematosus profundus develops from other patients with systemic lupus erythematosus. This variant of lupus erythematosus is rare in childhood.

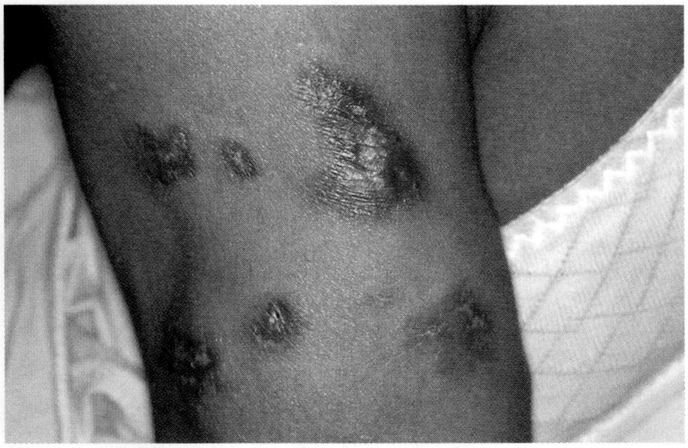

Figure 652-3 Deep nodule of lupus profundus with overlying hyperkeratotic lesion of discoid lupus erythematosus.

Clinical Manifestations

Lupus erythematosus profundus manifests as one to several firm, well-defined, purple plaques or nodules 1 to 3 cm in diameter, most commonly on the face, buttocks, or proximal extremities. This condition may occur in patients with systemic or discoid lupus erythematosus and may precede or follow the development of other cutaneous lesions. The overlying skin is usually normal but may be erythematous, atrophic, poikilodermatous, or hyperkeratotic (Fig. 652-3). Lesions may be painful and may ulcerate. On healing, a shallow depression generally remains or, rarely, soft pink areas of anetoderma result.

Histology

The histopathologic changes in lupus erythematosus profundus are distinctive and may allow the clinician to make the diagnosis in the absence of other cutaneous lesions of lupus erythematosus. The panniculitis is characterized by a mostly lobular dense infiltrate of lymphocytes and plasma cells. A dense perivascular and periappendigeal lymphocytic infiltrate is seen in the dermis. Lichenoid changes may be identified at the epidermal-dermal junction. Histopathologic differentiation from subcutaneous panniculitis–like T-cell lymphoma may be difficult. Results of lupus band and antinuclear antibody tests are usually positive.

Treatment

Nodules tend to be persistent. Hydroxychloroquine (2-5 mg/kg/day) is the **treatment of choice** for lupus erythematosus profundus. Intralesional corticosteroids may worsen the residual lipoatrophy. Immunosuppressive agents are indicated only for treatment of other severe manifestations of systemic lupus erythematosus. Avoidance of sun exposure and trauma is also important.

α_1-ANTITRYPSIN DEFICIENCY

Etiology/Pathogenesis

Individuals with α_1-antitrypsin deficiency have severe homozygous deficiency or, rarely, a partial deficiency of the protease inhibitor α_1-antitrypsin, which inhibits trypsin activity and the activity of elastase, serine proteases, collagenase, factor VIII, and kallikrein (Chapter 385). Panniculitis occurs with the Z subtype.

Clinical Manifestations

Cellulitis-like areas or tender, red nodules occur on the trunk or proximal extremities (Chapter 385). Nodules tend to ulcerate spontaneously and discharge an oily yellow fluid. Panniculitis may be associated with other manifestations of the disease, such as panacinar emphysema, noninfectious hepatitis, cirrhosis, persistent cutaneous vasculitis, cold contact urticaria, and acquired angioedema. Diagnosis can be substantiated by a decreased level of serum α_1-antitrypsin activity.

Histology
Extensive septal and lobular lymphocytic infiltrate with necrosis of the fat is observed.

Treatment
Treatment of the panniculitis in with α_1-antitrypsin deficiency is part of the overall treatment of the disease (Chapter 385).

PANCREATIC PANNICULITIS

Etiology/Pathogenesis
Pathogenesis of pancreatic panniculitis appears to be multifactorial, involving liberation of the lipolytic enzymes lipase, trypsin, and amylase into the circulation, causing adipocyte membrane damage and intracellular lipolysis. There is no correlation, however, between the occurrence of panniculitis and the serum concentration of pancreatic enzymes.

Clinical Manifestations
Pancreatic panniculitis manifests most commonly on the pretibial regions, thighs, or buttocks as tender, erythematous nodules that may be fluctuant and occasionally discharge an oily yellowish substance. It appears most often in males with alcoholism but may also occur in patients with pancreatitis as a result of cholelithiasis or abdominal trauma, with rupture of a pancreatic pseudocyst, with pancreatic ductal adenocarcinoma, or with pancreatic acinar cell carcinoma. Associated features may include polyarthritis (PPP [pancreatitis-panniculitis-polyarthritis] syndrome). In almost 65% of patients, abdominal signs are absent or mild, making the diagnosis difficult.

Histology
Microscopic changes consist of multiple foci of fat necrosis that contain ghost cells with thick, shadowy walls and no nuclei. A polymorphous inflammatory infiltrate surrounds the areas of fat necrosis.

Treatment
The primary pancreatic disorder must be treated. The arthritis may be chronic and responds poorly to treatment with nonsteroidal anti-inflammatory drugs and oral corticosteroids.

SUBCUTANEOUS FAT NECROSIS

Etiology/Pathogenesis
The cause of subcutaneous fat necrosis is unknown. The disease in infants may be due to ischemic injury under various circumstances, such as maternal preeclampsia, birth trauma, asphyxia, and prolonged hypothermia; in many affected infants, however, provocative factors are not identified. Susceptibility has been attributed to differences in composition between the subcutaneous tissue of young infants and that of older infants, children, and adults. Neonatal fat solidifies at a relatively high temperature because of its relatively greater concentration of high–melting point saturated fatty acids, such as palmitic and stearic acids.

Clinical Manifestations
This inflammatory disorder of adipose tissue occurs primarily in the first 4 wk of life in full-term or post-term infants. Typical lesions are asymptomatic, rubbery to firm, erythematous to violaceous plaques or nodules on the cheeks, buttocks, back, thighs, or upper arms (Fig. 652-4). Lesions may be focal or extensive and are generally asymptomatic, although they may be tender during the acute phase. Uncomplicated lesions involute spontaneously within weeks to months, usually without scarring or atrophy. Calcium deposition may occasionally occur within areas of fat necrosis, which may sometimes result in rupture and drainage of liquid material. A rare but potentially life-threatening complication is **hypercalcemia**. It manifests at 1-6 mo of age as lethargy, poor feeding, vomiting, failure to thrive, irritability, seizures, shortening of the QT interval on electrocardiography, or renal failure. The origin of the hypercalcemia is unknown.

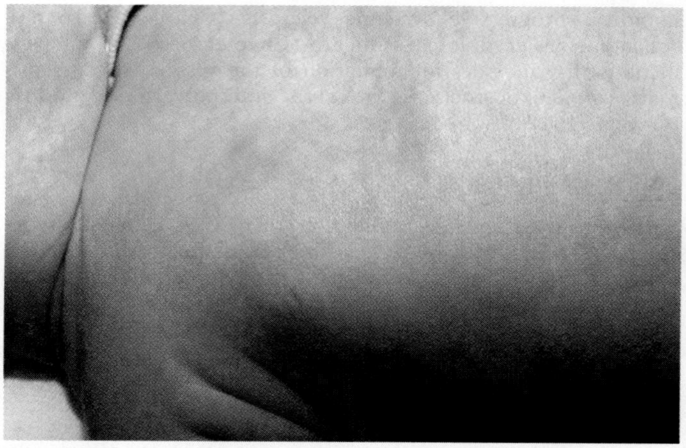

Figure 652-4 Red-purple nodular infiltration of the skin of the chest caused by subcutaneous fat necrosis.

Histology
Histopathologic changes in subcutaneous fat necrosis are diagnostic, consisting of: necrosis of fat; a granulomatous cellular infiltrate composed of lymphocytes, histiocytes, multinucleated giant cells, and fibroblasts; and radially arranged clefts of crystalline triglyceride within fat cells and multinucleated giant cells. Calcium deposits are commonly found in areas of fat necrosis.

Differential Diagnosis
Subcutaneous fat necrosis can be confused with sclerema neonatorum, panniculitis, cellulitis, and hematoma.

Treatment
Because the lesions are self-limited, therapy is not required for uncomplicated cases of subcutaneous fat necrosis. Needle aspiration of fluctuant lesions may prevent rupture and subsequent scarring but is rarely needed. Treatment of hypercalcemia is aimed at enhancing renal calcium excretion with hydration and furosemide (1-2 mg/kg/dose) and at limiting dietary calcium and vitamin D intake. Reduction of intestinal calcium absorption and alteration of vitamin D metabolism may be accomplished by administration of corticosteroids (0.5-1.0 mg/kg/day). Pamidronate (0.25-0.5 mg/kg/day) has been used in severe cases.

SCLEREMA NEONATORUM

Etiology/Pathogenesis
Although the cause remains unknown, four theories of pathogenesis for sclerema neonatorum have been proposed. It is theorized that sclerema neonatorum results from: hardening of the subcutaneous fat due to a decrease in body temperature as a consequence of circulatory shock; a defect in lipolytic enzymes or in lipid transport; association with an underlying severe disease; or a special form of edema affecting the connective tissue that supports the adipocytes.

Clinical Manifestations
This uncommon disorder of adipose tissue manifests abruptly in preterm, gravely ill infants as diffuse, yellowish white woody induration of the skin. Affected skin becomes stony in consistency, cold, and nonpitting. The face assumes a masklike expression, and joint mobility may be compromised because of inflexibility of the skin.

Histology
Histopathologic changes in sclerema neonatorum consist of increases in the size of fat cells and in the width of the fibrous connective tissue septa. In contrast to subcutaneous fat necrosis, with which this disorder is most apt to be confused, fat necrosis, inflammation, giant cells, and calcium crystals are generally absent.

Treatment
Sclerema neonatorum is almost always associated with serious illness, such as sepsis, congenital heart disease, multiple congenital anomalies, or hypothermia. The appearance of sclerema in a sick infant should be regarded as an ominous prognostic sign. The outcome depends on the response of the underlying disorder to treatment.

COLD PANNICULITIS

Etiology/Pathogenesis
The pathogenic mechanism of cold panniculitis may be similar to that of subcutaneous fat necrosis, involving a greater propensity of fat to solidify in infants than in that in older children and adults as a result of the higher percentage of saturated fatty acids in the subcutaneous fat of infants. Lesions occur in infants after prolonged cold exposure, especially on the cheeks, or after prolonged application of a cold object such as an ice cube, ice bag, or fruit ice pop to any area of the skin.

Clinical Manifestations
Ill-defined, erythematous to bluish, indurated plaques or nodules arise within hours to a couple days of exposure on exposed surfaces (face, arms, legs), persist for 2-3 wk, and heal without residua.

Histology
Histopathologic examination reveals an infiltrate of lymphoid and histiocytic cells around blood vessels at the dermal-subdermal junction and in the fat lobules; by the third day, some of the fat cells in the subcutis may have ruptured and coalesced into cystic structures.

Differential Diagnosis
Cold panniculitis may be confused with facial cellulitis caused by *Haemophilus influenzae* type b. Unlike in buccal cellulitis, the area may be cold to the touch, and the patient is afebrile and appears well.

Treatment
Treatment is unnecessary because cold panniculitis spontaneously resolves. Recurrence of the lesions is common, emphasizing the importance of parental education in treating affected patients.

CHILBLAINS (PERNIO)

Etiology/Pathogenesis
Vasospasm of arterioles due to damp cold exposure with resultant hypoxemia and localized perivascular mononuclear inflammation appears to be responsible for chilblains. The disease has been associated with cryoglobulins, lupus erythematosus with antiphospholipid antibodies, anorexia nervosa, and thin body habitus.

Clinical Manifestations
The condition is characterized by localized symmetric erythematous to purplish edematous plaques and nodules in areas exposed to cold, typically acral areas (distal hands and feet, ears, face; Chapter 69). Lesions develop 12-24 hr after cold exposure and may be associated with itching, burning, or pain. Blister formation and ulceration are rare.

Histology
Histopathologic examination reveals marked dermal edema and a perivascular and periappendigeal, predominantly T-cell lymphocytic infiltrate in the papillary and reticular dermis.

Differential Diagnosis
Raynaud phenomenon is more acute in nature than chilblains, with characteristic color changes and no chronic lesions. Frostbite due to extreme cold exposure is painful and involves freezing of the tissue with resultant tissue necrosis.

Treatment
Most cases of chilblains resolve spontaneously. Prevention is the treatment of choice. Nifedipine (0.25-0.5 mg/kg 3×/day, maximum 10 mg/dose) may be used in severe cases.

FACTITIAL PANNICULITIS

Etiology/Pathogenesis
Factitial panniculitis results from subcutaneous injection by the patient or a proxy of a foreign substance, the most common types of which are organic materials such as milk and feces; drugs such as the opiates and pentazocine; oily materials such as mineral oil and paraffin; and the synthetic polymer povidone.

Clinical Manifestations
Indurated plaques, ulcers, or nodules that liquefy and drain may be noted clinically in factitial panniculitis.

Histology
The histopathology is variable, depending on the injected substance, but may include the presence of birefringent crystals, oil cysts surrounded by fibrosis and inflammation, and an acute inflammatory reaction with fat necrosis. Vessels are characteristically spared.

Treatment
Treatment of factitial panniculitis must address the primary reason the patient is performing the self-destructive act.

BIBLIOGRAPHY
Please visit the Nelson Textbook of Pediatrics *website at www.expertconsult.com for the complete bibliography.*

652.2 Lipodystrophy

Joseph G. Morelli

Several rare conditions are associated with loss of fatty tissue in a partial or generalized distribution.

PARTIAL LIPODYSTROPHY

Partial lipodystrophy may be familial or acquired. Loss of adipose tissue is not preceded by an inflammatory phase, and histopathologic examination reveals only absence of subcutaneous fat.

There are 3 forms of familial partial lipodystrophy (FPLD):

Type I (FPLD1Köbberlingg) is characterized by loss of adipose tissue confined to the extremities and gluteal region. Fat distribution of the face, neck, and trunk may be normal or increased. Hyperlipidemia, insulin-resistant diabetes mellitus, and eruptive xanthomas may be seen. The gene is unknown, but only females are affected.

Type 2 (FPLD2–Dunnigan) is caused by mutations in the *laminin A/C* gene. Fat distribution is normal in childhood, but atrophy commences with puberty. Lipodystrophy is seen in the trunk, gluteal region, and extremities. Adipose tissue accumulates in the face and neck and may also be seen in the axillae, back, labia majora, and infra-abdominal region. Insulin-resistant diabetes mellitus and hypertriglyceridemia develop, but high-density lipoprotein and cholesterol levels are low. Both males and females are affected, but the diagnosis may be more difficult in males owing to body habitus.

Type 3 (FPLD3) is caused by mutations in the peroxisome proliferation–activated receptor gamma (*PPARG*) gene. Lipodystrophy is seen in the limbs and gluteal region. Insulin-resistant diabetes mellitus, primary amenorrhea, acanthosis nigricans, hypertension, and fatty infiltration of the liver are present.

AKT2* and *ZMPSTE24 mutations are newly recognized causes of partial lipodystrophy.

Acquired partial lipodystrophy (Barraquer-Simons syndrome) is caused by mutations in the *LMNB2* gene. Females are more commonly affected. Fat loss begins in childhood or adolescence and affects the face, neck, arms, thorax, and upper abdomen. Excess fat is seen in the hips and legs, especially in females. Low levels of complement C3 are almost universally seen. C3 nephritic factor is also present. C3 nephritic factor stabilizes C3 convertase, allowing for unopposed activation of the alternate complement pathway and the decreased level of C3. Membranous proliferative glomerulonephritis and other autoimmune diseases may develop. Insulin-resistant diabetes mellitus is rare.

GENERALIZED LIPODYSTROPHY

Generalized lipodystrophy may also be congenital or acquired.

Congenital generalized lipodystrophy is seen in 3 forms:

Type 1 (Berardinelli-Seip congenital lipodystrophy type 1 [BSCL1]) is an autosomal recessive disorder caused by mutations in the 1-acylglycerol-3-phosphate-O-acyltransferase (*AGPAT2*) gene.

Type 2 (Berardinelli-Seip congenital lipodystrophy type 2 [BSCL2]) is also autosomal recessive and caused by mutations in the seipin gene.

Type 3 (*CAV1*) is autosomal recessive and caused by mutations in the caveolin 1 gene.

Marked lipodystrophy occurs at birth or in early infancy. Diabetes mellitus, hypertriglyceridemia, hepatic steatosis, acanthosis nigricans, and muscular hypertrophy occur. BSCL2 is a more severe phenotype, with premature death occurring in ≈ 15% of cases.

Acquired generalized lipodystrophy is more common in females. The most common associated disorder is juvenile dermatomyositis (78%). Panniculitis is seen in 17%. More than half of the children may have other complications, including acanthosis nigricans, hyperpigmentation, hepatomegaly, hypertension, protuberant abdomen, and hyperlipidemia.

Localized lipoatrophy is an idiopathic condition that manifests as annular atrophy at the ankles; a bandlike semicircular depression 2-4 cm in diameter on the thighs, abdomen, and/or upper groin or as a centrifugally spreading, depressed, bluish plaque with an erythematous margin.

Insulin lipoatrophy usually occur approximately 6 mo-2 yr after initiation of relatively high doses of insulin. A dimple or well-circumscribed depression at the site of injection is typically seen, although loss of fat may extend beyond the site of injection, leading to an extensive, depressed plaque. Biopsy reveals a marked decrease or absence of subcutaneous tissue, without inflammation or fibrosis. In some patients, hypertrophy occurs clinically. In these cases, the mid-dermal collagen is replaced by hypertrophic fat cells on histopathologic sections. The mechanism of insulin lipoatrophy may be cross-reaction of insulin antibodies with fat cells; the incidence of this condition has decreased since the implementation of widespread use of highly purified insulins. Lesions may also be prevented by frequent alteration of injection sites.

BIBLIOGRAPHY

Please visit the Nelson Textbook of Pediatrics *website at* *www.expertconsult.com* *for the complete bibliography.*

Chapter 653
Disorders of the Sweat Glands

Joseph G. Morelli

Eccrine glands are found over nearly the entire skin surface and provide the primary means, through evaporation of the water in sweat, of cooling the body. These glands have no anatomic relationship to hair follicles and secrete a relatively large amount of odorless aqueous sweat. In contrast, apocrine sweat glands are limited in distribution to the axillae, anogenital skin, mammary glands, ceruminous glands of the ear, Moll glands in the eyelid, and selected areas of the face and scalp. Each apocrine gland duct enters the pilosebaceous follicle at the level of the infundibulum and secretes a small amount of a complex, viscous fluid that, on alteration by microorganisms, produces a distinctive body odor. Some disorders of these two types of sweat glands are similar pathogenetically, whereas others are unique to a given gland.

ANHIDROSIS

Neuropathic anhidrosis results from a disturbance in the neural pathway from the control center in the brain to the peripheral efferent nerve fibers that activate sweating. Disorders in this category, which are characterized by generalized anhidrosis, include tumors of the hypothalamus and damage to the floor of the 3rd ventricle. Pontine or medullary lesions may produce anhidrosis of the ipsilateral face or neck and ipsilateral or contralateral anhidrosis of the rest of the body. Peripheral or segmental neuropathies, caused by leprosy, amyloidosis, diabetes mellitus, alcoholic neuritis, or syringomyelia, may be associated with anhidrosis of the innervated skin. Various autonomic disorders are also associated with altered eccrine sweat gland function.

At the level of the sweat gland, anticholinergics (drugs such as atropine and scopolamine) may paralyze the sweat glands. Acute intoxication with barbiturates or diazepam has produced necrosis of sweat glands, resulting in anhidrosis with or without erythema and bullae. Eccrine glands are largely absent throughout the skin or are present in a localized area among patients with **anhidrotic ectodermal dysplasia** or **localized congenital absence** of sweat glands, respectively. Infiltrative or destructive disorders that may produce atrophy of sweat glands by pressure or scarring include scleroderma, acrodermatitis chronica atrophicans, radiodermatitis, burns, Sjögren syndrome, multiple myeloma, and lymphoma. Obstruction of sweat glands may occur in miliaria and in a number of inflammatory and hyperkeratotic disorders, such as the ichthyoses, psoriasis, lichen planus, pemphigus, porokeratosis, atopic dermatitis, and seborrheic dermatitis. Occlusion of the sweat pore may also occur with the topical agents aluminum and zirconium salts, formaldehyde, or glutaraldehyde.

Diverse disorders that are associated with anhidrosis by unknown mechanisms include dehydration; toxic overdose with lead, arsenic, thallium, fluorine, or morphine; uremia; cirrhosis; endocrine disorders such as Addison disease, diabetes mellitus, diabetes insipidus, and hyperthyroidism; and inherited conditions such as Fabry disease, Franceschetti-Jadassohn syndrome, which combines features of incontinentia pigmenti and anhidrotic ectodermal dysplasia, and familial anhidrosis with neurolabyrinthitis.

Anhidrosis may be complete, but in many cases, what appears clinically to be anhidrosis is actually **hypohidrosis** caused by anhidrosis of many but not all eccrine glands. Compensatory, localized hyperhidrosis of the remaining functional sweat glands may occur, particularly in diabetes mellitus and miliaria. The primary complication of anhidrosis is **hyperthermia**, seen primarily in anhidrotic ectodermal dysplasia or in otherwise normal preterm or full-term neonates who have immature eccrine glands.

HYPERHIDROSIS

Etiology/Pathogenesis

Hyperhidrosis is excessive sweating beyond what is physiologically necessary for temperature control and occurs in 3% of the population with about half having axillary hyperhidrosis. The numerous disorders that may be associated with increased production of eccrine sweat may also be classified into those with neural mechanisms involving an abnormality in the pathway from the neural regulatory centers to the sweat gland and those that are non-neurally mediated and occur by direct effects on the sweat glands (Table 653-1).

Table 653-1 CAUSES OF HYPERHIDROSIS

CORTICAL	
Emotional	
Familial dysautonomia	
Congenital ichthyosiform erythroderma	
Epidermolysis bullosa	
Nail-patella syndrome	
Jadassohn-Lewandowsky syndrome	
Pachyonychia congenita	
Palmoplantar keratoderma	
HYPOTHALAMIC	
Drugs:	Cardiovascular:
Antipyretics	Heart failure
Emetics	Shock
Insulin	Vasomotor
Meperidine	Cold injury
Exercise	Raynaud phenomenon
Infection:	Rheumatoid arthritis
Defervescence	Neurologic:
Chronic illness	Abscess
Metabolic:	Familial dysautonomia
Debility	Postencephalitic
Diabetes mellitus	Tumor
Hyperpituitarism	Miscellaneous:
Hyperthyroidism	Chédiak-Higashi syndrome
Hypoglycemia	Compensatory
Obesity	Phenylketonuria
Porphyria	Pheochromocytoma
Pregnancy	Vitiligo
Rickets	
Infantile scurvy	
MEDULLARY	
Physiologic gustatory sweating	
Encephalitis	
Granulosis rubra nasi	
Syringomyelia	
Thoracic sympathetic trunk injury	
SPINAL	
Cord transection	
Syringomyelia	
CHANGES IN BLOOD FLOW	
Maffucci syndrome	
Arteriovenous fistula	
Klippel-Trenaunay syndrome	
Glomus tumor	
Blue rubber-bleb nevus syndrome	

Clinical manifestations

The average age at onset of hyperhidrosis is 14-25 yr. The excess sweating may be continuous or may occur in response to emotional stimuli. In severe cases, sweat may be seen to drip constantly from the hands.

Treatment

Excessive sweating of the palms and soles (volar hyperhidrosis) and axillary sweating may respond to 20% aluminum chloride in anhydrous ethanol applied under occlusion for several hours, iontophoresis (palms and soles only), injection with botulinum toxin, therapy with oral anticholinergics, or in severe, refractory cases, cervicothoracic or lumbar sympathectomy.

MILIARIA

Etiology/Pathogenesis

Miliaria results from retention of sweat in occluded eccrine sweat ducts. The keratinous plug does not form until the later stages of the disease, and therefore, does not appear to be the primary cause of the sweat duct obstruction. The initial obstruction is postulated to be due to swelling of the ductal epidermal cells, perhaps from imbibition of water. Retrograde pressure may result in rupture of the duct and leakage of sweat into the epidermis and/or the dermis. The eruption is most often induced by hot, humid weather, but it may also be caused by high fever. Infants who are dressed too warmly may demonstrate this eruption indoors, even during the winter.

Clinical Manifestations

In **miliaria crystallina**, asymptomatic, noninflammatory, pinpoint, clear vesicles may suddenly erupt in profusion over large areas of the body surface, leaving brawny desquamation on healing (Fig. 653-1). This type of miliaria occurs most frequently in newborn infants because of the relative immaturity and delayed patency of the sweat duct and the tendency for infants to be nursed in relatively warm, humid conditions. It may also occur in older patients with hyperpyrexia.

Miliaria rubra is a less superficial eruption characterized by erythematous, minute papulovesicles that may impart a prickling sensation. The lesions are usually localized to sites of occlusion or to flexural areas, such as the neck, groin, and axillae, where friction may have a role in their pathogenesis. Involved skin may become macerated and eroded. Lesions of miliaria rubra, however, are extrafollicular.

Repeated attacks of miliaria rubra may lead to **miliaria profunda**, which is due to rupture of the sweat duct deeper in the skin, at the level of the dermal-epidermal junction. Severe, extensive miliaria rubra or miliaria profunda may result in

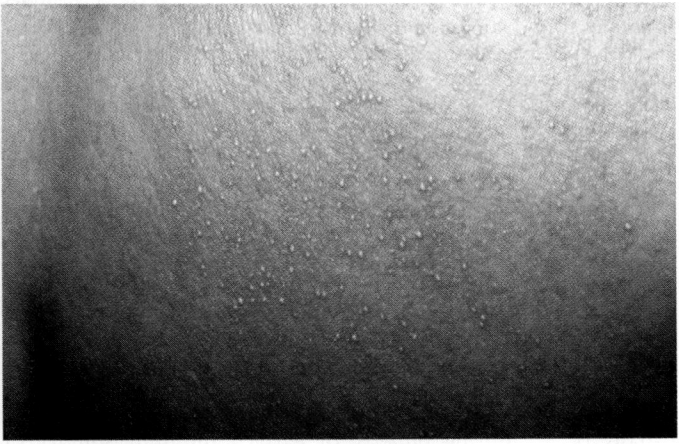

Figure 653-1 Superficial clear vesicles of miliaria crystallina.

disturbance of heat regulation. Lesions of miliaria rubra may become infected, particularly in malnourished or debilitated infants, leading to development of **periporitis staphylogenes**, which involves extension of the process from the sweat duct into the sweat gland.

Histology
Histologically, miliaria crystallina reveals an intracorneal or subcorneal vesicle in communication with the sweat duct, whereas in miliaria rubra, one sees focal areas of spongiosis and spongiotic vesicle formation in close proximity to sweat ducts that generally contain a keratinous plug.

Differential Diagnosis
The clarity of the fluid, superficiality of the vesicles, and absence of inflammation permit differentiation of miliaria crystalline from other blistering disorders. Miliaria rubra may be confused with or superimposed on other diaper area eruptions, including candidosis and folliculitis.

Treatment
All forms of miliaria respond dramatically to cooling of the patient by regulation of environmental temperatures and by removal of excessive clothing; administration of antipyretics is also beneficial to patients with fever. Topical agents are usually ineffective and may exacerbate the eruption.

BROMHIDROSIS

The excessive odor that characterizes bromhidrosis may result from alteration of either apocrine or eccrine sweat. Apocrine bromhidrosis develops after puberty as a result of the formation of short-chain fatty acids and ammonia by the action of anaerobic diphtheroids on axillary apocrine sweat. Eccrine bromhidrosis is caused by microbiologic degradation of stratum corneum that has become softened by excessive eccrine sweat. The soles of the feet and the intertriginous areas are the primary affected sites. Hyperhidrosis, warm weather, obesity, intertrigo, and diabetes mellitus are predisposing factors. **Treatments** that may be helpful include cleansing with germicidal soaps, topical clindamycin or erythromycin, or topical application of aluminum or zirconium. Treatment of any associated hyperhidrosis is mandatory.

HIDRADENITIS SUPPURATIVA

Etiology/Pathogenesis
Hidradenitis suppurativa is a disease of the apocrine gland–bearing areas of the skin. Pathogenesis of hidradenitis suppurativa is controversial. It is now believed that it is a primary inflammatory disorder of the hair follicle and not solely an alteration of apocrine glands. It is considered a part of the follicular occlusion tetrad, along with acne conglobata, dissecting cellulites of the scalp, and pilonidal sinus. Bacterial infection, particularly with *Staphylococcus aureus, Streptococcus milleri, Escherichia coli,* and, possibly, anaerobic streptococci, appears to be important in the progressive dilatation below the obstruction, leading to rupture of the duct, inflammation, sinus tract formation, and destructive scarring.

Clinical Manifestations
Hidradenitis suppurativa is a chronic, inflammatory, suppurative disorder of the apocrine glands in the axillae, the anogenital area, and, occasionally, the scalp, posterior aspect of the ears, female breasts, and periumbilical area. Onset of clinical manifestations is sometimes preceded by pruritus or discomfort and usually occurs during puberty or early adulthood. Solitary or multiple painful erythematous nodules, deep abscesses, and contracted scars are sharply confined to areas of skin containing apocrine glands. When the disease is severe and chronic, sinus tracts, ulcers, and thick, linear fibrotic bands develop. Hidradenitis suppurativa tends to persist for many years, punctuated by relapses and partial remissions. Complications include cellulitis, ulceration, and burrowing abscesses that may perforate adjacent structures, forming fistulas to the urethra, bladder, rectum, or peritoneum. Episodic inflammatory arthritis develops in some patients.

Histology
Early lesions are characterized by a keratinous plug in the apocrine duct or hair follicle orifice and by cystic distention of the follicle. The process generally but not necessarily extends into the apocrine gland. Later changes include inflammation within and around apocrine glands and the presence of groups of cocci within apocrine glands and in the adjacent dermis. Scarring may obliterate skin appendages.

Differential Diagnosis
Early lesions of hidradenitis suppurativa are often mistaken for infected epidermal cysts, furuncles, scrofuloderma, actinomycosis, cat-scratch disease, granuloma inguinale, or lymphogranuloma venereum. Sharp localization to areas of the body that bear apocrine glands, however, should suggest hidradenitis. When involvement is limited to the anogenital region, the condition may be difficult to distinguish from Crohn disease.

Treatment
Conservative management includes cessation of smoking, weight loss, and avoidance of irritation of the affected area. Warm compresses and topical antiseptic or antibacterial soaps may also be helpful. For mild, early, disease, topical clindamycin 1% is the treatment of choice. For more severe disease therapy may be initiated with tetracycline (500 mg bid), doxycycline (100 mg bid), or minocycline (100 mg bid). Some patients require intermittent or long-term antibiotic treatment. Oral retinoids (1 mg/kg/day) for 5-6 mo may also be effective. Oral contraceptive agents, which contain a high estrogen : progesterone ratio and low androgenicity of the progesterone, are another alternative. Surgical measures may be required for control or cure.

FOX-FORDYCE DISEASE

Etiology/Pathogenesis
The cause of Fox-Fordyce disease is unknown.

Clinical Manifestations
This disease is most common in females and manifests during puberty to the 3rd decade of life as pruritus in the axillae. Pruritus is exacerbated by emotional stress and stimuli that induce apocrine sweating. Dome-shaped, skin-colored to slightly hyperpigmented, follicular papules develop in the pruritic areas.

Histology
Histopathologically, one sees keratinous plugging of the distal apocrine duct, rupture of the intraepidermal portion of the apocrine duct, paraductal microvesicle formation, and paraductal acanthosis.

Treatment
Fox-Fordyce disease is difficult to treat. Oral contraceptive pills and topical corticosteroids or retinoic acid may help some patients.

BIBLIOGRAPHY
Please visit the Nelson Textbook of Pediatrics *website at www.expertconsult.com for the complete bibliography.*

Chapter 654
Disorders of Hair

Joseph G. Morelli

Disorders of hair in infants and children may be due to intrinsic disturbances of hair growth, underlying biochemical or metabolic defects, inflammatory dermatoses, or structural anomalies of the hair shaft. Excessive and abnormal hair growth is referred to as hypertrichosis or hirsutism. **Hypertrichosis** is excessive hair growth at inappropriate locations; hirsutism is an androgen-dependent male pattern of hair growth in women. **Hypotrichosis** is deficient hair growth. Hair loss, partial or complete, is called alopecia. Alopecia may be classified as nonscarring or scarring; the latter type is rare in children and, if present, is most often due to prolonged or untreated inflammatory conditions such as pyoderma and tinea capitis.

HYPERTRICHOSIS

Hypertrichosis is rare in children and may be localized or generalized and permanent or transient. Hypertrichosis has many causes, some of which are listed in Table 654-1.

HYPOTRICHOSIS AND ALOPECIA

Some of the disorders associated with hypotrichosis and alopecia are listed in Table 654-2. True alopecia is rarely congenital; it is more often related to an inflammatory dermatosis, mechanical factors, drug ingestion, infection, endocrinopathy, nutritional disturbance, or disturbance of the hair cycle. Any inflammatory condition of the scalp, such as atopic dermatitis or seborrheic dermatitis, if severe enough, may result in partial alopecia; hair growth returns to normal if the underlying condition is treated successfully, unless the hair follicle has been permanently damaged.

Hair loss in childhood should be divided into the following 4 categories: congenital diffuse, congenital localized, acquired diffuse, and acquired localized.

Acquired localized hair loss is the most common type of hair loss seen in childhood. Three conditions—traumatic alopecia, alopecia areata, tinea capitis—are predominantly seen (Tables 654-3 and 654-4).

TRAUMATIC ALOPECIA (TRACTION ALOPECIA, HAIR PULLING, TRICHOTILLOMANIA)

Traction Alopecia

Traction alopecia is common and is seen in almost 20% of African American schoolgirls. It is due to trauma to hair follicles from tight braids or ponytails, headbands, rubber bands, curlers, or rollers (Fig. 654-1). There is a greater risk of traction alopecia if hair trauma is combined with chemically relaxed hair. Broken hairs and inflammatory follicular papules in circumscribed patches at the scalp margins are characteristic and may be subtended by regional lymphadenopathy. Children and parents must be encouraged to avoid devices that cause trauma to the hair and, if necessary, to alter the hairstyle. Otherwise, scarring of hair follicles may occur.

Hair Pulling

Hair pulling in childhood is usually an acute reactional process related to emotional stress. It may also be seen in trichotillomania and as part of more severe psychiatric disorders.

TRICHOTILLOMANIA

Etiology/Pathogenesis The diagnostic criteria for trichotillomania include visible hair loss attributable to pulling; mounting tension preceding hair pulling; gratification or release of tension after hair pulling; and absence of hair pulling attributable to hallucinations, delusions, or an inflammatory skin condition.

Clinical Manifestations Compulsive pulling, twisting, and breaking of hair produces irregular areas of incomplete hair loss, most often on the crown and in the occipital and parietal areas of the scalp. Occasionally, eyebrows, eyelashes, and body hair are traumatized. Some plaques of alopecia may have a linear outline. The

Table 654-1 CAUSES OF AND CONDITIONS ASSOCIATED WITH HYPERTRICHOSIS

INTRINSIC FACTORS
Racial and familial forms such as hairy ears, hairy elbows, intraphalangeal hair, or generalized hirsutism
EXTRINSIC FACTORS
Local trauma
Malnutrition
Anorexia nervosa
Long-standing inflammatory dermatoses
Drugs: Diazoxide, phenytoin, corticosteroids, Cortisporin, cyclosporine, androgens, anabolic agents, hexachlorobenzene, minoxidil, psoralens, penicillamine, streptomycin
HAMARTOMAS OR NEVI
Congenital pigmented nevocytic nevus, hair follicle nevus, Becker nevus, congenital smooth muscle hamartoma, fawn-tail nevus associated with diastematomyelia
ENDOCRINE DISORDERS
Virilizing ovarian tumors, Cushing syndrome, acromegaly, hyperthyroidism, hypothyroidism, congenital adrenal hyperplasia, adrenal tumors, gonadal dysgenesis, male pseudohermaphroditism, non–endocrine hormone–secreting tumors, polycystic ovary syndrome
CONGENITAL AND GENETIC DISORDERS
Hypertrichosis lanuginosa, mucopolysaccharidosis, leprechaunism, congenital generalized lipodystrophy, de Lange syndrome, trisomy 18, Rubinstein-Taybi syndrome, Bloom syndrome, congenital hemihypertrophy, gingival fibromatosis with hypertrichosis, Winchester syndrome, lipoatrophic diabetes (Lawrence-Seip syndrome), fetal hydantoin syndrome, fetal alcohol syndrome, congenital erythropoietic or variegate porphyria (sun-exposed areas), porphyria cutanea tarda (sun-exposed areas), Cowden syndrome, Seckel syndrome, Gorlin syndrome, partial trisomy 3q, Ambra syndrome

Table 654-2 DISORDERS ASSOCIATED WITH ALOPECIA AND HYPOTRICHOSIS

Congenital total alopecia: Atrichia with papules, Moynahan alopecia syndrome
Congenital localized alopecia: Aplasia cutis, triangular alopecia, sebaceous nevus
Hereditary hypotrichosis: Marie-Unna syndrome, hypotrichosis with juvenile macular dystrophy, hypotrichosis–Mari type, ichthyosis with hypotrichosis, cartilage-hair hypoplasia, Hallermann-Streiff syndrome, trichorhinophalangeal syndrome, ectodermal dysplasia "pure" hair and nail and other ectodermal dysplasias
Diffuse alopecia of endocrine origin: Hypopituitarism, hypothyroidism, hypoparathyroidism, hyperthyroidism
Alopecia of nutritional origin: Marasmus, kwashiorkor, iron deficiency, zinc deficiency (acrodermatitis enteropathica), gluten-sensitive enteropathy, essential fatty acid deficiency, biotinidase deficiency
Disturbances of the hair cycle: Telogen effluvium
Toxic alopecia: Anagen effluvium
Autoimmune alopecia: Alopecia areata
Traumatic alopecia: Traction alopecia, trichotillomania
Cicatricial alopecia: Lupus erythematosus, lichen planopilaris, pseudopelade, morphea (en coup de saber) dermatomyositis, infection (kerion, favus, tuberculosis, syphilis, folliculitis, leishmaniasis, herpes zoster, varicella), acne keloidalis, follicular mucinosis, sarcoidosis
Hair shaft abnormalities: Monilethrix, pili annulati, pili torti, trichorrhexis invaginata, trichorrhexis nodosa, woolly hair syndrome, Menkes disease, trichothiodystrophy, trichodento-osseous syndrome, uncombable hair syndrome (spun-glass hair, pili trianguli et canaliculi)

Table 654-3 HELPFUL HISTORICAL CLUES IN DIAGNOSIS OF HAIR DISORDERS

HISTORICAL CONSIDERATIONS	TELOGEN EFFLUVIUM	TRICHOTILLOMANIA	TINEA CAPITIS	ALOPECIA AREATA
Are the spots itchy?	Negative	Negative	Positive	Usually negative
Do the spots come and go?	Negative	Sometimes positive	Negative	Sometimes positive
Is the hair falling out in clumps?	Positive	Negative	Negative	Usually negative
Are there any anxiety disorders or obsessive-compulsive tendencies?	Negative	Positive	Negative	Negative

From Lio PA: What's missing from this picture? An approach to alopecia in children, *Arch Dis Child Ed* 92:193–198, 2007.

Table 654-4 HELPFUL PHYSICAL EXAMINATION CLUES IN DIAGNOSIS OF HAIR DISORDERS

PHYSICAL FINDINGS	TELOGEN EFFLUVIUM	TRICHOTILLOMANIA	TINEA CAPITIS	ALOPECIA AREATA
Scarring?	Negative	Negative	Usually negative	Negative
Exclamation-point hairs?	Negative	Negative	Negative	Positive
Irregular pattern with mixed length and stubbly hairs?	Negative	Positive	Negative	Negative
Scaling, pustules or kerion?	Negative	Negative	Positive	Negative
Positive hair-pull test result?	Positive	Negative	Negative	Usually negative
Nail pitting or grooves?	Negative	Negative	Negative	Positive

From Lio PA: What's missing from this picture? An approach to alopecia in children, *Arch Dis Child Ed* 92:193–198, 2007.

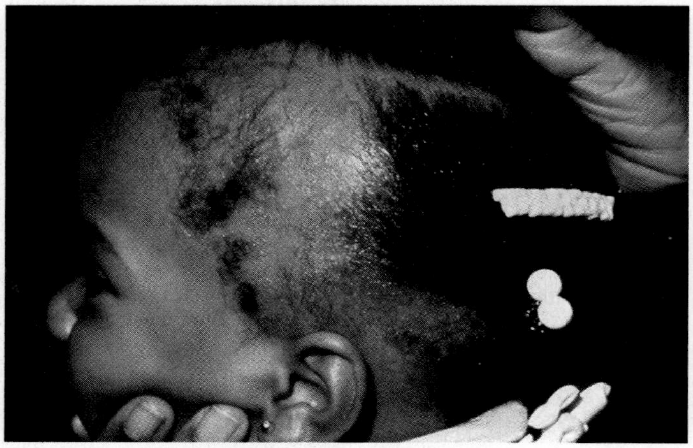

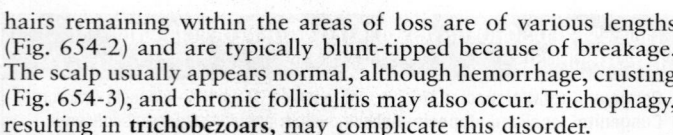

Figure 654-1 Traction alopecia.

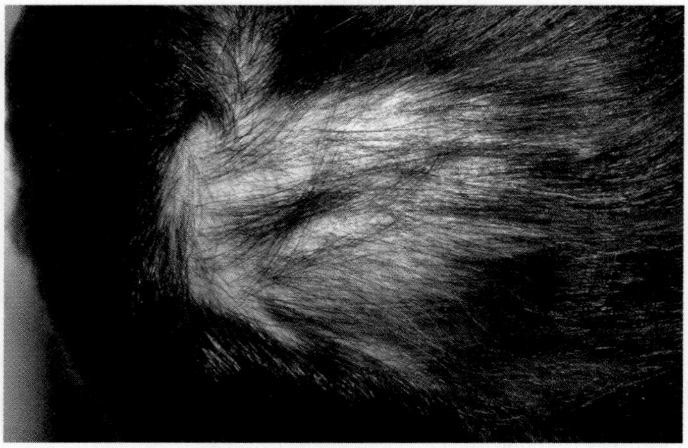

Figure 654-2 Hair pulling. Hairs are broken off at various lengths.

hairs remaining within the areas of loss are of various lengths (Fig. 654-2) and are typically blunt-tipped because of breakage. The scalp usually appears normal, although hemorrhage, crusting (Fig. 654-3), and chronic folliculitis may also occur. Trichophagy, resulting in **trichobezoars,** may complicate this disorder.

Differential Diagnosis Acute reactional hair pulling, tinea capitis, and alopecia areata must be considered in the differential diagnosis of trichotillomania (see Tables 654-3 and 654-4).

Histology Histologic changes include coexistent normal and damaged follicles, perifollicular hemorrhage, atrophy of some follicles, and catagen transformation of hair. In late stages, perifollicular fibrosis may occur. Long-term repeated trauma may result in irreversible damage and permanent alopecia.

Treatment Trichotillomania is closely related to obsessive-compulsive disorder and may be an expression of it for some children. When trichotillomania occur secondary to **obsessive-compulsive disorder,** clomipramine 50-150 mg/day or fluoxetine 40-80 mg/day may be helpful, particularly when combined with behavioral interventions (Chapter 22). N-Acetylcysteine may also be helpful.

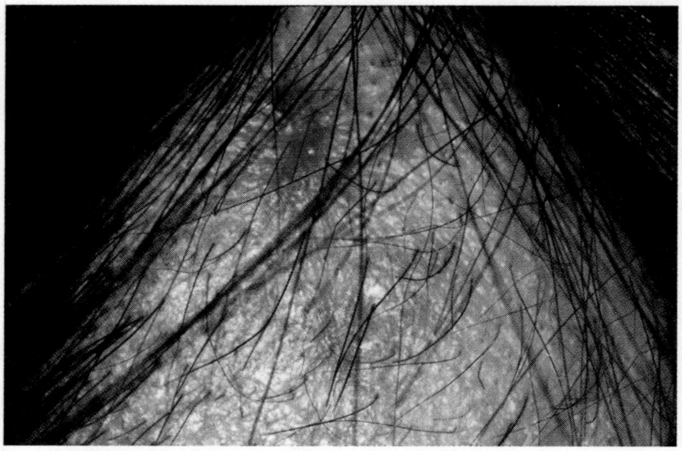

Figure 654-3 Hemorrhage and crusting secondary to hair pulling.

ALOPECIA AREATA

Etiology/Pathogenesis

Alopecia areata is an immune-mediated nonscarring alopecia. The cause is unknown. It is hypothesized that in genetically susceptible individuals, loss of immune privilege of the hair follicle allows for T-cell inflammation against anagen hairs follicles, leading to stoppage of hair growth.

Clinical Manifestations

Alopecia areata is characterized by rapid and complete loss of hair in round or oval patches on the scalp (Fig. 654-4) and on

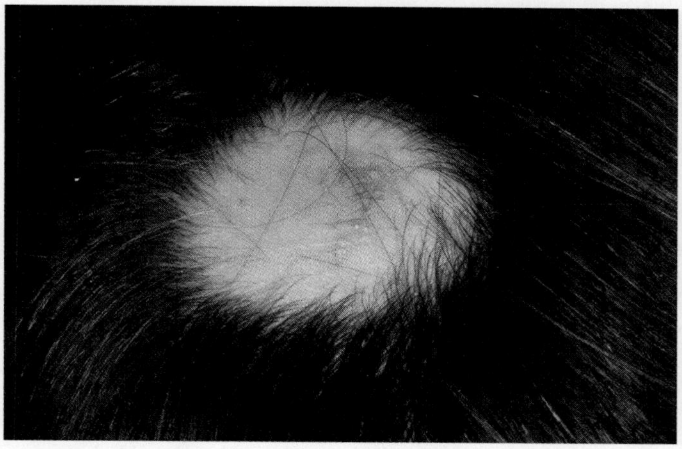

Figure 654-4 Circular patch of alopecia areata with normal-appearing scalp.

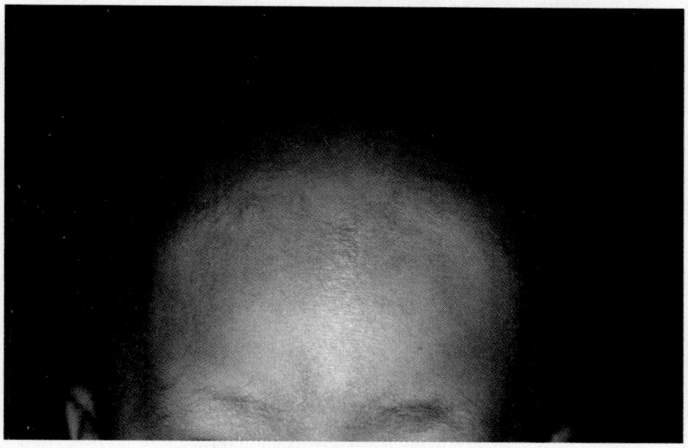

Figure 654-5 Alopecia totalis: total loss of scalp hair.

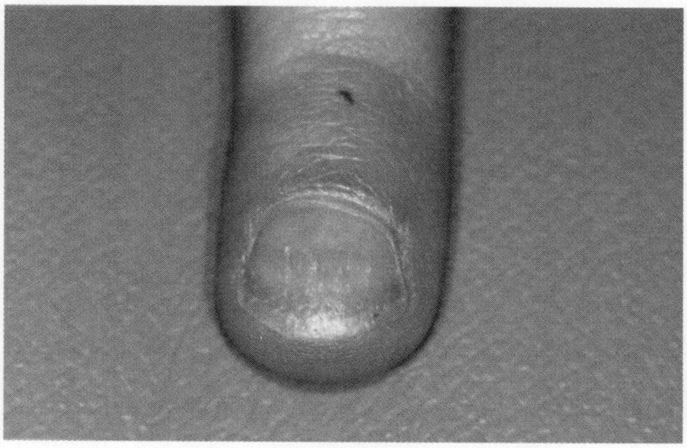

Figure 654-6 Multiple nail pits in alopecia areata.

other body sites. In alopecia totalis, all the scalp hair is lost (Fig. 654-5); alopecia universalis involves all body and scalp hair. The lifetime incidence of alopecia areata is 0.1% to 0.2% of the population. More than half of affected patients are younger than 20 yr.

The skin within the plaques of hair loss appears normal. Alopecia areata is associated with atopy and with nail changes such as pits (Fig. 654-6), longitudinal striations, and leukonychia. **Autoimmune diseases** such as Hashimoto thyroiditis, Addison

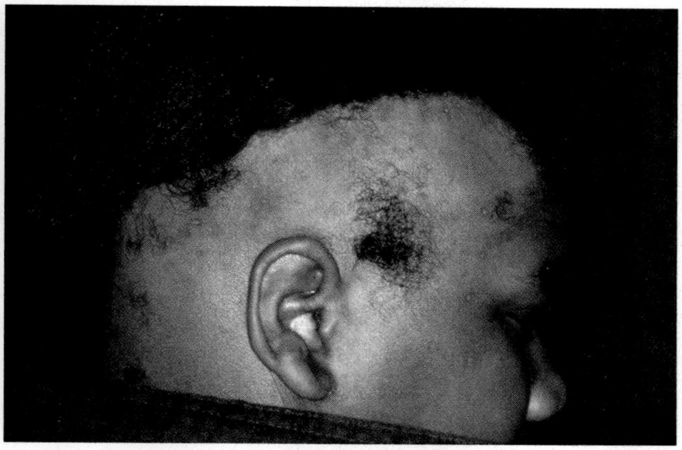

Figure 654-7 Ophiasis pattern of alopecia areata.

disease, pernicious anemia, ulcerative colitis, myasthenia gravis, collagen vascular diseases, and vitiligo may also be seen. An increased incidence of alopecia areata has been reported in patients with Down syndrome (5-10%).

Differential Diagnosis

Tinea capitis, seborrheic dermatitis, trichotillomania, traumatic alopecia, and lupus erythematosus should be considered in the differential diagnosis of alopecia areata (see Tables 654-3 and 654-4).

Histology

A perifollicular infiltrate of inflammatory round cells is found in biopsy specimens from active areas of alopecia areata.

Treatment

The course is unpredictable, but spontaneous resolution in 6-12 mo is usual, particularly when relatively small, stable patches of alopecia are present. Recurrences are common. Onset at a young age, extensive or prolonged hair loss, and numerous episodes are usually poor prognostic signs. Alopecia universalis, alopecia totalis, and alopecia ophiasis (Fig. 654-7)—a type of alopecia areata in which hair loss is circumferential—are also less likely to resolve. Therapy is difficult to evaluate because the course is erratic and unpredictable. The use of high- or superpotency topical corticosteroids is effective in some patients. Intradermal injections of steroid (triamcinolone 5 mg/mL) every 4-6 wk may also stimulate hair growth locally, but this mode of treatment is impractical in young children or in patients with extensive hair loss. Systemic corticosteroid therapy (prednisone 1 mg/kg/day) has been associated with good results; the permanence of cure is questionable, however, and the side effects of chronic oral corticosteroids are a serious deterrent. Additional therapies that are sometimes effective include short-contact anthralin, topical minoxidil, and contact sensitization with squaric acid dibutylester or diphencyprone. In general, parents and patients can be reassured that spontaneous remission of alopecia areata usually occurs. New hair growth may initially be of finer caliber and lighter color, but replacement by normal terminal hair can be expected.

ACQUIRED DIFFUSE HAIR LOSS

Telogen Effluvium

Telogen effluvium manifests as sudden loss of large amounts of hair, often with brushing, combing, and washing of hair. Diffuse loss of scalp hair occurs from premature conversion of growing, or anagen, hairs, which normally constitute 80-90% of hairs, to resting, or telogen, hairs. Hair loss is noted 6 wk-3 mo after the

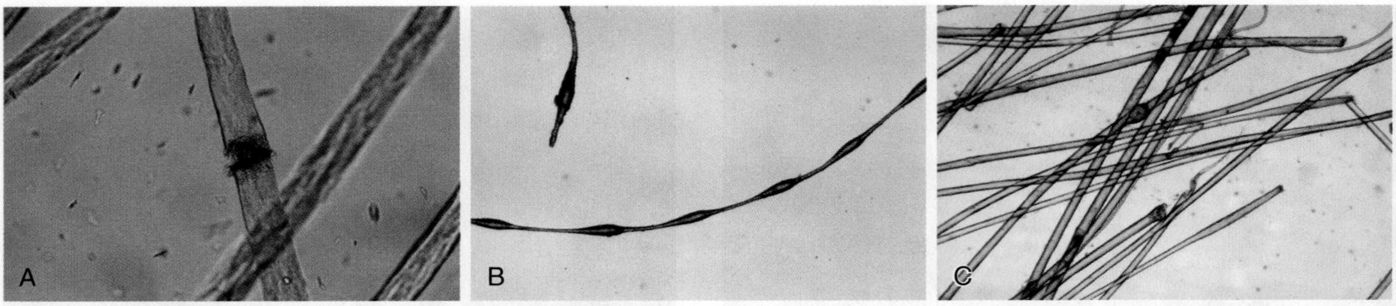

Figure 654-8 *A,* Microscopic hair fracture in trichorrhexis nodosa. *B,* Beading of hair in monilethrix. *C,* Cuplike abnormality of hair in Netherton syndrome.

precipitating cause, which may include childbirth; a febrile episode; surgery; acute blood loss, including blood donation; sudden severe weight loss; discontinuation of high-dose corticosteroids or oral contraceptives; and psychiatric stress. Telogen effluvium also accounts for the loss of hair by infants in the first few months of life; friction from bed sheets, particularly in infants with pruritic, atopic skin, may exacerbate the problem. There is no inflammatory reaction; the hair follicles remain intact, and telogen bulbs can be demonstrated microscopically on shed hairs. Because >50% of the scalp hair is rarely involved, alopecia is usually not severe. Parents should be reassured that normal hair growth will return within approximately 3-6 mo.

Toxic Alopecia (Anagen Effluvium)

Anagen effluvium is an acute, severe, diffuse inhibition of growth of anagen follicles, resulting in loss of >80-90% of scalp hair. Hairs become dystrophic, and the hair shaft breaks at the narrowed segment. Loss is diffuse, rapid (1-3 wk after treatment), and temporary, as regrowth occurs after the offending agent is discontinued. Causes of anagen effluvium include radiation; cancer chemotherapeutic agents such as antimetabolites, alkylating agents, and mitotic inhibitors; thallium; thiouracil; heparin; the coumarins; boric acid; and hypervitaminosis A.

CONGENITAL DIFFUSE HAIR LOSS

Congenital diffuse hair loss is defined as congenitally thin hair diffusely related to either hypoplasia of hair follicles or to structural defects in hair shafts.

Structural Defects of Hair

Structural defects of the hair shaft may be congenital, reflect known biochemical aberrations, or relate to damaging grooming practices. All the defects can be demonstrated by microscopic examination of affected hairs, particularly with scanning and transmission electron microscopy.

Trichorrhexis Nodosa

Congenital trichorrhexis nodosa is an autosomal dominant condition. The hair is dry, brittle, and lusterless, with irregularly spaced grayish white nodes on the hair shaft. Microscopically, the nodes have the appearance of two interlocking brushes (Fig. 654-8*A*). The defect results from a fracture of the hair shaft at the nodal points caused by disruption of the cells in the hair cortex. Trichorrhexis nodosa has also been observed in some infants with Menkes syndrome, trichothiodystrophy, citrullinemia, and argininosuccinic aciduria.

ACQUIRED TRICHORRHEXIS NODOSA Acquired trichorrhexis nodosa, the most common cause of hair breakage, occurs in two forms. Proximal defects are found most frequently in African-American children, whose complaint is not of alopecia but of failure of the hair to grow. The hair is short, and longitudinal splits, knots, and whitish nodules can be demonstrated in hair mounts. Easy breakage is demonstrated by gentle traction on the hair shafts. A history of other affected family members may be obtained. The problem may be caused by a combination of genetic predisposition and the cumulative mechanical trauma of rough combing and brushing, hair-straightening procedures, and "permanents." Patients must be cautioned to avoid damaging grooming techniques. A soft natural-bristle brush and a wide-toothed comb should be used. The condition is self-limited, with resolution in 2-4 yr if patients avoid damaging practices. Distal trichorrhexis nodosa is seen more frequently in white and Asian children. The distal portion of the hair shaft is thinned, ragged, and faded; white specks, sometimes mistaken for nits, may be noted along the shaft. Hair mounts reveal the paintbrush defect and the sites of excessive fragility and breakage. Localized areas of the moustache or beard may also be affected. Avoidance of traumatic grooming, regular trimming of affected ends, and the use of cream rinses to lessen tangling ameliorate this condition.

Pili Torti

Patients with pili torti present with spangled, brittle, coarse hair of different lengths over the entire scalp. There is a structural defect in which the hair shaft is grooved and flattened at irregular intervals and is twisted on its axis to various degrees. Minor twists that occur in normal hair should not be misconstrued as pili torti. Curvature of the hair follicle apparently leads to the flattening and rotation of the hair shaft. The genetic defect in isolated pili torti is unknown, and both autosomal dominant and recessive forms have been described. **Syndromes** in which the hair shaft abnormalities of pili torti are seen in association with other cutaneous and systemic abnormalities include Menkes kinky hair syndrome, Björnstad syndrome (pili torti with deafness; *BCS1L* gene), and multiple ectodermal dysplasia syndromes.

Menkes Kinky Hair Syndrome (Trichopoliodystrophy)

Males with Menkes kinky hair syndrome, an X-linked recessive trait, are born to an unaffected mother after a normal pregnancy. Neonatal problems include hypothermia, hypotonia, poor feeding, seizures, and failure to thrive. Hair is normal to sparse at birth but is replaced by short, fine, brittle, light-colored hair that may have features of trichorrhexis nodosa, pili torti, or monilethrix. The skin is hypopigmented and thin, cheeks typically appear plump, and the nasal bridge is depressed. Progressive psychomotor retardation is noted in early infancy. Mutations in the *ATP7A* gene, encoding a copper-transporting adenosine triphosphatase protein, cause Menkes kinky hair syndrome. It is due to maldistribution of the copper in the body. Copper uptake across the brush border of the small intestine is increased, but copper transport from these cells into the plasma is defective, resulting in low total body copper stores. Parenteral administration of copper-histidine is helpful if begun in the first 2 mo of life.

Monilethrix

The hair shaft defect known as monilethrix is inherited as an autosomal dominant trait with variable age of onset, severity, and course. Mutations in the hair keratins HBI, HB3, and HB6 have been identified. The hair appears dry, lusterless, and brittle, and it fractures spontaneously or with mild trauma. Eyebrows, lashes, body and pubic hair, and scalp hair may be affected. Monilethrix may be present at birth, but the hair is usually normal at birth and is replaced in the first few months of life by abnormal hairs; the condition is sometimes first apparent in childhood. Follicular papules may appear on the nape of the neck and the occiput and, occasionally, over the entire scalp. Short, fragile beaded hairs that emerge from the horny follicular plugs give a distinctive appearance. Keratosis pilaris and koilonychia of fingernails and toenails may also be present. Microscopically, a distinctive, regular beading pattern of the hair shaft is evident, characterized by elliptic nodes that are separated by narrower internodes (Fig. 654-8*B*). Not all hairs have nodes, and both normal and beaded hairs may break. Patients should be advised to handle the hair gently to minimize breakage. Treatment is generally ineffective.

Trichothiodystrophy
Hair in trichothiodystrophy is sparse, short, brittle, and uneven; the scalp hair, eyebrows, or eyelashes may be affected. Microscopically, the hair is flattened, folded, and variable in diameter; has longitudinal grooving; and has nodal swellings that resemble those seen in trichorrhexis nodosa. Under a polarizing microscope, distinctive alternating dark and light bands are seen. The abnormal hair has a cystine content that is <50% of normal because of a major reduction in and altered composition of constituent high-sulfur matrix proteins. Trichothiodystrophy may occur as an isolated finding or in association with various syndrome complexes that include intellectual impairment, short stature, ichthyosis, nail dystrophy, dental caries, cataracts, decreased fertility, neurologic abnormalities, bony abnormalities, and immunodeficiency (*TTDN1* gene). Some patients are photosensitive and have impairment of DNA repair mechanisms, similar to that seen in groups B and D xeroderma pigmentosum; the incidence of skin cancers, however, is not increased. Patients with trichothiodystrophy tend to resemble one another, with a receding chin, protruding ears, raspy voice, and sociable, outgoing personality. Trichoschisis, a fracture perpendicular to the hair shaft, is characteristic of the many syndromes that are associated with trichothiodystrophy. Perpendicular breakage of the hair shaft has also been described in association with other hair abnormalities, particularly monilethrix.

Trichorrhexis Invaginata (Bamboo Hair)
Short, sparse, fragile hair without apparent growth is characteristic of trichorrhexis invaginata, which is found primarily in association with Netherton syndrome (Chapter 649). It has also been reported in other ichthyosiform dermatoses. The distal portion of the hair is invaginated into the cuplike proximal portion, forming a fragile nodal swelling (Fig. 654-8*C*).

Pili Annulati
Alternate light and dark bands of the hair shaft characterize pili annulati. When viewed under the light microscope, the region of the hair shaft that appeared bright in reflected light instead appears dark in the transmitted light as a result of focal aggregates of abnormal air-filled cavities within the shaft. The hair is not fragile. The defect may be autosomal dominant or sporadic in inheritance. Pseudopili annulati is a variant of normal blond hair; an optical effect caused by the refraction and reflection of light from the partially twisted and flattened shaft creates the impression of banding.

Woolly Hair Disease
Woolly hair diseases manifest at birth as peculiarly tight, curly, abnormal hair in a non-black person. Autosomal dominant and recessive (*PKRY5* gene) types have been described. Woolly hair nevus, a sporadic form, involves only a circumscribed portion of the scalp hair. The affected hair is fine, tightly curled, and light colored, and it grows poorly. Microscopically, an affected hair is oval and shows twisting of 180 degrees on its axis.

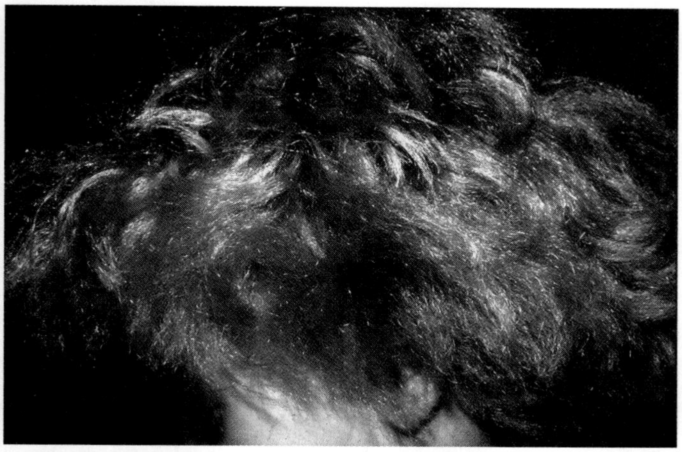

Figure 654-9 Disorderly, silvery blond hair in uncombable hair syndrome.

Uncombable Hair Syndrome (Spun-Glass Hair)
The hair of patients with uncombable hair syndrome appears disorderly, is often silvery blond (Fig. 654-9), and may break because of repeated, futile efforts to control it. The condition is probably autosomal dominant in inheritance. Eyebrows and eyelashes are normal. A longitudinal depression along the hair shaft is a constant feature, and most hair follicles and shafts are triangular (pili trianguli et canaliculi). The shape of the hair varies along its length, however, preventing the hairs from lying flat.

BIBLIOGRAPHY
Please visit the Nelson Textbook of Pediatrics *website at www.expertconsult.com for the complete bibliography.*

Chapter 655
Disorders of the Nails
Joseph G. Morelli

Nail abnormalities in children may be manifestations of generalized skin disease, skin disease localized to the periungual region, systemic disease, drugs, trauma, or localized bacterial and fungal infections (Table 655-1). Nail anomalies are also common in certain congenital disorders (Table 655-2).

ABNORMALITIES IN NAIL SHAPE OR SIZE
Anonychia is absence of the nail plate, usually a result of a congenital disorder or trauma. It may be an isolated finding or may be associated with malformations of the digits. **Koilonychia** is flattening and concavity of the nail plate with loss of normal contour, producing a spoon-shaped nail (Fig. 655-1). Koilonychia occurs as an autosomal dominant trait or in association with iron deficiency anemia, Plummer-Vinson syndrome, or hemochromatosis. The nail plate is relatively thin for the first year or two of life and, consequently, may be spoon-shaped in otherwise normal children.

Congenital nail dysplasia, an autosomal dominant disorder, manifests at birth as longitudinal streaks and thinning of the nail plate. There is platyonychia and koilonychia, which may overgrow the lateral folds and involve all nails of the toes and fingers.

Nail-patella syndrome is an autosomal dominant disorder in which the nails are 30-50% of their normal size and often have triangular or pyramidal lunulae. The thumbnails are always involved, although in some cases only the ulnar half of the nail may be affected or may be missing. The nails from the index

Table 655-1 WHITE NAIL OR NAIL BED CHANGES

DISEASE	CLINICAL APPEARANCE
Anemia	Diffuse white
Arsenic	Mees lines: transverse white lines
Cirrhosis	Terry nails: most of nail, zone of pink at distal end (see Fig. 655-3)
Congenital leukonychia (autosomal dominant; variety of patterns)	Syndrome of leukonychia, knuckle pads, deafness; isolated finding; partial white
Darier disease	Longitudinal white streaks
Half-and-half nail	Proximal white, distal pink azotemia
High fevers (some diseases)	Transverse white lines
Hypoalbuminemia	Muehrcke lines: stationary paired transverse bands
Hypocalcemia	Variable white
Malnutrition	Diffuse white
Pellagra	Diffuse milky white
Punctate leukonychia	Common white spots
Tinea and yeast	Variable patterns
Thallium toxicity (rat poison)	Variable white
Trauma	Repeated manicure: transverse striations
Zinc deficiency	Diffuse white

From Habif TP, editor: *Clinical dermatology,* ed 4, Philadelphia, 2004, Mosby, p 887.

Table 655-2 CONGENITAL DISEASES WITH NAIL DEFECTS

Large nails	Pachyonychia congenita, Rubinstein-Taybi syndrome, hemihypertrophy
Smallness or absence of nails	Ectodermal dysplasias, nail-patella, dyskeratosis congenita, focal dermal hypoplasia, cartilage-hair hypoplasia, Ellis–van Creveld, Larsen, epidermolysis bullosa, incontinentia pigmenti, Rothmund-Thomson, Turner, popliteal web, trisomy 13, trisomy 18, Apert, Gorlin-Pindborg, long arm 21 deletion, otopalatodigital, fetal alcohol, fetal hydantoin, elfin facies, anonychia, acrodermatitis enteropathica
Other	Congenital malalignment of the great toenails, familial dystrophic shedding of the nails

finger to the little finger are progressively less damaged. The patella is also smaller than usual, and this anomaly may lead to knee instability. Bony spines arising from the posterior aspect of the iliac bones, overextension of joints, skin laxity, and renal anomalies may also be present. Nail-patella syndrome is caused by mutations in the transcription factor *LMX1B* gene.

For a discussion of **pachyonychia congenita,** see Chapter 650.

Habit tic deformity consists of a depression down the center of the nail with numerous horizontal ridges extending across the nail from it. One or both thumbs are usually involved as a result of chronic rubbing and picking at the nail with an adjacent finger.

Clubbing of the nails (hippocratic nails) is characterized by swelling of each distal digit, an increase in the angle between the nail plate and the proximal nail fold (Lovibond angle) to >180 degrees, and a spongy feeling when one pushes down and away from the interphalangeal joint, because of an increase in fibrovascular tissue between the matrix and the phalanx (Fig. 655-2). The pathogenesis is not known. Nail clubbing is seen in association with diseases of numerous organ systems, including pulmonary, cardiovascular (cyanotic heart disease), gastrointestinal (celiac disease, inflammatory bowel disease), and hepatic (chronic hepatitis) systems, as well as in healthy individuals as an idiopathic or familial finding.

CHANGES IN NAIL COLOR

Leukonychia is a white opacity of the nail plate that may involve the entire plate or may be punctate or striate (see Table 655-1).

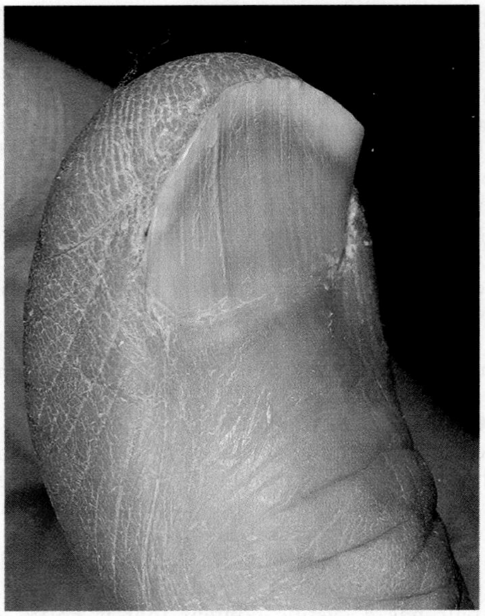

Figure 655-1 Spoon nails (koilonychia). Most cases are a variant of normal. (From Habif TP, editor: *Clinical dermatology,* ed 4, Philadelphia, 2004, Mosby, p 885.)

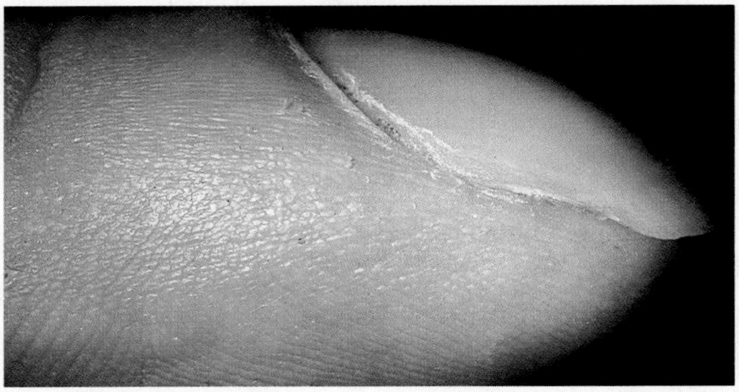

Figure 655-2 Finger clubbing. The distal phalanges are enlarged to a rounded bulbous shape. The nail enlarges and becomes curved, hard, and thickened. (From Habif TP, editor: *Clinical dermatology,* ed 4, Philadelphia, 2004, Mosby, p 885.)

The nail plate itself remains smooth and undamaged. Leukonychia can be traumatic or associated with infections such as leprosy and tuberculosis, dermatoses such as lichen planus and Darier disease, malignancies such as Hodgkin disease, anemia, and arsenic poisoning (Mees lines). Leukonychia of all nail surfaces is an uncommon hereditary autosomal dominant trait that may be associated with congenital epidermal cysts and renal calculi. Paired parallel white bands that do not change position with growth of the nail and thus reflect a change in the nail bed are associated with hypoalbuminemia and are called Muehrcke lines. When the proximal portion of the nail is white and the distal 20-50% of the nail is red, pink, or brown, the condition is called half-and-half nails or Lindsay nails; this is seen most commonly in patients with renal disease but may occur as a normal variant. White nails of **cirrhosis,** or Terry nails (Fig. 655-3), are characterized by a white ground-glass appearance of the entire or the proximal end of the nail and a normal pink distal 1-2 mm of the nail; this finding is associated with hypoalbuminemia.

Black pigmentation of an entire nail plate or linear bands of pigmentation (melanonychia striata) is common in black (90%) and Asian (10-20%) individuals but is unusual in white individuals (<1%). Most often, the pigment is melanin, which is produced by melanocytes of a junctional nevus in the nail matrix and nail bed and is of no consequence. Extension or alteration in the

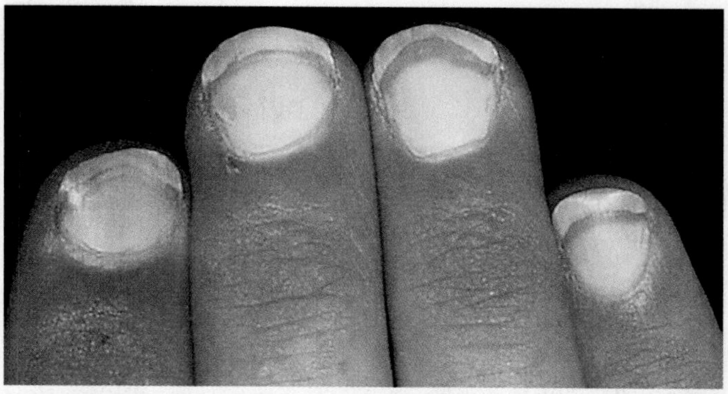

Figure 655-3 Terry nails. The nail bed is white with only a narrow zone of pink at the distal end. (From Habif TP, editor: *Clinical dermatology*, ed 4, Philadelphia, 2004, Mosby, p 885.)

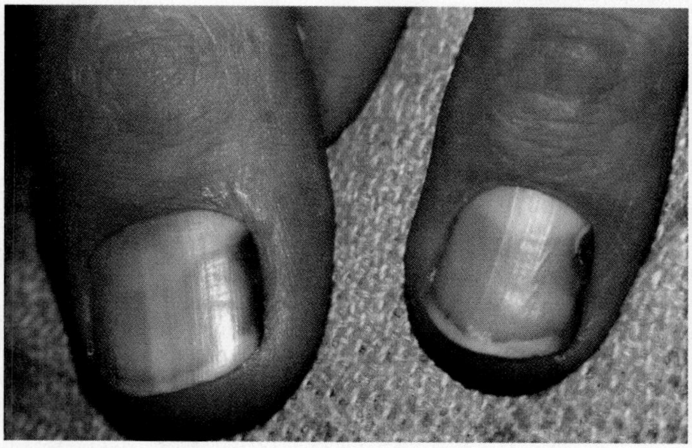

Figure 655-4 Green/black discoloration at the edge of the nails secondary to *Pseudomonas* infection.

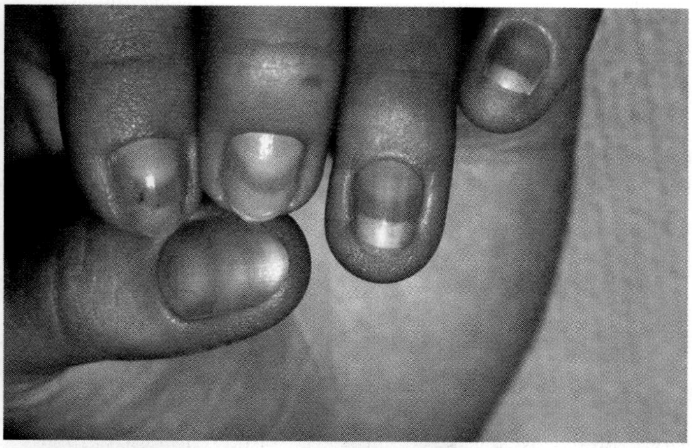

Figure 655-5 Distal onycholysis secondary to oral tetracycline usage and ultraviolet light exposure.

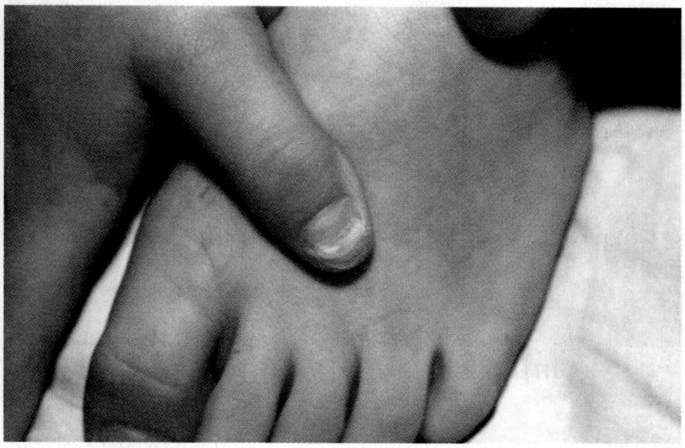

Figure 655-6 Beau lines. Longitudinal disruption of nail.

pigment should be evaluated by biopsy because of the possibility of malignant change.

Bluish black to greenish nails may be caused by *Pseudomonas* infection (Fig. 655-4), particularly in association with onycholysis or chronic paronychia. The coloration is due to subungual debris and pyocyanin pigment from the bacterial organisms.

Yellow nail syndrome manifests as thickened, excessively curved, slow-growing yellow nails without lunulae. All nails are affected in most cases. Associated systemic diseases include bronchiectasis, recurrent bronchitis, chylothorax, and focal edema of the limbs and face. Deficient lymphatic drainage, due to hypoplastic lymphatic vessels, is believed to lead to the manifestations of this syndrome.

Splinter hemorrhages most often result from minor trauma but may also be associated with subacute bacterial endocarditis, vasculitis, Langerhans cell histiocytosis, severe rheumatoid arthritis, peptic ulcer disease, hypertension, chronic glomerulonephritis, cirrhosis, scurvy, trichinosis, malignant neoplasms, and psoriasis.

NAIL SEPARATION

Onycholysis indicates separation of the nail plate from the distal nail bed. Common causes are trauma, long-term exposure to moisture, hyperhidrosis, cosmetics, psoriasis, fungal infection (distal onycholysis), atopic or contact dermatitis, porphyria, drugs (bleomycin, vincristine, retinoid agents, indomethacin, chlorpromazine [Thorazine]), and drug-induced phototoxicity from tetracyclines (Fig. 655-5) or chloramphenicol.

Beau lines are transverse grooves in the nail plate (Fig. 655-6) that represent a temporary disruption of formation of the nail plate. The lines first appear a few weeks after the event that caused the disruption in nail growth. A single transverse ridge appears at the proximal nail fold in most 4- to 6-wk-old infants and works its way distally as the nail grows; this line may reflect metabolic changes after delivery. At other ages, Beau lines are usually indicative of periodic trauma or episodic shutdown of the nail matrix secondary to a systemic disease such as hand-foot-and-mouth disease, measles, mumps, pneumonia, or zinc deficiency. **Onychomadesis** is an exaggeration of Beau lines leading to proximal separation of the nail bed (Fig. 655-7).

NAIL CHANGES ASSOCIATED WITH SKIN DISEASE

Nail changes may be particularly associated with various other diseases. Nail changes of **psoriasis** most characteristically include pitting, onycholysis, yellow-brown discoloration, and thickening. Nail changes in lichen planus include violaceous papules in the proximal nail fold and nail bed, leukonychia, longitudinal ridging, thinning of the entire nail plate, and pterygium formation, which is abnormal adherence of the cuticle to the nail plate or, if the plate is destroyed focally, to the nail bed. Postinfectious reactive arthritis syndromes may include painless erythematous induration of the base of the nail fold; subungual parakeratotic scaling; and thickening, opacification, or ridging of the nail plate. Dermatitis that involves the nail folds may produce dystrophy, roughening, and coarse pitting of the nails. Nail changes are more common in atopic dermatitis than in other forms of dermatitis

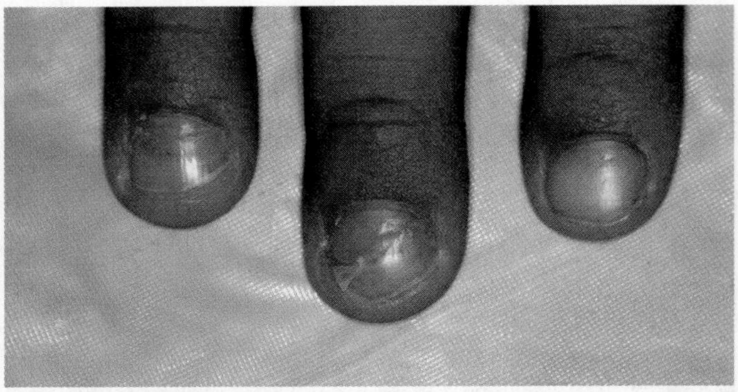

Figure 655-7 Onychomadesis. Proximal nail bed separation.

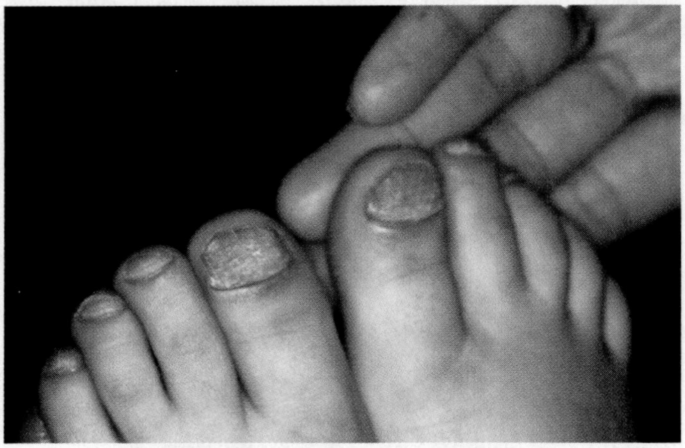

Figure 655-8 Dystrophy of all nails in trachyonychia.

that affect the hands. Darier disease is characterized by red or white streaks that extend longitudinally and cross the lunula. Where the streak meets the distal end of the nail, a V-shaped notch may be present. Total leukonychia may also occur. Transverse rows of fine pits are characteristic of alopecia areata. In severe cases, the entire nail surface may be rough. Patients with acrodermatitis enteropathica may have transverse grooves (Beau lines) and nail dystrophy as a result of periungual dermatitis.

TRACHYONYCHIA (20-NAIL DYSTROPHY)

Trachyonychia is characterized by longitudinal ridging, pitting, fragility, thinning, distal notching, and opalescent discoloration of all the nails (Fig. 655-8). Patients have no associated skin or systemic diseases and no other ectodermal defects. Its occasional association with alopecia areata has led some authorities to suggest that trachyonychia may reflect an abnormal immunologic response to the nail matrix, whereas histopathologic studies have suggested that it may be a manifestation of lichen planus, psoriasis, or spongiotic (eczematous) inflammation of the nail matrix. The disorder must be differentiated from fungal infections, psoriasis, nail changes of alopecia areata, and nail dystrophy secondary to eczema. Eczema and fungal infections rarely produce changes in all the nails simultaneously. The disorder is self-limited and eventually remits by adulthood.

NAIL INFECTION

Fungal infection of the nails has been classified into 4 types. *White superficial onychomycosis* manifests as diffuse or speckled white discoloration of the surface of the toenails. It is caused primarily by *Trichophyton mentagrophytes,* which invades the

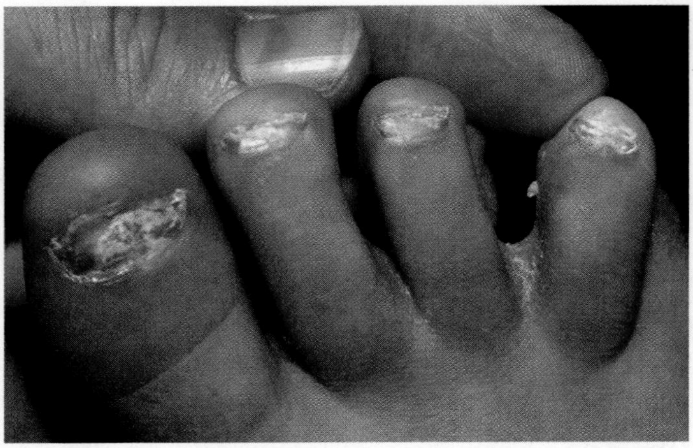

Figure 655-9 Discoloration, hyperkeratosis, and crumbling of nail secondary to dermatophyte infection.

nail plate. The organism may be scraped off the nail plate with a blade, but **treatment** is best accomplished by the addition of a topical azole antifungal agent. *Distal subungual onychomycosis* involves foci of onycholysis under the distal nail plate or along the lateral nail groove, followed by development of hyperkeratosis and yellow-brown discoloration. The process extends proximally, resulting in nail plate thickening, crumbling (Fig. 655-9), and separation from the nail bed. *Trichophyton rubrum* and, occasionally, *T. mentagrophytes* infect the toenails; fingernail disease is almost exclusively due to *T. rubrum,* which may be associated with superficial scaling of the plantar surface of the feet and often of one hand. The dermatophytes are found most readily at the most proximal area of the nail bed or adjacent ventral portion of the involved nail plates. **Topical therapies** such as ciclopirox 8% lacquer may be effective for solitary nail infection. Because of its long half-life in the nail, either terbinafine or itraconazole may be effective when given as pulse therapy (1 wk of each month for 3-4 mo). Dosage is weight dependent. Either agent is superior to griseofulvin, fluconazole, or ketoconazole. The risks, the most concerning of which is hepatic toxicity, and costs of oral therapy are minimized with the use of pulsed dosing.

Proximal white subungual onychomycosis occurs when the organism, generally *T. rubrum,* enters the nail through the proximal nail fold, producing yellow-white portions of the undersurface of the nail plate. The surface of the nail is unaffected. This occurs almost exclusively in immunocompromised patients and is a well-recognized manifestation of AIDS. Treatment includes oral terbinafine or itraconazole.

Candidal onychomycosis involves the entire nail plate in patients with chronic mucocutaneous candidiasis. It is also commonly seen in patients with AIDS. The organism, generally *Candida albicans,* enters distally or along the lateral nail folds, rapidly involves the entire thickness of the nail plate, and produces thickening, crumbling, and deformity of the plate. Topical azole antifungal agents may be sufficient for treatment of candidal onychomycosis in an immunocompetent host, but oral antifungal agents are necessary for treatment of patients with immune deficiencies.

PARONYCHIAL INFLAMMATION

Paronychial inflammation may be acute or chronic and generally involves 1 or 2 nail folds on the fingers. **Acute paronychia** manifests as erythema, warmth, edema, and tenderness of the proximal nail fold, most commonly as a result of pathogenic staphylococci or streptococci (Fig. 655-10). Warm soaks and oral antibiotics are generally effective; incision and drainage may be occasionally necessary. Development of chronic paronychia follows prolonged immersion in water (Fig. 655-11), such as occurs in finger or thumb sucking, exposure to irritating solutions, nail fold trauma, or diseases, including Raynaud phenomenon, collagen vascular diseases, and diabetes. Swelling of the proximal nail fold is followed by separation of the nail fold from the underlying nail plate and suppuration. Foreign material, embedded in the dermis of the nail fold, becomes a nidus for inflammation and infection with *Candida* species and mixed bacterial flora. A combination of attention to predisposing factors, meticulous drying of the hands, and long-term topical antifungal agents and topical potent corticosteroids may be required for successful treatment of chronic paronychia.

Ingrown nail occurs when the lateral edge of the nail, including spicules that have separated from the nail plate, penetrates the soft tissue of the lateral nail fold. Erythema, edema, and pain, most often involving the lateral great toes, are noted acutely; recurrent episodes may lead to formation of granulation tissue. Predisposing factors include (1) congenital malalignment (especially of the great toes); (2) compression of the side of the toe from poorly fitting shoes, particularly if the great toes are abnormally long and the lateral nail folds are prominent; and (3) improper cutting of the nail in a curvilinear manner rather than straight across. **Management** includes proper fitting of shoes; allowing the nail to grow out beyond the free edge before cutting it straight across; warm water soaks; oral antibiotics if cellulitis affects the lateral nail fold; and, in severe, recurrent cases, application of silver nitrate to granulation tissue, nail avulsion, or excision of the lateral aspect of the nail followed by matricectomy.

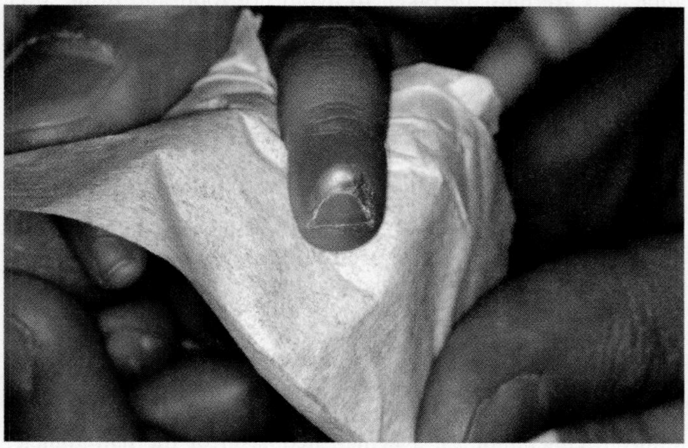

Figure 655-10 Acute paronychia secondary to *Staphylococcus aureus.*

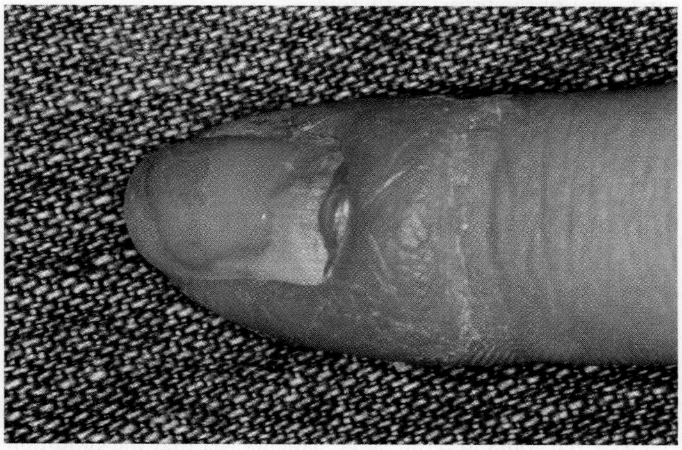

Figure 655-11 Chronic paronychia with erythema and lateral nail fold separation.

PARONYCHIAL TUMORS

Tumors in the paronychial area include pyogenic granulomas, mucous cysts, subungual exostoses, and junctional nevi. Periungual fibromas that appear in late childhood should suggest a diagnosis of tuberous sclerosis.

BIBLIOGRAPHY

Please visit the Nelson Textbook of Pediatrics *website at www.expertconsult.com for the complete bibliography.*

Chapter 656
Disorders of the Mucous Membranes

Joseph G. Morelli

The mucous membranes may be involved in developmental disorders, infections, acute and chronic skin diseases, genodermatoses, and benign and malignant tumors.

CHEILITIS

Inflammation of the lips (**cheilitis**) and angles of the mouth (**angular cheilitis** or **perlèche**) (Fig. 656-1) are most commonly due to dryness, chapping, and lip licking. Excessive salivation and drooling, particularly in children with neurologic deficits, may also cause chronic irritation. Lesions of oral thrush may occasionally extend to the angles of the mouth. Protection can be provided by frequent applications of a bland ointment such as petrolatum. Candidosis should be treated with an appropriate antifungal agent, and contact dermatitis of the perioral skin should be treated with a low-potency topical corticosteroid ointment preparation and frequent use of petrolatum or a similar emollient.

FORDYCE SPOTS

Fordyce spots are asymptomatic, minute, yellow-white papules on the vermilion border of the lips and buccal mucosa. These ectopic sebaceous glands may be found in otherwise normal individuals and require no therapy.

MUCOCELE

Mucus retention cysts are painless, fluctuant, tense, 2- to 10-mm, bluish papules on the lips (Fig. 656-2), tongue, palate, or buccal

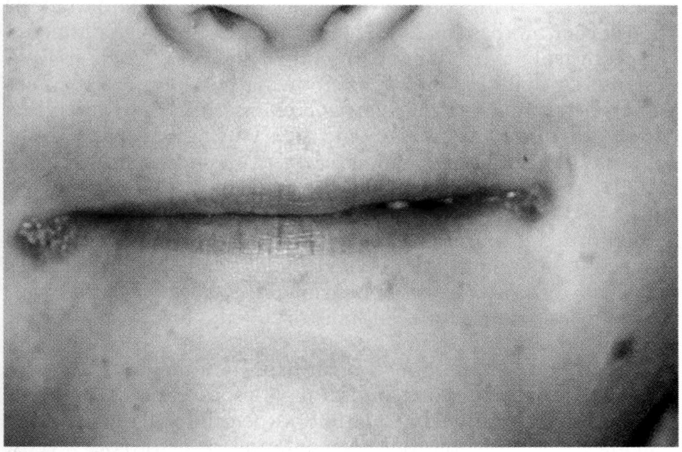

Figure 656-1 Angular cheilitis.

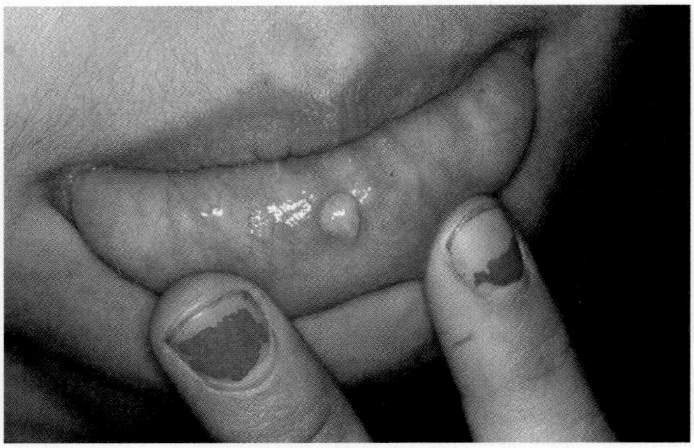

Figure 656-2 Mucocele on lower lip.

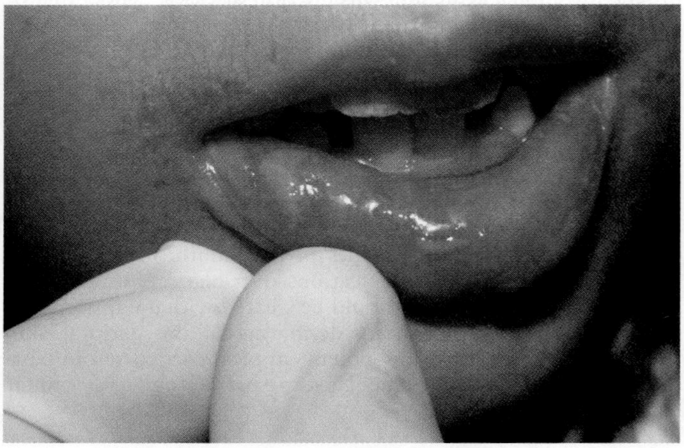

Figure 656-3 Aphthous ulceration on lower lip.

mucosa. Traumatic severance of the duct of a minor salivary gland leads to submucosal retention of mucus secretion. Those on the floor of the mouth are known as ranulas when the submaxillary or sublingual salivary ducts are involved. Fluctuations in size are usual, and the lesions may disappear temporarily after traumatic rupture. Recurrence is prevented by excision of the mucocele.

APHTHOUS STOMATITIS (CANKER SORES)

Aphthous stomatitis consists of solitary or multiple painful ulcerations occur on the labial (Fig. 656-3), buccal, or lingual mucosa and on the sublingual, palatal, or gingival mucosa (Chapter 307). Lesions may manifest initially as erythematous, indurated papules that erode rapidly to form sharply circumscribed, necrotic ulcers with a gray fibrinous exudate and an erythematous halo. Minor aphthous ulcers are 2-10 mm in diameter and heal spontaneously in 7-10 days. Major aphthous ulcers are >10 mm in diameter and take 10-30 days to heal. A third type of aphthous ulceration is herpetiform in appearance, manifesting as a few to numerous grouped 1- to 2-mm lesions that tend to coalesce into plaques that heal over 7-10 days. Approximately 30% of patients with recurrent lesions have a family history of the disorder (Chapter 307 for differential diagnosis).

The etiology of aphthous stomatitis is multifactorial; the condition probably represents an oral manifestation of a number of conditions. Altered local regulation of the cell-mediated immune system, after activation and accumulation of cytotoxic T cells, may contribute to the localized mucosal breakdown. It is a

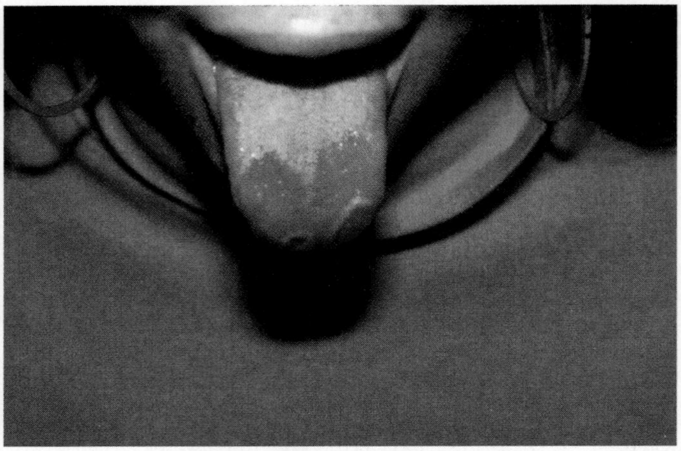

Figure 656-4 Geographic tongue.

common misconception that aphthous stomatitis is a manifestation of herpes simplex virus infection. Recurrent herpes infections remain localized to the lips and rarely cross the mucocutaneous junction; involvement of the oral mucosa occurs only in primary infections.

Treatment of aphthous stomatitis is palliative. The majority of mild cases do not require therapy. Relief of pain, particularly before eating, may be achieved with the use of a topical anesthetic such as viscous lidocaine or an oral rinse with a combined solution of elixir of diphenhydramine, viscous lidocaine, and an oral antacid. Care must be taken to avoid hot food and drink after the use of a topical anesthetic. A topical corticosteroid in a mucosa-adhering agent may help reduce inflammation, and topical tetracycline mouthwash may also hasten healing. In severe, debilitating cases, systemic therapy with corticosteroids, colchicine, cimetidine, or dapsone may be helpful.

COWDEN SYNDROME (MULTIPLE HAMARTOMA SYNDROME)

Cowden syndrome is an autosomal dominant condition that usually manifests in the 2nd or 3rd decade with smooth, pink or whitish papules on the palatal, gingival, buccal, and labial mucosae. Mutations in the tumor suppressor gene *PTEN* cause Cowden syndrome. The benign fibromas characteristic of the syndrome may coalesce into a cobblestone appearance. Numerous flesh-colored papules also develop on the face, particularly around the mouth, nose, and ears. These papules are most commonly trichilemmomas, a benign neoplasm of the hair follicle. Associated findings may include acral keratotic papules, thyroid goiter, gastrointestinal polyps, fibrocystic breast nodules, and carcinoma of the breast or thyroid.

EPSTEIN PEARLS (GINGIVAL CYSTS OF THE NEWBORN)

Epstein pearls are white keratin-containing cysts on the palatal or alveolar mucosa of approximately 80% of neonates. They cause no symptoms and are generally shed within a few weeks.

GEOGRAPHIC TONGUE (BENIGN MIGRATORY GLOSSITIS)

Geographic tongue consists of single or multiple sharply demarcated, irregular, smooth red plaques on the dorsum of the tongue caused by transient atrophy of the filiform papillae and the surface epithelium, often with elevated gray margins composed of intervening filiform papillae that are increased in thickness (Fig. 656-4). Symptoms of mild burning or irritation may occasionally be bothersome. Onset is rapid, and the pattern may change over hours to days. Some patients feel that the condition is exacerbated by stress or by hot or spicy foods. The histology of geographic tongue is similar to that of pustular psoriasis. No therapy other than reassurance is necessary.

SCROTAL (FISSURED) TONGUE

Approximately 1% of infants and 2.5% of children have many folds with deep grooves on the dorsal tongue surface, known as fissured tongue. These impart a pebbled or wrinkled appearance. Some cases are congenital, caused by incomplete fusion of the two halves of the tongue; others develop in association with infection, trauma, malnutrition, or low vitamin A levels. Many patients with fissured tongue also have geographic tongue. Food particles and debris may become trapped in the fissures, resulting in irritation, inflammation, and halitosis. Careful cleansing with a mouth rinse and soft-bristled toothbrush is recommended.

BLACK HAIRY TONGUE

Black hairy tongue is a dark coating on the dorsum of the tongue caused by hyperplasia and elongation of the filiform papillae; overgrowth of chromogenic bacteria and fungi and entrapped pigmented residues that adsorb to microbial plaque and desquamating keratin may contribute to the dark coloration. Changes often begin posteriorly and extend anteriorly on the dorsum of the tongue. The condition is most common in adults but may also manifest during adolescence. Poor oral hygiene and bacterial overgrowth, treatment with systemic antibiotics such as tetracycline (which promotes the growth of *Candida* spp.), and smoking are predisposing factors. Improved oral hygiene and brushing with a soft-bristled toothbrush may be all that is necessary for treatment.

ORAL HAIRY LEUKOPLAKIA

Oral hair leukoplakia occurs in approximately 25% of patients with AIDS but is rare in the pediatric population. It manifests as a mostly asymptomatic white thickening and accentuation of the normal vertical folds of the lateral margins of the tongue. The mucosa is white and irregularly thickened but remains soft. The condition may spread occasionally to the ventral tongue surface, the floor of the mouth, the tonsillar pillars, and the pharynx. The condition is due to Epstein-Barr virus, which is present in the upper layer of the affected epithelium. The plaques have no malignant potential. The disorder occurs predominantly in HIV-infected patients but may also be found in individuals who are immunosuppressed for other reasons, such as organ transplantation, leukemia, chemotherapy, and long-term use of inhaled steroids. The condition is generally asymptomatic and does not require therapy.

ACUTE NECROTIZING ULCERATIVE GINGIVITIS (VINCENT STOMATITIS, FUSOSPIROCHETAL GINGIVITIS, TRENCH MOUTH)

Acute necrotizing ulcerative gingivitis manifests as punched-out ulceration, necrosis, and bleeding of interdental papillae. A grayish white pseudomembrane may cover the ulcerations. Lesions may spread to involve the buccal mucosa, lips, tongue, tonsils, and pharynx and may be associated with dental pain, a bad taste, low-grade fever, and lymphadenopathy. It occurs most commonly in the 2nd or 3rd decade, particularly in the context of poor dental hygiene, scurvy, or pellagra.

NOMA

Noma is a severe form of fusospirillary gangrenous stomatitis that occurs primarily in malnourished children 2-5 yr of age who have had a preceding illness such as measles, scarlet fever, tuberculosis, malignancy, or immunodeficiency. It manifests as a painful, red, indurated papule on the alveolar margin, followed by ulceration and mutilating gangrenous destruction of tissue in the oronasal region. The process may also involve the scalp, neck, shoulders, perineum, and vulva. **Noma neonatorum** manifests in the first month of life as gangrenous lesions of the lips, nose, mouth, and anal regions. Affected infants are usually small for gestational age, malnourished, premature, and frequently ill, particularly with *Pseudomonas aeruginosa* sepsis. Care consists of nutritional support, conservative debridement of necrotic soft tissues, empirical broad-spectrum antibiotics such as penicillin and metronidazole, and, in the case of noma neonatorum, antipseudomonal antibiotics (Chapter 43).

BIBLIOGRAPHY

Please visit the Nelson Textbook of Pediatrics *website at www.expertconsult.com for the complete bibliography.*

Chapter 657 Cutaneous Bacterial Infections

657.1 Impetigo

Joseph G. Morelli

ETIOLOGY/PATHOGENESIS

Impetigo is the most common skin infection in children throughout the world. There are 2 classic forms of impetigo: nonbullous and bullous.

Staphylococcus aureus is the predominant organism of nonbullous impetigo in the USA; group A beta-hemolytic streptococci (GABHS) are implicated in the development of some lesions. The staphylococcal types that cause nonbullous impetigo are variable but are not generally from phage group 2, the group that is associated with scalded skin and toxic shock syndromes. Staphylococci generally spread from the nose to normal skin and then infect the skin. In contrast, the skin becomes colonized with GABHS an average of 10 days before development of impetigo. The skin serves as the source for acquisition of GABHS and the probable primary source for spread of impetigo. Lesions of nonbullous impetigo that grow staphylococci in culture cannot be distinguished clinically from those that grow pure cultures of GABHS.

Bullous impetigo is always caused by *S. aureus* strains that produce exfoliative toxins. The staphylococcal exfoliative toxins (ETA, ETB, ETD) blister the superficial epidermis by hydrolyzing human desmoglein 1, resulting in a subcorneal vesicle. This is also the target antigen of the autoantibodies in pemphigus foliaceus (Chapters 174 and 176).

CLINICAL MANIFESTATIONS

Nonbullous Impetigo

Nonbullous impetigo accounts for > 70% of cases. Lesions typically begin on the skin of the face or on extremities that have been traumatized. The most common lesions that precede nonbullous impetigo are insect bites, abrasions, lacerations, chickenpox, scabies pediculosis, and burns. A tiny vesicle or pustule forms initially and rapidly develops into a honey-colored crusted plaque that is generally <2 cm in diameter (Fig. 657-1). The infection may be spread to other parts of the body by the fingers, clothing, and towels. Lesions are associated with little to no pain or surrounding erythema, and constitutional symptoms are generally absent. Pruritus occurs occasionally, regional adenopathy is found in up to 90% of cases, and leukocytosis is present in about 50%.

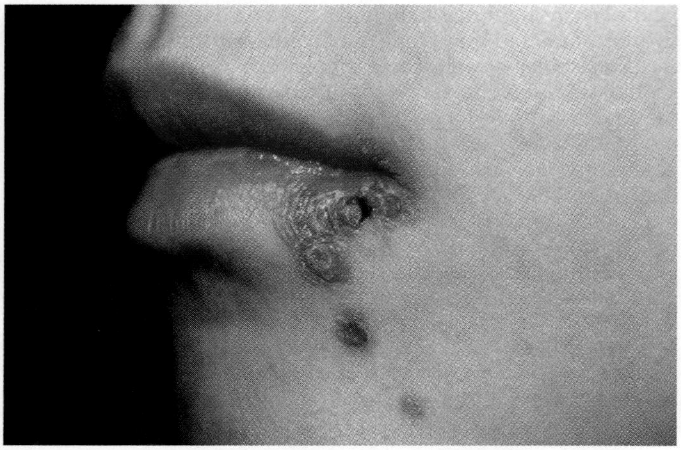

Figure 657-1 Multiple crusted and oozing lesions of impetigo.

Bullous Impetigo

Bullous impetigo is mainly an infection of infants and young children. Flaccid, transparent bullae develop most commonly on skin of the face, buttocks, trunk, perineum, and extremities. **Neonatal bullous impetigo** can begin in the diaper area. Rupture of a bulla occurs easily, leaving a narrow rim of scale at the edge of shallow, moist erosion. Surrounding erythema and regional adenopathy are generally absent. Unlike those of nonbullous impetigo, lesions of bullous impetigo are a manifestation of localized staphylococcal scalded skin syndrome and develop on intact skin.

Differential Diagnosis

The differential diagnosis of **nonbullous impetigo** includes viruses (herpes simplex, varicella-zoster), fungi (tinea corporis, kerion), arthropod bites, and parasitic infestations (scabies, pediculosis capitis), all of which may become impetiginized.

The differential diagnosis of **bullous impetigo** in neonates includes epidermolysis bullosa, bullous mastocytosis, herpetic infection, and early scalded skin syndrome. In older children, allergic contact dermatitis, burns, erythema multiforme, linear immunoglobulin (Ig) A dermatosis, pemphigus, and bullous pemphigoid must be considered, particularly if the lesions do not respond to therapy.

COMPLICATIONS

Potential but very rare complications of either nonbullous or bullous impetigo include osteomyelitis, septic arthritis, pneumonia, and septicemia. Positive blood culture results are very rare in otherwise healthy children with localized lesions. Cellulitis has been reported in up to 10% of patients with nonbullous impetigo and rarely follows the bullous form. Lymphangitis, suppurative lymphadenitis, guttate psoriasis, and scarlet fever occasionally follow streptococcal disease. There is no correlation between number of lesions and clinical involvement of the lymphatics or development of cellulitis in association with streptococcal impetigo.

Infection with nephritogenic strains of GABHS may result in **acute poststreptococcal glomerulonephritis** (Chapter 505.1). The clinical character of impetigo lesions is not predictive of the development of poststreptococcal glomerulonephritis. The most commonly affected age group is school-aged children, 3-7 yr old. The latent period from onset of impetigo to development of poststreptococcal glomerulonephritis averages 18-21 days, which is longer than the 10-day latency period after pharyngitis. Poststreptococcal glomerulonephritis occurs epidemically after either pharyngeal or skin infection. Impetigo-associated epidemics have been caused by M groups 2, 49, 53, 55, 56, 57, and 60. Strains of GABHS that are associated with endemic impetigo in the USA have little or no nephritogenic potential. Acute rheumatic fever does not occur as a result of impetigo.

TREATMENT

The decision on how to treat impetigo depends on the number of lesions and their locations. Topical therapy with mupirocin 2%, fusidic acid, and retapamulin 1% is acceptable for localized disease.

Systemic therapy with oral antibiotics should be prescribed for patients with widespread involvement; when lesions are near the mouth, where topical medication may be licked off; or in cases with evidence of deep involvement, including cellulitis, furunculosis, abscess formation, or suppurative lymphadenitis. Cephalexin, 25-50 mg/kg/day in two divided doses, is an excellent choice for initial therapy. No evidence suggests that a 10-day course of therapy is superior to a 7-day course. The emergence of methicillin-resistant *S. aureus* (MRSA) dictates that if a satisfactory clinical response is not achieved within 7 days, a culture should be performed and an appropriate antibiotic based on drug sensitivity should be given for an additional 7 days.

BIBLIOGRAPHY

Please visit the Nelson Textbook of Pediatrics *website at www.expertconsult.com for the complete bibliography.*

657.2 Subcutaneous Tissue Infections

Joseph G. Morelli

The principal determination for soft tissue infections is whether it is *nonnecrotizing* or *necrotizing*. The former responds to antibiotic therapy alone, whereas the latter requires prompt surgical removal of all devitalized tissue in addition to antimicrobial therapy. Necrotizing soft tissue infections are life-threatening conditions that are characterized by rapidly advancing local tissue destruction and systemic toxicity. Tissue necrosis distinguishes them from cellulitis. In cellulitis, an inflammatory infectious process involves subcutaneous tissue but does not destroy it. Necrotizing soft tissue infections characteristically manifest with a paucity of early cutaneous signs relative to the rapidity and degree of destruction of the subcutaneous tissues.

CELLULITIS

Etiology

Cellulitis is characterized by infection and inflammation of loose connective tissue, with limited involvement of the dermis and relative sparing of the epidermis. A break in the skin due to previous trauma, surgery, or an underlying skin lesion predisposes to cellulitis. Cellulitis is also more common in individuals with lymphatic stasis, diabetes mellitus, or immunosuppression.

Streptococcus pyogenes and *S. aureus* are the most common etiologic agents. In patients who are immunocompromised or have diabetes mellitus, a number of other bacterial or fungal agents may be involved, notably *Pseudomonas aeruginosa; Aeromonas hydrophila* and, occasionally, other Enterobacteriaceae; *Legionella* spp.; the Mucorales, particularly *Rhizopus* spp., *Mucor* spp., and *Absidia* spp.; and *Cryptococcus neoformans.* Children with relapsed nephrotic syndrome may experience cellulitis due to *Escherichia coli.* In children age 3 mo to 3-5 yr, *Haemophilus influenzae* type b was once an important cause of facial cellulitis, but its incidence has declined significantly since the institution of immunization against this organism.

Clinical Manifestations

Cellulitis manifests clinically as an area of edema, warmth, erythema, and tenderness. The lateral margins tend to be indistinct because the process is deep in the skin, primarily involving the subcutaneous tissues in addition to the dermis. Application of pressure may produce pitting. Although distinction cannot be made with certainty in any particular patient, cellulitis due to *S. aureus* tends to be more localized and may suppurate, whereas infections due to *S. pyogenes* (group A streptococci) tend to spread more rapidly and may be associated with lymphangitis. Regional adenopathy and constitutional signs and symptoms such as fever, chills, and malaise are uncommon. Complications of cellulitis are common but include subcutaneous abscess, bacteremia, osteomyelitis, septic arthritis, thrombophlebitis, endocarditis, and necrotizing fasciitis. Lymphangitis or glomerulonephritis can also follow infection with *S. pyogenes*.

Diagnosis

Aspirates from the site of inflammation, skin biopsy, and blood cultures allow identification of the causal organism in about 25% of cases of cellulitis. Yield of the causative organism is approximately 30% when the site of origin of the cellulitis is apparent, such as an abrasion or ulcer. An aspirate taken from the point of maximum inflammation yields the causal organism more often than a leading-edge aspirate. Lack of success in isolating an organism stems primarily from the low number of organisms present within the lesion.

Treatment

Empirical therapy for cellulitis should be directed by the history of the illness, the location and character of the cellulitis, and the age and immune status of the patient. Cellulitis in a neonate should prompt a full sepsis evaluation, followed by initiation of empirical intravenous therapy with a β-lactamase–stable antistaphylococcal antibiotic such as methicillin or vancomycin and an aminoglycoside such as gentamicin or a cephalosporin such as cefotaxime. Treatment of cellulitis in an infant or child younger than about 5 yr should provide coverage for *S. pyogenes* and *S. aureus* as well as *H. influenzae* type b and *S. pneumoniae*. The evaluation should include a blood culture, and if the infant is younger than 1 yr, if signs of systemic toxicity are present, or if an adequate examination cannot be carried out, a lumbar puncture should also be performed. In most cases of cellulitis on an extremity, regardless of age, *S. aureus* and *S. pyogenes* are the cause and bacteremia is highly unlikely in an otherwise well-appearing child. Blood cultures should be performed if sepsis is suspected.

If fever, lymphadenopathy, and other constitutional signs are absent (white blood cell count < 15,000), treatment of cellulitis on an extremity may be initiated orally on an outpatient basis with a penicillinase-resistant penicillin such as dicloxacillin or cloxacillin or a first-generation cephalosporin such as cephalexin or, if MRSA is suspected, with clindamycin. If improvement is not noted or the disease progresses significantly in the first 24-48 hr of therapy, parenteral therapy is necessary. If fever, lymphadenopathy, or constitutional signs are present, parenteral therapy should be initiated. Oxacillin or nafcillin is effective in most cases, although if systemic toxicity is significant, consideration should be given to the addition of clindamycin or vancomycin. Once the erythema, warmth, edema, and fever have decreased significantly, a 10-day course of treatment may be completed on an outpatient basis. Immobilization and elevation of an affected limb, particularly early in the course of therapy, may help reduce swelling and pain.

NECROTIZING FASCIITIS

Etiology

Necrotizing fasciitis is a subcutaneous tissue infection that involves the deep layer of superficial fascia but largely spares adjacent epidermis, deep fascia, and muscle.

Relatively few organisms possess sufficient virulence to cause necrotizing fasciitis when acting alone. The majority (55-75%) of cases of necrotizing fasciitis are polymicrobial in nature, with an average of 4 different organisms isolated. The organisms most commonly isolated in polymicrobial necrotizing fasciitis are *S. aureus*, streptococcal species, *Klebsiella* species, *E. coli*, and anaerobic bacteria.

The rest of the cases and the most fulminant infections, associated with toxic shock syndrome and a high case fatality rate, are usually caused by *S. pyogenes* (Chapter 176). Streptococcal necrotizing fasciitis may occur in the absence of toxic shock–like syndrome and is potentially fatal and associated with substantial morbidity. Necrotizing fasciitis can occasionally be caused by *S. aureus; Clostridium perfringens; Clostridium septicum; P. aeruginosa; Vibrio* spp., particularly *Vibrio vulnificus;* and fungi of the order Mucorales, particularly *Rhizopus* spp., *Mucor* spp., and *Absidia* spp. Necrotizing fasciitis has also been reported on rare occasions to result from non–group A streptococci such as group B, C, F, or G streptococci, *S. pneumoniae*, or *H. influenzae* type b.

Infections due to any one organism or combination of organisms cannot be distinguished clinically from one another, although development of **crepitance** signals the presence of *Clostridium* spp. or gram-negative bacilli such as *E. coli, Klebsiella, Proteus,* or *Aeromonas*.

Clinical Manifestations

Necrotizing fasciitis may occur anywhere on the body. Polymicrobial infections tend to occur on perineal and trunk areas. The incidence of necrotizing fasciitis is highest in hosts with systemic or local tissue immunocompromise, such as those with diabetes mellitus, neoplasia, or peripheral vascular disease as well as those who have recently undergone surgery, who abuse intravenous drugs, or who are undergoing immunosuppressive treatment, particularly with corticosteroids. The infection can also occur in healthy individuals after minor puncture wounds, abrasions, or lacerations; blunt trauma; surgical procedures, particularly of the abdomen, gastrointestinal or genitourinary tracts, or the perineum; or hypodermic needle injection.

Since the mid-1980s, there has been a resurgence of fulminant necrotizing soft tissue infections due to *S. pyogenes*, which may occur in previously healthy individuals. Streptococcal necrotizing cellulitis is classically located on an extremity. There may be a history of recent trauma to or operation in the area. Necrotizing fasciitis due to *S. pyogenes* may also occur after superinfection of varicella lesions. Children with this disease have tended to display onset, recrudescence, or persistence of high fever and signs of toxicity after the 3rd or 4th day of varicella. Common predisposing conditions in neonates are omphalitis and balanitis after circumcision.

Necrotizing fasciitis begins with acute onset of local swelling, erythema, tenderness, and heat. Fever is usually present, and pain, tenderness, and constitutional signs are out of proportion to cutaneous signs, especially with involvement of fascia and muscle. Lymphangitis and lymphadenitis may be absent. The infection advances along the superficial fascial plane, and initially there are few cutaneous signs to herald the serious nature and extent of the subcutaneous tissue necrosis that is occurring. Skin changes may appear over 24-48 hr as nutrient vessels are thrombosed and cutaneous ischemia develops. Early clinical findings include ill-defined cutaneous erythema and edema that extends beyond the area of erythema. Additional signs include formation of bullae filled initially with straw-colored and later bluish to hemorrhagic fluid, and darkening of affected tissues from red to purple to blue. Skin anesthesia and, finally, frank tissue gangrene and slough develop owing to the ischemia and necrosis. Vesiculation or bulla formation, ecchymoses, crepitus, anesthesia, and necrosis are ominous signs indicative of advanced disease. Children with varicella lesions may initially show no cutaneous signs of superinfection with invasive *S. pyogenes*, such as erythema or swelling. Significant systemic toxicity may accompany necrotizing fasciitis, including shock, organ failure, and death. Advance of the infection in this setting can be rapid, progressing to death within hours. Patients with involvement of the superficial or deep fascia and muscle tend to be more acutely and systemically ill and have more rapidly advancing disease than those with infection confined solely to subcutaneous tissues above the fascia. In an extremity, a **compartment syndrome** may develop, manifesting as tight edema, pain on motion, and loss of distal sensation and pulses; this is a surgical emergency.

Diagnosis

Definitive diagnosis of necrotizing fasciitis is made by surgical exploration, which should be undertaken as soon as the diagnosis is suspected. Necrotic fascia and subcutaneous tissue are gray and offer little resistance to blunt probing. Although MRI aids in delineating the extent and tissue planes of involvement, this procedure should not delay surgical intervention. Frozen-section incisional biopsy specimens obtained early in the course of the infection can aid management by decreasing the time to diagnosis and helping establish margins of involvement. Gram staining of tissue can be particularly useful if chains of gram-positive cocci, indicative of infection with *S. pyogenes,* are seen.

Treatment

Early supportive care, surgical debridement, and parenteral antibiotic administration are mandatory for necrotizing fasciitis. All devitalized tissue should be removed to freely bleeding edges, and repeat exploration is generally indicated within 24-36 hr to confirm that no necrotic tissue remains. This procedure may need to be repeated on several occasions until devitalized tissue has ceased to form. Meticulous daily wound care is also paramount.

Parenteral antibiotic therapy should be initiated as soon as possible with broad-spectrum agents against all potential pathogens. Initial empirical therapy should be instituted with vancomycin, linezolid, daptomycin, or quinupristin to cover gram-positive and quinolones to cover gram-negative organisms. Therapy should then be based on sensitivity of isolated organisms.

Prognosis

The combined case fatality rate among children and adults with necrotizing fasciitis and toxic shock–like syndrome due to *S. pyogenes* has been as high as 60%. Death is less common in children, however, and in cases not complicated by toxic shock–like syndrome.

BIBLIOGRAPHY

Please visit the Nelson Textbook of Pediatrics *website at www.expertconsult.com for the complete bibliography.*

657.3 Staphylococcal Scalded Skin Syndrome (Ritter Disease)

Joseph G. Morelli

ETIOLOGY AND PATHOGENESIS

Staphylococcal scalded skin syndrome is caused predominantly by phage group 2 staphylococci, particularly strains 71 and 55, which are present at localized sites of infection. Foci of infection include the nasopharynx and, less commonly, the umbilicus, urinary tract, a superficial abrasion, conjunctivae, and blood. The clinical manifestations of staphylococcal scalded skin syndrome are mediated by hematogenous spread, in the absence of specific antitoxin antibody of staphylococcal epidermolytic or exfoliative toxins A or B. The toxins have reproduced the disease in both animal models and human volunteers. Decreased renal clearance of the toxins may account for the fact that the disease is most common in infants and young children. Epidermolytic toxin A is heat stable and is encoded by bacterial chromosomal genes. Epidermolytic toxin B is heat labile and is encoded on a 37.5-kb plasmid. The site of blister cleavage is subcorneal. The epidermolytic toxins produce the split by binding to and cleaving desmoglein I. Intact bullae are consistently sterile, unlike those of bullous impetigo, but culture specimens should be obtained from all suspected sites of localized infection and from the blood to identify the source for elaboration of the epidermolytic toxins.

CLINICAL MANIFESTATIONS

Staphylococcal scalded skin syndrome, which occurs predominantly in infants and children younger than 5 yr, includes a range of disease from localized bullous impetigo to generalized cutaneous involvement with systemic illness. Onset of the rash may be preceded by malaise, fever, irritability, and exquisite tenderness of the skin. **Scarlatiniform erythema** develops diffusely and is accentuated in flexural and periorificial areas. The conjunctivae are inflamed and occasionally become purulent. The brightly erythematous skin may rapidly acquire a wrinkled appearance, and in severe cases, sterile, flaccid blisters and erosions develop diffusely. Circumoral erythema is characteristically prominent, as is radial crusting and fissuring around the eyes, mouth, and nose. At this stage, areas of epidermis may separate in response to gentle shear force (Nikolsky sign) (Fig. 657-2). As large sheets of epidermis peel away, moist, glistening, denuded areas become apparent, initially in the flexures and subsequently over much of the body surface (Fig. 657-3). This development may lead to secondary cutaneous infection, sepsis, and fluid and electrolyte disturbances. The desquamative phase begins after 2-5 days of cutaneous erythema; healing occurs without scarring in 10-14 days. Patients may have pharyngitis, conjunctivitis, and superficial erosions of the lips, but intraoral mucosal surfaces are spared. Although some patients appear ill, many are reasonably comfortable except for the marked skin tenderness.

DIFFERENTIAL DIAGNOSIS

A presumed **abortive** form of the disease manifests as diffuse, scarlatiniform, tender erythroderma that is accentuated in the flexural areas but does not progress to blister formation. In patients with this form, Nikolsky sign may be absent.

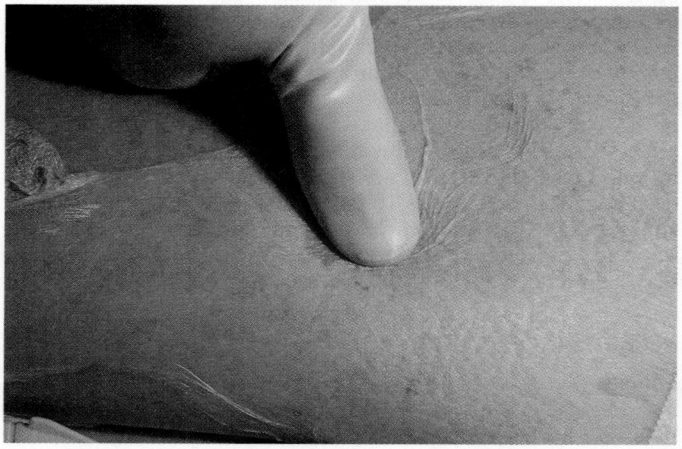

Figure 657-2 Nikolsky sign. With slight thumb pressure the skin wrinkles, slides laterally, and separates from the dermis. (From Habif TP, editor: *Clinical dermatology,* ed 4, Philadelphia, 2004, Mosby.)

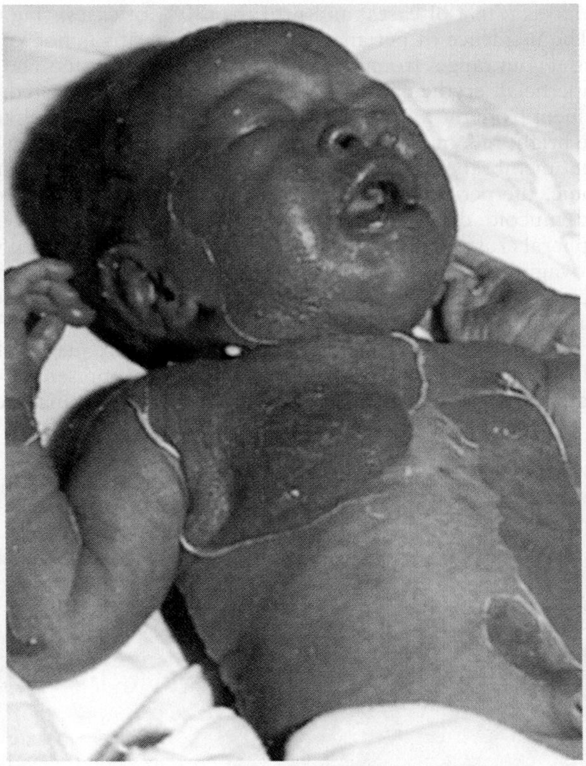

Figure 657-3 Infant with staphylococcal scalded skin syndrome.

Although the exanthem is similar to that of streptococcal scarlet fever, strawberry tongue and palatal petechiae are absent. Staphylococcal scalded skin syndrome may be mistaken for a number of other blistering and exfoliating disorders, including bullous impetigo, epidermolysis bullosa, epidermolytic hyperkeratosis, pemphigus, drug eruption, erythema multiforme, and drug-induced toxic epidermal necrolysis. Toxic epidermal necrolysis can often be distinguished by a history of drug ingestion, the presence of Nikolsky sign only at sites of erythema, absence of perioral crusting, full-thickness epidermal necrosis, and a blister cleavage plane in the lowermost epidermis.

HISTOLOGY

A subcorneal, granular layer split can be identified on skin biopsy. Absence of an inflammatory infiltrate is characteristic. Histology is identical to that seen in pemphigus foliaceus and subcorneal pustular dermatosis.

TREATMENT

Systemic therapy, given either orally in cases of localized involvement or parenterally with a semisynthetic penicillinase-resistant penicillin, should be prescribed, because the staphylococci are usually penicillin resistant. Clindamycin should be added to inhibit bacterial protein (toxin) synthesis. The skin should be gently moistened and cleansed. Application of an emollient provides lubrication and decreases discomfort. Topical antibiotics are unnecessary. Recovery is usually rapid, but complications such as excessive fluid loss, electrolyte imbalance, faulty temperature regulation, pneumonia, septicemia, and cellulitis may cause increased morbidity.

BIBLIOGRAPHY

Please visit the Nelson Textbook of Pediatrics *website at* www.expertconsult.com *for the complete bibliography.*

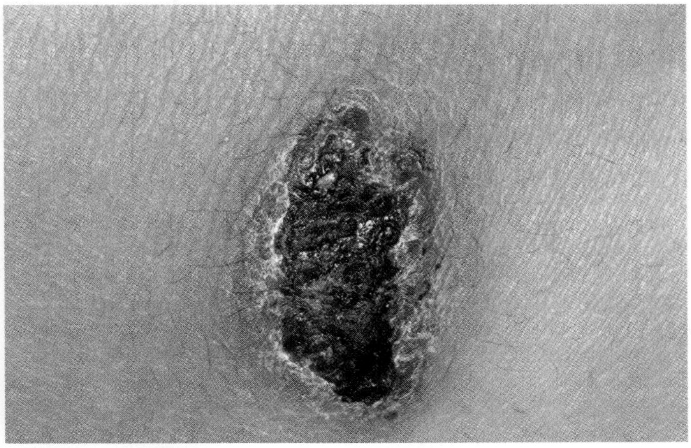

Figure 657-4 Dry, tightly adherent crust in ecthyma.

657.4 Ecthyma

Joseph G. Morelli

See also Chapters 182 and 202.

Ecthyma resembles nonbullous impetigo in onset and appearance but gradually evolves into a deeper, more chronic infection. The initial lesion is a vesicle or vesicular pustule with an erythematous base that erodes through the epidermis into the dermis to form an ulcer with elevated margins. The ulcer becomes obscured by a dry, heaped-up, tightly adherent crust (Fig. 657-4) that contributes to the persistence of the infection and scar formation. Lesions may be spread by autoinoculation, may be as large as 4 cm, and occur most frequently on the legs. Predisposing factors include the presence of pruritic lesions, such as insect bites, scabies, or pediculosis, that are subject to frequent scratching; poor hygiene; and malnutrition. Complications include lymphangitis, cellulitis, and, rarely, poststreptococcal glomerulonephritis. The causative agent is usually GABHS; *S. aureus* is also cultured from most lesions but is probably a secondary pathogen. Crusts should be softened with warm compresses and removed. Systemic antibiotic therapy, as for impetigo, is indicated; almost all lesions are responsive to treatment with penicillin.

Ecthyma gangrenosa is a necrotic ulcer covered with a gray-black eschar. It is usually a sign of *P. aeruginosa* sepsis and usually occurs in immunosuppressed patients. Ecthyma gangrenosum occurs in up to 6% of patients with systemic *P. aeruginosa* infection but can also occur as a primary cutaneous infection by inoculation. The lesion begins as a red or purpuric macule that vesiculates and then ulcerates. There is a surrounding rim of pink to violaceous skin. The punched-out ulcer develops raised edges with a dense, black, depressed, crusted center. Lesions may be single or multiple. Patients with bacteremia commonly have lesions in apocrine areas. Clinically similar lesions may also develop as a result of infection with other agents, such as *S. aureus, A. hydrophila, Enterobacter* spp., *Proteus* spp., *Burkholderia cepacia, Serratia marcescens, Aspergillus* spp., Mucorales, *E. coli,* and *Candida* spp. There is bacterial invasion of the adventitia and media of dermal veins but not arteries. The intima and lumina are spared. Blood and skin biopsy specimens for culture should be obtained, and empirical broad-spectrum, systemic therapy that includes coverage for *Pseudomonas* should be initiated as soon as possible.

BIBLIOGRAPHY

Please visit the Nelson Textbook of Pediatrics *website at* www.expertconsult.com *for the complete bibliography.*

657.5 Other Cutaneous Bacterial Infections

Joseph G. Morelli

BLASTOMYCOSIS-LIKE PYODERMA (PYODERMA VEGETANS)

Blastomycosis-like pyoderma is an exuberant cutaneous reaction to bacterial infection that occurs primarily in children who are malnourished and immunosuppressed. The organisms most commonly isolated from lesions are *S. aureus* and group A streptococcus, but several other organisms have been associated with these lesions, including *P. aeruginosa, Proteus mirabilis,* diphtheroids, *Bacillus* spp., and *C. perfringens.* Crusted, hyperplastic plaques on the extremities are characteristic, sometimes forming from the coalescence of many pinpoint, purulent, crusted abscesses (Fig. 657-5). Ulceration and sinus tract formation may develop, and additional lesions may appear at sites distant from the site of inoculation. Regional lymphadenopathy is common, but fever is not. Histopathologic examination reveals pseudoepitheliomatous hyperplasia and abscesses composed of neutrophils and/or eosinophils. Giant cells are usually lacking. The **differential diagnosis** includes deep fungal infection, particularly blastomycosis (Fig 657-6) and tuberculous and atypical mycobacterial infection. Underlying immunodeficiency should be ruled out, and the selection of antibiotics should be guided by susceptibility testing because the response to antibiotics is often poor.

BLISTERING DISTAL DACTYLITIS

Blistering distal dactylitis is a superficial blistering infection of the volar fat pad on the distal portion of the finger or thumb (Fig. 657-7). More than one finger may be involved, as may the volar surfaces of the proximal phalanges, palms, and toes. Blisters are filled with a watery purulent fluid that contains polymorphonuclear leukocytes and, usually, chains of gram-positive cocci. Patients commonly have no preceding history of trauma, and systemic symptoms are generally absent. Poststreptococcal glomerulonephritis has not occurred after blistering distal dactylitis. The infection is caused most commonly by group A streptococcus but has also occurred as a result of infection with *S. aureus.* If left untreated, blisters may continue to enlarge and extend to the paronychial area. The infection responds to incision and drainage and a 10-day course of systemic cephalosporin therapy.

PERIANAL INFECTIOUS DERMATITIS

Perianal infectious dermatitis presents most commonly in boys (70% of cases) between the ages of 6 mo and 10 yr as perianal dermatitis (90% of cases) and pruritus (80% of cases) (Fig 657-8). The incidence of perianal infectious dermatitis is not known precisely but ranges from 1/2,000 to 1/218 patient visits. The rash is superficial, erythematous, well marginated, nonindurated, and confluent from the anus outward. Acutely (<6 wk), the rash tends to be bright red, moist, and tender to touch. At this stage, a white pseudomembrane may be present. As the rash becomes more chronic, the perianal eruption may consist of painful fissures, a dried mucoid discharge, or psoriasiform plaques with yellow peripheral crust. In girls, the perianal rash may be associated with vulvovaginitis. In boys, the penis may be involved. Approximately 50% of patients have rectal pain, most commonly described as burning inside the anus during defecation, and 33% have blood-streaked stools. Fecal retention is a frequent behavioral response to the infection. Patients also have presented with guttate psoriasis. Although local induration or edema may occur,

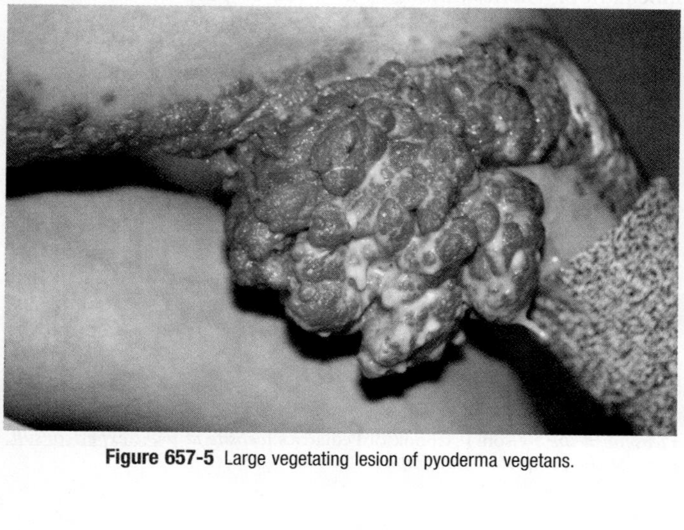

Figure 657-5 Large vegetating lesion of pyoderma vegetans.

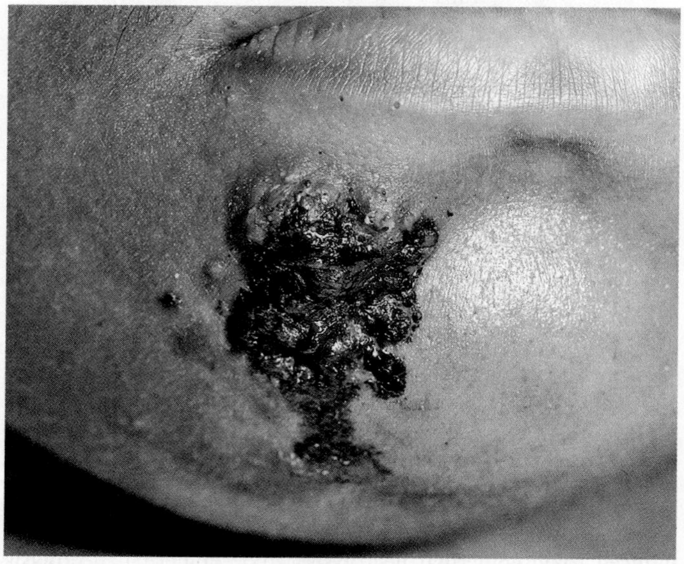

Figure 657-6 Cutaneous blastomycosis. Verrucous, crusted, erythematous plaque on the chin in a 15-year-old boy with respiratory symptoms and bone pain. (From Paller AS, Mancini AJ editors: *Hurwitz clinical pediatric dermatology,* ed 3, Philadelphia, 2006, Elsevier, p 471.)

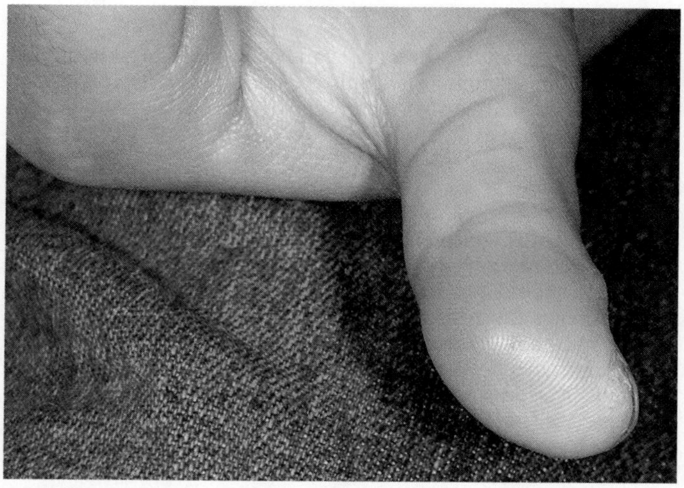

Figure 657-7 Blistering dactylitis. Edema and a tense bulla on the thumb of this 7 yr old girl. Culture of the blister fluid yielded *Staphylococcus aureus* rather than the more commonly seen group A β-hemolytic streptococcus (GABHS). (From Paller AS, Mancini AJ editors: *Hurwitz clinical pediatric dermatology,* ed 3, Philadelphia, 2006, Elsevier, p 372.)

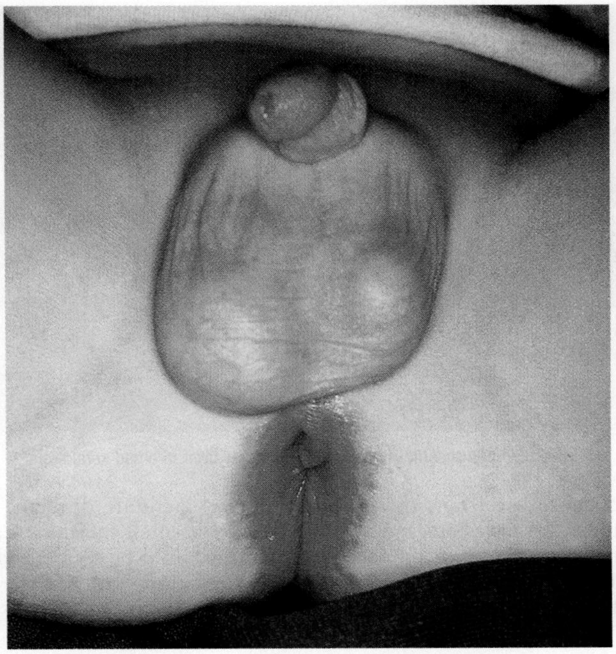

Figure 657-8 Perianal streptococcal dermatitis. Bright red erythema with a moist, tender surface. (From Paller AS, Mancini AJ editors: *Hurwitz clinical pediatric dermatology*, ed 3, Philadelphia, 2006, Elsevier, p 372.)

constitutional symptoms such as fever, headache, and malaise are absent, suggesting that subcutaneous involvement, as in cellulitis, is absent. Familial spread of perianal infectious dermatitis is common, particularly when family members bathe together or use the same water.

Perianal infectious dermatitis is usually caused by GABHS, but it may also be caused by *S. aureus*. The index case and family members should undergo culture; follow-up cultures to document bacteriologic cure after a course of treatment are recommended.

The **differential diagnosis** of perianal infectious dermatitis includes psoriasis, seborrheic dermatitis, candidosis, pinworm infestation, sexual abuse, and inflammatory bowel disease.

For GABHS perianal infectious dermatitis, treatment with a 7-day course of cefuroxime (20 mg/kg/day in 2 divided doses) is superior to treatment with penicillin. If *S. aureus* is cultured, treatment should be based on sensitivities.

ERYSIPELAS

See Chapter 176.

FOLLICULITIS

Folliculitis, or superficial infection of the hair follicle, is most often caused by *S. aureus* (Bockhart impetigo). The lesions are typically small, discrete, dome-shaped pustules with an erythematous base, located at the ostium of the pilosebaceous canals (Fig. 657-9). Hair growth is unimpaired, and the lesions heal without scarring. Favored sites include the scalp, buttocks, and extremities. Poor hygiene, maceration, drainage from wounds and abscesses, and shaving of the legs can be provocative factors. Folliculitis can also occur as a result of tar therapy or occlusive wraps. The moist environment encourages bacterial proliferation. In HIV-infected patients, *S. aureus* may produce confluent erythematous patches with satellite pustules in intertriginous areas and violaceous plaques composed of superficial follicular pustules in the scalp, axillae, or groin. The **differential diagnosis** include *Candida,* which may cause satellite follicular papules and pustules surrounding erythematous patches of intertrigo, and

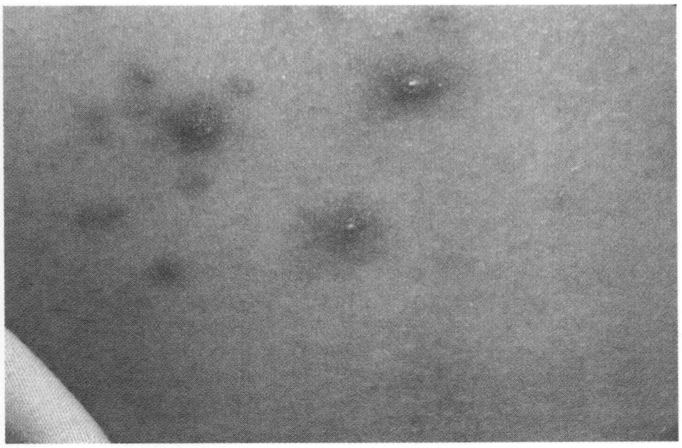

Figure 657-9 Folliculitis. Multiple follicular pustules.

Malassezia furfur, which produces 2- to 3-mm, pruritic, erythematous, perifollicular papules and pustules on the back, chest, and extremities, particularly in patients who have diabetes mellitus or are taking corticosteroids or antibiotics. Diagnosis is made by examining potassium hydroxide–treated scrapings from lesions. Detection of *Malassezia* may require a skin biopsy, demonstrating clusters of yeast and short, branching hyphae ("macaroni and meatballs") in widened follicular ostia mixed with keratinous debris.

Topical antibiotic therapy is usually all that is needed for mild cases, but more severe cases may require use of a systemic antibiotic such as dicloxacillin or cephalexin. Bacterial culture should be performed in treatment-resistant cases. In chronic recurrent folliculitis, daily application of a benzoyl peroxide 5% gel or wash may facilitate resolution.

Sycosis barbae is a deeper, more severe recurrent inflammatory form of folliculitis caused by *S. aureus* that involves the entire depth of the follicle. Erythematous follicular papules and pustules develop on the chin, upper lip, and angle of the jaw, primarily in young black males. Papules may coalesce into plaques, and healing may occur with scarring. Affected individuals are frequently found to be *S. aureus* carriers. **Treatment** with warm saline compresses and topical antibiotics such as mupirocin generally clears the infection. More extensive, recalcitrant cases may require therapy with β-lactamase–resistant systemic antibiotics and elimination of *S. aureus* from sites of carriage.

Hot tub folliculitis is attributable to *P. aeruginosa,* predominantly serotype O-11. The lesions are pruritic papules and pustules or deeply erythematous to violaceous nodules that develop 8-48 hr after exposure and are most dense in areas covered by a bathing suit (Fig. 657-10). Patients occasionally experience fever, malaise, and lymphadenopathy. The organism is readily cultured from pus. The eruption usually resolves spontaneously in 1-2 wk, often leaving postinflammatory hyperpigmentation. Consideration should be given to use of systemic antibiotics (ciprofloxacin) in adolescent patients with constitutional symptoms. Immunocompromised children are susceptible to complications of *Pseudomonas* folliculitis (cellulitis) and should avoid hot tubs.

FURUNCLES AND CARBUNCLES

Etiology

The causative agent in furuncles and carbuncles is usually *S. aureus,* which penetrates abraded perifollicular skin. Conditions predisposing to furuncle formation include obesity, hyperhidrosis, maceration, friction, and pre-existing dermatitis. Furunculosis is also more common in individuals with low serum iron levels, diabetes, malnutrition, HIV infection, or other

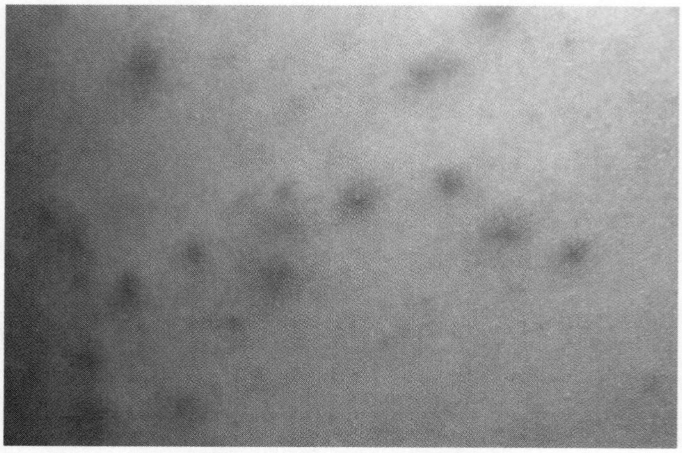

Figure 657-10 Papules and pustules in hot tub folliculitis.

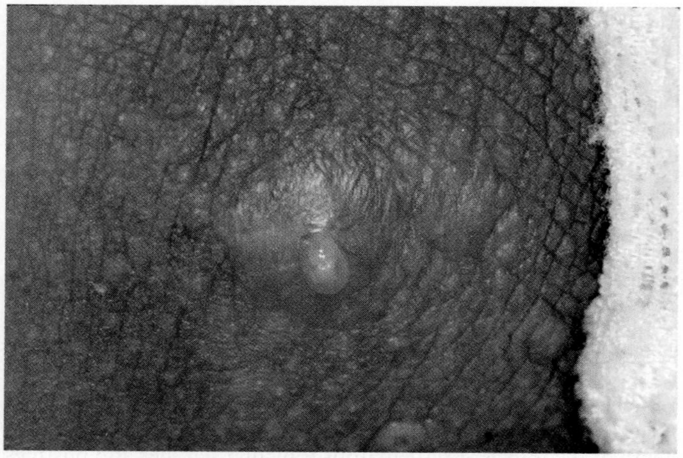

Figure 657-11 Rupture and discharge of pus in a furuncle.

immunodeficiency states. Recurrent furunculosis is frequently associated with carriage of *S. aureus* in the nares, axillae, or perineum or close contact with someone such as a family member who is a carrier. Other bacteria or fungi may occasionally cause furuncles or carbuncles.

Clinical Manifestations

This follicular lesion may originate from a preceding folliculitis or may arise initially as a deep-seated, tender, erythematous, perifollicular nodule. Although lesions are initially indurated, central necrosis and suppuration follow, leading to rupture and discharge of a central core of necrotic tissue and destruction of the follicle (Fig. 657-11). Healing occurs with scar formation. Sites of predilection are the hair-bearing areas on the face, neck, axillae, buttocks, and groin. Pain may be intense if the lesion is situated in an area where the skin is relatively fixed, such as in the external auditory canal or over the nasal cartilages. Patients with furuncles usually have no constitutional symptoms; bacteremia may occasionally ensue. Rarely, lesions on the upper lip or cheek may lead to cavernous sinus thrombosis. Infection of a group of contiguous follicles, with multiple drainage points, accompanied by inflammatory changes in surrounding connective tissue is a **carbuncle**. Carbuncles may be accompanied by fever, leukocytosis, and bacteremia.

Treatment

Treatment for furuncle and carbuncle includes regular bathing with antimicrobial soaps and wearing of loose-fitting clothing to minimize predisposing factors for furuncle formation. Frequent application of a hot, moist compress may facilitate drainage of lesions. Large lesions may be drained by a small incision. Carbuncles and large or numerous furuncles should be treated with systemic antibiotics chosen on the basis of culture and sensitivity testing results.

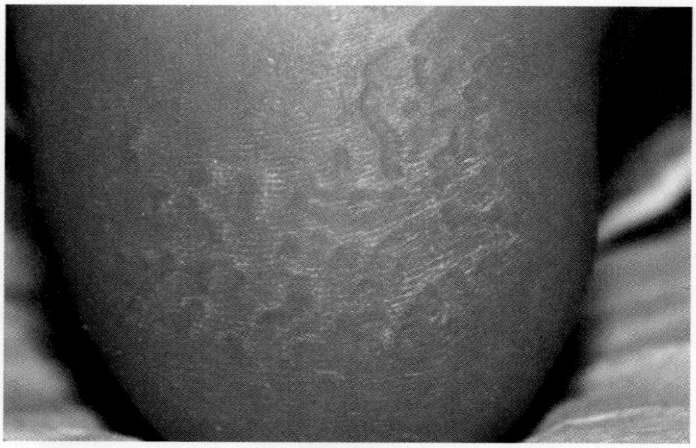

Figure 657-12 Superficial erosions of the horny layer in pitted keratolysis.

PITTED KERATOLYSIS

Pitted keratolysis occurs most frequently in humid tropical and subtropical climates, particularly in individuals whose feet are moist for prolonged periods, for example, as a result of hyperhidrosis, prolonged wearing of boots, or immersion in water. It occurs most commonly in young males from early adolescence to the late 20s. The lesions consist of 1- to 7-mm, irregularly shaped, superficial erosions of the horny layer on the soles, particularly at weight-bearing sites (Fig. 657-12). Brownish discoloration of involved areas may be apparent. A rare variant manifests as thinned, erythematous to violaceous plaques in addition to the typical pitted lesions. The condition is frequently malodorous, and is painful in about 50% of cases. The most likely etiologic agent is a species of *Corynebacterium*. *Dermatophilus congolensis* and *Kytococcus sedentarius* have also been isolated from lesions. Treatment of hyperhidrosis is mandatory. Avoidance of moisture and maceration produces slow, spontaneous resolution of the infection. Topical or systemic erythromycin and topical imidazole creams are standard therapy.

ERYTHRASMA

Erythrasma is a benign chronic superficial infection caused by *Corynebacterium minutissimum*. Predisposing factors include heat, humidity, obesity, skin maceration, diabetes mellitus, and poor hygiene. Approximately 20% of affected patients have involvement of the toe webs. Other frequently affected sites are moist, intertriginous areas such as the groin and axillae. The inframammary and perianal regions are occasionally involved. Sharply demarcated, irregularly bordered, slightly scaly, brownish red patches are characteristic of the disease. Mild pruritus is the only constant symptom. *C. minutissimum* is a complex of related organisms that produce porphyrins that fluoresce brilliant coral red under ultraviolet light. The diagnosis is readily made, and erythrasma is differentiated from dermatophyte infection and from tinea versicolor on Wood lamp examination. Bathing within 20 hr of Wood lamp examination, however, may remove the water-soluble porphyrins. Staining of skin scrapings with methylene blue or Gram stain reveals the pleomorphic, filamentous coccobacillary forms.

Effective **treatment** can be achieved with topical erythromycin, clindamycin, miconazole, or a 10- to 14-day course of oral erythromycin.

ERYSIPELOID

A rare cutaneous infection, erysipeloid is caused by inoculation of *Erysipelothrix rhusiopathiae* from contaminated animals, birds, fish, or their products. The localized cutaneous form is most common, characterized by well-demarcated diamond-shaped erythematous to violaceous patches at sites of inoculation. Local symptoms are generally not severe, constitutional symptoms are rare, and the lesions resolve spontaneously after weeks but can recur at the same site or develop elsewhere weeks to months later. The diffuse cutaneous form manifests as lesions at several areas of the body in addition to the site of inoculation. It is also self-limited. The systemic form, caused by hematogenous spread, is accompanied by constitutional symptoms and may include endocarditis, septic arthritis, cerebral infarct and abscess, meningitis, and pulmonary effusion. Diagnosis is confirmed by skin biopsy, which reveals the gram-positive organisms, and culture. The **treatment** of choice is parenteral penicillin or erythromycin.

TUBERCULOSIS OF THE SKIN (CHAPTERS 207 AND 209)

Cutaneous tuberculosis infection occurs worldwide, particularly in association with HIV infection, malnutrition, and poor sanitary conditions. Primary cutaneous tuberculosis is rare in the USA. All forms of cutaneous disease are caused by *Mycobacterium tuberculosis, Mycobacterium bovis,* and occasionally by the bacillus Calmette-Guérin (BCG), an attenuated vaccine form of *M. bovis.* The manifestations caused by a given organism are indistinguishable from one another. After invasion of the skin, mycobacteria either multiply intracellularly within macrophages, leading to progressive disease, or are controlled by the host immune reaction.

Primary cutaneous tuberculosis (tuberculous chancre) results when *M. tuberculosis* or *M. bovis* gains access to the skin or mucous membranes through trauma. Sites of predilection are the face, lower extremities, and genitals. The initial lesion develops 2-4 wk after introduction of the organism into the damaged tissue. A red-brown papule gradually enlarges to form a shallow, firm, sharply demarcated ulcer. Satellite abscesses may be present. Some lesions acquire a crust resembling impetigo, and others become heaped up and verrucous at the margins. The primary lesion can also manifest as a painless ulcer on the conjunctiva, gingiva, or palate and occasionally as a painless acute paronychia. Painless regional adenopathy may appear several weeks after the development of the primary lesion and may be accompanied by lymphangitis, lymphadenitis, or perforation of the skin surface, forming **scrofuloderma**. Untreated lesions heal with scarring within 12 mo but may reactivate, may form lupus vulgaris, or, rarely, may progress to the acute miliary form. Therefore, antituberculous therapy is indicated (Chapter 207).

M. tuberculosis or *M. bovis* can be cultured from the skin lesion and local lymph nodes, but acid-fast staining of histologic sections, particularly of a well-controlled infection, often does not reveal the organism. The **differential diagnosis** is broad, including a syphilitic chancre; deep fungal or atypical mycobacterial infection; leprosy; tularemia; cat-scratch disease; sporotrichosis; nocardiosis; leishmaniasis; reaction to foreign substances such as zirconium, beryllium, silk or nylon sutures, talc, and starch; papular acne rosacea; and lupus miliaris disseminatus faciei.

Scrofuloderma results from enlargement, cold abscess formation, and breakdown of a lymph node, most frequently in a cervical chain, with extension to the overlying skin. Linear or serpiginous ulcers and dissecting fistulas and subcutaneous tracts studded with soft nodules may develop. Spontaneous healing may take years, eventuating in cordlike keloid scars. Lupus vulgaris may also develop. Scrofuloderma of a cervical lymph node often originates in the larynx and was linked in the past to ingestion of milk containing *M. bovis.* Lesions may also originate from an underlying infected joint, tendon, bone, or epididymis. The **differential diagnosis** includes syphilitic gumma, deep fungal infections, actinomycosis, and hidradenitis suppurativa. The course is indolent, and constitutional symptoms are typically absent. Antituberculous therapy is indicated (Chapter 207).

Direct cutaneous inoculation of the tubercle bacillus into a previously infected individual with a moderate to high degree of immunity initially produces a small papule with surrounding inflammation. **Tuberculosis verrucosa cutis** (warty tuberculosis) forms when the papule becomes hyperkeratotic and warty, and several adjacent papules coalesce or a single papule expands peripherally to form a brownish red to violaceous, exudative, crusted verrucous plaque. Irregular extension of the margins of the plaque produces a serpiginous border. Children have the lesions most commonly on the lower extremities after trauma and contact with infected material such as sputum or soil. Regional lymph nodes are involved only rarely. Spontaneous healing with atrophic scarring takes place over months to years. Healing is also gradual with antituberculous therapy.

Lupus vulgaris is a rare, chronic, progressive form of cutaneous tuberculosis that develops in individuals with a moderate to high degree of tuberculin sensitivity induced by previous infection. The incidence is greater in cool, moist climates, particularly in females. Lupus vulgaris develops as a result of direct extension from underlying joints or lymph nodes; through lymphatic or hematogenous spread; or, rarely, by cutaneous inoculation with BCG vaccine. It most commonly follows cervical adenitis or pulmonary tuberculosis. Approximately 33% of cases are preceded by scrofuloderma, and 90% of cases manifest on the head and neck, most commonly on the nose or cheek. Involvement of the trunk is uncommon. A typical solitary lesion consists of a soft, brownish red papule that has an apple-jelly color when examined by diascopy. Peripheral expansion of the papule or, occasionally, the coalescence of several papules forms an irregular lesion of variable size and form. One or several lesions may develop, including nodules or plaques that are flat and serpiginous, hypertrophic and verrucous, or edematous in appearance. Spontaneous healing occurs centrally, and lesions characteristically reappear within the area of atrophy. Chronicity is characteristic, and persistence and progression of plaques over many years is common. Lymphadenitis is present in 40% of those with lupus vulgaris, and 10-20% has infection of the lungs, bones, or joints. Extensive deformities may be caused by vegetative masses and ulceration involving the nasal, buccal, or conjunctival mucosa; the palate; the gingiva; or the oropharynx. Squamous cell carcinoma, with a relatively high metastatic potential, may develop, usually after several years of the disease. After a temporary impairment in immunity, particularly after measles infection (lupus exanthematicus), multiple lesions may form at distant sites as a result of hematogenous spread from a latent focus of infection. The histopathology reveals a tuberculoid granuloma without caseation; organisms are extremely difficult to demonstrate. The **differential diagnosis** includes sarcoidosis, atypical mycobacterial infection, blastomycosis, chromoblastomycosis, actinomycosis, leishmaniasis, tertiary syphilis, leprosy, hypertrophic lichen planus, psoriasis, lupus erythematosus, lymphocytoma, and Bowen disease. Small lesions can be excised. Antituberculous drug therapy usually halts further spread and induces involution.

Orificial tuberculosis appears on the mucous membranes and periorificial skin after autoinoculation of mycobacteria from sites of progressive infection. It is a sign of advanced internal disease and carries a poor prognosis. Lesions appear as painful, yellowish or red nodules that form punched-out ulcers with inflammation and edema of the surrounding mucosa. **Treatment** consists of identification of the source of infection and initiation of antituberculous therapy.

Miliary tuberculosis (hematogenous primary tuberculosis) rarely manifests cutaneously and occurs most commonly in infants and in individuals who are immunosuppressed after chemotherapy or infection with measles or HIV. The eruption consists of crops of symmetrically distributed, minute, erythematous to purpuric macules, papules, or vesicles. The lesions may ulcerate, drain, crust, and form sinus tracts or may form subcutaneous gummas, especially in malnourished children with impaired immunity. Constitutional signs and symptoms are common, and a leukemoid reaction or aplastic anemia may develop. Tubercle bacilli are readily identified in an active lesion. A fulminant course should be anticipated, and aggressive antituberculous therapy is indicated.

Single or multiple metastatic tuberculous abscesses (**tuberculous gummas**) may develop on the extremities and trunk by hematogenous spread from a primary focus of infection during a period of decreased immunity, particularly in malnourished and immunosuppressed children. The fluctuant, nontender, erythematous subcutaneous nodules may ulcerate and form fistulas.

Vaccination with BCG characteristically produces a papule approximately 2 wk after vaccination. The papule expands in size, typically ulcerates within 2-4 mo, and heals slowly with scarring. In 1-2 per million vaccinations, a complication caused specifically by the BCG organism occurs, including regional lymphadenitis, lupus vulgaris, scrofuloderma, and subcutaneous abscess formation.

Tuberculids are skin reactions that exhibit tuberculoid features histologically but do not contain detectable mycobacteria. The lesions appear in a host who usually has moderate to strong tuberculin reactivity, has a history of previous tuberculosis of other organs, and usually shows a therapeutic response to antituberculous therapy. The cause of tuberculids is poorly understood. Most affected patients are in good health with no clear focus of disease at the time of the eruption. The most commonly observed tuberculid is the papulonecrotic tuberculid. Recurrent crops of symmetrically distributed, asymptomatic, firm, sterile, dusky-red papules appear on the extensor aspects of the limbs, the dorsum of the hands and feet, and the buttocks. The papules may undergo central ulceration and eventually heal, leaving sharply delineated, circular, depressed scars. The duration of the eruption is variable, but it usually disappears promptly after treatment of the primary infection. Lichen scrofulosorum, another form of tuberculid, is characterized by asymptomatic, grouped, pinhead-sized, often follicular pink or red papules that form discoid plaques, mainly on the trunk. Healing occurs without scarring.

Atypical mycobacterial infection may cause cutaneous lesions in children. *Mycobacterium marinum* is found in saltwater, freshwater, and diseased fish. In the USA, it is most commonly acquired from tropical fish tanks and swimming pools. Traumatic abrasion of the skin serves as a portal of entry for the organism. Approximately 3 wk after inoculation, a single reddish papule develops and enlarges slowly to form a violaceous nodule or, occasionally, a warty plaque (Fig. 657-13). The lesion occasionally breaks down to form a crusted ulcer or a suppurating abscess. Sporotrichoid erythematous nodules along lymphatics may also suppurate and drain. Lesions are most common on the elbows, knees, and feet of swimmers and on the hands and fingers in persons with aquarium-acquired infection. Systemic signs and symptoms are absent. Regional lymph nodes occasionally become slightly enlarged but do not break down. Rarely, the infection becomes disseminated, particularly in an immunosuppressed host. A biopsy specimen of a fully developed lesion demonstrates a granulomatous infiltrate with tuberculoid architecture. Treatment options include tetracycline, doxycycline, minocycline, clarithromycin, and rifampin plus ethambutol. Application of heat to the affected site may be a useful adjunctive therapy (Chapter 209).

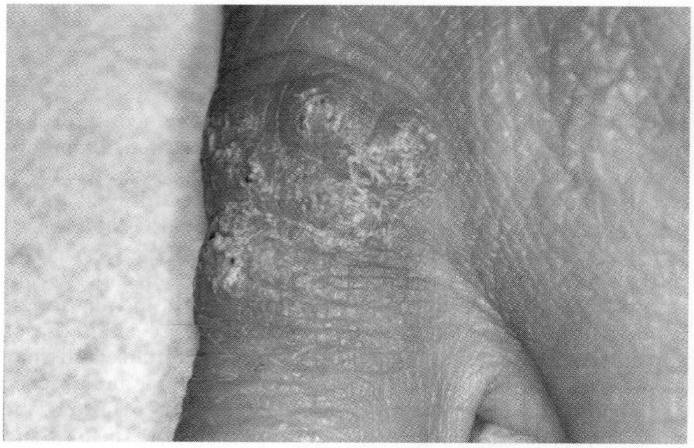

Figure 657-13 Violaceous, warty plaque of *Mycobacterium marinum* infection.

Mycobacterium kansasii primarily causes pulmonary disease; skin disease is rare, often occurring in an immunocompromised host. Most commonly, sporotrichoid nodules develop after inoculation of traumatized skin. Lesions may develop into ulcerated, crusted, or verrucous plaques. The organism is relatively sensitive to antituberculous medications, which should be chosen on the basis of susceptibility testing.

M. scrofulaceum causes cervical lymphadenitis (scrofuloderma) in young children, typically in the submandibular region. Nodes enlarge over several weeks, ulcerate, and drain. The local reaction is nontender and circumscribed, constitutional symptoms are absent, and there generally is no evidence of lung or other organ involvement. Other atypical mycobacteria may cause a similar presentation, including *Mycobacterium avium* complex, *Mycobacterium kansasii,* and *Mycobacterium fortuitum.* **Treatment** is accomplished by excision and administration of antituberculous drugs (Chapter 209).

Mycobacterium ulcerans (buruli ulcer) causes a painless subcutaneous nodule after inoculation of abraded skin. Most infections occur in children in tropical rain forests. The nodule usually ulcerates, develops undermined edges, and may spread over large areas, most commonly on an extremity. Local necrosis of subcutaneous fat, producing a septal panniculitis, is characteristic. Ulcers persist for months to years before healing spontaneously with scarring and sometimes with lymphedema. Constitutional symptoms and lymphadenopathy are absent. Diagnosis is made by culturing the organism at 32-33°C. **Treatment of choice** is early excision of the lesion. Local heat therapy and oral chemotherapy may benefit some patients.

M. avium complex, composed of >20 subtypes, most commonly causes chronic pulmonary infection. Cervical lymphadenitis and osteomyelitis occur occasionally, and papules or purulent leg ulcers occur rarely by primary inoculation. Skin lesions may be an early sign of disseminated infection. The lesions may take various forms, including erythematous papules, pustules, nodules, abscesses, ulcers, panniculitis, and sporotrichoid spread along lymphatics. For treatment, see Chapter 209.

M. fortuitum complex causes disease in an immunocompetent host principally by primary cutaneous inoculation after traumatic injury, injection, or surgery. A nodule, abscess, or cellulitis develops 4-6 wk after inoculation. In an immunocompromised host, numerous subcutaneous nodules may form, break down, and drain. **Treatment** is based on identification and susceptibility testing of the organism.

BIBLIOGRAPHY

Please visit the Nelson Textbook of Pediatrics *website at www.expertconsult.com for the complete bibliography.*

Chapter 658
Cutaneous Fungal Infections
Joseph G. Morelli

TINEA VERSICOLOR

A common, innocuous, chronic fungal infection of the stratum corneum, tinea versicolor is caused by the dimorphic yeast *Malassezia globosa*. The synonyms *Pityrosporum ovale* and *Pityrosporum orbiculare* were used previously to identify the causal organism.

Etiology
M. globosa is part of the indigenous flora, predominantly in the yeast form, and is found particularly in areas of skin that are rich in sebum production. Proliferation of filamentous forms occurs in the disease state. Predisposing factors include a warm, humid environment, excessive sweating, occlusion, high plasma cortisol levels, immunosuppression, malnourishment, and genetically determined susceptibility. The disease is most prevalent in adolescents and young adults.

Clinical Manifestations
The lesions of tinea versicolor vary widely in color. In white individuals, they are typically reddish brown, whereas in black individuals they may be either hypopigmented or hyperpigmented. The characteristic macules are covered with a fine scale. They often begin in a perifollicular location, enlarge, and merge to form confluent patches, most commonly on the neck, upper chest, back, and upper arms (Fig. 658-1). Facial lesions are common in adolescents; lesions occasionally appear on the forearms, dorsum of the hands, and pubis. There may be little or no pruritus. Involved areas do not tan after sun exposure. A papulopustular perifollicular variant of the disorder may occur on the back, chest, and sometimes the extremities.

Differential Diagnosis
Examination with a Wood lamp discloses a yellowish gold fluorescence. A potassium hydroxide (KOH) preparation of scrapings is diagnostic, demonstrating groups of thick-walled spores and myriad short, thick, angular hyphae resembling macaroni and meatballs. Skin biopsy, including culture and special stains for fungi (periodic acid–Schiff), are often necessary to make the diagnosis in cases of primarily follicular involvement. Microscopically, organisms and keratinous debris can be seen within dilated follicular ostia.

Figure 658-1 Hyperpigmented, sharply demarcated macules of varying sizes on the upper trunk characteristic of tinea versicolor.

Tinea versicolor must be distinguished from dermatophyte infections, seborrheic dermatitis, pityriasis alba, and secondary syphilis. Tinea versicolor may mimic nonscaling pigmentary disorders, such as postinflammatory pigmentary change, if a patient has removed the scales by scrubbing. *M. globosa* folliculitis must be distinguished from the other forms of folliculitis.

Treatment
Many therapeutic agents can be used to treat this disease successfully. The causative agent, a normal human saprophyte, is not eradicated from the skin, however, and the disorder recurs in predisposed individuals. Appropriate topical therapy may include one of the following: a selenium sulfide suspension applied overnight for 1 wk followed by 1 night per wk for 4 wk; an imidazole or terbinafine cream may be used twice daily for 2-4 wk. Oral therapy may be more convenient and may be achieved successfully with ketoconazole or fluconazole, 400 mg, repeated in 1 wk, or itraconazole, 200 mg/24 hr for 5-7 days. Recurrent episodes continue to respond promptly to these agents. Maintenance therapy with selenium sulfide applied overnight once a week may be used.

DERMATOPHYTOSES

Dermatophytoses are caused by a group of closely related filamentous fungi with a propensity for invading the stratum corneum, hair, and nails. The 3 principal genera responsible for infections are *Trichophyton, Microsporum,* and *Epidermophyton.*

Etiology
Trichophyton spp. cause lesions of all keratinized tissue, including skin, nails, and hair. *T Trichophyton rubrum* is the most common dermatophyte pathogen. *Microsporum* spp. principally invade the hair, and the *Epidermophyton* spp. invade the intertriginous skin. Dermatophyte infections are designated by the word **tinea** followed by the Latin word for the anatomic site of involvement. The dermatophytes are also classified according to source and natural habitat. Fungi acquired from the soil are called *geophilic*. They infect humans sporadically, inciting an inflammatory reaction. Dermatophytes that are acquired from animals are *zoophilic*. Transmission may be through direct contact or indirectly by infected animal hair or clothing. Infected animals are frequently asymptomatic. Dermatophytes acquired from humans are referred to as *anthropophilic*. These infestations range from chronic low-grade to acute inflammatory disease. *Epidermophyton* infections are transmitted only by humans, but various species of *Trichophyton* and *Microsporum* can be acquired from both human and nonhuman sources.

Epidemiology
Host defense has an important influence on the severity of the infection. Disease tends to be more severe in individuals with diabetes mellitus, lymphoid malignancies, immunosuppression, and states with high plasma cortisol levels, such as Cushing syndrome. Some dermatophytes, most notably the zoophilic species, tend to elicit more severe, suppurative inflammation in humans. Some degree of resistance to re-infection is acquired by most infected persons and may be associated with a delayed hypersensitivity response. No relationship has been demonstrated, however, between antibody levels and resistance to infection. The frequency and severity of infection are also affected by the geographic locale, the genetic susceptibility of the host, and the virulence of the strain of dermatophyte. Additional local factors that predispose to infection include trauma to the skin, hydration of the skin with maceration, occlusion, and elevated temperature.

Occasionally, a secondary skin eruption, referred to as a dermatophytid or "id" reaction, appears in sensitized individuals and has been attributed to circulating fungal antigens derived from the primary infection. The eruption is characterized by

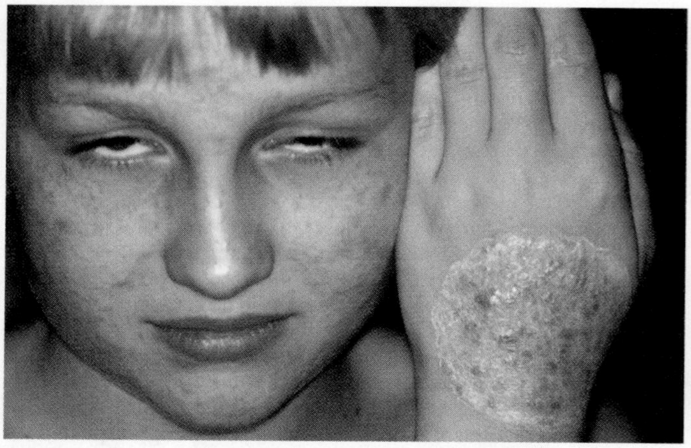

Figure 658-2 Id reaction. Papular eruption of the face associated with severe tinea infection of the hand.

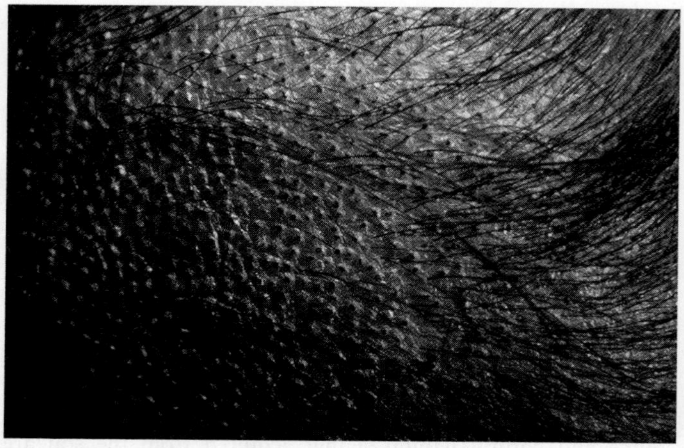

Figure 658-3 Black-dot ringworm with hairs broken off at the scalp.

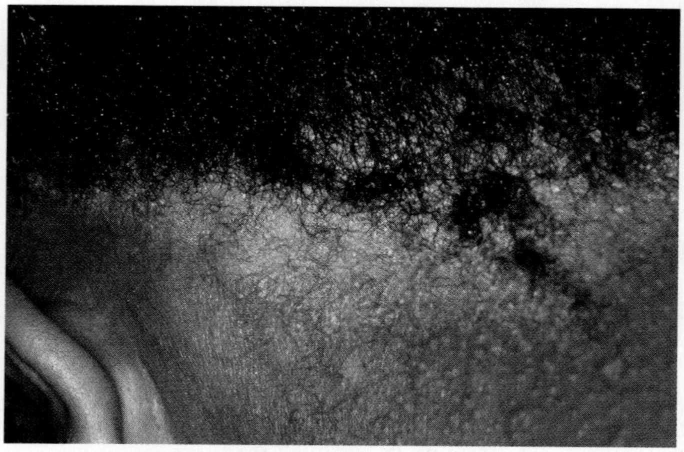

Figure 658-4 Tinea capitis mimicking seborrheic dermatitis.

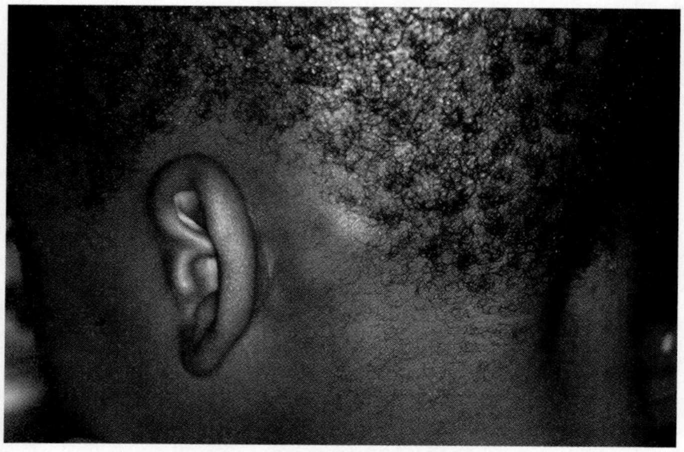

Figure 658-5 Lymphadenopathy associated with tinea capitis.

grouped papules (Fig. 658-2) and vesicles and, occasionally, by sterile pustules. Symmetric urticarial lesions and a more generalized maculopapular eruption also can occur. Id reactions are most often associated with tinea pedis but also occur with tinea capitis.

Tinea Capitis

CLINICAL MANIFESTATIONS Tinea capitis is a dermatophyte infection of the scalp most often caused by *Trichophyton tonsurans,* occasionally by *Microsporum canis*, and, much less commonly, by other Microsporum and *Trichophyton* spp. It is particularly common in black children age 4-14 yr. In *Microsporum* and some *Trichophyton* infections, the spores are distributed in a sheath-like fashion around the hair shaft (**ectothrix** infection), whereas *T. tonsurans* produces an infection within the hair shaft (endothrix). **Endothrix** infections may continue past the anagen phase of hair growth into telogen and are more chronic than infections with ectothrix organisms that persist only during the anagen phase. *T. tonsurans* is an anthropophilic species acquired most often by contact with infected hairs and epithelial cells that are on such surfaces as theater seats, hats, and combs. Dermatophyte spores may also be airborne within the immediate environment, and high carriage rates have been demonstrated in noninfected schoolmates and household members. *Microsporum canis* is a zoophilic species that is acquired from cats and dogs.

The clinical presentation of tinea capitis varies with the infecting organism. Endothrix infections such as those caused by *T. tonsurans* create a pattern known as "black-dot ringworm," characterized initially by many small circular patches of alopecia in which hairs are broken off close to the hair follicle (Fig. 658-3). Another clinical variant manifests as diffuse scaling, with minimal hair loss secondary. It strongly resembles seborrheic dermatitis, psoriasis, or atopic dermatitis (Fig. 658-4). *T. tonsurans* may also produce a chronic and more diffuse alopecia. Lymphadenopathy is common (Fig. 658-5). A severe inflammatory response produces elevated, boggy granulomatous masses (**kerions**), which are often studded with pustules (Fig. 658-6*A*). Fever, pain, and regional adenopathy are common, and permanent scarring and alopecia may result (Fig. 658-6*B*). The zoophilic organism *M. canis* or the geophilic organism *Microsporum gypseum* also may cause kerion formation. The pattern produced by *Microsporum audouinii*, the most common cause of tinea capitis in the 1940s and 1950s, is characterized initially by a small papule at the base of a hair follicle. The infection spreads peripherally, forming an erythematous and scaly circular plaque (**ringworm**) within which the infected hairs become brittle and broken. Numerous confluent patches of alopecia develop, and patients may complain of severe pruritus. *M. audouinii* infection is no longer common in the USA. **Favus** is a chronic form of tinea capitis that is rare in the USA and is caused by the fungus *Trichophyton schoenleinii.* Favus starts as yellowish red papules at the opening of hair follicles. The papules expand and coalesce to form cup-shaped, yellowish, crusted patches that fluoresce dull green under a Wood lamp.

DIFFERENTIAL DIAGNOSIS Tinea capitis can be confused with seborrheic dermatitis, psoriasis, alopecia areata, trichotillomania, and certain dystrophic hair disorders. When inflammation is pronounced, as in kerion, primary or secondary bacterial infection must also be considered. In adolescents, the patchy, moth-eaten

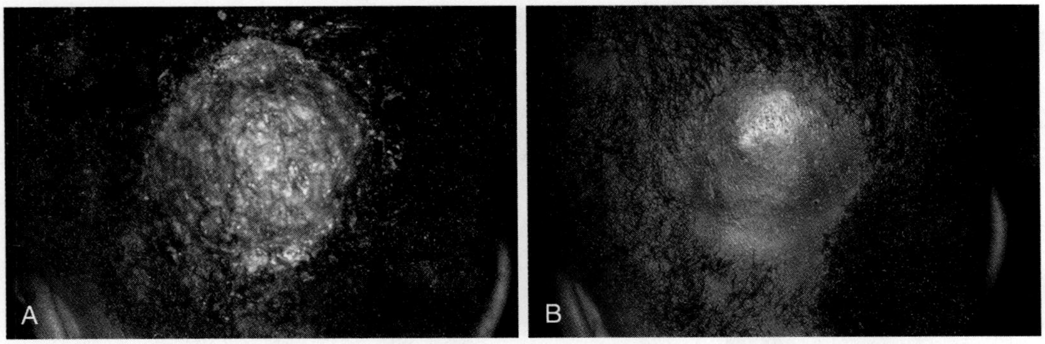

Figure 658-6 *A*, Kerion. Boggy granulomatous mass of the scalp. *B*, Scarring after kerion.

type of alopecia associated with secondary syphilis may resemble tinea capitis. If scarring occurs, discoid lupus erythematosus and lichen planopilaris must also be considered in the differential diagnosis.

The important diagnostic procedures for the various dermatophyte diseases include examination of infected hairs with a Wood lamp, microscopic examination of KOH preparations of infected material, and identification of the etiologic agent by culture. Hairs infected with common *Microsporum* spp. fluoresce a bright blue-green. Most *Trichophyton*-infected hairs do not fluoresce.

Microscopic examination of a KOH preparation of infected hair from the active border of a lesion discloses tiny spores surrounding the hair shaft in *Microsporum* infections and chains of spores within the hair shaft in *T. tonsurans* infections. Fungal elements are not usually seen in scales. A specific etiologic diagnosis of tinea capitis may be obtained by planting broken off infected hairs on Sabouraud medium with reagents to inhibit growth of other organisms. Such identification may require 2 wk or more.

TREATMENT Oral administration of griseofulvin microcrystalline (20 mg/kg/24 hr) is the recommended treatment for all forms of tinea capitis. It may be necessary for 8-12 wk and should be terminated only after fungal culture results are negative. Treatment for 1 month after a negative culture result minimizes the risk of recurrence. Adverse reactions to griseofulvin are rare but include nausea, vomiting, headache, blood dyscrasias, phototoxicity, and hepatotoxicity. Oral itraconazole is useful in instances of griseofulvin resistance, intolerance, or allergy. Itraconazole is given for 4-6 wk at a dosage of 3-5 mg/kg/24 hr with food. Capsules are preferable to the syrup, which may cause diarrhea. Terbinafine is also effective at a dosage of 3-6 mg/kg/24 hr for 4-6 wk or possibly in pulse therapy, although it has limited activity against *M. canis*. Neither itraconazole nor terbinafine is approved by the U.S. Food and Drug Administration (FDA) for treatment of dermatophyte infections in the pediatric population. Topical therapy alone is ineffective, but it may be an important adjunct because it may decrease the shedding of spores. Asymptomatic dermatophyte carriage in family members is common. One in 3 families have at least 1 member who is a carrier. Therefore, treatment of both patient and potential carriers with a sporicidal shampoo may hasten clinical resolution. Vigorous shampooing with a 2.5% selenium sulfide, zinc pyrithione, or ketoconazole shampoo is helpful. It is not necessary to shave the scalp.

Tinea Corporis

CLINICAL MANIFESTATIONS Tinea corporis, defined as infection of the glabrous skin, excluding the palms, soles, and groin, can be caused by most of the dermatophyte species, although *T. rubrum* and *Trichophyton mentagrophytes* are the most prevalent etiologic organisms. In children, infections with *M. canis* are also common. Tinea corporis can be acquired by direct contact with infected persons or by contact with infected scales or hairs

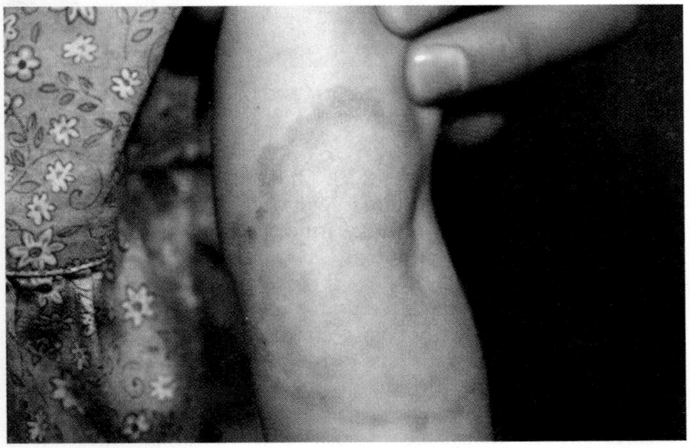

Figure 658-7 Annular plaque of tinea corporis with central clearing.

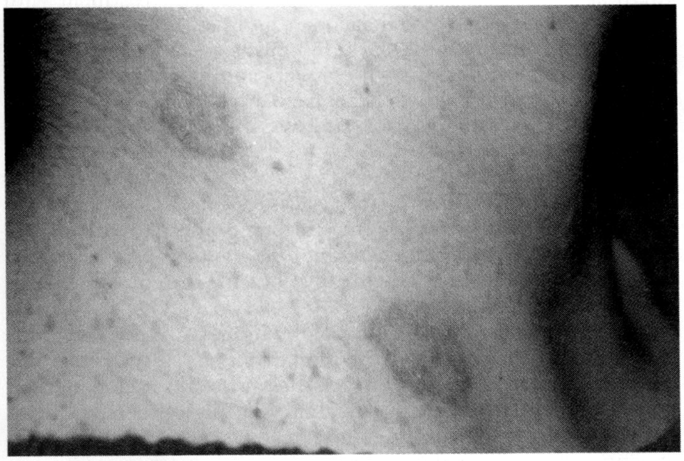

Figure 658-8 Minimal central clearing with tinea corporis.

deposited on environmental surfaces. *M. canis* infections are usually acquired from infected pets.

The most typical clinical lesion begins as a dry, mildly erythematous, elevated, scaly papule or plaque that spreads centrifugally and clears centrally to form the characteristic annular lesion responsible for the designation ringworm (Fig. 658-7). At times, plaques with advancing borders may spread over large areas. Grouped pustules are another variant. Most lesions clear spontaneously within several months, but some may become chronic. Central clearing does not always occur (Fig. 658-8), and differences in host response may result in wide variability in the clinical appearance—for example, granulomatous lesions called **Majocchi granuloma** due to penetration of organisms along the hair follicle to the level of the dermis, producing a fungal folliculitis

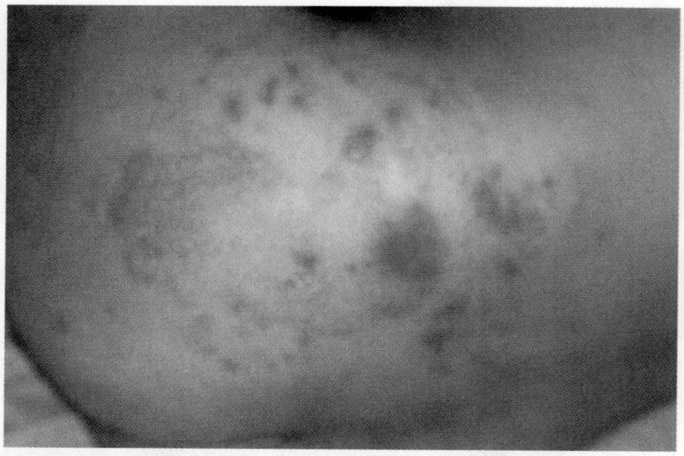

Figure 658-9 Follicular papule and pustule in Majocchi granuloma after use of a superpotent topical steroid.

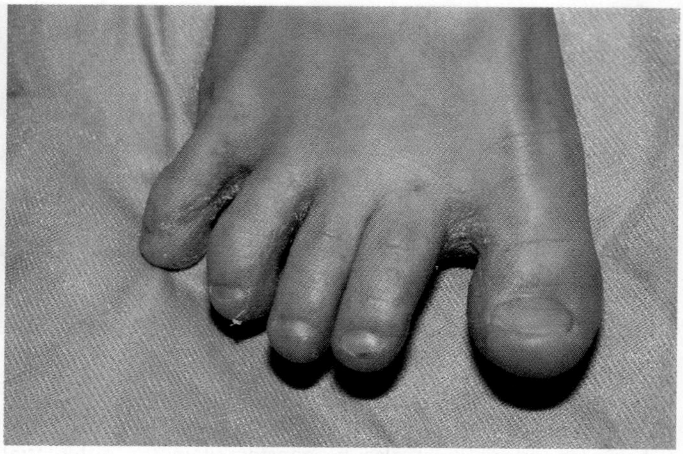

Figure 658-10 Interdigital tinea pedis.

and perifolliculitis (Fig. 658-9), and the kerion-like lesions referred to as tinea profunda. Majocchi granuloma is more common after inappropriate treatment with topical corticosteroids, especially the superpotent class.

DIFFERENTIAL DIAGNOSIS Many skin lesions, both infectious and noninfectious, must be differentiated from the lesions of tinea corporis. Those most frequently confused are granuloma annulare, nummular eczema, pityriasis rosea, psoriasis, seborrheic dermatitis, erythema chronicum migrans, and tinea versicolor. Microscopic examination of KOH wet mount preparations and cultures should always be performed when fungal infection is considered. Tinea corporis usually does not fluoresce with a Wood lamp.

TREATMENT Tinea corporis usually responds to treatment with one of the topical antifungal agents (e.g., imidazoles, terbinafine, naftifine) twice daily for 2-4 wk. In unusually severe or extensive disease, a course of therapy with oral griseofulvin microcrystalline may be required for 4 wk. Itraconazole has produced excellent results in many cases with a 1- to 2-wk course of oral therapy.

Tinea Cruris

CLINICAL MANIFESTATIONS Tinea cruris, or infection of the groin, occurs most often in adolescent males and is usually caused by the anthropophilic species *Epidermophyton floccosum* or *Trichophyton rubrum,* but occasionally by the zoophilic species *T. mentagrophytes.*

The initial clinical lesion is a small, raised, scaly, erythematous patch on the inner aspect of the thigh. This spreads peripherally, often developing numerous tiny vesicles at the advancing margin. It eventually forms bilateral, irregular, sharply bordered patches with hyperpigmented scaly centers. In some cases, particularly in infections with *T. mentagrophytes,* the inflammatory reaction is more intense and the infection may spread beyond the crural region. The penis is usually not involved in the infection, an important distinction from candidosis. Pruritus may be severe initially but abates as the inflammatory reaction subsides. Bacterial superinfection may alter the clinical appearance, and erythrasma or candidosis may coexist. Tinea cruris is more prevalent in obese persons and in persons who perspire excessively and wear tight-fitting clothing.

DIFFERENTIAL DIAGNOSIS The diagnosis of tinea cruris is confirmed by culture and by demonstration of septate hyphae on a KOH preparation of epidermal scrapings. The disorder must be differentiated from intertrigo, allergic contact dermatitis, candidosis, and erythrasma. Bacterial superinfection must be precluded when there is a severe inflammatory reaction.

TREATMENT Patients should be advised to wear loose cotton underwear. **Topical treatment** with an imidazole is recommended

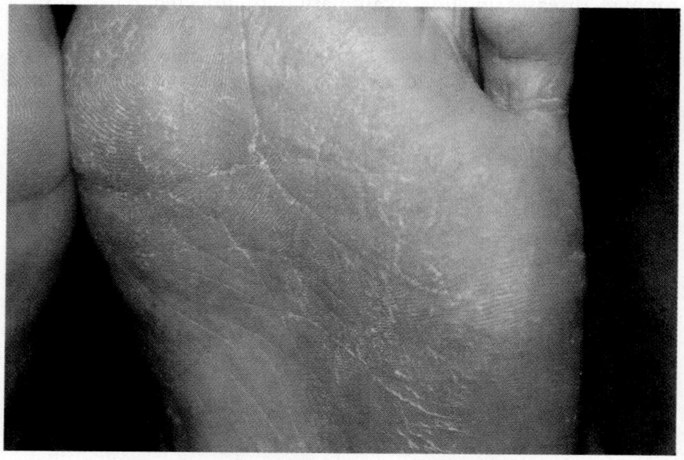

Figure 658-11 Diffuse, minimally erythematous tinea pedis.

for severe infection, especially because these agents are effective in mixed candidal-dermatophytic infections.

Tinea Pedis

CLINICAL MANIFESTATIONS Tinea pedis (athlete's foot), infection of the toe webs and soles of the feet, is uncommon in young children but occurs with some frequency in preadolescent and adolescent males. The usual etiologic agents are *T. rubrum, T. mentagrophytes,* and *E. floccosum.*

Most commonly, the lateral toe webs (3rd to 4th and 4th to 5th interdigital spaces) and the subdigital crevice are fissured, with maceration and peeling of the surrounding skin (Fig. 658-10). Severe tenderness, itching, and a persistent foul odor are characteristic. These lesions may become chronic. This type of infection may involve overgrowth by bacterial flora, including *Kytococcus sedantarius, Brevibacterium epidermidis,* and gram-negative organisms. Less commonly, a chronic diffuse hyperkeratosis of the sole of the foot occurs with only mild erythema (Fig. 658-11). In many cases, two feet and one hand are involved. This type of infection is more refractory to treatment and tends to recur. An inflammatory vesicular type of reaction may occur with *T. mentagrophytes* infection. This type is most common in young children. The lesions involve any area of the foot, including the dorsal surface, and are usually circumscribed. The initial papules progress to vesicles and bullae that may become pustular (Fig. 658-12). A number of factors, such as occlusive footwear and warm, humid weather, predispose to infection. Tinea pedis may be transmitted in shower facilities and swimming pool areas.

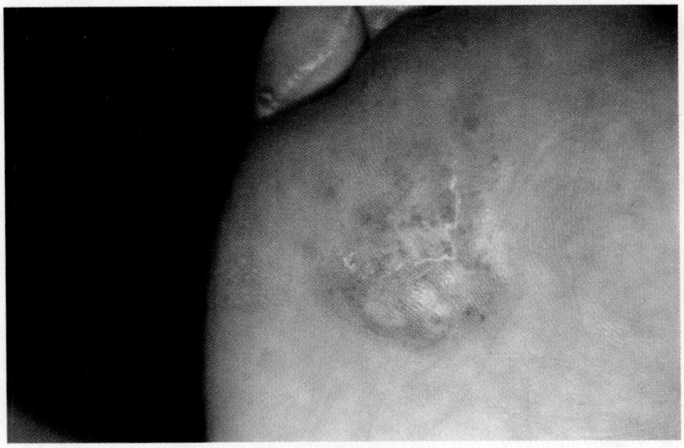

Figure 658-12 Vesicobullous tinea pedis.

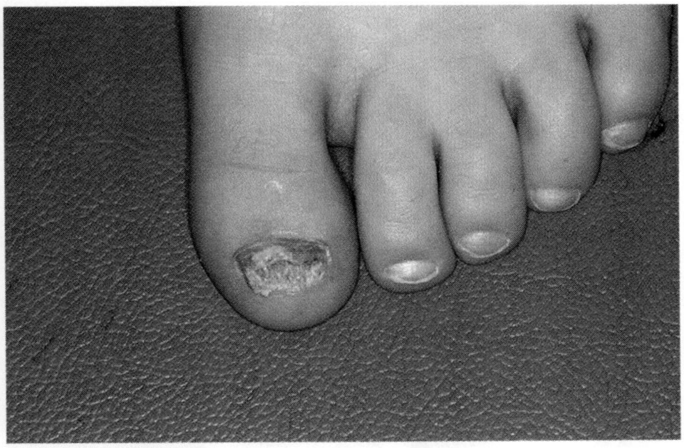

Figure 658-13 Hyperkeratotic nail in onychomycosis.

DIFFERENTIAL DIAGNOSIS Tinea pedis must be differentiated from simple maceration and peeling of the interdigital spaces, which is common in children. Infection with *Candida albicans* and various bacterial organisms (erythrasma) may cause confusion or may coexist with primary tinea pedis. Contact dermatitis, vesicular foot dermatitis, atopic dermatitis, and juvenile plantar dermatitis also simulate tinea pedis. Fungal mycelia can be seen on microscopic examination of a KOH preparation or by culture.

TREATMENT Treatment for mild infections includes simple measures such as avoidance of occlusive footwear, careful drying between the toes after bathing, and the use of an absorbent antifungal powder such as zinc undecylenate. Topical therapy with an imidazole is curative in most cases. Each of these agents is also effective against candidal infection. Several weeks of therapy may be necessary, and low-grade, chronic infections, particularly those caused by *T. rubrum*, may be refractory. In refractory cases, oral griseofulvin therapy may effect a cure, but recurrences are common.

Tinea Unguium

CLINICAL MANIFESTATIONS Tinea unguium is a dermatophyte infection of the nail plate. It occurs most often in patients with tinea pedis, but it may occur as a primary infection. It can be caused by a number of dermatophytes, of which *T. rubrum* and *T. mentagrophytes* are the most common.

The most superficial form of tinea unguium (i.e., white superficial onychomycosis) is due to *T. mentagrophytes*. It manifests as irregular single or numerous white patches on the surface of the nail unassociated with paronychial inflammation or deep infection. *T. rubrum* generally causes a more invasive, subungual infection that is initiated at the lateral distal margins of the nail and is often preceded by mild paronychia. The middle and ventral layers of the nail plate, and perhaps the nail bed, are the sites of infection. The nail initially develops a yellowish discoloration and slowly becomes thickened, brittle, and loosened from the nail bed (Fig. 658-13). In advanced infection, the nail may turn dark brown to black and may crack or break off.

DIFFERENTIAL DIAGNOSIS Tinea unguium must be differentiated from various dystrophic nail disorders. Changes due to trauma, psoriasis, lichen planus, eczema, and trachyonychia can all be confused with tinea unguium. Nails infected with *C. albicans* have several distinguishing features, most prominently a pronounced paronychial swelling. Thin shavings taken from the infected nail, preferably from the deeper areas, should be examined microscopically with KOH and cultured. Repeated attempts may be required to demonstrate the fungus. Histologic evaluation of nail clippings with special stains for dermatophytes can be diagnostic.

The long half-life of itraconazole in the nail has led to promising trials of intermittent short courses of therapy (double the normal dose for 1 wk of each month for 3-4 mo). Oral terbinafine is also used for the treatment of onychomycosis. Terbinafine once daily for 12 weeks is more effective than itraconazole pulse therapy. Griseofulvin and application of topical fungistatic agents to the nail bed are often ineffective and are not recommended.

Tinea Nigra Palmaris

Tinea nigra palmaris is a rare but distinctive superficial fungal infection that occurs principally in children and adolescents. It is caused by the dimorphic fungus *Phaeoannellomyces werneckii,* which imparts a gray-black color to the affected palm. The characteristic lesion is a well-defined hyperpigmented macule. Scaling and erythema are rare, and the lesions are asymptomatic. Tinea nigra is often mistaken for a junctional nevus, melanoma, or staining of the skin by contactants. Treatment is with an imidazole antifungal.

CANDIDAL INFECTIONS (CANDIDOSIS, CANDIDIASIS, AND MONILIASIS) (CHAPTER 226)

The dimorphic yeasts of the genus *Candida* are ubiquitous in the environment, but *C. albicans* usually causes candidosis in children. This yeast is not part of the indigenous skin flora, but it is a frequent transient on skin and may colonize the human alimentary tract and the vagina as a saprophytic organism. Certain environmental conditions, notably elevated temperature and humidity, are associated with an increased frequency of isolation of *C. albicans* from the skin. Many bacterial species inhibit the growth of *C. albicans,* and alteration of normal flora by the use of antibiotics may promote overgrowth of the yeast.

Oral Candidosis (Thrush)

See Chapter 226.

Vaginal Candidosis (Chapters 114 and 226)

C. albicans is an inhabitant of the vagina in 5-10% of women, and vaginal candidosis is not uncommon in adolescent girls. A number of factors can predispose to this infection, including antibiotic therapy, corticosteroid therapy, diabetes mellitus, pregnancy, and the use of oral contraceptives. The infection manifests as cheesy white plaques on an erythematous vaginal mucosa and a thick white-yellow discharge. The disease may be relatively mild or may produce pronounced inflammation and scaling of the external genitals and surrounding skin with progression to vesiculation and ulceration. Patients often complain of severe itching and burning in the vaginal area. Before treatment is initiated, the diagnosis should be confirmed by microscopic examination and/

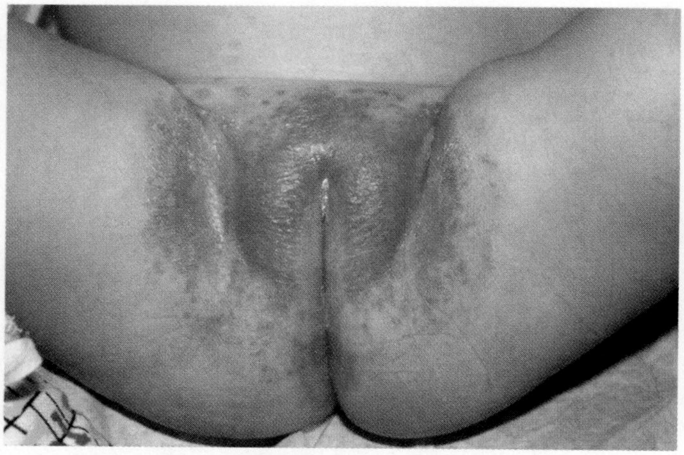

Figure 658-14 Erythematous confluent plaque caused by candidal infection.

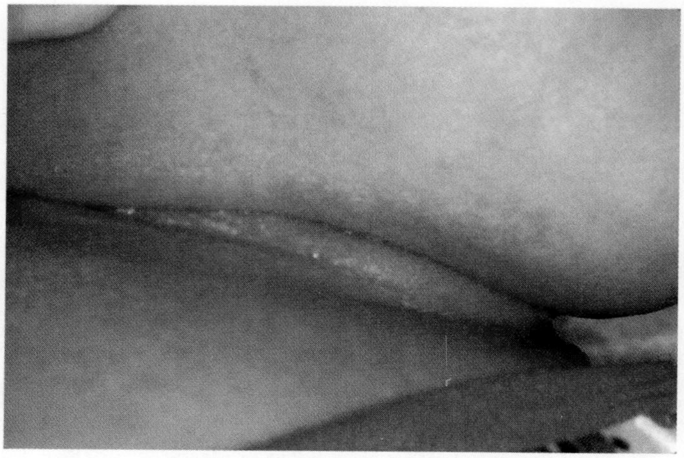

Figure 658-15 Intertriginous candidosis of the neck.

or culture. The infection may be eradicated by insertion of nystatin or imidazole vaginal tablets, suppositories, creams, or foam. If these products are ineffective, the addition of fluconazole 150 mg × 1 is effective.

Congenital Cutaneous Candidosis

See Chapter 226.

Candidal Diaper Dermatitis

Candidal diaper dermatitis is a ubiquitous problem in infants and, although relatively benign, is often frustrating because of its tendency to recur. Predisposed infants usually carry *C. albicans* in their intestinal tracts, and the warm, moist, occluded skin of the diaper area provides an optimal environment for its growth. A seborrheic, atopic, or primary irritant contact dermatitis usually provides a portal of entry for the yeast.

The primary clinical manifestation consists of an intensely erythematous, confluent plaque with a scalloped border and a sharply demarcated edge. It is formed by the confluence of numerous papules and vesicular pustules. Satellite pustules, those that stud the contiguous skin, are a hallmark of localized candidal infections. The perianal skin, inguinal folds, perineum, and lower abdomen are usually involved (Fig. 658-14). In males, the entire scrotum and penis may be involved, with an erosive balanitis of the perimeatal skin. In females, the lesions may be found on the vaginal mucosa and labia. In some infants, the process is generalized, with erythematous lesions distant from the diaper area. In some cases, the generalized process may represent a fungal id (hypersensitivity) reaction.

The **differential diagnosis** of candidal diaper dermatitis includes other eruptions of the diaper area that may coexist with candidal infection. For this reason, it is important to establish a diagnosis by means of KOH preparation or culture.

Treatment consists of applications of an imidazole cream 2 times daily. The combination of a corticosteroid and an antifungal agent may be justified if inflammation is severe but may confuse the situation if the diagnosis is not firmly established. Corticosteroid should not be continued for more than a few days. Protection of the diaper area by an application of thick zinc oxide paste overlying the anticandidal preparation may be helpful. The paste is more easily removed with mineral oil than with soap and water. Fungal id reactions gradually abate with successful treatment of the diaper dermatitis or may be treated with a mild corticosteroid preparation. When recurrences of diaper candidosis are frequent, it may be helpful to prescribe a course of oral anticandidal therapy to decrease the yeast population in the gastrointestinal tract. Some infants seem to be receptive hosts for *C. albicans* and may reacquire the organism from a colonized adult.

Intertriginous Candidosis

Intertriginous candidosis occurs most often in the axillae and groin, on the neck (Fig. 658-15), under the breasts, under pendulous abdominal fat folds, in the umbilicus, and in the gluteal cleft. Typical lesions are large, confluent areas of moist, denuded, erythematous skin with an irregular, macerated, scaly border. Satellite lesions are characteristic and consist of small vesicles or pustules on an erythematous base. With time, intertriginous candidal lesions may become lichenified, dry, scaly plaques. The lesions develop on skin subjected to irritation and maceration. Candidal superinfection is more likely to occur under conditions that lead to excessive perspiration, especially in obese children and in children with underlying disorders, such as diabetes mellitus. A similar condition, interdigital candidosis, commonly occurs in individuals whose hands are constantly immersed in water. Fissures occur between the fingers and have red denuded centers, with an overhanging white epithelial fringe. Similar lesions between the toes may be secondary to occlusive footwear. Treatment is the same as for other candidal infections.

Perianal Candidosis

Perianal dermatitis develops at sites of skin irritation as a result of occlusion, constant moisture, poor hygiene, anal fissures, and pruritus due to pinworm infestation. It may become superinfected with *C. albicans,* especially in children who are receiving oral antibiotic or corticosteroid medication. The involved skin becomes erythematous, macerated, and excoriated, and the lesions are identical to those of candidal intertrigo or candidal diaper rash. Application of a topical antifungal agent in conjunction with improved hygiene is usually effective. Underlying disorders such as pinworm infection must also be treated (Chapter 285).

Candidal Paronychia and Onychia

See Chapter 655.

Candidal Granuloma

Candidal granuloma is a rare response to an invasive candidal infection of skin. The lesions appear as crusted, verrucous plaques and hornlike projections on the scalp, face, and distal limbs. Affected patients may have single or numerous defects in immune mechanisms, and the granulomas are often refractory to topical therapy. A systemic anticandidal agent may be required for palliation or eradication of the infection.

BIBLIOGRAPHY

Please visit the Nelson Textbook of Pediatrics *website at* *www.expertconsult.com* *for the complete bibliography.*

Chapter 659
Cutaneous Viral Infections

Joseph G. Morelli

WART (VERRUCA)

Etiology

Human papillomaviruses (HPVs) cause a spectrum of disease from warts to squamous cell carcinoma of the skin and mucous membranes, including the larynx (Chapter 382.2). The human papillomaviruses are classified by genus, species, and type. More than 200 types are now known, and the entire genomes of about 100 are completely sequenced. The incidence of all types of warts is highest in children and adolescents. HPV is spread by direct contact and autoinoculation; transmission by fomites occurs. The clinical manifestations of infection develop ≥1 mo after inoculation and depend on the HPV type, the size of the inoculum, the immune status of the host, and the anatomic site.

Clinical Manifestations

Cutaneous warts develop in 5-10% of children. **Common warts** (verruca vulgaris), caused most commonly by HPV types 2 and 4, occur most frequently on the fingers, dorsum of the hands (Fig. 659-1), paronychial areas, face, knees, and elbows. They are well-circumscribed papules with an irregular, roughened, keratotic surface. When the surface is pared away, many black dots representing thrombosed dermal capillary loops are often visible. **Periungual warts** are often painful and may spread beneath the nail plate, separating it from the nail bed (Fig. 659-2). **Plantar warts,** although similar to the common wart, are caused by HPV type 1 and are usually flush with the surface of the sole because of the constant pressure from weight bearing. When plantar warts become hyperkeratotic (Fig. 659-3), they may be painful. Similar lesions (palmar) can also occur on the palms. They are sharply demarcated, often with a ring of thick callus. The surface keratotic material must sometimes be removed before the boundaries of the wart can be appreciated. Several contiguous warts (HPV type 4) may fuse to form a large plaque, the so-called mosaic wart. Flat warts (verruca plana), caused by HPV types 3 and 10, are slightly elevated, minimally hyperkeratotic papules that usually remain <3 mm in diameter and vary in color from pink to brown. They may occur in profusion on the face, arms, dorsum of the hands, and knees. The distribution of several lesions along a line of cutaneous trauma is a helpful diagnostic feature (Fig. 659-4). Lesions may be disseminated in the beard area and on the legs by shaving and from the hairline onto the scalp by combing the hair. **Epidermodysplasia verruciformis** (*EVER1*, *EVER2* genes), caused primarily by HPV types 5 and 8 (β-papillomaviruses, species 1), manifests as many diffuse verrucous papules. Wart types 9, 12, 14, 15, 17, 25, 36, 38, 47, and 50 may also be involved. Inheritance is thought to be primarily autosomal recessive, but an X-linked recessive form also has been postulated. Warts progress to **squamous cell carcinoma** in 10% of patients with epidermodysplasia verruciformis.

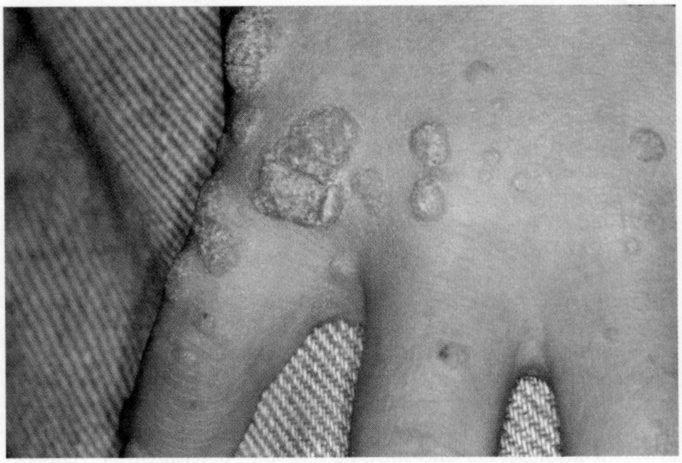

Figure 659-1 Verrucous papules on the back of the hand.

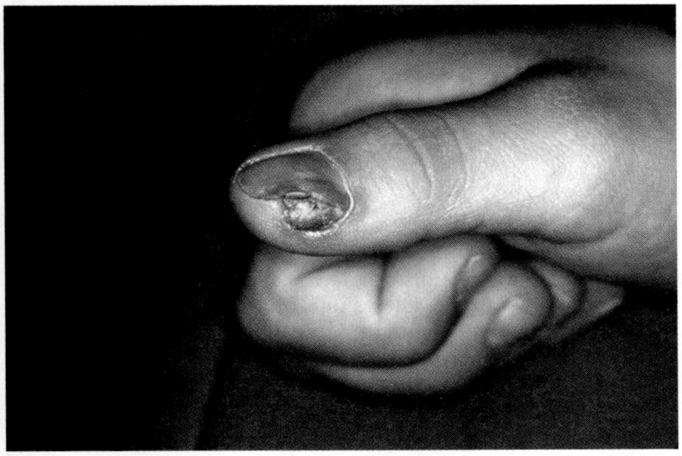

Figure 659-2 Periungual wart with disruption of nail growth.

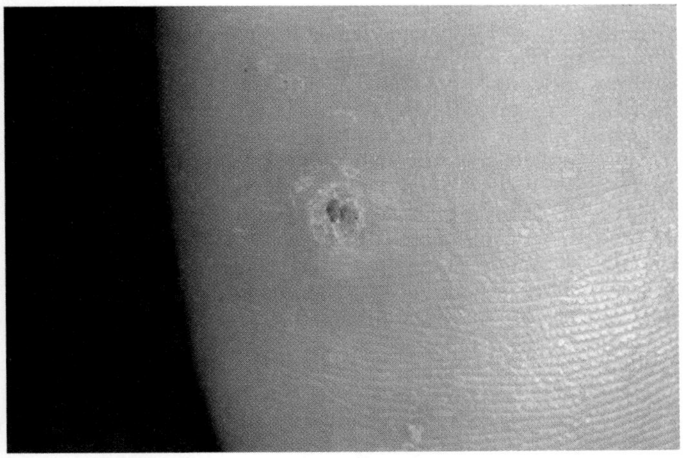

Figure 659-3 Hyperkeratotic plantar wart.

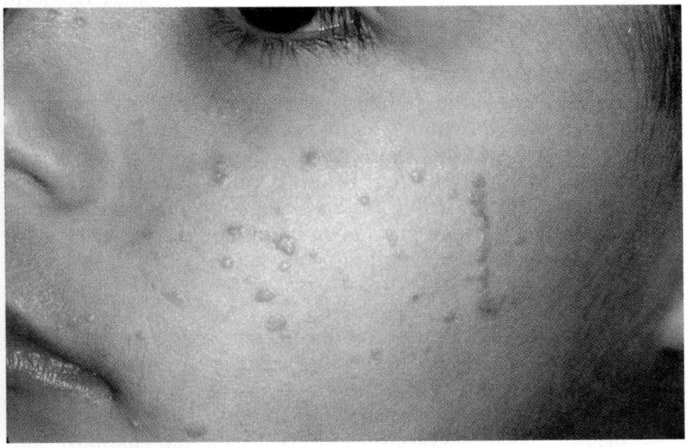

Figure 659-4 Multiple flat warts on the face with lesions in line of trauma.

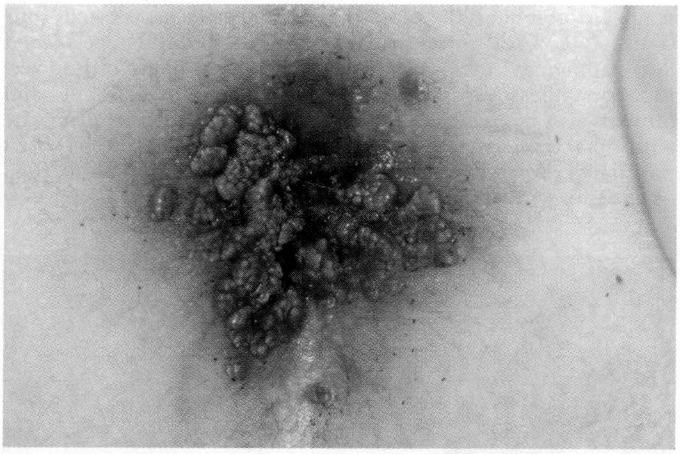

Figure 659-5 Condylomata acuminata in the perianal area of a toddler.

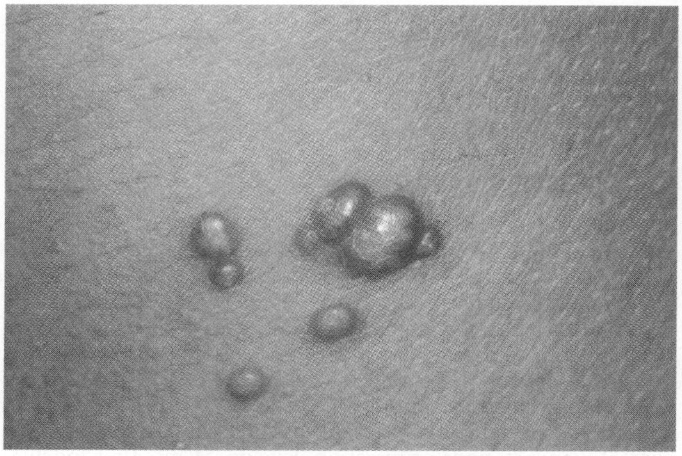

Figure 659-6 Grouped molluscum.

Genital HPV infection occurs in sexually active adolescents, most commonly as a result of infection with HPV types 6 and 11. **Condylomata acuminata** (mucous membrane warts) are moist, fleshy, papillomatous lesions that occur on the perianal mucosa (Fig. 659-5), labia, vaginal introitus, and perineal raphe and on the shaft, corona, and glans penis. Occasionally, they obstruct the urethral meatus or the vaginal introitus. Because they are located in intertriginous areas, they may become moist and friable. When untreated, condylomata proliferate and become confluent, at times forming large cauliflower-like masses. Lesions can also occur on the lips, gingivae, tongue, and conjunctivae. Genital warts in children may occur after inoculation during birth through an infected birth canal, as a consequence of sexual abuse, or from incidental spread from cutaneous warts. A significant proportion of genital warts in children contain HPV types that are usually isolated from cutaneous warts. HPV infection of the cervix is a major risk factor for development of carcinoma, particularly if the infection is due to HPV type 16, 18, 31, 33, 35, 39, 45, 52, 59, 67, 68, or 70. Immunization against types 6, 11, 16, and 18 is now available. Laryngeal (respiratory) papillomas contain the same HPV types as in anogenital papillomas. Transmission is believed to occur from mothers with genital HPV infection to neonates who aspirate infectious virus during birth.

Histology

The various types of warts share the basic changes of hyperplasia of the epidermal cells and vacuolation of the spinous keratinocytes, which may contain basophilic intranuclear inclusions (viral particles). Warts are confined to the epidermis and do not have "roots." Individuals with impaired cell-mediated immunity are particularly susceptible to HPV infection. Antibodies occur in response to infection but appear to have little protective effect.

Differential Diagnosis

Common warts are most often confused with molluscum contagiosum. Plantar and palmar warts may be difficult to distinguish from punctate keratoses, corns, and calluses. In contrast to calluses, warts obliterate normal skin markings. Juvenile flat warts mimic lichen planus, lichen nitidus, angiofibromas, syringomas, milia, and acne. Condylomata acuminata may resemble condylomata lata of secondary syphilis.

Treatment

Various therapeutic measures are effective in the treatment of warts. More than 65% of warts disappear spontaneously within 2 yr. Warts are epidermal lesions and do not produce scarring unless they are managed surgically or treated in an overly aggressive fashion. Hyperkeratotic lesions (common, plantar, and palmar warts) are more responsive to therapy if the excess keratotic debris is gently pared with a scalpel until thrombosed capillaries are apparent; further paring induces bleeding. Treatment is most successful when performed regularly and frequently (every 2-4 wk).

Common warts can be destroyed by applications of liquid nitrogen or by pulsed dye laser. Daily application of salicylic acid in flexible collodion or as a stick is a slow but painless method of removal that is effective in some patients. Plantar and palmar warts may be treated with 40% salicylic acid plasters. These should be applied for 5 days at a time with a 2-day rest period between applications. Following removal of the plaster and prolonged soaking in hot water, keratotic debris can be removed with an emery board or pumice stone. Condylomata respond best to weekly applications of 25% podophyllin in tincture of benzoin. The medication should be left on the warts for 4-6 hr and then removed by bathing. Keratinized warts near the genitalia (buttocks) do not respond to podophyllin. Imiquimod (5% cream) applied 3 times weekly is also beneficial. Imiquimod is indicated for genital warts but has also been used successfully to treat warts in other locations. For nongenital warts, imiquimod should be applied daily. Cimetidine 30-40 mg/kg/day has been used in children with multiple warts unresponsive to other treatments. Immunotherapy with squaric acid or intralesional candida antigen may also be employed. With all types of therapy, care should be taken to protect the surrounding normal skin from irritation.

MOLLUSCUM CONTAGIOSUM

Etiology

The poxvirus that causes molluscum contagiosum is a large double-stranded DNA virus that replicates in the cytoplasm of host epithelial cells. The three types cannot be differentiated on the basis of clinical appearance, location of lesions, or a patient's age or sex. Type 1 virus causes most infections. The disease is acquired by direct contact with an infected person or from fomites and is spread by autoinoculation. Children age 2-6 yr who are otherwise well and individuals who are immunosuppressed are affected most commonly. The incubation period is estimated to be ≥2 wk.

Clinical Manifestations

Discrete, pearly, skin-colored, smooth, dome-shaped, papules vary in size from 1 to 5 mm. They typically have a central umbilication from which a plug of cheesy material can be expressed. The papules may occur anywhere on the body, but the face, eyelids, neck, axillae, and thighs are sites of predilection (Fig. 659-6). They may be found in clusters on the genitals or in the groin of adolescents and may be associated with other venereal diseases in sexually active individuals. Lesions commonly involve

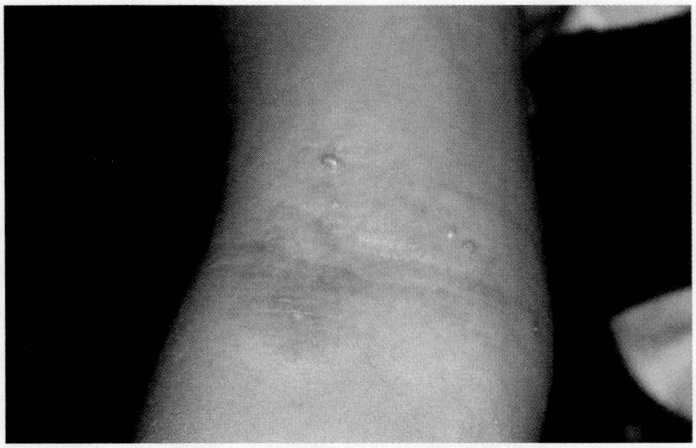

Figure 659-7 Molluscum with surrounding dermatitis.

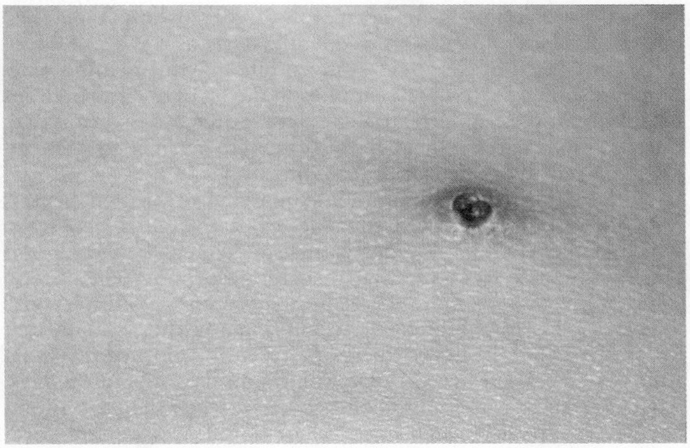

Figure 659-8 Inflamed molluscum. Crusted papule at site of previous molluscum.

the genital area in children but in most cases are not acquired by sexual transmission. Mild surrounding erythema or an eczematous dermatitis may accompany the papules (Fig. 659-7). Lesions on patients with AIDS tend to be large and numerous, particularly on the face. Exuberant lesions may also be found in children with leukemia and other immunodeficiencies. Children with atopic dermatitis are susceptible to widespread involvement in areas of dermatitis. A pustular eruption at the site of individual molluscum lesions is seen (Fig. 659-8). It is not a secondary bacterial infection, but an immunologic reaction to the molluscum virus and it should not be treated with antibiotics. Atrophic scars are often seen after this type of reaction.

Differential Diagnosis

Differential diagnosis of molluscum contagiosum includes trichoepithelioma, basal cell carcinoma, ectopic sebaceous glands, syringoma, hidrocystoma, keratoacanthoma, and warty dyskeratoma. In individuals with AIDS, cryptococcosis may be indistinguishable clinically from molluscum contagiosum. Rarely, coccidioidomycosis, histoplasmosis, or *Penicillium marneffei* infection masquerades as molluscum-like lesions in an immunocompromised host.

Histology

The epidermis is hyperplastic and hypertrophied, extending into the underlying dermis and projecting above the skin surface. The central plug of material, which is composed of virus-laden cells, may be shelled out from a lesion and examined under the microscope. The rounded, cup-shaped mass of homogeneous cells, often with identifiable lobules, is diagnostic. Specific antibody against molluscum contagiosum virus is detectable in most infected individuals but is of uncertain immunologic significance. Cell-mediated immunity is thought to be important in host defense.

Treatment

Molluscum contagiosum is a self-limited disease. The average attack lasts 6-9 mo. However, lesions can persist for years, can spread to distant sites, and may be transmitted to others. Affected patients should be advised to avoid shared baths and towels until the infection is clear. Infection may spread rapidly and produce hundreds of lesions in children with atopic dermatitis or immunodeficiency. In children old enough to tolerate a mild degree of pain, curettage is the **treatment of choice.** For younger children, cantharidin may be applied to the lesions and covered with adhesive bandages to prevent unwanted spread of the blistering agent. A blister forms at the site of application, and the molluscum is removed with the blister. Cantharidin should not be used on the face. Facial molluscum is more cosmetically upsetting to children and parents; imiquimod applied topically is beneficial if not excessively irritating. Molluscum is an epidermal disease and should not be overtreated such that scarring results.

BIBLIOGRAPHY

Please visit the Nelson Textbook of Pediatrics *website at* *www.expertconsult.com* *for the complete bibliography.*

Chapter 660
Arthropod Bites and Infestations

660.1 Arthropod Bites

Joseph G. Morelli

Arthropod bites are a common affliction of children and occasionally pose a problem in diagnosis. A patient may be unaware of the source of the lesions or may deny being bitten, making interpretation of the eruption difficult. In these cases, knowledge of the habits, life cycle, and clinical signs of the more common arthropod pests of humans may help lead to a correct diagnosis.

CLINICAL MANIFESTATIONS

The type of reaction that occurs after an arthropod bite depends on the species of insect and the age group and reactivity of the human host. Arthropods may cause injury to a host by various mechanisms, including mechanical trauma, such as the lacerating bite of a tsetse fly; invasion of host tissues, as in myiasis; contact dermatitis, as seen with repeated exposure to cockroach antigens; granulomatous reaction to retained mouthparts; transmission of systemic disease; injection of irritant cytotoxic or pharmacologically active substances, such as hyaluronidase, proteases, peptidases, and phospholipases in sting venom; and induction of anaphylaxis. Most reactions to arthropod bites depend on antibody formation to antigenic substances in saliva or venom. The type of reaction is determined primarily by the degree of previous exposure to the same or a related species of arthropod. When someone is bitten for the first time, no reaction develops. An immediate petechial reaction is occasionally seen. After repeated bites, sensitivity develops, producing a pruritic papule (Fig. 660-1) approximately 24 hr after the bite. This is the most common reaction seen in young children. With prolonged, repeated exposure, a wheal develops within minutes after a bite, followed 24 hr later by papule formation; this combination of reactions is seen commonly in older children. By adolescence or adulthood, only

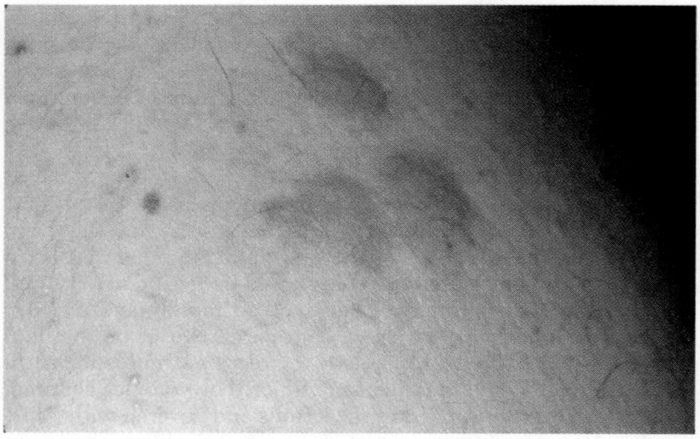

Figure 660-1 Pruritic papules after bedbug bites.

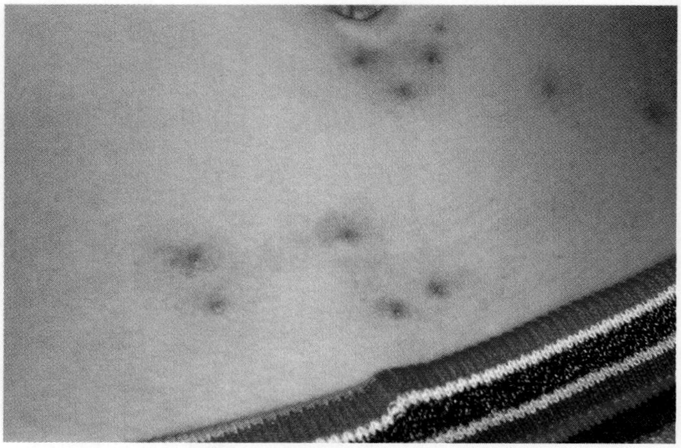

Figure 660-2 Red-brown papules in papular urticaria.

a wheal may form, unaccompanied by the delayed papular reaction. Thus, adults in the same household as affected children may be unaffected. Ultimately, as a person becomes insensitive to the bite, no reaction occurs at all. This stage of nonreactivity is maintained only as long as the individual continues to be bitten regularly. Individuals in whom papular urticaria develops are in the transitional phase between development of primarily a delayed papular reaction and development of an immediate urticarial reaction.

Arthropod bites may occur as solitary, numerous, or profuse lesions, depending on the feeding habits of the perpetrator. Fleas tend to sample their host several times within a small localized area, whereas mosquitoes tend to attack a host at more randomly scattered sites. Delayed hypersensitivity reactions to insect bites, the predominant lesions in the young and uninitiated, are characterized by firm, persistent papules that may become hyperpigmented and are often excoriated and crusted. Pruritus may be mild or severe, transient or persistent. A central punctum is usually visible but may disappear as the lesion ages or is scratched. The immediate hypersensitivity reaction is characterized by an evanescent, erythematous wheal. If edema is marked, a tiny vesicle may surmount the wheal. Certain beetles produce bullous lesions through the action of cantharidin, and various insects, including beetles and spiders, may cause hemorrhagic nodules and ulcers. Bites on the lower extremities are more likely to be severe or persistent or to become bullous than those located elsewhere. Complications of arthropod bites include development of impetigo, folliculitis, cellulitis, lymphangitis, and severe anaphylactic hypersensitivity reactions, particularly after the bite of certain hymenopterans. The histopathologic changes are variable, depending on the arthropod, the age of the lesion, and the reactivity of the host. Acute urticarial lesions tend to show central vesiculation in which eosinophils are numerous. Papules most commonly show dermal edema and a mixed superficial and deep perivascular inflammatory infiltrate, often including a number of eosinophils. At times, however, the dermal cellular infiltrate is so dense that a lymphoma is suspected. Many young children demonstrate extensive dermal but nonerythematous, nontender edema in response to mosquito bites ("skeeter" syndrome), which must be distinguished from cellulitis (painful, tender, red) and which responds to oral antihistamines. Retained mouthparts may stimulate a foreign body type of granulomatous reaction.

Papular urticaria occurs principally in the first decade of life. It may occur at any time of the year. The most common culprits are species of fleas, mites, bedbugs, gnats, mosquitoes, chiggers, and animal lice. Individuals with papular urticaria have predominantly transitional lesions in various stages of evolution between delayed-onset papules and immediate-onset wheals. The most characteristic lesion is an edematous, red-brown papule (Fig. 660-2). An individual lesion frequently starts as a wheal that, in turn, is replaced by a papule. A given bite may incite an id reaction at distant sites of quiescent bites in the form of erythematous macules, papules, or urticarial plaques. After a season or two, the reaction progresses from a transitional to a primarily immediate hypersensitivity urticarial reaction.

One of the most commonly encountered arthropod bites is that due to human, cat, or dog fleas (family *Pulicidae*). Eggs, which are generally laid in dusty areas and cracks between floorboards, give rise to larvae that then form cocoons. The cocoon stage can persist for up to 1 yr, and the flea emerges in response to vibrations from footsteps, accounting for the assaults that frequently befall the new owners of a recently reopened dwelling. Adult dog fleas can live without a blood meal for about 60 days. Attacks from fleas are more likely to occur when the fleas do not have access to their usual host; cat or dog fleas are more voracious and problematic when one visits an area frequented by the pet than when the pet is encountered directly. Flea bites tend to be grouped in lines or irregular clusters. Fleas are often not seen on the body of a pet. Diagnosis of flea bites is aided by examination of debris from the animal's bedding material. The debris is collected by shaking the bedding into a plastic bag and examining the contents for fleas or their eggs, larvae, or feces.

TREATMENT

Treatment is directed at alleviation of pruritus by oral antihistamines and cool compresses. Potent topical corticosteroids are helpful. Topical antihistamines are potent immunologic sensitizers and have no role in the treatment of insect bite reactions. A short course of systemic steroids may be helpful if many severe reactions occur, particularly around the eyes. Insect repellents containing diethyltoluamide (DEET) may afford moderate protection against mosquitoes, fleas, flies, chiggers, and ticks but are relatively ineffective against wasps, bees, and hornets. DEET must be applied to exposed skin and clothing to be effective. The most effective protection against mosquitoes, the human body louse, and other blood-feeding arthropods is use of DEET and permethrin-impregnated clothing. These measures are not effective, however, against the phlebotomine sand fly, which transmits leishmaniasis.

An effort should be made to identify and eradicate the etiologic agent. Pets should be carefully inspected. Crawl spaces, eaves, and other sites of the house or outbuildings frequented by animals and birds should be decontaminated, and baseboard crevices, mattresses, rugs, furniture, and animal sleeping quarters should be decontaminated. Agents that are effective for ridding the home of fleas include lindane, pyrethroids, and organic thiocyanates. Flea-infested pets may be treated with powders containing rotenone, pyrethroids, Malathion, or methoxychlor.

BIBLIOGRAPHY

Please visit the Nelson Textbook of Pediatrics *website at* *www.expertconsult.com* *for the complete bibliography.*

660.2 Scabies

Joseph G. Morelli

Scabies is caused by burrowing and release of toxic or antigenic substances by the female mite *Sarcoptes scabiei* var. *hominis*. The most important factor that determines spread of scabies is the extent and duration of physical contact with an affected individual. The children and sexual partner of an affected individual are most at risk. Scabies is transmitted only rarely by fomites because the isolated mite dies within 2-3 days.

ETIOLOGY AND PATHOGENESIS

An adult female mite measures approximately 0.4 mm in length, has 4 sets of legs, and has a hemispheric body marked by transverse corrugations, brown spines, and bristles on the dorsal surface. A male mite is approximately half her size and is similar in configuration. After impregnation on the skin surface, a gravid female exudes a keratolytic substance and burrows into the stratum corneum, often forming a shallow well within 30 min. She gradually extends this tract by 0.5-5 mm/24 hr along the boundary with the stratum granulosum. She deposits 10- 25 oval eggs and numerous brown fecal pellets (scybala) daily. When egg laying is completed, in 4-5 wk, she dies within the burrow. The eggs hatch in 3-5 days, releasing larvae that move to the skin surface to molt into nymphs. Maturity is achieved in about 2-3 wk. Mating occurs, and the gravid female invades the skin to complete the life cycle.

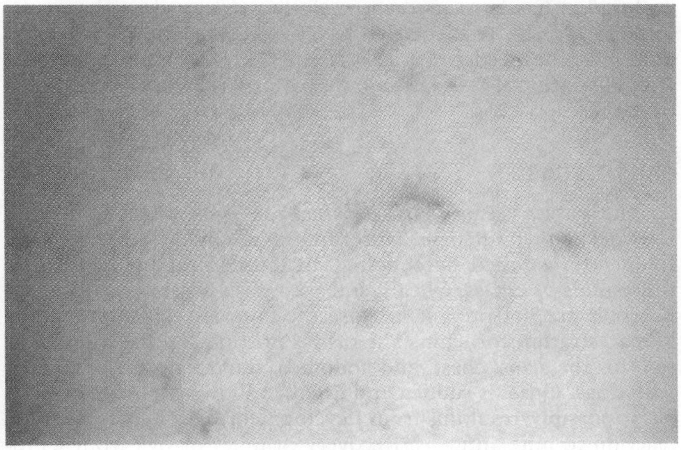

Figure 660-3 Classic scabies burrow.

CLINICAL MANIFESTATIONS

In an immunocompetent host, scabies is frequently heralded by intense pruritus, particularly at night. The first sign of the infestation often consists of 1- to 2-mm red papules, some of which are excoriated, crusted, or scaling. Threadlike burrows are the classic lesion of scabies (Fig. 660-3) but may not be seen in infants. In infants, bullae and pustules are relatively common. The eruption may also include wheals, papules, vesicles, and a superimposed eczematous dermatitis (Fig. 660-4). The palms, soles, and scalp are often affected. In older children and adolescents, the clinical pattern is similar to that in adults, in whom preferred sites are the interdigital spaces, wrist flexors, anterior axillary folds, ankles, buttocks, umbilicus and belt line, groin, genitals in men, and areolas in women. The head, neck, palms, and soles are generally spared. Red-brown nodules, most often located in covered areas such as the axillae, groin, and genitals, predominate in the less common variant called nodular scabies. Additional clues include facial sparing, affected family members, poor response to topical antibiotics, and transient response to topical steroids. Untreated, scabies may lead to eczematous dermatitis, impetigo, ecthyma, folliculitis, furunculosis, cellulitis, lymphangitis, and id reaction. Glomerulonephritis has developed in children from streptococcal impetiginization of scabies lesions. In some tropical areas, scabies is the predominant underlying cause of pyoderma. A latent period of about 1 mo follows an initial infestation. Thus, itching may be absent and lesions may be relatively inapparent in contacts who are asymptomatic carriers. On re-infestation, however, reactions to mite antigens are noted within hours.

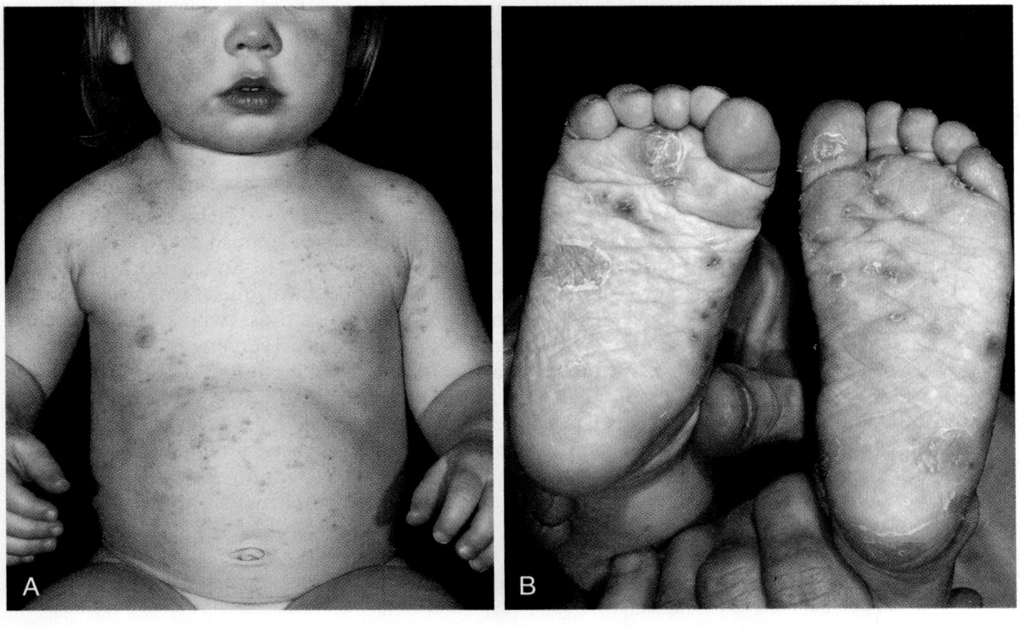

Figure 660-4 *A,* Diffuse scabies on an infant. The face is clear. The lesions are most numerous around the axillae, chest, and abdomen. *B,* Scabies. Infestation of the palms and soles is common in infants. The vesicular lesions have all ruptured. (From Habif TP, editor: *Clinical dermatology,* ed 4, Philadelphia, 2004, Mosby, pp 502–503.)

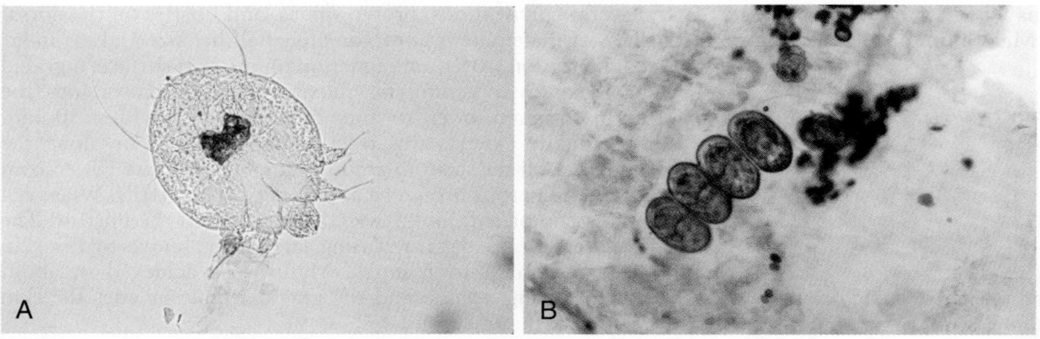

Figure 660-5 *A,* Human scabies mite obtained from scraping. *B,* Scabies ova and scybala.

DIFFERENTIAL DIAGNOSIS

Differential diagnosis of scabies can often be made clinically but is confirmed by microscopic identification of mites (Fig. 660-5*A*), ova, and scybala (Fig. 660-5*B*) in epithelial debris. Scrapings most often test positive when obtained from burrows or fresh papules. A reliable method is application of a drop of mineral oil on the selected lesion, scraping of it with a No. 15 blade, and transferring the oil and scrapings to a glass slide.

The differential diagnosis depends on the types of lesions present. Burrows are virtually pathognomonic for human scabies. Papulovesicular lesions are confused with papular urticaria, canine scabies, chickenpox, viral exanthems, drug eruptions, dermatitis herpetiformis, and folliculitis. Eczematous lesions may mimic atopic dermatitis and seborrheic dermatitis, and the less common bullous disorders of childhood may be suspected in infants with predominantly bullous lesions. Nodular scabies is frequently misdiagnosed as urticaria pigmentosa and Langerhans cell histiocytosis. The histopathologic appearance of nodular scabies, consisting of a deep, dense, perivascular infiltrate of lymphocytes, histiocytes, plasma cells, and atypical mononuclear cells, may mimic malignant lymphoid neoplasms.

TREATMENT

The treatment of choice for scabies is permethrin 5% cream (Elimite) applied to the entire body from the neck down, with particular attention to intensely involved areas, which is also standard therapy. Scabies is frequently found above the neck in infants, necessitating treatment of the scalp. The medication is left on the skin for 8-12 hr. If necessary, it may be reapplied in 1 wk for another 8- to 12-hr period. Additional therapies may include lindane 1% lotion or cream and oral ivermectin.

Transmission of mites is unlikely more than 24 hr after treatment. Pruritus, which is due to hypersensitivity to mite antigens, may persist for a number of days and may be alleviated by a topical corticosteroid preparation. If pruritus persists for >2 wk after treatment and new lesions are occurring, the patient should be reexamined for mites. Nodules are extremely resistant to treatment and may take several months to resolve. The entire family should be treated, as should caretakers of the infested child. Clothing, bed linens, and towels should be thoroughly laundered.

NORWEGIAN SCABIES

The Norwegian variant of human scabies is highly contagious and occurs mainly in individuals who are mentally and physically debilitated, particularly those who are institutionalized and those with Down syndrome; in patients with poor cutaneous sensation (leprosy, spina bifida); in patients who have severe systemic illness (leukemia, diabetes); and in immunosuppressed patients (HIV infection). Affected individuals are infested by myriad mites that inhabit the crusts and exfoliating scales of the skin and scalp. The nails may become thickened and dystrophic. The subungual debris is densely populated by mites. The infestation is often accompanied by generalized lymphadenopathy and eosinophilia. There is massive orthokeratosis and parakeratosis with numerous interspersed mites, psoriasiform epidermal hyperplasia, foci of spongiosis, and neutrophilic abscesses. Norwegian scabies is thought to represent a deficient host immune response to the organism. Management is difficult, requiring scrupulous isolation measures, removal of the thick scales, and repeated but careful applications of permethrin 5% cream. Ivermectin (200-250 μg/kg) has been used successfully as single-dose therapy in refractory cases, particularly in HIV-infected patients. A second dose may be needed a week later. The U.S. Food and Drug Administration (FDA) has not approved this agent for treatment of scabies.

CANINE SCABIES

Canine scabies is caused by *S. scabiei* var. *canis,* the dog mite that is associated with mange. The eruption in humans, which is most frequently acquired by cuddling an infested puppy, consists of tiny papules, vesicles, wheals, and excoriated eczematous plaques. Burrows are not present because the mite infrequently inhabits human stratum corneum. The rash is pruritic and has a predilection for the arms, chest, and abdomen, the usual sites of contact with dogs. Onset is sudden and usually follows exposure by 1-10 days, possibly resulting from development of a hypersensitivity reaction to mite antigens. Recovery of mites or ova from scrapings of human skin is rare. The disease is self-limited because humans are not a suitable host. Bathing and changing clothes are generally sufficient. Removal or treatment of the infested animal is necessary. Symptomatic therapy for itching is helpful. In rare cases in which mites are demonstrated in scrapings from an affected child, they can be eradicated by the same measures applicable to human scabies.

OTHER TYPES OF SCABIES

Other mites that occasionally bite humans include the chigger or harvest mite *(Eutrombicula alfreddugesi),* which prefers to live on grass, shrubs, vines, and stems of grain. Larvae have hooked mouthparts, which allow the chigger to attach to the skin, but not to burrow, to obtain a blood meal, most commonly on the lower legs. Avian mites may affect those who come into close contact with chickens or pet gerbils. Humans may occasionally be assaulted by avian mites that have infested a nest outside a window, an attic, heating vents, or an air conditioner. The dermatitis is variable, including grouped papules, wheals, and vesicular lesions on the wrists, neck, breasts, umbilicus, and anterior axillary folds. A prolonged investigation is often undertaken before the cause and source of the dermatitis are discovered.

BIBLIOGRAPHY

Please visit the Nelson Textbook of Pediatrics *website at www.expertconsult.com for the complete bibliography.*

660.3 Pediculosis

Joseph G. Morelli

Three types of lice are obligate parasites of the human host: body or clothing lice *(Pediculus humanus corporis)*, head lice *(Pediculus humanus capitis)*, and pubic or crab lice *(Phthirus pubis)*. Only the body louse serves as a vector of human disease (typhus, trench fever, relapsing fever). Body and head lice have similar physical characteristics. They are about 2-4 mm in length. Pubic lice are only 1-2 mm in length and are greater in width than length, giving them a crablike appearance. Female lice live for approximately 1 mo and deposit 3-10 eggs daily on the human host. Body lice, however, generally lay eggs in or near the seams of clothing. The ova or nits are glued to hairs or fibers of clothing but not directly on the body. Ova hatch in 1-2 wk and require another week to mature. Once the eggs hatch, the nits remain attached to the hair as empty sacs of chitin. Freshly hatched larvae die unless a meal is obtained within 24 hr and every few days thereafter. Both nymphs and adult lice feed on human blood, injecting their salivary juices into the host and depositing their fecal matter on the skin. Symptoms of infestation do not appear immediately but develop as an individual becomes sensitized. The hallmark of all types of pediculosis is pruritus.

Pediculosis corporis is rare in children except under conditions of poor hygiene, especially in colder climates when the opportunity to change clothes on a regular basis is lacking. The parasite is transmitted mainly on contaminated clothing or bedding. The primary lesion is a small, intensely pruritic, red macule or papule with a central hemorrhagic punctum, located on the shoulders, trunk, or buttocks. Additional lesions include excoriations, wheals, and eczematous, secondarily infected plaques. Massive infestation may be associated with constitutional symptoms of fever, malaise, and headache. Chronic infestation may lead to "vagabond's skin," which manifests as lichenified, scaling, hyperpigmented plaques, most commonly on the trunk. Lice are found on the skin only transiently when they are feeding. At other times, they inhabit the seams of clothing. Nits are attached firmly to fibers in the cloth and may remain viable for up to 1 mo. Nits hatch when they encounter warmth from the host's body when the clothes are worn again. Therapy consists of improved hygiene and hot water laundering of all infested clothing and bedding. A uniform temperature of 65°C, wet or dry, for 15-30 min kills all eggs and lice. Alternatively, eggs hatch and nymphs starve if clothing is stored for 2 wk at 75-85°F.

Pediculosis capitis is an intensely pruritic infestation of lice in the scalp hair. Fomites and head-to-head contact are important modes of transmission. In summer months in many areas of the USA and in the tropics at all times of the year, shared combs, brushes, or towels have a more important role in louse transmission. Translucent 0.5-mm eggs are laid near the proximal portion of the hair shaft and become adherent to one side of the shaft (Fig. 660-6). A nit cannot be moved along or knocked off the hair shaft with the fingers. Secondary pyoderma, after trauma due to scratching, may result in matting together of the hair and cervical and occipital lymphadenopathy. Hair loss does not result from pediculosis but may accompany the secondary pyoderma. Head lice are a major cause of numerous pyodermas of the scalp, particularly in tropical environments. Lice are not always visible, but nits are detectable on the hairs, most commonly in the occipital region and above the ears, rarely on beard or pubic hair. Dermatitis may also be noted on the neck and pinnae. An id reaction, consisting of erythematous patches and plaques, may develop, particularly on the trunk. For unknown reasons, head lice rarely infest African Americans.

Because of resistance of head lice to pyrethroids, malathion 0.5% in isopropanol is the treatment of choice for head lice and should be applied to dry hair until hair and scalp are wet, and left on for 12 hours. A second application 7-9 days after initial treatment may be necessary. This product is flammable, so care should be taken to avoid open flames. Malathion, like lindane shampoo, is not indicated for use in neonates and infants. Additional approved therapies include spinosad (if >4 yr old), benzyl alcohol lotion (if >6 mo), and ivermectin for difficult-to-treat head lice. All household members should be treated at the same time. Nits can be removed with a fine-toothed comb after application of a damp towel to the scalp for 30 min. Clothing and bed linens should be laundered in very hot water or dry-cleaned; brushes and combs should be discarded or coated with a pediculicide for 15 min and then thoroughly cleaned in boiling water. Children may return to school after the initial treatment.

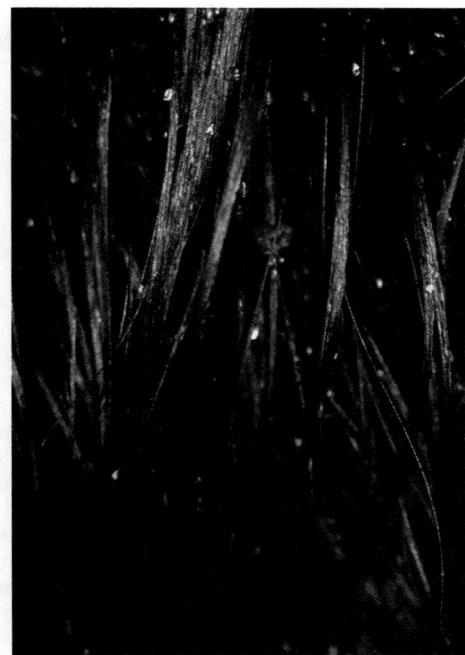

Figure 660-6 Intact nits on human hairs.

Pediculosis pubis is transmitted by skin-to-skin or sexual contact with an infested individual; the chance of acquiring the lice with one sexual exposure is 95%. The infestation is usually encountered in adolescents, although small children may occasionally acquire pubic lice on the eyelashes. Patients experience moderate to severe pruritus and may develop a secondary pyoderma from scratching. Excoriations tend to be shallower, and the incidence of secondary infection is lower than in pediculosis corporis. Maculae ceruleae are steel-gray spots, usually < 1 cm in diameter, which may appear in the pubic area and on the chest, abdomen, and thighs. Oval translucent nits, which are firmly attached to the hair shafts, may be visible to the naked eye or may be readily identified by a hand lens or by microscopic examination (see Fig. 660-6). Grittiness, as a result of adherent nits, may sometimes be detected when the fingers are run through infested hair. Adult lice are difficult to detect than head or body lice because of their lower level of activity and smaller, translucent bodies. Because pubic lice occasionally may wander or may be transferred to other sites on fomites, terminal hair on the trunk, thighs, axillary region, beard area, and eyelashes should be examined for nits. The coexistence of other venereal diseases should be considered. Treatment with a 10-min application of a pyrethrin preparation is usually effective. Re-treatment may be required in 7-10 days. The shampoo form of lindane, which requires a 10-min application time, is an alternative choice, but lindane cream and lotion are no longer recommended for treatment of pubic lice. Infestation of eyelashes is eradicated by petrolatum applied 3 to 5 times per 24 hr for 8-10 days. Clothing, towels, and bed linens may be contaminated with nit-bearing hairs and should be thoroughly laundered or dry-cleaned.

BIBLIOGRAPHY
Please visit the Nelson Textbook of Pediatrics *website at www.expertconsult.com for the complete bibliography.*

660.4 Seabather's Eruption

Joseph G. Morelli

Seabather's eruption is a severely pruritic dermatosis of inflammatory papules that develops within ≈ 12 hr of bathing in saltwater, primarily on body sites that were covered by a bathing suit. The eruption has been described primarily in connection with bathing in the waters of Florida and the Caribbean. Lesions, which may include pustules, vesicles, and urticarial plaques, are more numerous in individuals who keep their bathing suits on for an extended period after leaving the water. The eruption may be accompanied by systemic symptoms of fatigue, malaise, fever, chills, nausea, and headache; in one large series, ≈ 40% of children younger than 16 yr had fever. Duration of the pruritus and skin eruption is 1-2 wk. Lesions consist of a superficial and deep perivascular and interstitial infiltrate of lymphocytes, eosinophils, and neutrophils. The eruption appears to be due to an allergic hypersensitivity reaction to venom from larvae of the thimble jellyfish *(Linuche unguiculata)*. Treatment is largely symptomatic. Potent topical corticosteroids have been shown to provide relief to some patients.

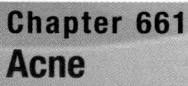

Chapter 661 Acne

Joseph G. Morelli

ACNE VULGARIS

Acne, particularly the comedonal form, occurs in 80% of adolescents.

Pathogenesis

Lesions of acne vulgaris develop in sebaceous follicles, which consist of large, multilobular sebaceous glands that drain their products into the follicular canals. The initial lesion of acne is a microcomedone, which progresses to a comedone. A comedone is a dilated epithelium-lined follicular sac filled with lamellated keratinous material, lipid, and bacteria. An open comedone, known as a **blackhead,** has a patulous pilosebaceous orifice that permits visualization of the plug. An open comedone becomes inflammatory less commonly than does a closed comedone or whitehead, which has only a pinpoint opening. An inflammatory papule or nodule develops from a comedone that has ruptured and extruded its follicular contents into the subadjacent dermis, inducing a neutrophilic inflammatory response. If the inflammatory reaction is close to the surface, a papule or pustule develops. If the inflammatory infiltrate develops deeper in the dermis, a nodule forms. Suppuration and an occasional giant cell reaction to the keratin and hair are the cause of nodulocystic lesions. These are not true cysts but liquefied masses of inflammatory debris.

The primary pathogenetic alterations in acne are (1) abnormal keratinization of the follicular epithelium, resulting in impaction of keratinized cells within the follicular lumen; (2) increased sebaceous gland production of sebum; (3) proliferation of *Propionibacterium acnes* within the follicle; and (4) inflammation. Comedonal acne (Fig. 661-1), particularly of the central face, is frequently the first sign of pubertal maturation. At puberty, the sebaceus gland enlarges and sebum production increases in response to the increased activities of androgens of primarily adrenal origin. Most patients with acne do not have endocrine abnormalities. Hyperresponsiveness of the sebocyte to androgens is likely involved in determining the severity of acne in a given individual. Sebocytes and follicular keratinocytes contain 5α-reductase and 3β- and 17β-hydroxyl-steroid dehydrogenase, which are capable of metabolizing androgens. A significant number of women with acne (25-50%), particularly those with relatively mild papulopustular acne, note that their acne flares about 1 wk before menstruation.

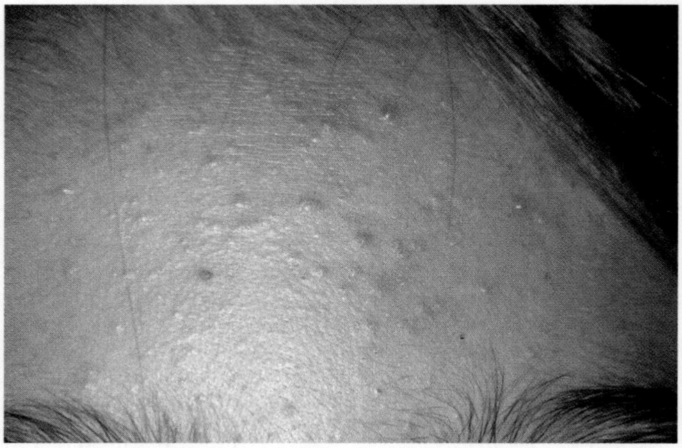

Figure 661-1 Primarily comedonal acne in a 7 yr old girl.

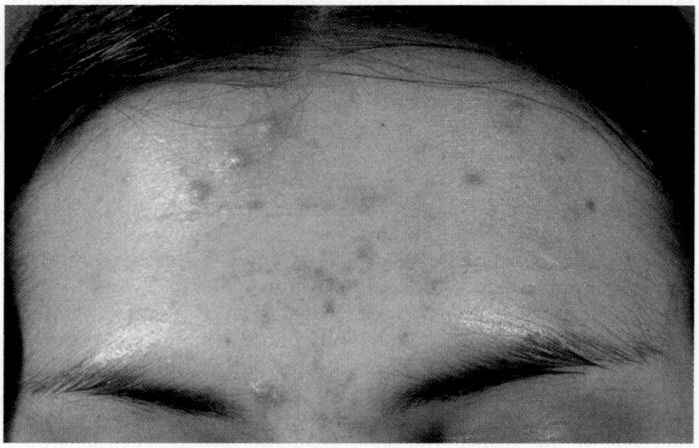

Figure 661-2 Inflammatory papules and pustules.

Freshly formed sebum consists of a mixture of triglycerides, wax esters, squalene, and sterol esters. Normal follicular bacteria produce lipases that hydrolyze sebum triglycerides to free fatty acids. Those of medium-chain length (C8-C14) may be provocative factors in initiating an inflammatory reaction. Sebum also provides a favorable substrate for proliferation of bacteria. *P. acnes* appears to be largely responsible for the formation of free fatty acids. Skin surface *P. acnes* counts do not correlate with the severity of acne. There is a correlation between reduction of *P. acnes* count and improvement in acne vulgaris. It is probable that bacterial proteases, hyaluronidases, and hydrolytic enzymes produce biologically active extracellular materials that increase the permeability of the follicular epithelium. Chemotactic factors released by the intrafollicular bacteria attract neutrophils and monocytes. Lysosomal enzymes from the neutrophils, released in the process of phagocytizing the bacteria, further disrupt the integrity of the follicular wall and intensify the inflammatory reaction.

Clinical Manifestations

Acne vulgaris is characterized by 4 basic types of lesions: open and closed comedones, papules, pustules (Fig. 661-2), and

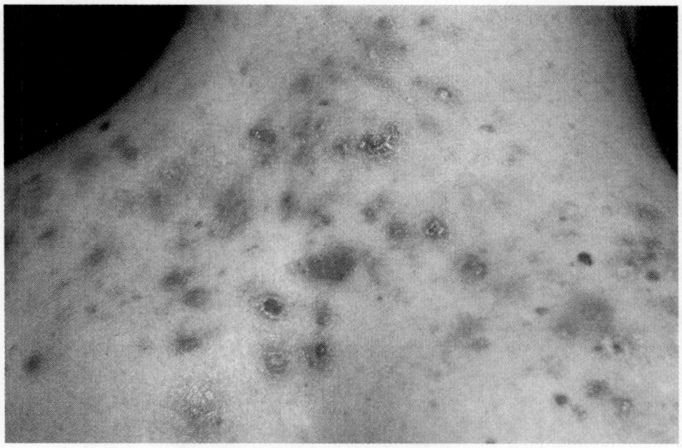

Figure 661-3 Severe nodulocystic acne.

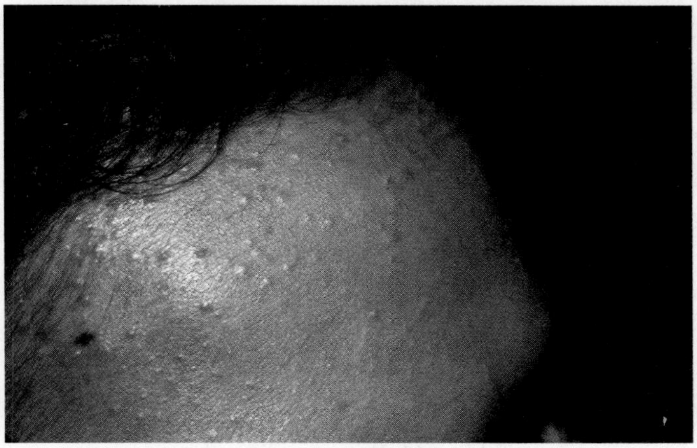

Figure 661-4 Pomade acne along the hairline.

Table 661-1 CLASSIFICATION OF ACNE

SEVERITY	DESCRIPTION
Mild	Comedones (noninflammatory lesions) are the main lesions. Papules and pustules may be present but are small and few in number (generally < 10).
Moderate	Moderate numbers of papules and pustules (10-40) and comedones (10-40) are present. Mild disease of the trunk may also be present.
Moderately severe	Numerous papules and pustules are present (40-100), usually with many comedones (40-100) and occasional larger, deeper nodular inflamed lesions (up to 5). Widespread affected areas usually involve the face, chest, and back.
Severe	Nodulocystic acne and acne conglobata with many large, painful nodular or pustular lesions are present, along with many smaller papules, pustules, and comedones.

From James WD: Clinical practice: acne, *N Engl J Med* 352:1463–1472, 2005.

nodulocystic lesions (Fig. 661-3 and Table 661-1). One or more types of lesions may predominate. In its mildest form, which is often seen early in adolescence, lesions are limited to comedones on the central area of the face. Lesions may also involve the chest, upper back, and deltoid areas. A predominance of lesions on the forehead, particularly closed comedones, is often attributable to prolonged use of greasy hair preparations (pomade acne) (Fig. 661-4). Marked involvement on the trunk is most often seen in males. Lesions often heal with temporary postinflammatory erythema and hyperpigmentation. Pitted, atrophic, or hypertrophic scars may be interspersed, depending on the severity, depth, and chronicity of the process. Diagnosis of acne is rarely difficult, although flat warts, folliculitis, and other types of acne may be confused with acne vulgaris.

Table 661-2 TYPICAL TREATMENT REGIMENS FOR ACNE

COMEDONAL ACNE
Topical retinoid *or* Azelaic acid
MILD PAPULOPUSTULAR ACNE
Topical retinoid *plus* Benzoyl peroxide *or* Benzoyl peroxide/topical antibiotic *or* Benzoyl peroxide/oral antibiotic
SEVERE PAPULOPUSTULAR OR NODULAR ACNE
Topical retinoid *plus* Benzoyl peroxide and oral antibiotic *or* Isotretinoin 1 mg/kg/day

Treatment

No evidence shows that early treatment, with the exception of isotretinoin, alters the course of acne. Acne can be controlled and severe scarring prevented by judicious maintenance therapy that is continued until the disease process has abated spontaneously. Therapy must be individualized and aimed at preventing microcomedone formation through reduction of follicular hyperkeratosis, sebum production, the *P. acnes* population in follicular orifices, and free fatty acid production. Initial control takes at least 6-8 wk, depending on the severity of the acne (Table 661-2 and Fig 661-5). It is also important to address the potentially severe emotional impact of acne on adolescents.

The pediatrician must be aware of the frequently poor correlation between acne severity and psychosocial impact, particularly in adolescents. As adolescents become preoccupied with their appearance, offering treatment even to the youngster whose acne is mild may enhance self-image.

DIET Little evidence shows that ingestion of particular foods can trigger acne flares. When a patient is convinced that certain dietary items exacerbate acne, it is prudent for him or her to omit those foods.

CLIMATE Climate appears to influence acne, in that improvement frequently occurs in summer and flares are more common in winter. Remission in summer may relate, in part, to the relative absence of stress. Emotional tension and fatigue seem to exacerbate acne in many individuals; the mechanism is unclear but has been proposed to relate to an increased adrenocortical response.

CLEANSING Cleansing with soap and water removes surface lipid and renders the skin less oily in appearance, but no evidence shows that surface lipid has a role in generating acne lesions. Only superficial drying and peeling are achieved by cleansing, and almost any mild soap or astringent is adequate. Repetitive cleansing can be harmful because it irritates and chaps the skin. Cleansing agents that contain abrasives and keratolytic agents, such as sulfur, resorcinol, and salicylic acid, may temporarily remove sebum from the skin surface. They exert a mild drying and peeling effect and suppress lesions to a limited degree. They do not prevent microcomedones from forming. No evidence shows that preparations containing alcohol or hexachlorophene decrease acne because surface bacteria are not involved in the pathogenesis. Greasy cosmetic and hair preparations must be discontinued because they exacerbate pre-existing acne and cause further plugging of follicular pores. Manipulation and squeezing of facial lesions only ruptures intact lesions and provokes a localized inflammatory reaction.

TOPICAL THERAPY All topical preparations must be used for 6-8 wk before their effectiveness can be assessed. Retinoids may be used alone for mild acne, but combination therapy is

Global Alliance Acne Treatment Algorithm

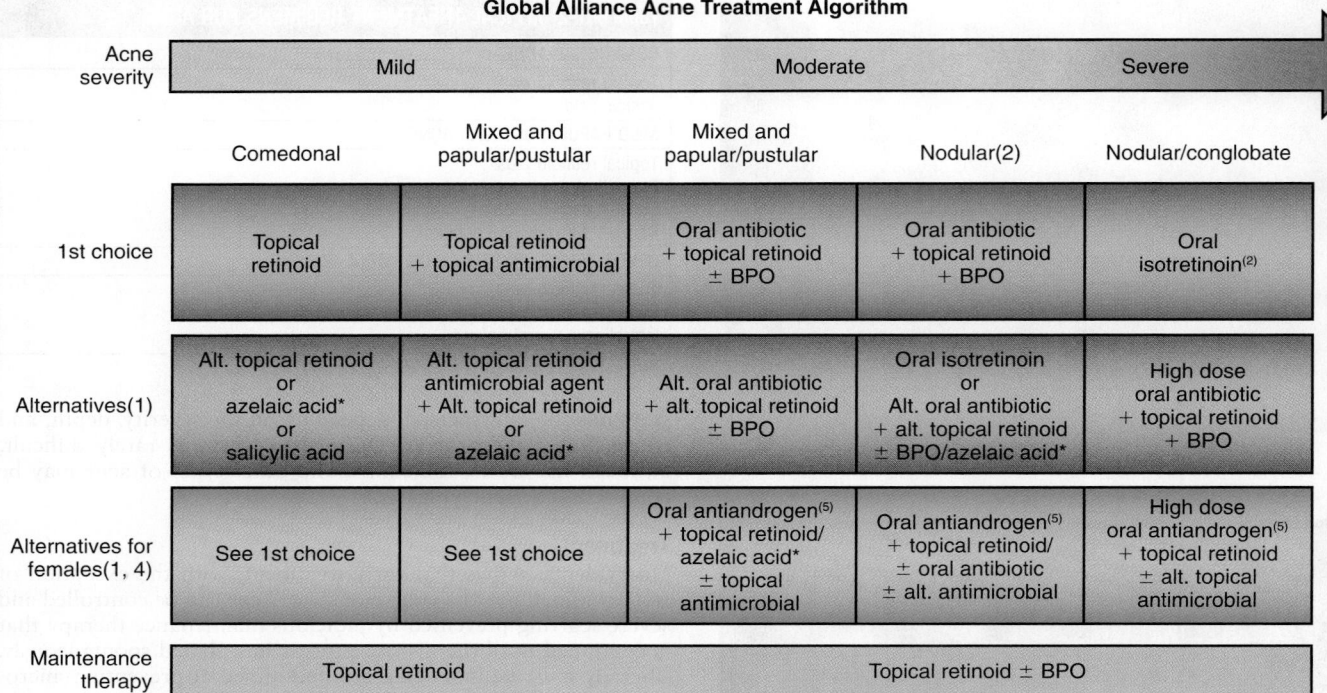

Acne severity	Mild	Mild	Moderate	Moderate	Severe
	Comedonal	Mixed and papular/pustular	Mixed and papular/pustular	Nodular(2)	Nodular/conglobate
1st choice	Topical retinoid	Topical retinoid + topical antimicrobial	Oral antibiotic + topical retinoid ± BPO	Oral antibiotic + topical retinoid + BPO	Oral isotretinoin(2)
Alternatives(1)	Alt. topical retinoid or azelaic acid* or salicylic acid	Alt. topical retinoid antimicrobial agent + Alt. topical retinoid or azelaic acid*	Alt. oral antibiotic + alt. topical retinoid ± BPO	Oral isotretinoin or Alt. oral antibiotic + alt. topical retinoid ± BPO/azelaic acid*	High dose oral antibiotic + topical retinoid + BPO
Alternatives for females(1, 4)	See 1st choice	See 1st choice	Oral antiandrogen(5) + topical retinoid/ azelaic acid* ± topical antimicrobial	Oral antiandrogen(5) + topical retinoid/ ± oral antibiotic ± alt. antimicrobial	High dose oral antiandrogen(5) + topical retinoid ± alt. topical antimicrobial
Maintenance therapy	Topical retinoid		Topical retinoid ± BPO		

1. Consider physical removal of comedones. 2. With small nodules (<0.5 cm). 3. Second course in case of relapse. 4. For pregnancy, options are limited. 5. For full discussion, see Gollnick H. et al. JAAD. 2003.49 (Suppl):1-37.

Figure 661-5 Acne treatment algorithm, BPO, benzoyl peroxide. (From Thiboutot D, Gollnick H; Global Alliance to Improve Acne, et al: New insights into the management of acne: an update from the global alliance to improve outcomes in acne, *J Am Acad Dermatol* 60:S1–S50, 2009.)

frequently more effective. A popular and effective combination is use of benzoyl peroxide gel in the morning and a retinoid at night.

Retinoids A topical retinoid should be the **primary treatment** for acne vulgaris. Topical retinoids have multiple actions, including inhibition of the formation and number of microcomedones, reduction of mature comedones, reduction of inflammatory lesions, and production of normal desquamation of the follicular epithelium. Retinoids should be applied daily to all the affected areas. The main side effects of retinoids are irritation and dryness. Not all patients initially tolerate daily use of a retinoid. It is prudent to begin therapy every other or every third day and slowly increase the frequency of application as tolerated. Tretinoin, adapalene, and tazarotene (Table 661-3) are the available retinoids. They are all approximately equal in efficacy, although adapalene is less irritating and tazarotene works slightly better for comedonal acne.

Benzoyl Peroxide Benzoyl peroxide is primarily an antimicrobial agent. It has an advantage over topical antibiotics in that it does not enhance antimicrobial resistance. It is available in multiple formulations and concentrations. The gel formulations are preferred, owing to better stability and more consistent release of the active ingredient. Washes and cleansers are useful for covering large surface areas such as the chest and back. As with retinoids, the main side effects are irritation and drying. Benzoyl peroxide can also bleach clothing.

Topical Antibiotics Topical antibiotics are indicated for the treatment of inflammatory acne. Clindamycin is the most commonly used. It is not as effective as oral antibiotics. It should not be used as monotherapy because it does not inhibit microcomedone formation and it has the potential to induce antimicrobial resistance. Irritation and dryness are generally less than with retinoids or benzoyl peroxide. Topical antibiotics are best used as combination products. The most common is benzoyl peroxide/clindamycin. A combination tretinoin/clindamycin product may also be used.

Azelaic Acid Azelaic acid (20% cream) has mild antimicrobial and keratolytic properties.

SYSTEMIC THERAPY Antibiotics, especially tetracycline and its derivatives (see Table 661-3), are indicated for treatment of patients whose acne has not responded to topical medications, who have moderate to severe inflammatory papulopustular and nodulocystic acne, and who have a propensity for scarring. Tetracycline and its derivatives act by reducing the growth and metabolism of *P. acnes.* They also have anti-inflammatory properties. For most adolescent patients, therapy may be initiated twice daily, for at least 6-8 wk, followed by a gradual decrease to the minimal effective dose. The drugs should always be administered in combination with a topical retinoid and topical benzoyl peroxide, but not topical antibiotics. Tetracycline absorption is inhibited by food, milk, iron supplements, aluminum hydroxide gel, and calcium-magnesium salts. It should be taken on an empty stomach 1 hr before or 2 hr after meals. Minocycline and doxycycline may be taken with food. Side effects of tetracycline and derivatives are rare. Side effects of tetracycline include vaginal candidosis, particularly in those who take tetracycline concurrently with oral contraceptives; gastrointestinal irritation; phototoxic reactions, including onycholysis and brown discoloration of nails; esophageal ulceration; inhibition of fetal skeletal growth; and staining of growing teeth, precluding its use during pregnancy and in those <8 yr. Doxycycline is the most photosensitizing of the tetracycline derivatives. Rarely, minocycline causes dizziness, intracranial hypertension, bluish discoloration of the skin and mucous membranes, hepatitis, and a lupus-like syndrome. A possible complication of prolonged systemic antibiotic use is proliferation of gram-negative organisms, particularly *Enterobacter, Klebsiella, Escherichia coli,* and *Pseudomonas aeruginosa,* producing severe, refractory folliculitis.

Women who have acne and hormonal abnormalities, whose acne is unresponsive to antibiotic therapy, or who are not candidates for isotretinoin therapy should be considered for

Table 661-3 MEDICATIONS FOR THE TREATMENT OF ACNE

DRUG	DOSE	SIDE EFFECT(S)	OTHER CONSIDERATIONS
TOPICAL AGENTS			
Retinoids			
Tretinoin	Applied once nightly; strengths of 0.025-0.1% available**	Irritation (redness and scaling)	Generics available
Adapalene	Applied once daily, at night or in the morning; 0.01%**	Minimal irritation	
Tazarotene*	Applied once nightly; 0.05, 0.1%	Irritation	Limited data suggest tazarotene more effective than alternatives
Antimicrobials			
Benzoyl peroxide, alone or with zinc, 2.5-10%	Applied once or twice daily	Benzoyl peroxide can bleach clothing and bedding	Available over the counter; 2.5-5% concentrations as effective as and less drying than 10% concentration
Clindamycin, erythromycin†	Applied once or twice daily	Propensity to resistance	Most effective for inflammatory lesions (rather than comedones); resistance a concern when used alone
Combination benzoyl peroxide and clindamycin or erythromycin Combination tretinoin and clindamycin	Applied once or twice daily		Combination more effective than topical antibiotics alone; limits development of resistance; use of individual products in combination less expensive and appears similarly effective
Other Topical Agents			
Azelaic acid, sodium sulfacetamide-sulfur, salicylic acid†	Applied once or twice daily	Well tolerated	Good adjunctive or alternative treatments
ORAL ANTIBIOTICS‡			
Tetracycline§	250-500 mg once or twice daily	Gastrointestinal upset, pseudomotor cerebri	Inexpensive; dosing limited by need to take on empty stomach
Doxycycline§	50-100 mg once or twice daily	Phototoxicity, pseudomotor cerebri	20 mg dose anti-inflammatory only; limited data on efficacy
Minocycline§	50-100 mg once or twice daily	Hyperpigmentation of teeth, oral mucosa, and skin; lupus-like reactions with long-term treatment, pseudomotor cerebri	
Trimethoprim-sulfamethoxazole	One dose (160 mg trimethoprim, 800 mg sulfamethoxazole) twice daily	Toxic epidermal necrolysis and allergic eruptions	Trimethoprim may be used alone in 300-mg dose twice daily; limited data available
Erythromycin†	250-500 mg twice ×daily	Gastrointestinal upset	Resistance problematic; consensus is that efficacy is limited
HORMONAL AGENTS¶			
Spironolactone§	50-200 mg in divided doses	Menstrual irregularities, breast tenderness	Higher doses more effective but cause more side effects; best given in combination with oral contraceptives
Estrogen-containing oral contraceptives	Daily	Potential side effects include thromboembolism	
ORAL RETINOID			
Isotretinoin‖	0.5-1.0 mg/kg/day in divided doses	Birth defects; adherence to pregnancy prevention program outlined by drug manufacturer, including two initial negative pregnancy tests, is essential; hypertriglyceridemia, elevated results on liver function tests, abnormal night vision, benign intracranial hypertension, dryness of the lips, ocular, nasal, and oral mucosa and skin, secondary staphylococcal infections, and arthralgias are possible common or important side effects; laboratory testing of lipid profiles and liver function tests monthly should be performed monthly until dose is stabilized	Relapse rate higher if patient is <16 yr at initial treatment, if acne is of high severity and involves the trunk, or if drug is used in adult women

*Tazarotene is in pregnancy category X: contraindicated in pregnancy.
†Clindamycin, erythromycin, and azelaic acid are in pregnancy category B: no evidence of risk in humans.
‡Oral antibiotics are indicated for moderate to severe disease; for the treatment of acne on the chest, back, or shoulders; and in patients with inflammatory disease in whom topical combinations have failed or are not tolerated.
§This drug is in pregnancy category D: positive evidence of risk in humans.
¶Hormonal agents are for use in women only.
‖Isotretinoin is in pregnancy category X: contraindicated in pregnancy. It should be used only in patients with severe acne that does not clear with combined oral and topical therapy.
**As cream or gel.
Modified from James WD: Clinical practice: acne, *N Engl J Med* 352:1463–1472, 2005.

a trial of hormonal therapy. Oral contraceptive pills are the primary form of hormonal therapy. Spironolactone has also shown effectiveness.

Isotretinoin (13-cis-retinoic acid; Accutane) is indicated for severe nodulocystic acne and moderate to severe acne that has not responded to conventional therapy. The recommended dosage is 0.5-1.0 mg/kg/24 hr. A standard course in the USA lasts 16-20 wk. At the end of one course of isotretinoin, 40% of patients are cured, 45% need conventional topical and/or oral medications to maintain adequate control, and 15% have relapses and need an additional course of isotretinoin. Dosages <0.5 mg/kg/24 hr, or a cumulative dose of <120 mg/kg, are associated with a significantly higher rate of treatment failure and relapse. If the disease process is not in remission 2 mo after the first course of isotretinoin, a second course should be considered. Isotretinoin reduces size and secretion of sebaceous glands, normalizes follicular keratinization, prevents new microcomedone formation, decreases the population of *P. acnes,* and exerts an anti-inflammatory effect.

Isotretinoin use has many side effects. It is highly **teratogenic** and is **absolutely contraindicated** in pregnancy. Pregnancy should be avoided for 6 wk after discontinuation of therapy. Two forms of birth control are required, as are monthly pregnancy tests. Concerns over cases of pregnancy despite warnings have prompted a manufacturer registration program, iPLEDGE (*www.ipledgeprogram.com*), which requires physician enrollment and careful patient pregnancy screening in order to prescribe isotretinoin. Many patients also experience cheilitis, xerosis, periodic epistaxis, and blepharoconjunctivitis. Increased serum triglyceride and cholesterol levels are also common. It is important to rule out pre-existing liver disease and hyperlipidemia before initiating therapy and to recheck laboratory values 4 wk after commencement of therapy. Less common but significant side effects include arthralgias, myalgias, temporary thinning of the hair, paronychia, increased susceptibility to sunburn, formation of pyogenic granulomas, and colonization of the skin with *Staphylococcus aureus,* leading to impetigo, secondarily infected dermatitis, and scalp folliculitis. Rarely, hyperostotic lesions of the spine develop after more than 1 course of isotretinoin. Concomitant use of tetracycline and isotretinoin is contraindicated because either drug, but particularly when they are used together, can cause benign intracranial hypertension. Although no cause-and-effect relationship has been established, drug-induced mood changes and depression and/or suicide have mandated close attention to psychiatric well-being before and during isotretinoin prescription.

SURGICAL THERAPY Intralesional injection of low-dose (3-5 mg/mL) mid-potency glucocorticoids (e.g., triamcinolone) with a 30-gauge needle on a tuberculin syringe may hasten the healing of individual, painful nodulocystic lesions. Dermabrasion or laser peel to minimize scarring should be considered only after the active process is quiescent. The management of scarring is described in Figure 661-6.

The role of pulsed dye laser in the treatment of inflammatory acne is controversial and inconclusive.

DRUG-INDUCED ACNE

Pubertal and postpubertal patients who are receiving systemic corticosteroid therapy are predisposed to steroid-induced acne. This monomorphous folliculitis occurs primarily on the face, neck, chest (Fig. 661-7), shoulders, upper back, arms, and rarely

Icepick (V)	Rolling (U)	Boxcar (M)	Keloids	Hypertrophic
Punch excision (deep bases) Elevation and grafting Laser resurfacing/ dermabrasion (many scars close together) Spot TCA peel	**Combined therapy** Micrograft and subcision + ± filler Resurfacing microdermabrasion Deep-spot TCA peel	**Shallow** ≤3 mm diameter-laser skin resurfacing >3 mm diameter-laser skin resurfacing ± punch elevation **Deep** ≤3 mm diameter-punch excision >3 mm diameter-punch excision or punch elevation Fractional thermolysis (deep or shallow) Dermabrasion CO_2 laser resurfacing	Intralesional corticosteroids Intralesional 5-FU Intralesional bleomycin Compression Imiquimod after intralesional excision Cryotherapy Pulsed-dye laser Excision + electrotherapy	Intralesional steroids Intralesional 5-FU Vascular laser Intralesional bleomycin Compression Imiquimod after intralesional excision
Adjunctive treatment: Topical retinoids 2 weeks prior to and following treatment, sunscreens, moisturizers				

Non-ablative lasers for mild disease; ablative and fractional lasers for moderate scarring

Figure 661-6 Treatment options for acne scars. CO_2, carbon dioxide; FU, fluorouracil; TCA, trichloroacetic acid. (From Thiboutot D, Gollnick H; Global Alliance to Improve Acne, et al: New insights into the management of acne: an update from the global alliance to improve outcomes in acne, *J Am Acad Dermatol* 60:S1–S50, 2009.)

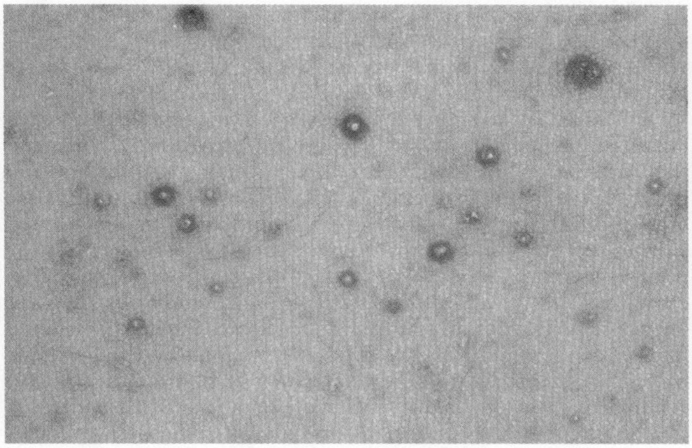

Figure 661-7 Monomorphous papular eruption of steroid acne.

on the scalp. Onset follows the initiation of steroid therapy by about 2 wk. The lesions are small, erythematous papules or pustules that may erupt in profusion and are all in the same stage of development. Comedones may occur subsequently, but nodulocystic lesions and scarring are rare. Pruritus is occasional. Although steroid acne is relatively refractory if the medication is continued, the eruption may respond to use of tretinoin and a benzoyl peroxide gel.

Other **drugs** that can induce **acneiform lesions** in susceptible individuals include isoniazid, phenytoin, phenobarbital, trimethadione, lithium carbonate, androgens (anabolic steroids), and vitamin B_{12}.

HALOGEN ACNE

Administration of medications containing iodides or bromides or, rarely, ingestion of massive amounts of vitamin-mineral preparations or iodine-containing "health foods" such as kelp may induce halogen acne. The lesions are often very inflammatory. Discontinuation of the provocative agent and appropriate topical preparations usually achieve reasonable therapeutic results.

CHLORACNE

Chloracne is due to external contact with, inhalation of, or ingestion of halogenated aromatic hydrocarbons, including polyhalogenated biphenyls, polyhalogenated naphthalenes, and dioxins. Lesions are primarily comedonal. Inflammatory lesions are infrequent but may include papules, pustules, nodules, and cysts. Healing occurs with atrophic or hypertrophic scarring. The face, postauricular regions, neck, axillae, genitals, and chest are most commonly involved. The nose is often spared. In cases of severe exposure, associated findings may include hepatitis, production of porphyrins, bulla formation on sun-exposed skin, hyperpigmentation, hypertrichosis, and palmar and plantar hyperhidrosis. Topical or oral retinoids may be effective; benzoyl peroxide and antibiotics are generally ineffective.

NEONATAL ACNE

Approximately 20% of normal neonates demonstrate at least a few comedones in the first mo of life. Closed comedones predominate on the cheeks and forehead (Fig. 661-8); open comedones and papulopustules occur occasionally. The cause of neonatal acne is unknown but has been attributed to placental transfer of maternal androgens, hyperactive neonatal adrenal glands, and a hypersensitive neonatal end-organ response to androgenic hormones. The hypertrophic sebaceous glands involute spontaneously over a few months, as does the acne. **Treatment** is usually unnecessary. If desired, the lesions can be treated effectively with topical tretinoin and/or benzoyl peroxide.

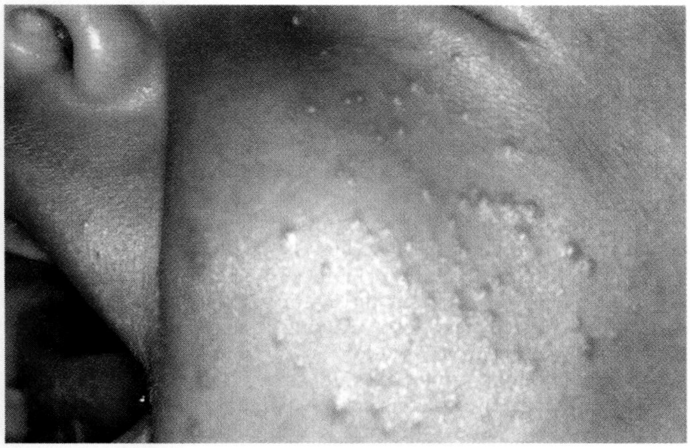

Figure 661-8 Comedonal acne in a neonate.

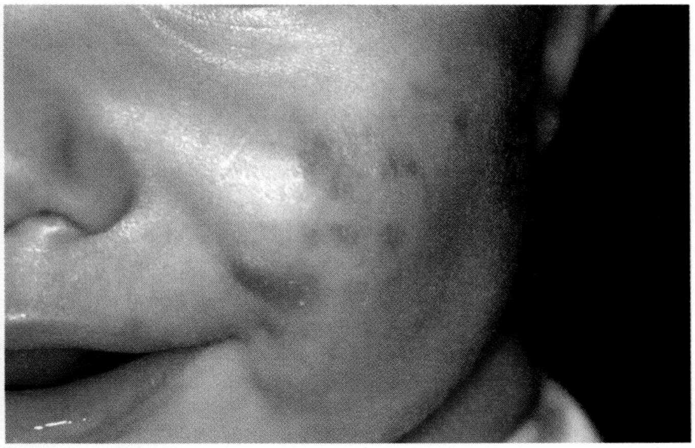

Figure 661-9 Inflammatory infantile acne.

INFANTILE ACNE

Infantile acne usually manifests after 1 yr of life, more commonly in boys than girls. Acne lesions are more numerous, pleomorphic, severe, and persistent than in neonatal acne (Fig. 661-9). Open and closed comedones predominate on the face. Papules and pustules occur frequently, but only occasionally do nodulocystic lesions develop. Pitted scarring is seen in 10-15%. The course may be relatively brief, or the lesions may persist for many months, although the eruption generally resolves by age 3 yr. Use of topical benzoyl peroxide gel and tretinoin usually clears the eruption within a few weeks. Oral erythromycin is occasionally necessary. A child with refractory acne warrants a search for an abnormal source of androgens, such as a virilizing tumor or congenital adrenal hyperplasia.

TROPICAL ACNE

A severe form of acne occurs in tropical climates and is believed to be due to the intense heat and humidity. Hydration of the pilosebaceous duct pore may accentuate blockage of the duct. Affected individuals tend to have an antecedent history of adolescent acne that is quiescent at the time of the eruption. Lesions occur mainly on the entire back, chest, buttocks, and thighs, with a predominance of suppurating papules and nodules. Secondary infection with *S. aureus* may be a complication. The eruption is refractory to acne therapy if the environmental factors are not eliminated.

ACNE CONGLOBATA

Acne conglobata is a chronic progressive inflammatory disease that occurs mainly in men, and more commonly in white than in black individuals, but it may begin during adolescence. Patients usually have a history of pre-existing acne vulgaris. The principal lesion is the nodule, although there is often a mixture of comedones with multiple pores, papules, pustules, nodules, cysts, abscesses, and subcutaneous dissection with formation of multichanneled sinus tracts. Severe scarring is characteristic. The face is relatively spared, but in addition to the back and chest, the buttocks, abdomen, arms, and thighs may be involved. Constitutional symptoms and anemia may accompany the inflammatory process. Coagulase-positive staphylococci and β-hemolytic streptococci are frequently cultured from lesions but do not appear to be primarily involved in the pathogenesis. Acne conglobata occasionally occurs in association with hidradenitis suppurativa and dissecting cellulitis of the scalp (as the follicular occlusion triad) and may be complicated by erosive arthritis and ankylosing spondyloarthritis. Endocrinologic studies are not revealing. Routine acne therapy is generally ineffective. Systemic therapy with a corticosteroid may be required to suppress the intense inflammatory activity. Isotretinoin is the most effective form of therapy for some patients but may produce a flare after its initiation.

ACNE FULMINANS (ACUTE FEBRILE ULCERATIVE ACNE)

Acne fulminans is characterized by abrupt onset of extensive inflammatory, tender ulcerative acneiform lesions on the back and chest of male teenagers. The distinctive feature is the tendency for large nodules to form exudative, necrotic, ulcerated, crusted plaques. Lesions often spare the face and heal with scarring. A preceding history of mild papulopustular or nodular acne is noted in most patients. Constitutional symptoms and signs are common, including fever, debilitation, arthralgias, myalgias, weight loss, and leukocytosis. Blood cultures are sterile. Lesions of **erythema nodosum** sometimes develop on the shins. **Osteolytic bone** lesions may develop in the clavicle, sternum, and epiphyseal growth plates; affected bones appear normal or have slight sclerosis or thickening on healing. Salicylates may be helpful for the myalgias, arthralgias, and fever. Corticosteroids (1.0 mg/kg of prednisone) are started first. Then 1 wk later, isotretinoin (0.5-1 mg/kg) is added. Dapsone may be effective if isotretinoin cannot be used. The corticosteroid dosage is tapered over approximately 6 wk. Antibiotics are not indicated unless there is evidence of secondary infection. Compared with acne conglobata, acne fulminans occurs in younger patients, is more explosive in onset, more commonly has associated constitutional symptoms and ulcerated crusted lesions, and less commonly has multiheaded comedones or involves the face.

BIBLIOGRAPHY

Please visit the Nelson Textbook of Pediatrics *website at www.expertconsult.com for the complete bibliography.*

Chapter 662 Tumors of the Skin

Joseph G. Morelli

See also Chapters 499 and 643.

EPIDERMAL INCLUSION CYST (EPIDERMOID CYST)

Epidermoid cysts are the nodules most commonly seen in children. Such a cyst is a sharply circumscribed, dome-shaped, firm, freely movable, skin-colored nodule (see Fig. 662-1 on the *Nelson Textbook of Pediatrics* website at www.expertconsult.com), often with a central dimple or punctum that is a plugged, dilated pore of a pilosebaceous follicle. Epidermoid cysts form most frequently on the face, neck, chest, or upper back and may periodically become inflamed and infected secondarily, particularly in association with acne vulgaris. The cyst wall may also rupture and induce an inflammatory reaction in the dermis. The wall of the cyst is derived from the follicular infundibulum. A mass of layered keratinized material that may have a cheesy consistency fills the cavity. Epidermoid cysts may arise from occlusion of pilosebaceous follicles, from implantation of epidermal cells into the dermis as a result of an injury that penetrates the epidermis, and from rests of epidermal cells. Multiple epidermoid cysts may be present in Gardner syndrome and the nevoid basal cell carcinoma syndrome. Excision of the cysts with removal of the entire sac and its contents is indicated, particularly if the cyst becomes recurrently infected. A fluctuant, infected cyst should be treated with an antibiotic effective against *Staphylococcus aureus.* After the inflammation subsides, the cyst should be removed.

For the full continuation of this chapter, please visit the Nelson Textbook of Pediatrics *website at www.expertconsult.com.*

Chapter 663 Nutritional Dermatoses

Joseph G. Morelli

ACRODERMATITIS ENTEROPATHICA

Acrodermatitis enteropathica is a rare autosomal recessive disorder caused by an inability to absorb sufficient zinc from the diet. The genetic defect is in the intestinal zinc specific transporter gene *SLC39A4*. Initial signs and symptoms usually occur in the first few months of life, often after weaning from breast milk to cow's milk. The cutaneous eruption consists of vesiculobullous, eczematous, dry, scaly, or psoriasiform skin lesions symmetrically distributed in the perioral, acral, and perineal areas (Fig. 663-1) and on the cheeks, knees, and elbows (Fig. 663-2). The hair often has a peculiar, reddish tint, and alopecia of some degree is characteristic. Ocular manifestations include photophobia, conjunctivitis, blepharitis, and corneal dystrophy detectable by slit-lamp examination. Associated manifestations include chronic diarrhea, stomatitis, glossitis, paronychia, nail dystrophy, growth retardation, irritability, delayed wound healing, intercurrent bacterial infections, and superinfection with *Candida albicans*. Lymphocyte function and free radical scavenging are impaired. Without treatment, the course is chronic and intermittent but often relentlessly progressive. When the disease is less severe, only growth retardation and delayed development may be apparent.

The **diagnosis** is established by the constellation of clinical findings and detection of a low plasma zinc concentration. Histopathologic changes in the skin are nonspecific and include parakeratosis and pallor of the upper epidermis. The variety of manifestations of the syndrome may be due to the facts that zinc has a role in numerous metabolic pathways, including those of copper, protein, essential fatty acids, and prostaglandins, and that zinc is incorporated into many zinc metalloenzymes.

Oral **therapy** with zinc compounds is the treatment of choice. Optimal doses range from 50 mg/24 hr of zinc sulfate, acetate, or gluconate daily for infants up to 150 mg/24 hr for children. Plasma zinc levels should be monitored, however, to individualize the dosage. Zinc therapy rapidly abolishes the manifestations of the disease. A syndrome resembling acrodermatitis enteropathica has been observed in patients with secondary zinc deficiency due to long-term total parenteral nutrition without supplemental zinc

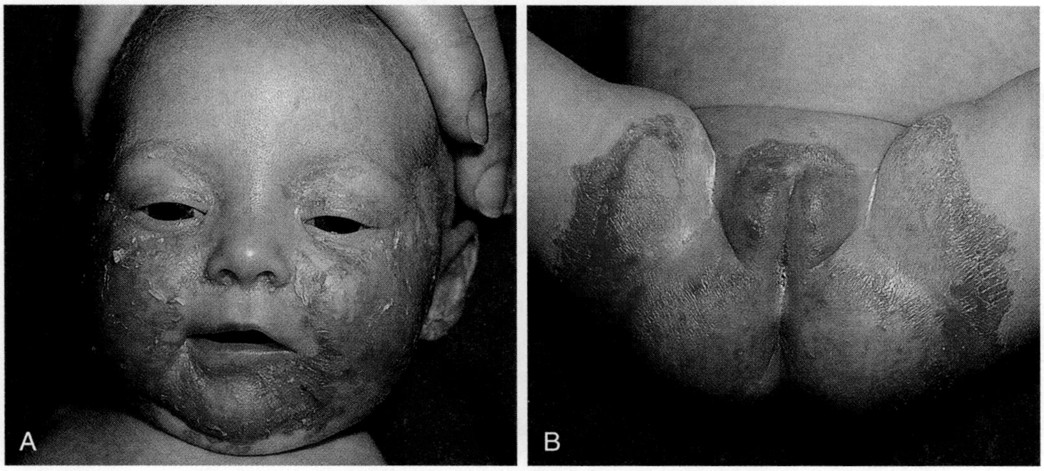

Figure 663-1 *A,* Periorificial eruption. *B,* Diaper rash. The skin findings are typical of zinc deficiency, in this case caused by low levels of zinc in breast milk. (From Eichenfield LF, Frieden IJ, Esterly NB: *Textbook of neonatal dermatology,* Philadelphia, 2001, WB Saunders, p 254.)

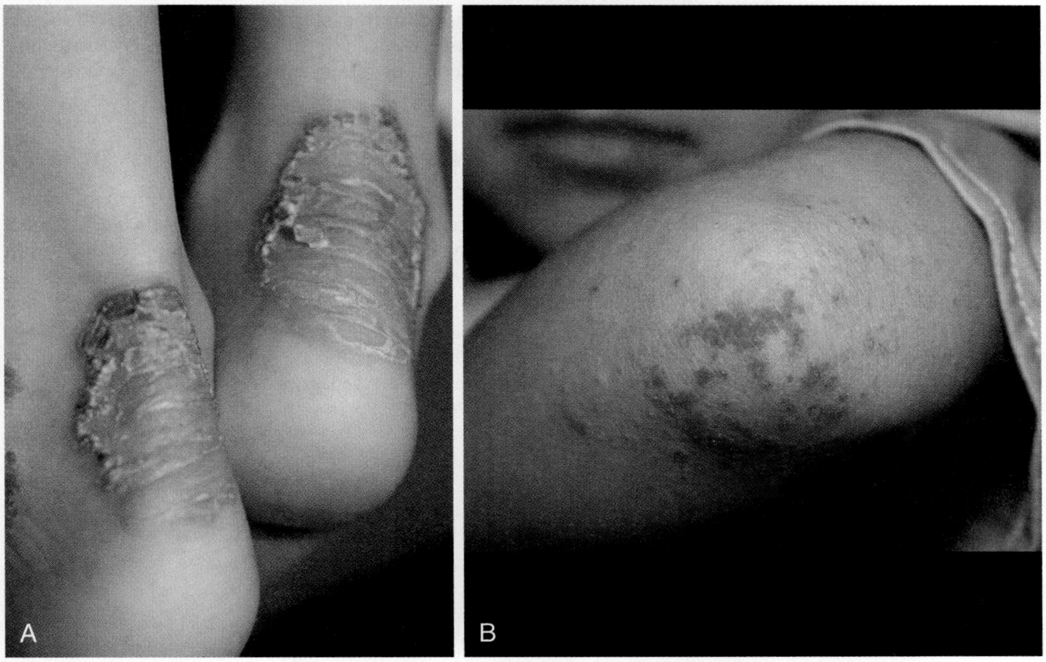

Figure 663-2 *A,* Psoriasiform lesion of zinc deficiency dermatitis on the ankles. *B,* Similar lesions on the elbows.

or to chronic malabsorption syndromes. A rash similar to that of acrodermatitis enteropathica has also been reported in infants fed breast milk that is low in zinc and in those with maple syrup urine disease, organic aciduria, methylmalonic acidemia, biotinidase deficiency, essential fatty acid deficiency, severe protein malnutrition (kwashiorkor), and cystic fibrosis.

ESSENTIAL FATTY ACID DEFICIENCY

Essential fatty acid deficiency causes a generalized, scaly dermatitis composed of thickened, erythematous, desquamating plaques. The eruption has been induced experimentally in animals fed a fat-free diet and has been observed in patients with chronic severe malabsorption, such as in short-gut syndrome, and in those sustained on a fat-free diet or fat-free parenteral alimentation. Linoleic acid (18:2 n-6) and arachidonic acid (20:4 n-6) are deficient, and an abnormal metabolite, 5,8,11-eicosatrienoic acid (20:3 n-9), is present in the plasma. Alterations in the triene:tetraene ratio are diagnostic. Additional manifestations of essential fatty acid deficiency include alopecia, thrombocytopenia, and failure to thrive. The horny layer of the skin contains microscopic cracks, the barrier function of the skin is disturbed, and transepidermal water loss is increased. Topical application of linoleic acid, which is present in sunflower seed and safflower oils, may ameliorate the clinical and biochemical skin manifestations. Appropriate nutrition should be provided.

KWASHIORKOR

Severe protein and essential amino acid deprivation in association with adequate caloric intake can lead to kwashiorkor, particularly at the time of weaning to a diet that consists primarily of corn, rice, or beans (Chapter 43). Diffuse fine reddish brown scaling (enamel/flaky paint sign) is the classic cutaneous finding. In severe cases, erosions and linear fissures develop (Fig. 663-3). Sun-exposed skin is relatively spared, as are the feet and dorsal aspects of the hands. Nails are thin and soft, and hair is sparse, thin, and depigmented, sometimes displaying a "flag sign" consisting of alternating light and dark bands that reflect alternating periods of adequate and inadequate nutrition. The cutaneous manifestations may closely resemble those of acrodermatitis enteropathica. The serum zinc level is often deficient, and in some cases, skin lesions of kwashiorkor heal more rapidly when zinc is applied topically.

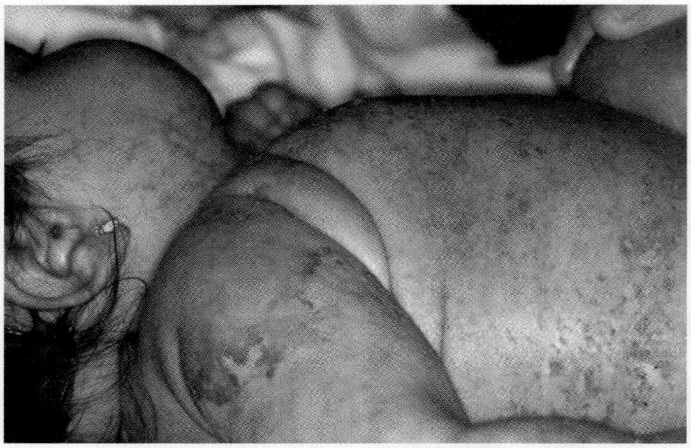

Figure 663-3 Erosions and scaling in kwashiorkor.

CYSTIC FIBROSIS (CHAPTER 395)

Protein-calorie malnutrition develops in 5-10% of patients with cystic fibrosis. Rash in infants with cystic fibrosis and malnutrition is rare but may appear by age 6 mo. The initial eruption consists of scaling, erythematous papules and progresses in 1-3 mo to extensive desquamating plaques. The rash is accentuated around the mouth and perineum and on the extremities (lower > upper). Alopecia may be present, but mucous membranes and nails are uninvolved.

PELLAGRA (CHAPTER 46)

Pellagra manifests as edema, erythema, and burning of sun-exposed skin on the face, neck, and dorsal aspects of the hands, forearms, and feet. Lesions of pellagra may also be provoked by burns, pressure, friction, and inflammation. The eruption on the face frequently follows a butterfly distribution, and the dermatitis encircling the neck has been termed "Casal's necklace." Blisters and scales develop, and the skin increasingly becomes dry, rough, thickened, cracked, and hyperpigmented. Skin infections may be unusually severe. Pellagra develops in patients with insufficient dietary intake or malabsorption of niacin and/or tryptophan. Administration of isoniazid, 6-mercaptopurine, or 5-fluorouracil may also produce pellagra. Nicotinamide supplementation and sun avoidance are the mainstays of therapy.

SCURVY (VITAMIN C OR ASCORBIC ACID DEFICIENCY) (CHAPTER 47)

Scurvy manifests initially as follicular hyperkeratosis and coiling of hair on the upper arms, back, buttocks, and lower extremities. Other features are perifollicular erythema and hemorrhage, particularly on the legs and advancing to involve large areas of hemorrhage; swollen, erythematous gums; stomatitis; and subperiosteal hematomas. The most common risk factors are alcoholism, low socioeconomic status, and psychiatric disease that results in poor nutrition. The best method of confirmation of a clinical diagnosis of scurvy is a trial of vitamin C supplementation.

VITAMIN A DEFICIENCY (CHAPTER 45.1)

Vitamin A deficiency manifests initially as impairment of visual adaptation to the dark. Cutaneous changes include xerosis and hyperkeratosis and hyperplasia of the epidermis, particularly the lining of hair follicles and sebaceous glands. In severe cases, desquamation may be prominent.

BIBLIOGRAPHY

Please visit the Nelson Textbook of Pediatrics *website at www.expertconsult.com for the complete bibliography.*

PART XXXII Bone and Joint Disorders

Section 1 ORTHOPEDIC PROBLEMS

Chapter 664
Growth and Development

Lawrence Wells, Kriti Sehgal, and John P. Dormans

Growth patterns and development in children are often unique to the individual child. Statistically, normal is defined as 95% of a population that falls within 2 standard deviations of the mean from any given measurement.

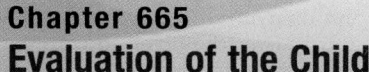

For the full continuation of this chapter, please visit the Nelson Textbook of Pediatrics *website at www.expertconsult.com.*

Chapter 665
Evaluation of the Child

Lawrence Wells, Kriti Sehgal, and John P. Dormans

A detailed history and thorough physical examination are invaluable in the evaluation of a child with an orthopedic problem. Often the child's family and acquaintances are important sources of information, especially in younger children and infants. Appropriate radiographic imaging and, occasionally, laboratory testing may be necessary to support the clinical diagnosis.

HISTORY

A comprehensive history should include details about the prenatal, perinatal, and postnatal periods. Prenatal history should include maternal health issues: smoking, prenatal vitamins, illicit use of drugs or narcotics, alcohol consumption, diabetes, rubella, and sexually transmitted infections. The child's prenatal and perinatal history should include information about the length of pregnancy, length of labor, type of labor (induced or spontaneous), presentation of fetus, evidence of any fetal distress at delivery, requirements of oxygen following the delivery, birth length and weight, Apgar score, muscle tone at birth, feeding history, and period of hospitalization. In older infants and young children, evaluation of developmental milestones for posture, locomotion, dexterity, social activities, and speech are important. Specific orthopedic questions should focus on joint, muscular, appendicular, or axial skeleton complaints. Information regarding pain or other symptoms in any of these areas should be appropriately elicited (Table 665-1). The family history can give clues to heritable disorders. It also can forecast expectations of the child's future development and allow appropriate interventions as necessary.

PHYSICAL EXAMINATION

The orthopedic physical examination includes a thorough examination of the musculoskeletal system along with a comprehensive neurologic examination. The musculoskeletal examination includes inspection, palpation, and evaluation of motion, stability, and gait. A basic neurologic examination includes sensory examination, motor function, and reflexes. The orthopedic physical examination requires basic knowledge of anatomy of joint range of motion, alignment, and stability. Many common musculoskeletal disorders can be diagnosed by the history and physical examination alone. One screening tool that has been useful in adults has now been adapted and evaluated for use in children, the pediatric gait, arms, legs, spine (pGALS) test, the components of which are listed in Figure 665-1.

Inspection

Initial examination of the child begins with inspection. The clinician should use the guidelines listed in Table 665-2 during inspection.

Palpation

Palpation of the involved region should include assessment of local temperature and tenderness; assessment for a swelling or mass, spasticity or contracture, and bone or joint deformity; and evaluation of anatomic axis of limb and of limb lengths.

Contractures are a loss of mobility of a joint from congenital or acquired causes and are caused by periarticular soft-tissue fibrosis or involvement of muscles crossing the joint. Congenital contractures are common in **arthrogryposis** (Chapter 674). Spasticity is an abnormal increase in tone associated with hyperreflexia and is common in cerebral palsy.

Deformity of the bone or joint is an abnormal fixed shape or position from congenital or acquired causes. It is important to assess the type of deformity, its location, and degree of deformity upon clinical examination. It is also important to assess whether the deformity is fixed or can be passively or actively corrected and whether there is any associated muscle spasm, local tenderness, or pain on motion. Classification of the deformity depends on the plane of deformity: **varus** (away from midline) or **valgus** (apex toward midline) (coronal plane), or **recurvatum** or **flexion** deformity (sagittal plane). In the axial skeleton, especially the spine, deformity can be defined as scoliosis, kyphosis, hyperlordosis, and kyphoscoliosis.

Range of Motion

Active and passive joint motion should be assessed, recorded, and be compared to the opposite side. Objective evaluation should be done with a goniometer and recorded.

Vocabulary for direction of joint motion is as follows:

Abduction: Away from the midline
Adduction: Toward the midline
Flexion: Movement of bending from the starting position
Extension: Movement from bending to the starting position
Supination: Rotating the forearm to face the palm upward
Pronation: Rotating the forearm to face the palm downward
Inversion: Turning the hindfoot inward
Eversion: Turning the hindfoot outward
Internal rotation: Turning inward toward the axis of the body
External rotation: Turning outward away from the axis of the body

Gait Assessment

Children typically begin walking between 8 and 16 mo of age. Early ambulation is characterized by short stride length, a fast

Table 665-1 CHARACTERIZATION OF PAIN AND PRESENTING SYMPTOM

Location: Whether pain is localized to a particular segment or involves a larger area.
Intensity: Usually on a pain scale of 1 to 10.
Quality: Tumor pain is often unrelenting, progressive, and often present during the night. Pain at night particularly suggests osteoid osteoma. Pain in inflammation and infection is usually continuous.
Onset: Was it acute and related to specific trauma or was it insidious? Acute pain and history of trauma are more commonly associated with fractures.
Duration: Whether transient, only lasting for minutes, or lasting for hours or days. Pain lasting for longer than 3-4 wk suggests a serious underlying problem.
Progress: Whether static, increasing, or decreasing.
Radiation: Pain radiating to upper or lower extremities or complaints of numbness, tingling, or weakness require appropriate work-up.
Aggravating factors: Relationship to any activities such as swimming or diving or any particular position.
Alleviating factors: Is the pain relieved by rest, heat, and/or medication? Conditions such as spondylolysis, Scheuermann disease, inflammatory spondyloarthropathy, muscle pulls, or overuse are improved by bed rest.
Gait and posture: Disturbances associated with pain.

Table 665-2 GUIDELINES DURING INSPECTION OF A CHILD WITH MUSCULOSKELETAL PROBLEM

- The patient should be *comfortable with adequate exposure and well-lit surroundings* (lest some important physical finding be missed). Infants or young children may be examined on their parent's lap so that they feel more secure and are more likely to be cooperative.
- It is important to inspect how the patient moves about in the room before and during the examination as well as during various maneuvers. *Balance, posture, and gait pattern* should also be checked.
- *General examination* findings should include inspection for skin rashes, café-au-lait spots, hairy patches, dimples, cysts, tuft of hair, or evidence of spinal midline defects that can indicate serious underlying problems that need review.
- *General body habitus,* including signs of cachexia, pallor, and nutritional deficiencies, should be noted.
- Note any obvious spinal asymmetry, axial or appendicular deformities, trunk decompensation, and evidence of muscle spasm or contractures. The *forward bending test* is valuable in assessing asymmetry and movement of the spine.
- It is essential to perform and document a *thorough neurologic examination.* Motor, sensory, and reflex testing should be performed and recorded.
- Any *discrepancies in limb lengths* as well as *muscle atrophy* should be recorded.
- The range of motion of all joints, their stability, and any evidence of hyperlaxity, peripheral pulsations, and lymphadenopathy should also be noted in all cases.

Table 665-3 CAUSES OF ABNORMAL GAIT

Limp
Pain
Torsional variations
Toe walking
Joint abnormalities
Leg-length discrepancy

cadence, and slow velocity with a wide-based stance. Gait cycle is a single sequence of functions that starts with heel strike, toe off, swing, and heel strike. The four events describe one gait cycle and include two phases: stance and swing. The stance phase is the period during which the foot is in contact with the ground. The swing phase is the portion of the gait cycle during which a limb is being advanced forward without ground contact (Chapter 664). Normal gait is a symmetric and smooth process. Deviation from the norm indicates potential abnormality and should trigger investigation.

Neurologic maturation is necessary for the development of gait and the normal progression of developmental milestones. A child's gait changes with neurologic maturation. Infants normally walk with greater hip and knee flexion, flexed arms, and a wider base of gait than older children. As the neurologic system continues to develop in the cephalocaudal direction, the efficiency and smoothness of gait increase. The gait characteristics of a 7 yr old child are similar to those of an adult. When the neurologic system is abnormal (cerebral palsy), gait can be disturbed, exhibiting pathologic reflexes and abnormal movements.

Deviations from normal gait occur in a variety of orthopedic conditions. Disorders that result in muscle weakness (e.g., spina bifida, muscular dystrophy), spasticity (e.g., cerebral palsy), or contractures (e.g., arthrogryposis) lead to abnormalities in gait. Other causes of gait disturbances include limp, pain, torsional variations (in-toeing and out-toeing), toe walking, joint abnormalities, and leg-length discrepancy (Table 665-3).

LIMPING

A thorough history and clinical examination are the first steps toward early identification of the underlying problem causing a limp. Limping can be considered as either **painful** (**antalgic**) or painless, with the differential diagnosis ranging from benign to serious causes (septic hip, tumor). In a painful gait, the stance phase is shortened as the child decreases the time spent on the painful extremity. In a painless gait, which indicates underlying proximal muscle weakness or hip instability, the stance phase is equal between the involved and uninvolved sides, but the child leans or shifts the center of gravity over the involved extremity for balance. A bilateral disorder produces a waddling gait. Trendelenberg gait is produced by weak abnormal hip abductors. In single leg stance, a Trendelenberg sign can often be elicited when abductors are weak.

Disorders most commonly responsible for an abnormal gait generally vary based on the age of the patient. The differential diagnosis of limping varies based on age group (Table 665-4) or mechanism (Table 665-5). Neurologic disorders, especially spinal cord or peripheral nerve disorders, can also produce limping and difficult walking. Antalgic gait is predominantly a result of trauma, infection, or pathologic fracture. Trendelenburg gait is generally due to congenital, developmental, or muscular disorders. Limping in some cases may also be due to nonskeletal causes such as testicular torsion, inguinal hernia, and appendicitis.

BACK PAIN

Children frequently have a specific skeletal pathology as the cause of back pain. The most common causes of back pain in children are trauma, spondylolysis, spondylolisthesis, and infection (see Table 671-2). Tumor and tumor-like lesions that cause back pain in children are likely to be missed unless a thorough clinical assessment and adequate work-up are performed when required. Nonorthopedic causes of back pain include urinary tract infections, nephrolithiasis, and pneumonia.

NEUROLOGIC EVALUATION

A careful neurologic evaluation is a part of every pediatric musculoskeletal examination (Chapter 584). The assessment should include evaluation of developmental milestones, muscle strength, sensory assessment, muscle tone, and deep tendon reflexes. The neurologic evaluation should also assess the spine and identify any deformity, such as scoliosis and kyphosis, or abnormal spinal mobility. Specific peripheral nerve examinations may be necessary.

As the nervous system matures, the developing cerebral cortex normally inhibits rudimentary reflexes that are often present at birth (Chapter 584). Therefore, persistence of these reflexes can indicate neurologic abnormality. The most commonly performed deep tendon reflex tests include biceps, triceps, quadriceps, and gastrocnemius and soleus tendons. Localized or diffuse weakness

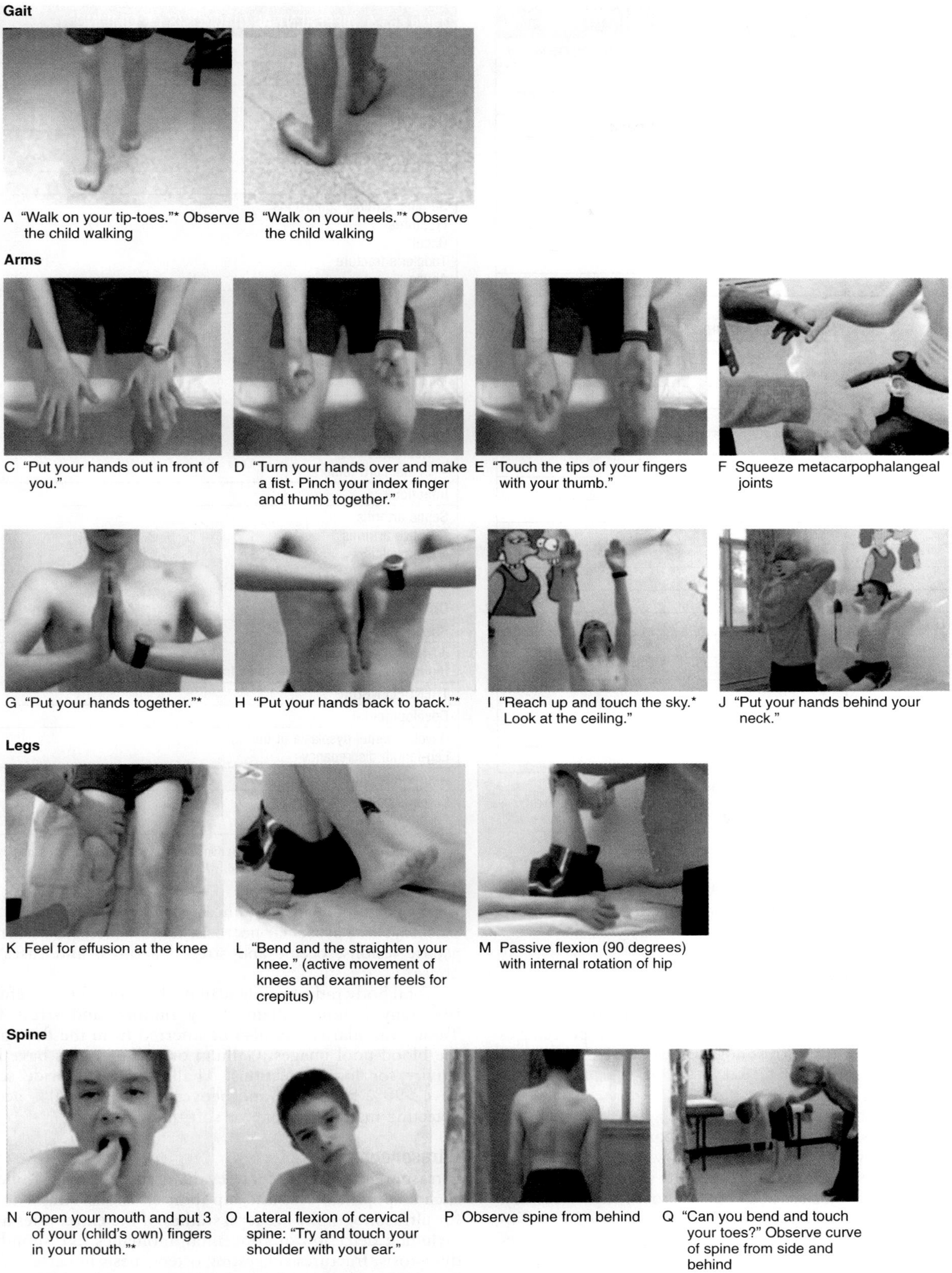

A "Walk on your tip-toes."* Observe the child walking
B "Walk on your heels."* Observe the child walking

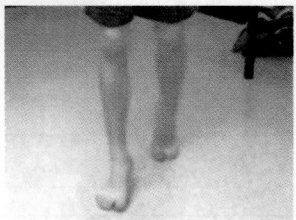

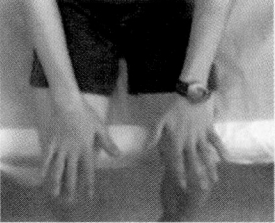

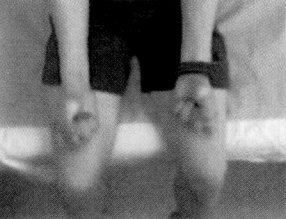

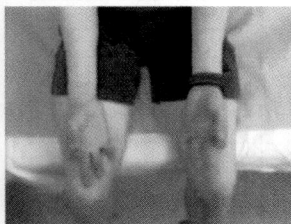

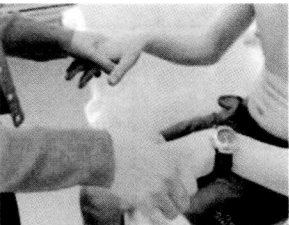

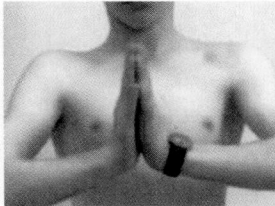

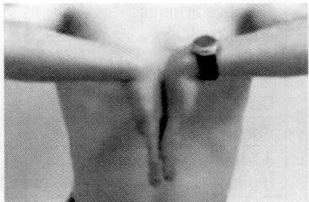

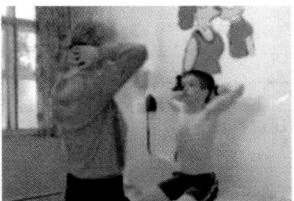

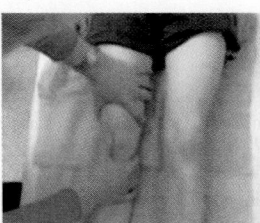

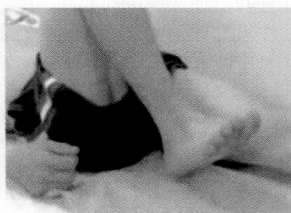

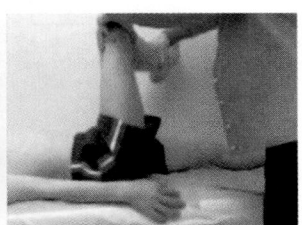

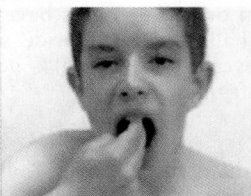

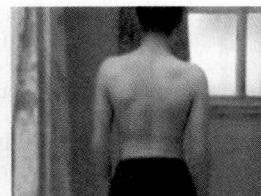

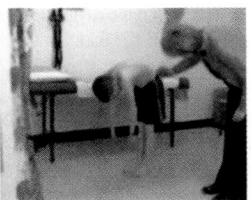

C "Put your hands out in front of you."
D "Turn your hands over and make a fist. Pinch your index finger and thumb together."
E "Touch the tips of your fingers with your thumb."
F Squeeze metacarpophalangeal joints
G "Put your hands together."*
H "Put your hands back to back."*
I "Reach up and touch the sky.* Look at the ceiling."
J "Put your hands behind your neck."

K Feel for effusion at the knee
L "Bend and the straighten your knee." (active movement of knees and examiner feels for crepitus)
M Passive flexion (90 degrees) with internal rotation of hip

N "Open your mouth and put 3 of your (child's own) fingers in your mouth."*
O Lateral flexion of cervical spine: "Try and touch your shoulder with your ear."
P Observe spine from behind
Q "Can you bend and touch your toes?" Observe curve of spine from side and behind

Figure 665-1 The components of pediatric gait, arms, legs, spine screen (pGALS), with illustration of movement. Screening questions: (1) Do you have any pain or stiffness in your joints, muscles, or back? (2) Do you have any difficulty getting yourself dressed without any help? (3) Do you have any difficulty going up and down stairs? *Additions and amendments to the original adult gait, arms, legs, spine screen. (From Foster HE, Kay LJ, Friswell M, et al: Musculoskeletal screening examination [pGALS] for school-age children based on the adult GALS screen, *Arthritis Rheum* 55:709–716, 2006.)

Table 665-4 COMMON CAUSES OF LIMPING ACCORDING TO AGE

ANTALGIC	TRENDELENBURG	LEG-LENGTH DISCREPANCY
TODDLER (1-3 YR)		
Infection	Hip dislocation (DDH)	–
Septic arthritis	Neuromuscular disease	
Hip	Cerebral palsy	
Knee	Poliomyelitis	
Osteomyelitis		
Diskitis		
Occult trauma		
Toddler's fracture		
Neoplasia		
CHILD (4-10 YR)		
Infection	Hip dislocation (DDH)	+
Septic arthritis	Neuromuscular disease	
Hip	Cerebral palsy	
Knee	Poliomyelitis	
Osteomyelitis		
Diskitis		
Transient synovitis, hip		
LCPD		
Tarsal coalition		
Rheumatologic disorder		
JRA		
Trauma		
Neoplasia		
ADOLESCENT (11+ YR)		
SCFE		+
Rheumatologic disorder		
JRA		
Trauma: fracture, overuse		
Tarsal coalition		
Neoplasia		

DDH, developmental dysplasia of the hip; JRA, juvenile rheumatoid arthritis; LCPD, Legg-Calvé-Perthes disease; SCFE, slipped capital femoral epiphysis; –, absent; +, present.
From Thompson GH: Gait disturbances. In Kliegman RM, editor: *Practical strategies of pediatric diagnosis and therapy,* Philadelphia, 1996, WB Saunders, pp 757–778.

Table 665-5 DIFFERENTIAL DIAGNOSIS OF LIMPING

ANTALGIC GAIT
Congenital
Tarsal coalition
Acquired
Legg-Calvé-Perthes disease Slipped capital femoral epiphysis
Trauma
Sprains, strains, contusions Fractures Occult Toddler's fracture Abuse
Neoplasia
Benign • Unicameral bone cyst • Osteoid osteoma Malignant • Osteogenic sarcoma • Ewing sarcoma • Leukemia • Neuroblastoma • Spinal cord tumors
Infectious
Septic arthritis Reactive arthritis Osteomyelitis • Acute • Subacute Diskitis
Rheumatologic
Juvenile rheumatoid arthritis Hip monoarticular synovitis (toxic transient synovitis)
TRENDELENBURG
Developmental
Developmental dysplasia of the hip Leg-length discrepancy
Neuromuscular
Cerebral palsy Poliomyelitis

From Thompson GH: Gait disturbances. In Kliegman RM, editor: *Practical strategies of pediatric diagnosis and therapy,* Philadelphia, 1996, WB Saunders, pp 757–778.

must be determined and documented. A thorough assessment and grading of muscle strength is mandatory in all cases of neuromuscular disorders.

RADIOGRAPHIC ASSESSMENT

Plain radiographs are the first step in evaluation of most musculoskeletal disorders. Advanced imaging includes special procedures such as nuclear bone scans, ultrasonography, CT, MRI, and positron emission tomography (PET).

Plain Radiographs

Routine radiographs are the first step and consist of anteroposterior and lateral views of the involved area with one joint above and below. Comparison views of the opposite side, if uninvolved, may be helpful in difficult situations but are not always necessary. It is important for the clinician to be aware of normal radiographic variants of the immature skeleton. Several synchondroses may be mistaken for fractures. A patient with "normal" plain radiographic appearance but having persistent pain or symptoms might need to be evaluated further with additional imaging studies.

Nuclear Medicine Imaging

A bone scan displays physiologic information rather than pure anatomy and relies on the emission of energy from the nucleotide injected into the patient. Indications include early septic arthritis, osteomyelitis, avascular necrosis, tumors (osteoid osteoma), metastatic lesions, occult and stress fractures, and cases of child abuse.

Total body radionuclide scan (technetium-99) is useful to identify bony lesions, inflammatory tumors, and stress fractures. Tumor vascularity can also be inferred from the flow phase and the blood pool images. Gallium or indium scans have high sensitivity for local infections. Thallium-201 chloride scintiscans have >90% sensitivity and between 80% and 90% accuracy in detecting malignant bone or soft-tissue tumors.

Ultrasonography

Ultrasonography is useful to evaluate suspected fluid-filled lesions such as popliteal cyst and hip joint effusions. Major indications for ultrasonography are fetal studies of the extremities and spine, including detection of congenital anomalies like spondylocostal dysostosis, fractures suggesting osteogenesis imperfecta, developmental dysplasia of the hip, joint effusions, occult *neonatal* spinal dysraphism, foreign bodies in soft tissues, and popliteal cysts of the knee.

Magnetic Resonance Imaging

MRI is the imaging modality of choice for defining the exact anatomic extent of most musculoskeletal lesions. MRI avoids ionizing radiation and doing does not produce any known harmful effects. It produces excellent anatomic images of the musculoskeletal system, including the soft tissue, bone marrow cavity, spinal cord, and brain. It is especially useful for defining the extent of soft-tissue lesions and injuries. Tissue planes are well delineated, allowing more accurate assessment tumor invasion into adjacent structures. Cartilage structures can be visualized (articular cartilage of the knee can be distinguished from the fibrocartilage of the meniscus). MRI is also helpful in visualizing unossified joints in the pediatric population including the shoulders, elbows, and hips of young infants.

Magnetic Resonance Angiography

Magnetic resonance angiography (MRA) has largely replaced routine angiography in the preoperative assessment of vascular lesions and bone tumors. MRA provides good visualization of peripheral vascular branches and tumor neovascularity in patients with primary bone tumors.

Computed Tomography

CT has enhanced the evaluation of multiple musculoskeletal disorders. Coronal, sagittal, and axial imaging is possible with CT including 3-dimensional reconstructions that can be beneficial in evaluating complex lesions of the axial and appendicular skeleton. It allows visualization of the detailed bone anatomy and the relationship of bones to contiguous structures. CT is useful to readily evaluate tarsal coalition, accessory navicular bone, infection, growth plate arrest, osteoid osteoma, pseudoarthrosis, bone and soft tissue tumors, spondylolysis, and spondylolisthesis.

CT is superior to MRI for assessing bone involvement and cortical destruction (even subtle changes), including calcification or ossification and fracture.

LABORATORY STUDIES

Laboratory tests are occasionally necessary in the evaluation of a child with musculoskeletal disorder. These may include a complete blood cell count; erythrocyte sedimentation rate; C-reactive protein assay; Lyme titers; and blood, wound, joint, periosteum, or bone cultures for infectious conditions such as septic arthritis or osteomyelitis. Rheumatoid factor, antinuclear antibodies, and human leukocyte antigen B27 may be necessary for children with suspected rheumatologic disorders. Creatine kinase, aldolase, aspartate aminotransferase, and dystrophin testing are indicated in children with suspected disorders of striated muscle such as Duchenne or Becker muscular dystrophy.

BIBLIOGRAPHY
Please visit the Nelson Textbook of Pediatrics *website at www.expertconsult.com for the complete bibliography.*

Chapter 666
The Foot and Toes

Harish S. Hosalkar, David A. Spiegel, and Richard S. Davidson

The foot may be divided into the **forefoot** (toes and metatarsals), the **midfoot** (cuneiforms, navicular, cuboid), and the **hindfoot** (talus and calcaneus). Although the tibiotalar joint (ankle) provides plantar flexion and dorsiflexion, the subtalar joint (between the talus and calcaneus) is oriented obliquely, providing inversion and eversion. Inversion represents a combination of plantar flexion and varus, and eversion involves dorsiflexion and valgus. The subtalar joint is especially important for walking on uneven surfaces. The talonavicular and calcaneocuboid joints connect the midfoot with the hindfoot.

Abnormalities affecting the osseous and articular structures of the foot may be congenital, developmental, neuromuscular, or inflammatory. Problems with the foot and/or toes may be associated with a host of connective tissue diseases and syndromes such as overuse syndromes, which are commonly observed in young athletes. Symptoms can include pain and abnormal shoe wear; cosmetic concerns are common.

666.1 Metatarsus Adductus

Harish S. Hosalkar, David A. Spiegel, and Richard S. Davidson

Metatarsus adductus is common in newborns and involves adduction of the forefoot relative to the hindfoot. When the forefoot is supinated and adducted, the deformity is termed *metatarsus varus* (Fig. 666-1). The most common cause is intrauterine molding, where the deformity is bilateral in 50% of cases. As with other intrauterine positional foot deformities, a careful hip examination should always be performed.

CLINICAL MANIFESTATIONS

The forefoot is adducted (occasionally supinated), whereas the midfoot and hindfoot are normal. The lateral border of the foot is convex, and the base of the 5th metatarsal appears prominent. Range of motion at the ankle and subtalar joints is normal. Both the magnitude and the degree of flexibility should be documented. When the foot is viewed from the plantar surface, a line through the midpoint of (and parallel to) the heel should normally extend through the 2nd toe. Flexibility is assessed by stabilizing the hindfoot and midfoot in a neutral position with one hand and applying pressure over the 1st metatarsal head with the other. In the walking child with an uncorrected metatarsus adductus deformity, an in-toe gait and abnormal shoe wear can occur. A subset of patients also have a dynamic adduction deformity of the great toe (hallux varus), which is often most noticeable during ambulation. This usually improves spontaneously and does not require treatment.

RADIOGRAPHIC EVALUATION

Radiographs are not performed routinely, but an anteroposterior (AP) and lateral weight-bearing or simulated weight-bearing radiographs are indicated in toddlers or older children with residual deformities. The AP radiographs demonstrate adduction of the metatarsals at the tarsometatarsal articulation and an increased intermetatarsal angle between the 1st and 2nd metatarsals.

TREATMENT

The treatment of metatarsus adductus is based on the rigidity of the deformity; most children respond to nonoperative treatment. Deformities that are flexible and overcorrect into abduction with

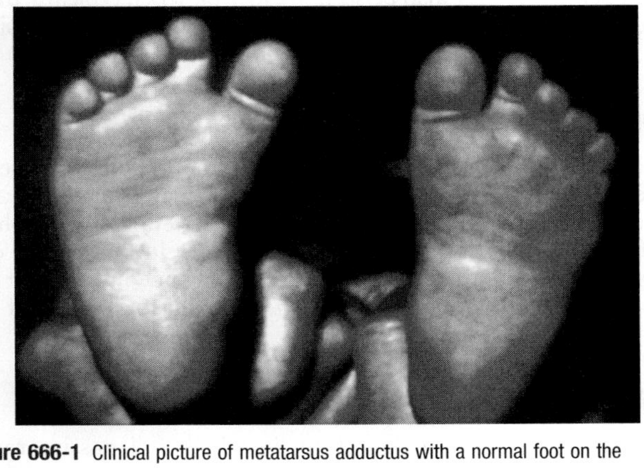

Figure 666-1 Clinical picture of metatarsus adductus with a normal foot on the opposite side.

passive manipulation may be observed. The feet that correct just to a neutral position can benefit from stretching exercises and retention in a slightly overcorrected position by a splint or reverse-last shoes. These are worn full time (22 hr/day), and the condition is re-evaluated in 4-6 wk. If improvement occurs, treatment can be continued. If there is no improvement, serial plaster casts should be considered. When stretching a foot with metatarsus adductus, care should be taken to maintain the hindfoot in neutral to slight varus alignment to avoid creating hindfoot valgus. Feet that cannot be corrected to a neutral position might benefit from serial casting; the best results are obtained when treatment is started before 8 mo of age. In addition to stretching the soft tissues, the goal is to alter physeal growth and stimulate remodeling, resulting in permanent correction. Once flexibility and alignment are restored, orthoses or corrective shoes are generally recommended for an additional period. A dynamic hallux varus usually improves spontaneously, and no active treatment is required.

Surgical treatment may be considered in the small subset of patients with symptomatic residual deformities that have not responded to previous treatment. Surgery is generally delayed until children are 4-6 yr of age. Cosmesis is often a concern, and pain and/or the inability to wear certain types of shoes occasionally leads patients to consider surgery. Options for surgical treatment include either soft-tissue release or osteotomy. An osteotomy (midfoot or multiple metatarsals) is most likely to result in permanent restoration of alignment.

BIBLIOGRAPHY

Please visit the Nelson Textbook of Pediatrics *website at www.expertconsult.com for the complete bibliography.*

666.2 Calcaneovalgus Feet

Harish S. Hosalkar, David A. Spiegel, and Richard S. Davidson

The calcaneovalgus foot is common in the newborn (30-50% of newborns have a mild version) and is secondary to in utero positioning. Excessive dorsiflexion and eversion are observed in the hindfoot, and the forefoot may be abducted. An associated external tibial torsion may be present.

CLINICAL MANIFESTATIONS

The infant typically presents with the foot dorsiflexed and everted, and occasionally the dorsum is in contact with the anterolateral surface of the lower leg. Plantar flexion and inversion are often restricted. As with other intrauterine positional deformities, a careful hip examination should be performed; if there is any concern, hip ultrasonography should be considered. The calcaneovalgus foot may be confused with a congenital vertical talus and is rarely associated with a posteromedial bow of the tibia. A calcaneovalgus deformity may also be seen in older patients, typically those with a neuromuscular imbalance involving weakness or paralysis of the gastrocnemius-soleus complex (polio, myelomeningocele).

RADIOGRAPHIC EVALUATION

Radiographs are usually not required, but they should be ordered if the deformity fails to correct spontaneously or with early treatment. AP and lateral radiographs, with a lateral radiograph of the foot in maximal plantar flexion, might help distinguish calcaneovalgus from a vertical talus. If a posteromedial bow of the tibia is suspected, anteroposterior and lateral radiographs of the tibia and fibula are necessary.

TREATMENT

Mild cases of calcaneovalgus foot, in which full passive range of motion is present at birth, require no active treatment. These usually resolve within the 1st weeks of life. A gentle stretching program, focusing on plantar flexion and inversion, is recommended for cases with some restriction in motion. For cases with a greater restriction in mobility, serial casts may be considered to restore motion and alignment. Casting is rarely required in the treatment of calcaneovalgus feet. The management for cases associated with a posteromedial bow of the tibia is similar.

666.3 Talipes Equinovarus (Clubfoot)

Harish S. Hosalkar, David A. Spiegel, and Richard S. Davidson

Talipes equinovarus (also known as *clubfoot*) describes a deformity involving malalignment of the calcaneotalar-navicular complex. Components of this deformity may be best understood using the mnemonic **CAVE** (cavus, adductus, varus, equinus). Although this is predominantly a hindfoot deformity, there are plantar flexion (cavus) of the 1st ray and adduction of the forefoot/midfoot on the hindfoot. The hindfoot is in varus and equinus. The clubfoot deformity may be positional, congenital, or associated with a variety of underlying diagnoses (neuromuscular or syndromic).

The **positional clubfoot** is a normal foot that has been held in a deformed position in utero and is found to be flexible on examination in the newborn nursery. The **congenital clubfoot** involves a spectrum of severity, while clubfoot associated with neuromuscular diagnoses or syndromes are typically rigid and more difficult to treat. Clubfoot is extremely common in patients with myelodysplasia and arthrogryposis (Chapter 674).

Congenital clubfoot is seen in approximately 1/1,000 births. Although numerous theories have been proposed, the etiology is multifactorial and likely involves the effects of environmental factors in a genetically susceptible host. The risk is approximately 1 in 4 when both a parent and one sibling have clubfeet. It occurs more commonly in males (2 : 1) and is bilateral in 50% of cases. The pathoanatomy involves both abnormal tarsal morphology (plantar and medial deviation of the head and neck of the talus) and abnormal relationships between the tarsal bones in all three planes, as well as associated contracture of the soft tissues on the plantar and medial aspects of the foot.

CLINICAL MANIFESTATIONS

A complete physical examination should be performed to rule out coexisting musculoskeletal and neuromuscular problems. The spine should be inspected for signs of occult dysraphism. Examination of the infant clubfoot demonstrates forefoot cavus and adductus and hindfoot varus and equinus (Fig. 666-2). The degree of flexibility varies, and all patients exhibit calf atrophy. Both internal tibial torsion and leg-length discrepancy (shortening of the ipsilateral extremity) are observed in a subset of cases.

RADIOGRAPHIC EVALUATION

Anteroposterior and lateral radiographs are recommended, often with the foot held in the maximally corrected position. Multiple radiographic measurements can be made to describe malalignment between the tarsal bones. The navicular bone does not ossify until 3-6 yr of age, so the focus of radiographic interpretation is the relationships between segments of the foot. A common radiographic finding is "parallelism" between lines drawn through the axis of the talus and the calcaneus on the lateral radiograph, indicating hindfoot varus. Many clinicians believe that radiographs are not required in the evaluation and treatment of clubfoot in infancy and reserve these studies for older children with persistent or recurrent deformities.

TREATMENT

Nonoperative treatment is initiated in all infants and should be started as soon as possible following birth. Techniques have included taping and strapping, manipulation and serial casting, and functional treatment. Historically, a significant percentage of patients treated by manipulation and casting required a surgical release, which was usually performed between 3 and 12 mo of age. Although many feet remain well aligned after surgical releases, a significant percentage of patients have required additional surgery for recurrent or residual deformities. Stiffness remains a concern at long-term follow-up. Pain is uncommon in childhood and adolescence, but symptoms can appear during adulthood. These concerns have led to considerable interest in less-invasive methods for treating the deformity.

The Ponseti method of clubfoot treatment involves a specific technique for manipulation and serial casting and may be best described as minimally invasive rather than nonoperative. The order of correction follows the mnemonic **CAVE**. Weekly cast changes are performed, and 5 to 10 casts are typically required. The most difficult deformity to correct is the hindfoot equinus, for which ~90% of patients require an outpatient percutaneous tenotomy of the heel cord. Following the tenotomy, a long leg cast with the foot in maximal abduction (70 degrees) and dorsiflexion is worn for 3 wk; the patient then begins a bracing program. An abduction brace is worn full time for 3 mo and then at nighttime for 3-5 yr. A subset of patients require transfer of the tibialis anterior tendon to the middle cuneiform for recurrence. Although most patients require some form of surgery, the procedures are minimal in comparison with a surgical release, which requires capsulotomy of the major joints (and lengthening of the muscles) to reposition the joints in space. The results of the Ponseti method are excellent at up to 40 yr of follow-up. Compliance with the splinting program is essential; recurrence is common if the brace is not worn as recommended. Functional treatment, or the French method, involves daily manipulations (supervised by a physical therapist) and splinting with elastic tape, as well as continuous passive motion (machine required) while the baby sleeps. Although the early results are promising, the method is labor intensive, and it remains unclear whether the technique will achieve greater popularity in the USA. These minimally invasive methods are most successful when treatment is begun at birth or during the first few months of life.

Surgical realignment has a definite role in the management of clubfeet, especially in the minority of congenital clubfeet that have failed nonoperative or minimally invasive methods, and for the neuromuscular and syndromic clubfeet that are characteristically rigid. In such cases, nonoperative methods such as the Ponseti technique are potentially of value in decreasing the magnitude of surgery required. Common surgical approaches include a release of the involved joints (realign the tarsal bones), a lengthening of the shortened posteromedial musculotendinous units, and usually pinning of the foot in the corrected position. The specific procedure is tailored to the unique characteristics of each deformity. For older children with untreated clubfeet or those in whom a recurrence or residual deformity is observed, bony procedures (osteotomies) may be required in addition to soft-tissue surgery. Triple arthrodesis is reserved as salvage for painful, deformed feet in adolescents and adults.

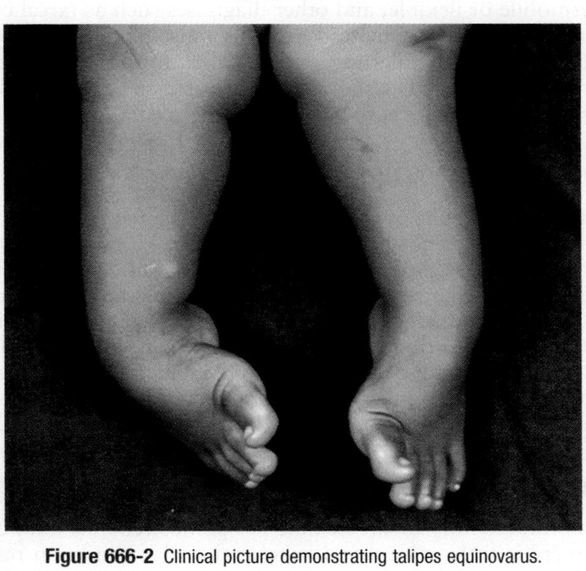

Figure 666-2 Clinical picture demonstrating talipes equinovarus.

BIBLIOGRAPHY

Please visit the Nelson Textbook of Pediatrics *website at www.expertconsult.com for the complete bibliography.*

666.4 Congenital Vertical Talus

Harish S. Hosalkar, David A. Spiegel, and Richard S. Davidson

Congenital vertical talus is an uncommon foot deformity in which the midfoot is dorsally dislocated on the hindfoot. Approximately 40% are associated with an underlying neuromuscular condition or a syndrome (Table 666-1); although the remaining 60% had been thought to be idiopathic, there is increasing evidence that some of these may be related to single gene defects. Neurologic causes include myelodysplasia, tethered cord, and sacral agenesis. Other associated conditions include arthrogryposis, Larsen syndrome, and chromosomal abnormalities (trisomy 13-15, 19). Depending on the age at diagnosis, the differential diagnosis might include a calcaneovalgus foot, oblique talus (talonavicular joint reduces passively), flexible flatfoot with a tight Achilles tendon, and tarsal coalition.

CLINICAL MANIFESTATIONS

Congenital vertical talus has also been described as a **rocker-bottom foot** (Fig. 666-3) or a Persian slipper foot. The plantar surface of the foot is convex, and the talar head is prominent along the medial border of the midfoot. The fore part of the foot is dorsiflexed (dorsally dislocated on the hindfoot) and abducted relative to the hindfoot, and the hindfoot is in equinus and valgus. There is an associated contracture of the anterolateral (tibialis anterior, toe extensors) and the posterior (Achilles tendon,

Table 666-1 ETIOLOGIES OF CONGENITAL VERTICAL TALUS

CENTRAL NERVOUS SYSTEM AND SPINAL CORD
Myelomeningocele Spinal muscular atrophy Diastematomyelia Sacral agenesis
MUSCLE
Distal arthrogryposis Arthrogryposis multiplex Neurofibromatosis
CHROMOSOMAL ABNORMALITY
Trisomy 18 Trisomy 15 Trisomy 13
KNOWN GENETIC SYNDROMES
Neurofibromatosis Prune-belly syndrome Rasmussen syndrome Split hand and split foot

From Alaee F, Boehm S, Dobbs M: A new approach to the treatment of congenital vertical talus, *J Child Orthop* 1:165–174, 2007.

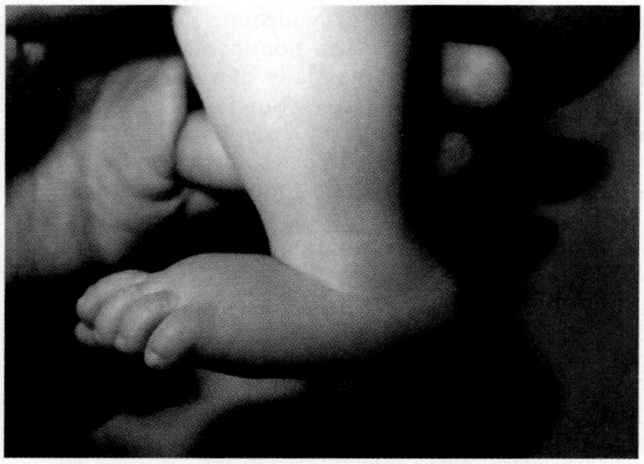

Figure 666-3 Rocker-bottom foot in congenital vertical talus.

peroneals) soft tissues. The deformity is typically rigid. A thorough physical examination is required to identify any coexisting neurologic and/or musculoskeletal abnormalities.

RADIOGRAPHIC EVALUATION

AP, lateral, and maximal plantar flexion radiographs should be obtained when the diagnosis is suspected. The plantar flexion view helps to determine whether the dorsal subluxation or dislocation of the midfoot on the hindfoot can be reduced passively. Although the navicular does not ossify until 3-6 yr of age, the relationship between the talus and the 1st metatarsal may be evaluated.

TREATMENT

The initial management consists of serial manipulation and casting, which is started shortly after birth. Initially, an attempt is made to reduce the dorsal dislocation of the forefoot and midfoot on the hindfoot. Once this has been achieved, attention can be directed toward stretching the hindfoot contracture. These deformities are typically rigid, and surgical intervention is required in the majority of cases. In such cases, casting helps to stretch out the contracted soft tissues. Surgery is generally performed between 6 and 12 mo of age; a soft-tissue release is performed as a one- or two-stage procedure. One component involves release and lengthening of the contracted anterior soft tissues in concert with an open reduction of the talonavicular joint, and the other involves a posterior release with lengthening of the contracted musculotendinous units. Fixation with Kirschner wires is commonly performed to maintain alignment. Postoperatively, casting is employed for a variable period; patients often use an orthosis for extended periods, depending on the underlying diagnosis. Salvage options for recurrent or residual deformities in older children include a subtalar or triple arthrodesis.

BIBLIOGRAPHY

Please visit the Nelson Textbook of Pediatrics *website at www.expertconsult.com for the complete bibliography.*

666.5 Hypermobile Pes Planus (Flexible Flatfeet)

Harish S. Hosalkar, David A. Spiegel, and Richard S. Davidson

Pes planus (also know as *flatfoot*) is a common diagnosis, with a prevalence of up to 23%, depending on the diagnostic criteria. Three types of flatfeet may be identified: a flexible flatfoot, a flexible flatfoot with a contracture of the Achilles tendon, and a rigid flatfoot. Flatfoot describes a change in foot shape, and there are several abnormalities in alignment between the tarsal bones. There is eversion of the subtalar complex. The hindfoot is aligned in valgus, and there is midfoot sag at the naviculocuneiform and/or the talonavicular joint. The forefoot is abducted relative to the hindfoot, and the head of the talus is uncovered and prominent along the plantar and medial border of the midfoot and hindfoot. Hypermobile or flexible pes planus is a common source of concern for parents, but these children are rarely symptomatic. Pes planus is common in neonates and toddlers and is associated with physiologic ligamentous laxity. Improvement may be seen when the longitudinal arch develops between 5 and 10 yr of age. Pes planus is less common in societies where shoes are not worn during infancy and childhood. A flexible-sole shoe is recommended. Flexible flatfeet persisting into adolescence and adulthood are usually associated with familial ligamentous laxity and can be identified in other family members.

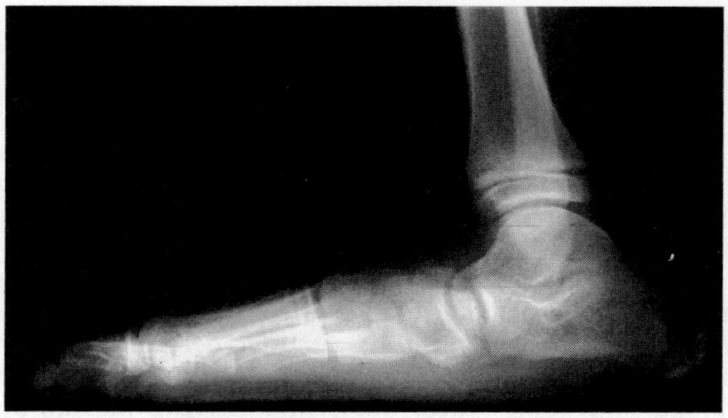

Figure 666-4 Lateral weight-bearing radiograph demonstrating features of flatfoot.

CLINICAL MANIFESTATIONS

Patients typically have a normal longitudinal arch when examined in a non–weight-bearing position, but the arch disappears when standing. The hindfoot collapses into valgus, and the midfoot sag becomes evident. Generalized ligamentous laxity is commonly observed. Range of motion should be assessed at both the subtalar and the ankle joints and will be normal in patients with a flexible flatfoot. When assessing range of motion at the ankle, the foot should always be inverted while testing dorsiflexion. If the foot is neutral or everted, spurious dorsiflexion can occur through the midfoot, masking a contracture of the Achilles tendon. If subtalar motion is restricted, then the foot is not hypermobile or flexible, and other diagnoses such as tarsal coalition and juvenile rheumatoid arthritis must be considered. On occasion, there is tenderness and/or callus formation under the talar head medially. The shoes should be assessed as well and can have evidence of excessive wear along the medial border.

RADIOGRAPHIC EVALUATION

Routine radiographs of asymptomatic flexible flatfeet are usually not indicated. Weight-bearing radiographs (AP and lateral) are required to assess the deformity. On the AP radiograph, there is widening of the angle between the longitudinal axis of the talus and the calcaneus, indicating excessive heel valgus. The lateral view shows distortion of the normal straight-line relationship between the long axis of the talus and the 1st metatarsal, with a sag either of the talonavicular or naviculocuneiform joint, resulting in flattening of the normal medial longitudinal arch (Fig. 666-4).

TREATMENT

The natural history of the flexible pes planus remains unknown, and there is little evidence to suggest that this condition results in long-term problems or disability. Thus, treatment is reserved for the small subset of patients who develop symptoms.

Patients with hindfoot pain or those with abnormal shoe wear might benefit from an orthosis, such as a medial arch support. Severe cases, often associated with an underlying connective tissue disorder such as Ehlers-Danlos syndrome or Down syndrome, might benefit from a custom orthosis such as the UCBL (University of California Biomechanics Laboratory) to better control the hindfoot and prevent collapse of the arch. Although an orthosis can relieve symptoms, there is no evidence for any permanent change in the shape of the foot or alignment of the tarsal bones.

Patients with a flexible flatfoot and a tight Achilles tendon should be treated by stretching exercises, and on occasion, the muscle needs to be lengthened surgically. For the few patients with persistent pain, surgical treatment may be considered.

There has been considerable interest in a lateral column lengthening, which addresses all components of the deformity. The procedure involves an osteotomy of the calcaneus, and a trapezoidal bone graft is placed. A lengthening of the Achilles tendon is required, and a plantar flexion osteotomy of the medial cuneiform is often performed. This procedure preserves the mobility of the hindfoot joints, in contrast to a subtalar or triple arthrodesis. A hindfoot arthrodesis can correct the deformity adequately, but the stress transfer to neighboring joints can result in late-onset, painful degenerative changes. Another option is to insert a spacer into the sinus tarsi to block eversion at the subtalar joint. These procedures may be complicated by synovitis or loosening of the implant.

BIBLIOGRAPHY

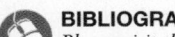

Please visit the Nelson Textbook of Pediatrics *website at* *www.expertconsult.com* *for the complete bibliography.*

666.6 Tarsal Coalition

Harish S. Hosalkar, David A. Spiegel, and Richard S. Davidson

Tarsal coalition (also known as *peroneal spastic flatfoot*) results from a congenital failure of segmentation of the primitive mesenchyme, leading to the union of two or more tarsal bones. The condition is characterized by a painful, rigid flatfoot deformity and peroneal (lateral calf) muscle spasm but without true spasticity. Any condition that alters the normal gliding and rotatory motion of the subtalar joint can produce the clinical appearance of a tarsal coalition. Thus, congenital malformations, arthritis or inflammatory disorders, infection, neoplasms, and trauma are possible causes.

The most common tarsal coalitions occur at the medial talocalcaneal (subtalar) facet and between the calcaneus and navicular (calcaneonavicular). Coalitions can be fibrous, cartilaginous, or osseous. Tarsal coalition occurs in approximately 1% of the general population and appears to be inherited as an autosomal dominant trait with nearly full penetrance. Approximately 60% of calcaneonavicular and 50% of medial facet talocalcaneal coalitions are bilateral.

CLINICAL MANIFESTATIONS

Approximately 25% of patients become symptomatic, typically during the 2nd decade of life. Although the flatfoot and a decrease in subtalar motion might have been present since early childhood, the onset of symptoms can correlate with the additional restriction in motion that occurs as a cartilaginous bar ossifies. The timing of ossification varies between the talonavicular (3-5 yr of age), the calcaneonavicular (8-12 yr), and the talocalcaneal (12-16 yr) coalitions. Hindfoot pain is commonly observed, especially in the region of the sinus tarsi and also under the head of the talus. Symptoms are activity related and are often increased with running or prolonged walking, especially on uneven surfaces. There may be tenderness over the site of the coalition and/or pain with testing of subtalar motion. The clinical appearance of a flatfoot is seen in both the weight-bearing and non–weight-bearing positions. There is a restriction in subtalar motion.

Table 666-2 RADIOGRAPHIC SECONDARY SIGNS ASSOCIATED WITH TARSAL CONDITIONS
Talar breaking
Posterior subtalar facet narrowing
Rounding and flattening of the lateral talar process
Hypoplasia of the talus, shortening of the talar neck
Anterior nose sign
Ball-and-socket ankle joint
Continuous C-sign
Flatfoot deformity
Altered navicular morphology (wide or laterally tapering)
Dysmorphic sustentaculum tali (enlarged and ovoid on lateral radiograph)

From Slovis TL, editor: *Caffey's pediatric diagnostic imaging*, ed 11, vol 2, Philadelphia, 2008, Mosby, p 2604.

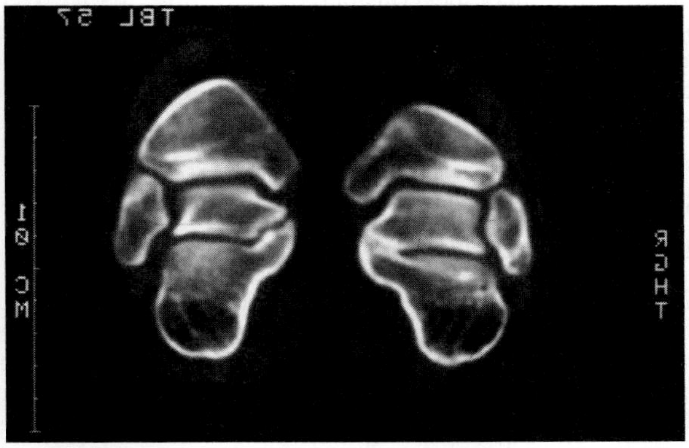

Figure 666-5 CT scan of the talocalcaneal complex demonstrating tarsal coalition.

RADIOGRAPHIC EVALUATION

AP and lateral weight-bearing radiographs and an oblique radiograph of the foot should be obtained (Table 666-2). A calcaneonavicular coalition will be seen best on the oblique radiograph. The lateral radiograph might show elongation of the anterior process of the calcaneus, known as the *anteater sign*. A talocalcaneal coalition may be seen on a Harris (axial) view of the heel. On the lateral radiograph, there may be narrowing of the posterior facet of the subtalar joint, or a C-shaped line along the medial outline of the talar dome and the inferior outline of the sustentaculum tali (C sign). Beaking of the anterior aspect of the talus on the lateral view is common and results from an alteration in the distribution of stress. This finding does not imply the presence of degenerative arthritis. Irregularity in the subchondral bony surfaces may be seen in patients with a cartilaginous coalition, in contrast to a well-formed bony bridge in those with an osseous coalition.

A fibrous coalition might require additional imaging studies to diagnose. Plain films may be diagnostic, but a CT scan is the imaging modality of choice when a coalition is suspected (Fig. 666-5). In addition to securing the diagnosis, this study helps to define the degree of joint involvement in patients with a talocalcaneal coalition. Coalitions are uncommon, but >1 tarsal coalition may be observed in the same patient.

TREATMENT

The treatment of symptomatic tarsal coalitions varies according to the type and extent of coalition, the age of the patient, and the presence and magnitude of symptoms. Treatment is required only for symptomatic coalitions, and the initial management consists of activity restriction and nonsteroidal anti-inflammatory medications, with or without a shoe insert. Immobilization in a short leg walking cast for 4-6 wk may be required in patients with more-pronounced symptoms.

For patients with chronic pain despite an adequate trial of nonoperative therapy, surgical treatment should be considered, and options include resection of the coalition, osteotomy, or arthrodesis. For the calcaneonavicular coalition, resection and interposition of the extensor digitorum brevis muscle have been successful. The surgical treatment of talocalcaneal coalitions is based on the degree of joint involvement, as defined by CT. For patients with <50% of the joint involved, resection of the coalition with interposition of fat or a split portion of the flexor hallucis tendon may be considered. For those with extensive involvement of the joint and/or degenerative changes, a triple arthrodesis may be the best option. The role of osteotomy in the management of tarsal coalition is currently under investigation.

666.7 Cavus Feet

Harish S. Hosalkar, David A. Spiegel, and Richard S. Davidson

Cavus is a deformity involving plantar flexion of the forefoot or midfoot on the hindfoot and can involve the entire forepart of the foot or just the medial column. The result is an elevation of the longitudinal arch (Fig. 666-6), and a deformity of the hindfoot often develops to compensate for the primary forefoot abnormality. Familial cavus can occur, but most patients with this deformity have an underlying neuromuscular etiology. The initial goal is to rule out (and treat) any underlying causes. These diagnoses can relate to abnormalities of the spinal cord (occult dysraphism, tethered cord, poliomyelitis, myelodysplasia, Friedrich ataxia) and peripheral nerves (hereditary motor and sensory neuropathies such as Charcot-Marie-Tooth disease, Dejerine-Sottas disease, Refsum disease). A unilateral cavus foot is most likely to result from an occult intraspinal anomaly, and bilateral involvement usually suggests an underlying nerve or muscle disease. Cavus is commonly observed in association with a hindfoot deformity. In cavovarus, which is the most common deformity in patients with the hereditary motor and sensory neuropathies, progressive weakness and muscle imbalance result in plantar flexion of the 1st ray or medial column. For the foot to land flat, the hindfoot must roll into varus. With equinocavus, the hindfoot is in equinus; in calcaneocavus (usually seen in polio or myelodysplasia), the hindfoot is in calcaneus (excessive dorsiflexion).

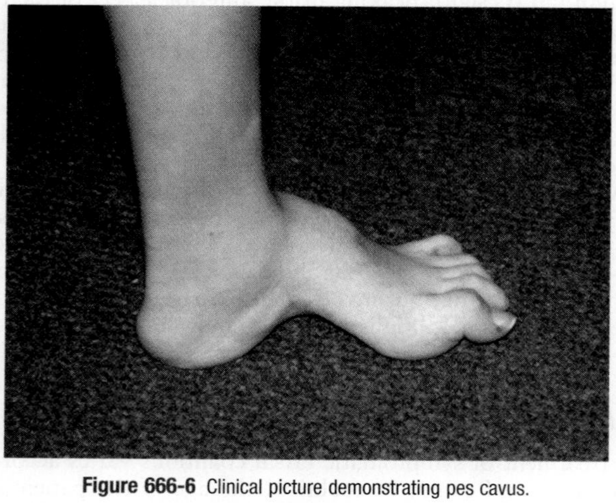

Figure 666-6 Clinical picture demonstrating pes cavus.

TREATMENT

The 1st step involves identifying any underlying diagnosis, because this knowledge helps to determine the specific management. With mild deformities, stretching of the plantar fascia and exercises to strengthen weakened muscles can help to delay progression. An ankle-foot orthosis may be necessary to stabilize the foot and improve ambulation.

Surgical treatment is indicated for progressive or symptomatic deformities that have failed to respond to nonoperative measures. The specific procedures recommended depend on the degree of deformity and the underlying diagnosis. In the case of a progressive neuromuscular condition, recurrence of deformity is commonly observed, and additional procedures may be required to maintain a plantigrade foot. Families should be counseled in detail regarding the disease process and the expected gains from the surgery. The goal of surgery is to restore motion and alignment and to improve muscle balance. For milder deformities, a soft-tissue release of the plantar fascia, often combined with a tendon transfer, might suffice. For patients with a fixed bony deformity of the forefoot and midfoot and/or the hindfoot, one or more osteotomies may be required for realignment. A triple arthrodesis (calcaneocuboid, talonavicular, and subtalar) may be required for severe or recurrent deformities in older patients.

666.8 Osteochondroses and Apophysitis

Harish S. Hosalkar, David A. Spiegel, and Richard S. Davidson

Osteochondroses are acquired focal disorders of ossification involving epiphyses, apophyses, and other epiphyseal equivalents. Idiopathic avascular necrosis is rarely observed in the tarsal navicular (**Köhler disease**) or the 2nd or 3rd metatarsal head (**Freiberg infraction**). Köhler disease (Fig. 666-7) typically appears

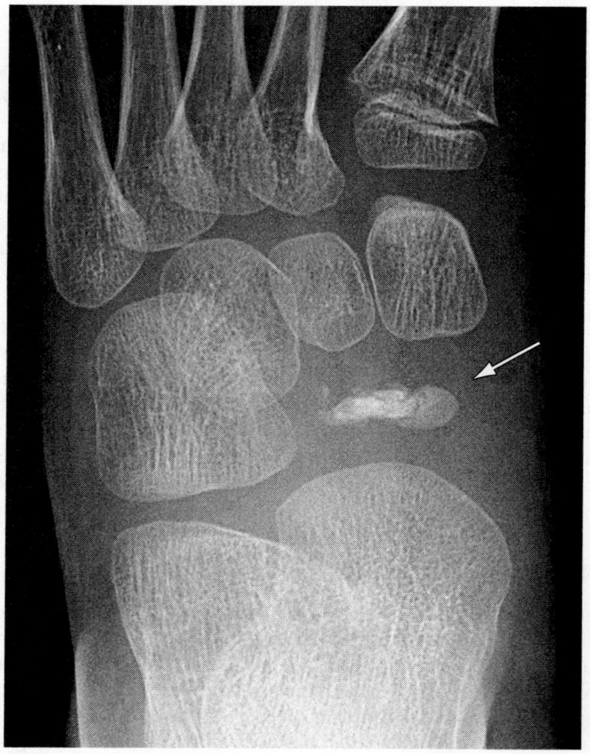

Figure 666-7 Köhler disease. Anteroposterior radiograph of a 7 yr old boy who presented with fever, pain, and swelling of the midfoot. The left foot reveals a small, fragmented, sclerotic navicular *(arrow)*. (From Slovis TL, editor: *Caffey's pediatric diagnostic imaging*, ed 11, vol 2, Philadelphia, 2008, Mosby.)

in children around age 5 or 6 yr and is 3-fold more common in boys than girls. Freiberg infraction is more common in girls and typically occur between ages 8 and 17 yr. Thess are generally self-limited conditions that commonly result in activity-related pain, which can at times be disabling. The treatment is based on the degree of symptoms and commonly includes restriction of activity. For patients with Köhler disease, a short leg cast (6-8 wk) can provide significant relief. Patients with Freiberg infraction can benefit from a period of casting and/or shoe modifications such as a rocker-bottom sole, a stiff-soled shoe, or a metatarsal bar. Degenerative changes occasionally occur following the gradual healing process, and surgical intervention is required in a subset of cases. Procedures have included joint debridement, bone grafting, redirectional osteotomy, subtotal or complete excision of the metatarsal head, and joint replacement.

Apophysitis represents inflammation at the insertion of a muscle group from repetitive tensile loading and is most commonly observed during periods of rapid growth. These stresses result in microfractures at the fibrocartilaginous insertion site, associated with inflammation. Calcaneal apophysitis (**Sever disease**) is the most common cause of heel pain in children; treatment includes activity modification, nonsteroidal anti-inflammatory medications, heel cord stretching exercises, and heel cushions or arch supports. **Iselin disease** represents an apophysitis at the 5th metatarsal base (peroneus brevis) and is less common. Radiographs should be considered when the symptoms are unilateral or with a failure to respond to treatment.

666.9 Puncture Wounds of the Foot

Harish S. Hosalkar, David A. Spiegel, and Richard S. Davidson

Most puncture wound injuries to the foot may be adequately managed in the emergency department. **Treatment** involves a thorough irrigation and a tetanus booster, if appropriate; many clinicians recommend antibiotics. Using this approach, most children heal without a complication. A subset of patients develop cellulitis, most often due to *Staphylococcus aureus* (Chapter 174), and require intravenous antibiotics with or without surgical drainage. Deep infection is uncommon and may be associated with septic arthritis, osteochondritis, or osteomyelitis. The most common organisms are *S. aureus* and *Pseudomonas* (Chapter 197); the treatment involves a thorough surgical debridement followed by a short (10-14 days) course of systemic antibiotics. Plain radiographs demonstrate any metallic fragments, but ultrasonography may be necessary to identify glass or wooden objects. Routine exploration and removal of foreign bodies is not required, but it may be necessary when symptoms are present, with recurrences, or when an infection is suspected. Pain and/or gait disturbance is more likely with superficial objects under the plantar surface of the foot. One special situation occurs when a puncture wound from a nail comes through an old sneaker. There is a high risk of a pseudomonal infection, and thorough irrigation and debridement under general anesthesia followed by systemic antibiotics for 10-14 days should be considered.

666.10 Toe Deformities

Harish S. Hosalkar, David A. Spiegel, and Richard S. Davidson

JUVENILE HALLUX VALGUS (BUNION)

Juvenile hallux valgus is 10-fold more common in girls and is typically associated with familial ligamentous laxity, and a positive family history is common. The etiology is multifactorial, and important factors include genetic factors, ligamentous laxity, pes planus, wearing shoes with a narrow toe box, and occasionally spasticity (cerebral palsy).

Clinical Manifestations

There is prominence of the 1st metatarsophalangeal (MTP) joint and often erythema from chronic irritation. The great toe is in valgus and is usually pronated, and there is splaying of the forefoot. Pes planus, with or without an associated heel cord contracture, is also observed commonly. Cosmesis is perhaps the most common concern, and some patients have pain in the region of the 1st MTP joint and/or difficulty with shoe wear.

Radiographic Evaluation

Weight-bearing AP and lateral radiographs of the feet are obtained. On the AP view, common measurements include the angular relationships between the 1st and 2nd metatarsals (intermetatarsal angle, <10 degrees is normal) and between the 1st metatarsal and the proximal phalanx (hallux valgus angle, <25 degrees is normal) (Fig. 666-8). The orientation of the 1st metatarsal-medial cuneiform joint is also documented. On the lateral radiograph, the angular relationship between the talus and the 1st metatarsal helps to identify a midfoot break associated with pes planus. Radiographs are more helpful in surgical planning than in establishing the diagnosis.

Treatment

Conservative management of adolescent bunions consists primarily of shoe modifications. It is important that footwear accommodate the width of the forefoot. Patients should avoid wearing shoes with a narrow toe box and/or a high heel. Shoe modifications such as a soft upper, bunion last, or heel cup may also be recommended. In the presence of a pes planus, an orthotic to restore the medial longitudinal arch may be beneficial. Stretching exercises are recommended to treat contracture of the Achilles tendon. The value of night splinting remains to be determined.

Surgical treatment is reserved for patients with persistent and disabling pain who have failed a course of nonoperative therapy. Surgery is not advised purely for cosmesis. Surgery is usually

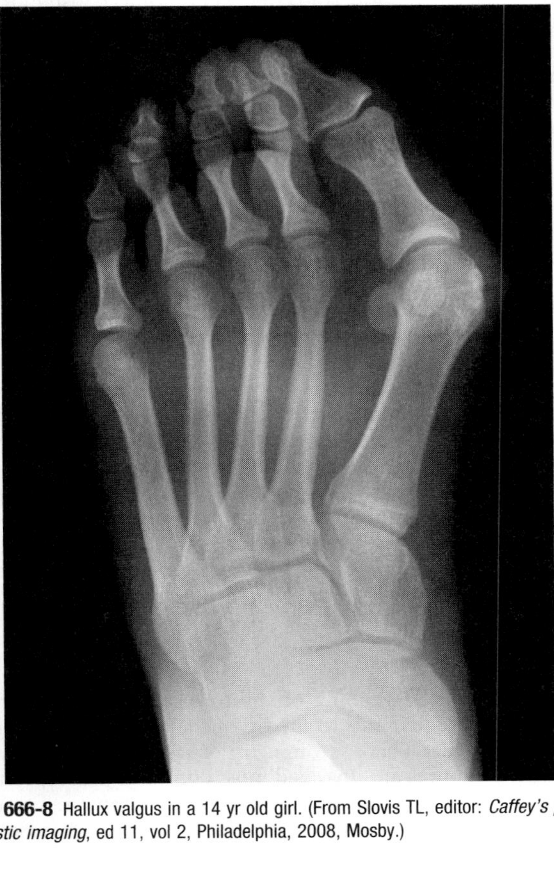

Figure 666-8 Hallux valgus in a 14 yr old girl. (From Slovis TL, editor: *Caffey's pediatric diagnostic imaging*, ed 11, vol 2, Philadelphia, 2008, Mosby.)

delayed until skeletal maturity to decrease the risk of recurrence. Radiographs are essential in preoperative planning to assess both the magnitude of deformity (hallux valgus angle, intermetatarsal angle, distal metatarsal articular angle) and associated features such as obliquity of the 1st metatarsal-medial cuneiform joint. Surgical treatment often involves a soft-tissue release and/or rebalancing procedure at the 1st MTP joint, and a single or double osteotomy of the 1st metatarsal to decrease foot width and realign the joints along the medial column of the forefoot. An arthrodesis of the 1st MTP joint may be indicated in patients with spasticity in order to prevent recurrence.

CURLY TOES

A curly toe is caused by contracture of the flexor digitorum longus, and there is flexion at the MTP and the interphalangeal (IP) joints associated with medial deviation of the toe. The toe usually lies underneath its neighbor, and the 4th and 5th toes are most commonly involved. The deformity rarely causes symptoms, and active treatment (stretching, splinting, or taping) is not required. Most cases improve over time, and a subset resolve completely. For the rare case in which there is chronic pain or skin irritation, release of the flexor digitorum longus muscle at the distal interphalangeal joint may be considered.

OVERLAPPING 5TH TOE

Congenital digitus minimus varus, or varus 5th toe, involves dorsiflexion and adduction of the 5th toe. The 5th toe typically overlaps the 4th. There is also a rotatory deformity of the toe, and the nail tends to point outward. The deformity is usually bilateral and might have a genetic basis. Symptoms are frequent and involve pain over the dorsum of the toe from shoe wear.

Nonoperative treatment has not been successful. For symptomatic patients, several different options for reconstruction have been described. Common features include releasing the contracted extensor tendon and the MTP joint capsule (dorsal, dorsomedial, or complete). A partial removal of the proximal phalanx and creation of a syndactyly between the 4th and 5th toes has been performed in conjunction with the release as well.

POLYDACTYLY

Polydactyly is the most common congenital toe deformity and is seen in approximately 2/1,000 births and is bilateral in 50% of cases. Polydactyly may be preaxial (great toe) or postaxial (5th toe), and occasionally one of the central toes is duplicated. Associated anomalies are found in approximately 10% of the preaxial and 20% of postaxial polydactyly. One third of patients also have polydactyly of the hand. Conditions that may be associated with polydactyly include Ellis-van Creveld (chondroectodermal dysplasia), longitudinal deficiency of the tibia, and Down syndrome. The extra digit may be either rudimentary or well formed, and plain radiographs of the foot help to define the anatomy and evaluate any coexisting bony anomalies.

Treatment is indicated for cosmesis and to allow fitting with standard shoes. This involves surgical removal of the extra digit, and the procedure is generally performed between 9 and 12 mo of age. Rudimentary digits may be surgically excised earlier but should not be "tied off."

SYNDACTYLY

Syndactyly involves webbing of the toes, which may be incomplete or complete (extends to the tip of the toes), and the toenails may be confluent. There is often a positive family history, and the 3rd and 4th toes are involved most commonly. Symptoms are extremely rare, and cosmetic concerns are uncommon. Treatment is only required for patients in whom there is an associated polydactyly (Fig. 666-9). In such cases, the border digit is excised, and the extra skin facilitates coverage of the wound. If the syndactyly does not involve the extra toe, then it can be observed. A complex syndactyly may be seen in patients with Apert syndrome.

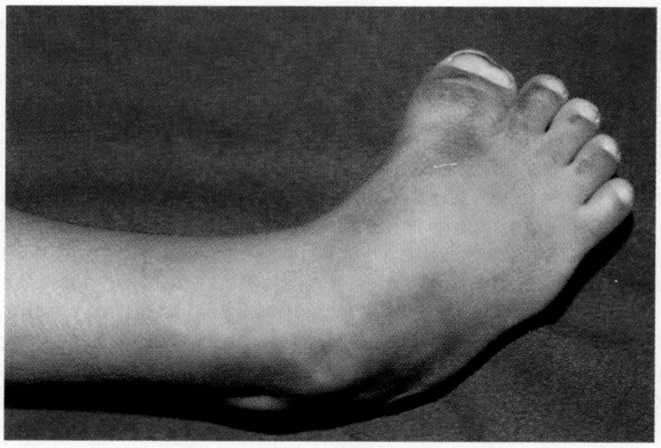

Figure 666-9 Clinical picture of polysyndactyly involving the great toe.

HAMMER TOE

A hammer toe involves flexion at the proximal IP (PIP) joint with or without the distal IP (DIP) joint, and the MTP joint may be hyperextended. This deformity may be distinguished from a curly toe by the absence of rotation. The 2nd toe is most commonly involved, and a painful callus can develop over the dorsum of the toe where it rubs on the shoe. Nonoperative therapy is rarely successful, and surgery is recommended for symptomatic cases. A release of the flexor tendons suffices in the majority of cases. Some authors have recommended a transfer of the flexor tendon to the extensor tendon. For severe cases with significant rigidity, especially in older patients, a partial or complete resection of the proximal phalanx and a PIP fusion may be required.

MALLET TOE

Mallet toe involves a flexion contracture at the DIP joint and results from congenital shortening of the flexor digitorum longus tendon. Patients can develop a painful callus on the plantar surface of the tuft. Because nonoperative therapy is usually unsuccessful, surgery is required for patients with chronic symptoms. For flexible deformities in younger children, release of the flexor digitorum longus tendon is recommended. For stiffer deformities in older patients, resection of the head of the middle phalanx, or arthrodesis of the DIP joint, may be considered.

CLAW TOE

A claw toe deformity involves hyperextension at the MTP joint and flexion at both the PIP and DIP joints, often associated with dorsal subluxation of the MTP joint. The majority are associated with an underlying neurologic disorder such as Charcot-Marie-Tooth disease. The etiology is usually muscle imbalance, and the extensor tendons are recruited to substitute for weakening of the tibialis anterior muscle. If treatment is elected, surgery is required. Transfer of the extensor digitorum (or hallucis) tendon to the metatarsal neck is commonly performed along with a dorsal capsulotomy of the MTP joint and fusion of the fusion of the PIP joint (IP joint of the great toe).

ANNULAR BANDS

Bands of amniotic tissue associated with amniotic disruption syndrome (early amniotic rupture sequence, congenital

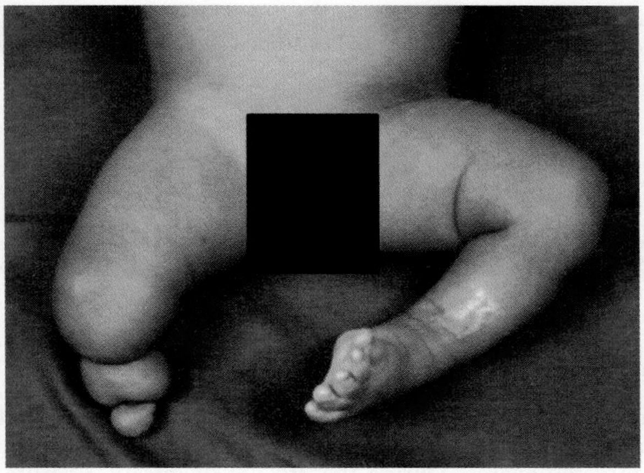

Figure 666-10 Constriction band syndrome with congenital amputation.

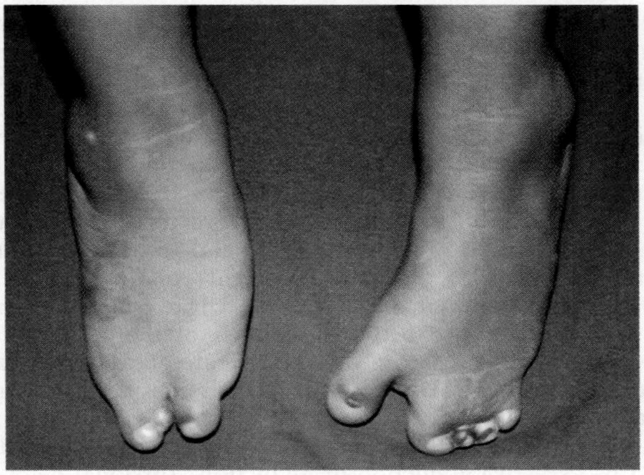

Figure 666-11 Constriction band syndrome with foot involvement.

constriction band syndrome, annular band syndrome) can become entwined along the extremities, resulting in a spectrum of problems from in utero amputation (Fig. 666-10) to a constriction ring along a digit (Fig. 666-11) (Chapter 102). These rings, if deep enough, can impair arterial or venous blood flow. Concerns regarding tissue viability are less common, but swelling from impairment in venous return is often a great problem. The treatment of annular bands usually involves observation; however, circumferential release of the band may be required emergently if arterial inflow is obstructed or electively to relieve venous congestion.

MACRODACTYLY

Macrodactyly represents an enlargement of the toes and can occur as an isolated problem or in association with a variety of other conditions such as Proteus syndrome (Fig. 666-12), neurofibromatosis, tuberous sclerosis, and Klippel-Trenaunay-Weber syndrome. This condition results from a deregulation of growth, and there is hyperplasia of one or more of the underlying tissues (osseous, nervous, lymphatic, vascular, fibrofatty). Macrodactyly of the toes may be seen in isolation (localized gigantism) or with enlargement of the entire foot. In addition to cosmetic concerns, patients might have difficulty wearing standard shoes.

The treatment is observation, if possible. This is a difficult condition to treat surgically, and complications are common. For involvement of a single toe, the best option may be a resection of the ray (including the metatarsal). For greater degrees of involvement, debulking of the various tissues is required. Often,

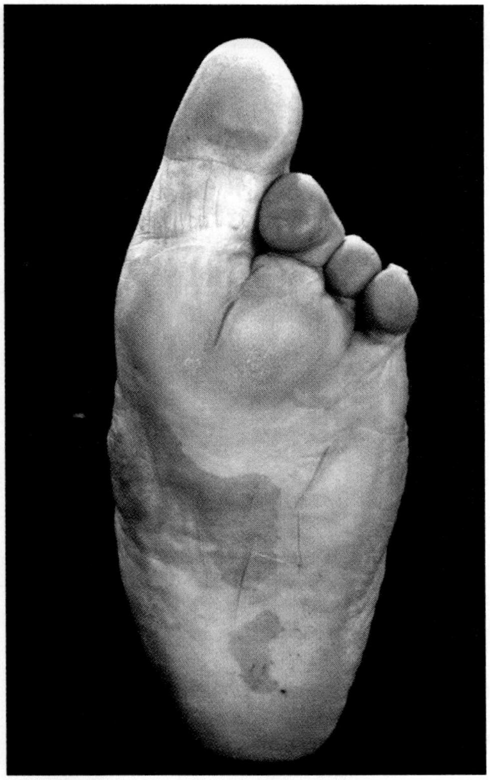

Figure 666-12 Macrodactyly of the great toe in a case of Proteus syndrome.

a growth arrest of the underlying osseous structures is performed. Stiffness and wound problems are common. The rate of recurrence is high, and more than one debulking may be required. Patients may elect to have an amputation if the process cannot be controlled by less extensive procedures.

SUBUNGUAL EXOSTOSIS

A subungual exostosis is a mass of normal bone tissue that projects out from the dorsal and medial surface of a toe, under the nail. The etiology is unknown but might relate to minor repetitive trauma. The great toe is involved most often. Patients present with discomfort, and the toenail may be elevated. The lesion may be demonstrated on plain radiographs and histologically involves normal bone with a fibrocartilaginous cap. The treatment for symptomatic lesions is excision, and the recurrence rate is in the range of 10%.

INGROWN TOENAIL

Ingrown toenails are relatively common in infants and young children and usually involve the medial or lateral border of the great toe. Symptoms include chronic irritation and discomfort; more advanced stages include drainage, infection, and granulations tissue. If conservative measures including shoe modifications, warm soaks, and appropriate nail trimming fail to control the symptoms, then surgical removal of a portion of the nail should be considered. Several surgical approaches are available, including avulsion of the ingrowing nail or avulsion with removal of the underlying germinal matrix. Chemical matrixectomy using NaOH is an alternative to surgery.

BIBLIOGRAPHY

Please visit the Nelson Textbook of Pediatrics *website at www.expertconsult.com for the complete bibliography.*

Table 666-3 DIFFERENTIAL DIAGNOSIS OF FOOT PAIN BY AGE

0-6 YEARS
Poorly fitting shoes Foreign body Fracture Osteomyelitis Leukemia Puncture wound Drawing of blood Dactylitis Juvenile rheumatoid arthritis (JRA)
6-12 YEARS
Poorly fitting shoes Sever disease Enthesopathy (JRA) Foreign body Accessory navicular Tarsal coalition Ewing sarcoma Hypermobile flatfoot Trauma (sprains, fractures) Puncture wound
12-20 YEARS
Poorly fitting shoes Stress fracture Foreign body Ingrown toenail Metatarsalgia Plantar fasciitis Osteochondroses (avascular necrosis) Freiberg Köhler Achilles tendinitis Trauma (sprains) Plantar warts Tarsal coalition

666.11 Painful Foot

Harish S. Hosalkar, David A. Spiegel, and Richard S. Davidson

A differential diagnosis for foot pain in different age ranges is shown in Table 666-3. In addition to the history and physical examination, plain radiographs are most helpful in establishing the diagnosis. Occasionally, more sophisticated imaging modalities are required.

666.12 Shoes

Harish S. Hosalkar, David A. Spiegel, and Richard S. Davidson

In toddlers and children, a shoe with a flexible sole is recommended. This recommendation is in part based on studies suggesting that the development of the longitudinal arch seems to be best in societies where shoes are not worn. With increased participation of children in sports on hard surfaces, well-cushioned, shock-absorbing shoes are helpful in the child and adolescent athlete to decrease the chances of developing an overuse syndrome. In small shoes, cushioning elements are often oversized. During school age the child's connective tissue gains stability. Cushioning for the school-age child must strike a balance between adequate cushioning and the growing child's need for adequate mechanical stimuli to help the muscles and bones develop. Connective tissue strength and joint flexibility reach adult levels by the age of 15 yr. Otherwise, shoe modifications are generally reserved for abnormalities in alignment between segments of the foot or symptoms from an underlying condition. Numerous modifications are available.

BIBLIOGRAPHY

Please visit the Nelson Textbook of Pediatrics *website at* www.expertconsult.com *for the complete bibliography.*

Chapter 667
Torsional and Angular Deformities

667.1 Normal Limb Development

Lawrence Wells and Kriti Sehgal

An understanding of normal limb development is essential for pediatricians to recognize pathologic conditions during routine and targeted exams. During the 7th wk of intrauterine life, the lower limb rotates medially to bring the great toe toward the midline. The hip joint forms by the 11th wk; the proximal femur and acetabulum continue to develop until physeal closure in adolescence. At birth, the femoral neck is rotated forward approximately 40 degrees. This forward rotation is referred to as anteversion (the angle between the axis of the femoral neck and the transcondylar axis). The increased anteversion increases the internal rotation of the hip. Femoral anteversion decreases to 15-20 degrees by 8-10 yr of age. The second source of limb rotation is found in the tibia. Infants can have 30 degrees of medial rotation of the tibia, and by maturity the rotation is between 5 degrees of medial rotation and 15 degrees of lateral rotation (Fig. 667-1). Excessive medial rotation of tibia is referred to as *medial tibial torsion.* The tibial torsion is the angular difference between the axis of the knee and the transmalleolar axis. The medial or lateral rotation beyond ±2 standard deviations (SDs) from the mean is considered abnormal rotation.

Limb rotation is also found in the foot. The abnormalities could be excessive adduction or abduction. Torsional deformity may be simple, involving a single segment, or complex, involving multiple segments. Complex deformities may be additive (internal tibial torsion and internal femoral torsion are additive) or compensatory (external tibial torsion and internal femoral torsion are compensatory).

The normal tibiofemoral angle at birth is 10-15 degrees of physiologic varus. The alignment changes to 0 degrees by 18 mo, and physiologic valgus up to 12 degrees is reached in between 3 and 4 yr of age. The normal valgus of 7 degrees is achieved by 5-8 yr of age (Fig. 667-2). Persistence of varus beyond 2 yr of age may be pathologic. Overall, 95% of developmental physiologic genu varum and genu valgum cases resolve with growth. Persistent genu valgum or valgus into adolescence is considered pathologic and deserves further evaluation.

BIBLIOGRAPHY

Please visit the Nelson Textbook of Pediatrics *website at* www.expertconsult.com *for the complete bibliography.*

667.2 Evaluation

Lawrence Wells and Kriti Sehgal

In evaluation of concerns relating to the limb, the pediatrician should obtain a history of the onset, progression, functional limitations, previous treatment, evidence of neuromuscular disorder, and any significant family history.

The examination should assess the exact torsional profile and include (1) foot progression angle, (2) femoral anteversion, (3) tibial version with thigh-foot angle, and (4) assessment of foot adduction and abduction.

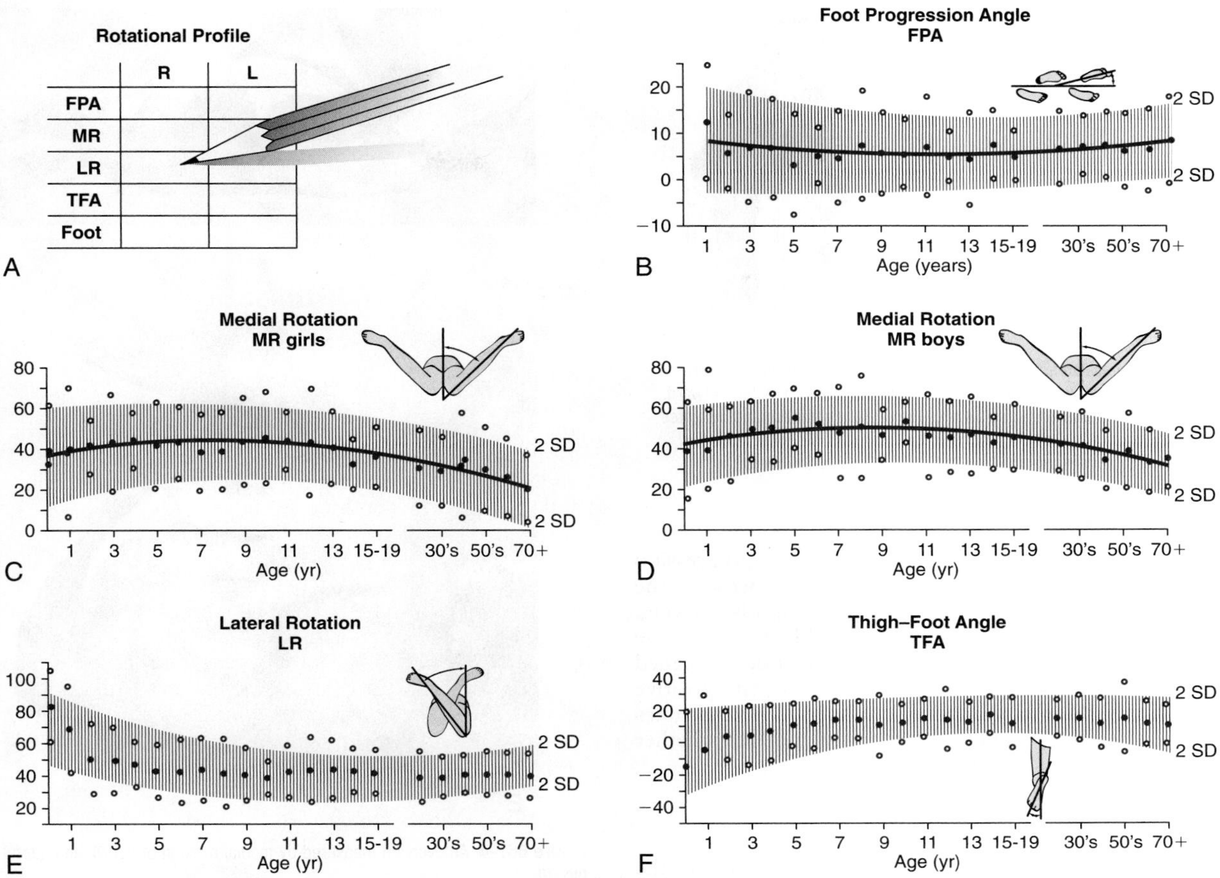

Figure 667-1 *A-F,* The rotational profile from birth to maturity is depicted graphically. All graphs include 2 standard deviations from the mean for the foot progression angle (FPA) for femoral medial rotation (MR) and lateral rotation (LR) (for boys and girls), and the thigh-foot angle (TFA). (From Morrissey RT, Weinstein SL, editors: *Lovell and Winter's pediatric orthopaedics,* ed 3, Philadelphia, 1990, Lippincott Williams & Wilkins.)

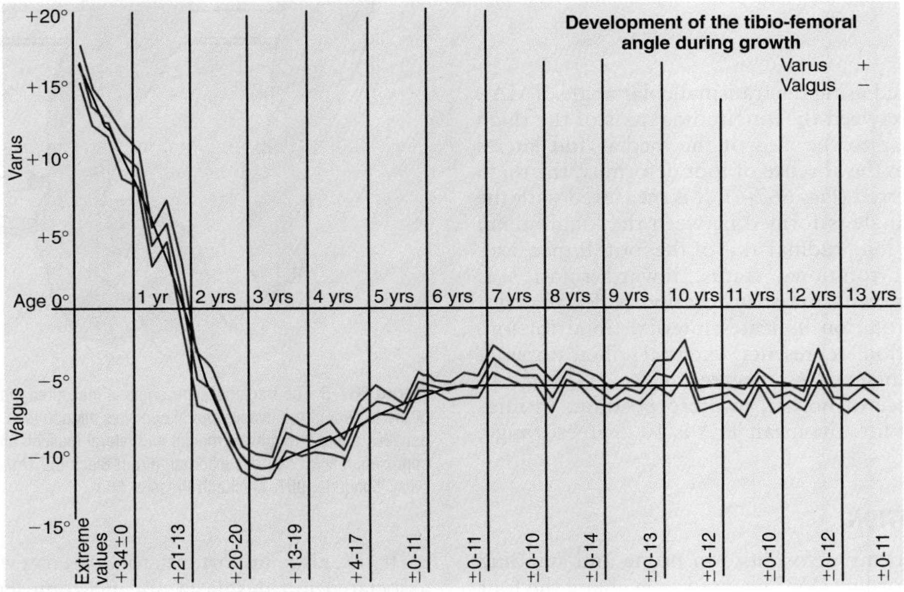

Figure 667-2 The normal coronal alignment of the knee plotted for age. (From Salenius P, Vanka E: The development of the tibiofemoral angle in children. *J Bone Joint Surg Am* 57:259–261, 1975.)

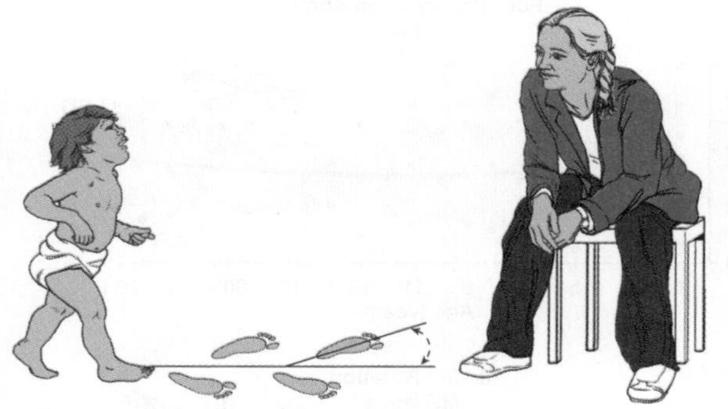

Figure 667-3 Foot progression angle. The long axis of the foot is compared with the direction in which the child is walking. If the long axis of the foot is directed outward, the angle is positive. If the foot is directed inward, the angle is negative and indicates in-toeing. (From Thompson GH: Gait disturbances. In Kliegman RM, editor: *Practical strategies in pediatric diagnosis and therapy.* Philadelphia, 2004, Saunders.)

FOOT PROGRESSION ANGLE

Limb position during gait is expressed as the foot progression angle (FPA) and represents the angular difference between the axis of the foot with the direction in which the child is walking. Its value is usually estimated by asking the child to walk in the clinic hallway (Fig. 667-3). Inward rotation of the foot is assigned a negative value, and outward rotation is designated with positive value. The normal FPA in children and adolescents is 10 degrees (range, −3 to 20 degrees). The FPA serves only to define whether there is an in-toeing or out-toeing gait.

FEMORAL ANTEVERSION

Measuring the hip rotation with the child in prone position, the hip in neutral flexion or extension, thighs together, and the knees flexed 90 degrees indirectly assesses the anteversion (Fig. 667-4). Both hips are assessed at the same time. As the lower leg is rotated ipsilaterally, this produces internal rotation of the hip, whereas contralateral rotation produces external rotation. Excessive anteversion increases internal rotation, and, retroversion increases the external rotation.

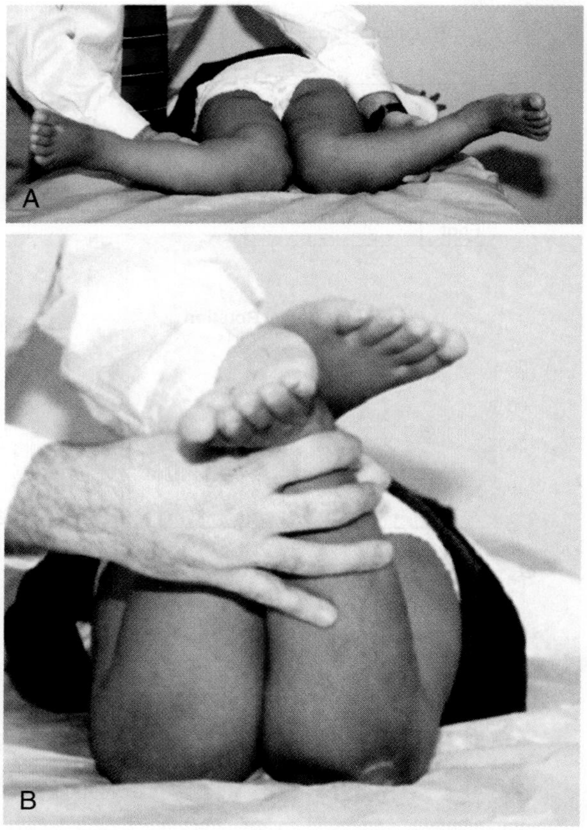

Figure 667-4 Anteversion measured by medial rotation of hip *(A)* and lateral rotation of hip *(B).*

TIBIAL ROTATION

Tibial rotation is measured using the transmalleolar angle (TMA). The TMA is the angle between the longitudinal axis of the thigh with a line perpendicular to the axis of the medial and lateral malleolus (Fig. 667-5). In the absence of foot deformity, the thigh foot angle (TFA) is preferred (Fig. 667-6). It is measured with the child lying prone. The angle is formed between the longitudinal axis of the thigh and the longitudinal axis of the foot. It measures the tibial and hindfoot rotational status. Inward rotation is assigned a negative value, and outward rotation is designated a positive value. Inward rotation indicates internal tibial torsion, whereas outward rotation represents external tibial torsion. Infants have a mean angle of −5 degrees (range, −35 to 40 degrees) as a consequence of normal in utero position. In mid-childhood through adult life, the mean TFA is 10 degrees (range, −5 to 30 degrees).

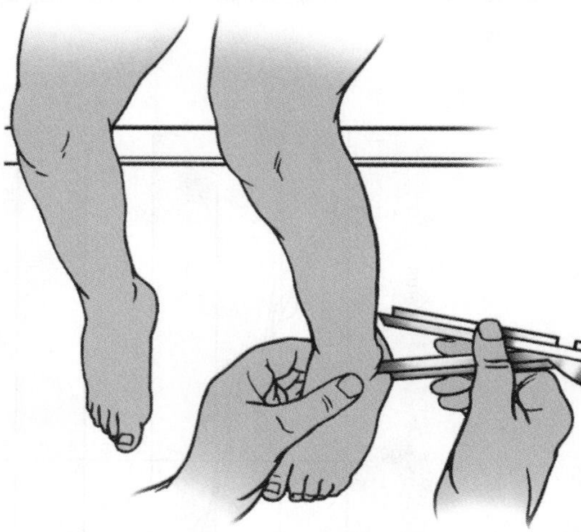

Figure 667-5 The transmalleolar angle is measured with the patient sitting at the edge of the table and the distal femoral condyles aligned with the side of the table. The angle between a line through the medial and lateral malleoli and edge of the table should be approximately 30 degrees external. (From Bleck EE: *Orthopaedic management in cerebral palsy,* London, 1987, MacKeith Press, p 55.)

FOOT SHAPE AND POSITION

The foot is observed for any deformities in prone and standing position. The heel bisector line (HBL) is used to evaluate the foot adduction and abduction deformities. The HBL is a line that divides the heel in two equal halves along the longitudinal axis (Fig. 667-7). It normally extends to the 2nd toe. When the HBL points medial to the 2nd toe, the forefoot is abducted, and when the HBL is lateral to the 2nd toe, the forefoot is adducted.

It is also important to screen every affected child for associated hip dysplasia and neuromuscular problems (cerebral palsy).

BIBLIOGRAPHY

Please visit the Nelson Textbook of Pediatrics *website at www.expertconsult.com for the complete bibliography.*

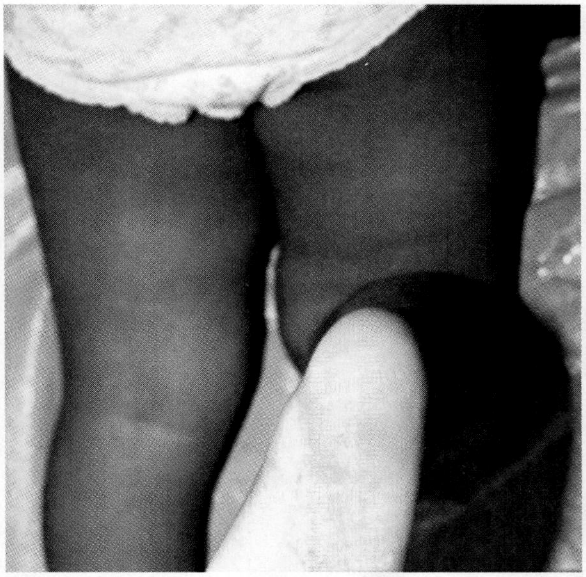

Figure 667-6 Thigh-foot angle.

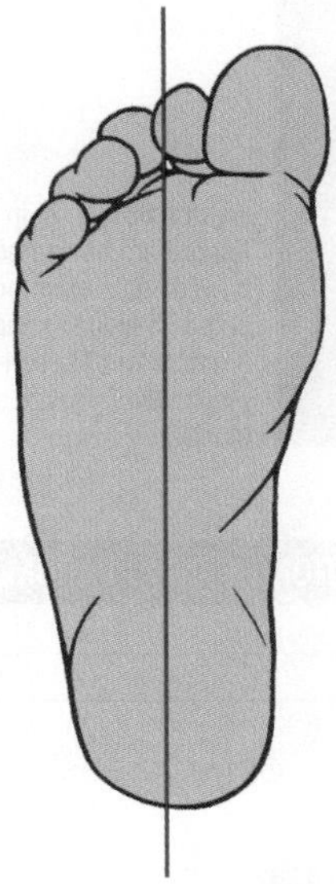

Figure 667-7 Schematic demonstration of heel bisector line.

667.3 Torsional Deformities

Lawrence Wells and Kriti Sehgal

INTERNAL FEMORAL TORSION

In-toeing gait most commonly results from excessive femoral anteversion. It occurs more commonly in girls than boys (2 : 1) in children 3-6 yr of age. The etiology of femoral torsion is controversial. Some believe that it is congenital and a result of persistent infantile femoral anteversion, whereas others believe it is acquired secondary to abnormal sitting habits. Some children are in habit of sitting in a W position or sleeping prone. On examination, most children with this condition have generalized ligamentous laxity. Gait examination reveals that entire leg is inwardly rotated. Internal hip rotation is increased beyond 70 degrees, and consequently the external rotation is restricted to 10-20 degrees. The patellas are pointing inward when the foot is straight, and compensatory external rotation of the tibia is demonstrated.

Diagnosis is made clinically on examination; CT can provide objective measurements but is rarely indicated. The treatment is predominantly observation and correction of abnormal sitting habits. The torsion usually corrects with growth by 8-10 yr of age. Persistent deformity, unacceptable cosmesis, functional impairment, anteversion >45 degrees, and no external rotation beyond neutral are some of the indications for operative intervention. Surgery involves derotation osteotomy of the femur.

INTERNAL TIBIAL TORSION

Medial tibial torsion manifests with **in-toeing gait** and is commonly associated with congenital metatarsus varus, genu valgum, or femoral anteversion. This condition is usually seen during the 2nd yr of life. Normally at birth, the medial malleolus lies behind the lateral malleolus, but by adulthood, it is reversed, with the tibia in 15 degrees of external rotation. The treatment is essentially observation and reassurance, because spontaneous resolution with normal growth and development can be anticipated. Significant improvement usually does not occur until the child begins to pull to stand and walk independently. Thereafter, correction can be seen as early as 4 yr of age and in some children by 8-10 yr of age. Persistent deformity with functional impairment is treated with supramalleolar osteotomy.

EXTERNAL FEMORAL TORSION

External femoral torsion can follow a slipped capital femoral epiphysis (SCFE); there is a low threshold to perform radiographs of the hips in children >10 yr of age. Femoral retrotorsion, when of idiopathic origin, is usually bilateral. The disorder is associated with an **out-toeing gait** and increased incidence of degenerative arthritis. The clinical examination of external femoral torsion shows excessive hip external rotation and limitation of internal rotation. The hip will externally rotate up to 70-90 degrees, whereas internal rotation is only 0-20 degrees. If SCFE is detected, it is treated surgically. Occasionally, persistent femoral retroversion after SCFE can produce functional impairment such as a severe out-toeing gait and difficulty opposing one's knees in the sitting position. The latter can be disabling to adolescent girls. Should this occur, a derotation osteotomy might be necessary.

EXTERNAL TIBIAL TORSION

Lateral tibial torsion is less common than medial rotation and is often associated with a calcaneovalgus foot. It can be compensatory to persistent femoral anteversion and idiopathic or secondary to a tight iliotibial band. The natural growth rotates the tibia externally, and hence external tibial torsion can become worse with time. Clinically, the patella faces outward when the foot is straight. The TFA and the TMA are increased. There may be associated patellofemoral instability with knee pain. Though some correction can occur with growth, extremely symptomatic children need supramalleolar osteotomy, which is usually done by 10-12 yr of age.

METATARSUS ADDUCTUS

Metatarsus adductus (Chapter 666.01) manifests with forefoot adduction and inversion of all metatarsals. Ten to 15% are associated with hip dysplasia. The prognosis is good, because the majority get better with nonoperative intervention. The feet, which are flexible and correctable up to neutral, are treated with stretching exercises. Those that are not completely correctable are treated with serial casting. Rigid deformities, which are not correctable by stretching, are treated with medial capsulotomy of the 1st metatarsal cuneiform joint and soft-tissue release by 2 yr of

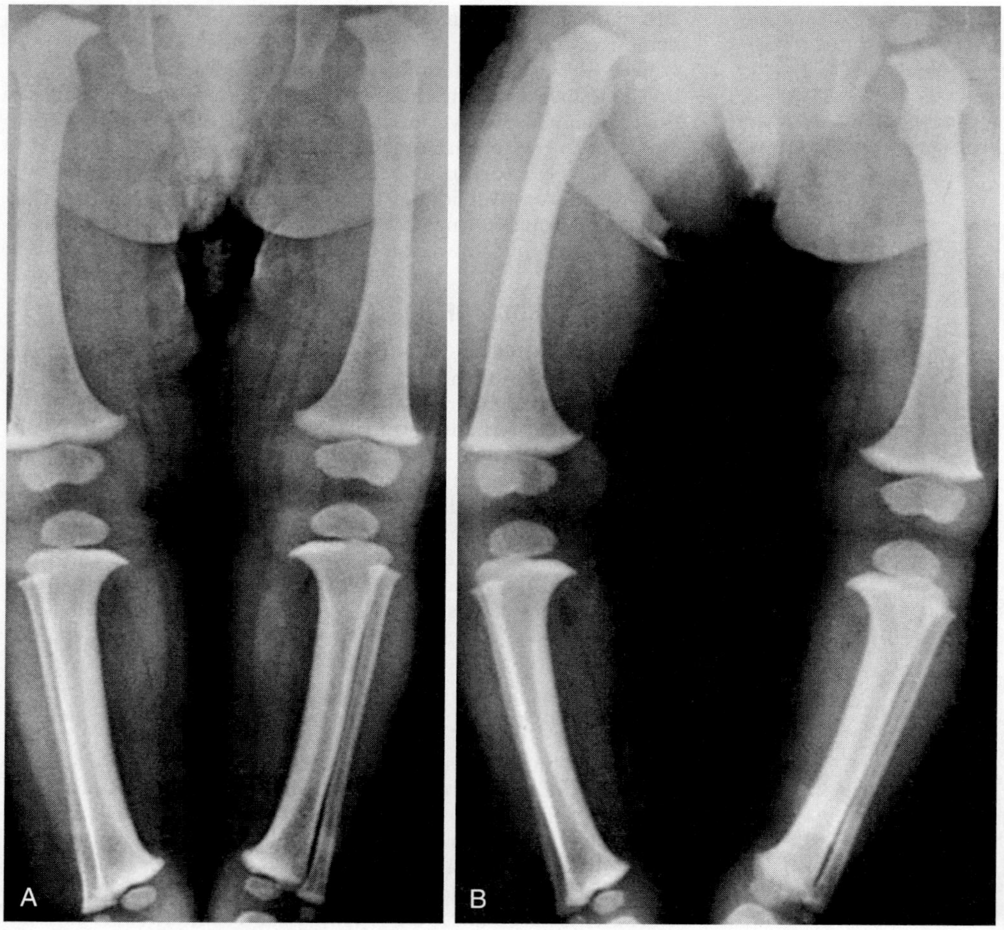

Figure 667-8 *A,* In recumbent position, tibia and femora are bowed but the legs do not appear bowed. *B,* In erect position during weight bearing and with ankles in apposition, the legs are bowed. (From Slovis TL, editor: *Caffey's pediatric diagnostic imaging,* ed 11, Philadelphia, 2008, Mosby.)

age. Osteotomies of the base of the metatarsal are usually done after 6 yr of age.

BIBLIOGRAPHY

Please visit the Nelson Textbook of Pediatrics *website at* *www.expertconsult.com* *for the complete bibliography.*

667.4 Coronal Plane Deformities

Lawrence Wells and Kriti Sehgal

Genu varum and genu valgum are common pediatric deformities of the knee. The age-appropriate normal values for knee angle are presented in Figure 667-2. Tibial bowing is common during the 1st year, bowlegs are common during the 2nd year, and knock-knees are most prominent between 3 and 4 yr of age.

GENU VARUM

Physiologic bowleg is a common torsional combination that is secondary to normal in utero positioning (Fig. 667-8). Spontaneous resolution with normal growth and development can be anticipated. Persistence of varus beyond 2 yr of age may be pathologic. The different causes are metabolic bone disease (vitamin D deficiency, rickets, hypophosphatasia), asymmetric growth arrest (trauma, infection, tumor, Blount), bone dysplasia (dwarfism, metaphyseal dysplasia), and congenital and neuromuscular disorders (Table 667-1). It is prudent to differentiate physiologic bowing from Blount disease (Table 667-2). Physiologic bowing should also be differentiated from rickets and skeletal dysplasia. Rickets has classic bone changes with trumpeting widening and fraying of the metaphysis and widening of the physis (Chapter 48).

Table 667-1 CLASSIFICATION OF GENU VARUM (BOWLEGS)

PHYSIOLOGIC
ASYMMETRIC GROWTH
Tibia vara (Blount disease) • Infantile • Juvenile • Adolescent Focal fibrocartilaginous dysplasia Physeal injury Trauma Infection Tumor
METABOLIC DISORDERS
Vitamin D deficiency (nutritional rickets) Vitamin D–resistant rickets Hypophosphatasia
SKELETAL DYSPLASIA
Metaphyseal dysplasia Achondroplasia Enchondromatosis

Modified from Thompson GH: Angular deformities of the lower extremities. In Chapman MW, editor: *Operative orthopedics*, ed 2, Philadelphia, 1993, JB Lippincott, pp 3131–3164.

TIBIA VARA

Idiopathic tibia vara, or **Blount disease,** is a developmental deformity resulting from abnormal endochondral ossification of the medial aspect of the proximal tibial physis leading to varus angulation and medial rotation of the tibia (Fig. 667-9). The incidence is greater in African-Americans and in toddlers who are overweight, have an affected family member, or started walking early in life. It has been classified into three types depending on the age at onset: infantile (1-3 yr), juvenile (4-10 yr), and adolescent (11 yr or older). The juvenile and adolescent forms are commonly combined as late-onset tibia vara. The exact cause of tibia vara remains unknown.

The infantile form of tibia vara is the most common; its characteristics include predominance in black girls, approximately 80% bilateral involvement, a prominent medial metaphyseal beak, internal tibial torsion, and leg-length discrepancy (LLD). The characteristics of the juvenile and adolescent forms (late onset) include predominance in black boys, normal or greater than normal height, approximately 50% bilateral involvement, slowly progressive genu varum deformity, pain rather than deformity as the primary initial complaint, no palpable proximal medial metaphyseal beak, minimal internal tibial torsion, mild medial collateral ligament laxity, and mild lower extremity length discrepancy. The infantile group has the greatest potential for progression.

An anteroposterior standing radiograph of both lower extremities with patellas facing forward and a lateral radiograph of the involved extremity should be obtained (Fig. 667-10). Weight-bearing radiographs are preferred and allow maximal presentation of the clinical deformity. The metaphyseal-diaphyseal angle can be measured and is useful in distinguishing between physiologic genu varum and early tibia vara (Fig. 667-11). Langenskiöld has six stages on radiographs (Fig. 667-12). The differentiation is based on fragmentation of the epiphysis, beaking of the medial tibial epiphysis, depression of the medial tibial

Table 667-2 DIFFERENTIATION OF LEG BOWING

PHYSIOLOGIC BOWING	BLOUNT DISEASE
Gentle and symmetric deformity	Asymmetric, abrupt, and sharp angulation
Metaphyseal-diaphyseal angle <11 degrees	Metaphyseal-diaphyseal angle >11 degrees
Normal appearance of the proximal tibial growth plate	Medial sloping of the epiphysis Widening of the physis Fragmentation of the metaphysis
No significant lateral thrust	Significant lateral thrust

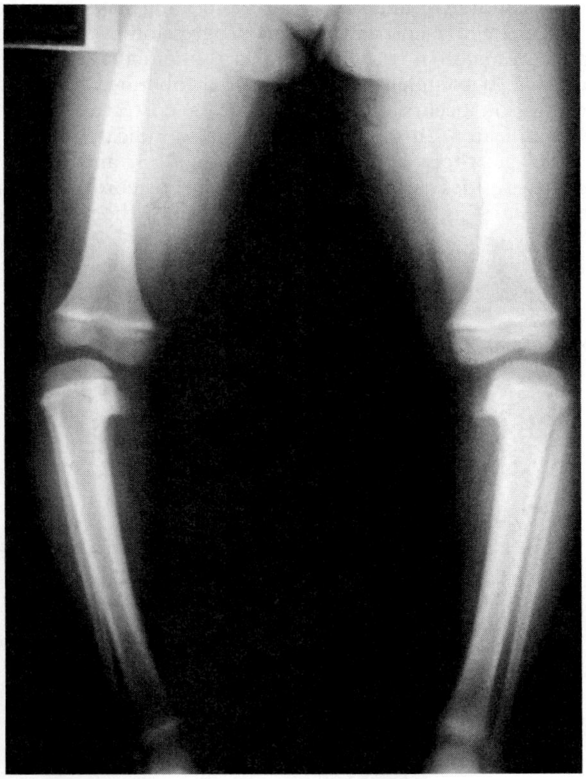

Figure 667-10 Anteroposterior radiograph of both knees in Blount disease.

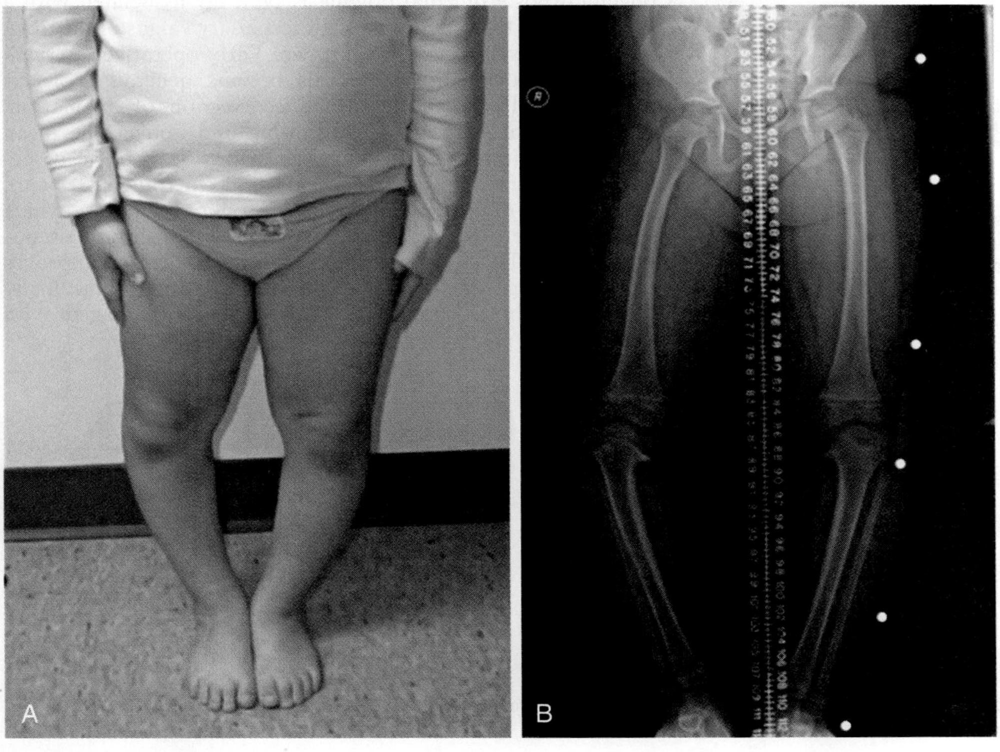

Figure 667-9 Clinical photograph *(A)* and standing anteroposterior radiograph *(B)* of a 5 yr old girl with bilateral early-onset Blount disease. (From Sabharwal S: Blount disease, *J Bone Joint Surg Am* 91:1758–1776, 2009.)

plateau, and formation of a bony bar. Occasionally, CT with three-dimensional reconstructions, or MRI, may be necessary to assess the meniscus, the articular surface of the proximal tibia including the posteromedial slope, or the integrity of the proximal tibial physis.

Management is based on the stage of the disease, the age of the child, and nature of presentation (primary or recurrent deformity). In children younger than 3 yr and Langenskiöld stage <3, bracing is effective and can prevent progression in 50% of these children. A maximal trial of 1 yr of orthotic management is recommended. If complete correction is not obtained after 1 yr or if progression occurs during this time, a corrective osteotomy may be indicated. Surgical treatment is also indicated in children >4 yr of age, those at Langenskiöld stage >3, and those with severe deformities. A proximal tibial valgus osteotomy and associated fibular diaphyseal osteotomy are usually the procedures of choice. In late-onset tibia vara, correction is also necessary to restore the mechanical axis of the knee. Hemiplateau elevation with correction of posteromedial slope has also been established as a treatment modality in relapsed cases.

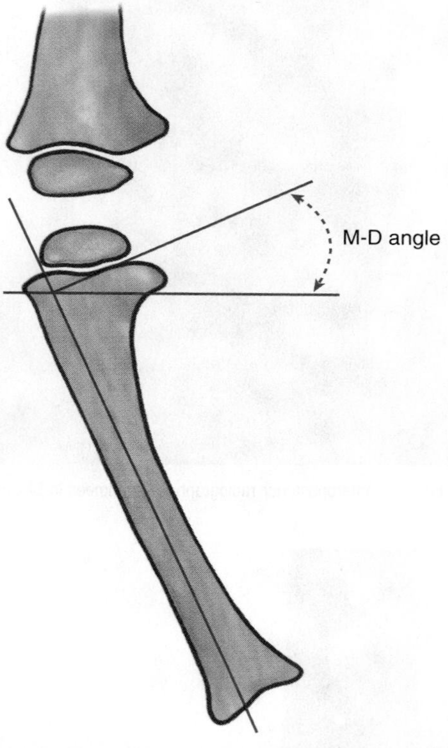

Figure 667-11 Metaphyseal-diaphyseal (M-D) angle. Draw a line on the radiograph through the proximal tibial physis. Draw another line along the lateral tibial cortex. Last, draw a line perpendicular to the shaft line as demonstrated in the diagram. (From Morrissey RT, Weinstein SL, editors: *Lovell and Winter's pediatric orthopaedics,* ed 3, Philadelphia, 1990, Lippincott Williams & Wilkins.)

GENU VALGUM (KNOCK-KNEES)

The normal valgus is achieved by 4 yr of age. Variation up to 15 degrees of valgus is possible until 6 yr of age, and thus physiologic valgus has a good chance of correction until this age. The intermalleolar distance with the knees approximated is normally <2 cm, and in a severe valgus deformity it could measure >10 cm. Pathologic conditions leading to valgus are metabolic bone disease (rickets, renal osteodystrophy), skeletal dysplasia, posttraumatic physeal arrest, tumors, and infection. The increased valgus at the knee causes lateral deviation of the mechanical axis with stretching of the medial aspect of the knee leading to knee pain. Deformities >15 degrees and occurring after 6 yr of age are unlikely to correct with growth and require surgical management. In the skeletally immature, medial tibial epiphyseal hemiepiphysiodesis or stapling (guided growth) is attempted for correction. In the skeletally mature, osteotomy is necessary at the center of rotation of angulation and is usually situated in the distal femur. Long-length anteroposterior radiographs of the leg in a weight-bearing stance are necessary for preoperative planning.

BIBLIOGRAPHY

Please visit the Nelson Textbook of Pediatrics *website at* www.expertconsult.com *for the complete bibliography.*

667.5 Congenital Angular Deformities of the Tibia and Fibula

Lawrence Wells and Kriti Sehgal

POSTEROMEDIAL TIBIAL BOWING

Congenital posteromedial bowing is typically associated with a calcaneovalgus foot and rarely with secondary valgus of the tibia, although the exact cause is unknown. Early operative intervention is not indicated because this bowing generally corrects with growth. However, despite the correction of angulation, there is residual shortening in the tibia and fibula. The mean growth inhibition is 12-13% (range, 5-27%). The mean leg-length-discrepancy (LLD) at maturity is 4 cm (range, 3-7 cm). The diagnosis of bowing is confirmed on radiographs, which show the posteromedial angulation without any other osseous abnormalities. The calcaneovalgus deformity of the foot improves with stretching or modified shoe wear and occasionally ankle-foot orthosis. Predicted LLD <4 cm is managed with

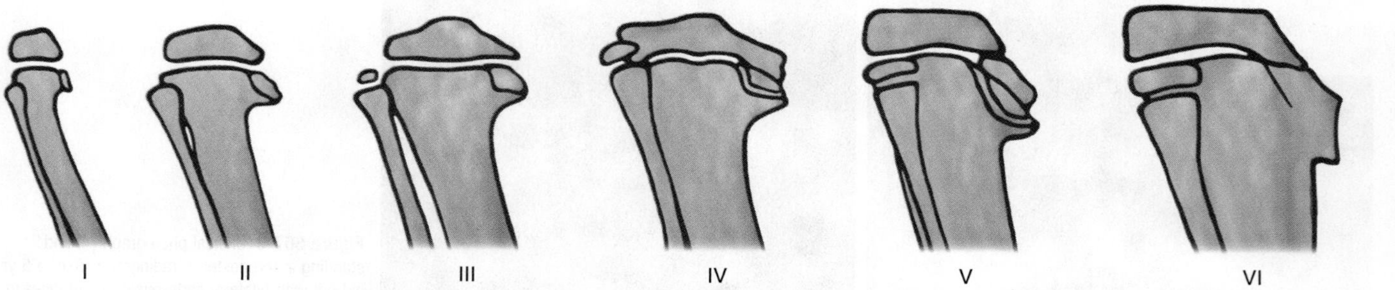

Figure 667-12 Depiction of the stages of infantile Blount disease. (From Langeskiöld A: Tibia vara [osteochondrosis deformans tibiae]: a survey of 23 cases, *Acta Chir Scand* 103:1, 1952.)

age-appropriate epiphysiodesis of the normal leg. LLD >4 cm is managed with combination of contralateral epiphysiodesis and ipsilateral lengthening. A corrective osteotomy for distal valgus may be required and can be done in the same setting while correcting LLD.

ANTEROMEDIAL TIBIAL BOWING (POSTAXIAL HEMIMELIA)

Fibular hemimelia is the most common cause of anteromedial bowing of the tibia. The fibular deficiency can occur with complete absence of fibula or a partial development both proximally and distally. It is associated with deformities of femur, knee, tibia, ankle, and foot. The femur is short and has lateral condylar hypoplasia, causing patellar instability and genu valgum deformity. The tibia has anteromedial bowing with reduced growth potential. The keys for management are the ankle stability and foot deformities. The ankle resembles a ball-and-socket joint with lateral instability. The foot deformities are characterized by the absence of lateral digits, equinocavovarus foot, and tarsal coalition.

Various surgical options have been described, and the treatment is tailored to the patient's needs and parents' acceptance. A severely deformed foot could be best managed with Syme or Boyd amputation, with prosthesis as early as 1 yr of age. In the salvageable foot, LLD can be treated with contralateral leg epiphysiodesis or ipsilateral limb lengthening.

ANTEROLATERAL TIBIAL BOWING

Anterolateral tibial bowing is associated with congenital pseudarthrosis of tibia. Fifty percent of the patients have neurofibromatosis, but only 10% of the neurofibromatosis patients have this lesion. The pseudarthrosis or site of nonunion is typically situated at the middle third and distal third of the tibia. Boyd has classified it in increasing severity depending on the presence of cystic and dysplastic changes. The treatment for this condition has been very frustrating, with poor results. Bracing has been recommended to prevent fracture early in the course; however, it has not been successful. Numerous surgical interventions have been attempted to achieve union such as single- and dual-onlay grafting with rigid internal fixation, intramedullary pinning with or without bone grafting, and an Ilizarov device. With the advent of microsurgery, live fibular grafts have been used with varying results. Due to the poor chances of successful union and considerable LLD, a below-knee amputation with early rehabilitation may be preferred. It is important not to attempt any osteotomy for correction of the tibial bowing.

TIBIAL LONGITUDINAL DEFICIENCY

Tibial longitudinal deficiency follows an autosomal dominant inheritance pattern and has been divided into four types depending on the deficient part of the tibia. The other associated anomalies are foot deformities, hip dysplasia, and symphalangism of the hand. The treatment revolves around presence of proximal tibial anlage and a functional quadriceps mechanism. In type Ia deformity, the proximal tibial anlage is absent and knee disarticulation with prosthesis is recommended. In types Ib and II, the tibial anlage is present and the management consists of an early Syme amputation, followed later by synostosis of the fibula with the tibia, and a below-knee prosthesis. Type III is rare and the principal management is with Syme amputation and a prosthesis. Type IV deformity is associated with ankle diastasis, which requires stabilization of the ankle and correction of LLD at a later stage.

BIBLIOGRAPHY

Please visit the Nelson Textbook of Pediatrics *website at www.expertconsult.com for the complete bibliography.*

Chapter 668
Leg-Length Discrepancy

Jared E. Friedman and Richard S. Davidson

Leg-length discrepancy (LLD), or anisomelia, in children can result from a variety of congenital or acquired conditions (see Table 668-1 on the *Nelson Textbook of Pediatrics* website at www.expertconsult.com). Congenital conditions include asymmetrical growth from hemihypertrophy, vascular and lymphatic anomalies, Beckwith-Wiedemann syndrome, hemiatrophy, bone dysplasias (proximal femoral focal deficiency [PFFD]), fibular and tibial hemimelia (see Fig. 668-1 on the *Nelson Textbook of Pediatrics* website at www.expertconsult.com), and Proteus syndrome. Associated acquired causes of limb length inequality include physeal fractures, infections involving the growth plate, fractures whose healing process stimulates growth, juvenile rheumatoid arthritis, and coxa vara. Neurologic diseases including spina bifida, cerebral palsy, head injury, and spinal dysraphisms, can also lead to LLD. These etiologies lead to structural limb length discrepancies, but soft tissue contractures of the lower extremity can also cause functional limb discrepancies even though the bones are of symmetrical length. Hip dysplasia can cause apparent limb length inequality of a functional type.

For the full continuation of this chapter, please visit the Nelson Textbook of Pediatrics *website at www.expertconsult.com.*

Chapter 669
The Knee

Lawrence Wells and Kriti Sehgal

NORMAL DEVELOPMENT OF THE KNEE

The knee is a major synovial joint and develops between the 3rd and 4th fetal mo. The secondary centers of ossification are formed between the 6th and 9th fetal mo for the distal femur and between the 8th fetal mo and the 1st postnatal mo for the upper tibia. The patellar ossification center appears between the 2nd and 4th yr in girls and the 3rd and 5th yr in boys.

NORMAL RANGE OF MOTION

The fully extended knee is normally in the neutral position. The normal range of motion extends from neutral to about 140 degrees, with most activities performed in the flexion arc of 0-70 degrees. Hyperextension of up to 10-15 degrees is considered normal in a child.

The knee is the largest joint in the body and is a modified hinge type of synovial joint that also permits some element of rotation. It consists of three joints merged into one: an intermediate one between the patella and the femur, and lateral and medial ones between the femoral and tibial condyles. The distal femur is cam shaped, allowing it to have a gliding, hinged motion. The major constraints of the knee are the medial and lateral collateral ligaments, the anterior and posterior cruciate ligaments, and the medial and lateral menisci. There are several bursae about the knee because most tendons around the knee run parallel to the bones and pull lengthwise across the knee joint.

Knee pain is one of the most common presenting complaints in older children and adolescents. This is commonly related to trauma but may also be insidious in onset. Knee effusion may be a common feature associated with knee pain. Depending on the etiology of the intra-articular process, the fluid collected in the knee may be blood (trauma- or hemophilia-induced hemarthrosis), inflammatory fluid (juvenile rheumatoid arthritis), or

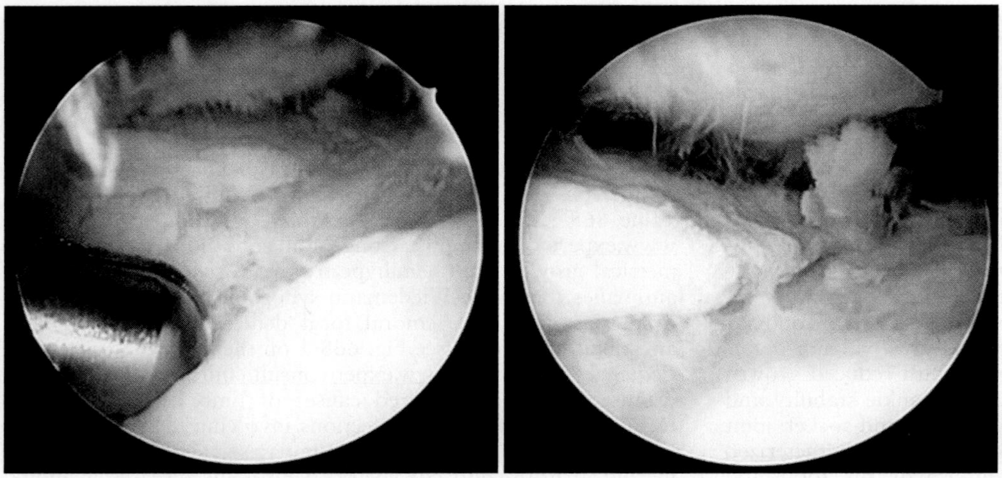

Figure 669-1 Arthroscopic image of discoid meniscus and arthroscopic shaving with meniscectomy.

purulent material (septic arthritis). The presence of fat globules in the blood aspirated from a hemarthrosis suggests an occult fracture. Recurrent effusions can indicate a chronic internal derangement such as a meniscal tear. Aspiration of the joint fluid is often necessary to establish the diagnosis as well as to offer relief of symptoms (Chapter 684).

669.1 Discoid Lateral Meniscus

Lawrence Wells and Kriti Sehgal

Discoid lateral meniscus (DLM) is an anatomic variation of the lateral meniscus that may be asymptomatic or can cause snapping or popping of the knee. There are three types of DLM. The first is the **Wrisberg ligament type** where the lateral meniscus has no attachment to the tibial plateau posteriorly but has a meniscofemoral ligament or ligament of Wrisberg that connects the posterior horn of the lateral meniscus to the lateral surface of the medial femoral condyle. The ligament prevents the gliding of the meniscus during knee extension, producing a snap with each excursion of the meniscus, leading to hypertrophy and irregularity. The second type is the **complete type,** which is characterized by a thickened lateral meniscus that does not move in and out of the center of the joint and has normal peripheral attachments. The third type is the **incomplete type,** which is smaller than the complete type and does not fill the lateral compartment.

CLINICAL MANIFESTATIONS AND DIAGNOSIS

The cause of discoid meniscus is not defined, but it may be a failure of an embryologic sequence of degeneration of the center of the meniscus. The normal meniscus is attached around its periphery and glides anteriorly and posteriorly with knee motion, but a discoid meniscus is less mobile and may be torn. Occasionally, there is no peripheral attachment around the posterolateral aspect of the meniscus, which can allow it to become displaced anteriorly with knee flexion, producing a loud click or clunk.

The usual presenting complaint is that of a popping or snapping of the knee that is both heard and felt by the child or parent. This is often noted in children >6 yr of age. Most often the snapping is not painful and the child is active. A second type of presentation is of a child who has had no knee symptoms but presents spontaneously or after an injury with pain, snapping, popping, or locking located along the lateral joint line. Physical examination might show a mild effusion and tenderness with fullness over the lateral joint line and crepitation with motion. The typical findings include a palpable snapping as the knee flexes and extends. Along the lateral joint line, the examiner feels a bulge, as the meniscus seems to protrude beyond the margin of the tibia. As the knee moves, the meniscus snaps into the intercondylar notch and the bulge disappears.

Anteroposterior radiography of the knee can show widening of the lateral aspect of the knee joint. Other findings include flattening of the lateral femoral condyle (giving a squared off appearance) and cupping of the lateral aspect of the tibial plateau. MRI or arthroscopy is required for definitive diagnosis.

TREATMENT

Many children with discoid menisci require no treatment. These children should be followed and treated only if pain or loss of motion occurs. Surgery may be considered when DLM leads to locking, swelling, loss of motion, inability to run, or inability to participate in sports. The treatment is to excise tears and reshape the meniscus arthroscopically (Fig. 669-1). Meniscal instability can occasionally be repaired or reconstructed. Complete excision may be necessary if other procedures are unsuccessful.

BIBLIOGRAPHY

Please visit the Nelson Textbook of Pediatrics *website at www.expertconsult.com for the complete bibliography.*

669.2 Popliteal Cysts (Baker Cysts)

Lawrence Wells and Kriti Sehgal

Popliteal cysts, or **Baker cysts,** common in children, are cystic masses filled with gelatinous material that develop in the popliteal fossa, are usually asymptomatic, and are not related to intra-articular pathology. They usually resolve spontaneously, although the process can take several years.

The usual presentation is that of a mass behind the knee that may be fairly large when first noted. There are usually no symptoms of internal derangement of the knee. Physical examination reveals a firm mass in the popliteal fossa, often medially located and usually distal to the popliteal crease. The mass is most prominent when the knee is extended and the patient is lying in prone position.

The most common site of origin is the bursa of the gastrocnemius and semimembranosus. Another common site of origin is a herniation through the posterior joint capsule of the knee. Histologically, the cysts are classified as fibrous, synovial, inflammatory, or transitional. Transillumination of the cyst on physical examination is a simple diagnostic test. Knee radiographs are normal and should be obtained to identify other lesions such as osteochondromas, osteochondritis dissecans, and malignancies.

The diagnosis may be confirmed by ultrasonography (to differentiate a solid mass from a cystic lesion) or aspiration. In most cases, these cysts should be left alone, because they often resolve spontaneously. Surgical excision of a popliteal cyst is indicated only when symptoms are severe and limiting and have not resolved after several months. The presence of a solid mass detected on examination or MRI requires exploration.

BIBLIOGRAPHY
Please visit the Nelson Textbook of Pediatrics *website at www.expertconsult.com for the complete bibliography.*

669.3 Osteochondritis Dissecans

Lawrence Wells and Kriti Sehgal

Osteochondritis dissecans occurs when an area of bone adjacent to the articular cartilage becomes avascular and ultimately separates from the underlying bone. The exact cause is unknown; however, causes of osteochondral fractures of the femoral condyle include impingement from a tall tibial spine, direct blows causing compaction, rotary forces, and joint compression forces. The juvenile form might represent a disturbance of epiphyseal development, with small accessory islets of bone being separated from the epiphysis. Familial predisposition has been suggested. Most lesions are located on the lateral portion of the medial femoral condyle, although they can also involve the lateral femoral condyle or the patella. Characteristic pathology of the lesion includes an area of avascular necrosis with a cleft on either side, with varying degrees of ischemia and fibrosis of the overlying hyaline cartilage.

CLINICAL MANIFESTATIONS AND DIAGNOSIS

The most common presenting complaint is vague knee pain. If the fragment becomes loose, there can be crepitation, popping, giving way, and occasionally locking of the knee with or without a mild effusion. Physical findings are minimal and can include parapatellar tenderness, quadriceps atrophy, and slight pain with range of motion. The Wilson test is noted to be a specific diagnostic sign. It is performed by flexing the knee to 90 degrees, fully rotating the tibia medially, and then gradually extending the knee. When the test is positive, there is pain at 30 degrees of flexion that is located over the medial femoral condyle anteriorly.

The lesion is usually noted on anteroposterior, lateral, and tunnel radiographs (notch view) of the knee. Early lesions manifest with a small radiolucency at the articular surface, and more advanced lesions have a well-demarcated segment of subchondral bone with a lucent line separating it from the condyle. In young children, small foci of ossification can appear beyond the margin of the main ossific nucleus. As revascularization occurs, the bone heals spontaneously. With increasing age, the risk increases for articular cartilage fracture and separation of the bony fragment, producing a loose body.

MRI is helpful in determining the integrity of the articular cartilage and stability of the lesion. Arthroscopy is the most reliable method of evaluating the status of the lesion (Fig. 669-2). Factors commonly associated with a good prognosis are younger age group, small lesion, non–weight-bearing location, and no displacement. Four stages are involved with the progression of osteochondritis dissecans. Stage I consists of a small area of subchondral compression; stage II consists of a partially detached fragment; in stage III, the fragment is completely detached but remains in the crater; and by stage IV, the fragment is loose in the joint.

TREATMENT

The initial management of osteochondritis dissecans in children with open growth plates includes observation with enough activity restrictions to allow the symptoms to resolve. Most stable lesions heal spontaneously over several months. Stage I and II lesions are managed with activity modification, isometric exercises, and a knee immobilizer. Healing can be confirmed by follow-up radiographs, at which point the patient can return to normal activity levels. Arthroscopy is indicated in patients in whom nonoperative treatment fails and in those with signs, symptoms, and other studies suggesting an unstable lesion. Stage III lesions are managed by drilling and stabilization with Kirschner wires or pins. Stage IV lesions, if small, are managed by excision, and large lesions or those involving the weight-bearing areas are either replaced or internally fixed. Bone and cartilage grafting may be necessary in very severe cases with loss of large fragments. After surgery, patients participate in a physical therapy program and may or may not be allowed to return to their preoperative activity levels. Treating osteochondritis dissecans early and effectively often prevents recurrent symptoms in adulthood, although some very severe lesions are symptomatic later in life.

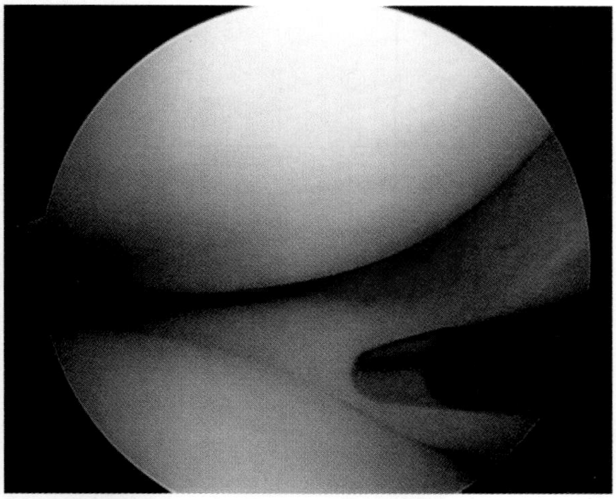

Figure 669-2 Classic arthroscopic image of osteochondritis dissecans lesion.

BIBLIOGRAPHY
Please visit the Nelson Textbook of Pediatrics *website at www.expertconsult.com for the complete bibliography.*

669.4 Osgood-Schlatter Disease

Lawrence Wells and Kriti Sehgal

Osgood-Schlatter disease manifests as pain over the tibial tubercle in a growing child. The patellar tendon inserts into the tibia tubercle, which is an extension of the proximal tibial epiphysis. Osgood-Schlatter disease is likely a traction apophysitis of the tibial tubercle growth plate and the adjacent patellar tendon. It occurs during late childhood or adolescence, especially in athletes, and is likely due to repetitive tensile microtrauma. It occurs between the ages of 10 and 15 yr; the onset in girls is about 2 yr before that in boys. It is more common in boys.

This disorder is self-limited in most patients and resolves with skeletal maturity. Pain directly over the tibial tubercle is the usual complaint, and swelling over the tubercle is often of concern. The pain is aggravated by activities but often persists even at rest. Physical examination reveals point tenderness over the tibial tubercle and the distal portion of the patellar tendon. There is often increased prominence of the tibia tubercle that is also firm.

Radiographs are usually the only diagnostic studies necessary (Fig. 669-3). Fragmentary ossification of the tibial tubercle is noted in some cases, which is often a normal variant. Some cases are associated with patella alta.

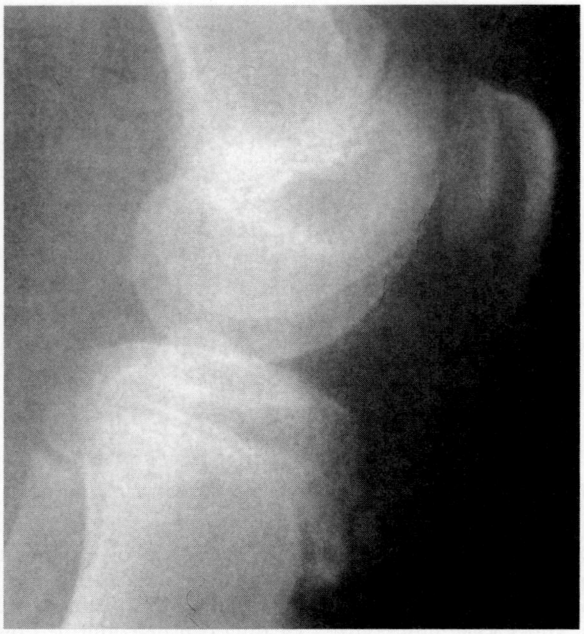

Figure 669-3 Lateral radiograph of the knee demonstrating apophysitis of the tibial tubercle in Osgood-Schlatter disease.

Rest, restriction of activities, and, occasionally, a knee immobilizer may be necessary, combined with an isometric and flexibility exercise program. Reassurance is important, because some patients and parents fear that the swollen tubercle may be a sign of malignancy. Complete resolution of symptoms through physiologic healing (physeal closure) of the tibia tubercle can require 12-24 mo. Removal of ossicles from the tubercle is rarely necessary in patients with persistent disabling symptoms. Complications are rare and include early closure of the tibial tubercle with recurvatum deformity and rarely patellar tendon rupture or avulsion of the tibial tubercle.

PATELLOFEMORAL DISORDERS

Patellofemoral joint stability depends on balance among the restraining ligaments, muscle forces, and the articular anatomy of the patellofemoral groove. The multiple factors that contribute to patellofemoral instability include quadriceps insufficiency, internal femoral torsion, external tibial torsion, the shallow sulcus, lateral tether, medial capsular attenuation, condylar hypoplasia, and genu valgum.

The patella has a V-shaped bottom that guides it through the sulcus in the distal femur. The force of the muscles pulling through the quadriceps mechanism and the patellar tendon do not act in a straight line because the patellar tendon inclines in a slightly lateral direction with respect to the line of the quadriceps. This is normally called the *Q angle*. This lateral movement, coupled with the movement of the restraining ligaments, tends to move the patella in a lateral direction. The vastus medialis muscle is necessary to counteract the laterally acting forces. An abnormality of any one or a group of these factors can make the patellofemoral joint function abnormally. Excessive instability of the patellofemoral joint can manifest as acute patellar dislocation, recurrent patellar subluxation or dislocation, habitual dislocation, and chronic dislocation.

BIBLIOGRAPHY

Please visit the Nelson Textbook of Pediatrics *website at www.expertconsult.com for the complete bibliography.*

669.5 Idiopathic Adolescent Anterior Knee Pain Syndrome

Lawrence Wells and Kriti Sehgal

Previously known as *chondromalacia patella*, idiopathic adolescent anterior knee pain syndrome or patellofemoral stress syndrome is common in adolescent girls, is often activity related and poorly localized, and can cause disability. It was originally thought to result from a deranged articular surface, and the name was changed with growing evidence that the articular surface is normal. The cause of the knee pain is unknown.

CLINICAL MANIFESTATIONS AND DIAGNOSIS

Symptoms are usually produced by vigorous physical activities such as running. There is usually no history of antecedent trauma. There are no mechanical symptoms associated such as locking, giving way, or recurrent effusion.

Active and passive range of motion of the knee, alignment of the lower extremity, knee stability, patellar tracking, areas of focal tenderness, and gait should be evaluated to identify any obvious causes of knee pain or instability. Routine radiographs, including anteroposterior, lateral, and tunnel views, are not particularly helpful in evaluating the cause of adolescent anterior knee pain, except that they can eliminate other etiologies. In the adolescent group, radiographs of the hip should be considered in suspected cases to rule out a slipped capital femoral epiphysis that can manifest as ill-defined knee pain.

TREATMENT

The natural history of anterior knee pain is one of spontaneous resolution over a period of years. The treatment is predominantly nonoperative and may include flexibility exercises, strengthening exercises (isometric quadriceps), contrast therapies (ice and heat), orthoses, and medications (nonsteroidal anti-inflammatory drugs). A success rate of 70-90% can be anticipated. Arthroscopic evaluation of the knee and patellofemoral joint is rarely necessary.

BIBLIOGRAPHY

Please visit the Nelson Textbook of Pediatrics *website at www.expertconsult.com for the complete bibliography.*

669.6 Patellar Subluxation and Dislocation

Lawrence Wells and Kriti Sehgal

Recurrent patellar dislocation is defined as >1 episode of dislocation of the patella documented by an observer or clearly described by the patient. **Recurrent patellar subluxation** describes the condition of >1 episode of patellar subluxation without frank dislocation. **Habitual dislocation of the patella** is defined as a dislocation that occurs every time the knee is flexed, and a **chronic dislocation of the patella** is one that never reduces throughout the arc of motion of the knee.

Traumatic patellar subluxation and dislocation can occur as a result of a direct trauma. Habitual subluxation or dislocation is usually due to a dysplastic knee with contracture of the lateral portion of the quadriceps mechanism. In this case, the patella displaces laterally whenever the knee is flexed. The most common etiologic factor in recurrent patellar dislocation is lateral malalignment of the quadriceps mechanism. A number of syndromes are associated with patellar instability, including Down syndrome, Turner syndrome, Kabuki make-up syndrome, and Rubinstein-Taybi syndrome.

CLINICAL MANIFESTATIONS AND DIAGNOSIS

The physical examination findings usually suggest the diagnosis. After an acute dislocation, there may be a hemarthrosis from capsular tearing or an osteochondral fracture. If the child is seen after a recent dislocation, there may be parapatellar tenderness and a mild effusion.

Examination of a child with a maltracking patella that is predisposed to dislocation often shows terminal subluxation of the patella when the knee is brought into full extension. There may be tenderness to palpation over the inferior surface of the lateral facet of the patella. Observe the tracking of the patella as the patient is allowed to flex the knee from full extension. In the patient with instability, the patella shifts laterally just as the knee begins to flex and then shifts medially with further flexion. This lateral displacement of the patella followed by medial movement is termed **J tracking.** The other classic physical sign is the **Fairbanks apprehension sign.** With the knee in 30 degrees of flexion, the examiner manually displaces the patella laterally and yields a subjective feeling of subluxation, resulting in the patient grabbing the examiner's hand to prevent manipulative dislocation.

It is important to assess the torsional profile of the patient to rule out possible rotational abnormalities of the femur or tibia or both.

Radiographic studies can help identify factors contributing to recurrent dislocation of the patella or after an acute dislocation. They should include anteroposterior, lateral, and skyline tangential views (obtained in full flexion) of the patella to assess for an osteochondral fracture from the lateral femoral condyle or the patella. Other views include the MacNab view (obtained with the knee in 40 degrees of flexion), which shows the relationship of the patella to the anterior part of the femoral intercondylar groove and might also demonstrate loose bodies and fractures of the patella or lateral condyle; the Merchant view obtained with the knee in 45 degrees of flexion; and the Laurin view with the knee in 20 degrees of flexion.

TREATMENT

An initial traumatic dislocation of the patella should be treated with a knee immobilizer for comfort. After a few days, the patient should begin isometric quadriceps-strengthening exercises, and more vigorous strengthening exercises can be done as the tenderness resolves. Once the immobilization is discontinued (~6 wk), the isometric exercise program should be continued until the knee is fully rehabilitated. Using this method, approximately 75% of patients do not have recurrent dislocations.

Initial management of recurrent dislocation of the patella should be nonoperative. If patellar subluxation is due to dynamic muscle imbalance, a specific muscle rehabilitation program, such as strengthening the vastus medialis, may be successful. Patellar stabilizing orthosis may be useful, although the mechanism of action and efficacy is uncertain.

Operative stabilization may be necessary with continued episodes of dislocation or failure of conservative management for patellar subluxation. The surgical approaches to growing children focus on realigning the quadriceps mechanism usually in combination with a lateral release and the creation of a medial patellar restraint. Realignment of the extensor mechanism may be accomplished by altering the muscle itself, changing its insertion into the patella, or altering the attachment of the patella to the tibia. Depending on the extent of involvement, an arthroscopic lateral release with or without a soft-tissue reconstruction with a realignment procedure may be performed. Torsional abnormalities of the femur or tibia may be addressed with rotational osteotomy of the distal femur or proximal tibia, or rarely both as deemed necessary.

BIBLIOGRAPHY

Please visit the Nelson Textbook of Pediatrics *website at www.expertconsult.com for the complete bibliography.*

Chapter 670
The Hip

Wudbhav N. Sankar, B. David Horn, Lawrence Wells, and John P. Dormans

The hip joint is a pivotal joint of the lower extremity, and its functional demands require both stability and flexibility. Anatomically, the hip joint is a ball-and-socket articulation between the femoral head and acetabulum.

GROWTH AND DEVELOPMENT

The hip joint begins to develop at about the 7th week of gestation, when a cleft appears in the mesenchyme of the primitive limb bud. These precartilaginous cells differentiate into a fully formed cartilaginous **femoral head** and **acetabulum** by the 11th week of gestation (Chapter 6.1). At birth, the neonatal acetabulum is completely composed of cartilage, with a thin rim of fibrocartilage called the **labrum.**

The very cellular hyaline cartilage of the acetabulum is continuous with the triradiate cartilages, which divide and interconnect the three osseous components of the pelvis (the **ilium, ischium,** and **pubis**). The concave shape of the hip joint is determined by the presence of a spherical femoral head.

Several factors determine acetabular depth, including interstitial growth within the acetabular cartilage, appositional growth under the perichondrium, and growth of adjacent bones (the ilium, ischium, and pubis). In the neonate, the entire proximal femur is a cartilaginous structure, which includes the femoral head and the greater and lesser trochanters. The three main growth areas are the physeal plate, the growth plate of the greater trochanter, and the femoral neck isthmus. Between the 4th and 7th mo of life, the proximal femoral ossification center (in the center of the femoral head) appears. This ossification center continues to enlarge, along with its cartilaginous anlage, until adult life, when only a thin layer of articular cartilage remains. During this period of growth, the thickness of the cartilage surrounding this bony nucleus gradually decreases, as does the thickness of the acetabular cartilage. The growth of the proximal femur is affected by muscle pull, the forces transmitted across the hip joint with weight bearing, normal joint nutrition, circulation, and muscle tone. Alterations in these factors can cause profound changes in development of the proximal femur.

VASCULAR SUPPLY

The blood supply to the capital femoral epiphysis is complex and changes with growth of the proximal femur. The proximal femur receives its arterial supply from intraosseous (primarily the medial femoral circumflex artery) and extraosseous vessels (Fig. 670-1). The **retinacular vessels** (extraosseous) lie on the surface of the femoral neck but are intracapsular because they enter the epiphysis from the periphery. This makes the blood supply vulnerable to damage from septic arthritis, trauma, thrombosis, and other vascular insults. Interruption of this tenuous blood supply can lead to avascular necrosis of the femoral head and permanent deformity of the hip.

BIBLIOGRAPHY

Please visit the Nelson Textbook of Pediatrics *website at www.expertconsult.com for the complete bibliography.*

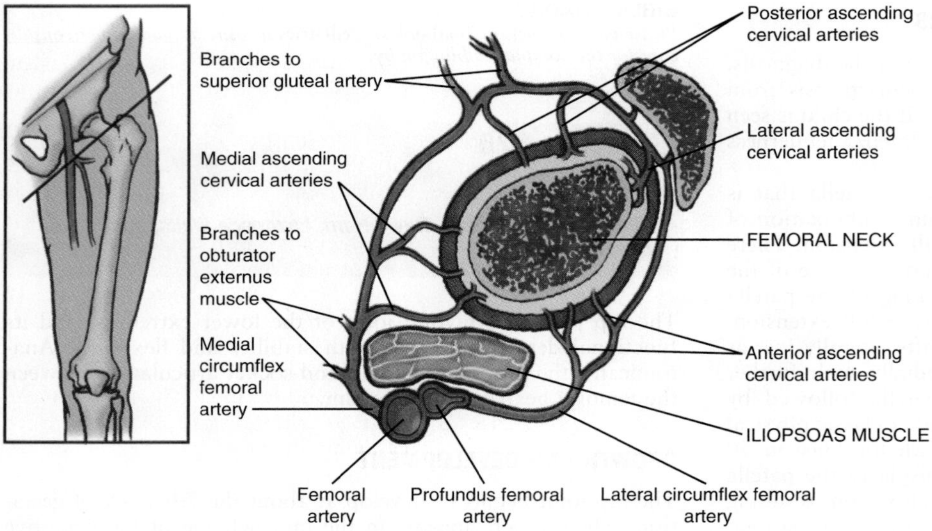

Figure 670-1 Diagrammatic illustration of vascular anatomy of the proximal femur.

670.1 Developmental Dysplasia of the Hip

Wudbhav N. Sankar, B. David Horn, Lawrence Wells, and John P. Dormans

Developmental dysplasia of the hip (DDH) refers to a spectrum of pathology in the development of the immature hip joint. The original term for the condition, congenital dislocation of the hip, was replaced by the current name to more accurately reflect the variable presentation of the disorder and to encompass mild dysplasias as well as frank dislocations.

CLASSIFICATION

Acetabular **dysplasia** refers to abnormal morphology and development of the acetabulum. Hip **subluxation** is defined as partial contact between the femoral head and acetabulum, whereas **dislocation** refers to a hip with no contact between the articulating surfaces of the hip. DDH is classified into two major groups: **typical** and **teratologic.** Typical DDH occurs in otherwise normal patients or those without defined syndromes or genetic conditions. Teratologic hip dislocations usually have identifiable causes such as arthrogyposis or a genetic syndrome and occur before birth.

ETIOLOGY AND RISK FACTORS

Although the exact etiology remains unknown, the final common pathway in the development of DDH is increased laxity of the hip capsule, which fails to maintain a stable femoroacetabular articulation. This increased laxity is probably the result of a combination of hormonal, mechanical, and genetic factors. A positive family history for DDH is found in 12-33% of affected patients. DDH is more common among female patients (80%). This is thought to be due to the greater susceptibility of female fetuses to maternal hormones such as relaxin, which increases ligamentous laxity. Although only 2-3% of all babies are born in breech presentation, the rate is 16-25% for patients with DDH.

Any condition that leads to a tighter intrauterine space and, consequently, less room for normal fetal motion may be associated with DDH. These conditions include oligohydramnios, large birth weight, and first pregnancy. The high rate of association of DDH with other intrauterine molding abnormalities, such as torticollis and metatarsus adductus, supports the theory that the "crowding phenomenon" has a role in the pathogenesis. The left hip is the most commonly affected hip; in the most common fetal position, this is the hip that is usually forced into adduction against the mother's sacrum.

EPIDEMIOLOGY

Although most newborn screening studies suggest that some degree of hip instability can be detected in 1/100 to 1/250 babies, actual dislocated or dislocatable hips are much less common, being found in 1-1.5 of 1000 live births.

There is marked geographic and racial variation in the incidence of DDH. The reported incidence based on geography ranges from 1.7/1,000 babies in Sweden to 75/1,000 in Yugoslavia to 188.5/1,000 in a district in Manitoba, Canada. The incidence of DDH in Chinese and African newborns is almost 0%, whereas it is 1% for hip dysplasia and 0.1% for hip dislocation in white newborns. These differences may be due to environmental factors, such as child-rearing practices, rather than to genetic predisposition. African and Asian caregivers have traditionally carried babies against their bodies in a shawl so that a child's hips are flexed, abducted, and free to move. This keeps the hips in the optimal position for stability and for dynamic molding of the developing acetabulum by the cartilaginous femoral head. Children in Native American and Eastern European cultures, which have a relatively high incidence of DDH, have historically been swaddled in confining clothes that bring their hips into extension. This position increases the tension of the psoas muscle-tendon unit and might predispose the hips to displace and eventually dislocate laterally and superiorly.

PATHOANATOMY

In DDH, several secondary anatomic changes can develop that can prevent reduction. Both the fatty tissue in the depths of the socket, known as the **pulvinar,** and the ligamentum teres can hypertrophy, blocking reduction of the femoral head. The transverse acetabular ligament usually thickens as well, which effectively narrows the opening of the acetabulum. In addition, the shortened iliopsoas tendon becomes taut across the front of the hip, creating an hourglass shape to the hip capsule, which limits access to the acetabulum. Over time, the dislocated femoral head places pressure on the acetabular rim and labrum, causing the labrum to infold and become thick.

The shape of a normal femoral head and acetabulum depends on a concentric reduction between the two. The more time that a hip spends dislocated, the more likely that the acetabulum will develop abnormally. Without a femoral head to provide a template, the acetabulum will become progressively shallow, with an oblique acetabular roof and a thickened medial wall.

CLINICAL FINDINGS

The Neonate

DDH in the neonate is asymptomatic and must be screened for by specific maneuvers. Physical examination must be carried out with the infant unclothed and placed supine in a warm, comfortable setting on a flat examination table.

The **Barlow** provocative maneuver assesses the potential for dislocation of a nondisplaced hip. The examiner adducts the flexed hip and gently pushes the thigh posteriorly in an effort to dislocate the femoral head (Fig. 670-2). In a positive test, the hip is felt to slide out of the acetabulum. As the examiner relaxes the proximal push, the hip can be felt to slip back into the acetabulum.

The **Ortolani** test is the reverse of Barlow test: The examiner attempts to reduce a dislocated hip (Fig. 670-3). The examiner grasps the child's thigh between the thumb and index finger and, with the 4th and 5th fingers, lifts the greater trochanter while simultaneously abducting the hip. When the test is positive, the femoral head will slip into the socket with a delicate clunk that is palpable but usually not audible. It should be a gentle, non-forced maneuver.

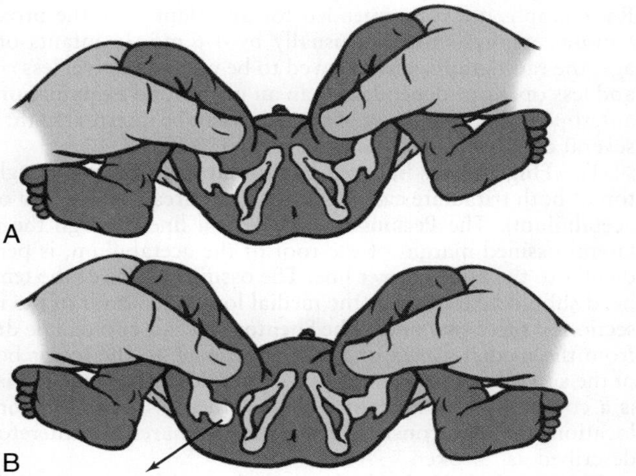

Figure 670-2 The Barlow provocative test is performed with the patient's knees and hips flexed. *A,* Holding the patient's limbs gently, with the thigh in adduction, the examiner applies a posteriorly directed force. *B,* This test is positive in a dislocatable hip.

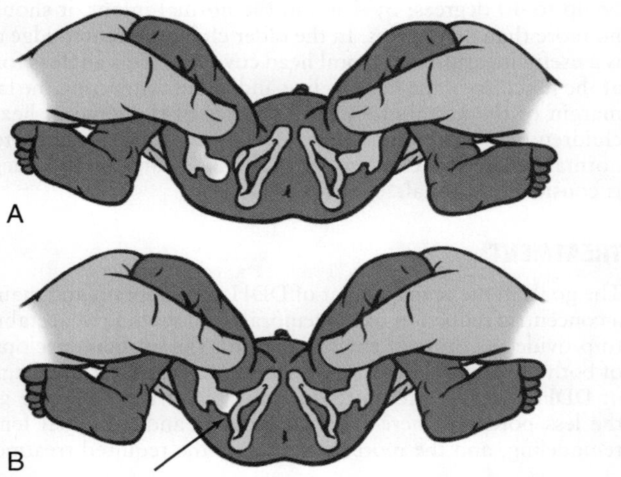

Figure 670-3 The Ortolani maneuver is the sign of the ball of the femoral head moving in and out of the acetabulum. *A,* The examiner holds the patient's thigh and gently abducts the hip while lifting the greater trochanter with two fingers. *B,* When the test is positive, the dislocated femoral head falls back into the acetabulum with a palpable clunk as the hip is abducted.

A **hip click** is the high-pitched sensation (or sound) felt at the very end of abduction during testing for DDH with Barlow and Ortolani maneuvers. Classically, a hip click is differentiated from a hip clunk, which is felt as the hip goes in and out of joint. Hip clicks usually originate in the ligamentum teres or occasionally in the fascia lata or psoas tendon and do not indicate a significant hip abnormality.

The Infant

As the baby enters the 2nd and 3rd months of life, the soft tissues begin to tighten and the Ortolani and Barlow tests are no longer reliable. In this age group, the examiner must look for other specific physical findings including limited hip abduction, apparent shortening of the thigh, proximal location of the greater trochanter, asymmetry of the gluteal or thigh folds (Fig. 670-4), and pistoning of the hip. Limitation of abduction is the most reliable sign of a dislocated hip in this age group.

Shortening of the thigh, the **Galeazzi sign,** is best appreciated by placing both hips in 90 degrees of flexion and comparing the height of the knees, looking for asymmetry (Fig. 670-5). Asymmetry of thigh and gluteal skin folds may be present in 10% of normal infants but suggests DDH. Another helpful test is the **Klisic test,** in which the examiner places the 3rd finger over the greater trochanter and the index finger of the same hand on the anterior superior iliac spine. In a normal hip, an imaginary line drawn between the two fingers points to the umbilicus. In the dislocated hip, the trochanter is elevated, and the line projects halfway between the umbilicus and the pubis (Fig. 670-6).

The Walking Child

The walking child often presents to the physician after the family has noticed a limp, a waddling gait, or a leg-length discrepancy. The affected side appears shorter than the normal extremity, and the child toe-walks on the affected side. The Trendelenburg sign is positive in these children, and an abductor lurch is usually observed when the child walks. As in the younger child, there is limited hip abduction on the affected side and the knees are at different levels when the hips are flexed (the Galeazzi sign). Excessive lordosis, which develops secondary to altered hip mechanics, is common and is often the presenting complaint.

DIAGNOSTIC TESTING

Ultrasonography

Because it is superior to radiographs for evaluating cartilaginous structures, ultrasonography is the diagnostic modality of choice for DDH before the appearance of the femoral head ossific

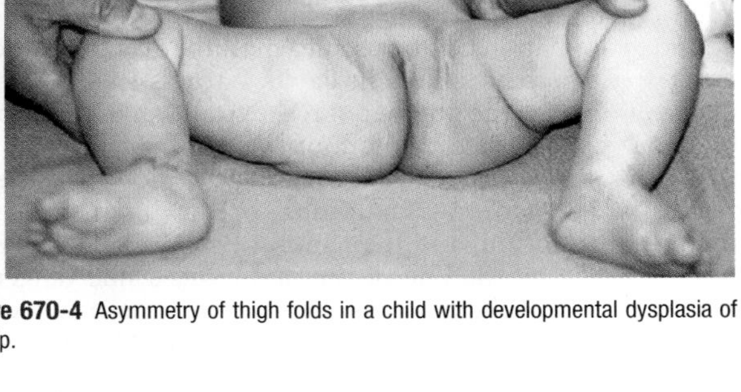

Figure 670-4 Asymmetry of thigh folds in a child with developmental dysplasia of the hip.

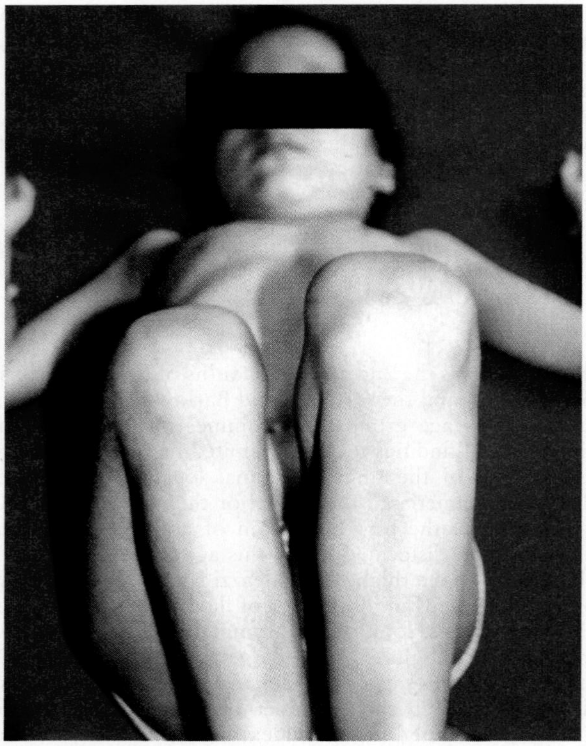

Figure 670-5 Positive Galeazzi sign noted in a case of untreated developmental dysplasia of the hip.

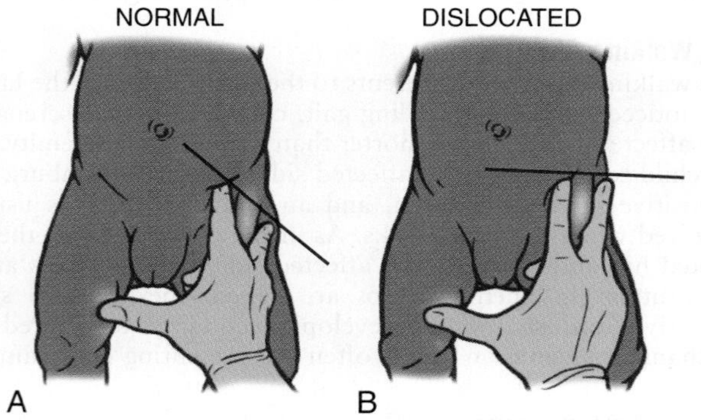

Figure 670-6 Klisic test. *A,* In a normal hip, an imaginary line drawn down through the tip of an index finger placed on the patient's iliac crest and the tip of the long finger placed on the patient's greater trochanter should point to the umbilicus. *B,* In a dislocated hip, this line drawn through the two fingertips runs below the umbilicus because the greater trochanter is abnormally high.

nucleus (4-6 mo). During the early newborn period (0-4 wk), however, physical examination is preferred over ultrasonography because there is a high incidence of false-positive sonograms in this age group. In addition to elucidating the static relationship of the femur to the acetabulum, ultrasonography provides dynamic information about the stability of the hip joint. The ultrasound examination can be used to monitor acetabular development, particularly of infants in Pavlik harness treatment; this method can minimize the number of radiographs taken and might allow the clinician to detect failure of treatment earlier.

In the Graf technique, the transducer is placed over the greater trochanter, which allows visualization of the ilium, the bony acetabulum, the labrum, and the femoral epiphysis (Fig. 670-7). The angle formed by the line of the ilium and a line tangential to the boney roof of the acetabulum is termed the α **angle** and represents the depth of the acetabulum. Values >60 degrees are considered normal, and those <60 degrees imply acetabular dysplasia. The β **angle** is formed by a line drawn tangential to the labrum and the line of the ilium; this represents the cartilaginous roof of the acetabulum. A normal β angle is <55 degrees; as the femoral head subluxates, the β angle increases. Another useful test is to evaluate the position of the center of the head compared to the vertical line of the ilium. If the line of the ilium falls lateral to the center of the head, the epiphysis is considered reduced. If the line falls medial to the center of the head, the epiphysis is undercovered and is either subluxated or dislocated.

Screening for DDH with ultrasound remains controversial. Although routinely performed in Europe, ultrasonographic screening has not been shown to be cost effective in the USA largely because of the cost associated with treating false-positive results. The current recommendations are that every newborn undergo a clinical examination for hip instability. Children who have findings suspicious for DDH should be followed up with ultrasound. Most authors agree that infants with risk factors for DDH (breech position, family history, torticollis) should be screened with ultrasound regardless of the clinical findings.

Radiography

Radiographs are recommended for an infant once the proximal femoral epiphysis ossifies, usually by 4-6 mo. In infants of this age, the radiographs have proved to be more effective, less costly, and less operator dependent than an ultrasound examination. An anteroposterior (AP) view of the pelvis can be interpreted through several classic lines drawn on it (Fig. 670-8).

The **Hilgenreiner line** is a horizontal line drawn through the top of both triradiate cartilages (the clear area in the depth of the acetabulum). The **Perkins line**, a vertical line through the most lateral ossified margin of the roof of the acetabulum, is perpendicular to the Hilgenreiner line. The ossific nucleus of the femoral head should be located in the medial lower quadrant of the intersection of these two lines. The **Shenton line** is a curved line drawn from the medial aspect of the femoral neck to the lower border of the superior pubic ramus. In a child with normal hips, this line is a continuous contour. In a child with hip subluxation or dislocation, this line consists of two separate arcs and therefore is described as "broken."

The **acetabular index** is the angle formed between the Hilgenreiner line and a line drawn from the depth of the acetabular socket to the most lateral ossified margin of the roof of the acetabulum. This angle measures the development of the osseous roof of the acetabulum. In the newborn, the acetabular index can be up to 40 degrees; by 4 mo in the normal infant, it should be no more than 30 degrees. In the older child, the **center-edge angle** is a useful measure of femoral head coverage. This angle is formed at the juncture of the Perkins line and a line connecting the lateral margin of the acetabulum to the center of the femoral head. In children 6-13 yr old, an angle >19 degrees has been reported as normal, whereas in children 14 yr and older, an angle >25 degrees is considered normal.

TREATMENT

The goals in the management of DDH are to obtain and maintain a concentric reduction of the femoral head within the acetabulum to provide the optimal environment for the normal development of both the femoral head and acetabulum. The later the diagnosis of DDH is made, the more difficult it is to achieve these goals, the less potential there is for acetabular and proximal femoral remodeling, and the more complex are the required treatments.

Newborns and Infants Younger Than 6 Months

Newborns hips that are Barlow positive (reduced but dislocatable) or Ortolani positive (dislocated but reducible) should generally be treated with a Pavlik harness as soon as the diagnosis is made. The management of newborns with dysplasia who are

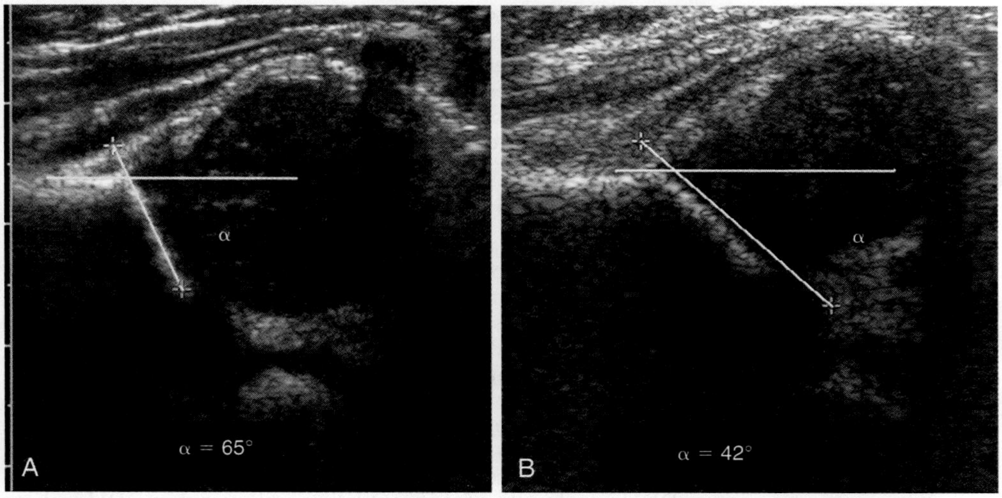

Figure 670-7 *A,* Normal ultrasonographic image of the hip in an infant. The alpha angle is >60 degrees. Note that a line drawn tangential to the ilium falls lateral to the center of the femoral head. *B,* In this child with developmental dysplasia of the hip, the left hip demonstrates an α angle of 42 degrees, and a line drawn tangential to the ilium shows that <50% of the femoral head is contained within the acetabulum.

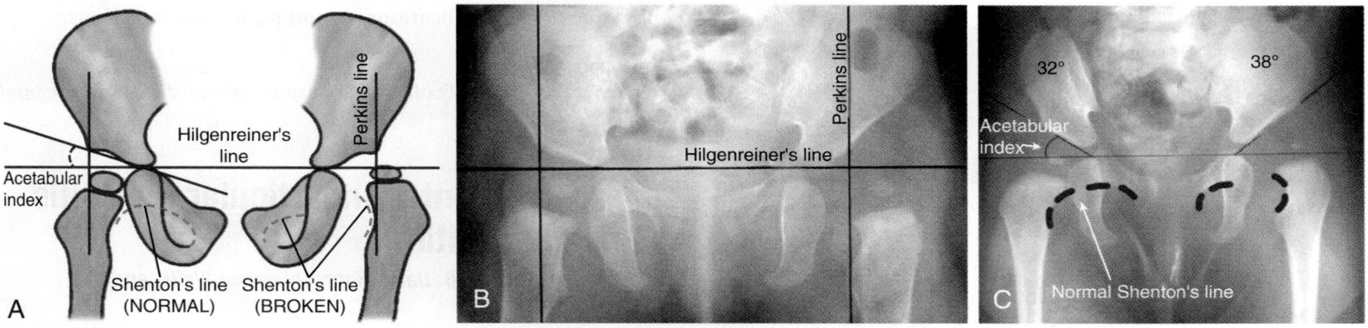

Figure 670-8 *A-C,* Radiographic measurements are useful in evaluating developmental dysplasia of the hip. The Hilgenreiner line is drawn through the triradiate cartilages. The Perkins line is drawn perpendicular to the Hilgenreiner line at the lateral edge of the acetabulum. The ossific nucleus of the femoral head should be located in the medial lower quadrant of the intersection of these two lines. The Shenton line curves along the femoral metaphysis and connects smoothly to the inner margin of the pubis. In a child with hip subluxation or dislocation, this line consists of two separate arcs and therefore is described as broken. The acetabular index is the angle between a line drawn along the margin of the acetabulum and the Hilgenreiner line; in normal newborns, it averages 27.5 degrees and decreases with age.

<4 wk of age is less clear. A significant proportion of these hips normalize within 3-4 wk; therefore, many physicians prefer to reexamine these newborns after a few weeks before making treatment decisions.

Triple diapers or abduction diapers have no place in the treatment of DDH in the newborn; they are usually ineffective and give the family a false sense of security. *Acetabular dysplasia, subluxation, or dislocation can all be readily managed with the Pavlik harness.* Although other braces are available (von Rosen splint, Frejka pillow), the Pavlik harness remains the most commonly used device worldwide (Fig. 670-9). By maintaining the Ortolani-positive hip in a Pavlik harness on a full-time basis for 6 wk, hip instability resolves in 95% of cases. After 6 mo of age, the failure rate for the Pavlik harness is >50% because it is difficult to maintain the increasingly active and crawling child in the harness. Frequent examinations and readjustments are necessary to ensure that the harness is fitting correctly. The anterior straps of the harness should be set to maintain the hips in flexion (usually ~100 degrees); excessive flexion is discouraged because of the risk of femoral nerve palsy. The posterior straps are designed to encourage abduction. These are generally set to allow adduction just to neutral, as forced abduction by the harness can lead to avascular necrosis of the femoral epiphysis.

If follow-up examinations and ultrasounds do not demonstrate concentric reduction of the hip after 3-4 wk of Pavlik harness treatment, the harness should be abandoned. Continued use of the harness beyond this period in a persistently dislocated hip can cause "Pavlik harness disease," or wearing away of the posterior aspect of the acetabulum, which can make the ultimate reduction less stable.

Children 6 Months to 2 Years of Age

The principal goals in the treatment of the late-diagnosed dysplasia are to obtain and maintain reduction of the hip without damaging the femoral head. **Closed reductions** are performed in the operating room under general anesthesia. The hip is moved to determine the range of motion in which it remains reduced. This is compared to the maximal range of motion to construct a "safe zone" (Fig. 670-10). An arthrogram obtained at the time of reduction is very helpful for evaluating the depth and stability of the reduction (Fig. 670-11). The reduction is maintained in a well-molded spica cast, with the "human position" of moderate flexion and abduction being the preferred position. After the procedure, single-cut CT or MRI may be used to confirm the reduction. Twelve weeks after closed reduction, the plaster cast is removed; an abduction orthosis is often used at this point to encourage further remodeling of the acetabulum. Failure to obtain a stable hip with a closed reduction indicates the need for an **open reduction.** In patients <2 yr of age, a secondary acetabular or femoral procedure is rarely required. The potential for acetabular development after closed or open reduction is excellent and continues for 4-8 yr after the procedure.

Children Older Than 2 Years

Children 2-6 yr of age with a hip dislocation usually require an open reduction. In this age group, a concomitant femoral

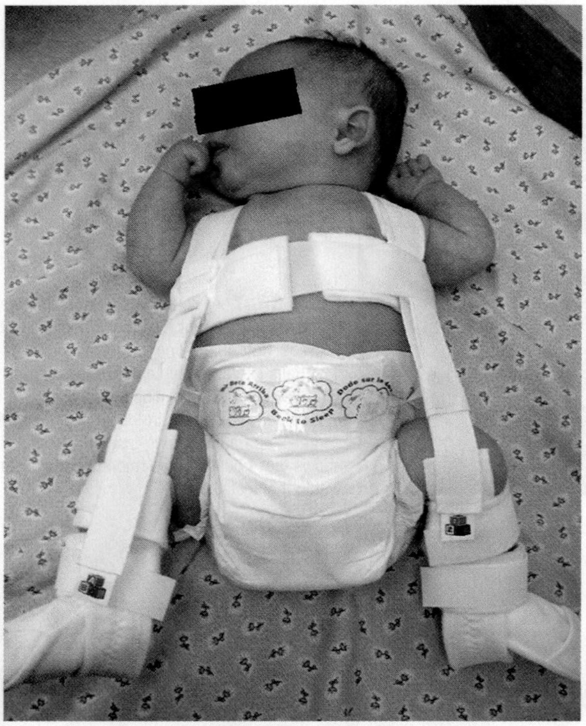

Figure 670-9 Photograph of a Pavlik harness.

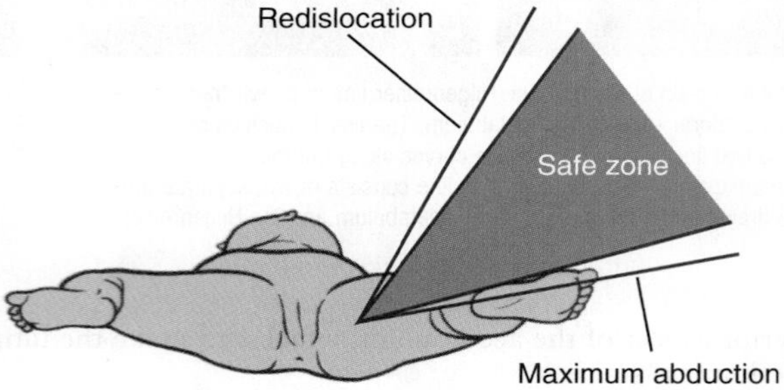

Figure 670-10 Diagrammatic illustration of the safe zone of Ramsey.

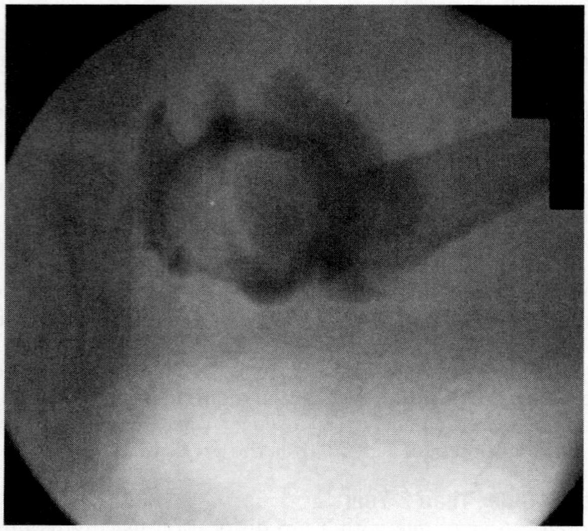

Figure 670-11 Arthrogram of a reduced hip for evaluating the stability of reduction.

shortening osteotomy is often performed to reduce the pressure on the proximal femur and minimize the risk of osteonecrosis. Because the potential for acetabular development is markedly diminished in these older children, a pelvic osteotomy is usually performed in conjunction with the open reduction. Postoperatively, patients are immobilized in a spica cast for 6-12 wk.

COMPLICATIONS

The most important complication of DDH is avascular necrosis of the femoral epiphysis. Reduction of the femoral head under pressure or in extreme abduction can result in occlusion of the epiphyseal vessels and produce either partial or total infarction of the epiphysis. Revascularization soon follows, but if the physis is severely damaged, abnormal growth and development can occur. The hip is most vulnerable to this complication before 4-6 mo, when the ossific nucleus appears. Management, as previously outlined, is designed to minimize this complication. With appropriate treatment, the incidence of avascular necrosis for DDH is reduced to 5-15%. Other complications in DDH include redislocation, residual subluxation, acetabular dysplasia, and postoperative complications, including wound infections.

BIBLIOGRAPHY

Please visit the Nelson Textbook of Pediatrics *website at* *www.expertconsult.com* *for the complete bibliography.*

670.2 Transient Monoarticular Synovitis (Toxic Synovitis)

Wudbhav N. Sankar, B. David Horn, Lawrence Wells, and John P. Dormans

Transient synovitis (toxic synovitis) is a reactive arthritis that characteristically affects the hip and is one of the most common causes of hip pain in young children.

ETIOLOGY

The cause of transient synovitis remains unknown. Most authors believe that transient synovitis is a nonspecific inflammatory condition. Others have suggested that the condition is a postviral immunologic synovitis because it tends to follow recent viral illnesses.

CLINICAL MANIFESTATIONS

Although transient synovitis can occur in all age groups, it is most prevalent in children between 3 and 8 yr of age, with a mean onset at age 6 yr. About 70% of all affected children have had a nonspecific upper respiratory tract infection 7-14 days before the onset of symptoms. Symptoms often develop acutely and usually consist of pain in the groin, anterior thigh, or knee, which may be referred from the hip. These children are usually ambulatory. The hip is not held flexed, abducted, or laterally rotated unless a significant effusion is present. Children with transient monoarticular synovitis walk with a painful, limping gait. They are often afebrile or have a low-grade fever <38°C.

DIAGNOSIS

Transient synovitis is a clinical diagnosis, but laboratory and radiographic tests can be useful to rule out other more serious conditions. In transient synovitis, infection labs (erythrocyte sedimentation rate [ESR], serum C-reactive protein [CRP], and white blood cell counts [WBC]) are relatively normal, but on occasion a mild elevation in the ESR is observed. AP and Lauenstein (frog-leg) lateral radiographs of the pelvis may be acquired and are also usually found to be normal. Ultrasonography of the hip is preferred to x-rays and often demonstrates a joint effusion.

The most important condition to exclude before confirming a diagnosis of toxic synovitis is septic arthritis. Children with septic arthritis usually appear more systemically ill than those with transient synovitis. The pain associated with septic arthritis is more severe, and children often refuse to walk or move their hip at all. High fever, refusal to walk, and elevations of the ESR, serum CRP, and WBC all point toward a diagnosis of septic arthritis. If the clinical scenario is suspicious for septic arthritis, an ultrasonography-guided aspiration of the hip joint should be performed to make the definitive diagnosis (Chapter 677).

TREATMENT

The treatment of transient monoarticular synovitis of the hip is symptomatic. Recommended therapies include activity limitation and relief of weight bearing until the pain subsides. Anti-inflammatory agents and analgesics can shorten the duration of pain. Most children recover completely within 3 wk.

BIBLIOGRAPHY

Please visit the Nelson Textbook of Pediatrics *website at www.expertconsult.com for the complete bibliography.*

670.3 Legg-Calvé-Perthes Disease

Wudbhav N. Sankar, B. David Horn, Lawrence Wells, and John P. Dormans

Legg-Calvé-Perthes disease (LCPD) is a hip disorder of unknown etiology that results from temporary interruption of the blood supply to the proximal femoral epiphysis, leading to osteonecrosis and femoral head deformity.

ETIOLOGY

Although the underlying etiology remains obscure, most authors agree that the final common pathway in the development of LCPD is disruption of the vascular supply to the femoral epiphysis, which results in ischemia and osteonecrosis. Infection, trauma, and transient synovitis have all been proposed as causative factors but are unsubstantiated. Factors leading to thrombophilia, an increased tendency to develop thrombosis and hypofibrinolysis, and a reduced ability to lyse thrombi have been identified. Factor V Leyden mutation, protein C and S deficiency, lupus anticoagulant, anticardiolipin antibodies, antitrypsin, and plasminogen activator might play a role in the abnormal clotting mechanism. These abnormalities in the clotting cascade are thought to increase blood viscosity and the risk for venous thrombosis. Poor venous outflow leads to increased intraosseous pressure, which in turn impedes arterial inflow, causing ischemia and cell death.

EPIDEMIOLOGY

The overall incidence of LCPD in the USA is about 1/1,200 children. LCPD is more common in boys than in girls by a ratio of 4 or 5 to 1. The peak incidence of the disease is between the ages of 4 and 8 yr. Bilateral involvement is seen in about 10% of the patients, but the hips are usually in different stages of collapse.

PATHOGENESIS

Early pathologic changes in the femoral head are the result of ischemia and necrosis; subsequent changes result from the repair process. Waldenstrom originally separated the course of the disease into 4 stages, though several modifications of his system have been described. The **initial** stage of the disease, which often lasts 6 months, is characterized by synovitis, joint irritability, and early necrosis of the femoral head. Revascularization then leads to osteoclastic-mediated resorption of the necrotic segment. The necrotic bone, however, is replaced by fibrovascular tissue and not new bone. This compromises the structural integrity of the femoral epiphysis. The second stage is the **fragmentation** stage, which typically lasts 8 mo. During this stage, the femoral epiphysis begins to collapse, usually laterally, and begins to extrude from the acetabulum. The **healing** stage, which lasts approximately 4 yr, begins with new bone formation in the subchondral region. Reossification begins centrally and expands in all directions. The degree of femoral head deformity depends on the severity of collapse and the amount of remodeling that occurs. The final stage is the **residual** stage, which begins after the entire head has reossified. A mild amount of remodeling of the femoral head still occurs until the child reaches skeletal maturity. LCPD often damages the proximal femoral physis leading to a short neck (coxa breva) and trochanteric overgrowth.

CLINICAL MANIFESTATIONS

The most common presenting symptom is a limp of varying duration. Pain, if present, is usually activity related and may be localized in the groin or referred to the anteromedial thigh or knee region. Failure to recognize that thigh or knee pain in a child may be secondary to hip pathology can cause further delay in the diagnosis. Less commonly, the onset of the disease may be much more acute and may be associated with a failure to ambulate. Parents often report that symptoms were initiated by a traumatic event.

Antalgic gait (a limp characterized by a shortening of gait phase on the injured side to alleviate weight-bearing pain) may be particularly prominent after strenuous activity at the end of the day. Hip motion, primarily internal rotation and abduction, is limited. Early in the course of the disease, the limited abduction is secondary to synovitis and muscle spasm in the adductor group; however, with time and the subsequent deformities that can develop, the limitation of abduction can become permanent. A mild hip flexion contracture of 10-20 degrees may be present. Atrophy of the muscles of the thigh, calf, or buttock from disuse secondary to pain may be evident. An apparent leg-length inequality may be caused by an adduction contracture or true shortening on the involved side from femoral head collapse.

DIAGNOSIS

Routine plain radiographs are the primary diagnostic tool for LCPD. AP and Lauenstein (frog-leg) lateral views are used to diagnose, stage, provide prognosis for, and follow the course of the disease and to assess results (Fig. 670-12). It is most important in following the course of the disease that all radiographs be viewed sequentially and compared with previous radiographs to assess the stage of the disease and to determine the true extent of epiphyseal involvement.

In the initial stage of LCPD, the radiographic changes include a decreased size of the ossification center, lateralization of the femoral head with widening of the medial joint space, a subchondral fracture, and physeal irregularity. In the fragmentation stage, the epiphysis appears fragmented, and there are scattered areas of increased radiolucency and radiodensity. During the reossification stage, the bone density returns to normal by new (woven) bone formation. The residual stage is marked by the reossification of the femoral head, gradual remodeling of head shape until skeletal maturity, and remodeling of the acetabulum.

In addition to these radiographic changes, several classic radiographic signs have been reported that describe a "head at risk" for severe deformity. Lateral extrusion of the epiphysis, a horizontal physis, calcification lateral to the epiphysis, subluxation of the hip, and a radiolucent horizontal V in the lateral

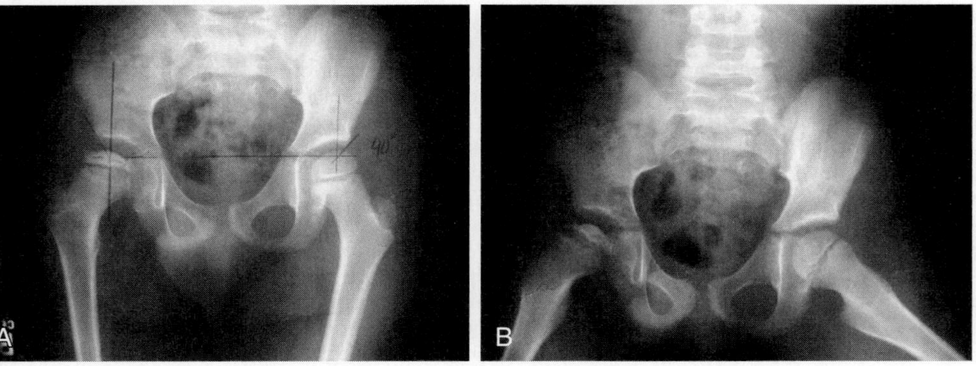

Figure 670-12 *A,* Anteroposterior radiograph of the pelvis shows epiphyseal fragmentation in the right hip, characteristic of the fragmentation phase of Legg-Calvé-Perthes disease. *B,* The frog-leg lateral view demonstrates subchondral fracture, increased density of the femoral head, and some collapse.

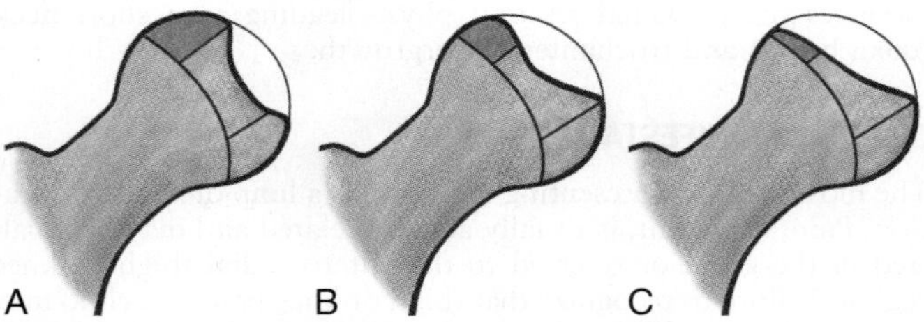

Figure 670-13 Lateral pillar classification for Legg-Calvé-Perthes disease. *A,* There is no involvement of the lateral pillar. *B,* More than 50% of the lateral pillar height is maintained. C, Less than 50% of the lateral pillar height is maintained.

aspect of the physis (Gage's sign) have all been associated with a poor prognosis.

In the absence of changes on plain radiographs, particularly in the early stages of the disease, radionuclide bone scanning with technetium-99m can reveal the avascularity of the femoral epiphysis. MRI is sensitive in detecting infarction but cannot accurately portray the stages of healing. Its role in the management of LCPD is not defined. Arthrography can be useful to dynamically assess the shape of the femoral head, demonstrate whether a hip can be contained, and diagnose hinge abduction.

CLASSIFICATION

Catterall proposed a four-group classification based on the amount of femoral epiphysis involvement and a set of radiographic "head at-risk" signs. Group I hips have anterior femoral head involvement of 25%, no sequestrum, and no metaphyseal abnormalities. Group II hips have up to 50% involvement and a clear demarcation between involved and uninvolved segments. Metaphyseal cysts may be present. Group III hips display up to 75% involvement and a large sequestrum. In group IV, the entire femoral head is involved. Use of the Catterall classification system has been limited because of a high degree of interobserver variability.

The **Herring lateral pillar classification** is the most widely used radiographic classification system for determining treatment and prognosis during the active stage of the disease (Fig. 670-13). Unlike the Catterral system, the Herring classification has been shown to have a high degree of interobserver reliability. Classification is based on several radiographs taken during the early fragmentation stage. The lateral pillar classification system for LCPD evaluates the shape of the femoral head epiphysis on AP radiograph of the hip. The head is divided into three sections or pillars. The lateral pillar occupies the lateral 15-30% of the head width, the central pillar is about 50% of the head width, and the medial pillar is 20-35% of the head width. The degree of involvement of the lateral pillar can be subdivided into three groups. In group A, the lateral pillar is radiographically normal. In group B, the lateral pillar has some lucency but >50% of the lateral pillar height is maintained. In group C, the lateral pillar is more lucent than in group B and <50% of the pillar height remains. Herring has added a B/C border group to the classification system to describe patients with ~50% collapse of the lateral pillar.

NATURAL HISTORY AND PROGNOSIS

The deformity and congruency at maturity and age at onset are the main prognostic factors for LCPD. Children who develop signs and symptoms before the age of 5 yr tend to recover without residual problems. Patients older than 9 yr of age at presentation usually have a poor prognosis. The reason for this difference is that the remodeling potential of the femoral head is higher in younger children. Greater extent of femoral head involvement and duration of the disease process are additional factors associated with a poor prognosis. Hips classified as Catterall groups III and IV and lateral pillar group C generally have a poor prognosis.

TREATMENT

The goal of treatment in LCPD is preservation of a spherical, well-covered femoral head and maintenance of hip range of motion that is close to normal. Although the treatment of LCPD remains controversial, most authors agree that the general approach to these patients should be guided by the principle of containment. This principle is predicated on the fact that while the femoral head is fragmenting and therefore in a softened condition it is best to contain it entirely within the acetabulum; by doing so, the acetabulum acts as a mold for the regenerating femoral head. Conversely, failure to contain the head permits it to deform, with resulting extrusion and impingement on the lateral edge of the acetabulum (hinge abduction). To be successful, containment must be instituted early while the femoral head is still moldable; once the head has healed, repositioning the femoral epiphysis will not aid remodeling and can in fact worsen symptoms.

Nonoperative treatment consists of activity limitation, protected weight-bearing, nonsteroidal anti-inflammatory medications, and physical therapy to maintain hip range of motion. Patients with severe pain might benefit from a short trial of bed rest and traction. Several different abduction devices have been used to achieve containment of the femoral head within the acetabulum. Petrie casts are two long-leg casts that are connected by a bar and can be helpful to keep the hips in abduction and internal rotation (the best position for containment). The most widely used abduction orthosis is the Atlanta Scottish Rite orthosis. These devices were thought to provide containment solely by abduction without fixed internal rotation. Recent studies, however, have not supported the efficacy of this brace.

Surgical containment may be approached from the femoral side, the acetabular side, or both sides of the hip joint. A varus osteotomy of the proximal femur is the most common procedure.

Pelvic osteotomies in LCPD are divided into three categories: acetabular rotational osteotomies, shelf procedures, and medial displacement or Chiari osteotomies. Any of these procedures can be combined with a proximal femoral varus osteotomy when severe deformity of the femoral head cannot be contained by a pelvic osteotomy alone.

After healing of the epiphysis, surgical treatment shifts from containment to managing the residual deformity. Patients with hinge abduction or joint incongruity might benefit from a valgus-producing proximal femoral osteotomy. Coxa breva and overgrowth of the greater trochanter can be managed by performing an advancement of the trochanter. This helps restore the length-tension relationship of the abductor mechanism and can alleviate abductor fatigue. Patients with femoroacetabular impingement from irregularity of the femoral head can often be helped with an osteoplasty or cheilectomy of the offending prominence.

BIBLIOGRAPHY

Please visit the Nelson Textbook of Pediatrics *website at* www.expertconsult.com *for the complete bibliography.*

670.4 Slipped Capital Femoral Epiphysis

Wudbhav N. Sankar, B. David Horn, Lawrence Wells, and John P. Dormans

Slipped capital femoral epiphysis (SCFE) is a hip disorder that affects adolescents, most often between 11 and 16 yr of age, and involves failure of the physis and displacement of the femoral head relative to the neck.

CLASSIFICATION

SCFEs may be classified temporally, according to onset of symptoms (acute, chronic, acute-on-chronic); functionally, according to patient's ability to bear weight (stable or unstable); or morphologically, as the extent of displacement of the femoral epiphysis relative to the neck (mild, moderate, or severe), as estimated by measurement on radiographic or CT images.

An **acute** SCFE has been characterized as one occurring in a patient who has prodromal symptoms for ≤3 weeks and should be distinguished from a purely traumatic separation of the epiphysis in a previously normal hip (a true Salter-Harris type I fracture; Chapter 675). The patient with an acute slip usually has some prodromal pain in the groin, thigh, or knee and usually reports a relatively minor injury (a twist or fall) that is not sufficiently violent to produce an acute fracture of this severity. Osteonecrosis is a significant and common complication of acute SCFE, with a reported incidence of 17-47%.

Chronic SCFE is the most common form of presentation. Typically, an adolescent presents with a few-month history of vague groin, thigh, or knee pain and a limp. Radiographs show a variable amount of posterior migration of the femoral epiphysis and remodeling of the femoral neck in the same direction; the upper end of the femur develops a bending of the neck.

Children with **acute-on-chronic** SCFE can have features of both acute and chronic conditions. Prodromal symptoms have been present for >3 wk with a sudden exacerbation of pain. Radiographs demonstrate femoral neck remodeling and further displacement of the capital epiphysis beyond the remodeled point of the femoral neck.

The stability classification separates patients based on their ability to ambulate and is more useful in predicting prognosis and establishing a treatment plan. The SCFE is considered **stable** when the child is able to walk with or without crutches. A child with an **unstable** SCFE is unable to walk with or without crutches. Patients with unstable SCFE have a much higher prevalence of osteonecrosis (up to 50%) compared to those with stable SCFE (nearly 0%). This is most likely due to the vascular injury caused at the time of initial displacement.

SCFE may also be categorized by the degree of displacement of the epiphysis on the femoral neck. The head-shaft angle difference is <30 degrees in mild slips, between 30 and 60 degrees in moderate slips, and >60 degrees in severe slips, compared to the normal contralateral side.

ETIOLOGY AND PATHOGENESIS

SCFEs are most likely caused by a combination of mechanical and endocrine factors. The plane of cleavage in most SCFEs occurs through the hypertrophic zone of the physis. During normal puberty, the physis becomes more vertically oriented, which converts mechanical forces from compression to shear. In addition, the hypertrophic zone becomes elongated in pubertal adolescents due to high levels of circulating hormones. This widening of the physis decreases the threshold for mechanical failure. Normal ossification depends on a number of different factors, including thyroid hormone, vitamin D, and calcium. It is therefore not surprising that SCFEs occur with increased incidence in children with medical disorders such as hypothyroidism, hypopituitarism, and renal osteodystrophy. Obesity, one of the largest risk factors for SCFE, affects both the mechanical load on the physis and the level of circulating hormones. The combination of mechanical and endocrine factors results in gradual failure of the physis, which allows posterior displacement of the femoral neck in relation to the head.

EPIDEMIOLOGY

The annual incidence of SCFE is 2/100,000 in the general population. Incidence has ranged from 0.2/100,000 in eastern Japan to 10.08/100,000 in the northeastern USA. The African-American and Polynesian populations have been reported to have an increased incidence of SCFE. Obesity is the most closely associated factor in the development of SCFE; about 65% of the patients are >90th percentile in weight-for-age profiles. There is a definite predilection for boys to be affected more often than girls and for the left hip to be affected more often than the right. Bilateral involvement has been reported in as many as 60% of cases, nearly half of which may be present at the time of initial presentation.

CLINICAL MANIFESTATIONS

The classic patient presenting with a SCFE is an obese, African-American boy between the ages of 11 and 16 yr. Girls present earlier, usually between 10 and 14 yr of age. Patients with chronic and stable SCFEs tend to present after weeks to months of symptoms. Patients usually limp to some degree and have an externally rotated lower extremity. Physical examination of the affected hip reveals a restriction of internal rotation, abduction, and flexion. Commonly, the examiner notes that as the affected hip is flexed, the thigh tends to rotate into progressively more external rotation (Fig. 670-14). Most patients complain of groin symptoms, but isolated thigh pain or knee pain is a common presentation from referred pain along the course of the obturator nerve. In fact, missed or delayed diagnosis often occurs in children who present with knee pain and do not receive appropriate imaging of the hip. Patients with unstable SCFEs usually present in an urgent fashion. Children typically refuse to allow any range of motion of the hip; much like a hip fracture, the extremity is shortened, abducted, and externally rotated.

DIAGNOSTIC STUDIES

Plain radiography including AP and frog-leg lateral views of both hips is usually the only imaging study needed to make the diagnosis. Because ~25% of patients have a contralateral slip on initial presentation, it is vital that both hips be carefully evaluated by the treating physician. Radiographic findings include widening and irregularity of the physis, a decrease in epiphyseal height in the center of the acetabulum, a crescent-shaped area of increased density in the proximal portion of the femoral neck, and the "blanch sign of Steel" corresponding to the double density created from the anteriorly displaced femoral neck overlying the femoral head. In an unaffected patient, the Klein line, a straight line drawn along the superior cortex of the femoral neck on the AP radiograph, should intersect some portion of the lateral capital femoral epiphysis. With progressive displacement of the epiphysis, the Klein line no longer intersects the epiphysis (Fig. 670-15). Although some of these radiographic findings can be subtle, most diagnoses can be readily made on the frog-leg lateral view, which reveals the characteristic posterior and inferior displacement of the epiphysis in relation to the femoral neck.

TREATMENT

Once the diagnosis is made, the patient should be admitted to the hospital immediately and placed on bed rest. Allowing the child to go home without definitive treatment increases the risk that a stable SCFE will become an unstable SCFE and that further displacement will occur. Children with atypical presentations (<10 yr of age, thin body habitus) should have screening labs sent to rule out an underlying endocrinopathy.

The goal of treatment is to prevent further progression of the slip and to stabilize (i.e., close) the physis. Although various forms of treatment have been used in the past, including spica casting, the current gold standard for the treatment of SCFE is in situ pinning with a single, large screw (Fig. 670-16). The term "in situ" implies that no attempt is made to reduce the displacement between the epiphysis and femoral neck because doing so increases the risk of osteonecrosis. Screws are typically placed percutaneously under fluoroscopic guidance. Postoperatively, most patients are allowed partial weight-bearing with crutches for 4-6 wk, followed by a gradual return to normal activities. Patients should be monitored with serial radiographs to be sure that the physis is closing and that the slip is stable. After healing from the initial stabilization, patients with severe residual deformity may be candidates for proximal femoral osteotomy to correct the deformity, reduce impingement, and improve range of motion.

Because 20-40% of children will develop a contralateral SCFE at some point, many orthopedists advocate prophylactic pin fixation of the contralateral (normal) side in patients with a unilateral SCFE. The benefits of preventing a possible slip must be balanced with the risks of performing a potentially unnecessary surgery. Several recent studies have attempted to analyze decision models for prophylactic pinning, but controversy remains regarding the optimal course of treatment.

COMPLICATIONS

Osteonecrosis and chondrolysis are the two most serious complications of SCFE. Osteonecrosis, or avascular necrosis, usually

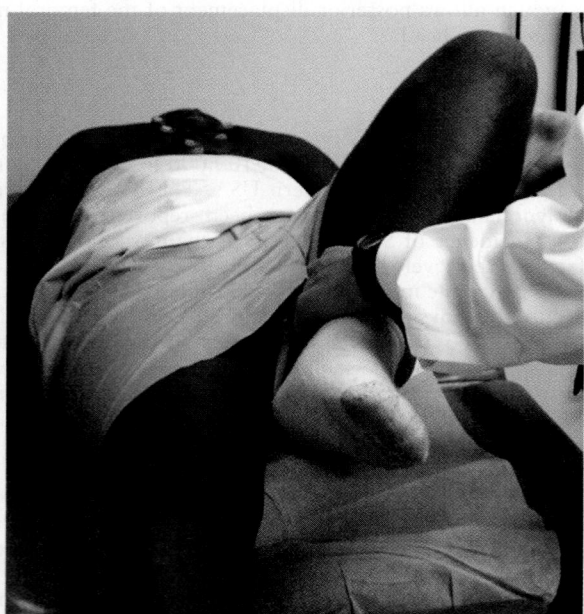

Figure 670-14 Progressive external rotation noted with flexion: the knee-axilla sign.

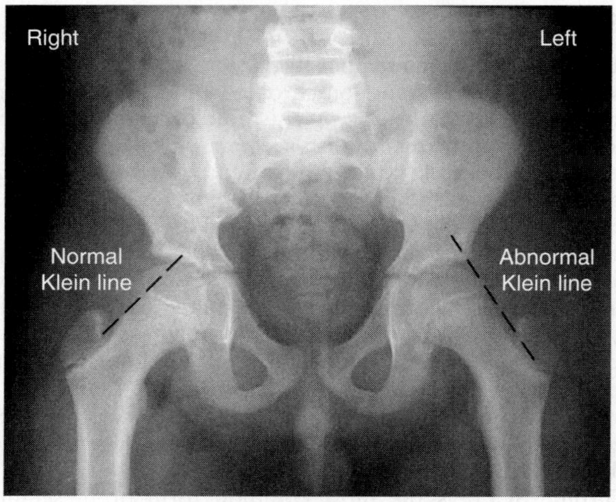

Figure 670-15 Illustration of the Klein line.

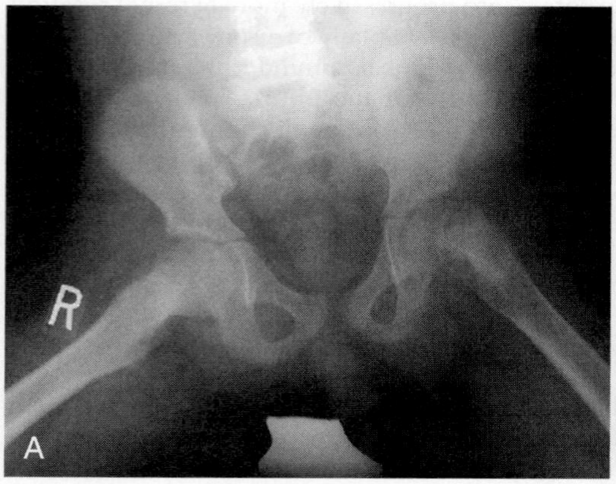

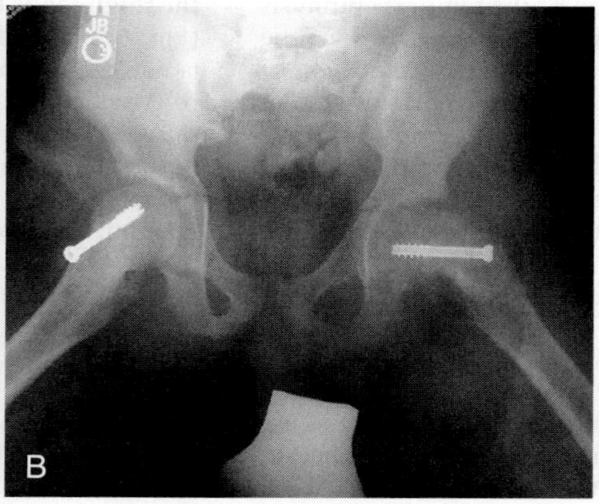

Figure 670-16 Preoperative *(A)* and postoperative *(B)* radiographs demonstrating the in situ pinning in a case of slipped capital femoral epiphysis.

occurs as a result of injury to the retinacular vessels. This can be caused by an initial force of injury, particularly in unstable slips, forced manipulation of an acute or unstable SCFE, compression from intracapsular hematoma, or as a direct injury during surgery. Partial forms of osteonecrosis can also appear following internal fixation; this can be caused by a disruption of the intraepiphyseal blood vessels. Chondrolysis, on the other hand, is an acute dissolution of articular cartilage in the hip. There are no clear causes of this complication, but it is believed to be associated with more-severe slips, to occur more commonly among African-Americans and girls, and to be associated with pins or screws protruding out of the femoral head.

BIBLIOGRAPHY

Please visit the Nelson Textbook of Pediatrics *website at* *www.expertconsult.com* *for the complete bibliography.*

Chapter 671 The Spine

David A. Spiegel and John P. Dormans

Abnormalities of the spine may be present at birth (congenital), can develop during childhood or adolescence, or can result from traumatic injuries. Alterations in spinal alignment are commonly of cosmetic concern to the patient and family. Sequelae from progressive spinal deformities include pain, cardiopulmonary dysfunction, and a loss of sitting balance (nonambulators). Early detection helps to facilitate treatment and to identify and address coexisting visceral and/or neurologic problems that may be associated with a spinal deformity. A classification of common spinal abnormalities is presented in Table 671-1.

Scoliosis is a complex three-dimensional deformity that is most commonly described as a lateral curvature of the spine in the frontal plane. Most cases of scoliosis have no demonstrable etiology, and are termed idiopathic. Scoliosis may be congenital or may be associated with a host of neuromuscular diseases or syndromes. Scoliosis may also be secondary to an infrapelvic deformity such as a leg-length discrepancy or a soft-tissue contracture around the hip (abduction or adduction).

In the lateral (sagittal) plane, the spine has normal curvatures in the cervical (lordotic or convex anteriorly), thoracic (kyphosis or convex posteriorly), and lumbar (lordosis) regions to maintain the relationships of body segments relative to the forces of gravity. Maintaining the center of gravity is important for balance and to minimize the amount of muscular activity (conserve energy) required to maintain upright posture. A vertical (gravity) line dropped from the 7th cervical vertebra should normally fall through the posterosuperior corner of the sacrum. Disorders of sagittal alignment include thoracic hyperkyphosis and lumbar hyperlordosis. **Thoracic hyperkyphosis** is seen most commonly in patients with **postural kyphosis** or with **Scheuermann disease.** Lumbar hyperlordosis may be associated with spondylolisthesis or may be secondary to hip flexion contractures.

Table 671-1 CLASSIFICATION OF SPINAL DEFORMITIES

SCOLIOSIS
Idiopathic
Infantile
Juvenile
Adolescent
Congenital
Failure of formation
Wedge vertebrae
Hemivertebrae
Failure of segmentation
Unilateral bar
Block vertebra
Mixed
Neuromuscular
Neuropathic diseases
Upper motor neuron
Cerebral palsy
Spinocerebellar degeneration (Friedreich ataxia, Charcot-Marie-Tooth disease)
Syringomyelia
Spinal cord tumor
Spinal cord trauma
Lower motor neuron
Poliomyelitis
Spinal muscular atrophy
Myopathies
Duchenne muscular dystrophy
Arthrogryposis
Other muscular dystrophies
Syndromes
Neurofibromatosis
Marfan syndrome
Compensatory
Leg-length discrepancy
KYPHOSIS
Postural kyphosis (flexible)
Scheuermann disease
Congenital kyphosis
Failure of formation
Failure of segmentation
Mixed

Adapted from the Terminology Committee, Scoliosis Research Society: A glossary of scoliosis terms, *Spine* 1:57, 1976.

671.1 Idiopathic Scoliosis

David A. Spiegel and John P. Dormans

ETIOLOGY AND EPIDEMIOLOGY

Scoliosis is a complex, 3-dimensional deformity of the spine, with abnormalities in the coronal, sagittal, and axial planes. The diagnosis is based on a coronal plane curvature of >10 degrees using the Cobb method. Idiopathic scoliosis is a diagnosis of exclusion; other causes must be ruled out (see Table 671-1). The etiology of idiopathic scoliosis remains unknown and is likely multifactorial, involving both genetic and environmental components. Major theories have been based on genetic factors, metabolic dysfunction (melatonin deficiency, calmodulin), neurologic dysfunction (craniocervical, vestibular and oculovestibular), and biomechanical factors (asynchrony in spinal growth, anterior spinal overgrowth, and others). With regard to genetic factors, although several different modes of inheritance have been suggested (autosomal dominant, multifactorial, X-linked), a single locus has yet to be identified. Abnormalities identified in connective tissue, muscle, and bone appear to be secondary. Melatonin and calmodulin might have indirect effects, and subtle abnormalities in vestibular, ocular, and proprioceptive function suggest that abnormal equilibrium might also play a role.

Idiopathic scoliosis is classified according to the age at onset, including infantile (rare, birth to 3 yr), juvenile (3-10 yr), and adolescent (≥11 yr). Adolescent idiopathic scoliosis (AIS) is most common (~70%). The prevalence of scoliosis (>10 degrees curvature) is ~2-3%; however, approximately 0.3% have a curve >30 degrees. The incidence is roughly equal in girls and boys for small curves (<10 degrees), but girls have 10 times the risk of developing a curvature >30 degrees.

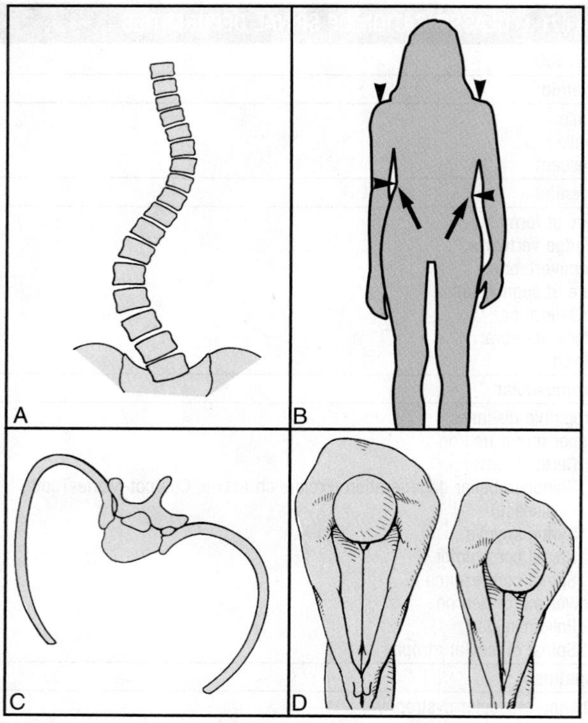

Figure 671-1 Structural changes in idiopathic scoliosis. *A,* As curvature increases, alterations in body configuration develop in both the primary and compensatory curve regions. *B,* Asymmetry of shoulder height, waistline, and elbow-to-flank distance are common findings. *C,* Vertebral rotation and associated posterior displacement of the ribs on the convex side of the curve are responsible for the characteristic deformity of the chest wall in scoliosis patients. *D,* In the school screening examination for scoliosis, the patient bends forward at the waist. Rib asymmetry of even a small degree is obvious (From Scoles PV: Spinal deformity in childhood and adolescence. In Behrman RE, Vaughn VC III, editors: *Nelson textbook of pediatrics, update 5,* Philadelphia, 1989, WB Saunders.)

CLINICAL MANIFESTATIONS

Patients usually present with a change in cosmetic appearance noted by family and/or friends or on a screening examination by a school nurse or primary care physician. The patient is evaluated in the standing position, from both the front and the side, to identify any asymmetry in the chest wall, trunk, and/or shoulders. Asymmetry of the posterior chest wall on forward bending (the Adams test) is the earliest abnormality (Fig. 671-1). Rotation of the vertebral bodies toward the convexity results in rotation and prominence of the attached ribs posteriorly. The anterior chest wall may be flattened on the concavity, due to inward rotation of the chest wall and ribs. Associated findings can include elevation of the shoulder, a lateral shift of the trunk, and an apparent leg-length discrepancy. The patient should also be evaluated from the side. The thoracic spine normally has a smooth, rounded kyphosis (20-50 degrees using the Cobb method from T3-T12) that extends down to the thoracolumbar junction, and the lumbar spine is normally lordotic (30-60 degrees using the Cobb method from T12-L5). Children normally have less cervical lordosis and more lumbar lordosis than do adults or adolescents. Typically, idiopathic scoliosis results in a loss of the normal thoracic kyphosis in the region of curvature (relative thoracic lordosis).

A careful neurologic examination should always be performed. A subset of curves are associated with an underlying neurologic diagnosis, especially in patients who present in the infant and juvenile years (20% have an associated intraspinal abnormality). The index of suspicion is raised in the presence of back pain or neurologic symptoms, café-au-lait spots, a sacral dimple or midline cutaneous abnormalities (hemangioma, hair patch or skin tag), unilateral foot deformity, or an atypical curve pattern. The examiner should always test the superficial abdominal reflex by lightly stroking the skin on both sides of the umbilicus. Normally, the umbilicus should deviate toward the side that was stroked. Asymmetry of the superficial abdominal reflex (or unilateral absence of this reflex) might suggest syringomyelia as an underlying diagnosis.

Screening for scoliosis facilitates earlier diagnosis and treatment, under the assumption that the natural history may be influenced by bracing, and that earlier identification of cases suitable for surgery reduces the complexity and risks of the surgery. Screening may be accomplished during primary care visits or as part of a school screening program. A consensus statement from professional societies (American Academy of Pediatrics, American Academy of Orthopaedic Surgeons, Pediatric Orthopaedic Society of North America, and the Scoliosis Research Society) states that if screening is to be carried out, this should be at 10 and 12 years of age for girls, and once at 13-14 years for boys. The Adams forward-bend test has been used to identify any asymmetry in the thoracic and/or lumbar region, and an inclinometer (scoliometer, Orthopaedic Systems Inc.) is also used to measure the degree of asymmetry. The number of degrees used for referral typically varies from 5 to 7, and the referral rate from these programs varies from 3% to 30%. School screening remains controversial, and less than half of the states in the USA have formal programs. The U.S. Preventive Services Task Force (USPSTF) has recently recommended against school screening in 2004, and further research is required to inform policy.

The **natural history** of idiopathic scoliosis varies considerably based on the age at diagnosis. Curvatures in excess of 80 degrees can result in restrictive pulmonary disease, and larger curves in excess of 100-120 degrees can result in a reduced life expectancy, due to cor pulmonale and cardiorespiratory failure. Scoliotic curves diagnosed in infancy through childhood are much more likely than adolescent curves to reach this magnitude. In general, adults with untreated AIS are expected to have similar life expectancy and similar functional activities, and no greater risk of cardiopulmonary complications, when compared with age-matched controls. Back pain may be more common, but it does not appear to be more disabling. Thoracolumbar or lumbar curves are more likely to cause pain during adulthood, particularly if there is an associated translational shift of the vertebrae. Dyspnea is common with thoracic curves of >80 degrees. Thoracic curves <30 degrees rarely progress after skeletal maturity, but those >45 or 50 degrees can continue to progress at approximately 1 degree per year through life. The cosmetic aspects of the deformity may be the most significant concern for the majority of patients with untreated AIS.

RADIOGRAPHIC EVALUATION

Standing high-quality posteroanterior (PA) and lateral radiographs of the entire spine are recommended at the initial evaluation for patients with clinical findings that suggest a spinal deformity. On the PA radiograph, the degree of curvature is determined by the Cobb method, in which the angle between the superior and inferior end vertebra (tilted into the curve) is measured (Fig. 671-2). A line is drawn across the superior end plate of each end vertebra, and the angle between perpendicular lines erected from each of these is measured. Although the indications for performing MRI are variable, this modality is helpful when an underlying cause for the scoliosis is suspected based on age (infantile, juvenile curves), abnormal findings on the history and physical examination, and atypical radiographic features (curve patterns and/or specific features). **Atypical radiographic** findings include uncommon curve patterns such as the left thoracic curve, double thoracic curves, high thoracic curves, widening of the spinal canal, and erosive or dysplastic changes in the vertebral body or ribs. On the lateral radiograph, an increase in thoracic

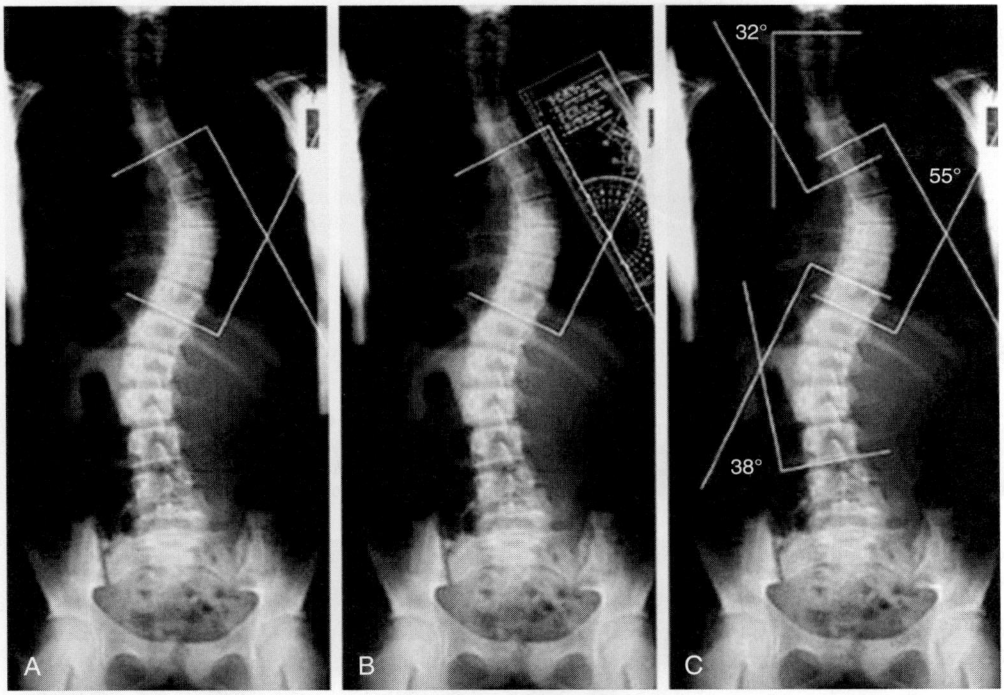

Figure 671-2 *A-C,* Cobb angles measurements. (From Morrissy, RT, Weinstein, SL: *Lovell & Winter's pediatric orthopaedics,* ed 6, Philadelphia, 2006, Lippincott Williams & Wilkins.)

kyphosis or an absence of segmental lordosis might suggest the presence of an underlying diagnosis.

TREATMENT

Options for treatment include observation, bracing, and surgical treatment. Treatment decisions are based on the natural history of each curvature, which relates to age (degree of skeletal maturity or growth remaining), the magnitude of the curve, and occasionally associated diagnoses and/or medical considerations. A positive family history does not help predict the behavior of an individual curve. Observation is always indicated for curvatures <20 degrees. Curves of larger magnitude may be treated by bracing or surgery. The risk of curve progression depends on the amount of growth remaining, the curve's magnitude, and gender. More than one parameter must be used when determining the amount of growth remaining, and both clinical (age, annual growth velocity, menarchal status, Tanner stage) and radiographic (Risser sign, skeletal age, maturation of olecranon apophysis) measures are available. Curves are more likely to progress if there is significant growth remaining (premenarchal, Tanner stage I or II, Risser 0 or 1). Premenarchal girls with curves between 20 and 30 degrees have a significantly higher risk of progression than do girls 2 yr after menarche with similar curves. Boys with curvature of the same magnitude appear to have similar risks of progression when judged by other maturation standards; however, the assessment of skeletal maturity in boys is more difficult.

Bracing

The goal of bracing is to prevent progression of the deformity, thereby reducing the need for surgery. The efficacy of bracing in AIS remains controversial, but most centers in North America offer a brace to selected patients with progressive curvatures. In AIS, the typical indications for bracing are a curve >30 degrees, or a curve from 20-25 degrees that has progressed >5 degrees, in a skeletally immature patient (Risser 0,1, or 2). Bracing is thought to be ineffective in curves >45 degrees. An "in brace" correction of 50% in Cobb angle is desirable.

The success of bracing is thought to increase with greater time spent in the brace, and the ideal program includes 23 hours in the brace per day. Protocols vary between 16 and 23 hours per day, recognizing that full compliance is difficult to achieve in the adolescent population. Bracing is commonly used as a temporizing measure for infantile and juvenile scoliosis given the high likelihood of significant progression, and the need to delay more definitive treatment. The success rate is much lower for infantile and juvenile curvatures, but the goal is to delay progression.

There are several options for braces (Fig. 671-3). The Milwaukee brace, employing longitudinal traction from the skull to the pelvis with lateral compression of the chest wall, can be adjusted for growth and thus is a good brace for patients with infantile or juvenile scoliosis. Underarm braces (the Boston or Wilmington braces) are less obvious and so are often preferred by adolescents. The Charleston brace provides a corrective force and is used only at night.

Surgery

Surgical treatment is indicated for the majority of patients with infantile or juvenile idiopathic scoliosis and in selected patients with AIS, when other methods of treatment have failed to control the deformity, and when further progression would be expected to result in unacceptable cosmesis and/or physiologic abnormalities. Such deformities are typically treated by a definitive spinal arthrodesis (fusion). The majority of progressive infantile and juvenile curves ultimately require a spinal arthrodesis, and the goal is to delay the definitive procedure until the pulmonary system and thoracic cage have matured and the trunk height has been maximized.

An alternative strategy is required for curvatures that progress despite bracing. In some centers, serial casting under general anesthesia is employed for selected infantile and juvenile curves to gain correction into a "braceable" range, followed by application of a spinal orthosis. The other option for progressive curvatures is a "growing rod" construct. A spinal rod (or 2 rods) is attached to anchors at the top and at the bottom of the curvature, and distraction forces are applied to achieve correction. The rods hold the spine in the corrected position, and they must then be lengthened every 6 months to maintain correction. Many curves have been controlled for years using such a protocol, and definitive fusion is delayed until a more optimal age.

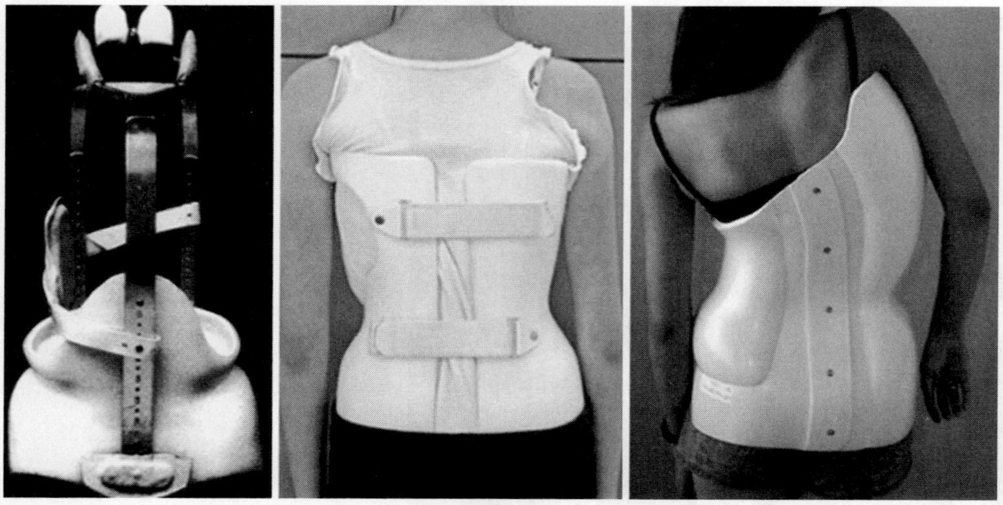

Figure 671-3 Various brace types. (From Morrissy, RT, Weinstein, SL: *Lovell & Winter's pediatric orthopaedics,* ed 6, Philadelphia, 2006, Lippincott Williams & Wilkins.)

With regard to AIS, surgical treatment is usually indicated for skeletally immature patients with progressive thoracic curves >45 degrees and skeletally mature patients with thoracic curves >50-55 degrees. Lumbar curves are more likely to progress, and surgical stabilization may be offered for curves as low as 35-40 degrees if there is a significant shift of the trunk relative to the pelvis and lower extremities. The goals of surgery are to arrest progression of the deformity, to improve cosmesis, and to minimize the number of vertebral segments that are stabilized. These are achieved through a spinal fusion or arthrodesis, and implants are used to apply mechanical forces to the bony elements to affect correction and to hold the spine in the corrected position until the spine fuses. Postoperative immobilization is usually not required. Options for bone grafting include autograft (iliac crest) or allograft, and in recent years most surgeons have used cancellous allograft with or without enhancers such as demineralized bone matrix.

The most common procedure is an instrumented posterior spinal fusion, and the typical spinal implant construct includes 2 rods anchored to the spine by hooks, wires, and/or screws (Fig. 671-4). In the last few years there has been significant interest in using a construct with pedicle screws at each level. Although correction of the axial deformity (rotation of the rib cage) is more pronounced with this technology, it remains unclear whether patient outcomes are improved. An anterior release and fusion, performed through a thoracotomy or thoracolumbar exposure, is indicated for isolated thoracolumbar and lumbar curves, to improve correctability of stiffer curves, and to prevent curve progression ("crankshaft") from continued anterior growth of the spine in selected patients with considerable growth remaining. A construct with multiple pedicle screws can allow the surgeon to avoid an anterior approach in many larger or stiffer curves (more powerful correction) and in younger patients (stiff enough to resist anterior spinal growth and prevent crankshaft). Thoracoscopic surgery has also been used to perform an anterior release with or without instrumentation and fusion, but this technique has been used much less often since the advent of thoracic pedicle screws. For idiopathic thoracolumbar and lumbar curves, an anterior fusion with instrumentation (usually screws in the vertebral body connected to 1 or 2 rods) can be done as an alternative to save lumbar motion segments.

There has been an interest in developing techniques to tether spinal growth, most commonly by placing metallic staples across each disk space on the convexity of a curvature. The goal is to slow or arrest growth on the convexity while allowing growth to proceed on the concavity, thereby preventing progression and possibly resulting in permanent correction without the need for an arthrodesis. The indications for this technique, and the long-term results, remain to be determined.

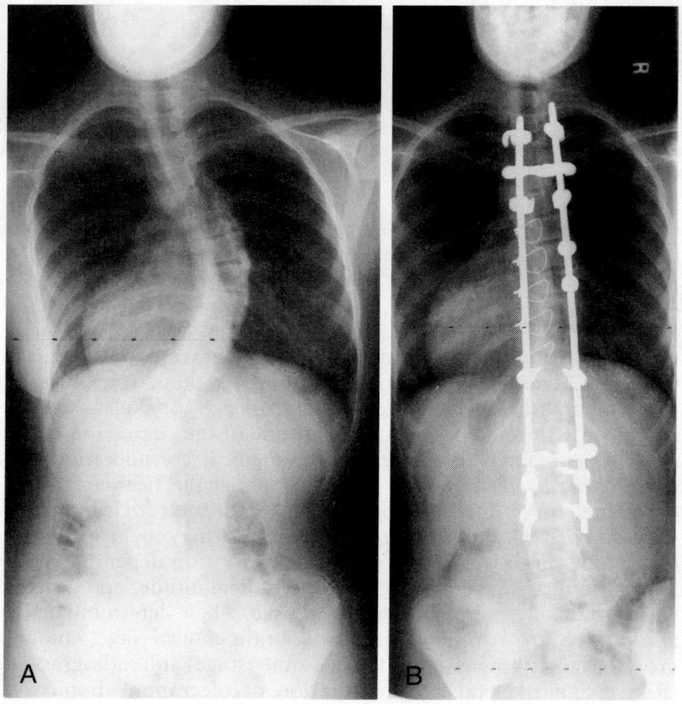

Figure 671-4 *A,* Preoperative standing posteroanterior radiograph of a 14 yr old girl who was skeletally immature and developed a 68-degree right thoracic and a 53-degree left lumbar scoliosis. Her trunk was shifted to the right, and the left shoulder was slightly depressed. *B,* Based on the risk of future progression, she was treated by an instrumented posterior spinal fusion from T3 to L3, with correction of the right thoracic curve to 20 degrees and the left lumbar curve to 10 degrees. Coronal spinal balance was restored, and shoulder height was maintained.

BIBLIOGRAPHY

Please visit the Nelson Textbook of Pediatrics *website at www.expertconsult.com for the complete bibliography.*

671.2 Congenital Scoliosis

David A. Spiegel and John P. Dormans

Congenital scoliosis results from abnormal growth and development of the vertebral column, likely due to intrauterine events at or about the 6th wk of gestation. There can be a partial or complete failure of formation (wedge vertebrae or hemivertebrae), a

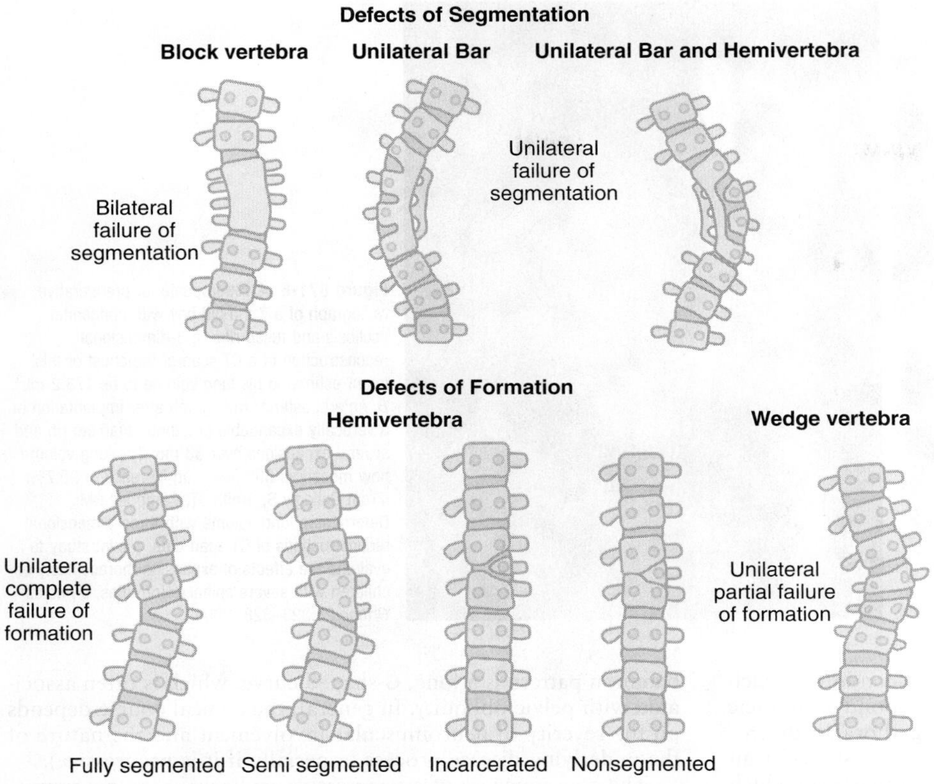

Figure 671-5 The defects of segmentation and formation that can occur during spinal development. (From McMaster MJ: Congenital scoliosis. In Weinstein SL, editor: *The pediatric spine: principles and practice,* ed 2, Philadelphia, 2001, Lippincott Williams & Wilkins, p 163.)

partial or complete failure of segmentation (unilateral unsegmented bars), or a combination of both (Fig. 671-5). One or more bony anomalies can occur in isolation or in combination.

As the spine (including the neural elements) and the viscera are formed around the 6th week in utero, patients with congenital scoliosis often have visceral and intraspinal anomalies as well. Once a congenital spinal anomaly is diagnosed, a priority is to rule out malformations in other organ systems. Genitourinary abnormalities are identified in 20-40% of children with congenital scoliosis and include unilateral renal agenesis, ureteral duplication, horseshoe kidney, and genital anomalies. Approximately 2% of these patients have a silent obstructive uropathy that may be life threatening. Renal ultrasonography should be performed early on in all children with congenital scoliosis, and other studies (CT, MRI) may also be required. Cardiac anomalies are identified in 10-25% of patients. A careful cardiac examination should be performed; some clinicians recommend routine echocardiography.

Approximately 20-40% of patients have an intraspinal anomaly. Infants with cutaneous abnormalities overlying the spine might benefit from ultrasonography to rule out an occult spinal dysraphic condition. MRI is usually recommended during the course of treatment. *Spinal dysraphism* is the general term applied to such lesions (Chapters 585 and 598). Examples include diastematomyelia, split cord malformations, intraspinal lipomas (intradural or extradural), arachnoid cysts, teratomas, dermoid sinuses, fibrous bands, and tight filum terminale. Cutaneous findings that may be seen in patients with closed spinal dysraphism include hair patches, skin tags or dimples, sinuses, and hemangiomas. Most of these lesions become clinically evident through tethering of the spinal cord, the symptoms of which include back and/or leg pain, calf atrophy, progressive unilateral foot deformity (especially cavovarus), and problems with bowel or bladder function.

The risk of progression depends on the growth potential of each anomaly, which can vary considerably, so close radiographic follow-up is required. Progression of these curves is most pronounced during periods of rapid growth, namely, the first 2-3 yr of life and during the adolescent growth spurt. The most severe form of congenital scoliosis is a unilateral unsegmented bar with a contralateral hemivertebra. In this anomaly, the spine is fused on 1 side (unsegmented bar) and has a growth center (hemivertebra) on the other side at the same level. A rapidly progressive curve is seen, and all patients usually require surgical stabilization. A unilateral unsegmented bar is also associated with significant progression and in most cases will require surgical intervention. An unsegmented bar might not be radiographically apparent, but the adjacent ribs on the concavity may be fused, providing a clue to the diagnosis. An isolated hemivertebra must be followed closely, and many of these will be associated with a progressive deformity that requires surgical intervention. In contrast, an isolated block vertebra has little growth potential and rarely requires treatment.

Early diagnosis and prompt treatment of progressive curves are essential. Bracing is not indicated for most congenital curves due to their structural nature, except in rare cases in which the goal is to control a flexible, compensatory curvature in another area of the spine. The treatment of progressive curves is preemptive spinal arthrodesis, and both anterior and posterior spinal fusion is often required. Other procedures that are employed in selected patients include an isolated posterior spinal fusion (sometimes an in situ fusion), convex hemiepiphysiodesis (only 1 side of the spine is fused to allow some correction of the deformity with growth), and partial or complete hemivertebra excision (usually in the lumbar spine). Spinal arthrodesis is ideally performed before a significant deformity has developed because intraoperative correction is difficult to achieve and the risk of neurologic complications is high.

When multiple levels of the thoracic spine are involved, especially in the presence of fused ribs, a progressive 3-dimensional deformity of the chest wall can impair lung development and function, resulting in a thoracic insufficiency syndrome. This syndrome is best described as the inability of the chest wall to support normal respiration. A thoracic insufficiency syndrome

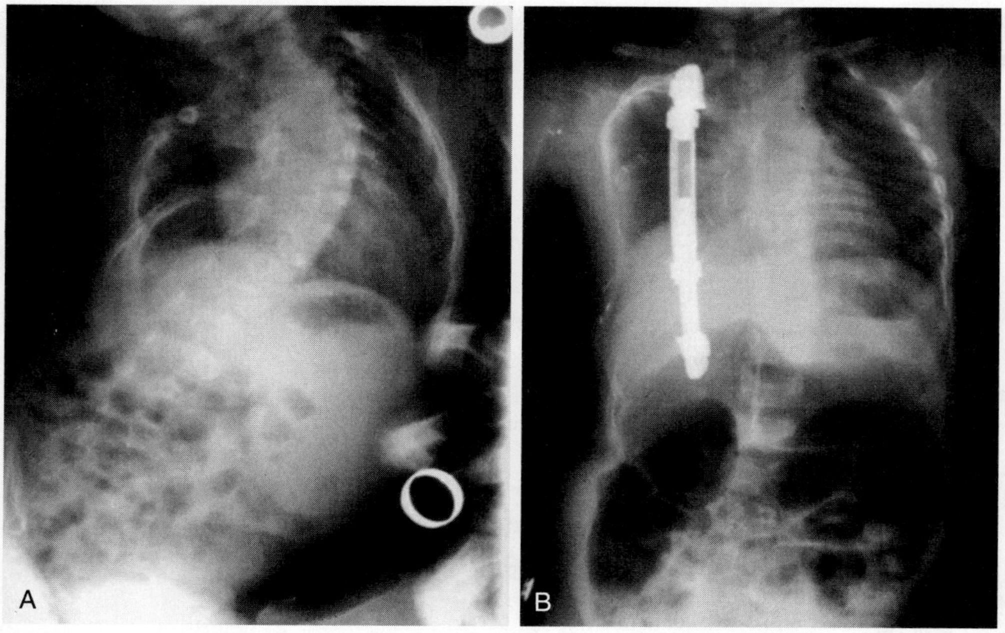

Figure 671-6 *A,* Anteroposterior preoperative radiograph of a 7 mo old boy with congenital scoliosis and fused ribs. A 3-dimensional reconstruction of a CT scan of the chest of this infant estimated his lung volume to be 173.2 mL^3. *B,* Anteroposterior radiograph after implantation of a vertically expandable prosthetic titanium rib and several expansions over 33 mo. The lung volume now measures 330.3mL^3, an increase of 90.7%. (From Gollogly S, Smith JT, Campbell RM: Determining lung volume with three-dimensional reconstructions of CT scan data: a pilot study to evaluate the effects of expansion thoracoplasty on children with severe spinal deformities, *J Pediatr Orthop* 23:323–328, 2004.)

may be seen in patients with several recognized conditions, such as Jarcho-Levin syndrome (spondylocostal or spondylothoracic dysplasia) and Jeune syndrome (asphyxiating thoracic dystrophy). There is interest in treating these difficult cases with an experimental technique called **expansion thoracoplasty,** in which the thoracic cage is gradually expanded over time by progressive lengthening of the chest wall on the concavity of the spinal deformity (or in some cases on both sides of the spine). The procedure involves an opening wedge thoracostomy, followed by placement of a vertical expandable titanium prosthetic rib. The implant is then distracted (lengthened) at regular intervals (Fig. 671-6). The primary goal is to gradually correct the chest wall deformity to improve pulmonary function, and a secondary goal is correction of an associated spinal deformity. This technique is currently not approved for the treatment of scoliosis in the absence of a thoracic insufficiency, and further study will help to refine (and possibly expand) the indications for the technique.

BIBLIOGRAPHY

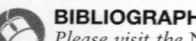

Please visit the Nelson Textbook of Pediatrics *website at* *www.expertconsult.com* *for the complete bibliography.*

671.3 Neuromuscular Scoliosis, Genetic Syndromes, and Compensatory Scoliosis

David A. Spiegel and John P. Dormans

NEUROMUSCULAR SCOLIOSIS

Scoliosis is often identified in children with neuromuscular diseases such as cerebral palsy, the muscular dystrophies and other myopathies, spinal muscular atrophy, Friedreich ataxia, myelomeningocele, polio, and arthrogryposis. The etiology and natural history differ from those seen in idiopathic and congenital scoliosis. Most cases result from weakness and/or imbalance of the trunk musculature, and spasticity plays a role in many patients as well. Coexisting congenital vertebral anomalies are seen in patients with myelomeningocele. Neuromuscular scoliosis is most common in the nonambulatory population and is diagnosed in up to 68% of nonambulatory patients with cerebral palsy and >90% of patients with Duchenne muscular dystrophy. The most common pattern is a long, C-shaped curve, which is often associated with pelvic obliquity. In general, the clinical course depends on the severity of neuromuscular involvement and the nature of the underlying disease process (especially if it is progressive).

The consequences of a progressive scoliosis in the neuromuscular population involve both function (sitting and standing balance) and ease of care; in some cases, visceral function is compromised. In patients who are wheelchair bound, one arm may be required for trunk support, which impairs upper extremity function. An associated pelvic obliquity results in asymmetric seating pressures, which can limit sitting endurance and possibly result in ischial decubiti. Severe curves may be associated with decreased pulmonary reserve, especially when the apex is in the thoracic spine, compounding pre-existing respiratory problems. Pain may be experienced from impingement of the rib cage on the iliac crest in large thoracolumbar curves. Marginal ambulators can lose the ability to ambulate as a result of scoliosis.

Diagnosis

The diagnosis is suspected on physical examination. Early detection is helpful because the results are optimal if treatment is completed before the magnitude and rigidity of the curve become severe. In patients who ambulate, the examination is as outlined in the section on idiopathic scoliosis. In nonambulators, the back is inspected with the patient sitting upright (with or without support) and any asymmetry is noted. These patients often need manual support to maintain an upright position. If any asymmetry is observed, then upright (sitting) PA and lateral radiographs are obtained.

Treatment

The **treatment** of neuromuscular scoliosis depends on the age of the patient, the underlying diagnosis, and the degree of progression. The goal is to achieve or maintain a straight spine over a level pelvis, especially in patients who are wheelchair bound, and to intervene early before curve magnitude and rigidity increase. In contrast to idiopathic and congenital scoliosis, neuromuscular curves can continue to progress after skeletal maturity. In general, curves of >40-50 degrees will continue to worsen over time.

Although brace treatment will not arrest progression in the long term, this strategy can help to slow the rate of progression until more definitive treatment can be carried out. Because the standard braces used for idiopathic scoliosis are poorly tolerated in neuromuscular patients, a soft spinal orthosis or seating modifications are often recommended. In addition to delaying progression, these orthoses improve sitting balance (upper extremity function), sitting tolerance, and ease of care.

In general, a spinal arthrodesis is offered to patients with progressive curvatures >40-50 degrees. The indications differ somewhat based on the underlying diagnosis. Patients with Duchenne muscular dystrophy are offered surgery when their curves progress beyond 20-30 degrees, before a significant decline in pulmonary or cardiac function preclude their ability to tolerate the surgery. There has been some controversy regarding the indications for spinal fusion in the patient with spastic quadriplegia, especially in patients with severe mental retardation. In this population, the indications must be individualized and typically involve a documented loss of function or ease of care or chronic discomfort. Patients with curves similar to those seen in idiopathic scoliosis are usually ambulatory and are managed by similar principles and surgical techniques. Patients who are nonambulatory, often with pelvic obliquity, are usually managed by a spinal fusion extending from the upper thoracic spine to the pelvis.

Segmental fixation is employed to maximize rigidity (each level in the curve serves as a point for fixation), and the typical construct includes sublaminar wires at each level, which are attached to 1 (unit rod) or 2 spinal rods. These rods extend down into the posterior ilium to achieve fixation across the lumbosacral joint. A brace is usually not required following this procedure. Although complications are relatively common in comparison with patients with non-neuromuscular curves, the available literature suggests that most patients benefit in terms of function and ease of care. This surgery should ideally be done at centers with significant experience (e.g., trained spine surgeons, anesthesia, intensive care unit).

SYNDROMES AND GENETIC DISORDERS

Syndromes and genetic diagnosis constitute a diverse group of diagnoses; representative examples include neurofibromatosis, osteogenesis imperfecta, connective tissue diseases (Marfan syndrome, Ehlers-Danlos syndrome), and Prader-Willi syndrome. Patients with these diagnoses should have their spine examined routinely during visits to their primary care physician. As for other types of scoliosis, the follow-up and treatment is based on the age of the patient, the degree of deformity, whether progression has been documented, and the underlying diagnosis.

COMPENSATORY SCOLIOSIS

Leg-length inequality is common and is usually associated with a small compensatory lumbar curvature (Chapter 668). This is 1 cause of false-positive screening examinations. Pelvic tilt toward the short side is associated with a lumbar curve (convexity away from the short leg). There is little evidence to suggest that a small compensatory lumbar curve places the patient at risk of progression or back pain. Because children with leg-length inequality can also have idiopathic or congenital scoliosis, a standing radiograph may be obtained with a block under the foot on the short side (to correct the leg-length discrepancy) to level the pelvis. If the curvature disappears when the limb-length discrepancy is corrected, then a diagnosis of a compensatory curve is made. An alternative is a PA radiograph with the patient seated. In neuromuscular disorders such as polio or cerebral palsy, an adduction or abduction contracture of the hip (fixed infrapelvic contracture) may be compensated for by a lumbar scoliosis to maintain standing or sitting balance. For patients who ambulate, a 10-degree fixed contracture will result in up to 3-cm apparent leg-length discrepancy.

BIBLIOGRAPHY

Please visit the Nelson Textbook of Pediatrics *website at www.expertconsult.com for the complete bibliography.*

671.4 Kyphosis (Round Back)

David A. Spiegel and John P. Dormans

The normal sagittal spinal contour is kyphotic in the thoracic spine and lordotic in the lumbar spine. The normal range for thoracic kyphosis is defined as 20-50 degrees of curvature between T3 and T12 using the Cobb technique, and hyperkyphosis is defined by a Cobb angle of >50 degrees. Patients with hyperkyphosis often present with cosmetic concerns and/or back pain, but neurologic dysfunction is rare. The terms *flexible* or *postural* are used to describe a curvature that can be corrected voluntarily. If full correction cannot be achieved with active or passive maneuvers, then a fixed or structural component is present. Such a structural hyperkyphosis is much more likely to be associated with an underlying diagnosis such as Scheuermann disease or congenital kyphosis.

A host of conditions may be associated with hyperkyphosis, most often owing to a compromise in the mechanical integrity or growth of the anterior elements of the spine. Examples include injuries (compression or burst fractures), infections (bacterial, tubercular, fungal), metabolic diseases (osteogenesis imperfecta, osteoporosis), neoplastic conditions (eosinophilic granuloma, leukemia), congenital conditions (failure of formation or segmentation), conditions associated with neuromuscular diseases, disorders of collagen (Marfan syndrome), and a number of bone dysplasias (neurofibromatosis, achondroplasia, mucopolysaccharidosis). A progressive kyphosis can also occur following laminectomy or radiation therapy.

Treatment is based on the severity of the deformity, the presence of symptoms (pain, neurologic compromise), and the natural history of the underlying disease process.

FLEXIBLE KYPHOSIS (POSTURAL KYPHOSIS)

Patients with postural kyphosis usually present with cosmetic concerns, and the deformity can be corrected voluntarily. There are no abnormalities of the vertebrae noted on the standing lateral radiograph. Postural kyphosis does not progress to a structural deformity, nor is there evidence to suggest that patients will have problems later in life. Any coexisting back pain is typically mild, is activity related, and occurs in the midthoracic region by the apex of the curvature. In addition to reassurance, activity modifications are used to treat any discomfort, and strengthening the extensor muscles of the spine is potentially beneficial as well. Neither bracing nor surgery plays a role in the management of this condition.

STRUCTURAL KYPHOSIS

Scheuermann Disease

Scheuermann disease is the most common form of structural hyperkyphosis and is defined by wedging (>5 degrees) of 3 or more consecutive vertebral bodies at the apex of the deformity on a standing lateral radiograph of the thoracolumbar spine. Associated radiographic findings include irregularities of the vertebral end plates, disk space narrowing, and Schmorls nodes (herniations of nuclear material through the end plate and into the vertebral body). The reported incidence varies from 0.4% to 10%, and boys are involved more than girls. Histologic specimens have shown a disordered pattern of endochondral ossification, but it remains unclear whether these findings are due to an underlying genetic or metabolic problem or repetitive mechanical stresses. The etiology is likely multifactorial, involving the influence of mechanical forces in a genetically susceptible patient. Patients with Scheuermann disease are taller, are heavier, and have a larger body mass index when compared with age-matched controls, but these findings have not been correlated with the magnitude of the curvature. Patients usually present during their adolescent growth spurt, and the curve is most likely to progress during this time. The incidence is 1-8%, and boys are more commonly affected.

Clinical Manifestations

In addition to hyperkyphosis of the thoracic spine, the apex of the deformity is typically in the lower thoracic spine rather than the mid-thoracic spine, and the curvature has a sharper contour at the apex. Patients are unable to correct the deformity voluntarily. Pain is a relatively common complaint and is typically mild, activity related, and located at the apex of the kyphosis. A recent study using the Scoliosis Research Society outcomes instrument found that higher magnitudes of kyphosis were associated with more pain, a lower self-image, and decreased function and activity. Neurologic symptoms are rare and are most commonly due to an associated thoracic disk herniation at or near the apex of the kyphosis.

The natural history of Scheuermann disease appears to be relatively benign, and whereas adults with untreated Scheuermann disease might have a greater intensity of back pain, the prevalence of back pain appears to be no different than in the general population. Patients might select more sedentary occupations, but their self-esteem, participation in activities of daily living and recreational activities, and level of education seem to be no different than in the general population.

Radiographic Evaluation

Standing PA and lateral radiographs are obtained (Fig. 671-7). The recommended technique for the lateral radiograph involves folding the arms across the chest. A vertical plumb line dropped from C7 should intersect the anterosuperior corner of the sacrum for maintenance of sagittal spinal balance. A coexisting spondylolisthesis is rarely identified on the lateral radiograph. The standing PA radiograph often reveals a mild scoliosis, which is rarely progressive. An MRI is indicated in the presence of neurologic symptoms, and some surgeons routinely obtain an MRI before correcting a kyphosis.

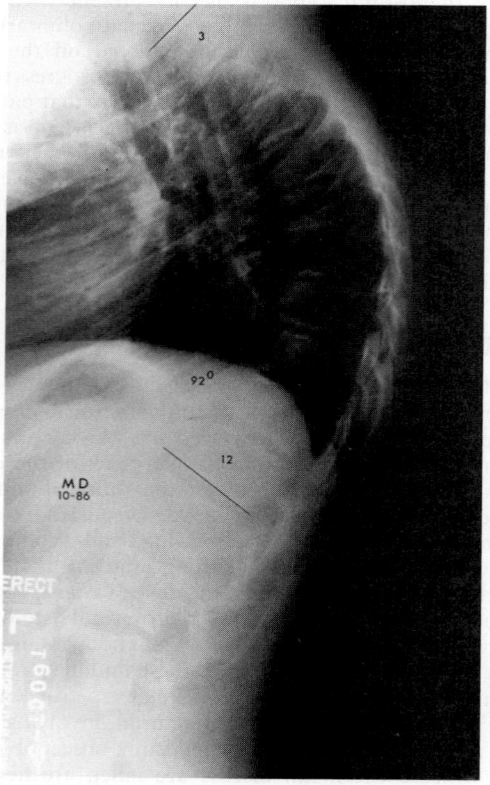

Figure 671-7 Standing lateral radiograph of a 14 yr old boy with severe Scheuermann kyphosis. This measures 92 degrees between T3 and T12. Note the wedging of the vertebrae at T6, T7, T8, and T9. The normal thoracic kyphosis is ≤40 degrees.

Treatment

Treatment is individualized and depends on the patient's degree of skeletal maturity, the magnitude of the deformity, and the presence of symptoms. Kyphotic deformities >90 degrees are more likely to be aesthetically unacceptable, symptomatic, and progressive. Deformities in excess of 100 degrees may be associated with pulmonary dysfunction, typically restrictive lung disease.

Skeletally immature patients with mild deformity might benefit from a hyperextension exercise program, but the effects of this strategy on the natural history remain to be documented. Patients with >1 yr of growth remaining and a kyphosis of >50-60 degrees might benefit from a bracing program. A Milwaukee brace (see Fig. 671-3) that extends up to the neck is recommended for curves with an apex above T7, but curves with a lower apex are often be treated by a thoracolumbar orthosis. The brace is recommended for 23 hr/day. On occasion, a serial casting (or stretching) program is instituted to gain flexibility before instituting the brace program. Although the goal of bracing is to prevent progression, a permanent improvement is observed in some patients. When bracing is effective in achieving permanent correction, radiographs show a reconstitution of anterior vertebral height (reversal of wedging). Skeletally mature patients with little or no pain and acceptable cosmesis are not treated.

Typical indications for surgery include progressive deformities >70-80 degrees in patients with persistent back pain despite nonoperative measures and/or dissatisfaction with their cosmetic appearance. The goal is to achieve a spinal arthrodesis while restoring the sagittal profile by correcting the thoracic kyphosis to within the normal range. Overcorrection can also impair sagittal balance, especially in patients with tight hamstrings. Formerly, an anterior release was typically performed before the posterior spinal fusion to improve flexibility, but there has been recent interest in performing an isolated posterior spinal fusion with multiple posterior osteotomies (removal of bone from the posterior elements), and the instrumentation and fusion typically extends from the upper thoracic to the upper lumbar spine.

CONGENITAL KYPHOSIS

Congenital kyphosis can result from either a failure of formation (more progressive and dangerous) or a failure of segmentation. In an anterior failure of formation (type I), there is an absence of a significant portion of the vertebra, resulting in a progressive kyphotic deformity or toppling over of the spine. This deformity results in neurologic dysfunction, if untreated, from compression of the spinal cord at the apex of the deformity. In type II congenital kyphosis there is an anterior failure of segmentation, with fusion of the involved vertebrae. Progression of kyphosis results from growth of the posterior elements of the spine and is typically slower and more variable than in type I deformities. There is a much lower chance of neurologic dysfunction. Patients must be followed closely, and treatment is required in a significant number of cases. As for congenital scoliosis, abnormalities of other organ systems (cardiac, renal, spinal cord) must be ruled out.

The treatment depends on the type of malformation, the degree of deformity, and whether neurologic symptoms are present. Bracing is ineffective for the primary curvature, but it is occasionally required to control compensatory curves. Surgery is the only effective treatment option for progressive curves or those with a poor natural history (type I), and it typically involves a spinal arthrodesis. Ideally, this can be performed before a significant deformity develops. Because the natural history is so poor for type I kyphoses, spinal fusion is usually performed shortly after the diagnosis is made. Depending on the degree of deformity and/or presence of neurologic dysfunction, excision of the vertebral remnant may be required to decompress the spinal cord and to restore alignment, in addition to a posterior spinal fusion. The vertebral remnant may be excised using an anterior approach before the posterior surgery or through the same posterior approach used for the spinal fusion. Surgical fusion can arrest progression, but deformity correction may be required to achieve a balanced spine. In patients with a mild deformity treated by a posterior spinal fusion, continued growth of the anterior column of the spine can result in some further improvement of the curvature over time. There is a significant risk of neurologic complications associated with surgery for congenital kyphosis, particularly the type I deformities.

BIBLIOGRAPHY

Please visit the Nelson Textbook of Pediatrics *website at www.expertconsult.com for the complete bibliography.*

671.5 Back Pain in Children

David A. Spiegel and John P. Dormans

Back pain is a relatively common complaint in children and adolescents, and the differential diagnosis is extensive (Table 671-2). Traditionally, it was thought that the majority of back pain in childhood and adolescence had an organic basis, suggesting the need for an extensive evaluation (including imaging studies) in all patients. Although back pain in infants and toddlers is often associated with underlying pathology, the likelihood of establishing a diagnosis in older children and adolescents is much less, roughly similar to that of the adult population. A definitive diagnosis may be established in 22-36%. The prevalence rate (5-75%) increases with age, approaching that of adults by the age of 18 yr, and most episodes of back pain resolve within 6 wk. Back pain can also be referred from the hip, the sacroiliac joint, or a visceral source. There is some evidence to suggest that back pain is more common with greater weights in backpacks. A thorough history and physical examination, often supplemented by imaging modalities, is required to rule out an underlying pathologic process. The treatment of back pain is tailored to the underlying diagnosis.

Table 671-2 DIFFERENTIAL DIAGNOSIS OF BACK PAIN
INFLAMMATORY OR INFECTIOUS
Diskitis
Vertebral osteomyelitis (pyogenic, tuberculous)
Spinal epidural abscess
Pyelonephritis
Pancreatitis
RHEUMATOLOGIC
Pauciarticular juvenile rheumatoid arthritis
Reiter syndrome
Ankylosing spondylitis
Psoriatic arthritis
DEVELOPMENTAL
Spondylolysis
Spondylolisthesis
Scheuermann disease
Scoliosis
TRAUMATIC (ACUTE VERSUS REPETITIVE)
Hip-pelvis anomalies
Herniated disk
Overuse syndromes
Vertebral stress fractures
Upper cervical spine instability
NEOPLASTIC
Vertebral Tumors
Benign
Eosinophilic granuloma
Aneurysmal bone cyst
Osteoid osteoma
Osteoblastoma
Malignant
Osteogenic sarcoma
Leukemia
Lymphoma
Metastatic Tumors
Spinal cord, ganglia, and nerve roots
Intramedullary spinal cord tumor
Sympathetic chain
Ganglioneuroma
Ganglioneuroblastoma
Neuroblastoma
OTHER
Intra-abdominal or pelvic pathology
Following lumbar puncture
Conversion reaction
Juvenile osteoporosis

CLINICAL EVALUATION

The history begins with the location, character, and duration of symptoms. Pain that is constant, unrelieved by rest, and wakes the patient from sleep is more likely to be secondary to an infection or neoplasm, as are systemic signs (fever) or symptoms (chills, weight loss, malaise). Symptoms of neurologic dysfunction also suggest that an underlying diagnosis is likely. The history must also uncover the presence of any radicular symptoms, gait disturbance, muscle weakness, alterations in sensation, and changes in bowel and/or bladder function.

The physical examination includes a complete musculoskeletal and neurologic assessment, and an abdominal exam should be performed. In appropriate cases, a gynecologic examination may also be helpful. The musculoskeletal examination begins in the standing position, noting any changes in alignment in the frontal or sagittal plane. Range of motion should be assessed in flexion, extension, and lateral bending. Flexion increases compression across the anterior elements of the spine (vertebral bodies and disks), and extension results in compression across the posterior elements (facet joints, pars interarticularis). Pain with flexion suggests an abnormality in the vertebral body or disk. Younger children should be asked to pick up an object off the floor, and pain is often due to diskitis. Pain with hyperextension (ask patient to hold the hyperextended position for 10-20 seconds) might have spondylolysis. Palpation will reveal any areas of tenderness and/or muscle spasm. Leg lengths are also assessed, by palpating the top of the iliac wings while the patient is standing. Because spinal pain may be referred, an abdominal examination should be performed, and in girls, a gynecologic evaluation may be necessary. The sacroiliac joint should be stressed by compression across the iliac wings or by forced external rotation with the hip and knee flexed to 90 degrees. The hamstring muscles should always be evaluated, because contracture is commonly associated with diagnoses such as Scheurmann disease, spondylolysis or spondylolisthesis, a herniated disk (or slipped vertebral apophysis), or other pathologies.

The neurologic examination includes manual muscle testing and an evaluation of sensation and proprioception. The superficial abdominal reflex should be tested by gently stroking the skin on each of the 4 quadrants surrounding the umbilicus. Normally, the umbilicus moves toward the area stimulated, and a normal examination is defined by a symmetric response (present or absent on both sides). Asymmetry suggests the presence of a subtle abnormality of spinal cord function, most commonly syringomyelia. The straight leg raise test is performed by raising up one leg with the knee extended. This test evaluates tension on the lower spinal nerve roots, and radicular symptoms (pain or tingling below the knee) will be reproduced. Possible causes of radiculopathy include a herniated disk, slipped vertebral apophysis, spondylolisthesis, tethered cord, and other causes. To further confirm the abnormal compression or stretch on the nerve root, the limb may be lowered to a position in which the symptoms are no longer present, and the foot is then dorsiflexed. Reproduction of the findings or symptoms with dorsiflexion of the foot further suggests the presence of nerve root compression or tension.

RADIOGRAPHIC AND LABORATORY EVALUATION

There are no specific guidelines for imaging in evaluating back pain in childhood and adolescence. For patients with any concerning signs or symptoms or for those with persistent symptoms, the initial study is commonly posteroanterior and lateral radiographs of the involved region of the spine. With lumbar back pain, some clinicians also obtain right and left oblique views. In patients with a normal neurologic examination, a bone scan can help to identify the location of pathology, and a bone scan with single-photon emission CT (SPECT) is more specific for the diagnosis of a stress reaction or spondylolysis, although an established stress fracture can have a negative scan. MRI is most helpful when neurologic symptoms or findings are present. CT is best at defining bony lesions, and a CT scan with thin cuts may be useful in the evaluation of spondylolysis.

Laboratory studies should also be considered, especially when systemic signs or constitutional symptoms are present, and may include a complete blood cell count with differential, erythrocyte sedimentation rate, C-reactive protein, and occasionally a rheumatoid factor, antinuclear antibody, Lyme, and/or HLA-B27.

BIBLIOGRAPHY

Please visit the Nelson Textbook of Pediatrics *website at www.expertconsult.com for the complete bibliography.*

671.6 Spondylolysis and Spondylolisthesis

David A. Spiegel and John P. Dormans

Spondylolysis is an acquired condition that involves a unilateral or bilateral defect in the pars interarticularis, the region of bone between the superior and inferior articular facets. Spondylolysis is identified in 4-6% of the adult population and is thought to result from repetitive hyperextension stresses, presumably resulting in mechanical impaction of the inferior articular facet of the superior vertebra against the pars interarticularis of the inferior vertebra. Repetitive tensile loading is also postulated in some cases, and abnormalities of the sacral growth plate have been implicated in some cases as well. The process can begin with a stress reaction, which can then lead to a stress fracture, and ultimately to an established pseudarthrosis (nonunion or "false joint") at the pars interarticularis. Spondylolysis is most common in athletes with activities involving repetitive spinal hyperextension, especially gymnasts, football players (especially interior linemen), weight lifters, and wrestlers. Persons with excessive lumbar lordosis may be at higher risk, and a genetic component has been suggested. The lesion is most common at L5, but it may also be identified at higher levels in the lumbar spine, and it rarely occurs at more than one level. The natural history is variable; many patients are asymptomatic, but a subset experiences mechanical low back pain that can limit activities and require treatment. Approximately 15-25% of patients develop a spondylolisthesis.

Spondylolisthesis involves slippage of 1 vertebra on another and is most common at L5 (85-95%). In children and adolescents, the most common types are dysplastic (congenital) and isthmic (results from a stress fracture). In a dysplastic spondylolisthesis, the posterior elements of the spine remain intact but are elongated. Progression of spondylolisthesis has been associated with a higher degree of slippage (>50%), lumbosacral kyphosis (slip angle > 40 degrees), and dome-shaped sacrum. It is more common in female and in younger patients.

CLINICAL MANIFESTATIONS

Symptomatic patients with spondylolysis or spondylolisthesis usually present with mechanical low back pain that can radiate to the buttocks and thigh but rarely below the knee. The pain is exacerbated by spinal hyperextension, which exerts compression on the posterior elements. A useful provocative test, with the patient standing, involves placing the spine in hyperextension and holding the position for up to 10-20 seconds. This compresses the posterior elements and might reproduce the symptoms. In contrast, pain emanating from disk space pathology is exacerbated by spinal flexion. Physical examination might also reveal tenderness over the spinous process of the involved vertebra. Hamstring spasm, with or without contracture, is commonly observed.

The physical findings may be more pronounced in patients with spondylolisthesis. The buttocks appear flattened (sacrum is more vertically inclined, lumbosacral kyphosis), and the abdomen might appear more protuberant (hyperlordosis above the lumbosacral kyphosis). There is often a palpable step off between the spinous processes at the involved levels, especially with a high-grade slip. Hamstring spasm or contracture is usually more pronounced than in spondylolysis. Gait disturbance is also observed, typically characterized by mild crouching, a short stride length, and an incomplete swing phase. A careful neurologic examination is required. In addition to back pain, neurologic symptoms (radiculopathy or bowel or bladder dysfunction) can result from compression of the cauda equina or nerve roots. Radicular symptoms or findings are uncommon except in high-grade spondylolisthesis, when there may be excessive tension (or mechanical compression) on the lower lumbar nerve roots. In contrast to lumbar disk herniations, which most commonly affect the lower root (L4-L5 disk herniation compresses the L5 nerve root), spondylolisthesis of L5 on S1 affects the L5 nerve root.

RADIOGRAPHIC EVALUATION

The initial evaluation of the lumbar region should include high-quality anteroposterior, lateral, and oblique radiographs. The pars is best visualized on the oblique radiographs, and a pars defect has been termed the Scotty dog sign. Standing PA and lateral radiographs are obtained if findings suggestive of scoliosis or hyperkyphosis are also present (Figs. 671-8 and 671-9). In patients with normal plain films, a bone scan with SPECT images can help to diagnose a spondylolysis during the early stages (stress reaction), before a fracture or an established pseudarthrosis develops. A CT scan with thin cuts can establish the presence of a pars defect or a pseudarthrosis. If the bone scan shows no increased uptake in the region, and a CT scan demonstrates a pars defect, then the potential for healing is felt to be limited. Although MRI is most commonly indicated in the presence of signs or symptoms of cauda equina or nerve root involvement, it has been used more and more during the diagnostic phase.

Spondylolisthesis is graded according to the degree of translation of the superior vertebra as follows: grade 1, <25%; grade 2, 25-50%; grade 3, 50-75%; grade 4, 75-100%; and grade 5, complete displacement or spondyloptosis. The degree of rotation of the upper vertebra on the lower (kyphosis) is also measured as the angle in between a line drawn along the posterior margin of the sacrum and a line drawn along the superior end plate of the L5 vertebra (slip angle). In patients with spondylolisthesis, flexion and extension films are occasionally performed to identify instability (excessive translation through this range of motion). Because progressive slippage can occur in a subset of skeletally

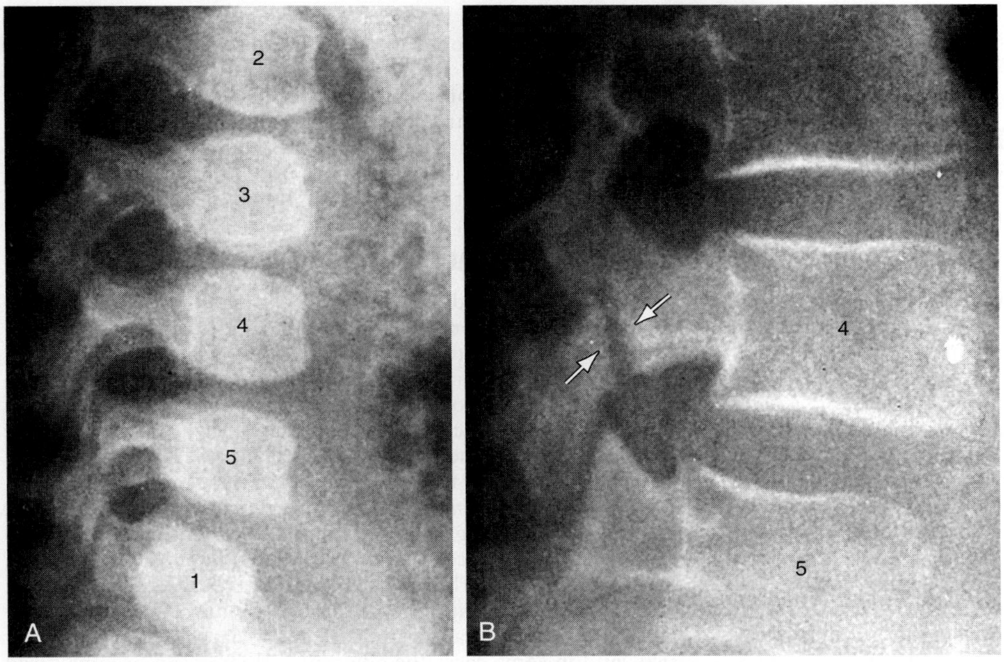

Figure 671-8 *A,* Normal spine at 9 mo of age. *B,* Spondylolysis in the L4 vertebra at 10 yr of age. (From Silverman FN, Kuhn JP: *Essentials of Caffrey's pediatric x-ray diagnosis,* Chicago, 1990, Year Book Medical Publishers, p 94.)

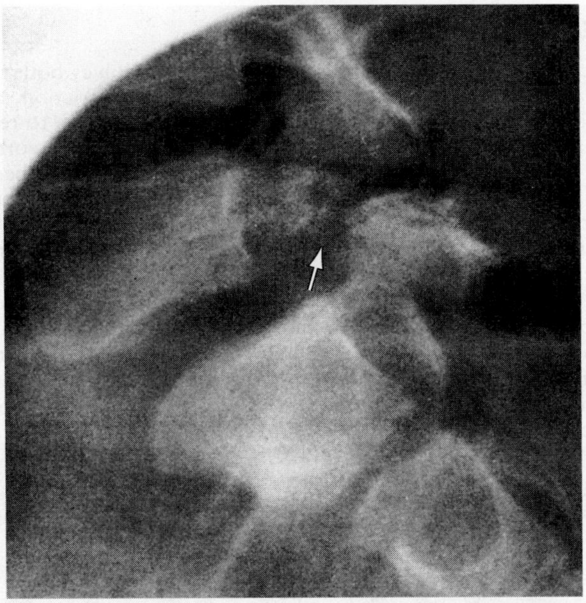

Figure 671-9 Defect in the pars interarticularis *(arrow)* of the neural arch of L5 (spondylolysis) that has permitted the body of L5 to slip forward (spondylolisthesis) on the body of S1. (From Silverman FN, Kuhn JP: *Essentials of Caffrey's pediatric x-ray diagnosis,* Chicago, 1990, Year Book Medical Publishers, p 95.)

immature patients, a standing lateral radiograph of the lumbar spine should be considered every 6-12 mo.

TREATMENT

Asymptomatic patients with spondylolysis require no active treatment, but those with pain are treated with rest and/or modification of activity, physical therapy (focusing on hamstring stretching and strengthening of the abdominal musculature), and non-narcotic analgesics. In patients with a stress reaction or early stress fracture without an established pseudarthrosis, healing may be achieved with nonoperative measures. Unilateral defects are more likely to heal when compared with bilateral defects, and the presence of high signal in the adjacent pedicle on MRI also implies a better chance of healing. A modified lumbosacral orthosis, which reduces lumbar lordosis (15 degrees of flexion of the lumbar spine) and immobilizes the spine, is typically recommended for 3-4 mo full time. For patients with an established pseudarthrosis, the goal is relief of symptoms rather than union. Overall, nonoperative measures are successful in the majority of patients, and a successful clinical outcome does not depend on healing of the lesion.

Surgery is offered when symptoms persist despite an adequate trial of nonoperative therapy. For spondylolysis, surgical options include repair of the pars defect versus spinal fusion. If the spondylolysis is at L5, then a posterior spinal fusion from L5 to S1 is most commonly performed. For the uncommon cases in which the defect is at L4 or at higher levels, techniques for repairing the defect should be considered. If successful, these procedures will avoid the need for surgical fusion. Some surgeons use an MRI to evaluate the disk space at that level and select a fusion rather than a pars repair if there are degenerative changes in the disk.

Recommendations for managing spondylolisthesis depend on the age of the patient, the presence of symptoms (pain and/or neurologic), the degree of deformity, and to a lesser extent cosmetic concerns. For low-grade lesions (<50% slippage) with chronic symptoms despite nonoperative treatment, a posterior spinal fusion alone, with or without instrumentation, may be successful. For skeletally immature patients with >50% slippage, with or without symptoms, surgery is offered given the risk of progression. The surgical approach for higher-grade slips varies among surgeons and institutions. The main principle is to stabilize the unstable segment of the spine through spinal fusion, either a posterior or an anterior and posterior spinal fusion with spinal instrumentation.

Whether or not to reduce the spondylolisthesis at the time of surgery remains a subject of controversy. A reduction may be achieved through gravity or intraoperative positioning or through direct realignment using the spinal implants. Although neurologic symptoms can resolve with stabilization, a decompression of the neural elements is commonly performed as a component of the stabilization procedure for high-grade spondylolisthesis.

BIBLIOGRAPHY
Please visit the Nelson Textbook of Pediatrics *website at www.expertconsult.com for the complete bibliography.*

671.7 Disk Space Infection

David A. Spiegel and John P. Dormans

Both diskitis and vertebral osteomyelitis may be considered as age-dependent variations of infectious spondylitis. Diskitis is generally seen in children <5 yr of age, and vertebral osteomyelitis occurs in older children and adolescents. This spectrum may be explained on the basis of anatomy; the vertebral column in infants and younger children has vascular channels that communicate between the vertebral end plate and the vascular disk space, allowing organisms to seed the disk space (Table 671-3). Once these channels have closed, the infection remains in the vertebra.

The available evidence suggests that diskitis is a low-grade bacterial infection rather than an inflammatory process. Cultures of either the blood or disk space are positive in only 50-60% of patients, and *Staphylococcus aureus* (Chapter 174) is the most common organism isolated. Cultures are more likely to be positive if the symptoms have been present for <6 wk. Other organisms include *Kingella kingae* (Chapter 676), group A streptococcus (Chapter 176), and *Escherichia coli* (Chapter 192).

The differential diagnosis includes infectious, inflammatory, neoplastic, and developmental conditions. Granulomatous infections, such as brucellosis and tuberculosis, and fungal infections typically involve the anterior elements of the spine and must always be considered under certain circumstances (immunocompromised host, history of travel to certain regions, immigrants from selected regions). Neoplastic diseases involving the anterior elements include eosinophilic granuloma, leukemia, and lymphoma. Inflammatory conditions such as juvenile idiopathic arthritis can also manifest with symptoms similar to diskitis. Back pain can also be referred from another source. Other conditions in the differential diagnosis include intra-abdominal conditions (appendicitis, pyelonephritis), septic arthritis of the sacroiliac joint, psoas abscess, or hip pathology (septic arthritis or other).

CLINICAL MANIFESTATIONS

A high index of suspicion is required to establish the diagnosis of diskitis, especially in younger patients. The differential includes vertebral osteomyelitis (see Table 671-3). In addition to back pain and/or fever, patients can experience malaise, and toddlers can develop a limp or refuse to walk or sit. Spinal motion is voluntarily reduced to alleviate pain, and paraspinal muscle spasm is common. Flexion of the spine compresses the anterior elements of the spine and should increase any discomfort. This may be tested by asking the child to pick up an object from the ground. There may a loss of the normal lumbar lordosis. Neurologic manifestations are rare. Patients may be afebrile, and although a complete blood count might remain normal, the erythrocyte sedimentation rate and the C-reactive protein are usually elevated. Older children might have fever and abdominal pain.

RADIOGRAPHIC EVALUATION

A PA and lateral radiograph of the thoracolumbar spine is the first imaging study ordered when the diagnosis is suspected, recognizing that characteristic findings of disk space narrowing and irregularity of the adjacent vertebral end plates often take 2-3 wk to develop after the onset of symptoms. Other changes noted on plain radiographs include demineralization, with erosions at the vertebral margins, and loss of vertebral height. The diagnosis may be established earlier using either a technetium bone scan or MRI. *MRI provides more information and is most helpful in identifying abscesses and ruling out vertebral osteomyelitis.* Plain radiographs during the course of follow-up might reveal sclerosis at the margins of the adjacent vertebral bodies after several months (remineralization), and although some restoration of vertebral body height can occur, disk space narrowing usually persists, and in some cases the adjacent vertebrae can become fused or enlarged.

TREATMENT

Once the diagnosis is established, treatment involves both treating symptoms and giving antibiotics. Activity restriction, analgesics, and immobilization in a spinal orthosis all help to relieve symptoms. Typically, a thoracolumbosacral orthosis is worn for 4-6 wk. Antibiotics effective against *S. aureus* are prescribed for 4-6 wk, and although treatment protocols vary, an intravenous route of administration is typically used for at least 1-2 wk. The treatment can then be converted to an oral regimen, assuming that the clinical response has been adequate in terms of both symptoms and inflammatory markers. A CT-guided needle biopsy of the disk space is reserved for children who fail to respond to these treatment measures and those in whom an alternative diagnosis is suspected. Surgical treatment is rarely required and involves either an open biopsy or drainage of an abscess.

BIBLIOGRAPHY
Please visit the Nelson Textbook of Pediatrics *website at www.expertconsult.com for the complete bibliography.*

Table 671-3 SPECTRUM OF NONTUBERCULOUS INFECTION OF THE SPINE

SIGNS, SYMPTOMS, AND DEMOGRAPHICS	DISKITIS	VERTEBRAL OSTEOMYELITIS
Most common age	Younger than 7 yr Peak at 3 yr	Older than 8 yr
Symptoms	Limp, back pain Refusal to walk	Same as for diskitis
Location of lesion	Lumbar	Anywhere along spine
Febrile	Less likely (28%)	More likely (79%)
Laboratory values (complete blood Count, sedimentation rate)	Nonspecific elevation	Nonspecific elevation
Plain radiograph	Early: normal>20 days: disk space abnormal	Early: normal 7-20 days: disk space and vertebrae abnormal
Magnetic resonance imaging	Localizes lesion	Localizes lesion Defined soft tissue involvement
Blood culture	Often negative	Often positive
Antibiotic therapy	Controversial	Yes

From Slovis TR, editor: *Caffey's pediatric diagnostic imaging,* ed 11, vol 1, Philadelphia, 2008, Elsevier.

671.8 Intervertebral Disk Herniation and Slipped Vertebral Apophysis

David A. Spiegel and John P. Dormans

Intervertebral disk herniation and slipped vertebral apophysis are extremely rare in children and uncommon in adolescents. The symptoms and physical findings are quite similar to those in adults. Although the etiology remains unknown, predisposing factors for both of these can include disk degeneration, congenital malformation (altered regional biomechanics), genetics, and environmental factors (trauma or repetitive stresses). *Herniated disk* is a term that reflects a spectrum of pathology from simple protrusion of the disk material with an intact annulus fibrosis to the herniation of a free fragment of disk material into the spinal canal. Both are space-occupying lesions, and symptoms are due to either direct mechanical compression of nerve roots (or cauda equina) or an inflammatory response in proximity to neural elements. Ossification of the ring apophysis begins around 6 years of age, and the apophysis fuses with the vertebral body at approximately 17 years of age. Slipped vertebral apophysis involves protrusion of a portion of the ring apophysis with or without an attached segment of bone. The symptoms are similar to that of a herniated disk; in one study the two entities coexisted in 28% of adolescent disk herniations.

CLINICAL MANIFESTATIONS

Symptoms of intervertebral disk herniation in adolescents are similar to those in adults; the major complaint is back pain, and radicular symptoms (if present) generally appear later in the course. The back pain is often made worse by coughing or straining. Although a history of acute injury is found in a subset of cases, many patients have a history of repetitive stresses, such as young elite athletes. Some patients have congenital anomalies of the lumbosacral spine. On physical examination, both paraspinal muscle spasm and a decrease in range of motion are common. Overt signs of neurologic involvement are absent in most patients, but the straight leg raise test is usually positive. With the positive straight leg test, the neurologic findings often do not correlate with the level of disk herniation. An intraspinal tumor should always be included in the differential diagnosis.

RADIOGRAPHIC EVALUATION

Radiographs often show loss of lumbar lordosis and a lumbar curvature (not a true scoliosis) that is due to muscle spasm. Degenerative changes and/or a loss of intervertebral disk height is occasionally noted on plain films; however, apophyseal fragments are usually not seen. MRI is the best study to establish the diagnosis, and CT is especially helpful to visualize a partially ossified fragment associated with a slipped apophysis. Types of slipped vertebral apophysis include an avulsion of the cortical margin with or without a fragment of cancellous bone, a lateral fracture, and a posterior wall fracture that extends from the superior vertebral endplate to the inferior vertebral endplate.

TREATMENT

The initial treatment is nonoperative in most patients and focuses on rest, activity modification, analgesics, and physical therapy. An orthosis can provide additional symptomatic relief. Complete bed rest is not recommended. The role of epidural steroids remains to be determined. Surgical treatment should be considered when nonoperative measures have failed or when a profound neurologic deficit or cauda equina syndrome is present either initially or as the clinical course evolves.

Unfortunately, children and adolescents respond less favorably to nonoperative therapy compared with adults, and a significant percentage require surgical intervention. The surgical technique involves laminotomy and subtotal disk excision to decompress the neural elements. In the case of a slipped vertebral apophysis, a similar approach is employed for decompression of the neural elements, but there is some controversy about whether or not to routinely remove the apophyseal fragment. Some surgeons remove the fragment when there are neurologic symptoms; one report suggested that an intraoperative assessment of the mobility of apophyseal fragments is helpful, and the authors only removed loose fragments. A bilateral laminotomy may be required in these cases to address the pathology.

Although the initial results are excellent in the majority of patients, the literature suggests that up to a third of patients have recurrent symptoms of back or leg pain at longer term follow-up. The reoperation rate is in the range of 15%, similar to that of the adult population. A spinal fusion may be required when clinical instability is present.

BIBLIOGRAPHY

Please visit the Nelson Textbook of Pediatrics *website at www.expertconsult.com for the complete bibliography.*

671.9 Tumors

David A. Spiegel and John P. Dormans

Back pain may be the most common presenting complaint in children who have a tumor involving the vertebral column or the spinal cord. Other associated symptoms can include weakness of the lower extremities, scoliosis, and loss of bowel or bladder function. The majority of tumors are benign (Chapter 495). Lesions that may be observed in the anterior elements of the spine include aneurysmal bone cyst, eosinophilic granuloma, leukemia, and lymphoma; common tumors involving the posterior elements include osteoid osteoma and osteoblastoma. Malignant tumors involving the vertebral column may be osseous (osteosarcoma or Ewing sarcoma) or rarely are due to metastatic disease. Lesions in the soft tissues surrounding the spine are most commonly neurogenic, involving the spinal cord and sympathetic nerves (ganglioneuroma, ganglioneuroblastoma, neuroblastoma). In addition to high-quality plain radiographs, modalities including a bone scan (localization, look for other lesions), MRI (soft-tissue extension, neurologic compression) and CT (excellent bony detail) are performed in most cases before making a treatment plan. A biopsy is usually required to establish the diagnosis, and the treatment of tumors of the spinal column can require a multidisciplinary approach and should ideally be done in centers with experience in managing these lesions.

Chapter 672 The Neck

672.1 Torticollis

David A. Spiegel and John P. Dormans

Torticollis is a symptom rather than a diagnosis, and describes the clinical findings of tilting of the head to the right or left side in combination with rotation of the head to the opposite side. Congenital muscular torticollis (CMT) is the most common etiology, but a variety of other conditions result in torticollis, and a detailed workup is often required to rule out other diagnoses in patients who lack the characteristic features of CMT (approximately 20%) (Fig. 672-1). The differential diagnosis includes trauma (clavicle fracture or brachial plexopathy), tumors or

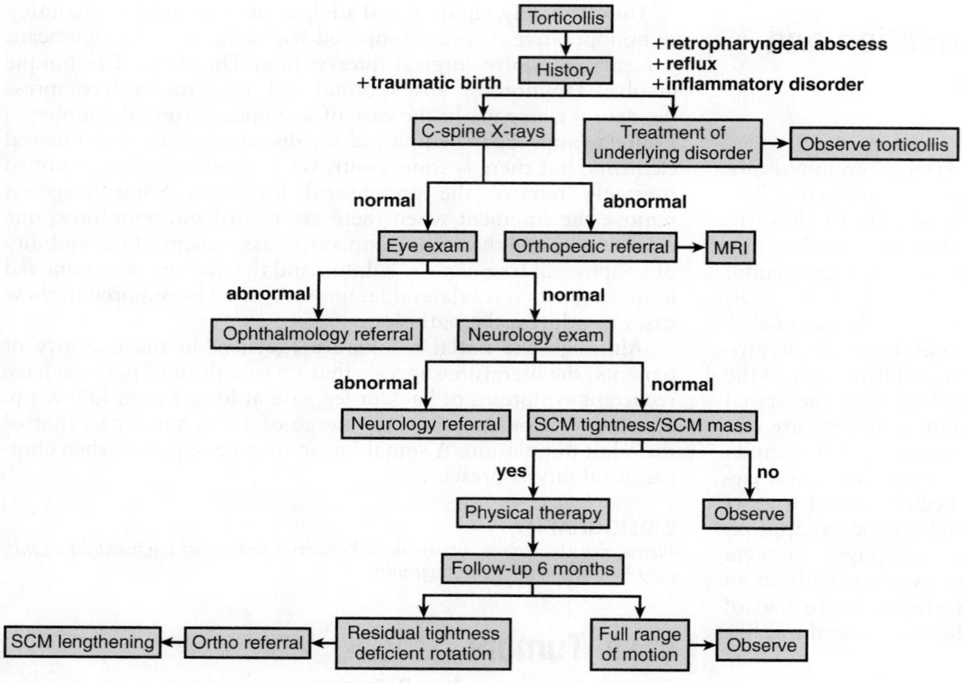

Figure 672-1 Algorithm for evaluation of muscular torticollis. SCM, sternocleidomastoid muscle. (From Do TT: Congenital muscular torticollis: current concepts and review of treatment, *Curr Opin Pediatr* 18:26–29, 2006.)

Table 672-1 DIFFERENTIAL DIAGNOSIS OF TORTICOLLIS

CONGENITAL
Osseous anomalies (Hemivertebra, unilateral atlanto-occipital fusion, Klippel-Feil syndrome)
Soft tissue abnormalities (unilateral absence of sternocleidomastoid, pterygium colli)
ACQUIRED
Positional deformation or congenital muscular torticollis
Trauma (muscular injury, fractures)
Cervical instability (atlanto-occipital subluxation, atlantoaxial subluxation, subaxial subluxation)
Atlantoaxial rotatory displacement
INFLAMMATION
Cervical lymphadenitis
Retropharyngeal abscess
Diskitis or vertebral osteomyelitis
Rheumatoid arthritis
NEUROLOGIC
Visual disturbances (nystagmus, superior oblique paresis)
Dystonic drug reactions (phenothiazines, haloperidol, metoclopramide)
Neoplasia (cervical spinal cord or posterior fossa tumor)
Chiari I malformation and/or syringomyelia
Wilson disease
Dystonia
Spasmus nutans (nystagmus, head bobbing, head tilting)
OTHER
Acute cervical disk calcification
Sandifer syndrome (gastroesophageal reflux, hiatal hernia)
Benign paroxysmal torticollis of infancy
Bone tumors (eosinophilic granuloma)
Soft tissue tumor
Hysteria

malformations of the central nervous system, ocular disorders, congenital bony abnormalities (Klippel-Feil syndrome), inflammatory conditions, and other diagnoses such as atlantoaxial rotatory displacement or Sandifer syndrome (Table 672-1).

The majority of cases discovered within the first few months of life represent **congenital muscular torticollis** (CMT), which occurs in up to 1/250 live births. In newborns, other diagnoses include clavicle fracture and/or brachial plexopathy. Although the etiology of CMT remains unknown, current evidence (muscle biopsies and MRI studies showing fibrosis) supports in utero muscular compression and/or stretch, possibly resulting in localized ischemia and an intramuscular compartment syndrome. CMT is more common in firstborn children and following difficult births.

A contracture of the left sternocleidomastoid muscle results in tilt of the head to the left and rotation to the right, and vice versa. A fibrotic mass is palpable within the substance of the sternocleidomastoid muscle in approximately 50% of patients, and it usually disappears within the first months of life, often being replaced by a fibrous band. CMT may be seen as part of a molded baby syndrome, occurring in combination with other findings thought to relate to intrauterine mechanical deformation such as developmental hip dysplasia, plagiocephaly, facial asymmetry, and foot deformities such as metatarsus adductus. A prospective study of 102 consecutive newborns demonstrated morphologic "asymmetries" in 73%, including torticollis (16%), mandibular asymmetry (13%), facial asymmetry (42%), and skull asymmetry (61%). Facial findings associated with CMT include flattening on the affected side, recessed eyebrow and zygoma, and inferior orbital displacement. There is also evidence to suggest that persistent sternocleidomastoid contracture can result in progressive deformation; although morphologic abnormalities of the cranium and cranial base may be observed in infancy, facial bone asymmetry develops at or later than 5 yr of age. Hip dysplasia occurs in ~3-9% of patients with CMT, and although guidelines for screening in patients with a normal hip examination have not been established, consideration should be given to obtaining either an ultrasound scan (1 mo of age) or a plain radiograph of the hip (4-5 mo of age). A delay in achieving early developmental milestones has been reported in babies with CMT, but this is most likely explained by a decrease in prone positioning while awake.

Torticollis can also result from congenital vertebral anomalies (including Klippel-Feil syndrome). Although there are no formal guidelines for when to order plain radiographs to rule out an underlying congenital osseous abnormality, radiographs of the cervical spine are suggested when the typical clinical features associated with congenital muscular torticollis are absent or if the deformity does not respond to treatment. This recommendation is supported by a study in which congenital vertebral anomalies were identified on screening radiographs in only 4 of 502 infants with torticollis in the absence of birth trauma; radiographic findings that would serve as a contraindication to a stretching program were only identified in a single patient.

The treatment of congenital muscular torticollis involves stretching, stimulation, and positioning measures, often supervised by a physical therapist. Resolution should be achieved in approximately 95% of cases, especially when the treatment is started during the first 4 mo of life. Intramuscular injection of botulinum toxin A (Botox) into the sternocleidomastoid may be considered in resistant cases of CMT, although further study is required to determine the effectiveness and indications for this modality. Complications include transient dysphagia and neck weakness.

For patients with a late diagnosis or those in whom the stretching program has failed to correct the deformity, surgical release of the sternocleidomastoid is considered. The optimal timing for surgery continues to be debated. Some authors have suggested that the procedure be performed at 12-18 mo of age to facilitate remodeling of craniofacial molding abnormalities, due to the greater growth potential in the younger patients. Others have suggested that outcomes are improved when the surgery is delayed until later, even to school age. Motion can be improved following surgical release even in teenagers. One study compared a cohort from 1-4 yr of age with another from 5-16 yr of age and concluded that although there were no significant differences in craniofacial asymmetry, residual contracture, and subjective measures, the older age group had less surgical scarring and head tilt. Surgical management results in adequate function and acceptable cosmesis in >90% of patients. With early diagnosis and treatment, surgery should be required in only a minority of cases.

The evaluation of torticollis becomes more complex when the typical findings associated with CMT are absent, the usual clinical response is not observed, or the deformity occurs at a later age. A careful history and physical examination is essential, supplemented by additional imaging studies and often consultation with an ophthalmologist, neurologist, or other specialists. Plain radiographs should be obtained to rule out an underlying congenital osseous abnormality, and an MRI of the brain and cervical spine are required in many cases to rule out a tumor (posterior fossa or brainstem) or a developmental condition such as a Chiari I malformation and/or syringomyelia.

Torticollis can result from congenital vertebral anomalies or congenital scoliosis, and progressive deformities can require surgical stabilization. **Ocular torticollis** can result from strabismus (weakness of the 4th cranial nerve) or a superior oblique muscle palsy. Sandifer's syndrome describes torticollis in association with gastroesophageal reflux. Atlantoaxial rotatory displacement represents a spectrum of rotational malalignment (subluxation to dislocation) between the atlas (C1) and the axis (C2), and may best be described as pathologic stickiness in the arc of joint motion. The malalignment may initially be reducible, but after weeks to months the deformity becomes fixed and irreducible. Thus, prompt diagnosis and treatment are essential.

A variety of conditions can lead to rotatory displacement, including infection or inflammation of the tissues of the upper airway, neck, and/or pharynx (Grisel syndrome). Traumatic injuries (usually minor) have been associated, and rotatory displacement occasionally complicates surgical procedures in the oropharynx, ear, or nose. The diagnosis is confirmed with a CT scan in which axial images are obtained from the occiput through C2 in neutral alignment and with maximal rotation to the right and to the left. The images essentially define the motion curve between the 2 vertebrae and determine whether any rotational malalignment is reducible, partially reducible, or fixed. Rotatory fixation exists when the relationship between C1 and C2 remains constant through the arc of motion.

The treatment varies based on the underlying pathology and the chronicity of symptoms. If the patient is seen within a few days of the onset of symptoms, then a trial of analgesics and a soft collar may be attempted. Patients with symptoms for >1 wk are often admitted to the hospital for analgesia, muscle relaxants, and a period of cervical traction. If this fails to restore normal anatomy and motion, then halo traction may be attempted. The amount of force transmitted is limited to 5-8 lb with cervical traction, due to pressure on the mandible. Much greater traction weights may be applied when a halo or Gardner Wells tongs are applied. If the malalignment is corrected and full cervical motion is restored, patients are typically immobilized for at least 6 wk in a halo vest. A pinless halo has been employed in some centers to immobilize these patients, because the device does not require pins to be placed into the skull and is better tolerated. Patients who fail to respond to traction, typically those with a fixed deformity, and those in whom the malalignment has recurred, may require a posterior atlantoaxial fusion to stabilize the articulation.

Paroxysmal torticollis of infancy is uncommon and may be due to vestibular dysfunction. Episodes can last for <1 wk, and the side of the deformity can alternate. The condition is self-limited, improves by 2 yr of age, and usually resolves by 3 yr of age. Gross and fine motor delays are identified in approximately 50% of patients, and there is a strong family history of migraines. Torticollis may also be seen in association with diskitis or vertebral osteomyelitis, juvenile rheumatoid arthritis, and cervical disk calcification.

BIBLIOGRAPHY

Please visit the Nelson Textbook of Pediatrics *website at www.expertconsult.com for the complete bibliography.*

672.2 Klippel-Feil Syndrome

David A. Spiegel and John P. Dormans

Klippel-Feil syndrome involves a congenital fusion (failure of segmentation) of one or more cervical motion segments, and the clinical triad of short neck, low hairline, and restriction of neck motion is seen in only about half of the patients. Most patients have associated congenital anomalies at the craniocervical junction (occiput-C2), the subaxial spine (below C2), or both (Fig. 672-2). A familial gene locus on the long arm of chromosome 8 has been identified. Abnormalities in other organ systems must be ruled out. Associated anomalies have been identified in the genitouríninary system (30-40%; unilateral renal agenesis, duplicated collecting systems, horseshoe kidney), auditory system, heart, neural axis, and the musculoskeletal system (Sprengel deformity in one third, scoliosis). Congenital cervical fusions or anomalies are also commonly seen in patients with Goldenhar syndrome, Mohr syndrome, VACTERL syndrome (*v*ertebral anomalies, *a*nal atresia, *c*ardiovascular anomalies, *t*racheoesophageal fistula, *e*sophageal atresia, *r*enal and/or radial anomalies, *l*imb defects), and fetal alcohol syndrome.

Characteristic physical findings include a low hairline and a short, webbed neck. Decreased cervical motion is often present, although the degree of restriction depends on both the location and the number of levels fused. Whereas a C1-C2 fusion restricts cervical rotation >50%, but an isolated fusion in the subaxial spine has negligible loss of motion. Patients are evaluated with posterior, anterior, lateral, and oblique views of the cervical spine. The characteristic finding is a congenital fusion of ≥2 vertebrae (failure of segmentation), and multiple vertebrae may be involved. Because congenital anomalies can exist in more than one region of the spine, radiographs of the thoracic and lumbosacral spine are routinely obtained. Approximately 75% of cases involve the upper 3 cervical vertebrae, and the most common level is C2-C3. Half of the patients will have involvement of <3 vertebrae.

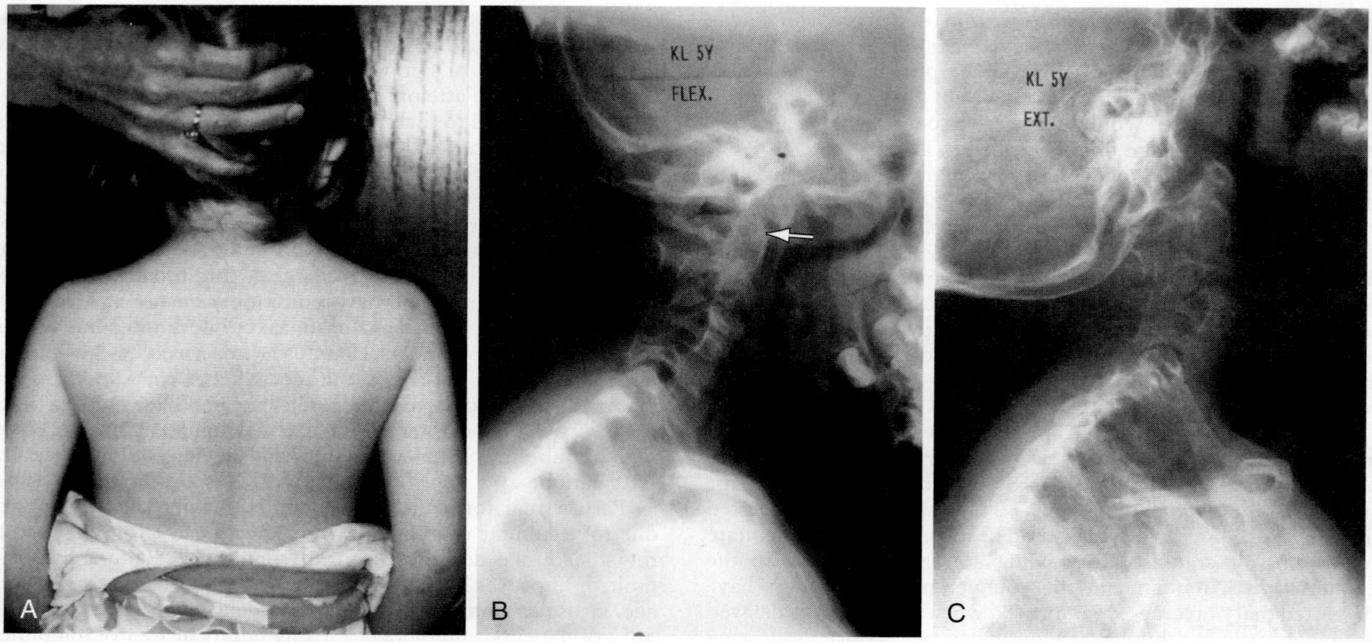

Figure 672-2 Clinical picture of a 5 yr old with Klippel-Feil syndrome. *A,* Note short neck and low hairline. Radiographs of the cervical spine (*B,* flexion; *C,* extension) demonstrate congenital fusion and evidence of spinal instability *(arrow).* (From Drummond DS: Pediatric cervical instability. In Weisel SE, Boden SD, Wisnecki RI, editors: *Seminars in spine surgery,* Philadelphia, 1996, WB Saunders, pp 292–309.)

Flexion and extension radiograph are commonly used to rule out hypermobility of instability, and an MRI with or without flexion and extension is also commonly obtained.

Symptoms are more common in adults than in children or adolescents and include pain and/or neurologic dysfunction. Excessive segmental motion can become clinically evident as radiculopathy or myelopathy, and brainstem compression can also occur. Spinal stenosis can also result in pain and/or neurologic compression. Degenerative changes in the disks and/or facet joints are likely due to the altered mechanical stresses, and segmental hypermobility (or instability) usually develops at the mobile segments adjacent to fused segments. The risk increases with the number of fused segments. MRI studies have demonstrated coexisting abnormalities in 85% of patients, including degenerative changes (disc protrusion, osteophytes, stenosis) and neural anomalies (syringomyelia, Chiari I malformation, diastematomyelia). A recent study found that there is a decrease in vertebral body width in the fused segments (likely due to interruption of appositional bone growth) and that the space available for the spinal cord was actually increased at these levels. Surgical treatments usually involve either decompression (with or without fusion) for stenosis associated with neural encroachment, and spinal fusion for instability. Occasionally a progressive cervicothoracic scoliosis requires stabilization to prevent deformity.

BIBLIOGRAPHY

Please visit the Nelson Textbook of Pediatrics *website at www.expertconsult.com for the complete bibliography.*

672.3 Cervical Anomalies and Instabilities

David A. Spiegel and John P. Dormans

Anomalies of the craniovertebral junction and/or the lower cervical spine may be seen in isolation or in association with other conditions such as genetic syndromes and skeletal dysplasias. Congenital anomalies can result from a mutation in the homeobox genes. Coexisting abnormalities in other organ systems (renal, cardiac, intraspinal) must be ruled out. The true incidence is unknown, because many of these anomalies remain asymptomatic and undiagnosed. A subset of these anomalies, whether symptomatic or asymptomatic, places the patient at risk of neurologic injury due to either cervical instability or spinal stenosis. There seems to be no difference between syndromic and nonsyndromic anomalies when considering symptoms, findings, or treatment. Cervical instabilities may be associated with certain congenital anomalies, or with a variety of other conditions predisposing to excessive laxity or mobility (connective tissue disorders, metabolic diseases). The host of cervical anomalies and instabilities are categorized in Table 672-2.

Patients present with a variety of complaints include headache, neck pain, or neurologic symptoms such as radicular pain or weakness (myelopathy). The spectrum of symptoms or physical findings associated with craniovertebral anomalies also includes failure to thrive, dysphagia, sleep apnea, torticollis, or scoliosis. The pathophysiology of neurologic dysfunction can involve neural compression (spinal cord or brainstem), vascular compression (vertebrobasilar symptoms), and/or altered cerebrospinal fluid (CSF) dynamics.

Physical findings include a restriction in cervical range of motion in some anomalies, with or without neurologic abnormalities. In the upper cervical spine, flexion and extension take place at the occiput-C1 articulation, and rotation occurs at the atlantoaxial (C1-C2) joint. Neither possesses inherent osseous stability and instead depends on the integrity of the ligaments and joint capsules to constrain motion. In addition to a comprehensive history and physical examination, imaging studies are required in all patients who are symptomatic, as well as in patients with disease processes known to be associated with cervical anomalies or instabilities.

The radiographic evaluation begins with anteroposterior, lateral, and open mouth (odontoid) views, which may be supplemented by dynamic (flexion and extension lateral of cervical spine) radiographs in most cases. Dynamic radiographs are used to evaluate the degree of translation between vertebrae, most

Table 672-2 CAUSES OF PEDIATRIC CERVICAL INSTABILITY

CONGENITAL
Vertebral (Bony Anomalies)
Cranio-occipital defects (occipital vertebrae, basilar impression, occipital dysplasias, condylar hypoplasia, occipitalized atlas) Atlantoaxial defects (aplasia of atlas arch, aplasia of odontoid process) Subaxial anomalies (failure of segmentation and/or fusion, spina bifida, spondylolisthesis)
Ligamentous or Combined Anomalies
Found at birth as an element of somatogenic aberration
Syndromic Disorders
Down syndrome Klippel-Feil syndrome 22q11.2 deletion syndrome Larsen syndrome Marfan syndrome Ehlers-Danlos syndrome
ACQUIRED
Trauma Infection (pyogenic, granulomatous) Tumor (including neurofibromatosis) Inflammatory conditions (e.g., juvenile rheumatoid arthritis) Osteochondrodysplasias (e.g., achondroplasia, diastrophic dysplasia, metatropic dysplasia, spondyloepiphyseal dysplasia) Storage disorders (e.g., mucopolysaccharidoses) Metabolic disorders (rickets) Miscellaneous (including osteogenesis imperfecta, sequela of surgery)

commonly C1 and C2, but also at the occipitocervical junction and in the subaxial spine. For a diagnosis of atlantoaxial instability, the atlanto-dens interval (ADI) should be <5 mm. Subaxial instability is suspected with translation of >3.5 mm and angulation of >11 degrees. Radiographic parameters for the diagnosis of occipitoatlantal instability are not well standardized. Computed tomography is used to define the bony anatomy of each anomaly, and MRI (including dynamic images in flexion and extension) is best for evaluating neurologic impingement.

Symptomatic treatment may be helpful, but patients with cervical instability and/or neurologic impingement often require surgical decompression and/or fusion. Fixed deformities with anterior compression require an anterior decompression prior to a posterior spinal fusion.

Pathologic conditions at the **craniovertebral junction** include occipitoatlantal fusion (occipitalization of the atlas), basilar impression and invagination, occipital vertebrae or condylar hypoplasia, and occipitoatlantal instability. These have been associated with conditions such as achondroplasia, diastrophic dysplasia, spondyloepiphyseal dysplasia, Morquio syndrome (mucopolysaccharidosis), and Larsen syndrome. Fusion between the occiput and C1 (occipitalization) is commonly associated with neurologic symptoms, often due to posterior compression at the level of the foramen magnum. Four morphologic types have been described, and patients with a coexisting fusion between C2 and C3 are at a higher risk (57%) of symptomatic atlantoaxial (C1-C2) instability. Basilar impression or invagination describes a situation in which the odontoid process migrates into the foramen magnum; it may be diagnosed in patients with rickets, skeletal dysplasias, osteogenesis imperfecta, and neurofibromatosis. Occipital condylar hypoplasia is a rare cause of upper cervical instability. Instability between the occiput and C1 may be associated with a variety of conditions associated with hyperlaxity (Down syndrome, Ehler-Danlos or other connective tissue disorders, post-traumatic) or with familial cervical dysplasia.

Atlantoaxial anomalies include hypoplasia (or aplasia) of the atlas, which often manifests with torticollis and may be associated with vertebral artery compression. Several variants have been reported. Hypoplasia (or aplasia) of the odontoid may be seen in Down syndrome, Morquio disease, and other skeletal dysplasias, and it is often associated with atlantoaxial instability. Familial cervical dysplasia is an autosomal dominant condition associated with a spectrum of anomalies involving C1 and C2. **Os odontoideum** represents a discontinuity in the midportion of the dens, and the upper portion of the dens moves along with the ring of C1, narrowing the space available for the spinal cord and often placing the spinal cord at risk of injury. The etiology of os odontoideum is still debated, and a traumatic origin is suspected in most cases, but one study found evidence for both post-traumatic and developmental variants.

The most common anomaly of the **lower cervical spine (subaxial)** is Klippel-Feil syndrome, and congenital fusions between vertebrae may also be seen in up to 50% of patients with fetal alcohol syndrome. Instabilities in this region are post-traumatic or develop from the abnormal stress distribution in the setting on congenital cervical fusions (Chapter 672.2).

DOWN SYNDROME

Ligamentous hyperlaxity is a characteristic feature of Down syndrome and can result in hypermobility or instability at the occipitoatlantal or the atlantoaxial joints (Chapter 76). Hypermobility or instability at C1-C2 is found in up to 40% of children with Down syndrome, with occipitoatlantal hypermobility in up to 61%. These patients can also have coexisting congenital or developmental anomalies of the cervical spine such as occipitalization of the atlas, atlantal arch hypoplasia, basilar invagination, os odontoideum, and odontoid hypoplasia. All patients require screening by history and physical examination (at regular intervals) and at least a single series of cervical spinal radiographs, including a lateral view in flexion and extension. The goal is to establish whether patients have normal mobility (normal radiographic parameters), hypermobility (excessive translation but not expected to be at neurologic risk), or instability (high risk of neurologic deterioration). Although the specific recommendations vary between states, both clinical and radiographic screenings are required before participation in Special Olympics.

The clinical diagnosis of neurologic dysfunction may be challenging in this population of patients, and subtle findings such as decreased exercise tolerance and gait abnormalities (increased tripping or falling) may be the earliest signs of myelopathy. Although formal neurologic testing may be impossible, clonus and hyperreflexia may be identified on physical examination. Imaging studies are commonly used to diagnose and follow patients with hypermobility or instability. With regard to the atlantoaxial joint, the atlanto-dens interval (ADI) is measured as the space between the dens and the anterior ring of C1 (ADI) on lateral radiographs in neutral, flexion, and extension (Fig. 672-3). A normal ADI in children with Down syndrome is <4.5 mm. Hypermobility is diagnosed with an ADI between 4.5 and 10 mm, and an ADI >10 mm represents instability and carries a significant risk of neurologic injury. An MRI with flexion and extension, usually performed under supervision, helps to further evaluate instability and neurologic compression. Although hypermobility at the occipitoatlantal joint is present in >50% of children with Down syndrome, most patients do not develop instability or neurologic symptoms. The relationships at this articulation are difficult to measure reliably on plain radiographs, and a dynamic MRI can help to clarify the significance of any questionable radiographic findings. Involvement of the subaxial spine is less common and is typically encountered in the adult population of patients with Down syndrome. Degenerative changes and/or instability can result in pain, radiculopathy, and myelopathy.

Recommendations for surveillance of potential cervical instability in children with Down syndrome vary, and no formal

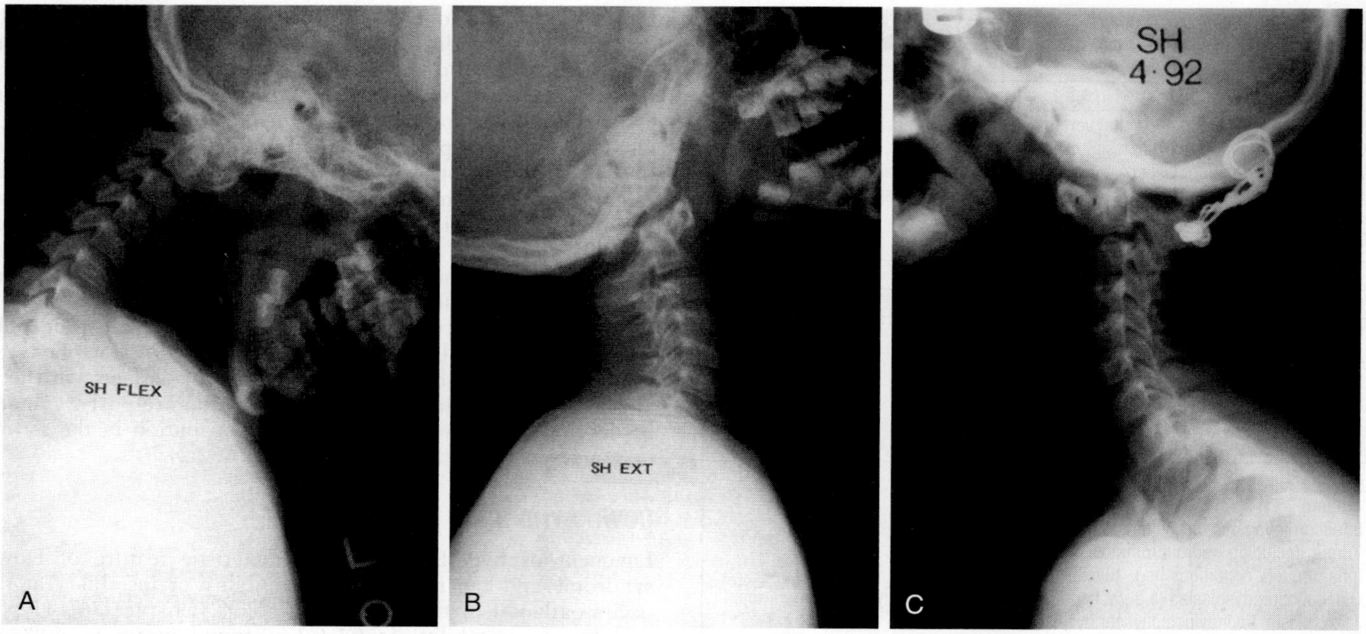

Figure 672-3 Flexion *(A)* and extension *(B)* radiographs of a case of Down syndrome demonstrating atlanto-occipital hypermobility and subluxation. *C,* Instability and symptoms were relieved by an occipitoaxial arthrodesis.

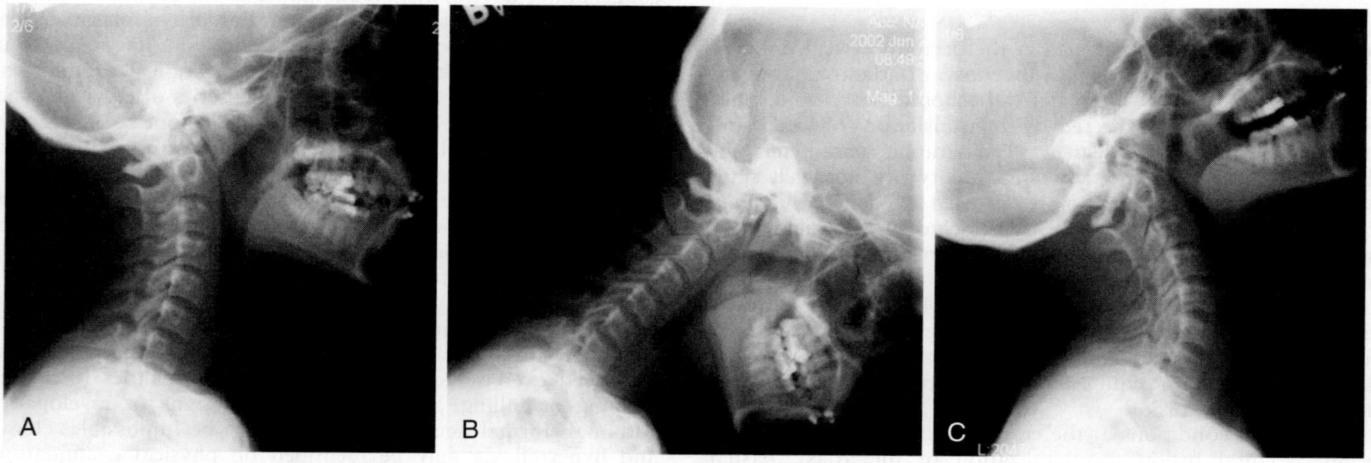

Figure 672-4 Radiographs of the cervical spine in a child with 22q11.2 deletion syndrome showing evidence of platybasia, occipitocervical, and atlantoaxial instability. *A,* Neutral radiograph. *B,* Flexion. *C,* Extension. (From Drummond DS: Pediatric cervical instability. In Weisel SE, Boden SD, Wisnecki RI, editors: *Seminars in spine surgery,* Philadelphia, 1996, WB Saunders, pp 292–309.)

guidelines have been established. An annual neurologic examination should be performed. It is reasonable to obtain plain radiographs of the cervical spine, including flexion-extension views, in all patients with Down syndrome. Flexion and extension radiographs are obtained every other year in those with a normal clinical exam. Those with abnormal findings or symptoms, or when neurologic compression is suspected, are sent for an MRI in flexion and extension. Patients with normal radiographs who are also neurologically normal may be allowed to participate in a full level of activities. Those in whom hypermobility is diagnosed should be restricted from contact sports and other high-risk activities that might increase the risk of trauma to the cervical spine. Only a small subset of patients with myelopathy or instability (ADI >10 mm) with impending neurologic injury are candidates for posterior atlantoaxial (or occipitocervical) fusion, because the risks of a major complication (death, neurologic dysfunction, nonunion of fusion) is significant in patients with Down syndrome.

22q11.2 DELETION SYNDROME

The chromosome abnormality deletion of 22q11.2 is a common genetic syndrome and encompasses a wide spectrum of abnormalities including cardiac, palate, and immunologic anomalies. At least one developmental anomaly of the occiput or cervical spine is noted in all patients (Fig. 672-4). The occipital variations observed include platybasia and basilar impression. Atlas variations include dysmorphic shape, open posterior arch, and occipitalization, and axis variations include a dysmorphic dens. A range of cervical vertebral fusions is noted in these patients, most commonly at C2 and C3. Increased segmental motion is observed on dynamic imaging in >50% of patients, often at more than one level. All patients should have screening radiographs, and many require follow-up for the cervical spine.

BIBLIOGRAPHY

Please visit the Nelson Textbook of Pediatrics *website at* *www.expertconsult.com* *for the complete bibliography.*

Chapter 673
The Upper Limb

Robert B. Carrigan

SHOULDER

The shoulder is a ball-and-socket joint that is similar to the hip; however, the shoulder has a greater range of motion than the hip. This is due to the size of the humeral head relative to the glenoid, as well as to the presence of scapulothoracic motion. The shoulder positions the hand along the surface of a theoretical sphere in space, with its center at the glenohumeral joint.

Brachial Plexus Birth Palsy

Injuries to the brachial plexus can occur in the peripartum time, usually as a result of a stretching mechanism. This palsy is often associated with large fetal size and shoulder dystocia. The incidence is 1-3/1,000 live births. The injury can range in severity from neurapraxia to complete rupture of the nerve root or avulsion of the nerve root from the spinal cord. More often, the upper roots (C5 and C6) are affected rather than a complete brachial plexus palsy. Rarely, in isolation, a lower plexus injury (C8 and T1) is observed. The clinical appearance of a C5-6 brachial plexus birth palsy is the waiter's tip position. The arm is held in a position of shoulder adduction and internal rotation, elbow extension, and wrist flexion. This is the classic Erb's palsy.

TREATMENT Occupational therapy for brachial plexus injuries should be instituted quickly to maintain passive range of motion of the limb and encourage use of the arm. If the biceps muscle does not demonstrate any recovery by 3 mo of age or shows persistent weakness at 5 mo of age, rupture or avulsion of the nerve roots is suspected. Surgical exploration and nerve grafting of the brachial plexus are then indicated. MRI and electrodiagnostic testing are not consistently reliable in this setting.

Shoulder dysplasia and dislocation (analogous to developmental dysplasia of the hip) can occur as a result of muscle imbalances in infants and older children and can require arthroscopic or open reduction and muscle balancing. Older children with residual weakness in shoulder abduction and external rotation can benefit from muscle transfers. Osteotomies are reserved for children with severely deformed glenohumeral joints and functional impairment from persistent shoulder internal rotation contracture.

Sprengel's Deformity

Sprengel's deformity, or congenital elevation of the scapula, is a disorder of development that involves a high scapula and limited scapulothoracic motion. The scapula originates in early embryogenesis at a level posterior to the 4th cervical vertebra, but it descends during development to below the 7th cervical vertebra. Failure of this descent, either unilateral or bilateral, is the Sprengel deformity. The severity of the deformity depends on the location of the scapula and associated anomalies. The scapula in mild cases is simply rotated, with a palpable or visible bump corresponding to the superomedial corner of the scapula in the region of the trapezius muscle. Function is generally good. In moderate cases, the scapula is higher on the neck and connected to the spine with an abnormal omovertebral ligament or even bone. Shoulder motion, particularly abduction, is limited. In severe cases, the scapula is small and positioned on the posterior neck, and the neck may be webbed. The majority of patients have associated anomalies of the musculoskeletal system, especially in the spine, making spinal evaluation important.

TREATMENT In mild cases, treatment is generally unnecessary, although a prominent and unsightly superomedial corner of the scapula can be excised. In more severe cases, surgical repositioning of the scapula with rebalancing of parascapular muscles can significantly improve both function and appearance.

ELBOW

The elbow is the most congruent joint in the body. The stability of the elbow is imparted via this bony congruity as well as through the medial and radial collateral ligaments. Where the shoulder positions the hand along the surface of a theoretical sphere, the elbow positions the hand within that sphere. The elbow allows extension and flexion through the ulnohumeral articulation and pronation and supination through the radiocapitellar articulation.

Panner's Disease

Panner's disease is a disruption of the blood flow to the articular cartilage and subchondral bone to the capitellum (Fig. 673-1). It typically occurs in boys between the ages of 5 and 13 yr. Presenting symptoms include lateral elbow pain, loss of motion, and, in advanced cases, mechanical symptoms of the elbow.

The mechanism of injury can be impaction or overloading of the joint, as seen with sports such as gymnastics and baseball. It can also be idiopathic. Radiographs of the elbow may be normal, but they can also show a small lucency within the capitellum. MRI is the study of choice to evaluate a suspected capitellar lesion. It can demonstrate the extent of the lesion as well as the integrity of the articular surface better than plain radiographs.

TREATMENT Treatment is typically conservative. Rest, activity modification, and patient education are initial treatment options. In cases where the articular cartilage fragments and loose bodies

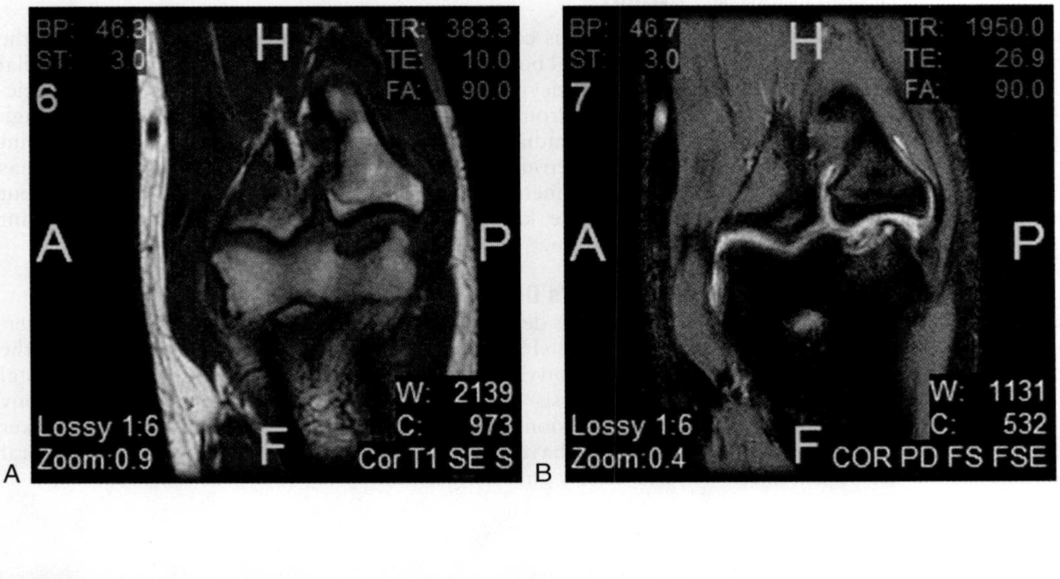

Figure 673-1 T1 *(A)* and T2 *(B)* coronal MRI images of the elbow depicting Panner disease of the elbow.

Table 673-1 SYNDROMES COMMONLY ASSOCIATED WITH RADIAL DEFICIENCY

SYNDROME	CHARACTERISTICS
Holt-Oram syndomre	Heart defects, most commonly atrial septal defects
Thrombocytopenia absent radius	Thrombocytopenia present at birth but improves over time
VACTERL association	Vertebral abnormalities, anal atresia, cardiac abnormalities, tracheoesophageal fistula, esophageal atresia, renal defects, radial dysplasia, lower limb abnormalities
Fanconi anemia	Aplastic anemia not present at birth, develops about 6 yr of age; fatal without bone marrow transplant; chromosomal breakage challenge test available for early diagnosis

From Trumble T, Budoff J, Cornwall R, editors: *Core knowledge in orthopedics: hand, elbow, shoulder*, Philadelphia, 2005, Elsevier, p 425.

Table 673-2 CLASSIFICATION OF RADIAL LONGITUDINAL DEFICIENCY

TYPE	CHARACTERISTICS
I	Short radius Minor radial deviation of the hand
II	Hypoplastic radius with abnormal growth at proximal and distal ends Moderate radial deviation of the hand
III	Partial absence of the radius Severe radial deviation of the hand
IV	Complete absence of the radius The most common type

Adapted from Bayne LG, Klug MS: Long-term review of the surgical treatment of radial deficiencies, *J Hand Surg Am* 12(2):169–179, 1987.

form, arthroscopy is warranted to remove the loose bodies and drill the lesion.

Radial Longitudinal Deficiency

Radial longitudinal deficiency of the forearm comprises a spectrum of conditions and diseases that have resulted in hypoplasia or absence of the radius (Table 673-1). This process was formerly referred to as *radial club hand*, but the name has been changed to *radial longitudinal deficiency*, which better characterizes the condition. Clinical characteristics consist of a small, shortened limb with the hand and wrist in excessive radial deviation.

Radial longitudinal deficiency can range in severity from mild to severe and has been classified into four types according to Bayne and Klug (Table 673-2). Radial longitudinal deficiency can be associated with other syndromes such as Holt-Oram and Fanconi's anemia.

TREATMENT The goals for the treatment of radial longitudinal deficiency include centralizing the hand and wrist on the forearm, balancing the wrist, and maintaining appropriate thumb and digital motion. Shortly after birth, parents are encouraged to passively stretch the wrist and hand to elongate the contracted radial soft tissues. Serial casting and splinting are ineffective at this time, due to the small size of the arm.

For surgical treatment, the preoperative plan begins with careful examination of the patient; considerations in regard to thumb and elbow function must be made before surgery. The surgery typically occurs when the child is 1 yr of age. Correction of the radial deviation as well as centralization of the wrist can be accomplished with a variety of different surgical techniques. These techniques include open release, capsular reefing, and tendon rebalancing. External fixation techniques have also been described.

Nursemaid Elbow

Nursemaid elbow is a subluxation of a ligament rather than a subluxation or dislocation of the radial head. The proximal end of the radius, or radial head, is anchored to the proximal ulna by the annular ligament, which wraps like a leash from the ulna, around the radial head, and back to the ulna. If the radius is pulled distally, the annular ligament can slip proximally off the radial head and into the joint between the radial head and the humerus (Fig. 673-2). The injury is typically produced when a longitudinal traction force is applied to the arm, such as when a falling child is caught by the hand, or when a child is pulled by the hand. The injury usually occurs in toddlers and rarely occurs in children >5 yr of age. Subluxation of the annular ligament produces immediate pain and limitation of supination. Flexion and extension of the elbow are not limited, and swelling is generally absent. The diagnosis is made by history and physical examination, as radiographs are typically normal.

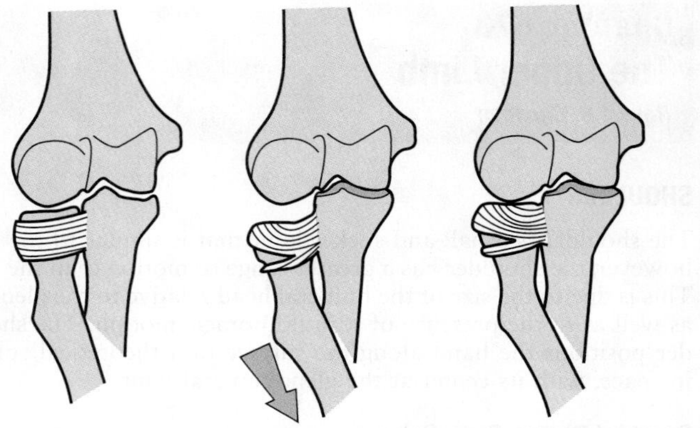

Figure 673-2 The pathology of nursemaid, or pulled, elbow. The annular ligament is partially torn when the arm is pulled. The radial head moves distally, and when traction is discontinued, the ligament is carried into the joint. (From Rang M: *Children's fractures*, ed 2, Philadelphia, 1983, JB Lippincott, p 193.)

TREATMENT The annular ligament is reduced by rotating the forearm into supination while holding pressure over the radial head. A palpable click or clunk can be felt. The child recovers active supination immediately and usually has immediate relief of discomfort. Immobilization is not required, but recurrent annular ligament subluxations can occur, and the parents should avoid activities that apply traction to the elbows. Parents can learn reduction maneuvers for recurrent episodes to avoid trips to the emergency department or pediatrician's office. Recurrent subluxation beyond 5 yr of age is rare. Irreducible subluxations tend to resolve spontaneously, with gradual resolution of symptoms over days to weeks; surgery is rarely indicated.

WRIST

The wrist is composed of the two forearm bones as well as the eight carpal bones. The wrist allows flexion, extension, and radial and ulnar deviation through the radiocarpal and midcarpal articulations. Pronation and supination occur, at the wrist, through the distal radial ulnar joint (DRUJ). The wrist is a complex joint with numerous ligamentous and soft tissue attachments. It has complex kinematics that allow its generous range of motion, but when these kinematics are altered they can cause significant dysfunction.

Madelung's Deformity

Madelung's deformity is a deformity of the wrist that is characterized as radial and palmar angulations of the distal aspect of the radius. Growth arrest of the palmar and ulnar aspect of the distal radial physis is the underlying cause of this deformity. Bony physeal lesions and an abnormal radiolunate ligament (Vicker ligament) have been implicated. The deformity can be bilateral and affects girls more than boys.

TREATMENT Treatment of Madelung's deformity is typically observation. Mild deformities can be observed until skeletal maturity. Moderate to severe deformities that either are painful or limit function may be candidates for surgical intervention. Surgical treatment for Madelung's deformity is motivated by appearance. Patients and their families are often concerned about the palmar angulation of the wrist as well as the resulting prominent distal ulna.

There are a multitude of surgical options for treating Madelung's deformity. For the skeletally immature patient, resection of the tethering soft tissue (Vicker ligament) and physiolysis (fat grafting of any bony lesion seen within the physis) is often the first option. When Madelung's deformity is encountered in skeletally mature patients, an osteotomy is often the treatment of choice. Dorsal closing wedge, dome, and ulnar shortening osteotomies may be used alone or in combination to achieve the desired result.

Long-term considerations of Madelung's deformity concern the incongruity of the DRUJ and resulting premature DRUJ arthritis.

Ganglion

As a synovial joint, the wrist articulation is lubricated with synovial fluid, which is produced by the synovial lining of the joint and maintained within the joint by the joint capsule. A defect in the capsule can allow fluid to leak from the joint into the soft tissues, resulting in a ganglion. The term *cyst* is a misnomer, because this extra-articular collection of fluid does not have its own true lining. The defect in the capsule can occur as a traumatic event, although trauma is rarely a feature of the presenting history. The fluid usually exits the joint in the interval between the scaphoid and lunate, resulting in a ganglion located at the dorsoradial aspect of the wrist. Ganglia can occur at other locations, such as the volar aspect of the wrist, or in the palm as a result of leakage of fluid from the flexor tendon sheaths. Pain is not commonly associated with ganglia in children, and when it is, it is unclear whether the cyst is the cause of the pain. The diagnosis is usually evident on physical examination, especially if the lesion transilluminates. Extensor tenosynovitis and anomalous muscles can mimic ganglion cysts, but radiography or MRI is not routinely required. Ultrasonography is an effective, noninvasive tool to support the diagnosis and reassure the patient and family.

TREATMENT Up to 80% of ganglia in children <10 yr of age resolve spontaneously within 1 yr of being noticed. If the ganglion is painful or bothersome and the child is >10 yr of age, treatment may be warranted. Simple aspiration of the fluid has a high recurrence rate and is painful for children given the large-bore needle required to aspirate the gelatinous fluid. Surgical excision, including excision of the stalk connecting the ganglion to its joint of origin, has a high success rate, although the ganglion can recur.

HAND

The hand and fingers allow complex and fine manipulations. An intricate balance among extrinsic flexors, extensors, and intrinsic muscles allow these complex motions to occur. Congenital anomalies of the hand and upper extremity rank just behind cardiac anomalies in incidence, and like cardiac anomalies, if they are not properly identified and remedied, they can have long-term consequences.

Camptodactyly

Camptodactyly is a nontraumatic flexion contracture of the proximal interphalangeal joint that is often progressive. The small and ring fingers are most often affected. Bilateralism is observed two thirds of the time. The etiology of camptodactyly is varied. Several different hypotheses have been offered as to the cause of this condition. Camptodactyly can be divided into three different types (Table 673-3).

Table 673-3 CLASSIFICATION OF CAMPTODACTYLY

TYPE	CHARACTERISTICS
I	Congenital no sex bias, small finger only
II	Acquired between 7-11 yr, typically progressive
III	Severe, significant contracture, bilateral and associated with other musculoskeletal syndromes

Adapted from Kozin SH: Pediatric hand surgery. In Beredjiklian PK, Bozentka DJ, editors: *Review of hand surgery,* Philadelphia, 2004, WB Saunders, pp 223–245.

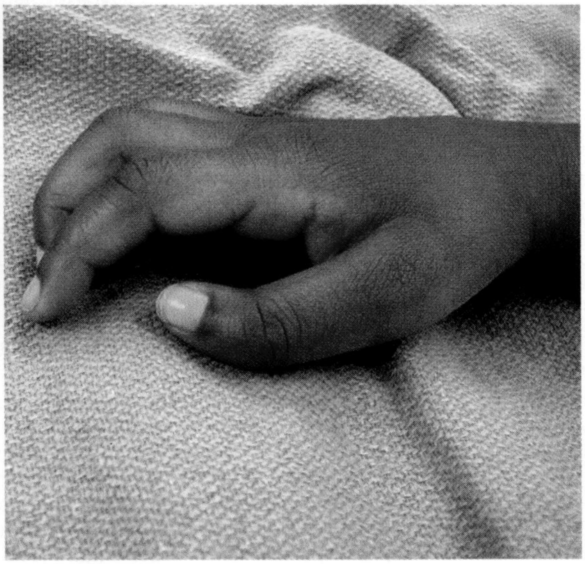

Figure 673-3 Clinodactyly of the thumb.

TREATMENT Nonsurgical treatment is the primary treatment of camptodactyly. Mild contractures of less than 30 degrees are usually well tolerated and do not need treatment. Serial casting and static and dynamic splinting are the treatments of choice for preventing progression of contractures. This should be performed until the child is skeletally mature.

Surgical treatment is limited to the treatment of severe contractures. At the time of surgery, all contracted and anomalous structures are released. Results of contracture release for camptodactyly are mixed; often a loss of flexion results from an attempt to improve extension.

Clinodactyly

Angular deformity of the digit in the coronal plane, distal to the metacarpophalangeal joint is clinodactyly. The most commonly observed finding is a mild radial deviation of the small finger at the level of the distal interphalangeal joint. This is often due to a triangular or trapezoidal middle phalanx. In some cases, a disruption of the physis at the middle phalanx produces a longitudinal epiphysial bracket. This bracket is thought to be the underlying cause for the formation the "delta phalanx" that is often observed in clinodactyly. Clinodactyly has been observed in other fingers, including the thumb (Fig. 673-3) and ring finger.

TREATMENT Often the treatment for clinodactyly is observation and not surgery. For severe deformities and for those affecting the thumb, surgery is often indicated. Surgery is technically demanding. Bracket resections, corrective osteotomies, and growth plate ablations are the most common procedures performed to correct the observed angular deformities. Results are good and recurrences are few when an appropriate procedure is performed.

Table 673-4 SYNDROMES ASSOCIATED WITH POLYDACTYLY

Carpenter syndrome
Ellis-van Creveld syndrome
Meckel-Gruber syndrome
Polysyndactyly
Trisomy 13
Orofaciodigital syndrome
Rubinstein-Taybi syndrome

Table 673-5 WASSEL CLASSIFICATION OF THUMB DUPLICATION

TYPE	CHARACTERISTICS
I	Bifid distal phalanx
II	Duplicate distal phalanx
III	Bifid proximal phalanx
IV	Duplicate proximal phalanx
V	Bifid metacarpal
VI	Duplicate metacarpal
VII	Triphalangeal component

Adapted from Wassel, HD: The results of surgery for polydactyly of the thumb. A review, *Clin Orthop* 125:175–193, 1969.

Polydactyly

Polydactyly or duplication of a digit can occur either as a preaxial deformity (involving the thumb) or as a post axial deformity (involving the small finger) (Table 673-4). Each has an inherited and genetic component. Duplication of the thumb occurs more in white children and is often unilateral, whereas duplication of the small finger occurs mainly in African-Americans and may be bilateral. Transmission is typically in an autosomal dominant pattern and has been linked to defects in genes localized to chromosome 2.

Duplication of the thumb was extensively studied by Wassel. Wassel subdivided thumb duplication on the basis of the degree of duplication. The seven types according to Wassel are listed in Table 673-5. Small finger duplication has been further subdivided into two types. Type A is a well-formed digit. Type B is a small, often underdeveloped supernumerary digit.

TREATMENT Thumb and small finger duplication is typically treated with ablation of the supernumerary digit. Treatment options vary based on the degree of involvement. Less well formed digits can be treated with suture ligation. Well-formed digits require reconstructive procedures that preserve important structures such as the collateral ligaments and nail folds.

Thumb Hypoplasia

Hypoplasia of the thumb is a challenging condition for both the patient and the doctor. The thumb represents ~40% of hand function. A less-than-optimal thumb can severely limit a patient's function as he or she grows and develops. Hypoplasia of the thumb can range from being mild with slight shortening and underdeveloped musculature to complete absence of the thumb (Fig. 673-4). Radiographs are useful to help determine osseous abnormalities. The most important finding on physical exam is the presence or absence of a stable carpometacarpal (CMC) joint. This finding helps guide surgical treatment.

TREATMENT If the thumb has a stable CMC joint, reconstruction is advised. Key elements of thumb reconstruction include rebuilding the ulnar collateral ligament of the metacarpophalangeal joint, tendon transfers to aid in abduction, and procedures to deepen the web space.

If a stable CMC joint is not present or the thumb is completely absent, **pollicization** (surgical construction of a thumb from a finger) is the definitive treatment. Pollicization is a complex procedure rotating the index finger along its neurovascular pedicle to form a thumb. This procedure is typically performed at around 1 yr of age and may be followed by subsequent procedures to deepen the web space or augment abduction (Fig. 673-5).

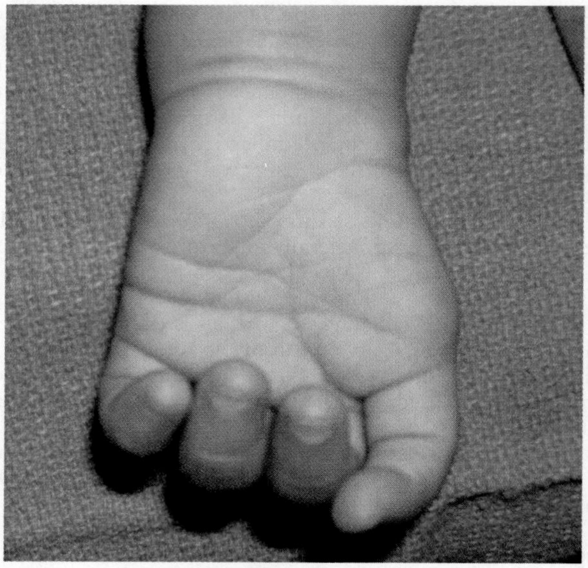

Figure 673-4 Congenital absence of the thumb.

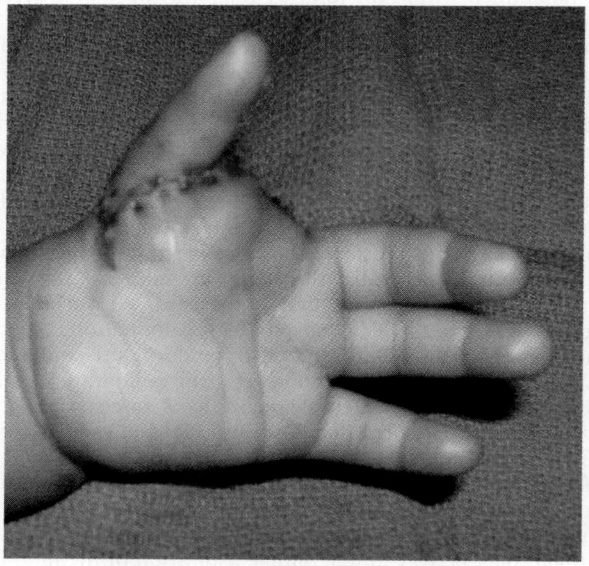

Figure 673-5 Postsurgical image after pollicization.

Syndactyly

Failure of the individual digits to separate during development produces syndactyly. Syndactyly is one of the more common anomalies observed in the upper limb (Table 673-6). It is seen in 0.5 of 1,000 live births. Syndactyly can be classified as simple (skin attachments only), complicated (bone and tendon attachments), complete (fusion to the tips, including the nail), or incomplete (simple webbing).

TREATMENT Division of the conjoined digits should be considered before the 2nd year of life. Border digits should be divided earlier (3-6 mo) because of concern over tethering effects of digits of unequal length. Digits of similar size, such as the ring and middle, may wait until the 12-18 mo age range. Reconstruction of the web space and nail folds as well as appropriate skin-grafting techniques must be used to ensure the best possible functional and cosmetic result.

Table 673-6 SYNDROMES ASSOCIATED WITH SYNDACTYLY
Apert syndrome
Carpenter syndrome
de Lange syndrome
Holt-Oram syndrome
Orofaciodigital syndrome
Polysyndactyly
Trisomy 21
Fetal hydantoin syndrome
Laurence-Moon-Biedl syndrome
Fanconi panctyopenia
Trisomy 13
Trisomy 18

Fingertip Injuries

Young children are fascinated with door-jambs or car doors and other tight spaces, making crush injuries to the fingertips quite common. Injury can range from a simple subungual hematoma to complete amputation of part or the entire fingertip. Radiographs are important to rule out fractures. Physeal fractures associated with nailbed injuries are **open fractures** with a high risk of osteomyelitis, growth arrest, and deformity if not treated promptly with formal surgical debridement and reduction. Tuft fractures involving the very distal portion of the distal phalanx are common and require little specific treatment other than that for the soft-tissue injury.

The treatment of the soft-tissue injury depends on the type of injury. For suture repairs, only absorbable sutures should be used, because suture removal from a young child's fingertip can require sedation or general anesthesia. If a subungual hematoma exists but the nail is normal and no displaced fracture exists, the nail need not be removed for nailbed repair. If the nail is torn or avulsed, the nail should be removed, the nail bed and skin should be repaired with absorbable sutures, and the nail (or a piece of foil if the nail is absent) should be replaced under the eponychial fold to prevent scar adhesion of the eponychial fold to the nail bed that can prevent nail regrowth.

If the fingertip is completely amputated, treatment depends on the level of amputation and the age of the child. Distal amputations of skin and fat in children <2 yr of age can be replaced as a composite graft with a reasonable chance of surviving. Similar amputations in older children can heal without replacing the skin as long as no bone is exposed and the amputated area is small. A variety of coverage procedures exist for amputations through the mid-portion of the nail. Amputations at or proximal to the proximal edge of the fingernail should be referred emergently to a replant center for consideration for microvascular replantation. When referring, all amputated parts should be saved, wrapped in saline-soaked gauze, placed in a watertight bag, and then placed in ice water. Ice should never directly contact the part, because it can cause severe osmotic and thermal injury.

Trigger Thumb and Fingers

The flexor tendons for the thumb and fingers pass through fibrous tunnels made up of a series of pulleys on the volar surface of the digits. These tunnels, for reasons that are not well understood, can become tight at the most proximal or 1st annular pulley. Swelling of the underlying tendon occurs, and the tendon no longer glides under the pulley. In children, the most common digit involved is the thumb. It has classically been thought to be a congenital problem, but prospective screening studies of large numbers of neonates have failed to find a single case in a newborn child. Trauma is rarely a feature of the history, and the condition is often painless. Overall function is rarely impaired. A trigger thumb typically manifests with the inability to fully extend the thumb interphalangeal joint. A palpable nodule can be felt in the flexor pollicis longus tendon at the base of the thumb. Other conditions can mimic trigger thumb, including the thumb-in-palm deformity of cerebral palsy. Similar findings in the fingers are much less common and can be associated with inflammatory conditions such as juvenile rheumatoid arthritis.

TREATMENT Trigger thumbs spontaneously resolve in up to 30% of children in whom they are diagnosed before 1 yr of age. Spontaneous resolution beyond that age is not common. Corticosteroid injections are effective in adults but are not effective in children and risk injury to the nearby digital nerves. Surgical release of the 1st annular pulley is curative and is generally performed between 1 and 3 yr of age. Treatment of trigger fingers other than the thumb in children involves evaluation and treatment of any underlying inflammatory process and in some cases surgical decompression of the flexor sheath.

BIBLIOGRAPHY

Please visit the Nelson Textbook of Pediatrics *website at www.expertconsult.com for the complete bibliography.*

Chapter 674
Arthrogryposis

Harish S. Hosalkar, Denis S. Drummond, and Richard S. Davidson

DEFINITION

Arthrogryposis multiplex congenita (AMC) is a congenital anomaly in the newborn involving multiple curved joints (see Fig. 674-1 on the *Nelson Textbook of Pediatrics* website at www.expertconsult.com). Arthrogryposis is a descriptive term and not an exact diagnosis, as there are as many as 300 possible underlying causes.

For the full continuation of this chapter, please visit the Nelson Textbook of Pediatrics *website at www.expertconsult.com.*

Chapter 675
Common Fractures

Lawrence Wells, Kriti Sehgal, and John P. Dormans

Trauma is a leading cause of death and disability in children >1 yr of age. Several factors make fractures of the immature skeleton different from those involving the mature skeleton. The anatomy, biomechanics, and physiology of the pediatric skeletal system are different from those of adults. This results in different fracture patterns (Fig. 675-1), diagnostic challenges, and management techniques specific to children to preserve growth and function.

Epiphyseal lines, rarefaction, dense growth lines, congenital fractures, and pseudofractures appear on radiographs, which could confuse the interpretation of a fracture. Most fractures in children heal well with indifferent treatment; that has led the unwary to neglect the fact that other fractures terminate disastrously if handled with inexpertise. The differences in the pediatric skeletal system predispose children to injuries different from those of adults. The important differences are the presence of periosseous cartilage, physes, and a thicker, stronger, more osteogenic periosteum that produces new bone, called *callus*, more rapidly and in greater amounts. The pediatric bone has low density and more porosity. The low density is due to lower mineral content and the increased porosity is due to increased number of haversian canals and vascular channels. These differences result in a comparatively lower modulus of elasticity and lower bending strength. The bone in children can fail either in tension or in compression; the fracture lines do not propagate as in adults, and hence there is less chance of comminuted fractures.

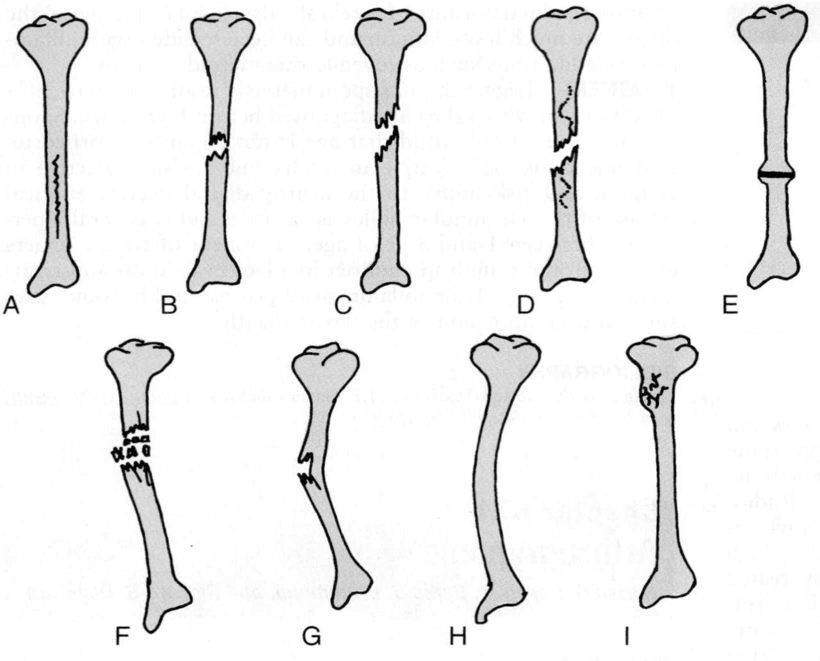

Figure 675-1 Illustration of fracture patterns. *A,* Longitudinal fracture line parallel to bony axis. *B,* Transverse fracture line perpendicular to bony axis. *C,* Oblique fracture line at angle to bony axis. *D,* Spiral fracture line runs a curvilinear course to the bony axis. *E,* Impacted fractured bone ends compressed together. *F,* Comminuted fragmentation of bone into three or more parts. *G,* Greenstick bending of bone with incomplete fracture of convex side. *H,* Bowing bone plastic deformation. *I,* Torus buckling fracture. (From White N, Sty R: Radiological evaluation and classification of pediatric fractures, *Clin Pediatr Emerg Med* 3:94–105, 2002.)

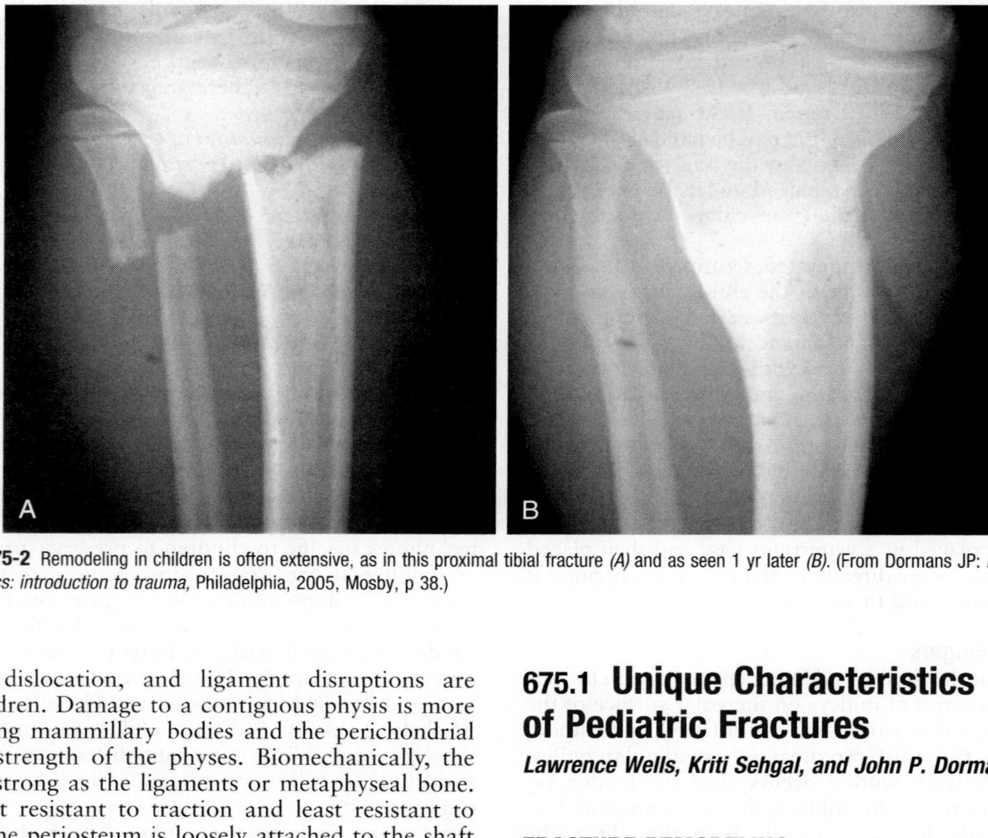

Figure 675-2 Remodeling in children is often extensive, as in this proximal tibial fracture *(A)* and as seen 1 yr later *(B).* (From Dormans JP: *Pediatric orthopedics: introduction to trauma,* Philadelphia, 2005, Mosby, p 38.)

Joint injuries, dislocation, and ligament disruptions are uncommon in children. Damage to a contiguous physis is more likely. Interdigitating mammillary bodies and the perichondrial ring enhance the strength of the physes. Biomechanically, the physes are not as strong as the ligaments or metaphyseal bone. The physis is most resistant to traction and least resistant to torsional forces. The periosteum is loosely attached to the shaft of bone and adheres densely to the physeal periphery. The periosteum is usually injured in all fractures, but it is less likely to have complete circumferential rupture, due to its loose attachment to the shaft. This intact hinge or sleeve of periosteum lessens the extent of fracture displacement and assists in reduction. The thick periosteum can also act as an impediment to closed reduction, particularly if the fracture has penetrated the periosteum, or in reduction of displaced growth plate.

675.1 Unique Characteristics of Pediatric Fractures

Lawrence Wells, Kriti Sehgal, and John P. Dormans

FRACTURE REMODELING

Remodeling is the 3rd and final phase in biology of fracture healing, preceded by the inflammatory and reparative phases. This occurs from a combination of appositional bone deposition on the concavity of deformity, resorption on the convexity, and asymmetric physeal growth. Thus, reduction accuracy is somewhat less important than it is in adults (Fig. 675-2). The 3 major factors that have a bearing on the potential for angular correction are skeletal age, distance to the joint, and orientation to the joint axis. The rotational deformity and angular deformity not in the axis of the joint motion are less likely to remodel. The amount of remaining growth provides the basis for remodeling; younger children have greater remodeling potential. Fractures adjacent to a physis undergo the greatest amount of remodeling, provided that the deformity is in the plane of the axis of motion for that joint. The fractures away from the elbow and closer to the knee joint have greater potential to remodel because this physis provides maximal growth to the bone. One can expect remodeling to occur over the next several months following injury throughout skeletal maturity. Skeletal maturity is reached in girls between 13 and 15 yr and in boys between 14 and 16 yr of age.

OVERGROWTH

Physeal stimulation from the hyperemia associated with fracture healing causes overgrowth. It is usually prominent in long bones such as the femur. The growth acceleration is usually present for 6 mo to 1 yr following the injury and does not present a continued progressive overgrowth unless complicated by a rare arteriovenous malformation. Femoral fractures in children <10 yr of age often overgrow by 1-3 cm. Bayonet apposition of bone is preferred to compensate for the expected overgrowth. This overgrowth phenomenon will result in equal or near equal limb lengths at the conclusion of fracture remodeling. After 10 yr of age, overgrowth is less of a problem and anatomic alignment is recommended. In physeal injuries, growth stimulation is associated with use of implants or fixation hardware that can cause chronic stimulus for longitudinal growth.

PROGRESSIVE DEFORMITY

Injuries to the physes can be complicated by progressive deformities with growth. The most common cause is complete or partial closure of the growth plate. As a consequence, angular deformity, shortening, or both, can occur. The partial arrest may be peripheral, central, or combined. The magnitude of deformity depends on the physis involved and the amount of growth remaining. CT and MRI are important for assessing partial arrests and formulating treatment (Fig. 675-3).

RAPID HEALING

Children's fractures heal quickly compared with those of adults. This is due to children's growth potential and thicker, more active periosteum. As children approach adolescence and maturity, the rate of healing slows and becomes similar to that of an adult.

BIBLIOGRAPHY

Please visit the Nelson Textbook of Pediatrics *website at www.expertconsult.com for the complete bibliography.*

675.2 Pediatric Fracture Patterns

Lawrence Wells, Kriti Sehgal, and John P. Dormans

The different pediatric fracture patterns are the reflection of a child's characteristic skeletal system. The majority of pediatric fractures can be managed by closed methods and heal well.

PLASTIC DEFORMATION

Plastic deformation is unique to children. It is most commonly seen in the ulna and occasionally the fibula. The fracture results from a force that produces microscopic failure on the tensile side of bone and does not propagate to the concave side (Fig. 675-4). The concave side of bone also shows evidence of microscopic failure in compression. The bone is angulated beyond its elastic limit, but the energy is insufficient to produce a fracture. Thus, no fracture line is visible radiographically (Fig. 675-5). The plastic deformation is permanent, and a bend in the ulna of <20 degrees in a 4 yr old child is expected to correct with growth.

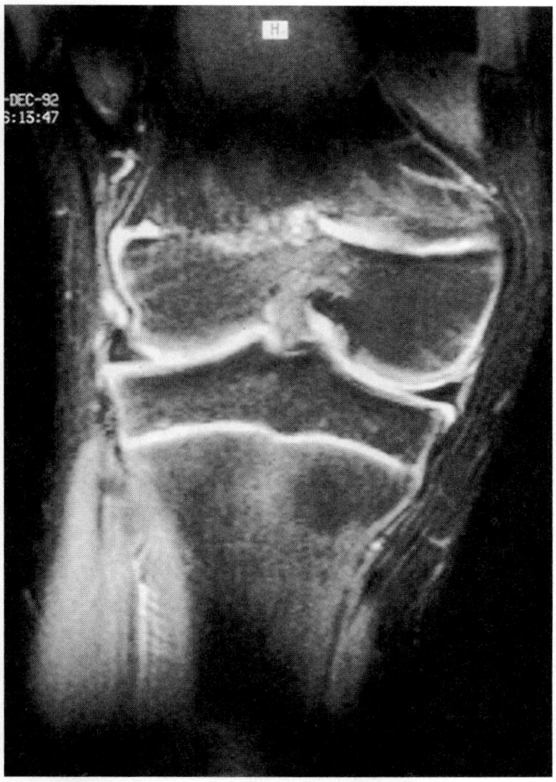

Figure 675-3 MRI with gradient echo sequence, illustrating distal femoral physeal bar. (From Dormans JP: *Pediatric orthopedics: introduction to trauma,* Philadelphia, 2005, Mosby, p 43.)

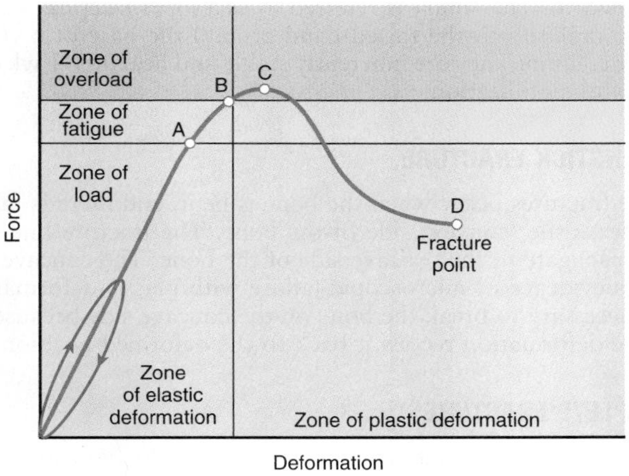

Figure 675-4 Graphic relation of bony deformation (bowing) and force (longitudinal compression) showing that the limit of an elastic response is not a fracture but plastic deformation. If the force continues, a fracture results. A, reversible bowing with stress; B, microfractures occur; C, point of maximal strength; between C and D, bowing fractures; D, linear fracture occurs. (Modified from Borden S IV: Roentgen recognition of acute plastic bowing of the forearm in children, *Am J Roentgenol Radium Ther Nucl Med* 125:524–530, 1975; from Slovis TL, editor: *Caffey's pediatric diagnostic imaging,* ed 11, vol 2, Philadelphia, 2008, Mosby, p 2777.)

BUCKLE OR TORUS FRACTURE

A compression failure of bone usually occurs at the junction of the metaphysis and diaphysis, especially in the distal radius

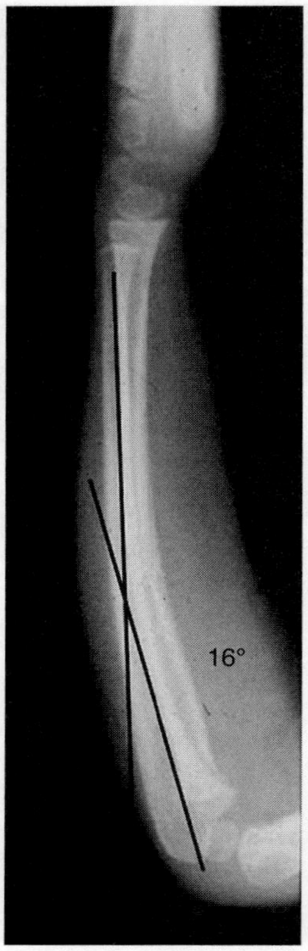

Figure 675-5 Plastic deformation is a microfailure in tension without a visible fracture line. (Courtesy of Dr. John Flynn, Children's Hospital, Philadelphia.)

(Fig. 675-6). This injury is referred to as a *torus fracture* because of its similarity to the raised band around the base of a classic Greek column. They are inherently stable and heal in 3-4 wk with simple immobilization.

GREENSTICK FRACTURE

These fractures occur when the bone is bent, and there is failure on the tensile (convex) side of the bone. The fracture line does not propagate to the concave side of the bone. The concave side shows evidence of microscopic failure with plastic deformation. It is necessary to break the bone on the concave side because the plastic deformation recoils it back to the deformed position.

COMPLETE FRACTURES

Fractures that propagate completely through the bone are called *complete fractures*. These fractures may be classified as spiral, transverse, or oblique, depending on the direction of the fracture lines. A rotational force usually creates the spiral fractures, and reduction is easy due to the presence of an intact periosteal hinge. Oblique fractures are in the diaphysis at 30 degrees to the axis of the bone and are inherently unstable. The transverse fractures occur following a 3-point bending force and are easily reduced by using the intact periosteum from the concave side.

EPIPHYSEAL FRACTURES

The injuries to the epiphysis involve the growth plate. There is always a potential for deformity to occur, and hence long-term observation is necessary. The distal radial physis is the most commonly injured physis. Salter and Harris (SH) classified epiphyseal injuries into 5 groups (Table 675-1 and Fig. 675-7). This classification helps to predict the outcome of the injury and offers guidelines in formulating treatment. SH type I and II fractures usually can be managed by closed reduction techniques and do not require perfect alignment, because they tend to remodel with growth. SH type II fractures of the distal femoral epiphysis need anatomic reduction. The SH type III and IV epiphyseal fractures involve the articular surface and require anatomic alignment to prevent any step off and realign the growth cells of the physis. SH type V fractures are usually not diagnosed initially. They manifest in the future with growth disturbance. Other injuries to the epiphysis are avulsion injuries of the tibial spine and muscle attachments to the pelvis. Osteochondral fractures are also defined as physeal injuries that do not involve the growth plate.

Table 675-1 SALTER-HARRIS CLASSIFICATION

SALTER-HARRIS TYPE	CHARACTERISTICS
I	Separation through the physis, usually through the zones of hypertrophic and degenerating cartilage cell columns
II	Fracture through a portion of the physis but extending through the metaphyses
III	Fracture through a portion of the physis extending through the epiphysis and into the joint
IV	Fracture across the metaphysis, physis, and epiphysis
V	Crush injury to the physis

CHILD ABUSE

The orthopedic surgeon sees 30-50% of physically abused children. Child abuse should be expected in nonambulatory children with lower extremity long bone fractures (Chapter 37). No fracture pattern or types are pathognomonic for child abuse; any type of fracture can result from nonaccidental trauma. The fractures that suggest intentional injury include femur fractures in nonambulatory children, distal femoral metaphyseal corner fractures, posterior rib fractures, scapular spinous process fractures, and proximal humeral fractures. A skeletal survey is essential in every suspected case of child abuse, because it can demonstrate other fractures in different stages of healing. Radiographically, some systemic diseases mimic signs of child abuse, such as osteogenesis imperfecta, osteomyelitis, Caffey disease, and fatigue fractures. Many hospitals have a multidisciplinary team to evaluate and treat patients who are victims of child abuse. It is mandatory to report these cases to social welfare agencies.

BIBLIOGRAPHY

Please visit the Nelson Textbook of Pediatrics *website at www.expertconsult.com for the complete bibliography.*

675.3 Upper Extremity Fractures

Lawrence Wells, Kriti Sehgal, and John P. Dormans

PHALANGEAL FRACTURES

The different phalangeal fracture patterns in children include physeal, diaphyseal, and tuft fractures. The mechanism of injury is a direct blow to the finger or typically a finger trapped in a door (Chapter 673). Crush injuries of the distal phalanx manifest with severe comminution of the underlying bone (tuft fracture), disruption of the nail bed, and significant soft-tissue injury. These injuries are best managed with antibiotics, tetanus prophylaxis, and irrigation. A mallet finger deformity is the inability to extend the distal portion of the digit and is caused by a hyperextension injury. It represents an avulsion fracture of the physis of the distal phalanx. The treatment is splinting the digit in extension for 3-4 wk. The physeal injuries of the proximal and middle phalanx are similarly treated with splint immobilization. Diaphyseal

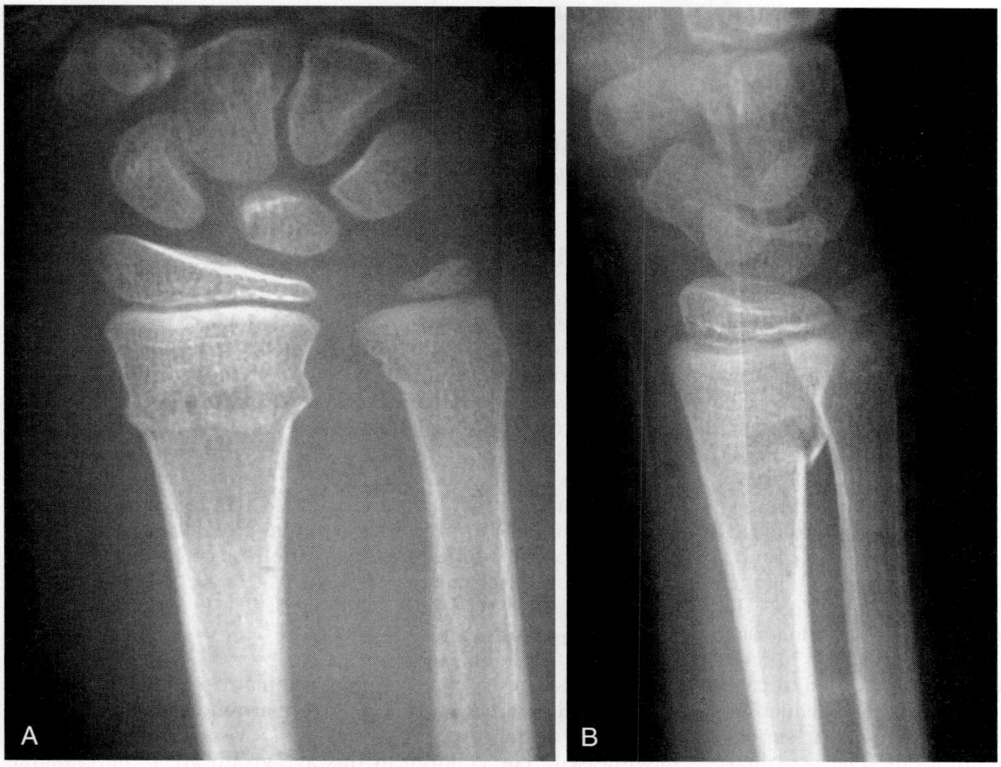

Figure 675-6 Buckle fracture is a partial failure in compression: anteroposterior *(A)* and lateral *(B)* radiographs of the distal radius. (From Dormans JP: *Pediatric orthopedics: introduction to trauma,* Philadelphia, 2005, Mosby, p 37.)

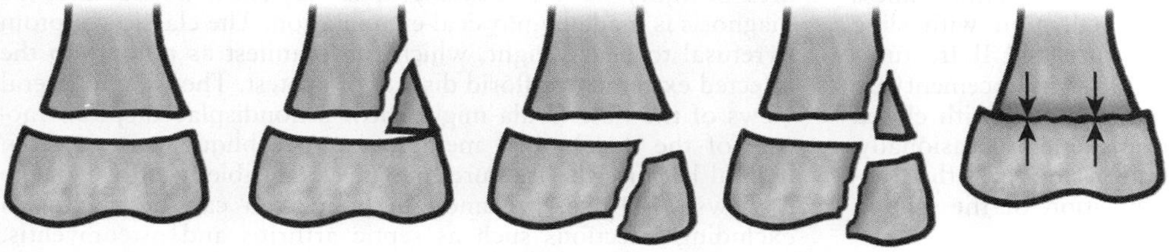

Figure 675-7 Salter-Harris classification of physeal fractures, types I-V.

fractures may be oblique, spiral, or transverse in fracture geometry. They are assessed for angular and rotational deformity with the finger in flexion. Any malrotation or angular deformity requires correction for optimal functioning of the hand. These deformities are corrected with closed reduction, and if unstable, they need stabilization.

FOREARM FRACTURES

Fractures of the wrist and forearm are very common fractures in children, accounting for nearly half of all fractures seen in the skeletally immature. The most common mechanism of injury is a fall on the outstretched hand. Eighty percent of forearm fractures involve the distal radius and ulna, 15% involve the middle third, and the rest are rare fractures of the proximal third of the radius or ulnar shaft. The majority of forearm fractures are torus or greenstick fractures. The torus fracture is an impacted fracture, and there is minimal soft-tissue swelling or hemorrhage. They are best treated in a short arm (below the elbow) cast and usually heal within 3-4 wk. Wrist buckle fractures have also been successfully treated with a removable splint. Impacted greenstick fractures of the forearm tend to be intrinsically stable (no cortical disruption) and may be managed with a soft bandage rather than casting.

Diaphyseal fractures could be more difficult to treat because the limits of acceptable reduction are much more stringent than for distal radial fractures. A significant malunion of a forearm diaphyseal fracture can lead to a permanent loss of pronation and supination, leading to functional difficulties. The physical examination focuses on soft-tissue injuries and ruling out any neurovascular involvement. The anteroposterior (AP) and lateral radiographs of the forearm and wrist confirm the diagnosis. Displaced and angulated fractures require manipulative closed reduction under general anesthesia. They are immobilized in an above-elbow cast for at least 6 wk. Loss of reduction and unstable fractures require open reduction and internal fixation.

DISTAL HUMERAL FRACTURES

Fractures around the elbow receive more attention because more aggressive management is needed to achieve a good result. Many injuries are intra-articular, involve the physeal cartilage, and can result in rare malunion or nonunion. As the distal humerus develops from a series of ossification centers, these ossification centers can be mistaken for fractures by inexperienced eyes. Careful radiographic evaluation is an essential part of diagnosing and managing distal humeral injuries. Common fractures include separation of the distal humeral epiphysis (transcondylar fracture), supracondylar fractures of the distal humerus, and epiphyseal fractures of the lateral or medial condyle. The mechanism of injury is a fall on an outstretched arm. The physical examination includes noting the location and extent of soft-tissue swelling, ruling out any neurovascular injury, specifically anterior interosseous nerve involvement or evidence of compartment syndrome. A transcondylar fracture in neonates should raise suspicion of child abuse. AP and lateral radiographs of the involved extremity are necessary for the diagnosis. If the fracture is not visible, but there is an altered relationship between the humerus and the radius and ulna or the presence of a posterior fat pad sign, a transcondylar fracture or an occult fracture should be suspected. Imaging studies such as CT, MRI, and ultrasonography may be required for further confirmation.

In general, distal humeral fractures need good restoration of anatomic alignment. This is necessary to prevent deformity and to allow for normal growth and development. Closed reduction alone, or in association with percutaneous fixation, is the preferred method. Open reduction is necessary for fractures that cannot be reduced by closed methods. Inadequate reductions can lead to cubitus varus, cubitus valgus, and rare nonunion or elbow instability.

PROXIMAL HUMERUS FRACTURES

Fractures of the proximal humerus account for <5% of fractures in children. They usually result from a fall onto an outstretched arm. The fracture pattern tends to vary with the age group. Children <5 yr of age have an SH I injury, those 5-10 yr of age have metaphyseal fractures, and children >11 yr have SH II injury. Examination includes a thorough neurologic evaluation, especially of the axillary nerve. The diagnosis is made on AP radiographs of the shoulder. An axillary view is obtained to rule out any dislocation. SH I injuries do not require reduction because they have excellent remodeling capacity, and simple immobilization in a sling for 2-3 wk is sufficient. The proximal humerus contributes 80% of the growth to the humerus. The metaphyseal fractures usually do not need reduction unless the angulation is >50 degrees. A closed reduction with sling immobilization adequately treats this fracture. SH II fractures with <30 degrees of angulation and <50% displacement are managed in a sling. Displaced fractures are treated with closed reduction and further stabilization if unstable. Occasionally, open reduction is required because of button-holing of the fracture spike through the deltoid or interposition of the tendon of biceps.

CLAVICULAR FRACTURES

Neonatal fractures occur as a result of direct trauma during birth, most often through a narrow pelvis or following shoulder dystocia. They can be missed initially and can appear with pseudoparalysis. Childhood fractures are usually the result of a fall on the affected shoulder or direct trauma to the clavicle. The most common site for fracture is the junction of the middle and lateral 3rd clavicle. Tenderness over the clavicle will make the diagnosis. A thorough neurovascular examination is important to diagnose any associated **brachial plexus injury.**

An AP radiograph of the clavicle demonstrates the fracture and can show overlap of the fragments. Physeal injuries occur through the medial or lateral growth plate and are sometimes difficult to differentiate from dislocations of the acromioclavicular or sternoclavicular joint. Further imaging such as a CT scan may be necessary to further define the injury. The treatment of most clavicle fractures consists of an application of a figure-of-eight clavicle strap. This will extend the shoulders and minimize the amount of overlap of the fracture fragments. For older adolescents with fracture fragments tinting the skin, operative management is increasingly more advised. The physeal fractures are treated with simple sling immobilization without any reduction attempt. Often, anatomic alignment is not achieved, nor is it necessary. The fractures heal rapidly usually in 3-6 wk. Usually a palpable mass of callus is visible in thin children. This remodels satisfactorily in 6-12 mo. Complete restoration of shoulder motion and function is uniformly achieved.

BIBLIOGRAPHY

Please visit the Nelson Textbook of Pediatrics *website at www.expertconsult.com for the complete bibliography.*

675.4 Fractures of Lower Extremity

Lawrence Wells, Kriti Sehgal, and John P. Dormans

HIP FRACTURE

Hip fractures in children account for <1% of all children's fractures. These injuries result from high-energy trauma and are often associated with injury to the chest, head, or abdomen. Treatment of hip fractures in children entails a complication rate of up to 60%, an overall avascular necrosis rate of 50%, and a malunion rate of up to 30%. The unique blood supply to the femoral head accounts for the high rate of avascular necrosis. Fractures are classified as transphyseal separations, transcervical fractures, cervicotrochanteric fractures, and intertrochanteric fractures. The management principle includes urgent anatomic reduction (either open or closed), stable internal fixation (avoiding the physis if possible), and spica casting.

TODDLER FRACTURE

Toddler fractures occur in young ambulatory children. The age range for this fracture is typically from around 1-4 yr. The injury often occurs after a seemingly harmless twist or fall and is often unwitnessed. The children in this age group are usually unable to articulate the mechanism of injury clearly or to describe the area of injury well. The radiographs may show no fracture; the diagnosis is made by physical examination. The classic symptom is refusal to bear weight, which can manifest as pulling up the affected extremity or florid display of protest. The AP and lateral views of the tibia-fibula might show a nondisplaced spiral fracture of the distal tibial metaphysis. An oblique view is often helpful because the fracture line may be visible in only 1 of the 3 views. A 3-phase technetium bone scan can be helpful in excluding infections such as septic arthritis and osteomyelitis. The fracture is treated with an above-knee cast for approximately 3 wk.

TIBIA AND FIBULA SHAFT FRACTURES

The tibia is the most commonly fractured bone of the lower limb in children. This fracture generally results from a direct injury. Most tibial fractures are associated with a fibular fracture, and the mean age of presentation is 8 yr. The child has pain, swelling, and deformity of the affected leg and is unable to bear weight. Distal neurovascular examination is important in assessment. The AP and lateral radiographs should include the knee and ankle. Closed reduction and immobilization are the standard method of treatment. Most fractures heal well, and children usually have excellent results. Open fractures need to undergo irrigation and debridement multiple times. The fractures with more-severe soft tissue injury are best treated with external fixation. The fracture healing in open fractures takes longer than closed injuries.

FEMORAL SHAFT FRACTURES

Fractures of the femur in children are common. All age groups, from early childhood to adolescence, can be affected. The mechanism of injury varies from low-energy twisting type injuries to high-velocity injuries in vehicular accidents. Femur fractures in children <2 yr should raise the concern for child abuse. A thorough physical examination is necessary to rule out other injuries and assess the neurovascular status. In the case of high-energy

Table 675-2 FEMORAL SHAFT FRACTURE: TREATMENT OPTIONS BY AGE

TREATMENT OPTIONS	0-2 YR	3-5 YR	6-10 YR	>11 YR
Spica cast	x	x		
Traction and spica cast		x	x	x
Intramedullary rod		x	x	x
External fixator		x*	x*	x*
Screw or plate		x	x	x

*Open fracture.
Modified from Wells L: Trauma related to the lower extremity. In Dormans JP, editor: *Pediatric orthopaedics: core knowledge in orthopaedics*, Philadelphia, 2005, Mosby, p 93.

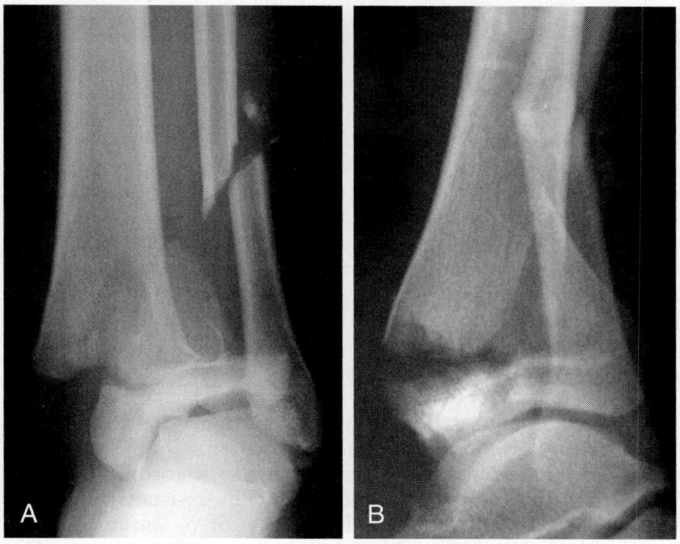

Figure 675-8 The triplane fracture is a transitional fracture: anteroposterior *(A)* and lateral *(B)* radiographs. (From Dormans JP: *Pediatric orthopedics: introduction to trauma,* Philadelphia, 2005, Mosby, p 38.)

trauma, any signs of hemodynamic instability should prompt the examiner to look for other sources of bleeding. AP and lateral radiographs of the femur demonstrate the fracture. An AP radiograph of the pelvis is obtained to rule out any associated pelvic fracture. Treatment of shaft fractures varies with the age group, as described in Table 675-2.

TRIPLANE AND TILLAUX FRACTURES

Triplane and Tillaux fracture patterns occur at the end of the growth period and are based on relative strength of the bone-physis junction and asymmetric closure of the tibial physis. The triplane fractures are so named because the injury has coronal, sagittal, and transverse components (Fig. 675-8). The Tillaux fracture is an avulsion fracture of the anterolateral aspect of the distal tibial epiphysis. Radiographs and further imaging with CT and 3-dimensional reconstructions are necessary to analyze the fracture geometry. The triplane fracture involves the articular surface and hence anatomic reduction is necessary. The reduction is further stabilized with internal fixation. The Tillaux fracture is treated by closed reduction. Open reduction is recommended if a residual intra-articular step off persists.

METATARSAL FRACTURES

Metatarsal fractures are common in children. They usually result from direct trauma to the dorsum of the foot. High-energy trauma or multiple fractures of the metatarsal base are associated with significant swelling. A high index for compartment syndrome of the foot must be maintained and compartment pressures must be measured if indicated. Diagnosis is obtained by AP, lateral, and oblique radiographs of the foot. Most metatarsal fractures can be treated by closed methods in a below-knee cast. Weight bearing is allowed as tolerated. Displaced fractures can require closed or open reduction with internal fixation. Percutaneous, smooth Kirschner wires generally provide sufficient internal fixation for these injuries. If the compartment pressure is increased, complete release of all compartments in the foot is necessary.

TOE PHALANGEAL FRACTURES

Fractures of the lesser toes are common and are usually secondary to direct blows. They commonly occur when the child is barefoot. The toes are swollen, ecchymotic, and tender. There may be a mild deformity. Diagnosis is made radiographically. Bleeding suggests the possibility of an open fracture. The lesser toes usually do not require closed reduction unless significantly displaced. If necessary, reduction can usually be accomplished with longitudinal traction on the toe. Casting is not usually necessary. Buddy taping of the fractured toe to an adjacent stable toe usually provides satisfactory alignment and relief of symptoms. Crutches and heel walking may be beneficial for several days until the soft-tissue swelling and the discomfort decrease.

BIBLIOGRAPHY

Please visit the Nelson Textbook of Pediatrics *website at www.expertconsult.com for the complete bibliography.*

675.5 Operative Treatment

Lawrence Wells, Kriti Sehgal, and John P. Dormans

Four to 5% of pediatric fractures require surgery. The common indications for operative treatment in children and adolescents include displaced physeal fractures, displaced intra-articular fractures, unstable fractures, multiple injuries, open fractures, failure to achieve adequate reduction in older children, failure to maintain an adequate reduction, and certain pathologic fractures.

The aim of operative intervention is to obtain anatomic alignment and relative stability. Rigid fixation is not necessary as it is in adults for early mobilization. The relatively stable construct can be supplemented with external immobilization. SH type III and IV injuries require anatomic alignment, and if they are unstable, internal fixation is used (smooth Kirschner wires, preferably avoiding the course across the growth plate). Multiple closed reductions of an epiphyseal fracture are contraindicated because they can cause permanent damage to the germinal cells of the physis.

SURGICAL TECHNIQUES

It is important to take great care with soft tissues and skin. The other indications for open reduction and internal fixation are unstable fractures of the spine, ipsilateral fractures of the femur, neurovascular injuries requiring repair, and, occasionally, open fractures of the femur and tibia. Closed reduction and minimally invasive fixation are specifically used for supracondylar fractures of the distal humerus, phalangeal fractures, and femoral neck fractures. Failure to obtain anatomic alignment by closed means is an indication for an open reduction.

The main indications for external fixation are summarized in Table 675-3. The advantages of external fixation include rigid immobilization of the fractures, access to open wounds for continued management, and easier patient mobilization for treatment of other injuries and transportation for diagnostic and

Table 675-3 COMMON INDICATIONS FOR EXTERNAL FIXATION IN PEDIATRIC FRACTURES

Grade II and III open fractures
Fractures associated with severe burns
Fractures with soft-tissue loss requiring free flaps or skin grafts
Fractures requiring distractions such as those with significant bone loss
Unstable pelvic fractures
Fractures in children with associated head injuries and spasticity
Fractures associated with vascular or nerve repairs or reconstruction

Table 675-4 COMPLICATIONS OF FRACTURE

ACUTE
Neurovascular injury
Hemorrhage
Fat embolism
Compartment syndrome
SUBACUTE OR CHRONIC
Premature growth plate fusion
Delayed union
Nonunion/pseudarthrosis
Malunion or deformity
Synostosis (cross union)
Heterotopic ossification or myositis ossificans
Osteomyelitis or septic arthritis
Post-traumatic osteolysis
Avascular necrosis
Post-traumatic cyst
Iatrogenic
Soft tissue infection
Hardware misplacement, migration, or infection
Casting complications
Hypocalcemia of immobilization
Superior mesenteric artery syndrome
Deep venous thrombosis or pulmonary embolism
Overgrowth
Refracture
Reflex sympathetic dystrophy syndrome
Premature degenerative joint disease (osteoarthritis)

From Slovis TL, editor: *Caffey's pediatric diagnostic imaging,* ed 11, vol 2, Philadelphia, 2008, Mosby, 2008, p 2781.

therapeutic procedures. The majority of complications with external fixation are pin tract infections, chronic osteomyelitis, and refractures after pin removal.

BIBLIOGRAPHY

Please visit the Nelson Textbook of Pediatrics *website at* www.expertconsult.com *for the complete bibliography.*

675.6 Complications of Fractures in Children

Lawrence Wells, Kriti Sehgal, and John P. Dormans

The complications specific to children are malalignment and correction by natural growth, physeal arrest, overgrowth, and refracture caused by rapid fracture healing (Table 675-4). The malalignment and late angulation is a common problem with fractures of the proximal tibial metaphysis. The physeal arrest can cause angular deformity or shortening. The angular deformities are treated by hemiepiphysiodesis or osteotomy. The shortening is treated with contralateral leg epiphysiodesis closer to skeletal maturity or lengthening of the short limb. Refractures cause more deformity and can necessitate open reduction. Other complications are reflex sympathetic dystrophy, ligamentous instability, malunion, nonunion, fat embolism, and neurovascular injuries.

675.7 Outcomes Assessment

Lawrence Wells, Kriti Sehgal, and John P. Dormans

Empirical and subjective assessment leads to erroneous conclusions and difficulty in comparison with outcome results from other studies. The 3 scales used to evaluate different modalities of treatment for musculoskeletal trauma are the Activities Scale for Kids, the Pediatric Functional Health Outcomes Instrument, and the Pediatric Outcome Data Collection Instruments. The American Academy of Orthopaedic Surgeons developed the Pediatric Functional Health Outcomes Instrument as an example of health status measure.

Chapter 676
Osteomyelitis

Sheldon L. Kaplan

Bone infections in children are relatively common and important because of their potential to cause permanent disability. Early recognition of osteomyelitis in young patients before extensive infection develops and prompt institution of appropriate medical and surgical therapy minimize permanent damage. The risk is greatest if the physis (the growth plate of bone) is damaged.

ETIOLOGY

Bacteria are the most common pathogens in acute skeletal infections. In osteomyelitis, *Staphylococcus aureus* (Chapter 174.1) is the most common infecting organism in all age groups, including newborns. Community-acquired methicillin-resistant *S. aureus* (CA-MRSA) isolates account for >50% of *S. aureus* isolates recovered from children with osteomyelitis in some reports. The USA300 clone of *S. aureus* is the most common among CA-MRSA isolates in the USA and is more likely to cause venous thrombosis in children with acute osteomyelitis than other *S. aureus* clones or other bacteria for reasons that are not known.

Group B streptococcus (Chapter 177) and gram-negative enteric bacilli (*Escherichia coli,* Chapter 192) are also prominent pathogens in neonates; group A streptococcus (Chapter 176) constitutes <10% of all cases. After 6 yr of age, most cases of osteomyelitis are caused by *S. aureus,* streptococcus, or *Pseudomonas aeruginosa* (Chapter 197). Cases of *Pseudomonas* infection are related almost exclusively to puncture wounds of the foot, with direct inoculation of *P. aeruginosa* from the foam padding of the shoe into bone or cartilage, which develops as osteochondritis. *Salmonella* species (Chapter 190) and *S. aureus* are the two most common causes of osteomyelitis in children with sickle cell anemia. *S. pneumoniae* (Chapter 175) most commonly causes osteomyelitis in children <24 mo of age or children with sickle cell anemia. *Bartonella henselae* (Chapter 201.2) can cause osteomyelitis of any bone but especially in pelvic and vertebral bones.

Kingella kingae may be the second most common cause of osteomyelitis in children <5 yr of age in some parts of the world. *K. kingae* is a slow-growing, gram-negative, β-hemolytic bacterium in pairs or short chains of short bacilli. The organism, once thought to be rare, is increasingly recognized as a cause of osteomyelitis, spondylodiskitis, septic arthritis and bacteremia, and, less commonly, in endocarditis. It has been identified as the causative agent in pneumonia and meningitis. Nearly 90% of identified *K. kingae* infections have been in young children.

Infection with atypical mycobacteria (Chapter 209), *S. aureus,* or *Pseudomonas* can occur after penetrating injuries. Fungal infections usually occur as part of multisystem disseminated disease; *Candida* (Chapter 226) osteomyelitis sometimes

Table 676-1 MICROORGANISMS ISOLATED FROM PATIENTS WITH OSTEOMYELITIS AND THEIR CLINICAL ASSOCIATIONS

MOST COMMON CLINICAL ASSOCIATION	MICROORGANISM
Frequent microorganism in any type of osteomyelitis	*Staphylococcus aureus* (susceptible or resistant to methicillin)
Foreign body–associated infection	Coagulase-negative staphylococci, other skin flora, atypical mycobacteria
Common in nosocomial infections	*Enterobacteriaceae, Pseudomonas aeruginosa, Candida* spp.
Decubitus ulcer	*S. aureus*, streptococci and/or anaerobic bacteria
Sickle cell disease	*Salmonella* spp., *S. aureus*, or *Streptococcus pneumoniae*
Exposure to kittens	*Bartonella henselae*
Human or animal bites	*Pasteurella multocida* or *Eikenella corrodens*
Immunocompromised patients	*Aspergillus* spp., *Candida albicans*, or *Mycobacteria* spp.
Populations in which tuberculosis is prevalent	*Mycobacterium tuberculosis*
Populations in which these pathogens are endemic	*Brucella* spp., *Coxiella burnetii*, fungi found in specific geographic areas (coccidioidomycosis, blastomycosis, histoplasmosis)

Modified From Lew DP, Waldvogel FA: Osteomyelitis, *Lancet* 364:369–379, 2004.

complicates fungemia in neonates with or without indwelling vascular catheters.

A microbial etiology is confirmed in ~60% of cases of osteomyelitis. Blood cultures are positive in ~50% of patients. Prior antibiotic therapy and the inhibitory effect of pus on microbial growth might explain the low bacterial yield.

EPIDEMIOLOGY

The median age of children with musculoskeletal infections is ~6 yr. The incidence of osteomyelitis in children is estimated to be 1 : 5,000. Bone infections are more common in boys than girls; the behavior of boys might predispose them to traumatic events. Except for the increased incidence of skeletal infection in patients with sickle cell disease, there is no predilection for osteomyelitis based on race.

The majority of osteomyelitis cases in previously healthy children are hematogenous. Minor closed trauma is a common preceding event in cases of osteomyelitis, occurring in ~30% of patients. Infection of bones can follow penetrating injuries or open fractures. Bone infection following orthopedic surgery is uncommon. Impaired host defenses also increase the risk of skeletal infection. Other risk factors are noted in Table 676-1.

PATHOGENESIS

The unique anatomy and circulation of the ends of long bones result in the predilection for localization of bloodborne bacteria. In the metaphysis, nutrient arteries branch into nonanastomosing capillaries under the physis, which make a sharp loop before entering venous sinusoids draining into the marrow. Blood flow in this area is thought to be "sluggish," predisposing to bacterial invasion. Once a bacterial focus is established, phagocytes migrate to the site and produce an inflammatory exudate (metaphyseal abscess). The generation of proteolytic enzymes, toxic oxygen radicals, and cytokines results in decreased oxygen tension, decreased pH, osteolysis, and tissue destruction. As the inflammatory exudate progresses, pressure increases spread through the porous metaphyseal space via the haversian system and Volkmann canals into the subperiosteal space. Purulence beneath the periosteum may lift the periosteal membrane of the bony surface, further impairing blood supply to the cortex and metaphysis.

In newborns and young infants, transphyseal blood vessels connect the metaphysis and epiphysis, so it is common for pus from the metaphysis to enter the joint space. This extension through the physis has the potential to result in abnormal growth and bone or joint deformity. During the latter part of the 1st year of life, the physis forms, obliterating the transphyseal blood vessels. Joint involvement, once the physis forms, can occur in joints where the metaphysis is intra-articular (hip, ankle, shoulder, and elbow), and subperiosteal pus ruptures into the joint space.

In later childhood, the periosteum becomes more adherent, favoring pus to decompress through the periosteum. Once the growth plate closes in late adolescence, hematogenous osteomyelitis more often begins in the diaphysis and can spread to the entire intramedullary canal.

CLINICAL MANIFESTATIONS

The earliest signs and symptoms of osteomyelitis, often subtle and nonspecific, are generally highly dependent on the age of the patient. Neonates might exhibit **pseudoparalysis** or pain with movement of the affected extremity (e.g., diaper changes). Half of neonates do not have fever and might not appear ill. Older infants and children are more likely to have fever, pain, and localizing signs such as edema, erythema, and warmth. With involvement of the lower extremities, limp or refusal to walk is seen in approximately half of patients.

Focal tenderness over a long bone can be an important finding. Local swelling and redness with osteomyelitis can mean that the infection has spread out of the metaphysis into the subperiosteal space, representing a secondary soft-tissue inflammatory response. Pelvic osteomyelitis can manifest with subtle findings such as hip, thigh, or abdominal pain. Back pain with or without tenderness to palpation overlying the vertebral processes is noted in vertebral osteomyelitis.

Long bones are principally involved in osteomyelitis (Table 676-2); the femur and tibia are equally affected and together constitute almost half of all cases. The bones of the upper extremities account for one fourth of all cases. Flat bones are less commonly affected.

There is usually only a single site of bone or joint involvement. Several bones are infected in <10% of cases; the exception is osteomyelitis in neonates, in whom two or more bones are involved in almost half of the cases. Children with subacute symptoms and focal finding in the metaphyseal area (usually of tibia) might have a **Brodie abscess,** with radiographic lucency and surrounding reactive bone.

DIAGNOSIS

The diagnosis of osteomyelitis is clinical; blood cultures should be performed in all suspected cases. Depending on the results of imaging studies (see later) aspiration or biopsy of bone or subperiosteal abscess for Gram stain, culture, and possibly bone histology provides the optimal specimen for culture to confirm the diagnosis. These specimens are often obtained by the interventional radiologist or at the time of surgical drainage by the orthopedic surgeon. Direct inoculation of clinical specimens into aerobic blood culture bottles can improve the recovery of *K. kingae,* particularly if held for 1 wk. Polymerase chain reaction appears to be the most sensitive technique to detect *K. kingae,* with detection up to 6 days after antibiotics are initiated.

There are no specific laboratory tests for osteomyelitis. The white blood cell count and differential, erythrocyte sedimentation rate (ESR), or C-reactive protein (CRP) are generally elevated in children with bone infections but are nonspecific and not helpful in distinguishing between skeletal infection and other

Table 676-2 SITES OF OSTEOMYELITIS IN CHILDREN

BONE	%
Femur	23-28
Tibia	20-24
Humerus	5-13
Radius	5-6
Phalanx	3-5
Pelvis	4-8
Calcaneus	4-8
Ulna	4-8
Metatarsal	~2
Vertebrae	~2
Sacrum	~2
Clavicle	~2
Skull	~1
Carpal bone	<1
Rib	<1
Metacarpal	<1
Cuboid	<1
Cuneiform	<1
Pyriform aperture	<1
Olecranon	<1
Maxilla	<1
Mandible	<1
Scapula	<1
Sternum	<1
Foot	1

Modified from Gafur OA, Copley LA, Hollmig ST, et al: The impact of the current epidemiology of pediatric musculoskeletal infection on evaluation and treatment guidelines, *J Pediatr Orthop* 28(7):777–785, 2008.

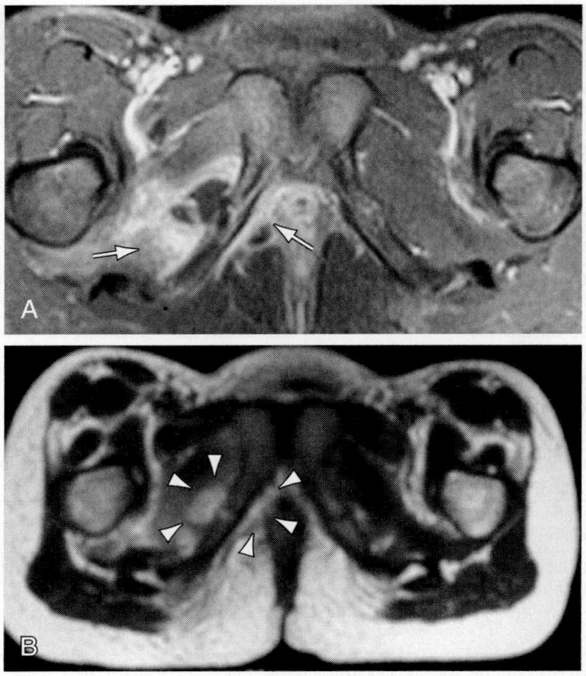

Figure 676-1 MRI of an 8 yr old girl with acute pelvic hematogenous osteomyelitis. *A,* Axial T1-weighted contrast-enhanced MRI with fat saturation reveals a nonenhancing fluid collection adjacent to the inflamed pubic synchondrosis. *B,* The fluid collection appears hyperintense on the corresponding T2-weighted image *(arrowheads).* In addition, a contrast enhancement within the adjacent internal obturator muscle is seen *(arrow),* indicating pelvic acute pelvic hematogenous osteomyelitis with complicating adjacent abscess formation and soft tissue inflammation. (From Weber-Chrysochoou C, Corti N, Goetschel P, et al: Pelvic osteomyelitis: a diagnostic challenge in children, *J Pediatr Surg* 42:553–557, 2007.)

inflammatory processes. The leukocyte count and ESR may be normal during the first few days of infection, and normal test results do not preclude the diagnosis of skeletal infection. However, most children with acute hematogenous osteomyelitis have elevations in the ESR and/or CRP. Monitoring elevated ESR and CRP may be of value in assessing response to therapy or identifying complications.

RADIOGRAPHIC EVALUATION

Radiographic studies play a crucial role in the evaluation of osteomyelitis. Conventional radiographs, ultrasonography, CT, MRI, and radionuclide studies can all contribute to establishing the diagnosis. Plain radiographs are often used for initial evaluation to exclude other causes such as trauma and foreign bodies. MRI has emerged as the most sensitive and specific test and is widely used for diagnosis. The sequence of radionuclide studies or MRI is often determined by age, site, and clinical presentation.

Plain Radiographs

Within 72 hr of onset of symptoms of osteomyelitis, plain radiographs of the involved site using soft-tissue technique and compared to the opposite extremity, if necessary, can show displacement of the deep muscle planes from the adjacent metaphysis caused by deep-tissue edema. Lytic bone changes are not visible on radiographs until 30-50% of the bony matrix is destroyed. Tubular long bones do not show lytic changes for 7-14 days after onset of infection. Infection in flat and irregular bones can take longer to appear.

Computed Tomography and Magnetic Resonance Imaging

CT can demonstrate osseous and soft-tissue abnormalities and is ideal for detecting gas in soft tissues. In selected children who cannot remain still or tolerate sedation, CT is a valuable imaging modality. **MRI is more sensitive than CT or radionuclide imaging in acute osteomyelitis and is the best radiographic imaging technique for identifying abscesses and for differentiating between bone and soft-tissue infection.** MRI provides precise anatomic detail of subperiosteal pus and accumulation of purulent debris in the bone marrow and metaphyses for possible surgical intervention. In acute osteomyelitis, purulent debris and edema appear dark, with decreased signal intensity on T1-weighted images, with fat appearing bright (Fig. 676-1). The opposite is seen in T2-weighted images. The signal from fat can be diminished with fat-suppression techniques to enhance visualization. Gadolinium administration can also enhance MRI. Cellulitis and sinus tracts appear as areas of high signal intensity on T2-weighted images. MRI can also demonstrate a contiguous septic arthritis, pyomyositis, or venous thrombosis.

Radionuclide Studies

Radionuclide imaging can be valuable in suspected bone infections, especially early in the course of infection and/or if multiple foci are suspected or an unusual site is suspected, as in the pelvis. Technetium-99 methylene diphosphonate (^{99m}Tc), which accumulates in areas of increased bone turnover, is the preferred agent for radionuclide bone imaging (three-phase bone scan). Osteomyelitis causes increased vascularity, inflammation, and increased osteoblastic activity, resulting in an increased concentration of ^{99m}Tc. Any areas of increased blood flow or inflammation can cause increased uptake of ^{99m}Tc in the first and second phases, but osteomyelitis causes increased uptake of ^{99m}Tc in the third phase (4-6 hr). Three-phase imaging with ^{99m}Tc has excellent sensitivity (84-100%) and specificity (70-96%) in hematogenous osteomyelitis and can detect osteomyelitis within 24-48 hr after onset of symptoms. The sensitivity in neonates is much lower, due to poor bone mineralization. Advantages include infrequent need for sedation, lower cost, and the ability to image the entire skeleton for detection of multiple foci.

DIFFERENTIAL DIAGNOSIS

Distinguishing osteomyelitis from cellulitis or trauma (accidental or abuse) is the most common clinical circumstance. Myositis or pyomyositis can also appear similar to osteomyelitis with fever, warm and swollen extremities, and limping; tenderness to palpation of the affected soft tissue area is generally more diffuse than noted in acute osteomyelitis. Nevertheless, distinguishing myositis and pyomyositis from osteomyelitis clinically may be difficult. Myositis and pyomyositis often are found adjacent to an osteomyelitis on MRI. Pyomyositis is often caused by *S. aureus* or group A streptococcus. The pelvic muscles are a common site of infection and can mimic a pelvic osteomyelitis. MRI is the definitive study to identify and localize pelvic pyomyositis. An iliopsoas abscess can manifest with thigh pain, limp, and fever and must be considered in the differential diagnosis of osteomyelitis. The iliopsoas abscess may be primary (hematogenous: *S. aureus*) or secondary to infection in adjacent bone (*S. aureus*), kidney (*E. coli*) or intestine (*E. coli*, *Bacteroides* spp.). *M. tuberculosis* has been reported in patients with HIV infection.

Appendicitis, urinary tract infection, and gynecologic disease are among the conditions in the differential diagnosis of pelvic osteomyelitis. Children with leukemia commonly have bone pain or joint pain as an early symptom. Neuroblastoma with bone involvement may be mistaken for osteomyelitis. Primary bone tumors need to be considered, but fever and other signs of illness are generally absent except in Ewing sarcoma. In patients with sickle cell disease, distinguishing bone infection from infarction may be challenging. Chronic recurrent multifocal osteomyelitis (CRMO) and synovitis, acne, pustulosis, hyperostosis, and osteitis syndrome are rare noninfectious conditions in children characterized by recurrent osteoarticular inflammation and different skin conditions, palmoplantar pustulosis, psoriasis, severe acne, neutrophilic dermatosis (Sweet syndrome, Chapter 163), and pyoderma gangrenosum.

TREATMENT

Optimal treatment of skeletal infections requires collaborative efforts of pediatricians, orthopedic surgeons, and radiologists. Obtaining material for culture (blood, periosteal abscess, bone) before antibiotics are given is essential. Because most patients with osteomyelitis have an indolent, non–life-threatening condition, cultures should be obtained even if there is a delay of a few hours in initiating antibiotics.

Antibiotic Therapy

The initial empirical antibiotic therapy is based on knowledge of likely bacterial pathogens at various ages, the results of the Gram stain of aspirated material, and additional considerations. In neonates, an antistaphylococcal penicillin, such as nafcillin or oxacillin (150-200 mg/kg/24 hr divided q6h IV), and a broad-spectrum cephalosporin, such as cefotaxime (150-225 mg/kg/24 hr divided q8h IV), provide coverage for the *S. aureus,* group B streptococcus, and gram-negative bacilli. If methicillin-resistant *Staphylococcus* is suspected, vancomycin is substituted for nafcillin. If the neonate is a small premature infant or has a central vascular catheter, the possibility of nosocomial bacteria (*Pseudomonas* or coagulase-negative staphylococci) or fungi *(Candida)* should be considered. In older infants and children, the principal pathogens are *S. aureus* and streptococcus.

A major factor influencing the selection of empirical therapy is the rate of methicillin resistance among community *S. aureus* isolates. If MRSA accounts for ≥10% of community *S. aureus* isolates, including an antibiotic effective against CA-MRSA in the initial empirical antibiotic regimen is suggested. Vancomycin (45 mg/kg/24 hr divided q8h or 60 mg/kg/24 hr divided q6h IV) is the gold standard agent for treating invasive MRSA infections, especially when the child is critically ill. Clindamycin (30-40 mg/kg/24 hr q8hr) is also recommended when the rate of clindamycin resistance is ≤10% among community *S. aureus* isolates and the child is not severely ill. Cefazolin (100 mg/kg/24 hr divided q8h IV) or nafcillin (150-200 mg/kg/24 hr divided q6h) is the agent of choice for parenteral treatment of osteomyelitis caused by methicillin-susceptible *S. aureus*. Penicillin is first-line therapy for treating osteomyelitis due to susceptible strains of *S. pneumoniae* as well as all group A streptococcus. Cefotaxime or ceftriaxone is recommended for pneumococcal isolates with resistance to penicillin or for most *Salmonella* spp.

Special situations dictate deviations from the usual empirical antibiotic selection. In patients with sickle cell disease with osteomyelitis, gram-negative enteric bacteria *(Salmonella)* are common pathogens as well as *S. aureus,* so a broad-spectrum cephalosporin such as cefotaxime (150-225 mg/kg/24 hr divided q8h) is used in addition to vancomycin or clindamycin. Clindamycin (40 mg/kg/24 hr divided q6h IV) is a useful alternative drug for patients allergic to β-lactam drugs. In addition to good antistaphylococcal activity, clindamycin has broad activity against anaerobes and is useful for treating infections secondary to penetrating injuries or compound fractures. For immunocompromised patients, combination therapy is usually initiated, such as with vancomycin and ceftazidime, or with piperacillin-tazobactam and an aminoglycoside. *K. kingae* usually responds to β-lactam antibiotics, including cefotaxime. Although the efficacy of treating osteomyelitis caused by *B. henselae* is uncertain, azithromycin plus rifampin may be considered.

When the pathogen is identified and antibiotic susceptibilities are determined, appropriate adjustments in antibiotics are made as necessary. If a pathogen is not identified and a patient's condition is improving, therapy is continued with the initially selected antibiotic. This selection is more complicated currently owing to the presence of MRSA isolates in the community. If a pathogen is not identified and a patient's condition is not improving, reaspiration or biopsy and the possibility of a noninfectious condition should be considered.

Duration of antibiotic therapy is individualized depending on the organism isolated and clinical course. For most infections including those caused by *S. aureus*, the minimal duration of antibiotics is 21-28 days, provided that the patient shows prompt resolution of signs and symptoms (within 5-7 days) and the CRP and ESR have normalized; a total of 4-6 wk of therapy may be required. For group A streptococcus, *S. pneumoniae,* or *H. influenzae* type b, treatment duration maybe shorter. A total of 7-10 postoperative days of treatment is adequate for *Pseudomonas* osteochondritis when thorough curettage of infected tissue has been performed. Immunocompromised patients generally require prolonged courses of therapy, as do patients with mycobacterial or fungal infection.

Changing antibiotics from the intravenous route to oral administration when a patient's condition clearly has improved and the child is afebrile for ≥48-72 hr, may be considered. For the oral antibiotic regimen with β-lactam drugs for susceptible staphylococcal or streptococcal infection, cephalexin (80-100 mg/kg/24 hr q8h) or oral clindamycin (30-40 mg/kg/24 hr q8h) can be used to complete therapy for children with clindamycin-susceptible CA-MRSA or for patients who are seriously allergic or cannot tolerate β-lactam antibiotics. The oral regimen decreases the risk of complications related to prolonged intravenous therapy, is more comfortable for patients, and permits treatment outside the hospital if adherence to treatment can be ensured. Outpatient intravenous antibiotic therapy via a central venous catheter can be used for completing therapy at home, as an alternative; however, catheter-related complications, including infection or mechanical problems, can lead to readmission or emergency department visits.

In children with venous thrombosis complicating osteomyelitis, anticoagulants generally are administered under the supervision of a hematologist until the thrombus has resolved.

Surgical Therapy

When frank pus is obtained from subperiosteal or metaphyseal aspiration or is suspected based on MRI findings, a surgical drainage procedure is usually indicated. Surgical intervention is also often indicated after a penetrating injury and when a retained foreign body is possible. In selected cases, catheter drainage performed by an interventional radiologist is adequate.

Treatment of chronic osteomyelitis consists of surgical removal of sinus tracts and sequestrum, if present. Antibiotic therapy is continued for several months or longer until clinical and radiographic findings suggest that healing has occurred. Monitoring the CRP or ESR is not helpful in most cases of chronic osteomyelitis.

Physical Therapy

The major role of physical medicine is a preventive one. If a child is allowed to lie in bed with an extremity in flexion, limitation of extension can develop within a few days. The affected extremity should be kept in extension with sandbags, splints, or, if necessary, a temporary cast. Casts are also indicated when there is a potential for pathologic fracture. After 2-3 days, when pain is easing, passive range of motion exercises are started and continued until the child resumes normal activity. In neglected cases with flexion contractures, prolonged physical therapy is required.

PROGNOSIS

When pus is drained and appropriate antibiotic therapy is given, the improvement in signs and symptoms is rapid. Failure to improve or worsening by 72 hr requires review of the appropriateness of the antibiotic therapy, the need for surgical intervention, or the correctness of the diagnosis. Acute-phase reactants may be useful as monitors. The serum CRP typically normalizes within 7 days after start of treatment, whereas the ESR typically rises for 5-7 days, and then falls slowly, dropping sharply after 10-14 days. Failure of either of these acute-phase reactants to follow the usual course should raise concerns about the adequacy of therapy. Recurrence of disease and development of chronic infection after treatment occur in <10% of patients.

Because children are in a dynamic state of growth, sequelae of skeletal infections might not become apparent for months or years; therefore, long-term follow-up is necessary with close attention to range of motion of joints and bone length. Although firm data about the impact of delayed treatment on outcome are not available, it appears that initiation of medical and surgical therapy within 1 wk of onset of symptoms provides a better prognosis than delayed treatment.

BIBLIOGRAPHY

Please visit the Nelson Textbook of Pediatrics *website at www.expertconsult.com for the complete bibliography.*

Chapter 677
Septic Arthritis

Sheldon L. Kaplan

Septic arthritis in infants and children has the potential to cause permanent disability. Early recognition of septic arthritis in young patients before extensive infection develops and prompt institution of appropriate medical and surgical therapy minimize further damage to the synovium, adjacent cartilage, and bone.

ETIOLOGY

Historically, *Haemophilus influenzae* type b (Chapter 186) accounted for more than half of all cases of bacterial arthritis in infants and young children. Since the development of the conjugate, it is now a rare cause; *Staphylococcus aureus* (Chapter 174.1) has emerged as the most common infection in all age groups. Methicillin-resistant *S. aureus* accounts for a high proportion (>25%) of community *S. aureus* isolates in many areas of the USA and throughout the world. Group A streptococcus (Chapter 176) and *Streptococcus pneumoniae* (pneumococcus) (Chapter 175) historically cause 10-20%; *S. pneumoniae* is most likely in the first 2 years of life. *Kingella kingae* is recognized as a relatively common etiology with improved culture and polymerase chain reaction (PCR) methods in children <5 yr old (Chapter 676). In sexually active adolescents, gonococcus (Chapter 185) is a common cause of septic arthritis and tenosynovitis, usually of small joints or as a monoarticular infection of a large joint (knee). *Neisseria meningitidis* (Chapter 184) can cause either a septic arthritis that occurs in the first few days of illness or a reactive arthritis that is typically seen several days after antibiotics have been initiated. Group B streptococcus (Chapter 177) is an important cause of septic arthritis in neonates.

Fungal infections usually occur as part of multisystem disseminated disease; *Candida* arthritis can complicate systemic infection in neonates with or without indwelling vascular catheters. Primary viral infections of joints are rare, but arthritis accompanies many viral (parvovirus, mumps, rubella live vaccines) syndromes, suggesting an immune-mediated pathogenesis.

A microbial etiology is confirmed in about 65% of cases of septic arthritis. Prior antibiotic therapy and the inhibitory effect of pus on microbial growth might explain the low bacterial yield. Additionally, some cases treated as bacterial arthritis are actually postinfectious (gastrointestinal or genitourinary) reactive arthritis (Chapter 151) rather than primary infection. Lyme disease produces an arthritis more like a rheumatologic disorder and not typically suppurative.

EPIDEMIOLOGY

Septic arthritis is more common in young children. Half of all cases occur by 2 yr of age and three fourths of all cases occur by 5 yr of age. Adolescents and neonates are at risk of gonococcal septic arthritis.

The majority of infections in otherwise healthy children are of hematogenous origin. Infection of joints can follow penetrating injuries or procedures such as trauma, arthroscopy, prosthetic joint surgery, intra-articular steroid injection, and orthopedic surgery, although this is uncommon. Immunocompromised patients and those with rheumatologic joint disease are also at increased risk of joint infection.

PATHOGENESIS

Septic arthritis primarily occurs as a result of hematogenous seeding of the synovial space. Less often, organisms enter the joint space by direct inoculation or extension from a contiguous focus. The synovial membrane has a rich vascular supply and lacks a basement membrane, providing an ideal environment for hematogenous seeding. The presence of bacterial products (endotoxin or other toxins) within the joint space stimulates cytokine production (tumor necrosis factor-α, interleukin-1) within the joint, triggering an inflammatory cascade. The cytokines stimulate chemotaxis of neutrophils into the joint space, where proteolytic enzymes and elastases are released by neutrophils, damaging the cartilage. Proteolytic enzymes released from the synovial cells and chondrocytes also contribute to destruction of cartilage and synovium. Bacterial hyaluronidase breaks down the hyaluronic acid in the synovial fluid, making the fluid less viscous

Table 677-1 ANATOMIC DISTRIBUTION OF SEPTIC ARTHRITIS

BONE	%
Knee	~40
Hip	22-40
Ankle	4-13
Elbow	8-12
Wrist	1-4
Shoulder	~3
Interphalangeal	<1
Metatarsal	<1
Sacroiliac	<1
Acromioclavicular	<1
Metacarpal	<1
Toe	~1

Modified from Gafur OA, Copley LA, Hollmig ST, et al: The impact of the current epidemiology of pediatric musculoskeletal infection on evaluation and treatment guidelines, *J Pediatr Orthop* 28:777–785, 2008.

and diminishing its ability to lubricate and protect the joint cartilage. Damage to the cartilage can occur through increased friction, especially for weight-bearing joints. The increased pressure within the joint space from accumulation of purulent material can compromise the vascular supply and induce pressure necrosis of the cartilage. Synovial and cartilage destruction results from a combination of proteolytic enzymes and mechanical factors.

CLINICAL MANIFESTATIONS

Most septic arthritides are monoarticular. The signs and symptoms of septic arthritis depend on the age of the patient. Early signs and symptoms may be subtle, particularly in neonates. Septic arthritis in neonates and young infants is often associated with adjacent osteomyelitis caused by transphyseal spread of infection, although osteomyelitis contiguous with an infected joint can be seen at any age (Chapter 676).

Older infants and children might have fever and pain, with localizing signs such as swelling, erythema, and warmth of the affected joint. With involvement of joints of the pelvis and lower extremities, limp or refusal to walk is often seen.

Erythema and edema of the skin and soft tissue overlying the site of infection are seen earlier in septic arthritis than in osteomyelitis, because the bulging infected synovium is usually more superficial, whereas the metaphysis is located more deeply. Septic arthritis of the hip is an exception because of the deep location of the hip joint.

Joints of the lower extremity constitute 75% of all cases of septic arthritis (Table 677-1). The elbow, wrist, and shoulder joints are involved in about 25% of cases, and small joints are uncommonly infected. Suppurative infections of the hip, shoulder, elbow, and ankle in older infants and children may be associated with an adjacent osteomyelitis of the proximal femur, proximal humerus, proximal radius, and distal tibia because the metaphysis extends intra-articularly.

DIAGNOSIS

Blood cultures should be performed in all cases of suspected septic arthritis. Aspiration of the joint fluid for Gram stain and culture when the history and physical findings indicate septic arthritis remains the definitive diagnostic technique and provides the optimal specimen for culture to confirm the diagnosis. Most large joint spaces are easy to aspirate, but the hip can pose technical problems; ultrasound guidance facilitates aspiration. Aspiration of joint pus provides the best specimen for bacteriologic culture of infection. If gonococcus is suspected, cervical, anal, and

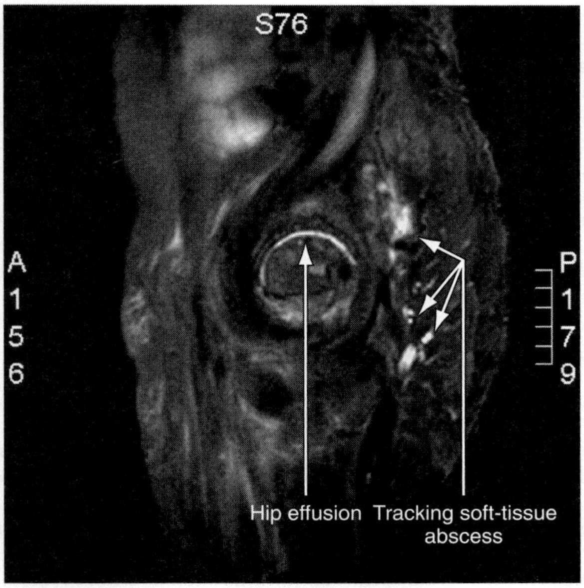

Figure 677-1 MRI of staphylococcal septic arthritis of left hip, with fluid collections between planes of gluteal muscles. *Arrows* indicate fluid collection. (From Matthews CJ, Weston VC, Jones A, et al: Bacterial septic arthritis in adults, *Lancet* 375:846–854, 2010.)

throat cultures should also be obtained. In addition to prompt inoculation onto solid media, inoculation of the specimen in blood culture bottles can increase recovery of *K. kingae*. PCR appears to be the most sensitive method for detecting *K. kingae* in joint fluid.

Synovial fluid analysis for cell count, differential, protein, and glucose has limited usefulness because noninfectious inflammatory diseases, such as rheumatic fever and rheumatoid arthritis, can also cause exuberant reaction with increased cells and protein and decreased glucose. Nevertheless, cell counts >50,000-100,000 cells/mm^3 generally indicate an infectious process. Synovial fluid characteristics of septic arthritis can suggest infection but are not sufficiently specific to exclude infection.

The white blood cell count and differential, erythrocyte sedimentation rate (ESR), and C-reactive protein (CRP) are generally elevated in children with joint infections but are nonspecific and might not be helpful in distinguishing between infection and other inflammatory processes. The leukocyte count and ESR may be normal during the first few days of infection, and normal test results do not preclude the diagnosis of septic arthritis. Monitoring elevated ESR and CRP may be of value in assessing response to therapy or identifying complications.

Radiographic Evaluation

Radiographic studies play a crucial role in evaluating septic arthritis. Conventional radiographs, ultrasonography, CT, MRI, and radionuclide studies can all contribute to establishing the diagnosis (Fig. 677-1).

PLAIN RADIOGRAPHS Plain films of septic arthritis can show widening of the joint capsule, soft-tissue edema, and obliteration of normal fat lines. Plain films of the hip can show medial displacement of the obturator muscle into the pelvis (the obturator sign), lateral displacement or obliteration of the gluteal fat lines, and elevation of the Shenton line with a widened arc.

ULTRASONOGRAPHY Ultrasonography is particularly helpful in detecting joint effusion and fluid collection in the soft tissue and subperiosteal regions. Ultrasonography is highly sensitive in detecting joint effusion, particularly for the hip joint, where plain radiographs are normal in >50% of cases of septic arthritis of the hip. Ultrasonography can serve as an aid in performing hip aspiration.

COMPUTED TOMOGRAPHY AND MAGNETIC RESONANCE IMAGING CT and MRI may be useful in confirming the presence of joint fluid in patients with suspected osteoarthritis infections. MRI may be useful in excluding adjacent osteomyelitis.

RADIONUCLIDE IMAGING Radionuclide imaging compared to radiographs is more sensitive in providing supportive evidence of the diagnosis of septic arthritis; a scan may be positive within 2 days of the onset of symptoms. Three-phase imaging with technetium-99 methylene diphosphonate shows symmetric uptake on both sides of the joint, limited to the bony structures adjacent to the joint. Radionuclide imaging is also useful for evaluating the sacroiliac joint.

DIFFERENTIAL DIAGNOSIS

The differential diagnosis of septic arthritis depends on the joint or joints involved and the age of the patient. For the hip, toxic synovitis, Legg-Calvé-Perthes disease, slipped capital femoral epiphysis, psoas abscess, and proximal femoral, pelvic, or vertebral osteomyelitis as well as diskitis should be considered. For the knee, distal femoral or proximal tibial osteomyelitis, pauciarticular rheumatoid arthritis, and referred pain from the hip should be considered. Other conditions such as trauma, cellulitis, pyomyositis, sickle cell disease, hemophilia, and Henoch-Schönlein purpura can mimic purulent arthritis. When several joints are involved, serum sickness, collagen vascular disease, rheumatic fever, and Henoch-Schönlein purpura should be considered. Arthritis is one of the extraintestinal manifestations of inflammatory bowel disease. Reactive arthritis following a variety of bacterial (gastrointestinal or genital) and parasitic infections, streptococcal pharyngitis, or viral hepatitis can resemble acute septic arthritis (Chapter 151).

TREATMENT

Optimal treatment of septic arthritis requires cooperation of pediatricians, orthopedic surgeons, and radiologists to benefit the patient.

Antibiotic Therapy

The initial empirical antibiotic therapy is based on knowledge of likely bacterial pathogens at various ages, the results of the Gram stain of aspirated material, and additional considerations. In neonates, an antistaphylococcal penicillin, such as nafcillin or oxacillin (150-200 mg/kg/24 hr divided q6h IV), and a broad-spectrum cephalosporin, such as cefotaxime (150-225 mg/kg/24 hr divided q8h IV), provide coverage for the *S. aureus,* group B streptococcus, and gram-negative bacilli. If MRSA is a concern, vancomycin is selected in favor of nafcillin or oxacillin. If the neonate is a small premature infant or has a central vascular catheter, the possibility of nosocomial bacteria (*Pseudomonas aeruginosa* or coagulase-negative staphylococci) or fungi *(Candida)* should be considered.

In older infants and children with septic arthritis, empirical therapy to cover for *S. aureus*, streptococci, and *K. kingae* includes cefazolin (100-150 mg/kg/24 hr divided q8h) or nafcillin (150-200 mg/kg/24 hr divided q6h).

In areas where methicillin resistance is noted in ≥10% of community *S. aureus* strains (CA-MRSA), including an antibiotic that is effective against CA-MRSA isolates is suggested. Clindamycin (30-40 mg/kg divided q8h) and vancomycin (15 mg/kg q6-8h IV) are alternatives when treating CA-methicillin-resistant *S. aureus* infections. For immunocompromised patients, combination therapy is usually initiated, such as with vancomycin and ceftazidime or with extended-spectrum penicillins and β-lactamase inhibitors with an aminoglycoside. Adjunct therapy with dexamethasone for 4 days with antibiotic therapy appeared to benefit children with septic arthritis in one study but has not been studied in children with CA-MRSA septic arthritis.

When the pathogen is identified, appropriate changes in antibiotics are made, if necessary. If a pathogen is not identified and a patient's condition is improving, therapy is continued with the antibiotic selected initially. If a pathogen is not identified and a patient's condition is not improving, re-aspiration or the possibility of a noninfectious condition should be considered.

Duration of antibiotic therapy is individualized depending on the organism isolated and the clinical course. Ten to 14 days is usually adequate for streptococci, *S. pneumoniae*, and *K. kingae;* longer therapy may be needed for *S. aureus* and gram-negative infections. Normalization of ESR and CRP in addition to a normal examination supports discontinuing antibiotic therapy. In selected patients, obtaining a plain radiograph of the joint before completing therapy can provide evidence (typically periosteal new bone) of a previously unappreciated contiguous site of osteomyelitis that would likely prolong antibiotic treatment. Oral antibiotics can be used to complete therapy once the patient is afebrile for 48-72 hr and is clearly improving.

Surgical Therapy

Infection of the hip is generally considered a surgical emergency because of the vulnerability of the blood supply to the head of the femur. For joints other than the hip, daily aspirations of synovial fluid may be required. Generally, one or two subsequent aspirations suffice. If fluid continues to accumulate after 4-5 days, arthrotomy or video assisted arthroscopy is needed. At the time of surgery, the joint is flushed with sterile saline solution. Antibiotics are not instilled because they are irritating to synovial tissue, and adequate amounts of antibiotic are achieved in joint fluid with systemic administration.

PROGNOSIS

When pus is drained and appropriate antibiotic therapy is given, the improvement in signs and symptoms is rapid. Failure to improve or worsening by 72 hr requires review of the appropriateness of the antibiotic therapy, the need for surgical intervention, and the correctness of the diagnosis. Acute-phase reactants may be useful as monitors. Failure of either of these acute-phase reactants to follow the usual course should raise concerns about the adequacy of therapy. Recurrence of disease and development of chronic infection after treatment occur in <10% of patients.

Because children are in a dynamic state of growth, sequelae of skeletal infections might not become apparent for months or years; therefore, long-term follow-up is necessary, with close attention to range of motion of joints and bone length. Although firm data about the impact of delayed treatment on outcome are not available, it appears that initiation of medical and surgical therapy within 1 wk of onset of symptoms provides a better prognosis than delayed treatment.

BIBLIOGRAPHY

Please visit the Nelson Textbook of Pediatrics *website at www.expertconsult.com for the complete bibliography.*

Section 2 SPORTS MEDICINE

Chapter 678 Epidemiology and Prevention of Injuries

Gregory L. Landry

The Centers for Disease Control and Prevention recommend moderate to vigorous physical activity on a regular basis for all adolescents. Physical activity has favorable effects on hypertension, obesity, and serum lipid levels in youths. In adults, physical activity is associated with lower rates of cardiovascular disease, type 2 diabetes mellitus, osteoporosis, and colon and breast cancer.

Pediatricians should promote physical activity to their patients, especially those with lower rates of physical activity and sports participation, including children with special health care needs and those from lower socioeconomic groups. Coincident with promoting sports participation and physical activity, physicians have the responsibility of providing medical clearance for participation in physical activity and sports and for diagnosis and rehabilitation of injuries.

Approximately 30 million children and adolescents participate in organized sports in the USA. Approximately 3 million injuries occur annually if injury is defined as time lost from the sport. Deaths in sports are rare, with the majority of nontraumatic deaths caused by cardiac diseases (Chapter 430). Overall, injury rates and injury severity in sports increase with age and pubertal development, related to the greater speed, strength, and intensity of competition.

Recognizing mechanisms of injury and enforcing rules that reduce the likelihood of that mechanism of injury, including penalizing dangerous play, have reduced catastrophic injury rates. Injury rates have also been reduced by removing environmental hazards, such as trampolines in gymnastics and stationary (vs breakaway) bases in softball, and by modifying heat injury rates in soccer tournaments by adding water breaks and reducing the playing time. Wearing equipment such as mouth guards can reduce dental injuries. A common reason for reinjury is lack of rehabilitation of old injuries; appropriate rehabilitation reduces injury rates. Preseason training for high school athletes, with an emphasis on speed, agility, jump training, and flexibility, is associated with lower injury rates in soccer and fewer serious knee injuries in female athletes. Traditional stretching maneuvers or massage might not reduce the risk of injury or muscle soreness, but ankle taping is helpful particularly to prevent reinjury of the ankle. One setting for implementing some of these prevention strategies and for detecting unrehabilitated injuries and medical problems that could affect participation in sports is the preparticipation sports examination (PSE).

PREPARTICIPATION SPORTS EXAMINATION

The PSE is performed with a directed history and a directed physical examination, including a screening musculoskeletal examination. It identifies possible problems in 1-8% of athletes and excludes <1% from participation. The PSE is not a substitute for the recommended comprehensive annual evaluation, which looks at behaviors that are potentially harmful to teens, such as sexual activity, drug use, and violence, and assesses for depression and suicidal ideation. The purposes of the PSE include detecting medical conditions that delay or disqualify athletic participation owing to a risk of injury or death, detecting previously undiagnosed medical conditions, detecting medical conditions that need further evaluation or rehabilitation before participation, providing guidance for sports participation for patients with health conditions, and meeting legal and insurance obligations. If possible, the PSE should be combined with the comprehensive annual health visit with emphasis on preventive health care (Chapters 5 and 14).

State requirements for how often a youth needs a PSE differ, ranging from annually to entry to a new school level (middle school, high school, college). At a minimum, a focused, annual interim evaluation should be done on an otherwise healthy young athlete. The PSE is optimally performed 3-6 wk before the start of practice.

History and Physical Examination

The essential components of the PSE are the history and focused medical and musculoskeletal screening examinations. Identified problems require more investigation (Tables 678-1 and 678-2). In the absence of symptoms, no screening laboratory tests are required.

Seventy-five percent of significant findings are identified by the history; a standardized questionnaire given to the parent and athlete is important because the young athlete might not know or might forget important aspects of his or her history. The questionnaire should include questions about previous medical, surgical, cardiac, pulmonary, neurologic, dermatologic, visual, psychologic, musculoskeletal, and menstrual problems, as well as about heat illness, medications, allergies, immunizations, and diet. The most common identified problems are **unrehabilitated injuries.** An investigation of previous injuries including diagnostic tests, treatment, and present functional status is indicated.

Sudden death during sports can result from undetected cardiac disease such as hypertrophic or other cardiomyopathies, anomalous coronary vessels, or a ruptured aorta in Marfan syndrome (Chapter 693). In many cases, the underlying heart disease is not suspected, and death is the first sign of heart disease (Chapter

Table 678-1 PREPARTICIPATION SPORTS EXAMINATION

COMPONENT OF THE PHYSICAL EXAMINATION	CONDITION TO BE DETECTED
Vital signs	Hypertension, cardiac disease, brady- or tachycardia
Height and weight	Obesity, eating disorders
Vision and pupil size	Legal blindness, absent eye, anisocoria, amblyopia
Lymph node	Infectious diseases, malignancy
Cardiac (performed standing and supine)	Heart murmur, prior surgery, dysrhythmia
Pulmonary	Recurrent and exercise-induced bronchospasm, chronic lung disease
Abdomen	Organomegaly, abdominal mass
Skin	Contagious diseases (impetigo, herpes, staphylococcal, streptococcal)
Genitourinary	Varicocele, undescended testes, tumor, hernia
Musculoskeletal	Acute and chronic injuries, physical anomalies (scoliosis)

Table 678-2 MEDICAL CONDITIONS AND SPORTS PARTICIPATION

CONDITION	MAY PARTICIPATE	EXPLANATION
Atlantoaxial instability (instability of the joint between cervical vertebrae 1 and 2)	Qualified yes	Athlete (particularly if he or she has Down syndrome or juvenile rheumatoid arthritis with cervical involvement) needs evaluation to assess the risk of spinal cord injury during sports participation, especially when using a trampoline
Bleeding disorder	Qualified yes	Athlete needs evaluation
Diabetes mellitus	Yes	All sports can be played with proper attention and appropriate adjustments to diet (particularly carbohydrate intake), blood glucose concentrations, hydration, and insulin therapy Blood glucose concentrations should be monitored before exercise, every 30 min during continuous exercise, 15 min after completion of exercise, and at bedtime
Eating disorders	Qualified yes	Athlete with an eating disorder needs medical and psychiatric assessment before participation
Fever	No	Elevated core temperature can indicate a pathologic medical condition (infection or disease) that is often manifest by increased resting metabolism and heart rate. Accordingly, during the athlete's usual exercise regimen, fever can result in greater heat storage, decreased heat tolerance, increased risk of heat illness, increased cardiopulmonary effort, reduced maximal exercise capacity, and increased risk of hypotension because of altered vascular tone and dehydration. On rare occasions, fever accompanies myocarditis or other conditions that can make usual exercise dangerous
Heat illness, history of	Qualified yes	Because of the likelihood of recurrence, the athlete needs individual assessment to determine the presence of predisposing conditions and behavior and to develop a prevention strategy that includes sufficient acclimatization (to the environment and to exercise intensity and duration), conditioning, hydration, and salt intake, as well as other effective measures to improve heat tolerance and to reduce heat injury risk (e.g., protective equipment and uniform configurations)
HIV infection	Yes	Because of the apparent minimal risk to others, all sports may be played as athlete's state of health allows (especially if viral load is undetectable or very low) For all athletes, skin lesions should be covered properly, and athletic personnel should use universal precautions when handling blood or body fluids with visible blood Certain sports (such as wrestling and boxing) can create a situation that favors viral transmission (likely bleeding plus skin breaks); if viral load is detectable, then athletes should be advised to avoid such high-contact sports
Malignant neoplasm	Qualified yes	Athlete needs individual assessment
Musculoskeletal disorders	Qualified yes	Athlete needs individual assessment
Myopathies	Qualified yes	Athlete needs individual assessment
Obesity	Yes	Because of the increased risk of heat illness and cardiovascular strain, obese athletes particularly need careful acclimatization (to the environment and to exercise intensity and duration), sufficient hydration, and potential activity and recovery modifications during competition and training.
Organ transplant recipient (and those taking immunosuppressive medications)	Qualified yes	Athlete needs individual assessment for contact, collision, and limited-contact sports In addition to potential risk of infections, some medications (e.g., prednisone) increase tendency for bruising
Skin infections, including herpes simplex, molluscum contagiosum, verrucae (warts), staphylococcal and streptococcal infections (furuncles [boils], carbuncles, impetigo, methicillin-resistant *Staphylococcus aureus* [cellulitis and/or abscesses]), scabies, and tinea	Qualified yes	During contagious periods, participation in gymnastics or cheerleading with mats, martial arts, wrestling, or other collision, contact, or limited-contact sports is not allowed
Spleen, enlarged	Qualified yes	If the spleen is acutely enlarged, then participation should be avoided because of risk of rupture If the spleen is chronically enlarged, then individual assessment is needed before collision, contact, or limited-contact sports are played
CARDIOVASCULAR		
Carditis (inflammation of the heart)	No	Carditis can result in sudden death with exertion
Hypertension (high blood pressure)	Qualified yes	Those with hypertension >5 mm Hg above the 99th percentile for age, sex, and height should avoid heavy weightlifting and power lifting, bodybuilding, and high-static component sports Those with sustained hypertension (>95th percentile for age, sex, and height) need evaluation The National High Blood Pressure Education Program Working Group report defined prehypertension and stage 1 and stage 2 hypertension in children and adolescents <18 yr of age
Congenital heart disease (structural heart defects present at birth)	Qualified yes	Consultation with a cardiologist is recommended Those who have mild forms may participate fully in most cases; those who have moderate or severe forms or who have undergone surgery need evaluation The 36th Bethesda Conference defined mild, moderate, and severe disease for common cardiac lesions
Heart murmur	Qualified yes	If the murmur is innocent (does not indicate heart disease), full participation is permitted; otherwise, athlete needs evaluation (see structural heart disease, especially hypertrophic cardiomyopathy and mitral valve prolapse)
Dysrhythmia (Irregular Heart Rhythm)		
Long-QT syndrome	Qualified yes	Consultation with a cardiologist is advised. Those with symptoms (chest pain, syncope, near-syncope, dizziness, shortness of breath, or other symptoms of possible dysrhythmia) or evidence of mitral regurgitation on physical examination need evaluation; all others may participate fully
Malignant ventricular arrhythmias	Qualified yes	
Symptomatic Wolff-Parkinson-White syndrome	Qualified yes	
Advanced heart block	Qualified yes	
Family history of sudden death or previous sudden cardiac event	Qualified yes	
Implantation of a cardioverter-defibrillator	Qualified yes	

Table 678-2 MEDICAL CONDITIONS AND SPORTS PARTICIPATION—cont'd

CONDITION	MAY PARTICIPATE	EXPLANATION
Structural or Acquired Heart Disease		
Hypertrophic cardiomyopathy	Qualified no	Consultation with a cardiologist is recommended. The 36th Bethesda Conference provided detailed recommendations. Most of these conditions carry a significant risk of sudden cardiac death associated with intense physical exercise. Hypertrophic cardiomyopathy requires thorough and repeated evaluations, because disease can change manifestations during later adolescence. Marfan syndrome with an aortic aneurysm also can cause sudden death during intense physical exercise. An athlete who has ever received chemotherapy with anthracyclines may be at increased risk for cardiac problems owing to the cardiotoxic effects of the medications, and resistance training in this population should be approached with caution; strength training that avoids isometric contractions may be permitted. Athlete needs evaluation
Coronary artery anomalies	Qualified no	
Arrhythmogenic right ventricular cardiomyopathy	Qualified no	
Acute rheumatic fever with carditis	Qualified no	
Ehlers-Danlos syndrome, vascular form	Qualified no	
Marfan syndrome	Qualified yes	
Mitral valve prolapse	Qualified yes	
Anthracycline use	Qualified yes	
Vasculitis, vascular disease	Qualified yes	
Kawasaki disease (coronary artery vasculitis)	Qualified yes	Consultation with a cardiologist is recommended. Athlete needs individual evaluation to assess risk on the basis of disease activity, pathologic changes, and medical regimen
Pulmonary hypertension	Qualified yes	
EYES		
Functionally 1-eyed athlete	Qualified yes	A functionally 1-eyed athlete is defined as having best-corrected visual acuity worse than 20/40 in the poorer-seeing eye. Such an athlete would suffer significant disability if the better eye were seriously injured, as would an athlete with loss of an eye. Specifically, boxing and full-contact martial arts are not recommended for functionally 1-eyed athletes, because eye protection is impractical and/or not permitted. Some athletes who previously underwent intraocular eye surgery or had a serious eye injury may have increased risk of injury because of weakened eye tissue. Availability of eye guards approved by the American Society for Testing and Materials and other protective equipment might allow participation in most sports, but this must be judged on an individual basis
Loss of an eye	Qualified yes	
Detached retina or family history of retinal detachment at young age	Qualified yes	
High myopia	Qualified yes	
Connective tissue disorder, such as Marfan or Stickler syndrome	Qualified yes	
Previous intraocular eye surgery or serious eye injury	Qualified yes	
Conjunctivitis, infectious	Qualified no	Athlete with active infectious conjunctivitis should be excluded from swimming
GASTROINTESTINAL		
Malabsorption syndromes (celiac disease or cystic fibrosis)	Qualified yes	Athlete needs individual assessment for general malnutrition or specific deficits resulting in coagulation or other defects; with appropriate treatment, these deficits can be treated adequately to permit normal activities
Short-bowel syndrome or other disorders requiring specialized nutritional support, including parenteral or enteral nutrition	Qualified yes	Athlete needs individual assessment for collision, contact, or limited-contact sports Central or peripheral indwelling venous catheter might require special considerations for activities and emergency preparedness for unexpected trauma to the device(s)
Hepatitis, infectious (primarily hepatitis C)	Yes	All athletes should receive hepatitis B vaccination before participation. Because of the apparent minimal risk to others, all sports may be played as the athlete's state of health allows For all athletes, skin lesions should be covered properly, and athletic personnel should use universal precautions when handling blood or body fluids with visible blood
Liver, enlarged	Qualified yes	If the liver is acutely enlarged, participation should be avoided because of risk of rupture If the liver is chronically enlarged, individual assessment is needed before collision, contact, or limited-contact sports are played Patients with chronic liver disease can have changes in liver function that affect stamina, mental status, coagulation, or nutritional status
Diarrhea, infectious	Qualified no	Unless symptoms are mild and athlete is fully hydrated, no participation is permitted, because diarrhea can increase risk of dehydration and heat illness (see fever)
GENITOURINARY		
Kidney, absence of one	Qualified yes	Athlete needs individual assessment for contact, collision, and limited-contact sports Protective equipment can reduce risk of injury to the remaining kidney sufficiently to allow participation in most sports, providing such equipment remains in place during the activity
Ovary, absence of one	Yes	Risk of severe injury to remaining ovary is minimal
Pregnancy and postpartum period	Qualified yes	Athlete needs individual assessment As pregnancy progresses, modifications to usual exercise routines become necessary; activities with high risk of falling or abdominal trauma should be avoided Scuba diving and activities posing risk of altitude sickness should also be avoided during pregnancy After the birth, physiologic and morphologic changes of pregnancy take 4-6 wk to return to baseline
Testicle, undescended or absence of one	Yes	Certain sports require a protective cup
NEUROLOGIC		
Cerebral palsy	Qualified yes	Athlete needs evaluation to assess functional capacity to perform sports-specific activity
History of serious head or spine trauma or abnormality, including craniotomy, epidural bleeding, subdural hematoma, intracerebral hemorrhage, second-impact syndrome, vascular malformation, and neck fracture	Qualified yes	Athlete needs individual assessment for collision, contact, or limited-contact sports

Continued

Table 678-2 MEDICAL CONDITIONS AND SPORTS PARTICIPATION—cont'd

CONDITION	MAY PARTICIPATE	EXPLANATION
History of simple concussion (mild traumatic brain injury), multiple simple concussions, and/or complex concussion	Qualified yes	Athlete needs individual assessment Research supports a conservative approach to concussion management, including no athletic participation while symptomatic or when deficits in judgment or cognition are detected, followed by graduated return to full activity
Recurrent headaches	Yes	Athlete needs individual assessment
Seizure disorder, well controlled	Yes	Risk of seizure during participation is minimal
Seizure disorder, poorly controlled	Qualified yes	Athlete needs individual assessment for collision, contact, or limited-contact sports The following noncontact sports should be avoided: archery, riflery, swimming, weightlifting, power lifting, strength training, and sports involving heights; in these sports, a seizure during activity can pose a risk to self or others
Recurrent plexopathy (burner or stinger) and cervical cord neuropraxia with persistent defects	Qualified yes	Athlete needs individual assessment for collision, contact, or limited-contact sports; regaining normal strength is an important benchmark for return to play
RESPIRATORY		
Pulmonary compromise, including cystic fibrosis	Qualified yes	Athlete needs individual assessment but, generally, all sports may be played if oxygenation remains satisfactory during graded exercise test Athletes with cystic fibrosis need acclimatization and good hydration to reduce risk of heat illness
Asthma	Yes	With proper medication and education, only athletes with severe asthma need to modify their participation For those using inhalers, recommend having a written action plan and using a peak flowmeter daily Athletes with asthma might encounter risks when scuba diving
Acute upper respiratory infection	Qualified yes	Upper respiratory obstruction can affect pulmonary function Athlete needs individual assessment for all except mild disease (see Fever)
RHEUMATOLOGIC		
Juvenile rheumatoid arthritis	Qualified yes	Athletes with systemic or polyarticular juvenile rheumatoid arthritis and history of cervical spine involvement need radiographs of C1 and C2 to assess risk of spinal cord injury Athletes with systemic or HLA-B27–associated arthritis require cardiovascular assessment for possible cardiac complications during exercise For those with micrognathia (open bite and exposed teeth), mouth guards are helpful If uveitis is present, risk of eye damage from trauma is increased; ophthalmologic assessment is recommended In visually impaired athletes, guidelines for functionally 1-eyed athletes should be followed
Juvenile dermatomyositis, idiopathic myositis	Qualified yes	Athlete with juvenile dermatomyositis or systemic lupus erythematosis with cardiac involvement requires cardiology assessment before participation. Athletes receiving systemic corticosteroid therapy are at higher risk for osteoporotic fractures and avascular necrosis, which should be assessed before clearance; those receiving immunosuppressive medications are at higher risk for serious infection. Sports activities should be avoided when myositis is active. Rhabdomyolysis during intensive exercise can cause renal injury in athletes with idiopathic myositis and other myopathies. Because of photosensitivity with juvenile dermatomyositis and systemic lupus erythematosus, sun protection is necessary during outdoor activities. With Raynaud phenomenon, exposure to the cold presents risk to hands and feet
Systemic lupus erythematosus	Qualified yes	
Raynaud phenomenon	Qualified yes	
SICKLE CELL		
Sickle cell disease	Qualified yes	Athlete needs individual assessment In general, if illness status permits, all sports may be played; however, any sport or activity that entails overexertion, overheating, dehydration, or chilling should be avoided Participation at high altitude, especially when not acclimatized, also poses risk of sickle cell crisis
Sickle cell trait	Yes	Athletes with sickle cell trait generally do not have increased risk of sudden death or other medical problems during athletic participation under normal environmental conditions; however, when high exertional activity is performed under extreme conditions of heat and humidity or increased altitude, such catastrophic complications have occurred rarely Athletes with sickle cell trait, like all athletes, should be progressively acclimatized to the environment and to the intensity and duration of activities and should be sufficiently hydrated to reduce the risk of exertional heat illness and/or rhabdomyolysis According to National Institutes of Health management guidelines, sickle cell trait is not a contraindication to participation in competitive athletics, and there is no requirement for screening before participation More research is needed to fully assess potential risks and benefits of screening athletes for sickle cell trait

This table is intended for use by medical and nonmedical personnel. "Needs evaluation" means that a physician with appropriate knowledge and experience should assess the safety of a given sport for an athlete with the listed medical condition. Unless otherwise noted, this need for special consideration is because of variability in the severity of the disease, the risk of injury for the specific sports, or both.

From Rice SG; the Council on Sports Medicine and Fitness, American Academy of Pediatrics: Medical conditions affecting sports participation, *Pediatrics* 121:841–848, 2008.

Increasing dynamic component →

Increasing static component ↑	A. Low (<40% Max O_2)	B. Moderate (40-70% Max O_2)	C. High (>70% Max O_2)
III. High (>50% MVC)	**IIIA (Moderate)** Bobsledding/luge[a, b] Field events (throwing) Gymnastics[a, b] Martial arts[a] Sailing Sport climbing Water skiing[a, b] Weight lifting[a, b] Wind surfing[a, b]	**IIIB (High moderate)** Body building[a, b] Downhill skiing[a, b] Skateboarding[a, b] Snowboarding[a, b] Wrestling[a]	**IIIC (High)** Boxing[a, c] Canoeing/kayaking Cycling[a, b] Decathlon Rowing Speed skating[a, b] Triathlon[a, b]
II. Moderate (20-50% MVC)	**IIA (Low moderate)** Archery Auto racing[a, b] Diving[a, b] Equestrian[a, b] Motorcycling[a, b]	**IIB (Moderate)** American football[a] Field events (jumping) Figure skating[a] Rodeoing[a, b] Rugby[a] Running (sprint) Surfing[a, b] Synchronized swimming[b]	**IIC (High moderate)** Basketball[a] Ice hockey[a] Cross-country skiing (skating technique) Lacrosse[a] Running (middle distance) Swimming Team handball
I. Low (<20% MVC)	**IA (Low)** Billiards Bowling Cricket[d] Curling Golf Riflery	**IB (Low moderate)** Baseball/softball[a] Fencing Table tennis Volleyball	**IC (Moderate)** Badminton Cross-country skiing (classic technique) Field hockey[a] Orienteering Race walking Racquetball/squash Running (long distance) Soccer[a] Tennis

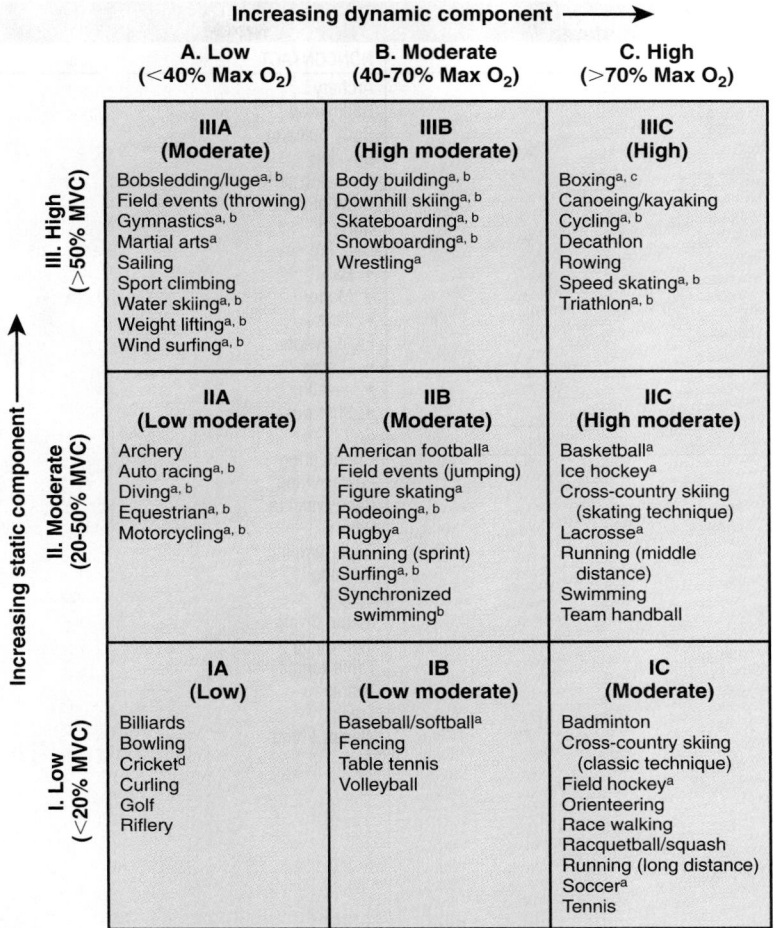

Figure 678-1 Classification of sports according to cardiovascular demands (based on combined static and dynamic components). This classification is based on peak static and dynamic components achieved during competition. The higher values may be reached during training. The increasing dynamic component is defined in terms of the estimated percentage of maximal oxygen uptake (Max O_2) achieved and results in increasing cardiac output. The increasing static component is related to the estimated percentage of maximal voluntary contraction (MVC) reached and results in increasing blood pressure load. Activities with the lowest total cardiovascular demands (cardiac output and blood pressure) are shown in box IA, and those with the highest demands are shown in box IIIC. Boxes IIA and IB depict activities with low to moderate total cardiovascular demands; boxes IIIA, IIB, and IC depict activities with moderate total cardiovascular demands; and boxes IIIB and IIC depict high-moderate total cardiovascular demands. These categories progress diagonally across the graph from lower left to upper right. [a]Danger of bodily collision. [b]Increased risk if syncope occurs. [c]Participation is not recommended by the American Academy of Pediatrics. [d]The American Academy of Pediatrics classifies cricket in the IB box (low static component and moderate dynamic component). (From Mitchell JH, Haskell W, Snell P, et al: 36th Bethesda conference. Task force 8: classification of sports. *J Am Coll Cardiol* 45:1364–1367, 2005.)

430). Chest radiographs, electrocardiograms (ECGs), and echocardiograms are not recommended as routine screening tests. If there is a **suspicion** of heart disease, such as a history of syncope, presyncope, palpitations, or excessive dyspnea with exercise, or a family history of a condition such as hypertrophic cardiomyopathy or prolonged QT or Marfan syndrome, the evaluation should be complete and include a 12-lead ECG, an echocardiogram, Holter or event-capture monitoring, and a stress test with electrocardiographic monitoring. Recommendations for participation with identified cardiac disease should be made in consultation with a cardiologist.

Disqualification and limitations for sports participation among various medical conditions are available from the American Academy of Pediatrics (see Table 678-2). Sports may also be classified by intensity (Fig. 678-1) and contact (Table 678-3). Athletes may seek to participate in sports against medical advice and have done so successfully for professional sports. Section 504(a) of the Rehabilitation Act of 1973 prohibits discrimination against disabled athletes if they have capabilities or skills required to play a competitive sport. This was reinforced through the Americans with Disabilities Act of 1990. An amateur athlete has no absolute right to decide whether to participate in competitive sports. Participation in competitive sports is considered a privilege, not a right. *Knapp* v *Northwestern University* established that "difficult medical decisions involving complex medical problems can be made by responsible physicians exercising prudent judgment (which will be necessarily conservative when definitive scientific evidence is lacking or conflicting) and relying on the recommendations of specialist consultants or guidelines established by a panel of experts."

Table 678-3 CLASSIFICATION OF SPORTS BY CONTACT

CONTACT OR COLLISION	NONCONTACT
Basketball	Archery
Boxing*	Badminton
Diving	Body building
Field hockey	Bowling
Football, tackle	Canoeing or kayaking (flat water)
Ice hockey†	Crew or rowing
Lacrosse	Curling
Martial arts	Dancing
Rodeo	• Ballet
Rugby	• Modern
Ski jumping	• Jazz
Soccer	Field events
Team handball	• Discus
Water polo	• Javelin
Wrestling	• Shot put
LIMITED CONTACT	Golf
Baseball	Orienteering‡
Bicycling	Power lifting
Cheerleading	Race walking
Canoeing or kayaking (white water)	Riflery
Fencing	Rope jumping
Field events	Running
• High jump	Sailing
• Pole vault	Scuba diving
Floor hockey	Swimming
Football, flag	Table tennis
Gymnastics	Tennis
Handball	Track
Horseback riding	Weight lifting
Racquetball	
Skating	
• Ice	
• Inline	
• Roller	
Skiing	
• Cross-country	
• Downhill	
• Water	
Skateboarding	
Snowboarding	
Softball	
Squash	
Ultimate Frisbee	
Volleyball	
Windsurfing or surfing	

*Participation not recommended by the American Academy of Pediatrics.
†The American Academy of Pediatrics recommends limiting the amount of body checking allowed for hockey players ≤15 yr to reduce injuries.
‡A race (contest) in which competitors use a map and compass to find their way through unfamiliar territory.
From the American Academy of Pediatrics, Committee on Sports Medicine and Fitness: Medical conditions affecting sports participation, *Pediatrics* 107:1205, 2001.

BIBLIOGRAPHY
Please visit the Nelson Textbook of Pediatrics *website at www.expertconsult.com for the complete bibliography.*

Chapter 679
Management of Musculoskeletal Injury
Gregory L. Landry

MECHANISM OF INJURY

Acute Injuries

Sprains, strains, and contusions account for the majority of musculoskeletal injuries. A **sprain** is an injury to a ligament or joint capsule. A **strain** is an injury to a muscle or tendon. A **contusion** is a crush injury to any soft tissue. The history of the injury can be unclear, but it is especially helpful in assessing knee and shoulder injuries. More severe injuries, indicating structural derangement, can have acute signs and symptoms such as immediate swelling, deformity, numbness or weakness, inability to continue playing, inability to walk without a limp, a loud painful pop, mechanical locking of the joint, or the sensation of instability. Most sprains are graded 1-3, with *grade 1* meaning that some fibers have been torn with no evidence of laxity of the ligament when tested on physical examination. A *grade 2* means more fibers are torn resulting in some laxity of the ligament but a good end point, meaning not all fibers are torn. A *grade 3* sprain means all the fibers are torn, and testing of the ligaments results in a "mushy" endpoint on physical examination. Strains are also graded 1-3, with a *grade 1* causing mild pain with testing the muscle and very little weakness. *Grade 2* injuries cause more pain and moderate weakness with testing the muscle. *Grade 3* muscle strains are complete rupture of the muscle or tendon and result in marked weakness and sometimes a palpable defect in the muscle or tendon.

Overuse Injuries

Overuse injuries are caused by repetitive microtrauma that exceeds the body's rate of repair. This occurs in muscles, tendons, bone, bursae, cartilage, and nerves. Overuse injuries occur in all sports but more commonly in sports emphasizing repetitive motion (swimming, running, tennis, gymnastics). Factors can be categorized into extrinsic (training errors, poor equipment or workout surface) and intrinsic (athlete's anatomy or medical conditions). Training error is the most commonly identified factor. At the beginning of the workout program, athletes might violate the 10% rule: Do not increase the duration or intensity of workouts more than 10% per week. Intrinsic factors include abnormal biomechanics (leg-length discrepancy, pes planus, pes cavus, tarsal coalition, valgus heel, external tibial torsion, femoral anteversion), muscle imbalance, inflexibility, and medical conditions (deconditioning, nutritional deficits, amenorrhea, obesity). The athlete should be asked about the specifics of training. Runners should be asked about their shoes, orthotics, running surface, weekly mileage or time spent running per week, speed or hill workouts, and previous injuries and rehabilitation. When causative factors are identified, they can be eliminated or modified so that after rehabilitation the athlete does not return to the same regimen and suffer reinjury.

For athletes engaged in excessive training that causes an overuse injury, curtailing all exercise is not usually necessary. Treatment is a reduction of training load (relative rest) combined with a rehabilitation program designed to return athletes to their sport as soon as possible while minimizing exposure to reinjury. Early identification of an overuse injury requires less alteration of the workout regimen.

The goals of treatment are to control pain and spasm to rehabilitate flexibility, strength, endurance, and proprioceptive deficits (Table 679-1). In many overuse injuries, the role of inflammation in the process is minimal. For most injuries to tendons, the term *tendinitis* is obsolete because there is little or no inflammation on histopathology of tendons. Instead, there is evidence of microscopic trauma to the tissue. Most of these entities are now more appropriately called **tendinosis** and, when the tendon tissue is scarred and very abnormal, **tendinopathy**. There is little role for anti-inflammatory medication in the treatment except as an analgesic.

INITIAL EVALUATION OF THE INJURED EXTREMITY

Initially, the examiner should determine the quality of the peripheral pulses and capillary refill rate as well as the gross motor and sensory function to assess for neurovascular injury. The first priorities are to maintain vascular and skeletal stability.

Criteria for immediate attention and rapid orthopedic consultation include vascular compromise, nerve compromise, and open fracture. The exposed wound should be covered with sterile saline-soaked gauze, and the injured limb should be padded and splinted. Pressure should be applied to any site of bleeding. Additional criteria include deep laceration over a joint, unreducible dislocation, grade III (complete) tear of a muscle-tendon unit, and displaced, significantly angulated fractures (depends on the bone involved, the degree of displacement and angulation, and neurovascular status of the extremity).

Table 679-1 STAGING OF OVERUSE INJURIES

GRADE	GRADING SYMPTOMS	TREATMENT
I	Pain only after activity Does not interfere with performance or intensity Generalized tenderness Disappears before next session	Modification of activity, consider cross-training, home rehabilitation program
II	Minimal pain with activity Does not interfere with performance More localized tenderness	Modification of activity, cross-training, home rehabilitation program
III	Pain interferes with activity and performance Definite area of tenderness Usually disappears between sessions	Significant modification of activity, strongly encourage cross-training, home rehabilitation program, and outpatient physical therapy
IV	Pain with activities of daily living Pain does not disappear between sessions Marked interference with performance and training intensity	Discontinue activity temporarily, cross-training only, oral analgesic, home rehabilitation program, and intensive outpatient physical therapy
V	Pain interferes with activities of daily living Signs of tissue injury (e.g., edema) Chronic or recurrent symptoms	Prolonged discontinuation of activity, cross-training only, oral analgesic, home rehabilitation program, and intensive outpatient physical therapy

TRANSITION FROM IMMEDIATE MANAGEMENT TO RETURN TO PLAY

Rehabilitation of a musculoskeletal injury should begin on the day of the injury.

Phase 1

Limit further injury, control swelling and pain, and minimize strength and flexibility losses. This requires the use of an appropriate device such as crutches or a sling, ice, compression, elevation, and analgesia. Crutches, air stirrups for ankle sprains, slings for arm injuries, and elastic wraps (4-8 in) for compression are a reasonable inventory of office supplies. Ice in a plastic bag is placed directly on the skin for 20 min continuously, 3 to 4 times per day until the swelling resolves. Compression limits further bleeding and swelling but should not be so tight that it limits perfusion. Elevation of the extremity promotes venous return and limits swelling. A nonsteroidal anti-inflammatory drug (NSAID) or acetaminophen is indicated for analgesia.

Pain-free isometric strengthening and range of motion should be initiated as soon as possible. Pain inhibits full muscle contraction; deconditioning results if the pain and resultant nonuse persist for days to weeks, thus delaying recovery. Education about the nature of the injury and the specifics of rehabilitation exercises, including handouts with written instructions and drawings demonstrating the exercises, are helpful.

Phase 2

Improve strength and range of motion (i.e., flexibility) while allowing the injured structures to heal. Protective devices are removed when the patient's strength and flexibility improve and activities of daily living are pain free. Flexibility can then be improved by a program of specific stretches, held for 15-30 sec for 3 to 5 repetitions, once or twice daily. A physical therapist or athletic trainer is invaluable in guiding the athlete through this process. Protective devices might need to be used for months during sports participation. Swimming, water jogging, and stationary cycling are good aerobic exercises that can allow the injured extremity to get relative rest or be used pain free while maintaining cardiovascular fitness.

Phase 3

Achieve near normal strength and flexibility of the injured structures and further improve or maintain cardiovascular fitness. Strength and endurance are improved under controlled conditions using elastic bands and eventually free weights or exercise equipment. Proprioceptive training allows the athlete to redevelop a kinesthetic sense, which is critical to joint function and stability.

Phase 4

Return to exercise or competition without restriction. When the athlete has reached nearly normal flexibility, strength, proprioception, and endurance, he or she can start sports-specific exercises. The athlete will make the transition from the rehabilitation program to functional rehabilitation appropriate for the sport.

Substituting sports participation for rehabilitation is inappropriate; rather, there should be progressive stepwise functional return to a full activity or play program. For instance, a basketball player recovering from an ankle injury might begin a walk-run-sprint-cut program before returning to competition. At any point in this progression, if pain is experienced, the athlete needs to stop, apply ice, avoid running for 1-2 days, continue to do ankle exercises, and then resume running at a lower intensity and progress accordingly.

Relative Rest and Return-to-Play Guidelines

Relative rest means that the athlete can do whatever he or she wants as long as the injured structures do not hurt during or within 24 hr of the activity. Exercising beyond the pain threshold delays recovery.

DIFFERENTIAL DIAGNOSES OF MUSCULOSKELETAL PAIN

Traumatic, rheumatologic, infectious, hematologic, psychologic, and oncologic processes can cause the presenting complaint of musculoskeletal pain. Symptoms such as fatigue, weight loss, rash, multiple joint complaints, fever, chronic or recent illness, and persistence of pain suggest diagnoses other than sports-related trauma. Incongruity between the patient's history and physical examination findings should lead to further evaluation. A negative review of systems with an injury history consistent with the physical findings suggests a sports-related etiology.

BIBLIOGRAPHY

Please visit the Nelson Textbook of Pediatrics *website at www.expertconsult.com for the complete bibliography.*

679.1 Growth Plate Injuries

Gregory L. Landry

About 20% of pediatric sports injuries seen in the emergency department are fractures, and 25% of those fractures involve an epiphyseal growth plate or physis (Chapter 675). Growth in long bones occurs in 3 areas and is susceptible to injury. Immature bone can be acutely injured at the **physis** (Salter-Harris fractures), the **articular surface** (osteochondritis dissecans), or the **apophysis** (avulsion fractures). Boys suffer about twice as many physeal fractures as girls; the peak incidence of fracture is during peak height velocity (girls, 12 ± 2.5 yr; boys, 14 ± 2 yr). The physis is a pressure growth plate and is responsible for longitudinal growth in bone. The apophysis is a bony outgrowth at the attachment of a tendon and is a traction physis. The epiphysis is the end of a long bone, distal or proximal to the long bone, and contains articular cartilage at the joint.

The most common **physeal injuries** are to the distal radius, followed by phalangeal and distal tibial fractures. About 94% of forearm fractures in skateboarding, roller skating, and scooter riding involve the distal radius. Physeal injuries at the knee (distal femur, proximal tibia) are rare. Growth disturbance following a growth plate injury is a function of location and the part of the physis fractured. These factors influence the probability a physeal bar will form, resulting in growth arrest. The areas making the largest contribution to longitudinal growth in the upper extremities are the proximal humerus and distal radius and ulna; in the lower extremities, they are the distal femur and the proximal tibia and fibula. Injuries to these areas are more likely to cause growth disturbance compared with physeal injuries at the other end of these long bones. The type of the physis fracture relative to risk of growth disturbance is described by the Salter-Harris classification system (see Table 675-1). A grade I injury is least likely to result in growth disturbance, and grade V is the most likely fracture to result in growth disturbance.

Osteochondritis dissecans (OCD) affects the subchondral bone and overlying articular surface (Chapter 669.3). With avascular necrosis of subchondral bone, the articular surface can flatten, soften, or break off in fragments. The etiology is unknown but may be related to repetitive stress injury in some patients. In children and adolescents, 51% of lesions occur on the lateral aspect of the medial femoral condyle, 17% occur on the lateral condyle, and 7% occur on the patella. Bilateral involvement is reported in 13-30% of cases. Other joints where OCD lesions are also seen are the ankle (talus), elbow (usually involving the capitellum), and radial head. OCD classically affects athletes in their 2nd decade. The most common presentation is poorly localized vague knee pain. There is rarely a history of recent acute trauma. Some OCD lesions are asymptomatic (diagnosed on "routine" radiographs), whereas others are manifested as joint effusion, pain, decreased range of motion, and mechanical symptoms (locking, popping, catching). Activity usually worsens the pain.

Physical examination might show no specific findings. Sometimes tenderness over the involved condyle can be elicited by deep palpation with the knee flexed. Diagnosis is usually made with plain radiographs (Fig. 679-1). A tunnel view radiograph should be obtained to better view the posterior two thirds of the femoral condyle. Patients with OCD should be referred to an orthopedic surgeon for further evaluation.

Avulsion fractures occur when a forceful muscle contraction dislodges the apophysis from the bone. They occur most commonly around the hip (Fig. 679-2) and are treated nonsurgically. Acute fractures to other apophyses (knee and elbow) require urgent orthopedic consultation. Chronically increased traction at the muscle-apophysis attachment can lead to repetitive microtrauma and pain at the apophysis. The most common areas affected are the knee (Osgood-Schlatter and Sindig-Larsen-Johannson disease), the ankle (Sever disease) (Fig. 679-3), and

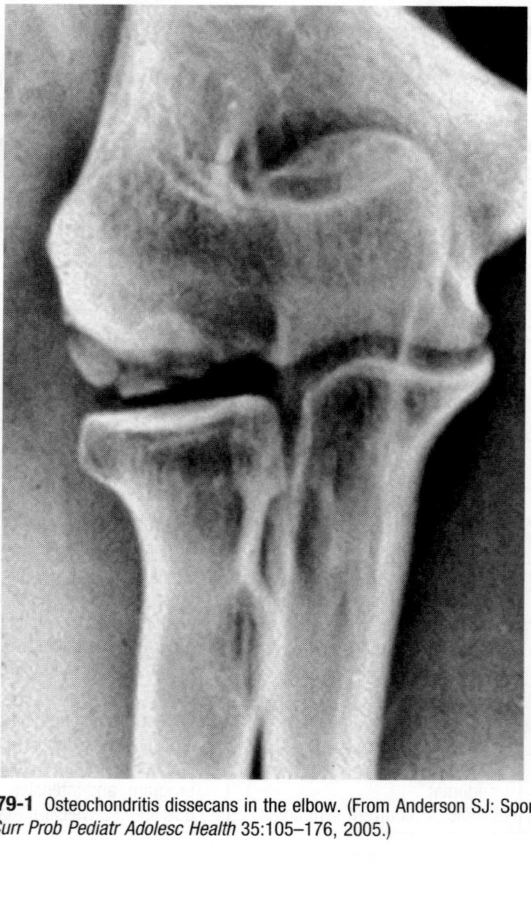

Figure 679-1 Osteochondritis dissecans in the elbow. (From Anderson SJ: Sports injuries, *Curr Prob Pediatr Adolesc Health* 35:105–176, 2005.)

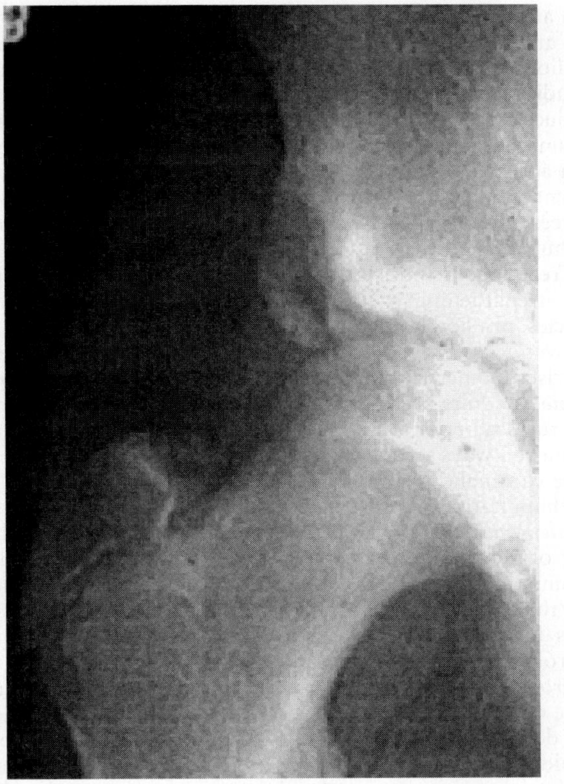

Figure 679-2 Anterior inferior iliac spine avulsion. (From Anderson SJ: Lower extremity injuries in youth sports, *Pediatr Clin North Am* 49:627–641, 2003.)

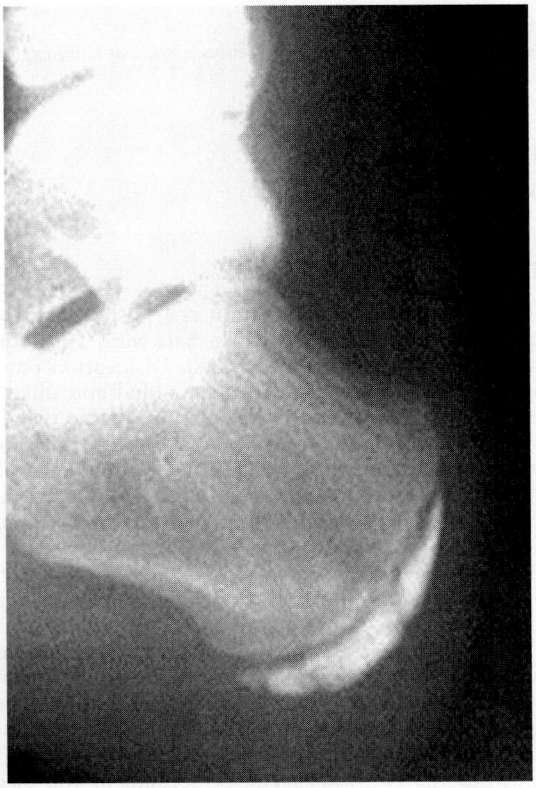

Figure 679-3 Calcaneal apophysitis (Sever disease). (From Anderson SJ: Sports injuries, *Curr Prob Pediatr Adolesc Health* 35:105–176, 2005.)

the medial epicondyle (Little League elbow). Traction apophysitis of the knee and ankle can potentially be treated in a primary care setting. The main goal of treatment is to minimize the intensity and incidence of pain and disability. Exercises that increase the strength, flexibility, and endurance of the muscles attached at the apophysis, using the relative rest principle, are appropriate. Symptoms can last for 12-24 mo if untreated. As growth slows, symptoms abate.

BIBLIOGRAPHY

Please visit the Nelson Textbook of Pediatrics *website at* *www.expertconsult.com* *for the complete bibliography.*

679.2 Shoulder Injuries

Gregory L. Landry

Shoulder pain associated with radiating symptoms down the arm should suggest the possibility of a neck injury. Neck pain and tenderness or limitation of cervical range of motion requires that the cervical spine be immobilized and that the athlete be transferred for further evaluation. If there is no neck pain or tenderness or limitation of motion of the cervical spine, then the shoulder is the site of the primary injury.

CLAVICLE FRACTURES

One of the most common shoulder injuries is a clavicle fracture. Injury is usually sustained by a fall on the lateral shoulder, on an outstretched hand, or by direct blow. About 80% of fractures occur in the middle third of the clavicle. They are treated with an arm sling. Nondisplaced medial and lateral 3rd fractures are usually treated conservatively. If displaced, medial and lateral 3rd fractures require orthopedic consultation, due to a higher incidence of acromioclavicular osteoarthritis (lateral) and physeal involvement (medial).

ACROMIOCLAVICULAR SEPARATION

An acromioclavicular (AC) separation most commonly occurs when an athlete sustains a direct blow to the acromion with the humerus in an adducted position, forcing the acromion inferiorly and medially. Patients have discrete tenderness at the AC joint and can have an apparent step off between the distal clavicle and the acromion (Fig. 679-4).

Type I AC injuries involve the AC ligament, have no visible deformity, and have normal radiographs. Cross-chest maneuver of the arm causes sharp pain at the AC joint. **Type II** injuries, which involve the acromioclavicular ligament and the coracoclavicular ligament, have a slightly more prominent distal clavicle on examination, but radiographs are usually normal (might show slight widening of the AC joint). Type I and II injuries are treated nonoperatively. A sling and analgesic are useful for pain control. Range-of-motion exercises are initiated after pain is controlled. As the pain-free range improves, strengthening of the rotator cuff, deltoid, and trapezius muscles can start. Usual return to play is 1-2 wk for type I and 2-4 wk for type II. When the AC joint is nontender, the shoulder has full range of motion and the patient has sufficient strength to be functionally protected from a collision or fall and perform the maneuvers required for the sport, return to play is allowed.

Type III injury has worsened ligamentous tearing with deltotrapezial fascial detachment from the distal clavicle. Type III injuries should be treated surgically only in rare cases and mostly for cosmetic reasons. The majority can be treated in a similar fashion as grade I and II injuries. **Types IV, V, and VI** AC injuries have progressive worsening of ligamentous and fascial disruption with worsened clavicular displacement. Fortunately, these injuries are rare but require surgical repair.

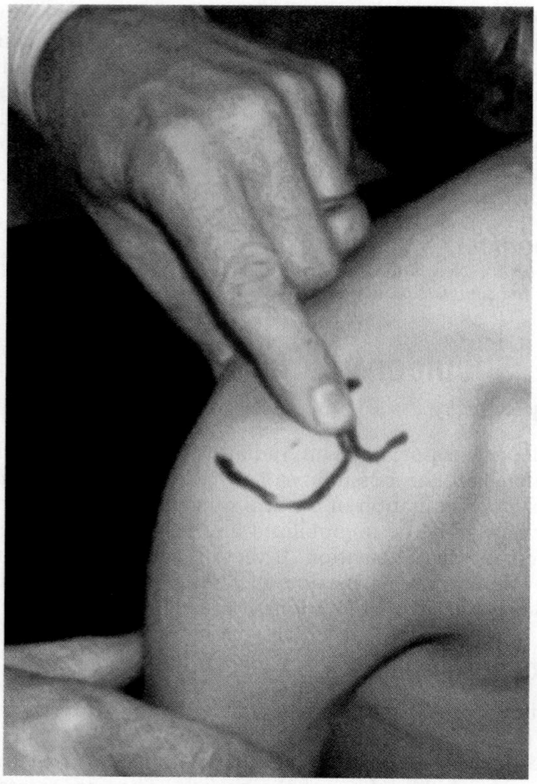

Figure 679-4 Palpitation of acromioclavicular joint. (From Anderson SJ: Sports injuries, *Curr Prob Pediatr Adolesc Health* 35:105–176, 2005.)

ANTERIOR DISLOCATION

The most common mechanism of injury is making contact with another player with the shoulder abducted to 90 degrees and forcefully rotated externally. A common example of the latter is a football player tackling another player only with the arm. Patients complain of severe pain and that their shoulder "popped out of place" or "shifted." Patients with an unreduced anterior dislocation have a hollow region inferior to the acromion and a bulge in the anterior portion of the shoulder caused by anterior displacement of the humeral head. Abnormal sensation of the lateral deltoid region (axillary nerve) and the extensor surface of the proximal forearm (musculocutaneous nerve) should be noted.

An attempt to reduce the anterior dislocation is indicated, assuming no crepitance is present. Once the dislocation is reduced and radiographs show a normal position, immobilization for a few days for comfort is indicated. The period of immobilization is controversial, but most sports medicine practitioners believe that early range-of-motion and strengthening exercises are important. As the rotator cuff muscles strengthen, progressive strengthening occurs at greater degrees of abduction and external rotation. Patients can return to play when strength, flexibility, and proprioception are equal to that of the uninvolved side so that they can protect the shoulder and perform the sports-specific activities without pain. In most cases, surgery is not recommended unless the shoulder has been dislocated at least 3 times. Earlier repair may be considered for athletes in high-risk collision sports, because the recurrence rate is very high in those sports.

ROTATOR CUFF INJURY

The rotator cuff is formed by the supraspinatus, infraspinatus, teres minor, and subscapularis. The supraspinatus is most commonly injured. *Rotator cuff tendinosis* is manifested as shoulder pain at the top of the arc of motion. Pain is usually poorly localized and may be referred to the deltoid area. The onset may be insidious. Pain is worse with activity but is often present at rest, including nighttime pain. Strength testing of the cuff muscles produces pain and can demonstrate some weakness compared to the uninjured shoulder. Supraspinatus tendinosis produces pain with active abduction in the "empty can" position in which the patient abducts the arm to 90 degrees, forward flexes it to 30 degrees anterior to the parasagittal plane, and internally rotates the humerus.

Treatment includes ice, modification of technique, rest, stretching, strengthening of the rotator cuff and scapular stabilizer muscles, physiotherapy, and analgesic. Prevention includes avoiding overwork, proper technique, and strengthening and stretching exercises. Sometimes this is called *rotator cuff impingement syndrome* in adults because of impingement of the cuff by the bony structures superior to the cuff. Rotator cuff pain in young athletes is almost always secondary to glenohumeral instability. Stretching alone can make the pain worse, and the most important aspect of rehabilitation is strengthening of the cuff muscles.

Glenoid labrum tears can appear like rotator cuff tendinosis. One of the most common lesions, the **SLAP** lesion (superior *l*abrum *a*nterior and *p*osterior), is difficult to diagnose clinically. Pain that occurs with clicking or catching in the shoulder is suspicious for a labrum tear. Radiographs are usually normal. MR arthrography is the best study to identify lesions.

Proximal humeral stress fracture (epiphysiolysis) is a rare cause of proximal shoulder pain and is suspected when shoulder pain does not respond to routine measures. Gradual onset of deep shoulder pain occurs in a young (open epiphyseal plates) athlete involved in repetitive overhead motion, such as in baseball or tennis, but with no history of trauma. Tenderness is noted over the proximal humerus; the diagnosis is confirmed by detecting a widened epiphyseal plate on plain radiographs, increased uptake on nuclear scan, or edema of the physis on MRI. Treatment is total rest from throwing for 6-8 wk.

BIBLIOGRAPHY

Please visit the Nelson Textbook of Pediatrics *website at* *www.expertconsult.com* *for the complete bibliography.*

679.3 Elbow Injuries

Gregory L. Landry

ACUTE INJURIES

The most common elbow dislocation is a posterior dislocation. The mechanism of injury is falling backward onto the outstretched arm with the elbow extended. Dislocation potentially compromises the brachial artery. Intact radial and ulnar pulses are the best indicators of vascular integrity of the distal upper extremity. An obvious deformity is noted, with the olecranon process displaced prominently behind the distal humerus. Reduction is performed by gently applying longitudinal traction to the forearm with gentle upward pressure on the distal humerus. If reduction is not possible, the arm should be padded and placed in a sling and the patient transferred to an emergency facility. Elbow injuries can compromise the radial, median, and ulnar nerves.

Supracondylar humeral fractures can result from the same mechanism of injury as elbow dislocations and can be complicated by coexisting injury to the brachial artery and, to a lesser extent, the median, radial, and ulnar nerves. An acute compartment syndrome can develop after these fractures (Fig. 679-5).

A blow to the elbow can cause bleeding in the olecranon bursa, resulting in *olecranon bursitis*. These rarely require aspiration and can be managed with ice, analgesia, and compression

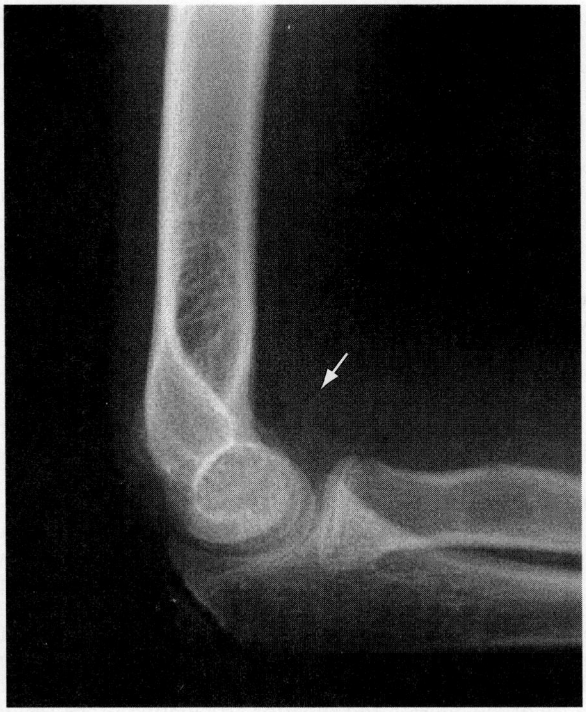

Figure 679-5 Deflection of the coronoid fat pad with a joint effusion (fat pad sign) showing evidence of a fracture. (From Gomez JE: Upper extremity injuries in youth sports, *Pediatr Clin North Am* 49:593–626, 2002.)

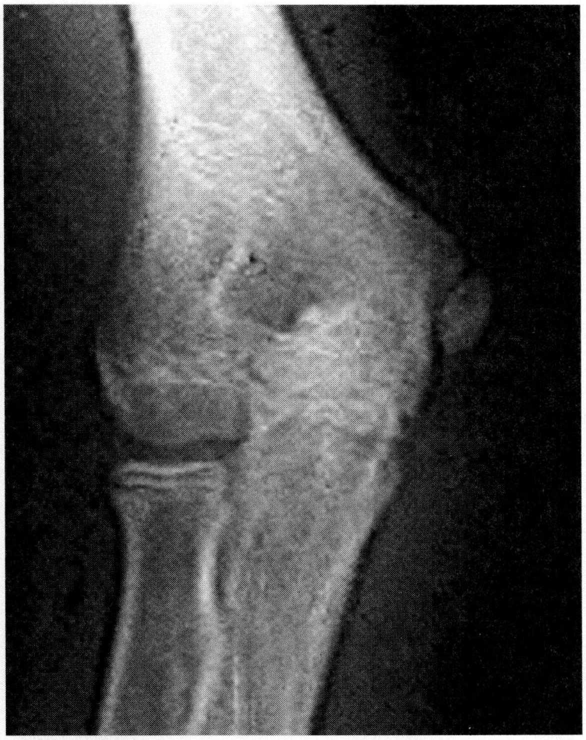

Figure 679-6 Medial epicondylitis. (From Anderson SJ: Sports injuries, *Curr Prob Pediatr Adolesc Health* 35:105–176, 2005.)

dressings. An appropriate pad provides comfort and helps prevent reinjury.

Chronic Injuries

Overuse injuries occur primarily in throwing sports and sports that require repetitive wrist flexion or extension or demand weight bearing on hands (gymnastics). "Little League elbow" is a broad term for several different elbow problems.

Throwing overhand creates valgus stress to the elbow with medial opening of the joint and lateral compressive forces.

Medial elbow pain is a common complaint of young throwers, resulting from repetitive valgus overload of the wrist flexor-pronator muscle groups and their attachment on the medial apophysis. In preadolescents who still have maturing secondary ossification centers, *traction apophysitis of the medial epicondyle* is likely. Patients have tenderness along the medial epicondyle; this is exacerbated by valgus stress or resisted wrist flexion and pronation. Treatment includes no throwing for 4-6 wk, pain-free strengthening, and stretching of the flexor-pronator group, followed by 1-2 wk of a progressive functional throwing program with accelerated rehabilitation. This problem has to be treated with rest because of the risk of nonunion of the apophysis and chronic pain. If pain occurs acutely, *avulsion fracture of the medial epicondyle* must be considered. Radiographs should be taken in any thrower with acute elbow pain (Fig. 679-6). If the medial epicondyle is avulsed, orthopedic consultation is indicated.

In older adolescents and young adults with a fused apophysis, the vulnerable structure is the *ulnar collateral ligament* (UCL). UCL tears are usually seen in pitchers but can be seen in any throwing athlete. Laxity may be appreciated with valgus stress of the elbow with it flexed to 30 degrees. MRI arthrography or ultrasonography is often necessary to assess the integrity of the UCL. If there is a complete tear, surgical repair is indicated if the athlete wants to continue a pitching career. Ulnar nerve dysfunction can be a complication of valgus overload and can occur with any of the diagnoses previously discussed.

Lateral elbow pain can be caused by compression during the throwing motion at the radiocapitellar joint. *Panner disease* is osteochondrosis of the capitellum that occurs between ages 7 and 12 yr (Fig. 679-7). *OCD* of the capitellum occurs at age 13-16 yr (see Fig. 679-1). These two entities might represent a continuum of the same disease. Although patients with both conditions present with insidious onset of lateral elbow pain exacerbated by throwing, patients with OCD have mechanical symptoms (popping, locking) and, more commonly, decreased range of motion. Patients with Panner disease have no mechanical symptoms and often have normal range of motion. The prognosis of Panner disease is excellent, and treatments consist of relative rest (no throwing), brief immobilization, and repeat radiographs in 6-12 wk to assess bone remodeling. OCD requires orthopedic consultation.

Lateral epicondylitis, or tennis elbow, is the most common overuse elbow injury in adults. It is rare in children and adolescents. It is tendinosis of the extensor muscle origin on the lateral epicondyle. Tenderness is elicited over the lateral epicondyle, and pain is felt with passive wrist flexion and resisted wrist extension. Treatment includes relative rest, analgesia, and specific stretching and strengthening exercises. Functional rehabilitation, such as returning to playing tennis, should be gradual and progressive.

Elbow injuries might not be prevented by preseason stretching and strengthening exercises. The most important consideration for preventing elbow injuries in throwers is limitation of the number of pitches and advising players, coaches, and athletes that they should stop immediately when they experience elbow pain. If it persists, they need medical evaluation. It has been recommended that a young pitcher have age-specific limits on pitch counts. A good rule of thumb is the maximal number of pitches per game should be approximately 6 times the pitcher's age in years. For more information, consult the Little League Baseball website at *www.littleleague.org/media/newsarchive/03_2006/06pitch_count_08-25-06.htm.*

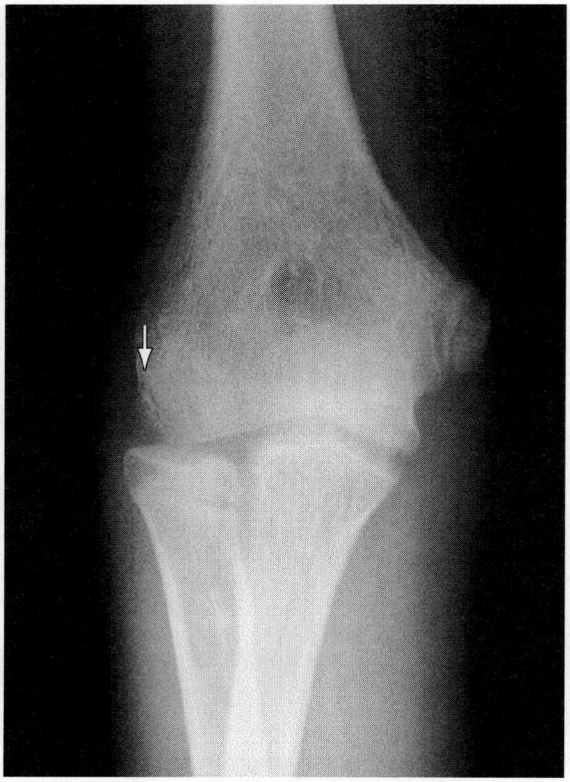

Figure 679-7 Panner disease. Note fragmentation of the humeral capitellum and flattening of the articular surface *(arrow)*. (Courtesy of Ralph J. Curtis, MD. From Gomez JE: Upper extremity injuries in youth sports, *Pediatr Clin North Am* 49:593–626, 2002.)

Other, less common problems that cause elbow pain are ulnar neuropathy, triceps tendinitis and olecranon apophysitis, and loose bodies.

BIBLIOGRAPHY

Please visit the Nelson Textbook of Pediatrics *website at* www.expertconsult.com *for the complete bibliography.*

679.4 Low Back Injuries

Gregory L. Landry

SPONDYLOLYSIS, SPONDYLOLISTHESIS, AND FACET SYNDROME

Spondylolysis

Spondylolysis, a common cause of back pain in athletes, is a stress fracture of the pars interarticularis (Chapter 671.6). It can occur at any vertebral level but is most likely at L4 or L5. Prevalence in adolescent athletes evaluated for low back pain is 13-47%. Besides acute hyperextension that causes an acute fracture, the mechanism of injury is either a congenital defect or hypoplastic pars, which is exacerbated by lumbar extension loading, or a stress fracture due to repetitive extension loading. Ballet, weight lifting, gymnastics, and football are examples of sports in which repetitive extension loading of the lumbar spine occurs; it occurs in any activity in which there is repetitive extension loading, including swimming.

Patients often present with pain of insidious onset. However, there may be a precipitating injury such as a fall or single episode of hyperextension. The pain is worse with extension, can radiate to the buttocks, and can eventually affect activities of daily living. Rest or supine positioning usually alleviates the pain.

On examination, the pain is reproduced with lumbar extension while standing, especially when standing on 1 leg *(single-leg hyperextension test)*. Limited forward spinal flexion and tight hamstrings may be seen. Neurologic examination should be normal. There is well-localized tenderness to deep palpation just lateral to the spinous process on the affected side and is usually at L4 or L5.

The diagnosis is confirmed by finding a pars defect on an oblique lumbar spine radiograph. The defect is rarely seen on anteroposterior (AP) and lateral views. Bone single-photon emission CT (SPECT) is needed to confirm diagnosis if radiographs are normal. A plain CT scan can help to identify the degree of bony involvement and is sometimes used to assess healing.

Treatment includes pain relief and activity restriction. Rehabilitation consisting of trunk strengthening, hip flexor stretching, and hamstring stretching is important in most cases. Antilordotic bracing is controversial and is probably most effective for the stress fracture type of spondylolysis.

Spondylolisthesis and Facet Syndrome

Spondylolysis, spondylolisthesis, and facet syndrome are injuries posterior to vertebral bodies. *Spondylolisthesis* occurs when bilateral pars defects exist and forward displacement or slippage of a vertebra occurs on the vertebra inferior to it (Chapter 671.6). *Facet syndrome* has a similar history and physical examination findings as spondylolysis. It is caused by instability or injury to the facet joint, posterior to the pars interarticularis and at the interface of the inferior and superior articulating processes. Facet syndrome can be established by identifying facet abnormalities on CT or by exclusion, requiring a nondiagnostic radiograph and nuclear scan to rule out spondylolysis.

Treatment of posterior element injuries is conservative, directed at reducing the extension-loading activity, often for 2-3 mo. Walking, swimming, and cycling are appropriate exercises during rehabilitation.

LUMBAR DISK HERNIATION, STRAIN, AND CONTUSION

Lumbar disk herniation manifests as back pain that is worse with forward flexion, lateral bending, and prolonged sitting, especially in an automobile. It is less likely to produce sciatica in children and adolescents compared to adults (Chapter 671.8). Physical examination findings may be minimal but usually include pain with forward flexion and lateral bending. It is unusual to have a positive straight leg test or any neurologic deficit in young athlete with an injured disk. There may be tenderness of the vertebral spinous process at the level of the disk. MRI usually confirms the clinical diagnosis. Assuming the herniation is not large and the pain is not intractable, the treatment of choice is analgesia and physical therapy. Bed rest or surgery is rarely necessary.

Acute lumbar strain or contusion occurs after a precipitating event. Physical examination reveals diffuse tenderness lateral to the spine.

Treatment includes analgesia, massage, and physical therapy, as tolerated. The natural history of acute back strain in adults is that 50% are better in 1 wk, 80% in 1 mo, and 90% in 2 mo, regardless of therapy. The course of back pain in young athletes is probably similar.

SACROILIITIS

Sacroiliitis manifests as lumbar pain that is usually chronic but occasionally is associated with a history of trauma. Patients have a positive result with the **Patrick test,** which includes resting the foot of the affected side on the opposite knee (hip flexed 90 degrees), stabilizing the opposite iliac crest, and externally rotating the hip on the affected side (pushing the knee down and lateral). A radiograph of the sacroiliac joints is indicated, and if results are positive, exploration for a rheumatologic disease (ankylosing spondylitis, juvenile rheumatoid arthritis, ulcerative colitis) is warranted.

Treatment is with relative rest, NSAIDs, and physical therapy. Ankylosing spondylitis is more likely if the onset of lower back pain is before age 40 yr, if there is morning stiffness that is associated with improvement with activity, and if the pain has a gradual onset and has lasted >3 mo.

OTHER CAUSES

Other causes of lower back pain include infection (osteomyelitis, diskitis) and neoplasia. These should be considered in patients with fever, weight loss, other constitutional signs, or lack of response to initial therapy. Osteomyelitis of the lower back or pelvis is often, but not always, associated with fever.

BIBLIOGRAPHY

Please visit the Nelson Textbook of Pediatrics *website at* *www.expertconsult.com* *for the complete bibliography.*

679.5 Hip and Pelvis Injuries

Gregory L. Landry

Hip and pelvis injuries represent a small percentage of sports injuries, but they are potentially severe and require prompt diagnosis. Hip pathology can manifest as knee pain and normal findings on knee examination.

In children, *transient synovitis* is the most common cause. It usually manifests with acute onset of a limp, with the child refusing to use the affected leg and having painful range of motion on examination. There may be a history of minor trauma. This is a self-limiting condition that usually resolves in 48-72 hr.

Legg-Calvé-Perthes disease (avascular necrosis of the femoral head) also manifests in childhood with insidious onset of limp and hip pain (Chapter 670.3).

Until the skeleton matures (Table 679-2), younger athletes are susceptible to apophyseal injuries (e.g., the anterior superior iliac spine). *Apophysitis* develops from overuse or from direct trauma. *Avulsion fractures* occur in adolescents playing sports requiring sudden, explosive bursts of speed (Fig. 679-8). Large muscles contract and create force greater than the strength of the attachment of the muscle to the apophysis. The most common sites of avulsion fractures (and the attaching muscles) are the anterior superior iliac spine (sartorius), anterior inferior iliac spine (rectus femoris), lesser femoral trochanter (iliopsoas), and ischial tuberosity (hamstrings). Symptoms include localized pain and swelling, with decreased strength and range of motion. Radiographs are required. Initial **treatment** includes ice, analgesics, rest, and pain-free range-of-motion exercises. Crutches are usually needed for ambulation. Surgery is usually not indicated because most of these fractures—even large or displaced ones—heal well. Contact to the bone around the hip and pelvis causes exquisitely tender subperiosteal hematomas called *hip pointers.* Symptomatic care includes rest, ice, analgesia, and protection from reinjury.

Slipped capital femoral epiphysis usually occurs in the 11-15 yr age range during the time of rapid linear bone growth (Chapter 670.4).

A *femoral neck stress fracture* can manifest as vague progressive hip pain in an endurance athlete. Girls with the female athlete triad are especially at risk. This diagnosis should always be kept in mind in the running athlete with vague anterior thigh pain. On examination, there may be pain with passive stretch of the hip flexors and pain with hip rotation. If radiographs do not demonstrate a periosteal reaction consistent with a stress fracture, a bone scan or MRI may be required. Orthopedic consultation is necessary in femoral neck stress fractures because of their predisposition to nonunion and displacement with minor trauma or continued weight bearing. These fractures carry increased risk of avascular necrosis of the femoral head.

Osteitis pubis is an inflammation at the pubic symphysis that may be caused by excessive side-to-side rocking of the pelvis. It can be seen in an athlete in any running sport and is more common in sports requiring more use of the adductor muscles such as ice hockey, soccer, and inline skating. Athletes typically present with vague groin pain that may be unilateral or bilateral. On physical examination, there is tenderness over the symphysis and sometimes over the proximal adductors. Adduction strength testing causes discomfort. Radiographic evidence (irregularity, sclerosis, widening of the pubic symphysis with osteolysis) might not be present until symptoms are present for 6-8 wk; a bone scan and MRI are more sensitive to early changes. Relative rest for 6-12 wk may be required. Some patients require corticosteroid injection as adjunctive therapy.

Table 679-2 AGE OF APPEARANCE AND FUSION OF APOPHYSES IN HIP AND PELVIS

APOPHYSIS	APPEARANCE (yr)	FUSION (yr)	RELATED MUSCLE GROUP(S)
AIIS	13-15	16-18	Quadriceps
ASIS	13-15	21-25	Sartorious
Lesser trochanter	11-12	16-17	Iliopsoas
Greater trochanter	2-3	16-17	Gluteal
Ischial tuberosity	13-15	20-25	Hamstrings
Iliac crest	13-15	21-25	Abdominal obliques Latissimus dorsi

AIIS, anterior inferior iliac spine; ASIS, anterior superior iliac spine.
From Waite BL, Krabak BJ: Examination and treatment of pediatric injuries of the hip and pelvis, *Phys Med Rehabil Clin North Am* 19:305–318, ix, 2008.

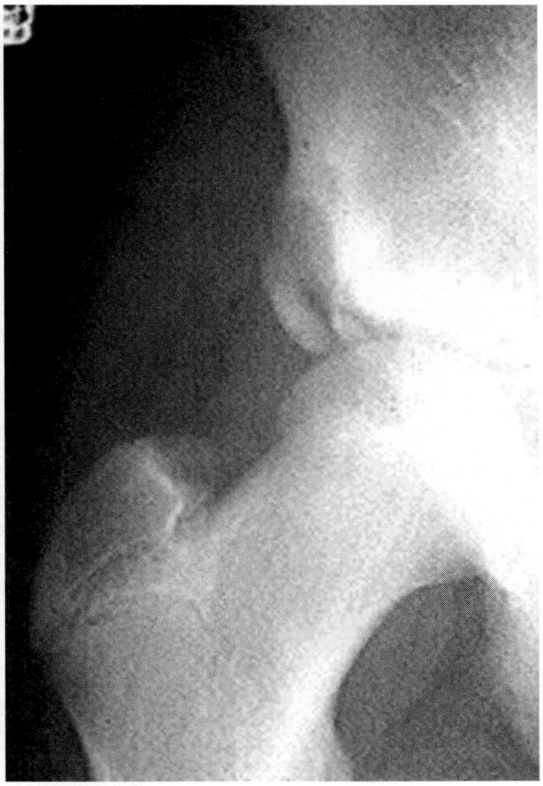

Figure 679-8 Apophyseal avulsion, pelvis. (From Anderson SJ: Sports injuries, *Curr Prob Pediatr Adolesc Health* 35:105–176, 2005.)

Acetabular labrum tears can occur in the hip, similar to glenoid labrum tears in the shoulder. Athletes might have a history of trauma and complain of sharp anterior hip pain associated with a clicking or catching sensation. Clinical diagnosis is difficult; magnetic resonance arthrography is useful for diagnosis.

Snapping hip syndrome is caused by the iliopsoas tendon's riding over the anterior hip capsule or the iliotibial band over the greater trochanter. It is commonly seen in ballet dancers and runners; it can occur as an acute or overuse injury (more common). Athletes present with either a painful or painless click or snap in the hip, usually located lateral or anterior and deep in the joint. Examination often reproduces the symptoms. Radiographs are not usually needed in the work-up. **Treatment** involves an analgesia, relative rest, biomechanical assessment, and core flexibility and strengthening. The athlete may return to activity as tolerated.

BIBLIOGRAPHY

Please visit the Nelson Textbook of Pediatrics *website at www.expertconsult.com for the complete bibliography.*

679.6 Knee Injuries

Gregory L. Landry

The knee is the most common musculoskeletal site for complaints among adolescents; some youth may be more prone to such injuries (Table 679-3). Acute knee injuries that cause immediate disability are likely to be due to fracture, patellar dislocation, anterior cruciate ligament (ACL) injury, or meniscal tear. The mechanism of injury is usually a weight-bearing event. After injury, if a player cannot bear weight within a few minutes, a fracture or significant internal derangement is more likely. If a player is able to bear weight and return to play after the injury, a serious injury is less likely to have occurred. If the knee swells within several hours of the injury, the swelling is likely due to a hemarthrosis and a more severe injury.

The injury most likely to occur with a hemarthrosis is an **ACL** injury. The ACL is usually injured from being hit directly, landing off balance from a jump, quickly changing direction while running, or hyperextension. Significant swelling and instability are often present. The majority of athletes with an ACL injury need orthopedic consultation and an ACL reconstruction. Functional bracing without ACL reconstruction increases the risk of meniscal injury and recurrent instability.

Posterior cruciate ligament injury occurs from a direct blow to the region of the proximal tibia, such as might occur with a dashboard injury or a fall to the knees in volleyball. Posterior cruciate ligament injuries are rare and are usually treated nonsurgically.

Medial collateral ligament (MCL) injuries result from a valgus blow to the outside of the knee. Isolated *lateral collateral ligament* injuries are uncommon and result from significant varus knee stress. Because they are extra-articular, isolated collateral injuries should not produce much of a knee effusion or disability. Regardless of severity, isolated medial and lateral collateral injuries are managed nonsurgically with aggressive rehabilitation.

Meniscal tears occur by the same mechanisms as ACL injuries. They are associated with hemarthrosis, joint line pain, and often

Table 679-3 SUMMARY OF MODIFIABLE AND NONMODIFIABLE INTRINSIC RISK FACTORS RELATED TO INCREASED RISK OF INJURY OF THE ANTERIOR CRUCIATE LIGAMENT

MODIFIABLE RISK FACTORS	NONMODIFIABLE RISK FACTORS	POTENTIAL CONTROL OR TREATMENT TECHNIQUE
ANATOMIC		
	BMI	Monitor and control relative body mass
	Femoral notch index (ACL size)	NM training targeted to decrease other risk factors
	Knee recurvatum	NM training targeted to improve dynamic knee flexion
	General joint laxity	NM training targeted to improve joint stiffness
	Family history (genetic predisoposition)	NM training targeted to decrease other risk factors
	Prior injury history	Full physical rehabilitation following injury
DEVELOPMENTAL AND HORMONAL		
	Sex, female	NM training prior to onset of risk factors
	Pubertal and post-pubertal maturation status	NM training during pre-puberty
	Preovulatory menstrual status	Oral contraceptives in female patients*
	ACL tensile strength	NM training targeted to decrease other risk factors
	Neuromuscular shunt	NM training targeted to improve neuromuscular control
BIOMECHANICAL		
Knee abduction		NM training targeted to improve coronal plane loads
Anterior tibial shear		NM training targeted to improve dynamic knee flexion
Lateral trunk motion		NM training targeted to improve trunk strength and control
Tibial rotation		NM training targeted to control transverse motions and influence sagittal plane deceleration mechanics
Dynamic foot pronation		Foot orthoses
Fatigue resistance		Strength and conditioning training
Ground reaction forces		NM training targeted to improve force absorption strategies
NEUROMUSCULAR		
Relative hamstring recruitment		NM training targeted to improve hamstring strength and recruitment
Hip abduction strength		NM training targeted to improve high strength and recruitment
Trunk proprioception		NM training targeted to improve trunk strength and control

ACL, anterior cruciate ligament; BMI, body mass index; NM, neuromuscular.

*Pilot evidence indicates it might be a potential control strategy.

From Alentorn-Geli E, Myer GD, Silvers HJ, et al: Prevention of non-contact anterior cruciate ligament injuries in soccer players. Part 1: mechanisms of injury and underlying risk factors, *Knee Surg Sports Traumatol Arthrosc* 7:705–709, 2009.

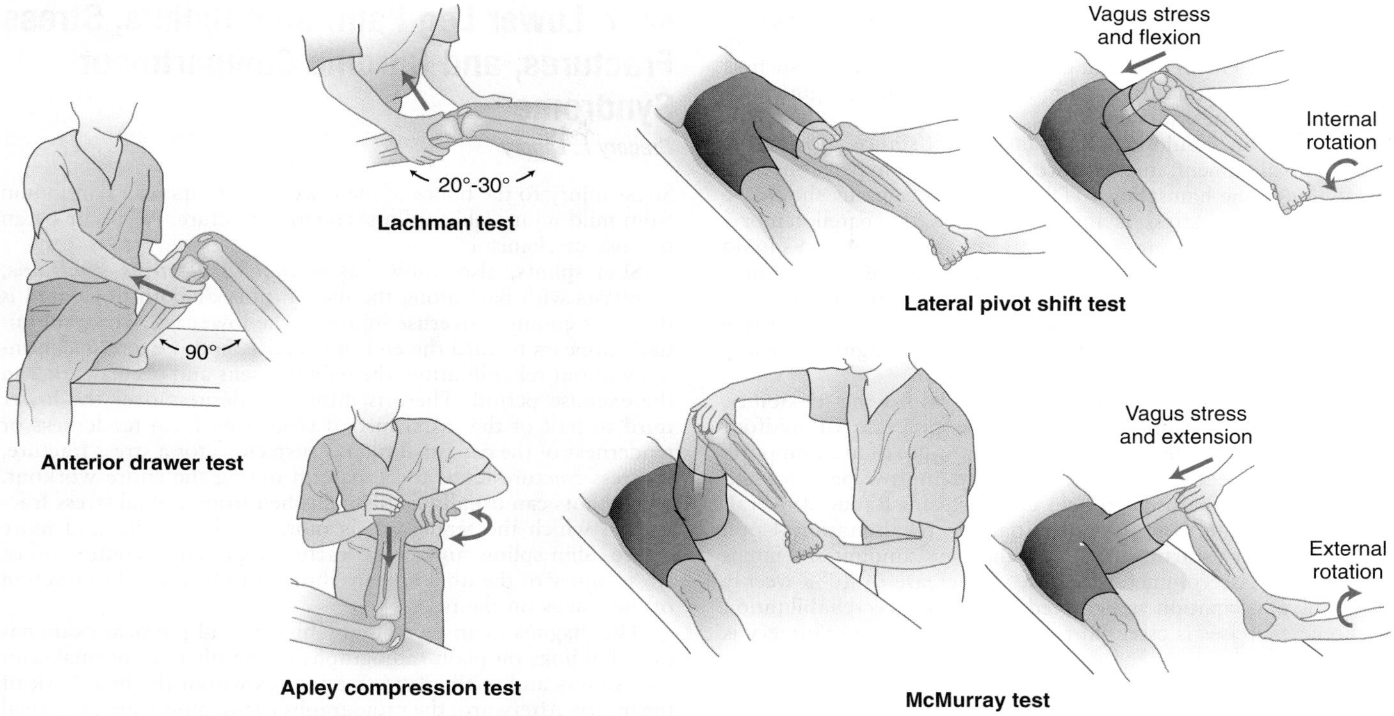

Figure 679-9 Examination maneuvers include the Lachman, anterior drawer, lateral pivot shift, Apley compression, and McMurray tests; the right knee is shown. The Lachman test, performed to detect anterior cruciate ligament (ACL) injures, is conducted with the patient supine and the knee flexed 20-30 degrees. The anterior drawer test detects ACL injuries and is performed with the patient supine and the knee in 90 degrees of flexion. The lateral pivot shift test is performed with the patient supine, the hip flexed 45 degrees, and the knee in full extension. Internal rotation is applied to the tibia while the knee is flexed to 40 degrees under a valgus stress (pushing the outside of the knee medially). The Apley compression test, used to assess meniscal integrity, is performed with the patient prone and the examiner's knee over the patient's posterior thigh. The tibia is externally rotated while a downward compressive force is applied over the tibia. The McMurray test, used to assess meniscal integrity, is performed with the patient supine and the examiner standing on the side of the affected knee.

pain in full flexion. Orthopedic consultation is indicated when a meniscal tear is suspected.

Patellar dislocation occurs most often as a noncontact injury when the quadriceps muscles forcefully contract to extend the knee while the lower leg is externally rotated. Patellar dislocation is the second most common cause of hemarthrosis. The patella is almost always dislocated laterally, and this motion tears the medial patellar retinaculum, causing bleeding in the joint. Recurrent episodes of patellar instability are associated with less swelling. Patellar instability is usually treated nonsurgically with a patella-stabilizing sleeve and an aggressive rehabilitation program. Recurrent instability can require surgical intervention.

INITIAL TREATMENT OF ACUTE KNEE INJURIES

The physician should inspect for an effusion and obvious deformities; if any deformity is present, the physician should assess neurovascular status and transfer the patient for emergency care. If no gross deformities are present and neurovascular integrity is intact, initial maneuvers include full passive extension and gentle valgus stress to the knee while it is in extension. If there is laxity of the knee with valgus stress in full extension, both the ACL and MCL have been injured. The patient's ability to contract the quadriceps muscles should be noted. Pain occurring with quadriceps contraction or inability to contract the quadriceps muscle implies an injury to the extensor mechanism. Tenderness over the medial patella, medial retinaculum, and/or above the adductor tubercle is associated with a patellar dislocation. Point tenderness is consistent with fracture or injury to the underlying structure; a medial meniscal tear can manifest as tenderness along the medial joint line, but medial joint line tenderness is not specific for a medial meniscus tear. Pain or limitation in either passive flexion or extension while rotating the tibia implies a meniscal injury, as do other maneuvers (Fig. 679-9). Ligament injury is manifested as pain or laxity with the appropriate maneuver.

If a patient cannot bear weight pain free or has clinical signs of instability, the knee should be immobilized, crutches given, and plain radiographs obtained. If the patella is dislocated, reduction can be achieved with knee extension. Developed as the **Ottawa knee rules,** radiographs are required for pediatric patients with knee injury who have any of these findings: isolated tenderness of patella, fibular head tenderness, inability to flex 90 degrees, and inability to bear weight both immediately and in the emergency department for 4 steps (regardless of limping). Straight-leg immobilizers offer no structural support and are only used for comfort. If any brace is used, a hinged brace is indicated for stabilization such as an injury when both ACL and MCL might have been injured. The leg should be elevated, and elastic wrap can be applied for compression.

CHRONIC INJURIES

Patellofemoral Stress Syndrome

Patellofemoral stress syndrome (PFSS) is the most common cause of anterior knee pain. PFSS is also known as *patellofemoral pain syndrome* or *patellofemoral dysfunction* (Chapter 669.5). It is a diagnosis of exclusion used to describe anterior knee pain that has no other identifiable pathology. Pain is usually difficult to localize. Patients indicate a diffuse area over the anterior knee as the source, or they might feel as if the pain is coming from behind the patella. Bilateral pain is common, and pain is often worse going up stairs, after sitting for prolonged periods, or after squatting or running. There should be negative history for significant swelling, which would indicate a more serious injury. History of change in activity is common, such as altered training surface or terrain, increased training regimen, or performance of new tasks.

Examination should include evaluation of stance and gait for lower limb alignment, musculature, and midfoot hyperpronation. Flexibility of the hamstrings, ITB, and gastrocnemius should be assessed, because stress is increased across the patellofemoral joint when these structures are tight. Hip range of motion should be assessed to rule out hip pathology. Medial patellar tenderness or pain with compression of the patellofemoral joint confirms the diagnosis in the absence of an effusion and no other positive findings on the examination. PFSS is a clinical diagnosis usually managed without imaging.

Treatment focuses on assessing and improving flexibility, strength, and gait abnormalities. In the presence of midfoot hyperpronation (ankle valgus), new shoes or use of arch supports can improve patellofemoral mechanics and improve pain. Ice and an analgesic can be used to help control pain. Reduced overall activity or training is important initially in rehabilitation. Upon return to activity, starting at 50% of the usual amount and intensity of work is recommended, with an increase of 10% weekly until full participation is achieved. Maintenance rehabilitation via home exercises is essential to prevent recurrences. Surgery is rarely indicated.

Osgood-Schlatter Disease

Osgood-Schlatter disease is a traction apophysitis occurring at the insertion of the patellar tendon on the tibial tuberosity (Chapter 669.4). Because it is also related to overuse of the extensor mechanism, Osgood-Schlatter disease is **treated** like PFSS. A protective pad to protect the tibial tubercle from direct trauma can be used. The most common complication is cosmetic; the tibial tubercle on the affected side (or both if bilateral) may be slightly more prominent. Patients only need to take time from sports if they are limping.

Other Chronic Injuries

Sinding-Larsen-Johansson disease is a traction apophysitis occurring at the inferior pole of the patella. It occurs most often in volleyball and basketball athletes. **Treatment** is similar to that of PFSS and Osgood-Schlatter disease.

Patellar tendinosis (jumper's knee) is due to repetitive microtrauma of the patellar tendon, usually at the inferior pole of the patella. In about 10% of the cases, the quadriceps tendon above the patella is affected. It is associated with jumping sports but occurs in runners as well. **Treatment** is similar to that for PFSS. Relative rest is more important in patellar tendinosis because chronic pain is associated with irreversible changes in the tendon.

ITB friction syndrome is the most common cause of chronic lateral knee pain. Generally it is not associated with swelling or instability. It is due to friction of the ITB along the lateral knee, resulting in bursitis. Tenderness is elicited along the ITB as it courses over the lateral femoral condyle or at its insertion at the Gerdy tubercle, along the lateral tibial plateau. Tightness of the ITB is also noted using the Ober test. To perform an Ober test, the athlete lies on one side and the superior hip is extended with the knee flexed. The examiner holds the ankle in midair, and if the knee moves inferiorly, it implies a flexible ITB and a negative Ober test. If the knee and leg stay in midair, the ITB is tight and the Ober test is positive. **Treatment** principles follow those for PFSS, except emphasis is on improving flexibility of the ITB.

BIBLIOGRAPHY

Please visit the Nelson Textbook of Pediatrics *website at www.expertconsult.com for the complete bibliography.*

679.7 Lower Leg Pain: Shin Splints, Stress Fractures, and Chronic Compartment Syndrome

Gregory L. Landry

Stress injury to the bones of the lower leg occurs on a continuum from mild injury (shin splints) to stress fracture. All occur by an overuse mechanism.

Shin splints, also known as *medial tibial stress syndrome,* manifests with pain along the medial tibia or both tibiae and is the most common overuse injury of the lower leg. The pain initially appears toward the end of exercise, and if exercise continues without rehabilitation, the pain worsens and occurs earlier in the exercise period. There is diffuse tenderness over the lower third to half of the distal medial tibia. Any focal tenderness or tenderness of the proximal tibia is suspicious for a stress fracture. A stress fracture tends to be painful during the entire workout. Shin splints can usually be distinguished from a **tibial stress fracture** in which the tenderness is more focal (2-5 cm) and more severe. Shin splints and stress fracture represent a continuum of stress injury to the tibia and are thought to be related to traction of the soleus on the tibia.

The diagnosis can be made by history and physical examination. Findings on plain radiographs of the tibia are normal with shin splints and in tibial stress fractures within the first 2 wk of the injury. Afterward, the radiographs can demonstrate periosteal reaction if a stress fracture is present. Sensitivity of plain radiographs may be increased by obtaining 4 views of the tibia: AP, lateral, and both oblique views. A bone scan is the most sensitive test to diagnose stress fractures; it demonstrates discrete tracer uptake at the site(s) of the stress fracture. Increased uptake may be noted in the presence of shin splints, but in a fusiform pattern along the periosteal surface. If results of the bone scan are normal, the diagnosis is likely to be shin splints or chronic compartment syndrome (CCS). MRI has replaced bone scan as the most sensitive tool for diagnosing stress fractures in long bones in many medical centers.

The **treatment** of shin splints and tibial stress fractures is similar, involving relative rest, correcting training errors and kinetic chain dysfunction, and often the use of better running shoes. Fitness can be maintained with non–weight-bearing activities such as swimming, cycling, and water jogging. With shin splints, after 7-10 days, patients can usually start on the walk-jog program. If pain worsens, 2-3 pain-free days are required before resuming the walk-jog program. Ice should be used daily and an analgesic should be used for pain control. Orthotics or new shoes may be useful in patients who hyperpronate. Stretching the plantar flexors and strengthening the ankle dorsiflexors can be useful. Being pain free for 7-10 days is recommended before exercise is commenced.

CCS occurs in an athlete in a running sport, usually during a period of heavy training. It is due to muscle hypertrophy and increased intracompartmental pressure with exercise. There is typically a pain-free period of about 10 min at the beginning of a workout before onset of constant throbbing pain that is difficult to localize. It lasts for minutes to hours after exercise and is relieved by ice and elevation. In a classic case, there is numbness of the foot associated with high pressure within the corresponding muscle compartment. The most common compartment affected is the anterolateral compartment with compression of the peroneal nerve. The physical examination in the office is often normal, but weakness of the extensor hallucis longus and decreased sensation in the web space between the 1st and 2nd toe may be present.

If CCS is suspected, referral to an appropriate surgeon (orthopedic or vascular) to measure the intracompartmental pressure is indicated. Treatment is surgical and requires fasciotomy to relieve the pressure.

BIBLIOGRAPHY

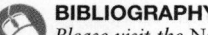

Please visit the Nelson Textbook of Pediatrics *website at* *www.expertconsult.com* *for the complete bibliography.*

679.8 Ankle Injuries

Gregory L. Landry

Ankle injuries are the most common acute athletic injury. About 85% of ankle injuries are sprains, and 85% of those are inversion injuries (foot planted with the lateral fibula moving toward the ground), 5% are eversion injuries (foot planted with the medial malleolus moving toward the ground), and 10% are combined.

EXAMINATION AND INJURY GRADING SCALE

In obvious cases of fracture or dislocation, evaluating neurovascular status with as little movement as possible is the priority. If no deformity is obvious, the next step is inspection for edema, ecchymosis, and anatomic variants. Key sites to palpate for tenderness are the entire length of the fibula; the medial and lateral malleoli; the base of the 5th metatarsal; the anterior, medial, and lateral joint lines; and the navicular and the Achilles tendon complex. Assessment of active range of motion (patient alone) in dorsiflexion, plantar flexion, inversion, and eversion and of resisted range of motion is indicated.

Provocative testing attempts to evaluate the integrity of the ligaments. In a patient with a markedly swollen, painful ankle, provocative testing is difficult because of muscle spasm and involuntary guarding. It is more useful on the field before much bleeding and edema have occurred. The anterior drawer test assesses for anterior translation of the talus and competence of the anterior talofibular ligament. The inversion stress test examines the competence of the anterior talofibular and calcaneofibular ligaments (Fig. 679-10). In the acute setting, the integrity of the tibiofibular ligaments and syndesmosis is examined by the syndesmosis squeeze test. Pain with squeezing the lower leg implies injury to the interosseous membrane and syndesmosis between the tibia and fibula, making a severe injury more suspicious. Athletes with this injury cannot bear any weight and also have severe pain with external rotation of the foot. Occasionally the peroneal tendon dislocates from the fibular groove simultaneously with an ankle sprain. To assess for peroneal tendon instability, the examiner applies pressure from behind the peroneal tendon with resisting eversion and plantar flexion, and the tendon pops anteriorly. If either a syndesmotic injury or an acute peroneal dislocation is suspected, orthopedic consultation should be sought.

RADIOGRAPHS

AP, lateral, and mortise views of the ankle are obtained when patients have pain in the area of the malleoli, are unable to bear weight, or have bone tenderness over the posterior distal tibia or fibula. The Ottawa ankle rules help define who requires radiographs (Fig. 679-11). A foot series (AP, lateral, and oblique views) should be obtained when patients have pain in the area of the midfoot or bone tenderness over the navicular or 5th metatarsal. It is important to differentiate an avulsion fracture of the proximal 5th metatarsal from the Jones fracture of the proximal 5th metatarsal (a lucency about 2 cm from the proximal end). The former is treated as an ankle sprain; the latter fracture has an increased risk of nonunion and requires orthopedic consultation. The *talar dome fracture* is manifested as an ankle sprain that does

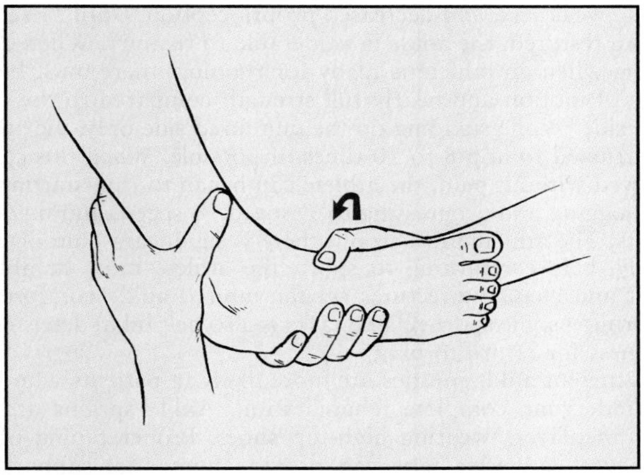

Figure 679-10 Inversion stress tilt test for ankle instability. (From Hergenroeder AC: Diagnosis and treatment of ankle sprains. A review, *Am J Dis Child* 144:809–814, 1990.)

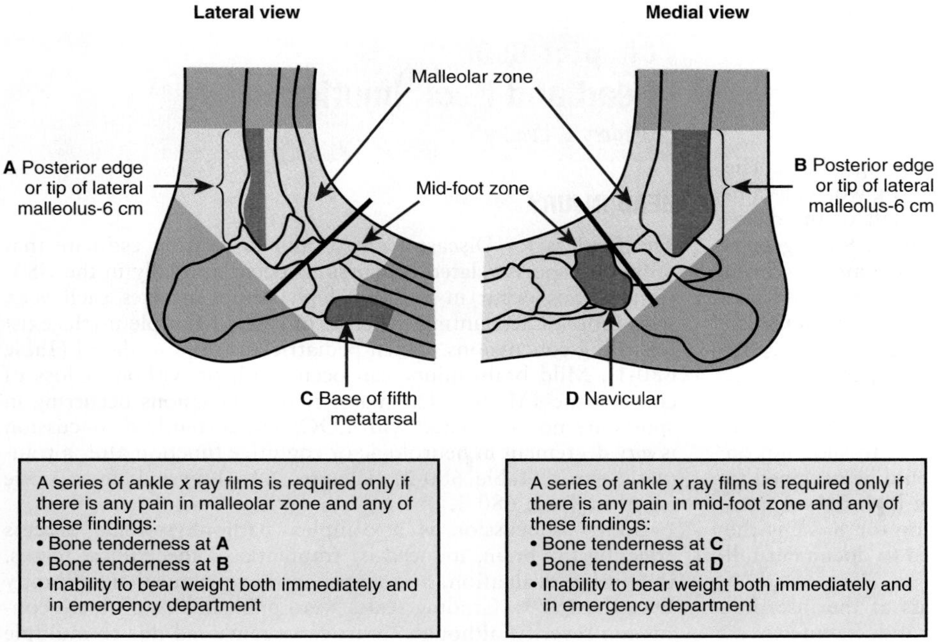

Medial view
Malleolar zone
Mid-foot zone

A series of ankle *x* ray films is required only if there is any pain in malleolar zone and any of these findings:

Figure 679-11 Ottawa ankle rules. (From Bachmann LM, Kolb E, Koller MT, et al: Accuracy of Ottawa ankle rules to exclude fractures of the ankle and mid-foot; systematic review, *BMJ* 326:417–419, 2003.)

not improve. Radiographs on initial presentation can have subtle abnormalities. Any suspicion on the initial radiographs of a talar dome fracture warrants orthopedic consultation and further imaging. In the early adolescent, always look carefully at the tibial epiphysis. Nondisplaced Salter III fractures can be subtle and need to be recognized early and referred to an orthopedic surgeon promptly.

INITIAL TREATMENT OF ANKLE SPRAINS

Ankle sprains need to **treated** with RICE: rest, ice, compression, and elevation. This should be followed for the first 48-72 hr after the injury to minimize bleeding and edema. For an ankle injury, this consists of crutches and an elastic wrap, although other compression devices such as an air stirrup splint work quite well. This allows early weight bearing with protection and can be removed for rehabilitation. It is important to start a rehabilitation program as soon as possible.

Rehabilitation

Rehabilitation should begin the day of injury; for patients who have pain with movement, isometric strengthening can be started. Important deficits to correct include loss of dorsiflexion, peroneal muscle weakness, and decreased proprioception. Until these deficits are restored, the ankle is vulnerable to reinjury. When determining when an athlete is ready for running, there must be full range of motion and nearly full strength compared to the uninjured side. While standing on the uninjured side only, the athlete is instructed to hop 8 to 10 times, if possible. When this can be achieved without pain, the athlete can began to run, starting out with jogging and progressing to ½ speed, ¾ speed, and finally to sprints. The athlete must stop if there is significant pain or limp. Finally, before returning to sport, the athlete must be able to sprint and change directions off the injured ankle comfortably. Performing some sport-related tasks is also helpful in determining readiness for return to play.

Recurrent ankle injuries are more likely in patients who have not undergone complete rehabilitation. Ankle sprains are less likely in players wearing high-top shoes. Proper taping of the ankle with adhesive tape can provide functional support but loosens with use and is unavailable to most athletes. Lace-up ankle braces are useful for preventing recurrences. They are more supportive than tape and can be tightened repeatedly during the course of a practice or a game. Most sports physicians recommend their use indefinitely to help prevent further sprains.

679.9 Foot Injuries

Gregory L. Landry

Metatarsal stress fractures can occur in any running athlete. The history is insidious pain with activity that is getting worse. Examination reveals point tenderness over the midshaft of the metatarsal, most commonly the 2nd or 3rd metatarsal. Radiographs might not show the periosteal reaction before pain has been present for 2 wk or more. **Treatment** is relative rest for 6-8 wk. Shoes with good arch supports reduce stress to the metatarsals.

Vague dorsal foot pain in an athlete in a running sport can represent a **navicular stress fracture.** Unlike other stress fractures, it might not localize well on examination. If there is any tenderness around the navicular, a stress fracture should be suspected. This stress fracture can take many weeks to show up on plain radiographs, so a bone scan or MRI should be obtained to make the diagnosis. Because this fracture is at high risk of nonunion, immobilization and non–weight bearing for 8 wk is the usual **treatment.** A CT scan should be obtained to document full healing after the period of immobilization.

Sever disease (calcaneal apophysitis) occurs at the insertion of the Achilles tendon on the calcaneus and manifests as activity-related pain (see Fig. 679-3). It is more common in boys (2 : 1), is often bilateral, and usually occurs between ages 8 and 13 yr. Tenderness is elicited at the insertion of the Achilles tendon into the calcaneus, especially with squeezing the heel (positive squeeze test). Sever disease is associated with tight Achilles tendons and midfoot hyperpronation that puts more stress on the plantar flexors of the foot. **Treatment** includes relative rest, ice, massage, stretching, and strengthening the Achilles tendon. Correcting the midfoot hyperpronation with orthotics, arch supports, or better shoes is important in most athletes with Sever disease. If the foot is neutral or there is mild hyperpronation, ¼-in heel lifts will be helpful to unload the Achilles tendon and its insertion. With optimal management, symptoms improve in 4-8 wk. Generally, if there is no limp during the athletic activity, young athletes with Sever disease should be allowed to play.

Plantar fasciitis is an overuse injury resulting in degeneration of the plantar aponeurosis. Rare in prepubertal children, this diagnosis is more likely in an adolescent or young adult. Athletes report heel pain with activity that is worse with first steps of the day or after several hours of non–weight bearing. Tenderness is elicited on the medial calcaneal tuberosity. Relative rest from weight-bearing activity is helpful. Athletes get plantar fasciitis when shoes are worn with inadequate arch supports. New shoes or use of semirigid arch supports often lessen the pain. Stretching the calves and plantar fascia helps. Some patients benefit from night splints even though they can make sleep difficult. As long as there is no limping with athletic activity, the athlete may continue participation. Complete recovery is usually seen at 6 mo. Corticosteroid and extracorporeal shock-wave therapy are reserved for severe, chronic cases.

Calcaneal stress fracture is seen in the older adolescent or young adult involved in a running sport. There is heel pain with any weight-bearing activity. The physical examination reveals pain with squeezing the calcaneus. Sclerosis can show up on the AP and lateral radiographs after 2-3 wk of pain. A bone scan or MRI needs to be performed to clinch the diagnosis in some cases. The calcaneus is an uncommon location for a stress fracture; it is associated with osteopenia (amenorrheic girls). **Treatment** is rest from running and other weight-bearing activity for at least 8 wk. Immobilization is rarely necessary.

BIBLIOGRAPHY

Please visit the Nelson Textbook of Pediatrics *website at www.expertconsult.com for the complete bibliography.*

Chapter 680
Head and Neck Injuries

Gregory L. Landry

HEAD INJURY

The Centers for Disease Control and Prevention estimate that ~300,000 sports-related concussions occur annually in the USA. Concussions occur in >62,000 high school athletes each year, with football accounting for 63% of cases. Multiple myths exist regarding concussions, which pediatricians need to dispel (Table 680-1). Mild brain injury can occur with or without a loss of consciousness (LOC). The majority of concussions occurring in sports are not associated with LOC, and currently a concussion is *any* decrement in neurologic or cognitive function after a traumatic event (Table 680-2) (Chapter 63). Low-risk factors are noted in Table 680-3.

Sports concussion is a complex pathophysiologic process affecting the brain, induced by traumatic biomechanical forces. Definition, evaluation, and treatment have evolved significantly since the 1970s. Grading scales were published to evaluate concussion severity, although controversy remained due to multiple

Table 680-1 IMPORTANT FACTS REGARDING CONCUSSIONS AND CHILDREN

- High school athletes are more vulnerable to concussions than older athletes and can take longer to recover.
- Failure to properly manage a concussion can lead to long-term cumulative consequences.
- Loss of consciousness is not an appropriate marker for the presence or absence of concussion.
- High school athletes are 3 times more likely to experience a second concussion if concussed once during a season
- More than 5% of high school athletes are concussed each year while participating in collision sports.

Adapted from Theye F, Mueller KA: "Heads up": concussions in high school sports, *Clin Med Res* 2(3):165–171, 2004.

Table 680-2 CONCUSSION SIGNS AND SYMPTOMS

CONCUSSION SYMPTOMS
Headache or "pressure" in head
Nausea or vomiting
Balance problems or dizziness
Double or blurry vision
Sensitivity to light
Sensitivity to noise
Feeling sluggish, hazy, foggy, or groggy
Concentration or memory problems
Confusion
Does not "feel right" or is "feeling down"
CONCUSSION SIGNS
Appears dazed or stunned
Is confused about assignment or position
Forgets an instruction
Is unsure of game, score, or opponent
Moves clumsily
Answers questions slowly
Loses consciousness *(even briefly)*
Shows mood, behavior, or personality changes
Can't recall events *before* hit or fall (retrograde amnesia)
Can't recall events *after* hit or fall (antegrade amnesia)

Adapted from the Centers for Disease Control Heads Up Concussion Campaign; From Grady MF, Goodman A: Concussion in the adolescent athlete, *Curr Prob Pediatr Adolesc Health Care* 40:153–169, 2010.

Table 680-3 LOW-RISK CHARACTERISTICS FOR CLINICALLY IMPORTANT BRAIN INJURIES

Normal mental status
No loss of consciousness
No vomiting
Nonsevere injury mechanism
No signs of basilar skull fracture
No severe headache

From Grady MF, Goodman A: Concussion in the adolescent athlete, *Curr Prob Pediatr Adolesc Health Care* 40:153–169, 2010.

guidelines. In November 2008, the 3rd International Symposium on Concussion in Sport confirmed that injury-grading scales should no longer be used. The participants also abandoned the simple vs complex classification suggested in the 2nd symposium in 2005. Instead, individual response should guide evaluation and return-to-play decisions. When a concussion is suspected, the athlete should be removed from the activity and medically evaluated. Regular monitoring over the initial few hours following injury is important. The group suggested use of an assessment tool called SCAT (Sport Concussion Assessment Tool) to assist the clinician in assessing the athlete.

Concussions usually resolve over 7-10 days and do not involve complications. In a large-scale study among college athletes, balance deficits resolved in 3-5 days, baseline cognitive functioning returned in 5-7 days, and other symptoms resolved by 7 days; it is not known if high school athletes respond similarly. The athlete is held out of activity until he or she is asymptomatic, after which return to activity is gradual. "Cognitive rest," during which young athletes limit exertion during routine daily tasks as well as with schoolwork, is important in recovery as well.

Table 680-4 GRADUATED RETURN-TO-PLAY PROTOCOL

1. No activity: Complete physical and *cognitive* rest until asymptomatic at rest. Once an athlete is symptomatic at rest, progress through following stages. Each stage should take a minimum of 24 hours to complete.
   Progress to the next stage only if asymptomatic with the new activities.
   If the new stage provokes symptoms, return to the previous stage for at least 24 hours.
2. Low levels of physical exertion as tolerated (symptoms do not get worse or come back during or after the activity).
   This includes walking, light jogging, light stationary biking.
3. Moderate levels of physical exertion as tolerated.
   This includes sport-specific exercises such as skating drills in ice hockey, running drills in soccer, but no head-impact activities.
4. Noncontact sport specific-training drills including passing drills in football and ice hockey; may start progressive weight training.
5. Full contact practice following medical clearance, participate in normal training activities.
6. Normal game play.

In general, the athlete progresses from 1 step to the next as long as he or she remains asymptomatic for 24 hours at each step. If the athlete becomes symptomatic during 1 of these steps, he or she returns to the previous step for at least 24 hours. Athletes must be off any medications that are being used to treat symptoms to be considered symptom-free at rest.

From Grady MF, Goodman A: Concussion in the adolescent athlete, *Curr Prob Pediatr Adolesc Health Care* 40:153–169, 2010.

Return to play should progress through a system of tasks, with the athlete advancing only if asymptomatic (Table 680-4):

1. Rest until asymptomatic
2. Light aerobic exercise; no resistance training
3. Sport-specific training
4. Noncontact drills
5. Full-contact drills
6. Game play

If the athlete exhibits any of the symptoms of concussion (see Table 680-2), he or she should not return to the task for at least 24 hr. The athlete should not be using medications to treat symptoms during the return-to-play program.

Athletes who have symptoms from multiple concussions might need to be handled more conservatively. Persistent symptoms of cognitive impairment include poor attention or concentration, memory dysfunction, irritability, anxiety, depressed mood, sleep disturbances, persistent low-grade headache, lightheadedness, and/or intolerance of bright lights or loud noises. Exertion typically exacerbates concussion symptoms. Work-up is more extensive in the athletes with recurrent injuries. Physicians who specialize in treating this injury should manage these patients.

In concussion, CT and MRI are usually normal. For most concussions, neuroimaging is usually not necessary. However, neuroimaging should be used when there is suspicion of intracranial structural pathology, due to a focal finding on neurologic examination or symptoms that are worsening. The risk of intracranial pathology is increased in the presence of continued emesis, prolonged headache, persistent antegrade amnesia (poor short-term memory), seizures, Glasgow Coma Scale score <15, and signs of basal skull fracture or depressed skull fracture.

NECK INJURIES

The most common injuries to the neck are soft tissue injuries (contusions, muscle strains, ligament sprains). However, when an athlete complains of midline cervical pain or neck pain on range of motion, has focal neurologic deficits, or has lost consciousness, a neck fracture must be assumed. The cervical spine should be immobilized, and anteroposterior, lateral, oblique, and open-mouth views should be obtained before the immobilizer is removed. If active flexion and extension cannot be performed, CT should be performed (Chapter 598.5).

There is often overlap among cervical sprain, strain, and contusion. Several radiographic signs indicate instability: interspinous widening, vertebral subluxation, vertebral compression fracture, loss of cervical lordosis. MRI is very sensitive and should be used to diagnose and define ligamentous and spinal cord injuries. After a negative radiographic examination for fracture and a normal neurologic examination, the neck can be immobilized in a soft collar for comfort. Rest and anti-inflammatory medications benefit minor injuries. The collar is gradually withdrawn, and range-of-motion exercises are instituted. The athlete may return to play once full strength range of motion is restored and sport-specific neck function is present. It is important to maintain a cervical conditioning program to help prevent recurrence.

Cervical disk injuries in sports usually result from uncontrolled lateral bending or flexion. Cervical injuries are less common than lumbar disk injuries, and they are uncommon in pediatric patients. Most cervical disk problems resolve over several months with initial rest, immobilization, anti-inflammatory medications, activity modification, and cervical traction. Range-of-motion and subsequent strength training are instituted after symptoms improve.

BRACHIAL PLEXUS INJURIES

The brachial plexus includes nerves originating from C5-T1 and emerging from the spinal column in the deep triangle of the neck. The upper trunk (C5-C6) can be contused or stretched during football when tackling with the shoulder or having the head forcefully flexed laterally. The brachial plexus can also be injured from a direct blow to the anterior chest. Manifestations include unilateral burning (known as a *burner* or *stinger*), paresthesias, and weakness in the arm, usually in a C5-C6 distribution manifested as the inability to forward flex or abduct the shoulder. These symptoms often resolve spontaneously within minutes. Bilateral symptoms, such as transient quadriplegia, are an indication to curtail participation until the patient is evaluated by MRI. If a patient has recurrent "stingers," an MRI of the cervical spine is indicated to look for disk pathology.

BIBLIOGRAPHY

Please visit the Nelson Textbook of Pediatrics *website at www.expertconsult.com for the complete bibliography.*

Chapter 681
Heat Injuries
Gregory L. Landry

Heat illness is the 3rd leading cause of death in U.S. high school athletes. It is a continuum of clinical signs and symptoms that can be mild (heat stress) to fatal (heatstroke) (Chapter 64). Children are more vulnerable to heat illness than adults. They have greater ratio of surface area to body mass than adults and produce greater heat per kilogram of body weight than adults during activity. The sweat rate is lower in children and the temperature at which sweating occurs is higher. Children can take longer to acclimatize to warmer, more humid environments (typically 8-12 near-consecutive days of 30-45 min exposures). Children also have a blunted thirst response compared to adults and might not consume enough fluid during exercise to prevent dehydration.

Three categories for heat illness are generally used: **heat cramps, heat exhaustion,** and **heat stroke.** However, symptoms of heat illness overlap and advance as the core temperature rises. **Heat cramps** are the most common heat injury and usually occur in mild dehydration and or salt depletion, usually affecting the calf and hamstring muscles. They tend to occur later in activity, as muscle fatigue is reached and water loss and sodium loss worsen. They respond to oral rehydration with electrolyte solution and with gentle stretching. The athlete can return to play when ability to perform is not impaired. **Heat syncope** is fainting after prolonged exercise attributed to poor vasomotor tone and depleted intravascular volume, and it responds to fluids, cooling, and supine positioning. **Heat edema** is mild edema of the hands and feet during initial exposure to heat; it resolves with acclimatization. **Heat tetany** is carpopedal tingling or spasms caused by heat-related hyperventilation. It responds to moving to a cooler environment and decreasing respiratory rate (or rebreathing by breathing into a bag).

Heat exhaustion is a moderate illness with core temperature 100-103°F (37.7-39.4°C). Performance is obviously affected, but central nervous system (CNS) dysfunction is mild, if present. It is manifested as headache, nausea, vomiting, dizziness, orthostasis, weakness, piloerection, and possibly syncope. **Treatment** includes moving to a cool environment, cooling the body with fans, removing excess clothing, and placing ice over the groin and axillae. If a patient is not able to tolerate oral rehydration, IV fluids are indicated. Patients should be monitored, including rectal temperature, for signs of heat stroke. If rapid improvement is not achieved, transport to an emergency facility is recommended.

Heat stroke is a severe illness manifested by CNS disturbances and potential tissue damage. It is a medical emergency; the mortality rate is 50%. Sports-related heat stroke is characterized by profuse sweating and is related to intense exertion, whereas "classic" heatstroke with dry, hot skin is of slower onset (days) in elderly or chronically ill persons. Rectal temperature is usually >104°F (40°C). Significant damage to the heart, brain, liver, kidneys, and muscle occurs with possible fatal consequences if untreated. **Treatment** is immediate whole-body cooling via cold water immersion. Airway, breathing, circulation, core temperature, and CNS status should be monitored constantly. Rapid cooling should be ceased when core temperature is ~101-102°F (38.3-38.9°C). IV fluid at a rate of 800 mL/m^2 in the first hour with normal saline or lactated Ringer solution improves intravascular volume and the body's ability to dissipate heat. Immediate transport to an emergency facility is necessary. Physician clearance is required before return to exercise.

Dehydration is common to all heat illness; therefore, measures to prevent dehydration can also prevent heat illness. Thirst is not an adequate indicator of hydration status because it is initiated at 2-3% dehydration. Athletes are advised to be well hydrated before exercise and should drink every 20 min during exercise (5 oz for those weighing 40 kg, 9 oz for 60 kg, and 10-12 oz for those >60 kg). Free access to cold water should be advocated to coaches. During a football practice, scheduled breaks every 20-30 min with helmets off to get out of the heat can decrease the cumulative amount of heat exposure. Practices and competition should be scheduled in the early morning or late afternoon to avoid the hottest part of the day. Guidelines have been published about modifying activity related to temperature and humidity (Fig. 681-1). Proper clothing such as shorts and t-shirts without helmets can improve heat dissipation. Prepractice and postpractice weight can be helpful in determining the amount of fluid necessary to replace (8 oz for each pound of weight loss).

Heat index °F (°C)													
	Relative humidity (%)												
Temperature °F (°C)	40	45	50	55	60	65	70	75	80	85	90	95	100
110 (47)	136 (58)												
108 (43)	130 (54)	137 (58)											
106 (41)	124 (51)	130 (54)	137 (58)										
104 (40)	119 (48)	124 (51)	131 (55)	137 (58)									
102 (39)	114 (46)	119 (48)	124 (51)	130 (54)	137 (58)								
100 (38)	109 (43)	114 (46)	118 (48)	124 (51)	129 (54)	136 (58)							
98 (37)	105 (41)	109 (43)	113 (45)	117 (47)	123 (51)	128 (53)	134 (57)						
96 (36)	101 (38)	104 (40)	108 (42)	112 (44)	116 (47)	121 (49)	126 (52)	132 (56)					
94 (34)	97 (36)	100 (38)	103 (39)	106 (41)	110 (43)	114 (46)	119 (48)	124 (51)	129 (54)	135 (57)			
92 (33)	94 (34)	96 (36)	99 (37)	101 (38)	105 (41)	108 (42)	112 (44)	116 (47)	121 (49)	126 (52)	131 (55)		
90 (32)	91 (33)	93 (34)	95 (35)	97 (36)	100 (38)	103 (39)	106 (41)	109 (43)	113 (45)	117 (47)	122 (50)	127 (53)	132 (56)
88 (31)	88 (31)	89 (32)	91 (33)	93 (34)	95 (35)	98 (37)	100 (38)	103 (39)	106 (41)	110 (43)	113 (45)	117 (47)	121 (49)
86 (30)	85 (29)	87 (31)	88 (31)	89 (32)	91 (33)	93 (34)	95 (35)	97 (36)	100 (38)	102 (39)	105 (41)	108 (42)	112 (44)
84 (29)	83 (28)	84 (29)	85 (29)	86 (30)	88 (31)	89 (32)	90 (32)	92 (33)	94 (34)	96 (36)	98 (37)	100 (38)	103 (39)
82 (28)	81 (27)	82 (28)	83 (28)	84 (29)	84 (29)	85 (29)	86 (30)	88 (31)	89 (32)	90 (32)	91 (33)	93 (34)	95 (35)
80 (27)	80 (27)	80 (27)	81 (27)	81 (27)	82 (28)	82 (28)	83 (28)	84 (29)	84 (29)	85 (29)	86 (30)	86 (30)	87 (31)

Category	Heat index	Possible heat disorders for people in high risk groups
Extreme danger	130°F or higher (54°C or higher)	Heat stroke or sunstroke likely.
Danger	105 - 129°F (41 - 54°C)	Sunstroke, muscle cramps, and/or heat exhaustion likely. Heatstroke possible with prolonged exposure and/ or physical activity.
Extreme caution	90 - 105°F (32 - 41°C)	Sunstroke, muscle cramps, and/or heat exhaustion possible with prolonged exposure and/ or physical activity.
Caution	80 - 90°F (27 - 32°C)	Fatigue possible with prolonged exposure and/or physical activity.

Heat index reference chart provided by the National Weather Service, Tulsa, Oklahoma.
Note: Exposure to full sunshine can increase Heat Index values by up to 15°F

Figure 681-1 Heat stroke index. (From Jardine DS: Heat illness and heat stroke, *Pediatr Rev* 28:249–258, 2007.)

Water is adequate for most persons who exercise <1 hr, although there is evidence that children drink more water when it is flavored. Fluids with electrolyte and carbohydrate are more important for persons who exercise for >1 hr. Salt pills should not be used by most people because of their risk of causing hypernatremia and delayed gastric emptying. They may be useful in a person with a high sweat rate or recurrent heat cramps. Prolonged exercise (marathon running) with only water replacement places the athlete at risk of hyponatremia.

BIBLIOGRAPHY

Please visit the Nelson Textbook of Pediatrics *website at www.expertconsult.com for the complete bibliography.*

Chapter 682
Female Athletes: Menstrual Problems and the Risk of Osteopenia

Gregory L. Landry

Overtraining in young women can be associated with its effect on reproductive function and bone mineral status especially when combined with calorie restriction (Chapters 26 and 110).

The majority of bone mass is acquired by the end of the 2nd decade (Chapter 698). About 60-70% of adult bone mass is genetically determined, and the remaining is influenced by 3 controllable factors: exercise, calcium intake, and sex steroids, primarily estrogen. Exercise promotes bone mineralization in the majority of young women and is to be encouraged. In girls with eating disorders and those who exercise to the point of excessive weight loss with amenorrhea or oligomenorrhea, exercise can be detrimental to bone mineral acquisition, resulting in reduced bone mineral content, or **osteopenia.**

Specifically, bone mineralization is negatively affected by amenorrhea (absence of menstruation for ≥3 consecutive months). This may be influenced by abnormal eating patterns, or "disordered eating." When occurring together, disordered eating, amenorrhea, and osteoporosis form the **female athlete triad.** At health supervision visits and the preparticipation physical examination, special attention should be given to screening for any features of the triad.

Menstrual abnormalities (including **amenorrhea**) results from suppression of the spontaneous hypothalamic pulsatile secretion of gonadotropin-releasing hormone. It is believed that the amenorrhea results from reduced energy availability, defined as energy intake minus expenditure. Energy availability below a threshold of 30 kcal/kg/day lean body mass (LBM) is thought to result in menstrual disturbances. Negative energy balance also appears to lower levels of leptin, which affects both nutritional state and the reproductive system. Other causes to be ruled out are pregnancy, pituitary tumors, thyroid abnormalities, polycystic ovary syndrome, anabolic-androgenic steroid use, and other medication side effects.

The low estrogen state of amenorrhea predisposes the female athlete to osteopenia and puts her at risk for stress fractures, especially of the spine and lower extremity. If left unchecked, bone loss is partially irreversible despite resumed menses, estrogen replacement, or calcium supplements. Routine bone mineral density screening is not recommended but can help guide treatment and return to activity in severe cases.

Normal ovulation and menses can be recovered in athletes with amenorrhea. This usually involves decreasing exercise amount and/or increasing caloric intake. However, many athletes are resistant to decrease their training, and other methods, such as hormone supplementation, should be discussed. Nutritional counseling is important to help the athlete develop a plan for increasing calories. Calcium intake should be addressed, with the goal being at least 1,500 mg daily. If amenorrhea is present for ≥6 mo, hormone supplementation is recommended.

Three eating disorders can occur in the context of amenorrhea: anorexia nervosa, manifesting as weight <85% of estimated ideal body weight with evidence of starvation manifesting as bradycardia, hypothermia, and orthostatic hypotension or orthostatic tachycardia; bulimia nervosa, manifesting as reduced or normal weight with wider fluctuations of weight than would be expected based on the reported caloric intake and exercise; and eating disorder not otherwise specified, with some of the features of either anorexia or bulimia nervosa, yet not meeting all criteria from the *Diagnostic and Statistical Manual of Mental Disorders,* 4th edition, for diagnosis of either (Chapter 26). The third type of eating disorder is sometimes diagnosed as an atypical eating disorder. Multiple symptoms and methods can occur together, from unhealthy caloric or fat restriction to bingeing and purging. Clues to the problem are weight loss, food restriction, depression, fatigue and worsened athletic performance, and preoccupation with calories and weight. The athlete might avoid events surrounding food consumption or might hide and discard food. Signs and symptoms include fat depletion, muscle wasting, bradycardia worsened from baseline, orthostatic hypotension, constipation, cold intolerance, hypothermia, gastric motility problems, and, in some cases, lanugo. Electrolyte abnormalities can lead to cardiac dysrhythmias. Psychiatric problems (depression, anxiety, suicide risk) are of higher incidence in this population.

For **treatment** of eating disorders, control of the symptoms is a central theme. The first step is confronting the athlete about the abnormal behavior and unhealthy weight. Generally, exercise is not recommended if the body weight is <85% of estimated ideal body weight, although there are exceptions, especially if the athlete is eumenorrheic. If the athlete is unable to gain weight with nutrition and medical counseling alone, then psychologic consultation is sought.

Most athletes will not initially admit a problem, and many are unaware of the serious physical consequences. A helpful technique in talking to these athletes is to sensitively point out performance issues. Education about decreased strength, endurance, and concentration can be a motivating factor for treatment. Often, the athlete's family needs to be involved, and the athlete should be encouraged to reveal necessary information to them. Psychology or psychiatry referral is important in the multidisciplinary approach to treatment of disordered eating. It is important for the physician to monitor the athlete's physical health while the mental health professional is caring for the mental aspects of the eating disorder.

BIBLIOGRAPHY

Please visit the Nelson Textbook of Pediatrics *website at www.expertconsult.com for the complete bibliography.*

Chapter 683
Performance-Enhancing Aids

Gregory L. Landry

Performance-enhancing drugs have been used by athletes since at least since 776 BCE. Ergogenic aids are substances used for performance enhancement, most of which are unregulated supplements (Table 683-1). The 1994 Dietary Supplement and Health Education Act limited the ability of the U.S. Food and Drug Administration to regulate any product labeled as a supplement. Many agents have significant side effects without proven ergogenic properties. In 2005, the American Academy of Pediatrics published a policy statement strongly condemning their use in children and adolescents. The US 2004 Controlled Substance Act outlawed the purchase of steroidal supplements such as tetrahydrogestrione (THG), and androstenedione (Andro), with the exception of dehydroepiandrosterone (DHEA).

The prevalence of lifetime steroid use is highest among boys and in the USA (5.1%); The European School Survey Project on Alcohol and Other Drugs found that 1% of European youth reported any use of steroids. Trends indicate that use of steroids declined by half from 2006-2010. Steroids in oral, injectable, and skin cream form are taken in various patterns. *Cycling* describes taking multiple doses of steroids for a period, ceasing, and then starting again. *Stacking* refers to the use of different types of steroids in both oral and injectable forms. *Pyramiding* involves slowly increasing the steroid dose to a peak amount and then gradually tapering down.

Anabolic-androgenic steroids (**AAS**) have been used in supraphysiologic doses for their ability to increase muscle size and strength and decrease body fat. The evidence of increased muscle mass and strength is controversial but is supported by objective data. The effects appear to be related to the myotrophic action at androgen receptors as well as competitive antagonism at catabolism-mediating corticosteroid receptors. They have significant endocrinologic side effects, such as decreased sperm count and testicular atrophy in men and menstrual irregularities and virilization in women. Hepatic problems include elevated aminotransaminases and γ-glutamyl transferase, cholestatic jaundice, peliosis hepatitis, and a variety of tumors, including hepatocellular carcinoma. There is evidence that AAS might cause

Table 683-1 ERGOGENIC DRUGS

ERGOGENIC DRUG	CATEGORY	GOALS OF USE	ATHLETIC EFFECT	ADVERSE EFFECTS
Anabolic-androgenic steroids	Controlled substance	Gain muscle mass, strength	Increase muscle mass, strength	Multiple organ systems: infertility, gynecomastia, female virilization, hypertension, atherosclerosis, physeal closure, aggression, depression
Androstenedione	Controlled substance	Increase testosterone to gain muscle mass, strength	No measurable effect	Increase estrogens in men; overlaps systemic risks with steroids
Dehydroepiandrosterone (DHEA)	Nutritional supplement	Increase testosterone to gain muscle mass, strength	No measurable effect	Increase estrogens in men; impurities in preparation
Growth hormone	Controlled substance	Increase muscle mass, strength, and definition	Decreases subcutaneous fat; no performance effect	Acromegaly effects: increased lipids, myopathy, glucose intolerance, physeal closure
Creatine	Nutritional supplement	Gain muscle mass, strength	Increase muscle strength gains; performance benefit in short, anaerobic tasks	Dehydration, muscle cramps, gastrointestinal distress, compromised renal function
Ephedra alkaloids	Possibly returning as nutritional supplement	Increase weight loss, delay fatigue	Increases metabolism; no clear performance benefit	Cerebral vascular accident, arrhythmia, myocardial infarction, seizure, psychosis, hypertension, death

From Calfee R, Fadale P: Popular ergogenic drugs and supplements in young athletes, *Pediatrics* 117:e577–e589, 2006.

cardiovascular problems as well, including higher blood pressure, lower high-density lipoprotein, higher low-density lipoprotein, higher homocysteine, and decreased glucose tolerance. The psychologic effects include aggression, several personality disorders, and a variety of other psychologic problems (anxiety, paranoia, mania, depression, psychosis). Physical findings include gynecomastia, testicular shrinkage, jaundice, acne, and marked striae. Women can develop hirsutism, voice deepening, and male-pattern baldness.

Testosterone precursors (also known as *prohormones*) include androstenedione and DHEA. Their use in the adolescent population has increased markedly in conjunction with reports of high-profile athletes' use. They are androgenic but have not been proved to be anabolic. If they are anabolic at all, they work by increasing the production of testosterone. They also increase production of estrogenic metabolites. The side effects are similar to those of AAS and far outweigh any ergogenic benefit. Since January 2005, these substances cannot be sold without prescription.

Creatine is an amino acid mostly stored in skeletal muscle. Its key feature is ability to rephosphorylate adenosine diphosphate to adenosine triphosphate, therefore increasing muscle performance. Its use has increased, especially since other supplements have been withdrawn from the market. Thirty percent of high school football players have used creatine. There is evidence that creatine, as a source of increased energy, enhances strength and maximal exercise performance when used during training. There is no evidence that creatine affects hydration or temperature regulation. Concerns about nephritis in case reports have not been supported by controlled studies. However, there are few long-term studies evaluating creatine use.

BIBLIOGRAPHY

Please visit the Nelson Textbook of Pediatrics *website at* *www.expertconsult.com* *for the complete bibliography.*

Chapter 684
Specific Sports and Associated Injuries

Gregory L. Landry

GYMNASTICS

Gymnastics participants are beginning the sport at 5-6 yr of age and achieving the highest level of competition in the mid-teens, often retiring by age 20 yr. Boys tend to have more upper extremity injuries, and girls have more lower extremity injuries. In addition to mechanical or traumatic injuries, female gymnasts tend to have delayed menarche and can have hypothalamic amenorrhea or oligomenorrhea, associated with low body weight. The typical body habitus of the elite gymnast manifest as reduced weight for height, coupled with amenorrhea or oligomenorrhea, suggests that reduced bone density is a problem for female gymnasts. In most gymnasts, bone density tends to be high. It is speculated that this is secondary to the repetitive high-impact activities. In spite of this increased bone density, stress fractures are a significant problem. The short stature associated with male and female gymnasts is probably caused by selection bias and not the result of gymnastics training.

Common problems include acute traumatic injuries, such as an ankle sprain, and chronic overuse injuries, such as wrist and spine stress fractures. The incidence of injury increases with the level of skill and is greatest in the floor exercise. Wrist pain due to chronic upper extremity weight bearing can be caused by a distal radial stress Salter I fracture, which typically occurs on the radial dorsal aspect of the wrist and is worsened by passive extension and palpation. Other wrist injuries include triangular fibrocartilage complex tears, scaphoid fractures, dorsal ganglions, and carpal ligament injuries.

Treatment in almost all cases involves immobilization for some period, application of ice, and administration of analgesic drugs. If pain persists, the correct diagnosis can be made by MRI or arthroscopic examination to rule out intra-articular tears, loose bodies, or ligamentous instability. The pediatrician should have a low threshold for referral to a hand specialist in a wrist injury that is not improving with rest. Ligamentous laxity can predispose to elbow or shoulder dislocation and ankle sprains. Spine problems include spondylolysis (pars interarticularis stress fracture) and spondylolisthesis (Chapter 671.6) due to repetitive extension loading.

For the full continuation of this chapter, please visit the Nelson Textbook of Pediatrics *website at* *www.expertconsult.com*.

Section 3 THE SKELETAL DYSPLASIAS

Chapter 685
General Considerations

William A. Horton and Jacqueline T. Hecht

The genetically and clinically heterogeneous group of disorders of skeletal development and growth are referred to as **skeletal dysplasias, bone dysplasias,** and **osteochondrodysplasias**. Their prevalence is estimated to be about 1/4,000 births. They can be divided into the osteodysplasias typified by osteogenesis imperfecta (Chapter 692) and the chondrodysplasias. The latter result from mutations of genes that are essential for skeletal development and growth. The clinical picture is dominated by skeletal abnormalities. The manifestations may be restricted to the skeleton, but in most cases nonskeletal tissues are also involved. The disorders may be lethal in utero or mild with features that go undetected.

For the full continuation of this chapter, please visit the Nelson Textbook of Pediatrics *website at* *www.expertconsult.com*.

Chapter 686
Disorders Involving Cartilage Matrix Proteins

William A. Horton and Jacqueline T. Hecht

Functional disturbances of cartilage matrix proteins result in several bone and joint disorders. They fall into five groups corresponding primarily to the defective proteins: three collagens and the noncollagenous proteins COMP (cartilage oligomeric matrix protein), matrilin 3, and aggrecan. The clinical phenotypes differ between and within the groups, especially the spondyloepiphyseal dysplasia (SED) group. In some groups, there is substantial variation in clinical severity.

SPONDYLOEPIPHYSEAL DYSPLASIAS

The term *spondyloepiphyseal dysplasia* refers to a heterogeneous group of disorders characterized by shortening of the trunk and, to a lesser extent, the limbs. Severity ranges from achondrogenesis type II to the slightly less severe hypochondrogenesis (these two types are lethal in the perinatal period) to SED congenita and its variants, including Kniest dysplasia (which are apparent at birth and are usually nonlethal), to late-onset SED (which might not be detected until adolescence or later). The radiographic hallmarks are abnormal development of the vertebral bodies and of epiphyses, the extent of which corresponds to the clinical severity. Most of the SEDs result from heterozygous mutations of *COL2A1;* they are autosomal dominant disorders. The mutations are dispersed throughout the gene; there is a poor correlation between the mutation's location and the resultant clinical phenotype. For familial cases, prenatal diagnosis is possible if the mutation is identified. Schimke immuno-osseous dysplasia may be an exception because it is an autosomal recessive disorder characterized by short stature, hyperpigmented macules, unusual facies, proteinuria and progressive renal failure, cerebral ischemia, and a T-cell defect with lymphopenia and recurrent infections.

Lethal Spondyloepiphyseal Dysplasias

Achondrogenesis type II (OMIM 200610) is characterized by severe shortening of the neck and trunk and especially the limbs and by a large, soft head. Fetal hydrops and prematurity are common; infants are stillborn or die shortly after birth. Hypochondrogenesis (OMIM 200610) refers to a clinical phenotype intermediate between achondrogenesis type II and SED congenita. It is typically lethal in the newborn period.

The severity of radiographic changes correlates with the clinical severity (Fig. 686-1). Both conditions produce short, broad tubular bones with cupped metaphyses. The pelvic bones are hypoplastic, and the cranial bones are not well mineralized. The vertebral bodies are poorly ossified in the entire spine in achondrogenesis type II and in the cervical and sacral spine in hypochondrogenesis. The pedicles are ossified in both.

Spondyloepiphyseal Dysplasia Congenita

The phenotype of this group, SED congenita (OMIM 183900), is apparent at birth. The head and face are usually normal, but a cleft palate is common. The neck is short and the chest is barrel shaped (Fig. 686-2). Kyphosis and exaggeration of the normal lumbar lordosis are common. The proximal segments of the limbs are shorter than the hands and feet, which often appear normal. Some infants have clubfoot or exhibit hypotonia.

Skeletal radiographs of the newborn reveal short tubular bones, delayed ossification of vertebral bodies, and proximal limb bone epiphyses (Fig. 686-3). Hypoplasia of the odontoid

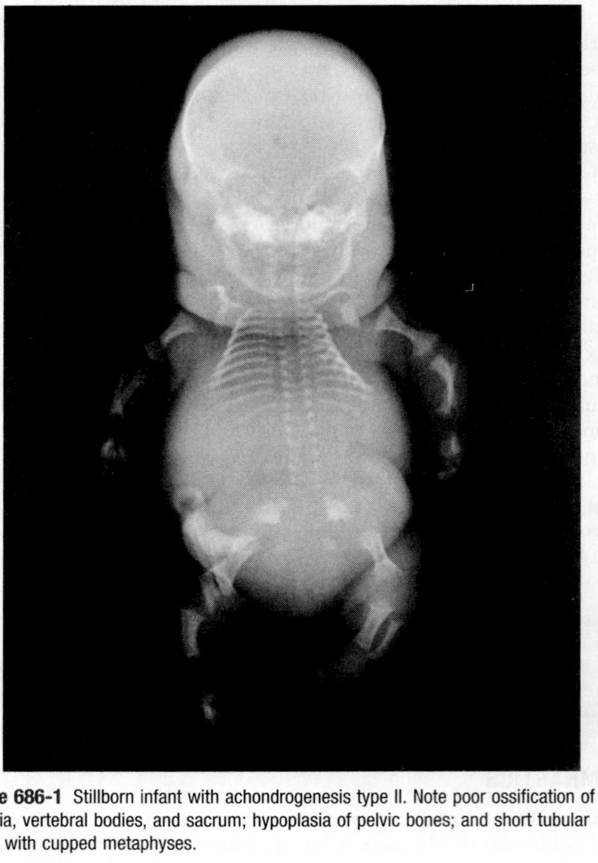

Figure 686-1 Stillborn infant with achondrogenesis type II. Note poor ossification of calvaria, vertebral bodies, and sacrum; hypoplasia of pelvic bones; and short tubular bones with cupped metaphyses.

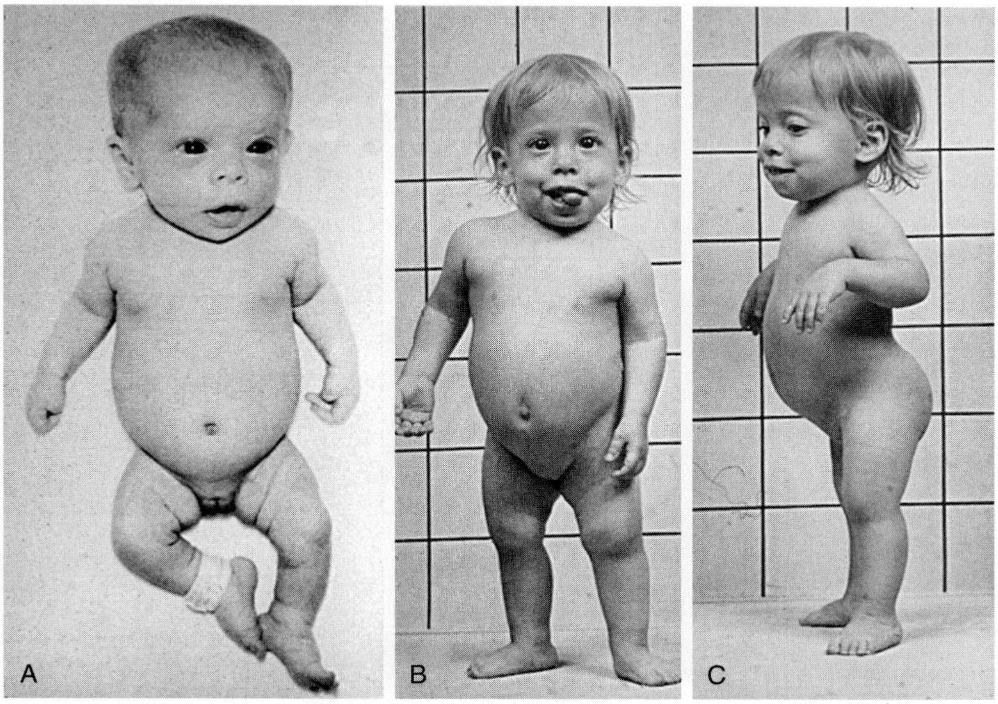

Figure 686-2 Spondyloepiphyseal dysplasia congenita is shown in infancy *(A)* and early childhood *(B, C)*. Note the short extremities, relatively normal hands, flat facies, and exaggerated lordosis.

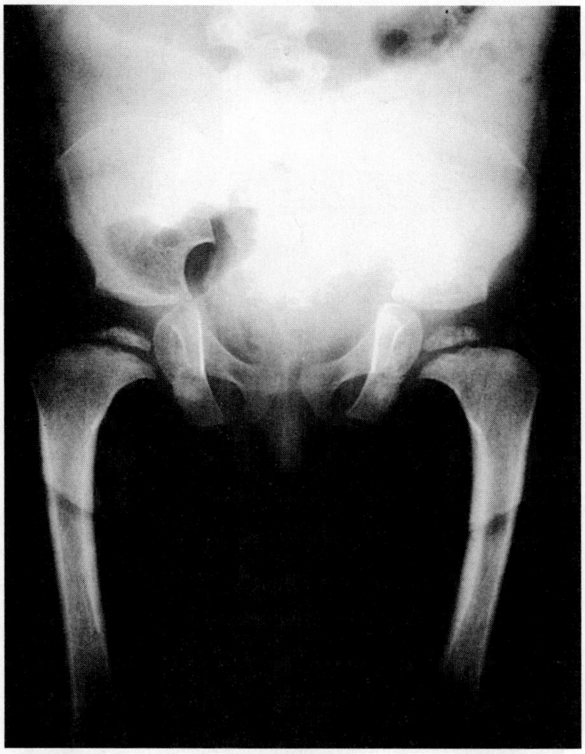

Figure 686-3 Radiograph of spondyloepiphyseal dysplasia congenita pelvis demonstrating squared pelvis, hypoplastic capital femoral epiphyses, and femoral necks that are wide and short.

process, a short, square pelvis with a poorly ossified symphysis pubis, and mild irregularity of metaphyses are apparent.

Infants usually have normal developmental milestones; a waddling gait typically appears in early childhood. Childhood complications include respiratory compromise from spinal deformities and spinal cord compression due to cervicomedullary instability. The disproportion and shortening become progressively worse with age, and adult heights range from 95 to 128 cm. Myopia is typical; adults are predisposed to retinal detachment. Precocious osteoarthritis occurs in adulthood and requires surgical joint replacement.

KNIEST DYSPLASIA

The Kniest dysplasia variant of SED (OMIM 156550) manifests at birth with a short trunk and limbs associated with a flat face, prominent eyes, enlarged joints, cleft palate, and clubfoot. Radiographs show vertebral defects and short tubular bones with epiphyseal irregularities and metaphyseal enlargement that gives rise to a dumbbell appearance.

Motor development is often delayed because of the joint deformities, although intelligence is normal. Hearing loss and myopia commonly develop during childhood, and retinal detachment can occur as a late complication. Joint enlargement progresses during childhood and becomes painful; it is accompanied by flexion contractures and muscle atrophy, which may be incapacitating by adolescence.

LATE-ONSET SPONDYLOEPIPHYSEAL DYSPLASIA

Late-onset spondyloepiphyseal dysplasia is a mild to very mild clinical phenotype characterized by slightly short stature associated with mild epiphyseal and vertebral abnormalities on radiographs. It is typically detected during childhood or adolescence but can go unrecognized until adulthood when precocious osteoarthritis appears. This designation is nosologically distinct from SED tarda, which is clinically similar but results from mutation of the X-linked gene *SEDL*.

AGGRECAN-RELATED SPONDYLOEPIPHYSEAL DYSPLASIAS

Mutations of aggrecan have been detected in two SED-like conditions. SED-Kimberley is relatively mild, with short stature, stocky build, and early onset osteoarthritis of weight-bearing joints. A more severe and generalized clinical phenotype with characteristic radiographic changes including widened metaphyses is observed in SEMD-Aggrecan type.

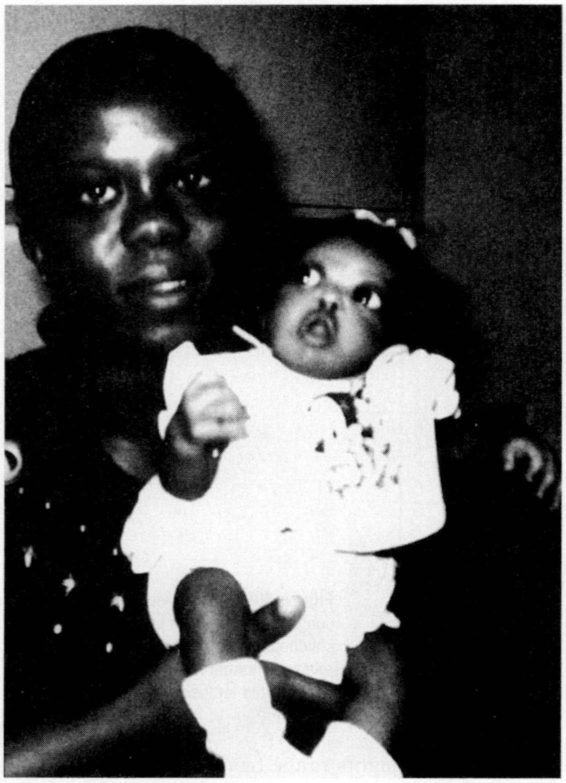

Figure 686-4 Stickler syndrome in mother and child. The facies are flat and the eyes are prominent.

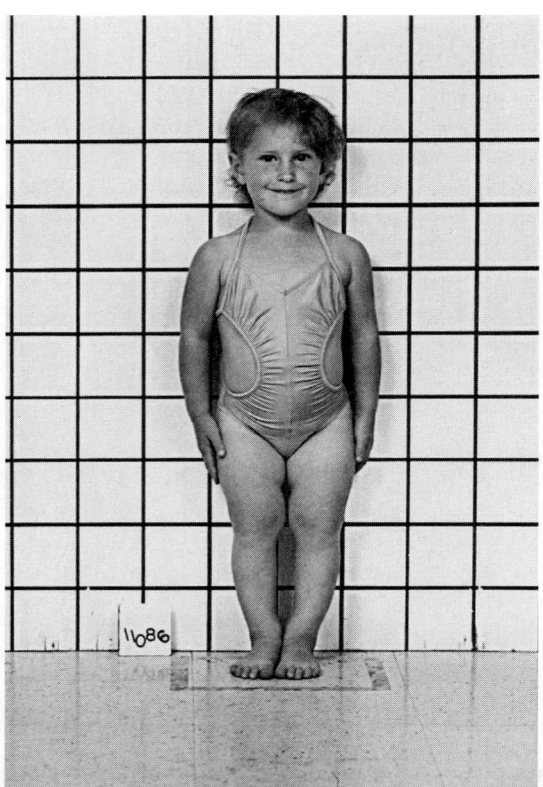

Figure 686-5 Female patient with metaphyseal dysplasia, type Schmid. The facies are normal and stature is mildly reduced. Mild tibia vara is present.

STICKLER DYSPLASIA (HEREDITARY OSTEOARTHRO-OPHTHALMOPATHY)

Short stature is not a feature of Stickler dysplasia (OMIM 184840). It resembles SED because of its joint and eye manifestations. Mutations of genes encoding type XI collagen, which functionally interacts with type II collagen, have been identified in Stickler-like disorders (OMIM 184840, OMIM 215150). Stickler dysplasia is often identified in the newborn because of cleft palate and micrognathia (Pierre Robin anomaly, Chapter 303). Infants typically have severe myopia and additional ophthalmologic complications, including choroidoretinal and vitreous degeneration; retinal detachment is common during childhood (Fig. 686-4). Sensorineural hearing loss can arise during adolescence, which is when symptoms of osteoarthritis can also begin. Special attention must be given to the eye complications even in childhood.

SCHMID METAPHYSEAL DYSPLASIA

Schmid metaphyseal dysplasia (OMIM 156500) is one of several chondrodysplasias in which metaphyseal abnormalities dominate the radiographic features. It typically manifests in early childhood with mild short stature, bowing of the legs, and a waddling gait (Fig. 686-5). Joints, such as the wrist, may be enlarged. Radiographs show flaring and irregular mineralization of the metaphyses of tubular bones of the proximal limbs (Fig. 686-6). Coxa vara is usually present and can require surgical correction. Short stature becomes more evident with age and affects the lower extremities more than the upper extremities; the manifestations are limited to the skeleton.

Schmid metaphyseal chondrodysplasia is due to heterozygous mutations of the gene encoding type X collagen; it is an autosomal dominant trait. The distribution of type X collagen is restricted to the region of growing bone in which cartilage is

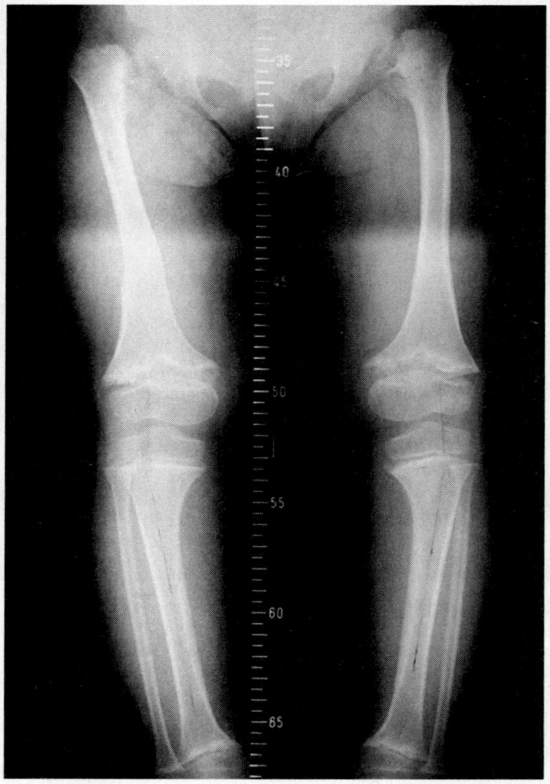

Figure 686-6 Radiograph of lower extremities in Schmid metaphyseal dysplasia showing short tubular bones and metaphyseal flaring and irregularities, abnormal capital femoral epiphyses, and femoral necks. The epiphyses are normal. Coxa vara is present.

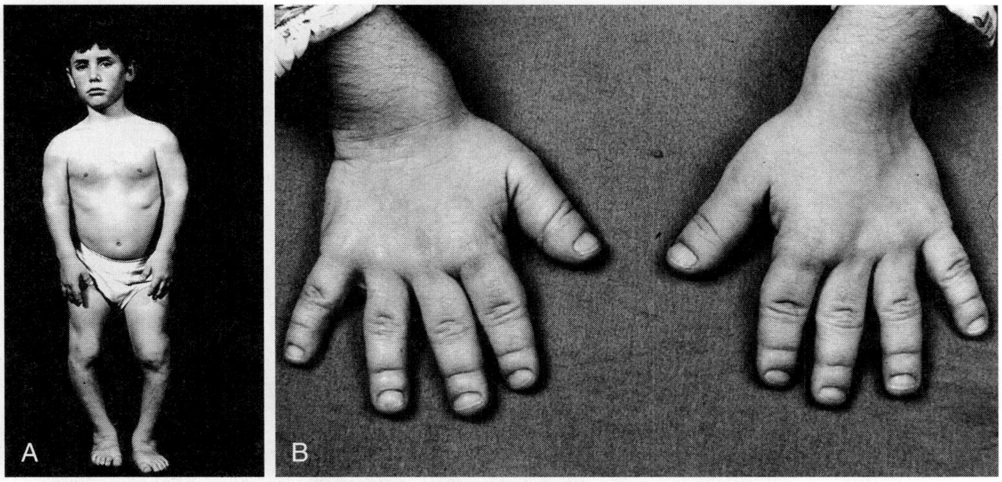

Figure 686-7 *A,* Pseudoachondroplasia in an adolescent boy. The facies and head circumference are normal. There is shortening of all extremities and bowing of the lower extremities. *B,* Photograph of hands, demonstrating short stubby fingers.

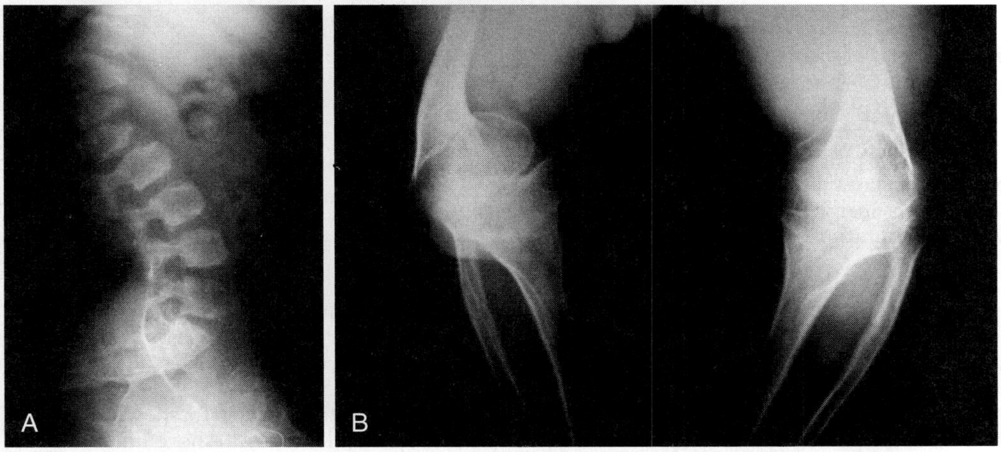

Figure 686-8 *A,* Lateral thoracolumbar spine radiograph of a patient with pseudoachondroplasia showing central protrusion (tonguing) of the anterior aspect of upper lumbar and lower thoracic vertebrae. Note reduced vertebral body heights (platyspondyly) and secondary lordosis. *B,* Lower extremity radiograph of patient with pseudoachondroplasia showing large metaphyses, poorly formed epiphyses, and marked bowing of the long bones.

converted into bone. This might explain why radiographic changes are confined to the metaphyses.

PSEUDOACHONDROPLASIA AND MULTIPLE EPIPHYSEAL DYSPLASIA

Pseudoachondroplasia (OMIM 177170) and multiple epiphyseal dysplasia (MED) (OMIM 600969) are two distinct phenotypes that are grouped together because they result from mutations of the gene encoding COMP. The mutations are heterozygous in both; they are autosomal dominant traits. The clinical phenotypes are restricted to skeletal tissues.

Newborns with pseudoachondroplasia are average in size and appearance. Gait abnormalities and short stature mainly affect the limbs and become apparent in late infancy. The short stature becomes marked as the child grows and is associated with generalized joint laxity (Fig. 686-7). The hands are short, broad, and deviated in an ulnar direction; the forearms are bowed. Developmental milestones and intelligence are usually normal. Lumbar lordosis and deformities of the knee develop during childhood; the latter often requires surgical correction. Pain is common in weight-bearing joints during childhood and adolescence, and osteoarthritis develops late in the 2nd decade of life. Adults range in height from 105 to 128 cm.

Skeletal radiographs show distinctive abnormalities of vertebral bodies and of both epiphyses and metaphyses of tubular bones (Fig. 686-8).

The MED phenotype has skeletal abnormalities that predominantly affect the epiphyses as noted on radiographs. Two classic forms are a severe Fairbank type and a mild Ribbing type. Because of overlap in clinical features and because COMP mutations are found in both types, they may be considered clinical variants.

The more severe clinical phenotype has its onset during childhood, with mild short-limbed short stature, pain in weight-bearing joints, and a waddling gait. Radiographs show delayed and irregular ossification of epiphyses. In more mildly affected patients the disorder might not be recognized until adolescence or adulthood. Radiographic changes may be limited to the capital femoral epiphyses. In the latter case, mild MED must be distinguished from bilateral Legg-Calvé-Perthes disease (Chapter 670.3). Precocious osteoarthritis of hips and knees is the major complication in adults with MED. Adult heights range from 136 to 151 cm.

There are families with clinical and radiographic manifestations of MED that are not due to mutations of COMP. Some are linked to the gene encoding one of the type IX collagen chains. It has been suggested that COMP and type IX collagen interact functionally in cartilage matrix, thus explaining why mutations of different genes produce similar pictures. Mutations of the genes coding for another cartilage matrix protein, matrilin 3, and the diastrophic dysplasia sulfate transporter have also been found in patients with MED. For familial cases of pseudoachondroplasia and MED resulting from mutation in COMP, prenatal diagnosis is available.

BIBLIOGRAPHY

Please visit the Nelson Textbook of Pediatrics *website at www.expertconsult.com for the complete bibliography.*

Chapter 687
Disorders Involving Transmembrane Receptors

William A. Horton and Jacqueline T. Hecht

Disorders involving transmembrane receptors result from heterozygous mutations of genes encoding *FGFR3* (fibroblast growth factor receptor 3) and *PTHR* (parathyroid hormone receptor). The mutations cause the receptors to become activated in the absence of physiologic ligands, which accentuates normal receptor function of negatively regulating bone growth. The mutations act by gain of negative function. In the *FGFR3* mutation group, in which the clinical phenotypes range from severe to mild, the severity appears to correlate with the extent to which the receptor is activated. *PTHR* and especially *FGFR3* mutations tend to recur in unrelated individuals.

ACHONDROPLASIA GROUP

The achondroplasia group represents a substantial percentage of patients with chondrodysplasias and contains thanatophoric dysplasia (TD), the most common lethal chondrodysplasia, with a birth prevalence of 1/35,000 births; achondroplasia, the most common nonlethal chondrodysplasia, with a birth prevalence of 1/15,000 to 1/40,000 births; and hypochondroplasia. All three have mutations in a small number of locations in the *FGFR3* gene. There is a strong correlation between the mutation site and the clinical phenotype.

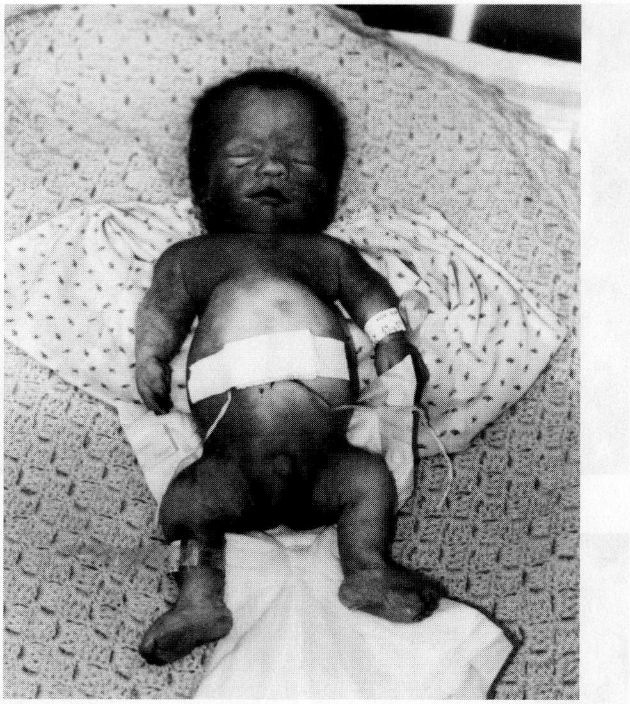

Figure 687-1 Stillborn infant with thanatophoric dysplasia. Limbs are very short, with upper limbs extending only two thirds of the way down the abdomen. The chest is narrow, exaggerating the protuberance of the abdomen. The head is relatively large.

Thanatophoric Dysplasia

TD (OMIM 187600, 187610) manifests before or at birth. In the former situation, ultrasonographic examination in midgestation or later reveals a large head and very short limbs; the pregnancy is often accompanied by polyhydramnios and premature delivery. Very short limbs, short neck, long narrow thorax, and large head with midfacial hypoplasia dominate the clinical phenotype at birth (Fig. 687-1). The cloverleaf skull deformity known as **kleeblattschädel** is sometimes found. Newborns have severe respiratory distress because of their small thorax. Although this distress can be treated by intense respiratory care, the long-term prognosis is poor.

Skeletal radiographs distinguish two slightly different forms called TD I and TD II. In the more common TD I, radiographs show large calvariae with a small cranial base, marked thinning and flattening of vertebral bodies visualized best on lateral view, very short ribs, severe hypoplasia of pelvic bones, and very short and bowed tubular bones with flared metaphyses (Fig. 687-2). The femurs are curved and shaped like a telephone receiver. TD II differs mainly in that there are longer and straighter femurs.

The TD II clinical phenotype is associated with mutations that map to codon 650 of *FGFR3*, causing the substitution of a glutamic acid for the lysine. This activates the tyrosine kinase activity of a receptor that transmits signals to intracellular pathways. Mutation of lysine 650 to methionine is associated with a clinical phenotype intermediate between TD and achondroplasia, referred to as severe achondroplasia with developmental delay and acanthosis nigricans (SADDAN). Mutations of the TD I phenotype map mainly to two regions in the extracellular domain of the receptor, where they substitute cysteine residues for other amino acids. Free cysteine residues are thought to form disulfide bonds promoting dimerization of receptor molecules, leading to activation and signal transmission.

TD I and TD II represent new mutations to normal parents. The recurrence risk is low. Because the mutated codons in TD are mutable for unknown reasons and because of the theoretical risk of germ cell mosaicism, parents are offered prenatal diagnosis for subsequent pregnancies.

Achondroplasia

Achondroplasia (OMIM 100800) is the prototype chondrodysplasia. It typically manifests at birth with short limbs, a long narrow trunk, and a large head with midfacial hypoplasia and prominent forehead (Fig. 687-3). The limb shortening is greatest in the proximal segments, and the fingers often display a trident configuration. Most joints are hyperextensible, but extension is restricted at the elbow. A thoracolumbar gibbus is often found. Usually, birth length is slightly less than normal but occasionally plots within the low-normal range.

DIAGNOSIS Skeletal radiographs confirm the diagnosis (Figs. 687-3 and 687-4). The calvarial bones are large, whereas the cranial base and facial bones are small. The vertebral pedicles are short throughout the spine as noted on a lateral radiograph. The interpedicular distance, which normally increases from the 1st to the 5th lumbar vertebra, decreases in achondroplasia. The iliac bones are short and round, and the acetabular roofs are flat. The tubular bones are short with mildly irregular and flared metaphyses. The fibula is disproportionately long compared with the tibia.

CLINICAL MANIFESTATIONS Infants usually exhibit delayed motor milestones, often not walking alone until 18-24 mo. This is due to hypotonia and mechanical difficulty balancing the large head on a normal-sized trunk and short extremities. Intelligence is normal unless central nervous system complications develop. As the child begins to walk, the gibbus usually gives way to an exaggerated lumbar lordosis.

Infants and children with achondroplasia progressively fall below normal standards for length and height. They can be plotted against standards established for achondroplasia. Adult heights typically are 118-145 cm for men and 112-136 cm for women. Surgical limb lengthening and human growth hormone treatment have been used to increase height; both are controversial.

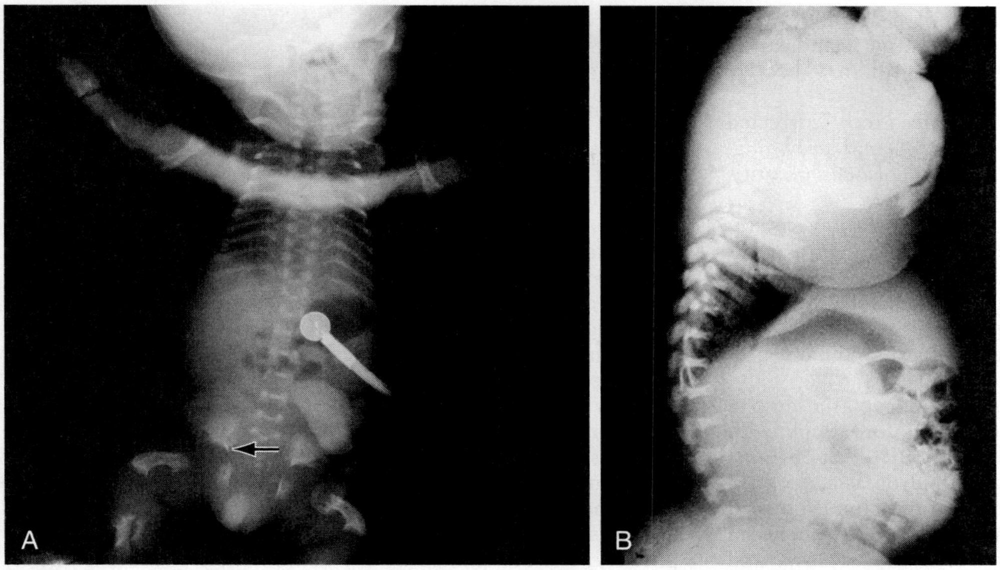

Figure 687-2 *A*, Neonatal radiograph of a child with thanatophoric dysplasia. Note medial acetabular spurs (*arrow*), hypoplastic iliac bones, bowed femora with rounded protrusion of proximal femurs, hypoplastic thorax, and wafer-thin vertebral bodies. *B*, Lateral radiograph of the thoracolumbar spine in thanatophoric dysplasia, showing marked vertebral flattening and short ribs. Ossification defect of the central portion of the vertebral bodies is present.

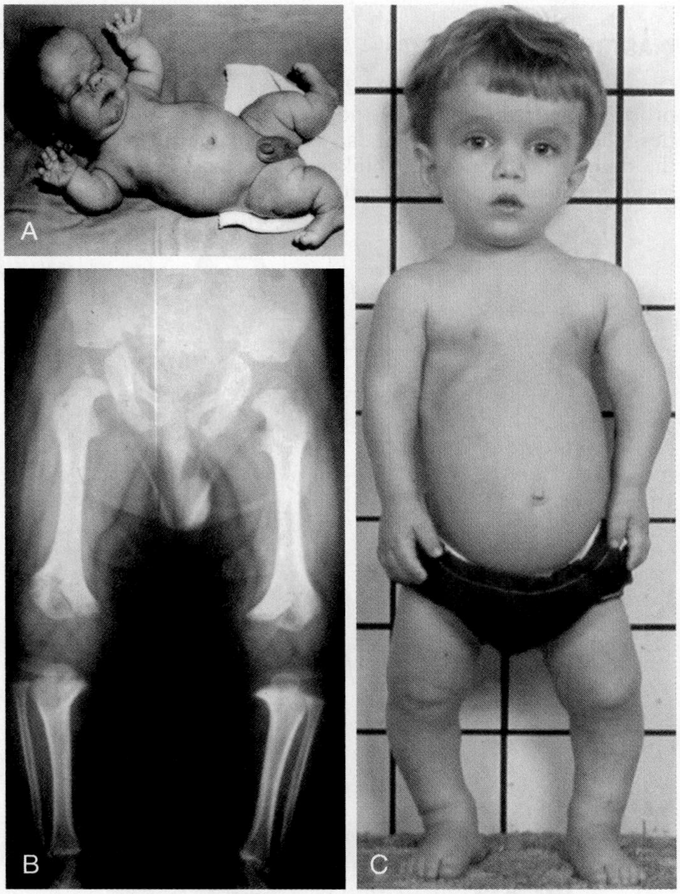

Figure 687-3 Achondroplasia phenotype at different ages. *A*, Infant with achondroplasia with macrocephaly, frontal bossing, midface hypoplasia, small chest, rhizomelic shortening of all the limbs, redundant skin folds, and extreme joint laxity. Note the trident hand with short fingers and abducted hips. *B*, Typical radiographic findings from a child with achondroplasia. All of the tubular bones are short, but the fibula is relatively long compared to the tibia. There is protrusion of the epiphysis into the metaphysis of the distal femur, creating the chevron deformity, and to a lesser extent of the proximal tibia. The iliac bones are rounded, the acetabular roof is horizontal, and the sacrosciatic notches are small. *C*, A 3 yr old with achondroplasia with the typical features shown in *A*. Note that the redundant skin folds are no longer present and that joint laxity has improved. Rhizomelic shortening of the extremities is more pronounced and accompanied by tibial bowing. (From Horton WA, Hall JG, Hecht JT: Achondroplasia, *Lancet* 370:162–172, 2007.)

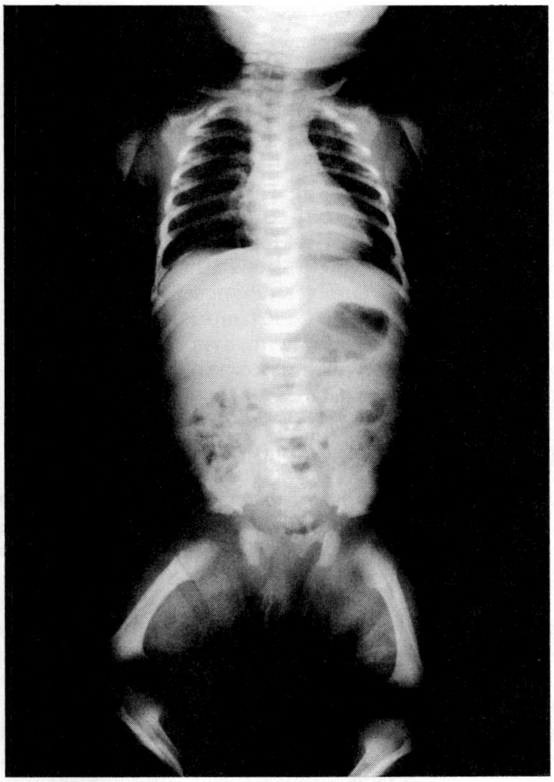

Figure 687-4 Radiograph of infant with achondroplasia, demonstrating interpedicular narrowing of the 1st through 5th lumbar vertebrae, short round iliac bones, and flat acetabular roofs. The tubular bones are short and show mild irregularities of the metaphyses.

Virtually all infants and children with achondroplasia have large heads, although only a fraction have true hydrocephalus. Head circumference should be carefully monitored using standards developed for achondroplasia, as should neurologic function in general. The spinal canal is stenotic, and spinal cord compression can occur at the foramen magnum and in the lumbar spine. The former usually occurs in infants and small children; it may be associated with hypotonia, failure to thrive, quadriparesis, central and obstructive apnea, and sudden death. Surgical correction may be required for severe stenosis. Lumbar spinal stenosis usually does not occur until early adulthood. Symptoms include paresthesias, numbness, and claudication in the legs. Loss of bladder and bowel control may be late complications.

Bowing of the legs is common and might need to be corrected surgically. Other common problems include dental crowding, articulation difficulties, obesity, and frequent episodes of otitis media, which can contribute to hearing loss.

GENETICS All patients with typical achondroplasia have mutations at *FGFR3* codon 380. The mutation maps to the transmembrane domain of the receptor and is thought to stabilize receptor dimers that enhance receptor signals, the consequences of which inhibit linear bone growth. Achondroplasia behaves as an autosomal dominant trait; most cases arise from a new mutation to normal parents.

Because of the high frequency of achondroplasia among dwarfing conditions, it is relatively common for adults with achondroplasia to marry. Such couples have a 50% risk of transmitting their condition, heterozygous achondroplasia, to each offspring, as well as a 25% risk of **homozygous achondroplasia.** The latter condition exhibits intermediate severity between thanatophoric dysplasia and heterozygous achondroplasia and is usually lethal in the newborn period. Prenatal diagnosis is available and has been used to diagnose homozygous achondroplasia.

Hypochondroplasia

Hypochondroplasia (OMIM 146000) resembles achondroplasia but is milder. Usually, it is not apparent until childhood, when mild short stature affecting the limbs becomes evident. Children have a stocky build and slight frontal bossing of the head. Learning disabilities may be more common in this condition. Radiographic changes are mild and consistent with the mild achondroplastic phenotype. Complications are rare; in some patients the condition is never diagnosed. Adult heights range from 116 to 146 cm. An *FGFR3* mutation at codon 540 has been found in many patients with hypochondroplasia. Genetic heterogeneity exists in hypochondroplasia, and other genetic loci are expected to be identified.

JANSEN METAPHYSEAL DYSPLASIA

Jansen metaphyseal chondrodysplasia (OMIM 156400) is a rare, dominantly inherited chondrodysplasia characterized by severe shortening of limbs associated with an unusual facial appearance. Sometimes it is accompanied by clubfoot and hypercalcemia. At birth, a diagnosis can be made from these clinical findings and radiographs that show short tubular bones with characteristic metaphyseal abnormalities that include flaring, irregular mineralization, fragmentation, and widening of the physeal space. The epiphyses are normal.

The joints become enlarged and limited in mobility with age. Flexion contractures develop at the knees and hips, producing a bent-over posture. Intelligence is normal, although there may be hearing loss.

Jansen metaphyseal chondrodysplasia is caused by activating mutations of *PTHR1*. This G protein–coupled transmembrane receptor serves as a receptor for both PTH and PTHrP. Signaling through this receptor serves as a brake on the terminal differentiation of cartilage cells at a critical step in bone growth. Because the mutations activate the receptor, they enhance the braking effect and thereby slow bone growth. Loss of function mutations of *PTHR1* are observed in Blomstrand chondrodysplasia, whose clinical features are the mirror image of Jansen metaphyseal chondrodysplasia.

BIBLIOGRAPHY

Please visit the Nelson Textbook of Pediatrics *website at* *www.expertconsult.com* *for the complete bibliography.*

Chapter 688
Disorders Involving Ion Transporters

William A. Horton and Jacqueline T. Hecht

In order of decreasing severity, the disorders involving ion transporters include achondrogenesis type 1B, atelosteogenesis type II, and diastrophic dysplasia. They result from the functional loss of the sulfate ion transporter called *diastrophic dysplasia sulfate transporter* (DTDST), which is also referred to as *SLC26A2* (solute carrier family 26, member 2). This protein transports sulfate ions into cells and is important for cartilage cells that add sulfate moieties to newly synthesized proteoglycans destined for cartilage extracellular matrix. Matrix proteoglycans are responsible for many of the properties of cartilage that allow it to serve as a template for skeletal development. The clinical manifestations result from defective sulfation of cartilage proteoglycans.

A number of mutant alleles have been found for the *DTDST* gene; they variably disturb transporter function. The disorders are recessive traits requiring the presence of 2 mutant alleles. The phenotype is determined by the combination of mutant alleles; some alleles are present in more than one disorder.

DIASTROPHIC DYSPLASIA

Diastrophic dysplasia (OMIM 22600) is a well-characterized disorder recognized at birth by the presence of very short extremities, clubfoot, and short hands, with proximal displacement of the thumb producing a hitchhiker appearance (Fig. 688-1). The hands are usually deviated in an ulnar direction. Bony fusion of

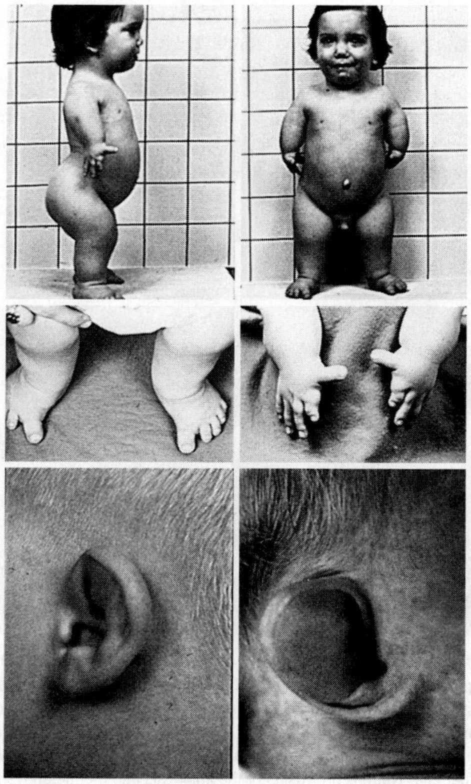

Figure 688-1 Child with diastrophic dysplasia. The extremities are dramatically shortened (*top*). Clubfoot is commonly observed (*middle left*). The fingers are short, especially the index finger; the thumb characteristically is proximally placed and has a hitchhiker appearance (*middle right*). The upper helix of the ears becomes swollen 3-4 wk postnatally (*lower left*), and this inflammation spontaneously resolves, leaving a cauliflower deformity of the pinnae (*lower right*).

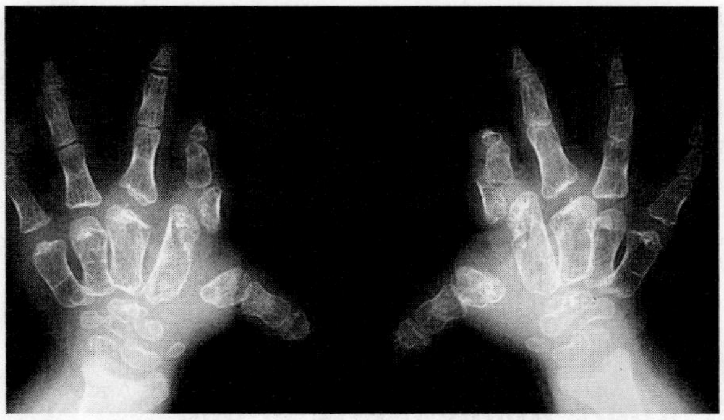

Figure 688-2 Radiograph of hands in diastrophic dysplasia. The metacarpals and phalanges are irregular and short. The first metacarpal is ovoid.

the metacarpophalangeal joints (symphalangism) is common, as is restricted movement of many joints, including hips, knees, and elbows. The external ears often become inflamed soon after birth. The inflammation resolves spontaneously but leaves the ears fibrotic and contracted (cauliflower ear deformity). Many newborns have a cleft palate.

Radiographs reveal short and broad tubular bones with flared metaphyses and flat, irregular epiphyses (Fig. 688-2).

The capital femoral epiphyses are hypoplastic, and the femoral heads are broad. The ulnas and fibulas are disproportionately short. Carpal centers may be developmentally advanced; the first metacarpal is typically ovoid, and the metatarsals are twisted medially. There may be vertebral abnormalities, including clefts of cervical vertebral lamina and narrowing of the interpedicular distances in the lumbar spine.

Complications are primarily orthopedic and tend to be severe and progressive. The clubfoot deformity in the newborn resists usual treatments, and multiple corrective surgeries are common. Scoliosis typically develops during early childhood. It often requires multiple surgical procedures to control, and it sometimes compromises respiratory function in older children. Despite the orthopedic problems, patients typically have a normal life span and reach adult heights in the 105-130 cm range, depending on the severity of scoliosis. Growth curves are available for diastrophic dysplasia.

Some patients are mildly affected and exhibit slight short stature and joint contractures, no clubfoot or cleft palate, and correspondingly mild radiographic changes. The mild phenotype tends to recur within families. The recurrence risk of this autosomal recessive condition is 25%. Ultrasonographic examination can be employed for prenatal diagnosis, but if *DTDST* mutations can be identified in the patients or parents, molecular genetic diagnosis is possible.

ACHONDROGENESIS TYPE 1B AND ATELOSTEOGENESIS TYPE II

Achondrogenesis type 1B (OMIM 600972) and atelosteogenesis type II (OMIM 256050) are rare recessive lethal chondrodysplasias. The most serious is achondrogenesis type 1B, which demonstrates a severe lack of skeletal development usually detected in utero or after a miscarriage. The limbs are extremely short, and the head is soft. Skeletal radiographs show poor to missing ossification of skull bones, vertebral bodies, fibulas, and ankle bones. The pelvis is hypoplastic, and the ribs are short. The femurs are short and exhibit a trapezoid shape with irregular metaphyses.

Infants with atelosteogenesis type II are stillborn or die soon after birth; prematurity is common. They exhibit very short limbs, especially the proximal segments. Clubfoot and dislocations of the elbows and knees may be detected. Hypoplasia of vertebral bodies, especially in the cervical and lumbar spine, is found on radiographs. The femora and humeri are hypoplastic and display a club-shaped appearance. The distal limb bones, including the ulna and fibula, are poorly ossified.

Both disorders carry a 25% recurrence risk and are potentially detectable in utero by mutation analysis if the mutant alleles are identified in the parents. Prenatal diagnosis is possible with fetal imaging.

BIBLIOGRAPHY

Please visit the Nelson Textbook of Pediatrics *website at* *www.expertconsult.com* *for the complete bibliography.*

Chapter 689 Disorders Involving Transcription Factors

William A. Horton and Jacqueline T. Hecht

There are three disorders involving transcription factors that result in bone dysplasias. One, campomelic dysplasia, is historically considered a chondrodysplasia. The other two, cleidocranial dysplasia and nail-patella syndrome, have been regarded as dysostoses, or abnormalities of single bones. The mutant genes that encode these transcription factors are *SOX9, RUNX2 (CBFA1)*, and *LMX1B*, respectively, and are members of much larger gene families. For instance, *SOX9* is a member of the *SOX* family of genes related to the *SRY* (sex-determining region of the Y chromosome) gene; *RUNX2 (CBFA1)* belongs to the runt family of transcription factor genes, and *LMX1B* is one of the LIM homeodomain gene family. All three disorders are due to haploinsufficiency of the respective gene products; the disorders are dominant traits. For familial cases of cleidocranial dysplasia and nail-patella syndrome, prenatal diagnosis is possible if the mutations are identified. Campomelic dysplasia results from new mutational events and has a low risk of recurrence in subsequent pregnancies.

CAMPOMELIC DYSPLASIA

Apparent in newborn infants, campomelic dysplasia (OMIM 114290) is characterized by bowing of long bones (especially in the lower legs), short bones, respiratory distress, and other anomalies that include defects of the cervical spine, central nervous system, heart, and kidneys. Several cases of sex reversal of XY males have been reported. Radiographs confirm the bowing and often show hypoplasia of the scapulae and pelvic bones (Fig. 689-1). Affected infants usually die of respiratory distress in the neonatal period. Complications in children and adolescents who survive include short stature with progressive kyphoscoliosis, recurrent apnea and respiratory infections, and learning difficulties.

CLEIDOCRANIAL DYSPLASIA

Cleidocranial dysplasia (OMIM 114290) is recognized in infants because of drooping shoulders, open fontanelles, prominent forehead, mild short stature, and dental abnormalities (Fig. 689-2). Radiographs reveal hypoplastic or absent clavicles, delayed ossification of the cranial bones with multiple ossification centers (wormian bones), and delayed ossification of pelvic bones. The course is usually uncomplicated except for dislocations, especially of the shoulders, and dental anomalies (numerous teeth) that require therapy.

NAIL-PATELLA SYNDROME

Dysplasia of the nails, absence or hypoplasia of the patella, abnormalities of the elbow, and spurs or "horns" extending from

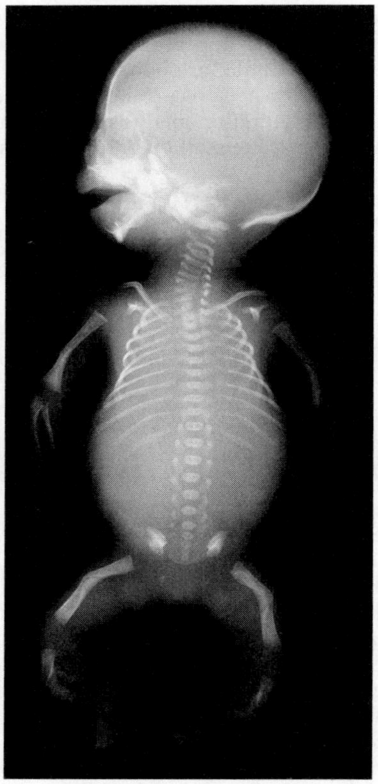

Figure 689-1 Radiograph in a fetus of 21 weeks' gestation with campomelic dysplasia. Findings include a large skull with a small face; hypoplastic/absent scapular bodies; 11 ribs; poorly ossified thoracic pedicles; tall, narrow iliac wings; and short extremities with proportionately long, bowed femurs. (From Slovis TL, editor: *Caffey's pediatric diagnostic imaging*, ed 11, vol 2, Philadelphia, 2008, Mosby.)

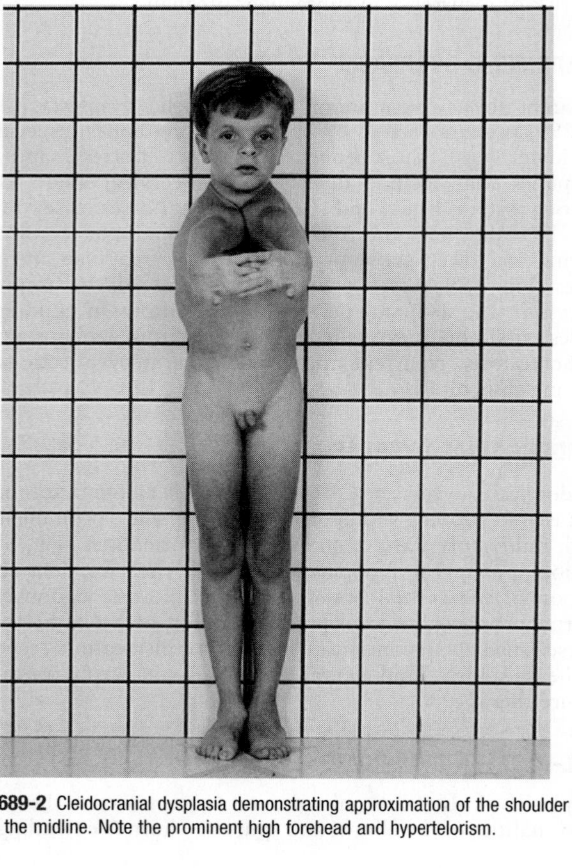

Figure 689-2 Cleidocranial dysplasia demonstrating approximation of the shoulder girdle in the midline. Note the prominent high forehead and hypertelorism.

the iliac bones characterize the nail-patella syndrome (OMIM 119600), which is also called *osteo-onychodysostosis.* Some patients have nephritis that resembles chronic glomerulonephritis. There is a wide spectrum of severity; some patients present in early childhood, whereas others are asymptomatic as adults.

BIBLIOGRAPHY

Please visit the Nelson Textbook of Pediatrics *website at* *www.expertconsult.com* *for the complete bibliography.*

Chapter 690
Disorders Involving Defective Bone Resorption

William A. Horton and Jacqueline T. Hecht

Bone dysplasias displaying increased bone density are rare. Osteopetrosis, which has many subtypes, and pyknodysostosis result from defective bone resorption.

OSTEOPETROSIS

Two main forms of osteopetrosis have been delineated: a severe autosomal recessive form (OMIM 259700) with an incidence of ~1/250,000 births and a mild autosomal dominant form (OMIM 166600) with an incidence of ~1/20,000 births. Disturbances of osteoclast function due to mutations in a gene encoding an osteoclast-specific subunit of the vacuolar proton pump (*TCIRG1*) are found in most patients with the recessive form. Mutations of the gene encoding the chloride channel protein, *CLCN7*, are observed in the dominant form of osteopetrosis. Both types of mutations lead to disturbances of acidification needed for normal osteoclast function.

The severe form is usually detected in infancy or earlier because of macrocephaly, hepatosplenomegaly, deafness, blindness, and severe anemia. Radiographs reveal diffuse bone sclerosis. Later films show the characteristic bone-within-bone appearance (Fig. 690-1). With time, infants typically fail to thrive and show psychomotor delay and worsening of cranial neuropathies and anemia. Dental problems, osteomyelitis of the mandible, and pathologic fractures are common. The most severely affected patients die during infancy; less severely affected patients rarely survive beyond the 2nd decade. Those who survive beyond infancy usually have learning disorders but might have normal intelligence despite hearing and vision loss.

Clinical Manifestations

Most of the manifestations are due to failure to remodel growing bones. This leads to narrowing of cranial nerve foramina and encroachment on marrow spaces, which results in secondary complications, such as optic and facial nerve dysfunction, and anemia accompanied by compensatory extramedullary hematopoiesis in the liver and spleen. The unusually dense bones are weak, leading to increased risk of fractures.

The autosomal dominant form of osteopetrosis (Albers-Schönberg disease, osteopetrosis tarda, or marble bone disease) usually manifests during childhood or adolescence with fractures and mild anemia and, less often, as cranial nerve dysfunction, dental abnormalities, or osteomyelitis of the mandible. Skeletal radiographs reveal a generalized increase in bone density and clubbing of metaphyses. Alternating bands of lucent and dense bands produce a sandwich appearance to vertebral bodies. The radiographic changes are sometimes incidental findings in otherwise asymptomatic adolescents and adults.

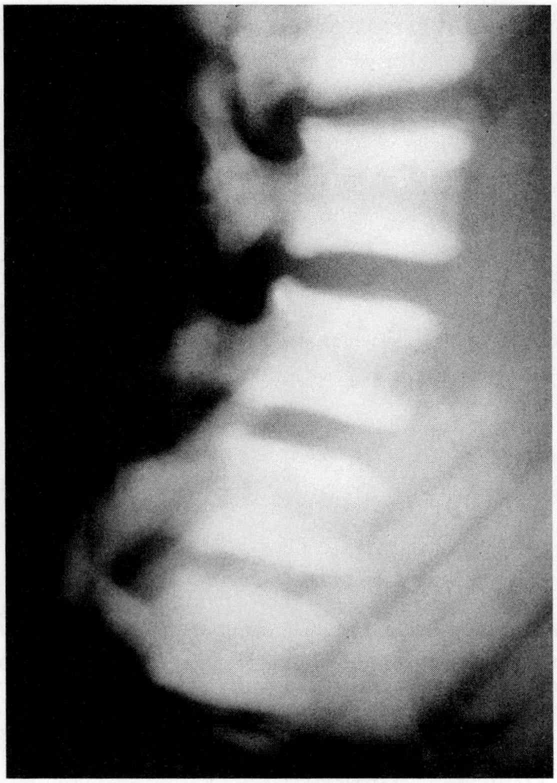

Figure 690-1 Lateral radiograph showing bone-in-bone appearance that is characteristic of osteopetrosis.

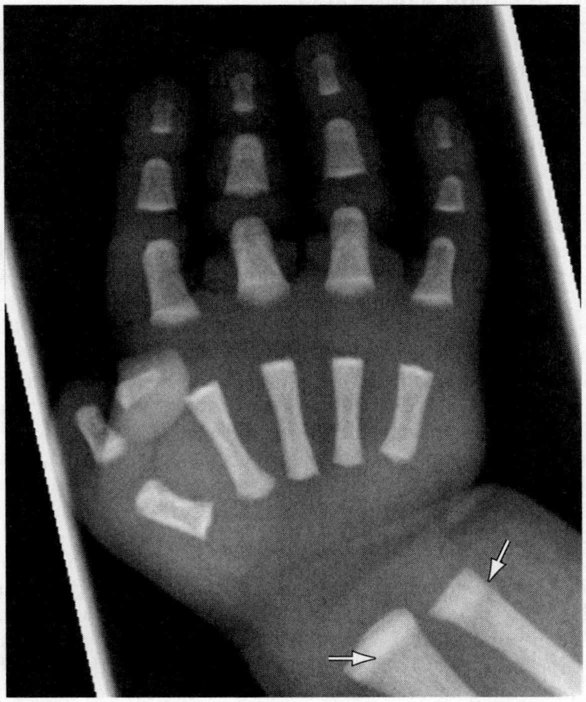

Figure 690-2 Right hand radiograph, age 2 wk. Note metaphyseal lucent bands in the distal ulna and radius (*arrows*) and short tubular bones. (From Stark Z, Savarirayan R: Osteopetrosis, *Orphanet J Rare Dis* 4:5, 2009.)

Treatment

Some patients with severe osteopetrosis have responded to bone marrow transplantation. Calcitriol and interferon-γ have also been used with equivocal results. Symptomatic care, such as dental care, transfusions for anemia, and antibiotic treatment of infections, is important for patients who survive infancy.

PYKNODYSOSTOSIS

An autosomal recessive bone dysplasia, pyknodysostosis (OMIM 265800) manifests in early childhood with short limbs, characteristic facies, an open anterior fontanel, a large skull with frontal and occipital bossing, and dental abnormalities. The hands and feet are short and broad, and the nails may be dysplastic. The sclerae may be blue. Minimal trauma often leads to fractures. Treatment is symptomatic and focused mainly on the management of dental problems and fractures. The prognosis is generally good, and patients typically reach heights of 130-150 cm.

Skeletal radiographs show a generalized increase in bone density. In contrast to many disorders in this group, the metaphyses are normal. Other changes include wide sutures and wormian bones in the skull, a small mandible, and hypoplasia of the distal phalanges (Fig. 690-2).

Several mutations have been found in the gene encoding cathepsin K, a cysteine protease that is highly expressed in osteoclasts. The mutations predict loss of enzyme function, suggesting that there is an inability of osteoclasts to degrade bone matrix and remodel bones.

BIBLIOGRAPHY

Please visit the Nelson Textbook of Pediatrics *website at www.expertconsult.com for the complete bibliography.*

Chapter 691
Disorders for Which Defects Are Poorly Understood or Unknown

William A. Horton and Jacqueline T. Hecht

There are many chondrodysplasias, or chondrodysplasia clinical phenotypes, for which the genetic cause or basic mechanism is poorly understood or not known. Many illustrate features not found in other disorders and have historical significance in the evolution of chondrodysplasia nomenclature and classification.

ELLIS–VAN CREVELD SYNDROME

The Ellis-van Creveld syndrome (OMIM 225500), also known as **chondroectodermal dysplasia**, is a skeletal and an ectodermal dysplasia. The skeletal dysplasia presents at birth with short limbs, especially the middle and distal segments, accompanied by postaxial polydactyly of the hands and sometimes of the feet. Nail dysplasia and dental anomalies (including neonatal, absent, and premature loss of teeth and upper lip defects) constitute the ectodermal dysplasia. Common manifestations also include atrial septal defects and other congenital heart defects.

Skeletal radiographs reveal short tubular bones with clubbed ends, especially the proximal tibia and ulna (Fig. 691-1). Carpal bones display extra ossification centers and fusion; cone-shaped epiphyses are evident in the hands. A bony spur is often noted above the medial aspect of the acetabulum.

Ellis-van Creveld syndrome is an autosomal recessive trait that occurs most often in the Amish. Mutations have been identified in one of two genes, *EVC (EVC1)* and *EVC2*, which map in a head-to-head configuration to chromosome 4p. The functions of the gene products are unknown. About 30% of patients die of

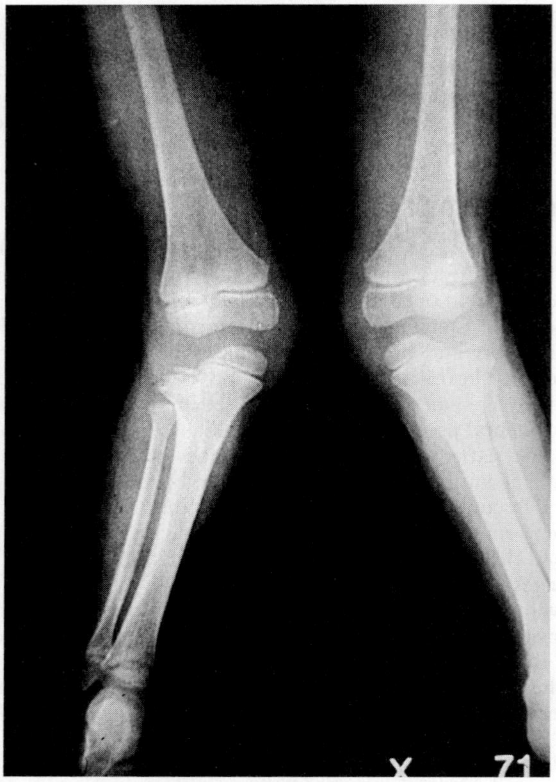

Figure 691-1 Radiograph of lower extremities in Ellis-van Creveld syndrome. Tubular bones are short, and proximal fibula is short. Ossification is retarded in lateral tibia epiphyses, causing a knock-knee deformity.

cardiac or respiratory problems during infancy. Life span is otherwise normal; adult heights range from 119 to 161 cm.

ASPHYXIATING THORACIC DYSTROPHY

Asphyxiating thoracic dystrophy (OMIM 208500), or Jeune syndrome, is an autosomal recessive chondrodysplasia that resembles Ellis-van Creveld syndrome. Newborn infants present with a long, narrow thorax and respiratory insufficiency associated with pulmonary hypoplasia. Neonates often die. Other neonatal manifestations include slightly short limbs and postaxial polydactyly. Mutations have been identified in the gene encoding cytoplasmic dynein 2 heavy chain 1 (*DYNC2H1*), which maps to chromosome 11q14.3-q23.1.

Skeletal radiographs show very short ribs with anterior expansion. Tubular limb bones are short with bulbous ends; cone-shaped epiphyses occur in hand bones. The iliac bones are short and square with a spur above the medial aspect of the acetabulum.

If infants survive the neonatal period, respiratory function usually improves as the rib cage grows. Surgery that produces lateral thoracic expansion improves rib growth and enhances chest wall dimensions. Progressive renal dysfunction often develops during childhood. Intestinal malabsorption and hepatic dysfunction have also been reported.

SHORT-RIB POLYDACTYLY SYNDROMES

Four types of short-rib polydactyly syndrome (types I-IV) (OMIM 263530, 263520, 263510, 269860) have been described. All are lethal in the newborn period. Neonates present with respiratory distress, an extremely small thorax, very short extremities, polydactyly, and a variety of nonskeletal defects. Radiographs demonstrate very short ribs and tubular bones with changes characteristic for each type. All four types are autosomal recessive

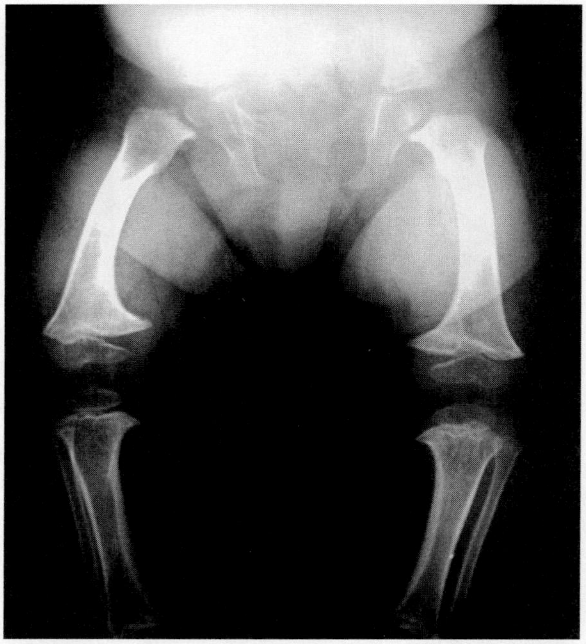

Figure 691-2 Radiograph of lower extremities in cartilage-hair hypoplasia. The tubular bones are short and the metaphyses are flared and irregular. The fibula is disproportionately long compared with the tibia. The femoral necks are short.

traits. Mutations of *DYNC2H1* have been detected in short-rib polydactyly syndrome type III, making it allelic to asphyxiating thoracic dystrophy.

CARTILAGE-HAIR HYPOPLASIA

Cartilage-hair hypoplasia (CHH) (OMIM 250250) is also known as **metaphyseal chondrodysplasia—McKusick type.** It is recognized during the 2nd year because of growth deficiency affecting the limbs, accompanied by flaring of the lower rib cage, a prominent sternum, and bowing of the legs. The hands and feet are short, and the fingers are very short with extreme ligamentous laxity. The hair is thin, sparse, and light colored, and nails are hypoplastic. The skin is hypopigmented.

Radiographs show short tubular bones with flared, irregularly mineralized, and cupped metaphyses (Fig. 691-2). The knees are more affected than are the hips, and the fibula is disproportionately longer than the tibia. The metacarpals and phalanges are short and broad. Spinal radiographs reveal mild platyspondyly.

Nonskeletal manifestations associated with CHH include immunodeficiency (T-cell abnormalities, neutropenia, leukopenia, and susceptibility to chickenpox; children also may have complications from smallpox and polio vaccinations), malabsorption, celiac disease, and Hirschsprung disease. Adults are at risk for malignancy, especially non-Hodgkin lymphoma and skin tumors. Adults reach heights of 107-157 cm.

CHH shows autosomal recessive inheritance. Although rare, its highest prevalence is in the Amish and Finnish populations. It results from mutations of a gene coding for a large untranslated RNA component of an enzyme complex involved in processing mitochondrial RNA (RMRP). Loss of this gene product interferes with processing of both mRNA and rRNA. Loss of rRNA processing correlates with the extent of bone dysplasia, whereas loss of mRNA processing correlates with degree of hair hypoplasia, immunodeficiency, and hematologic abnormality. RMRP mutations are occasionally detected in patients with mild metaphyseal dysplasia lacking the extraskeletal features characteristic of CHH. Prenatal diagnosis is available if the mutation is identified either in the patient or parents.

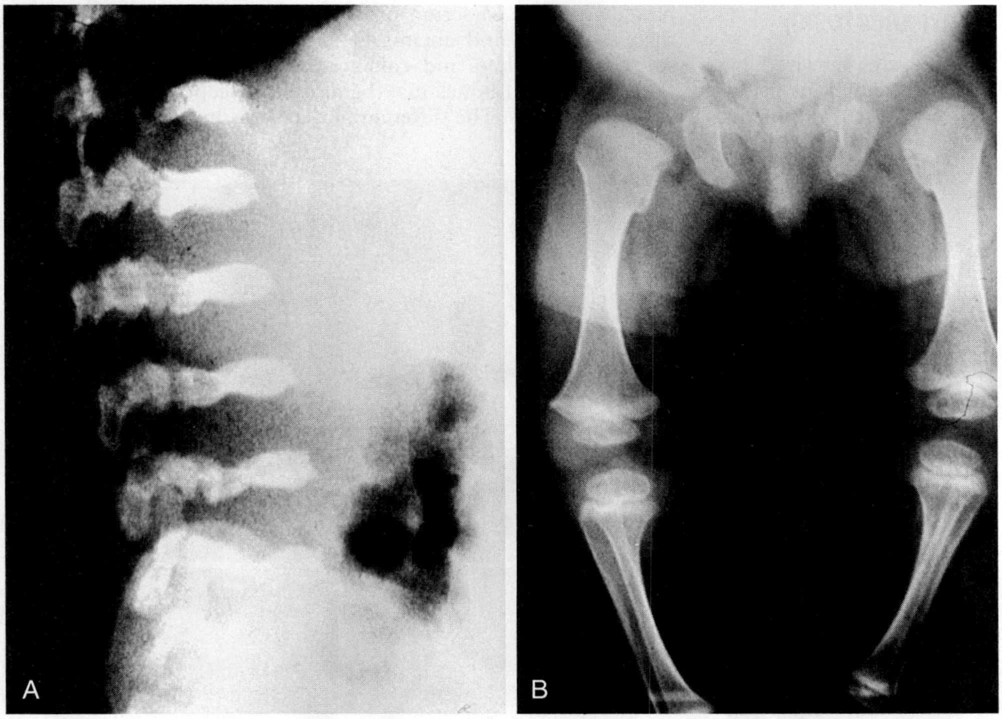

Figure 691-3 *A,* Radiograph of the lateral thoracolumbar spine in metatropic dysplasia showing severe platyspondyly. *B,* Radiograph of lower extremities in metatropic dysplasia showing short tubular bones with widened metaphyses. The femurs have a dumbbell appearance.

METATROPIC DYSPLASIA

There are two recognized forms of metatropic dysplasia (OMIM 156530, 250600), an autosomal dominant and an autosomal recessive form, although the existence of a recessive form has been questioned. Heterozygous mutations of *TRPV4* (transient receptor potential vanilloid family 4), which encodes a calcium-permeable cation channel, have been identified in the dominant form.

Newborn infants present with a long narrow trunk and short extremities. A tail-like appendage sometimes extends from the base of the spine. Odontoid hypoplasia is common and may be associated with cervical instability. Kyphoscoliosis appears in late infancy and progresses through childhood, often becoming severe enough to compromise cardiopulmonary function. The joints are large and become progressively restricted in mobility, except in the hands. Contractures often develop in the hips and knees during childhood. Although severely affected infants can die at a young age from respiratory failure, patients usually survive, although they can become disabled as adults from the progressive musculoskeletal deformities. Adult heights range from 110 to 120 cm.

Skeletal radiographs show characteristic changes dominated by severe platyspondyly and short tubular bones with expanded and deformed metaphyses that exhibit a dumbbell appearance (Fig. 691-3). The pelvic bones are hypoplastic and exhibit a halberd appearance because of a small sacrosciatic notch and a notch above the lateral margin of the acetabulum.

SPONDYLOMETAPHYSEAL DYSPLASIA, KOZLOWSKI TYPE

The Kozlowski type of spondylometaphyseal dysplasia (SMDK) (OMIM 184252) is an allelic disorder to autosomal dominant metatropic dysplasia as mutations of *TRPV4* have been detected. Mutations of *TRPV4* have also been identified in autosomal dominant brachyolmia, whose phenotype is dominated by progressive scoliosis and platyspondyly on x-rays.

SMDK manifests in early childhood with mild short stature involving mostly the trunk and a waddling gait. The hands and feet may be short and stubby. Radiographs show flattening of vertebral bodies. The metaphyses of tubular bones are widened and irregularly mineralized, especially at the proximal femur. The pelvic bones manifest mild hypoplasia.

Scoliosis can develop during adolescence. The disorder is otherwise uncomplicated, and manifestations are limited to the skeleton. Adults reach heights of 130-150 cm. The Kozlowski type of spondylometaphyseal dysplasia is an autosomal dominant trait.

DISORDERS INVOLVING FILAMINS

Mutations of genes encoding filamin A and filamin B proteins have been detected in diverse disorders of skeletal development: filamin A mutations in otopalatodigital syndromes type 1 and 2 frontometaphyseal dysplasia and Melnick-Needles syndrome (OMIM 311300, 304120, 305620, 309350) and filamin B mutations in Larsen syndrome and perinatal lethal ateosteogenesis types I and III (OMIM 150250, 108720, 108721). Filamins functionally connect extracellular to intracellular structural proteins, thereby linking cells to their local microenvironment, which is essential for skeletal development and growth.

JUVENILE OSTEOCHONDROSES

The juvenile osteochondroses are a heterogeneous group of disorders in which regional disturbances in bone growth cause noninflammatory arthropathies. They are summarized in Table 691-1. Some have localized pain and tenderness (Freiberg disease, Osgood-Schlatter disease, osteochondritis dissecans), whereas others present with painless limitation of joint movement (Legg-Calvé-Perthes disease, Scheuermann disease). Bone growth may be disrupted, leading to deformities. The diagnosis is usually confirmed radiographically, and treatment is symptomatic. The pathogenesis of these disorders is believed to involve ischemic necrosis of primary and secondary ossification centers. Although familial forms have been reported, these disorders usually occur sporadically.

CAFFEY DISEASE (INFANTILE CORTICAL HYPEROSTOSIS)

This is a rare disorder of unknown etiology characterized by cortical hyperostosis with inflammation of the contiguous fascia and muscle. It is often sporadic, but both autosomal dominant and autosomal recessive inheritance have been reported. In three unrelated families with autosomal dominant inheritance, a linkage to mutations of the *COL1A1* gene (codes for the α_1 chain of type I collagen) has been reported.

Prenatal and more often postnatal onset have been described. Prenatal onset may be mild (autosomal dominant) or severe (autosomal recessive). Severe prenatal disease is characterized by typical bone lesions, polyhydramnios, hydrops fetalis, severe respiratory distress, prematurity, and high mortality. Onset in infancy (<6 mo; average, 10 wk) is most common; manifestations include the sudden onset of irritability, swelling of contiguous soft tissue that precedes the cortical thickening of the underlying bones, fever, and anorexia. The swelling is painful with a woodlike induration but with minimal warmth or redness; suppuration is absent. There are unpredictable remissions and relapses; an episode can last 2 wk to 3 mo. The most common bones involved include the mandible (75%) (Fig. 691-4), the clavicle, and the ulna. If swelling is not prominent or visible, the diagnosis might not be evident.

Laboratory features include elevated erythrocyte sedimentation rate and serum alkaline phosphatase as well as, in some patients, increased serum prostaglandin E levels. There may be thrombocytosis and anemia. The **radiographic features** include soft-tissue swelling and calcification and cortical hyperostosis (Fig. 691-5). All bones may be affected except the phalanges or vertebral bodies. The **differential diagnosis** includes other causes

TABLE 691-1 JUVENILE OSTEOCHONDROSES

EPONYM	AFFECTED REGION	AGE AT PRESENTATION
Legg-Calvé-Perthes disease	Capital femoral epiphysis	3-12 yr
Osgood-Schlatter disease	Tibial tubercle	10-16 yr
Sever disease	Os calcaneus	6-10 yr
Freiberg disease	Head of second metatarsal	10-14 yr
Scheuermann disease	Vertebral bodies	Adolescence
Blount disease	Medial aspect of proximal tibial epiphysis	Infancy or adolescence
Osteochondritis dissecans	Subchondral regions of knee, hip, elbow, and ankle	Adolescence

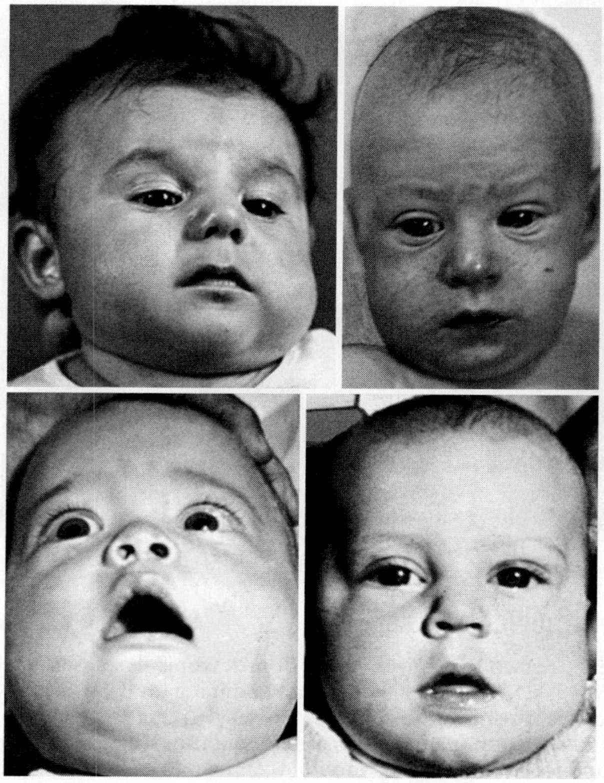

Figure 691-4 Facies in infantile cortical hyperostosis. In almost all cases, the changes have appeared before the 5th month of life. Unilateral swelling of the left cheek and left side of the jaw in an infant 12 wk of age. (From Kuhn JP, Slovis TL, Haller JO: *Caffey's pediatric diagnostic imaging*, ed 10, vol 2, Philadelphia, 2004, Mosby.)

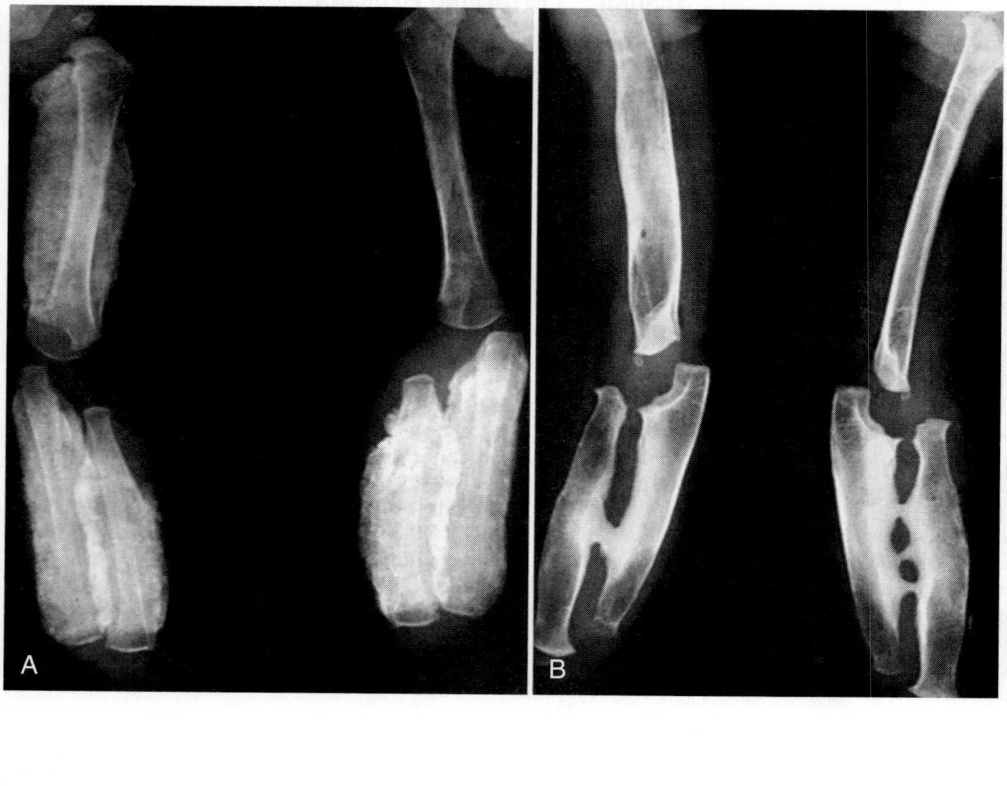

Figure 691-5 Residual bony bridges between each radius and ulna in infantile cortical hyperostosis. *A*, Massive cortical thickenings of the radii and ulnas at 4½ mo of age. Pressure from the external thickenings has forced the radial heads laterad out of the elbows. *B*, At 12½ mo, 9 mo after onset, all affected bones are still greatly swollen, owing largely to expansion of the medullary cavities, although there are still residues of the earlier cortical thickening. The radial heads are still dislocated, and the radial diaphyses are now anchored in this ectopic position by solid bony bridges between them and the ulnar diaphyses, a single bridge on the right and three on the left. At 32 mo, these bridges were still intact, although they had diminished slightly in caliber. It is possible that these bony bridges represent ossification of parts of the interosseous membrane. (From Kuhn JP, Slovis TL, Haller JO: *Caffey's pediatric diagnostic imaging*, ed 10, vol 2, Philadelphia, 2004, Mosby.)

of hyperostosis such as chronic vitamin A intoxication, prolonged prostaglandin E infusion in children with ductal dependent congenital heart disease, primary bone tumors, and scurvy.

Complications are unusual but include pseudoparalysis with limb or scapula involvement, pleural effusions (rib), torticollis (clavicle), mandibular asymmetry, bone fusion (ribs or ulna and radius), and bone angulation deformities (common with severe prenatal onset).

Treatment includes indomethacin and prednisone if there is a poor response to indomethacin.

BIBLIOGRAPHY

Please visit the Nelson Textbook of Pediatrics *website at www.expertconsult.com for the complete bibliography.*

Chapter 692
Osteogenesis Imperfecta

Joan C. Marini

Osteoporosis, a feature of both inherited and acquired disorders, classically demonstrates fragility of the skeletal system and a susceptibility to fractures of the long bones or vertebral compressions from mild or inconsequential trauma. **Osteogenesis imperfecta (OI)** (brittle bone disease), the most common genetic cause of osteoporosis, is a generalized disorder of connective tissue. The spectrum of OI is extremely broad, ranging from forms that are lethal in the perinatal period to a mild form in which the diagnosis may be equivocal in an adult.

ETIOLOGY

Structural or quantitative defects in type I collagen cause the full clinical spectrum of OI. Type I collagen is the primary component of the extracellular matrix of bone and skin. Ten percent of cases clinically indistinguishable from OI do not have a molecular defect in type I collagen. Some of these cases have biochemically normal collagen and unknown genetic defects. Other cases have overmodified collagen and severe or lethal OI-like bone dysplasia. These cases are caused by recessive null mutations in a collagen-modifying enzyme, prolyl 3-hydroxylase 1 (coded by the *LEPRE1* gene on chromosome 1p34.1) or its associated protein, CRTAP.

EPIDEMIOLOGY

The autosomal dominant forms of OI occur equally in all racial and ethnic groups, and recessive forms occur predominantly in ethnic groups with consanguineous marriages. The West African founder mutation for type VIII OI has a carrier frequency of 1/200-300 among African Americans. The incidence of OI detectable in infancy is about 1/20,000. There is a similar incidence of the mild form OI type I.

PATHOLOGY

The collagen structural mutations cause OI bone to be globally abnormal. The bone matrix contains abnormal type I collagen fibrils and relatively increased levels of types III and V collagen. Several noncollagenous proteins of bone matrix are also reduced. The hydroxyapatite crystals deposited on this matrix are poorly aligned with the long axis of fibrils.

PATHOGENESIS

Type I collagen is a heterotrimer composed of two $\alpha 1(I)$ chains and one $\alpha 2(I)$ chain. The chains are synthesized as procollagen molecules with short globular extensions on both ends of the central helical domain. The helical domain is composed of uninterrupted repeats of the sequence Gly-X-Y, where Gly is glycine, X is often proline, and Y is often hydroxyproline. The presence of glycine at every 3rd residue is crucial to helix formation because its small side chain can be accommodated in the interior of the helix. The chains are assembled at their carboxyl ends; helix formation then proceeds linearly in a carboxyl to amino direction. Concomitant with helix assembly and formation, helical proline and lysine residues are hydroxylated by prolyl 4-hydroxylase and lysyl hydroxylase and some hydroxylysine residues are glycosylated.

Collagen structural defects are predominantly of two types: 80% are point mutations causing substitutions of helical glycine residues or crucial residues in the C-propeptide by other amino acids, and 20% are single exon splicing defects. The clinically mild OI type I has a quantitative defect, with null mutations in one $\alpha 1(I)$ allele leading to a reduced amount of normal collagen.

The glycine substitutions in the two α chains have distinct genotype-phenotype relationships. One third of mutations in the $\alpha 1$ chain are lethal, and those in $\alpha 2(I)$ are predominantly nonlethal. Two lethal regions in $\alpha 1(I)$ align with major ligand binding regions of the collagen helix. Lethal mutations in $\alpha 2(I)$ occur in 8 regularly spaced clusters along the chain that align with binding regions for matrix proteoglycans in the collagen fibril.

Classic OI is an autosomal dominant disorder. Some familial recurrences of OI are caused by parental mosaicism for dominant collagen mutations. Recessive OI (types VII and VIII) accounts for 5-7% of new OI in North America. These types are caused by null mutations in the genes coding for two of the components of the collagen prolyl 3-hydroxylation complex in the endoplasmic reticulum, *LEPRE1*, which encodes P3H1, or *CRTAP*. This complex is responsible for post-translational modification of a single proline residue, P986, on the $\alpha 1(I)$ chains. It is not yet clear whether absence of the complex or the modification is the crucial feature of recessive OI.

CLINICAL MANIFESTATIONS

OI has the triad of fragile bones, blue sclerae, and early deafness. OI was once divided into "congenita," the forms detectable at birth, and "tarda," the forms detectable later in childhood; this did not account for the variability of OI. The Sillence classification divides OI into four types based on clinical and radiographic criteria. Additional types have been proposed based on histologic distinctions.

Osteogenesis Imperfecta Type I (Mild)

OI type I is sufficiently mild that it is often found in large pedigrees. Many type I families have blue sclerae, recurrent fractures in childhood, and presenile hearing loss (30-60%). Both types I and IV are divided into A and B subtypes, depending on the absence (A) or presence (B) of **dentinogenesis imperfecta**. Other possible connective tissue abnormalities include easy bruising, joint laxity, and mild short stature compared with family members. Fractures result from mild to moderate trauma and decrease after puberty.

Osteogenesis Imperfecta Type II (Perinatal Lethal)

Infants with OI type II may be stillborn or die in the 1st yr of life. Birthweight and length are small for gestational age. There is extreme fragility of the skeleton and other connective tissues. There are multiple intrauterine fractures of long bones, which have a crumpled appearance on radiographs. There are striking micromelia and bowing of extremities; the legs are held abducted at right angles to the body in the frog-leg position. Multiple rib fractures create a beaded appearance, and the small thorax contributes to respiratory insufficiency. The skull is large for body

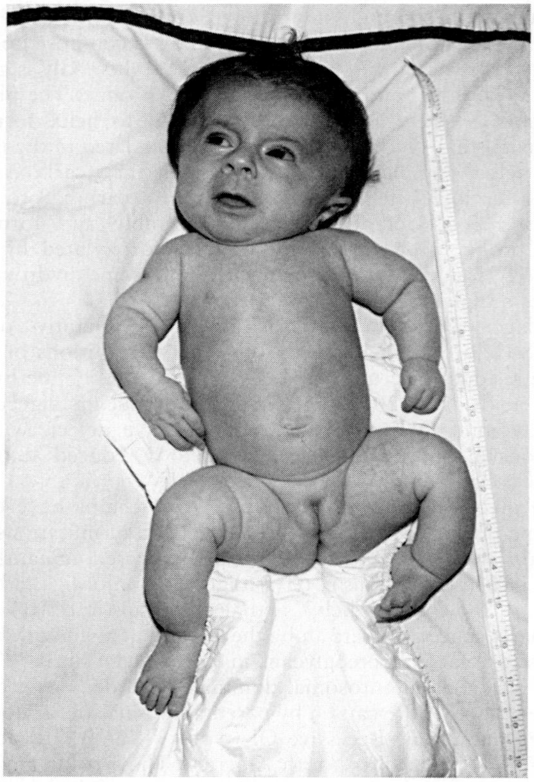

Figure 692-1 Infant with type III osteogenesis imperfecta displays shortened bowed extremities, thoracic deformity, and relative macrocephaly.

size, with enlarged anterior and posterior fontanels. Sclerae are dark blue-gray.

Osteogenesis Imperfecta Type III (Progressive Deforming)

OI type III is the most severe nonlethal form of OI and results in significant physical disability. Birthweight and length are often low normal. Fractures usually occur in utero. There is relative macrocephaly and triangular facies (Fig. 692-1). Postnatally, fractures occur from inconsequential trauma and heal with deformity. Disorganization of the bone matrix results in a "popcorn" appearance at the metaphyses (Fig. 692-2). The rib cage has flaring at the base, and pectal deformity is frequent. Virtually all type III patients have scoliosis and vertebral compression. Growth falls below the curve by the 1st year; all type III patients have extreme short stature. Scleral hue ranges from white to blue.

Osteogenesis Imperfecta Type IV (Moderately Severe)

Patients with OI type IV can present at birth with in utero fractures or bowing of lower long bones. They can also present with recurrent fractures after ambulation. Most children have moderate bowing even with infrequent fractures. Children with OI type IV require orthopedic and rehabilitation intervention, but they are usually able to attain community ambulation skills. Fracture rates decrease after puberty. Radiographically, they are osteoporotic and have metaphyseal flaring and vertebral compressions. Patients with type IV have moderate short stature. Scleral hue may be blue or white.

Osteogenesis Imperfecta Type V (Hyperplastic Callus) and Type VI (Mineralization Defect)

Types V and VI OI patients clinically have OI type IV, but they have distinct findings on bone histology. Type V patients also

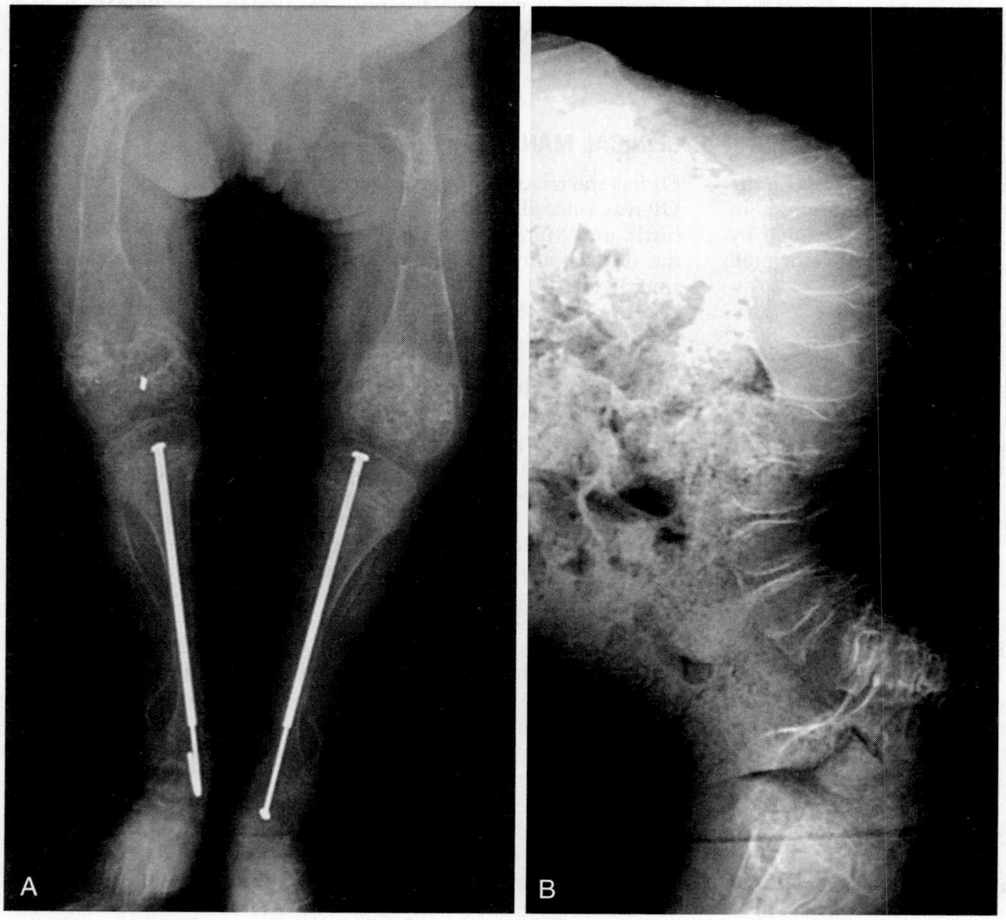

Figure 692-2 Typical features of type III osteogenesis imperfecta radiographs in a 6 yr old child. *A*, Lower long bones are osteoporotic, with metaphyseal flaring, "popcorn" formation at growth plates, and placement of intramedullary rods. *B*, Vertical bodies are compressed and osteoporotic.

have hyperplastic callus, calcification of the interosseous membrane of the forearm, and a radiodense metaphyseal band. The absence of a collagen defect supports the distinct grouping; the genetic etiology is unknown. They constitute <5% of OI populations.

Osteogenesis Imperfecta Types VII and VIII (Recessive Form)

Types VII and VIII patients have null mutations in *P3H1* and *CRTAP*, respectively. Clinically they overlap types II and III OI but have distinct features including white sclerae, rhizomelia, and small to normal head circumference. Surviving children have severe osteochondrodysplasia with extreme short stature and dual energy x-ray absorptiometry (DEXA) L1-L2 z-score in the −6 to −7 range.

LABORATORY FINDINGS

The diagnosis of types I-IV and VII/VIII is confirmed by collagen biochemical studies using cultured dermal fibroblasts. Both dominant and recessive types have a positive biochemical test (over modified collagen on gel electrophoresis), although dominant cases caused by collagen defects in the amino third of the chains have a false negative biochemical test. In OI type I, the reduced amount of type I collagen results in an increase in the ratio of type III to type I collagen on gel electrophoresis. DNA sequencing to identify mutations in *COL1A1, COL1A2, LEPRE1,* or *CRTAP* is useful to distinguish types and to facilitate family screening and prenatal diagnosis.

Severe OI can be detected prenatally by level II ultrasonography as early as 16 wk of gestation. OI and thanatophoric dysplasia may be confused. Fetal ultrasonography might not detect OI type IV and rarely detects OI type I. For recurrent cases, chorionic villus biopsy can be used for biochemical or molecular studies. Amniocytes produce false-positive biochemical studies but can be used for molecular studies in appropriate cases.

In the neonatal period, the normal to elevated alkaline phosphatase levels present in OI distinguish it from hypophosphatasia.

COMPLICATIONS

The morbidity and mortality of OI are cardiopulmonary. Recurrent pneumonias and declining pulmonary function occur in childhood, and cor pulmonale is seen in adults.

Neurologic complications include basilar invagination, brainstem compression, hydrocephalus, and syringohydromyelia. Most children with OI types III and IV have basilar invagination, but brainstem compression is uncommon. Basilar invagination is best detected with spiral CT of the craniocervical junction (Fig. 692-3).

TREATMENT

There is no cure for OI. For severe nonlethal OI, active physical rehabilitation in the early years allows children to attain a higher functional level than orthopedic management alone. Children with OI type I and some with type IV are spontaneous ambulators. Children with types III and IV OI benefit from gait aids and a program of swimming and conditioning. Severely affected patients require a wheelchair for community mobility but can acquire transfer and self-care skills. Teens with OI can require psychologic support with body image issues. Growth hormone improves bone histology in growth-responsive children (usually types I and IV).

Orthopedic management of OI is aimed at fracture management and correction of deformity to enable function. Fractures should be promptly splinted or cast; OI fractures heal well, and cast removal should be aimed at minimizing immobilization osteoporosis. Correction of long bone deformity

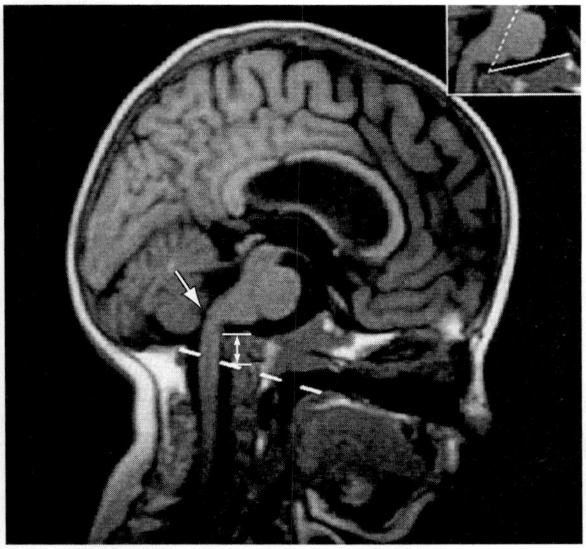

Figure 692-3 Typical feature of basilar invagination shown in the sagittal MRI of an asymptomatic child with type III osteogenesis imperfecta. There is invagination of the odontoid above the Chamberlain line, causing compression and kinking at the pontomedullary junction (*arrow*).

requires an osteotomy procedure and placement of an intramedullary rod.

A several-year course of treatment of children with OI with bisphosphonates (IV pamidronate or oral olpadronate) confers some benefits. Bisphosphonates decrease bone resorption by osteoclasts; OI patients have increased bone volume that still contains the defective collagen. Bisphosphonates are more beneficial for vertebrae (trabecular bone) than long bones (cortical bone). Treatment for 1-2 yr results in increased L1-4 DEXA and, more importantly, improved vertebral compressions and area, which can prevent or delay the scoliosis of OI. Relative risk of long bone fractures is modestly decreased. However, the material properties of long bones are weakened by prolonged treatment and nonunion after osteotomy is increased. There is no effect of bisphosphonates on mobility scores, muscle strength, or bone pain. Limiting treatment duration to 2-3 yr in mid-childhood can maximize benefits and minimize detriment to cortical material properties. Benefits appear to persist several years after the treatment interval. Side effects include abnormal long bone remodeling, increased incidence of fracture non-union, and osteopetrotic-like brittleness to bone.

PROGNOSIS

OI is a chronic condition that limits both life span and functional level. Infants with OI type II usually die within months to a year of life. An occasional child with radiographic type II and extreme growth deficiency survives to the teen years. Persons with OI type III have a reduced life span with clusters of mortality from pulmonary causes in early childhood, the teen years, and the 40s. OI types I and IV are compatible with a full life span.

Individuals with OI type III are usually wheelchair dependent. With aggressive rehabilitation, they can attain transfer skills and household ambulation. OI type IV children usually attain community ambulation skills either independently or with gait aids.

GENETIC COUNSELING

For autosomal dominant OI, the risk of an affected individual passing the gene to his or her offspring is 50%. An affected child usually has about the same severity of OI as the parent; however, there is variability of expression, and the child's condition can be either more or less severe than that of the parent. The empirical recurrence risk to an apparently unaffected couple of having a second child with OI is 5-7%; this is the statistical chance that one parent has germ line mosaicism. The collagen mutation in the mosaic parent is present in some germ cells and may be present in somatic tissues. If a parent is a mosaic carrier, the risk of recurrence may be as high as 50%. For recessive OI, the recurrence risk is 25% per pregnancy. No known individual with severe nonlethal recessive OI has had a child.

BIBLIOGRAPHY

Please visit the Nelson Textbook of Pediatrics *website at www.expertconsult.com for the complete bibliography.*

Chapter 693
Marfan Syndrome

Jefferson Doyle and Harry Dietz III

Marfan syndrome (MFS) is an autosomal dominant disorder caused by mutations in the gene encoding the extracellular matrix (ECM) protein fibrillin-1. It is primarily associated with skeletal, cardiovascular, and ocular pathology, displaying near-complete penetrance but variable expression. Diagnosis is based on clinical findings, some of which are age dependent.

EPIDEMIOLOGY

The incidence of this disorder is about 1/5,000-10,000 births. About 30% of cases are sporadic, due to de novo mutations; new mutations often associate with advanced paternal age.

PATHOGENESIS

MFS is associated with abnormal biosynthesis of fibrillin-1, a 350-kd ECM protein that is the major constituent of microfibrils. The fibrillin-1 *(FBN1)* locus resides on the long arm of chromosome 15 (15q21), and the gene is composed of 65 exons. More than 1,000 mutations distributed throughout *FBN1* have been identified, many being unique to a given family. With the exception of an early-onset and severe presentation of MFS associated with some mutations in exons 26-27 and 31-32, no clear phenotype-genotype correlation has been identified. There is considerable intrafamily variability, suggesting that epigenetic, modifier gene, environmental, or other unidentified factors might influence expression of the disease.

MFS was traditionally considered to result from a structural deficiency of connective tissues. Reduced fibrillin-1 was thought to lead to a primary derangement of elastic fiber deposition, because both skin and aorta from affected patients show decreased elastin, along with elastic fiber fragmentation. In response to stress (such as hemodynamic forces in the proximal aorta), affected organs were thought to manifest this structural insufficiency with accelerated degeneration. However, it was difficult to reconcile certain manifestations of the disease with this structural deficiency model (i.e., bony overgrowth is more suggestive of excess cell proliferation than structural insufficiency).

Additional research has identified a cytokine-regulatory role for fibrillin-1 that appears to have important implications for MFS. Fibrillin-1 shares significant homology with the latent transforming growth factor β (TGF-β) binding proteins (LTBPs). TGF-β is secreted from cells as part of a large latent complex (LLC) that includes the mature cytokine (TGF-β), a dimer of its processed amino-terminal pro-peptide called *latency associated peptide* (LAP), and one of three LTBPs. Mice heterozygous for a mutation in the fibrillin-1 gene typical of those that cause MFS in humans (C1039G) display many of the classic features of MFS, including progressive aortic root dilatation. TGF-β signaling has been shown to be increased in the aortas of these mice, as well as the aortic wall from patients with MFS, suggesting that failed ECM sequestration of the LLC by fibrillin-1 leads to increased TGF-β signaling in MFS. Neutralizing antibodies to TGF-β have been shown to reduce the aortic size and improve the aortic wall architecture in these mice.

Aberrant TGF-β signaling might also play a role in the wider spectrum of manifestations of MFS. Increased TGF-β signaling has been observed in many tissues in MFS mice, including the developing lung, skeletal muscle, mitral valve, and dura. Treatment of these mice with agents that antagonize TGF-β signaling attenuates or prevents pulmonary emphysema, skeletal muscle myopathy, and myxomatous degeneration of the mitral valve. Patients with heterozygous mutations in TGF-β receptors 1 and 2 *(TGFβR1* and *TGFβR2)* have MFS-like manifestations yet normal fibrillin-1. Paradoxically, these mutations also appear to result in increased TGF-β signaling in tissues of these patients. The resulting Loeys-Dietz syndrome (LDS) has much phenotypic overlap with MFS, but it also has many discriminating features (see Differential Diagnosis).

CLINICAL MANIFESTATIONS

MFS is a multisystem disorder, with cardinal manifestations in the skeletal, cardiovascular, and ocular systems.

Skeletal System

Disproportionate overgrowth of the long bones is often the most striking and immediately evident manifestation of MFS. Anterior chest deformity is caused by overgrowth of the ribs, pushing the sternum anteriorly (pectus carinatum) or posteriorly (pectus excavatum). Overgrowth of arms and legs can lead to an arm span >1.05 times the height or a reduced upper to lower segment ratio (in the absence of severe scoliosis). Arachnodactyly (overgrowth of the fingers) is generally a subjective finding. The combination of long fingers and loose joints leads to the characteristic Walker-Murdoch or wrist sign: full overlap of the distal phalanges of the thumb and fifth finger when wrapped around the contralateral wrist (Fig. 693-1). The Steinberg or thumb sign is present when the distal phalanx of the thumb fully extends beyond the ulnar border of the hand when folded across the palm (Fig. 693-2), with or without active assistance by the patient or examiner.

Thoracolumbar scoliosis is commonly present and can contribute to the systemic score of the diagnosis (Table 693-1). Protrusio acetabuli (inward bulging of the acetabulum into the pelvic cavity), which is generally asymptomatic in young adults, is best identified with radiographic imaging. Pes planus (flat feet) is commonly present and varies from mild and asymptomatic to severe deformity, wherein medial displacement of the medial malleolus results in collapse of the arch and often reactive hip and knee disturbances. Curiously, a subset of patients with the disorder present with an exaggerated arch (pes cavus). Although joint laxity or hypermobility is often identified, joints can be normal or even develop contractures. Reduced extension of the elbows is common and can contribute to the systemic score of the diagnosis (see Table 693-1). Contracture of the fingers (camptodactyly) is commonly observed, especially in children with severe and rapidly progressive MFS. Several craniofacial manifestations are often present and can contribute to the diagnosis (Fig. 693-3). These include a long narrow skull (dolicocephaly), recession of the eyeball within the socket (enophthalmos), recessed lower mandible (retrognathia) or small chin (micrognathia), malar hypoplasia (malar flattening), and downward-slanting palpebral fissures.

Cardiovascular System

Manifestations of MFS in the cardiovascular system are conveniently divided into those affecting the heart and those affecting

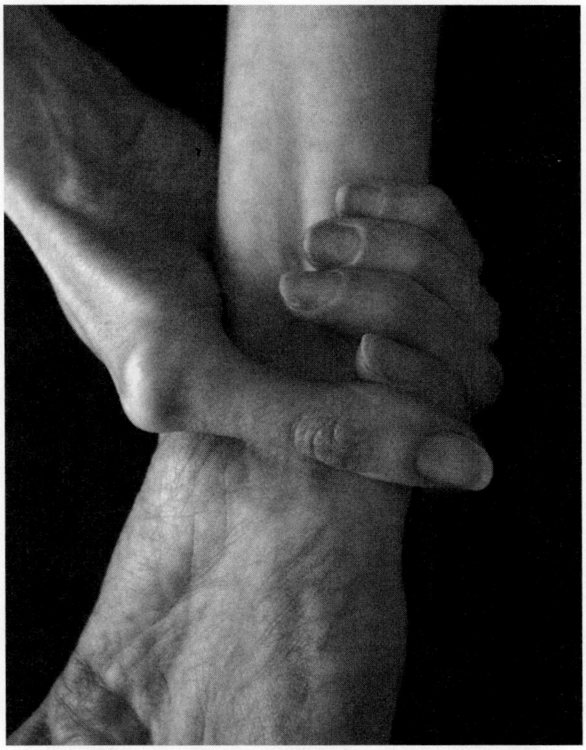

Figure 693-1 Wrist sign. When the wrist is grasped by the contralateral hand, the thumb overlaps the terminal phalanx of the 5th digit. (From McBride ART, Gargan M: Marfan syndrome, *Curr Orthop* 20:418–423, 2006.)

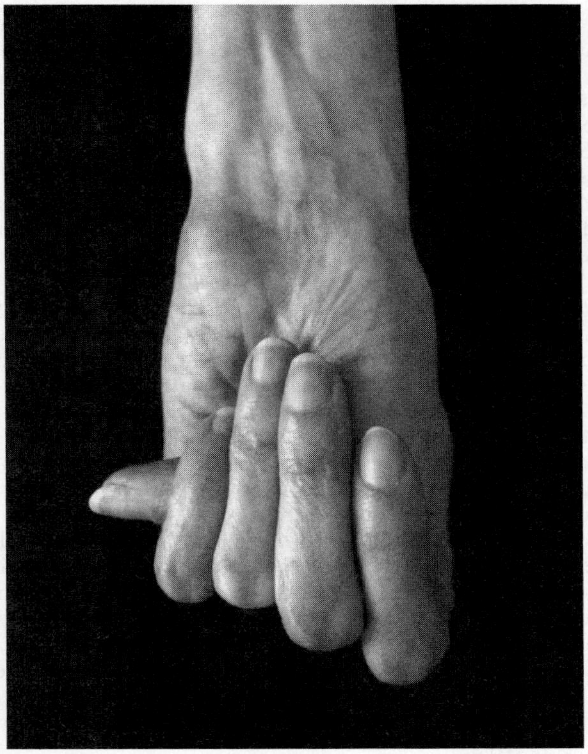

Figure 693-2 Thumb sign. When the hand is clenched without assistance, the entire thumbnail projects beyond the border of the hand. (From McBride ART, Gargan M: Marfan syndrome, *Curr Orthop* 20:418–423, 2006.)

the vasculature. Within the heart, the atrioventricular (AV) valves are most often affected. Thickening of the AV valves is common and often associated with prolapse of the mitral and/or tricuspid valves. Variable degrees of regurgitation may be present. In children with early onset and severe MFS, insufficiency of the mitral valve can lead to congestive heart failure, pulmonary hypertension, and death in infancy; this manifestation represents the leading cause of morbidity and mortality in young children with the disorder (Chapter 422.3). Aortic valve dysfunction is generally a late occurrence, attributed to stretching of the aortic annulus by an expanding root aneurysm. Both the aortic and AV valves seem to be more prone to calcification in persons with MFS.

Ventricular dysrhythmia has been described in children with MFS (Chapter 429). In association with mitral valve dysfunction, supraventricular arrhythmia (e.g., atrial fibrillation or supraventricular tachycardia) may be seen. There is also an increased prevalence of prolonged QT interval on electrocardiographic surveys of patients with MFS. Dilated cardiomyopathy, beyond that explained by aortic or mitral valve regurgitation, seems to occur with increased prevalence in patients with MFS, perhaps implicating a role for fibrillin-1 in the cardiac ventricles. However, the incidence seems to be low, and the occurrence of mild to moderate ventricular systolic dysfunction is often attributed to mitral or aortic insufficiency or to the use of β-adrenergic receptor blockade.

Aortic aneurysm and dissection remain the most life-threatening manifestations of MFS. This finding is age dependent, prompting life-long monitoring by echocardiography or other imaging modalities. Dilatation at the sinuses of Valsalva can begin in utero in severe cases, although some unequivocally affected persons never reach an aortic size that requires surgical intervention. In contrast to atherosclerotic aneurysms and some other forms of ascending aortic aneurysms, dilatation in MFS is generally greatest at (and often restricted to) the aortic root. Normal aortic dimensions vary with both age and body size, hence proper interpretation of aortic dimensions mandates comparison to age-dependent nomograms. The two most important determinants of risk of dissection of the aorta are the maximal dimension and a family history of dissection.

Surgical repair of the aorta is recommended when its greatest diameter reaches about 50 mm in adults. Early intervention is considered in those with a family history of early dissection. There are no definitive methods to guide the timing of surgery in childhood. The observation that dissection is extremely rare in this age group, irrespective of aortic size, has prompted many centers to adopt the adult criterion of 50 mm. Early surgery is often undertaken given a rapid rate of growth (>10 mm in a year) or the emergence of significant aortic regurgitation. Most patients with acute aortic dissection have classic symptoms, including severe chest pain, often radiating along the path of dissection. This path almost invariably begins at the aortic root (type A), and dissection can remain isolated (type II) or can propagate along the length of the descending aorta (type I). Acute-onset congestive heart failure typically indicates severe aortic valve insufficiency, complicating the aortic dissection. Depending on the involvement of the carotid arteries, some patients can have neurologic sequelae, due to cerebrovascular injury. Involvement of the coronary arteries can lead to myocardial infarction or sudden cardiac death. The mechanism of death usually includes rupture into the pericardial sac with subsequent pericardial tamponade. Chronic aortic dissection and intimal tears usually occur more insidiously, often without chest pain. Dilatation of the main pulmonary artery or descending thoracic or abdominal aorta can also occur, although relatively rarely.

Ocular System

Ectopia lentis (dislocation of the ocular lens) of any degree constitutes a major part of the diagnostic criteria for Marfan

Table 693-1 Diagnostic Criteria for Marfan Syndrome (MFS)

In the absence of a family history of MFS, a diagnosis can be reached in 1 of 4 scenarios:
1. Aortic diameter at Sinuses of Valsalva Z-score ≥2 AND Ectopia Lentis = MFS* 2. Aortic diameter at Sinuses of Valsalva Z-score ≥2 AND *FBN1* mutation = MFS 3. Aortic diameter at Sinuses of Valsalva Z-score ≥2 AND Systemic Score ≥7 = MFS* 4. Ectopia Lentis AND *FBN1* mutation known to associate with aortic aneurysm = MFS
In the absence of a family history of MFS, alternative diagnoses to MFS include:
1. Ectopia Lentis ± Systemic Score AND *FBN1* mutation not known to associate with aortic aneurysm or no *FBN1* mutation = Ectopia Lentis syndrome 2. Aortic diameter at Sinuses of Valsalva Z-score <2 AND Systemic Score ≥5 (with at least one skeletal feature) without Ectopia Lentis = MASS phenotype 3. Mitral Valve Prolapse AND Aortic diameter at Sinuses of Valsalva Z-score <2 AND Systemic Score <5 without Ectopia Lentis = Mitral Valve Prolapse syndrome
In the presence of a family history of MFS, a diagnosis can be reached in 1 of 3 scenarios:
1. Ectopia Lentis AND Family History of MFS = MFS 2. Systemic Score ≥7 AND Family History of MFS = MFS* 3. Aortic diameter at Sinuses of Valsalva Z-score ≥2 if older than 20 yr or ≥3 if younger than 20 yr AND Family History of MFS = MFS*
SCORING OF SYSTEMIC FEATURES (IN POINTS)†
Wrist AND thumb sign = 3 (wrist OR thumb sign = 1) Pectus carinatum deformity = 2 (pectus excavatum or chest asymmetry = 1) Hindfoot deformity = 2 (plain pes planus = 1) Pneumothorax = 2 Dural ectasia = 2 Protrusio acetabuli = 2 Reduced US/LS AND increased arm/height AND no severe scoliosis = 1 Scoliosis or thoracolumbar kyphosis = 1 Reduced elbow extension = 1 Facial features (3/5) = 1 (dolichocephaly, enophthalmos, downslanting palpebral fissures, malar hypoplasia, retrognathia) Skin striae = 1 Myopia >3 diopters = 1 Mitral valve prolapse (all types) = 1
CRITERIA FOR CAUSAL *FBN1* MUTATION
Mutation previously shown to segregate in a Marfan family Any one of the following *de novo* mutations (with proven paternity and absence of disease in parents): Nonsense mutation In-frame and out-of-frame deletion/insertion Splice site mutations affecting canonical splice sequence or shown to alter splicing on mRNA/cDNA level Missense mutation affecting/creating cysteine residues Missense mutation affecting conserved residues of the EGF consensus sequence [(D/N)X(D/N)(E/Q)Xm(D/N)Xn(Y/F), with m and n representing variable number of residues; D, aspartic acid; N, asparagine; E, glutamic acid; Q, glutamine; Y, tyrosine; F, phenylalanine] Other missense mutations: segregation in family, if possible, + absence in 400 ethnically matched control chromosomes; if no family history, absence in 400 ethnically matched control chromosomes Linkage of haplotype for n≥6 meioses to the *FBN1* locus

US/LS, upper segment/lower segment ratio.
*Without discriminating features of SGS, LDS, or vEDS (as defined in Table 693-2) *and* after TGFBR1/2, collagen biochemistry, COL3A1 testing if indicated. Other conditions/genes will emerge with time.
†Maximum total: 20 points; score ≥7 indicates systemic involvement.
From Loeys BL, Dietz HC, Braverman AC, et al: The revised Ghent nosology for the Marfan syndrome, *J Med Genet* 47:476–485, 2010.

syndrome (see Table 693-1), although it is not unique to the disorder. Ectopia lentis occurs in around 60-70% of patients with the disorder. When identified, it should prompt further assessment for MFS, although homocystinuria, Weill-Marchesani, and familial ectopia lentis are also associated with this condition. Other manifestations include early and severe myopia, flat cornea, increased axial length of the globe, hypoplastic iris, and ciliary muscle hypoplasia, causing decreased miosis. Patients with MFS can also have retinal detachment and a predisposition for early cataracts or glaucoma.

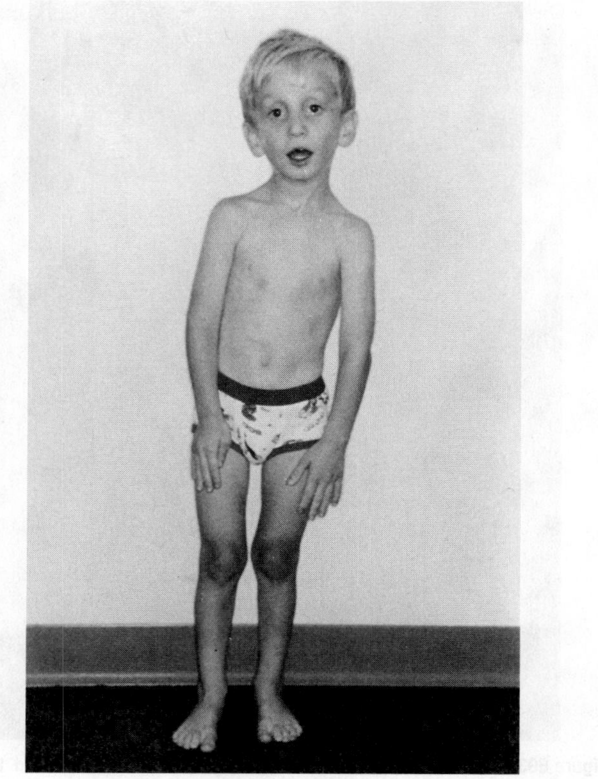

Figure 693-3 Marfan syndrome. Note the elongated facies, droopy lids, apparent dolichostenomelia, and mild scoliosis.

Pulmonary System

Several factors can result in pulmonary disease in patients with MFS. Pectus excavatum or progressive scoliosis can contribute to a restrictive pattern of lung disease. Widening of the distal airspaces with or without discrete bullae or (often apical) blebs can predispose to spontaneous pneumothorax, which occurs in up to 15% of patients. During assessment of pulmonary volumes and function, one should recognize that long-bone overgrowth affecting the lower extremities can lead to a reduction in the normalized forced vital capacity and total lung capacity. However, if normalized to thoracic size or sitting height, pulmonary function testing is often normal in patients with the disorder.

Skin and Integument

In contrast with other connective tissue disorders (e.g., Ehlers-Danlos syndrome), patients with MFS typically have normal skin texture and elasticity. The most common manifestation in the skin is striae atrophicae, which occurs in about two thirds of patients. In contrast to striae in those without a connective tissue disorder, stretch marks tend to occur in patients with MFS in the absence of obesity, rapid gain in muscle mass, or pregnancy, and at sites not associated with increased skin distention (e.g., the anterior shoulder or lower back). Another common manifestation is inguinal hernia, either occurring at birth or acquired in adolescence. There is an increased risk of surgical and recurrent hernias in MFS.

Dural Ectasia

Widening of the dural sac or root sleeves (dural ectasia) is present in 63-92% of MFS patients. Although dural ectasia can result in lumbar back pain, it is often asymptomatic and should be assessed by lumbosacral imaging with CT or MRI. When present, it contributes to the systemic score of the diagnostic criteria, although the specificity and predictive value of this criterion are unknown. Incidence of dural ectasia in other connective tissue disorders has not been rigorously assessed, although roughly 24% of patients with Ehlers-Danlos syndrome and many patients with LDS also show it.

FAMILY AND GENETIC HISTORY

The current criteria established for the diagnosis of MFS emphasize the need for a first-degree relative to independently meet the criteria before including family history as a major criterion for diagnosis. The criteria that are required to meet a causal mutation in a patient with MFS are described in Table 693-1.

DIAGNOSIS

Given the complexity of the diagnostic evaluation for MFS and the differential diagnosis, the evaluation should be coordinated by an individual or team with extensive experience in the diagnosis of connective tissue disorders. Diagnosis is based on criteria that include both clinical and molecular analyses (see Table 693-1).

In the absence of a conclusive family history of MFS, the diagnosis can be established in 4 distinct scenarios:

1. The presence of aortic root dilatation (Z-score ≥2 when standardized to age and body size) or dissection, as well as ectopia lentis, allows the unequivocal diagnosis of MFS, irrespective of the presence or absence of systemic features, except when there are signs indicative of Shprintzen-Goldberg syndrome (SGS), Loeys-Dietz syndrome (LDS), or vascular Ehlers-Danlos syndrome (vEDS) (see Table 693-2).
2. The presence of aortic root dilatation (Z-score ≥2) or dissection, and the identification of a bona fide *FBN1* mutation, is sufficient to establish the diagnosis, even when ectopia lentis is absent. An overview of criteria that enhance confidence in the pathogenetic potential of *FBN1* mutations is provided in Table 693-1. These include missense mutations that substitute or create cysteine residues, alter one of the conserved residues important for calcium binding in epidermal growth factor–like (EGF) domains, create a premature termination codon (nonsense mutations), delete or insert coding sequence, or disrupt the consensus sequence for pre-mRNA splicing. Evidence for pathogenicity of other types of missense mutations would include absence in at least 400 ethnically matched control chromosomes and co-segregation with disease in the family, or *de novo* occurrence in a sporadic case (with confirmation of paternity). Definitive evidence of linkage to a predisposing *FBN1* haplotype can substitute for an *FBN1* mutation for diagnostic purposes, but this linkage analysis requires at least 6 informative meioses in the patient's family to confirm the MFS-associated *FBN1* allele.
3. Where aortic root dilatation (Z-score ≥2) or dissection is present but ectopia lentis is absent and the *FBN1* status is either unknown or negative, a diagnosis of MFS is confirmed by the presence of sufficient systemic findings (≥7 points; see Table 693-1). However, features suggestive of SGS, LDS, or vEDS must be excluded, and appropriate alternative genetic testing (for mutations in TGFBR1/2, COL3A1, and other newly discovered genes, as well as collagen biochemistry) should be performed.
4. In the presence of ectopia lentis but absence of aortic root dilatation/dissection, the identification of an *FBN1* mutation previously associated with aortic disease is sufficient to make the diagnosis of MFS. If the *FBN1* mutation is not unequivocally associated with cardiovascular disease in either a related or unrelated proband, the patient should be classified as "ectopia lentis syndrome."

In an individual with a positive family history of MFS (where a family member has been independently diagnosed using the above criteria), the diagnosis can be established:

1. In the presence of ectopia lentis
2. With a systemic score ≥7 points (as per Table 693-1)
3. In the presence of aortic root dilatation (Z-score ≥2 in individuals ≥20 yr old, or Z-score ≥3 in individuals <20 yr old)

In the case of scenarios 2 and 3 (i.e., a systemic score ≥7 or aortic root dilatation), features suggestive of SGS, LDS, or vEDS must again be excluded and appropriate alternative genetic testing should be performed (as above).

Special consideration should be given to young individuals (<20 yr old) without a positive family history of MFS, who may not fit into one of the 4 proposed scenarios. In the absence of an *FBN1* mutation, if insufficient systemic features (<7) and/or borderline aortic root measurements (Z-score <3) are present, the term "nonspecific connective tissue disorder" should be used until follow-up echocardiographic evaluation shows aortic root dilation (Z-score ≥3). If the presence of an *FBN1* mutation is identified in a sporadic or familial case, but aortic root measurements are still below a Z-score of 3, the term "potential MFS" should be used until the aorta reaches threshold. Neonatal MFS is not considered as a separate category, but rather represents the severe end of the disease spectrum.

In adults (>20 yr), there are 3 main categories of alternative diagnoses: ectopia lentis syndrome (ELS), MASS phenotype (myopia, mitral valve prolapse, borderline [Z<2] aortic root enlargement, skin and skeletal findings), and mitral valve prolapse syndrome (MVPS).

Finally, some patients will remain difficult to classify due to overlap of phenotypes from different entities, the evolving nature of these connective tissue diseases, the absence of a mutation after screening of the appropriate genes, or divergence between the phenotype and the genotype. However, these patients should be uncommon and will hopefully benefit from better definition of still unrecognized conditions in the future.

DIFFERENTIAL DIAGNOSIS

Several disorders are included in the differential diagnosis of MFS on the basis of similar skeletal, cardiac, or ophthalmologic manifestations (Table 693-2). Many patients referred for possible MFS are found to have evidence of a systemic connective tissue disorder, including long limbs, deformity of the thoracic cage, striae atrophicae, mitral valve prolapse, and mild and nonprogressive dilatation of the aortic root, but do not meet diagnostic criteria for MFS. This constellation of features not fulfilling the diagnostic requirements of MFS is referred to by the acronym MASS phenotype, emphasizing the mitral, aortic, skin, and skeletal manifestations. The MASS phenotype can segregate in large pedigrees and remain stable over time. This diagnosis is most challenging in the context of an isolated and young patient. In this setting, careful follow-up is needed to distinguish MASS phenotype from emerging MFS, especially in children.

Other fibrillinopathies, such as familial mitral valve prolapse (MVP) syndrome and familial ectopia lentis, also include subdiagnostic manifestations and can be due to mutations in the gene encoding fibrillin-1. Also included in the differential diagnosis of the disorder is homocystinuria, caused by a deficiency of cystathionine β-synthase. Patients with homocystinuria often have tall stature, long-bone overgrowth, and ectopia lentis, but they do not typically have aortic enlargement or dissection. By contrast with MFS, the inheritance of homocystinuria (Chapter 79.3) is autosomal recessive, and affected persons often have mental retardation, a predisposition to thromboembolism, and a high incidence of coronary artery atherosclerosis. Observation of severely elevated concentrations of plasma homocystine is an efficient mechanism to distinguish homocystinuria from MFS.

Table 693-2 DIFFERENTIAL DIAGNOSIS OF MARFAN SYNDROME

DIFFERENTIAL DIAGNOSIS	OMIM NUMBER	CARDIAC FEATURES	VASCULAR FEATURES	SYSTEMIC FEATURES
MASS	604308	Mitral valve prolapse	Borderline or nonprogressive	Non-specific skin and skeletal findings, myopia
Familial thoracic aortic aneurysm	132900	Generally none Rare forms with PDA	Sinus of Valsalva, ascending aortic aneurysm	Generally none Rare livedo reticularis and iris flocculi with *ACTA2* mutations
BAV with AoA	109730	Bicuspid aortic valve	Sinus of Valsalva, ascending aortic aneurysm	None
Familial ectopia lentis	129600	None	None	Lens dislocation, nonspecific skeletal features
Ehlers-Danlos syndrome, type IV	130050	Mitral valve prolapse	Aneurysm and rupture of any medium to large muscular artery No predisposition for aortic root enlargement	Joint hypermobility, atrophic scars, translucent skin, easy bruising, hernias, rupture of hollow organs
Homocystinuria	236200	Mitral valve prolapse	Intravascular thrombosis	Tall stature, ectopia lentis, long-bone overgrowth, mental retardation
Loeys-Dietz syndrome	609192	Patent ductus arteriosus; atrial septal defect, bicuspid aortic valve	Sinus of Valsalva aneurysm, arterial tortuosity, or aneurysms in other arteries Vascular dissection at relatively young ages and small aortic dimensions	Hypertelorism, cleft palate, broad or bifid uvula, exotropia, craniosynostosis, malar hypoplasia, blue sclerae, arachnodactyly, pectus deformity, scoliosis, joint laxity, easy bruising, dystrophic scars, translucent skin, cervical spine instability, club foot, rare developmental delay
Shprintzen-Goldberg syndrome	182212	None	Rare sinus of Valsalva aneurysm	Hypertelorism, craniosynostosis, arched palate, arachnodactyly, pectus deformity, scoliosis, joint laxity, developmental delay

AoA, ascending aortic aneurysm; BAV, bicommissural aortic valve; MASS, mitral, aortic, skin, and skeletal manifestations; OMIM, Online Mendelian Inheritance in Man; PDA, patent ductus arteriosus.
From Judge DP, Dietz HC: Marfan's syndrome, *Lancet* 366:1965–1976, 2005.

Familial thoracic aortic aneurysm (FTAA) syndrome segregates as a dominant trait and can show vascular disease identical to MFS, including aortic root aneurysm and dissection. However, these persons generally do not show any of the systemic manifestations of MFS. Other families show an association between bicommissural aortic valve and ascending aortic aneurysm, which can also segregate as a dominant trait. Here, maximum dilatation often occurs further up in the ascending aorta, beyond the sinotubular junction. There is emerging evidence that bicommissural aortic valve and aneurysm both represent primary manifestations of a single gene defect, and that family members of a proband can have aneurysm without accompanying valve disease. These patients typically do not show any systemic features of a connective tissue disorder.

Unlike with MFS, many families with both FTAA syndrome and with bicommissural aortic valve and ascending aortic aneurysm show reduced penetrance. Although a number of genetic loci and genes have been described for thoracic aortic aneurysm syndrome, they do not account for a significant percentage of cases to allow efficient molecular testing, mandating ongoing clinical follow-up of at-risk family members. In most cases, the management principles that have been generated for MFS have proved effective for these other forms of familial aortic aneurysm.

Important to the differential is Loeys-Dietz syndrome (LDS). As in MFS, patients with LDS show malar hypoplasia, arched palate, retrognathia, pectus deformity, scoliosis, joint laxity, dural ectasia, and aortic root aneurysms and dissection. Although their fingers tend to be long, overgrowth of the long bones is subtle or absent, and they do not show ectopia lentis. Unique features of LDS include a high incidence of hypertelorism, broad or bifid uvula, arterial tortuosity in large and medium-sized vessels (predominantly neck vessels) and a high risk of aneurysm and dissection throughout the arterial tree. Aortic root aneurysms tend to dissect at younger ages and smaller dimensions than in MFS, often leading to death in early childhood. In view of the severe nature of vascular disease in LDS, correct diagnosis and aggressive management is essential in these patients.

Less-consistent features of LDS include blue sclerae, translucent skin, easy bruising, craniosynostosis, cleft palate, Chiari type I malformation of the brain, learning disability, congenital heart disease (patent ductus arteriosus, atrial septal defect, bicommissural aortic valve), and clubfoot deformity. There is significant overlap between LDS and the Shprintzen-Goldberg syndrome that includes craniosynostosis, hypertelorism, arched palate, learning disability, bone overgrowth, pectus deformity, and scoliosis. In contrast to LDS, vascular disease is a rare manifestation of Shprintzen-Goldberg syndrome.

LABORATORY FINDINGS

Laboratory studies should document a negative urinary cyanide nitroprusside test or specific amino acid studies to exclude cystathionine synthase deficiency (homocystinuria). Although it is estimated that most, if not all, people with classic MFS have an *FBN1* mutation, the large size of this gene and the extreme allelic heterogeneity in MFS have frustrated efficient molecular diagnosis. The yield of mutation screening varies based on technique and clinical presentation. Recent experience suggests that >95% of people with typical MFS will have an identifiable *FBN1* mutation. It remains unclear whether the "missing" mutations are simply atypical in character or location within *FBN1* or occur in another gene. Some reports suggest that mutations in *TGFβR2* are occasionally seen in classic MFS; whether or not these patients have discriminating features of LDS remains to be determined.

Other diseases in the differential such as MVP syndrome, MASS phenotype, familial ectopia lentis, Weill-Marchesani syndrome, and Shprintzen-Goldberg syndrome have all been associated with mutations in the *FBN1* gene. It is often difficult or impossible to predict the phenotype from the nature or location of a *FBN1* mutation in MFS. Hence, molecular genetic techniques can contribute to the diagnosis, but they do not substitute for comprehensive clinical evaluation and follow-up. The absence or presence of an *FBN1* mutation is not sufficient to exclude or establish the diagnosis, respectively.

TREATMENT

Management focuses on preventing complications and genetic counseling. In view of the potential complexity of management required by some patients, referral to a multidisciplinary center with experience in MFS is advisable. The pediatrician should work in concert with pediatric subspecialists to coordinate a rational approach to monitoring and treatment of potential complications. Yearly evaluations for cardiovascular disease, scoliosis, or ophthalmologic problems are imperative.

CURRENT AND FUTURE THERAPIES

Most therapies currently available or under investigation aim to diminish aortic complications. They can be categorized as activity restrictions, surgeries, endocarditis prophylaxis, current pharmacologic approaches and emerging or experimental strategies.

Activity Restrictions

Physical therapy can improve neuromuscular tone in infancy, and aerobic exertion in moderation is recommended during childhood and adulthood. Strenuous physical exertion, competitive athletics, and particularly isometric activities such as weight lifting are associated with an increased risk of aortic complications or ocular problems such as retinal detachment and should be discouraged. Consensus guidelines have been developed for activity limitations.

Surgery for Aortic Aneurysm

Successful surgical repair of aortic root aneurysms may be the single most important cause of improvement in life expectancy for patients with MFS to date. Surgical outcome is more favorable if undertaken on an elective rather than an urgent or emergent basis. Therefore, aortic root surgery in MFS should be recommended for patients with an aortic root diameter ≥50 mm and considered for those with a rapid rate of enlargement (>5-10 mm/yr) or a family history of early aortic dissection. Preserving the native aortic valve at the time of repair is desirable to avoid the need for lifelong anticoagulation with warfarin, although the long-term durability of the native aortic valve in MFS remains to be fully elucidated. Replacing the aortic root with a pulmonary root autograft (Ross procedure) is not recommended, due to the observations of progressive enlargement of the pulmonary root when exposed to systemic pressure and eventual autograft failure.

Endocarditis Prophylaxis

The American Heart Association (AHA) no longer routinely recommends the use of antibiotic prophylaxis for persons with structural or valvular heart disease, but exceptions are made for select groups at the greatest risk for bad outcomes from infectious endocarditis. The Professional Advisory Board of the National Marfan Foundation believes that patients with MFS (as well as other patients with certain connective tissue disorders who are at high risk for severe and rapidly progressive degeneration and dysfunction of multiple heart valves and for early and recurrent cardiovascular surgeries) should continue to receive prophylaxis for subacute bacterial endocarditis (SBE). SBE prophylaxis is especially important because it remains unknown but possible that the myxomatous valves typical of MFS represent a preferred substrate for endocarditis.

Current Pharmacologic Approaches

Based on the putative role of hemodynamic stress in aortic dilatation in MFS, β-blockers have traditionally been considered the standard of care, due to their negative inotropic and chronotropic effects. While multiple small observational studies have supported a protective effect of β-blockers in MFS, and a reduced rate of aortic growth was seen in MFS mice treated with propanolol, other analyses have concluded that there is insufficient evidence to support their routine use. Calcium channel antagonists (e.g., verapamil) and angiotensin converting enzyme (ACE) inhibitors (e.g., enalapril) offer alternative therapeutic options. However, there is again no conclusive evidence supporting the use of either of these classes of agent in the treatment of MFS.

Emerging and Experimental Strategies

There is extensive evidence linking angiotensin II signaling to TGF-β activation and signaling. In addition, direct activation of TGF-β-responsive signaling cascades by angiotensin II (independent of TGF-β ligands) has been reported. In a mouse model of MFS, the angiotensin II receptor type 1 blocker (ARB) losartan has been shown to completely prevent pathologic aortic root growth and to normalize both aortic wall thickness and architecture, findings that were absent in placebo-treated and propanolol-treated mice. These data suggest the potential for productive aortic wall remodeling in MFS after TGF-β inhibition. Remarkably, improvements in pulmonary and skeletal muscle pathology in these mice also occurred with losartan, further supporting the conclusion that this treatment works by decreasing TGF-β signaling rather than by simply reducing hemodynamic stress on structurally predisposed tissues.

In support of its relevance to humans, a study assessing the effect of ARBs in a small cohort of pediatric patients with MFS who had severe aortic root enlargement despite previous alternate medical therapy, showed that ARBs significantly slowed the rate of aortic root and sinotubular junction dilatation (both of which occur in MFS), whereas the distal ascending aorta (which does not normally become dilated in MFS) remained unaffected. In light of this growing body of evidence, a multicenter prospective clinical trial to assess the potential therapeutic benefit of ARBs in patients with MFS is under way.

TGF-β Neutralizing Antibodies

Several studies have shown the ability of antibodies that antagonize TGF-β to modulate the manifestations of MFS in mice, including defective pulmonary alveolar septation, myxomatous atrioventricular valves, skeletal muscle myopathy, and aortic root aneurysms. Currently, therapeutic delivery of TGF-β neutralizing antibody is not available for humans. However, a humanized anti–TGF-β1 monoclonal antibody (CAT-192) is currently under investigation for treatment of other TGF-β-related disorders, and its use remains a potential strategy for treating MFS.

Other FDA-Approved Agents

It has been proposed that ACE inhibitors might prove as effective as, or more effective than, ARBs in treating MFS. By limiting the production of angiotensin II, ACE inhibitors effectively limit signaling through the type 1 and type 2 angiotensin receptors (AT1R and AT2R, respectively). By contrast, ARBs selectively block the AT1R and might actually increase signaling through the AT2R. Given that AT2R signaling can promote cell death but also can limit TGF-β signaling, the relative benefit of the two approaches remains controversial. Several small studies suggest there is some protection afforded by ACE inhibitors in MFS, but this issue will only be definitively resolved with additional experimentation and clinical experience.

Other work has suggested that doxycycline might improve aortic root pathology in MFS. Matrix metalloproteinases (MMPs) 2 and 9 are extracellular TGF-β-responsive proteinases that cause elastic fiber damage. Doxycycline, through its broad inhibition of MMPs, has been shown to reduce aortic root growth and rupture in mouse models of MFS.

PROGNOSIS

Although prognosis is highly variable, the average life expectancy for people with MFS approaches normal, particularly in those who underwent aortic root surgery after 1980. However, there is still morbidity and early mortality associated with the disorder, placing both physical and mental stresses on patients and their families. Awareness of these issues and referral for support services can facilitate a positive perspective toward the condition.

GENETIC COUNSELING

The heritable nature of MFS makes recurrence risk (genetic) counseling mandatory. Approximately 30% of cases are the first affected individuals in their families. Fathers of these sporadic cases are, on average, 7 to 10 years older than fathers in the general population. This paternal age effect suggests that these cases represent new dominant mutations with minimal recurrence risk to the future offspring of the normal parents. Due to rare reports of gonadal mosaicism in a phenotypically normal parent, the recurrence risk for parents of a sporadic case can be reported as low but not zero. Each child of an affected parent, however, has a 50% risk of inheriting a number 15 chromosome with the MFS mutation and thus being affected. Recurrence risk counseling is best accomplished by professionals with expertise in the issues surrounding the disorder.

BIBLIOGRAPHY

Please visit the Nelson Textbook of Pediatrics *website at www.expertconsult.com for the complete bibliography.*

Section 4 METABOLIC BONE DISEASE

Chapter 694
Bone Structure, Growth, and Hormonal Regulation

Russell W. Chesney

Also see Chapters 48 and 564.

Bone is constantly being formed **(modeling)** and re-formed **(remodeling)**. It is a dynamic organ capable of rapid turnover, bearing weight, and withstanding the stresses of various physical activities. Bone is the major body reservoir for calcium, phosphorus, and magnesium. Disorders that affect this organ and the process of mineralization are designated **metabolic bone diseases.**

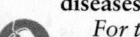

For the full continuation of this chapter, please visit the Nelson Textbook of Pediatrics *website at www.expertconsult.com.*

Chapter 695
Primary Chondrodystrophy (Metaphyseal Dysplasia)

Russell W. Chesney

Skeletal dysplasias fall under 3 major subgroupings: **osteodysplasias, chondrodysplasias,** and **dysostoses.** The osteodysplasias affect bone density and often lead to osteopenia. The chondrodysplasias are genetic disorders of cartilage and result in deficient linear growth. The dysostoses affect a single bone.

For the full continuation of this chapter, please visit the Nelson Textbook of Pediatrics *website at www.expertconsult.com.*

Chapter 696
Hypophosphatasia

Russell W. Chesney

Hypophosphatasia is defined by low serum alkaline phosphatase activity and radiographically resembles rickets. This autosomal recessive disorder, affecting mainly the skeleton and teeth, is an inborn error of metabolism in which activity of the tissue-nonspecific (liver, bone, kidney) alkaline phosphatase isoenzyme (TNSALP) is deficient, although activity of the intestinal and placental isoenzymes is normal. Single point mutations of the gene prevent expression of the activity of this enzyme in vitro and indicate its necessity for normal skeletal mineralization. A large proportion of the >100 mutations of the gene identified to date are missense mutations, although splice-site mutations, small deletions, and frame-shift mutations also have been found. The only phenotype associated with these mutations is hypophosphatasia. Some patients have a regulatory defect involving this enzyme rather than a mutation.

For the full continuation of this chapter, please visit the Nelson Textbook of Pediatrics *website at www.expertconsult.com.*

Chapter 697
Hyperphosphatasia

Russell W. Chesney

Hyperphosphatasia is characterized by excessive elevation of the bone isoenzyme of alkaline phosphatase in serum and significant growth failure. Osteoid proliferation in the subperiosteal portion of bone results in separation of the periosteum from the bone cortex. Bowing and thickening of the diaphyses are common, along with osteopenia (see Fig. 697-1 on the *Nelson Textbook of Pediatrics* website at www.expertconsult.com). The disease usually has its onset by 2-3 yr of age, when painful deformity developing in the extremities leads to abnormal gait and sometimes fractures. Other common findings include pectus carinatum, kyphoscoliosis, and rib fraying. The skull is large, and the cranium is thickened (widened diploë) and may be deformed. Skull involvement can lead to progressive and profound hearing loss. Radiographically, the bony texture is variable; dense areas (showing a teased cotton-wool appearance) are interspersed with radiolucent areas and general demineralization. Long bones appear cylindrical, lose metaphyseal modeling, and contain pseudocysts that show a dense, bony halo.

For the full continuation of this chapter, please visit the Nelson Textbook of Pediatrics *website at www.expertconsult.com.*

Chapter 698
Osteoporosis

Russell W. Chesney

Osteoporosis is relatively uncommon in children even though it is the most common bone disorder in adults. Bone volume is diminished and the incidence of fractures is greatly increased in this condition. In contrast to osteomalacia, which shows under-mineralization and normal bone volume, histologic sections of bone in all forms of osteoporosis reveal a normal degree of

Table 698-1 RISKS FOR OSTEOPOROSIS
ENDOCRINE DISORDERS
Female Hypogonadism
Turner syndrome
Hypothalamic amenorrhea (athletic triad)
Anorexia nervosa
Premature and primary ovarian failure
Depot medroxyprogesterone acetate therapy
Estrogen receptor α *(ESR1)* mutations
Hyperprolactinemia
Male Hypogonadism
Primary gonadal failure (Klinefelter syndrome)
Secondary gonadal failure (idiopathic hypogonadotropic hypogonadism)
Delayed puberty
Hyperthyroidism
Hyperparathyroidism
Hypercortisolism (therapeutic or Cushing disease)
Growth hormone deficiency
Thyrotoxicosis
INFLAMMATORY DISORDERS
Dermatomyositis
Chronic hepatitis
Systemic lupus erythematosus
GASTROINTESTINAL DISORDERS
Malabsorption syndromes (cystic fibrosis, celiac disease, biliary atresia)
True or perceived milk intolerance
Inflammatory bowel disease
Chronic obstructive jaundice
Primary biliary cirrhosis and other cirrhoses
Alactasia
Subtotal gastrectomy
BONE MARROW DISORDERS
Bone marrow transplant
Lymphoma
Leukemia
Hemolytic anemias (sickle cell anemia, thalassemia)
Systemic mastocytosis
CONNECTIVE TISSUE/BONE DISORDERS
Juvenile osteoporosis
Osteogenesis imperfecta
Ehler-Danlos syndrome
Marfan syndrome
Homocystinuria
Fibrous dysplasia
Previous or recurrent low impact fractures
DRUGS
Alcohol
Heparin
Glucocorticosteroids
Thyroxine
Anticonvulsants
Gonadotropin-releasing hormone agonists
Cyclosporine
Chemotherapy
Cigarettes
MISCELLANEOUS DISORDERS
Immobilization (cerebral palsy, spinal muscular atrophy, Duchenne dystrophy)
Rheumatoid arthritis
Renal disease
Glycogen storage disease type 1
Chronic hepatitis
Low calcium dietary intake
Gaucher disease
Severe congenital neutropenia

mineralization but a reduction in the volume of bone, especially trabecular bone (vertebral bone). In osteoporosis, by definition, there is also a reduced amount of bone tissue (termed *osteopenia*), which is associated with atraumatic (pathologic) fractures. Osteoporosis in children may be primary or secondary (Table 698-1). The primary osteoporoses can be divided into heritable disorders of connective tissue, including osteogenesis imperfecta, Bruck syndrome, osteoporosis-pseudoglioma syndrome, Ehlers-Danlos syndrome, Marfan syndrome, homocystinuria, and idiopathic juvenile osteoporosis. Secondary forms of osteoporosis include various neuromuscular disorders, chronic illness, endocrine disorders, and drug-induced and inborn errors of metabolism, including lysinuric protein intolerance and Gaucher disease.

When no obvious primary or secondary cause can be detected, **idiopathic juvenile osteoporosis** should be considered, especially if the following clinical features are evident: onset before puberty, long-bone and lower back pain, vertebral fractures, long-bone and metatarsal fractures, a washed-out appearance of the spine and appendicular skeleton, and improvement after puberty. Trabecular bones such as the spine and metatarsals are particularly affected by atraumatic fractures.

In general, blood values of minerals, vitamin D metabolites, alkaline phosphatase, and parathyroid hormone are normal. Evaluation of bone mineral content and bone density by dual-energy x-ray absorptiometry or, less often, quantitative CT shows markedly reduced values. Several modes of therapy (including oral calcium supplements, calcitriol, bisphosphonates, and calcitonin) have been used with some success in individual conditions, but the effect of these treatments is difficult to gauge because spontaneous recovery occurs after the onset of puberty in >75% of cases.

Osteoporosis-pseudoglioma is an autosomal recessive disorder manifested by variable age at onset, low bone mass, fractures in childhood, and abnormal eye development, and the defective gene has been mapped to chromosome 11q12-13. The mutation is a loss of function in the gene for low-density lipoprotein receptor-related protein 5. Interestingly, gain-of-function mutations result in a gene product that increases bone density.

The life cycle implications of either significant demineralization or osteoporosis in childhood need to be stressed. Events in childhood influence peak bone mass, and late adolescence is a period of rapid bone mineral accretion. Peak bone mass is achieved by 20-35 yr of age (depending on the bone measured), and the contribution during childhood is considerable. A number of measures have been shown to influence bone mass: vitamin D (400-800 IU daily), calcium intake (≥1,200 mg/day in adolescents), and weight-bearing exercise throughout childhood. Weight-bearing exercise enhances bone formation and reduces bone resorption. Other factors that can prevent acquisition of peak bone mass include use of alcohol and tobacco. Excellent sources of dietary calcium include mainly dairy products but also bony fish, green vegetables, and calcium-supplemented drinks (e.g., orange juice). Yogurt and cheeses can be used in lactase-deficient children. Because it appears that adult-onset osteoporosis is the result of a number of genetic factors, thus forming a complex trait interaction, specific interventions during childhood to influence bone mass are not available.

The treatment of secondary osteoporosis is best achieved by treating the underlying disorder when feasible. Hypogonadism should be treated with hormone replacement therapy, especially in thin athletic women. Calcium intake should be increased to 1,500-2,000 mg/day. In glucocorticoid-induced osteoporosis, an emphasis on the lowest possible dose to prevent disease activity (inflammatory bowel disease) with alternate-day or topical therapy and the use of inhaled glucocorticoids in asthma is essential. Special diets for inborn errors of metabolism are also appropriate. Celiac disease may be overrepresented in adults with osteoporosis and should be screened for and treated appropriately (Chapter 330.2). Treatment with bisphosphonates that inhibit bone resorption in certain secondary (glucocorticoid-induced) and adult-onset osteoporosis has been successful. Bisphosphonate therapy is also beneficial in osteogenesis imperfecta and cerebral palsy.

BIBLIOGRAPHY

Please visit the Nelson Textbook of Pediatrics *website at www.expertconsult.com for the complete bibliography.*

PART XXXIII Environmental Health Hazards

Chapter 699
Biologic Effects of Radiation on Children

Thomas L. Slovis

BASIC PRINCIPLES

Radiation exposure may be natural (50%) or environmental (man-made) (50%). Radon gas accounts for the majority (37%) of natural radiation. The contribution of man-made radiation has dramatically increased to 50% from 15% in the mid-1980s. CT now is responsible for 24% of all radiation exposure and almost half of man-made radiation (see Fig. 699-1 on the *Nelson Textbook of Pediatrics* website at www.expertconsult.com). Though it has been estimated that as high as 2% of all cancers in the USA may be attributable to radiation from CT studies, 75% of radiologists and emergency department physicians underestimate the radiation dose from CT. Some imaging procedures do not produce radiation (see Table 699-1 on the *Nelson Textbook of Pediatrics* website at www.expertconsult.com), and not all radiation-producing modalities expose a child to the same amount of radiation (see Table 699-2 on the *Nelson Textbook of Pediatrics* website at www.expertconsult.com).

For the full continuation of this chapter, please visit the Nelson Textbook of Pediatrics *website at www.expertconsult.com.*

Chapter 700
Chemical Pollutants

Philip J. Landrigan and Joel A. Forman

As many as 80,000 synthetic chemicals have been developed worldwide since World War II, assuring that children everywhere face certainty of chemical exposure. Children are especially likely to be exposed to the nearly 3,000 high-production-volume (HPV) chemicals that are produced in amounts of 1 million pounds or more per year and are most widely dispersed in the environment. Biomonitoring data on blood and urine levels of over 200 synthetic chemicals obtained by the Centers for Disease Control and Prevention (CDC) in a sample of the U.S. population through the National Health and Nutrition Examination Survey (NHANES) document that American children are exposed to a broad array of synthetic chemicals. In some cases, children carry a greater body burden than adults. The 2006 World Health Organization (WHO) publication *Preventing Disease through Healthy Environments: Towards an Estimate of the Environmental Burden of Disease* estimates that approximately one third of deaths among children 0 to 1 yr of age can be attributed to environmental factors. Southeast Asia and the Western Pacific house half of the world's children and are among the most rapidly industrializing regions of the globe, often with limited controls in place to reduce environmental exposures for children.

For the full continuation of this chapter, please visit the Nelson Textbook of Pediatrics *website at www.expertconsult.com.*

Chapter 701
Heavy Metal Intoxication

Prashant V. Mahajan

The main threats to humans from heavy metals are associated with exposure to lead (Chapter 702), cadmium, mercury, and arsenic. The most prevalent of these exposures is lead. This chapter discusses mercury and arsenic.

The general population is exposed to mercury primarily via food; fish is a major source of methyl mercury exposure. Arsenic exposure can occur from contaminated food or water; globally, more than 100 million people are estimated to be chronically exposed to drinking water containing high arsenic levels. Heavy metal intoxication results in diverse multiorgan toxicity through widespread disruption of vital cellular functions. A meticulous history of environmental exposure may be necessary to correctly identify heavy metals as the source of the protean manifestations associated with such exposure.

For the full continuation of this chapter, please visit the Nelson Textbook of Pediatrics *website at www.expertconsult.com.*

Chapter 702
Lead Poisoning

Morri Markowitz

Lead is a metal that exists in four isotopic forms. Chemically, its low melting point and ability to form stable compounds have made it useful in the manufacture of hundreds of products. Clinically, it is purely a toxicant; no organism has an essential function that is lead-dependent. Nevertheless, its commercial attractiveness has resulted in the processing of millions of tons of lead ore, leading to widespread dissemination of lead in the human environment.

The threshold level at which lead causes biochemical, subclinical, or clinical disturbance has been redefined many times during the past 50 yr. The blood lead level (BLL) is the gold standard for determining health effects. The U.S. Centers for Disease Control and Prevention (CDC), the American Academy of Pediatrics (AAP), and numerous other national and international organizations (e.g., Global Lead Network—Alliance to End Childhood Lead Poisoning, and The National Referral Centre for Lead Poisoning in India) consider a BLL of 10 µg/dL or greater as a level of concern for public health purposes. However, lead toxicity occurs below this threshold, and no safe level has been identified. Current recommendations by the CDC address this gap.

PUBLIC HEALTH HISTORY

Between 1976 and 1980, more than 85% of preschool children in the USA had BLLs of 10 µg/dL or higher; 98% of African-American preschoolers fulfilled this criterion. Over the next 25 yr, government regulations resulted in the significant reduction of three main contributors to lead exposure by means of (1) the elimination of the use of tetraethyl leaded gasoline, (2) the banning of lead-containing solder to seal food- and beverage-containing cans, and (3) the application of a federal rule that limited the amount of lead allowed in paint intended for household use to less than 0.06% by weight. Surveillance by the CDC has shown that the prevalence of elevated BLLs *(≥ 10 μg/dL)* has declined markedly, and by *2004 it was below 1.5%* in all preschoolers. However, an additional 6% had a level between 5 and 10 μg/dL, and 23.6% had levels between 2.5 and 5 μg/dL. In sum, nearly a third of U.S. preschool children continued to have measurable BLLs as measured by currently available clinical laboratory methodologies. Thus, nearly 6 million children continue to have evidence of lead exposure and nearly 300,000 have values that reach the CDC level of concern. Fortunately, children with levels high enough to be life-threatening are only rarely seen, although deaths continue to occur. Factors that indicate increased risk of lead poisoning, in addition to preschool age, include low socioeconomic status; living in older housing, built primarily before 1960; urban location; and African-American race. Another high-risk group that has been identified consists of recent immigrants from less wealthy countries, including adoptees.

Progress is also being made globally. In Mexico, the introduction of unleaded gasoline in 1990 was associated with a decline in BLLs among first-grade students, from 17 μg/dL in 1990 to 6.2 μg/dL in 1997. By 2009, all but 17 countries had completely phased out leaded gasoline usage, with the remaining countries that continue to use leaded gasoline being primarily from the former Soviet Union and in North Africa. In Malta, after the import of red lead paint was banned and the use of lead-treated wood for fuel in bakeries was prohibited, mean BLLs of pregnant women and newborns decreased by 45%. After it was documented that children living in the neighborhood of a battery factory in Nicaragua had a mean BLL of 17.2 μg/dL, whereas children in the control community had a mean BLL of 7.4 μg/dL, the factory was closed. Despite these advances, the World Health Organization (WHO) estimates that nearly a quarter billion people have BLLs above 5 μg/dL; of those that are children, 90% live in developing countries, where in some regions BLLs may be 10- to 20-fold higher than in developed countries.

Unfortunately, lead-related disasters continue to occur. In 2010, the CDC identified numerous lead-contaminated villages in northern Nigeria. The grinding of ore to extract gold caused widespread leaded dust dissemination. It is likely that hundreds of children died as a consequence of this activity, and all remaining children in the villages assessed to date were lead poisoned, with 97% having a blood lead level ≥45 μg/dL.

SOURCES OF EXPOSURE

Lead poisoning may occur in utero, because lead readily crosses the placenta from maternal blood. The spectrum of toxicity is similar to that experienced by children after birth. The source of maternal blood lead content is either redistribution from endogenous stores (i.e., the mother's skeleton) or lead newly acquired from ongoing environmental exposure.

Several hundred products contain lead, including batteries, cable sheathing, cosmetics, mineral supplements, plastics, toys (Table 702-1), and traditional medicines (Table 702-2). Major sources of exposure vary among and within countries; the major source of exposure in the USA remains old lead-based paint. About 38 million homes, mainly built before 1950, have lead-based paint (2000 estimate). As paint deteriorates, it chalks, flakes, and turns to dust. Improper rehabilitation work of painted surfaces (e.g., sanding) can result in dissemination of lead-containing dust throughout a home. The dust can coat all surfaces, including children's hands. All of these forms of lead can be ingested. If heat is used to strip paint, then lead vapor concentrations in the room can reach levels sufficient to cause lead poisoning via inhalation.

Table 702-1 SOURCES OF LEAD

Paint chips
Dust
Soil
Parent's or older child's occupational exposure (auto repair, smelting, construction, remodeling, plumbing, gun/bullet exposure, painting)
Glazed ceramics
Herbal remedies (e.g., Ayurvedic medications)
Home remedies, including antiperspirants, deodorants (litargirio)
Jewelry (toys or parents')
Stored battery casings (or living near a battery smelter)
Lead-based gasoline
Moonshine alcohol
Mexican candies; Ecuadorian chocolates
Indoor firing ranges
Imported spices (*swanuri marili, zafron, kozhambu*)
Lead-based cosmetics (kohl, surma)
Lead plumbing (water)
Imported foods in lead-containing cans
Imported toys
Home renovations
Antique toys or furniture

Table 702-2 CASES OF LEAD ENCEPHALOPATHY ASSOCIATED WITH TRADITIONAL MEDICINES BY TYPE OF MEDICATION

TRADITIONAL MEDICAL SYSTEM	CASES OF LEAD ENCEPHALOPATHY N (%)	N (%) PEDIATRIC CASES WITHIN CAM SYSTEM OR MEDICATION
Ayurveda	5 (7)	1(20)
Ghasard	1 (1)	1 (100)
Traditional Middle Eastern practices	66 (87)	66 (100)
Azarcon and Greta	2 (3)	2 (100)
Traditional Chinese medicine	2 (3)	2 (100)
Total	76 (100)	72 (95)

CAM, complementary and alternative medicines.
From Karri SK, Saper RB, Kales SN: Lead encephalopathy due to traditional medicines, *Curr Drug Safety* 3:54–59, 2008.

METABOLISM

The nonnutritive hand-to-mouth activity of young children is the most common pathway by which lead enters the body. In nearly all cases, lead is ingested, either as a component of dust licked off of surfaces or in swallowed paint chips, through water contaminated by its flow through lead pipes or brass fixtures, or from food or liquids contaminated by contact with lead-glazed ceramic ware. Cutaneous contamination with inorganic lead compounds, such as those found in pigments, does not result in a substantial amount of absorption. Organic lead compounds such as tetraethyl lead may penetrate through skin, however.

The percentage of lead absorbed from the gut depends on several factors: particle size, pH, other material in the gut, and nutritional status of essential elements. Large paint chips are difficult to digest and are mainly excreted. Fine dust can be dissolved more readily, however, especially in an acid medium. Lead eaten on an empty stomach is better absorbed than that taken with a meal. The presence of calcium and iron may decrease lead absorption by direct competition for binding sites; iron (and probably calcium) deficiency results in enhanced lead absorption, retention, and toxicity.

After absorption, lead is disseminated throughout the body. Most retained lead accumulates in bone, where it may reside for years. It circulates bound to erythrocytes; about 97% in blood is bound on or in the red blood cells. The plasma fraction is too small to be measured by conventional techniques; it is presumably the plasma portion that may enter cells and induce toxicity.

Thus, clinical laboratories report the blood lead level, not the serum or plasma lead level.

Lead has multiple effects in cells. It binds to enzymes, particularly those with available sulfhydryl groups, changing the contour and diminishing function. The heme pathway, present in all cells, has three enzymes susceptible to lead inhibitory effects. The last enzyme in this pathway, ferrochelatase, enables protoporphyrin to chelate iron, thus forming heme. Protoporphyrin is readily measurable in red blood cells. Levels of protoporphyrin higher than 35 µg/dL are abnormal and are consistent with lead poisoning, iron deficiency, or recent inflammatory disease.

Lack of heme affects multiple metabolic pathways. The accumulation of excess amounts of protoporphyrin and other heme precursors also is toxic. Measurement of the **erythrocyte protoporphyrin** (EP) level is, therefore, a useful tool for monitoring biochemical lead toxicity. EP levels begin to rise several weeks after BLLs have reached 20 µg/dL in a susceptible portion of the population and are elevated in nearly all children with BLLs higher than 50 µg/dL. A drop in EP levels also lags behind a decline in BLLs by several weeks, because it depends on both cell turnover and cessation of further overproduction by marrow red blood cell precursors.

A second mechanism of lead toxicity works via its competition with calcium. Many calcium-binding proteins have a higher affinity for lead than for calcium. Lead bound to these proteins may alter function, resulting in abnormal intracellular and intercellular signaling. Neurotransmitter release is, in part, a calcium-dependent process that is adversely affected by lead.

Although these two mechanisms of toxicity may be reversible, a third mechanism prevents the development of the normal tertiary brain structure. In immature mammals the normal neuronal pruning process that results in elimination of multiple intercellular brain connections is inhibited by lead. Failure to construct the appropriate tertiary brain structure during the first few years of life may result in a permanent abnormality. It is tempting to extrapolate from these anatomic findings to the clinical correlate of attention-deficit/hyperactivity disorder observed in lead-poisoned children.

CLINICAL EFFECTS

The BLL is the best-studied measure of the lead burden in children. Although subclinical and clinical findings correlate with BLLs in populations, there is considerable interindividual variability in this relationship. Lead encephalopathy is more likely to be observed in children with BLLs higher than 100 µg/dL; however, one child with a BLL of 300 µg/dL may have no symptoms, whereas another with the same level may be comatose. Susceptibility may be associated with polymorphisms in genes coding for lead-binding proteins, such as delta-aminolevulinic acid dehydratase, an enzyme in the heme pathway.

Several subclinical effects of lead have been demonstrated in cross-sectional epidemiologic studies. Hearing and height are inversely related to BLLs in children; in neither case, however, does the lead effect reach a level that would bring an individual child to medical attention. As BLLs increased in the study population, more sound (at all frequencies) was needed to reach the hearing threshold. Children with higher BLLs are slightly shorter than those with lower levels; for every 10-µg increase in the BLL, the children are 1 cm shorter. Chronic lead exposure also may delay puberty.

Several longitudinal studies have followed cohorts of children from birth for as long as 20 yr and examined the relationship between BLLs and cognitive test scores over time. In general, there is agreement that BLLs, expressed as either a level obtained at around 2 yr of age or a measure that integrates multiple BLLs drawn from a subject over time, are inversely related to cognitive test scores. On average, for each 1-µg/dL elevation in BLL the cognitive score is approximately 0.25-0.50 points lower. Because the BLLs from early childhood are predictors of the cognitive test results performed years later, this finding implies that the effects of lead can be permanent. Concurrent testing of lead levels and cognition sometimes also shows an association.

The effect of in utero lead exposure is less clear. Scores on the Bayley Scale of Mental Development were obtained repeatedly every 6 mo for the first 2 yr of life in a cohort of infants born to middle-class families. Results correlated inversely with cord BLL, a measure of in utero exposure, but not with BLLs obtained concurrently at the time of developmental testing. However, after 2 yr of age, all other cognitive tests performed on the cohort over the next 10y r correlated with the BLLs at age 2 yr but not with cord BLLs, indicating that the effects of prenatal lead exposure on brain function were superseded by early childhood events and later BLLs. Later studies performed in cohorts of Mexican children monitored from the prenatal period confirms the association between in utero lead exposure and later cognitive outcomes. No threshold for BLL was identified in these studies; maternal blood lead levels between 0 and 10 µg/dL even as early as the first trimester were associated with about a 6-point drop in cognitive test score results when the children were tested up to age 10 yr.

An intervention study, in which moderately lead-poisoned children with initial BLLs 20-55 µg/dL were aggressively managed over 6 mo, addressed the issue of the effects of treatment on cognitive development. Components of treatment included education regarding sources of lead and its abatement, nutritional guidance, multiple home and clinic visits, and, for a subset, chelation therapy. Average BLLs declined and cognitive scores were inversely related to the change in BLL. For every 1-µg/dL fall in BLL, cognitive scores were 0.25 point higher.

Behavior also is adversely affected by lead exposure. Hyperactivity is noted in young school-aged children with histories of lead poisoning or with concurrent elevations in BLL. Older children with higher bone lead content are more likely to be aggressive and to have behaviors that are predictive of later juvenile delinquency. One report supports the concept of long-term effects of early lead exposure. In this longitudinal study, the mothers of a cohort were enrolled during their pregnancies. BLLs were obtained early in pregnancy, at birth, and then multiple times in the offspring during the first 6 years. The investigators report that the relative rate of arrests, especially for violent crimes, increased significantly in relationship to the BLLs. For every 5-µg/dL increase in BLL the adjusted arrest rate was 1.40 (95% confidence interval [CI], 1.07–1.85) for prenatal BLLs and 1.27 (95% CI, 1.03–1.57) for 6-yr BLLs.

Whether the behavioral effects of lead are reversible is unclear. In one small, short-term study, 7 yr old hyperactive children with BLLs in the 20s were randomly allocated to receive a chelating agent (penicillamine), methylphenidate, or placebo. Teacher and parent ratings of behavior improved for the first two groups but not the placebo group. BLLs declined only in the chelated group. Two year old lead-poisoned children enrolled in a placebo-controlled trial of the chelating agent succimer showed no mean difference in behavior at 4 or 7 yr of age.

These studies support the concept that early exposure to lead can result in long-term deficits in cognition and behavior; they also hold out the possibility that reductions in lead burden may be associated with improvement in cognitive test scores.

CLINICAL SYMPTOMS

Gastrointestinal Tract and Central Nervous System

GI symptoms of lead poisoning include anorexia, abdominal pain, vomiting, and constipation, often occurring and recurring over a period of weeks. Children with BLLs higher than 20 µg/dL are twice as likely to have GI complaints as those with lower BLLs. **CNS symptoms** are related to worsening cerebral edema and increased intracranial pressure. Headaches, change in

Table 702-3 MINIMUM PERSONAL RISK QUESTIONNAIRE

1. Does the child live in or visit regularly a house that was built before 1950? (Include settings such as daycare, babysitter's or relative's home.)
2. Does the child live in or regularly visit a house built before 1978 with recent (past 6 months) or ongoing renovations or remodeling?
3. Does the child have a sibling or playmate who has or did have lead poisoning?

From *Screening young children for lead poisoning: guidance for state and local public health officials,* Atlanta, 1997, Centers for Disease Control and Prevention.

mentation, lethargy, papilledema, seizures, and coma leading to death are rarely seen at levels lower than 100 µg/dL but have been reported in children with a BLL as low as 70 µg/dL. The last-reported death directly attributable to lead toxicity in the USA was in 2006 in a child with a BLL of 180 µg/dL. There is no clear cutoff BLL value for the appearance of hyperactivity, but it is more likely to be observed in children who have levels higher than 20 µg/dL.

Other organs also may be affected by lead toxicity, but symptoms usually are not apparent in children. At high levels (>100 µg/dL), **renal tubular dysfunction** is observed. Lead may induce a reversible Fanconi syndrome (Chapter 523). In addition, at high BLLs, **red blood cell survival** is shortened, possibly contributing to a hemolytic anemia, although most cases of anemia in lead-poisoned children are due to other factors, such as iron deficiency and hemoglobinopathies. Older patients may develop a peripheral neuropathy.

DIAGNOSIS

Screening

It is estimated that 99% of lead-poisoned children are identified by screening procedures rather than through clinical recognition of lead-related symptoms. Until 1997 universal screening by blood lead testing of all children at ages 12 mo and 24 mo was the standard in the USA. Given the national decline in the prevalence of lead poisoning, the recommendations have been revised to target blood lead testing of high-risk populations. High risk is based on an evaluation of the likelihood of lead exposure. Departments of health are responsible for determining the local prevalence of lead poisoning as well as the percentage of housing built before 1950, the period of peak leaded paint use. When this information is available, informed screening guidelines for practitioners can be issued. For instance, in the state of New York, where a large percentage of housing was built pre-1950, the Department of Health mandates that all children be tested for lead poisoning via blood analyses. In the absence of such data the practitioner should continue to test all children at both 12 mo and 24 mo. In areas where the prevalence of lead poisoning and old housing is low, targeted screening may be performed on the basis of a risk assessment. Three questions form the basis of a questionnaire (Table 702-3), and items that are pertinent to the locale or individual may be added. If there is a lead-based industry in the child's neighborhood, the child is a recent immigrant from a country that still permits use of leaded gasoline, or the child has pica or developmental delay, blood lead testing would be appropriate. All Medicaid-eligible children should be screened. Venous sampling is preferred to capillary sampling because the chances of false-positive and false-negative results are less with the former.

Interpretation of Blood Lead Levels

The threshold for lead effects and the level of concern for risk management purposes are not the same. Laboratory issues make the interpretation of values between 0 and 5 µg/dL more difficult. Some labs certified as proficient by the CDC or other testing programs can accurately measure BLLs to 2 µg/dL; others only to 5 µg/dL. A screening value at or above 2 µg/dL is consistent with exposure and requires a second round of testing for a diagnosis and to determine the appropriate intervention. The timing for the "repeat" evaluation depends on the initial value (Table 702-4). If the diagnostic (second) test confirms that the BLL is elevated, then further testing is required by the recommended schedule (Table 702-5). A confirmed venous BLL of 45 µg/dL or higher requires prompt chelation therapy.

Table 702-4 FOLLOW-UP OF BLOOD LEAD LEVEL SCREENING TEST

IF SCREENING BLOOD LEAD LEVEL (µg/dL) IS:	*CDC:* REPEAT DIAGNOSTIC VENOUS BLOOD LEAD TESTING BY:	*AAP:* REPEAT DIAGNOSTIC VENOUS BLOOD LEAD TESTING BY:
<10	Not defined; < 1 year	Not defined
10-19	3 mo	1 mo
20-44	1 wk-1 mo (sooner the higher the lead)	1 wk
45-59	48 hr	48hr
60-69	24 hr	48 hr
≥70	Immediately	Immediately

AAP, American Academy of Pediatrics; CDC, Centers for Disease Control and Prevention.
Adapted from *Screening young children for lead poisoning: guidance for state and local public health officials,* Atlanta, 1997, Centers for Disease Control and Prevention; and American Academy of Pediatrics, Committee on Environmental Health: Screening for elevated blood lead levels, *Pediatrics* 101:1072–1078, 1998.

Other Tools for Assessment

BLL determinations remain the gold standard for evaluating children. Techniques are available to measure lead in other tissues and body fluids. Experimentally, the method of x-ray fluorescence (XRF) allows direct and noninvasive assessment of bone lead stores. XRF methodology was used to evaluate a population that had long-term exposure to lead from a polluting battery-recycling factory. The study found that the school-aged children had elevated lead levels in bone but not in venous blood, a finding that is consistent with our understanding of the slow turnover of lead in bone, which is measurable in years, in contrast to that in blood, which is measurable in weeks. It also indicates that children may have substantial lead in their bodies that is not detected by routine blood lead testing. This stored lead may be released to toxic levels if bone resorption rates suddenly increase, as occurs with prolonged immobilization of longer than a week and during pregnancy. Thus, children with histories of elevated BLLs are potentially at risk for recrudescence of lead toxicity long after ingestion has stopped and may pass this lead to the next generation. XRF methodology is not available for clinical use in children.

Lead also can be measured in urine. Spontaneous excretion, even in children with high BLLs, is usually low. Lead excretion may be stimulated by treatment with chelating agents, and this property of these drugs forms the basis of their use as a component of lead treatment. It also has been used to develop a test that differentiates children with lead burdens responsive to chelation therapy, the **lead mobilization test**. In this test, a timed urine collection follows one or two doses of chelating agent and the lead content is determined. However, this test is no longer recommended.

Lead in hair also is measurable but has problems of contamination and interpretability. Further research is required before indications for hair testing are established. Other tests are used as indirect assessments of lead exposure and accumulation. Radiographs of long bones may show dense bands at the metaphyses, which may be difficult to distinguish from growth arrest lines but, if caused by lead, are indicative of months to years of exposure. For children with acute symptoms, when a BLL result is not immediately available, a kidneys-ureters-bladder (KUB) radiograph may reveal radiopaque flecks in the intestinal tract, a

Table 702-5 SUMMARY OF RECOMMENDATIONS FOR CHILDREN WITH CONFIRMED (VENOUS) ELEVATED BLOOD LEAD CONCENTRATIONS

BLOOD LEAD CONCENTRATION (μg/dL)	RECOMMENDATIONS
<10	As levels approach 10 μg/dL use the 10-14 μg/dL recommendations
10-14	Lead education (sources, route of entry):
	Dietary counseling (calcium and iron)
	Environmental (methods for hazard reduction)
	Follow-up blood lead monitoring in 1-3 mo
15-19	Lead education:
	Dietary
	Environmental
	Follow-up blood lead monitoring in 1-2 mo
	Proceed according to actions for 20-24 μg/dL if:
	A follow-up blood lead concentration is in this range at least 3 mo after initial venous test *or*
	Blood lead concentration increases
20-44	Lead education:
	Dietary
	Environmental
	Follow-up blood lead monitoring in 1 wk-1 mo (sooner if value is higher)
	Complete history and physical examination
	Laboratory studies:
	Hemoglobin or hematocrit
	Iron status
	Environmental investigation
	Lead hazard reduction
	Neurodevelopmental monitoring
	Abdominal radiography (if particulate lead ingestion is suspected) with bowel decontamination if indicated
45-69	Lead education:
	Dietary
	Environmental
	Follow-up blood lead monitoring
	Complete history and physical examination
	Laboratory studies:
	Hemoglobin or hematocrit
	Iron status
	Free erythrocyte protoporphyrin (EP) or zinc protoporphyrin (ZPP)
	Environmental investigation
	Lead hazard reduction
	Neurodevelopmental monitoring
	Abdominal radiography with bowel decontamination if indicated
	Chelation therapy
≥70	Hospitalize and commence chelation therapy
	Proceed according to actions for 45-69 μg/dL
NOT RECOMMENDED AT ANY BLOOD LEAD CONCENTRATION	
Searching for gingival lead lines	
Evaluation of renal function (except during chelation with $CaNa_2EDTA$ [ethylenediaminetetraacetic acid])	
Testing of hair, teeth, or fingernails for lead	
Radiographic imaging of long bones	
X-ray fluorescence of long bones	

From American Academy of Pediatrics: Lead exposure in children: prevention, defection, and management, *Pediatrics* 116:1036–1046, 2005.

finding that is consistent with recent ingestion of lead-containing plaster or paint chips. The absence of radiographic findings does not rule out lead poisoning, however.

Because BLLs reflect recent ingestion or redistribution from other tissues but do not necessarily correlate with the body burden of lead or lead toxicity in an individual child, tests of lead effects also may be useful. After several weeks of lead accumulation and a BLL higher than 20 μg/dL, increases in EP values to more than 35 μg/dL may occur. An elevated EP value that cannot be attributed to iron deficiency or recent inflammatory illness is both an indicator of lead effect and a useful means of assessing the success of the treatment; the EP level will begin to fall a few weeks after successful interventions that reduce lead ingestion and increase lead excretion. Because EP is light sensitive, whole blood samples should be covered in aluminum foil (or equivalent) until analyzed.

TREATMENT

Once lead is in bone, it is released only slowly and is difficult to remove even with chelating agents. Because the cognitive/behavioral effects of lead may be irreversible, the main effort in treating lead poisoning is to **prevent** it from occurring and to **prevent** further ingestion by already-poisoned children. The main components in the effort to eliminate lead poisoning are universally applicable to all children (and adults), as follows: (1) identification and elimination of environmental sources of lead exposure, (2) behavioral modification to reduce nonnutritive hand-to-mouth activity, and (3) dietary counseling to ensure sufficient intake of the essential elements calcium and iron. For the small minority of children with more severe lead poisoning, drug treatment is available that enhances lead excretion.

During health maintenance visits a limited risk assessment is warranted, which includes questions pertaining to the most common sources of lead exposure: the condition of old paint, secondary occupational exposure via an adult living in the home, or proximity to an industrial source of pollution. If such a source is identified, its elimination usually requires the assistance of public health and housing agencies as well as education for the parents. The family should move out of a lead-contaminated apartment until repairs are completed. During repairs, repeated washes of surfaces and the use of high-efficiency particle accumulator (HEPA) vacuum cleaners help reduce exposure to lead-containing dust. Careful selection of a contractor who is certified to perform lead abatement work is necessary. Sloppy work can cause dissemination of lead-containing dust and chips throughout a home or building and result in further elevation of a child's BLL. After the work is completed, dust wipe samples should be collected from floors and windowsills or wells to verify that the risk from lead has abated.

A single case of lead poisoning is often discovered in a household with multiple family members, including other young children, even in a household with a common source of exposure such as peeling lead-based paint. The mere presence of lead in an environment does not produce lead poisoning. Parental efforts at **reducing the hand-to-mouth activity** of the affected child are necessary to reduce the risk of lead ingestion. Handwashing effectively removes lead, but in a home with lead-containing dust, lead rapidly begins to reaccumulate on the child's hands after washing. Therefore, handwashing is best limited to the period immediately before nutritive hand-to-mouth activity occurs.

Because there is competition between lead and essential minerals, it is reasonable to promote a healthy diet that is sufficient in calcium and iron. The recommended daily intakes of these metals vary somewhat with age. In general, for children 1 yr of age and up a calcium intake of about 1 g per day is sufficient and convenient to remember (roughly the calcium content of a quart of milk [≈1,200 mg/qt] or calcium-fortified orange juice). Calcium

Table 702-6 CHELATION THERAPY

NAME	SYNONYM	DOSE	TOXICITY
Succimer	Chemet, 2,3-dimercaptosuccinic acid (DMSA)	350 mg/m² body surface area/dose (***not 10 mg/kg***) q8h, PO for 5 days, then q12h for 14 days	Gastrointestinal distress, rashes; elevated LFTs, depressed white blood cell count
Edetate*	$CaNa_2EDTA$ (calcium disodium edetate), versenate	1,000-1,500 mg/m² body surface area/d; IV infusion—continuous or intermittent; IM divided q6h or q12h for 5 days	Proteinuria, pyuria, rising blood urea nitrogen/creatinine—all rare Hypercalcemia if too rapid an infusion Tissue inflammation if infusion infiltrates
British antilewisite (BAL)	Dimercaprol, British antilewisite	300-500 mg/m² body surface area/ day; **IM only** divided q4h for 3-5 days. Only for BLL ≥ 70 µg/dL	GI distress, altered mentation; elevated LFTs, hemolysis if glucose-6-phosphate dehydrogenase deficiency; no concomitant iron treatment
D-Pen	Penicillamine	10 mg/kg/d for 2 wk increasing to 25-40 mg/kg/d; oral, divided q12h. For 12-20 wk	Rashes, fever; blood dyscrasias, elevated LFTs, proteinuria Allergic cross-reactivity with penicillin

*Always given as the calcium salt; never as the sodium salt without calcium.
G6PD,LFT, liver function test.
From Markowitz ME: Lead poisoning, *Pediatr Rev* 21:327–335, 2000.

absorption is vitamin D–dependent; milk is vitamin D–fortified, but other nutritional sources of calcium often are not. A multivitamin containing vitamin D may be prescribed for children who do not drink sufficient milk or who have inadequate sunlight exposure. Iron requirements also vary with age, ranging from 6 mg/day for infants to 12 mg/day for adolescents. For children identified biochemically as being iron-deficient, therapeutic iron at a daily dose of 5-6 mg/kg for 3 mo is appropriate. Iron absorption is enhanced when ingested with ascorbic acid (citrus juices). Giving additional calcium or iron above the recommended daily intakes to mineral-sufficient children has not been shown to be of therapeutic benefit in the treatment of lead poisoning.

Drug treatment to remove lead is lifesaving for children with lead encephalopathy. In nonencephalopathic children, it prevents symptom progression and further toxicity. Guidelines for chelation are based on the BLL. A child with a venous BLL 45 µg/dL or higher should be treated. Four drugs are available in the USA: 2,3-dimercaptosuccinic acid (DMSA [succimer]), $CaNa_2EDTA$ (versenate), British antilewisite (BAL [dimercaprol]), and penicillamine. DMSA and penicillamine can be given orally, whereas $CaNa_2EDTA$ and BAL can be administered only parenterally. The choice of agent is guided by the severity of the lead poisoning, the effectiveness of the drug, and the ease of administration (Table 702-6). Children with BLLs of 44-70 µg/dL may be treated with a single drug, preferably DMSA. Those with BLLs of 70 µg/dL or greater require two-drug treatment: $CaNa_2EDTA$ in combination with either DMSA or BAL for those without evidence of encephalopathy, or $CaNa_2EDTA$ and BAL for those with encephalopathy. Data on the combined treatment with $CaNa_2EDTA$ and DMSA for children with BLLs higher than 100 µg/dL are very limited.

Drug-related toxicities are minor and reversible. These include gastrointestinal distress, transient elevations in transaminases, active urinary sediment, and neutropenia. These types of events are least common for $CaNa_2EDTA$ and DMSA and more common for BAL and penicillamine. All of the drugs are effective in reducing BLLs when given in sufficient doses and for the prescribed time. These drugs also may increase lead absorption from the gut and should be administered to children in lead-free environments. Some authorities also recommend the administration of a cathartic immediately prior to or concomitant with the initiation of chelation to eliminate any lead already in the gut.

None of these agents removes all lead from the body. Within days to weeks after completion of a course of therapy the BLL rises, even in the absence of new lead ingestion. The source of this rebound in the BLL is believed to be bone. Serial examinations of bone lead content by XRF have shown that chelation with $CaNa_2EDTA$ is associated with a decline in bone lead levels but that residual bone lead remains detectable even after multiple courses of treatment.

Repeat chelation is indicated if the BLL rebounds to 45 µg/dL or higher. Children with initial BLLs higher than 70 µg/dL are likely to require more than one course. A minimum of 3 days between courses is recommended to prevent treatment-related toxicities, especially in the kidney.

The indication for chelation therapy for children with BLLs less than 45 µg/dL is less clear. Use of these drugs in children with BLLs from 20-44 µg/dL will result in transiently lowered BLLs, and in some case this lowering will be accompanied by reversal of lead-induced enzyme inhibition. However, few children increase their excretion of lead significantly during chelation, raising the question of whether any long-term benefit is achieved. A study of 2 yr old children with BLLs of 20-44 µg/dL who were randomized to receive either DMSA or placebo found that the drop in BLLs was greater in the first 6 mo after enrollment in the DMSA-treated group, but the levels converged by 1 yr of follow-up. *Mean* cognitive test scores obtained at 4 and 7 yr of age were not statistically different between the groups. Chelation with DMSA (and $CaNa_2EDTA$) is not recommended for all children with BLLs from 20-44 µg/dL. Further work needs to be done to determine whether there are subgroups of children with BLLs lower than 45 µg/dL who might benefit from chelation. For example, if children are selected for chelation after demonstrating responsiveness to a test dose of a chelating agent with an enhanced lead diuresis—an indication that the drug is effective at removing lead permanently from the body—will there be better clinical/subclinical outcomes? It also remains to be demonstrated whether other chelating agents available in the USA or elsewhere are effective at either substantially reducing body stores (bone) of lead or at reversing the cognitive deficits attributable to lead at these BLLs.

With successful intervention, BLLs decline, with the greatest fall in BLL occurring in the first 2 mo after therapy is initiated. Subsequently the rate of change in BLL declines slowly so that by 6-12 mo after identification, the BLL of the average child with moderate lead poisoning (BLL >20 µg/dL) will be 50% lower. Children with more markedly elevated BLLs may take years to reach the CDC threshold of concern, 10 µg/dL, even if all sources of lead exposure have been eliminated, behavior has been modified, and nutrition has been maximized. Early screening remains the best way of avoiding and therefore obviating the need for the treatment of lead poisoning.

BIBLIOGRAPHY

Please visit the Nelson Textbook of Pediatrics *website at www.expertconsult.com for the complete bibliography.*

Chapter 703 Nonbacterial Food Poisoning

703.1 Mushroom Poisoning

Denise A. Salerno and Stephen C. Aronoff

Mushrooms are a great source of nutrition. They are low in calories, fat free, and high in protein, making them an ideal food except for the fact that some are highly toxic if ingested. Picking and consumption of wild mushrooms are increasingly popular in the USA. This rise in popularity has led to increased reports of severe and fatal mushroom poisonings.

For the full continuation of this chapter, please visit the Nelson Textbook of Pediatrics *website at* *www.expertconsult.com*.

703.2 Solanine Poisoning

Denise A. Salerno and Stephen C. Aronoff

Solanine is a mixture of several related toxins found in greened and sprouted potatoes. Potatoes exposed to light and allowed to sprout produce a number of alkaloid glycosides containing the cholesterol derivative solanidine. Two of these glycosides, α-solanine and α-chaconine, are found in highest concentration in the peels of greened potatoes and in the sprouts. Some solanine can be removed by boiling but not by baking. The major effect of α-solanine and α-chaconine is inhibition of cholinesterase. Cardiotoxic and teratogenic effects have also been reported.

For the full continuation of this chapter, please visit the Nelson Textbook of Pediatrics *website at* *www.expertconsult.com*.

703.3 Seafood Poisoning

Denise A. Salerno and Stephen C. Aronoff

CIGUATERA FISH POISONING

Ciguatera fish poisoning is the most frequently reported seafood-toxin illness in the world. Major outbreaks of ciguatera fish poisoning have been reported in Florida, Hawaii, French Polynesia, the Marshall Islands, the Caribbean, the South Pacific, and the Virgin Islands. With modern methods of transportation, the illness now occurs worldwide. Grouper is the most commonly identified source of the toxin, followed by snapper, kingfish, amberjack, dolphin, eel, and barracuda. Poisoning has also been associated with farm-raised salmon.

For the full continuation of this chapter, please visit the Nelson Textbook of Pediatrics *website at* *www.expertconsult.com*.

703.4 Melamine Poisoning

Denise A. Salerno and Stephen C. Aronoff

Melamine (1,3,5-triazine-2,4,6-triamine, or $C_3H_6N_6$), a compound developed in the 1830s, is found in many plastics, adhesives, laminated products, cement, cleansers, fire retardant paint, and more. Melamine poisoning from food products was unheard of until 2007, when melamine-tainted pet food caused the death of many dogs and cats in the USA. In 2008, feeding of melamine-tainted infant formula to more than 300,000 children resulted in kidney injuries, 50,000 hospitalizations, and 6 deaths in China. This was the first reported epidemic of melamine-tainted milk products.

For the full continuation of this chapter, please visit the Nelson Textbook of Pediatrics *website at* *www.expertconsult.com*.

Chapter 704 Biologic and Chemical Terrorism

Theodore J. Cieslak and Fred M. Henretig

Events of the last decade across the globe remind us that terrorists can strike at any time utilizing any number of unconventional weapons, including biologic and chemical agents. Children will not be spared in these attacks on civilians, and indeed, schools and daycare sites may be the targets of these actions. Pediatricians must be familiar with the clinical manifestations of diseases induced by biologic and chemical agents, many of which can be treated successfully if the diagnosis is made early, therapy is initiated promptly, and preventive measures are instituted.

For the full continuation of this chapter, please visit the Nelson Textbook of Pediatrics *website at* *www.expertconsult.com*.

Chapter 705 Animal and Human Bites

Charles M. Ginsburg

Besides dogs and cats, many animals inflict bites, including large cats (tigers, lions, leopards) wild dogs, hyenas, wolves, crocodiles, and other reptiles. The profile of bites varies by country and region. Among an estimated 3-6 million animal bites per year in the USA, approximately 80-90% are from dogs, 5-15% from cats, 2-5% from rodents, and the remainder from rabbits, ferrets, farm animals, monkeys, and reptiles. Approximately 1% of dog bite wounds and 6% of cat bite wounds require hospitalization, with an annual cost of $100 million in health care expenses and lost income. Bites from dogs are also most common in Bangladesh, India, Pakistan, and Myanmar, whereas in Nepal, cattle and buffalo account for more than half of bites, followed by dogs, pigs, and horses.

EPIDEMIOLOGY

During the past 3 decades, there have been approximately 20 deaths per year in the USA from dog-inflicted injuries; 65% of these occurred in children younger than 11 yr. The breed of dog involved in attacks on children varies; Table 705-1 depicts the risk index by breed from one study of 341 dog bites. Rottweilers, pit bulls, and German shepherds accounted for more than 50% of all fatal bite-related injuries. Unaltered male dogs account for approximately 75% of attacks; nursing dams often inflict injury to humans when children attempt to handle one of their puppies.

The majority of **dog-related** attacks occur in children between the ages of 6 and 11 yr. Boys are attacked more often than girls (1.5 : 1). Approximately 65% of the attacks occur around the home, 75% of the biting animals are known by the children, and almost 50% of the attacks are said to be unprovoked. Similar statistics apply in Canada, where 70% of all bites reported in one study were sustained by children between 2 and 14 yr; 65% of the dogs involved in the biting were part of the family or extended family and occurred in someone's home.

Of the approximately 450,000 reported **cat bites** per year occurring in the USA, nearly all are inflicted by known household animals. Because rat bites and gerbil bites are not reportable conditions, little is known about the epidemiology of these injuries or the incidence of infection after rodent-inflicted bites or scratches.

Few data exist on the incidence and demographics of **human bite** injuries in pediatric patients; however, preschool and early school-aged children appear to be at greatest risk of sustaining

Table 705-1 RISK OF DOG BITES AMONG CHILDREN IN THE USA, BY DOG BREED

DOG BREED	NO. DOG BITES (%)	DOG POPULATION (%)	RISK INDEX
German shepherd	105 (34)	12	2.83
Doberman	8 (3)	1.1	2.71
Spitz	5 (2)	1.1	1.81
Pekingese	10 (3)	1.9	1.56
Dachshund	22 (7)	5.2	1.35
Schnauzer	5 (2)	1.5	1.33
Collie	10 (3)	2.3	1.30
Hound dog	15 (5)	3.9	1.29
Poodle	10 (3)	3.1	0.98
Rottweiler	3 (1)	1.1	0.92
Beagle	3 (1)	1.2	0.80
Terrier	15 (5)	8.1	0.61
Bernese dog	3 (1)	1.7	0.58
Labrador retriever	11 (4)	8.2	0.49
Cross-breed	39 (13)	28	0.46
Spaniel	5 (2)	6.5	0.31
Shi tzu	1 (0.3)	1.2	0.26
Maltese	0 (0.0)	1.1	0.00

Data about the distribution of the dog population were collected from the local community dog register. The risk index was calculated by dividing the representation of a dog breed among the total dog population by the representation of this breed among all evaluated dog bites.
From Schalamon J, Ainoedhofer H, Singer G, et al: Analysis of dog bites in children who are younger than 17 years, *Pediatrics* 117:e374–e379, 2006.

an injury from a bite by a human. Human bites are a common cause of injury in daycare centers in the USA, although in some series the proportion of human bites is highest among adolescents. In adolescents, fist-to-mouth (tooth) injuries are associated with fights.

CLINICAL MANIFESTATIONS

Dog bite–related injuries can be divided into three, almost equal categories: abrasions, puncture wounds, and lacerations with or without an associated avulsion of tissue. Dog bites may be crush injuries. The most common type of injury from cat and rat bites is a puncture wound. Cat bites often penetrate to deep tissue. Human bite injuries are of two types: an occlusion injury that is incurred when the upper and lower teeth come together on a body part and, in older children and young adults, a clenched-fist injury that occurs when the injured fist, usually on the dominant hand, comes in contact with the tooth of another individual.

DIAGNOSIS

Management of the bite victim should begin with a thorough history and physical examination. Careful attention should be paid to the circumstances surrounding the bite (e.g., type of animal [domestic or sylvatic], whether the attack was provoked or unprovoked, location of the attack); a history of drug allergies; and the immunization status of the child (tetanus) and animal (rabies). During physical examination, meticulous attention should be paid to the type, size, and depth of the injury; the presence of foreign material in the wound; the status of underlying structures; and, when the bite is on an extremity, the range of motion of the affected area. A diagram of the injury should be recorded in the patient's medical record. A radiograph of the affected part should be obtained if there is likelihood that a bone or joint could have been penetrated or fractured or if foreign material is present. The possibility of a fracture or penetrating injury of the skull should be considered in individuals, particularly infants, who have sustained dog bite injuries to the face or head.

COMPLICATIONS

Infection is the most common complication of bite injuries, regardless of the species of biting animal. The decision to obtain material for culture from a wound depends on the species of the biting animal, the length of time that has elapsed since the injury, the depth of the wound, the presence of foreign material contaminating the wound, and whether there is evidence of infection. Although potentially pathogenic bacteria have been isolated from up to 80% of dog bite wounds that are brought to medical attention within 8 hr after the bite, the infection rate for wounds receiving medical attention in <8 hr is small (2.5-20%). Thus, unless they are deep and extensive, dog bite wounds that are less than 8 hr old do not need to be cultured unless there is evidence of contamination or early signs of infection or the patient is immunocompromised. Species of *Capnocytophaga canimorsus,* uncommon pathogens in bite-inflicted injuries, have been isolated from nearly 5% of infected wounds in immunocompromised patients. The infection rate in **cat bite** wounds that receive early medical attention is at least 50%; therefore, it is prudent to obtain material for culture from all but the most trivial cat-inflicted wounds and from all other animal bite wounds that are not brought to medical attention within 8 h, regardless of species of the biting animal.

The rate of infection after **rodent bite** injuries is not known. Most of the oral flora of rats is similar to that of other mammals; however, approximately 50% and 25% of rats harbor strains of *Streptobacillus moniliformis* and *Spirillum minus,* respectively, in their oral flora. Each of these agents has the potential to cause infection (Chapter 705.1).

All **human bite** wounds, regardless of the mechanism of injury, should be regarded as carrying high risk for infection and should be cultured. Because of the high incidence of anaerobic infection after bite wounds, it is important to obtain material for anaerobic as well as aerobic cultures.

Common causes of soft tissue bacterial infections after dog, cat, or human bites are noted in Table 705-2. High risk for infection after a bite is associated with wounds in the hand, foot, or genitals, penetration of bone or tendons, human or cat bites, delay in treatment longer than 24 hr, presence of foreign material, immunosuppression (asplenia), and crush or deep puncture wounds.

TREATMENT (TABLE 705-3)

After the appropriate material has been obtained for culture, the wound should be anesthetized, cleaned, and vigorously irrigated with copious amounts of normal saline. Irrigation with antibiotic-containing solutions provides no advantage over irrigation with saline alone and may cause local irritation of the tissues. Puncture wounds should be thoroughly cleansed and gently irrigated with a catheter or blunt-tipped needle; high-pressure irrigation should not be employed. Avulsed or devitalized tissue should be debrided and any fluctuant areas incised and drained.

There is much controversy about, and few data exist to determine, whether bite wounds should undergo primary closure or delayed primary closure (3-5 days) or should be allowed to heal by secondary intention. Factors to be considered are the type, size, and depth of the wound; the anatomic location; the presence of infection; the time since the injury; and the potential for cosmetic disfigurement. Surgical consultation should be obtained for all patients with deep or extensive wounds; wounds involving the face or bones and joints; and infected wounds that require open drainage. Although there is general agreement that infected wounds and those that are older than 24 hr should not be sutured, there are disagreement about and varying clinical experience with the efficacy and safety of closing wounds that are less than 8 hr old with no evidence of infection. Because all **hand wounds** are at high risk for infection, particularly if there has been disruption of the tendons or penetration of the bones,

Table 705-2 MICROORGANISMS ASSOCIATED WITH BITES

DOG BITES
Staphylococcus species *Streptococcus* species *Eikenella* species *Pasteurella* species *Proteus* species *Klebsiella* species *Haemophilus* species *Enterobacter* species DF-2 or *Capnocytophaga canimorsus* *Bacteroides* species *Moraxella* species *Corynebacterium* species *Neisseria* species *Fusobacterium* species *Prevotella* species *Porphyromonas* species
CAT BITES
Pasteurella species *Actinomyces* species *Propionibacterium* species *Bacteroides* species *Fusobacterium* species *Clostridium* species *Wolinella* species *Peptostreptococcus* species *Staphylococcus* species *Streptococcus* species
HERBIVORE BITES
Actinobacillus lignieresii *Actinobacillus suis* *Pasteurella multocida* *Pasteurella caballi* *Staphylococcus hyicus* subsp *hyicus*
SWINE BITES
Pasteurella aerogenes *Pasteurella multocida* *Bacteroides* species *Proteus* species *Actinobacillus suis* *Streptococcus* species *Flavobacterium* species *Mycoplasma* species
RODENT BITES—RAT BITE FEVER
Streptobacillus moniliformis *Spirillum minus*
PRIMATE BITES
Bacteroides species *Fusobacterium* species *Eikenella corrodens* *Streptococcus* species *Enterococcus* species *Staphylococcus* species Enterobacteriaceae Simian herpes virus
LARGE REPTILE (CROCODILE, ALLIGATOR) BITES
Aeromonas hydrophila *Pseudomonas pseudomallei* *Pseudomonas aeruginosa* *Proteus* species *Enterococcus* species *Clostridium* species

Adapted from Perkins Garth A, Harris NS: *Animal bites* (website). http://emedicine.medscape.com/article/768875-overview. Accessed December 3, 2010. Reprinted with permission from eMedicine.com, 2009.

delayed primary closure is recommended for all but the most trivial bite wounds of the hands. **Facial lacerations** are at smaller risk for secondary infection because of the more luxuriant blood supply to this region. Many plastic surgeons advocate primary closure of facial bite wounds that have been brought to medical attention within 6 hr and have been thoroughly irrigated and debrided.

Table 705-3 PROPHYLACTIC MANAGEMENT OF HUMAN OR ANIMAL BITE WOUNDS TO PREVENT INFECTION

CATEGORY OF MANAGEMENT	MANAGEMENT
Cleansing	Sponge away visible dirt. Irrigate with a copious volume of sterile saline solution by high-pressure syringe irrigation.*
	Do not irrigate puncture wounds. Standard precautions should be used.
Wound culture	No for fresh wounds, unless signs of infection exist.
	Yes for wounds more than 8-12 hr old and wounds that appear infected.†
Radiographs	Indicated for penetrating injuries overlying bones or joints, for suspected fracture, or to assess foreign body inoculation.
Debridement	Remove devitalized tissue.
Operative debridement and exploration	Yes for one of the following conditions: • Extensive wounds (devitalized tissue) • Involvement of the metacarpophalangeal joint (closed-fist injury) • Cranial bites by large animal
Wound closure	Yes for selected fresh, nonpuncture bite wounds (see text)
Assess tetanus immunization status	Yes
Assess risk of rabies from animal bites	Yes
Assess risk of hepatitis B virus infection from human bites	Yes
Assess risk of human immunodeficiency virus from human bites	Yes
Initiate antimicrobial therapy	Yes for any of the following: • Moderate or severe bite wounds, especially if edema or crush injury is present • Puncture wounds, especially if penetration of bone, tendon sheath, or joint has occurred • Facial bites • Hand and foot bites • Genital area bites • Wounds in immunocompromised and asplenic people • Wounds with signs of infection
Follow-up	Inspect wound for signs of infection within 48 hr

*Use of 18-gauge needle with a large-volume syringe is effective. Antimicrobial or anti-infective solutions offer no advantage and may increase tissue irritation.
†Both aerobic and anaerobic bacterial culture should be performed.
Modified from American Academy of Pediatrics. Bite wounds. In Pickering LK, Baker CJ, Long SS, et al, editors: *Red book: 2006 report of the committee on infectious disease,* ed 27, Elk Grove Village, IL, 2006, AAP, pp 191–195.

Few studies unequivocally demonstrate the efficacy of antimicrobial agents for **prophylaxis** of bite injuries. There is general consensus that antibiotics should be administered to all victims of human bites and all but the most trivial of dog, cat, and rat bite injuries, regardless of whether there is evidence of infection. The bacteriology of bite wound infections is primarily a reflection of the oral flora of the biting animal and, to a lesser extent, of the skin flora of the victim (see Table 705-2). Because each of the multitudes of aerobic and anaerobic bacterial species that colonize the oral cavity of the biting animal has the potential to invade local tissue, multiply, and cause tissue destruction, most bite wound infections are polymicrobial. Evidence suggests that as many as five different species may be isolated from infected dog bite wounds.

Despite the large degree of homology in the bacterial flora of the oral cavity among humans, dogs, and cats, important differences exist between the biting species, and they are reflected in the type of wound infections that occur. The predominant bacterial species isolated from infected dog bite wounds are *Staphylococcus aureus* (20-30%), *Pasteurella multocida* (20-30%), *Staphylococcus intermedius* (25%), and *C. canimorsus;* approximately one half of dog bite wound infections contain mixed anaerobes. Similar species are isolated from infected cat bite wounds; however, *P. multocida* is the predominant species in at least 50% of cat bite wound infections. At least 50% of rats harbor strains of *Streptobacillus moniliformis* in the oropharynx, and approximately 25% harbor *Spirillum minor,* an aerobic gram-negative organism. In human bite wounds, nontypable strains of *Haemophilus influenzae, Eikenella corrodens, S. aureus,* α-hemolytic streptococci, and β-lactamase–producing aerobes (about 50%) are the predominant species. Clenched-fist injuries are particularly prone to infection by *Eikenella* spp. (25%) and anaerobic bacteria (50%).

The choice between oral and parenteral antimicrobial agents should be based on the severity of the wound, the presence and degree of overt infection, signs of systemic toxicity, and the patient's immune status. Amoxicillin-clavulanate is an excellent choice for empirical oral therapy for human and animal bite wounds because of its activity against most of the strains of bacteria that have been isolated from infected bite injuries. Similarly, ticarcillin-clavulanate or ampicillin and sulbactam are preferred for patients who require empirical parenteral therapy. Procaine penicillin remains the drug of choice for prophylaxis and treatment of rat-inflicted injuries. First-generation cephalosporins have limited activity against *P. multocida* and *E. corrodens* and, therefore, should not be used for prophylaxis or empirical initial therapy of bite wound infections. The therapeutic alternatives for penicillin-allergic patients are limited, because the traditional alternative agents are generally inactive against one or more of the multiple pathogens that cause bite wound infections. Although erythromycin is commonly recommended as an alternative agent for penicillin-allergic patients who have suffered dog and cat bites, it has incomplete activity against strains of *P. multocida* and *S. moniliformis* and is not effective against *E. corrodens.* Similarly, clindamycin and the combination trimethoprim-sulfamethoxazole have limited activity against strains of *P. multocida* and anaerobic bacteria, respectively. Azithromycin and the ketolide antibiotics may be considered because they have activity against aerobic and anaerobic bacteria that are present in infected bite wounds. Tetracycline is the drug of choice for penicillin-allergic patients who have sustained rat bite injuries.

Although **tetanus** occurs only rarely after human or animal bite injuries, it is important to obtain a careful immunization history and to provide tetanus toxoid to all patients who are incompletely immunized or those in whom it has been longer than 10 yr since the last immunization. The need for postexposure rabies vaccine in victims of dog and cat bites depends on whether the biting animal is known to have been vaccinated and, most importantly, on local experience with rabid animals in the community (Chapter 266). In developing countries, bites from dogs, cats, foxes, skunks, and raccoons carry a high risk of rabies. Annually worldwide, animal bites result in more than10 million postexposure treatments. An estimated 55,000 deaths due to rabies occur each year, although this number probably represents an underestimation. Most deaths occur in low-income families in developing countries. The local health department should be consulted for advice in all instances in which the vaccination status of the biting animal is unknown and whether there is known endemic rabies in the community. Postexposure prophylaxis for hepatitis B should be considered in the rare instance in which an individual has sustained a human bite from an individual who is at high risk for hepatitis B (Chapter 350).

All but the most trivial bite wounds of the hand should be immobilized in position of function for 3-5 days, and patients with bite wounds of an extremity should be instructed to keep the affected extremity elevated for 24-36 hr or until the edema has resolved. All bite wound victims should be reevaluated within 24-36 hr after the injury.

Table 705-4 CODE OF BEHAVIOR WHEN HANDLING A DOG

DOG CHARACTERISTICSS	RECOMMENDED HUMAN BEHAVIOR
Dogs sniff as a means of communication.	Before petting a dog, let it sniff you.
Dogs like to chase moving objects.	Do not run past dogs.
Dogs run faster than humans.	Do not try to outrun a dog.
Screaming may incite predatory behavior.	Remain calm if a dog approaches.
The order of precedence needs to be in evidence.	Do not hug or kiss a dog.
Direct eye contact may be interpreted as aggression.	Avoid direct eye contact.
Dogs tend to attack extremities, face, and neck.	If attacked, stand still (feet together) and protect neck and face with arms and hands.
Lying on the ground provokes attacks.	Stand up. If attacked while lying, keep face down and cover the ears with the hands. Do not move.
Fighting dogs bite at anything that is near.	Do not try to stop 2 fighting dogs.

From Schalamon J, Ainoedhofer H, Singer G, et al: Analysis of dog bites in children who are younger than 17 years, *Pediatrics* 117:e374–e379, 2006.

PREVENTION

It is possible to reduce the risk of injury with anticipatory guidance. Parents should be routinely counseled during prenatal visits and routine health maintenance examinations about the risks of having potentially biting pets in the household. All patients should be cautioned against harboring exotic animals for pets. Additionally, parents should be made aware of the proclivity of certain breeds of dogs to inflict serious injuries and the protective instincts of nursing dams. All young children should be closely supervised, particularly when in the presence of animals, and from a very early age should be taught to respect animals and to be aware of their potential to inflict injury (Tables 705-4 and 705-5).

Reduction of the rate of human bite injuries, particularly in daycare centers and schools, can be achieved by good surveillance of the children and adequate supervisory personnel-to-child ratios.

BIBLIOGRAPHY

Please visit the Nelson Textbook of Pediatrics *website at* www.expertconsult.com *for the complete bibliography.*

705.1 Rat Bite Fever

Charles M. Ginsburg

ETIOLOGY

Rat bite fever is a generic term that has been applied to at least two distinct clinical syndromes, each caused by a different microbial agent.

Rat bite fever due to *Streptobacillus moniliformis* is most commonly reported in the USA as well as Brazil, Canada, Mexico, Paraguay, Great Britain, and France; it has been identified elsewhere in Europe and in Australia. *S. moniliformis* is a gram-negative bacillus that is present in the nasopharyngeal flora of approximately 10-100% of healthy laboratory rats and 50-100% of healthy wild rats. Infection with *S. moniliformis*

Table 705-5 MEASURES FOR PREVENTING DOG BITES

- Realistically evaluate environment and lifestyle and consult with a professional (e.g., veterinarian, animal behaviorist, or responsible breeder) to determine suitable breeds of dogs for consideration.
- Dogs with histories of aggression are inappropriate in households with children.
- Be sensitive to cues that a child is fearful or apprehensive about a dog and, if so, delay acquiring a dog.
- Spend time with a dog before buying or adopting it. Use caution when bringing a dog or puppy into the home of an infant or toddler.
- Spay/neuter virtually all dogs (this frequently reduces aggressive tendencies).
- Never leave infants or young children alone with any dog.
- Properly socialize and train any dog entering the household. Teach the dog submissive behaviors (e.g., rolling over to expose abdomen and relinquishing food without growling).
- Immediately seek professional advice (e.g., from veterinarians, animal behaviorists, or responsible breeders) if the dog develops aggressive or undesirable behaviors.
- Do not play aggressive games with your dog (e.g., wrestling).
- Teach children basic safety around dogs and review regularly:
  - Never approach an unfamiliar dog.
  - Never run from a dog and scream.
  - Remain motionless when approached by an unfamiliar dog (e.g., "be still like a tree").
  - If knocked over by a dog, roll into a ball and lie still (e.g., "be still like a log").
  - Never play with a dog unless supervised by an adult.
  - Immediately report stray dogs or dogs displaying unusual behavior to an adult.
  - Avoid direct eye contact with a dog.
  - Do not disturb a dog who is sleeping, eating, or caring for puppies.
  - Do not pet a dog without allowing it to see and sniff you first.
  - If bitten, immediately report the bite to an adult.

From Centers for Disease Control and Prevention: Dog bite-related fatalities—United States, 1995-1996, *MMWR Morb Mortal Wkly Rep* 46:463–467, 1997.

most commonly occurs following the bite of a rat; however, infection has also been reported in individuals who have been scratched by rats, in those who have handled dead rats, and in those who have ingested milk contaminated with the bacterium (Haverhill fever). Rat bite fever may also be transmitted by bites from wild mice. Although there have been occasional reports of the disease due to bites from other animals, these reports have not been confirmed.

Rat bite fever caused by *Spirillum minus,* called **sodoku,** is most commonly reported in Asia. *S. minus* is a small spiral, aerobic gram-negative organism. The incubation period of sodoku is longer (14-21 days) than that of the streptobacillary form of disease, and myalgia and arthritis are less common manifestations.

Reports of rat bite fever from Africa are rare, probably reflecting underrecognition rather than absence of the disease.

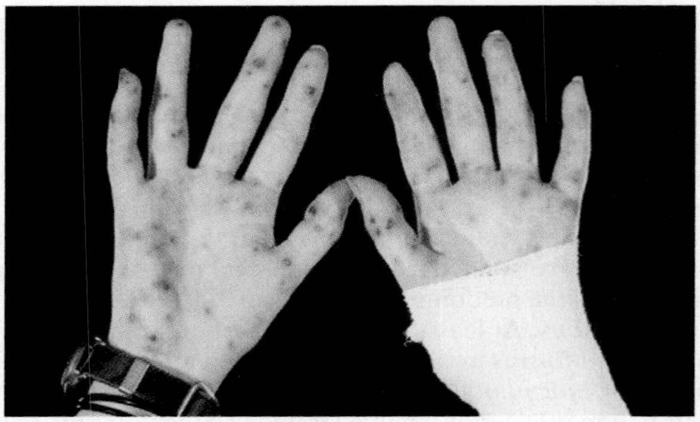

Figure 705-1 Maculopapular rash with small dark red eruptions on hand of person with rat-bite fever. (From Van Nood E, Peters SH: Rat-bite fever, *Neth J Med* 63:319–321, 2005.)

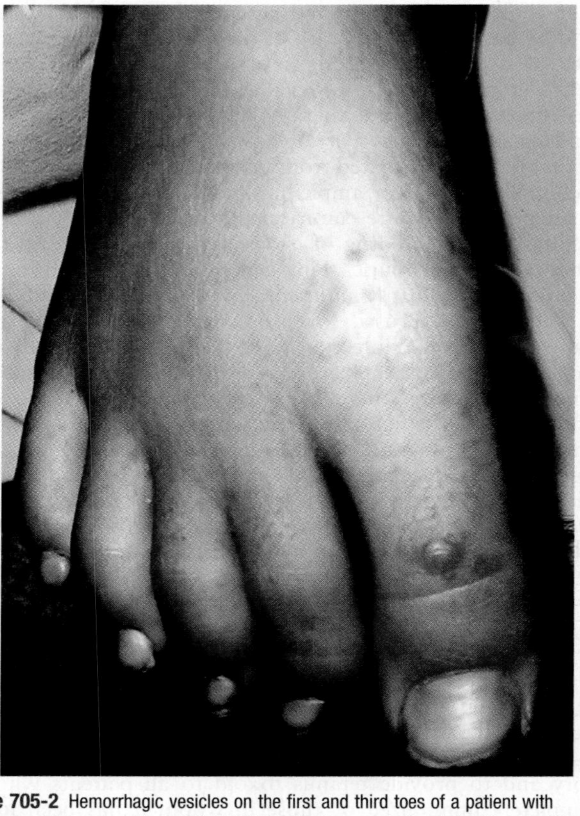

Figure 705-2 Hemorrhagic vesicles on the first and third toes of a patient with advanced rat bite fever. (From Elliott SP: Rat bite fever and *Streptobacillus moniliformis, Clin Microbiol Rev* 20:13–22, 2007.)

CLINICAL COURSE

The incubation period for the streptobacillary form of rat bite fever is variable, ranging from 3-10 days. The illness is characterized by an abrupt onset of fever up to 41°C (fever occurring in >90% of reported cases), severe throbbing headache, intense myalgia, chills, and vomiting. In virtually all instances, the lesion at the cutaneous inoculation site has healed by the time the systemic systems first appear. Shortly after the onset of the fever, a polymorphic rash occurs in up to 75% of patients. In most patients, the rash consists of blotchy, red maculopapular lesions that often have a petechial component; the distribution of the rash is variable, but it usually is most dense on the extremities (Fig. 705-1). Hemorrhagic vesicles may develop on the hands and feet, and are very tender to palpation (Fig. 705-2).

Approximately 50% of patients have arthritis, which first manifests toward the end of the first week of disease; early on, the arthritis may be migratory. If untreated, the fever, rash and arthritis last from 14-21 days; often, there is a biphasic pattern to the fever and arthritis. A wide range of complications have been reported in patients with rat bite fever, the most common being pneumonia, persistent arthritis, brain and soft tissue abscesses, and, less commonly, myocarditis or endocarditis. The mortality rate of untreated rat bite fever is estimated to be about 13%.

The hallmark of *Spirillum*-induced disease is fever associated with an indurated, often suppurative, nonhealing lesion at the bite site. Lymphadenitis and lymphadenopathy invariably are present in the regional nodes that drain the inoculation site, and many patients have a generalized macular rash that is most prominent when fever is present. In untreated patients, sodoku has a relapsing course; symptoms abate after 5-7 days of chills and fever but recur 7-10 days later. There may be multiple cycles if the disease is not recognized and treated.

DIAGNOSIS

Diagnosis of the streptobacillary form of rat bite fever is difficult, because the disease is uncommon and is often confused with Rocky Mountain spotted fever (Chapter 220) or, less commonly, meningococcemia (Chapter 184). Furthermore, *S. moniliformis* is difficult both to isolate and to identify with classic bacteriologic techniques. The organism is fastidious, requires enriched media for growth, and is inhibited by sodium polyanetholsulfonate, an additive present in most commercial blood culture bottles. A definitive diagnosis is made when the organism is recovered from blood or joint fluid or is identified in human samples with molecular technology such as polymerase chain reaction (PCR) analysis, which has been used successfully with humans and laboratory animals.

Diagnosis of sodoku is made on clinical grounds, because there are no diagnostic serologic tests and *S. minus* has not been cultured on artificial media. Rarely, the organism may be identified in gram-stained smears of pus from the infected inoculation site.

TREATMENT

Penicillin is the drug of choice for both forms of rat bite fever. Intravenous penicillin G is recommended for 7-10 days, followed by oral penicillin V for an additional 7 days. If the patient has had a prompt response and has improved in 5-7 days without evidence of endocarditis, the transition to oral penicillin can be made at that time. Tetracycline or streptomycin is an effective alternative for penicillin-allergic patients. Patients with endocarditis due to *S. moniliformis* require high-dose penicillin G and streptomycin or gentamicin.

BIBLIOGRAPHY

Please visit the Nelson Textbook of Pediatrics *website at www.expertconsult.com for the complete bibliography.*

705.2 Monkeypox

Charles M. Ginsburg

ETIOLOGY

Monkeypox virus, causing the disease monkeypox, is the most important member for humans of the genus Orthopoxvirus since the eradication of smallpox, caused by variola virus. The disease was first described in monkeys in a zoo in Denmark more than a half century ago. Monkeys are the predominant host for the virus; however, it appears to be endemic in African squirrels in the rain forest and is present in African rats, mice, domestic pigs, hedgehogs, and opossums. It also has been identified in and transmitted by prairie dogs in the USA and has affected elephants in zoos. The severity varies by strain and by host; it is relatively mild in *Cynomolgus* monkeys but severe in orangutans.

Monkeypox virus was first observed in humans from West and Central Africa in the 1970s at the time that smallpox had been eradicated from the area. In the 1970s, the secondary attack rate was around 3%, much lower than the 80% seen in unvaccinated smallpox contacts. Few cases were observed over the next two decades; however, during a subsequent outbreak in the 1990s when smallpox titers were no longer present in the population, the secondary attack rate exceeded 75%. Monkeypox outbreaks have also been reported in the Sudan. Monkeypox was accidently introduced into the USA in 2003, presumably through rodents from Ghana that infected prairie dogs who were distributed as pets. More than 70 humans were infected, typically members of the households of the infected prairie dogs and workers in the pet stores or animal hospitals caring for the pets. Primary transmission of the disease from infected animal to human is by bite or by human contact with an infected animal's blood, wound discharge, or body fluid. Human-to-human transmission of infection is uncommon but is believed to have been an important source for transmission of new cases during the U.S. outbreak.

CLINICAL COURSE

The clinical signs, symptoms, and course of monkeypox are similar to those of smallpox, although usually milder. After a 10- to 14-day incubation period during which the virus replicates in lymphoid tissues, humans experience an abrupt onset of malaise, fever, myalgia, headache, and severe backache. A nonproductive cough, nausea, vomiting, and abdominal pain may be present. Generalized lymphadenopathy, a rare finding in smallpox, is invariably present during the acute stages of the illness. After a 2- to 4-day prodrome, an exanthem appears in cephalad-to-caudal progression. As the rash progresses, the high spiking fever begins to abate. The initial rash generally first appears on the face and consists of erythematous macules. Within hours of first appearance, the macules transform into firm papules that rapidly vesiculate and become pustular over 2-3 days. Unlike smallpox lesions, but similar to chickenpox lesions, the lesions of monkeypox tend to occur in crops. Late into the second week of illness, the lesions begin to desiccate, crust, scab, and fall off.

Monkeypox should be suspected in any child who has the characteristic prodrome associated with an atypical form of chickenpox and a history of contact with prairie dogs or exotic mammals such as Gambian rats and rope squirrels. Any one of the following criteria establishes a definitive diagnosis:

1. Isolation of monkeypox virus in culture.
2. Demonstration of monkeypox DNA by PCR testing in a clinical specimen.
3. Demonstration of virus morphologically consistent with an Orthopoxvirus by electron microscopy in the absence of exposure to another Orthopoxvirus.
4. Demonstration of the presence of Orthopoxvirus in tissue using immunohistochemical testing methods in the absence of exposure to another Orthopoxvirus.

TREATMENT

There is no proven effective therapy for monkeypox. In spite of evidence that preexposure administration of smallpox vaccine is 85% effective in preventing or attenuating the disease, the rarity of the disease does not warrant universal vaccination. In instances of known exposure or in epidemic situations, there may be an indication for administering the vaccine. Consideration should be given to vaccinating close family contacts and health care workers who provide care to infected individuals. Vaccine is said to be preventative if given within 2 wk of exposure. Individuals with a compromised immune system and those who have had life-threatening allergies to latex or to smallpox vaccine or any of its components (polymyxin B, streptomycin, chlortetracycline, neomycin) also should not receive the smallpox vaccine.

Although there are data that indicate that cidofovir has in vitro virocidal activity against monkeypox virus and has also been effective in preventing monkeypox infection in animals, there are no data to support its effectiveness in humans.

Careful attention should be paid to skin hygiene, maintenance of adequate nutrition and hydration, and prompt implementation of local or systemic therapy of secondary bacterial infection that may occur. To prevent human-to-human spread of disease, a combination of the Centers for Disease Control and Prevention guidelines for droplet and airborne infection control should be implemented.

BIBLIOGRAPHY
Please visit the Nelson Textbook of Pediatrics *website at www.expertconsult.com for the complete bibliography.*

Chapter 706
Envenomations

Bill J. Schroeder and Robert L. Norris

Few experiences are more frightening for patients than being bitten or stung by a venomous animal or insect. Most bites and stings by spiders, snakes, scorpions, and other venomous animals cause little more than local pain and do not require medical attention. There are thousands of species of potentially harmful or deadly venomous creatures worldwide, and each country/region has its own array of medically important organisms.

An important concept that is commonly confused in this topic is the terms *venomous* and *poisonous*. Venom is produced in specialized glands of the host and is usually injected by means of a bite or sting. *Poisonous* refers to detrimental effects from consuming or touching a plant, animal, or insect. One major difference is that poison is generally found throughout the animal and venom is isolated to the specialized glands.

Another important concept is that not every bite from a venomous creature is harmful. In many cases no venom is injected, so-called dry bites. A dry bite may occur for many reasons, including failure of the venom delivery mechanism and depletion of venom. Up to 20% of pit viper, 80% of coral snake, and approximately 50% of all venomous snake bites are dry.

In the 2007 report of the American Association of Poison Control Centers, 70,833 consultations were related to bites and stings of various creatures, with approximately one third involving victims younger than 19 years. There were 3 deaths, all in adult males, 2 by snakes and 1 by a stinging insect.

GENERAL APPROACH TO THE ENVENOMATED CHILD

Children may be bitten or stung as they play and explore their environment. The evaluation may be hampered by an unclear history of the circumstances and the possible offending organism, particularly with preverbal children. The overall effects of some venomous bites and stings may be relatively more severe in children than in adults, because children generally receive a similar venom load from the offending animal yet have less circulating blood volume to dilute its effects.

General Management

When faced with an envenomated child, the treating physician should anticipate a dynamic clinical syndrome that may progress with time. A high level of diligence should be maintained so that important, potentially subtle findings are not missed. As with any disease process, treatment of an envenomated child should start with assessing and managing as necessary the airway, breathing, and circulation (ABCs). Most envenomations require little more than local wound care, pain control, reassurance, and possibly observation. The severely envenomated child may need airway and respiratory protection and support (e.g., high-concentration oxygen administration and endotracheal intubation) and adequate IV access in an unaffected extremity if possible. Early hypotension tends to be related to vasodilatation and should be treated with volume expansion using appropriate infusion of physiologic saline solutions (normal saline boluses of 20 mL/kg body weight; repeated as needed up to 3 times). Shock unresponsive to volume repletion may require addition of a vasoactive pharmacologic agent such as epinephrine or dopamine (in addition to antivenom administration as appropriate—see later).

The affected body part should be immobilized in a position of function and any areas of edema should be marked, measured and monitored. If antivenom (AV) is available for the envenomation, efforts should be initiated to locate and secure an adequate amount to treat the patient (at least a starting dose). In the USA, regional poison control centers can facilitate this effort and are especially helpful if the offending species is exotic. Guidance in dosing the appropriate AV can generally be found in the package insert that accompanies the agent, although the advice in inserts for some products from developing countries may contain inaccurate and incorrect recommendations. Physicians who do not regularly treat venomous bites and stings should consult local or regional experts for assistance.

Antivenom Administration

Specific AVs are available for many venomous creatures of the world, particularly snakes, spiders, and scorpions. These products essentially impart passive immunity to the victim and should be given in cases of significant envenomation as early in the process as possible, because AV is capable of neutralizing only circulating, unbound venom components in the blood.

Antivenoms may be either in liquid form or lyophilized (requiring reconstitution prior to administration). Most AVs are given intravenously. There is no benefit to giving any AV locally at the bite site. As soon as the need for AV is established, it should be placed into solution (generally diluted in a quantity of normal saline equivalent to 20 mL/kg body weight, up to 250-1000 mL total).

As heterologous serum products, AVs carry some variable risk of inducing nonallergic or allergic anaphylactic reactions. Therefore, the patient should be closely monitored, and a physician should be present during the infusion, with access to all the appropriate equipment and medications needed to reverse such a reaction. Skin tests, often recommended by AV manufacturers, are unreliable and should be omitted.

Intravenous AV should be started slowly, and the rate gradually increased as tolerated by the patient, with a goal to administer the entire dose in approximately 1 hr.

If the victim experiences a reaction to the product, it should be temporarily stopped. Intramuscular epinephrine and intravenous antihistamines and steroids should be given. Then the AV should be restarted, possibly at a slower rate and in more dilute solution. If the reaction is severe, the decision must be made as to whether the benefits of the AV outweigh the risks of anaphylaxis on the basis of the patient's clinical condition.

AV can also cause delayed immunoglobulin G and M–mediated serum sickness in some patients. Serum sickness occurs 1-2 weeks after AV administration, manifesting as fever, myalgias, arthralgias, urticaria, and potential renal and neurologic involvement. It is easily treated with oral steroids, antihistamines, and acetaminophen.

General Wound Care

As with all other breaks in the skin, bites and stings require basic wound care, including copious tap water or normal saline irrigation under pressure when possible. Tetanus immunization should be updated as needed. Blisters should be left intact to act as natural bandages and help prevent infection. Exposed tissue should be covered with wet to dry dressings. Necrotic wounds, such as those that might follow some snake and spider bites, should be judiciously debrided, with removal of only clearly necrotic tissue. Reconstructive surgery with skin grafts or muscle/tendon grafts may be necessary. In general, prophylactic antibiotics are not necessary except, perhaps, in cases in which an ill-informed "rescuer" cut into the bite and applied mouth suction.

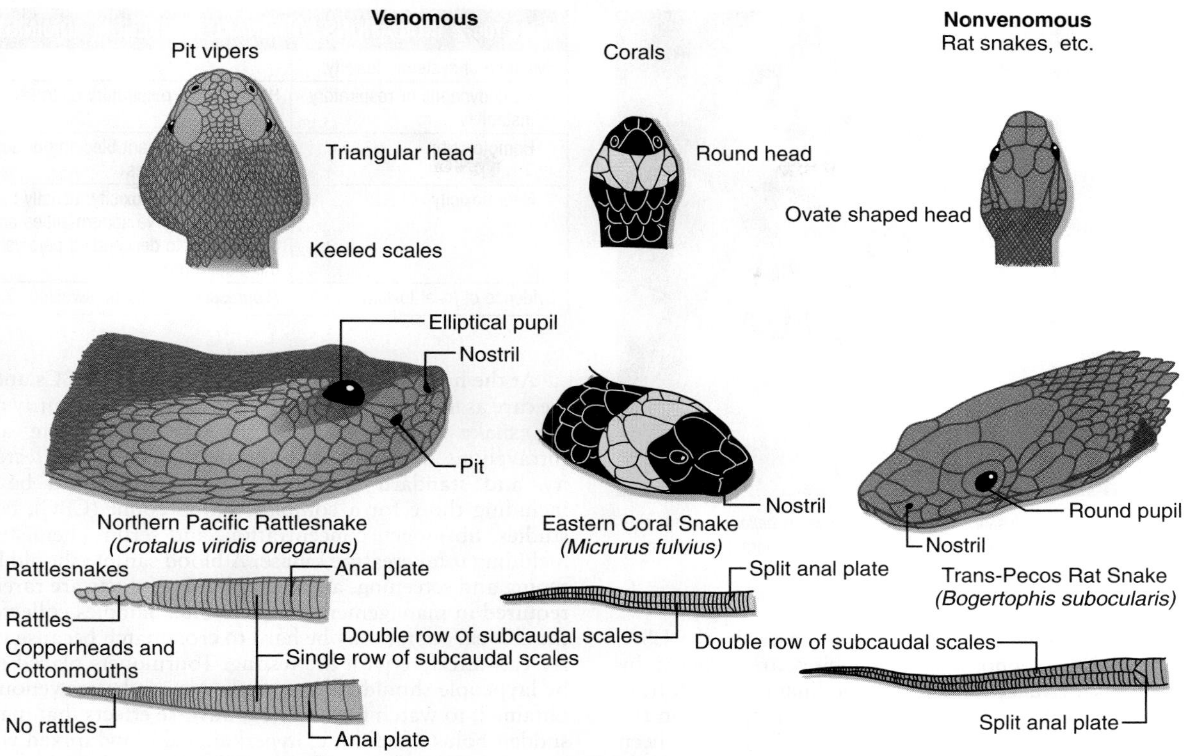

Figure 706-1 Anatomic comparison of pit vipers, coral snakes, and nonvenomous snakes of the USA. (Note: the northern Pacific rattlesnake is now classified as *Crotalus oreganus oreganus*.) (Modified from Adams JG, et al, editors: *Emergency medicine,* Philadelphia, 2008, Saunders/Elsevier. © Elsevier, drawing by Marlin Sawyer.)

Table 706-1 MEDICALLY IMPORTANT SNAKE FAMILIES

FAMILY	VENOMOUS?	LOCATION	EXAMPLES	TOXIN EFFECTS/OTHER COMMENTS
Colubridae	Some species	Most parts of the world	Garter snakes (*Thamnophis* spp), king snakes and milk snakes (*Lampropeltis* spp)	Largest family of snakes; most are considered harmless to humans; a few species are dangerously toxic (e.g., African boomslang [*Dispholidus typus*])
Boidae	None	Most parts of the world	*Boa* species, *Python* species	Constrictors; unsupervised children should not be allowed access to large constrictors
Viperidae				
Subfamily Crotalinae (pit vipers)	All	Americas, Asia	Rattlesnakes (*Crotalus* spp), cottonmouths and copperheads (*Agkistrodon* spp), Lancehead pit vipers (*Bothrops* spp)	Heat-sensing "pit" between each eye and nostril
Subfamily Viperinae (true vipers)	All	Europe, Africa, Middle East, Asia	Puff adder (*Bitis arietans*), Gaboon viper (*Bitis gabonica*)	No heat-sensing pits
Elapidae	All	Americas, Africa, Middle East, Asia	Cobras (*Naja* spp), mambas (*Dendroaspis* spp), kraits (*Bungarus* spp), coral snakes (*Micrurus* spp), and the venomous snakes of Australia	Highly variable venom effects—some largely neurotoxic, others causing severe local tissue damage
Hydrophiidae	All	Warm waters of the Pacific Ocean, Indian Ocean, and Oceana (none in the Atlantic Ocean)	Sea snakes including the pelagic sea snake (*Pelamis platurus*)	Neurotoxins and myotoxins; rarely bite humans unless provoked

Antibiotics should generally be reserved for signs of established secondary infection.

SNAKE BITES

Most snake bites are inflicted by nonvenomous species and are of no more consequence than a potentially contaminated puncture wound (Fig. 706-1). Venomous snakes, however, kill many tens of thousands of people in the world each year. The precise number is difficult to ascertain, because the toll in human suffering is far greatest in developing nations. Developed nations, with established medical care systems, have relatively few fatalities each year.

Most of the world's medically significant venomous snakes belong to one of two families—Viperidae and Elapidae (Table 706-1). In developing nations, most snake envenomations occur in agricultural workers who inadvertently contact snakes while in the fields. Many victims of snake envenomation in developed nations are adolescent or young adult males, frequently intoxicated, who are attempting to handle or catch the snake. Bites

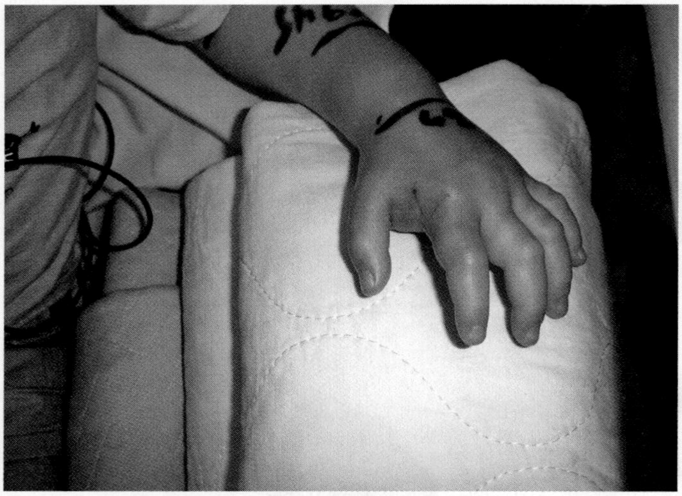

Figure 706-2 Southern Pacific rattlesnake bite (*Crotalus oreganus helleri)* in a 2 yr old boy. Note the fang marks, swelling, and bruising of the tissues (photograph taken 2 hr following the bite). (Courtesy of Sean Bush, MD.)

are located on an extremity in over 95% of cases. In the USA, approximately 98% of venomous snake bites are inflicted by pit vipers (family Viperidae; subfamily Crotalinae). A small fraction of bites are caused by coral snakes (family Elapidae) in the South and Southwest, and by exotic snakes that have been imported.

Venoms and Effects

Snake venoms are complex mixtures of proteins including large enzymes that cause local tissue destruction and low molecular weight polypeptides that have the more lethal systemic effects. The symptoms and severity of an envenomation vary according to the type of snake, the amount of venom injected, and the location of the bite. The fear caused by a snake bite can result in nausea, vomiting, diarrhea, cold/clammy skin, and even syncope regardless of whether or not venom was injected. In general, viper venoms can have deleterious effects on almost any organ system. Most viper bites cause significant local pain, swelling, ecchymosis, and variable necrosis of the bitten extremity (Fig. 706-2). The pain and swelling typically begin quickly after the bite and progress over hours to days. Serious envenomations may result in a consumptive coagulopathy, hypotension, and respiratory distress. In contrast, venoms from the Elapidae tend to be more neurotoxic with little or no local tissue damage. These bites cause variable local pain and the onset of systemic effects can be delayed for hours. Manifestations of neurotoxicity generally begin with cranial nerve palsies such as ptosis, dysarthria, and dysphagia and may progress to respiratory failure and complete paralysis. There are exceptions; some members of the Elapidae family cause little or no neurotoxicity but rather severe tissue necrosis (e.g., African spitting cobras). Some vipers cause significant neurotoxicity (e.g., some populations of the Mohave rattlesnake [*Crotalus scutulatus*]). Physicians should proactively learn the important species in their regions, including how the species can be identified, the expected effects of their venoms, and proper approaches to management.

Management

Prehospital care should focus on immobilization and rapid transport to the emergency department. Constrictive clothing, jewelry, and watches should be removed, and the injured body part should be immobilized in a position of function at the level of the heart. All proposed field treatments for snake bites, such as tourniquets, ice, electric-shock, incision, and suction, have proven problematic, with most being ineffective and deleterious.

Table 706-2 INDICATIONS FOR SNAKE ANTIVENOM ADMINISTRATION

Evidence of systemic toxicity:	
Hemodynamic or respiratory instability	Hypotension, respiratory distress
Hemotoxicity	Clinically significant bleeding or abnormal coagulation studies
Neurotoxicity	Any evidence of toxicity: usually beginning with cranial nerve abnormalities and progressing to descending paralysis including the diaphragm
Evidence of local toxicity	*Progressive* soft tissue swelling

At the hospital, attention is directed to the ABCs and supportive care as needed. An effort should be made to identify the offending snake and then to secure the appropriate antivenom. Intravenous access should be established in an unaffected extremity, and standard laboratory specimens should be obtained, including those for a complete blood count (CBC), coagulation studies, fibrinogen concentration, and serum chemistry analysis including total creatine kinase. A blood sample should be sent for typing and screening, although blood products are rarely actually required in management of snake bite. Samples collected later in the clinical course may be hard to crossmatch because venom and AV can interfere with the testing. Tourniquets placed in the field by laypeople should be cautiously removed after venous access is obtained, to watch for and treat adverse effects that may follow a sudden bolus of acidotic, hyperkalemic blood mixed with venom into the systemic circulation. The bitten extremity should be marked at 2 or more sites proximal to the bite, and the circumferences at these locations should be assessed every 15 min to monitor for progressive edema—indicative of ongoing venom effects.

AVs are relatively specific for the snake species against which they are designed to protect. There is no benefit to administering an AV for an unrelated species, and doing so certainly involves unacceptable risk (e.g., anaphylaxis) and expense. If it is determined that the child requires AV, a search for the appropriate product should begin as soon as possible—checking the hospital pharmacy, regional poison control center, and perhaps local zoos and museums that keep captive snakes.

Indications for administering antivenom can be found in Table 706-2.

Occasionally the sharp, recurved teeth of snakes, including nonvenomous snakes, are left behind in wounds; they should be identified (using soft tissue radiographs or ultrasound as needed) and removed.

Disposition

Any child with a potential venomous snake bite should be admitted to a closely observed setting for at least 24 hr, regardless of whether evidence of envenomation exists or AV has been given.

SPIDER BITES

More than 20,000 venomous spiders have been identified, but most lack either potent venom or fangs long enough to penetrate human skin, and are therefore of no medical significance. No spiders can be considered truly deadly, meaning that an untreated bite in a human would be expected to cause death. The spiders of medical significance can be broadly divided into 2 major groups: those that cause a neurotoxic syndrome and those that cause tissue necrosis. In the USA, the only significant morbidities are caused by one genus of spider from each group: *Lactrodectus* (the widow spiders) and *Loxosceles* (the fiddleback or recluse spiders).

Neurotoxic Spiders

The major neurotoxic spiders are the widow spiders (*Latrodectus* spp), the funnel web spiders (*Atrax* and *Hydranyche* spp—found

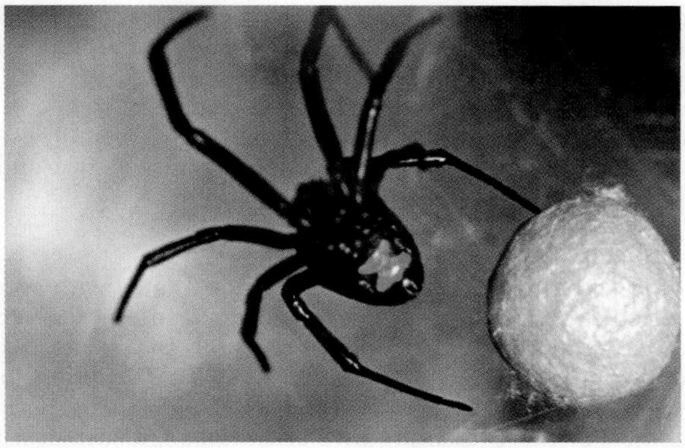

Figure 706-3 This "black widow" spider, *Latrodectus mactans*, was photographed during a study of migrant labor camp disease vectors. Though spiders are "mostly" harmless to man, two genera, *Latrodectus spp*, the "black widow" spiders, and *Loxosceles spp*, including the "brown recluse" spider, *Loxosceles reclusa*, produce bites that are poisonous to humans. (From The Centers for Disease Control and Prevention Public Health Image Library, Image #5449.)

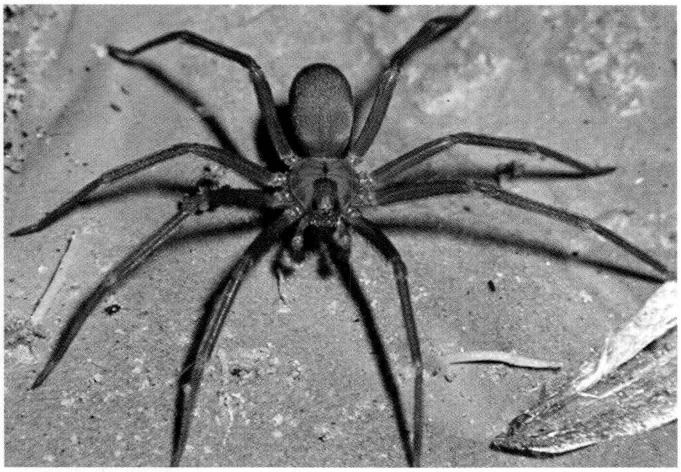

Figure 706-4 Male recluse spider (*Loxosceles* sp). Note the distinct violin-shaped marking on the dorsum of the cephalothorax. (Courtesy of Michael Cardwell/Extreme Wildlife Photography.)

in Australia), and the banana spiders (*Phoneutria* spp—indigenous to Latin America).

VENOMS AND EFFECTS. Neurotoxic spiders all possess venoms that act at neural synapses, both at neuromuscular junctions and at autonomic nervous system junctions. All of the widow spiders (*Latrodectus* spp, including the well-studied black widow [*Latrodectus mactans;* Fig. 706-3)] and the Australian red-back spider [*Latrodectus hasseltii*]) possess very similar venoms, with the most important neurotoxin being α-latrotoxin. The neurotoxin of the Sydney funnel web spider (*Atrax robustus*) is robustoxin.

Bites by the neurotoxic spiders tend to be very painful, and the offending spider is often seen. Systemic effects may include hypertension, tachycardia, bradycardia, hypersalivation, diaphoresis, and diffuse muscle spasms.

MANAGEMENT. Management of neurotoxic spider envenomation centers on sound supportive care. Several *Latrodectus* AVs are available, and each appears to be effective regardless of which species of widow spider was responsible for the bite. There is also an AV for the Sydney funnel web spider, the only species of funnel web that has caused human fatalities (none since the introduction of the AV), and a polyspecific AV for the banana spider in South America. These AVs should be used in significant bites with potentially serious systemic effects. The package insert for the appropriate product is used to guide therapy.

In the USA, *Latrodectus* AV is administered to reverse serious systemic effects of widow spider envenomation. One vial is given either intramuscularly (IM) or IV. Efficacy is usually noted within 1 hr of administration, reversal of systemic toxicity and relief of pain being noted. Occasionally, a second vial is necessary. There have been deaths related to acute nonallergic anaphylactic reactions to the U.S. AV, so its administration should be undertaken with due caution and close monitoring.

If AV is to be withheld or is not available, generous doses of opioid analgesics and benzodiazepines may be used to ease symptoms (though this may require up to 72 hr of therapy).

DISPOSITION. Most neurotoxic spider bite victims, even those requiring AV, can be discharged from the emergency department if they have a satisfactory response to therapy. Parents should be warned to bring their child back for any recurrence of venom effects. Children with more severe cases should be admitted for 24 hr of monitoring.

Necrotizing Spiders

VENOMS AND EFFECTS. Although many spiders may cause a small amount of local tissue damage after their bites, the spiders most notorious for their dermonecrotic potential are the violin or recluse spiders of the genus *Loxosceles*. The best known member of this genus is the brown recluse (*Loxosceles reclusa*) (Fig. 706-4), found in the midwestern and southern portions of the USA. The venom of *Loxosceles* spiders contains a phospholipase enzyme, sphingomyelinase D, which attacks cell membranes and can cause local tissue damage that can occasionally be severe. The bite of this spider is generally painless and initially goes unnoticed. A few hours after the bite, pain related to focal ischemia begins at the site. Within a day, the site may have a central clear or blood-filled vesicle with surrounding ecchymosis and a rim of pale ischemia. The lesion may gradually expand over a period of days to weeks until necrotic tissue sloughs and healing begins.

Rare cases of systemic loxoscelism appear to be more common in young children than adults. They present with systemic toxicity, including fever, chills, nausea, malaise, diffuse macular rash, and petechiae, and may experience hemolysis, coagulopathy, and/or renal failure.

MANAGEMENT. For necrotizing spider bites, management of the wound involves sound supportive care, including intermittent local ice therapy for the first 72 hr and administration of antibiotics if there is any question of secondary bacterial infection. Daily wound cleansings, combined with splinting of the bitten area, should be performed until the wound is healed.

Nothing has been definitively proven effective in limiting the extent of necrosis following a spider bite. There is no role for steroids in managing necrotic arachnidism. Dapsone, though used anecdotally in managing *Loxosceles* bites in adults, is not approved for use in children and should not be prescribed.

Children appearing systemically unwell should be admitted and undergo laboratory evaluation (CBC, coagulation studies, and urinalysis). Systemic loxoscelism is managed with intravenous hydration, management of renal failure as needed, and a brief course of systemic steroids to stabilize red blood cell membranes. Though there are documented fatalities following bites by the South American violin spider (*Loxosceles laeta*), there has never been a definitively proven fatality following a brown recluse bite in the USA. No AV is commercially available in the USA for management of necrotizing spider bites such as those from *Loxosceles* species.

DISPOSITION. Victims with potentially necrotic bites should be monitored for a few days with daily wound checks. Local, intermittent cooling therapy should be continued for approximately 72 hr. Any child with a probable necrotizing spider bite and evidence of systemic involvement should be admitted to be watched for hemolysis and coagulopathy.

SCORPION STINGS

Of the more than 1,200 species of scorpions worldwide, only a few cause more than a painful sting. In the USA, there is one medically significant scorpion, the bark scorpion (*Centruroides sculpturatus* [formerly *Centruroides exilicauda*]). Though this scorpion has caused death in children in the past, such an outcome is exceedingly rare. It is found only in Arizona and small areas of immediately surrounding states. In other regions of the world, especially Latin America, Africa, the Middle East, and Asia, a number of scorpions regularly cause fatalities, particularly in small children.

Venoms and Effects

The major components of important scorpion venoms are neurotoxins that alter neural membrane ionic channels, causing autonomic and cardiovascular dysfunction through the release of acetylcholine and catecholamines. Manifestations of scorpion stings in children vary from mild to severe and may include pain, paresthesias, roving eye movements, cranial nerve dysfunction, opisthotonos/emprosthotonos, seizures, hypertensive crisis, cardiovascular collapse, and respiratory failure.

Management

Most stings require only pain control and respond well to ice, immobilization, and analgesics. Management of severe stings should begin with the ABCs. Opioid analgesics may have some synergy with scorpion neurotoxins and should be used with caution. Benzodiazepines may be more useful, especially for severe muscle spasms or sedation of the agitated child. Approximately 20 different scorpion AVs are available worldwide, but their use is controversial, due to variable efficacy and the risk of potential nonallergic anaphylaxis. Practitioners should be familiar with the local standard of care for treating the stings of their indigenous scorpions and should consult a local or regional expert for assistance as necessary. In the USA, there are currently no commercially available AVs for the bark scorpion, but clinical experience is growing with the experimental use of a Mexican antivenom (Alacramyn) in certain Arizona hospitals. The practitioner should contact the Arizona Poison Control for details and assistance (520-626-6016). In some regions of the world, prazosin is used in severe scorpion stings to ameliorate acute cardiovascular effects.

Disposition

The child with evidence of systemic toxicity following a scorpion sting should be admitted for at least 24 hr of monitoring (including cardiac monitoring) and, if envenomation is severe, should be monitored in a pediatric intensive care unit. In the absence of systemic toxicity and with adequate pain control, children older than 1 yr can be discharged home with a responsible adult.

HYMENOPTERA STINGS

The insect order Hymenoptera includes the stinging ants, bees, and wasps, which are characterized by the presence of a modified ovipositor (stinger) at the end of the abdomen through which venom is injected. Various members of the order can be found throughout the world.

Venoms and Effects

Hymenoptera venoms, mixtures of proteins and vasoactive substances, are not very potent. Most stings result in only local pain, redness, and swelling, followed by itching and resolution. Some patients experience a large local reaction in which swelling progresses beyond the sting site, possibly involving the entire extremity. Approximately 0.4-0.8% of children are at risk for acute, life-threatening reactions due to hymenoptera venom sensitivity. Each year, an estimated 50-150 people in the USA die of allergic anaphylaxis caused by hymenoptera stings (Chapter 64). Rare cases of delayed serum sickness can follow hymenoptera stings. Finally, with the spread of Africanized honey bees (*Apis mellifera scutellata*), massive stinging episodes resulting in systemic venom toxicity (hypotension, respiratory failure, shock, hemolysis, and renal failure) appear to be increasing in Latin America and the southwestern U.S. states.

Management

Children with typical local reactions can be treated with application of cold compresses and with analgesics and antihistamines as needed. Children with large local reactions should also receive a 5-day course of oral corticosteroids and a prescription for an epinephrine autoinjection kit (and instructions in its use) prior to discharge. Patients presenting with urticaria, angioedema, wheezing, or hypotension should be treated aggressively for an immediate hypersensitivity reaction with intramuscular epinephrine (0.01 mg/kg, up to 0.3-0.5 mg of 1:1000 formulation), airway management as needed, oxygen, intravenous fluids, antihistamines, and corticosteroids. Children suffering massive stinging episodes should undergo treatment similar to that for allergic anaphylaxis.

Disposition

Children with local reactions (limited or large local) can be discharged with continued care as outlined previously and instructions for wound precautions. More difficult disposition decisions are involved for children with systemic manifestations. Children with only diffuse urticaria, who are stable after a period of observation, can be discharged in the care of a responsible adult to continue antihistamines and steroids and to carry an epinephrine self-administration kit. These children seem to be at little risk for progressing to systemic anaphylaxis with future stings. Children suffering more than simple hives (e.g., wheezing, evidence of laryngeal edema or cardiovascular instability) should be admitted for 24 hr of observation and should receive a referral to an allergist for testing for hymenoptera venom sensitivity and possible immunotherapy. Immunotherapy reduces the risk of systemic anaphylaxis from future stings in high-risk patients from somewhere between 30 and 60% to less than 5%.

MARINE ENVENOMATION

The most commonly encountered venomous marine creatures are the jellyfish (Cnidaria), stingrays (Chondricthyes), and members of the family Scorpaenidae—the lionfish, scorpionfish, and stonefish. Although most injuries occur when a child ventures into the animal's natural environment, lionfish (*Pterois* spp.) are commonly kept in private aquariums and children may be stung if they attempt to handle these beautiful fish.

Venoms and Effects

All jellyfish have unique stinging cells called **nematocysts**. These cells contain a highly folded tubule that everts on contact and injects venom. The venom is antigenic and can be dermonecrotic, hemolytic, cardiotoxic, or neuropathic, depending on the species. The nematocysts can sting even after the tentacle is severed from the body and after the jellyfish is dead. The Pacific box jellyfish *(Chironex fleckeri)* of Australia, with its cardiotoxic venom, is known to cause rapidly fatal stings. Although fatal anaphylaxis to jellyfish stings has been reported in coastal waters of the USA, these events are rare. For clinicians in the Americas, the primary concern with jellyfish stings is localized pain that may be associated with paresthesias or pruritus. Rarely, jellyfish victims may have systemic symptoms such as nausea, vomiting, headache, and chills.

Stingrays have a sharp, retro-serrated spine and associated venom gland at the base of the tail. Stings tend to occur when the victim steps on the animal hidden in the surf. Injuries involve jagged lacerations from the spine, and the venom has vasoconstrictive properties that can result in tissue necrosis and poor wound healing. Stingray envenomations are noteworthy for immediate and intense pain at the site of injury that lasts 24-48 h. Some patients experience nausea, vomiting, and muscle cramps, and, rarely, hypotension or seizures.

The Scorpaenidae have venomous dorsal, pelvic, and anal spines that become erect when threatened. The glands associated with these spines contain venoms that result in direct myotoxicity leading to paralysis of cardiac, involuntary, and skeletal muscles. Envenomation causes immediate pain that may persist for hours or days. Victims may experience intense local tissue destruction in which superinfections are common. Systemic symptoms include vomiting, abdominal pain, headache, delirium, seizures, and respiratory failure.

Management

Treatment of jellyfish stings begins in the ocean. The involved skin should be quickly rinsed in seawater (fresh water may stimulate further nematocyst firing). Dousing the sting site with vinegar or rubbing alcohol can inhibit nematocyst discharge. Visible tentacle fragments should be removed with a gloved hand or forceps, and microscopic fragments may be removed by gently shaving the affected area. Folk remedies such as rubbing the sting with sand and applying urine are not helpful and cause more irritation. Meat tenderizer is not effective. Antihistamines and corticosteroids are indicated for swelling and urticaria. Antibiotics are not needed.

Treatment of stingray and Scorpaenidae stings is similar. These toxins are heat labile, and immersion in hot water (approximately 42°C) for 30-60 min denatures the protein constituents and decreases pain significantly. The wounds should be thoroughly cleaned and explored with use of local or regional anesthesia to rule out retention of spine or integument fragments. Stingray spines are radiopaque and may be seen on plain films of the wounded area. Lacerations should be treated with delayed primary closure or allowed to heal by secondary intention. Systemic analgesia should be provided as needed. Due to the risk of secondary bacterial infection, there should be a low threshold for administering prophylactic antibiotics to cover *Staphylococcus*, *Streptococcus*, and *Vibrio* species, and wounds should be rechecked daily for a few days.

Disposition

After wound care, most victims can be discharged home with responsible adults. If there are significant systemic effects after pain control is achieved, the child should be admitted for monitoring and further care as needed.

Bites and stings by venomous creatures are common occurrences in children, but they uncommonly cause major morbidity or mortality. The majority of such injuries do very well with sound supportive care. In serious cases, aggressive management of the ABCs combined with specific interventions (such as AVs when available) maximize the potential for an optimal outcome. A low threshold should be maintained for consulting specialists in envenomation medicine as needed.

BIBLIOGRAPHY

Please visit the Nelson Textbook of Pediatrics *website at www.expertconsult.com for the complete bibliography.*

PART XXXIV Laboratory Medicine

Chapter 707
Laboratory Testing in Infants and Children
Stanley F. Lo

Reference intervals, more commonly known as normal values, are difficult to establish within the pediatric population. Differences in genetic composition, physiologic development, environmental influences, and subclinical disease are variables that need to be considered when developing reference intervals. Other considerations for further defining reference intervals include partitioning based on sex and age. The most commonly used reference range is generally given as the mean of the reference population ±2 standard deviations (SD). This is acceptable when the distribution of results for the tested population is essentially gaussian. The serum sodium concentration in children, which is tightly controlled physiologically, has a distribution that is essentially gaussian; the mean value ±2 SD gives a range very close to that actually observed in 95% of children (see Table 707-1 on the *Nelson Textbook of Pediatrics* website at www.expertconsult.com). However, not all analytes have a gaussian distribution. The serum creatine kinase level, which is subject to diverse influences and is not actively controlled, does not show a gaussian distribution, as evidenced by the lack of agreement between the range actually observed and that predicted by the mean value ±2 SD. In these cases, a reference interval defining the 2.5-97.5th percentiles are typically used.

Reference cutoffs are typically established from large studies with a large reference population. Examples of these cutoffs are illustrated by reference cutoffs established for cholesterol, lipoproteins, and neonatal bilirubin. Patient results exceeding these cutoffs have a future risk of acquiring disease. A final modification needed for reporting reference intervals is referencing the Tanner stage of sexual maturation, which is most useful in assessing pituitary and gonadal function.

The establishment of common reference intervals remains an elusive target. While some patient results are directly comparable between laboratories and methods, most are not. Careful interpretation of patient results must consider when testing was performed and what method was used. Higher order methods, methods that are more accurate and precise, continue to be slowly developed. These will be critical to the standardization of tests and the establishment of common reference intervals.

For the full continuation of this chapter, please visit the Nelson Textbook of Pediatrics *website at www.expertconsult.com.*

Chapter 708
Reference Intervals for Laboratory Tests and Procedures
Stanley F. Lo

In Tables 708-1 through 708-6 (found on the *Nelson Textbook of Pediatrics* website at www.expertconsult.com), the reference intervals apply to infants, children, and adolescents when possible. For many analyses, however, separate reference intervals for children and adolescents are not well delineated. When interpreting a test result, the reference interval supplied by the laboratory performing the test should always be used as these intervals are instrument and/or method dependent. See Figures 708-1 to 708-3 (also located on the *Nelson Textbook of Pediatrics* website at www.expertconsult.com) for estimations related to dosages.

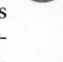

Index

Web entries can be found by visiting the Nelson Textbook of Pediatrics *website at* www.expertconsult.com

A
AA amyloidosis, 857-858, *see also website*
AADC. *See* Aromatic amino acid decarboxylase deficiency (AADC); Aromatic L-amino acid decarboxylase (AADC) deficiency
Aagenaes syndrome, 1382
AAIDD. *See* American Association on Intellectual and Developmental Disabilities (AAIDD)
A-ao_2. *See* Alveolar-arterial oxygen (A-ao_2) gradient
AAP. *See* American Academy of Pediatrics (AAP)
AAS. *See* Anabolic-androgenic steroids (AAS)
ABA. *See* Applied behavior analysis (ABA)
Abacavir
  adverse reaction to, 826
  for HIV infection, 1168t-1171t
Abatacept
  for juvenile idiopathic arthritis, 838t
  for rheumatic disease, *see website*
Abbreviations in laboratory testing, *see website*
ABCA3 gene defect, 1497-1498, *see also website*
ABCB4 gene defect, 1383t
ABCB11 gene defect, 1383t
ABCC2 gene defect, 1383t
ABCD. *See* Amphotericin B colloid dispersion (ABCD)
ABCDE assessment in pediatric emergency, 279
ABCD rule in melanoma assessment, 2232-2233
ABCs of resuscitation, 575
ABC transporters, *see website*
Abdomen
  eating disorders effects on, 93t
  malnutrition effects on, 175t
  newborn assessment of, 535-536
  protuberant, *see website*
  traumatic injury to, 338-339, 338t-339t, 339f
    due to child abuse, 140
Abdominal actinomyces, *see website*
Abdominal distention, 1249
  in Hirschsprung disease, 1285, 1285t
  in malabsorption syndromes, 1305, 1306f
  in newborn, 535-536, *see also website*
  nondigestive causes of, 1241t
Abdominal epilepsy, 1247t
Abdominal mass(es), 1249
  in newborn assessment, 535
  nondigestive causes of, 1241t
  as sign of cancer, 1728
  in Wilms tumor, 1758
Abdominal migraine, 1346t, 2042
Abdominal pain, 1247-1248, 1247t-1248t
  in acute intermittent porphyrias, *see website*
  in acutely ill child, 276
  of appendicitis, 1350
  in *Campylobacter* infection, 969
  exclusion from day care due to, *see website*
  functional, 1346-1349, 1346t-1348t
  in hyperparathyroidism, 1921
  nondigestive causes of, 1241t
  in pancreatitis, 1371
  of peptic ulcer disease, 1292
  in Wilms tumor, 1758
Abdominal palpation
  in acutely ill child evaluation, 276-277
  in appendicitis, 1350
  in intussusception, 1288
Abdominal tenderness in appendicitis, 1350
Abdominal thrusts
  for airway obstruction, 282-283, 283f
  drowning and, 344
Abdominal tuberculosis, 1006
Abdominal tumors, 1758t
Abdominal undescended testis, 1859
Abdominal visceral nerve block, 372
Abdominal wall defects, 578
  in newborn, 535-536
Abducens nerve
  neurologic examination of, *see website*
  palsy of, 2160
Abduction, 2331
Abetalipoproteinemia, 477-478, 1312-1313
Abilify. *See* Arpiprazole
Ablation
  catheter, for supraventricular tachycardia, 1614-1615
  nerve, 373
ABLC. *See* Amphotericin B lipid complex (ABLC)
ABO incompatibility, 619
Abortive poliomyelitis, 1083, 1086
ABP. *See* American Board of Pediatrics (ABP)
ABPA. *See* Allergic bronchopulmonary aspergillosis (ABPA)
ABPM. *See* Ambulatory blood pressure monitoring (ABPM)
ABR. *See* Auditory brainstem evoked response (ABR)
Abrasions, 341
  corneal, 2184
Abscess
  Bezold, 2210-2211
  brain, 2098-2099, 2099f
    due to anaerobes, *see website*
    cerebrospinal fluid findings in, 2088t
    imaging studies in, *see website*
    with tetralogy of Fallot, 1576
  Brodie, 2395
  with Crohn disease, 1300-1301
  dental, 1255, 1256f
  epidural, poliovirus infection *versus*, 1085t
  fever of unknown origin in, 900t
  liver, 1404-1405, 1404f-1405f
    amebic, 1179
  muscle, 905
  pelonidal, 1362
  perianal, 1360, 1360f
  peritoneal, 1417-1418
  peritonsillar, 1440, 1442
    croup *versus*, 1447
  pharyngeal, lateral, 1440-1442, 1441f
  psoas, 1300-1301
  pulmonary, 1480-1481
    clinical manifestations of, 1480
    diagnosis of, 1480, 1480f-1481f
    pathology and pathogenesis of, 1480
    prognosis for, 1481
    treatment of, 1480-1481
  renal, 1830, 1832
  retropharyngeal, 1440-1442, 1441f
  tubo-ovarian, 1871, *see website*
Absence seizure, 2019, 2023
  atypical, 2023
  treatment of, 2028
Absolute bioavailability in drug therapy, *see website*
Absolute eosinophilia count, 739-740
Absolute neutrophil count (ANC)
  in fever of unknown origin, 901
  in immunocompromised patient, *see website*
  in leukopenia, 746
Absorption, *see also website*
  of drugs, *see website*
  malabsorption due to defects of, 1304-1305
  of vitamin A, 188
Abstinence, neonatal, 623-625, 624t
Abstinence-only sex education, 701-702
Abuse
  defined, 135
  psychological, 136
  sexual, 135-136, 142-146, 144f
    assessment and management of, 143-144, 143f
    defined, 135-136, 142
    genital *Chlamydia trachomatis* due to, 1036
    physical examination in, 144-145, 144f-145f
    presentation of, 142-143
    prevention of, 144-145
    sexually transmitted disease due to, 145, 145t, 935
    of special needs girls, 1874
    trichomoniasis due to, 1185
    vulvovaginitis and, 1865
  substance (*See* Substance abuse)
Abuse and neglect, 135-147
  assessment of, 141
  clinical manifestations of, 137-140, 137f-139f, 138t-139t
  definitions associated with, 135-136
  etiology of, 136-137, 136t
  eye injuries due to, 2186, 2186f
  factitious disorder by proxy as, 146-147
  foster and kinship care and, *see website*
  fractures due to, 2390
  as global situation, 136
  head trauma due to, 301
  interventions for, 141
  outcomes of, 141-142
  prevention of, 142
  sexual (*See* Sexual abuse)
  traumatic retinopathy related to, 2180, 2181f
  United States situation, 136
Abusive head trauma (ABH), 139-140, 139f, 298f-299f, 301
  hemorrhagic stroke due to, 2084
ABVD regimen for Hodgkin lymphoma, 1742, 1743t
ABVE-PC regimen for Hodgkin lymphoma, 1742, 1743t
AC. *See* Acromioclavicular (AC) separation; Assist-control (AC) mode
Academic disabilities, *see also website*
Acanthamoeba, 1178, *see also website*
Acanthocytosis, 1661f, *see also website*
Acanthosis nigricans, 185, 185f, 2266-2267, 2266f, 2428
Acarbose, 1992t
Acardiac fetus, 554
$ACAT_2$. *See* Acetoacetyl CoA thiolase deficiency ($ACAT_2$)
Accelerated junctional ectopic tachycardia (JET), 1615
Acceleration of fetal heart rate, 543-544
Acceptable macronutrient distribution range (AMDR), *see website*
Access in food security, 170-171
Accessory nerve, neurologic examination of, *see website*
Accessory nipple, 2221, *see also website*
Accessory tragus, 2221, 2221f
Access to care
  for adolescent, 662-663, 663f
  international, *see website*
Accident prevention. *See* Injury control

Page numbers followed by f indicate figures and t indicate tables.

Accident-prone child, 19
Accommodation
 for neurodevelopmental dysfunction, *see website*
 ocular
  abnormalities of, 2152
  in hyperopia, 2151
Accommodative esotropia, 2158-2159, 2159f
Accountable Care Organizations, *see website*
Accreditation, child care, *see website*
Accreditation Council for Graduate Medical Education (ACGME), *see website*
Accuracy of laboratory tests, *see website*
Accutane. *See* Isotretinoin
ACD. *See* Anemia of chronic disease (ACD)
ACE. *See* Angiotensin-converting enzyme (ACE); Antegrade continence enema procedure (ACE)
ACEIs. *See* Angiotensin-converting enzyme inhibitors (ACEIs)
Acetabular index, 2358
Acetabular labrum tear, 2414
Acetabulum, 2355
Acetadote. *See N*-Acetylcysteine
Acetalotrauma, 321f
Acetaminophen
 drug interactions with, *see website*
 for fever, *see website*
 for migraine, 2044t
 for pain management, 363, 364t
  in palliative care, 155t-156t
 poisoning with, 253-254, 258-260, 259f, 259t
  antidote for, 256t-257t
 for typhoid fever, 957
Acetaxolamide-responsiveness myotonia, 2125t
Acetazolamide
 adverse effects of, 2031t
 dosages, 2030t
Acetoacetyl CoA thiolase deficiency ($ACAT_2$), 433-434
 cytosolic, 434-435
 mitochondrial, 433-434, 434f
Acetohexamide, 1992t
Acetylcholine (ACh), myasthenia gravis and, 2132, 2133t
Acetylcholine (ACh) inhibitors for myasthenia gravis, 2135t
N-Acetylcysteine for acetaminophen poisoning, 256t-257t, 259
ACG1 gene, *see website*
aCGH. *See* Array comparative genomic hybridization (aCGH)
ACGME. *See* Accreditation Council for Graduate Medical Education (ACGME)
ACh. *See* Acetylcholine (ACh), myasthenia gravis and
Achalasia, 1264-1265
 cricopharyngeal, 1264
Achondrogenesis type 1B, 2431
Achondroplasia, 1517-1518, 2428-2430, 2429f
 gain-of-function mutation in, *see website*
Achromic nevus, 2234, 2234f
Acid-base balance, 1808, 1808f, *see also website*
Acid-base disorders
 clinical assessment of, 229-231, 230t, 231f
 metabolic acidosis as, 231-235, 231t
 metabolic alkalosis as, 235-238, 235t
 mixed, 230
 respiratory acidosis as, 238-240, 239t
 respiratory alkalosis as, 240-242, 241t
 simple, 230
 terminology associated with, 229-230
Acidemia(s), 229-230
 fetal therapy for, 551t
 isovaleric, 431-432
 methylmalonic, 437-438
  homocystinuria with, 438
 organic, 430-438
 propionic, 436-437
 pyroglutamic, 443-444
Acid-fastness of mycobacteria, 996
Acidosis
 cardiac arrest due to, 289t
 following open heart surgery, 1604
 lactic, 232
  carbohydrate metabolism defects with, 503-509, 504f-505f, 507t-509t, 508f
  in type I glycogen storage disease, 492-493
 metabolic, 230t-231t, 231-235
  in acute renal failure, 1820-1821
  in chronic kidney disease, 1824
  as complication of enterocystoplasty, *see website*
  in dehydration, 247
  hypophosphatemia and, 227
  in respiratory distress syndrome, 586
  in tetralogy of Fallot, 1574
 renal tubular, 1808-1811, 1809t
  distal (type I), 1810
  hyperkalemic (type IV), 1810-1811, 1811f
  metabolic acidosis and, 232
  nephrotoxins in, 1817t
  proximal (type II), 1808-1810, 1809t
  rickets due to, 208, 1811
 respiratory, 230t, 238-240, 239t
Acid(s). *See also* Acid-base balance; Acid-base disorders
 household
  conjunctivitis due to, 2168
  ingestion of, 266, 1272-1273, 1272t
 secretion of in peptic ulcer disease, 1291-1294
Aciduria
 argininosuccinic, 448f, 452
 glutaric type I, 454-455
 D-glyceric acid, 440
 hereditary orotic, *see website*
 γ-hydroxybutyric, 447
 3-hydroxy-3-methylglutaric, 435
 3-methylglutaconic, 433
 mevalonic, 435-436
 N-carbamyl-β-amino, *see website*
Acinus, 1368, *see also website*
ACIP. *See* Advisory Committee on Immunization Practices (ACIP)
ACL. *See* Anterior cruciate ligament (ACL) injuries
Acne, 2322-2328
 chlor-, 2327
 conglobata, 2328
 drug-induced, 2326-2327, 2327f
 fulminans, 2328
 halogen, 2327
 infantile, 2327, 2327f
 neonatal, 2327, 2327f
 in PAPA syndrome, 858-859
 tropical, 2327-2328
 vulgaris, 2322-2326
  classification of, 2323t
  clinical manifestations of, 2322-2326, 2322f-2323f
  pathogenesis of, 2322, 2322f
  treatment of, 2323-2326, 2323t, 2324f, 2325t, 2326f
Acneiform drug eruption, *see website*
Aconitum, potential toxicity of, 272t-273t
Acoustic immittance testing, 2194-2195, 2194f, 2194t, 2204
Acoustic reflectometry, 2195-2196
Acoustic reflex test (ART), 2195
Acoustic trauma, *see website*
Acquaintance rape, 703
Acquired immunity, *see website*
Acquired immunodeficiency syndrome. *See* HIV/AIDS
Acridine orange stain, *see website*
Acrocyanosis in newborn, 533
Acrodermatitis enteropathica, 1321, 2328-2329, 2329f
 in maple syrup urine disease, 431
Acrodynia, *see website*
Acromegaly, *see website*
Acromioclavicular (AC) separation, 2409, 2410f
Acropustulosis, infantile, 2220
ACS. *See* Acute chest syndrome (ACS)
ACTG1 gene, 2190t
ACTH. *See* Adrenocorticotropic hormone (ACTH)
Actinic prurigo, 2257, 2257f
Actinobacillus bacteria in periodontitis, 1257
Actinomyces, 929, *see also website*
Actinomyces israelii, *see website*
Actinomycin D
 for cancer therapy, *see website*
 for Wilms tumor, 1759
Actinomycosis, 929
Action signs, mental health, 57, 57t
Action tremor, 2056-2057
Activated charcoal for poisoning, 257-258, 257t
Activated partial thromboplastin time (APTT), 1697
 reference values for, 1698t
Activation-induced cytidine deaminase (AICDA), mutations in, 726-727
Active immunization, 883-884, 884t. *See also* Vaccine(s)
Active muscle tone, 2109
Active sleep behavioral state, *see website*
Activin in testicular function, *see website*
Activity restriction
 due to chronic illness, *see website*
 for Marfan syndrome, 2445
Actonitum species toxicity, 269t
ACTs. *See* Adrenocortical tumors (ACTs)
Acular. *See* Ketolorac tromethamine
Acupuncture, 273-274
 for pain management, 371
Acute chest syndrome (ACS), in sickle cell disease, 1667-1668
Acute disseminated encephalomyelitis (ADEM), 2079, 2079f, 2080t
Acute generalized exanthematous pustulosis (AGEP), *see website*
Acute genital ulcer (AGU), 708, 709t
Acute hemorrhagic edema (AHE), 870
Acute idiopathic pulmonary hemorrhage (AIPH), 1503, 1504f
Acute illness
 anesthesia in (*See* Anesthesia)
 burn injury as, 349-357
 cold injury as, 357-359
 disposition and, 277-278
 drowning and submersion injury as, 341-348
 emergency medical services for, 278, *see also website*
 history taking in, 275-276
 management of, 277
 mechanical ventilation for, 321-329
  long-term, 329-333
 neurologic emergency and, 296-304
  abusive head trauma, 301
  brain death, 304, *see also website*
  care principles, 296-297, 297f
  hypoxic-ischemic insult and encephalopathy, 301-303
  intracerebral hemorrhage, 303-304
  status epilepticus, 303
  stroke, 303-304
  traumatic brain injury, 297-301, 298f-301f
 pain management in, 360-375
 perioperative care in (*See* Perioperative care)
 physical examination in, 276-277
 respiratory distress and failure as, 314-333
 risk factors for, 277
 sedation in (*See* Sedation)
 shock as, 305-314
 traumatic injury as, 333-341
Acute inflammatory upper airway obstruction, 1445-1450
 bacterial tracheitis as, 1449-1450, 1449f
 infectious, 1445-1449, 1446f-1447f
Acute intermittent porphyrias (AIP), 1247t, *see also website*

Acute liver failure (ALF), 1412-1415, 1414t
with hepatitis A, 1395-1396
with hepatitis B, 1397-1398
Acute lung injury, 316, 317f, 317t
Acute lymphocytic leukemia (ALL), 1732-1737
arthralgia and, *see website*
cellular classification of, 1732-1733, 1733f, 1733t
clinical manifestations of, 1733-1734
diagnosis of, 1734
differential diagnosis of, 1734
epidemiology of, 1732
etiology of, 1732, 1732t
hematopoietic stem cell transplantation for, 757, 758f
incidence and survival rates for, 1726t
prognosis for, 1736-1737
risk factors for, 1727t
secondary, due to radiation therapy, *see website*
supportive care for, 1736
treatment of, 1734-1736, 1735f-1736f
Acute myeloid leukemia (AML), 748t, 1737-1738, 1737t-1738t
hematopoietic stem cell transplantation for, 757-758
incidence and survival rates for, 1726t
risk factors for, 1727t
Acute otitis media (AOM), 2199-2201
complications of, 2210-2211
definitions of, 2199t
in influenza, 1124
Moraxella catarrhalis in, *see website*
otitis media with effusion *versus*, 2203-2204, 2203f
with parainfluenza viruses, 1125t
treatment of, 2205, 2205t, 2206f-2207f, 2207t
Acute poststreptococcal glomerulonephritis (APSGN), 1783-1785, 1783f-1784f, 1785t
Acute promyelocytic leukemia (APL), 1737-1738
Acute radiation syndrome, *see website*
Acute renal failure (ARF), 1818-1822, 1818t
clinical manifestations and diagnosis of, 1819
laboratory findings in, 1819-1820, 1820t
nephrotoxins in, 1817t
pathogenesis of, 1818-1819, 1819t
prognosis for, 1822
treatment of, 1820-1822, 1821t
Acute respiratory distress syndrome (ARDS), 316
Acute respiratory failure
chronic severe, 1519-1526
due to congenital central hypoventilation syndrome, 1520-1522
in cystic fibrosis, 1494
infections associated with, 1525
mechanical ventilation for, 1524-1526
due to metabolic disease, 1523-1524
due to myelomeningocele with Arnold-Chiari type II malformation, 1522
due to neuromuscular diseases, 1520t
due to obesity hypoventilation syndrome, 1522-1523
due to obstructive sleep apnea, 1523
due to spinal cord injury, 1523
Acute tubular necrosis (ATN), 1819
Acyanotic congenital heart disease
absence of pulmonary valve as, 1571
in adults, contraception and, 1609
aortic stenosis as, 1565-1567, 1565f-1566f
aorticopulmonary window defect as, 1561
atrial septal defect as, 1551
atrioventricular septal defects as, 1554-1556, 1554f-1555f
coarctation of the aorta, 1567-1570, 1567f, 1569f
with ventricular septal defect, 1570
coronary-cameral fistula as, 1561
evaluation of, 1549-1550
mitral stenosis as, 1570, *see also website*
mitral valve insufficiency as, 1571-1572, 1571t
mitral valve prolapse as, 1572
Acyanotic congenital heart disease *(Continued)*
ostium secundum defect as, 1551-1553, 1551f-1553f
partial anomalous pulmonary venous return as, 1553-1554
patent ductus arteriosus as, 1559-1561, 1560f
pulmonary valve stenosis
infundibular and double chamber right ventricle as, 1564
with intact ventricular septum, 1561-1563, 1562f-1564f
intracardiac shunt with, 1564
peripheral, 1564-1565
pulmonary valvular insufficiency as, 1571
pulmonary venous hypertension as, 1570-1571
sinus venosus atrial septal defect, 1553
supracristal ventricular septal defect with aortic insufficiency as, 1559
tricuspid regurgitation as, 1572
ventricular septal defect as, 1556-1558, 1556f-1557f
Acyclovir, *see also website*
drug interactions with, *see website*
for herpes simplex virus infection, 1102-1103
for herpes zoster, 1108-1109
for sexually transmitted infection, 713t
for varicella-zoster virus, 1108
Acyl CoA dehydrogenase deficiency
hypoglycemia in, 529
medium-chain, 459-460
short-chain, 460
very long chain, 460
AD. *See* Advance directive (AD); Atopic dermatitis (AD); Autistic disorder (AD)
ADA. *See* Adenosine deaminase (ADA)
Adalimumab
for Crohn disease, 1303
for juvenile idiopathic arthritis, 838t
for rheumatic disease, *see website*
Adams test, 2366
ADAMTS 13 deficiency, 1792-1793
Adapalene for acne, 2325t
Adaptive immunity, *see website*
ADCC. *See* Antibody-dependent cellular cytotoxicity (ADCC)
Adderall. *See* Amphetamine combination
Addison disease, autoimmune, 1926-1927
Adduction, 2331
Adductor response, crossed, *see website*
Adefovir, 1399, *see also website*
ADEM. *See* Acute disseminated encephalomyelitis (ADEM)
Adenine phosphoribosyltransferase (APRT) deficiency, *see website*
Adenitis in PFAPA syndrome, 859-860
Adenocarcinoma
of colon and rectum, 1773, *see also website*
pancreatic, *see website*
Adenoid cystic carcinoma, 1504
Adenoidectomy, 1444-1445, 1444t
for otitis media, 2213
Adenoids
anatomy of, 1442
disorders of, 1443-1445
normal function of, 1442
Adenoma
aldosterone-secreting, *see website*
bronchial, 1504, *see also website*
islet cell, 527
prolactin-secreting pituitary, *see website*
Adenosine
for arrhythmias, 1611t-1612t
for pediatric resuscitation and arrhythmias, 294t
Adenosine deaminase (ADA)
deficiency of, 732
prenatal diagnosis of, *see website*
Adenosine triphosphate (ATP)
in *Chlamydophila pneumoniae*, 1033-1034
hyperinsulinemia and, 522-523
Adenosylcobalamin deficiency, *see website*
Adenotonsillectomy, 51
Adenoviruses (AdVs), 1131-1133, 1132t
gastroenteritis due to, 1326t
Kawasaki disease *versus*, 865
in pneumonia, 1475t
after stem cell transplantation, *see website*
Adenylosuccinate lyase (ADSL) deficiency, *see website*
Adequate intake (AI), *see website*
ADHD. *See* Attention deficit/hyperactivity disorder (ADHD)
Adherence
in diabetes mellitus therapy, 1986
drug therapy, *see also website*
in asthma management, 788
in HIV infection, 1171-1172
in tuberculosis, 1009
after renal transplantation, *see website*
Adhesions, intestinal, 1287
Adhesive otitis media, 2212
ADHR. *See* Autosomal dominant hypophosphatemic rickets (ADHR)
Adie syndrome, 2156
Adie tonic pupil, 2152
Adiponectin, 183-184
Adipose tissue, insulin level effects on, 1975t
Adiposity rebound, 179
Adjustment to chronic illness, *see website*
Adjuvants agents in immunizing agents, 883
ADM. *See* Antroduodenal manometry (ADM)
Adnexal torsion of ovary, 1871
Adolescence, defined, 649
Adolescent
aggressive periodontitis in, 1257
appendicitis diagnosis in female, 1353
assent and consent of, *see website*
atopic dermatitis in, 804
bariatric surgery for, 186
birthrates for, *see website*
breast development in, 685, *see also website*
breast masses in, *see website*
causes of limping in, 2334t
chronic fatigue syndrome in, 714, *see also website*
congenital heart disease in, 1609-1610, 1609t
contraception in, 692-699, 695t
barrier methods, 694
combination methods, 696
counseling regarding, 694
emergency, 698-699, 698t
epidemiology of, 692-694, 693f-694f, 693t
hormonal methods, 696-698, 696t-697t, 697f
intrauterine devices, 699
spermicides, 694
disruptive behavioral disturbances in, 99-100
driving of car by, 22
drowning or submersion injury to, 342
epidemiology of health problems in, 660-663, 660f-661f, 661t
ethics in health care of, *see website*
feeding of, 166-167, 166f, 167t
in foster care, *see website*
gonococcal infection in, 938-939
growth and development of, 650t
charts for assessment of, *see website*
during early adolescence, 649-653, 650t-652t, 651f-652f
during late adolescence, 654
during middle adolescence, 653-654
gynecological examination of, *see website*
health care access for, 662-663, 663f
health care delivery to, 663-667, 664t
legal issues in, 664-665, *see also website*
health enhancement for, 667
HIV/AIDS in, 1158-1159
homosexual, 658-659
idiopathic anterior knee pain syndrome in, 2354
injury risk factors for, 20
intellectual disability in, 125

Adolescent *(Continued)*
interviewing of, 665-666, 666t
iron deficiency-anemia in, 1656
leading causes of death for, 5t
lipoprotein patterns in, 479, 479t
male disorders in, *see website*
menstruation problems in, 685-692, 686t
abnormal uterine bleeding, 688-690, 689t-690t
amenorrhea, 686-688, 687f, 687t-688t
dysmenorrhea, 690-691, 691t
premenstrual syndrome, 691-692, 692t
pertussis in, 945
physical examination of, 666-667
pregnancy of, 699-702, *see also website*
characteristic of teen parent in, 700-701
clinical manifestations of, 700
counseling and initial management of, 700
diagnosis of, 700, 700t
epidemiology of, 699, 699t
etiology of, 699-700
health care for parents and children in, 702t
medical complications of mothers and babies in, 701
prevention of, 701-702
psychosocial outcomes/risk for mother and child in, 701-702
repeat, 701
psychosocial assessment of, 56, 666, 666t
rape of, 702-705, 703t-704t
recommended immunization schedule for, 889
as research subject, *see website*
response to death of, *see website*
response to divorce of, *see website*
scoliosis in, 1518
screening procedures for, 665-667
sexual identity development in, 654-658
factors that influence, 655
gender variance/gender role nonconformity in, 655-656
gender variant identity/transgender children in, 656-658, 657t
terms and definitions in, 654-655
sexually transmitted diseases in, 705-714
definitions, etiology, and clinical manifestations of, 707-709, 707f-708f, 709t
diagnosis of, 709-711, 709t-711t, 710f
epidemiology of, 705-714, 706f
etiology of, 705, 705t
pathogenesis of, 706, 707f
prevention of, 714
screening for, 706-707, 707t
treatment of, 711-714, 712t-713t
sleep changes in, 47t
sleep hygiene for, 49t
substance abuse by, 671-685, 671f
of alcohol, 678-679, 678t-679t
of amphetamines, 683-684, 684t
clinical manifestations of, 673-674, 676t
of cocaine, 683
complications of, 677
diagnosis of, 677, 677t
epidemiology of, 672-673, 673t, 675t
etiology of, 671-672, 672t-673t
of hallucinogens, 682-683
of inhalants, 681-682, 681t-682t
of marijuana, 680-681, 680t
motor vehicle accidents and, 22
of opiates, 684-685
prevention of, 677, 677t
prognosis for, 677
screening for, 674-677, 676t
of tobacco, 679-680, 680t
treatment of, 677
transition to adult care, 667, *see also website*
21 critical health objectives for, 662t, 663
violent behavior in, 667-671, 667t-670t, 668f
well child care for, 16
X-linked adrenoleukodystrophy in, 468
Adolescent-limited offenders, 669
Adoption, 130-134, 131t
Adoption and Safe Families Act, *see website*
ADP. *See* δ-Aminolevulinic acid dehydratase porphyria (ADP)
ADPKD. *See* Autosomal dominant polycystic kidney disease (ADPKD)
ADPLD. *See* Autosomal dominant polycystic liver disease (ADPLD)
Adrenal androgens
actions of, *see website*
excess of in congenital adrenal hyperplasia, 1933
regulation of, *see website*
Adrenal cortex, 1923, *see also website*
Adrenal crisis, 1927
treatment of vomiting associated with, 1244t
Adrenal gland
calcification within, 1943, *see also website*
disorders of
due to cancer and its therapy, *see website*
Cushing syndrome as, 1939-1941
with hypoglycemia, 527
pheochromocytoma as, 1941-1943
primary aldosteronism as, 1941
hemorrhage into, 1927
as delivery room emergency, 578
histology and embryology of, 1923
masses of, 1943
steroid biosynthesis in, 1923, *see also website*
X-linked adrenoleukodystrophy and dysfunction, 468
Adrenal hyperplasia
congenital, 1930-1939, 1931f
adrenocortical insufficiency due to, 1924, 1925t
due to 11β-hydroxylase deficiency, 1935-1936
due to 3β-hydroxysteroid dehydrogenase deficiency, 1936
diagnosis and treatment of, 1931f, 1932t
due to 17-hydroxylase deficiency, 1936-1937
due to 21-hydroxylase deficiency, 1930-1935
hypokalemia in, 223-224
metabolic alkalosis in, 236
lipoid, 1937, 1964
Adrenal hypoplasia congenita (AHC), 1924
Adrenalin
for anaphylaxis, 818t
for asthma exacerbations, 797t-798t
Adrenal insufficiency, 1924-1930
in critical care setting, 1929-1930, *see also website*
hypothyroidism-associated, 1903t
primary, 1924-1928, 1925t
secondary, 1929-1930
Adrenalitis
autoimmune, 1925t
tuberculous, 1925t
Adrenal medulla, 1923-1924, *see also website*
dysfunction of in congenital adrenal hyperplasia, 1933
Adrenal rests, testicular, *see website*
Adrenal tumors, 1773, *see also website*
Adrenarche, premature, 1894
α-Adrenergic agents
for allergic disease, 770-773
for heart failure, *see website*
for psychiatric disorders, 63
for systemic hypertension, 1645t
β-Adrenergic agonists
for allergic disease, 770-773
for asthma
long-acting, 791-792, 794-795
short-acting, 792t, 796, 797t-798t
for heart failure, *see website*
α-Adrenergic blockers for urinary lithiasis, 770-773
β-Adrenergic receptor blockers. *See* β-blockers
Adrenocortical insufficiency, 1924-1930
in critical care setting, 1929-1930, *see also website*
primary, 1924-1928, 1925t
secondary, 1929-1930
Adrenocortical tumors (ACTs), 1941, *see also website*
Adrenocorticotropic hormone (ACTH), *see also website*
in cortisol regulation, 1923, *see also website*
in Cushing syndrome, 1939
insensitivity syndromes of, 1925t
for seizures, 2032
for West syndrome, 2027
Adrenoleukodystrophy, 466t, 1925t, 2073-2074
X-linked, 467-470, 469f
Adrenoleukodystrophy (ALD), 1924
Adrenomyeloneuropathy (AMN), 467-468, 1925t, 2074
Adriamycin. *See* Doxorubicin
ADRs. *See* Adverse drug reactions (ADRs)
ADSL. *See* Adenylosuccinate lyase (ADSL) deficiency
Adult care, adolescent transition to, 667, *see also website*
Adult(s)
gonococcal infection in, 938-939
Adult tapeworm infection, 1232-1234, 1232t, 1233f-1234f
Adult T-cell leukemia/lymphoma (ATL), *see website*
Advanced airway management techniques
bag-valve-mask positive pressure ventilation in, 284-285, 284f-285f
endotracheal intubation in, 285, 286f, 287t
Advanced care planning in palliative care, 151-159
Advance directive (AD), *see website*
Advanced life support
for bradycardia, 288f
for pulseless arrest, 293f
for tachycardia, 290f
Adverse drug events (ADEs), *see website*
Adverse drug reactions (ADRs), *see website*
Advisory Committee on Immunization Practices (ACIP), 885
Advocacy
in abuse and neglect management, 142
for emergency medical services for children, *see website*
in gender variance, 655-656
in intellectual disability management, 129
AdVs. *See* Adenoviruses (AdVs)
Aedes aegypti, 1147
AEDs. *See* Antiepileptic drugs (AEDs); Automated external defibrillation (AEDs)
aEEG. *See* Amplitude integrated electroencephalography (aEEG)
Aeroallergens, 764
atopic dermatitis and, 806
Aeromonas, 974, *see also website*
inflammatory bowel disease *versus*, 1298t
in traveler's diarrhea, 1338t
Aerosolized therapy for cystic fibrosis, 1492
Affordability of health care for adolescents, 663
A fibers in abdominal pain, 1247-1248
Afibrinogenemia, congenital, 1704
African American population
asthma in, 781
cultural values associated with, *see website*
death rates for, 3t-4t
home remedies for fever, colic and teething among, *see website*
infant mortality rates for, *see website*
injuries in, 20
red cell counts for, 1648, 1650f
as special needs population, 7
African Burkitt lymphoma, 1111, 1112t
Africanized honeybee, allergic responses to, 807f
African tick-bite fever, 1039t-1040t
African trypanosomiasis, 1190-1193, 1192f

Afrin. *See* Oxymetazoline
Afterload reducers, 313t, *see also website*
Agammaglobulinemia
B cell immunodeficiency screening and, 720
X-linked, 723-724
malignancy susceptibility associated with, *see website*
Aganglionic megacolon, 1283t, 1284-1287
Agar disk diffusion antimicrobial susceptibility testing, *see website*
AGAT. *See* Arginine:glycine amidinotransferase (AGAT) deficiency
Age
causes of death by, 5t
gestational
assessment of, 557, 558f
eye examination schedule based on, 2175t
large-for, *see website*
maternal, high-risk pregnancies and, *see website*
mortality rates by, 3t
pain scales and, 361, 362f, 363t
percentile curves for weight and length/stature by, *see website*
Age factors
in allergic disease, 764
in cancer diagnosis of, 1728-1729
in cancer rates, 1726f
in childhood injuries, 20
in chronic diarrhea, 1343t
in drug disposition, *see website*
in homicide, 667t
in neonatal infection, 633-636, 634t
in otitis media, 2200
in pharmacodynamics, *see website*
in pneumonia, 1476t
in typhoid fever, 955
Agenesis
cerebellar vermis, 2054
corpus callosum, 2005-2006, 2005f
cranial nerve, 2006-2007
pancreatic, 1368, *see also website*
penile, 1857
renal, 1827, 1828f
sacral, 2118
sacral, neuropathic bladder and, *see website*
AGEP. *See* Acute generalized exanthematous pustulosis (AGEP)
Ages and Stages Questionnaire-3 (ASQ-3), 41t-43t
Agglutination, labial, 1867t-1868t
Agglutination test
in brucellosis, 981
in group A streptococci infection, 918
in leptospirosis, 1024-1025
in toxoplasmosis, 1213-1214
in tuberculosis, 1019-1020
in tularemia, 979
Aggrecan-related spondyloepiphyseal dysplasias, 2425
Aggregatibacter bacteria in periodontitis, 1257
Aggressive behavior, 100
Agitation
psychopharmacologic management of, 61t
treatment of in palliative care, 155t-157t
Agminated lentigine
Agonists, receptor binding by, *see website*
AGU. *See* Acute genital ulcer (AGU); Aspartylglucosaminuria (AGU)
Agyria, 2003
AHA. *See* American Heart Association (AHA)
AHC. *See* Adrenal hypoplasia congenita (AHC)
AHE. *See* Acute hemorrhagic edema (AHE)
AHR. *See* Airway hyperresponsiveness (AHR)
AI. *See* Adequate intake (AI)
AICA. *See* 5-Amino-4-imidazolecarboxamide (AICA) riboside deficiency
Aicardi-Goutieres syndrome, 2060t
Aicardi syndrome, 2005, 2035-2036
AICDA. *See* Activation-induced cytidine deaminase (AICDA)
Aichi virus, 1135
AIDS. *See* HIV/AIDS
AIH. *See* Autoimmune hepatitis (AIH)
AIP. *See* Acute intermittent porphyrias (AIP)
AIPH. *See* Acute idiopathic pulmonary hemorrhage (AIPH)
Airborne isolation, *see website*
Air-conduction signals in audiometry, 2193
Air crescent in aspergillosis, 1060
AIRE. *See* Autoimmune regulator gene (AIRE)
Air embolism, pulmonary, 597
Air leaks, extrapulmonary, 597-599, 598f-599f
Air pollutants, *see also website*
wheezing and bronchitis and, 1460
Air transport, *see website*
Airway
artificial
for epiglottitis, 1448
for respiratory distress and failure, 319
bronchoscopy of, *see website*
difficult, general anesthesia and, *see website*
disorders of in mucopolysaccharidoses, 515t
dynamics of in health and disease, 1420, *see also website*
foreign bodies in, 1453-1454, 1453f
laryngoscopy of, *see website*
narrowing of, 283-284
in pediatric emergency assessment, 279-281
preanesthetic evaluation of, *see website*
radiography of, *see website*
respiratory acidosis due to disease of, 239t
in trauma survey, 335
Airway clearance treatment
for atelectasis, *see website*
for respiratory insufficiency, 1525
Airway conductance, *see website*
Airway hyperresponsiveness (AHR), 780
Airway management
bag-valve-mask positive pressure ventilation for, 284-285, 284f-285f
endotracheal intubation for, 285, 286f, 287t
Airway obstruction
acute inflammatory upper, 1445-1450
bacterial tracheitis as, 1449-1450, 1449f
infectious, 1445-1449, 1446f-1447f
in asthma, 782, 784
critical high airway obstruction syndrome (CHAOS), 577, 578f
management of, 282-283, 282f-283f
neonatal, 577, 578f
respiratory distress due to, 315t
in respiratory syncytial virus infection, 1127-1128
due to tonsil and adenoid pathology, 1443, 1445
in traumatic injury, 335
Airway pressure release ventilation (APRV), 326
Airway resistance, *see website*
AIS. *See* Arterial ischemic stroke (AIS)
AISs. *See* Androgen insensitivity syndromes (AISs)
Akinesia, as goal of anesthesia, *see website*
AKR1D1 gene defect, 1383t
AL. *See* Argininosuccinate lyase (AL) deficiency
ALA. *See* α-Linolenic acid (ALA); δ-Aminolevulinic acid (ALA)
Alacrima, 1925, 2165-2166
ALAD. *See* δ-Aminolevulinic acid dehydratase (ALAD) deficiency
Alagille syndrome, 408t, 1383t, 1385
congenital heart disease with, 1531t, 1561-1562, 1564
Alanine aminotransferase (ALT)
in autoimmune hepatitis, 1409
in liver disease, 1378
in obesity, 185t
reference values for, *see website*
in viral hepatitis, 1394-1395
Alavert. *See* Loratadine
Albendazole, *see also website*
for ascariasis, 1217-1218
for cysticercosis, 1236
Albendazole *(Continued)*
for echinococcosis, 1239
for enterobiasis, 1222
for filariasis, 1225
for giardiasis, 1182, 1182t
for *Gnathostoma spinigerum*, 1227
for infectious diarrhea, 1337t
for toxocariasis, 1228-1229
for trichinosis, 1229
for vulvovaginitis, 1868t
Albenza. *See* Albendazole
Albinism, 424-425, 424t, 2238-2239, 2238t
Albright hereditary osteodystrophy, 1919-1920
Albumin
drug binding and, *see website*
infusion for burn injury, 353
in malnutrition with chronic diarrhea, 1343t
for nephrotic syndrome, 1805
reference values for, *see website*
Albuterol
for anaphylaxis, 818t
for asthma, 796, 797t-798t
ALCAPA. *See* Anomalous origin of coronary arteries (ALCAPA)
Alcaptonuria, 423
ALCL. *See* Anaplastic large cell lymphoma (ALCL)
Alcohol
drug interactions with, *see website*
effects of, *see website*
neonatal withdrawal from, 624
poisoning with, 267-268
in adolescents, 676t
hypoglycemia in, 529
porphyria cutanea tarda and, *see website*
Alcoholism, hypophosphatemia due to, 228
Alcohol use
in adolescents, 672, 673t, 678-679, 678t-679t
drowning due to, 24
motor vehicle accidents and, 22
urine screening for, 676t
breast-feeding and, 161t
drowning or submersion injury associated with, 342
maternal
fetal alcohol syndrome due to, 625-626
as sudden infant death syndrome risk factor, 1424
Alcohol Use Disorders Identification Test (AUDIT), 678-679, 678t
ALD. *See* Adrenoleukodystrophy (ALD)
Aldosterone, *see also website*
deficiency of in congenital adrenal hyperplasia, 1931-1933
regulation of, *see website*
synthase deficiency, 1938
Aldosteronism
glucocorticoid-remediable, 236
primary, 1941
Alemtuzumab, *see website*
Alert, Verbal, Pain, Unresponsive (AVPU) Pediatric Response Scale, 281
Alert state, *see website*
Alexander anomaly, 2189-2190
Alexander disease, 2074-2075
ALF. *See* Acute liver failure (ALF)
Alfentanil, 367t
Algid malaria, 1206
Alice in Wonderland syndrome, 1114, *see also website*
α-Linolenic acid (ALA), *see website*
Alkalemia, 229-230, 237
Alkaline phosphatase
deficiency of, rickets due to, *see website*
reference values for, *see website*
Alkalinization urinary, for poisoning, 258
with salicylates, 260
Alkalis, households
conjunctivitis due to, 2168
ingestion of, 266
ocular burns with, 2186

Alkalosis, 229-230
forced, for persistent pulmonary hypertension of the newborn, 593
hypochloremic, in cystic fibrosis, 1487
metabolic, 230t, 235-238, 235t
clinical manifestations of, 237
diagnosis of, 237-238
etiology and pathophysiology of, 235-237, 235t
treatment of, 238
respiratory, 230t, 240-242, 241t
compensatory, 230
ALL. *See* Acute lymphocytic leukemia (ALL)
Allegra. *See* Fexofenadine
Allele, *see website*
Allelic heterogeneity, *see website*
Allergen immunotherapy
for allergic disease, 773-775
for atopic dermatitis, 805
Allergens, *see website*
Allergic bronchopulmonary aspergillosis (ABPA), 1474
Aspergillus in, 1059
immunoglobulin E levels in, 766
Allergic cluck, 764
Allergic conjunctivitis, 765, 809-810, 810f, 2167t, 2168
Allergic contact dermatitis, 2251
Allergic disease, 764
anaphylaxis as, 816-819
Aspergillus in, 1058-1062
in cystic fibrosis, 1494
asthma as, 780-801
atopic dermatitis as, 801-807
diagnosis of, 764-768
history in, 764-765
physical examination in, 765
testing in, 765-768, 766t
drug reactions as, 824-828
HIV-related, 1166
in eosinophilia, 740
food reactions as, 820-824, 820t-821t, 823f, 823t
insect allergy as, 807-809, 807f, 809t
key elements of, *see website*
mechanism of tissue inflammation in, *see website*
ocular, 809-811, 810f, 811t
in otitis media, 2202
rhinitis as, 775-780, 776t-780t, 777f
serum sickness as, 819-820
treatment of, 768-775
allergen immunotherapy for, 773-775
environmental control measures in, 768-770, 769t
pharmacologic, 770-773
urticaria (hives) and angioedema as, 811-816
Allergic granulomatosis, 868t
Allergic rhinitis (AR), 775-780, 776t-780t, 777f
allergen immunotherapy for, 774-775
Allergic salute, 764
Allergic shiner, 765
Allergy
acute laryngeal swelling due to, 1448
contact, involving eyes, 810
cow's milk protein, 821, 1340
drug, 824-828
food, 820-824, 820t-821t, 823f, 823t
atopic dermatitis and, 806
latex, neuropathic bladder and, *see website*
ocular, 809-811
wheezing in, 1457
Allgrove syndrome, 1264
adrenal insufficiency with, 1925, 1925t
autonomic neuropathy with, 2142
Allium cepa, 271t
Allogenic stem cell transplantation, 757, 758t
from HLA-identical sibling, 757-760
Alloimmune neonatal neutropenia, 749-750
Alloimmune thrombocytopenic purpura, neonatal, 1720
Alloiococcus otitidis, 2201
Allopurinol, drug interactions with, *see website*
All-terrain vehicle (ATV) accident, 22
Almotriptan for migraine, 2044t
Alopecia
areata, 2290-2291, 2291f
disorders associated with, 2289t
hypertrichosis and, 2289, 2289t
toxic, 2292
traction, 2289, 2290f
traumatic, 2289-2290
Alpers disease, 1406, *see also website*
α-Adrenergic agents
for allergic disease, 770-773
for attention deficit/hyperactivity disorder, 111t
for heart failure, *see website*
for psychiatric disorders, 63
for psychosis and agitation, 64t
for systemic hypertension, 1645t
α-Adrenergic blockers for urinary lithiasis, 770-773
α-Fetoprotein concentration, 543t
in brain tumors, 1747-1748
in CNS germ cell tumors, 1752-1753
in germ cell tumors, 1770
in ovarian carcinomas, 1872t
α-Thalassemia(s), 1674, 1674t, 1676-1677
Alpha-linolenic acid (ALA), *see website*
Alpha toxin, *see website*
Alport syndrome, 1782-1783, 1782f
Alprazolam, 692t
ALPS. *See* Autoimmune lymphoproliferative syndrome (ALPS)
Alstrom syndrome, 182t
ALT. *See* Alanine aminotransferase (ALT)
ALTE. *See* Apparent life-threatening event (ALTE)
Alternating attention, *see website*
Alternating hemiplegia of childhood, 2060t, 2061, *see also website*
stroke like events *versus*, 2086
Alternative medicine. *See* Complementary and alternative medicine
Alternative pathway of complement system, *see also website*
deficiencies of, 754t
Alveolar air equation, *see website*
Alveolar alveolitis, *Aspergillus* in, 1059
Alveolar-arterial oxygen (A-ao_2) gradient, 318, *see also website*
Alveolar compartment, pulmonary edema and, 1468
Alveolar gas composition, 316
Alveolar gas exchange, *see website*
Alveolar hemorrhage, 1498-1500, 1498t
Alveolar hypoventilation, 1523
Alveolar macrophages, *see website*
Alveolar microlithiasis, *see website*
Alveolar partial pressure of carbon dioxide ($Paco_2$), 1521, *see also website*
Alveolar partial pressure of oxygen (Pao_2), *see website*
Alveolar proteinosis, 1497, *see also website*
Alveolar rhabdomyosarcoma, 1760
Alveolar soft part sarcoma, 1762t
Alveolar ventilation, 316-317, *see also website*
Alveolitis, extrinsic alveolar, 1059
Alzheimer's disease, familial, *see website*
Amanita poisoning, *see website*
Amantadine, 1123-1124, *see also website*
Amastigotes, in trypanosomiasis, 1193, 1193f
Amaurosis, 2153-2154
Ambiguous genitalia, 1958-1968, 1960f
diagnosis of, 1959t, 1961
etiologic classification of, 1959t
inguinal hernia with, 1365
ovotesticular, 1968
revised nomenclature in, 1958-1959, 1959t
sex differentiation and, 1958-1959, 1960f
surgical management of, 1935
46,XX, 1959t
46,XY, 1962
Amblyopia, 2152, 2158
with ptosis, 2163
Ambulance, ground *versus* air, *see website*
Ambulatory blood pressure monitoring (ABPM), 1639-1640
AMC. *See* Arthrogryposis multiplex congenita (AMC)
AMDR. *See* Acceptable macronutrient distribution range (AMDR)
Amebiasis, 1178-1180, 1179f, 1180t, *see also website*
liver abscess due to, 1404, 1405f
Amebic meningoencephalitis, 1178, *see also website*
cerebrospinal fluid findings in, 2088t
Amegakaryoctic thrombocytopenia, 1689, 1719-1720
Amelogenesis imperfecta, 1250, 1250f
Amenorrhea, 686-688, 686t-688t, 687f
sports-related, 2422
Ameobapores, 1178
Ameobapore A, 1178-1179
American Academy of Pediatrics (AAP), 12
on complementary feeding, 164
on genetic testing, 382-383
model for quality improvement from, *see website*
American Association on Intellectual and Developmental Disabilities (AAIDD), 122-124
American Board of Pediatrics (ABP), 12
American College of Medical Genetics, on neonatal screening, *see website*
American Heart Association (AHA)
on infective endocarditis, 1626, 1626t
step I diet of, 480
American nightshade, potential toxicity of, 272t-273t
American trypanosomiasis, 1193-1198, 1193f-1194f, 1195t, *see also website*
Ametropia, 2150-2151
Ametropic amblyopia, 2152
AMH. *See* Antimüllerian hormones (AMH)
AMH gene, *see website*
AMH-receptor gene, *see website*
Amides, 367t
Amikacin, *see also website*
for bacterial meningitis, 2093t
for cystic fibrosis lung infection, 1492t
for neonatal infection, 645t
for tuberculosis, 1008t
Amikin. *See* Amikacin
Amiloride for systemic hypertension, 1645t
Aminata poisoning, *see website*
Amino acids
defects in metabolism of (*See* Amino acid metabolism defects)
dietary reference intakes for, *see website*
indispensable, dispensable, and conditionally dispensable, *see website*
malabsorption of, 1305t
in protein, *see website*
Amino acid formula, 164
Amino acid metabolism defects, 418-456
of arginine, citrulline, and ornithine, 418-421, 448f-449f, 448t, 450t
of aspartic acid, 455-456, 456f
of cysteine/cystine, 429
of glutamic acid, 443-445, 444f
of glycine, 438-441, 439f, 441f
of histidine, 453
liver effects of, 1389t
of lysine, 453-455, 454f
malabsorption due to, 1318
of methionine, 425-429, 426f
neonatal seizures due to, 2034-2035
of neurotransmitters, 445-447
newborn screening for, 416, 417t
odors associated with, 418t
of phenylalanine, 418-422, 419f, 421f
of proline, 442-443, 442f

Amino acid metabolism defects *(Continued)*
of serine, 442
of tryptophan, 429-430, 429f
of tyrosine, 422-425
of valine, leucine, isoleucine, and related organic acidemias, 430-438, 430f
α-Aminoadipic semialdehyde dehydrogenase deficiency, 453-454
γ-Aminobutyric acid (GABA)
deficiency of, 445t, 447
in seizures, 2025
drug therapy and, 2025-2026
neonatal, 2033
in status epilepticus, 2038
Aminoglycoside-modifying agents, *see website*
Aminoglycosides, 563t, *see also website*
5-Amino-4-imidazolecarboxamide (AICA) riboside deficiency, *see website*
δ-Aminolevulinic acid (ALA), *see website*
δ-Aminolevulinic acid dehydratase (ALAD) deficiency, *see website*
δ-Aminolevulinic acid dehydratase porphyria (ADP), *see website*
Aminophylline for neonatal apnea, 581
5-Aminosalicylate (5-ASA), 1298-1299
Amiodarone
goiter due to, 1908
hypothyroidism due to, 1901
for pediatric resuscitation and arrhythmias, 294t
Amiodarone for arrhythmias, 1611t-1612t
Amiodipine, 1645t
Amitriptyline
for functional abdominal pain, 1348t
for migraine prophylaxis, 2044, 2044t
for pain management, 364t
for vomiting prophylaxis, 1244t
AML. *See* Acute myeloid leukemia (AML)
Ammaglobulinemia, enterovirus and, 1089
Ammonia, reference values for, *see website*
AMN. *See* Adrenomyeloneuropathy (AMN)
Amnesia
as goal of anesthesia, *see website*
due to shellfish poisoning, *see website*
Amniocentesis, 543t, 548-549
in erythroblastosis fetalis, 617
Amnion nodosum, 552
Amniotic constriction bands, 533, 2220-2221, 2343, *see website*
Amniotic fluid
in biophysical profile, 543t
diagnostic testing of, 548
high-risk pregnancies and, *see website*
Amoxicillin, *see also website*
for acute cystitis, 1832
for cystic fibrosis lung infection, 1492t
for group A streptococci infection, 918
for *Helicobacter pylori* gastritis, 1293t
for infective endocarditis prophylaxis, 1626t
for Lyme disease, 1028t
for otitis media, 2206-2208, 2207t
for pharyngitis, 1439-1440
for sinusitis, 1437-1438
for *Staphylococcus aureus*, 907-908
for typhoid fever, 957, 958t
for vulvovaginitis, 1868t
Amoxicillin-clavulanate, *see also website*
for cystic fibrosis lung infection, 1492t
for otitis media, 2207t, 2208
for sinusitis, 1437-1438
for *Staphylococcus aureus*, 907-908
for vulvovaginitis, 1868t
Amoxil. *See* Amoxicillin
Amphetamine combination for attention deficit/hyperactivity disorder, 62t
Amphetamines, adolescent use of, 683-684, 684t
urine screening for, 676t
Amphetamine salts, for attention deficit/hyperactivity disorder, 111t
Amphotericin B, *see also website*
for coccidioidomycosis, 1067
for histoplasmosis, 1063-1064
Amphotericin B *(Continued)*
for *Leishmania*, *see website*
for parasitic infection, *see website*
possible adverse reactions to in premature infant, 563t
Amphotericin B colloid dispersion (ABCD), *see also website*
for candidiasis, 1054t, 1056t
Amphotericin B deoxycholate
for blastomycosis, 1065
for candidiasis, 1054t, 1056t
for coccidioidomycosis, 1067
for leishmaniasis, 1190
for zygomycosis, *see website*
Amphotericin B lipid complex (ABLC), *see also website*
for candidiasis, 1054t, 1056t
for leishmaniasis, 1190
for zygomycosis, *see website*
Ampicillin, *see also website*
for bacterial meningitis, 2093t
for group B streptococci, 927
for infectious diarrhea, 1337t
for listeriosis, *see website*
for meningococcal disease, 933t
for neonatal infection, 645t
for pyelonephritis, 1832
for *Salmonella* gastroenteritis, 953t
for *Shigella* infection, 961
for *Staphylococcus aureus*, 907t
for typhoid fever, 958t
"Ampicillin rash," 1112-1113
Ampicillin-sulbactam, 907t, *see also website*
Amplification in proto-oncogene activation, *see website*
Amplitude integrated electroencephalography (aEEG), 571t
Amputation
fingertip, 2387
for leg-length discrepancy, *see website*
Amrinone for heart failure, *see website*
Amylase, *see also website*
disorders associated with elevation of, 1371, 1371t
in pancreatitis, 1371
reference values for, *see website*
Amylase isoenzymes, reference values for, *see website*
Amylin adjunct therapy for type 1 diabetes mellitus, 1979
Amyl nitrate, as inhalant, 681t
Amylo-1,6-glucosidase deficiency, 528
Amyloidosis, 860, *see also website*
Amylopectinosis, 497
Amyoplasia, 2118
in arthrogryposis, *see website*
Amyopoathic juvenile dermatomyositis, 848
AN. *See* Anorexia nervosa (AN)
ANA. *See* Antinuclear antibodies (ANAs)
Anabolic-androgenic steroids (AAS), 2422-2423, 2423t
Anaerobic bacterial infections
botulism as, 987-991
Clostridium difficile infection as, 994-995
due to other organisms, 995, *see also website*
pneumonia as, 1475t
tetanus as, 991-994
Anafranil. *See* Clomipramine
Anagen effluvium, 2292
Anakinra
for juvenile idiopathic arthritis, 838t
for rheumatic disease, *see website*
Anal canal, anatomy of, 1360f
Anal fissure, 1359
Analgesia/analgesics. *See also* Pain management
acetaminophen, aspirin, and nonsteroidal antiinflammatory drugs as, 363-364, 364t
for anesthesia, *see website*
for cyclic vomiting syndrome, 1244t
epidural, *see website*
in general anesthesia, *see website*
Analgesia/analgesics *(Continued)*
for intubation, 321t
for migraine, 2044t
opioids, 364-367, 365t-367t, 367f
adverse reaction to, 828
patient-controlled
for pain management, 365-367, 367f
postoperative, *see website*
pharmacokinetics and pharmacodynamics of, 362-363
poisoning with, 258-261
in rapid sequence intubation, 287t
in serotonin syndrome, 265t
Anal stenosis, 1357
Analytical validity, 376
Analytic testing, *see website*
Anaphase of mitosis, 394-395
Anaphylactoid reaction, 816
Anaphylaxis, 816-819, 816t-818t
biphasic, 817
exercise-induced, 814
after Hymenoptera sting, 808
after vaccine, 892
Anaplasma phagocytophilum, 1026, 1039t-1040t
Anaplasmosis, 1048-1050, 1050f
Anaplastic astrocytoma, 1750
Anaplastic large cell lymphoma (ALCL), 1739-1740, 1744t
Anastia, *see website*
Anastrozole, 1893
Anatomic dead space, 316-317
ANC. *See* Absolute neutrophil count (ANC)
ANCA. *See* Antineutrophil cytoplasmic antibody (ANCA)
Ancef. *See* Cefazolin
Ancylostoma, 1218-1221
Ancylostoma caninum, *see website*
Ancylostoma duodenale, *see website*
Andersen disease, 494t-495t, 497, *see also website*
Andersen-Tawil syndrome, 2130
Anderson disease, 1313
Anderson syndrome, 2125t
Androgens, adrenal
actions of, *see website*
defects in, 1965-1967
excess of in congenital adrenal hyperplasia, 1933
regulation of, *see website*
Androgenic drugs, administration during pregnancy, 1962-1963
Androgenic lesion of ovary, 1958
Androgen insensitivity in amenorrhea, 687t
Androgen insensitivity syndromes (AISs), 1966, 1966f
Androgen receptor, *see website*
Androstenedione, 2423, 2423t
Anemia of chronic disease (ACD), 1653, *see also website*
Anemia(s), 1648-1650, 1648t
acquired pure red blood cell, 1652-1653
of acute renal failure, 1821
anesthesia and, *see website*
aplastic, 748t, 1690-1691
hematopoietic stem cell transplantation for, 759, 759f
cardiac arrest due to, 289t
of chronic disease, 1653
chronic hemolysis as, 1653
in chronic kidney disease, 1823t, 1825
congenital
Diamond-Blackfan, 1650-1651
dyserythropoietic, 1654, *see also website*
hypoplastic, 1650-1651
Pearson's syndrome as, 1652
Cooley, 1675-1676
differential diagnosis of, 1649-1650, 1649f-1650f
Fanconi, 759, 1684-1686, 1685f, 1685t
malignancy susceptibility associated with, *see website*

Anemia(s) *(Continued)*
fetal therapy for, 551t
hemolytic (*See* Hemolytic anemia)
history and physical examination in, 1648-1649
HIV-related, 1166
iron-deficiency, 1655-1658, 1656t-1658t, 1657f
with celiac disease, 1309
due to hookworm, 1219
in kala-azar, 1189
laboratory studies in, 1649
in malaria, 1199-1200
malarial, 1206
in malnutrition, 172
megaloblastic, 1655, *see also website*
folic acid deficiency in, 1655
thiamine-responsiveness, 191
vitamin B_{12} (cobalamin) deficiency in, 1655
microcytic, 1658, *see also website*
in newborn, 612-615, 613f, 613t-614t
as oncologic emergency, *see website*
parvovirus B19 infection in red cell aplasia as, 1652-1653
physiologic of infancy, 1654-1655
of prematurity, 614
of renal disease, 1653
renal transplantation and, *see website*
respiratory signs and symptoms of, *see website*
retinopathy due to, 2180
sickle cell (*See* Sickle cell disease (SCD))
sideroblastic, 1658, *see also website*
transient erythroblastopenia of childhood as, 1652-1653, 1652t
Anencephaly, 2003
Anesthesia
general, 359, *see also website*
local
adverse reaction to, 827
for pain management, 367-368, 367t-368t
toxicity, neonatal seizures due to, 2034, 2036
regional, *see also website*
for pain management, 371
Anetoderma, 2277
Aneuploid cells, 399-400
Aneuploidy, 399-400, 400t, 404t
sex chromosome, 408-410, 409t
47,XYY as, 410
Klinefelter syndrome as, 410
Noonan syndrome as, 410, 410t
overgrowth in, *see website*
Turner syndrome as, 409-410
Aneurysm, 1638-1639
aortic, in Marfan syndrome, 2441, 2445
cerebral
hemorrhagic stroke due to, 2084-2085
imaging studies in, *see website*
coronary artery, in Kawasaki disease, 864, 865f
ventricular septal, 1557
Angel dust, 683
Angelman syndromes, 391-392, 408t, 412-413
Angina, Vincent, *see website*
Angiocardiography, 1548
in atrioventricular defect, 1555
Angioedema, 811-816
chronic idiopathic, 813
croup *versus*, 1447
diagnosis of, 812t, 813-814
drug eruptions in, *see website*
etiology and pathogenesis of, 811-812
due to food allergy, 822
hereditary, 753, 755, 815-816
physical, 812-813
pressure-induced, 813
treatment of, 814-815, 815t
Angiofibroma, juvenile nasopharyngeal, 1432-1433
Angiography
catheter, *see website*
computed tomography
in neurologic examination, *see website*
in Takayasu arteritis, 872, 872f
in liver dysfunction, 1379
magnetic resonance
in abusive head trauma, 139-140
in cardiovascular disease, 1545-1546, 1546f
computer processing of, 1546
in neurologic examination, *see website*
in orthopedic problems, 2335
in osteomyelitis, 2396, 2396f
in rheumatic disease, *see website*
in septic arthritis, 2400
radionuclide, 1546
Angiokeratoma
circumscriptum, 2224
in Fabry disease, 489, 489f
in GM_1 gangliosidosis, 483
of Mibelli, 2229
Angiokeratoma corporis diffusum, 2139, 2230-2231
Angioma
spider, as manifestation of liver disease, 1376
tufted, 2228, 2229f
Angiomatosis, bacillary, 983t, 986
Angioplasty, balloon, 1569
Angiosarcoma, 1762t
Angiostrongyliasis, *see website*
Angiostrongylus cantonensis, 1226-1227, 1327t-1328t
Angiotensin-converting enzyme (ACE), 861
Angiotensin-converting enzyme inhibitors (ACEIs)
for heart failure, *see website*
for hypertension
of chronic kidney disease, 1825
systemic, 1645t
for Marfan syndrome, 2445
Angiotensin II receptor blockers (ARBs)
for heart failure, *see website*
for systemic hypertension, 1645t
Angiotensin in aldosterone regulation, *see website*
Angle Classification of Malocclusion, *see website*
Angular cheilitis, 2297, 2297f
candidal, 1055
due to riboflavin deficiency, 193, 193f
Angular deformities, 2344-2351
Anhidrosis, 2286-2287
congenital insensitivity to, 2143
Anhidrotic ectodermal dysplasia, 2223, 2223f, 2223t
ANI. *See* Autoimmune neutropenia of infancy (ANI)
Anicteric leptospirosis, 1024
Anidulafungin, *see also website*
for candidiasis, 1054t, 1056t
Animal antisera preparations, 882-883
Animal bites, 2454-2460
clinical manifestations of, 2455
complications of, 2455, 2456t
diagnosis of, 2455
epidemiology of, 2454-2455, 2455t
monkeypox due to, 2459-2460
prevention of, 2457, 2457t-2458t
rat bite fever due to, 2457-2459, 2458f
treatment of, 2455-2457, 2456t
Animal-borne infection
hemorrhagic fevers, 1150t
hookworm, 1220t
leptospirosis, 1023-1024
psittacosis, *see website*
rabies, 1154-1157
Rocky Mountain spotted fever, 1041
Salmonella, 949, 953-954
toxoplasmosis, 1208-1216
during travel, *see website*
tularemia, 978
Yersinia, 971-972
Animal dander allergens, 769, 769t
Animal filariae infection, 1226
Anion gap, 234f
in hyperkalemic renal tubular acidosis, 1811
in metabolic acidosis, 233-234
in poisonings, 254t
normal, 234
reference values for, *see website*
Anions in total body water, *see website*
Aniridia, 2154-2155, 2154f
Anisakiasis, *see website*
Anise tea, potential toxicity of, 272t-273t
Anisocoria, 2155
Anisomelia. *See* Leg-length discrepancy (LLD)
Anisometropia, 2151
Anisometropic amblyopia, 2152
Ankle
avulsion fracture of, 2408-2409
sports injury to, 2417-2418, 2417f
Ankle jerk in neurologic examination, *see website*
Ankle sprain, 2418
in basketball and volleyball, *see website*
Ankyloglossia, 534, 1261
Ankylosing spondylitis (AS), 839, *see also website*
Ann Arbor Conference staging of Hodgkin lymphoma, 1741, 1741t
Annular constriction bands, 533, 2220-2221, 2343, *see website*
Annular pancreas, *see website*
Anodontia, 1250
Anomalies. *See* Congenital anomalies
Anomalous origin of coronary arteries (ALCAPA), 1598-1599, 1599f
Anonychia, 2293
Anorchia, congenital, 1944
Anorectal disorders, 1355-1362
anal fissure as, 1359
hemorrhoids as, 1360, 1361f
malformations as, 1355-1356, 1356f, 1357t, 1359t
perianal abscess and fistula as, 1360, 1360f
pilonidal sinus and abscess as, 1362
rectal mucosal prolapse as, 1361
Anorectal manometry (ARM)
in congenital intestinal pseudo-obstruction, 1283t
in Hirschsprung disease, 1286
Anorectoplasty, posterior sagittal, 1358
Anorexia, 1241-1242
nondigestive causes of, 1241t
treatment of in palliative care, 155t-157t
Anorexia nervosa (AN), 90, 90t. *See also* Eating disorders
eating and weight control habits in, 92t
in female athlete, 2422
hypokalemia in, 223
symptoms commonly reported in, 93t
Anosmia, 1948-1949, *see also website*
neurologic examination of, *see website*
Anotia, *see website*
Anovulatory menstrual cycle, 653
abnormal uterine bleeding due to, 688, 689t-690t
Anoxia, due to drowning, 343
Antacids
drug interactions with, *see website*
for gastroesophageal reflux disease, 1268
hypophosphatemia and, 227
Antagonists, receptor binding by, *see website*
Antegrade continence enema procedure (ACE), 1359
Antegrade pressure-perfusion flow study, 1841
Antegrade pyelogram, 1841
Anterior chamber
development of, *see website*
examination of, 2150
Anterior cruciate ligament (ACL) injuries, 2414, 2414t
Anterior dislocation of shoulder, 2410
Anterior drawer test, 2415f
Anterior knee pain syndrome, 2354

Anterior lenticonus, 2172
Anterior uveitis, 2167t
Anterolateral tibial bowing, 2351
Anteromedial tibial bowing, 2351
Anteversion, femoral, 2344, 2346
Anthracycline use, sports participation and, 2402t-2404t
Anthrax
  terrorism and, 891, *see website*
  vaccine for, 884t, 891
Anthropometric evaluation in chronic diarrhea, 1343
Anti-acetylcholine (ACh) antibodies, 2134
Antiadrenal cytoplasmic antibodies, 1926
Antiandrogens
  for familial male gonadotropin-independent precocious puberty, 1893
  gynecomastia due to, *see website*
  for polycystic ovary syndrome, *see website*
Antiarrhythmic agents, 1610, 1611t-1612t
  pharmacokinetics of, *see website*
Antibiotic-associated diarrhea, 994-995
Antibiotic prophylaxis. *See* Prophylaxis
Antibiotics/antibiotic therapy, 903, *see also website*. See also *specific types*
  for acne
    systemic, 2324-2326, 2324f, 2325t
    topical, 2324, 2324f
  age- and risk-specific use of, *see website*
  aminoglycosides in, *see website*
  for appendicitis, 1355
  for bacterial meningitis, 2091-2094
  carbapenems in, *see website*
  cephalosporins in, *see website*
  for cystic fibrosis, 1491-1492, 1492t
  daptomycin in, *see website*
  for fever in neutropenic patient, *see website*
  for fever without localizing signs, 898
  glycopeptides in, *see website*
  for group A streptococci infection, 918
  gynecomastia due to, *see website*
  for immunocompromised and hospitalized patients, *see website*
  for infectious diarrhea, 1337, 1337t
  for infective endocarditis, 1624, 1625t
  intrapartum, 633-634
  lincosamides in, *see website*
  macrolides in, *see website*
  for medical devices-associated infections, *see website*
  for neonatal infection, 644-646, 645t, *see also website*
  for osteomyelitis, 2397-2398
  for otitis media, 2206-2207
  penicillins in, *see website*
  for pertussis, 946, 947t
  principles of, *see website*
  quinolones in, *see website*
  resistance to (*See* Antimicrobial resistance)
  for rheumatic fever, 923-924
  for septic arthritis, 2400
  in serotonin syndrome, 265t
  for *Shigella* infection, 961
  for skin disorders, 2217
  for *Staphylococcus aureus* infection, 906-908
  streptogramins and oxazolidinones in, *see website*
  sulfonamides in, *see website*
  tetracyclines in, *see website*
  for vulvovaginal infections, 1868t
Antibodies
  autoimmune hemolytic anemia associated with
    "cold," 1682-1683
    "warm," 1680-1682
  monoclonal, 883
  in rheumatic disease, *see website*
Antibodies to infliximab (ATI), 1303
Antibody deficiency(ies), 721t, 722-728, 724f
  common variable immunodeficiency as, 724-725, 724t
  enteroviral meningoencephalitis with, 1092
Antibody deficiency(ies) *(Continued)*
  genetics of, 723t
  hyper-immunoglobulin M syndrome as, 726-727
  immunoglobulin A deficiency as, 725
  immunoglobulin G subclass deficiencies as, 725-726
  immunoglobulin heavy- and light-chain deletions as, 726
  infection in, *see website*
  X-linked agammaglobulinemia as, 723-724, 724f
  X-linked lymphoproliferative disease as, 727
Antibody-dependent cellular cytotoxicity (ADCC), *see website*
Antibody testing
  in cytomegalovirus, 1116
  in Epstein-Barr virus, 1113-1114, 1114f
  in toxoplasmosis, 1213
  in varicella-zoster virus infection, 1108
Anticholinergic agents
  for allergic disease, 770
  for asthma, 796, 797t-798t
  for motion sickness, 1244t
  poisoning with
    antidote for, 256t-257t
Anticholinergic poison syndrome, 253t
Anticholinergic syndromes, 676t
Anticipatory guidance
  for foster care children, *see website*
  for health eating habits, 188t
  in injury prevention, 19t
  in palliative care, 151-159
  in well child care, 14
Anticoagulants, 1711-1712
  lupus, 844
Anticoagulation therapy
  for cerebral sinovenous thrombosis, 2083-2084
  for pulmonary embolism, 1502
Anticonvulsants. *See* Antiepileptic drugs (AEDs)
Anti-deoxyribonuclease B titer, reference values for, *see website*
Antidepressants
  for migraine prophylaxis, 2044t
  for neuropathic pain, 368t
  for pain management, 368-369
  poisoning with, 263-266, 264f
  for psychiatric disorders, 61-62, 63t
  in serotonin syndrome, 265t
  tricyclic
    for attention deficit/hyperactivity disorder, 111t
    for neuropathic pain, 368t
    toxicity of, 251t
Anti-D gamma globulin, 615
Antidiuresis, nephrogenic syndrome of inappropriate, 1884
Antidiuretic hormone (ADH), *see website*
  arginine (*See* Growth hormone (GH))
  for central diabetes insipidus, 1883
  maintenance fluids and hyponatremia and, 243-244
  in osmolality regulation, *see website*
  for portal hypertension, *see website*
  reference values for, *see website*
  syndrome of inappropriate, 1884, 1886
  in water balance, 1881-1882, 1882f
Antidotes for poisoning, 256t-258t, 258
Antidromic conduction, 1613-1614
Antiemetics
  for nausea and vomiting with migraine, 2043
  in serotonin syndrome, 265t
Antiepileptic drugs (AEDs)
  choice of, 2026-2029, 2029t
  initiating and monitoring of, 2029-2032, 2030t-2031t
  mechanisms of action of, 2025-2026
  for migraine prophylaxis, 2044-2045, 2044t
  for neuropathic pain, 368t
  for pain management, 369-370
  in serotonin syndrome, 265t
Antifungal agents, 1053, 2217, *see also website*
Antigen-dependent stages of B-cell development, *see website*
Antigen detection
  in bacterial and fungal infection diagnosis, *see website*
  in coccidioidomycosis, 1066
  in group A streptococci infection, 917-918
  in HIV, *see website*
  in office, *see website*
  in parainfluenza viruses, 1125t
  in viral infection diagnosis, *see website*
Antigenic drift, 1122
Antigen-presenting cells (APCs), *see website*
Antigen-specific immunoglobulin, *see website*
Anti-glomerular basement membrane disease, *see website*
Antihemophilic factor, 1696t
Anti-hepatitis A virus, 1395, 1396t
Antihistamines
  for allergic disease, 770-771, 771t
  for allergic rhinitis, 777-779, 777t-778t
  for atopic dermatitis, 805
  for common cold, 1435
  for cyclic vomiting syndrome, 1244t
  for migraine prophylaxis, 2044t
  for motion sickness, 1244t
  for urticaria and angioedema, 814-815, 815t
Antihypertensives, 1645f, 1645t-1646t
  gynecomastia due to, *see website*
  for migraine prophylaxis, 2044t
Anti-immunoglobulin E
  for allergic disease, 772
  for asthma, 794t, 796
  for atopic dermatitis, 805
Antiinflammatory cytokines, *see website*
Antiinflammatory therapy
  for cystic fibrosis, 1493
  for rheumatic fever, 923
Anti-interleukin-4 drugs, 773
Anti-interleukin-5 drugs, 773
Antimalarials, toxicity of, 251t
Antimetabolites for atopic dermatitis, 805
Antimicrobial resistance, *see also website*
  in child care setting, *see website*
  Haemophilus influenzae, 941
  mechanism of, *see website*
  Mycobacterium tuberculosis, 1008-1009
  in neonatal infection, 644
  nocardiosis, *see website*
  in otitis media, 2205-2206
  Pseudomonas aeruginosa, *see website*
  Streptococcus pneumoniae, 913
  tuberculosis, 998, 1008-1009
Antimicrobial susceptibility testing, *see website*
Antimony, gastroenteritis due to, 1328t-1329t
Antimotility agents, 1337, *see also website*
Antimüllerian hormones (AMH), 1946, *see also website*
Antineutrophil cytoplasmic antibody (ANCA)
  in inflammatory bowel disease, 1295
  in pulmonary hemosiderosis, 1499
  in rheumatic disease, *see website*
  in vasculitis, 874-876, 874t, 875f
Antinuclear antibodies (ANAs)
  in juvenile idiopathic arthritis, 836
  in rheumatic disease, *see website*
  in spondyloarthritides, *see website*
  in systemic lupus erythematosus, 844
Antioxidants, porphyria cutanea tarda and, *see website*
Antiparasitic therapy, 1177, *see also website*
Antiphospholipid antibody syndrome (APS), 1709
Antiplasmin
  deficiency, 1704
  reference values for, 1698t
Antipsychotics
  for pain management, 370
  for psychiatric disorders, 62-63, 64t
  toxicity of, 266

Antiquitin deficiency, 453-454
Antireflux therapy, 1267-1268
Antiretroviral therapy
  highly active, 1159
  for HIV infection, 1167-1174, 1168t-1171t
  hypersensitivity to, 826
Antirheumatics, *see website*
Antiseptic skin care of newborn, 537
Antisera preparations, 882t
  hyperimmune animal, 882-883
Antistreptolysin O assay, 918
Antithrombin-III, reference values for, 1698t
Antithrombotic agents, 1710t
Antithymocyte globulin (ATG)
  for pancytopenia, 1692
  in renal transplantation, *see website*
Antithyroid drugs, 1912t
  adverse reactions to, 1911-1912
Antitoxin
  botulism, 882-883
  diphtheria, 882-883, 882t, *see also website*
  tetanus, 992-993
α-Antitrypsin
  deficiency of, 1393
    emphysema and, 1462-1463, *see also website*
    subcutaneous tissue disease due to, 2283-2284
  measurement of
    in chronic diarrhea, 1344t
    in protein losing enteropathy, 1307
Antivenom administration, 2460
  for snake bites, 2462, 2462t
Antiviral therapy, 1069, *see also website*
  for common cold, 1435
  drug interactions with, *see website*
  for fever in neutropenic patient, *see website*
  for herpesviruses, *see website*
Antley-Bixler syndrome, 1937-1938, 1962, 2012t
Antroduodenal manometry (ADM), 1283t
Anus
  candidal infection of, 2314
  ectopic, 1357
  imperforate, 1356, 1356f-1357f
    neuropathic bladder and, *see website*
  infectious dermatitis of, 2304-2305, 2305f
  newborn assessment of, 536
Anxiety
  psychopharmacologic management of, 61t, 63t
  respiratory signs and symptoms of, *see website*
  separation, 32
  stranger, 30, 33
  treatment of in palliative care, 155t-157t, 158
  in type 1 diabetes mellitus, 1986
Anxiety attack, seizure *versus*, *see website*
Anxiety disorders, 77-82, 78t-82t
  attention deficit/hyperactivity disorder *versus*, 110
Anxiolytic agents, 62
  for anesthesia, *see website*
  for cyclic vomiting syndrome, 1244t
  for depression and anxiety symptoms, 63t
AOM. *See* Acute otitis media (AOM)
Aorta
  coarctation of, 1567-1570, 1567f, 1569f
    in adults, 1608
    with ventricular septal defect, 1570
  fetal development of, 1527, *see also website*
Aortic aneurysm in Marfan syndrome, 2441
  surgery for, 2441, 2445
Aortic arch
  anomalies of, 1597f-1598f, 1597t
    coarctation with disease of, 1570
    embryonic development of, *see website*
  development of, 1527-1528, *see also website*
  double, 1452, 1596-1597, 1597f
  interrupted, 1570
Aortic insufficiency, 1628
Aorticopulmonary (AP) window defect, 1561
Aorticopulmonary window defect, 1560-1561
Aortic stenosis
  critical, 1565
  sudden death due to, 1619
Aortic valve
  coarctation with disease of, 1570
  replacement of, 1566-1567
Aortic valve stenosis, 1565-1567, 1565f-1566f
  in adults, 1608-1609
Aortogram, pulmonary, *see website*
Aortopulmonary translocation, 1566-1567
APCs. *See* Antigen-presenting cells (APCs)
APECED. *See* Autoimmune polyendocrinopathy-candidiasis ectodermal dysplasia (APECED)
Apert syndrome, 1531t, 2012t, 2013
Apgar score, 536, 536t-537t
  hypoxic-ischemic encephalopathy and, 570t
Aphthous stomatitis, 2298, 2298f
  in PFAPA, 859-860
Aphthous ulcer
  genital, 1866, 1866f
  oral, 1260, 1260t
Apical pulse, assessment of, 1533
APL. *See* Acute promyelocytic leukemia (APL)
Aplasia
  Leydig cell, 1964
  lung, 1463
  muscle, 2118
  optic nerve, 2181
  parathyroid gland, 1917
  red blood cell, 1652-1653
    parvovirus B19 infection in, 1095-1097, 1653
Aplasia cutis congenita, 2221-2222, 2221f
Aplastic anemia, 748t, 1690-1691
  hematopoietic stem cell transplantation for, 759, 759f
Aplastic crisis
  due to parvovirus B19, 1095-1096
Apley compression test, 2415f
APL-RARα oncogene, *see website*
Apnea
  brain death and, *see website*
  congenital myasthenic syndrome with episodic, 2133, 2133t
  as delivery room emergency, 575
  in factitious disorder by proxy, 146
  due to gastroesophageal reflux disease, 1269-1270
  neonatal, 580-581, 580t
  in newborn, *see website*
  obstructive sleep
    with Down syndrome, 403t
    obesity with, 184t
  postoperative, *see website*
  of prematurity, 580-581
  seizures and, *see website*
  sleep
    enuresis with, 72
    general anesthesia and, *see website*
    obstructive, 49-51, 49t-50t, 1523
    with type 2 diabetes mellitus, 1993t
  sudden death syndrome and, 581
Apnea test, *see website*
Apneustic center, *see website*
APOA-1. *See* Apolipoprotein A-1 (APOA-1)
Apocrine glands, morphology of, *see website*
APOL1. *See* Apolipoprotein L-1 (APOL1)
Apolipoprotein A-1 (APOA-1) deficiency, 477
Apolipoprotein L-1 (APOL1), 1191
Apolipoproteins, 471
Apophysis
  age of appearance and fusion of, 2413t
  slipped vertebral, 2377
  sports injuries involving, 2408
Apophysitis, 2340-2341
  calcaneal, 2418
  sports-related, 2413
Apoptosis, *see website*
Apparent life-threatening event (ALTE), 1428
Apparent volume of distribution, *see website*
Appearance of newborn, 532-533
Appendageal structures of skin, *see website*
Appendectomy, 1354-1355
  actinomycosis following, *see website*
Appendicitis, 1349-1355
  abdominal pain of, 1247t-1248t
  Angiostrongylus costaricensis versus, 1227
  clinical features of, 1349-1350
  Clostridium, *see website*
  in cystic fibrosis, 1495
  diagnostic studies in, 1351-1353, 1351f-1352f, 1351t
  differential diagnosis of, 1353-1354
  pathology of, 1349
  physical examination in, 1350
  treatment of, 1354-1355
Appendix testis, torsion of, 1862, 1862f
Appetite, control of, 183f
Appetite suppressants, cardiac manifestations of, 1531t
Apple allergy, 821, 821t
Apple juice, diarrhea and, 1335t
Applied behavior analysis (ABA), *see website*
Apraxia
  oculomotor, 2161, *see also website*
  verbal, 119
APRT. *See* Adenine phosphoribosyltransferase (APRT) deficiency
APRV. *See* Airway pressure release ventilation (APRV)
APS. *See* Antiphospholipid antibody syndrome (APS); Autoimmune polyendocrinopathy (APS)
APS-1. *See* Autoimmune polyendocriniopathy, type I (APS-1)
APS-2. *See* Autoimmune polyendocrinopathy type II(APS-2)
APSGN. *See* Acute poststreptococcal glomerulonephritis (APSGN)
Aptivus. *See* Tipanavir
APTT. *See* Activated partial thromboplastin time (APTT)
APVs. *See* Avian pneumoviruses (APVs)
AQP2 gene, 1812
Aquagenic urticaria, 813
Aqueous vasopressin for central diabetes insipidus, 1883-1884
AR. *See* Allergic rhinitis (AR)
ARA. *See* Arachidonic acid (ARA)
ARA-A. *See* Vidarabine
Ara-A. *See* Vidarabine
Ara-C. *See* Cytarabine
Arachidonic acid (ARA), *see also website*
  deficiency, cutaneous manifestations of, 2329
Arachnoid cysts, 2006
Arboviral encephalitis
  in North America, 1141-1144, 1142f-1143f
  outside North America, 1144-1147, 1145t
Arboviruses in viral meningoencephalitis, 2095-2096
ARBs. *See* Angiotensin II receptor blockers (ARBs)
Arcuate uterus, *see website*
ARDS. *See* Acute respiratory distress syndrome (ARDS)
Area under the curve (AUC), *see website*
Argentine hemorrhagic fever, 1151-1152
Arginase deficiency, 448f, 452
Arginine, defects in metabolism of, 418-421, 448f-449f, 448t, 450t
Arginine:glycine aminotransferase (AGAT) deficiency, 441
Arginine vasopressin. *See* Growth hormone (GH)
Argininosuccinate lyase (AL) deficiency, 448f, 452
Argininosuccinate synthetase (AS) deficiency, 451-452
ARH. *See* Autosomal recessive hypercholesterolemia (ARH)

Arhinia, 1430
ARHR. *See* Autosomal recessive hypophosphatemic rickets (ARHR)
ARM. *See* Anorectal manometry (ARM)
Arm. *See* Upper extremity(ies)
Arnold Chiari malformations, 1264
  myelomeningocele with, 1522
  respiratory insufficiency due to, 1522
Aromatase deficiency, 1962
Aromatherapy for pain management, 371
Aromatic amino acid decarboxylase deficiency (AADC), 2060t
Aromatic L-amino acid decarboxylase (AADC) deficiency, 445-446
Arousal
  confusional, 51-52
  newborn, *see website*
Arousal disorders, non-REM partial, *see website*
Arpiprazole
  for mood stabilization, 64t
  for psychosis and agitation, 64t
ARPKD. *See* Autosomal recessive polycystic kidney disease (ARPKD)
Array comparative genomic hybridization (aCGH), 376, 377t, 396-398, 400f
Arrhythmias. *See* Cardiac arrhythmias
Arrhythmogenic right ventricular cardiomyopathy (ARVC), 1629t-1630t, 1633-1634
ARSA gene, 2072
Arsenic poisoning, *see also website*
  gastroenteritis due to, 1328t-1329t
ART. *See* Acoustic reflex test (ART)
Artemether, *see also website*
  for malaria, 1202, 1203t-1205t
Artemis deficiency, 733
Artemisia absinthium, potential toxicity of, 272t-273t
Arterial access for emergencies, 292-294, 296f
Arterial baroceptors in respiration regulation, *see website*
Arterial blood gases (ABGs), *see also website*
  in acid-base disorders, 230
  interpretation of, *see website*
  normal values, 230t
Arterial dissection, 2080
Arterial ecchymotic Ehlers-Danlos syndrome, 2278
Arterial ischemic stroke (AIS), 2080-2082, 2081f-2082f, 2081t-2082t
Arterial oxygen content (Cao_2), *see website*
Arterial partial pressure of carbon dioxide ($Paco_2$), *see website*
Arterial switch procedure
  Jatene, 1586, 1587f
  Mustard or Senning, 1586-1587
Arteriography, pulmonary, *see website*
Arteriomesenteric duodenal compression syndrome, 1287
Arteriovenous fistula, 1638, *see also website*
  hepatic, *see website*
  pulmonary, 1599, *see also website*
Arteriovenous malformations (AVMs), 2225, 2226f
  hemorrhagic stroke due to, 2084-2085
  imaging studies in, *see website*
  spinal, 2107-2108
Arteritis
  mesenteric, postoperative, 1569
  Takayasu, 868t, 871-872
Artesunate, *see also website*
  for malaria, 1202
Arthralgia
  in acute rheumatic fever, 922
  with parvovirus B19 infection, 1095
  in rheumatic disease, *see website*
Arthritis. *See also* Rheumatic disease
  in acute rheumatic fever, 921-922
  in alcaptonuria, 423
  conditions causing, 836t
  enteroviruses in, 1091-1092
Arthritis *(Continued)*
  enthesitis-related, 831t, *see website*
  following meningococcal disease, 933
  following rubella, 1077
  gonococcal, 937-938
  inflammatory bowel disease with, *see website*
  juvenile idiopathic, 829-839
    arthralgia in, *see website*
    cardiac manifestations of, 1532t
    classification of, 829t-831t
    clinical manifestations of, 831-835, 832f-834f, 833t, 835t
    diagnosis of, *see website*
    differential diagnosis of, 835, 836t
    epidemiology of, 829
    etiology of, 829-831
    fever of unknown origin in, 899
    laboratory findings in, 835-836, 837f
    pathogenesis of, 831, 831f-832f
    prognosis for, 838-839, 839f
    sports participation and, 2402t-2404t
    treatment of, 837-838
  due to Lyme disease, 1027, 1028t
  due to mumps, 1080
  due to parvovirus B19, 1095
  with parvovirus B19 infection, 1095
  psoriatic, *see website*
  reactive and postinfection, 839-841, 840f, 840t, 1333t
    Campylobacter, 919
    streptococcal, 919
  in rheumatic disease, *see website*
  septic, 2398-2400, 2399f, 2399t
    Pseudomonas aeruginosa, 976t
    toxic synovitis *versus*, 2361
  suppurative, *Haemophilus influenzae* in, 942
Arthrochalasia, 2278
Arthrochalasis multiplex congenita, 2278
Arthrodesis for arthrogryposis, *see website*
Arthrogryposis, 2387
  associated etiologies of, *see also website*
Arthrogryposis multiplex congenita (AMC), *see also website*
Arthropathy, human T-lymphocyte-associated, *see website*
Arthropod bites, 2317-2319, 2318f
Arthropod vectors in trypanosomiasis, 1194f, 1195
Artificial airway
  for epiglottitis, 1448
  for respiratory distress and failure, 319
Artificial sweeteners, 1982
Art therapy for pain management, 371
ARVC. *See* Arrhythmogenic right ventricular cardiomyopathy (ARVC)
ARX gene, 2060t, *see also website*
Arylamine *N*-acetyltransferases, drug biotransformation and, *see website*
AS. *See* Ankylosing spondylitis (AS); Argininosuccinate synthetase (AS)
ASA. *See* Aspirin (ASA)
5-ASA. *See* 5-Aminosalicylate (5-ASA)
Asbestos exposure, *see website*
Ascariasis, 1217, 1217f
Ascending bacterial infection, neonatal, 630, 630f-631f
Ascending undescended testis, 1859
Ascites, 1416, *see also website*
  management of in cholestasis, 1388
  as manifestation of liver disease, 1376
Ascorbic acid, 194t, 198
  deficiency of, 198-200, 199f-200f
    skin manifestations of, 2330
  dietary needs and sources of, 198
  dietary reference intakes for, *see website*
  for methemoglobin, 1673
  toxicity of, 200
ASCUS. *See* Atypical squamous cells of undetermined significance (ASCUS)
ASD. *See* Atrial septal defect (ASD)
Aseptic technique, *see website*
Ashkenazi Jews
  essential pentosuria in, *see website*
  persistent hyperinsulinemic hypoglycemia of infancy in, 523
  Tay-Sachs disease in, 485-487, 2070
Asian population
  cultural values associated with, *see website*
  death rates for, 3t-4t
Askin tumor, 1765
Ask-Upmark kidney, 1828
L-Asparaginase for cancer therapy, *see website*
Aspartate aminotransferase (AST)
  in liver disease, 1378
  in obesity, 185t
  reference values for, *see website*
  in viral hepatitis, 1394-1395
Aspartic acid, defects in metabolism of, 455-456, 456f
Aspart insulin analogs, 1976, 1977f
Aspartylglucosaminuria (AGU), 484t, *see also website*
Asperger's disorder, 101t, 105t, 106
  language disorders of, 118
Aspergilloma, pulmonary, 1059
  chronic, 1059
  invasive, 1060
Aspergillosis, allergic bronchopulmonary, 1474
  immunoglobulin E levels in, 766
Aspergillus, 1058-1062
  allergic disease due to, 1058
    in cystic fibrosis, 1494
  allergic reaction to, 769-770
  after hematopoietic stem cell transplantation, 762-763
  invasive, 1060-1061
  noninvasive, 1059
  in pneumonia, 1475t
Asphyxia
  birth, cerebral palsy with, 2063-2064
  multiorgan systemic effects of, 569t
Asphyxiating thoracic dystrophy, 1517, 2434
Aspiration, 1469-1471
  diagnostic tests of, 1472t
  due to drowning, 343
  duodenal in exocrine pancreatic function, 1307
  foreign body, 1453-1454
    croup *versus*, 1447
    neonatal, 590, 591f
    wheezing in, 1457
  of gastric contents, 1470
  of hydrocarbon, 1470-1471, 1470f
  joint, in septic arthritis, 2399
  meconium, 590-592
  nasotracheal, *see website*
  pulmonary, in drowning, 343
  recurrent, 1471-1473, 1471t, 1473f
  sinus, 1437
  splenic, in leishmaniasis, 1189
  of vomitus, 1243t
Aspiration pneumonia
  due to hydrocarbon toxicity, 267
  neonatal, 590, 591f
Aspirin (ASA)
  for acute rheumatic fever, 923
  adverse reaction to, 828
  gastric ulcer due to, 1293
  for Kawasaki disease, 866-867, 867t
  for pain management, 363, 364t
Asplenia
  abnormal position of the heart and, 1589t, 1595-1596
  congenital heart disease with, 1531t
  fever without a focus in, 896t
  infections and, *see website*
ASQ-3. *See* Ages and Stages Questionnaire-3 (ASQ-3)
Assassin bugs in trypanosomiasis, 1195
Assent
  adolescent, *see website*
  child, *see website*

Assist-control (AC) mode in mechanical ventilation, 324
Association studies, genetic, *see website*
ASST. *See* Autologous skin test (ASST)
AST. *See* Aspartate aminotransferase (AST)
Astatic epilepsy, myoclonic, 2024
Astatic seizure, 2019
Astelin. *See* Azelastine
Asthma, 780-801
  allergen immunotherapy for, 774-775
  allergic rhinitis with, 776, 777f
  Aspergillus as trigger of, 1059
  child care and, *see website*
  clinical manifestations and diagnosis of, 782-783, 784t
  common cold and, 1436
  differential diagnosis of, 783, 785t
  environmental factors in, 781
  epidemiology of, 781-782
  etiology of, 781, 781f
  gastroesophageal reflux disease with, 1269-1270
  general anesthesia and, *see website*
  genetics of, 781
  herbs for, 271t
  laboratory findings in, 783-785, 785t, 786f-787f
  obesity with, 184t
  pathogenesis of, 782, 783t
  physical examination in, 765
  prevalence of, 4
  prevention of, 801
  prognosis for, 801
  respiratory syncytial virus infection and, 1129
  risk factors for, 782, 782t
  risk factors for morbidity and mortality associated with, 799t
  sports participation and, 2402t-2404t
  treatment of, 785-801, 788f
    adherence to regimen in, 788
    anticholinergic agents for, 796
    anti-immunoglobulin E (Omalizumab) for, 796
    control of factors contributing to, 788-791, 791t
    corticosteroids for
      inhaled, 793, 795t
      systemic, 793-794
    delivery devices and inhalation techniques for, 796-798
    for exacerbations, 798-801
    in infants and young children, 800-801
    inhaled β-agonists for
      long-acting, 794-795
      short-acting, 001, 796
    leukotriene-modifying agents for, 795-796
    long-term controller medications for, 793-796, 794t
    nonsteroidal antiinflammatory drugs for, 796
    patient education in, 788, 791t
    in pregnancy, 801
    principles of pharmacology for, 791-793
    quick-reliever medications for, 796, 797t-798t
    referral to specialist for, 793
    regular assessment and monitoring in, 785-788, 789t-790t
    stepwise approach to, 792-793, 792t
    during surgery, 801
    theophylline for, 796
  triggers for, 783t
    Aspergillus as, 1059
  types of, 782, 782t
  wheezing in, 1457
Asthma masqueraders, 785
Astigmatism, 2150-2151
Astrakhan fever, 1043-1044
Astrocytoma, 1748-1750, 1749f
Astrovirus, 1134-1137, 1326t
Asymmetry, breast, *see website*
Asymptomatic bacteriuria, 1830
Asystole, cardiac, 1521
Atarax. *See* Hydroxyzine
Ataxia, 2054t, 2055
  cerebellar
    gait of, *see website*
    varicella-zoster virus in, 1109
  episodic, *see website*
  Friedreich, 2055
  in neurologic examination, *see website*
  sensory, gait of, *see website*
  strokelike events *versus*, 2086
Ataxia-telangiectasia, 735, 2055, 2057t
  cutaneous manifestations of, 2230
  infections in, *see website*
  malignancy susceptibility associated with, *see website*
  ovarian defects with, 1956
Ataxia with isolated vitamin E deficiency (AVED), *see website*
Atazanavir
  drug interactions with, *see website*
  for HIV infection, 1168t-1171t
Atelectasis, 1504, *see also website*
  in cystic fibrosis, 1493
  postanesthetic, *see website*
  of tympanic membrane, 2212
Atelosteogenesis type II, 2431
Atenolol
  for arrhythmias, 1611t-1612t
  for systemic hypertension, 1645t
ATG. *See* Antithymocyte globulin (ATG)
α-Thalassemia, 1676-1677
Atherosclerosis, 470-471, 471f
Athetoid cerebral palsy, 2063-2064
Athetosis, 2056, 2058
Athlete. *See* Sports
Athlete's foot, 2312-2313, 2312f
ATI. *See* Antibodies to infliximab (ATI)
Ativan. *See* Lorazepam
ATL. *See* Adult T-cell leukemia/lymphoma (ATL)
Atlantoaxial anomalies, 2381
Atlantoaxial instability, sports participation and, 2402t-2404t
ATN. *See* Acute tubular necrosis (ATN)
Atomoxetine, 61
  for attention deficit/hyperactivity disorder, 62t, 110, 111t
Atonic seizure, 2019
  evaluation of, 2015-2016
Atopic dermatitis (AD), 801-807
  avoiding triggers for, 805-806
  clinical manifestations of, 802, 802f-803f, 803t
  complications of, 806
  diagnosis and differential diagnosis of, 803-804, 803t
  etiology of, 801
  of external ear canal, 2199
  due to food allergy, 822
  laboratory findings in, 803
  pathogenesis of, 802
  pathology of, 801
  prevention of, 807
  prognosis for, 806-807
  treatment of, 804-805, 804t
  vulvar, 1867t-1868t
Atopic keratoconjunctivitis, 810
Atovaquone, *see website*
Atovaquone-proguanil for malaria treatment and chemoprophylaxis, 1202, 1203t-1205t, 1207, 1207t, *see also website*
  in HIV infection, 1175t-1176t
ATP. *See* Adenosine triphosphate (ATP)
ATP1A2 gene, 2016t
ATP7B gene, 1383t
ATP8b1 gene, 1383t
Atresia
  auditory canal, *see website*
  biliary, 1385-1387, 1386f-1387f
    jaundice due to, 607
    liver transplantation for, *see website*
Atresia *(Continued)*
  choanal, 575, 1430, 1430f, *see also website*
  duodenal, 1277-1278
  esophageal, 1262-1263, 1262f
  intestinal, 1277-1281
  jejunal, 1278-1280, 1279f
  laryngeal, 1451
  pulmonary valve
    with intact ventricular septum, 1578-1580, 1579f
    with tetralogy of Fallot, 1573-1574, 1578
  rectal, 1358
  tracheal, 1452
  tricuspid, 1580-1582, 1580f-1581f
  urethral, 1846
Atrial contraction, premature, 1612, 1612f
Atrial ectopic tachycardia, 1615
Atrial fibrillation, 1615-1616, 1616f, *see also website*
Atrial flutter, 1615, 1615f, 1616t
Atrial natriuretic peptide (ANP), 1882, *see also website*
Atrial pacemaker, wandering, 1612, 1612f
Atrial septal defect (ASD), 1551
  in adults, 1605-1606
  familial secundum, *see website*
  ostium secundum, 1551-1553
  sinus venosus, 1553
Atrial septostomy, Rashkind balloon, 1586, 1586f
Atrial tachycardia, 1615, 1616t
Atrioventricular (AV) block, 1618-1619, 1618f
Atrioventricular (AV) canal defects, 1554-1556
  in adult, 1607
  embryonic development of, *see website*
Atrioventricular (AV) septal defects, 1554-1556, 1554f-1555f
  in adults, 1607
Atrioventricular (AV) valves, defects in Marfan syndrome, 2440-2441
Atrioventricular node reentry tachycardia (AVNRT), 1613-1615
Atrioventricular reciprocating tachycardia (AVRT), 1613
Atripla. *See* Tenofovir
Atriple. *See* Emtricitabine
At-risk populations. *See* Special risk populations
Atrium
  embryonic development of, *see website*
  enlargement, electrocardiography of, 1539, 1539f
  in fetal circulation, *see website*
Atropa belladonna toxicity, 269t, 272t-273t
Atrophy
  assessment in neurologic examination, *see website*
  corticosteroid-induced
    dermal, 2274
    subcutaneous, 2282, 2282f
  macular, 2277
  optic, *see website*
  spinal muscular, 2136-2138, 2136t, 2137f
Atropine
  for cholinesterase-inhibiting insecticides poisoning, 256t-257t, 267
  for pediatric resuscitation and arrhythmias, 294t
  in rapid sequence intubation, 287t
Atrovent nasal spray. *See* Ipratropium bromide
ATRX gene, *see website*
Attachment
  development and, *see website*
  maternal-infant, *see website*
  parent-infant, 538-540
Attack, dog-related, 2454
Attention deficit/hyperactivity disorder (ADHD), 108
  clinical manifestations of, 108-109
  diagnosis and differential diagnosis of, 109-110, 109t
  epidemiology of, 108

Attention deficit/hyperactivity disorder (ADHD) *(Continued)*
etiology of, 108
neurodevelopmental function and, *see website*
pathogenesis of, *see website*
prevalence of, 4
prevention of, 112
prognosis for, 112
sudden death and medications for, 1621
treatment of, 110-112, 111t
medications in, 62t
Attention dysfunction, *see website*
ATV. *See* All-terrain vehicle (ATV) accident
Atypical absence seizure, 2023
Atypical antidepressant toxicity, 265
Atypical pneumonia, 1477
Atypical squamous cells of undetermined significance (ASCUS), 1139-1140
Atypical teratoid/rhabdoid tumor, 1752
AUC. *See* Area under the curve (AUC)
Audiometry, 2193, 2193f
for adolescents, 666
behavioral observation, 2194
play, 2193-2194
referral for, 2193t
visual reinforcement, 2194
AUDIT. *See* Alcohol Use Disorders Identification Test (AUDIT)
Auditory brainstem evoked response (ABR), 2192, 2195
Auditory canal
clearing of, 2202-2203
congenital stenosis or atresia of, *see website*
foreign body in, *see website*
traumatic injury to, 2213-2214, *see also website*
tumors of, 2214
Auditory processing disorders, 2188
Augmentation, breast, *see website*
Augmentation cystoplasty, *see website*
Augmentin. *See* Amoxicillin-clavulanate
Aura
migraine with, 2041-2042
with seizures, 2015-2016, 2019
Auramine-rhodamine stain, *see website*
Auricle trauma, 2213-2214, *see also website*
Auscultation
of heart sounds
in acutely ill child evaluation, 276
in cardiac examination, 1533
of lungs
in acutely ill child evaluation, 276
in assessment of respiratory pathology, *see website*
of skill, *see website*
Auspitz sign, 829
Authoritative aspect of eating disorder treatment, 93
Authority gradients for patient safety, *see website*
Autistic disorder (AD), 100-106, 101t
clinical manifestations of, 100-101, 101t
diagnosis of, 101, 102t
differential diagnosis, 101
early identification of, 102, 103f-104f
epidemiology of, 101-102
etiology of, 102
intellectual disability *versus*, 126
language disorders in, 118, 118f
pathology of, 102
prognosis for, 105-106
treatment of, 102-105, 105t
Autoantibodies
in autoimmune hepatitis, 1408t, 1409
diabetes mellitus and, 1974
in systemic lupus erythematosus, 842-843
Autoimmune Addison disease, 1926-1927
Autoimmune adrenalitis, 1925t
Autoimmune disease
diabetes mellitus with, 1996-1997
pulmonary manifestations of, *see website*
Autoimmune enteropathy, 1305-1306, 1341
Autoimmune hemolytic anemia, 1680-1683, 1681t, *see also website*
associated with "cold" antibodies, 1682-1683
associated with "warm" antibodies, 1680-1682
Autoimmune hepatitis (AIH), 1408-1410, 1408t, 1410f
fulminant hepatic failure due to, 1413
with inflammatory bowel disease, *see website*
Autoimmune hypoparathyroidism, 1918
Autoimmune lymphoproliferative syndrome (ALPS), 737-738, 737t, 738f
Autoimmune neuropsychiatric disorders associated with *Streptococcus pyogenes*, 81, 919
movement disorders associated with, 76
Autoimmune neutropenia, 750
Autoimmune neutropenia of infancy (ANI), 750
Autoimmune ovarian failure, 1956
Autoimmune pancreatitis, 1373
Autoimmune polyendocrinopathy, type I (APS-1), 1926
autoimmune thyroiditis with, 1904
Autoimmune polyendocrinopathy (APS), 1925t, 1969
Autoimmune polyendocrinopathy-candidiasis ectodermal dysplasia (APECED), 730
Autoimmune polyendocrinopathy type II (APS-2), 1926-1927
Autoimmune regulator gene (AIRE), 1409
Autoimmune thrombocytopenic purpura, 1714-1718
Autoimmune thyroiditis, 1903-1905
hypothyroidism due to, 1901
with Turner syndrome, 1953
Autoimmune urticaria, 812t, 814
Autoimmunity in type 1 diabetes mellitus, 1970, 1973-1974, 1973f
Autoinflammatory syndrome, familial cold, 855t, 858
Autologous skin test (ASST), 813
Autologous stem cell transplantation, 757, *see also website*
Automated external defibrillation (AEDs), 1621
Automatic control of respiration, *see website*
Automatisms in seizures, 2021
Autonomic instability, *see website*
Autonomic nervous system (ANS)
congenital central hypoventilation syndrome and dysfunction of, 1521
in hypoglycemia, 519t
mushroom poisoning effects on, *see website*
Neonatal Intensive Care Unit Neurobehavioral Scale and, 624t
Autonomic neuropathies, 2141-2143, 2141t-2142t
Autonomic storms, *see website*
Auto-positive end-expiratory pressure, 328-329
Autoresuscitation, sudden infant death syndrome and, 1428
Autosomal dominant hearing loss, 2189
Autosomal dominant hypoparathyroidism, 1917-1918
Autosomal dominant hypophosphatemic rickets (ADHR), 202t, 207
Autosomal dominant inheritance, 383-385, 387f
Autosomal dominant polycystic kidney disease, 1798, 1798f
Autosomal dominant polycystic kidney disease (ADPKD), *see website*
Autosomal dominant polycystic liver disease (ADPLD), *see also website*
congenital heart disease with, 1531t
Autosomal dominant recurrent fever, 858
Autosomal liver and muscle phosphorylase kinase deficiency, 498
Autosomal liver phosphorylase kinase deficiency, 498
Autosomal recessive dopa-responsive dystonia, 445
Autosomal recessive hearing loss, 2189
Autosomal recessive hypercholesterolemia (ARH), 473t, 475
Autosomal recessive hyper-immunoglobulin M syndrome, 726-727
Autosomal recessive hypoparathyroidism with dysmorphic features, 1917
Autosomal recessive hypophosphatemic rickets (ARHR), 202t
Autosomal recessive inheritance, 385-388, 388f
Autosomal recessive polycystic kidney disease (ARPKD), *see also website*
hematuria due to, 1796-1798, 1797f, 1797t
Autosomal recessive proximal renal tubular acidosis, 1808
Autosomal recessive severe combined immunodeficiency, 732-733
Autumn crocus toxicity, 269t
AV. *See* Atrioventricular (AV)
Availability in food security, 170-171
AVED. *See* Ataxia with isolated vitamin E deficiency (AVED)
Avian influenza, *see website*
Avian mite bite, 2320
Avian pneumoviruses (APVs), 1129-1130
Avidity test in toxoplasmosis, 1214
AVMs. *See* Arteriovenous malformations (AVMs)
AVNRT. *See* Atrioventricular node reentry tachycardia (AVNRT)
AVPR2 gene, 1812
AVPU. *See* Alert, Verbal, Pain, Unresponsive (AVPU) Pediatric Response Scale
AVRT. *See* Atrioventricular reciprocating tachycardia (AVRT)
Avulsion fracture, sports-related, 2408-2409, 2409f
of medial epicondyle, 2411, 2411f
pelvic, 2413
Awareness during general anesthesia, *see website*
Axenfeld-Rieger syndrome, 408t
Axillary hair development, *see website*
Axonal neuropathy, giant, 2140
Axonal peroneal muscular atrophy, 2139
Ayurvedic herbal remedies, potential toxicity of, 272t-273t
Azactam. *See* Aztreonam
Azaspiracid poisoning, *see website*
Azathioprine
for atopic dermatitis, 805
for autoimmune hepatitis, 1410
for Crohn disease, 1303
for lupus nephritis, 1788
for rheumatic disease, *see website*
Azelaic acid for acne, 2324, 2325t
Azelastine
for allergic conjunctivitis, 811t
for allergic disease, 771
for allergic rhinitis, 779, 780t
Azithromycin, *see also website*
for babesiosis, *see website*
for to cat-scratch disease, 985
for chancroid, *see website*
for *Chlamydia trachomatis*, 1036-1037
for *Chlamydophila pneumoniae*, 1035
for cryptosporidiosis, 1184
for cystic fibrosis lung infection, 1492t
for infectious diarrhea, 1337t
for *Legionella* infection, *see website*
for Mediterranean spotted fever, 1044
for nongonococcal urethritis, 1033
for nontuberculous mycobacterial prophylaxis, 1015-1016
for otitis media, 2207t
for pertussis, 947t
for pharyngitis, 1440
for sexually transmitted infections in adolescents, 712t
for *Shigella* infection, 961
for traveler's diarrhea, *see website*
for typhoid fever, 958t
Azoles, *see website*
Azotemia, prerenal, 1818-1819

Aztreonam, *see also website*
  for cystic fibrosis lung infection, 1492t
  for neonatal infection, 645t

B

BA. *See* Biliary atresia (BA)
BAAT gene defect, 1383t
Babesia microti, 1026
Babesiosis, 1207, *see also website*
Babinski sign, *see website*
Baby Doe Regulations, *see website*
Baby foods, nutritive value of, *see website*
Bacillary angiomatosis, 983t, 986
Bacillary dysentery, *Shigella*, 959-961
Bacillary peliosis, 986
Bacille Calmette-Guérin (BCG) vaccine, 884t, 1010-1011
  for immigrant children, 133
  international, 894
  tuberculin skin testing and, 1001
Bacillus anthracis, 1324t-1325t
Bacillus cereus, 1324t-1325t
Back
  low, sports injury to, 2412-2413
  rickets and, 201t
  round, 2371-2373
Back blows for airway obstruction, 282, 283f
Back pain, 2332, 2373-2374, 2373t
  in rheumatic disease, *see website*
  in spondyloarthritides, *see website*
Back to Sleep campaign, 1429
Baclofen
  for muscle spasm, in palliative care, 155t-156t
  for spasticity of cerebral palsy, 2064-2065
BACNS. *See* Benign angiitis of central nervous system (BACNS)
Bacteremia
  Aeromonas, *see website*
  anaerobic, *see website*
  Bartonella, 983t, 987
  blood culture for, *see website*
  Campylobacter, 969
  coagulase-negative staphylococci, 909-910
  fever without a focus and, 897-898
  Haemophilus influenzae, 943
  meningococcal, 931-932, 932f
  Moraxella catarrhalis, *see website*
  Pseudomonas aeruginosa, 975
  Salmonella, 950-952
  in sickle cell disease, 1663, 1663t
  Staphylococcus aureus, 905
  Staphylococcus epidermis, 910
Bacteria
  in breast milk, 540t
  in dental caries, 1255
  rapid antigen detection of, *see website*
Bacterial colonization in neonate, 630
Bacterial dysentery, 1331-1332, 1332t
Bacterial infection(s)
  anaerobic
    botulism as, 987-991
    Clostridium difficile infection as, 994-995
    due to other organisms, 995, *see also website*
    tetanus as, 991-994
  in childcare setting, *see website*
  congenital heart disease and, 1603
  of conjunctiva, 2167t
  cutaneous, 2299-2308
    blastomycosis-like pyoderma, 2304, 2304f
    blistering distal dactylitis as, 2304, 2304f
    ecthyma as, 2303, 2303f
    erysipeloid as, 2307
    erythrasma as, 2306
    folliculitis as, 2305, 2305f-2306f
    furuncles and carbuncles as, 2305-2306, 2306f
    impetigo as, 2299-2300, 2300f
    perianal dermatitis as, 2304-2305, 2305f
    pitted keratolysis as, 2306
    staphylococcal scaled skin syndrome as, 2302-2303, 2302f
Bacterial infection(s) *(Continued)*
    of subcutaneous tissue, 2300-2302
    tuberculous, 2307-2308, 2308f
  fever of unknown origin in, 900t
  following organ transplantation, *see website*
  food-borne, 1324t-1325t
  gram-negative
    due to *Aeromonas*, 974, *see also website*
    due to *Bartonella*, 982-987
    Brucella, 980-982
    due to *Burkholderia*, 975, *see also website*
    due to *Campylobacter*, 968-970
    chancroid as, 944, *see also website*
    cholera as, 965-968
    due to *Escherichia coli*, 961-965
    due to *Haemophilus influenzae*, 940-943
    due to *Legionella*, 982, *see also website*
    due to *Moraxella catarrhalis*, 944, *see also website*
    due to *Neisseria gonorrhoeae*, 935-940
    due to *Neisseria meningitidis*, 929-935
    pertussis as, 944-948
    due to *Plesiomonas shigelloides*, 974, *see also website*
    due to *Pseudomonas aeruginosa*, 975-977
    due to *Salmonella*, 948-958
    due to *Stenotrophomonas*, 976, *see also website*
    tularemia as, 978-980
    due to *Yersinia*, 971-974
  gram-positive
    Actinomyces, 929, *see also website*
    due to diphtheria, 929, *see also website*
    due to enterococcus, 928, *see also website*
    due to group A streptococcus, 914-925
      rheumatic fever as, 920-925
    due to group B streptococcus, 925-928
    due to *Listeria monocytogenes*, 929, *see also website*
    Nocardia, 929, *see also website*
    due to non-group A or B streptococci, 928, *see also website*
    staphylococcal, 903-910
    due to *Streptococcus pneumoniae*, 910-914
  HIV-related, *see website*
  laboratory diagnosis of, *see website*
  meningitis as, 2087-2095
  myocarditis as, 1634-1635
  neonatal, 632t
    diagnosis of, 638t, 642-644
    manifestations of, 638t
    pathogenesis of ascending, 630, 630f-631f
    septic, 636-637, 637t-638t, 643t
  in osteomyelitis, 2394-2395
  in pneumonia, 1475t, 1476-1477
  predisposition to due to immunodeficiency, 716t
  respiratory syncytial virus infection with, 1128
  secondary to varicella-zoster virus, 1109
  sinusitis as, 1436-1437
  stem cell transplantation and, *see website*
  tracheitis as, 1449-1450, 1449f
    croup *versus*, 1447
  traveler's diarrhea due to, 1338t
Bacterial meningitis, 2087-2095
  cerebrospinal fluid findings in, 2088t
  clinical manifestations of, 2090
  complications of, 2094
  diagnosis of, 2090-2091, 2092t-2093t
  epidemiology of, 2087
  etiology of, 2087
  Haemophilus influenzae type b in, 2089
  hearing loss due to, *see website*
  Neisseria meningitidis in, 2087-2089
  neonatal, 646
  pathogenesis of, 2089-2090
  pathology and pathophysiology of, 2089
  prevention of, 2095
  prognosis for, 2095
  Streptococcus pneumoniae in, 2087
  treatment of, 2091-2094, 2093t
Bacterial overgrowth, intestinal, 1283-1284, 1313, 1340
Bacterial resistance, *see also website*
  in child care setting, *see website*
  Haemophilus influenzae, 941
  mechanism of, *see website*
  Mycobacterium tuberculosis, 1008-1009
  nocardiosis, *see website*
  Pseudomonas aeruginosa, *see website*
  Streptococcus pneumoniae, 913
  tuberculosis, 998, 1008-1009
Bacterial vaginosis
  prophylaxis following rape, 704t
  sexual abuse and, 145t
Bacteriuria, asymptomatic, 1830
Bacteroides fragilis, *see website*
Bactrim. *See* Trimethoprim-sulfamethoxazole (TMP-SMX)
BAD-1. *See Blastomyces* adhesion-1 (BAD-1)
Baere-Stevenson syndrome, 2012t
BAERs. *See* Brainstem auditory-evoked responses (BAERs)
Bag-valve-mask positive pressure ventilation, 284-285, 284f-285f
Bailler-Gerold syndrome, 2012t
Baker cyst, 2353
BAL. *See* British antilewisite (BAL); Bronchoalveolar lavage (BAL)
Balamuthia mandrillaris, 1178, *see also website*
Balanitis xerotica obliterans, 1854f, 1857
Balantidium coli, 1183, *see website*
Bald-faced hornet, allergic responses to, 807f
Ballard scoring system, 557
Ballet, injuries in, *see website*
Balloon angioplasty, 1569
Balloon atrial septostomy, Rashkind, 1586, 1586f
Balloon valvuloplasty
  for aortic stenosis, 1566
  for pulmonary valve stenosis, 1563
Bamboo hair, 2293
Bancroftian filariasis, 1224-1225
Bannayan-Ruvalcaba-Riley syndrome, *see website*
Banti syndrome, *see website*
Barbiturates
  adverse effects of, 2031t
  for anesthesia, *see website*
  drug interactions with, *see website*
  urine screening for adolescent use of, 676t
Bardet-Biedl syndrome, 182t
Bare lymphocytic syndrome, 734
Bariatric surgery, 186
Barium enema
  in Hirschsprung disease, 1285f-1286f, 1286
  in ulcerative colitis, 1297, 1299f
Barium fluoroscopy, *see also website*
  in achalasia, 1264-1265, 1265f
Barium radiography in gastroesophageal reflux disease, 1267, 1267f
Barium swallow, *see website*
"Barking" cough of croup, 1446
Barlow provocative maneuver, 2357, 2357f
Baroceptors in respiration regulation, *see website*
Barraquer-Simons syndrome, 2286
Barrett esophagus, 1269
Barrier methods for contraception, 694
Barth syndrome, 433, 748t
Bartonella, 982-987, 983t
  in infective endocarditis, 1624t
Bartonella bacilliformis, 982, 983f
Bartonella henselae, 983, 984f-985f, 986, 2168
Bartonella quintana, 986
Bartonellosis, 982, 983f
Bartter syndrome, 221, 223, 236-237, 551t, 1813-1814, 1813t
  renal magnesium loss in, *see website*
Basal cell carcinoma, *see also website*
  nevoid, 1747t
Basal cell nevus syndrome, *see website*
Basal layer, 2215

BASD. *See* Bile acid synthetic defect (BASD)
Base. *See also* Acid-base balance
excessive intake of in metabolic alkalosis, 237
in oral rehydration solutions, 1335t
Baseball, injuries in, *see website*
Base excess, reference values for, *see website*
Basement membrane, *see website*
Base therapy for metabolic acidosis, 234
"Basic helix-loop-helix" (bHLH) proteins, 2112
Basic life support algorithm, 280f
Basilar-type migraine, 2042
Basiliximab, *see website*
Basketball, injuries in, *see website*
Basophilia, *see website*
Basophils
in food allergy, 816
reference values for, *see website*
Bassinet, 538
"Bathing suit" melanocyte nevus, 2232f
Bath oil for skin disorders, 2216
Bathtub drowning, 24, 343
Batten disease, 2073
Battery
in ear canal, *see website*
ingestion of, 1290
Battle sign, *see website*
Bauer-Kirby method, *see website*
Bayley Scales of Infant Development (BSID-II), 126-127
Baylisascariasis, *see website*
B-cell lymphoma, 1739-1740, 1744t
B cells, 722
abnormalities of
evaluation of, 715-720, 720t
immunizations in, 892t
infection with, *see website*
inheritance in development of, *see website*
parvovirus B19, 1095
screening for, 718t, 719
treatment of, 727-728
fetal development and differentiation of, *see website*
in Graves disease, 1909-1910
in HIV infection, 1161
interaction with other immune cells, *see website*
postnatal, *see website*
in systemic lupus erythematosus, 843
BCG. *See* Bacille Calmette-Guérin (BCG)
BCR-ABL gene, *see website*
cancer therapy specific to, *see website*
BDRD2 gene, 2016t
BEACOPP regimen for Hodgkin lymphoma, 1742, 1743t
Beals syndrome, *see website*
BEARS Sleep Screening Algorithm, 54t
Beau lines, 2295, 2295f
Becker disease, 2125t
Becker muscular dystrophy (BMD), 2119-2123
clinical manifestations of, 2113t, 2119-2120
diagnosis of, 2120-2121, 2121f
dilated cardiomyopathy with, 1630
genetic etiology and pathogenesis of, 2121-2122, 2122f
laboratory findings in, 2120
treatment of, 2123
Becker nevus, 2235, 2235f
Beckwith-Wiedemann syndrome, 522t, 523, 525-526, 527f
malignancy susceptibility associated with, *see website*
overgrowth in, *see website*
Beclomethasone
for allergic rhinitis, 778t-779t
for asthma, 795t
Beconase. *See* Beclomethasone
BED. *See* Binge eating disorder (BED)
Bedbug bite, 2318f
Bedding, sudden infant death syndrome and, 1425
Bed sharing, sudden infant death syndrome and, 1425
Bed-wetting, 71-73, 72t-73t
Beef tapeworm, 1232-1233, 1232t, *see website*
Bee pollen for asthma, 271t
Behavior
child health and, 2-3
Down syndrome and, 401
effects of malnutrition on, 175t
emerging patterns of from 1 to 5 years of age, 32t
health risk, in adolescents, 661f
high-risk pregnancies and, *see website*
lead poisoning effects on, 2450
sexual, 655
violent, in adolescent, 667-671, 667t-670t, 668f
Behavioral development
during first year of life, 28t
prenatal, *see website*
Behavioral disorders/issues. *See also* Psychiatric disorders
assessment and interviewing for, 56-60
in children born to teen mothers, 701
in chronic illness, *see website*
disruptive, 96-100, 97t
in childhood and adolescence, 99-100
in infancy and toddlerhood, 99
in obesity, 184t
office intervention for, 16
postoperative, *see website*
treatment of, 60-66
hospitalization in, 66
psychopharmacology, 60-65
psychotherapy in, 65-66
in type 1 diabetes mellitus, 1986
Behavioral insomnia of childhood
limit setting type, 48
sleep onset association type, 48
Behavioral observation audiometry (BOA), 2194
Behavioral screening and surveillance, 39-40, 41t-45t
Behavioral staring, *see website*
Behavioral states, newborn, *see website*
Behavioral syndrome, due to selective serotonin reuptake inhibitors, 625, 625f
Behavioral theories of development, *see website*
Behavioral therapy
for attention deficit/hyperactivity disorder, 110
based on behavioral theories, *see website*
Behavior rating scale, in attention deficit/ hyperactivity disorder, 110
Behçet disease, 853-854
cutaneous manifestations of, *see website*
oral ulceration in, 1260t
Behr optic atrophy, *see website*
Bejel, 1023, *see also website*
Belladona toxicity, 269t
Bell clapper deformity, 1861
Bell palsy, 2146-2147, 2146t, 2147f
Benadryl. *See* Diphenhydramine
Benazepril, 1645t
Benign angiitis of central nervous system (BACNS), 876
Benign congenital hypotonia, 2119
Benign generalized seizures, 2023
treatment of, 2028
Benign paroxysmal torticollis of infancy, 2060t, 2061, *see also website*
Benign recurrent intrahepatic cholestasis (BRCI), 1383-1384, 1383t
Benign sleep myoclonus, *see website*
Benzathine penicillin, 645t
for acute rheumatic fever prophylaxis, 924t
for diphtheria, *see website*
for group A streptococci infection, 918
for neonatal infection, 645t
for pharyngitis, 1439-1440
for sexually transmitted infections in adolescents, 712t
for tuberculosis, 1021t-1022t
Benzene, as inhalant, 681t
Benznidazole for trypanosomiasis, 1197
Benzocaine toxicity, 251t
Benzodiazepines
adverse effects of, 2031t
for anesthesia, *see website*
antidote for poisoning with, 256t-257t
for pain management, 370
pharmacokinetics of, *see website*
urine screening for adolescent use of, 676t
Benzoyl peroxide for acne, 2324, 2325t
Benzyl alcohol, 563t
Berardinelli-Seip congenital lipodystrophy type 1 (BSCL1), 2286
berardinelli-seip congenital lipodystrophy type 2 (BSCL2), 2286
Bereavement, 45, *see also website*
Bernard-Soulier syndrome, 1721
Best vitelliform degeneration, 2178
β-Adrenergic receptor blockers. *See* β-blockers
β-Adrenergic agonists
for allergic disease, 770-773
for asthma
long-acting, 791-792, 794-795
short-acting, 792t, 796, 797t-798t
for bronchopulmonary dysplasia, *see website*
for heart failure, *see website*
β-blockers
for arrhythmias, 1611t-1612t
for Graves disease, 1912
for heart failure, *see website*
for long Q-T syndromes, 1618
for Marfan syndrome, 2445
for migraine prophylaxis, 2045
pharmacokinetics of, *see website*
poisoning with, 251t, 261
antidote for, 256t-257t
for systemic hypertension, 1645t
β-cells
diabetes mellitus and
type 1, 1972-1974, 1973f
type 2, 1990
genetic defects of, 1993-1995
hyperplasia in hyperinsulinemia, 521-522
microadenoma in hyperinsulinemia, 521-522
β-Ketothiolase deficiency, 433-434, 434f
β-Thalassemia(s), 1674t, 1675-1676
Beta-lactams
hypersensitivity, 825-826
mechanism of resistance to, *see website*
Beta toxin, *see website*
Bethesda system, 1138t
Bevacizumab, *see website*
common medications implicated in, 257t
salicylates in formation of, 260
Bezold abscess, 2210-2211
BFU-MK. *See* Burst-forming unit-megakaryocytes (BFU-MK)
BH_4 deficiency, 446
hyperphenylalaninemia with, 420-421, 421f
bHLH. *See* "Basic helix-loop-helix" (bHLH) proteins
3β-HSD. *See* 3β-Hydroxy C_{27}-steroid dehydrogenase (3β-HSD) deficiency
Biaxin. *See* Clarithromycin
Bicarbonate (HCO_3^-)
in acid-base balance, 1808, *see website*
metabolic alkalosis and, 237
reference values for, *see website*
in respiratory acidosis, 238
Bicarbonate (HCO_3) buffer system, *see website*
Bicillin. *See* Penicillin G, benzathine
Bicornuate uterus, *see website*
Bicycle injuries, 22-23
Bidirectional Glenn shunt, 1581, 1581f
Biemond syndrome, 182t
Bier block, 372
Bifunctional enzyme defect, 466t
Big "d," 682
Bigeminy, 1612-1613
Bigender, 655
Biguanide, 1992t
Bile acid CoA ligase deficiency, 1385

Bile acids
  disorders of transport, secretion, conjugation, and biosynthesis of, 1383-1384, *see also website*
  liver effects of, 1389t
  malabsorption of, 1306t, 1312
    chronic diarrhea with, 1341
Bile acid synthetic defect (BASD), 1383t
Bile ducts, cystic dilatation of, *see website*
Bile flow, cholestasis and functional abnormalities of, 1381
Bile salt export pump (BSEP) deficiency, 1383t, 1384
Bilevel continuous positive airway pressure (BiPAP)
  at home, 332, 1524-1525
  for obstructive sleep apnea, 51
  for respiratory distress and respiratory failure, 320
Biliary atresia (BA), 1385-1387, 1386f-1387f
  jaundice due to, 607
  liver transplantation for, *see website*
Biliary cirrhosis
  in cystic fibrosis, 1485, 1496
  as manifestation of liver disease, 1374
Biliary dyskinesia, *see website*
Biliary system
  disease of
  (*See also* Liver disease)
    cystic, 1415, *see also website*
    due to cystic fibrosis, 1487
    embryogenesis disorders as, 1385
    evaluation of, 1379, 1380f
    malabsorption due to, 1318
  in drug absorption, *see website*
  morphogenesis of, 1374, *see also website*
Bilious vomiting in intestinal malrotation, 1280-1281
Bilirubin
  assessment in risk of jaundice, 605-606
  in congenital dyserythropoietic anemia, *see website*
  conjugated, 1375
    elevation of (*See* Cholestasis)
  δ fraction, 1375
  drug binding and, *see website*
  free, 1375
  in graft *versus* host disease, 761t
  indirect, 605-606
  inherited deficient conjugation of, 1389-1390
  in jaundice, 1374-1375
  neonatal metabolism of, 603-604, 604f
  normal neonatal values of, 605
  reference values for, *see website*
  unconjugated, 603-604
Bilirubin encephalopathy. *See* Kernicterus
Biltricide. *See* Praziquantel
Binary toxin, 994
BinaxNOW Malaria test, 1201-1202
Binax urinary test, *see website*
Binge eating disorder (BED), 90. *See also* Eating disorders
Binge-purge type anorexia nervosa, 90
Binocular vision, 2150
Bioavailability in drug therapy, *see website*
Biobehavioral therapy for migraine, 2045
Biochemical testing in liver disease, 1379-1381
Bioequivalence of drug, *see website*
Biofeedback for pain management, 371
Biologic agents
  adverse reactions to, 826-827
  for cancer, *see website*
  for juvenile idiopathic arthritis, 838t
Biologic development. *See* Physical development
Biologic disease-modifying antirheumatic drugs, *see website*
Biologic influences on development, *see website*
Biologic terrorism, 2454, *see also website*
Biomarkers in pharmacodynamics, *see website*
Biomicroscopy, 2150
Biophysical profile (BPP), 542, 543t
Biopsy
  in chronic diarrhea, 1344
  in fever of unknown origin, 902
  in giardiasis, 1182
  liver, 1381
    fetal, 543t
    in neonatal cholestasis, 1385-1386
  lung, *see website*
  muscle, 2111-2112
    in Duchenne and Becker muscular dystrophy, 2120, 2120f
    in myasthenia gravis, 2134
    in neuromuscular disorders, 2110t
  myocardial, in heart transplantation monitoring, *see website*
  of nerves, 2112
  rectal suction, in Hirschsprung disease, 1285-1286
  in renal transplantation, *see website*
  skin, *see website*
    fetal, 543t
    in urticarial vasculitis, 814
  small bowel, 1306
Biopsychosocial formulation in psychiatric diagnostic evaluation, 60
Biopsychosocial models
  of development, *see website*
  for eating disorder treatment, 94
Bioterrorism. *See* Terrorism
Biotin, 194t, 196
  defects in utilization of, 432-433
  dietary deficiency of, 433
  dietary reference intakes for, *see website*
  for holocarboxylase synthetase deficiency, 432
Biotinidase deficiency, 432-433
  secondary to pyruvate carboxylase deficiency, 506
Biotransformation, drug, *see website*
BiPAP. *See* Bilevel continuous positive airway pressure (BiPAP)
Biphasic anaphylaxis, 817
Bipolar disorder, 85-87, 85t
Birbeck granule, 1773-1774
Bird fancier or breeder lung, *see website*
Birth asphyxia, cerebral palsy with, 2063-2064
Birth defects, 629, *see also website*. *See also* Congenital anomalies
Birth history
  in neurologic evaluation, *see website*
  in wheezing, 1458
Birth injury
  brachial plexus palsy due to, 2383
  facial palsy as, 2147
  fractures as, 578-579
  of peripheral nerves, 573-574
  of spine and spinal cord, 573
  visceral, 578
Birthmarks, child abuse bruising *versus*, 137
Birthrates
  adolescent, 699, 699t, *see also website*
  preterm, *see website*
Birthweight
  high-risk infant and, 552-553, 553f
  low (*See* Low birthweight (LBW))
  very low (*See* Very low birthweight (VLBW))
Bisacodyl suppositories, 74t
Bisexuality, 658
Bismuth subsalicylate, *see website*
Bisoprolol, 1645t
Bitemporal aplasia cutis congenita, 2222
Bites
  due to abuse and neglect, 138
  animal and human, 2454-2460
    clinical manifestations of, 2455
    complications of, 2455, 2456t
    diagnosis of, 2455
    epidemiology of, 2454-2455, 2455t
    monkeypox due to, 2459-2460
    prevention of, 2457, 2457t-2458t
    rat bite fever due to, 2457-2459, 2458f
    treatment of, 2455-2457, 2456t
Bites *(Continued)*
  arthropod, 2317-2319, 2318f
  snake, 2461-2462, 2461f-2462f, 2461t-2462t
  spider, 2462-2463, 2463f
Bithionol, *see website*
Biting insect allergy, 807-809
Bitot spots, 189-190, 189f
BK virus, 1157, *see also website*
BL. *See* Burkitt lymphoma (BL)
Black-dot ringworm, 2310, 2310f
Blackfoot disease, *see website*
Black hairy tongue, 2299
Blackhead, 2322
"Black measles," 1072
Black pigmentation of nails, 2294-2295
Black spot poison ivy, 2251
Bladder
  congenital anomalies, 1847, *see also website*
  congenital intestinal pseudo-obstruction and, 1283
  control during preschool years, 33
  neurogenic, 1849-1850, 1849f
  neuropathic, 1847, *see also website*
    reflux with, 1835
  overactive, 1847-1849, 1849f
  pediatric unstable, 73
Bladder diverticulum, *see website*
Bladder exstrophy, 1847, *see also website*
Bladder neck obstruction, 1845
Bladder outlet obstruction, 1839t
Blalock-Taussig shunt, 1577
Blastocystis hominis, 1337t, *see also website*
Blastomyces adhesion-1 (BAD-1), 1064
Blastomyces dermatitidis, 1064-1065
  in pneumonia, 1475t
Blastomycosis, 1064-1065
Blastomycosis-like pyoderma, 2304, 2304f
Blastospores, 1053
Blau syndrome, 858-860
Bleeding. *See* Hemorrhage/bleeding
Bleeding disorders, 1699-1704
  sports participation and, 2402t-2404t
Bleeding time (BT)
  in hemostatic disorders, 1697
  reference values for, 1698t
Blenoxane. *See* Bleomycin
Bleomycin
  for cancer therapy, *see website*
  drug interactions with, *see website*
Blepharitis, 2164, 2167t
Blepharospasm, 2164
Blindness
  causes of, 2153t
  due to *Chlamydia trachomatis*, 1035
  night, 2154
    due to vitamin A deficiency, 189
  river, 1225, *see also website*
"Blistering agents," *see website*
Blistering cutaneous porphyria, *see website*
Blistering distal dactylitis, 2304, 2304f
Blister(s). *See also* Vesiculobullous disorders
  disorders of, 2241t
  fever, 901, 1099-1100
  in hand-foot-and-mouth disease, 1090f
  in porphyria cutanea tarda, *see website*
  sucking, 2218
BLL. *See* Blood lead level (BLL)
Block, heart
  atrioventricular, 1618-1619, 1618f
  bundle branch, electrocardiographic assessment of, 1540
  complete, 1618-1619, 1618f
    genetics of, *see website*
  electrocardiography of first degree, 1540
  familial secundum atrial septal defect with, *see website*
  fetal therapy for, 551t
  sinoatrial, 1618
Blocking therapy for internal radiation contamination, *see website*

Blood
fetal
scalp sampling of, 544
umbilical cord sampling, 544, 549, 617
multiple organ dysfunction syndrome and, 312t
shock-related dysfunction of, 307t
Blood-borne infections in child care setting, *see website*
Blood cholesterol screening, 479-480
Blood culture, *see also website*
in brucellosis, 981
in candidiasis, 1054
in fever of unknown origin, 902
in nontuberculous mycobacteria, 1015
in septic arthritis, 2399
in typhoid fever, 956-957
Blood disorders
anemia(s) as, 1648-1650, 1648t
acquired pure red blood cell, 1652-1653
of chronic disease, 1653, *see also website*
chronic hemolysis as, 1653
congenital dyserythropoietic, 1654, *see also website*
congenital hypoplastic anemia as, 1650-1651
Diamond-Blackfan anemia as, 1650-1651
differential diagnosis of, 1649-1650, 1649f-1650f
hemolytic (*See* Hemolytic anemia)
history and physical examination in, 1648-1649
iron-deficiency, 1655-1658, 1656t-1658t, 1657f
laboratory studies in, 1649
megaloblastic, 1655
microcytic, 1658, *see also website*
in newborn, 612-615
parvovirus B19 infection-associated red cell aplasia as, 1652-1653
Pearson's syndrome as, 1652
physiologic of infancy, 1654-1655
of renal disease, 1653, *see also website*
retinopathy due to, 2180
sideroblastic, 1658, *see also website*
transient erythroblastopenia of childhood as, 1652-1653, 1652t
blood transfusions for
of neutrophils (granulocytes), 1693, *see also website*
of plasma, 1693, *see also website*
of platelets, 1693, *see also website*
of red blood cells, 1692-1693, *see also website*
risks of, 1693, *see also website*
cardiac manifestations of, 1531t
with Down syndrome, 403t
fetal therapy for, 551t
general anesthesia and, *see website*
hematuria due to, 1795-1796
hemorrhagic and thrombotic
acquired inhibitors of coagulation in, 1712-1713
clinical and laboratory evaluation of, 1696-1699
clinical manifestations of, 1709-1710
complications of, 1711
diagnosis of, 1710, 1710f
disseminated intravascular coagulation as, 1713-1714, 1713t
epidemiology of, 1709-1711, 1709t
hemostasis and, 1693-1699
due to hereditary clotting factor deficiencies, 1699-1704
hereditary predisposition to, 1707-1708, 1708t
laboratory testing in, 1710
due to liver disease, 1712, *see also website*
platelet and blood vessel disorders as, 1714-1722
postnatal vitamin K deficiency as, 1712
Blood disorders *(Continued)*
treatment of, 1710-1712, 1710t
von Willebrand disease as, 1704-1707, 1705f
hemorrhagic stroke due to, 2084-2085, 2085t
HIV-related, 1166
liver disease due to, *see website*
lymphatic, 1724, *see also website*
in newborn
anemia as, 612-615, 613f, 613t-614t
hemolytic disease as, 615-619, 616t, 620t
hemorrhage as, 620-621, 621t
plethora as, 619-620
as oncologic emergency, *see website*
in palliative care, 158
pancytopenia as
acquired, 1691-1692, 1691t
inherited, 1684-1690, 1684t
polycythemia as, 1683, *see also website*
secondary, 1683, *see also website*
in premature infants, 559t
splenic, 1723, *see also website*
in systemic lupus erythematosus, 843t
Blood flow
cerebral perfusion pressure and, 297f
fetal, *see website*
hepatic, *see website*
in fetal circulation, *see website*
pulmonary, cyanotic congenital heart disease associated with, 1573-1596, *see also website*
splenic, *see website*
in transitional circulation, 1529, *see also website*
Blood gases, *see also website*
in acid-base disorders, 230
interpretation of, *see website*
normal values, 230t
Blood glucose monitoring, 1976-1977, 1983, 1983t
Blood group incompatibility
ABO, hemolytic disease of newborn due to, 619
Rh, in newborn, 615-619
Blood in stool, exclusion from day care due to, *see website*
Blood lead level (BLL), 2448-2451, 2451t-2452t
Blood lipids
atherogenesis and, 470-471, 471f
cardiovascular disease and, 470
Blood loss
fetal, 552
gastrointestinal, *see website*
iron deficiency-anemia due to, 1656
in traumatic injury, 336t
Blood manifestations
due to cat-scratch disease, 985
in mitochondrial encephalomyopathy, 2065t
Blood pressure (BP)
adolescent assessment of, 666
age-specific percentiles for, 1534f-1535f
ambulatory monitoring of, 1639-1640
in cardiac physical examination, 1533
in coarctation of the aorta, 1568
measurement of children, 1639-1640
monitoring in respiratory distress syndrome, 586
in newborn examination, 535, 535f
normal, 280t
in pediatric emergency assessment, 279
in primary hypertension, 1639-1640
Blood smear
in Chagas disease, 1196-1197
in congenital dyserythropoietic anemia, *see website*
in iron deficiency-anemia, 1657f
in malaria, 1201
Blood studies in febrile seizure, 2018, 2036
Blood supply
to capital femoral epiphysis, 2356
to kidney, *see website*
Blood transfusion(s)
for anemia in newborn, 613t, 614
for β-thalassemia, 1675
Blood transfusion(s) *(Continued)*
for erythroblastosis fetalis, 617-618
erythropoietin therapy in (*See* Blood transfusion(s))
exchange
for erythroblastosis fetalis, 618
for hyperbilirubinemia, 611f, 612, 612t
fetal, 549-552
for erythroblastosis fetalis, 617
HIV transmission through, 1159
iron overload due to, 1675
of neutrophils (granulocytes), 1693, *see also website*
of plasma, 1693, *see also website*
of platelets, 1693, *see also website*
of red blood cells, 1692-1693, *see also website*
risks of, 1693, *see also website*
Blood urea nitrogen (BUN)
in dehydration, 246
in plasma osmolality, *see website*
reference values for, *see website*
Blood vessel disorders, 1638-1639, 1722
Bloody diarrhea, *Shigella* in, 959
Bloody discharge from nipple, *see website*
Bloom syndrome, 2258
malignancy susceptibility associated with, *see website*
Blotters, 682
Blount disease, 2350, 2436t
obesity with, 184t
Blown pupil, 2155-2156
Blow-out orbital fracture, 2186
Blue cell tumor, 1754, 1761
Blue diaper syndrome, 1319
Blue nevus, 2234
Blue rubber bleb nevus, 2230
"Blue spells" in tetralogy of Fallot, 1574
BMD. *See* Becker muscular dystrophy (BMD)
BMI. *See* Body mass index (BMI)
BN. *See* Bulimia nervosa (BN)
BNP. *See* Brain natriuretic peptide (BNP); B-type natriuretic peptide (BNP)
BO. *See* Bronchiolitis obliterans (BO)
BOA. *See* Behavioral observation audiometry (BOA)
Bobbing, ocular, 2162t
Bochdalek hernia, 594-596, 595f-596f
Bockhart impetigo, 2305
Body fluids, 212, *see also website*
Body image, eating disorders and, 93t
Body louse, 986
Body mass index (BMI), 180f-181f
for age percentiles, *see website*
in nutrition assessment, 172
in obesity, 179, 184-185, *see also website*
Body proportions, *see website*
Body surface area (BSA)
drug dosages based on, *see website*
estimation for burn injury, 351-352, 352f
Body temperature. *See* Temperature
Body weight. *See* Weight
Bodywork therapies, 273
Boerhaave syndrome, *see website*
Bohn nodules, 1260
Bolivian hemorrhagic fever, 1151-1152
Bolus feedings for premature infant, 560
Bonding. *See* Attachment
Bone(s)
anatomic locations of, *see website*
cystic fibrosis and, 1494
dysplasias of (*See* Skeletal dysplasias)
effects of malnutrition on, 175t
glucocorticoid effect on, *see website*
growth and development of, 2331, *see also website*
hormones and peptides of metabolism of, 1916
long, *see website*
maturation of, *see website*
orthopedic problems of (*See* Orthopedic problems)

Bone(s) *(Continued)*
structure, growth, and hormonal regulation of, 2446, *see also website*
in congenital hypothyroidism, 1899-1900, 1900f
typhoid fever and, 957t
Bone disease. *See also* Orthopedic problems
adynamic, in chronic kidney disease, 1825
due to bacillary angiomatosis, 986
dysplasias as (*See* Skeletal dysplasias)
malignant tumors as, 1763-1766, 1763t, 1764f
Ewing sarcoma as, 1765-1766, 1765f
incidence and survival rates for, 1726t
osteosarcoma as, 1763-1764, 1764f
risk factors for, 1727t
secondary, due to radiation therapy, *see website*
work-up of, 1731t
metabolic
hyperphosphatemia as, 2446, *see also website*
hypophosphatemia as, 2446, *see also website*
in newborn, 623
osteoporosis as, 2446-2447, 2447t
primary chondrodystrophy (metaphyseal dysplasia) as, 2446, *see also website*
in progeria, *see website*
Bone infection, 2394-2398
Aspergillus in, 1061
nontuberculous mycobacterial, 1013
Staphylococcus aureus, 905
tuberculous, 1006
Bone marrow. *See also* Pancytopenia
cellular, 1684
failure of, 1690, 1690t
(*See also* Pancytopenia)
in acute myeloid leukemia, 1737
hypocellular, 1684
infiltration, 1684
neutropenia in disorders of, 749
Bone marrow culture in brucellosis, 981
Bone marrow transplantation. *See* Hematopoietic stem cell transplantation (HSCT)
Bone resorption, disorders of, 2432-2433
Bone widows, 300f
Bony labyrinth disease, 2213, *see also website*
BOOP. *See* Bronchiolitis obliterans organizing pneumonia (BOOP)
Booster seat, 22
Borderline lepromatous leprosy, *see website*
Borderline leprosy, *see website*
Bordetella parapertussis, 944-948
Bordetella pertussis, 944-948
Bornholm disease, 1090
Borrelia, 1025, *see also website*
Borrelia burgdorferi, 1025-1029
maternal, *see website*
Bosentan for pulmonary hypertension, 1602t
Botanical medicine, nutritional aspects of, 169
Bothria, 1233
Botryoid rhabdomyosarcoma, 1760
Bottle, Mead Johnson, 1253
Bottle-feeding of premature infant, 560-562
Botulinum toxin, 987-988
for achalasia, 1265
for spasticity of cerebral palsy, 2064-2065
Botulism, 987-991
clinical manifestations of, 988-989, 989f
complications of, 990-991, 991t
diagnosis of, 989-990, 989t
differential diagnosis of, 989-990, 990t
epidemiology of, 987-988
etiology of, 987
immune globulin for, 882t
pathogenesis of, 988
prevention of, 991
prognosis for, 991
supportive care for, 990
in terrorism, *see website*
treatment of, 990
Botulism antitoxin, 258t, 882-883
Botulism immune globulin (BIG), 990
Boutonneuse fever, 1039t-1040t
Bowel control during preschool years, 33
Bowel resection
for Crohn disease, 1303-1304
short bowel syndrome due to, 1314
Bowing, tibial
anterolateral, 2351
anteromedial, 2351
posteromedial, 2351
Bowleg, 2348-2350, 2348t-2349t
Bowman's space, *see website*
Boys
first sign of puberty in, 649
growth curves for, *see website*
percentile growth curves for, *see website*
BP. *See* Blood pressure (BP); Bullous pemphigoid (BP)
BPD. *See* Bronchopulmonary dysplasia (BPD)
BPP. *See* Biophysical profile (BPP)
Brachial plexus
birth injury to, 573-574, 574f, 2383
sports injury to, 2420
Brachial plexus block for pain management, 371-372
Brachycephaly, *see website*
Brachydactyly, *see website*
Bracing
for Scheuermann disease, 2372
for scoliosis, 2367, 2368f
Bradyarrhythmias, emergency management of, 287, 288f
Bradycardia
in cardiac physical examination, 1531-1532
fetal, 542
during fever, *see website*
neonatal, 580t
sinus, 1610-1612
Bradypnea in pediatric emergency assessment, 280-281
Brain. *See also* Neurologic *entries*
herniation of, 297
prenatal development of, *see website*
reading systems in, 113, 113f
Brain abscess, 2098-2099, 2099f
due to anaerobes, *see website*
cerebrospinal fluid findings in, 2088t
imaging studies in, *see website*
with tetralogy of Fallot, 1576
Brain death, 304, *see also website*
after neonatal hypoxic-ischemic encephalopathy, 572-573
Brain hemorrhage, due to hypernatremia, 214
Brain injury
in newborn, 568-569, 568f
traumatic, 297-301, 298f-301f
due to abuse, 301
attention deficit/hyperactivity disorder following, 108
due to child abuse, 139-140, 139f, 301
mild, 301
sports-related, 2418-2419, 2419t
due to football, *see website*
in trauma survey, 337, 337f
Brain lesion, precocious puberty due to, 1889-1890, 1889f-1890f
Brain malformations
muscle development and, 2118
neonatal seizures due to, 2034
Brain natriuretic peptide (BNP), 1469
Brainstem
congenital anomalies of, 2006-2007
multiple sclerosis effects on, 2077t
respiratory distress due to lesion of, 315t
tumors of, 1753, 1753f
Brainstem auditory-evoked responses (BAERs), 2192, *see also website*
Brain stem glioma, 1748t
Brainstem reflexes, brain death and, *see website*
Brain tumor(s), 1746-1753
astrocytoma as, 1748-1750, 1749f
ataxia with, 2055
Brain tumor(s) *(Continued)*
of brainstem, 1753, 1753f
choroid plexus, 1750-1751
clinical manifestations of, 1747
complications and long-term management of, 1753
craniopharyngioma as, 1752
diagnosis of, 1747-1748
embryonal, 1751-1752, 1751f
ependymal, 1750, 1750f
epidemiology of, 1746
etiology of, 1746, 1747t
germ cell, 1752-1753
incidence and survival rates for, 1726t
metastatic, 1753
pathogenesis of, 1746-1747, 1747f-1748f, 1748t
pineal parenchymal, 1752
precocious puberty due to, 1889-1890, 1889f-1890f
risk factors for, 1727t
secondary, due to radiation therapy, *see website*
work-up of, 1731t
Branched-chain ketonuria, 528
Branchial cleft cysts and sinuses, 2221
Branching enzyme deficiency, 497
BRAT diet, 1136
Brazilian blastomycosis, 1068, *see also website*
BRCA1 gene defect, *see website*
BRCA2 gene defect, *see website*
"Breakthrough varicella," 1105-1106
Breast
development of, 651f, 685, *see also website*
abnormal, *see website*
in central precocious puberty, 1887
examination of
in adolescent, 666, *see also website*
newborn, 536
infections of, *see website*
masses in, *see website*
mastalgia of, *see website*
nipple discharge from, *see website*
self examination of, *see website*
surgical alterations to, *see website*
trauma and inflammation of, *see website*
Breast bud, *see website*
Breast cancer, *see website*
male, 1947
Breast-feeding, 160
benefits of, 161t
collection of breast milk, 162
complementary feeding and, 164-165
contraindications to, 161t
drugs and, 539t-540t, 540
engorgement and, 160
exclusive, for gastroenteritis prevention, 1338
growth of infant and, 162
HIV transmission through, 1159
inadequate milk intake, 161
jaundice and, 162, 607, 607f
mastitis during, 160
medical contraindications to, 540, 540t
milk leakage in, 160
of newborn, 539-540, 539t
nipple pain due to, 160
otitis media and, 2200
patterns of milk supply and, 160, 162t
of premature infant, 560-562
steps to encourage, 161t
sudden infant death syndrome and, 1425
ten steps to successful, 539t
type 1 diabetes mellitus and, 1972
Breath, first, 580
Breath-holding spells, 99, *see also website*
Breath hydrogen test, 1306
Breathing
in newborn assessment, 535
in pediatric emergency assessment, 279-281
rescue, 282-283, 282f

Breathing *(Continued)*
sleep-disordered, 49
in cystic fibrosis, 1494
in trauma survey, 336, 336t
work of, *see website*
Breathing movements, fetal, 543t
Breathing patterns in newborn, 580
Breathlessness in asthma, 784t
Breath sounds in newborn, 535
Breech deformation sequence, *see website*
Brethine for asthma, 797t-798t
Bright Futures Guidelines for Health Supervision of Infants, Children, and Adolescents, 14, 15f
Brill-Zinsser disease, 1039t-1040t, 1047-1048
Bristol Stool Form Score, 1848, 1849f
British antilewisite (BAL), 2453, 2453t, *see also website*
Brittle diabetes, 1985-1986
Brodie abscess, 2395
Brody disease, 2125t
Bromhidrosis, 2288
Bromide
adverse effects of, 2031t
dosages of, 2030t
Bromocriptine, *see website*
Brompheniramine, 777t-778t
Bronchi
foreign body in, 1453f, 1454
neoplasms of, *see website*
Bronchial adenoma, 1504
Bronchial carcinoid, 1504
Bronchial obstruction in tuberculosis, 998, 1000f, 1002
Bronchial provocation testing in allergic disease, 768
Bronchiectasis, 1479, *see also website*
in asthma, 785
in cystic fibrosis, 1485
Bronchiolectasis in cystic fibrosis, 1485
Bronchiolitis, 1456-1459
in cystic fibrosis, 1485
parainfluenza virus, 1125t
respiratory syncytial virus, 1127-1129
treatment of, 1459
wheezing with, 1458-1459
Bronchiolitis obliterans (BO), 1463, *see also website*
in cystic fibrosis, 1485
in heart-lung or lung transplantation rejection, *see website*
Bronchiolitis obliterans organizing pneumonia (BOOP), *see website*
Bronchitis, 1459-1460
follicular, 1463
Bronchoalveolar lavage (BAL), *see also website*
in aspiration syndromes, 1472t
for cystic fibrosis, 1493
Bronchobiliary fistula, 1467
Bronchodilators
for bronchiolitis, 1459
for cystic fibrosis, 1493
Bronchogenic cyst, 1466, 1466f
Bronchomalacia, 1452, 1455, 1524, *see also website*
Bronchoprovocation challenge, 784
Bronchopulmonary aspergillosis, allergic
Aspergillus in, 1059
immunoglobulin E levels in, 766
Bronchopulmonary dysplasia (BPD), 1516, *see also website*
general anesthesia and, *see website*
due to mechanical ventilation for respiratory distress syndrome, 585, 587-590, 588f, 589t
Bronchoscopic aspiration for atelectasis, *see website*
Bronchoscopy, *see website*
Bronchospasm
exercise-induced, 784
during induction of anesthesia, *see website*
Bronze baby syndrome, 611
Broviac catheter, infection with, *see website*
Brown oculocutaneous albinism, 2238
Brown-Séquard syndrome, 2105
Brown syndrome, 2160-2161, 2160f
Brucella, 980-982, 981t
in infective endocarditis, 1624t
Brucella abortus, 1324t-1325t
Brucella melitensis, 1324t-1325t
Brucella suis, 1324t-1325t
Brudzinski sign, 2090
Brugada syndrome, *see website*
Brugia malayi, 1224-1225, *see also website*
Brugia timori, 1224-1225, *see also website*
Bruising, due to child abuse, 137-138, 137f
Bruits, cranial, *see website*
Brushfield spots, *see website*
Bruton agammaglobulinemia, 723-724
Bruton tyrosine kinase (Btk), 723, 724f
Bruxism, 75
BSAP, infant botulism and, 989
BSCL1. *See* Berardinelli-Seip congenital lipodystrophy type 1 (BSCL1)
BSCL2. *See* Berardinelli-Seip congenital lipodystrophy type 2 (BSCL2)
BSEP. *See* Bile salt export pump (BSEP) deficiency
BSID-II. *See* Bayley Scales of Infant Development (BSID-II)
B symptoms in Hodgkin lymphoma, 1741
BT. *See* Bleeding time (BT)
β-thalassemia, 1675-1676, 1675f
Btk gene. *See* Bruton tyrosine kinase (Btk)
B-type natriuretic peptide (BNP), *see website*
Bubonic plague, 973
Buckle fracture, 2390, 2391f
Budd-Chiari syndrome, *see website*
Budesonide
for allergic rhinitis, 778t-779t, 779-780
for asthma, 794t-795t
Buffers, *see website*
Bulbar involvement in Guillain-Barré syndrome, 2143-2144
Bulbar palsies, due to botulism, 988, 989f
Bulbar poliomyelitis, 1083-1084, 1086
Bulimia nervosa (BN), 90, 90t. *See also* Eating disorders
eating and weight control habits in, 92t
in female athlete, 2422
symptoms commonly reported in, 93t
Bulk, muscle, assessment in neurologic examination, *see website*
Bullae
examination of, *see website*
of Stevens-Johnson syndrome, 2243f
Bullous congenital ichthyosiform erythroderma, 2270, 2270f
Bullous dermatosis of childhood, 2249, 2249f
Bullous emphysema, 1462, 1462f
Bullous impetigo, 2299-2300
group A streptococci in, 917
Bullous myringitis, 2199
Bullous pemphigoid (BP), 2248
immunofluorescence of, *see website*
Bullying, 100, 135, 669t, *see also website*
Bumetanide
for acute renal failure, 1820
for heart failure, *see website*
BUN. *See* Blood urea nitrogen (BUN)
Bundle branch block, 1540
Bunion, 2341, 2341f
Buprenorphine, 367t
Bupropion
for attention deficit/hyperactivity disorder, 111t
for depression and anxiety symptoms, 63t
poisoning with, 265
for weight loss in adults, 187t
Buried penis, 1856
Burkholderia cepacia, 975, *see also website*
in cystic fibrosis infections, 1482, 1492t
Burkholderia mallei, *see website*
Burkholderia pseudomallei, *see website*
Burkitt lymphoma (BL), 1743, 1744t
Epstein-Barr virus-associated, 1111, 1112t
of small intestine, 1314-1315
Burner, 2402t-2404t, 2420, *see website*
Burn(s), 349-357
body surface area estimation for, 351-352, 352f
due to child abuse, 137f-138f, 138
as childhood injury, 23-24
classification of, 351, 351f, 351t
complement system dysfunction in, 756
death due to, 18
electrical, 356, 357t
emergency care for, 350-351, 350f, 350t
encephalopathy associated with, 2068
epidemiology of, 349
first aid measures for, 350
fluid resuscitation for, 352-353
general anesthesia and, *see website*
hemolytic anemia secondary to, *see website*
indications for hospitalization for, 349-350, 349t
infections of
herpes simplex virus, 1103
prevention of, 353-354, 353t
Pseudomonas aeruginosa in, 975-976
inhalation injury with, 354-355
long-term outcomes for, 355-356, 356t
nutritional support for, 354
ocular, 2185-2186
oral ulceration due to, 1260t
outpatient management of, 352, 352f, 352t
pain relief for, 355
prevention of, 349, 349t
psychologic adjustment to, 355
reconstruction and rehabilitation for, 355
school reentry after, 355-356
surgical management of, 353-354
topical therapy for, 354
Burst-forming unit-megakaryocytes (BFU-MK), *see website*
Buruli ulcer disease, 1012-1013, 1015
BuSpar. *See* Buspirone
Buspirone, 63t
Butane, as inhalant, 681t
1,4-Butanediol, adolescent abuse of, 675t
Butorphanol, 367t
Butyl nitrate, as inhalant, 681t
γ-Butyrolactone, adolescent abuse of, 675t
Byler disease, 1383, 1383t
Bypass strategies for neurodevelopmental dysfunction, *see website*

C
C1, *see website*
deficiency of, 753, 754t, *see also website*
C1 inhibitor, *see website*
deficiency of, 755
in hereditary angioedema, 815-816
C1q, *see website*
C1q deficiency, 753, 754t
partial, 755
in systemic lupus erythematosus, 841
C2, *see website*
C2 deficiency, 753-754, 754t
in systemic lupus erythematosus, 841
C3, *see also website*
in acute poststreptococcal glomerulonephritis, 1784
in membranoproliferative glomerulonephritis, 1787
C3b, *see website*
C3 deficiency, 753-754, 754t
C4, 1426-1427, *see also website*
C4 deficiency, 753-754, 754t
in systemic lupus erythematosus, 841
C5, *see website*
C5b, *see website*
C5 deficiency, 754, 754t
C6 deficiency, 754, 754t
C7 deficiency, 754, 754t

C8 deficiency, 753-754, 754t
C9, *see website*
C9 deficiency, 754t
CA-125, 1872t
Cachexia treatment in palliative care, 157t
CACT. *See* Carnitine acylcarnitine translocase (CACT) deficiency
Cadmium, gastroenteritis due to, 1328t-1329t
Café-au-lait spots, 2237, 2237f, 2237t
  in neurofibromatosis, 2046-2047, 2047f
Caffeine, for neonatal apnea, 581
Caffey disease, 2436-2437, 2436f
CAH. *See* Congenital adrenal hyperplasia (CAH)
Calabar swellings, 1225-1226, 1226f
Calcaneal apophysitis, 2418
Calcaneal stress fracture, 2418
Calcaneovalgus feet, 2336
Calciferol, dietary reference intakes for, *see website*
Calcification
  adrenal, 1943, *see also website*
  in juvenile dermatomyositis, 847, 848f, 849
  of teeth, 1249-1250, 1250t
Calcineurin inhibitors, 2217
  in renal transplantation, *see website*
  topical, for atopic dermatitis, 804-805
Calcitonin, *see website*
Calcitriol
  for hypoparathyroidism, 1919
  for renal osteodystrophy, 1824-1825
Calcium, *see also website*
  conversion factors for, *see website*
  glucocorticoid effect on, *see website*
  in hyperparathyroidism, 1921
  in hypoparathyroidism, 1918-1919
  malabsorption of, 1321
  parathyroid gland in homeostasis of, 1916
  reference values for, *see website*
  renal tubular regulation of, *see website*
  rickets due to deficiency of, 201t-202t, 206, *see also website*
  in vegetarian diet, 168
Calcium channel blockers (CCBs)
  pharmacokinetics of, *see website*
  poisoning with, 251t, 261-262
    antidote for, 256t-257t
  for pulmonary hypertension, 1602t
  for systemic hypertension, 1645t
Calcium channelopathies, 2125t
Calcium chloride for pediatric resuscitation and arrhythmias, 294t
Calcium disodium for poisoning, 256t-257t
Calcium gluconate for hypoparathyroidism, 1919
Calcium oxalate calculi, *see website*
Calcium phosphate calculi, *see website*
Calcium salts
  as poisoning antidote, 256t-258t
  possible adverse reactions to in premature infant, 563t
Calcium stones, *see website*
Calcofluor white stain, *see website*
Calculi
  gallbladder, *see website*
  urinary, 1864, *see also website*
    abdominal pain of, 1248t
    as complication of enterocystoplasty, *see website*
Calicivirus, 1134-1137, 1326t
California encephalitis, 1142-1143
Caloric intake
  in bronchopulmonary dysplasia, *see website*
  in burn injury, 354
  in chronic kidney disease, 1824
  for eating disorder treatment, 95
  with "fast food" meal, 182
  growth and, *see website*
  for obese child, 186, 186t
  in type 1 diabetes mellitus, 1981-1982, 1982t
Caloric testing in neurologic examination, *see website*
Calprotectin concentration in chronic diarrhea, 1344t
Campath-1H. *See* Alemtuzumab
CAMP factor, 925
Camphor toxicity, 251t
Campomelic syndrome, 1963, 2431, 2432f
Camptodactyly, 2385, 2385t, *see website*
Campylobacter, 968-970
  clinical manifestations of, 969-970
  complications of, 970
  diagnosis of, 970
  epidemiology of, 968-969
  etiology of, 968, 968t
  gastroenteritis due to, 1324t-1325t
    treatment of, 1337t
  inflammatory bowel disease *versus*, 1298t
  neonatal, 632t
  pathogenesis of, 969
  prevention of, 970
  prognosis for, 970
  in traveler's diarrhea, 1338t
  treatment of, 970
CAMT. *See* Congenital amegakaryocytic thrombocytopenia (CAMT)
Canadian C-spine rule, 337-338, 338f
Canadian immunization schedule, 895
Canakinumab, *see website*
Canal, atrioventricular, 1554-1556
  in adults, 1607
Canavan disease, 455-456, 456f
Cancer. *See* Malignancy
Cancer antigen-125, 1872t
Candesartan for systemic hypertension, 1645t
Candida, 1053-1056
  chronic mucocutaneous, 1056
  in diaper dermatitis, 1055, 1866, 2250, 2314, 2314f
  after hematopoietic stem cell transplantation, 762
  in HIV infection, 1055
  in immunocompromised patients, 1055-1056, 1056t
  maternal, *see website*
  mucocutaneous, 1056, *see website*
  neonatal, 1053-1054, 1054t
    sepsis due to, 635t
  oral, 1054-1055, 1259-1260
    HIV-related, 1164
  oropharyngeal, 1259-1260
  predisposition to infection due to immunodeficiency, 716t
  in septic arthritis, 2398
  in skin infections, 2313-2314
  in ungual and periungual infections, 1055
  in vulvovaginitis, 1055
Candida skin test, 720
Candidosis
  interiginous, 2314, 2314f
  perianal, 2314
  vaginal, 2313-2314
Canine scabies, 2320
Canker sore, 1260, 1260t, 2298
Cannabinoids
  for neuropathic pain, 368t
  urine screening for adolescent use of, 676t
Cao_2. *See* Arterial oxygen content (Cao_2)
Cao gio, 137-138
Cap, cervical, 694
Capillariasis, *see website*
Capillaries, renal, *see website*
Capillary hemangioma, eyelid, 2164-2165, 2164f
Capillary hydrostatic pressure, pulmonary edema and, 1468
Capillary malformations, 2224, 2225f
Capillary wedge pressure, 311t
Capnocytophaga canimorsus, *see website*
Capnography, 318
Capreomycin, *see also website*
  for tuberculosis, 1008t
Capsular polysaccharide
  group B streptococci, 926
  Neisseria meningitidis, 932
Captopril
  for heart failure, *see website*
  for systemic hypertension, 1645t
Caput succedaneum, 565
Carbamates poisoning, 266-267
Carbamazepine
  adverse effects of, 2031t
  drug interactions with, *see website*
  for pain management, 369-370
  for seizures
    dosages of, 2030t
Carbamyl phosphate synthetase (CPS) deficiency, 448f, 449-451
Carbapenems, *see also website*
  adverse reactions to, 826
Carbenicillin, *see also website*
  for cystic fibrosis lung infection, 1492t
Carbohydrates
  adequate macronutrient distribution range for, *see website*
  dietary reference intakes for, *see website*
  digestion of, *see website*
  malabsorption of, 1305t, 1306-1307, 1315-1317
    chronic diarrhea with, 1341
  metabolism of
    defects of (*See* Carbohydrate metabolism, defects of)
    hepatic, *see website*
  in oral rehydration solutions, 1335t
  type 1 diabetes mellitus and intake of, 1981, 1982t
Carbohydrate-deficient glycoprotein syndrome, 1311
Carbohydrate loading for acute intermittent porphyrias, *see website*
Carbohydrate metabolism, defects of, 492-509, 493f, 494t-495t
  of fructose, 503
  of galactose, 502-503
  glycogen storage diseases as, 492-501
    Fanconi-Bickel syndrome as, 499, 1318
    glycogen synthetase deficiency as, 498
    mimicking hypertrophic cardiomyopathy, 500
    type I, 492-496
    type II, 499-500, 500f
    type III, 496-497, 496f
    type IV, 497
    type IX, 497-498
    type V, 500-501
    type VI, 497
    type VII, 501
  of glycoprotein, 509, *see also website*
  with lactic acidosis, 503-509, 504f-505f, 507t-509t, 508f
  liver effects of, 1389t
  malabsorption due to, 1318
  of pentose, 509, *see also website*
Carbon dioxide (CO_2)
  in acid-base balance, *see website*
  lack of responsiveness to in bronchopulmonary dysplasia, 1521
  partial pressure of, *see website*
    in asthma, 784t
    in brain death, *see website*
    normal values of, 230t
    reference values for, *see website*
    in respiratory acidosis, 238-239
    in respiratory failure, 316
Carbon monoxide (CO)
  diffusing capacity for, *see website*
  poisoning with, 269-270
    antidote for, 256t-257t
  reference values for, *see website*
Carbon tetrachloride poisoning, 267
Carboplatin and cisplatin for cancer therapy, *see website*
Carboxylase deficiencies, 432-433
Carbuncle, 2305-2306
Carcinogenesis, radiation, *see website*

Carcinogens, environmental, *see website*
Carcinoid
 bronchial, 1504
 cardiac manifestations of, 1531t
Carcinoid tumor, *see website*
Carcinoma
 adenoid cystic, 1504
 basal cell, *see website*
 bronchogenic, *see website*
 choroid plexus, 1750-1751
 colorectal, 1773, *see also website*
 hepatocellular, 1772
  in type II glycogen storage disease, 496
 medullary, diarrhea caused by, *see website*
 mucoepidermoid, 1504, *see also website*
 nevoid basal cell, 1747t, *see website*
 ovarian, 1871-1872, 1872t
 pancreatic, *see website*
 renal cell, 1760
 thyroid, 1914-1916
  medullary, 1915-1916
Card agglutination trypanosomiasis test (CATT), 1192
Cardiac arrest
 emergency management of, 289-292, 291f-293f, 294t
 potentially treatable conditions associated with, 289t
Cardiac arrhythmias
 AV block as, 1618-1619, 1618f
 due to cancer and its therapy, *see website*
 Corynebacterium diphtheriae-associated toxic cardiomyopathy with, *see website*
 emergency management of, 287-289, 288f, 290f
  medications for, 294t
 extrasystoles as, 1610-1613
 genetics of heritable, *see website*
 long Q-T syndrome as, 1616-1618, 1617t
 with Marfan syndrome, 2441
 due to metabolic alkalosis, 237
 due to poisonings, 255t
 sinus, 1610-1613, 1612f-1613f
 sinus node dysfunction as, 1618, 1618f
 sports participation and, 2402t-2404t
 sudden death due to, 1620-1621, 1620f-1621f
 supraventricular tachycardia as, 1613-1616, 1614f-1616f
 therapy for, 1610, 1611t-1612t
 ventricular tachyarrhythmias, 1616, 1616t
Cardiac asystole, 1521
Cardiac catheterization, 1546-1549, 1547f-1548f
 in atrioventricular defect, 1555
 diagnostic, 1547
 interventional, 1548-1549
 for pulmonary valve stenosis, 1563
Cardiac compressions in cardiopulmonary resuscitation, 291, 291f-292f
Cardiac cycle, 1536f
Cardiac death, *see website*
Cardiac differentiation, 1528, *see also website*
Cardiac examination, 1533-1536, 1536f
Cardiac function, developmental changes in, 1528, *see also website*
Cardiac glycoside-containing plants, toxicity with, 269t
Cardiac looping, 1527, *see also website*
Cardiac morphogenesis, 1527, *see also website*
Cardiac output (CO)
 heart failure and, *see website*
 medications to maintain, 294t
 neonatal, *see website*
 in shock, 311t
 thermodilution measurement of, 1547-1548
 total fetal, *see website*
Cardiac pacing
 for AV heart block, 1619
 for supraventricular tachycardia, 1614-1615
Cardiac septation, 1527
Cardiac syncope, *see website*
Cardiac tamponade
 cardiac arrest due to, 289t
 as life-threatening injury, 336t
Cardiac teratogenic effects, 1527
Cardiac valves, disease of, 1626-1628
Cardiogenic shock, 285, 307t, 1638, *see also website*
 defined, 305
 hemodynamic variables in, 311t
 pathophysiology of, 305-306
 treatment of, 312-313
Cardiomegaly in infants of diabetic mothers, 628
Cardiomyopathy
 arrhythmogenic right ventricular, 1633-1634
 in Becker muscular dystrophy, 2119
 due to cancer and its therapy, *see website*
 Chagas disease-related, 1196
 in chronic kidney disease, 1823t
 dilated, 1629f, 1630-1631
  genetics of, *see website*
  sudden death due to, 1620
 in Duchenne muscular dystrophy, 2119
 endocardial fibroelastosis as, 1633-1634
 evaluation of, 1550
 fetal development of, *see website*
 hypertrophic, 1631-1632, 1632f
  genetics of, *see website*
  glycogen storage diseases mimicking, 500
  sports participation and, 2402t-2404t
  sudden death due to, 1619-1620
 in plasma membrane carnitine transport defect, 460
 restrictive, 1633, 1633f
 sudden death due to, 1619-1620
 toxic, due to diphtheria, *see website*
 X-linked, 433
Cardiopulmonary resuscitation (CPR), 289-292, 291f-293f, 294t
 care following, 296
  medications in, 294t
 for drowning, 344-345
  hypothermic, 346
 equipment for office emergencies, *see website*
 infection protection and control in, *see website*
 medications for, 294t
 withholding of, *see website*
Cardiothoracic ratio, 1537
Cardiovascular disease
 blood lipids and, 470-471, 471f
 due to cancer and its therapy, *see website*
 cardiac arrhythmias as
  AV block as, 1618-1619, 1618f
  extrasystoles as, 1610-1613
  long Q-T syndrome as, 1616-1618, 1617t
  sinus, 1610-1613, 1612f-1613f
  sinus node dysfunction as, 1618, 1618f
  supraventricular tachycardia as, 1613-1616, 1614f-1616f
  therapy for, 1610, 1611t-1612t
  ventricular tachyarrhythmias, 1616, 1616f, 1616t
 cardiogenic shock for, 1638, *see also website*
 congenital (*See* Congenital heart disease (CHD))
 evaluation of, 1529-1536
  cardiac catheterization in, 1546-1549, 1547f
  cardiac examination in, 1533-1536, 1536f
  computed tomography in, 1545-1546, 1547f
  echocardiographic, 1541-1545, 1542f-1544f
  electrocardiographic, 1537, 1538f-1541f
  exercise testing in, 1545
  general physical examination in, 1530-1533, 1532t, 1534f-1535f
  history in, 1530, 1530t-1532t
  magnetic resonance angiography in, 1545-1546, 1545f-1546f
  magnetic resonance imaging in, 1545-1546
  radiologic, 1537, 1537f
  radionuclide studies in, 1545-1546
 failure to thrive in, 148t
 general anesthesia and, *see website*
Cardiovascular disease *(Continued)*
 heart failure due to, 1638, *see also website*
 HIV-related, 1165
 infective endocarditis as, 1622-1626, 1622t-1626t
 liver disease with, *see website*
 mucopolysaccharidoses and, 515t
 myocardial, 1628-1635, 1630t
  arrhythmogenic right ventricular cardiomyopathy as, 1633-1634
  dilated cardiomyopathy as, 1629f, 1630-1631
  endocardial fibroelastosis as, 1633-1634
  etiology of, 1629t
  hypertrophic cardiomyopathy as, 1631-1632, 1632f
  left ventricular noncompaction as, 1633-1634, 1634f
  myocarditis as, 1634-1635, 1634t
  restrictive cardiomyopathy as, 1633, 1633f
 with obesity, 184t
 pericardial, 1635-1637, 1636t, 1637f
 of peripheral vascular system
  arteriovenous fistula as, 1638, *see also website*
  Kawasaki disease as, 1638, *see also website*
  primary hypertension as, 1639-1647
 phosphorylase kinase deficiency as, 498
 in premature infants, 559t
 psychopharmacology and, 65
 renal transplantation and, *see website*
 respiratory distress and, 315-316, 315t
 respiratory signs and symptoms of, *see website*
 rheumatic, 1626-1628
 sports participation and, 2402t-2404t
 sudden death due to, 1619-1621, 1620f-1621f
 transplantation for, 1638, *see also website*
 tuberculous, 1004
 tumors of heart as, 1637, *see also website*
 with Turner syndrome, 1952-1953
Cardiovascular manifestations, 1532t
 in eating disorders, 91-92, 93t
 in food adverse reactions, 820-821
 in Kawasaki disease, 864
 in Lyme disease, 1027, 1028t
 in lysosomal storage disorders, 485t
 in malnutrition, 175t
 in Marfan syndrome, 2440-2441
 in mitochondrial encephalomyopathy, 2065t
 in poisoning, 252t
 in systemic inflammatory response syndrome, 309t
 in systemic lupus erythematosus, 843t
 in tuberous sclerosis, 2050, 2050f
 in typhoid fever, 957t
Cardiovascular medication poisoning, 261-263
Cardiovascular system
 development of, 1527
 inhalation anesthetic effects on, *see website*
 management of in drowning, 345
 newborn assessment of, 535, 535f
 preanesthetic assessment of, *see website*
 shock-related dysfunction of, 307t
 transition from fetal to neonatal circulation in, 1529, *see also website*
Cardioversion, synchronized, 288-289
Carditis
 in acute rheumatic fever, 922
 enlarged, sports participation and, 2402t-2404t
Care. *See* Health care; Medical care
Care planning, advanced, in palliative care, 151-159
Care settings for palliative care, 151
Caries, dental, 1254-1256, 1255f-1256f
Carmustine, *see website*
Carney complex, 1939-1940
Carnitine acylcarnitine translocase (CACT) deficiency, 457t, 461
Carnitine cycle, 458
 defects in, 460-461

Carnitine deficiency
 cardiac manifestations of, 1531t
 myopathies with, *see website*
Carnitine palmitoyltransferase (CPT) deficiency, *see website*
Carnitine palmitoyltransferase -IA (CPT-IA) deficiency, 461
Carnitine palmitoyl transferase-I (CPT-I) deficiency, 457t
Carnitine palmitoyltransferase-II (CPT-II) deficiency, 457t, 461
Carnitine transporter deficiency, 457t
Caroli disease and syndrome, *see website*
Carotid bodies in respiration regulation, *see website*
Carpal bones, centers of ossification appearance in, 29t
Carpenter syndrome
 congenital heart disease with, 1531t
 craniosynostosis in, 2012t, 2013
 obesity due to, 182t
Carrier detection in immunodeficiencies, *see website*
Carrión disease, 982
Carrot allergy, 821, 821t
Car seats, 21-22, 21f, 21t
Cartilage hair hypoplasia (CHH), 733-734, 748t, 1690, 2434
Cartilage matrix proteins, skeletal dysplasias of, 2424-2427
 spondyloepiphyseal, 2424-2425, 2424f
Carvedilol
 for heart failure, *see website*
 for systemic hypertension, 1645t
Caspofungin, *see also website*
 for candidiasis, 1054t, 1056t
Casting, serial, for clubfoot, 2337
Castleman disease, 1724, *see also website*
 HIV-related, *see website*
 multicentric, 1121
Cast syndrome, 1287
Catabolic losses in diabetes mellitus, 1980
Catalase, *Staphylococcus aureus* production of, 904
Catalase-positive organism, 745
Cat allergens, 769
Catamenial pneumothorax, 1509
Cataplexy, 53
Cataracts, 2169-2172, 2170f-2172f, 2170t
 due to congenital rubella syndrome, 1077-1078, 1077f
 with Down syndrome, 403t
 due to hypoparathyroidism, 1918
 with myotonic muscular dystrophy, 2124
 due to radiation exposure, *see website*
 due to total body irradiation, *see website*
Catarrhal stage of pertussis, 945
Cat bite, 2454-2460
CATCH 22 syndrome, 728-729
 congenital heart disease with, 1531t, 1576
 genetics of, *see website*
Catch-up immunization schedule, 889, 890f
Catecholamines, 1923-1924, *see also website*
 in neuroendocrine tumor-associated diarrhea, *see website*
 in pheochromocytoma, 1942
Cat eye syndrome, 1531t
Cat flea typhus, 1039t-1040t
Cathepsin C gene, 2273
Catheter ablation for supraventricular tachycardia, 1614-1615
Catheter angiography, *see website*
Catheter infection
 Candida, 1055
 due to coagulase-negative staphylococci, 910
 nontuberculous mycobacterial, 1012t, 1013
Catheter-related bloodstream infection (CRBSI), *see website*
Catheters/catheterization
 cardiac, 1546-1549, 1547f-1548f
  in atrioventricular defect, 1555
  for pulmonary valve stenosis, 1563
 central venous
  fever without a focus in, 896t
  infection with, due to coagulase-negative staphylococci, 910
 peritoneal dialysis, infection associated with, *see website*
 umbilical artery
  in respiratory distress syndrome, 586
  risks associated with, 587
 urethral, infection associated with, *see website*
Cations in total body water, *see website*
Cat roundworm, 1227-1229
Cat-scratch disease (CSD), 983, 983t, 984f-985f
 ocular, 2168
CATT. *See* Card agglutination trypanosomiasis test (CATT)
Caudal anesthesia, 373
Caudal regression syndrome, 1356
Caustics ingestion and/or poisoning, 266, 1272-1273, 1272t-1273t
CAVE, 2336-2337
Cavus feet, 2340, 2340f
CBF. *See* Cerebral blood flow (CBF)
CBG. *See* Corticosteroid-binding globulin deficiency (CBG)
CBL. *See* Cobalamin (CBL)
CBS. *See* Cystathionine β-synthase (CBS) deficiency
CBT. *See* Cognitive-behavioral therapy (CBT)
CCAM. *See* Congenital cystic adenomatoid malformation (CCAM)
CCBs. *See* Calcium channel blockers (CCBs)
CCDD. *See* Congenital cranial nerve dysinnervation disorders (CCDD)
CCHS. *See* Congenital central hypoventilation syndrome (CCHS)
CCK. *See* Cholecystokinin (CCK)
CCR5 gene, 1159-1161
CCS. *See* Chronic compartment syndrome (CCS)
CCSK. *See* Clear cell sarcoma of kidney (CCSK)
CD2, development and differentiation of, *see website*
CD3
 deficiencies of, 729, 733
 development and differentiation of, *see website*
 flow cytometry testing of, 720-722
CD4
 in amyloidosis, 860-861
 development and differentiation of, *see website*
 flow cytometry testing of, 720-722
 in HIV/AIDS, 1157-1161
 interaction with other immune cells, *see website*
CD4CD25, *see website*
CD7, development and differentiation of, *see website*
CD8
 development and differentiation of, *see website*
 in Epstein-Barr virus, 1111
 flow cytometry testing of, 720-722
 interaction with other immune cells, *see website*
CD8 lymphocytopenia, 730
CD10, development and differentiation of, *see website*
CD19, development and differentiation of, *see website*
CD22, development and differentiation of, *see website*
CD23, development and differentiation of, *see website*
CD34, development and differentiation of, *see website*
CD40
 development and differentiation of, *see website*
 interaction with other immune cells, *see website*
 mutations in, 727
CD40 ligand, mutations in, 726
CD45
 deficiency of, 733
 interaction with other immune cells, *see website*
CD54, interaction with other immune cells, *see website*
CD58, interaction with other immune cells, *see website*
CD73, development and differentiation of, *see website*
CD154, interaction with other immune cells, *see website*
CDA. *See* Congenital dyserythropoietic anemia (CDA)
CD classification, *see website*
CDGs. *See* Congenital disorders of glycosylation (CDGs)
CDH. *See* Congenital diaphragmatic hernia (CDH)
CDI. *See Clostridium difficile* infection (CDI)
C_{DYN}. see dynamic compliance (C_{DYN}) assessment in mechanical ventilation
Ceclor. *See* Cefaclor
Cefaclor, *see website*
Cefadroxil, *see website*
Cefalexin for osteomyelitis, 2397-2398
Cefazolin, *see also website*
 for infective endocarditis, 1625t
 for infective endocarditis prophylaxis, 1626t
 for neonatal infection, 645t
 for septic arthritis, 2400
 for *Staphylococcus aureus*, 907t
Cefdinir, *see also website*
 for otitis media, 2207t, 2208
Cefepime, *see also website*
 for cystic fibrosis lung infection, 1492t
 for neonatal infection, 645t
Cefixime, *see also website*
 for gonococcal disease, 938-939
 for pyelonephritis, 1832
 for *Salmonella* gastroenteritis, 953t
 for sexually transmitted infections in adolescents, 712t
 for *Shigella* infection, 961
 for typhoid fever, 958t
Cefizox. *See* Ceftiaoxime
Cefobid. *See* Cefoperazone sodium
Cefoperazone sodium, *see website*
Cefotan. *See* Cefotetan
Cefotaxime, *see also website*
 for bacterial meningitis, 2091, 2093t
 for gonococcal conjunctivitis, 2166-2167
 for meningococcal disease, 933t
 for neonatal infection, 645t
 for osteomyelitis, 2397
 for pneumococcal meningitis, 913
 for pyelonephritis, 1832
 for *Salmonella* gastroenteritis, 953t
 for septic arthritis, 2400
Cefotetan, *see also website*
 for gonococcal disease, 939
Cefoxitin, *see also website*
 for gonococcal disease, 939
 for nontuberculous mycobacteria, *see website*
Cefpodoxime
 for gonococcal disease, 938-939
 for otitis media, 2207t
Cefpodoxime proxetil, *see website*
Cefprozil, *see website*
Ceftazidime, *see also website*
 for bacterial meningitis, 2093t
 for cystic fibrosis lung infection, 1492t
 for neonatal infection, 645t
 Pseudomonas aeruginosa, *see website*
Ceftin. *See* Cefuroxime
Ceftizoxime, 938-939, *see also website*
Ceftriaxone, *see also website*
 for bacterial meningitis, 2091
 for chancroid, *see website*
 for gonococcal conjunctivitis, 2166-2167

Ceftriaxone *(Continued)*
for gonococcal disease, 938-939
for infectious diarrhea, 1337t
for infective endocarditis, 1625t
for infective endocarditis prophylaxis, 1626t
for Lyme disease, 1028t
for meningococcal disease, 933t
for *Neisseria meningitidis* prophylaxis, 934t
for neonatal infection, 645t
for otitis media, 2207t, 2208
for pyelonephritis, 1832
for *Salmonella* gastroenteritis, 953t
for sexually transmitted infections in adolescents, 712t
for *Shigella* infection, 961
for typhoid fever, 958t
Ceftriaxone for bacterial meningitis, 2093t
Cefuroxime, *see also website*
for Lyme disease, 1028t
for otitis media, 2207t, 2208
for vulvovaginitis, 1868t
Cefzil. *See* Cefprozil
"C-E" grip, 284, 284f
CEHD. *See* Congenital enterocyte heparin deficiency (CEHD)
Celecoxib
for pain management, 364t
for rheumatic disease, *see website*
Celexa. *See* Citalopram
Celiac disease, 1306f, 1308-1311, 1308f, 1309t-1310t, 1310f
with Down syndrome, 403t
sports participation and, 2402t-2404t
type 1 diabetes mellitus with, 1996
Celiac plexus nerve block, 372
Cell-mediated immunity
in HIV infection, 1161
in tuberculosis, 1000-1001
Cellular immunodeficiencies, 728-730, 728t
autoimmune polyendocrinopathy-candidiasis ectodermal dysplasia as, 730
CD8 lymphocytopenia as, 730
defective cytokine production as, 729
defective expression of T-cell receptor-CD3 complex as, 729, 729f
infection with, *see website*
treatment of, 736-737, 737t
Cellular marrow, 1684
Cellulitis, 2300-2301
of auricle and external auditory canal, 2198
Haemophilus influenzae in, 942
orbital, 2167t, 2183-2184, 2183t, 2184f
due to sinusitis, 1438
peritonsillar, 1440, 1442
preseptal, 2183
Center-edge angle, 2358
Centers of ossification, 29t, *see also website*
Central auditory processing disorders, 2188
Central chemoreceptors in respiration regulation, *see website*
Central cord syndrome, 2103
Central core myopathy, 2113t, 2115t, 2117-2118
Central diabetes insipidus, 1883
hypernatremia due to, 213, 213t
Central giant cell granuloma of jaw, *see website*
Central hearing loss, 2188
Central nervous system (CNS). *See also* Neurologic *entries*
glucocorticoid effect on, *see website*
inhalant abuse and, 681t
lead poisoning effects on, 2450-2451
mushroom poisoning effects on, *see website*
in Neonatal Intensive Care Unit Neurobehavioral Scale, 624t
of premature infants, 559t
prenatal development of, *see website*
respiration regulation by, *see website*
Central nervous system (CNS) disorders, 565
angiitis as, 876
associated with otitis media, 2211-2212
Central nervous system (CNS) disorders *(Continued)*
brain tumor(s) as, 1746-1753
astrocytoma as, 1748-1750, 1749f
ataxia with, 2055
of brainstem, 1753, 1753f
choroid plexus, 1750-1751
clinical manifestations of, 1747
complications and long-term management of, 1753
craniopharyngioma as, 1752
diagnosis of, 1747-1748
embryonal, 1751-1752, 1751f
ependymal, 1750, 1750f
epidemiology of, 1746
etiology of, 1746, 1747t
germ cell, 1752-1753
incidence and survival rates for, 1726t
metastatic, 1753
pathogenesis of, 1746-1747, 1747f-1748f, 1748t
pineal parenchymal, 1752
precocious puberty due to, 1889-1890, 1889f-1890f
risk factors for, 1727t
secondary, due to radiation therapy, *see website*
congenital anomalies as, 1998-2013
agenesis of corpus callosum as, 2005-2006, 2005f
agenesis of cranial nerves, 2006-2007
anencephaly as, 2003
craniosynostosis as, 2011-2013, 2012t
disorders of neuronal migration as, 2003-2005, 2003f-2004f
dysgenesis of posterior fossa, 2006-2007
encephalocele as, 2002-2003
holoprosencephaly as, 2005-2006, 2006f
hydrocephalus as, 2008-2011, 2008t, 2009f-2011f
meningocele as, 1999
microcephaly as, 2007-2008, 2007t
muscle development and, 2118
myelomeningocele as, 2000-2002, 2001f
neural tube defects as, 1998-1999, 1999f
spina bifida occulta as, 1999, 2000f, 2001t
cranial, 565-566, 565f
demyelinating, 2076-2080, 2076t
acute disseminated encephalomyelitis as, 2079, 2079f, 2080t
multiple sclerosis as, 2076, 2077t, 2078f
neuromyelitis optica as, 2077
HIV-related, 1164-1165
hypoxic-ischemic encephalopathy as, 298f-299f, 301-303, 302f, 569-573, 570t
infection as, 2086-2098
anaerobic, *see website*
Aspergillus in, 1061
bacterial meningitis as, 2087-2095
Blastomyces dermatitidis, 1064
eosinophilic meningitis as, 2097-2098
Listeria monocytogenes, *see website*
neonatal seizures due to, 2034
Pseudomonas aeruginosa, 976t
Rocky Mountain spotted fever, 1042
Staphylococcus aureus, 905
stroke-like events *versus*, 2085
tuberculous, 1005-1006
viral meningoencephalitis as, 2095-2097
intracranial hemorrhage as, 566-568, 567f, 568t
pulmonary manifestations of, *see website*
respiratory acidosis due to, 239, 241t
respiratory distress due to, 315t, 316
of spine and spinal cord
due to birth, 573
Central nervous system (CNS) manifestations
in candidiasis, 1054
in childhood cancers, 1728, 1730f
Central nervous system (CNS) manifestations *(Continued)*
in eating disorders, 92
in hemolytic-uremic syndrome, 1793
in HIV infection, 1162
in mitochondrial encephalomyopathy, 2065t
in pertussis, 947
in poisoning, 252t
in poliovirus, 1082
in toxoplasmosis, 1212-1213, 1212f
in typhoid fever, 957t
Central nervous system (CNS) therapy for acute lymphocytic leukemia, 1735
Central pontine myelinolysis (CPM), 218
Central venous catheter (CVC)
fever without a focus in, 896t
infection with, *see website*
due to coagulase-negative staphylococci, 910
Central venous pressure in shock, 311t
Centromere antibody in rheumatic disease, *see website*
Centronuclear myopathy, 2113-2114
CEP. *See* Congenital erythropoietic porphyria (CEP)
Cephalexin, *see also website*
for cystic fibrosis lung infection, 1492t
for *Staphylococcus aureus*, 907-908
for vulvovaginitis, 1868t
Cephalic tetanus, 992
Cephalic vein, venous access in, 292, 295f
Cephalohematoma, 565, 565f
Cephalometric radiograph, *see website*
Cephalosporins, *see also website*
adverse reactions to, 826, *see also website*
classification of, *see website*
for group A streptococci infection, 918
for pyelonephritis, 1832
for sexually transmitted infections in adolescents, 712t
third-generation for neonatal infection, 644
Cephalostat, *see website*
Cephalothin for neonatal infection, 645t
Cephaloxin for impetigo, 2300
Cephamycins, *see website*
Cephradine, *see website*
Ceptaz. *See* Ceftazidime
CeraLyte, 1335t
Cereal-based oral rehydration, 1334
Cerebellar astrocytoma, 1748t
Cerebellar ataxia, 2054
gait of, *see website*
varicella-zoster virus in, 1109
Cerebellar hypoplasia, 2118
Cerebellar pathways, multiple sclerosis effects on, 2077t
Cerebellar vermis agenesis, 2054
Cerebellum
congenital anomalies of, 2006-2007
coordination assessment in disorders of, *see website*
multiple sclerosis effects on, 2077t
Cerebral aneurysm
hemorrhagic stroke due to, 2084-2085
imaging studies in, *see website*
Cerebral blood flow (CBF), cerebral perfusion pressure and, 297f
Cerebral edema
with fulminant hepatic failure, 1414
due to type 1 diabetes mellitus, 1981
Cerebral gigantism, *see website*
Cerebral herniation, 297, 299-300
Cerebral malaria, 1206
Cerebral necrosis, due to radiation therapy, *see website*
Cerebral palsy (CP), 2061-2065
clinical manifestations of, 2062-2064, 2062t, 2063f
diagnosis of, 2064
epidemiology and etiology of, 2061-2062
intellectual disability *versus*, 126
as movement disorder, 2059-2060

Cerebral palsy (CP) *(Continued)*
neuropathic bladder in, *see website*
sports participation and, 2402t-2404t
treatment of, 2064-2065, 2064f
Cerebral perfusion pressure (CPP), 296
cerebral blood flow and, 297f
Cerebral salt wasting, 1884t
hyponatremia due to decreased, 1885-1886
Cerebral sinovenous thrombosis (CSVT), 1709, 2082-2084, 2083f, 2083t
Cerebral thrombosis, with tetralogy of Fallot, 1576
Cerebrohepatorenal syndrome (CHRS), 1382-1383, 2069
Cerebrospinal fluid (CSF)
hydrocephalus and, 2008-2011
increased volume of, 297
latex agglutination testing on, *see website*
Cerebrospinal fluid (CSF) examination, *see also website*
in bacterial meningitis, 2088t, 2090
in brain abscess, 2098-2099
in central nervous system infections, 2088t
in coccidioidomycosis, 1066
in *Cryptococcus neoformans*, 1057-1058
in enteroviral meningitis, 1091
in meningococcal meningitis, 932
in neurologic evaluation, *see website*
in poliovirus infection, 1084
in tuberculosis, 1006
Cerebrospinal fluid (CSF) shunts
infections associated with, *see website*
coagulase-negative staphylococci, 910
Cerebrotendinous xanthomatosis, 478-479, 1312
Cerebrum, multiple sclerosis effects on, 2077t
Ceroid lipofuscinosis, infantile, 484t
Certification of pediatricians, 12
Cerubidine. *See* Daunorubicin
Cerumen, *see website*
Cervical cap, 694
Cervical culture in gonococcal disease, 938
Cervical lymphadenopathy
Corynebacterium diphtheriae, *see website*
as sign of childhood cancers, 1730f
Cervical spine
anomalies and instabilities of, 2380-2382, 2381t, 2382f
in Down syndrome, 2381-2382
sports participation and, 2402t-2404t
juvenile idiopathic arthritis involvement in, 832, 834f
in trauma survey, 335
traumatic injury to, 337-338, 338f
in drowning victim, 344
Cervicitis, 708, 708f
abnormal uterine bleeding due to, 689t-690t
Cervicofacial actinomycosis, *see website*
Cervix
anomalies of, *see website*
maternal testing of, 543t
neoplasm of, 1873-1874, 1873t
abnormal uterine bleeding due to, 689t-690t
human papillomavirus and, 1139-1140, 1729
maternal, *see website*
Cesarean section, *see also website*
maternal HIV infection and, 1159
CESD. *See* Cholesterol ester storage disease (CESD)
Cestodes, 1232-1234, 1232t
Cetirizine
for allergic rhinitis, 777-779, 777t-778t
for anaphylaxis, 818t
for urticaria and angioedema, 815t
CETP. *See* Cholesteryl ester transfer protein (CETP) deficiency
Cetuximab, *see website*
CFB gene, 1792t
CFEOM. *See* Congenital fibrosis of extraocular muscles (CFEOM)
CF1 gene, 1792t
CFH gene, 1792t
CFHr1/3 gene, 1792t
C fibers in abdominal pain, 1247-1248
CFRD. *See* Cystic fibrosis-related diabetes (CFRD)
CFS. *See* Chronic fatigue syndrome (CFS)
CFTR. *See* Cystic fibrosis transmembrane conductance regular protein (CFTR)
CFU-MK. *See* Colony-forming unit-megakaryocytes (CFU-MK)
CGD. *See* Chronic granulomatous disease (CGD)
CGH. *See* Comparative genomic hybridization (CGH)
CGM. *See* Continuous glucose monitoring (CGM)
CGMS. *See* Continuous glucose monitoring system (CGMS)
CH_{50}. *See* Total hemolytic complement activity (CH_{50})
Chadwick's sign, 700
Chagas disease, 1193-1198, 1193f-1194f, 1195t, *see also website*
Chagoma, 1194f, 1195-1196
Chamomile, German, 271t
CHAMP, 1471
Chanarin-Dorfman syndrome, 2272
Chancre, 1016, 1191
Chancroid, 708, 709t, 944, *see also website*
Changes disease, *see website*
Channelopathies, 2125t
in long and short Q-T syndrome, 1617t
strokelike events *versus*, 2086
sudden infant death syndrome and, 1423t, 1426
CHAOS. *See* Critical high airway obstruction syndrome (CHAOS)
Chaotic atrial tachycardia, 1615
Charcoal, activated, 257t
for poisoning, 257
Charcot-Marie-Tooth (CMT) disease, 2138-2139, 2138t
CHARGE association, 729, 1262, 1430
congenital heart disease with, 1531t
Char syndrome, *see website*
Chédiak-Higashi syndrome (CHS), 425, 742t, 744-745, 748t, 751, 2238t, 2239
Cheilitis, 1261, 2297, 2297f
angular, 2297, 2297f
candidal, 1055
due to riboflavin deficiency, 193, 193f
candidal, 1055
Chelation therapy
for arsenic and mercury intoxication, *see website*
for internal radiation contamination, *see website*
for Wilson disease, 1392
Chemet. *See* Dimercaptosuccinic acid (DMSA)
Chemical burn
of eye, 2185-2186
oral ulceration due to, 1260t
Chemical conjunctivitis, 2168
Chemical dependence, 677
Chemical pleurodesis for pneumothorax, 1511-1512
Chemical pollutants, 2448, *see also website*
Chemical terrorism, 2454, *see also website*
Chemoprophylaxis
acute rheumatic fever, 924t
group B streptococcus, 927-928
during pregnancy, 927-928
influenza virus, 1125
malarial, 1207, 1207t, *see also website*
Chemoreceptors in respiration regulation, *see website*
Chemotaxis, 741
Chemotherapy, *see also website*
breast-feeding and, 161t
as cancer risk factor, 1727t
common agents used in, *see website*
for Hodgkin lymphoma, 1741-1742, 1743t
hypersensitivity to agents used in, 826
hypogonadism due to, 1945
Chemotherapy *(Continued)*
infections associated with, *see website*
malabsorption due to, 1314
neutropenia associated with, 1055
for osteosarcoma, 1764
toxic effects of, *see website*
vomiting with, therapy for, 1244t
Cherry red spot, 2178
in Tay-Sachs disease, 485, 2069, 2072f
Chest
computed tomography and magnetic resonance imaging of, *see website*
examination of
in allergic disease, 765
in newborn, 535
funnel, 1516-1517, 1516f
life-threatening injuries to, 336, 336t
rickets and, 201t
transillumination of, *see website*
Chest compressions in cardiopulmonary resuscitation, 291, 291f-292f
Chester porphyria, *see website*
Chest pain
differential diagnosis of, 1530t
history of, 1530
as manifestation of extrapulmonary disease, 1526, *see also website*
in rheumatic disease, *see website*
Chest radiography
in aspiration syndromes, 1472-1473, 1472t, 1473f
in cardiac assessment, 1537
in coccidioidomycosis, 1067, 1067f
in congenital diaphragmatic hernia, 594-595, 595f
in pneumonia, 1477, 1477f-1478f
in pulmonary abscess, 1480, 1480f-1481f
in pulmonary edema, 1469, 1469t
in respiratory disease diagnosis, *see website*
in tetralogy of Fallot, 1574-1575, 1575f
in total anomalous pulmonary venous return, 1589, 1590f
in tuberculosis, 999f-1000f
in ventricular septal defect, 1557, 1557f
Chest tube for emergencies, 295
Chest wall, *see website*
Cheyne-Stokes respirations, *see website*
CHH. *See* Cartilage hair hypoplasia (CHH)
Chiari malformations, 2006, 2009, 2009f
myelomeningocele in, 2001-2002
syringomyelia in, 2103-2104, 2104f
Chickenpox. *See* Varicella-zoster virus (VZV)
Chief complaint in neurologic evaluation, *see website*
Chigger bite, 2320
scrub typhus due to, 1045
Chilblains, 358, 2285
Child abuse. *See* Abuse and neglect
Child care, 45, *see also website*
communicable disease and, 895
giardiasis, 1181
eating in setting of, 165
facilities for, 895
Childhood disintegrative disorder, 106, *see also website*
Child Protective Services (CPS), 141
Child-rearing practices, 2-3
Children's Oncology Group (COG), *see also website*
on Wilms tumor treatment, 1759
Children's Yale-Brown Obsessive-Compulsive Scale (C-YBOCS), 80
Child restraint in motor vehicles, 21, 21f, 21t
CHILD syndrome, 1531t, 2234-2235, 2268t, 2272, 2272f
CHIME syndrome, 2268t
Chinese herbal medications for atopic dermatitis, 805
Chinese liver fluke, *see website*
Chin trembling, *see website*
Chiropractic treatment, 273

CHL. *See* Conductive hearing loss (CHL)
Chlamydia trachomatis, 1035-1038
adolescent, 706f, 712t
in conjunctivitis, 1037, 2166
fetal therapy for, 551t
genital culture of, *see website*
genital tract infections due to, 1035-1036
gonococcal disease with, 938-939
lymphogranuloma venereum due to, 1038
maternal, *see website*
in pneumonia, 1037, 1475t
prophylaxis following rape, 704, 704t
sexual abuse and, 145t
trachoma due to, 1035
in vulvovaginitis, 1865
Chlamydophila pneumoniae, 1033-1035, 1034f
pneumonia due to, 1475t
Chlamydophila psittaci, 1038, *see also website*
pneumonia due to, 1475t
Chlamydospores, 1053
Chlazaion, 2164
Chloramphenicol, *see also website*
for *Bartonella* infection, 983
for cystic fibrosis lung infection, 1492t
for louse-borne typhus, 1048
for meningococcal disease, 933t
for murine typhus, 1047
for neonatal infection, 645t
possible adverse reactions to in premature infant, 563t
for scrub typhus, 1045
for typhoid fever, 957, 958t
Chloride
dietary reference intakes for, *see website*
metabolic alkalosis and, 235-237, 235t
in oral rehydration solutions, 1335t
reference values for, *see website*
in total body water, *see website*
Chloride channelopathies, 2125t
Chloride diarrhea, 1306t, 1320-1321, 1341
Chloride-losing diarrhea, congenital, 223
Chlorinated hydrocarbon exposure, *see website*
Chlorine, in terrorism, *see website*
Chloroma in acute myeloid leukemia, 1737
Chloromycetin. *See* Chloramphenicol
Chloroquine
malaria resistant to, travel and, 1207t, *see also website*
for malaria treatment and chemoprophylaxis, 1202, 1203t-1205t, 1207, 1207t, *see also website*
for porphyria cutanea tarda, *see website*
toxicity of, 251t
Chlorosis, 1219
Chlorothiazide for heart failure, *see website*
Chlorothiazide for systemic hypertension, 1645t
Chlorpheniramine for allergic rhinitis, 777t-778t
Chlorpromazine
for chemotherapy-associated vomiting, 1244t
for pain management, 364t
toxicity of, 251t
Chlorpropamide, 1992t
Chlorthalidone for systemic hypertension, 1645t
Chlor-Trimeton. *See* Chlorpheniramine
Choanal atresia, 575, 1430, 1430f, *see also website*
Cholangiocytes, fetal development of, *see website*
Cholangiography
in liver dysfunction, 1379
magnetic resonance, in sclerosing cholangitis, *see website*
Cholangiopancreatography, endoscopic retrograde, 1379
Cholangitis
liver disease with, 1378
sclerosing, with inflammatory bowel disease, *see website*
Cholecystitis, *see website*
Cholecystokinin (CCK), *see website*
Choledochal cyst, *see also website*
abdominal pain of, 1247t
Cholelithiasis, *see also website*
abdominal pain of, 1247t
Cholera, 965-968
clinical manifestations of, 966, 967f
complications of, 967
diagnosis and differential diagnosis of, 967
epidemiology of, 965, 966f
etiology of, 965
laboratory findings in, 966
pathogenesis of, 966
prevention of, 967-968
travel and, *see website*
treatment of, 967, 967t
Cholera gravis, 966
Cholera toxin, 1330, 1331f
Cholera vaccine, 967-968, 968t
travel and, *see website*
Cholestasis
differential diagnosis of, 1377t
as manifestation of liver disease, 1374
maternal, *see website*
neonatal, 1381-1388, 1381f
evaluation of, 1382, 1382t
intrahepatic, 452, 1382-1384, 1383t-1384t
management of, 1387-1388, 1387t
mechanism of, 1381-1382
prognosis for, 1388
types of, 1382t
in older child, 1388
with total parenteral nutrition, *see website*
in viral hepatitis, 1395
Cholesteatoma
as complication of otitis media, 2211, 2211f
congenital, 2211, 2212f, *see also website*
Cholesterol
dietary reference intakes for, *see website*
disorders of intracellular metabolism of, 478-479
adrenocortical insufficiency due to, 1926
high-density lipoproteins and reverse transport of, 473
laboratory testing of
in obesity, 185t
for screening, 479-480
low, conditions associated with, 477-478, 478t
in steroid biosynthesis, 1923, *see also website*
Cholesterol ester storage disease (CESD), 479, 491
Cholesterol gallstones, *see website*
Cholesterol granuloma of tympanic membrane, 2212
Cholesteryl ester transfer protein (CETP) deficiency, 477
Choline, dietary reference intakes for, *see website*
Choline magnesium salicylate for pain management, 364t
Cholinergic poison syndrome, 253t
Cholinergic syndromes, 676t
Cholinergic urticaria, 812-813
Cholinesterase-inhibiting insecticides, poisoning with, 266-267
Cholinesterase inhibitors, 2134-2135
Chondritis, 2198
Chondrodysplasia, Jansen-type metaphyseal, 1923
Chondrodysplasia punctata (CPD), 2272
Chondrodystrophy, primary, 2446, *see also website*
Chondroectodermal dysplasia, 2433-2434
Chondrolysis in slipped capital femoral epiphysis, 2365
Chondromalacia, tracheal, 1455
Chondromalacia patella, 2354
Chordee
with hypospadias, 1852
without hypospadias, 1854, 1854f
Chorea, 2056t-2058t, 2058
in acute rheumatic fever, 922, 924
obsessive compulsive disorder and, 919
Sydenham, 2055-2056
Chorea-acanthocytosis, 2057t
Chorea gravidarum, 2056
Choreoathetoid cerebral palsy, 2063-2064
Choreoathetosis, 2056
Chorioamnionitis, 551t, 630, 630f
Chorioangioma, 552
Chorioepithelioma, 1957
Chorionic gonadotropin, human
in brain tumors, 1747-1748
in germ cell tumors, 1770
of central nervous system, 1752-1753
in ovarian carcinomas, 1872t
Chorionic villus sampling, 543t
Chorioretinitis, 2172-2174, 2173t
candidiasis, 1057
Toxoplasmosis gondii, 1210, 1210f, 1213-1215
Choroid
gyrate atrophy of, 453
in tuberculosis, 1004
Choroiditis, 2173, 2173f
Choroid plexus
fetal cysts, ultrasound of, 550t
tumor, 1750-1751
Chotzen syndrome, 2013
Christmas factor, 1696t
Christmas tree pattern, 2262
CHRNA4 gene, 2016t
CHRNB2 gene, 2016t
Chromium, *see website*
Chromones for allergic disease, 771-772
Chromosomal disorders, 381
in acute lymphocytic leukemia, 1732-1733, 1733t
in acute myeloid leukemia, 1738t
cataracts due to, 2171
chromosome instability syndromes as, 412
dysmorphology due to, *see website*
fragile chromosome sites as, 411-412, 411t
mosaicism as, 412
of numbers, 399-403
aneuploidy and polyploidy as, 399-400, 400t
Down syndrome as, 400-403
trisomy 13 as, 405f
trisomy 18 as, 405f
severe intellectual disability in, 123t
sex chromosome aneuploidy as, 408-410, 409t
Klinefelter syndrome as, 410
Noonan syndrome as, 410, 410t
Turner syndrome as, 409-410
47,XYY as, 410
of structure, 404-408
deletions and duplications as, 406-407, 406t, 407f, 408t-409t
insertions as, 407
inversions as, 405-406
isochromosomes as, 407
marker and ring chromosomes as, 408
translocations as, 404-405, 406f
uniparental disomy and imprinting as, 412-414, 413f-414f
Chromosomal translocation, 404-405, 406f
in Down syndrome, 402-403
in listeriosis, *see website*
in proto-oncogene activation, *see website*
Chromosome(s)
analysis of, 394-399, 395f-400f, 397t
marker, 408
mitochondrial, *see website*
ring, 408
study of (*See* Cytogenetics)
Chromosome paints, 396
Chromosome 11p deletion, *see website*
Chromosome 13q deletion, *see website*
Chromosome 22q11.2 deletion, 2382
Chronic compartment syndrome (CCS), 2416-2417
Chronic disease
adolescent, ethical considerations regarding, *see website*
anemias of, 1653
in childhood, 149, *see also website*

Chronic disease *(Continued)*
Crohn disease appearance as, 1302
in foster care children, *see website*
Chronic fatigue syndrome (CFS), 714, *see also website*
Chronic granulomatous disease (CGD), 742t, 745-746, 745f
aspergillosis with, 1061
fetal therapy for, 551t
infections and, *see website*
phagocytic killing defects in, *see website*
Chronic infantile neurologic cutaneous and articular disease (CINCA), 855t, 858
Chronic kidney disease (CKD), 1822-1825
etiology of, 1822
maternal, 545
pathogenesis of, 1822, 1823t
treatment of, 1823-1825
Chronic myelogenous leukemia (CML), 748t, 1738-1739
hematopoietic stem cell transplantation for, 758
Chronic progressive external ophthalmoplegia (CPEO), 391t, 2131-2132
Chronic renal failure, rickets due to, 205-206
Chronic respiratory failure, 1519
in cystic fibrosis, 1494
Chronic suppurative otitis media (CSOM), 2210
CHRS. *See* Cerebrohepatorenal syndrome (CHRS)
CHS. *See* Chédiak-Higashi syndrome (CHS)
Churg-Strauss syndrome (CSS), 868t, 874-876, 874t, 1474
Chylomicronemia, familial, 473t, 476, 476f
Chylomicron retention disease, 1313
Chylothorax, 1514-1515, 1514f-1515f
Chylous ascites, 1416, *see also website*
Chymotrypsin, 1344t, 1369-1370, *see also website*
Ciclesonide, 778t-779t, 779-780
Cicuta species toxicity, 269t
CID. *See* Combined immunodeficiency (CID)
Cidofovir, 1116-1117, *see also website*
Cigarette smoking
adolescent, 672, 673t, 679, 680t
allergic reaction to, 769
breast-feeding and, 161t
fires due to, 24
porphyria cutanea tarda and, *see website*
as sudden infant death syndrome risk factor, 1424
wheezing and bronchitis and, 1460
Ciguatera fish poisoning, 1328t-1329t, 2454, *see also website*
Cilastatin, *see website*
Ciliary, respiratory, 1497, *see also website*
Ciliary dyskinesia, primary, 1497, *see also website*
Cimetidine
drug interactions with, *see website*
for *Helicobacter pylori* gastritis, 1293t
for urticaria and angioedema, 815t
CINCA. *See* Chronic infantile neurologic cutaneous and articular disease (CINCA)
Cipro. *See* Ciprofloxacin
Ciprofloxacin, *see also website*
for anthrax, *see website*
for chancroid, *see website*
for infectious diarrhea, 1337t
for meningococcal disease, 933t
for neonatal infection, 645t
for plague, *see website*
for *Shigella* infection, 961
Circadian rhythm in sleep, 46
Circulation
fetal, 1529, *see also website*
persistent, 592-594, 592f
glucocorticoids in, *see website*
neonatal, 1529, *see also website*
in pediatric emergency assessment, 281
renal, *see website*
Circulation *(Continued)*
transitional, 1529, *see also website*
in trauma survey, 336-337, 336t
Circulatory collapse, malarial, 1206
Circumcision, 1854-1856, 1855f, *see also website*
CIRH1A gene defect, 1383t
Cirrhosis
biliary
in cystic fibrosis, 1485, 1496
as manifestation of liver disease, 1374
Indian childhood, 1392
as manifestation of liver disease, 1374
portal hypertension with, *see website*
Cisapride, 563t
Cisatracurium, 321t
Cis-regulatory genomic sequences, *see website*
Citalopram
for depression and anxiety symptoms, 63t
for premenstrual dysphoric disorder, 692t
Citrobacter, neonatal, 632t
Citrulline, defects in metabolism of, 447-453, 448f-449f, 448t, 450t
Citrullinemia, 448f, 451-452
CJD. *See* Creutzfeldt-Jakob disease (CJD)
CK. *See* Creatine kinase (CK)
CKD. *See* Chronic kidney disease (CKD)
CLA. *See* Cutaneous lymphocyte-associated antigen (CLA)
Claforan. *See* Cefotaxime
Clarinex. *See* Desloratadine
Clarithromycin, *see also website*
for *Chlamydophila pneumoniae*, 1035
for *Helicobacter pylori* gastritis, 1293t
for infective endocarditis prophylaxis, 1626t
for *Legionella* infection, *see website*
for Mediterranean spotted fever, 1044
for *Mycobacterium avium* complex prophylaxis, 1175t-1176t
for *Mycoplasma pneumoniae*, 1031
for nontuberculous mycobacterial prophylaxis, 1015-1016
for otitis media, 2207t
for pertussis, 947t
for pharyngitis, 1440
for vulvovaginitis, 1868t
Claritin. *See* Loratadine
Clasp-knife phenomenon, *see website*
Classical pathway of complement system, *see website*
deficiencies of, 753-755, 754t
Class III malocclusion, *see website*
Class II malocclusion, *see website*
Class I occlusion, *see website*
Clavicular fracture, 2392
as birth injury, 578-579
as delivery room emergency, 578-579
as sports injury, 2409
Clavulanate, *see website*
Claw toe, 2342-2343
CLCN2 gene, 2016t
CLCN7 gene, 2432
CLDN1 gene, 1383t
CLE. *See* Congenital lobar emphysema (CLE)
Clean-contaminated wound, perioperative prophylaxis and, *see website*
Cleansing, acne and, 2323
Clean wound, perioperative prophylaxis and, *see website*
Clearance, *see website*
Clear cell sarcoma of kidney (CCSK), 1760
Cleft(s)
branchial, 2221
laryngeal, 1452
laryngotracheoesophageal, 1263, 1452
lip and palate, 1252-1253, 1252f
dental problems associated with, 1251t
mitral valve, 1554
sternal, 1517
Cleidocranial dysplasia, 2431, 2432f
oral manifestations of, 1254
Cleocin. *See* Clindamycin
CLIA. *See* Clinical Laboratory Improvement Amendments (CLIA) of 1988
Climate, acne and, 2323
Clindamycin, *see also website*
for acne, 2325t
for anthrax, *see website*
for babesiosis, *see website*
for cystic fibrosis lung infection, 1492t
for gonococcal disease, 939
for group A streptococci infection, 919
for infective endocarditis prophylaxis, 1626t
for malaria, 1203t-1205t, *see website*
for neonatal infection, 645t
for osteomyelitis, 2397-2398
for penicillin-allergic patients, 918-919
for pharyngitis, 1440
for *Pneumocystis jiroveci*, *see website*
for *Staphylococcus aureus*, 907-908, 907t
Clinical diagnosis, *see website*
Clinical geneticist, 382t
Clinical interview. *See* Interviewing
Clinical Laboratory Improvement Amendments (CLIA) of 1988
HIV testing and, *see website*
on office bacteriology, *see website*
Clinical pyelonephritis, 1829-1830, 1830f
Clinical Risk Index for Babies (CRIB), 563
Clinical trials
for childhood cancer, *see website*
for vaccine development, 884-885
Clinical utility, 377
Clinical validity, 376
Clinodactyly, 2385, 2385f, *see also website*
Clitoris
abnormalities of, *see website*
newborn assessment of, *see website*
Cloaca
anomalies of, *see website*
persistent, 1358
Cloacal exstrophy, 1847, *see also website*
Clobamaz, 2030t
Clofazimine, *see website*
Clomipramine
for depression and anxiety symptoms, 63t
for premenstrual dysphoric disorder, 692t
Clonazepam
for depression and anxiety symptoms, 63t
dosages of, 2030t
for neuroirritability in palliative care, 155t-156t
Clonic seizure
neonatal, 2034
treatment of, 2028
Clonidine
for attention deficit/hyperactivity disorder, 111t
epidural, 373
for neuroirritability in palliative care, 155t-156t
poisoning with, 262
for systemic hypertension, 1645t
toxicity of, 251t
Clonorchis sinensis, *see website*
Clonus, *see website*
Closed bite, *see website*
Closed-loop intestinal obstruction, 1287-1289
Closed reduction for developmental dysplasia of hip, 2359-2360, 2360f
Clostridium, 632t, *see also website*
Clostridium botulinum, 987-991
clinical manifestations of, 988-989, 989f
complications of, 990-991, 991t
diagnosis of, 989-990, 989t
differential diagnosis of, 989-990, 990t
epidemiology of, 987-988
etiology of, 987
gastroenteritis due to, 1324t-1325t
treatment of, 1337t
pathogenesis of, 988
poliovirus infection *versus*, 1085t
prevention of, 991

Clostridium botulinum (Continued)
prognosis for, 991
supportive care for, 990
treatment of, 990
Clostridium difficile infection (CDI), 994-995
inflammatory bowel disease *versus*, 1297, 1298t
treatment of, 1337t
Clostridium difficile toxin, 1313
Clostridium perfringens, 1324t-1325t, 1331-1332
Clostridium tetani, 991-994, 994t
Clothes, work, chemical pollutants in, *see website*
Clotting cascade, 1694f
Clotting factor(s), 1696-1697, 1696t
in hemostasis, 1694
hereditary deficiencies of, 1699-1704
reference values for, 1698t
Clotting factor assay, 1697-1698, 1698t
Clouston syndrome, 2223
Cloxacillin, *see website*
Clubbing
digital, *see website*
of nails, 2294, 2294f
"Club drugs," 675t, 682
Clubfoot, 2336, 2337f
Cluck, allergic, 764
Clusters of differentiation, *see website*
Clutton joint, 1017t, 1018
CMFTD. *See* Congenital muscle fiber-type disproportion (CMFTD)
CML. *See* Chronic myelogenous leukemia (CML)
CMS-EA. *See* Congenital myasthenic syndrome with episodic apnea (CMS-EA)
CMT. *See* Charcot-Marie-Tooth (CMT) disease; Congenital muscular torticollis (CMT)
CMV. *See* Cytomegalovirus (CMV)
CMV-IG. *See* Cytomegalovirus immune globulin (CMV-IG)
CMYC oncogene, *see website*
CNLDO. *See* Congenital nasolacrimal duct obstruction (CNLDO)
CNS. *See* Central nervous system (CNS)
CNVs. *See* Copy number variations (CNVs)
CO. *See* Carbon monoxide (CO)
CO_2. *See* Carbon dioxide (CO_2)
COACH syndrome, *see website*
Coagulase, *Staphylococcus aureus* production of, 904
Coagulase-negative staphylococci (CONS), 909-910
neonatal, 635, 635t
sepsis due to, 636t
Coagulation
acquired inhibitors of, 1712-1713
disseminated intravascular, 1713-1714, 1713t, *see also website*
with meningococcus, 930-931
in newborn, 621
Coagulation factors. *See* Clotting factor(s)
Coagulation factor assay, 1697-1698, 1698t
Coagulation proteins, 1694
Coagulopathy
abnormal uterine bleeding due to, 689t-690t
with fulminant hepatic failure, 1414
hematuria associated with, 1796
hypothyroidism-associated, 1903t
Coalescent mastoiditis, 2210-2211, 2210f
Coal tar preparations, 805
Coarctation of the aorta, 1567-1570, 1567f, 1569f
in adults, 1608
with ventricular septal defect, 1570
Coartem, 1202, 1203t-1205t
Coats disease, 2179, 2179f
Cobalamin (CBL), 194t, 197
defects in metabolism of, 437-438, 1320
deficiency of, 197-198
anemia due to, 1655
dietary reference intakes for, *see website*
Cobblestoning in vernal conjunctivitis, 810, 810f
Cobb method, 2365-2366, 2367f
Coca Cola, diarrhea and, 1335t
Cocaine
adolescent use of, 683
urine screening for, 676t
maternal abuse of, 624
Cocci anaerobic, *see website*
Coccidioides, 1065-1068
Coccidioidomycosis, 1065-1068, 1065f-1067f, 1066t, 1068t
pneumonia due to, 1475t
Cochlear implant, 2196, 2196t
Cockayne syndrome, 2257-2258, *see also website*
cardiac manifestations of, 1531t
Cockroach allergens, 769, 769t
Codeine
equianalgesic doses and half-life of, 367t
for pain management, 365t
urine screening for adolescent abuse of, 676t
Coefficient of variation (CV), *see website*
Coffee for asthma, 271t
COG. *See* Children's Oncology Group (COG)
Cogan syndrome, 876, *see also website*
Cognition
assessment in communication disorder, 120
social, *see website*
Cognitive-behavioral therapy (CBT), 66
for anxiety disorder, 78
for chronic fatigue syndrome, *see website*
for eating disorders, 95
for functional abdominal pain, 1348, 1348t
for obsessive-compulsive disorder, 80-81
Cognitive complications
of cancer and its treatment, *see website*
of congenital diaphragmatic hernia, 596
in sickle cell disease, 1669
Cognitive development, *see website*
during adolescence, 650t
early, 649-651
middle, 653
age 0-2 months, 27
age 2-6 months, 30
age 6-12 months, 30
age 12-18 months, 31, 32t
age 18-24 months, 32
during first 2 years, 27t
during middle childhood, 37-38, 37t
during preschool years, 34
Cognitive distortions, suicide and, 88
Cognitive function
elementary school success and, 37-38, 37t
in type 1 diabetes mellitus, 1986
Cognitive impairment
due to cancer and its treatment, *see website*
malarial, 1206
pain assessment and, 361
Cognitive Mapping, *see website*
Cognitive theories of development, *see website*
Cohen syndrome, 182t, 748t
COID. *See* Committee on Infectious Diseases (COID)
Coining, 137-138, *see website*
COLA1A gene, 2278
COL1A1 gene, 2278, 2439
COL1A2 gene, 2278, 2439
COL2A1 gene, *see website*
COL3A1 gene, 2278
COL4A3 gene, 1782
COL4A4 gene, 1782
COL4A5 gene, 1782
COL4A6 gene, 1782
COL5A1 gene, 2278
COL5A2 gene, 2278
COL9A2 gene, *see website*
COL9A3 gene, *see website*
COL10A1 gene, *see website*
COL11A1 gene, *see website*
COL11A2 gene, 2190t, *see also website*
Colchicine, 857
Colchicum autumnale toxicity, 269t
Cold, common, 1434-1436, 1434t-1435t
Cold agglutinin disease, 1682-1683
"Cold" antibodies, autoimmune hemolytic anemia associated with, 1682-1683, *see also website*
Cold-induced fat necrosis, 358
Cold injuries, 357-359
neonatal, 622
Cold panniculitis, 2285
Cold sore, 1099-1100
Cold urticaria, 812
Cold water immersion, 343-344
Colectomy, 1300
Coleus forskohlii, 271t
Colic, home remedies among African Americans for, *see website*
Co-lipase, *see website*
deficiency, diarrhea due to, 1306t
Colitis
amebic, 1179
fulminant, 1297
granulomatous (*See* Crohn's disease)
pseudomembranous, 994-995
ulcerative, 1295-1300
clinical manifestations of, 1297
Crohn disease *versus*, 1295, 1295t
diagnosis of, 1297-1298, 1299f
differential diagnosis of, 1297, 1298t
prognosis for, 1300
treatment of, 1298-1300
Collagen, type I, defects in, 2437
Collagenosis, reactive perforating, 2279, 2279f
Collapse-consolidation in tuberculosis, 998, 1000f
Collateral ligament injury, 2414
Collective violence, 668-669
Collodion baby, 2267, 2268t, 2269f
Colloid goiter, 1908
Colloid milium, 2256
Colloids
for anaphylaxis, 818t
for skin disorders, 2216
Coloboma
eyelid, 2164
fundus, 2181
iris, 2155
optic nerve, *see website*
Colocasia toxicity, 269t
Colon
cancer of (*See* Colorectal cancer (CRC))
digestion and absorption in, *see website*
duplication of, 1281
mega-, in Chagas disease, 1196
Colonization
bacterial, neonatal, 630
by group B streptococci, 925-926
during pregnancy, 925-928
Moraxella catarrhalis, *see website*
Colonoscopy, 1297-1298
Colony-forming unit-megakaryocytes (CFU-MK), *see website*
Color
nail, changes in, 2294-2295
of stools, *see website*
Colorado tick fever, 1142-1144
Color Doppler echocardiography, 1568
Colorectal cancer (CRC), 1297, 1773, *see also website*
Color vision testing, 2149
Colpocephaly, 2005
Coma
brain death and, *see website*
due to drowning, 345-346
malarial, 1201
nonketotic hyperosmolar, 1981
pentobarbital, for status epilepticus, 2039t
due to poisonings, 255t
in traumatic brain injury, 298
Combavir. *See* Lamivudine
Combination vaccines, 889

Combined immunodeficiency (CID), 730-738, 731t
  enteroviral meningoencephalitis with, 1092
  infection with, *see website*
  severe, 730-733, 731t, 732f
    autosomal recessive, 732-733
    reticular dysgenesis as, 733
    X-linked, 732, 732f
  treatment of, 736-737, 737t
Comedonal acne, 2322-2323, 2322f
  neonatal, 2327, 2327f
"Coming out" by transgender adolescents, 656-657
Comitant strabismus, 2158-2159
Comminuted fracture, 2388f
Committee on Infectious Diseases (COID), on vaccine policy, 885
Committees, pediatric ethics, *see website*
Common cold, 1434-1436, 1434t-1435t
Common innocent murmur, 1536
Common variable immunodeficiency (CVID), 720, 724-725, 724t, 748t
  malabsorption with, 1314
Common wart, 2315
Commotio cordis, 1621
Communicable disease, child care and, 895, *see also website*
Communication
  about life-threatening or life-altering illness, 151-152, *see also website*
  in autistic disorder, 100
  cerebral palsy and, 2065
  during first 2 years, 27t
  during 2-6 months, 30
  during 6-12 months, 31
  in palliative care, 151-159
  for patient safety, *see website*
  in post-resuscitation care, 296
  in transport medicine, *see website*
Communication disorders, 114-122
  in Asperger's syndrome, 118
  in autism and pervasive developmental disorders, 118
  classification of, 117, 117t
  clinical manifestations of, 117
  comorbid psychiatric disorders, 121
  diagnostic evaluation of, 120-121
  dysfluency (stuttering, stammering) as, 122, 122t
  epidemiology of, 116
  etiology of, 116
  isolated expressive language disorder as, 118
  in mental retardation, 118
  motor speech disorders as, 118-119
  non-causes of, 120
  pathogenesis of, 116-117
  pragmatic language disorder as, 118
  prognosis for, 121
  rare causes of, 119
  screening for, 119-120, 120t
  selective mutism as, 118
  specific language impairment as, 117-118
  treatment of, 121
Community
  chronic illness and, *see website*
  obesity prevention in, 187t
  well child care and, 16-17
Community-acquired pneumonia, 1474-1479
Community violence, 668-669, *see website*
Comparative genomic hybridization (CGH), 376, 377t, 396
Compartment(s)
  in pharmacokinetics, *see website*
  pulmonary edema and, 1468
  of total body water, *see website*
Compartment syndrome
  chronic, 2416-2417
  with necrotizing fasciitis, 2301-2302
Compassionate care for foster care children, *see website*
Compavir. *See* Zidovudine (ZDV)
Compazine. *See* Prochlorperazine
Compensated shock, 285, 305
Compensatory overinflation, 1460-1461
Compensatory respiratory alkalosis, 230
Compensatory scoliosis, 2371
Competence, cultural, *see website*
COMP gene, *see website*
Complaints, psychosomatic illness and, 68
Complementary and alternative medicine, 270-274
  acupuncture, 273-274
  for cancer, *see website*
  dietary supplements, 270-273, 271t-272t
    toxicity of, 272t-273t
  massage and other bodywork therapies, 273
  nutritional aspects of, 169
  in palliative care, 158
  Spanish-English botanical name translation chart, 274t
Complementation, 1684
Complement fixation (CF) test, *see website*
Complement system, 753
  alternative pathway of, *see website*
  classical and lectin pathway of, *see website*
  constituents of, *see website*
  control mechanisms of, *see website*
  disorders of
    evaluation of, 720t, 722
    fever without a focus in, 896t
    genetic, 753-755, 754t
    immunizations in, 892t
    infection with, *see website*
    meningococcus and, 931, 933
    of plasma, membrane, or serosal control proteins, 755
    screening for, 718t
    secondary, 755-756
    treatment of, 756
  evaluation of, 753
  in host defense, *see website*
  membrane attack complex in, *see website*
  in neonatal immunity, 631
  in serum sickness, 819
Complete blood count (CBC)
  in appendicitis, 1351
  in immunodeficiency screening, 718t
  in malabsorption, 1306
  reference intervals for, *see website*
Complete fracture, 2390
Complete heart block, 1618-1619, 1618f
  genetics of, *see website*
Complex febrile seizure, 2017
Complex partial seizure, 2021
Complex regional pain syndrome (CRPS), 374-375, 879-880, 879t, 2060t, 2061
Compliance. *See also* Adherence
  chest wall, *see website*
  respiratory, 322, *see also website*
    assessment in mechanical ventilation, 328
    diseases associated with decreased, 323
Composite graft in intestinal transplantation, *see website*
Compressions, chest, in cardiopulmonary resuscitation, 291, 291f-292f
Compulsions, 80
Computed tomography angiography (CTA)
  in neurologic examination, *see website*
  in Takayasu arteritis, 872, 872f
Computed tomography (CT)
  in abdominal trauma, 338-339, 339f
  in amebiasis, 1179, 1179f
  in appendicitis, 1351-1352, 1352f
  in aspiration syndromes, 1472t, 1473f
  in bronchiectasis, *see website*
  in cardiovascular disease, 1545-1546, 1547f
  chest, *see website*
  in cystic fibrosis, 1488, 1490f
  in fever of unknown origin, 902
  in genitourinary trauma, *see website*
  Haller index on chest, 1516
  in interstitial lung disease, *see website*
Computed tomography (CT) *(Continued)*
  in liver abscess, 1404, 1404f
  in liver dysfunction, 1379
  in lymphocytic choriomeningitis virus infection, *see website*
  in neurologic examination, *see website*
  in orthopedic problems, 2335
  in osteomyelitis, 2396
  in pancreatitis, 1371-1372, 1372f
  in pork tapeworm, 1235, 1236f
  radiation exposure with, *see website*
    reduction of, *see website*
  in retropharyngeal abscess, 1441, 1441f
  in rhabdomyosarcoma, 1761, 1761f
  in septic arthritis, 2400
  spiral reconstruction, *see website*
  in toxoplasmosis, 1212-1213, 1212f
  in traumatic brain injury, 298f-299f
  in tuberculosis, 1006
  in urinary tract obstruction, 1841
  in Wilms tumor, 1758-1759, 1759f
  in X-linked adrenoleukodystrophy, 468, 469f
Computed tomography venography (CTV), 2083, 2083f
Concerta. *See* Methylphenidate
Concrescence, tooth, 1250
Concussion. *See also* Traumatic brain injury (TBI)
  periodontal ligament, 1258
  sports-related, 2402t-2404t, 2418-2419, 2419t
    in soccer players, *see website*
Conditioning therapy for nocturnal incontinence, 1852
Condoms, 694f, 695t
Conduct disorder, 97-98, 97t. *See also* Disruptive behavioral disorders
  adolescent violence and, 669, 670t
Conduction
  antidromic, 1613-1614
  orthodromic, 1613-1614
Conduction disorder, following tetralogy of Fallot repair, 1577-1578
Conductive hearing loss (CHL), 2188. *See also* Hearing impairment or loss
Condylomata acuminata, 1867t-1868t, 2316, 2316f
  sexual abuse and, 145t
Condylomata lata, 1016-1017
Confidentiality of adolescent medical information, *see website*
Conformal irradiation, *see website*
Confusional arousal, 51-52
Congenital adrenal hyperplasia (CAH), 1930-1939, 1931f
  adrenocortical insufficiency due to, 1924, 1925t
  due to 11β-hydroxylase deficiency, 1935-1936
  due to 3β-hydroxysteroid dehydrogenase deficiency, 1936
  diagnosis and treatment of, 1931f, 1932t
  disorders of sex development due to, 1962
  due to 17-hydroxylase deficiency, 1936-1937
  due to 21-hydroxylase deficiency, 1930-1935
  hypokalemia in, 223-224
  metabolic alkalosis in, 236
Congenital aganglionic megacolon, 1283t, 1284-1287, 1285f-1286f
Congenital amegakaryocytic thrombocytopenia (CAMT), 1689, 1719-1720, 1719f
Congenital anemia, 1650-1652
Congenital anomalies, *see website*
  anorectal, 1355-1356, 1356f, 1357t, 1359t
  ataxia with, 2054
  of bladder, 1847
  of central nervous system, 1998-2013
    agenesis of corpus callosum as, 2005-2006, 2005f
    agenesis of cranial nerves, 2006-2007
    anencephaly as, 2003
    craniosynostosis as, 2011-2013, 2012t

Congenital anomalies *(Continued)*
disorders of neuronal migration as, 2003-2005, 2003f-2004f
dysgenesis of posterior fossa, 2006-2007
encephalocele as, 2002-2003
holoprosencephaly as, 2005-2006, 2006f
hydrocephalus as, 2008-2011, 2008t, 2009f-2011f
meningocele as, 1999
microcephaly as, 2007-2008, 2007t
muscle development and, 2118
myelomeningocele as, 2000-2002, 2001f
neural tube defects as, 1998-1999, 1999f
spina bifida occulta as, 1999, 2000f, 2001t
of cervical spine, 2380-2382, 2381t
congenital heart disease with, 1531t
deviation terms in, *see website*
of ears, 2196, *see website*
esophageal, 1262-1263
fetal therapy for, 551t
gallbladder, 1415
hearing loss due to, 2189-2190
in infants of diabetic mothers, 628
of kidney, 1827-1829, 1828f-1829f
hematuria due to, 1796
of larynx, trachea, and bronchi, 1450-1452, 1450f-1452f
of lung, 1463-1467
agenesis and aplasia as, 1463
bronchobiliary fistula as, 1467
bronchogenic cysts as, 1466, 1466f
cystic adenomatoid malformation as, 1464, 1465f
hernia as, 1467
lymphangiectasia as, 1467
sequestration as, 1465, 1466f
of nose, 1429-1431, 1430f-1431f
otitis media with, 2200
pancreatic, 1368, *see also website*
of penis and urethra, 1852-1858
of peritoneum, 1416
of respiratory tract, wheezing due to, 1457
of ribs, 1518-1519
with skeletal dysplasias, *see website*
of skin, 2221-2222, 2221f
of stomach, 1274-1276
of teeth, 1250-1251, 1250f-1251f
teratogens in, 547-548
vulvovaginal and müllerian, 1874, *see also website*
Congenital anorchia, 1944
Congenital central hypoventilation syndrome (CCHS), 1520-1522, *see also website*
Congenital cholesteatoma, *see website*
Congenital cranial nerve dysinnervation disorders (CCDD), 2006
Congenital cystic adenomatoid malformation (CCAM), 1464, 1465f
Congenital cytomegalovirus (CMV), 1116-1117
Congenital diaphragmatic hernia (CDH), 594-596, 595f-596f
Congenital disorders of glycosylation (CDGs), *see website*
Congenital dyserythropoietic anemia (CDA), 1654, *see also website*
Congenital enterocyte heparin deficiency (CEHD), 1311
Congenital erythropoietic porphyria (CEP), 2256, 2256f, *see also website*
Congenital fibrosis of extraocular muscles (CFEOM), 2006
Congenital glutamine deficiency, 445
Congenital goiter, 1905-1906, 1906f
Congenital heart disease (CHD)
acyanotic
absence of pulmonary valve as, 1571
aorticopulmonary window defect as, 1561
aortic stenosis as, 1565-1567, 1565f
atrial septal defect as, 1551
atrioventricular septal defects as, 1554-1556, 1554f-1555f

Congenital heart disease (CHD) *(Continued)*
coarctation of the aorta, 1567-1570, 1567f, 1569f
coronary-cameral fistula as, 1561
left-to-right-shunt lesions as, 1551-1561
mitral stenosis as, 1570, *see also website*
mitral valve insufficiency as, 1571-1572, 1571t
mitral valve prolapse as, 1572
obstructive, 1561-1571
ostium secundum defect as, 1551-1553, 1551f-1553f
partial anomalous pulmonary venous return as, 1553-1554
patent ductus arteriosus as, 1559-1561, 1560f
pulmonary valve stenosis as, 1561-1565, 1562f-1564f
pulmonary valvular insufficiency as, 1571
pulmonary venous hypertension as, 1570-1571
regurgitation lesions as, 1571
sinus venosus atrial septal defect, 1553
supracristal ventricular septal defect with aortic insufficiency as, 1559
tricuspid regurgitation as, 1572
ventricular septal defect as, 1556-1558, 1556f-1557f
in adolescents, 1609-1610, 1609t
anomalous origin of coronary arteries as, 1598-1599, 1599f
aortic arch anomalies as, 1596-1598, 1597f-1598f, 1597t
auscultation in, 1536
cyanotic
abnormal position of heart and heterotaxy syndromes as, 1595-1596
associated with decreased pulmonary blood flow, 1573-1585
associated with increased pulmonary blood flow, 1585-1596
double-outlet right ventricle as, 1582, 1588-1589
Ebstein anomaly of the tricuspid valve as, 1583-1585, 1584f
evaluation of, 1572-1573
heterotaxy syndromes as, 1589t, 1595-1596
hypoplastic left heart syndrome as, 1592-1595, 1593f-1595f
pulmonary atresia as, 1578-1580, 1579f
single ventricle as, 1592
tetralogy of Fallot, 1573-1578, 1573f, 1575f, 1577f
total anomalous pulmonary venous return as, 1589-1590, 1589t, 1590f
transposition of the great arteries as, 1582-1583, 1583f, 1585-1588, 1585f-1586f, 1588f
tricuspid atresia as, 1580-1582, 1580f-1581f
truncus arteriosus as, 1590-1592, 1591f
diverticulum of left ventricle as, 1599-1600
with Down syndrome, 403t
ectopia cordis as, 1599
Eisenmenger syndrome as, 1601-1602
etiology of, *see website*
evaluation of, 1549-1551
fever without a focus in, 896t
genetic counseling in, *see website*
genetics of, *see website*
infective endocarditis and, 1622
medical history in, 1530
pregnancy, 1609
prevalence of, 1549, *see also website*
pulmonary arteriovenous fistula as, 1599, *see also website*
pulmonary hypertension as, 1600-1602, 1600t, 1601f, 1602t
respiratory signs and symptoms of, *see website*
sports participation and, 2402t-2404t
sudden death due to, 1619

Congenital heart disease (CHD) *(Continued)*
surgical treatment of, 1602-1610, 1605t
long-term management following, 1604-1605
postoperative management following, 1603-1604
Turner syndrome with, 1952-1953
Congenital hepatic fibrosis, *see website*
Congenital hyperthyroidism, 1913, 1913f
Congenital hypomyelinating neuropathy, 2140, *see also website*
Congenital hypopituitarism, 1876-1879
Congenital hypothyroidism, 1895-1901
Congenital hypotonia, benign, 2119
Congenital ichthyosiform erythroderma
bullous, 2270, 2270f
nonbullous, 2267-2268, 2269f
Congenital insensitivity to pain and anhidrosis, 2143
Congenital lip pits, *see website*
Congenital lobar emphysema (CLE), 1461
Congenital Lyme disease, 1027
Congenital lymphocytic choriomeningitis virus, *see website*
Congenital malaria, 1201
Congenital melanocytic nevi, 2232, 2232f
Congenital muscle fiber-type disproportion (CMFTD), 2115
Congenital muscular dystrophy, 2113t, 2123-2126, 2128f
Congenital muscular torticollis (CMT), 2377-2379
Congenital myasthenic syndrome with episodic apnea (CMS-EA), 2133, 2133t
Congenital mydriasis, 2155
Congenital nasolacrimal duct obstruction (CNLDO), 2165
Congenital nephrotic syndrome, 1806, 1807t
Congenital neutropenia, severe, 750
Congenital ocular motor apraxia, 2161
Congenital omphalocele, *see website*
Congenital phlebectasia, 2224-2225, 2226f
Congenital rubella syndrome, 1077-1078, 1077f, 1077t
congenital heart disease with, 1531t
in type 1 diabetes mellitus development, 1971
vaccine for, 881t
Congenital scoliosis, 1518, 2368-2370, 2369f
in arthrogryposis, *see website*
Congenital secondary polycythemia, *see website*
Congenital sideroblastic anemia, *see website*
Congenital subglottic hemangioma, *see website*
Congenital syphilis, 1016-1018, 1016f-1017f, 1017t
clinical manifestations of, 1017-1018, 1017f-1019f, 1017t
diagnosis of, 1020f, 1021, 1021t
hearing loss due to, *see website*
prevention of, 1023
treatment of, 1022
Congenital toxoplasmosis, 1208-1211, 1210f, 1214-1215
Congenital tuberculosis, 1000, 1007
Congenital varicella-zoster virus, 1106-1107, 1107f
Congenital vertical talus, 2337-2338, 2337t, 2338f
Congenital vitamin D deficiency, 205
Congestive heart failure. *See* Heart failure
Congestive splenomegaly, *see website*
Conium maculatum toxicity, 269t
Conjoined twins, 553
Conjugated bilirubin, 1375
elevation of (*See* Cholestasis)
Conjugated vaccine, 883
Conjunctiva
disorders of, 2166-2169
examination of, 2150
foreign body in, 2185
Conjunctivitis, 2166-2169, 2167t, 2168f-2169f
adenovirus, 1132
allergic, 765, 809-810, 810f, 2168

Conjunctivitis *(Continued)*
Chlamydia trachomatis, 1035, 1037
exclusion from day care due to, *see website*
giant papillary, 810
gonococcal, 712t, 939
Haemophilus influenzae in, 943
hemorrhagic, due to enterovirus, 1091
herpes simplex virus, 1101
in Kawasaki disease, 863, 864f
sports participation and, 2402t-2404t
tularemia inoculation, 978
vernal, 2168, 2168f
viral, 2168
Conjunctivitis otitis media syndrome, 2205
Connective tissue disease
cardiac manifestations of, 1531t
mixed, evaluation of, *see website*
skin manifestations of, *see website*
Connective tissue nevus, 2235
Conn syndrome, 2129
Conotruncal heart defects, *see website*
Conradi-Hünermann syndrome, 1531t, 2268t
CONS. *See* Coagulase-negative staphylococci (CONS)
Consanguinity, 385, *see also website*
Consent of adolescent, *see website*
Consolidation treatment for acute lymphocytic leukemia, 1735
Constipation, 1245-1247, 1246t
abdominal pain of, 1247t
due to anogenital malformation, 1359t
with Down syndrome, 403t
functional, 1284, 1284t
in Hirschsprung disease, 1285, 1285t
maintenance therapy for, 74t
neonatal, 600
neuropathic bladder and, *see website*
nondigestive causes of, 1241t
due to opioids, 366t
treatment of in palliative care, 155t-157t, 158
Constitutional growth delay, 1880
Constriction bands, amniotic, 533, 2220-2221, 2343, *see also website*
Constrictive pericarditis, 1637
Consultation, ethics, *see website*
Contact allergy involving eyes, 810
Contact dermatitis, 804, 2250-2252, 2250f-2251f
allergic, 2251
of external ear canal, 2199
vulvar, 1867t-1868t
Contact factors deficiency, 1703
Contact isolation, *see website*
Contact lenses for hyperopia, 2151
Contaminated wound, perioperative prophylaxis and, *see website*
Contamination, internal radiation, *see website*
Contiguous gene deletion syndrome, 406
Contiguous gene disorders, 381
Contingent responses, development and, *see website*
Continuing education for emergency medical services for children, *see website*
Continuity of care, *see website*
Continuous gene deletion syndrome, 2269
Continuous glucose monitoring (CGM), real-time, 1983-1984
Continuous glucose monitoring system (CGMS), 1983
Continuous heart murmur, 1535
Continuous positive airway pressure (CPAP)
at home, 332, 1524-1525
for neonatal apnea, 581
for obstructive sleep apnea, 51
for respiratory distress and respiratory failure, 320, 585
Continuous renal replacement therapy (CRRT), 1822
Continuous subcutaneous insulin infusion (CSII), 1977
Continuum of care model in emergency medical services for children, *see website*
Contraception, 692-699, 695t
barrier methods for, 694
combination methods for, 696
counseling regarding, 694
emergency, 698-699, 698t, 704t
epidemiology of, 692-694, 693f-694f, 693t
hormonal methods for, 696-698, 696t-697t, 697f
intrauterine devices for, 699
minors right to consent for, *see website*
special needs girls and, 1875
spermicides for, 694
for women with congenital heart disease, 1609
Contraceptive patch, for special needs girls, 1875
Contraceptive ring, 697
special needs girls and, 1875
Contraceptives, oral, 695t-696t, 696-698
for acne, 2325t
for amenorrhea, 688t
drug interactions with, *see website*
for dysmenorrhea, 691t
for emergency contraception, 698t
missed pills and, 696, 697f, 697t
for polycystic ovary syndrome, *see website*
special needs girls and, 1875
Contraction stress test (CST), 542, 543t
Contractures
assessment of, 2331
in Becker muscular dystrophy, 2119
congenital, orthopedic management of, *see website*
in Duchenne muscular dystrophy, 2119
in neuromuscular disorders, 2109
Contrast enema, 1297, 1299f
Contrast radiography, 1267, 1267f
Control, preschoolers need for, 35-36
Controllers in respiration regulation, *see website*
Control proteins, complement, deficiencies of, 754t, 755
Control variable in mechanical ventilation, 324-325
Contusion
lumbar disk, as sports injury, 2412
as sports injury, 2406
due to football, *see website*
Convalescent stage of pertussis, 945
Convective heart loss in newborn, 536-537
Conventions, international, for protection of children from effects of war, *see website*
Convergent retractorius, 2161
Conversion disorder, 68t, 69
Convex lenses for hyperopia, 2151
Cooley anemia, 1675-1676
Coordination, neurologic examination of, *see website*
Copegus. *See* Ribavirin
Coping styles
psychosomatic illness and, 68
in type 1 diabetes mellitus, 1986
Copper-histadine therapy, 2075
Copper toxicity, *see website*
gastroenteritis due to, 1328t-1329t
in Wilson disease, 1391, 1391f
COPP regimen for Hodgkin lymphoma, 1742, 1743t
Coprine ingestion, *see website*
Coprolalia, 77
Coproporphyria, hereditary, *see website*
Coproporphyrinogen oxidase (CPO), *see website*
Copy number variations (CNVs), 399, *see also website*
Cord. *See* Umbilical cord
Cordocentesis, 543t, 544, 549
Corectopia, 2155
Cornea
chemical burns of, 2185-2186
development of, *see website*
disorders of, 2169, *see also website*
Cornea *(Continued)*
open globe injury and, 2185
superficial abrasions of, 2184
Corneal manifestations of system disease, *see website*
Corneal reflex
brain death and, *see website*
in strabismus diagnosis, 2157
Cornelia de Lange syndrome, 2007t
Cornification, disorders of, 2267-2272, 2268t
Cornstarch for type I glycogen storage disease, 495
Coronal plane deformities, 2348
Coronary artery(ies)
aneurysm of in Kawasaki disease, 864, 865f
anomalous origin of, 1598-1599, 1599f
disease of, 459
graft, *see website*
sports participation and anomalies of, 2402t-2404t
sudden death and anomalies of, 1619
Coronary-cameral fistula, 1561
Coronary sinusoidal channel, 1578-1579
Coronaviruses, 1134, *see also website*
in pneumonia, 1475t
Corporal punishment, abuse *versus*, 135
Cor pulmonale, *see website*
Corpus callostomy for seizures, 2032-2033
Corpus callosum agenesis, 2005-2006, 2005f
Cortex
adrenal, 1923, *see also website*
renal, 1778
Cortical dysplasian focal, 2004
Cortical hyperostosis, infantile, 2436-2437, 2436f
Cortical necrosis, renal, 1818
Corticosteroid-binding globulin deficiency (CBG), 1926
Corticosteroids
adrenal insufficiency due to abrupt cessation of, 1929
adverse effects of, 795t
for allergic rhinitis, intranasal inhaled, 778t-780t, 779-780
for anaphylaxis, 818t
for asthma
inhaled, 791-793, 794t-795t
systemic, 793-794, 794t, 797t-798t, 800
for atopic dermatitis
systemic, 805
topical, 804, 804t
atrophy due to
epidermal, 2274
subcutaneous tissue, 2282, 2282f
for bacterial meningitis, 2092-2094
for chronic granulomatous disease, 746
for Crohn disease, 1303
for croup, 1448
for Diamond-Blackfan anemia, 1651
for Hansen disease, *see website*
immunizations and, 891
for juvenile dermatomyositis, 849
for pulmonary hemosiderosis, 1500
in renal transplantation, *see website*
for respiratory distress syndrome, 586
antenatal, for prevention of, 584
for scleroderma, 853
for skin disorders, 2217, 2217t
for systemic lupus erythematosus, 844
for tuberculosis, 1009
for wheezing, 1459
Corticotropin deficiency, 1929
Corticotropinoma, *see website*
Corticotropin-releasing hormone (CRH), *see website*
Cortinarius poisoning, *see website*
Cortisol
in adrenal insufficiency, 1928
in Cushing syndrome, 1940
decreased binding affinity of, 1926
deficiency of

Cortisol *(Continued)*
in congenital adrenal hyperplasia, 1931-1933
hypoglycemia in, 527-528
reference values for, *see website*
regulation of, 1923, *see also website*
Corynebacterium diphtheria, 929, *see also website*
poliovirus infection *versus*, 1085t
Corynebacterium minutissimum, 2306
Corynebacterium ulcerans, 929, *see also website*
Costeff optic atrophy syndrome, 433
Costs
of antiseizure therapy, 2028
of chronic illness in childhood, *see website*
of health care, 11
Cotrim. *See* Trimethoprim-sulfamethoxazole (TMP-SMX)
Cough
in asthma, 782, 782t
in common cold, 1435
of croup, 1446
in cystic fibrosis, 1485-1486
habit, *see website*
as manifestation of extrapulmonary disease, 1526
of pertussis, 945-946
as prominent finding in disorders, 1460t
recurrent or persistent, *see website*
in respiratory syncytial virus infection, 1128
Cough etiquette, *see website*
Cough reflex, brain death and, *see website*
Coumarin, 1711
Councilman bodies, *see website*
Counseling
contraceptive, 694
in dysmorphology, *see website*
genetic, 377-379, 378t
in acute intermittent porphyrias, *see website*
in chronic granulomatous disease, 746
in congenital heart disease, *see website*
in erythropoietic protoporphyria, *see website*
in hearing loss, 2196
in Marfan syndrome, 2446
in neurofibromatosis, 2048
in osteogenesis imperfecta, 2439-2440
in peroxisomal disorders, 467
in transmissible spongiform encephalopathies, *see website*
in X-linked adrenoleukodystrophy, 470
in intellectual disability management, 129
for neurodevelopmental dysfunction, *see website*
nutrition, 169-170
in seizures, 2025, 2026t
teen pregnancy, 700
Counter-regulatory hormones, 518
deficiency of, 520t
Cover tests for strabismus, 2157-2158
Cowden syndrome, 1747t, 2298
Cow's milk
allergy to, 821, 821t
pulmonary hemosiderosis with, 1498-1499
type 1 diabetes mellitus and, 1972
Cow's milk protein-based formula, 163
COX-2. *See* Cyclo-oxygenase 2 (COX-2) inhibitors
Coxiella burnetii, 1039t-1040t, 1051-1053
in breast milk, 540t
in pneumonia, 1475t
COX inhibitors. *See* Cyclo-oxygenase (COX) inhibitors poisoning
Coxsackie, 1088t
in hand-foot-and-mouth disease, 1090, 1090f
maternal, *see website*
in myocarditis and pericarditis, 1091
neonatal, 1092
in orchitis, 1091
in pharyngitis, 1439
CP. *See* Cerebral palsy (CP)
CPAP. *See* Continuous positive airway pressure (CPAP)
CPB coactivator, *see website*
CPD. *See* Chondrodysplasia punctata (CPD)
CPE. *See* Cytopathic effect (CPE)
CPEO. *See* Chronic progressive external ophthalmoplegia (CPEO)
CPM. *See* Central pontine myelinolysis (CPM)
CPO. *See* Coproporphyrinogen oxidase (CPO)
CPP. *See* Cerebral perfusion pressure (CPP)
CPR. *See* Cardiopulmonary resuscitation (CPR)
CPS. *See* Carbamyl phosphate synthetase (CPS) deficiency; Child Protective Services (CPS)
CPT. *See* Carnitine palmitoyltransferase (CPT) deficiency
CPT-IA. *See* Carnitine palmitoyltransferase-IA (CPT-IA) deficiency
CPT-II. *See* Carnitine palmitoyltransferase-II (CPT-II) deficiency
Crackles
in asthma, 783
auscultation of, *see website*
Cradle cap, 2253-2254, 2253f
CRAFFT mnemonic, 674-677, 676t
Cranial bruits, *see website*
Cranial disorders in newborn, 565-566, 565f
Cranial nerves
agenesis of, 2006-2007
Lyme disease and, 1026, 1028t
neurologic examination of, *see website*
Cranial synostosis, 533-534
Cranial ultrasonography, *see website*
Craniofrontonasal dysplasia, 2012t
Craniopharyngioma, 1752
Craniosynostosis, 2011-2013, 2012t
neurologic examination and, *see website*
skull palpation in assessment of, *see website*
Craniotabes, 200, 533-534
skull palpation in assessment of, *see website*
Craniovertebral junction, pathologic conditions at, 2381
CRBSI. *See* Catheter-related bloodstream infection (CRBSI)
CRC. *See* Colorectal cancer (CRC)
C-reactive protein
in appendicitis, 1351
reference values for, *see website*
Creams, 2216
Creatine
deficiency of, 441, 441f
for performance enhancement, 2423, 2423t
Creatine kinase (CK)
in Duchenne muscular dystrophy, 2120-2121
in neuromuscular disorders, 2110
reference values for, *see website*
Creatinine in posterior urethral valves, 427
CREB-binding protein, *see website*
Creeping eruption, 1220, *see also website*
Crepitance, 2301
Crescent formation in Bowman's space, *see website*
Crescentic progressive glomerulonephritis, 1789-1790
Cretinism, 1895, 1906-1908
Creutzfeldt-Jakob disease (CJD), 1177, *see also website*
maternal, *see website*
CRH. *See* Corticotropin-releasing hormone (CRH)
CRIB. *See* Clinical Risk Index for Babies (CRIB)
Cri-du-chat syndrome, 2007t
Crigler-Najjar syndrome, 604-605, 1390
Crimean-Congo hemorrhagic fever, 1151-1152
Critical aortic stenosis, 1565
Critical high airway obstruction syndrome (CHAOS), 577, 578f
Critical illness. *See also* Acute illness
adrenal insufficiency in, 1929-1930, *see also website*
ethics in treatment of, *see website*
Critical illness *(Continued)*
polyneuropathy in, poliovirus infection *versus*, 1085t
"Critical sample" in hyperinsulinemia, 521, 522t
Crixivan. *See* Indinavir
Crohn's disease, 1300-1304
abdominal pain of, 1247t
clinical manifestations of, 1300-1301, 1301f
cutaneous, *see website*
diagnosis of, 1302
differential diagnosis of, 1301-1302, 1302t
liver disease associated with, *see website*
malabsorption in, 1322, *see also website*
metastatic, *see website*
oral ulcerations in, 1260t
prognosis for, 1304
treatment of, 1302-1304
ulcerative colitis *versus*, 1295, 1295t
Crolom. *See* Cromolyn sodium
Cromolyn sodium
for allergic conjunctivitis, 811t
for allergic disease, 771-772
for allergic rhinitis, 780t
for asthma, 794t, 796
Cross bite, *see website*
Cross-dresser, 655
Crossed adductor response, *see website*
Cross-gender roles, 655
Crossing over, genetic, 395
Cross-Kusick-Breen syndrome, 2239
Crotalidae-specific Fab antibodies, 258t
Croup, 1446-1447, 1446f
in parainfluenza viruses, 1125t, 1126
spasmodic, 1447
Crouzonomesodermoskeletal syndrome, 2012t
Crouzon syndrome, 1531t, 2012t, 2013
Crowding, dental, *see website*
Crown
completion of, 1250t
injuries to, 1258, 1258t
CRPS. *See* Complex regional pain syndrome (CRPS)
CRRT. *See* Continuous renal replacement therapy (CRRT)
CRTAP gene, 2439
Cruciate ligament injuries, 2414, 2414t
Crush injury of phalanx, 2391
Crusts, examination of, *see website*
Crying during age 0-2 months, 27
Cryohydrocytosis, *see website*
Cryoproteins, 812
Cryotherapy
for retinopathy of prematurity, 2175-2176
for sexually transmitted infection, 713t
Cryptococcoma, 1056
Cryptococcus neoformans, 1056-1058
in pneumonia, 1475t
Cryptogenic epilepsy, 2013
Cryptorchidism, 1858-1860, 1860f, 1944
after inguinal repair, 1367
Cryptorchid testis, 1859
Cryptosporidium, 1183-1184, *see also website*
gastroenteritis due to, 1327t-1328t
treatment of, 1337t
inflammatory bowel disease *versus*, 1298t
Crystalloids for anaphylaxis, 818t
Crysticillin. *See* Penicillin G, procaine
CSD. *See* Cat-scratch disease (CSD)
CSF. *See* Cerebrospinal fluid (CSF)
CSII. *See* Continuous subcutaneous insulin infusion (CSII)
CSOM. *See* Chronic suppurative otitis media (CSOM)
CSS. *See* Churg-Strauss syndrome (CSS)
CST. *See* Contraction stress test (CST)
C_{STAT}. *See* Static compliance (C_{STAT}) assessment in mechanical ventilation
CSVT. *See* Cerebral sinovenous thrombosis (CSVT)
CTSK gene, *see website*
Cubital vein, venous access in, 292, 295f

Cued recall, *see website*
Cuff, blood pressure, 1533
Cuirasse, 1524
Cullen sign, 1371
Cultural competence, *see website*
Cultural desire, *see website*
Cultural encounters, *see website*
Cultural factors/issues, 13
in high-risk pregnancies, *see website*
in nutrition and feeding, 167-168
in objections to treatment, *see website*
in psychosomatic illness, 67
in suicide, 88
Cultural groups, newly recognized, *see website*
Cultural knowledge, *see website*
Cultural practices, bruises caused by, 137-138
Cultural skill, *see website*
Culture
in anaerobic infection, *see website*
blood, *see website*
in brucellosis, 981
in *Campylobacter* infection, 970
in candidiasis, 1054
cerebrospinal fluid, *see website*
in *Clostridium difficile* infection, 995
in enterovirus infection, 1092-1093
in Epstein-Barr virus, 1113
in fever of unknown origin, 902
genital, *see website*
in genital *Chlamydia trachomatis*, 1036
in gonococcal disease, 938
in *Haemophilus influenzae*, 941
in HIV infection, 1166t
importance of to medical practice, *see website*
in infectious enteritis, 1334
of medical profession, *see website*
in nontuberculous mycobacteria, 1014-1015
in parainfluenza viruses, 1125t
in pertussis, 945-946
respiratory, *see website*
of safety, *see website*
in septic arthritis, 2399
in *Shigella* infection, 960
in sinusitis, 1437
throat, *see website*
in toxoplasmosis, 1213
in tuberculosis, 1003, 1006
in typhoid fever, 956-957
in urinary tract infection, 1831-1832
urine, *see website*
Cupping, 137-138, 202, 203f
Curly toes, 2342
Curosurf, 585
Currarino triad, 1285
Cushing syndrome, 1939-1941, 1939t
corticotropinoma with, *see website*
metabolic alkalosis in, 236
myopathies with, 2129
obesity due to, 182t
Cushion defect, endocardial, 1554
Cutaneous defects, 2220-2222
Cutaneous diphtheria, *see website*
Cutaneous hydration for atopic dermatitis, 804
Cutaneous larva migrans, 1220, 1220f, 1220t, *see also website*
Cutaneous leishmaniasis
diffuse, 1188
localized, 1187
Cutaneous lymphocyte-associated antigen (CLA), 802
Cutaneous polyarteritis nodosa, 872-874
Cutis laxa, 1531t, 2277-2278, 2277f
Cutis marmorata, 2218
Cutis marmorata telangiectatica congenita, 2224-2225, 2226f
Cutis verticis gyrata, 2222
Cuts, 340-341
CV. *See* Coefficient of variation (CV)
CVID. *See* Common variable immunodeficiency (CVID)
CXCR-4, 1157-1158
Cyanide poisoning, 270, *see also website*
antidote for, 256t-257t
Cyanosis
abnormal hemoglobins causing, 1672
history of, 1530
as manifestation of extrapulmonary disease, 1526, *see also website*
in newborn, 533, *see also website*
physical examination of, 1531
Cyanotic congenital heart disease
abnormal position of heart and heterotaxy syndromes as, 1595-1596
in adults, 1607
associated with decreased pulmonary blood flow, 1573-1585
associated with increased pulmonary blood flow, 1585-1596
double-outlet right ventricle as, 1582
with malposition of great arteries, 1588-1589
with pulmonary stenosis, 1588
Ebstein anomaly of the tricuspid valve as, 1583-1585, 1584f
evaluation of, 1550-1551, 1572-1573
extracardiac complications of, 1603t
heterotaxy syndromes as, 1589t, 1595-1596
hypoplastic left heart syndrome as, 1592-1595, 1593f-1595f
pulmonary atresia as, 1578-1580, 1579f
respiratory distress syndrome *versus*, 583-584
single ventricle as, 1592
tetralogy of Fallot, 1573-1578, 1573f, 1575f, 1577f
with pulmonary atresia, 1578
total anomalous pulmonary venous return as, 1589-1590, 1589t, 1590f
transposition of the great arteries as
d-, 1585-1587, 1585f-1586f
with intact ventricular septum, 1585-1587, 1586f
l-, 1587-1588, 1588f
with ventricular septal defect, 1587
with ventricular septal defect and pulmonary stenosis as, 1574, 1583f
tricuspid atresia as, 1580-1582, 1580f-1581f
truncus arteriosus as, 1590-1592, 1591f
C-YBOCS. *See* Children's Yale-Brown Obsessive-Compulsive Scale (C-YBOCS)
Cyclic neutropenia, 750
Cyclic vomiting, 1242, 1243t-1244t
with migraine, 2042
Cyclitis, 2172-2174
Cyclo-oxygenase 2 (COX-2) inhibitors for rheumatic disease, *see website*
Cyclo-oxygenase (COX) inhibitors poisoning, 260
Cyclophosphamide
for cancer therapy, *see website*
for lupus nephritis, 1788
for nephrotic syndrome, 1805
for rheumatic disease, *see website*
Cycloserine, 1008t, *see also website*
Cyclospora cayetanensis, 1184, 1327t-1328t, *see also website*
in traveler's diarrhea, 1338t
treatment of, 1337t
Cyclosporine
for atopic dermatitis, 805
diabetes associated with, 1997
drug interactions with, *see website*
gingival overgrowth due to, 1257
for nephrotic syndrome, 1805
for pancytopenia, 1692
for rheumatic disease, *see website*
for urticaria and angioedema, 815t
Cyclothymic disorder, 85
CYP1A2 gene, *see website*
CYP3A4 gene, 1411, *see also website*
CYP3A5 gene, *see website*
CYP3A7 gene, *see website*
CYP11A1 gene, *see website*
CYP11B1 gene, *see website*
CYP27B1 gene, 1971
CYP7BI gene, 1383t
CYP2C9 gene, *see website*
CYP2C19 gene, *see website*
CYP2D6 gene, *see website*
CYP17 gene, *see website*
CYP19 gene, *see website*
Cyproheptadine
for Cushing syndrome, 1941
for migraine prophylaxis, 2044t
for urticaria, 814
for vomiting prophylaxis, 1244t
CYPs, *see also website*
in adrenal biosynthesis, *see website*
in aldosterone synthase deficiency, 1938
in congenital adrenal hyperplasia, 1930
in glucocorticoid-suppressible hyperaldosterone, 1938
in P450 oxidoreductase deficiency, 1937
CYPS1A2 gene, *see website*
Cyst(s)
arachnoid, 2006
Baker, 2353
branchial cleft and thyroglossal, 2221
breast, *see website*
bronchogenic, 1466, 1466f
choledochal, *see website*
abdominal pain of, 1247t
dental lamina, 1260
dentigerous, *see website*
epidermal inclusion, *see website*
eruption, *see website*
esophageal
duplication, 1263-1264
neuroenteric, 1264
follicular, 1957-1958
foregut, 1452
Giardia, 1181
gingival of newborn, 2298
hydatid, *see website*
laryngeal, 1451-1452, 1452f
neuroenteric, 1281
ovarian, 1871-1872
paraurethral urethral, 1858, 1858f
pilar, *see website*
popliteal, 2353
trichilemmal, *see website*
urachal, *see website*
urethral, 1857-1858
Cystadenoma
ovarian, 1871
pancreatic, *see website*
Cystathionine β-synthase (CBS) deficiency, 425-427
Cystathioninemia, 428-429
Cystathioninuria, 428-429
Cysteine/cystine, defects in metabolism of, 429
Cystic abdominal masses, 535
Cystic adenomatoid malformation, 1464, 1465f
Cystic anomalies of kidney, 1827-1828, 1828f
Cystic disease of liver and biliary tract, 1415, *see also website*
Cystic dysplasia, renal, 1827
Cysticercosis, 1234-1237, 1237t
Cysticercus, 1233-1235
Cystic fibrosis (CF), 1481-1497
clinical manifestations of, 1485-1487, 1486f-1487f, 1486t
complications of, 1482t
dental problems associated with, 1251t
diabetes related to, 1996
diagnosis and assessment of, 1487-1490, 1488t, 1489f-1490f
general anesthesia and, *see website*
genetics of, 1481-1482, 1483f, 1483t, *see also website*
liver disease due to, *see website*
meconium ileus in, 601, 601f
metabolic alkalosis due to, 236
neonatal screening for, *see website*
newborn screening for, 1490

Cystic fibrosis (CF) *(Continued)*
pancreatic insufficiency in, 1369
pathogenesis of, 1482-1485, 1484f-1485f
pathology of, 1485
prognosis for, 1497
Pseudomonas aeruginosa in, 976
skin manifestations in, 2330
treatment in, 1490-1493
antibiotic, 1491-1492, 1492t
anti-inflammatory, 1493
bronchodilator, 1493
emerging therapies in, 1493
endoscopy and lavage in, 1493
general approach to, 1490-1491, 1491t
of intestinal complications, 1495-1496
pulmonary, 1491-1493
of pulmonary complications, 1493-1495
urinary lithiasis with, *see website*
Cystic fibrosis-related diabetes (CFRD), 1996
Cystic fibrosis transmembrane conductance regular protein (CFTR)
cystic fibrosis and, 1481-1485
liver disease and, 1383t
Cystic hygroma, 1724, 1772, *see also website*
Cystine calculi, *see website*
Cystinosis, 1808-1809
hypothyroidism due to, 1901
Cystinuria, 1319, 1814
Cystitis, 1830
hemorrhagic, 1799
adenovirus in, 1132
infectious causes of, 1799
treatment of, 1832-1833
Cystography, vesicoureteral reflux, 1836
Cystoplasty, augmentation, *see website*
Cystosarcoma phylloides, *see website*
Cystourethrogram, voiding
in urinary tract infection, 1833, 1833f
in urinary tract obstruction, 1840
in vesicoureteral reflux, 1836, 1837f
Cytarabine, *see website*
Cytochrome-*c* oxidase, 1406
Cytochrome C oxidase deficiency myopathy, reversible infantile, 2066-2067
Cytochrome P450 system
in adrenal biosynthesis, *see website*
drugs and, *see website*
hepatic injury and, 1411
porphyria cutanea tarda and, *see website*
Cytogenetics, 394-414
abnormalities of chromosomal number in, 399-403
aneuploidy and polyploidy as, 399-400, 400t
Down syndrome as, 400-403
trisomy 13 as, 405f
trisomy 18 as, 405f
abnormalities of chromosomal structure in, 404-408
deletions and duplications as, 406-407, 406t, 407f, 408t-409t
insertions as, 407
inversions as, 405-406
isochromosomes as, 407
marker and ring chromosomes as, 408
translocations as, 404-405, 406f
chromosome instability syndromes in, 412
fragile chromosome sites in, 411-412, 411t
methods of chromosome analysis in, 394-399, 395f-400f, 397t
mosaicism in, 412
sex chromosome aneuploidy in, 408-410, 409t
Klinefelter syndrome as, 410
Noonan syndrome as, 410, 410t
Turner syndrome as, 409-410
47,XYY as, 410
uniparental disomy and imprinting in, 412-414, 413f-414f
Cytokine receptor γ chain, mutations in gene encoding, 732, 732f
Cytokines, *see also website*
in allergic disease, *see website*
in atopic dermatitis, 802
classification of, *see website*
defective production of, 729
fetal, *see website*
in HIV infection, 1161
meningococcus and, 930
in *Mycoplasma pneumoniae*, 1030
in neonatal immunity, 632
in systemic lupus erythematosus, 843
Cytomegalic inclusion disease, 1116
Cytomegalovirus (CMV), 1115-1117
antivirals for, *see website*
in child care setting, *see website*
clinical manifestations of, 1115-1116
congenital, 1116-1117
diagnosis of, 1116
epidemiology of, 1115
etiology of, 1115
fetal therapy for, 551t
ganciclovir for, *see website*
hearing loss due to, 2188-2189
HIV-related, *see website*
prophylaxis for, 1175t-1176t
immune globulin for, 882t
in immunocompromised patient, 1116-1117
inflammatory bowel disease *versus*, 1297, 1298t
maternal
breast-feeding and, 161t, 540t
fetal and neonatal effects of, *see website*
in microcephaly, 2007t
pathogenesis of, 1115
perinatal, 1116
in pneumonia, 1475t
prevention of, 1117
transfusion-associated, *see website*
after transplantation, *see also website*
intestinal, *see website*
kidney, *see website*
stem cell, 762-763, *see also website*
treatment of, 1116-1117
vaccine for, 1117
Cytomegalovirus immune globulin (CMV-IG), *see website*
Cytopathic effect (CPE), *see website*
Cytosine arabinoside. *See* Cytarabine
Cytosolic acetoacetyl CoA thiolase deficiency, 434-435
Cytosolic 5'-nucleotidase, overactive, *see website*
Cytotoxics
for juvenile idiopathic arthritis, 838t
for rheumatic disease, *see website*
Cytotoxic T cells
development and differentiation of, *see website*
flow cytometry testing of, 720-722
interaction with other immune cells, *see website*
Cytotoxic T lymphocyte-associated 4 gene, 1971
Cytotoxin
A, 975
tracheal, 944-945
Cytovene. *See* Ganciclovir
Cytoxan. *See* Cyclophosphamide

D

Daclizumab, *see website*
Dacryoadenitis, 2167t, 2182-2183
Dacryocystitis, 2167t, 2183
with congenital nasolacrimal duct obstruction, 2165
Dacryocystocele, 2165
Dacryostenosis, 2165, 2165f
Dactinomycin
for cancer therapy, *see website*
for Wilms tumor, 1759
Dactylitis
blistering distal, 2304, 2304f
in sickle cell disease, 1663-1664, 1664f
DAEC. *See* Diffusely adherent *Escherichia coli* (DAEC)
DAH. *See* Diffuse alveolar hemorrhage (DAH)
Dalfopristin, *see website*
Dalfopristin-quinupristin, *see website*
Dalrymple sign, 2163
Danazol for endometriosis, 690-691
Dance therapy or pain management, 371
Dandy-Walker malformation, 2006, 2010, 2010f
Danon disease, 494t-495t, 500, *see also website*
D antigen, isoimmune hemolytic disease from, 615
Dantrolene, 2064
Dapsone, *see website*
Daptomycin, 907t, *see also website*
Darier disease, 2263, 2263f
Darier sign, 814
Dark-field microscopy, 1020-1021
Darunavir, 1168t-1171t
Dasatinib, *see website*
Data, quality, *see website*
Database, *see website*
Date rape, 703
Date registry, *see website*
Dating of fetus, 541
Datura stramonium toxicity, 269t
Daunorubicin, *see website*
Davidenkow syndrome, 2138
DAX1 gene, 1924, *see also website*
Day care. *See* Child care
Daydreaming, seizures and, *see website*
Daytime frequency syndrome of childhood, 1851
Daytime incontinence, 73
DBA. *See* Diamond-Blackfan anemia (DBA)
DBNC. *See* Death by neurologic criteria (DBNC)
DBT. *See* Dialectical behavior therapy (DBT)
DC. *See* Dyskeratosis congenita (DC)
DCL. *See* Diffuse cutaneous leishmaniasis (DCL)
DCM. *See* Dilated cardiomyopathy (DCM)
DCs. *See* Dendritic cells (DCs)
DDAVP. *See* Desmopressin acetate (DDAVP)
DDE. *See* Doctrine of double effect (DDE)
DDEB. *See* Dominant dystrophic epidermolysis bullosa (DDEB)
DDH. *See* Developmental dysplasia of hip (DDH)
ddI. *See* Didanosine (ddI)
D-dimer, 1697
DDT exposure, *see website*
"Deadly nightshade" toxicity, 269t, 272t-273t
Dead space ventilation, 316-318, *see also website*
in mechanical ventilation, 329
Deafness. *See also* Hearing impairment or loss
due to congenital rubella syndrome, 1077-1078
familial, cardiac manifestations of, 1531t
genetics of, 391t
maternally inherited diabetes and, 1994-1995
Death, 1-2
due to acute rheumatic fever, 920
brain, 572-573
cancer-related, 1725
reduction in, *see website*
cardiac, *see website*
causes of, 3t, 5t, 18f
developmental perspective on, *see website*
ethics in declaration of, *see website*
due to injury, 17-18, 17t
leading causes of by age, 18f
major causes of, *see website*
due to maltreatment, 136t
due to measles, 1072t
overview of, 532
palliative care and (*See* Palliative care)
of parent or sibling, *see website*
of patient, health care provider and, *see website*
perinatal, *see website*
pneumonia, 1474, 1475t
postneonatal, *see website*

Death *(Continued)*
poverty and, 6, 6f
of preterm and low birthweight infants, 563
racial factors in, 4t
reduction of, 2f
due to sepsis syndrome, 646, 647t
sudden, 1619-1621, 1620f-1621f, 1620t-1621t
associated with stimulants, 61
during sports, 2401-2405
sudden infant (*See* Sudden infant death syndrome (SIDS))
due to undernutrition, 173
worldwide indicators of, 3t
Death by neurologic criteria (DBNC), *see website*
Death rates
birthweight categories in, *see website*
for children, 1-2, 2f
fetal and neonatal, *see website*
infant, *see website*
from neonatal bacterial meningitis, 646
racial and ethnic factors in, *see website*
for selected years, *see website*
by sex, race, and, age, 3t
worldwide indicators of, 3t
"Death rattle," 157
DEB. *See* Dystrophic epidermolysis bullosa (DEB)
Debrancher deficiency, 496-497, 496f, 528
Decadron. *See* Dexamethasone
Deceleration of fetal heart rate, 543-544, 544f, 545t
Decimal factors, prefixes denoting, *see website*
Decision-making in palliative care, 153
Declomycin. *See* Demeclocycline
Decompensated shock, 285, 305, 307f
Decontamination for poisonings, 254-257, 257t
Deep sedation, *see website*
Deep tendon reflexes assessment
in neurologic examination, *see website*
in neuromuscular disorders, 2109, 2110t
Deep vein thrombosis (DVT), 1709
estrogen contraceptives and, 1875
pulmonary embolism with, 1500-1501, 1501t
DEET. *See* N,N-diethyl-*m*-toluamide (DEET)
Deferasirox, 1675-1676
Deferoxamine, 1675-1676
for iron poisoning, 256t-257t, 263
Defibrillation
automated external, 1621
emergency, 291-292, 293f
Deficit therapy, 245-247, 247t. *See also* Dehydration
for hyponatremic dehydration, 247-248
monitoring and adjustment of, 247, 247t
Deformations, congenital, *see website*
Deformity, *see website*
Degenerative diseases, ataxia with, 2055
Dehydration
calculation of fluid deficit in, 246
due to cholera, 965-968
clinical manifestations of, 246, 246t
deficit therapy for, 245-249, 247t
in diabetes mellitus, 1979-1980
due to gastroenteritis, 1333, 1333t-1334t
hypernatremic, 214, 248-249, 248t
hyponatremic, 247-248, 1884-1885
laboratory findings in, 246
with malnutrition, 1316-1317
management of, 247, 247t
in protein-energy malnutrition, 178t
due to *Shigella* infection, 960
sports-related, 2420
symptoms associated with, 1333t
due to traveler's diarrhea, *see website*
Dehydroepiandrosterone (DHEA)
in ovarian carcinomas, 1872t
for performance enhancement, 2423, 2423t
in puberty, *see website*
Dehydroepiandrosterone sulfate (DHEAS), 686
Deiodination defects, 1896
Déjerine-Sottas disease, 2139, *see also website*
de Lange syndrome, 1531t
Delayed eruption of teeth, *see website*
Delayed sleep phase disorder (DSPD), 53-54
Del Castillo syndrome, 1945
Deletions, genetic, 406-407, 406t, 407f, 408t, *see also website*
congenital heart disease with, 1531t
Deletion 11p, *see website*
Deletion 9q34, 182t
Deletion 13q, *see website*
Deletion 22q11.2, 2382
Delirium
emergence, *see website*
hypothyroidism-associated, 1903t
Delivery
birth injury due to
fractures as, 578-579
of peripheral nerves, 573-574
of spine and spinal cord, 573
visceral, 578
cesarean section for, *see website*
high-risk pregnancy and, *see website*
Delivery room
care of newborn in, 536-538
antiseptic skin and cord care in, 537
maintenance of body heat in, 536-537
emergencies in, 575-579
abdominal wall defects as, 578
airway obstruction as, 577, 578f
birth injury as, 578-579
failure to initiate or sustain respiration as, 575
meconium staining as, 577
neonatal resuscitation as, 575-577, 576f-577f, 576t
pneumothorax as, 577, 578f
respiratory distress and failure as, 575
shock as, 577
δ Fraction bilirubin, 1375
δ-Thalassemia, 1676
Demeclocycline, *see website*
Demerol
De Morsier syndrome, 2006
Demyelinating disorders of central nervous system, 2076-2080, 2076t
acute disseminated encephalomyelitis as, 2079, 2079f, 2080t
multiple sclerosis as, 2076, 2077t, 2078f
neuromyelitis optica as, 2077
stroke-like events *versus*, 2085
Denavir. *See* Penciclovir
Dendritic cells (DCs), 739, *see also website*
Dendritic keratitis, *see website*
Dengue fever, 1147-1150, 1147t
Dengue hemorrhagic fever, 1147-1150, 1147t
Dengue shock syndrome, 1148
Dennie lines, 765
Dennie-Morgan folds, 765
Dense body syndrome, 1722
Dental abscess, 1255, 1256f
Dental caries, 1254-1256, 1255f-1256f
Dental crowding, *see website*
Dental development, *see website*
Dental lamina, 1249
Dental lamina cyst, 1260
Dental procedures, infective endocarditis prophylaxis for, 1626t
Dental radiology, 1261, *see also website*
Dental sealant, 1256
Dental trauma, 1258-1259, 1258f-1259f, 1258t
Dentatorubropallidoluysian atrophy, 2057t
Dent disease, 227, 1814
hypophosphatemia due to, 207
Dentigerous cyst, *see website*
Dentin, injuries to, 1258t
Dentinogenesis imperfecta, 1250, 1251f, 1253-1254
Denys-Drash syndrome, 1962-1963
renal transplantation and, *see website*
WT1 gene mutation in, *see website*
11-Deoxycortisol, *see website*
Deoxyguanosine kinase (dGK), 1406
Depakote. *See* Divalproex
Dependence, chemical, 677
Depo-Medrol. *See* Methylprednisolone
Depo-Provera. *See* Medroxyprogesterone acetate
Depot medroxyprogesterone acetate (DMPA), 1875
Depression
attention deficit/hyperactivity disorder *versus*, 110
major, 82-85, 83t-84t
maternal, child adjustment and, *see website*
postpartum, *see website*
in adolescents, 701
psychopharmacologic management of, 61t, 63t
treatment of in palliative care, 157t, 158
in type 1 diabetes mellitus, 1986
Deprivation amblyopia, 2152
Dermacentor andersoni, 1041
Dermacentor variabilis, 1041
Dermatitis
atopic, 801-807
avoiding triggers for, 805-806
clinical manifestations of, 802, 802f-803f, 803t
complications of, 806
diagnosis and differential diagnosis of, 803-804, 803t
etiology of, 801
of external ear canal, 2199
due to food allergy, 822
laboratory findings in, 803
pathogenesis of, 802
pathology of, 801
prevention of, 807
prognosis for, 806-807
treatment of, 804-805, 804t
vulvar, 1867t-1868t
contact, 804, 2250-2252, 2250f-2251f
of external ear canal, 2199
vulvar, 1867t-1868t
diaper, 1866, 2250, 2250f
Candida in, 1055, 2314, 2314f
of external auditory canal, 2198-2199
human T-lymphocyte-associated, *see website*
due to niacin deficiency, 193-195, 195f
perianal, 2304-2305, 2305f
group A streptococcus in, 917
seborrheic, 2253-2254, 2253f-2254f
of external ear canal, 2198
vulvar, 1867t-1868t
vesicular hand and foot, 2253, 2253f
Dermatitis herpetiformis (DH), 2248-2249, 2248f
immunofluorescence of, *see website*
Dermatofibroma, *see website*
Dermatographism, 813
Dermatomal distribution in herpes zoster, 1107, 1107f
Dermatomegaly, 2277-2278
Dermatomyositis
cardiac manifestations of, 1531t
juvenile, 846-850, 847f-849f, 848t
arthralgia in, *see website*
cutaneous manifestations of, *see website*
evaluation of, *see website*
Dermatophagoides farinae, 768
Dermatophagoides pteronyssinus, 768
Dermatophytoses, 2309-2313, 2310f
tinea capitis as, 2310-2311, 2310f-2311f
tinea corporis as, 2311-2312, 2311f-2312f
tinea cruris as, 2312
tinea nigra palmaris as, 2313
tinea pedis, 2312-2313, 2312f-2313f
tinea unguium as, 2313, 2313f
Dermatospraxis, 2278
Dermis
disorders of, 2273-2282
corticosteroid-induced atrophy as, 2274
cutis laxa as, 2277-2278, 2277f
Ehlers-Danlos syndrome as, 2278
elastosis perforans serpiginosa as, 2279, 2279f

Dermis *(Continued)*
focal hypoplasia as, 2222
granuloma annulare as, 2274-2275, 2274f
keloid as, 2273-2274, 2273f
lichen sclerosus as, 2275, 2275f
lipoid proteinosis as, 2276-2277
macular atrophy as, 2277
mastocytosis as, 2280-2282, 2280f-2281f, 2280t-2281t
morphea as, 2275-2276, 2276f
in mucopolysaccharidoses, 2280, 2280f
necrobiosis lipoidica as, 2275, 2275f
pseudoxanthoma elasticum as, 2278-2279, 2278f
reactive perforating collagenosis as, 2279, 2279f
scleredema as, 2276
striae cutis distensae as, 2274, 2274f
morphology of, *see website*
Dermoids
nasal, 1431
ocular, 2169, *see also website*
Dermolipoma, 2169
DES. *See* Diethylstilbestrol (DES); Discreet Event Stimulation (DES)
Desensitization
drug, 825
systematic for phobias, 81
Desert herb, 272t-273t
Desert rheumatism, 1065-1068
Desferal. *See* Deferoxamine
Desflurane for anesthesia, *see website*
Desipramine
for attention deficit/hyperactivity disorder, 111t
for pain management, 364t
Desire, cultural, *see website*
Desloratadine
for allergic rhinitis, 777t-778t, 779
for urticaria and angioedema, 815t
Desmoplastic small round cell tumor (DSRCT), 1773
Desmopressin acetate (DDAVP)
for central diabetes insipidus, 1883
for nocturnal enuresis, 72-73, 73t
for nocturnal incontinence, 1852
for platelet dysfunction, 1722
Desquamation in Kawasaki disease, 863, 864f
Deterministic effects of radiation, *see website*
Detrusor-sphincter dyssynergia, 1849
Development. *See also* Growth and development
assessment of in neurologic evaluation, *see website*
child care and, *see website*
loss, separation, and grief and, *see website*
Developmental delay, 39
in Down syndrome, 401, 402t
in foreign-born adoptee, 131
in foster care children, *see website*
screening and surveillance of, 39-40, 41t-45t, *see also website*
Developmental disorders
of muscle, 2112-2119
pervasive, 100, 101t-102t
Asperger's disorder, 105t, 106
autistic disorder, 100-106, 101t, 103f-104f, 105t
childhood disintegrative disorder, 106, *see also website*
language disorders of, 118
Developmental dysphasia, 117
Developmental dysplasia of hip (DDH), 2356
classification of, 2356
clinical findings in, 2357, 2357f-2358f
complications of, 2360
diagnostic testing of, 2358, 2359f
epidemiology of, 2357
etiology and risk factors for, 2356-2357
pathoanatomy of, 2357
treatment of, 2359, 2360f
Developmental history in psychiatric diagnostic evaluation, 60
Developmental Milestones (DM), 41t-43t
Developmental phenotypes, *see website*
Developmental plasticity, *see website*
Developmental risk, *see website*
Developmental screening and surveillance, 39-40, 41t-45t
Developmental therapy for neurodevelopmental dysfunction, *see website*
Devic disease, 2077
Deworming, 1219-1220
Dexamethasone
for asthma, 746
for bacterial meningitis, 2094
for chemotherapy-associated vomiting, 1244t
for croup, 1448
myopathies due to, 2129
for nausea in palliative care, 155t-156t
possible adverse reactions to in premature infant, 563t
for typhoid fever, 958
Dexamethasone suppression test, 1940
Dexedrine. *See* Dextroamphetamine
Dexmedetomidine, *see website*
Dexmethylphenidate, 62t, 111t
Dextroamphetamine, 62t, 111t
Dextroposition, 1596
Dextrose for oral hypoglycemic poisoning, 263
DFA. *See* Direct fluorescent-antibody (DFA)
DGCR. *See* DiGeorge chromosomal region (DGCR)
DGI. *See* Disseminated gonococcal infection (DGI)
dGK. *See* Deoxyguanosine kinase (dGK)
DH. *See* Dermatitis herpetiformis (DH)
DHA. *See* Docosahexaenoic acid (DHA)
DHCR7 gene, *see website*
DHEA. *See* Dehydroepiandrosterone (DHEA)
DHEAS. *See* Dehydroepiandrosterone sulfate (DHEAS)
DHH gene, *see website*
DHS. *See* Drug hypersensitivity syndrome (DHS)
DI. *See* Diabetes insipidus (DI)
Diabetes, lipoatrophic, 1995
Diabetes insipidus (DI), 1881-1884, 1882f, 1882t
central, 1883
hypernatremia due to, 213, 213t
nephrogenic, 1812, 1883-1884
nephrotoxins in, 1817t
vasopressin-resistant, 1882
Diabetes mellitus (DM), 1968-1997
autoimmune diseases with, 1996-1997
cystic fibrosis-related, 1996
general anesthesia and, *see website*
genetic defects of insulin action in, 1995-1996
impaired glucose tolerance as, 1993
introduction and classification of, 1968, *see also website*
maternal, 545, *see website*
congenital heart disease with, 1531t
fetal therapy for, 551t
maternally inherited diabetes and deafness as, 1994-1995
maturity-onset diabetes of youth as, 1993-1994, 1994t
necrobiosis lipoidica with, 2275
of newborn, 1995
type 1 (*See* Type 1 diabetes mellitus (T1DM))
type 2 (*See* Type 2 diabetes mellitus (T2DM))
Diabetic ketoacidosis (DKA), 1976
classification of, 1976t
treatment of, 1979, 1979t, 1981
Diabetic mothers, infants born to, 521, 627-629, 627f-628f
Diabetic nephropathy, 1988, 1988t
Diabetic neuropathy, 1989
Diabetic retinopathy, 1987, 1988t, 2179-2180, 2180f
Diagnostic microbiology, 881, *see also website*
Diagnostic otoscope head, 2202
Diagnostic testing
genetic, 376-377, 377f
molecular, *see website*
prenatal (*See* Prenatal diagnosis)
respiratory, 1421, *see also website*
serologic, *see website*
Dialectical behavior therapy (DBT), 95
Dialysis
for acute renal failure, 1821-1822, 1821t
for end-stage renal disease, 1826, 1826t
for poisoning, 258
with toxic alcohols, 268
Dialysis catheters, infection associated with, *see website*
Diamond-Blackfan anemia (DBA), 1650-1651
transient erythroblastopenia of childhood *versus*, 1652t
Diamorphine, 367t
Diaper changing in nursery, 538
Diaper dermatitis, 1866, 2250, 2250f
Candida in, 1055, 2314, 2314f
DIAPH1 gene, 2190t
Diaphragm
contraceptive, 694
eventration of, 597
Diaphragmatic hernia, 594-596, 594f
congenital (Bochdalek), 594-596, 595f-596f
as delivery room emergency, 575
Diaphragm pacing, 332-333, 1524-1525
in congenital central hypoventilation syndrome, 1522
Diaphyseal fracture, 2391-2392
Diarrhea, 1243-1245, 1245t. *See also* Gastroenteritis; Malabsorption
adenovirus, 1132
antibiotic-associated, 994-995
Campylobacter, 969
in childcare setting, *see website*
chloride, 236, 1306t, 1320-1321, 1341
chloride-losing, congenital, 223
due to cholera, 965-968
chronic, 1339-1346
assessment of, 1340-1341, 1343f, 1343t-1345t
definition and epidemiology of, 1339-1346
etiology of, 1339, 1340t, 1342t
due to neuroendocrine tumor, 1346, *see also website*
pathophysiology of, 1339, 1339f-1340f
treatment of, 1342-1344
Clostridium difficile, 994-995
differential diagnosis of, 1246t
Escherichia coli, 961-965
exclusion from day care due to, *see website*
Giardia, 1181-1182
hemolytic-uremic syndrome following, 1791, 1791t
infectious, 1333t
clinical manifestations of, 1331-1332, 1332t
complications of, 1333-1334, 1333t
diagnosis of, 1333-1334, 1333t
epidemiology of, 1323, 1326f
pathogenesis of, 1323-1330, 1330f-1331f, 1330t
prevention of, 1337-1338
risk factors for, 1330-1331
sports participation and, 2402t-2404t
treatment of, 1334-1337, 1334t-1335t, 1335f-1336f, 1337t
inflammatory, 1330
in Kawasaki disease, 864f
maintenance water for, 244-245, 245t
malnutrition with, 1316
due to measles, 1072, 1072t
metabolic acidosis due to, 232
neonatal diseases of, 1306t
in newborn, *see website*
nondigestive causes of, 1241t
noninflammatory, 1330
osmotic, 1245, 1339, 1339f
persistent, 1331, 1336f
phenotypic, 1311-1312, 1341, 1343f

Diarrhea *(Continued)*
Plesiomonas shigelloides, *see website*
postinfection, 1313
rotavirus, calcivirus, and astrovirus, 1134-1137
secretory, 1245, 1339, 1339f
due to shellfish poisoning, *see website*
Shigella in, 959-960
sodium, 1321, 1341
syndromic, 1311-1312
toddler's, *see website*
traveler's, 1338-1339, 1338t, *see website*
treatment of in palliative care, 157t
in typhoid fever, 956, 956t
watery
in microvillus inclusion disease, 1305
in tufting enteropathy, 1311
Diastematomyelia, 2102, 2103f
Diastolic blood pressure, 1534f-1535f
Diastolic murmur auscultation, 1535-1536
Diastolic overload pattern, 1539
Diastrophic dysplasia, 2430-2431, 2430f-2431f
Diastrophic dysplasia sulfate transporter (DTDST), loss of, 2430-2431
Diazepam
for muscle spasm in palliative care, 155t-156t
for seizures
dosages of, 2030t
febrile, 2018
neonatal, 2037
in palliative care, 155t-156t
for spasticity of cerebral palsy, 2064
for status epilepticus, 2038, 2039t
for tetanus, 993
DIC. *See* Disseminated intravascular coagulation (DIC)
Dicarboxylic aminoaciduria, 1319
Dichotomous trait, *see website*
Dicloxacillin, *see also website*
for cystic fibrosis lung infection, 1492t
for *Staphylococcus aureus*, 907-908
for vulvovaginitis, 1868t
Didanosine (ddI), 1167, 1168t-1171t
DIDMOAD, 1994
Diencephalic seizure, *see website*
Dientamoeba fragilis, *see website*
Diet
acne and, 2323
acute gastroenteritis and, 1334-1336
BRAT, 1136
in cystic fibrosis, 1495
dental caries development and, 1256
for eosinophilic esophagitis, 1270
F57, 176-177, 177t-178t
F100, 176-177, 177t-178t
gluten-free, 1310-1311
habits regarding in eating disorders, 92t
heart failure and, *see website*
for hyperlipidemia, 480-481
ketogenic, for seizures, 2032
for obese child, 186, 186t
pesticide exposure through, *see website*
"traffic light," 186, 186t
type 1 diabetes mellitus and, 1981-1983, 1982t
development of, 1972
Dietary analysis, short method, *see website*
Dietary fiber
for functional abdominal pain, 1348t
reference intakes for, *see website*
Dietary lipids, transport of, 471
Dietary reference intakes (DRI), *see website*
Dietary supplements, 270-273, 271t-272t
nutritional aspects of, 169
Spanish-English botanical name translation chart, 274t
toxicity of, 272t-273t, 1412t
Diethylcarbamazine, *see also website*
for filariasis, 1225
for loiasis, 1225-1226
Diethylpropion for weight loss in adults, 187t
Diethylstilbestrol (DES), *see website*
Diffenbachia toxicity, 269t
Differential, reference values for, *see website*
Differential agglutination test, in toxoplasmosis, 1214
Differential diagnosis, testing for refining of, *see website*
Diffuse alveolar hemorrhage (DAH), 1498-1500, 1498t
Diffuse cutaneous leishmaniasis (DCL), 1188
Diffuse cutaneous mastocytosis, 2281, 2281f
Diffuse hemangiomatosis, 2228, 2228f
Diffuse large B-cell lymphoma (DLBCL), 1739-1740, 1744t
Diffusely adherent *Escherichia coli* (DAEC), 962t, 964
Diffusing capacity for carbon monoxide (DLCO), *see website*
Diffusion, pulmonary, 318
Digenic inheritance, 389, 390f
DiGeorge chromosomal region (DGCR), 728-729
congenital heart disease and, *see website*
DiGeorge syndrome, 408t, 728-729, 1531t, 1576
psychosis with, *see website*
Digestion, *see also website*
malabsorption due to defects of, 1304-1305
Digestive system
disorders of (*See* Digestive system disorders)
in drug absorption, *see website*
maintenance water and, 244, 244t
manifestations of non-digestive tract disease in (*See* Digestive system manifestations)
normal phenomena of, 1240, *see also website*
Digestive system disorders
adenovirus in, 1132
anaerobic organisms in, *see website*
due to cancer and its therapy, *see website*
chest pain in, 1530t
child care and, *see website*
coronaviruses in, *see website*
cutaneous manifestations of, *see website*
disorders of in mucopolysaccharidoses, 515t
of esophagus
clinical manifestations of, *see website*
congenital anomalies as, 1262-1263
diagnosis of, *see website*
dysmotility as, 1264-1265, 1265f
eosinophilic esophagitis as, 1270
gastroesophageal reflux disease, 1266-1270, 1267f-1268f
hiatal hernia as, 1265, 1265f-1266f
infective esophagitis as, 1270
due to ingestion, 1271-1273, 1272f-1273f, 1272t-1273t
obstructing and motility disorders as, 1263-1264
perforation as, 1271, *see also website*
"pill" esophagitis as, 1270
varices as, 1271, *see also website*
of exocrine pancreas
anatomic abnormalities as, 1368, *see also website*
associated with pancreatic insufficiency, 1369-1370
pancreatic function tests in, 1369, *see also website*
pancreatitis as, 1370-1373, 1370t-1371t, 1372f-1373f
pseudocyst as, 1373
tumor as, 1374, *see also website*
failure to thrive in, 148t
due to food allergy, 821-822
of gallbladder, 1415, *see also website*
general anesthesia and, *see website*
hypomagnesemia due to, *see website*
intestinal
acute appendicitis as, 1349-1355
adhesions as, 1287
anal fissure as, 1359
anorectal malformations as, 1355-1356, 1356f, 1357t, 1359t
Digestive system disorders *(Continued)*
atresia, stenosis, and malrotation as, 1277-1281, 1278f-1280f
bezoars as, 1291
chronic diarrhea as, 1339-1346
closed-loop obstruction as, 1287-1289
duplication as, 1281
eosinophilic gastroenteritis as, 1304
foreign bodies as, 1290, 1290f
functional abdominal pain as, 1346-1349, 1346t-1348t
functional constipation as, 1284, 1284t
gastroenteritis as, 1323-1339
(*See also* Gastroenteritis)
hemorrhoids as, 1360, 1361f
Hirschsprung disease as, 1283t, 1284-1287, 1285f-1286f
ileus as, 1287
inflammatory bowel disease as, 1294-1304, 1295t-1296t
inguinal hernia as, 1362-1368
intestinal neuronal dysplasia as, 1287, *see also website*
intussusception as, 1287-1289, 1289f
malabsorption as, 1304-1322
Meckel diverticulum and other remnants of omphalomesenteric duct as, 1281-1282, 1282f
motility disorders as, 1283-1287
peptic ulcer disease as, 1291-1294, 1291t, 1292f-1293f, 1293t
perianal abscess and fistula as, 1360, 1360f
pilonidal sinus and abscess as, 1362
pseudo-obstruction as, 1283-1284, 1283t
rectal mucosal prolapse as, 1361
superior mesenteric artery syndrome, 1287
of liver and biliary system
autoimmune hepatitis as, 1408-1410, 1408t, 1410f
biliary atresia as, 1385-1387, 1386f-1387f
cholestasis as, 1381-1388
cystic, 1415, *see also website*
drug- and toxin-induced injury as, 1410-1412, 1412t
evaluation of, 1379, 1380f
fulminant hepatic failure as, 1412-1415, 1414t
liver abscess as, 1404-1405, 1404f-1405f
liver transplantation for, 1415, *see also website*
manifestations of, 1374-1381, 1375t
metabolic, 1388-1393
mitochondrial hepatopathies as, 1405-1408, 1406t-1407t
portal hypertension and varices as, 1415, *see also website*
with systemic disorders, 1405, *see also website*
viral hepatitis as, 1393-1404
of newborn, 600-612
constipation as, 600
jaundice and hyperbilirubinemia as, 603-608
kernicterus as, 608-612
meconium ileus in cystic fibrosis as, 601, 601f
meconium peritonitis as, 601
meconium plugs as, 600-601, 600f
neonatal necrotizing enterocolitis as, 601-603, 602f, 602t
vomiting as, 600-601
with obesity, 184t
of oral cavity
associated with other conditions, 1251, 1251t, 1252f, 1253-1254
cleft lip and palate, 1252-1253, 1252f
dental caries, 1254-1256, 1255f-1256f
dental trauma, 1258-1259, 1258f-1259f, 1258t
diagnostic radiology in, 1261, *see also website*
malocclusion, 1252, *see also website*

Digestive system disorders *(Continued)*
periodontal, 1257-1258
of salivary glands and jaw, 1261, see also website
soft tissue lesions, 1259-1261, 1260f, 1260t
syndromes with manifestations in, 1252f, 1253-1254
of peritoneum
ascites as, 1416, see also website
chylous ascites as, 1416, see also website
epigastric hernia as, 1418, see also website
malformations as, 1416
peritonitis as, 1416-1418
in premature infants, 559t
psychopharmacology and, 65
signs and symptoms of
abdominal distention and abdominal masses, 1249
abdominal pain, 1247-1248, 1247t-1248t
anorexia, 1241-1242
constipation, 1245-1247, 1246t
diarrhea, 1243-1245, 1245t-1246t
dysphagia, 1240-1241, 1241t-1242t
gastrointestinal bleeding, 1248-1249, 1248t
regurgitation, 1241, 1242t
vomiting, 1242-1243, 1243t-1245t
sports participation and, 2402t-2404t
of stomach
bezoars as, 1291
eosinophilic gastroenteritis as, 1304
foreign bodies as, 1290
gastric duplication as, 1276
gastric outlet obstruction as, 1275-1276
gastric volvulus as, 1276
hypertrophic gastropathy as, 1276
peptic ulcer disease as, 1291-1294, 1291t, 1292f-1293f, 1293t
pyloric stenosis as, 1274-1275, 1274f-1275f
of teeth, 1249-1251, 1251t, 1254-1256
tuberculous, 1006
tumors as, 1362, see also website
due to whole-body irradiation, see website
Digestive system manifestations, 1241t
in celiac disease, 1309t
in Chagas disease, 1196
in chronic kidney disease, 1823t
in congenital disorders of glycosylation, see website
in cystic fibrosis, 1486-1487, 1487f
in factitious disorder by proxy, 146
in food adverse reactions, 820-821, 820t
in food allergy, 821-822
in multiple organ dysfunction syndrome, 312t
in mushroom poisoning, see website
in Neonatal Intensive Care Unit Neurobehavioral Scale, 624t
in oral cavity, 1251, 1251t, 1252f, 1253-1254
in poisoning, 252t
lead, 2450-2451
in systemic inflammatory response syndrome, 309t
with Turner syndrome, 1953
Digiband. *See* Digoxin-specific Fab antibodies
DigiFab. *See* Digoxin-specific Fab antibodies
Digit
fracture of, 2391
herpes simplex virus infection of, 1100, 1100f
infantile fibroma of, see website
sucking of, see website
trigger, 2387
Digital clubbing, see website
Digitalis
for heart failure, see website
poisoning with, 256t-257t
Digitalis purpurea, 272t-273t
Digits, centers of ossification appearance in, 29t
Digitus minimus varus, 2342
Digoxin
for arrhythmias, 1611t-1612t
for heart failure, see website
poisoning with, 262-263
Digoxin-specific Fab antibodies, 256t-257t, 262-263
Dihydrolipoyl dehydrogenase deficiency, 431
Dihydropyrimidinase (DPH) deficiency, see website
Dihydropyrimidine dehydrogenase (DPD) deficiency, see website
1,25Dihydroxycholecalciferol$_2$D$_3$ (1,25(OH)$_2$D$_3$), 1922, see also website
Dilated cardiomyopathy (DCM), 1629f, 1629t-1630t, 1630-1631
genetics of, see website
sudden death due to, 1620
Dilated fixed pupil, 2155-2156
Diloxanide furoate, 1180, 1180t, see also website
Diltiazem for pulmonary hypertension, 1602t
Dilution testing, see website
Dilution therapy for internal radiation contamination, see website
DIMD. *See* drug-induced movement disorders (DIMD)
Dimenhydrinate for motion sickness, 1244t
Dimension of Quality, see website
Dimercaprol
for arsenic and mercury intoxication, see website
for lead poisoning, 2453, 2453t
Dimercaptosuccinic acid (DMSA), 256t-257t, see also website
Dimercaptosuccinic acid (DMSA) renal scan, 1833, 1833f
Dimetapp. *See* Brompheniramine
Dimetapp Children's ND. *See* Loratadine
Dimorphous leprosy, see website
Dimples, skin, 2220
Dioxin exposure, see website
Diphallia, 1857
Diphenhydramine
for allergic rhinitis, 777t-778t
for anaphylaxis, 818t
for cyclic vomiting syndrome, 1244t
for pruritus in palliative care, 155t-156t
for urticaria, 814
Diphenoxylate, see website
Diphtheria, 929, see also website
testing for antibodies to, 719-720
Diphtheria, tetanus, pertussis (DPT) vaccine, see website
Diphtheria acellular pertussis (DTaP) vaccine, 884t, 947-948, 993
with *Haemophilus influenzae* type b vaccine (DTaP/Hib), 884t
hepatitis B-inactivated polio vaccine (DTaP-HepB-IPV), 884t
HIV infection and, 1173f
with inactivated polio vaccine and *Haemophilus influenzae* type b vaccine (DTaP-IPV/Hib), 884t
with inactivated polio vaccine (DTaP-IPV), 884t
recommended schedule for, 886, 887f
for travel, 891t, see also website
Diphtheria antitoxin, 882-883, 882t
Diphtheria toxoid, 884t
Diphtheria vaccine, 881t
Diphyllobothrium latum, 1232t, 1233-1234, 1234f, see also website
Diplegia, spastic, in cerebral palsy, 2062-2063, 2062t, 2063f
Diploid cells, 395, see also website
Diplopia, 2152
in neurologic examination, see website
Dipstick urinary test, 1799-1800
Dipylidium caninum, 1232t, 1234, see also website
Direct DNA-based mutation testing, 376, 377t
Direct fluorescent-antibody (DFA), see also website
in pertussis, 945-946
Directly observed therapy, 1007, see website
Dirty wound, perioperative prophylaxis and, see website
Disability in pediatric emergency assessment, 281
Disabled newborn, ethics in care of, see website
Disasters
humanitarian, see website
natural, drowning during, 343
preparedness for, see website
Disc edema, see website
Discharge
from hospital of premature or low birthweight infant, 563-564, 564t
nipple, see website
from nursery, 538, 538t
vaginal
pathologic, 711t
in vulvovaginitis, 1866
Discharge examination of newborn, 532
Discharge planning
for long-term mechanical ventilation, 331, 1525-1526
for psychiatric hospitalization, 66
Discipline for preschoolers, 36
Discoid lateral meniscus (DLM), 2352
Discoid lupus erythematosus (DLE), see website
Discoid rash in systemic lupus erythematosus, 842, 842f
Discourse problems, see website
Discreet Event Stimulation (DES), see website
Discrimination, chronic illness and, see website
Disease detection in well child care, 14
Disease-modifying antirheumatic drugs (DMARDs)
for juvenile idiopathic arthritis, 837, 838t
for rheumatic disease, see website
Disease prevention in well child care, 14
Disequilibrium syndrome, see website
Disimpaction, fecal, 74, 74t
Disintegrative disorder, 106, see also website
Disk herniation, 2377
as sports injury, 2412
Diskitis, 2376, 2376t
Disk space infection, 2376, 2376t
Dislocation
hip, with arthrogryposis, see website
patellar, 2355, 2415
of shoulder, 2410
Disomy, uniparental, 412-413, 413f
Disopyramide, 1611t-1612t
Disorders of sex development (DSD), 1958-1968, 1960f
diagnosis of, 1959t, 1961
etiologic classification of, 1959t
genetics of, see website
ovotesticular, 1968
revised nomenclature in, 1958-1959, 1959t
sex differentiation and, 1958-1959, 1960f
undescended testis in, 1859
46,XX, 1959t
46,XY, 1962
Dispatch center in transport medicine, see website
Disposition in pharmacokinetics, see website
Disruption birth defects, see website
Disruptive behavioral disorders, 96-100, 97t
in childhood and adolescence, 99-100
in infancy and toddlerhood, 99
Disseminated gonococcal infection (DGI), 937, 939
Disseminated intravascular coagulation (DIC), 1713-1714, 1713t, see also website
with meningococcus, 930-931
in newborn, 621
as oncologic emergency, see website
Disseminated tuberculosis, 998, 1004
Distal arthrogryposis, see website
Distal humeral fracture, 2392
Distal renal tubular acidosis, 208
Distention, abdominal, 1249
in Hirschsprung disease, 1285, 1285t
in malabsorption syndromes, 1305, 1306f

Distention, abdominal *(Continued)*
in newborn, 535-536, *see website*
nondigestive causes of, 1241t
Distraction for pain management, 370-371
Distress, fetal, 541-545, 542f, 543t, 544f, 545t
Distribution, drug, *see website*
Distributive shock, 285, 307t
clinical manifestations of, 308
defined, 305
hemodynamic variables in, 311t
pathophysiology of, 305
treatment of, 312
Diuretics
for acute renal failure, 1820
for heart failure, *see website*
for hypertension
of chronic kidney disease, 1825
systemic, 1645t
metabolic alkalosis due to, 236-237
Diurnal enuresis, 71
Diurnal incontinence, 73, 1847-1848, 1848f-1849f, 1848t
Divalproex, 64t
Diverticulitis, 1282
Diverticulum
bladder, *see website*
left ventricle, 1599-1600
Meckel, 1281-1282, 1282f
abdominal pain of, 1247t
urethral, 1847
Zenker, 1264
Divided attention, *see website*
Divorce, *see website*
Dizygotic twins, 553-554
Dizziness in ear disorders, *see website*
DKA. *See* Diabetic ketoacidosis (DKA)
DLBCL. *See* Diffuse large B-cell lymphoma (DLBCL)
DLCO. *See* Diffusing capacity for carbon monoxide (DLCO)
DLE. *See* Discoid lupus erythematosus (DLE)
DLM. *See* Discoid lateral meniscus (DLM)
DM. *See* Developmental Milestones (DM)
DMARDs. *See* Disease-modifying antirheumatic drugs (DMARDs)
DMD. *See* Duchenne muscular dystrophy (DMD)
DM gene, 2124
DMPA. *See* Medroxyprogesterone acetate (DMPA)
DMRT1 gene, *see website*
DMSA. *See* Dimercaptosuccinic acid (DMSA)
DNA
aCGH testing of, 376
in HIV infection, 1158
malignancy susceptibility associated with defects in repair of, *see website*
mitochondrial
(*See* Mitochondrial *entries*)
mitochondrial encephalomyopathy due to mutations of, 2066
in molecular genetics, *see website*
radiation injury to, *see website*
replication of, *see website*
in sudden infant death syndrome, 1427
transcription of, *see website*
DNA-based mutation testing, direct, 376, 377t
DNA11 gene, *see website*
DNAH5 gene, *see website*
DNA markers in neuromuscular disorders, 2110
DNA probes, *see website*
DNAR. *See* do-not-attempt-resuscitation (DNAR) order
DNA testing. *See* Genetic testing
Dobutamine
for cardiac output maintenance and post-resuscitation stabilization, 294t
for heart failure, *see website*
in neonatal resuscitation, 577
for shock, 313t
Docosahexaenoic acid (DHA), *see website*
Doctrine of double effect (DDE), *see website*
Documentation of female genital examination, *see website*
Docusate, 155t-156t
Dog allergens, 769
Dog bites, 2454-2460, 2455t-2456t
Dog heartworm, 1226
Dog-related attack, 2454
Dog roundworm, 1227-1229
Dog tapeworm, 1234, *see also website*
Doll's eyes reflex, *see website*
Domestic violence, *see website*
Dominant dystrophic epidermolysis bullosa (DDEB), 2246, 2246f
Dominant inheritance, autosomal, 383-385, 387f
Donor
for heart transplantation, *see website*
for hematopoietic stem cell transplantation, *see website*
haploidentical, *see website*
sibling, 757-760, 758t
unrelated, *see website*
for intestinal transplant, *see website*
for renal transplantation, *see website*
Do-not-attempt-resuscitation (DNAR) order, 153-154, *see website*
Dopamine, 1923-1924, *see also website*
for acute renal failure, 1820
for cardiac output maintenance and post-resuscitation stabilization, 294t
genetic disorders of, 445t
for heart failure, *see website*
in neonatal resuscitation, 577
for shock, 313t
Dopamine antagonists for vomiting, 1244t
Dopamine β-hydroxylase deficiency, 421f, 446
Dopamine hypothesis in attention deficit/hyperactivity disorder, *see website*
Dopamine 4 receptor gene, 108
Dopamine transfer gene, 108
Dopa-responsive dystonia (DRD), 445, 2059, 2060t
Doppler echocardiography, 1542-1543, 1544f
in coarctation of the aorta, 1568
in ventricular septal defect, 1557
Doribax. *See* Doripenem
Doripenem, *see website*
Dorsal hood, 1852, 1854
DORV. *See* Double-outlet right ventricle (DORV)
Dosages, *see also website*
for antiepileptics, 2029-2031, 2030t
chronic renal disease and, *see website*
radiation, *see website*
Doss porphyria, *see website*
Double aortic arch, 1596-1597, 1597f
fetal development of, 1528
"Double bubble" sign in duodenal obstruction, 1278, 1278f
Doublecortin, 2003
Double elevator palsy, 2160, 2160f
Double helix, *see website*
Double heterozygotes, 389
Double-inlet ventricle, 1592
Double-outlet right ventricle (DORV), 1582
with malposition of great arteries, 1588-1589
with pulmonary stenosis, 1588
Double quotidian fever, *see website*
Double vision, 2152
Doula, *see website*
Dowling-Meara, 2244, 2245f, 2245t
Down syndrome, 400-403, 401f
cervical spine abnormalities in, 2381-2382, 2382f
clinical features of, 402t
congenital heart disease with, 1531t, 1554, *see also website*
developmental milestones in, 402t
general anesthesia and, *see website*
genetics of, 400-403, 404t
health supervision in, 403t
hypothyroidism with, 1901
Down syndrome *(Continued)*
intellectual function in, 403f
leukemias with, 1738, 1738f
malformations in, *see website*
maternal age and, *see website*
microcephaly with, 2007t
obesity due to, 182t
pancytopenia in, 1689-1690
prenatal screening for, *see website*
self-help skills and, 403t
Doxazosin, 1645t
Doxorubicin
for cancer therapy, *see website*
for Wilms tumor, 1759
Doxtrocardia, 1596
Doxy. *See* Doxycycline
Doxycycline, *see also website*
for acne, 2325t
for brucellosis, 981t
for *Chlamydia trachomatis*, 1036
for cholera, 967t
for ehrlichioses, 1050
for gonococcal disease, 939
for louse-borne typhus, 1048
for Lyme disease, 1028t
for lymphogranuloma venereum, 1038
for malaria treatment and chemoprophylaxis, 1203t-1205t, 1207, 1207t, *see also website*
for murine typhus, 1047
for nontuberculosis mycobacteria, *see website*
for psittacosis, *see website*
for Q fever, 1052
for rickettsial disease, 1039t-1040t
for Rocky Mountain spotted fever, 1043
for scrub typhus, 1045
for sexually transmitted infections in adolescents, 712t
DPD. *See* Dihydropyrimidine dehydrogenase (DPD) deficiency
DPH. *See* Dihydropyrimidinase (DPH) deficiency
DPI. *See* Dry powder inhaler (DPI)
DPP10, *see website*
DQ molecules, 846, 1308-1309
in celiac disease, 1308
in type 1 diabetes mellitus, 1970-1971
Dracunculiasis, 1227, *see also website*
Drag queens and kings, 655
Dramamine. *See* Dimenhydrinate
Dravet syndrome, 2017, 2027-2028
DRD. *See* Dopa-responsive dystonia (DRD)
Dressings
for burn injury, 352, 352t
wet, 2216
DRESS syndrome, 827-828, 2244, *see also website*
DRI. *See* Dietary reference intakes (DRI)
Dronabinol in palliative care, 155t-156t
Drop attack, 2019
Droplet isolation, *see website*
Drowning, 341-348
as childhood injury, 24
epidemiology of, 342-343
etiology of, 341-342
as leading cause of death, 24
management of, 344-347
pathophysiology of, 343-344
prevention of, 347-348, 348t, *see also website*
prognosis for, 347
resuscitation for, 344-345
Drowsy state, *see website*
Drug(s)
absorption of, *see website*
acne induced by, 2326-2327, 2327f
acute intermittent porphyrias and, *see website*
adherence and compliance in, *see website*
administration and formulation of, *see website*
adverse reactions to, 824-828, *see also website*
acute liver failure due to, 1413
anaphylactic, 816-819, 816t
cutaneous manifestatations of, *see website*

Drug(s) *(Continued)*
HIV-related, 1166
in immunosuppressed patient, *see website*
urticaria in, 812t, 814
for allergic disorders, 568-569
for anesthesia, *see website*
for asthma, 791-798
for attention deficit/hyperactivity disorder, 110-112, 111t, 112f
autoimmune hemolytic anemias due to, 1681, 1681t
bioequivalence of, *see website*
breast-feeding and, 539t-540t, 540
cataracts due to, 2171
clearance of, *see website*
definitions of terms associated with, *see website*
diabetes mellitus associated with, 1986
distribution of, *see website*
dosages and regimens in, *see website*
chronic renal disease and, *see website*
drug absorption and, *see website*
drug distribution and, *see website*
drug-drug interactions in, *see website*
drug formulation and administration in, *see website*
drug metabolism and, *see website*
dystonias induced by, 2059
for fetal treatment, 550-552
for grief and loss, *see website*
gynecomastia due to, *see website*
for hyperlipidemia, 481-482, 481t
hypothyroidism due to, 1901
maternal use of, 546-547, 546t
metabolism of, *see website*
in premature and low birthweight infants, 353-354, 563t
migraine secondary to overuse of, 2046
monitoring drug levels in, *see website*
for mycobacterial infection, 996, *see also website*
neutropenia due to, 748-749, 749t
newborn brain injury due to, 568-569
for office emergencies, *see website*
ontogenic effects on, *see website*
for pain management, 362-370
performance enhancing, 2422-2423, 2423t
personalized medicine and, *see website*
pharmacodynamics in, *see website*
pharmacogenetics of (*See* Pharmacogenetics)
pharmacogenomics of (*See* Pharmacogenomics)
plasma concentration of, *see website*
poisoning with, 258-266
(*See also* Poisoning)
principles of, 250, *see also website*
for psychiatric disorders, 60-65
renal drug elimination and, *see website*
renal elimination of, *see website*
for respiratory distress syndrome, 586
for rheumatic disease, *see website*
surrogate endpoints and biomarkers in, *see website*
used in anesthesia, *see website*
for weight loss, 186, 187t
Drug abuse. *See* Substance abuse
Drug allergy, 824-828
Drug biotransformation, *see website*
Drug dosages, *see website*
Drug-drug interactions, *see website*
Drug eruptions, *see website*
Drug fever, HIV-related, *see website*
Drug hypersensitivity syndrome (DHS), 827t
Drug-induced adrenocortical insufficiency, 1927
Drug-induced hypersensitivity syndrome, 827-828, 827t
Drug-induced liver injury, 1410-1412, 1412t
Drug-induced lupus, 843-844, 844t, *see website*
Drug-induced movement disorders (DIMD), 2059
Drug-induced precocious puberty, 1894
Drug-induced thrombocytopenia, 1718
Drug monitoring, therapeutic, *see website*
Drug rash, *see website*
Drug receptors, *see website*
Drug regimen, *see website*
Drug transporters, *see website*
Drug withdrawal ,neonatal seizures due to, 2035
Drummond syndrome, 1319
Drusen of optic nerve, *see website*
"Dry crab yaws," *see website*
"Dry eye," 2165-2166
Dry mouth, *see website*
Dry powder inhaler (DPI), 796-798
DSD. *See* Disorders of sex development (DSD)
DSPD. *See* Delayed sleep phase disorder (DSPD)
DSRCT. *See* Desmoplastic small round cell tumor (DSRCT)
d4T. *See* Stavudine (d4T)
DTaP. *See* Diphtheria acellular pertussis (DTaP) vaccine
DTDST. *See* Diastrophic dysplasia sulfate transporter (DTDST), loss of
DTDST gene, *see website*
D-test, 913
d-TGA. *See* D-transposition of the great arteries (d-TGA)
D-transposition of the great arteries (d-TGA), 1585, 1585f
with intact ventricular septum, 1585-1587, 1586f
Dual oxidase maturation factor 2 (DUOXA2), *see website*
Dual porphyria, *see website*
Duane retraction syndrome, 2006
Duane syndrome, 2160
Dubin-Johnson syndrome, 1383t, 1391
Dubowitz syndrome, 1690
Duchenne muscular dystrophy (DMD), 2119-2123
chronic severe respiratory insufficiency with, 1519
clinical manifestations of, 2119-2120
cardiac, 1531t
diagnosis of, 2120-2121, 2120f-2121f
dilated cardiomyopathy with, 1630
genetic etiology and pathogenesis of, 2113t, 2121-2122, 2122f
laboratory findings in, 2120
treatment of, 2123
Ductal plate malformation, *see website*
Ductus arteriosis, *see also website*
fetal development of, 1527-1528
in neonatal circulation, 1527-1528
Duke criteria, 1624
Dulcolax for constipation, 155t-156t
DUMBBELS, 266
"Dumb" rabies, 1155
Duncan disease, 727
Epstein-Barr virus and, 1112
malignancy susceptibility associated with, *see website*
Dunnigan-type lipodystrophy, 2286
Duodenal aspirate in exocrine pancreatic function, 1307
Duodenal obstruction, 1277-1278, 1278f
DUOXA2. *See* Dual oxidase maturation factor 2 (DUOXA2)
Duplication
gastric, 1276
genetic, 406-407, 409t, *see also website*
congenital heart disease with, 1531t
intestinal, 1281
upper urinary tract, 1834-1835, 1835f
urethral, 1857-1858
vulvar, *see website*
Duplication cysts, esophageal, 1263-1264
Dural ectasia in Marfan syndrome, 2442-2443
Duration of pain, 2332t
Duricef. *See* Cefadroxil
Dust mite allergens, 768-769, 769t
Dutch fever, 857-858
DVT. *See* Deep vein thrombosis (DVT)
Dwarfism
cardiac manifestations of, 1531t
neonatal, *see website*
pituitary, 627
short-limbed, 733
Dwarf tapeworm, 1234, *see also website*
Dye studies in aspiration syndromes, 1472t
Dynamic compliance (C_{DYN}) assessment in mechanical ventilation, 328
Dynapen. *See* Dicloxacillin
DYNC2H1 gene, *see website*
Dyneins, *see website*
Dysarthria, 118-119
Dysautonomia, familial, 2142
fever of unknown origin due to dysfunction of, 901
Dysbetalipoproteinemia, familial, 473t, 476
Dyscalculia, *see website*
Dyschondrosteosis, Leri-Weil, 388-389
Dyscoria, 2155
Dysdiadochokinesia, *see website*
Dysentery
bacterial, 1331-1332, 1332t
Plesiomonas shigelloides, *see website*
Shigella, 959-961
DYSF gene, 2126
Dysfibrinogenemia, 1704
Dysfluency (stuttering, stammering), 34, 122, 122t
Dysfunction Voiding Symptom Score, 1848, 1848f
Dysgenesis
mixed gonadal, 1954-1955
muscular, 2119
posterior fossa, 2006-2007
renal, 1827-1828
testicular, 1945
thyroid, 1895-1896
Dysgerminoma, 1770, 1872t
Dysgraphia, *see website*
Dyshidrotic eczema, 2253, 2253f
Dyshidrotic pompholyx, 2253
Dyshormonogenesis, 1896
Dyskeratosis congenita (DC), 748t, 1687-1689, 1688f, 2222, 2222f
stem cell transplantation for, 759
Dyskinesia
biliary, *see website*
paroxysmal, *see website*
primary ciliary, 1497, *see also website*
Dyskinetic cerebral palsy, 2063-2064
Dyslexia, 112-114, 113f
Dyslipidemia
with obesity, 184t
with type 2 diabetes mellitus, 1993t
Dysmenorrhea, 690-691, 691t
Dysmetria, *see also website*
ocular motor, 2162
Dysmorphology, 629, *see also website*. *See also* Congenital anomalies
in lysosomal storage disorders, 485t
Dysmotility, esophageal, 1264-1265, 1265f
Dysostosis multiplex, 511, 513f
Dyspepsia
abdominal pain of, 1247t
functional, 1346t
Dysphagia, 1240-1241, 1241t-1242t, *see also website*
neurologic examination of, *see website*
due to obstructing and motility disorders of esophagus, 1263
treatment of in palliative care, 157t
Dysphagia lusoria, 1264
Dysphasia, developmental, 117
Dysplasia, *see website*
bronchopulmonary, 1516, *see also website*
general anesthesia and, *see website*
due to mechanical ventilation for respiratory distress syndrome, 585, 587-588
chondroectodermal, 2433-2434

Dysplasia *(Continued)*
cleidocranial, 2431, 2432f
oral manifestations of, 1254
congenital nail, 2293
developmental of hip, 2356, 2357f-2359f
ectodermal, 2222-2223, 2223f, 2223t
oral manifestations of, 1254
focal cortical, 2004
focal facial ectodermal, 2222
intestinal epithelial, 1341
intestinal neuronal, 1286
lymphatic, 1724
polyostotic fibrous, precocious puberty due to, 1892, 1892f
renal, 1827-1828
Schimke immunoosseous, 1690
septo-optic, 527
diabetes insipidus with, 1883
skeletal (*See* Skeletal dysplasias)
Dysplexia, 2154
Dyspnea
as manifestation of extrapulmonary disease, 1526, *see also website*
in palliative care, 157
nonpharmacologic treatment of, 157t
pharmacologic treatment of, 155t-156t
Dyspraxia, 116, *see website*
Dysthymic disorder, 87, 87t
Dystonia, 2058-2059, 2060t
autosomal recessive dopa-responsive, 445
Dystonia musculorum deformans, 2059
Dystrophic epidermolysis bullosa (DEB), 2246, 2246f-2247f
Dystrophin in Duchenne and Becker muscular dystrophy, 2121, 2121f-2122f
DYT1 gene, 2059

E
EA. *See* Esophageal atresia (EA)
EAEC. *See* Enteroaggregative *Escherichia coli* (EAEC)
Eagle-Barrett syndrome, 1845
E2A-PBX1 oncogene, *see website*
EAR. *See* Estimated average requirement (EAR)
Ear
low-set, *see website*
newborn assessment of, 534
Ear disorders
clinical manifestations of, 2188, *see also website*
congenital malformations as, 2196, *see also website*
external otitis as, 2196-2199, 2198f
facial paralysis due to, *see website*
hearing loss as, 2188-2196
clinical audiologic evaluation of, 2193-2196
effects of, 2190-2192, 2191t
etiology of, 2188-2190, 2189t-2191t, 2191f
genetic counseling in, 2196
identification of, 2192, 2193t
incidence and prevalence of, 2188
screening for, 2192, 2192f
treatment of, 2196, 2196t
types of, 2188
of inner ear and bony labyrinth, 2213, *see also website*
in mucopolysaccharidoses, 515t
nontuberculous mycobacterial infection, 1012t
otitis media as, 2199-2213
adenoidectomy for, 2213
clinical manifestations of, 2202
definition of, 2199t
developmental sequelae of, 2213
diagnosis of, 2203-2204, 2203f-2204f
epidemiology of, 2200-2201
etiology of, 2201
examination of eardrum in, 2202-2205
Haemophilus influenzae in, 943
intracranial complications of, 2211-2212
Moraxella catarrhalis in, *see website*
pathogenesis of, 2201-2202
Ear disorders *(Continued)*
physical sequelae of, 2212-2213
prevention of, 2213
treatment of, 2205-2209, 2205t, 2206f-2207f, 2207t, 2209t
otitis media with effusion as
complications of, 2210-2211, 2210f-2212f, 2210t
etiology of, 2201
management of, 2209-2211, 2209t
tympanometry in, 2194-2195
physical examination in, *see website*
Toxoplasmosis gondii in, 1213
traumatic injury as, 2213-2214, *see also website*
tumors as, 2214, *see also website*
Eardrum
examination of, 2202-2205
retraction of, *see website*
Early adolescence
growth and development during, 649-653, 650t
biologic, 649, 650t-652t, 651f-652f
cognitive and moral, 649-651
implications for pediatricians and parents, 653
relationships with family, peers, and society, 652-653
self-concept, 651-652
sexuality, 653
Early childhood, well child care in, 16
Early childhood caries (ECC), 1255, 1255f
Early epileptic infantile encephalopathy (EEIE), 2023
Early exfoliation in dental development, *see website*
Early myoclonic infantile encephalopathy (EMIE), 2023
East African trypanosomiasis, 1190-1193, *see also website*
Eastern equine encephalitis (EEE), 1141, 1143-1144
EAST syndrome, 223, 237, *see also website*
Eating
foreign-born adoptees and, 131
at home, 166-167, 167t
at school, 167
Eating disorders, 90-96
clinical manifestations of, 91, 92t-94t
complications of, 91-93
definitions associated with, 90, 90t
differential diagnosis, 91
epidemiology of, 90-91
in female athlete, 2422
laboratory findings in, 91
pathology and pathogenesis of, *see website*
prevention of, 96
prognosis for, 96
sports participation and, 2402t-2404t
treatment of, 93-96, 95t
in type 1 diabetes mellitus, 1986-1987
Eating out, 167
Eaton-Lambert syndrome, 2133
EB. *See* Epidermolysis bullosa (EB)
Ebola hemorrhagic fever, 1151-1152
EBS. *See* Epidermolysis bullosa simplex (EBS)
Ebstein anomaly of the tricuspid valve, 1583-1585, 1584f
embryonic development of, 1527
EBV. *See* Epstein-Barr virus (EBV)
ECC. *See* Early childhood caries (ECC)
Ecchymosis, 2184
Eccrine sweat glands
disorders of, 2286-2288, 2287f, 2287t
morphology of, *see website*
ECF. *See* Extracellular fluid (ECF)
ECG. *See* Electrocardiography (ECG)
Echinacea, 1436
Echinocandins, *see website*
Echinococcus granulosus, 1232t, 1237-1239, 1238f, *see also website*
Echinococcus multilocularis, 1232t, 1237-1239, *see also website*
Echocardiography, 1541-1545
in atrioventricular defect, 1555, 1555f
in coarctation of the aorta, 1568, 1569f
Doppler, 1542-1543, 1544f
fetal, 1544-1545, 1544f
genetic counseling and, *see website*
in heart failure, *see website*
in Kawasaki disease, 865
M-mode, 1541, 1542f
in ostium secundum defect, 1552, 1552f
in patent ductus arteriosus, 1559-1560, 1560f
in pulmonary valve stenosis, 1562-1563, 1563f
in tetralogy of Fallot, 1575, 1575f
three-dimensional, 1543, 1544f
in total anomalous pulmonary venous return, 1589-1590, 1590f
transesophageal, 1541, 1543-1544
in tricuspid atresia, 1580, 1581f
two-dimensional, 1541-1542, 1542f-1543f, 1573
in ventricular septal defect, 1556f, 1557
Echovirus, 1088t
Eclampsia, *see also website*
maternal diabetes mellitus and, 545
ECMO. *See* Extracorporeal membrane oxygenation (ECMO)
Ecologic model of development, *see website*
Economic factors. *See* Socioeconomic factors
ECP. *See* Eosinophil cationic protein (ECP)
Ecstasy, 682
Ecthyma, 2303, 2303f
Ecthyma gangrenosum, 2303
Pseudomonas aeruginosa, 975, 976t
Ectodermal dysplasia (ED), 2222-2223, 2223f, 2223t
of face, 2222
oral manifestations of, 1254
Ectopia cordis, 1599
Ectopia lentis, 2171-2172, 2172f
homocystinuria, 425-426
Ectopic anus, 1357
Ectopic kidney, 1828, 1829f
Ectopic pancreatic rests, *see website*
Ectopic tachycardia
atrial, 1615
junctional, 1615, 1616t
Ectopic undescended testis, 1859
Ectopic ureter, 1842-1843, 1842f
incontinence due to, 1850-1851, 1850f-1851f
Ectopic ureterocele, 1843, 1843f
prolapsed, 1858, 1858f
Ectropion, 2163-2164
Eczema
atopic, 801-807
dyshidrotic, 2253, 2253f
immunodeficiency with thrombocytopenia and, 734-735
nummular, 2252, 2252f
Eczema herpeticum, 1100, 1100f, 1103
atopic dermatitis with, 806
Eczematous disorders, 2249-2254
contact dermatitis as, 2250-2252, 2250f-2251f
of external ear canal, 2199
lichen simplex chronicus as, 2252, 2253f
nummular, 2252, 2252f
pityriasis alba as, 2252, 2252f
seborrheic dermatitis as, 2253-2254, 2253f-2254f
vesicular hand and foot dermatitis as, 2253, 2253f
Eczema vaccinatum, atopic dermatitis with, 806
ED. *See* Ectodermal dysplasia (ED); Emergency department (ED)
Edema
acute hemorrhagic, 870
cerebral
with fulminant hepatic failure, 1414
due to type 1 diabetes mellitus, 1981

Edema *(Continued)*
disc, *see website*
eyelid, traumatic, 2184
heat, 2420
laryngeal in hereditary angioedema, 815
in nephrotic syndrome, 1802, 1804-1805
in newborn, 532-533, 622
peripheral, physical examination of, 1531
pulmonary, 1468-1469, 1468t-1469t
Edematous malnutrition, 175
Edinburgh Postnatal Depression Scale, *see website*
Edrophonium chloride, in myasthenia gravis diagnosis, 2134
EDS. *See* Ehlers-Danlos syndrome (EDS); Excessive daytime sleepiness (EDS)
Education
abstinence-only sex, 701-702
children born to teen mothers and, 701
continuing, for emergency medical services for children, *see website*
foster care children and, *see website*
for injury prevention, 20, 20t
in intellectual disability, 128
patient and family (*See* Patient and family education)
sexual, for special needs girls, 1874
Educational diagnostician, *see website*
Educational outreach in transport medicine, *see website*
Edwardsiella tarda, 1298t
Edward syndrome, 2007t
EEE. *See* Eastern Equine encephalitis (EEE)
EEG. *See* Electroencephalography (EEG)
EEIE. *See* Early epileptic infantile encephalopathy (EEIE)
EER. *See* Estimated energy requirement (EER)
EF. *See* Executive functioning (EF)
Efavirenz
drug interactions with, *see website*
for HIV infection, 1168t-1171t
EFE. *See* Endocardial fibroelastosis (EFE)
Effective dose, radiation, *see website*
Effectiveness in quality of care, *see website*
Effectors of respiration, *see website*
Effexor. *See* Venlafaxine
Efficiency in quality of care, *see website*
Effusion
middle-ear, 2199-2200
otitis media with, 2199-2200
complications of, 2210-2211, 2210f-2212f, 2210t
etiology of, 2201
management of, 2209-2211, 2209t
tympanometry in, 2194-2195
pericardial tuberculous, 1009
pleural
with pneumonia, 1479, 1479t
tansudative, 1513
tuberculous, 1003-1004, 1004f
EFHC1 gene, 2016t
Eflornithine, *see website*
EGFR gene, *see website*
Egg allergy, 821, 821t
Egocentrism, 34
EHEC. *See* Enterohemorrhagic *Escherichia coli* (EHEC)
Ehlers-Danlos syndrome (EDS), 1722, 2278
cardiac manifestations of, 1532t
sports participation and, 2402t-2404t
Ehrlichiosis, 1039t-1040t, 1048-1050, 1050f
maternal, *see website*
EhROM1. *See Entamoebe histolytica* rhomboid protease 1 (EhROM1)
Eicosapentaenoic acid (EPA), *see website*
EIEC. *See* Enteroinvasive *Escherichia coli* (EIEC)
8 Millennium Development Goals (MDGs), 1, 173-174
Eisenmenger syndrome, 1601-1602
EITB. *See* Enzyme-linked immunotransfer blot (EITB)
Ejection clicks, 1533-1535
Ekiri syndrome, 960
EKV. *See* Erythrokeratoderma variabillis (EKV)
Elastance, respiratory, 322
Elastase, fecal, 1307, 1369
Elastase concentration in chronic diarrhea, 1344t
Elastic recoil, pulmonary, *see website*
Elastic work, *see website*
Elastolysis, generalized, 2277-2278
Elastosis perforans serpiginosa (EPS), 2279, 2279f
Elavil. *See* Amitriptyline
Elbow
arthrogryposis involving, *see website*
fracture around, 2392
musculoskeletal pain syndrome of, 877t
orthopedic disorders of, 2383-2384, 2383f-2384f, 2384t
sports injury to, 2410-2412, 2411f-2412f
Electrical burns, 356, 357t
Electrocardiography (ECG), 1537
in atrioventricular defect, 1555, 1555f
in brain death diagnosis, *see website*
in congenital hypothyroidism, 1900
in congenital intestinal pseudo-obstruction, 1283t
developmental changes on, 1537-1539, 1538f-1539f
exercise, 1545
follow open heart surgery, 1604
in hypokalemia, 224
in neuromuscular disorders, 2112
in poisonings, 254, 254t
with tricyclic antidepressants, 251t, 264
P-R and Q-T intervals on, 1540, 1540f
in pulmonary atresia, 1579
in pulmonary embolism, 1502
P waves on, 1539, 1539f
QRS complex on, 1539-1540, 1540f
rate and rhythm on, 1539
ST segment and T-wave abnormalities on, 1540, 1541f
in tetralogy of Fallot, 1575
twenty-four hour recordings in supraventricular tachycardia, 1614-1615
in Wolff-Parkinson-White syndrome, 1613-1614, 1614f
Electroencephalography (EEG)
in febrile seizure, 2018
in hypoxic-ischemic encephalopathy, 571, 571t
in intellectual disability, 127t
in neurologic assessment, *see website*
in seizures, 2021, 2022f
neonatal, 2035
Electrolytes
absorption disorders of, 1319
composition of in fluid compartments, *see website*
for diarrheagenic *Escherichia coli*, 964
magnesium as, 224-225, *see also website*
in maintenance fluids, 243, 243t
for chronic kidney disease, 1823-1824
variations in, 244
measurement of in intravenous rehydration, 247
phosphorus as, 225-229
disorders of, 226-229
metabolism of, 225-226
potassium as, 219-224
disorders of, 219-224
metabolism of, 219
sodium as, 212-219
disorders of, 212-219
metabolism of, 212
Electromyography (EMG)
in botulism, 989
in juvenile dermatomyositis, 848
in neuromuscular disorders, 2110t, 2111
Electron transfer flavoprotein dehydrogenase (ETF-DH) deficiency, 461
Electron transfer flavoprotein (ETF) deficiency, 461
Electrophysiology studies in heart failure management, *see website*
Elemental mercury exposure, *see website*
"Elephant ear" toxicity, 269t
Eletriptan, 2044t
Elfornithine, 1192
ELIFA. *See* Enzyme-linked immunofiltration test (ELIFA)
Elimination. *See* Excretion
Elimination half-life ($T_{1/2}$) of drug, *see website*
ELISA. *See* Enzyme-linked immunosorbent assay (ELISA)
ELISPOT. *See* Enzyme-linked immunospot (ELISPOT) assay
Elliptocytosis, hereditary, 1661f, 1662
Ellis-van Creveld syndrome, 2433-2434, 2434f
congenital heart disease with, 1531t, *see website*
EM. *See* Erythema multiforme (EM)
Emancipated youth, 664-665
Embolism, pulmonary, 1500-1502, 1501t, 1709
air, 597
cardiac arrest due to, 289t
Embryonal brain tumor, 1751-1752, 1751f
Embryonal rhabdomyosarcoma, 1760
Embryonic development, *see website*
Embryonic hemoglobins, *see website*
Embryonic testicular regression syndrome, 1963
Embryoscopy, 543t
EMC-1 gene, 2276
Emedastine difumarate, 811t
Emergence from anesthesia, *see website*
Emergency contraception, 698-699, 698t, 704t
Emergency defibrillation, 291-292, 293f
Emergency department (ED)
asthma and, 781, 799
care of children in, *see website*
transport of child from, *see website*
visits by adolescents, 663
visits due to injury, 19, 19f
Emergency(ies), 279-296
airway management techniques for, 284-285
airway narrowing as, 283-284
airway obstruction as, 282-283, 282f-283f
bradyarrhythmias and tachyarrhythmias as, 287-289, 288f, 290f
burn injury as, 350-351, 350f, 350t
cardiac arrests as, 289-292
cardiopulmonary resuscitation for, 289-292, 291f-293f, 294t
delivery room, 575-579
general assessment in, 279, 280f
humanitarian, *see website*
hypertensive, 1646t
hyponatremia as, 1886
neurologic, 296-304
abusive head trauma as, 301
brain death as, 304, *see website*
care principles in, 296-297, 297f
hypoxic-ischemic insult and encephalopathy as, 301-303, 302f
intracerebral hemorrhage as, 303-304
status epilepticus as, 303
stroke as, 303-304
traumatic brain injury as, 297-301, 298f-301f
oncologic, *see website*
parenchymal lung disease as, 284
pericardiocentesis for, 295-296
post-resuscitation care after, 296
primary assessment in, 279-281, 280t-281t
secondary assessment in, 281
shock as, 285-286
tertiary assessment in, 281-282
thoracentesis and chest tube placement for, 295
vascular access for, 292-294, 295f-296f
Emergency medical services for children (EMSC), 278, *see also website*

Emergency medical technicians (EMTs), *see website*
Emergency Triage Assessment and Treatment (ETAT), *see website*
Emery-Dreifuss muscular dystrophy, 2113t, 2123
Emesis. *See* Vomiting
EMG. *See* Electromyography (EMG)
EMIE. *See* Early myoclonic infantile encephalopathy (EMIE)
EMLA. *See* Eutectic mixture of local anesthetics (EMLA)
Emmetropia, 2150-2151
Emotional development, *see also website*
  age 0-2 months, 27-28
  age 2-6 months, 30
  age 6-12 months, 30-31
  age 12-18 months, 31
  age 18-24 months, 32
  in foreign-born adoptees, 131
  during middle childhood, 38
  during preschool years, 35-36
Emotion-focused coping, 1985-1986
Empacho, *see website*
Emphysema, 1460-1462, 1507-1509
  α-antitrypsin deficiency and, 1462-1463, *see also website*
  bullous, 1462, 1462f
  congenital lobar, 1461, 1461f
  neonatal pulmonary interstitial, 597-599, 598f
  overinflation and, 1460-1462
Empirical antireflux therapy, 1267-1268
Empirical use of antibacterial agents, *see website*
Employee. *See* Health care providers
EMSC. *See* Emergency medical services for children (EMSC)
EMT-P. *See* Paramedics (EMT-P)
Emtricitabine, 1168t-1171t
Emtriva. *See* Emtricitabine
EMTs. *See* Emergency medical technicians (EMTs)
E-Mycin. *See* Erythromycin
Enalapril
  for heart failure, *see website*
  for systemic hypertension, 1645t
Enamel, injuries to, 1258t
Encephalitic rabies, 1154-1155
Encephalitis
  arboviral
    in North America, 1141-1144, 1142f-1143f
    outside North America, 1144-1147, 1145t
  California, 1142-1143
  Eastern equine, 1141, 1143-1144
  enteroviral, 1091
  following rubella, 1077
  herpes, 1101, 1103
  imaging studies in, *see website*
  Japanese, 1145
    vaccine for, 891t, *see website*
  La Crosse, 1142-1144
  measles, 1072, 1072t
  microcephaly with, 2007t
  Rasmussen's, 2023
  St. Louis, 1141, 1143-1144
  tick-borne, 1146
  varicella-zoster virus, 1109
  Venezuelan equine, 1144-1147
  Western equine, 1141, 1143-1144
  West Nile, 1142-1144, 1142f-1143f
Encephalitozoon cuniculi, *see website*
Encephalitozoon hellem, *see website*
Encephalocele, 2002-2003
  intranasal, 1431
Encephalomyelitis, acute disseminated, 2079, 2079f, 2080t
Encephalomyelopathy, subacute necrotizing, 506-509
Encephalomyopathy, subacute necrotizing, 2067
Encephalopathy, 2061-2069
  burn, 2068
  due to cat-scratch disease, 985
  cerebral palsy as, 2061-2065
Encephalopathy *(Continued)*
  early epileptic infantile, 2023
  early myoclonic infantile, 2023
  epileptic, 2013
  glycine, 439-440
  hepatic, 1376-1377, 1414t
  HIV, 1164, 2068
  hypertensive, 2068
    strokelike events *versus*, 2086
  hypoxic-ischemic, 298f-299f, 301-303, 302f, 569-573, 569t-570t
    microcephaly with, 2007t
    seizure due to, 2034
    strokelike events *versus*, 2085
  lethal toxic, 960
  Lyme, 1027
  mitochondrial, 2065-2068, 2065t
  radiation, 2068-2069
  transmissible spongiform, 1177, *see also website*
  vaccine, febrile seizures with, 2017
  Wernicke, 192
  Zellweger syndrome as, 2069
Encopresis, 73-75, 74f, 74t
Encounters, cultural, *see website*
En coup de sabre, 851t, 852f, 2276
Endemic Burkitt lymphoma, 1111, 1112t
Endemic cretinism, 1907
Endemic goiter
  cretinism and, 1906-1908
  maternal, *see website*
Endemic syphilis, 1023, *see also website*
End-gaze nystagmus, *see website*
Endocardial cushion defect, 1554-1556
  in adults, 1607
Endocardial fibroelastosis (EFE), 1566, 1633-1634
Endocarditis
  in acute rheumatic fever, 922
  Bartonella, 983t, 987
  due to coagulase-negative staphylococci, 910
  infective, 1622-1626
    acute rheumatic fever *versus*, 923, 923t
    clinical manifestations of, 1623, 1623t
    congenital heart disease and, 1609
    diagnosis of, 1623-1624, 1624t
    epidemiology of, 1622-1623
    etiology of, 1622, 1622t
    prevention of, 1626, 1626t
    prognosis and complications of, 1624
    retinopathy associated with, 2180
    in tetralogy of Fallot, 1576
    treatment of, 1624-1626, 1625t
  prophylaxis, 1609
    in Marfan syndrome, 2445
  Pseudomonas aeruginosa, 976t
  Staphylococcus aureus, 905
Endochondral ossification, *see website*
Endocrine disorders
  of adrenal glands
    adrenocortical insufficiency as, 1924-1930
    adrenocortical tumors as, 1941
    congenital adrenal hyperplasia and related disorders as, 1930-1939
    Cushing syndrome as, 1939-1941, 1939t
    masses as, 1943
    pheochromocytoma as, 1941-1943
    primary aldosteronism as, 1941
  cardiac manifestations of, 1531t
  diabetes mellitus as (*See* Diabetes mellitus (DM))
  disorders of sex development as, 1958-1968
  failure to thrive in, 148t
  fetal therapy for, 551t
  general anesthesia and, *see website*
  gonadal
    gynecomastia as, 1950-1951
    hypofunction of ovaries as, 1951-1957
    hypofunction of testes as, 1943-1950
    pseudoprecocity resulting from ovarian lesions as, 1957-1958
Endocrine disorders *(Continued)*
    pseudoprecocity resulting from testicular tumors as, 1950, *see also website*
  hypoglycemia associated with, 527-528
  of hypothalamus and pituitary gland
    diabetes insipidus as, 1881-1884
    hyperpituitarism, tall stature, and overgrowth syndromes as, 1886, *see also website*
    hyponatremia as, 1884-1886
    hypopituitarism as, 1876-1881
    pubertal development disorders as, 1886-1894
  liver disease with, 1377
  in myotonic muscular dystrophy, 2124
  in newborn, 627-629
  obesity and, 182t, 184t, 185
  of parathyroid gland
    hyperparathyroidism as, 1920-1923
    hypoparathyroidism as, 1916-1919
    pseudohypoparathyroidism (Albright hereditary osteodystrophy) as, 1919-1920
  in premature infants, 559t
  systemic inflammatory response syndrome and, 309t
  of thyroid gland
    carcinoma of thyroid as, 1914-1916
    goiter as, 1905-1909
    hyperthyroidism as, 1909-1913
    hypothyroidism as, 1895-1903
    thyroiditis as, 1903-1905
    thyroxine-binding globulin defects as, 1894-1895, *see also website*
  due to toxoplasmosis, 1211-1212
Endocrine myopathy, 2129-2130
Endocrine system
  chemical pollutants effect on, *see website*
  hormones of hypothalamus and pituitary gland in, 1876, *see also website*
  lysosomal storage disorders and, 485t
  multiple organ dysfunction syndrome and, 312t
  overweight and obesity and, 183, 183f
  in physiology of puberty, 1886, *see also website*
Endodermal sinus tumor, vaginal, 1873
Endodontic therapy, 1258
Endometrial polyps, 689t-690t
Endometrial stroma sarcoma, 1873
Endometrioma, 1871
Endometriosis, 690-691, 691t
Endometritis, 690
Endometrium, amenorrhea and, 688
Endophthalmitis, 2167t
  in candidiasis, 1054
  Pseudomonas aeruginosa, 976t
Endoscopic repair of vesicoureteral reflux, 1837f, 1838
Endoscopic retrograde cholangiopancreatography (ERCP), 1379
Endoscopy
  in cystic fibrosis treatment, 1493
  in esophageal varices, *see website*
  in gastroesophageal reflux disease, 1267, 1268f
  in sinusitis, 1437
  in ulcerative colitis, 1297-1298
Endotoxin, *Neisseria meningitidis*, 930
Endotracheal intubation
  aspirate diagnostic microbiology, *see website*
  for asthma exacerbation, 800
  complications of in newborn, 586-587
  for congenital diaphragmatic hernia, 595
  in infant botulism, 990
  for infectious acute upper airway obstruction, 1448
  manual ventilation before and after, 320-321
  medications for placement of, 321t
  in neonatal resuscitation, 575-576, 576t
  placement of, 285, 286f, 287t

Endotracheal intubation *(Continued)*
for respiratory distress and failure, 320
size and depth dimensions for, 320t
End-stage renal disease, 1825-1826, 1826t
due to diabetic nephropathy, 1988
kidney transplantation for (*See* Kidney transplantation)
Enema
barium
in Hirschsprung disease, 1285f-1286f, 1286
in ulcerative colitis, 1297, 1299f
for constipation in palliative care, 155t-156t
for constipation maintenance therapy, 74t
for fecal disimpaction, 74t
Energy requirements, *see website*
Enfalyte, 1335t
Enfuvirtide, 1168t-1171t
ENL. *See* Erythema nodosum leprosum (ENL) reactions
Enlargement of cardiac chambers, 1537
ENPP1 gene mutation, 182t
Entamoebe histolytica, 1178-1180, *see also website*
gastroenteritis due to, 1327t-1328t
treatment of, 1337t
inflammatory bowel disease *versus*, 1298t
in traveler's diarrhea, 1338t
Entamoebe histolytica rhomboid protease 1 (EhROM1), 1178-1179
Enteral feeding
for acute gastroenteritis, 1334-1336
for Crohn disease, 1303
Enteric adenoviruses, 1135
Enteric anendocrinosis, 1306t, 1311
Enteric fever, 954-958
clinical features of, 955-956, 956f, 956t
complications of, 956, 957t
diagnosis of, 956-957
differential diagnosis of, 957
epidemiology of, 954
etiology of, 954
pathogenesis of, 954-955, 955f
prevention of, 958
treatment of, 957-958, 958t
Enteric hyperoxaluria, 440
urinary lithiasis with, *see website*
Enteric infection, chronic diarrhea due to, 1340
Enteric string test, 1223-1224
Enteritis. *See* Gastroenteritis regional (*See* Crohn's disease)
Enteritis necroticans, *see website*
Enteroaggregative *Escherichia coli* (EAEC), 962t, 963-964
Enterobacter, neonatal, 632t
sepsis due to, 635t-636t
Enterobiasis, 1222, 1222f, *see also website*
Enterobius vermicularis, 1222, 1222f, *see also website*
in vulvovaginitis, 1868t
Enterococcus, 928, *see also website*
neonatal, 632t
sepsis due to, 635t
vancomycin-resistant, *see website*
Enterocolitis
neonatal necrotizing, 569, 601-603, 602f, 602t
Staphylococcus aureus in, 905-906
Enterocolonic fistula with Crohn disease, 1300-1301
Enterocystoplasty, *see website*
Enterocyte defects, chronic diarrhea due to, 1341
Enterocyte heparin sulfate deficiency, 1311
Enterocytozoon species, *see website*
Enteroenteric fistula with Crohn disease, 1300-1301
Enterohemorrhagic *Escherichia coli* (EHEC), 1324t-1325t
Enteroinvasive *Escherichia coli* (EIEC), 962, 962t, 1337t
Enterokinase deficiency, 1306t, 1317-1318
Enteropathogenic *Escherichia coli* (EPEC), 962-963, 962t, 1337t
Enteropathy
autoimmune, 1305-1306, 1341
food protein-induced, 821
gluten-sensitivity, 1308-1311, 1308f, 1309t-1310t, 1310f
protein-losing, 1307, 1312t
due to malrotation, 1280-1281
tufting, 1306t, 1311
Enteropeptidase deficiency, 1317-1318
Entero-Test, 1223-1224
Enterotoxigenic *Escherichia coli* (ETEC), 962, 962t, 1324t-1325t, 1330
in traveler's diarrhea, 1338t
treatment of, 1337t
Enterotoxin
Bacillus cereus, 1324t-1325t
in infectious diarrhea, 1330-1332, 1331f
shiga, 959
Staphylococcus aureus, 904, 1324t-1325t
Enteroviruses, 1088-1094
clinical manifestations of, 1089-1092, 1090f
complications and prognosis for, 1094
diagnosis of, 1092-1093
differential diagnosis of, 1093, 1093t
epidemiology of, 1088
etiology of, 1088, 1088t
pathogenesis of, 1088-1089
in pneumonia, 1475t
poliovirus *versus*, 1085t
prevention of, 1094
treatment of, 1093-1094
in type 1 diabetes mellitus development, 1971
in viral meningoencephalitis, 2095
Enthesitis-related arthritis (ERA), 839, *see also website*
in juvenile idiopathic arthritis, 831t
in reactive arthritis, 840, 840f
Entropion, 2163-2164
Entry inhibitors for HIV infection, 1168t-1171t
Enuresis, 71-73, 72t-73t
nocturnal, 1851-1852, 1851t
Envenomations, 2460-2465
general approach to, 2460-2461
hemolytic anemia secondary to, *see website*
due to hymenoptera sting, 2464
marine, 2464-2465
due to scorpion sting, 2464
due to snake bite, 2461-2462, 2461f-2462f, 2461t-2462t
due to spider bite, 2462-2463, 2463f
Environment
food, 167, 168f
modification for injury prevention, 20, 20t
in trauma survey, 337
Environmental control measures
for allergic disease, 768-770, 769t
for asthma, 788-789, 791t
for infection prevention, *see website*
Environmental exposures in childhood cancers, 1725
Environmental factors
in acute lymphocytic leukemia, 1732t
in allergic disease, 764-765
in asthma, 781
in childhood injuries, 21
in genetics, *see website*
in inflammatory bowel disease, 1295
in overweight and obesity, 182
in psychosomatic illness, 67-68
in puberty, *see website*
in sudden infant death syndrome, 1424, 1424t
genetic factors interaction in, 1427, 1427f
in suicide, 88
in systemic lupus erythematosus, 841
in type 1 diabetes mellitus, 1971-1972
in type 2 diabetes mellitus, 1991
Environmental health hazards
animal and human bites as, 2454-2460
biologic and chemical terrorism as, 2454, *see also website*
chemical pollutants as, 2448, *see also website*
Environmental health hazards *(Continued)*
envenomations as, 2460-2465
general approach to, 2460-2461
due to hymenoptera sting, 2464
marine, 2464-2465
due to scorpion sting, 2464
due to snake bite, 2461-2462, 2461f-2462f, 2461t-2462t
due to spider bite, 2462-2463, 2463f
heavy metals as, 2448, *see also website*
lead as, 2448-2453
nonbacterial food poisoning as, 2454, *see also website*
radiation exposure as, 2448, *see also website*
Environmental tobacco smoke. *See* Second-hand smoke
ENV region, 1157
Enzyme deficiencies
anemias due to, 1677-1680, 1678f-1680f, 1679t
Hypoglycemia In, 524t
malabsorption due to, 1317-1319
pancreatic, 1369
cystic fibrosis and, 1495
Enzyme-linked immunofiltration test (ELIFA), 1214
Enzyme-linked immunosorbent assay (ELISA)
in arboviral encephalitis, 1144
in *Clostridium difficile* infection, 995
in coccidioidomycosis, 1066
in giardiasis, 1182
in histoplasmosis, 1063
in Lyme disease, 1028
in toxoplasmosis, 1213-1214
in tuberculosis, 1020
Enzyme-linked immunospot (ELISPOT) assay, *see website*
Enzyme-linked immunotransfer blot (EITB), 1235
Enzyme multiplicity, *see website*
Enzyme replacement therapy (ERT)
for genetic disorders, 380
for mucopolysaccharidoses, 514
Enzymes
muscle-derived in juvenile dermatomyositis, 848, 848t
in neuromuscular disorders, 2110
pancreatic, *see also website*
deficiencies of, 1369
replacement of, 1369-1370
EoE. *See* Eosinophilic esophagitis (EoE)
Eosinophil cationic protein (ECP), 739
Eosinophil count, 739-740
in allergic disease, 766
in intestinal pathogens in immigrant children, 133
Eosinophilia
allergic disease and, 740, 766
causes of, 740t
diseases associated with, 739-741
drug rash with, *see website*
infectious disease and, 740
pulmonary infiltrates with, 1474
in strongyloidiasis, 1223
in toxicariasis, 1228
tropical pulmonary, 1224, *see also website*
Eosinophilic cystitis, 1830
Eosinophilic esophagitis (EoE), 1264, 1270
Eosinophilic gastroenteritis, 1304
chronic diarrhea in, 1340-1341
due to hookworm, 1219
malabsorption due to, 1321, *see also website*
Eosinophilic lung disease, 1474, *see also website*
Eosinophilic meningitis, 2097-2098
Eosinophilic pustular folliculitis (EPF), 2220
Eosinophils, 739-741
in allergic disease, *see website*
reference values for, *see website*
EP. *See* Erythrocyte protoporphyrin (EP)
EPA. *See* Eicosapentaenoic acid (EPA)
EPEC. *See* Enteropathogenic *Escherichia coli* (EPEC)

Ependymal tumor, 1750, 1750f
Ependymoma, 1748t
EPF. *See* Eosinophilic pustular folliculitis (EPF)
Ephedra alkaloids for performance enhancement, 2423t
Ephedra sinica
  for asthma, 271t
  potential toxicity of, 272t-273t
Ephedrine
  adolescent abuse of, 675t
  for myasthenia gravis, 2135t
Ephelides (freckles), 2236
EPHX1 gene defect, 1383t
Epiblepharon, 2163-2164, 2164f
Epicanthal folds, 2163
Epicondylitis, lateral, 2411
Epidemic dengue-like disease, 1147
Epidemic keratoconjunctivitis, 2168
Epidemic typhus, 1039t-1040t, 1047-1048
Epidermal inclusion cyst, 2328
Epidermal necrolysis, toxic, 2243-2244
Epidermal nevus syndrome, rickets due to, 207
Epidermis
  diseases of, 2259-2267
    acanthosis nigricans as, 2266-2267, 2266f
    Darier disease as, 2263, 2263f
    Gianotti-Crosti syndrome as, 2266, 2266f
    keratosis pilaris as, 2261, 2261f
    lichen nitidus as, 2263-2264, 2264f
    lichen planus as, 2264-2265, 2265f
    lichen spinulosus as, 2261-2262
    lichen striatus as, 2264
    pityriasis lichenoides as, 2260-2261, 2260f-2261f
    pityriasis rosea as, 2262, 2262f
    pityriasis rubra pilaris as, 2262-2263, 2263f
    porokeratosis as, 2265-2266, 2265f
    psoriasis as, 2259-2260, 2259f
  morphology of, 2215, *see also website*
  nevi of, 2234-2235, 2234f
Epidermodysplasia verruciformis, 2315f
Epidermoid cyst, 2328
Epidermolysis bullosa (EB), 2221-2222, 2244, 2245t
Epidermolysis bullosa simplex (EBS), 2244, 2245f
Epidermolytic hyperkeratosis, 2268t, 2270, 2270f
Epidermophyton skin infections, 2309-2313
Epididymitis, 707-708, 1862-1863
Epidural abscess, poliovirus infection *versus*, 1085t
Epidural anesthesia, 373, *see also website*
Epidural hemorrhage in newborn, 566
Epigastric hernia, 1418, *see also website*
Epigenetic modification, 391-392
Epiglottitis, 1446-1447, 1447f
  Haemophilus influenzae in, 942
  treatment of, 1448
Epilepsia partialis continua, 2019
Epilepsy, 2013. *See also* Seizures
  abdominal, 1247t
  classification of syndromes, 2014t-2015t
  genetics of, 2016t
  imaging studies in, *see website*
  photoparoxysmal, 2023
  psychosis associated with, 106, *see also website*
  pyridoxine-dependent, 453-455
  treatment of, 2025-2033
Epileptic encephalopathy, 2013
Epileptic syndrome, 2013
  by age of onset, 2020t
  family history of, 2019
  with generally good prognosis, 2016t
Epileptogenesis, 2024-2025
Epileptogenic zone, 2032
Epimastigotes, in trypanosomiasis, 1193, 1193f
Epimerase deficiency, 503
Epinastine hydrochloride for allergic conjunctivitis, 811t
Epinephrine, 1923-1924, *see also website*
  for anaphylaxis, 817, 818t
  for asthma exacerbations, 797t-798t
  for cardiac output maintenance and post-resuscitation stabilization, 294t
  for croup, 1448
  for heart failure, *see website*
  hypoglycemia due to deficiency of, 528
  in neonatal resuscitation, 576-577
  for pediatric resuscitation and arrhythmias, 294t
  in pheochromocytoma, 1942
  release of in hypoglycemia, 518-519, 519t
  self-injectable
    for anaphylaxis, 817
    for insect allergy, 809
  for shock, 313t
Epi-Pen. *See* Self-injectable epinephrine
Epiphyseal dysplasias, multiple, 2427
Epiphyseal fracture, 2390, 2390t, 2391f
  as delivery room emergency, 579
Epiphysiodesis for leg-length discrepancy, *see website*
Epiphysis, *see website*
Episcleritis, 2167t
Episodic ataxias, *see website*
Epispadias, 1847, *see also website*
Epistaxis, 1432-1433, 1432t
Epitaxy in urinary lithiasis, *see website*
Epithelial cancer, 1726t
Epithelial cells
  Chlamydophila pneumoniae in, 1034f
  Epstein-Barr virus in, 1111
  Salmonella in, 950, 952f
  Shigella in, 959
Epithelial dysplasia, intestinal, 1341
Epithelial ovarian cancer, 1872, 1872t
Epithelioid cell nevus, 2233, 2233f
Epithelioma, basal cell, *see website*
Epivir. *See* Lamivudine
EPO. *See* Erythropoietin (EPO)
Epoprostenol for pulmonary hypertension, 1602t
EPP. *See* Equal pressure point (EPP); Erythropoietic protoporphyria (EPP)
EPS. *See* Elastosis perforans serpiginosa (EPS)
Epsilon toxin, *see website*
Epstein-Barr virus (EBV), 1110-1115
  clinical manifestations of, 1112-1113, 1113f
  complications of, 1114
  diagnosis of, 1113
  epidemiology of, 1110-1111
  etiology of, 1110
  following organ transplantation, *see website*
  Hodgkin lymphoma and, 1740
  laboratory testing in, 1113-1114, 1114f
  malignancy susceptibility associated with, *see website*
  maternal
    breast-feeding and, 540t
    fetal and neonatal effects of, *see website*
  oncogenesis of, 1111-1112
  pathogenesis of, 1111
  predisposition to infection due to immunodeficiency, 716t
  prevention of, 1115
  prognosis for, 1114
  after transplantation
    hematopoietic stem cell transplantation, 763
    intestinal, *see website*
    kidney, *see website*
  treatment of, 1114
Epstein pearls, 534, 2218, 2298
EPT. *See* Expedited partner therapy (EPT)
Epzicom. *See* Abacavir
Equal pressure point (EPP), *see website*
Equation of motion, 321-322, 322f
Equine encephalitis
  Eastern, 1141, 1143-1144
  Venezuelan, 1144-1147
  Western, 1141, 1143-1144
Equipment
  for home mechanical ventilation, 1524-1525
  in international pediatric emergency medicine, *see website*
  personal protective, *see website*
  resuscitation for office emergencies, *see website*
Equity in quality of care, *see website*
ERA. *See* Enthesitis-related arthritis (ERA)
ERBB2/HER-2 oncogene, *see website*
Erb-Duchenne paralysis, 573-574
ERCP. *See* Endoscopic retrograde cholangiopancreatography (ERCP)
Ergocalciferol
  in bone formation, *see website*
  for renal osteodystrophy, 1824-1825
Ergogenic drugs, 2422, 2423t
Erikson theory, *see website*
Erlenmeyer flask, 1636
Erosion, examination of, *see website*
Errors, medical, *see website*
ERT. *See* Enzyme replacement therapy (ERT)
Ertapenem, *see website*
Eruption of teeth, 1250, 1250t, *see also website*
  cyst associated with, *see website*
  delayed, 1251
Eruptive vellus hair cyst, *see website*
ERV. *See* Expiratory reserve volume (ERV)
Ery-C. *See* Erythromycin
Erysipelas, 917
Erysipeloid, 2307
Ery-Tab. *See* Erythromycin
Erythema
  necrolytic migratory, *see website*
  palmar, as manifestation of liver disease, 1376
Erythema infectiosum, 1094-1097, 1095f-1096f. *See also* Parvovirus B19
Erythema marginatum, 922, 922f
Erythema migrans in Lyme disease, 1026, 1027f, 1028t
Erythema multiforme (EM), 1103, 2241-2242, 2242f
  in Lyme disease, 1031f
Erythema nodosum, 2282-2285, 2282f, 2282t
  enteric infection and, 1333t
Erythema nodosum leprosum (ENL) reactions, *see website*
Erythematous rash of scarlet fever, 916f
Erythema toxicum, 2219, 2219f
  in newborn, 533
Erythrasma, 2306
Erythroblastosis fetalis, 615-619, 620t
  due to ABO incompatibility, 619
  fetal therapy for, 551t
  hyperinsulinemia in, 521
  due to Rh incompatibility, 615-619, 616t
Erythrocyte protoporphyrin (EP), 2450
Erythrocytes, *see website*
Erythrocyte sedimentation rate (ESR)
  in fever of unknown origin, 901
  in immunodeficiency screening, 718t
Erythrocytic phase of malaria, 1199, 1199f
Erythrogenic toxin in scarlet fever, 916
Erythrokeratoderma, symmetric progressive, 2270-2271
Erythrokeratoderma variabillis (EKV), 2270, 2271f
Erythromelalgia, 375, 880, 880f
Erythromycin, *see also website*
  for acne, 2325t
  for chancroid, *see website*
  for *Chlamydia trachomatis*, 1036-1037
  for *Chlamydophila pneumoniae*, 1035
  for cystic fibrosis lung infection, 1492t
  for diphtheria, *see website*
  drug interactions with, *see website*
  for gonococcal conjunctivitis, 2166-2167
  for infectious diarrhea, 1337t
  for *Legionella* infection, *see website*
  for lymphogranuloma venereum, 1038
  for neonatal infection, 645t

Erythromycin *(Continued)*
for pertussis, 947t
for pharyngitis, 1440
possible adverse reactions to in premature infant, 563t
for relapsing fever, *see website*
for vulvovaginitis, 1868t
Erythropoiesis, fetal, *see website*
Erythropoietic porphyria, congenital, 2256, 2256f
Erythropoietic protoporphyria (EPP), 2256, 2256f, *see website*
Erythropoietin (EPO)
fetal, *see website*
in physiologic anemia of infancy, 1654
transfusion of, *see website*
Erythropoietin therapy, 1692-1693, *see also website*
Escherichia coli, 961-965, 962t
diagnosis of, 964
diffusely adherent, 964
enteroaggregative, 963-964
enterohemorrhagic, 1324t-1325t
enteroinvasive, 962, 1337t
enteropathogenic, 962-963, 1337t
enterotoxigenic, 962, 1324t-1325t, 1330
in traveler's diarrhea, 1338t
treatment of, 1337t
hemolytic-uremic syndrome following, 1791
maternal
breast-feeding and, 540t
fetal and neonatal effects of, *see website*
neonatal, 632t
sepsis due to, 635t-636t
prevention of, 965
Shiga toxin-producing, 963
in child-care setting, *see website*
in traveler's diarrhea, 1338t
treatment of, 964-965
in urinary tract infection, 1829-1831
Escherichia coli 0157:H7
in diarrhea-associated hemolytic-uremic syndrome, 1791-1792
inflammatory bowel disease *versus*, 1298t
Escitalopram, 63t
Eskalith. *See* Lithium
Esodeviations, 2158
Esophageal atresia (EA), 1262-1263, 1262f
Esophageal bleeding, *see website*
Esophageal duplication cysts, 1263-1264
Esophageal dysphagia, 1240, 1242t
Esophageal motility, *see also website*
congenital intestinal pseudo-obstruction and, 1283t
Esophageal pH monitoring in aspiration syndromes, 1472t
Esophageal sphincter, *see also website*
dysfunction of, 1264-1265
gastroesophageal reflux disease and, 1266
Esophageal varices, 1415, *see also website*
Esophagitis
abdominal pain of, 1247t
allergic eosinophilic, 822
candidal, 1055
eosinophilic, 1264, 1270
due to gastroesophageal reflux disease, 1269
infective, 1270
"pill," 1270
due to vomiting, 1243t
Esophagus
Barrett, 1269
disorders of
clinical manifestations of, *see website*
congenital anomalies as, 1262-1263
diagnosis of, *see website*
dysmotility as, 1264-1265, 1265f
eosinophilic esophagitis as, 1270
esophageal atresia as, 1262-1263, 1262f
gastroesophageal reflux disease, 1266-1270, 1267f-1268f
general anesthesia and, *see website*
Esophagus *(Continued)*
hiatal hernia as, 1265, 1265f-1266f
infective esophagitis as, 1270
due to ingestion, 1271-1273, 1272f-1273f, 1272t-1273t
laryngotracheoesophageal clefts as, 1263
obstructing and motility disorders as, 1263-1264
perforation as, 1271, *see also website*
"pill" esophagitis as, 1270
tracheoesophageal fistula as, 1262-1263, 1262f-1263f
varices as, 1271, 1415, *see also website*
embryology, anatomy, and function of, 1261, *see also website*
foreign bodies in, 1271-1272
mega-, in Chagas disease, 1196
Esotropia, 2158, 2158f-2159f
Espundia, 1188
ESR. *See* Erythrocyte sedimentation rate (ESR)
Essential fatty acid deficiency, *see also website*
dermatoses due to, 2329
Essential hypertension, 1639-1647
Essential pentosuria, *see website*
Essential tremor (ET), 2057-2058
Esters, 367t
Estimated average requirement (EAR), *see website*
Estimated energy requirement (EER), *see website*
Estradiol in ovarian carcinomas, 1872t
Estrogen contraceptives
for acne, 2325t
for special needs girls, 1875
Estrogenic lesion of ovary, 1957-1958
Estrogen(s)
gynecomastia due to exogenous sources of, 1950
ovarian production of, *see website*
for overgrowth syndrome, *see website*
porphyria cutanea tarda and, *see website*
for Turner syndrome, 1954
vaginal bleeding due to exposure to, 1870
E_3 subunit deficiency, 431
ET. *See* Essential tremor (ET)
Etanercept
for juvenile idiopathic arthritis, 838t
for rheumatic disease, *see website*
ETAT. *See* Emergency Triage Assessment and Treatment (ETAT)
ETEC. *See* Enterotoxigenic *Escherichia coli* (ETEC)
E test, 2148, *see also website*
ETF. *See* Electron transfer flavoprotein (ETF) deficiency
ETF-DH. *See* Electron transfer flavoprotein dehydrogenase (ETF-DH) deficiency
Ethambutol, 1008t, *see also website*
Ethanol. *See* Alcohol
Ethanolamines, 771t
Ethics/ethical factors, 13
in adolescent health care, *see website*
assent and parenteral permission in, *see website*
in balancing maternal and fetal interests, *see website*
in care of disabled newborns, *see website*
committees on, *see website*
consultations regarding, *see website*
in declaring death, *see website*
emerging issues associated with, *see website*
justice and, *see website*
in long-term mechanical ventilation, 330-331
in newborn screening and genetic testing, 382-383, *see also website*
in organ donation, *see website*
in red cell counts, 1648, 1650f
in religious or cultural objections to treatment, *see website*
in research, *see website*
in suicide, 87
in treatment of critically ill children, *see website*
Ethionamide, 1008t, *see also website*
Ethmoidal sinuses, 1436, 1436f
Ethnic factors. *See* Racial and ethnic factors
Ethosuximide dosages, 2030t
Ethylenediamines, 771t
Ethylene glycol poisoning, 267-268
antidote for, 256t-257t
metabolic acidosis due to, 233
Etodolac. *See* Nonsteroidal antiinflammatory drugs (NSAIDs)
Etomidat, *see website*
Etoposide, *see website*
Etravirine intelence, 1168t-1171t
Eulenberg disease, 2125
Eunuchoid habitus, 1954
Euroglyphus maynei, 768
Europe, pediatricians per population in, 12f
European hornet, allergic responses to, 807f
European immunization schedule, 895
Eustachian tube anatomy, otitis media and, 2201
Eutectic mixture of local anesthetics (EMLA), 367
Euthyroidism, 1905
Euvolemic hyponatremia, 216
Evans syndrome, 1679
Evaporation heat loss in newborn, 536-537
EVC1 gene, 2433-2434
EVC2 gene, 2433-2434
Eventration of diaphragm, 597
Eversion, 2331
Evidence-based practice in well child care, 16
Evoked potentials in neurologic assessment, *see website*
Ewengii ehrlichiosis, 1039t-1040t
Ewing sarcoma, 1763t, 1765-1766, 1765f
risk factors for, 1727t
work-up of, 1731t
Exanthematous pustulosis, acute generalized, *see website*
Excessive daytime sleepiness (EDS), 53
Exchange programs, international, *see website*
Exchange transfusion
for erythroblastosis fetalis, 618
for hyperbilirubinemia, 611f, 612, 612t
Excimer laser correction for myopia, 2151
Excitability in seizures, 2025
Excoriation, examination of, *see website*
Excretion
of drugs, *see website*
enhanced for poisonings, 257-258
hepatic, *see website*
of magnesium, *see website*
of phosphorus, 226
of potassium, 219
of sodium, 212, *see also website*
Excretory urogram, 1841
Executive functioning (EF), *see website*
Exercise
habits regarding in eating disorders, 92t
hematuria due to vigorous, 1799
hyperinsulinemia induced by, 527
Kegel, 1849
Exercise electrocardiography, 1545
Exercise-induced anaphylaxis, 814
Exercise-induced bronchospasm, 784
Exercise intolerance, as manifestation of extrapulmonary disease, 1526, *see also website*
Exercise testing
in asthma, 784, 785t
in cardiovascular disease, 1545
in respiratory disease, *see website*
Exercise therapy for chronic fatigue syndrome, *see website*
Exfoliatins A and B, 904
Exfoliation in dental development, *see website*
Exhaled nitric oxide in asthma, 784-785
Exhaled tidal volume (VTE) in mechanical ventilation, 328
Exhaustion, heat, 2420
EXIT procedure. *See* Ex utero intrapartum treatment procedure (EXIT procedure)

Exit site infection. *See* Catheter-related bloodstream infection (CRBSI)
Exjade. *See* Deferasirox
Exocrine pancreas
  disorders of
    anatomic abnormalities as, 1368, *see also website*
    associated with pancreatic insufficiency, 1369-1370
    pancreatic function tests in, 1369, *see also website*
    pancreatitis as, 1370-1373, 1370t-1371t, 1372f-1373f
    pseudocyst as, 1373
    tumor as, 1374, *see also website*
  embryology, anatomy, and physiology of, 1368, *see also website*
  malabsorption and, 1307-1308, 1307f, 1317
Exodeviations, 2159
Exoerythrocytic phase of malaria, 1199, 1199f
Exons, genetic, *see website*
Exopolysaccharide biofilm of coagulase-negative staphylococci, 909
Exostoses
  of ear canal, 2199
  subungual, 2343
Exosurf, 585
Exotoxins, pyrogenic
  in scarlet fever, 916
  streptococcal, 915
Exotropia, 2159
Expansile skeletal hyperplasia, *see website*
Expansion thoracoplasty, 2369-2370, 2370f
Expedited partner therapy (EPT), 714
Experimental strategies in Marfan syndrome, 2445
Expiratory reserve volume (ERV), *see website*
Expiratory time constant in mechanical ventilation, 323
Expiratory time in mechanical ventilation, 327
Explicit memory, *see website*
Exposure
  in pediatric emergency assessment, 281
  in trauma survey, 337
Expression proteomics, *see website*
Expressive language
  development of, 115-116
  dysfunction of, 117t, 118, *see also website*
Exstrophy, bladder, 1847, *see also website*
Extension, 2331
Extensively drug resistant (XDR), 1009
External auditory canal
  clearing of, 2202-2203
  congenital stenosis or atresia of, *see website*
  foreign body in, *see website*
  traumatic injury to, 2213-2214, *see also website*
  tumors of, 2214
External ear, malformations of, 2196, *see also website*
External fixation
  for fracture, 2394, 2394t
  for leg-length discrepancy, *see website*
External genitalia. *See* Genitalia
External jugular vein, venous access in, 295f
External otitis, 2196-2199, 2198f
  examination of, *see website*
  Pseudomonas aeruginosa, 976t
External rotation, 2331
External tibial torsion, 2347
Extracellular fluid (ECF), *see website*
Extracorporeal membrane oxygenation (ECMO)
  for congenital diaphragmatic hernia, 595-596
  for persistent pulmonary hypertension of the newborn, 593-594
  for shock, 314
Extrahepatic cholestasis, 1381
Extraocular muscles
  congenital fibrosis of, 2006
  weakness of in neuromuscular disorders, 2115t
Extrapulmonary air leaks, 597-599, 598f-599f
Extrapulmonary sequestration, 1466
Extrapyramidal cerebral palsy, 2062t, 2063-2064
Extrasystoles, 1610-1613
Extrathoracic airway, *see website*
  obstruction of, *see website*
Extravascular drug absorption, *see website*
Extremity(ies)
  conditions causing arthritic pain in, 836t
  effects of eating disorders on, 93t
  fracture of
    as birth injury, 579
    as delivery room emergency, 579
  newborn assessment of, 536
  orthopedic problems with, 2383-2387
  rickets and, 201t
  trauma to, 339-340
Extrinsic alveolar alveolitis, *Aspergillus* in, 1059
Extrusion injury, dental, 1259
Exudates
  in empyema, 1507
  in serofibrous pleurisy, 1506-1507
Ex utero intrapartum treatment procedure (EXIT procedure), 577, 578f
EYA4 gene, 2190t
Eyes
  growth and development of, 2148, *see also website*
  newborn assessment of, 534
Eye disorders
  conjunctival, 2166-2169, 2167t, 2168f-2169f
  corneal, 2169, *see also website*
  glaucoma as, 2181, *see also website*
  infection as
    adenovirus, 1132
    Aspergillus, 1061
    cryptococcus neoformans, 1057
    enteroviruses, 1091
    gonococcal, 937
    Haemophilus influenzae, 942
    herpes simplex virus, 1101
    microsporidiosis, *see website*
    newborn prophylaxis against, 537
    Toxoplasmosis gondii, 1210, 1210f, 1213-1215
  of lacrimal system, 2165-2166, 2165f
  larva migrans as, 1227-1229, 1228t
  of lens, 2169-2172, 2170f-2172f, 2170t
  of lid, 2163-2165, 2164f
  in Marfan syndrome, 2441-2442
  of movement and alignment, 2157-2162
    congenital ocular motor apraxia as, 2161
    non-nystagmus as, 2162, 2162t
    nystagmus as, 2161-2162, 2161t, 2162f
    strabismus as, 2157-2161, 2158f-2160f
  in mucopolysaccharidoses, 515t
  neuromyelitis optica as (*See* Neuromyelitis optica (NMO))
  ocular allergies as, 809-811, 810f, 811t
  of optic nerve, 2181, *see also website*
  optic neuropathy
    Leber hereditary, 2067
  of orbit, 2181-2184, 2182f
  of pupil and iris, 2154-2157, 2157f
  of refraction and accommodation, 2150-2152
  of retina and vitreous, 2174-2181
    Best vitelliform degeneration as, 2178
    with blood disorders, 2180
    cherry red spot as, 2178
    Coats disease as, 2179, 2179f
    coloboma of the fundus as, 2181
    diabetic retinopathy as, 2179-2180, 2180f
    familial exudative vitreoretinopathy as, 2179
    hypertensive retinopathy as, 2179, 2179f
    myelinated nerve fibers as, 2181
    persistent fetal vasculature as, 2176
    phakomas as, 2178, 2178f
    retinal detachment as, 2179
    retinitis pigmentosa as, 2177-2178, 2177f
    retinoblastoma, 2176-2177
    retinoblastoma as, 2176f
Eye disorders *(Continued)*
    retinopathy of prematurity as, 2174-2176, 2175f, 2175t
    retinoschisis as, 2178
    Stargardt disease as, 2178
    with subacute bacterial endocarditis, 2180
    trauma-related, 2180, 2181f
  sports participation and, 2402t-2404t
  traumatic injury as, 2184-2187, 2184f-2186f
  of uveal tract, 2172-2174, 2173f-2174f, 2173t
  of vision, 2152-2154, 2153t
Eye examination, 2148-2150, 2149t
  based on gestational age at birth, 2175t
  fever of unknown origin and, 901
  in juvenile idiopathic arthritis, 833t, 2173t
Eyegrounds examination, 2016
Eyelid
  abnormalities of, 2163-2165, 2164f
  ecchymosis and swelling of, 2184
  lacerations of, 2184
Eye manifestations
  in albinism, 424
  in Behçet disease, 854
  in childhood cancers, 1728
  in eating disorders, 93t
  in Graves disease, 1910, 1911f, 1913
  in malnutrition, 175t
  in mitochondrial encephalomyopathy, 2065t
  in poisoning, 252t
  in systemic lupus erythematosus, 843t
  in tyrosinemia type II, 422-423
Eye protection, *see website*
Ezetimibe for hyperlipidemia, 481t, 482

F

FAB. *See* French-American-British (FAB) classification
Fab antibodies, digoxin-specific, 256t-257t, 262-263
Fabric, nonflammable, 23
Fabry crisis, 489
Fabry disease, 484t, 488-489, 489f, 2139-2140
  cardiac manifestations of, 1531t
  cutaneous manifestations of, 2230-2231
Face
  effects of malnutrition on, 175t
  newborn assessment of, 534t
Face shield, *see website*
FACES scale, 363t
Facet syndrome, 2412
  due to sports injury, 2412
Facial cold autoinflammatory syndrome (FCAS), 814
Facial ectodermal dysplasia, 2222
Facial nerve
  neurologic examination of, *see website*
  palsy of, 574
  paralysis of, due to ear disorders, 2211, *see also website*
Facial phenotype in congenital central hypoventilation syndrome, 1521
Facial weakness
  in myotonic muscular dystrophy, 2123f
  in neuromuscular disorders, 2115t
Facioscapulohumeral muscular dystrophy, 2113t, 2126
Factitial panniculitis, 2285
Factitious disorder, 69, 69t
Factitious disorder by proxy (FDP), 146-147
Factor 1 deficiency, 755
Factor D deficiency, 754, 754t
Factor H deficiency, 754t, 755
Factor I deficiency, 1704
Factor II
  deficiency of, 1703
  reference values for, 1698t
Factor IX deficiency, 1699-1702, 1700f, 1701t
Factor V
  deficiency of, 1703-1704
    factor VIII deficiency combined with, 1704
  reference values for, 1698t

Factor VII
deficiency, 1703
reference values for, 1698t
Factor VIII
deficiency, 1699-1702, 1701t
factor V deficiency combined with, 1704
in hemostasis, 1694
increased concentrations of, 1708
Factor V Leiden, 1698, 1708
Factor X
deficiency, 1703
reference values for, 1698t
Factor XI
deficiency, 1702-1703
reference values for, 1698t
Factor XII
deficiency, 1703
reference values for, 1698t
Factor XIII
deficiency, 1704
reference values for, 1698t
Facultative anaerobes, 995
Failure to thrive (FTT), 147-149
due to cardiac disease, 1530-1531
clinical manifestations of, 147
differential diagnosis of, 147f, 148t
epidemiology of, 147
etiology and diagnosis of, 147-148, 148t-149t
growth charts in assessment of, *see website*
HIV-related, 1165
prognosis for, 149
treatment of, 148-149
Fairbanks apprehension sign, 2355
Falls, injury due to, 25
False-negative results, 376-377, *see also website*
False-positive results, 376, *see also website*
proteinuria, 1800
Famciclovir, *see also website*
for herpes simplex virus infection, 1102-1103
for sexually transmitted infection, 713t
Familial adenomatous polyposis (FAP), *see website*
Familial aplastic anemia, 1690
Familial apolipoprotein A-1 deficiency, 477
Familial chylomicronemia, 473t, 476, 476f
Familial clustering, genetic, 389-390
Familial cold autoinflammatory syndrome (FCAS), 855t, 858
Familial combined hyperlipidemia (FCHL), 473t, 475
Familial defective APOB-100 (FDB), 473t, 475
Familial dysalbuminemic hyperthyroxinemia, *see website*
Familial dysautonomia, 2142
fever of unknown origin due to dysfunction of, 901
Familial dysbetalipoproteinemia (FDBL), 473t, 476
Familial exudative vitreoretinopathy (FEVR), 2179
Familial glucocorticoid deficiency, 1924-1925
Familial hemiplegic migraine, *see website*
Familial hemophagocytic lymphohistiocytoses (FHLH), 1774-1776
Familial Hibernian fever, 858
Familial hypercalciuric hypercalcemia, 1922-1923
Familial hypercholanemia (FHC), 1384
Familial hypercholesterolemia (FH), 473, 473t, 475t
heterozygous, 474
homozygous, 473-474, 473f-474f
Familial hypertriglyceridemia (FHGT), 473t, 476-477
Familial hypobetalipoproteinemia, 478
Familial lecithin-cholesterol acyltransferase (LCAT) deficiency, 477
Familial male gonadotropin-independent precocious puberty, 1893
Familial Mediterranean fever (FMF), 855t, 856-857, 857f
abdominal pain of, 1247t
Familial nonhemolytic unconjugated hyperbilirubinemia, 1389-1390
Familial partial lipodystrophy, 2285-2286
Familial peeling skin, 2268t
Familial protein intolerance, 455
Familial rectal pain syndrome, *see website*
Familial secundum atrial septal defect, *see website*
Family
adolescence and, 652-654
adoption and, 131-132
communication with in post-resuscitation care, 296
discussion of cancer treatment with, *see website*
education of (*See* Patient and family education)
impact of chronic illness on, *see website*
move or relocation of, *see website*
obesity prevention in, 187t
well child care and, 16-17
Family-centered care
of foster care children, *see website*
during transport, *see website*
Family child-care, 895
Family counseling
in intellectual disability management, 129
for neurodevelopmental dysfunction, *see website*
Family factors in psychosomatic illness, 68
Family history
as cancer risk factor, 1727t
of cardiovascular disease, 1530
in dyslexia, 112
in genetic transmission, 383
in hematuria, 1779
in Marfan syndrome, 2443
in microcephaly, 2007-2008
in neurologic evaluation, *see website*
in obesity, 185
in persistent hyperinsulinemic hypoglycemia, 522t
in skeletal dysplasias, *see website*
of type 2 diabetes mellitus, 1991
in wheezing, 1458
Family Psychosocial Screening (FPS), 41t-43t
Family systems, development and, *see website*
Family therapy for psychiatric disorders, 66
Famotidine
for functional abdominal pain, 1348t
for *Helicobacter pylori* gastritis, 1293t
for urticaria and angioedema, 815t
Famvir. *See* Famciclovir
Fanconi anemia, 1684-1686, 1685f, 1685t
malignancy susceptibility associated with, *see website*
stem cell transplantation for, 759
Fanconi-Bickel syndrome, 494t-495t, 499, 1319
Fanconi syndrome
hypophosphatemia in, 227
nephrotoxins in, 1817t
renal tubular acidosis with, 1808-1810
rickets due to, 202t, 207
FAO. *See* Food and Agriculture Organization (FAO)
FAP. *See* Familial adenomatous polyposis (FAP)
Farber disease, 484t, 491, 491f
Farmer's lung, *see website*
Farsightedness, 2150-2151
of newborn, *see website*
FAS. *See* Fetal alcohol syndrome (FAS)
Fasciculation of muscle in neuromuscular disorders, 2109
Fasciitis, necrotizing, 2301-2302
anaerobic, *see website*
group A streptococcal, 919
Fasciola hepatica, *see website*
Fasciolopsis buski, *see website*
FAST. *See* Focused assessment with sonography in trauma (FAST)
"Fast food," 182
Fasting, preoperative, *see website*
Fasting glucose, *see website*
Fasting time to hypoglycemia, 521t
Fatal familial insomnia (FFI), 1177, *see also website*
Fatigue
in palliative care, 155t-156t, 157
in rheumatic disease, *see website*
Fat necrosis
cold-induced, 358
subcutaneous, 2284, 2284f
hypercalcemia with, 1922
Fat(s). *See also* Lipids
absorption of, *see website*
adequate macronutrient distribution range for, *see website*
dietary reference intakes for, *see website*
intake in type 1 diabetes mellitus, 1982, 1982t
malabsorption of, 1305t, 1307, 1318-1319
transport disorders of, 1318-1319
Fatty acids
free, neonatal transient hypoglycemia and, 520-521, 522t
metabolic disorders of, 417t
oxidation disorders of, 456-462, 457t, 458f-459f
hypoglycemia in, 524t, 529
polyunsaturated, dietary reference intakes for, *see website*
saturated and *trans*, dietary reference intakes for, *see website*
in vegetarian diet, 168
very long chain, disorders of, 462-470, 462t-464t, 464f-465f, 466t, 469f
Fatty liver disease
nonalcoholic, 184t, *see website*
with type 2 diabetes mellitus, 1993t
FAVS syndrome, 1531t
FBMs. *See* Fetal breathing movements (FBMs)
FBN1 gene, 2012t, 2440, 2443
FCA. *See* Focal cerebral arteriopathy (FCA)
FCAS. *See* Familial cold autoinflammatory syndrome (FCAS)
FcεRI, *see website*
FcεRII, *see website*
FCHL. *See* Familial combined hyperlipidemia (FCHL)
F1C1 protein, 1383-1384, 1383t
FDB. *See* Familial defective APOB-100 (FDB)
FDBL. *See* Familial dysbetalipoproteinemia (FDBL)
FDCs. *See* Follicular dendritic cells (FDCs)
F57 diet, 176-177, 177t-178t
F100 diet, 176-177, 177t-178t
FDP. *See* Factitious disorder by proxy (FDP)
Fear of self-injecting (FSI), 1986
Feasibility in quality measurement, *see website*
Febrile seizure, 2013, 2017-2019, 2017t, 2018f
in measles, 1072
Febrile status epilepticus, 2017
Febrile ulcerative acne, 2328
Fecal elastase, 1307, 1369
Fecal incontinence, 73-74
Fecal leukocytes in chronic diarrhea, 1344t
Fecal occult blood in chronic diarrhea, 1344t
Fecal reducing substances in chronic diarrhea, 1344t
Fecal testing for parasitic infection, *see website*
Federal funding for health care, 10
Feeding
with cleft lip or palate, 1252
cultural considerations in, 167-168
emotional development and, 27-28
enteral, for acute gastroenteritis, 1334-1336
failure to in newborn, *see website*
during first year of life
breast-feeding, 160
(*See also* Breast-feeding)

Feeding *(Continued)*
complementary feeding, 164-165
formula feeding, 162-164, 162f
of foreign-born adoptees, 131
nasogastric tube, in infant botulism, 990
nasojejunal tube, in infant botulism, 990
otitis media and, 2200
in palliative care, 158
of premature and low birthweight infants, 560-562, 561f
of school-age children and adolescents, 166-167, 166f, 167t
sudden infant death syndrome and care practices and exposures in, 1425
of toddlers and preschool-age children, 165, 165t
FEES. *See* Fiberoptic endoscopic evaluation of swallowing (FEES)
FEF max. *See* Maximum forced expiratory flow (FEF max)
Felbamate
adverse effects of, 2031t
dosages of, 2030t
Fel d 1, 769
Felodipine for systemic hypertension, 1645t
Female athlete, 2421-2422
Female athlete triad, 686, 2422
Female condom, 695t
Feminizing adrenal tumor, 1941
Femoral anteversion, 2346
Femoral head, 2355
Femoral neck
normal development of, 2344
stress fracture of, 2413
Femoral pulse, assessment of, 1532-1533
Femoral shaft fracture, 2393, 2393t
Femoral torsion, 2347
Femoral vein, venous access in, 292, 295f
Fentanyl
for anesthesia, *see website*
equianalgesic doses and half-life of, 367t
for intubation, 321t
for pain management, 365t
in palliative care, 155t-156t
transdermal patch, 155t-156t
possible adverse reactions to in premature infant, 563t
Ferritin
in congenital dyserythropoietic anemia, *see website*
in iron deficiency-anemia, 1656t
reference values for, *see website*
in systemic-onset juvenile idiopathic arthritis, 836
Ferrochelatase (FETCH), *see website*
Ferrous sulfate, 52
Fertility
female, impact of cancer therapy on, 1870-1871
male, inguinal hernia repair and, 1368
Fetal alcohol syndrome (FAS), 625-626, 626f, 626t, *see website*
congenital heart disease with, 1531t
microcephaly with, 2007t
Fetal aspiration syndrome, 590, 591f
Fetal breathing movements (FBMs), 543t
Fetal circulation, 1529, *see also website*
congenital heart disease and, *see website*
persistent, 592-594, 592f
transition to neonatal circulation, 1529, *see also website*
Fetal disease
intrauterine diagnosis of, 548-550, 549f, 550t
treatment and prevention of, 550-552, 551t
Fetal distress, 541-545, 542f, 543t, 544f, 545t
diagnosis of, 550
therapy for, 551t
Fetal heart rate
acceleration of, 543-544
in biophysical profile, 543t
deceleration of, 543-544, 544f
Fetal heart rate *(Continued)*
monitoring of, 542, 543t
variability of, 545t
Fetal hemoglobin (Hbf), *see also website*
syndromes of hereditary persistence of, 1673-1674
Fetal hydantoin syndrome, microcephaly with, 2007t
Fetal programming, *see website*
Fetal thyroid hormones, *see website*
Fetal tissue analysis, 543t
Fetal transfusion syndrome, 554
α-Fetoprotein concentration, 543t
in brain tumors, 1747-1748
in CNS germ cell tumors, 1752-1753
in germ cell tumors, 1770
in ovarian carcinomas, 1872t
Fetoscopy, 543t
Fetus, 541-552
assessment of anatomy of, 549f
cardiac catheterization, interventional in, 1548
dating of, 541
death of, *see website*
echocardiography of, 1544-1545, 1544f
ethical considerations in balancing maternal interests and interests of, *see website*
growth, development, and maturity of, 26, 541, 541f, *see also website*
hematopoietic system development in, 1648, *see also website*
infections associated with, 543t, 547-548
Campylobacter in, 970
congenital lymphocytic choriomeningitis, 548
cytomegalovirus, 1116
herpes simplex virus, 1101, 1102f, 1103
parvovirus B19, 1095-1096
tuberculous, 1007, 1011
lymphopoiesis in, *see website*
maternal disease and, 545
maternal medication and toxin exposure and, 546-547, 546t-547t
overgrowth of, *see website*
prenatal diagnosis of, 380t, 381, *see also website*
of cystic fibrosis, 1490
genetic counseling in, 378
and prevention, 379, 548-550
radiation exposure to, 548
respiration regulation in, *see website*
steroid biosynthesis in, *see website*
teratogen exposure to, 547-548
FEV_1. *See* Forced expiratory volume in 1 sec (FEV_1)
Fever
in bacterial meningitis, 2094
in common cold, 1435
in croup, 1446
sports participation and, 2402t-2404t
Fever blister, 901, 1099-1100
Fever of unknown origin (FUO), 898-902
diagnosis of, 899-902, 900t-901t
etiology of, 898-899, 899t
in HIV, diseases associated with, *see website*
prognosis for, 902
treatment of, 898t, 902
Fever(s), 896
in acutely ill child, 275-276
in acute rheumatic fever, 922
in appendicitis, 1351t
in babesiosis, *see website*
clinical features of, *see website*
Colorado tick, 1142-1144
defined, 896
definition of, *see website*
dengue, 1147-1150
in dengue-like disease, 1148
double quotidian, *see website*
in drowning, 346
drug, HIV-related, *see website*
in enterovirus infection, 1089-1090
Fever(s) *(Continued)*
etiology of, *see website*
evaluation of, *see website*
exclusion from day care due to, *see website*
glandular, 1110
hemorrhagic, 1150-1153, 1150t
dengue, 1147-1150, 1147t
with renal syndrome, 1151-1153
in herpangina, 1090
home remedies among African Americans for, *see website*
with hyperimmunoglobulinemia D, 436
in immunocompromised patient, *see website*
intermittent, *see website*
in Kawasaki disease, 863, 864f
Lassa, 1151-1152, 1152t
maintenance water and electrolytes and, 244
in malaria, 1200-1202
Mediterranean spotted, 1043-1044
in neonatal infection, 637-639
neutropenia and, *see website*
in newborn, *see website*
parrot, 1038, *see also website*
pathogenesis of, *see website*
Q, 1039t-1040t, 1051-1053
rat bite, 2457-2459
relapsing, 1025, *see also website*
in returning travelers, *see website*
rheumatic, 920-925
in rheumatic disease, *see website*
Rift Valley, 1151-1152
Rocky Mountain spotted, 1038-1043, 1041f-1042f
Kawasaki disease *versus*, 865-866
Rocky Mountain spotted fever, 1042
in roseola, 1118
scarlet, 916, 916f
seizures due to, 2017-2019, 2017t, 2018f
in sickle cell disease, 1663, 1663t
in systemic-onset juvenile idiopathic arthritis, 832-834, 834f
treatment of, *see website*
trench, 986
tsutsugamushi, 1045
typhoid, 954-958
valley, 1065-1068
without localizing signs, 896-898, 896t-898t
Haemophilus influenzae in, 943
yellow, 1150, *see also website*
Fever syndromes, hereditary, 855-860, 855t-856t
Blau syndrome as, 858-859
chronic infantile neurologic cutaneous and articular disease as, 858
familial cold autoinflammatory syndrome as, 858
familial Mediterranean fever as, 856-857, 857f
hyperimmunoglobulinemia D syndrome as, 857-858
Muckle-Wells syndrome as, 858
periodic fever, aphthous stomatitis, pharyngitis, and adenitis as, 859-860
pyogenic arthritis, pyoderma gangrenosum, and acne syndrome as, 858-859
tumor necrosis factor receptor-associated periodic syndrome as, 858, 859f
FEVR. *See* Familial exudative vitreoretinopathy (FEVR)
Fexofenadine
for allergic rhinitis, 777t-778t, 779
for urticaria and angioedema, 815t
FFAs. *See* Free fatty acids (FFAs)
FFI. *See* Fatal familial insomnia (FFI)
FGFR. *See* Fibroblast growth factor receptor (FGFR)
FGFR3 gene, 2428, 2430, *see website*
FGIDs. *See* Functional gastrointestinal disorders (FGIDs)
FGR2 gene, 2012t
FGR3 gene, 2012t
FH. *See* Familial hypercholesterolemia (FH)
FHA. *See* Filament hemagglutinin (FHA)

FHC. *See* Familial hypercholanemia (FHC)
FHGT. *See* Familial hypertriglyceridemia (FHGT)
FHLH. *See* Familial hemophagocytic lymphohistiocytoses (FHLH)
Fiber, dietary
for functional abdominal pain, 1348t
reference intakes for, *see website*
in type 1 diabetes mellitus, 1982, 1982t
Fiberoptic endoscopic evaluation of swallowing (FEES), *see also website*
in aspiration syndromes, 1472-1473, 1472t
Fibrillary infiltrating astrocytoma, 1748-1749
Fibrillation
atrial, 1615-1616, 1616f
familial, genetics of, *see website*
ventricular, 1616
Fibrillin-1, abnormal biosynthesis of, 2440
Fibrinogen, 1696t
deficiency, 1704
reference values for, 1698t
Fibrinolytic system, tests of, 1699
Fibrinopurulent stage of empyema, 1507
Fibrin-stabilizing factor, 1696t
deficiency of, 1704
Fibroadenoma, breast, *see website*
Fibroblast growth factor receptor (FGFR), mutations in, 2013
Fibroids, uterine, 689t-690t
Fibroma
cardiac, *see website*
infantile digital, *see website*
ossifying of jaw, *see website*
Fibromyalgia, 375, 878-879, 879f, *see also website*
Fibrosarcoma, 1762t
Fibrosis
congenital hepatic, *see website*
tubulointerstitial, *see website*
Fibula
congenital and angular deformities of, 2350-2351
fracture of, 2392-2393
Fibular hemimelia, 2351
Fictitious hyperkalemia, 219
Field triage, 333t, 334f
Fifth day fits, 2035
Fifth disease, 1095, 1095f-1096f. *See also* Parvovirus B19
50% inhibitory dose (ID_{50}), *see website*
Filament hemagglutinin (FHA), 944-945
Filamins, disorders involving, 2435
Filariasis, 1224-1225, 1225f, *see also website*
Financial costs. *See* Costs
Financing, vaccine, 885
Fine motor development, *see also website*
during first 2 years, 27t
Finger. *See* Digit
Fingertip injury, 2387
FIO_2. *See* Fraction of inspired oxygen (FIO_2)
Fire ant, allergic responses to, 807f
Firearm injuries, 24-25
Fire-related injury, 18, 23-24. *See also* Burn(s)
Fire setting, 100
Fireworks-related injury, 23
ocular, 2186
First aid measures for burn injury, 350
First breath, 580
First-degree burn, 351, 351t
First-degree heart block, 1618
electrocardiography of, 1540
First-degree relative, 383
First-generation antihistamines, 771, 771t
First-generation cephalosporins, *see website*
First heart sound, auscultation of, 1533
First-pass effect of drug, *see website*
FISH. *See* Fluorescence in situ hybridization (FISH)
Fish allergy, 821, 821t, 823t
Fish poisoning, 2454, *see also website*
Fish tank granuloma, 1013
Fish tapeworm, 1233-1234, *see website*
Fissure
anal, 1359
examination of, *see website*
Fissured tongue, 1261, 2299
FISTS mnemonic, 669-670, 670t
Fistula
arteriovenous, 1638, *see also website*
bronchobiliary, 1467
coronary-cameral, 1561
with Crohn disease, 1300-1301
hepatic arteriovenous, *see website*
perianal, 1360, 1360f
perilymphatic, *see website*
pulmonary arteriovenous, 1599, *see also website*
rectobulbarurethral, 1357
rectoprostaticurethral, 1357
tracheoesophageal, 1262-1263, 1262f-1263f, *see website*
urethral, 1857-1858
Fitz-Hugh-Curtis syndrome, 936, 939, 1036
"Five Wishes," 151
Five-year survival rates, cancer, 1726f
Fixation, external
for fracture, 2394, 2394t
for leg-length discrepancy, *see website*
Flaccid paralysis
due to botulism, 988-990
differential diagnosis of, 1084-1086, 1085t
in neuromuscular disorders, 2109-2110, 2112t
Flagyl. *See* Metronidazole
Flail chest as life-threatening injury, 336t
Flame-retardant sleepwear, 23
Flatfoot
flexible, 2338, 2338f
peroneal spastic, 2339-2340
Flavivirus, 1147t
Flea bites, 2318
Flecainide for arrhythmias, 1611t-1612t
Fleet enema, hypophosphatemia due to, 228-229
"Flesh-eating bacteria," *see website*
Flexible kyphosis, 2371
Flexion, 2331
Flonase. *See* Fluticasone
Flow cytometry
in B cell deficiency screening, 720
in leukocyte adhesion deficiency, 744
in T cell deficiency screening, 720-722
in X-linked agammaglobulinemia, 724
Flower cells, *see website*
Flow study, antegrade pressure-perfusion, 1841
Flow volume loop, *see website*
Fluconazole, *see also website*
for candidiasis, 1054t, 1056t
for coccidioidomycosis, 1067
for *Cryptococcus neoformans*, 1058
for leishmaniasis, 1190
for neonatal infection, 644
for *Paracoccidioides brasiliensis*, *see website*
Fluency, 114
Fluid deficit. *See also* Dehydration
calculation of, 246
Fluid intake
for premature and low birthweight infants, 559-560
sports and, 2421
Fluid management in kidney transplantation, *see website*
Fluid replacement, intraoperative, *see website*
Fluid resuscitation
for burn injury, 352-353
for shock, 336-337
Fluids, body. *See* Body fluids
Fluid therapy, 242, 242t
for bacterial meningitis, 2094
for chronic kidney disease, 1823-1824
for dehydration, 245-249, 247t
for diabetes insipidus, 1883-1884
for diarrheagenic *Escherichia coli*, 964
for drowning victim, 345
Fluid therapy *(Continued)*
glucose in, 243
for hypernatremia, 214-215
hyponatremia and, 243-244
intravenous solutions for, 243, 243t
maintenance, 242, 242t
glucose in, 243
hyponatremia and, 243-244
intravenous solutions for, 243, 243t
selection of, 243
variations in, 244, 244t
water in, 242-243, 243t
replacement, 242, 244-245, 245t
selection of solutions for, 243
water in, 242-243, 243t
variations in, 244, 244t
Flukes, 1231-1232, *see also website*
Flumadine. *See* Rimantadine
Flumazenil, 256t-257t
Flunarizine, 2044, 2044t
Flunisolide
for allergic rhinitis, 778t-779t
for asthma, 795t
Flunitrazepam, adolescent abuse of, 675t
Fluorescence in situ hybridization (FISH), 395-396, 397f-398f
in intellectual disability, 125
Fluorescent treponemal antibody absorption (FTA-ABS) test, 1019-1020
Fluoride, *see website*
for dental caries prevention, 1256, 1256t
5-Fluorocytosine (5-FU), *see website*
Fluoroquinolones, *see also website*
drug interactions with, *see website*
for *Staphylococcus aureus*, 907t
for typhoid fever, 957-958, 958t
Fluoroscopy
barium, *see also website*
in achalasia, 1264-1265, 1265f
in respiratory disease diagnosis, *see website*
Fluorosis, 1251
Fluoxetine
for depression and anxiety symptoms, 63t
for pain management, 364t
for premenstrual dysphoric disorder, 692t
for weight loss in adults, 187t
Flutamide for familial male gonadotropin-independent precocious puberty, 1893
Fluticasone
for allergic rhinitis, 778t-779t
for asthma, 794t-795t
Fluticasone propionate, 779-780
Flutter, atrial, 1615, 1615f, 1616t
Flutter-like oscillations of eye, 2162
Flying squirrel typhus, 1039t-1040t
Fly-through imaging, 1546, 1546f
FMF. *See* Familial Mediterranean fever (FMF)
FMR1 gene, 411, 411t
fMRI. *See* Functional magnetic resonance imaging (fMRI)
Foam cells, 1782
Focal cerebral arteriopathy (FCA), 2080
Focal cortical dysplasia, 2004
Focal dermal hypoplasia, 2222
Focal facial ectodermal dysplasia, 2222
Focalin. *See* Dexmethylphenidate
Focal segmental glomerulosclerosis (FSGS), 1803t, 1804
renal transplantation in, *see website*
Focal seizure, 2013
evaluation of, 2015-2016
Foci in tuberculosis, 998, 1002-1003
Focused assessment with sonography in trauma (FAST), 339
Fogo selvagem, 2247
Folate, 196-197
deficiency of, 197, 748t, 1655, *see also website*
megaloblastic anemia due to, 1655
dietary reference intakes for, *see website*

Folate *(Continued)*
for folate deficiency-related anemia, *see website*
malabsorption of, 1320
myelomeningocele and, 2001
neural tube defects and, 1998
reference values for, *see website*
toxicity of, 197
Folate receptors, autoantibody against, maternal, *see website*
Folic acid, 194t
supplementation during pregnancy, 2001
supplementation for neural tube defect prevention, 552
Folinic acid, as poisoning antidote, 258t
Follicle-stimulating hormone (FSH), *see also website*
in amenorrhea, 686
in hypogonadism, 1945-1946
Follicular bronchitis, 1463
Follicular conjunctivitis, 1035
Follicular cyst, 1957-1958
Follicular dendritic cells (FDCs), *see website*
Folliculitis, 2305, 2305f
eosinophilic pustular, 2220
hot tub, 2305, 2306f
Follistatin in testicular function, *see website*
Fomepizole for toxic alcohol poisoning, 256t-257t, 268
Fomivirsen, *see website*
Fontanels
in neurologic examination, *see website*
newborn examination of, 533-534, 534t
Fontan procedure
modified, for tricuspid atresia, 1581-1582
for pulmonary atresia, 1579-1580
Food. *See also* Feeding; Nutrition
adverse reaction to, 820-824, 820t-821t, 823f, 823t
anaphylaxis due to, 816-817, 816t
atopic dermatitis and, 806
challenge testing in, 768
chronic diarrhea due to, 1341
urticaria due to, 812t, 814
chemical pollutants in, *see website*
composition of for short method of dietary analysis, *see website*
drug interaction with, *see website*
functional, 169
habits regarding in eating disorders, 92t
organic, 169
ready to use therapeutic, 177, 177f
as reward, 167
Food and Agriculture Organization (FAO), 171
Food and Drug Administration (FDA), on teratogens, 547
Food assistance programs, 170
Food-borne illness
bacterial, 1324t-1325t
botulism, 987-991
Campylobacter, 968-969
Clostridium, *see website*
listeriosis as, *see website*
noninfectious, 1328t-1329t, 2454, *see also website*
due to melamine poisoning, 2454, *see also website*
due to mushroom poisoning, 2454, *see also website*
due to seafood poisoning, 2454, *see also website*
due to solanine poisoning, 2454
parasitic, 1327t-1328t
Salmonella, 949-950
Shigella, 959
Staphylococcus aureus in, 906
toxoplasmosis, 1208-1216
during travel, *see website*
viral, 1326t
Food challenges in allergic disease, 768
Food environment, 167, 168f
Food insecurity, 170-171
Food intolerance, 820, 820t
Food safety, 169
Food security, 170
Foot
arthrogryposis involving, *see website*
calcaneovalgus, 2336
cavus, 2340, 2340f
immersion, 358
limb rotation in, 2344
musculoskeletal pain syndrome of, 877t
painful, differential diagnosis for, 2344t
palmoplantar keratodermas of, 2272-2273
sports injury to, 2417f
venous access in, 292, 295f
vesicular dermatitis of, 2253
Football, injuries in, *see website*
Foot disorders
calcaneovalgus feet as, 2336
cavus feet as, 2340, 2340f
congenital vertical talus as, 2337-2338, 2337t, 2338f
hypermobile pes planus (flatfoot) as, 2338, 2338f
metatarsus adductus as, 2335, 2335f
osteochondroses/apophysitis as, 2340-2341, 2340f
painful foot in, 2344, 2344t
puncture wounds as, 2341
shoes and, 2344
talipes equinovarus (clubfoot) as, 2336, 2337f
tarsal coalition as, 2339-2340, 2339f, 2339t
toe deformities as, 2341-2342
Foot progression angle (FPA), 2345f-2346f, 2346
Foramen of Morgagni hernia, 597, 597f
Foramen ovale in neonatal circulation, *see website*
Forced expiratory volume in 1 sec (FEV_1), *see also website*
in asthma, 784, 785t, 786f, 789t-790t
in pulmonary function testing, *see website*
Forced expiratory volume in 1 sec (FEV_1)/forced vital capacity (FVC) ratio, 784, 785t, 786f, 789t-790t, *see also website*
Forced vital capacity (FVC), *see also website*
in asthma, 784, 785t, 786f, 789t-790t
in pulmonary function testing, *see website*
Forchheimer spots, 1075-1076
Fordyce spots, 1260-1261, 2297
Forearm fracture, 2391-2392
Forefoot, 2335
Foregut, 1273
Foregut cyst, 1452
Foreign body(ies)
airway, 1453-1454, 1453f
aspiration of
croup *versus*, 1447
management of, 282-283
neonatal, 590, 591f
wheezing in, 1457
bronchial, 1453f, 1454
esophageal, 1271-1272, 1272f-1273f
external ear canal, *see website*
in eye, 2167t, 2185, 2185f
laryngeal, 1454
nose, 1431-1432
in stomach and intestine, 1290, 1290f
tracheal, 1454
uterine
abnormal uterine bleeding due to, 689t-690t
dysmenorrhea due to, 690
vaginal, 1866f, 1867
abnormal uterine bleeding due to, 689t-690t
bleeding due to, 1869
dysmenorrhea due to, 690
Foreign-born children. *See* Immigrant children
Forensic evidence collection following rape, 704
Formeterol, 794t
Formula feeding, 162-164, 162f
human milk *versus*, 161t
otitis media and, 2200
of premature infant, 560
Fortaz. *See* Ceftazidime
Fosamprenavir, 1168t-1171t
Foscarnet, *see also website*
for cytomegalovirus infection, 1116-1117
for varicella-zoster virus, 1108
Foscavir. *See* Foscarnet
Fosinopril for systemic hypertension, 1645t
Fosphenytoin
for seizures, neonatal, 2037
for status epilepticus, 2038-2039
Foster care, 134, *see also website*
Foster Care Independence Act of 1999, *see website*
Fostering Connections to Success and Increasing Adoptions Act, *see website*
Founder effect, 381
Fournier gangrene, *see website*
Fourth-generation cephalosporins, *see website*
Fourth Geneva Convention, *see website*
Fourth heart sound, auscultation of, 1533
Fourth nerve palsy, 2159-2160
Fox-Fordyce disease, 2288
Foxglove toxicity, 269t, 272t-273t
FOXP3 gene, *see website*
FPA. *See* Foot progression angle (FPA)
FPS. *See* Family Psychosocial Screening (FPS)
Fraction of inspired oxygen (FIO_2)
in mechanical ventilation, 327
oxygen administration and, 319
partial pressure of carbon dioxide divided into, 319
Fracture(s), 2387-2394, 2388f
avulsion, sports-related, 2408-2409, 2409f
as birth injury, 578-579
buckle or torus, 2390, 2391f
due to child abuse, 138-139, 2390
clavicular, 2392
as birth injury, 578-579
as delivery room emergency, 578-579
as sports injury, 2409
complete, 2390
complications of, 2394t
epiphyseal, 2390, 2390t, 2391f
as delivery room emergency, 579
of extremities, 579
femoral shaft, 2393, 2393t
forearm, 2391-2392
greenstick, 2390
healing of, 2389
hip, 2392
humeral
distal, 2392
proximal, 2392
as sports injury, 2410
supracondylar, 2410
lower extremity, 2392
metatarsal, 2393
of nose, as delivery room emergency, 579
orbital, 2186
outcomes of, 2394
overgrowth after, 2389
patterns of, 2389
pelvic, 339
phalangeal, 2391
plastic deformation, 2389-2390, 2389f-2390f
progressive deformity after, 2389, 2389f
remodeling of, 2388f, 2389
ribs
due to child abuse, 138
traumatic, 338
skull, in newborn, 565-566
stress, 2416-2417
calcaneal, 2418
femoral neck, 2413
humeral, 2410
metatarsal, 2418
navicular, 2418
in runners, *see website*
tibial, 2416
surgical treatment of, 2393-2394, 2394t
temporal bone, *see website*
tibial and fibular, 2392-2393
Tillaux, 2393

Fracture(s) *(Continued)*
timetable of radiologic changes in, 139t
toe, 2393
tooth, 1258, 1258f
triplane, 2393, 2393f
types of, 2388f
upper extremity, 2390-2391
Fragile chromosome sites, 411-412, 411t
Fragile X gene, 411
Fragile X syndrome, 411-412, *see also website*
congenital heart disease with, 1531t
intellectual disability and, 127t
Fragmentation hemolysis, 1661f, 1683, *see also website*
Frameshift, genetic, *see website*
Framework for well child care, 16
Franceschetti syndrome, 1254
Francisella tularensis, 978-980, 978f, 978t-979t
in pneumonia, 1475t
Frank-Starling curves, *see website*
Fraser syndrome, *see website*
Fraying in rickets, 202, 203f
FRC. *See* Functional residual capacity (FRC)
Freckles, 2236
in neurofibromatosis, 2046-2047
Free bilirubin, 1375
Free fatty acids (FFAs), 520-521, 522t
Free recall, *see website*
Free water clearance, hyponatremia due to decreased, 1885
Freiberg disease, 2436t
Freiberg infraction, 2340-2341
French-American-British (FAB) classification
of acute lymphocytic leukemia, 1732
of acute myeloid leukemia, 1737, 1737t
Frenulum, lingual, short, *see website*
Freon, as inhalant, 681t
Freudian theory, *see website*
Friedreich ataxia, 2055
cardiac manifestations of, 1531t
Frisen scale, *see website*
Frohlich syndrome, 182t
Frontal plagiocephaly, 2012
Frontal sinuses, 1436
Frostbite, 358
of auricle, *see website*
Frostnip, 357-358
Frovatriptan for migraine, 2044t
Fructokinase deficiency, 503
Fructose, defects in metabolism of, 503-504
Fructose-1,6-diphosphatase deficiency, 524t, 529
Fructose intolerance
hereditary, 494t-495t, 503, 524t
hypoglycemia in, 529
Fructose malabsorption, 1316-1317
FSGS. *See* Focal segmental glomerulosclerosis (FSGS)
FSGS1 gene, 1803t
FSGS2 gene, 1803t
FSH. *See* Follicle-stimulating hormone (FSH)
FSI. *See* Fear of self-injecting (FSI)
FTA-ABS. *See* Fluorescent treponemal antibody absorption (FTA-ABS) test
FTT. *See* Failure to thrive (FTT)
5-FU. *See* 5-Fluorocytosine (5-FU)
Fucosidosis, 484t, 489-490
Fukuda stepping test, *see website*
Fukuyama congenital muscular dystrophy, 2127
Full-thickness burn, 351, 351t
Fulminant colitis, 1297
Fulminant hepatic failure, 1412-1415, 1414t. *See also* Acute liver failure (ALF)
Fumagillin, *see website*
Functional abdominal pain, 1346-1349
Functional constipation, 1284, 1284t
Functional foods, 169
Functional gastrointestinal disorders (FGIDs), 1346-1349, 1346t-1348t
Functional magnetic resonance imaging (fMRI), *see website*
Functional proteomics, *see website*
Functional residual capacity (FRC), *see also website*
abnormalities of, *see website*
chest wall compliance and, *see website*
decreased, *see website*
first breath and, 580
in mechanical ventilation, 322, 323f
Fundoplication
for gastroesophageal reflux disease, 1268-1269
Nissen, 527
Fundus
coloboma of, 2181
development of, *see website*
examination of, 2150
Fundus flavimaculatus, 2178
Fungal infections
due to *Aspergillus*, 1058-1062
due to *Blastomyces dermatitidis*, 1064-1065
due to *Candida*, 1053-1056
chronic mucocutaneous, 1056
in immunocompromised patients, 1055-1056, 1056t
neonatal, 1053-1054, 1054t
due to *Coccidioides*, 1065-1068
due to *Cryptococcus neoformans*, 1056-1058
cutaneous, 2309-2314
atopic dermatitis with, 806
candidal, 2313-2314
dermatophytoses as, 2309-2313, 2310f
tinea versicolor as, 2309, 2309f
fever of unknown origin in, 900t
following organ transplantation, *see website*
due to *Histoplasma capsulatum*, 1062-1064
HIV-related, *see website*
due to *Malassezia*, 1058, *see also website*
maternal, *see website*
of nails, 2296
neonatal
diagnosis of, 642-644
sepsis due to, 635t-636t
due to *Paracoccidioides brasiliensis*, 1068, *see also website*
due to *Pneumocystis jiroveci*, 1069, *see also website*
in pneumonia, 1475t
predisposition to due to immunodeficiency, 716t
due to *Sporothrix schenckii*, 1068, *see also website*
therapy for, 1053, *see also website*
zygomycosis as, 1069, *see also website*
Fungemia, *see website*
Fungus
allergic reaction to, 769-770
rapid antigen detection of, *see website*
Funnel chest, 1516-1517, 1516f
FUO. *See* Fever of unknown origin (FUO)
Furadantin. *See* Nitrofurantoin
Furan. *See* Nitrofurantoin
Furazolidone, *see also website*
for giardiasis, 1182, 1182t
for infectious diarrhea, 1337t
"Furious" rabies, 1154-1155
Furosemide
for acute renal failure, 1820
for heart failure, *see website*
for hypertensive emergencies, 1646t
for nephrotic syndrome, 1805
possible adverse reactions to in premature infant, 563t
for subcutaneous fat necrosis, 2284
for systemic hypertension, 1645t
Furuncle, 2305-2306, 2306f
external otitis *versus*, 2197
Furunculosis, 2198
Fusion, tooth, 1250
Fusion genes, cancer associated with, *see website*
Fusion inhibitors for HIV infection, 1168t-1171t
Fusobacterium, *see website*
Fusobacterium necrophorum, *see website*
Fusospirochetal gingivitis, 2299
Futility, life-sustaining medical treatment and, *see website*
Fuzeion. *See* Enfuvirtide
FVC. *See* Forced vital capacity (FVC)
FWT1 oncogene, 1757-1758
FWT2 oncogene, 1757-1758

G
GABA. *See* γ-Aminobutyric acid (GABA)
Gabapentin
adverse effects of, 2031t
for migraine prophylaxis, 2044t
for neuroirritability in palliative care, 155t-156t
for pain management, 364t, 369-370
neuropathic, 368t
in palliative care, 155t-156t
for seizures, 2030t
GABHS. *See* Group A beta-hemolytic streptococci (GABHS)
GABRA1 gene, 2016t
GABRG2 gene, 2016t
GAD. *See* Generalized anxiety disorder (GAD); Glutamic acid decarboxylase (GAD) deficiency
GAG. *See* Glycosaminoglycan (GAG)
Gag reflex, *see website*
brain death and, *see website*
GAG region, 1157
Gain-of-function gene mutation, *see website*
Gait
assessment of, 2331-2332, 2332t, 2333f
causes of abnormal, 2332t
in-toeing, 2347
of Legg-Calvé-Perthes disease, 2361
maturation of, *see website*
neurologic examination of, *see website*
Gait, arms, legs, spine screen (GALS), 2331, 2333f
Galactokinase deficiency, 502
cataracts with, 2171
Galactorrhea, *see website*
Galactose, defects in metabolism of, 494t-495t, 502-503
Galactosemia, 524t
cataracts with, 2170-2171
fetal therapy for, 551t
malignancy susceptibility associated with, *see website*
ovarian damage due to, 1956
transferase deficiency, 502-503
Galactosialidosis, 484t, *see website*
Galerina poisoning, *see website*
Gallbladder
disorders of, 1415, *see also website*
with obesity, 184t
normal size of, 1387
Gallstones, *see website*
Gambian trypanosomiasis, 1190-1193
Gambierdiscus toxicus, *see website*
Gammaglobulin, intravenous, 866-867, 867t
γ-Thalassemia, 1676
GAMT. *See* Guanidinoacetate methyltransferase (GAMT) deficiency
Ganciclovir, 1116-1117, *see also website*
Ganglion, 2385
Ganglioneuroblastoma, diarrhea caused by, *see website*
Ganglioneuroma, diarrhea caused by, *see website*
Gangliosidosis, 2069-2072
GM_1, 483-491, 2069-2070, 2072f
GM_2, 484-487, 2070-2071
Gang rape, 703
Gangrene, *see website*
Gantamicin, 644
Gantanol. *See* Sulfamethoxazole
Gantrisin. *See* Sulfisoxazole
Garamycin. *See* Gentamicin
Gardner syndrome, *see website*
GAS. *See* Group A streptococcus (GAS)

Gases. *See also* Oxygen administration
inhaled
in neonatal resuscitation, 576
for respiratory distress and failure, 319-320
toxic, 269-270
Gases composition
alveolar, 316
inspired, 316
Gas exchange, *see website*
Gas gangrene, *see website*
Gasping, sudden infant death syndrome and, 1428
Gastric content aspiration, 1470
Gastric duplication, 1276
Gastric emptying, drug absorption and, *see website*
Gastric fluid, loss of, 245
Gastric lavage for poisoning, 255-257
Gastric mucosa, *see also website*
malabsorption due to defects of, 1305t
peptic ulcer disease and, 1291-1292
Gastric outlet obstruction, 1275-1276
Gastric volvulus, 1276
Gastrin in neuroendocrine tumor-associated diarrhea, *see website*
Gastrinoma, diarrhea caused by, *see website*
Gastroenteritis, 1323-1339
Aeromonas, *see website*
appendicitis *versus*, 1353
bacterial, 1324t-1325t
Campylobacter, 968-970
reactive arthritis due to, 970
clinical manifestations of, 1331-1332, 1332t
complications of, 1333-1334, 1333t
diagnosis of, 1333-1334, 1333t
eosinophilic, 1304
chronic diarrhea in, 1340-1341
due to hookworm, 1219
malabsorption due to, 1321
epidemiology of, 1323, 1326f
Escherichia coli, 961-965
etiology of, 1323
global trends in, 1326f
noninfectious, 1328t-1329t
parasitic, 1327t-1328t
pathogenesis of, 1323-1330, 1330f-1331f, 1330t
Plesiomonas shigelloides, 974, *see also website*
prevention of, 1337-1338
risk factors for, 1330-1331
rotavirus, calcivirus, and astrovirus, 1134-1137
Salmonella, 951-953, 953t
Shigella, 959-961
traveler's diarrhea as, 1338-1339, 1338t
treatment of, 1334-1337, 1334t-1335t, 1335f-1336f, 1337t
viral, 1326t
Gastroesophageal junction (GEJ), *see website*
Gastroesophageal reflux disease (GERD), 1266-1270
aspiration due to, 1471
asthma and, 783, 791
bronchopulmonary dysplasia with, *see website*
clinical manifestations of, 1267
complications of, 1269-1270
due to congenital diaphragmatic hernia, 596
in cystic fibrosis, 1496
diagnosis of, 1267-1268, 1267f-1268f
epidemiology and natural history of, 1266
epilepsy *versus*, *see website*
management of, 1268-1269
pathophysiology of, 1266
reactive airway disease, 1263
respiratory signs and symptoms of, *see website*
wheezing in, 1458
Gastrointestinal bleeding, 1248-1249, 1248t
in acute renal failure, 1821
Gastrointestinal decontamination for poisoning, 255
Gastrointestinal disorders. *See* Digestive system disorders
Gastrointestinal obstruction
causes of, 1243t
vomiting due to, 1242
Gastrointestinal stromal cell tumor (GIST), *see website*
Gastropathy, hypertrophic, 1276
Gastrostomy feeding, 560
GATA3 gene, 1917
Gatifloxacin, *see website*
Gaucher disease, 484t, 487-488, 487f
cardiac manifestations of, 1531t
cutaneous manifestations of, 2268t
Gay men, 658
GBM. *See* Glomerular basement membrane (GBM)
GBS. *See* Gram-positive bacterial infection; Guillain-Barré syndrome (GBS)
GCAD. *See* Graft coronary artery disease (GCAD)
GCS. *See* Glasgow Coma Scale (GCS)
GCTs. *See* Germ cell tumors (GCTs)
Gefitinib, *see website*
GEFS+. *See* Generalized epilepsy with febrile seizures plus (GEFS+)
GEJ. *See* Gastroesophageal junction (GEJ)
Gell and Coombs classification, 824
Gemifloxacin, *see website*
Gemination, tooth, 1250
Gender consistency, 655
Gender constancy, 655
Gender factors
in childhood injuries, 20
in otitis media, 2200
Gender identity, 655
Gender identity disorder, 656, 657t
Gender labeling, 655
Gender queen, 655
Gender role, 655
Gender role nonconformity, 655-656
Gender variance, 655-656
Gender variant, 655
Gender variant identity, 656-658
Gene(s)
fusion, cancer associated with, *see website*
modifier, *see website*
in oncogenesis, *see website*
Gene amplification in proto-oncogene activation, *see website*
Gene polymorphism
defined, *see website*
effects on drug response, *see website*
General anesthesia, 359, *see also website*
General appearance
of newborn, 532-533
in pediatric emergency assessment, 279
General assessment in pediatric emergency, 279, 280f
Generalized anxiety disorder (GAD), 80, 80t
Generalized epilepsy with febrile seizures plus (GEFS+), 2017
Generalized lipodystrophy, 2286
Generalized motor seizure, 2023
Generalized seizure, 2013, 2023-2024
benign, 2023
treatment of, 2028
secondary, 2021, 2022f
severe, 2023-2024
treatment of, 2028
Generation, skipped, 383-385
Gene-replacement therapies, 381
Genetic approach in pediatric medicine, 380-383
Genetic association, *see website*
Genetic counseling, 377-379, 378t
in acute intermittent porphyrias, *see website*
in chronic granulomatous disease, 746
in congenital heart disease, *see website*
in erythropoietic protoporphyria, *see website*
in hearing loss, 2196
in Marfan syndrome, 2446
Genetic counseling *(Continued)*
in neurofibromatosis, 2048
in osteogenesis imperfecta, 2439-2440
in paroxysmal disorders, 467
in transmissible spongiform encephalopathies, *see website*
in X-linked adrenoleukodystrophy, 470
Genetic counselor, 382t
Genetic disorders
aneuploidy and polyploidy as, 399-400, 400t
burden of, 380-381
diabetes mellitus associated with, 1986
failure to thrive in, 148t
genotype-phenotype correlation's in, *see website*
hypomelanosis of Ito, 412
management and treatment of, 379-380
of neurotransmitters, 445-447, 445t
obesity due to, 182t, 185
severe intellectual disability in, 123t
vascular, 2230-2231
Genetic epidemiology, *see website*
Genetic factors
in childhood cancers, 1727t
in development, *see website*
in drug response (*See* Pharmacogenetics)
in febrile seizures, 2017
in high-risk pregnancy, *see website*
in immunodeficiencies, *see also website*
antibody, 723t, 724-725, 724f
combined, 731t
in inflammatory bowel disease, 1294-1295
in meningococcus, 931
in otitis media, 2200
in psychosomatic illness, 68
in puberty, *see website*
in sudden infant death syndrome, 1423t, 1425-1427, 1426f
environmental factors interaction in, 1427, 1427f
Genetic heterogeneity, 376
Genetic imprinting, 391-393, 393f
Geneticists, 382t
Genetic professionals, 382, 382t
Genetic recombination, 376, 395, *see website*
Genetics
of acute lymphocytic leukemia, 1732-1733, 1732t-1733t
of allergic disease, *see website*
of antibody deficiency disorders, 723t
of asthma, 781
of attention deficit/hyperactivity disorder, 108
of autistic disorder, 102
of cancer, 1728, *see also website*
changing paradigm of, 381-382
of Chédiak-Higashi syndrome, 744
of chorea, 2057t
of chronic granulomatous disease, 745-746
of combined immunodeficiency disorders, 731t
of common disorders, 414-415, 415f, *see also website*
of congenital central hypoventilation syndrome, 1520-1521
of congenital diarrheal disease, 1342t
of congenital heart disease, *see website*
of congenital muscle fiber-type disproportion, 2116
of craniosynostosis, 2012t
of cystic fibrosis, 1481-1482, 1483f, 1483t
cyto- (*See* Cytogenetics)
of developmental disorders of muscle, 2112-2113, 2113t
of diabetes mellitus
type 1, 1970-1971, 1970f, 1974
type 2, 1991
of DiGeorge syndrome, 728-729
of Down syndrome, 404t
of Duchenne and Becker muscular dystrophy, 2121-2122, 2122f
of embryonic gonadal differentiation, *see website*

Genetics *(Continued)*
environment and, *see website*
of epilepsy, 2016t
ethical considerations, 382-383
of febrile seizures, 2017
fundamentals of molecular, *see website*
of gluten-sensitivity enteropathy, 1308-1309
of hearing loss, 2189, 2190t
of hemolytic-uremic syndrome, 1792t
of hemophilia, 1700-1701
of hereditary spherocytosis, 1659t
human genome in, 383, *see website*
Human Genome Project in, 383, *see also website*
of 21-hydroxylase deficiency, 1930
of hyperphenylalaninemia, 418
of hypopigmentation, 2238t
of inguinal hernia, 1363
internet reference sites associated with, 380t
of language and communication disorders, 116
of leukocyte adhesion deficiency as, 741
of maple syrup urine disease, 431
of Marfan syndrome, 2443
of multiple pituitary hormone deficiency, 1876-1878
of myeloperoxidase deficiency, 745
of myotonic muscular dystrophy, 2123f
of myotubular myopathy, 2115
of nemaline rod myopathy, 2117
of nephrotic syndrome, 1803t
of neuroblastoma, 1755t
of neuromuscular disorders, 2110
of overweight and obesity, 182-183, 182t
pharmaco- (*See* Pharmacogenetics)
of primary ciliary dyskinesia, *see website*
of skeletal dysplasias, *see website*
of spinal muscular atrophy, 2137
of surfactant disorders, *see website*
types of professions associated with, 382, 382t
of tyrosinemia, 422
variations and mutations in, *see website*
of von Willebrand disease, 1706
of Wilms tumor, 1757-1758, 1757t
of Wiskott-Aldrich syndrome, 734
Genetic testing
in arthrogryposis, *see website*
in celiac disease, 1309
in cystic fibrosis, 1488
diagnostic, 376-377, 377f, 381-382
ethics of, 382-383, *see website*
fetal, 543t
in intellectual disability, 125, 127t
pharmacogenetic, 377
predicative, 377
predispositional, 377
in seizure therapy, 2029
Genetic transmission, 383-394
digenic inheritance in, 389, 390f
family history and pedigree notation in, 383, 384f-387f
genetic imprinting in, 391-393, 393f
mendelian inheritance in, 383-388
autosomal dominant, 383-385, 387f
autosomal recessive, 385-388, 388f
pseudodominant, 388, 388f
X-linked, 388, 388f-389f
mitochondrial inheritance, 390-391, 390f-391f, 391t
multifactorial and polygenic inheritance in, 393-394, 393f
pseudogenetic inheritance and familial clustering in, 389-390
in triplet repeat expansion disorders, 391, 392t, 393f
Y-linked inheritance in, 388-389, 390f
Genital culture, *see website*
Genital herpes, 708, 709t, 1100-1101, 1103
maternal, 1103-1104
sexual abuse and, 145t
treatment of, 713t
Genitalia
ambiguous (*See* Ambiguous genitalia)
aphthous ulcers of, 1866, 1866f
examination of, female, *see also website*
following rape, 704
following sexual abuse, 144-145, 144f
newborn assessment of, 536
preschooler curiosity regarding, 35
Genital tuberculosis, 1007
Genital ulcer syndromes, 708
Genital warts, 1138-1139, 1139f, 2316, 2316f
sexual abuse and, 145, 145t
treatment in adolescents, 713t
Genitourinary disorders
anaerobic infection as, *see website*
Chlamydia trachomatis infection as, 1035-1036
due to cystic fibrosis, 1487
enteroviruses in, 1091
mycoplasmal infection as, 1032-1033
sports participation and, 2402t-2404t
tuberculous infection as, 1006-1007
due to typhoid fever, 957t
Genitourinary system of newborn, 621, *see also website*
Genitourinary trauma, 339, 1864, *see also website*
Genome-wide association studies (GWAS), *see website*
Genomic disorders, 381
Genomic imprinting, 391-393, 393f
in cancer development, *see website*
in oncogenesis, *see website*
Genomics, pharmacology with. *See* Pharmacogenomics
Genotype
of acute lymphocytic leukemia, 1733f
defined, *see website*
of dysmorphology, *see website*
Genotype-phenotype correlations in genetic disorders, *see website*
Gentamicin, *see also website*
for bacterial meningitis, 2093t
for brucellosis, 981t
for gonococcal disease, 939
for infective endocarditis, 1625t
for neonatal infection, 645t
for plague, *see website*
possible adverse reactions to in premature infant, 563t
for pyelonephritis, 1832
for *Staphylococcus aureus*, 907t
for tularemia, 979
Genu valgum, 2350
Genu varum, 2348-2350, 2348f, 2348t-2349t
Geocillin. *See* Carbenicillin
Geodon. *See* Ziprasidone
Geographic factors
in adolescent health, 660, 660f
in arboviral encephalitis, 1141-1143, 1142f-1143f
outside of U.S., 1145t
in dengue-like disease, 1147t
in developmental dysplasia of the hip, 2356
in echinococcosis, 1237, 1237f
in hantavirus pulmonary syndrome, *see website*
in insect allergy, 807f
in Lyme disease, 1025, 1025f
in malaria, 1198-1199, 1198f
in poliovirus infection, 1081, 1082f
in porphyria cutanea tarda, *see website*
in tuberculosis, 996f-997f
in worldwide death rates, 3-4, 3t
Geographic tongue, 1261, 2298-2299, 2298f
Geopen injection. *See* Carbenicillin
GERD. *See* Gastroesophageal reflux disease (GERD)
German chamomile for sedation, 271t
German measles. *See* Rubella
Germ cell tumors (GCTs), 1769-1771, 1770f
of central nervous system, 1752-1753
incidence and survival rates for, 1726t
ovarian, 1871-1872
risk factors for, 1727t
in undescended testis, 1859
work-up of, 1731t
Germinoma, 1770
Germline mosaicism, 383-385
Germ line stat 1 mutation, 735
Germ tube test in candidiasis, 1053
Gerstmann-Sträussler-Scheinker syndrome (GSS), 1177, *see also website*
Gestational age
assessment of, 557, 558f
eye examination schedule based on, 2175t
large-for, *see website*
GFGR2 gene, 2012t
GFR. *See* Glomerular filtration rate (GFR)
GGT. *See* γ-Glutamyl transpeptidase (GGT)
GH1 gene, 1878
Ghon complex in tuberculosis, 998
GHRH. *See* Growth hormone-releasing hormone (GHRH)
Gianotti-Crosti syndrome, 2266, 2266f
Epstein-Barr virus and, 1112-1113
Giant axonal neuropathy, 2140
Giant cell arteritis, 868t
Giant cell granuloma of jaw, *see website*
Giant cell pneumonia, 1071
Giant cells, in response to hepatic injury, 1394
Giant papillary conjunctivitis, 810
Giardia duodenalis, *see website*
Giardia lamblia, 1180-1183, 1181t-1182t
gastroenteritis due to, 1327t-1328t
treatment of, 1337t
inflammatory bowel disease *versus*, 1298t
in traveler's diarrhea, 1338t
Giemsa stain, *see website*
Gigantism, *see website*
Giggle incontinence, 1851
Gilbert syndrome, 606
abdominal pain of, 1247t
Gingival cysts of newborn, 2298
Gingival lesions, due to vitamin C deficiency, 198, 199f
Gingival overgrowth, cyclosporine- or phenytoin-induced, 1257
Gingivitis, 1257
necrotizing ulcerative, 1257-1258, 1260t, 2299, *see also website*
Gingivostomatitis herpetic, 1102, 1260, 1260f, 1260t
Ginkgo biloba for asthma, 271t
Girls
first sign of puberty in, 649
growth curves for, *see website*
percentile growth curves for, *see website*
GIST. *See* Gastrointestinal stromal cell tumor (GIST)
Gitelman syndrome, 223, 1813t, 1814, *see also website*
GJB2 gene, 2190t
GJB6 gene, 2190t
GKB3 gene, 2190t
Gla-containing proteins, 210
Glanders, *see website*
Glandular disease, *Francisella tularensis*, 979
Glandular fever, 1110
Glanzmann thrombasthenia, 1721-1722
Glargine insulin, 1976
Glasgow Coma Scale (GCS)
in drowning victim, 347
in pediatric emergency, 281, 281t
in traumatic brain injury, 298, 337
Glaucoma, 2181, *see also website*
Gleevec. *See* Imatinab mesylate
Glenn cavopulmonary anastomosis, *see website*
Glenn procedure, 1579-1580
Glenn shunt, bidirectional, 1581
Glenoid labrum tear, 2410

Gliding undescended testis, 1859
Glimepride, 1992t
Glioma
brain stem, 1748t
environmental carcinogens and, *see website*
intranasal, 1431
optic nerve, *see website*
in neurofibromatosis, 2047f
Glipizide, 1992t
Glitinides, 1992t
GLL. *See* Graduated licensing law (GLL)
Global abuse and neglect, 136
Global childhood injuries, 19
Global developmental delay, 124
Global hypoxic-ischemic insult, 301-303
Global impact of drowning, 342-343
Globin genes, *see website*
Globoid cell leukodystrophy, 490-491, 2071-2072
Globulins
drug binding and, *see website*
serum, liver disease and, 1378
Globus, 1240
Glomerular basement membrane (GBM), *see website*
Glomerular disease, 1778, *see also website*
isolated with recurrent gross, 1781-1783
Glomerular filtration, 1778, *see also website*
Glomerular filtration rate (GFR), *see website*
Glomerular proteinuria, 1801, 1801t
Glomerular tubular balance, *see website*
Glomerulonephritis, 1778, *see also website*
acute, 1785t
poststreptococcal, 1783-1785, 1783f-1784f, 1785t
associated with infection, 1333t, 1783-1786
associated with systemic lupus erythematosus, 1788-1789
due to leprosy, *see website*
membranoproliferative, 1787-1788
rapidly progressive, 1785t, 1789-1790, 1790f, 1790t
Glomerulopathy, membranous, 1786-1787
Glomerulosclerosis, focal segmental, 1803t, 1804
Glomerulus, anatomy of, 1778, *see also website*
Glossitis
benign migratory, 2298-2299
migratory, 1261
due to riboflavin deficiency, 193f
Glossopharyngeal nerve, neurologic examination of, *see website*
Gloves, *see website*
Glucagon
for hypoglycemia, 1985
as poisoning antidote, 256t-257t
Glucagonoma syndrome, *see website*
Glucocorticoid receptor, *see also website*
in steroid hormone regulation, *see website*
Glucocorticoid-remediable aldosteronism, 236
Glucocorticoids
actions of, *see also website*
for allergic disease, 772
familial deficiency of, 1924-1925
for 21-hydroxylase deficiency, 1934-1935
receptor gene mutation, 1962
regulation of secretion of, 1923
for rheumatic disease, *see website*
Glucocorticoid-suppressible hyperaldosteronism, 1938-1939
Glucocorticosteroids, topical, 2217t
Gluconeogenesis, disorders of, 504, 529
Glucose. *See also* Hyperglycemia; Hypoglycemia
cerebral, 517
cerebrospinal fluid
in CNS infection, 2088t
normal, *see website*
in tuberculosis, 1006
homeostasis of
in infants and children, 518
in newborn, 518
in hyperinsulinism, 521t
Glucose *(Continued)*
impaired tolerance of (*See* Impaired glucose tolerance (IGT))
intolerance of in chronic kidney disease, 1823t
laboratory testing of
in diabetes mellitus, 1975-1976, *see website*
in obesity, 185t
in maintenance fluid therapy, 243
monitoring of in type 1 diabetes mellitus, 1976-1977, 1983-1984, 1983t
for pediatric resuscitation and arrhythmias, 294t
in plasma osmolality, *see website*
as poisoning antidote, 258t
reference values for, *see website*
Glucose-galactose malabsorption, 1306t, 1317-1319
chronic diarrhea with, 1341
Glucose-6-phosphatase dehydrogenase (G6PD)
deficiency of, 492-496, 504
hemolytic anemia due to, 1678-1680, 1679f-1680f, 1679t, *see website*
hypoglycemia in, 528
primaquine therapy and, *see website*
Rocky Mountain spotted fever and, 1042
reference values for, *see website*
Glucose tolerance test, 1993
reference values for, *see website*
Glucose transporter 1 (GLUT-1) defects, 529
Glucose transporter 2 (GLUT-2) defects, 499, 529
α-Glucosidasie inhibitors, 1992t
Glucuronosyl transferase (UGT)
deficiency, 1390
partial, 1390
drug biotransformation and, *see website*
drug metabolism and, *see website*
GLUT-1. *See* Glucose transporter 1 (GLUT-1) defects
GLUT-2. *See* Glucose transporter 2 (GLUT-2) defects
Glutamate pyruvate in liver dysfunction evaluation, 1378
Glutamic acid, defects in metabolism of, 442f, 444f
Glutamic acid decarboxylase (GAD) deficiency, 447
Glutamic acid decarboxylase (GAD) transaminase deficiency, 447
Glutamic oxaloacetic transaminase in liver dysfunction evaluation, 1378
Glutamine
in acid-base balance, *see website*
congenital deficiency of, 445
γ-Glutamylcysteine synthetase deficiency, 444
γ-Glutamyl transpeptidase (GGT)
deficiency of, 444-445
reference values for, *see website*
Glutaric aciduria, 454-455, 2060t
Glutathionemia, 444-445
Glutathione synthetase deficiency, 443-445, 444f, 742t
GLUT2 deficiency, 1319
Gluten, type 1 diabetes mellitus and early exposure to, 1972
Gluten-free diet, 1310-1311
Gluten-sensitivity enteropathy, 1308-1311, 1308f, 1309t-1310t, 1310f
Glycemic control in type 1 diabetes mellitus, 1984
long-term complications associated with, 1988-1989, 1988t
Glycemic index, *see website*
D-Glyceric acid aciduria, 440
Glycerin enema, 74t
Glycerin suppositories, 74t
Glycerol for bacterial meningitis, 2094
Glycine
defects in metabolism of, 438-441, 439f, 441f, 1319
genetic disorders of, 445t
Glycine encephalopathy, 439-440
Glycogenoses, 494t-495t, 2113t, 2131, *see also website*
Glycogenosis type II, 1523-1524
Glycogen storage diseases (GSDs), 492-501, 493f, 494t-495t, 748t, 751
cardiac manifestations of, 1531t
Fanconi-Bickel syndrome as, 499
glycogen synthetase deficiency as, 498
hypoglycemia in, 528
mimicking hypertrophic cardiomyopathy, 500
type I, 492-496, 504
malignancy susceptibility associated with, *see website*
type II, 499-500, 500f
type III, 496-497, 496f
type IV, 497
type IX, 497-498
type V, 500-501
type VI, 497
type VII, 501
Glycogen synthetase deficiency, 494t-495t, 498
hypoglycemia in, 528
Glycolytic enzyme deficiencies, 1677-1678
Glycopeptides, *see website*
Glycoprotein(s)
degradation and structure, disorders of, 509, *see also website*
Rhesus-associated, *see website*
variant surface, 1191
Glycoprotein syndrome, carbohydrate-deficient, 1311
Glycopyrrolate for respiratory secretions, 155t-156t
Glycosaminoglycan (GAG), 509, 514
Glycosylated hemoglobin (HbA_{1A}), 1984
Glycosylation, congenital disorders of, 1311, *see website*
Glycyrrhize glabra for asthma, 271t
GM-CSF. *See* Granulocyte macrophage-colony-stimulating factor (GM-CSF)
GM_1 gangliosidosis, 483-491, 484t, 2060t, 2069-2070, 2072f
GM_2 gangliosidosis, 484-487, 484t, 2070-2071
Gnathostoma species, 1220t, 1227, *see website*
GnRH. *See* Gonadotropin-releasing hormone (GnRH)
Goiter, 1905-1909
acquired, 1908-1909
congenital, 1905-1906, 1906f
endemic
cretinism and, 1906-1908
maternal, *see website*
fetal therapy for, 551t
intratracheal, 1906
due to iodine-deficiency, 1907f
iodine-deficiency endemic, 1897
in lymphocytic thyroiditis, 1903-1904
Goitrogens, 1908t
Goltz syndrome, 2222
Gonadal tumors, 1769-1771
non-germ cell, 1770
Gonadoblastoma, 1770, 1955, 1958
Gonadotropin deficiency
female, 1956
male, 1949
Gonadotropin-independent precocious puberty, familial male, 1893
Gonadotropin-releasing hormone (GnRH)
for growth hormone deficiencies, 1881
in precocious puberty diagnosis, 1888
in puberty, *see website*
Gonadotropin-releasing hormone (GnRH) agonists
for endometriosis, 690-691
for precocious puberty, 1889
Gonadotropin-secreting tumors, 1891
Gonads
development and function of, 1943, *see also website*
diagnostic aids, *see website*

Gonads *(Continued)*
dysfunction of due to cancer and its therapy, *see website*
effects of eating disorders on, 92-93
gynecomastia as, 1950-1951
ovaries as
function of, *see website*
hypofunction of, 1951-1957
pseudoprecocity resulting from lesions of, 1957-1958
testes as
function of, *see website*
hypofunction of, 1943-1950
pseudoprecocity resulting from tumors of, 1943-1950
see website
therapeutic aids, *see website*
Gongylonemiasis, *see website*
Gonococcus. *See* Gonorrhea
Gonorrhea, 935-940
clinical manifestations of, 937
complications of, 939
in conjunctivitis, 2166-2167
diagnosis of, 710t, 937-938
epidemiology of, 935-936
etiology of, 935
maternal, *see website*
neonatal, 632t
pathogenesis and pathology of, 936-937
prevention of, 939-940
prognosis for, 939
prophylaxis following rape, 704, 704t
sexual abuse and, 145t
treatment of, 938-939
in adolescent, 712t
Goodell sign, 700
Goodpasture disease, 1499, 1785t, 1790-1791, 1791f
Gordon syndrome, 221, 1814
Gorlin-Goltz syndrome, *see website*
Gorlin syndrome, 408t, *see also website*
Goserelin acetate for precocious puberty, 1889
Gottron papules
in juvenile dermatomyositis, 846-847, 847f, *see website*
in rheumatic disease, *see website*
Gout, *see website*
Gower's sign, *see website*
Gown, *see website*
G6PD. *See* Glucose-6-phosphatase dehydrogenase (G6PD)
gp 41 protein, 1157-1158, 1158f
gp 120 protein, 1157-1158, 1158f
Graded exercise therapy for chronic fatigue syndrome, *see website*
Gradenigo syndrome, 2210-2211
Graduated licensing law (GLL), 22
Graft(s)
failure, stem cell transplantation, 762
intestinal, *see website*
liver, *see website*
Graft coronary artery disease (GCAD), *see website*
Graf technique, 2358
Graft thrombosis, renal transplantation, *see website*
Graft *versus* host disease (GVHD)
cutaneous manifestations of, 760-761, *see also website*
in hematopoietic stem cell transplantation, 760-762, 761f-762f, 761t
liver involvement in, *see website*
in intestinal transplantation, *see website*
malabsorption due to, 1314
as oncologic emergency, *see website*
Grain allergy, 823t
Gram-negative bacterial infections
due to *Aeromonas*, 974, *see also website*
due to *Bartonella*, 982-987
breast-feeding and, 540t
Gram-negative bacterial infections *(Continued)*
due to *Brucella*, 980-982
due to *Burkholderia*, 975, *see also website*
due to *Campylobacter*, 968-970
chancroid as, 944, *see also website*
cholera as, 965-968
due to *Escherichia coli*, 961-965
due to *Haemophilus influenzae*, 940-943
due to *Legionella*, 982, *see also website*
due to *Moraxella catarrhalis*, 944, *see also website*
due to *Neisseria gonorrhoeae*, 935-940
due to *Neisseria meningitidis*, 929-935
neonatal, 632t
sepsis due to, 635t-636t
pertussis as, 944-948
due to *Plesiomonas shigelloides*, 974, *see also website*
pneumonia as, 1475t
due to *Pseudomonas aeruginosa*, 975-977
due to *Salmonella*, 948-958
enteric (typhoid) fever due to, 954-958
nontyphoidal, 949-954
due to *Shigella*, 959-961
due to *Stenotrophomonas*, 976, *see also website*
tularemia as, 978-980
due to *Yersinia*, 971-974
Gram-positive bacterial infection
Actinomyces, 929, *see also website*
due to diphtheria, 929, *see also website*
due to enterococcus, 928, *see also website*
due to group A streptococcus, 914-925
rheumatic fever as, 920-925
due to group B streptococcus, 925-928
due to *Listeria monocytogenes*, 929, *see also website*
malignancy-related, *see website*
neonatal, 632t
sepsis due to, 635t-636t
Nocardia, 929, *see also website*
due to non-group A or B streptococci, 928, *see also website*
due to staphylococci, 903-910
coagulase-negative, 909-910
Staphylococcus aureus, 904-908
toxic shock syndrome, 908-909
due to *Streptococcus pneumoniae*, 910-914
Gram stain, *see website*
Granisetron for vomiting, 1244t
Granular cells, 2215
Granule(s)
Birbeck, 1773-1774
deficiency of, 742t
sorting disorders of, 748t, 751
Granulocyte colony-stimulating factor (G -CSF)
in allergic disease, *see website*
for Fanconi anemia, 1686
fetal, *see website*
Granulocyte macrophage-colony-stimulating factor (GM-CSF), *see website*
Granulocytes, *see website*
Granulocyte transfusion (GTX), 1693, *see also website*
Granulocytopoiesis
fetal, *see website*
primary disorders of, 750
Granuloma
in brucellosis, 980
candidal, 2314
caseating in nontuberculous mycobacteria, 1012
cholesterol, of tympanic membrane, 2212
coccidioidal, 1065-1068
fish tank, 1013
giant cell of jaw, *see website*
pyogenic, 2229, 2229f
swimming pool, 1013
umbilical, *see website*
Granuloma annulare, 2274-2275, 2274f
Granulomatosis
allergic, 868t
Wegener's, 868t, 874-876, 874t, *see also website*
alveolar hemorrhage with, 1499
Granulomatous amebic meningoencephalitis, 1178, *see also website*
Granulomatous colitis. *See* Crohn's disease
Granulomatous disease
chronic, 742t, 745-746, 745f
aspergillosis with, 1061
fetal therapy for, 551t
infections and, *see website*
fever of unknown origin in, 900t
hypercalcemia in, 1922
Granulomatous thyroiditis, subacute, 1905
Granulomatous vasculitis, 868t
Granulosa cell tumor, juvenile, ovarian, 1957-1958
Graphomotor function, *see website*
Grasp response in neurologic examination, *see website*
"Grass," 680-681
Graves disease, 1909-1913, 1909t, 1911f, 1912t
cardiac manifestations of, 1531t
maternal, *see website*
Gray baby syndrome, *see website*
Gray (Gy), *see website*
Gray platelet syndrome, 1722
Great arteries
malposition of with double-outlet right ventricle, 1588-1589
transposition of the
(*See* Transposition of great arteries (TGA))
Great saphenous vein, venous access in, 292, 295f
Green and Anderson method, *see website*
Greenstick fracture, 2388f, 2390
Grey Turner sign, 1371
Grief, *see website*
Griscelli syndrome type II, 748t, 751
Griseofulvin
drug interactions with, *see website*
for tinea capitis, 2311
Gross motor development during first 2 years, 27t
Gross motor incoordination, *see website*
Ground transport, *see website*
Group A beta-hemolytic streptococci (GABHS)
glomerulonephritis development after, 1783-1785
in impetigo, 2299
in pharyngitis, 1439
in pharyngotonsillitis, 1443
Group A streptococcus (GAS), 914-925
clinical manifestations of, 916-917, 916f, 917t
complications of, 919
diagnosis of, 917-918
differential diagnosis of, 918
epidemiology of, 915
etiology of, 915
glomerulonephritis associated with, 1783-1785, 1783f-1784f, 1785t
obsessive-compulsive disorder associated with, 81
pathogenesis of, 915-916
in pneumonia, 1475t
prevention of, 920
prognosis for, 920
in rheumatic fever, 920-925
severe, 917, 917t
in toxic shock syndrome, 909
treatment of, 918-919
with varicella-zoster virus, 1109
in vulvovaginitis, 1868t
Group B streptococcus (GBS), 925-928
clinical manifestations of, 926-927, 926t
diagnosis of, 927
epidemiology of, 925-926, 925f
etiology of, 925

Group B streptococcus (GBS) *(Continued)*
fetal therapy for, 551t
laboratory findings in, 927
maternal
breast-feeding and, 540t
fetal and neonatal effects of, *see website*
neonatal, 632t
in meningitis, 646
prophylaxis for, 640, 640f, 640t
sepsis due to, 635t
in osteomyelitis, 2394
pathogenesis of, 926
in pneumonia, 1475t
prevention of, 927-928
prognosis for, 927
treatment of, 927, 927t
Group C streptococci, 928, *see also website*
in pharyngitis, 1439
Group G streptococci, 928, *see also website*
Group therapy for eating disorders, 95
Growing pains, 878, 878t, *see website*
Growth and development, 26
adolescent, 649-659, 650t
during early adolescence, 649-659, 650t-652t, 651f
during late adolescence, 654
during middle adolescence, 653-654
assessment of, 39, *see also website*
attachment and contingency and, *see website*
behavioral, *see also website*
during first year of life, 28t
biologic influences on, *see website*
biopsychosocial models of, *see website*
breast-feeding and, 162
caloric requirements for, *see website*
centers of ossification in, 29t
child care and, *see website*
cognitive
during adolescence, 649-651, 653
age 0-2 months, 27
age 2-6 months, 30
age 6-12 months, 30
age 12-18 months, 31-32
age 18-24 months, 32
during middle childhood, 37-38, 37t
during preschool years, 34
communication
ages 2-6 months, 30
ages 6-12 months, 31
cystic fibrosis and, 1496
domains of, *see website*
with Down syndrome, 403t
ecologic model of, *see website*
effects on drug disposition, *see website*
effects on pharmacodynamics, *see website*
embryonic, *see website*
emotional
age 0-2 months, 27-28
age 2-6 months, 30
age 6-12 months, 30-31
age 12-18 months, 31, 32t
age 18-24 months, 32
during middle childhood, 38
during preschool years, 35-36
family systems and, *see website*
fetal
assessment of, 26, *see also website*
restriction of (*See* Intrauterine growth restriction (IUGR))
during first year, 26-31
age 0-2 months, 26-29
age 2-6 months, 29-30
age 6-12 months, 30-31
developmental milestones in, 27t
glucocorticoids and, *see website*
linguistic
age 12-18 months, 31
age 18-24 months, 33
during preschool years, 34
loss, separation, and grief and, *see website*
during middle childhood, 36-39
Growth and development *(Continued)*
moral
during adolescence, 649-651, 653
during middle childhood, 38
during preschool years, 35-36
neurologic, *see website*
newborn, 26
maternal-infant attachment in, *see website*
pediatrician's role in, *see website*
physical
adolescent, 649, 650t-652t, 651f-652f, 653-654
age 0-2 months, 27, 29f
age 2-6 months, 29-30
age 6-12 months, 30
age 12-18 months, 31-32
age 18-24 months, 32-33
during middle childhood, 36-37
percentile curves for, *see website*
during preschool years, 33-34
of play
during preschool years, 34-35
of premature infant, 562
during preschool years, 33-36
psychologic influences on, *see website*
resilience and, *see website*
risk factors in, *see website*
during second year, 31-33
developmental milestones in, 27t
in skeletal dysplasias, *see website*
social
during adolescence, 652-654
during middle childhood, 38
social factors in, *see website*
somatic, *see website*
statistics used in describing, *see website*
theories of emotion and cognition in, *see website*
transactional model of, *see website*
Growth charts, *see also website*
derivation and interpretation of, *see website*
in obesity assessment, 179, 180f-181f, 184-185
Growth factor
deficiency of due to cancer and its therapy, *see website*
for Fanconi anemia, 1686
hematopoietic, for fever in neutropenic patient, *see website*
insulin-like, *see website*
oncogenes code for, *see website*
vascular endothelial
in ovarian carcinomas, 1872t
in retinopathy of prematurity, 2174
in sudden infant death syndrome, 1422, 1427
Growth hormone (GH), *see also website*
deficiency and insensitivity of
abnormalities of growth hormone receptor in, 1879
classification of, 1876-1878
clinical manifestations of, 1879
combined with other pituitary hormone deficiencies, 1876-1878, 1876t
complications and adverse effects of, 1881
diabetes insipidus due to, 1881-1884
differential diagnosis of, 1880-1881
genetic forms of, 1878
hypoglycemia in, 527-528
laboratory findings in, 1879-1880
obesity due to, 182t
post-receptor forms of, 1879
radiologic findings in, 1880
treatment of, 1881
excess secretion of, *see website*
myopathies with, 2129-2130
human, 1880-1881
for Turner syndrome, 1954
hyponatremia due to disorders of, 1884-1886
for performance enhancement, 2423t
underproduction of (*See* Hypopituitarism)
Growth hormone (GH) receptor, *see website*
abnormalities of, 1879
Growth hormone-releasing hormone (GHRH), *see website*
Growth hormone-releasing hormone (GHRH) receptor, mutations in, 1878
Growth impairment
in chronic kidney disease, 1823t, 1824
in congenital hypothyroidism, 1898
constitutional, 1880
in Crohn disease, 1300-1302
in cystic fibrosis, 1496
in failure to thrive, 147
fetal, 541, 541f
therapy for, 551t
in foreign-born adoptee, 131
after hematopoietic stem cell transplantation, *see website*
in hypothyroidism, 1901, 1902f
due to immunosuppression therapy, *see website*
due to inhaled corticosteroids, 793
in 3-methylglutaconic aciduria, 433
with Turner syndrome, 1952, 1952f
Growth plate
sports injury to, 2408-2409, 2408f-2409f
widening of in rickets, 200, 202, 203f
Growth-remaining charts, epiphysiodesis and, *see website*
Growth restriction, intrauterine, 555-564
definitions associated with, 555
factors related to, 557t
fetal therapy for, 551t
gestational age at birth assessment in, 557, 558f
incidence of, 555-556
nursery care in, 558-562
prognosis for, 562-563, 563t
spectrum of disease in, 558, 559t
type 2 diabetes mellitus and, 1990
Grunting
during expiration in newborn, 535
as sign of respiratory pathology, *see website*
GSDs. *See* Glycogen storage diseases (GSDs)
GSS. *See* Gerstmann-Sträussler-Scheinker syndrome (GSS)
GTX. *See* Granulocyte transfusion (GTX)
Guanfacine, 111t
Guanidinoacetate methyltransferase (GAMT) deficiency, 441
Guidance, anticipatory
health eating habits, 188t
in injury prevention, 19t
in palliative care, 151-159
in well child care, 14
Guillain-Barré syndrome (GBS), 2143-2146, 2144t, 2145f-2146f
botulism *versus*, 989-990
Campylobacter and, 919, 969, 1333t
poliovirus infection *versus*, 1084, 1085t
Gum boil, 1261
Gun injuries, 24-25
Günther disease, 2256, *see also website*
Gut, fetal development of, 1273
Guttate psoriasis, 2259
GVHD. *See* Graft *versus* host disease (GVHD)
GWAS. *See* Genome-wide association studies (GWAS)
Gy. *See* Gray (Gy)
Gymnastics, injuries in, 2423t
Gynecological care for special needs girls, 1874-1875
Gynecological examination, *see website*
of special needs girls, 1874
Gynecological problems
of breast, 1870, *see also website*
hirsutism as, *see website*
history and physical examination in, 1865, *see also website*

Gynecological problems *(Continued)*
neoplasms as, 1870-1874
cervical, 1873-1874, 1873t
impact of cancer therapy on fertility and, 1870-1871
ovarian, 1870-1871, 1872t
uterine, 1872-1873
vaginal, 1873
vulvar, 1873
polycystic ovary syndrome, 1870, *see also website*
vaginal bleeding as, 1869-1870
vulvovaginal and müllerian anomalies of, 1874, *see also website*
vulvovaginitis as, 1865-1869, 1865f-1866f, 1867t-1868t, 1868f
Gynecomastia, 1950-1951
due to drugs, *see website*
Gyrate atrophy of retina and choroid, 453
Gyromitra poisoning, *see website*

H

H^+. *See* Hydrogen ions (H^+)
HAART. *See* Highly active antiretroviral therapy (HAART)
Habit cough, *see website*
Habit disorders, 75-76
Habit tic deformity, 2294
Habituation, fetal, *see website*
HACEK group, *see website*
HAE. *See* Hereditary angioedema (HAE)
Haemophilus ducreyi, 712t, 944, *see also website*
Haemophilus influenzae, 940-943
antibiotic resistance by, 941
in bacterial meningitis, 2087
clinical manifestations and treatment of, 941-943
in cystic fibrosis infections, 1482, 1492t
diagnosis of, 941
epidemiology of, 940
etiology of, 940
immunity to, 941, 941t
neonatal, 632t
in otitis media, 2201, *see also website*
pathogenesis of, 940-941
prevention of, 943
testing for antibodies to, 719-720
vaccine for, 943
Haemophilus influenzae type b
in child-care setting, *see website*
epidemiology of, 940
hearing loss due to, 2188-2189
immunity to, 941
in meningitis, 941-942, 2087, 2089
prevention of, 2095
in pneumonia, 1475t
prophylaxis for, 943
in septic arthritis, 2398
Haemophilus influenzae type b vaccine (Hib), 881t, 941t, 943
diphtheria acellular pertussis (DTaP) vaccine with (DTaP/Hib), 884t
with hepatitis B vaccine (Hip-HepB), 884t
HIV infection and, 1173f
international, 894
recommended schedule for, 886, 887f
for travel, *see website*
Hageman factor, 1696t
Hair
axillary, development of, *see website*
bamboo, 2293
disorders of, 2289-2293, 2289t-2290t
effects of eating disorders on, 93t
effects of malnutrition on, 175t
over lumbosacral area in newborn, 533
pubic, sexual maturity ratings of changes in, 651f
repetitive pulling of, 75
spun-glass, 2293, 2293f
structural defects of, 2292
HAIR-AN syndrome, 686
Hair follicles, morphology of, *see website*
Hair loss. *See also* Alopecia
acquired diffuse, 2291-2292
congenital diffuse, 2292-2293
Hair pulling, 2289-2290, 2290f
Haldol. *See* Haloperidol
Half-life of drug, *see website*
Haller index on chest computed tomography, 1516
Hallopeau-Siemens epidermolysis bullosa, 2245t, 2246
Hallucinations, 106-107, 107f
hypnagogic/hypnopompic, 53
Hallucinogens, 682-683
Hallux valgus, 2341, 2341f
Halogen acne, 2327
Halo nevus, 2233, 2233f
Haloperidol, 63
for agitation in palliative care, 155t-156t
for pain management, 364t
for psychosis and agitation, 64t
Halo sign, 1060
Haltia-Santavuori disease, 2073
Hamartoma
connective tissue, 2235
hypothalamus, precocious puberty due to, 1890
intestinal, *see website*
in iris, due to neurofibromatosis, 2046-2047, 2047f
multiple, 2298
smooth muscle, 2235-2236
Hamartoma syndrome, overgrowth in, *see website*
Hamman sign, 1512
Hammer toe, 2342
Ham test, *see website*
Hand
arthrogryposis involving, *see website*
orthopedic problems of, 2385-2387, 2385f-2386f, 2385t-2387t
palmoplantar keratodermas of, 2272-2273, 2273f
venous access in, 292, 295f
vesicular dermatitis of, 2253, 2253f
Handedness, 33
Hand-foot-mouth disease, 1090, 1090f, 1260t
Hand-foot syndrome, 1663-1664
Handguns, 24-25, 667-668, 670t
Hand hygiene, *see website*
Hand-Schüller-Christian disease, 1773-1774
Handwashing, 647
Hansen disease, 1011, *see also website*
Hantavirus in pneumonia, 1475t
Hantavirus pulmonary syndrome (HPS), 1154, *see also website*
HAPE. *See* High-altitude pulmonary edema (HAPE)
Haplo-hematopoietic stem cell transplantation (HSCT), *see website*
Haploid cells, 395, *see website*
Haploinsufficiency, *see website*
Haplotypes, *see website*
HapMap, *see website*
Haproglobin in congenital dyserythropoietic anemia, *see website*
Harderoporphyrinogen, *see website*
Hardy-Weinberg formula, 388
Harlequin color change, 2218
in newborn, 533
Harlequin ichthyosis, 2267, 2268t
Harness, Pavlik, 2359, 2360f
Harrison groove in rickets, 200, 202f
Hartnup disorder, 429-430, 1319, 2258
Harvest mite bite, 2320
"Hash," 680-681
Hashimoto thyroiditis, 1903-1905
myasthenia gravis with, 2133
type 1 diabetes mellitus with, 1996
Hassall's corpuscles, *see website*
HAT. *See* Human African trypanosomiasis (HAT)
Havrix, *see website*
Hawkinsinuria, 423
Hb. *See* Hemoglobin (Hb)
HbA_{1A}. *See* Glycosylated hemoglobin (HbA_{1A})
Hb AS. *See* Hemoglobin AS
Hb C. *See* Hemoglobin C (Hb C)
HBeAg. *See* Hepatitis B e antigen (HBeAg)
Hbf. *See* Fetal hemoglobin (Hbf)
HBIG. *See* Hepatitis B immunoglobulin (HBIG)
Hb S. *See* Hemoglobin S (Hb S)
HBsAg. *See* Hepatitis B s antigen (HBsAg)
HCM. *See* Hypertrophic cardiomyopathy (HCM)
HCO_3^-. *See* Bicarbonate (HCO_3^-)
HCoV-229E. *See* Human coronavirus 229E (HCoV-229E)
HCoV-HKU1. *See* Human coronavirus HKU1 (HCoV-HKU1)
HCoV-NL63. *See* Human coronavirus NL63 (HCoV-NL63)
HCoV-OC43. *See* Human coronavirus OC43 (HCoV-OC43)
HCP. *See* Hereditary coproporphyria (HCP)
HCS. *See* Holocarboxylase synthetase (HCS) deficiency
HD. *See* Huntington's disease (HD)
HDL. *See* High-density lipoproteins (HDL)
HDR syndrome, 1917
Head
centers of ossification appearance in, 29t
examination of in neurologic evaluation, *see website*
newborn assessment of, 533-534, 534t
positioning of for bag-valve-mask ventilation, 284-285, 285f
rickets and, 201t
Headache, 2039-2046
in brain tumors, 1747
migraine
familial hemiplegic, *see website*
syncope induced by, *see website*
recurrent, sports participation and, 2402t-2404t
in Rocky Mountain spotted fever, 1042
secondary, 2045-2046, 2045t
sinus, 2045-2046
tension-type, 2046
thunderclap, 2084
Head and neck block for pain management, 371
Head circumference
in autistic disorder, 101-102
in neurologic examination, *see website*
percentile curves for, *see website*
Head drop, 2019
Head injury. *See* Traumatic brain injury (TBI)
Head lice. *See* Pediculosis
HEADS/SF/FIRST mnemonic, 666, 666t
HEADSS screening interview, 57, 57t
Head-tilt/chin-lift maneuver, 282, 282f, 291f
Head trauma. *See also* Traumatic brain injury (TBI)
abusive, 139-140, 139f
hemorrhagic stroke due to, 2084
Healing of fracture, 2389
Health
among postinfancy children, 2-4
child care and, *see website*
genetic contribution to, 414-415, 415f
homosexuality and, 659
worldwide, 3t
Health Belief Model, *see website*
Health care
access to
for adolescent, 662-663, 663f
international, *see website*
adolescent, delivery of, 663-667, 664t
for at-risk populations, 10-11
costs of, 11
evaluation of, 11

Health care (Continued)
foster and kinship care and, see website
medical errors in, see website
patterns of, 9
prenatal, see website
preventive (See Preventive health care)
quality of (See Quality, of health care)
Health-care associated infection. See Nosocomial infection
Health care providers
death of patient and, see website
infection control and prevention for, see website
obesity prevention and, 187t
palliative care and, 153
training of for emergencies, see website
Health care reform, effects on quality, see website
Health information technology (HIT), see website
Health insurance
for adolescents, 663, 664f
travel and, see website
Health Insurance Portability and Accountability Act of 1996 (HIPPA), see website
Health InterNetwork Access to Research Initiative (HINARI), see website
Health promotion
in community, 17
in well child care, 14
Health risk behaviors in adolescents, 661f
Health services. See Health care
Hearing impairment or loss, 2188-2196
due to cancer and its therapy, see website
in cleft lip and palate, 1253
clinical audiologic evaluation of, 2193-2196, 2193f
conductive, 2188
due to congenital rubella syndrome, 1077-1078
with Down syndrome, 403t
effects of, 2190-2192, 2191t
etiology of, 2188-2190, 2189t-2191t, 2191f
familial, cardiac manifestations of, 1531t
genetic counseling in, 2196
genetics of, 391t
identification of, 2192, 2193t
incidence and prevalence of, 2188
infectious causes of, 2191t, see also website
language disorders due to, 119
maternally inherited diabetes and, 1994-1995
screening for, 2192, 2192f
in adolescent, 666
in intellectual disability, 127t
in neurologic examination, see website
in newborn, 538
sensorineural, 2188
due to toxoplasmosis, 1213
treatment of, 2196, 2196t
types of, 2188
in X-linked adrenoleukodystrophy, 468
Heart. See also Cardiac entries; Cardiovascular entries
abnormal position of, 1595-1596
development of, 1527, see also website
examination of, 1533-1536, 1536f
mumps virus in, 1080
newborn assessment of, 535, 535f
radiologic assessment of, 1537
transition from fetal to neonatal circulation in, 1529, see also website
tumors of, 1637, see also website
following transplantation, see website
Heart block
atrioventricular, 1618-1619, 1618f
bundle branch, 1540
complete, 1618-1619, 1618f
genetics of, see website
electrocardiography of first degree, 1540
familial secundum atrial septal defect with, see website
Heart block (Continued)
fetal therapy for, 551t
sinoatrial, 1618
Heartburn, 1261
Heart disease. See also Cardiovascular disease
congenital (See Congenital heart disease (CHD))
failure to thrive in, 148t
phosphorylase kinase deficiency as, 498
psychopharmacology and, 65
renal transplantation and, see website
rheumatic, 1626-1628
tuberculous, 1004
with Turner syndrome, 1952-1953
Heart failure, 1550, 1638
cardiogenic shock for, 1638, see also website
in cystic fibrosis, 1494-1495
follow open heart surgery, 1604
history of, 1530
hypothyroidism-associated, 1903t
physical examination of, 1531
total body water regulation and, see website
Heart-lung transplantation, 1638, see also website
Heart murmur
auscultation of, 1535-1536
infective endocarditis and, 1623
of mitral insufficiency, 1571-1572
sports participation and, 2402t-2404t
Heart rate
assessment of, 1531-1532, 1532t
fetal
acceleration of, 543-544
in biophysical profile, 543t
deceleration of, 543-544, 544f
monitoring of, 542, 543t
neonatal resuscitation and, 575-576
normal, 280t
Heart sounds
in acutely ill child evaluation, 276
in cardiac examination, 1533
Heart transplantation, 1638, see also website
for hypoplastic left heart syndrome, 1595
Heart tube, embryonic, 1527
Heartworm, dog, 1226
Heat cramps, 2420
Heat edema, 2420
Heat exhaustion, 2420
Heat injury, sports-related, 2402t-2404t, 2420-2421, 2421f
Heat stroke, 2420, 2421f
Heat syncope, 2420
Heat tetany, 2420
Heavy metal intoxication, 2448, see also website
Heel bisector line (HBL), 2346, 2347f
Hegar sign, 700
Height. See also Length
for age, in nutrition assessment, 172
growth charts for assessment of, see website
Heimlich maneuver, 282-283, 283f
Heiner syndrome, 1498-1499
Heinz bodies, 1670-1671, 1678, see also website
Helicobacter pylori, 1292, 1292f-1293f, 1293t, 1294
Heliotrope rash of juvenile dermatomyositis, 846-847
Heliox. See Helium-oxygen mixture
Helium-oxygen mixture, 319-320
Helmet for bicycle injury prevention, 22-23
Helminthic disease
adult tapeworm, 1232-1234, 1232t, 1233f-1234f
Angiostrongylus cantonensis, 1226-1227
animal filariae, 1226
ascariasis, 1217
cysticercosis, 1234-1237, 1236f, 1237t
dracunculiasis, 1227
echinococcosis, 1237-1239, 1238f
enterobiasis, 1222, 1222f
flukes, 1231-1232, see also website
Gnathostoma spinigerum, 1227
Helminthic disease (Continued)
hookworms, 1218-1221
loiasis, 1225-1226, 1226f
lymphatic filariasis, 1224-1225, 1225f
Onchocera volvulus, 1225
schistosomiasis, 1230-1231, 1230f-1231f
strongyloidiasis, 1223-1224, 1223f
toxocariasis, 1227-1229, 1228t
treatment of, see website
trichinosis, 1229-1230
trichuriasis, 1221-1222, 1221f
Helper T cells
in allergic disease, see website
in amyloidosis, 860-861
development and differentiation of, see website
in Epstein-Barr virus, 1111
flow cytometry testing of, 720-722
in HIV/AIDS, 1157-1161
interaction with other immune cells, see website
Hemagglutinin protein in influenza virus, 1122
Hemangioendothelioma, 1762t
kaposiform, 2229
Hemangioma, 1772, 2226-2228, 2227f, 2227t-2228t, see also website
abnormal uterine bleeding due to, 689t-690t
capillary eyelid, 2164-2165, 2164f
hepatic, hypothyroidism due to, 1901
nasal, 1431
noninvoluting congenital, 2229
orbital, 2182, 2182f
rapidly involuting congenital, 2229
subglottic, see website
vascular malformations *versus*, 2225t
Hemangiomatosis, diffuse, 2228, 2228f
Hemangiopericytoma, 1762t
Hematemesis, 1248
Hematochezia, 1248
Hematocrit
in abnormal uterine bleeding, 688-690
in anemia, 1648t
fetal, see website
in polycythemia, see website
reference intervals for, see website
Hematologic disorders. See Blood disorders
Hematoma
subcapsular, 578
subdural, due to child abuse, 139, 139f
Hematopoietic growth factor, see website
Hematopoietic stem cell transplantation (HSCT), 757
for acute lymphocytic leukemia, 757, 758f
for acute myeloid leukemia, 757-758
for aplastic anemia, 759, 759f
autologous, see website
for β-thalassemia, 1676
for Chédiak-Higashi syndrome, 744-745
for chronic myelogenous leukemia, 758
for Diamond-Blackfan anemia, 1651
donors and sources for, 760
children as, see website
haploidentical, see website
HLA-compatible sibling, 757-760, 758t
umbilical cord, see website
unrelated, see website
donor *versus* recipient NK-cell alloreactivity in, see website
for Fanconi anemia, 1686
fungal infection associated with, 1055
graft *versus* host disease and rejection of, 760-762, 761f-762f, 761t
for Hodgkin disease, 759
for immunodeficiency disorders, 760
infectious complications of, 762-763
enteroviruses in, 1092
for juvenile myelomonocytic leukemia, 758
late effects of, 763, see also website
for Lesch-Nyhan disease, see website
for leukocyte adhesion deficiency, 744
liver disease due to, see website
for mucopolysaccharidoses, 514

Hematopoietic stem cell transplantation (HSCT) *(Continued)*
for myelodysplastic syndromes, 758-759
for non-Hodgkin lymphoma, 759
pancytopenia caused by, 1692
for sickle cell disease, 759-760
for thalassemia, 759, 760f
for X-linked adrenoleukodystrophy, 468-469
Hematopoietic syndrome, due to whole-body irradiation, *see website*
Hematopoietic system, *see website*. See Blood disorders
Hematuria
in Alport syndrome, 1782-1783, 1782f
anatomic abnormalities associated with, 1796-1799
due to autosomal dominant polycystic kidney disease, 1798, 1798f
due to autosomal recessive polycystic kidney disease, 1796-1798, 1797f, 1797t
benign familial, 1783
clinical evaluation of, 1778-1781, 1779t-1780t, 1780f
in glomerulonephritis associated with systemic lupus erythematosus, 1788-1789
in Goodpasture disease, 1790-1791, 1791f
hematologic diseases causing, 1795-1796
in hemolytic-uremic syndrome, 1791-1794, 1791t-1792t
in Henoch-Schönlein purpura nephritis, 1789
due to idiopathic hypercalciuria, 1795
in immunoglobulin A nephropathy, 1781-1782, 1781f
isolated glomerular disease with recurrent gross, 1781-1783
lower urinary tract causes of, 1799
in membranoproliferative glomerulonephritis, 1787-1788
in membranous glomerulopathy, 1786-1787
in rapidly progressive glomerulonephritis, 1789-1790, 1790f, 1790t
due to renal vein thrombosis, 1794-1795
in thin basement membrane disease, 1783
due to trauma, 1799
due to vascular abnormalities, 1794
due to vigorous exercise, 1799
Heme biosynthetic pathway, *see website*
Heme synthetase deficiency, *see website*
Hemiconvulsion, hemiplegia, epilepsy (HHE) syndrome, 2038
Hemifacial microsomia, 1254
Hemimelia, fibular, 2351
Hemin, for acute intermittent porphyrias, *see website*
Hemiparesis, with seizures, 2016-2017
Hemiparetic gait, *see website*
Hemiplegia
alternating of childhood, 2060t, 2061, *see also website*
strokelike events *versus*, 2086
in cerebral palsy, 2062, 2062t
Hemiplegic migraine, 2042
Hemispherectomy for seizures, 2032-2033
Hemlock toxicity, 269t
Hemochromatosis
cardiac manifestations of, 1531t
malignancy susceptibility associated with, *see website*
neonatal, 1383, 1393
type 4, 1321
Hemodialysis
for end-stage renal disease, 1826
for metabolic acidosis, 235
osmolality during, *see website*
for poisoning with toxic alcohols, 268
Hemodynamics of ventricular septal defect, 1557-1558
Hemoglobin A_{1C} in obesity, 185t
Hemoglobin AS (Hb AS), 1670, 1670t-1671t
Hemoglobin C (Hb C), 1663-1670
Hemoglobin Eβ, 1670
Hemoglobin F, 1675
Hemoglobin (Hb)
in abnormal uterine bleeding, 688-690
adult, *see website*
alterations of by disease, *see website*
in anemia, 1648t
of chronic disease, *see website*
neonatal, 612, 614-615
in congenital dyserythropoietic anemia, *see website*
development of, *see website*
embryonic, *see website*
fetal, *see website*
in erythroblastosis fetalis, 617
syndromes of hereditary persistence of, 1673-1674
glycosylated, 1984
in hereditary spherocytosis, 1660
in iron deficiency-anemia, 1656t-1657t
in polycythemia, *see website*
reference intervals for, *see website*
in systemic-onset juvenile idiopathic arthritis, 836
Hemoglobin M, 1672
Hemoglobinopathies, 1662-1677
abnormal hemoglobins causing cyanosis as, 1672
abnormal hemoglobins with increased oxygen affinity as, 1671
hemoglobin C as, 1663-1670
hemoglobin Eβ as, 1670
hereditary methemoglobinemia as, 1672-1673, 1673f
sickle cell disease as, 1663-1670
clinical manifestations of, 1663-1669, 1663t, 1665t, 1666f, 1668t
diagnosis of, 1669, 1669t
sickle cell trait as, 1663-1670, 1670t-1671t
syndromes of hereditary persistence of fetal hemoglobin as, 1673-1674
thalassemia syndromes as, 1674-1677, 1674t, 1675f
unstable hemoglobin disorders as, 1670-1671
Hemoglobin S (Hb S), 1663
Hemoglobinuria
paroxysmal cold, 1683
paroxysmal nocturnal, 748t, 755, 1662, *see also website*
Hemolysis
chronic, 1653
in congenital erythropoietic porphyria, *see website*
defined, 1659
fragmentation, 1661f, 1683, *see also website*
Hemolytic anemia
acanthocytosis as, *see website*
autoimmune, 1680-1683, 1681t
due to bartonellosis, 982
definitions and classification of, 1659, *see also website*
enteric infection and, 1333t
enzymatic defects in, 1677-1680, 1678f-1680f, 1679t
after Epstein-Barr virus infection, 1114
due to extracellular factors, 1683, *see also website*
hemoglobinopathies as, 1662-1677
abnormal hemoglobins causing cyanosis as, 1672
abnormal hemoglobins with increased oxygen affinity as, 1671
hemoglobin C as, 1663-1670
hemoglobin Eβ, 1670
hereditary methemoglobinemia as, 1672-1673, 1673f
sickle cell disease as, 1663-1670
sickle cell trait as, 1663-1670, 1670t-1671t
syndromes of hereditary persistence of fetal hemoglobin as, 1673-1674
Hemolytic anemia *(Continued)*
thalassemia syndromes as, 1674-1677, 1674t, 1675f
unstable, 1670-1671
hereditary elliptocytosis as, 1662, *see also website*
hereditary spherocytosis as, 1659-1662, 1659t, 1660f-1662f
hereditary stomatocytosis as, 1662, *see also website*
paroxysmal nocturnal hemoglobinuria as, 1662, *see also website*
parvovirus B19 infection and, 1095
Hemolytic disease of newborn, 615-619, 620t
due to ABO incompatibility, 619
due to Rh incompatibility, 615-619, 616t
Hemolytic-uremic syndrome (HUS), 1718, 1791-1794, 1791t-1792t
enteric infection and, 1333t
Hemophagocytic lymphohistiocytosis (HLH), 744, 1774-1776, 1776t
Hemophilia A, 1699-1702, 1701t
Hemophilia B, 1699-1702, 1700f, 1701t
Hemophilia C, 1702-1703
Hemoptysis
as manifestation of extrapulmonary disease, *see website*
pulmonary, 1503-1504, 1503t, 1504f
in cystic fibrosis, 1493
Hemorrhage/bleeding
into adrenal glands, 1927
as delivery room emergency, 578
alveolar, diffuse, 1498-1500, 1498t
cardiac arrest due to, 289t
into chest cavity, 1513-1514
in chronic kidney disease, 1823t
endobronchial, in cystic fibrosis, 1493
epistaxis as, 1432-1433
esophageal, *see website*
gastrointestinal, 1248-1249, 1248t
in acute renal failure, 1821
due to hemangioma, 2227t
intracranial, 303-304
cerebral palsy and, 2061-2062
due to child abuse, 139, 139f
due to hypernatremia, 214
imaging studies in, *see website*
in newborn, 566-568, 567f, 568t
in high-risk pregnancy, *see website*
in newborn, 620-621, 621t
from nose, 1432-1433, 1432t
peptic ulcer, 1293
perifollicular, due to vitamin C deficiency, 198-199, 199f
pulmonary, 1503-1504, 1503t, 1504f
neonatal, 599
retinal
due to child abuse, 139-140, 140f, 2186, 2186f
neurologic examination of, *see website*
in newborn, 534, 566, *see website*
due to vomiting, 1243t
subarachnoid
emergency management of, 304
in newborn, 566
subconjunctival, 2168-2169
in newborn, 566
subgaleal, 565
transplacental, anemia due to, 612-613
umbilical, *see website*
uterine, abnormal, 686t, 688-690, 689t-690t
vaginal, 1869-1870
variceal, 1376, 1415, *see also website*
vitamin K-deficiency, 210
Hemorrhagic conjunctivitis, due to enterovirus, 1091
Hemorrhagic corpus luteum, 1871
Hemorrhagic cystitis, 1799
adenovirus in, 1132
Hemorrhagic cystitis, acute, 1830

Hemorrhagic disorders
acquired inhibitors of coagulation in, 1712-1713
clinical and laboratory evaluation of, 1696-1699
disseminated intravascular coagulation as, 1713-1714, 1713t
hemostasis and, 1693-1699
hereditary clotting factor deficiencies as, 1699-1704
due to liver disease, 1712, *see also website*
of newborn, 620-621, 621t
platelet and blood vessel disorders as, 1714
megakaryopoiesis as, 1714, 1715f
thrombocytopenia as, 1714, 1716t
postnatal vitamin K deficiency as, 1712
thrombotic, hereditary predisposition to, 1707-1708, 1708t
von Willebrand disease as, 1704-1707, 1705f
Hemorrhagic edema, acute, 870
Hemorrhagic fever(s), 1150-1153, 1150t
dengue, 1147-1150, 1147t
Hemorrhagic fever with renal syndrome (HFRS), 1151-1153, *see also website*
Hemorrhagic measles, 1072
Hemorrhagic stroke (HS), 2084-2085, 2084f, 2085t
Hemorrhagic telangiectasia, hereditary, 2230
Hemorrhoids, 1360, 1361f
Hemosiderin, 1499
Hemosiderinuria, *see website*
Hemosiderosis, pulmonary, 1498-1500, 1498t
Hemostasis, 1693-1699
clinical and laboratory evaluation of, 1695-1696
developmental, 1695
pathology of, 1695
process of, 1694, 1694f-1695f
Hemothorax, 1513-1514, 1514f
as life-threatening injury, 336t
HEMPAS, *see website*
Henderson-Hasselbalch equation, *see website*
Henoch-Schönlein purpura (HSP), 868-871, 868t, 869f-870f, 870t, 874t, 1722, *see also website*
abdominal pain of, 1247t
alveolar hemorrhage with, 1499
cutaneous manifestations of, *see website*
immunofluorescence in, *see website*
nephritis associated with, 1789
scrotal involvement in, 1863
Hen's egg allergy, 821, 821t
HEP. *See* Hepatoerythropoietic porphyria (HEP)
HEPA. *See* High-efficiency particulate air (HEPA) filter
HepA. *See* Hepatitis A vaccine (HepA)
Heparin
deficiency of, 1311
degradation of, 509, 510f
low molecular weight, 1711
possible adverse reactions to in premature infant, 563t
for pulmonary embolism, 1502
unfractioned, 1710t, 1711
Hepatic arteriovenous fistula, *see website*
Hepatic crisis in tyrosinemia, 422
Hepatic disease. *See* Liver disease
Hepatic encephalopathy, 1414t
Hepatic fibrosis, *see website*
Hepatic lipase deficiency, 473t, 477
Hepatic tumor, precocious puberty due to, 1891
Hepatitis
antivirals for, *see website*
autoimmune, 1408-1410, 1408t, 1410f
with inflammatory bowel disease, *see website*
in child-care setting, *see website*
congenital alloimmune, 1393
neonatal, biliary atresia *versus*, 1385-1386
peliosis, 987
psychopharmacology and, 64-65
Hepatitis *(Continued)*
sports participation and, 2402t-2404t
viral, 1393-1404, 1393t
acute renal failure with, 1413
approach to, 1403-1404, 1403f
biochemical profiles in, 1394-1395
causes and differential diagnosis of, 1394, 1394t
pathogenesis of, 1394
Hepatitis A, 1395-1396, 1395f, 1396t
breast-feeding and, 540t
in child care setting, *see website*
gastroenteritis with, 1326t
in immigrant children, 133
malignancy susceptibility associated with, *see website*
Hepatitis A vaccine (HepA), 884t, 1396
with hepatitis B vaccine (HepA-HepB), 884t
HIV infection and, 1173f
recommended schedule for, 886-889, 887f-888f
for travel, *see website*
Hepatitis B, 1397-1400, 1398f
acute renal failure with, 1413
in adolescent, 709
in child-care setting, *see website*
maternal, 132-134
breast-feeding and, 161t, 540t
fetal and neonatal effects of, *see website*
prophylaxis following rape, 704t
Hepatitis B arthritis-dermatitis syndrome, 840
Hepatitis B e antigen (HBeAg), 1397
Hepatitis B immunoglobulin (HBIG), 882t, 1399, 1399t
Hepatitis B s antigen (HBsAg), 1397
Hepatitis B vaccine (HepB), 884t, 1399-1400, 1399t
with diphtheria acellular pertussis vaccine and inactivated polio vaccine (DTaP-HepB-IPV), 884t
with *Haemophilus influenzae* type b vaccine (Hib-HepB), 884t
with hepatitis A vaccine (HepA-HepB), 884t
HIV infection and, 1173f
in newborn, 537
recommended schedule for, 886, 887f-888f
for travel, 891t, *see also website*
as universal vaccine, 1399-1400
Hepatitis C, 1400-1402, 1400f
in child-care setting, *see website*
hypothyroidism due to, 1901
in immigrant children, 133
maternal
breast-feeding and, 161t, 540t
fetal and neonatal effects of, *see website*
in porphyria cutanea tarda, *see website*
sports participation and, 2402t-2404t
Hepatitis D, 1402
Hepatitis E, 1402-1403
breast-feeding and, 540t
Hepatobiliary tract disorders
in cystic fibrosis, 1496
HIV-related, 1165
due to typhoid fever, 957t
Hepatoblastoma, 1771-1772, 1771f
incidence and survival rates for, 1726t
precocious puberty with, 1891
risk factors for, 1727t
Hepatocellular carcinoma, 1772
in type II glycogen storage disease, 496
Hepatocytes, *see website*
Hepatoerythropoietic porphyria (HEP), *see website*
Hepatomegaly, 524t, 1375, 1375t
Hepatopathies, mitochondrial, 1405-1408, 1406t-1407t
Hepatoportoenterostomy procedure, 1387
Hepatopulmonary syndrome, 1376
Hepatorenal syndrome (HRS), 1376
Hepatorenal tyrosinemia, 422-425
Hepatosplenomegaly, due to cat-scratch disease, 985, 985f
Hepatotoxicity, 1410-1412
fulminant hepatic failure due to, 1413
HepB. *See* Hepatitis B vaccine (HepB)
Hepsera. *See* Adefovir
Herald patch, 2262
Herbal medicine, 270-273, 271t-272t
for atopic dermatitis, 805
drug interaction with, *see website*
nutritional aspects of, 169
Spanish-English translation chart, 274t
toxicity of, 272t-273t, 1412t
Herbivore bite, 2454-2460
Herculin gene, 2112
Hereditary angioedema (HAE), 753, 755, 815-816
Hereditary clotting factor deficiencies, 1699-1704
Hereditary coproporphyria (HCP), *see website*
Hereditary elliptocytosis, 1661f, 1662, *see also website*
Hereditary fructose intolerance (HFI), 494t-495t, 503
Hereditary hemorrhagic telangiectasia (HHT), 2230
Hereditary hypophosphatemic rickets with hypercalciuria (HHRH), 207
Hereditary methemoglobinemia, 1672-1673, 1673f
Hereditary motor-sensory neuropathies (HMSNs), 2138-2140
Hereditary nonpolyposis colon cancer (HNPCC), 1773
Hereditary orotic aciduria, *see website*
Hereditary osteoarthro-ophthalmopathy, 2426, 2426f
Hereditary periodic fever syndromes, 855-860, 855t-856t
Blau syndrome as, 858-859
chronic infantile neurologic cutaneous and articular disease as, 858
familial cold autoinflammatory syndrome as, 858
familial Mediterranean fever as, 856-857, 857f
hyperimmunoglobulinemia D syndrome as, 857-858
Muckle-Wells syndrome as, 858
periodic fever, aphthous stomatitis, pharyngitis, and adenitis as, 859-860
pyogenic arthritis, pyoderma gangrenosum, and acne syndrome as, 858-859
tumor necrosis factor receptor-associated periodic syndrome as, 858, 859f
Hereditary spherocytosis, 1659-1662, 1659t, 1660f-1662f
Hereditary stomatocytosis, 1662, *see also website*
Hereditary tyrosinemia, 422-425
Hereditary xanthinuria, *see website*
Hering-Breuer inflation index, *see website*
Heritability, *see website*
Herlitz junctional epidermolysis bullosa, 2244-2246, 2245t
Herlyn-Werner-Wunderlich syndrome (HWWS), *see website*
Hermansky-Pudlak syndrome, 425, 748t, 2238t
Hernia/hernation
cerebral, 297, 299-300
diaphragmatic, 594-596, 594f
congenital (Bochdalek), 594-596, 595f-596f, *see website*
as delivery room emergency, 575
epigastric, 1418
foramen of Morgagni, 597, 597f
hiatal, 1265, 1265f-1266f
incisional, *see website*
inguinal, 1362-1368
abdominal pain of, 1247t
clinical presentation of, 1364

Hernia/hernation *(Continued)*
complications after surgical repair of, 1367-1368
direct, 1366-1367
embryology and pathogenesis of, 1362-1363, 1363f
evaluation of, 1364-1365
femoral, 1367
genetics of, 1363
incarcerated, 1365
incarceration of, 1367
incidence of, 1364
management of, 1365-1366, 1367f
pathology of, 1363-1364, 1364t
internal, 1289
intervertebral disk, 2377
as sports injury, 2412
lung, 1467
paraesophageal, 597
strangulated, 1365
umbilical, *see website*
Heroin
adolescent use of, 684-685
urine screening for, 676t
maternal addiction to, 623-624
Herpangina, 1090, 1260t
Herpes
genital, 708, 709t, 1100-1101, 1103
maternal, 1103-1104
sexual abuse and, 145t
treatment of, 713t
Herpes gladiatorum, 1100, 1102, *see also website*
Herpes labialis, 1099-1100, 1102, 1260, 1260t
Herpes simplex virus (HSV), 1097-1104
acyclovir for, *see website*
antivirals for, *see website*
atopic dermatitis and, 806
in Bell palsy, 2147f
in child care setting, *see website*
clinical manifestations of, 1099-1101
cutaneous, 1100, 1100f
diagnosis of, 1102
in encephalitis, 1101
epidemiology of, 1098
in erythema multiforme, 2241, 2242f
etiology of, 1098
exclusion from day care due to, *see website*
of external ear, 2199
genital, 1100-1101
sexual abuse and, 145t
in gingivostomatitis, 1260, 1260f
in herpes labialis, 1099-1100, 1260
in immunocompromised patients, 1101
immunofluorescent-antibody testing of, *see website*
laboratory findings in, 1102
maternal
breast-feeding and, 161t, 540t
fetal and neonatal effects of, *see website*
ocular, 1101
oropharyngeal, 1099, 1099f
pathogenesis of, 1098-1099
perinatal, 1101, 1102f
in pneumonia, 1475t
predisposition to infection due to immunodeficiency, 716t
prevention of, 1103-1104
prognosis for, 1103
treatment of, 1102-1103
in viral meningoencephalitis, 2096
vulvar, 1867t-1868t
Herpesviruses
antiviral therapy for, *see website*
in child care setting, *see website*
human herpesvirus 6, 1117-1120
breast-feeding and, 540t
human herpesvirus 7, 1117-1120
breast-feeding and, 540t
Herpes zoster, 1104-1105, 1107-1109, 1107f-1108f
exclusion from day care due to, *see website*
vaccine for, 1110
Herpetic gingivostomatitis, 1260, 1260f, 1260t
Herpetic whitlow, 1100, 1100f, 1102
Herplex. *See* Idoxuridine
Herring lateral pillar classification, 2362, 2362f
Hers disease, 494t-495t, 497
HESX1 gene, 1876t, 1877
Heterochromia, 2156
Heterogeneity, 376
allelic, *see website*
locus, *see website*
Heterophile antibody test, 1113
Heterophoria, 2157
Heterophyes heterophyes, *see website*
Heterotaxy syndromes, cardiosplenic, 1589t, 1595-1596
Heterotopic heart transplantation, *see website*
Heterotropia, 2003, 2003f, 2157
neuronal, 2004
Heterozygotes
detection in cystic fibrosis, 1490
double, 389
Heterozygous familial hypercholesterolemia (FH), 474
Hexachlorophene, 563t
Hexane, as inhalant, 681t
Hexose monophosphate pathway, deficiencies of enzymes of, 1678
HFE. *See* Human factors engineering (HFE)
HFI. *See* Hereditary fructose intolerance (HFI)
HFjV. *See* High-frequency jet ventilation (HFjV)
HFO. *See* High-frequency oscillation (HFO)
HFRS. *See* Hemorrhagic fever with renal syndrome (HFRS)
HFV. *See* High-frequency ventilation (HFV)
HGE. *See* Human granulocytic ehrlichiosis (HGE)
hGH. *See* Human growth hormone (hGH)
HGPS. *See* Hutchinson-Gilford progeria syndrome (HGPS)
HH. *See* Hypogonadotropic hypogonadism (HH)
HHE. *See* Hemiconvulsion, hemiplegia, epilepsy (HHE) syndrome
HHH. *See* Hyperammonemia-hyperornithinemia-homocitrullinemia (HHH) syndrome
HHRH. *See* Hereditary hypophosphatemic rickets with hypercalciuria (HHRH)
HHT. *See* Hereditary hemorrhagic telangiectasia (HHT)
HHV-6. *See* Human herpesvirus 6 (HHV-6)
HHV-7. *See* Human herpesvirus 7 (HHV-7)
HHV-8. *See* Human herpesviruses 8 (HHV-8)
Hiatal hernia, 1265, 1265f-1266f
Hib. *See Haemophilus influenzae* type b vaccine (Hib)
Hibernian fever, familial, 858
Hickman catheter, infection with, *see website*
Hidden penis, 1856
Hidradenitis suppurativa, 2288
Hidrotic ectodermal dysplasia, 2223
HIE. *See* Hypoxic-ischemic encephalopathy (HIE)
High-altitude pulmonary edema (HAPE), 1469
High-density lipoproteins (HDL), 471, 472f, 472t, 479t
disorders of metabolism of, 477
laboratory testing of in obesity, 185t
reverse cholesterol transport and, 473
High-efficiency particulate air (HEPA) filter, 769
High endothelial venules, *see website*
High-frequency jet ventilation (HFjV), 326-327
High-frequency oscillation (HFO), 326
High-frequency ventilation (HFV), 326-327
High-grade squamous intraepithelial lesion (HSIL), 1138t
Highly active antiretroviral therapy (HAART), 1159
High molecular weight kininogen (HMWK)
deficiency of, 1703
reference values for, 1698t
High-production-volume (HPV) chemicals, 2448
High-quality child care, *see website*
High-risk infant, 552-564, 552t, 553f
large-for-gestational-age, *see website*
multiple gestation pregnancy and, 553-555, 554t, 555f
post-term, *see website*
prematurity and intrauterine growth restriction and, 555-564
transport of, 564, *see also website*
High-risk pregnancy, 540-541, *see also website*
High-tension electrical wire burn, 356
Hilgenreiner line, 2358
HINARI. *See* Health InterNetwork Access to Research Initiative (HINARI)
Hindfoot, 2335
Hindgut, 1273
Hinman syndrome, 1849-1850, 1849f
Hip
arthrogryposis involving, *see website*
centers of ossification appearance in, 29t
dislocation of, with arthrogryposis, *see website*
disorders of, 2355-2365
developmental dysplasia as, 2356, 2357f-2359f
Legg-Calvé-Perthes disease as, 2361, 2362f
slipped capital femoral epiphysis as, 2363, 2364f
transient monoarticular synovitis as, 2360
fracture of, 2392
growth and development of, 2355
musculoskeletal pain syndrome of, 877t
normal development of, 2344
sports injury to, 2407t, 2413-2414
subluxation of, 2356
vascular supply to, 2356, 2356f
Hip click, 2357
HIPPA. *See* Health Insurance Portability and Accountability Act of 1996 (HIPPA)
Hirschberg corneal reflex, 2157
Hirschsprung disease, 1283t, 1284-1287, 1285f-1286f, *see also website*
congenital central hypoventilation syndrome with, 1520
intestinal atresia and meconium ileus *versus*, 1279
neonatal, 600
Hirsutism, *see website*
Hispanic population
cultural values associated with, *see website*
death rates for, 3t-4t
disease beliefs or practices of, *see website*
empacho and, *see website*
infant mortality rates in, *see website*
Histamine
genetic disorders of, 445t
in neuroendocrine tumor-associated diarrhea, *see website*
Histamine-2 receptor antagonists (H2RAs)
for gastroesophageal reflux disease, 1268
for peptic ulcer disease, 1294
Histamine$_1$-type antihistamines, 771, 771t
Histerlin for precocious puberty, 1889
Histidine, defects in metabolism of, 453
Histidine decarboxylase deficiency, 447
Histidinuria, 1319
Histiocytic necrotizing lymphadenitis, 1724, *see also website*
Histiocytoma, *see website*
Histiocytoma, malignant fibrous, 1762t
Histiocytosis, 1773-1777
class I, 1775-1776, 1775f
classification and pathology of, 1773-1774, 1774t
class II, 1774-1776, 1776t
class III, 1776-1777
infections associated with, 1774t
Langerhans cell, 1773-1774

Histiocytosis *(Continued)*
diabetes insipidus with, 1883
seborrheic dermatitis with, 2253-2254
Histiocytosis X, 1773-1774
Histone antibody in rheumatic disease, *see website*
Histoplasma capsulatum, 1062-1064
in pneumonia, 1475t
Histoplasmosis, 1062-1064
HIV-related, *see website*
oral ulcerations in, 1260t
History
in acute illness, 275-276
in allergic disease, 764-765
in anemia, 1648-1649
in attention deficit/hyperactivity disorder, 109-110
in cardiovascular disease, 1530, 1530t-1532t
in dysmorphology, *see website*
in fever, *see website*
in fever of unknown origin, 899-901
in gynecological problems, 1865
in hemostatic disorders, 1696-1699
in intellectual disability, 127t
in neurologic evaluation, *see website*
in orthopedic problems, 2331, 2332t
perinatal, 532
in poisonings, 251-253, 252t
in preanesthetic, *see website*
in preparticipation sports examination, 2401-2405, 2402t-2404t, 2405f
in respiratory disease, *see website*
in seizures, 2019
in skin disorders, 2215, *see also website*
in wheezing, 1458, 1458t
History of pediatrics, 1-5
HIT. *See* Health information technology (HIT)
HIV/AIDS, 1157-1177
in adolescent, 709
adrenal insufficiency with, 1925t
amebiasis with, 1179
bacillary angiomatosis in, 986
cardiovascular system involvement, 1165
central nervous system involvement in, 1164-1165
in child-care setting, *see website*
classification of, 1162, 1162t-1163t
clinical manifestations of, 1162-1166, 1162t-1163t
diagnosis of, 1166-1167, 1166t
predictive value theory and serologic testing for, *see website*
encephalopathy in, 2068
epidemiology of, 1158-1159
etiology of, 1157-1158, 1158f
fetal therapy for, 551t
fever of unknown origin in, 899t, *see also website*
fever without a focus in, 896t
gastrointestinal and hepatobiliary tract involvement in, 1165
hematologic and malignant disease due to, 1166
in immigrant children, 134
infections with, 1162-1164, 1164t, *see website*
Candida, 1055
coccidioidomycosis, 1065-1068
Cryptococcus neoformans, 1058
histoplasmosis, 1063-1064
Pneumocystis jiroveci, *see website*
toxoplasmosis, 1210
tuberculosis, 1007-1008
varicella-zoster virus, 1106, 1108-1109
inflammatory bowel disease *versus* enteropathy of, 1298t
malabsorption with, 1314
maternal
breast-feeding and, 161t, 540t
fetal and neonatal effects of, *see website*
nutrition in, 174
pathogenesis of, 1159-1162, 1160f
HIV/AIDS *(Continued)*
in porphyria cutanea tarda, *see website*
prevention of, 1174-1177
prognosis for, 1174
prophylaxis following rape, 704, 704t
renal disease due to, 1165-1166
respiratory tract involvement in, 1165
seborrheic dermatitis with, 2253-2254
sexual abuse and, 145t
skin manifestations of, 1166
sports participation and, 2402t-2404t
syphilis with, 1022
as threat to homosexual youth, 659
transmission of, 1159
treatment of, 1167-1174
adherence to, 1171-1172
antiretrovirals in, 1167-1172, 1168t-1171t
combination therapy in, 1167-1171
dosing in, 1172
initiation of, 1172
monitoring of, 1172-1173
supportive care in, 1173-1174, 1173f, 1174t-1176t
Hives, 811-816, 812t
HLA. *See* Human leukocyte antigen (HLA)
HLH. *See* Hemophagocytic lymphohistiocytosis (HLH)
HLHS. *See* Hypoplastic left heart syndrome (HLHS)
HMB. *See* Hydroxymethylbilane (HMB)
HME. *See* Human monocytic ehrlichiosis (HME)
HMG. *See* 3-Hydroxy-3-methylglutaryl (HMG) CoA synthase deficiency
HMG CoA. *See* β-Hydroxy-β-methylglutaryl CoA (HMG CoA) synthase deficiency
HMPV. *See* Human metapneumovirus (HMPV)
HMSNs. *See* Hereditary motor-sensory neuropathies (HMSNs)
HMWK. *See* High molecular weight kininogen (HMWK)
H1N1 influenza, 1121-1122
H5N1 influenza, 1122
HNPCC. *See* Hereditary nonpolyposis colon cancer (HNPCC)
Hoarseness, due to gastroesophageal reflux disease, 1269
Hockey, injuries in, *see website*
Hodgkin lymphoma, 1739-1743
diagnosis of, 1741, 1741t, 1742f
epidemiology of, 1740
Epstein-Barr virus-associated, 1112
hematopoietic stem cell transplantation for, 759
incidence and survival rates for, 1726t
pathogenesis of, 1740-1741, 1740f-1741f, 1741t
prognosis for, 1743, 1744t
relapse of, 1743, 1744t
risk factors for, 1727t
treatment of, 1741-1742, 1743t
work-up of, 1731t
Holocarboxylase synthetase (HCS) deficiency, 432
secondary to pyruvate carboxylase deficiency, 506
Holoprosencephaly, 2005-2006, 2006f, *see website*
Holosystolic murmur, 1535
Holter recordings in supraventricular tachycardia, 1614-1615
Holt-Oram syndrome, 1531t, *see also website*
Home care
of asthma exacerbations, 799
of child with life-threatening illness, 151
of premature or low birthweight infant, 564
Homeless children, 7-8
health services for, 10
Home mechanical ventilation, 1524-1526
equipment for, 1524-1525
noninvasive, 332
Home mechanical ventilation *(Continued)*
team approach to, 331-332, 331t
through tracheostomy interface, 332-333
Home monitoring
in congenital central hypoventilation syndrome, 1522
for sudden infant death syndrome prevention, 1428-1429
Homeostatic process in sleep, 46
Homes tremor, 2058
Homicide, 18
by age and type, 667t
with firearms, 25
Homocysteine testing, 1699
Homocystinemia, 425-429
Homocystinuria, 425-429, 428f, 1708
cardiac manifestations of, 1531t
methylmalonic acidemia with, 438
tall stature in, *see website*
Homophobia, 658
Homosexuality, adolescent, 658-659
Homozygous familial hypercholesterolemia (FH), 473-474, 473f-474f
Homozygous hypobetalipoproteinemia, 1313
Homozygous variegate porphyria, *see website*
Honeybee, allergic responses to, 807f
Hookworm, 1218-1221
clinical manifestations of, 1219
cutaneous larva migrans as, 1220, 1220f, 1220t
diagnosis of, 1219-1220, 1219f
dog and cat, *see website*
epidemiology of, 1219
etiology of, 1218, 1218f
maternal, *see website*
pathogenesis of, 1219
prevention of, 1220
treatment of, 1220, *see website*
Hops for sedation, 271t
Hordeolum, 2164
Horizontal suspension test, *see website*
Horizontal transmission, 385
Hormones
of adrenal glands, 1923, *see also website*
for amenorrhea, 688t
in bone regulation, 2446, *see also website*
for contraception, 696-698, 696t-697t, 697f (*See also* Oral contraceptives (OCs))
gynecomastia due to, *see website*
of hypothalamus and pituitary gland, 1876, *see also website*
of parathyroid gland, 1916
of thyroid gland, *see website*
for undescended testis, 1860
Horner syndrome, 2155
eye manifestations in, *see website*
neuroblastoma associated with, 1754, 1754t
Hornet, allergic responses to, 807f
Horseshoe kidney, 1828-1829, 1829f
Hospital
emergency care in, in developing world, *see website*
international resources associated with care in, *see website*
referring, responsibility of in transport medicine, *see website*
Hospitalization
of adolescents, 663, 663f
for asthma, 781, 799-801
for burn injury, 349-350, 349t
for eating disorders, 95t
for Kawasaki disease, 863
due to measles, 1072t
in patterns of health care, 9
for pertussis, 946
for pneumonia, 1478, 1478t
psychiatric, 66
separation due to, *see website*
Host factors
in *Neisseria meningitidis*, 931
in otitis media, 2201-2202

Hot tub folliculitis, 2305, 2306f
Household products poisoning with, 266-268
Howell-Jolly bodies, see website
HP. See Hypersensitivity pneumonia (HP)
HPRT. See Hypoxanthine-guanine phosphoribosyltransferase (HPRT) deficiency
HPS. See Hantavirus pulmonary syndrome (HPS)
HPV. See High-production-volume (HPV) chemicals; Human papillomavirus (HPV)
H2RAs. See Histamine-2 receptor antagonists (H2RAs)
HRS. See Hepatorenal syndrome (HRS)
HRVs. See Human rhinoviruses (HRVs)
HS. See Hemorrhagic stroke (HS)
HSCT. See Hematopoietic stem cell transplantation (HSCT)
HSD3B2 gene, see website
HSD3B7 gene, 1383t
HSIL. See High-grade squamous intraepithelial lesion (HSIL)
HSP. See Henoch-Schönlein purpura (HSP)
HSV. See Herpes simplex virus (HSV)
5-HT_{1A}. See Serotonin 1A (5-HT_{1A})
HTLV. See Human T-lymphotropic virus (HTLV)
5-HTT gene, SIDS and, 1426
Huffing, 681-682
Human African trypanosomiasis (HAT), 1190-1193
Human bite, 2454-2460
Human chorionic gonadotropin
  in brain tumors, 1747-1748
  in CNS germ cell tumors, 1752-1753
  in germ cell tumor, 1770
  in ovarian carcinomas, 1872t
Human coronavirus 229E (HCoV-229E), see website
Human coronavirus HKU1 (HCoV-HKU1), see website
Human coronavirus NL63 (HCoV-NL63), see website
Human coronavirus OC43 (HCoV-OC43), see website
Human factors engineering (HFE), see website
Human genome, 383, see also website
Human Genome Project, 383, see also website
Human granulocytic ehrlichiosis (HGE), 1039t-1040t, 1048-1050
Human growth hormone (hGH), 1880-1881
  for Turner syndrome, 1954
Human herpesviruses 8 (HHV-8), 1121
  malignancy susceptibility associated with, see website
Human herpesvirus 6 (HHV-6), 1117-1120, 1119f
  breast-feeding and, 540t
Human herpesvirus 7 (HHV-7), 1117-1120, 1119f
  breast-feeding and, 540t
Human immunodeficiency virus. See HIV/AIDS
Humanitarian disasters, see website
Humanitarian efforts for protection of children from effects of war, see website
Human leukocyte antigen (HLA), see also website
  type 1 diabetes mellitus and, 1970-1971, 1970f
Human leukocyte antigen (HLA)-B27
  in reactive arthritis, 839
  in spondyloarthritides, see website
Human leukocyte antigen (HLA)-B51, 854
Human leukocyte antigen (HLA)-DQ2, 1308-1309
Human leukocyte antigen (HLA)-DQ8, 1308-1309
Human leukocyte antigen (HLA)-DQA1*05, 1308
Human leukocyte antigen (HLA)-DQA1*0501, 846
Human leukocyte antigen (HLA)-DQB1*02, 1308
Human leukocyte antigen (HLA)-DRB*0301, 846, 1308
Human leukocyte antigen (HLA)-DRB*0302, 1308
Human leukocyte antigen (HLA) matching for stem cell transplantation, 757
  from sibling, 757-760
  from unrelated donor, see website
Human metapneumovirus (HMPV), 1129-1131, 1130f, 1131t
  in pneumonia, 1475t
Human milk. See also Breast-feeding
  collection of, 162
  inadequate intake of, 161
  infant formula *versus*, 161t
  leakage of, 160
  patterns of supply of, 162t
  protective effects of, 161t
Human monocytic ehrlichiosis (HME), 1039t-1040t, 1048-1050
Human papillomavirus (HPV), 1137-1141
  in adolescent, 709, 713t
  antivirals for, see website
  clinical manifestations of, 1139, 1139f
  complications of, 1140
  cutaneous infection due to, 2315-2316
  diagnosis of, 1139-1140
  differential diagnosis of, 1140
  epidemiology of, 1137-1139, 1138t
  etiology of, 1137
  malignancy susceptibility associated with, see website
  predisposition to infection due to immunodeficiency, 716t
  prevention of, 1140-1141
  prognosis for, 1140-1141
  prophylaxis following rape, 704t
  treatment of, 1140
  vaccine for, 884t, 888f, 891t, 1141
Human recombinant DNase for cystic fibrosis, 1491
Human rhinoviruses (HRVs), 1133-1134
Human T-lymphotropic virus (HTLV), 1177, see also website
  breast-feeding and, 161t, 540t
Humeral fracture
  distal, 2392
  proximal, 2392
    as sports injury, 2410
  supracondylar, 2410
Humerus, centers of ossification appearance in, 29t
Humidifier hypersensitivity pneumonia, see website
Humidity, thermoregulation in premature infant and, 559
Humoral immunodeficiencies. See B-cells, abnormalities of
Humulus lupulus for sedation, 271t
Hungry bone syndrome, 226-227, see also website
Hunter disease, 511-512, 511f, 512t
  cardiac manifestations of, 1531t
Huntington's disease (HD), 391, 2060t
Hurler disease, 510-511, 511f, 513f
  cardiac manifestations of, 1531t
Hurler-Scheie disease, 511, 512t
HUS. See Hemolytic-uremic syndrome (HUS)
Hutchinson-Gilford progeria syndrome (HGPS), see website
Hutchinson syndrome, 1754t
Hutchinson teeth, 1017t, 1019f
HWWS. See Herlyn-Werner-Wunderlich syndrome (HWWS)
Hyaline membrane disease, 581-590, 583f
Hyalinosis cutis et mucosae, 2276-2277
Hyaluronidase deficiency, 512t
Hybridization
  comparative genomic, 396
    array, 376, 377t, 396-398, 400f
  fluorescence in situ, 395-396, 397f-398f
    in intellectual disability, 125
    multicolor, 396
Hydatid cyst, see website
Hydatid disease, 1237-1239
Hydatidosis, 1237-1239
Hydatid sand, 1238
Hydoxocalamin, as poisoning antidote, 256t-257t
Hydralazine
  for heart failure, see website
  for hypertensive emergencies, 1646t
  for systemic hypertension, 1645t
Hydranencephaly, 2011, 2011f
Hydration
  cutaneous, for atopic dermatitis, 804
  in palliative care, 158
  withholding of artificial, see website
Hydroa aestivale, see website
Hydroa vacciniforme, 2256-2257
Hydrocalycosis, 1841
Hydrocarbons
  aspiration of, 1470-1471, 1470f
  poisoning with, 267
Hydrocele, 1863-1864, 1863f
  hernia and, 1363-1364, 1363f
Hydrocephalus, 2008-2011, 2008t, 2009f-2011f
  in bacterial meningitis, 2089
  imaging studies in, see website
  language disorders due to, 119
  with myelomeningocele, 2001-2002
  otitic, 2212
  due to pork tapeworm, 1235
  posthemorrhage, 567-568
  with primary ciliary dyskinesia, see website
  Toxoplasmosis gondii, 1212
Hydrochlorothiazide, 1645t
Hydrocodone, 365t
Hydrocortisone, see also website
  for shock, 313
  for thyroid storm, 1912t
Hydrocytosis, see website
Hydrogen cyanide poisoning, 270
Hydrogen ions (H^+) in acid-base balance, see website
Hydrometrocolpos, 536
Hydromorphone
  equianalgesic doses and half-life of, 367t
  for pain management, 365t
    in palliative care, 155t-156t
Hydronephrosis
  abdominal pain of, 1247t
  with urinary tract obstruction, 1839-1840, 1840t
Hydrops fetalis
  edema in, 622
  nonimmune, in congenital erythropoietic porphyria, see website
  parvovirus B19 infection and, 1095, 1653
  Rh incompatibility and, 615-616
Hydrops of gallbladder, see website
Hydrothorax, 1513
Hydroxocobalamin for cyanide poisoning, 270, see also website
3-Hydroxyacyl CoA dehydrogenase deficiency
  long-chain, 460
  short-chain, 460
β-Hydroxy-β-methylglutaryl CoA (HMG CoA) synthase deficiency, 461-462
γ-Hydroxybutyrate, adolescent abuse of, 675t
γ-Hydroxybutyric aciduria, 447
Hydroxychloroquine
  for juvenile dermatomyositis, 849
  for lupus erythematosus profundus, 2283
  for malaria, 1203t-1205t
  for porphyria cutanea tarda, see website
  for rheumatic disease, see website
  for systemic lupus erythematosus, 844
3β-Hydroxy C_{27}-steroid dehydrogenase (3β-HSD) deficiency, 1384
11β-Hydroxylase deficiency, 1932t, 1935-1936
  adrenal insufficiency with, 1925t
17-Hydroxylase deficiency, 1936-1937, 1964
  adrenal insufficiency with, 1925t

21-Hydroxylase deficiency, 1930-1935, 1932t
  adrenal insufficiency with, 1925t
  fetal therapy for, 551t
β-Hydroxylase deficiency, 421f, 446
Hydroxylase deficiency, tyrosine, 445
Hydroxymethylbilane (HMB), *see website*
3-Hydroxy-3-methylglutaric aciduria, 435
3-Hydroxy-3-methylglutaryl (HMG) CoA synthase deficiency, 435
4-Hydroxyphenylpyruvate dioxygenase deficiency, 423
17-hydroxypregenolone, *see website*
Hydroxyproline malabsorption, 1319
3β-Hydroxysteroid dehydrogenase (3β-HSD) deficiency, 1925t, 1932t, 1936, 1964
17β-Hydroxysteroid dehydrogenase deficiency, 1959-1961
Hydroxyurea for sickle cell disease pain, 1665
Hydroxyzine
  for depression and anxiety symptoms, 63t
  for pruritus in palliative care, 155t-156t
  for urticaria, 814
Hygiene
  for gastroenteritis prevention, 1338
  hand, *see website*
    in child-care setting, *see website*
    waterless, *see website*
  for herpes simplex virus prevention, 1103
  oral, for dental caries prevention, 1256
  sleep, 48t-49t
Hygroma, cystic, 1772, *see also website*
Hymen
  abnormalities of, *see website*
  polyps of, 1869
  sexual abuse examination and, 144, 144f-145f
Hymenolepiasis, 1232t, 1234, *see also website*
Hymenoptera, allergic responses to, 807-809, 807f
Hyoscyamine sulfate for respiratory secretions, 155t-156t
Hyperactivity, psychopharmacologic management of, 61t. *See also* Attention deficit/hyperactivity disorder (ADHD)
Hyperacusis in Tay-Sachs disease, 485
Hyperacute rejection of renal transplantation, *see website*
Hyperaldosteronism
  glucocorticoid-suppressible, 1938-1939
  myopathies with, 2129
Hyperammonemia, 447-453, 448f-449f, 448t, 450t
  with persistent hyperinsulinemic hypoglycemia of infancy, 525
Hyperammonemia-hyperornithinemia-homocitrullinemia (HHH) syndrome, 453
Hyperamylasemia, 1371, 1371t
Hyperargininemia, 448f, 452
Hyperbaric oxygen (HBO), 270
Hyperbilirubinemia
  familial nonhemolytic unconjugated, 1389-1390
  inherited conjugated, 1390
  neonatal, 603-608, 607t
    due to biliary atresia, 607
    breast-feeding associated, 607, 607f
    clinical manifestations of, 604, 604t
    differential diagnosis of, 604-605, 605f, 606t
    etiology of, 603-608, 604f, 604t
    kernicterus due to, 608-612
    pathologic, 606-607
    physiologic, 605-606, 606f
    treatment of, 610-612, 610f-611f, 611t-612t
  nomogram for risk assessment of, *see website*
  pyloric stenosis with, 1274
  unconjugated, differential diagnosis of, 1376t
Hypercalcemia
  causes of, 1921-1922
  differential diagnosis of, 1921-1922
  etiologic classification of, 1921t
  due to hyperparathyroidism, 1921
Hypercalcemia *(Continued)*
  as oncologic emergency, *see website*
  with subcutaneous fat necrosis, 2284
Hypercalciuria
  hematuria in, 1795
  hereditary hypophosphatemic rickets with, 207
  in urinary lithiasis, *see website*
Hypercapnia
  permissive, in mechanical ventilation for respiratory distress syndrome, 585
  due to surfactant deficiency, 582
Hypercarbia, chronic, respiration regulation in, *see website*
Hypercholanemia, familial, 1384
Hypercholesterolemia, 473-475, 473f-474f, 475t
  autosomal recessive, 475
  hypertriglycerides with, 475-476
  polygenic, 473t, 475
HyperCKemia, 2126
Hypercoagulable states, renal transplantation and, *see website*
Hypercyanotic attacks in tetralogy of Fallot, 1574
"Hyperdynamic pulmonary hypertension," 1557
Hyperekplexia, *see website*
Hypereosinophilic syndrome, 740
Hyperfiltration injury in chronic kidney disease, 1822
Hypergammaglobulinema in HIV infection, 1161
Hyperglobulinemia in kala-azar, 1189
Hyperglycemia
  in cystic fibrosis, 1496
  in diabetes mellitus, 1979-1980
  hyponatremia with, 1885
  neonatal, 439
  plasma osmolality and, 212, *see also website*
Hyperglycinemia, 438-441
  ketotic, 436
  nonketotic, 439-440
Hypergonadotropic hypogonadism
  female, 1951-1956
  gynecomastia with, 1950-1951
  male, 1944-1945
Hyperhidrosis, 2287, 2287t
Hyperimmune animal antisera preparations, 882-883
Hyperimmune globulin preparations, 882
Hyperimmunoglobulinemia D syndrome, 855t, 857-858
  fever with, 436
  infection and, *see website*
Hyper-immunoglobulin E syndrome, 736, 736t, 742t
Hyper-immunoglobulin M syndrome, 726-727, 748t
Hyperinfection syndrome of strongyloidiasis, 1223
Hyperinsulinema, 521-527, 521t-524t, 525f-527f
  in infants of diabetic mothers, 627-628
  obesity due to, 182t
Hyperinsulinemic state, 518
Hyperkalemia, 219-222
  in acute renal failure, 1820
  cardiac arrest due to, 289t
  in chronic kidney disease, 1823t
  clinical manifestations of, 221
  diagnosis of, 221
  electrocardiogram of, 1541f
  etiology and pathophysiology of, 219-221, 220t
  fictitious, 219
  as oncologic emergency, *see website*
  spurious, 219
  treatment of, 221-222
Hyperkalemic periodic paralysis, 220, 2113t, 2125t, 2130
Hyperkalemic renal tubular acidosis, 1810-1811
Hyperkeratosis, epidermolytic, 2268t, 2270, 2270f
Hyperleukocytosis as oncologic emergency, *see website*
Hyperlexia, 119
Hyperlipidemia
  in chronic kidney disease, 1823t
  familial combined, 473t, 475
  secondary causes of, 477t
Hyperlipoproteinemias, 473-482, 473t
  blood cholesterol screening for, 479-480
  conditions associated with low cholesterol as, 477-478, 478t
  high-density lipoproteins metabolism disorders as, 477
  hypercholesterolemia as, 473-475, 473f-474f, 475t
    hypertriglycerides with, 475-476
  hypertriglyceridemias as, 476, 476f, 477t
  intracellular cholesterol metabolism disorders as, 478-479
  risk assessment and treatment of, 480-482, 480f, 481t-482t
  type III, 476
  type IV, 476-477
Hyperlucent lung, unilateral, 1461
Hypermagnesemia, 623, *see also website*
Hypermenorrhea, 686t
Hypermethioninemia, 427-428
Hypermobile Ehlers-Danlos syndrome, 2278
Hypermobile pes planus (flatfoot), 2338, 2338f
Hypermobility syndrome, benign, *see website*
Hypermyelinating neuropathy, 2140
Hypernasality, *see website*
Hypernatremia, 212-215
  causes of, 1883
  clinical manifestations of, 213-214
  in diabetes insipidus, 1882-1883
  diagnosis of, 214
  etiology and pathophysiology of, 213, 213t
  treatment of, 214-215, 214f
Hypernatremic dehydration, 248-249, 248t
Hyperopia, 2150-2151
  of newborn, *see website*
Hyperostosis, 190, 191f, 2436-2437, 2436f
Hyperoxaluria, 440-441
  in urinary lithiasis, *see website*
Hyperoxia test, 1573
Hyperparathyroidism, 1920-1923
  hypercalcemia *versus*, 1921-1922, 1921t
  hypophosphatemia in, 227
  maternal, *see website*
  myopathies with, 2129
Hyperparathyroidism-jaw tumor syndrome, 1921
Hyperphenylalaninemia, 418-420
  due to deficiency of BH_4, 420-421, 421f
  maternal, 420
Hyperphosphatemia, 228-229, 228t, 2446, *see also website*
  in chronic kidney disease, 1822
  as oncologic emergency, *see website*
Hyperpigmented lesions, 2236-2238, 2236f-2237f
Hyperpituitarism, 1886, *see also website*
Hyperplasia
  β-cell in hyperinsulinemia, 521-522
  congenital adrenal, 1930-1939, 1931f
    adrenocortical insufficiency due to, 1924
    due to 11β-hydroxylase deficiency, 1935-1936
    due to 3β-hydroxysteroid dehydrogenase deficiency, 1936
    diagnosis and treatment of, 1931f, 1932t
    due to 17-hydroxylase deficiency, 1936-1937
    due to 21-hydroxylase deficiency, 1930-1935
    hypokalemia in, 223-224
    metabolic alkalosis in, 236
  gingival, 1257
  lipoid adrenal, 1937, 1964
  nodular lymphoid, *see website*
  sebaceous, 2218

Hyperprolactinemia
in BH_4 deficiency, 421
delayed puberty due to, 1949
Hyperprolinemia, 442-443, 447, 454
Hypersensitivity
in adverse drug reactions, 824
cow's milk, 1498
cutaneous manifestations of, *see website*
drug, 824-828
fever of unknown origin in, 900t
to food, 820t
to inhaled materials, 1473, *see also website*
serum sickness as, 819
in tuberculosis pathogenesis, 998
vaccine, 827
to vaccine, 892
Hypersensitivity angitis, 868t
Hypersensitivity pneumonia (HP), 1473, *see also website*
Hypersensitivity syndrome, drug-induced, 827-828, 827t
Hypersensitivity vasculitis, 876, 876t
Hypersomnia, 53
Hypersplenism, *see website*
Hypertelorism, 2181-2182
Hypertension
in acute renal failure, 1821
in chronic kidney disease, 1823t, 1825
due to immunosuppression therapy, *see website*
maternal, 545
with obesity, 184t
persistent pulmonary of the newborn, 592-594, 592f, *see also website*
portal, 1415, *see also website*
as manifestation of liver disease, 1376
primary (essential), 1639-1647
blood pressure measurement in, 1639-1640
clinical manifestations of, 1641-1642
diagnosis of, 1642, 1642f, 1643t-1644t
etiology and pathophysiology of, 1640-1641, 1641t
prevalence of, 1639
treatment of, 1642-1647, 1644f-1646f, 1645t-1646t
pulmonary, 1570-1571, 1600-1602, 1600t, 1601f, 1602t, *see website*
"hyperdynamic," 1557
sports participation and, 2402t-2404t
in systemic scleroderma, 851
"rebound," 1569
renovascular, 1642, 1644f, 1646f
sports participation and, 2402t-2404t
with type 2 diabetes mellitus, 1993t
white coat, 1639
in Wilms tumor, 1758
Hypertensive encephalopathy, 2068
strokelike events *versus*, 2086
Hypertensive retinopathy, 2179, 2179f
Hyperthermia
with anhidrosis, 2287
malignant, 2130-2131
hyperkalemia and, 220
postoperative, *see website*
microcephaly with, 2007t
in newborn, 622
Hyperthyroidism, 1909-1913
causes of, 1909, 1909t
congenital, 1913, 1913f
in Graves disease, 1909-1913, 1909t, 1911f, 1912t
maternal, 545
myopathies with, 2129
Hyperthyroxinemia, familial dysalbuminemic, *see website*
Hypertonic saline for cystic fibrosis, 1491
Hypertrichosis, 2289, 2289t
alopecia and, 2289, 2289t
Hypertriglyceridemias, 473t, 476-477, 476f, 477t
Hypertriglycerides, hypercholesterolemia with, 475-476
Hypertrophic cardiomyopathy (HCM), 1629t-1630t, 1631-1632, 1632f
genetics of, *see website*
glycogen storage diseases mimicking, 500
sports participation and, 2402t-2404t
sudden death due to, 1619-1620
Hypertrophic gastropathy, 1276
Hypertrophic osteoarthropathy, *see website*
Hypertrophic pyloric stenosis, 1274-1275, 1274f-1275f
Hypertrophy
assessment in neurologic examination, *see website*
breast, *see website*
ventricular
electrocardiography of, 1538, 1538f
radiographic assessment of, 1537
systemic hypertension with, 1642
Hyperuricemia as oncologic emergency, *see website*
Hyperventilation
for persistent pulmonary hypertension of the newborn, 593
respiratory alkalosis and, 241
Hyperventilation spell, *see website*
Hyperviscosity in plethora, 619
Hypervitaminosis A, 190-191, 191f
Hypervitaminosis D, 208-209
hypercalcemia with, 1923
Hypervolemic hyponatremia, 216, 218
Hyphema, 2185
Hypnagogic/hypnopompic hallucinations, 53
Hypnosis as goal of anesthesia, *see website*
Hypnotherapy for pain management, 371
Hypnotics
for anesthesia, *see website*
poisoning with, 253t
Hypoalbuminemia in protein losing enteropathy, 1307
Hypoalphalipoproteinemia, 477
Hypobetalipoproteinemia
familial, 478
homozygous, 1313
Hypocalcemia
in acute renal failure, 1821
etiologic classification of, 1917t
hypomagnesemia with secondary, *see website*
due to hypoparathyroidism, 1916-1917
in newborn, 623
in poisonings, 254t
Hypocalcification of tooth, 1250-1251
Hypocellular marrow, 1684
Hypochloremic alkalosis in cystic fibrosis, 1487
Hypochondroplasia, 2430
Hypochromic microcytic anemia, *see website*
Hypocitraturia, *see website*
Hypocomplementemic urticarial vasculitis, 876
Hypodysplasia, renal, 1827
Hypogammaglobulinemia
acquired, 724-725
enterovirus and, 1089
HIV-related, 1175t-1176t
Hypoglossal nerve, neurologic examination of, *see website*
Hypoglycemia, 517-531
with adrenal insufficiency, 1927
classification of, 519-521, 520t
clinical manifestations of, 518-519, 519f, 519t, 521t, 524t
definition of, 517
diagnosis and differential diagnosis of, 524t, 530
endocrine deficiency and, 527-528
factitious, 521
in infants of diabetic mothers, 628
intraoperative, *see website*
ketotic, 524t, 528
leucine-sensitive, 525
malarial, 1206
Hypoglycemia *(Continued)*
management of in protein-energy malnutrition, 178t
neonatal seizures due to, 2034
in newborn, 518
persistent or recurrent, 521-530, 522t-523t, 525f-527f
in poisonings, 254t
prognosis for, 531
significance and sequelae of, 517-518
stroke-like events *versus*, 2085
treatment of, 530-531
in type 1 diabetes mellitus, 1985
in type I glycogen storage disease, 492-493
Hypoglycemics
oral, 1992-1993, 1992t
poisoning with, 251t, 263
Hypoglycinemia, 438-441
Hypogonadism
female
primary, 1951-1956
secondary, 1956-1957
gynecomastia with, 1950-1951
male, 1943-1950, 1944t
primary, 1944-1945
secondary, 1948-1949
Hypogonadotropic hypogonadism (HH)
female, 1956-1957
male, 1944-1945
Hypohidrotic ectodermal dysplasia, 2223, 2223f, 2223t
Hypokalemia, 222-224
cardiac arrest due to, 289t
clinical manifestations of, 224
diagnosis of, 224, 225f
electrocardiogram of, 1540f
etiology and pathophysiology of, 222-224, 222t
with primary aldosteronism, *see website*
treatment of, 224
Hypokalemic periodic paralysis, 222-223, 2125t, 2130
poliovirus infection *versus*, 1085t
Hypolactasia, primary adult type, 1317
Hypomagnesemia, *see also website*
cardiac arrest due to, 289t
neonatal seizures due to, 2034
in newborn, 623
Hypomania, 85
Hypomastia, *see website*
Hypomelanosis of Ito, 412, 2237f, 2239-2240, 2239f-2240f, 2240t
Hypomenorrhea, 686t
Hypomyelinating neuropathy, congenital, 2140, *see also website*
Hyponatremia
in acute intermittent porphyrias, *see website*
in acute renal failure, 1821
causes of, 1884-1885
in diabetes insipidus, 215-219
clinical manifestations of, 217
diagnosis of, 217-218
etiology and pathophysiology of, 215-217, 215t, 217t
treatment of, 218-219
differential diagnosis of, 1884t
emergency treatment of, 1886
hypothyroidism-associated, 1903t
maintenance fluids and, 243-244
neonatal seizures due to, 2034
as oncologic emergency, *see website*
runner's, 1885
treatment of, 1885-1886
Hyponatremic dehydration, 247-248
Hypoparathyroidism, 1916-1919, 1917t
maternal, 1917
Hypophosphatasia, 454, 1922
Hypophosphatemia, 226-228, 227t, 2446, *see also website*
Hypophosphatemic rickets, 202t
autosomal dominant, 207
autosomal recessive, 202t

Hypophosphatemic rickets *(Continued)*
due to Fanconi syndrome, 207
hereditary with hypercalciuria, 207
X-linked, 206-207
Hypopigmentation
in albinism, 424
genes associated with, 2238t
Hypopigmented lesion, 2237f-2240f, 2238-2240, 2238t, 2240t
Hypopituitarism, 1876-1881
abnormalities of growth hormone receptor in, 1879
acquired forms, 1878-1879
causes of, 1877t
classification of, 1876t-1877t
clinical manifestations of, 1879
congenital, 1878-1879
differential diagnosis of, 1880-1881
genetics of, 1876-1878
hypoglycemia with, 518
hypogonadotropic hypogonadism with, 1956
laboratory findings in, 1879-1880
primary, 1880-1881
psychosocial causes of, 1881
radiologic findings in, 1880
treatment of, 1881
complications and adverse effects of, 1881
Hypoplasia
adrenal, 1924
cartilage hair, 733-734, 1690, 2434
cerebellar, 2118
focal dermal, 2222
lipoid adrenal, 1925t
lymphoid in X-linked agammaglobulinemia, 724
of mandible, as delivery room emergency, 575
nasal, 1430
optic nerve, *see website*
parathyroid gland, 1917
pontocerebellar, 2007
pulmonary, 1464
with congenital diaphragmatic hernia, 594
due to oligohydramnios, *see website*
renal, 1827-1828
thumb, 2386, 2386f
thymic, 728-729
tooth, 1250-1251
urethral, 1846-1847, 1857-1858
Hypoplastic anemia, congenital, 1650-1651
Hypoplastic left heart syndrome (HLHS), 1592-1595, 1593f-1595f
Hypoplastic nail, *see website*
Hypopyon, 2156
Hyposmia, 1948
Hypospadias, 1852-1854, 1853f
Hyposplenism, 1723
Hypotelorism, 2181-2182
Hypotension
during induction of anesthesia, *see website*
in newborn, *see website*
orthostatic, *see website*
Hypothalamus. *See Also* Pituitary gland disorders
fever of unknown origin due to dysfunction of, 901
hamartoma of, precocious puberty with, 1890
hormones of, 1876, *see also website*
hypothyroidism due to disease of, 1901
puberty physiology and, 1886, *see also website*
Hypothermia
cardiac arrest due to, 289t
as cold injury, 358, 359f
due to drowning or submersion injury, 343-344, 346-347
hypothyroidism-associated, 1903t
induced
for hypoxic-ischemic encephalopathy, 302, 571
in post-resuscitation care, 296
management of in protein-energy malnutrition, 178t
Hypothermia *(Continued)*
in newborn, *see website*
postoperative, *see website*
Hypothyroidism, 1895-1903
acquired
clinical manifestations of, 1901-1902, 1902f, 1903t
diagnostic studies of, 1902-1903
epidemiology of, 1901
etiology of, 1901, 1901t
treatment and prognosis for, 1903, 1903t
amenorrhea due to, 686
due to cancer and its therapy, *see website*
cardiac manifestations of, 1531t
classification of, 1895t
congenital, 1895-1901
clinical manifestations of, 1898-1899, 1898f
epidemiology of, 1895
etiology of, 1895-1897
laboratory findings in, 1899-1900, 1899t, 1900f
in preterm babies, 1897
prognosis for, 1900-1901
thyroid hormone unresponsiveness as, 1897
treatment of, 1900
with Down syndrome, 403t
due to iodine deficiency, *see website*
maternal, 545
myopathies with, 2129
obesity due to, 182t, 185
precocious puberty and, 1891
due to total body irradiation, *see website*
Hypothyroxinemia of prematurity, 627
Hypotonia
assessment in neurologic examination, *see website*
benign congenital, 2119
in neuromuscular disorders, 2109-2110, 2115t
Hypoventilation, alveolar, acquired, 1523
Hypoventilation syndrome
congenital central, 1520-1522
obesity, 1522-1523
Hypovolemia
cardiac arrest due to, 289t
with fulminant hepatic failure, 1414
Hypovolemic hyponatremia, 215-218
Hypovolemic shock, 285, 307t
clinical manifestations of, 308
defined, 305
hemodynamic variables in, 311t
pathophysiology of, 305
Hypoxanthine-guanine phosphoribosyltransferase (HPRT) deficiency, *see website*
Hypoxemia, *see also website*
permissive in mechanical ventilation for respiratory distress syndrome, 585
respiratory alkalosis due to, 240-242, 241t
Hypoxia
cardiac arrest due to, 289t
chronic, respiration regulation in, *see website*
fetal, 550
therapy for, 551t
respiratory alkalosis due to, 240, 241t
due to surfactant deficiency, 582
Hypoxic-ischemic encephalopathy (HIE), 298f-299f, 301-303, 302f, 569-573, 569t-570t
in drowning, 346
microcephaly with, 2007t
seizure due to, 2034
stroke-like events *versus*, 2085
Hypoxic-ischemic insult, global, 301-303
Hypsarrhythmia, 2024

I
IAHS. *See* Infection-associated hemophagocytic syndrome (IAHS)
IAR. *See* Intermittent allergic rhinitis (IAR)
Iatrogenic cryptorchidism after inguinal repair, 1367
IBD. *See* Inflammatory bowel disease (IBD)
Ibuprofen
for dysmenorrhea, 691t
for juvenile idiopathic arthritis, 838t
for migraine, 2043, 2044t
for pain management, 364t
poisoning with, 260-261
for rheumatic disease, *see website*
IC. *See* Inspiratory capacity (IC)
"Ice," 683-684
Ice hockey, injuries in, *see website*
I-cell disease, 491-492
I-cell disease mucolipidosis type II, 1523
ICF. *See* Intracellular fluid (ICF)
Ichthyosiform dermatoses, 2271-2272
Ichthyosiform erythroderma, 2268t
Ichthyosis, 2267-2272, 2268t
follicularis, 2268t
harlequin, 2267
hystrix, 2234, 2268t
lamellar, 2267-2268, 2269f
vulgaris, 2269, 2269f
X-linked, 2269-2270, 2270f
ICP. *See* Intracranial pressure (ICP)
ICs. *See* Inhaled corticosteroids (ICs)
Ictal-induced psychosis, *see website*
Icteric leptospirosis, 1024
Icteropyloric syndrome, 1274
Icterus. *See* Jaundice
Icterus neonatorum, 605-606, 606f
ID_{50}. *See* 50% inhibitory dose (ID_{50})
Idamycin. *See* Idarubicin
Idarubicin for cancer therapy, *see website*
IDDM2 gene locus, 1971
IDEA. *See* Individuals with Disabilities Education Act (IDEA)
Identification, microbial, *see website*
Identity
adolescent formation of, 650t
gender, 655
Idiogenic osmoles, 214
Idiopathic pulmonary hemorrhage (IPH), 1498-1500
Idiopathic thrombocytopenic purpura (ITP), 1714-1718, 1717f
maternal, *see website*
IDL. *See* Intermediate density lipoproteins (IDL)
Idoxuridine, *see website*
IEP. *See* Individualized education program (IEP)
IF. *See* Intestinal failure (IF); Intrinsic factor (IF)
IFA. *See* Immunofluorescent-antibody (IFA) technique
Ifex. *See* Ifosfamide
IFN-γ. *See* Interferon-γ (IFN-γ)
Ifosfamide for cancer therapy, *see website*
IFSP. *See* Individualized family service plan (IFSP)
IgA. *See* Immunoglobulin A (IgA)
IGF-1. *See* Insulin-like growth factor 1 (IGF-1)
IGF2. *See* Insulin-like growth factor receptor 2 (IGF2) gene inactivation
IGFBP. *See* Insulin-like growth factor-binding protein (IGFBP)
IgG. *See* Immunoglobulin G (IgG)
IgG-IFA. *See* Immunoglobulin G indirect fluorescent-antibody (IgG-IFA) testing
IgM. *See* Immunoglobulin M (IgM)
IgM-ELISA. *See* Immunoglobulin M enzyme-linked immunosorbent assay (IgM-ELISA), in toxoplasmosis
IgM-IFA. *See* Immunoglobulin M indirect fluorescent-antibody (IgM-IFA) testing,
IGT. *See* Impaired glucose tolerance (IGT)
IL. *See* Indeterminate leprosy (IL)
IL-1. *See* Interleukin-1 (IL-1)
IL-3. *See* Interleukin-3 (IL-3)
IL-4. *See* Interleukin-4 (IL-4)
IL-5. *See* Interleukin-5 (IL-5)
IL-6. *See* Interleukin-6 (IL-6)
IL-9. *See* Interleukin-9 (IL-9)
IL-12. *See* Interleukin-12 (IL-12)
IL-13. *See* Interleukin-13 (IL-13)

ILAR. *See* International League of Association for Rheumatology (ILAR)
IL-1β. *See* Interleukin-1β (IL-1β)
ILD. *See* Interstitial lung disease (ILD)
Ileal atresia and obstruction, 1278-1280, 1279f
Ileitis, regional. *See* Crohn's disease
Ileoileal intussusception, 1289
Ileus, 1277-1281, 1287
  abdominal pain of, 1248t
  closed-loop, 1287-1289
  congenital, *see website*
  in cystic fibrosis, 1495
  duodenal, 1277-1278
  hypothyroidism-associated, 1903t
  intrinsic *versus* extrinsic, 1277
  jejunal and ileal, 1278-1280
  due to malrotation, 1280-1281
  meconium, 601, 601f, 1279
    in cystic fibrosis, 1486, 1487f, 1495
Iliohypogastric nerve block, 372
Ilioingual nerve block, 372
Iliotibial band syndrome, 2416, *see also website*
Ilium, 2355
Ilizarov device, *see website*
Illicium anisatum, potential toxicity of, 272t-273t
Illness
  exclusion from day care due to, *see website*
  integrated management of childhood, 1334, 1335f
Iloprost for pulmonary hypertension, 1602t
Ilopsoas muscle, blood into, 1699-1700, 1700f
IM. *See* Intramuscular (IM) drug administration
IMAGe syndrome, 1925t
Imaging studies
  in acute disseminated encephalomyelitis, 2079
  in cancer, *see website*
  in chronic diarrhea, 1344
  in coccidioidomycosis, 1067, 1067f
  in febrile seizures, 2018
  fetal, 543t
  hepatic, 1381
  in intellectual disability, 127t
  in malabsorption disorders, 1308
  in migraine, 2042, 2043t
  in neurologic assessment, *see website*
  in neurologic disorders, *see website*
  in neuromuscular disorders, 2111
  in orthopedic problems, 2334
  radiation exposure and, *see website*
  in rheumatic disease, *see website*
  in urinary tract infection, 1833, 1833f
  in urinary tract obstruction, 1839-1841, 1839f-1841f, 1840t
Imatinib, 1739, *see also website*
IMCI. *See* Integrated Management of Childhood Illness (IMCI)
Imerslund-Grasbeck syndrome, 1320
I231-MIBG studies. *See* Iodine-123 meta-iodobenzylguanidine (I231-MIBG) studies
IMIG. *See* Intramuscular immunoglobulin (IMIG)
Iminoglycinuria, 1319
Imipenem, 645t, *see also website*
Imipenem-cilastin, 1492t
Imipramine
  for attention deficit/hyperactivity disorder, 111t
  for depression and anxiety symptoms, 63t
  for nocturnal incontinence, 1852
Imiquimod
  for genital warts, 713t
  for human papillomavirus, 1140
Imitres. *See* Sumatriptan
Immersion, cold water, 343-344
Immersion burn, due to child abuse, 138
Immersion foot, 358
Immigrant children, 6-7
  adoption of, 130-134
  effects of relocation on, *see website*
  medical evaluation of, 132-134
Immobility as goal of anesthesia, *see website*
Immobilization, hypercalcemia due to prolonged, 1923
Immotile cilia syndrome, 1497, *see also website*
Immune complexes
  in adverse drug reactions, 824
  in glomerular disease, *see website*
  in hepatitis B, 1397
  in serum sickness, 819
Immune dysregulation, polyendocrinopathy, enteropathy, X-linked (IPEX) syndrome, 738, 1312, 1341, 1969, 1995
Immune neutropenia, 749
Immune reconstitution inflammatory syndrome (IRIS), 1162
Immune response
  to immunizations, 883
  in influenza virus, 1122-1123
  of lung to injury, *see website*
  in tuberculosis, 998, 999f
Immune system
  complement in, 753, *see also website*
  evaluation of, 715-722
  fetal development of, *see website*
  glucocorticoids and, *see website*
  malignancy susceptibility associated with, *see website*
  phagocytic
    disorders of, 741-746, 742t
    eosinophils in, 739-741
    monocytes, macrophages, and dendritic cells in, 739, *see also website*
    neutrophils in, 739, *see also website*
  postnatal development of, *see website*
  T cells, B cells, and natural killer cells in, 722, *see also website*
Immunity
  acquired, *see website*
  to group B streptococci, 926
  to Haemophilus influenzae, 941, 941t
  immune cell interaction in, *see website*
  innate, *see website*
  to meningococcus, 931
  in newborns, 631-632
  after *Plasmodium*, 1200
  to *Shigella*, 959
  to tuberculosis, 1000-1001
  to varicella, 1109, 1109t
Immunization(s), 881-895, 881t. *See also* Vaccine(s)
  active, 883-884, 884t
  for adolescents, 664
  chronic kidney disease and, 1825
  congenital heart disease and, 1603
  HIV infection and, 1173, 1173f
  for homosexual youth, 659
  immigrant children and, 132, 134
  immunodeficiencies and, 889-891, 892t
  improving coverage of, 893, 893t
  international practices on, 893-895
  maternal, group B streptococcus, 928
  National Immunization Days and, 1087
  parental refusal of, 893, *see website*
  passive, 881-883
  precautions and contraindications for, 892-893
  recommended schedule for, 886, 887f-888f, 890f
    catch-up, 889, 890f
  renal transplantation and, *see website*
  safety monitoring of, 886, 886t
  in special circumstances, 889-891
  sudden infant death syndrome and, 1425
  for travel, 889, 891t, *see website*
  type 1 diabetes mellitus and, 1972
  vaccination system in USA and, 884-886, 885f
  websites and resources associated with, 894t
Immunocompromised patient
  bacillary angiomatosis in, 986
  candidiasis in, 1055-1056
  Cryptosporidium in, 1184
  fever without a focus in, 896t
Immunocompromised patient *(Continued)*
  infections in, 902, *see also website*
    with acquired immunodeficiencies, *see website*
    adenovirus in, 1132
    with B cell defects (humoral immunodeficiencies), *see website*
    blastomycosis, 1064-1065
    Cryptococcus neoformans, 1056-1057
    cytomegalovirus, 1116-1117
    with defective splenic function, opsonization, and complement activity, *see website*
    with fever and neutropenia, *see website*
    herpes simplex virus, 1101, 1103
    histoplasmosis, 1063
    with malignancies, *see website*
    parvovirus B19, 1096
    with phagocytic defects, *see website*
    Pneumocystis jiroveci, *see website*
    prevention of, *see website*
    with primary immunodeficiencies, *see website*
    Pseudomonas aeruginosa, 976
    with T cell defects (cell-mediated immunodeficiencies), *see website*
    Toxoplasmosis gondii, 1208, 1210, 1215
    with transplantation, *see website*
    Trypanosoma cruzi, 1196
    varicella-zoster virus, 1107
  vaccine recommendations for, 889-891, 892t
Immunodeficiency(ies), 715-722, 716t, 721t
  acquired (*See also* HIV/AIDS)
    infection with, *see website*
  antibody, 722-728, 724f
    common variable immunodeficiency as, 724-725, 724t
    genetics of, 723t
    hyper-immunoglobulin M syndrome as, 726-727
    immunoglobulin A deficiency as, 725
    immunoglobulin G subclass deficiencies as, 725-726
    immunoglobulin heavy- and light-chain deletions as, 726
    X-linked agammaglobulinemia as, 723-724, 723f
    X-linked lymphoproliferative disease as, 727
  atopic dermatitis *versus*, 803-804, 803t
  autoimmune lymphoproliferative syndrome as, 737-738, 737t, 738f
  B cell
    evaluation of, 715-720
    infection with, *see website*
    treatment of, 727-728
  cellular, 728-729, 728t
    autoimmune polyendocrinopathy-candidiasis ectodermal dysplasia as, 730
    CD8 lymphocytopenia as, 730
    defective cytokine production as, 729
    defective expression of T-cell receptor-CD3 complex as, 729, 729f
    thymic hypoplasia as, 728-729
    treatment of, 736-737, 737t
  classification of, 721t
  clinical manifestations of, 716t-718t
  combined, 730-738
    genetic basis of, 731t
    infection with, *see website*
    severe, 730-733, 731t, 732f
    treatment of, 736-737, 737t
  common variable, 724-725
  complement system, 722
  dysregulation, 737-738
  evaluation of, 715, 718t, 719f, 720t
  hematopoietic stem cell transplantation for, 760
  immunization and, 889-891, 892t
  infections with, *see website*
  inheritance in development of, *see website*
  in innate immunity, 735-736

Immunodeficiency(ies) *(Continued)*
malabsorption with, 1313-1314
malignancy susceptibility associated with, *see website*
maternal, 545
neutropenia in, 751-752
NK cells, 722
phagocytic
evaluation of, 722
infection with, *see website*
prenatal diagnosis and carrier detection in, *see website*
pulmonary manifestations of, *see website*
red blood cell aplasia in, 1653
T cell
evaluation of, 720-722
infection with, *see website*
with thrombocytopenia and eczema, 734-735
Immunofluorescence studies
in *Chlamydophila pneumoniae*, 1034-1035
in parainfluenza viruses, 1125t
in skin disorders, *see website*
in toxoplasmosis, 1213
Immunofluorescent-antibody (IFA) technique, *see website*
Immunoglobulin(s), 882t
administered with measles vaccine, 1074, 1074t
botulism, 990
for chronic diarrhea therapy, 1345-1346
cytomegalovirus, 882t
development and differentiation of, *see website*
for enterovirus infection, 1093-1094
heavy- and light-chain deletions of, 726
hepatitis A, 1396, 1396t
hepatitis B, 882t, 1399, 1399t
intramuscular, 882, 882t
intravenous, 882t
for antibody deficiencies, *see website*
for B-cell defects, 727-728
for cytomegalovirus prophylaxis, 1117
for hepatitis A virus, 1396, 1396t
for hepatitis B virus, 1399, 1399t
for hyperbilirubinemia, 611-612
for idiopathic thrombocytopenic purpura, 1717
for myasthenia gravis, 2135
for rheumatic disease, *see website*
for seizures, 2032
specific preparations of, 882, 882t
for tetanus, 992-993
for urticaria and angioedema, 815t
for viral infection, *see website*
in neonatal immunity, 631
postnatal, *see website*
rabies, 882t
subclasses of, *see website*
subcutaneous for B-cell defects, 727-728
tetanus, 882t, 992
vaccinia, 882t
varicella-zoster, 882t, 1106, 1110, *see website*
Immunoglobulin A (IgA)
deficiency of, 725, 748t
celiac disease and, 1309
infection and, *see website*
malabsorption with, 1314
development and differentiation of, *see website*
in Henoch-Schönlein purpura, 868-869
postnatal, *see website*
reference values for, *see website*
in screening for B cell defects, 719
subclasses of, *see website*
Immunoglobulin A (IgA) dermatosis, linear, 2249, 2249f
immunofluorescence of, *see website*
Immunoglobulin A (IgA) nephropathy, 1781-1782, 1781f, 1785t
Immunoglobulin D (IgD), reference values for, *see website*
Immunoglobulin E (IgE)
in adverse drug reactions, 824
in allergic disease, 766, *see website*
radioallergosorbent testing of, 766-767, 767t
allergic rhinitis, 775-777
anti-, for allergic disease, 772
in atopic dermatitis, 802
development and differentiation of, *see website*
in food adverse reactions, 820-822, 823t
hyper-, 736, 736t
in insect allergy, 807-808
in nonallergic disease, 767t
reference values for, *see website*
in urticaria and angioedema, 811
Immunoglobulin G (IgG), *see also website*
in adverse drug reactions, 824
antibody testing for, *see website*
in cytomegalovirus, 1116
deficiencies of
in common variable immunodeficiency, 725
infection and, *see website*
development and differentiation of, *see website*
in hepatitis A, 1395, 1396t
in Lyme disease, *see website*
in neonatal immunity, 631
postnatal, *see website*
reference values for, *see website*
in screening for B cell deficiencies, 720
subclasses of, *see website*
deficiencies of, 725-726, *see website*
Immunoglobulin G indirect fluorescent-antibody (IgG-IFA) testing, in toxoplasmosis, 1213
Immunoglobulin M enzyme-linked immunosorbent assay (IgM-ELISA), in toxoplasmosis, 1213-1214
Immunoglobulin M (IgM)
in adverse drug reactions, 824
antibody testing for, *see website*
in arboviral encephalitis, 1144
in cytomegalovirus, 1116
development and differentiation of, *see website*
hyper-, 726-727
in Lyme disease, 1028, *see website*
in measles, 1071
postnatal, *see website*
reference values for, *see website*
of rubella, 1076-1077
Immunoglobulin M indirect fluorescent-antibody (IgM-IFA) testing, in toxoplasmosis, 1213
Immunoproliferative small intestinal disease (IPSID), 1314-1315
Immunoprophylaxis. *See also* Prophylaxis
cytomegalovirus, 1117
otitis media, 2213
respiratory syncytial virus, 1129
Immunosorbent agglutination test (ISAGA), in toxoplasmosis, 1214
Immunosuppression
complications of, *see website*
cutaneous manifestations in setting of, *see website*
dental problems associated with, 1251t
for heart transplantation, *see website*
for intestinal transplantation, *see website*
for kidney transplantation, *see website*
for liver transplantation, *see website*
pharmacokinetics and, *see website*
Immunotherapy
allergen, 773-775
for atopic dermatitis, 805
venom, for insect allergy, 808-809, 809t
Imodium. *See* Loperamide
Impacted fracture, 2388f
Impaired glucose tolerance (IGT), 1993, *see also website*
Impending status epilepticus, 2037-2038
Imperforate anus, 1356, 1356f-1357f
neuropathic bladder and, *see website*
Impetigo, 2299-2300, 2300f
Bockhart, 2305
bullous, group A streptococci in, 917
in child-care setting, *see website*
exclusion from day care due to, *see website*
group A streptococcus in, 916-917
streptococcal, 915
Impiramine for nocturnal enuresis, 73t
Implant
cochlear, 2196, 2196t
progestin for special needs girls, 1875
Implicit memory, *see website*
Imprinting, genetic, 391-393, 393f
in cancer development, *see website*
Imprinting disorders, 413-414, 414f
Impulsivity, psychopharmacologic management of, 61t
IMRT. *See* Intensity modulated radiation therapy (IMRT)
IMV. *See* Intermittent mandatory ventilation (IMV)
Inactivated polio vaccine (IPV), 884t, 1087-1088
with diphtheria acellular pertussis vaccine and hepatitis B vaccine (DTaP-HepB-IPV), 884t
with diphtheria acellular pertussis vaccine (DTaP-IPV), 884t
with diphtheria acellular pertussis vaccine *Haemophilus influenzae* type b vaccine (DTaP-IPV/Hib), 884t
HIV infection and, 1173f
recommended schedule for, 886-889, 887f-888f
for travel, *see website*
Inamrinone, 294t
Inattention, psychopharmacologic management of, 61t
Inborn errors of metabolism, 416-418
of amino acids, 418-456
of arginine, citrulline, and ornithine, 447-453, 448f-449f, 448t, 450t
of aspartic acid, 455-456, 456f
of cysteine/cystine, 429
of glutamic acid, 443-445, 444f
of glycine, 438-441, 439f, 441f
of histidine, 453
of lysine, 453-455, 454f
malabsorption due to, 1318
of methionine, 425-429, 426f
of neurotransmitters, 445-447
newborn screening for, 416, 417t
of phenylalanine, 418-422, 419f, 421f
of proline, 442-443, 442f
of serine, 442
of tryptophan, 429-430, 429f
of tyrosine, 422-425
of valine, leucine, isoleucine, and related organic acidemias, 430-438, 430f
of carbohydrates, 492-509, 493f, 494t-495t, *see website*
of fructose, 503
of galactose, 502-503
glycogen storage diseases as, 492-501, 496f, 500f
of glycoprotein, 509, *see also website*
with lactic acidosis, 503-509, 504f-505f, 507t-509t, 508f
malabsorption due to, 1318
of pentose, 509, *see also website*
cardiac manifestations of, 1531t
clinical manifestations of, 416-418, 417f, 418t
common characteristics of, 416
hepatic, 1388-1393, 1389t
α-antitrypsin deficiency, 1393
inherited deficient conjugation of bilirubin as, 1389-1390
neonatal iron storage disease as, 1393
Wilson disease, 1391, 1391f

Inborn errors of metabolism *(Continued)*
of lipids, 456-492
of lipoprotein metabolism and transport, 470-482, 471f-474f, 472t-473t, 476f, 477t-479t, 480f, 481t-482t
lysosomal storage disorders as, 482-491, 483f, 484t-485t, 486f-487f, 489f, 491f
of mitochondrial fatty acid β-oxidation, 456-462, 457t, 458f-459f
mucolipidoses as, 491-492
of very long chain fatty acids, 462-470, 462t-464t, 464f-465f, 466t, 469f
liver effects of, 1389t
metabolic acidosis due to, 233
myocardial disease with, 1629t
neonatal seizures due to, 2036
newborn screening for, 416, 417t
physiologic therapies for, 379
of purine and pyrimidine, 516, *see also website*
severe intellectual disability in, 123t
strokelike events *versus*, 2086
treatment of, 418
Incarcerated inguinal hernia, 1365
Incidentalomas, *see website*
Incisional hernia, *see website*
Incomplete penetrance, genetic, 383-385, 387f
Inconspicuous penis, 1856, 1856f
Incontinence
diurnal, 73
fecal, 73-74
giggle, 1851
urinary, 1848t, 1850-1851, 1850f
diurnal, 1847-1848, 1848f-1849f
due to neuropathic bladder, *see website*
Incontinentia pigmenti, 2052-2053, 2053f
Incoordination
cricopharyngeal, 1264
gross motor, *see website*
Increased intracranial pressure (ICP), 297
in bacterial meningitis, 2089, 2094
in brain tumors, 1747
general anesthesia and, *see website*
migraine secondary to, 2046
as oncologic emergency, *see website*
Incubated osmotic fragility test, 1660-1661
IND. *See* Intestinal neuronal dysplasia (IND)
Inderal. *See* Propranolol
Indeterminate leprosy (IL), *see website*
India Ink stain, *see website*
Indian childhood cirrhosis, 1392
Indian Health Service, 10
Indian tick typhus, 1043-1044
Indicanuria, 1319
Indinavir
drug interactions with, *see website*
for HIV infection, 1168t-1171t
Indinavir calculi, *see website*
Indirect bilirubin, 605-606
Indirect cystography, 1836
Indirect fluorescent-antibody testing, in toxoplasmosis, 1213
Individualized education program (IEP), *see also website*
in intellectual disability, 128
Individualized family service plan (IFSP), *see also website*
in intellectual disability, 128
Individuals with Disabilities Education Act (IDEA), 122-123, *see also website*
Indole intoxication, *see website*
Indomethacin
possible adverse reactions to in premature infant, 563t
for prevention of intraventricular hemorrhage, 568
Indoor air pollution, *see website*
Induction of general anesthesia, *see also website*
adverse reactions to agents used for, 827
Infant
acne in, 2327, 2327f
asthma in, 800-801
behavioral and psychosocial assessment of, 56
born to diabetic mother, 545, *see website*
congenital heart disease with, 1531t
fetal therapy for, 551t
hypoglycemia in, 521
botulism in, 987-991
child restraint in motor vehicles for, 21t
developmental dysplasia of hip in, 2357-2360, 2357f-2358f, 2360f
digital fibroma in, *see website*
disruptive behavioral disturbances in, 99
drowning or submersion injury to, 342
feeding of
breast-feeding, 160
(*See also* Breast-feeding)
complementary feeding, 164-165
formula feeding, 162-164, 162f
fever without a focus in, 896t
fever without localizing signs in, 897-898, 897t
gonococcal infection in, 939
growth and development of, 26-31, 28t-29t
age 0-2 months, 26-29
age 2-6 months, 29-30
age 6-12 months, 30-31
breast-feeding and, 162
charts for assessment of, *see website*
cognitive, 27, 30
communication, 30-31
developmental milestones in, 27t
emotional, 27-28, 30-31
physical, 27, 29-31, 29f
gynecological examination of, *see website*
hypoglycemia in, 518-521, 520t
intellectual disability in, 125t
leading causes of death for, 5t
leukemia in, 1739
pain assessment in, 361
perception and effects of pain on, 373-375
pertussis in, 945
respiration regulation in, *see website*
sleep changes in, 47t
well child care for, 16
Infant formula, 162-164, 162f
human milk *versus*, 161t
otitis media and, 2200
Infantile acropustulosis, 2220
Infantile cortical hyperostosis, 2436-2437, 2436f
Infantile encephalopathy, early epileptic, 2023
Infantile parkinsonism, 445
Infantile polyarteritis nodosa, 862-867
Infantile Refsum disease, 464, 466t
Infant mortality rates, *see website*
Infarction
periventricular hemorrhage, 566
pulmonary, 1500-1502, 1501t
Infasurf, 585
Infected wound, perioperative prophylaxis and, *see website*
Infection-associated hemophagocytic syndrome (IAHS), 1774, 1774t
Infection prevention and control, 895, *see also website*
Infection prevention and control committee, *see website*
Infection preventionists, *see website*
Infection(s)
adrenocortical insufficiency due to, 1927
anaerobic
botulism as, 987-991
Clostridium difficile infection as, 994-995
due to other organisms, 995, *see also website*
tetanus as, 991-994
antibiotic therapy for, 903, *see also website*
in arthritis development, 839-841, 840f, 840t
ataxia due to, 2054
atopic dermatitis and, 806
Infection(s) *(Continued)*
bacterial (*See* Bacterial infection(s))
due to bites, 2455
bone, 2394-2398
central nervous system, 2086-2098
anaerobic, *see website*
Aspergillus in, 1061
bacterial meningitis as, 2087-2095
eosinophilic meningitis as, 2097-2098
neonatal seizures due to, 2034
Staphylococcus aureus, 905
stroke-like events *versus*, 2085
tuberculous, 1005-1006
viral meningoencephalitis as, 2095-2097
due to chemotherapy, *see website*
in child care setting, 895, *see also website*
chlamydial
Chlamydia trachomatis, 1035-1038
Chlamydophila pneumoniae, 1033-1035
psittacosis as, 1038, *see also website*
in cystic fibrosis, 1484
disk space, 2376, 2376t
eosinophilia and, 740
failure to thrive in, 148t
fetal therapy for, 551t
fungal (*See* Fungal infections)
glomerulonephritis associated with, 1783-1786, 1783f-1784f, 1785t
gram-positive (*See* Gram-positive bacterial infection)
hearing loss due to, 2188-2189, 2191t, *see also website*
hematopoietic stem cell transplantation-related, 762-763
in immigrant children, 131t, 132-134
in immunocompromised patient, 902, *see also website*
with acquired immunodeficiencies, *see website*
adenovirus in, 1132
with B cell defects (humoral immunodeficiencies), *see website*
Candida, 1055-1056, 1056t
cytomegalovirus, 1116-1117
with defective splenic function, opsonization, and complement activity, *see website*
with fever and neutropenia, *see website*
herpes simplex virus, 1101, 1103
with malignancies, *see website*
parvovirus B19, 1096
with phagocytic defects, *see website*
prevention of, *see website*
with primary immunodeficiencies, *see website*
Pseudomonas aeruginosa, 976
with T cell defects, *see website*
Toxoplasmosis gondii, 1208, 1210, 1215
with transplantation, *see website*
Trypanosoma cruzi, 1196
international health care and, *see website*
international prevention of, *see website*
intestinal, 1313
(*See also* Gastroenteritis)
Aeromonas in, *see website*
Campylobacter in, 969-970
eosinophilic, 1304, 1321
in immigrant children, 133
salmonellosis, 951
juvenile idiopathic arthritis and, 835
malnutrition and, 173, 178t
maternal, 545
medical device-associated, 903, *see also website*
molecular diagnosis of, *see website*
mycobacterial
Hansen disease as, 1011, *see also website*
nontuberculous, 1011-1016
treatment of, 996, *see also website*
tuberculosis as, 996-1011

Infection(s) *(Continued)*
mycoplasmal
genital, 1032-1033
Mycoplasma pneumoniae, 1029-1032
of nails, 2296, 2296f
neonatal, 629-648
bacterial, 630, 630f-631f, 636-637, 638t, 642-644
brain injury due to, 568-569
clinical manifestations of, 636-639, 637t-638t
complications and prognosis for, 646, 647t
diagnosis of, 639-644
early-onset, 633-636, 634t
Enterococcus, *see website*
enterovirus in, 1092
epidemiology of, 629, 633-636
etiology of, 632-633, 633t
evaluation of, 643t
fungal, 642-644
Haemophilus influenzae in, 943
immunity and, 631-632
intrauterine, 629-630, 630f, 636-642, 637t
late-onset, 631, 633-636, 634t-635t
listeriosis, *see website*
modes of transmission of, 629-631
nosocomial, 634-636, 635t-636t, 647-648
pathogenesis of, 629-631, 630f-631f
postnatal, 631
prematurity and low birth weight and, 634, 634f-635f
prevention of, 647-648, 647t
prophylaxis for, 640f-642f, 640t
systemic inflammatory response syndrome due to, 637-639
treatment of, 644-646, 645t
varicella-zoster virus, 1106
with nephrotic syndrome, 1805
neutropenia associated with, 747-748, 749t
nosocomial
fever of unknown origin in, 899t
Legionella, *see website*
neonatal, 632-636, 635t-636t, 647-648, 647t
prevention and control of, 647-648, 647t, 895, *see also website*
Pseudomonas aeruginosa in, 976
respiratory syncytial virus, 1127
Salmonella, 950
orbital, 2182-2184
parasitic (*See* Parasitic infections)
perinatal, 543t, 547-548
Campylobacter in, 970
congenital lymphocytic choriomeningitis, 548
cytomegalovirus, 1116
herpes simplex virus, 1101, 1102f, 1103
tuberculous, 1007, 1011
predisposition to, 716t
prevention of
(*See also* Infection prevention and control)
in burn injury, 353-354, 353t
in child care setting, *see website*
immunizations for, 881-895, 881t-882t
in premature and low birthweight infants, 353-354
as protection against type diabetes mellitus, 1972
renal transplantation and, *see website*
rickettsial, 1038, 1039t-1040t
due to *Anaplasmosis*, 1048-1050
ehrlichioses as, 1048-1050
Mediterranean spotted fever as, 1043-1044
Q fever as, 1051-1053
Rocky Mountain spotted fever as, 1038-1043
scrub typhus as, 1045-1046
typhus group rickettsiae as, 1046-1048
serologic diagnosis of, *see website*
Infection(s) *(Continued)*
spirochetal
bejel as, 1023, *see also website*
leptospirosis as, 1023-1025
Lyme disease as, 1025-1029
pinta as, 1023, *see also website*
relapsing fever as, 1025, *see also website*
syphilis as, 1016-1023
yaws as, 1023, *see also website*
systemic inflammatory response syndrome and, 309t
after transplantation
heart, *see website*
intestinal, *see website*
kidney, *see website*
travel and, 896, *see also website*
immunizations prior to, 889, 891t
in type 1 diabetes mellitus, 1987, 1987t
umbilical, *see website*
urinary tract, 1829-1834
alternate recommendations for, 1833-1834
clinical manifestations and classification of, 1829-1830, 1830f
coagulase-negative staphylococci in, 910
diagnosis of, 1831-1832
hematuria in, 1791-1795, 1799
imaging studies of, 1833, 1833f
pathogenesis and pathology of, 1830-1831, 1831f, 1831t
prevalence and history of, 1829
treatment of, 1832-1833, 1832f
viral (*See* Viral infections)
Infectious mononucleosis, 1110-1115
Infectious mononucleosis-like illness, 1110
Infective endocarditis, 1622-1626
acute rheumatic fever *versus*, 923, 923t
clinical manifestations of, 1623, 1623t
congenital heart disease and, 1609
dental procedures prophylaxis, 1626t
diagnosis of, 1623-1624, 1624t
epidemiology of, 1622-1623
etiology of, 1622, 1622t
prevention of, 1626, 1626t
prognosis and complications of, 1624
in tetralogy of Fallot, 1576
treatment of, 1624-1626, 1625t
Infergen. *See* Interferon-α
Infertility, due to cancer and its therapy, 1870-1871, *see also website*
Infestation
pediculosis, 2321-2322, 2321f
scabies, 2319-2320, 2319f-2320f
seabather's eruption, 2322
Infiltrates, lung
in acute lung injury, 317f
in amyloidosis, 861, 861f
in eosinophilic lung disease, 1474
recurrent or persistent, *see website*
Infiltration, bone marrow, 1684
Inflammation
breast, *see website*
chronic, obesity and, 183-184
cutaneous, pigmentary changes due to, 2238
cytokines in regulation of, *see website*
newborn brain injury due to, 568-569, 568f
orbital, 2182
paronychial, 2296-2297, 2297f
systemic inflammatory response syndrome and, 307, 309t, 310f, 637-639, 639t
Inflammatory bowel disease (IBD), 1294-1304, 1295t-1296t
arthritis with, *see website*
Crohn's disease as, 1300-1304
cutaneous manifestations of, *see website*
juvenile idiopathic arthritis and, 835
liver disease with, *see website*
malabsorption due to, 1322, *see also website*
ulcerative colitis as, 1295-1300
Inflammatory diarrhea, 1330
Inflammatory mediators in neonatal immunity, 632
Inflammatory pseudotumor, tracheal, *see website*
Inflammatory response
in allergic disease, *see website*
genetic basis of, *see website*
phagocytic, 739, *see also website*
Infliximab
antibodies to, 1303
for Crohn disease, 1303
for juvenile idiopathic arthritis, 838t
for rheumatic disease, *see website*
Influenza vaccine, 884t
HIV infection and, 1173f
recommended schedule for, 886-889, 887f-888f
for travel, *see website*
Influenza viruses, 1121-1125, 1123t-1124t
antivirals for, *see website*
in pneumonia, 1475t
Information explosion of 21st century, 11-12
Information technology, quality improvement and, *see website*
Infrequent voiding, 1850
Infundibular pulmonary valve stenosis, 1564
ventricular septal defect with, 1558
Infundibular stenosis, 1841
Ingestion
caustic, 1272-1273, 1272t
of foreign bodies, 1271-1272, 1272f-1273f
Ingrown nail, 2297
Inguinal hernia, 1362-1368
abdominal pain of, 1247t
clinical presentation of, 1364
complications after surgery for, 1367-1368
direct, 1366-1367
embryology and pathogenesis of, 1362-1363, 1363f
evaluation of, 1364-1365
femoral, 1367
genetics of, 1363
incarcerated, 1365, 1367
incidence of, 1364
management of, 1365-1366, 1367f
pathology of, 1363-1364, 1364t
Inguinal swelling, evaluation of, 1364-1365
Inguinal undescended testis, 1859
INH. *See* Isoniazid (INH)
Inhalants abuse, 673t, 681-682, 681t-682t
Inhalation anesthetics, *see website*
Inhalation botulism, 987-991
Inhalation injury, 354-355
Inhaled β-agonists for asthma
long-acting, 794-795
short-acting, 792t, 796, 797t-798t
Inhaled corticosteroids (ICs)
for asthma, 791-793, 794t-795t
for wheezing, 1459
Inhaled gases
for respiratory distress and failure, 319-320
Inhaled insulin therapy, 1977-1979
Inhaled materials, hypersensitivity to, 1473, *see also website*
Inhaled nitric oxide (iNO)
for anesthesia, *see website*
for congenital diaphragmatic hernia, 595
for persistent pulmonary hypertension of the newborn, 593
for respiratory distress and failure, 319, 586
Inhaler, dry powder, 796-798
Inherent strengths in special risk populations, 8-9
Inheritance
digenic, 389, 390f
in immunodeficiency development, *see website*
mendelian, 383-388
autosomal dominant, 383-385, 387f
autosomal recessive, 385-388, 388f
pseudodominant, 388, 388f
X-linked, 388, 388f-389f
mitochondrial, 390-391, 390f-391f, 391t
multifactorial and polygenic, 393-394, 393f

Inheritance *(Continued)*
pseudogenetic, 389-390
Y-linked, 388-389, 390f
Inherited conjugated hyperbilirubinemia, 1390
Inherited deficient conjugation of bilirubin as, 1389-1390
Inherited pancytopenia, 1684-1690, 1684t
Inherited primary dystonias, 2059
Inhibin
in ovarian carcinomas, 1872t
in testicular function, *see website*
Inhibition control, *see website*
Initial examination of newborn, 532
Injection, contraceptive, 695t, 697-698
Injury(ies), 333-341. *See also* Emergency(ies)
abdominal, 338-339, 338t-339t, 339f
due to child abuse, 140
abrasions as, 341
in adolescents, 661-662
bicycle, 22-23
birth
brachial plexus palsy due to, 2383
facial palsy as, 2147
fractures as, 578-579
of peripheral nerves, 573-574
of spine and spinal cord, 573
visceral, 578
breast, *see website*
burns as, 349-357
cold, 357-359
neonatal, 622
cutaneous, warts with, 2315, 2315f
death due to, 17-18, 17t
dental, 1258-1259, 1258f-1259f, 1258t
drowning, 24
of ear, 2213-2214, *see also website*
early childhood, foster and kinship care and, *see website*
epidemiology of, 333
eye, 2184-2187, 2184f-2186f
cataracts due to, 2171
falls, 25
fingertip, 2387
fire- and burn-related, 23-24
firearm, 24-25
genitourinary, 1864, *see also website*
global, 19
inhalation injury as, 354-355
international health care and, *see website*
international pediatric emergency medicine and, *see website*
international prevention of, *see website*
to kidney, 1799
lacerations and cuts as, 340-341
leading causes of, 18f
mechanism of, 21-25
migraine secondary to, 2045
motor vehicle, 21-22, 21f, 21t
nonfatal, 19, 19f
optic nerve, *see website*
overuse, 2406-2407, 2407t
pedestrian, 23
peripheral nerve, 573-574, 574f
poisoning, 24
primary survey of, 333-337
airway/cervical spine, 335
breathing, 336, 336t
circulation, 336-337, 336t
exposure and environmental control, 337
neurologic deficit, 337
psychological and social support for, 340
psychosocial consequences of, 25
puncture wounds of foot, 2341
regionalization and trauma teams for, 333, 333t, 334f-335f, 335t
retinopathy due to, 2180, 2181f
risk factors for, 20-21
secondary survey, 337-340
abdominal trauma, 338-339, 338t-339t, 339f
cervical spine trauma, 337-338, 338f
extremity trauma, 339-340
Injury(ies) *(Continued)*
head trauma, 337, 337f
lower genitourinary trauma, 339
pelvic trauma, 339
radiologic and laboratory evaluation, 340
thoracic trauma, 335t, 338
ski- and snow board-related, 23
spinal and spinal cord, 2106
during birth, 573
respiratory insufficiency due to, 1523
to spleen, *see website*
sports
acute, 2406
of ankle, 2417-2418, 2417f
differential diagnosis of, 2408
of elbow, 2410-2412, 2411f-2412f
epidemiology and prevention of, 2401-2406
of foot, 2418
of growth plate, 2408-2409, 2408f-2409f
of head and neck, 2418-2420
due to heat, 2420-2421, 2421f
of hip and pelvis, 2407t, 2413-2414, 2413f
initial evaluation of, 2407
of knee, 2414-2416, 2414t, 2415f
of low back, 2412-2413
of lower leg, 2416-2417
mechanism of, 2406-2407
ocular, 2186-2187
overuse, 2406-2407, 2407t
return to play following, 2407-2408
of shoulder, 2409-2410, 2410f
of temporal bone, *see website*
transport following, *see website*
traumatic brain, 297-301, 298f-301f
attention deficit/hyperactivity disorder following, 108
due to child abuse, 139-140, 139f, 301, 2181f
mild, 301
sports-related, 2418-2419, 2419t
in trauma survey, 337
during travel, *see website*
violence, 25
vulvar or vaginal, 1869
Injury control, 17, 18f
principles of, 19-20, 19t-20t
Innate immunity, *see also website*
immunodeficiencies in, 735-736
to *Shigella*, 959
Inner ear
congenital malformations of, 2196, *see also website*
diseases of, 2213, *see also website*
iNO. *See* Inhaled nitric oxide (iNO)
Inocybe poisoning, *see website*
Inorganic mercury salts, *see website*
Inpatient services in international pediatric emergency medicine, *see website*
INR. *See* International normalized ratio (INR)
Insect allergens, 769
Insect allergy, 807-809, 807f, 809t
Insect-borne infection, during travel, *see website*
Insecticides poisoning, 266-267
Insect repellent
for malaria prevention, 1207
for travelers, *see website*
for tularemia prevention, 980
Insertion, genetic, 407, *see also website*
Insomnia, 47-48, 48t-49t. *See also* Sleep disorders
fatal familial, 1177, *see also website*
treatment of in palliative care, 155t-156t
Inspection in orthopedic problems, 2331, 2332t
Inspiratory capacity (IC), *see website*
Inspiratory flow pattern in mechanical ventilation, 327-328
Inspiratory flow waveform, 326
Inspiratory time constant in mechanical ventilation, 323
Inspiratory time in mechanical ventilation, 325-327
Inspired gas, composition of, 316
Inspissated bile syndrome, 618
Instability
autonomic, *see website*
cervical spine, 2380-2382
in Down syndrome, 2381-2382, 2382f
sports participation and, 2402t-2404t
Institute of Medicine (IOM)
on quality of care, *see website*
on vaccine safety, 886
Institutional review boards (IRBs), *see website*
Insulin
adverse reaction to, 827
diabetes mellitus and
type 1, 1971
type 2, 1990
genetic defects of action of, 1995-1996
as poisoning antidote, 256t-258t
resistance to in polycystic ovary syndrome, *see website*
Insulin gene, abnormalities of, 1995
Insulin levels
in hyperinsulinism, 521, 521t-522t
in hypoglycemia, 521t
in obesity, 185t
Insulin-like growth factor-binding protein (IGFBP), 521
Insulin-like growth factor 1 (IGF-1), 1881, *see also website*
Insulin-like growth factor receptor 2 (IGF2) gene inactivation, *see website*
Insulin lipodystrophy, 2286
Insulinoma, *see website*
Insulin pump therapy, 1977
Insulin resistance in diabetes mellitus, 1972
Insulin resistance syndrome, *see website*
Insulin therapy
continuous subcutaneous infusion for, 1977
current intensive regimens for, 1984-1985
fear of self-injecting and self-testing in, 1986
inhaled or oral, 1977-1979
for type 1 diabetes mellitus, 1976-1979, 1977f-1978f, 1979t
during surgery, 1987, 1987t
Insurance, health
for adolescents, 663, 664f
travel and, *see website*
Integrase inhibitors for HIV infection, 1168t-1171t
Integrated Management of Childhood Illness (IMCI), 1334, 1335f, *see also website*
Integrative medicine, 270-274. *See also* Complementary and alternative medicine
Intellectual disability, 122-129
in Becker muscular dystrophy, 2120
clinical manifestations of, 124-125, 125t
complications of, 127
diagnosis of, 122-124, 123t
diagnostic psychologic testing in, 126-127
differential diagnosis of, 125-126
in Duchenne muscular dystrophy, 2119
epidemiology of, 124
etiology of, 123t, 124
with homocystinuria, 425-426
laboratory findings in, 125, 126f, 127t
language disorders of, 118, 118f
in myotonic muscular dystrophy, 2124
pathology and pathogenesis of, *see website*
prevalence of, 4
prevention of, 127-128
prognosis for, 129, 129t
supportive care and management of, 128-129
treatment of, 128
Intellectual function, *see website*
Intelligent quotient (IQ)
in intellectual disability, 123
intellectual functioning and, *see website*
risk factors and, *see website*
Intensification treatment for acute lymphocytic leukemia, 1735
Intensity modulated radiation therapy (IMRT), *see website*

Intensity of pain, 2332t
Intention tremor, 2056-2057
Interactional abilities of newborn, *see website*
Intercostal block, 372
Interdisciplinary management of intellectual disability, 128
Interferon-α, *see website*
Interferon-α 2a plus ribavirin, *see website*
Interferon-α 2b
  for hepatitis B, 1399
  for hepatitis C, 1401
  plus ribavirin, *see website*
Interferons for hepatitis and human papillomavirus, *see website*
Interferon-γ (IFN-γ)
  for atopic dermatitis, 805
  for chronic granulomatous disease, 746
  in Rocky Mountain spotted fever, 1041
Interferon-γ-interleukin-12 axis deficiency, *see website*
Interferon-γ receptor 1 mutations, 735
Interferon-γ receptor 2 mutations, 735
Interferon-γ release assay, *see also website*
  for tuberculosis, 1001, 1002t
Interferon-induced helicase gene, 1971
Interferon signature in systemic lupus erythematosus, 843
Interiginous candidosis, 2314, 2314f
Interleukin-1β (IL-1β), *see website*
Interleukin-1 (IL-1) antagonists
  for juvenile idiopathic arthritis, 838t
  for rheumatic disease, *see website*
Interleukin-1 (IL-1) receptor, type 1 diabetes mellitus and, 1971
Interleukin-1 (IL-1) receptor antagonists, deficiency of, 858
Interleukin-2 (IL-2) receptor
  α chain mutation, 733
  type 1 diabetes mellitus and, 1971
Interleukin-2 (IL-2) receptor antibodies, *see website*
Interleukin-3 (IL-3), *see website*
Interleukin-4 (IL-4)
  in allergic disease, *see website*
  in atopic dermatitis, 802
Interleukin-5 (IL-5), *see website*
Interleukin-6 (IL-6), 1427
Interleukin-6 (IL-6) antagonist, *see website*
Interleukin-7(IL-7) Rα deficiency, 732
Interleukin-9 (IL-9), *see website*
Interleukin-12 (IL-12)
  for allergic disease, 773
  defects of, *see website*
  Salmonella and, 951
Interleukin-12 (IL-12) receptor β1 mutation, 735
Interleukin-13 (IL-13)
  in allergic disease, *see website*
  in atopic dermatitis, 802
Interleukins (ILs), *see also website*
  in allergic disease, *see website*
  celiac disease, 1308
  fetal, *see website*
  in HIV infection, 1161
  interaction with other immune cells, *see website*
  in systemic lupus erythematosus, 843
Interleukin-1R-associated kinase 4 (IRAK4) deficiency, 735-736
Intermediate density lipoproteins (IDL), 471-473, 472f, 472t
Intermittent acute porphyria, *see website*
Intermittent allergic rhinitis (IAR), 775
Intermittent dialysis for acute renal failure, 1821, 1821t
Intermittent fever, *see website*
Intermittent mandatory ventilation (IMV), 324, 324f
Internal femoral torsion, 2347
Internal jugular vein, venous access in, 295f
Internal radiation contamination, *see website*
Internal rotation, 2331
Internal tibial torsion, 2347
International Association for Medical Assistance to Travelers, *see website*
International Classification of Headache Disorders, 2040, 2040t-2041t
International conventions for protection of children from effects of war, *see website*
International efforts for quality improvement, *see website*
International immunization practices, 893-895
International League of Association for Rheumatology (ILAR), 829, 830t
International Neuroblastoma Staging System, 1755t, 1756
International normalized ratio (INR), 1696
  in fulminant hepatic failure, 1412-1415
  in liver disease, 1378-1379
International pediatric emergency medicine (IPEM), *see website*
International Union of Pharmacology (IUPHAR), *see website*
Internet
  harassment on, 668
  resources on, 11
    for genetic disorders, 380t
    for pharmacogenetics and pharmacogenomics, *see website*
    for vaccines, 894t
Internuclear ophthalmoplegia, *see website*
Interpersonal violence, 668-669
Interphase of mitosis, 394-395
Interpheron alpha-2a for Behçet disease, 854
Interstitial compartment, pulmonary edema and, 1468
Interstitial cystitis, 1830
Interstitial fluid, *see website*
Interstitial keratitis, *see website*
Interstitial lung disease (ILD), 1497, *see also website*
Interstitial nephritis, 1814-1816
  nephrotoxins in, 1817t
Interstitial pneumonia
  lymphocytic, HIV-related, 1165
  in lysinuric protein intolerance, 455
Intervertebral disk herniation, 2377
Intervertebral disk space infection, 2376t
Interviewing
  of adolescent, 665-666, 666t
    following rape, 704
  for attention deficit/hyperactivity disorder, 109-110
  for psychologic disorders, 56-58, 57t
Intestinal disorders
  acute appendicitis as, 1349-1355
    clinical features of, 1349-1350
    diagnostic approach to, 1353-1354
    diagnostic studies in, 1351-1353, 1351f-1352f, 1351t
    differential diagnosis of, 1353
    pathology of, 1349
    physical examination in, 1350
  adhesions as, 1287
  anorectal, 1355-1362
    anal fissure as, 1359
    hemorrhoids as, 1360, 1361f
    malformations as, 1355-1356, 1356f, 1357t, 1359t
    perianal abscess and fistula as, 1360, 1360f
    pilonidal sinus and abscess as, 1362
    rectal mucosal prolapse as, 1361
  atresia, stenosis, and malrotation as, 1277-1281, 1279f-1280f
  bezoars as, 1291
  chronic diarrhea as, 1339-1346
    assessment of, 1340-1341, 1343f, 1343t-1345t
    definition and epidemiology of, 1339-1346
    etiology of, 1339, 1340t, 1342t
    due to neuroendocrine tumor, 1346, *see also website*
Intestinal disorders *(Continued)*
    pathophysiology of, 1339, 1339f-1340f
    treatment of, 1342-1344
  clinical approach to, 1305-1306
  closed-loop obstruction as, 1287-1289
  in cystic fibrosis, 1486-1487, 1487f
    treatment of, 1495-1496
  duodenal obstruction, 1277-1278, 1278f
  duplication as, 1281
  eosinophilic gastroenteritis as, 1304
  foreign bodies as, 1290, 1290f
  functional abdominal pain as, 1346-1349, 1346t-1348t
  functional constipation as, 1284, 1284t
  gastroenteritis as, 1323-1339
    bacterial, 1324t-1325t
    clinical manifestations of, 1331-1332, 1332t
    complications of, 1333-1334, 1333t
    diagnosis of, 1333-1334, 1333t
    etiology of, 1323
    global trends in, 1326f
    noninfectious, 1328t-1329t
    parasitic, 1327t-1328t
    pathogenesis of, 1323-1330, 1330f-1331f, 1330t
    prevention of, 1337-1338
    risk factors for, 1330-1331
    traveler's diarrhea as, 1338-1339, 1338t
    treatment of, 1334-1337, 1334t-1335t, 1335f-1336f, 1337t
    viral, 1326t
  Hirschsprung disease as, 1283t, 1284-1287, 1285f-1286f
  ileus as, 1287
    in cystic fibrosis, 1495
  in immigrant children, 133
  inflammatory bowel disease as, 1294-1304, 1295t-1296t
  inguinal hernia as, 1362-1368
    clinical presentation of, 1364
    complications after surgical repair of, 1367-1368
    direct, 1366-1367
    embryology and pathogenesis of, 1362-1363, 1363f
    evaluation of, 1364-1365
    femoral, 1367
    genetics of, 1363
    incarcerated, 1365
    incidence of, 1364
    management of, 1365-1366, 1367f
    pathology of, 1363-1364, 1364t
  intestinal neuronal dysplasia as, 1287, *see also website*
  intussusception as, 1287-1289, 1289f
  malabsorption as, 1304-1322, 1305t
    of bile acid, 1312
    of carbohydrates, 1306-1307
    classification of, 1305t
    clinical approach to, 1305-1306, 1306f, 1306t
    due to enzyme deficiencies, 1317-1319
    in eosinophilic gastroenteritis, 1321, *see also website*
    evaluation of, 1306-1308
    exocrine pancreatic function and, 1307-1308, 1307f
    of fat, 1307
    due to gluten-sensitivity enteropathy, 1308-1311, 1308f, 1309t-1310t, 1310f
    with immunodeficiency disorders, 1313-1314
    due to immunoproliferative small intestinal disease, 1314-1315
    in inflammatory bowel disease, 1322, *see also website*
    due to intestinal infections and infestations, 1313
    due to intestinal mucosal disorders, 1308
    due to liver and biliary disorders, 1318
    due to malnutrition, 1315

Intestinal disorders *(Continued)*
other syndromes of, 1311-1313
of protein, 1307
rare inborn defects causing, 1317
due to short bowel syndrome, 1314, 1315t, 1316f
Meckel diverticulum and other remnants of omphalomesenteric duct as, 1281-1282, 1282f
motility disorders as, 1283-1287
chronic diarrhea due to, 1341
peptic ulcer disease as, 1291-1294, 1291t, 1292f-1293f, 1293t
pseudo-obstruction as, 1283-1284, 1283t
superior mesenteric artery syndrome, 1287, *see also website*
transplantation for, 1322-1323, *see also website*
tumors as, 1362, *see also website*
Intestinal epithelial dysplasia, 1341
Intestinal failure (IF), transplantation for, 1322-1323, *see also website*
Intestinal flukes, *see website*
Intestinal lymphangiectasia, 1311
Intestinal microsporidiosis, *see website*
Intestinal mucosal disorders, 1308
Intestinal myopathy, 1283
Intestinal neuronal dysplasia (IND), 1286
Intestinal neuropathy, 1283
Intestinal obstruction. *See* Ileus
Intestine
digestion and absorption in, *see website*
disorders of (*See* Intestinal disorders)
in drug absorption, *see website*
normal development, structure, and function of, 1273, *see also website*
transplantation of, 1322-1323, *see also website*
In-toeing gate, 2347
Intoxication. *See* Poisoning
Intracellular fluid (ICF), *see website*
Intracerebral hemorrhage, 303-304
cerebral palsy and, 2061-2062
Intracranial hemorrhage
due to child abuse, 139, 139f
in newborn, 565f, 566-568
in high-risk pregnancy, *see website*
Intracranial pressure (ICP), 296
drowning and, 345-346
increased, 297
in bacterial meningitis, 2089, 2094
in brain tumors, 1747
general anesthesia and, *see website*
migraine secondary to, 2046
as oncologic emergency, *see website*
monitoring of, 297
traumatic brain injury and, 298-300, 301f, 337
Intractable diarrhea syndrome, 1341, 1342t
Intrahepatic cholestasis, 452, 1381-1384, 1382t-1384t
Intraluminal impedance, 1267, *see also website*
Intramembranous ossification, *see website*
Intramuscular (IM) drug administration, *see website*
Intramuscular (IM) epinephrine for anaphylaxis, 817
Intramuscular immunoglobulin (IMIG), 882, 882t
Intranasal inhaled corticosteroids, 778t-780t, 779-780
Intraoral dental radiographs, *see website*
Intraosseous (IO) access for emergencies, 292, 296f, 336
Intraosseous (IO) drug administration, *see website*
Intrapulmonary airway, *see website*
Intrapulmonary sequestration, 1466
Intrapulmonary shunt, 317-318
Intrathecal analgesia, 373
Intrathoracic-extrapulmonary airway, *see website*
Intrauterine devices (IUDs), 695t, 699
actinomycosis with, *see website*
for special needs girls, 1875
Intrauterine diagnosis of fetal disease, 548-550, 549f, 550t
Intrauterine growth restriction (IUGR), 555-564
definitions associated with, 555
factors related to, 557t
fetal therapy for, 551t
gestational age at birth assessment in, 557, 558f
incidence of, 555-556
nursery care in, 558-562
prognosis for, 562-563, 563t
spectrum of disease in, 558, 559t
type 2 diabetes mellitus and, 1990
Intrauterine infection
clinical manifestations of, 636-639, 637t
diagnosis of, 640-642
pathogenesis of, 629-630, 630f
Intravascular access device, infections associated with, *see website*
Intravascular stent, 1548, 1548f
for coarctation of the aorta, 1569
Intravenous anesthetics, *see website*
Intravenous gammaglobulin for Kawasaki disease, 866-867, 867t
Intravenous immunoglobulin (IVIG), 882, 882t
for antibody deficiencies, *see website*
for B-cell defects, 727-728
for cytomegalovirus prophylaxis, 1117
for erythroblastosis fetalis, 618
hepatitis A, 1396, 1396t
for hyperbilirubinemia, 611-612
for idiopathic thrombocytopenic purpura, 1717
for myasthenia gravis, 2135
for rheumatic disease, *see website*
for seizures, 2032
for tetanus, 992-993
for urticaria and angioedema, 815t
Intravenous (IV) drug administration, *see website*
Intravenous (IV) maintenance solutions, 243, 243t
glucose in, 243
hyponatremia and, 243-244
for office emergencies, *see website*
selection of, 243
Intravenous regional block (IVRA), 372
Intraventricular hemorrhage (IVH), 566-568, 567f, 568t
Intrinsic factor (IF), 1320
megaloblastic anemias due to deficiency of, *see website*
Intrinsic renal acute renal failure, 1819
Intro-A. *See* Interferon-α
Introns, genetic, *see website*
Intrusion injury, dental, 1259
Intubation
endotracheal
for asthma exacerbation, 800
for congenital diaphragmatic hernia, 595
in infant botulism, 990
for infectious acute upper airway obstruction, 1448
manual ventilation before and after, 320-321
medications for placement of tube in, 321t
placement of, 285, 286f, 287t
placement of tube in, 285, 286f, 287t
for respiratory distress and failure, 320
selection of tube for, 285
size and depth dimensions of tube for, 320t
rapid sequence, 285, 287t
Intussusception, 1287-1289, 1289f
abdominal pain of, 1247t-1248t
In utero positioning, orthopedic problems and, *see website*
Inversion
chromosomal, 405-406
musculoskeletal, 2331
Inversion stress test for ankle, 2417, 2417f
Invirase. *See* Saquinavir
Involuntary movement assessment in neurologic examination, *see website*
IO. *See* Intraosseous (IO)
Iodide(s)
defect of transport of, 1896
goiter due to, 1908
Iodine, *see website*
deficiency of, *see website*
goiter or cretinism due to, 1906-1908
hypothyroidism due to exposure to, 1897
intake of, *see website*
radioactive for Graves disease, 1912t
Iodine-deficiency endemic goiter, 1897
Iodine-deficiency goiter and cretinism, 1906-1908
Iodine-123 meta-iodobenzylguanidine (I231-MIBG) studies, 1754-1756
Iodoquinol
for amebiasis, 1180t
for balantidiasis, 1183, *see also website*
for infectious diarrhea, 1337t
IOM. *See* Institute of Medicine (IOM)
Ion channels
pharmacogenetics and, *see website*
strokelike events *versus* mutations of, 2086
Ionized calcium, reference values for, *see website*
Ion transporters, skeletal dysplasias involving, 2430-2431
Iota toxin, *see website*
IPEM. *See* International pediatric emergency medicine (IPEM)
IPEX syndrome, 738, 1312, 1341, 1969, 1995
IPH. *See* Idiopathic pulmonary hemorrhage (IPH)
Ipratropium bromide
for allergic disease, 770
for allergic rhinitis, 779, 780t
for asthma, 796, 797t-798t
for wheezing, 1459
IPSID. *See* Immunoproliferative small intestinal disease (IPSID)
IPV. *See* Inactivated polio vaccine (IPV)
IQ. *See* Intelligent quotient (IQ)
IRAK4. *See* Interleukin-1R-associated kinase 4 (IRAK4) deficiency
Irbesartan for systemic hypertension, 1645t
IRBs. *See* Institutional review boards (IRBs)
Iridocyclitis, 2173
IRIS. *See* Immune reconstitution inflammatory syndrome (IRIS)
Iris
abnormalities of, 2154-2157, 2154f
development of, *see website*
hamartomas in, due to neurofibromatosis, 2046-2047, 2047f
neurologic examination of, *see website*
Iritis, 2172-2174
Iron
dietary reference intakes for, *see website*
in malnutrition with chronic diarrhea, 1343t
poisoning with, 263
antidote for, 256t-257t
reference values for, *see website*
as trace element, *see website*
vegetarian diets and, 168
Iron-deficiency anemia, 1655-1658
with celiac disease, 1309
clinical manifestations of, 1656
differential diagnosis of, 1657, 1658t
etiology of, 1656
due to hookworm, 1219
laboratory findings in, 1656-1657, 1656t-1657t, 1657f
prevention of, 1657-1658
treatment of, 1658, 1658t
Iron lung, 1524
Iron overload
due to blood transfusions, 1675-1676
in sickle cell disease, 1667

Iron storage disease, neonatal, 1383, 1393
Irradiation. *See also* Radiation exposure; Radiation therapy
conformal, *see website*
Irreversible shock, 285
Irrigation
of laceration, 341
whole-bowel, for poisoning, 257
Irritability in newborn, *see website*
Irritable bowel syndrome (IBS), 1348-1349
abdominal pain of, 1247t, 1346t, 1348-1349
Campylobacter and, 969
chronic diarrhea with, 1341
Irritant contact dermatitis, 2250
Irritant receptors in respiration regulation, *see website*
Irritants, avoidance of for atopic dermatitis, 806
ISAGA. *See* Immunosorbent agglutination test (ISAGA), in toxoplasmosis
Ischemia
due to drowning, 343
encephalopathy due to, 298f-299f, 301-303, 302f, *569-573*, *569t-570t*
in drowning, 346
microcephaly with, 2007t
seizure due to, 2034
stroke-like events *versus*, 2085
Ischemic stroke, arterial, 2080-2082, 2081f-2082f, 2081t-2082t
Ischium, 2355
Iselin disease, 2341
Islet cells
adenoma of, 527
transplantation of, 1989-1990
Isochromosomes, 407
Isoenzymes, reference values for, *see website*
Isoflurane, *see website*
Isohemagglutinins, 719
Isolation for infection prevention and control, *see also website*
for pertussis, 946
Isolation techniques, *see website*
Isoleucine, defects in metabolism of, 430-438
Isoniazid (INH), *see also website*
drug interactions with, *see website*
poisoning with, antidote for, 256t-257t
for tuberculosis, 1007, 1008t, *see website*
prophylaxis in HIV infection, 1175t-1176t
Isopropyl alcohol poisoning, 267-268
Isoproterenol for heart failure, *see website*
Isospora belli, 1184, *see also website*
inflammatory bowel disease *versus*, 1298t
treatment of, 1337t
Isotonic fluids, 243
Isotretinoin
for acne, 2325t, 2326
for cancer therapy, *see website*
Isovaleric acidemia, 431-432
Isovolumic hyponatremia, 218
Isoxazole intoxication, *see website*
Isradipine for systemic hypertension, 1645t
Israeli spotted fever, 1043-1044
ITP. *See* Idiopathic thrombocytopenic purpura (ITP)
Itraconazole, *see also website*
for blastomycosis, 1065
for chronic granulomatous disease, 746
for coccidioidomycosis, 1067
for *Cryptococcus neoformans*, 1058
for *Paracoccidioides brasiliensis*, *see website*
for tinea capitis, 2311
IUDs. *See* Intrauterine devices (IUDs)
IUGR. *See* Intrauterine growth restriction (IUGR)
IUPHAR. *See* International Union of Pharmacology (IUPHAR)
IV. *See* Intravenous (IV)
Ivemark syndrome type 2, *see website*
Ivermectin, 1224, *see also website*
IVH. *See* Intraventricular hemorrhage (IVH)
IVIG. *See* Intravenous immunoglobulin (IVIG)
IVRA. *See* Intravenous regional block (IVRA)
Ixodes scapularis, 1026
Iyengar yoga, 371

J
Jacksonian march, 2021
Jackson-Weiss syndrome, 2012t
Jacobsen syndrome, 408t
Jactatio capitis nocturna, *see website*
Jadassohn-Lewandowski syndrome, 2273
JAG1 gene defect, 1383t
Jak3 deficiency, 732
JAK2 mutation, *see website*
Jamaican vomiting syndrome, 529
Janeway lesion, 1623
Jansen metaphyseal dysplasia, 2430
Jansen-type metaphyseal chondrodysplasia, 1923, *see also website*
Jansky-Bielschowsky disease, 2073
Janz syndrome, 2023
Japanese encephalitis, 1145
poliovirus infection *versus*, 1085t
Japanese encephalitis vaccine, 884t, 894, 1146, *see also website*
for travel, 891t, *see also website*
Japanese immunization schedule, 895
Japanese star, potential toxicity of, 272t-273t
Jarisch-Herxheimer reaction, 1021-1022, 1029
JAS. *See* Juvenile ankylosing spondylitis (JAS)
Jatene procedure, 1586, 1587f
Jaundice, *see also website*. See also Cholestasis
breast-feeding, 162
in cystic fibrosis, 1496
as manifestation of liver disease, 1375, 1376t-1377t
neonatal, 603-608, 607t, *see also website*
due to biliary atresia (*See* Biliary atresia (BA))
breast-feeding associated, 607, 607f
clinical manifestations of, 604, 604t
differential diagnosis of, 604-605, 605f, 606t
etiology of, 603-608, 604f, 604t
pathologic, 606-607
physiologic, 605-606, 606f
due to Rh incompatibility, 616
treatment of, 610-612, 610f-611f, 611t-612t
Jaw
disorders of, 1261, *see also website*
hyperparathyroidism-jaw tumor syndrome, 1921
lumpy, *see website*
Jaw-thrust/spine stabilization maneuver, 291f
JC virus, 1157, *see also website*
JDM. *See* Juvenile dermatomyositis (JDM)
JEB. *See* Junctional epidermolysis bullosa (JEB)
Jejunal atresia, 1278-1280, 1279f
Jejunum, short bowel syndrome and, 1315, 1316f
Jequirity bean toxicity, 269t
Jervell and Lange-Nielsen syndrome
cardiac manifestations of, 1531t
genetics of, *see website*
JET. *See* Junctional ectopic tachycardia (JET)
Jeune syndrome, *see website*
JIA. *See* Juvenile idiopathic arthritis (JIA)
Jimsonweed toxicity, 269t, 272t-273t
Jitteriness *versus* seizures, 2034, *see also website*
JMML. *See* Juvenile myelomonocytic leukemia (JMML)
Joint(s)
Clutton, 1017t, 1018
orthopedic problems of (*See* Orthopedic problems)
Joint complications
in cystic fibrosis, 1494
in typhoid fever, 957t
Joint infection. *See also* Septic arthritis
nontuberculous mycobacterial, 1013
tuberculous, 1006
Jones criteria, 921, 921t
Joubert syndrome, 1816, 2006, 2054, *see also website*
JPFS. *See* Juvenile primary fibromyalgia syndrome (JPFS)
JPS. *See* Juvenile polyposis syndrome (JPS)
JRA. *See* Juvenile rheumatoid arthritis (JRA)
J receptors in respiration regulation, *see website*
J tracking, 2355
Judgment in adolescent, 649-651
Jugular vein, venous access in, 292, 295f
Jugular venous pulse, assessment of, 1533
Jumper's knee, 2416, *see also website*
Junctional ectopic tachycardia (JET), 1615, 1616t
Junctional epidermolysis bullosa (JEB), 2244-2246, 2246f
Justice, pediatric ethics and, *see website*
Just right phenomenon, 78
Juvenile ankylosing spondylitis (JAS), 660, *see also website*
Juvenile dermatomyositis (JDM), 846-850, 847f-849f, 848t
arthralgia in, *see website*
cutaneous manifestations of, *see website*
evaluation of, *see website*
Juvenile granulosa cell tumor, ovarian, 1957-1958
Juvenile hallux valgus, 2341, 2341f
Juvenile idiopathic arthritis (JIA), 829-839, 831t
arthralgia in, *see website*
cardiac manifestations of, 1532t
classification of, 829t-830t
clinical manifestations of, 831-835, 832f-834f, 833t, 835t
diagnosis of, 835, *see website*
differential diagnosis of, 835, 836t
epidemiology of, 829
etiology of, 829-831
eye examinations in, 2173t
fever of unknown origin in, 899
laboratory findings in, 835-836, 837f
pathogenesis of, 831, 831f-832f
prognosis for, 838-839, 839f
sports participation and, 2402t-2404t
treatment of, 837-838, 838t
Juvenile myelomonocytic leukemia (JMML), 1739
hematopoietic stem cell transplantation for, 758
Juvenile myoclonic epilepsy, 2023
Juvenile nasopharyngeal angiofibroma, 1432-1433
Juvenile osteochondroses, 2435, 2436t
Juvenile plantar dermatosis, 2250-2251, 2251f
Juvenile polyposis syndrome (JPS), *see website*
Juvenile primary fibromyalgia syndrome (JPFS), 878-879
Juvenile rheumatoid arthritis (JRA), 829
Juvenile xanthogranuloma, *see website*
ocular lesion of, 2156

K
Kala-azar, 1188-1189, 1189f
Kaletra. *See* Lopinavir/ritonavir
KAL gene, 1948
Kallmann syndrome, 1948, 2269
Kanamycin, 1008t, *see also website*
Kangaroo mother care, 559
Kaposiform hemangioendothelioma, 2229
Kaposi's sarcoma (KS)
HIV-related, *see website*
human herpesvirus 8 in, 1121
Kaposi varicelliform eruption, 806
Kartagener triad, *see also website*
congenital heart disease with, 1531t
Karyotyping
in dysmorphology, *see website*
spectral, 396
Kasabach-Merritt syndrome, 1719, 2227t, 2229, *see also website*
Kasai procedure, 1387

Katayama syndrome, 1230-1231
Kava kava for sedation, 271t
Kawasaki disease (KD), 862-867, 868t
  aneurysms in, 1638, *see also website*
  clinical manifestations of, 863-864, 863t, 864f-865f
    cardiac, 1531t
    cutaneous, *see website*
  complications of, 867
  cutaneous manifestations of, *see website*
  diagnosis of, 865, 866f
  differential diagnosis of, 865-866, 866t
  epidemiology of, 863
  etiology of, 862-863
  laboratory findings in, 865
  pathology of, 863
  prognosis for, 867
  sports participation and, 2402t-2404t
  treatment of, 866-867, 867t
Kayser-Fleischer ring, 1391, 1391f
KCNE2 gene, 1425-1426
KCNH2 gene, 1425-1426
KCNJ11 gene, 1995
KCNQ1 gene, 1425-1426
KCNQ2 gene, 2016t
KCNQ3 gene, 2016t
KCNQ4 gene, 2190t
KD. *See* Kawasaki disease (KD); Krabbe disease (KD)
Kearns-Sayre syndrome (KSS), 391t, 2067-2068
  adrenal insufficiency with, 1925t
  cardiac manifestations of, 1531t
  myopathies with, 2131
Keflex. *See* Cephalexin
Keftab. *See* Cephalexin
Kefurox. *See* Cefuroxime
Kefzol. *See* Cefazolin
Kegel exercise, 1849
Kelley-Seegmiller syndrome, *see website*
Keloid, 2273-2274, 2273f
Kenya tick typhus, 1043-1044
Keratinization, disorders of, 2267-2273
Keratinocytes, 2215
Keratitis, 2167t
  Acanthamoeba, *see website*
  dendritic, *see website*
  with ichthyosis and deafness, 2268t
  interstitial, *see website*
  Pseudomonas aeruginosa, 976t
Keratoconjunctivitis
  atopic, 806, 810
  epidemic, 2168
  herpes simplex virus, 1101
  vernal, 810, 810f
Keratoconus, *see also website*
  in allergic disease, 765
  in atopic dermatitis, 806
Keratoderma blennorrhagica, 840, 840f
Keratodermas, palmoplantar, 2272-2273, 2273f
Keratolysis, pitted, 2306
Keratolytic agents for skin disorders, 2216
Keratosis follicularis, 2263, 2263f
Keratosis pilaris, 2261, 2261f
Kerion, 2310, 2311f
Kerner-Morrison syndrome, 1754t
Kernicterus
  dystonia with, 2060t
  in newborn, 608-612
    clinical manifestations of, 608-612, 608t
    incidence and prognosis for, 608
    prevention of, 608-610, 609f
    treatment of, 610-612, 610f-611f, 611t-612t
Kernig sign, 2090
Ketamine
  adolescent abuse of, 675t
  for anesthesia, *see website*
  for intubation, 321t
Keto acid accumulation, in type diabetes mellitus, 1980-1981
Ketoacidosis
  diabetic, 1975
    treatment of, 1979, 1979t
  starvation, 232
Ketoconazole
  adrenal insufficiency due to, 1927
  drug interactions with, *see website*
  for familial male gonadotropin-independent precocious puberty, 1893
Ketogenic diet, 2032
Ketolorac tromethamine, 811t
Ketone
  defects in synthesis of, 461-462
  defects in utilization of, 462
Ketonuria, branched-chain, 528
Ketorolac
  for pain management, 363, 364t
  for vomiting, 1244t
17-Ketosteroid reductase deficiency, 1964-1967
β-Ketothiolase deficiency, 433-434, 434f
Ketotic hyperglycinemia, 436
Ketotic hypoglycemia, 524t, 528
Ketotifen fumarate, 811t
Kidneys
  in acid-base balance, *see website*
  anatomy of, 1778, *see also website*
  Ask-Upmark, 1828
  congenital anomalies of, 1827-1829
  in drug elimination, *see website*
  ectopic, 1828, 1829f
  embryonic development of, *see website*
  glucocorticoids and, *see website*
  glucocorticoids role in, *see website*
  horseshoe, 1828-1829, 1829f
  medullary sponge, 1810
  shock-related dysfunction of, 307t
  sodium regulation in, *see website*
  traumatic injury to, 1864, *see also website*
Kidney biopsy in renal transplantation, *see website*
Kidney disease. *See also* Urologic disorders
  Alport syndrome as, 1782-1783, 1782f
  anemia of, 1653, *see also website*
  due to cancer and its therapy, *see website*
  end-stage, 1825-1826, 1826t
    due to diabetic nephropathy, 1988
  failure to thrive in, 148t
  glomerulonephritis as
    associated with infection, 1783-1786, 1783f-1784f, 1785t
    associated with systemic lupus erythematosus, 1788-1789
    membranoproliferative, 1787-1788
    rapidly progressive, 1789-1790, 1790f, 1790t
  Goodpasture disease as, 1790-1791, 1791f
  hematuria in
    anatomic abnormalities associated with, 1796-1799
    clinical evaluation of, 1778-1781, 1779t-1780t, 1780f
    due to congenital anomalies, 1796
    hematologic diseases causing, 1795-1796
    due to idiopathic hypercalciuria, 1795
    isolated glomerular disease with recurrent gross, 1781-1783
    lower urinary tract causes of, 1799
    membranous glomerulopathy as, 1786-1787
    due to renal vein thrombosis, 1794-1795
    in thin basement membrane disease, 1783
    due to trauma, 1799
    upper urinary tract causes of, 1794-1795
    due to vascular abnormalities, 1794
    due to vigorous exercise, 1799
  hemolytic anemia secondary to, *see website*
  hemolytic-uremic syndrome as, 1791-1794, 1791t-1792t
  Henoch-Schönlein purpura nephritis as, 1789
  HIV-related, 1165-1166
  hypomagnesemia due to, *see website*
Kidney disease *(Continued)*
  immunoglobulin A nephropathy as, 1781-1782, 1781f
  maternal, 545
  neoplasms as, 1757-1760, 1757t-1759t, 1759f
  nephrotic syndrome as, 1801-1807, 1803t, 1806t
    congenital, 1807, 1807t
    etiology of, 1802, 1802f, 1802t
    idiopathic, 1803t, 1804-1806, 1804f
    pathophysiology of, 1802-1804
    secondary, 1806
  polycystic
    autosomal dominant, 1531t, 1798, 1798f, *see website*
    autosomal recessive, 1796-1798, 1797f, 1797t, *see website*
  in premature infants, 559t
  proteinuria and, 1799-1800
    fixed, 1800-1801, 1801t
    orthostatic, 1800
    transient, 1800
  psychopharmacology and, 65
  renal failure as, 1818-1826
    acute, 1818-1822, 1818t-1821t
    chronic, 1822-1825, 1823t
    cortical necrosis in, 1818
  rickets due to, 203, 205-206
  in sickle cell disease, 1668-1669
  toxic nephropathy as, 1816-1818, 1817t
  transplantation for, 1826, *see also website*
  tuberculous, 1006-1007
  tubular
    Bartter syndrome as, 1813-1814, 1813t
    Gitelman syndrome as, 1814
    inherited transport disorders of, 1813-1814
    nephrogenic diabetes insipidus as, 1812
    renal tubular acidosis as, 1808-1811, 1809t, 1811f
    tubulointerstitial nephritis as, 1814-1816, 1815t
  in type I glycogen storage disease, 495
  uromodulin-associated, *see website*
Kidney manifestations
  in multiple organ dysfunction syndrome, 312t
  in mushroom poisoning, *see website*
  in systemic lupus erythematosus, 843t
  in Turner syndrome, 1953
Kidney stones, 1864, *see also website*
  abdominal pain of, 1248t
  as complication of enterocystoplasty, *see website*
Kidney transplantation, 1826, *see also website*
  maternal, *see website*
KID syndrome, 2268t, 2272
Kikuchi-Fujimoto disease, 1724, *see also website*
Kindler syndrome, 2244
Kindling, 2024-2025
Kinetic tremor, simple, 2056-2057
Kingella kingae, 2394
Kininogen, high molecular weight
  deficiency of, 1703
  reference values for, 1698t
Kinky hair disease, 2075
Kinship care, 134, *see also website*
Kinyoun stain, *see website*
Kippel-Feil syndrome, 2379-2380, 2380f
Kissing bugs in trypanosomiasis, 1195
Kiwi allergy, 821, 821t
Klebsiella, neonatal, 632t
  sepsis due to, 635t-636t
Kleeblattschädel deformity, 2012, 2428
Kleihauer-Betke test, 612-613
Klein line, 2364, 2364f
Klein-Waardenburg syndrome, 2239
Klinefelter syndrome, 409t, 410, 1946
  gynecomastia with, 1950-1951
  malignancy susceptibility associated with, *see website*
  tall stature in, *see website*

Klippel-Trenaunay syndrome, 2225-2226, 2226f
Klippel-Trenaunay-Weber syndrome, 2225-2226
Klisic test, 2357, 2358f
Klonopin. *See* Clonazepam
Klotho gene, *see website*
Klumpke paralysis, 573-574
Knee
arthrogryposis involving, *see website*
avulsion fracture of, 2408-2409
centers of ossification appearance in, 29t
musculoskeletal pain syndrome of, 877t
normal coronal alignment of, 2345f
normal development of, 2351-2352
orthopedic disorders of, 2351-2355
discoid lateral meniscus as, 2352, 2352f
idiopathic adolescent anterior knee pain syndrome as, 2354
Osgood-Schlatter disease as, 2354, 2354f
osteochondritis dissecans as, 2353, 2353f
patellar subluxation and dislocation, 2355
popliteal cyst as, 2353
range of motion of, 2352
sports injury to, 2414-2416, 2414t, 2415f
runner's knee as, *see website*
in wrestlers, *see website*
Knee pain, 2351-2352
Kniest dysplasias, 2425
Knock-knees, 2350
Knowledge, cultural, *see website*
Köbberlingg-type lipodystrophy, 2285-2286
Kocher-Debré-Sémèlaigne syndrome, 1898-1899, 2129
Koebner phenomenon
Gianotti-Crosti syndrome, 2266
in psoriasis, 829, 2244
in systemic-onset juvenile idiopathic arthritis, 832-834
KOH. *See* Potassium hydroxide (KOH) preparation
Kohlberg theory, *see website*
Köhler disease, 2340-2341, 2340f
Koilonychia, 2293, 2294f
Koplik spots, 1070, 1070f
Kostmann syndrome, 748t, 750
Krabbe disease (KD), 484t, 490-491, 2071-2072
KS. *See* Kaposi's sarcoma (KS)
KSS. *See* Kearns-Sayre syndrome (KSS)
Kugelberg-Welander disease, 2136
Kupffer cells, *see website*
Kuru, 1177, *see also website*
Kveim-Siltzbach test, 862
Kwashiorkor, 175, 175f-176f, 2329
Kyasanur Forest disease, 1150, 1152
Kyphoscoliosis, 1518, 2278
Kyphosis, 2371-2373, 2372f
congenital, 2372-2373
flexible, 2371
Kytril. *See* Granisetron

L
LA. *See* Latex agglutination (LA) test; Linoleic acid (LA)
LABAs. *See* Long-acting inhaled β-adrenergic agents (LABAs)
Labetalol, 1645t-1646t
Labial agglutination, 1867t-1868t
Labial asymmetry and hypertrophy, *see website*
Labile factor, 1696t
Labor, premature
group B streptococci prophylaxis in, 640f
therapy for, 551t
Laboratory geneticist, 382t
Laboratory test(s), 2466, *see also website*
reference intervals for, *see website*
Labor history in neurologic evaluation, *see website*
Labrum, 2355
Labyrinthitis, 2211, *see also website*
ataxia *versus*, 2054
Lacerations, 340-341
of eyelid, 2184
Lachman test, 2415f
Lacrimal apparatus, examination of, 2150
Lacrimal system disorders, 2165-2166, 2165f
La Crosse encephalitis, 1142-1144
Lactase deficiency, 1306t, 1317
Lactate dehydrogenase (LDL)
in congenital dyserythropoietic anemia, *see website*
in ovarian carcinomas, 1872t
reference values for, *see website*
Lactic acidosis, 232
carbohydrate metabolism defects with, 503-509, 504f-505f, 507t-509t, 508f
in type I glycogen storage disease, 492-493
Lactobacillus rhamnosus
for atopic dermatitis, 805
for functional abdominal pain, 1348t
for infectious diarrhea, 1336-1337
Lactobezoars, 1291
Lactose, resumption of intake following gastroenteritis, 1336
Lactose-free diet, 1348t
Lactose intolerance
abdominal pain of, 1247t
chronic diarrhea with, 1341
secondary, 1317
Lactulose
for constipation in palliative care, 155t-156t
for constipation maintenance therapy, 74t
for fecal disimpaction, 74t
LAD. *See* Leukocyte adhesion deficiency (LAD)
Ladd bands, 1280
Lafora body disease, 2024
Lagophthalmos, 2163
LAIV. *See* Live-attenuated influenza vaccine (LAIV)
Lambert-Eaton myasthenia gravis (LEMS), 2133t
LAMB2 gene, 1807
LAMB syndrome, 2236
Lamellar ichthyosis, 2267-2268, 2268t, 2269f
Lamictal. *See* Lamotrigine
Lamivudine, *see also website*
for hepatitis B, 1399
for HIV infection, 1168t-1171t
Lamotrigine
for mood stabilization, 64t
for neuropathic pain, 368t
for seizures
adverse effects of, 2031t
dosages of, 2030t
LAMP2. *See* Lysosomal-associated membrane protein 2 (LAMP2) deficiency
Lamuvidine, *see website*
Lancefield carbohydrate C, 910
Landau-Kleffner syndrome, 119, 2023-2024
Landouzy-Dejerine disease, 2126
Landry ascending paralysis, 2143
Langer-Giedion syndrome, 408t
Langerhans cell histiocytosis (LCH), 1773-1774
diabetes insipidus with, 1883
seborrheic dermatitis with, 2253-2254
Langerhans cells, *see website*
Language
chronically ill child and, *see website*
cultural skill by health care worker and, *see website*
development of, 115t
age 12-18 months, 31
age 18-24 months, 33
during first 2 years, 27t
during preschool years, 34
development of in foreign-born adoptee, 131
elementary school success and, 37t
expressive, 115-116
receptive, 114-116
speech *versus*, 34
Language disorders
in Asperger's syndrome, 118
in autism and pervasive developmental disorders, 118
classification of, 117, 117t
Language disorders *(Continued)*
due to cleft lip and palate, 1253
clinical manifestations of, 117
comorbid psychiatric disorders, 121
diagnostic evaluation of, 120-121
dysfluency (stuttering, stammering) as, 122, 122t
epidemiology of, 116
etiology of, 116
isolated expressive language disorder as, 118
in mental retardation, 118
motor speech disorders as, 118-119
as neurodevelopmental dysfunction, *see website*
non-causes of, 120
pathogenesis of, 116-117
pragmatic language disorder as, 118
prognosis for, 121
rare causes of, 119
screening for, 119-120, 120t
selective mutism as, 118
specific language impairment as, 117-118
treatment of, 121
due to velopharyngeal dysfunction, 1253
Lansoprazole
CYP2C19 gene in metabolism of, *see website*
for *Helicobacter pylori* gastritis, 1293t
Lanugo, *see website*
Laparoscopic surgery
for appendicitis, 1355
in contralateral inguinal exploration, 1366, 1367f
for inguinal hernia, 1366
Lap belt restraint, 22
Large-for-gestational-age (LGA) infant, *see website*
Larva currens, 1223
Larva migrans
cutaneous, 1220, 1220f, 1220t, *see also website*
ocular, 1227-1229, 1228t
Laryngeal actinomycosis, *see website*
Laryngeal cleft, posterior, 1452
Laryngeal diphtheria, *see website*
Laryngeal edema in hereditary angioedema, 815
Laryngeal foreign body, 1454
Laryngeal swelling, allergic, 1448
Laryngeal *website*s and atresia, 1451, 1451f
Laryngitis
acute infectious, 1447
reflux, 1269
Laryngocele, 1451-1452
Laryngomalacia, 1450, 1450f
Laryngoscopy, 1450, 1450f, *see also website*
Laryngospasm during induction of anesthesia, *see website*
Laryngotracheal stenosis, 1454-1455
Laryngotracheitis, 1446
Laryngotracheobronchitis, 1446-1447, 1446f
Laryngotracheobronchoscopy, 1267
Laryngotracheoesophageal cleft (LTEC), 1263, 1452
Larynx
congenital anomalies of, 1450-1452
neoplasms of, *see website*
papillomatosis of, 1139
tuberculosis of, 1004-1005
Laser photocoagulation for retinopathy of prematurity, 2175-2176
Laser therapy for skin disorders, 2218
LASIK, 2151
Lassa fever, 1151-1152, 1152t
Late adolescence, growth and development during, 654
Late deceleration of fetal heart rate, 543-544, 545t
Latency, 36
Latent syphilis, 1016-1017
Latent tuberculosis infection (LTBI), 996-997
Late-onset central hypoventilation syndrome with hypothalamic dysfunction (LO-CHS), 1521-1522

Lateral epicondylitis, 2411
Lateral meniscus, discoid, 2352, 2352f
Lateral penile curvature, 1857
Lateral pivot shift test, 2415f
Latex agglutination (LA) test, *see website*
Latex allergy
anaphylactic reaction to, 816, 816t
neuropathic bladder and, *see website*
Latino population
cultural values associated with, *see website*
death rates for, 3t-4t
disease beliefs or practices of, *see website*
empacho and, *see website*
as special needs population, 7
Latrodectus antivenin, 258t
Laundry, infection protection and control and, *see website*
Lavage
Bronchoalveolar, *see also website*
in aspiration syndromes, 1472t
for cystic fibrosis, 1493
gastric, for poisoning, 255-257
Lavandula for sedation, 271t
Lavender for sedation, 271t
Laxatives, habits regarding in eating disorders, 92t
Lazarus sign, *see website*
LBW. *See* Low birthweight (LBW)
LBWC. *See* Limb-body wall complex (LBWC)
LCA. *See* Leber congenital retinal amaurosis (LCA)
LCAT. *See* Lecithin-cholesterol acyltransferase (LCAT) deficiency
LCH. *See* Langerhans cell histiocytosis (LCH)
LCHAD. *See* Long-chain 3-hydroxyacyl CoA dehydrogenase (LCHAD) deficiency
LCL. *See* Localized cutaneous leishmaniasis (LCL)
LCMV. *See* Lymphocytic choriomeningitis virus (LCMV)
LCPD. *See* Legg-Calvé-Perthes disease (LCPD)
LCT gene, 1317
l2,3-Dimercaptosuccinic acid (DMSA), 2453, 2453t
LDL. *See* Low-density lipoproteins (LDL)
Lead, reference values for, *see website*
Lead exposure/poisoning, *see website*
abdominal pain of, 1247t
δ-aminolevulinic acid dehydratase deficiency due to, *see website*
antidote for, 256t-257t
clinical effects of, 2450
clinical symptoms of, 2450-2451
diagnosis of, 2451-2452, 2451t-2452t
intellectual disability and, 127t
metabolism in, 2449-2450
public health history of, 2448-2449
sources of, 2449, 2449t
treatment of, 2452-2453, 2453t
Lead mobilization test, 2451
Lead pipe, *see website*
LEAN Methodology, *see website*
Learning disorders, *see also website*. *See also* Neurodevelopmental dysfunction
attention deficit/hyperactivity disorder as, 108
clinical manifestations of, 108-109
diagnosis and differential diagnosis of, 109-110, 109t
epidemiology of, 108
etiology of, 108
pathogenesis of, *see website*
prevention of, 112
prognosis for, 112
treatment of, 110-112, 111t, 112f
dyslexia as, 112-114, 113f
intellectual disability as, 122-129
clinical manifestations of, 124-125, 125t
complications of, 127
diagnosis of, 122-124, 123t
diagnostic psychologic testing in, 126-127
differential diagnosis of, 125-126
Learning disorders *(Continued)*
epidemiology of, 124
etiology of, 123t, 124
laboratory findings in, 125, 126f, 127t
pathology and pathogenesis of, *see website*
prevention of, 127-128
prognosis for, 129, 129t
supportive care and management of, 128-129
treatment of, 128
language and communication disorders as, 114-122
in Asperger's syndrome, 118
in autism and pervasive developmental disorders, 118
classification of, 117, 117t
clinical manifestations of, 117
comorbid psychiatric disorders, 121
diagnostic evaluation of, 120-121
dysfluency (stuttering, stammering) as, 122, 122t
epidemiology of, 116
etiology of, 116
isolated expressive language disorder as, 118
in mental retardation, 118
motor speech disorders as, 118-119
non-causes of, 120
pathogenesis of, 116-117
pragmatic language disorder as, 118
prognosis for, 121
rare causes of, 119
screening for, 119-120, 120t
selective mutism as, 118
specific language impairment as, 117-118
treatment of, 121
neurodevelopmental dysfunction as, 108, *see also website*
Leber congenital retinal amaurosis (LCA), 2177
Leber hereditary optic neuropathy (LHON), 391t, 2067, *see also website*
Lecithin, amniotic fluid, 548
Lecithin-cholesterol acyltransferase (LCAT) deficiency, 477
Lecithin-sphingomyelin (L:S) ratio, 548-549
Lectin pathway of complement system, *see website*
deficiencies of, 754t
Leflunomide, 838t, *see also website*
Left shift, *see also website*
in appendicitis, 1351
Left-to-right-shunt
in adults, 1605-1606
cardiac lesions of, 1551-1561
evaluation of, 1549-1550
in neonatal circulation, *see website*
Left ventricular assist device (LVAD), *see website*
Left ventricular diverticulum, 1599-1600
Left ventricular hypertrophy
electrocardiographic assessment of, 1539-1540, 1540f
systemic hypertension with, 1642
Left ventricular noncompaction (LVNC), 1629t-1630t, 1633-1634, 1634f
Leg. *See* Lower extremity(ies)
Legal issues in adolescent health care, 664-665, *see also website*
Legg-Calvé-Perthes disease (LCPD), 2361, 2362f, 2436t
Legionella, 982, *see also website*
in infective endocarditis, 1624t
in pneumonia, 1475t
Legislation
foster and kinship care, *see website*
registration, Evaluation, Authorization, and restriction to Chemicals (REACH), *see website*
Leg-length discrepancy (LLD), 2351, *see also website*
in posteromedial tibial bowing, 2351
Legume allergy, 823t
Leigh disease, 391t, 506-509, 2067, 2132
Leiomyoma, 1873, *see also website*
Leiomyosarcoma, 1762t, 1873
risk factors for, 1727t
Leishmaniasis, 1186-1190
diagnosis of, 1189
differential diagnosis of, 1189
etiology of, 1186-1187
laboratory findings in, 1189
mucosal, 1188
pathogenesis of, 1187-1189, 1188f
pathology of, 1187
predisposition to due to immunodeficiency, 716t
prevention of, 1190
treatment of, 1189-1190, *see website*
visceral, 1188-1189
Leisure and recreational activities in intellectual disability management, 128-129
Lemierre syndrome, 1439, 1442, 1442f, *see website*
Lemon balm for sedation, 271t
LEMS. *See* Lambert-Eaton myasthenia gravis (LEMS)
Lenalidomide, *see website*
Length, percentile curves for, *see website*
Lennox-Gastaut syndrome, 2022-2024
treatment of, 2027
Lens
development of, *see website*
disorders of, 2169-2172, 2170f-2172f, 2170t
Lente insulin, 1976, 1977f
Lenticonus, 2172
Lentigines, 2236-2237, 2236f
Lentiginosis profusa, 2236
Lentiginous nevus
speckled, 2233, 2233f
zosteriform, 2233
LEOPARD syndrome
cardiac manifestations of, 1531t
cutaneous manifestations of, 2236, 2236f
Lepra reaction, *see website*
Leprechaunism, 1995-1996
LEPRE1 gene, 2439
Lepromatous leprosy (LL), *see website*
Leprosy, 1011, *see also website*
Leprosy patient, *see website*
Leptin deficiency, obesity due to, 182t
Leptin receptor gene deficiency, obesity due to, 182t
Leptospira, 1023-1025, 1024f
Leptospira biflexa, 1023
Leptospira interrogans, 1023
Leptospiruric leptospirosis, 1024
Leri-Weil dyschondrosteosis, 388-389
LES. *See* Lower esophageal sphincter (LES)
Lesbian, 658
Lesch-Nyhan disease (LND), 2057t, *see also website*
Lethal neonatal dwarfism, *see website*
Lethal spondyloepiphyseal dysplasias, 2424, 2424f
Lethal toxic encephalopathy, 960
Lethargy in newborn, *see website*
Letrozole, 1893
Letterer-Siwe disease, 1773-1774
Leucine, defects in metabolism of, 430-438
Leucine-sensitive hypoglycemia, 525
Leukemia, 1732-1739
acute lymphocytic, 1732-1737
arthralgia and, *see website*
cellular classification of, 1732-1733, 1733f, 1733t
clinical manifestations of, 1733-1734
differential diagnosis of, 1734
epidemiology of, 1732
etiology of, 1732, 1732t
hematopoietic stem cell transplantation for, 757, 758f
incidence and survival rates for, 1726t
prognosis for, 1736-1737
risk factors for, 1727t

Leukemia *(Continued)*
secondary, due to radiation therapy, *see website*
supportive care for, 1736
treatment of, 1734-1736, 1735f-1736f
acute myelogenous, 1737-1738, 1737t-1738t
acute myeloid, 748t, 1737-1738, 1737t-1738t
hematopoietic stem cell transplantation for, 757-758
incidence and survival rates for, 1726t
risk factors for, 1727t
adult T-cell, *see website*
chromosomal translocation in, *see website*
chronic myelogenous, 748t, 1738-1739
hematopoietic stem cell transplantation for, 758
in Down syndrome, 1738, 1738f
environmental carcinogens and, *see website*
infant, 1739
juvenile idiopathic arthritis *versus*, 835
juvenile myelomonocytic, 1739
hematopoietic stem cell transplantation for, 758
of temporal bone, *see website*
treatment of, *see website*
work-up of, 1731t
Leukemia cutis, 1739
Leukemoid reaction, *see website*
Leukocoria, 1768-1769, 1768f, 2157, 2157f
Leukocystoclastic vasculitis, 868t, 876
due to cat-scratch disease, 985
Leukocyte adhesion deficiency (LAD), 741-744, 742t, *see also website*
Leukocyte differential
in immunodeficiency screening, 718t
reference values for, *see website*
Leukocytes
in chronic diarrhea, 1344t
in CNS infection, 2088t
fetal, *see website*
polymorphonuclear, 2220
Leukocytosis, 752
in eosinophilic pustular folliculitis, 2220
in Epstein-Barr virus infection, 1113
in hantavirus pulmonary syndrome, *see website*
monocytosis as, *see website*
neutrophilia as, *see website*
as oncologic emergency, *see website*
in pertussis, 945
Leukodystrophy, 2075, 2140
adrenal insufficiency with, 1924, 1925t
globoid cell, 490-491, 2071-2072
metachromatic, 484t, 490
Leukodystrophy, metachromatic, 2072
Leukokoria in newborn, 534
Leukomalacia, periventricular, 566-568
cerebral palsy and, 2061-2063
optic nerve hypoplasia with, *see website*
Leukonychia, 2294
Leukopenia, 746-752, 747t
due to ehrlichiosis, 1049
HIV-related, 1166
infections with, *see website*
in kala-azar, 1189
neutropenia as, 746-750
in varicella-zoster virus, 1108
Leukoplakia, oral hairy, 2299
Leukorrhea, physiologic, 1866
Leukotriene-modifying agents (LTRAs)
for allergic disease, 772
for asthma, 794t, 795-796
for urticaria and angioedema, 815t
Leukovorin, 1215
Leuprolide
for endometriosis, 690-691
for premenstrual dysphoric disorder, 692t
Leuprolide acetate, 1889
Levalbuterol for asthma, 796, 797t-798t
Levamisole, 1805
Levatiracetam, 2044t
Level of consciousness (LOC) in hypoxic-ischemic encephalopathy, 571t
Levetiracetam
adverse effects of, 2031t
dosages of, 2030t
Levocabastine hydrochloride, 811t
Levocardia, 1596
Levocetirizine, 777t-778t, 779
Levodopa, 2064
Levofloxacin, *see also website*
for *Chlamydia trachomatis*, 1036
for tuberculosis, 1008t
Levorphanol for neuropathic pain, 368t
Levothyroxine for hypothyroidism
acquired, 1903
congenital, 1900
Lewisite, in terrorism, *see website*
Lexapro. *See* Escitalopram
Lexiva. *See* Fosamprenavir
Leydig cell aplasia, 1964
Leydig cell tumor, testicular, *see website*
LGA. *See* Large-for-gestational-age (LGA) infant
LGAs. *See* Low-grade astrocytomas (LGAs)
LGI1 gene, 2016t
L-glyceric aciduria, 441
LGMD. *See* Limb-girdle muscular dystrophy (LGMD)
LH. *See* Luteinizing hormone (LH)
Lhermitte's sign, *see website*
LHGCR gene, *see website*
LHON. *See* Leber hereditary optic neuropathy (LHON)
LHRH. *See* Luteinizing hormone-releasing hormone (LHRH)
LHX3 gene, 1876t, 1877
LHX4 gene, 1876t, 1877-1878
Lice. *See* Pediculosis
Licensing, child care, *see website*
Lichenification
in atopic dermatitis, 802, 803f
examination of, *see website*
Lichen nitidus, 2263-2264, 2264f
Lichenoid eruption in graft *versus* host disease, *see website*
Lichen planus, 2264-2265, 2265f
Lichen sclerosus, 1867t-1868t, 1868f, 2275, 2275f
vaginal bleeding due to, 1869
Lichen simplex chronicus, 2252, 2253f
Lichen spinulosus, 2261-2262
Lichen striatus, 2264
Licorice for asthma, 271t
Liddle syndrome, 223-224, 236, 1814
Lidocaine
for arrhythmias, 1611t-1612t
for pediatric resuscitation and arrhythmias, 294t
in rapid sequence intubation, 287t
Lid(s)
abnormalities of, 2163-2165, 2164f
due to trauma, 2184
examination of, 2150
Life course-limited offenders, 669
Lifestyle
polycystic ovary syndrome and, *see website*
type 2 diabetes mellitus and, 1991
Life-sustaining medical treatment (LSMT), *see website*
Li-Fraumeni syndrome, 1747t, 1750-1751, 1763, *see also website*
Lightning burns, 356
Light reflex, pupillary, 2157, 2157f
brain death and, *see website*
in newborn, 534
in retinoblastoma, 1768-1769, 1768f
as sign of cancer, 1730f
Light sedation, *see website*
Light sensitivity in migraine, 2041
Likert Scale, 363t
Lily of the valley toxicity, 269t
Limb
deformities of, evaluation of, 2346
normal development of, 2344, 2345f-2346f
Limb-body wall complex (LBWC), 2221
Limb-girdle muscular dystrophy (LGMD), 2113t, 2126, 2126t
Limb lengthening for leg-length discrepancy, *see website*
Limit dextrinosis, 496-497, 496f
Limp
assessment of, 2332, 2334t
of Legg-Calvé-Perthes disease, 2361
Lincosamides, *see website*
Lindane toxicity, 251t
Linear immunoglobulin A dermatosis, 2249, 2249f
immunofluorescence of, *see website*
Linear nevus syndrome, 2052
Linear nondose threshold (LNT), *see website*
Linear scleroderma, 850, 851f
Linens, infection protection and control and, *see website*
Line sepsis, 910
Linezolid, *see also website*
for cystic fibrosis lung infection, 1492t
for neonatal infection, 645t
for *Staphylococcus aureus*, 907t
for vancomycin-resistant *Enterococcus*, *see website*
Lingual frenulum, short, *see website*
Linguistic development
age 12-18 months, 31
age 18-24 months, 33
during preschool years, 34
Linkage testing, 376, 377t, *see also website*
Linoleic acid (LA), *see also website*
deficiency, cutaneous manifestations of, 2329
LIP. *See* Lymphocytic interstitial pneumonia (LIP)
Lip(s)
assessment of in allergic disease, 765
cleft, 1252-1253, 1252f
dental problems associated with, 1251t
congenital pits of, *see website*
Lipase, *see also website*
deficiency of, 1369-1370
diarrhea due to, 1306t
hepatic, 473t, 477
in pancreatitis, 1371
reference values for, *see website*
replacement of, 1370
Lipids
atherogenesis and, 470-471, 471f
cardiovascular disease and, 470
metabolism and transport of, 471-473, *see also website*
storage disorders of, 484t
Lipid metabolism, defects in, 456-492
of lipoprotein metabolism and transport, 470-482, 471f-474f, 472t-473t, 476f, 477t-479t, 480f, 481t-482t
liver effects of, 1389t
lysosomal storage disorders as, 482-491, 483f, 484t-485t, 486f-487f, 489f, 491f
of mitochondrial fatty acid β-oxidation, 456-492, 457t, 458f-459f
mucolipidoses as, 491-492
of very long chain fatty acids, 462-470, 462t-464t, 464f-465f, 466t, 469f
Lipid myopathies, 2132, *see also website*
Lipidoses, 482-491, 483f, 486f
cholesterol ester storage disease as, 491
clinical findings in, 484t
Fabry disease as, 488-489, 489f
Farber disease as, 491, 491f
fucosidosis as, 489-490
Gaucher disease as, 487-488, 487f
GM_1 gangliosidosis as, 483-491
GM_2 gangliosidosis as, 484-487
Krabbe disease as, 490-491
metachromatic leukodystrophy as, 490

Lipidoses *(Continued)*
multiple sulfatase deficiency as, 490
Neimann-Pick disease as, 488
Schindler disease as, 490
symptoms of, 485t
Wolman disease as, 491
Lipoatrophic diabetes, 1995
Lipodystrophy, 2285-2286
juvenile dermatomyositis, 847
Lipofuscinoses, neuronal ceroid, 2073, 2073t
Lipoid adrenal hyperplasia, 1937, 1964
Lipoid adrenal hypoplasia, 1925t
Lipoid proteinosis, 2276-2277
Lipoma, *see website*
Lipophosphoglycan (LPG), 1186-1187
Lipoprotein a, 1708
Lipoproteins
atherogenesis and, 470-471, 471f
cardiovascular disease and, 470
characteristics of, 472t
disorders of, 473-482, 473f-474f, 473t, 475t, 476f, 477t-479t, 480f
blood cholesterol screening for, 479-480
risk assessment and treatment of, 480f, 481-482, 481t-482t
high-density, 471, 472f, 472t, 479t
disorders of metabolism of, 477
laboratory testing of in obesity, 185t
reverse cholesterol transport and, 473
low-density, 471-473, 472f, 472t, 479t
laboratory testing of in obesity, 185t
metabolism and transport of, 471-473, 472f
patterns of in children and adolescents, 479, 479t
Liposarcoma, 1762t
Liposomal amphotericin B, *see also website*
for candidiasis, 1054t, 1056t
for *Leishmania* infection, *see website*
for leishmaniasis, 1190
5-Lipoxygenase inhibitor for asthma, 794t
Lisch nodules, 2156
in neurofibromatosis, 2046-2047, 2047f
Lisinopril for systemic hypertension, 1645t
Lispro insulin analogs, 1976, 1977f
Lissencephaly, 2003, 2004f, *see also website*
Listeria monocytogenes, 929, *see also website*
in bacterial meningitis, 2091
gastroenteritis due to, 1324t-1325t
maternal
breast-feeding and, 540t
fetal and neonatal effects of, *see website*
neonatal, 632t
sepsis due to, 636t
Listeriolysin, *see website*
Lithiasis
gallbladder, *see website*
urinary, 1864, *see also website*
abdominal pain of, 1248t
Lithium
goiter due to, 1908
for mood stabilization, 63, 64t
Lithobid. *See* Lithium
Lithotripsy, *see website*
Live-attenuated influenza vaccine (LAIV), 883-884, 884t
Liver
birth injury to, 578
enlarged, sports participation and, 2402t-2404t
excretory function of, *see website*
hepatocytic function in, *see website*
insulin level effects on, 1975t
metabolic functions of, *see website*
morphogenesis of, 1374, *see also website*
newborn assessment of, 535
porphyria cutanea tarda and, *see website*
shock-related dysfunction of, 307t
transport of lipids from, 471-473
Liver biopsy, 1381
fetal, 543t
in neonatal cholestasis, 1385-1386
Liver disease
abscess as, 1404-1405, 1404f-1405f
amebic, 1179
autoimmune hepatitis as, 1408-1410, 1408t, 1410f
biliary atresia as, 1385-1387, 1386f-1387f
due to cancer and its therapy, *see website*
cholestasis as, 1381-1388, 1381f
evaluation of, 1382, 1382t
intrahepatic, 1382-1384, 1383t-1384t
management of, 1387-1388, 1387t
mechanism of, 1381-1382
in older child, 1388
prognosis for, 1388
types of, 1382t
chronic diarrhea with, 1341
cystic, 1415, *see also website*
drug- and toxin-induced injury as, 1410-1412, 1412t
in erythropoietic protoporphyria, *see website*
evaluation of, 1379, 1380f
fulminant hepatic failure as, 1412-1415, 1414t
general anesthesia and, *see website*
glycogen storage disease as, 492-499
hemolytic anemia secondary to, *see website*
hemorrhagic disorders due to, 1712, *see also website*
due to intestinal failure, *see website*
liver transplantation for, 1415, *see also website*
malabsorption due to, 1318
manifestations of, 1374-1381, 1375t-1377t
hepatomegaly as, 1375t
metabolic, 1388-1393, 1389t
α-antitrypsin deficiency, 1393
Indian childhood cirrhosis, 1392
inherited deficient conjugation of bilirubin as, 1389-1390
neonatal iron storage disease as, 1393
Wilson disease, 1391, 1391f
mitochondrial hepatopathies as, 1405-1408, 1406t-1407t
neoplastic, 1771-1772, 1771f
in porphyria cutanea tarda, *see website*
portal hypertension and varices as, 1415, *see also website*
propylthiouracil and, 1911-1912
psychopharmacology and, 64-65
pulmonary manifestations of, *see website*
with systemic disorders, 1405, *see also website*
viral hepatitis as, 1393-1404, 1393t
approach to, 1403-1404, 1403f
biochemical profiles in, 1394-1395
causes and differential diagnosis of, 1394, 1394t
due to hepatitis A virus, 1395-1396, 1395f, 1396t
due to hepatitis B virus, 1397-1400, 1398f, 1399t
due to hepatitis C virus, 1400-1402, 1400f
due to hepatitis D virus, 1402
due to hepatitis E virus, 1402-1403
pathogenesis of, 1394
Liver failure, 1412-1415, 1414t
with hepatitis A, 1395-1396
with hepatitis B, 1397-1398
Liver flukes, *see website*
Liver-kidney microsomal (LKM) antibody, 1409
Liver phosphorylase deficiency, 497
hypoglycemia in, 528
Liver phosphorylase kinase deficiency, 498
Liver transplantation, 1415, *see also website*
for acute liver failure, 1414
for type I glycogen storage disease, 495
Liver tumor
precocious puberty due to, 1891
work-up of, 1731t
Livostin. *See* Levocabastine hydrochloride
LKM. *See* Liver-kidney microsomal (LKM) antibody
LL. *See* Lepromatous leprosy (LL); Lymphoblastic lymphoma (LL)
LLD. *See* Leg-length discrepancy (LLD)
L/L genotype, 1426
LMNA gene mutations, *see website*
LMW. *See* Low molecular weight (LMW) heparin
LMX1B gene, 1803t, 2431, *see website*
LND. *See* Lesch-Nyhan disease (LND)
LNT. *See* Linear nondose threshold (LNT)
Loading dose for antiepileptics, 2029-2031
Loa loa, 1225-1226, 1226f, *see website*
Lobar nephronia, acute, 1830, 1830f
Lobar panniculitis, 2282-2283
Lobelia inflata, potential toxicity of, 272t-273t
Lobular capillary hemangioma, 2229
Local anesthesia
adverse reaction to, 827
definition of, *see website*
for pain management, 367-368, 367t-368t
toxicity, neonatal seizures due to, 2034, 2036
Localized cutaneous leishmaniasis (LCL), 1187-1188
Location of pain, 2332t
LO-CHS. *See* Late-onset central hypoventilation syndrome with hypothalamic dysfunction (LO-CHS)
Loci of developmental disorders of muscle, 2113-2114, 2113t
Lockjaw, 991
Locus heterogeneity, *see website*
Lodoquinol, *see website*
Lodoxamide tromethamine
for allergic conjunctivitis, 811t
for allergic disease, 772
Loeffler syndrome, 1223
Loeys-Dietz syndrome, 2444t, *see also website*
Löffler syndrome, *see website*
Logical thinking in adolescent, 649-651
Logistic access in chronic illness, *see website*
Loiasis, 1225-1226, 1226f
Lomotil toxicity, 251t
Lone star tick, 1048-1049
Long-acting inhaled β-adrenergic agents (LABAs)
for allergic disease, 770
for asthma, 791-792, 794-795
Long bones, *see also website*
osteomyelitis in, 2395
Long-chain fatty acid transporter deficiency, 457t
Long-chain 3-hydroxyacyl CoA dehydrogenase (LCHAD) deficiency, 457t, 460
Longdan xieganwan, potential toxicity of, 272t-273t
Longitudinal deficiency
radial, 2384, 2384t
tibial, 2351
Longitudinal vaginal septa, *see website*
Long Q-T syndrome (LQTS), 1616-1618, 1617t
electrocardiogram of, 1540f
genetics of, *see website*
genotype-phenotype correlation in, *see website*
seizures *versus*, *see website*
sports participation and, 2402t-2404t
sudden death due to, 1620, 1620f
sudden infant death syndrome and, 1425-1426, 1426f
Long terminal repeats, 1157
Long-term memory (LTM), *see website*
Long-term survivors (LTSs), HIV, 1161
Long-term video electroencephalography monitoring, *see website*
Loop diuretics, metabolic alkalosis due to, 236
Looping, cardiac, 1527, *see also website*
Loop of Henle, *see website*
Loose folds of skin, 2220
Loperamide, 1337, *see also website*
Lopinavir/ritonavir for HIV infection, 1168t-1171t
Lorabid. *See* Loracarbef
Loracarbef, *see website*

Loratadine
for allergic rhinitis, 777t-778t, 779
for urticaria and angioedema, 815t
Lorazepam
for anxiety
in burn injury, 355
in palliative care, 155t-156t
for cyclic vomiting syndrome, 1244t
for depression and anxiety symptoms, 63t
for hypoxic-ischemic encephalopathy, 571
for intubation, 321t
for nausea in palliative care, 155t-156t
for pain management in palliative care, 155t-156t
for seizures
dosages of, 2030t
neonatal, 2037
in palliative care, 155t-156t
for sleep disturbance/insomnia in palliative care, 155t-156t
for status epilepticus, 2038, 2039t
Lorenzo's oil therapy, 469
Losartan for systemic hypertension, 1645t
Loss, 45, *see also website*
Lotions, 2216
Louse-borne disease
relapsing fever, *see website*
typhus, 1039t-1040t
epidemic, 1047-1048
Lovenorgestrel, 698
Low back sports injury, 2412-2413
Low birthweight (LBW), *see website*. *See also* Prematurity/premature infant
dental problems associated with, 1251t
incidence of, 555
prenatal nutrition and, *see website*
rates of, *see website*
spectrum of disease in, 558, 559t
type 2 diabetes mellitus and, 1990
Low-density lipoproteins (LDL), 471-473, 472f, 472t, 479t
laboratory testing of in obesity, 185t
Lower body segment, body proportions and, *see website*
Lower esophageal sphincter (LES), *see website*
dysmotility of, 1264-1265, 1265f
gastroesophageal reflux disease and, 1266
Lower extremity(ies)
arthrogryposis involving, *see website*
assessment of, 2333f
fractures of, 2392, 2393t
as delivery room emergency, 579
growth and development of, *see website*
musculoskeletal pain syndrome of, 877t
septic arthritis in, 2399
sports injury to, 2416-2417
venous access in, 295f
Lower extremity nerve block, 372
Lower inflection point, 323-324
Lower respiratory tract infection (LRTI)
anaerobic, *see website*
human metapneumovirus, 1130-1131
respiratory culture in, *see website*
wheezing and, 1456-1457
Lowe syndrome, 1809-1810
Low-grade astrocytomas (LGAs), 1748-1750
Low-grade squamous intraepithelial lesion (LSIL), 1137-1138, 1138t
Low molecular weight (LMW) heparin, 1710t, 1711
for pulmonary embolism, 1502
LP. *See* Lumbar puncture (LP)
LPG. *See* Lipophosphoglycan (LPG)
LPI. *See* Lysinuric protein intolerance (LPI)
LQTS. *See* Long Q-T syndrome (LQTS)
LRTI. *See* Lower respiratory tract infection (LRTI)
LSD. *See* Lysergic acid diethylamide (LSD)
LSIL. *See* Low-grade squamous intraepithelial lesion (LSIL)
LSMT. *See* Life-sustaining medical treatment (LSMT)
L:S ratio. *See* Lecithin-sphingomyelin (L:S) ratio
LTBI. *See* Latent tuberculosis infection (LTBI)
LTEC. *See* laryngotracheoesophageal cleft (LTEC)
l-TGA. *See* L-transposition of the great arteries (l-TGA)
LTM. *See* Long-term memory (LTM)
L-transposition of the great arteries (l-TGA), 1587-1588, 1588f
LTRAs. *See* Leukotriene-modifying agents (LTRAs)
Lubricants for skin disorders, 2216
Lugol iodine stain, *see website*
Lujan syndrome, *see website*
Lumbar anesthesia, 373
Lumbar disk herniation, strain, and contusion, 2412
Lumbar plexus block, 372
Lumbar puncture (LP)
in bacterial meningitis, 2090-2091
in febrile seizure, 2018, 2036
in neurologic evaluation, *see website*
Lumbar sympathetic block, 373
Lumefantrine, 1203t-1205t, *see also website*
Lumpy-bumpy deposits, glomerular, *see website*
in acute poststreptococcal glomerulonephritis, 1783, 1783f
Lumpy jaw, *see website*
Lungs. *See also* Respiratory system
in acid-base balance, *see website*
auscultation of in acutely ill child evaluation, 276
immune response of, *see website*
iron, 1524
maintenance water and, 244t
skeletal diseases influencing function of, 1516-1519
unilateral hyperlucent, 1461
vasculature of, *see website*
ventilator-induced injury to, 329
work of breathing in, *see website*
Lung biopsy, *see website*
Lung capacities, *see website*
Lung compliance, *see website*
Lung disease. *See also* Respiratory disease
abscess as, 1480-1481
due to anaerobes, *see website*
clinical manifestations of, 1480
diagnosis of, 1480, 1480f-1481f
pathology and pathogenesis of, 1480
prognosis for, 1481
treatment of, 1480-1481
due to cancer and its therapy, *see website*
coccidioidomycosis, 1065-1068
congenital, 1463-1467
agenesis and aplasia as, 1463
bronchobiliary fistula as, 1467
bronchogenic cysts as, 1466, 1466f
cystic adenomatoid malformation as, 1464, 1465f
hernia as, 1467
hypoplasia as, 1464
lymphangiectasia as, 1467
sequestration as, 1465, 1466f
eosinophilic lung disease as, 1474, *see also website*
failure to thrive in, 148t
interstitial, 1497, *see also website*
nontuberculous mycobacterial infection of, 1012t, 1013-1015, 1014f
obesity with, 184t
parenchymal
emergency airway management in, 284
hypersensitivity to inhaled materials as, 1473, *see also website*
paraquat lung as, 1474, *see also website*
silo filler disease as, 1474, *see also website*
respiratory acidosis due to, 239, 239t
Lung disease *(Continued)*
respiratory alkalosis and, 241
in sickle cell disease, 1667-1668, 1668f, 1668t
Lung flukes, *see website*
Lung infiltrates
in acute lung injury, 317f
in amyloidosis, 861, 861f
in eosinophilic lung disease, 1474
recurrent or persistent, *see website*
Lung injury
acute, 316, 317f, 317t
ventilator-induced, 329
Lung percussion, *see website*
Lung sounds
in acutely ill child evaluation, 276
in assessment of respiratory pathology, *see website*
Lung tap, *see website*
Lung transplantation, 1638, *see also website*
for cystic fibrosis, 1494
Lung volumes, *see website*
Lungworm, rat, 1226-1227
Luphocin. *See* Vancomycin
Lupus
drug-induced, 843-844, 844t, *see website*
neonatal, 845-846, 845f
cutaneous manifestations of, *see website*
Lupus anticoagulant, 844
fetal therapy for, 551t
Lupus erythematosus, discoid, *see website*
Lupus erythematosus (LE)
arthralgia in, *see website*
cutaneous manifestations of, *see website*
immunofluorescence of, *see website*
maternal, *see website*
neonatal, 845-846, 845f
systemic (*See* Systemic lupus erythematosus (SLE))
Lupus erythematosus panniculitis, 2283, 2283f
Lupus erythematosus profundus, 2283, 2283f
Lupus nephritis, 1788-1789
Lupus vulgaris, 2307
Luteinizing hormone (LH), *see also website*
in amenorrhea, 686
in hypogonadism, 1945-1946
in polycystic ovary syndrome, *see website*
in precocious puberty, 1888
in puberty, 1886
in testicular function, *see website*
Luteinizing hormone-releasing hormone (LHRH), 1860
Lutz-Splendore-Almeida disease, 1068
LVAD. *See* Left ventricular assist device (LVAD)
LVNC. *See* Left ventricular noncompaction (LVNC)
17,20 Lyase deficiency, 1964
Lying, 99
Lyme disease, 1025-1029
clinical manifestations of, 1026-1028, 1026t, 1027f
cardiac, 1531t
congenital, 1027
diagnosis of, 1028
epidemiology of, 1025, 1025f
etiology of, 1025
fetal therapy for, 551t
juvenile idiopathic arthritis *versus*, 835
pathology and pathogenesis of, 1026
prevention of, 1029
prognosis for, 1029
serology of, 1028, *see website*
transmission of, 1025-1026
treatment of, 1028-1029, 1028t
Lymphadenitis
histiocytic necrotizing, 1724, *see also website*
impetigo in, 916-917
nontuberculous mycobacterial, 1012-1013, 1012f-1013f, 1012t, 1015
tuberculous, 1002, 1005

Lymphadenopathy, 1724, *see also website*
with cat-scratch disease, 984, 984f
with chancroid, *see website*
Corynebacterium diphtheriae, *see website*
Epstein-Barr virus, 1112
as sign of childhood cancers, 1730f
sinus histiocytosis massive, 1724, *see also website*
with tinea capitis, 2310, 2310f
Lymphangiectasia, 1724
congenital pulmonary, 1467
intestinal, 1311
Lymphangioma, 1724, 1772, *see also website*
Lymphangioma circumscriptum, *see website*
Lymphangiomatosis, 1724
Lymphangitis, *see website*
Lymphatic compartment, pulmonary edema and, 1468
Lymphatic dysplasia, 1724
Lymphatic filariasis, 1224-1225, 1225f
Lymphatic system
abnormalities of, 1724, *see also website*
anatomy and function of, 1723, *see also website*
in total body water regulation, *see website*
Lymphedema, *see also website*
familial, 2224t
Lymphedema praecox, *see website*
Lymph node disease
Cryptococcus neoformans infection as, 1057
tuberculous, 998, 1005, 1005f
Lymph node syndrome, mucocutaneous, 862-867
Lymphoblastic lymphoma (LL), 1743, 1744t
Lymphocyte blastogenesis to *Toxoplasmosis* antigens, 1214
Lymphocyte count
in adenosine deaminase deficiency, 732
normal values for, 719f
in roseola, 1119
in severe combined immunodeficiency, 731
whole-body irradiation and, *see website*
Lymphocytes, *see also website*. *See also* B cells; Natural killer (NK) cells; T cells
cytokines in regulation of, *see website*
in pertussis, 945
reference values for, *see website*
Lymphocytic choriomeningitis virus (LCMV), 1153, *see also website*
maternal, *see website*
Lymphocytic interstitial pneumonia (LIP), 1165
Lymphocytic leukemia. *See* Acute lymphocytic leukemia (ALL)
Lymphocytic thyroiditis, 1903-1905
type 1 diabetes mellitus with, 1996
Lymphocytosis, *see website*
Lymphogranuloma venereum (LGV), 1038
Lymphohematogenous (disseminated) tuberculosis, 1004
Lymphohistiocytosis, 1775-1776, 1775t
hemophagocytic, 744, 1774-1776, 1776t
Lymphoid hypoplasia in X-linked agammaglobulinemia, 724
Lymphoid organs, development of, *see website*
Lymphoid tyrosine phosphatase (SNP), 1971
Lymphoma, 1739-1746
adult T-cell, *see website*
anaplastic large cell, 1739-1740, 1744t
Burkitt, 1743, 1744t
Epstein-Barr virus-associated, 1112t
of small intestine, 1314-1315
of gastrointestinal tract, *see website*
HIV-related, 1164-1165, *see website*
Hodgkin, 1739-1743, 1740f-1742f, 1741t, 1743t
incidence and survival rates for, 1726t
risk factors for, 1727t
work-up of, 1731t
late effects in children and adolescents with, 1746
lymphoblastic, 1743, 1744t
Lymphoma *(Continued)*
Mediterranean of small intestine, 1314-1315
mucosa associated lymphoid tissue, 1315
non-Hodgkin, 1730f, 1743-1746, 1744f-1745f, 1745t
hematopoietic stem cell transplantation for, 759
of small intestine, 1314-1315
of temporal bone, *see website*
work-up of, 1731t
primary effusion based, 1121
Lymphopenia, 752, 752t
in adenosine deaminase deficiency, 732
due to ehrlichiosis, 1049
in severe combined immunodeficiency, 731
Lymphopoiesis, *see website*
Lymphoproliferation, human T-lymphocyte-associated, *see website*
Lymphoproliferative disease, 721t
autoimmune, 737-738, 737t, 738f
post-transplantation, *see website*
X-linked, 727
Epstein-Barr virus and, 1112
Lynch syndrome, *see website*
Lysergic acid diethylamide (LSD), 682
Lysine, defects in metabolism of, 453-455, 454f
Lysinuric protein intolerance (LPI), 455, 1320
Lysosomal acid α-1,4-glucosidase deficiency, 499-500, 500f
Lysosomal-associated membrane protein 2 (LAMP2) deficiency, 500
Lysosomal storage disorders, 482-491, 483f, 486f
cholesterol ester storage disease as, 491
clinical findings in, 484t
Fabry disease as, 488-489, 489f
Farber disease as, 491, 491f
fucosidosis as, 489-490
Gaucher disease as, 487-488, 487f
genetic therapies for, 381
GM_1 gangliosidosis as, 483-491
GM_2 gangliosidosis as, 484-487
Krabbe disease as, 490-491
metachromatic leukodystrophy as, 490
multiple sulfatase deficiency as, 490
Neimann-Pick disease as, 488
Schindler disease as, 490
symptoms of, 485t
Wolman disease as, 491
Lysyl hydroxylase deficiency, 2278

M

MAC. *See* Minimal alveolar concentration (MAC); Mycobacterium avium complex (MAC)
Machado-Joseph disease (MJD), 2057t
Macleod syndrome, 1461
Macroadenoma, insulin-secreting, 522-523
Macrocephaly
in neurologic examination, *see website*
in Tay-Sachs disease, 485
Macrodactyly, 2343, 2343f
Macrodantin. *See* Nitrofurantoin
Macrodontia, 1250
Macrolides, *see website*
Macromastia, *see website*
Macronutrients, *see website*
Macrophage activation syndrome (MAS), 832-834, 835t
Macrophage-colony-stimulating factor (M-CSF), fetal, *see website*
Macrophages, 739
abnormalities of, *see website*
in allergic disease, *see website*
in amyloidosis, 860-861
Coxiella burnetii in, 1051
development of, *see website*
fetal, *see website*
functional activities of, *see website*
in neonatal immunity, 632
Salmonella interaction with, 950
in tuberculosis, 999f
Macrosomia, 522t
Macular atrophy, 2277
Macular red cherry spot, 483
Macule, examination of, *see website*
Madelung deformity, 2384-2385
Mafenide acetate for burn injury, 353, 353t
Maffucci syndrome, 2230
MAG-3. *See* Mercaptoacetyl triglycine (MAG-3) diuretic renogram
Magical thinking, 34-35
Magnesium, 224-225, *see also website*
Magnesium sulfate for pediatric resuscitation and arrhythmias, 294t
Magnetic resonance angiography (MRA)
in abusive head trauma, 139-140
in cardiovascular disease, 1545-1546, 1546f
computer processing of, 1546
in neurologic examination, *see website*
in orthopedic problems, 2335
in osteomyelitis, 2396, 2396f
in rheumatic disease, *see website*
in septic arthritis, 2400
Magnetic resonance cholangiography (MRC), *see website*
Magnetic resonance imaging (MRI)
in appendicitis, 1352-1353
in arterial ischemic stroke, 2080, 2081f
in attention deficit/hyperactivity disorder, *see website*
in Canavan disease, 456, 456f
in cardiovascular disease, 1545-1546, 1545f
chest, *see website*
fetal, 543t
in fever of unknown origin, 902
functional in neurologic examination, *see website*
in generalized seizures, 2021, 2022f
in hypoxic-ischemic encephalopathy, 302, 302f, 570, 571f-573f
in juvenile idiopathic arthritis, 837f
of Müllerian anomalies, *see website*
in neurologic examination, *see website*
in orthopedic problems, 2334-2335
in osteomyelitis, 2396
in pork tapeworm, 1235, 1236f
in septic arthritis, 2399f, 2400
in sickle cell disease, 1666-1667, 1666f
in tuberculosis, 1006
in X-linked adrenoleukodystrophy, 468, 469f
Magnetic resonance spectroscopy (MRS), 1545-1546
Magnetic resonance urography, 1841, 1841f
Magnetic resonance venography (MRV), *see website*
Magnet ingestion, 1290, 1290f
Ma huang
for asthma, 271t
potential toxicity of, 272t-273t
Maintenance of Certification (MOC), *see website*
Maintenance therapy, 242, 242t
glucose in, 243
hyponatremia and, 243-244
intravenous solutions for, 243, 243t
selection of solutions for, 243
water in, 242-243, 243t
variations in, 244, 244t
Major aortopulmonary collateral arteries (MAPCAs), 1573-1575, 1578
Major basic protein (MBP), neutrophil, 739
Major depression, 82-85, 83t-84t
Major histocompatibility complex (MHC), *see also website*
defective expression of, 734
type 1 diabetes mellitus and, 1970
Major outer membrane protein (MOMP), 1033-1034
Malabsorption, 1304-1322, 1305t
bile acid, 1312
of carbohydrates, 1306-1307, 1315-1317
classification of, 1305t
clinical approach to, 1305-1306, 1306f, 1306t

Malabsorption *(Continued)*
in eosinophilic gastroenteritis, 1321, *see also website*
evaluation of, 1306-1308
exocrine pancreatic function and, 1307-1308, 1307f
of fat, 1307
of fructose, 1316-1317
due to gluten-sensitivity enteropathy, 1308-1311, 1308f, 1309t-1310t, 1310f
with immunodeficiency disorders, 1313-1314
due to immunoproliferative small intestinal disease, 1314-1315
in inflammatory bowel disease, 1322, *see also website*
due to intestinal infections and infestations, 1313
due to intestinal mucosal disorders, 1308
due to liver and biliary disorders, 1318
due to malnutrition, 1315
due to malrotation, 1280-1281
other syndromes of, 1311-1313
of protein, 1307
rare inborn defects causing, 1317
due to short bowel syndrome, 1314, 1315t, 1316f
sports participation and, 2402t-2404t
Malaria, 1198-1207
cerebral, 1206
clinical manifestations of, 1200-1201, 1201t
complications of, 1206
congenital, 1201
diagnosis of, 1201-1202
differential diagnosis of, 1202
etiology of, 1198-1199, 1198f
maternal, *see website*
pathogenesis of, 1199-1200, 1199f-1200f
predisposition to due to immunodeficiency, 716t
prevention of, 1206-1207, 1207t
prophylaxis
in HIV infection, 1175t-1176t
for travel, *see website*
returning traveler with fever and, *see website*
treatment of, 1202, 1203t-1205t, *see website*
Malarone. *See* Atovaquone-proguanil
Malar rash, *see website*
Malassezia, 1058, 2253, 2305, 2309, *see also website*
Malathion, 2321, *see also website*
Malayan filariasis, 1224-1225
Mal de Meleda, 2272
Male breast cancer, 1947
Male disorders in adolescent, *see website*
Male fertility, inguinal hernia repair and, 1368
Male rape, 703
Malformations, *see website*. *See* Congenital anomalies
Malignancy
adenoid cystic, 1504
adrenal, 1773, *see also website*
basal cell, *see website*
bone, 1763-1768, 1763t, 1764f-1765f
brain tumors as, 1746-1753
astrocytoma as, 1748-1750, 1749f
of brainstem, 1753, 1753f
choroid plexus, 1750-1751
clinical manifestations of, 1747
complications and long-term management of, 1753
craniopharyngioma as, 1752
diagnosis of, 1747-1748
embryonal, 1751-1752, 1751f
ependymal, 1750, 1750f
epidemiology of, 1746
etiology of, 1746, 1747t
germ cell, 1752-1753
metastatic, 1753
pathogenesis of, 1746-1747, 1747f-1748f, 1748t
pineal parenchymal, 1752

Malignancy *(Continued)*
breast, *see website*
male, 1947
bronchogenic, *see website*
Candida infections with, 1055
cervical, 1873-1874, 1873t
abnormal uterine bleeding due to, 689t-690t
human papillomavirus and, 1139-1140, 1729
choroid plexus, 1750-1751
colorectal, 1773, *see also website*
inherited syndromes of, *see website*
ulcerative colitis and risk for, 1297
as complication of enterocystoplasty, *see website*
cutaneous manifestations of, *see website*
desmoplastic small round cell tumor as, 1773
diagnosis of, 1728-1731
age-related manifestations of, 1728-1729
early detection in, 1729-1731
ensuring the, 1731, 1731t
physical examination in, 1728
signs and symptoms in, 1728, 1728t-1729t
staging in, 1731
diarrhea caused by, *see website*
epidemiology of, 1725-1727, 1726f-1727f, 1726t
Epstein-Barr virus associated, 1111-1112, 1112t
fever without a focus in, 896t
general anesthesia and, *see website*
gonadal and germ cell neoplasms as, 1769-1771, 1770f
gynecologic, 1870-1874
hematopoietic stem cell transplantation for (*See* Hematopoietic stem cell transplantation (HSCT))
hepatocellular, 1772
in type II glycogen storage disease, 496
histiocytosis syndromes of childhood as, 1773-1777, 1774t-1776t, 1775f
HIV-related, 1166
hypercalcemia due to, 1922
immunizations and, 891
impact of cancer therapy on fertility and, 1870-1871
incidence rates for, 1727f
infections with, *see website*
influencing the incidence of, 1725-1727
of kidney, 1757-1760, 1757t-1759t, 1759f
of larynx, trachea, and bronchi, *see website*
leukemias as, 1732-1739
of liver, 1771-1772, 1771f
lymphoma as, 1739-1746
manifestations of, 1729t
melanoma as, 1772-1773, *see also website*
molecular and cellular biology of, 1728, *see also website*
mucoepidermoid, 1504, *see also website*
nasopharyngeal, 1773, *see also website*
Epstein-Barr virus-associated, 1111, 1112t
neuroblastoma as, 1753-1757, 1754t-1755t, 1756f
nevoid basal cell, 1747t, *see website*
ovarian, 1871-1873, 1872t
pain management in, 374, 374t
pancreatic, 1374, *see also website*
pulmonary embolism with, 1500
renal cell, 1760
retinoblastoma as, 1768-1769, 1768f
risk factors for, 1727t
secondary, *see website*
signs and symptoms of, 1728, 1728t-1729t
soft tissue sarcoma as, 1760-1762, 1761f, 1761t-1762t
sports participation and, 2402t-2404t
syndromes predisposing to, *see website*
thyroid, 1772, 1914-1916, *see also website*
medullary, 1915-1916
tonsillar, 1443
treatment of, 1731-1732, *see also website*

Malignancy *(Continued)*
acute toxic effects of and supportive care for, *see website*
chemotherapy in, *see website*
diagnosis and staging in, *see website*
discussion of with patient and family in, *see website*
impact on fertility, 1870-1871
late adverse effects of, *see website*
multimodal, multidisciplinary approach to, *see website*
palliative care in, *see website*
radiation therapy in, *see website*
surgery in, *see website*
"two-hit" model of development of, *see website*
uterine, 1872-1873
abnormal uterine bleeding due to, 689t-690t
vaginal, 1873
vulvar, 1873
Malignant external otitis, 2197
Malignant hyperthermia, 2130-2131
hyperkalemia and, 220
postoperative, *see website*
Malignant melanoma, maternal, *see website*
Malingering, 69, *see also website*
Mallet finger deformity, 2391
Mallet toe, 2342
Mallory-Weiss tear, 1243t
Malnutrition, 170
with chronic diarrhea, 1343t
common causes of in early life, 148t
definitions of, 172t
due to enzyme deficiencies, 1317-1319
food insecurity and, 170-171
malabsorption due to, 1315
protein-energy, 174-179, *see also website*
clinical manifestations of, 175, 175f-176f, 175t
pathophysiology of, 175-176
treatment of, 176-179, 176t-179t, 177f-178f
undernutrition in, 171-174, 171f, 171t
consequences of, 173-174
interventions for, 174, 174f
measurement of, 171-172
prevalence of, 172-173
Malone antegrade continence enema procedure, *see website*
Malone procedure, 1359
Malrotation, intestinal, 1280-1281, 1280f
MALT. *See* Mucosa associated lymphoid tissue (MALT) lymphoma
Maltreatment. *See* Abuse and neglect
Management sciences (MS), *see website*
Mandible, hypoplasia of, as delivery room emergency, 575
Mandibulofacial dysostosis, 1254
Manganese, *see website*
Mania
in bipolar disorder, 86
psychopharmacologic management of, 61t
Mannan-binding lectin-associated serine protease 2 (MASP-2) deficiency, 754-755, 754t
Mannan-binding lectin (MBL) deficiency, 754-755, 754t
Mannitol, 1820
α-Mannosidosis, 484t
β-Mannosidosis, 484t
βS-Mannosidosis, *see website*
Manometry
in congenital intestinal pseudo-obstruction, 1283t
esophageal, *see website*
in achalasia, 1264-1265
in Hirschsprung disease, 1286
Mansonella ozzardi, *see website*
Mansonella perstans, *see website*
Mansonella streptocerca, *see website*
Mantoux tuberculin skin test, 1001
MAO. *See* Monoamine oxidase (MAO) deficiency

MAOIs. *See* Monoamine oxidase inhibitors (MAOIs)
MAP. *See* Mean arterial pressure (MAP)
MAPCAs. *See* Major aortopulmonary collateral arteries (MAPCAs)
Maple syrup urine disease (MSUD), 430-438
  hypoglycemia in, 528
  neonatal seizures due to, 2036
Mapping, linkage, 376, 377t, *see also website*
Marasmic kwashiorkor, 175
Marasmus, 175
Maraviroc for HIV infection, 1168t-1171t
Marburg disease, 1151-1152
Marcus Gunn jaw-winking ptosis, 2163
Marcus Gunn phenomenon, 2006
Marcus Gunn pupil, 2156
Marden-Walker syndrome, 2138
Marenostrin, 856
Marfan syndrome (MFS), 2440-2446
  clinical manifestations of, 2440-2443, 2441f-2442f
    cardiac, 1531t
  current and future therapies for, 2445
  diagnostic criteria for, 2442t
  differential diagnosis of, 2443-2444, 2444t
  epidemiology of, 2440
  family and genetic history in, 2443
  genetic counseling in, 2446
  genetics of, *see website*
  genetics of congenital heart disease with, *see website*
  laboratory findings in, 2444
  overgrowth in, *see website*
  pathogenesis of, 2440
  prognosis for, 2445
  sports participation and, 2402t-2404t
  treatment of, 2444-2445
Marijuana, 672, 673t, 680-681, 680t
Marine envenomation, 2464-2465
Marker chromosome, 408
Marnier-Kuhn syndrome, *see website*
Maroteaux-Lamy disease, 511f, 512t, 514
Marshall syndrome, 859-860
MAS. *See* Macrophage activation syndrome (MAS)
Masculinization, *see website*
Mask
  for infection protection and control, *see website*
  oxygen administration through, 319
MASP-2. *See* Mannan-binding lectin-associated serine protease 2 (MASP-2) deficiency
Masquerade syndromes, 2174
Massage, 273
  for pain management, 371
Mass(es)
  abdominal, 1249
    in newborn assessment, 535
    nondigestive causes of, 1241t
    as sign of cancer, 1728
    in Wilms tumor, 1758
  adrenal, 1943
  breast, *see website*
  mediastinal
    anesthesia and, *see website*
    in Hodgkin lymphoma, 1741, 1742f
  nasal, midline congenital, 1431, 1431f
Mastalgia, *see website*
Mast cells
  in allergic disease, *see website*
  in food allergy, 816
Mastitis, *see also website*
  breast-feeding and, 160, 540t
Mastocytoma, diarrhea caused by, *see website*
Mastocytosis, 814, 2280-2282, 2280f-2281f, 2280t-2281t
Mastoiditis, 2210-2211, 2210f, 2210t
  Pseudomonas aeruginosa, 976t
Masturbation, seizure *versus*, *see website*
Maternal disease, 545
Maternal factors
  in attention deficit/hyperactivity disorder, 108
  in high-risk pregnancies, *see website*
  in sudden infant death syndrome, 1424
Maternal-infant attachment, *see website*
Maternal infection, 545
Maternal interests, fetal interests *versus*, *see website*
Maternally inherited diabetes and deafness (MIDD), 1994-1995
Maternal phenylketonuria (PKU), *see also website*
  congenital heart disease with, 1531t
  fetal therapy for, 551t
Maternal radiation exposure, *see website*
Maternal serum α-fetoprotein concentration, 543t
Maternal substance abuse
  neonatal metabolic disturbances due to, 623-625, 624t
  sudden infant death syndrome and, 1424
Maternal tetanus, 991
Maternal thyroiditis, postpartum, 1904t
Mathematics disorder, *see website*
MATN3 gene, *see website*
Matrix, urinary stone, *see website*
Mature minor, 664-665, *see website*
Maturity
  assessment of, 557, 558f
  fetal, 541
Maturity-onset diabetes of the young (MODY), 1993-1994, 1994t, *see also website*
Mauric syndrome, 1988
Maxillary sinuses, 1436, 1436f
Maximal midexpiratory flow rate, *see website*
Maximum forced expiratory flow (FEF max), *see website*
Maximum urine osmolality, *see website*
Maxipime. *See* Cefepime
Mayer-Rokitansky-Küster-Hauser syndrome (MRKH), 1827, *see website*
MBC. *See* Minimum bactericidal concentration (MBC)
MBL. *See* Mannan-binding lectin (MBL) deficiency
MBP. *See* Major basic protein (MBP), neutrophil
MCAD. *See* Medium-chain acyl CoA dehydrogenase (MCAD) deficiency
McArdie disease, 494t-495t, 500-501, *see also website*
McCune-Albright syndrome, 207, 1892, 1908-1909, 1940, 1957-1958, *see website*
MCDK. *See* Multicystic dysplastic kidney (MCDK)
MCH. *See* Erythrocytes
M-CHAT. *See* Modified Checklist for Autism in Toddlers (M-CHAT)
MCHC. *See* Mean corpuscular hemoglobin concentration (MCHC)
MCKD. *See* Medullary cystic kidney disease complex (MCKD)
McKinney-Vento Act, 10
McKusick Metaphyseal chondrodysplasia, 2434
MCL. *See* Medial collateral ligament (MCL) injury
McLeod syndrome, 2057t
McMurray test, 2415f
MCNS. *See* Minimal change nephrotic syndrome (MCNS)
MCP. *See* Medical control physician (MCP)
MCP gene, 1792t
M-CSF. *See* Macrophage-colony-stimulating factor (M-CSF)
MCTD. *See* Mixed connective tissue disease (MCTD)
MCV. *See* Mean corpuscular volume (MCV); Meningococcal conjugate vaccine (MCV)
MDAC. *See* Multi-dose activated charcoal (MDAC)
MDGs. *See* Millennium Development Goals (MDGs)
MDI. *See* Metered-dose inhaler (MDI)
MDMA. *See* Methylenedioxymethamphetamine (MDMA)
MDR3 mutations, 1383t, 1384
MDS. *See* Mitochondrial DNA depletion syndrome (MDS)
Mead Johnson bottle, 1253
Mean arterial pressure (MAP), 311t
Mean corpuscular hemoglobin concentration (MCHC), reference values for, *see website*
Mean corpuscular hemoglobin (MCH), reference values for, *see website*
Mean corpuscular volume (MCV)
  in anemia, 1648t, 1649, 1649f
  in congenital dyserythropoietic anemia, *see website*
  fetal, *see website*
  in iron deficiency-anemia, 1656t-1657t
  in megaloblastic anemias, *see website*
  reference values for, *see website*
Measles, 1069-1075
  atypical, 1071
  in child-care setting, *see website*
  clinical manifestations of, 1070-1071, 1070f-1071f
  complications of, 1071-1073, 1072t
  diagnosis of, 1071
  differential diagnosis of, 1071
  epidemiology of, 1069-1070, 1070f
  etiology of, 1069
  exclusion from day care due to, *see website*
  hemorrhagic, 1072
  in immigrant children, 134
  inapparent, 1071
  Kawasaki disease *versus*, 865-866
  laboratory findings in, 1071
  maternal, *see website*
  pathogenesis of, 1070
  pathology of, 1070
  pneumonia with, 1475t
  prevention of, 1073-1075
  prognosis for, 1073
  transmission of, 1070
  treatment of, 1073
  vaccine for, 881t, 895, 1073-1075, 1074t
    for travel, 891t
  vitamin A deficiency and, 1073, 1073t
Measles, mumps, rubella, varicella (MMRV) vaccine, 884t, 1078
Measles, mumps, rubella (MMR) vaccine, 884t, 1073-1075, 1074t, 1078, 1081
  adverse reaction to, 827
  HIV infection and, 1173
  recommended schedule for, 886-889, 887f-888f
  for travel, *see website*
Measurements in growth assessment, accurate, *see website*
Mebendazole, *see also website*
  for ascariasis, 1217-1218
  for enterobiasis, 1222
  for trichinosis, 1229
  for trichuriasis, 1221-1222
  for vulvovaginitis, 1868t
Mechanical ventilation, 321-329, 321f-322f
  airway pressure release, 326
  assist control mode in, 324
  for asthma exacerbation, 800
  basic concepts of, 321-324
  bronchopulmonary dysplasia due to, 585, 587-590, 588f, 589t
  for congenital diaphragmatic hernia, 595
  control variable mode in, 324-325, 325f
  conventional settings for, 327
  equation of motion in, 321-322, 322f
  expiratory phase maneuvers in, 326
  functional residual capacity in, 322, 323f
  high-frequency, 326-327
  initiation of inspiration in, 324
  inspiratory phase characteristics in, 325-326

Mechanical ventilation *(Continued)*
intermittent mandatory ventilation mode in, 324, 324f
long-term, 329-333, 1524-1526
goals of, 330
in-hospital management and discharge planning for, 331, 1525-1526
methods of, 332-333
patient selection and ethical considerations in, 330-331, 330t
team approach to home, 331-332, 331t
lung injury due to, 329
monitoring of respiratory mechanics in, 328-329, 328f
opening pressure in, 323-324, 324f
patient-ventilator asynchrony in, 327-328
for persistent pulmonary hypertension of the newborn, 593
in pertussis management, 947
phases of, 324-326
PHOX2B gene and dependence on, 1520
for respiratory distress syndrome, 584-585
support modes in, 325, 328
termination of inspiration cycle in, 326
time constant in, 322-323, 323f
weaning from, 329, 586
Mechanobullous disorders, 2244-2246, 2245f-2247f, 2245t
Meckel diverticulum, 1281-1282, 1282f
abdominal pain of, 1247t
Meckel-Gruber syndrome, 1531t
encephalocele with, 2003
Meckel syndrome, *see website*
Meconium aspiration, 590-592
Meconium ileus, 601, 601f, 1279
in cystic fibrosis, 1486, 1487f, 1495
Meconium peritonitis, 601
in cystic fibrosis, 1487f
Meconium plugs, 600-601, 600f
in cystic fibrosis, 1487f
Meconium staining, 577
fetal therapy for, 551t
high-risk infant due to, 552
in hypoxic-ischemic encephalopathy, 570
Mectizan. *See* Ivermectin
MED. *See* Multiple epiphyseal dysplasias (MED)
Media, radiocontrast, adverse reaction to, 828
Media coverage of war, *see website*
Medial collateral ligament (MCL) injury, 2414
Median, statistical, *see website*
Median cubital vein, venous access in, 292, 295f
Mediastinal "crunch," 1512
Mediastinal disease in Hodgkin lymphoma, 1741, 1742f
Mediastinal masses, anesthesia and, *see website*
Mediastinum, air or gas in, 1512
Media violence, *see website*
Medicaid, 10
Medical biochemical geneticist, 382t
Medical care
coordination of for foster care children, *see website*
of critically ill child, *see website*
of disabled newborns, *see website*
Medical control, *see website*
Medical control physician (MCP), *see website*
Medical device-associated infection, 903, *see also website*
Medical errors, *see website*
Medical history. *See* History
Medical home, *see website*
Medical profession, culture of, *see website*
Medical records
adolescent confidentiality of, *see website*
preadoption review of, 130
Medication. *See* Drug(s)
Mediterranean fever, familial, 855t, 856-857, 857f
abdominal pain of, 1247t
Mediterranean lymphoma of small intestine, 1314-1315
Mediterranean spotted fever (MSF), 1039t-1040t, 1043-1044
Medium-chain acyl CoA dehydrogenase (MCAD) deficiency, 457t, 459-460
Medroxyprogesterone acetate (DMPA), 697-698, 1875
Medulla, renal, 1778
Medullary carcinoma, diarrhea caused by, *see website*
Medullary cystic kidney disease complex (MCKD), 1816
Medullary sponge kidney, 1810
Medullary thyroid carcinoma (MTC), 1915-1916
Medulloblastoma, 1748t, 1751-1752, 1751f
MEE. *See* Middle-ear effusion (MEE)
Mees lines, 2294, *see website*
Mefenamic acid for dysmenorrhea, 691t
Mefloquine, 1202, 1203t-1205t, 1207, 1207t, *see website*
in HIV infection, 1175t-1176t
Mefoxin. *See* Cefoxitin
Megacolon
in Chagas disease, 1196
congenital aganglionic, 1283t, 1284-1287, 1285f-1286f
toxic, 1297-1298
Megacystis-megaureter syndrome, 1834, 1835f
Megaesophagus in Chagas disease, 1196
Megakaryocytes, fetal, *see website*
Megakaryopoiesis, 1714, 1715f
Megalencephaly, 2010-2011
Megaloblastic anemias, 1655, *see also website*
folic acid deficiency in, 1655, *see also website*
thiamine-responsiveness, 191
vitamin B_{12} (cobalamin) deficiency in, 1655, *see also website*
Megalocorneal, 2169, *see also website*
Megalourethra, 1857-1858
Megameatal variant, 1852
Megaureter, 1844-1845, 1844f, 1844t
Megestrol acetate for anorexia, 155t-156t
Meglumine antimonate, *see website*
Meige disease, *see website*
Meiosis, 395
Melamine exposure/poisoning, 2454, *see also website*
Melanin deficiency, 424-425
Melanoblast migration abnormalities, 2239-2240
Melanocortin 4 receptor gene deficiency, 182t
Melanocytes, *see website*
Melanocytic nevi
acquired, 2231, 2231f
atypical, 2231-2232
congenital, 2232, 2232f
Melanoma, 1772-1773, 2232-2233, *see also website*
nevi associated with, 2231
Melanosis
Becker, 2235, 2235f
pustular in newborn, 533
transient neonatal pustular, 2219-2220, 2219f
Melarsoprol, 1192, *see also website*
MELAS. *See* Mitochondrial myopathy, encephalopathy, lactic acidosis, and strokelike episodes (MELAS)
Melatonin for delayed sleep phase disorder, 53-54
Melioidosis, *see website*
Melissa officinalis for sedation, 271t
Meloxicam, 838t, *see also website*
Membrane attack complex, *see website*
Membrane cofactor protein, 1792t
Membrane complement control protein deficiency, 755
Membranoproliferative glomerulonephritis (MPGN), 1787-1788, 1803t
renal transplantation in, *see website*
Membranous conjunctivitis, 2168
Membranous nephropathy (MN), 1786-1787, 1803t
Memory, *see website*
MEN. *See* Multiple endocrine neoplasia (MEN)
Menaquinones, 210
Menarche, 653, 685
premature, 1894
Mendelian inheritance, 383-388
autosomal dominant, 383-385, 387f
autosomal recessive, 385-388, 388f
of cataracts, 2170
pseudodominant, 388, 388f
X-linked, 388, 388f-389f
Menelaus method, *see website*
Meningitis
amebic, *see website*
bacterial, 2087-2095
cerebrospinal fluid findings in, 2088t
clinical manifestations of, 2090
complications of, 2094
diagnosis of, 2090-2091, 2092t-2093t
epidemiology of, 2087
etiology of, 2087
Haemophilus influenzae type b in, 2089
hearing loss due to, *see website*
Neisseria meningitidis in, 2087-2089
neonatal, 646
pathogenesis of, 2089-2090
pathology and pathophysiology of, 2089
prevention of, 2095
prognosis for, 2095
Streptococcus pneumoniae in, 2087
treatment of, 2091-2094, 2093t
cerebrospinal fluid findings in, 2088t
as cerebrospinal fluid shunt infection, *see website*
in child-care setting, *see website*
coccidioidal, 1068
Cryptococcus neoformans in, 1057
Enterococcus, *see website*
enteroviral, 1091-1092
eosinophilic, 2097-2098
group B streptococcal, 927
Haemophilus influenzae in, 941-942
herpes simplex virus, 1101
imaging studies in, *see website*
Listeria monocytogenes, *see website*
Lyme disease, 1026, 1028t
lymphocytic choriomeningitis virus, 1153, *see also website*
meningococcal, 931-932
microcephaly with, 2007t
due to mumps, 1080
pneumococcal, 913
Pseudomonas aeruginosa, *see website*
Salmonella, 952
Staphylococcus aureus in, 905
tuberculous, 1005-1006, 1009
"Meningitis belt," *see website*
Meningocele, 1999
Meningococcal conjugate vaccine (MCV), 884t
recommended schedule for, 887f, 889
for special circumstances, 889
for travel, 891t, *see website*
Meningococcal polysaccharide vaccine (MPSV4), 884t, 934, *see also website*
Meningococcemia, 931-932, 932f
Meningococcus, 929-935
clinical manifestations of, 931-932, 932f
diagnosis of, 932
differential diagnosis of, 932
epidemiology of, 930
etiology of, 929-930
host factors in, 931
immunity to, 931
pathogenesis of, 930-931
prevention of, 933-935, 934t
prognosis for, 933
treatment of, 932-933, 933t
vaccine for, 884t, 888f, 934-935, 934t
Meningococcus vaccine for travel, *see website*

Meningoencephalitis
  amebic, *see website*
    cerebrospinal fluid findings in, 2088t
  enteroviral, 1092
  due to human monocytic ehrlichiosis, 1049
  due to mumps, 1080
  trypanosomal, 1191-1192
  viral, 2095-2097
    cerebrospinal fluid findings in, 2088t
Meniscal tear in knee, 2414-2415
Meniscus, discoid lateral, 2352, 2352f
Menkes disease, 1321, 2075, *see website*
Menkes kinky hair syndrome, 2292
Menometrorrhagia, 686t
Menopause, premature, due to cancer and its therapy, *see website*
Menorrhagia, 686t, 688-690
Menstrual cramps, painful, 690-691
Menstruation
  irregularities of, 685-686, 686t
    abnormal uterine bleeding, 688-690, 689t-690t
    amenorrhea, 686-688, 687f, 687t-688t
    dysmenorrhea, 690-691, 691t
    premenstrual syndrome, 691-692, 692t
  normal, 685
  special needs girls and, 1874-1875
  sports participation and, 2421-2422
  toxic shock syndrome and, 908-909
Mental health action signs, 57, 57t
Mental health issues. *See also* Psychiatric disorders
  in foster care children, *see website*
  in homosexuality, 658-659
  office intervention for, 16
Mental health services
  minors right to consent for, *see website*
  referral to in eating disorders, 95-96
Mental retardation. *See* Intellectual disability
Mental status
  of acutely ill child, 275
  bacterial meningitis and, 2090
  effects of eating disorders on, 93t
  evaluation of, *see website*
    in psychiatric diagnostic evaluation, 60
Mentha pulegium, potential toxicity of, 272t-273t
Meperidine
  for cyclic vomiting syndrome, 1244t
  equianalgesic doses and half-life of, 367t
  for pain management, 365t
Mephenytoin hydroxylase deficiency, *see website*
Mercaptoacetyl triglycine (MAG-3) diuretic renogram, 1839f-1840f, 1840-1841
6-Mercaptopurine
  for autoimmune hepatitis, 1410
  for cancer therapy, *see website*
  for Crohn disease, 1303
Mercury exposure/poisoning, 1328t-1329t, *see also website*
Merkel cell polyomavirus, 1157
Merkel cells, *see website*
Meropenem, *see website*
  for bacterial meningitis, 2093t
  for cystic fibrosis lung infection, 1492t
  for meningococcal disease, 933t
  for neonatal infection, 645t
Merozoites, 1199
Merrem. *See* Meropenem
MERRF. *See* Myoclonus epilepsy and ragged red fibers (MERRF)
Mesangial proliferation in idiopathic nephrotic syndrome, 1804
Mesenteric arteritis, postoperative, 1569
Mesenteric artery syndrome, superior, 1287, *see also website*
Mesial temporal sclerosis, 2023
Mesoblastic nephroma, 1760
Mesonephric duct, *see website*
Messenger DNA in sudden infant death syndrome, 1427
Messenger RNA, *see website*
Mestinon. *See* Pyridostigmine bromide
Metabolic acidosis, 230t, 231-235
  in acute renal failure, 1820-1821
  in chronic kidney disease, 1824
  clinical manifestations of, 233
  as complication of enterocystoplasty, *see website*
  in dehydration, 247
  diagnosis of, 233-234, 234f
  etiology and pathophysiology of, 231-233, 231t
  hypophosphatemia and, 227
  in poisonings, 254t
  in respiratory distress syndrome, 586
  in tetralogy of Fallot, 1574
  treatment of, 234-235
Metabolic alkalosis, 230t, 235-238
  clinical manifestations of, 237
  diagnosis of, 237-238
  etiology and pathophysiology of, 235-237, 235t
  treatment of, 238
Metabolic bone disease
  hyperphosphatemia as, 2446, *see also website*
  hypophosphatemia as, 2446, *see also website*
  in newborn, 623
  osteoporosis as, 2446-2447, 2447t
  primary chondrodystrophy (metaphyseal dysplasia) as, 2446, *see also website*
Metabolic disorders, 416-418, 417f, 418t
  of amino acids, 418-456
    of arginine, citrulline, and ornithine, 447-453, 448f-449f, 448t, 450t
    of aspartic acid, 455-456, 456f
    of cysteine/cystine, 429
    of glutamic acid, 443-445, 444f
    of glycine, 438-441, 439f, 441f
    of histidine, 453
    of lysine, 453-455, 454f
    malabsorption due to, 1318
    of methionine, 425-429, 426f
    of neurotransmitters, 445-447, 445t
    of phenylalanine, 418-422, 419f, 421f
    of proline, 442-443, 442f
    of serine, 442
    of tryptophan, 429-430, 429f
    of tyrosine, 422-425
    of valine, leucine, isoleucine, and related organic acidemias, 430-438, 430f
  ataxia with, 2055
  of carbohydrates, 492-509, 493f, 494t-495t, *see website*
    of fructose, 503
    of galactose, 502-503
    glycogen storage diseases as, 492-501, 496f, 500f
    of glycoprotein, 509, *see also website*
    with lactic acidosis, 503-509, 504f-505f, 507t-509t, 508f
    malabsorption due to, 1318
    of pentose, 509, *see also website*
  cataracts due to, 2170-2171
  dystonia due to, 2060-2061
  failure to thrive in, 148t
  fetal therapy for, 551t
  hypoglycemia as, 517-531
    classification of, 519-521, 520t
    clinical manifestations of, 518-519, 519f, 519t, 521t, 524t
    definition of, 517
    diagnosis and differential diagnosis of, 524t, 530
    endocrine deficiency and, 527-528
    in newborn, 518
    persistent or recurrent, 521-530, 522t-523t, 525f-527f
    prognosis for, 531
    significance and sequelae of, 517-518
    treatment of, 530-531
Metabolic disorders *(Continued)*
  language disorders due to, 119
  of lipids, 456-492
    of lipoprotein metabolism and transport, 470-482, 471f-474f, 472t-473t, 476f, 477t-479t, 480f, 481t-482t
    lysosomal storage disorders as, 482-491, 483f, 484t-485t, 486f-487f, 489f, 491f
    of mitochondrial fatty acid β-oxidation, 456-462, 457t, 458f-459f
    mucolipidoses as, 491-492
    of very long chain fatty acids, 462-470, 462t-464t, 464f-465f, 466t, 469f
  of liver, 1388-1393, 1389t
    α-antitrypsin deficiency, 1393
    Indian childhood cirrhosis, 1392
    inherited deficient conjugation of bilirubin as, 1389-1390
    neonatal iron storage disease as, 1393
    Wilson disease, 1391, 1391f
  mucopolysaccharidoses as, 509-516, 510f-511f, 511t-512t, 513f, 515t-516t
  multiple organ dysfunction syndrome and, 312t
  neutropenia in, 751
  newborn screening for, 416, 417t
  physiologic therapies for, 379
  porphyrias as, 517, *see also website*
  in premature infants, 559t
  progeria as, 516, *see also website*
  of purine and pyrimidine, 516, *see also website*
  respiratory distress due to, 315t, 316
  respiratory insufficiency due to, 1523-1524
  severe intellectual disability in, 123t
  strokelike events *versus*, 2086
  systemic inflammatory response syndrome and, 309t
Metabolic disturbances
  in newborn, 418-456
    cold injury as, 622
    edema as, 622
    fetal alcohol syndrome as, 625-626, 626f, 626t
    hypermagnesemia as, 623
    hyperthermia as, 622
    hypomagnesemia as, 623
    due to maternal substance abuse, 623-625, 624t
    metabolic bone disease as, 623
    seizures due to, 2034-2035
    due to selective serotonin reuptake inhibitors, 625, 625f
  as oncologic emergency, *see website*
Metabolic myopathies, 2130-2132, 2130t
  glycogenoses as, 2131, *see also website*
  lipid, 2132, *see also website*
  malignant hyperthermia as, 2130-2131
  mitochondrial, 2132
  periodic paralyses as, 2130
  vitamin E deficiency, 2132
Metabolic syndrome, 183, 184t
Metabolism
  of calcium and bone, 1916, *see also website*
  of drugs, *see also website*
    adverse reactions and, 824
    in premature and low birthweight infants, 353-354, 563t
  effects of eating disorders on, 93t
  effects of vomiting on, 1243t
  glucocorticoids in, *see website*
  hepatic, *see website*
  of lead, 2449-2450
  of lipoproteins, 471-473
  of magnesium, *see website*
  of phosphorus, 225-226, 226t
  of potassium, 219
  of sodium, 212
  surfactant, inherited disorders of, 1497-1498, *see also website*
  of vitamin A, 188

Metabolomics, *see website*
Metabonomics, *see website*
Metacarpal bones, centers of ossification
 appearance in, 29t
Metachromatic leukodystrophy (MLD), 484t, 490, 2072
Metacyclic trypomastigotes, 1193f
Metadate CD. *See* Methylphenidate
Metadate ER. *See* Methylphenidate
Metagonimus yokogawai, *see website*
Metalinguistic difficulties, *see website*
Metalloporphyrins, 612
Metal metabolism, defects of, 1389t
Metanephric blastema, *see website*
Metanephrines
 in neuroendocrine tumor-associated diarrhea, *see website*
 in pheochromocytoma, 1942
Metaphase of mitosis, 394-395
Metaphyseal chondrodysplasia
 Jansen-type, 1923
 McKusick type, 2434
Metaphyseal dysplasia, 2446, *see also website*
 Jansen, 2430
 Schmid, 2426-2427, 2426f
Metaphyseal fracture, due to child abuse, 138, 139f
Metaphysis, *see website*
Metapneumovirus, human, 1129-1131, 1130f, 1131t
Metastases, brain, 1753
Metastatic Crohn disease, *see website*
Metatarsal fracture, 2393
 stress, 2418
Metatarsus adductus, 2335, 2335f, 2348
Metatarsus varus, 2335
Metatropic dysplasias, 2435, 2435f
Metered-dose inhaler (MDI), 796-798, *see also website*
Metformin, 1992, 1992t
 for polycystic ovary syndrome, *see website*
Methacholine challenge testing, 768
Methadone
 equianalgesic doses and half-life of, 367t
 maternal addiction to, 624
 for pain management, 365t
  in palliative care, 155t-156t
 poisoning with, 251t, 261
Methamphetamine abue, 683-684
Methanol poisoning, 267-268
 antidote for, 256t-257t
Methaqualone, adolescent use of, 676t
Methemoglobin, 1672
Methemoglobinemia
 acquired, 1673t
 antidote for poisoning with, 256t-257t
 hereditary, 1672-1673, 1673f
 respiratory signs and symptoms of, *see website*
Methenamine silver stain, *see website*
Methicillin, 645t
Methicillin-resistant *Staphylococcus aureus* (MRSA), 907t
 osteomyelitis and, 2397
Methicillin-susceptible *Staphylococcus aureus* (MSSA), 906-907, 907t
Methimazole, 1911-1912
Methionine, defects in metabolism of, 425-429, 426f, 428f, 1319
Methotrexate (MTX)
 for atopic dermatitis, 805
 for cancer therapy, *see website*
 for Crohn disease, 1303
 drug interactions with, *see website*
 for juvenile dermatomyositis, 849
 for juvenile idiopathic arthritis, 837, 838t
 for psoriasis, 2260
 for rheumatic disease, *see website*
 for scleroderma, 853
Methsuximide, dosages for, 2030t
2-Methylacyl CoA racemase deficiency, 465, 466t
Methylcobalamin
 deficiency of, *see website*
 homocystinuria due to defects of, 427, 428f
3-Methylcrotonyl CoA carboxylase deficiency, 433
Methyldopa, 1645t
Methylene blue for poisoning, 256t-257t
Methylene chloride, as inhalant, 681t
Methylene chloride poisoning, 267
Methylenedioxymethamphetamine (MDMA), 675t, 682
Methylenetetrahydrofolate reductase (MTHFR) deficiency, 427
3-Methylglutaconic aciduria, 433
3-Methylglutaconyl CoA hydratase deficiency, 433
Methylin. *See* Methylphenidate
Methylmalonic acidemia, 437-438
 homocystinuria with, 438
Methyl mercury, *see website*
Methylphenidate
 for attention deficit/hyperactivity disorder, 62t, 111t
 for fatigue in palliative care, 155t-156t
Methylprednisolone
 for anaphylaxis, 818t
 for juvenile dermatomyositis, 849
 for rheumatic disease, *see website*
 for systemic lupus erythematosus, 844
Methylprednisone
 for asthma, 746, 794t, 797t-798t
 for multiple sclerosis, 2077
Methyl salicylates toxicity, 251t
Metoclopramide, 155t-156t
 for chemotherapy-associated vomiting, 1244t
 drug interactions with, *see website*
Metoprolol
 for heart failure, *see website*
 for systemic hypertension, 1645t
Metorchis conjunctus, *see website*
Metro-IV. *See* Metronidazole
Metronidazole, *see also website*
 for amebiasis, 1180t, *see also website*
 for balantidiasis, 1183, *see also website*
 for *Clostridium difficile* infection, 995
 for dracunculiasis, 1227
 for giardiasis, *see website*
 for *Helicobacter pylori* gastritis, 1293t
 for infectious diarrhea, 1337t
 for neonatal infection, 645t
 for tetanus, 993
 for trichomoniasis, 1186
 for vulvovaginitis, 1868t
Metrorrhagia, 686t
Mevalonic aciduria, 435-436
Mexican tea, 272t-273t
Mexiletine
 for arrhythmias, 1611t-1612t
 for neuropathic pain, 368t
Meziocillin, *see website*
Mezlin. *See* Meziocillin
Mezlocillin for neonatal infection, 645t
M-FISH. *See* Multicolor fluorescence in situ hybridization (M-FISH)
MFS. *See* Marfan syndrome (MFS)
MGRS. *See* Multicenter Growth Center Study (MGRS)
MHC. *See* Major histocompatibility complex (MHC)
MIC. *See* Minimum inhibitory concentration (MIC)
Micafungin, 1054t, 1056t, *see also website*
Michel anomaly, 2189-2190
Michelis-Castrillo syndrome, *see website*
Microadenoma in hyperinsulinemia, 521-522
Microalbuminuria, 1800
 with type 2 diabetes mellitus, 1993t
Microangiopathy, thrombotic, 1713-1714
Microarray technology, *see website*
Microbiology, diagnostic, 881, 903, *see also website*
 pulmonary, *see also website*
  in cystic fibrosis, 1490
Microcephaly, 2007-2008, 2007t
 in neurologic examination, *see website*
Microcoria, 2155
Microcornea, *see website*
Microcytic anemia, 1658, *see also website*
 iron-deficiency, 1655-1658
 megaloblastic, 1655, *see also website*
Microdeletion, 406, 408t, *see website*
Microdeletion syndrome, 396
Microdontia, 1250
Microduplication, genetic, 406, *see also website*
Micrognathia in juvenile idiopathic arthritis, 832
Microimmunofluorescence (MIF)
 in *Chlamydophila pneumoniae*, 1034-1035
 in psittacosis, *see website*
Microlithiasis, pulmonary alveolar, 1463, *see also website*
Micronutrients
 deficiencies of, 211, *see also website*
  in malnutrition, 172
 dietary reference intakes for, *see website*
 management of in protein-energy malnutrition, 178t
 supplementation for chronic diarrhea, 1345
Micropenis, 1856-1857, 1857f
Microphthalmia with linear defects (MLS), 408t
Microscopic polyangiitis (MPA), 874-876, 874t
Microscopy in bacterial and fungal infection diagnosis, *see website*
Microspherophakia, 2172
Microsporidia, 1185, *see website*
Microsporum skin infections, 2309-2313
Microtia, *see website*
Microvillus inclusion disease, 1306t, 1311
 chronic diarrhea with, 1341, 1342f
Midazolam
 for anesthesia, *see website*
 for burn injury, 355
 for intubation, 321t
 for neonatal seizures, 2037
 for status epilepticus, 303, 2038-2039, 2039t
MIDD. *See* Maternally inherited diabetes and deafness (MIDD)
Middle adolescence, growth and development during, 653-654
Middle childhood. *See* School-age child
Middle ear
 congenital malformations of, 2196, *see also website*
 traumatic injury to, *see website*
 tuberculosis of, 1004-1005
Middle-ear effusion (MEE), 2199-2200
 acute otitis media *versus* otitis media with effusion and, 2203-2204
Midget, 2335
Midgut, 1273
 incomplete rotation of, 1280-1281, 1280f
Midline nasal masses, congenital, 1431, 1431f
Mid-upper arm circumference (MUAC), in nutrition assessment, 172
Mid ureteral obstruction, 1842
MIF. *See* Microimmunofluorescence (MIF)
Mifepristone, 699
Miglitol, 1992t
Migraine, 2039-2046
 abdominal, 1346t, 2042
 classification and clinical manifestations of, 2040-2042, 2040t-2041t
 diagnosis and differential diagnosis of, 2042-2043, 2043t
 epidemiology of, 2040
 familial hemiplegic, *see website*
 strokelike events *versus*, 2085
 syncope induced by, *see website*
 treatment of, 2043-2045, 2044t
 vomiting prophylaxis for, 1244t

Migrant children, 7
effects of relocation on, *see website*
health services for, 10
Migrant Health Program, 10
Migrating partial epilepsy, 2022-2023
Migratory glossitis, 1261, 2298-2299
Migratory polyarthritis in acute rheumatic fever, 921-922
MII. *See* Multichannel intraluminal impedance (MII)
Milaria crystallina, 2287, 2287f
Milaria profunda, 2287-2288
Milaria rubra, 2287
Miliaria, 2287-2288, 2287f
Miliary tuberculosis, 1002, 1003f, 1004, 1009, 2308
Milium, 2218, *see website*
Milk
cow's
allergy to, 821, 821t
hypersensitivity, 1498-1499
type 1 diabetes mellitus and, 1972
human
formula *versus*, 161t
protective effects of, 161t
Milk allergy, 821, 821t
Milk line, *see website*
Milkmaid's grip, 922
Milk of magnesia
for constipation maintenance therapy, 74t
for fecal disimpaction, 74t
Milk of molasses enema, 74t
Millard rotation-advancement technique, 1252-1253
Millennium Development Goals (MDGs), 1, 173-174
Miller-Dieker syndrome, 408t
Miller-Fisher syndrome, 2143-2144
Milligrams to milliequivalents per liter conversions, *see website*
Milrinone
for cardiac output maintenance and post-resuscitation stabilization, 294t
for cardiogenic shock, 313t
for heart failure, *see website*
Miltefosine, 1190
Milwaukee brace
for Scheuermann disease, 2372
for scoliosis, 2367
Milwaukee Protocol, 1155
Minamata disease, *see website*
Mineralocorticoid receptors, 1923, *see also website*
Mineralization in dental development, *see website*
Mineralocorticoids
actions of, *see website*
for 21-hydroxylase deficiency, 1934
Mineral oil
for constipation maintenance therapy, 74t
for fecal disimpaction, 74t
Minerals
absorption disorders of, 1305t, 1319
deficiency in metabolic bone disease, *see website*
supplemental in cystic fibrosis, 1495
Miner's tea, 272t-273t
Minicore myopathy, 2117-2118
Minimal alveolar concentration (MAC), of inhalation anesthetic, *see website*
Minimal change nephrotic syndrome (MCNS), 1803t, 1804
Minimal residual disease (MRD), 1737
Minimum bactericidal concentration (MBC), *see website*
Minimum inhibitory concentration (MIC), *see website*
Minimum urine osmolality, *see website*
Minocycline, *see also website*
for acne, 2325t
for Hansen disease, *see website*
Minor, mature, 664-665, *see website*
Minor consent laws, *see website*
Minority children, 6-7
Minoxidil
for hypertensive emergencies, 1646t
for systemic hypertension, 1645t
Minute volume (V_T), 316-317, *see also website*
Miosis, congenital, 2155
Miracidia, 1230
Miralax, 155t-156t
Miscarriage, parvovirus B19 infection and, 1653
Missense mutation, genetic, *see website*
Missense mutations of *MPL*, 1689
Mistletoe, potential toxicity of, 272t-273t
Mitochondrial acetoacetyl CoA thiolase deficiency, 433-434, 434f
Mitochondrial chromosome, *see website*
Mitochondrial disease, 506, 507t-509t, 508f
diabetes mellitus due to, 1994-1995
hypoparathyroidism associated with, 1918
Mitochondrial DNA depletion syndrome (MDS), 1406, 2132
Shwachman-Diamond syndrome with, 1687
Mitochondrial encephalopathies, 2065-2068, 2065t
Mitochondrial fatty acid β-oxidation disorders, 456-492, 457t, 458f-459f
Mitochondrial hepatopathies, 1405-1408, 1406t-1407t
Mitochondrial 3-hydroxy-3-methylglutaryl CoA synthase deficiency, 435
Mitochondrial inheritance, 390-391, 390f-391f, 391t
Mitochondrial myopathy, 1630, 2113t, 2132
Mitochondrial myopathy, encephalopathy, lactic acidosis, and strokelike episodes (MELAS), 391, 391t, 2066, 2113t, 2131
Mitochondrial respiratory chain defects, 506, 507t-509t, 508f
Mitochondrial trifunctional protein (TFP) deficiency, 457t, 460
Mitosis, 394-395
Mitral valve
cleft in anterior leaflet of, 1554
coarctation with disease of, 1570
Mitral valve insufficiency, 1571-1572, 1571t
of rheumatic origin, 1627
Mitral valve prolapse, 1572
Mitral valve regurgitation, 1571, 1571t
Mitral valve stenosis, 1570, *see also website*
of rheumatic origin, 1627-1628
Mitral valvuloplasty, 1572
Mitrofanoff procedure, *see website*
Mixed amphetamine salts, 111t
Mixed connective tissue disease (MCTD), *see website*
Mixed gonadal dysgenesis, 1954-1955
Mixed hearing loss, 2188
Mixed venous oxygen saturation, in shock, 309-310
MJD. *See* Machado-Joseph disease (MJD)
ML. *See* Mucosal leishmaniasis (ML)
MLC. *See* Myosin light chain (MLC)
MLD. *See* Metachromatic leukodystrophy (MLD)
MLS. *See* Microphthalmia with linear defects (MLS)
M-mode echocardiography, 1541, 1542f
MMR. *See* Measles, mumps, rubella (MMR) vaccine
MMRV. *See* Measles, mumps, rubella, varicella (MMRV) vaccine
MN. *See* Membranous nephropathy (MN)
Mobility, tympanic membrane, *see website*
Mobitz type 1 heart block, 1618
Möbius syndrome, 534, 2006, 2160
MOC. *See* Maintenance of Certification (MOC)
Model for Improvement, *see website*
Modeling, bone, 2446
Modified Checklist for Autism in Toddlers (M-CHAT), 41t-43t
Modifier gene, *see website*
MODS. *See* Multiple organ dysfunction syndrome (MODS)
MODY. *See* Maturity-onset diabetes of the young (MODY)
Mold allergens, 769t
Molding of skull, assessment of, *see website*
Molecular defects
liver disease caused by, 1383t
in persistent hyperinsulinemic hypoglycemia, 522t
Molecular diagnostics, *see website*
Molecular genetics, fundamentals of, *see website*
Molecularly targeted therapy for cancer, *see website*
Mollaret meningitis, 1101
Molluscum contagiosum, 1867t-1868t, 1868f, 2316-2317, 2316f-2317f
Molybdenum, *see website*
Molybdenum cofactor deficiency, 429, *see website*
Mometasone
for allergic rhinitis, 778t-779t, 779-780
for asthma, 795t
MOMP. *See* Major outer membrane protein (MOMP)
Monamine neurotransmitter metabolism, disorders of, 2059
Mondini anomaly, 2189-2190, 2191f
Mongolian spots, 2219, 2219f
child abuse bruising *versus*, 137
in newborn, 533
Monilethrix, 2292-2293, 2292f
Moniliformis moniliformis, *see website*
Monitoring, home
in mechanical ventilation, 1525
for sudden infant death syndrome prevention, 1428-1429
in type 1 diabetes mellitus, 1983, 1983t
Monkeypox, 2459-2460
Monkshood toxicity, 269t, 272t-273t
Monoamine oxidase inhibitors (MAOIs)
poisoning with, 251t, 265-266
in serotonin syndrome, 265t
Monoamine oxidase (MAO) deficiency, 447
Monochorionic twins, 554, 554t
Monoclonal antibodies, 882t, 883
for cancer therapy, *see website*
in renal transplantation, *see website*
Monocular elevation deficiency, 2160, 2160f
Monocytes, 632, 739, *see also website*
reference values for, *see website*
Monocytosis, *see website*
Monogenic type 1 diabetes mellitus, 1970
Monomethylhydrazine intoxication, *see website*
Mononeuritis multiplex, 2140
Mononuclear phagocyte system, *see website*
Mononucleosis, 1110-1115
Mononucleosis-like illness, 1110
Monophonic wheeze, 1456
Monosomy, 381, 399-400
malignancy susceptibility associated with, *see website*
Monozygotic twins, 553-554
Montelukast
for asthma, 794t, 795-796
for urticaria and angioedema, 815t
Montenegro skin test, 1187
Mood disorders, 82
bipolar disorder as, 85-87, 85t
dysthymic disorder as, 87, 87t
major depression as, 82-85, 83t-84t
Mood stabilizers, 63, 64t
Moral development
during adolescence, 649-651, 650t
during middle childhood, 38
during preschool years, 35-36
Moral thinking, 35-36
in adolescent, 649-651

Moraxella catarrhalis, 944, 2201, *see also website*
in pneumonia, 1475t
Morbidity(ies)
among children, 4-5
overview of, 532, *see also website*
perinatal and neonatal, *see website*
Morbillivirus, 1069
Morning glory disc anomaly, *see website*
Moro reflex
in hypoxic-ischemic encephalopathy, 571t
in neurologic examination, *see website*
Morphea, 850, 851f, 851t, 2275-2276, 2276f
Morphine
equianalgesic doses and half-life of, 367t
for intubation, 321t
for pain management, 365t
in burn injury, 355
in palliative care, 155t-156t
possible adverse reactions to in premature infant, 563t
urine screening for adolescent abuse of, 676t
Morquio disease, 511f, 512t, 514
Morquio-Ullrich syndrome, 1531t
Mortality. *See* Death
Mortality rates. *See* Death rates
Morula, 1048
Mosaicism, 381, 383-385, 412
with Turner syndrome, 1953
45,X/46,XY, 409-410, 410t
Moseley straight-line graph, *see website*
Mosquitoes
in arboviral encephalitis transmission, 1141-1142
avoidance during travel, *see website*
in dengue fever transmission, 1147
in hemorrhagic fevers transmission, 1150t
in yellow fever transmission, *see website*
Mossy fibers, 2024-2025
"Mother yaw," *see website*
Motility
esophageal, *see website*
congenital intestinal pseudo-obstruction and, 1283t
ocular, 2150
Motility disorders
diarrhea with, 1245, 1245t
esophageal, 1263-1264
intestinal, 1283-1287
chronic diarrhea due to, 1341
Motion, equation of, 321-322, 322f
Motion sickness, 1244t
Motivational therapy for nocturnal incontinence, 1852
Motor apraxia, congenital ocular, 2161
Motor dysmetria, ocular, 2162
Motor function, *see also website*
development of during first 2 years, 27t
effects of cancer and its therapy, *see website*
neurologic examination of, *see website*
Motor neuron disorders, 2132-2138
Motor neuropathies, hereditary, 2138-2140
Motor nystagmus, 2161
Motor seizure, 2019
generalized, 2023
Motor speech disorders, 118-119
Motor tic, 76, *see website*
Motor unit, disorders of. *See* Neuromuscular disorders
Motor vehicle injuries, 21-22, 21f, 21t
as leading cause of death, 18
prevention of, *see website*
MOTT. *See* Mycobacteria other than tuberculosis (MOTT)
Mouse mite, 1044
Mouth
effects of malnutrition on, 175t
newborn assessment of, 534
trench, 2299, *see website*
ulcers of in rheumatic disease, *see website*
Mouth-to-mouth ventilation, 282, 282f
Move/family relocation, *see website*
Movement disorders, 2053-2061
ataxias as, 2054t, 2055
chorea, athetosis, tremor as, 2056t-2058t, 2058
dystonia as, 2058-2059, 2060t
seizures and, *see website*
sleep-related, 52-53
Movements, involuntary, assessment in neurologic examination, *see website*
Movement therapy for pain management, 371
Moxifloxacin, *see website*
Moyamoya disease, 2080, 2082f, 2082t
MPA. *See* Microscopic polyangiitis (MPA)
MPGN. *See* Membranoproliferative glomerulonephritis (MPGN)
MPL, missense mutations of, 1689
MPO. *See* Myeloperoxidase (MPO)
M protein antigen in group A streptococci, 910-911, 915
MPS. *See* Mucopolysaccharidoses (MPS)
MPSV. *See* Meningococcal polysaccharide vaccine (MPSV)
MPV17 mutation, 1406-1407
MRA. *See* Magnetic resonance angiography (MRA)
MRC. *See* Magnetic resonance cholangiography (MRC)
MRD. *See* Minimal residual disease (MRD)
MRKH. *See* Mayer-Rokitansky-Küster-Hauser syndrome (MRKH)
MRS. *See* Magnetic resonance spectroscopy (MRS)
MRSA. *See* Methicillin-resistant *Staphylococcus aureus* (MRSA)
MS. *See* Management sciences (MS); Multiple sclerosis (MS)
MSF. *See* Mediterranean spotted fever (MSF)
MS/MS. *See* Tandem mass spectrometry (MS/MS)
MSSA. *See* Methicillin-susceptible *Staphylococcus aureus* (MSSA)
MSUD. *See* Maple syrup urine disease (MSUD)
MTC. *See* Medullary thyroid carcinoma (MTC)
MTHFR. *See* Methylenetetrahydrofolate reductase (MTHFR) deficiency
MTM1 gene, 2115
MTX. *See* Methotrexate (MTX)
MUAC. *See* Mid-upper arm circumference (MUAC), in nutrition assessment
Mucha-Habermann disease, 2260-2261, *see also website*
Muckle-Wells syndrome (MWS), 814, 855t, 858
Mucocele, 2297-2298, 2298f, *see also website*
Mucocutaneous candidiasis, 1056, *see also website*
Mucocutaneous lymph node syndrome, 862-867
Mucocutaneous rash in congenital syphilis, 1017-1018, 1018f
Mucoepidermoid carcinoma, 1504, *see also website*
Mucolipidoses, 484t, 491-492
Mucomyst. *See* *N*-Acetylcysteine
Mucopolysaccharidoses (MPS), 509-516, 510f-511f, 511t-512t
clinical entities of, 510-514, 513f
diagnosis and differential diagnosis of, 514
respiratory insufficiency due to, 1523
skin disorders associated with, 2280, 2280f
treatment of, 514-516, 515t-516t
Mucormycosis, 1069, *see also website*
in pneumonia, 1475t
Mucosa
gastric, *see website*
malabsorption due to defects of, 1305t
peptic ulcer disease and, 1291-1292
nasal, 1429-1430
rectal, prolapse of, 1361
Mucosa associated lymphoid tissue (MALT) lymphoma, 1315
Mucosal disorders
intestinal, 1308, 1311
rectal, 1361
Mucosal leishmaniasis (ML), 1187-1188, *see also website*
Mucosal neuroma syndrome, 1916, *see website*
Mucous membrane disorders, 2297-2299
Muenke syndrome, 2012t
Mulibrey nanism, 1531t
Müllerian anomalies, 1874, *see also website*
amenorrhea due to, 686, 687t
Müllerian duct syndrome, persistent, 1964-1965
Müllerian inhibiting substance, 1872t, *see also website*
Multicenter Growth Center Study (MGRS), *see website*
Multicentric Castleman disease, 1121
Multichannel cochlear implant, 2196, 2196t
Multichannel intraluminal impedance (MII), *see website*
in gastroesophageal reflux disease, 1267
Multicolor fluorescence in situ hybridization (M-FISH), 396
Multicore myopathy, 2117-2118
Multicystic dysplastic kidney (MCDK), 1827-1828, 1828f
Multidisciplinary team. *See* Team approach
Multi-dose activated charcoal (MDAC), 257-258
Multifactorial inheritance, 381, 393-394, 393f
Multiple endocrine neoplasia (MEN), type 1, 527
hyperparathyroidism with, 1920-1921
malignancy susceptibility associated with, *see website*
Zollinger-Ellison syndrome with, 1294
Multiple endocrine neoplasia (MEN), type 2A, 1916
pheochromocytoma with, 1942
thyroid tumors and, *see website*
Multiple endocrine neoplasia (MEN), type 2B, 1916, *see also website*
Multiple epiphyseal dysplasias (MED), 2427
Multiple gestation pregnancy, 553-555, 554t, 555f
Multiple hamartoma syndrome, 2298
Multiple organ dysfunction syndrome (MODS) in shock, 305, 311t-312t
Multiple physician model for emergency care, *see website*
Multiple sclerosis (MS), 2076, 2077t, 2078f
Multiple sulfatase deficiency, 490
Multivisceral graft in intestinal transplantation, *see website*
Mumps, 1078-1081, 1079f-1080f
in child-care setting, *see website*
exclusion from day care due to, *see website*
type 1 diabetes mellitus development and, 1971
in viral meningoencephalitis, 2096
Mumps vaccine, 881t, 884t, 1081
Munchausen syndrome by proxy, 146-147, 527
Munro-Kellie doctrine, 297f
Mupirocin, *see website*
Murine typhus, 1039t-1040t, 1046-1047
Murmur, heart
auscultation of, 1535-1536
of mitral insufficiency, 1571-1572
sports participation and, 2402t-2404t
Muromonab CD-3 in renal transplantation, *see website*
Muscarine poisoning, *see website*
Muscle(s)
brain malformations and development of, 2118
congenital hypothyroidism and, 1898-1899
developmental disorders of, 2112-2119
drug absorption in, *see website*
effects of malnutrition on, 175t
glycogenoses disorders of, 494t-495t, 499-501, 500f
imaging of, 2111

Muscle(s) *(Continued)*
insulin level effects on, 1975t
mitochondrial encephalomyopathy and, 2065t
neuromuscular disorders of (*See* Neuromuscular disorders)
phosphorylase kinase deficiency in, 498
Staphylococcus aureus abscess in, 905
Muscle adenosine monophosphate deaminase deficiency, *see website*
Muscle atrophy, assessment in neurologic examination, *see website*
Muscle biopsy, 2111-2112
in Duchenne and Becker muscular dystrophy, 2120, 2120f
in myasthenia gravis, 2134
in neuromuscular disorders, 2110t
Muscle bulk assessment in neurologic examination, *see website*
Muscle-derived enzymes in juvenile dermatomyositis, 848, 848t
Muscle-eye-brain disease of Santavuori, 2127
Muscle fibers, respiratory, *see website*
Muscle glycogen synthase deficiency, 498
Muscle pain in neuromuscular disorders, 2109
Muscle phosphofructokinase deficiency, 501
Muscle phosphorylase deficiency, 500-501
Muscle receptors in respiration regulation, *see website*
Muscle relaxants
for anesthesia, *see website*
in rapid sequence intubation, 287t
Muscle rigidity assessment in neurologic examination, *see website*
Muscle spasm, treatment of in palliative care, 155t-156t
Muscle spasticity assessment in neurologic examination, *see website*
Muscle strength assessment in neurologic examination, *see website*
Muscle tone
assessment
in neurologic examination, *see website*
in neuromuscular disorders, 2109
in hypoxic-ischemic encephalopathy, 571t
Muscle wasting in malabsorption syndromes, 1305, 1306f
Muscle weakness
in Becker muscular dystrophy, 2119
in Duchenne muscular dystrophy, 2119
in Guillain-Barré syndrome, 2143
in juvenile dermatomyositis, 847, 848t, 849
in myotonic muscular dystrophy, 2123, 2123f
in neuromuscular disorders, 2110t-2111t, 2115t
Muscular atrophy, spinal, 2136-2138, 2136t, 2137f
chronic severe respiratory insufficiency with, 1519-1520, 1520t
Muscular dysgenesis (proteus syndrome myopathy), 2119
Muscular dystrophy(ies), 2119-2129
Becker, 2119-2123
dilated cardiomyopathy with, 1630
congenital, 2123-2126, 2128f
Duchenne, 2119-2123, 2120f-2121f
cardiac manifestations of, 1531t
chronic severe respiratory insufficiency with, 1519
dilated cardiomyopathy with, 1630
Emery-Dreifuss, 2123
facioscapulohumeral, 2126
limb-girdle, 2126, 2126t
myotonic, 2123, 2123f
maternal, *see website*
Muscular relaxation as goal of anesthesia, *see website*
Muscular torticollis, congenital, 2377-2379
Musculoskeletal disorders
orthopedic (*See* Orthopedic problems)
due to sports injury (*See* Sports injuries)
Musculoskeletal pain syndromes, 876-880, 877t-878t
complex regional pain syndrome as, 879-880, 879t
erythromelalgia as, 880, 880f
fibromyalgia as, 878-879, 879f
growing pains as, 878
Mushroom poisoning, 2454, *see also website*
gastroenteritis due to, 1328t-1329t
Music therapy for pain management, 371
Muslim population
cultural values associated with, *see website*
disease beliefs or practices of, *see website*
Mustard, in terrorism, *see website*
Mustard procedure, 1586-1587
Mutations, genetic, *see website*
Mutilating keratoderma, 2273
Mutism, selective, 79, 118
MVK gene mutations, 857-858
MWS. *See* Muckle-Wells syndrome (MWS)
Myalgia in neuromuscular disorders, 2109
Myasthenia gravis, 2132-2136, 2133t
clinical manifestations of, 2132-2133
complications of, 2135
laboratory findings and diagnosis of, 2133-2134
maternal, *see website*
poliovirus infection *versus*, 1085t
prognosis for, 2135
treatment of, 2135, 2135t
Mycetoma, *see website*
Mycifradin. *See* Neomycin
MYCN oncogene, 1754, 1757
Mycobacterial infection
DNA probes in, *see website*
Hansen disease as, 1011, *see also website*
HIV-related, 1163-1164
nontuberculous, 1011-1016
in cystic fibrosis, 1494
predisposition to due to immunodeficiency, 716t
treatment of, 996, *see also website*
tuberculosis as, 996-1011
Mycobacteria other than tuberculosis (MOTT), 1011-1016
Mycobacterium abscessus, 1014
in cystic fibrosis infection, 1494
treatment of, *see website*
Mycobacterium avium complex (MAC), 1011-1014, 1014f
cutaneous, 2308
in cystic fibrosis infection, 1494
HIV-related, 1163-1164
prophylaxis for, 1174, 1175t-1176t
treatment of, *see website*
Mycobacterium bovis
cutaneous, 2307-2308
Mycobacterium chelonae, *see website*
Mycobacterium fortuitum group, 2308, *see also website*
Mycobacterium genavense, *see website*
Mycobacterium haemophilus, *see website*
Mycobacterium kansasii
in cutaneous infection, 2308
in cystic fibrosis infection, 1494
treatment of, *see website*
Mycobacterium lentiflavum, *see website*
Mycobacterium leprae, 1011, *see also website*
predisposition to infection due to immunodeficiency, 716t
treatment of, *see website*
Mycobacterium marinum
in skin infection, 2308, 2308f
treatment of, *see website*
Mycobacterium scrofulaceum skin infection, 2308
Mycobacterium tuberculosis, 996-1011, 996f-997f. *See also* Tuberculosis (TB)
clinical manifestations and diagnosis of, 1002-1007, 1003f
cutaneous, 2307-2308
Mycobacterium tuberculosis (Continued)
epidemiology of, 996-998, 998t
etiology of, 996
HIV-related, *see website*
prophylaxis for, 1175t-1176t
immunity to, 1000-1001
inflammatory bowel disease *versus*, 1298t
maternal, 1000
breast-feeding and, 540t
fetal and neonatal effects of, *see website*
neonatal, 632t
in newborn, 1000
pathogenesis of, 998-1001, 999f-1000f
in pneumonia, 1475t
prevention of, 1010-1011
transmission of, 998
treatment of, 1007-1010, 1008t, *see website*
tuberculin skin testing for, 1001, 1002t
vaccine for travel, *see website*
Mycobacterium ulcerans, 1013
cutaneous, 2308
treatment of, *see website*
Mycophenolate, *see also website*
for atopic dermatitis, 805
for nephrotic syndrome, 1805
for rheumatic disease, *see website*
Mycoplasma genitalium, 1032-1033
Mycoplasma hominis, 1032-1033
maternal, *see website*
Mycoplasmal infections
genital, 1032-1033
in infective endocarditis, 1624t
Mycoplasma pneumoniae, 1029-1032, 1031f
in pneumonia, 1475t, 1476
in Stevens-Johnson syndrome, 2242
MYC proto-oncogene, *see website*
Mydriasis, congenital, 2155
Myelination
during age 0-2 months, 26-27
of optic nerve fibers, 2181
Myelitis
radiation, *see website*
transverse, 2107, 2107t
poliovirus infection *versus*, 1085t
Myelocytes, reference values for, *see website*
Myelodysplastic syndromes, 748t
hematopoietic stem cell transplantation for, 758-759
Myelogenous leukemia, chronic, 748t, 1739
hematopoietic stem cell transplantation for, 758
Myeloid cells, acquired disorders of, 747, 748t
Myeloid leukemia, acute. *See* Acute myeloid leukemia (AML)
Myeloid precursor cells, intrinsic disorders of, 747, 748t
Myelomeningocele, 2000-2002, 2001f
with Arnold-Chiari type II malformation, 1522
Myelomonocytic leukemia, juvenile, 758
Myelopathy, human T-lymphotropic virus in, *see website*
Myeloperoxidase (MPO), *see website*
deficiency of, 742t, 745
Myelopoiesis, ineffective, 750-751
Myeloproliferative disorders, Down syndrome with, 1738
Myelosuppression, due to chemotherapy, *see website*
Myenteric plexus neuropathies, 2143
Myf5 gene, 2112
MYF6 gene, 2112
MYH9-related thrombocytopenia, 1720
Myoadenylate deaminase deficiency, *see website*
Myocardial biopsy in heart transplantation monitoring, *see website*
Myocardial disease, 1628-1635, 1630t
arrhythmogenic right ventricular cardiomyopathy as, 1633-1634
dilated cardiomyopathy as, 1629f, 1630-1631
etiology of, 1629t

Myocardial disease *(Continued)*
hypertrophic cardiomyopathy as, 1631-1632, 1632f
left ventricular noncompaction as, 1633-1634, 1634f
myocarditis as, 1634-1635, 1634t
restrictive cardiomyopathy as, 1633, 1633f
Myocarditis, 1629t, 1634-1635, 1634t
in acute rheumatic fever, 922
enterovirus, 1089, 1091
in Kawasaki disease, 864
measles, 1072
due to mumps, 1080
parvovirus B19 in, 1096
sudden death due to, 1620
Myoclonic astatic epilepsy, 2024
Myoclonic seizure, neonatal, 2034
Myoclonus
benign sleep, *see website*
epilepsy and ragged red fibers (MERRF), 2067
in hypoxic-ischemic encephalopathy, 571t
neonatal sleep, *see website*
in newborn, 532-533
in seizure evaluation, 2015-2016
Myoclonus dystonia, 2059
Myoclonus epilepsy and ragged red fibers (MERRF), 391, 391t, 2067, 2113t
Myoclonus of early infancy, benign, *see website*
Myocytes in cardiac development, 1528
MYOD1 gene, 2112
Myofascial pain disorders, 375
Myofibrillar myopathies, 2118, 2118f
Myogenic factor 5 gene, 2112
Myogenic regulatory genes, 2112-2113, 2113t
Myogenin gene, 2112
Myomosphorylase deficiency, *see website*
Myonecrosis, *see website*
Myopathic gait, *see website*
Myopathy
central core, 2117-2118
endocrine, 2129-2130
intestinal, 1283
lipid, 2132, *see also website*
metabolic, 2130-2132
mitochondrial, 2132
myofibrillar, 2118, 2118f
myotubular, 2114, 2114f, 2115t
nemaline rod, 2116-2117, 2116f-2117f
proteus syndrome, 2119
reversible infantile cytochrome C oxidase deficiency, 2066-2067
sports participation and, 2402t-2404t
steroid-induced, 2129-2130, 2129t
thyroid, 2129
toxic, 2129-2130, 2129t
Myopia, 2150-2151
sports participation and, 2402t-2404t
Myosin light chain (MLC), *see website*
Myositis, enteroviruses in, 1092
Myostatin gene, 2112-2113
Myotina in myotonic muscular dystrophy, 2123-2124
Myotonia congenita, 2113t, 2125, 2125t
Myotonia fluctuans, 2125t
Myotonia permanens, 2125t
Myotonic chondrodystrophy, 2125
Myotonic muscular dystrophy, 2123, 2123f
maternal, *see website*
Myotubular myopathy, 2114, 2114f, 2115t
MyPyramid, 166, 166f
Myringitis, bullous, 2199
Myringotomy, 2208
insertion of tympanostomy tubes with, 2208-2210, 2213
"My Wishes," 151
Myxedematous syndrome, 1907
Myxoma, cardiac, *see website*

N
Na^+. *See* Sodium
NAAT. *See* Nucleic acid amplification testing (NAAT)
Nabilone. *See* Tetrahydrocannabinol (THC)
N-Acetylglutamate (NAG) synthetase deficiencies, 448f, 449-451
NADH cytochrome B5 reductase deficiency, 1673
NADPH. *See* Nicotinamide-adenine dinucleotide phosphate (NADPH)
Naegleria meningoencephalitis, 1178, *see also website*
NAEYC. *See* National Accreditation for the Education of Young Children (NAEYC)
Nafarelin, 690-691
Nafcil. *See* Nafcillin
Nafcillin, *see website*
for bacterial meningitis, 2093t
for cystic fibrosis lung infection, 1492t
for infective endocarditis, 1625t
for neonatal infection, 645t
for osteomyelitis, 2397
for septic arthritis, 2400
for *Staphylococcus aureus*, 907t
NAFLD. *See* Nonalcoholic fatty liver disease (NAFLD)
NAG. *See* N-Acetylglutamate (NAG) synthetase deficiencies
Nagayama spots, 1118
Nail(s)
disorders of, 2293-2297, 2294t
changes in nail color as, 2294-2295, 2295f
due to infection, 2296, 2296f
ingrown toenail as, 2343
paronychial inflammation as, 2296-2297, 2297f
separation as, 2295, 2295f-2296f
in size or shape, 2293-2294, 2294f
with skin disease, 2295-2296
trachyonychia as, 2296
effects of malnutrition on, 175t
hypoplastic, *see website*
ingrown, 2297
juvenile dermatomyositis and, 847, 847f
morphology of, *see website*
spoon, 2294f
Nail color, changes in, 2294-2295, 2295f
Nail-patella syndrome, 2293-2294, 2431-2432
Nail pitting
in alopecia areata, 2291, 2291f
in psoriatic arthritis, *see website*
Nail separation, 2295, 2295f-2296f
NAIP gene, 2137
Na^+,K^+-ATPase. *See* Sodium-potassium adenosine triphosphatase (Na^+,K^+-ATPase)
Nalbuphine, 367t
Nalidixic acid, *see website*
Naloxone
in neonatal resuscitation, 576
for pediatric resuscitation and arrhythmias, 294t
for poisoning, 256t-257t
Nanophyetus salmincola, *see website*
Naphazoline hydrochloride for allergic conjunctivitis, 811t
Naphcon-A. *See* Naphazoline hydrochloride
Naprosyn for pain management, 364t
Naproxen
for dysmenorrhea, 691t
for juvenile idiopathic arthritis, 838t
for rheumatic disease, *see website*
for spondyloarthritides, *see website*
Naproxen sodium for migraine, 2043
Naratriptan for migraine, 2044t
Narcolepsy, 53
Narcolepsy-cataplexy syndrome, *see website*
Narcosis as delivery room emergency, 575
Narcotics
adverse reaction to, 828
pharmacokinetics of, *see website*
NARP syndrome, 391t, 2067
Narrative therapy, 66
Narrow complex tachycardia, 288-289
Nasacort. *See* Triamcinolone
Nasal cannula oxygen, 319
Nasal continuous positive airway pressure (CPAP), 51
Nasalcrom. *See* Cromolyn sodium
Nasal hypoplasia, 1430
Nasal inhaled corticosteroids, 778t-780t, 779-780
Nasal masses, midline congenital, 1431, 1431f
Nasal obstruction in common cold, 1435
Nasal polyps, 1433, 1433f
in cystic fibrosis, 1496
Nasal septum, congenital defects of, 1430
Nasarel. *See* Flunisolide
Nasogastric tube feeding, 990
Nasojejunal tube feeding, 990
Nasolacrimal duct obstruction, 2165
Nasonex. *See* Mometasone
Nasopharyngeal airway for respiratory distress and failure, 319
Nasopharynx
angiofibroma of, 1432-1433
cancer of, 1773
Epstein-Barr virus-associated, 1111, 1112t
Neisseria meningitidis in, 929-930
Nasotracheal aspiration, *see website*
Natal teeth, 1251
Nateglinide, 1992t
National Accreditation for the Education of Young Children (NAEYC), *see website*
National Cancer Institute cancer trials, *see website*
National Cholesterol Education Program (NCEP), 479-480
National Cooperative Group Program, cancer mortality rate reduction due to, *see website*
National Hansen's Disease Program, *see website*
National Immunization Days (NIDs), 1087
National Institutes of Health (NIH)
on anaphylaxis diagnosis, 817, 817t
on asthma management, 785-786, 789t-790t, 791-792, 792t
National organizations involved in quality improvement, *see website*
National Vaccine Injury Compensation Program (NVICP), 886
Native American population
actinic prurigo in, 2257
cultural values associated with, *see website*
death rates for, 3t
disease beliefs or practices of, *see website*
health services for, 10
injuries in, 20
as special risk population, 6-7
NAT2 polymorphism, *see website*
Natriuretic peptide
atrial, 1882, *see website*
brain, in pulmonary edema, 1469
B-type, in heart failure, *see website*
Natural disaster, drowning during, 343
Natural immunity, *see website*
Natural killer (NK) cells, 722
abnormalities of
evaluation of, 722
inheritance in, *see website*
fetal development of, *see website*
in hematopoietic stem cell transplantation alloreactivity, *see website*
interaction with other immune cells, *see website*
in neonatal immunity, 632
postnatal, *see website*
Nausea
in appendicitis, 1350, 1351t
due to opioids, 366t
postoperative, *see website*
treatment in palliative care, 155t-157t, 158
Navajo neurohepatopathy (NNH), 1406-1407
Navicular stress fracture, 2418
NBAS. *See* Newborn Behavior Assessment Scale (NBAS)
N-carbamyl-β-amino aciduria, *see website*
NCEP. *See* National Cholesterol Education Program (NCEP)

NCLs. *See* Neuronal ceroid lipofuscinoses (NCLs)
NCV. *See* Nerve conduction velocity (NCV)
NDI. *See* Nephrogenic diabetes insipidus (NDI)
Nearsightedness, 2150-2151
Nebcin. *See* Tobramycin
Nebulizer
  for anaphylaxis drug delivery, 818t
  for asthma drug delivery, 797t-798t, 798
  for croup therapy, 1448
NEC. *See* Neonatal necrotizing enterocolitis (NEC)
Necator americanus, 1218-1221, *see website*
Neck
  newborn assessment of, 534-535
  orthopedic problems of, 2377-2382
    cervical anomalies and instabilities as, 2380-2382, 2381t
    in Down syndrome, 2381-2382, 2382f
    Kippel-Feil syndrome as, 2379-2380, 2380f
    in 22q11.2 deletion syndrome, 2382, 2382f
    torticollis in, 2377-2379, 2378f, 2378t
  sports injuries of, 2419-2420
    due to football, *see website*
  webbed, with Turner syndrome, 1952-1953
Necrobiosis lipoidica, 2275, 2275f
Necrolysis, toxic epidermal, 826, 827t, 2243-2244
Necrolytic migratory erythema (NME), *see website*
Necrosis
  acute tubular, 1819
  cerebral, due to radiation therapy, *see website*
  cold-induced fat, 358
  renal cortical, 1818
  subcutaneous fat, 2284, 2284f
    hypercalcemia with, 1922
Necrotizing encephalomyopathy, subacute, 506-509, 2067
Necrotizing enterocolitis, neonatal, 569, 601-603, 602f, 602t
Necrotizing external otitis, 2197
Necrotizing fasciitis, 2301-2302
  anaerobic, *see website*
  group A streptococcal, 919
Necrotizing periodontal disease, 1257-1258
Necrotizing pneumonia, *Staphylococcus aureus* in, 905
Necrotizing ulcerative gingivitis, 1260t, 2299, *see also website*
Nedocromil sodium
  for allergic conjunctivitis, 811t
  for allergic disease, 771-772
  for asthma, 794t, 796
Needle exposure, infections via, *see website*
Needle length for vaccine, 886
NeF. *See* Nephritic factor (NeF)
NegGram. *See* Nalidixic acid
Neglect, 135-136, 140. *See also* Abuse and neglect
Neisseria
  Moraxella catarrhalis versus, *see website*
  predisposition to infection due to immunodeficiency, 716t
Neisseria gonorrhoeae, 935-940
  clinical manifestations of, 937
  complications of, 939
  in conjunctivitis, 2166
  diagnosis of, 937-938
  epidemiology of, 935-936
  etiology of, 935
  genital culture of, *see website*
  maternal, *see website*
  neonatal, 632t
  pathogenesis and pathology of, 936-937
  prevention of, 939-940
  prognosis for, 939
  prophylaxis following rape, 704, 704t
  treatment of, 712t, 938-939
  in vulvovaginitis, 1865, 1868t
Neisseria meningitidis, 929-935
  in child-care setting, *see website*
  clinical manifestations of, 931-932, 932f
  complications of, 933
  diagnosis of, 932
  differential diagnosis of, 932
  epidemiology of, 930
  etiology of, 929-930
  host factors in, 931
  immunity to, 931
  in meningitis, 2087-2089
    prevention of, 2095
  neonatal, 632t
  pathogenesis of, 930-931
  in pneumonia, 1475t
  prevention of, 933-935, 934t
  prognosis for, 933
  in septic arthritis, 2398
  treatment of, 932-933, 933t
  vaccine for, 934-935
Nelfinavir for HIV infection, 1168t-1171t
Nelson syndrome, 1941
Nemaline rod myopathy, 2113t, 2115t, 2116-2117, 2116f-2117f
NEMO. *See* Nuclear factor κB (NF-κB) essential modulator (NEMO)
Neomycin, *see website*
Neonatal acne, 2327, 2327f
Neonatal behavioral syndrome, 625, 625f
Neonatal cholestasis, 1381-1388
Neonatal circulation, 1529, *see also website*
  transition from fetal to, 1529, *see also website*
Neonatal Intensive Care Unit Neurobehavioral Scale (NNNS), 624, 624t
Neonatal iron storage disease (NISD), 1383, 1393
Neonatal lupus, 845-846, 845f, *see also website*
Neonatal mortality, *see website*
Neonatal necrotizing enterocolitis (NEC), 601-603, 602f, 602t
Neonatal seizures, 2033-2037
Neonatal seizure syndrome, 2035
Neonatal sleep myoclonus, *see website*
Neonatal teeth, 1251
Neonatal tetanus, 991-992
Neonate. *See* Newborn
Neorickettsia sennetsu, 1039t-1040t, 1048
Neo-synephrine. *See* Phenylephrine
Nephritic factor (NeF), 755-756
  in membranoproliferative glomerulonephritis, 1787
Nephritic features, 1804
Nephritic syndrome, acute, 1779-1780
  acute poststreptoccocal glomerulonephritis as, 1783-1785
Nephritis
  acute lobar, 1830, 1830f
  Henoch-Schönlein purpura, 1789
  lupus, 1788-1789
  tubulointerstitial, 1814-1816, 1815t
Nephroblastoma, incidence and survival rates for, 1726t
Nephrocalcinosis, *see website*
Nephrogenic diabetes insipidus (NDI), 1812, 1883-1884
  hypernatremia due to, 213, 213t
  nephrotoxins in, 1817t
Nephrogenic syndrome of inappropriate antidiuresis, 216, 1884
Nephrology. *See also* Urologic disorders
  Alport syndrome in, 1782-1783, 1782f
  cortical necrosis in, 1818
  end-stage renal disease in, 1825-1826, 1826t
  glomerular disease in, 1778, *see also website*
  glomerular filtration in, 1778, *see also website*
  glomerulonephritis in
    associated with infection, 1783-1786, 1783f-1784f, 1785t
    associated with systemic lupus erythematosus, 1788-1789
    membranoproliferative, 1787-1788
Nephrology *(Continued)*
    rapidly progressive, 1789-1790, 1790f, 1790t
  glomerulus anatomy in, 1778, *see also website*
  Goodpasture disease in, 1790-1791, 1791f
  hematuria in
    anatomic abnormalities associated with, 1796-1799
    clinical evaluation of, 1778-1781, 1779t-1780t, 1780f
    due to congenital anomalies, 1796
    hematologic diseases causing, 1795-1796
    due to idiopathic hypercalciuria, 1795
    isolated glomerular disease with recurrent gross, 1781-1783
    lower urinary tract causes of, 1799
    due to renal vein thrombosis, 1794-1795
    in thin basement membrane disease, 1783
    due to trauma, 1799
    upper urinary tract causes of, 1794-1795
    due to vascular abnormalities, 1794
    due to vigorous exercise, 1799
  hemolytic-uremic syndrome in, 1791-1794, 1791t-1792t
  Henoch-Schönlein purpura nephritis in, 1789
  immunoglobulin A nephropathy in, 1781-1782, 1781f
  membranous glomerulopathy in, 1786-1787
  nephrotic syndrome in, 1801-1807, 1803t, 1806t
    congenital, 1807, 1807t
    etiology of, 1802, 1802f, 1802t
    idiopathic, 1803t, 1804-1806, 1804f
    pathophysiology of, 1802-1804
    secondary, 1806
  polycystic kidney disease in
    autosomal dominant, 1798, 1798f
    autosomal recessive, 1796-1798, 1797f, 1797t
  proteinuria in, 1799-1800
    fixed, 1800-1801, 1801t
    orthostatic, 1800
    transient, 1800
  renal failure in, 1818-1826
    acute, 1818-1822, 1818t-1821t
    chronic, 1822-1825, 1823t
  toxic nephropathy in, 1816-1818, 1817t
  transplantation for, 1826, *see also website*
  tubular disorders in
    Bartter syndrome as, 1813-1814, 1813t
    Gitelman syndrome as, 1814
    inherited transport disorders of, 1813-1814
    nephrogenic diabetes insipidus as, 1812
    renal tubular acidosis as, 1808-1811, 1809t, 1811f
    tubulointerstitial nephritis as, 1814-1816, 1815t
Nephroma, mesoblastic, 1760
Nephrons, *see website*
Nephropathy
  diabetic, 1988, 1988t
  HIV-related, 1165-1166
  immunoglobulin A, 1781-1782, 1781f, 1785t
  membranous, 1786-1787
  polyomavirus, *see website*
  post-infection, 1333t
  reflux, 1834-1838
  sickle cell, 1795-1796
  toxic, 1816-1818, 1817t
Nephrotic syndrome, 1801-1807, 1803t, 1806t
  congenital, 1806, 1807t
  etiology of, 1802, 1802f, 1802t
  idiopathic, 1803t, 1804-1806, 1804f
  nephrotoxins in, 1817t
  pathophysiology of, 1802-1804
  secondary, 1806
Nephrotoxicity, 1816-1818
  amphotericin B, *see website*
Nerve ablation and destruction, 373
Nerve agents for terrorism, *see website*
Nerve biopsy, 2112
Nerve blocks. *See* Regional anesthesia

Nerve conduction velocity (NCV), 2110-2111
Nesprin gene, 2123
Netherton disease, *see website*
Netherton syndrome, 2268t, 2271, 2271f-2272f
Netilmicin, *see also website*
  for cystic fibrosis lung infection, 1492t
  for neonatal infection, 645t
Nettleship-Falls ocular albinism, 425
Neural crest tumors, 1520-1521
Neural tube defects (NTDs), 1998-1999, *see website*
  fetal therapy for, 551t, 552
  genetic and environmental factors in, 394
  neuropathic bladder with, *see website*
Neuraminidase inhibitors for influenza, 1123
Neuraminidase protein in influenza virus, 1122
Neuritis
  optic, *see website*
  sciatic, acute traumatic, poliovirus infection, 1085t
Neuroacademic problems, *see website*
Neuroblastoma, 1753-1757
  arthralgia and, *see website*
  clinical manifestations of, 1754, 1756f
  diagnosis of, 1754-1756, 1756f
  diarrhea caused by, *see website*
  epidemiology of, 1753
  incidence and survival rates for, 1726t
  juvenile idiopathic arthritis *versus*, 835
  pathogenesis of, 1754, 1754t-1755t
  pathology of, 1754
  risk factors for, 1727t
  treatment of, 1757
  work-up of, 1731t
Neurocardiogenic syncope, *see website*
Neurocristopathy syndrome, 1754t
Neurocutaneous syndromes, 2046-2053
  incontinentia pigmenti as, 2052-2053, 2053f
  linear nevus syndrome as, 2052
  neurofibromatosis as, 2046-2048, 2047f-2048f, 2048t
  PHACE syndrome as, 2052
  Sturge-Weber syndrome as, 2051-2052, 2051f
  tuberous sclerosis complex as, 2049-2051, 2049f-2050f, 2049t
  von Hippel-Lindau disease as, 2052
Neurocysticercosis, 1234-1237
Neurodegeneration, pantothenate kinase-associated, 2057t, 2060
Neurodegenerative disorders, 2069-2076, 2070t
  adrenoleukodystrophy as, 2073-2074
  Alexander disease as, 2074-2075
  Menkes disease as, 2075
  neuronal ceroid lipofuscinoses as, 2073, 2073t
  Pelizaeus-Merzbacher disease as, 2074
  Rett syndrome as, 2075
  sialidosis as, 2074
  sphingolipidoses as, 2069-2072, 2071f-2072f
  subacute sclerosing panencephalitis as, 2075-2076
Neurodermatitis of external ear canal, 2199
Neurodevelopmental dysfunction, 108, *see also website*
Neurodevelopmental function, 108
Neurodevelopmental variation, 108
Neuroendocrine tumor, chronic diarrhea due to, 1346, *see also website*
Neuroenteric cyst, 1264, 1281
Neuroferritinopathy, 2057t
Neurofibromatosis, 2046-2048, 2047f-2048f, 2048t
  brain tumors associated with, 1747t
  Café-au-lait spots with, 2237
  laryngeal, *see website*
  malignancy susceptibility associated with, *see website*
  pheochromocytoma with, 1942
Neurofibrosarcoma, 1762t
Neurogenic bladder, 1849-1850, 1849f
Neuroirritability treatment of in palliative care, 155t-156t, 157-158
Neuroleptic malignant syndrome (NMS), 65, 2059
Neurologic deficit
  in sickle cell disease, 1667
  in trauma survey, 337
Neurologic disorders, 565-574
  brain abscess as, 2098-2099, 2099f
  central nervous system infections as, 2086-2098
  congenital anomalies of central nervous system as, 1998-2013
    agenesis of corpus callosum as, 2005-2006, 2005f
    agenesis of cranial nerves, 2006-2007
    anencephaly as, 2003
    craniosynostosis as, 2011-2013, 2012t
    disorders of neuronal migration as, 2003-2005, 2003f-2004f
    dysgenesis of posterior fossa, 2006-2007
    encephalocele as, 2002-2003
    holoprosencephaly as, 2005-2006, 2006f
    hydrocephalus as, 2008-2011, 2008t, 2009f-2011f
    meningocele as, 1999
    microcephaly as, 2007-2008, 2007t
    myelomeningocele as, 2000-2002, 2001f
    neural tube defects as, 1998-1999, 1999f
    spina bifida occulta as, 1999, 2000f, 2001t
  coronavirus in, *see website*
  cranial, 565-566, 565f
  demyelinating of central nervous system, 2076-2080, 2076t
    acute disseminated encephalomyelitis as, 2079, 2079f, 2080t
    multiple sclerosis as, 2076, 2077t, 2078f
    neuromyelitis optica as, 2077
  encephalopathies as, 2061-2069
    burn, 2068
    cerebral palsy as, 2061-2065
    HIV, 2068
    hypertensive, 2068
    hypoxic-ischemic, 298f-299f, 301-303, 302f, 569-573
    mitochondrial, 2065-2068, 2065t
    radiation, 2068-2069
    Zellweger syndrome as, 2069
  enteroviruses in, 1091-1092
  evaluation of, 1998, *see also website*
  failure to thrive in, 148t
  general anesthesia and, *see website*
  headaches as, 2039-2046
    migraine, 2040-2045
    secondary, 2045-2046, 2045t
    tension-type, 2046
  intracranial hemorrhage as, 566, 567f, 568t
  manifesting as respiratory distress, 316
  of movement, 2053-2061
    ataxias as, 2054t, 2055
    chorea, athetosis, tremor as, 2056t-2058t, 2058
    dystonia as, 2058-2059, 2060t
  in mucopolysaccharidoses, 515t
  neurocutaneous, 2046-2053
    incontinentia pigmenti as, 2052-2053, 2053f
    linear nevus syndrome as, 2052
    neurofibromatosis as, 2046-2048, 2047f-2048f, 2048t
    PHACE syndrome as, 2052
    Sturge-Weber syndrome as, 2051-2052, 2051f
    tuberous sclerosis complex as, 2049-2051, 2049f-2050f, 2049t
    von Hippel-Lindau disease as, 2052
  neurodegenerative, 2069-2076, 2070t
    adrenoleukodystrophy as, 2073-2074
    Alexander disease as, 2074-2075
    Menkes disease as, 2075
    neuronal ceroid lipofuscinoses as, 2073, 2073t
    Pelizaeus-Merzbacher disease as, 2074
    Rett syndrome as, 2075
Neurologic disorders *(Continued)*
    sialidosis as, 2074
    sphingolipidoses as, 2069-2072, 2071f-2072f
    subacute sclerosing panencephalitis as, 2075-2076
  obesity with, 184t
  peripheral nerve injuries as, 573-574, 574f
  pseudotumor cerebri as, 2099-2101, 2100f, 2100t
  psychopharmacology and, 65
  seizures as, 2013-2039
    conditions that mimic, 2039, *see also website*
    epileptic syndrome and, 2013, 2014t-2016t
    evaluation of, 2015-2017
    febrile, 2017-2019, 2017t, 2018f
    generalized, 2023-2024
    genetic factors in, 2016t
    mechanisms of, 2024-2025
    neonatal, 2033-2037, 2035t
    partial, 2021-2023, 2022f
    status epilepticus due to, 2037-2039, 2039t
    treatment of, 2018, 2025-2033
    types of, 2014t
    unprovoked, 2019-2021, 2020t
  of spinal cord, 2101-2108
    diastematomyelia as, 2102, 2103f
    spinal arteriovenous malformations as, 2107-2108
    syringomyelia as, 2103, 2104f
    tethered cord, 2101-2102, 2101f-2102f
    transverse myelitis as, 2107, 2107t
    traumatic, 2106
    tumors as, 2105, 2105f
  of spine and spinal cord, due to birth, 573
  sports participation and, 2402t-2404t
  stroke syndromes as, 2080-2086
    arterial ischemic stroke as, 2080-2082, 2081f-2082f, 2081t-2082t
    cerebral sinovenous thrombosis as, 2082-2084, 2083f, 2083t
    differential diagnosis of, 2085-2086, 2086t
    hemorrhagic, 2084-2085, 2084f, 2085t
Neurologic emergency(ies), 296-304
  abusive head trauma as, 301
  brain death as, 304, *see website*
  care principles in, 296-297, 297f
  hypoxic-ischemic insult and encephalopathy as, 301-303
  intracerebral hemorrhage as, 303-304
  status epilepticus as, 303
  stroke as, 303-304
  traumatic brain injury as, 297-301, 298f-301f
    due to abuse, 301
    mild, 301
Neurologic examination
  in back pain, 2373-2374
  of coordination, *see website*
  of cranial nerves, *see website*
  general examination in, *see website*
  of head, *see website*
  of mental status, *see website*
  of motor function, *see website*
  of newborn, 536
  in orthopedic problems, 2332-2334
  in pediatric emergency, 281, 281t
  of reflexes, *see website*
  in scoliosis, 2366
  of sensory function, *see website*
  of station and gait, *see website*
Neurologic manifestations and complications
  in acute intermittent porphyrias, *see website*
  in acute renal failure, 1821
  after cardiopulmonary bypass, 1604
  due to cat-scratch disease, 985
  in congenital disorders of glycosylation, *see website*
  in eating disorders, 93t, 1212f
  in endemic goiter, 1907
  in Epstein-Barr virus infection, 1114

Neurologic manifestations and complications (Continued)
in hypernatremia, 213-214
due to immunosuppression therapy, see website
in lead poisoning, 2450-2451
in Lyme disease, 1031
in lysosomal storage disorders, 485t
in malnutrition, 175t
in mushroom poisoning, see website
in Neonatal Intensive Care Unit Neurobehavioral Scale, 624t
in neurofibromatosis, 2047-2048, 2047f
in *Shigella* infection, 960
due to sickle cell disease, 1666-1667, 1666f
in sickle cell disease, 1666-1667, 1666f
systemic inflammatory response syndrome and, 309t
in systemic lupus erythematosus, 843t
in toxoplasmosis, 1212-1213, 1212f
Neurologic system
management of in drowning, 345-346
overweight and obesity and, 183, 183f
preanesthetic assessment of, see website
prenatal development of, see website
shock-related dysfunction of, 307t
in trauma survey, 337
Neuroma, plexiform, of eyelid, 2165
Neuroma syndrome, mucosal, 1916
Neuromotor function, language disorders due to impairment of, 119
Neuromuscular blocking agents
analgesia and sedation with, see website
reversal of, see website
for intubation, 321t
Neuromuscular disorders
atelectasis with, see website
autonomic neuropathies as, 2141-2143, 2141t-2142t
Bell palsy as, 2146-2147, 2146t, 2147f
due to botulism, see website
clinical manifestations of, 2109-2110, 2110f, 2110t-2111t
cardiac, 1531t
pulmonary, see website
developmental, 2112-2119
amyoplasia as, 2118
arthrogryposis as, 2113
benign congenital hypotonia as, 2119
brain malformations and, 2118
central core, minicore, and multicore myopathies as, 2117-2118
congenital muscle fiber-type disproportion as, 2115
genetics of, 2112-2113, 2113t
muscular dysgenesis (proteus syndrome myopathy) as, 2119
myofibrillar myopathies as, 2118, 2118f
myotubular myopathy as, 2114, 2114f, 2115t
nemaline rod myopathy as, 2116-2117, 2116f-2117f
differential diagnosis of, 2111t-2112t
endocrine and toxic myopathies as, 2129-2130
evaluation and investigation of, 2109-2112
general anesthesia and, see website
Guillain-Barré syndrome as, 2143-2146, 2144t, 2145f-2146f
hereditary motor-sensory neuropathies as, 2138-2140
laboratory findings in, 2110-2112
metabolic myopathies as, 2130-2132, 2130t
muscular dystrophies as, 2119-2129
Becker, 2119-2123, 2121f-2122f
congenital, 2123-2126, 2128f
Duchenne, 2119-2123, 2120f-2122f
Emery-Dreifuss, 2123
fascioscapulohumeral, 2126
limb-girdle, 2126, 2126t
myotonic, 2123, 2123f
Neuromuscular disorders (Continued)
myocardial disease with, 1629t
due to nerve agents, see website
of neuromuscular transmission and motor neurons, 2132-2138
poliovirus infection *versus*, 1085t
respiratory distress due to, 315t
respiratory insufficiency due to, 1519-1520, 1520t
toxic neuropathies as, 2140-2141, 2141t
Neuromuscular scoliosis, 2370-2371
Neuromuscular symptoms, terrorism and, see website
Neuromuscular transmission disorders, 2132-2138
Neuromyelitis optica, see website
Neuromyelitis optica (NMO), 2077
Neuromyopathy of severe illness, 1524
Neuronal apoptosis inhibitory gene, 2137
Neuronal ceroid lipofuscinoses (NCLs), 2073, 2073t
Neuronal dysplasia, intestinal, 1286, see also website
Neuronal heterotopias, 2004
Neuronal injury in seizures, 2025
Neuronal migration, disorders of, 2003-2005, 2003f-2004f
Neuronal plasticity, see website
Neuropathic bladder, 1847, see also website
reflux with, 1835
Neuropathic pain, 360t, 367-368, 368t, 374
Neuropathy
autonomic, 2141-2143, 2141t-2142t
of Chédiak-Higashi syndrome, 744
congenital hypomyelinating, 2140, see also website
diabetic, 1989
hereditary motor-sensory, 2138-2140
hypermyelinating, 2140
intestinal, 1283
myenteric plexus, 2143
optic
Leber, 2067, see website
traumatic, see website
peripheral
due to cancer and its therapy, see website
in tyrosinemia, 422
poliovirus infection *versus*, 1085t
tomaculous, 2140
toxic, 2140-2141, 2141t
due to diphtheria, see website
Neuropsychiatric disorders associated with *Streptococcus pyogenes*, 81, 919
movement disorders associated with, 76
Neurotoxicity, anesthesia-induced, 360, see also website
Neurotoxic shellfish poisoning, see website
Neurotoxin, botulism, 987
Neurotransmitter precursors for BH_4 deficiency, 421
Neurotransmitters
genetic disorders of, 445-447, 445t
in respiratory control, see website
sudden infant death syndrome and, 1422
Neutral lipid storage disease, 2268t
Neutral Protamine Hagedorn (NPH) insulin, 1976, 1977f
Neutropenia, 746-750
associated with cancer therapy, see website
autoimmune, 750
of infancy, 750
maternal, see website
neonatal passive, 750
in bone marrow disorders, 749
due to cancer therapy, see website
cyclic, 750
drug-induced, 748-749, 749t
etiology of, 747-749, 747t-748t
fever and, see website
in granule sorting disorders, 751
immune, 749
Neutropenia (Continued)
in immune function disorders, 751-752
in immunocompromised patient, see website
ineffective myelopoiesis, 750-751
infectious causes of, 747-748, 749t
lymphopenia as, 752, 752t
in metabolic disorders, 751
in 3-methylglutaconic aciduria, 433
neonatal, 631-632
alloimmune, 749-750
passive autoimmune, 750
as oncologic emergency, see website
severe congenital, 750
in Shwachman-Diamond syndrome, 750-751
in splenic disease, 749
in type I glycogen storage disease, 493
Neutrophil count
in acutely ill child evaluation, 277
in fever of unknown origin, 901
in immunocompromised patient, see website
in leukopenia, 746
in roseola, 1119
Neutrophilia, see website
Neutrophils, 739
fetal, see website
function of, see website
hematopoiesis, see website
in human granulocytic ehrlichiosis, 1050f
maturation and kinetics of, see website
in neonatal immunity, 631-632
oral ulceration due to defects of, 1260t
in phagocytic inflammatory response, see website
reference values for, see website
transfusion of, 1693, see also website
Never Events, see website
Nevirapine
drug interactions with, see website
for HIV infection, 1168t-1171t
Nevoid basal cell carcinoma, 1747t, see also website
Nevoid telangiectasia, unilateral, 2230
Nevus, 2231-2236
Becker, 2235, 2235f
blue, 2234
blue rubber bleb, 2230
comedonicus, 2235
conjunctival, 2169
connective tissue, 2235
depigmentosus (achromic), 2234, 2234f
epidermal, 2234-2235, 2234f
eyelid, 2164
halo, 2233, 2233f
of Ita, 2233-2234
melanocytic
acquired, 2231, 2231f
atypical, 2231-2232
congenital, 2232, 2232f
melanoma as, 2232-2233
of Ota, 2233-2234
sebaceus (Jadassohn), 2235
smooth muscle hamartoma as, 2235-2236
spilus, 2233, 2233f
Spitz (spindle and epithelioid cell), 2233, 2233f
zosteriform lentiginous, 2233
Nevus anemicus, 2226
Nevus basal cell carcinoma syndrome, see website
Nevus simplex, 2218-2219
Nevus syndrome, 2052
malignancy susceptibility associated with, see website
rickets due to, 207
Newborn
acne in, 2327, 2327f
antibiotic therapy for, see website
Apgar evaluation of, 536, 536t-537t
blood disorders in, 612-621
anemia as, 612-615, 613f, 613t-614t
hemolytic disease as, 615-619, 616t, 620t

Newborn *(Continued)*
hemorrhage as, 620-621, 621t
plethora as, 619-620
thrombocytopenia as, 1720
breast abnormalities in, *see website*
breast-feeding of, 539-540, 539t
breathing patterns in, 580
circumcision of, *see website*
clinical manifestations of diseases in, 564-565, *see also website*
complement system reductions in, 756
congenital anomalies in (*See* Congenital anomalies)
corneal opacities in, *see website*
death of (*See* Death; Death rates)
delivery room emergencies of, 575-579
abdominal wall defects as, 578
airway obstruction as, 577, 578f
birth injury as, 578-579
failure to initiate or sustain respiration as, 575
meconium staining as, 577
neonatal resuscitation as, 575-577, 576f-577f, 576t
pneumothorax as, 577, 578f
respiratory distress and failure as, 575
shock as, 577
developmental dysplasia of hip in, 2357, 2359-2360, 2360f
diabetes mellitus of, 1995
of diabetic mother, 627-629, 627f-628f
digestive system disorders of, 600-612
constipation as, 600
jaundice and hyperbilirubinemia as, 603-608
kernicterus as, 608-612
meconium ileus in cystic fibrosis as, 601, 601f
meconium peritonitis as, 601
meconium plugs as, 600-601, 600f
neonatal necrotizing enterocolitis as, 601-603, 602f, 602t
vomiting as, 600-601
disabled, ethics in care of, *see website*
dysmorphology in, 629, *see also website*
endocrinopathies in, 627-629
fever without a focus in, 896t
fever without localizing signs in, 896-897
genitourinary system of, 621, *see also website*
gingival cysts of, 2298
growth and development of, 26, 29t, *see also website*
age 0-2 months, 26-29
cognitive, 27
developmental milestones in, 27t
emotional, 27-28
maternal-infant attachment in, *see website*
pediatrician's role in, *see website*
physical, 27, 29f
restriction of (*See* Intrauterine growth restriction (IUGR))
gynecological examination of, *see website*
high-risk, 552-564, 552t, 553f
large-for-gestational-age, *see website*
multiple gestation pregnancy and, 553-555, 554t, 555f
post-term, *see website*
prematurity and intrauterine growth restriction and, 555-564
transport of, 564, *see also website*
hyperthyroidism in, 1913f
hypoglycemia in, 518-521, 520t
infections of, 629-648
bacterial, 630, 630f-631f, 636-637, 638t, 642-644
Candida, 1053-1054, 1054t
clinical manifestations of, 636-639, 637t
complications and prognosis for, 646, 647t
diagnosis of, 639-644
early-onset, 633-636, 634t
Enterococcus, *see website*

Newborn *(Continued)*
enterovirus, 1092
epidemiology of, 629, 633-636
etiology of, 632-633, 632t-633t
evaluation of, 643t
fungal, 642-644
genital mycoplasma as, 1033
gonococcal, 936
Haemophilus influenzae in, 943
herpes simplex virus, 1098, 1101, 1102f
intrauterine, 629-630, 630f, 636-642, 637t
late-onset, 631, 633-636, 634t-635t
listeriosis, *see website*
modes of transmission of, 629-631
nosocomial, 634-636, 635t-636t, 647-648, 647t
pathogenesis of, 629-631, 630f-631f
prematurity and low birth weight and, 634, 634f-635f
prevention of, 647-648, 647t
prophylaxis for, 640f-642f, 640t
systemic inflammatory response syndrome due to, 637-639
toxoplasmosis, 1208-1211, 1210f, 1214-1215
treatment of, 644-646, 645t
tuberculosis as, 1000
varicella-zoster virus, 1106-1107
intellectual disability in, 125t
lupus in, 845-846, 845f
metabolic disturbances in, 622-626
cold injury as, 622
edema as, 622
fetal alcohol syndrome as, 625-626, 626f, 626t
hypermagnesemia as, 623
hyperthermia as, 622
hypomagnesemia as, 623
due to maternal substance abuse, 623-625, 624t
metabolic bone disease as, 623
due to selective serotonin reuptake inhibitors, 625, 625f
neurologic disorders of, 565-574
cranial, 565-566, 565f
hypoxic-ischemic encephalopathy as, 298f-299f, 569-573, 569t-570t
due to inflammation, infection, and medications, 568-569, 568f
intracranial hemorrhage as, 566-568, 567f, 568t
peripheral nerve injuries as, 573-574, 574f
of spine and spinal cord, 573
neutropenia in
alloimmune, 749-750
passive autoimmune, 750
nursery care of, 538, 538t
overgrowth of, *see website*
pain assessment in, 361
parent-infant attachment/bonding and, 538-540, *see also website*
perception and effects of pain on, 373-375
physical examination of, 532-536
abdomen in, 535-536
anus in, 536
chest in, 535
extremities in, 536
face in, 534
general appearance in, 532-533
genitals in, 536
growth and behavior, *see website*
heart in, 535, 535f
neck in, 534-535
neurologic assessment in, 536
(*See also* Neurologic examination)
skin in, 533, 533f
skull in, 533-534, 534t
premature (*See* Prematurity/premature infant)
red blood cell life span in, *see website*
respiration regulation in, *see website*
respiratory tract disorders of, 579-599, 579f

Newborn *(Continued)*
apnea as, 580-581, 580t
diaphragmatic hernia as, 594-596
eventration as, 597
extrapulmonary air leaks as, 597-599, 598f-599f
foramen of Morgagni hernia as, 597, 597f
foreign material aspiration as, 590, 591f
meconium aspiration as, 590-592
paraesophageal hernia as, 597
persistent pulmonary hypertension of the newborn as, 592-594, 592f
pulmonary hemorrhage as, 599
respiratory distress syndrome as, 581-590
transient tachypnea as, 590
routine delivery room and initial care of, 536-538
antiseptic skin and cord care in, 537
maintenance of body heat in, 536-537
screening and genetic testing of, *see also website*
for cystic fibrosis, 1490
ethical considerations in, 382-383, *see website*
for genetic metabolic conditions, 416, 417t
for 21-hydroxylase deficiency, 1934
for hyperphenylalaninemia, 419-420
seizures in, 2033-2037
skin diseases in, 2218-2220, 2218f-2219f
sleep changes in, 47t
syphilis in, 1016, 1016f-1017f
tetanus in, 991-992
transition of to pulmonary respiration in, 579-580
tuberculosis in, 1000, 1007
umbilicus of, 622, *see also website*
Newborn Behavior Assessment Scale (NBAS), *see website*
New-onset refractory status epilepticus (NORSE), 2038
NF-κB. *See* Nuclear factor κB (NF-κB)
NGU. *See* Nongonococcal urethritis (NGU)
NHBD. *See* Non-heart-beating donor (NHBD)
NHL. *See* Non-Hodgkin lymphoma (NHL)
Niacin, 193, 194t
deficiency of, 193-195, 195f
dietary reference intakes for, *see website*
toxicity of, 195
NICH. *See* Noninvoluting congenital hemangioma (NICH)
Nickel dermatitis, 2251, 2251f
Niclosamide, *see website*
Nicotinamide-adenine dinucleotide phosphate (NADPH), 745
Nicotinamide for Hartnup syndrome, 430
Nicotine dependence, 679, 680t
Nicotinic acid, 481t, 482
Niemann-Pick disease (NPD), 484t, 488
Nifedipine
for chilblains, 2285
drug interactions with, *see website*
for hypertensive emergencies, 1646t
for pulmonary hypertension, 1602t
Nifurtimox, 1197, *see also website*
Night blindness, 2154
due to vitamin A deficiency, 189
Nigh terrors, seizure *versus*, *see website*
Nightmares, 52t
seizure *versus*, *see website*
Nikolsky sign, 2244, 2247, 2302, 2302f
Nilotinib, *see website*
911 system, *see website*
Nipple, supernumerary, 2221, *see website*
Nipple discharge, *see website*
Nipple pain due to breast-feeding, 160
NISD. *See* Neonatal iron storage disease (NISD)
Nissen fundoplication, 527
Nitazoxanide, *see also website*
for ascariasis, 1217-1218
for giardiasis, 1182, 1182t
for trichuriasis, 1221-1222

Nitisinone (NTBC), 422
Nitrazepam for seizures
  dosages of, 2030t
  febrile, 2018
Nitric oxide (NO)
  adolescent huffing of, 681t
  exhaled, in asthma, 784-785
  inhaled
    for anesthesia, *see website*
    for congenital diaphragmatic hernia, 595
    for persistent pulmonary hypertension of the newborn, 593
    for respiratory distress and failure, 319, 586
  in rectal dialysate, 1344t
Nitrites
  adolescent abuse of, 675t
  for cyanide poisoning, *see website*
  gastroenteritis due to, 1328t-1329t
Nitrofurantoin, 1832, *see also website*
Nitroglycerin
  for cardiogenic shock, 313t
  for heart failure, *see website*
Nitroprusside
  for cardiogenic shock, 313t
  for heart failure, *see website*
  for hypertensive emergencies, 1646t
Nizatidine, 1293t
NK. *See* Natural killer (NK) cells
NKH. *See* Nonketotic hyperglycinemia (NKH)
NKX2.1 gene, 1895
NKX2.5 gene, 1895
NKX2.5 mutations, *see website*
NLH. *See* Nodular lymphoid hyperplasia (NLH)
NME. *See* Necrolytic migratory erythema (NME)
NMO. *See* Neuromyelitis optica (NMO)
NMS. *See* Neuroleptic malignant syndrome (NMS)
NMYC oncogene, *see website*
N,N-diethyl-*m*-toluamide (DEET)
  for malaria prevention, 1207
  for travelers, *see website*
  for tularemia prevention, 980
NNH. *See* Navajo neurohepatopathy (NNH)
NNNS. *See* Neonatal Intensive Care Unit Neurobehavioral Scale (NNNS)
NNRTIs. *See* Non-nucleoside reverse transcriptase inhibitors (NNRTIs)
NO. *See* Nitric oxide (NO); Nitrous oxide (NO)
Nocardia, 929, *see also website*
  in pneumonia, 1475t
Nocardiosis, 929
Nociception, 360, 361f
Nocturnal enuresis, 71-73, 72t, 1851-1852, 1851t
Nocturnal hemoglobinuria, paroxysmal, 748t, 755, 1662, *see also website*
Nodes, with cat-scratch disease, 984
NOD2 gene, 1294-1295
Nodular lymphoid hyperplasia (NLH), *see website*
Nodule(s)
  in acne, 2322-2323, 2323f
  in autoimmune thyroiditis, 1905
  Bohn, 1260
  examination of, *see website*
  Lisch, 2047f, 2156
    in neurofibromatosis, 2046-2047
  rheumatoid, 832
  subcutaneous
    in acute myeloid leukemia, 1737
    in acute rheumatic fever, 922
  thyroid, 1915, 1915t
  of thyroid carcinoma, 1914
  vocal, *see website*
Noma, 175, 176f, 2299
Nonadherence. *See* Adherence
Nonalcoholic fatty liver disease (NAFLD), 184t, *see also website*
Nonallelic homologous recombination, *see website*
Nonbacterial food poisoning, 2454, *see also website*
Nonbicarbonate buffers, *see website*
Nonbiologic disease-modifying antirheumatic drugs, *see website*
Noncomitant strabismus, 2159
Nondiscrimination, chronic illness and, *see website*
Nondisjunction, chromosomal, 400
Nonedematous malnutrition, 175
Nonfatal injuries, 19, 19f
Nonflammable fabric, 23
Non-germ cell gonadal tumors, 1770
Nongonococcal urethritis (NGU)
  Trichomonas vaginalis in, 1186
  Ureaplasma in, 1032-1033
Non-group A or B streptococci, 928, *see also website*
Non-heart-beating donor (NHBD), *see website*
Non-Herlitz junctional epidermolysis bullosa, 2244-2246, 2245t
Non-Hodgkin lymphoma (NHL), 1730f, 1743-1746, 1744f-1745f, 1745t
  hematopoietic stem cell transplantation for, 759
  of small intestine, 1314-1315
  of temporal bone, *see website*
  work-up of, 1731t
Noninflammatory diarrhea, 1330
Noninvoluting congenital hemangioma (NICH), 2229
Nonketotic hyperglycinemia (NKH), 439-440
Nonketotic hyperosmolar coma, 1981
Nonmenstrual toxic shock syndrome and, 908
Non-neurogenic neurogenic bladder, 1849-1850, 1849f
Non-nucleoside reverse transcriptase inhibitors (NNRTIs), 1162t
Nonnutritive sweeteners, 1982
Nonpalpable testis, 1859
Nonparalytic poliomyelitis, 1083, 1086
Non-polyanaline repeat expansion mutation (NPARM), 1520-1521
Nonpolyposis colon cancer syndrome (NHPCC), *see website*
Non-rapid eye movement (NREM), *see website*
Nonrebreather mask, 319
Non-REM partial arousal disorders, *see website*
Nonsteroidal antiinflammatory drugs (NSAIDs)
  adverse reaction to, 828, *see also website*
  for asthma, 796
  for dysmenorrhea, 691t
  gastric ulcer due to, 1293
  for juvenile idiopathic arthritis, 837, 838t
  for migraine, 2043
  for pain management, 363
  poisoning with, 260-261
  pseuoporphyria due to, *see website*
  for rheumatic disease, *see website*
  topical, for skin disorders, 2217
Nonstress test (NST), 542, 543t
Nontherapeutic research, *see website*
Nontreponemal test, 1019, 1019f
Nontuberculous mycobacteria (NTM), 1011-1016
  clinical manifestations of, 1012-1014, 1012f-1014f, 1012t
  diagnosis of, 1014-1015
  epidemiology of, 1012
  etiology of, 1011-1012
  pathogenesis of, 1012
  treatment of, 1015-1016
Nonvenereal treponemal infections, 1023, *see also website*
Noonan syndrome, 410, 410t, 1690, 1946, 1955-1956
  congenital heart disease with, 1531t, 1561-1562, *see also website*
  embryonic development of, *see website*
  malignancy susceptibility associated with, *see website*
Norepinephrine, 1923, *see also website*
  for cardiac output maintenance and post-resuscitation stabilization, 294t
  genetic disorders of, 445t
  for heart failure, *see website*
  in pheochromocytoma, 1942
  for shock, 313t
Norfloxacin for traveler's diarrhea, *see website*
Normal, statistical, *see website*
Normal saline (NS), 243, 243t
  for anaphylaxis, 818t
Normethsuximide dosages, 2030t
Noroviruses, 1326t
Nor-plant. *See* Lovenorgestrel
NORSE. *See* New-onset refractory status epilepticus (NORSE)
North American liver fluke, *see website*
Nortriptyline
  for attention deficit/hyperactivity disorder, 111t
  for pain management, 364t
    in palliative care, 155t-156t
Norvir. *See* Ritonavir
Norwalk virus, 1134, 1136
Norwegian scabies, 2320
Norwood procedure, 1593-1595, 1594f
Nose
  birth injury to, 579
  congenital disorders of, 1429-1431, 1430f-1431f
  epistaxis of, 1432-1433, 1432t
  examination of
    in allergic disease, 765
    in newborn, 534
  foreign body in, 1431-1432
  fracture of, as delivery room emergency, 579
  normal, 1429
  physiology of, 1429-1430
  polyps in, 1433, 1433f
  radiography of, *see website*
  saddle deformity
    in congenital syphilis, 1017t, 1018, 1019f
    in Wegener's granulomatosis, 874, 875f
Nosebleed, 1432-1433, 1432t
Nosema corneum, *see website*
Nosocomial infection
  fever of unknown origin in, 899t
  Legionella, *see website*
  neonatal, 632-636, 635t-636t
    prevention of, 647-648, 647t
  prevention and control of, 895, *see also website*
  Pseudomonas aeruginosa in, 976
  respiratory syncytial virus, 1127
  Salmonella, 950
Nostrilla. *See* Oxymetazoline
Notching of inferior border of ribs, 1568
NovaRing. *See* Vaginal contraceptive ring
Novobiocin, 563t
NO_x. *See* Oxides of nitrogen (NO_x)
NPARM. *See* Non-polyanaline repeat expansion mutation (NPARM)
NPD. *See* Niemann-Pick disease (NPD)
NPH insulin, 1976, 1977f
NPHS1 gene, 1803t, 1807
NPHS2 gene, 1803t, 1807
NR5A1 gene, *see website*
NRAS gene, *see website*
NREM. *See* Non-rapid eye movement (NREM)
NROB1 gene, *see website*
NRS. *See* Numerical Rating Scale (NRS) for pain assessment
NRTIs. *See* Nucleoside/nucleotide reverse transcriptase inhibitors (NRTIs)
NS. *See* Normal saline (NS)
NSAIDs. *See* Nonsteroidal antiinflammatory drugs (NSAIDs)
NST. *See* Nonstress test (NST)
NTBC. *See* Nitisinone (NTBC)
NTDs. *See* Neural tube defects (NTDs)
NTM. *See* Nontuberculous mycobacteria (NTM)

Nuclear factor κB (NF-κB) essential modulator (NEMO) mutations, 726
Nuclear medicine imaging
in aspiration syndromes, 1472t
in congenital hypothyroidism, 1900
esophageal, *see website*
in fever of unknown origin, 902
hepatic, 1379
in Meckel diverticulum, 1282, 1282f
in neonatal cholestasis, 1385
in orthopedic problems, 2334
in osteomyelitis, 2396-2397
pulmonary, *see website*
in pulmonary embolism, 1502
radiation exposure from, *see website*
in septic arthritis, 2400
thyroid, *see website*
in urinary tract obstruction, 1840-1841
Nucleic acid amplification testing (NAAT), *see also website*
in *Chlamydia trachomatis*, 1036-1037
in gonococcal disease, 938
in *Mycobacterium tuberculosis*, 996
in sexually transmitted disease, 709
Nucleoside/nucleotide analogs for hepatitis B, 1399
Nucleoside/nucleotide reverse transcriptase inhibitors (NRTIs), 1167, 1168t-1171t
Numerical Rating Scale (NRS) for pain assessment, 361
Nummular eczema, 2252, 2252f
Nurse-geneticist, 382t
Nursemaid elbow, 2384, 2384f
Nursery care
of newborn, 538, 538t
of premature infant, 558-562
Nursing. *See* Breast-feeding
Nut allergy, 821, 821t, 823t
Nutrition. *See also* Diet; Malnutrition
acute intermittent porphyrias and, *see website*
in acute renal failure, 1821
assessment of before renal transplantation, *see website*
in burn management, 354
chronic diarrhea and, 1344-1345
in chronic kidney disease, 1824
dietary reference intakes in, *see website*
in eating disorders treatment, 94-95
effects of vomiting on, 1243t
ethics of withholding, *see website*
feedings in
during first year of life, 160-165
of school-age children and adolescents, 166-167
of toddlers and preschool-age children, 165
home mechanical ventilation and, 1525-1526
issues associated with
complementary and alternative medicine, 169
cultural considerations, 167-168
food assistance programs, 170
food environment, 167, 168f
food safety, 169
in gastroesophageal reflux disease, 1269
nutritional programming, 169
organic foods, 169
preventive nutrition counseling, 169-170
using food as reward, 167
vegetarianism, 168
maternal, *see website*
measuring adequacy of, *see website*
overweight and obesity and, 179-188
body mass index and, 179, 180f-181f
comorbidities of, 183-184, 184t
endocrine and neural physiology of, 183
environmental factors in, 182
epidemiology of, 179
etiology of, 179-183
evaluation of, 184-185, 185f, 185t
genetics in, 182-183, 182t
identification of, 184
Nutrition *(Continued)*
interventions for, 185-186, 186t-187t
prevention of, 186-188, 187t-188t
parenteral
cholestasis associated with, *see website*
for premature and low birthweight infants, 559-560
for short bowel syndrome, 1316
prenatal, birth weight and, *see website*
requirements for, 160, *see also website*
in *Shigella* treatment, 961
three myths about, 170t
in type 1 diabetes mellitus, 1981-1983, 1982t
vitamin A deficiencies and excess in, 188-191
vitamin B complex deficiency and excess in, 191-198
Nutritional dermatoses, 2328-2330, 2329f-2330f
Nutritive value of baby foods, *see website*
NVICP. *See* National Vaccine Injury Compensation Program (NVICP)
Nyctalopia, 2154
Nystagmus, 2161-2162, 2161t, 2162f
with Down syndrome, 403t
in ear disorders, *see website*
end-gaze, *see website*
in neurologic examination, *see website*
Nystagmus retractorius, 2161

O
OAE. *See* Otoacoustic emissions (OAE) testing
Oasthouse urine disease, 1319
OATPs. *See* Organic anion transporting polypeptides (OATPs)
Obesity, 179-188
body mass index and, 179, 180f-181f, *see also website*
due to cancer and its therapy, *see website*
comorbidities of, 183-184, 184t
endocrine and neural physiology of, 183
environmental factors in, 182
epidemiology of, 179
etiology of, 179-183
evaluation of, 184-185, 185f, 185t
genetics in, 182-183, 182t
growth charts for assessment of, *see website*
identification of, 184
interventions for, 185-186, 186t-187t
liver disease and, *see website*
maternal, *see website*
with polycystic ovary syndrome, *see website*
prevention of, 186-188, 187t-188t
pulmonary manifestations of, *see website*
sleep-disordered breathing and, 49
slipped capital femoral epiphysis and, 184t, 2363-2364
sports participation and, 2402t-2404t
type 2 diabetes mellitus and, 1990-1991
Obesity hypoventilation syndrome, 1522-1523
Object, transitional, 31-32
Object permanence, 30
Obligate anaerobes, 995
Oblique fracture, 2388f, 2390
Observation
in acutely ill child evaluation, 276
in appendicitis, 1354
in brain death diagnosis, *see website*
Obsessions, 80
Obsessive-compulsive disorder (OCD), 80-81, 81t
group A streptococci infection and, 919
trichotillomania as, 2290
Obstruction
airway
acute inflammatory upper, 1445-1450, 1446f
in asthma, 782, 784
critical high airway obstruction syndrome (CHAOS), 577, 578f
extrathoracic, *see website*
intrapulmonary, *see website*
intrathoracic-extrapulmonary, *see website*
Obstruction *(Continued)*
management of, 282-283, 282f-283f
neonatal, 577, 578f
respiratory distress due to, 315t
in respiratory syncytial virus infection, 1127-1128
due to tonsil and adenoid pathology, 1443, 1445
in traumatic injury, 335
bronchial in tuberculosis, 998, 1000f, 1002
congenital nasolacrimal duct, 2165
duodenal, 1277-1278, 1278f
esophageal, *see website*
Eustachian tube, 2201
gastric outlet, 1275-1276
gastrointestinal
causes of, 1243t
vomiting due to, 1242
intestinal (*See* Ileus)
midureteral, 1842
nasal in common cold, 1435
ureteropelvic junction, 1841-1842
of urinary tract, 1838-1847, 1839t
Obstructive congenital heart disease, 1561-1571
in adults, 1608
Obstructive disorders of esophagus, 1263-1264
Obstructive jaundice in cystic fibrosis, 1496
Obstructive shock, 285, 305, 307t
clinical manifestations of, 308
hemodynamic variables in, 311t
treatment of, 313
Obstructive sleep apnea (OSA), 49-51, 49t-50t, 1523
with Down syndrome, 403t
obesity with, 184t
Obstructive uropathy, nephrotoxins in, 1817t
OCA. *See* Oculocutaneous albinism (OCA)
Occipital bone fracture
Occipital horn syndrome, 1321, 2075
Occipital plagiocephaly, 2012
Occult bacteremia, fever without a focus and, 897-898
Occult blood, fecal, 1344t
Occult spinal dysraphism, 1999, 2000f, 2001t
neuropathic bladder, *see website*
Occupants in motor vehicle accident, 21-22
Occupational therapy
for juvenile dermatomyositis, 849
for respiratory insufficiency, 1525
OCD. *See* Obsessive-compulsive disorder (OCD); Osteochondritis dissecans (OCD)
Ochronosis in alcaptonuria, 423
OCs. *See* Oral contraceptives (OCs)
Octopia lentis, in Marfan syndrome, 2441-2442
Octreotide
for chemotherapy-associated vomiting, 1244t
for sulfonylurea poisoning, 256t-257t, 263
OCTs. *See* Organic cation transporters (OCTs)
Ocuflox. *See* Ofloxacin
Ocular allergies, 809-811, 810f, 811t
Ocular bobbing, 2162t, *see website*
Ocular larva migrans (OLM), 1227-1229, 1228t
Ocular motility, 2150
Ocular motor apraxia, congenital, 2161
Ocular motor dysmetria, 2162, 2162t
Ocular torticollis, 2379
Oculocephalic reflex, brain death and, *see website*
Oculocerebral renal syndrome of Lowe, 2171
Oculocerebrorenal syndrome of Lowe, 1809-1810
Oculocutaneous albinism (OCA), 2238-2239
Oculocutaneous tyrosinemia, 422-423
Oculoglandular tularemia, 979
Oculomotor apraxia type Cogan, 1816
Oculomotor nerve
neurologic examination of, *see website*
palsy of, 2159, 2159f
seizures and abnormalities of, *see website*
Oculosympathetic paresis, 2155

Oculovestibular reflex, brain death and, *see website*
Odansetron for vomiting, 1244t
Odor
inborn errors of amino acid metabolism associated with, 418t
in poisonings, 252t
Odynophagia, 1240, 1262
Oesophagostomum bifurcum, *see website*
Office
isolation techniques for, *see website*
microbiologic testing in, *see website*
preparedness for emergencies, *see website*
Ofloxacin, 1036, *see also website*
1,25$(OH)_2D_3$. *See* 1,25Dihydroxycholecalciferol$_2D_3$ (1,25$(OH)_2D_3$)
Ohtahara syndrome, 1164
OI. *See* Osteogenesis imperfecta (OI)
Oil spill hazards, *see website*
Ointments, 2216
OIs. *See* Opportunistic infections (OIs)
OKT3. *See* Muromonab CD-3
Olanzapine, 64t
Oleander toxicity, 269t
Olecranon bursitis, 2410-2411
Olfactory nerve, neurologic examination of, *see website*
Oligoarthritis in juvenile idiopathic arthritis, 831t, 832, 832f, 837
Oligodendroglioma, 1750
Oligohydramnios
fetal therapy for, 551t
high-risk infant due to, 552
in high-risk pregnancies, *see website*
in renal agenesis, 1827
Oligomeganophronia, 1828
Oligomenorrhea, 686t
Oligosaccharidoses, 484t
Oliguria, fluid therapy adjustments and, 245, 245t
OLM. *See* Ocular larva migrans (OLM)
Olopatadine
for allergic conjunctivitis, 811t
for allergic disease, 771-772
OLT. *See* Orthotopic liver transplantation (OLT)
OM. *See* Otitis media (OM)
Omalizumab
for allergic disease, 772
for asthma, 794t, 796
for atopic dermatitis, 805
OME. *See* Otitis media with effusion (OME)
Omen syndrome, 732-733
Omeprazole, 1293t
Omnaris. *See* Ciclesonide
Omnicef. *See* Cefdinir
Omnipen. *See* Ampicillin
Omphalitis, 639, *see also website*
in newborn, 535-536
Omphalocele, congenital, *see website*
Omphalomesenteric duct, remnants of, 1281-1282
Omsk hemorrhagic fever, 1151-1152
Onchocera volvulus, 1225, *see website*
Oncogenes, *see website*
Oncogenesis, 1728, *see also website*
of Epstein-Barr virus, 1111-1112, 1112t
Oncosphere, 1234-1235
Oncovin. *See* Vincristine
Ondansetron
for chemotherapy-associated vomiting, 1244t
for nausea in palliative care, 155t-156t
Onions for asthma, 271t
Online harassment, 668
Onset of pain, 2332t
Ontogency
drug disposition and, *see website*
pharmacodynamics and, *see website*
Onycholysis, 2295, 2295f
Onychomadesis, 2295, 2296f
Onychomycosis, 2296
candidal, 1055
Oocyst in toxoplasmosis, 1208
Oophoritis, due to mumps, 1080
Opa adhesins, 930
Opacities, neonatal corneal, *see website*
OPC. *See* Oropharyngeal candidiasis (OPC)
Opc adhesins, 930
Opcon-A. *See* Naphazoline hydrochloride
Open bite, *see website*
Open globe, 2185
Open pneumothorax, 336t
Operating otoscope head, 2202
Operations Management, *see website*
Ophthalmia neonatorum, 2166
Ophthalmitis, gonococcal, 937
Ophthalmologic examination, 2148-2150, 2149t
fever of unknown origin and, 901
in juvenile idiopathic arthritis, 833t
Ophthalmopathy, thyroid-related, 2182
Ophthalmoplegia
chronic progressive external, 391t, 2131-2132
internuclear in neurologic examination, *see website*
progressive external, 2067-2068
Ophthalmoscopy, 2150
Opiates
adolescent use of, 684-685
urine screening for, 676t
intoxication, 676t
Opioids
adverse reaction to, 366t, 828
for anesthesia, *see website*
for neuropathic pain, 368t
for pain management, 364-367, 365t-367t, 367f
pharmacokinetics of, *see website*
poisoning with, 251t, 253t, 261
antidote for, 256t-257t
Opisthorchiasis, *see website*
Opisthorchis viverrini, *see website*
Opisthotonos
assessment in neurologic examination, *see website*
with tetanus, 992
Opportunistic infections (OIs)
chronic diarrhea due to, 1340
following organ transplantation, *see website*
HIV-related, 1162-1163
prophylaxis for, 1174, 1175t-1176t
Pseudomonas aeruginosa, 975, *see also website*
Oppositional defiant disorder, 96-98, 97t. *See also* Disruptive behavioral disorders
adolescent violence and, 669, 670t
Opsoclonus, 2162, 2162t
in neurologic examination, *see website*
Opsoclonus myoclonus syndrome, 1754t, *see also website*
Opsonins, *see website*
Opsonization defects, infection with, *see website*
Optic atrophy, *see website*
Optic disc, *see also website*
Optic nerve
abnormalities of, 2181, *see also website*
glaucoma as, 2181, *see also website*
drusen of, *see website*
hypoplasia of, 2006
multiple sclerosis effects on, 2077t
myelination of fibers of, 2181
neurologic examination of, *see website*
traumatic injury to, 2185
Optic nerve aplasia, 2181
Optic nerve coloboma, *see website*
Optic nerve glioma, *see also website*
in neurofibromatosis, 2047f
Optic nerve hypoplasia, *see website*
Optic neuritis, *see website*
Optic neuropathy
Leber, 2067, *see also website*
Leber hereditary, 2067
traumatic, *see website*
Opticrom. *See* Cromolyn sodium
Optokinetic nystagmus (OKN), 2148, *see also website*
OPV. *See* Oral polio vaccine (OPV)
Oral allergy syndrome, 822
Oral candidiasis, 1054-1055
HIV-related, 1164
Oral cavity
diagnostic radiology in dental assessment of, 1261, *see also website*
disorders of
associated with other conditions, 1251, 1251t
cleft lip and palate, 1252-1253, 1252f
dental caries as, 1254-1256, 1255f-1256f
dental trauma, 1258-1259, 1258f-1259f, 1258t
malocclusion, 1252, *see also website*
periodontal, 1257-1258
of salivary glands and jaw, 1261, *see also website*
soft tissue lesions, 1259-1261, 1260f, 1260t
syndromes with manifestations in, 1252f, 1253-1254
Oral contraceptives (OCs), 695t-696t, 696-698
for acne, 2325t
for amenorrhea, 688t
drug interactions with, *see website*
for dysmenorrhea, 691t
for emergency contraception, 698t
missed pills and, 696, 697f, 697t
for polycystic ovary syndrome, *see website*
special needs girls and, 1875
Oral hairy leukoplakia, 2299
Oral hygiene in dental caries prevention, 1256
Oral hypoglycemics, 1992-1993, 1992t
poisoning with, 251t, 263
Oralin insulin, 1977
Oral manifestations, 1253-1254
Oral polio vaccine (OPV), 894, 1087-1088
for travel, *see website*
Oral rehydration therapy
for acute gastroenteritis, 1334, 1335t
for cholera, 967
for malnutrition, 176-177
Oral solutions, composition of, *see website*
Orbit
abnormalities of, 2181-2182
complications of due to sinusitis, 1438
penetrating wounds of, 2186
Orbital cellulitis, 2167t, 2183-2184, 2183t, 2184f
Haemophilus influenzae in, 942
due to sinusitis, 1438
Orbital fracture, 2186
Orbital inflammation, 2182
Orbital pseudotumor, 2182
Orbital tumors, 2182, 2182f
Orchiopexy, scrotal, 1861-1862
Orchitis
due to Coxsackie, 1091
due to mumps, 1080
Orellanine poisoning, *see website*
Organ donation. *See* Transplantation
Organ dysfunction in shock, 305, 307t
Organic acidemias, 430-438, 430f
Organic anion transporting polypeptides (OATPs), *see website*
Organic cation transporters (OCTs), *see website*
Organic foods, 169
Organic mercury exposure, *see website*
Organizational stage of empyema, 1507
Organization skills, *see website*
Organophosphate poisoning, 266-267
antidote for, 256t-257t
Organ transplantation. *See* Transplantation
Oriental sore, 1188

Orientia tsutsugamushi, 1039t-1040t, 1045-1046
Orificial tuberculosis, 2307
Orlistat for weight loss in adults, 187t
Ornithine, defects in metabolism of, 447-453, 448f-449f, 448t, 450t
Ornithine transcarbamylase (OTC) deficiency, 448f, 451
Ornithosis, 1038, *see also website*
Oropharyngeal airway for respiratory distress and failure, 319
Oropharyngeal candidiasis (OPC), 1259-1260
Oropharyngeal dysphagia, 1240, 1241t
Oropharyngeal infections
  Francisella tularensis, 979
  herpes simplex virus in, 1099, 1099f
Oroticaciduria, 1655
Orotic aciduria, hereditary, *see website*
Oroya fever, 982
Orthodromic conduction, 1613-1614
Orthographic problems, *see website*
Orthopedic management of arthrogryposis, *see website*
Orthopedic problems
  arthrogryposis as, 2387, *see also website*
  chest pain in, 1530t
  deformation birth defects as, *see website*
  disorders of in mucopolysaccharidoses, 515t
  of elbow, 2383-2384, 2383f-2384f, 2384t
  evaluation of, 2331-2335
    of back pain, 2332
    history in, 2331, 2332t
    laboratory studies in, 2335
    of limp, 2332, 2334t
    neurologic, 2332-2334
    physical examination in, 2331-2332, 2332t, 2333f
    radiographic, 2334-2335
  of foot and toes, 2335-2344
    calcaneovalgus feet as, 2336
    cavus feet as, 2340, 2340f
    congenital vertical talus as, 2337-2338, 2337t, 2338f
    hypermobile pes planus (flatfoot) as, 2338, 2338f
    metatarsus adductus as, 2335, 2335f
    osteochondroses/apophysitis as, 2340-2341, 2340f
    painful foot in, 2344, 2344t
    puncture wounds as, 2341
    shoes and, 2344
    talipes equinovarus (clubfoot) as, 2336, 2337f
    tarsal coalition as, 2339-2340, 2339f, 2339t
    toe deformities as, 2341-2342
  fractures as, 2387-2394, 2388f
    buckle or torus, 2390
    due to child abuse, 2390
    complete, 2390
    complications of, 2394, 2394t
    epiphyseal, 2390, 2390t, 2391f
    greenstick, 2390
    healing of, 2389
    lower extremity, 2392, 2393t
    outcomes of, 2394
    overgrowth after, 2389
    patterns of, 2389
    plastic deformation, 2389-2390, 2389f-2390f
    progressive deformity after, 2389, 2389f
    remodeling of, 2388f, 2389
    surgical treatment of, 2393-2394, 2394t
    upper extremity, 2390-2391
  growth and development and, 2331, *see also website*
  of hand, 2385-2387, 2385f-2386f, 2385t-2387t
  of hip, 2355-2365
    developmental dysplasia as, 2356, 2357f-2359f
    Legg-Calvé-Perthes disease as, 2361, 2362f
Orthopedic problems *(Continued)*
    slipped capital femoral epiphysis as, 2363, 2364f
    transient monoarticular synovitis as, 2360
  in juvenile idiopathic arthritis, 838-839
  of knee, 2351-2355
    discoid lateral meniscus as, 2352, 2352f
    idiopathic adolescent anterior knee pain syndrome as, 2354
    Osgood-Schlatter disease as, 2354, 2354f
    osteochondritis dissecans as, 2353, 2353f
    patellar subluxation and dislocation, 2355
    popliteal cyst as, 2353
  leg-length discrepancy as, 2351, *see also website*
  of neck, 2377-2382
    cervical anomalies and instabilities as, 2380-2382, 2381t
    in Down syndrome, 2381-2382, 2382f
    Kippel-Feil syndrome as, 2379-2380, 2380f
    in 22q11.2 deletion syndrome, 2382, 2382f
    torticollis in, 2377-2379, 2378f, 2378t
  obesity with, 184t
  osteomyelitis as, 2394-2398, 2395t-2396t, 2396f
  in progeria, *see website*
  septic arthritis as, 2398-2400, 2399f, 2399t
  of shoulder, 2383
  of spine, 2365-2377, 2365t
    back pain as, 2373-2374, 2373t
    disk space infection as, 2376, 2376t
    intervertebral disk herniation and slipped vertebral apophysis as, 2377
    kyphosis as, 2371-2373, 2372f
    scoliosis as
      compensatory, 2371
      congenital, 2368-2370, 2369f
      idiopathic, 2365-2368, 2366f, 2368f
      neuromuscular, 2370-2371
    spondylolysis and spondylolisthesis as, 2374-2376, 2375f
    syndromes and genetic disorders, 2371
    tumors as, 2377
  due to sports injury (*See* Sports *entries*)
  in systemic lupus erythematosus, 843t
  torsional and angular, 2344-2351
  of wrist, 2384-2385
Orthopedic prostheses, infection associated with, *see website*
Orthophoria, 2157
Orthostatic hypotension, *see website*
Orthostatic intolerance, *see website*
Orthostatic proteinuria, 1800
Orthotopic liver transplantation (OLT), 1414
Orthotopic ureterocele, 1843-1844, 1843f
Ortolani test, 2357, 2357f
OSA. *See* Obstructive sleep apnea (OSA)
Oseitis pubis, 2413
Oseltamivir, 1123, 1123t-1124t, *see also website*
Osgood-Schlatter disease, 2354, 2354f, 2436t
  sports-related, 2416
Osler nodes, 1623
Osler-Weber-Rendu syndrome, 1531t, 1599, 2230
Osmolal gap, 254t, *see also website*
Osmolality, *see also website*
  in acute renal failure, 1819, 1820t
  in diabetes insipidus, 1882
  of intravenous solutions, 217, 243
  in nephrogenic diabetes insipidus, 1812
  reference values for, *see website*
  regulation of, 212
Osmolarity of oral rehydration solutions, 1335t
Osmoles
  idiogenic, 214
  unmeasured, *see website*
Osmotic diarrhea, 1245, 1245t, 1339, 1339f
Osmotic diuresis, *see website*
Osmotic equilibrium, *see website*
Osmotic fragility test, 1660-1661, 1662f
Os odontoideum, 2381
Ossification
  centers of, 29t, *see website*
  endochondral, *see website*
  intramembranous, *see website*
Ossifying fibroma of jaw, *see website*
Osteoarthropathy
  in cystic fibrosis, 1494
  hypertrophic, *see website*
Osteochondritis dissecans (OCD), 2353, 2353f, 2436t
  as sports injury, 2408, 2408f
Osteochondritis in congenital syphilis, 1017-1018, 1018f
Osteochondrodysplasias. *See* Skeletal dysplasias
Osteochondroses, 2340-2341, 2340f
  juvenile, 2435, 2436t
Osteodystrophy
  Albright hereditary, 1919-1920
  renal in chronic kidney disease, 1823t, 1824-1825
Osteogenesis imperfecta (OI), 2437-2440
  clinical manifestations of, 2437-2439, 2438f
    cardiac, 1532t
    oral, 1253-1254
  complications of, 2439, 2439f
  dentinogenesis imperfecta with, 1250
  epidemiology of, 2437
  etiology of, 2437
  genetic counseling in, 2439-2440
  laboratory findings in, 2439
  middle ear and inner ear involvement in, *see website*
  pathogenesis of, 2437
  pathology of, 2437
  prognosis for, 2439
  treatment of, 2439
Osteoma of ear canal, 2199
Osteomyelitis, 2394-2398
  clinical manifestations of, 2395, 2396t
  diagnosis of, 2395-2396
  differential diagnosis of, 2397
  epidemiology of, 2395, 2395t
  etiology of, 2394-2395
  pathogenesis of, 2395
  prognosis for, 2398
  Pseudomonas aeruginosa, 976t
  radiographic evaluation of, 2396-2397, 2396f
  treatment of, 2397-2398
  vertebral, 2376, 2376t
Osteonecrosis in slipped capital femoral epiphysis, 2365
Osteopathia striata, 2222
Osteopenia, 2446-2447
  in female athlete, 2421-2422
Osteopetrosis, 2432-2433, 2433f
Osteoporosis, 2446-2447, 2447t
  due to inhaled corticosteroids, 793
  with osteogenesis imperfecta, 2437
Osteoporosis-pseudoglioma, 2447
Osteosarcoma, 1763-1766, 1763t, 1764f
  Ewing sarcoma as, 1765-1766, 1765f
  incidence and survival rates for, 1726t
  risk factors for, 1727t
  telangiectatic, 1763
  work-up of, 1731t
Ostium primum defects, 1554-1556
  in adults, 1607
Ostium secundum defect, 1551-1553, 1551f-1553f
Ostomastoiditis, nontuberculous mycobacterial, 1013
Otalgia, *see website*
OTC. *See* Ornithine transcarbamylase (OTC) deficiency; Over-the-counter (OTC) preparations
Otitic hydrocephalus, 2212
Otitis externa, 2196-2199, 2198f
  examination of, *see website*
  Pseudomonas aeruginosa, 976t

Otitis media (OM), 2199-2213
adenoidectomy for, 2213
adhesive, 2212
bacterial causes of, *see website*
in child-care setting, *see website*
in cleft lip and palate, 1253
clinical manifestations of, 2202
as complication of common cold, 1436
definition of, 2199t
developmental sequelae of, 2213
diagnosis of, 2203-2204, 2203f-2204f
epidemiology of, 2200-2201
etiology of, 2201
examination of eardrum in, 2202-2205
external otitis *versus*, 2197
Haemophilus influenzae in, 943
in influenza, 1124
intracranial complications of, 2211-2212
due to measles, 1071-1072, 1072t
Moraxella catarrhalis in, *see website*
nontuberculous mycobacterial, 1013
otitis media with effusion *versus*, 2203-2204, 2203f
in parainfluenza viruses, 1125t
pathogenesis of, 2201-2202
physical sequelae of, 2212-2213
prevention of, 2213
treatment of, 2205-2209, 2205t, 2206f-2207f, 2207t
with Turner syndrome, 1953
Otitis media with effusion (OME), 2199-2200
acute otitis media *versus*, 2203-2204, 2203f
complications of, 2210-2211, 2210f-2212f, 2210t
etiology of, 2201
management of, 2209-2211, 2209t
tympanometry in, 2194-2195
Otitis prone, *see website*
Otoacoustic emissions (OAE) testing, 2192, 2195
Otomycosis, 2197-2198
Aspergillus in, 1060
Otorrhea
purulent, *see website*
tube, 2208-2209
Otosclerosis, *see website*
Otoscopy, 2202, *see also website*
Ottawa ankle rules, 2417-2418, 2417f
Outcome measures in emergency medical services for children, *see website*
Out-toeing gate, 2347
Ovalocytes, *see website*
Ovary(ies)
autoimmune failure of, 1956
development of, *see website*
function of, *see website*
hypofunction of, 1951-1957, 1951t
primary, 1951-1956, 1952f
secondary, 1956-1957
neonatal assessment of, *see website*
neoplasms of, 1871-1872, 1872t
pseudoprecocity resulting from, 1957-1958
polycystic syndrome of, 1870, *see also website*
amenorrhea due to, 686
with type 2 diabetes mellitus, 1993t
in type I glycogen storage disease, 493-495
Overactive bladder, 73, 1847-1849, 1849f
Overdose syndrome, opiate, 685
Overgrowth syndromes, *see website*
Overinflation, 1460-1462, 1461f-1462f
Overlapping 5th toe, 2342
Overlap syndrome, *see website*
Overriding sutures, cranial, *see website*
Over-the-counter (OTC) preparations
for common cold, 1435
drug interaction with, *see website*
Overuse injury, 2406-2407, 2407t
elbow, 2411-2412
Overweight, 36t, 179-188
body mass index and, 179, 180f-181f
comorbidities of, 183-184, 184t
Overweight *(Continued)*
endocrine and neural physiology of, 183
environmental factors in, 182
epidemiology of, 179
etiology of, 179-183
evaluation of, 184-185, 185f, 185t
genetics in, 182-183, 182t
identification of, 184
interventions for, 185-186, 186t-187t
prevention of, 186-188, 187t-188t
sleep-disordered breathing and, 49
systemic hypertension and, 1641
type 1 diabetes mellitus and, 1982
Ovotesticular disorders of sex development (DSD), 1968
Oxacillin, *see also website*
for infective endocarditis, 1625t
for neonatal infection, 645t
for osteomyelitis, 2397
for septic arthritis, 2400
for *Staphylococcus aureus*, 907t
Oxalate-containing plants toxicity, 269t
Oxalosis, 440-441
Oxamniquine, *see website*
Oxandrolone for Turner syndrome, 1954
Oxazolidinones, *see website*
Oxcarbazepine
adverse effects of, 2031t
dosages of, 2030t
Oxidative phosphorylation (OCPHOS) disease, 506, 507t-509t, 508f, 1405-1406
Oxides of nitrogen (NO_x), *see website*
5-Oxoprolinuria, 443-444
3-Oxothiolase deficiency, 433-434, 434f
Oxotoxin, 904
Oxybutynin for nocturnal incontinence, 1852
Oxycodone
equianalgesic doses and half-life of, 367t
for pain management, 365t
in palliative care, 155t-156t
Oxycontin, 155t-156t
Oxygen
fraction of inspired
in mechanical ventilation, 327
oxygen administration and, 319
partial pressure of carbon dioxide divided into, 319
hyperbaric for carbon monoxide poisoning, 270
partial pressure of, *see also website*
in asthma, 784t
divided into fraction of inspired oxygen, 319
in fetal circulation, *see website*
in respiratory alkalosis, 240
in respiratory failure, 316
in transitional circulation, 1529, *see also website*
as poisoning antidote, 256t-257t
Oxygen administration
for anaphylaxis, 818t
for asthma exacerbation, 797t-798t, 800
for bronchopulmonary dysplasia, *see website*
in neonatal resuscitation, 576
in premature infant, 559
possible adverse reactions to, 563t
for respiratory distress and failure, 319, 584
Oxygenation assessment in respiratory distress and failure, 318-319
Oxygen delivery, *see website*
Oxygen-hemoglobin dissociation curve, *see website*
Oxygen index (QI), 319
Oxygen saturation, mixed venous, in shock, 309-310
Oxygen saturation (Sao_2) in asthma, 784t
Oxyhemoglobin (So_2), *see website*
Oxymetazoline, 780t
Oxysterol 7α-hydroxylase deficiency, 1384
Oxytocin, *see website*
Ozone pollutants, *see website*

P

PA. *See* Pilocytic astrocytoma (PA)
PAC. *See* Premature atrial contraction (PAC)
Pachyonychia congenita, 2273
Pacifiers
otitis media and, 2200
sudden infant death syndrome and, 1425
Pacing
cardiac
for AV heart block, 1619
for supraventricular tachycardia, 1614-1615
diaphragm, 332-333, 1524-1525
in congenital central hypoventilation syndrome, 1522
PACNS. *See* Primary angiitis of central nervous system (PACNS)
$PaCO_2$. *See* Alveolar partial pressure of carbon dioxide ($Paco_2$)
PACU. *See* Postanesthesia care unit (PACU)
Pagophagia, 1656
Pain
abdominal, 1247-1248, 1247t-1248t
of appendicitis, 1350
in *Campylobacter* infection, 969
exclusion from day care due to, *see website*
in hyperparathyroidism, 1921
nondigestive causes of, 1241t
nonorganic chronic, 1346-1349, 1346t-1348t
in pancreatitis, 1371
of peptic ulcer disease, 1292
in Wilms tumor, 1758
assessment and measurement of, 360-361, 362f, 363t
back, 2332, 2373-2374, 2373t
in rheumatic disease, *see website*
in spondyloarthritides, *see website*
categories of, 360, 360t
chest
differential diagnosis of, 1530t
history of, 1530
as manifestation of extrapulmonary disease, 1526, *see also website*
in rheumatic disease, *see website*
due to chronic illness, *see website*
congenital insensitivity to, 2143
definition of, 360
esophageal, 1261
in Fabry disease, 489
foot, 2344, 2344t
growing, 878, 878t, *see also website*
knee, 2351-2352
muscle in neuromuscular disorders, 2109
musculoskeletal, assessment of, 2331, 2332t
neuropathic, 360t, 367-368, 368t, 374
in newborn, *see website*
nociception in, 360, 361f
not result of identifiable or diagnosable conditions, 375
perception and effects of on newborns and infants, 373-375
in sickle cell disease, 1664-1665, 1665t
somatic, 1248
due to sports injury, 2408
syndromes, 374-375
treatment of (*See* Pain management)
visceral, 1248
Pain disorder
diagnostic criteria for, 68t, 69
paroxysmal extreme, *see website*
Pain management, 360-375
for advanced disease, 374
in burn injury, 355
for cancer, 374, 374t, *see also website*
invasive interventions for, 371-373
nonpharmacologic, 370-371
in palliative care, 154-157, 154t-156t
nonpharmacologic, 157t
pharmacologic, 362-370, 368f

Pain management (Continued)
acetaminophen, aspirin, and nonsteroidal antiinflammatory drugs for, 363-364, 364t
antidepressants for, 368-369
antiepileptic drugs for, 369-370
antipsychotics and major sedatives for, 370
benzodiazepines for, 370
local anesthetics for, 367-368, 367t-368t
opioids, 364-367, 365t-367t, 367f
pharmacokinetics and pharmacodynamics of analgesics in, 362-363
serotonin and selective serotonin reuptake inhibitors for, 369
unconventional medications for, 368-370, 368f
postoperative, *see website*
Pain receptors in respiration regulation, *see website*
Pain syndrome(s)
arthralgia and, *see website*
complex regional, 374-375
erythromelalgia, 375
musculoskeletal, 876-880, 877t-878t
complex regional pain syndrome as, 879-880, 879t
erythromelalgia as, 880, 880f
fibromyalgia as, 878-879, 879f
growing pains as, 878
myofascial pain disorders and fibromyalgia, 375
PAIR, 1238-1239
Palate, cleft, 1252-1253, 1252f
dental problems associated with, 1251t
Palatine tonsil, 1442
Paley multiplier method, *see website*
Palivizumab, 882t, 883, *see also website*
for respiratory syncytial virus prophylaxis, 1129
Palliative care, 149-159, 150f
care settings for, 151
communication, advanced care planning, and anticipatory guidance, 151-159
for child, 152, 153t
for parents, 151-152
for pediatrician, 159
for siblings, 152-153
for staff, 153
conditions appropriate for, 149-150, 149t
decision-making in, 153
resuscitation status in, 153-154
symptoms management in, 154-158, 154t-157t
during terminal phase, 158-159
Palliative sedation, 158
Pallister-Hall syndrome (PHS), *see also website*
adrenal insufficiency with, 1925t
congenital heart disease with, 1531t
Pallister-Killian syndrome, 412
Pallor
in iron deficiency-anemia, 1656
in newborn, 533, *see website*
Palmar erythema as manifestation of liver disease, 1376
Palmaris longus muscle aplasia, 2118
Palmoplantar keratodermas (PPKs), 2272-2273, 2273f
Palpation
abdominal
in acutely ill child evaluation, 276-277
in appendicitis, 1350
in intussusception, 1288
of skull in neurologic examination, *see website*
Palsy(ies)
Bell, 2146-2147, 2146t, 2147f
brachial, as birth injury, 573-574, 574f, 2383
bulbar due to botulism, 988, 989f
facial nerve, 574
sixth nerve, 2160
third nerve, 2159, 2159f
PAM. *See* Pulmonary alveolar microlithiasis (PAM)
2PAM. *See* Pralidoxime
PAMPs. *See* Pathogen-associated molecular patterns (PAMPs)
PAN. *See* Polyarteritis nodosa (PAN)
pANCA. *See* Perinuclear antineutrophil cytoplasmic antibody (pANCA)
Pancreas
annular, *see website*
disorders of
anatomic abnormalities as, 1368, *see also website*
associated with pancreatic insufficiency, 1369-1370
chronic diarrhea with, 1340-1341
due to cystic fibrosis, 1487-1488
in cystic fibrosis, 1485
pancreatic function tests in, 1369, *see also website*
pancreatitis as, 1370-1373, 1370t-1371t, 1372f-1373f
pseudocyst as, 1373
tumor as, 1374, *see also website*
embryology, anatomy, and physiology of, 1368, *see also website*
malabsorption and, 1307-1308, 1317
transplantation of, 1989-1990
Pancreas divisum, *see website*
Pancreatic agenesis, 1368, *see also website*
Pancreatic β-cells
genetic defects of, 1993-1995
loss of function in diabetes mellitus, 1973-1974, 1973f
Pancreatic enzymes, *see also website*
deficiencies of, 1369
replacement of, 1369-1370
in cystic fibrosis, 1495
Pancreatic function tests, 1369, *see also website*
Pancreatic insufficiency, 1369
treatment of, 1369-1370
Pancreatic panniculitis, 2284
Pancreatitis, 1370-1373
abdominal pain of, 1247t-1248t
acute, 1370-1372, 1370t-1371t
chronic, 1372-1373, 1373f
in cystic fibrosis, 1496
with hyperparathyroidism, 1921
due to mumps, 1080
in type I glycogen storage disease, 493-495
Pancreato-blastoma, *see website*
Pancuronium, *see website*
Pancytopenia
acquired, 1691-1692, 1691t
inherited, 1684-1690, 1684t
amegakaryocytic thrombocytopenia as, 1689
dyskeratosis congenita as, 1687-1689, 1688f
Fanconi anemia as, 1684-1686, 1685f, 1685t
Shwachman-Diamond syndrome as, 1686-1687
PANDAS. *See* Pediatric autoimmune neuropsychiatric disorders associated with *Streptococcus pyogenes* (PANDAS)
Panencephalitis, subacute sclerosing, 1072-1073, 2075-2076
Panic attack, 79, 79t
seizure *versus*, *see website*
Panic disorder, 79-80, 79t
respiratory signs and symptoms of, *see website*
Panner disease, 2383-2384, 2383f, 2411, 2412f
Panniculitis, 2282-2285
cold, 358, 2285
factitial, 2285
lupus erythematosus, 2283, 2283f
pancreatic, 2284
post-steroid, 2283
Panniculus, *see website*
Panophthalmitis, 2173
Panoramic radiograph, *see website*
Pansystolic murmur, 1535
Panton-Valentine leukocidin (PVL), 904
Pantoprazole, 1293t
Pantothenate kinase-associated neurodegeneration, 2057t, 2060
Pantothenic acid, 194t
dietary reference intakes for, *see website*
Pao_2. *See* Alveolar partial pressure of oxygen (Pao_2)
PAP. *See* Pulmonary alveolar proteinosis (PAP)
PAPA. *See* Pyogenic arthritis, pyoderma gangrenosum, and acne (PAPA) syndrome
Papanicolaou (Pap) test, 1873-1874
Paper wasp, allergic responses to, 807f
Papilledema, *see also website*
of optic nerve, *see website*
as sign of cancer, 1728, 1730f
in pseudomotor cerebri, 2100-2101, 2100f
Papillitis, disc edema *versus*, *see website*
Papilloma, choroid plexus, 1750-1751
Papillomatosis, recurrent respiratory, *see website*
Papillomavirus, 1137-1141
antivirals for, *see website*
clinical manifestations of, 1139, 1139f
complications of, 1140
diagnosis of, 1139-1140
differential diagnosis of, 1140
epidemiology of, 1137-1138, 1138t
etiology of, 1137
pathogenesis of, 1138-1139
prevention of, 1141
prognosis for, 1140-1141
treatment of, 1140
Papillon-Lefèvre syndrome, 2273
Pap test. *See* Papanicolaou (Pap) test
Papular acrodermatitis of childhood, 2266, 2266f
Papular-purpuric "gloves and socks" syndrome (PPGSS), 1096-1097, 1096f
Papular urticaria, 2318, 2318f
Papule(s)
of acne, 2322-2323, 2322f
in cat-scratch disease, 984, 984f
of dracunculiasis, 1227
of erythema multiforme, 2241, 2242f
examination of, *see website*
Gottron
in juvenile dermatomyositis, 846-847, 847f, *see website*
in rheumatic disease, *see website*
in syphilis, 1016
PAR. *See* Perennial allergic rhinitis (PAR)
Para-aminosalicylic acid (PAS), 1008t, *see also website*
Paracentric chromosomal inversion, 405-406
Parachute reflex, *see website*
Paracoccidioides brasiliensis, 1068, *see also website*
Paradoxical pupil reaction, 2156
Paradoxical respiration, *see website*
Paraesophageal hernia, 597, 1265, 1265f
Paragonimiasis, *see website*
Paragonimus westermani, *see website*
Parahemophilia, 1703
Parainfluenza viruses (PIVs), 1125-1126, 1125t
in pneumonia, 1475t
Paraldehyde for status epilepticus, 2039t
Paralysis
Corynebacterium diphtheriae, *see website*
Erb-Duchenne, 573-574
facial, due to ear disorders, 2211, *see also website*
flaccid
due to botulism, 988-990
differential diagnosis of, 1084-1086, 1085t
in neuromuscular disorders, 2109-2110, 2112t
due to poliovirus infection, 1083-1084
hyperkalemic periodic, 220, 2113t, 2125t, 2130

Paralysis *(Continued)*
hypokalemic periodic, 222-223, 2125t, 2130
poliovirus infection *versus*, 1085t
Klumpke, 573-574
Landry ascending, 2143
oculosympathetic, 2155
periodic, 2130
hyperkalemic, 220
hypokalemic, 222-223
thyrotoxic, 222-223
pharmacologic in mechanical ventilation, 328
phrenic nerve, 574
due to poliovirus infection, 1082-1084
sleep, 53
seizure *versus*, *see website*
with tetanus, 992-993
tick, 2135-2136
vocal cord, 1451
Paralytic poliomyelitis, 1081-1088
Paralytic rabies, 1155
Paralytic scoliosis in arthrogryposis, *see website*
Paralytic shellfish poisoning, 1328t-1329t, *see website*
Parameatal urethral cyst, 1857-1858
Paramedics (EMT-P), *see website*
Paramyotonia, 2125
Paramyotonia congenita, 2113t, 2125t
Paranasal sinuses, 1436
cystic fibrosis and, 1485, 1488
Paraphimosis, 1854, 1854f
Paraquat lung, 1474
Parasitic infections
abdominal pain of, 1247t
fever of unknown origin in, 900t
food-borne, 1326t
helminthic
adult tapeworm, 1232-1234
Angiostrongylus cantonensis, 1226-1227
animal filariae, 1226
ascariasis, 1217-1218
cysticercosis, 1234-1237
dracunculiasis, 1227
echinococcosis, 1237-1239
enterobiasis, 1222
flukes, 1231-1232, *see also website*
Gnathostoma spinigerum, 1227
hookworms, 1218-1221
loiasis, 1225-1226
lymphatic filariasis, 1224-1225
Onchocera volvulus, 1225
schistosomiasis, 1230-1231
strongyloidiasis, 1223-1224
toxocariasis, 1227-1229
treatment of, *see website*
trichinosis, 1229-1230
trichuriasis, 1221-1222
HIV-related, *see website*
in immigrant children, 133
laboratory diagnosis of, *see website*
maternal
breast-feeding and, 540t
fetal and neonatal effects of, *see website*
in pneumonia, 1475t
predisposition to due to immunodeficiency, 716t
protozoan
African trypanosomiasis, 1190-1193
amebiasis, 1178-1180
American trypanosomiasis, 1193-1198
babesiosis, 1207, *see also website*
Balantidium coli, 1183
Cryptosporidium, 1183-1184
Cyclospora cayetanensis, 1184
Giardia lamblia, 1180-1183
Isospora belli, 1184
leishmaniasis, 1186-1190
malaria, 1198-1207
microsporidia, 1185
primary amebic meningoencephalitis, 1178, *see also website*
toxoplasmosis, 1208-1216
Parasitic infections *(Continued)*
treatment of, *see website*
Trichomonas vaginalis, 1185-1186
therapy for, 1177, *see also website*
traveler's diarrhea due to, 1338t
Parasomnias, 51-52, 52t
Parathyroid hormone (PTH)
in calcium homeostasis and bone metabolism, *see website*
disorders of
hyperparathyroidism as, 1920-1923
hypoparathyroidism as, 1916-1919
pseudohypoparathyroidism (Albright hereditary osteodystrophy), 1919-1920
Parathyroid hormone-related peptides (PTHrP), *see website*
Paraurethral urethral cyst, 1858, 1858f
Paravertebral block, 372
Parenchymal lung disease
emergency airway management in, 284
eosinophilic lung disease as, 1474, *see also website*
hypersensitivity to inhaled materials as, 1473, *see also website*
paraquat lung as, 1474
silo filler disease as, 1474, *see also website*
Parental permission, *see website*
Parenteral drug administration, *see website*
Parenteral nutrition for short bowel syndrome, 1316
Parenteral solutions, composition of, *see website*
Parent-infant bonding/attachment, 538-540, *see also website*
Parent(s)
death of, *see website*
genetic counseling and, 378
immunization refusal by, 893, *see website*
palliative care and, 151-152
presence during induction of anesthesia, *see website*
psychologic changes in during pregnancy, *see website*
role in maternal-infant attachment, *see website*
teen, characteristics of, 700-701
Parents' Evaluation of Developmental Status (PEDs), 41t-43t
Parinaud syndrome, 979, 984-985, 984f, 2161, 2168, 2169f
Parkinsonism, infantile, 445
PARM. *See* Polyanaline repeat expansion mutation (PARM)
P arm, 395
Paromomycin, *see also website*
for amebiasis, 1180, 1180t
for giardiasis, 1182, 1182t
for infectious diarrhea, 1337t
Paronychia, candidal, 1055
Paronychial inflammation, 2296-2297, 2297f
Paronychial tumors, 2297
Parotitis, *see also website*
in mumps, 1079, 1079f-1080f
Paroxetine for premenstrual dysphoric disorder, 692t
Paroxysmal cold hemoglobinuria, 1683
Paroxysmal depolarization shift (PDS), 2025
Paroxysmal dyskinesias, *see website*
Paroxysmal extreme pain disorder, *see website*
Paroxysmal hypercyanotic attacks in tetralogy of Fallot, 1574
Paroxysmal kinesigenic choreoathetosis (PKC), 2057t
Paroxysmal nocturnal hemoglobinuria (PNH), 1662, *see also website*
Paroxysmal stage of pertussis, 945
Paroxysmal tonic upgaze of childhood, *see website*
Paroxysmal torticollis of infancy, 2379
Paroxysms
in malaria, 1200-1201
seizures and, *see website*
Parrot fever, 1038, *see also website*
Parry Romberg syndrome, 851t
Partial agonists, receptor binding by, *see website*
Partial hospital program (PHP) for eating disorders, 96
Partial lipodystrophy, 2285-2286
Partial liquid ventilation (PLV), 596
Partial pressure of carbon dioxide (P_{CO_2}), *see also website*
arterial, *see website*
in asthma, 784t
in brain death, *see website*
reference values for, 230t, *see also website*
in respiratory acidosis, 238-239
in respiratory failure, 316
Partial pressure of oxygen in inspired gas (P_{IO_2}), *see website*
Partial pressure of oxygen (P_{O_2}), *see also website*
alveolar, *see website*
in asthma, 784t
divided into fraction of inspired oxygen, 319
in fetal circulation, *see website*
interpretation of, *see website*
in respiratory alkalosis, 240
in respiratory failure, 316
in transitional circulation, 1529, *see also website*
Partial rebreather mask, 319
Partial seizure, 2013, 2021-2023, 2022f
benign epilepsy syndromes with, 2021-2022
severe epilepsy syndromes with, 2022-2023
treatment of, 2028
Partial thromboplastin time, 1697
Partial trisomy, 403
Parulis, 1261
Parvovirus B19, 1094-1097, 1095f-1096f
arthritis associated with, 840
fetal therapy for, 551t
maternal, *see website*
red cell aplasia due to, 1652-1653
sickle cell disease and, 1663
PAS. *See Para*-aminosalicylic acid (PAS)
Passiflora alata for sedation, 271t
Passionflower for sedation, 271t
Passive immunity, immunization for, 881-883
Passive muscle tone, 2109
Pastes for skin disorders, 2216
Patellar dislocation, 2415
Patellar subluxation and dislocation, 2355
Patellar tendinosis, 2416
in basketball and volleyball, *see website*
Patellofemoral disorders, 2354
arthralgia and, *see website*
Patellofemoral stress syndrome (PFSS), 2415-2416
Patent ductus arteriosus (PDA), 1559-1561, 1560f
in adults, 1607
prevalence of, 1549
pulmonary atresia and, 1578-1579
respiratory distress syndrome and, 587
Patent foramen ovale (PFO), 1551
Patent urachus, *see website*
Pathocil. *See* Dicloxacillin
Pathogen-associated molecular patterns (PAMPs), 855
Pathogenicity islands, group B streptococci, 926
Patient, discussion of cancer treatment with, *see website*
Patient and family education
in asthma management, 788, 791t
for child abuse prevention, 142
in diabetes mellitus management, 1979
in functional abdominal pain, 1348
in pain management, 371
in pelvic examination, *see website*
in psychosomatic illness, 70
in seizures, 2025, 2026t
Patient-centered care in quality of care, *see website*

Patient-controlled analgesia (PCA)
for pain management, 365-367, 367f
postoperative, *see website*
Patient positioning
for ear examination or procedures, *see website*
for female genital examination, 1425
in gastroesophageal reflux disease, 1268
in infant botulism, 990
sudden infant death syndrome and, 1425
Patient safety, *see website*
Patrick test, 2412-2413
Pattern recognition receptors (PRRs), 855
Pausinystalia yohimbe, potential toxicity of, 272t-273t
Pavlik harness, 2359, 2360f
PAX3 gene, 2112-2113
PAX6 gene, 2154-2155
PAX7 gene, 2112-2113
PBD. *See* Peroxisomal biogenesis disorders (PBD)
PBG. *See* Porphobilinogen (PBG)
PBGD. *See* Porphobilinogen deaminase (PBGD) deficiency
PCA. *See* Patient-controlled analgesia (PCA)
PCD. *See* Primary ciliary dyskinesia (PCD)
PCO_2. *See* Partial pressure of carbon dioxide (Pco_2)
PCOS. *See* Polycystic ovary syndrome (PCOS)
PCP. *See* Phencyclidine (PCP); Primary care physician (PCP), role in emergency medical services
PCT. *See* Porphyria cutanea tarda (PCT)
PCV 13. *See* Pneumococcal conjugate vaccine (13 valent) (PCV 13)
PD. *See* Phenotypic diarrhea (PD)
PDA. *See* Patent ductus arteriosus (PDA)
PDD. *See* Pervasive developmental disorders (PDD)
PDF. *See* Personal flotation device (PDF)
PDGFRα. *See* Platelet-derived growth factor receptor α (PDGFRα)
PDGFRβ. *See* Platelet-derived growth factor receptor β (PDGFRβ)
PDS. *See* Paroxysmal depolarization shift (PDS)
PDSA. *See* Plan-Do-Study-Act (PDSA) cycle
"Peace pill," 683
Peach allergy, 821, 821t
Peak admittance in tympanometry, 2194-2195, 2194t
Peak expiratory flow (PEF)
assessment of, *see website*
in asthma, 784t, 785, 787f
Peak inspiratory pressure (PIP) in mechanical ventilation, 328
Peanut allergy, 821, 821t
Pearson syndrome, 391t, 748t, 1369, 1652
Pectus carinatum, 1517
Pectus excavatum, 1516-1517, 1516f
Pedestrian injuries, 23
Pedialyte, 1335t
Pediarix, 889
Pediatric Appendicitis score, 1351, 1351t
Pediatric autoimmune neuropsychiatric disorders associated with *Streptococcus pyogenes* (PANDAS), 81, 919
movement disorders associated with, 76
Pediatric emergency medicine (PEM), international, *see website*. *See* Emergency medical services for children (EMSC)
Pediatric gait, arms, legs, spine screen (pGALS), 2331
Pediatrician. *See* Health care worker
Pediatric Rhinoconjunctivitis Quality of Life Questionnaire (PRQLQ), 776
Pediatric Risk of Admission II (PRISA II), *see website*
Pediatric Risk of Mortality (PRISM) scoring system, *see website*
Pediatrics, 1-13
child mortality and, 1-2, 2f, 3t, 5t
genetics and, 382, 382t
growth of specialization of, 12-13
Pediatrics *(Continued)*
health among postinfancy children and, 2-4
health care costs and, 11
information explosion of 21st century and, 11-12
morbidities and, 4-5
organization of the profession, 12-13
patterns of health care in, 9
planning and implementing a system of care in, 9-11
scope and history of, 1-5
special risk populations in, 5-9
Pediatric Symptoms Checklist (PSC), 41t-43t, 58, 59f
Pediatric transport medicine, *see website*
Pediatric unstable bladder, 73
Pediculosis
head, 2321-2322, 2321f
in child-care setting, *see website*
pubic, 712t, 2321
treatment of, *see website*
Pediculosis capitis, 2321
Pediculosis corporis, 2321
Pediculosis pubis, 2321
Pediculus humanus var. *corporis*, 986
Pedigree, 383, 384f-387f
autosomal dominant, 387f
autosomal recessive, 388f
Pedigree notation in genetic transmission, 383, 384f-387f
PEDs. *See* Parents' Evaluation of Developmental Status (PEDs)
Peeling skin, familial, 2268t
PEEP. *See* Positive end-expiratory pressure (PEEP)
Peeping undescended testis, 1859
Peers, adolescent development of relationships with, 650t, 652-654
PEF. *See* Peak expiratory flow (PEF)
Pegaspar. *See* Pegaspargase
Pegaspargase for cancer therapy, *see website*
Peginterferon
for hepatitis B, 1399
for hepatitis C, 1401
PEG-Intron. *See* Pegylated interferon
Peg-shaped lateral teeth, 1250
Pegvisomant for growth hormone excess, *see website*
Pegylated interferon, *see website*
Pegylation, *see website*
PEL. *See* Primary effusion based lymphoma (PEL)
Peliosis, bacillary, 983t, 986
Peliosis hepatitis, 987
Pelizaeus-Merzbacher disease (PMD), 2074
Pelkan spur, 199
Pellagra, 2330
due to niacin deficiency, 195, 195f
Pelodera strongyloides, 1220t
Pelvic actinomyces, *see website*
Pelvic examination, *see website*. *See* Gynecological examination
Pelvic inflammatory disease (PID), 708, 939, 1871
abnormal uterine bleeding due to, 689t-690t
anaerobic, *see website*
dysmenorrhea due to, 691t
evaluation for, 710-711, 711t
gonococcal, 936
Pelvis
fetal ultrasound of, 550t
musculoskeletal pain syndrome of, 877t
sports injury to, 2407t, 2413-2414, 2413f
traumatic injury to, 339
urinary tract obstruction of, 1839t
PEM. *See* Pediatric emergency medicine (PEM); Protein-energy malnutrition (PEM)
Pemirolast potassium, 811t
Pemphigus, 2247-2248
immunofluorescence of, *see website*
Pemphigus foliaceus, 2247-2248, 2247f
Pemphigus vulgaris (PV), 2247
Pena-Shokeir syndrome, 2138
Penciclovir, *see website*
Pendred syndrome, 1896, 1906, 2190t
Penetrance, genetic, *see website*
incomplete, 383-385, 387f
Penetrating wounds of orbit, 2186
D-Penicillamine, *see also website*
for lead poisoning, 2453, 2453t
Penicillins, *see also website*
adverse reactions to, 825-826, *see also website*
allergy to, 918
for group A streptococci infection, 918
resistance to (*See* Antimicrobial resistance)
for vulvovaginitis, 1868t
Penicillin G, *see also website*
for actinomycosis, *see website*
for bacterial meningitis, 2093t
for diphtheria, *see website*
for group A streptococci infection, 918
for group B streptococci, 927
for infective endocarditis, 1625t
for meningococcal disease, 933t
for neonatal infection, 645t
for tetanus, 993
for tuberculosis, 1021-1022, 1021t-1022t
Penicillin G, benzathine, 645t
for acute rheumatic fever prophylaxis, 924t
for diphtheria, *see website*
for group A streptococci infection, 918
for neonatal infection, 645t
for pharyngitis, 1439-1440
for sexually transmitted infections in adolescents, 712t
for tuberculosis, 1021t-1022t
Penicillin G, procaine, 645t
for diphtheria, *see website*
for neonatal infection, 645t
for tuberculosis, 1021t
Penicillin V, *see also website*
for actinomycosis, *see website*
for acute rheumatic fever prophylaxis, 924t
for group A streptococci infection, 918
for pharyngitis, 1439-1440
for post-splenectomy prophylaxis, *see website*
Penis
agenesis of, 1857
circumcision and, 1854-1856, 1855f
disorders of
chordee without hypospadias as, 1854, 1854f
inconspicuous penis as, 1856, 1856f
micropenis as, 1856-1857, 1857f
phimosis and paraphimosis as, 1854, 1855f
priapism, 1857
torsion as, 1856
lateral curvature of, 1857
traumatic injury to, *see website*
Pennyroyal, potential toxicity of, 272t-273t
Pentacel, 889
Pentalogy of Cantrell, 1599
Pentamidine, 1192, *see also website*
Penta X, 1531t
Pentazocine, 367t
Pentobarbital
for anesthesia, *see website*
for traumatic brain injury, 300
Pentobarbital coma for status epilepticus, 2039t
Pentose, defects in metabolism of, 494t-495t, 495, *see also website*
Pentosuria, essential, *see website*
Pen VK. *See* Penicillin V
PEO. *See* Progressive external ophthalmoplegia (PEO)
PEPCK. *See* Phosphoenolpyruvate carboxykinase (PEPCK) deficiency
Peppermint oil for functional abdominal pain, 1348t
Pepper syndrome, 1754t

Peptic ulcer disease, 1291-1294, 1291t, 1292f-1293f, 1293t
abdominal pain of, 1247t
Peptide absorption disorders, 1318
Peptostreptococcus, *see website*
Percentile, statistical, *see website*
Percentile curves for growth, *see website*
Perceptual functioning, *see also website*
elementary school success and, 37t
Percussion, lung, *see website*
Percutaneous drug administration, *see website*
Percutaneous umbilical blood sampling (PUBS), 543t, 544, 549
in erythroblastosis fetalis, 617
Perennial allergic conjunctivitis, 809-810
Perennial allergic rhinitis (PAR), 775
Perforation
of augmented bladder, *see website*
esophageal, 1271, *see also website*
nasal septum, 1430
tympanic membrane, 2210, 2212
traumatic, *see website*
Performance enhancing drugs, 2422-2423, 2423t
Performance Improvement (PI), *see website*
Performance management, *see website*
Performance measure, *see website*
Perfusion, shock-related decrease of, 308t
Perfusion pressure, cerebral, 296
cerebral blood flow and, 297f
Periactin. *See* Cyproheptadine
Perianal abscess and fistula, 1360, 1360f
Perianal candidosis, 2314
Perianal dermatitis, 917
Perianal infectious dermatitis, 2304-2305, 2305f
Perianal pruritus in enterobiasis, 1222
Pericardial disease, 1635-1637, 1636t, 1637f
Pericardial effusion, tuberculous, 1009
Pericardiocentesis for emergencies, 295-296
Pericarditis
with acute rheumatic fever, 922
with chronic kidney disease, 1823t
enteroviruses in, 1091
Haemophilus influenzae in, 942
in Kawasaki disease, 864
tuberculous, 1004, 1009
Pericentric chromosomal inversion, 405-406
Perichondritis, 2198
Pericoronitis, 1257
Perifollicular petechiae, due to vitamin C deficiency, 198-199, 199f
Perihepatitis. *See* Fitz-Hugh-Curtis syndrome
Perilymphatic fistula (PLF), *see website*
Perinatal history, 532
in dysmorphology, *see website*
Perinatal infections, 543t, 547-548
Campylobacter in, 970
congenital lymphocytic choriomeningitis, 548
cytomegalovirus, 1116
herpes simplex virus, 1101, 1102f, 1103
tuberculous, 1007, 1011
Perinatal mortality, *see website*
Perinatal stroke, 2082
Perinaud syndrome in brain tumors, 1747
Perineal pruritus in enterobiasis, 1222
Perinuclear antineutrophil cytoplasmic antibody (pANCA), 1295
Periodic breathing pattern in newborn, 580
Periodic fever, aphthous stomatitis, pharyngitis, and adenitis (PFAPA), 859-860
Periodicity Schedule, 14, 15f
Periodic limb movement disorder (PLMD), 52-53
Periodic paralysis, 2130
hyperkalemic, 220, 2113t, 2125t, 2130
hypokalemic, 222-223, 2125t, 2130
poliovirus infection *versus*, 1085t
thyrotoxic, 222-223
Periodontal disease, 1257-1258
Periodontal injury, 1258-1259, 1259f
Perioperative care, 359, *see also website*
Periostitis in congenital syphilis, 1017-1018, 1018f
Peripartum influences on maternal-infant attachment, *see website*
Peripheral blood smear
in Chagas disease, 1196-1197
in iron deficiency-anemia, 1657f
in malaria, 1201
Peripheral chemoreceptors in respiration regulation, *see website*
Peripheral edema, physical examination of, 1531
Peripheral nerve injuries in newborn, 573-574, 574f
Peripheral neuropathy
due to cancer and its therapy, *see website*
in tyrosinemia, 422
Peripheral vascular resistance (PVR), 592, 592f
Peripheral vascular system disease
arteriovenous fistula as, 1638, *see also website*
Kawasaki disease as, 1638, *see also website*
primary hypertension as, 1639-1647
blood pressure measurement in, 1639-1640
clinical manifestations of, 1641-1642
definition of, 1639
diagnosis of, 1642, 1642f, 1643t-1644t
etiology and pathophysiology of, 1640-1641, 1641t
prevalence of, 1639
treatment of, 1642-1647, 1644f-1646f, 1645t-1646t
Peritoneal dialysis
for acute renal failure, 1821-1822, 1821t
catheters for, infection associated with, *see website*
for end-stage renal disease, 1826, 1826t
Peritoneum disorders
ascites as, 1416, *see also website*
chylous, 1416, *see also website*
epigastric hernia as, 1418, *see also website*
malformations as, 1416
peritonitis as, 1416-1418
Peritonitis, 1416-1418
meconium, 601
in cystic fibrosis, 1487f
with nephrotic syndrome, 1805
due to peritoneal dialysis catheterization, *see website*
tuberculous, 1006
Peritonsillar cellulitis/abscess, 1440, 1442
croup *versus*, 1447
Periungual infection with *Candida*, 1055
Periungual wart, 2315, 2315f
Periventricular leukomalacia (PVL), 566-568
cerebral palsy and, 2061-2063
optic nerve hypoplasia with, *see website*
Perkins line, 2358
Perlèche, 2297
Perlman syndrome, *see website*
Permanent neonatal diabetes mellitus (PNDM), 1995
Permethrin, 2320, *see also website*
Permission, parental, *see website*
Permissive hypercapnia in mechanical ventilation for respiratory distress syndrome, 585
Permissive hypoxemia in mechanical ventilation for respiratory distress syndrome, 585
Pernio, 358, 2285
Peroneal muscular atrophy, 2138-2139
axonal type, 2139
Peroneal spastic flatfoot, 2339-2340
Peroral drug absorption, *see website*
Peroral drug administration, *see website*
Peroxisomal biogenesis disorders (PBD), 462-463, 463t-464t, 464f
Peroxisomal disorders, 462-467
complications of, 467
diagnosis of, 466-467
epidemiology of, 462
etiology of, 462, 462t-463t
genetic counseling in, 467
laboratory findings in, 465-466, 466t
Peroxisomal disorders *(Continued)*
pathogenesis of, 462-465, 463t-464t, 464f-465f
pathology of, 462
treatment of, 467
Persistent diarrhea, 1331, 1336f
Persistent fetal vasculature, 2176
Persistent hyperinsulinemic hypoglycemia of infancy (PHHI), 522-523
Persistent Müllerian duct syndrome, 1964-1965
Persistent pulmonary hypertension of the newborn (PPHN), 592-594, 592f, *see also website*
Persistent pupillary membrane, 2156
Persistent rhinitis (PR), 775
Personal flotation device (PDF), 24
Personalized medicine, *see website*
Personal protective equipment (PPE), *see website*
Pertussis, 944-948
in child-care setting, *see website*
clinical manifestations of, 945
complications of, 947
diagnosis of, 945-946
epidemiology of, 944
etiology of, 944
pathogenesis of, 944-945
prevention of, 947-948
re-infection, 944
treatment of, 946-947, 946t
vaccines for, 881t, 947-948
Pertussis toxin (PT), 944-945
Pervasive developmental disorders (PDD), 100, 101t-102t
Asperger's disorder, 105t, 106
autistic disorder, 100-106, 101t, 103f-104f, 105t
childhood disintegrative disorder, 106, *see also website*
language disorders of, 118
Pes planus (flatfoot), 2338, 2338f
Pest allergens, 769
Pesticide exposure, *see website*
gastroenteritis due to, 1328t-1329t
Pet dander allergens, 769, 769t
Petechiae
fever with, 896t
perifollicular, due to vitamin C deficiency, 198-199, 199f
due to vomiting, 1243t
Peters anomaly, *see website*
Petit mal seizure, 2023
Pet therapy for pain management, 371
Peutz-Jeghers syndrome (PJS), *see website*
cutaneous manifestations of, 2236-2237
malignancy susceptibility associated with, *see website*
PFAPA. *See* Periodic fever, aphthous stomatitis, pharyngitis, and adenitis (PFAPA)
Pfaundler-Hurler disease, 512t
Pfeiffer syndrome, 2012t, 2013
PFIC. *See* Progressive familial intrahepatic cholestasis (PFIC)
PFO. *See* Patent foramen ovale (PFO)
PFSS. *See* Patellofemoral stress syndrome (PFSS)
pGALS. *See* Pediatric gait, arms, legs, spine screen (pGALS)
PGD. *See* Preimplantation genetic diagnosis (PGD)
P-glycoprotein transporter, *see website*
pH, 230t, *see also website*
in acid-base disorders, 230
esophageal, in aspiration syndromes, 1472t
of fetal scalp blood, 544
PHACE syndrome, 2052
congenital heart disease with, 1531t, 1569
Phagocyte disorders, 721t, 741-746, 742t, 743f
Chédiak-Higashi syndrome as, 744-745
chronic granulomatous disease as, 745-746, 745f
evaluation of, 720t, 722
immunizations in, 892t

Phagocyte disorders *(Continued)*
infections with, *see website*
leukocyte adhesion deficiency as, 741-744
leukocytosis as, 752, *see also website*
leukopenia as, 746-752
myeloperoxidase deficiency as, 745
screening for, 718t
Phagocytic inflammatory response, *see website*
Phagocytic system
eosinophils in, 739-741
monocytes, macrophages, and dendritic cells in, 739, *see also website*
neutrophils in, 739, *see also website*
Phagosomes, *see website*
Phakomas, retinal, 2178, 2178f
Phakomatosis pigmentovascularis, 2226
Phalangeal fracture, 2391
Pharmacobetabonomics, *see website*
Pharmacodynamics, *see also website*
of analgesics, 362-363
ontogenic effects on, *see website*
Pharmacogenetic polymorphisms, *see website*
Pharmacogenetics, 250, *see also website*
Pharmacogenetic testing in acute lymphocytic leukemia, 1736
Pharmacogenomics, 250, *see also website*
Pharmacokinetics, *see also website*
of analgesics, 362-363
Pharmacoproteomics, *see website*
Pharyngeal abscess, 1440-1442, 1441f
Pharyngeal culture in gonococcal disease, 938
Pharyngitis, 1439-1440
in child-care setting, *see website*
Epstein-Barr virus, 1112, 1113f
gonococcal, 937
in PFAPA, 859-860
streptococcal, 914-925
acute rheumatic fever and, 921, 923
Pharyngotonsillitis, 1443-1444, 1443f
Phasic sinus arrhythmia, 1610, 1612f
Phencyclidine (PCP), 676t, 683
Pheniramine maleate, 811t
Phenobarbital
adrenal insufficiency due to, 1927
adverse effects of, 2031t
for chorea, 924
for hypoxic-ischemic encephalopathy, 571
neonatal withdrawal from, 624
possible adverse reactions to in premature infant, 563t
for seizures
dosages of, 2030t
febrile, 2018
neonatal, 2037
for status epilepticus, 2038-2039, 2039t
for vomiting prophylaxis, 1244t
Phenocopy, *see website*
Phenomic awareness, 114
Phenothiazines
toxicity of, 251t
for vomiting, 1244t
Phenotypes, *see website*
Phenotypic diarrhea (PD), 1311-1312, 1341, 1343f
Phentermine for weight loss in adults, 187t
Phenylalanine, defects in metabolism of, 418-422, 419f, 421f
Phenylephrine
for allergic rhinitis, 780t
for shock, 313t
Phenylketonuria (PKU), 418-422, 419f, 421f
maternal, *see website*
congenital heart disease with, 1531t
fetal therapy for, 551t
Phenytoin
adrenal insufficiency due to, 1927
adverse effects of, 2031t
for arrhythmias, 1611t-1612t
drug interactions with, *see website*
gingival overgrowth due to, 1257
for hypoxic-ischemic encephalopathy, 571
Phenytoin *(Continued)*
for seizures
dosages of, 2030t
neonatal, 2037
PHEO. *See* Pheochromocytoma (PHEO)
Pheochromocytoma, 1941-1943
cardiac manifestations of, 1531t
diarrhea caused by, *see website*
Pheochromocytoma (PHEO), 1773
PHH. *See* Posthemorrhage hydrocephalus (PHH)
PHHI. *See* Persistent hyperinsulinemic hypoglycemia of infancy (PHHI)
Philadelphia chromosome, 1738-1739, *see also website*
Philodendron toxicity, 269t
Phimosis, 1854, 1855f
PHKG2 gene, 498
Phlebectasia, congenital, 2224-2225, 2226f
Phlebotomy for porphyria cutanea tarda, *see website*
Phlyctenules, *see website*
pH monitoring, esophageal, 1267
Phobias, 78t, 81
social, 78, 79t
Phobic hallucinations, acute, 106-107
Phonemes, 112
Phonics, 114
Phonologic disorder, 117t, 119, *see website*
Phonologic processing, *see website*
Phonology, 114
Phonophobia in migraine, 2041
Phosgene, in terrorism, *see website*
Phosphate, renal tubular regulation of, *see website*
Phosphate and tension homolog (PTEN), *see website*
Phosphate enema, 74t
Phosphatonin, 206, *see also website*
overproduction of, 207
Phosphodiesterase inhibitors, *see website*
Phosphoenolpyruvate carboxykinase (PEPCK) deficiency, 504
hypoglycemia in, 529
Phosphofructokinase deficiency, 1677
muscle, 501
Phosphoglycerate deficiency, 442, 1677-1678
Phosphoribosylpyrophosphate (PRPP) synthetase superactivity, *see website*
Phosphorus, 225-229
conversion factors for, *see website*
disorders of
hyperphosphatemia as, 228-229
hypophosphatemia as, 226-228, 227t
excretion of, 226
intake of, 226
metabolism of, 225-226, 226t
reference values for, *see website*
rickets due to deficiency of, 201t-202t, 206-207, *see website*
Phosphorylase deficiency
liver, 497
hypoglycemia in, 528
muscle, 500-501
thymidine, *see website*
Phosphorylase kinase deficiency, 494t-495t, 497-498
Phosphorylation disease, oxidative, 506, 507t-509t, 508f
Phosphoserine aminotransferase deficiency, 442
Photoallergic reaction, 2255
Photocoagulation, laser, 2175-2176
Photodermatitis, 2256
Photoparoxysmal epilepsy, 2023
Photophobia in migraine, 2041
Photopsia, 2041-2042
Photosensitivity, 2254-2259, *see also website*
Phototherapy
for atopic dermatitis, 805
for hemolytic disease of newborn due to ABO blood group incompatibility, 619
Phototherapy *(Continued)*
for hyperbilirubinemia, 610-611, 610f, 612t
for psoriasis, 2260
Photoxic reactions, 2255-2256
PHOX2B gene
congenital central hypoventilation syndrome and, 1520-1521
ventilator dependence and, 1520
PHP. *See* Partial hospital program (PHP); Pseudohypoparathyroidism (PHP)
Phrenic nerve injury in newborn, 574
PHS. *See* Pallister-Hall syndrome (PHS)
Phthirus pubis, 712t
Physeal injury, 2408
Physical abuse, 135. *See also* Abuse and neglect
Physical activity
in eating disorders treatment, 94-95
energy requirements and, *see website*
overweight and obesity and, 182, 186
Physical development
adolescent
during early adolescence, 649, 650t-652t, 651f-652f
during late adolescence, 654
during middle adolescence, 653
age 0-2 months, 27, 29f
age 2-6 months, 29-30
age 6-12 months, 30
age 12-18 months, 31
age 18-24 months, 32-33
assessment of, 39, *see also website*
during middle childhood, 36-37, 36t
of premature infant, 562
during preschool years, 33-34
Physical education, congenital heart disease and, 1603
Physical examination
in acute illness, 276-277
of adolescent, 666-667
following rape, 704
in allergic disease, 765
in anemia, 1648-1649
in appendicitis, 1350
in attention deficit/hyperactivity disorder, 110
of breast, *see website*
self-examination, *see website*
in cancer, 1728, 1730f
in cardiovascular disease, 1530-1533, 1532t
in communication disorder, 121
in dysmorphology, *see website*
of ear, *see website*
in failure to thrive, 149t
in fever of unknown origin, 901, 901t
of foreign-born adoptees, 132-134
in genetic metabolic disease, 416-417
gynecological, *see website*
of special needs girls, 1874
in hemostatic disorders, 1696
in intellectual disability, 127t
in mucopolysaccharidoses, 515t-516t
neurologic, *see website*
of newborn, 532-536
abdomen in, 535-536
anus in, 536
chest in, 535
extremities in, 536
face in, 534
general appearance in, 532-533
genitals in, 536
growth and behavior, *see website*
heart in, 535, 535f
neck in, 534-535
neurologic assessment in, 536
(*See also* Neurologic examination)
skin in, 533, 533f
skull in, 533-534, 534t
in orthopedic problems, 2331-2332, 2332t, 2333f
in poisonings, 253
preparticipation sports, 2401-2405, 2401t-2404t, 2405f

Physical examination *(Continued)*
in respiratory disease, *see website*
in seizures, 2019
in skin disorders, *see website*
in systemic hypertension, 1642, 1643t
in wheezing, 1458
Physical therapy
for juvenile dermatomyositis, 849
for osteomyelitis, 2398
for pain management, 371
for respiratory insufficiency, 1525
Physiologic anemia of infancy, 1654-1655
Physiologic buffers, *see website*
Physiologic dead space, 316-317
Physiologic jaundice, 605-606, 606f
Physiologic studies, sudden infant death syndrome and, 1428
Physiotherapy for Duchenne and Becker muscular dystrophy, 2122
Physis, *see website*
Physostigmine as poisoning antidote, 256t-257t
Phytobezoars, 1291
Phytolacca americana, potential toxicity of, 272t-273t
Phytosterolaemia, *see website*
PI. *See* Performance Improvement (PI)
Piaget theory, *see website*
Pica, 71
PID. *See* Pelvic inflammatory disease (PID)
PIE. *See* Pulmonary interstitial emphysema (PIE)
Piebaldism, 425, 2238t, 2239, 2239f
Pierre Robin syndrome, 1254, 1254f, *see also website*
Pierson syndrome, 1807
Pigbel, *see website*
Pigeon fancier or breeder lung, *see website*
Pigmentation, McCune-Albright syndrome in abnormal, 1892, 1892f
Pigment disorders
hyper-, 2236-2238, 2236f-2237f
hypo-, 2237f-2240f, 2238-2240, 2238t, 2240t
of nails, 2294-2295
Pilar cyst, *see website*
Pili annulati, 2293
Pili tori, 2292
"Pill" esophagitis, 1270
Pilocytic astrocytoma (PA), 1748, 1749f
Pilomatricoma, *see website*
Pilomyxoid astrocytoma, 1749
Pilonidal disease, 1362
Pineal parenchymal tumor, 1752
Pinguecula, 2169
Pinhole effect, 2151
Pink disease, *see website*
Pinna
malformations of, *see website*
pits and sinus tracts anterior to, 2221
PINT. *See* Premature Infants in Need of Transfusion (PINT) study
Pinworm, 1222, *see also website*
in vulvovaginitis, 1866, 1868t
Pio_2. *See* Partial pressure of oxygen in inspired gas (Pio_2)
PIP. *See* Peak inspiratory pressure (PIP)
Piperacillin, *see also website*
for cystic fibrosis lung infection, 1492t
for neonatal infection, 645t
for *Pseudomonas aeruginosa*, *see website*
Piperacillin-tazobactam, *see also website*
for cystic fibrosis lung infection, 1492t
for neonatal infection, 645t
Pseudomonas aeruginosa, *see website*
Piperazines, 771t, 1217-1218
Piper methysticum for sedation, 271t
Pipracil. *See* Piperacillin
Pirbuterol, 796
PIT1 gene, 1876t, 1877
Pits
preauricular, 2221
splenic, *see website*
Pitted keratolysis, 2306
Pituitary dwarfism, 627
Pituitary gland
hormones of, 1876, *see also website*
puberty physiology and, 1886, *see also website*
Pituitary gland disorders
corticotropinoma as, *see website*
diabetes insipidus as, 1881-1884
excess growth hormone secretion as, *see website*
fetal and neonatal overgrowth as, *see website*
gigantism as, *see website*
hyperpituitarism, 1886, *see also website*
hyponatremia as, 1884-1886
hypopituitarism as, 1876-1881
hypothyroidism due to disease of, 1901
prolactinoma as, *see website*
pubertal development disorders as, 1886-1894
tall stature as, *see website*
tumors of, adrenal insufficiency due to, 1926t
Pityriasis alba, 2252, 2252f
Pityriasis lichenoides, 2260-2261, 2260f-2261f
Pityriasis lichenoides chronica (PLC), 2260-2261
Pityriasis lichenoides et varioliformis acuta (PLEVA), *see website*
Pityriasis rosea, 2262, 2262f
Pityriasis rubra pilaris, 2262-2263, 2263f
PIVKA. *See* Proteins induced by vitamin K absence (PIVKA)
PIVs. *See* Parainfluenza viruses (PIVs)
PiZZ defect, 1461-1462
PJS. *See* Peutz-Jeghers syndrome (PJS)
PK. *See* Prekallikrein (PK)
PKC. *See* Paroxysmal kinesigenic choreoathetosis (PKC)
PKDL. *See* Post-kala-azar dermal leishmaniasis (PKDL)
PKHD1 gene defect, 1383t, 1796, 1798
PKU. *See* Phenylketonuria (PKU)
Placenta
chemical pollutants crossing, *see website*
in fetal circulation, 1529, *see also website*
infections crossing, 636-639, 637t
listeriosis of, *see website*
separation of, *see website*
twinning and, 554, 554t
vascular anastomoses in monochorionic twins, 554
Plagiocephaly, *see also website*
frontal, 2012
occipital, 2012
Plague, 973-974, *see also website*
Plan-Do-Study-Act (PDSA) cycle, *see website*
Plantar dermatosis, juvenile, 2250-2251, 2251f
Plantar fasciitis, 2418, *see website*
Plantar keratodermas, 2272-2273, 2273f
Plantar response assessment in neurologic examination, *see website*
Plantar wart, 2315, 2315f
"Plant-based diet," 168
Plants, toxicity of, 268-269, 268t-269t
Plaque, examination of, *see website*
Plasma anion gap, 233-234
Plasma complement control protein deficiency, 755
Plasma concentration of drug, *see website*
Plasmalogen synthesis, isolated defects of, 464-465
Plasma membrane carnitine transport defect, 460-461
Plasma membrane in cardiac development, *see website*
Plasmapheresis, 2135
Plasma thromboplastin antecedent, 1696t
Plasma transfusion, 1693, *see also website*
Plasma volume, hyponatremia due to decreased, 1885
Plasma water, *see website*
Plasminogen, reference values for, 1698t
Plasminogen activator inhibitor, reference values for, 1698t
Plasminogen activator inhibitor deficiency, 1704
Plasmodium. See Malaria
Plasticity
developmental, *see website*
neuronal, *see website*
Platelets
disorders of, 1714-1722
fetal, *see website*
transfusion of, 1693, *see also website*
Platelet adhesion, 1713
Platelet aggregation, 1698
Platelet count
in dengue fever, 1149
fetal, *see website*
in hemolytic-uremic syndrome, 1793
in hemostatic disorders, 1696-1697
normal, 1714
reference values for, *see website*
in Rocky Mountain spotted fever, 1042
Platelet-derived growth factor receptor α (PDGFRα), *see website*
Platelet-derived growth factor receptor β (PDGFRβ), *see website*
Platelet function analyzer, 1697
Platinol. *See* Carboplatin and cisplastin
Play
in autistic disorder, 100
during preschool years, 34-35
Play audiometry, 2193-2194
PLC. *See* Pityriasis lichenoides chronica (PLC); Posterior laryngeal cleft (PLC)
Pleocytosis in enteroviral meningitis, 1091
Pleomorphic rhabdomyosarcoma, 1760
Plesiomonas shigelloides, 974, *see also website*
in infectious diarrhea, 1337t
inflammatory bowel disease *versus*, 1298t
in traveler's diarrhea, 1338t
Plethora in newborn, 619-620
Plethysmography, *see website*
Pleural cavity
accumulation of blood in, 1513-1514
visualization of, *see website*
Pleural effusion
with pneumonia, 1479, 1479t
transudative, 1513
tuberculous, 1003-1004, 1004f
Pleural fluid examination
in pneumonia, 1479t
in serofibrinous pleurisy, 1506-1507
in tuberculosis, 1003-1004
Pleurisy, 1505-1509
dry or plastic, 1505, 1505f-1506f
purulent, 1507-1509, 1508f
serofibrinous or serosanguineous, 1506-1507
Pleurisy effusion, 1505-1509, 1505f-1506f
Pleurodesis, chemical, 1511-1512
Pleurodynia, due to enterovirus, 1090
PLEVA. *See* Pityriasis lichenoides et varioliformis acuta (PLEVA)
Plexiform neurofibromas, 2046-2047
Plexiform neuroma of eyelid, 2165
PLF. *See* Perilymphatic fistula (PLF)
PLMD. *See* Periodic limb movement disorder (PLMD)
PLOD gene, 2278
Plumboporphyria, *see website*
Plummer disease, 1915
Pluripotential stem cells, *see website*
Plus disease, 2175
PLV. *See* Partial liquid ventilation (PLV)
PMD. *See* Pelizaeus-Merzbacher disease (PMD)
PMS. *See* Premenstrual syndrome (PMS)
PNDM. *See* Permanent neonatal diabetes mellitus (PNDM)
PNET. *See* Primitive neuroectodermal tumor (PNET)
Pneumatic otoscope head, 2202
Pneumococcal conjugate vaccine (13 valent) (PCV 13), 884t, 889, 914t
Pneumococcus. *See Streptococcus pneumoniae*

Pneumococcus vaccine, 884t, 913-914, 914t, 2095
cochlear implants and, 2196t
HIV infection and, 1173f
in nephrotic syndrome, 1805
otitis media and, 2200, 2201f
pneumonia hospitalization and, 1479
recommended schedule for, 887f-888f
for travel, *see website*
Pneumocystis jiroveci, 1069, *see also website*
Pneumocystis jiroveci pneumonia, HIV-related, 1162-1163, *see website*
prophylaxis for, 1173-1174, 1174t-1176t
Pneumomediastinum, 1512-1513, 1512f-1513f
neonatal, 597-599, 599f
due to vomiting, 1243t
Pneumonia, 1474-1479
adenovirus, 1132-1133
due to anaerobes, *see website*
aspiration
due to hydrocarbon toxicity, 267
neonatal, 590, 591f
atypical, 1477
Blastomyces dermatitidis, 1064
bronchiolitis obliterans organizing, *see website*
in child-care setting, *see website*
Chlamydia trachomatis, 1037
Chlamydophila pneumoniae, 1033-1035
clinical manifestations of, 1476-1477
Coccidioides, 1066-1068
complications of, 1479, 1479f, 1479t
diagnosis of, 1477-1478, 1477f-1478f
differential diagnosis of, 1477t
empyema with, 1507-1508, 1508f
epidemiology of, 1474, 1474f, 1475t
etiology of, 1475-1476, 1475t-1476t
Francisella tularensis, 979
giant cell, 1071
Haemophilus influenzae in, 942
hypersensitivity, 1473, *see also website*
in influenza, 1124
interstitial in lysinuric protein intolerance, 455
Legionella, *see website*
lymphocytic interstitial, HIV-related, 1165
due to measles, 1071, 1072t
Mycoplasma pneumoniae in, 1030
neonatal, 633, 633t, 639
respiratory distress syndrome *versus*, 583-584
treatment of, 644-646
nosocomial, *Pseudomonas aeruginosa* in, 976
in parainfluenza viruses, 1125t
pathogenesis of, 1476
Pneumocystis jiroveci, 1069, *see also website*
HIV-related, 1162-1163, 1173-1174, 1175t-1176t, *see website*
prevention of, 1479
prognosis for, 1478-1479
Pseudomonas aeruginosa, 976t
respiratory syncytial virus, 1127-1128
Staphylococcus aureus, 905-906
Streptococcus pneumoniae, 912f
treatment of, 1478, 1478t
varicella, 1106, 1109
ventilator-associated, 329
Pneumonic plague, 973
Pneumopericardium, 597-599
Pneumotaxic center, *see website*
Pneumothorax, 1509-1512, 1509t, 1510f-1511f
in cystic fibrosis, 1494
neonatal, 577, 578f, 597-599, 598f
open, 336t
tension, 289t, 336, 336t
due to vomiting, 1243t
PNH. *See* Paroxysmal nocturnal hemoglobinuria (PNH)
PNP. *See* Purine nucleoside phosphorylase (PNP) deficiency
Po_2. *See* Partial pressure of oxygen (Po_2)
Pocket infection. *See* Catheter-related bloodstream infection (CRBSI)
Podofilox
for genital warts, 713t
for human papillomavirus, 1140
Poikiloderma, 2258, 2258f
Point mutation in proto-oncogene activation, *see website*
Poiseuille's law, *see website*
Poison control center
Poison hemlock toxicity, 269t
Poisoning, 250-270
acetaminophen, 258-260, 259f, 259t
amphotericin B, *see website*
analgesics, 258-261
anesthesia, *see website*
antidepressants, 263-266, 264f
antipsychotics, 266
arsenic, *see website*
ascorbic acid, 200
β-blockers, 261
calcium channel blockers, 261-262
cancer treatment, *see website*
carbon monoxide, 269-270
cardiac arrest due to, 289t
cardiovascular medications, 261-263
caustics, 266
as childhood injury, 24
cholinesterase-inhibiting insecticides, 266-267
clonidine, 262
common nontoxic and minimally toxic products and, 251t
diagnostic testing in, 254, 254t
digoxin, 262-263
ethylene glycol, 268
folate, 197
food-borne (*See* Food-borne illness)
gastroenteritis due to, 1328t-1329t
herb, 270, 272t-273t
historical and physical findings in, 251-253, 252t
household products, 266-268
hydrocarbons, 267
hydrogen cyanide, 270
ibuprofen and other nonsteroidal antiinflammatory drugs, 260-261
initial evaluation in, 251-254
iron, 263
laboratory evaluation in, 253-254, 254t
lead, 2448-2453
δ-aminolevulinic acid dehydratase deficiency due to, *see website*
major modes of presentation, drugs associated with, 255t
management of, 254
antidotes, 256t-258t, 258
decontamination, 254-257, 257t
enhanced elimination, 257-258
supportive care, 258
mercury, *see website*
methamphetamine, 684t
methanol, 267-268
mushroom, 2454, *see also website*
niacin, 195
oral hypoglycemic, 263
oral opioids, 261
plant, 268-269, 268t-269t
psychiatric medications, 263-266
pyridoxine, 196
recognizable syndromes of, 253t
respiratory distress due to, 316
respiratory signs and symptoms of, *see website*
riboflavin, 193
salicylates, 260
salt
hypernatremia and, 214
plasma osmolality in, *see website*
seafood, 2454, *see also website*
selective serotonin reuptake inhibitors, 264-265, 265f, 265t
small dose medications, 251t
solanine, 2454, *see also website*
thiamine, 192
Poisoning *(Continued)*
toxic alcohols, 267-268
vitamin A, 190
Poison ivy, 2251, 2251f
Pokeweed toxicity, 269t, 272t-273t
Policy(ies)
for emergency departments, *see website*
vaccine, 885
Policy of pay per performance (P4P), *see website*
Polioencephalitis, 1084
Poliomyelitis
abortive, 1083, 1086
in child-care setting, *see website*
maternal, *see website*
nonparalytic, 1083, 1086
paralytic, 1083-1084, 1086
Polio vaccine, 881t, 884t, 894, 1087-1088
HIV infection and, 1173f
international, 894
recommended schedule for, 886-889, 887f-888f
for travel, *see website*
Polioviruses, 1081-1088
clinical manifestations of, 1082-1084
complications of, 1086-1087
diagnosis of, 1084
differential diagnosis of, 1084-1086, 1085t
epidemiology of, 1081, 1082f
etiology of, 1081
pathogenesis of, 1081-1082
prevention of, 1087-1088
prognosis for, 1087
transmission of, 1081
treatment of, 1086
Poliovirus receptor, 1081
Pollakiuria, 1851
Pollen allergens, 769t
Pollen-food syndrome, 822
Pollicization, 2386, 2386f
Pollutants
chemical, 2448, *see also website*
wheezing and bronchitis due to, 1460
POL region, 1157
Polyanaline repeat expansion mutation (PARM), 1520-1521
Polyangiitis, microscopic, 874-876, 874t
Polyarteritis nodosa (PAN), 868t, 872-874, 873f
infantile, 862-867, 868t
Polyarthritis
in juvenile idiopathic arthritis, 831t, 832, 833f
migratory, in acute rheumatic fever, 921-922
Polychlorinated biphenyl exposure, *see website*
Polychondritis, relapsing, 880, *see also website*
Polycillin. *See* Ampicillin
Polycystic kidney disease
autosomal dominant, *see website*
congenital heart disease with, 1531t
hematuria due to, 1798, 1798f
autosomal recessive, *see website*
hematuria due to, 1796-1798, 1797f, 1797t
Polycystic liver disease, autosomal dominant, *see website*
Polycystic ovary syndrome (PCOS), 1870, *see also website*
amenorrhea due to, 686
with obesity, 184t
with type 2 diabetes mellitus, 1993t
in type I glycogen storage disease, 493-495
Polycythemia, 1683, *see also website*
in cyanotic patient, 1541, 1603
plethora in newborn due to, 619-620
secondary, 1683, *see also website*
Polycythemia rubra vera, *see website*
Polydactyly, 2342, 2386, 2386t
Polydactyly syndromes, short-rib, 2434
Polydipsia
in diabetes insipidus, 1881-1882
differential diagnosis of, 1882t
due to hypokalemia, 224
osmolality and, *see website*
primary, hyponatremia due to, 1885

Polyendocrinopathy (APS), 1925t
Polyenes, *see website*
Polyethylene glycol
  for constipation maintenance therapy, 74t
  for fecal disimpaction, 74t
Polygenic hypercholesterolemia, 473t, 475
Polygenic inheritance, 393-394
Polyglucosan body disease, 497
Polyhydramnios
  esophageal functioning and, *see website*
  fetal therapy for, 551t
  in high-risk pregnancies, *see website*
Polymastia, *see website*
Polymenorrhea, 686t
Polymerase chain reaction (PCR), 376, *see also website*
  in Duchenne and Becker muscular dystrophy, 2120
  in enterovirus infection, 1093
  in hepatitis A, 1396t
  in HIV infection, 1166-1167, 1166t
  in parainfluenza viruses, 1125t
  in pertussis, 945-946
  in Q fever, 1052
  in rabies, 1155
  in respiratory syncytial virus infection, 1128
  in roseola, 1119
  in toxoplasmosis, 1214
  in trichomoniasis, 1186
Polymicrogyrias, 2004
Polymorphism, *see website*
Polymorphonuclear leukocytes, 2220
Polymorphous light eruption, 2257
Polymox. *See* Amoxicillin
Polymyositis-scleroderma antibody, *see website*
Polyneuropathy
  Corynebacterium diphtheriae, *see website*
  critical illness, poliovirus infection *versus*, 1085t
Polyomavirus, 1157, *see also website*
Polyomavirus nephropathy (PVN), *see website*
Polyostotic fibrous dysplasia, 1892
Polyploidy, 399-400, 400t
Polypoid cells, 399
Polyposis, familial adenomatous, *see website*
Polyp(s)
  cervical, abnormal uterine bleeding due to, 689t-690t
  endometrial, abnormal uterine bleeding due to, 689t-690t
  juvenile polyposis syndrome, *see website*
    malignancy susceptibility associated with, *see website*
  nasal, 1431, 1433, 1433f
    in cystic fibrosis, 1496
  umbilical, *see website*
Polysomnogram (PSG), 50-51
Polysplenia, 1531t, 1589t, 1595-1596
Polysyllabic jargoning, 31
Polythelia, *see website*
Polyunsaturated fatty acids (PUFAs), *see website*
Polyuria
  in diabetes insipidus, 1881-1882
  differential diagnosis of, 1882t
  fluid therapy adjustments and, 245, 245t
  due to hypokalemia, 224
Pomade acne, 2322-2323, 2323f
Pompe disease, 494t-495t, 499-500, 500f
  cardiac manifestations of, 1531t
  myopathy with, *see website*
Ponseti method for clubfoot treatment, 2337
Pontocerebellar hypoplasia, 2007
PONV. *See* Postoperative nausea and vomiting (PONV)
Popliteal angle measurement, *see website*
Popliteal cyst, 2353
Population stratification, *see website*
POR. *See* P450 oxidoreductase (POR) deficiency
Porencephaly, 2004-2005
POR gene, *see website*
Pork tapeworm, 1232-1235, 1232t, *see also website*
Porokeratosis, 2265-2266, 2265f
Porphobilinogen deaminase (PBGD) deficiency, *see website*
Porphobilinogen (PBG), *see website*
Porphyria cutanea tarda (PCT), *see website*
Porphyrias, 517, *see also website*
  abdominal pain of, 1247t
  photosensitivity in, 2256, 2256f
Portal hypertension, 1415, *see also website*
  as manifestation of liver disease, 1376
Portal vein thrombosis, *see website*
Port-wine stain, 2224, 2225f
Posaconazole, *see website*
Position 57 in DQB1, type 1 diabetes mellitus and, 1970-1971
Positioning
  for ear examination or procedures, *see website*
  for female genital examination, 1425
  in gastroesophageal reflux disease, 1268
  in infant botulism, 990
  sudden infant death syndrome and, 1425
Positive end-expiratory pressure (PEEP), 327, *see also website*
  expiratory phase maneuvers in, 326
  lung injury and, 329
  for pulmonary edema, 1469
Positive pressure ventilation
  bag-valve-mask, 284-285, 284f-285f
  for home care, 1525
  for respiratory distress and failure, 320
Positron emission tomography (PET), *see website*
Postanesthesia care unit (PACU), *see website*
Postcoarctectomy syndrome, 1569
Postconcussive syndrome, 301
Postenteritis syndrome, 1340
Posterior cruciate ligament injuries, 2414
Posterior fossa dysgenesis, 2006-2007
Posterior fossa tumors, 1748t
Posterior laryngeal cleft (PLC), 1452
Posterior lenticonus, 2172
Posterior sagittal anorectoplasty (PSARP), 1358
Posteromedial tibial bowing, 2351
Posthemorrhagic hydrocephalus (PHH), 567-568
Postictal psychosis, *see website*
Postinfection arthritis, 839-841, 840f, 840t
Postinfection diarrhea, 1313
Post-kala-azar dermal leishmaniasis (PKDL), 1189
Postneonatal mortality, *see website*
Postoperative nausea and vomiting (PONV), *see website*
Postoperative pain management, *see website*
Postpartum depression, *see website*
Postpartum thyroiditis, 1904t
Postpericardiotomy syndrome, 1604
Postpolio syndrome, 1087
Postrenal acute renal failure, 1819
Post-streptococcal arthritis, 840
Post-term infant, *see website*
Post-transplantation lymphoproliferative disorder (PTLD), *see website*
Post-traumatic stress disorder (PTSD), 81-82, 82t
  associated with war, *see website*
  following injury, 25
  prevalence of, 4-5
Postural kyphosis, 2371
Postural proteinuria, 1800
Postural tachycardia syndrome, *see website*
Postural tremor, 2056-2057
Posture in hypoxic-ischemic encephalopathy, 570t-571t
"Pot," 680-681
Potassium, 219-224, *see also website*
  in acute renal failure, 1820
  dietary reference intakes for, *see website*
  disorders of
    hyperkalemia as, 219-222
    hypokalemia as, 222-224
  excretion of, 219
Potassium *(Continued)*
  intake of, 219
  measurement of in intravenous rehydration, 247
  metabolism of, 219
  in oral rehydration solutions, 1335t
  periodic paralysis related to, 2130
  reference values for, *see website*
  renal tubular regulation of, *see website*
  in total body water, *see website*
  urinary wasting of, hypokalemia in, 223
Potassium-aggravated myotonia, 2125t
Potassium channel autoantibodies, syndrome of, *see website*
Potassium channel genes, sudden infant death syndrome and, 1425-1426
Potassium chloride in intravenous solutions, 243
Potassium hydroxide (KOH) preparation, *see website*
Potassium iodine for internal radiation contamination, *see website*
Potocki-Shaffer syndrome, 408t
Pot puffy tumor, 1438
Pott disease, 1006
Potter facies, 1828f
Potter syndrome, 1827
Pouchitis, 1300
POU1F1 gene, 1876-1877, 1876t
POU3F4 gene, 2190t
POU4F3 gene, 2190t
Poverty, 6, 6f
  childhood injury and, 20-21
  developmental risk due to, *see website*
  health services children in, 10-11
  malnutrition and, 173-174
Powders for skin disorders, 2216
P450 oxidoreductase (POR) deficiency, 1937
P4P. *See* Policy of pay per performance (P4P)
PPE. *See* Personal protective equipment (PPE)
PPGSS. *See* Papular-purpuric "gloves and socks" syndrome (PPGSS)
PPHN. *See* Persistent pulmonary hypertension of the newborn (PPHN)
PPIs. *See* Proton pump inhibitors (PPIs)
PPKs. *See* Palmoplantar keratodermas (PPKs)
PPNAD. *See* Primary pigmented nodular adrenocortical disease (PPNAD)
PPO. *See* Protoporphyrinogen oxidase (PPO)
PR. *See* Persistent rhinitis (PR)
Practitioners in international pediatric emergency medicine, *see website*
Prader-Willi syndrome, 412-413, 413f
  adrenal insufficiency with, 1929
  genetics of, 391-392, 408t
  obesity due to, 182t
Pragmatic language disorder, 118
Pragmatic language skills, 114, *see also website*
Pralidoxime, 256t-257t, 267
Pramlinitide acetate, 1977
Praziquantel, *see also website*
  for clonorchiasis, *see website*
  for cysticercosis, 1236
  for intestinal flukes, *see website*
  for paragonimiasis, *see website*
  for schistosomiasis, 1231
  for tapeworms, 1233
Prazosin
  for heart failure, *see website*
  for systemic hypertension, 1645t
Prealbumin
  in malnutrition with chronic diarrhea, 1343t
  reference values for, *see website*
Preanesthetic evaluation, *see website*
Preauricular sinuses and pits, 2221
Pre-B cells, *see website*
preBotC. *See* Pre-Botzinger complex (preBotC)
Pre-Botzinger complex (preBotC), *see website*
Prebronchiectasis, *see website*
Precipitation-crystallization in urinary lithiasis, *see website*
Precision of laboratory tests, *see website*

Precocious puberty, 1886-1894, 1887t, *see also website*
due to brain irradiation, 1890
due to cancer and its therapy, *see website*
central, 1887, 1888f
familial male gonadotropin-independent, 1893
due to gonadotropin-secreting tumors, 1891
hypothyroidism and, 1891
incomplete, 1893
due to McCune-Albright syndrome, 1892, 1892f
medicational, 1894
due to organic brain lesions, 1889-1890, 1889f-1890f
pseudohypoparathyroidism with, 1920
tall stature in, *see website*
vaginal bleeding with, 1869
Precordial bulge, 1533
Precursor B-cell acute lymphocytic leukemia, 1733t, 1734
Predictive genetic testing, 377
Predictive value (PV), *see website*
Predispositional genetic testing, 377
Prednisolone
for amyloidosis, 862
for asthma, 794t, 797t-798t
Prednisone, *see also website*
for acute rheumatic fever, 923
for amyloidosis, 862
for asthma, 793, 794t, 797t-798t
for autoimmune hepatitis, 1410
for Bell palsy, 2147
for chronic granulomatous disease, 746
and dexamethasone for cancer therapy, *see website*
for Duchenne and Becker muscular dystrophy, 2122
for Henoch-Schönlein purpura, 870
for hypersensitivity pneumonia, *see website*
for idiopathic thrombocytopenic purpura, 1717
for inflammatory bowel disease, 1299
for lupus nephritis, 1788
for nephrotic syndrome, 1804-1805
for rheumatic disease, *see website*
for systemic lupus erythematosus, 844
Preeclampsia, 545, *see also website*
Prefixes denoting decimal factors, *see website*
Pregabalin
for neuropathic pain, 368t
for pain management, 370
Pregnancy
abnormal uterine bleeding during, 689t-690t
acute intermittent porphyrias and, *see website*
adolescent, 699-702, *see also website*
characteristic of teen parent in, 700-701
clinical manifestations of, 700
counseling and initial management of, 700
diagnosis of, 700, 700t
epidemiology of, 699, 699t
etiology of, 699-700
health care for parents and children in, 702t
medical complications of mothers and babies in, 701
prevention of, 701-702
psychosocial outcomes/risk for mother and child in, 701-702
repeat, 701
amenorrhea in, 686
androgen administration during, 1962-1963
asthma treatment during, 801
congenital heart disease and, 1609
dysmenorrhea during, 691t
folic acid supplementation during, 2001
group B streptococci colonization during, 925-926
chemoprophylaxis for, 927-928
high-risk, 540-541, *see also website*
isotretinoin contraindication during, 2325
listeriosis in, *see website*
Pregnancy *(Continued)*
medication use during, 546-547, 546t-547t
multiple gestation, 553-555, 554t, 555f
obesity prevention during, 187t
prenatal diagnosis and prevention during, 379
psychologic changes in parents during, *see website*
psychologic stress during, *see website*
radiation exposure during, 548
sports participation and, 2402t-2404t
syphilis in, 1022
(*See also* Congenital syphilis)
toxoplasmosis in, 1215-1216
tuberculosis in, 1000
in women with hyperphenylalaninemia, 420
Pregnancy-associated plasma protein-A (PAPP-A), 402-403
Pregnancy-related factors in sudden infant death syndrome, 1424-1425
Pregnenolone, *see website*
Prehospital care, *see website*
Prehypertension, 1639
Preimplantation genetic diagnosis (PGD), 381
Prekallikrein (PK)
deficiency of, 1703
reference values for, 1698t
Premature atrial contraction (PAC), 1612, 1612f
Premature Infants in Need of Transfusion (PINT) study, 614
Premature labor, therapy for, 551t
Premature rupture of membrane (PROM), 551t, *see website*
group B streptococci prophylaxis in, 641f
Premature ventricular contractions (PVCs), 1612-1613, 1613f
Prematurity/premature infant, 555-564
anemia of, 614
birthrates for, *see website*
blood transfusions in, *see website*
cataract of, 2170
definitions associated with, 555
discharge from hospital of, 563-564, 564t
drug metabolism immaturity in, 562, 563t
electrocardiography of, 1539f
factors related to, 556-557, 557t
feeding of, 560
initiation of, 561-562, 561f
fluid requirements for, 559-560
gestational age at birth assessment in, 557, 558f
growth charts and, *see website*
in high-risk pregnancies, *see website*
home care of, 564
hypoglycemia in, 519-521
hypothyroidism in, 1897
hypothyroxinemia of, 627
idiopathic apnea of prematurity, 580-581
incidence of, 555-556, 555f-556f
infection prevention in, 562
neonatal infection and, 634, 634f-635f, 635t
nursery care in, 558-562
pain perception and effects of pain in, 373
physiologic anemia of, 1654
predicting mortality of, 563
prognosis for, 562-563, 563t
retinopathy of, 2151, 2174-2176, 2175f, 2175t
rickets of, 208
skin of, 533, 533f
spectrum of disease in, 558, 559t
sudden infant death syndrome in, 1428
in teenage pregnancy, 701
thermal control and, 559
total parenteral nutrition for, 560
transpiration of in motor vehicles, 22
vaccination of, 891
very low birthweight due to (*See* Very low birthweight (VLBW) infant)
vitamin E deficiency in, *see website*
vitamin requirements for, 562
Premenstrual dysphoric disorder, 691, 692t
Premenstrual syndrome (PMS), 691-692, 692t
Premutation
Premyocardial cells, 1527
Prenatal care, *see website*
Prenatal development, *see website*
Prenatal diagnosis, 380t, 381, *see also website*
of cystic fibrosis, 1490
of erythroblastosis fetalis, 617
genetic counseling in, 378
and prevention, 379, 548-550
Prenatal factors in maternal-infant attachment, *see website*
Preoperative preparation, *see website*
Preparticipation sports examination (PSE), 2401-2405, 2401t-2404t, 2405f
Prepuce, newborn assessment of, 536, 536t
Prerenal acute renal failure, 1818-1819
Presbyopia, 2152
Preschool child
antibiotic therapy for, *see website*
asthma in, 165
behavioral and psychosocial assessment of, 56
child restraint in motor vehicles for, 21t
developmental dysfluency in, 122, 122t
drowning or submersion injury to, 342
feeding of, 165, 165t
growth and development of, 33-36
emotional and moral, 35-36
language, cognition, and play, 34-35
physical, 33-34
intellectual disability in, 125t
leading causes of death for, 5t
response to death by, *see website*
sleep changes in, 47t
Prescription drug abuse, adolescent, 673t
Presenting in psychiatric diagnostic evaluation, 58
Preseptal cellulitis, 2183
Haemophilus influenzae in, 942
Preservatives in immunizing agents, 883
Pressure-controlled ventilation (PCV), 325, 325f, 325t
Pressure gradient in breathing, *see website*
Pressure-induced urticaria and angioedema, 813
Pressure load, cardiac lesions in increased, 1550
Pressure-regulated volume control mechanical ventilation, 325-326
Pressure support ventilation (PSV), 325
Preventive health care, 13-25
adolescent, 663, 664t
in behavioral and mental health issues, 16
in chronic illness, *see website*
evidence and, 16
family and community in, 16-17
guidelines for, 14
in infancy and early childhood, 16
for injury control, 17-25
international, *see website*
in middle childhood and adolescence, 16
nutrition counseling in, 169-170
periodicity of, 14
prenatal, 379, 550-552, 551t
quality improvement of, 16
strength-based approaches and framework for, 16
tasks of, 14-16
Prevotella, *see website*
Prezista. *See* Darunavir
Priapism, 1857
in sickle cell disease, 1665-1666
Prick skin test in food adverse reactions, 822
PRIFLE criteria, 1818, 1818t
Primaquine, 1203t-1205t, *see also website*
Primary angiitis of central nervous system (PACNS), 876
Primary care physician (PCP), role in emergency medical services, *see website*
Primary ciliary dyskinesia (PCD), 1497, *see also website*
Primary complex in tuberculosis, 998, 1002

Primary effusion based lymphoma (PEL), 1121
Primary hypertension, 1639-1647
Primary pigmented nodular adrenocortical disease (PPNAD), 1939-1940
Primate bite, 2454-2460
Primaxin. *See* Impenem-cilastatin
Primidone
  adverse effects of, 2031t
  dosages of, 2030t
Primitive neuroectodermal tumor (PNET), 1751, 1765
Primitive reflexes assessment in neurologic examination, *see website*
P-R intervals, 1540, 1540f
  prolonged in poisonings, 254t
Prion in transmissible spongiform encephalopathies, *see website*
PRISA II. *See* Pediatric Risk of Admission II (PRISA II)
PRISM. *See* Pediatric Risk of Mortality (PRISM) scoring system
PRKAR1A, 1939-1940
PRKCSH gene defect, 1383t
PRL. *See* Prolactin (PRL)
PRNP gene, *see website*
Proaccelerin, 1696t
Proarrhythmia, 1614
Probiotics
  for atopic dermatitis, 805
  for infectious diarrhea, 1336-1337
  for inflammatory bowel disease, 1299
Problem-focused coping, 1985-1986
Procainamide
  for arrhythmias, 1611t-1612t
  for pediatric resuscitation and arrhythmias, 294t
Procaine penicillin G, 645t
  for diphtheria, *see website*
  for neonatal infection, 645t
  for tuberculosis, 1021t
Procedural memory, *see website*
Procedures for emergency departments, *see website*
Process improvement, *see website*
Prochlorperazine
  for chemotherapy-associated vomiting, 1244t
  for migraine, 2044t
Procoagulants, 1698t
  reference values for, 1698t
Proconvertin, 1696t
Proctitis
  infectious, 1332t
  ulcerative, 1295, 1297
Proctocolitis, food protein-induced, 821
Produce-associated salmonellosis, 949-950
Product modification for injury prevention, 19-20, 20t
Product multiplicity, *see website*
Professional organizations, 12
  international pediatric emergency medicine, *see website*
Progeria, 516, *see also website*
  cardiac manifestations of, 1531t
Progesterone contraceptives for special needs girls, 1875
Progesterone intrauterine devices (IUDs) for special needs girls, 1875
Progestin for amenorrhea, 688t
Progestin implant for special needs girls, 1875
Progestin-only contraceptives, 695t, 697-698
  for special needs girls, 1875
Proglottids, 1232
Prognostic subgroups in cancer diagnosis and staging, *see website*
Programming, fetal, *see website*
Progressive external ophthalmoplegia (PEO), 2067-2068
Progressive familial intrahepatic cholestasis (PFIC), 1383-1384, 1384t
Progressive rubella panencephalitis (PRP), 1077
Progressive systemic sclerosis, cutaneous manifestations of, *see website*
Progress of pain, 2332t
Proguanil, 1203t-1205t, *see also website*
Prohormones for performance enhancement, 2423
Prokinetic agents for gastroesophageal reflux disease, 1268
Prolactinoma, 686, *see also website*
Prolactin (PRL), *see website*
Prolapse
  ectopic ureterocele, 1858, 1858f
  mitral valve, 1572
  rectal, 1361
    in cystic fibrosis, 1496
  urethral, 1858, 1858f
    vaginal bleeding due to, 1869
Prolidase deficiency, 443
Proline
  defects in metabolism of, 442, 442f, 1319
  genetic disorders of, 445t
Proloprim. *See* Trimethoprim
PROM. *See* Premature rupture of membrane (PROM)
Promyelocytic leukemia, acute, 1737-1738
Pronation, 2331
Prone positioning, sudden infant death syndrome and, 1425
Pro-opiomelanocortin deficiency, 182t
Propafenone, 1611t-1612t
Propamidine, *see website*
Propane, as inhalant, 681t
Properdin deficiency, 754t, 755
  fever without a focus in, 896t
Prophase of mitosis, 394-395
Prophylaxis
  acute rheumatic fever, 924, 924t-925t
  animal and human bite, 2456t
  bacterial meningitis, 2095
  candidal, *see website*
  cytomegalovirus, 1117
  diphtheria, *see website*
  endocarditis, 1609, 1626, 1626t
    in Marfan syndrome, 2445
  epiglottitis, 1448
  following splenectomy, *see website*
  graft *versus* host disease, 760-761
  group B streptococcus, 927-928
  Haemophilus influenzae type B, 943
  hemophilia, 1702
  hepatitis B, 1400
  HIV, 1173
    for opportunistic infections with, 1173-1174
  malarial, 1207, 1207t
    for travel, *see website*
  measles, postexposure, 1075
  migraine, 2043-2045, 2044t
  neonatal gonococcal, 1037
  neonatal group B streptococcus, 640, 640f, 640t
  neonatal infection, 640f-642f, 640t
  nontuberculous mycobacterial, 1015-1016
  otitis media, 2213
  preexposure chemical, *see website*
  preoperative, *see website*
  rabies, 1155-1157, 1156f, 1156t
  rape victim, 704, 704t
  respiratory syncytial virus, 1129
  surgical, *see website*
  tetanus, 993-994
  ureteropelvic junction obstruction, 1841-1842
  varicella, 1110
  vesicoureteral reflux, 1836-1838
Propionibacterium acnes, 2322
Propionic acidemia, 436-437
Propionyl CoA carboxylase deficiency, 436-437
PROP1 mutations, 1876-1877, 1876t
Propofol, 321t, 2039, 2039t, *see also website*
Propranolol
  for arrhythmias, 1611t-1612t
  for congenital hypothyroidism, 1913
  for Graves disease, 1912
Propranolol *(Continued)*
  for migraine prophylaxis, 2044t
  for systemic hypertension, 1645t
  for tetralogy of Fallot, 1576
  for thyroid storm, 1912t
Proprotein convertase 1/3 deficiency, 1312
Propylthiouracil (PTU)
  for congenital hypothyroidism, 1913
  for Graves disease, 1911-1912
  for thyroid storm, 1912t
Prospective memory, *see website*
Prostaglandins
  in neuroendocrine tumor-associated diarrhea, *see website*
  possible adverse reactions to in premature infant, 563t
Prostaglandin E_1
  for cardiogenic shock, 313t
  for coarctation of the aorta, 1568-1569
  for pulmonary atresia, 1579-1580
  for tetralogy of Fallot, 1576
  for transposition of great arteries with ventricular septal defect and pulmonary stenosis, 1582-1583
  for tricuspid atresia, 1581
Prostaphlin. *See* Oxacillin
Prosthesis
  orthopedic
    after amputation for leg-length discrepancy, *see website*
    infection associated with, *see website*
  testicular, 1860, 1860f
Prostigmine methylsulfate, in myasthenia gravis diagnosis, 2134
Protamine, as poisoning antidote, 258t
Pro-T cells, *see website*
Protease inhibitors
  for HIV infection, 1167, 1168t-1171t
  pharmacokinetics of, *see website*
Protease-resistant proteins (PrP), *see website*
Protective factors for abuse and neglect, 136-137
Protein(s)
  in acute renal failure, 1820t
  adequate macronutrient distribution range for, *see website*
  cerebrospinal fluid
    in CNS infection, 2088t
    normal values of, *see website*
  dietary reference intakes for, *see website*
  digestion and absorption of, *see website*
  drug binding to, *see website*
  familial intolerance of, 455
  gla-containing, 210
  metabolism of
    disorders of, 1389t
    hepatic, *see website*
  pleural, in tuberculosis, 1003-1004
  reference values for, *see website*
Protein A, *Staphylococcus aureus* production of, 904
Protein AT deficiency, 1708
Protein C
  deficiency of, 1708
  reference values for, 1698t
Protein-energy malnutrition (PEM), 174-179, *see also website*
  clinical manifestations of, 175, 175f-176f, 175t
  pathophysiology of, 175-176
  treatment of, 176-179, 176t-179t, 177f-178f
Protein hydrolysate formula, 164
Protein-losing enteropathy, 1307, 1312t
  causes of, 1312t
  due to malrotation, 1280-1281
Proteinosis, pulmonary alveolar, 1497, *see also website*
Protein S
  deficiency of, 1708
  reference values for, 1698t
Proteins induced by vitamin K absence (PIVKA), 210

Protein tyrosine inhibitors for cancer, *see website*
Proteinuria, 1799-1800
  in chronic kidney disease, 1822
  fixed, 1800-1801
  glomerular, 1801, 1801t
  in immunoglobulin A nephropathy, 1781-1782
  in nephrotic syndrome, 1801
  orthostatic, 1800
  transient, 1800
  tubular, 1801
Proteomic studies, *see website*
Proteus, neonatal, 632t
Proteus syndrome myopathy, 2119
Prothrombin, 1696t
  deficiency of, 1703
Prothrombin gene mutation, 1698, 1708
Prothrombin time (PT)
  in hemostatic disorders, 1697
  in liver disease, 1378-1379
  reference values for, 1698t
Protocols for emergency departments, *see website*
Protoheme ferrolyase deficiency, *see website*
Proton magnetic resonance spectroscopy (MRS), *see website*
Proton pump inhibitors (PPIs)
  for gastroesophageal reflux disease, 1268
  for *Helicobacter pylori* gastritis, 1293t
  for peptic ulcer disease, 1294
Proto-oncogenes, *see website*
Protoporphyria, erythropoietic, 2450, *see also website*
Protoporphyrinogen oxidase (PPO), *see website*
Protoscolex, 1234-1235, 1237-1238
Protozoan disease
  amebiasis, 1178-1180
  babesiosis, 1207, *see also website*
  Balantidium coli, 1183
  Cryptosporidium, 1183-1184
  Cyclospora cayetanensis, 1184
  Giardia lamblia, 1180-1183
  Isospora belli, 1184
  leishmaniasis, 1186-1190
  malaria, 1198-1207
  microsporidia, 1185
  primary amebic meningoencephalitis, 1178, *see also website*
  toxoplasmosis, 1208-1216
  treatment of, *see website*
  Trichomonas vaginalis, 1185-1186
  trypanosomiasis
    African, 1190-1193
    American, 1193-1198
Provitamins A, 188, 189t
Provocation paralysis, due to poliovirus infection, 1083
Provocation testing in allergic disease, 768
Proximal humeral fracture, 2392
Prozac. *See* Fluoxetine
Prozone effect, 1019
PRP. *See* Progressive rubella panencephalitis (PRP); Recurrent respiratory papillomatosis (RPR)
PrP. *See* Protease-resistant proteins (PrP)
PRPP. *See* Phosphoribosylpyrophosphate (PRPP) synthetase superactivity
PRQLQ. *See* Pediatric Rhinoconjunctivitis Quality of Life Questionnaire (PRQLQ)
PRRs. *See* Pattern recognition receptors (PRRs)
PRSS1 gene mutation, 1372-1373
Prune-belly syndrome, 1844f-1845f
Pruritus
  in atopic dermatitis, 802
  due to cholestasis, 1388
  in enterobiasis, 1222
  as manifestation of liver disease, 1377t
  due to opioids, 366t
  treatment of in palliative care, 155t-157t
Prussian blue for internal radiation contamination, *see website*
PSARP. *See* Posterior sagittal anorectoplasty (PSARP)
PSC. *See* Pediatric Symptoms Checklist (PSC)
PSE. *See* Preparticipation sports examination (PSE)
pseudoachlasia, 1264
Pseudoachondroplasia, 2427, 2427f
Pseudocyst
  of Chagas disease, 1196
  pancreatic, 1373
Pseudodominant inheritance, 388, 388f
Pseudoephedrine for allergic rhinitis, 777t-778t, 779
Pseudoesotropia, 2158
Pseudogenetic inheritance, 389-390
Pseudo-Hurler polydystrophy, 491-492
Pseudohyperparathyroidism, 1920
Pseudohypertrophy assessment in neurologic examination, *see website*
Pseudohyphae, 1053
Pseudohypoaldosteronism type 1, 221
Pseudohypoaldosteronism type 2, 221
Pseudohyponatremia, 1885, *see also website*
Pseudohypoparathyroidism (PHP), 1919-1920
  obesity due to, 182t
Pseudo Lennox-Gastaut syndrome, 2022-2023
Pseudomembranous colitis, 994-995
Pseudomembranous conjunctivitis, 2168
Pseudomonas
  in conjunctivitis, 2166
  neonatal, 632t
    sepsis due to, 635t-636t
    treatment of, 644
  in osteomyelitis, 2394
  in pyelonephritis, 1832
Pseudomonas aeruginosa, 975-977
  clinical manifestations of, 975-976, 976t
  in cystic fibrosis-related infections, 1482, 1484-1485, 1492t
  diagnosis of, 976
  epidemiology, 975
  etiology of, 975
  pathogenesis of, 975
  pathology of, 975
  prevention of, 977
  prognosis for, 977
  supportive care for, 977
  treatment of, 976-977
Pseudomonas maltophilia, 977, *see also website*
Pseudomycelium, 1053
Pseudo-obstruction, intestinal, 1283-1284, 1283t
Pseudoparalysis due to osteomyelitis, 2395
Pseudoparalysis in newborn, 579, *see also website*
Pseudoparalysis of Parrot, 1018
Pseudoporphyria, *see website*
Pseudoporphyria, due to nonsteroidal antiinflammatory drugs, *see website*
Pseudoprecocity
  resulting from ovarian lesions, 1957-1958
  resulting from testicular tumor, 1943-1950
Pseudopseudohypoparathyroidism, 1919-1920
Pseudosplenomegaly, *see website*
Pseudo-status epilepticus, 2038
Pseudostrabismus, 2158
Pseudotumor, orbital, 2182
Pseudotumor cerebri, 190-191, 2099-2101, 2100f, 2100t
  otitic hydrocephalus as, 2212
Pseudoxanthoma elasticum (PXE), 2278-2279, 2278f
  cardiac manifestations of, 1532t
PSG. *See* Polysomnogram (PSG)
Psilocybe poisoning, *see website*
Psittacosis, 1038, *see also website*
Psoas abscess with Crohn disease, 1300-1301
Psoriasis, 2259-2260, 2259f
  nail changes of, 2295-2296
  vulvar, 1867t-1868t
Psoriatic arthritis, *see also website*
  in juvenile idiopathic arthritis, 831t, 835
PSV. *See* Pressure support ventilation (PSV)
Psychiatric disorders, 57t
  anxiety disorders as, 77-82, 78t-82t
  assessment and interviewing for, 56-60, 57t, 59f
  disruptive behavioral disorders as, 96-100, 97t
  eating disorders as, 90-96
    clinical manifestations of, 91, 92t-94t
    complications of, 91-93
    definitions associated with, 90, 90t
    differential diagnosis, 91
    epidemiology of, 90-91
    laboratory findings in, 91
    pathology and pathogenesis of, *see website*
    prevention of, 96
    prognosis for, 96
    treatment of, 93-96, 95t
  encopresis as, 73-75, 74f, 74t
  enuresis (bed-wetting) as, 71-73, 72t-73t
  general anesthesia and, *see website*
  habit disorders as, 75-76
  hallucinations as, 106-107, 107f
  language disorders as risk factor for, 121
  mood disorders as, 82
    bipolar disorder, 85-87, 85t
    dysthymic disorder, 87, 87t
    major depression, 82-85, 83t-84t
  office intervention for, 16
  pervasive developmental disorders as, 100, 101t-102t
    Asperger's disorder, 105t, 106
    autistic disorder, 100-106, 101t, 103f-104f, 105t
    childhood disintegrative disorder, 106, *see also website*
  pica as, 71
  presenting problems, 56
  psychosis associated with epilepsy, 106, *see also website*
  psychosomatic illness as, 67-70, 67f, 67t-70t
  referral for, 58
  rumination disorder as, 70-71
  schizophrenia as, 106, *see also website*
  suicide and attempted suicide as, 87-89, 88f, 89t
  tic disorders as, 76
  Tourette's syndrome as, 77
  treatment of, 60-66
    hospitalization in, 66
    psychopharmacology in, 60-65, 61t
    psychotherapy in, 65-66
Psychiatric hospitalization, 66
Psychoanalytical theories of development, *see website*
Psychodynamic psychotherapy, 66
Psychogenic eye disturbances, 2154
Psychogenic movement disorders, 2061
Psychogenic nonepileptic seizures, *see website*
Psychogenic tremor, 2058
Psychologic adjustment to burn injury, 355
Psychological abuse, 136
Psychological complications
  of drowning, 346
  of general anesthesia, *see website*
  of obesity, 184t
  of sickle cell disease, 1669
  of type 1 diabetes mellitus, 1986
Psychological factors affecting general medicine conditions, 67
"Psychological First Aid," *see website*
Psychological support following traumatic injury, 340
Psychologic disorders, seizures and, *see website*
Psychologic evaluation
  in communication disorders, 120
  in renal transplantation, *see website*
Psychologic impact of war, *see also website*
Psychologic influences
  on development, *see website*
  on neurodevelopmental dysfunction, *see website*

Psychologic stress
  during pregnancy, *see website*
  in psychosomatic illness, 68
  type 1 diabetes mellitus development and, 1972
Psychopharmacology, 60-65, 61t
  α-adrenergic agents, 63
  antidepressants, 61-62, 63t
  antipsychotics, 62-63, 64t
  mood stabilizers, 63, 64t
  for physical illness, 63-65
  stimulants, 61, 62t
  toxicity, 263-266
Psychosis
  associated with epilepsy, 106, *see also website*
  due to glucocorticoid excess, *see website*
  psychopharmacologic management of, 61t
Psychosocial assessment of adolescent, 666, 666t
Psychosocial causes of hypopituitarism, 1881
Psychosocial consequences
  of injuries, 25
  of teen pregnancy, 701-702
Psychosocial development during adolescence, 654
Psychosocial issues
  in juvenile idiopathic arthritis, 839
  in Turner syndrome, 1953
Psychosomatic illness, 67-70, 67f, 67t-70t
Psychotherapy, 65-66
  for bipolar disorder, 86
  for grief and loss, *see website*
  for neurodevelopmental dysfunction, *see website*
  for pain management, 371
PT. *See* Pertussis toxin (PT); Prothrombin time (PT)
PTC124 for cystic fibrosis, 1493
PTCH1 gene, *see website*
PTCH2 gene, *see website*
PTEN. *See* Phosphate and tension homolog (PTEN)
Pteroylglutamic acid, 196-197
Pterygium, 2169
  with arthrogryposis, *see website*
PTHR1 gene, 2430, *see also website*
PTHrP. *See* Parathyroid hormone-related peptides (PTHrP)
PTLD. *See* Post-transplantation lymphoproliferative disorder (PTLD)
Ptosis, 2163
  in neuromuscular disorders, 2115t
PTPN11 gene, 1946
PTPN22 gene, 1971
PTSD. *See* Post-traumatic stress disorder (PTSD)
PTU. *See* Propylthiouracil (PTU)
P53 tumor suppressor gene, mutations, 1914, *see website*
PTX2 gene, 1876t, 1878
Pubarche, *see website*
Pubarche, premature, 1894
Puberty. *See also* Adolescent, growth and development of
  defined, 649
  physiology of, 1886, *see also website*
  precocious, 1886-1894, 1887t, *see also website*
    due to brain irradiation, 1890
    due to cancer and its therapy, *see website*
    central, 1887, 1888f
    familial male gonadotropin-independent, 1893
    due to gonadotropin-secreting tumors, 1891
    hypothyroidism and, 1891
    incomplete, 1893
    due to McCune-Albright syndrome, 1892f
    medicational, 1894
    due to organic brain lesions, 1889-1890, 1889f-1890f
    pseudohypoparathyroidism with, 1920
Puberty *(Continued)*
    tall stature in, *see website*
    vaginal bleeding with, 1869
  timing of onset, 649
    secular trend for decreasing age of, 649
Pubic hair, sexual maturity ratings of changes in, 651f
Pubis, 2355
PUBS. *See* Percutaneous umbilical blood sampling (PUBS)
"Puddle sign," *see website*
PUFAs. *See* Polyunsaturated fatty acids (PUFAs)
Puffer fish toxicity, 1328t-1329t
Pulicidae, 2318
Pulling of hair, 2289-2290, 2290f
Pulmonary abscess, 1480-1481
  clinical manifestations of, 1480
  diagnosis of, 1480, 1480f-1481f
  pathology and pathogenesis of, 1480
  prognosis for, 1481
  treatment of, 1480-1481
Pulmonary actinomyces, *see website*
Pulmonary agenesis and aplasia, 1463
Pulmonary air embolism, 597
Pulmonary alveolar microlithiasis (PAM), 1463, *see also website*
Pulmonary alveolar proteinosis (PAP), 1497, *see also website*
Pulmonary arteriography, *see website*
Pulmonary arteriovenous fistula, 1599, *see also website*
Pulmonary artery
  absence of branch, with tetralogy of Fallot, 1576
  in fetal circulation, *see website*
  fetal development of, 1527, *see also website*
Pulmonary artery sling, 1452
Pulmonary aspiration due to drowning, 343
Pulmonary blood flow
  decreased, cyanotic congenital heart disease associated with, 1573-1585
  increased, cyanotic congenital heart disease associated with, 1576-1577, 1585-1596
Pulmonary edema, 1468-1469, 1468t-1469t
Pulmonary embolism, 1500-1502, 1501t, 1709
  cardiac arrest due to, 289t
Pulmonary function tests, *see also website*
  in asthma, 783-785, 785t, 786f-787f
  in cystic fibrosis, 1488-1490
  in interstitial lung disease, *see website*
  in pulmonary hemosiderosis, 1500
Pulmonary hemoptysis, 1503-1504, 1503t, 1504f
  in cystic fibrosis, 1493
Pulmonary hemorrhage, 1503-1504, 1503t, 1504f
  neonatal, 599
Pulmonary hemosiderosis, 1498-1500
Pulmonary hypertension, 1600-1602, 1600t, 1601f, 1602t, *see website*
  "hyperdynamic," 1557
  sports participation and, 2402t-2404t
  in systemic scleroderma, 851
Pulmonary hypoplasia, 1464
  with congenital diaphragmatic hernia, 594
  due to oligohydramnios, *see website*
  with pneumothorax, 597
Pulmonary infarction, 1500-1502, 1501t
Pulmonary infection
  aspergilloma as, 1059
    chronic, 1059
    invasive, 1060
  Coccidioides in, 1066-1068
  tuberculosis as, 1002-1003, 1003f (*See also* Tuberculosis (TB))
Pulmonary infiltrates with eosinophilia (PIE), 1474
Pulmonary interstitial emphysema (PIE), 597-599, 598f
Pulmonary lymphangiectasia, congenital, 1467
Pulmonary lymphatic compartment, pulmonary edema and, 1468
Pulmonary sequestration, 1465, 1466f
  in partial anomalous pulmonary venous return, 1553-1554
Pulmonary therapy for cystic fibrosis, 1491-1493
Pulmonary tumors, 1504, *see also website*
Pulmonary valve
  congenital absence of, 1571
    with tetralogy of Fallot, 1576
  rheumatic disease of, 1628
Pulmonary valve atresia
  with intact ventricular septum, 1578-1580, 1579f
  with tetralogy of Fallot, 1573-1574, 1578
Pulmonary valve stenosis
  in adults, 1608
  double-outlet right ventricle with, 1588
  infundibular
    and double chamber right ventricle, 1564
    ventricular septal defect with, 1558
  with intact ventricular septum, 1561-1563, 1562f-1564f
  intracardiac shunt with, 1564
  peripheral, 1564-1565
  in tetralogy of Fallot, 1573-1578
  transposition of the great arteries and ventricular septal defect with, 1574, 1583f
Pulmonary valvular insufficiency, 1571
Pulmonary vascular disease, 1601-1602
Pulmonary vascular pressure, pulmonary edema and, 1468
Pulmonary vascular resistance (PVR), *see website*
  in neonatal circulation, 1529
Pulmonary vasculature, *see website*
Pulmonary venous hypertension, 1570-1571
Pulmonary venous return, partial anomalous, 1553-1554
Pulmonary venous return, total anomalous, 1589-1590, 1589t, 1590f
Pulp, splenic, 1723
Pulpitis, 1255
Pulseless arrest, management of, 291-292, 293f
Pulseless disease, 871-872
Pulse oximetry
  fetal, 544
  in respiratory distress and respiratory failure, 318
Pulse rate in asthma, 784t
Pulses
  assessment of, 1532-1533
  in coarctation of the aorta, 1568
  in newborn, 535
Pulsus paradoxus, 765, 784t
Pulvinar, 2356-2357
Puncture wounds of foot, 2341
Pupil
  abnormalities of, 2154-2157
  blown, 2155-2156
  dilated fixed, 2155-2156
  examination of, 2149-2150
    in neurologic assessment, *see website*
  Marcus Gunn, 2156
  tonic, 2156
Pupillary light reflex, 2157, 2157f
  brain death and, *see website*
  in newborn, 534
  in retinoblastoma, 1768-1769, 1768f
  as sign of cancer, 1730f
Pupillary membrane, *see website*
Purine catabolism disorders, *see website*
Purine metabolism disorders, 516, *see also website*
Purine nucleoside phosphorylase (PNP) deficiency, 733
  prenatal diagnosis of, *see website*
Purine nucleotide synthesis disorders, *see website*
Purine salvage abnormalities, *see website*
Purinethol. *See* 6-Mercaptopurine

Purpura
Henoch-Schönlein, 868-871, 869f-870f, 870t, 874t, 1722, *see website*
cutaneous manifestations of, *see website*
immunofluorescence in, *see website*
nephritis associated with, 1789
idiopathic thrombocytopenic, 1714-1718, 1717f
maternal, *see website*
thrombotic thrombocytopenic, 1718-1719
Purpura fulminans, 931-932
Purpuric rash in rheumatic disease, *see website*
Purtscher retinopathy, 2180
Purulent conjunctivitis, 2167-2168
exclusion from day care due to, *see website*
Purulent otorrhea, *see website*
Purulent pericarditis, 1636
Purulent pleurisy, 1507-1509, 1508f
Pustular folliculitis, eosinophilic, 2220
Pustular melanosis
in newborn, 533
transient neonatal, 2219-2220, 2219f
Pustule(s)
of acne, 2322-2323, 2322f
in drug eruption, *see website*
examination of, *see website*
Pustulosis, acute generalized exanthematous, *see website*
PU.1 transcription factor, *see website*
PV. *See* Pemphigus vulgaris (PV); Predictive value (PV)
PVCs. *See* Premature ventricular contractions (PVCs)
PVL. *See* Panton-Valentine leukocidin (PVL); Periventricular leukomalacia (PVL)
PVN. *See* Polyomavirus nephropathy (PVN)
PVR. *See* Peripheral vascular resistance (PVR); Pulmonary vascular resistance (PVR)
P wave, 1539, 1539f
in supraventricular tachycardia, 1613, 1614f
PXE. *See* Pseudoxanthoma elasticum (PXE)
Pyelitis, 1829-1830
Pyelogram, antegrade, 1841
Pyelonephritis, 1829-1830
clinical, 1829-1830, 1830f
imaging of, 1833
treatment of, 1832
Pyelonephritis scarring, 1829-1830
Pyknodysostosis, 2433, 2433f
Pyle disease, *see website*
Pyloric stenosis, 1274-1275, 1274f-1275f
Pyloromyotomy, 1275
Pyoderma, streptococcal, 915-917
Pyoderma gangrenosum in PAPA syndrome, 858-859
Pyoderma vegetans, 2304, 2304f
Pyogenic arthritis, pyoderma gangrenosum, and acne (PAPA) syndrome, 858-859
Pyogenic granuloma, 2229, 2229f
Pyomyositis, *Staphylococcus aureus* in, 905
Pyrantel pamoate, 1217-1218, *see also website*
Pyrazinamide
for tuberculosis, 1007, 1008t
Pyrazinamide (PZA), *see website*
Pyridostigmine bromide, 2135t
Pyridoxal phosphate, 2028
Pyridoxine, 194t, 195-196
deficiency of, 196
neonatal seizures due to, 2035
for epilepsy, 2028
as poisoning antidote, 256t-257t
for mushroom poisoning, *see website*
toxicity of, 196
Pyridoxine dependency, 2036
Pyridoxine-dependent epilepsy, 453-455, 2028
Pyriform aperture stenosis, 1431
Pyrimethamine
for *Pneumocystis jiroveci*, *see website*
for toxoplasmosis, 1215, *see also website*
Pyrimidine metabolism disorders, 516, *see also website*
Pyrimidine 5'-nucleotidase deficiency, *see website*
Pyrimidines, *see website*
Pyrin, 856
Pyrin domain (PYD), 856
Pyrogenic exotoxins
in scarlet fever, 916
streptococcal, 915
Pyrogens in fever, *see website*
Pyroglutamic acidemia, 443-444
Pyropoikilocytosis, hereditary, 1661f, *see website*
Pyrroloporphyria, *see website*
Pyruvate, disorders of metabolism of, 494t-495t, 505-509
Pyruvate carboxylase deficiency, 494t-495t, 506
secondary to holocarboxylase synthetase or biotinidase, 506
Pyruvate dehydrogenase complex deficiency, 494t-495t, 505-506
Pyruvate kinase deficiency, hemolytic anemia due to, 1677, 1678f, *see also website*
Pyuria
in Kawasaki disease, 863, 864f
in urinary tract infection, 1831
PZA. *See* Pyrazinamide (PZA)

Q
Q arm, 395
Q fever, 1039t-1040t, 1051-1053
Q fever vaccine, 1052-1053
QI. *See* Oxygen index (QI); Quality improvement (QI)
QRS complex, 1537-1540, 1540f
prolonged in poisonings, 254t
with antipsychotics, 266
with atypical antidepressants, 265
with tricyclic antidepressants, 264, 264f
in supraventricular tachycardia, 1613, 1614f
in tachycardias, 288-289
in Wolff-Parkinson-White syndrome, 1613-1614
QRS frontal-plane axis, 1538
Q-T intervals, 1540, 1540f
prolonged, 1540
in long Q-T syndrome, 1540f
in poisonings, 254t
sudden infant death syndrome and, 1428
Q-T syndrome
long, 1616-1618, 1617t
genetics of, *see website*
genotype-phenotype correlation in, *see website*
sports participation and, 2402t-2404t
sudden death due to, 1620, 1620f
sudden infant death syndrome and, 1425-1426, 1426f
short, 1617t, 1618
sudden infant death syndrome and, 1426
Quadriceps myopathy, 2121
Quadriplegia, spastic, in cerebral palsy, 2063
Qualitative quality data, *see website*
Quality
of child care, *see website*
of health care, *see also website*
for adolescents, 663
Quality improvement (QI), 13, *see also website*
of well child care, 16
Quality initiative, *see website*
Quality of pain, 2332t
QuantiFERON-TB, 1000-1001
Quantitative quality data, *see website*
Quantitative trait, *see website*
Query fever, 1051-1053
Quetiapine
for pain management, 364t
for psychosis and agitation, 64t
Quinacrine, 1182, 1182t, *see also website*
Quinapril, 1645t
Quinidine, 1611t-1612t, *see also website*
Quinidine sulfate
for myasthenia gravis, 2135t
Quinine
for babesiosis, *see website*
for malaria, 1203t-1205t, *see website*
toxicity of, 251t
Quinolones, 961, *see also website*
Quinupristin/dalfopristin, *see also website*
for *Staphylococcus aureus*, 907t
for vancomycin-resistant *Enterococcus*, *see website*

R
RA. *See* Retinoic acid (RA)
Rabeprazole, 1293t
Rabies, 1154-1157, 1156f, 1156t
poliovirus infection *versus*, 1085t
Rabies immune globulin (RIG), 882t, *see also website*
Rabies vaccine, 884t, 1155
for travel, 891t, *see also website*
Rabson-Mendenhall syndrome, 1996
RAC-2 deficiency, 742t, 743-744
Rachitic rosary, 200, 203f
Racial and ethnic factors
in adolescent drug use, 672
in childhood cancers, 1727t
in childhood injuries, 20
in child mortality, 2f, 3t-4t
in cleft lip and palate, 1252
in cystic fibrosis, 1481-1482, 1483f, 1483t
in developmental dysplasia of the hip, 2356
in Familial Mediterranean fever, 856
in infant mortality rates, *see website*
in neonatal jaundice, 605-606
in otitis media, 2200
in sexually transmitted disease, 705, 706f
Racial minority children, 6-7
Rad, *see website*
Radial artery, cannulation of, 292-294, 296f
Radial-femoral delay, 1532-1533
in coarctation of the aorta, 1568
Radial longitudinal deficiency, 2384, 2384t
Radial pulse, assessment of, 1532-1533
Radiation carcinogenesis, *see website*
Radiation contamination, internal, *see website*
Radiation exposure
acute and late effects of, *see website*
basic principles of, 2448, *see also website*
biologic effects of, *see website*
as cancer risk factor, 1727t
in thyroid carcinoma, 1914
decreasing unnecessary, *see website*
due to external contamination, *see website*
fetal, 548
due to internal contamination, *see website*
maternal, *see website*
microcephaly due to, 2007t
whole-body, *see website*
Radiation heat loss in newborn, 536-537
Radiation myelitis, *see website*
Radiation pain, 2332t
Radiation sickness, *see website*
Radiation syndrome, acute, *see website*
Radiation therapy
acute and late effects of, *see website*
to brain, precocious puberty due to, 1890
for cancer, *see website*
as cancer risk factor, 1727t
in thyroid carcinoma, 1914
encephalopathy due to, 2068-2069
for Hodgkin lymphoma, 1741-1742
hypogonadism due to, 1945
hypothyroidism due to, 1901
intensity modulated, *see website*
total body, late effects of, *see website*
Radioactive iodine for Graves disease, 1912t
Radioallergosorbent test (RAST), 766-767, 767t
Radiocontrast media, adverse reaction to, 828
Radiography
in aspiration syndromes, 1472-1473, 1472t, 1473f
in asthma, 785, 787f

Radiography *(Continued)*
in back pain, 2374
cephalometric, *see website*
in coccidioidomycosis, 1067, 1067f
in congenital diaphragmatic hernia, 594-595, 595f
in congenital vertical talus, 2338
contrast, in gastroesophageal reflux disease, 1267, 1267f
in croup, 1446, 1446f
in dental assessment, 1261, *see also website*
in developmental dysplasia of hip, 2358-2359, 2359f
in disk space infection, 2376
in esophageal foreign body, 1271, 1272f
in fever of unknown origin, 902
in hallux valgus, 2341-2342, 2341f
intraoral dental, *see website*
in jejeunoileal atresia, 1279-1280, 1279f
in juvenile dermatomyositis, 848-849, 849f
in juvenile idiopathic arthritis, 836, 837f
in kyphosis, 2372, 2372f
in leg-length discrepancy, *see website*
in liver dysfunction, 1379
in metatarsus adductus, 2335-2336
in neonatal necrotizing enterocolitis, 602, 602f
in orthopedic problems, 2334-2335
in osteomyelitis, 2396-2397, 2396f
panoramic, *see website*
in pes planus, 2338-2339, 2338f
in pneumonia, 1477, 1477f-1478f
in pneumothorax, 1510, 1510f-1511f
in pulmonary abscess, 1480, 1480f-1481f
in pulmonary edema, 1469, 1469t
in pulmonary embolism, 1502
in respiratory disease diagnosis, *see website*
in respiratory distress syndrome, 582, 583f
in rheumatic disease, *see website*
in rickets, 203f
in scoliosis, 2366-2367, 2367f
in septic arthritis, 2399-2400, 2399f
in skeletal dysplasias, *see website*
in spondylolysis and spondylolisthesis, 2374-2375, 2375f
in sports-related ankle injury, 2417-2418, 2417f
in talipes equinovarus, 2337
in tetralogy of Fallot, 1574-1575, 1575f
in total anomalous pulmonary venous return, 1589, 1590f
in tracheoesophageal fistula, 1262-1263, 1262f-1263f
in tuberculosis, 999f-1000f, 1006
in ventricular septal defect, 1557, 1557f
in vitamin C deficiency, 199, 199f
Radioiodine administration
for Graves disease, 1912
hypothyroidism due to, 1896
Radioisotope studies in urinary tract obstruction, 1840-1841
Radionuclide studies
in aspiration syndromes, 1472t
esophageal, *see website*
in fever of unknown origin, 902
hepatic, 1379
in Meckel diverticulum, 1282, 1282f
in osteomyelitis, 2396-2397
pulmonary, *see website*
in pulmonary embolism, 1502
in septic arthritis, 2400
thyroid, *see website*
Radon gas exposure, *see website*
RAEB. *See* Refractory anemia with excess of blasts (RAEB)
RAEs. *See* Retinol activity equivalents (RAEs)
RAG-1. *See* Recombinase activating genes 1 *(RAG-1)*
RAG-2. *See* Recombinase activating genes 2 *(RAG-2)*
Rage attack, seizure *versus*, *see website*
Ragged red fibers, myoclonus epilepsy and, 2067
Rales
in asthma, 783
auscultation of, *see website*
Raltegravir for HIV infection, 1168t-1171t
Ramipril, 1645t
Ramsay Hunt syndrome, 2055, 2199
Random variation, *see website*
Range of motion (ROM)
arthrogryposis and, *see website*
assessment of, 2331
of knee, 2352
Ranitidine
for anaphylaxis, 818t
for *Helicobacter pylori* gastritis, 1293t
for urticaria and angioedema, 815t
Ranula, *see website*
Rape, adolescent, 702-705, 703t-704t
"Rape kit," 143
Rapid antigen detection
in bacterial and fungal infection diagnosis, *see website*
in group A streptococci infection, 917-918
in HIV, *see website*
in office, *see website*
in parainfluenza viruses, 1125t
in viral infection diagnosis, *see website*
Rapid eye movement (REM), *see website*
Rapidly involuting congenital hemangioma (RICH), 2229
Rapidly progressive glomerulonephritis, 1785t, 1789-1790, 1790f, 1790t
Rapid-onset with hypothalamic dysfunction, hypoventilation, and autonomic dysregulation (ROHHAD), 1521-1522
Rapid plasma reagin (RPR) test, 1019, 1019f
Rapid sequence intubation (RSI), 285, 287t
gastric content and, *see website*
Rash
in congenital syphilis, 1017-1018, 1018f
drug, *see website*
of Epstein-Barr virus, 1112-1113
of Henoch-Schönlein purpura, 869, 869f
of juvenile dermatomyositis, 846-847, 847f, 848t
of Kawasaki disease, 863, 864f
in Lyme disease, 1026, 1027f
of measles, 1070-1071, 1070f-1071f
due to neonatal infection, 639
of neonatal lupus, 845, 845f
of parvovirus B19 infection, 1095-1097, 1095f-1096f
in rheumatic disease, *see website*
road, 341
of Rocky Mountain spotted fever, 1042, 1042f
of roseola, 1118, 1119f
of rubella, 1075-1076, 1076f
of scarlet fever, 916, 916f
of systemic lupus erythematosus, 842, 842f, *see website*
of systemic-onset juvenile idiopathic arthritis, 832-834, 834f
of varicella-zoster virus infection, 1105, 1105f
Rashkind balloon atrial septostomy, 1586, 1586f
RAS-MARK pathway, 1946
Rasmussen's encephalitis, 2023
RAST. *See* Radioallergosorbent test (RAST)
Rastelli operation, 1582
Rat bite fever, 2457-2459, 2458f
Rating scales, mental health, 57, 57t
Rat lungworm, 1226-1227
"Raves," 682
Raynaud disease, 852
Raynaud phenomenon (RP), 852, 852t
in rheumatic disease, *see website*
sports participation and, 2402t-2404t
RBCs. *See* Red blood cells (RBCs)
RBP. *See* Retinol-binding protein (RBP)
RB tumor suppressor gene, inactivation of, *see website*
RCC. *See* Renal cell carcinoma (RCC)
RCDP. *See* Rhizomelic chondrodysplasia punctata (RCDP)
RCM. *See* Restrictive cardiomyopathy (RCM)
RDA. *See* Recommended dietary allowance (RDA)
RDEB. *See* Recessive dystrophic epidermolysis bullosa (RDEB)
RDS. *See* Respiratory distress syndrome (RDS)
RDW. *See* Red cell distribution width (RDW)
Re. *See* Reynolds number (Re)
REACH. *See* Registration, Evaluation, Authorization, and restriction to Chemicals (REACH) legislation
Reactivation tuberculosis, 998-1000, 1003
Reactive airway disease, gastroesophageal reflux disease with, 1263
Reactive arthritis, 839-841, 840f, 840t
post-*Campylobacter* enteritis, 970
post-infection, 1333t
poststreptococcal, 919
Reactive fetal heart rate (FHR), 543t
Reactive perforating collagenosis (RPC), 2279, 2279f
Reading
to child, 34-35
dyslexia and, 112-114
Reading disorders, *see website*
Ready to use therapeutic foods (RUFTs), 177, 177f
Real-time continuous glucose monitoring (RT-CGM), 1983-1984
Real-time polymerase chain reaction (RT-PCR), *see website*
in enterovirus infection, 1093
in respiratory syncytial virus infection, 1128
Reasoning in adolescent, 649-651
Rebetol. *See* Ribavirin
"Rebound" hypertension, 1569
Recall
cued, *see website*
free, *see website*
recognition, *see website*
Receptive language
development of, 114-116
dysfunction of, 117t, *see also website*
Recessive dystrophic epidermolysis bullosa (RDEB), 2246, 2247f
Recessive inheritance, autosomal, 385-388, 388f
Recessive X-linked ichthyosis, 2268t
Reciprocal translocations, 404-405
Recognition recall, *see website*
Recombinant growth factor
for Fanconi anemia, 1686
for Turner syndrome, 1954
Recombinant insulin-like growth factor-1, 1881
Recombinant tissue plasminogen activator (rTPA), 304, 1712
Recombinase activating genes 1 *(RAG-1)*
deficiency of, 732-733
Recombinase activating genes 2 *(RAG-2)*, *see website*
deficiency of, 732-733
Recombination, genetic, 376, 395, *see also website*
Recommendations for Preventive Pediatric Health Care, 14, 15f
Recommended dietary allowance (RDA), *see website*
Reconstruction for burn injury, 355
Recreational activity, drowning during, 342
Recrudescence in malaria, 1201
Recruitment, alveolar, 323
Rectal atresia, 1358
Rectal cancer, 1773
Rectal examination
in fever of unknown origin, 901
in Hirschsprung disease, 1285, 1285t
Rectal mucosal prolapse, 1361
Rectal prolapse, 1361
in cystic fibrosis, 1496

Rectal suction biopsy in Hirschsprung disease, 1285-1286
Rectal swab culture
in *Campylobacter* infection, 970
in *Shigella* infection, 960
Rectobulbarurethral fistula, 1357
Rectoprostaticurethral fistula, 1357
Rectum. *See also* Anorectal disorders
drug absorption in, *see website*
Recurrence risk, 383
Recurrent respiratory papillomatosis (RPR), *see website*
Recurrent seizures, 2019-2020
Red blood cells (RBCs)
aplasia of, 1653
parvovirus B19 infection in, 1095-1097, 1653
development of, *see website*
life span of in fetus and neonate, *see website*
morphologic abnormalities of, 1650f
neonatal, *see website*
parvovirus B19 infection in aplasia of, 1652-1653
premature destruction of (*See* Hemolytic anemia)
reduction of hemoglobin concentration of (*See* Anemia(s))
transfusion of, 1692-1693, *see also website*
in urine (*See* Hematuria)
Red blood cells (RBCs) count
in iron deficiency-anemia, 1656t
from 18 weeks of gestation to 14 weeks of life, 613t
Red cell distribution width (RDW)
in congenital dyserythropoietic anemia, *see website*
in iron deficiency-anemia, 1656t
Red cherry spot, macular, 483
Red eye, differential diagnosis of, 2167t
Red glass test, *see website*
Red man syndrome, 828
Red pulp, splenic, 1723
Red reflex test, *see website*
Red Spitz nevus, 2233f
5α-Reductase deficiency, 1965-1966, 1965f
Reduction for developmental dysplasia of hip, 2359-2360, 2360f
Redundant skin, 2220
Red urine, 1779, 1779t
in congenital erythropoietic porphyria, *see website*
Reduviid insects in trypanosomiasis, 1195
Reed-Sternberg (RS) cell, 1740
Refeeding syndrome, 91-92, 178-179, 178f, 179t, 226
Reference intervals, 2466, *see also website*
Referral
asthma, 793
chronic illness, *see website*
genetic disorders, 379
hearing loss, 2193t
homosexuality, 659
psychiatric disorders, 58
eating disorders, 95-96
sexual abuse, 143
to specialized facility, *see website*
Reflex(es)
brain death and, *see website*
corneal, 2157, *see also website*
deep tendon, 2109, 2110t, *see website*
doll's eyes, *see website*
gag, *see website*
moro, 571t
in neurologic examination, *see website*
neurologic examination of, *see website*
oculocephalic, *see website*
oculovestibular, *see website*
parachute, *see website*
primitive, *see website*
pupillary light, 2157, 2157f, *see also website*
brain death and, *see website*
Reflex(es) *(Continued)*
in newborn, 534
in retinoblastoma, 1768-1769, 1768f
as sign of cancer, 1730f
tendon, 2109
in hypoxic-ischemic encephalopathy, 571t
tonic clonic, *see website*
Reflex sympathetic dystrophy, 2143
Reflex test
acoustic, 2195
red, *see website*
Reflux
gastroesophageal (*See* Gastroesophageal reflux disease (GERD))
infant, 1266-1267
vesicoureteral, 1834-1838
Reflux laryngitis, 1269
Reflux-related renal injury, 1834
Refraction
abnormalities of, 2150-2152
testing of, 2150
Refractory anemia with excess of blasts (RAEB), 758-759
Refractory status epilepticus, 2038
Refsum disease, 464-465, 466t
cardiac manifestations of, 1531t
cutaneous manifestations of, 2139, 2271-2272
Refugee children, 6
Regional anesthesia, 371, *see also website*
Regional enteritis/ileitis. *See* Crohn's disease
Registration, Evaluation, Authorization, and restriction to Chemicals (REACH) legislation, *see website*
Reglan. *See* Metoclopramide
Regular insulin, 1976, 1977f
Regulation, child care, *see website*
Regurgitation, 1241, 1242t, *see also website*
cardiac, 1571
mitral, 1571, 1571t
tricuspid, 1572
Rehabilitation
for burn injury, 355
following heart transplantation, *see website*
for sports-related ankle injury, 2418
Rehabilitation model in psychosomatic illness, 70
Rehydralyte, 1335t
Rehydration therapy
for acute gastroenteritis, 1334, 1335t
for cholera, 967
for malnutrition, 176-177
for rotavirus, calcivirus, and astrovirus gastroenteritis, 1136
Rejection
of heart transplant, *see website*
of hematopoietic stem cell transplantation, 760-762
of intestinal transplantation, *see website*
of renal transplantation, *see website*
Relapsing
of acute lymphocytic leukemia, 1736
of Hodgkin lymphoma, 1743
of nephrotic syndrome, 1805
of polychondritis, 880, *see also website*
Relapsing fever, 1025, *see also website*
Relationships, adolescent development of, 652-654
Relative bioavailability in drug therapy, *see website*
Relative rest following sports injury, 2408
Relaxation
muscular, as goal of anesthesia, *see website*
for pain management, 370
transient lower esophageal sphincter, *see website*
gastroesophageal reflux disease and, 1266
Relenza. *See* Zanamivir
Reliability
in patient safety, *see website*
in quality measurement, *see website*
Religious objections to treatment, *see website*
REM. *See* Rapid eye movement (REM)
Remifentanil, *see website*
Remission induction, 1734
Remodeling, fracture, 2388f, 2389
Remote symptomatic seizure, 2013
REM sleep disorders, *see website*
Renal abscess, 1830, 1832
Renal agenesis, 1827, 1828f
Renal artery, *see website*
Renal biopsy
in renal transplantation, *see website*
in systemic lupus erythematosus, 842
Renal calculi, 1248t, 1864, *see also website*
Renal capillaries, *see website*
Renal cell carcinoma (RCC), 1760
Renal circulation, *see website*
Renal cortex, 1778
Renal dysfunction
due to immunosuppression therapy, *see website*
liver disease with, 1377
Renal dysgenesis, 1827-1828
Renal failure, 1818-1826
acute, 1818-1822, 1818t-1820t
clinical manifestations and diagnosis of, 1819
laboratory findings in, 1819-1820, 1820t
nephrotoxins in, 1817t
pathogenesis of, 1818-1819, 1819t
prognosis for, 1822
treatment of, 1820-1822, 1821t
chronic, 1822-1825, 1823t
vitamin D deficiency due to, 205-206
cortical necrosis in, 1818
dental problems associated with, 1251t
metabolic acidosis in, 232
rickets due to, 202t, 203, 205-206
Renal medulla, 1778
Renal osteodystrophy, 1823t, 1824-1825
Renal scan, dimercaptosuccinic acid, 1833, 1833f
Renal scintigraphy, 1840-1841
Renal solute loads, for premature infant, 559
Renal transplantation, 1826, *see also website*
maternal, *see website*
Renal tubular acidosis (RTA), 1808-1811
distal (type I), 1810
hyperkalemic (type IV), 1810-1811, 1811f
metabolic acidosis and, 232
nephrotoxins in, 1817t
proximal (type II), 1808-1810, 1809t
rickets due to, 208, 1811
urinary lithiasis with, *see website*
Renal tubules
acid-base balance and, *see website*
disorders of
Bartter syndrome as, 1813-1814, 1813t
Gitelman syndrome as, 1814
hyperkalemia and, 221
inherited transport disorders of, 1813-1814
nephrogenic diabetes insipidus as, 1812
renal tubular acidosis as, 1811f
tubulointerstitial nephritis as, 1814-1816, 1815t
function of, 1807, *see also website*
Renal ultrasonography, 1839-1840, 1839f
Renal vasculitis, nephrotoxins in, 1817t
Renal vein thrombosis (RVT), 1709
hematuria due to, 1794-1795
in newborn assessment, 535
Rendu-Osler-Weber syndrome, 1530, 1531t
Renin-angiotensin system, *see website*
Renogram, mercaptoacetyl triglycine (MAG-3) diuretic, 1839f-1840f, 1840-1841
Renovascular hypertension, 1642, 1644f, 1646f
Repaglinide, 1992t
RePEAT. *See* Revised Pediatric Emergency Assessment Tool (RePEAT)
Repeat expansion disorders, 391, 392t, 393f

Replacement fluid therapy, 242, 244-245, 245t
Replacement therapy for genetic disorders, 379-380
Replantation of tooth, 1259
Replication, *see also website*
enterovirus, 1089
Epstein-Barr virus, 1111
herpes simplex virus, 1098-1099
Reporting, quality, *see website*
Reproductive factors in high-risk pregnancies, *see website*
Reproductive history in skeletal dysplasias, *see website*
Reproductive system, effects of cancer and its therapy on, *see website*
Reptilase time, 1697
Reptile bite, 2454-2460
Rescue breathing, 282-283, 282f
Research, *see website*
Reserpine
possible adverse reactions to in premature infant, 563t
for spasticity of cerebral palsy, 2064
Residency Review and Redesign in Pediatrics (R3P), 11
Residual volume (RV), *see website*
Resilience, development and, *see website*
Resistance, pulmonary, 322, *see also website*
Resistive work, *see website*
Resorption, bone, disorders involving defective, 2432-2433
Resources, *see also website*
child care information, *see website*
developmental-behavioral screening and surveillance, 40
international, for pediatric emergency medicine, 894t
internet
for genetic disorders, 379, 380t
for pharmacogenetics and pharmacogenomics, *see website*
for vaccines, 894t
for vaccines, 894t
Respiration(s)
Cheyne-Stokes, *see website*
in newborn
failure to initiate or sustain, 575
transition to pulmonary respiration in, 579-580
paradoxical, *see website*
pulmonary mechanics in, *see website*
regulation of, *see website*
Respiratory acidosis, 230t, 238-240, 239t
Respiratory alkalosis, 230t, 240-242, 241t
compensatory, 230
Respiratory chain defects, 494t-495t
mitochondrial, 506, 507t-509t, 508f
Respiratory culture, *see website*
Respiratory depression
due to opioids, 366t
postanesthetic, *see website*
Respiratory disease
acute inflammatory upper airway obstruction as, 1445-1450
bacterial tracheitis as, 1449-1450, 1449f
infectious, 1445-1449, 1446f-1447f
airway dynamics in, *see website*
alveolar hemorrhage, diffuse in, 1498-1500, 1498t
aspiration as, 1469-1471
due to drowning, 343
of gastric contents, 1470
of hydrocarbon, 1470-1471, 1470f
meconium, 590-592
neonatal foreign body, 590, 591f
recurrent, 1471-1473, 1471t-1472t, 1473f
atelectasis as, 1504, *see also website*
blood gases interpretation in, *see website*
bronchiectasis as, 1479, *see also website*
bronchiolitis as, 1456-1459
Respiratory disease *(Continued)*
bronchiolitis obliterans as, 1463, *see also website*
bronchitis as, 1459-1460
follicular, 1463
bronchomalacia as, 1455, *see also website*
bronchopulmonary dysplasia as, 1516, *see also website*
due to cancer and its therapy, *see website*
chest pain in, 1530t
child care and infections of, *see website*
chronic or recurrent symptoms in, 1445, *see also website*
chronic severe respiratory insufficiency as, 1519-1526
chylothorax as, 1514-1515, 1514f-1515f
clinical signs interpretation in, *see website*
coccidioidomycosis, 1065-1068
common cold as, 1434-1436, 1434t-1435t
congenital anomalies as
of larynx, trachea, and bronchi, 1450-1452, 1450f-1452f
of lung, 1463-1467, 1465f-1466f
of nose, 1429-1431
cystic fibrosis as, 1481-1497
diagnosis of, 1421, *see also website*
emphysema as, 1460-1462, 1461f-1462f, 1507-1509
α-antitrypsin deficiency and, 1462-1463, *see also website*
failure to thrive in, 148t
due to food allergy, 822
foreign body
airway, 1453-1454, 1453f
esophageal, 1271-1272, 1272f-1273f
nasal, 1431-1432
neonatal aspiration, 590, 591f
gas exchange in, *see website*
general anesthesia and, *see website*
hemothorax as, 1513-1514, 1514f
histoplasmosis as, 1062-1064
human papillomavirus, 1138
hydrothorax as, 1513
immune response of lung in, *see website*
interstitial lung disease as, 1497, *see also website*
laryngotracheal stenosis as, 1454-1455
lateral pharyngeal abscess as, 1440-1442, 1441f
manifesting as respiratory distress, 314-315, 315t
neoplasms of larynx, trachea, and bronchi as, *see website*
of newborn, 579-599
apnea as, 580-581, 580t
diaphragmatic hernia as, 594-596
eventration as, 597
extrapulmonary air leaks as, 597-599, 598f-599f
foramen of Morgagni hernia as, 597, 597f
foreign material aspiration as, 590, 591f
meconium aspiration as, 590-592
paraesophageal hernia as, 597
persistent pulmonary hypertension of the newborn as, 592-594, 592f
pneumonia as, 639
pulmonary hemorrhage as, 599
respiratory distress syndrome as, 581-590
transient tachypnea as, 590
of nose
congenital, 1429-1431
epistaxis as, 1432-1433, 1432t
foreign body as, 1431-1432
nasal polyps as, 1433, 1433f
obesity with, 184t
overinflation as, 1460-1462, 1461f-1462f
parenchymal
emergency airway management in, 284
eosinophilic lung disease as, 1474, *see also website*
Respiratory disease *(Continued)*
hypersensitivity to inhaled materials as, 1473, *see also website*
paraquat lung as, 1474, *see also website*
silo filler disease as, 1474, *see also website*
peritonsillar cellulitis/abscess as, 1440, 1442
pharyngitis as, 1439-1440
pleurisy and pleural effusions as, 1505-1509, 1505f-1506f, 1508f
pneumomediastinum as, 1512-1513, 1512f-1513f
pneumonia as, 1474-1479, 1474f, 1475t-1479t, 1477f-1479f
(*See also* Pneumonia)
in newborn, 639
pneumothorax as, 1509-1512, 1509t, 1510f-1511f
in premature infants, 559t
primary ciliary dyskinesia as, 1497, *see also website*
psychopharmacology and, 65
pulmonary abscess as, 1480-1481, 1480f-1481f
pulmonary alveolar microlithiasis as, 1463, *see also website*
pulmonary alveolar proteinosis as, 1497, *see also website*
pulmonary edema as, 1468-1469, 1468t-1469t
pulmonary embolism and infarction as, 1500-1502, 1501t
pulmonary hemorrhage and hemoptysis as, 1503-1504, 1503t, 1504f
pulmonary mechanics and work of breathing in, *see website*
pulmonary tumors as, 1504, *see also website*
pulmonary vasculature in, *see website*
retropharyngeal abscess as, 1440-1442, 1441f
in sickle cell disease, 1667-1668, 1668f, 1668t
sinusitis as, 1436-1438, 1436f-1438f
sports participation and, 2402t-2404t
sublottic stenosis as, 1454
sudden infant death syndrome as, 1421-1429
surfactant metabolism, inherited disorders as, 1497-1498, *see also website*
of tonsils and adenoids, 1442-1445, 1443f
tracheomalacia as, 1455, *see also website*
ventilation-perfusion relationship in, *see website*
wheezing in, 1456-1460, 1457t
Respiratory distress, 314
in acutely ill child, 275
advanced airway management techniques for
bag-valve-mask positive pressure ventilation in, 284-285, 284f-285f
endotracheal intubation in, 285, 286f, 287t
due to airway narrowing, 283-284
due to airway obstruction, 282-283, 282f-283f
cardiovascular disease manifesting as, 315-316, 315t
in congenital diaphragmatic hernia, 595
as delivery room emergency, 575
in malaria, 1206
management of, 282-285, 319-321
mechanical ventilation for, 321-329
monitoring in, 318-319
neurologic disease manifesting as, 316
nonpulmonary causes of, 315-316, 315t
due to parenchymal lung disease, 284
respiratory disease manifesting as, 314-315, 315t
toxic-metabolic states manifesting as, 316
Respiratory distress syndrome (RDS), 581-590
clinical manifestations of, 582
complications of, 586-590, 588f, 589t
diagnosis of, 582-584, 583f
etiology and pathophysiology of, 581-582, 582f-583f
incidence of, 581
prevention of, 584
prognosis for, 590
treatment of, 584-586

Respiratory failure, 316, 317f, 317t, *see also website*
advanced airway management techniques for
bag-valve-mask positive pressure ventilation in, 284-285, 284f-285f
endotracheal intubation in, 285, 286f, 287t
due to airway narrowing, 283-284
due to airway obstruction, 282-283, 282f-283f
due to congenital central hypoventilation syndrome, 1520-1522
in cystic fibrosis, 1494
as delivery room emergency, *575*
follow open heart surgery, 1604
management of, 282-285, 319-321
mechanical ventilation for, 321-329
monitoring in, 318-319
due to neuromuscular diseases, 1519-1520, 1520t
due to parenchymal lung disease, 284
pathophysiology of, 316-318
in pediatric emergency, 282-285
presentation profiles of, 317f
Respiratory insufficiency
chronic severe, 1519-1526
due to congenital central hypoventilation syndrome, 1520-1522
infections associated with, 1525
mechanical ventilation for, 1524-1526
due to metabolic disease, 1523-1524
due to myelomeningocele with Arnold-Chiari type II malformation, 1522
due to neuromuscular diseases, 1520t
due to obesity hypoventilation syndrome, 1522-1523
due to obstructive sleep apnea, 1523
due to spinal cord injury, 1523
Respiratory manifestations, 1526, *see also website*
in asthma, 782
in chemical terrorism, *see website*
cystic fibrosis, 1485-1486
in enteroviruses, 1090
in food adverse reactions, 820-821
in food allergy, 822
in gastroesophageal reflux disease, 1269
in liver disease, 1377-1378
in lysosomal storage disorders, 485t
in Marfan syndrome, 2442
in multiple organ dysfunction syndrome, 312t
in Niemann-Pick disease, 488
in poisoning, 252t
in setting of terrorism, *see website*
in systemic inflammatory response syndrome, 309t
in systemic lupus erythematosus, 843t
in systemic scleroderma, 851
in typhoid fever, 957t
Respiratory rate
in asthma, 784t
in newborn, 535
normal, 280t
in respiratory distress, 315t
Respiratory secretions, treatment of in palliative care, 155t-156t, 157
Respiratory signs
extrapulmonary disease with, 1526, *see also website*
interpretation of, *see website*
Respiratory symptoms, chronic or recurrent, 1445, *see also website*
Respiratory syncytial virus (RSV), 1126-1129
antivirals for, *see website*
in bronchiolitis, 1456
in common cold, 1434, 1434t
HIV-related, 1164
in otitis media, 2201
palivizumab for, 883
in pneumonia, 1475t
vaccine for, 1129
Respiratory system
airway dynamics in, *see website*
blood gases and, *see website*
Respiratory system *(Continued)*
chest wall in, *see website*
gas exchange in, *see website*
immune response of, *see website*
inhalation anesthetic effects on, *see website*
lung volumes and capacities in, *see website*
management of in drowning, 345
poliovirus infection effects on, 1084
pulmonary mechanics and work of breathing in, *see website*
pulmonary vasculature in, *see website*
respiration regulation in, *see website*
shock-related dysfunction of, 307t
ventilation-perfusion relationship in, *see website*
Respiratory tract infections
actinomyces in, *see website*
adenovirus in, 1132
anaerobic, *see website*
antivirals for, *see website*
aspergilloma as, 1059
Coccidioides in, 1066-1068
coronaviruses in, *see website*
diphtheria in, *see website*
group A streptococcus in, 916
HIV-related, 1165
Staphylococcus aureus, 905
Staphylococcus aureus in, 905
tuberculosis as, 1002-1003, 1003f
(*See also* Tuberculosis (TB))
Rest following sports injury, 2408
Restless legs syndrome (RLS), 52-53
Restless leg syndrome (RSL)
seizure *versus*, *see website*
Restraint
child motor vehicle, 21-22, 21f, 21t
for ear examination or procedures, *see website*
Restrictive cardiomyopathy (RCM), 1629t-1630t, 1633, 1633f
Restrictive dermopathy, *see website*
Rest tremor, 2056-2057
Resuscitation
cardiopulmonary, 289-292, 291f-293f, 294t
for drowning, 344-345
withholding of, 153-154, *see website*
care following, 296
medications in, 294t
equipment for in office emergencies, *see website*
fluid, for burn injury, 352-353
infection protection and control in, *see website*
medications for, 294t
neonatal, *575-577*, *576f-577f*, *576t*
in palliative care, 153-154
Retentive encopresis, 73
RET gene, 1916, *see website*
Reticular dysgenesis, 733
pancytopenia in, 1690
Reticulocyte count
in anemia, 1649f
reference values for, *see website*
Reticulocyte hemoglobin content, 1656t-1657t
Reticulocyte index, 1659
Reticulocytes in congenital dyserythropoietic anemia, *see website*
Reticuloendothelial sequestration, 749
Retina
gyrate atrophy of, 453
neurologic examination of, *see website*
Retinal cherry red spot, 485, 2069, 2072f
Retinal detachment, 2179
sports participation and, 2402t-2404t
Retinal disorders, 2174-2181
Best vitelliform degeneration as, 2178
with blood disorders, 2180
cherry red spot as, 2178
Coats disease as, 2179, 2179f
coloboma of the fundus as, 2181
diabetic retinopathy as, 2179-2180, 2180f
familial exudative vitreoretinopathy as, 2179
hypertensive retinopathy as, 2179, 2179f
Retinal disorders *(Continued)*
myelinated nerve fibers as, 2181
persistent fetal vasculature as, 2176
phakomas as, 2178, 2178f
retinal detachment as, 2179
retinitis pigmentosa as, 2177-2178, 2177f
genetics of, 389
retinoblastoma as, 2176-2177, 2176f
retinopathy of prematurity as, 2174-2176, 2175f, 2175t
retinoschisis as, 2178
Stargardt disease as, 2178
with subacute bacterial endocarditis, 2180
trauma-related, 2180, 2181f
Retinal hemorrhage
due to child abuse, 139-140, 140f, 2186, 2186f
neurologic examination of, *see website*
in newborn, *534*, *566*, *see website*
due to vomiting, 1243t
Retinitis pigmentosa, 1816
with primary ciliary dyskinesia, *see website*
Retinoblastoma, 1768-1769, 1768f, 2176-2177, 2176f
bone tumors associated with, 1763
incidence and survival rates for, 1726t
malignancy susceptibility associated with, *see website*
risk factors for, 1727t
work-up of, 1731t
Retinoblastoma gene, 1768
Retinoblastoma protein, 1768
Retinoic acid embryopathy, *see website*
Retinoic acid (RA), 189
Retinoids
for acne, 2324, 2324f, 2325t
for pityriasis rubra pilaris, 2263
for psoriasis, 2260
Retinol activity equivalents (RAEs), 190, *see also website*
Retinol-binding protein (RBP), 188, 1343t
Retinopathy
due to cat-scratch disease, 985
diabetic, 1987, 1988t, 2179-2180, 2180f
hypertensive, 2179, 2179f
salt-and-pepper, due to congenital rubella syndrome, 1077-1078
in subacute bacterial endocarditis, 2180
trauma-related, 2180
Retinopathy of prematurity (ROP), 2151, 2174-2176
Retinoschisis, 2178
RET oncogene, *see website*
Retractile testis, 1859
Retractions in respiratory distress, 315t
Retrocaval ureter, 1842
Retrocochlear hearing loss, 2188
Retrograde pyelogram in urinary tract obstruction, 1841
Retropharyngeal abscess, 1440-1442, 1441f
Retropharyngeal space infection, 1444
Retrovir. *See* Zidovudine (ZDV)
Rett syndrome (RS), 101t, 2075
Return-to-play, 2407-2408
following head injury, 2419, 2419t
Reunion, child's response to, *see website*
Reverse transcriptase inhibitors, non-nucleoside, 1162t
Reverse transcriptase inhibitors, nucleoside/nucleotide, 1167, 1168t-1171t
Reverse transcription polymerase chain reaction (RT-PCR), 1155
Reversible infantile cytochrome C oxidase deficiency myopathy, 2066-2067
Review of systems, laboratory screening for, *see website*
Revised Pediatric Emergency Assessment Tool (RePEAT), *see website*
Reward, food as, 167
Reyataz. *See* Atazanavir
Reye syndrome, 1407, 1407t, 2068
Reynolds number (Re), *see website*

RF. *See* Rheumatoid factor (RF)
Rhabdoid tumor of kidney (RTK), 1760
Rhabdomyolysis
  due to hypophosphatemia, 228
  in poisonings, 254t
Rhabdomyoma, cardiac, *see website*
Rhabdomyosarcoma, 1760-1762, 1761f, 1761t
  diagnosis of, 1728
  laryngeal, *see website*
  of middle ear or ear canal, *see website*
  pancreatic, *see website*
  risk factors for, 1727t
  uterine, 1872
  vaginal, 1869
  work-up of, 1731t
Rh deficiency syndrome, *see website*
Rhesus, maternal, *see website*
Rhesus-associated glycoprotein (RHAG), *see website*
Rheumatic disease
  amyloidosis as, 860, *see also website*
  ankylosing spondylitis and other spondyloarthritides as, 839, *see also website*
  Behçet disease as, 853-854
  diagnosis of, 829, *see also website*
  fever of unknown origin in, 900t
  hereditary periodic fever syndromes as, 855-860, 855t-856t
    Blau syndrome as, 858-859
    chronic infantile neurologic cutaneous and articular disease as, 858
    familial cold autoinflammatory syndrome as, 858
    familial Mediterranean fever as, 856-857, 857f
    hyperimmunoglobulinemia D syndrome as, 857-858
    Muckle-Wells syndrome as, 858
    periodic fever, aphthous stomatitis, pharyngitis, and adenitis as, 859-860
    pyogenic arthritis, pyoderma gangrenosum, and acne syndrome as, 858-859
    tumor necrosis factor receptor-associated periodic syndrome as, 858, 859f
  hypertrophic osteoarthropathy as, *see website*
  juvenile dermatomyositis as, 846-850
  juvenile idiopathic arthritis as, 829-839
  Kawasaki disease as, 862-867
  Mucha-Habermann disease as, *see website*
  musculoskeletal pain syndromes as, 876-880, 877t-878t
    complex regional pain syndrome as, 879-880
    erythromelalgia as, 880
    fibromyalgia as, 878-879
    growing pains as, 878
  neonatal lupus as, 845-846
  Raynaud phenomenon as, 852
  reactive and postinfection arthritis as, 839-841
  relapsing polychondritis as, 880, *see also website*
  sarcoidosis as, 860-862, 861f
  scleroderma as, 850-853
  Sjögren syndrome as, 854, *see also website*
  sports participation and, 2402t-2404t
  Sweet syndrome as, *see website*
  systemic lupus erythematosus as, 841-846
  treatment of, 829, *see also website*
  vasculitis syndromes as, 867-876, 868t, 876t
    antineutrophil cytoplasmic antibodies (ANCA)-associated vasculitis as, 874-876
    classification of, 868t
    Henoch-Schönlein purpura as, 868-871, 869f-870f, 870t
    polyarteritis nodosa and cutaneous polyarteritis nodosa as, 872-874
    Takayasu arteritis as, 871-872, 871t, 872f
Rheumatic fever, 920-925
  clinical manifestations and diagnosis of, 921-923, 921t, 922f
Rheumatic fever *(Continued)*
  complications of, 924
  differential diagnosis of, 923, 923t
  epidemiology of, 920-921
  etiology of, 920
  pathogenesis of, 921
  prevention of, 924-925, 924t-925t
  prognosis for, 924
  sports participation and, 2402t-2404t
  treatment of, 923-924
Rheumatic heart disease, 1626-1628
Rheumatoid arthritis, acute rheumatic fever *versus*, 923, 923t
Rheumatoid factor (RF), 831t, 832
Rheumatoid nodules, 832
Rh incompatibility, 550
Rh incompatibility, hemolytic disease of newborn due to, 615-619, 616t
Rhinitis
  allergic, 775-780, 776t-780t, 777f
    allergen immunotherapy for, 774-775
  with asthma, 791
  common cold as, 1434-1436
Rhinitis medicamentosa, 1435
Rhinitis pigmentosa (RP), 2177-2178, 2177f
Rhinoconjunctivitis, food-induced, 822
Rhinocort AQ. *See* Budesonide
Rhinorrhea
  in common cold, 1435
  in respiratory syncytial virus infection, 1128
Rhinosinusitis in cystic fibrosis, 1496
Rhinoviruses, 1133-1134
  in common cold, 1434, 1434t
  in pneumonia, 1475t
Rhizomelic chondrodysplasia punctata (RCDP), 464, 465f, 466t, 2272
Rhizotomy procedure for spastic diplegia, 2064, 2064f
Rhodesian trypanosomiasis, 1190-1193
Rhododendron toxicity, 269t
RhoGAM, 615
Rhombencephalitis, enteroviral, 1091-1092
Rhombencephalosynapsis, 2006-2007
Rhonchi, auscultation of, *see website*
Rhus dermatitis, 2251, 2251f
Rhythm disturbances, cardiac, 1610-1619
Rhythmic movements, sleep-related, 52-53
Ribavirin, *see also website*
  for parainfluenza viruses, 1126
  for respiratory syncytial virus infection, 1129
Riboflavin, 192, 194t
  deficiency of, 192-193, 193f
  dietary reference intakes for, *see website*
  toxicity of, 193
Ribose-5-phosphate isomerase deficiency, 494t-495t, *see website*
Ribosome disorders, 748t, 750-751
Ribs
  congenital anomalies of, 1518-1519
  fracture of
    due to child abuse, 138
    traumatic, 338
  notching of inferior border of, 1568
RICE treatment for ankle sprains, 2418
RICH. *See* Rapidly involuting congenital hemangioma (RICH)
Richner-Hanhart syndrome, 422-423, 2273
Rickets, *see also website*
  autosomal dominant hypophosphatemic, 207
  due to calcium deficiency, 206
  clinical evaluation of, 202-204
  clinical manifestations of, 200-202, 201t-202t, 202f
  congenital, 205
  due to Dent disease, 207
  diagnosis of, 202
  etiology of, 200, 201t
  due to Fanconi syndrome, 207
  hereditary hypophosphatemic with hypercalciuria, 207
  overview of, 200, 201t
  due to phosphorous deficiency, 206-207
Rickets *(Continued)*
  of prematurity, 208
  radiology in, 202, 203f
  due to renal tubular acidosis, 208, 1811
  vitamin D-dependent
    dental problems associated with, 1251t
    type 1, 205
    type 2, 205
  due to vitamin D disorders, 204-206
  X-linked hypophosphatemic, 206-207
Rickettsia africae, 1039t-1040t
Rickettsia akari, 1039t-1040t, 1043-1044
Rickettsia conorii, 1039t-1040t, 1043-1044
Rickettsia felis, 1039t-1040t, 1046
Rickettsial infections, 1038, 1039t-1040t
  due to *Anaplasmosis*, 1048-1050
  ehrlichioses as, 1048-1050
  Mediterranean spotted fever as, 1043-1044
  in pneumonia, 1475t
  Q fever as, 1051-1053
  rickettsialpox as, 1044-1045
  Rocky Mountain spotted fever as, 1038-1043
  scrub typhus as, 1045-1046
  typhus group rickettsiae as, 1046-1048
Rickettsialpox, 1039t-1040t, 1044-1045
Rickettsia prowazekii, 1039t-1040t, 1047-1048
Rickettsia rickettsii, 1038-1043, 1039t-1040t, 1041f-1042f
  in pneumonia, 1475t
Rickettsia slovaca, 1039t-1040t
Rickettsia typhi, 1039t-1040t, 1046-1047
Riedel's thyroiditis, 1904t
Rifabutin, *see website*
Rifampin, *see also website*
  adrenal insufficiency due to, 1927
  for asthma, 746
  for bacterial meningitis, 2093t
  for brucellosis, 981t
  drug interactions with, *see website*
  for epiglottitis prophylaxis, 1448
  for Hansen disease, *see website*
  for *Neisseria meningitidis* prophylaxis, 934t
  for neonatal infection, 645t
  for *Staphylococcus aureus*, 907t
  for tuberculosis, 1007, 1008t, *see also website*
    prophylaxis in HIV infection, 1175t-1176t
Rifamycins, *see website*
Rifapentine, *see website*
RIFLE criteria, 1818, 1818t
Rift Valley fever, 1151-1152
RIG. *See* Rabies immune globulin (RIG)
Riga-Fede disease, 1251
Right aortic arch, 1596
  fetal development of, 1528
Right-to-left shunt in neonatal circulation, *see website*
Right ventricle
  double-chamber, 1564
  double-outlet, 1582
    with malposition of great arteries, 1588-1589
    with pulmonary stenosis, 1588
Right ventricular cardiomyopathy, arrhythmogenic, 1633-1634
Right ventricular hypertrophy, 1539, 1540f
Rigid endoscopy in sinusitis, 1437
Rigidity, muscle, assessment in neurologic examination, *see website*
Riley-Day syndrome
  cardiac manifestations of, 1531t
  genetics of, 2113t
Rimantadine, 1123-1124, *see also website*
Rim nevi, 2231, 2231f
Ring, vaginal contraceptive, 697
  special needs girls and, 1875
Ring chromosome, 408
Ringer lactate (RL), 243, 243t
  for anaphylaxis, 818t
Ring form of *Plasmodium*, 1199
RING3 gene, 2016t
Rings, vascular, 1596-1598, 1597f-1598f, 1597t

Ringworm
black-dot, 2310, 2310f
in child-care setting, *see website*
Rippling muscle disease, 2125t, 2126
Risk, developmental, *see website*
Risk adjustment, *see also website*
in emergency medical services for children, 278
Risk factors
for abuse and neglect, 136
screening of, 142
for acute illness, 277
for adolescent drug use and abuse, 672
for adverse drug reactions, 825
for asthma, 782-783, 782t
for childhood cancers, 1727t
for childhood injuries, 20-21
for developmental dysplasia of hip, 2356-2357
for disruptive behavioral disorders, 98
for gastroenteritis, 1330-1331
for HIV infection, 1159
in intelligent quotient (IQ), *see website*
for major depression, 83-84
prenatal, for attachment, *see website*
for psychosomatic illness, 67-68
for school violence, *see website*
for sudden infant death syndrome, 1423t-1424t, 1424-1427
for suicide, 88
for tuberculosis, 997-998, 998t
for type 1 diabetes mellitus, 1971-1972
for type 2 diabetes mellitus, 1991
for urinary tract infection, 1830-1831, 1831t
Risperdal. *See* Risperidone
Risperidone, 64t
for pain management, 364t
for psychosis and agitation, 64t
Risus sardonicus, 992
Ritalin. *See* Methylphenidate
Ritonavir, 1168t-1171t, *see also website*
Ritter disease, 2302-2303, 2302f
Rituximab
for juvenile idiopathic arthritis, 838t
for rheumatic disease, *see website*
River blindness, 1225, *see website*
Rizatriptan, 2044t
RL. *See* Ringer lactate (RL)
RLS. *See* Restless legs syndrome (RLS)
R-mix, *see website*
RMPR gene, *see website*
RMSF. *See* Rocky Mountain spotted fever (RMSF)
RNA
in enterovirus, 1089
in HIV infection, 1158
in influenza virus, 1122
messenger, in molecular genetics, *see website*
"Road rash," 341
Robertsonian translocation, 402-403, 405
Robinow syndrome, 1856-1857
Rocaltrol. *See* Calcitriol
Rocephin. *See* Ceftriaxone
Rocker bed, 1524
Rocker-bottom foot, 2338, 2338f
Rocky Mountain spotted fever (RMSF), 1038-1043, 1039t-1040t, 1041f-1042f
Kawasaki disease *versus*, 865-866
Rocuronium for intubation, 321t
Rodent
bite, 2455
hantavirus pulmonary syndrome due to, *see website*
Roferon-A. *See* Interferon-α
ROHHAD. *See* Rapid-onset with hypothalamic dysfunction, hypoventilation, and autonomic dysregulation (ROHHAD)
Role(s)
gender, 655
nonconformity to, 655-656
social sex, 655
ROM. *See* Range of motion (ROM)
Rome III criteria for diagnosis of functional abdominal pain, 1346, 1347t
Rome Statute of the International Criminal Court, *see website*
Root canal, 1258
ROP. *See* Retinopathy of prematurity (ROP)
Rope sign, 1084
Rosai-Dorfman disease, 1724, *see also website*
Rosary
in rickets, 200, 203f
due to vitamin C deficiency, 198, 199f
Rosenthal fibers, 1748
Roseola, 1117-1120, 1119f
Roseola infantum, 1117-1118
Roseola subitum, 1117-1118
Rosiglitazone, 1992t
Ross procedure, 1566-1567
Rotarix, 889
RotaTeq, 889
Rotation, 2331
limb, normal, 2344, 2345f
tibial, 2346
Rotator cuff impingement syndrome, 2410
Rotator cuff injury, 2410
Rotavirus, 1134-1137, 1135f
in child-care setting, *see website*
gastroenteritis with, 1326t, 1330f
in traveler's diarrhea, 1338t
Rotavirus vaccine, 884t, 1137
in gastroenteritis prevention, 1338
HIV infection and, 1173, 1173f
immunocompetence and, 891
recommended schedule for, 887f, 889
for travel, 891t
Rothmund-Thompson syndrome, 2258, 2258f, *see also website*
bone tumors associated with, 1763
malignancy susceptibility associated with, *see website*
Rotor syndrome, 1391
Round back, 2371-2373
Roundworm
cat, 1227-1229
dog, 1227-1229
Roussy-Lévy syndrome, 2055, 2139
RP. *See* Raynaud phenomenon (RP); Rhinitis pigmentosa (RP)
R3P. *See* Residency Review and Redesign in Pediatrics (R3P)
RPC. *See* Reactive perforating collagenosis (RPC)
RPR. *See* Rapid plasma reagin (RPR) test
RS. *See* Reed-Sternberg (RS) cell; Rett syndrome (RS)
RSI. *See* Rapid sequence intubation (RSI)
RSV. *See* Respiratory syncytial virus (RSV)
RTA. *See* Renal tubular acidosis (RTA)
RT-CGM. *See* Real-time continuous glucose monitoring (RT-CGM)
RTK. *See* Rhabdoid tumor of kidney (RTK)
rTPA. *See* Recombinant tissue plasminogen activator (rTPA)
RT-PCR. *See* Real-time polymerase chain reaction (RT-PCR); Reverse transcription polymerase chain reaction (RT-PCR)
RU-486. *See* Mifepristone
Rubella, 1075-1078
arthritis associated with, 840
in child-care setting, *see website*
clinical manifestations of, 1075-1076, 1076f
complications of, 1077-1078, 1077f, 1077t
congenital heart disease with, 1531t
diagnosis of, 1076-1077
differential diagnosis of, 1077
epidemiology of, 1075, 1075f
etiology of, 1075
exclusion from day care due to, *see website*
laboratory findings in, 1076
maternal
breast-feeding and, 540t
fetal and neonatal effects of, *see website*
Rubella *(Continued)*
in microcephaly, 2007t
pathogenesis of, 1075, 1076f
pathology of, 1075, 1076t
prevention of, 1078
prognosis for, 1078
supportive care for, 1078
in type 1 diabetes mellitus development, 1971
vaccine for, 881t, 884t, 1078
Rubeola. *See* Measles
Rubinstein-Taybi syndrome, 408t, *see also website*
congenital heart disease with, 1531t
microcephaly with, 2007t
Rufinamide
adverse effects of, 2031t
dosages of, 2030t
Rufous albinism, 425, 2238
RUFTs. *See* Ready to use therapeutic foods (RUFTs)
Rumack-Matthew nomogram for acetaminophen poisoning, 259, 259f
Rumination disorder, 70-71
Runaway and thrown-away children, 8
health services for, 10
Runner's hyponatremia, 1885
Runner's knee, *see website*
Running, injuries in, *see website*
Running away, 99-100
RUNX2 gene, 2431, *see website*
Rupture, esophageal, spontaneous, *see website*
Rural-urban location, childhood injuries and, 20-21
Rush immunotherapy, 774
Rutuximab, *see website*
RV. *See* Residual volume (RV)
RVT. *See* Renal vein thrombosis (RVT)
RYR1 gene, 2117

S
Sabin-Feldman dye test, 1213
Saccadic intrusions, *see website*
Saccharin, 1982
Saccharomyces boulardii, 1336-1337
Saccular cyst of larynx, 1451-1452, 1452f
Sacral agenesis, 2118
Sacral agenesis, neuropathic bladder and, *see website*
Sacroiliitis
in spondyloarthritides, *see website*
as sports injury, 2412-2413
SAD. *See* Separation anxiety disorder (SAD)
SADDAN. *See* Severe achondroplasia with developmental delay and acanthosis nigricans (SADDAN)
Saddle nose deformity
in congenital syphilis, 1017t, 1018, 1019f
in Wegener's granulomatosis, 874, 875f
Saethre-Chotzen syndrome, 2012t
Safety
food, 169
patient, *see website*
in quality of care, *see website*
transport, *see website*
travel, *see website*
vaccine, 886, 886t
water, 347-348, 348t
Safety World Inventory and Literacy Screener (SWILS), 41t-43t
Safe zone of Ramsey, 2360f
Saiboku-to, 271t
Salicylates
for acute rheumatic fever, 923
poisoning with, 253t, 260
antidote for, 256t-257t
hypoglycemia in, 529
metabolic acidosis due to, 233
Saline
normal, 243, 243t
for anaphylaxis, 818t

Saline, hypertonic
  for cystic fibrosis, 1491
Saliva, HIV in, 1159
Salivary glands
  disorders, 1261, *see also website*
  effects of eating disorders on, 93t
Salmeterol, 794t
Salmonella enterica serovar Typhi, 954-958
Salmonellosis, 948-958, 949t
  in child-care setting, *see website*
  enteric (typhoid) fever due to, 954-958
    clinical features of, 955-956, 956f, 956t
    complications of, 956, 957t
    diagnosis of, 956-957
    differential diagnosis of, 957
    epidemiology of, 954
    etiology of, 954
    pathogenesis of, 954-955, 955f
    prevention of, 958
    prognosis for, 958
    treatment of, 957-958, 958t
  gastroenteritis due to, 1324t-1325t
    treatment of, 1337t
  inflammatory bowel disease *versus*, 1298t
  neonatal, 632t
    sepsis due to, 636t
  nontyphoidal, 949-954
    clinical manifestations of, 951-952
    complications of, 952-953
    diagnosis of, 953
    epidemiology of, 949-950
    etiology of, 949
    pathogenesis of, 950-951, 951f, 952t, 955f
    prevention of, 953-954, 953t
    prognosis for, 953
    treatment of, 953, 953t
  traveler's diarrhea due to, 1338t
Salmon patch, 2218-2219
Salpingitis, due to genital *Chlamydia trachomatis*, 1036
Salt-and-pepper retinopathy, due to congenital rubella syndrome, 1077-1078
Salt depletion in cystic fibrosis, 1487, 1496
Salter-Harris classification of epiphyseal injury, 2390, 2390t, 2391f
Salter-Harris fracture, 2408
Salt loss, hyponatremia due to, 1885
Salt poisoning
  hypernatremia and, 214
  plasma osmolality in, *see website*
Salt wasting
  cerebral, 1884t
    hyponatremia due to, 1885-1886
  renal, hyponatremia due to, 216
Salute, allergic, 764
Sandhoff disease, 484-487
Sandifer syndrome, 1267, *see also website*
Sandoff disease, 2070-2071
Sandostatin. *See* Octreotide
Sanfilippo disease, 511f, 512, 512t, 513f
Sanition, 1338
San Joaquin fever, 1065-1068
Sano procedure, 1593-1594
Santmyer swallow, *see website*
SAO. *See* Southeastern Asian ovalocytes (SAO)
Sao_2. *See* Oxygen saturation (Sao_2)
Saphenous vein, venous access in, 292, 295f
Sapoviruses, 1326t
Sappinia diploidea, *see website*
Saprophytic *Aspergillus* syndromes, 1059
Saquinavir
  drug interactions with, *see website*
  for HIV infection, 1168t-1171t
SAR. *See* Seasonal allergic rhinitis (SAR)
Sarcoidosis, 860-862, 861f
  cardiac manifestations of, 1531t
  cerebrospinal fluid findings in, 2088t
Sarcolemma in cardiac development, *see website*
Sarcoma
  clear cell, of the kidney, 1760
  Ewing, 1763t, 1765-1766, 1765f
Sarcoma *(Continued)*
    risk factors for, 1727t
    work-up of, 1731t
  Kaposi's
    HIV-related, *see website*
    human herpesvirus 8 in, 1121
  soft tissue, 1760-1762, 1761f, 1761t-1762t
    secondary, due to radiation therapy, *see website*
Sarcoma botrypoides, 1761, 1873
Sarcoplasmic reticulum (SR), in cardiac development, *see website*
Sarcoptes scabiei var. *canis*, 2320
Sarcoptes scabiei var. *hominis*, 2319
Sarcosinemia, 440
Sardonic smile of tetanus, 992
Sarin, in terrorism, *see website*
SARS-CoV. *See* Severe acute respiratory syndrome -associated coronavirus (SARS-CoV)
SAT. *See* Serum agglutination test (SAT)
Saturated fatty acids, *see website*
SBDS gene mutation, 1686-1687
SBT. *See* Spontaneous breathing trial (SBT)
SCA. *See* Spinocerebellar ataxia (SCA)
Scabies, 2319-2320, 2319f-2320f, *see also website*
  canine, 2320
  in child-care setting, *see website*
  genital, 712t
  Norwegian, 2320
SCAD. *See* Short-chain acyl CoA dehydrogenase (SCAD) deficiency
Scald burns, 23, 352, 352f
  due to child abuse, 138
Scales, examination of, *see website*
Scalp blood, fetal sampling of, 544
Scaphocephaly, *see website*
Scapular winging, 2127
Scapulohumeral muscular dystrophy, 2123
Scarf sign, *see website*
Scarlatiniform erythema, 2302
Scarlet fever, 916, 916f, 1439
Scars
  acne, 2326f
  examination of, *see website*
  pyelonephritis, 1829-1830
SCD. *See* Sickle cell disease (SCD)
SCF. *See* Stem cell factor (SCF)
SCFAs. *See* Short-chain fatty acids (SCFAs)
SCFE. *See* Slipped capital femoral epiphysis (SCFE)
SCHAD. *See* Short-chain 3-hydroxyacyl CoA dehydrogenase (SCHAD) deficiency
Scheibe anomaly, 2189-2190
Scheie disease, 511, 512t
  cardiac manifestations of, 1531t
Schema, 30
Scheuermann disease, 2371-2372, 2436t
Schimke immunoosseous dysplasia, 748t, 1690
Schindler disease, 484t, 490
SCHIP. *See* State Children's Health Insurance Program (SCHIP)
Schistosomiasis, 1230-1231, 1230f-1231f, *see also website*
  predisposition to due to immunodeficiency, 716t
Schizencephaly, 2003-2004, 2004f
Schizophrenia, 106, *see also website*
Schmid metaphyseal dysplasia, 2426-2427, 2426f, *see also website*
School
  chemical pollutants in, *see website*
  chronic illness and, *see website*
  eating at, 167
  obesity prevention in, 187t
  perceptual, cognitive, and language processes required for success in elementary, 37-38, 37t
  reentry after burn injury, 355-356
School *(Continued)*
  refusal to attend due to social phobia, 79
  violence in, 135, 668, *see also website*
School-age child
  behavioral and psychosocial assessment in, 56
  causes of limping in, 2334t
  child restraint in motor vehicles for, 21t
  disruptive behavioral disturbances in, 99-100
  drowning or submersion injury to, 342
  feeding of, 166-167, 166f, 167t
  growth and development during, 36-39
    cognitive, 37-38, 37t
    physical, 36-37, 36t
    social, emotional, and moral, 38-39
  injury risk factors for, 20
  intellectual disability in, 125t
  leading causes of death of, 5t
  lying of, 99
  pain assessment of, 361
  response to death by, *see website*
  response to divorce by, *see website*
  shoes for, 2344
  sleep changes in, 47t
  well child care for, 16
"School readiness," 37
Schwartz-Jampel disease, 2125, 2125t
SCI. *See* Severe combined immunodeficiency (SCI); Spinal cord injury (SCI)
Sciatic nerve block, 372
Sciatic neuritis, acute traumatic, poliovirus infection, 1085t
SCIDX1. *See* X-linked severe combined immunodeficiency (SCIDX1)
SCIG. *See* Subcutaneous immunoglobulin (SCIG)
Scimitar syndrome, 1531t, 1553-1554, 1596
Scintigraphy
  in aspiration syndromes, 1472t
  in congenital hypothyroidism, 1900
  in neonatal cholestasis, 1385
  in urinary tract obstruction, 1840-1841
SCIWORA. *See* Spinal cord injury without radiographic abnormalities (SCIWORA)
Sclera, development of, *see website*
Scleredema, 2276
Scleredema adultorum, 2276
Scleredema of Buschke, 2276
Sclerema neonatorum, 2284-2285
Scleritis, 2167t
Sclerocornea, *see website*
Sclerodactyly, 850-851, 852f
Scleroderma, 850-853
  classification of, 850, 851t
  clinical manifestations of, 850-852
    cardiac, 1532t
  diagnosis of, 852, 853t
  differential diagnosis of, 852-853
  epidemiology of, 850
  etiology and pathogenesis of, 850
  laboratory findings in, 853
  localized, 851f-852f
  prognosis for, 853
  Raynaud phenomenon and, 852, 852t
  systemic, 850-852, 852f
  treatment of, 853
Sclerosing cholangitis, with inflammatory bowel disease, *see website*
Sclerosing panencephalitis, subacute, 1072-1073, 2075-2076
Sclerosis
  mesial temporal, 2023
  progressive systemic, cutaneous manifestations of, *see website*
  tuberous, 2049-2051, 2049f-2050f, 2049t
    brain tumors associated with, 1747t
    cardiac manifestations of, 1531t
    malignancy susceptibility associated with, *see website*
SCM. *See* Sternocleidomastoid (SCM) muscle
SCN1A gene, 2016t
SCN2A gene, 2016t

SCN5A gene, 1425-1426, 1426f
SCN1B gene, 2016t
Scolex, 1232
Scoliosis
in arthrogryposis, *see website*
associated with pelvic obliquity, *see website*
compensatory, 2371
congenital, 2368-2370
idiopathic
clinical manifestations of, 2366, 2366f
etiology and epidemiology of, 2365
radiographic evaluation of, 2366-2367, 2367f
screening for, 666
treatment of, 2367-2368, 2368f
neuromuscular, 2370-2371
Scombroid fish poisoning, 1328t-1329t, *see website*
Scopolamine
for motion sickness, 1244t
patch
for nausea in palliative care, 155t-156t
for respiratory secretions in palliative care, 155t-156t
Scorbutic rosary, due to vitamin C deficiency, 198, 199f
Score for Neonatal Acute Physiology (SNAP), 563t
Scorpion sting, 2464
SCOT. *See* Succinyl CoA:3-ketoacid CoA transferase (SCOT) deficiency
Scotty dog sign, 2374
Screening
in acutely ill child evaluation, 277
for adolescent drug use, 674-677, 676t
of adolescents, 665-667
of adoptees, 131t
antenatal, *see website*
autistic disorder, 102, 103f-104f
cancer, 1730-1731
for child abuse risk factors, 142
communication and language disorders, 119-120, 120t
cystic fibrosis, *see website*
defined, *see website*
developmental and behavioral, 39-40, 41t-45t
developmental delay, *see website*
of diabetic child, 1987, 1988t
Down syndrome, 401-402
for foreign-born adoptees, 130-131, 131t
hearing loss, 2192, 2192f
for immunodeficiencies, 715, 718t, 719
laboratory for review of systems, *see website*
lead poisoning, 2451-2452, 2451t
major depressive disorders, 84t
newborn, 537-538, *see website*
for cystic fibrosis, 1490
ethics of, 382-383, *see website*
for genetic conditions, 416, 417t
for 21-hydroxylase deficiency, 1934
for hyperphenylalaninemia, 419-420
scoliosis, 2366
sexually transmitted disease, 706-707, 707t
substance abuse, 674-677, 676t
toxicology, 253, 254t
in type 1 diabetes mellitus, 1988-1989, 1988t
vision, 2148, 2149t
Scrofula, 1005
Scrofuloderma, 2307
Scrotal contents, disorders and anomalies of, 1858-1864, 1860f
Scrotal orchiopexy, 1861-1862
Scrotal swelling, 1860-1861, 1860t-1861t
evaluation of, 1364-1365
Scrotal tongue, 2299
Scrotum
newborn assessment of, 536
shawl, *see website*
Scrotum examination of adolescent, 666
Scrub typhus, 1039t-1040t, 1045-1046
Scrumpox, 1100
Scurvy, 198-200, 199f-200f
skin manifestations of, 2330
SD. *See* Standard deviation (SD); Syndromic diarrhea (SD)
SDB. *See* Sleep-disordered breathing (SDB)
SDS. *See* Shwachman-Diamond syndrome (SDS)
Seabather's eruption, 2322
Seafood poisoning, 2454, *see also website*
Seasonal allergic conjunctivitis, 809-810
Seasonal allergic rhinitis (SAR), 775
Seasonal factors
in the common cold, 1434
in otitis media, 2200
in rotavirus, 1135f, 1136-1137
Seat belt restraint, 22
Sebaceous hyperplasia, 2218
Seborrheic blepharitis, 2164
Seborrheic dermatitis, 2253-2254, 2253f-2254f
of external ear canal, 2198
vulvar, 1867t-1868t
Seckel syndrome, 1690
Secondary generalized seizure, 2021, 2022f
Secondary headache, 2045-2046, 2045t
Secondary malignancy, *see website*
Secondary syphilis, 1016-1017, 1017f
Second-degree burn, 351, 351t
Second-degree heart block, 1618
Second-generation antihistamines, 771, 771t
for allergic rhinitis, 777-779
for urticaria and angioedema, 815t
Second-generation cephalosporins, *see website*
Second-hand smoke
otitis media and, 2200
sudden infant death syndrome and, 1424
Second heart sound, auscultation of, 1533
Secretions, pulmonary
examination of, *see website*
treatment of in palliative care, 155t-156t, 157
Secretory diarrhea, 1245, 1245t, 1339, 1339f
SED. *See* Spondyloepiphyseal dysplasias (SED)
Sedation, 359, *see also website*
herbs for, 271t
in mechanical ventilation, 328
for pain management, 370
palliative, 158
for persistent pulmonary hypertension of the newborn, 593
in rapid sequence intubation, 287t
Sedatives
for anesthesia, *see website*
for intubation, 321t
poisoning with, 253t
in adolescents, 676t
SEDL gene, *see website*
SEER. *See* Survival Epidemiology and End Results (SEER)
Segregation analysis, *see website*
Seizure disorder, 2013
Seizures, 2013-2039
absence, 2023
in acute intermittent porphyrias, *see website*
with bacterial meningitis, 2094
conditions that mimic, 2039, *see also website*
dental problems associated with, 1251t
diencephalic, *see website*
epileptic syndrome and, 2013, 2014t-2016t
evaluation of, 2015-2017
in factitious disorder by proxy, 146
febrile, 2017-2019, 2017t, 2018f
in measles, 1072
general anesthesia and, *see website*
generalized, 2023-2024
benign, 2023
motor, 2023
severe, 2023-2024
genetic factors in, 2016t
in hypoxic-ischemic encephalopathy, 571t
jitteriness *versus*, 2034, *see also website*
in malaria, 1206
Seizures *(Continued)*
mechanisms of, 2024-2025
in newborn, 2033-2037, 2035t, *see website*
nocturnal, 52t
partial, 2021-2023, 2022f
benign epilepsy syndromes with, 2021-2022
severe epilepsy syndromes with, 2022-2023
due to poisonings, 255t
due to pork tapeworm, 1235
psychogenic nonepileptic, *see website*
with roseola, 1120
secondary generalized, 2021, 2022f
sports participation and, 2402t-2404t
status epilepticus due to, 2037-2039, 2039t
strokelike events *versus*, 2085
due to tetanus, 992-993
treatment of, 2018, 2025-2033
choice of drug for, 2026-2029, 2029t
counseling in, 2025, 2026t
deciding on long-term therapy for, 2025, 2026f
discontinuation of, 2033
initiating and monitoring of, 2029-2032, 2030t-2031t
mechanisms of action of antiepileptic drugs for, 2025-2026
in palliative care, 155t-156t, 157-158
surgery for, 2032-2033
types of, 2014t
unprovoked, 2019-2021, 2020t
in X-linked adrenoleukodystrophy, 468
Selective attention, *see website*
Selective mutism, 79, 118
Selective serotonin reuptake inhibitors (SSRIs), 61
for anxiety disorder, 78
for attention deficit/hyperactivity disorder, 62t
for depression and anxiety symptoms, 63t, 84
for eating disorders, 95
maternal use of, neonatal behavioral syndromes due to, 625, 625f
for pain management, 369
neuropathic, 368t
poisoning with, 264-265, 265f, 265t
for premenstrual dysphoric disorder, 692t
safety and efficacy concerns about, 82
in serotonin syndrome, 265, 265t
for tic disorders, 76
Selenium, *see website*
Self-concept, development of, 650t, 651-653
Self examination of breast, *see website*
Self-help skill in Down syndrome, 403t
Self-injectable epinephrine
for anaphylaxis, 817
for insect allergy, 809
Self-injury in Lesch-Nyhan disease, *see website*
Self-monitoring of blood glucose (SMBG), 1982-1983
Sellick maneuver, 287t
Selzentry. *See* Maraviroc
Semantics, 114
Semantic deficit, *see website*
SEM disease, 1101
Seminoma, 1770
Senior-Løken syndrome, 1816
Senna
for constipation in palliative care, 155t-156t
for constipation maintenance therapy, 74t
Sennetsu ehrlichiosis, 1039t-1040t
Senning procedure, 1586-1587
Sensitivity of laboratory tests, *see website*
Sensitization phase of allergy, *see website*
Sensorineural hearing loss (SNHL), 2188. *See also* Hearing impairment or loss
infectious causes of, 2191t, *see also website*
sudden, 2188
syndromic, 2190t
Sensors in respiration regulation, *see website*
Sensory ataxia, gait of, *see website*
Sensory function, *see website*
Sensory neuropathies, hereditary, 2138-2140

Sensory nystagmus, 2161
Sensory testing (ST) of esophagus, *see website*
Separation, 45, *see also website*
Separation anxiety, 32
Separation anxiety disorder (SAD), 77-78
Separation of nails, 2295, 2295f-2296f
Sepiapterin reductase deficiency, 446
Sepsis
  due to anaerobes, *see website*
  cardiac manifestations of, 1532t
  Enterococcus, *see website*
  infant botulism *versus*, 989
  international consensus definitions of, 311t
  liver disease and, *see website*
  neonatal, 635t-638t, 636-637, 643t
    respiratory distress syndrome *versus*, 583-584
    treatment of, 646
  postanginal, *see website*
  recurrent, in factitious disorder by proxy, 146
  respiratory distress due to, 315t
  Staphylococcus aureus, 905
Sepsis syndrome, *Cryptococcus neoformans* in, 1057
Septal defect
  atrial, 1551
    in adults, 1605-1606
    familial secundum, with heart block, *see website*
    ostium secundum, 1551-1553
    sinus venosus, 1553
  atrioventricular, 1554-1556, 1554f-1555f
    in adults, 1607
  uterine, *see website*
  ventricular, 1556-1558, 1556f-1557f
    in adults, 1606-1607
    coarctation of the aorta, 1570
    embryonic development of, *see website*
    supracristal, with aortic insufficiency, 1559
    transitional circulation and, *see website*
    transposition of the great arteries, 1587
    with transposition of the great arteries and pulmonary stenosis, 1574, 1583f
Septate uterus, *see website*
Septic arthritis, 2398-2400, 2399f, 2399t
  Pseudomonas aeruginosa, 976t
  toxic synovitis *versus*, 2361
Septicemia
  Aeromonas, 974, *see also website*
  Pseudomonas aeruginosa, 976-977
  Staphylococcus aureus, 908
Septicemic leptospirosis, 1024
Septicemic plague, 973
Septic shock, 307t
  clinical manifestations of, 309
  defined, 305
  hemodynamic variables in, 311t
  pathophysiology of, 306-307, 310f
  treatment of, 312
Septo-optic dysplasia, 527
  adrenal insufficiency with, 1929
  of de Morsier, *see website*
  diabetes insipidus with, 1883
Septostomy, Rashkind balloon atrial, 1586, 1586f
Septra. *See* Trimethoprim-sulfamethoxazole (TMP-SMX)
Sequestration
  pulmonary, 1465, 1466f
  splenic, 1719
Serial casting for clubfoot, 2337
Serine
  defects in metabolism of, 442
  genetic disorders of, 445t
Serology, *see also website*
  in aspergillosis, 1060
  in celiac disease, 1309
  in *Chlamydophila pneumoniae*, 1034-1035
  in coccidioidomycosis, 1066-1067
  in congenital toxoplasmosis, 1214-1215
  in dengue-like disease, 1148-1149
  for differential diagnosis, *see website*
Serology *(Continued)*
  in enterovirus infection, 1093
  in fever of unknown origin, 902
  in hepatitis C, 1401
  in Lyme disease, 1028
  in parvovirus B19 infection, 1097
  in pneumonia, 1477-1478
  in pork tapeworm, 1235
  in roseola, 1119-1120
  in toxoplasmosis, 1213-1214
Seroquel. *See* Quetiapine
Serosal complement control protein deficiency, 755
Serotonin
  genetic disorders of, 445t
  in neuroendocrine tumor-associated diarrhea, *see website*
  for pain management, 369
Serotonin 1A (5-HT_{1A}), in sudden infant death syndrome, 1422-1424, 1423t
Serotonin discontinuation syndrome, 625
Serotonin syndrome, 65, 253t, 265, 265f, 265t, 625
Seroverters, 1166
Serratai, 632t, 635t
Sertoli Cell-only syndrome, 1945
Sertraline
  for depression and anxiety symptoms, 63t
  for premenstrual dysphoric disorder, 692t
  for weight loss in adults, 187t
Serum α-fetoprotein concentration, 543t
Serum agglutination test (SAT)
  in brucellosis, 981
  in group A streptococci infection, 918
  in tularemia, 979
Serum enzymes in neuromuscular disorders, 2110
Serum sickness, 819-820
Serum-sickness like reaction (SSLR), *see website*
SET-C. *See* Social effectiveness therapy for children (SET-C)
Setleis syndrome, 2222
Settings of care for palliative care, 151
Sever disease, 2408-2409, 2418, 2436t
Severe achondroplasia with developmental delay and acanthosis nigricans (SADDAN), 2428
Severe acute malnutrition, 174-179
  clinical manifestations of, 175, 175f-176f, 175t
  pathophysiology of, 175-176
  treatment of, 176-179, 176t-179t, 177f-178f
Severe acute respiratory syndrome -associated coronavirus (SARS-CoV), 1134, *see also website*
Severe combined immunodeficiency (SCI), 721t, 730-733, 731t, 732f, 748t
  autosomal recessive, 732-733
  fetal therapy for, 551t
  flow cytometry testing in, 720-722
  infections in, *see website*
  malignancy susceptibility associated with, *see website*
  Pneumocystis jiroveci pneumonia with, *see website*
  reticular dysgenesis as, 733
  X-inked, 732, 732f
Severe congenital neutropenia, 750
Severe generalized seizures, 2023-2024
Sevoflurane for anesthesia, *see website*
Sex
  assigned at birth, 655
  disorders of development of (*See* Disorders of sex development (DSD))
  mortality rates by, 3t
  types and definitions, 654
Sex chromosome aneuploidy, 408-410, 409t
  Klinefelter syndrome as, 410
  Noonan syndrome as, 410, 410t
  Turner syndrome as, 409-410
  47,XYY as, 410
Sex cord tumor, *see website*
Sex development, disorders of, 1958-1968, 1960f
  diagnosis of, 1959t, 1961
  etiologic classification of, 1959t
  ovotesticular, 1968
  revised nomenclature in, 1958-1959, 1959t
  sex differentiation and, 1958-1959, 1960f
  undescended testis in, 1859
  46,XX, 1959t
  46,XY, 1962
Sex differentiation, 1958-1959, 1960f
Sex-hormone binding globulin (SHBG), *see website*
Sex partner treatment for *Chlamydia trachomatis*, 1036-1037
Sexual abuse, 135-136, 142-146, 144f
  assessment and management of, 143-144, 143f
  defined, 135-136, 142
  genital *Chlamydia trachomatis* due to, 1036
  physical examination in, 144-145, 144f-145f
  presentation of, 142-143
  prevention of, 144-145
  sexually transmitted disease due to, 145, 145t, 935
  of special needs girls, 1874
  trichomoniasis due to, 1185
  vulvovaginitis and, 1865
Sexual activity by adolescents, 692-693, 693f, 693t
  contraceptive use during, 693-694, 694f
Sexual behavior, 655
  trends in prevalence of, 693t
Sexual development, 649
  delayed due to total body irradiation, *see website*
  Turner syndrome and, 1953
Sexual differentiation, 1958-1959, 1960f
Sexual education for special needs girls, 1874
Sexual identity
  defined, 654
  development of, 654-658
    factors that influence, 655
    gender variance/gender role nonconformity in, 655-656
    gender variant identity/transgender children in, 656-658, 657t
    terms and definitions in, 654-655
Sexuality
  adolescent development of, 650t, 653-654
  special needs girls and, 1874
Sexually transmitted infections (STIs), 705-714
  chancroid as, 944
  Chlamydia trachomatis in, 1035-1036
  definitions, etiology, and clinical manifestations of, 707-709, 707f-708f, 709t
  diagnosis of, 709-711, 709t-711t, 710f
  epidemiology of, 705-714, 706f
  etiology of, 705, 705t
  human papillomavirus, 1137
  lymphogranuloma venereum as, 1038
  maternal, 639-640
  pathogenesis of, 706, 707f
  prevention of, 714
  screening for, 144-145, 706-707, 707t
    in adolescent, 667
  sexual abuse and, 144-145, 145t
  as threat to homosexual youth, 659
  treatment of, 711-714, 712t-713t
Sexual maturity rating (SMR), 649, 650t, 651f, 652t
Sexual orientation, 655, 658
SF1 gene, *see website*
SFTPA1 gene, 1497-1498
SFTPA2 gene, 1497-1498
SFTPB gene, 1497-1498, *see also website*
SFTPC gene, 1497-1498, *see also website*
SFTPD gene, 1497-1498
SGA. *See* Small for gestational age (SGA) newborn
Shagreen patch, 2050

Shake lotions for skin disorders, 2216
Shaken baby syndrome, 2181f
Shampoo for skin disorders, 2216
Shape of head in neurologic examination, *see website*
Shawl scrotum, *see website*
SHBG. *See* Sex-hormone binding globulin (SHBG)
SH2D1A mutation, 727
Sheat allergy, 823t
Sheep liver fluke, *see website*
"Sheets," 683
Shellfish allergy, 821, 821t, 823t
Shellfish poisoning, 1328t-1329t, *see also website*
Shenton line, 2358
SHH. *See* Sonic hedgehog (SHH) pathway
Shiga toxin, 959
Shiga toxin-producing *Escherichia coli* (STEC), 962t, 963
Shiga toxin-producing *Escherichia coli* (STEC), 963
  in child-care setting, *see website*
Shigella, 959-961
  clinical manifestations and complications of, 960
  diagnosis of, 960
  differential diagnosis of, 960
  epidemiology of, 959
  etiology of, 959
  gastroenteritis due to, 1324t-1325t, 1330, 1332f
    treatment of, 1324t-1325t
  immunity to, 959
  inflammatory bowel disease *versus*, 1298t
  pathogenesis of, 959
  prevention of, 961
  treatment of, 960-961
  in vulvovaginitis, 1865-1866, 1868t
Shiner, allergic, 765
Shingles. *See* Herpes zoster
Shinipi-to for asthma, 271t
Shin splints, 2416-2417, *see website*
Shock, 305-314. *See also specific types*
  cardiogenic, 305
  clinical manifestations of, 308-309, 311t
  compensated, 285, 305
  decompensated, 285, 305, 307f
  defined, 305
  diagnosis of, 309
  distributive, 305
  epidemiology of, 305, 306f
  hypovolemic, 305
  laboratory findings in, 309-310
  management of, 285-286
  neonatal, 577
  obstructive, 305
  pathophysiology of, 305-308, 307f-308f, 307t-309t, 310f
  prognosis for, 314
  recognition of, 285-286
  in traumatic injury, 336-337
  treatment of, 310-314, 312t-313t
  types of, 305, 307t
  vasodilatory, 305, 308f
  due to vomiting, 1243t
Shoe dermatitis, 2251-2252
Shoes, 2344
Shone syndrome, 1565, 1570
Short-acting inhaled β-adrenergic agents (SABAs), 792t, 796, 797t-798t
Short bowel syndrome, 1314, 1315t, 1316f
  chronic diarrhea with, 1341
  sports participation and, 2402t-2404t
Short-chain acyl CoA dehydrogenase (SCAD) deficiency, 457t, 460
Short-chain fatty acids (SCFAs), *see website*
Short-chain 3-hydroxyacyl CoA dehydrogenase (SCHAD) deficiency, 457t, 460
Short Q-T syndrome (SQTS), 1617t, 1618
  sudden infant death syndrome and, 1426
Short-rib polydactyly syndromes, 2434
Short stature
  due to hypothyroidism, 1902f
  due to skeletal dysplasia, *see website*
  with Turner syndrome, 1952, 1952f
Short-term memory (STM), *see website*
Shoulder
  arthrogryposis involving, *see website*
  musculoskeletal pain syndrome of, 877t
  orthopedic disorders of, 2383
  sports injury to, 2409-2410, 2410f
SHOX mutations, 388-389
Shprintzen-Goldberg syndrome, 2012t
Shprintzen syndrome, 1576, *see website*
Shuddering attacks, *see website*
Shunt(s)
  Blalock-Taussig, 1577
  cerebrospinal fluid, infections associated with, *see also website*
    coagulase-negative staphylococci, 910
  Glenn, bidirectional, 1581
  intrapulmonary, 317-318
  transjugular intrahepatic portosystemic, *see website*
Shwachman-Diamond syndrome (SDS), 748t, 750-751, 1318, 1369, 1686-1687
SIADH. *See* Syndrome of inappropriate antidiuretic hormone (SIADH)
Sialidosis, 484t, 2074, *see website*
Siamese twins, 553
Sibling
  death of, *see website*
  hematopoietic stem cell transplantation from, 757-760, 758t
  palliative care and, 152-153
  sudden infant death syndrome in, 1428
Sibutramine, 187t
Sickle cell crisis
  abdominal pain of, 1247t
  hepatic, *see website*
Sickle cell disease (SCD), 1663-1670
  clinical manifestations of, 1663-1669
    cardiac, 1531t
    cognitive and psychological complications, 1669
    dactylitis, 1663-1664, 1664f
    fever and bacteremia, 1663, 1663t
    iron overload, 1667
    kidney disease, 1668-1669
    lung disease, 1667-1668, 1668f, 1668t
    neurologic, 1666-1667, 1666f
    pain, 1664-1665, 1665t
    priapism, 1665-1666
    splenic sequestration, 1664
  complement system dysfunction in, 756
  diagnosis of, 1669, 1669t
  fever without a focus in, 896t
  gain-of-function mutation in, *see website*
  general anesthesia and, *see website*
  hematopoietic stem cell transplantation for, 759-760
  hepatic dysfunction with, *see website*
  maternal, *see website*
  nephropathy due to, 1795-1796
  osteomyelitis and, 2397
  sports participation and, 2402t-2404t
Sickle cell syndromes, 1669-1670
Sickle cell trait, 1663-1670, 1670t-1671t
  nephropathy due to, 1795-1796
  sports participation and, 2402t-2404t
Sick sinus syndrome, 1618
Sideroblastic anemia, 1658, *see also website*
SIDS. *See* Sudden infant death syndrome (SIDS)
Signal transducers in oncogenesis, *see website*
Silage gas poisoning, *see website*
Sildenafil for pulmonary hypertension, 1602t
"Silk glove" sign, 1364
Silo filler disease, 1474, *see also website*
Silver nitrate solutions for burn injury, 353, 353t
Silver sulfadiazine for burn injury, 353, 353t
Silybin, *see website*
Simian virus 40, 1750-1751
Simon foci, 1003
Simple partial seizure, 2021
Simpson-Golabi-Behmel syndrome, *see website*
Sinding-Larsen-Johansson disease, 2416
Sinecatechins
  for genital warts, 713t
  for human papillomavirus, 1140
Single-gene disorders, 380-381
Single-nucleotide polymorphism (SNP), *see website*
Single-photon emission computed tomography (SPECT), *see website*
Single ventricle, 1592
Sinoatrial block, 1618
Sinus
  branchial cleft and thyroglossal, 2221
  pilonidal, 1362
  preauricular, 2221
  radiography of, *see website*
Sinus arrest, 1618
Sinus arrhythmias, 1610-1613, 1612f-1613f
Sinus bradycardia, 1610-1612
Sinus headache, 2045-2046
Sinus histiocytosis massive lymphadenopathy, 1724, *see also website*
Sinusitis, 1436-1438, 1436f-1438f
  allergic *Aspergillus*, 1059
  Aspergillus in, 1059-1060
    invasive, 1061
  in child-care setting, *see website*
  as complication of common cold, 1436
  in cystic fibrosis, 1496
  Haemophilus influenzae in, 943
  imaging studies of, *see website*
  migraine secondary to, 2045
  Moraxella catarrhalis in, *see website*
Sinus node dysfunction, 1618, 1618f
Sinus tachycardia, 1616t
  supraventricular tachycardia *versus*, 1613
Sinus venosus atrial septal defect (ASD), 1553
Sipple syndrome, *see website*
SIRS. *See* Systemic inflammatory response syndrome (SIRS)
Sitosterolemia, 473t, 475, 1320
Situs inversus totalis, *see website*
Six Sigma, *see website*
Sixth disease, 1117-1118
Sixth nerve palsy, 2160
Sjögren-Larsson syndrome, 2268t, 2271
Sjögren syndrome, 854, *see also website*
Skeletal disease, pulmonary function influenced by, 1516-1519
Skeletal dysplasias
  achondrogenesis type 1B as, 2431
  achondroplasia as, 2428-2430, 2429f
  asphyxiating thoracic dystrophy as, 2434
  associated anomalies in, *see website*
  atelosteogenesis type II, 2431
  Caffey disease as, 2436-2437, 2436f
  campomelic, 2431, 2432f
  cartilage-hair hypoplasia as, 2434
  of cartilage matrix proteins, 2424-2427
  cleidocranial, 2431, 2432f
  clinical manifestations of, *see website*
  of defective bone resorption, 2432-2433
  diagnosis of, *see website*
  diastrophic, 2430-2431, 2430f-2431f
  Ellis-van Creveld syndrome as, 2433-2434, 2434f
  general considerations in, 2424, *see also website*
  genetics of, *see website*
  hypochondroplasia as, 2430
  infantile cortical hyperostosis as, 2436-2437, 2436f
  involving filamins, 2435
  of ion transporters, 2430-2431
  juvenile osteochondroses as, 2435, 2436t
  Kniest, 2425

Skeletal dysplasias *(Continued)*
major problems associated with, *see website*
Marfan syndrome as, 2440-2446
metaphyseal, 2446, *see also website*
Jansen, 2430
Schmid, 2426-2427, 2426f
metatropic, 2435, 2435f
multiple epiphyseal, 2427
nail-patella syndrome as, 2431-2432
osteogenesis imperfecta as, 2437-2440, 2438f-2439f
osteopetrosis as, 2432-2433, 2433f
pathophysiology of, *see website*
pseudoachondroplasia, 2427, 2427f
pyknodysostosis as, 2433, 2433f
short-rib polydactyly syndromes as, 2434
spondyloepiphyseal, 2424-2425, 2424f-2425f
aggrecan-related, 2425
late-onset, 2425
spondylometaphyseal, Kozlowski type, 2435
Stickler, 2426, 2426f
thanatophoric, 2428-2430, 2428f-2429f
of transcription factors, 2431-2432
of transmembrane receptors, 2428-2430
treatment of, *see website*
Skeletal infection
Cryptococcus neoformans in, 1057
nontuberculous mycobacterial, 1012t
Skeletal injuries, due to child abuse, 138, 138t
Skeletal manifestations
in homocystinuria, 425-426
in Marfan syndrome, 2440, 2441f-2442f
Skeletal maturation, *see website*
Skeleton
effects of malnutrition on, 175t
growth considerations, *see website*
Skew deviation in neurologic examination, *see website*
Skiing, injuries in, *see website*
Skill, cultural, *see website*
Skin
congenital absence of, 2221-2222, 2221f
disinfection for blood culture, *see website*
drug absorption in, *see website*
glucocorticoid effect on, *see website*
maintenance water and, 244t
morphology of, 2215, *see also website*
newborn assessment of, 533, 533f
redundant, 2220
Skin biopsy, *see website*
fetal, 543t
in urticarial vasculitis, 814
Skin care
in newborn, 537
in palliative care, 158
Skin dimples, 2220
Skin disorders
acne as, 2322-2328
chlor-, 2327
conglobata, 2328
drug-induced, 2326-2327, 2327f
fulminans, 2328
halogen, 2327
infantile, 2327, 2327f
neonatal, 2327, 2327f
tropical, 2327-2328
vulgaris, 2322-2326
due to arthropod bites, 2317-2319, 2318f
atopic dermatitis as, 801-807
in child-care setting, *see website*
cutaneous defects as, 2220-2222, 2221f-2222f
of dermis, 2273-2282
corticosteroid-induced atrophy as, 2274
cutis laxa as, 2277-2278, 2277f
Ehlers-Danlos syndrome as, 2278
elastosis perforans serpiginous as, 2279, 2279f
granuloma annulare as, 2274-2275, 2274f
keloid as, 2273-2274, 2273f
lichen sclerosus as, 2275, 2275f
lipoid proteinosis as, 2276-2277
Skin disorders *(Continued)*
macular atrophy as, 2277
mastocytosis as, 2280-2282, 2280f-2281f, 2280t-2281t
morphea as, 2275-2276, 2276f
in mucopolysaccharidoses, 2280, 2280f
necrobiosis lipoidica, 2275, 2275f
pseudoxanthoma elasticum as, 2278-2279, 2278f
reactive perforating collagenosis as, 2279, 2279f
scleredema as, 2276
striae cutis distensae as, 2274, 2274f
ectodermal dysplasia as, 2222-2223, 2223f, 2223t
eczematous, 2249-2254
contact dermatitis as, 2250-2252, 2250f-2251f
lichen simplex chronicus as, 2252, 2253f
nummular, 2252, 2252f
pityriasis alba as, 2252, 2252f
seborrheic dermatitis as, 2253-2254, 2253f-2254f
vesicular hand and foot dermatitis as, 2253, 2253f
of epidermis, 2259-2267
acanthosis nigricans as, 2266-2267, 2266f
Darier disease as, 2263, 2263f
Gianotti-Crosti syndrome as, 2266, 2266f
keratosis pilaris as, 2261, 2261f
lichen nitidus as, 2263-2264, 2264f
lichen planus as, 2264-2265, 2265f
lichen spinulosus as, 2261-2262
lichen striatus as, 2264
pityriasis lichenoides as, 2260-2261, 2260f-2261f
pityriasis rosea as, 2262, 2262f
pityriasis rubra pilaris as, 2262-2263, 2263f
porokeratosis as, 2265-2266, 2265f
psoriasis as, 2259-2260, 2259f
evaluation of, 2215, *see also website*
due to food allergy, 822
of hair, 2289-2293
herbs for, 272t
HIV-related, 1166
hyperpigmented lesion as, 2236-2238, 2236f-2237f
hypopigmented lesion as, 2238-2240, 2238f-2240f, 2238t, 2240t
infections as (*See* Skin infections)
due to infestation
pediculosis as, 2321-2322, 2321f
scabies as, 2319-2320, 2319f-2320f
seabather's eruption, 2322
of keratinization, 2267-2273
as manifestation of systemic disease, *see website*
of mucous membranes, 2297-2299
due to multisystem drug reactions, 2215, *see also website*
nail changes associated with, 2295-2296
of nails, 2293-2297
neonatal, 2218-2220, 2218f-2219f
neurocutaneous, 2046-2053
incontinentia pigmenti as, 2052-2053, 2053f
linear nevus syndrome as, 2052
neurofibromatosis as, 2046-2048, 2047f-2048f, 2048t
PHACE syndrome as, 2052
Sturge-Weber syndrome as, 2051-2052, 2051f
tuberous sclerosis complex as, 2049-2051, 2049f-2050f, 2049t
von Hippel-Lindau disease as, 2052
nevi as, 2231-2236
nutritional dermatoses as, 2328-2330
of photosensitivity, 2254-2259
smooth muscle hamartoma as, 2235-2236
of subcutaneous tissue, 2282-2286, 2282f-2284f, 2282t
of sweat glands, 2286-2288, 2287f, 2287t
Skin disorders *(Continued)*
therapy for, 2215-2218
tumors as, 2328, *see also website*
vascular, 2223-2231, 2224t
arteriovenous malformations as, 2225, 2226f
benign acquired, 2229-2230, 2229f-2230f
birthmarks as, 2223
capillary malformations (port-wine stain) as, 2224, 2225f
genetic, 2230-2231
Klippel-Trenaunay and Klippel-Trenaunay-Weber syndromes as, 2225-2226, 2226f
malformations as, 2224
nevus anemicus as, 2226
phakomatosis pigmentovascularis as, 2226
tumors as, 2226-2231, 2227f-2229f, 2227t-2228t
vascular malformations as, 2224t-2225t
venous malformations as, 2224-2225, 2225f-2226f
vesiculobullous, 2241-2249, 2241t
dermatitis herpetiformis as, 2248-2249, 2248f
erythema multiforme as, 2241-2242, 2242f
linear immunoglobulin A dermatosis as, 2249, 2249f
mechanobullous, 2244-2246, 2245f-2247f, 2245t
pemphigus as, 2247-2248, 2247f
Stevens-Johnson syndrome as, 2242-2243, 2243f
toxic epidermal necrolysis as, 2243-2244
Skin infections
Aeromonas in, 974, *see also website*
anaerobic, *see website*
aspergillosis as, 1061
bacterial, 2299-2308
blastomycosis-like pyoderma, 2304, 2304f
blistering distal dactylitis as, 2304, 2304f
ecthyma as, 2303, 2303f
erysipeloid as, 2307
erythrasma as, 2306
folliculitis as, 2305, 2305f-2306f
furuncles and carbuncles as, 2305-2306, 2306f
impetigo as, 2299-2300, 2300f
perianal dermatitis as, 2304-2305, 2305f
pitted keratolysis as, 2306
staphylococcal scaled skin syndrome as, 2302-2303, 2302f
of subcutaneous tissue, 2300-2302
tuberculous, 2307-2308, 2308f
Blastomyces dermatitidis, 1064
in child care setting, *see website*
Cryptococcus neoformans in, 1057
diphtheria in, *see website*
fungal, 2309-2314
atopic dermatitis with, 806
candidal, 2313-2314
dermatophytoses as, 2309-2313, 2310f
tinea versicolor as, 2309, 2309f
group A streptococcal, 916-917
herpes simplex virus, 1100, 1100f, 1102-1103
human T-lymphocyte-associated, *see website*
in immigrant children, 134
leishmaniasis, 1188, 1188f
nocardiosis as, *see website*
nontuberculous mycobacterial, 1012t, 1013
parvovirus B19 in, 1096-1097, 1096f
Pseudomonas aeruginosa, 976t
sporotrichosis, *see website*
sports participation and, 2402t-2404t
Staphylococcus aureus in, 905
in child-care setting, *see website*
viral, 2315-2317
atopic dermatitis with, 806
Skin lesions
in atopic dermatitis, 802, 802f-803f
human papillomavirus, 1138-1139, 1139f, 2315-2316, 2315f

Skin lesions *(Continued)*
of leprosy, *see website*
in tuberculosis, 1004
in tuberous sclerosis complex, 2050, 2050f
Skin manifestations, *see also website*
in allergic disease, 765
in chemical terrorism, *see website*
in connective tissue disease, *see website*
in eating disorders, 93t
in enterovirus, 1090
hand-foot-and-mouth disease, 1088, 1090f
in factitious disorder by proxy, 146
in food adverse reactions, 820-821
in food allergy, 822
in gastrointestinal disease, *see website*
in graft *versus* host disease, 760-761, 761f, *see also website*
chronic, 761-762, 762f
in insect allergy, 808
in Lyme disease, 1026, 1027f
in malignancy, *see website*
in malnutrition, 175t
in Marfan syndrome, 2442
in measles, 1070-1071, 1070f-1071f
in Neonatal Intensive Care Unit Neurobehavioral Scale, 624t
in parvovirus B19 infection, 1095-1097, 1095f-1096f
in poisoning, 252t
in porphyria cutanea tarda, *see website*
in radiation exposure, *see website*
in serum sickness, 819
in setting of immunosuppression, *see website*
in systemic lupus erythematosus, 842, 842f, 843t
in systemic scleroderma, 852f, 850-851
in toxoplasmosis, 1211
in vasculitis, *see website*
Skin testing
allergic, 767-768, 767t
autologous, 813
Candida, in T-cell function assessment, 720
Montenegro, 1187
prick, in food adverse reactions, 822
tuberculin, 1001, 1002t
in fever of unknown origin, 902
in HIV infection, 1174
Skin-to-skin contact for maintenance of newborn body heat, 537
Skipped generation, 383-385
Ski-related injuries, 23
Skull
auscultation of in neurologic examination, *see website*
fracture of, in newborn, 565-566
newborn assessment of, 533-534, 534t
palpation in neurologic examination, *see website*
Skull roentgenogram, *see website*
SKY. *See* Spectral karyotyping (SKY)
SLAP lesion, 2410
"Slapped cheek" appearance of fifth disease, 1095, 1095f
SLC26A4 gene, 2190t
SLD. *See* Specific learning disabilities (SLD)
SLE. *See* St. Louis encephalitis (SLE); Systemic lupus erythematosus (SLE)
Sleep
foreign-born adoptees and, 131
introduction to, 46
normal developmental changes in, 47t
overweight and obesity and, 182
requirements of, 29f
during 2-6 months of age, 30
respiration regulation during, *see website*
sudden infant death syndrome and environment of, 1425
Sleep apnea
enuresis with, 72
general anesthesia and, *see website*
obstructive, 49-51, 49t-50t, 1523
Sleep apnea *(Continued)*
Down syndrome with, 403t
obesity with, 184t
with type 2 diabetes mellitus, 1993t
"Sleep attack," 53
Sleep debt, 46
Sleep-disordered breathing (SDB), 49
in cystic fibrosis, 1494
Sleep disorders, 46-54
attention deficit/hyperactivity disorder *versus*, 110
delayed sleep phase disorder as, 53-54
evaluation of, 54-55
health supervision of, 54, 54t
insomnia as, 47-48, 48t-49t
narcolepsy as, 53
obstructive sleep apnea as, 49-51, 49t-50t
parasomnias, 51-52, 52t
restless legs syndrome, periodic limb movement disorder, and rhythmic movement as, 52-53
seizures and, *see website*
treatment of in palliative care, 155t-156t
Sleep hygiene, 48t-49t
Sleeping sickness, 1190-1193, 1192f, *see also website*
Sleep loss, 46
Sleep paralysis, 53
seizure *versus*, *see website*
Sleep studies in respiratory disease, *see website*
Sleep terrors, 51-52
Sleep transition disorders, *see website*
Sleepwalking, 51-52
Sleepwear, flame-retardant, 23
SLI. *See* Specific language impairment (SLI)
Sliding hiatal hernia, 1265, 1265f
Slime layer
of coagulase-negative staphylococci, 909
of *Staphylococcus aureus*, 904
Slipped capital femoral epiphysis (SCFE), 2363, 2364f
obesity with, 184t
Slipped vertebral apophysis, 2377
SLIT. *See* Sublingual immunotherapy (SLIT)
Slit-lamp examination, 2150
SLOS. *See* Smith-Lemli-Opitz syndrome (SLOS)
Slow learner, *see website*
SLURP-1 gene, 2272
Sly syndrome, 512t, 514
SMA. *See* Spinal muscular atrophy (SMA)
Small bowel
bacterial overgrowth in, 1340
biopsy of, 1306
digestion and absorption in, *see website*
disease of
(*See also* Intestinal disorders)
immunoproliferative, 1314-1315
Small for gestational age (SGA) newborn
as high-risk infant, 552-553
hypoglycemia in, 519-521
problems associated with, 557t
Smallpox
in terrorism, 891, *see also website*
vaccine for, 881t, 884t, 891
Small vessel vasculitis, with hepatitis C, 1401
SMARCAL1 gene, 1803t
SMBGS. *See* Self-monitoring of blood glucose (SMBG)
Smell, loss of. *See* Anosmia
Smile, sardonic, of tetanus, 992
Smith antibody, *see website*
Smith-Lemli-Opitz syndrome (SLOS), 478, 478t, 1967, *see website*
adrenal insufficiency with, 1925t, 1926
congenital heart disease with, 1531t
microcephaly with, 2007t
Smith-Magenis syndrome, 408t
Smith-Strang disease, 1319
SMN gene, 2136-2137
Smoke, second-hand
otitis media and, 2200
sudden infant death syndrome and, 1424
Smoke detector, 24
Smokeless tobacco, 680
Smoking. *See* Cigarette smoking
Smooth muscle antibody in rheumatic disease, *see website*
Smooth muscle hamartoma, 2235-2236
SMR. *See* Sexual maturity rating (SMR)
Snail fever, 1230-1231
Snake bite, 2461-2462, 2461f-2462f, 2461t-2462t
SNAP. *See* Score for Neonatal Acute Physiology (SNAP)
Snapping hit syndrome, 2414
SNHL. *See* Sensorineural hearing loss (SNHL)
Sn-mesoporphyrin (SnMP), for hyperbilirubinemia, 612
SnMP. *See* Sn-mesoporphyrin (SnMP), for hyperbilirubinemia
Snoring, 49
Snow board-related injuries, 23
SNP. *See* Lymphoid tyrosine phosphatase (SNP); Single-nucleotide polymorphism (SNP)
Snuffles in congenital syphilis, 1017-1018
So_2. *See* Oxyhemoglobin (So_2)
Soap for skin disorders, 2216
SOAP MM, 285
Soccer, injuries in, *see website*
Social anxiety disorder, 78
Social behavior evaluation, 120
Social cognition, *see website*
Social Cognitive Theory, *see website*
Social development
in foreign-born adoptees, 131
during middle childhood, 38
Social effectiveness therapy for children (SET-C), 79
Social factors
in child health, 2-3
in development, *see website*
in suicide, 88
Social history
in neurologic evaluation, *see website*
in poisonings, 253
in wheezing, 1458
Social issues
in children born to teen mothers, 701
regarding homosexuality, 658
Social phobia (SP), 78, 79t
Social sex role, 655
Social support
following traumatic injury, 340
during pregnancy, *see website*
Society, adolescent development of relationships with, 652-654
Socioeconomic factors
in childhood injuries, 20
in chronic illness, *see website*
in *Haemophilus influenzae* type b, 940
in high-risk pregnancies, *see website*
in malnutrition, 173
in otitis media, 2200
in psychosomatic illness, 67
Sodium (Na^+), 212-219, *see website*
in acute renal failure, 1819, 1820t
dietary reference intakes for, *see website*
disorders of
hypernatremia as, 212-215
hyponatremia as, 215-219
excretion of, 212, *see also website*
hypernatremia due to deficits of, 213, 213t
in hyponatremia, 1884
intake of, 212
metabolism of, 212
in oral rehydration solutions, 1335t
reference values for, *see website*
renal tubular regulation of, *see website*
resorption of, *see website*

Sodium (Na^+) *(Continued)*
retention of, *see also website*
in chronic kidney disease, 1823t
supplementation for burn injury, 353
in total body water, *see website*
Sodium bicarbonate
for metabolic acidosis, 234-235
in neonatal resuscitation, 576-577
for pediatric resuscitation and arrhythmias, 294t
for tricyclic antidepressants poisoning, 256t-258t, 264
Sodium channel genes, sudden infant death syndrome and, 1425-1426
Sodium channelopathies, 2125t
Sodium cromoglycate for allergic rhinitis, 779
Sodium diarrhea, 1321, 1341
Sodium fluoride, gastroenteritis due to, 1328t-1329t
Sodium iodide for thyroid storm, 1912t
Sodium nitroprusside
for cardiac output maintenance and post-resuscitation stabilization, 294t
for hypertensive emergencies, 1646t
Sodium-potassium adenosine triphosphatase (Na^+,K^+-ATPase), 219
Sodium stibogluconate, 1189-1190, *see also website*
Sodium wasting in chronic kidney disease, 1823t
Sodoku, 2458
Soft bedding, sudden infant death syndrome and, 1425
Soft tissue infection
Aeromonas in, 974, *see also website*
anaerobic, *see website*
nontuberculous mycobacterial, 1013
due to typhoid fever, 957t
Soft tissue lesions of oral cavity, 1259-1261, 1260f, 1260t
Soft tissue sarcoma, 1760-1762
incidence and survival rates for, 1726t
rhabdomyosarcoma as, 1760-1762, 1761f, 1761t
secondary, due to radiation therapy, *see website*
Solanine poisoning, 2454, *see also website*
Solar urticaria, 813, 2257, 2257f
Soles, palmoplantar keratodermas of, 2272-2273
Solu-Medrol. *See* Methylprednisolone
Soman, in terrorism, *see website*
Somatic development, *see website*
Somatic mutation, 383-385
Somatic pain, 360t, 1248
Somatoform disorders, 67, 68t
diagnostic criteria for, 68t, 69
undifferentiated, 68t
Somatosensory amplification, 68
Somatosensory-evoked potentials (SSEPs), *see website*
Somatostatin analogs for growth hormone excess, *see website*
Somatostatin in neuroendocrine tumor-associated diarrhea, *see website*
Somatostatinoma, diarrhea caused by, *see website*
Somogyi phenomenon, 1985-1986
Sonic hedgehog (SHH) pathway, *see website*
Sorbitol, 1982
for constipation maintenance therapy, 74t
for fecal disimpaction, 74t
Sore throat in common cold, 1435
Sotos syndrome, 408t, *see also website*
South African genetic porphyria, *see website*
South American blastomycosis, 1068
Southeast Asian liver fluke, *see website*
Southeast Asian population, cultural values associated with, *see website*
Southeastern Asian ovalocytes (SAO), *see website*
SOX9 gene, 2431, *see also website*
Soybean allergy, 821, 821t
Soy formula, 163-164
SP. *See* Social phobia (SP)
Spaghetti and meatballs appearance of *Malassezia*, *see website*
Spanish-English translation of botanical names, 274t
Spasmodic croup, 1447
Spasm(s)
esophageal, diffuse, 1265
neonatal, 2034
with seizures, 2019
Spasmus nutans, 2161-2162, *see website*
Spastic diplegia in cerebral palsy, 2062-2063, 2062t, 2063f
treatment of, 2064, 2064f
Spastic hemiplegia in cerebral palsy, 2062, 2062t
Spasticity, muscle, assessment in neurologic examination, *see website*
Spastic quadriplegia in cerebral palsy, 2063
Spatial functioning, *see website*
SP-B. *See* Surfactant protein B (SP-B)
SP-C. *See* Surfactant protein C (SP-C)
Special cause variation, *see website*
Specialist referral
asthma, 793
chronic illness, *see website*
genetic disorders, 379
homosexuality, 659
psychiatric disorders, 58
eating disorders, 95-96
sexual abuse, 143
Specialization of pediatrics, 12-13
Special needs children, 5-9
abused and neglected children, 135-147
assessment of, 141
clinical manifestations of, 137-140, 137f-139f, 138t-139t
definitions associated with, 135-136
etiology of, 136-137, 136t
factitious disorder by proxy as, 146-147
foster and kinship care and, *see website*
as global situation, 136
interventions for, 141
outcomes of, 141-142
prevention of, 142
sexual (*See* Sexual abuse)
United States situation, 136
adopted children, 130-134, 131t
child care and, *see website*
children affected by war, 8, 135, *see also website*
children impacted by violence (*See* Violence)
children in foster and kinship care, 134, *see also website*
children in poverty, 6, 6f
children of immigrants and racial minority groups, 6-7
children of migrant workers, 7
chronic illness in childhood, 149, *see also website*
failure to thrive, 147-149
clinical manifestations of, 147
differential diagnosis of, 147f, 148t
epidemiology of, 147
etiology and diagnosis of, 147-148, 148t-149t
prognosis for, 149
treatment of, 148-149
goals of pediatricians regarding, 9
gynecological care for, 1874-1875
health services for, 10-11
homeless children, 7-8
inherent strengths in, 8-9
palliative care for, 149-159, 150f
communication, advanced care planning, and anticipatory guidance in, 151-159, 153t
conditions appropriate for, 149-150, 149t
decision-making in, 153
resuscitation status in, 153-154
settings for, 151
Special needs children *(Continued)*
symptoms management in, 154-158, 154t-157t
during terminal phase, 158-159
runaway and thrown-away children, 8
Special Supplemental Nutrition Program for Women, Infants, and Children (WIC), 170
Specialty care. *See* Referral
Specific airway resistance, *see website*
Specific gravity, pleural, in tuberculosis, 1003-1004
Specific language impairment (SLI), 116-118
Specific learning disabilities (SLD), *see website*. *See also* Neurodevelopmental dysfunction
Speckled lentiginous nevus, 2233, 2233f
SPECT. *See* Single-photon emission computed tomography (SPECT)
Spectral karyotyping (SKY), 396
Spectrometry, tandem mass, *see website*
Spectroscopy, magnetic resonance, 1545-1546, *see also website*
Speculum pelvic examination, *see website*
Speech
language *versus*, 34
in myotonic muscular dystrophy, 2124
Speech disorders. *See* Language disorders
Speech-language therapy, 121
Speech-recognition threshold (SRT) in audiometry, 2193
Speech therapy in respiratory insufficiency, 1525
Spelling and writing impairments, *see website*
Spermatic cord torsion, 1861-1862
Spermatocele, 1863
Spermicides, 694, 695t
Sphenoidal sinuses, 1436
Spherocytosis, hereditary, 1659-1662, 1659t, 1660f-1662f, *see website*
Sphingolipid metabolism, 482-483, 483f
Sphingolipidoses, 484t, 2069-2072, 2071f-2072f
Sphrintzen-Goldberg syndrome, 2444t
Sphygmomanometer, 1533
Spider angioma, 2229-2230, 2230f
as manifestation of liver disease, 1376
Spider bite, 2462-2463, 2463f
Spielmeyer-Vogt disease, 2073
Spina bifida occulta, 1999, 2000f, 2001t
Spinal arteriovenous malformations, 2107-2108
Spinal cord
compression of as oncologic emergency, *see website*
diastematomyelia as, 2102, 2103f
respiratory distress due to, 315t
spinal arteriovenous malformations as, 2107-2108
syringomyelia as, 2103, 2104f
tethered cord, 2101-2102, 2101f-2102f
transverse myelitis as, 2107, 2107t
traumatic (*See* Spinal cord injury (SCI))
tumors as, 2105, 2105f
multiple sclerosis effects on, 2077t
Spinal cord injury (SCI), 2106
during birth, 573
poliovirus infection *versus*, 1085t
respiratory insufficiency due to, 1523
Spinal cord injury without radiographic abnormalities (SCIWORA), 337, 2106
Spinal disorders, 2365-2377, 2365t
back pain as, 2373-2374, 2373t
disk space infection as, 2376, 2376t
intervertebral disk herniation and slipped vertebral apophysis as, 2377
kyphosis as, 2371-2373, 2372f
scoliosis as
compensatory, 2371
congenital, 2368-2370, 2369f
idiopathic, 2365-2368, 2366f-2368f
neuromuscular, 2370-2371
spondylolysis and spondylolisthesis as, 2374-2376, 2375f
syndromes and genetic disorders of, 2371
tumors as, 2377

Spinal dysraphism
  congenital scoliosis with, 2369
  occult, neuropathic bladder and, *see website*
Spinal fusion for scoliosis
  idiopathic, 2368, 2368f
  neuromuscular, 2371
Spinal muscular atrophy (SMA), 2136-2138, 2136t, 2137f
  chronic severe respiratory insufficiency with, 1519-1520, 1520t
  long-term mechanical ventilation for, 1524
Spinal paralytic poliomyelitis, 1083
Spindle nevus, 2233, 2233f
Spine
  arthrogryposis involving, *see website*
  assessment of, 2333f
  birth injuries to, 573
  cervical
    juvenile idiopathic arthritis involvement in, 832, 834f
    in trauma survey, 335
    traumatic injury to, 337-338, 338f
  infection of, 2376, 2376t
  musculoskeletal pain syndrome of, 877t
SPINK5, *see website*
SPINK gene mutation, 1373
Spinocerebellar ataxia (SCA), 2057t
Spiral fracture, 2388f, 2390
Spiral reconstruction computed tomography, *see website*
Spiramycin, 1215
Spirillum minus, 2458
Spiritual issues, grief and, *see website*
Spirochetal infection
  bejel as, 1023, *see also website*
  leptospirosis as, 1023-1025
  Lyme disease as, 1025-1029
  pinta as, 1023, *see also website*
  relapsing fever as, 1025, *see also website*
  syphilis as, 1016-1023
  yaws as, 1023, *see also website*
Spirometra mansonoides, 1232t
Spirometry
  in asthma, 783-784, 785t, 786f
  in pulmonary function testing, *see website*
Spironolactone, 1645t
  for acne, 2325t
  for familial male gonadotropin-independent precocious puberty, 1893
  for heart failure, *see website*
Spitz nevus, 2233, 2233f
Splash burn, due to child abuse, 138
Spleen
  anatomy and function of, 1723, *see also website*
  disorders of
    abnormal position of the heart and, 1589t, 1595-1596
    hyposplenism as, 1723, *see also website*
    infection with, *see website*
    neutropenia due to, 749
    splenomegaly as, 1723, *see also website*
  enlarged, sports participation, 2402t-2404t
  trauma to, *see website*
Splenectomy, *see website*
Splenic aspiration in leishmaniasis, 1189
Splenic sequestration in sickle cell disease, 1664
Splenomegaly, 1723, *see also website*
  malarial, 1206
  in Niemann-Pick disease, 488
  in portal hypertension, *see website*
Splinter hemorrhages of nails, 2295
Splinting for clubfoot, 2337
Split cord malformation, 2102, 2103f
Splitting of 2nd heart sound, 1533
SPNETs. *See* Supratentorial primitive neuroectodermal tumors (SPNETs)
Spondyloarthritides, 839, *see also website*
Spondylocostal dysostosis syndromes, *see website*
Spondyloepiphyseal dysplasias (SED), 2424-2425, 2424f
  aggrecan-related, 2425
  Kniest dysplasia as variant of, 2425
  late-onset, 2425
Spondyloepiphyseal dysplasias (SED) congenita, 2424-2425, 2425f
Spondylolisthesis, 2374-2376
  due to sports injury, 2412
Spondylolysis, 2374-2376
  due to sports injury, 2412
Spondylometaphyseal dysplasia, Kozlowski type, 2435
Spongiosis in atopic dermatitis, 801
Spontaneous breathing trial (SBT), 329
Spontaneous pneumothorax, 1509
Spoon nails, 2293, 2294f
Sporothrix schenckii, 1068, *see also website*
Sporotrichoid nocardiosis, *see website*
Sports
  classification by contact, 2406t
  drowning during, 342
  female athlete triad and, 686
  herpes simplex virus infection associated with, 1100
  herpes simplex virus infection related to, 1102
  performance-enhancing aids, 2422-2423, 2423t
  sickle cell trait and, 1671t
Sports examination, preparticipation, 2401-2405, 2401t-2404t, 2405f
Sports injuries
  acute, 2406
  of ankle, 2417-2418, 2417f
  in ballet, *see website*
  in baseball, *see website*
  in basketball and volleyball, *see website*
  differential diagnosis of, 2408
  of elbow, 2410-2412, 2411f-2412f
  epidemiology and prevention of, 2401-2406
  of foot, 2418
  in football, *see website*
  of growth plate, 2408-2409, 2408f-2409f
  in gymnastics, *see website*
  of head and neck, 2418-2420, 2419t
  due to heat, 2420-2421, 2421f
  of hip and pelvis, 2407t, 2413-2414, 2413f
  in ice hockey, *see website*
  initial evaluation of, 2407
  of knee, 2414-2416, 2414t, 2415f
  of low back, 2412-2413
  of lower leg, 2416-2417
  mechanism of, 2406-2407
  ocular, 2186-2187
  overuse, 2406-2407, 2407t
  return to play following, 2407-2408
  in running, *see website*
  of shoulder, 2409-2410, 2410f
  in skiing, *see website*
  in soccer, *see website*
  in swimming, *see website*
  in tennis, *see website*
  in wrestling, *see website*
Sports medicine
  menstrual problems and osteopenia in, 2421-2422
  performance-enhancing aids, 2422-2423, 2423t
  sports injuries in (*See* Sports injuries)
Sports participation, examination prior to, 2401-2405, 2401t-2404t, 2405f
Sprain
  ankle, 2418
    in basketball and volleyball, *see website*
  as sports injury, 2406
Sprengel deformity, 2383
Sprue, tropical, 1313-1314
Spun-glass hair, 2293, 2293f
Spurious hyperkalemia, 219
Sputum culture in tuberculosis, 1003
SQTS. *See* Short Q-T syndrome (SQTS)
Squamous intraepithelial lesion
  high-grade, 1138t
  low-grade, 1137-1138
SR. *See* Sarcoplasmic reticulum (SR), in cardiac development
SRD5A2 gene, *see website*
SRT. *See* Speech-recognition threshold (SRT)
SRY gene, *see website*
SSEPs. *See* Somatosensory-evoked potentials (SSEPs)
S/S genotype, 1426
SSLR. *See* Serum-sickness like reaction (SSLR)
SSPE. *See* Subacute sclerosing panencephalitis (SSPE)
SSRIs. *See* Selective serotonin reuptake inhibitors (SSRIs)
ST. *See* Sensory testing (ST)
St. Louis encephalitis (SLE), 1141, 1143-1144
Stabilizers in immunizing agents, 883
Stable factor, 1696t
Staff. *See* Health care providers
Staging
  of cancer, 1731
    Hodgkin lymphoma, 1741, 1741t
    neuroblastoma, 1755t, 1756
    non-Hodgkin lymphoma, 1743-1744, 1745t
    treatment and, *see website*
    Wilms tumor, 1759t
  of graft *versus* host disease, 761t
Stains, for microscopic examination, *see website*
Stammering, 122
Standard deviation (SD), *see website*
Standard precautions, *see website*
Standard value on growth charts, *see website*
Staphylococcal scaled skin syndrome, 2302-2303, 2302f
Staphylococci, 903-910
  in blepharitis, 2164
  coagulase-negative, 909-910
  in toxic shock syndrome, 905, 908-909, 909t
Staphylococcus aureus, 904-908
  atopic dermatitis and, 806
  in breast milk, 540t
  in cellulitis, 2300
  in child-care setting, *see website*
  clinical manifestations of, 905-906
  in cystic fibrosis infections, 1482, 1492t
  diagnosis of, 906-908
  differential diagnosis of, 906, 906f
  epidemiology of, 904
  etiology of, 904
  in folliculitis, 2305
  in furuncles and carbuncles, 2305-2306
  in furunculosis, 2198
  gastroenteritis due to, 1324t-1325t
  in hordeolum, 2164
  in impetigo, 2299
  in infective endocarditis, 1622
  in mastitis, *see website*
  methicillin-resistant, 907t
  methicillin-susceptible, 906-907
  neonatal, 632t
    sepsis due to, 635t-636t
  in osteomyelitis, 2394
  in otitis media, 2201
  pathogenesis of, 904-905, 904f
  in pneumonia, 1475t, 1476
  prevention of, 908
  prognosis for, 908
  in septic arthritis, 2398
  slime layer of, 904
  in toxic shock syndrome, 905, 908-909, 909t
  treatment of, 906-908, 907t
  with varicella-zoster virus, 1109
  in vulvovaginitis, 1868t
Staphylococcus epidermis, 909-910
Stargardt disease, 2178
StAR gene, *see website*
Staring, behavioral, *see website*
Starvation ketoacidosis, 232
State child care licensing, *see website*

State Children's Health Insurance Program (SCHIP), 10
States, behavioral, *see website*
Static compliance (C_{STAT}) assessment in mechanical ventilation, 328
Station, neurologic examination of, *see website*
Stature, percentile curves for, *see website*
  derivation and interpretation of, *see website*
Status asthmaticus, 797t-798t, 798-799
Status epilepticus, 303, 2037-2039, 2039t
  febrile, 2017
  due to traumatic brain injury, 300
Status marmoratus, 2063-2064
Status migrainosus, 2040-2041
Statutory rape, 703
Stavudine (d4T)
  drug interactions with, *see website*
  for HIV infection, 1167, 1168t-1171t
Steady state in drug therapy, *see website*
Stealing, 99
Steatocrit in chronic diarrhea, 1344t
Steatocystoma multiplex, *see website*
Steatohepatitis, nonalcoholic, 1408
STEC. *See* Shiga toxin-producing *Escherichia coli* (STEC)
Steinburg sign, 2440, 2441f
Stellae ganglion block, 373
Stellate macular retinopathy, 985
Stellwag sign, 2163
Stem cell factor (SCF), fetal, *see website*
Stem cells
  differentiation into cardiac cells, *see website*
  transplantation of (*See* Hematopoietic stem cell transplantation (HSCT))
Stenotrophomonas, 976, *see also website*
Stent, intravascular, 1548, 1548f
  for coarctation of the aorta, 1569
Stepping gait, *see website*
Stepwise approach to asthma management, 792-793, 792t
Sterile pyuria in urinary tract infection, 1831-1832
Sternal clefts, 1517
Sternal fracture, due to child abuse, 138
Sternocleidomastoid (SCM) muscle, *see also website*
  aplasia of, 2118
Steroids
  acne due to, 2326-2327, 2327f
  cataracts due to, 2171
  diabetes associated with, 1997
  panniculitis due to, 2283
  performance-enhancing, 2422-2423
  pharmacokinetics of, *see website*
  for seizures, 2032
Steroid hormone
  actions of, 1923, *see also website*
  adrenal gland biosynthesis of, 1923, *see also website*
Steroid-induced myopathy, 2129-2130, 2129t
Steroid-sparing immunosuppressive drugs
  for systemic lupus erythematosus, 844-845
Stevens-Johnson syndrome, 826, 827t, 1031, 1031f, 2242-2243, 2243f
Stewart-Prower factor, 1696t
Stickler dysplasia, 1254, 2426, 2426f
Stiff-Person syndrome, 1995-1996
Stigma of gender variance, 655-656
Stimulants
  adolescent abuse of, 683-684
  for attention deficit/hyperactivity disorder, 62t, 111-112
  cardiac evaluation before administration of, 112f
  for psychiatric disorders, 61, 62t
Sting
  hymenoptera, 807-809
  scorpion, 2464
Stinger, 2402t-2404t, 2420, *see also website*
Stinging insect allergy, 807-809, 807f, 809t
Stinging papule of dracunculiasis, 1227
STIs. *See* Sexually transmitted infections (STIs)
STM. *See* Short-term memory (STM)
Stochastic effects of radiation, *see website*
Stomach
  congenital anomalies of, 1274-1276
  digestion and absorption in, *see website*
  disorders of
    bezoars as, 1291
    eosinophilic gastroenteritis as, 1304
    foreign bodies as, 1290
    gastric duplication as, 1276
    gastric outlet obstruction as, 1275-1276
    hypertrophic gastropathy as, 1276
    peptic ulcer disease as, 1291-1294, 1291t, 1292f-1293f, 1293t
    pyloric stenosis as, 1274-1275, 1274f-1275f
    volvulus as, 1276
  in drug absorption, *see website*
  fetal ultrasound of, 550t
  normal development, structure, and function of, 1273, *see also website*
Stomatitis
  aphthous, 2298, 2298f
    in PFAPA, 859-860
  Vincent, 2299
Stomatocytosis, hereditary, 1661f, *see also website*
Stones. *See* Lithiasis
Stool(s), *see also website*
  blood in, exclusion from day care due to, *see website*
  diarrhea and, 1243-1244
  frequency of, *see website*
  rapid antigen detection of, *see website*
Stool culture, *see also website*
  in *Campylobacter* infection, 970
  in *Clostridium difficile* infection, 995
  in gastroenteritis, 1334
  in *Shigella* infection, 960
  in typhoid fever, 956-957
Stoplight zone system, 786-788
Storage disease
  cholesterol ester, 491
  neonatal iron, 1393
Storage of vitamin A, 188
Strabismic amblyopia, 2152
Strabismus, 2157-2161, 2158f-2160f
  with Down syndrome, 403t
  in neurologic examination, *see website*
Strain
  lumbar disk, as sports injury, 2412
  as sports injury, 2406
Stramonium folium, potential toxicity of, 272t-273t
Stranger anxiety, 30, 33
Stranger rape, 703
Strangulated hernia, 1365
Strattera. *See* Atomoxetine
Strawberry tongue in Kawasaki disease, 863, 864f
Strength, muscle, assessment in neurologic examination, *see website*
Strength-based approaches to well child care, 16
Strengths, inherent, in special risk populations, 8-9
Streptobacillus moniliformis, 2457-2458
Streptococcal toxic shock syndrome, 909, 919
Streptococci
  arthritis associated with, 840
  group A, 914-925
    clinical manifestations of, 916-917, 916f, 917t
    complications of, 919
    diagnosis of, 917-918
    differential diagnosis of, 918
    epidemiology of, 915
    glomerulonephritis associated with, 1783-1785, 1783f-1784f, 1785t
    in impetigo, 2299
    pathogenesis of, 915-916
Streptococci *(Continued)*
    in pneumonia, 1475t
    prevention of, 920
    prognosis for, 920
    in rheumatic fever, 920-925
    severe, 917, 917t
    in toxic shock syndrome, 909
    treatment of, 918-919
    with varicella-zoster virus, 1109
    in vulvovaginitis, 1868t
  group B, 925-928
    in breast milk, 540t
    clinical manifestations of, 926-927, 926t
    diagnosis of, 927
    epidemiology of, 925-926, 925f
    etiology of, 925
    fetal therapy for, 551t
    laboratory findings in, 927
    maternal, *see website*
    neonatal, 632t
    in osteomyelitis, 2394
    pathogenesis of, 926
    in pneumonia, 1475t
    prevention of, 927-928
    prognosis for, 927
    treatment of, 927, 927t
  group C, 928, *see also website*
    in pharyngitis, 1439
  group G, 928, *see also website*
  non-group A or B, 928, *see also website*
  in pharyngitis, 1439
  viridans
    in infective endocarditis, 1622, 1625t
    neonatal, 632t
      sepsis due to, 636t
Streptococcus agalactiae. See Group B streptococci
Streptococcus mutans in dental caries, 1255
Streptococcus pneumoniae, 910-914
  antibiotic resistant, 2205-2206
  in bacterial meningitis, 2087
  in child-care setting, *see website*
  clinical manifestations of, 912-913, 912f
  diagnosis of, 913
  in diarrhea-associated hemolytic-uremic syndrome, 1791-1793
  in empyema, 1507-1508
  epidemiology of, 911, 911f, 911t
  etiology of, 910-911
  hearing loss due to, 2188-2189
  neonatal sepsis due to, 636t
  in otitis media, 2201, *see website*
  pathogenesis of, 912
  in pneumonia, 1475t, 1476
  predisposition to infection due to immunodeficiency, 716t
  prevention of, 913-914, 914t
  prognosis for, 913
  rapid antigen detection of, *see website*
  testing for antibodies to, 719-720
  treatment of, 913
  vaccine for
  (*See* Pneumococci vaccine)
  in vulvovaginitis, 1868t
Streptococcus pyogenes
  in cellulitis, 2300-2301
  in necrotizing fasciitis, 2301
Streptogramins, *see website*
Streptokinase, 1509
Streptomycin, 979, *see also website*
  for brucellosis, 981t
  for tuberculosis, 1008t
Streptozyme test, 918
Stress, psychologic
  during pregnancy, *see website*
  type 1 diabetes mellitus development and, 1972
Stress fracture
  calcaneal, 2418
  navicular, 2418

Stress fracture *(Continued)*
sports-related, 2416-2417
femoral neck, 2413
humeral, 2410
metatarsal, 2418
in runners, *see website*
tibial, 2416
Stress ulcer, 1293
Stretch marks, 2274, 2274f
Stretch receptors in respiration regulation, *see website*
Striae cutis distensae, 2274, 2274f
Strictures, urethral, 1847
Stridor
auscultation of, *see website*
due to gastroesophageal reflux disease, 1269-1270
in laryngomalacia, 1450
postanesthetic, *see website*
recurrent or persistent, *see website*
at rest, croup and, 1448
as sign of respiratory pathology, *see website*
Stroke, 303-304
arterial ischemic, 2080-2082, 2081f
heat, 2420, 2421f
hemorrhagic, 2084-2085, 2084f, 2085t
perinatal, 2082
sickle cell disease and, 1667
Stroke syndromes, 2080-2086
arterial ischemic stroke as, 2080-2082, 2081f-2082f, 2081t-2082t
cerebral sinovenous thrombosis as, 2082-2084, 2083f, 2083t
differential diagnosis of, 2085-2086, 2086t
hemorrhagic, 2084-2085, 2084f, 2085t
Stromectol. *See* Ivermectin
Strongyloides stercoralis, 1220t, 1223-1224, 1223f, *see also website*
Strongyloidiasis, 1223-1224, 1223f
Structural growth, *see website*
Struvite calculi, *see website*
Struvite stones, *see website*
ST segment abnormalities, 1540
Sturge-Weber syndrome (SWS), 2051-2052, 2051f, 2224
Stuttering, 34, 117t, 122, 122t
Subaceous glands, morphology of, *see website*
Subacute necrotizing encephalomyelopathy, 506-509
Subacute sclerosing panencephalitis (SSPE), 1072-1073, 2075-2076
Subaortic stenosis, 1565
Subarachnoid hemorrhage (SAH)
emergency management of, 304
in newborn, 566
Subcapsular hematoma, 578
Subconjunctival hemorrhage, 2168-2169
in newborn, 566
Subcutaneous emphysema, 1462
Subcutaneous fat necrosis, 2284, 2284f
hypercalcemia with, 1922
Subcutaneous immunoglobulin (SCIG) for B-cell defects, 727-728
Subcutaneous nodules
in acute myeloid leukemia, 1737
in acute rheumatic fever, 922
Subcutaneous tissue
bacterial infection of, 2300-2302
diseases of, 2282-2286, 2282f-2284f
morphology of, *see website*
Subdural hematoma, due to child abuse, 139
Subdural hemorrhage in newborn, 566
Subgaleal hemorrhage, 565
Sublingual immunotherapy (SLIT), 774
Sublottic hemangioma, *see website*
Sublottic stenosis, 1454
Subluxation
dental, 1259
hip, 2356
patellar, 2355
Submersion injury, 341-348
epidemiology of, 342-343
etiology of, 341-342
management of, 344-347
pathophysiology of, 343-344
prevention of, 347-348, 348t
prognosis for, 347
resuscitation for, 344-345
Suboxone poisoning, 251t, 261
Substance abuse
adolescent, 671-685, 671f
of alcohol, 678-679, 678t-679t
of amphetamines, 683-684, 684t
clinical manifestations of, 673-674, 676t
of cocaine, 683
complications of, 677
diagnosis of, 677, 677t
drowning due to, 24
epidemiology of, 672-673, 673t, 675t
etiology of, 671-672, 672t-673t
of hallucinogens, 682-683
homosexuality and, 658-659
of inhalants, 681-682, 681t-682t
of marijuana, 680-681, 680t
of opiates, 684-685
pregnancy and, 701
of prescription drugs, 673t
prevention of, 677, 677t
prognosis for, 677
screening for, 674-677, 676t
of tobacco, 679-680, 680t
treatment of, 677
attention deficit/hyperactivity disorder *versus*, 110
of hydrocarbons, 267
maternal
fetal and neonatal effects of, *see website*
neonatal metabolic disturbances due to, 623-625, 624t
sudden infant death syndrome and, 1424
serotonin syndrome and, 265t
systemic hypertension due to, 1640-1641
Substernal thrust, 1533
Substitution, genetic, *see website*
Substrate specificity, *see website*
Subtle neonatal seizure, 2034
Subungual exostosis, 2343
Subvalvular stenosis, 1565
Succimer
for arsenic and mercury intoxication, *see website*
for lead poisoning, 2453, 2453t
for poisoning, 256t-257t
Succinic semialdehyde dehydrogenase deficiency, 447
Succinimides, adverse effects of, 2031t
Succinylcholine for anesthesia, *see website*
Succinyl CoA:3-ketoacid CoA transferase (SCOT) deficiency, 435, 462
Sucking
of digits, *see website*
of thumb, 75
Sucking blister, 2218
Sucking chest wound, 336t
Sucralfate, 1293t
Sucrase-isomaltase deficiency, 1318
Sucrose for pain management, 364t
Sudafed. *See* Pseudoephedrine
Sudden death, 1619-1621, 1620f-1621f, 1620t-1621t
associated with stimulants, 61
during sports, 2401-2405
Sudden infant death syndrome (SIDS), 1421-1429
apnea and, 581
in child-care settings, *see website*
clinical strategies for prevention of, 1428-1429
differential diagnosis of, 1422t-1423t
epidemiology of, 1422
infant groups at increased risk for, 1428
pathology of, 1422-1424
Sudden infant death syndrome (SIDS) *(Continued)*
risk factors for
environmental, 1424, 1424t
genetic, 1423t, 1425-1427, 1426f
genetic and environmental interactions in, 1427, 1427f
modifiable, 1424-1425
nonmodifiable, 1424
Sufentanil, 367t
Suffocation, 18
Sugammadex, *see website*
Suglottic stenosis, 1451
Suicide and attempted suicide, 18, 87-89, 88f, 89t
among homosexual youth, 658-659
with firearms, 24-25
Sulbactam, *see website*
Sulfadiazine, *see also website*
for acute rheumatic fever prophylaxis, 924t
for toxoplasmosis, 1215, *see also website*
Sulfamethoxazole, *see website*
Sulfasalazine
for inflammatory bowel disease, 1298-1299
for juvenile idiopathic arthritis, 838t
for rheumatic disease, *see website*
for spondyloarthritides, *see website*
for urticaria and angioedema, 815t
Sulfatase, multiple deficiency of, 490
Sulfate ion transporter, loss of, 2430-2431
Sulfatrim. *See* Trimethoprim-sulfamethoxazole (TMP-SMX)
Sulfisoxazole, *see also website*
for acute rheumatic fever prophylaxis, 924t
possible adverse reactions to in premature infant, 563t
Sulfite oxidase deficiency, 429
Sulfonamides, 826, *see also website*
Sulfonylureas, 1992, 1992t
poisoning with, 263
antidote for, 256t-257t
Sulfur granules in actinomycosis, *see website*
Sulthiame, 2030t
Sumatriptan
for migraine, 2044t
for vomiting, 1244t
Sunburn reaction, acute, 2254-2255, 2254f, 2254t-2255t
Sunburst pattern of osteosarcoma, 1763-1764, 1764f
Sunlight, cutaneous reactions to, 2254-2255, 2254f, 2254t-2255t
Sunscreen, 2217-2218
Superfecundation, 553
Superficial nerves, thickening of in leprosy, *see website*
Superior mesenteric artery syndrome, 1287, *see also website*
Superior vena cava syndrome, *see website*
Supernumerary nipples, 2221, *see also website*
Supernumerary teeth, 1430
Supination, 2331
Supine positioning, sudden infant death syndrome and, 1425
Supplements
dietary, 270-273, 271t-272t
nutritional aspects of, 169
Spanish-English botanical name translation chart, 274t
toxicity of, 272t-273t
vitamin, nutritional aspects of, 169
Support, social
following traumatic injury, 340
during pregnancy, *see website*
Support groups
chronic illness, *see website*
genetic disorders, 379
Supportive psychotherapy, 66
Suppositories, 74t
for constipation maintenance therapy, 74t
Suppression as eye disorder, 2152-2153

Suppurative arthritis
Haemophilus influenzae in, 942
Suppurative parotitis, *see website*
Suppurative thyroiditis, 1904t, 1905
Supracristal ventricular septal defect with aortic insufficiency, 1559
Supraglottitis, 1446-1447, 1447f
Haemophilus influenzae in, 942
Supratentorial primitive neuroectodermal tumors (SPNETs), 1752
Supravalvular stenosis, 1565
Supraventricular tachycardia (SVT), 1613-1616, 1614f-1616f
emergency management of, 288-289
fetal therapy for, 551t
Suprax. *See* Cefixime
Suramin, 1192, *see also website*
Surface area estimation, *see website*
Surfactant
composition of, 581, 582f
inherited disorders of, 1497-1498, *see also website*
respiratory distress syndrome due to, 581-582, 585
prophylactic administration of, 585
replacement of, 585-586
Surfactant protein A (SP-A), 1497-1498
Surfactant protein B (SP-B) deficiency, *see website*
Surfactant protein C (SP-C) disease, *see website*
Surfactant protein D (SP-D), *see website*
Surgery
for achalasia, 1265
for acne, 2326
for ambiguous genitalia, 1935
for anorectal malformations, 1358-1359, 1359t
antibiotic prophylaxis for, *see website*
for aortic aneurysm in Marfan syndrome, 2445
for appendicitis, 1354-1355
asthma management during, 801
bariatric, 186
for biliary atresia, 1387
for breast alterations, *see website*
for burn management, 353-354
for cancer, *see website*
for cleft lip or palate, 1252-1253
for coccidioidomycosis, 1068
complications of, 2394
for congenital diaphragmatic hernia, 596, 596f
for congenital heart disease, 1602-1610, 1605t
coarctation of the aorta, 1569
d-transposition of the great arteries, 1586-1587, 1587f
hypoplastic left heart syndrome, 1593-1595, 1594f
long-term management following, 1604-1605
ostium primum defects, 1555-1556
postoperative management following, 1603-1604
tetralogy of Fallot, 1576-1577, 1577f
ventricular septal defect, 1558
contraceptive, special needs girls and, 1875
for Crohn's disease, 1303-1304
in cystic fibrosis management, 1496-1497
diabetes mellitus management during, 1987, 1987t
for empyema, 1509
evaluation before, *see website*
fluid maintenance during, *see website*
for fractures, 2393-2394, 2394t
for gastroesophageal reflux disease, 1268-1269
general anesthesia during (*See* General anesthesia)
for Graves disease, 1912t
for Hirschsprung disease, 1285-1286
Surgery *(Continued)*
hypothyroidism due to, 1912-1913
for inguinal hernia, 1365-1366, 1367f
for intestinal malrotation, 1281
intestinal transplantation, *see website*
for neonatal necrotizing enterocolitis, 603
for nontuberculous mycobacterial lymphadenitis, 1015
for osteomyelitis, 2398
pain management following, *see website*
for patent ductus arteriosus, 1560-1561
for peptic ulcer disease, 1294
for pneumothorax, 1511-1512
postanesthesia care following, *see website*
preparation for, *see website*
for pyloric stenosis, 1275
for scoliosis, 2367-2368, 2368f
for seizures, 2032-2033
for septic arthritis, 2400
for tricuspid atresia, 1581-1582, 1581f
for ulcerative colitis, 1300
for urinary lithiasis, *see website*
for vesicoureteral reflux, 1836-1838, 1837f-1838f
Surgical otoscope head, 2202
SUR1 mutations, 523
Surrogate endpoints in pharmacodynamics, *see website*
Survanta, 585
Surveillance
autistic disorder, 103f-104f
developmental and behavioral, 39-40, 41t-45t
Survival Epidemiology and End Results (SEER), 1727f
Survival rates, cancer, 1726f, 1726t
for acute lymphocytic leukemia, 1735f-1736f
Susceptibility testing, antimicrobial, *see also website*
in nontuberculous mycobacteria, 1015
Suspending fluids in immunizing agents, 883
Sustained attention, *see website*
Sustiva. *See* Efavirenz
Sutures
cranial
in neurologic examination, *see website*
newborn examination of, 533-534
premature closure of, 2011-2013
for laceration closure, 341
SVT. *See* Supraventricular tachycardia (SVT)
Swallowed blood syndrome, 621
Swallowing, 1240, *see also website*
difficulty in (*See* Dysphagia)
dysmotility and, 1264-1265
fetal, *see website*
fiberoptic endoscopic evaluation of, *see website*
pain during (*See* Odynophagia)
Swallowing studies in aspiration syndromes, 1472t
Sweat glands
cystic fibrosis and, 1487
disorders of, 2286-2288, 2287f, 2287t
morphology of, *see website*
Sweat testing in cystic fibrosis, 1487-1488
Swedish porphyria, *see website*
Sweet syndrome, *see website*
SWILS. *See* Safety World Inventory and Literacy Screener (SWILS)
Swim, learning to, 348
Swimmer's ear, 2197. *See also* External otitis
Swimmer's itch, 1231
Swimming, injuries in, *see website*
Swimming pool granuloma, 1013
Swine bite, 2454-2460
SWS. *See* Sturge-Weber syndrome (SWS)
Swyer-James syndrome, 1461
Swyer syndrome, 1963-1964
Sycosis barbae, 2305
Sydenham chorea, 2055-2056
Sylvian aqueduct syndrome, 2161
Symblepharon, 2169
Symbols in laboratory testing, *see website*
Symmetrel. *See* Amantadine
Symmetric progressive erythrokeratoderma, 2270-2271
Sympathetic nerve block, 372-373
Sympathetic ophthalmia, 2173-2174
Sympathomimetic poison syndrome, 253t
Sympathomimetic syndromes, 676t
Symptomatic seizure, 2013
Symptom review in psychiatric diagnostic evaluation, 58
Synapses, development and, *see website*
Synchronized cardioversion, 288-289
Syncope, *see also website*
heat, 2420
Syndactyly, 2342, 2342f, 2386, 2387t, *see also website*
Syndrome of inappropriate antidiuretic hormone (SIADH)
diagnostic criteria for, 217t
hyponatremia due to, 216, 218-219, 1884
plasma osmolality and, *see website*
treatment of, 1886
Syndromic diarrhea (SD), 1311-1312
Synercid. *See* Quinupristin/dalfopristin
Synergistic gangrene, *see website*
Synophrys, *see website*
Synostosis, cranial, 533-534
Synovial fluid analysis, 2399
Synovial sarcoma, 1762t
Synovitis
toxic, 840
transient, 840
monoarticular, 2360
as sports injury, 2413
Syntax difficulties, *see website*
Syphilis, 1016-1023
cerebrospinal fluid findings in, 2088t
clinical manifestations and laboratory findings in, 1016-1018
congenital, 1016-1018, 1017f-1020f, 1017t, 1021-1023, 1021t
diagnosis of, 1018-1021, 1019f
endemic, 1023, *see also website*
epidemiology of, 1016, 1016f-1017f
etiology of, 1016
fetal therapy for, 551t
genital ulcers due to, 708, 709t
hearing loss due to, *see website*
in immigrant children, 133
maternal
Breast-feeding and, 540t
fetal and neonatal effects of, *see website*
oral ulcerations in, 1260t
in pregnancy, 1022
prevention of, 1022-1023
secondary, 1016-1017, 1017f
sexual abuse and, 145t
treatment of, 1021-1022, 1021t-1022t
SYR gene, *see website*
Syringoma, *see website*
Syringomyelia, 2103, 2104f
Syrup of ipecac, 255
Systematic desensitization for phobias, 81
Systemic inflammatory response syndrome (SIRS), 307, 309t, 310f, 311t, 637-639, 639t
anesthesia and, *see website*
Systemic lupus erythematosus (SLE), 841-846
alveolar hemorrhage with, 1499
arthralgia in, *see website*
cerebrospinal fluid findings in, 2088t
chorea in, 2056
clinical manifestations of, 843, 843t
cardiac, 1532t
cutaneous, *see website*
complications of, 845, 845t
diagnosis of, 843, 843t, *see website*
differential diagnosis of, 843-844, 844t
epidemiology of, 841-842
etiology of, 841
fever of unknown origin in, 899

Systemic lupus erythematosus (SLE) *(Continued)*
glomerulonephritis associated with, 1788-1789
immunofluorescence in, *see website*
insulin receptors autoantibody development in, 1996
laboratory findings in, 844, 844t
maternal, *see website*
myocardial disease with, 1629t
oral ulceration in, 1260t
pathogenesis of, 842-843
pathology of, 842, 842f
prognosis for, 845
sports participation and, 2402t-2404t
treatment of, 844-845
Systemic-onset juvenile idiopathic arthritis, 832-834, 836, 838
Systemic vascular resistance, 311t
System of care, planning and implementing
Systems approach in patient safety, *see website*
Systolic blood pressure
age-specific percentiles for, 1534f-1535f
assessment of, 1639
Systolic ejection murmur, 1535
Systolic overload pattern, 1539

T
$T_{1/2}$. *See* Elimination half-life ($T_{1/2}$) of drug
T_2. *See* Thiolase (T_2) deficiency
T_3. *See* Triiodothyronine (T_3)
T_4. *See* Thyroxine (T_4)
TA. *See* Takayasu arteritis (TA)
Tabun, in terrorism, *see website*
TAC. *See* Tetracaine, epinephrine, and cocaine (TAC)
Tache noire, 1044
Tachyarrhythmias
emergency management of, 287-289, 290f
ventricular, 1616, 1616f, 1616t
"Tachy-brady syndrome," 1618, 1618f
Tachycardia
in acute intermittent porphyrias, *see website*
in cardiac physical examination, 1531-1532
with *Corynebacterium diphtheriae*-associated toxic cardiomyopathy, *see website*
fetal, 542
during fever, *see website*
sinus, 1616t
supraventricular tachycardia *versus*, 1613
supraventricular, 1613-1616, 1614f-1616f
fetal therapy for, 551t
Tachycardia syndrome, postural, *see website*
Tachypnea
in acutely ill child, 275
maintenance water and electrolytes and, 244
as manifestation of extrapulmonary disease, 1526
transient of newborn, 590
respiratory distress syndrome *versus*, 583-584
Tacrolimus
diabetes associated with, 1997
intestinal transplantation and, *see website*
for nephrotic syndrome, 1805
Taenia asiatica, 1232t
Taenia multiceps, 1232t
Taenia saginata, 1232-1233, 1232t, *see also website*
Taenia solium, 1232-1233, 1232t, *see also website*
Takayasu arteritis (TA), 868t, 871-872, 871t, 872f
Talar dome fracture, 2417-2418
Talipes equinovarus (clubfoot), 2336, 2337f
Tall stature, *see website*
Tamiflu. *See* Oseltamivir
Tamponade, cardiac, 336t
Tandem mass spectrometry (MS/MS), *see website*
Tangier disease, 477, 1320
Tanner stages, 649
Tantrum, 35
Tapeworm infection, 1232-1234, 1232t, 1233f-1234f, *see also website*
TAPVR. *See* Total anomalous pulmonary venous return (TAPVR)
TAR. *See* Thrombocytopenia-absent radius (TAR) syndrome
Tardive dyskinesia, drug-induced, 2059
Targeted array comparative genomic hybridization (aCGH), 398
Target serum levels in antibacterial therapy, *see website*
Target sign in aspergillosis, 1060
Tar preparations, 2216-2217
for atopic dermatitis, 805
Tarsal coalition, 2339-2340, 2339f, 2339t
Tarui disease, 494t-495t, 501, *see website*
TAT. *See* Tetanus antitoxin (TAT)
Taussig-Bing malformation, 1582
Taxis, 1365-1366
Taxus species toxicity, 269t
Tay-Sachs disease, 484-487, 2070
Tazarotene, 2325t
Tazicer. *See* Ceftazidime
Tazidime. *See* Ceftazidime
Tazobactam, *see website*
Tazobactam/piperacillin, 645t
TB. *See* Tuberculosis (TB)
TBE. *See* Tick-borne encephalitis (TBE)
TBG. *See* Thyroxine-binding globulin (TBG)
TBI. *See* Total body irradiation (TBI); Traumatic brain injury (TBI)
TBMD. *See* Thin basement membrane disease (TBMD)
TC. *See* Time constant (TC)
TCAs. *See* Tricyclic antidepressants (TCAs)
TCD. *See* Transcranial Doppler (TCD) assessment
T cell antibodies in renal transplantation, *see website*
T-cell mitogens, *see website*
T-cell receptor-CD3 complex (Ti-CD3), defective expression of, 729, 729f
T-cell receptor recombination excision circles (TRECs), *see website*
T-cell receptors (TCRs), 720-722, *see website*
T cells, 722
abnormalities of
of activation, 729-730
evaluation of, 720-722, 720t
immunizations in, 892t
infection with, *see website*
inheritance in development of, *see website*
screening for, 718t
in adverse drug reactions, 824
in allergic disease, *see website*
in atopic dermatitis, 802
celiac disease, 1308
Cytotoxic (*See* Cytotoxic T cells)
fetal development and differentiation of, *see website*
in Graves disease, 1909-1910
helper (*See* Helper T cells)
interaction with other immune cells, *see website*
in juvenile idiopathic arthritis, 831, 831f
postnatal, *see website*
subsets of, *see website*
in systemic lupus erythematosus, 843
in tuberculosis, 999f
TC1RG1 gene, 2432
TCS1 gene, 2049
TCS2 gene, 2049
Tdap. *See* Tetanus toxoid, reduced diphtheria toxoid and acellular pertussis (Tdap) vaccine
T1DM. *See* Type 1 diabetes mellitus (T1DM)
T2DM. *See* Type 2 diabetes mellitus (T2DM)
TDT. *See* Transmission disequilibrium test (TDT)
TE. *See* Thromboembolic event (TE)
Tea
for asthma, 271t
potential toxicity of, 272t-273t
Team
transport, *see website*
trauma, 333, 335f
Team approach
in home mechanical ventilation, 331-332, 331t
in rheumatic disease, *see website*
Teamwork for patient safety, *see website*
Tear film, 2165
Tears
in newborn, *see website*
reduced or absent secretion of, 2165-2166
TEC. *See* Transient erythroblastopenia of childhood (TEC)
Technetium-99m scan. *See also* Radionuclide studies
in liver dysfunction, 1379
in lung pathology, *see website*
in osteomyelitis, 2396-2397
Technology, health information, *see website*
Teenager. *See* Adolescent
Teeth
anomalies of, 1250-1251, 1250f-1251f
avulsion of, 1259
calcification of, 1249-1250, 1250t
congenital erythropoietic porphyria effects on, *see website*
development of, 1249
discolored, 1251
disorders of
associated with other conditions, 1251, 1251t
dental caries as, 1254-1256, 1255f-1256f
eruption cyst, *see website*
malocclusion, 1252, *see also website*
teething as, 1257
effects of eating disorders on, 93t
effects of malnutrition on, 175t
eruption of, 1250, 1250t
delayed, 1251
grinding of, 75
Hutchinson, 1017t, 1019f
intruded, 1259
during middle childhood, 36
natal, 1251
neonatal, 1251
radiology in assessment of, 1261, *see also website*
replantation of, 1259
subluxation of, 1259
supernumerary, 1430
traumatic injury to, 1258, 1258f-1259f, 1258t
Teething, 1257
home remedies among African Americans for, *see website*
TEF. *See* Tracheoesophageal fistula (TEF)
Tegopen. *See* Cloxacillin
Teichoic acid, 904
Teicoplanin, *see website*
Telangiectasia
hereditary benign, 2230
hereditary hemorrhagic, 2230
spider, 2230f
unilateral nevoid, 2230
Telangiectasia macularis eruptiva perstans, 2281
Telangiectatic osteosarcoma, 1763
Telecanthus, *see website*
Teleoroentgenogram in leg-length discrepancy, *see website*
Telithromycin, *see website*
Telogen effluvium, 2291-2292
Telomerase in oncogenesis, *see website*
Telomere mutations, 406
Telophase of mitosis, 394-395
Temperament, *see also website*
psychosomatic illness and, 68
Temperature
Celsius and Fahrenheit equivalents, *see website*
in hyperthermia, 622
maintenance of for low birthweight infant, 559
maintenance of in newborn, 536-537

Temperature receptors in respiration regulation, see website
Temper tantrum, 99
Temporal arteritis, 868t
Temporal bone
 fracture of, see website
 otitis media complications within, 2210
 tumors of, 2214, see also website
Temporomandibular joint (TMJ) disease in juvenile idiopathic arthritis, 832
TEN. *See* Toxic epidermal necrolysis (TEN)
Tendinopathy as sports injury, 2407
Tendinosis
 patellar, 2416
 rotator cuff, 2407
 as sports injury, 2407
Tendon reflexes
 in hypoxic-ischemic encephalopathy, 571t
 in neuromuscular disorders, 2109
Tennis, injuries in, see website
Tennis elbow, 2411, see website
Tenofovir, 1168t-1171t, see also website
Tenosynovitis-dermatitis syndrome, gonococcal, 937
TENS. *See* Transcutaneous electrical nerve stimulation (TENS)
Tension pneumothorax, 336, 336t, 1510-1511
 cardiac arrest due to, 289t
Tension-type headache (TTH), 2046
Teratogens, 547-548
 antiepileptics as, 2029, 2029t
 cardiac, 1527
 development and, see website
 isotretinoin as, 2325
Teratoid/rhabdoid tumor, 1752
Teratoma, 1770
 ovarian, 1871, 1872t
Terazosin, 1645t
Terbinafine, 2311
Terbutaline, 796, 797t-798t
Terminal hair, see website
Terminal illness
 in adolescents, see website
 palliative care for (*See* Palliative care)
Terrorism
 biological and chemical, 2454, see also website
 impact on children, see website
 vaccines and, 891
Terry nails, 2294, 2295f
Tertiary syphilis, 1016-1017
Testicular adrenal rests, see website
Testicular dysgenesis syndrome, 1945
Testicular feminization syndrome, 1365
Testicular prosthesis, 1860, 1860f
Testicular regression syndrome, 1944
Testicular torsion, 1861-1862, 1861f-1862f
Testicular tumor, 1864
Testis
 defects in differentiation of, 1962
 defects in hormones of, 1963-1964
 development of, see website
 embryonic regression syndrome of, 1963
 function of, see website
 hypofunction of, 1943-1950, 1944t
  primary, 1944-1945
  secondary, 1948-1949
 newborn assessment of, 536
 nonpalpable, 1859
 pseudoprecocity resulting from tumors of, 1943-1950
 puberty and, see website
  central precocious, 1887
 retractile, 1859
 traumatic injury to, see website
 tumors of, 1864
 undescended, 1858-1860, 1860f
  in neuromuscular disorders, 2109
  sports participation and, 2402t-2404t
 vanishing, 1859
Testosterone
 in ovarian carcinomas, 1872t
 in testicular function, see website
Testosterone precursors for performance enhancement, 2423
Tetanospasmin, 991
Tetanus, 991-994, 994t
 after animal or human bite, 2457
 due to nasal foreign body, 1432
 neonatal, 639
 testing for antibodies to, 719-720
Tetanus and diphtheria toxoid (Td), 884t
Tetanus antitoxin (TAT), 992-993
Tetanus immunoglobulin (TIG), 882t, 992
Tetanus toxin, 991-992
Tetanus toxoid, reduced diphtheria toxoid and acellular pertussis (Tdap) vaccine, 884t, 948, 993
 recommended schedule for, 888f
 for travel, see website
Tetanus vaccine, 881t, 993
Tetany
 heat, 2420
 in newborn, 623
 in pseudohypoparathyroidism, 1919
Tethered cord, 2101-2102, 2101f-2102f
Tetracaine, epinephrine, and cocaine (TAC), 367-368
Tetracycline, see also website
 for acne, 2324, 2325t
 for balantidiasis, 1183, see also website
 for cholera, 967t
 for *Dientamoeba fragilis*, see website
 discolored teeth due to, 1251
 for ehrlichioses, 1050
 for louse-borne typhus, 1048
 for malaria, 1203t-1205t, see also website
 for murine typhus, 1047
 possible adverse reactions to in premature infant, 563t
 for psittacosis, see website
 for relapsing fever, see website
 for Rocky Mountain spotted fever, 1043
 for scrub typhus, 1045
Tetrahydrobiopterin (BH_4) deficiency, 446
 hyperphenylalaninemia with, 420-421, 421f
Tetrahydrocannabinol (THC), 680-681, 1244t
Tetralogy of Fallot, 1573-1578, 1573f
 in adults, 1607-1608
 associated anomalies, 1576
 clinical manifestations of, 1574
 complications of, 1576
 diagnosis of, 1574-1576, 1575f
 pathophysiology of, 1573-1574
 treatment of, 1576-1577, 1577f
"Tet spells" in tetralogy of Fallot, 1574
Textiles, infection protection and control and, see website
TFA. *See* Thigh-foot angle (TFA)
TFP. *See* Mitochondrial trifunctional protein (TFP) deficiency
TGA. *See* Transposition of the great arteries (TGA)
TGF-β. *See* Transforming growth factor-β (TGF-β)
TG2 in celiac disease, 1308
Thalassemia(s), 1674-1677
 α-, 1676-1677
 β-, 1675-1676
 δ-, 1676
 epidemiology of, 1674
 fetal therapy for, 551t
 γ-, 1676
 hematopoietic stem cell transplantation for, 759, 760f
 major, 1675-1676, 1675f
  cardiac manifestations of, 1531t
 pathophysiology of, 1674, 1674t
Thalidomide, 2257, see also website
Thallium, gastroenteritis due to, 1328t-1329t
Thanatophoric dysplasia, 2428, 2428f-2429f
THBD gene, 1792t
THC. *See* Tetrahydrocannabinol (THC)
THE. *See* Tricho-hepato-enteric (THE) syndrome
Thelarche, see website
 premature, 1893-1894, see also website
Theophylline
 for allergic disease, 772
 for asthma, 794t, 796
 drug interactions with, see website
 for neonatal apnea, 581
 toxicity of, 251t
Theories of emotion and cognition, see website
Theory of Planned Behavior, see website
Theory of Reasoned Action, see website
The patch, 695t, 696-697
"The pill," 696-698
Therapeutic drug monitoring, see website
Therapeutic range, see website
Thermal amplitude, 1679
Thermodilution measurement of cardiac output, 1547-1548
Thermoregulation
 during anesthesia, see website
 of newborn, 536-537
  low birthweight, 559
 postoperative, see website
Thiabendazole, 1224, see also website
Thiamine, 191, 194t
 deficiency of, 191-192
 dietary reference intakes for, see website
 toxicity of, 192
Thiamine-responsive maple syrup urine disease, 431
Thiamine-responsiveness megaloblastic anemia (TRMA), 191, see also website
Thiazide diuretics
 for hypertension of chronic kidney disease, 1825
 metabolic alkalosis due to, 236
Thiazolidinedione, 1992, 1992t
Thick blood smear in malaria, 1201
Thienamycin, see website
Thigh-foot angle (TFA), 2345f, 2346, 2347f
Thimerosal exposure, see website
Thin basement membrane disease (TBMD), 1783
Thin blood smear in malaria, 1201
Thinking
 logical, in adolescent, 649-651
 magical, 34-35
 moral, 35-36
  in adolescent, 649-651
Thiolase (T_2) deficiency, 433-435, 434f
Thiopental
 for anesthesia, see website
 for intubation, 321t
 for status epilepticus, 2039t
Thiopurine *S*-methyltransferase (TPMT), see website
Thioridazine toxicity, 251t
Third-degree burn, 351, 351t
Third-degree heart block, 1618
Third-generation cephalosporins, see also website
 for neonatal infection, 644
 for pyelonephritis, 1832
Third heart sound, auscultation of, 1533
Third nerve palsy, 2159, 2159f
Thirst, regulation of, 1882
Thombosis, cerebral, 1576
Thomsen disease, 2113t, 2125, 2125t
Thoracentesis, see also website
 for emergencies, 295
Thoracic anesthesia, 373
Thoracic dystrophy, asphyxiating, 2434
Thoracic-pelvic-phalangeal dystrophy, 1517
Thoracic trauma, 335t, 338
Thoracoplasty, expansion, 2369-2370, 2370f
Thoracoscopic surgery, video-assisted
 for empyema, 1509
 for pneumothorax, 1511-1512
Thoracoscopy, see website
Thorazine. *See* Chlorpromazine

3-day measles. *See* Rubella
Three-dimensional echocardiography, 1543, 1544f
317 Discretionary Federal Grant Program, 885
3D reconstruction of computed tomography, 1546, 1547f
Thrills, 1533
 in tetralogy of Fallot, 1574
Throat culture, *see website*
 in group A streptococci infection, 917
Thrombin time, 1697
Thrombocytopenia, 1714
 due to acquired disorders causing decreased production, 1721
 amegakaryoctic, 1689
 classification of, 1716t
 congenital amegakaryocytic, 1719-1720, 1719f
 differential diagnosis of, 1716t, 1717f
 drug-induced, 1718
 due to ehrlichiosis, 1049
 fetal therapy for, 551t
 following rubella, 1077
 hematuria associated with, 1796
 in hemolytic-uremic syndrome, 1793
 HIV-related, 1166
 idiopathic thrombocytopenic purpura in, 1714-1718, 1717f
 immunodeficiency with eczema and, 734-735
 maternal, *see website*
 neonatal, 1720
 as oncologic emergency, *see website*
 in Rocky Mountain spotted fever, 1042
Thrombocytopenia-absent radius (TAR) syndrome, 1531t, 1719
Thrombocytopenic purpura
 idiopathic, 1717f
  maternal, *see website*
 thrombotic, 1718-1719
Thrombocytosis in pertussis, 945
Thromboembolic event (TE), 1709-1712
 in nephrotic syndrome, 1805-1806
Thromboemolism, venous, 1709
Thrombolytic therapy, 1710t, 1712
 for pulmonary embolism, 1502
Thrombopoiesis, fetal, *see website*
Thrombopoietin, 1714, *see also website*
Thrombosis
 cerebral sinovenous, 1709, 2082-2084, 2083f, 2083t
 deep vein, 1709
  estrogen contraceptives and, 1875
  pulmonary embolism with, 1500-1501, 1501t
 portal vein, *see website*
  due to exchange transfusion, 618
 renal transplantation and, *see website*
 renal vein, 1709
  hematuria due to, 1794-1795
  in newborn assessment, 535
Thrombotic disease, 1709-1712
 clinical manifestations of, 1709-1710
 complications of, 1711
 diagnosis of, 1710, 1710f
 epidemiology of, 1709-1711, 1709t
 hereditary predisposition to, 1707-1708, 1708t
 laboratory testing in, 1710
 treatment of, 1710-1712, 1710t
Thrombotic microangiopathy, 1713-1714
Thrombotic predisposition, testing for, 1699
Thrombotic thrombocytopenic purpura (TTP), 1718-1719
Thrown-away children, 8
Thrush, 1054-1055
 HIV-related, 1164
Thumb
 hypoplasia of, 2386, 2386f
 sucking of, 75
 trigger, 2387
Thumb method of chest compressions, 291, 292f
Thumb sign in Marfan syndrome, 2440, 2441f
Thunderclap headache, 2084
Thymectomy for myasthenia gravis, 2135
Thymic hypoplasia, 728-729
Thymidine kinase in congenital dyserythropoietic anemia, *see website*
Thymidine kinase 2 (TK2), 1406
 deficiency of, *see website*
Thymidine phosphorylase deficiency, *see website*
Thymoglobulin in renal transplantation, *see website*
Thyroglobulin, *see also website*
 measurement of, *see website*
 reference values for, 1899t
 synthesis defects of, 1896
Thyroglossal cysts and sinuses, 2221
Thyroidal peroxidase, *see website*
 defects of, 1896
Thyroid antiperoxidase antibodies (TPOAbs)
 in lymphocytic thyroiditis, 1903
 in Turner syndrome, 1953-1954
Thyroid cancer, secondary, due to radiation therapy, *see website*
Thyroid crisis, 1910
Thyroid dysgenesis, 1895-1896
Thyroidectomy, hypothyroidism due to, 1912-1913
Thyroid function tests, 1899t
Thyroid gland
 carcinoma as, 1914-1916
  medullary, 1915-1916
 development and physiology of, 1894, *see also website*
 disorders of
  arthralgia and, *see website*
  autoimmune, 1901
  goiter as, 1905-1909
  hormone studies of, 1894, *see also website*
  hyperthyroidism as, 1909-1913
  hypothyroidism as, 1895-1903
  thyroiditis as, 1903-1905
  thyroxine-binding globulin defects as, 1894-1895
  transport defects and, 1896
 solitary nodule of, 1915, 1915t
Thyroiditis, 1903-1905, 1904t
 granulomatous, subacute, 1905
 lymphocytic (Hashimoto, autoimmune), 1903-1905
  hypothyroidism due to, 1901
  myasthenia gravis with, 2133
  with Turner syndrome, 1953
  type 1 diabetes mellitus with, 1996
 due to mumps, 1080
 suppurative, 1904t, 1905
Thyroid myopathies, 2129
Thyroid-related ophthalmopathy, 2182
Thyroid-stimulating hormone (TSH), *see also website*
 in hypothyroidism
  acquired, 1901
  congenital, 1895, 1899
 measurement of, *see website*
 reference values for, 1899t, *see website*
 testing of in intellectual disability, 127t
 in thyroid hormone unresponsiveness, 1897
 in thyroid regulation, *see website*
Thyroid storm, 1910
 management of, 1912t
Thyroid tumors, 1772
Thyrotoxicosis, myopathies due to, 2129
Thyrotoxic periodic paralysis, 222-223
Thyrotropin
 deficiency of, 1896-1897
 unresponsiveness of, 1897
Thyrotropin receptor-blocking antibody, 1896
Thyrotropin receptor-stimulating antibody (TRSAb)
 in congenital hypothyroidism, 1913
 in Graves disease, 1909-1911
Thyrotropin-releasing hormone (TRH)
 deficiency of, 1896-1897
 reference values for, *see website*
Thyrotropin-releasing receptor abnormalities, 1897
Thyroxine, reference values for, *see website*
Thyroxine-binding globulin (TBG)
 defects of, 1894-1895, *see also website*
 serum, *see website*
Thyroxine (T_4), *see also website*
 in congenital hypothyroidism, 1899
 defective synthesis of, 1896
 fetal, *see website*
 in preterm infant, 1897
 testing of, *see website*
  in intellectual disability, 127t
 in thyroid hormone unresponsiveness, 1897
Thyroxine (T_4) binding globulin in congenital hypothyroidism, 1899
Tiagabine
 adverse effects of, 2031t
 dosages of, 2030t
TIBC. *See* Total iron-binding capacity (TIBC), reference values for
Tibia
 bowing of
  anterolateral, 2351
  anteromedial, 2351
  posteromedial, 2351
 congenital and angular deformities of, 2350-2351
 fracture of, 2392-2393
  stress, 2416
 normal development of, 2344
Tibial longitudinal deficiency, 2351
Tibial rotation, 2346, 2346f
Tibial torsion
 external, 2347
 internal, 2347
 normal, 2344
Tibia vara, 2349f-2350f, 2350
 obesity with, 184t
Tibiofemoral angle, 2344
TIBOLA. *See* Tick-borne lymphadenopathy (TIBOLA)
Tic, motor, 76, *see also website*
Ticar. *See* Ticarcillin
Ticarcillin, *see also website*
 for cystic fibrosis lung infection, 1492t
 for neonatal infection, 645t
Ticarcillin-clavulanate, *see also website*
 for cystic fibrosis lung infection, 1492t
 for neonatal infection, 645t
Ti-CD3. *See* T-cell receptor-CD3 complex (Ti-CD3)
Tic disorders, 76
 group A streptococci infection and, 919
Ticks, removal of attached, 1043
Tick-borne encephalitis (TBE), 1146
Tick-borne illness
 babesiosis, 1207, *see also website*
 Colorado tick fever, 1142-1144
 ehrlichioses, 1048-1049
 hemorrhagic fevers, 1150t
 Lyme disease, 1025-1026
 Mediterranean spotted fever, 1044
 relapsing fever, 1025, *see also website*
 Rocky Mountain spotted fever, 1041, 1041f
 tularemia, 978
Tick-borne lymphadenopathy (TIBOLA), 1039t-1040t
Tick paralysis, 2135-2136
Tidal recruitment, 323-324
Tidal volume (V_T), *see also website*
 in mechanical ventilation, 327-328
TIG. *See* Tetanus immunoglobulin (TIG)
Tigecycline, *see website*
Tillaux fracture, 2393
Tilted optic disc, *see website*
Time constant (TC), *see website*
 in mechanical ventilation, 322-323, 323f

Timeliness in quality of care, *see website*
Timentin. *See* Ticarcillin-clavulanate
TIN. *See* Tubulointerstitial nephritis (TIN)
Tin, gastroenteritis due to, 1328t-1329t
Tindamax. *See* Tinidazole
Tinea capitis, 2310-2311, 2310f-2311f
Tinea corporis, 2311-2312, 2311f-2312f
Tinea cruris, 2312
Tinea in child-care setting, *see website*
Tinea nigra palmaris, 2313
Tinea pedis, 2312-2313, 2312f-2313f
Tinea unguium, 2313, 2313f
Tinea versicolor, 2309, 2309f, *see also website*
Tinidazole, *see also website*
  for amebiasis, 1180, 1180t
  for giardiasis, 1182, 1182t
  for trichomoniasis, 1186
  for vulvovaginitis, 1868t
Tinnitus, *see website*
TIP. *See* Tubularized incised plate (TIP)
Tipanavir for HIV infection, 1168t-1171t
TIPS. *See* Transjugular intrahepatic portosystemic shunt (TIPS)
Tissue analysis, fetal, 543t
Tissue culture cytotoxicity assay in *Clostridium difficile* infection, 995
Tissue factor in hemostasis, 1694
Tissue hypoxia, respiratory alkalosis due to, 240, 241t
Tissue plasminogen activator (TPA), recombinant, 304, 1712
Tissue type plasminogen activator (TPA), reference values for, 1698t
Titmus test, 2150
TJP2 gene defect, 1383t
TK2. *See* Thymidine kinase 2 (TK2)
TL. *See* Tuberculoid leprosy (TL)
TLC. *See* Total lung capacity (TLC)
TLESR. *See* Transient lower esophageal sphincter relaxation (TLESR)
TLRs. *See* Toll-like receptors (TLRs)
TLS. *See* Tumor lysis syndrome (TLS)
T lymphocyte-dependent vaccine, 883
T-lymphotropic virus, 1177, *see also website*
  breast-feeding and, 161t
TM. *See* Tympanic membrane (TM)
TMA. *See* Transcription-mediated amplification (TMA)
TMJ. *See* Temporomandibular joint (TMJ) disease
TMP-SMX. *See* Trimethoprim-sulfamethoxazole (TMP-SMX)
TNDM. *See* Transient neonatal diabetes mellitus (TNDM)
TNF-α. *See* Tumor necrosis factor α (TNF-α)
Tobacco
  adolescent use of, 679-680, 680t
  toxicity of, 269t
Tobacco smoke, exposure to, *see website*
Tobramycin, *see also website*
  for bacterial meningitis, 2093t
  for cystic fibrosis infection, 1492, 1492t
  for neonatal infection, 645t
Tocilizumab, *see website*
Tocopherol, dietary reference intakes for, *see website*
Toddler
  antibiotic therapy for, *see website*
  behavioral and psychosocial assessment of, 56
  causes of limping in, 2334t
  child restraint in motor vehicles for, 21t
  disruptive behavioral disturbances in, 99
  drowning or submersion injury to, 342
  feeding of, 165, 165t
  fever without localizing signs in, 897-898, 898t
  growth and development of, 31-33
  injury risk factors for, 20
  intellectual disability in, 125t
  leading causes of death for, 5t
Toddler *(Continued)*
  lower extremity fracture of, 2392
  response to death by, *see website*
  shoes for, 2344
  sleep changes in, 47t
Toddler's diarrhea, 1341, *see website*
Toe
  deformities of, 2341-2342
  fracture of, 2393
Toenail, ingrown
Tofranil. *See* Imipramine
Togavirus, 1147t
Toilet training, 71, 1847
Tolazoline, 563t
Tolbutamide, 1992t
Tolerable upper intake level (UL), *see website*
Tolerance, bacterial, *see website*
Toll-like receptors (TLRs), 855
  in *Neisseria meningitidis*, 930-931
Tolterodine, 1852
Toluene, as inhalant, 681, 681t
Tomaculous neuropathy, 2140
Tomography, positron emission, *see website*
Tone, muscle
  assessment in neurologic examination, *see website*
Tone, muscle, assessment in neuromuscular disorders, 2109
Tongue
  black hairy, 2299
  fissured, 1261, 2299
  geographic, 1261, 2298-2299, 2298f
  hypoglossal nerve in function of, *see website*
  of newborn, 534
  oral hairy leukoplakia of, 2299
  scrotal, 2299
  strawberry in Kawasaki disease, 863, 864f
Tongue-tied, 534, 1261, *see website*
Tonic clonic reflex in neurologic examination, *see website*
Tonic pupil, 2156
Tonic seizure, 2019
  evaluation of, 2015-2016
  neonatal, 2034
  treatment of, 2028
Tonic upgaze of childhood, paroxysmal, *see website*
Tonometry, 2150
Tonsillectomy
  for pharyngotonsillitis, 1443-1445, 1444t
  for recurrent pharyngitis, 1440
Tonsillitis, 1443-1444, 1443f
  Corynebacterium diphtheriae, *see website*
  Epstein-Barr virus, 1112, 1113f
Tonsils
  anatomy of, 1442
  disorders of, 1443-1445, 1443f
  normal function of, 1442
Topical therapy
  for acne, 2323-2324, 2324f, 2325t
  for atopic dermatitis, 804, 804t
  for burns, 353t, 354
  for skin disorders
    antibiotics, 2217
    corticosteroids, 2217, 2217t
    nonsteroidal antiinflammatory drugs, 2217
Topiramate
  adverse effects of, 2031t
  for migraine prophylaxis, 2044t, 2045
  for pain management, 370
  for seizures, 2030t
  for weight loss in adults, 187t
Toradol. *See* Ketorolac
TORCH, 640-641
Torsades de pointes, 1620, 1621f
Torsion
  of appendix testis, 1862, 1862f
  femoral internal, 2347
  ovarian, adnexal, 1871
  penile, 1856
  testicular, 1861-1862, 1861f-1862f
Torsion *(Continued)*
  tibial
    external, 2347
    internal, 2347
    normal, 2344
Torsional deformities, 2344-2351
Torticollis, 2377-2379, 2378f, 2378t
  benign paroxysmal of infancy, 2060t, 2061, *see also website*
  in newborn, 534-535
Torus buckling fracture, 2388f, 2390, 2391f
Torus fracture, 2390
Total anomalous pulmonary venous return (TAPVR), 1589-1590, 1589t, 1590f
  genetics of congenital heart disease with, *see website*
Total body irradiation (TBI), late effects of, *see website*
Total body water (TBW), 212
  compartments of, *see website*
  drug distribution and, *see website*
  electrolytes in, *see website*
  hypervolemic hyponatremia and, 216
  osmolality of, *see website*
    regulation of, *see website*
  regulation of volume of, *see website*
  sodium in, 212
Total cholesterol in obesity, 185t
Total dead space, 316-317
Total hemolytic complement activity (CH_{50}), 753
Total iron-binding capacity (TIBC), reference values for, *see website*
Total lung capacity (TLC), *see website*
Total parenteral nutrition (TPN), 559-560
  cholestasis associated with, *see also website*
Tourette's syndrome (TS), 76-77
  group A streptococci infection and, 919
Toxic alopecia, 2292
Toxic cardiomyopathy, due to diphtheria, *see website*
Toxic epidermal necrolysis (TEN), 826, 827t, 2242-2244
Toxicity. *See* Poisoning
Toxic megacolon, 1297-1298
Toxic myopathy, 2129-2130, 2129t
Toxic neuropathy, 2140-2141, 2141t, *see also website*
Toxicology screen, 253, 254t
Toxic shock syndrome toxin-1 (TSST-1), 904
Toxic shock syndrome (TSS)
  staphylococcal, 905, 908-909, 909t
  streptococcal, 915, 917t
Toxic synovitis, 840
  of hip, 2360
Toxigenic *Corynebacterium diphtheriae*, *see website*
Toxin(s)
  A, 994
  alpha, *see website*
  B, 994
  Bacillus cereus, 1324t-1325t
  beta, *see website*
  binary, 994
  botulinum, 987-988
    for achalasia, 1265
    for spasticity of cerebral palsy, 2064-2065
  cataracts due to, 2171
  cholera, 1330
  Clostridium, *see website*
  Clostridium botulinum, 1324t-1325t
  Clostridium difficile, 1313
  Clostridium perfringens, 1324t-1325t
  epsilon, *see website*
  erythrogenic in scarlet fever, 916
  fetal exposure to, 546-547
  hemolytic anemia secondary to, *see website*
  in infectious diarrhea, 1330-1332, 1331f
  in liver injury, 1410-1412, 1412t
  nephropathy due to, 1816-1818, 1817t
  pertussis, 944-945
  in respiratory distress, 316

Toxin(s) *(Continued)*
shiga, 959
Staphylococcus aureus, 904, 1324t-1325t
tetanus, 991-992
Vibrio cholerae, 1324t-1325t
Toxocariasis, 1227-1229, 1228t
Toxoid, 883
diphtheria, 884t
tetanus, 884t
Toxoplasmosis, 1208-1216
clinical manifestations of, 1209-1210, 1210f, 1211t, 1212f
congenital, 1208-1211, 1214-1215
diagnosis of, 1213-1215
epidemiology of, 1208
etiology of, 1208, 1209f
fetal therapy for, 551t
gastroenteritis due to, 1327t-1328t
in hearing loss, *see website*
HIV-related, 1164-1165
prophylaxis for, 1175t-1176t
maternal, 1215-1216, *see website*
in microcephaly, 2007t
pathogenesis of, 1208-1209
prevention of, 1216
prognosis for, 1216
systemic signs of, 1211-1213
treatment of, 1215-1216, *see website*
Toxoplasmosis gondii, 1208-1216, *see also website*
in breast milk, 540t
gastroenteritis due to, 1327t-1328t
TPA. *See* Tissue type plasminogen activator (TPA)
TPHA. *See Treponema pallidum* hemagglutination assay (TPHA)
TPI. *See* Triose phosphate isomerase (TPI) deficiency
TPMT. *See* Thiopurine *S*-methyltransferase (TPMT)
TPN. *See* Total parenteral nutrition (TPN)
TPOAbs. *See* Thyroid antiperoxidase antibodies (TPOAbs)
TPPA. *See Treponema pallidum* particle agglutination test (TPPA)
Trace elements, *see website*
Trachea
collapse of, *see website*
compression of as oncologic emergency, *see website*
foreign body in, 1454
goiter within, 1906
intubation of (*See* Endotracheal intubation)
neoplasms of, *see website*
stenosis, *website*s, and atresia of, 1452
Tracheal cytotoxin, 944-945
Tracheitis
bacterial, 1449-1450, 1449f
croup *versus*, 1447
Staphylococcus aureus in, 905
Tracheobronchitis, acute, 1459
Tracheoesophageal fistula, *see website*
Tracheoesophageal fistula (TEF), 1262-1263, 1262f-1263f, *see also website*
Tracheomalacia, 1452, 1455, 1524, *see also website*
Tracheostomy, home mechanical ventilation through, 332-333
Tracheotomy for infectious acute upper airway obstruction, 1448
Trachoma, 1035-1038
Traction alopecia, 2289, 2290f
Traction response, *see website*
Trafficking in children, 136
"Traffic light" diet, 186, 186t
Tragus, accessory, 2221, 2221f
Training for emergencies, *see website*
Tramadol, 367t
Transactional model of development, *see website*
Transaldolase deficiency, 494t-495t, *see website*
Transcatheter closure of patent ductus arteriosus, 1560f, 1561
Transcondylar fracture, 2392
Transcranial Doppler (TCD) assessment in sickle cell disease, 1667
Transcription, *see also website*
HIV, 1157-1158
Transcription factors, 2431-2432, *see also website*
Transcription-mediated amplification (TMA) in *Chlamydia trachomatis*, 1036
Transcriptome, *see website*
Transcutaneous electrical nerve stimulation (TENS), 371
Transdermal fentanyl patch, 155t-156t
Transdermal patch for contraception, 695t, 696-697
Transderm Scop. *See* Scopolamine
Transesophageal echocardiography, 1541, 1543-1544
Transesophageal pacing, 1614-1615
Trans fats, *see website*
Transferase deficiency, 502-503
Transfer dysphagia, 1240
Transferrin
in iron deficiency-anemia, 1656t-1657t
in malnutrition with chronic diarrhea, 1343t
Transferrin receptors in iron deficiency-anemia, 1657t
Transforming growth factor-β (TGF-β)
Marfan syndrome and, 2440
neutralizing antibodies, 2445
Transfusion(s). *See* Blood transfusion(s)
Transgender, 655-658
Transglutaminase deficiency, 1704
Transient erythroblastopenia of childhood (TEC), 1652-1653, 1652t
Transient hyperammonemia of newborn, 452-453
Transient lower esophageal sphincter relaxation (TLESR), *see website*
gastroesophageal reflux disease and, 1266
Transient monoarticular synovitis of hip, 2360
Transient neonatal diabetes mellitus (TNDM), 1995
Transient neonatal pustular melanosis, 2219-2220, 2219f
Transient synovitis of hip, 2413
Transient tachypnea of newborn (TTN), 590
Transillumination
in acute inguinal-scrotal swelling, 1364-1365
of chest, *see website*
of sinuses, 1437
Transitional circulation, *see website*
congenital heart disease and, *see website*
Transitional object, 31-32
Transjugular intrahepatic portosystemic shunt (TIPS), *see website*
Translation, *see also website*
HIV, 1158
Translocase deficiency, 492-496
Translocation, 404-405, 406f
in Down syndrome, 402-403
in listeriosis, *see website*
in proto-oncogene activation, *see website*
Transmalleolar angle, 2346, 2346f
Transmembrane receptors, skeletal dysplasias involving, 2428-2430
Transmissible spongiform encephalopathies (TSEs), 1177, *see also website*
Transmission disequilibrium test (TDT), *see website*
Transplacental chemical exposure, *see website*
Transplacental hemorrhage, anemia due to, 612-613
Transplacental intrauterine infection, 636-639, 637t
Transplantation
candidal infections associated with, 1055
for genetic disorders, 380
Transplantation *(Continued)*
heart, 1638, *see also website*
for hypoplastic left heart syndrome, 1595
heart-lung, 1638, *see also website*
hematopoietic stem cell (*See* Hematopoietic stem cell transplantation (HSCT))
infections associated with, *see website*
intestinal, 1322-1323, *see also website*
of islet cells, 1989-1990
liver, 1415, *see also website*
for acute liver failure, 1414
for type I glycogen storage disease, 495
lung, for cystic fibrosis, 1494
of pancreas, 1989-1990
renal, 1826, *see also website*
maternal, *see website*
sports participation and, 2402t-2404t
umbilical cord blood, *see website*
Transport
of acutely ill child, 278, *see also website*
of chronically ill child, *see website*
of folate, congenital abnormalities of in anemia, *see website*
of high-risk newborn, 564, *see also website*
of lipoproteins, 471-473
tubular, inherited disorders of, 1813-1814
of vitamin A, 188
of vitamin B_{12}, congenital abnormalities of in anemia, *see website*
Transporters
drug, *see also website*
ion, skeletal dysplasias involving, 2430-2431
Transport team, *see website*
Transposition of the great arteries (TGA)
in adults, 1608
d-, 1585, 1585f
with intact ventricular septum, 1585-1587, 1586f
l-, 1587-1588, 1588f
with ventricular septal defect, 1587
and pulmonary stenosis, 1574, 1583f
Transsexual, 655
Transtheoretical Model, *see website*
Transthyretin, reference values for, *see website*
Transtubular potassium gradient (TTKG), 221
Transverse fracture, 2388f, 2390
Transverse myelitis, 2107, 2107t
Transvestite, 655
TRAP. *See* Twin reversed arterial perfusion (TRAP) syndrome
Trapped penis, 1856, 1856f
TRAPS. *See* Tumor necrosis factor receptor-associated periodic syndrome (TRAPS)
Trastuzumab, *see website*
Trauma. *See* Injury(ies)
Trauma score, 335t
Trauma team, 333, 335f
Traumatic alopecia, 2289-2290
Traumatic brain injury (TBI), 297-301, 298f-301f
attention deficit/hyperactivity disorder following, 108
due to child abuse, 139-140, 139f, 301
mild, 301
sports-related, 2418-2419
due to football, *see website*
in trauma survey, 337, 337f
Traumatic intracranial hemorrhage in newborn, 566
Travel, 896, *see also website*
arboviral encephalitis and, 1144-1147
immunizations for, 889, 891t
malaria prevention and, 1207, 1207t
Traveler's diarrhea, 1338-1339, 1338t, *see also website*
Trazodone
for depression and anxiety symptoms, 63t
for sleep disturbance/insomnia in palliative care, 155t-156t

Treacher Collins syndrome
congenital heart disease with, 1531t
oral manifestations of, 1254
Treatment, religious objections to, see website
Treatment plan in psychiatric diagnostic evaluation, 60
TRECs. See T-cell receptor recombination excision circles (TRECs)
Tree nut allergy, 821, 821t, 823t
Treg cells, see website
T regulatory cells, see website
Tremor(s), 2056-2058, 2058t
Trench fever, 983t, 986
Trench foot, 358
Trench mouth, 2299, see website
Treponema carateum, 1023, see also website
Treponemal tests, 1019-1020
Treponema pallidum
neonatal, 632t
in syphilis, 1016
(See also Syphilis)
adolescent treatment of, 712t
Treponema pallidum hemagglutination assay (TPHA), 1019-1020
Treponema pallidum particle agglutination test (TPPA), 1019-1020
Treponema pallidum subspecies *endemicum*, 1023, see also website
Treponema pertenue, 1023, see also website
Treprostinil for pulmonary hypertension, 1602t
Tretinoin
for acne, 2325t
for cancer therapy, see website
TRH. See Thyrotropin-releasing hormone (TRH)
Triad syndrome, 1845
Triage
in international pediatric emergency medicine, see website
in multiple trauma, 333t, 334f
Triage officer model for emergency care, see website
Triamcinolone
for allergic rhinitis, 778t-779t
for asthma, 795t
Triamterene, 1645t
Triatomines in trypanosomiasis, 1195
Trichilemmal cyst, see website
Trichinella spiralis, 1229-1230, 1327t-1328t, see also website
Trichinosis, 1229-1230
Trichlorethylene, as inhalant, 681t
Trichloroacetic acid, 713t
Trichloroethylene exposure, see website
Trichobezoars, 1291
Trichoepithelioma, see website
Tricho-hepato-enteric (THE) syndrome, 1311-1312
Trichomonas vaginalis, 1185-1186, 1185f, see also website
adolescent treatment of, 712t
prophylaxis following rape, 704t
sexual abuse and, 145t
treatment of, 712t
in vulvovaginitis, 1868t
Trichophyton rubrum, 806
Trichophyton spp. in skin infection, 2309-2313
Trichopoliodystrophy, 2292
Trichorrhexis invaginata, 2293
Trichorrhexis nodosa, 1312, 2292, 2292f
Trichostrongylus, see website
Trichothiodystrophy, 2268t, 2272, 2293
Trichotillomania, 75, 2289-2290
Trichrome stain, see website
Trichuriasis, 1221-1222, 1221f, see website
Triclabendazole, see website
Tricuspid atresia, 1580-1582, 1580f-1581f
Tricuspid regurgitation, 1572
Tricuspid valve
disease of, 1628
Ebstein anomaly of the, 1583-1585, 1584f
Tricyclic antidepressants (TCAs)
for attention deficit/hyperactivity disorder, 111t
for depression and anxiety symptoms, 63t
heart disease and, 65
for neuropathic pain, 368t
for pain management, 369
poisoning with, 251t, 264, 264f
antidote for, 256t-257t
in psychopharmacology, 62
Trientine, 1392
Trifluridine, see website
Trifunctional protein (TFP), mitochondrial, deficiency of, 460
Trigeminal nerve, neurologic examination of, see website
Trigeminy, 1612-1613
Triggers
for asthma, 783t
Aspergillus as, 1059
for atopic dermatitis, 805-806
Trigger thumb and fingers, 2387
Triglycerides, 479t
laboratory testing of in obesity, 185t
Trigonecephaly, 2012
Trihexyphenidyl, 2064
Triiodothyronine (T_3), see also website
in congenital hypothyroidism, 1899
fetal, see website
measurement of, 1894
reference values for, 1899t, see also website
in thyroid hormone unresponsiveness, 1897
Triiodothyronine (T_3) resin uptake test, reference values for, 1899t
Trilisate, 155t-156t
Trimethoprim, see website
Trimethoprim-sulfamethoxazole (TMP-SMX), see also website
for acute cystitis, 1832
for brucellosis, 981t
for cyclosporiasis, see website
for cystic fibrosis lung infection, 1492t
for diarrheagenic *Escherichia coli*, 964-965
drug interactions with, see website
for infectious diarrhea, 1337t
for isosporiasis, 1184, see website
for nontuberculosis mycobacteria, see website
for *Paracoccidioides brasiliensis*, see website
for pertussis, 947t
for *Pneumocystis jiroveci*, see website
HIV-related, 1163, 1173-1174, 1175t-1176t
for *Shigella* infection, 961
for *Staphylococcus aureus*, 907t
for *Toxoplasmosis gondii* prophylaxis in HIV infection, 1168t-1171t
for vulvovaginitis, 1868t
Trimethylaminuria, 440
Trimpex. See Trimethoprim
Triose phosphate isomerase (TPI) deficiency, 1677
Triplane fracture, 2393, 2393f
Triple A syndrome, 1925, 1925t
Triplet repeat expansion disorders, 391, 392t, 393f
Triplets, 553
Triploid cells, 399
Triploidy, 1531t
Triptan, 2043, 2044t
Trismus, tetanus in, 992
Trisomy, 400, 400t
partial, 403
Trisomy 8, 404t
malignancy susceptibility associated with, see website
Trisomy 9, 404t
congenital heart disease with, 1531t
Trisomy 13, 404t, 405f
congenital heart disease with, 1531t
Trisomy 16, 404t
Trisomy 18, 404t, 405f
congenital heart disease with, 1531t
microcephaly with, 2007t
Trisomy 21, 400-403. See also Down syndrome
congenital heart disease with, 1531t, 1554, see also website
malignancy susceptibility associated with, see website
microcephaly with, 2007t
Trisomy by trisomy rescue, 413
Trisomy 12p, 404t
congenital heart disease with, 1531t
Trisomy X, 409t
Trizavir. See Zidovudine (ZDV)
Trizivir. See Abacavir
TRMA. See Thiamine-responsiveness megaloblastic anemia (TRMA)
Trochlear nerve
neurologic examination of, see website
palsy of, 2159-2160
Trombiculid mite, 1045
Tropheryma whipplei, 1314
in infective endocarditis, 1624t
Trophic feeding of premature infant, 561
Trophozoite, in malaria, 1199, 1199f
Tropical acne, 2327-2328
Tropical pancreatitis, 1373
Tropical pulmonary eosinophilia, 1224, see website
Tropical splenomegaly syndrome, 1206
Tropical sprue, 1313-1314
TRPV4 gene, 2435, see website
TRSAb. See Thyrotropin receptor-stimulating antibody (TRSAb)
Truancy, 99-100
Trumerfeld zone, 199
Truncal ataxia in neurologic examination, see website
Truncal nerve block, 372
Truncus arteriosus, 1590-1592, 1591f
Truvada. See Emtricitabine; Tenofovir
Trychophyton, 2296
Trypanosoma brucei complex, 1190-1193, 1192f, see also website
Trypanosoma cruzi, 1193-1198, 1193f-1194f, 1195t, see also website
Trypanosomiasis
African, 1190-1193, 1192f, see website
maternal, see website
Trypomastigotes, 1193, 1193f
Trypsin, see website
Trypsinogen
deficiency of, 1306t, 1318
in exocrine pancreatic function, 1307
Tryptophan, defects in metabolism of, 429-430, 429f, 1319
TS. See Tourette's syndrome (TS)
TSC. See Tuberous sclerosis complex (TSC)
TSEs. See Transmissible spongiform encephalopathies (TSEs)
Tsetse fly, in trypanosomiasis, 1190
TSH. See Thyroid-stimulating hormone (TSH)
T-SPOT.TB, 1000-1001
TSS. See Toxic shock syndrome (TSS)
TST. See Tuberculin skin testing (TST)
Tsutsugamushi fever, 1045
TTH. See Tension-type headache (TTH)
TTKG. See Transtubular potassium gradient (TTKG)
TTN. See Transient tachypnea of newborn (TTN)
TTP. See Thrombotic thrombocytopenic purpura (TTP)
TTSS-1. See Type II secretion system (TTSS-1)
TTSS-3. See Type III secretion system (TTSS-3)
Tube feeding in infant botulism, 990
Tuberculids, 2308
Tuberculin skin testing (TST), 1001, 1002t
in fever of unknown origin, 902
in HIV infection, 1174
of immigrant children, 133
Tuberculoid leprosy (TL), see website
Tuberculoma

Tuberculosis (TB), 996-1011, 996f-997f
abdominal and gastrointestinal, 1006
of bone and joints, 1006
breast-feeding and, 161t
of central nervous system, 1005-1006
in child care setting, *see website*
clinical manifestations and diagnosis of, 1002-1007, 1003f
congenital, 1000
cutaneous, 1006, 2307-2308, 2308f
drug-resistance, 1008-1009
epidemiology of, 996-998, 998t
etiology of, 996
fetal therapy for, 551t
with HIV infection, 1007
prophylaxis for, 1175t-1176t
in immigrant children, 133
immunity to, 1000-1001
inflammatory bowel disease *versus*, 1298t
of lymph nodes, 1005, 1005f
lymphohematogenous (disseminated), 1004
miliary, 2308
in newborn, 1000
orificial, 2307
pathogenesis of, 998-1001, 999f-1000f
perinatal, 1007, 1011
pleural, 1003-1004, 1004f
in pregnancy, 1000
prevention of, 1010-1011
reactivation, 998-1000, 1003
respiratory culture in, *see website*
transmission of, 998
treatment of, 1007-1010, 1008t, *see also website*
tuberculin skin testing for, 1001, 1002t
Tuberculosis vaccine for travel, *see website*
Tuberculosis verrucosa cutis, 2307
Tuberculous adrenalitis, 1925t
Tuberculous gummas, 2308
Tuberous sclerosis complex (TSC), 2049-2051, 2049f-2050f, 2049t
brain tumors associated with, 1747t
cardiac manifestations of, 1531t
malignancy susceptibility associated with, *see website*
retinal phakoma of, 2178f
Tubes
chest, for emergencies, 295
endotracheal
manual ventilation before and after, 320-321
medications for placement of, 321t
placement of, 285, 286f, 287t
for respiratory distress and failure, 320
size and depth dimensions for, 320t
tympanostomy, 2208-2210, 2213
Tubo-ovarian abscess, 1871, *see website*
Tubularized incised plate (TIP), 1853-1854
Tubular proteinuria, 1801
Tubules, renal
disorders of
Bartter syndrome as, 1813-1814, 1813t
Gitelman syndrome as, 1814
inherited transport disorders of, 1813-1814
nephrogenic diabetes insipidus as, 1812
renal tubular acidosis as, 1811f
tubulointerstitial nephritis as, 1814-1816, 1815t
function of, 1807, *see also website*
Tubulointerstitial fibrosis, *see website*
Tubulointerstitial nephritis (TIN), 1814-1816, 1815t
Tufted angioma, 2228, 2229f
Tufting enteropathy, 1306t, 1311
Tularemia, 978-980, 978f, 978t-979t
in terrorism, *see website*
Tumor(s). *See also specific types*
adrenal, 1773
adrenocortical, 1941, *see also website*
bone, 1763-1768, 1763t, 1764f-1765f
brain, 1746-1753
Tumor(s) *(Continued)*
(*See also* Brain tumor(s))
carcinoid, *see website*
cutaneous, examination of, *see website*
desmoplastic small round cell, 1773
of digestive tract, 1362, *see also website*
of ear and temporal bone, 2214, *see also website*
of eyelid, 2164-2165, 2164f
germ cell, 1769-1771, 1770f
of central nervous system, 1752-1753
gonadotropin-secreting, precocious puberty due to, 1891
of heart, 1637, *see also website*
following transplantation, *see website*
hepatic
precocious puberty due to, 1891
incidence and survival rates for, 1726t
of jaw, *see website*
neural crest, congenital central hypoventilation syndrome with, 1520-1521
neuroendocrine, chronic diarrhea due to, 1346, *see also website*
orbital, 2182, 2182f
ovarian, 1871-1872, 1872t
pseudoprecocity resulting from, 1957-1958
pancreatic, 1374, *see also website*
paronychial, 2297
porphyria due to, *see website*
pot puffy, 1438
pulmonary, 1504, *see also website*
rhabdoid of kidney, 1760
rickets due to, 202t, 207
risk factors for, 1727t
of skin, 2328, *see also website*
spinal, 2377
of spinal cord, 2105, 2105f
testicular, 1864
pseudoprecocity due to, 1950, *see also website*
thyroid, 1772, *see also website*
of umbilicus, *see website*
vascular, 1772, *see also website*
cutaneous, 2226-2231, 2227f-2229f, 2227t-2228t
gastrointestinal, *see website*
Wilms, 1757-1760, 1757t-1759t, 1759f
Tumor lysis syndrome (TLS), 1819, *see also website*
Tumor markers, 1731, 1731t
in ovarian carcinoma, 1872t
Tumor necrosis factor α (TNF-α)
in lung injury, *see website*
in Rocky Mountain spotted fever, 1041
in sudden infant death syndrome, 1427
Tumor necrosis factor α (TNF-α) antagonists
for Behçet disease, 854
for juvenile idiopathic arthritis, 838t
for rheumatic disease, *see website*
for spondyloarthritides, *see website*
Tumor necrosis factor receptor-associated periodic syndrome (TRAPS), 855t, 858, 859f
Tumor suppressor genes, alterations in regulation of, *see website*
Tunnel tract infection. *See* Catheter-related bloodstream infection (CRBSI)
Turbulence air flow, *see website*
Turcot syndrome, 1747t, *see website*
Turf toe, *see website*
Turner syndrome, 409-410, 409t, 1951-1954, 1952f
clinical findings in, 410f
congenital heart disease with, 1531t, 1567
genetics of, 409-410
hypothyroidism with, 1901
obesity due to, 182t
signs associated with, 409t
Turricephaly, 2012
T-wave, 1537-1538
abnormalities of, 1540, 1541f
21st century, information explosion of, 11-12
Twenty-four hour electrocardiography (Holter) recordings, 1614-1615
20-nail dystrophy, 2296
Twinject. *See* Self-injectable epinephrine
Twinning, tooth, 1250
Twin reversed arterial perfusion (TRAP) syndrome, 554
fetal therapy for, 551t
Twins
conjoined, 553
etiology of, 553
incidence of, 553
monozygotic *versus* dizygotic, 553-554
placenta and, 554, 554t
problems with, 554
prognosis for, 554-555, 555f
Twin-twin transfusion syndrome, 554
fetal therapy for, 551t
TWIST heterogenous, 2012t
Two-dimensional echocardiography, 1541-1542, 1542f-1543f, 1573
in coarctation of the aorta, 1568, 1569f
in tetralogy of Fallot, 1575, 1575f
in ventricular septal defect, 1557
"Two-hit" model of cancer development, *see also website*
in retinoblastoma, 1768
22q11.2 deletion syndrome, 2382, 2382f
congenital heart disease and, *see website*
2-step command, 33
Tygacil. *See* Tigecycline
Tylophora indica for asthma, 271t
Tympanic membrane (TM)
atelectasis of, 2212
cholesterol granuloma of, 2212
examination of, *see website*
mobility of, *see website*
in otitis media, 2203-2204, 2203f
in otitis media with effusion, 2204f
perforation of, 2210, 2212
traumatic, *see website*
traumatic injury to, *see website*
Tympanocentesis, 2208, *see website*
Tympanogram, 2204, 2204f
Tympanometry, 2194, 2194f, 2194t
in otitis media, 2204-2205, 2204f
with effusion, 2194-2195
in otitis media with effusion, 2194-2195
Tympanosclerosis, 2212
Tympanostomy tubes, 2208-2210, 2213
Type 1 diabetes mellitus (T1DM), 1969-1990
anxiety and depression in, 1986
autoimmune, 1970
behavioral/psychologic aspects of, 1986
brittle, 1985-1986
catabolic losses in, 1980
cataracts with, 2171
cerebral edema in, 1981
clinical manifestations of, 1975
cognitive function and, 1986
coping styles in, 1986
dawn phenomenon in, 1985-1986
dental problems associated with, 1251t
diagnosis of, 1975-1976
eating disorders in, 1986-1987
environmental factors in, 1971-1972
epidemiology of, 1969-1970, 1969f
fear of self-injecting and self-testing in, 1986
genetics of, 1970-1971, 1970f
hyperglycemia and dehydration in, 1979-1980
hypoglycemia in, 1985
hypothyroidism with, 1901
infections in, 1987, 1987t
keto acid accumulation in, 1980-1981
ketoacidosis in, 1979, 1979t, 1981
long-term complications of, 1988-1989, 1988t
management of during surgery, 1987, 1987t
metabolic acidosis in, 232
monogenic, 1970
neuropathy in, 1989

Type 1 diabetes mellitus (T1DM) *(Continued)*
nonketotic hyperosmolar coma in, 1981
pancreas and islet transplantation and regeneration for, 1989-1990
pathogenesis and natural history of, 1972, 1972f-1973f
pathophysiology of, 1975, 1975t
prediction and prevention of, 1974-1975
prognosis for, 1989
Somogyi phenomenon in, 1985-1986
treatment of, 1976-1986
amylin based adjunct therapy for, 1979
education in, 1979
glycemic control in, 1984
insulin therapy for, 1976-1979, 1977f-1978f, 1979t, 1984-1985
monitoring in, 1983, 1983t
of new-onset diabetes without ketoacidosis, 1976
nonadherence in, 1986
nutritional, 1981-1983
real-time continuous glucose monitoring in, 1983-1984
Type 2 diabetes mellitus (T2DM), 1990-1993
clinical features of, 1991-1992, 1991t
complications of, 1993, 1993t
environmental and lifestyle-related risk factors in, 1991
epidemiology of, 1990-1991
epigenetics and fetal programming in, 1991
genetics of, 1991
natural history of, 1990
obesity in, 184t, 185, 185f
prevention of, 1993
treatment of, 1992-1993, 1992t
Type I collagen, defects in, 2437
Type III secretion system (TTSS-3), *Shigella*, 959
Type II secretion system (TTSS-1), *Salmonella*, 950
Typhlitis, *see website*
Typhoidal tularemia, 979
Typhoid fever, 954-958
clinical features of, 955-956, 956f, 956t
complications of, 956, 957t
diagnosis of, 956-957
differential diagnosis of, 957
epidemiology of, 954
etiology of, 954
pathogenesis of, 954-955, 955f
prevention of, 958
treatment of, 957-958, 958t
Typhoid vaccine, 884t, 958
for travel, 891t, *see website*
Typhus
cat flea, 1039t-1040t
epidemic, 1039t-1040t, 1047-1048
flying squirrel, 1039t-1040t
murine, 1039t-1040t, 1046-1047
scrub, 1039t-1040t, 1045-1046
Typhus group rickettsiae, 1046-1048
Tyrosine, defects in metabolism of, 422-425, 424t
Tyrosine hydroxylase deficiency, 445
Tyrosinemia
malignancy susceptibility associated with, *see website*
transient of newborn, 423
type I, 422-425
type II, 422-423
type III, 423
Tyrosinosis, 422-425
Tzanck smear, 1108, *see also website*

U
UAKD. *See* Uromodulin-associated kidney disease (UAKD)
UBE3A gene, 391-393
UBOs. *See* "Unidentified bright objects" (UBOs)
UES. *See* Upper esophageal sphincter (UES)
UGT. *See* Glucuronosyl transferase (UGT)
UL. *See* Tolerable upper intake level (UL)
Ulcerative colitis, 1295-1300
clinical manifestations of, 1297
Crohn disease *versus*, 1295, 1295t
diagnosis of, 1297-1298, 1299f
differential diagnosis of, 1297, 1298t
liver disease associated with, *see website*
malabsorption in, 1322, *see also website*
prognosis for, 1300
treatment of, 1298-1300
Ulcerative gingivitis, necrotizing, 1260t, *see website*
Ulceroglandular tularemia, 979
Ulcer/ulceration
aphthous
genital, 1866, 1866f
oral, 1260, 1260t
Buruli ulcer disease, 1012-1013, 1015
corneal, *see website*
examination of, *see website*
genital, 708
hemangioma and, 2227t
oral, 1260t
in rheumatic disease, *see website*
peptic, 1291-1294, 1291t, 1292f-1293f, 1293t
abdominal pain of, 1247t
stress, 1293
Ulnar artery, cannulation of, 292-294
Ultracef. *See* Cefadroxil
Ultralene insulin, 1976
Ultrasound
in acute inguinal-scrotal swelling, 1364-1365
in appendicitis, 1351, 1352f
cranial, *see website*
in developmental dysplasia of hip, 2358-2360
of fetus, 541, 543t
diagnostic, 548, 549f, 550t
in erythroblastosis fetalis, 617
in intussusception, 1288, 1289f
in liver abscess, 1404, 1405f
in liver dysfunction, 1379
in neonatal cholestasis, 1385, 1387f
in orthopedic problems, 2334
in pyloric stenosis, 1274, 1275f
in septic arthritis, 2399
of thyroid, *see website*
in urinary tract obstruction, 1839-1840, 1839f
Ultraviolet A (UVA) radiation, 2254-2255
Ultraviolet B (UVB) radiation, 2254-2255
Umbilical artery, *see also website*
catheterization of
in respiratory distress syndrome, 586
risks associated with, 587
Umbilical cord, *see also website*
blood sampling from, 543t, 544, 549
in erythroblastosis fetalis, 617
care of, 537
delayed clamping of for prevention of anemia, 614
Umbilical cord blood transplants (UCBT), *see website*
Umbilical tetanus, 991
Umbilicus, 622, *see also website*
Unbound bilirubin, 1375
Uncombable hair syndrome, 2293, 2293f
Unconjugated bilirubin, 603-604
Unconjugated hyperbilirubinemia, 1376t
Undernutrition, 170-174, 171f, 171t. *See also* Malnutrition
consequences of, 173-174
food insecurity and, 170-171
interventions for, 174, 174f
measurement of, 171-172
prevalence of, 172-173
Undescended testis, 1858-1860, 1860f
in neuromuscular disorders, 2109
sports participation and, 2402t-2404t
Undifferentiated somatoform disorders, 68t
Unfractioned heparin, 1710t, 1711
UNG. *See* Uracil DNA glycosylase (UNG), mutations in
Ungual infection, with *Candida*, 1055
UNICEF. *See* United Nations Children's Fund (UNICEF)
Unicornuate uterus and rudimentary horns, *see website*
"Unidentified bright objects" (UBOs), 2047-2048, 2048f
Unilateral hyperlucent lung, 1461
Uninhibited bladder, 73
Uniparental disomy (UPD), 412-413, 413f
Unipen. *See* Nafcillin
United Nations Children's Fund (UNICEF)
on breast-feeding, 160, 161t, 539t
on injury prevention, *see website*
Integrated Management of Childhood Illness guidelines from, *see website*
United Nations Convention on the Rights of the Child, *see website*
Unit-megakaryocytes, *see website*
Univentricular heart, 1592
Universal precautions. *See* Standard precautions
Unmeasured osmoles, *see website*
Unna-Thost palmoplantar keratodermas, 2272, 2273f
Unprovoked seizure, 2013, 2019-2021, 2020t
Unstable bladder, 73
Unstable hemoglobin disorders, 1670-1671
Unvericht Lundborg disease, 2024
UP. *See* β-Ureidopropionase (UP) deficiency
UPD. *See* Uniparental disomy (UPD)
Upgaze of childhood, paroxysmal tonic, *see website*
UPJ. *See* Ureteropelvic junction obstruction (UPJ)
Upper airway
acute inflammatory obstruction of, 1445-1450
bacterial tracheitis as, 1449-1450, 1449f
infectious, 1445-1449, 1446f-1447f
obstruction of, 283
respiratory acidosis due to disease of, 239t
Upper airway film, *see website*
Upper body segment, body proportions and, *see website*
Upper esophageal sphincter (UES), *see also website*
dysmotility of, 1264-1265
Upper extremity block, 371
Upper extremity(ies)
arthrogryposis involving, *see website*
assessment of, 2333f
fractures of, 2390-2391
growth and development of, *see website*
musculoskeletal pain syndrome of, 877t
orthopedic disorders of, 2383-2387
venous access in, 295f
Upper intake level (UL), *see website*
Upper respiratory tract infection
anaerobic, *see website*
anesthesia and, *see website*
HIV-related, 1165
sports participation and, 2402t-2404t
tuberculous, 1004-1005
Upper urinary tract, duplication of, 1834-1835, 1835f
Urachal anomalies, *see website*
Uracil DNA glycosylase (UNG), mutations in, 727
Urbach-Wiethe disease, 2276-2277
Urban-rural location, childhood injuries and, 20-21
Urea cycle, defects in, 447-453
Urea in plasma osmolality, *see website*
Urea nitrogen
dehydration, 246
in plasma osmolality, *see website*
reference values for, *see website*
Ureaplasma urealyticum, 1032-1033
maternal, *see website*
β-Ureidopropionase (UP) deficiency, *see website*
Uremia, *see website*

Ureter
ectopic, 1842-1843, 1842f
obstruction of, 1839, 1839t
retrocaval, 1842
Ureteral bud, *see website*
Ureteral octopia, incontinence due to, 1850-1851, 1850f-1851f
Ureterocele, 1843-1844, 1843f
ectopic, 1843, 1843f
prolapsed, 1858, 1858f
Ureteropelvic junction obstruction (UPJ), 1839t, 1841-1842
Urethral anomalies, 1857-1858
Urethral atresia, 1846
Urethral catheters, infection associated with, *see website*
Urethral cyst, parameatal, 1857-1858
Urethral diverticula, 1847
Urethral duplication, 1857-1858
Urethral fistula, 1857-1858
Urethral hypoplasia, 1846-1847, 1857-1858
Urethral injury, *see website*
Urethral lesions, female, 1858, 1858f
Urethral obstruction, 1839t
Urethral prolapse, 1858, 1858f
vaginal bleeding due to, 1869
Urethral strictures, 1847
Urethral valves
anterior, 1847
posterior, 1845-1846, 1846f
Urethritis, 707, 707f, 709
gonococcal, 937-938
nongonococcal
Trichomonas vaginalis in, 1186
Ureaplasma in, 1032-1033
Urgent care for chronic illness, *see website*
Uric acid, *see website*
Uric acid calculi, *see website*
Uridine diphosphate galactose-4-epimerase deficiency, 503
Uridine monophosphate hydrolase 1 deficiency, *see website*
overactive cytosolic 5'-nucleotidase and, *see website*
Uridine monophosphate synthase type I deficiency, *see website*
Uridyl transferase deficiency, 502-503
Urinalysis in acute renal failure, 1819, 1820t
Urinary acidification, normal, 1808, 1808f
Urinary alkalinization for poisoning, 258
with salicylates, 260
Urinary concentrating defect in chronic kidney disease, 1823t
Urinary incontinence, 1850-1851, 1850f
causes of, 1848t
diurnal, 1847-1848, 1848f-1849f
giggle, 1851
due to neuropathic bladder, *see website*
Urinary lithiasis, 1864, *see also website*
abdominal pain of, 1248t
as complication of enterocystoplasty, *see website*
Urinary retention, due to opioids, 366t
Urinary test, Binax, *see website*
Urinary tract
congenital intestinal pseudo-obstruction and, 1283
traumatic injury to, *see website*
Urinary tract infection (UTI), 1829-1834
abdominal pain of, 1247t-1248t
alternate recommendations for, 1833-1834
circumcision and, 1855
clinical manifestations and classification of, 1829-1830, 1830f
coagulase-negative staphylococci in, 910
as complication of enterocystoplasty, *see website*
diagnosis of, 1831-1832
Enterococcus, *see website*
hematuria in, 1794-1795, 1799
imaging studies of, 1833, 1833f
Urinary tract infection (UTI) *(Continued)*
pathogenesis and pathology of, 1830-1831, 1831f, 1831t
prevalence and history of, 1829
Pseudomonas aeruginosa, 976t
treatment of, 1832-1833, 1832f
Urinary tract obstruction, 1838-1847, 1839t
anterior urethral valves in, 1847
bladder neck, 1845
clinical manifestations of, 1839
diagnosis of, 1839-1841, 1839f-1841f, 1840t
ectopic ureter in, 1842-1843, 1842f
etiology of, 1838-1839
hydrocalycosis in, 1841
megaureter in, 1844-1845, 1844f, 1844t
midureteral, 1842
posterior urethral valves in, 1845-1846, 1846f
prune-belly syndrome in, 1844f-1845f
ureterocele in, 1843-1844, 1843f
ureteropelvic junction, 1841-1842
urethral atresia in, 1846
urethral diverticula in male in, 1847
urethral hypoplasia in, 1846-1847
urethral strictures in, 1847
Urinary wasting potassium, 223
Urine
fetal, testing of, 543t
red, 1779, 1779t
in congenital erythropoietic porphyria, *see website*
red blood cells in (*See* Hematuria)
screening, for adolescent drug use, 676t
Urine alarm treatment for nocturnal enuresis, 72
Urine culture, *see also website*
in urinary tract infection, 1831-1832
Urine osmolality, *see website*
Urine output, fluid therapy and, 245, 245t
UROD. *See* Uroporphyrinogen decarboxylase (UROD)
Urography in urinary tract obstruction, 1841, 1841f
Urologic disorders
congenital anomalies of
of bladder, 1847, *see also website*
of kidney, 1827-1829, 1828f-1829f
of penis and urethra, 1852-1858
genitourinary trauma as, 1864, *see also website*
neuropathic bladder as, 1847, *see also website*
obstructive, 1838-1847
renal agenesis as, 1827, 1828f
renal dysgenesis as, 1827-1828
renal transplantation and, 1826, *see also website*
of scrotal contents, 1858-1864
traumatic, 1864
urinary lithiasis as, 1864, *see also website*
urinary tract infections as, 1829-1834
vesicoureteral reflux as, 1834-1838
voiding dysfunction as, 1847-1852
Uromodulin-associated kidney disease (UAKD), *see website*
Uropathy
obstructive
nephrotoxins in, 1817t
Uroporphyrinogen decarboxylase (UROD), *see website*
deficiency of, *see website*
Uroporphyrinogen III synthase (UROS), *see website*
deficiency of, *see website*
UROS. *See* Uroporphyrinogen III synthase (UROS)
Urticaria (hives), 811-816
aquagenic, 813
cholinergic, 812-813
chronic idiopathic, 813
cold, 812
diagnosis of, 812t, 813-814, 813f-814f
drug eruptions in, *see website*
etiology and pathogenesis of, 811-812, 812t
Urticaria (hives) *(Continued)*
due to food allergy, 822
papular, 2318, 2318f
physical, 812-813
pressure-induced, 813
solar, 813, 2257, 2257f
treatment of, 814-815, 815t
Urticaria pigmentosa, 814, 2280-2281, 2281f
Usability in quality measurement, *see website*
Usher syndrome, 2190t
Uterine bleeding, abnormal, 686t, 688-690, 689t-690t
Uterine compression, deformations due to, *see website*
Uterine didelphys, *see website*
Uterine fibroids, 689t-690t
Uterus
anomalies of, *see website*
neoplasm of, 1872-1873
UTI. *See* Urinary tract infection (UTI)
Utilization in food security, 170-171
UVA. *See* Ultraviolet A (UVA) radiation
UVB. *See* Ultraviolet B (UVB) radiation
Uveal tract disorders, 2172-2174, 2173f-2174f, 2173t
Uveitis, 2172-2174, 2173f, 2173t
anterior, 2167t
enteroviral, 1091
human T-lymphocyte-associated, *see website*
in juvenile idiopathic arthritis, 838, 839f
tubulointerstitial nephritis with, 1816

V
VA. *See* Ventriculoatrial (VA) shunt
VABS. *See* Vineland Adaptive Behavior Scale (VABS)
Vaccine Adverse Event Reporting System (VAERS), 885
Vaccine-associated paralytic poliomyelitis (VAPP), 1082, 1084
Vaccine encephalopathy, febrile seizures with, 2017
Vaccine(s), 883-884, 884t
for adolescents, 664
adverse reactions to, 827
anthrax, 884t
Bacille Calmette-Guérin, 884t, 1010-1011
bioterrorism and, 891
cancer therapy and, *see website*
cholera, 967-968, 968t
chronic kidney disease and, 1825
combination, 889
congenital heart disease and, 1603
conjugated, 883
cytomegalovirus, 1117
delivery of, 886
development of, 884-885, 885f
diphtheria, *see website*
diphtheria acellular pertussis, 884t, 947-948
financing for, 885
group B streptococcus, 928
Haemophilus influenzae type B, 943
hepatitis A, 884t, 1396
for immigrant children, 133
hepatitis B, 1399-1400, 1399t
for immigrant children, 132-133
in newborn, 537
as universal vaccine, 1399-1400
herpes zoster, 1110
HIV infection and, 1173, 1173f
for homosexual youth, 659
human papillomavirus, 884t, 888f, 891t, 1141
immigrant children and, 132, 134
immunodeficiencies and, 889-891, 892t
improving coverage of, 893, 893t
influenza, 884t
international practices on, 893-895
Japanese encephalitis, 884t, 1146
for measles, 1073-1075, 1074t
measles, mumps, rubella, 884t, 1073-1075, 1074t

Vaccine(s) *(Continued)*
adverse reaction to, 827
recommended schedule for, 886-889, 887f-888f
for travel, *see website*
meningococcal, 884t, 934-935, 934t
mumps, 1081
parental refusal of, 893, *see website*
for pertussis, 947-948
pneumococcus, 884t, 2095
otitis media and, 2200, 2201f
pneumonia hospitalization and, 1479
policy on, 885
polio, 1087-1088
precautions and contraindications for, 892-893
production of, 885
Q fever, 1052-1053
rabies, 884t, 1155
recommended schedule for, 886, 887f-888f, 890f
catch-up, 889, 890f
renal transplantation and, *see website*
respiratory syncytial virus, 1129
rotavirus, 884t, 1137
in gastroenteritis prevention, 1338
rubella, 1078
safety monitoring of, 886, 886t
smallpox, 884t
in special circumstances, 889-891
sudden infant death syndrome and, 1425
tetanus, 993
T lymphocyte-dependent, 883
for travel, 889, 891t, *see website*
type 1 diabetes mellitus and, 1972
typhoid, 884t, 958
varicella, 1109-1110
"breakthrough varicella" due to, 1105-1106
websites and resources associated with, 894t
yellow fever, 884t, *see website*
Vaccine Safety Datalink (VSD), 886
Vaccines for Children (VFC) program, 885
Vaccinia immune globulin, 882t
VACTERL anomalad, 1356
VACTREL syndrome, 1262
VAD. *See* Ventricular assist device (VAD)
VAERS. *See* Vaccine Adverse Event Reporting System (VAERS)
Vagal nerve stimulation for seizures, 2032-2033
Vagal syncope, *see website*
Vagina
abnormal uterine bleeding from, 689t-690t
anomalies of, *see website*
neoplasm of, 1873
bleeding due to, 689t-690t, 1869
traumatic injury to, vaginal bleeding due to, 1869
Vaginal bleeding, 1869-1870
abnormal, 688-690, 689t-690t
Vaginal candidosis, 2313-2314
Vaginal contraceptive ring, 697
special needs girls and, 1875
Vaginal discharge
pathologic, 711t
in vulvovaginitis, 1866
Vaginal foreign body, 1866f, 1867
Vaginal orifice, neonatal examination of, *see website*
Vaginal voiding, 1850, 1850f
Vaginitis, 708, 1865
group A streptococcus in, 917
Vaginosis, bacterial
prophylaxis following rape, 704t
sexual abuse and, 145t
Vagovagal syncope, *see website*
Vagus nerve, neurologic examination of, *see website*
Valacyclovir, 1102-1103, *see also website*
Valcyte. *See* Valganciclovir
Valeriana officinalis for sedation, 271t
Valerian for sedation, 271t
Valganciclovir, 1175t-1176t, *see also website*
Validity
analytical, 376
clinical, 376
in quality measurement, *see website*
Valine, defects in metabolism of, 430-438
Valley fever, 1065-1068
Valproate
drug interactions with, *see website*
for neuropathic pain, 368t
for seizures, 2030t
for status epilepticus, 2039t
Valproic acid
adverse effects of, 2031t
for Landau-Kleffner syndrome, 2024
for migraine prophylaxis, 2044t, 2045
as mood stabilizer, 63
Valsalva, compulsive, *see website*
Valtrex. *See* Valacyclovir
Valvular heart disease. *See also specific valves*
due to acute rheumatic fever, 922
Valvuloplasty
balloon
for aortic stenosis, 1566
for pulmonary valve stenosis, 1563
mitral, 1572
Vancocin. *See* Vancomycin
Vancomycin, *see also website*
for bacterial meningitis, 2091, 2093t
for brain abscess, 2099
for *Clostridium difficile* infection, 995
for cystic fibrosis lung infection, 1492t
for infective endocarditis, 1625t
for meningococcal disease, 932
for neonatal infection, 644, 645t
for pneumococcal meningitis, 913
for *Staphylococcus aureus*, 906-907, 907t
Vancomycin-resistant *Enterococcus* (VRE), *see website*
Van den Bergh reaction, 603
Vanishing testis, 1859, 1944
Vanishing twin syndrome, 553
Vantin. *See* Cefpodoxime proxetil
VAPP. *See* Vaccine-associated paralytic poliomyelitis (VAPP)
Vaqta, *see website*
Varapamil, 1611t-1612t
Variability of fetal heart rate, 542-544, 545t
Variable expression, 383-385
Variable expressivity, 380-381
Variant surface glycoproteins (VSG), 1191
Variceal hemorrhage, 1376
Varicella vaccine, 884t, 1109-1110
"breakthrough varicella" due to, 1105-1106
HIV infection and, 1173f
recommended schedule for, 887f-888f
for travel, 891t, *see website*
Varicella-zoster virus immune globulin (VariZIG), 882t, 1110, *see also website*
in HIV infection, 1175t-1176t
for neonatal varicella, 1106
Varicella-zoster virus (VZV), 1104-1110, 1105f, 1107f, 1109t
acyclovir for, *see website*
antivirals for, *see website*
in Bell palsy, 2147f
in child care setting, *see website*
HIV-related, 1164
prophylaxis for, 1175t-1176t
immunofluorescent-antibody testing of, *see website*
maternal
breast-feeding and, 161t, 540t
fetal and neonatal effects of, *see website*
in pneumonia, 1475t
poliovirus infection *versus*, 1085t
in viral meningoencephalitis, 2096
Varices, esophageal, 1271, *see also website*
portal hypertension and, 1415, *see also website*
Varicocele, 1863, 1863f
Variegate porphyria (VP), *see website*
VariZIG. *See* Varicella-zoster virus immune globulin (VariZIG)
Varus 5th toe, 2342
VAS. *See* Visual analog pain scales (VAS)
Vascular abnormalities
hematuria due to, 1794
laryngeal, 1264, *see also website*
in progeria, *see website*
Vascular access, 292-294, 295f
office emergencies and, *see website*
Vascular compartment, pulmonary edema and, 1468
Vascular disorders
hemorrhagic stroke due to, 2084-2085, 2085t
pulmonary, 1601-1602
sports participation and, 2402t-2404t
Vascular endothelial growth factor (VEGF)
in ovarian carcinomas, 1872t
in retinopathy of prematurity, 2174
in sudden infant death syndrome, 1422, 1427
Vascular events, seizures due to, 2034
Vascular lesions of skin, 2224t, *see also website*
arteriovenous malformations as, 2225, 2226f
benign acquired, 2229-2230, 2229f-2230f
birthmarks as, 2223
capillary malformations (port-wine stain) as, 2224, 2225f
genetic, 2230-2231
Klippel-Trenaunay and Klippel-Trenaunay-Weber syndromes as, 2225-2226, 2226f
malformations as, 2224
nevus anemicus as, 2226
phakomatosis pigmentovascularis as, 2226
vascular malformations as, 2224t-2225t
venous malformations as, 2224-2225, 2225f-2226f
Vascular resistance
pulmonary, *see website*
in neonatal circulation, 1529, *see also website*
systemic in shock, 311t
Vascular ring, 1452, 1596-1598, 1597f-1598f, 1597t
Vascular system
of hip, 2356, 2356f
pulmonary, *see website*
Vascular tumors, 1772, *see also website*
cutaneous, 2226-2231, 2227f-2229f, 2227t-2228t
gastrointestinal, *see website*
Vasculitis
drug eruptions in, *see website*
hypersensitivity, 876, 876t
hypocomplementemic urticarial, 876
leukocytoclastic, 876
due to cat-scratch disease, 985
in meningococcus, 930-931
renal, nephrotoxins in, 1817t
small vessel, with hepatitis C, 1401
sports participation and, 2402t-2404t
urticarial, 814
Vasculitis syndromes, 867-876, 868t, 876t
antineutrophil cytoplasmic antibodies (ANCA)-associated vasculitis as, 874-876
classification of, 868t
cutaneous manifestations of, *see website*
Henoch-Schönlein purpura as, 868-871, 869f-870f, 870t
polyarteritis nodosa and cutaneous polyarteritis nodosa as, 872-874, 873f
Takayasu arteritis as, 871-872, 871t, 872f
Vas deferens, injury to related to inguinal hernia repair, 1368
Vasoactive intestinal polypeptide (VIP), *see website*
Vasodilators
for cardiogenic shock, 313, 313t
for systemic hypertension, 1645t
Vasodilatory shock, 305, 308f
Vasopressin. *See* Antidiuretic hormone (ADH)
Vasopressin-resistant diabetes insipidus, 1882

Vasovagal syncope, *see website*
VATERR syndrome, 1356
VATER syndrome, 1262
  congenital heart disease with, 1531t
VATS. *See* Video-assisted thoracoscopic surgery (VATS)
VC. *See* Vital capacity (VC)
VCD. *See* Vocal cord dysfunction (VCD)
V-Cillin K. *See* Penicillin V
VCUG. *See* Voiding cystourethrogram (VCUG)
VCV. *See* Volume-controlled ventilation (VCV)
VDJ segments, *see website*
VDRL. *See* Venereal Disease Research Laboratory (VDRL) test
Vecuronium
  for anesthesia, *see website*
  for intubation, 321t
VEE. *See* Venezuelan equine encephalitis (VEE)
Vegetarianism, 168
Vegetative cells, 1185
VEGF. *See* Vascular endothelial growth factor (VEGF)
VEGFR-1, 2, *see website*
Veillonella, *see website*
Vein of Galen malformation, 1639
Velban. *See* Vinblastine
Vellus hair, *see website*
Velocardiofacial syndrome (VCFS), 407f, *see also website*
Velopharyngeal dysfunction (VPD), due to cleft lip and palate, 1253
Velosef. *See* Cephradine
Venereal Disease Research Laboratory (VDRL) test, 1019, 1019f, 1021
Venezuelan equine encephalitis (VEE), 1144-1147
Venezuelan hemorrhagic fever, 1151-1152
Venlafaxine
  for depression and anxiety symptoms, 63t
  poisoning with, 265
Venography
  computed tomography, in cerebral sinovenous thrombosis, 2083, 2083f
  magnetic resonance, in neurologic examination, *see website*
Venom immunotherapy (VI), 808-809, 809t
Venom(s), 2460-2465
  general approach to, 2460-2461
  hemolytic anemia secondary to, *see website*
  hymenoptera, 2464
  insect, 807-809
  marine, 2464-2465
  scorpion, 2464
  snake, 2461-2462, 2461f-2462f, 2461t-2462t
  spider, 2462-2463, 2463f
Veno-occlusive disease (VOD), of liver, *see website*
Venous access, 292, 295f
Venous admixture, 317-318
Venous malformations, 2224-2225, 2224t, 2225f-2226f
Venous patterns, assessment in neurologic examination, *see website*
Venous return, pulmonary
  partial anomalous, 1553-1554
  total anomalous, 1589-1590, 1589t, 1590f
Venous thromboembolism (VTE), 1500-1502, 1501t, 1709
Venous thrombosis, renal transplantation and, *see website*
Ventilation
  alveolar, 316-317, *see also website*
  dead space, 316-318, *see also website*
    in mechanical ventilation, 329
  insufficiency of, due to paralytic poliomyelitis, 1084, 1086
  manual
    bag-valve-mask positive pressure as, 284-285, 284f-285f
    in preintubation and postintubation periods, 320-321
Ventilation *(Continued)*
  mechanical (*See* Mechanical ventilation)
  mouth-to-mouth, 282, 282f
  partial liquid, for congenital diaphragmatic hernia, 596
Ventilation deficit assessment in respiratory distress and failure, 318-319
Ventilation index (VI), 319
Ventilation-perfusion (V/Q) mismatch, 317-318
Ventilation-perfusion (V/Q) radionuclide scan, 1502
Ventilation-perfusion (V/Q) ratio, *see website*
Ventilator dependence, *PHOX2B* gene and, 1520
Ventilatory failure, hypothyroidism-associated, 1903t
Ventilatory support in congenital central hypoventilation syndrome, 1522
Ventricle
  diverticulum of, 1599-1600
  double-outlet right, 1582
    with malposition of great arteries, 1588-1589
    with pulmonary stenosis, 1588
  embryonic development of, *see website*
  in fetal circulation, *see website*
  noncompaction, 1633-1634, 1634f
  single, 1592
  in transitional circulation, *see website*
Ventricular accelerated rhythm, 1616
Ventricular assist device (VAD), 314
Ventricular contractions, premature, 1612-1613, 1613f
Ventricular fibrillation, 1616
Ventricular hypertrophy
  electrocardiography of, 1538-1540, 1538f, 1540f
  radiographic assessment of, 1537
  systemic hypertension with, 1642
Ventricular inversion, 1595
Ventricular septal aneurysm, 1557
Ventricular septal defect (VSD), 1556-1558, 1556f-1557f
  in adults, 1606-1607
  coarctation of the aorta, 1570
  embryonic development of, *see website*
  supracristal, with aortic insufficiency, 1559
  in teratology of Fallot, 1573-1578
  transitional circulation and, *see website*
  transposition of the great arteries, 1587
  with transposition of the great arteries and pulmonary stenosis, 1574, 1583f
  tricuspid atresia and, 1580, 1580f
Ventricular tachyarrhythmias (VT), 1616, 1616f, 1616t
  with Marfan syndrome, 2441
Ventriculoatrial (VA) shunt infection, *see website*
Ventriculography in tetralogy of Fallot, 1575, 1575f
Ventriculoperitoneal (VP) shunt infection, *see website*
Venturi mask, 319
VePesid. *See* Etoposide
VEPs. *See* Visual-evoked potentials (VEPs)
Veramyst. *See* Fluticasone
Verbal apraxia, 119
Verbal auditory agnosia, 119
Vericonazole, 1065
Vermont Oxford Network (VON), *see website*
Vernal conjunctivitis, 2168, 2168f
Vernal keratoconjunctivitis, 810, 810f
Verotoxin in hemolytic-uremic syndrome, 1791-1792
Verruca, 2315-2316, 2315f
Verruca peruana, 982, 983f
Versenate for lead poisoning, 2453
Vertebral apophysis, slipped, 2377
Vertebral osteomyelitis, 2376, 2376t
Vertical suspension test, *see website*
Vertical talus, 2337-2338, 2337t, 2338f
Vertical transmission of HIV, 1158-1159
Vertigo, *see website*
Very long chain acyl CoA dehydrogenase (VLCAD) deficiency, 457t, 460
Very long chain fatty acids (VLCFA) disorders, 462-470
  adrenoleukodystrophy (X-linked) as, 467-470
  paroxysmal, 462-467, 462t-464t, 464f-465f, 466t
Very low birthweight (VLBW), 556. *See also* Prematurity/premature infant
  factors related to, 556-557
  rates of, *see website*
Very low density lipoproteins (VLDL), 471-473, 472f, 472t
Vesicle, examination of, *see website*
Vesicoureteral reflux, 1834-1838, 1834f
  classification of, 1834-1836, 1834f-1835f
  clinical manifestations of, 1836
  diagnosis of, 1836, 1836f
  natural history of, 1836, 1837f
  treatment of, 1836-1838, 1837f-1838f
Vesicular hand and foot dermatitis, 2253, 2253f
Vesiculobullous disorders, 2241-2249, 2241t
  dermatitis herpetiformis as, 2248-2249, 2248f
  erythema multiforme as, 2241-2242, 2242f
  linear immunoglobulin A dermatosis as, 2249, 2249f
  mechanobullous, 2244-2246, 2245f-2247f, 2245t
  pemphigus as, 2247-2248, 2247f
  Stevens-Johnson syndrome as, 2242-2243, 2243f
  toxic epidermal necrolysis as, 2243-2244
Vestibulocochlear nerve, neurologic examination of, *see website*
Vestibulopathy, strokelike events *versus*, 2086
VFC. *See* Vaccines for Children (VFC) program
VHL. *See* von Hippel-Lindau disease (VHL)
VI. *See* Venom immunotherapy (VI); Ventilation index (VI)
Vibramycin. *See* Doxycycline
Vibrio cholerae, 965-968
  gastroenteritis due to, 1324t-1325t, 1330
Vibrio parahaemolyticus, 1324t-1325t
Vibrio vulnificus, 1324t-1325t
Vidarabine, *see website*
Video-assisted thoracoscopic surgery (VATS)
  for empyema, 1509
  for pneumothorax, 1511-1512
Videofluoroscopic swallow study (VSS), 1472t
Videx. *See* Didanosine (ddI)
Vigabatrin
  adverse effects of, 2031t
  for West syndrome, 2027
Vinblastine, *see website*
Vincent angina, *see website*
Vincent's curtsy, 1848-1849
Vincent stomatitis, 2299
Vincristine, 1759, *see also website*
Vineland Adaptive Behavior Scale (VABS), 127
Violence, 25, 135, *see also website*
  due to bullying, 135, *see also website*
  school, 668, *see also website*
  teen pregnancy and, 701
  due to war, 8, 135, *see also website*
Violent behavior, adolescent, 667-671, 667t-670t, 668f
VIP. *See* Vasoactive intestinal polypeptide (VIP)
VIRA-A. *See* Vidarabine
Viracept. *See* Nelfinavir
Viral infections
  adenovirus, 1131-1133
  arboviral encephalitis
    in North America, 1141-1144
    outside North America, 1144-1147, 1145t
  arthritis associated with, 840, 840t
  astrovirus, 1134-1137
  calicivirus, 1134-1137
  cancer therapy and, *see website*

Viral infections *(Continued)*
in common cold, 1434
of conjunctiva, 2167t, 2168, 2168f
coronavirus, 1134, *see also website*
cutaneous, 2315-2317
cytomegalovirus, 1115-1117
dengue fever and dengue hemorrhagic fever as, 1147-1150
Epstein-Barr virus, 1110-1115
fever in, *see website*
fever of unknown origin in, 900t
following organ transplantation, *see website*
food-borne, 1326t
hantavirus pulmonary syndrome, 1154, *see also website*
hearing loss due to, *see website*
hemorrhagic fevers as, 1150-1153
hepatitis as, 1393-1404, 1393t
acute renal failure with, 1413
approach to, 1403-1404, 1403f
biochemical profiles in, 1394-1395
causes and differential diagnosis of, 1394, 1394t
due to hepatitis A virus, 1395-1396, 1395f, 1396t
due to hepatitis B virus, 1397-1400, 1398f, 1399t
due to hepatitis C virus, 1400-1402, 1400f
due to hepatitis D virus, 1402
due to hepatitis E virus, 1402-1403
pathogenesis of, 1394
herpes simplex virus, 1097-1104
HIV-related, 1164, *see website*
human herpesvirus 6 and 7, 1117-1120
human herpesviruses 8, 1121
human immunodeficiency virus, 1157-1177 (*See also* HIV/AIDS)
human metapneumovirus as, 1129-1131
human papillomavirus, 1137-1141
human T-lymphotropic virus, 1177, *see also website*
influenza virus, 1121-1125
laboratory diagnosis of, *see website*
lymphocytic choriomeningitis virus, 1153, *see also website*
maternal, *see website*
measles as, 1069-1075
in meningoencephalitis, 2095-2097
cerebrospinal fluid findings in, 2088t
mumps as, 1078-1081
myocarditis as, 1634
neonatal, 635-636
neutropenia in, 747-748
nonpolio enterovirus, 1088-1094
otitis media as, 2202
parainfluenza virus, 1125-1126
parvovirus B19, 1094-1097
pharyngitis as, 1439
in pneumonia, 1475t, 1476-1477
polioviruses, 1081-1088
polyomavirus, 1157, *see also website*
predisposition to due to immunodeficiency, 716t
rabies as, 1154-1157
respiratory syncytial virus, 1126-1129
rhinovirus, 1133-1134
roseola as, 1117-1120
rotavirus, 1134-1137
rubella as, 1075-1078
stem cell transplantation and, *see website*
therapy for, 1069, *see also website*
transmissible spongiform encephalopathies as, 1177, *see also website*
traveler's diarrhea due to, 1338t
in type 1 diabetes mellitus development, 1971
varicella-zoster virus, 1104-1110
yellow fever as, 1150, *see also website*
Viral load in HIV infection, 1161
Viramune. *See* Nevirapine
Virazole. *See* Ribavirin
Viread. *See* Tenofovir
Viremia, herpes simplex virus, 1099
Virginal breast hypertrophy, *see website*
Virgin B cell, *see website*
Viridans streptococci
in infective endocarditis, 1622, 1625t
neonatal, 632t
sepsis due to, 636t
Virilizing adrenocortical tumor, 1941, *see also website*
maternal, 1962
Virologic assay for hepatitis C virus, 1401
Viroptic. *See* Trifluridine
Virus(es)
in breast milk, 540t
in oncogenesis, *see website*
Visceral larva migrans (VLM), 1227-1229, 1228t, *see also website*
Visceral leishmaniasis (VL), 1187-1189, 1189f
Visceral pain, 360t, 1248
Visceroatrial situs, 1595
Viscum album, potential toxicity of, 272t-273t
Vision
disorders of, 2152-2154, 2153t, *see website*
due to *Chlamydia trachomatis*, 1035
due to vitamin A deficiency, 189
function of, *see website*
Neonatal Intensive Care Unit Neurobehavioral Scale and, 624t
testing of, 2149t
for adolescents, 666
in intellectual disability, 127t
in neurologic examination, *see website*
Vistaril. *See* Hydroxyzine
Vistide. *See* Cidofovir
Visual acuity, 2148
assessment in neurologic examination, *see website*
of newborn, *see website*
during preschool years, 33
in vision screening, 2149t
Visual analog pain scales (VAS), 361, 363t
Visual-evoked potentials (VEPs), *see website*
Visual field assessment, 2148-2149
in neurologic examination, *see website*
Visual reinforcement audiometry (VRA), 2194
Vital capacity (VC), *see website*
Vital signs in pediatric emergency assessment, 279, 280t
Vitamins
absorption disorders of, 1305t, 1319
dietary reference intakes for, *see website*
overview of, 188
for premature and low birthweight infants, 562
supplemental
for chronic diarrhea, 1345
in cystic fibrosis, 1495
nutritional aspects of, 169
water-soluble, 194t
Vitamin A
absorption, transport, metabolism, and storage of, 188
deficiency of, 189-190, 189f-190f
due to malabsorption, 1319
malnutrition and, 172
measles with, 1073, 1073t
skin manifestations of, 2330
dietary reference intakes for, *see website*
excess of, 190-191, 191f
function and mechanism of action of, 189
overview of, 188, 189t
supplementation, 190
for neonatal cholestasis, 1387
for respiratory distress syndrome, 586
Vitamin B_1, 191, 194t
deficiency of, 191-192
dietary reference intakes for, *see website*
toxicity of, 192
Vitamin B_2, 192-193, 194t
deficiency of, 192-193, 193f
dietary reference intakes for, *see website*
Vitamin B_3, 193, 194t
deficiency of, 193-195, 195f
toxicity of, 195
Vitamin B_5, 194t
dietary reference intakes for, *see website*
Vitamin B_6, 194t, 195-196
deficiency of, 196
dietary reference intakes for, *see website*
for homocystinuria, 426-427
toxicity of, 196
Vitamin B_6-dependent epilepsy, 453-455
Vitamin B_{12}, 194t, 197
defects in metabolism of, 437-438, 1320
deficiency of, 197-198, 748t
anemia due to, 1655, *see also website*
dietary reference intakes for, *see website*
in vegetarian diet, 168
Vitamin B complex, 191
Vitamin B_6 dependence syndrome, 196
Vitamin C, 194t, 198
deficiency of, 198-200, 199f-200f
skin manifestations of, 2330
dietary needs and sources of, 198
dietary reference intakes for, *see website*
for methemoglobin, 1673
for premature and low birthweight infants, 560
toxicity of, 200
Vitamin D, *see also website*
in bone formation, *see website*
deficiency of
calcium deficiency and, 206
due to chronic renal failure, 205-206
congenital, 205
hypophosphatemia and, 227-228
due to malabsorption, 1318
nutritional, 204-205
rickets due to, 200-206, 202t
secondary, 205
dietary reference intakes for, *see website*
excess of, 208-209
physical and metabolic properties and food sources of, 201t
physiology of, 204
supplementation, 165
for premature and low birthweight infants, 560
for renal osteodystrophy, 1824-1825
Vitamin D-dependent rickets
dental problems associated with, 1251t
type 1, 205
type 2, 205
Vitamin E
deficiency of, 209, *see also website*
in cystic fibrosis, 1486-1487
due to malabsorption, 1318-1319
myopathy associated with, 2132
dietary reference intakes for, *see website*
physical and metabolic properties and food sources of, 201t
for premature and low birthweight infants, 560
in premature infant, possible adverse reactions to, 563t
supplementary for neonatal cholestasis, 1387-1388
Vitamin K, *see website*
deficiency of, 209-211
in cystic fibrosis, 1486-1487
due to malabsorption, 1319
postneonatal, 1712
dietary reference intakes for, *see website*
injection of in newborn, 537
physical and metabolic properties and food sources of, 201t
possible adverse reactions to in premature infant, 563t
Vitamin K-deficiency bleeding (VKDB), 210
Vitamin K-dependent factors, deficiency of, 620-621
Vitelliform degeneration, Best, 2178

Vitiligo, 2240, 2240f, 2240t
Vitravene. *See* Fomivirsen
Vitreoretinopathy, familial exudative, 2179
Vitreous seeding, 1768
Vittaforma cornea, *see website*
VKBD. *See* Vitamin K-deficiency bleeding (VKDB)
VL. *See* Visceral leishmaniasis (VL)
VLBW. *See* Very low birthweight (VLBW)
VLCAD. *See* Very long chain acyl CoA dehydrogenase (VLCAD) deficiency
VLCFA. *See* Very long chain fatty acids (VLCFA)
VLDL. *See* Very low density lipoproteins (VLDL)
VLM. *See* Visceral larva migrans (VLM)
V3 loop, 1157-1158
Vocal cord dysfunction (VCD), asthma *versus*, 783
Vocal cord paralysis, 1451
Vocal nodules, *see website*
Vocal tic, 76
VOD. *See* Veno-occlusive disease (VOD)
Vogt-Koyanagi-Harada syndrome, 2240
Vohwinkel palmoplantar keratoderma, 2273
Voiding, normal, 71, 1847
Voiding cystourethrogram (VCUG)
  in urinary tract infection, 1833, 1833f
  in urinary tract obstruction, 1840
  in vesicoureteral reflux, 1836, 1837f
Voiding dysfunction, 1847-1852
  diurnal incontinence in, 73
  enuresis in, 71-73
  Hinman syndrome as, 1849-1850, 1849f
  incontinence as, 1850-1851, 1850f-1851f
    diurnal, 1847-1848, 1848f-1849f, 1848t
  infrequent voiding as, 1850
  nocturnal enuresis as, 1851-1852, 1851t
  overactive bladder as, 1848-1849, 1849f
  due to urinary tract infection, 1832-1833
  vaginal voiding as, 1850, 1850f
  without incontinence, 1851
Volatile substance abuse (VSA), 681-682
Volleyball, injuries in, *see website*
Volume-controlled ventilation (VCV), 325-326, 325f, 325t
Volume depletion, *see also website*
  metabolic alkalosis and, 235
Volume of distribution, *see website*
Volume overload, *see also website*
  congenital heart disease in, 1549-1550
Volume regulation, *see website*
Volume support ventilation (VSV), 325
Voluntary control of respiration, *see website*
Volvulus, gastric, 1276
  with malrotation, 1281
Vomiting, 1242-1243
  in acutely ill child, 275
  in appendicitis, 1350, 1351t
  due to cholera, 966
  complications of, 1243t
  cyclic, 1242, 1243t
  differential diagnosis of, 1242t
  exclusion from day care due to, *see website*
  habits regarding in eating disorders, 92t
  in intestinal malrotation, 1280-1281
  in intestinal obstruction, 1242, 1243t
  Jamaican vomiting syndrome, 529
  maintenance water for, 245, 245t
  with migraine, 2042
    antiemetics for, 2043
  neonatal, 600-601
  in newborn, *see website*
  nondigestive causes of, 1241t
  due to opioids, 366t
  in palliative care, 157t, 158
  postoperative, *see website*
  in pyloric stenosis, 1274
  therapy for
    nonpharmacologic and supportive, 1245t
    pharmacologic, 1244t
Vomitoxin, 1328t-1329t
VON. *See* Vermont Oxford Network (VON)
von Gierke disease, 492-496, 494t-495t
  malignancy susceptibility associated with, *see website*
  myopathy with, 2131
von Graefe sign, 2163
von Hippel-Lindau disease (VHL), 1942, 2052
  brain tumors associated with, 1747t
  cardiac manifestations of, 1531t
  malignancy susceptibility associated with, *see website*
von Meyenburg complexes, *see website*
von Recklinghausen disease, 2237
von Willebrand disease (VWD), 1704-1707, 1705f
von Willebrand factor
  in hemostasis, 1694
  reference values for, 1698t
Voriconazole, 1056t, *see also website*
Vorner palmoplantar keratodermas, 2273f
VP. *See* Variegate porphyria (VP); Ventriculoperitoneal (VP) shunt
VPD. *See* Velopharyngeal dysfunction (VPD)
VPS33B gene defect, 1383t
V/Q. *See* Ventilation-perfusion (V/Q)
VRA. *See* Visual reinforcement audiometry (VRA)
VRE. *See* Vancomycin-resistant *Enterococcus* (VRE)
VSA. *See* Volatile substance abuse (VSA)
VSD. *See* Vaccine Safety Datalink (VSD); Ventricular septal defect (VSD)
VSG. *See* Variant surface glycoproteins (VSG)
VSS. *See* Videofluoroscopic swallow study (VSS)
VSV. *See* Volume support ventilation (VSV)
VT. *See* Ventricular tachyarrhythmias (VT)
VT. *See* Tidal volume (VT)
V_T. *See* Minute volume (V_T); Tidal volume (V_T)
VTE. *See* Venous thromboembolism (VTE)
Vulva
  anomalies of, *see website*
  neoplasm of, 1873
    vaginal bleeding due to, 1869
  traumatic injury to, vaginal bleeding due to, 1869
Vulvitis, 1865
Vulvovaginal anomalies, 1874, *see also website*
Vulvovaginitis, 1865-1869, 1868f
  with *Candida*, 1055
  clinical manifestations of, 1866, 1866f
  diagnosis and differential diagnosis of, 1866-1867, 1866f
  epidemiology of, 1865-1866
  etiology of, 1865, 1865f, 1867t-1868t
  gonococcal, 937-938
  treatment and prevention of, 1867-1869, 1868t
  vaginal bleeding in, 1869
VURD syndrome, 1846
VWD. *See* von Willebrand disease (VWD)
VX, in terrorism, *see website*
VX-770 for cystic fibrosis, 1493

W

Waardenburg syndrome, 425, 2156, 2190t, 2238t, 2239, *see also website*
Wada test, 2032
Waddling gait, *see website*
WAGR syndrome, 408t, 1963
Waived tests, *see website*
Waldeyer ring, 1442
Walker criteria for mitochondrial disease, 508t
Walker-Murdoch sign, 2440, 2441f
Walker-Warburg syndrome, 2127
Walking
  learning to, 31
  during preschool years, 33
Wandering atrial pacemaker, 1612, 1612f
Wandering raphe, 1855-1856
War, 8, 135, *see also website*
Warfarin, 1710t, 1711
"Warm" antibodies, autoimmune hemolytic anemia associated with, 1680-1682, *see also website*
Warthin-Finkeldey giant cells, 1070
Warts
  cutaneous, 1138, 1139f, 2315-2316, 2315f
  genital, 1138-1139, 1139f, 2316, 2316f
    sexual abuse and, 145, 145t
    treatment in adolescents, 713t
Wasp, allergic responses to, 807f
Wassel classification of thumb duplication, 2386, 2386t
Water
  chemical pollutants in, *see website*
  dietary reference intakes for, *see website*
  hyponatremia due to excess ingestion of, 217
  maintenance, 242-243, 243t
    variations in, 244, 244t
  physiology of balance of, 1881-1884, 1882f
  sources of loss of, 244t
  sports and intake of, 2421
  total body, 212, *see also website*
    hypervolemic hyponatremia and, 216
    sodium in, 212
  travel and, *see website*
Water-borne illness
  Aeromonas, *see website*
  dracunculiasis, 1227
  Legionella, *see website*
  Plesiomonas shigelloides, *see website*
Water deficit
  hypernatremia due to, 213-214, 213t
  maintenance water and electrolytes and, 244
  sources of loss in, 244t
Water deprivation test, 214
Water hemlock toxicity, 269t
Waterless hand hygiene, *see website*
Water lily sign, 1239
Water safety, 347-348, 348t
Water-soluble vitamins, 194t
Watery diarrhea
  in microvillus inclusion disease, 1305
  in tufting enteropathy, 1311
Watery diarrhea-hypokalemia-acidosis syndrome, 1370
Ways to Enhance Children's Activity and Nutrition (WECAN), 187
WBC. *See* White blood cell (WBC)
WBI. *See* Whole-bowel irrigation (WBI)
Weakness
  in Becker muscular dystrophy, 2119
  in Duchenne muscular dystrophy, 2119
  in Guillain-Barré syndrome, 2143
  in juvenile dermatomyositis, 847, 848t, 849
  in myotonic muscular dystrophy, 2123, 2123f
  in neuromuscular disorders, 2110t-2111t, 2115t
  in rheumatic disease, *see website*
Weaning
  breast-feeding, 164-165, 164t
  mechanical ventilation, 329, 586
Weapon carrying by adolescents, 669t
Weaver syndrome, *see website*
Webbed neck, with Turner syndrome, 1952-1953
Webbed penis, 1856
Weber-Cockayne syndrome, 2244
Webs
  laryngeal, 1451, 1451f
  tracheal, 1452
Websites. *See* Internet
WECAN. *See* Ways to Enhance Children's Activity and Nutrition (WECAN)
Wechsler Scales, 127
WEE. *See* Western equine encephalitis (WEE)
"Weed," 680-681
Weeping lesion, treatment of, 2215
Wegener's granulomatosis, 868t, 874-876, 874t, *see also website*
  alveolar hemorrhage with, 1499

Weight
for age, in nutrition assessment, 172
at birth (*See* Birthweight)
drug dosages based on, *see website*
ideal, *see website*
in maintenance water calculations, 243t
percentile curves for, *see website*
Weight gain in premature infants, 561, 561f
Weill-Marchesani syndrome, 1531t
Weil syndrome, 1024
Wellbutrin. *See* Bupropion
Well child care, 13-25
in behavioral and mental health issues, 16
evidence and, 16
family and community in, 16-17
guidelines for, 14
in infancy and early childhood, 16
for injury control, 17-25
in middle childhood and adolescence, 16
periodicity of, 14
quality improvement of, 16
strength-based approaches and framework for, 16
tasks of, 14-16
Well syndrome, 1024
Wenckebach heart block, 1618
Werdnig-Hoffman disease, 2136, 2137f
Wermer syndrome, 527
malignancy susceptibility associated with, *see website*
Werner syndrome, 1531t, *see also website*
Wernicke encephalopathy, 192
West African trypanosomiasis, 1190-1193, 1192f, *see also website*
Western equine encephalitis (WEE), 1141, 1143-1144
Western immunoblot
in Lyme disease, 1028
in toxoplasmosis, 1214
Westfall variant, 2056
West Nile encephalitis (WNE), 1142-1144, 1142f-1143f
poliovirus infection *versus*, 1084, 1085t
West Nile virus, maternal, *see website*
West syndrome, 2024
treatment of, 2014, 2027
Wet dressing, 2216
WFS1 gene, 2190t
Wheals, examination of, *see website*
Wheat allergy, 821, 821t
Wheeze/wheezing
in allergic disease, 765
in asthma, 782, 782t, 784t
auscultation of, *see website*
in bronchiolitis, 1456-1459
in bronchitis, 1459-1460, 1460t
clinical manifestations in, 1458-1459
definitions and general pathophysiology of, 1456
differential diagnosis of, 1457t
etiology of, 1456-1458
history and physical examination in, 1458, 1458t
as manifestation of extrapulmonary disease, *see website*
monophonic, 1456
prevention of, 1459
prognosis for, 1459
recurrent or persistent, *see website*
in respiratory syncytial virus infection, 1127-1129
as sign of respiratory pathology, *see website*
treatment of, 1459
WHIM syndrome, 748t
Whipple disease, 1314
Whipworm, 1221-1222, *see website*
Whitaker test, 1841
White blood cell (WBC) count, 752. *See also* Leukocytosis
in acutely ill child evaluation, 277
White blood cell (WBC) count *(Continued)*
in acute lymphocytic leukemia treatment, 1734
in appendicitis, 1351, 1351t
in dengue fever, 1149
in Epstein-Barr virus infection, 1113
in hantavirus pulmonary syndrome, *see website*
in leukemoid reaction, *see website*
in leukopenia, 746
in Lyme disease, 1028
monocytosis as, *see website*
neutrophilia as, *see website*
in pertussis, 945
in pneumonia, 1477
reference values for, 1656t
in roseola, 1119
in *Shigella* infection, 960
White coat hypertension, 1639
White line of Fränkel, 199, 199f
White nails, 2294, 2294t
White pulp, splenic, 1723
White pupillary reflex, 2157, 2157f
brain death and, *see website*
in newborn, 534
in retinoblastoma, 1768-1769, 1768f
as sign of cancer, 1730f
White spot lesion, 1254, 1255f
WHO. *See* World Health Organization (WHO)
Whole-body irradiation, *see website*
Whole-bowel irrigation (WBI) for poisoning, 257
Whole-genome array, 398
Whooping cough, 944
WIC. *See* Special Supplemental Nutrition Program for Women, Infants, and Children (WIC)
Widal test, 957
Widow's peak, *see website*
Wiedemann-Rautenstrauch syndrome, *see website*
Wigglesworthia glossinidia, 1193
Wild bedbugs in trypanosomiasis, 1195
Wilkie syndrome, 1287, *see also website*
Williams-Campbell syndrome, *see website*
Williams syndrome, 408t
congenital heart disease with, 1531t, 1564-1565, 1565f, *see website*
hypercalcemia with, 1922-1923
hypothyroidism with, 1901
Wilms tumor, 1757-1760, 1757t-1759t, 1759f
incidence and survival rates for, 1726t
risk factors for, 1727t
work-up of, 1731t
Wilson disease, 1383t, 1391, 1391f
chorea with, 2057t
dystonia with, 2060
hemolytic anemia secondary to, *see website*
Wimberger's lines, 1018
Windsock *website*, 1277-1278
Wiskott-Aldrich syndrome, 734-735, 1720
malignancy susceptibility associated with, *see website*
Withdrawal, 253t
marijuana, 680
methamphetamine, 684t
neonatal, 623-625, 624t
opiates in adolescent, 684-685
Withholding and withdrawing life-sustaining treatment, *see website*
Witnessing violence, *see website*
WM. *See* Working memory (WM)
WNE. *See* West Nile encephalitis (WNE)
WNT4 gene, *see website*
WOB. *See* Work of breathing (WOB)
Wolffian duct, *see website*
Wolff-Parkinson-White syndrome, 1584
genetics of, *see website*
sports participation and, 2402t-2404t
sudden death due to, 1620, 1620f
supraventricular tachycardia in, 1613-1614, 1614f
Wolfram syndrome, 1883
Wolfsbane, potential toxicity of, 272t-273t
Wolman disease, 479, 484t, 491, 1313, 1926
Wood lamp, *see website*
Woolly hair disease, 2293
Wool-sorters disease, *see website*
Work clothes, chemical pollutants in, *see website*
Working memory (WM), *see website*
Work of breathing (WOB), *see website*
World Health Organization (WHO)
on breast-feeding, 160, 161t, 539t
on cancer pain management, 374, 374t
on complementary feeding, 164
growth charts of, *see website*
on growth of breast-fed infants, 162
Health InterNetwork Access to Research Initiative from (*See* Health InterNetwork Access to Research Initiative)
on injury prevention, *see website*
Integrated Management of Childhood Illness guidelines from, *see website*
lupus nephritis classification from, 1789
lymphoid neoplasm classification from, 1740-1741, 1741t
on polio vaccination, 1087
on pulmonary hypertension, 1600t
on sever malaria, 1201t
Wormwood, 272t-273t
Wound botulism, 987-991
Wound closure for laceration, 341
Wound infection
following inguinal surgery repair, 1367
prophylaxis for prevention of, *see website*
Wound management
in envenomations, 2460-2461
tetanus prophylaxis in, 993-994
Wound membranes for burn injury, 352, 352t
Wrestling
herpes simplex virus infection in, 1100, 1102
injuries in, *see website*
Wright stain, *see website*
Wrisberg ligament type, 2352
Wrist
arthrogryposis involving, *see website*
disorders of, 2384-2385
fracture of, 2391-2392
Wrist sign in Marfan syndrome, 2440, 2441f
Writing impairment, *see website*
graphomotor function and, *see website*
WT1 gene, 1758, 1803t, 1807, 1962, *see website*
Wuchereria bancrofti, 1224-1225, *see website*
WU virus, 1157, *see also website*

X

"X," 682
X-ALD. *See* X-linked adrenoleukodystrophy (X-ALD)
Xanthine oxidoreductase deficiency (XOR), *see website*
Xanthochromia, *see website*
Xanthogranuloma, juvenile, *see also website*
ocular lesion of, 2156
Xanthogranulomatous pyelonephritis, 1830
Xanthoma as manifestation of liver disease, 1376
Xanthomatosis, cerebrotendinous, 478-479, 1312
Xanthomonas maltophilia, 977, *see also website*
45,X chromosome, in Turner syndrome, 1952-1953
X chromosome inactivation, 388
XDR. *See* Extensively drug resistant (XDR)
Xerocytosis, *see website*
Xeroderma pigmentosum, 2258, 2258f
malignancy susceptibility associated with, *see website*
Xerophthalmia, due to vitamin A deficiency, 189-190, 190f
Xerostoma, *see website*
XLA. *See* X-linked agammaglobulinemia (XLA)

XLH. *See* X-linked hypophosphatemic rickets (XLH)
X-linked adrenoleukodystrophy (X-ALD), 466t, 467-470, 469f
X-linked agammaglobulinemia (XLA), 723-724, 724f
  malignancy susceptibility associated with, *see website*
X-linked Alport syndrome, 1782-1783
X-linked cardiomyopathy, 433, *see also website*
X-linked dominance, 388, 389f
X-linked growth hormone deficiency, 1878
X-linked hyper-immunoglobulin M syndrome, 726
X-linked hypophosphatemic rickets (XLH), 202t, 206-207
X-linked ichthycosis, 2269-2270, 2270f
X-linked ichthyosis, 2268t, 2269-2270
X-linked immunodeficiency, malignancy susceptibility associated with, *see website*
X-linked inheritance, 388, 388f-389f
X-linked lissencephaly, *see website*
X-linked liver phosphorylase kinase deficiency, 498
X-linked lymphoproliferative disease (XLP), 727
  Epstein-Barr virus and, 1112
X-linked protoporphyria, *see website*
X-linked recessive hypoparathyroidism, 1917
X-linked severe combined immunodeficiency (SCIDX1), 732, 732f
XLP. *See* X-linked lymphoproliferative disease (XLP)
45,X males, 1948
XOR. *See* Xanthine oxidoreductase deficiency (XOR)
46-,XX, 1959t, *see also website*
XX gonadal dysgenesis, 1954
XX males, 409t, 1948, *see website*
XXX females, 1955
47,XXX males, 1948, *see also website*
XXXX females, 1955
XXXXX females, 1955
49-XXXXY, 1947
48-XXXY, 1947
45,X/46,XY gonadal dysgenesis, 1954-1955
45,X/46,XY mosaicism, 409-410
47,XXY syndrome, 1946, *see also website*. *See also* Klinefelter syndrome
XXYY, 1947
46,XY disorders of sex development, 1959t, 1962
XY female, 409t, *see also website*
XY gonadal agenesis syndrome, 1963
Xylitol, 1982
XY pure gonadal dysgenesis, 1963-1964
47,XYY, 410
XYY syndrome, 409t, *see also website*
Xyzal. *See* Levocetirizine

Y
Yaws, 1023, *see also website*
Y chromosome, mosaicism of, Turner syndrome and, 1953
Yeast cells, candidal, 1053
Yellow fever, 1150, *see also website*
Yellow fever vaccine, 884t, *see also website*
  international, 894
Yellow fever vaccine-associated viscerotropic disease, *see website*
Yellow jacket, allergic responses to, 807f
Yellow nail syndrome, 2295, *see website*
Yellow oleander toxicity, 269t
Yersinia, 971-974
  Crohn disease *versus*, 1301
  in infectious diarrhea, 1337t
  inflammatory bowel disease *versus*, 1298t
  in vulvovaginitis, 1865-1866
Yersinia enterocolitica, 971-972, 1324t-1325t
Yersinia pestis, 973-974
  in pneumonia, 1475t
Yersinia pseudotuberculosis, 972-973, 1324t-1325t
Yew toxicity, 269t
Y-linked inheritance, 388-389, 390f
YMSM. *See* Young men who have sex with men (YMSM)
Yoga for pain management, 371
Yohimbe, potential toxicity of, 272t-273t
Young men who have sex with men (YMSM), 659
Yuzpe method, 699

Z
Zafirlukast
  for asthma, 795-796
  for urticaria and angioedema, 815t
Zanamivir, *see also website*
  for influenza, 1123, 1123t
ZAP-70. *See* Zeta-associated protein 70 (ZAP-70)
ZDV. *See* Zidovudine (ZDV)
Zebra bodies, 2139
Zeitgebers, 46
Zellweger syndrome, 463, 464f, 464t, 466t, 1382-1383, 2069, 2132
Zenker diverticulum, 1264
Zerit. *See* Stavudine (d4T)
Zeta-associated protein 70 (ZAP-70), 730
Ziagen. *See* Abacavir
Zidovudine (ZDV)
  drug interactions with, *see website*
  for HIV infection, 1167-1171, 1168t-1171t
    prophylactic, 1173
Ziehl-Neelsen stain, *see website*
Zileuton for asthma, 795
Zinacef. *See* Cefuroxime
Zinc, *see website*
  deficiency, *see website*
    in acrodermatitis enteropathica, 2328-2329, 2329f
  dietary reference intakes for, *see website*
  gastroenteritis due to, 1328t-1329t
  supplementation of
    for acrodermatitis enteropathica, 2328-2329
    for cholera, 967
    common cold and, 1436
    for infectious diarrhea, 1336
    for malnutrition, 172
    for Wilson disease, 1392
  in vegetarian diet, 168
Zinc protoporphyrin (ZPP), 1657t
Zinnser-Engman-Cole syndrome, 2222, 2222f
Ziprasidone, 64t
Zithromax. *See* Azithromycin
Zofran. *See* Ondansetron
Zollinger-Ellison syndrome, 1294
  diarrhea caused by, *see website*
Zolmitriptan, 2044t
Zoloft. *See* Sertraline
Zona fasciculata, *see website*
Zona glomerulosa, *see website*
Zona reticularis, *see website*
Zonisamide
  adverse effects of, 2031t
  for seizures, 2030t
  for weight loss in adults, 187t
Zoonotic disease. *See* Animal-borne infection
Zosteriform lentiginous nevus, 2233
Zosyn. *See* Piperacillin-tazobactam
Zovirax. *See* Acyclovir
ZPP. *See* Zinc protoporphyrin (ZPP)
Z score, *see website*
Zygomycosis, 1069, *see also website*
Zyprexa. *See* Olanzapine
Zyrtec. *See* Cetirizine
Zyvox. *See* Linezolid